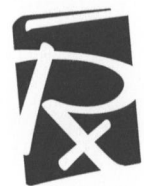

21ST EDITION

Remington

The Science and Practice of Pharmacy

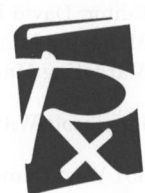

21ST EDITION

Remington

The Science and Practice
of Pharmacy

LIPPINCOTT WILLIAMS & WILKINS
A **Wolters Kluwer** Company

Philadelphia • Baltimore • New York • London
Buenos Aires • Hong Kong • Sydney • Tokyo

Editor: David B. Troy
Managing Editor: Matthew J. Hauber
Marketing Manager: Marisa A. O'Brien

Lippincott Williams & Wilkins

351 West Camden Street
Baltimore, Maryland 21201-2436 USA

530 Walnut Street
Philadelphia, PA 19106

To purchase additional copies of this book call our customer service department at **(800) 638-3030** or fax orders to **(301) 824-7390.** International customers should call **(301) 714-2324.**

Remington: The Science and Practice of Pharmacy . . . *A treatise on the theory and practice of the pharmaceutical sciences, with essential information about pharmaceutical and medicinal agents; also, a guide to the professional responsibilities of the pharmacist as the drug information specialist of the health team . . . A textbook and reference work for pharmacists, physicians, and other practitioners of the pharmaceutical and medical sciences.*

Twenty-first Edition—2005

Published in the 185th year of the
PHILADELPHIA COLLEGE OF PHARMACY AND SCIENCE

Remington Historical/Biographical Data

The following is a record of the editors and the dates of publication of successive editions of this book, prior to the 13th Edition known as Remington's Practice of Pharmacy and subsequently as Remington's Pharmadeutical Sciences trhough the 20th edition.

First Edition, 1886
Second Edition, 1889
Third Edition, 1897
Fourth Edition, 1905
 Joseph P. Remington

Fifth Edition, 1907
Sixth Edition, 1917
 Joseph P. Remington

Assisted by
 E. Fullerton Cook

Seventh Edition, 1926
 Editors
 E. Fullerton Cook
 Charles H. LaWall

Eighth Edition, 1936
 Editors
 E. Fullerton Cook
 Charles H. LaWall

Associated Editors
 Ivor Griffith
 Adley B. Nichols
 Arthur Osol

Ninth Edition, 1948
Tenth Edition, 1951
 Editors
 E. Fullerton Cook
 Eric W. Martin

Eleventh Edition, 1956
 Editors
 Eric W. Martin
 E. Fullerton Cook

Associated Editors
 E. Emerson Leuallen
 Arthur Osol
 Linwood F. Tice
 Clarence T. Van Meter

Twelfth Edition, 1961
 Editors
 Eric W. Martin
 E. Fullerton Cook
 E. Emerson Leuallen
 Arthur Osol
 Linwood F. Tice
 Clarence T. Van Meter

Assistant to the Editors
 John E. Hoover

Thirteenth Edition, 1965
 Editor-in-Chief
 Eric W. Martin
 Editors
 Grafton D. Chase
 Herald R. Cox
 Richard A. Deno
 Alfonso R. Gennaro
 Stewart C. Harvey

Managing Editor
 John E. Hoover

 Robert E. King
 E. Emerson Leuallen
 Author Osol
 Ewart A. Swinyard
 Clarence T. Van Meter

Fourteenth Edition, 1970
 Chairman, Editorial Board
 Arthur Osol
 Editors
 Grafton D. Chase
 Richard A. Deno
 Alfonso R. Gennaro
 Melvin R. Gibson
 Stewart C. Harvey

Managing Editor
 John E. Hoover

 Robert E. King
 Alfred N. Martin
 Ewart A. Swinyard
 Clarence T. Van Meter

Fifteenth Edition, 1975
 Chairman, Editorial Board
 Arthur Osol
 Editors
 John T. Anderson
 Cecil L. Bendush
 Grafton D. Chase
 Alfonso R. Gennaro
 Melvin R. Gibson

Managing Editor
 John E. Hoover

 C. Boyd Granberg
 Stewart C. Harvey
 Robert E. King
 Alfred N. Martin
 Ewart A. Swinyard

Sixteenth Edition, 1980
 Chairman, Editorial Board
 Arthur Osol
 Editors
 Grafton D. Chase
 Alfonso R. Gennaro
 Melvin R. Gibson

 C. Boyd Granberg
 Stewart C. Harvey
 Robert E. King
 Alfred N. Martin
 Ewart A. Swinyard
 Gilbert L. Zink

Seventeenth Edition, 1985
 Chairman, Editorial Board
 Alfonso R. Gennaro
 Editors
 Grafton D. Chase
 Ara H. DerMarderosian
 Stewart C. Harvey
 Daniel A. Hussar
 Thomas Medwick

Managing Editor
 John E. Hoover

 Edward G. Rippie
 Joseph B. Schwartz
 Ewart A. Swinyard
 Gilbert L. Zink

Eighteenth Edition, 1990
 Chairman, Editorial Board
 Alfonso R. Gennaro

 Editors
 Grafton D. Chase
 Ara H. DerMarderosian
 Stewart C. Harvey
 Daniel A. Hussar
 Thomas Medwick

Managing Editor
 John E. Hoover
Editorial Assistant
 Bonnie Packer

 Edward G. Rippie
 Joseph B. Schwartz
 Ewart A. Swinyard
 Gilbert L. Zink

Editorial Board

Authors

Marie Abate, BS, PharmD / Professor of Clinical Pharmacy and Director, West Virginia Center for Drug and Health Information, School of Pharmacy, West Virginia University. Chapter 9, *Clinical Drug Literature*

Steven R Abel, PharmD, FASHP / Professor and Head, Department of Pharmacy Practice, Purdue University School of Pharmacy and Pharmacal Sciences. Chapter 100, *Professional Communications*

Bradley L Ackermann, PhD / Research Advisor, Lilly Research Laboratories, Eli Lilly & Co. Chapter 34, *Instrumental Methods of Analysis*

Mignon S Adams, MSLS / Associate Professor of Information Science; Chair of the Department of Information Science; Director of Library and Information Services, University of the Sciences in Philadelphia. Chapter 8, *Information Resources in Pharmacy and the Pharmaceutical Sciences*

Michael J Akers, PhD / Director of Pharmaceutical Research and Development, Baxter Pharmaceutical Solutions, LLC. Chapter 41, *Parenteral Solutions*

Adam W G Alani, MSc / Research Assistant, School of Pharmacy, University of Wisconsin-Madison. Chapter 47, *Extended-Release and Targeted Drug Delivery Systems*

Loyd V Allen, Jr, PhD / Professor Emeritus, Department of Medicinal Chemistry and Pharmaceutics, College of Pharmacy, University of Oklahoma and Editor-In-Chief, International Journal of Pharmaceutical Compounding. Chapter 105, *Extemporaneous Prescription Compounding*

Heidi M Anderson, PhD / Professor and Assistant Dean, Education Innovation, College of Pharmacy, University of Kentucky. Chapter 97, *Patient Communication*

Howard Y Ando, PhD / Director of Candidate Enabling and Development, Pfizer Global Research and Development. Chapter 38, *Property-Based Drug Design and Preformulation*

R Jayachandra Babu, PhD / Research Associate, College of Pharmacy, Florida A&M University. Chapter 33, *Chromatography*

Thomas A Barbolt, PhD, DABT / Senior Research Fellow, ETHICON, Somerville, NJ. Chapter 109, *Surgical Supplies*

Kenneth N Barker, PhD / Distinguished Sterling Professor and Director, Center for Pharmacy Operations and Design, Harrison School of Pharmacy, Auburn University. Chapter 95, *Technology and Automation*

Sara J Beis, MS, RPh / Consultant, Akron, OH. Chapter 112, *Re-Engineering Pharmacy Practice*

Robert W Bennett, MS, RPh / Associate Professor of Clinical Pharmacy; Director, Pharmacy Continuing Education, Department of Pharmacy Practice, Purdue University School of Pharmacy. Chapter 112, *Re-Engineering Pharmacy Practice*

Paul M Beringer, PharmD / Associate Professor of Clinical Pharmacy, School of Pharmacy, University of Southern California. Chapter 59, *Clinical Pharmacokinetics and Pharmacodynamics*

Richard J Bertin, PhD, RPh / Executive Director, Board of Pharmaceutical Specialties, Washington, DC. Chapter 120, *Specialization in Pharmacy Practice*

Lawrence H Block, PhD / Professor of Pharmaceutics, Mylan School of Pharmacy, Duquesne University. Chapter 23, *Rheology* and Chapter 44, *Medicated Topicals*

Allan D Bokser, PhD / Associate Director of Analytical Development, Neurocrine Biosciences, Inc. Chapter 52, *Stability of Pharmaceutical Products*

Sanford Bolton, PhD / Visiting Professor, College of Pharmacy, University of Arizona. Chapter 12, *Statistics*

Michael R Borenstein, RPh, PhD / Associate Professor and Chairman, Department of Pharmaceutical Sciences, Temple University School of Pharmacy. Chapter 78, *General Anesthetics*; Chapter 85, *Central Nervous System Stimulants*

Joseph I Boullata, PharmD, BCNSP / Professor of Pharmacy Practice, Temple University School of Pharmacy. Chapter 92, *Nutrients and Associated Substances*

Bill J Bowman, PhD, RPh / Assistant Professor of Pharmaceutical Sciences, College of Pharmacy–Glendale, Midwestern University. Chapter 21, *Colloidal Dispersions*; Chapter 26, *Natural Products*

Leslie Ann Bowman, AMLS / Associate Professor of Information Science and Coordinator of Instructional Services, Joseph W England Library, University of the Sciences in Philadelphia. Chapter 8, *Information Resources in Pharmacy and the Pharmaceutical Sciences*

Cynthia A Burman, BS, PharmD / Medical Information Scientist, GlaxoSmithKline, Philadelphia, PA. Chapter 75, *Diuretic Drugs*

Paul M Bummer, PhD / Associate Professor of Pharmaceutical Sciences, College of Pharmacy, University of Kentucky. Chapter 20, *Interfacial Phenomena*

Daniel J Canney, PhD / Associate Professor of Medicinal Chemistry, Department of Pharmaceutical Sciences, Temple University School of Pharmacy. Chapter 71, *Cholinomimetic Drugs* and Chapter 73, *Antimuscarinic and Antispasmodic Drugs*

Bradley C Cannon, PharmD / Clinical Assistant Professor, University of Illinois at Chicago, College of Pharmacy. Chapter 122, *Development of a Pharmacy Care Plan and Patient Problem Solving*

F Lee Cantrell, PharmD / Assistant Clinical Professor of Pharmacy, School of Pharmacy, University of California, San Francisco, San Diego Program; Assistant Director, San Diego Division, California Poison Control System, University of California San Diego Medical Center. Chapter 103, *Poison Control*

Ajai Chaudhary, MPharm, PhD / Head, Drug Disposition, Lilly Research Laboratories, Eli Lilly & Co. Chapter 34, *Instrumental Methods of Analysis*

Amy Christopher, MS / Assistant Professor of Information Science and Web Manager, University of the Sciences in Philadelphia. Chapter 8, *Information Resources in Pharmacy and the Pharmaceutical Sciences*

Michael M Crowley, PhD / Vice President, Drug Delivery Technology and Manufacturing Services, PharmaForm, LLC. Chapter 39, *Solutions, Emulsions, Suspensions, and Extracts*

Ara H DerMarderosian, PhD / Professor of Pharmacognosy; Research Professor of Medicinal Chemistry, University of the Sciences in Philadelphia. Chapter 7, *Pharmacists and Public Health*; Chapter 49, *Biotechnology and Drugs*; Chapter 93, *Pesticides*; Chapter 132, *Complementary and Alternative Medical Health Care*

Xuan Ding, PhD / School of Pharmacy, University of Wisconsin-Madison. Chapter 47, *Extended-Release and Targeted Drug Delivery Systems*

Clarence A Discher, PhD / Deceased. Chapter 24, *Inorganic Pharmaceutical Chemistry*

William R Doucette, PhD / Associate Professor, Director for the Center to Improve Medication Use in the Community, College of Pharmacy, The University of Iowa. Chapter 116, *Marketing Pharmaceutical Care Services*

Teresa Pete Dowling, PharmD / Director, Promotional Regulatory Affairs, AstraZeneca LP. Chapter 5, *Pharmacists in Industry*

G L Drusano, MD / Co-Director, Ordway Research Institute. Chapter 63, *Pharmacokinetics/Pharmacodynamics in Drug Development*

John E Enders, PhD, MBA / Director of Quality Assurance, Delmont Laboratories, Swarthmore, PA. Chapter 51, *Quality Assurance and Control*

Sharon Murphy Enright, MBA, RPh / President, Envision Change, LLC, New Berlin, WI. Chapter 102, *Providing a Framework for Ensuring Medication Use Safety*

Donald O Fedder, DrPH, FAPhA, BOCO / Professor, Pharmaceutical Health Services Research and Epidemiology and Preventive Medicine, University of Maryland Schools of Pharmacy and Medicine. Chapter 110, *Health Accessories*

Bill G Felkey, MS / Professor, Pharmacy Care Systems, Harrison School of Pharmacy, Auburn University. Chapter 95, *Technology and Automation*

Linda A Felton, PhD / Associate Professor of Pharmaceutics, College of Pharmacy, University of New Mexico Health Sciences Center. Chapter 37, *Powders;* Chapter 48, *The New Drug Approval Process and Clinical Trial Design*

Joseph L Fink III, BS Pharm, JD / Vice President for Corporate Relations and Economic Outreach; Professor of Pharmacy, College of Pharmacy, University of Kentucky. Chapter 1, *Scope of Pharmacy;* Chapter 111, *Laws Governing Pharmacy*

Michael R Franklin, PhD / Professor, Department of Pharmacology and Toxicology, University of Utah. Chapter 57, *Drug Absorption, Action, and Disposition;* Chapter 91, *Enzymes*

Donald N Franz, PhD / Professor Emeritus, Department of Pharmacology and Toxicology, University of Utah. Chapter 57, *Drug Absorption, Action, and Disposition*

Raymond E Galinsky, PharmD / Professor of Pharmaceutics, School of Pharmacy and Pharmacal Sciences, Purdue University. Chapter 58, *Basic Pharmacokinetics and Pharmacodynamics*

Daniele K Gelone, PharmD / Assistant Professor of Clinical Pharmacy, Department of Pharmacy Practice and Pharmacy Administration, Philadelphia College of Pharmacy, University of the Sciences in Philadelphia. Chapter 87, *Immunoactive Drugs*

Steven P Gelone, PharmD / Consultant, AGE Consultants, Wyndmoor, PA. Chapter 88, *Parasiticides;* Chapter 89, *Immunizing Agents;* Chapter 90, *Anti-Infectives*

Alfonso R Gennaro, PhD / Emeritus Professor, Department of Chemistry and Biochemistry, University of the Sciences in Philadelphia. Chapter 25, *Organic Pharmaceutical Chemistry*

Doug Geraets, PharmD, FCCP, BCPS / Clinical Pharmacy Specialist-Ambulatory Care, Iowa City VA Medical Center; Adjunct Associate Professor, Clinical and Administrative Pharmacy, College of Pharmacy, The University of Iowa. Chapter 121, *Pharmacists and Disease State Management*

Steven J Gilbert, RPh, PharmD(c) / excelleRx Inc., Philadelphia, PA. Chapter 4, *The Practice of Community Pharmacy*

Martin C Gregory, BM, BCh, DPhil / Professor of Medicine, Division of Nephrology, University of Utah School of Medicine. Chapter 56, *Diseases: Manifestations and Pathophysiology*

Pardeep K Gupta, PhD / Associate Professor, Philadelphia College of Pharmacy, University of the Sciences in Philadelphia. Chapter 16, *Solutions and Phase Equilibria;* Chapter 27, *Drug Nomenclature USAN*

Amy Marie Haddad, PhD / Professor, School of Pharmacy and Health Professions, Creighton University. Chapter 84, *Application of Ethical Principles to Practice Dilemmas*

Dennis D Hager, RPh, PharmD(c) / excelleRx Inc., Philadelphia, PA. Chapter 4, *The Practice of Community Pharmacy*

Donald E Hagman PhD / Vice President, Scientific Affairs, CardinalHealth, Inc. Chapter 40, *Sterilization*

William A Hess, BSc Pharm / Captain and Pharmacist Director, FDA Center Consultant, United States Public Health Service. Chapter 6, *Pharmacists in Government*

Gregory J Higby, PhD / Director, American Institute of the History of Pharmacy, School of Pharmacy, University of Wisconsin-Madison. Chapter 2, *Evolution of Pharmacy*

James R Hildebrand III, BS, PharmD / Director of Clinical Pharmacy, Alfred I du Pont Hospital for Children. Chapter 9, *Clinical Drug Literature*

William B Hladik III, MS, FASHP, FAPhA / Associate Professor of Pharmacy Practice, College of Pharmacy, University of New Mexico and Director, Australian Radiopharmacy Network, Bristol-Myers Squibb Medical Imaging, Melbourne, Victoria, Australia. Chapter 29, *Fundamentals of Medical Radionuclides*

Marlon Honeywell, PharmD / Associate Professor of Pharmacy Practice, College of Pharmacy, Florida A&M University. Chapter 125, *Diagnostic Self-Care*

John E Hoover, BSc Pharm, RPh / Consultant, Biomedical Communications. Chapter 66, *Gastrointestinal and Liver Drugs;* Chapter 69, *Respiratory Drugs;* Chapter 74, *Skeletal Muscle Relaxants;* Chapter 76, *Uterine and Antimigraine Drugs;* Chapter 81, *Antiepileptic Drugs;* Chapter 84, *Histamine and Antihistaminic Drugs*

Daniel A Hussar, PhD / Remington Professor of Pharmacy, Philadelphia College of Pharmacy, University of the Sciences in Philadelphia. Chapter 98, *Patient Compliance* and Chapter 104, *Drug Interactions*

Michael F Imperato, PharmD / excelleRx Inc., Philadelphia, PA. Chapter 4, *The Practice of Community Pharmacy*

Matthew K Ito, PharmD, FCCP, BCPS / Professor and Vice Chair of Pharmacy Practice, TJ Long School of Pharmacy and Health Sciences, University of the Pacific; Director, Cardiac Rehabilitation Cholesterol Clinic, San Diego VA Healthcare System. Chapter 121, *Pharmacists and Disease State Management*

Timothy J Ives, PharmD, MPH, BCPS, FCCP / Associate Professor of Pharmacy and Medicine, School of Pharmacy, University of North Carolina at Chapel Hill. Chapter 7, *Pharmacists and Public Health*

Rajni Jani, PhD / Senior Director, Department of Pharmaceutics, Alcon Research, Ltd. Chapter 43, *Ophthalmic Preparations*

Tara M Jenkins, MS, PharmD / Assistant Professor of Pharmacy Practice, School of Pharmacy, Hampton University. Chapter 125, *Diagnostic Self-Care*

Steven B Johnson, PharmD / Division of Pharmaceutical Evaluation II, Food and Drug Administration, Rockville, MD. Chapter 53, *Bioavailability and Bioequivalency Testing*

Robert Jordan, PharmD Candidate / College of Pharmacy–Glendale, Midwestern University. Chapter 26, *Natural Products*

Calvin H Knowlton, RPh, MDiv, PhD, FACA / excelleRx Inc., Philadelphia, PA. Chapter 4, *The Practice of Community Pharmacy*

David J Kroll, PhD / Senior Research Pharmacologist, Natural Products Laboratory, Research Triangle Institute (RTI). Chapter 49, *Biotechnology and Drugs*

Vijay Kumar, MS, MBA / Chief Operating Officer, Acura Pharmaceuticals. Chapter 35, *Dissolution*

John C Lang, PhD / Director of Emerging Technologies, Alcon Research, Ltd. Chapter 43, *Ophthalmic Preparations*

Arthur J Lawrence, PhD, RPh / Rear Admiral and Assistant Surgeon General, Deputy Assistant Secretary for Health Operations, United States Public Health Service. Chapter 6, *Pharmacists in Government*

Eric J Lien, PhD / Professor of Pharmacy/Pharmaceutics and Biomedicinal Chemistry, School of Pharmacy, University of Southern California. Chapter 13, *Molecular Structure, Properties, and States of Matter*

Hetty A Lima, RPh, FASHP / Vice President, Marketing, Caremark, Inc. Chapter 130, *Aseptic Processing for Home Infusion Pharmaceuticals*

Sylvia H Liu, BVM, DACVP / Vice President, Research and Development, ETHICON, Somerville, NJ. Chapter 109, *Surgical Supplies*

Stan G Louie, PharmD / Associate Professor of Pharmacy, University of Southern California. Chapter 60, *Principles of Immunology*

Eva Lydick, PhD / Chief Research Officer, Lovelace Clinic Foundation. Chapter 118, *Pharmaceutical Risk Management*

Elaine Mackowiak, PhD, RPh / Professor of Pharmaceutical Chemistry (School of Pharmacy) and Clinical Associate Professor of Diagnostic Imaging (School of Medicine), Temple University. Chapter 64, *Diagnostic Drugs and Reagents*

Henry J Malinowski, PhD / Division of Pharmaceutical Evaluation II, Food and Drug Administration, Rockville, MD. Chapter 53, *Bioavailability and Bioequivalency Testing*

Michael A Mancano, PharmD / Associate Professor of Clinical Pharmacy, Temple University School of Pharmacy. Chapter 77, *Hormones and Hormone Antagonists*

Laura A Mandos, BS, PharmD / Associate Professor of Clinical Pharmacy, Philadelphia College of Pharmacy, University of the Sciences in Philadelphia. Chapter 80, *Antianxiety Agents and Hypnotic Drugs*

Anthony S Manoguerra, PharmD / Professor of Clinical Pharmacy, School of Pharmacy, University of California, San Francisco, San Diego Program; Director, San Diego Division, California Poison Control System, University of California San Diego Medical Center. Chapter 103, *Poison Control*

Robert W Martin III, MD / Chairman, Department of Dermatology; Chief, Division of Dermatopathology, Arnett Clinic, Lafayette, Indiana; Clinical Assistant Professor, Department of Dermatology, Indiana University School of Medicine. Chapter 133, *Chronic Wound Care*

Robert L McCarthy, PhD / Dean and Professor, School of Pharmacy, University of Connecticut. Chapter 3, *Ethics and Professionalism*

Michael R McConnell, RPh / Founder and Consultant, National Notification Center. Chapter 115, *Product Recalls and Withdrawals*

Randal P McDonough, PharmD, MS / Associate Professor (Clinical), Director of Practice Development and Educational Programs, College of Pharmacy, The University of Iowa. Chapter 116, *Marketing Pharmaceutical Care Services*

William F McGhan, PharmD, PhD / Professor of Pharmacy and Health Policy, Department of Pharmacy Practice and Pharmacy Administration, Philadelphia College of Pharmacy, University of the Sciences in Philadelphia. Chapter 113, *Pharmacoeconomics*

Howard L McLeod, PharmD / Associate Professor, Department of Medicine, Washington University School of Medicine. Chapter 62, *Pharmacogenomics*

Mary Lynn McPherson, PharmD / Associate Professor, Pharmacy Practice and Science Department, School of Pharmacy, University of Maryland. Chapter 110, *Health Accessories*

Thomas Medwick, PhD / Emeritus Professor of Pharmaceutical Chemistry, School of Pharmacy, Rutgers University. Chapter 24, *Inorganic Pharmaceutical Chemistry*

Robert Middleton, PharmD / Department of Pharmacy, Beebe Medical Center, Lewes, DE. Chapter 61, *Adverse Drug Reactions Clinical Toxicology*

Michael Montagne, PhD / Professor of Social Pharmacy, Massachusetts College of Pharmacy—Boston. Chapter 3, *Ethics and Professionalism* and Chapter 99, *Drug Education*

Louis A Morris, PhD / President, Louis A Morris and Associates, Inc. Chapter 118, *Pharmaceutical Risk Management*

Michael D Murray, PharmD, MPH / Professor and Chair, Pharmaceutical Policy and Evaluative Sciences, School of Pharmacy, The University of North Carolina at Chapel Hill. Chapter 108, *Pharmacoepidemiology*

Gail D Newton, PhD, RPh / Associate Professor of Pharmacy Practice, School of Pharmacy and Pharmacal Sciences, Purdue University. Chapter 123, *Ambulatory Patient Care*

Jeffrey P Norenberg, MS, PharmD, BCNP, FASHP, FAPhA / Associate Professor and Director, Radiopharmaceutical Sciences, College of Pharmacy, University of New Mexico Health Sciences Center. Chapter 29, *Fundamentals of Medical Radionuclides*

Robert E O'Connor, PhD / Senior Director, European Technical Operations, Janssen Pharmaceutica. Chapter 37, *Powders*

Judith A O'Donnell, MD / Associate Professor of Medicine and Public Health, Drexel University Schools of Medicine and Public Health. Chapter 90, *Anti-Infectives*

Patrick B O'Donnell, PhD / Associate Director of Product Development, Neurocrine Biosciences, Inc. Chapter 52, *Stability of Pharmaceutical Products*

Clyde M Ofner III, PhD / Associate Professor and Director, Graduate Program in Pharmaceutics, Philadelphia College of Pharmacy, University of the Sciences in Philadelphia. Chapter 21, *Colloidal Dispersions*

Carol Ott, PharmD, BCPP / Affiliate Assistant Professor of Pharmacy Practice, School of Pharmacy, Purdue University. Chapter 129, *Long-Term Care*

James A Palmieri, PharmD / Assistant Professor of Pharmacy Practice, TJ Long School of Pharmacy and Health Sciences, University of the Pacific; Clinical Pharmacy Specialist, Cardiovascular Disease Management, The Mercy Heart Institute, Sacramento, CA. Chapter 121, *Pharmacists and Disease State Management*

Susie H Park, PharmD / Assistant Professor of Clinical Pharmacy, University of Southern California. Chapter 60, *Principles of Immunology*

John H Parker, PhD / President, Tech Manage Associates, Clarks Summit, PA. Chapter 51, *Quality Assurance and Control*

Payal Patel, BSc (Pharm), PharmD / Evidence-Based Pharmacy Consultant, London Health Sciences Centre, London, Ontario, Canada. Chapter 128, *Emergency Medicine Pharmacy Practice*

Garnet E Peck, PhD / Professor Emeritus of Industrial and Physical Pharmacy, School of Pharmacy and Pharmacal Sciences, Purdue University. Chapter 36, *Separation*

Thomas G Pettinger, BSP, BOCO / Staff Orthotist, Great Plains Health Company, Fargo, North Dakota. Chapter 110, *Health Accessories*

Peggy Piascik, PhD / Associate Professor of Pharmacy - Practice, University of Kentucky. Chapter 97, *Patient Communication*

James A Ponto, MS, BCNP / Chief Nuclear Pharmacist and Professor (Clinical), University of Iowa Hospitals & Clinics and College of Pharmacy University of Iowa. Chapter 106, *Nuclear Pharmacy Practice*

Cathy Y Poon, PharmD / Associate Professor of Clinical Pharmacy Philadelphia College of Pharmacy, University of the Sciences in Philadelphia. Chapter 18, *Tonicity, Osmoticity, Osmolality, and Osmolarity*; Chapter 32, *Clinical Analysis*

Stuart C Porter, PhD / President, PPT, Hatfield, PA. Chapter 46, *Coating of Pharmaceutical Dosage Forms*

W Steven Pray, BS (Pharm), MPH, PhD / Bernhardt Professor of Nonprescription Drugs and Devices, College of Pharmacy, Southwestern Oklahoma State University. Chapter 124, *Self-Care*

Shelly J Prince, PhD / Associate Professor of Pharmaceutics, College of Pharmacy, Southwestern Oklahoma State University. Chapter 11, *Metrology and Pharmaceutical Calculations*

Barrett E Rabinow, PhD / Senior Director, Strategic Technical Development, Baxter Healthcare Corporation, Round Lake, IL. Chapter 54, *Plastic Packaging Materials*

Galen W Radebaugh, PhD / Vice President of Analytical Development, Schering-Plough Research Institute. Chapter 38, *Property-Based Drug Design and Preformulation*

Robert B Raffa, PhD / Professor of Pharmacology, Temple University School of Pharmacy. Chapter 83, *Analgesic, Antipyretic, and Anti-Inflammatory Drugs*

Dennis W Raisch, RPh, PhD / Associate Center Director, Scientific Affairs, VA Cooperative Studies Program Clinical Research Pharmacy Coordinating Center, Albuquerque. Chapter 48, *The New Drug Approval Process and Clinical Trial Design*

William J Reilly, Jr, RPh, MBA / Managing Consultant, Tunnell Consulting, King of Prussia, PA. Chapter 55, *Pharmaceutical Necessities*

June E Riedlinger, RPh, PharmD / Adjunct Associate Professor, Southwest College of Naturopathic Medicine and Adjunct Associate Professor of Pharmacy Practice, School of Pharmacy—Boston, Massachusetts College of Pharmacy and Health Sciences. Chapter 132, *Complementary and Alternative Medical Health Care*

Joseph R Robinson, PhD / Professor of Pharmacy and Ophthalmology, School of Pharmacy, University of Wisconsin-Madison. Chapter 47, *Extended-Release and Targeted Drug Delivery Systems*

Mark G Robson, PhD, MPH / Chairman, Environmental and Occupational Health, UMDNJ School of Public Health. Chapter 93, *Pesticides*

Robert E Roehrs, PhD / Vice President (Retired), Department of Drug Regulatory Affairs, Alcon Research, Ltd. Chapter 43, *Ophthalmic Preparations*

Lisa Cencia Rohan, PhD / Assistant Professor of Pharmaceutical Sciences, School of Pharmacy, University of Pittsburgh. Chapter 23, *Rheology*

Theodore J Roseman, PhD / Vice President, Scientific Affairs, Baxter Healthcare Corporation, Round Lake, IL. Chapter 54, *Plastic Packaging Material*

Joseph T Rubino, PhD / Principal Research Scientist, Chemical and Pharmaceutical Development, Wyeth Research. Chapter 22, *Coarse Dispersions*

Orapin P Rubino, PhD / Group Leader, Formulation Development, Glatt Air Techniques, Inc. Chapter 22, *Coarse Dispersions*

Charles Ruchalski, PharmD / Assistant Professor of Clinical Pharmacy, School of Pharmacy, Temple University. Chapter 77, *Hormones and Hormone Antagonists*

Maria I Rudis, PharmD / Director, Emergency Medicine/Critical Care Pharmacy Residency Program; Assistant Professor of Clinical Pharmacy and Emergency Medicine, University of Southern California. Chapter 128, *Emergency Medicine Pharmacy Practice*

Edward M Rudnic, PhD / President and Chief Executive Officer, Advancis Pharmaceutical Corp. Chapter 45, *Oral Solid Dosage Forms*

Michael T Rupp, PhD, RPh / Professor of Pharmacy Administration, College of Pharmacy, Midwestern University–Glendale. Chapter 117, *Documenting, Billing, and Reimbursement for Pharmaceutical Care Services*

Mandip Singh Sachdeva, PhD / Professor of Pharmaceutics, College of Pharmacy, Florida A&M University. Chapter 33, *Chromatography*

Roger Schnaare, PhD / Professor Emeritus of Pharmacy, Philadelphia College of Pharmacy, University of the Sciences in Philadelphia; Senior Pharmaceutics Fellow, Biosyn Inc. Chapter 11, *Metrology and Pharmaceutical Calculations* and Chapter 23, *Rheology*

Jean M Scholtz, BS, PharmD, BCPS / Associate Professor of Clinical Pharmacy, Department of Pharmacy Practice, Philadelphia College of Pharmacy, University of the Sciences in Philadelphia. Chapter 86, *Antineoplastic Drugs*

Hans Schott, PhD / Professor Emeritus of Pharmaceutics and Colloidal Chemistry, Temple University. Chapter 21, *Colloidal Dispersions*

Joseph B Schwartz, PhD / Burroughs-Wellcome Fund Professor of Pharmaceutics, Director of Industrial Pharmacy Research, Philadelphia College of Pharmacy, University of

the Sciences in Philadelphia. Chapter 37, *Powders;* Chapter 45, *Oral Solid Dosage Forms*

Christopher J Sciarra, MS (Industrial Pharmacy) / Vice President, Sciarra Laboratories, Inc, Chapter 50, *Aerosols*

John J Sciarra, PhD / President, Sciarra Laboratories, Inc. Chapter 50, *Aerosols*

Bruce E Scott, MS / Chief Operating Officer, McKesson Medication Management, Brooklyn Park, MN. Chapter 127, *Hospital Pharmacy Practice*

Steven A Scott, PharmD / Associate Professor of Pharmacy Practice, School of Pharmacy, Purdue University. Chapter 101, *The Prescription*

Bonnie L Senst, MS / Director of Pharmacy, Mercy and Unity Hospitals, Fridley, MN. Chapter 127, *Hospital Pharmacy Practice*

Nancy L Shapiro, PharmD, BCPS / Clinical Assistant Professor and Pharmacotherapist in Ambulatory Care, Department of Pharmacy Practice, University of Illinois at Chicago College of Pharmacy. Chapter 126, *Preventive Care*

Stanley M Shaw, PhD / Professor and Head, Division of Nuclear Pharmacy, School of Pharmacy and Pharmacal Sciences, Purdue University. Chapter 106, *Nuclear Pharmacy Practice*

Amy Heck Sheehan, PharmD / Associate Professor of Pharmacy Practice, Purdue University School of Pharmacy and Pharmacal Sciences. Chapter 100, *Professional Communications*

Joel Shuster, PharmD, BCPP / Professor of Clinical Pharmacy, Temple University School of Pharmacy. Chapter 82, *Psychopharmacologic Agents*

Gurkeerat Singh, MPharm, PhD / Principle Research Scientist, Lilly Research Laboratories, Eli Lilly & Co. Chapter 34, *Instrumental Methods of Analysis*

Dara Bultman Sitter, PhD, RPh / Staff Pharmacist, Consumer Prescription Center, Appleton, WI. Chapter 96, *The Patient: Behavioral Determinants*

Raymond D Skwierczynski, PhD / Director of Formulation Science, Millennium Pharmaceuticals, Cambridge, MA. Chapter 30, *Analysis of Medicinals*

Karen E Smith, MS, RPh, CPHQ / Envision Change, LLC, New Berlin, WI. Chapter 102, *Providing a Framework for Ensuring Medication Use Safety*

Gail Goodman Snitkoff, PhD / Associate Professor, Division of Basic and Pharmaceutical Sciences, Albany College of Pharmacy. Chapter 31, *Biological Testing*

Gregory A Stephenson, PhD / Research Advisor, Lilly Research Laboratories, Eli Lilly & Co. Chapter 34, *Instrumental Methods of Analysis*

Michael B Strong, MD / Assistant Professor of Medicine, University of Utah Hospital. Chapter 56, *Diseases: Manifestations and Pathophysiology*

Bonnie L Svarstad, PhD / Professor Emerita of Social Pharmacy, School of Pharmacy, University of Wisconsin–Madison. Chapter 96, *The Patient: Behavioral Determinants*

Craig K Svensson, PharmD, PhD / Lyle & Sharon Bighley Professor in Pharmaceutical Sciences, College of Pharmacy, The University of Iowa. Chapter 58, *Basic Pharmacokinetics and Pharmacodynamics*

James Swarbrick, DSc, PhD / President, PharmaceuTech. Chapter 22, *Coarse Dispersions*

Timothy W Synold, PharmD / Assistant Professor, Department of Medical Oncology, City of Hope Comprehensive Cancer Center. Chapter 62, *Pharmacogenomics*

Robert L Talbert, PharmD, BCPS, FCCP / Professor and Division Head, Division of Pharmacotherapy, College of Pharmacy, The University of Texas at Austin; Professor of Pharmacology and Medicine, The University of Texas Health Science Center at San Antonio. Chapter 120, *Specialization in Pharmacy Practice*

Mathew Thambi, PharmD, BCPS / Clinical Assistant Professor, College of Pharmacy, University of Illinois at Chicago. Chapter 133, *Chronic Wound Care*

Mark Thomas, MS / Director of Pharmacy, Children's Hospitals and Clinics, Minneapolis, MN. Chapter 127, *Hospital Pharmacy Practice*

Mark A Touchette, PharmD, BCPS / Sr. Manager, Inpatient Pharmacy Services, Henry Ford Hospital, Detroit, MI. Chapter 119, *Integrated Health Care Delivery Systems*

Salvatore J Turco, PharmD, FASHP / Professor of Pharmacy, Temple University School of Pharmacy. Chapter 42, *Intravenous Admixtures*

Deepika Vadher, PharmD, BCPS / Assistant Professor of Clinical Pharmacy, Philadelphia College of Pharmacy and Science, University of the Sciences in Philadelphia. Chapter 122, *Development of a Pharmacy Care Plan and Patient Problem Solving*

Jesse C Vivian, BS Pharm, JD / Professor of Pharmacy Law, Department of Pharmacy Practice, Eugene Applebaum College of Pharmacy and Health Sciences, Wayne State University. Chapter 111, *Laws Governing Pharmacy*

Ronnie A Weathermon, PharmD / Clinical Education Consultant, Pfizer Inc. Chapter 131, *The Pharmacist's Role in Substance Use Disorders*

Maria L Webb, PhD / VP Drug Discovery, Pharmacopeia, Inc. Chapter 10, *Research*

Timothy S Wiedmann, PhD / Professor of Pharmaceutics, College of Pharmacy, University of Minnesota. Chapter 15, *Thermodynamics*

Rodney J Wigent, PhD / Professor of Chemistry, Research Professor of Pharmaceutics; Dean, College of Graduate Studies, University of the Sciences in Philadelphia. Chapter 19, *Chemical Kinetics*

Lori A Wilken, PharmD, CDE, AE-C / Clinical Assistant Professor, College of Pharmacy, University of Illinois at Chicago. Chapter 131, *The Pharmacist's Role in Substance Use Disorders*

Susan R Winkler, PharmD, BCPS / Clinical Associate Professor, College of Pharmacy, University of Illinois at Chicago. Chapter 131, *The Pharmacist's Role in Substance Use Disorders*

Michael E Winter, PharmD / Professor of Clinical Pharmacy, School of Pharmacy, University of California San Francisco. Chapter 59, *Clinical Pharmacokinetics and Pharmacodynamics*

Anna M Wodlinger, PharmD, BCPS / Assistant Professor of Clinical Pharmacy, Temple University School of Pharmacy. Chapter 68, *Cardiovascular Drugs*

Olivia Bennett Wood, MPH, RD / Associate Professor of Foods and Nutrition, School of Consumer and Family Sciences, Purdue University. Chapter 107, *Nutrition in Pharmacy Practice*

Barbara J Zarowitz, PharmD, FCCP, BCPS / Vice President, Pharmacy Care Management, Henry Ford Health System, Detroit, MI. Chapter 119, *Integrated Health Care Delivery Systems*

Randy J Zauhar, PhD / Associate Professor of Biochemistry, Department of Chemistry & Biochemistry, University of the Sciences in Philadelphia. Chapter 28, *Structure–Activity Relationship and Drug Design*

Preface to the Twenty-First Edition

For over 100 years and throughout 20 previous editions, *Remington: The Science and Practice of Pharmacy* has stood as the definitive text and reference source of all aspects of the science and practice of pharmacy. In this new edition, you will find a text that is practice-oriented while maintaining its traditionally reliable coverage of scientific aspects. The 21st edition keeps pace with the changes in pharmacy curriculum and professional pharmacy practice in general.

In the years since the first publication of *Remington's Pharmaceutical Sciences*, there have been many changes in the field of pharmacy and pharmacy practice. Although this edition of *Remington* maintains the general philosophy of previous editions, several changes have been made to present fresh and new information and to take advantage of the advances made in recent years. Each section of the book has been critically reviewed and revised to reflect the emerging trends in the field. The overall organization of the book is the same as the previous editions.

The biggest change in the 21st edition is in the *Pharmacy Practice* section. This section has been reorganized and expanded to reflect the changing realities of comtemporary practice. The integration of new scientific information into clinical practice is often difficult, and one of the key purposes of this section is to help clinicians translate these scientific advances into clinical practice and care of patients. This section brings the reader up to date on the latest trends and approaches. New chapters have been added that cover the areas of:

- The application of ethical principles to practice dilemmas
- Statistics applied to pharmacy practice
- Technology and automation
- Professional communication
- Medication errors
- Re-engineering pharmacy practice
- Management of special risk medicines
- Specialization of pharmacy practice
- Disease state management
- Emergency patient care
- Wound care

The *Pharmaceutical and Medicinal Agents* section is the most very useful part of the book in terms of core drug information. For this edition, we've added more than 100 new drug monographs, and the previously existing material has been up-dated. We realize that this is a section that is nearly impossible to keep current, and we've tried to include as many new drugs as possible. Because of space constraints, we were limited to the most important or most widely used drugs.

Another significant addition to this edition is the expansion of the *Pharmacodynamics and Pharmacokinetics* section to include the new, growing area of Pharmacogenomics. This chapter highlights many of the important advances including: practical applications and technological considerations, molecular diagnostics for optimizing drug therapy, and pharmacogenomics and drug development.

Many people were involved in creating this edition. I am grateful to all the Section Editors and authors for their skillful review of the literature and for incorporating their own unique perspectives and experience into their chapters. With this edition, we welcome five new Section Editors. They represent a wide geographic diversity and spectrum of experience. We also have approximately 100 new authors who represent over 32 universities as well as positions in governmental agencies and private industry.

I also gratefully acknowledge the extensive contributions of the authors and Section Editors of previous editions of *Remington* for laying the foundation for the current volume. I recognize that we all stand upon the shoulders of giants and are supported by those leaders who taught and inspired many previous generations.

I especially thank Alfonso R Gennaro, PhD for his continued support. Dr. Gennaro was *Remington* editor for the past four editions. No one is more familiar with *Remington* than he is. Dr. Gennaro has been instrumental in the creation and review of the drug monographs. Ensuring scientific accuracy is critical in a book such as *Remington*, and he has been very generous with his time and expertise in this area.

A heartfelt thanks also goes to Mr. John Hoover, author and indexer, who has been involved with *Remington* since the 1960s and has provided editorial guidance at every step of the process.

It is a pleasure and honor to work on a book with such a long and rich tradition.

Randy Hendrickson
Editor

Preface to 1st Edition

The rapid and substantial progress made in Pharmacy within the last decade has created a necessity for a work treating of the improved apparatus, the revised processes, and the recently introduced preparations of the age.

The vast advances made in theoretical and applied chemistry and physics have much to do with the development of pharmaceutical science, and these have been reflected in all the revised editions of the Pharmacopoeias which have been recently published. When the author was elected in 1874 to the chair of Theory and Practice of Pharmacy in the Philadelphia College of Pharmacy, the outlines of study which had been so carefully prepared for the classes by his eminent predecessors, Professor William Proctor, Jr, and Professor Edward Parrish, were found to be not strictly in accord, either in their arrangement of the subjects or in their method of treatment. Desiring to preserve the distinctive characteristics of each, an effort was at once made to frame a system which should embody their valuable features, embrace new subjects, and still retain that harmony of plan and proper sequence which are absolutely essential to the success of any system.

The strictly alphabetical classification of subjects which is now universally adopted by pharmacopoeias and dispensatories, although admirable in works of reference, presents an effectual stumbling block to the acquisition of pharmaceutical knowledge through systematic study; the vast accumulation of facts collected under each head arranged lexically, they necessarily have no connection with one another, and thus the saving of labor effected by considering similar groups together, and the value of the association of kindred subjects, are lost to the student. In the method of grouping the subjects which is herein adopted, the constant aim has been to arrange the latter in such a manner that the reader shall be gradually led from the consideration of elementary subjects to those which involve more advanced knowledge, whilst the groups themselves are so placed as to follow one another in a natural sequence.

The work is divided into six parts. Part I is devoted to detailed descriptions of apparatus and definitions and comments on general pharmaceutical processes.

The Official Preparations alone are considered in Part II. Due weight and prominence are thus given to the Pharmacopoeia, the National authority, which is now so thoroughly recognized.

In order to suit the convenience of pharmacists who prefer to *weigh solids* and *measure liquids*, the official formulas are expressed, in addition to parts by weight, in *avoirdupois weight* and *apothecaries' measure.* These equivalents are printed in *bold type* near the margin, and arranged so as to fit them for quick and accurate reference.

Part III treats of Inorganic Chemical Substances. Precedence is of course given to official preparation in these. The descriptions, solubilities, and tests for identity and impurities of each substance are systematically tabulated under its proper title. It is confidently believed that by this method of arrangement the valuable descriptive features of the Pharmacopoeia will be more prominently developed, read reference facilitated, and close study of the details rendered easy. Each chemical operation is accompanied by equations, whilst the reaction is, in addition, explained in words.

The Carbon Compounds, or Organic Chemical Substances, are considered in Part IV. These are naturally grouped according to the physical and medical properties of their principal constituents, beginning with simple bodies like cellulin, gum, etc, and progressing to the most highly organized alkaloids, etc.

Part V is devoted to Extemporaneous Pharmacy. Care has been taken to treat of the practice which would be best adapted for the needs of the many pharmacists who conduct operations upon a moderate scale, rather than for those of the few who manage very large establishments. In this, as well as in other parts of the work, operations are illustrated which are conducted by manufacturing pharmacists.

Part VI contains a formulary of Pharmaceutical Preparations which have not been recognized by the Pharmacopoeia. The recipes selected are chiefly those which have been heretofore rather difficult of access to most pharmacists, yet such as are likely to be in request. Many private formulas are embraced in the collection; and such of the preparations of the old Pharmacopoeias as have not been included in the new edition, but are still in use, have been inserted.

In conclusion, the author ventures to express the hope that the work will prove an efficient help to the pharmaceutical student as well as to the pharmacist and the physician. Although the labor has been mainly performed amidst the harassing cares of active professional duties, and perfection is known to be unattainable, no pains have been spared to discover and correct errors and omissions in the text. The author's warmest acknowledgments, are tendered to Mr A B Taylor, Mr Joseph McCreery, and Mr George M Smith for their valuable assistance in revising the proof sheets, and to the latter especially for his work on the index. The outline illustrations, by Mr John Collins, were drawn either from the actual objects or from photographs taken by the author.

Philadelphia, October, 1885   JPR

Contents

PART 1

Orientation

Ara DerMarderosian, PhD
Professor of Pharmacognosy
Research Professor of Medicinal Chemistry
University of the Sciences in Philadelphia
Philadelphia, PA

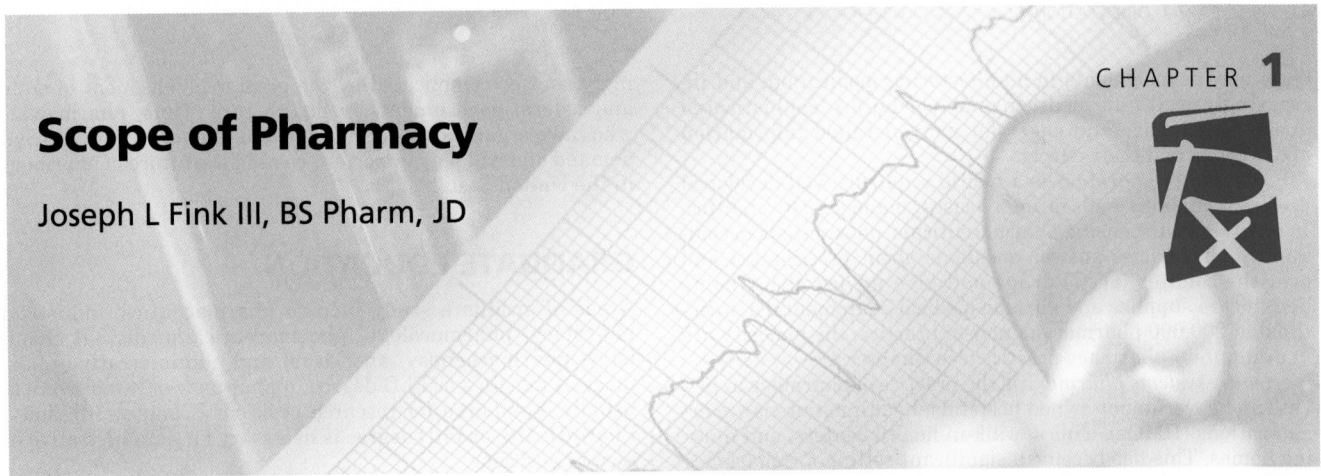

CHAPTER 1

Scope of Pharmacy

Joseph L Fink III, BS Pharm, JD

Pharmacy is the art and science of preparing and dispensing medications and the provision of drug-related information to the public. It involves the interpretation of prescription orders; the compounding, labeling, and dispensing of drugs and devices; drug product selection and drug utilization reviews; patient monitoring and intervention; and the provision of cognitive services related to use of medications and devices. The American Pharmacists Association describes the mission of pharmacy as serving society as "the profession responsible for the appropriate use of medications, devices, and services to achieve optimal therapeutic outcomes." The Report of the Commission of Pharmacy, *Pharmacists for the Future* (often referred to as the Millis Report), states that "pharmacy should be conceived basically as a knowledge system that renders a health service by concerning itself with understanding drugs and their effects." Thus, pharmaceutical care is a necessary element of total health care.

The current philosophy or approach to professional practice in pharmacy is designated as *pharmaceutical care*. This concept holds that the important role of the pharmacist is "the responsible provision of drug therapy for the purpose of achieving definite outcomes that improve a patient's quality of life." Pharmacists, then, are those who are educated and licensed to dispense drugs and to provide drug information—they are experts on medications. They are the most accessible member of today's health care team, and often are the first source of assistance and advice on many common ailments and health care matters.

EDUCATION

There is currently one professional degree in pharmacy: the doctorate (PharmD). The PharmD curriculum usually requires 6 academic years to complete the degree requirements. Pharmacists who hold the baccalaureate in pharmacy degree (BSPharm or BPharm) may be admitted to a doctor of pharmacy program, in which instance the combined period of study may be longer than 6 academic years. There are 87 colleges and schools of pharmacy in the United States (see www.aacp.org).

In 1992, the American Association of Colleges of Pharmacy (AACP) house of delegates voted "to support a single entry-level educational program at the doctoral level (PharmD)." The vote of the deans and faculty delegates affirmed their support of an entry-level program of at least 6 years. Perhaps even more importantly, the Accreditation Council for Pharmaceutical Education (ACPE), the national organization that accredits professional degree programs in pharmacy, has adopted that position as well. The transition from a two-degree approach (BSPharm and PharmD) to the current sole degree is now complete.

GENERAL EDUCATION—Courses in the social sciences, humanities, arts, history, and literature provide the broad general education required of a professional in today's society.

PREREQUISITE COURSES—Mathematics and the physical and biological sciences teach the principles, the application of which find their way into many of the upper-level professional pharmacy courses.

PROFESSIONAL COURSES—Basic to most pharmacy curricula are courses in pharmacology, medicinal chemistry, pharmaceutics, biopharmaceutics, and the clinical-pharmacy externships. Courses in social and administrative pharmacy as well as pharmacy law also are found in this sequence.

Opportunities for students to specialize or minor in certain professional areas have become more available and increasingly popular. Most prominent are hospital/institutional pharmacy, nuclear pharmacy, management, and various research specialties.

LICENSURE REQUIREMENTS

The practice of pharmacy in any given state is regulated by that state and the Board of Pharmacy within that state. The law in all states, including the District of Columbia and Puerto Rico, requires applicants for licensure to be of good moral character; have graduated from an Accreditation Council for Pharmaceutical Education (ACPE) accredited first professional degree program; have passed an examination given by the Board of Pharmacy; and be 21 years of age.

All states require that candidates for licensure have a record of practical experience or internship training acquired under the supervision and instruction of a licensed practitioner. Some jurisdictions grant licensure by licensure transfer, known colloquially as reciprocity. Requirements vary from state to state.

The vast majority of jurisdictions have established continuing education/competency requirements for relicensure. The types of programs that are recognized and the prescribed range of acceptable content matter are fairly uniform. The ACPE also has responsibility for accrediting providers of professional continuing education programming.

A list of the governmental agencies that license pharmacists in the various states is available from the National Association of Boards of Pharmacy, 700 Busse Highway, Park Ridge, IL 60068-2402 (see www.nabp.org).

CAREERS

Job opportunities for pharmacists are expected to grow about as fast as the average for all occupations, mainly due to the increased pharmaceutical needs of a larger and older population. Other factors likely to increase demand for pharmacists include the likelihood of scientific advances that will provide more drug products for the prevention, diagnosis, and treatment of disease; new developments in administering medication; and increasingly well-informed consumers who are sophisticated about health care and eager for more detailed information about drugs and their effects.

Community pharmacy is a hybrid requiring well-developed professional skills and, in many cases, management abilities. In addition to dispensing pharmaceuticals, pharmacists in community pharmacies answer questions about prescription and over-the-counter (OTC) drugs and give advice about home health care supplies and durable medical equipment. Of an estimated 200,000 pharmacists now in practice, the majority are in community pharmacy practice (see Chapter 4).

Health-systems pharmacy is the practice of pharmacy in private and government-owned hospitals, health maintenance organizations (HMOs), clinics, walk-in health centers, and nursing homes. This has become a significant setting for pharmacy practice over the past 50 years or so. In these settings, pharmacists dispense medication, prepare sterile solutions, advise other professionals and patients on the use of drugs, monitor drug regimens, and evaluate drug use. They advise other professionals on the selection and effects of drugs and, in some cases, make patient rounds with them or provide direct patient care (see Chapters 123, 127, and 129).

Nuclear pharmacy applies the principles and practices of pharmacy and nuclear chemistry to produce radioactive drugs used for diagnosis and therapy (see Chapters 29 and 106).

Industrial pharmacy offers opportunities to pharmacists of all educational levels. The largest number of pharmacists are involved in marketing and administration. Some pharmaceutical manufacturers employ pharmacists as their professional service representatives, to educate physicians and pharmacists about the manufacturer's products. This can be a rewarding career for persons with the right personality and motivation, and it is often a stepping-stone to supervisory positions in sales and a path toward integration into the administrative and sales structure of a pharmaceutical firm. Pharmacists with master's degrees in business or additional degrees in law find additional opportunities in the pharmaceutical industry in the marketing, sales, and legal departments. Pharmacists can also serve the industry as professional communications managers and clinical research scientists; research and development personnel often have advanced degrees, although this is not always the case. Production and quality-control (or quality-assurance) supervisory positions often are held by pharmacists (see Chapters 5 and 10).

Government service offers opportunities to pharmacists in various capacities. They may serve as noncommissioned or commissioned officers in the Army, Navy, Air Force, and Coast Guard. They also serve as commissioned officers in the United States Public Health Service, which furnishes pharmacists for the Food and Drug Administration, Bureau of Prisons, and the Indian Health Service. Appointments are available for pharmacists in the Drug Enforcement Administration of the Department of Justice, and in the National Institutes of Health, the Center for Medicare and Medicaid Services, the Health Resources and Services Administration, and various other agencies (see Chapter 6).

Pharmaceutical education offers opportunities to pharmacists with advanced degrees in any of the professional specialties. Expanding enrollments and changes in the curricula at colleges to meet the employment needs of the future result in an increased need for college-level instructors. Potentially higher salaries, more freedom for research and writing, independence of action, and the cultural surroundings in pharmaceutical education make teaching attractive.

Pharmaceutical journalism offers rewarding experiences for a limited number of pharmacists with writing and editing skills.

Organizational management careers are available for those with pharmacy education who wish to serve in national and state associations and on boards of pharmacy. The increasing number of pharmacists and the interface of pharmacy with insurance carriers and health and welfare agencies mean the responsibilities of associations and boards must expand accordingly, and be complicated by the greater involvement of state and federal governments in health care. Thus, pharmacists who have organizational interests and talents will be in great demand and will play important roles in the future of pharmacy in the United States.

GRADUATE EDUCATION

Areas of graduate study include pharmaceutics, industrial pharmacy, pharmacology, pharmaceutical/medicinal chemistry, pharmacognosy, and social and administrative pharmacy. A master's or PhD degree in pharmacy or a related field usually is required for research positions (Chapter 10), and a PharmD, MS, or PhD degree is necessary for administrative or faculty positions.

Although a number of graduates pursue advanced degrees in pharmacy, some enter a 1- or 2-year residency program or fellowship. A pharmacy residency is an organized, directed, postgraduate training program in a defined area of pharmacy practice.

ORGANIZATIONS

AMERICAN PHARMACISTS ASSOCIATION (APhA)— The APhA is the national professional organization of pharmacists representing pharmacy practitioners, and pharmaceutical scientists and students. Since its founding in 1852, APhA has been a leader in the professional and scientific advancement of pharmacy. Membership in one of the three academies of the APhA—the Academy of Pharmacy Practice and Management (APPM), the Academy of Pharmaceutical Research and Science (APRS), and the Academy of Students of Pharmacy (ASP)—offers members specialized benefits and the opportunity to influence their practice areas.

AMERICAN SOCIETY OF HEALTH-SYSTEM PHARMACISTS (ASHP)—The ASHP is the professional association of pharmacists who practice in organized health care settings. The ASHP endeavors to create an environment in which pharmacists can focus the full potential of their knowledge and expertise on patient care. The mission of ASHP is to represent its more than 25,000 members, providing leadership that will enable pharmacists in organized health-care settings to provide high-quality pharmaceutical services that foster the efficacy, safety, and cost-effectiveness of drug use; contribute to programs and services that emphasize the health needs of the public and the prevention of disease; and promote pharmacy as an essential component of the health care team.

AMERICAN SOCIETY OF CONSULTANT PHARMACISTS (ASCP)—The ASCP promotes the development and advancement of pharmaceutical care activities directed at patients in long-term care institutions.

NATIONAL COMMUNITY PHARMACISTS ASSOCIATION (NCPA)—Membership in NCPA, formerly known as the National Association of Retail Druggists (NARD), is open to independent community pharmacy owners, managers, and employees, as well as pharmacy students and corporations. NCPA is dedicated to the continuing growth and prosperity of the independent community pharmacy in the United States.

AMERICAN ASSOCIATION OF PHARMACEUTICAL SCIENTISTS (AAPS)—The AAPS serves an advocacy role for the pharmaceutical sciences, promotes the economic viability of the pharmaceutical sciences and its scientists, and represents scientific interests within academia, industry, government, and other research institutions. AAPS members are eligible for membership in one of several disciplinary sections: Analysis and Pharmaceutical Quality; Biotechnology; Clinical Sciences; Economic, Marketing, and Management Sciences; Medicinal and Natural Products Chemistry; Pharmaceutical Technology; Pharmaceutics and Drug Delivery; Pharmacokinetics, Pharmacodynamics, and Drug Metabolism; and Regulatory Affairs.

PHARMACY PROFESSIONAL DEGREE PROGRAMS

The following colleges and schools offering professional degree programs in pharmacy hold membership in the AACP.

Alabama	Auburn University, Harrison School of Pharmacy, Auburn University, AL 36849
	Samford University, McWhorter School of Pharmacy, Birmingham, AL 35229
Arizona	Midwestern University, College of Pharmacy-Glendale, Glendale, AZ 85308
	University of Arizona, College of Pharmacy, Tucson, AZ 85721
Arkansas	University of Arkansas for Medical Sciences, College of Pharmacy, Little Rock, AR 72205
California	University of California, San Francisco, School of Pharmacy, San Francisco, CA 94143
	University of the Pacific, Thomas J. Long School of Pharmacy and Health Sciences, Stockton, CA 95211
	University of Southern California, School of Pharmacy, Los Angeles, CA 90089
	Western University of the Health Sciences, College of Pharmacy, Pomona, CA 91766
	Loma Linda University, School of Pharmacy, Loma Linda, CA 92350
	University of California, San Diego, School of Pharmacy and Pharmaceutical Sciences, La Jolla, CA 92093
Colorado	University of Colorado, Health Sciences Center, School of Pharmacy, Denver, CO 80262
Connecticut	University of Connecticut, School of Pharmacy, Storrs, CT 06269
District of Columbia	Howard University, College of Pharmacy, Nursing and Allied Health Sciences, Washington, DC 20059
Florida	Florida Agricultural and Mechanical University, College of Pharmacy and Pharmaceutical Sciences, Tallahassee, FL 32307
	Nova Southeastern University, College of Pharmacy, Fort Lauderdale, FL 33328
	Palm Beach Atlantic University, School of Pharmacy, West Palm Beach, FL 33416
	University of Florida, College of Pharmacy, Gainesville, FL 32610
Georgia	Mercer University, Southern School of Pharmacy, Atlanta, GA 30341
	University of Georgia, College of Pharmacy, Athens, GA 30602
Idaho	Idaho State University, College of Pharmacy, Pocatello, ID 83209
Illinois	Midwestern University, Chicago College of Pharmacy, Downers Grove, IL 60515
	University of Illinois at Chicago, College of Pharmacy, Chicago, IL 60612
Indiana	Butler University, College of Pharmacy and Health Sciences, Indianapolis, IN 46208
	Purdue University School of Pharmacy and Pharmacal Sciences, West Lafayette, IN 47907
Iowa	Drake University, College of Pharmacy and Health Sciences, Des Moines, IA 50311
	University of Iowa, College of Pharmacy, Iowa City, IA 52242
Kansas	University of Kansas, School of Pharmacy, Lawrence, KS 66045
Kentucky	University of Kentucky, College of Pharmacy, Lexington, KY 40536
Louisiana	University of Louisiana at Monroe, School of Pharmacy, Monroe, LA 71209
	Xavier University of Louisiana, College of Pharmacy, New Orleans, LA 70125
Maryland	University of Maryland, School of Pharmacy, Baltimore, MD 21201
Massachusetts	Massachusetts College of Pharmacy and Health Sciences-Boston Campus, Boston, MA 02115
	Massachusetts College of Pharmacy and Health Sciences-Worcester Campus, Worcester, MA 01610
	Northeastern University, School of Pharmacy, Boston, MA 02115
Michigan	Ferris State University, College of Pharmacy, Big Rapids, MI 49307
	University of Michigan, College of Pharmacy, Ann Arbor, MI 48109
	Wayne State University, Eugene Applebaum College of Pharmacy and Health Sciences, Detroit, MI 48202
Minnesota	University of Minnesota, College of Pharmacy, Minneapolis, MN 55455
Mississippi	University of Mississippi, School of Pharmacy, University, MS 38655
Missouri	St Louis College of Pharmacy, St Louis, MO 63110
	University of Missouri-Kansas City, School of Pharmacy, Kansas City, MO 64110
Montana	University of Montana, School of Pharmacy and Allied Health Sciences, Missoula, MT 59812
Nebraska	Creighton University, School of Pharmacy and Health Professions, Omaha, NE 68178
	University of Nebraska Medical Center, College of Pharmacy, Omaha, NE 68198
Nevada	University of Southern Nevada, Henderson, NV 89014
New Jersey	Rutgers, the State University of New Jersey, Ernest Mario College of Pharmacy, Piscataway, NJ 08854
New Mexico	University of New Mexico, College of Pharmacy, Albuquerque, NM 87131
New York	Union University, Albany College of Pharmacy, Albany, NY 12208
	Long Island University, Arnold and Marie Schwartz College of Pharmacy and Health Sciences, Brooklyn, NY 11201
	St John's University, College of Pharmacy and Allied Health Professions, Jamaica, NY 11439
	State University of New York at Buffalo, School of Pharmacy and Pharmaceutical Sciences, Amherst, NY 14260
North Carolina	Campbell University, School of Pharmacy, Buies Creek, NC 27506
	University of North Carolina at Chapel Hill, School of Pharmacy, Chapel Hill, NC 27599
North Dakota	North Dakota State University, College of Pharmacy, Fargo, ND 58105
Ohio	Ohio Northern University, R.H. Raabe College of Pharmacy, Ada, OH 45810
	The Ohio State University, College of Pharmacy, Columbus, OH 43210
	University of Cincinnati, College of Pharmacy, Cincinnati, OH 45267
	University of Toledo, College of Pharmacy, Toledo, OH 43606
Oklahoma	Southwestern Oklahoma State University, School of Pharmacy, Weatherford, OK 73096
	University of Oklahoma, College of Pharmacy, Oklahoma City, OK 73190
Oregon	Oregon State University, College of Pharmacy, Corvallis, OR 97331
Pennsylvania	Duquesne University, Mylan School of Pharmacy, Pittsburgh, PA 15282
	Lake Erie College of Osteopathic Medicine, School of Pharmacy, Erie, PA 16509
	Temple University, School of Pharmacy, Philadelphia, PA 19140
	University of Pittsburgh, School of Pharmacy, Pittsburgh, PA 15261
	University of the Sciences in Philadelphia, Philadelphia College of Pharmacy, Philadelphia, PA 19104
	Wilkes University, Nesbitt School of Pharmacy, Wilkes-Barre, PA 18766
Puerto Rico	University of Puerto Rico, School of Pharmacy, San Juan, PR 00936

Rhode Island	University of Rhode Island, College of Pharmacy, Kingston, RI 02881	Utah	University of Utah, College of Pharmacy, Salt Lake City, UT 84112
South Carolina	Medical University of South Carolina, College of Pharmacy, Charleston, SC 29425	Virginia	Hampton University, School of Pharmacy, Hampton, VA 23668
	University of South Carolina, College of Pharmacy, Columbia, SC 29208		Shenandoah University, Bernard J Dunn School of Pharmacy, Winchester, VA 22601
South Dakota	South Dakota State University, College of Pharmacy, Brookings, SD 57007		Virginia Commonwealth University, School of Pharmacy, Richmond, VA 23298
Tennessee	University of Tennessee, Memphis, College of Pharmacy, Memphis, TN 38163	Washington	University of Washington, School of Pharmacy, Seattle, WA 98195
Texas	Texas Southern University, College of Pharmacy and Health Sciences, Houston, TX 77004		Washington State University, College of Pharmacy, Pullman, WA 99164
	Texas Tech University Health Sciences Center, School of Pharmacy, Amarillo, TX 79106	West Virginia	West Virginia University, School of Pharmacy, Morgantown, WV 26506
	University of Houston, College of Pharmacy, Houston, TX 77204	Wisconsin	University of Wisconsin-Madison, School of Pharmacy, Madison, WI 53705
	The University of Texas at Austin, College of Pharmacy, Austin, TX 78712	Wyoming	University of Wyoming, School of Pharmacy, Laramie, WY 82071

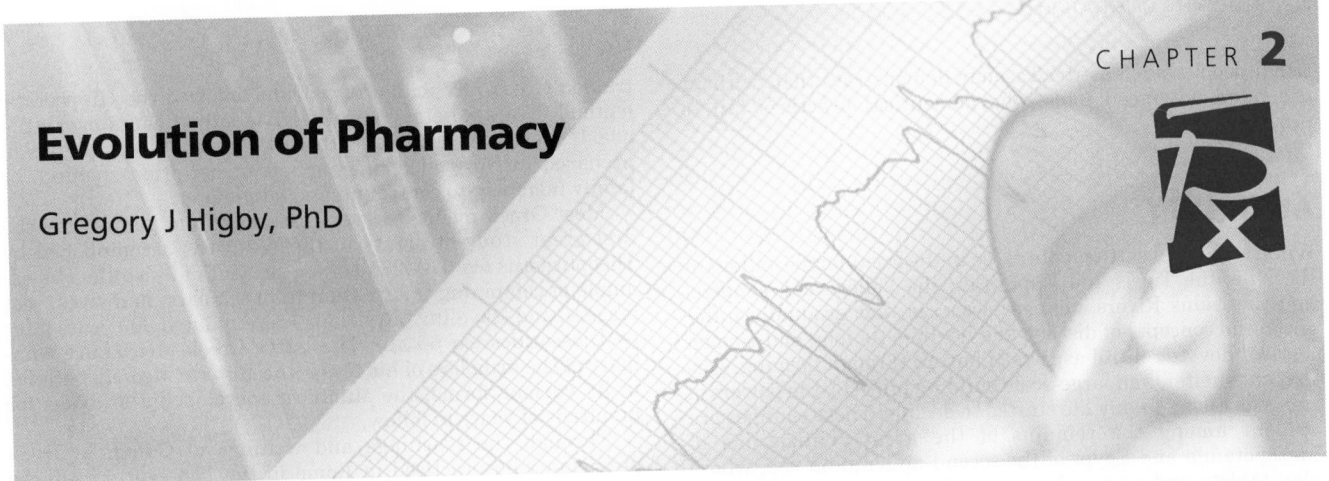

CHAPTER 2

Evolution of Pharmacy

Gregory J Higby, PhD

THE DRUG-TAKING ANIMAL

Among the several characteristics unique to *Homo sapiens* is our propensity to treat ailments, physical and mental, with medicines. From archeological evidence, this urge to soothe the burdens of disease is as old as humanity's search for other tools. Like the nodules of flint used to make knives and axes, medicines rarely occur in nature in their most useful (or palatable) form. First, the active ingredients or *drugs* must be collected, processed, and prepared for incorporation into medicaments. This activity, done since the dawn of humanity, is still the central focus of the practice of *pharmacy*. Put another way, pharmacy is, and has been, the art (and later science) of fashioning one of our most important tools—medicines.

For today's pharmacists it is imperative that this deep-seated role of medicines in human history is understood. As with other tools, drugs have been used to gain increased control over our lives, to make them better and longer. Over the millennia the understanding of how drugs work has changed dramatically, in part influencing how they are used (and abused). As is often the case with knowledge, however, common wisdom about medicines is a mixture of myth and science, folklore, and demonstrated fact. Old ideas meld with new concepts to produce a faulty jumble that can lead patients into trouble.

A basic introduction to the development of ideas concerning drugs, as well as the evolution of the profession, increases the ability of pharmacists to adjust to the challenges presented as our professional roles expand. As the dispensers of medicine, we have much to gain from a basic appreciation of the complex role that drugs and medicines have played in the past and of pharmacy's part in this development.

A complete world history of how increased drug knowledge, medical progress, commerce, technology, and professional development came together to produce modern pharmacy would fill this entire volume. Instead, this short chapter will tell two parallel stories: how the concept of *drug* evolved over time and how a separate profession arose to prepare drugs into medicines in the West.

Throughout history, drugs have held a special fascination. Beyond the sensational stories of the part drugs have played in exploration, commerce, political intrigue, scientific discovery, and the arts, they have directly influenced the lives of millions. Drugs such as insulin have kept thousands alive, and antibiotics and chemotherapeutic agents have saved thousands more. The simple fact that all medicines become useful through pharmacy bears repeating, and the safe and effective use of such medicines has developed recently into a primary concern for this relatively young profession. Although pharmacy as a skill is perhaps as old as the making of stone implements, the practice of this singular art by a recognized specialist is only about 1000 years old. For this specialization to occur a need had to arise—but that is getting a bit ahead of the story.

PREHISTORIC PHARMACY

Since humanity's earliest past, pharmacy has been a part of everyday life. Excavations of some of mankind's oldest settlements, such as Shanidar (*ca* 30,000 BCE), support the contention that prehistoric peoples gathered plants for medicinal purposes. By trial and error, the folk knowledge of the healing properties of certain natural substances grew. Although tribal healers or *shamans* often guarded this healing knowledge closely, the recognition of medicinal plants, which were sometimes used as food, spices, or charms, apparently was so widespread that it hindered any necessity for a special class of drug gatherers and keepers. The arts of primitive pharmacy probably were mastered by all who practiced the domestic medicine of the household.

When healers at Shanidar or other prehistoric settlements approached disease, they placed it within the context of their general understanding of the world around them, which was alive with good and evil spirits. Early peoples explained illness in supernatural terms, as they did the other changes and disasters surrounding them. Treatments followed suit, in that beneficial medicines worked through supernatural means. The spells of sorcerers, sometimes cast with the aid of magical substances, could be combated with the same remedies.

The magical potions for curing were part of the duty of the shaman. Usually in charge of all or most things supernatural in a tribe, the shaman diagnosed and treated most serious or chronic illness. He or she compounded the remedies needed to stave off the influences of evil spells or spirits. This basic pattern, common among ancient peoples, held sway over nearly all of the span of human existence. The substances of healing potions, connected for thousands of years with the supernatural world, continue to hold a special place, a fascination for all. Thus, out of these origins a dual heritage has been derived: drugs as both simple tools and special substances with nearly supernatural powers.

The discovery that certain natural substances could ease the suffering of human existence, however, should not be trivialized. Even though early peoples discovered only a small number of effective drugs, the very concept of influencing bodily functions via an outside force must be considered one of humanity's greatest advances. The further development of this concept required the environment of civilization. To flourish, rational medical therapy needed the tools provided by settled cultures—writing, systems of exchange, and weights and measures. Contemporary tribal peoples such as the Tasaday demonstrate that, without the more advanced tools, pharmaceutical practices fail to progress.

ANTIQUITY

When organized settlements arose in the great fertile valleys of the Nile, the Tigris and Euphrates, the Yellow and Yangtze, and the Indus Rivers, changes occurred that gradually influenced the concepts of disease and healing. As men and women learned how to control aspects of nature through farming, permanent shelter, and large-scale building projects, the powers of the gods in day-to-day life started to decline. These changes are evident among the remains of the great civilizations of Mesopotamia and Egypt of the second millennium BCE, whose clay tablets and papyri document the beginnings of rational drug use in the West.

An examination of these ancient records reveals a gradual separation of empirical healing (based on experience) from the purely spiritual. For the Babylonians, medical care was provided by two classes of practitioners: the *asipu* (magical healer) and the *asu* (empirical healer). The *asipu* relied more heavily on spells and used magical stones far more than plant materials; the *asu* drew upon a large collection of drugs and manipulated them into several dosage forms that are still basic today, such as suppositories, pills, washes, enemas, and ointments. The *asipu* and the *asu* were not in direct competition and sometimes cooperated on difficult cases. Apparently the ill often went back and forth between the two types of healers looking for a cure.

The extensive records that survive of Egyptian medical practices demonstrate even greater pharmaceutical sophistication, with more dosage forms compounded from more detailed formulas. The Egyptian medical texts, like those from Babylon, show a close connection between supernatural and empirical healing. Suggested recipes usually began with a prayer or incantation. Plant drugs, of which laxatives and enemas were the most prominent, were the main vehicle of healing power. As was the case with healing practices in Mesopotamia, certain individuals specialized in the preparation and sale of drugs. Were these early medicine makers the forebears of today's pharmacists? No, because physicians and other healers again took on the duties of medicine preparation as these two great river civilizations declined. A fully separate pharmaceutical calling would be centuries away.

During the millennium that followed, the roots of the modern medical profession in the West arose out of the flowering of Greek civilization in the basin of the Aegean Sea. In the earliest records of ancient Greece, one finds a similar mixed concept of drug or *pharmakon*, a word that meant magic spell, remedy, or poison. In the *Odyssey*, Homer (*ca* 800 BCE) refers to the esteemed medical wisdom of Egypt, thus illustrating the ebb and flow of ancient knowledge long before the printed word. The early Greek physicians described by Homer, the *demiourgoi*, had advanced to where they diagnosed *natural* causes for illness, while still not rejecting the use of supernatural healing in conjunction with empirical remedies. Some people beset with persistent afflictions traveled to a temple of the god Asklepios, where they would sleep with the hope of being visited during the night by the god or his daughter Hygeia, who carried a magical serpent and a bowl of healing medicine.

The rational tradition within Greek medicine that was evident in Homer's work was refined and codified in the body of literature connected with the name of Hippocrates of Cos (*ca* 425 BCE). Building on the foundations laid by previous natural philosophers such as Thales (*ca* 590 BCE), Anaximander (*ca* 550 BCE), Parmenides (*ca* 470 BCE), and Empedocles (*ca* 450 BCE), the Hippocratic writers constructed a rational explanation of illness. They accomplished this by forging a conceptual link between the environment and humanity by connecting the four elements of earth, air, fire, and water to four governing humors of the body: black bile, blood, yellow bile, and phlegm. The

trained Greek physician (*iatros*) who followed the Hippocratic method favored dietary and life-style adjustments over drug use. If these conservative methods failed, the Greek physician prepared his own medicines or left prescriptions behind for family members to compound and administer.

Most Greek medicines were prepared from plants, and the first great study of plants in the West was accomplished by Theophrastus (*ca* 370–285 BCE), a student of Aristotle. His example of combining information from scholars, midwives, root diggers, and traveling physicians was emulated 300 years later by Dioscorides (*ca* 65 AD). The latter Greek physician's summary of the drug lore of his times, the *Materia Medica*, became, in its various forms, the standard encyclopedia of drugs for hundreds of years to follow.

Through the teachings and writings of Galen, a Greek physician who practiced in Rome in the 2nd century AD, the humoral system of medicine gained ascendancy for the next 1500 years. Setting aside the conservative drug use of the orthodox Hippocratics, Galen devised an elaborate system that attempted to balance the humors of an ill individual by using drugs of a supposedly contrary nature. For example, to treat an external inflammation, a follower of Galen might apply cucumber, a cool and wet drug. The same Galenist also might have tried bleeding, a favorite treatment to remove the apparent excess of blood that caused the illness. In addition to the questionable practice of bleeding, Galen advocated the use of polypharmaceutical preparations (what would be termed "shotgun prescriptions" today). He argued that the patient's body would pull out of a complex prescription the substances that it needed to restore its humoral balance.

Medicine in classic antiquity reached its pinnacle with Galen, and the writers who followed tended to be compilers and commentators on his work, not original thinkers. Galen's influence was so pervasive among medical practitioners that the basics of his healing approach—the balance of the body's four humors through contrary drugs—mixed with folklore and superstition to guide common people in their own treatment of ailments. In the Western half of the Roman Empire, such medical knowledge became especially valuable as civilization crumbled in the years following 400 AD.

THE MIDDLE AGES

Traditionally, the Middle Ages are defined as the period from the first fall of Rome (*ca* 400 AD) to the fall of Constantinople (1453). The first half of this millennium was once referred to as the "Dark Ages" by historians because of the political and social chaos that existed in the lands that had once been part of the western half of the Roman Empire. Modern historians have revealed, however, that many advances were made during the centuries between 400 and 900 AD, including a new, independent calling that emerged out of the flourishing Islamic civilization—pharmacy.

The story of how Greco-Roman philosophy, science, and art returned to western Europe and sparked the creative period known as the Renaissance is one of the most fascinating of human history. It began with the crumbling of civil authority in the western half of the Roman Empire during the 4th and 5th centuries. Greco-Roman culture survived in the Eastern (Byzantine) half of the empire, but with considerably less creative energy. With Roman authority gone in the West, the Church became the stabilizing cultural force, and local feudalism arose to replace centralized government.

The use of drugs to treat illness underwent another shift, as pagan temples, some of which had operated in conjunction with Greco-Roman healing methods, were closed. Rational drug therapy declined in the West, to be replaced by the Church's teaching that sin and disease were related intimately. The cult surrounding the healing saints of Cosmas and Damian exemplifies this attitude. Monasteries became centers for healing, both spiritual and corporal, because the two were not viewed as essentially separate. Cast to their own devices, monks put together their own short versions of classical medical texts (epitomes) and planted gardens to grow the medicinal herbs that were no longer available after the collapse of trade and commerce. Strong in their faith, these amateur healers tended to ascribe their cures to the will of God, rather than to their meager medical resources.

As Western Europe struggled, a new civilization arose among those who followed the teachings of Mohammed (570–632). The formerly nomadic peoples who united into the nations of Islam conquered huge areas of the Middle East and Africa, eventually expanding into Spain, Sicily, and Eastern Europe. Because their faith taught them to respect the written word and those who studied it, they tolerated the scholarship of the Christian sectarians who had fled persecution in the Eastern Roman Empire; the Nestorians, for example, established a famous school in Gondeshapur in the 6th century.

Among the Islamic nations, Greek writings, including those dealing with medicine, were translated into Arabic. At first the Arabs accepted the authority of Greek medical writings totally, especially those of Galen and Dioscorides. But as their sophistication grew, Islamic medical men like Rhazes (860–932) and Avicenna (980–1063) added to the writings of the Greeks. The far-flung trading outposts of the conquering Arabs also brought new drugs and spices to the centers of learning. Moreover, Arab physicians rejected the old idea that foul-tasting medicines worked best. Instead, they devoted a great deal of effort to making their dosage forms elegant and palatable, through the silvering and gilding of pills and the use of syrups.

The new, more sophisticated medicines required elaborate preparation. In the cosmopolitan city of Baghdad of the 9th century, this work was taken over by specialists, the occupational ancestors of today's pharmacists. In places such as Spain and southern Italy where the Islamic world interacted most with recovering western Europe, several of the institutions and developments of the more highly developed Arabic culture— such as the separation of pharmacy and medicine—passed over to the West.

By the mid-13th century, when Frederick II, the ruler of the Kingdom of the Two Sicilies, codified the separate practice of pharmacy for the first time in Europe, public pharmacies had become relatively common in southern Europe. Practitioners of pharmacy had joined together within guilds, which sometimes included dealers in similar goods, such as spicers or grocers, or physicians.

Arabic culture had returned classical scientific and medical knowledge to Europe. At centers such as Toledo and Salerno, the writings of the Greeks, which had been translated into Arabic centuries before on the fringes of the old eastern half of the Roman Empire, were translated into Latin for the use of European scholars. Thus, at the emerging universities of Europe such as Paris (1150), Oxford (1167), and Salerno (1180), scholars discussed the works of the great medical authorities such as Dioscorides, Galen, and Avicenna.

However, the debates on medicine among European academics were based on speculation, not observation. Theirs was a philosophical pursuit, with no great impact on medical practice. For significant change to occur in the use of drugs, the scholastic approach had to be set aside and a more skeptical, observational methodology adopted. This new, experimental age we now call the Renaissance.

THE RENAISSANCE AND EARLY MODERN EUROPE

The Renaissance, simply put, was the beginning of the modern period. Changes that had begun during the European Middle Ages, and were stimulated further by contacts with other cultures, gained momentum. The burst of creative energy that would result in our present shared culture of the West stemmed not from a single episode, but from a series of events.

In 1453 Constantinople (Istanbul) fell to the conquering Turks, and the remnants of the Greek scholarly community there fled west, carrying their books and knowledge with them. About that same time, Johann Gutenberg began printing with movable type, starting an information revolution. Within a half century, Columbus discovered the New World, Vasco da Gama found the sea route to India that Columbus had sought, commerce based on money and banking was established, and syphilis raged through Europe. It was a time for new ideas through reinterpretation of the old classical themes, and through exploration on the high sea and in the laboratory.

The time was ripe for casting off the old concepts of diseases and drugs of Galen. The new drugs that were arriving from far-off lands were unknown to the ancients. Printers, after fulfilling the demand for religious books such as bibles and hymnals, turned to producing medical and pharmaceutical works, especially those that could benefit from profuse and detailed illustrations. On the medical side, for example, this trend is exemplified in the anatomical masterworks of Andres Vesalius (1514–1564).

For pharmacy, printing had a profound effect on the study of plant drugs, because illustrations of the plants could be reproduced easily. Medical botanists such as Otto Brunfels (1500–1534), Leonhart Fuchs (1501–1566), and John Gerard (1545–1612) illustrated their works with realistic renditions of plants, allowing readers to do serious field work or find the drugs needed for their practices. Among the most gifted of these investigators was Valerius Cordus (1515–1544), who also wrote a work in another popular genre—formula books. His *Dispensatorium* (1546) became the official standard for the preparation of medicines in the city of Nuremberg and generally is considered the first pharmacopeia.

Although they were critical to the advancement of medical science, the nearly modern, precise works of Fuchs and Vesalius did not influence the treatment of disease as much as the speculative, mystically tinged writings of an itinerant Swiss surgeon who dubbed himself "Paracelsus." Born Philippus Aureolus Theophrastus Bombastus von Hohenheim in 1493, the year Columbus went on his second trip, this medical rebel represents well the combined attitudes of the common man, the scholarly physician, the practical surgeon, and the alchemist. The battles of Paracelsus against the static ideas of Galen, Avicenna, and other traditional authorities opened a window into the complicated mind of the Renaissance. As Erwin Ackerknecht observed in *A Short History of Medicine,*

> "Paracelsus is one of the most contradictory figures of a contradictory age. He was more modern than most of his contemporaries in his relentless and uncompromising drive for the new and in his opposition to blind obedience to authoritarianism and books. On the other hand, he was more medieval than most of his contemporaries in his all-pervading mystic religiosity. His writings are a strange mixture of intelligent observation and mystical nonsense, of humble sincerity and boasting megalomania."

Paracelsus was the most important advocate of chemically prepared drugs from crude plant and mineral substances, yet he believed firmly that the collection of those substances should be determined by astrology. He stated, again and again, his total faith in observation while at the same time preaching the "doctrine of signature," a belief that God had placed a sign on healing substances indicating their use against disease (eg, liverwort resembles a liver, so it must be good for liver ailments).

An outspoken enemy of university-educated physicians, Paracelsus denigrated their scholasticism and wrote his own works in his native language rather than in the traditional Latin. He harshly criticized pharmacy practitioners as well, even though his advocacy of chemically prepared medicines was to spark the growth of the modern pharmaceutical sciences. Chemical processes, especially distillation, empowered the follower of Paracelsus to isolate the healing principles of a drug, its *quintessence*. Eventually, as the efficacy of some of these drugs became known, they entered professional medical practice and appeared in books on medicines. Thus, a great leap in the history of pharmacy, the preparation of medicines, emerged when a tool of science, chemistry, was adopted to make one of humanity's most ancient of tools, drugs.

Paracelsus and his followers, who chastised practitioners of pharmacy, soon took a position on the forefront of chemistry during the 16th century. The apothecary Johann Hartmann (1568–1631), for example, was the first professor of chemistry at a European university. This trend continued through the 17th, 18th, and into the beginning of the 19th century as chemistry emerged as a separate profession. For a period of about 300 years, a small minority of practicing pharmacists made significant investigations into the chemistry of drugs, and along the way isolated many drugs that are still used today and contributed much to general chemical knowledge. During that same period, when men and their ships sailed the seas looking for new lands, and returned with new drugs, practitioners of pharmacy explored a much smaller, but equally exciting, world in their laboratories.

Much of the stimulation for the early research came out of the discovery of drugs in recently explored lands. Just as Galen did not know all the diseases in the world, Dioscorides and his Arab elaborators did not know all the drugs in the world. Tobacco, guaiac, cascara sagrada, ipecac, and cinchona bark were among the scores of new plant drugs from the New World.

Cinchona bark, from which quinine was extracted in 1820, first came to Europe around 1640, at which point it created a crisis within scholastic medicine. Galen's elaborate system of balancing humors by using drugs of opposite qualities could not explain cinchona bark's efficacy against malaria. Not only did the bark cure malarial fevers, but also it had little effect on other fevers. Here was something Galen said could *not* exist, but Paracelsus insisted *must* exist—a specific remedy for a disease. This conceptual crisis, plus the efforts of those advocating chemical medicines, displaced the therapeutic agreement of Galenism, which had lasted nearly 1500 years. The following period, about 250 years, was a time of therapeutic chaos that lasted until the present era of modern pharmacology.

During the time of turmoil for therapeutics while the followers of Paracelsus and Galen argued, the calling of pharmacy established the legal and scientific foundations of the modern profession. Out of the medieval complex of guilds on the European continent grew organizations that represented pharmacy.

As the occupational division from medicine spread north, pharmacy practitioners joined together or aligned themselves with similar groups, such as the sellers of spices or physicians and surgeons. The guilds of the late Middle Ages and early Renaissance wielded considerable power, setting up training requirements, examinations, and restrictions on the number and locations of shops. Conflicts within guilds that held pharmacists and near competitors often led to government intervention and new laws that clarified the professional role of pharmacy. Eventually, however, interprofessional friction would lead to the separation of pharmacists into their own organizations, often under governmental authority (eg, the French Collége de Pharmacie in 1777).

The cooperation between pharmaceutical guilds and governmental bodies also led to the standardization of medicines through the publication of books called *pharmacopeias*. Because of greater pharmaceutical sophistication, the increased number of herbals and distillation books, and the availability of new drugs, physicians wanted assurance that their prescriptions would be prepared uniformly within their city or state. To this end, in 1499 the guild of physicians and pharmacists of Florence sanctioned the *Nuovo receptario* as their book of standards. Historians, however, generally credit the *Dispensatorium* of Valerius Cordus as the first pharmacopeia, which was adopted by the government of Nuremberg, Germany, in 1546.

It is a bit ironic that from the mid-1600s to the mid-1800s, when controversy raged within medicine regarding the proper use of drugs, pharmacy made its greatest contribution to science as well as becoming firmly established as a profession on the European continent. As chemical medicines became more prevalent in medical practice, pharmacists were forced to learn the new methods of preparation and manipulation. To do so they turned to the most popular textbooks on chemistry, which were composed by pharmacists such as Nicaise LeFebvre (*Traité de chymie*, 1660) and Nicolas Lemery (*Cours de chymie*, 1675).

The volume of chemical discoveries made by pharmacists would fill a chapter twice this size. Carl Wilhelm Scheele (1742–1786), for example, discovered oxygen in 1773, a year before Priestley, as well as chlorine, glycerin, and several inorganic acids. Martin Klaproth (1743–1817) was a pharmacist who pioneered the field of analytical chemistry. Like Scheele, he made his discoveries using the equipment of the pharmacy in which he worked. Other pharmacists, such as Andreas Marggraf (1709–1782), became such proficient chemists that they pursued chemical work full-time. Along the way pharmacists contributed much to the development of chemical apparatus, especially analytical chemists such as Klaproth, Marggraf, Antoine Baumé (1728–1804), Carl Freidrich Mohr (1806–1879), and Henri Moissan (1852–1907). Moissan, a French pharmacist, received the Nobel prize in chemistry in 1906 for his isolation of fluorine.

Since most drugs before 1900 were derived from the plant kingdom, it is not surprising that pharmacists dominated the investigation of botanical drugs during the 1700s and 1800s. In collaboration with interested physicians, pharmacists documented the sources of plant drugs around the globe, making significant contributions to the nascent science of botany. Combining this proficiency with their skills in manipulative chemistry, pharmacists continued the search begun by the Paracelsians to find pure healing principles within medicinal plants.

Approaching pharmacy with a more modern viewpoint, these men sought to isolate pure, crystalline chemicals that could be measured accurately and identified chemically. Medicinal preparations of crude drugs, no matter how carefully made, fluctuated considerably in potency because of the natural variation of active constituents in botanicals. Thus, the pursuit of active principles was no easy task, and it fascinated pharmaceutical investigators for nearly 300 years. To search, separate, characterize, and identify the scores of chemicals contained in the simplest plant drug was a challenge as great as any exploration.

Discoveries came gradually through hit and miss research until the late 1700s, when Scheele, for example, extracted several plant acids including citric acid (1784). The single, most important breakthrough occurred during the first decade of the 19th century when the pharmacist Friedrich Sertürner extracted morphine from crude opium. The announcement of his method opened up the era of alkaloidal chemistry, which resulted in the isolation of several pure drugs from crude preparations. The French pharmacists Joseph Pelletier and Joseph Caventou isolated several alkaloids, notably quinine in 1820. Not only were these new, pure drugs rapidly adopted by physicians because their potency was assured, but their existence allowed physiologists to administer drugs accurately during their research, which became the wellspring for modern pharmacology.

Much later, after 1850 or so, the scientific disciplines of pharmacy began to become more professionalized in colleges and manufacturing concerns with a subsequent decline in *drug shop science*. Pharmacists interested in research left the shop behind for the institutional laboratory.

Despite the impressive achievements of a few pharmacy practitioners, most pharmacists of the early modern period viewed science as secondary to professional and financial success. European pharmacists achieved these goals through strict internal controls on the profession and relatively cordial relations with physicians. In some states on the European continent, the number and location of pharmacies were limited by law, as were the requirements for education and licensure. Lists of standard prices softened competition. By the 19th century, the combination of the fame generated by scientific contributions and solid upper-middle-class credentials had elevated pharmacists throughout much of Europe to a social position similar to that of physicians.

Such conditions did not hold for Britain, however, where the position of the pharmaceutical profession within the hierarchy of healing did not become established firmly until the mid-19th century. The original class of pharmacy practitioners, the apothecaries, had evolved during the 1600s and 1700s into a second group of medical practitioners, servicing those who could not afford the high fees demanded by the small cadre of university-educated physicians.

As apothecaries became more and more like general practitioners of medicine, *chemists* and *druggists* (ie, those who manufactured and sold drugs and medicines for the apothecaries) rose up to take over the open pharmaceutical niche. Conflicts and court cases erupted during these years, and the boundaries between the physicians, apothecaries, chemists, and druggists shifted accordingly. It was during this period of confusion within the British health community that the British settled what would become the United States of America, a situation that contributed to the development of the unique American profession of pharmacy.

AMERICAN PHARMACY

The exceptional character of American pharmacy* arises out of its remarkable history. When settlers came to the shores of North America, there was little to attract trained or established medical personnel. Unlike the lands of Central and South America, there were no treasures to confiscate or spices to export. This was a land for toil, not spoils. As the frontier was pushed back slowly, most of the populace relied on domestic or "kitchen" medicine guided by home medical books (if the settler could read). When this failed, the colonist often turned to a nearby figure of authority such as a clergyman or government official to provide medical advice or guidance.

As the colonies grew more prosperous during the early 18th century, they attracted ambitious businessmen from England, including apothecaries. In the New World, British apothecaries continued to combine pharmaceutical and medical practice, serving the large segment of the public who could not afford university-trained physicians. In North America, the boundaries between medicine and pharmacy were even cloudier, with most physicians having some sort of shop practice. Most apothecary shops were run either by an attending physician or his apprentice, or by an apothecary hired by the owner-physician. In other words, most men who practiced medicine for their livelihood also practiced their own pharmacy, either out of their homes or in *doctor shops*.

A few 18th-century chemists and druggists—practitioners who limited themselves to drug-selling and medicinal preparation—did practice in the larger cities on the Atlantic coast. These forerunners of today's pharmacists had two main areas of sales. As *druggists* they served as wholesalers of the drugs and medicines used by apothecaries, surgeons, midwives, and physicians. They also undersold the apothecaries in the marketing of patent medicines (secret remedies of unknown composition), which became increasingly popular up through the Revolutionary War. There were very few laws that directly involved Anglo-American pharmacy during the colonial period, and no effective laws restricted the practice of American pharmacy until the 1870s. Anyone with luck, pluck, and sufficient capital could open up an apothecary or druggist shop.

The hardships imposed by the Revolutionary War proved to be critical in the development of a separate pharmaceutical occupation in America. Britain had been the source of almost all

of the drugs dispensed by physicians and apothecaries. In order to meet the demand, American druggists, the wholesale distributors of drugs, had to learn how to manufacture their own chemically based drugs and how to make common preparations of the crude drugs previously obtained from Britain. In addition, these druggists had to learn how to imitate the popular British patent medicines that were so much in demand by the public. To meet war needs druggists, such as the Marshalls in Philadelphia, greatly expanded their production capabilities. Out of the war came a network for the production, packaging, and distribution of drugs and medicines.

But a profession of pharmacy, at least as we know it, was not spawned during the period of the Revolutionary War. Pharmacy—the compounding of medicines—still was done almost completely by physicians in their own shops or offices (continuing to practice according to the model of the British apothecary) or by their apprentices. Aside from those wholesale druggists who also had an *out front* business—that is, a retail store that sold their products and filled occasional prescriptions—nonmedical practitioners of pharmacy were rare and without any sort of group identity. Many of those who did practice pharmacy solely were either immigrants from the European continent or former employees in doctor shops who bought businesses from their old physician-employers.

To succeed, of course, these chemists needed prescriptions to dispense. Back in the 1760s, in his famous *Discourse* on medical education, Dr John Morgan, a pioneer in American medical education, had advocated the separation of medicine and pharmacy with physicians writing prescriptions. A few physicians did follow Morgan's lead, but the practice did not become common until well into the 19th century. Morgan himself returned to operating a shop to make ends meet.

The years surrounding the War of 1812 brought significant changes in American business and health care that strongly influenced pharmacy's professional development. It was not until the early years of the 19th century that American physicians began to view the special service of an apothecary as distinct and essential. The first hospitals of the young republic, for instance, employed medical apprentices as staff apothecaries. As described in the *Brief Account of the New-York Hospital* (1804), a "house Surgeon and Apothecary constantly reside in the Hospital—these offices are filled by the students of the Physicians and Surgeons belonging to the Hospital, which affords an excellent school for the young men appointed to those places." The staff apothecary practiced both pharmacy and medicine in a manner analogous to the British apothecary of the 18th century, going on rounds and treating patients.

By 1811, however, the position of apothecary at the New-York Hospital had changed. The person chosen was a full-time pharmaceutical practitioner who was tested, before hiring, on his prowess as a compounder of medicines. Instead of being obligated to go on rounds, he was required to stay in his *shop* at all times. By 1819 the services of the New-York Hospital apothecary were so critical that he was required to put up a $250 bond to guarantee that he would not leave his position with less than a 2-month notice.

The war with England cut off trade with the largest suppliers of drugs and medicines to the US. In contrast with the stopgap measures used during the Revolutionary War to meet military and domestic demands, during the War of 1812 the American drug trade developed its own resources for the production of basic pharmaceuticals, including patent medicines. When peace returned, some American firms faltered under English pressure, but others continued and formed the basis for the future American drug industry.

The years following the War of 1812 were transitional. More and more physicians gained their clinical experience in hospitals and dispensaries instead of with preceptors, learning to write prescriptions, rather than compound them. After graduation some of these young physicians continued to write out prescriptions, thereby stimulating the growth of pharmacy. As physicians began writing prescriptions for apothecaries to

_____
*The discussion on American pharmacy is based in part on data from "Professionalism and the Nineteenth-Century American Pharmacist," *Pharm Hist* 1986; 28: 115.

dispense, concern arose over the consistency with which these medicines were being compounded. In 1808 the Massachusetts Medical Society published a state guide to drug standards, with a national convention of physicians approving a *Pharmacopoeia of the United States of America* (USP) in 1820. Although the USP was not recognized as official by the federal government for years to come, it rapidly became accepted nationally as the primary guide to drugs.

The appearance of these books reflected both the growing amount of prescription writing and the medical profession's increasing reliance on pharmacists. The number of pharmacy practitioners in urban areas reached the critical mass necessary for the establishment of local pharmaceutical societies such as the Philadelphia College of Pharmacy (1821) and the Massachusetts College of Pharmacy (1823). These *colleges* (the term being used in the sense of associated colleagues) established night schools for the instruction of apprentices and discussion groups on scientific pharmacy. The small class of retail apothecaries and wholesale druggists presented no particular threat to urban physicians in the first decades of the 19th century, and the situation provided them with several conveniences.

ANTEBELLUM AMERICA: PHARMACY FINDS ITS NICHE

The years prior to the American Civil War were to be the most critical for American practitioners of pharmacy; the boundaries of practice between physicians and pharmacists that were drawn during this period still exist relatively unchanged today. During the 1820s and 1830s, East Coast apothecary shops became more standardized in their appearance and in the stock they carried. Pharmacy followed the trend of specialty retailing and concentrated on drugs, medicines, surgical supplies, artificial teeth and limbs, dyestuffs, essences, and chemicals. Grocers took over the selling of exotic dietary items such as figs, raisins, and citrus fruits. Drugstores in small cities and towns, however, tended to keep in stock more general articles such as glass, paints, varnishes, and oils. Above all, apothecary shops became the main distributors of patent medicines, one of the most profitable lines of merchandise in the history of American business.

The educated elite of Atlantic coast physicians fostered the development of a well-trained, yet subservient, pharmaceutical profession. They welcomed the early pharmaceutical associations and served as faculty for the first American pharmacy schools. Physicians voiced support for the growth of an independent profession of pharmacy as a "necessity for a division of labor" to meet the "growing demands" of their communities. As the quality of drugs imported from Europe declined, physicians began to rely on the expertise of pharmacy practitioners to detect adulterated or low-potency drugs.

The relationship between the physician and the druggist began to sour in the 1840s. Feeling more confident of their social standing, apothecaries began shifting their efforts from pleasing physicians to attending the ills of customers. Consequently, American apothecaries took to refilling prescriptions without physician authorization or directly treating customers, a practice called *counter-prescribing*. In the large cities, doctor's shops were back on the rise after a decline of two decades. Medical schools continued to turn out graduates by the hundreds, most of whom sought their fortunes in urban areas, where they would *open shop*.

As the 1850s progressed, the growth of American pharmacy accelerated. The US Census figures for druggists and apothecaries in 1850 and 1860 illustrate the dramatic growth in the profession, especially when compared with physicians. In 1850 and 1860, respectively, the *per capita* number of physicians did not change significantly (1:572 to 1:576), while the number of druggists grew by nearly 25% (from 1:3778 to 1:2850). This trend continued, at a slightly lower rate, through the rest of the 19th century.

American pharmacy was caught up both in developments within the health-care sector and in the larger changes occurring in American commerce. As mass-manufacturers began producing drug preparations in the late 1850s, less-skilled men entered the ranks of pharmacy. With large firms doing much of the complicated work, these *mere shopkeepers* flooded the marketplace. Physicians had supported the growth of the pharmaceutical profession largely because it served their own interests, releasing them from the drudgery of compounding medicines and stocking a shop. Moreover, physicians came to depend upon the expertise of the best druggists and apothecaries. With the development of the pharmaceutical industry, however, this relationship changed. As one physician put it in 1860, "It is an admitted and lamentable fact that many of those now practicing pharmacy are totally incompetent to fulfill the responsibilities of the true apothecary. They know nothing of the science of preparing medicines."

By the late 1850s, while the general economy was in crisis and secession strife was imminent, physicians and pharmacists indulged in a great deal of finger-pointing in both the professional and popular arenas. Both groups blamed each other for the continued popularity of patent medicines. Moreover, competition had reached such a high level that it threatened the integrity of the boundaries that had developed to separate the two professions. Pharmacists were convinced that dispensing physicians and doctor's shops were the cause of much of their difficulties, while physicians complained about *counter-prescribing*. With no legal restrictions on medical or pharmaceutical practice, the lines of separation between medicine and pharmacy were growing hazy. The onset of the Civil War ended much of the bickering between apothecaries and physicians. After the War, the boundaries between the professions were drawn more clearly, aided in part by new approaches to professionalization.

THE SEARCH FOR PROFESSIONALISM

In part to raise the stature of their rapidly growing calling, a small group of elite druggists and apothecaries met in Philadelphia in 1852 to found the American Pharmaceutical Association (APhA). They saw the gains made by pharmacy in the 1830s and 1840s being swept away by a rising tide of destructive competition. For American pharmacists of the mid-19th century, organizations like the Philadelphia College of Pharmacy or the APhA held the promise of increasing their professional stature by fostering individual improvement, not by winning the favor of physicians or government bureaucrats.

The crux of this independent achievement was the mastery of prescription compounding. The growth of large-scale pharmaceutical manufacturing during the Civil War years struck fear in the hearts of pharmacy leaders. As William Procter Jr stated (1869),

"Pharmacy may be defined to be the art of preparing and dispensing medicines, and embodies the knowledge and skill requisite to carry them out in practice. But if the preparation of medicines is taken from the apothecary and he becomes merely the dispenser of them his business is shorn of half its dignity and importance, and he relapses into a simple shopkeeper."

Most American pharmacists, undereducated and underskilled, took advantage of the growing number of ready-made preparations offered by large firms. This was in spite of the arguments put forth by the leaders of pharmacy since the 1830s that the special ability to produce official preparations successfully in-house was what made the individual pharmacist more than a mere merchant. Moreover, this expertise only could be learned through experience, under the watchful eye of a preceptor. As fewer basic ingredients for compounding were made in the shop, however, apprentices would become preceptors and pass along their ignorance.

Pharmacists, at the conclusion of the Civil War, initially rejected the notion that formal educational requirements would solve the problem. They had no interest in any measures that interfered with their freedom to practice. Moreover, some immigrants from the Continent, where states often restricted pharmaceutical practice, expressed opposition to the legal control of pharmacies. Many had come to North America to open their own shops, rather than wait years in their native lands for permission.

In the late 1860s the academic model of professionalism being worked out by other so-called "new professions" such as engineering attracted the attention of some pharmaceutical leaders. Using university degrees, plus state licensing or institutional certification, these new professions set themselves apart from other occupations as "communities of the competent." They sought to avoid the ordeals of the marketplace by putting a cognitive gap between their work and the public's understanding. Theoretically, by controlling admissions to professional schools and raising examination standards, destructive competition could be reduced or even eliminated.

LEGISLATION

The APhA responded to the movement of the late 1860s toward increased public protection and occupational security through law by publishing a model pharmacy act. Physicians and others concerned with the safe use of poisons and potent drugs had petitioned state legislatures for laws governing pharmacy. Initially, pharmacists took a negative view, reacting to the idea that physicians or bureaucrats would gain authority over pharmacy practice via state inspectors or licensing boards. To ensure that the profession's best interests would be protected, the APhA empowered a committee to draw up a model law. Reflecting the ambivalent attitude of many pharmacists toward legal regulation, the APhA published and distributed their model law without endorsement. As small businessmen, pharmacists did not want outside restriction on their trade.

During the 1870s state legislatures began considering in earnest pharmacy bills sponsored by nonpharmacists. Reacting to this trend, pharmacists organized statewide associations to coordinate support for their own bills, which were often versions of the APhA model. Although not enthusiastic at first about regulation of their businesses, pharmacists wanted a voice in the process. The eventual success of their efforts in the 1870s, 1880s, and 1890s evinced a changing attitude toward the pursuit of professionalism from the 1860s.

The boundary between masters of the pharmaceutical art and mere store clerks, which had always been flimsy, was disintegrating. Pharmacists sought new ways to demonstrate their competence and to separate themselves from ignorant drug sellers and quacks. The evidence for this expertise, however, shifted away from individual achievement in the marketplace toward group identification and institutional certification.

TRANSITION TO A MODERN PROFESSION

The period between 1870 and 1920 was transitional for both pharmacy and pharmaceutical education. Before the Civil War perhaps only 1 in 20 American pharmacists had finished formal schooling in pharmacy, which had consisted of night courses to supplement apprenticeship training. With the passage of state laws requiring the examination and registration of pharmacists from the 1870s on, pharmacy became part of the wave of professionalization sweeping across American society. The new professionals based their claims of status on their diplomas and licenses, not their products.

Pharmacy got caught up in this trend, and even though state laws did not require a pharmacy school diploma for licensure until the early 20th century, the prestige attached to the sheepskin attracted students to the burgeoning number of schools, as public expectations increased and "professional" became a coveted title.

Pharmaceutical education around the turn of the century was related closely to practice as pharmacist-educators such as Joseph Remington replaced the physicians and other nonphar-

macy practitioners who had dominated the earlier schools. Students also had a wide range of possible educational experiences.

- Short-term cram schools were available for those who just wanted to pass a state board exam.
- Small, local schools sprang up in medium size cities offering basic instruction and large diplomas for display.
- The old-line schools, affiliated with local pharmaceutical organizations, provided students with excellent practical education, plus an opportunity to explore specialty areas, depending on the college's faculty.
- Starting with the University of Michigan in 1868, schools of pharmacy affiliated themselves with state colleges and universities, a trend that altered the direction of American pharmaceutical education.

As part of larger university communities, these pharmacy schools aspired to the high standards of scholarship exhibited by established disciplines and other professions. The leaders of the university faculties helped transform pharmaceutical education from a vocational to a scientific orientation through pharmacy programs that emphasized full-time coursework and laboratory study.

During this period pharmacy's part in health care solidified, as the dispensing of medicines by physicians declined. However, the rise of the cut-rate drugstore and, more importantly, the chain drugstore, also occurred during these 50 years, which further increased economic pressure on the profession.

Still, most pharmacists worked in their own *corner drugstore,* which became a fixture in American life with its shelves of patent medicines for all ills and a soda fountain for delightful beverages; the proprietor, often called *doc,* attended to the minor aches and pains of customers or made chocolate sodas with equal skill. Although the pharmacist relied on prescription compounding for his professional identity, this provided only a small fraction of his income. To protect this independent and uniquely American style of practice from the incursion of larger retailers, the National Association of Retail Druggists (NARD) was founded in 1898. At first the APhA welcomed and cooperated with the new national organization, but the split that eventually developed between the APhA, which was oriented to scientific and professional advancement, and NARD, which concentrated on the individual commercial success of owners, weakened the profession's voice in national affairs in the years to come.

It was an exciting time in medicine, with therapeutics undergoing a transformation. The germ theory of disease, championed by laboratory scientists such as Louis Pasteur and Robert Koch, resulted in significant immunological advances in the 1880s and 1890s. Pasteur's rabies vaccine and Emil von Behring's diphtheria antitoxin demonstrated that cures for infectious diseases could arise from the laboratory. Paul Ehrlich transcended the biological efforts of his predecessors when he introduced Salvarsan in 1910, the first chemotherapeutic agent. Although it fell short of Ehrlich's ideal of a *magic bullet,* which could destroy microorganisms selectively without damaging the patient, Salvarsan did inspire others to search for drugs with chemotherapeutic potential. Aside from the biologicals, however, few of the drugs discovered during the late 19th and early 20th centuries had a significant impact on the prevention or cure of disease.

Industrial research on drugs produced several new agents, such as the analgesic and antipyretic aspirin or the sedative chloral hydrate, that reduced the pain and suffering associated with illness. Even though pharmacies served as important outlets for sera, antitoxins, and vaccines, most of the medicines compounded or sold by pharmacists around the turn of the century eased symptoms, rather than treated root illnesses.

As scientific pharmacology explained how drugs worked on a cellular and organ system level, the concept of drugs and their actions held by professionals and laypeople diverged. The public clung to outdated ideas of humoralism augmented by a modicum of germ theory. Such beliefs made consumers susceptible to patent medicine advertising, which misled them into equating the effects of strong laxatives and analgesics with the cure of disease. With far greater understanding of the nature of disease, health professionals joined together with muckraking journalists and politicians of the Progressive Era to attack patent medicine *cure-alls*. The 1906 Food and Drugs Act, passed mainly in response to poor food-production methods, also addressed problems in the drug trade. Even though it proved ineffectual against patent medicine fakery, the 1906 act did establish the *United States Pharmacopeia* as well as the *National Formulary* of the APhA as official compendia, providing the US with truly national drug standards for the first time.

It was during these years that pharmacists finally abandoned the in-shop manufacturing of the ingredients of their prescriptions. The pharmaceutical industry had progressed to the point where they could produce basic preparations of crude drugs more cheaply and reliably than could the individual practitioner. Moreover, industry was the source for the new synthetic drugs such as antipyrine and aspirin that resulted from developments in organic chemistry. As compounding, not the making of stock preparations, always had been the crux of pharmacy practice, this change was lamented only by a few of the profession's old guard. The hands of pharmacists still fashioned the essential tools of medicine.

Pharmacy education adapted gradually to the change. Coursework shifted away from the identification of crude plant drugs and their various preparations to a greater emphasis on the chemical compatibility of the ingredients within each prescription. The professional credentials of American pharmacists were strengthened in 1932 when a 4-year BSc degree became standard for licensure. For the next three decades pharmacy schools graduated pharmacists who could claim to be *chemists on the corner*. Yet at the same time that the profession achieved the goal of a scientifically trained workforce fully capable of carrying out all the steps involved in the making of medicines, the technology of the pharmaceutical industry assumed that responsibility.

THE ERA OF COUNT AND POUR

The middle third of the 20th century was a time of dramatic change for all of medical care including pharmacy. In therapeutics, many of the great scourges of humanity were conquered through the introduction of antibiotics. Although the phenomenon of antibiosis had been observed by Pasteur in the 1870s, the first significant antibiotic substance was not discovered until Alexander Fleming noticed the effects of a colony of *penicillium* mold on a misplaced petri dish in 1928. Development of penicillin did not occur, however, until a decade later when the threat of war in Europe inspired a British team to pursue the scaled-up production of the drug. Other antibiotics followed shortly, as did new classes of therapeutic agents, such as the corticosteroids, tranquilizers, antidepressants, antihypertensives, radioactive isotopes, and oral contraceptives. The pharmacy, which had served as an outpost for the relief of suffering and the treatment of minor ailments, came to hold preventives and cures for serious disease.

Following World War II American pharmaceutical firms applied high technology to the production of medicines and rapidly became one of the most advanced industries in the world. New drugs, new dosage forms, and new marketing methods reinforced a trend evident from the early 1900s of physicians shifting away from prescribing complex mixtures of ingredients toward ready-made, single-entity medicines mass-manufactured by large companies. In the 1930s about 75% of prescriptions required some compounding by a pharmacist; by 1950 that figure had dropped to about 25%. The movement away from prescriptions "tailor-made" for each individual patient accelerated so that by 1960 only about 1 in 25 prescriptions needed the compounding skills of a pharmacist, with the trend leveling out around 1970 at about 1 in 100.

Pharmacists, however, were not at a loss for work. The number of prescriptions grew even faster as new, effective drugs came onto the market. In community pharmacies the income from the sale of prescription drugs increased faster than *out-front* sales of over-the-counter medicines, cosmetics, and other traditional *drugstore* goods. Chain stores and other large retailers rushed into the drug business, displacing the independent corner drugstore as the typical purveyor of pharmaceutical services, especially in urban areas.

Modifications in pharmaceutical legislation and education reflected these dramatic changes in therapeutics and practice, to varying degrees. Federal laws regulating the production of drugs and pharmacy practice were modernized in 1938, 1952, and 1962, the last set of amendments requiring that medicines be judged both safe and effective to be on the market. Laws regulating drugs of high abuse potential were updated through the Drug Abuse Act of 1970, which was subsequently enforced through the Drug Enforcement Agency. In contrast to the law, educational reform came more slowly.

Proposals for 6-year Doctor of Pharmacy degrees to raise the professional standing of pharmacy gained interest in a few places, with the first such program initiated at the University of Southern California in 1950. But, as a whole, pharmaceutical educators compromised and selected a 5-year bachelor of science in pharmacy as the standard degree beginning in 1960. The pharmacy curriculum continued to emphasize the physical sciences that underlie the making of medicines, however, ignoring the fact that compounding was disappearing from American pharmacy practice.

Because of the large growth of prescribing, community pharmacists of the 1950s and 1960s stepped back from soda fountains and cigar counters to practice pharmacy nearly full time. Yet, for all of their education, they did little more than routinely fill prescriptions—placing a small number of dosage units from a large bottle into a smaller, properly labeled one. Despite the added responsibility of distributing the hundreds of new and potent medicines coming on the market, pharmacists had little opportunity to use their 4, 5, or 6 years of higher education. The restricted role of the pharmacist is exemplified by the following statement from the Code of Ethics of the APhA, which was in effect from its adoption in 1952 until its revision in 1969:

> "The pharmacist does not discuss the therapeutic effects or composition of a prescription with a patient. When such questions are asked, he suggests that the qualified practitioner (ie, physician or dentist) is the proper person with whom such matters should be discussed."

In 1969 the APhA revamped its Code of Ethics in the face of the large changes occurring in pharmacy. Instead of deferring to physicians, the APhA advanced this statement as the first section of its Code: "A pharmacist should hold the health and safety of patients to be of first consideration; he should render to each patient the full measure of his ability as an essential health practitioner." This dramatic reversal resulted from a new idea that swept through pharmacy during the mid- to late-1960s called clinical pharmacy.

THE EMERGENCE OF CLINICAL PHARMACY

The concept of *clinical pharmacy* sprang from a combination of factors, including the development of the subdiscipline of hospital pharmacy since the 1920s, the growth of clinical pharmacology since the 1940s, innovative teaching programs, and the decline of pharmacology instruction in medical schools. To some extent, pharmacy took over an aspect of medical care that had been partially abandoned by physicians. Overburdened by patient loads and the explosion of new drugs, physicians turned to pharmacists more and more for drug information, especially within institutional settings.

Viewed historically, however, the expansion of pharmacy's role to include patient instruction on proper drug use seems a logical extension of the pharmacist's role as toolmaker. Moreover, clinical pharmacy practice bridged the gap between professional and lay understanding of drug action. During the past century medical science far surpassed the public's comprehension of physiology and disease. The concept of how the tool of medicine works, once shared by both doctor and patient, had been lost. The public's trust in medical practitioners subsequently has declined. Pharmacists, by sharing insights into the workings of medicines, have become trusted professionals in American society.

Aside from recent innovations in the relationship between pharmacist and patient, several other notable changes have occurred within American pharmacy that have gone relatively unnoticed by the public. Outwardly, the practice of pharmacy today differs little in appearance from that of 60 years ago. An individual hands over a small slip of paper received from a physician to a pharmacist who then retreats into a work area and appears later with a container of medicine. But on closer examination, the changes seem revolutionary. For example, women, who made up only 4% of the profession in 1950, entered the field rapidly starting in the 1970s. By the year 2000 they were approximately 40% of the pharmaceutical workforce and will be the majority in the near future.

Pharmacists, traditionally conservative in the face of technological innovation, adapted computer technology to their work as quickly as any other profession of the late 20th century. Institutional practice, once viewed as the lowest rung on the profession's ladder, became the work area of choice for graduates during the 1970s and 1980s, a period of unprecedented hospital growth. Just as the division of labor opened up a niche for pharmacists in the early 1800s, pharmaceutical specialties such as radiopharmacy, clinical pharmacotherapy, and nutritional support practice have demonstrated the maturity of the American pharmaceutical profession. Once relegated to counting and pouring, pharmacists headed institutional reviews of drug utilization and served as consultants to all types of health-care facilities. A comparison of Part I of this current edition of this text with previous editions will reveal the unprecedented expansion of opportunities for pharmacists in recent times.

THE CONFLICTING PARADIGMS OF PHARMACEUTICAL CARE AND MANAGED CARE

The 1990s in American pharmacy begin with a clarion call for a paradigm shift to Pharmaceutical Care, a practice model described by Charles D. Hepler and Linda Strand as "the responsible provision of drug therapy for the purpose of achieving definite outcomes that improve a patient's quality of life." The diverse organizations of American pharmacy rallied to this expanded vision of practice. Established schools of pharmacy shifted in earnest to all-PharmD programs to better prepare graduates for the expected challenges. Governmental regulations, such as those connected with the Omnibus Budget Reconciliation Act of 1990 (OBRA 90), pushed pharmacy in the direction of greater responsibility. OBRA 90 requires pharmacists to provide counseling to Medicaid patients and to participate in prospective and retrospective drug use review (DUR) programs. Eventually, states added rules calling for more pharmacy services. This new path to a greater professional role for pharmacist seemed assured.

As the 1990s moved ahead, it soon became clear that the supposed decade of pharmaceutical care was turning into a decade of confusion, conflict, and controversy. The Clinton Administration tackled the difficult task of reforming the complex American health care system. This effort failed, but it did inspire a raft of consolidations throughout the pharmaceutical enterprise, which resulted in a leaner and meaner industry. Third-parties turned to the principles of managed care to cut costs. Important new classes of drugs appeared, which when combined with an aging population, led to a rapid rise in prescription volume. Prescribing further increased under the pressure of direct-to-consumer advertising, which was given relatively free rein by the late 1990s. The emergence of Internet pharmacies, building on the established mail-order business of earlier years, added to the turmoil of the pharmaceutical marketplace. Independently owned drugstores closed across the nation, replaced in many localities by pharmacies tucked inside mass merchandisers or grocery stores. As the decade ended with the distractions of the Y2K non-event, far more pharmacists found themselves acting as arbiters of managed care squabbles than as advanced care providers.

THE FUTURE

It is too soon for historians to judge the long-term influence of the pharmaceutical care concept. Two full generations of pharmacists have been educated and trained after the general adoption of the aims of clinical pharmacy. Present day-to-day practice reflects this important shift from the product orientation of previous decades to an orientation concerned with patients receiving necessary drug information. In the midst of a harsh economic and regulatory climate, only time will tell if the often divided and divisive pharmaceutical profession will unite and continue its progress toward greater societal responsibility for the ancient tool we call medicines.

HISTORY AS A DISCIPLINE

Like the other fields of pharmacy described in this textbook, the history of pharmacy is a distinct discipline that produces a body of research. The following bibliography and chronology, updated from the previous editions by Glenn Sonnedecker, is provided for those interested in pursuing some specific aspect of pharmaceutical history. Readers interested in learning more about important figures in the history of American pharmacy should consult *RPS-13*, page 20. Additional guidance can be obtained from the American Institute of the History of Pharmacy, University of Wisconsin at Madison, 777 Highland Avenue, Madison, WI 53705. Links to useful websites pertinent to the field are found at www.aihp.org.

BIBLIOGRAPHIC NOTES

Besides giving recognition to sources on which the above historical essay is based, these references suggest further readings and reference materials. English-language publications are cited unless there is no approximate counterpart of a foreign-language publication. For those with deeper historical interests, bibliographies in some of the publications mentioned will lead to more specialized and often more meaningful literature.

The book with the most comprehensive scope in English is *Kremers and Urdang's History of Pharmacy,* revised by Glenn Sonnedecker (Philadelphia: Lippincott, 1976; AIHP reprint, 1986); see the glossary, Appendix 6, as well as the notes and references for bibliographic material. Hermann Schelenz, *Geschichte der Pharmazie* (Berlin: J. Springer, 1904; republished Hildesheim: Gg Olms, 1965) is a monumental reference work; although it is now outdated in many details, it richly documents the earlier literature. Erwin H Ackerknecht, *Therapeutics from the Primitives to the 20th Century* (New York: Hafner [1973]; German edition, 1970) is a general overview. Another overview is Ronald D Mann, *Modern Drug Use: An Enquiry on Historical Principles* (Lancaster; Boston: MTP Press, 1984). See also GJ Higby and EC Stroud, editors, *The Inside Story of Medicines: A Symposium* (Madison, WI: American Institute of the History of Pharmacy, 1997). A valuable short synthesis is John Parascandola, "A Brief History of Drug Use," in *Perspectives on Medicines in Society,* Albert I Wertheimer and P Bush, editors (Drug Intell, 1977). For illustrations, see particularly W-H Hein and DA Wittop Koning, *Bildkatalog zur Geschichte der Pharmazie* (ns Bd 33), *Veroffentlichungen der Internationalen Gesellschaft fur Geschichte der Pharmazie* (Stuttgart, 1969). For an excellent survey with scores of fine historical images, see DL Cowen and WH Helfand, *Pharmacy: An Illustrated History* (New York: Abrams, 1990).

A few general guides to the historical literature are GJ Higby and EC Stroud, editors, *The History of Pharmacy: A Selected, Annotated Bibliography* (New York: Garland, 1995); Glenn Sonnedecker, JH Hoch, and Wolfgang Schneider, *Some Pharmaco-Historical Guidelines to the Literature* (Madison, WI: American Institute of the History of Pharmacy, 1959; reprinted from *Am J Pharm Educ* 1959; 23: 143); *Index-Catalogue of the Library of the Surgeon-General's Office* (Washington, DC: US Army, 4 series, 1880–1936); E-H Guitard, *Manuel d'histoire de la littérature pharmaceutique* (Paris, 1942); *Bibliography of the History of Medicine* (Bethesda, MD: National Library of Medicine, USPHS, No. 1, 1965, et seq.; annual that includes pharmacy); *Current Work in the History of Medicine*, a quarterly from The Wellcome Historical Medical Library, London, since 1954 (includes pharmacy internationally), most recently collated in 1986; "Bibliography of the History of Medicine of the United States and Canada," published annually, 1939–1966, in the *Bulletin of the History of Medicine,* which includes a pharmacy section; E-H Guitard, *Index des travaux d'histoire de la pharmacie de 1913 à 1963* (Paris: Société d'Histoire de la Pharmacie [1968]); "Pharmazie Geschichtliche Rundschau," GE Dann, editor, vol 1 (1954–1957, et seq) is historical abstracts, a periodic supplement to the *Pharmazeutische Zeitung*; Glenn Sonnedecker and Alex Berman, *Some Bibliographic Aids for Historical Writers in Pharmacy* (Madison, WI: American Institute of the History of Pharmacy, 1958); and David L Cowen, *America's Pre-Pharmacopeial Literature* (Madison, WI: American Institute of the History of Pharmacy, 1961). Nydia M King's *A Selection of Primary Sources for the History of Pharmacy in the United States* (Madison, WI: American Institute of the History of Pharmacy, 1987) describes in detail 89 key works that document American pharmacy from 1720 to 1940 (microform or photoduplicated copies of 85 of the 89 works are available from University Microfilms International of Ann Arbor, MI.) For the scientific aspects of pharmacy see the *ISIS Cumulative Bibliography* (London: Mansell, 1971) and its continuations, which includes pharmacy. Useful World Wide Web resources include HISTLINE from the National Library of Medicine (http://igm.nlm.nih.gov/) and the Pharmaziehistorischen Bibliographie or PhB (http://www.ubka.uni-karlsruhe. de/pharm/phb.html). Some general information about the history of pharmacy can be obtained from the website of the American Institute of the History of Pharmacy (http:// www. aihp. org).

On Antiquity: The most definitive paper of general scope on Egypt is by Frans Jonckheere, *Le 'Préparateur de Remédes' dans l'organisation de la pharmacie égyptienne* (Veroffentlichung Nr 29; Berlin: Deutsche Akademie der Wissenschaften zu Berlin, Institut fur Orientforschung, 1955; Sonderdruck aus "Aegyptologische Studien . . ."). CD Leake, *The Old Egyptian Medical Papyri* (Lawrence: University of Kansas Press, 1952) gives an overview of the documents; for a first-hand impression of the papyrus most important pharmaceutically, see Bendix Ebbell's translation, *The Papyrus Ebers: The Greatest Egyptian Medical Document* (Copenhagen: Levin & Munksgaard; London: H. Milford, Oxford University Press, 1937). Henry Sigerist, *A History of Medicine, Vol 1: Primitive and Archaic Medicine* (New York: Oxford University Press, 1951–1961) is the best general survey. See also J. Worth Estes, *The Medical Skills of Ancient Egypt* (Canton, MA: Science History/USA, 1989), and Lise Manniche, *An Ancient Egyptian Herbal* (Austin: University of Texas Press, 1989). On Mesopotamia, an excellent book of breadth, relevant to pharmacy, is Martin Levey's, *Chemistry and Chemical Technology in Ancient Mesopotamia* (Amsterdam; New York: Elsevier, 1959); on Assyria, see monographs by Reginald C Thompson. The best sociohistorical review in English is Henry E Sigerist, *A History of Medicine, Vol II: Early Greek, Hindu and*

Persian Medicine (New York: Oxford University Press, 1961); works more specifically on pharmacy are J Berendes, *Die Pharmacie bei den alten Culturvolkern,* 2 vols (Halle aS, 1891), and Alfred Schmidt, *Drogen und Drogenhandel im Altertum* (Leipzig: JA Barth, 1924). The Hippocratic treatises have been translated into English by WHS Jones and ET Withington, *Hippocrates,* 4 vols (London, 1923–1931); a compilation on Hippocratic drugs was published by Johann H Dierbach, *Die Arzneimittel des Hippokrates . . .* (Heidelberg, 1824). For modern scholarship, from a different viewpoint, see Jerry Stannard, "Hippocratic Pharmacology" (*Bull Hist Med* 1961; 35: 497); see also his article "Materia Medica and Philosophical Theory in Aretaeus" (*Sudhoffs Arch Gesch Med Naturw* 1964; 48: 27). The foundation of western drug lore, the Materia Medica of Dioscorides, is reinterpreted by John Riddle in *Dioscorides on Pharmacy and Medicine* (Austin: University of Texas Press, 1985). Those interested in texts from the ancient period should check "Texts and Sources in Ancient Pharmacy," by John Scarborough (*Pharm Hist* 1987; 29: 81, 133). Common dealers in drugs are discussed by Vivian Nutton, "The Drug Trade in Antiquity" (*J Roy Soc Med* 1985; 78: 138). On Greek temple medicine, see Ch Kerenyi, *Le Medecin divin* (Basle, 1948), and EJ Edelstein and L Edelstein, *Asclepius, A Collection and Interpretation of the Testimonies,* 2 vols (Baltimore, 1945; reprinted New York: Arno Press, 1975). The first volume of a projected series by the late Rudolf Schmitz, *Geschichte der Pharmazie* (Eschborn: Govi-Verlag, 1998), covers the ancient period up to the start of the Middle Ages.

On the Middle Ages: For a general survey of *medieval Islam* and its influence, see Lucien Leclerc, *Histoire de la médecine Arabe,* 2 vols (Paris: E Leroux, 1876); also see Donald Campbell, *Arabian Medicine and Its Influence on the Middle Ages,* 2 vols (London: K. Paul, Trench, Trubner, 1926), and Cyril Elgood, *A Medical History of Persia and the Eastern Caliphate from the Earliest Times until the Year A.D. 1932* (Cambridge, England: Cambridge University Press, 1951). Much has been translated or written about Arabic materia medica and drug therapy, to which the principal key is Sami K Hamarneh's *Bibliography on Medicine and Pharmacy in Medieval Islam* (Stuttgart: Wissenschaftliche Verlagsgesellschaft, 1964), a part of the Internationale Gesellschaft für Geschichte der Pharmazie series. Among Hamarneh's other publications, see especially *Origins of Pharmacy and Therapy in the Near East* (Tokyo: Naito Foundation, 1973); also of much general interest is "The Rise of Professional Pharmacy in Islam" (*Med Hist* 1962; 6: 59). For a detailed view into 10th-century Spain (with a useful bibliography), see SK Hamarneh and G Sonnedecker, *A Pharmaceutical View of Abulcasis al-Zahrawi in Moorish Spain* (Leiden: EJ Brill, 1963). Important works by Max Meyerhof include several on materia medica, such as his monograph *The Abridged Version of "The Book of Simple Drugs" of Ahmad ibn Muhammad al-Ghâfiqî* (Publication no 4, Cairo: The Egyptian University Faculty of Medicine/Government Press, 1932), on al-Beruni in *Studien zur Geschichte des Naturwissenschaften und der Medizin,* vol 3 (Berlin, 1943, pp 159–208); and his four articles in the Ciba Symposia (vol 6, Nos 5 and 6, 1944). See likewise the writings of Martin Levey, such as *The Medical Formulary, or Agrabadhin of al-Kindi* (Madison: University of Wisconsin Press, 1966).

On Medieval Europe: A volume still not superseded (although outdated in details) is George F Fort, *Medical Economy During the Middle Ages* (New York, 1883; reprinted New York: AM Kelley, 1970); see also David Riesman, *The Story of Medicine in the Middle Ages* (New York: PB Hoeber, 1935). A valuable guide and commentary is Henry E Sigerist's, "The Latin Medical Literature of the Early Middle Ages" (*J Hist Med* 1958; 13: 127). Four papers contained in the *Symposium on Byzantine Medicine* (Washington, DC: Dumbarton Oaks Research Library and Collection, 1985), edited by John Scarborough, relate to the history of pharmacy. Works of more specifically pharmaceutical interest must include the definitive study on the renowned pharmacomedical edicts in the Kingdom of the Two Sicilies by Wolfgang-Hagen Hein and Kurt Sappert, *Die*

Medizinalordnung Friedrichs II. Eine pharmaziehistorische Studie (Eutin: Internationale Gesellschaft für Geschichte der Pharmazie, 1957). In the periodical literature, note particularly the writings of Alfons Lutz, such as "Der verschollene frühsalernitanische Antidotarius magnus . . ." and its rich bibliography (new series, vol 16; Stuttgart: Veröffentlichungen der Internationalen Gesellschaft für Geschichte der Pharmazie, 1960, pp 97–133); also see the works of Rudolf Schmitz, such as ". . . Apothekerstandes im Hoch und Spät-Mittelalter" (vol 13; Stuttgart: Veröffentlichungen der Internationalen Gesellschaft für Geschichte der Pharmazie, 1958, pp 157–165) and "Ueber deutsche mittelalterliche Quellen zur Geschichte von Pharmazie und Medizin" (*Deut Apotheker-Ztg* 1960; 100: 980). English language studies of unusual value and clarity include articles by GE Trease, such as "The Spicers and Apothecaries of the Royal Household in the Reigns of Henry III, Edward I and Edward II" (*Nottingham Mediaeval Studies* 1959; 3: 19; abridged in *Pharm J*, 4 April 1949, pp 246–248). A uniquely useful work is Sister Mary Francis Xavier [Welhoefer], "Statutes of the Guild of Physicians, Apothecaries and Merchants in Florence (1313–1316): A Brief Commentary, with an Introduction and Translation," (unpublished PhD dissertation, University of Wisconsin, 1935), even though it is dated as to many details. On medieval European materia medica, see Henry E Sigerist, "Materia Medica in the Middle Ages" (*Bull Hist Med* 1939; 7: 417), and his "Studien und Texte zur frühmittelalterlichen Rezeptliteratur" (vol 13; Leipzig: Studien zur Geschichte der Medizin, 1923, pp 187ff). Probably the earliest pharmacist's textbook and manual has been translated into German by Leo Zimmermann, *Saladini de Asculo . . . Compendium aromatariorum* (Leipzig, 1919); for a Hebrew translation, see Suessmann Muntner, editor, *Sefer ha-rokhim* (Tel-Aviv: np, 1953).

On Modern Europe: For a reliable and concise medical overview, see Erwin Ackerknecht, *A Short History of Medicine* (New York: Ronald Press, 1955); for detailed references, supplement it with Fielding H Garrison, *An Introduction to the History of Medicine*, 4th ed (Philadelphia; London: WB Saunders, 1929; republished 1960), noting especially the bibliographic essays of Appendix III. Some international survey volumes on pharmacy, with particular reference to the modern period, are listed in Sonnedecker and Berman's *Some Bibliographic Aids for Historical Writers in Pharmacy* (Madison, WI: American Institute of the History of Pharmacy, 1958). A gap has been closed, meanwhile, by Leslie G Matthews, *History of Pharmacy in Britain* (Edinburgh and London: E & S Livingstone, 1962) and Cecil Wall, HC Cameron, and EA Underwood, *A History of the Worshipful Society of Apothecaries of London, Vol I: 1617–1815* (London: Oxford University Press, 1963). For those contemplating research in British archives, see L Richmond, J Stevenson & A Turton, eds., *The Pharmaceutical Industry: A Guide to Historical Records* (Burlington, VT: Ashgate, 2003). There is not yet a comprehensive, up-to-date history that deals with European pharmacy; bibliographies, such as those cited in the earlier section on general literature guides, will yield books and monographs from particular topical and national viewpoints. For an example of a specialized topic, see Richard Palmer, "Pharmacy in the Republic of Venice," in *The Medical Renaissance of the Sixteenth Century*, A Wear, editor (New York: Cambridge University Press, 1985); see also R Pötzsch, editor, *The Pharmacy: Windows on History* (Roche, 1996). A specialized book of note is M. S. Conroy, *In Health and Sickness: Pharmacy, Pharmacists, and the Pharmaceutical Industry in Late Imperial, Early Soviet Russia* (New York, Columbia University Press, 1994). Especially rich in European history are the publications, 1927 to the present, of the International Society for the History of Pharmacy; a partial key has been published by Herbert Hugel, Die "Veroffentlichungen der Internationalen Gesellschaft für Geschichte der Pharmazie 1953–1965: Eine Bibliographie" (new series Bd 29; Stuttgart: Veröffentlichungen der Internationalen Gesellschaft für Geschichte der Pharmazie, 1967).

On the US: The standard volume in English, *Kremers and Urdang's History of Pharmacy*, revised by Glenn Sonnedecker

(Philadelphia: Lippincott, 1976), devotes approximately two-thirds of the main text to the United States, and its bibliographies open up a wide range of other American literature. Noteworthy are the anniversary issues of *Druggists Circular* (vol 51, January 1907) and *Pharmaceutical Era* (vol 16, no 27, 31 December 1896). See also Glenn Sonnedecker, "Structure and Stress of American Pharmacy" (*Pharm J*, 14 April 1956, pp 3–8). A series of 18 historical articles on American pharmacy were published in *J APhA* during 2000, 2001, and 2002. Four papers covering a wide variety of American topics are contained in GJ Higby & EC Stroud, eds., *Apothecaries and the Drug Trade* (Madison: American Institute of the History of Pharmacy, 2001). The story of American pharmacy's umbrella organization is told by George Griffenhagen, *150 Years of Caring: A Pictorial History of the American Pharmaceutical Association* (Washington, DC: APhA, 2002). Pharmaceutical education is explored in depth by Robert A. Buerki, "In Search of Excellence: The First Century of the American Association of Colleges of Pharmacy," *Am J Pharm Ed* 63 (Fall Supplement 1999): 1–210. A useful look at certain aspects of colonial American pharmacy can be found in Renate Wilson, *Pious Traders in Medicine: a German Pharmaceutical Network in Eighteenth-Century North America* (University Park, PA: Pennsylvania State University Press, 2000). Several different aspects of 19th-century practice are considered by Gregory Higby, *In Service to American Pharmacy: The Professional Life of William Procter, Jr* (Tuscaloosa: University of Alabama Press, 1992). A solid biography of a 20th-century American pharmacist is James Madison, *Eli Lilly: A Life, 1885–1977* (Indianapolis: Indiana Historical Society, 1989). Other valuable biographies include Michael A Flannery, *John Uri Lloyd: The Great American Eclectic* (Carbondale: Southern Illinois University Press, 1998) and Sabine Knoll-Schütze, *Friedrich Hoffmann (1832–1904) and the 'Pharmaceutische Rundschau'* (New York: Peter Lang, 2003). Changes in the use and production of drugs are explored by John Harley Warner, *The Therapeutic Perspective: Medical Practice, Knowledge, and Identity in America, 1820–1885* (Cambridge: Harvard University Press, 1986) and John P Swann, *Academic Scientists and the Pharmaceutical Industry: Cooperative Research in Twentieth-Century America* (Baltimore: Johns Hopkins University Press, 1988). See also John Parascandola, *The Development of American Pharmacology: John J. Abel and the Shaping of a Discipline* (Baltimore: Johns Hopkins University Press, 1992) and Harry M Marks, *The Progress of Experiment: Science and Therapeutic Reform in the United States, 1900–1990* (Cambridge, UK; New York: Cambridge University Press, 1997). Short histories of individual drugs are provided by Walter Sneader, *Drug Prototypes and Their Exploitation* (New York: John Wiley, 1996). For a contemporary use of historical arguments in policy analysis, see a series of articles written by RW Holland & CM Nimmo on "Transitions in Pharmacy Practice," that appear in the *Amer J Health-System Pharm* 56 (1999): 1758–64, 1981–7, 2234–41, 2458–62, 57 (2000): 64–72. A useful bibliography that is still in print is by George Griffenhagen, *Bibliography of Papers Published by the American Pharmaceutical Association that were presented before the Association's Section on Historical Pharmacy, 1904–1967* (Madison, WI: American Institute of the History of Pharmacy, nd), which includes subject and author indexes; although it emphasizes American history, it is by no means restricted to it. The "Pharmacy" section of the annual bibliography in the *Bulletin of the History of Medicine* at one time offered an important key to the literature, which was cumulated in *Bibliography of the History of Medicine of the United States and Canada, 1939–1960,* Genevieve Miller, editor (Baltimore: Johns Hopkins University Press, 1964). See also other bibliographies listed earlier in the section on general literature guides. Also noteworthy is the "Bookshelf" section of *Pharmacy in History*, a quarterly of the American Institute of the History of Pharmacy (Madison, WI); and the sections on "History and Ethics," "Sociology and Economics," and "Literature" in the ongoing *International Pharmaceutical Abstracts* (Washington, DC: American Society of Hospital Pharmacists).

A CHRONOLOGY FOR PHARMACISTS

The dating of events often involves uncertainties, approximations, and questions of meaning that are not apparent in a concise table such as that below. Particularly, dates before the 18th century often are unverifiable or estimated.

BCE

2000?	**Earliest formulary** known in history (Sumerian).
1500	**Ebers Papyrus,** Egyptian manuscript pertaining to pharmacy and therapy.
460	**Hippocrates,** famous Greek physician, is born.
350	**Diocles** writes an important treatise on materia medica.
372	**Theophrastus** (372–285), the "father of botany," is born.

AD

50	**Dioscorides** writes an important book on materia medica.
130	**Galen,** a Roman physician who experimented with compounded drugs, is born.
303	**Cosmas and Damian,** patron saints of pharmacy and medicine, are martyred.
857	**Johann Mesue Senior** (777–857), Arabian physician, dies.
925	**Rhazes** (865–925), Persian physician, dies.
1035	**Avicenna** (980–1035), physician and philosopher, dies.
1178	**Pharmacists are mentioned in French records.**
1180	**Guild of Pepperers** is already active in London.
1225	**Apothecary shop** is established at Cologne.
1297	**Guild of Pharmacists** is organized in Bruges (Flanders).
1345	**Apothecary shops** have been established in London.
1348	**The Black Death** (bubonic plague) strikes Europe.
1480	**Poison law** is enacted by James I of Scotland.
1499	**Guild pharmacopoeia** is published in Florence, Italy.
1529	**Paracelsus** (1493–1541) publishes his first treatise.
1546	**The Nuremberg Pharmacopoeia** (Dispensatory of Valerius Cordus) is perhaps the first to become "official."
1589	**Galileo Galilei** demonstrates the law of falling bodies.
1604	**Louis Hébert** becomes first pharmacist to settle in North America.
1617	**Society of Apothecaries** in London is organized.
1618	**First London pharmacopoeia** is published.
1620	**Pilgrims** settle at Plymouth, Massachusetts.
1628	**William Harvey** publishes his book on the **circulation of the blood.**
1646	**William Davis** operates an apothecary shop, possibly one of the first in America (Boston).
1665	**Sir Isaac Newton** describes the law of gravitation.
1680	**Antonie van Leeuwenhoek** discovers **yeast** plants.
1703	**English apothecaries are authorized to prescribe** as well as dispense.
1715	**Bartram's Botanical Gardens** established at Philadelphia.
1718	**E-Fr Geoffroy,** French pharmacist, establishes the first tabulation of relationships between chemical substances.
1736	**First law related to pharmacy** in America is enacted in Virginia.
1752	**First hospital pharmacy** in America is established at Pennsylvania Hospital in Philadelphia; Jonathan Roberts is the apothecary.
1762	**Antoine Baumé** publishes his *Élémens de pharmacie* in France.
1765	**John Morgan,** American medical education pioneer, advocates **prescription writing** in US.
1773	**Karl Wilhelm Scheele isolates oxygen** about 1773; **Joseph Priestley** independently isolates oxygen by 1774.
1774	**Scheele** discovers **chlorine.**

1776	**Declaration of Independence** is written, and the position of Apothecary General is created for the Continental Army.
	Christopher Marshall, famous American pharmacist, makes medicines for wounded soldiers.
1777	**Collége de Pharmacie** is established in Paris.
1783	**Pilâtre de Rozier,** a pharmacist, makes **first human flight** in a balloon accompanied by the Marquis d'Arlandes.
1785	**William Withering** publishes his treatise on **digitalis.**
	Thomas Fowler introduces **Fowler's Solution** (potassium arsenite solution).
1787	**Ergot** introduced in obstetrics by **Paullitzsky.**
1790	**First US patent law passed.** Elisha Perkins takes out first medical patent in 1796.
1793	**Yellow fever epidemic** strikes Philadelphia.
	Trommsdorff's *Journal der pharmacie* is founded, the first professional-scientific journal devoted to pharmacy.
1798	**Edward Jenner** publishes his work on **vaccination.**
1805	German pharmacist **Friedrich Sertürner** reports isolation of **morphine.**
1809	*Journal de pharmacie et de chimie* founded; first published as *Bulletin de pharmacie.*
1811	**Bernard Courtois,** a French pharmacist, discovers **iodine.**
1818	French pharmacist-chemists **Joseph Caventou** and **Pierre Pelletier** isolate **strychnine.**
1820	**Pelletier** and **Caventou** isolate **quinine.**
	First edition of *United States Pharmacopoeia* is published.
1821	**Philadelphia College of Pharmacy** is founded as the first local association and school of pharmacy in the United States.
1823	**Massachusetts College of Pharmacy** founded.
1825	**First American professional journal of pharmacy published,** the *American Journal of Pharmacy.*
1826	**Antoine Balard,** French pharmacist, discovers **bromine.**
	Hennel synthesizes **ethyl alcohol.**
1828	**Friedrich Wöhler** synthesizes **urea,** thus bridging gulf between organic and inorganic chemistry.
1829	**New York College of Pharmacy** is founded.
1831	**Chloroform** is prepared independently by **Justus von Liebig** and by **Eugene Soubeiran.**
1832	**Pierre Robiquet,** French pharmacist, isolates **codeine.**
1834	**Friedlieb Ferdinand Runge,** German pharmacist, prepares **carbolic acid** and **aniline.**
1842	**Crawford Long** performs the first **operation using ether anesthesia.**
1843	**Oliver Wendell Holmes** points out that puerperal fever is contagious.
1848	**First American code of pharmaceutical ethics** prepared by Philadelphia College of Pharmacy.
	First drug import law enacted by Congress to curb adulterations.
1852	**American Pharmaceutical Association** is founded as the first national organization.
	Charles Darwin publishes his *Origin of Species.*
1865	**First international pharmaceutical conference** is held in Brunswick, Germany.
1868	**University of Michigan** opens pharmacy course that will have far-reaching influence in modernizing American pharmaceutical education.
1883	**First National Retail Druggists Association** founded.
1888	**First National Formulary** issued by American Pharmaceutical Association.
1890	**Emil von Behring** and **Shibasaburo Kitasato** introduce **serum therapy.**
1893	**Felix Hoffmann** and **Arthur Eichengrün** discover **aspirin.**
1895	**Wilhelm Roentgen** discovers **x-rays.**
1898	**Marie** and **Pierre Curie** discover **radium.**

National Association of Retail Druggists is founded in the US.

1899 **Walter Reed** proves mosquitoes carry **yellow fever**.

1900 **American Association of Colleges of Pharmacy** is founded.

1902 **First International Pharmacopeial Conference** held at Brussels, Belgium.

First American PhD supervised in pharmacy granted at University of Wisconsin.

1906 **Federal Food and Drugs Act** passed in the US.

1910 **Paul Ehrlich** and **Sahachiro Hata** introduce **arsphenamine** (also known as Salvarsan or "606") in widespread clinical trial for the treatment of syphilis.

1912 **First** Assembly of **International Pharmaceutical Federation** (The Hague, Netherlands).

1922 **Sir Frederick Banting** and **Charles Best** isolate **insulin**.

1928 **Sir Alexander Fleming** discovers **penicillin**, the first antibiotic.

1935 **Gerhard Domagk** introduces **prontosil**, the first sulfa drug.

1937 *American Journal of Pharmaceutical Education* is founded, the first periodical devoted to **pharmaceutical education**.

1938 **League of Nations Commission on International Pharmacopeial Standards** holds conferences.

Important revision of Federal Pure Food and Drugs Act (US).

1940 **Howard Florey** and **Ernst Chain** hold the first **clinical trials of penicillin**.

1942 **American Society of Hospital Pharmacists** is founded.

1944 Antibiotic activity of **streptomycin** is announced.

1945 **Atomic energy** released for use in warfare and medicine.

1947 **Medical Service Corps** created in US Army, with pharmacy represented by special group of commissioned officers.

1948 **First Pan-American Congress of Pharmacy and Biochemistry**.

1949 **Cortisone** and **ACTH** are introduced for rheumatic arthritis.

Influence for change initiated by analysis and suggested reforms from **Pharmaceutical Survey** (US).

1951 **First International Pharmacopoeia** of the World Health Organization.

1952 **Chlorpromazine** is introduced into psychiatry, thus opening the field of psychopharmacology.

1955 **Salk poliomyelitis vaccine** is released for general use.

1959 **Synthetic modifications of natural penicillin** introduced.

American Society of Pharmacognosy founded.

1962 Important amendments of the **US Food, Drug, and Cosmetic Act**.

1969 American Society of **Consultant Pharmacists** (ASCP) established.

1973 US Supreme Court decision (No 72-1176) holds that states may require that licensed pharmacists have **ownership-control of pharmacies**.

Congress enacts **Health Maintenance Organization** Act.

1975 Official **drug standardization program** is unified by US Pharmacopeia absorbing National Formulary.

Report by Study Commission on Pharmacy (AACP) gives impetus to trend toward drug information and **counseling role** of pharmacists.

1977 Clinical trials of **adenine arabinoside** against herpes raise prospect of **controlling viral diseases**.

1979 **American College of Clinical Pharmacy** is founded.

1982 **Specialty certification** begins in American pharmacy with the board certification of 63 pharmacists in the field of nuclear pharmacy.

1984 Drug Price Competition and Patent Term Restoration Act encourages **growth of generics**.

1986 **American Association of Pharmaceutical Scientists** is founded.

1989 **American Council on Pharmaceutical Education** (ACPE) announces intent to develop accreditation standards for **Doctor of Pharmacy** programs only.

1990 Omnibus Budget Reconciliation Act (OBRA) requires that **pharmacists counsel Medicaid patients** (effective 1993).

1995 **Pharmacy Technician** Certification Board formed.

1996 National Association of Retail Druggists (f. 1898) **changes name** to National Community Pharmacists Association.

1997 **National Association of Boards of Pharmacy** (NABP) proposes **regular competency tests** for pharmacists.

2003 After 150 years, the APhA changes its name to the **American Pharmacists Association**.

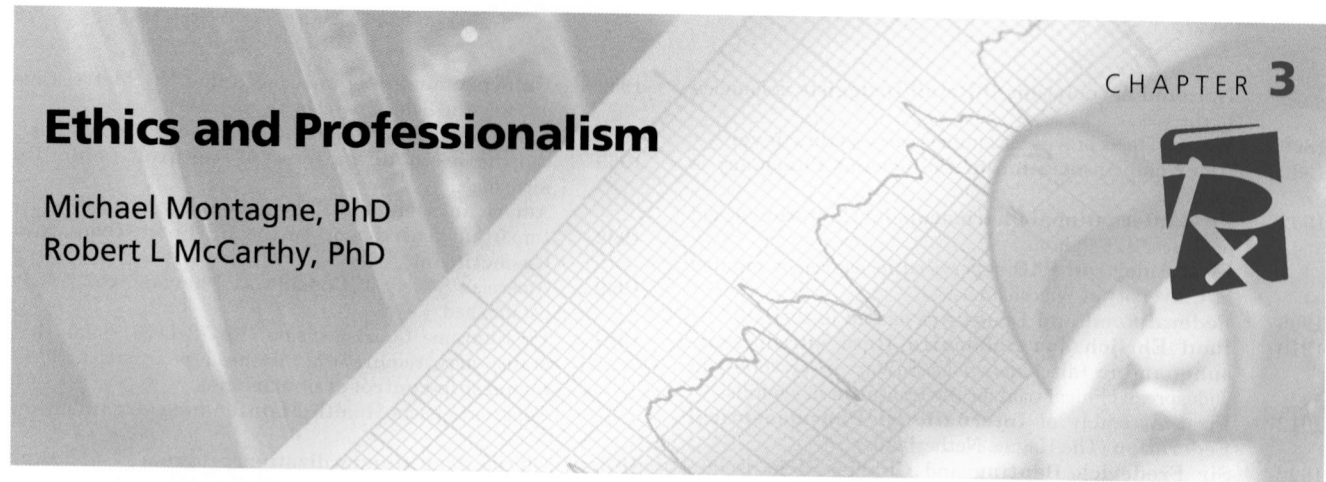

CHAPTER 3

Ethics and Professionalism

Michael Montagne, PhD

Robert L McCarthy, PhD

The quest to construct systematically an ethical framework for Western civilization was begun over 2000 years ago by Socrates. He approached ethics as a science, as being "governed by principles of universal validity, so that what was good for one was good for all, and what was my neighbor's duty was my duty also."[1] However, acceptance of the Socratic approach has proved burdensome. After 2000 years of effort, humankind universally adheres to not even one ethical principle.

No set of ethical principles, no matter how carefully thought out or how well constructed, can provide the individual professional with guidance for each decision about clients, peers, or society. There are people who believe that because each situation is different, each decision requires separate analysis of possible outcomes from different actions and the weighing of right and wrong. Regardless of one's stance or approach, however, the health professional in today's society needs continual self-examination of professional duties and ethical principles to be prepared for the conflicts and dilemmas they will face.

BEING PROFESSIONAL

In this discussion, professional ethics is used only to denote "the profession's interpretation of the will of society for the conduct of the members of that profession augmented by the special knowledge that only the members of the profession possess."[2] In other contexts, the term might be used to denote those ethical principles to which society believes any individual claiming professional status should subscribe. What is to be gained by development of a set of ethical principles, or a code of ethics (Fig 3-1), by a profession to which it expects its members to abide?

First, a code of ethics makes the decision-making process more efficient. In opposition to situational ethicists, Veatch claims:

> "Yet if those who must resolve the ever-increasing ethical dilemmas in medicine—including patients, family members, physicians, nurses, hospital administrators, and public policy-makers—treat every case as something entirely fresh, entirely novel, they will have lost perhaps the best way of reaching solutions: to understand the general principles of ethics and face each new situation from a systematic ethical stance."[3]

Clinical practice predisposes pharmacists to a situationalist approach to ethics through its emphasis on individual differences in response to therapeutic regimens. Some guidelines, however, exist for adjusting drug therapy in patients with compromised renal or hepatic function, electrolyte or hormonal imbalance, and other pathological abnormalities. Therapeutic guidelines give us a place to begin solving a clinical problem. Rules of morality serve the same purpose:

> "They may at least act as rules-of-thumb for handling easy cases. They may at least summarize ethical reasoning that has gone before by others who have found themselves in somewhat similar situations. They may at least serve as guidelines for formulating thinking about the problem at hand."[4]

Second, individual professionals occasionally may need guidelines for directing their professional behavior. Each decision made by a professional requires calling upon a store of technological information as well as the individual's own sense of right and wrong. Almost assuredly, all professionals will be confronted with situations that they have never considered in great detail. Where one can find no apparent theological or personal ethical principles to apply, one might turn to professional ethics for guidance.

Finally, professional ethics establish a pattern of behavior that clients come to expect from members of the profession. Once a consistent pattern of behavior is discerned by clients, they expect that behavior to remain constant, and their expectations become part of the relationship they establish with the professional. To better understand the role of and necessity for ethics in professions, one must first look at the characteristics of professions.

PROFESSIONAL CHARACTERISTICS

The first characteristic of a professional is possession of a specialized body of knowledge; using this body of knowledge enables the practitioner to perform a highly useful social function. All lawful occupations provide some positive benefit to society and are based on specialized knowledge. The professions generally are more socially useful than many other occupations, but social utility alone does not make an occupation a profession.

An applied body of knowledge may be composed of knowledge of a manual skill or intellectual knowledge. The latter is of primary significance as a criterion for professions. The pharmacist is not considered a professional because of good typing skills. Rather, he or she possesses the relevant professional knowledge about drugs and patients that permits the pharmacist to advise patients and prescribers concerning drug therapy, detect drug interactions, select appropriate product sources, and exercise professional judgment.

The exercise of proper judgment is a key element in this first professional characteristic. Professional services traditionally are rendered to an individual rather than to a group. Using the specialized body of knowledge of the profession and the intellectual abilities of the professional, the practitioner makes a judgment as to the best course of treatment for each individual.

Code of Ethics

American Pharmacists Association

Preamble

Pharmacists are health professionals who assist individuals in making the best use of medications. This Code, prepared and supported by pharmacists, is intended to state publicly the principles that form the fundamental basis of the roles and responsibilities of pharmacists. These principles, based on moral obligations and virtues, are established to guide pharmacists in relationships with patients, health professionals, and society.

I. A pharmacist respects the covenantal relationship between the patient and pharmacist.

Considering the patient-pharmacist relationship as a covenant means that a pharmacist has moral obligations in response to the gift of trust received from society. In return for this gift, a pharmacist promises to help individuals achieve optimum benefit from their medications, to be committed to their welfare, and to maintain their trust.

II. A pharmacist promotes the good of every patient in a caring, compassionate, and confidential manner.

A pharmacist places concern for the well-being of the patient at the center of professional practice. In doing so, a pharmacist considers needs stated by the patient as well as those defined by health science. A pharmacist is dedicated to protecting the dignity of the patient. With a caring attitude and a compassionate spirit, a pharmacist focuses on serving the patient in a private and confidential manner.

III. A pharmacist respects the autonomy and dignity of each patient.

A pharmacist promotes the right of self-determination and recognizes individual self-worth by encouraging patients to participate in decisions about their health. A pharmacist communicates with patients in terms that are understandable. In all cases, a pharmacist respects personal and cultural differences among patients.

IV. A pharmacist acts with honesty and integrity in professional relationships.

A pharmacist has a duty to tell the truth and to act with conviction of conscience. A pharmacist avoids discriminatory practices, behavior or work conditions that impair professional judgment, and actions that compromise dedication to the best interests of patients.

V. A pharmacist maintains professional competence.

A pharmacist has a duty to maintain knowledge and abilities as new medications, devices, and technologies become available and as health information advances.

VI. A pharmacist respects the values and abilities of colleagues and other health professionals.

When appropriate, a pharmacist asks for the consultation of colleagues or other health professionals or refers the patient. A pharmacist acknowledges that colleagues and other health professionals may differ in the beliefs and values they apply to the care of the patient.

VII. A pharmacist serves individual, community, and societal needs.

The primary obligation of a pharmacist is to individual patients. However, the obligations of a pharmacist may at times extend beyond the individual to the community and society. In these situations, the pharmacist recognizes the responsibilities that accompany these obligations and acts accordingly.

VIII. A pharmacist seeks justice in the distribution of health resources.

When health resources are allocated, a pharmacist is fair and equitable, balancing the needs of patients and society.

Figure 3-1. Code of ethic (Originally published in "Code of Ethics for Pharmacists." *Am J Health-Syst Pharm* 1995; 52: 2131. © 1995, American Society of Health-System Pharmacists, Inc. All rights reserved. Reprinted wiith permission.)

The second characteristic of a professional is a set of specific attitudes that influence professional behavior. The basic component of this set of attitudes is altruism, an unselfish concern for the welfare of others:

"The professional man, it has been said, does not work in order to be paid: he is paid in order that he may work. Every decision he makes in the course of his career is based on his sense of what is right, not on his estimate of what is profitable."[5]

Professionals are concerned with matters that are vital to the health or well-being of their clients. The practitioner employs highly specialized technical knowledge, which the patient or client does not possess. Both the client's lack of knowledge and the vital nature of professional services provide the professional with an opportunity to exploit the client. The consequences of such exploitation are severe. The smooth functioning of the professions requires that the practitioner must consider the needs of the patient as paramount, relegating his or her own material needs to an inferior position.

Social sanction, the third characteristic of a professional, is a resultant effect of the two characteristics already discussed. Whether an occupation is considered to be a profession depends, to a large degree, on whether society views it as such.

One measure of social sanction is the granting of exclusive rights of practice through the licensing power of the state.

Licensing not only attempts to protect the public from incompetent practitioners, but also frequently creates a relationship of trust between society and the professionals, because within the sphere of professional activities, the professional exercises an authoritative power over patients. As explained by Greenwood,

"[T]he professional dictates what is good or evil for the client, who has no choice but to accede to professional judgment. Here the premise is that, because he [or she] lacks the requisite theoretical background, the client cannot diagnose his [or her] own needs or discriminate among the range of possibilities for meeting them."[6]

The extent of the public's trust is a measure of the degree of social sanction, and this is evident in society's permitting the exercise of sovereign power over professional matters. Given the legal monopoly inherent in professional licensing, the failure of society to impose further controls on the profession is sanctioning, by implication, the profession's performance and self-regulation. Thus, professions have evolved as occupations connected with high status. The functional relationship of professions to

Oath of a Pharmacist

American Association of Colleges of Pharmacy

At this time, I vow to devote my professional life to the service of all humankind through the profession of pharmacy. I will consider the welfare of humanity and relief of human suffering my primary concerns. I will apply my knowledge, experience, and skills to the best of my ability to assure optimal drug therapy outcomes for the patients I serve.

I will do my best to keep abreast of developments and maintain professional competency in my profession of pharmacy. I will maintain the highest principles of moral, ethical, and legal conduct. I will embrace and advocate change in the profession of pharmacy that improves patient care. I take these vows voluntarily with the full realization of the responsibility with which I am entrusted by the public.

Figure 3-2. Oath of a pharmacist. (From http://www. aacp.org/site/ tertiary.asp? TRACKID 5 & VID 5 2 & CID 5 686 & DID 5 4339. Accessed May 14, 2004.)

society reinforces their status position, and the status itself acts as a motivating factor in the drive of any occupation to gain recognition as a profession.

Several studies have attempted to identify which occupations qualify as professions. The most prominent study was done by Carr-Saunders and Wilson in 1933.[7] Primarily because of the commercial elements inherent in modern pharmacy practice, the study reached no definitive conclusion as to pharmacy's professional status. More recent studies have produced similar results. Montague,[8] Smith,[9] Smith and Knapp,[10] and Denzin and Mettlin[11] consistently found pharmacy to fall short of full professional status. The key issues include a lack of autonomy (eg, pharmacists follow orders, fill prescriptions, decided by others, the prescriber) and potential or real conflicts regarding professional compensation based more so on products than on services (eg, pharmacists counsel patients on non-prescription products without charging a fee, but compensation comes through the sale of that product).

All professions, however, can be found to fall short of being a complete profession in at least a few respects. Pharmacy has a legitimate claim to a theoretical body of knowledge, to a growing degree of socially sanctioned decision-making authority, and to a commitment of service functions as articulated by a code of ethics and an oath (Fig 3-2) that is sworn by individuals entering the profession.

ETHICAL DECISIONMAKING

Pharmacy ethics has received a great deal of recent attention, but the study of ethics, ethical questions, and codes of ethics has been an integral component of pharmacy and medical practice for centuries. The first code of ethics for medicine was credited to Hippocrates in the 4th century BC. In many ways, the Hippocratic code is timeless. For example, his direction that no physician should "give a deadly drug to anybody if asked for it, nor . . . make a suggestion to this effect"[12] provides one moral perspective on the contemporary issue of assisted suicide.

Over the past decade or so, the attention given to pharmacy ethics in the professional and scientific literature, and in schools and colleges of pharmacy, has changed a great deal.

Only 2 of the 52 schools that responded to a 1980 survey required a formal, separate course in ethics; 32 schools offered no course, required or elective, of which ethics was an explicit part.[13] Today, however, most pharmacy schools require some instruction in ethics. A 1991 survey of ethics instruction at pharmacy schools found that, "while the quantity of ethics instruction has not increased, there are encouraging signs that the quality and depth of ethics education is improving."[14]

Several factors appear responsible for the heightened attention given to the study of ethics in pharmacy, including the explosion of biotechnology and the rapidly rising cost of health care in the US, of which drugs are an important component.

Macro Ethical Issues versus Micro Ethical Situations

Ethical situations in pharmacy can be divided into two broad categories: macro and micro.

Macro ethical issues are issues that are not specific to a given pharmacist, but rather are those that must be addressed by all pharmacists and by society in general. These include abortion, assisted suicide, genetic engineering, rationing of and access to health care, organ transplantation, and *in vitro* fertilization.

Micro situations are those issues that may confront individual pharmacists in the course of their daily practice. They include the use of placebos, patient confidentiality (eg, revealing information about a patient's medications to members of the family), and informed consent (eg, what and how much information about a medication should be disclosed to a patient).

Sometimes, *macro* issues are manifested in *micro* situations. This is especially true with socially controversial issues. For example, a pharmacist may receive a prescription for a drug and know that it is intended for use in an assisted suicide. Not only must the pharmacist deal with the legal issues involved, but also with the ethical responsibility as a health care professional. A further complication in such situations is the influence of the pharmacist's personal beliefs in choosing the course of action.

Competence, Trustworthiness, and Caring

Any examination of pharmacy ethics must begin with a discussion of the basic moral responsibilities that all health care practitioners have toward their patients. Berger[15] has attempted to describe the characteristics that a pharmacist should possess:

1. Pharmacists must be competent. They must possess a knowledge base that at least minimally allows them to carry out their functions as reliable therapeutic experts.
2. Pharmacists must be trustworthy. Patients must know that they can seek the confidential advice and assistance of their pharmacist and that their wishes will be carried out.
3. Pharmacists must care for and about their patients. As the 1995 American Pharmaceutical (now Pharmacists) Association (APhA) Code of Ethics directs, "A pharmacist places concern for the well-being of the patient at the center of professional practice."[16]

Pharmacists, unfortunately, do not always effectively communicate their concern for the welfare of their patients. All too often patients perceive just the opposite. Busy practitioners who fail to spend adequate time interacting with their patients do little to alter this perception. Conversely, pharmacists who do spend time with their patients and attempt to understand their concerns are much more likely to be viewed as caring.

Health Professional–Patient Relationship: Consumerism Versus Paternalism

It was not long ago that when a patient was instructed by their physician or pharmacist to take a medication, they did so without question. Medical paternalism—the belief that the health care professional knew best—was accepted as standard practice by most health care professionals and their patients. The medical rights of patients were not as widely recognized as other rights they held, such as suffrage or due process. Today, patients have become true consumers of medical care. Patients wish, and have a right, to be informed and asked for their consent. For a health care professional to do otherwise would not only be unprofessional and unethical, but also have potential legal ramifications.

Patients also expect a certain level of service. As with sellers of other goods and services, health professionals who fail to meet the demands of medical consumers for care will quickly find themselves without customers and, sometimes, with legal problems.[17]

Moral Rights Versus Legal Rights to Health Care

Any discussion of pharmacy ethics must be clear about what is meant by the term *right*. In this society, one frequently refers to the legal rights of individuals. *Legal rights* are either guaranteed fundamentally in the US Constitution (eg, the rights of free speech and assembly) or are provided by laws and regulations promulgated at the federal, state, or local level. We sometimes confuse what are really legal rights with our moral obligations.

Moral rights are quite different from legal rights. Granted, these rights may be reinforced by laws, but their basis lies not in law but in ethical principles. Such rights might include the right to live without fear of harm and the right to food and adequate shelter. More recently, Americans have grappled with the question of health care as a moral right.

As one might expect, moral rights and legal rights may conflict. There is disagreement, for example, over whether issues such as abortion involve moral rights or legal rights.

Patient's Rights

When a patient seeks the care of a pharmacist, what rights do they have? What can they reasonably expect from pharmacists? Patients can expect that pharmacists will employ their knowledge and experience in caring for them. They can expect that, as autonomous individuals, pharmacists will respond to their wishes about their treatment.

The American health care system seems fundamentally based upon ensuring the rights of patients. Patients generally choose their own physician, pharmacy, and hospital. Patients are allowed to choose from multiple options of treatment when they exist. Patients must give their approval, through the process of informed consent, prior to the initiation of care. All of the preceding presupposes that treatment is available and that the patient has the economic wherewithal to pay for that treatment. For patients who are uninsured or lack the ability to pay, the right to choose the nature of their health care is meaningless.

Patients also have a right to treatment that is both safe and effective within given parameters. The fundamental question that must be posed prior to considering any medical or surgical treatment for a patient is, Is the treatment safe and effective? Such a legal standard for drugs has been in effect since the passage of federal legislation in the early part of the 20th century.[18] Not only must a drug be shown to be effective—that is, able to produce the effect for which it was administered—it must work with a certain degree of safety.

Medical Practitioners' Duty to Their Patients

What is the responsibility of medical practitioners? Some might argue that health care providers have a Hippocratic responsibility to their patients, and that this responsibility focuses solely on what is best for the patient, irrespective of the consequences to others. This view is supported by the Code of Ethics of the APhA (American Pharmaceutical Association, now called the American Pharmacists Association), which states in part that "a pharmacist promotes the good of every patient in a caring, compassionate, and confidential manner."[16]

The Code appears to suggest that pharmacists have a moral obligation to do whatever they deem necessary in the interest of their patients. But the Code goes on to state that "a pharmacist serves individual, community and societal needs."[16] What then is the extent of the pharmacist's duty to his or her patients? Is it the pharmacist's moral obligation to care for them without exception?

Legal Responsibility Versus Moral Obligation

Rem Edwards provides an example of a radical interpretation of the Hippocratic oath insofar as he asserts that medical professionals have an obligation to do whatever is necessary to relieve the pain and suffering of their patients.[19] Edward's contention, however laudatory, has serious flaws when applied to pharmacists. All pharmacists practice under the practical constraints of law that may limit their doing *whatever is necessary*. Consequently, although they have a moral obligation to care for their patients, this obligation is constrained by law.

Thus, patient rights and practitioner responsibility may sometimes be in conflict, not on ethical grounds but on legal ones. Directing a pharmacist to assume an individualistic approach and take an illegal, yet ethical, action for a patient despite legal consequences is asking the pharmacist to subjugate his or her own interests to that of the patient.

ETHICAL RESPONSIBILITY

In traditional pharmacy practice, both the legal and ethical obligations of pharmacists centered around ensuring that the proper medication as ordered by the prescriber was delivered to the patient. Physicians, not pharmacists, were the health care professionals who held ultimate responsibility for monitoring the progress of a patient and ensuring that the desired outcome was achieved.

The concept of "pharmaceutical care," however, directs that this responsibility is to be a shared obligation between the prescriber and the pharmacist.[17] According to the Commission to Implement Change in Pharmaceutical Care, the mission of pharmacy practice is to render pharmaceutical care. Pharmaceutical care focuses pharmacists' attitudes, behaviors, commitments, concerns, ethics, functions, knowledge, responsibilities, and skills on the provision of drug therapy with the goal of achieving definite outcomes toward the improvement of the quality of life of the patient.[20] Pharmaceutical care forces pharmacy practitioners to change their focus, broaden their professional responsibility.

VEATCH'S FRAMEWORK FOR ETHICAL ANALYSIS

Robert Veatch[21] has suggested a framework for ethical analysis that can be used by pharmacists to determine the ethical course of action to follow in a given situation. His four-step approach involves (1) ensuring adequate knowledge of all the pertinent facts involved in a given situation, and the application of (2) moral rules, (3) ethical principles, and (4) ethical theories.

Veatch contends that some ethical situations can be solved without the application of moral rules, ethical principles, or ethical theories. Sometimes an ethical dilemma can be solved by simply ensuring all the facts are known about a case (step 1). For example, a question of whether to break patient confidentiality might be moot if the patient has already agreed to allow the health professional to divulge such information.

If step 1 does not provide an answer, the professional may proceed to step 2, the application of moral rules. The rules of confidentiality and/or consent (informed consent) may offer some guidance. If a dilemma still exists, ethical principles may be employed (step 3). These include autonomy, beneficence, nonmaleficence, veracity, fidelity, and justice. Ethical theories, Veatch suggests, are the ultimate arbiter of ethical dilemmas (step 4).

ETHICAL THEORIES

Although many approaches to ethics (such as virtue-based and feminist theories) have applicability to the biomedical field, the majority of contemporary biomedical texts focus on two prominent types: teleological (consequentialist) theories and deontological (nonconsequentialist) theories.

Teleological theories, such as utilitarianism, state that the rightness or wrongness of an action depends on the consequences produced. As Beauchamp and Childress suggest, "Consequentialism is the moral theory that actions are right or wrong according to their consequences rather than any intrinsic features they may have, such as truthfulness or fidelity."[22] Utilitarianism, as a consequentialist theory, directs that the most appropriate course of action is that which will produce the *greatest good for the greatest number* when the consequences of all action alternatives in a given situation are weighed.

Conversely, deontological theories, such as Kantian ethical theory, argue that the rightness or wrongness of an action is independent of the actions produced. As Beauchamp and Childress point out, "Deontologists maintain that the concepts of obligation and right are independent of the concept of good and the right actions are not determined exclusively by the production of good consequences."[23] Deontologists maintain that factors such as integrity and truth must be included when determining the ethical acceptability of a given action.

ETHICAL PRINCIPLES AND MORAL RULES

Pharmacists have an ethical obligation to care for their patients. Moral rules and ethical principles, rather than ethical theories, are more likely to be the *tools* used by pharmacists on a daily basis as they face ethical situations. Ethical principles and moral rules provide guidance for practitioners about what the commitments of patient care entail.

Autonomy

The principle of autonomy states that an individual's liberty of choice, action, and thought is not to be interfered with. As Beauchamp and Childress have noted, "Autonomy has . . . been used to refer to a set of diverse notions including self-governance, liberty rights, privacy, individual choice, liberty to follow one's will, causing one's own behavior, and being one's own person."[24]

In health care, we think of autonomy as the right of individuals to make decisions about what will happen to their bodies, what choices will be made among competing options, and what they choose to take, or not take, into their bodies. We also allude to questions of autonomy when we refer to choice among health care providers, and the choice of refusing medical treatment.[25] There are two ethically justifiable exceptions to the principle of autonomy: weak paternalism and the harm principle.

The concept of medical paternalism is in direct conflict with the principle of autonomy. Medical paternalism suggests that pharmacists and other health care professionals—because of their education and training—know what is best for their pa-

tients. As a result, health care professionals believe they are justified in overriding the autonomy of a patient. Medical paternalism dominated Western medical practice until the last several decades, when the primacy of patient rights and the concept of medical consumerism became recognized.

A form of medical paternalism, weak paternalism, still allows the autonomy of an individual to be violated if that individual is not or does not appear to be autonomous, or if minimal intervention is necessary to determine whether the patient is autonomous. Some have argued that weak paternalism isn't paternalism: if one lacks the ability to make an autonomous decision, then how can his or her autonomy be overridden? Weak paternalism has remained generally accepted as a justifiable exception to the principle of autonomy.

Strong paternalism—the violation of the autonomy of another person because you believe they are either making the wrong decision or a decision that will cause harm to themselves—is not considered an ethically justifiable reason to override a patient's autonomy. However, under the harm principle, one is justified in overriding the autonomy of another if, in the exercise of that autonomy, harm may come to others.

Informed Consent

The principle of autonomy is a vital component of informed consent. For example, when one provides informed consent to an individual contemplating participation in a clinical research trial, one respects the right of that individual to make an autonomous decision. The rule of informed consent directs that patients must be fully *informed* about the *benefits* and *risks* of their participation in a clinical trial, taking a medication, or electing to have surgery, and this disclosure must be followed by their autonomous consent.

For legal and ethical reasons, informed consent is always obtained formally in situations such as clinical research and surgery through an informed consent form. In the case of clinical research, these documents are usually drafted by the investigator or pharmaceutical manufacturer and subsequently are approved by the institutional review board (IRB) where the research will take place. The role of the IRB will be discussed later in this chapter.

Informed consent is also obtained informally in some instances. For example, whenever a pharmacist counsels a patient and dispenses a medication to a patient, a type of informal informed consent occurs. The patient is informed about the benefits and any risks of the drug, and then decides whether to take it. Informed consent is composed of five elements: disclosure, understanding, voluntariness, competence, and consent.[25]

Disclosure directs that all the pertinent information that is necessary for an informed decision must be made available to the patient. *Understanding* requires that patients fully understand what they are consenting to, including any benefits or hazards. *Voluntariness* instructs that patients who choose to enroll in a research endeavor or be compliant in taking medication must be free from coercion. *Competence* requires that patients be autonomous individuals, who have the functioning ability to make decisions for themselves. *Consent* provides the patient with a point of decision, and is the final legal and moral criterion to be met in ensuring that informed consent has been obtained.

Confidentiality

The rule of *confidentiality,* like informed consent, is an application of the principle of patient autonomy. When pharmacists keep information private from others, unless the patient gives permission to release it, they respect the autonomous decision of the individual. Medical confidentiality need not be requested explicitly by patients; all medical information, by nature, is generally considered to be confidential, unless the patient grants approval for its release. Confidentiality and privacy have received a great deal of attention recently with the passage and implementation of the Health Insurance Portability and Accountability (HIPAA) Act.

Though often used interchangeably, the terms *confidentiality* and *privacy* do differ. A violation of privacy occurs in situations where personal information is obtained/revealed by an individual who has not been granted access to such information. A computer hacker would be an example. Conversely, a violation of confidentiality results from the inappropriate release of personal information to others by a person, such as a health care professional, who has been granted access to such information.

In health care, it is sometimes unclear which members of the health care team may have access to confidential medical records without the express consent of the patient. Should a pharmacist or physical therapist caring for a patient have the same access to medical records that is afforded the patient's physician or hospital nurse? Another difficult ethical situation involves a patient who explicitly expresses a desire not to have information divulged to a member of the health care team. For example, a patient may tell a pharmacist of her decision to alter her prescribed therapeutic regimen, but request that the pharmacist not disclose this information to her physician.

Confidentiality has the same two ethically justifiable exceptions as does the principle of autonomy, the harm principle, and weak paternalism. As with autonomy, a pharmacist may be ethically justified in violating the confidentiality of a patient when keeping information private may harm others (harm principle) or when the patient lacks autonomy (weak paternalism).

Beneficence/Nonmaleficence

Beneficence and nonmaleficence are ethical principles that are, in a sense, complimentary to one another. Beneficence indicates that you act in a manner to *do good*. Nonmaleficence refers to *taking due care or avoiding harm*. Beauchamp and Childress compare these related principles:

The word nonmaleficence is sometimes used more broadly to include the prevention of harm and the removal of harmful conditions. However, because prevention and removal require positive acts to assist others, we include them under beneficence along with the provision of benefit. Nonmaleficence is restricted . . . to the noninfliction of harm.[26]

Fidelity

Fidelity requires that pharmacists act in such a way as to demonstrate loyalty to their patients. A type of bond or promise is established between the practitioner and the patient. This professional relationship places on the pharmacist the burden of acting in the best interest of the patient. Pharmacists have an obligation of fidelity to all their patients, regardless of the length of the professional relationship. In community pharmacy, for example, practitioners have the same obligation to show fidelity to an occasional patient as they have for a *regular* customer.[17]

The depth of the fidelity relationship between the pharmacist and patient is a topic of ongoing discussion among pharmacy ethicists. Two forms of fidelity are frequently alluded to: covenantal and contractual. Covenantal fidelity is often described as an intimate and spiritual commitment between individuals. Examples would include the fidelity of marriage and the fidelity between a member of the clergy and his or her congregation. Conversely, contractual fidelity does not involve a level of commitment beyond that owed another as the result of a binding agreement. An example of this form of fidelity would be the relationship one might have with a contractor such as a plumber or electrician. What remains in dispute is where the

pharmacist–patient relationship lies along the continuum between covenant and contract.

Veracity

Veracity is the ethical principle that instructs pharmacists to be honest in their dealings with patients. There may be times when the violation of veracity may be ethically justifiable (as with the use of placebos), but the violation of this principle for non-patient-centered reasons would appear to be unethical. In a professional relationship based upon professional fidelity, patients have a right to expect that their pharmacist will be forthright in dealings with them.[17]

Distributive Justice

Distributive justice refers to the equal distribution of the benefits and burdens of society among all members of this society. We often think of distributive justice in terms of our health care delivery system. This principle is frequently used as a justification for providing health care as a right to all Americans.

Even though justice instructs that pharmacists demonstrate an equivalent amount of care, pharmacists do not always provide care with equal fervor to all patients. Sadly, issues such as the patient's socioeconomic status often impact the level and intensity of care provided by health care professionals. Medicaid patients are sometimes provided a much lower quality of care than a patient who is a cash-paying customer or who has a full-coverage drug benefits plan. All too often, the care provided by a health care professional is viewed in terms of the personal reward for the professional, such as the level of reimbursement the care is likely to reap. Justice demands that the focus be on patients and their medical needs, not on the financial impact on the health care professional.[17]

ETHICAL CODES

Ethical principles and rules that apply to medical practice and research, such as autonomy, beneficence, and justice, have long served as the basis for a system or code of ethical conduct. Western medical ethics is primarily based on the Hippocratic code attributed to the Greek philosopher Hippocrates, 5th century BC Medicine (American Medical Association) and pharmacy (Philadelphia College of Pharmacy) developed codes of conduct for their respective practitioners in 1848. As Montagne notes, "the guiding principles of these codes were a respect for human life and service to humanity."[27] The Holocaust during World War II, and the subsequent Nuremberg trials, would prompt the first major development of a code dealing specifically with experimentation on human subjects.

Subsequent to Nuremberg, several other codes of medical ethics were established. In 1949, the World Medical Association drafted the Geneva Convention Code of Medical Ethics, a contemporary version of the Hippocratic oath. In the 1960s, the same organization established an ethical code on clinical research. In 1964, the Declaration of Helsinki was adopted based upon the Nuremberg principles, and it was further revised in 1975. In 1972, the American Hospital Association issued a *Statement on a Patient's Bill of Rights*. In 1977, the Declaration of Hawaii provided ethical guidelines for clinical research in psychiatry.[27]

Ethical codes provide health care professionals with ethical principles and standards by which to guide their practice. However, ethical principles and codes cannot hope to provide health care professionals with answers to every moral question that may arise in the course of their practice. Ethical questions in health care involve decision-making that is usually situation-specific. The purpose of such principles and codes is not to provide practitioners with right and wrong answers, but to offer them a framework to use when faced with ethical questions. As

Montagne points out, "the formulation of an oath or ethical code does not remove the moral choices and the need to carefully consider in each situation and the alternative actions or decisions that can be made."[28]

APhA Code of Ethics

The Code of Ethics of the APhA is the only code of ethics that specifically guides the practice of pharmacy. A careful examination of the evolution of the Code since its inception in 1852 shows both a greater degree of responsibility to the patient expected of the pharmacist and a greater respect for the autonomy of patients.

The first APhA Code in 1852 seemed to reflect the wide acceptance of medical paternalism, the attitude that the *physician knows best*. Amazingly, the code seems to suggest that errors by physicians or pharmacists, unless done with malice, need not—in fact should not—be revealed to patients!

The 1952 version of the Code clearly outlined the duties of a pharmacist, and these were quite in conflict with what is accepted practice today. The 1952 Code instructs, seemingly in direct conflict with what we see as pharmaceutical care today, that "the pharmacist does not discuss the therapeutic effects or composition of a prescription with a patient."[29]

The 1994 Code (see Fig 3-1), much less prescriptive than earlier versions, speaks to the "covenantal relationship between the patient and the pharmacist" and the obligation of pharmacists to promote "the good of every patient in a caring . . . manner."[16] The elements of pharmaceutical care appear throughout, and the Code is consistent with the new mission of pharmacy.

ETHICAL CONFLICTS AND ISSUES IN HEALTH CARE

The conflict between the personal interests of the professional and the duty to subordinate these interests to the benefit of the patient presents one of the major unresolved problems of the professions. In addition, changing patterns in pharmacy and health care delivery present additional ethical conflicts.

The traditional focus of professional service has been on the individual. Professional services have not been mass-produced, but rather each rendering of a service is specifically tailored to the individual needs of a specific patient. In general, the ethics of professions have evolved on the basis of primacy of the individual.

Within the health professions, the impairment of physical or mental functioning as a result of drug use or other factors has become a very important issue. While some studies have indicated that the level of social/recreational drug use among physicians and pharmacists does not differ much from that of general society, the extent of drug-use problems in the health professions is great enough to warrant the development of prevention programs and referral groups.[30] Regardless of the appropriateness or inappropriateness of such drug-taking in general, the professional ethics of the pharmacist should dictate that any degree of impairment while practicing pharmacy is unacceptable. The impact of such impairment on the ability to perform one's professional duties, especially the delivery of patient care, is considerable. Such cases affect the image of pharmacy, the trust of the patient, and impact many other ethical and interpersonal aspects of professional practice.

Innovative uses for old and new drug products have created a number of ethical dilemmas.[31–33] Conflicts continue to occur for many pharmacists when they find themselves faced with dispensing placebogenic agents, oral contraceptives, drugs for lethal injections, and drugs for controlling certain types of behavior (see the bibliography for some representative references in this area). The whole process of modern drug development probably will continue to generate a wide variety of ethical concerns. In a way, these activities might represent the most important type of emerging conflicts for society and for pharmacy,

which is viewed as the profession responsible for monitoring and controlling drug use.

Law and Ethics

Many of the laws, regulations, and other rules that govern our daily life are an outgrowth of our morality and ethics. Those laws that prevent homicide, robbery, and other offenses are simply a codification of the values we share as members of society. Unfortunately, laws and regulations cannot be promulgated to cover every eventuality, nuance, condition, or situation. They are created in such a way as to provide legal guidelines for the *usual* or *most common* situation. What should be done, therefore, when such a situation (eg, committing homicide in self-defense) arises, especially if the legal course of action is inconsistent with the ethical course of action?

Conflicts can and will emerge with changes in the laws relating to the practice of pharmacy, in the evolution of new problems and developments in both the profession and the population it serves, and in the roles and functions of drug use in our society. The conflict often might be between a certain law or regulation and an ethical principle held by the profession. Many pharmacists have faced dispensing decisions in which the act of providing the drug would be in the best interests of the patient, but it also would violate a specific law or regulation related to the practice of pharmacy, or it would be contrary to his or her own beliefs and ethical stances.

These conflicts occur fairly routinely in pharmacy. For example, what should a pharmacist do when a patient's prescription for heart medicine has been depleted, no refills remain, and the prescriber is unavailable? Clearly, most pharmacists would do the ethical thing and provide such patients with a few doses to hold them over until a new prescription can be obtained, even though this course of action is illegal. To follow the example a bit farther, what if the medication is a controlled substance used for pain control in a terminally ill patient? The potential for legal action from drug enforcement authorities might make a pharmacist reluctant to dispense extra doses, even though the patient might be in just as much need.

Rationing of Health Care Services

As the cost of providing health care services continues to grow, some have suggested and even attempted to implement a system that would ration the availability of health care. American health care policy makers have tried to avoid this approach because it represents a contradiction with a long-standing implicit belief that all that can be done for each patient ought to be done. Medical insurance, both publicly and privately funded, has attempted to support this ideal. But, in the absence of cost-containment, rising insurance rates have resulted, thereby driving individuals out of the health insurance system and threatening the viability of governmental programs.

The consequence of this policy is seen in both increasing numbers of individuals who are unable to afford health insurance and increasing restrictions on who qualifies for public programs. Therefore, fewer people have access to health care, or at the very least many have decreased choices of where they can receive health care (eg, municipal hospitals, free clinics). As McDermott points out,

> "Approximately 15% of our people [Americans] have no health insurance coverage at any one time, and at least 57 million nonelderly Americans lack health insurance for some part of the year. This does not even include the underinsured and those on Medicaid whose coverage cannot begin to provide them with access that is consistent with good health care."[34]

For at least the present, most American health care planners have determined that rationing of care, in any manner, is not a viable alternative for dealing with our present crisis, current facts not withstanding.[35–37] At the same time, there is a shared determination by the government and the public at large that reform is essential and, further, that whatever changes are made, they must ensure universal access to health care while controlling costs and reducing fraud.[38,39] As Friedman notes, "high health care costs breed medical indigence; if one is to be fixed, so must the other."[40]

Assisted Suicide

Although medical euthanasia (*mercy killing*) has long been an ethical issue, it has only been in recent years that the question of assisted suicide has been examined. The activities of assisted suicide advocate Dr Jack Kevorkian spurred a great deal of public and professional discussion of this issue.[41–44] Several states have considered the legality of assisted suicide; some have rejected it, while others have accepted it within strict guidelines.[45] The US Supreme Court decided that there is no constitutionally guaranteed right to assisted suicide. This decision has not ended the legal debate, but rather has shifted it to the states, who must decide the legality of assisted suicide on their own.

From an ethical perspective, the key issue remains whether assisted suicide violates the Hippocratic responsibilities of health care practitioners to *do no harm*. Those who advocate its availability to patients suggest that allowing a patient to continue to experience unrelenting pain is doing harm.[46,47] They suggest that patients have the right to make an autonomous decision to end their life; their opponents worry that legal assisted suicide would be abused.

Human Drug Experimentation

Several ethical codes deal with research on human subjects, including the testing of drugs.[48–50] Two important ethical aspects of human drug experimentation are the role of the institutional review board (IRB) and the use of placebos.

The IRB is the body responsible for overseeing all clinical research conducted within a given institution.[51] Traditionally, most clinical drug research was conducted in hospital settings; however, with the shift in the locus of health care delivery from the inpatient to the ambulatory setting, IRBs are now found in managed-care organizations and other ambulatory facilities.

The IRB has two primary responsibilities. The first is to ensure the integrity and scientific rigor of the proposed research study. The risk versus benefit ratio for the study's participants is evaluated. Should the risks outweigh the benefits, the IRB would likely reject the research. The board acts as somewhat of a *subject advocate*, making sure that the rights and welfare of the patient-subject are protected.[52] The IRB's second major responsibility is to evaluate and approve informed consent forms used in conjunction with the research. Such forms should be drafted consistent with the elements of informed consent discussed previously.

IRBs vary in their size and representation. Their membership may include physicians, nurses, other allied health professionals (including pharmacists), institutional administrators, attorneys, clergy, medical ethicists, and community members.[25]

Placebos have generally had two roles in medicine: (1) in clinical drug research, as part of the research methodology; and (2) as a means for providing a therapeutic response in selected patient situations.[53–55] The use of placebos has long been an integral component of clinical drug research. Whether the drug being tested is a new drug compound or an existing drug under study for a new indication, placebos have served as a point of comparison for determining therapeutic efficacy. Although the use of placebos in some instances has been shown to provide therapeutic usefulness (eg, pain control), placebos, by definition, are agents devoid of pharmacologic activity.

Patient-subjects who receive placebos as a component of their participation in a clinical drug study generally cannot hope to derive any benefit (beneficence) from these substances. This raises the question of whether the use of placebos in drug research, despite the obvious scientific advantages, is ethical. The question is further complicated by the expectation that placebos will be employed in clinical research. An FDA regulator has stated, "it is desirable to include some placebo controlled studies unless it is considered unethical to do so."[56] This suggests that the use of placebos is ethical in certain instances, but unethical in others.[25]

The use of placebos to address genuine or perceived therapeutic outcomes is even more ethically problematic. The belief that the health care practitioner *knows best* and, therefore, is justified in practicing medical paternalism has been a long-standing component of the so-called *medical authority* model of practice. Under this model, the perceptions/desires of the patient are subjugated to the judgment of the health care professional. It would be used, for example, as justification for a practitioner to place a patient on a placebo without the knowledge of the patient. In current medical ethic, however, this use of placebos in the absence of the patient's knowledge and consent might be judged to be unethical—a direct violation of patient autonomy and informed consent.

Drug Formularies

Drug formularies are a list of drugs that are approved for use either within an institution or for reimbursement by a third-party payer. Their purpose is to eliminate therapeutic duplication and provide patients with the best drug at the lowest cost.

In the early days of formularies, they were used by hospitals to control drug inventories and provide prescribers with a list of *drugs of choice* for various conditions. However, the absence of a drug from the formulary was not usually a great barrier to a prescriber obtaining it for the patient. A special request could be made by the prescriber to a member of the pharmacy and therapeutics committee of the hospital, and usually the drug would be obtained.

When managed-care organizations (MCOs) and pharmacy benefit management companies (PBMs) began to employ formularies, circumventing them became much more difficult. This restrictive use of formularies has led to a number of important ethical questions. For example, does the use of generic and/or therapeutic substitution violate the autonomy of the patient and/or prescriber? Is the use of such substitution a violation of informed consent? Does the use of formularies violate the ethical principles of beneficence (*do good*) and nonmaleficence (*avoid harm*)?[57]

CONCLUSION

The ethics of pharmacy in the US has experienced a continuous evolution as the profession itself has changed. Pharmacy practice is far different today than it was when APhA issued its first code of ethics in 1852. The current changes that pharmacy (and indeed all of health care) is experiencing makes the existence of an ethical framework and personal ethic even more vital today than it was in the past. The pharmacists of the mid-19th century could not imagine the medical innovations and technological wonders that have occurred, and the financial questions that have been raised and debated in the last quarter of the 20th century.

As the concept of pharmaceutical care expands to an ever-growing number of practice sites, pharmacists must be schooled not only in their expanding ethical responsibilities as independent practitioners, but also in their traditional moral obligations to patients. The APhA Code of Ethics and the profession at large must remain responsive to an ever-changing environment.

In spite of the deficiencies of self-regulation, there remains much that can be done within pharmacy to increase the service contribution of pharmacists through ethics. The situation was summarized by Dean LaWall when, 85 years ago, he described pharmacy as "[a] highly specialized calling, which may rise to the dignity of a true profession or sink to the level of the lowest commercialism, according to the ideals, the ability, and the training of the one who practices it."[58]

REFERENCES

1. Tomlin EWF. *The Western Philosophers: An Introduction.* New York: Harper & Row, 1963, p 26.
2. Smith MC. In Wertheimer AI, Smith MC, eds. *Pharmacy Practice: Social and Behavioral Aspects,* 2nd ed. Baltimore: University Park Press, 1981, p 305.
3. Veatch RM. *Case Studies in Medical Ethics.* Cambridge: Harvard University Press, 1977, p 1.
4. Veatch RM. *A Theory of Medical Ethics.* New York: Basic Books, 1981.
5. Marshall TH. *Can J Econ Political Sci* 1939; 5:325.
6. Greenwood E. In Noscow S, Form WH, eds. *Man, Work and Society.* New York: Basic Books, 1962, p 210.
7. Carr-Saunders AM, Wilson PA. *The Professions.* New York: Oxford University Press, 1933, p 141.
8. Montague JB. *J APhA* 1968; NS8:228.
9. Smith MC. *Am J Pharm Educ* 1970; 34:16.
10. Smith MC, Knapp DA. *Pharmacy, Drugs and Medical Care,* 4th ed. Baltimore: Williams & Wilkins, 1987.
11. Denzin NR, Mettlin CJ. *Soc Forces* 1968; 46:357.
12. Edelstein L. In Temkin O, Temkin CL, eds. *Ancient Medicine: Selected Papers of Ludwig Edelstein.* Baltimore: Johns Hopkins University Press, 1967, p 6.
13. Smith MC, Smith MD. *Am J Pharm Educ* 1981; 45:14.
14. Haddad M et al. *Am J Pharm Educ* 1993; 57:34S.
15. Berger BA. *Am J Hosp Pharm* 1993; 50:2399.
16. "Code of Ethics for Pharmacists." *Am J Health-Sys Pharm* 1995; 52:2131.
17. McCarthy RL. In Haddad AM, Buerki, RA, eds. *Ethical Dimensions of Pharmaceutical Care.* Binghamton, NY: Pharmaceutical Products Press, 1996.
18. Musto DF. *The American Disease: Origins of Narcotic Control.* New York: Oxford University Press, 1987.
19. Edwards RB. *Soc Sci Med* 1984; 18:515.
20. American Association of Colleges of Pharmacy. *What is the Mission of Pharmaceutical Education?* Background Paper I, Commission to Implement Change in Pharmaceutical Education, 1991.
21. Veatch RM. *Am J Hosp Pharm* 1989; 46:109.
22. Beauchamp TL, Childress JF. *Principles of Biomedical Ethics,* 3rd ed. New York: Oxford University Press, 1989, p 25.
23. Beauchamp TL, Childress JF. *Principles of Biomedical Ethics,* 3rd ed. New York: Oxford University Press, 1989, p 26.
24. Beauchamp TL, Childress JF. *Principles of Biomedical Ethics,* 3rd ed. New York: Oxford University Press, 1989, pp 67–68.
25. McCarthy RL. In Bleidt B, Montagne M, eds. *Clinical Research in Pharmaceutical Development.* New York: Dekker, 1996.
26. Beauchamp TL, Childress JF. *Principles of Biomedical Ethics,* 3rd ed. New York: Oxford University Press, 1989, p 194.
27. Montagne M. In Swarbrick J, Boylan JC, eds. *Encyclopedia of Pharmaceutical Technology,* vol 5. New York: Dekker, 1992, p 303.
28. Montagne M. In Swarbrick J, Boylan JC, eds. *Encyclopedia of Pharmaceutical Technology,* vol 5. New York: Dekker, 1992, p 304.
29. "Code of Ethics of the American Pharmaceutical Association." *J APhA* 1952; 13:721.
30. McAuliffe WE, et al. *Am J Hosp Pharm* 1987; 44:311.
31. Montagne M, ed. *J Drug Issues* 1988; 18:139.
32. Montagne M, ed. *J Drug Issues* 1992; 22:195.
33. McCarthy RL, Montagne M. *Am J Hosp Pharm* 1993; 50:992.
34. McDermott J. *JAMA* 1994; 271:782.
35. Butler J. *The Ethics of Healthcare Rationing.* Herndon, VA: Cassell Academic, 2000.
36. Hunter DJ. *Desperately Seeking Solutions: Rationing Health Care.* Reading, MA: Addison-Wesley, 1998.
37. Ubel PA. *Pricing Life: Why It's Time for Health Care Rationing.* Cambridge, MA: MIT Press, 1999.
38. Hall MA. *Making Medical Spending Decisions: The Law, Ethics, and Economics of Rationing Mechanisms.* New York: Oxford University Press, 1997.
39. Strosberg MA, Wiener JM, Baker R, et al, eds. *Rationing America's Medical Care: The Oregon Plan and Beyond.* Washington DC: The Brookings Institution, 1992.
40. Friedman E. *JAMA* 1993; 269:2437.
41. Dworkin G, Frey RG, Bok S. *Euthanasia and Physician-Assisted Suicide.* New York: Cambridge University Press, 1998.
42. Battin MP, Rhodes R, Silvers A, eds. *Physician Assisted Suicide: Expanding the Debate.* London: Routledge, 1998.
43. Snyder L, Caplan AL. *Assisted Suicide: Finding Common Ground.* Bloomington, IN: Indiana University Press, 2001.
44. Torr J, ed. *Euthanasia: Opposing Viewpoints.* San Diego, CA: Greenhaven Press, 2000.
45. Haley K, Lee M, eds. *The Oregon Death with Dignity Act: A Guidebook for Health Care Providers.* Portland, OR: Center for Ethics in Health Care, 1988.
46. Humphry D. *Final Exit: The Practicalities of Self-Deliverance and Assisted Suicide for the Dying,* 3rd ed. Reno, NV: Delta, 2002.
47. Palmer LI. *Endings and Beginnings: Law, Medicine, and Society in Assisted Life and Death.* New York: Praeger, 2000.
48. Vanderpool HY, ed. *The Ethics of Research Involving Human Subjects: Facing the 21st Century.* Frederick, MD: University Publishing Group, 1996.
49. Shamoo AE, Resnik DB. *Responsible Conduct of Research.* New York: Oxford University Press, 2003.
50. Brody BA. *Ethical Issues in Drug Testing, Approval, and Pricing: The Clot-Dissolving Drugs.* New York: Oxford University Press, 1995.
51. Amdur RJ. *Institutional Review Board Member Handbook.* Sudbury, MA: Jones & Bartlett, 2002.
52. Gallelli JF, Hiranaka PK, Grimes GJ Jr. In Brown TR, Smith MC, eds. *Handbook of Institutional Pharmacy Practice,* 2nd ed. Baltimore: Williams & Wilkins, 1986.
53. Harrington A, ed. *The Placebo Effect: An Interdisciplinary Exploration.* Cambridge, MA: Harvard University Press, 1999.
54. Shapiro AK, Shapiro E. *The Powerful Placebo: From Ancient Priest to Modern Physician.* Baltimore: Johns Hopkins University Press, 2001.
55. Moerman DE. *Meaning, Medicine and the Placebo Effect.* New York: Cambridge University Press, 2002.
56. Freedman B. *IRB* 1990; 12:1.
57. McCarthy RL. *J Managed Care Pharm* 1996; 2(2):76.
58. LaWall CH. *Four Thousand Years of Pharmacy.* Philadelphia: Lippincott, 1920: p v.
59. http://www.aacp.org/site/tertiary.asp? TRACKID = &VID = 2&CID = 686 & DID = 4339. Accessed May 14, 2004.

BIBLIOGRAPHY

Asbury CH. *Orphan Drugs: Medical Versus Market Value.* Lexington, MA: Lexington Books, 1985.
Bakalar JB, Grinspoon L. *Drug Control in a Free Society.* London: Cambridge University Press, 1984.
Basara LR, Montagne M. *Searching for Magic Bullets: Orphan Drugs, Consumer Activism, and Pharmaceutical Development.* New York: Haworth, 1994.
Bezold C. *The Future of Pharmaceuticals.* New York: Wiley, 1981.
Boyce E, et al. *DICP Ann Pharmacother* 1989; 23:590.
Brody H. *Placebos and Philosophy of Medicine: Clinical, Conceptual, and Ethical Issues.* Chicago: University of Chicago Press, 1977.
Buerki RA, Vottero LD. *Ethical Responsibility in Pharmacy Practice.* Madison, WI: American Institute of the History of Pharmacy, 1994.
Cook RJ, Dickens BM, Fathalla MF. *Reproductive Health and Human Rights: Integrating Medicine, Ethics, and Law.* New York: Oxford University Press, 2003.
Coombs RH. *Drug-Impaired Professionals.* Cambridge: Harvard University Press, 1997.
Goodman KW. *Ethics and Evidence-Based Medicine: Fallibility and Responsibility in Clinical Science.* New York: Cambridge University Press, 2003.
Haddad A. *Teaching and Learning Strategies in Pharmacy Ethics.* New York: Pharmaceutical Products Press, 1997.
Heifetz MD. *Easier Said Than Done: Moral Decisions in Medical Uncertainty.* Buffalo, NY: Prometheus Books, 1992.
Humber JM, Almeder RF, eds. *Mental Illness and Public Health Care.* Totowa, NJ: Humana Press, 2002.
Jonsen AR, Siegler M, Winslade WJ. *Clinical Ethics: A Practical Approach to Ethical Decisions in Clinical Medicine.* New York: McGraw-Hill, 1998.
Lennard HL. *Mystification and Drug Misuse.* San Francisco: Jossey-Bass, 1971.

Lock S, Wells F, Farthing M, eds. *Fraud and Misconduct in Biomedical Research,* 3rd ed. London: BMJ Books, 2001.

Montagne M, Pugh CB, Fink JL. *Am J Hosp Pharm* 1988; 45:1509.

Murray TH, Gaylin W, Macklin R, eds. *Feeling Good and Doing Better: Ethics and Nontherapeutic Drug Use.* Clifton, NJ: Humana Press, 1984.

Salek S, Edgar A, eds. *Pharmaceutical Ethics.* New York: J Wiley, 2002.

Sechzer JA, ed. *The Role of Animals in Biomedical Research.* New York: New York Academy of Science, 1983.

Silverman M, Lee PR, Lydecker M. *Prescriptions for Death: The Drugging of the Third World.* Berkeley: University of California Press, 1982.

Smith MC, et al. *Pharmacy Ethics.* New York: Pharmaceutical Products Press, 1991.

Smith T. *Ethics in Medical Research: A Handbook of Good Practice.* New York: Cambridge University Press, 1999.

Temin P. *Taking Your Medicine: Drug Regulation in the United States.* Cambridge: Harvard University Press, 1980.

Veatch RM. *J Drug Issues* 1977; 7:253.

Veatch RM, Haddad A. *Case Studies in Pharmacy Ethics.* New York: Oxford University Press, 1999.

Weinstein B. *Ethical Issues in Pharmacy.* Vancouver, WA: Applied Therapeutics, 1996.

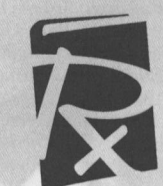

CHAPTER 4

The Practice of Community Pharmacy

Calvin H Knowlton, RPh, MDiv, PhD

Steven J Gilbert, RPh, PharmD(c)

Dennis D Hager, RPh, PharmD(c)

Michael F Imperato, PharmD

Community Pharmacy Practice: The Context of the System

While few may take the time to look back to past editions of *Remington*, if you were to do so what you would find is an ongoing pilgrimage of change for community pharmacists. The direction clearly has been, and continues to be, a path toward increasing a patient care focus. The scenery and contextual landscape have changed dramatically. Polemics formerly surrounding the commercialization of community practice—the separation of professional and business functions—continue; however, the accretion of US health care in general from professionalism and autonomy toward a business structure has tended to mitigate the view of pharmacists as the singular 'sore thumbs' entrenched in an obvious commercial backdrop, as compared to other players in the diverse health care arena.

As this pilgrimage continues toward asserting a role in optimizing the medication use process (ie, pharmaceutical care), community pharmacy is not yet there in its nascent measure of success. Progress has been made in cognitive service remuneration and some score carding based upon improvement in economic, clinical, and humanistic patient outcomes; however, the customary success metrics for community pharmacy remain focused upon the processing of Rxs rather than the outcome associated with appropriate medication management by pharmacists. Continuing in the classical metric tradition, in 2002 the 54,000 community pharmacies processed, on average, 56,550 Rxs per pharmacy at an average price of $54.[1] For the first time in recent history, the 2002 Rx market sagged compared to previous years. While a decade earlier Rx volume (both number of Rxs and revenue from Rxs) rose unabated at 8% to 10% per year, 2002 was flat with 2001.

The community pharmacy workforce continues to gain in sophistication. In spite of the uptake of the PharmD degree, which entices practitioners to an array of non-community pharmacy based clinical opportunities, the surge of certified pharmacy technicians and technology has enabled community pharmacy to dispense these 3.1 billion Rxs. These same workforce enhancers have also provided community pharmacists with time to initiative various patient care services that have started to demonstrate the value of pharmaceutical care in the community setting. The leading of these studies were the Asheville Project and Project ImPACT.

The Asheville Project (12 pharmacies, 85 patients with diabetes) found that patients with pharmaceutical care interventions faired better than a comparison group. The Asheville Project started in March 1997. The services performed by pharmacists include patient education and training, clinical assessment, monitoring, follow-up, and referral. Participating patients had lower overall health costs, missed fewer days of work or school, and required less intensive health care interventions.[2,3,4]

Project ImPACT focus on community pharmacists' interventions (26 pharmacies) with patients suffering dyslipidemias (397 patients). With this pre-post comparison group design, rates of persistence, compliance, and attainment of clinical goals was demonstrated using pharmaceutical care.[5]

Distribution and Control of Medications

The classical paradigm in community pharmacy was that the community pharmacist must assess all of the following:

- Appropriateness of dose for this patient
- Patient allergy to the medication or similar medication
- Potential interactions with other prescribed and non-prescription medications
- Contraindications of the medication with other known diseases the patient may have
- Appropriate dose scheduling to maximize effect and minimize adverse events
- Appropriateness of this medication for this patient for this health condition

The pharmacist also is, and has been, required to:

- Assure accuracy of dispensing and labeling
- Provide the patient with information on proper storage of the medication
- Advise the patient on potential risks and benefits
- Advise the patient on how to deal with missed doses and adverse events and
- Assess the patient's understanding of the prescription instructions to maximize compliance and adherence to the instructions.

The contemporary thrust includes an expansion of responsibility to:

- Consider the appropriateness of the entire pharmacotherapy care plan
- Consider the inherited parameters that may affect medication transport, receptor activity, and metabolism (eg, pharmacogenomics)
- Monitor the results of the pharmacotherapy care plan (eg, pertinent clinical endpoints and quality of life outcomes secondary to the medication regimen)

Preparation of Compounded Pharmaceuticals

The vast majority of prescriptions dispensed are for dosage forms manufactured by the Food and Drug Administration (FDA)-approved manufacturers. These standardized dosages meet the needs for most patients and are produced under the Good Manufacturing Practices established by the FDA. Many patients, however, need custom-made dosages to solve specific problems. For these unique needs many community pharmacists offer specialized compounding services. Patients may need extremely small doses for pediatric or geriatric use. They may also need preservative-free products, liquids with special flavors or delivery systems that are not commercially available. Additionally some medications may not have sufficient shelf life to withstand the commercial distribution process and therefore need to be prepared at the time of dispensing. For all of these reasons, compounding of finished dosage forms is a valuable service offered in thousands of community pharmacies across the nation.

Compounding has always been the art and science unique to pharmacists and continues to be a part of contemporary pharmacy practice. Those community pharmacists who continue to offer these services do so under *Good Compounding Practices* established by the United States Pharmacopoeia.[6] The array of dosage forms possible through compounding is far wider than those available from manufacturers. It is more economical to compound specialized prescriptions since the market demand for each product is not sufficient to justify creation of a manufactured product.

Forces of Change in Community Pharmacy Practice

There are a number of external forces at work encouraging change in pharmacy practice. The five most definitive forces are (1) the demand for prescription drugs, (2) pharmaceutical innovation, (3) health care cost containment initiatives, (4) the need for improved medication safety, and (5) the Health Insurance Portability and Accountability Act of 1996 (HIPAA).

Demand for prescription drugs has increased through two modes. The evolution of third-party payment cards has removed some of the economic barriers to drug therapy. The conversion of many indemnity and major medical plans to direct insurance coverage has increased prescription volume 20% to 35% among those patients. With financial barriers removed, many prescriptions are now dispensed that previously were not. Additionally the number of people over 65 years old is significantly increasing in the US population. This age group uses 33% of prescription drugs and 40% of non-prescription drugs while they represent only 12% of the population.[7] By the year 2020 the number of people over the age of 65 will double. These two factors alone will contribute to a 35% increase in prescriptions dispensed. Legislative proposals to include coverage of prescription drug within the Medicare benefit may increase this pressure as well.

Pharmaceutical innovation has further accelerated the growth in the prescription drug market. The continued introduction of new, more powerful, more potent, more useful and more toxic drug entities continues to increase the number of patients for whom drug treatment replaces surgery, hospitalization, or other treatment modes. Dramatic new entries that do not replace existing drugs but do replace other treatment modes drive an expanding market for prescription medications and pharmacy services. The combination of these two forces has given rise to the third trend, which are health care cost containment initiatives.

The health financing system in the US has experienced cost increases in excess of the Consumer Price Index (CPI) for more than two decades. As a result insurers and employers who pay the insurance bills have demanded that controls be applied to these rising costs.[8] Insurers, pharmacy benefit managers (PBMs), and governmental agencies have applied various strategies to prescription drug benefit plans in an effort to control costs. Many now use generic incentive policies, prior authorization programs, therapeutic formularies, and competitive bidding procedures to reduce the total cost of prescription drugs.

Community pharmacists now spend a significant amount of time administering these cost-controlling strategies for insurers. It is estimated that 20% of the time spent by pharmacists in the fulfillment of these tasks can be delegated to non-licensed personnel.[9] These three forces drive community pharmacy practice in new directions creating a need for continued automation, a need for more technical support, and opportunities for alternate pharmacist roles.

The pace of pharmaceutical innovation combined with the increasing use of medications has exposed a major public health problem—the need for improved medication safety. Medications are only effective when taken properly, yet medication compliance is very poor in the US[10–12] This failure to take drugs as prescribed results in drug misadventuring or increased drug-related problems. Drug-related problems can also be caused by issues other than compliance as described below[13]

- Indication issues (eg, untreated indication, unnecessary drug therapy)
- Effectiveness issues (eg, wrong drug, dosage too low)
- Safety issues (eg, adverse drug reactions, dosage too high)
- Adherence issues (eg, inappropriate compliance)

Clearly, these issues warrant a need for more assessment and monitoring of medication use.[10,13] This need is magnified as one investigates those increases in unnecessary morbidity and mortality associated with drug misadventuring.

The literature provides significant evidence that drug misadventuring, whether intentional or unintentional, is associated with increased costs and negative patient outcomes. Johnson and Bootman published one of the most alarming studies in 1995.[14] The study results suggest that drug-related morbidity and mortality in the US ambulatory care population was estimated to cost $76.6 billion in 1994. These costs are attributed mainly to an increased number of hospital admissions, long-term care admissions, physician visits, and prescription drug use, as shown below:

- Hospitalizations: 8.7 million admissions at a cost of $47 billion
- Long-term care facilities: 3.15 million admissions at a cost of $14.4 billion
- Physician visits: 115 million visits at a cost of $7.5 billion
- Prescriptions to resolve treatment failures and new medical problems: $1.93 billion

As evidenced by this study, drug-related morbidity and mortality represent a serious public health problem. The problem is becoming more visible as public policy makers, employers, and managed care administrators attempt to understand health care resource utilization. They are illuminating the magnitude of the drug-related morbidity and mortality problem and affirming the need for improvement in medication management. Furthermore, they are emphasizing disease prevention and patient education as ways to reduce overall medical and prescription costs.

Community pharmacists are in a position to fulfill this societal need and provide pharmaceuticals and pharmaceutical services with the intention of improving patient health outcomes. They have the education and ability to manage drug therapy and provide prevention and education services to patients. Moreover, pharmacists are the most accessible and trusted health care professionals. The 1995 Report of the Pew Health Professions Commission supports pharmacists fulfilling these alternate roles and recommends that pharmacists, in particular, engage in activities related to comprehensive drug therapy management such as selecting appropriate drug therapies, educating and monitoring patients, and continually assessing therapy outcomes.[15]

The Health Insurance Portability and Accountability Act of 1996 went into effect in April 2003. It is a far-reaching piece of legislation. Its intent is to secure patient records containing individually identifiable health information so that they are not readily available to those who do not need them. All community pharmacies manage personal health information (PHI) as a routine part of doing business. Pharmacies are required to train all personnel who may handle PHI in how to maintain PHI security and document employee competency. Systems for maintaining the security of PHI must be in place as well. Patient consultation areas need to be designed to insure complete confidentiality of the conversation between patient and pharmacist. The full impact of HIPAA on the practice of community pharmacy is yet to be fully determined.

Shifting Responsibilities

The many data elements to be evaluated at every prescription processing, combined with the variety of formularies and insurance variables, have created a distribution system that requires automation. Today virtually every community pharmacy in the country uses computers, on-line claims processing, and various other forms of automation. Some pharmacies also use automated dispensing systems to count doses, fill bottles, and print patient information and labels. The next decade will see a rapidly expanding use of automated filling systems to reduce the technical functions performed by pharmacists.

In addition to automation, pharmacy technicians are performing many clerical and technical tasks. Technicians have been increasing in numbers and assuming more responsibility over the past 20 years, and today they play a very important role in freeing pharmacists for more patient-focused activities such as counseling and disease state management. Allowing technicians to perform many distributive functions provides time for pharmacists to perform patient care activities. Four pharmacy organizations created the Pharmacy Technician Certification Board to develop, administer, and review a national certification program for technicians.[16] As of April 2003, 131,562 pharmacy technicians across the nation had passed the Pharmacy Technician Certification Examination, and approximately 30% to 40% of certified technicians worked in a community pharmacy setting.[17] Training and certifying pharmacy technicians expands their role, which ultimately allows the pharmacist to spend more time delivering pharmaceutical care services.

As the number of prescriptions dispensed continues to rise and the demand for cost containment remains strong, it is extremely important that community pharmacists focus their limited time on those aspects of practice that make the most effective use of their education and training. First and foremost among these are promoting appropriate drug therapy and avoidance of drug misadventuring. The potential health care cost savings associated with these aspects of practice are enormous. In order to deliver this level of care at community pharmacy sites, it is essential for increases in the use of automation and technical personnel to occur.

Pharmaceutical Care in Community Practice

With the influx of new medication classes, as well as the aging of the American population, the role of the pharmacist in providing effective medication therapy for their patients is more vital than ever. The only method for providing this vital service is in performing pharmaceutical care. This is the same pharmaceutical care that was defined by Hepler and Strand in 1989 as being "the responsible provision of drug therapy and other patient care services for the purpose of achieving outcomes related to the prevention or cure of disease, the elimination or reduction of a patient's symptoms, or the prevention, arrest, or slowing of a disease process."[18] There are several ways in which community practice is performing pharmaceutical care every day, from counseling and prospective drug utilization review at the time of dispensing all the way to disease state management and collaborative practice agreements. While counseling and prospective DUR are requirements of every prescription dispensed, it is disease state management and collaborative practice that are the leading edge of pharmacy practice in the community.

OBRA 90 requires that a minimum amount of pharmaceutical care be performed with each prescription dispensed. All medications must undergo a prospective DUR during which a comprehensive review of the patient's prescription order is performed as well as an evaluation of the appropriateness of the medication for the patient.[19] This application of pharmaceutical care provides for "the responsible provision of drug therapy" but fails to address the patient's outcomes. This level of pharmaceutical care requires a patient history and allergy information and the willingness of the patient to talk about their medications.

Disease state management addresses therapeutic outcomes. In this application of pharmaceutical care pharmacists monitor disease progression as well as problems with medication regimens. Pharmacists in community practice settings offer screening or wellness clinics where screenings tests and monitoring or certain disease states occur. Blood pressure and blood glucose are screening tests that are easily performed with an inexpensive piece of equipment and a little training. However, the technology now exists to perform hemoglobin A1C in diabetics as well as PT/INR and lipid testing in cardiac patients. At this point the results are relayed back to the prescriber who would then make adjustments in the drug regimen. Along with the monitoring, pharmacists can also make recommendations on nutritional support, immunization and OTC preparations, which should and should not be used in conjunction with the patient's drug regimen. This level of pharmaceutical care in addition requires the requisite equipment as well as physician support in the form of referrals and willingness to accept outside suggestions.

Collaborative practice takes disease state management and makes the pharmacist the driving force in medication planning decisions. The practice model that exists in this type of pharmaceutical care is one where a physician refers a patient with a specific condition to a pharmacist run clinic. This pharmacist would then do all medication care planning under the limits of the collaborative agreement and be responsible for all follow up and monitoring required. This level of pharmaceutical care requires the pharmacist to have an intimate knowledge of all the patient's medical history.

If collaborative practice and disease state management are the most advanced form of pharmaceutical care then pharmacogenomics is the next natural evolution. The ability to predict drug therapy outcomes before initiation by studying a patient's genetic profile will improve mediation efficacy, patient safety and quality of life while decreasing adverse reactions as well as help contain cost. Pharmacogenomics analyzes a patient's genetic profile to ascertain which medication will provide the best possibility of efficacy with the least risk adverse reactions. This genetic profile can assess receptor affinity as well as polymorphic pathways in the metabolic pathways of medications, thus allowing the provider to "predict" the outcome of drug therapy before initiation.

Embracing these new practice standards is not without problems and disadvantages. In an age of ever-increasing prescription volume it is difficult to divert pharmacists from their primary role. Also this new level of practice requires increased access to patient records as well as more advanced equipment, training, and floor space for the clinic area.[20] Physician involvement is not easy with the perception being that pharmacy is impinging on what has traditionally been the physician's role. And lastly there is a need for increased education of the existing population of pharmacists for this increased role.[21]

Economic Issues of Pharmaceutical Care

Community pharmacists have been hesitant to provide comprehensive pharmaceutical care primarily due to economic constraints. These economic issues, as we will see in the following discussion, are a key component in the evolution of the community pharmacy practice model. With little compensation for pharmaceutical services, there was little incentive for pharmacists to invest in advanced education, the restructuring of their pharmacy, the hiring of more technical help, and the purchasing of technology to support advanced patient care. However, as stated previously, because of the diminishing margins for medications it is imperative that pharmacists broaden their practice model to include reimbursement for cognitive services. Therefore, it became necessary to convince patients, payers, and regulators that pharmaceutical care is of value. Let us further explore the primary challenge of this task.

There are three primary models for health insurance currently employed in the US: risk pooling, cost containment and demand. Of these, the demand model has the greatest potential for the development of a successful platform from which pharmacists may receive direct reimbursement for pharmaceutical care. The cornerstone of a successful demand model is the establishment of the value of the service(s) provided in the mind of the consumer. In essence, the consumer must perceive a sufficient value of the service provided, be willing to initially pay for it out-of-pocket, and demand payment for these services from third party payers. The third party carriers must in turn establish a uniform fee schedule upon which to base this reimbursement. Rather than wait for consumers to make the demand on insurance carriers to cover these cognitive services, pharmacist must initiate the process by establishing a private pay basis from which the private and public insurance carriers would draw.[22] There has been recent progress in this area to render this process more than an academic discussion.

The inpatient pharmacists at a large east-coast teaching hospital had been providing cognitive services (eg, in the areas of pharmacokinetic consultation, patient and family medication education, nutritional assessment for patients receiving metabolic support, adjustment of parenteral nutrient regimens and drug regimen reviews) for years without receiving direct compensation for same. A decision was made by pharmacy administration to discontinue the practice of pro bono care and charge private insurance carriers for pharmacist interventions. The fee schedule was based on the "charge level" system used by AMA and is based on the acuity of the illness or injury and the relative complexity of the issues (not based on the amount of time necessarily spent on intervention). All interventions are documented in a uniform format (SOAP) in patients' progress notes and no charge may be generated unless this entry completed. Specific software package developed specifically for this process for the purposes of establishing both audit trails for the interventions and tracking of successful reimbursements from private insurers. Audited results indicate that reimbursement by private insurance carriers was at 59% of the charged rate. Because of the success of this program, it has been expanded to included diabetes and asthma management for employees of the health system.[23] There has also been some progress in the area of cognitive services reimbursement at the federal level.

Medicare presently does not compensate the health care system for therapy (i.e. cognitive) services provided by pharmacists. A recently introduced bill (the "Medicare Pharmacist Services Coverage Act") would for the first time, recognize pharmacists as health care "providers" under Medicare and permit compensation for "high level drug therapy."[24] The areas proposed for inclusion in this program are anticoagulation, diabetes, asthma and hypertension management. Again, the impetus for this significant modification to the Medicare program has been driven on two primary fronts:

1. Clients of privately funded pharmacist managed programs value the service as an integral and previously missing component of their overall disease management and decreased levels of reimbursement and;
2. Decreased levels of reimbursement and managed care imposed algorithms have drastically decreased the amount of physician time before patients with the net result that medication matters related to various disease states are not addressed with patients.

To convince payers that pharmaceutical care has value and can save enormous amounts of money, numerous studies have been conducted.[25, 26] In a recent study at the University of Kansas,

direct savings from community pharmacist interventions averaged $27.63 for each therapeutic substitution, $35.55 per drug discontinuation, $32.36 for drugs deemed not necessary to dispense, and $21.98 for each generic substitution.[27] To further demonstrate how pharmacists can reduce total health care costs and improve patient health, Project ImPACT (Improve Persistence and Compliance with Therapy): Hyperlipidemia was established.[28] Community pharmacists participating in this project offered cholesterol tests and regular counseling to patients with hyperlipidemia, a form of high blood cholesterol. Participating pharmacists spent up to 30 minutes per visit with patients, explaining laboratory test results, suggesting lifestyle changes, and stressing the importance of staying on their prescribed medication. According to preliminary results, 84 percent of the 469 enrolled patients are still taking their medicine as prescribed and about 50 percent of those patients have achieved their cholesterol-lowering goals. As a result of these findings, payers, both public and private, and patients are realizing that pharmaceutical care leads to improved patient health and offers substantial savings in health care costs. In other words, pharmaceutical care provided by community pharmacists is of value.

As payers and patients realize the value of pharmaceutical care, they are more willing to reimburse pharmacists for their pharmaceutical care services and disease management activities.[29] Financially, it is better to pay the pharmacist a fee to prevent a drug therapy complication than to pay for an emergency room visit or hospitalization due to a drug therapy complication. Therefore, programs are slowly being implemented to reimburse pharmacists for pharmaceutical care. An established program is the Mississippi Medicaid Waiver Program. The Health Care Financing Administration (HCFA) has approved a Medicaid Waiver in Mississippi to pay for pharmaceutical care in four disease states: asthma, diabetes, hyperlipidemia, and anticoagulation.[30] The waiver allows for licensed, credentialed pharmacists to receive reimbursement for disease management activities. Programs like this provide continuing evidence that payers as a direct result of patient advocacy are recognizing the value of pharmaceutical care and are reimbursing pharmacists for their services.

Community pharmacists are encouraged to provide pharmaceutical care as they are compensated for their services. Moreover, there is less economic risk involved in investing in the delivery of pharmaceutical care when reimbursement programs are in place. As the practice and business platforms for community pharmacy practice evolve from the predominant fee-for-dispensed-medication model to one of evidence-based pharmacotherapy, direct payment for cognitive services will become an even more critical component. This is especially true as the community pharmacist becomes more regarded as a healthcare resource for both medication and education in the evolution to a practice of true medication management.

REFERENCES

1. Gebhart F. *Drug Topics* 2003; 147(6):38.
2. Cranor CW, Christensen DB. *J Am Pharm Assoc* 2003; 43:149.
3. Cranor CW, Christensen DB. *J Am Pharm Assoc* 2003; 43:160.
4. Cranor CW, Bunting BA, Christensen DB. *J Am Pharm Assoc* 2003; 43:173.
5. Bluml BM, McKenney JM, Cziraky MJ. *J Am Pharm Assoc* 2000; 40:155.
6. Pharmacy Compounding Practices & Sterile Drug Products For Home Use, United States Pharmcopeia National Formulary, USP Rockville, MD, 1996.
7. Duncker A, Greenberg S. *A Profile of Older Americans*, AARP, Washington DC, 1997 (available at http://research.aarp.org/general/profile97.html)
8. The Third Strategic Planning Conference for Pharmacy Practice Report, Supplement to American Pharmacy, APhA, Washington DC, October 7–10, 1994.
9. Hepler CD, Strand LM. *Am J Hosp Pharm* 1990; 47(3):533.

10. Hatoum HT, Valuck RJ: Drug use and the health care system. In: Knowlton CH, Penna RP, eds. *Pharmaceutical Care*, 1996.

11. Manasse HR. *Am J Hosp Pharm* 1989; 46:929.

12. Strand LM. *Report at Podium Presentation, Pharmaceutical Care Outcomes Research Conference*, University of Georgia, Athens, AT, Sept 1996.

13. Maine LL, Penna RP. Pharmaceutical care: an overview. In: Knowlton CH, Penna RP, eds. *Pharmaceutical Care*, 1996.

14. Johnson JA, Bootman JL. *Arch Intern Med* 1995; 155:1949.

15. Pew Health Professions Commission Report: *Critical Challenges Revitalizing the Health Professions for the Twenty-First Century*. CA-UCSF Center for Health Professions, San Francisco, CA, 1995.

16. Knowlton HL. *J Am Pharmaceut Assoc* 1997; 38:12

17. Harteker LR. *The Pharmacy Technician Companion*, APhA, Washington DC, 1998.

18. Hepler CD, Strand LM. *Am J Hosp Pharm* 1990; 47:533.

19. Abood RR, Brushwood DB. *Pharmacy Practice and the Law*, 2nd ed, 1997.

20. Isett JI, McKone BJ. Practice changes facilitated by pharmaceutical care. In: Knowlton CH, Penna RP, eds. *Pharmaceutical Care*, 1996.

21. Amsler MR, Murray MD, Tierney WM. *J Am Pharm Assoc* 2001; 41:850.

22. Ganther JM. *J Am Pharm Assoc* 2002; 42:875.

23. Michalets EL, Williams E. *Am J Health-Syst Pharm* 2001; 58:164.

24. Young D. *Am J Health-Syst Pharm* 2002, 59:811.

25. Huffman DC (ed). Washington DC: NARD, 1996.

26. Johnson JA, Bootman JL. *Am J Health-Syst Pharm* 1997; 54:554.

27. Bochamer C (ed). *NCPA Newsletter* 1997; 119:1.

28. Bluml BM et al. *J Am Pharm Assoc* 1998; 38:529.

29. Knowlton CH. *J Am Pharm Assoc* 1997; 37:361.

30. Stevens WL (ed). *MS State Board of Pharmacy Newsletter* 1998; 4(4): June.

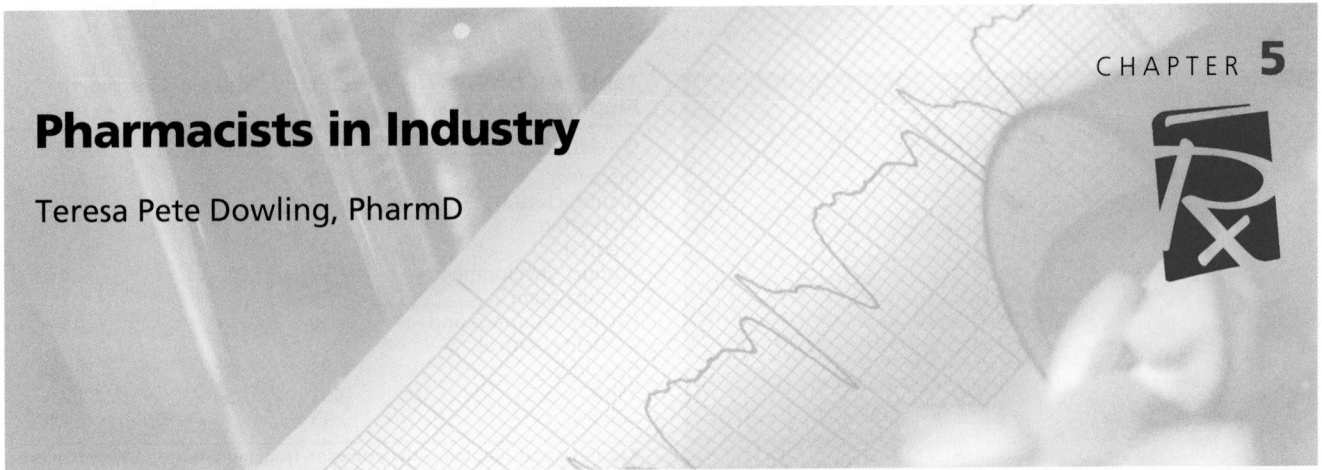

CHAPTER 5

Pharmacists in Industry

Teresa Pete Dowling, PharmD

The pharmaceutical industry in the United States is a for-profit environment. Its goal is to bring value to its shareholders, and it does this by doing good for people (Fig 5-1). Integral to the mission of a pharmaceutical company involved in research is the discovery of new chemical entities (NCEs), their toxicological testing, the development of these entities into dosage forms, clinical trials in humans of these investigational drugs or biologics, regulatory review and approval of the new products, and marketing of the products for appropriate use by health care professionals and consumers.

In 2003, the industry invested an estimated $33.2 billion in discovering and developing new medicines.[1] Hundreds of employees are involved as a new chemical entity moves through the stages of product development. Hundreds to thousands of people become subjects in the clinical trials depending on the proposed indications.

Many of the NCEs died on the road of discovery and testing. On average it takes 10 to 15 years and costs more than $800 million to advance a potential new medicine from a research idea to a treatment approved by the FDA.[2] When one of your company's NCEs is approved by FDA, the feelings of achievement and success are great among the product team members.

Pharmacists may choose many environments to practice pharmacy and to apply their knowledge and skills to the improvement of patient care. One area is the pharmaceutical industry where major advances in patient care, research to improve patient's lives, and education for health care professionals and patients are happening every day. The input into patient care is indirect rather than direct, and the products and programs have the potential to touch numerous patients' lives.

OPPORTUNITIES FOR PHARMACISTS

As of June 1996, the US pharmaceutical industry employed a total of 367,871 people worldwide. Of this total, 203,009 were employed in the US, and 164,862 were employed abroad.[3] Among those working in the US, 60,163 were involved in production; 58,082 worked in marketing; 50,802 were involved in medical R&D; and 28,642 worked in administration. The remaining 5321 were responsible for distribution activities. The Pharmaceutical Research and Manufacturers of America, the organiza-

tion that collected these data, do not have it available as of 2004. It would be very interesting to see the impact on the number of employees in the US pharmaceutical industry when one considers the mergers, acquisitions, down-sizing, and growth (eg, in the biotechnology area) that has occurred over the last 8 years. However, the 1996 data can be used to give an estimate of number of positions within certain divisions of the industry.

It is difficult to obtain the percent of pharmacists that work in the pharmaceutical industry. Approximately 2.7% of pharmacists practice in the industry, according to the *National Pharmacist Workforce Study: 2000*.[4] It is estimated that there are 257,256 licensed pharmacists with in-state addresses based upon census data as of June 30, 2003.[5] If the percentage of pharmacists in industry stayed about the same, there would be approximately 7000 pharmacists working in the pharmaceutical industry.

Riggins and Plowman reported a survey of pharmacists employment and satisfaction trends at one pharmaceutical company (Table 5-1) that found pharmacists employed in many areas of the company.[6] These included drug discovery, manufacturing, marketing, medical information, product development, quality assurance, sales, and regulatory. A follow-up survey in 2001 revealed project management, health outcomes research, legal, information technology, training and development, and scientific communications as additional areas of employment for pharmacists.[7] These listings should not be considered complete. For example, one additional area is drug surveillance or safety; also, pharmacists move into other departments once they enter the industry, based upon their interests and skills.

Most of these positions would start at an entry level; however some, such as medical liaison and account representative, would require some years of clinical or sales experience. The entry-level salaries are often competitive with other areas of pharmacy practice, and the opportunities for long-range advancement, earnings, and fringe benefits are good in industry. Industry pharmacists are able to use their pharmacy training and skills and at the same time, experience professional growth, personal satisfaction, and a challenging environment.

Most companies are lean on full-time staff, and an individual will find that job responsibilities will be more than one full-time equivalent at times of peak team activity. The Career Pathways Evaluation Program, Pharmacist Profile Survey, formerly the Glaxo Pharmacy Specialty Survey, is maintained by the American Pharmaceutical Association and provides information about 17 career paths for pharmacists. The survey was administered in spring 2002 and included pharmacists in industry. One of the questions concerned work schedules. On average, the industry respondents stated that they work 49 hours/week. Flexible working arrangements and telecommuting help to bring some work-life balance to the job.

T. P. Dowling is an employee of AstraZeneca. All opinions expressed in this chapter are those of the author and do not represent those of AstraZeneca. The author acknowledges and thanks Jack Robbins, Maryann Brennan, Bernard J Hark, and Nancy Pettineo. Sections of this chapter were reproduced as written by Jack Robbins, PhD, who authored this chapter for a previous edition of the text. M Brennan, BJ Hark, PharmD, and N Pettineo, PharmD were instrumental in searching the literature for updated references.

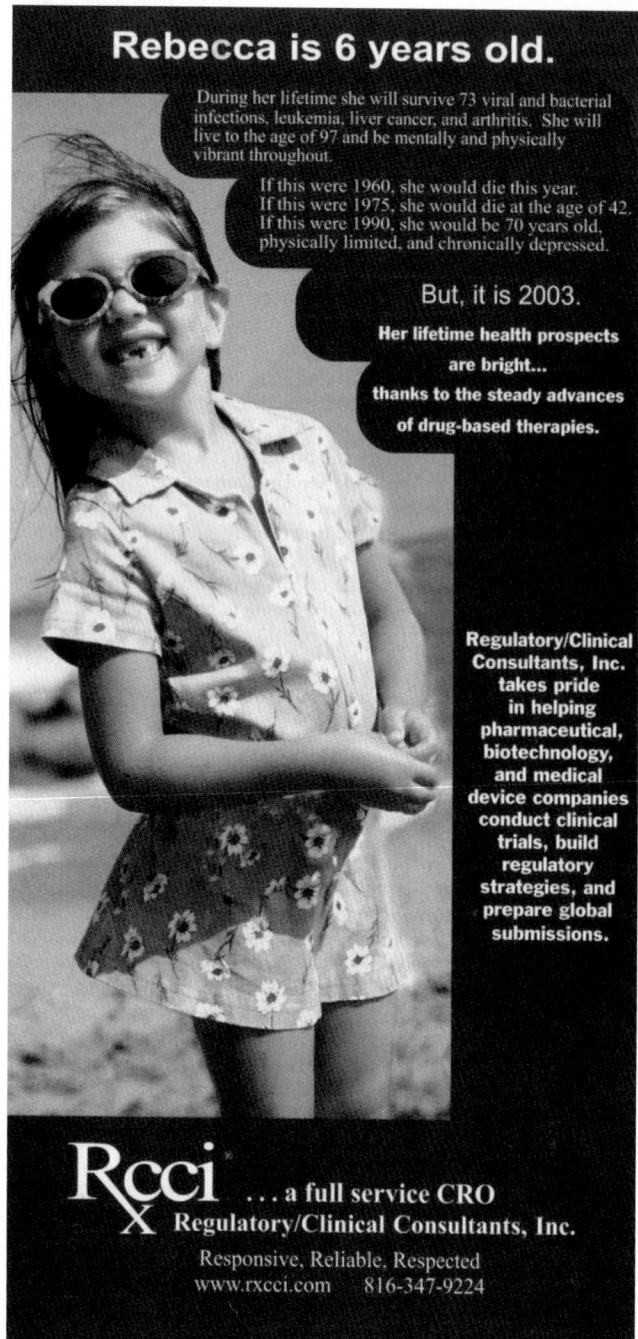

Figure 5-1. An example of the impact of pharmaceuticals to patients' lives. *Copyright 2004, Regulatory/Clinical Consultants, Inc. Used with permission. All rights reserved.* Regulatory/Clinical Consultants, Inc. used this ad to promote their services to the industry. The ad drew worldwide attention and was recognized for its strongly positive message about the progress of pharmaceuticals over the past 50 years.

Table 5-1. Division in Which Lilly Pharmacists were Employed in 1998

DIVISION	NO. OF PHARMACISTS	PERCENTAGE
Discovery	18	2.7%
Manufacturing	25	3.7%
Marketing	52	7.7%
Medical	72	10.6%
Product development	37	5.4%
Product team	35	5.2%
Quality assurance and quality control	10	1.5%
Regulatory	35	5.2%
Sales	402	59.2%
Other	19	2.8%

Reprinted and adapted with permission from Riggins JL and Plowman BH: Pharmacists employment and satisfaction trends at Eli Lilly and Company. *Drug Information Journal.* 2000;34:1223–9, Table 5.© 2000, Drug Information Association.

duction and quality control, legal, regulatory affairs, and management and administration.

Potential Positions within the Industry Sales

The sales area is one of the ways for pharmacists to get into the pharmaceutical industry. The sales representative (also called professional services representative, professional sales representative, or professional sales specialist) usually call upon physicians, pharmacists, nurses, and, in some cases, dentists and veterinarians with details on the products of their companies. The objective of these calls is to provide the various professional audiences with enough comprehensive information on a product to encourage the product's appropriate use by the health care providers.

Many companies prefer that candidates for a sales position have a science background, and thus they favor applications with pharmacy training. Equally important in being considered for a sales position are the personal traits and attitudes of the applicant, such as a congenial personality, effective oral communication skills, and a strong interest in selling.

Entry-level salaries for sales positions in most areas of the country generally are competitive with other pharmacy practice positions. In addition, most pharmaceutical companies offer excellent benefits packages such as company cars, expense reimbursement, travel to medical and pharmacy conventions, comprehensive medical insurance for the family, and reimbursement for education programs.

Marketing

The marketing department is responsible for developing and implementing marketing plans to promote the company's products to the appropriate audiences. Every company in the industry has, over time, developed its own unique marketing organization. In some firms, the department is organized by category, such as prescription-products marketing and OTC-products marketing. In other firms, marketing is divided into therapy areas, such as cardiovascular or respiratory products. In still others, brand teams are formed to drive the activities for the product. Whatever their structure, most marketing departments include:

- *Marketing Research*, which analyzes business trends, sales histories of the company's products, competitive information, prescribing and recommendation habits of practitioners, and new business opportunities within the market.
- *Marketing Strategy/Planning*, which is responsible for anticipating and developing products and services to meet the needs of the market place in the long term.

When presenting potential roles within the industry, authors often select specific divisions within the company. Each company has developed its own titles for positions. It is often frustrating to realize that the same position can have many titles; however, this is important to remember when looking at positions within the industry. Also, these positions may be placed within different reporting divisions when comparing one company to another. The areas that will be highlighted within this chapter are sales, marketing, medical affairs (headquarters- and field-based positions), research and development, pro-

- *Product Management*, which oversees the overall marketing plan for a specific product, and is responsible for the profits or losses generated by that product.
- *Life Cycle Management*, which evaluates new uses for the product and supports research to study these uses, leading to new indications or to publications.
- *Promotion/ePromotion*, which develops the promotional pieces for the product.

A degree in pharmacy may be helpful but generally is not a requirement for a marketing position. Experience in the industry, usually gained in the sales department, plus an understanding of the health-care delivery system, general business principles, and a basic knowledge of R&D, manufacturing, quality assurance, and distribution are helpful in obtaining a position in the marketing department of a pharmaceutical company. The MBA would be an appropriate advanced degree, and many obtain the degree while in sales or in the marketing department.

Medical Affairs, Headquarters-based and Field-based Personnel

Within the company, a department provides information and services to health care practitioners in response to unsolicited inquiries, fosters research, gives presentations to practitioners, does sales training, and obtains the input of thought leaders. Most members of this department are health care providers and pharmacists are excellent for positions in Medical Affairs. A group of industry employees, most of who are pharmacists, published a supplement to discuss and describe this practice area.[9]

HEADQUARTERS-BASED PERSONNEL— MEDICAL COMMUNICATIONS GROUPS, MEDICAL INFORMATION MANAGERS

Health care providers recognize that the pharmaceutical company knows the most about its products. When the providers have questions about the products, they call the company and expect rapid, concise, accurate, and scientifically-balanced answers to their questions. These questions come to the Medical Communications group within Medical Affairs. Although previously staffed by physicians, this area has been a primary entrance position for clinical pharmacists in industry since the 1980s. It is a "spin-off" of the drug information center in the hospital setting.

Each company provides avenues for health care practitioners to ask questions and report adverse events. In industry, pharmacists are excellent for this position. They staff the company's 1-800 drug information telephone inquiry center, also staffed by nurses, responding to inquiries and capturing adverse events. Pharmacists with a Doctor of Pharmacy degree are often hired to develop the databases utilized by the company to answer these unsolicited inquiries. The responses in these databases are scientifically rigorous and balanced. Many of these pharmacists also teach the sales force, respond to questions from the marketing team, and review promotional pieces used by the company. Technology is a key requirement to aiding the company in responding to unsolicited inquiries. Managers in Medical Affairs develop an understanding of telephone response systems, fax-back programs, web-based information, and inquiry tracking and response systems.

FIELD-BASED PERSONNEL—MEDICAL LIAISONS, PRODUCT DEVELOPMENT SCIENTISTS, MEDICAL INFORMATION SCIENTISTS

Most pharmaceutical companies have deployed highly trained personnel to the field to provide support and information to opinion leaders, clinical investigators, and decision makers in health care organizations. Pharmacists with a Doctor of Phar- macy degree constitute the majority of pharmaceutical company personnel in these positions. The position requires the application of scientific and product knowledge to disease management in response to inquiries from health care professionals. Individuals are expected to develop working relationships with opinion leaders and to foster research. Good people skills and excellent presentation skills help these individuals succeed. Physicians and PhDs are also among the individuals utilized by this group. These teams are regionally located throughout the country.

Field-based personnel are aligned with the product teams or therapeutic areas and share information directly with these marketing teams. They also develop and deliver scientific training programs to the sales force.

Research and Development

Pharmacists in the industry are engaged in R&D of new drugs or new indication or dosage forms for existing products. This area of the industry is stimulating and challenging and is suited especially to pharmacists with strong scientific backgrounds.

PhDs are often required to progress in the area of dosage form development. PharmDs are becoming more involved with clinical research and protocol development, along with nurses and PhDs in biological sciences.

Individuals in research must be willing to move to new areas of research in the company as a project come to completion or is killed when the investigational drug does not preform as expected or desired. They work on tight timelines to conduct clinical trials in a timely manner with rapid enrollment and strict attention to *Good Clinical Practices*. When the study is completed, they draft the clinical study report for filing with regulatory agencies. Project management of the clinical trials program is an exciting opportunity for research-oriented pharmacists.

Health economics research is another area where pharmacists with specialized training are evaluating the cost-effectiveness of new medicines. These data are especially important to a company in its discussion with managed care plans. Research on patient-reported outcomes, what was grouped more into health-related quality of life, is also very important to companies as they evaluate their products.

Production and Quality Control

Pharmacists working in production often serve in managerial positions. They are responsible for anticipating the company's needs and planning for the plant facilities, equipment, and personnel who will be needed to meet the company's production goals. They are also responsible for establishing and administering manufacturing procedures and controls to ensure the production of high-quality products that will meet rigid company and FDA standards.

Pharmaceutical manufacturing is changing constantly by developing new technologies. Equipment often becomes obsolete in as short a time as 3 to 5 years. Thus, pharmacists and other production employees constantly must learn and adapt to new technology and procedures. Pharmacists who want to advance in careers in manufacturing usually will need advanced degrees beyond their entry-level pharmacy diplomas.

Research-intensive pharmaceutical companies constantly conduct thousands of assays and quality assurance (QA) tests each year to maintain the quality of their products. QA activities begin while the safety and efficacy of a new product are being established. The R&D, manufacturing, and QA departments of the company jointly establish final production and QA specifications for a new product.

The QA department establishes sampling and testing procedures to make certain that each lot of a product meets both company and FDA specifications. The system also ensures the potency, purity, and dose-to-dose uniformity of the product, in addition to the chemical, physical, and biological data; stability of the finished trade package; and appropriate expiration dates. The QA department also checks not only for the quality and quantity of the active ingredients, but also for the uniformity and predictability of the nonactive ingredients. Pharmacists can work in many QA areas.

Legal Department or Regulatory Affairs Department

Some pharmacists decide to pursue a law degree. With this additional credential, they can consider positions as lawyers in the legal departments within companies. While there are many areas of law that are of value to the company, patent lawyers and lawyers that work with the product teams to provide legal consul on the laws and regulations for marketing pharmaceuticals within the US are very important. Pharmacists as lawyers understand the science behind the product and can fill both of these roles. Companies may want the lawyers that they hire to have legal experience prior to entering the company.

Regulatory Affairs is the department within the pharmaceutical company that handles the interactions between the company and the medicines regulatory body of the country in which the company is located. In the US, this regulatory body would be the Food and Drug Administration. Individuals within the company learn the regulations and processes that must be following for submitting an Investigational New Drug application (IND), a New Drug Application (NDA), and many other special documents including post-marketing surveillance reports. Regulatory Affairs individuals work within the company with all groups that have input into these documents. Many interactions are with R&D staff as the IND and NDA documents and other reports are developed and also with Marketing as the materials for promotion are developed. Regulatory Affairs will work with a cross-functional team to develop the draft Prescribing Information for submission to the FDA.

Pharmacists with their science background in drugs, diseases, and patient care can understand these documents as drafted by team members and work to improve them to the guidance of the regulations. They also can understand the regulatory agencies during the interactions that occur and help to establish regulatory strategy with the product teams.

Management and Administration

As pharmacists in the industry perform successfully at their positions, they move up within the department and within the company to positions in management and administration. Here, they ensure that the department functions smoothly and achieves its objectives. In some companies, managers are still involved with aspects of daily staff functions.

Bendis commented that a pharmacist's career path in management might span well over 10 to 15 years.[10] Using the sales and marketing area as an example, she outlined the following succession of positions illustrated by rank that may be achieved:

- Professional sales representative
- Coordinator, sales training
- District sales manager
- Product manager
- Regional sales director
- Vice president of sales
- Vice president of marketing
- President

While it doesn't happen often that people progress to president of the company, it does happen.

Pharmacy training provides a good basis for management and administration, but on-the-job experience is usually the key to success in management. Many of the people in management positions in the industry began their careers at entry-level positions and learned the organization from the inside. Qualities of discipline, hard work, and dedication go a long way in helping a pharmacist advance into a management position.

Selecting a Pharmaceutical Company

Not all pharmaceutical companies are the same. When deciding to investigate the pharmaceutical industry as a career choice, it is important to study the companies as well as the type of positions that you want (Table 5-2). *The Pink Sheet* may be a source of the information that you need. There is the potential for movement among the companies in the pharmaceutical industry as clinical research in one area is completed and is growing elsewhere or as a sales force ramps down in one area and expands in another. Here are questions that you may want to ask yourself and the individuals with whom you interview.

- How large is this company? The size of the company can be obtained from it Annual Report, usually posted on its corporate web site. Large companies usually have very defined job descriptions. Small companies will provide more opportunity to do a variety of jobs in a given area. You will be able to know most of the people at headquarters or the business unit where you work.
- What is the company's mission and shared values? The company mission statement will be found in its annual report and usually is posted on its Web site.
- Is this a US-based company or is its global headquarters based in Europe or Japan? There are cultural differences that come into play when you work for a European-based or Japanese-based company. Teams in the US may need to work differently to influence the global brand team and to understand their international colleagues. There may be the opportunity for international travel to team meetings. Also, there is the benefit of exposure to other cultures.
- How much travel is involved with this position? There are positions in clinical research and in field-based Medical Affairs that are 60% travel. How does this fit into your plans right now?
- Is relocation necessary?
- What are the company's major products? How many do they have? Are any of these products going off patent soon?
- What does the company have in its pipeline? How does its pipeline compare to other companies? Articles are published yearly in journals such as *Fortune* or *Medical Advertising News* that rank different aspects of pharmaceutical companies. It would be important to look at these over a few years to see improvements or declines. Ask about the trends that you see when you interview or with your faculty and preceptors.
- How does this company's sales force compare to others?
- What legal actions or investigations, if any, are underway concerning this company? Have they just finished any notable legal settlements? Many pharmaceutical companies have come under scrutiny of the States Attorneys General's Offices and the Plaintiffs' bar. This increased legal activity probably will continue for some time.
- What is the career progression for individuals who take this position? Where have individuals in the department moved within the company? Has the department attracted any staff from other departments within the company?
- How was this company ranked by Working Mother's Magazine? Are there lactation rooms? Is there a sponsored day care facility on site or close by?

Table 5-2. Potential Sources for Pharmaceutical Industry News

Drug Information Journal
Fortune
First Word (daily global e-news letter)
Medical Advertising News
Pharmaceutical Executive
The Pink Sheet
Science (check the Companies of Choice listing)
Scrip
Working Mothers (check the 100 Best Companies listing)

- Which degree programs does the company support if you wish to go back to school?
- What are your goals and desires? Do they match what this company offers?
- Is there any opportunity for you to do a summer internship, clerkship, residency or fellowship in the industry?

CONCLUSION

In 1995, Gmerek et al stated that "the pharmacist who will succeed in the pharmaceutical industry is the one who has a strong scientific background, is research-oriented, understands the business needs of the organization, and works well in a collaborative, or team situation."[11] The education that a pharmacist receives in the sciences, pharmacology, pharmacy, and therapeutics fosters success at many industry positions. No degree promises you success in your position. Hard work, dedication to quality, and having fun are drivers to success at any position. The pharmaceutical industry lets pharmacists apply their training in a team environment and grow with the company.

REFERENCES

1. www.phrma.org/whoweare, accessed March 31, 2004
2. DiMasi JA, Hansen RW, Grabowski HG. *J Health Econ* 2003; 22:151.
3. *PhRMA Industry Profile*, Washington, DC: Pharmaceutical Research and Manufacturers of America, March 1997.
4. The Midwest Pharmacy Workforce Research Consortium. *Final report of the national pharmacist workforce survey:2000*; Table 4.1. www.accp.org/DOC/MainNavigation/Resources/Section_4_PDF.pdf, accessed April 9, 2004.
5. *Survey of Pharmacy Law–2003–2004*. Park Ridge, IL: National Association of Boards of Pharmacy, 2003.
6. Riggins JL, Plowman BH. *Drug Information J* 2000; 34:1223.
7. Riggins JL. Data on file. Eli Lilly and Company, Indianapolis, 2001: file no. RSRiggs501.
8. Category 14. Pharmaceutical Industry. *Career Pathways Evaluation Program*. Washington, DC: American Pharmaceutical Association. 2002. www.aphanet.org/pathways/Pathways.html accessed on March 25, 2004.
9. DePew CC (guest editor). *Drug Information J* 2000; 34:991.
10. Bendis I. *Pharmacy Times* 1997; 63:86.
11. Gmerek AM, Bakker-Arkema RG, Texter MJ, et al. *Int Pharm J* 1995; 9:150.

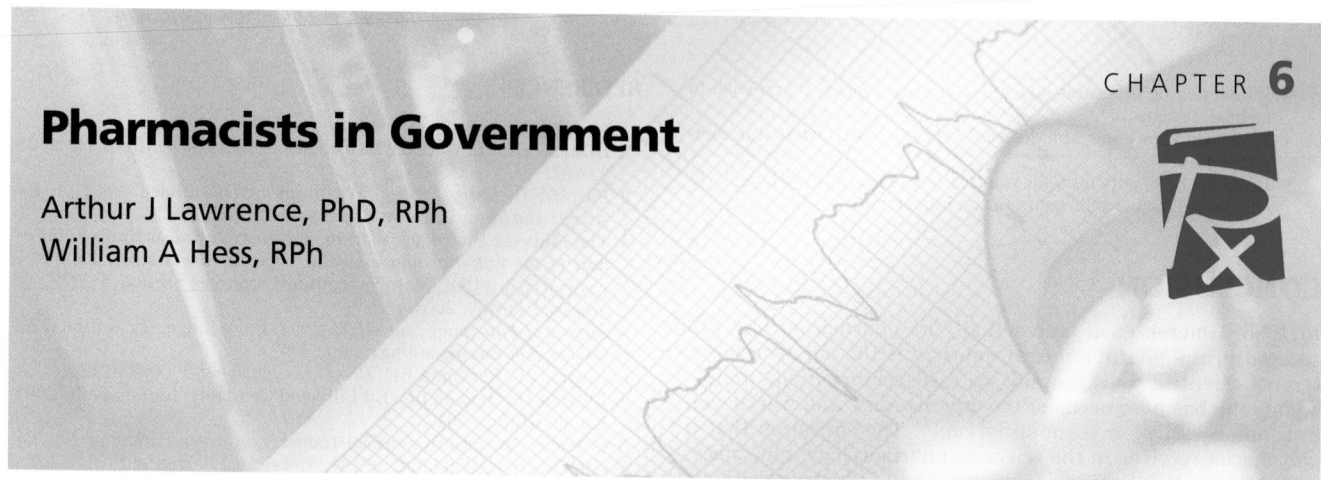

CHAPTER 6

Pharmacists in Government

Arthur J Lawrence, PhD, RPh

William A Hess, RPh

The emphasis on effective and efficient health care services for the population of the United States, and the recent terrorist attacks upon its populace, are increasing the importance of pharmaceutical managed patient-care services and pharmacist participation in complex health programs. New and exciting possibilities for adaptive pharmacy practice and careers are offered in government sectors, with the federal sector offering the broadest range of opportunities.

The trend toward systems of managed care administration has set into motion several initiatives that have already reformed the provision of health care in the US. While commitments and action steps at the end of the last century sought to reduce the overall size of the federal establishment, it became abundantly clear at the beginning of this century that certain parts of that establishment that had been designed to protect against terrorism actually needed to be expanded. Both the form and effect of changes in the federal sector will be spread over several years. It can be anticipated that federal-sector health systems will be extremely dynamic through the turn of the century and beyond.

Pharmacists and the profession of pharmacy are at the crossroads of health care. Opportunities for the creation of new forms of practice abound. Nowhere is this truer than in the federal sector, which offers numerous opportunities for innovation through novel clinical delivery systems, research, and in policy and regulatory mechanisms. While it used to be true that pharmacists practicing within the several federal services were not the highest paid practitioners in the profession, changes due to federal legislation providing for an accession bonus, special pay, loan repayment, and board certified pay for pharmacist officers have made it more competitive with the private sector. Pharmacist officers and federal civilian pharmacists also enjoy a benefits package that is highly competitive with the private sector. In addition, pharmacists desiring to practice advanced forms of clinical activities usually find greater fulfillment in federal practice than in most of the private sector. Federal uniformed service also offers the unique opportunity to pursue a career in which one's seniority and retirement program remains intact throughout one's career moves. Those pharmacists who are not product-oriented, but rather hold values and educational backgrounds oriented toward patient care and public health, find a particularly rewarding form of practice in federal service. Finally, even if pharmacists do not choose a full-time federal career, there are ample opportunities for intermittent federal service throughout the nation.

PHARMACISTS AND GOVERNMENT SERVICE

Pharmacists and their predecessors, the apothecaries and druggists, have served their country and government with distinction since the founding of the colonies. Although direct employment of large numbers of pharmacists is a relatively recent phenomenon, more subtle and indirect assistance has been provided for centuries. Pharmacists, apothecaries, and druggists have responded uniformly to the call of their country to perform critical tasks in support of causes ranging from defense to improving national social equity.

As health care and medical technologies have advanced and become increasingly complex, pharmacists have been called upon to perform tasks that are pivotal to the achievement of improving the health of the individual patient as well as the collective health of the nation. Paradoxically, most of the demands placed on the profession and its practitioners are expanding the pharmacist's role into new and different institutional and consulting territories, while at the same time intensifying demands for those performing in the more traditional community dispensing and distributive role. The ability of the pharmacist to be the health professional uniquely equipped to respond to these changing needs and demands rests with the nature of pharmacy and, to a large extent, the educational system that has evolved from the traditions of the apothecaries.

Pharmacy education and practice rests on a foundation of a synthesis of sciences. Pharmacists enter the practice world with a background and education that prepares them to be highly skilled and expert in several different intellectual and practical areas. This training and experience allows the pharmacist to move farther into the generalist role or choose to pursue a specialist role. Whichever role is chosen, the pharmacist remains a broadly educated member of society, offering a flexibility of performance of functions that is unseen in any other health profession. Pharmacists have gone to extraordinary measures to reach out to other disciplines in the health care team, and this has invariably opened up new opportunities for pharmacists and has led to a deeper reliance upon a pharmacist's expertise. It is precisely this high level of flexibility that makes the pharmacist an exceptionally valuable resource in government practice. Today, given the rapidly changing social and political environments into which government is interwoven, such flexibility is an essential element in adding value to the health system.

CAREER OPPORTUNITIES

Opportunities in the federal sector are not merely employment opportunities, but are truly career opportunities. Federal service offers more variety and differentiation in the types of positions that a pharmacist may fill than does the private sector. In addition, the federal sector offers the pharmacist opportunities for which there is no comparison in the private sector. In the federal sector, it is not unusual to find a pharmacist in a position that neither calls for the specific expertise of a pharmacist nor is normally filled with a pharmacist. Federal pharmacists often occupy important positions of this nature because of their greater level of understanding of health care; this is the culmination of the skills they possess along with the on-the-job and federally funded training that they receive.

For most pharmacists, entry into federal service is through the traditional roles of dispensing and preparation of pharmaceuticals, then advancing to greater responsibilities in scope and magnitude. At some point in their career, most federal pharmacists must choose between accepting more distribution-oriented supervisory duties, or branching into a less traditional, more management and administrative path. For many pharmacists occupying high-level positions, advancement removes them entirely from traditional dispensing and other direct patient-oriented tasks. These posts generally are upper management or policy-making positions, where the specific requirement for experience in pharmacy practice is indirect or nonexistent.

In many respects, this pattern is similar to that which can be expected in some forms of multi-unit and chain-type community stores and in larger institutional practice in the private sector. Pharmacists in federal leadership positions have considerably greater, more far-reaching impact than do their peers in the private sector. The practice profile probably more closely resembles the events of a career in industry. The functional difference between federal and industry/multi-unit practice is that the federal climate offers the broadest range of types of practice, spanning the entire continuum from staff pharmacist functions through high-level management, administration, and policy making.

The federal agencies that offer career opportunities for pharmacists are the Department of Veterans Affairs (DVA), which employs the greatest number; the U.S. Public Health Service (PHS); and the Department of Defense (DOD), through the Army, Navy, and Air Force. The PHS and the three services within the DOD offer positions as either civil service or commissioned officers. The DVA and other federal agencies have primarily focused upon civil service appointments, but there are some PHS commissioned officer pharmacists who have been detailed to these agencies, and one needs to fully investigate such possibilities when job-hunting.

In the PHS, and in the Army, Navy, and Air Force, commissioned officers are used as rapidly mobile professional experts. Civil service is used as an ancillary method of recruitment, and offers significantly more geographic stability. Within the PHS, pharmacist officers of the Commissioned Corps provide the majority of pharmacy services; civil service recruitment is used in limited instances.

UNIFORMED SERVICE REQUIREMENTS

Of the seven uniformed services, four provide commissioned officer opportunities for pharmacists. The Air Force commissions pharmacists as members of the Biomedical Service Corps. The Army categorizes pharmacists as officer members of the Medical Service Corps. The Navy commissions pharmacists as members of the Medical Service Corps, and assigns some members of their health professional staffs as support for the Marine Corps. The Commissioned Corps of the PHS commissions pharmacists as members of a distinct pharmacist category, and these pharmacists primarily serve in Department of Health and Human Services agencies such as the National Institutes of Health, the Centers for Disease Control and Prevention, the Food and Drug Administration, and the Indian Health Service. PHS commissioned officer pharmacists are also assigned to several other federal Departments, such as the Department of Justice, where they provide medical and health support to the Bureau of Prisons, and the Department of Homeland Security, where they provide medical and health support for the Coast Guard and National Disaster Medical System. PHS commissioned officer pharmacists similarly provide medical and health support for the National Oceanic and Atmospheric Administration in afloat and ashore establishments.

It is important for the pharmacist applicant to understand that accepting a commission as a member of one of the uniformed services obligates the individual to a higher order of service. Anyone seeking a career as a health professional and commissioned officer must keep in mind that professional pharmaceutical knowledge and expertise do not by themselves characterize a good officer. The individual must possess other qualifications and skills as required of any commissioned officer, whether serving in a health corps or in a combat arms corps. These qualifications include dedication to a larger cause; excellent judgment, leadership, efficiency, and effectiveness; and devotion to organizational purpose. These qualifications also include the willingness to take certain risks, such as working in a theatre of combat operations, pre-positioning in an area about to be devastated by a hurricane, or venturing into a contaminated area after a bioterrorist attack. The extent to which an officer exhibits and activates these attributes is carefully considered by promotion boards in addition to the skillful application of professional prowess.

Most successful applicants can expect to be commissioned as an extended duty reserve officer when first called to active duty. Applicants must possess a baccalaureate degree in pharmacy from an institution accredited by the American Council on Pharmaceutical Education (ACPE) and be licensed by exam to practice in one of the states or territories of the US or the District of Columbia. Generally, the licensure that is claimed must have been earned by examination, and not by reciprocity.

All applicants must be of good moral character, at least 21 years of age, and physically qualified. All applicants are required to undergo a government-provided, comprehensive physical examination prior to commissioning. In all cases, applicants must provide adequate information for a complete background and security check and be willing to undergo a credentialing process. In most cases, appointees with advanced degrees and/or specialized training and education are awarded added credit for rank purposes, in recognition of their attainment.

US ARMY

The Continental Congress established a hospital for the care of wounded and disabled in 1775 and simultaneously established the position of "Apothecary" as a member of its officer complement. In 1776, Congress created the office of "Druggist," whose duty it was to "receive and deliver all medicines, instruments and shop furniture of the United States." The Medical Department was reorganized in 1777 and the country divided into four districts. Congress provided that there would be one Apothecary General for each district. Each district Apothecary General was charged to "receive, prepare and deliver medicines and other articles of his department to the hospitals and Army, as shall be ordered by the director general."

During the Revolutionary War, a central laboratory was established for the manufacture of various pharmaceuticals needed to support the operations of the Continental Army. The first Apothecary General, Andrew Craigie, manufactured the majority of these products. His shop in Carlisle, Pennsylvania, was one of the first large-scale manufacturing operations in the colonies.

Professional recognition of the Apothecary, Druggist, and Pharmacist in the Army has been varied, but has improved over the past two centuries. During the Civil War, medical officers controlled the acquisition and preparation of medicinals in both the Union and Confederate Armies. Druggists frequently were found in supporting roles, especially among Union volunteer regiments, but they did not occupy commissioned positions. Between the end of the Civil War and the period immediately after World War II, pharmacists served in capacities for which some received commissions; others were assigned to the enlisted ranks. During World War I, several pharmacists served in support roles in the Army's Sanitary Corps.

Most recently, active and reserve Army pharmacists have risen to numerous challenges in supporting the Army War Fighter ensuring the projection and sustainment of a healthy and medically fit force. Army pharmacists have deployed both home and abroad in support of our nation's global war on terrorism for Operation Enduring Freedom (OEF) and Operation Iraqi Freedom (OIF) in addition to other worldwide deployments.

Army Pharmacy

The degree of professional recognition of pharmacists, as well as pharmacy practice, is radically different in today's Army. Pharmacists are vital members of the Medical Service Corps and serve throughout the world in support of the mission of the Army Medical Department, which is to ensure the health of the soldier during times of peace and war. To accomplish this mission, the Army operates 106 ambulatory care clinics, 20 general hospitals, and 8 medical centers, as well as several fixed and mobile ambulatory-care medical activities.

There currently are approximately 153 commissioned pharmacist officers on active duty and approximately 260 Reserve pharmacist officers. The reserve officers are comprised of Reserve Troop Program Unit Members (TPU), Individual Ready Reserve (IRR), and Individual Mobilization Augmentee's (IMA). The Reserve officers are used to supplement the active duty force and are available for deployment on very short notice. Reserve officers can be called to active duty as part of an entire unit or as an individual to fill a specific vacancy.

Most pharmacist officers, active duty or reserve, are assigned to Army medical centers and general hospitals in the US. Army general hospitals have all the characteristics of the modern community hospital, but restrict their operations to providing for the care of active duty and retired personnel and their dependent beneficiaries. All eight of the medical centers conduct advanced education, training, and research programs and are equipped with much of the same sophisticated technology to be found in university-affiliated teaching hospitals.

Service as a pharmacist officer in the Army provides the opportunity for international travel and service. The Army has pharmacist officers stationed outside the US in hospitals in Germany, Korea, Panama, Japan, Italy, Belgium, and Southwest Asia. Career-status pharmacists can anticipate having the opportunity for a foreign-duty assignment at least once during their career. During an armed conflict, active duty pharmacists join ranks with their reserve counterparts in being assigned to and deploying with combat support hospitals (CSH), mobile army surgical hospitals (MASH), field hospitals (FH), medical logistics battalions, and medical logistics centers that are located in the theatre of operations.

An active pharmacy technician program supports pharmacist officers. The Army conducts pharmacy technician training at the Academy of Health Sciences at Fort Sam Houston, Texas, via a program of studies accredited with the American Society of Health-System Pharmacists (ASHP). A total of more than 600 pharmacy technicians are now on duty. Army pharmacists and technicians dispense in excess of 75,000 ambulatory-care prescriptions and 55,000 inpatient medication orders daily.

Army medical activities also use the civil service system to employ pharmacists. The Army employs some 400 civilian pharmacists in a variety of General Schedule (GS) grades, plus an additional 300 civilian technicians. Most of these civilian pharmacists are employed within the continental US and can expect geographic stability.

The Army provides several opportunities for advanced education, training, and research. Each of its medical centers conducts research programs. Four medical centers (Brooke AMC, Madigan AMC, Tripler AMC, and Walter Reed AMC) operate hospital pharmacy residency programs that are fully ASHP-accredited. In addition, a hematology–oncology and nuclear pharmacy residency is offered at Walter Reed Army Medical Center. Continuing education courses and opportunities are offered through military-provided programs of study, as well as attendance at civilian pharmacy programs; the expenses are covered under military reimbursement.

The Army is active in providing external education opportunities for its pharmacists. Each year, highly motivated officers are selected for Army-sponsored graduate studies in civilian institutions and Army-sponsored Training with Industry opportunities with national pharmaceutical organizations. Officers customarily pursue graduate education in institutional pharmacy leading to either a Master of Science or Doctor of Pharmacy degree. There is a limited opportunity for officers to pursue studies directed at earning a PhD degree in pharmacology. Officers selected for the training with the industry program are offered fellowship-learning opportunities within the healthcare community, including the pharmaceutical industry, regulatory agencies, and professional organizations. After training, Army pharmacists are positioned in key leadership roles to apply their knowledge and skills to advance the practice of pharmacy within the Army Medical Department. While attending sponsored education, officers receive full pay and allowances as well as tuition assistance.

The career path for all pharmacist officers extends from the rank of Second Lieutenant (O–1 grade) through Colonel (O–6 grade). It is possible for officers to be promoted through these ranks over a career of 21 years, based upon the promotion methods now in effect. All promotions are competitive.

Army pharmacy practice presents several unique opportunities. The Army Medical Material Development Activity manages and directs the development of pharmaceuticals and particularized delivery systems. The functions of the pharmacist assigned to duty in this activity are the assurance of program performance in terms of cost, schedule, logistics, quality, and adherence to specifications. Many, if not most, of the projects within this activity are unique to the military and are not seen in civilian practice. Delivery systems for combat casualty care, chemical warfare pretreatment, treatment devices and antiparasitic agents are examples of some of the areas in which the pharmacist would be expected to work.

As mentioned previously, the Army trains pharmacy technicians at their own school. The school offers an 18-week program, conducted on a rotating basis, approximately six times a year; the class size averages 40 to 60 students. Classes provide interservice education for active Army, Reserve, and National Guard components, and foreign military services. The school is supervised by a pharmacist officer and has a staff of an additional eight pharmacist officers and more than 20 senior enlisted military pharmacy technicians. This staff offers other more specialized courses of study in sterile products preparation and therapy and drug distribution. A course orienting all newly commissioned pharmacist officers to the organization and operation of Army pharmacy services, career opportunities, and expectations of performance is presented periodically by the staff.

Army pharmacists continue to provide value every day as contributing members of the Army and Department of Defense Health Care Team. With the implementation of futuristic initiatives such as pharmacy informatics, a pharmacist-lead Department of Defense Military Vaccine office, and the continued quality care improvements in the delivery of clinical services that ensure medication-use safety for all patients, Army pharmacists will continue to be a vital link between the Medical Service Corps and the Army Medical Department in conserving the fighting strength and compassionately and effectively managing the medication-use aspects of the health of our Soldiers and Army family.

US AIR FORCE

Today's US Air Force (USAF) was preceded by the Army Air Corps. The Air Force Medical Service (AFMS) was authorized and activated on July 1, 1949. In March 1965, the Medical Service Corps (MSC) was reorganized into two distinct corps. The component including officers who conduct medical administration, supply, and non-clinical patient support activities remained in the MSC. The new added corps, the Biomedical Service Corps (BSC), consists of officers representing 17 areas of health practice who carry out clinically oriented functions. Pharmacists were transferred into the BSC, and this is the service in which they are now commissioned.

The mission of the AFMS and the BSC is to provide the medical support needed to maintain the highest possible degree of readiness of Air Force combat forces. The general mission is quite similar to that of the Army and the Navy, but differs in the methods and locations of delivery of services. As is the case with all other uniformed services facilities, during peacetime the Air Force provides health services to retired and active-duty service members and their dependents.

The Air Force operates 78 pharmacist-staffed medical facilities worldwide. In the US, these range from small ambulatory clinics to large medical centers. The service has additional hospitals and major clinics located overseas. The service also provides supplemental health services to beneficiaries in smaller support operations throughout the Air Force system. The Air Force operates a global network of aircraft and professionals for the purpose of aeromedical evacuation of members of all services. There are four aeromedical staging units in the continental US and another one located overseas.

Air Force hospitals range in size from 10- to 500-bed facilities, whose character depends upon the nature of the mission of the command in which they are located. The size and range of services are determined by the composition and quantity of those requiring support. Each of the major commands administers hospitals and clinics of the full range of sizes. The Air Force Medical Center is the largest and provides a full range of general, specialist, and tertiary support. Medical centers sponsor internships and residencies in most medical specialties and also offer broad integration of pharmacy services into the teaching mission. Research occupies an important focus in the day-to-day activities of most medical centers. There are five medical centers located in the continental US; the largest is Wilford Hall at the USAF Medical Center in San Antonio, Texas, with a full clinical teaching program.

Medium-sized hospitals of the USAF tend to be smaller than 100 beds and are designed to provide a full range of community-oriented care to beneficiaries within a geographically circumscribed area. Patients with conditions that cannot be handled at a USAF hospital commonly are referred to a multi-specialty civilian facility in the area or, in many cases, referred to other uniformed treatment facilities. Although they are geographically separated from the medical-center class of hospitals, these medium-sized hospitals remain linked to medical centers through parallel programs of patient care, medical education, and research. There are nine hospitals of this class in the US, plus two overseas facilities.

Air Force Pharmacy

As one would expect, given the varying characteristics of the different facilities of the Air Force, the specific qualities of pharmacy practice are variable from command to command and location to location. All treatment facilities offer ambulatory-care services, so pharmacy practice is a combination of inpatient institutional and outpatient dispensing. Workload statistics show that 23 facilities dispense more than 1000 ambulatory-care prescriptions a day; of these, 8 dispense over 2000 prescriptions per day, and one processes and dispenses in excess of 4000 prescriptions a day.

Pharmacist officers supervise, review, and monitor all functions of the dispensing activity. To deal with this volume and to provide the pharmacist with professional tools such as an up-to-date patient profile on each patient, the Air Force service is heavily computerized. Currently all DOD, retail network, and mail order pharmacies are linked through a centralized screening system that allows monitoring of patient medication profiles regardless of where the patient accesses the system. Additional automation, in development and testing, will also integrate inpatient pharmaceuticals, giving the pharmacist a complete spectrum of patient-specific drug information. Prescription digital imagery and barcode technology are currently utilized for outpatient prescriptions in all Air Force facilities to further improve patient safety.

Larger facilities employ specialist pharmacists. Most medical centers use pharmacists as drug information specialists who provide consultative services to medical and allied support staffs. In other large facilities, some pharmacist specialists devote a portion of their time to distributive functions. In all cases, pharmacists serve as active members of the pharmacy and therapeutics committees, which possess more far-reaching authority than in the civilian community. The pharmacist's role in selecting therapeutic alternatives and substitutable pharmacologically active entities is broader than in civilian practice.

The BSC currently has on active duty approximately 255 pharmacist commissioned officers, supported by approximately 1100 enlisted highly trained technicians. Additional pharmacy support is provided by pharmacists and technicians employed under the civil service system. Technician support spans several roles, from basic pharmacy administration to the supervised preparation of intravenous additives and solutions.

The career path for Air Force pharmacist officers is similar to that of the Army and Navy. Pharmacists serve as commissioned officers in grades from Second Lieutenant (O–1) through, and including, Colonel (O–6). With completion of the entry-level PharmD degree, direct commissioned pharmacists will enter active duty in the grade Captain (O–3). All new officers are provided a formalized orientation program upon entry. This 4-week program orients the pharmacist to the Air Force and to the Air Force medical community. Additional instruction in military courtesies, career development, and the operation of readiness programs also is provided.

Within the first 2 years of service, all pharmacists are required to return for advanced training. A 3-week course in management, concentrating on the finer skills of managing a clinical administrative career, serves as the foundation for future advancements in position and rank.

Sometime after the initial 2 years of service, pharmacist officers may be selected to attend the Squadron Officers School, which offers a full 7-week course in leadership. During the course, the pharmacist officer is integrated with other mixed-skills officers and receives information that helps build understanding of the Air Force mission, how it integrates with national objectives, and the roles and requirements of the career officer in the Air Force.

Air Force pharmacist officers are expected not only to maintain their skills, but also to improve them by constantly engaging in knowledge-enhancing activities. All pharmacists in the Air Force must achieve a minimum number of continuing education hours that reflect customary state requirements for the maintenance of licensure. All forms of ACPE-approved continuing education are supported through paid attendance.

Advanced academic education is encouraged by the Air Force. Under the sponsorship of the Air Force Institute of Technology program, highly motivated pharmacists are selected for attendance at several different types of civilian institutions. The Air Force sets aside funds for advanced education specifically for the purpose of personnel earning advanced credentials, including specialty training, graduate degrees, certificates of proficiency, and ASHP-accredited residencies. While in attendance at an approved program of study, pharmacists remain active-duty officers and receive full pay and allowances.

US NAVY

The organization and mission of health care in the Navy is very different from that of the Army and the Air Force. All three share the common element of being a part of the armed forces, but the basic requirements of supporting a naval and marine force on land and on sea change central elements in providing support to the active and reserve establishments. Services on ships of the line, in amphibious forces, and on fully deployable hospital ships and fleet hospitals give Navy practice a character all its own.

The status of pharmacists in the Navy has been, in much the same fashion as in the Army and Air Force, variable over the years; there have been significant improvements since the 1960s. For many years proceeding the turn of the century, pharmacists were a component of the Hospital Corps. In 1898, Congress provided for the appointment of pharmacists within the Hospital Corps and for their rank to be equal to that of warrant officers, and a total of 25 pharmacist warrant officers were authorized. Since the passage of the Medical Service Corps Act in 1947, pharmacists have been commissioned members of the Navy.

The mission of the Naval Medical Department is Force Health Protection. In order to fulfill that mission, the Naval Medical Department strives to create a healthy and fit force and deploy along with that force to protect them, restore the health of the deployed and non-deployed force, and support the DOD TRICARE for Life initiative.

Naval facilities in San Diego, California; Bethesda, Maryland; Pensacola, Florida; Jacksonville, Florida; Camp Pendleton, California; and Portsmouth, Virginia, conduct active teaching programs. All hospitals, regardless of size, operate active ambulatory-care dispensing programs, which prepare and deliver from 100 to more than 4500 prescriptions a day and provide a full range of medication management consultative services. All hospitals operate unit-dose dispensing and distribution systems and intravenous admixture services.

Unique to the Navy in combat support is the operation of hospital ships. Two hospital ships operated by Military Sealift Command are designed to provide emergency, on-site care for US combatant forces deployed in war or other operations. USNS Mercy (T-AH 19) and USNS Comfort (T-AH 20) each contain 12 fully-equipped operating rooms, a 1000-bed hospital facility, radiological services, medical laboratory, a pharmacy, an optometry lab, a cat scan, and two oxygen producing plants. Both vessels have a helicopter deck capable of landing large military helicopters, as well as side ports to take on patients at sea. Both hospital ships are converted San Clemente-class super tankers. Mercy was delivered in 1986 and Comfort in 1987. Normally, the ships are kept in a reduced operating status in Baltimore, Maryland and San Diego, California, by a small crew of civilian mariners and active duty Navy medical and support personnel. Each ship can be fully activated and crewed within 5 days

Unique to the Navy is Fleet Hospitals. Fleet Hospitals are re-locatable, self-contained facilities designed to provide medical, surgical, and acute care services in support of the fleet and the fleet marine forces engaged in combat operations. A Fleet Hospital has the capability of a 250- to 500-bed hospital and is fully equipped with ward facilities, operating rooms, and an intensive care unit. They are different from a traditional Army MASH unit in that they are able to give the patient a wider range of care, from trauma surgery to physical therapy to pharmacy services.

Navy Pharmacy

The Navy currently has 160 pharmacist officers who serve primarily within hospitals. Navy pharmacist officers are augmented by nearly 120 pharmacists who are employed under the civil service system or by contracts, and slightly more than 900 technicians. Over 50% of Navy pharmacists possess advanced degrees, have completed an ASHP-accredited residency program, or both. Career officers are afforded the opportunity to apply for postgraduate education. The Navy annually sponsors officers for postgraduate education to earn a Master degree in one of the following: Hospital Pharmacy, Pharmacoeconomics, Health Policy, or Pharmacy Systems or a Post Doctor of Pharmacy degree. Officers selected for postgraduate education remain on active duty and receive full pay and allowances for up to 2 years of study. Additionally, the Navy operates ASHP-accredited residency programs at San Diego and Bethesda.

Navy pharmacist officers also have the opportunity to attend specialized schools, which are service-oriented or train with industry leaders in pharmacy benefit management to enhance their knowledge and value as a professional officer. They may apply for Director's Training with Industry; the Navy War College at Newport, Rhode Island; the Naval Postgraduate School at Monterey, California; or most any of the schools operated by the Department of Defense. Most of these ancillary schools offer year-long programs and prepare the Navy pharmacist for assignments and responsibilities over and above those of the customary practice of pharmacy.

The career path for Navy pharmacist officers is similar to that of the other Department of Defense services. Pharmacists serve in grades from Ensign (O–1) through Captain (O–6). Almost all officers enter as a Lieutenant (O–3), unless the person does not have a PharmD degree. If this is the case, they may enter as either an Ensign (O–1) or Lieutenant Junior Grade (O–2). Professional degree and years of experience determine entry grade. All new pharmacist officers attend Officer Indoctrination School at Newport, Rhode Island. Here, basic instruction is given in military courtesy, organization of the Navy, and other military indoctrination subjects. Pharmacy opportunities differ from other services basically in the nature and location of the usual Navy duty station.

The Navy offers several nontraditional opportunities for the pharmacist. Pharmacist officers serve as staff officers, at the Naval School of Health Sciences, the DOD Pharmacoeconomic Center and the TRICARE Management Activity. It is also possible for Navy pharmacist officers to expand their horizons into a more administrative roles through appointment as Chief of Ancillary Services where they are responsible for multiple services, including pharmacy, laboratory, radiology, and social work. All pharmacist officers who achieve the rank of Captain are asked to screen for executive leadership positions; these include Executive Officers and Commanding Officers of Medical Treatment Facilities.

The operational nature of the Navy gives rise to a concern with methods of supply and logistics. Pharmacists, who are familiar with storage standards and are additionally equipped with a Navy education, serve in several joint-command situations. Opportunities in medical supply and logistics are available at the Defense Supply Center Philadelphia and the Joint Readiness Clinical Advisory Board, at Fort Detrick, Maryland. In addition, medication management needs require pharmacist officer staffing on the hospital ships and in the fleet hospital units.

US PUBLIC HEALTH SERVICE

The US Public Health Service (PHS) of the Department of Health and Human Services (DHHS) is the oldest health arm of the federal government. It is the successor to the US Marine Hospitals Service, which was established by Congress in 1798 to provide services to "merchant seamen, naval and marine officers, and naval and marine enlisteds." The progenitors to today's pharmacists were employed in the Marine Hospitals system from its very beginnings. All varieties of practitioners and titles (Apothecaries, Chemists, Druggists, and Pharmacists) have been employed. An unusual aspect of the employment of these Apothecaries was that, even in earlier periods, they were dedicated to the preparation and dispensing duties that are now associated with the operation of a contemporary pharmacy; Apothecaries in most other federal services had to do "double duty," tending to patients as well as preparing pharmaceuticals. Pharmacy practice has been a respected specialty in the PHS service since its very beginning.

The US Marine Hospitals Service was reorganized in 1871, placed under the supervision of a centralized office, and given leadership in the form of the "Supervising Surgeon." The Service was fully moved administratively within the Department of the Treasury. In 1875, the Office of the Supervising Surgeon was changed to that of Supervising Surgeon General, and his official title similarly changed. This second reorganization added the requirements that the Supervising Surgeon General be appointed by the President, with the advice and consent of the Senate.

In 1871, Dr John M Woodworth, Supervising Surgeon General, made the establishment of a mobile corps of health professionals to respond to health needs and crises within the US a top priority. He established rules, regulations, appointment standards, and examination requirements that paralleled those of military organizations, except that the standards relating to professional practice were set higher. Just as military officers were expected to display the highest level of military professionalism, Woodworth expected and demanded a commensurate level of excellence and dedication targeted specifically to patient care. A system of ranks and promotions was established; officers were appointed with the understanding that they would serve at the pleasure of, and for the good of, the service. Woodworth clearly established the Commissioned Corps as a meritocracy. As a battle-tested veteran—a Union surgeon of the Civil War—he understood the benefits of military-style discipline and organization, and gave them special meaning in the requirements for organized health care.

On January 4, 1889, Congress statutorily established the Commissioned Corps of the Marine Hospitals Service, legally organizing it with rank, benefits, obligations, and management methods parallel to Army and Navy officer corps. Additional statutory changes in 1902 and 1912 strengthened the position of the Commissioned Corps as the fundamental professional personnel system for the service. Statutory changes made during these periods changed the focus of the service from a hospital and health service for the Merchant Marine to a true preventive health and research organization of national scope.

For career and grade purposes, the Parker Act of 1930 provided for the appointment and promotion of pharmacists up to the grade of a Naval Lieutenant (O–3); all rank restrictions were subsequently removed by the PHS Act of 1944. Since 1944, pharmacists have been able to compete for all grades within the Commissioned Corps, up to and including Rear Admiral, Upper Half (O–8), with the title Assistant Surgeon General. By current statutory requirement, one Commissioned Corps pharmacist officer serves as an Assistant Surgeon General, Rear Admiral, Lower Half (O–7), and functions as the service's Chief Pharmacist Officer.

Organization

The PHS is the principal health agency of the Federal Government. Its mission is to protect and advance the health of the American people. The service is directed and overseen by the Secretary of Health and Human Services, with the consultation of both the Assistant Secretary for Health and the Surgeon General, who provide leadership and guidance on all health-related activities including research and development, education and training, and the organizing and financing of healthcare delivery services. The Assistant Secretary for Health also serves as a convener of various cross-departmental working groups. The Assistant Secretary for Health is the statutory chairperson for many of these working groups. The Assistant Secretary for Health can also hold the position of Surgeon General, or each position may be filled by a different official.

The PHS is organized into line-operating divisions, each with its own particular mission and focus. The PHS consists of the Office of Public Health and Science, with Regional Health Administrators located in PHS regional offices geographically dispersed throughout the US; the Administration for Children and Families (ACF); Agency for Healthcare Research and Quality (AHRQ); the Administration on Aging (AoA); the Agency for Toxic Substances and Disease Registry (ATSDR); the Centers for Disease Control and Prevention (CDC); the Centers for Medicare and Medicaid Services (CMS); the Food and Drug Administration (FDA); the Health Resources and Services Administration (HRSA); the Indian Health Service (IHS); the National Institutes of Health (NIH); the Program Support Center (PSC); and the Substance Abuse and Mental Health Services Administration (SAMHSA). Opportunities are available to the pharmacist in most of these agencies. Both civil servants and commissioned officers staff the PHS. Approximately 845 pharmacist officers and 250 civil servant pharmacists are employed in the service, and Figure 6-1 shows the relative distribution of those 845 pharmacist officers.

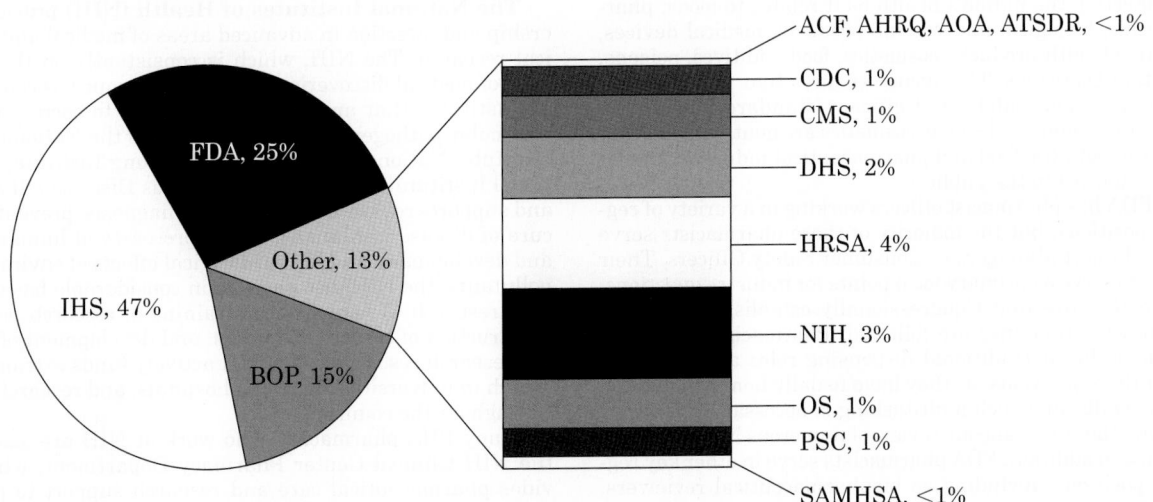

Figure 6-1. Distribution of USPHS Pharmacist Officers.

The Administration for Children and Families (ACF) is responsible for federal programs that promote the economic and social well-being of families, children, individuals, and communities.

The Agency for Health Research and Quality (AHRQ) identifies strategies to improve health care access, foster appropriate use, and reduce unnecessary expenditures, and is the federal government's principal agency for the conduct of health services research. The agency conducts broad-based outcomes and quality research, mainly through the awarding of grants to qualified researchers. The agency also issues periodic authoritative statements on treatment modalities and their effectiveness. The agency focuses heavily on the dissemination of the results of its research.

The Administration on Aging (AoA) is one of the nation's largest providers of home- and community-based care for older persons and their caregivers. Their mission is to promote the dignity and independence of older people and to help society prepare for an aging population.

The Agency for Toxic Substances and Disease Registry (ATSDR) implements the health-related provisions of Superfund (the Comprehensive Environmental Response, Compensation and Liability Act of 1980). ATSDR is charged with assessing health hazards at specific hazardous waste sites, helping to prevent or reduce exposure and the illnesses that result, and increasing knowledge and understanding of the health effects that may result from exposure to hazardous substances.

The Centers for Disease Control and Prevention (CDC) provides leadership in the control and prevention of diseases and monitors the immunization status of the population. It develops advanced methods for testing and preventing communicable and vector-borne diseases and conducts a substantial program for improving the performance of clinical laboratories. The CDC is extremely active in assisting state governments and local health authorities in preventing and controlling diseases within their respective jurisdictions. Through its National Institute of Occupational Safety and Health (NIOSH), the CDC monitors and researches safety standards in the workplace.

CDC has the responsibility for managing the Strategic National Stockpile Program (formerly called the National Pharmaceutical Stockpile Program) to ensure the availability and rapid deployment of life-saving pharmaceuticals, antidotes, other medical supplies, and equipment necessary to counter the effects of nerve agents, biological pathogens, and chemical agents. The Strategic National Stockpile Program employs pharmacist officers who stand ready for immediate deployment to any US location in the event of a terrorist attack using a biological toxin or chemical agent directed against a civilian population.

The Food and Drug Administration (FDA) is charged with protecting the nation's health as it relates to foods, pharmaceuticals, biological and vaccine products, medical devices, radioactive health products, cosmetics, food additives, poisons, and certain pesticides. The agency ensures that pharmaceutical products meet safety and efficacy standards, foods are unadulterated and wholesome, cosmetics are nontoxic, and that products in both the food and pharmaceutical industries do not present a hazard to the public.

The FDA has pharmacist officers working in a variety of regulatory positions, but the majority of these pharmacists serve as either Project Managers or Consumer Safety Officers. Their roles are to serve as primary focal points for industry questions, and to make sure that Congressionally established drug approval process timelines are followed. Pharmacists who have been successful at traditional dispensing roles are especially adept at these positions, as they have usually honed their multitasking skills, and such multitasking is necessary when they coordinate the simultaneous review of numerous New Drug Applications. In addition, FDA pharmacists serve in other key regulatory positions, including as biopharmaceutical reviewers, drug safety experts, drug information experts, and as inspectors at pharmaceutical plants. Some FDA pharmacists work with national and international standards-setting organizations in order to streamline the drug approval process and to simplify drug labeling.

FDA pharmacist officers have formalized appointments as preceptors for schools of pharmacy throughout the nation and have established an extremely dynamic integrated program in order to maximize the exposure of pharmacy students to the regulatory process. One goal of this program is to attract pharmacy students to the PHS as a career goal. In the past, PHS pharmacist officers were likely to take a position with the FDA only after first serving in some other PHS agency (eg, IHS or NIH), but this paradigm is rapidly changing. However, most FDA supervisors still believe that in order to be truly effective at an FDA position, several years' worth of traditional pharmacist experience is necessary, and such pharmacist officers usually have the competitive edge in both FDA job placement and PHS promotions.

FDA pharmacist officers are afforded a substantial amount of continuing education, both to help them to be highly effective in their regulatory position, and to help them maintain their clinical skills. This includes courses in regulatory law, biotechnology, and data management, as well as in disease state management. FDA has supported its pharmacist officers in their pursuits of advanced degrees, especially the Masters in Public Health degree that is offered through the Uniformed Services University of the Health Sciences, which is available at no cost and which equips the pharmacist officer to manage regulatory health care issues. In addition, because of the non-clinical nature of most positions, FDA pharmacist officers are usually encouraged to practice clinical pharmacy for several hours each week and are often allowed time away from their job in order to accomplish this professional development.

The Health Resource and Services Administration (HRSA) provides leadership in the identification and deployment of health personnel and in the educational, physical, financial, and organizational resources necessary to achieve optimal health services for all persons in the nation. As such, many of the agency's programs are targeted specifically to serve populations who are disadvantaged. The agency contains a component that is concerned specifically with issues of maternal and child health. The HRSA also participates in initiatives and studies that address the integration of public and private resources to improve the responsiveness of the health system to various populations of the country. The HRSA supports service delivery programs through grants and contracts and provides for improved access to health-care systems in both rural and urban environments. An arm of the agency provides the health-care personnel who serve as the medical and health support cadre for the Bureau of Citizenship and Immigration Services, which is under the Department of Homeland Security.

The National Institutes of Health (NIH) provides leadership and direction in advanced areas of medical and biomedical research. The NIH, which is consistently on the leading edge of medical discoveries and new techniques, is composed of 19 institutes that are arranged topically to correspond with particular pathogenetic concerns (such as the National Cancer Institute; National Heart, Blood and Lung Institute; and National Institute of Allergy and Infectious Diseases). It conducts and supports research in the causes, diagnosis, prevention, and cure of disease in humans, in the processes of human growth and development, and in the biological effects of environmental pollutants; the NIH also engages in considerable basic life-science research. It supports the training of research personnel, construction of research facilities, and development of promising research resources. The NIH actively funds extramural research in universities, teaching hospitals, and research centers throughout the country.

Many PHS pharmacists who work at NIH are assigned to the NIH Clinical Center Pharmacy Department, which provides pharmaceutical care and research support to patients, health care providers, and investigators. Pharmacy staff members conduct and participate in research programs that enhance knowledge regarding optimal dosing and appropriate use of investigational and commercially available agents. Pharmacists at the NIH Clinical Center manage commercially available and investigational drugs in approximately 1000 drug protocols. This includes managing the equivalent of a small pharmaceutical production plant where oral and parenteral investigational drug products are manufactured.

In order to keep PHS pharmacists who work at the NIH Clinical Center Pharmacy Department on the cutting edge of medicine, they must take annual performance improvement training and must take an annual competency examination. Since the professional atmosphere on the NIH campus closely mimics that of a large university, there is ample opportunity to attend highly specialized lectures on a wide variety of medical topics. As a result, NIH pharmacists are looked upon as highly knowledgeable, integral members of the health care team; they perform drug utilization reviews, and routinely participate on patient medical team rounds, as blinded investigators for drug protocols, and on institutional review boards. In addition, NIH pharmacists are greatly encouraged to publish in the refereed medical and pharmaceutical journals. One publication in particular led to the adoption of national standards for personal protective equipment for health care workers that handled chemotherapeutic drugs.

NIH Clinical Center Pharmacy Department has a robust drug information center and highly trained staff of clinical specialists who answer thousands of drug information questions each year. It also has a highly competitive ASHP-accredited Residency Program, where one can focus upon Pharmacy Practice, Drug Information and Pharmacotherapy, Oncology, and Primary Care.

The Substance Abuse and Mental Health Services Administration (SAMHSA) focuses its efforts on substance abuse prevention and treatment and provides funding for programs which have interlinkages between drug treatment activities and primary-care programs. A major concern of SAMHSA programming is injection drug use as a cofactor in the transmission of HIV. Several SAMHSA programs seek to use the treatment of substance abusers as an opportunity to provide both primary and secondary prevention counseling. Pharmacist officers who have been detailed by SAMHSA to the District of Columbia Government usually practice at St. Elizabeth's Hospital, which is a psychiatric hospital.

The Indian Health Service (IHS) provides direct health services to 1.5 million American Indians and native Alaskans who are members of approximately 557 federally recognized tribes in 35 states.

The IHS operates the largest health maintenance organization (HMO) in the US. The IHS cares for most of the American Indians and native Alaskans who live primarily on or near Indian reservations and lands.

Pharmacy practice in the IHS is the one of the primary entry points for new PHS pharmacists, and its form of practice is very advanced and unique among all of the federal services. Although the original focus of the IHS was to promote the elimination of infectious diseases such as tuberculosis, great strides in the IHS' programs have nearly solved that issue; thus, the focus now is on comprehensive care, prevention, and rehabilitation.

The IHS direct-care establishment consists of 49 general hospitals, 155 service units, and 545 ambulatory facilities. Although the service population is spread across 35 states, the concentration of beneficiaries resides in the western half of the nation and in Alaska.

The IHS facilities are small compared to the average size of the DVA or military hospitals. Of the 49 hospitals, 33 have less than 50 beds, 12 have between 50 and 99 beds, and 4 have more than 100 beds. The largest facility operates 170 beds. All IHS hospitals operate unit-dose or modified unit-dose programs and provide central intravenous admixture services. The larger of the IHS hospitals have drug information services staffed by pharmacists who have formalized appointments with colleges of pharmacy and serve actively as preceptors. All IHS hospitals

provide both ambulatory and inpatient care. The care activity associated with a patient's inpatient and ambulatory history is documented in a single record system that readily is accessible to the pharmacist. Pharmacists routinely monitor drug therapy and have all the necessary information to render clinical judgments on a patient's drug therapy and other clinical issues. All prescriptions are filled directly from entries in the patient's permanent health record. The nature of the IHS system creates a situation where the pharmacist usually is the last health-care professional to see the patient before discharge and frequently is the only professional regularly seen in an ambulatory environment. The IHS pharmacists have virtually total responsibility to ensure that patients understand their diagnosis, treatment, and follow-up requirements. Compliance with treatment plans is reviewed with the patient during each pharmacist consultation.

In most IHS settings, pharmacists provide primary-care services to patients and many pharmacists are certified with prescribing authority as an integral part of their practice. In most IHS facilities, there are formalized programs under which an appropriately educated and trained pharmacist is authorized to assess and treat patients with selected acute and chronic conditions, obtain patient histories, evaluate vital signs, order laboratory tests, and perform physical assessment techniques. These pharmacists are expected to exercise independent judgment in modifying, initiating, or otherwise altering drug therapies.

Pharmacists entering the IHS will find that practice differs significantly from traditional practice and that added training is necessary to accommodate the new roles. To develop these skills, a comprehensive clinical pharmacy training program has been developed, which is an integral portion of the IHS pharmacist's career development pathway.

Added educational opportunities are offered through service-sponsored attendance at professional meetings and continuing education seminars. Annually, all officers who are interested in further formal training are asked to complete a request for training out of service, which is granted based upon the anticipated needs of the service and funds available. There is no fixed limit on the number of pharmacists who may be sponsored. While officers pursue sponsored education, they remain on active duty and receive full pay and allowances. A commitment to serve twice the number of years of training accrues to the sponsored officer.

Commissioned Corps Readiness Force (CCRF) pharmacist officers are from most of the DHHS operating divisions. The CCRF is a cadre of US Public Health Service (PHS) officers, uniquely qualified by education and skills, who can be mobilized in times of extraordinary need during disaster, strife, or other public health emergencies and in response to domestic or international requests, to provide leadership and expertise by directing, enhancing, and supporting the services of the PHS and other DHHS Operational Divisions (OPDIVs), other US government agencies, and/or other respondents. CCRF pharmacist officers deploy to both natural disasters and to terrorist attacks and are therefore held to much higher readiness and proficiency standards than the average PHS pharmacist officer. They receive specialized training in emergency preparedness and response, including mass vaccinations, responding to weapons of mass destruction, and the management of the National Strategic Stockpile Program. CCRF pharmacists are often consulted upon, and routinely recommend, therapeutic substitution because of the very limited and ever changing formulary during an emergency. Recently, CCRF pharmacists have deployed in response to the terrorist attacks upon the World Trade Center, and in response to the bioterrorist anthrax attacks that quickly followed.

PHS Agreements with Other Departments

The PHS provides pharmacists for the health-care programs of the Bureau of Prisons (BOP) and US Marshals Service under agreement with the Attorney General and the Department of Justice. The pharmacist officers in the BOP program are assigned to most of the intermediate- and large-size federal prisons and operate both inpatient and ambulatory services. Pharmacy operations within the BOP are unique and offer challenges not seen in other components of government. All pharmacists serving in this program are provided specially tailored training and education in the psychology of working within the prison environment. Additionally, all officers assigned to BOP, including pharmacists, are required to participate in firearms training and must establish a qualifying level of proficiency; periodic retraining sessions are required.

The PHS provides pharmacists for the health-care programs of Department of Homeland Security, and this is particularly noteworthy since it houses both the Coast Guard and the National Disaster Medical System (NDMS), the latter which had been under DHHS until 2003. NDMS is a joint partnership with PHS, DHHS, DOD, and the Department of Veterans Affairs. Many PHS pharmacists serve under NDMS, both in the Commissioned Corps, and as civil servant intermittent appointees. Most of these pharmacists assist the nation in responding to natural disasters and acts of terrorism through Disaster Medical Assistance Teams and are integral to the overall federal medical response.

Pharmacist officers in the PHS also can serve in international assignments with the World Health Organization, the Pan-American Health Organization, the Agency for International Development, and as support to the government of Micronesia.

PHS Pharmacy

The PHS offers the most variegated forms of pharmacy practice of any of the federal services. Pharmacists have the opportunity to practice in a traditional manner, engage in regulatory affairs, or compete for high-level policy and planning positions. Because the PHS is the prime supplier of health personnel to the DHHS, it is possible for pharmacists to access opportunities up to the departmental level.

The PHS offers unique opportunities for training and education. The pharmacist corps of the PHS offers pharmacy students as well as graduate pharmacists opportunities to learn. Pharmacy students may apply for participation in the Commissioned Officer Student Training and Externship Program (COSTEP). The junior COSTEP offers the pharmacy student a paid externship experience lasting from 30 to 120 days in one of the DHHS operating divisions, during which the student serves as, and is paid as, a commissioned officer holding the rank of Ensign (O–1). The senior COSTEP also offers the pharmacy student a commission as an Ensign, but not a short-term assignment. Instead, the pharmacy student receives pay while attending their sixth year of pharmacy school, and in return, is automatically promoted to the rank of Lieutenant (O–3) upon graduation and is obligated to remain on active duty for an additional 2 years.

Pharmacist officers customarily are eligible for transfer to other positions after the completion of an initial 2-year tour of duty. Although pharmacist officers in the PHS are not limited to positions of traditional pharmacy practice, it is the service's philosophy that pharmacist officers must clearly evidence that they are highly competent pharmacists prior to the service considering any reassignment into a nontraditional position.

The potential career pattern for commissioned officer pharmacists differs markedly from other uniformed services as all ranks from the entry level of Ensign (O–1) through Rear Admiral, Upper Half (O–8) are available. Pharmacists who graduate with a Doctor of Pharmacy degree are first commissioned at the rank of a Lieutenant (O–3 grade) and can progress through the rank of Captain (O–6 grade). One pharmacist is selected to serve a 4-year term as the service's Chief Pharmacist Officer and holds the rank of Rear Admiral, Lower Half

(O–7 grade). Pharmacist officers succeeding in attainment of the rank of Rear Admiral, Upper Half (O–8 grade), normally do so by competing successfully for high-level program management or policy-making positions, either in the service or the department.

DEPARTMENT OF VETERANS AFFAIRS

The roots of the Department of Veterans Affairs (DVA) health-care system, as is true of many other federal health-care programs, are to be found in the PHS. In November 1918, PHS Surgeon General Rupert Blue was wrestling with two pressing issues. The first, and most immediate, was that a serious, virulent influenza was taking its toll in the American population. This strain, termed the Spanish Flu, gave rise to severe symptoms and took essential war material workers off the production lines for extended periods. Blue was also an exceptional strategic planner, and by mid-1918 he sensed that the war was drawing to a close, and knew that significant numbers of disabled and injured veterans would require care. He was concerned for the health of those who had served and would need additional care. He actively promoted legislative action to ensure that appropriate assistance would be available to the war-disabled upon their return home.

On March 3, 1919, Congress passed legislation empowering the Surgeon General of the PHS to provide for "discharged sick and disabled soldiers, sailors and marines; Army and Navy nurses, male and female." The Hospitals Division of the service expanded dramatically to meet the needs of these added beneficiaries; several existing Army hospitals and facilities were absorbed into the system. The PHS was given complete charge of veterans' health, including what would later be provided under the War Risk Insurance program.

In accordance with provisions of the Sweet Act, which established a distinct Veterans Bureau in the Department of the Treasury, a presidential executive order was issued directing that, effective May 1, 1922, all hospitals and outpatient facilities that had been opened or operated under the Surgeon General for the purpose of treating veterans were to be transferred to the new bureau. The Surgeon General transferred 57 hospitals; 17,000 beds; 13,000 inpatients; 9 additional new hospitals under construction; and in excess of 2300 physicians, pharmacists, nurses, and other health professionals to the health operations of the Veterans Bureau.

In 1946, the successor to the Veterans Bureau, the Veterans Administration (VA), underwent a major reorganization. The importance of pharmacy practice was recognized and the position of Chief Pharmacist of the VA's Bureau of Medicine and Surgery was established. This position continues today as the Director of Pharmacy Services, with a Central Office Pharmacy Staff. The DVA now operates the largest multi-institutional system of pharmacy services in the US.

In 1989 the Veterans Administration, through an act of Congress, became the Department of Veterans Affairs. The old Department of Medicine and Surgery became the Veterans Health Administration (VHA).

The mission of the VHA is to provide medical care to its statutory beneficiary population. Its largest beneficiary population consists of veterans of US uniformed services; however, certain dependents of veterans also comprise a substantial number of beneficiaries.

Veterans who were discharged from one of the uniformed services, under conditions other than dishonorable, are eligible to receive services. Beneficiary classes are broken down into "primary" and "other." The primary classification consists of veterans who were discharged or retired because of an injury or disability incurred or aggravated in the performance of their duties. Ex-service members who seek care for treatment of a disease or injury incurred in the line of duty are given first priority.

DVA Pharmacy

Pharmacy service in the DVA operates under the VHA. The VHA administers the largest multi-treatment facility health-care system in the United States. Pharmacy services, available in nearly all of these facilities, represent the largest multi-site pharmacy system in the United States. The treatment facility system encompasses 163 medical centers, which provide comprehensive, full-service inpatient care as well as ambulatory care; over 800 ambulatory-care centers and 131 nursing-care facilities; and 33 domiciliaries that offer a range of services from custodial to extended care for the neurologically disabled. These are organized into 21 distinct health care networks that comprise the DVA's health enterprise. There are approximately 8600 full-time pharmacy staff members and an additional 600 who serve part time. Of the full-time staff, approximately 4,600 are pharmacists, representing 55% of the full-time staff; an equal proportion of part-time staff are pharmacists as well.

Of major significance, especially to those interested in practicing pharmacy in a creative, research-based environment, is that the DVA operates the largest health professional training effort in the US. Nearly 110,000 health professional students receive clinical education in a DVA facility. The DVA offers nearly 3000 medical residency positions, representing virtually all medical specialties dealing with adult and geriatric medicine. Opportunities for part-time experience through affiliated rotations are made available to approximately 30,000 medical residents and 24,000 medical students. Over the past several years DVA pharmacy services have made a successful effort to integrate pharmacy operations and investigations into the overall medical research effort. Consequently, new and exciting vistas, especially in the practice of clinical pharmacy, have been opened.

Education and training possibilities in DVA pharmacy correspond with the extensive potential in the DVA system in general. Most schools of pharmacy have established formal relationships with pharmacies and pharmacists in DVA facilities. The DVA offers approximately 256 ASHP-accredited residency positions in 66 locations. DVA pharmacies routinely provide training to over 2000 pharmacy students annually. The DVA staff dispensed over 120 million ambulatory-care prescriptions in fiscal year 2002. DVA continues to provide comprehensive IV admixture services but does not tabulate the data nationally. Clinical pharmacy activities continue to grow significantly and 1400 clinical pharmacists have some form of prescriptive authority and expanded Scope of Practice Statement approved by the medical staff.

Pharmacists perform a full range of professional tasks and, with a professional to support ratio of almost 1:1, are provided with adequate time to discharge the professional duties. DVA pharmacists are exceptionally active in the areas of clinical pharmacy practice and quality assurance. The policies of the DVA pharmacy services central office encourage all pharmacists, regardless of their functional duties or their particular educational background, to practice in a highly patient-oriented manner. Pharmacists increasingly are becoming providers of technical information and consultative services to medical and dental staffs.

DVA has developed comprehensive automated systems to provide care to veterans. DVA has established 7 highly automated Consolidated Mail Outpatient Pharmacies (CMOP) that can fill up to 15 million prescriptions per site with significant reduction in staffing and improvements in medication errors. The dispensing accuracy of DVA CMOPs approached 99.997% in 2002. During this time, the CMOP program dispensed 75 million of the 120 million prescriptions filled that year.

In addition to the CMOP system the DVA automated pharmacy system provides Electronic Order entry for physicians as well as a comprehensive electronic medical record. DVA physicians use electronic order entry for approximately 95% of all medication orders and prescriptions. On the wards, the VA has implemented a Bar Code Medication Administration System (BCMA) to document medications and reduce medication errors.

DVA medical centers have implemented comprehensive quality assurance programs that involve pharmacists. The DVA uses several different quality assessment formats, including a systematic internal review along with a paralleling systematic external review procedure. The former is conducted by each individual institution as a self-assessment technique, whereas the latter involves peer assessments. DVA pharmacists are heavy contributors to assessments and policy-making processes in the selection of drugs, patient profiles, drug interactions, and adverse drug experience detection and prevention.

Veterans Affairs Employment

Unlike the uniformed services, the Veterans Health Administration uses civilian employees only. Since December 1989, all VHA pharmacists are appointed under a Hybrid Title 38 personnel classification system. This is a system by which positions are graded in accordance with the functions of the position as defined by applicable criteria. Hybrid Title 38 provided VHA pharmacists the opportunity to have non-supervisory, clinical roles with appropriate grades.

Generally, pharmacists occupy positions graded as GS-11 through GS-14. Most entry- and staff-level professional staff are graded at GS-11. Supervisory Pharmacists, Clinical Pharmacists/Pharmacy Specialists, and Assistant Chief Pharmacists generally are graded at GS-12 through GS-14, depending upon the size and type of medical facility and scope of pharmacy services. Pharmacy Directors range from GS-12 to GS-15 grade. All sites currently have special pay authorized for the staff pharmacist level and DVA may offer recruitment, retention, or relocation bonuses as well. Other incentives include a loan repayment plan as well as tuition support of second clinical and management degrees.

As described above, Hybrid Title 38 provides the vehicle to enable VHA pharmacy practice to transform from a purely distributive role to one that recognizes the pharmacist's place in quality patient care. Career progression within the DVA health-care system can now be achieved through administrative and clinical means. The opportunity to remain at one facility or relocate to other VHA health-care facilities is very attractive to many young professionals.

VHA pharmacy practice offers the pharmacist interested in all facets of professional practice an opportunity to experience many varieties of personal-career patterns. Growing, dynamic programs in ambulatory care and geriatrics, as well as acute medicine, provide practitioners a multitude of practice opportunities and the ability to contribute to a continuum of care wherever they choose to practice.

STATE, COUNTY, AND MUNICIPAL GOVERNMENT AGENCIES

In addition to employment in federal government agencies dealing with regulation of the distribution of drugs, numerous opportunities exist for similar service with state departments of health, state boards of pharmacy, state bureaus of controlled drugs, state and county welfare administration departments, and similar agencies. This applies also to the larger municipalities.

The coordination of municipal, state, and federal drug enforcement procedures, especially for regulation of controlled drugs and dangerous drugs and poisons, opens a great opportunity for pharmacists who are especially interested in regulatory activities. Very often those who start in federal positions and acquire considerable experience at that level have the opportunity to take over administrative functions of a similar nature in state and municipal agencies, where their coordination efforts are enhanced greatly by past experience at the federal level.

The administrative functions of state, county, and local organizations that enforce health and welfare regulations frequently include specific duties that require a background of pharmaceutical training.

Many of these agencies deal with such matters as disease prevention and medical care. State governments have increasingly assumed the administration of welfare medical-care programs. In carrying out this function state and local appropriations are being augmented or matched by federal appropriations. In such instances, pharmacists frequently are employed to supervise the administration of pharmaceutical services in welfare medical-care programs, especially those involving what has become known as "vendor payments" for prescription drugs and pharmaceutical services. These agencies usually appoint advisory committees that consist of representatives of the various health professions, including pharmacists, to aid in developing and enforcing their programs.

Some pharmacists are employed by these agencies on a full-time basis and usually are designated as Pharmacy Advisors or Consultants. State welfare agencies, which are called on to pay for the millions of prescriptions that are supplied annually to indigent or medically indigent and aging patients, will employ such consultants on a full- or part-time basis or will create positions under the civil service for pharmacists. These positions provide an expert review of the pricing of prescriptions to keep them within the range of payment prescribed by the agency. These pharmacists are expected to give advice on the best methods of reducing drug costs to the welfare agency. They also are expected to work with medical consultants and members of the medical profession in devising limitations and extensions of medical-care services as may be indicated.

Although government service does not pay as well as employment in the private sector, it has compensations in the form of retirement benefits, medical services, and annual and sick leave benefits that are very attractive. In recent years, government agencies have also tended to provide time for formal education in various specialties, enabling the incumbents of these positions to improve their status.

LOCATING CURRENT INFORMATION

The information presented in this chapter is accurate as of the time of its publication, but the nature of the governmental system changes rapidly. Those interested in pursuing a career in federal or other government service should seek current information. The best way to do this is to discuss one's interest with the personnel responsible for placement at a college of pharmacy. Placement officers invariably know how to access recent information. When a pharmacist desires to proceed further than the information stage, college personnel can offer referrals to government agency representatives for detailed, in-depth information and discussion.

ACKNOWLEDGMENTS—The authors gratefully acknowledge the assistance of the following individuals for their role in the preparation of this chapter: RADM Richard S Walling, CAPT Robert E Pittman, CAPT Elizabeth Nolan, COL Ardis Meier, COL W Michael Heath, LTC Jasper Watkins, Dr Virginia Torrise, Dr Jeff Ramirez, and ENS Kristen M Albright.

BIBLIOGRAPHY

A History of the Hospital Corps and The Dental Technician Rating, Naval School of Health Sciences, Portsmouth, Virginia, NAVEDTRA 13130, 2003, https://www-nshspts.med.navy.mil/Courses/History/manual/intro.htm

USNS Mercy T-AH 19, 2003, http://www.mercy.navy.mil/

USNS Comfort T-AH 20, 2003, http://www.comfort.navy.mil/

Babb J, Tosatto R, Hayslett J. *J Am Pharm Assoc (Wash)* 2002; 42(5 suppl 1):S50–1

Bayles BC, Hall GE, Hostettler C, et al. *Am J Health-Syst Pharm* 1997; 54:778.

Carmona RH. *Preparedness and Pharmacy Science.* American Pharmaceutical Association (APhA) Conference - Academy of Students of Pharmacy (ASP) Opening Session, New Orleans, Louisiana, 2003, http://www.surgeongeneral.gov/news/speeches/pharmaconf032903.htm

Floyd D. Spence National Defense Authorization Act for Fiscal Year 2001 (aka HR 4205, which later became Public Law No: 106-398), SEC. 628.

Furman B. *A Profile of the United States Public Health Service, 1798–1948.* Publ No NIH 73-369. Washington, DC: Department of Health, Education, and Welfare, 1973.

Gill H. *The Apothecary in Colonial Virginia.* Williamsburg, VA: Colonial Williamsburg Fund, 1972.

Herrier RN, Boyce RW, Apgar DA. *Hosp Formul* 1990; 25(1):67–8, 76–8, 80.

Huntzinger PE. *Mil Med* 2000; 165(11):855.

Kremers E, Urdang G, Sonnedecker G. *Kremers and Urdang's History of Pharmacy,* 4th ed., reprinted by the American Institute of the History of Pharmacy, Madison, WI, 1986.

Montello MJ, Ames T. *Am J Health-Syst Pharm* 1999; 56:236.

Mullan F., *Plagues and Politics: The Story of the United States Public Health Service.* New York: Basic Books, 1989.

Normark JW, Williams RF, Hostettler CF, et al. *Am J Health-Syst Pharm* 1999; 56:568.

Ogden JE, Muniz A, Patterson AA, et al. *Am J Health-Syst Pharm* 1997; 54:761.

Paavola FG, Dermanoski KR, Pittman RE. *Am J Health-Syst Pharm* 1997; 54:766.

Spain J. *Mil Med* 1999; 164:693.

Williams RF, Moran EL, Bottaro SD 2nd, et al. *Am J Health-Syst Pharm* 1997; 54:773.

Young JH. *Am J Health-Syst Pharm* 1997; 54:783.

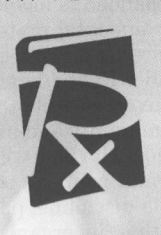

CHAPTER 7

Pharmacists and Public Health

Timothy J Ives, PharmD, MPH, BCPS, FCCP

Ara H DerMarderosian, PhD

Public health is a societal effort to protect, promote, and restore the public's health.[1] It is a combination of sciences, skills, and beliefs that are directed to the prevention, maintenance, and improvement of the health of all the people through collective or social actions. The programs, services, and institutions involved emphasize the prevention of disease and the health needs of the population as a whole. Public health activities change with changing technology and social values, but the goals remain the same: to reduce the amount of disease, premature death, and disease-produced discomfort and disability in the population. Public health is thus a social institution, a discipline, and a practice. The Institute of Medicine defines the mission of public health as "fulfilling society's interest in assuring conditions in which people can be healthy."[2]

Public health programs in the US were established initially to handle the epidemics of communicable diseases and high levels of infant and maternal mortality that were prevalent during the late 1800s and early 1900s. Much of the problem related to a lack of sanitation, overcrowding, and a failure to adhere to appropriate hygienic measures; by the 1960s, most of these problems were under control.

HISTORY

The first public health organizations in America developed in the late 18th century in the port cities along the Eastern coastline, largely in response to early infectious disease threats such as the 1793 yellow fever epidemic in Philadelphia. By the middle of the 19th century, reformers advocated the collection of vital statistics, birth/death registrations, and more comprehensive data on the health of the population, especially as communicable disease outbreaks continued. One such reformer, Lemuel Shattuck, a schoolteacher, publisher, and bookseller, was primarily responsible for instituting a vital statistics registry in Massachusetts.

The *Report of the Sanitary Commission of Massachusetts, 1850* is a classic and comprehensive document of recommendations for organizing public health.[2] In 1872, the American Public Health Association (APHA) was formed to "advance sanitary science and promote the practical application of personal hygiene."[3] By 1880, permanent state and local health departments and boards had been formed; their financial backing, and hence their impact, was very limited. After 1912, when the US Public Health Service (PHS) was increased in size and responsibilities, a network of federal, state, and county/city health departments began to emerge. The primary unit to administer programs was the city or county health department with its team of a physician, nurse, sanitarian, and administrative staff.

The PHS, originally named the Marine Hospital Service, was created on July 16, 1798, when President John Adams signed the Act for the Relief of Sick and Disabled Seamen. From the beginning, the PHS has been at the forefront of addressing the public health issues facing this country, from curtailing the spread of contagious diseases in 19th century, to providing health care to those with special needs. Today, PHS activities include not only regulation of food, drugs, and toxic substances, but also supporting disease control and prevention, biomedical research, health care to underserved populations, mental health, substances abuse prevention, health promotion, and international health.

Prior to World War II, traditional programs formed the bulk of public health work: disposal of sewage, provision of pure water, communicable disease control, and the care of mothers and infants. Health education was the main weapon of attack. This changed, however, with the advent of antibiotics and the expanded development of vaccines, both of which reduced the danger of infections.

As chronic diseases began to assume a major role in morbidity and mortality, hospital care replaced care in the home. Comparable changes in public health accelerated as federal funding increased; health departments provided an increasing amount of direct patient care in the clinic and in the home. Funding shifts at the national and state levels have reversed this trend somewhat, but trends continue to point to the emergence of an organized medical care service with an emphasis on keeping people well, a forerunner of a national health service.

The first permanent county health department in America was not formed until the early years of the 20th century. At that time, the primary aim of public health services was to control communicable disease by enforcing sanitary codes that eliminated contamination of food, water, and milk by human excreta. With the advent of immunization, communities instituted programs for disease prevention with vaccines; gradually, more personal health services were added, such as maternal and child health. In many areas of the country, the primary provider of these community-based services has been the public health nurse. Pharmacists should become acquainted with local public health nurses and the variety of services they provide to their patients.

Since the 1970s, new public health issues have emerged. These include infectious disease outbreaks such as AIDS, West Nile virus, or Severe Acute Respiratory Syndrome (SARS); access to quality health care for all Americans; environmental problems such as exposure to and disposal of toxic chemicals and wastes, nuclear wastes, and smog and air pollution; and societal problems such as care of a growing elderly population, teenage pregnancy, and substance abuse. The health of the public has been and continues to be influenced by governmental policies and Medicare; discussions continue to call for overall reform of the health-care system in the United States. Over the past 50 years, the public health infrastructure has expanded to include everything from occupational safety to environmental protection; however, worldwide socioeconomic issues have created an enormous public health problem worldwide. Public health is at a major crossroads because of the convergence of problems related to social and biological factors, community and individual problems, and widespread economic and social policy issues. In the face of world problems of an economic, political, population control, and environmental nature, as a discipline, public health continues to experience changes, both in its organization and accomplishments. American pharmacy and medicine have diminished or eliminated teaching public health as an entity.

During the past few decades, because traditional acute health-care services have had a limited effect on improving the overall national health status, health professionals have initiated health promotion and disease prevention (wellness) strategies in their respective practices. Pharmacists, with a renewed emphasis on the clinical care of the patient,[5] have been encouraged to use pharmaceutical care strategies to uphold the health of the patients that they serve. Prevention is a major component of that philosophy. Pharmacists, in a unique position to promote public health because of their easy access and good communication skills, remain the most trusted health profession.

HEALTH GUIDELINES

The first set of national health targets was published in 1979 as *Healthy People: The Surgeon General's Report on Health Promotion and Disease Prevention.*[6] The series of Department of Health and Human Services (DHHS) *Healthy People 1990, 2000* and *2010* reports (www.healthypeople.gov) put a strong emphasis upon comprehensive preventative programs that are office, community, or population based,[7] serving to improve the health of the people of this country. With a growing influence, national pharmacy organizations, and the pharmacy leadership in the US Public Health Service submitted new objectives for consideration in the development of the *Healthy People 2010* report (Table 7-1).

The *Guide to Clinical Preventive Services*, developed by the United States Preventive Services Task Force (USPSTF),[8] is an evidence-based review of over 100 interventions to prevent 60 different medical conditions. The guide offers some of the most comprehensive, evidence-based, graded prevention recommendations that pharmacists or other clinicians can provide to patients. The USPSTF grades its recommendations according

Table 7-1. Pharmacy-Oriented Objectives in Healthy People 2010

1. Reduce by 50% Medicare admissions to short stay acute hospitals due to drug therapy management problems.
2. Increase to 75% the proportion of Medicare enrollees with diabetes receiving appropriate educational and preventive services.
3. Increase to 25% the proportion of pharmacies providing administration of influenza and pneumococcal immunizations to adults.
4. Decrease the number of pharmacies who sell tobacco and tobacco-related products to no more than 20% and increase the number of pharmacists who provide tobacco cessation counseling, support, and referrals to smokers to 90%.
5. Substance abuse: add prescription medications to alcohol and other drugs that contribute to substance abuse.
6. Increase the number of pharmacies that offer patient counseling on diabetes and other chronic diseases.
7. Reduce by 50% the number of courses of antibiotics prescribed for the common cold per population.
8. Increase the number of medical, nursing, public health, pharmacy, dentistry and allied health academic training programs that include a unit on the prevention and control of emerging, re-emerging and drug-resistant infectious diseases.

to one of five classifications (www.ahrq.gov/clinic/3rduspstf/ratings.htm) which reflect the strength of available evidence and the magnitude of the net benefit.[9] Some of these conditions are routinely seen, triaged, or managed by pharmacists, including cardiovascular conditions; infectious and sexually transmitted diseases; various forms of cancer, trauma, and injuries; and alcohol, tobacco, and other substance abuse. Pharmacists in primary care settings have frequent opportunities to screen for many of these conditions, educate patients, and encourage them to attempt to change their health behaviors.[10]

Pharmacists can utilize two excellent sources of evidence-based health care information, the National Guidelines Clearinghouse (NGC; www.guideline.gov), a comprehensive database of evidence-based clinical practice guidelines, and the National Quality Measures Clearinghouse (NQMC; www.qualitymeasures.ahrq.gov). The NGC, a comprehensive database of evidence-based clinical practice guidelines and related documents, provides health care providers, health plans, integrated delivery systems, and others an accessible mechanism for obtaining objective, detailed information on clinical practice guidelines and to further their dissemination, implementation, and use. Key components of NGC include structured abstracts about specific guidelines and their development, links to full-text guidelines, where available; a Guideline comparison utility that gives users the ability to generate side-by-side comparisons for any combination of two or more guidelines, guideline comparisons (aka Guideline Syntheses) which compare guidelines covering similar topics, highlighting areas of similarity and difference. These syntheses often provide a comparison of guidelines developed in different countries, providing insight into commonalities and differences in international health practices; and an annotated bibliography database where users can search for citations for publications and resources about guidelines, including guideline development and methodology, structure, evaluation, and implementation

The National Quality Measures Clearinghouse (NQMC; www.qualitymeasures.ahrq.gov), is sponsored by the Agency for Healthcare Research and Quality (AHRQ), for information on specific evidence-based health care quality measures and measure sets to promote widespread access to quality measures to health care practitioners. Its mission is to provide practitioners, health care providers, health plans, integrated delivery systems, purchasers and others an accessible mechanism for obtaining detailed information on quality measures, and to further their dissemination, implementation, and use in order to inform health care decisions. Key components of NQMC include a structured, standardized abstracts (summaries) containing information about measures and their development; a utility for comparing attributes of two or more quality measures in a side-by-side comparison; and links to full-text quality measures.

Similarly, the Centers for Disease Control and Prevention (CDC) in Atlanta, GA, offers *CDC Recommends*, quick access to documents containing CDC recommendations for the prevention, control, treatment, and detection of infectious and chronic diseases, environmental hazards, natural or human-generated disasters, occupational diseases and injuries, intentional and unintentional injuries and disabilities, and other public health conditions. This compendium of documents allows public health practitioners and others to quickly access CDC recommendations from a single point, independent of where they were originally published. Presently, there are over 400 documents containing recommendations and 80 documents archived for research or historical purposes maintained in the system.

Healthy People (www.healthypeople.gov) is the national prevention initiative designed to improve the health of all Americans. It identifies three national public health goals: increase the span of healthy life, reduce health disparities among Americans, and achieve access to preventive services for all Americans. Detailed in the latest report are 300 specific objectives for health promotion and disease prevention programs in 22 separate priority areas (Table 7-2), with quantitative targets

Table 7-2. Healthy People 2010 Priority Areas

1. Physical Activity and Fitness
2. Nutrition
3. Tobacco
4. Substance Abuse: Alcohol and Other Drugs
5. Family Planning
6. Mental Health and Mental Disorders
7. Violent and Abusive Behavior
8. Educational and Community-Based Programs
9. Unintentional Injuries
10. Occupational Safety and Health
11. Environmental Health
12. Food and Drug Safety
13. Oral Health
14. Maternal and Infant Health
15. Heart Disease and Stroke
16. Cancer
17. Diabetes and Chronic Disabling Conditions
18. HIV Infection
19. Sexually Transmitted Diseases
20. Immunization and Infectious Diseases
21. Clinical Preventative Services
22. Surveillance and Data Systems

to be achieved by the year 2010. The mission of public health is defined further as being directed on four fronts: optimizing public health service delivery, protecting the community against environmental hazards, assisting and reinforcing the community health-care provider system, and assisting individuals (consumers) to achieve optimal health status through promoting medical self-help principles.

In 1981, a policy statement of the APHA focused on the role of the pharmacist in public health and the importance and need for increased involvement of pharmacists in public health settings.[11] The report states the problem, underutilization of the patient-oriented pharmacist; gives the purpose, the need to maximize the use of existing health-care professionals and facilities; and provides positions and recommendations, to identify current and future roles for pharmacists in public health, provide essential background information about these roles, and describe means of implementing or maximizing these functions. This policy statement identifies the need for public health pharmacists to become public health educators and role models, and it also provides detailed suggestions for pharmacist public health activities. These activities are to be achieved not only at the *micro* level, such as speaking to community groups on drug topics and providing hypertension screening, but also at the *macro* level (ie, with managerial level health planning, evaluation, and administration).

Few pharmacists have asserted themselves and established a functional and visible role in public health. The average community pharmacist, however, does not participate on a regular basis in community health-promoting activities. The APHA policy statement emphasizes that community pharmacists are an underused source of health data that could assist health planners in these areas.

In general and individual disease prevention and health promotion programs, the public health activities of the pharmacist could include community preventive health care, primary care, referral, health education, drug information, toxicology, and health planning. Pharmacists should consider increased involvement with immunization programs, substance abuse education and monitoring, sexually transmitted disease education, family planning, fluoridation, poison prevention, disaster preparedness, environmental protection, workplace safety, peer review, and health data collection. With program targeted to individual patients, activities suggested for improvement are increased patient education, screening and referral, medication maintenance, compliance counseling, patient monitoring, and family counseling.

A particular set of functions for pharmacy services in public health settings include planning for health care for wide geographic areas or communities; managing, administering, and evaluating health-care programs, systems, and facilities; providing direct-person health-care service (eg, education and maternal and child care) and environmental health; developing and promoting legislation and deriving regulations pertaining to the public's health; and training health-care workers needed to carry out these functions. Community pharmacists are both knowledgeable in and can easily embrace community-oriented activities, such as speaking to groups on health-related matters, referring patients to community agencies, and participating in community-based programs on sexually transmitted diseases, mental health, substance abuse, poisoning, and cancer signals.

Regional or state health planning boards should use community pharmacists to provide epidemiological data on prescribing patterns, local illness patterns and various socioeconomic factors related to prevalent disease states. Finally, the position paper encourages more exposure of pharmacists to public health in their training and to promote the pursuit of advanced degrees (ie, Master of Public Health [MPH] or Doctor of Public Health [DrPH]) in schools of public health.

Advocates have urged pharmacists to document their roles in several specific practice areas and have provided data where pharmacists have shown leadership and significant contributions to the field of community health.[12, 13] Most pharmacists are employed in the community setting where they have a significant impact on the health status of the population, however, there is an ongoing need to focus both education and incentives in the direction of public health. At the *macro* level, pharmacists usually are salaried, and work in private and public institutions, agencies, and organizations that focus health care on defined population groups. This type of pharmacist requires a wide breadth and depth of knowledge, usually administrative and organizational skills (eg, health planning, monitoring state Medicaid drug programs, providing in-service education, developing health-promotional materials, and planning community health campaigns).

In 1972, Gibson,[14–16] in a review of public health instruction in colleges of pharmacy, found uniform deficiencies in the following: a definition of public health in pharmacy, a perceived relevance of public health to pharmacy, textbook(s) focusing upon the role of pharmacy in public health, faculty qualified to teach the subject, and sites where students could become involved with public health projects and personnel. In 1985, this issue was addressed by an Ad Hoc Committee on Public Health within the American Association of Colleges of Pharmacy (AACP).[17]

Pharmacy educators should develop community practitioners who can interface between the profession of pharmacy and community health planning agencies. Currently, these pharmacists frequently provide health promotion and disease prevention (HPDP) activities such as providing drug and nutrition counseling, screening for hypertension and diabetes, providing weight control programs, counseling on the appropriate use of prescribed and/or over-the-counter (OTC) medications, referring patients to specific health-care providers, and performing drug and medical histories. Having the majority of pharmacy practitioners involved in these types of programs continues to evolve through federal legislation such as the Omnibus Budget Reconciliation Act (OBRA) of 1990, which mandated pharmacists to consult and counsel patients on drug and health matters.

While most reimbursement for pharmacists remains product-related, pharmacists have been getting more involved in providing cognitive services that are now becoming reimbursable from third-party beneficiaries. These services include innovative disease management arrangements, intensive patient counseling and education, and physician-initiated pharmacotherapeutic consultations.

Involvement can be initiated directly with local health departments and with assistance from national pharmacy organizations such as the American Pharmacists Association (APhA),

American Society of Health-System Pharmacists (ASHP), American College of Clinical Pharmacy (ACCP), or their state affiliates. Pharmacists can volunteer their services, share their ideas, perspectives, and knowledge, and be available for collaborative community health efforts. Initial involvement of a minor nature often leads to greater potential for future mutually beneficial public health endeavors.

Through the National Center for Health Statistics (NCHS), pharmacists can become aware of sources of health data (eg, Vital Statistics System (www.cdc.gov/nchs/nvss.htm); National Notifiable Disease Surveillance System (www.cdc.gov/epo/dphsi/nndsshis.htm), Morbidity and Mortality Weekly Report (www.cdc.gov/mmwr), and National Health Interview Survey (NHIS; www.cdc.gov/nchs/nhis.htm) and how epidemiology plays an important part in overall public health strategies. Health services must be viewed on all levels, from international to local. With increasingly shorter travel times and an increasing number of people traveling, it is vital to have a global awareness of health and disease.

In addressing the challenges of public health for the 21st century, Frenk proposed an effort to integrate tradition and progress with new directions, including research to provide scientifically validated information relevant to the problems of decision-makers at all levels, support of continued academic education in public health to promote excellence and broaden university milieu, application of the population approach to all related fields of health on a multinational level, and a greater openness to concepts from the social, biological, and behavioral sciences.[18] A review of the public health literature of the last 10 years demonstrates some of the major public health concerns:

- The epidemiologic and biostatistics studies associated with infectious diseases - HIV disease, AIDS, tuberculosis, SARS, etc.
- The appropriate amount of physical activity for good health, and diet, hormones, and cancer.
- Environmental and occupational health (eg, health effects of low-level ionizing radiation, occupational health concerns, worksite drug testing, and hazardous waste generation and safe disposal).
- Global change (eg, ozone depletion, greenhouse warming and public health policy toward toxic or nuclear waste disposal).
- Public health practice: global immunization, polio eradication from the Western Hemisphere, health issues for college students, mortality of Native American infants, the public health practice of tobacco control and lessons learned, the changing epidemiology of asthma morbidity and mortality, mammography use and cost-effectiveness.
- Behavioral aspects of health: depression and public health, obesity, poverty and cultural diversity challenges for health promotion among the medically underserved or non-English speaking members of the community, smoking in pregnancy, and heterosexual transmission of HIV.
- Health services: unnecessary surgery, low pre-school immunization coverage, access and cost implications of state limitations on Medicaid reimbursement for pharmaceuticals, containing costs while improving quality of care, the insurance gap, retiree health benefits, emergency medical services, improper use of antibiotics, aging, and national health systems throughout the world.
- Bioterrorism, with its growing influence of viral, bacterial, biochemical, and nuclear toxins (eg, anthrax, botulism), and its management/prevention across all sectors of the health care field.
- The exponential growth in the interest in and practice of complementary/alternate medicine, nutrition, and lifestyle.

HEALTH SERVICES PROGRAMS

Federal health legislation is based upon the federal government's constitutional right to "promote the general welfare," but the states retain sovereign rights in guarding the health of their inhabitants. Within the states, health departments provide a wide spectrum of services to the community under the rubric of public health.

Usually, local health departments are affiliated with their state's health department. In the more sparsely settled states with adequate local coverage, the state health department acts in a consultant capacity; in states with inadequate local

services, personnel from the state central office often provide direct services. The state may, in turn, call upon federal health consultants for advice and assistance.

A health director, usually with an advanced degree in public health, is responsible for the overall management of a health department. As a part of the health department team, public health nurses provide the bulk of the personal health services, both in clinics and in the home; they deal with the care of people ranging from newborn infants to elderly patients with multiple medical conditions. Their primary concern is to apply the principles of prevention to the patients, to promote health or to retard the progress of a disease where a return to health is not possible. Environmental health specialists are responsible for the control of disease by environmental techniques. Animal control officers serve to control endemics within a broad number of animal species.

Public health has often been popularly regarded as a health care service for the financially, socially, or geographically disadvantaged, but in reality, public health services are for all members of the community (eg, epidemics, or post-natural disaster care such as after hurricanes, tornadoes, or blizzards), as they are supported by the county or state tax base. Pharmacists should become acquainted with their local health department and its wide range of services and avail themselves of these services whenever the need arises. Further, pharmacists can get involved locally in public health, as many county boards of health are required by state or local statutes to have a pharmacist on the Board.

EPIDEMIOLOGY

Epidemiology is the study of the distribution and determinants of health-related events in specific populations and the applications of this field in the control of these events. Epidemiology relates to the interaction of hosts and their environment, with attention to those particular agents in the environment that are causal factors of disease. Originating in the investigation of outbreaks of communicable disease in the 19th century, epidemiology is being applied increasingly to those non-communicable, chronic diseases that are of the most significance in today's aging population such as cardiovascular disease, cancer, and stroke. The alert pharmacist who can apply the basic principles of epidemiology in their community will become a significant member of the health team.

In the US, a longer lifespan can be achieved by direct measures that are initiated early in childhood and sustained throughout adulthood, especially with the current recognition of the contribution of psychosocial and behavioral risk factors to the prevalence of disease. To this end, a 1979 report of the Surgeon General[6] recommended action in the following areas, many of which can actively involve pharmacists: family planning, pregnancy and infant care, immunizations, sexually transmissible diseases, control of toxic agents, occupational health and safety, control of accidental injuries, fluoridation of community water supplies, reduction in the spread of communicable and infectious diseases, tobacco cessation, reduction of drug/alcohol use/abuse, improved nutrition, and exercise and fitness and stress modification. The continued and remarkable decrease in the number of smokers during the past quarter century is an example of what can be accomplished if a sufficient percentage of the community get involved in a coordinated plan.

Pharmacists should fulfill not only a referral role for patients suspected of having a particular illness, but also can collaborate with the local health departments or health planning agencies in epidemiology. Through their daily and multiple interactions with many patients, pharmacists can contribute to the knowledge base of disease patterns prevalent in the community. More than any professional group, pharmacists become aware of community-based epidemic infectious diseases in its earliest stages. The arrival of an unusual number of people with diarrheal disease for OTC products may be the result of an outbreak of food-borne disease. The monitoring of numbers and types of prescriptions often points to an epidemic, and the focused pharmacist can set up a systematic monitoring system for more scientific validity.

Pharmacoepidemiology, a subspecialty of epidemiology that is pertinent to pharmacy, involves the safety or risk assessment of a new drug, starting with its early use and continuing through its longer use cycle. It involves generating information about pharmaceutical outcomes and monitoring associated risks, particularly in the postmarketing environment. There are three major parts to these studies: a knowledge base, a conceptual framework, and an interpretive framework. With these perspectives, a pharmacoepidemiologist can establish a surveillance system, understand a posed research question, select strategies, apply methodologies, and interpret the results of purposeful investigations. Population-based studies are designed in an unbiased manner to include all patients (or a representative sample of patients) who may have been exposed to a common risk factor, have an identified disease, or a medical condition in a given population during a given time period. This type of study of a population is expected to provide an unbiased view of the examined medical condition/disease in the population as a whole.[19]

The ready availability of statistical software packages has made multivariate analysis more available to public health researchers. Further, there are numerous sources for public health statistics on the Internet (eg, http://www.lib.umich.edu/govdocs/sthealth.html or www.lib.berkeley.edu/PUBL/stats.html). Public health research studies focus on generalized linear models, so that the types of outcomes common in public health (eg, continuous measures binary indicators of disease counts, times to events) can be handled in a uniform manner.

DISEASE PREVENTION

Three levels of prevention exist: primary, secondary, and tertiary:

Primary prevention is helping people maintain their health or improve the quality of their lives through a healthy lifestyle. An example of primary prevention is the control of infections through immunization. Also, adopting healthy lifestyle practices may lead to increased longevity as well, for example, eating foods low in saturated fat, salt, and simple sugars; refraining from tobacco use; limiting alcohol consumption; controlling weight; sleeping 7 to 8 hours a night; being physically active; and eating in moderation. The aim of primary prevention is to modify lifestyles to the benefit of the individual and, ultimately, to the community.

Secondary prevention is the early diagnosis and treatment of an already existing disease. For example, the use of penicillin in the treatment of a streptococcal infection prevents the onset of rheumatic fever. Thus, a pharmacist can perform a vital service by advising patients who present a febrile illness characterized by a sore throat to see a physician.

Tertiary prevention largely consists of rehabilitation. Most chronic diseases cannot be cured, but their progress can be retarded with maximum benefit to the patient. Much can be done, for instance, with rheumatoid arthritis to make patients more comfortable and more productive in their daily lives.

HEALTH MEASUREMENT

The pharmacist is the health professional in most frequent contact with the general public, and this function as a community health educator makes the pharmacist's role unique. By staying abreast of local health statistics, pharmacists can function as a valuable resource person to researchers conducting epidemiological studies in the community.

All events that are measurable must be related to the population in which they occur, usually known as the *population at risk*. Events to be measured must be reduced to a common factor of population.

The *crude birth rate* is only a crude measurement of births because the population at risk includes all the men, women, and children in the geographical area of concern; most of this population cannot bear children. A more accurate measurement would be to confine the population at risk to women, a sex-specific rate. Including only the women of child-bearing age who can conceive would be a further refinement of the group, an age/gender-specific rate. The *fertility rate* is a far more accurate measurement of births.

Death rates follow the same pattern as birth rates, ranging from the crude death rate to age and sex-specific rates. The most commonly used indicator of health services is the *infant death, or mortality, rate*. This age-specific rate, which measures the number of deaths occurring in infants below the age of one year, is often used as an indicator of the effectiveness of a nation's health services; the implication is that the care of the mother and baby reflects the availability and efficiency of medical care. *Incident rates* show the number of new cases of a disease that occur in a population during a period of time, usually one year. *Prevalence rates* provide the number of new and old cases that are present in a community at a particular point in time.

HEALTH EDUCATION

The objective of health education is to provide the individualized information necessary for patients to modify their behavior, all in an effort to live a healthier life. Pharmacists actively promote good health practices through their own personal example, and by reaching out to provide professional information to the public. Many pharmacies participate in patient health education through the use of pamphlets and bulletins that cover every medical subject imaginable, including all the major chronic diseases, drug classes, drugs of abuse, drug and food interactions, sexually transmitted diseases, immunizations, family planning, health promotion, fluoridation, poison prevention, alternative therapies, disaster preparedness, environmental protection, and workplace safety.

The Internet serves as a primary site for review and receipt of health information. Occasionally, the material received through this medium may be misleading and is usually generalizible without the ability to be put into a patient's specific context. Pharmacists can offer an invaluable service by refuting misinformation or by reframing the information into the patient's specific situation.

Participation of pharmacists in community health education programs must be recommended, but it is in the everyday person-to-person contact that the pharmacist serves most effectively. To display pamphlets with health information is admirable, but it is substantially better to augment this with verbal instruction. People can always benefit from a few words of advice or direction on health matters, and the greater availability of the pharmacist in the community is a vital link to the health of individuals, or of the community in general.

The primary emphasis of the health education activities of the pharmacist is awareness of the early signs and symptoms of the major diseases within their community, and a willingness to provide those citizens who may require such information, often in association with various health agencies, both official and voluntary. These groups have basic differences in governance, financial support, legal responsibilities, and primary focus. In general, official agencies are governed by appointed officials, and supported by taxes to provide direct services to the public, while the scope of activities are dictated via legislative fiat. Voluntary and philanthropic agencies have greater flexibility to support new programs than do state or federal agencies, with no legal authority to enforce health rules and regulations. Pharmacists need to understand the basic origins and differences of these agencies to derive the greatest benefits for the patients and populations that they serve.

The following sections illustrate examples of areas of health care where pharmacists can have a positive impact on the health outcomes of their communities:

COMMUNICABLE DISEASE CONTROL

During the 20th century, control of infectious diseases has been accomplished in large measure by the environmental control of food, milk, water, and sewage. Although some serious communicable diseases have been practically eradicated, others such as tuberculosis (TB) and syphilis are still common and are now appearing in drug-resistant forms.[20] The estimated number of cases of sexually transmitted diseases (STDs), hospital-acquired infections, influenza, and other acute respiratory illnesses number in the millions. The most common STD, *chlamydia*, has reached epidemic proportions. Certain viral diseases, including acquired immunodeficiency syndrome (AIDS), West Nile virus, and Severe Acute Respiratory Syndrome (SARS), remain resistant to eradication, or sufficient treatment modalities have not been identified, to date.[21,22] Further, the threat of bioterrorism, with smallpox and its high rate of transmission and potential mortality, requires a new level of planning, training, monitoring, and vaccination practices.[23]

In some areas of the US, such as inner cities, and the world (such as Third World countries), greater than 9 out of 10 individuals are either at risk of being infected, or are currently infected with HIV. Pharmacists can become involved in educational programs promoting safer sexual practices, particularly the use of condoms. Many pharmacies have prominent displays that offer ready accessibility to condoms, all in an effort to minimize barriers to their purchase and use.

As a part of developing a comprehensive national HIV prevention strategy, federal agencies and professional health-care organizations have recommended that injection drug users (IDUs) be given greater access to clean syringes and drug treatment programs. The once-only use of sterile needles and syringes remains the safest and most effective approach to limit the transmission of HIV among IDUs who cannot or will not stop injecting drugs.

The CDC, the Health Resources and Services Administration (HRSA), the Substance Abuse and Mental Health Services Administration (SAMHSA), and the National Institute on Drug Abuse (NIDA) jointly have published the *HIV Prevention Bulletin: Medical Advice for Persons Who Inject Illicit Drugs* (http://www.cdc.gov/idu/pubs/hiv_prev.htm). The primary recommendation of this document was to provide counseling to IDUs to stop using and injecting drugs, if possible by entering and completing a substance abuse treatment program that includes relapse prevention. For those who continue to inject drugs, HIV prevention strategies include not reusing or sharing syringes, water, or drug preparation equipment; using only syringes that come from a reliable source, such as pharmacies; using a new, sterile syringe to prepare and inject drugs; and safely disposing of the syringe after one use. While politically volatile, numerous states have passed legislation to address the availability of syringes to reduce the spread of HIV transmission. As the absolute number of individuals worldwide who are HIV-infected has not reached a plateau, use of highly active antiretroviral therapy (ie, a combination of double or triple combination antiretroviral drug regimens) continues to improve outcomes in this country, and worldwide, provided that adequate public health resources (ie, the medications, and the means to deliver them) are available in sufficient supply.

The role of the pharmacist in the control of communicable diseases consists of an awareness of the natural history of these diseases in both the individual and the community, and referral of patients to health care facilities, when indicated. The pharmacist is in a position to dispel much of the ignorance and myths attached to these diseases, especially STDs, particularly in high-risk sectors of the population (eg, youth). In this aspect of community disease control, pharmacists can have their greatest impact, and one of the best opportunities for health education, via written, visual, oral, or via audio or video, is when a patient is waiting to be seen in a clinic, or waiting for a prescription to be filled.

The pharmacist's role in educating the public about effective health measures cannot be overemphasized, but it is vital that the pharmacist has the most current information to carry it out. The control of communicable diseases is based upon adequate case finding and the supervision and prophylactic treatment of close contacts. As community health educators, pharmacists can remove barriers to care by involving themselves with sociosexual and psychosocial problems as they relate to public health, understanding their patients' subcultures, and knowing how sexual activities and other social behavior vary from one group to another. Patients should be counseled freely and advised on STD prevention methods, available methods of treatment, and the necessity for receiving the treatment.

Immunization has controlled the childhood infections of measles, mumps, rubella, poliomyelitis, diphtheria, and whooping cough. New changes in recommended regimens should be expected as new products are developed. Pharmacists should remain up-to-date with immunization schedules and advise parents, particularly those who have infants or young children, of the importance of adhering to the recommended times.

Independent of those times when vaccines are in short supply or back order, the pharmacist often will have many vaccines in stock for immediate or urgent administration by private physicians that local health departments need only on an occasional basis and, therefore, do not stock routinely. Where mass community immunization clinics (eg, at local health departments) are used to immunize the public, the pharmacist is the primary health care professional responsible for obtaining, storing, preparing, and administering the vaccine.

An increasing number of states and within the PHS, pharmacists are acquiring the knowledge and the requisite skills to administer the vaccines directly, pursuant to an order from another health-care practitioner who is licensed to prescribe. This can provide increased access to immunizations. The information necessary for a vaccination program can be found in *Epidemiology & Prevention of Vaccine-Preventable Diseases,* available from the CDC, an excellent first step for acquiring these skills. *The Report of the Committee on Infectious Diseases,* published periodically by the American Academy of Pediatrics, provides a sensible immunization schedule.

The Control of Communicable Diseases Manual, published by APHA,[24] concisely summarizes all known communicable diseases with the etiology, treatment, and control of each disease. Pharmacists who wish to keep current on communicable disease patterns should subscribe to the CDC's *Morbidity and Mortality Weekly Report* (MMWR; www.cdc.gov/mmwr). The MMWR contains epidemiologic notes, reports of disease outbreaks, and current statistics by disease and geographical location at home and abroad.

UNIVERSAL PRECAUTIONS FOR PREVENTION OF TRANSMISSION OF HIV AND OTHER BLOOD BORNE INFECTIONS

Universal precautions, as defined by the CDC (www.cdc.gov/mmwr/preview/mmwrhtml/00000039.htm), are a set of precautions designed to prevent the transmission of HIV, hepatitis B virus (HBV), hepatitis C virus (HCV), and other blood borne pathogens to first-aid or health-care providers. Under universal precautions, all blood and certain body fluids are considered potentially infectious.

Universal precautions apply to blood, other body fluids containing visible blood, semen, and vaginal secretions, as well as to tissues and to the following fluids: cerebrospinal, synovial, pleural, peritoneal, pericardial, and amniotic. These precautions do not apply to feces, nasal secretions, sputum, sweat, tears, urine, and vomitus unless they contain visible blood. Further, these precautions do not apply to saliva except when it is visibly contaminated with blood or in the dental setting where blood contamination of saliva is predictable.

Universal precautions involve the use of protective barriers such as gloves, gowns, aprons, masks, or protective eyewear, which can reduce the risk of exposure of the clinician's skin or mucous membranes to potentially infective materials. In addition, it is recommended that all clinicians take precautions to prevent injuries caused by syringes, scalpels, and other sharp instruments or devices.

Pregnant health-care practitioners are not known to be at greater risk of contracting HIV infection than are clinicians who are not pregnant; however, if a clinician develops HIV infection during pregnancy, the infant is at risk of infection by perinatal transmission. Because of this risk, pregnant health practitioners should be especially familiar with, and strictly adhere to, precautions to minimize the risk of HIV transmission.

Even though universal precautions took the place of and eliminated the need for the isolation category "Blood and Body Fluid Precautions" in the *CDC Guidelines for Isolation Precautions in Hospitals* (www.cdc.gov/ncidod/hip/isolat/isolat.htm),[25] implementing universal precautions does not eliminate the need for other types of isolation precautions. These guidelines (standard precautions) include isolation in hospitals, droplet precautions for influenza, airborne isolation for pulmonary tuberculosis, and contact isolation for drug-resistant *Staphylococcus aureus*. Standard precautions were developed for use in hospitals and may not necessarily be indicated in other settings where universal precautions are used, such as child-care settings and schools.

INTERNATIONAL/GLOBAL HEALTH

Globalization has decreased the distinctions between the issues of community or domestic health, and international health.[26,27] Pharmacists should have an understanding of the complexity of diseases encountered in international travel. When considering or suspecting an infectious disease in a patient, pharmacists should ask them if they have traveled nationally or abroad within the past 2 weeks, and if so, where. The epidemic of Severe Acute Respiratory Syndrome (SARS) provides an excellent example of how global transmission of a virus can occur.

The World Health Organization (WHO; www.who.int), with 192 member nations, is the only official international health organization. Apart from reporting disease trends, WHO controls many aspects of international health. By international agreement, there are only three diseases to which quarantine regulations still apply: cholera, plague, and yellow fever. One WHO program that is of particular significance to pharmacy is the international standardization of immunological agents, vaccines, and toxoids.

Pharmacists can be of invaluable assistance to international travelers in advising them what to take in the way of medications, especially for infectious conditions such as malaria and traveler's diarrhea. Referral to the local health department may be easier for those pharmacists who lack the facilities or knowledge base, but they should retain some degree of interest in travelers' requirements, if only as a public service. Information on creating a traveler's medical chest is available in several publications; generally included are a broad-spectrum oral antibiotic, adhesive bandages, remedies for travel sickness, acetaminophen/ibuprofen/aspirin, a thermometer, and antibiotic cream or ointment. Immunizations also must be up to date. Annually, several of the professional pharmacy journals update travelers' needs in the areas of immunizations and emergency drugs for trips. The CDC provides this information at the

National Center for Infectious Diseases Traveler's Health web page (www.cdc.gov/travel/)

CHRONIC DISEASE MANAGEMENT

Patterns of diseases over the past 100 years have been shaped by the improvements in diagnosis, treatment, and prevention in health care. Because the control of infectious diseases has resulted in a longer life expectancy, chronic diseases have become the primary causes of mortality in this country. Accidents and cardiovascular, oncologic, and neurovascular conditions are the current primary causative factors of mortality. With no readily foreseeable solution to the control of chronic conditions, pharmacists should still encourage patients to avail themselves of the few proven techniques for chronic disease prevention, and they can recommend methods of preventing disease, particularly cardiovascular disease.[28]

The pharmacist's role in the control of chronic disease[29] can range from the support of proven community programs such as screening and disease management clinics for diabetes,[28] to surveillance for the first signs of diseases associated with an occupational hazard (eg, environmental toxin spill). The pharmacist is unique in having a basic understanding of disease processes and in being in daily contact with the public. The pharmacist's ability to prevent or to intervene in the initial stages of illness in chronic disease is unparalleled.

In economic terms, cancer remains the most important health problem in the US, followed by affordability of health care, AIDS/HIV disease, obesity, and heart disease.[30] In 2000, the CDC reported that, according to the *Annual Report to the Nation on the Status of Cancer, 1975–2000* (www.cdc.gov/cancer), death rates from the four leading cancers (lung, breast, prostate, and colorectal) show a decline nationally and in most states during the late 1990s. For certain cancers such as stomach cancer, an appropriate diet can help in prevention, although in general these conditions must be dealt with by early diagnosis and treatment. Techniques such as the Pap smear serve as specific preventive methods as well, although secondary prevention is the main point of attack.

Pharmacists should be acquainted with the warning signals of cancer and advise any patient who exhibits them to seek medical advice immediately. Pharmacists can encourage patients to obtain routine physical examinations, pap smears, mammograms, colorectal examinations, or other tests. Further, patients can be taught self-performed techniques such as breast or testicular examinations. Local cancer societies can provide health education literature for professional and public education.

The mortality rates for both heart disease and stroke have decreased for the past 10 years, probably as a result of such well-promoted measures as stopping tobacco use, controlling hypertension, lowering cholesterol (including saturated and trans-fat) intake, increasing physical activity, and having a good overall health awareness.[31–33] Stroke prevention, in particular, is correlated primarily with the control of hypertension and associated risk factors.

With secondary and tertiary prevention, early diagnosis, and treatment and rehabilitation, respectively, are the primary measures in chronic disease management. Pharmacotherapeutic innovations within the past 10 years have had a positive impact, resulting in the lower mortality rates from cardiovascular and cerebrovascular disease. As medications comprise the basis of modalities for hypertension, pharmacists should be at the forefront of monitoring, especially in encouraging compliance with prescribed regimens. Because they are in a unique position to measure their patients' blood pressure and advise them about its normal variations, pharmacists are becoming more involved in hypertension screening and referral.[34] Pharmacists should be well acquainted with the community-based services that offer diagnosis, treatment, and rehabilitation.[33] As appropriate, local medical societies and heart associations should be consulted as pharmacists become involved in blood pressure screening and monitoring programs.

Guidelines for the involved pharmacist can be found in the Seventh Report of the Joint National Committee on Prevention, Detection, Evaluation, and Treatment of High Blood Pressure (JNC VII), released in May 2003 by the National Heart, Lung, and Blood Institute. This report was developed using evidence-based medicine and consensus to make clinical decisions.[35] An update to the Sixth Report (JNC VI, published in 1997), it provides a contemporary approach to hypertension prevention and control, including data from the second phase of the third National Health and Nutrition Examination Survey (NHANES), updated information on the US government's Healthy People 2010 objectives, a discussion of new pharmacotherapies including combination agents, the role of managed care in hypertension treatment, and information from recent randomized controlled trials on hypertension prevention and treatment.

The report also provides a guide to assist in risk stratification into three stages of blood pressure ranges, in an effort to individualize treatment. Strategies for individualizing treatment in special populations are provided in a revised treatment algorithm. Of particular interest are the new recommendations for lifestyle changes independent of risk group: diet, weight reduction, alcohol limitation, smoking cessation, and regular physical activity.

The fourth most common cause of death in the US today is accidents. Injuries are the leading cause of death for children and young adults. Accident prevention relies on a few specific actions, such as the use of automobile seat belts. With accidental poisonings, the pharmacist should be a leader in control and prevention. In small communities, the pharmacist should be considered as the prime consultant for advice in poisoning cases and should be able to refer the caller to the nearest poison control or information center when unable to deal with the matter personally. Pharmacists must be aware of the dangers arising from industrial toxins and be alert to their manifestations in patients who seek relief in OTC medicines.

As a part of community educational services, the pharmacist should be viewed as a leader in disseminating information about poisoning and its prevention, especially during National Poison Prevention Week in the third week of March. Many pharmacists run poison control centers nationally, usually within larger regional hospitals or academic medical centers.

MATERNAL AND CHILD HEALTH

Mother and child health was the first public health program of the 20th century. Infant and child mortality rates were exceptionally high, largely because of diarrhea and respiratory diseases; many of the latter were propagated by non-pasteurized milk, an ideal medium for bacterial proliferation. The first move to combat this form of infant mortality came in the form of milk stations, where purified milk was provided to mothers and their children. Gradually, the concept of maternal and child health expanded to the formation of direct patient care and health education programs aimed at both the mother and child (or fetus), provided both in clinic settings and at home. Since the end of World War II, maternal mortality has declined some 45%, and infant mortality has been reduced by about 75%, thus demonstrating the utility of these programs. One of the major programs in America that has had a positive impact on outcomes is the Special Supplemental Nutrition Program for Women, Infants, and Children, also known as the WIC program (www.fns.usda.gov/wic/aboutwic/default.htm). The WIC target population are low-income, nutritionally at risk: Pregnant women (through pregnancy and up to 6 weeks after birth or after pregnancy ends), breastfeeding women (up to an infant's first birthday), non-breastfeeding postpartum women (up to 6 months after the birth of an infant or after pregnancy ends), infants (up to their first birthday), and children up to their fifth

birthday. WIC serves 45% of all infants born in the US. WIC participants receive supplemental nutritious foods, nutrition education and counseling at WIC clinics, and screening/referrals to other health, welfare, and social services.

The basic premise behind maternal and child health is to assist the mother and her child through the time when they are exposed to the greatest risks of disease and mortality: during pregnancy, the puerperium (the first 6 weeks after birth), and through the first year of life. The prognosis and overall health of the infant are directly influenced by its care *in utero*. The earlier that prenatal care is initiated, even in the pre-conception phase, the more beneficial is the effect, not only to the mother but also to the child. Pharmacists who understand the normal course of pregnancy and infancy, and all of the attendant health-care issues, are in constant demand.

Mothers can be instructed on simple matters of diet, hygiene, and overall management of their pregnancy and infant. This is of particular importance with mothers who have an incomplete understanding of the importance of receiving coordinated and continuous prenatal care. Pharmacists who are able to discuss the various available contraceptive methods in an intelligent and professional manner are important, especially in the postpartum period. Before delivery, parents can be advised to obtain an infant car seat, and instructed on its proper instruction within the car and the correct method of seating and securing the child into the seat. Many city/county health departments have infant car seat loan programs for a nominal fee. Based upon the immunologic and nutritional benefits supplied, breast-feeding is still the best option for the baby, and pharmacists should encourage breast-feeding, whenever possible.

A primary aspect of disease control in the infant is childhood immunizations. All infants should be immunized fully to avoid the dangerous diseases associated with the first years of childhood. Primary immunization should begin at birth (with hepatitis B vaccine) and must continue until the fourth dose of triple vaccine (ie, diphtheria, tetanus, pertussis) is given at 12 months, with a follow-up dose at 4 to 6 years (www.cdc.gov/nip/recs/child-schedule.pdf, or www.cispimmunize.org).

Mortality from sudden infant death syndrome (SIDS) continues to decrease at a steady rate. The SIDS rate for 1995 was 0.87 deaths per 1000 live births. One measure contributing to the decline is the implementation of prevention recommendations that are based upon the best available evidence. SIDS has long been associated with women who smoke during pregnancy. Infants who were in the presence of second-hand smoke in the home after birth were twice as likely to die from SIDS, and constant smoke exposure both during and after pregnancy triples a baby's risk for SIDS. Also, babies who died of SIDS were less likely to been breast-fed.

The American Academy of Pediatrics recommends that healthy infants sleep on their backs or sides to reduce the risk for SIDS (www.healthychildcare.org/section_SIDS.cfm). These recommendations are considered to be primarily important during the first 6 months of age, when a baby's risk of SIDS is greatest. The US Public Health Service, American Academy of Pediatrics, SIDS Alliance, and the Association of SIDS Program Professionals jointly sponsor the *Back-to-Sleep Campaign*, a program to reduce the risk of SIDS. In this program, parents are advised to place their babies on their back or side to sleep when being put down for a nap or to bed for the night.

Worldwide, overpopulation is the most serious public health problem. *Family planning,* as population control is alternatively called in the Western countries, consists not only in spacing births by deliberate contraceptive use, but also in helping women who cannot conceive to bear children. Contraceptives, both prescription and OTC, are available in community pharmacies, and pharmacists should be at the vanguard of family planning.

In addition to family planning, other programs that have received much attention recently are lead poisoning prevention for children, infant, and preschool child health-care services, services for handicapped children, and nutritional education and support for children. The increase in working mothers in this country and the concomitant increase in use of child-care centers has focused interest in these programs.

NUTRITION

Good nutrition, including a diet that is low in saturated fats and contains five or more servings of fruits and vegetables each day, plays a key role in maintaining good health. Improvements in the American diet have the potential to extend the productive lifespan of Americans, and reduce their risk of chronic diseases (eg, heart disease, stroke, various types of cancers, diabetes mellitus, and osteoporosis. A direct relationship between obesity and morbidity is well established, as well as an inverse one with both length and quality of life. For this reason, pharmacists should be aware of normal nutritional requirements and the problem of malnutrition or poor nutrition among the patient population that they serve. Pharmacists can make significant contributions in nutrition by advising patients about basic food needs; helping to correct improper food habits, especially in children; advising on special requirements for nutrients during prenatal and maternal periods, suggesting special dietary instructions for patients with diabetes and people with food allergies; and participating in supporting school lunch programs and food stamp plans.

Sufficient data exist regarding dietary risk factors for chronic diseases, providing an excellent opportunity to promote specific healthy behaviors to the US population (www.cdc.gov/NCCdphp/burdenbook2002/03_nutriadult.htm). Generally, these include such simple measures as lowering the fat intake in the diet (especially saturated fat), using less salt, and increasing green and yellow vegetables and whole grain cereals/fiber in the diet (www.nutrition.gov). For maximum benefit, these measures should be coupled with maintaining body weight within recommended limits, avoiding obesity, keeping good physical activity, and avoiding both alcohol and tobacco.

Over 20% of Americans greater than 20 years of age are at least 10% over their ideal body weight, putting them at increased risk of developing diabetes, digestive system diseases, and cardiovascular disease (www.ahrq.gov/clinic/3rduspstf/obesity/obesrr.htm).[37] Many people who lose weight when in good health, regain this weight. The popular notion that there are magic drugs to control weight has been dispelled with the removal of products containing ephedra (OTC), fenfluramine (Pondimin) and dexfenfluramine (Redux) from the market over the last decade.

Pharmacists can recommend nutritional education and guidance offered through the many materials available from voluntary health organizations and local and state health departments. As people lose weight better in peer support groups, pharmacists can become acquainted with the local organizations aimed at helping people of all ages lose weight, such as Weight Watchers, TOPS (Take Off Pounds Sensibly), and YMCA and YWCA programs.

ORAL HEALTH

A large proportion of Americans suffer from tooth decay or periodontal disease. Untreated tooth decay remains a problem. About one-third of persons across all age groups have untreated decay. Among adults aged 35 to 44, 48% have gingivitis, and 22 percent have destructive gum disease. Tobacco use increases the risk of gum disease. In the US, 30,000 people are diagnosed with mouth and throat cancer each year, and 8,000 die of these cancers. *A National Call to Action to Promote Oral Health* marks the latest in an ongoing effort to address the country's oral health needs in the 21st century. Reflecting the work of a partnership of public and private organizations, the *Call to Action* builds on *Oral Health in America: A Report of the Surgeon General* (May 2000) and the *Healthy People 2010* focus

area on Oral Health. The *Call to Action* seeks to expand on these efforts by enlisting the expertise of individuals, health researchers and care providers, communities, and policymakers at all levels of society (www.nidcr.nih.gov/sgr/nationalcalltoaction.htm). Pharmacists have numerous opportunities on a daily basis to positively affect this trend. Most oral conditions are preventable by appropriate self-care and use of fluoridated toothpastes, oral fluoride supplements, dental sealants, flossing, avoidance of tobacco use (especially oral tobacco products such as chewing tobacco or snuff), and regular dental visits.

The American Dental Association has published pamphlets for dentists and pharmacists that cover oral structures and diseases, prevention of caries, OTC and prescription dental drugs, and how these two professions can collaborate. The American Dental Hygienists Association's Oral Health Information page (www.adha.org/oralhealth/index.html) has numerous pieces of information and publications on preventive oral care. Presently, patients should be counseled to visit a dentist at least annually (if not more frequently for more high-risk patients), and to floss daily, brush their teeth daily with a fluoride-containing dentifrice, and use fluoride for caries prevention and chemotherapeutic mouth rinses for reduction of plaque.

In 2003, 65.8% of the US population on public water supplies has access to fluoridated water systems population; the objective for the year 2010 is to increase that number to at least 75%. Fluoride supplementation is recommended for children living in areas with inadequate water fluoridation. Resistance to water fluoridation began in 1950 and continues to raise controversy in some segments of the population. The charges raised by opponents tend to be more sophisticated variations on themes used since the inception of fluoridation, namely the alleged adverse health consequences (eg, cancer or AIDS) and infringement on freedom of choice. Although various anti-fluoride advocacy groups have gained much publicity in their attempt to create the illusion of a scientific controversy about fluoridation, claims of a health hazard from water fluoridation remain unfounded. The American Dental Association cites extensive research demonstrating that fluoridation does not increase the incidence or mortality rate of any chronic condition, including cancer, heart disease, intra-cranial lesions, nephritis, cirrhosis, and Down syndrome. No correlation between fluoride in the water supply and cancer in human beings has been demonstrated by studies to date. Fluoridation of drinking water supplies at a level of 1 ppm (part per million) protects against dental caries, and in such concentrations is not associated with any known adverse health effects. Fluoride toxicity from water sources would be improbable because of the large quantities of water that would need to be consumed at any one time.

ENVIRONMENTAL HEALTH

All elements of the natural environment can be altered, sometimes with harmful results. Air, food, water, and the earth can all become sources of illness, in the home, public, or work environments. With increased industrialization, air, in Western, as well as developing countries, now contains noxious substances that are either direct results of combustion or produced by photochemical change. *Smog* (a term first coined from "smoke" and "fog" in 1905) is the classic example of the latter; it results from the interaction of the ultraviolet rays in sunshine and the unburned hydrocarbons of automobile engines or factories and smokestacks. These products, when trapped by the thermal inversion engendered by local topography, cause damage to mucous membranes and lungs when inhaled. There is a close correlation of such diseases with age, especially in persons whose heart, lungs, and immune system may already be compromised. Acute episodes of air pollution have been found to exacerbate illness and even cause death in people who already have respiratory and cardiovascular diseases. Supporting evidence exists demonstrating that second-hand tobacco smoke increases the risk of cardiovascular diseases or cancer as well.

Food remains a significant vehicle of disease organisms. Although pasteurization has eliminated milk as a medium for disease distribution, the same cannot be said for other foods. Food-borne disease, more commonly but often incorrectly called "food poisoning," is grossly underreported: the 400 to 500 outbreaks comprising some 5000 to 10,000 persons per year probably can be increased by a factor of 10 to represent its true magnitude. In most instances the illness produced by contaminated food is mild and of short duration, but more severe outbreaks (such as hepatitis A, most commonly seen in public restaurants) can occur. Epidemics of food-borne disease are dramatic and sudden, and most people become sick within 6 to 24 hours after consuming the contaminated foodstuffs. The epidemic pattern of food-borne disease presents differently from the gastrointestinal symptoms (eg, nausea, vomiting, and diarrhea) induced by intestinal enteroviruses. When pharmacists note a sudden increase in OTC sales of anti-nausea and anti-diarrhea agents, the local health department should be notified immediately so that they can initiate a rapid case investigation to prevent further spread.

Water-borne infectious disease is uncommon today, but this does not mean that all public water supplies are pure and potable. Many complaints about the taste, appearance, and physical qualities of locally supplied water have led to a brisk US trade in bottled water. A modern concern of many citizens is the presence of chemical toxins in the environment and in the diet. Well-documented data exist documenting cancer development in animals from ingested materials, but there also is little proof that many of these substances ever produce human cancer. Host factors may have a significant and vital role in disease of any type, and pharmacists, especially those in the community, should stay aware of developments pertaining to toxic and carcinogenic substances. Water contamination with ground-source chemicals (eg, pesticides, fertilizers) remains an ongoing possibility, and pharmacists should remain aware of outbreaks and refer patients to local health departments for assistance, when necessary.

Occupational illnesses provide evidence that the workplace can play an immense role in disease occurrence. For example, for hundreds of years, pneumoconioses in the form of silicosis have been known to occur in miners as black lung disease; more recently byssinosis, brown lung disease, was observed in textile workers. Asbestos exposure has been associated with cancer. All occupations that expose workers to dust are hazardous to a degree, depending on the size of the dust particles and their consequent ability to penetrate into the lung substance, combined with their concentration and the length of the workers' exposure time.

Pharmacists should be aware of the local occupations, companies, and factories and to be cognizant of the initial symptoms of disease. Again, pharmacists should become acquainted with the local community and to adapt the principles of health and medical care to the particular situations encountered. The pharmacist's continuing education requirements should include watching the local pattern of society and its diseases, and changing the emphasis toward evolving disease patterns and their control.

Included in the current environmental issues are the workplace and the future of occupational safety and health regulations, hazards of local ambient environments, such as hazardous and other waste dumps, radioactive waste from weapons production, air emissions, and groundwater contamination of unknown magnitude; the Clean Air act and other regulatory initiatives; waste reduction and minimization, and radioactive waste and weapons production; global pollution, chlorofluorocarbons and the land ozone layer, the greenhouse effect, and global climate change; and conserving the tropical forest and biological diversity.[38]

With constant change to the physical, biological, cultural, social, and economic environment, both pharmacists and citizens should cultivate an informed awareness of these changes, and pharmacists should adapt their methods of health education, disease prevention, and disease control to the changes in each community.[38] This is especially true of air and water pollution, which require concerted community action for their control, but pharmacists may play a much more fundamental and personal role in controlling food-borne diseases; often, the first indication of an outbreak of food-borne disease is time-limited, with an unusually large number of people seeking relief from nausea, vomiting, and diarrhea. The pharmacist's role in environmental health is related primarily to being alert to the conditions prevailing in the community and of working with others to adequately control any of the attendant hazards.

MENTAL HEALTH

The topic of mental illness and its causation, manifestations, and control is vast. It is estimated that there are an approximate equivalent number of beds in this country for patients with mental health conditions as for all other ailments combined. It has been estimated that approximately 10% of the population in this country are affected with some form of emotional disorder requiring treatment. An estimated 2.4 million chronically mentally ill individuals have been identified in the US (excluding the mentally retarded and chronic substance abusers). Out of this number, about half (1.1 million) live at home, some 700,000 are residents of nursing homes, 450,000 live in single rooms or congregate-care facilities, and at least 150,000 are found in psychiatric hospitals. Of the 450,000 homeless persons, an estimated one-third of them have a serious mental illness. Pharmacists should be aware of their local community mental health services, especially those catering to ambulatory patients. The timely referral of patients exhibiting unusual behavior to these facilities may be life saving, especially in those persons who demonstrate suicidal tendencies.

Suicide is the one outcome of a mental illness that can be measured directly. Fortunately, many suicide attempts are merely gestures, but this does not negate the importance of prevention whenever possible. Suicide has been demonstrated to occur most commonly in older, unmarried, and affluent males. Although women attempt to commit suicide more often than men, they are not as successful. The agents used in suicide vary with their availability. In the US, firearms figure most prominently, as they are readily available; in the United Kingdom where there are stringent gun-control laws, medications such as acetaminophen are the primary etiologic agents.

With these and other epidemiological facts at their disposal, pharmacists can be alert to potential suicide victims among patients and should do everything possible to bring aid to them. An individual's quiet plea for help, potentially offered in the form of overt or covert references to low personal self-esteem and to the uselessness of life, should never be neglected. Even a solitary phrase expressing self-disgust with the implication that the best way out is to end it all should never be ignored, as it may be a clue to contemplation of suicide. Depression, whose cardinal symptoms are as readily recognizable to observant laypeople as they are to health professionals, can be the forerunner of attempted suicide. Pharmacists should never be reluctant to ask patients directly whether they have ever considered, or are now considering, committing suicide or harming themselves or others. Whenever a pharmacist detects a potentially suicidal patient, he or she should talk to the patient and seek aid from family and community mental health services— no patient's plea for help should be ignored. Pharmacists who have interest in this area of practice should become familiar with any of the depression scales (eg, the Zung Self-Rating Depression Scale) that can be used for screening for depression.

ALCOHOL/SUBSTANCE ABUSE

Abuse of alcohol, tobacco, and other substances, in general, is a worldwide public health problem of enormous dimensions.[36] In the US, between 450,000 and 600,000 premature deaths annually are related to these substances, representing nearly one-third of all deaths. Substance abuse has become a common in American society, and the societal need to stay informed has never been greater. Again, the expert knowledge of the pharmacist should be used to good advantage in both an individual and community context.

Alcoholism is estimated to affect millions of men and women in the US. Alcoholism is a biopsychosocial disorder with many causes and many ramifications. Alcoholics Anonymous (AA) is a voluntary organization founded by a recovering alcoholic for individuals suffering from and recovering from alcoholism. The organization has branches for the spouses of alcoholics (Al-Anon) and their children (Ala-Teen) as well. AA groups exist in nearly all cities and many smaller towns, and individuals in recovery are always ready to help. Other types of clinics and treatment centers are available through government agencies' health, social services, mental health services, or public assistance departments.

Abuse of other agents has received more acceptance among younger people. Particularly in younger people, marijuana has been implicated as a gateway drug, such that harder drugs such as crack cocaine, amphetamines, or controlled prescription medications may follow the use of the milder ones. The trend of misuse/abuse of prescription medications (eg, opiates (OxyContin), benzodiazeines (alprazolam, Xanax), or stimulants (methylphenidate, Ritalin)) continues to rise. Again, the pharmacist is in the unparalleled position of being the most competent professional member of the community who can advise local agencies about substance abuse (including prescription, OTC, social, and illicit drugs) and its effects. The knowledge and participation of pharmacists adds to their professional reputation.

For general information on substance abuse, the Federal government and professional health organizations are often a valuable resource. The National Institute on Drug Abuse (NIDA; www.nida.nih.gov) has produced a science-based guide to drug addiction treatment, *Principles of Drug Addiction Treatment: A Research-Based Guide* (www.nida.nih.gov/PODAT/PODATindex.html). Based upon a comprehensive review of 25 years of treatment research findings, it describes the conditions required for truly effective drug abuse treatment. It also delineates the most common types of drug addiction treatment, identifies treatment approaches for which there is strong scientific evidence of efficacy, and answers the questions about treatment that are asked most frequently by providers, policy makers, patients, and the public.

The National Clearinghouse for Alcohol and Drug Information's PREVLINE (Prevention Online, www.health.org) contains the most current information on alcohol and drug use and abuse, with searchable bibliographic research databases, web pages especially designed for children, and an on-line catalog of substance abuse education materials.

Dealing with the diseases of alcoholism and substance abuse are peculiarly within the purview of the pharmacist. No other disease entities, with the possible exception of poison control, lend themselves more readily to intervention by pharmacists. Pharmacists have many opportunities to help individuals who become dependent upon alcohol, even though many will resist help. All community agencies, professional and voluntary, should be called into play, including church, voluntary, and government groups.

PUBLIC HEALTH RESEARCH

If the pharmacist evinces a sincere interest in community health programs, there may be opportunities to participate in public health research programs, especially those concerned with drugs and their control. In general, investigation of community disease is based on two methods, retrospective and prospective surveys.

Retrospective studies, based upon historical data, are readily obtained by asking questions of the population under investigation. Prospective studies actually observe the events that occur in the population over time. The retrospective method is inexpensive, takes little time, deals with a stable population, and requires a minimum amount of work, however, it relies on memory (recall bias), is difficult to conduct with a control group, and because the investigator knows what to look for, the introduction of observer bias is an issue. Conversely, prospective studies may take years to complete, are more expensive, contend with shifting populations, and require a vast amount of resources; but they are easy to use with a control group, do not rely on memory, and can minimize observer bias.

A classic example of the use of these methods comes from an observation by an Australian ophthalmologist in 1941 who saw an unusually large number of congenital cataracts in infants.[39] A retrospective investigation revealed that all the women concerned had had rubella (German measles) during their pregnancies, a retrospective discovery. This finding caused some women to obtain medically supervised abortions when they revealed to their physicians that they had had rubella during their pregnancies and were afraid of having a baby with a congenital deformity. Although rubella epidemics have largely been eliminated because of vaccination programs, it still exists in the US population, and therefore, pregnant women may be at risk if their immunization status is not current. The incidence of congenital rubella syndrome has increased since 1986, and in at least half of cases, the cause was determined to be missed opportunities for vaccination.[40] Pharmacists should offer their preventative services in the investigation of disease patterns in their community, especially with those of an infectious etiology, in the management of pharmacotherapy and its outcomes.

SUMMARY

Pharmacists are the most accessible and highly trusted health-care professionals. The pharmacist routinely sees the patient at the time of a prescription refill, which can be an opportune time to discuss public health issues; pharmacists can also use this time to identify early signs and symptoms of disease, if counseling and patient assessment are performed. New opportunities in this venue include provision of immunizations and performing smoking/tobacco cessation programs.

The role of the pharmacist has been and continues to undergo change. Early in the new millennium, this profession has some unique opportunities to acquire roles in the public health arena and to build partnerships with health departments, other health-care providers, and the community at large.

The availability of information such as the *Healthy People* reports, the *Guide to Clinical Preventive Services,* and the CDC Guideline Database, provide opportunities for pharmacists to take a more active role in preventive services and health promotion activities. Issues presented in the 1981 APHA statement on the role of the pharmacist in public health still exist, such as the underuse of patient-oriented pharmacists and the need to use existing health-care professionals and facilities. Thus, the pharmacist's role in public health remains unfulfilled. At this point in the professional evolution of the practice of pharmacy, it is time to address seriously the public health issues that affect everyone through the inclusion of the pharmacist as an engaged primary care member of the health care team.

REFERENCES

1. Last JM. *A Dictionary of Epidemiology,* 4th ed. New York: Oxford University Press, 2001.
2. Institute of Medicine, Committee for the Study of the Future of Public Health. *The Future of Public Health.* Washington, DC: National Academy Press, 1988.
3. Shattuck L. *A General Plan for the Promotion of Public and Personal Health, Devised, Prepared, and Recommended by the Commissioners*

Appointed under a Resolve of the Legislature of the State. Report of the Sanitary Commission of Massachusetts, 1850. Cambridge: Harvard University Press, 1948.

4. Cavins HM. *Bull Hist Med* 1943; 13:419–425.
5. Hepler CD, Strand LM. Opportunities and responsibilities in pharmaceutical care. *Am J Hosp Pharm* 1990; 47:533–543.
6. *Healthy People: The Surgeon General's Report on Health Promotion and Disease Prevention.* Washington, DC: Department of Health and Human Services/Public Health Service, 1979.
7. U.S. Department of Health and Human Services. *Healthy People 2010: Understanding and Improving Health. 2nd ed.* Washington, DC: U.S. Government Printing Office, November 2000.
8. U.S. Preventive Services Task Force. *Guide to Clinical Preventive Services: An Assessment of the Effectiveness of 169 Interventions: Report of the U.S. Preventive Services Task Force.* Baltimore: Williams & Wilkins, 1989.
9. U.S. Preventive Services Task Force Ratings: Strength of Recommendations and Quality of Evidence. *Guide to Clinical Preventive Services,* 3rd ed. *Periodic Updates,* 2000–2003. Agency for Healthcare Research and Quality, Rockville, MD.
10. Calis KA, Hutchison L, Elliott ME, et al. American College of Clinical Pharmacy *White Paper: Healthy People 2010: Challenges, Opportunities, and a Call to Action for America's Pharmacists,* 2003.
11. Pharmacists formally recognized for their role in public health. *Am Pharm* 1981; NS21: 9.
12. Cain RM, Kahn JS. *Am J Public Health* 1971; 61:2223–2228.
13. Bush PJ, Johnson KW. *Am J Pharm Educ* 1979; 43:249–253.
14. Gibson MR. *Am J Pharm Educ* 1972; 36:189–200.
15. Gibson MR. *Am J Pharm Educ* 1972; 36:561–570.
16. Gibson MR. *Am J Pharm Educ* 1973; 37:1–27.
17. Beardsley RS, Bootman JL, Christensen DB, et al. *Am J Pharm Educ* 1985; 49:413–417.
18. Frenk J. *Annu Rev Pub Health* 1993; 14:469–490.
19. Choi BCK. *Chronic Diseases in Canada* 1998; 19:145–151.
20. Cohen ML. *Nature* 2000; 406:762–767.
21. Morse DL. *N Engl J Med* 2003; 348:2173–2174.
22. Varia M, Wilson S, Sarwal S, et al. *CMAJ* 2003; 169:285–292.
23. Ferguson NM, Keeling MJ, Edmunds WJ, et al. *Nature* 2003; 425:681–685.
24. Chin J, ed. *Control of Communicable Diseases Manual,* 17th ed. Washington, DC: American Public Health Association, 2000.
25. Garner JS. *Infect Control Hosp Epidemiol* 1996; 17:53–80.
26. Frenk J, Gómez-Dantés O. *Lancet* 2002; 325:95–97.
27. Board on International Health, Institute of Medicine. *America's vital interest in global health: protecting our people, enhancing our economy, and advancing our international interests.* Washington, DC: National Academy Press, 1997:1.
28. Rothman R, Malone R, Bryant B, et al. *Am J Med Qual* 2003; 18: 51–58.
29. Wagner EH. *Br Med J* 2000; 320:569–572.
30. Health Pulse of America 2003 Survey. The Roper Center for Public Opinion Research, University of Connecticut, for the Henry J. Kaiser Family Foundation, July 2003.
31. Fletcher GF. *Circulation* 1997; 96:355–357.
32. Whelton PK. *J Human Hypertens* 1996; 10 (suppl 1):S47–S50.
33. Carter BL, Zillich AJ, Elliott WJ. *J Clin Hypertens* 2003; 5:31–37.
34. Grundy SM, et al. *Circulation* 1997; 95:2329–2331.
35. The seventh report of the Joint National Committee on Prevention, Detection, Evaluation, and Treatment of High Blood Pressure. *JAMA* 2003; 289:2560–2572.
36. Giovino GA. *Oncogene* 2002; 21:7326–7340.
37. U.S. Preventive Services Task Force. *Screening for Obesity in Adults: Recommendations and Rationale.* November 2003. Agency for Healthcare Research and Quality, Rockville, MD.
38. Bloom BR. *Nature* 1999; 402 (suppl):C63–64.
39. Gregg NM. *Trans Ophthalmol Soc Aust* 1942; 3:35.
40. Lee SH, Ewert DP, Frederick PD, et al. *JAMA* 1992; 267:2616–2620.

BIBLIOGRAPHY

General Public Health

Baker EL, et al. *JAMA* 1994; 272:1276–1272.
Brown ER. *Am J Public Health* 1997; 87:554–557.
Garrett L. *The Coming Plague: Newly Emerging Diseases in a World Out of Balance.* New York: Farrar, Strauss, & Giroux, 1994.
Ibrahim MA, House RH, Levine RH. *Fam Commun Health* 1995; 18:17–25.
Institute of Medicine, Committee for the Study of the Future of Public Health. *The Future of Public Health.* Washington, DC: National Academy Press, 1988.
Institute of Medicine, Committee on Public Health. *Healthy Communities: New Partnerships for the Future of Public Health.* Washington, DC: National Academy Press, 1996.
Kondratas R. *Images from the History of the Public Health Service.* Washington, DC: Department of Health and Human Services/Public Health Service, 1994.
Scutchfield FD, Keck CW. *Principles of Public Health Practice.* Albany, NY: Delmar, 1997.
Pew Health Professions Commission. *Critical Challenges: Revitalizing the Health Professions for the Twenty-First Century.* University of California at San Francisco, 1995.

Epidemiology

Bailar JC III, et al, eds. *Assessing Risks to Health: Methodological Approaches.* Westport, CT: (www.greenwood.com), Auburn House, 1993.
Cook RJ, Sackett DL. *Br Med J* 1995; 310:452–454.
Gehlbach SN. *Interpreting the Medical Literature: Practical Epidemiology for Clinicians,* 4th ed. New York: McGraw-Hill, 2002.
Hartzema AG, Porta MS, Tilson HH, eds. *Pharmacoepidemiology: An Introduction,* 3rd ed. Cincinnati, OH: Harvey Whitney, 1998.
Sackett DL. *Br Med J* 1996; 312:71–72.
Sackett DL, et al. *Clinical Epidemiology: A Basic Science for Clinical Medicine,* 2nd ed. Boston: Little, Brown, 1991.
Strom BL. *Pharmacoepidemiology,* 3rd ed. West Sussex: John Wiley & Sons, 2000.

Public Health and Pharmacy

Bush PJ. *The Pharmacist Role in Disease Prevention and Health Promotion.* Bethesda, MD: ASHP Research & Education Foundation, 1983.
Lambert RL, Wertheimer AI, Dobbert DJ, et al. *Am J Public Health* 1977; 67:252–253.

Environmental Health

Bingham E, Meader WV. Governmental regulation of environmental hazards in the 1990s. *Annu Rev Pub Health* 1990; 11:419–434.
DiBerardinis LJ, ed. *Handbook of Occupational Safety and Health,* 2nd ed. New York: Wiley–Interscience, 1998.
Greenberg M. *Public Health and the Environment.* New York: Guilford Press, 1987.
Levy BS, Wegman DH, eds. *Occupational Health.* Boston: Little, Brown, 1983.
Zuckerman B, Jefferson D, eds. *Human Population and the Environmental Crisis.* Sudbury, MA: Jones & Bartlett, 1996.

Administration

Brown RE, et al. *National Expenditures for Health Promotion and Disease Prevention Activities in the United States.* Washington, DC: Medical Technology Assessment and Policy Research Center, Battelle, 1991.
Ware JE Jr. *Annu Rev Public Health* 1995; 16:327–354.
Roper WL, Thacker SB. *Ann NY Acad Sci* 1993; 703:33–39.

Prevention

Cardiology

Dajani AS, et al. *Circulation* 1997; 96:358–366.
Gomel M, et al. *Am J Public Health* 1993; 83:1231–1238.
Hennekens CH, Dyken ML, Fuster V. *Circulation* 1997; 96:2751–2753.
Jeffery RW, et al. *Am J Public Health* 1993; 83:395–401.
Joint WHO/ISFC Meeting on Rheumatic Fever/Rheumatic Heart Disease, with Emphasis on Primary Prevention. Strategy for controlling rheumatic fever/rheumatic heart disease, with emphasis on primary prevention (Memorandum). *Bull WHO* 1995; 73:583–587.
Jones PH, Gotto AM Jr. *Am J Cardiol* 1995; 76:118–121C.
Maron DJ. *Clin Cardiol* 1996; 19:419–423.
Ramsay LE, et al. *Lancet* 1996; 348:387–388.
Rimm EB, et al. *JAMA* 1998; 279:359–364.
The Medical Research Council's General Practice Research Framework. *Lancet* 1998; 351:233–241.

Endocrine

ABTC Cancer Prevention Study Group. *Ann Epidemiol* 1994; 4:1–10.
American College of Physicians. *Ann Intern Med* 1992; 117:1038–1041.
Engelgau MM, Narayan KM, Saaddine JB, et al. *J Am Soc Nephrol* 2003; 14 (suppl 2): S88–S91.

Hosking D, et al. *N Engl J Med* 1998; 338:485–492.

Kelsey JL, Bernstein L. *Annu Rev Public Health* 1996; 17:47–67.

Kerlikowske K, et al. *JAMA* 1995; 273:149–154.

Manson JE, Spelsberg A. *Am J Prev Med* 1994; 10:172–184.

Newton KM, et al. *J Women Health* 1997; 6:459–465.

The Expert Committee on the Diagnosis and Classification of Diabetes Mellitus. *Diabetes Care* 2002; 26:S5–S20.

Smith-Warner SA, et al. *JAMA* 1998; 279:535–540.

Worden JK, et al. *Prev Med* 1990; 19:254–269.

Infectious Diseases

Ameratunga SN, Lennon DR, Martin D. *N Zeal Med J* 1994; 107:193–194.

Cooper ER, et al. *J Infect Dis* 1996; 174:1207–1211.

Lobel HO, Kozarsky PE. *JAMA* 1997; 278:1767–1771.

Mant D. *Lancet* 1994; 344:1343–1346.

Patel R, Kinsinger L. *Am J Prev Med* 1997; 13:74–77.

Prevention

Butler-Jones D. *Can J Public Health* 1996; 87(suppl 2): S75–S78.

Simpson JM, Klar N, Donner A. *Am J Public Health* 1995; 85:1378–1393.

Wall S. *Int J Epidemiol* 1995; 24:655–664.

Dietary and Other Lifestyle Issues

American Academy of Pediatrics. *Pediatrics* 1995; 95:777.

Boushey CJ, et al. *JAMA* 1995; 274:1049–1057.

Byers R. *N Engl J Med* 1995; 333:723–724.

Cushman R, James W, Waclawik H. *Am J Public Health* 1991; 81:1044–1046.

Fletcher GF, et al. Statement on exercise. *Circulation* 1996; 94:857–862.

Heart Protection Study Collaborative Group. *Lancet* 2003; 361:2005–2016.

Jeffery RW, French SA. *Am J Public Health* 1998; 88:277–280.

Kleinman DV, Hickey DJ, Lipton JA. *J Am Coll Dent* 2003; 70:16–21.

Kuczmarski RJ, et al. *JAMA* 1994; 272:205–211.

Kujala UM, et al. *JAMA* 1998; 279:440–444.

Rimm EB, et al. *JAMA* 1998; 279:359–364.

Robinson JK, et al. *Prev Med* 1997; 26:364–372.

Task Force on Infant Positioning and SIDS, American Academy of Pediatrics. Positioning and SIDS. *Pediatrics* 1992; 89:1120–1126.

Vivekananthan DP, Penn MS, Sapp SK, et al. *Lancet* 2003; 361:2017–2023.

Pulmonary

DiFranza JR, Lew RA. *Pediatrics* 1996; 97:560–568.

The Health Benefits of Smoking Cessation: A Report of the Surgeon General. Publication CDC 90-8416. Rockville, MD: Department of Health and Human Services, 1990.

Jonas MA, et al. *Circulation* 1992; 86:1664–1669.

Lando HA, et al. *Am J Public Health* 1990; 80:554–559.

Substance Abuse

Aguirre-Molina M, Dorman DM. *Ann Rev Public Health* 1996; 17:337–358.

Department of Health and Human Services. Preventing Tobacco Use among Young People: A Report of the Surgeon General. Publication S/N 017-01-00491-0. Washington, DC: US Government Printing Office, 1994.

Ellickson PL, Bell RM, McGuigan K. *Am J Public Health* 1993; 83:856–861.

Perry CL, et al. *Am J Public Health* 1992; 82:1210–1216.

Yesalis CE, et al. *Arch Pediatr Adolesc Med* 1997; 151:1197–1206.

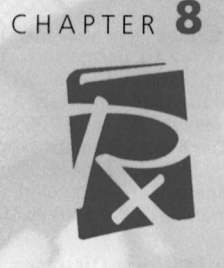

Information Resources in Pharmacy and the Pharmaceutical Sciences

Leslie Ann Bowman, AMLS

Mignon S Adams, MSLS

Amy Christopher, MS

Pharmacists and pharmaceutical scientists have a constant need for reliable and current information, and in the modern world information is everywhere. It is presented on television and radio, sent from computer to computer over the Internet, and passed from person to person using telephones and fax machines. The great challenge is sorting out the current information from the dated, the reliable from the questionable, the actual from the imagined. Practitioners and scientists must be able to find and identify different types of information in a variety of formats and media. In addition to meeting their own information needs, pharmacists must also be able to assist patients in meeting their information needs with regard to drugs, therapies, and diseases. This chapter will discuss primary and secondary literature and how to find each, the specialized reference sources in pharmacy and the pharmaceutical sciences, and the use of the Internet. The primary focus is on the literature and the information it contains. For a discussion of the critical evaluation of literature see Chapter 9.

TYPES OF LITERATURE AND HOW TO FIND THEM

Primary Literature

As with other sciences, the primary literature of the pharmaceutical sciences is the scientific journal. For more than three centuries, the scholarly journal has been the channel through which scientific research has been reported, evaluated, and disseminated.

Scientific research enters the primary literature by a prescribed route. When researchers have concluded a study, they usually write the results in a standard format that includes an abstract or summary, a review of past research in the area, a description of the methodology used, the results, a discussion of what the results mean, and a list of references. The finished article is then submitted to a scholarly journal, which may be published by a professional organization or by a commercial scientific publisher. The journal editor then sends the manuscript to be peer-reviewed by one or more researchers in the same field as the authors. Usually the reviewers are unaware of the authors' identities. Manuscripts that are found to meet criteria of sound research are accepted for publication and are published in the journal.

Nearly all scientific journals are now produced in digital form as well as in print. Because of the high costs of printing and mailing, and the dwindling number of subscribers to many specialized journals, research publications of the near future may exist only online.

Several different types of professional journals may contain primary literature of interest to those in pharmacy. Pharma-

ceutical scientists read and publish in basic science journals such as

European Journal of Pharmacology (Amsterdam, Netherlands: Elsevier Science)
Journal of Natural Products (Columbus, OH: American Chemical Society)
Pharmaceutical Research (New York: Kluwer/ Plenum)

Clinical pharmacists use major medical journals such as

Annals of Internal Medicine (Philadelphia: American College of Physicians)
JAMA: Journal of the American Medical Association (Chicago: AMA)
New England Journal of Medicine (Boston: Massachusetts Medical Society)

or journals that specialize in a particular disease or in drug therapy, such as

American Journal of Cardiology (Amsterdam, Netherlands: Elsevier Science)
American Journal of Health-System Pharmacy (Bethesda, MD: American Society of Health-System Pharmacists)
Annals of Pharmacotherapy (Cincinnati, OH: Harvey Whitney Books)
Diabetes (Alexandria, VA: American Diabetes Association)

Researchers in pharmacy administration have available to them such journals as

Journal of Pharmaceutical Marketing and Management (Binghamton, NY: Pharmaceutical Products Press)
Pharmacoeconomics (Auckland, New Zealand: Adis International)
Social Science and Medicine (Amsterdam, Netherlands: Elsevier Science)

Finally, those who teach pharmacy have

American Journal of Pharmaceutical Education (Alexandria, VA: AACP)
Journal of Pharmacy Teaching (Binghamton, NY: Pharmaceutical Products Press)

These journals are only a few of the thousands of scientific journals published worldwide. Finding articles on one particular area of interest requires more effort than scanning the issues of a few journal titles regularly.

Not long ago, someone researching a topic would be urged to begin with a standard bibliography, and to follow this by using printed indexes and abstracts that could be consulted only in a library. Advances in computer technology have made most printed finding tools obsolete. Printed sources are outdated the day they are published and, in the opinion of most, are much less convenient to use than online tools. Most online indexes can be accessed from desktop computers using the Internet. Many indexes link to the full text articles themselves, thus obviating many steps (both logically and geographically).

Researchers may also subscribe to table-of-contents alerting services, whereby the tables of content of selected journals are e-mailed to the researcher at the time of the publication of the issue. Some are services that must be purchased, such as those through companies like Ingenta. Or, publishers may offer the service as part of an individual or institutional subscription.

Finally, there are "packaged" medical collections that allow users to search across collections of textbooks, databases, and other materials. Collections such as Stat!Ref, MDConsult, and UpToDate are discussed under "textbooks."

Databases

Online databases, because of their convenience and ubiquity, are now the first choice to consult for locating pharmaceutical literature. For clinical literature, the databases of choice are *MEDLINE*, *EMBASE*, evidence-based medicine databases, the *Iowa Drug Information Service* (*IDIS*), and *International Pharmaceutical Abstracts*. For drug development, *Chemical Abstracts* and *BIOSIS Previews* are the most comprehensive. Each of these is available in print, through the World Wide Web ("the web"), on magnetic tape to be loaded on a local mainframe, or through commercial vendors such as Dialog or Ovid. Educational institutions and corporations often provide access for their researchers to one or more of these databases. An individual also can purchase access through a subscription or per-search arrangement with database providers or vendors.

Searching online databases appears to be easy—deceptively so—but doing a successful search can require a great deal of skill and prior experience. Novice searchers are often too impatient to learn proper searching techniques and may either miss many relevant items or retrieve a large number of irrelevant ones. Attending a class, consulting a manual, or working with a librarian can much improve a researcher's ability to do a comprehensive and highly relevant search.

MEDLINE

MEDLINE is produced by the US National Library of Medicine (Bethesda, MD). Its coverage of 4600 highly regarded clinical journals makes it the preeminent biomedical database. It is subsidized by the US government, with one search engine, PubMed, available at no cost all over the world. The resulting low or no cost to its users means that it is often the first and only choice of those seeking medical information. Its coverage is strongest in clinical and therapeutic topics.

The National Library of Medicine produces *MEDLINE* and makes it available directly to the public, but a number of other vendors make the database available as well. Each of these vendors has its own set of searching protocols, usually called *search engines*; each is a little different from the others, and each has a somewhat different way of indexing the files. The same search done with different *MEDLINE* search engines may yield different results.

PubMed (http://pubmed.gov), the *MEDLINE* search engine provided free to the world over the Internet by the National Library of Medicine, is a very easy to use and powerful search engine. Included as part of its website are excellent tutorials. Those who learn to use PubMed well get excellent results, but it is very easy to do a bad search in PubMed. The commercial vendor Ovid provides a search engine that forces its users to do better searches, so many institutions and corporations purchase access to it. Finally, there are several other free Internet-accessible versions of *MEDLINE*. Their search engines are considered to be less powerful than PubMed or Ovid and they should not be used.

PubMed also provides links to the articles it cites that are available in fulltext on the Internet. However, the articles must be free or part of their library's subscription in order for users to access them. Another feature of PubMed, Loansome Doc, lets unaffiliated searchers set up accounts with a medical library and order articles directly from them (at a cost). Institutions with subscriptions to Ovid may also choose to subscribe to electronic journals so that their users can connect directly to the articles they find in *MEDLINE*.

EMBASE

Another highly regarded medical database is *EMBASE*, produced and provided by Elsevier, a commercial publisher based in Amsterdam, Netherlands. Although its coverage of 4000 journals is comparable to *MEDLINE*, there is surprisingly little overlap between the two. In one 2000 study[1], a search for controlled clinical trials for 3 medical conditions, done in both *MEDLINE* and *EMBASE*, yielded a total of 4111 citations, but only 30% of these citations appeared in both databases.

EMBASE covers European literature in much more depth than does *MEDLINE*. It also is considered to be somewhat stronger in drug information and in areas of biological science related to human medicine. Because of its European focus and its high cost as compared to *MEDLINE*, *EMBASE* is searched less often in the US than perhaps it should be.

EMBASE is available through online vendors such as Dialog and Ovid, and through the web. A recent product, EMBASE.com, includes not only *EMBASE*, but also unique *MEDLINE* records so that both databases are searched simultaneously. EMBASE.com also includes links to articles from some major medical journals. Subsets on specific topics such as drug information or cardiology are available separately.

Evidence-Based Medicine (EBM) Databases

Increasingly health professionals are asked to base their decisions on evidence as demonstrated in randomized controlled trials (RCT's). In both PubMed and Ovid, *MEDLINE* searches can be limited to RCT's. However, strong proponents of EBM feel that only RCT's that meet vigorous standards of methodology should be used. They prefer "systematic reviews": reviews in which all RCT's on a particular topic are collected and analyzed, a meta-analysis is performed (if possible), and that evidence is then used to come to a clinical decision.

PubMed allows the searcher to limit his or her results to systematic reviews. There are also several efforts to collect and make available systematic reviews.

The *Cochrane Library*, the best-known such collection, is a volunteer effort begun in Great Britain. International teams donate their time to identify all published and nonpublished RCT's on a particular topic and then to prepare a systematic review with implications for practice. Abstracts of the systematic reviews are available free on the Internet. The reviews themselves may be purchased from the *Cochrane Library* organization or searched through subscription to Ovid, Dialog, and other vendors.

A major drawback to the *Cochrane Library* is the amount of time it takes for volunteers to complete their projects. Similar commercial products finish their reviews somewhat faster. These include *Clinical Evidence* (*BMJ*), PIER (American College of Physicians), and Infopoems (Infopoems). Also, the American College of Physicians, through its *ACP Journal Club*, monitors major internal medicine journals and selects for review those articles with the most significance for therapeutic practice.

IOWA DRUG INFORMATION SYSTEM

Iowa Drug Information System (*IDIS*) is produced by the College of Pharmacy of the University of Iowa. *IDIS* is a handy self-contained product that allows the user to search for drug therapy articles selected from 200 clinical journals and to access the fulltext of the articles. Access is provided on the web, by CD-ROM, or on microfiche. This product is especially useful for drug information centers and HMO's that may not otherwise be able to access a large collection of electronic journals.

INTERNATIONAL PHARMACEUTICAL ABSTRACTS

The scope of the *International Pharmaceutical Abstracts (IPA)* is different from either *MEDLINE* or *EMBASE*. *IPA* is produced by the American Society of Health-System Pharmacists (ASHP) and covers 850 pharmacy periodicals. It is a small database, but it covers publications not indexed elsewhere, including pharmacy trade magazines, state pharmacy journals, and the meeting abstracts of pharmacy-related associations.

Some drug therapy journals that are indexed in *MEDLINE* also are indexed by *IPA*. However, because *IPA*'s indexing rules are somewhat different from *MEDLINE*'s, a researcher may sometimes turn up materials in *IPA* that were missed in *MEDLINE* searches.

Many pharmacy and pharmaceutical science topics are much better searched in *IPA* than in any other database. This is the best database to use to find large numbers of articles on pharmacy administration, drug laws and legislation, and pharmacy ethics. Pharmaceutical manufacturing is covered as well. Ovid, Dialog, and the American Society of Health-System Pharmacists make *IPA* available through the web and on CD-ROM. Links from *IPA* to the indexed fulltext articles are not available as of this writing.

CHEMICAL ABSTRACTS

Chemical Abstracts (sometimes called *CAplus* or *CA Search*) covers areas of interest to pharmaceutical scientists. Perhaps the world's largest scientific database, *Chemical Abstracts* is produced by the American Chemical Society's Chemical Abstracts Service (CAS) in Columbus, Ohio. It contains 17 million abstracts from journals, patents, technical reports, books, conference proceedings, and dissertations. It is the most important database for those interested in drug development.

An important adjunct to *Chemical Abstracts* is the CAS Registry System that assigns code numbers to chemical substances, providing a unique identifier for each substance no matter how many names the chemical may have worldwide. This CAS registry number is so valuable that other databases use it to make sure that searchers can find all literature relating to a particular chemical. The CAS Registry System may be searched separately in some database systems.

A special type of searching that can be done in *Chemical Abstracts* is structure searching. It allows the user to draw the chemical structure of a substance and to search from that.

There are links from a *Chemical Abstracts* search to full-text articles available on the web, but to access them the searcher or the searcher's institution must subscribe to the journal that contains the article.

Vendors of *Chemical Abstracts* include Ovid, Dialog, and STN. Some subsets of the database are available on CD-ROM. Some institutions and corporations subscribe to SciFinder (or its academic equivalent, SciFinder Scholar), a user-friendly web interface that allows unlimited searching. Otherwise, *Chemical Abstracts* is very expensive to search and should be accessed only by those trained to do so. Classes are offered around the country by CAS. Academic chemistry or science librarians can often direct a researcher to an experienced freelance literature researcher.

BIOSIS PREVIEWS

Another important scientific database is *BIOSIS Previews*, the online version of *Biological Abstracts* and the *BioResearch Index*. It is produced by BIOSIS (Philadelphia, PA). *BIOSIS Previews* covers the literature of the life sciences, including preclinical toxicity and carcinogenicity studies. Among the many

ways it can be searched are by keywords, broad subject areas, and codes representing taxonomic groups. Vendors include BIOSIS, Ovid, Dialog, and STN. Ovid provides links to fulltext articles.

Other Databases

In addition to the major online databases described above, there are many specialized databases that might be of use in the study of pharmacy. Some of these are available on standalone CD-ROMs, but most are accessible only through one of the two major database vendors, Dialog and Ovid.

ADIS LMS Drug Alerts (Langhorne, PA, ADIS International): Evaluates key articles from 2300 journals. Includes an evaluation score for clinical trials.

Adis Newsletters (Langhorne, PA: Adis International): Contains articles from the publications *Inpharma, Reactions*, and *Pharmacoeconomics*.

Adis Clinical Trials (Langhorne, PA: Adis International). Evaluates "key papers" from 1600 international clinical journals.

Adis R&D Insight (Langhorne, PA: Adis International). Reports on drugs under development, including clinical and marketing information.

ESPICom Pharmaceutical and Medical Device News (Chichester, UK: ESPICOM Business Intelligence). Fulltext of articles from *Pharma-Company Insight* and *Medical Industry Week*.

AMED: Allied and Complementary Medicine Database (London: British Library). Index to 596 journals, mostly European, Its coverage of complementary medicine is the most useful aspect for pharmacists. Document delivery system available.

Derwent Drug File (London: Derwent Information): Covers 1150 pharmaceutical journals on drug development and manufacture. Much more highly focused on drugs than is *Chemical Abstracts*.

Derwent Drug Registry File (London: Derwent Information): Retrieves groups of drugs with common structural features.

DIOGENES FDA Regulatory Updates (Gaithersburg, MD: Diogenes): News stories and unpublished documents relating to US regulation.

Drug Data Report (Barcelona: Prous Science): Continuously updated information on more than 65,000 bioactive compounds.

F-D-C Reports (Chevy Chase, MD: F-D-C Reports): Complete text of F-D-C Reports' industry newsletters including *Prescription Pharmaceuticals & Biotechnology* (*Pink Sheet*) and *Nonprescription Pharmaceuticals and Nutritionals* (*Tan Sheet*).

IMSWorld (London: IMS Global Services): Collection of databases that profile pharmaceutical companies, the pharmaceutical industry by country, and new drug launches.

NDA Pipeline: New Drugs (Chevy Chase, MD: F-D-C Reports): Tracks drugs through discovery, clinical trials, New Drug Application, and approval or disapproval by the FDA.

Pharmaceutical and Healthcare Industry News (Richmond, Surrey, England: PJB Publications): Complete text of PJB's industry newsletters: *SCRIP: World Pharmaceutical News*; *Clinica: World Medical Device and Diagnostic News*; *Animal Pharm* and others.

Pharmaceutical News Index (*PNI*) (Ann Arbor, MI: ProQuest): Indexes a number of major pharmaceutical industry newsletters.

Pharmaprojects (Richmond, Surrey, England: PJB Publications): Reports on worldwide progress of new pharmaceutical products.

SciSearch (Philadelphia: Institute for Scientific Information): If one knows of a pertinent article, one can locate subsequent articles that have cited the original publication.

SEDBASE: Side Effects of Drugs (Amsterdam, Netherlands: Elsevier Science): Analysis of published drug side-effects literature.

Toxfile (Bethesda, MD: National Library of Medicine): Compiles toxicity information from several online databases.

Searching of these databases can be expensive and require skill and experience. Science librarians and freelance literature researchers have the requisite abilities to get the best and most cost-effective results.

Secondary Literature

Compilations, commentaries, and digests of the primary scientific literature are referred to as *secondary literature*. A *review article* summarizes the research that has been done on a particular topic. While EBM supporters downplay the traditional review article, it is still a useful secondary source. Usually written by invitation, the review article can serve as an excellent introduction to an area of research. Review articles are found in scholarly journals and also in special book collections with titles that begin *Annual Review of . . .*, *Progress in . . .* or something similar. Review articles in both journals and books can be found by using online or print indexes.

Other secondary sources include drug monographs, treatises, and various books written for a professional audience. They can be identified by using standard bibliographies, such as those found in a textbook, or in such compilations as the *AACP Basic Resources List for Pharmaceutical Education* (see "Sources for Further Reference" below). Once titles of interest are identified, a researcher should use library catalogs to locate the works themselves.

Almost all library catalogs are accessible from the web. From a desktop computer, a researcher can consult the catalog of the National Library of Medicine or large pharmacy school collections, such as that of the Philadelphia College of Pharmacy at the University of the Sciences in Philadelphia. Books unavailable in a local library usually can be obtained through interlibrary loan.

Textbooks

Textbooks are usually thought of as being written for students, but they can also serve as a state-of-the-art summation for a particular area. In medicine, certain textbooks are held in such high regard that editions continue to be produced long after the original authors are gone. *Remington: The Science and Practice of Pharmacy* (21st ed., Baltimore: Lippincott Williams & Wilkins, 2005) and *Goodman and Gilman's The Pharmacologic Basis of Therapeutics* (Hardman JG, Limbird LL, Gilman, AG, eds, 10th ed., New York: McGraw-Hill, 2001) are examples of works known by the names of those who first wrote them and which are considered to be the standard of practice. Textbooks can serve as an introduction to a new area, and reading new editions is a way to keep up to date.

Textbook Collections

Increasingly, standard textbooks are being made available online, primarily as part of packages. Stat!Ref (Jackson, WY: Teton Data Systems) and MDConsult (Amsterdam: Elsevier Science) are examples of products that allow the researcher to search across a number of textbooks and other materials at once. In addition to textbooks, MDConsult includes the fulltext of 50 journals and a thousand clinical practice guidelines. UpToDate (Wellesley, MA: UpToDate) is still yet another way of packaging online information. It includes topic reviews on hundreds of topics with links to *MEDLINE* abstracts. These packages can be purchased as web subscriptions, CD-ROMs or DVDs.

Trade Literature

In addition to scholarly literature, both pharmacists and pharmaceutical scientists can benefit from accounts of good practice and expressions of opinion. Periodicals such as *Journal of the American Pharmaceutical Association* (Washington, DC: APhA), *Drug Topics* (Montvale, NJ: Medical Economics), or *Pharmaceutical Executive* (Eugene, OR: Advanstar Communications) contain this kind of information. Articles on a particular topic can be found by using the *IPA* database.

SPECIAL INFORMATION SOURCES IN PHARMACY AND THE PHARMACEUTICAL SCIENCES

A variety of reference works are published on drugs and their uses. Many people call all such sources *pharmacopeias,* but a modern pharmacopeia is a very specialized reference work used mostly by pharmaceutical scientists and manufacturers. Reference works containing information on the therapeutic use of drugs such as the well-known *Physicians' Desk Reference* (*PDR*) are more properly called *drug compendia.* Pharmacists and other professionals in the pharmaceutical and health-care professions need to know the different types of drug reference works, what types of information can be found in them, and examples of each.

We will outline some of the major types of pharmacy and pharmaceutical science reference works available and give brief descriptions of important titles in each category. This is not a comprehensive bibliography but it does include references to bibliographies at the end. Almost all of the works described are available in print format. Notable exceptions are the *DRUGDEX System*, the *IDENTIDEX System*, and the *POISINDEX System*. These three titles are all produced by MICROMEDEX, and are available only in electronic formats.

Many of the other titles mentioned below are also available online or in other electronic formats. Since information about the various formats and their availability changes so rapidly, it is not included here. However, publishers' Internet addresses (URLs) have been included for the reader's convenience in obtaining information on the availability of other versions.

Numbers in brackets in the following text refer to references at the end of each section.

Pharmacopeias

In the past, pharmacopeias included information on the therapeutic uses of drugs, but modern pharmacopeias present official standards for purity, strength, quality, and analysis of drugs. Pharmacopeias are issued or authorized by governments or by international agencies. Most pharmacopeias are kept up-to-date through regular supplements.

The Federal Food, Drug, and Cosmetic (FDC) Act recognizes the *United States Pharmacopeia/National Formulary* (*USP/NF*) [1] as the official pharmacopeia of the United States. The *USP/NF* actually consists of two separate titles published in one volume. It does not include all the drugs approved for use in the United States (see *Approved Drug Products with Therapeutic Equivalence Evaluations* below); rather, it includes only those drugs and excipients for which standards have been developed and accepted by the members of the United States Pharmacopeial Convention, a representative organization of physicians, pharmacists, and others in the pharmaceutical and health-care communities. The *USP* is the larger of the two titles in the *USP/NF* and contains monographs on drugs and other substances with therapeutic uses. Standards for many dietary supplements, including some from botanical sources, are included in the *USP*. The *NF* includes monographs for excipients, the nontherapeutic additives used in pharmaceuticals (see Chapter 45 for more information about excipients).

After the *USP/NF*, the best-known national pharmacopeia is probably the *British Pharmacopoeia* (*BP*) [2], authorized by the government of the United Kingdom. The *European Pharmacopoeia* [3], published by the Council of Europe, sets standards for the use of the Council's members. The standards in the World Health Organization's (WHO) *International Pharmacopoeia* [4] are recommendations for the consideration of individual countries rather than requirements.

1. *United States Pharmacopeia/National Formulary.* Rockville, MD: United States Pharmacopeial Convention (http://www.usp.org), annual.
2. *British Pharmacopoeia 2003.* London: Her Majesty's Stationery Office (http://www.hmso.gov.uk). 6 volumes.
3. *European Pharmacopoeia,* 4th ed. Strasbourg, France: Council of Europe (http://www.coe.int), 2002.
4. *International Pharmacopoeia,* 3rd ed. Geneva: WHO (http://www.who.int/en), 1979–2003. 5 volumes.

Formularies and Related Lists

In the past, formularies were recipe books for making drugs, but now they are usually lists of drugs approved for use by a particular hospital, health plan, or government. Many hospitals and health plans have committees to consider which drugs should be included in the institution's formulary. In the United States, these committees are usually called pharmacy and therapeutics committees (P&T committees). Most P&T committees are composed of members of the institution's medical staff and include one or more representatives from the pharmacy. Chapter 127 discusses P&T committees and their roles.

In the United States, the Food and Drug Administration (FDA) has the responsibility to determine that marketed drugs are safe and effective. The FDA produces *Approved Drug Products with Therapeutic Equivalence Evaluations* [5], an annual publication that is popularly called the *Orange Book* after the color of its cover. The *Orange Book* lists both the drugs that have been approved by the FDA, and the FDA's evaluations of the therapeutic equivalence of different manufacturers' preparations of approved drugs. The *Orange Book* does not include drugs that were on the market prior to 1938, nor does it list drugs approved only on the basis of safety. Lists of products on the market before 1938 along with the complete *Orange Book* may be found in *USP DI, Volume III, Approved Drug Products and Legal Requirements* [6]. The *National Formulary* published with the *USP* is not a true formulary (see "Pharmacopeias" above).

5. *Approved Drug Products with Therapeutic Equivalence Evaluations.* Rockville, MD: Food and Drug Administration, US Department of Health and Human Services (www.fda.gov), annual.
6. *USP DI, Volume III, Approved Drug Products and Legal Requirements.* Englewood, CO: Thomson MICROMEDEX (http://www.micromedex.com), annual.

Nomenclature

Every drug has at least two names, its full chemical name and its generic drug name. A drug may also have other names including variant chemical names, proprietary trade names, and variant generic names. Additionally, drug names sometimes differ between countries. Table 8-1 lists some of the names used for the drug acetaminophen. For more information on drug names, see Chapter 27.

The *USP Dictionary of USAN and International Drug Names* [7] is the authoritative list of the United States adopted names (USANs) for drugs. As the title indicates, this work is published by the publisher of the *USP*, the United States Pharmacopeial Convention, as part of its standards-setting responsibilities. The World Health Organization establishes international nonproprietary names (INNs) and publishes them in *International Nonproprietary Names (INN) for Pharmaceutical Substances* [8].

Two other important sources for verifying drug names, especially those used outside of the United States, are *Index Nominum* [9] and the *Merck Index* [10].

Index Nominum is edited by the Swiss Pharmaceutical Society and includes drug names from around the world. Most *Index Nominum* monographs include chemical names and structures, generic names, proprietary names, therapeutic uses, and manufacturers.

The *Merck Index* has over 10,000 monographs on drugs, common organic chemicals, and a variety of other substances used in the pharmaceutical and chemical industries. Each *Merck Index* monograph includes the substance's various names (including chemical, generic, and proprietary), physical constants, chemical formula and structure, patent information, therapeutic category, and literature citations.

7. *USP Dictionary of USAN and International Drug Names.* Rockville, MD: US Pharmacopeial Convention (http://www.usp.org), annual.
8. *International Nonproprietary Names (INN) for Pharmaceutical Substances,* Cumulative List No. 10. Geneva: WHO (http://www.who.int/en), 2002. Available as CD-ROM only.

9. Swiss Pharmaceutical Society, ed. *Index Nominum: International Drug Directory,* 18th ed. Stuttgart, Germany: Medpharm (distributed in the US by CRC Press, http://www.crcpress.com), 2004.
10. O'Neil MJ, Smith A, Heckelman PE, eds. *Merck Index: an Encyclopedia of Chemicals, Drugs, and Biologicals,* 13th ed. Whitehouse Station, NJ: Merck (http://www.merck.com), 2001.

US Drug Compendia: Prescription Products

For concise information on the therapeutic use of drugs (including dosage, contraindications, adverse effects, and pharmacokinetics), there are a variety of drug compendia. Probably the best-known one is the *Physicians' Desk Reference* [11], commonly referred to as the *PDR*. Other titles often found in pharmacies and pharmacy libraries in the United States are *AHFS Drug Information* [12] (sometimes called the *American Hospital Formulary Service*); *Drug Facts and Comparisons* [13]; *Mosby's Drug Consult* [14]; and *USP DI, Volume I, Drug Information for the Health Care Professional* [15]. Each of these works is arranged slightly differently with its own criteria for inclusion, but all include monographs for drugs with details on their therapeutic use.

The *PDR* lists only those drugs sold under a trade name, and the monographs it publishes are the FDA-approved labeling for those drugs. All of the other compendia contain information from the FDA-approved labeling as well as additional data from other sources, such as journal articles and textbooks. They also include descriptions of so-called *off-label uses,* therapeutic uses of a drug that do not appear on the FDA-approved labeling. Except for the *PDR*, these compendia are written or edited by pharmacists or other health-care professionals. The criteria for inclusion in these compendia vary from title to title; for example, *Drug Facts and Comparisons* includes some nonprescription products. All of these titles, including the *PDR*, are issued annually and most are updated by supplements throughout the year. A notable exception is *Drug Facts and Comparisons,* which is published both as a loose-leaf service updated monthly and as an annual volume.

By virtue of its electronic format, the *DRUGDEX System* [16] contains much more information than can fit into any one-volume printed compendium. *DRUGDEX*'s drug monographs are longer and more detailed than those found in the above compendia, and each monograph includes extensive references to the medical literature. In addition to monographs about individual drug products, *DRUGDEX* includes Drug Consults,

Table 8-1. Selected Names of a Drug

TYPE OF NAME	NAME
United States Approved Name (USAN)	Acetaminophen
United States Pharmacopeia (USP)	Acetaminophen
Recommended International Nonproprietary Name (Rec.INN)	Paracetamol
European Pharmacopoiea	Paracetamol
Chemical names	N-(4-Hydroxyphenyl)acetamide 4'-Hydroxyacetanilide p-Acetaminophenol
Proprietary names (country)	Asomal (Turkey) Becetamol (Switzerland) Dristancito (Argentina) Progesic (Indonesia; Hong Kong) Tylenol (United States and others)

Data from O'Neil, MJ; Smith, A; Heckelman, PE, eds. *Merck Index: an Encyclopedia of Chemicals, Drugs, and Biologicals,* 13th ed. Whitehouse Station, NJ: Merck, 2001, and Swiss Pharmaceutical Society, ed. *Index Nominum: International Drug Directory,* 18th ed. Stuttgart, Germany: Medpharm, 2004.

which answer questions about specific drugs and drug therapies. In addition to prescription drugs, the Drug Consults cover such topics as investigational drugs, herbal medications, and drugs of abuse. *DRUGDEX* monographs are written by drug information specialists. The *DRUGDEX* database is updated quarterly, but the individual monographs in it are not updated as frequently. Each monograph includes the date of its latest revision and its author's name.

11. *Physicians' Desk Reference.* Montvale, NJ: Thomson PDR (http://www.pdr.net), annual.
12. *AHFS Drug Information.* Bethesda, MD: ASHP (http://www.ashp.org), annual.
13. *Drug Facts and Comparisons.* St Louis, MO: Facts and Comparisons (http://www.factsandcomparisons.com), loose-leaf updated monthly or annual bound volume.
14. *Mosby's Drug Consult.* St Louis, MO: Mosby (http://www.us.elsevierhealth.com), annual.
15. *USP DI, Volume I, Drug Information for the Health Care Professional.* Englewood, CO: Thomson MICROMEDEX (http://www.micromedex.com), annual.
16. *DRUGDEX System.* Englewood, CO: MICROMEDEX (http://www.micromedex.com), quarterly.

US Drug Compendia: Nonprescription Products

The number of nonprescription drugs and the market for them continues to grow. There are several drug compendia dedicated to these products and their proper use.

The *Handbook of Nonprescription Drugs* [17] is organized by symptom or disorder. Each chapter includes a description of the symptom/disorder and available treatments. The book includes tables of available drugs and their ingredients, and extensive decision trees to aid health professionals in consulting with patients about nonprescription therapies. Chapters include literature references.

Nonprescription Drug Therapy [18] is also arranged by symptom/disorder. While it covers the same topics as the *Handbook of Nonprescription Drugs*, it is much more concise. It is available as a loose-leaf service updated quarterly or as an annual bound volume.

The *Physicians' Desk Reference for Nonprescription Drugs and Dietary Supplements* [19] includes participating manufacturers' label information for nonprescription products.

17. Berardi, RR, ed. *Handbook of Nonprescription Drugs: An Interactive Approach to Self-Care,* 14th ed. Washington, DC: APhA (http://www.aphanet.org), 2004.
18. Covington, TR, ed. *Nonprescription Drug Therapy: Guiding Patient Self-Care.* St. Louis: Facts and Comparisons (http://www.factsandcomparisons.com), loose-leaf service updated quarterly or annual volume.
19. *Physicians' Desk Reference for Nonprescription Drugs and Dietary Supplements.* Montvale, NJ: Thomson PDR (http://www.pdr.net), annual.

US Drug Compendia: Parenterals

Parenteral drugs are those that are injected directly into the body and not absorbed through the gastrointestinal system.

Trissel's *Handbook on Injectable Drugs* [20] has dosage, stability, and compatibility information. The *Handbook* also includes monographs for some investigational drugs and for some foreign drugs. The *King Guide to Parenteral Admixtures* [21] is a comprehensive reference on the compatibility of parenterals. This work is in tabular format and includes information on the compatibility of both drug-drug and drug-infusion fluid mixtures.

20. Trissel LA. *Handbook on Injectable Drugs,* 12th ed. Bethesda, MD: ASHP (http://www.ashp.org), 2003.
21. Catania PA, ed. *King Guide to Parenteral Admixtures.* St Louis, MO: King Guide Publications (http://www.kingguide.com), loose-leaf updated quarterly or annual bound volume.

US Drug Compendia: Catalogs

The major catalog of products commonly found in US drugstores and pharmacies is the *Drug Topics Red Book* [22]. This catalog lists average wholesale prices and manufacturers for both prescription and nonprescription products, including a variety of health and beauty aids. It includes generic drug information that is often difficult to find elsewhere. The *Red Book* also includes other information of use to a practicing pharmacist, such as lists of the top-selling prescription drugs, and directories of poison control centers and state boards of pharmacy.

22. *Drug Topics Red Book.* Montvale, NJ: Thomson PDR (http://www.pdr.net), annual.

US Drug Compendia: Physical Identification

Several of the drug compendia described above include color photographs of tablets, capsules, and other dosage forms to aid in their identification. However, the most useful sources for the physical identification of drugs are ones that include an index of the codes imprinted on the dosage forms. Both *Ident-A-Drug Reference for Drug Tablet and Capsule Identification* [23] and the *IDENTIDEX System* [24] include such an index. The *IDENTIDEX System* also indexes the physical description (color and shape) of the dosage form and includes street drugs. In addition, the *IDENTIDEX System* includes monographs on the toxicology of the substances indexed.

23. *Ident-A-Drug Reference for Drug Tablet and Capsule Identification.* Stockton, CA: Therapeutic Research Center (http://www.therapeuticresearch.com), annual.
24. *IDENTIDEX System.* Englewood, CO: MICROMEDEX (http://www.micromedex.com), quarterly.

US Drug Compendia: Consumer Drug Information

Drug information for consumers can be found in a variety of publications including books, newspapers, magazines, and pamphlets as well as at many websites on the Internet. This section will consider only two types of books: guides sold to consumers by trade publishers, and compendia sold to pharmacists and other health-care professionals by organizations better known for their professional publications.

Among the most popular of the consumer guides are: Griffith's *Complete Guide to Prescription and Nonprescription Drugs* [25]; Rybacki's *Essential Guide to Prescription Drugs* [26]; and *The Pill Book* [27]. All of these books include basic information about drugs including the conditions they are used to treat, their safe use and their possible adverse effects.

Patient Drug Facts [28] and *USP DI, Volume II, Advice for the Patient* [29] are both marketed to pharmacists and other health-care professionals to assist them in their patient counseling activities. *Patient Drug Facts* includes both a quarterly loose-leaf update service and computer software. The loose-leaf is for use by the pharmacist in patient counseling, and the software provides customized printouts for patients. *USP DI, Volume II, Advice for the Patient* is published annually with supplements issued during the year. Pharmacists are given permission to make copies of individual monographs for patients when filling prescriptions for the drugs. *USP DI, Volume II, Advice for the Patient* is also sold directly to consumers by Consumer Reports under the title *Consumer Drug Reference*. Its monographs are available free on the Internet at various sites including the National Library of Medicine's consumer health site, MedlinePlus <http://www.medlineplus.gov>.

25. Griffith HW. *Complete Guide to Prescription & Nonprescription Drugs.* New York: Perigee (http://penguinputnam.com), annual.
26. Rybacki JJ. *The Essential Guide to Prescription Drugs.* New York: HarperCollins (http://www.harpercollins.com), annual.

27. Silverman, HM, ed. *The Pill Book*. New York: Bantam (http://www.randomhouse.com), biennial.
28. *Patient Drug Facts*. St. Louis, MO: Facts and Comparisons (http://www.factsandcomparisons.com), loose-leaf updated quarterly or bound volume.
29. *USP DI, Volume II, Advice for the Patient*. Englewood, CO: Thomson MICROMEDEX (http://www.micromedex.com), annual. Also published as *Complete Drug Reference*. Yonkers, NY: Consumer Reports, annual.

Foreign Drug Compendia

Martindale: The Complete Drug Reference [30] is one of the preeminent international drug compendia. It is a compendium of therapeutic and other information on drugs and medicines from around the world. Its monographs include synopses and citations of published literature. *Martindale* also includes lists of proprietary products and manufacturers, making it an invaluable reference for identifying foreign drugs.

Most developed countries have at least one drug compendium with information about the drugs available there. Examples include the *CPS: Compendium of Pharmaceutical Specialties* [31] (Canada), *Diccionario de Especialidades Farmaceuticas* [32] (Mexico), *Rote Liste* [33] (Germany), and *Vidal* [34] (France).

30. Sweetman SC, ed. *Martindale: The Complete Drug Reference*, 33rd ed. London; Chicago: Pharmaceutical Press (http://www.pharmpress.com), 2002.
31. *CPS: Compendium of Pharmaceutical Specialties*. Ottawa, Canada: Canadian Pharmacists Association (http://www.pharmacists.ca), annual.
32. *Diccionario de Especialidades Farmaceuticas*. Mexico City: Ediciones PLM (distributed in the US by Thomson PDR, http://www.pdr.net), annual.
33. *Rote Liste*. Aulendorf, Germany: Editio Cantor Verlag (http://www.ecv.de/), annual.
34. *Vidal: Le Dictionnaire*. Paris: Vidal (http://www.vidal.fr), annual.

Herbal Medicines and Natural Products

In recent years, interest in herbal medicines and medicines from other natural products has grown among health-care professionals, scientists, and the general public.

The Review of Natural Products [35] is a monthly loose-leaf service that covers both herbal and other natural products (for example, charcoal and shark derivatives). Its monographs are written for health-care professionals, and each includes a brief overview of the chemistry, pharmacology, and toxicology of the product. Because it is updated every month, the *Review* often has information on products of current popular interest. *Herbal Medicines* [36] is written for health-care professionals, particularly those in the United Kingdom. Each of the monographs includes a 'Pharmaceutical Comment' with a recommendation on whether the herbal medicine should be used.

Pharmacognosy, Phytochemistry, Medicinal Plants [37] by Jean Bruneton is written for scientists working in the areas of pharmacognosy and phytochemistry. Each chapter describes a class of phytochemicals and the plants from which the chemicals may be isolated.

Tyler's Honest Herbal: A Sensible Guide to the Use of Herbs and Related Remedies [38] is written for the layperson. Each monograph includes a review of the literature and recommendations from the author.

35. *The Review of Natural Products*. St Louis, MO: Facts and Comparisons (http://www.factsandcomparisons.com), loose-leaf updated monthly or annual bound volume.
36. Barnes J, Anderson LA, Phillipson JD. *Herbal Medicines: A Guide for Healthcare Professionals*, 2nd ed. London: Pharmaceutical Press (http://www.pharmpress.com), 2002.
37. Bruneton J. *Pharmacognosy, Phytochemistry, Medicinal Plants*, 2nd ed. Paris: Lavoisier (distributed in the US by Springer, http://www.springeronline.com), 1999.

38. Foster S, Tyler VE. *Tyler's Honest Herbal: A Sensible Guide to the Use of Herbs and Related Remedies*. 4th ed. Binghamton, NY: Haworth Herbal (http://www.haworthpressinc.com), 1999.

Drug Interactions and Adverse Drug Reactions

Three loose-leaf titles monitor and report on the clinical literature about drug interactions: Hansten and Horn's *Drug Interactions: Analysis and Management* [39]; *Drug Interaction Facts* [40]; and *Evaluations of Drug Interactions* [41]. Each of these is updated several times a year. All include information on the drugs (or drug classes) involved in an interaction, the clinical significance of the interaction, the mechanism of the interaction, and the published evidence of the interaction.

As herbal medicines have become more popular with consumers, there has been increasing concern about the interactions they may have with other medications. *Drug Interaction Facts: Herbal Supplements and Food* [42] reviews the literature on these interactions and those between medications and food. It is updated quarterly.

Meyler's Side Effects of Drugs: an Encyclopedia of Adverse Reactions and Interactions [43] is a comprehensive review of the literature on adverse drug reactions and interactions. Between editions, it is supplemented by the *Side Effects of Drugs Annual* [44]. Both of these titles make extensive references to their own earlier editions and volumes as well as to the clinical literature.

In addition, all of the titles that were listed above in the section "US Drug Compendia: Prescription Products" contain information on possible drug interactions and adverse drug reactions.

39. Hansten PD, Horn JR. *Drug Interactions: Analysis and Management*. St. Louis: Facts and Comparisons (http://www.factsandcomparisons.com), loose-leaf updated quarterly.
40. *Drug Interaction Facts*. St Louis, MO: Facts and Comparisons (http://www.factsandcomparisons.com), loose-leaf updated quarterly or annual bound volume.
41. *Evaluations of Drug Interactions*. St Louis, MO: First DataBank (http://www.firstdatabank.com), loose-leaf updated 6 times per year.
42. *Drug Interaction Facts: Herbal Supplements and Food*. St Louis, MO: Facts and Comparisons (http://www.factsandcomparisons.com), loose-leaf updated quarterly.
43. Dukes MNG, ed. *Meyler's Side Effects of Drugs: an Encyclopedia of Adverse Reactions and Interactions*, 14th ed. Amsterdam, Netherlands: Elsevier (http://www.elsevier.com), 2000.
44. *Side Effects of Drugs Annual*. Amsterdam, Netherlands: Elsevier (http://www.elsevier.com), annual.

Poisoning and Toxicology

The field of toxicology is a large and diverse one that encompasses the laboratory research specialty as well as the clinical management of poisoning, including forensics and occupational (and home) health and safety issues.

One of the most comprehensive works on poisons and poisoning is the *POISINDEX System* [45] from MICROMEDEX. The *POISINDEX System* database includes product and substance information for household and industrial chemicals, pharmaceuticals, plants, and animals. It includes protocols for treating poisoning from all the listed substances.

The Poisoning & Toxicology Handbook [46] provides its user with a quick guide to toxicology, poisons, and poisoning. In *Sax's Dangerous Properties of Industrial Materials* [47], the emphasis is on the substances themselves. Each monograph includes chemical and physical data on the substance as well as toxicological data and literature citations.

Clarke's Analysis of Drugs and Poisons [48] provides methods of analysis used to determine the presence of specific drugs in biological samples. In addition, its drug monographs include ultraviolet and infrared spectra, and information on the fate of the drug and its metabolites in the body.

45. *POISINDEX System*. Englewood, CO: MICROMEDEX (http://www.micromedex.com); quarterly.
46. Leikin, JB; Paloucek, FP. *Poisoning & Toxicology Handbook*, 3rd ed. Hudson, OH: Lexi-Comp (http://www.lexi.com), 2002.
47. Lewis RJ. *Sax's Dangerous Properties of Industrial Materials*, 10th ed. New York, Wiley (http://www.wiley.com), 2000. 3 volumes.
48. Moffat, HC. *Clarke's Analysis of Drugs and Poisons: in Pharmaceuticals, Body Fluids and Post-Mortem Material*. 3rd ed. London: Pharmaceutical Press (http://www.pharmpress.com), 2003. 2 volumes.

Cosmetics and Toiletries

The *International Cosmetic Ingredient Dictionary and Handbook* [49] contains information on the chemical class, composition, function, and label requirements of ingredients used in cosmetics manufactured in the US, the European Union, and elsewhere. The series *Cosmetic and Toiletry Formulations* [50] contains industrial recipes for making a variety of cosmetics and toiletries. Each formulation includes the raw materials needed and the amount of each, suggestions of how to formulate the product, and the source of the formulation.

49. *International Cosmetic Ingredient Dictionary and Handbook*, 8th ed. Washington, DC: Cosmetic, Toiletry and Fragrance Association (http://www.ctfa.org), 2000. 3 volumes.
50. Flick EW. *Cosmetic and Toiletry Formulations*, 2nd ed. Park Ridge, NJ: Noyes (http://www.williamandrew.com/), 1989– Multiple volumes.

Other Sources for Pharmaceutical Scientists

In addition to the above sources, pharmaceutical scientists often need information sources on the development and manufacture of pharmaceutical products including the excipients used in them.

The *Pharmaceutical Dictionary* [51] provides translations to and from English, French, German and Spanish for terms commonly used by pharmaceutical scientists and those employed in pharmaceutical manufacturing. The *Encyclopedia of Pharmaceutical Technology* [52] contains signed articles about the materials, methods, and processes used in producing drugs and dosage forms. It also includes articles on the development and regulation of pharmaceuticals.

The series *Profiles of Drug Substances, Excipients and Related Methodology* [53] began as *Analytical Profiles of Drug Substances* [54] in 1972. Its purpose was to supplement the monographs published in various compendia by providing information on the physical and chemical properties, methods of synthesis, and other biochemical data of drug substances. Twenty years later, the series increased its coverage to include excipients and changed its title to *Analytical Profiles of Drug Substances and Excipients* [55]. In 2003, the series changed its title once again to the current one, *Profiles of Drug Substances, Excipients and Related Methodology*. The volumes are not cumulative but each volume includes a cumulative index.

The *Handbook of Pharmaceutical Excipients* [56] describes the uses and the chemical and physical properties of excipients used in the manufacture of pharmaceutical dosage forms. Most of its monographs include illustrations. The monographs in the *Fiedler Encyclopedia of Excipients* [57] are much briefer than those of the *Handbook of Pharmaceutical Excipients*, but it includes many more entries and is a particularly good source for tradenames.

51. Maas A, Brawley J. *Pharmaceutical Dictionary: English, Deutsch, Français, Español*. 4th ed., rev. and expanded. Aulendorf, Germany: Editio Cantor Verlag (http://www.ecv.de/), 2002.
52. Swarbrick J, Boylan JC, eds. *Encyclopedia of Pharmaceutical Technology*, 2nd ed. New York: Dekker (http://www.dekker.com), 2003. 3 volumes.
53. *Profiles of Drug Substances, Excipients and Related Methodology*, volume 30. Amsterdam, Boston: Elsevier (http://www.elsevier.com), 2003.
54. Florey K, ed. *Analytical Profiles of Drug Substances*, volumes 1–20. New York: Academic Press (http://us.elsevierhealth.com), 1972–1991.
55. *Analytical Profiles of Drug Substances and Excipients*, volumes 21–29. San Diego, CA: Academic Press (http://us.elsevierhealth.com), 1992–2002.
56. Rowe, RC, Sheskey, PJ, Weller PJ, eds. *Handbook of Pharmaceutical Excipients*, 4th ed. Washington, DC: APhA (http://www.aphanet.org), 2003.
57. Hoepfner E-MH, Reng A, Schmidt PC, eds. *Fiedler Encyclopedia of Excipients: for Pharmaceuticals, Cosmetics and Related Areas*, 5th ed. Aulendorf, Germany: Editio Cantor Verlag (http://www.ecv.de/), 2002. 2 volumes.

Sources For Further Reference

This chapter has presented some of the major pharmacy and pharmaceutical science reference works in brief. Bonnie Snow, in her book *Drug Information: A Guide to Current Resources* [58], considers the universe of such works in greater depth. The Library/Educational Resources Section of the American Association of Colleges of Pharmacy (AACP) maintains the *AACP Basic Resources List for Pharmaceutical Education* [59]. This list is arranged by subject and includes current textbooks and treatises as well as reference works recommended for inclusion in pharmacy college libraries. The list is available at the AACP's website.

58. Snow B. *Drug Information: A Guide to Current Resources*, 2nd ed. Lanham, MD: Medical Library Association and Scarecrow Press (http://www.scarecrowpress.com/), 1999.
59. *AACP Basic Resources List for Pharmaceutical Education*. Alexandria, VA: AACP, irregular. Accessible via http://www.aacp.org/

RESOURCES ON THE INTERNET

The Internet has revolutionized information and communications for all professions. Internet resources are available 24 hours a day, worldwide, to virtually anyone with a computer and telecommunications capability. Pharmacists and pharmaceutical scientists are well represented on the Internet. Resources are available to help these professionals communicate with each other, address patient needs, and keep informed about drug developments. We will discuss the types of pharmacy-related resources available on the Internet, giving special emphasis to resources available through the web.

Electronic Mail and Discussion Groups

Electronic mail, or *e-mail*, was one of the first Internet resources available to pharmacists and is used daily by many professionals. E-mail allows the pharmacist to communicate quickly with patients, physicians, and colleagues around the world. The sender posts a message to a specific Internet e-mail address. The message is delivered via the Internet and stored in the receiver's inbox until it is read. The receiver of the message may reply to the message, forward it to another e-mail user, print the message, delete it, or store it for future reference. Electronic attachments such as document files, pictures, and sound or video clips may also be sent via e-mail.

Several e-mail discussion groups, or *mailing lists,* have developed for the pharmacist. These forums allow groups of pharmacists with common interests or specialties to share information and ideas. The mailing list's software allows a user to subscribe to a discussion group and post messages to a central address. These messages are then automatically distributed to all of the subscribers to the list. Mailing lists exist for students, members of professional organizations, and individuals interested in specific topics (eg, geriatric pharmacotherapy, immunology-transplants, or hypertension).

Some e-mail mailing lists are moderated, restricted in membership, or both. In a *moderated list,* messages are first routed to an individual who determines whether the message fits within the scope of the discussion group. The message is then either forwarded on to the group or rejected. Some mailing lists, maintain an *archive* of past messages that is available on the web. Lists of pharmacy related mailing lists may be found on the web at the Virtual Pharmacy Library (http://www.pharmacy.org) and at PharmWeb (http://www.pharmweb.com).

Pharmacists also communicate via *Usenet newsgroups.* These discussion forums allow individuals to post a new message or to reply to a message. Newsgroups are accessed through an *Internet service provider* (ISP) using software called a *newsreader.* Common newreaders include Microsoft Outlook Express and Netscape Messenger. Newsgroups differ from mailing lists in that the messages are stored centrally, not redistributed to individual subscribers. At any time, an individual may access newsgroup files to read the accumulation of recent newsgroup messages or the archive of older messages. Groups.google.com offers a web interface to newsgroups and other Internet discussion groups. Sci.med.pharmacy is a pharmacy-related newsgroup for patients and professionals.

The World Wide Web

The World Wide Web is the fastest growing and best-known component of the Internet. Information is presented in pages that contain *hyperlinks,* electronic links to other web pages. Every web page has an individual URL (uniform resource locator), which is the page's address for retrieval. The pages are retrieved and displayed by *browser* software such as Netscape Navigator and Microsoft Internet Explorer. When a *web page* is displayed, the viewer can click on the links, usually represented by underlined or highlighted words or images. This instructs the computer to retrieve and display the linked web page.

Search Engines and Directories

There are several ways to find pharmacy and pharmaceutical information on the web. *Search engines* and *directories* allow users to search for websites, e-mail addresses, messages posted to newsgroups or mailing lists, and images or sound files. They may also allow access by browsing categories such as drug information, clinical resources, pharmaceutical companies, employment opportunities, societies and associations, consumer-oriented sites, and research sites.

The *engine* portion of these services employ *natural language searching*—users simply ask their question in a search box: "What are the adverse effects of alcohol consumption?" Users may enter words or phrases such as "fetal alcohol syndrome" or use Boolean operators (*and, or,* and *not*) in their query. Power track interfaces are available on most search engines for the experienced searcher. Advanced query forms allow users to refine their searches (ie, specify the language of the web site or a date range, use Boolean operators, or search specific fields including URLs). Popular search engines include Google (http://www.google.com), All the Web (http://www.alltheweb.com) and MSN Search (http://www.search.msn.com).

Meta-search engines such as MetaCrawler.com, Dogpile.com, and Search.com afford the opportunity to query multiple search engines simultaneously. Search results are organized in a uniform format, listing the search engines in which the query terms were found.

The *directory* portions of these services are maintained by human indexers who organize links to websites into categories. The best services are selective in their listings and organize, annotate, and evaluate the included sites. Yahoo! (http://www.yahoo.com/) includes a search directory that allows browsing by clicking on various categories organized in a hierarchical structure. For example, online pharmacy journals may be found by navigating first to the health menu, then to pharmacy and finally to the journals category. This navigation scheme is useful when the searcher does not know the title of a particular website. Users may also search Yahoo! by entering a word or phrase into a search box that appears on every page. Many users combine the two strategies by first browsing to a section and then searching that category for more specific information.

Major Pharmacy Websites

The web offers a wealth of information for the pharmacist and pharmaceutical scientist. Sites have evolved that allow professionals to gain immediate drug information. Commercial, government, and educational sites provide access to a variety of information. Two major pharmacy-related web sites are PharmWeb and the Virtual Pharmacy Library.

PharmWeb (http://www.pharmweb.net/) is a structured website providing worldwide pharmaceutical and health-related information. This site provides a wide range of services including computer space where pharmaceutical and health-related organizations may house their own web pages. PharmWeb provides pharmacists with several communication mechanisms. The site sponsors moderated discussion groups and mailing lists. Users may link to real-time chat forums or arrange a virtual meeting with colleagues in a discussion room. PharmWeb maintains a searchable directory of people working in the health-care professions. The PharmWeb Yellow Pages is a directory of pharmaceutical information on the Internet. It lists and links to companies, pharmacies, hospitals, and other organizations. This resource also links to pharmacy schools, government and regulatory bodies around the world.

The Virtual Pharmacy Library (http://www.pharmacy.org) is part of the broader World Wide Web Virtual Library (http://www.vlib.org/) that has been in existence since 1994. The Virtual Pharmacy Library is updated and maintained by David W.A. Bourne, of the University of Oklahoma College of Pharmacy. It is a comprehensive directory providing organized lists of links to pharmacy related databases, government web sites, pharmaceutical company, community pharmacy and hospital pages, and job information.

Professional Development

Several major pharmacy-related professional organizations have a presence on the web. These sites allow the pharmacist to learn about the benefits of membership, register online for conferences, and order publications and materials. Members can easily communicate with organization staff. Some organizations provide table of contents listings or limited full text access to their journals and news publications.

The ASHP's website (http://www.ashp.org/) has a drug product shortages management resource center, provides job listings and online continuing education, and online updates to the publication *AHFS Drug Information.* The professional advocacy section reports on ASHP actions in legislative and regulatory affairs, and the site provides the ASHP practice standards online.

The American Pharmacists Association (APhA) also provides a wealth of information through the Internet (http://www.aphanet.org). In addition to member services, this site provides science and research news, government affairs and consumer information.

The American Association of Colleges of Pharmacy (AACP) website (http://www.aacp.org/) is a very good source of information for pharmacy educators and students. It also includes the AACP *Basic Resources List for Pharmaceutical Education,* described above.

The web supports continuing education for practicing pharmacists. The source for finding accredited programs is the American Council on Pharmaceutical Education (http://www.acpe-accredit.org). Their web site contains a comprehensive list with links to web sites of providers.

Libraries and Educational Organizations

Librarians and information professionals have been active in selecting and organizing links to resources on the Internet. Librarians at several academic medical centers in the Midwest have cooperatively developed HealthWeb (http://www.health-web.org), which provides access to evaluated health-related Internet resources, including sections for pharmacy and pharmacology resources. Emory University's Robert W Woodruff Health Sciences Center Library supports MedWeb (http://www.medweb.emory.edu/MedWeb/. This site organizes health science resources into over 100 categories. The Pharmacy and Pharmacology section contains approximately eight subcategories. This organized hierarchy helps a user to find needed resources.

Pharmacy schools and colleges are also good sources for links to web-based information. The University of Oklahoma College of Pharmacy (http://www.pharmacy.ouhsc.edu/) maintains a comprehensive website providing information about the college's programs and links to appropriate Internet resources, including links to instructional, multimedia, pharmacokinetics, and toxicology resources.

David J. Temple, with the support of the Welsh School of Pharmacy at Cardiff University in Wales, edits a complete world list of schools of pharmacy (http://www.fip.org/education/). This listing includes Doctorate of Pharmacy programs and nontraditional educational programs.

Government Websites

A wealth of government information on the Internet is available to the pharmacist. The FDA home page (http://www.fda.gov/) is an umbrella site linking to the units of the agency, including the Center for Drug Evaluation and Research (CDER) and the Center for Biologics Evaluation and Research (CBER). The CDER site contains the full text of several publications, including the *Approved Drug Products with Therapeutic Equivalence Evaluations* (also known as the *Orange Book*), *National Drug Code Directory,* and the latest new and generic drug approval information in the *FDA Drug Approvals List.* MedWatch is the FDA's safety information and adverse event reporting program, and can be accessed from their site. The site contains drug shortage information, a searchable database of inactive ingredients, and major drug information pages. Regulatory guidance information, top drug news, consumer health information, and public health advisories are also provided.

Electronic Publications

Electronic publishing has boomed on the web. The literature of pharmacy and pharmaceutical sciences is becoming available online. The full text of many publications is available only to paid subscribers, but many publishers allow individuals to view tables of contents or abstracts at no fee. For example, viewers may browse the table of contents of *Pharmaceutical Research,* published for the American Association of Pharmaceutical Scientists by Kluwer/Plenum Press. The *Medical Letter on Drugs and Therapeutics,* a newsletter specializing in new drug evaluations, maintains a website with a table of contents archive and sample issues (http://www.medletter.com/). *Drugtopics.com* is an online publication associated with the trade magazine, *Drug Topics.* Emory University's MedWeb site maintains a comprehensive list of pharmacy-related electronic publications.

On-Line Community Pharmacies

Many community pharmacies have expanded their services to Internet customers. These online pharmacies allow consumers to fill prescriptions and purchase over-the-counter products online. These services usually require the patient to mail in a written prescription, or provide the name and phone number of the prescribing physician. Most of these services will bill third-party insurance. The National Association of Boards of Pharmacy developed the Verified Internet Pharmacy Practice Sites (VIPPS) program (http://www.nabp.net/vipps) in response to a growing concern of the safety of Internet pharmacies. VIPPS-certified pharmacies comply with criteria such as overall quality control, security and authorization of prescriptions, privacy rights of patients and adequate patient/pharmacist consultation. These pharmacies also must comply with the licensing requirements of their state and other states that they do business in.

Health Information for the Consumer

In addition to resources for the professional pharmacist, the web is a source for health information for the consumer. Several pharmacy organizations provide unbiased drug and health-related information to consumers. The University of Maryland Drug Information Service maintains such a website (http://www.pharmacy.umaryland.edu/UMDI/). Consumers may ask questions concerning pharmaceuticals or health-related topics. Visitors also may browse an archive of frequently asked questions. The FDA maintains a Consumer Drug Information web site (http://www.consumerdruginformation.com) providing information sheets about newly approved prescription drugs. DrugDigest (http://www.drugdigest.org) is a noncommercial, evidence-based, consumer health and drug information site. PDRHealth (http://www.pdrhealth.com/) from the publishers of the PDR provides disease overviews, health and wellness information, drug information and information about clinical trials.

Site Evaluations

The pharmacist must evaluate health information found on the Internet as thoroughly as any other type of medical information. Websites should identify sources, present unbiased and complete information, clearly state the authors' names and credentials, and keep information up to date. Good health-related websites present a mission statement and a disclaimer that encourages individuals to seek the advice of their own physicians. The Health on the Net Foundation (http://www.hon.ch/) is a nonprofit organization dedicated to building and supporting the international health and medical community on the Internet. The foundation's HONcode Principles provide a recommended code of conduct for medical and health websites.

ACKNOWLEDGMENT—The authors wish to thank Laura B Spencer for her assistance in preparing this chapter.

REFERENCE

1. Suarez-Almazor ME, Belseck E, Homik J, et al. *Control Clin Trials* 2000; 21:476.

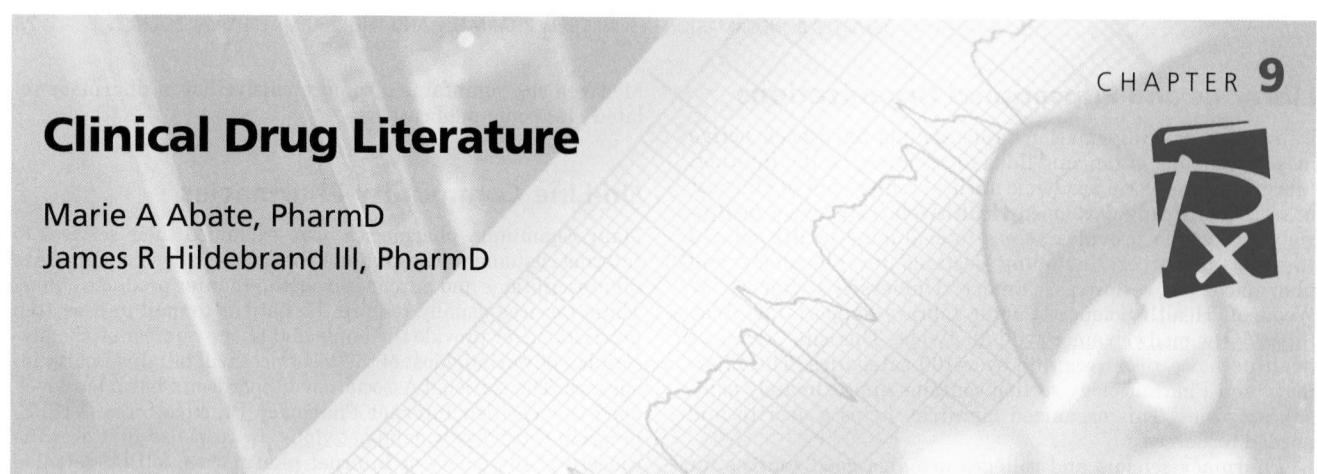

CHAPTER **9**

Clinical Drug Literature

Marie A Abate, PharmD
James R Hildebrand III, PharmD

Accessing, reviewing, analyzing, evaluating, and interpreting the clinical drug literature are important responsibilities of health-care practitioners; this is particularly true for pharmacists, who are the "drug experts." Pharmacists have been using and providing drug information for years, focusing initially on drug product compounding and dispensing information; however, the need for drug information has continued to expand along with the expansion of pharmacists' roles. The 1975 report of the Study Commission on Pharmacy concluded that the pharmacy profession was not effective in developing, organizing, and distributing knowledge and information about drugs. In fact, they felt that pharmacy's greatest deficiency was its inadequacy as an information transmitting system to patients, physicians, and other health-care practitioners.[1]

Although more work needs to be done to fully realize the pharmacist's potential in all practice settings, the profession has certainly made great strides forward since the Study Commission's report with regard to providing enhanced drug information to patients, physicians, and other health-care professionals. This is evidenced by the continual growth and development of patient-oriented pharmacy services across practice settings. Also, the establishment of the entry-level Doctor of Pharmacy degree program will better prepare future practitioners to assume their proper role as information specialists on the health-care team.

The types of drug information needed by practicing pharmacists and other health-care professionals are varied and include, but are not limited to, information about side/adverse effects, drug interactions, uses, teratogenicity, stability, and compatibility; product identification and availability; dosages and administration; toxicity, pharmacokinetics, pharmacodynamics, pharmacogenomics, health-related quality of life, and pharmacoeconomics; and efficacy, including the comparative efficacy among drugs in the same chemical or pharmacological class as well as among drugs from different classes. Health professionals must be knowledgeable about not only the variety of information resources available and how and why to use them, but importantly, must be able to critically analyze, evaluate, and interpret the information they retrieve.

The advances in computer technology, the continual growth of the Internet, and the widespread availability of free MEDLINE and other database-searching capabilities have placed unprecedented amounts of information readily within an individual's grasp. In particular, patients and health-care providers are increasingly turning to the Internet as an information resource, despite the unregulated and variable quality of information provided there.[2] It has been estimated that about 100 million Americans seek online health-related information. Key responsibilities of pharmacists and other health professionals include differentiating good from poor quality information, identifying the strengths and limitations of the

available information, appropriately applying the information they obtain to patient care, and recommending to patients high quality web sites.

This chapter provides introductory information about the roles of the pharmacist in the area of drug information, and defines tertiary and secondary information resources and their uses. The discussion then focuses on the primary literature and its evaluation. The quality of pharmaceutical manufacturers' and Internet information are also discussed.

THE PHARMACIST AND DRUG INFORMATION

Pharmacists are involved with many aspects of drug related information, including literature retrieval and analysis, adverse drug events, drug use decisions, educational activities, and clinical research. A primary role of the pharmacist as a pharmaceutical care provider is to respond to drug information questions from other health-care professionals and patients and to help resolve drug therapy related problems. Thus, a key activity of modern pharmacy practitioners is conducting literature searches to locate complete, up-to-date information upon which patient-care decisions can be made. Selecting the proper database and search strategy is an important consideration when searching for information. Medical *informatics* has been defined as the rapidly developing science that deals with the storage, retrieval, and optimal use of biomedical information, data, and knowledge for problem-solving and decision-making.[3] Once acceptable sources of information are identified and retrieved, the pharmacist must analyze and evaluate the published literature and develop recommendations based on the best available data. An understanding of searching techniques, research design, and biostatistics is important to the critical evaluation of literature. Once evidence from published clinical research is obtained, pharmacists should also apply evidence-based medicine (EBM) principles to their drug therapy related decisions. Two fundamental principles of EBM involve: (1) using consideration of benefits/risks, inconvenience, costs, and patient values together with evidence in making clinical recommendations, and 2) considering the hierarchy of evidence (eg, observations, strength of published study designs) when making clinical decisions.[4] Since EBM is being increasingly taught to and applied by health care practitioners, pharmacists should be knowledgeable about this process. The Evidence-Based Medicine Working Group has published a book that reviews the essentials for applying EBM to clinical practice, and this resource is recommended to readers wishing to learn more about this area.[4] Many of the principles discussed are included in the "Primary Literature and its Evaluation" section later in this chapter.

Adverse drug events/experiences/reactions not only result in patient morbidity and mortality, but also increase health-care costs by millions of dollars annually. Pharmacists play an active role in preventing, detecting, and reporting adverse events. Pharmacists are one of the major groups of health-care professionals who report adverse drug events to the Food and Drug Administration (FDA) via MedWatch (phone 800-FDA-1088; online at www.accessdata.fda.gov/scripts/medwatch; fax 800-FDA-0178). Pharmacists can also implement systems to prevent drug misadventures (such as errors in the prescribing, dispensing, and administration of medications) and to enhance patient compliance. Pharmacists can report medication errors to the US Pharmacopoeia (USP) via the Medication Errors Reporting (MER) Program (800-23-ERROR; via the web at www.usp.org/mer).

Another important role that pharmacists perform is actively participating in pharmacy and therapeutics committees that make decisions concerning rational drug use within health-care institutions. Through the design and conduct of drug utilization reviews and drug usage evaluations, pharmacists can contribute to continual improvement in the manner in which drugs are used.

Pharmacists are involved in many different drug information educational activities that are conducted for other health-care professionals and patients. Since the practice of medicine and pharmacy involves lifelong learning about the ongoing advances in pharmacotherapeutics, pharmacists can contribute to the continuing education of health-care professionals through the preparation and dissemination of newsletters and by providing seminars and lectures. Pharmacists also can provide verbal and written information to patients about their medications.

Participation in clinical research trials is another application of the drug information skills of pharmacists, allowing them to improve their understanding of how drugs work and ultimately enhance patient care. Their familiarity with the research process also makes them especially well suited to serve on institutional review boards, which are established to protect the rights of study subjects.

Drug information centers were established in the mid-1960s,[5,6] and they are staffed by pharmacists who review, collect, organize, and analyze drug information and disseminate it to health-care professionals and consumers.[7,8] Drug information centers or services often exist as functioning departments within health-care institutions, within the pharmaceutical industry, in academic settings, or as independent centers serving health-care professionals and the public.[9–12] The activities of drug information centers or services have increased dramatically since they were first established. Drug information centers or services are an excellent resource for health-care practitioners when assistance is required in handling a difficult clinical problem or when significant time or resource constraints exist.

TYPES OF LITERATURE

The types of literature can be divided into tertiary, secondary, and primary sources. *Tertiary sources* consist of general reference works and textbooks. When basic information on topics such as pharmacotherapeutics, toxicology, or drug interactions is required, a tertiary literature source may be the best means of starting the learning process and often provide references to more in-depth information if needed.

Secondary sources, literature used to identify and locate primary and other resources, consist of bibliographies, abstracting services, and indexing services. Pharmacists should use a secondary literature source when extensive or detailed information is needed, when a topic is new enough that it is not likely to be included in standard reference sources, when newly published data are needed to augment older information, when the most recent information concerning a topic is required, or whenever primary literature is needed.

The advantages of secondary literature sources are that several are now available to anyone with a computer and Internet access, they are generally current and up-to-date, and they are the best method for identifying primary literature sources. Some secondary literature sources contain a full text version of articles, making it possible to review the information available without going to a library or requesting copies from literature retrieval services or libraries. The disadvantages of secondary literature sources include that several are costly, they can require specific training on their use, and accessing the articles they retrieve can be difficult or time-consuming if one is not located near a medical library. When selecting a specific secondary resource, one must also consider the scope of primary literature and topics covered and the lag time from the date of publication of articles until they appear in the secondary source, which can be considerable in some cases.

Primary sources consist of original studies and reports in journals, monographs, and published conference proceedings and symposia. The primary literature should be consulted when making recommendations concerning the optimal therapy for disease states, when searching for recent reports of adverse events or drug interactions, when looking for information about new or investigational drugs or uses, or any time the tertiary literature does not provide needed information.

PRIMARY LITERATURE AND ITS EVALUATION

An understanding of basic study designs is important when assessing the validity of the results from clinical trials. Researchers may use the wrong study design, use the right methods incorrectly, misinterpret their results, report their results selectively, reference other studies selectively or incorrectly, or draw unjustified conclusions from their research.[13] Health-care professionals must critically evaluate study methods and results to ensure they are sufficiently valid to produce useful information. Pharmacists should be familiar with the methodologies employed in safety and efficacy trials as well as trials designed to evaluate pharmacokinetics, pharmacodynamics, pharmacoeconomics, patient outcomes, and quality of life. Special care must be exercised when reviewing promotional literature and using pharmaceutical sales representatives as sources of drug and drug-related information.[14,15]

Recent efforts on the part of biomedical journal editors, researchers, statisticians, and authors to improve the quality of reports of clinical trials resulted in the development and subsequent revision of the Consolidated Standards of Reporting Trials (CONSORT) statement.[16] The standards proposed by the CONSORT group have resulted in content suggestions and checklists for authors to use when submitting manuscripts of randomized controlled trials to medical journals. These standards have been adopted by such prestigious journals as the *British Medical Journal, JAMA,* the *Lancet,* and *Annals of Internal Medicine.* An initiative to improve the quality of reporting of diagnostic accuracy studies, the Standards for Reporting of Diagnostic Accuracy (STARD) is also underway.[17] A checklist of the types of information that should be provided in such studies has been prepared. However, the reader must realize that the CONSORT and similar processes have limitations, and thus should not assume that the articles published following these processes are automatically free of bias.[18] For example, the CONSORT recommendations cannot prevent authors from misrepresenting their research. The successful pharmacy practitioner must have the skills necessary to critically evaluate primary literature and to draw their own conclusions based on a study's merits, rather than simply relying upon the authors' conclusions.

In general, medical studies can be divided into two broad general types, descriptive and explanatory. *Descriptive studies* simply record data from observations, whereas *explanatory studies* use comparisons as a basis for deriving conclusions about cause and effect.

Table 9-1. Strength of Design of Clinical Trials

STRENGTH	STUDY TYPE
Strongest	Randomized experimental
	Cohort
	Case-control
	Case series
Weakest	Case report

Each study type has advantages and disadvantages, and these should be considered by researchers when selecting the design to use. Factors such as the number of patients required to obtain meaningful results, the study's complexity, the amount of time required to conduct the study, and the cost of study completion are important considerations when selecting a design. The critical reader should be aware of these factors when deciding how much credence to give to the findings from trials employing a given study type. The relative strength and weakness of each of these study types is shown in Table 9-1.

Descriptive Studies

A descriptive study can be used to document and communicate experiences that the author feels are important to bring to the attention of the medical community. The investigator simply records data from observations made and draws conclusions as to possible reasons for the events witnessed. Alternatively, descriptive studies may describe unusual or new events, such as the occurrence of sudden infant death syndrome (SIDS) in several siblings within a single family.

Descriptive studies fall into two main types: (1) case reports or (2) case series. *Case reports* are based on the observations of individual patients. They are often used to describe an adverse event following the use of a particular drug or group of drugs, or to report a possible drug interaction. Case reports frequently generate hypotheses to serve as the basis for more rigorous studies to examine the relationship between drug administration and the outcomes observed.

Case series document observations from a group or series of patients, all of whom have been exposed to a particular drug or group of drugs. The outcomes are observed and recorded. Case series are also used to examine the prior histories of patients with the same outcome in hopes of identifying a possible cause and effect relationship. Case series are useful for estimating the incidence of an adverse event of a newly marketed drug when there is limited information available about that particular event. Conversely, case series can be employed to help ensure that a certain adverse event is not associated with the use of a drug, for example, suicidal ideation following haloperidol use.

A major limitation of descriptive studies is that they do not provide definitive explanations, determine causes, or supply evidence that one drug is superior to another. Indeed, the outcome observed might not even be related to the drug. For these reasons, readers must exercise a great deal of caution when interpreting the results of case reports or case series and should not draw conclusions about causality from them.

Explanatory Studies

Explanatory studies use a more rigorous design to identify answers to questions that arise in clinical medicine. Investigators employ these designs to determine the efficacy of medications or identify whether there is a true relationship between the use of a drug and the occurrence of an outcome (eg, whether oral contraceptives cause an increased incidence of breast cancer, or what role the eradication of *Helicobacter pylori* plays in the prevention of peptic ulcer disease recurrence). Explanatory studies can be divided into two main designs: (1) observational and (2) experimental.

OBSERVATIONAL STUDIES: CASE-CONTROL, COHORT, CROSS-SECTIONAL

When conducting *observational studies,* the investigators are bystanders to the events under study. They examine the natural course of health events, gather data about the subjects included, and then classify and sort the data. The investigators employ comparisons to provide insights into the cause of diseases or the risk factors associated with disease occurrence.

When evaluating the relationship between drugs and the occurrence of specific outcomes, there are two basic approaches an investigator can take: work from the effect or outcome back to the cause or exposure (case-control studies), or proceed from the cause or exposure to the effect or outcome (cohort studies). Cross-sectional studies collect data simultaneously from the comparison groups.

Case-Control Studies

In *case-control studies,* one group of patients with a target condition or disease (the cases) are selected and compared with another group of individuals without the condition or disease (the controls). Cases and controls are compared with respect to existing or past characteristics or exposures that are thought to be relevant to the development of the disease or condition under evaluation.

A case-control study design has several advantages. Case-control studies take little time to design, initiate, and conduct because the outcomes have already been experienced. They are useful for the study of rare diseases or conditions that take many years to develop because they require fewer patients than other study designs. Additionally, since case-control studies use patients who have already developed the disease of interest, there is no need to wait for time to elapse between an exposure and the manifestation of diseases with long latency periods.

From an ethical perspective, case-control studies have an advantage in areas of investigation where neither experimental nor follow-up observational studies can be sanctioned (eg, the incidence of HIV-positive tests following injuries with needles contaminated with HIV-positive blood, drug teratogenicity). Further, case-control studies are ideal for initiating exploratory studies (so-called "fishing expeditions") of disease etiology so that a specific hypothesis can be formulated and sufficiently supported to justify a detailed investigation. There is no risk to the patients involved in case-control studies because they have already experienced the outcome under evaluation. Finally, when compared to other types of explanatory study designs, case-control studies are inexpensive, since existing records can often be used to collect the necessary data.

There are several disadvantages associated with the case-control study design. A detailed study of mechanism is rarely possible with this design. The case-control method is not suited to the evaluation of therapy because there is no comparison to other drugs, nor is it suited to study disease prophylaxis. In these situations, experimental trials should be used.

A major problem with the case-control design is the reliance on patient recall or on existing medical records for information. Sufficiently accurate information may not be available from medical records. Likewise, information concerning the dose, duration, or drug administration in relation to the event under evaluation may be inadequately recorded and imperfectly remembered. Validation of information collected is difficult or sometimes impossible to accomplish.

The case-control design has incomplete control of extraneous variables that may affect the cause and effect relationship. Case-control studies are subject to antecedent-consequent relationships (the chicken-and-egg phenomenon)—one cannot be sure whether the characteristic really led to the effect or disease, or if the outcome in some way predisposed people to acquire factors or characteristics that appear to be predictive of the disease.

Case-control studies are also subject to numerous types of bias. An exhaustive discussion of biases associated with case-control trials is beyond the scope of this chapter, but several types can be highlighted. Case-control study design may be affected by *recall bias* (selective recall). Patients who have unpleasant experiences or diseases may recall the past quite differently from those in a comparison, nondiseased group. Other important biases to consider when evaluating case-control studies include *reporting bias,* which occurs when publicity concerning a disease results in an increase in the disease's reporting; and *surveillance bias,* which can occur when a disease or condition under study is asymptomatic, mild, or otherwise liable to escape routine attention. With surveillance bias, the condition is likely to go unreported in the control group and is more likely to be detected in the patients under frequent medical surveillance in the case group.

The appropriate selection of cases is important to the reporting of valid results in case-control studies. Who patients are, where they come from, and what spectrum of disease they represent are important considerations. However, selection of an appropriate control group is difficult when conducting case-control studies because it is almost impossible to find a comparison group identical to the cases. A sampling procedure is intended to avoid over- or under-representation of exposed cases and exposed controls in the study, thus avoiding biased selection. Each eligible case in the target population, irrespective of exposure, should ideally have an equal chance of appearing in the study. Methods have been developed to help manage the problems associated with the proper selection of a control group in case-control studies, although they cannot eliminate the problems. One such method is through the selection of *multiple controls,* wherein more than one control group is selected for comparison. Another method employed is *matching,* which uses the selection of control subjects who share particular characteristics with the cases.

Cohort Studies (Follow-up Studies)

Cohort studies begin with patients who have not yet experienced the outcome; these patients are then followed over time, looking for differences in the outcome's development. The characteristics that are thought to influence the development of the disease of interest are catalogued and measured, and comparisons of patient groups with (exposed) or without (nonexposed) the various characteristics are made to identify the causes of the outcome of interest. The cohort study represents the best observational study design strategy when there are no time or financial limitations.

Historical (or retrospective) cohort studies can be conducted using data contained in large medical databases. The cohorts (those with characteristics/exposed and those without characteristics/nonexposed) are established and their experience is assessed from existing records. The main feature of a historical cohort study is that all outcomes have occurred before the start of the investigation. The key element is that individuals are identified for inclusion in either the study or control group without knowledge by the investigators of whether the disease has later developed.

A cohort study design has several advantages over the case-control study. This design allows for the complete description of experience subsequent to exposure, including rates of progression, staging of disease, and natural history. The cohort design offers greater assurance that the characteristics under study preceded the outcome under study. It also permits the study of multiple potential effects of a given exposure, thereby obtaining information on potential benefits as well as risks. The cohort design allows for the calculation of rates of disease in exposed and unexposed individuals after the cohorts are established and their experience is assessed. In addition, this design permits flexibility in choosing the variables to be systematically recorded. Cohort studies can delineate various types of consequences that may be produced by a single risk factor.

In contrast to the case-control design, the cohort design (with the exception of the historical cohort) has few problems associated with incomplete medical records, and there is no recall bias. Another advantage of the cohort study design over the case-control design is that the cohort design is not associated with antecedent-consequent relationship problems.

Cohort studies do have disadvantages. Cohort studies are subject to patient selection problems. Every effort must be made to identify independently each characteristic affecting the disease or outcome under study and to ensure an even distribution of these factors. The external validity (discussed later in this chapter) of cohort studies may be difficult to determine, because clinicians may not know how closely the subjects described in the cohort study mirror their patients.

The major problem of the cohort study design is maintaining patient follow-up over time. As time goes on, patients move, fail to respond to questionnaires, or decide to quit the study, which can result in an uneven distribution of patients between groups. Reports of cohort studies should identify the attempts made by the investigators to track down subjects and minimize the number lost to follow-up. The investigators should identify the rate of follow-up losses and explore for the possibility of biased attrition. By examining the characteristics of dropouts, the investigator may identify reasons for subject loss that are related to the outcomes under study, and compensate for any differences identified. The more similar the dropouts are to those in the study group, the less chance there is for attrition bias. Finally, if possible, investigators should contact a representative sample of the dropouts to identify the reasons for discontinuation and take any differences into account when analyzing the study results.

Another disadvantage associated with cohort studies is that current practice, usage, or exposure to study factors may change over time, making the findings of the study irrelevant. Cohort studies are also subject to surveillance bias due to an unequal examination or scrutiny of the subjects under evaluation. Since cohort studies follow patients over time, they may require a potentially long duration of follow-up when a long lag time exists between cause and effect. Cohort studies are relatively expensive to conduct because they require an expenditure of resources over long time periods. Finally, like case-control studies, a detailed study of mechanism is rarely possible with cohort studies.

Cross-Sectional Studies (Prevalence Studies)

The *cross-sectional study* also gathers data from both study and control groups, but it makes simultaneous assessments of both the outcome and potential predictors at the same (ie, present) time. The cross-sectional design is suited for studies designed to evaluate a new laboratory test or a new application of an existing test, to evaluate the receiver-operator characteristics of diagnostic procedures, to identify risk factors and etiological agents of a disease or condition, and to determine the prevalence of a disease or condition at a specific point in time.

Advantages of the cross-sectional design include the efficiencies and time-savings that result from all of the information being collected at the same time. Investigators do not have to wait for outcomes to develop when conducting cross-sectional studies.

As cross-sectional studies compare a desired study group with a control group, they are subject to selection problems. The type of patients selected for the study group has a major influence on the results. External validity is a concern, since the findings can only be applied to other patients to the extent that they exhibit similar characteristics to the study subjects. Selection methods must define the characteristics of subjects who will be included in the analysis. Sampling rules must be formulated to avoid bias in the study results. Methods such as *systematic sampling* (selecting the *n*th individual who is eligible for the study), *random sampling* (where each possible individual has a fixed and determinate probability of selection), and *matched sampling* (the pairing of one or more controls to each study subject on the basis of specified variables to eliminate their effects on the comparison) are frequently employed in the cross-sectional design.

An additional disadvantage of this design is the existence of antecedent-consequent relationships (the chicken-and-egg phenomenon), as described earlier.

EXPERIMENTAL STUDIES

Experimental studies are prospective trials in which *intervention,* an attempt to regulate the variables in a study, occurs on the part of the investigators.[19] There are two types of experimental studies, controlled and noncontrolled. *Controlled studies,* in contrast to noncontrolled studies, use a comparison group(s) in addition to the group receiving the drug being investigated. This allows the investigator to help account for the possible influence that other outside factors (eg, environmen-

tal) could have on a study's outcomes independent of the drug being evaluated.

Since the controlled study is the strongest type of experimental study, the remainder of the discussion will focus on the controlled design. Several guides and checklists have been published to assist readers in evaluating the quality of experimental clinical studies.[20] Table 9-2 lists the criteria usually included in such checklists, and can be used as a guide for the evaluation of published clinical drug studies.

Journals/Authors

The quality of the journal an article is published in can be used as a preliminary, indirect measure of the potential quality of the article itself. An *editorial board* is one method that helps to ensure the quality of the information that a particular journal publishes. *Peer review* is another method employed for helping ensure the quality of articles published. This is a process in which a journal sends out a received manuscript to

Table 9-2. Criteria for the Evaluation of Published Experimental Drug Studies

AREA/STUDY SECTION	CRITERIA
I. Journal/authors	Editorial board present.
	Peer review used.
	Author(s) has/have expertise in subject.
	Potential conflicts of interest absent.
II. Introduction/background	Background and rationale clear.
	Relevant previous work cited.
	Objective(s) clearly stated.
	Objective(s) described in sufficient detail.
III. Methods	
A. Patients/subjects	Inclusion and exclusion criteria clearly defined.
	Inclusion and exclusion criteria appropriate for objective(s).
	Inclusion and exclusion criteria complete.
	Number of patients/subjects adequate.
	Source and selection of patients/subjects described.
	Appropriate study setting.
B. Study design	Type(s) of control(s) used appropriate.
	Design appropriate to address study objective(s).
	Randomization process described and followed.
	Type of blinding used adequate and employed successfully.
C. Treatment considerations	Dosages of study and control drugs adequate and comparable.
	Dosage frequency appropriate.
	Route(s) of administration and dosage forms appropriate.
	Duration of therapy adequate.
	If measured, plasma/serum/blood concentrations adequate.
	Any concurrent medications accounted for.
D. Outcome measures	Efficacy and safety measures included.
	End points defined clearly.
	Measurements valid, reliable.
	Known confounders accounted for.
	Measure(s) clinically important.
	Compliance measured.
E. Data analysis	Power analysis performed and power adequate.
	Types of statistical tests and analyses described clearly and appropriate.
IV. Results	Statistical tests and analyses used for key outcome measures.
	Measures of variability provided with measures of central tendency.
	P values or confidence intervals reported.
	Size of treatment effect important clinically.
	Actual numbers included with percentages.
	Side/adverse effects reported.
	Text/tables/graphs clear and consistent.
	Reason(s) for patient/subject dropout provided; handling of dropout data described.
V. Discussion	Data obtained consistent with conclusions.
	Study limitations addressed.
	Significance of findings discussed.
	Extrapolation of findings consistent with study design.

"peers," other individuals with expertise in the area, who review and comment on the quality of the manuscript and the work undertaken in addition to providing suggestions for revision, prior to a decision being made regarding publishability. Based upon the peer reviewers' comments and the editors' opinions, a decision is made to return the manuscript to the author(s) for revision, reject the manuscript, or publish the manuscript. Although the best approach for the peer review process has been debated and peer review does not guarantee the quality of work described,[21] it is another important method for providing the reader with some measure of confidence in the information published.

Many journals ask authors to describe any potential *conflicts of interest* when they submit their manuscript for publication consideration. According to the International Committee of Medical Journal Editors, "Conflict of interest for a given manuscript exists when a participant in the peer review and publication process-author, reviewer, and editor-has ties to activities that could inappropriately influence his or her judgment, whether or not judgment is in fact affected."[22] These potential conflicts of interest include serving as a consultant for or an employee of the manufacturer of one or more of the drugs being investigated, obtaining a grant from the manufacturer to fund the study undertaken, or holding stock in a company that manufacturers one or more of the study drugs. The problem faced is how to perform research studies that might be translated into marketable products in a way that will hold all sponsors, investigators, authors, and journals involved in the publication of clinical trials to objective, honest, scientific, and ethical behavior uninfluenced by financial considerations. The existence of a potential conflict of interest does not automatically invalidate the findings reported; rather, the reader should keep this possible conflict in mind when analyzing the study's results and the author's interpretation and discussion of the findings, particularly if biased or unsupported statements appear to exist.[23]

Introduction/Background

Several points should be covered by the author in the introduction or background portion of a published study. The rationale for the study should be clearly described and pertinent previous work in the area, with both positive and negative findings if they exist, should be summarized and cited. The specific study objective or hypothesis should be described in sufficient detail to enable the reader to determine if it actually addresses the problem explored and whether it can be reasonably accomplished by the study.

METHODS

The methods or methodology section includes several important areas to review and analyze in order to assess the overall quality of a study: patients/subjects, study design, treatments used, outcome measures, and the data analyses used. Particular attention should be devoted to the methods employed by the investigators in conducting the study. Flawed methods produce results that yield incorrect conclusions, and patients may suffer harm from either ineffective or toxic therapy.

Patients/Subjects

It is important to examine the types of patients or subjects included in a clinical study to determine whether the study sample is representative of the desired study population and the extent to which the study's results can be extrapolated to others outside the study sample. The study's inclusion and exclusion criteria are key to making these determinations.

The *inclusion criteria* define the characteristics a patient or subject must have to be included in a specific study. The *exclu-*

sion criteria include those characteristics that, if present, would prevent a patient or subject from being enrolled. The inclusion and exclusion criteria should be defined clearly. This is crucial for determining the extent to which a study's results can be applied or extrapolated to patients outside the study. For example, if patients with "renal dysfunction" are excluded from study participation, then its meaning should be clear to the reader (eg, what the exact creatinine clearance values are that constituted "renal dysfunction").

The study sample should also be representative of the population that the authors are interested in examining as part of their study objective; that is, the characteristics of the patients enrolled in the study should be similar to other patients likely to be found in the population of interest, and this population should be appropriate for the study's objective.

Finally, whether any other inclusion or exclusion criteria should have been incorporated to strengthen the study must be considered. For example, it might be appropriate to exclude concurrent medications known to increase blood pressure in a study of a new antihypertensive medication.

An important consideration when analyzing a study's results is the *sample size,* or number of subjects included. Sample size is one of the factors affecting a study's power, the extent to which a statistical test can detect a significant difference among treatments if such a difference really exists (ie, appropriately rejecting the *null hypothesis,* no difference among treatments, when it is false).

As sample size increases, *power* increases as well. Thus, the smaller the number of patients enrolled in a study and the lower the power, the greater the likelihood of a type II error, also referred to as beta. A *type II error* is, by definition, failing to reject the null hypothesis when it is actually false—that is, concluding that there is no statistically significant difference among treatments when there actually is. Ideally, power should be calculated by the investigators prior to study initiation and reported for the reader.[24] By convention, an acceptable degree of power in a study is considered to be at least 0.8 or 80%.

When reading a study that concludes there was no significant difference present among treatments, consider whether the power was adequate. If the power was not reported, consider the number of patients involved (the larger the better) and the actual magnitude of the difference found.[24] For example, a difference in mean serum cholesterol concentrations of only 1.5 mg/100 mL between two antilipidemic drug groups is unlikely to be clinically relevant even if a large number of patients were enrolled; a difference of 1.5 mg/100 mL might be found to be statistically significant if a very large number of patients were studied.

More information regarding sample size and how to determine an appropriate number of subjects to enroll is beyond the scope of this chapter and can be found in other articles.[25,26]

The *source* of the patients/subjects enrolled in a study should be considered with regard to the potential ability to extrapolate the results, as well as the manner in which they were selected for inclusion. For example, if a study examined subjects who were selected from among nursing home residents, the results might not be applicable to relatively healthy, active elderly persons.

The *setting* of the study should also be appropriate for the study's objective; if the objective is geared toward active outpatients, then the study should best be conducted in the outpatient setting. If the subjects were randomly selected from the population of interest, as opposed to nonrandom techniques such as convenience or consecutive sampling, the method used should be described.

Investigators conducting randomized clinical trials are required to follow Good Clinical Practices (GCPs) in the design, conduct, analysis, and reporting of studies.[27] Good clinical practice sets ethical and scientific standards for all research involving human participants. The FDA in conjunction with the European Union and Japan has developed a series of guidances to facilitate the mutual acceptance of clinical data by the regulatory authorities of all countries involved (see http://www.fda.gov/cder/guidance/959fnl.pdf). Compliance with GCP ensures that the rights, safety, and well being of study participants are protected, consistent with the principles that have their origin in the *Declaration of Helsinki*. A primary tenet of GCP is the submission of research protocols to an Ethics Committee (EC) or Institutional Review Board (IRB). Research is generally not accepted for publication without assurance that the study was reviewed by an IRB and that informed consent was obtained from research participants prior to their participation in the clinical study.

Study Design

Several design aspects warrant consideration when analyzing the quality of a published experimental study. The first involves the type of control employed. An *active control* uses a drug with proven efficacy for the treatment of a condition as a comparison to the drug being evaluated. For example, in a study of a new nonsteroidal anti-inflammatory agent that compares its efficacy to a group of patients receiving naproxen, the naproxen group would constitute the active control. A *placebo control* incorporates a group of subjects receiving placebo as the comparison group. A *no treatment control* incorporates a group of subjects receiving no therapy as the comparison group. A *historical control* uses as the comparison group individuals who received the intervention previously as part of a different study or as part of a different evaluation.

An active control can only provide information about the relative efficacy of drugs—whether one was more efficacious, less efficacious, or the same as another. However, it is possible that neither the active control nor the drug being evaluated were truly efficacious for the patient groups being studied. In contrast, a placebo control allows one to determine the true efficacy of a drug for treatment of a certain condition.

Placebo controls are preferable to no treatment controls because they minimize possible bias introduced by the patient as a result of knowing what they are receiving. Either placebo or no treatment controls can pose an ethical dilemma, however, for studies involving serious illnesses in which patients should receive active therapy.

Historical controls should only be used in special circumstances, such as when the disease being treated has known high mortality and it would be easy to identify a new efficacious therapy. In many studies, both active and placebo controls are employed to allow for determinations of both the actual and comparable efficacies of a given agent.

Another consideration involves the type of design used in a controlled experimental study. The controlled experimental designs include concurrent control (parallel treatment), crossover, and time series (before and after). Of these, the concurrent control design is generally preferred.

In the *concurrent control design*, patients are divided into at least two groups: control versus experimental. They only receive the intervention of the one group they were assigned to. Results obtained from the experimental group(s) are then compared with those from the control group. With this design, it is important that the experimental and control group patients are as similar as possible to help ensure comparability of the results.

In a *crossover design*, the patients are initially assigned to either the control or experimental groups; after completion, they are then placed in the other group(s) so that each patient eventually receives each intervention. The crossover design generally includes a *washout* period between each intervention to allow the treatment and its effects to be eliminated from the body prior to beginning the next study phase. Since the patients are the same in the control and experimental groups in a crossover design, it is easier to eliminate differences in patient characteristics as being responsible for any differences identified between groups. A smaller sample size can also be used for

the crossover design as compared to the concurrent control. Disadvantages of the crossover as compared to the concurrent control design include a longer study duration, the effects of time itself on the results, and the possibility of carryover effects occurring (ie, effects from the previous intervention persisting and affecting the results from the subsequent intervention, such as when an inadequate or no washout period was employed). More complex analyses are required because differences might be identified among groups depending on the order in which they received the interventions. For example, patients who received the control first might be found to respond differently than patients who received the control last.

In the *time series design*, each patient also receives each study intervention except, in contrast to the crossover design, they receive each intervention at the same time. This makes analyses of the results easier compared to the crossover design, but the time series design cannot control for the effects that time itself might have on the outcomes.

Randomization is the process of randomly assigning the enrolled patients/subjects to study groups (eg, control versus treatment groups) using a technique such as random numbers. This is a very important procedure for ensuring a study's quality. It helps to eliminate subjective factors and bias when assigning subjects to treatment groups, and reduces the likelihood that differences in subject characteristics (either identified or unidentified) are actually responsible for the outcomes observed rather than the treatment itself.[28] It is important to recognize that randomization does not guarantee that a study's groups will be identical; through chance alone the groups could be different with regard to one or more important criteria.

Studies will usually compare the study groups after randomization with regard to characteristics that might influence outcomes (eg, age, sex, race, number of years with a certain condition) to ensure that they are indeed comparable. If baseline differences exist, these can often be accounted for later using statistical methods.[29] When a study refers to itself as a "randomized controlled" trial, the word "randomized" is referring to assignment, not selection. The actual process used for randomization to study groups should be reported in a study. A reader should consider whether the process was indeed truly random and whether the investigators adhered to the process they described.

Blinding, or *masking*, is a process in which the identity of the control and experimental groups in a study is not known to the subjects and/or investigators; that is, the subjects and observers do not know who is receiving the control or experimental treatments.

In an *unblinded study*, also referred to as *open label*, both the subjects and investigators are aware of the group assignments. There is a risk of bias introduction by either the subjects or investigators with this type of design.

In a *single-blind study*, the subjects are unaware of the intervention they are receiving but the investigators know. This type of blinding might be acceptable when the measures employed in the study are all objective (eg, blood concentrations). In the *double-blind study*, neither the subjects nor investigators are aware of the intervention each subject is receiving. This type of blinding is preferred for studies to minimize the likelihood of bias introduced by the subjects or investigators and is an important part of the "gold standard" study design—controlled, randomized, double-blind. The term *triple-blind* has been used for studies in which an individual other than the investigator analyzes the data, and the subjects, investigators, and data analyzers are unaware of the group assignments.

When blinding is used in a study, it is important for the investigators to describe the means by which this was accomplished (eg, identical appearing/smelling/tasting capsules, tablets, or liquids) as well as any evidence as to whether the blinding was successful.[16]

There is always a danger of *unblinding* (unmasking) occurring in a blinded study. This is when the subjects or investigators can successfully guess or identify the intervention given. Unblinding is more likely when the drug involved has an odor or taste that is difficult to disguise, or when characteristic side effects or laboratory test alterations occur that would alert the subjects or investigators to the true identify of the treatment. For example, the headache from nitroglycerin or the red-orange urine discoloration from rifampin could likely lead to unblinding, even in a double-blind study. The investigators should provide evidence either supporting or negating the success of the blinding employed.

Treatment Considerations

When evaluating the quality of clinical studies, pharmacists in particular should pay close attention to the appropriateness of the treatment regimens employed. Characteristics of the treatment regimens to examine include the dosage, dosing frequency, route of administration, dosage form, and duration of therapy for each drug used, any drug concentrations obtained, and the use of any concurrent medications.

With regard to the *dosages* of the experimental drug and any active controls, they should be appropriate and comparable. For example, if the active control is being dosed at the high end of its usual dosage range, the experimental drug should generally be dosed comparably. Also, if the dosage of a drug is usually adjusted based on an individual's response in clinical practice, it might be inappropriate to employ a fixed dose of that drug for all the patients in a study.

The dosing *frequency* should be consistent with the pharmacokinetics and pharmacodynamics of the drug. If a drug has an established therapeutic serum, plasma, or blood concentration range, then the study should measure drug *concentrations* in the patients and ensure that they are appropriate. Likewise, the concentrations should be taken at the correct times in relation to the doses and at steady state for efficacy studies.

Some studies allow patients to take other nonexperimental medications concurrently with the drug in the study. For example, a study of the effects of zinc capsules on flu symptoms might allow patients to also take acetaminophen as needed. If *concurrent medications* are allowed in a study, it is important for the reader to consider whether these medications could interact with the study drug or affect the disease state or symptoms being studied. If the concurrent medication could affect the study outcomes, it is important that the study record and quantitate the amounts taken in both the control and experimental groups and analyze whether these quantities were comparable or could have otherwise influenced the study's findings.

Outcome Measures

The outcomes of interest to be measured in a clinical study should be derived from the study's objective. In an efficacy study, the outcome measures should include not only determinations of efficacy but of safety as well. For example, in a study of a new antihypertensive medication, determining the systolic and diastolic blood pressures would be important, as would recording the drug's adverse effects or effects on blood lipids or glucose.

The *desired end point(s)* of the study, the key measures that will support or refute the study's hypothesis,[30] should be clearly specified to the reader and should be identified by the investigators at the beginning of the study. In the antihypertensive example mentioned earlier, the main or primary end point might be the ability of the drug to decrease systolic and diastolic blood pressures to the normal ranges.

A study might also have *secondary end points,* meaning other measures of interest but not of primary concern. For example, the effect of an antihypertensive drug on serum triglycerides might be an important secondary end point but not the major reason for performing the specific trial. The investigators should specify the minimum differences between the control and experimental groups that they feel are of importance.[16] As

the reader, you should also ensure that these differences are of clinical importance.

The techniques or methods used to measure or determine whether the study's outcome was achieved should be valid. *Validity* refers to whether the measurement is really measuring what the investigators would like to measure or think they are measuring.[31] Types of validity include, but are not limited to, internal, external, and construct validity:

Internal validity refers to the extent that, within the study, the tests, measurements, results, and interpretation were appropriate and accurate.[32]

External validity is generalizability, the extent to which the results can be extrapolated or applied to other nonstudy individuals and across settings or times.[31,32] External validity is important to clinicians who are interested in the degree to which they can apply the results from an individual study to their patients. Readers should examine factors such as the study's inclusion and exclusion criteria, how subjects were selected, and the study setting to assist them in determining the generalizability of its results.

Construct validity refers to the extent to which a measure actually reflects what it purports to measure. This can be determined by the extent to which it agrees or converges with other methods established to measure the same variable, and the extent to which it disagrees with or diverges from other methods used to measure different effects.[31]

In addition to being valid, measures in a study should also be reliable, specific, and sensitive.

Reliability refers to the extent to which a measure provides similar results when used on different occasions—that is, its reproducibility.[33]

Specificity refers to the degree to which a measure can accurately detect only the disease or effect of interest. Stated another way, it refers to the degree to which a measure can accurately classify as negative those people who lack the disease or effect.

Sensitivity indicates the extent to which a measure can identify the presence of the effect or disease.[34]

Confounding variables, or confounders, are factors that could affect the outcome being measured (in addition to the characteristic of interest), thereby confusing the interpretation of the results.[35,36] For example, if a study was examining the effect of age on ulcer relapse rate and several of the ulcer subjects also smoked (a known factor influencing relapse), smoking could be a confounder when analyzing the results. If a study has known confounding variables present, the investigators should account for their presence either in the study design (methods section) or in the analysis of the results.[37]

Finally, it is important that clinical drug studies assess the degree of patient *compliance* with their therapy, as noncompliance with one of the drug regimens in a study could make that drug erroneously appear less efficacious than another.[37] Studies should make an effort to determine the extent of patient compliance by using a variety of methods (eg, pill counts, patient self-report, diaries, or drug concentrations) and report this information for the reader.

Data Analysis

The methods section of a study should generally include a discussion of power (sometimes found in the results section) and the type of statistical tests or analyses performed on the data collected. (Power was referred to earlier in the discussion of sample size.) A common reason for the failure to detect significant differences among treatment groups in a study is a lack of statistical power, often a result of too small a number of patients enrolled or actually completing the study. As a reader, check to see whether the investigators performed a power analysis and reported this information. If so, determine whether the power was appropriate. If not, consider whether a lack of power might have been responsible for any negative finding reported.

As a reader, determine whether the statistical tests or analyses employed are described in sufficient detail to allow for their replication.[38] The tests or analyses used should also be appropriate for the variables of interest.

Results

The results section of a published study is of obvious importance to the reader. There are several areas to focus on within this section and key questions to ask. These areas include the statistical tests and analyses performed and the specific findings reported, side or adverse effects, the presentation of the data, and patient dropouts. The topic of statistics is covered in more detail in Chapter 12. However, important statistics-related points that the reader should consider when critically analyzing studies will be discussed here.

The first consideration is that statistical tests and analyses should have been performed on all the key outcome measures. There are primarily two types of statistics involved: descriptive statistics and inferential statistics.

Descriptive statistics, numerical or graphical summaries of data, include measures of central tendency (eg, mean, median, mode), measures of variability (eg, range, standard deviation, variance, standard error), and measures of precision for effect estimates (eg, confidence intervals).

Most *inferential statistics,* methods to generalize from the data obtained from the study sample to the entire population of interest, involve the tests and analyses (eg, parametric tests, nonparametric tests) performed to test hypotheses and determine whether statistically significant differences exist among study groups. Other statistical procedures include correlation and regression analyses (to describe and quantify the association among study variables) and estimates of risk associated with developing a disease, condition, or adverse event (eg, relative risk, odds ratio).

Next, readers should consider whether the statistical method employed in a study is appropriate for the type of variable being examined. For example, parametric tests (such as *t* tests or ANOVA, analysis of variance) should be used only when certain criteria are met, such as normally or near-normally distributed data, continuous level data, or variances of the populations from which the samples are drawn being nearly equal. If these criteria do not apply, then nonparametric tests (eg, Chi-square test, Fisher's exact test, or Mann-Whitney *U* test) should be employed, taking into account whether the data are *nominal* (data without numerical qualities that can be placed into mutually exclusive categories) or *ordinal* (data that can be rank ordered on a scale, but differences between rankings cannot be precisely measured).

It is also important that information about the variability of study data be provided in addition to information about the central tendency of that data. For example, the mean is commonly used to illustrate the "average" or representative value in a group of data. However, the mean can be affected significantly by a small number of outlying data points (extreme high or low values) and therefore might not represent accurately where most of the individual data values lie. Also, the mean might have the same value regardless of whether all the individual data points cluster very closely or widely around it.

Because clinicians are interested in applying the results from studies to their individual patients, an indication of the variability of the individual data points in a study is valuable. For example, suppose two studies report the same mean plasma concentrations of 50 mg/mL in response to drug administration. However, the individual patients' drug levels in the two different studies are as follows (in mg/mL): 48, 49, 50, 51, 52 and 1, 5, 50, 95, 99. Although the mean values are identical, the patients in the latter study exhibit much more variability in response to the drug. Thus, studies that report values such as means for their outcome measures should also include corresponding ranges or standard deviations.[38]

Further, the results from statistical analyses performed should include exact *P* values or confidence intervals.[37,38] The *P* value indicates the *probability* of a type I error (ie, rejecting the null hypothesis when it is in fact true). Stated another way, it means concluding that a statistically significant difference exists among treatments when there actually isn't one and the results are due to chance. The probability of a type I error is also referred to as the alpha level. The smaller the *P* value, the less the likelihood that a type I error was responsible for the difference observed (or the less the likelihood that chance was responsible for the difference observed). Thus, a *P* value of 0.001 indicates that the likelihood of a type I error, or that chance alone was responsible for the difference observed, is only 1 out of 1000. By convention, $P < 0.05$ is generally considered statistically significant.

However, since *P* values only indicate the risk of type I error and do not provide information about the magnitude of the clinical effect, the *confidence interval* (CI) is increasingly being reported. The CI is calculated using the study sample data and provides the likelihood or confidence that the true population value is included within the range of values reported.[29] For example, if a study reports a difference in the response rates between two treatments of 35% with a 95% CI of 30–40%, this means that there is a 95% likelihood that the true difference in the response rates if the population as a whole were studied would fall between 30% and 40%. Although the 95% CI is generally calculated, the reader may also see 90% or 99% CIs reported in studies. The CI provides health practitioners with useful data for predicting how their patients would likely respond to the same treatment (assuming that their patients had similar characteristics as those in the study sample, ie, are part of the population the study sample represented).

The size of the actual treatment effects reported in studies should be clinically useful.[29] Further, when reporting results in studies, actual numbers should be included with any percentage change data.[38] For example, large percentages can be misleading when small numbers are involved, and the reader should be aware of this.

It is difficult to determine the clinical utility of a treatment without considering safety as well as efficacy. This includes not only the risk of adverse reactions from the drug regimen employed, but also the risk to the patient of an adverse event if he or she is not treated. The reader should assess the side or adverse effects reported in a study when determining how to incorporate the results into clinical practice. A "number needed to harm" can be calculated, representing the number of patients that need to be treated to cause one adverse effect, in a manner similar to the "number needed to treat" approach.[39]

When presenting data in a study, any tables or graphs used should be clear and not misleading. Also, the text description should be consistent with the information illustrated in the tables or graphs. Finally, the reason for any patient/subject losses (dropouts) should be provided as they could influence the interpretation of the clinical usefulness of the treatment employed. For example, patients could drop out of a study because the therapy was ineffective or intolerable side effects developed. Two approaches used for handling the data from dropouts include the intent-to-treat (or intention-to-treat) and exclusion of subjects (or per protocol) methods.

With the *intention-to-treat analysis,* the data from all patients are analyzed together with the rest of the data from the group they were originally assigned to, regardless of whether they completed the entire treatment (ie, it evaluates the treatment as originally offered to the patients). The advantage of this method is that it better reflects normal clinical practice with regard to drug therapy; however, if large numbers of subjects dropout from non–drug-related causes (eg, subjects move away or simply don't want to bother with follow-up study visits), the true efficacy of a drug can be obscured. For example, suppose 10 patients are enrolled in a study and only 5 complete it, with the remainder dropping out for non–therapy-related reasons. If the drug is efficacious in four of the five patients, the efficacy with the intention-to-treat method would be reported as only 40% (4 of the 10 patients originally assigned to treatment).

The *exclusion of subjects* or *per protocol method* excludes the data from subjects who do not complete the therapy as assigned (ie, it evaluates the treatment as actually taken by the patients). This method does not underestimate the efficacy of treatment, but it also does not take into account those reasons for dropout that affect the clinical usefulness of a drug (eg, side effects or lack of efficacy).

In some studies, the reader will see the data reported by using both methods. This provides the best way in which to evaluate the results of a study.

Discussion

Considerations when evaluating the final discussion section of a published study include whether the conclusions of the investigators are consistent with the data obtained and reported; whether the investigators explored the potential limitations of their study and its design (eg, small study size, the occurrence of "unblinding," or large dropout rate); and whether any extrapolation of their findings, or discussion of the study's external validity, was consistent with the study's original objectives and design, particularly the inclusion/exclusion criteria employed. The discussion should provide an honest synopsis of the significance of the findings in light of all other available evidence.

The significance of the findings should include a statement about the clinical relevance of the results, not simply the statistical significance. It is possible for very small differences between study groups to obtain statistical significance (ie, low risk of type I error), but the differences could be too small to be of clinical usefulness. Also, the significance of the findings should include an assessment of the benefit versus risk from the therapy employed. The "number needed to treat" provides an estimate of the number of patients that would need to receive the treatment in order to prevent one adverse event. Finally, published studies should also relate their findings to previous work in that area. For example, an analysis of 26 published randomized controlled trials found that only two of the studies discussed their results in the context of a systematic review of earlier work, and four additional articles referred to relevant systematic reviews but did not update these reviews with the addition of their results.[40]

Electronic communications are dramatically impacting the way study information is exchanged among the healthcare community. The World Wide Web offers researchers the opportunity to present data that support their published findings, describe their methods in greater detail, illustrate their recent presentations, allow others to comment on work in preliminary stages and to have those comments available to be viewed by other readers, and the web also provides important sources of specialized information and links to other Web sites and citations. The Internet provides a means to publish scientific work and to distribute it widely without major barriers to access; however, it is important that quality assurance (eg, peer review) is still maintained. Many medical journals have already instituted the dissemination of important studies by presenting the data at their web sites prior to publication in their journal. Other journals provide access to their issues via the Internet at no charge. Electronic biomedical publishing is beginning to change the face of the medical literature and how it is accessed.

REFERENCES

One of the International Committee of Medical Journal Editors' requirements for publishing manuscripts is that the references cited in the article must be verified by the author. Whenever possible, authors should cite results obtained from a clinical trial rather than relying on the accuracy of another author's reporting of the results in a review article. Readers should be cautious when references cited are over-represented by papers authored by one of the study authors.

SUMMARIES OF THE LITERATURE

Clinicians are often interested in obtaining a comprehensive summary of the available information on a specific topic instead of individual studies. *Review articles* constitute one type of publication, a systematic overview, used for summarizing the medical literature on a certain subject. These reviews generally compile published information on broad aspects of a topic and offer recommendations or conclusions based upon the author's opinions. Authors of review articles should specify the methods they used to identify the relevant literature (eg, databases and search terms used) as well as how they selected the articles included in order to avoid a biased sampling (ie, selection of only articles that support a given hypothesis). One advantage of a review article is that it provides a healthcare practitioner who might know little about a specific subject with a summary of much of the published information on that topic. This can allow the practitioner to become fairly up-to-date on a topic relatively quickly. A review article's bibliography can also be used as a source for clinical studies of interest on a subject.

Unlike a qualitative review article, a meta-analysis (another type of systematic overview) is a summary article that provides quantitative data. A *meta-analysis* uses formal statistical techniques to sum a body of separate, but similar, original research studies in order to formulate a conclusion.[28] Meta-analyses have been reported to an increasing extent in the medical literature. Meta-analyses can be used to increase statistical power for end points and subgroup analyses, to improve estimates of effect size, to address questions not posed at the start of individual trials, to provide preliminary data regarding sample sizes and hypotheses needed for large definitive clinical studies, to help resolve uncertainties when individual trials disagree, and to generalize conclusions to a more varied range of patients and treatment protocols.[28,41–44]

Despite the convenience and proposed advantages of review articles and meta-analyses, several problems or pitfalls exist. Review articles often are not based upon a focused clinical question, might not include the criteria used by the authors in locating relevant material or in selecting the articles to include, might not assess the validity of the studies included, and can reflect subjective and inaccurate opinions of the authors.[45] Potential problems with meta-analyses are summarized in Table 9-3 and should be kept in mind when reading them. A published

Table 9-3. Issues and Problems with Meta-Analyses

Which studies should be included in the analysis?
Could selection bias be present in the studies included?
What should be done with poorly designed trials?
Should the studies included be weighted using predetermined criteria?
Have all the relevant studies been retrieved? Publication bias (the tendency of journals to publish studies with positive findings) could influence the results if only published studies are sought; however, obtaining all the relevant published and unpublished literature could be difficult.
Were tests of homogeneity done to minimize the likelihood that significant heterogeneous trials were combined?
Were the adverse effects in each study that were included in the analysis appropriately considered?
Were differences in the treatment interventions present? Differences in the treatment interventions (eg, drug dosages, dosing intervals or duration of administration) could make it difficult to combine study results.

users' guide for how to use review articles includes several important questions to ask about these articles, such as are the results valid, what are the results, and how can the results apply to patient care?[45]

Studies have reported that discrepancies can exist between meta-analyses and subsequent large well-controlled trials.[44,47,48] The results of meta-analyses were found to disagree 10–35% of the time with subsequent large clinical trials.[47,48] It has been suggested that meta-analyses should be used primarily to generate hypotheses for further study in large controlled trials rather than to test hypotheses, and to help understand and predict discrepancies in the findings of different trials.[44,48] However, in the absence of definitive studies, a well-performed meta-analysis can provide valuable guidance with regard to therapeutic recommendations.

When searching the secondary information source MEDLINE, it is easy to identify and retrieve literature summaries by limiting the search to publication types such as review article or meta-analysis. Once these types of articles are retrieved, however, the reader should also conduct a critical analysis of them.

PHARMACEUTICAL INDUSTRY AND PUBLISHED INFORMATION

The pharmaceutical industry represents a rich source of information concerning the medicines it produces. By some accounts, the pharmaceutical industry spends more time and resources on generating, analyzing, and disseminating medical information than it does on manufacturing its medications.[49] Most of the data generated during the discovery phase of new drugs remains confidential. In order to obtain approval to market a drug, drug manufacturers must compile an application containing results from clinical trials conducted for the indications sought. Pharmaceutical marketing is aimed mainly at physicians, although it has been increasingly targeting consumers as well, and has been criticized because it may lead to inappropriate physician prescribing and thereby potentially increase costs while leading to a worsening in health. Drug companies realize the value of publications of studies of their drugs as a means of influencing medical practice. There is a preponderance of positive studies sponsored by pharmaceutical manufacturers that are published in the medical literature. Reasons for this include the use of protocols that employ inappropriate doses of comparator drugs, selective publication of studies that have significant findings, selective reporting of studies using the more favorable per protocol analysis, and multiple publications from the same studies.[50,51] The income for the medical journals themselves from the publication of clinical trials may also play a role in the overrepresentation of positive studies in the medical literature.

Promotional Information

Although the main reason that journals publish drug advertisements is to earn money, advertisements may have educational value as well. The Federal Food, Drug, and Cosmetic Act requires that all drug advertisements contain (among other things) information in brief summary relating to side effects, contraindications, and effectiveness. Typically, print advertisements include a reprinting of the risk-related sections of the product's approved labeling (also called full prescribing information or the package insert). The FDA encourages sponsors to write this risk information in language appropriate for the targeted audience. In addition to the specific disclosure requirements, advertisements cannot be false or misleading or omit material facts. They also must present a fair balance between effectiveness and risk information.

Pharmacists, health care professionals and consumers alike should be cautious when assessing information concerning efficacy, safety, convenience, or economics that is contained in pharmaceutical advertisements. The FDA through the Division of Drug Marketing Advertising and Communications (DDMAC) has authority over the publication of promotional information. However, it lacks the resources to ensure that all promotional information is accurate, truthful and well balanced. Journal editors likewise lack the appropriate resources to carefully review all advertisements submitted for publication in their journal. One thing editors can do is to ensure that advertisements are easily distinguishable from other articles by the use of color and placement within the journal.[52] Advertisers have been criticized for their use of false or misleading claims, extension of the indications, making exaggerated claims, and application of one standard for developed countries and another for the developing countries.[14] Use of terms such as "Drug of Choice" or "New" carry connotations that can be misleading and the FDA has prescribed definitions of such terms to help ensure that promotional language is not misleading.

INTERNET MEDICAL INFORMATION

There are estimated to be over 167 million US Internet users, a figure that has increased steadily. Over 63% of adults were reported to have online access, with more than 100 million Americans looking online at least once for health/medical information.[53] The Health On the Net Foundation conducted an Internet survey in 2001 to characterize Internet use for medical and health related purposes. Of 3,325 respondents, 70% were $\geq$ 40 years of age. Ninety-two percent browsed web sites; the majority searched for medical literature (83%), drug information (81%), or disease descriptions (67%). Only about 63% of persons discussed the search results with their care provider(s).[54] The more recent 2002 survey reported similar findings, with about 28% of patients indicating that accuracy was the most critical issue facing medical information on the Internet (the highest percentage for any issue).[55]

Web sites have been found to provide incomplete or incorrect information on various health topics such as complementary medicine for inflammatory bowel disease or emergency contraception. Only a minority (20%) of Internet information from traditional medical sites discussing childhood diarrhea treatment were found to actually conform to American Academy of Pediatrics guidelines.[56] Of 19 web pages providing information about the home management of cough in children, their quality scores ranged from −5 to 5 (maximum of 6 points), with only three sites scoring 3 or above. Ten of the 19 received negative scores, indicating they provided more incorrect than correct information.[57] In one study, the investigators developed a rating scale, based upon clinical practice guidelines published by the Agency for Health Care Research and Quality, for determining the quality of web-based information on depression treatment. Of 21 web sites evaluated, the mean quality score was only 4.7 out of a maximum of 43 points.[58] In another study, of 10 sites providing English language depression information, only 44% supplied more than minimal coverage and completely accurate information. For childhood asthma and obesity, only 36% and 37% of sites, respectively, provided more than minimal coverage and completely correct information.[59] Internet information about St. John's Wort, an herbal product, was found to be of predominantly poor quality.[60] Additional analysis found that citing professional sources and a lack of financial interest were significantly associated with providing correct information, although content quality was still found to be fairly low in such sites. A recent review of studies examining web site quality found that most concluded that quality was a problem, although the methodology employed by the individual studies was variable.[61] Given widespread, increasing public use of the Internet, it is critical that its medical information be accurate and reliable. This is particularly true since most people do not appear to actually use rigorous criteria when determining a web site's accuracy and credibility, even when claiming to do so.[62]

Pharmacists and other health care professionals should be knowledgeable about key points to look for and criteria to use to help determine the quality of Internet information, and they should assist patients in locating reputable web sites that will meet the patients' medical information needs.

A wide range of organizations have developed or are in the process of developing methods or tools for evaluating and rating web site quality that can be used by web site developers or consumers. These methods/tools include codes of conduct, quality labels, user guides, filters, and third party certification.[63] Codes of conduct consist of quality criteria for the content of Internet sites for use by developers and consumers. However, the extent to which oversight is provided with regard to implementation of the code is variable and can be nonexistent. A quality label or award is included on a web site to indicate the developer's commitment to adhere to a code of conduct. The degree to which this is enforced and the criteria upon which the label is assigned can be unclear. While user guides can help consumers perform their own evaluation of a web site, the time, effort, and expertise required on the part of consumers to rate web sites can make these of limited benefit. Filters are used to accept or reject web sites based on preestablished criteria, and serve a "gateway" function. These can be very useful to consumers although high in cost to maintain due to the expertise required to review web sites. Third party accreditation labels are awarded to web sites that meet the criteria established by a third party organization or accrediting body. These are not yet in existence on a large-scale basis.

One study reviewed rating instruments that have been used to assess web site quality and provide site awards, with 98 instruments identified from 1997 to 2002.[64] Of these, many were not functioning at the end of that 5-year period. Many more were not eligible for review in the study because they did not provide a description of their rating criteria used. A total of 11 rating instruments were ultimately reviewed. Of these, none appeared to have been validated. A number of initiatives have been underway to identify or to help consumers identify high quality Internet health information sites.[64,65] These include government organizations such as Medline Plus from the National Library of Medicine, Healthfinder from the US Department of Health and Human Services, and HealthInsite from the Australia Department of Health and Aging,[64,65] as well as two initiatives from the United Kingdom, the Electronic Quality Information for Patients (EQUIP) and the Organising Medical Networked Information (OMNI),[65] among several others. Readers are urged to refer to these latter two references for additional information and the web site addresses for these initiatives.

REFERENCES

1. *Pharmacists for the Future: The Report of the Study Commission on Pharmacy.* Ann Arbor, MI: Health Administration Press, 1975, p 48.
2. Karp S, Monroe AF. *Manag Care Quart* 2002; 10(2):3–8.
3. Blois MS, Shortliffe EH. The computer meets medicine: emergence of a discipline. In Shortliffe EH, Perreault LE, Wiederhold G, et al, eds. *Medical Informatics: Computer Applications in Health Care.* Reading, MA: Addison-Wesley, 1990, p 20.
4. The Evidence-Based Medicine Working Group. *Users' guides to the medical literature. Essentials of evidence-based clinical practice.* Guyatt G, Rennie D, eds. Chicago, IL: AMA Press, 2002, pp 8–14.
5. Grace M, Wertheimer AI. *Am J Hosp Pharm* 1975; 32:903–904.
6. Pearson RE, Lauper RD, Davis LJ. *Am J Hosp Pharm* 1975; 32:31–34.
7. Price KO, Goldwire MA. *Am Pharm* 1994; NS34:30–39.
8. Gong SD, Millares M, VanRiper KB. *Am J Hosp Pharm* 1992; 49:1121–1130.
9. Russello CM, Peterson AM. *Am Pharm* 1993; NS33(11):49–52.
10. Martin S. *Am Pharm* 1991; NS31(2):25–26.
11. Justice J. *Am Pharm* 1993; NS33(11):53–57
12. Colvin C. *Am J Hosp Pharm* 1990; 47:1989–1990.
13. Altman DG. *BMJ* 1994; 308:283–284.
14. Villaneuva P, Peiro S, Libero J, et al. *Lancet* 2003; 361:27–32.
15. Ziegler MG, Lew P, Singer BC. *JAMA* 1995; 273:1296–1298.
16. Moher D, Schulz KF, Altman D for the CONSORT Group. *JAMA* 2001;285:1987–1991 http://www.consort-statement.org/revised-statement.htm, Accessed July 28, 2003.
17. Bossuyt PM, Reitsma JB, Gatsonis CA, et al. *BMJ* 2003; 326:41–44.
18. Moher D. *JAMA* 1998; 279:1489–1491.
19. Gehlbach SH, ed. *Interpreting the Medical Literature.* New York: McGraw-Hill, 2002, p 17.
20. Moher D, Jadad AR, Nichol G, et al. *Control Clin Trials* 1995; 16:62–73.
21. Altman LK. *Lancet* 1996; 347:1382–1386.
22. Uniform Requirements for Manuscripts Submitted to Biomedical Journals. Available at http://www.icmje.org/index.html#conflict. Accessed July 28, 2003.
23. Alpert JS, Furman S, Smaha L. *Arch Intern Med* 2002; 162:635–637.
24. Gehlbach, *Interpreting the Medical Literature,* p 156.
25. Young MJ, Bresnitz EA, Strom BL. *Ann Intern Med* 1983; 99:248–251.
26. Stolley PD, Strom BL. *Clin Pharmacol Ther* 1986; 39:489–490.
27. Expert Working Group (Efficacy) of the International Conference on Harmonisation. Guidance for Industry: E6 Good Clinical Practice: Consolidated Guidance. April 1996. http://www.fda.gov/cder/guidance/959fnl.pdf. Accessed July 28, 2003.
28. Berger VW, Bears JD. *Vaccine* 2003; 21:468–472.
29. Guyatt GH, Sackett DL, Cook DJ. *JAMA* 1993; 270:2598–2601.
30. Adam A, Posner J, eds. *A Guide to Clinical Drug Research.* Dordrecht: Kluwer Academic, 1995, p 7.
31. Motheral BR. *J Managed Care Pharm* 1998; 4:382–390.
32. Gehlbach, *Interpreting the Medical Literature,* p 84.
33. Gehlbach, *Interpreting the Medical Literature,* p 130.
34. Gehlbach, *Interpreting the Medical Literature,* p 181.
35. Gehlbach, *Interpreting the Medical Literature,* p 226.
36. Basskin L. *Formulary* 1997; 32: 279–280,283–286.
37. Cho MK, Bero LA. *JAMA* 1994; 272:101–104.
38. The Asilomar Working Group on Recommendations for Reporting of Clinical Trials in the Biomedical Literature. *Ann Intern Med* 1996; 124:741–743.
39. Guyatt et al. *Users' Guides to the Medical Literature,* pp 378–380.
40. Clarke M, Chalmers I. *JAMA* 1998; 280:280–282.
41. Egger M, Smith GD. *BMJ* 1998; 316:61–66.
42. Egger M, Smith GD. *BMJ* 1997; 315:1371–1374.
43. Egger M, Smith GD, Phillips AN. *BMJ* 1997; 315:1533–1537.
44. Borzak S, Ridker PM. *Ann Intern Med* 1995; 123:873–877.
45. Guyatt et al. *Users' Guides to the Medical Literature,* pp 243–266.
46. Gibaldi M. *Drugs* 1993; 46:805–815.
47. LeLorier J, Gregoire G, Benhaddad A, et al. *N Engl J Med* 1997; 337:536–542.
48. Ioannidis JP, Cappelleri JC, Lau J. *JAMA* 1998; 279:1089–1093.
49. Collier J, Iheanacho I. *Lancet* 2002; 360:1405–1409.
50. Melander H, Ahlqvist-Rastad J, Meijer G, et al. *BMJ* 2003; 326:1171–1175.
51. Lexchin J, Bero LA, Djulbegovic B, et al. *BMJ* 2003; 326:1167–1176.
52. Fletcher RH, Fletcher SW. *Ann Intern Med* 1992; 116:951–952.
53. Harris Interactive. 100 million U.S. net users are 'cyberchondriacs' (April 25, 2001). http://www.nua.ie/surveys. Accessed October 2003.
54. Health on the Net Foundation. Evolution of Internet use for health purposes. www.hon.ch/Survey/FebMar2001/survey.html. Accessed October 2003.
55. Health on the Net Foundation. Excerpt of the 8th HON's survey of health and medical internet users. www.hon.ch/Survey/8thHONresults.html. Accessed October 2003.
56. McClung HJ, Murray RD, Heitlinger LA. *Pediatrics* 1998; 101(6):1–4. (Pediatrics online) http://www.pediatrics.org/cgi/content/full/101/6/e2
57. Pandolfini C, Impicciatore P, Bonati M. *Pediatrics* 2000;105(1): 1–8. (Pediatrics online) http://www.pediatrics.org/cgi/content/full/105/1/e1
58. Griffiths KM, Christensen H. *BMJ* 2000; 321:1511–1515.
59. Berland GK, Elliott MN, Morales LS, et al. *JAMA* 2001; 285:2612–2621.
60. Martin-Facklam M, Kostrzewa M, Schubert F, et al. *Am J Med* 2002; 113:740–745.
61. Eysenbach G, Powell P, Kuss O, et al. *JAMA* 2002; 287:2691–2700.
62. Eysenbach G, Kohler C. *BMJ* 2002; 324:573–577.
63. Wilson P. *BMJ* 2002;324:598–602.
64. Gagliardi A, Jadad AR. *BMJ* 2002; 324:569–573.
65. Huang QR. *Aust Fam Physician* 2003; 32:335–341.

APPENDIX Selected Journals of Interest to Pharmacy

ACP Journal Club (American College of Physicians)
AJHP: American Journal of Health-System Pharmacy
American Family Physician
American Heart Journal
American Journal of Cardiology
American Journal of Clinical Nutrition
American Journal of Emergency Medicine
American Journal of Medicine
American Journal of Obstetrics and Gynecology
American Journal of Psychiatry
American Journal of Respiratory and Critical Care Medicine
Anesthesiology
Annals of Allergy, Asthma, and Immunology
Annals of Emergency Medicine
Annals of Internal Medicine
Annals of Neurology
Annals of Pharmacotherapy
Archives of Dermatology
Archives of General Psychiatry
Archives of Internal Medicine
Archives of Neurology
Archives of Pediatrics and Adolescent Medicine
Arthritis and Rheumatism
BMJ: British Medical Journal
Cancer
Chest
Circulation
Clinical Infectious Diseases
Clinical Obstetrics and Gynecology
Clinical Orthopaedics and Related Research
Clinical Pediatrics
Clinical Pharmacokinetics
Clinical Pharmacology and Therapeutics
Clinics in Sports Medicine
CMAJ/Canadian Medical Association Journal
Critical Care Medicine
Diabetes
Diabetes Care

Digestive Diseases and Sciences
Disease-a-Month
Diseases of the Colon & Rectum
Drugs
Endocrinology
Emergency Medicine Clinics of North America
Fertility and Sterility
Gastroenterology
Geriatrics
Gut
JAMA: The Journal of the American Medical Association
Journal of Allergy and Clinical Immunology
Journal of Alternative and Complementary Medicine
Journal of Clinical Endocrinology and Metabolism
Journal of Family Practice
Journal of Infectious Diseases
Journal of Pediatrics
Journal of Substance Abuse Treatment
Journal of the American Academy of Dermatology
Journal of the American College of Cardiology
Journal of the American Dietetic Association
Journal of the American Geriatrics Society
Journal of the National Cancer Institute
Lancet
Medical Clinics of North America
Medical Letter on Drugs and Therapeutics
Medicine
Neurology
New England Journal of Medicine
Obstetrics and Gynecology
Pediatric Clinics of North America
Pediatrics
PharmacoEconomics
Pharmacotherapy
Postgraduate Medicine
Rheumatology
Sports Medicine
Therapeutic Drug Monitoring

Data from Hill DR, Stickell H, Crow SJ. Brandon/Hill selected list of print books and journals for the small medical library. http://www.mssm.edu/library/brandon-hill/small_medical/pdf/brandon4.pdf. Accessed January 2004.

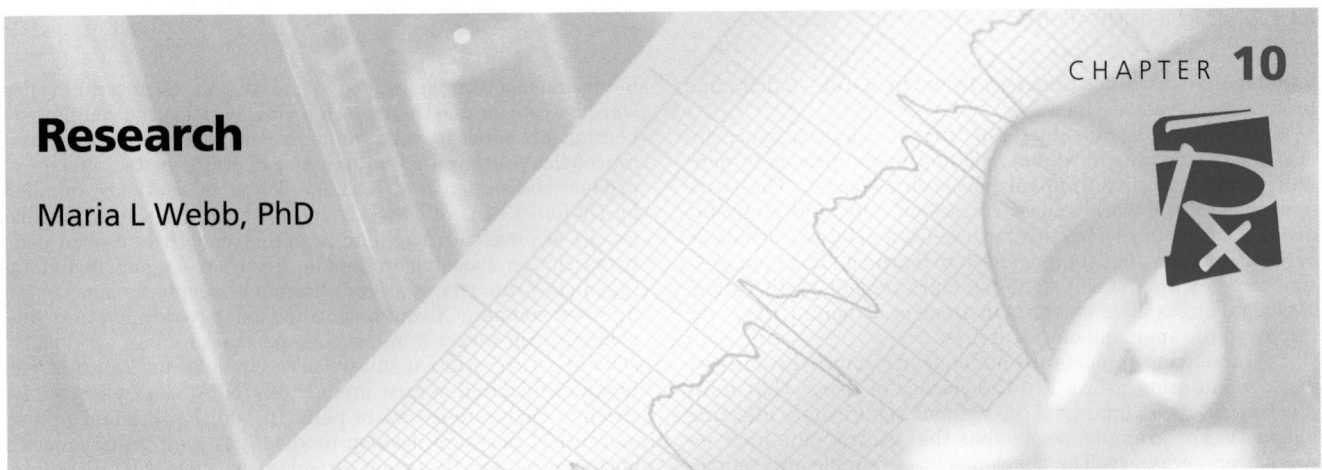

CHAPTER 10

Research

Maria L Webb, PhD

Medical and pharmaceutical research provide a basis for the development of new therapeutic approaches to human and animal disease. This process of drug discovery research can be basic (seeking an understanding of biological phenomena that are unknown) or applied (using principals that are known to produce a desired new product or effect). In either case, drug discovery research results from an unmet clinical need, a recognized deficit in treatment options. The outcome of a successful drug discovery program is the generation of a therapeutic where none previously existed, or the replacement of established therapies in favor of a newer modality that is safer and more efficacious.[1]

The main function of the pharmaceutical industry is to create products (ie, drugs, that have an impact on health care). Products of this type can be foreseen to some extent through knowledge and study and thus are amenable to planned research and development (R&D). For example, if the cause of a disease has been identified as an infection by a microorganism, a search can be undertaken for an agent that will prevent or cure the infection. However, in some instances, the etiology of a disease is unknown despite intensive investigation. In the latter situation, the pathway to a satisfactory cure or method of prevention cannot be foreseen or forecast. In such cases, products may only be developed after application of careful investigations, from a revolutionary new approach, or perhaps from a serendipitous finding.

Although much of the drug discovery research in the United States is carried out by major pharmaceutical manufacturers and biotechnology companies, this research is dependent on a vast and growing background of scientific knowledge generated by diverse organizations. Universities, private institutes, governmental laboratories, and industrial research all play significant roles in developing new technologies and knowledge that provides the basis for discovery and the ultimate generation of a new product. This new knowledge may involve development of a new technology, improved scientific methodology and instrumentation, or increased understanding of the basic molecular or cell biology underlying a disease.

The major objective of research in the pharmaceutical industry is to produce safe drugs that prevent, cure, or ameliorate disease. Interim research goals that lead to this major objective are to:

- Understand the molecular basis of biological mechanisms in health and disease.
- Develop new biological testing procedures relevant to human medicine.
- Develop a quantitative understanding of the interaction of drugs with key biological systems, leading to the more rational design of drugs.
- Understand the absorption, transport, and mode of action of drugs.

- Develop drugs of low toxicity, reproducible delivery, and high specificity for a given pathological state.

This chapter will touch on the above points to illustrate how drug discovery research is used to develop new products that fulfill clinical needs.

EVOLUTION OF 20TH CENTURY PHARMACEUTICAL RESEARCH

The search for medicines to treat disease began with natural products. Up to the early part of the 20th century, pharmaceuticals derived almost entirely from natural products such as menthol, which was derived from peppermint and used for treating coughs and colds. The practice of gathering and preparing dried herbs was commonplace. Boneset tea reduced fevers, peppermint relieved an aching tooth or a colicky baby, and foxglove could revive a failing heart. Early challenges were to develop and manufacture drugs of uniform strength and quality, as the quality often varied with the raw materials or the skill of the pharmacist. Current challenges for natural products relate more to mining natural biodiversity[2] and meeting the synthetic challenges.[3]

Until World War I, most synthetic drugs and chemicals used in the United States were discovered and produced in Europe. When supplies were curtailed by the war, the impetus was provided for the establishment of an independent US chemical and pharmaceutical industry. Accordingly, production of chemicals and drugs was undertaken and was the stimulus for the development of industrial research. In the following years, the US pharmaceutical industry made major contributions through discovery and development of new drugs, and it assumed a place of leadership in the world.

Toward the mid-20th century, chemical research on the isolation, identification, and synthesis of drugs began to yield many important drug substances. During this time the synthesis and manufacture of vitamins was a major focus of companies such as Roche and Merck. Discovery and development of the sulfonamides, antibiotics, and other anti-infective agents dramatically reduced the death rates from a number of infectious diseases. Among the major drugs discovered and/or developed in the United States during this period were insulin, sulfonamides, penicillin and broad-spectrum antibiotics, cortisone and other steroid compounds, isoniazid for the treatment of tuberculosis, diuretics, and the tranquilizers. Principally through the use of drugs like isoniazid, the tuberculosis death rate between 1945 and 1978 declined from 39 per 100,000 people to 1 per 100,000 people. As a large proportion of the deaths from these diseases had occurred prior to adulthood, these drugs allowed more individuals than ever before to mature and assume productive roles in society.

Since the 1980s, new classes of drugs that impact hypertension and lipidemias have emerged and made inroads to morbidity and mortality from cardiovascular disease. These are now some of the world's most efficacious, safe, and profitable drugs. Cancer medicines are moving from cytotoxic agents to cytostatic agents, but there is much to learn and do to progress this complex area of cell signaling and rampant proliferation. New challenges have emerged in areas of dementia given our improved life span and our awareness.

Of increasing importance as longevity improves and the world population grows are the classes of drugs that have marked effects on quality of life without significantly affecting longevity. For example, compounds that control pain have always been necessary. The development of reliable oral contraceptive therapy made intelligent family planning possible. Tranquilizers and other central nervous system drugs made an important contribution to the treatment of mental illness and restoration to normal activities. Newer life style drugs as we head into the 21st century are those that impact addictive behaviors such as smoking, weight control, sexual dysfunction.

PHARMACEUTICAL RESEARCH ORGANIZATIONS

The pharmaceutical and biotechnology industries are leaders among all US industries in the support of R&D. The industry finances almost all of its R&D with its own funds; no other industry spends as high a percentage of R&D funds for basic and applied research. A significant portion of every sales dollar is devoted to drug research activities (Table 10-1). For instance, in 2001, US pharmaceutical companies devoted 12–20% of their sales revenues to R&D.[4] The average R&D spending for the top 20 pharma companies was US 1.9 billion or 16.3% of sales. This expenditure in part underlies the cost of prescription drugs.[5]

Technological advances have led to an explosion of small biotechnology companies that specialize in one or more steps in the preclinical and clinical processes. Often large pharmaceutical companies contract to the smaller outside companies as a way of extending their internal resources. The trend toward outsourcing among large pharmaceuticals companies has led to the growth of many companies such as Covance that contract production of biopharmaceuticals.[6]

The academic community plays a vital role in the development of new drugs. Its role includes, but is not limited to, research on a basic understanding of disease states, development of biochemical or physiological rationale for drug targets, the initial evaluation of new drugs, consultantships with companies to use their academic and scientific expertise to guide pharmaceutical research, and certainly not least, the training of scientists. During the late 1980s and early 1990s, scientists at universities made many basic discoveries toward identification of enabling technologies, which led to the founding of many

biotechnology companies. Over time, the platform technologies were used to enable the biotech technology-focused company to become a product-focused company, the true endpoint of pharmaceutical research. Examples of a platform technology to product conversion are: (1) Ligand Pharmaceuticals, founded by Dr Ron Evans of the Salk Institute, was based on the discovery of novel intracellular receptors and their role in gene transcription, focusing on the identification of agonists and antagonists primarily of steroid hormone receptors. Ligand and its sister company X-ceptor continue today to work on these important drug target families. Ligand markets four products—ONTAK, Targretin capsules, Targretin gel, and Panretin gel. Ligand's fifth and newest product, AVINZA, is a treatment for chronic, moderate-to-severe pain. In addition, Ligand's pharmaceutical partners develop products for men's and women's hormone-related diseases, osteoporosis, metabolic disorders, and cardiovascular and inflammatory diseases. (2) Vertex was founded by Dr Joshua Boger, using the structure-based design that relies on the high-resolution molecular image of the active site of a disease molecule. Vertex has several major pharmaceutical partnerships including with GlaxoSmithKline for the development and marketing of Agenerase (amprenavir) for HIV, and with Kissei for p38 MAP Kinase inhibitors for use in inflammatory disease. (3) In contrast to the target-family focus brought by Ligand and X-ceptor or the structure-based desing brought by Vertex, Pharmacopeia, founded by Drs Michael Wigler and Clark Still, a combinatorial chemistry company employs chemical and biological diversity and high-throughput screening approaches to lead and drug discovery. Pharmacopeia has a drug pipeline based on its collaborations with key pharmaceutical partners such as Schering-Plough, Bristol-Myers Squibb, Daiichi, and Berlex Laboratories. Thus, partnerships between academia and biotechnology, as well as between biotechnology and large pharma, have propelled both the genesis and evolution of biotech. It is likely that change will continue to occur at a faster pace in the smaller and more opportunistic biotech area than in its large pharma partners.

Clinicians and clinical scientists often lead the discovery of new uses for drugs and new directions for research based on observations made in the clinical setting. Chlorpromazine was originally synthesized as an antihistamine but found to be useful as a tranquilizer. The clinical use of this compound, and of other central nervous system drugs, has resulted in a marked reduction in the number of the mentally ill needing hospitalization.

Research in the academic community has been supported to a major extent by agencies of the US government, such as the Public Health Service (PHS), the National Institutes of Health (NIH), the Center for Disease Control (CDC), and the National Science Foundation (NSF). The pharmaceutical industry also contributes financial support to academic laboratories where research of general or specific interest to the industry is conducted. Institutes established by private endowment such as the Sloan-Kettering Institute, Shriner Children's Hospitals, the Institute for the Study of Aging, and the Gates Foundation all pursue basic and applied research in many fields related to the public health. Many hospitals also maintain research clinics and/or privately or publicly endowed foundations to pursue causes and treatment of specific diseases, a related group of diseases, diseases endemic to a certain geographical area, or groups of diseases affecting a certain organ of the body. Because research does not depend on the vending of items or services, it is not immediately self-supportive and necessarily must be supported by public as well as private funds.

Interest in pharmaco-epidemiological research has prompted the development and need for review criteria in this area. The Hartzema guide[7] makes use of case-controlled and cohort studies as major methodologies in this field. Generally, the evaluation criteria for case-controlled and cohort studies address proper sample-frame definition, compatibility of cases and controls, drug-exposure validations, unintended-effect ascertainment procedures, and related considerations. Although these

Table 10-1. Leading Pharmaceutical Companies Ranked by R&D Spending (US$ in millions) in 2001

COMPANY	R&D SPENDING	PHARMA SALES	R&D AS % OF SALES
Pfizer	4,847	25,518	19
GlaxoSmithKline	3,694	24,791	14.9
AstraZeneca	2,687	16,183	16.6
Aventis	2,574	14,879	17.3
Johnson & Johnson	2,465	14,851	16.6
Merck & Co	2,456	19,732	12.4
Eli Lilly	2,235	10,856	20.6
Pharmacia	2,085	11,970	17.4
Bristol-Myers Squibb	2,066	15,300	13.5
Novartis	2,046	11,963	17.1

From Charish P. *Scrip Magazine* 2003; (February):41.

can be confusing, Hartzema provides interpretation of the statistics used in reporting case-controlled and cohort studies and gives review criteria for meta-analysis, an approach to integrating the pharmaco-epidemiological literature.

THE SEARCH FOR NEW DRUGS

Until the early 20th century, most useful drugs, such as morphine, quinine, digitalis, ergot, and atropine to name a few, were derived from plant sources, and their therapeutic uses were based on serendipitous discoveries. As the science of medicinal chemistry evolved, screening of natural products has become more methodical. Screening of natural products is based on the concept that evolution favors molecular conservation. However, the future of natural products screening for drug discovery is presently limited by speed and compound diversity.

In the mid-20th century, useful drugs were derived from natural products, chemical syntheses, or combinations of both sources. The approaches used to identify lead molecules that evolved to drugs covered the spectrum between molecular diversity to rational design. Rational, or structure-based, drug design refers to a process that begins with a high-resolution map to the active site of a disease target. With an x-ray crystal structure or a nuclear magnetic resonance image, medicinal and protein chemists can engineer molecules to fit, or better fit, the active site. This approach is appealing, has been applied by biotechnology companies in a more high-throughput fashion, and has been successful in the field of human immunodeficiency virus (HIV) protease inhibitors, and many protein kinases.

Structure-based design is not currently applicable to all classes of drug targets, however. Guanine nucleotide-coupled receptors (GPCRs), which have proven to be one of the most feasible classes of drug targets, intertwine between the extra- and intracellular surface seven times. Because of their architecture in the lipid bilayer of the cell membrane, the structure of these "heptahelical receptors" has not been solved. However, using processes described below, many successful drugs have been found that work through GPCRs.

The advent of combinatorial chemistry in the 1980s and 1990s greatly impacted drug discovery. This technology refers to the generation of compounds in sets, or libraries, that are typically chemically related and made by combining sets of reactions such that the chemical steps are efficiently conducted. Combinatorial chemistry was initially applied to amino acids and nucleotides by Affymax and NeXagen, respectively. Since then, several companies predominantly Pharmacopeia and Arqule, have applied this technology to small molecules. Having large numbers of compounds allows for increases in subtle alterations in chemical relatedness as well as chemical diversity. This point is critical since the biological target is the true measure of a successful chemical interaction and attempts to use descriptors to capture chemical diversity will not discriminate in the relevant ways that biology does. This point was well made by Jurgen Drewes[8] when he wrote that "It is, however, by no means certain to what extent molecular diversity as viewed by chemists and as calculated by structural descriptors resembles diversity as 'seen' by a biological target molecule."

Collections of compounds can be designed to be "drug-like" in that they have favorable physicochemical properties in common with known drugs. These properties were first elucidated by Dr Chris Lipinski of Pfizer and have become known as the "Lipinski Rule of 5". Based on his analysis of drugs developed predominantly at Pfizer, Dr. Lipinski described key traits for a molecule to have suitability as a drug.[9] These traits are less than 5 hydrogen-bonds, less that 10 hydrogen-bond acceptors, an octanol-water partition coefficient less than 5, and a molecular weight less than 5. It is important to note, however, that approximately 25% of the drugs in the Comprehensive Medical Chemistry (CMC) data base do not follow the "Rule of Five." Typically, these exceptions are antibacterials, antineoplastics,

or CNS drugs. The large percentage of exceptions would advise against overly strict adherence to these guidelines as rules. Indeed, it is rare to identify a drug in a HTS and best to think of compound collections as sources of leads that can be optimized by medicinal chemists, biologists, and pharmacologists to drugs.

The testing of compound collections in high-throughput screens (HTS) is another area where key advancement has occurred in the last 25 years of the pharmaceutical industry. HTS allows scientists to devise biochemical assays around a molecular target using new technologies. With more sensitive high-throughput technologies focused on identification of activity at a precise molecular target, the likelihood that a compound will be identified in a high-throughput screen (HTS) also increases. One of the primary impacts of combinatorial chemistry and its HTS counterpart has been the identification of leads from chemical libraries more efficiently.

Chemical Libraries and Sample Collections

Prior to the advent of combinatorial chemistry, organic chemists in the pharmaceutical industry synthesized new compounds one at a time. The collection of these compounds was not particularly diverse but led to hundreds of thousands of compounds in a company's sample collection. Combinatorial chemistry has greatly increased the efficiency of compound synthesis leading to significantly larger compound collections. For example, at present Pharmacopeia has 7 million drug-like compounds. The explosion in synthesis of chemical libraries necessitated more efficient testing of biological activity.

Initial screening of thousands of compounds is accomplished rapidly by use of in vitro enzymatic or receptor screens. Typically, several unique active lead compounds emerge, which are studied in a variety of secondary assays, either confirming or refuting the original hypothesis.

The small molecular weight of compounds in a chemical library favors the chance of their oral availability. The Lipinski guideline that is applied for oral absorption across the gastrointestinal tract is that a compound should be about 500 daltons.[9] Other guidelines are polar surface area and hydrophobicity measures.[10] Orally available drugs are highly desirable, and that is why small molecule drug discovery remains the focus of pharmaceuticals over their biological counterparts.

Whether a molecular diversity or rational design approach was followed to identify the lead molecule, drug discovery tends to proceed thereafter through an iterative process of chemical modification and biological testing. Teams of scientists improve the characteristics of their lead compound in an optimization process. If successful in building the appropriate characteristics, this process results in a drug candidate.

Natural Product Sources

In addition to compound collections, organic chemists and biochemists derive leads from natural product sources. Natural products can derive from plant and animal sources; in the latter category microbial and marine organisms often are considered separately from ordinary domestic animals. Digitalis glycosides, such as digitalis and digoxin, derive from the foxglove plant and are powerful cardiac stimulants. The poppy plant has provided opium alkaloids (morphine, codeine) used in analgesia; and the belladonna plant provided the belladonna alkaloids (atropine and scopolamine) used as parasympathetic blockers. In addition to the plant alkaloids mentioned earlier, some important natural products include antibiotics, steroid and peptide hormones, vitamins, enzymes, prostaglandins, and pheromones.

Although serendipity plays a relatively large role in the search for natural products, rational biological inputs based on deficiency syndromes, replacement therapy, or known biological effects clearly influence the development of these drugs. Nutritionists, endocrinologists, pharmacologists, microbiologists, biochemists, and physiologists all play a vital role in understanding the underlying biological mechanisms. Antibiotics, steroids, and prostaglandins provided fertile new fields for chemical modification, leading, in all three cases, to drugs that are more useful than the parent compounds. Much research is being undertaken by the NIH and private companies on unique natural products that have anticancer properties. For example, Taxol (paclitaxel), which derives from the bark of a Pacific yew tree (*Taxus brevifolia*), was developed for the treatment of ovarian cancer by Bristol-Myers Squibb. As mentioned earlier, current challenges for natural products research relate to mining natural biodiversity[2] and meeting the synthetic challenges.[3]

FUNCTIONS OF RESEARCH SCIENTISTS

The pharmaceutical industry is an outstanding example of successful collaboration between scientists of biological and physical sciences disciplines. Chemists and other physical scientists predominantly have been responsible for synthesis, isolation, and characterization of medicinal agents. However, biological scientists have played an equally essential role in originating meaningful screening and testing models and in the overall evaluation of new agents. Qualified specialists in many fields including pharmacy, physics, statistics, chemistry, biology, engineering, pharmacology, physiology, medicine, and many others take part in the tremendous research effort in pharmaceuticals. Cooperation is a major feature of today's scientific investigations. Multidisciplinary teams are essential in industrial research requiring collaboration and effective communication as frequently a hundred or more scientists may be involved in discovering and developing a compound into a useful drug.

Some industrial research laboratories are organized according to scientific disciplines, such as departments of organic chemistry or pharmacology. Other companies may use a project-team style wherein chemists, biologists, and pharmacologists are organized into a project unit for the purpose of discovering drugs useful for a particular disease state. Frequently the latter organizational approach is focused on therapeutic areas such as diseases of the cardiovascular, immunological, or central nervous systems. Irrespective of the organizational style, problems in drug discovery and development have become so complex that a multidisciplinary approach to research nearly always is used. For the sake of simplicity, this section will outline the functions of scientists with particular backgrounds who play leading roles in pharmaceutical research; however, the reader should understand that drug development is a cooperative venture among all scientists.

Organic Chemistry

As noted previously, organic chemists synthesize new drug candidates as well as isolate and characterize natural products, such as alkaloids. In each case, there is interest in the complex relationships between chemical structure and pharmacological action. These structure-activity-relationships (SARs) are fundamental to drug discovery. Once synthesized, compounds are evaluated for numerous types of biological and pharmacological action. Observation of interesting and repeatable biological activity opens pathways for additional chemical research effort in the expansion of the series and often leads to significant new medicinal products. Determination of the pharmacological activity of a compound is an involved process with very small changes in structure frequently yielding profound changes in the pharmacological effect. Many of the currently used antispasmodics, anticonvulsants, local anesthetics, non-narcotic analgesics, chemotherapeutic agents, and hypnotics have been products of this approach.

Another research approach is to identify, isolate, and purify compounds from biologically active mixtures. The determination of the structure of a biologically active molecule provides a twofold benefit to pharmacy and medicine. It makes possible research leading to synthesis and modification of the structure. Changes in structure usually are accompanied with changes in biological activity, and occasionally vast improvement is accomplished. For example, our present knowledge of adrenal corticosteroids began with the study of the various components in an extract of the adrenal cortex. The components were characterized structurally and biological activities were assessed. Eventually, cortisone was synthesized from bile acids. Today, some synthetic analogs of cortisone are available that are superior therapeutically to the naturally occurring steroids.

A second example comes from the tetracyclines, a clinically important group of antibiotics. The first of these, 7-chlorotetracycline, was isolated in 1948 from *Streptomyces aureofaciens*. Shortly thereafter, a group of scientists isolated 5-hydroxytetracycline from *Streptomyces rimosus,* and in 1953 its structure was established. Once the chemical structure of this antibiotic was known, the way was opened for systematic variation of the basic nucleus to obtain new drugs with improved properties. Specifically, the catalytic removal of chlorine from 7-chlorotetracycline gave tetracycline itself, which proved to be superior to either of the above-mentioned antibiotics, and has replaced them to a large extent. Although tetracycline subsequently has been isolated from a Streptomyces species, this useful antibiotic is prepared more readily by the semisynthetic method.

Studies on the structure and synthesis of penicillins led to the development of the semisynthetic penicillins and later to cephalosporins and monobactams. These new compounds have made possible major improvements in antibiotic therapy. Total synthesis is made possible by knowledge of chemical structures and, in many instances, is important economically in reducing the cost of the drug. Chloramphenicol, which can be obtained from cultures of *Streptomyces venezuelae*, combats bacteria-produced typhoid dysentery and Rocky Mountain spotted fever. A commercially feasible chemical synthesis has replaced the fermentation process for production of the antibiotic.

Microbiology

Since the discovery and development of penicillin during World War II, the search for new antibiotics among the metabolic products of microorganisms has constituted a major research effort in the pharmaceutical industry. The proven clinical usefulness of antibiotics in treating many bacterial infections has fully justified this effort. Microbiologists have searched among a wide variety of fungi and bacteria looking for antibiotic substances. In this search, microorganisms from plant tissues, animal sources, the sea, many types of soil, and from many other ecological niches have been examined. More than 1000 antibiotic substances have been detected and at least partially characterized. A combination of microbiological and chemical methods is required to distinguish the new antibiotics from the host of older ones that already have been discovered.

After a culture has been found to produce a new antibiotic, microbiologists then turn their attention to the biosynthesis of the compound, seeking to improve yields in order to produce quantities of the compound for testing and evaluation. An effort also is made to understand biosynthetic pathways, improve yields further, and facilitate the biosynthetic production of the isotope-labeled antibiotic for pharmacological and toxicological evaluation.

New antibiotics are being evaluated for application in an increasing number of disease conditions. Tests are conducted to determine activity of new antibiotics against a variety of yeasts, molds, and protozoa, as well as against normal and antibiotic-resistant bacterial pathogens. The antibacterial drugs have contributed to major advances in the control of bacterial and other microbial diseases. However, impetus for continued research is provided by problems of drug resistance, patient sensitivity, and the inability to control certain infections.

Microbiologists are concerned not only with the microorganisms that produce antibiotics, but also with the microbial pathogens that the antibiotics are expected to control. The mode of transmission of disease and the pathogenicity, virulence, and invasiveness of the infectious microorganisms are under investigation. A serious problem in drug resistance involves the transfer of drug resistance among gram-negative bacteria by means of an episome bearing one or more antibiotic resistance factors. Agents that prevent the emergence of the resistance factor, or that prevent its transfer, have been sought. Current research is being directed toward agents that enhance host resistance.

Integration of microbiological research and organic chemical research resulted in the production of a series of semisynthetic penicillins and cephalosporins. These antibiotics are chemically modified derivatives of biosynthetically produced antibiotics, which possess improved spectra of action or other advantageous chemical and biological properties.

Biochemistry, Cell Biology, and Molecular Biology

Pharmaceutical research in biochemistry, cell biology and molecular biology has exploded in the past 20 years. These areas include investigations of specific action of substances affecting cellular processes such as the mode of action of biologically active compounds. Biochemistry and cell biology are focused on understanding the underlying biochemical and cellular processes that are involved in the wonderfully complex mechanism of living things: the signal transduction processes, the energy-yielding systems, and the synthetic systems for generation of proteins, nucleic acids, and other macromolecules. Normal cellular communication and metabolic patterns are determined, and efforts are made to define the abnormal conditions that occur in various disease states. Biochemists also are involved in the isolation, purification, and characterization of small and large biologically active molecules.

The increasing sophistication of research demands that an understanding of the molecular bases of diseases emerge as a primary goal. This knowledge has strongly influenced both the methodology of testing new drugs and the choice or design of compounds to be tested. Biological targets (ie, the molecular locations where drugs act) are identified, isolated, and characterized. Usually this involves the cloning and expression of the target from human tissue as well as from various other species that may serve as model systems in drug testing. Some of the receptor systems for which drugs have been developed include those for catecholamines, opiates and steroids, and various peptide hormones such as bradykinin, angiotensin II, and endothelin. The discovery of the enkephalins, natural brain polypeptides that bind the opiate receptor, has opened new horizons in CNS pharmacology. This information has been useful in acquiring new knowledge of the interaction between drugs and their receptor sites and in understanding the requirements for specific spatial orientation of essential structural features of drugs. Drug design also makes provision for those characteristics that will assure absorption, transport to the receptor site and elimination of the therapeutic agent.

Biochemists and cell biologists develop the biomedical rationale to guide medicinal chemists in the design of drugs that are more selective for specific aspects of disease. For example, knowledge of the structure and biochemical function of coenzymes stimulated chemists to synthesize a large number of analogs of coenzymes, some of which have proven to be useful compounds in the chemotherapy of cancer.

Increasing emphasis is being placed on studies of enzymatic processes such as those related to the biosynthesis of cholesterol, fatty acids, and triglycerides; regulation and control of protein and nucleic acid synthesis; absorption processes; and

biochemical mechanisms in central nervous processes and ischemia. The significance of elevated blood levels of cholesterol and certain other lipids in atherosclerosis has focused attention on drugs affecting cholesterol metabolism. Several of these drugs, such as Pravachol, Lipitor, and Crestor are now available. These drugs have had a dramatic impact in reducing serum cholesterol, and more may be expected.

Acute problems associated with atherosclerosis often are caused by thrombi. Current antithrombolytic approaches are directed at inhibiting platelet aggregation through warfarin (Coumadin); heparins; aspirin; Integrilin (eptifibatide) or ReoPro (abciximab)—inhibitors of gpIIb/IIIa; or ticlopidine. The direct inhibition of the clotting enzyme, thrombin is also a drug target. This approach involves the investigation of thrombin receptor inhibition. Enzymes that are capable of dissolving a recently formed blood clot, such as streptokinase, tissue plasminogen activator (tPA), and urokinase, have been approved and are useful under specific primary care circumstances in the treatment of stroke.

Major advances have been made in the field of gastrointestinal physiology; many new gastrointestinal polypeptide hormones have been isolated and characterized, and their primary functions have been determined. Evidence for many years pointed to the existence of gastric receptors for histamine in addition to the vascular receptors. Recently, new drugs have been designed to block specifically the H2 receptor and have been very successful in the treatment of peptic ulcer.

Molecular biological research has impacted every area of drug discovery. Molecular biology provides insight into the organism's fundamental genetic composition.

Of note to pharmaceutical research is the use of recombinant expression as a source of scarce or valuable human proteins such as growth hormone, antibodies, interferon, and insulin. This science also allows dissection of cell pathways and the generation of reagents for better assays. A major objective of research is the design of satisfactory model systems in animals, cell culture, and other innovative means to give reliable predictions of the safety and efficacy of new drugs in humans. Molecular biology has advanced the reduction in the numbers of animals used in drug research. Tests for biological activity at the molecular level are done first, after which animal tests using standardized, controlled experiments are conducted.

Virology and Immunology

The search for antiviral agents, which has depended on the development of methodology for propagation and assaying of viruses in tissue culture, has led to more precise procedures of testing compounds for antiviral activity. Tissue-culture techniques have made possible the production of large quantities of viruses for vaccine manufacture. New and improved vaccines represent a major objective of biologic research. New separation methods developed in biochemistry and physical chemistry have been applied to the isolation and purification of viruses, and have led to preparation of highly purified and concentrated vaccines. Such vaccines are more effective and produce markedly fewer side effects.

The discovery of HIV and its epidemiological implications has opened new avenues of research to develop suitable therapies. In combinations with cocktails of other drugs, HIV protease inhibitors are the main avenue of therapeutic approach for controlling HIV today. The discovery that chemokines and chemokine receptors are involved as co-receptors for HIV defined new pharmaceutical strategies toward small-molecule drug discovery.

New viral threats will surely emerge. Currently, the world is working to understand a new corona virus which has led to the SARS threat. New viruses will threaten the world due to global travel and could be used in bioterrorism. Advances in virology will add new understanding, disease controls through treatement, and eventually cures.

Recent immunological research has focused attention on a number of important diseases with an autoimmune component such as arthritis, Lupus, IBD, and multiple sclerosis. These diseases continue to be poorly treated over time. Suppression of immune phenomena or induction of immune tolerance may be of great importance. A more detailed knowledge of the molecular basis of B and T differentiation, signal transduction, and leukocyte trafficking is needed to search for drugs that either enhance or inhibit these immune responses. In addition, a clearer picture of the molecular basis of immune disease is required to improve the probability that additional drugs will be found to alleviate allergic reactions.

Immunological research also has been directed toward cancer. The existence of tumor-specific antigens in both virus- and chemical-induced tumors, as well as new evidence for host reactions to the tumor, increase the possibility of useful immunological approaches to cancer. One of the most important developments in the past decade has been the isolation and production of monoclonal antibodies. These agents can be used to identify tumor-specific antigens and thus serve as powerful in vitro diagnostic and therapeutic tools. The technique can be applied to other antigens as well. These substances are being developed as carrier systems for drugs by virtue of their ability to deliver the antibody-drug complex directly to the antigen-producing cell or tissue.

Pharmacology

The role of pharmacological research in drug discovery continues to evolve. Initially, the pharmacologist was a whole animal biologist who developed animal models of disease to the extent possible, and tested compounds in animals to measure efficacy. Classical pharmacology contributed in two major areas[11]: (1) The design and operation of animal model for detecting and evaluating the activity of compounds, and (2) Determination of the dosage, toxicity, mode of action, metabolism, and fate of a drug candidate in the body. More recently, the molecular pharmacologist is involved in the discovery and validation of new targets for drug discovery, as well as the generation of new assays, both in vitro and in vivo. Classic pharmacological methods using intact animals, whole organs, and isolated tissues tended to be used 10 years ago. These have evolved to more automated and molecular oriented methods where purified or recombinant enzyme and receptor systems are used in initial phases of discovery pharmacology, with in vivo testing following as needed. Potential drug candidates are examined early on for specificity against other unrelated molecules, a means of reducing side effects in individuals. Safety assessments are done earlier in the discovery process and allow the physician and clinical pharmacologist to work together to set the starting points for dosing drugs with minimal side effects and to monitor what form of toxicity might appear, or what conditions in the patient would contraindicate use of the drug.

The study of drug absorption, distribution, metabolism, and excretion is frequently referred to as ADME. Drug therapy requires an elaborate and thorough knowledge of the kinetics of these processes after intravenous and/or oral administration of the drug. Initial studies are often conducted using in vitro experimental systems such as Caco cell permeability to determine the likelihood of oral absorption, or stability to human liver microsomes to determine the likelihood of metabolic stability. Common next steps are to test suitable compounds in animals to determine if the experimental systems are accurate for a particular chemical series and to extend the data set to a whole organism. Experiments are often performed with radioactive forms of the drug to determine the amounts of drug and its metabolites that appear in blood, urine, and tissues. Animals can be used to determine the manner in which a living organism assimilates a drug; however, human pharmacokinetic studies are essential to determine the fate of the compound in man:

Is it accumulated in specific organs, is it excreted into bile or urine, and is it metabolized?

To determine the concentration of drugs in biological fluids or tissues requires special separation techniques as well as sensitive, accurate, and precise instrumental measurements. Accurate quantitation and identification of the drug and its metabolites usually requires the use of chromatographic techniques coupled with the mass spectrometry. These sensitive LC/MS methods provide powerful data on early drug candidate molecules that influence the direction of new chemical synthesis.

Toxicology

To be certain that a new drug is safe, detailed studies are made of the effects of varying doses and prolonged administration of that drug. The pharmacologist provides acute toxicity data; however, the toxicologist then must refine the acute toxicity measurement in laboratory animals and begin subacute and chronic studies. The latter are conducted in a variety of species, at several dosage levels of the drug and over periods of time ranging from 3 months up to 30 months. During the test period, animals are observed carefully for all adverse symptoms. At the end of this period, and occasionally during its progress, the animals are killed, and their vital tissues (such as liver, heart, kidney, intestine, or brain) are removed and studied grossly and microscopically by a pathologist.

In addition to gross and microscopic pathology, biochemical and physiological responses are measured as an indication of liver function, kidney function, or endocrine function. During recent years, metabolic investigations have become more sophisticated and have been brought to bear on the comparative effects of drugs on various animals and on humans. In some instances, the metabolism of drugs or the therapeutic effects of drugs vary from species to species. Such variability can be the basis for differences in toxicity as well as differences in efficacy. For these reasons, increasing emphasis is being given to studies of comparative metabolism in man and animals to determine which laboratory animal handles the drug in a manner similar to humans. Selection of that species for extensive toxicity testing increases confidence that the toxic reactions that may occur in man will have been predicted by the animal tests.

Reproductive studies to determine the potential effects of the new drug on the reproductive processes and on subsequent generations are performed. Teratological studies are done to determine whether the new drug affects the fetus. Special toxicity tests have been designed to detect specific toxic reactions, such as nerve damage resulting in hearing loss.

Carcinogenicity trials, which are lifelong studies in animals carried out at doses approximating the maximum (tolerated) human dose, provide evidence of a new drug's ability to potentially produce human cancer. Several newer methods of toxicity are evolving in the biotech industry using gene activation methodology whereby one can evaluate if a candidate drug is transcriptionally active at a number of genes involved in liver metabolism or stress responses. These methods are likely to transform toxicological testing in the future.

In 1992 a global effort aimed at establishing uniform standards for toxicology testing of new drugs began, under the auspices of the International Conference on Harmonization (ICH). Guidelines were published on toxicology testing in late 1992 for drugs. Biologicals were not covered by those guidelines. Product-specific toxicology programs normally are required for biologicals. Toxicological studies are assuming increasing importance in the world of pharmacy and medicine. As knowledge and skills increase, and ability to measure toxic reactions improves, the greater safety and efficacy of new drugs may be ensured.

During the 1990s significant progress has been achieved in the concept of replacing animals in toxicology/safety assessment with numerous in vitro systems. These are attempts to reduce the number of animals used and to refine the manner in which they are used. A review of annual reports of testing in the United States, United Kingdom, and Japan showed that the number of animals used was being reduced continuously for all species.[12] Overall, multiple in vitro systems have been developed for screening and testing for eye and skin irritation, skin sensitization, teratology, and other endpoints; and a scientific consensus has been reached on requirements and processes for validation. However, the use of these newer test systems in place of existing in vivo tests is not yet a reality. Much progress and dialog has continued in the decade of the 1990s on modification of both US and international requirements and guidelines for testing, and for defining an approval process for alternatives and innovations.

Physical Chemistry

Modern research in pharmacy and medicine is supported and expedited by instrumentation. Modern instruments make possible the rapid and accurate measurement of physical and chemical properties of molecules. Separation and characterization of molecules are sometimes possible today in a matter of hours or days; only a decade or two ago, such work often required days, weeks, or even months. Examples of specialized physicochemical and computational methods that are applicable to structural research are electron microscopy, nuclear magnetic resonance (NMR) spectroscopy, and crystallography.

NMR spectra identify chemical groups and indicate the nature of neighboring chemical groups in the molecule. Mass spectrometry permits determination of the molecular weight and empiric formula of an organic molecule, and of the major fragments of the molecule. With this information, it is often possible to deduce the entire structure of a molecule rapidly and precisely. X-ray crystallographic analysis enables the physical chemist to determine the precise position of each atom of a molecule as it exists in the crystalline form. Structures of both the drug target and a potential drug in the active site of an enzyme have been critical to the discovery of HIV protease inhibitors.

Physicochemical studies are directed at the chemical groups and stereochemical configuration of biologically active molecules; these studies can describe molecules in terms of energy and electron distributions, and approximate the influence of the chemical environment on these distributions. The spatial and electronic conformation of drugs and the changes in conformation that occur in various environments govern the absorption, transport, distribution, and reaction with the receptor site. If description of molecules in these functional terms is achieved, correlation of electronic structure with function may be possible, and the design of safer, specific, and more effective drugs on a rational basis may occur.

Information Science

The information sciences (IS) have spearheaded a great amount of data generation, assimilation, and scientific communication. IS departments are now commonplace in academic, government, and industrial settings. The amount and sophistication of chemical and biological information has led to the critical role of bench-top and desktop computers in assimilating data. Computer-assisted chemistry, computer graphics, and relational databases have added a new dimension in structure and activity relationships. The computer-based monitoring and analysis of animal studies is routine. On-line signal processing allows investigators to interact more fully with their experiments. Computer-assisted automation permits collection of more data, with a resulting increase in accuracy; sophisticated software packages are available commercially or may be developed in-house.

Communication between scientists and the literature also has evolved with the explosion of IS technologies and access to the Internet. Attention and access to the scientific and patent literature has accelerated. Formerly, the individual scientist subscribed personally to a few journals and depended on a scientific library for coverage of additional new scientific findings. With the tremendous growth of the scientific and patent literature and the emergence of interdisciplinary investigations, desktop searches are conducted by individual scientists to stay abreast of the literature. Despite increasing use is being made of various kinds of alerting services and facilities, many of them computer-based, for retrieval or retrospective search of pertinent information, personal perusal of literature remains critical and ability to initiate desktop searches are fundamental to independent scientific research.

DRUG DEVELOPMENT

Before a new drug candidate can proceed to toxicological or clinical evaluation, considerable analytical chemical development is required to lay the groundwork for subsequent quality control and stability studies. Drug standards are established and analytical methods for the bulk drug and the proposed final product are devised. Tentative chemical, physical, and biological specifications of the candidate drug are established. Simultaneously with analytical development, pharmaceutical chemists begin formulation studies toward the goal of a stable, highly acceptable product that delivers the correct amount of drug in a reproducible, effective manner. Sometimes a new drug must be modified chemically via esterification to a prodrug in order to provide a form that is pharmaceutically acceptable and effective. Accelerated and long-term stability studies are started to estimate the conditions in which the product will be stable.

If a compound has desirable activity in an experimental testing system and appears to be safe upon toxicological examination, it becomes a candidate for clinical trial. Two additional tasks must be accomplished before a clinical trial can be undertaken. First, the drug candidate must be in a suitable, stable dosage form, and the candidate compound must be available for absorption and transport to the site of action. The stabilization of a drug candidate must preclude physical or chemical change (discoloration, precipitation, or decomposition). These components, or excipients, must often meet the standards outlined in the US Pharmacopeia/National Formulary (USP/NF), European pharmacopeias, or other national compendia. Because of the many physical forms in which pharmaceuticals are presented, the research necessary is broad in scope, and not only involves the principles of physical pharmacy but also requires the application of principles from the allied fields of chemistry and biology.

The second task at this stage is to file an Investigational New Drug (IND) application with the FDA. The IND is, in fact, a document that gives a full description of the new drug, where and how it is manufactured, all quality control information and standards, stability, analytical methods, pharmacology, toxicology, documentation of efficacy in animals, and the physicians (and their qualifications) who will be doing the clinical studies with complete protocols of the proposed clinical studies.

A new drug is administered to humans for the first time by a physician or clinical pharmacologist. These Phase I studies are carried out most often in healthy male volunteers in order to study the safety and pharmacokinetics of a new drug. The first trial of a drug in humans is done with great caution and on a very limited basis.

When dosing limits have been established and are found acceptable, the drug made is available to a larger number of practicing specialists for the Phase II study, which principally is concerned with the determination of safety and efficacy in patients having the primary disease for which the drug is to be tested. The minimum effective dose, the maximum tolerated dose, and the dose response (intermediate doses) also must be determined.

If, after Phase II, the drug still looks promising, it is distributed more widely to selected practicing physicians in the Phase III study. The purpose of the Phase III stage is to secure data from a larger number of patients on efficacy and incidence of side effects.

Finally, before the new drug can be marketed, a New Drug Application (NDA) is filed with the FDA and approval obtained. The NDA contains most of the information included in the IND, revised and updated, as well as all the results of the clinical studies proving safety and efficacy. Most all clinical, laboratory, and patient history data are processed on computers. These medical data are updated in computerized retrieval systems and are designed to provide timely information during the FDA review. These systems also provide an additional information resource for premarketing and postmarketing queries. Only after FDA approval of the NDA can distribution and marketing of the new drug begin.

Depending on the nature of the disease, and the clinical endpoints that are monitored, some drugs require long-ranging and expensive clinical trials. Some trials by necessity monitor mortality rates. Clinical trials are carefully designed with the input of statisticians to determine numbers of patients and duration of the studies. Trials cost hundreds of million of dollars (Fig 10-1) over multi-year periods, and they demand careful monitoring throughout.

Figure 10-1 also depicts the clinical research effort on a new drug represents the culmination of many years of effort by large numbers of scientists of many disciplines and skills. It is the proving ground where the intelligence, creativity, and perseverance of laboratory researchers come to fruition. Of the candidate drugs that come to clinical research, only a few survive as safe and efficacious and are added to the portfolio of therapeutics. Indeed, the 2002 reports from the Pharmaceutical Manufacturers of America (PhRMA) titled Increased Length and Complexity of the Research and Development Process[13] and Incentives to Discover New Medicines: Pharmaceutical Patents[14] revealed the following information on the drug discovery research process:

- One in 5000 compounds screened is approved for patient use
- The average cost of one new medicine is $500 million
- It takes an average of 12–15 years to develop a new medicine.
- Only 3 in 10 prescription drugs generate revenue that meet or exceed the average R&D costs
- The time that companies have to recoup their investment is decreasing due to generic competition

Together with the cost of conducting R&D (Table 10-1), the above data explains the rising costs of prescription drugs. In National Institute for Health Care Management (NIHCM) Report of "Prescription Drug Expenditures in 2001", the top 50 selling drugs are listed.[15] The top 10 of these are "blockbusters" (ie, over $1 billion in sales(Table 10-2)[15] and account for $27 bil-

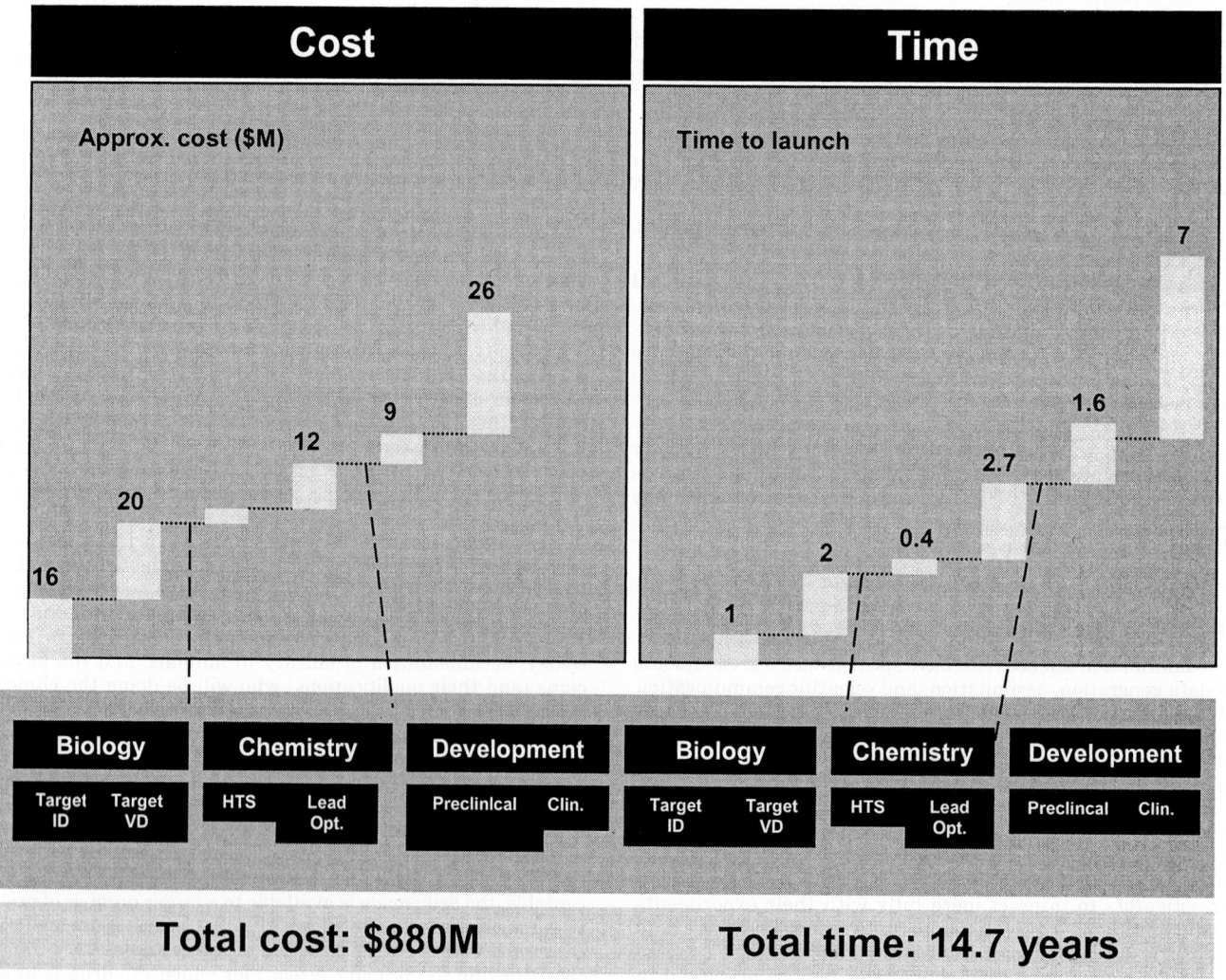

Figure 10-1. The cost and time from target identification to clinical trials. (From the Boston Consulting Group, 2001.)

Table 10-2. The Top-Selling Drugs in 2001

RANK	DRUG	COMPANY	TYPE OF DRUG	2001 SALES(BILLIONS)
1	Lipitor	Pfizer	Cholesterol reducer	4.5
2	Prilosec	AstraZeneca	Antiulcer	4.0
3	Prevacid	Takeda-Abbott Pharma	Antiulcer	3.2
4	Zocor	Merck	Cholesterol reducer	2.7
5	Celebrex	Pfizer	Anti-arthritic	2.4
6	Zoloft	Pfizer	Anti-depressant	2.2
7	Paxil	GlaxoSmithKline	Anti-depressant	2.1
8	Vioxx	Merck	Anti-arthritic	2.0
9	Prozac	Lilly	Anti-depressant	2.0
10	Augmentin	GlaxoSmithKline	Enhanced antibiotic	1.9

From the National Institute for Health Care Management Research and Educational Foundation. *Prescription Drug Expenditures in 2001: Another Year of Escalating Costs.* Washington DC, 2002.

lion of sales in a $155 billion market, or 17% of the market). Another factor in rising costs that cannot be discounted is the view that overall research productivity and investment in innovative research for new approaches and new medicines in the large pharma tier of companies has declined.[16] This may in part be attributable to merger and acquisition (M&A) consolidation in the industry. Of the top 10 companies, all are the result of M&A (Table 10-3).[15,16]

The drug discovery research effort represents the culmination of, on average, 12 to 15 years of research and development by many scientists from multiple disciplines. It is the proving ground where the intelligence, creativity, and perseverance of researchers come to fruition. Of the candidate drugs that come

to clinical research, only ~20% survive as safe and efficacious and are added to the portfolio of therapeutics. The great investment in pharmaceutical research in the early part of the 20th century that has led to advancements in pharmaceutical therapies needs to be remade in the 21st century.

REFERENCES

1. Spilker B, ed. *Multinational Pharmaceutical Companies: Principles and Practices*, 2nd ed. New York: Raven, 1994.
2. Tulp M, Bohlin L. *Trends Pharmacol Sci* 2002; 23:225.
3. Schreiber SL, Nicolaou KC, Davies K. *Chemistry & Biology* 2002; 9:1.
4. Charish P. *Scrip Magazine* 2003; (February):41.
5. Pharmaceutical Manufacturer's Association. 2002 Annual Report. *Why Prescription Drugs Cost So Much.* Washington, DC, 2002.
6. McCoy M. *Chem Eng News* 1998(July): 27.
7. Hartzema AG. *Ann Pharmacother* 1992; 26(1):96.
8. Drews J. *Science* 2000; 287:1960.
9. Lipinski CA. *Pharmaceutical News* 2002; 9:195.
10. Egan WJ Merz KM Jr, Baldwin JJ. *J Med Chem* 43:3867.
11. Frenkel JK. *Fed Proc* 1969; 28(1):160.
12. Gad SC. *Fundam Appl Toxicol* 1990; 15(1):8.
13. Pharmaceutical Manufacturer's Association. 2002 Report: *Increased Length and Complexity of the Research and Development Process.* Washington, DC, 2002.
14. Pharmaceutical Manufacturer's Association. 2002 Report: *Incentives to Discover New Medicines: Pharmaceutical Patents.* Washington, DC, 2002.
15. National Institute for Health Care Management Research and Educational Foundation. *Prescription Drug Expenditures in 2001: Another Year of Escalating Costs.* Washington DC, 2002.
16. Drews J. *Drug Discovery Today* 8:411.

Table 10-3. Top 10 Pharmaceutical Companies Worldwide in Prescription Sales (US$ in millions) for the First Six Months of 2002

RANK	COMPANY	PHARMA SALES	INCREASE (%)
1	Pfizer	13,131	9.1
2	GlaxoSmithKline	12,968	8.1
3	Merck & Co	10,053	−2.3
4	AstraZeneca	8,635	8.7
5	Johnson & Johnson	8,439	14.8
6	Aventis	7,910	9.8
7	Novartis	6,456	8.8
8	Bristol-Myers Squibb	6,408	−30.1
9	Hoffman-La Roche	5,807	1.3
10	Wyeth	5,803	11.2

From Charish P. *Scrip Magazine* 2003; (February):41.

PART 2

Pharmaceutics

William J. Reilly, Jr, RPh, MBA
K.W. Tunnell Consulting
King of Prussia, PA

CHAPTER **11**

Metrology and Pharmaceutical Calculations

Roger L Schnaare, PhD
Shelly J Prince, PhD

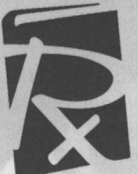

One of the first technical operations that the student of pharmacy must learn is the manipulation of balances, weights, and measures of volume. This entails a study of the various systems of weights and measures, their relationships, and a mastery of the mathematics involved. This chapter considers the fundamental principles of metrology underlying the testing, manufacturing, and compounding of pharmaceutical preparations:

Weights and Measures—An accumulation of facts concerning the various systems, with tables of conversion factors and practical equivalents. The relationships among the various systems of weights and measures are clarified.

Weighing and Measuring—A discussion of the various types of balances, particularly prescription balances and methods of using, testing, and protecting them; also of various devices and methods for measuring large or small volumes of fluids.

Density and Specific Gravity—A consideration of the mass/volume ratio of a substance (density), and the ratio of the weight (mass) of one substance to the weight (mass) of another substance taken as the standard (specific gravity).

Pharmaceutical Calculations—A review of basic mathematical principles and their use in solving pharmaceutical problems.

WEIGHTS AND MEASURES

Weight is a measure of the gravitational force acting on a body; weight is directly proportional to the body's mass. The latter, being a constant based on inertia, never varies, whereas weight varies slightly with latitude, altitude, temperature, and pressure. The effect of these factors usually is not considered unless very precise weighing and large quantities are involved.

Measure is the determination of the volume or extent of a body. Temperature and pressure have a pronounced effect, especially on gases or liquids. These factors, therefore, are considered when making precise measurements.

All standard weights and measures in the US are derived from or based on the United States National Prototype Standards of the Meter and the Kilogram. The standards are made of platinum-iridium, and are in the custody of the National Institute of Standards and Technology (NIST) in Washington, DC.

History

A brief outline of the origin of the many systems of weights and measures may help clarify the essential distinctions between them. The sense of the weight of a body cannot be conveyed intelligibly to the mind unless a means of comparison is chosen. As weight is the measure of the gravitational force of a body, this force is expressed in terms of standards of resistance, which exactly balance the body and keep it in equilibrium when used with a mechanical device constructed for this specific purpose. Such standards are termed *weights* and the mechanical devices are called *balances* or *scales*.

The standards that have been chosen by various nations are arbitrary, and instances are common where different standards are in use at the same time in the same country. Many of the ancient standards clearly are referable to variable parts of the human body, such as nail, foot, span, pace, cubit (length of

the forearm), and fathom or faethm (stretch of the arms). In the history of metrology three periods may be traced:

1. The *Ancient* period, during which the old classical standards originated, terminated with the decline of the Roman Empire. The unit of distance used by all nations for maritime measurements, the *nautical* or *meridian* mile (1/60 of a degree of the earth's equatorial circumference) is exactly equal to 1000 Egyptian fathoms or 4000 Egyptian cubits. These Egyptian measurements, which have persisted for more than 4000 years, were based on astronomical or meridian measurements that were recorded imperishably in the great Pyramid at Ghizeh, whose perimeter is exactly 500 of these fathoms, or 1/2 nautical mile.

2. The *Medieval* period extended to the 16th century. During this period the old standards were lost, but their names were preserved, and European nations adopted various independent standards.

3. The *Modern* period extends from the 16th century to the present. Since the 17th century, the efforts of most enlightened nations have been directed toward scientific accuracy and simplicity, and during the present century toward international uniformity.

Historical metrology, also referred to as *documentary metrology*, is concerned with the study of monuments and records of ancient periods. *Inductive metrology* is concerned with the accumulation of data concerning the measurement of large numbers of objects that have been referred to as standards but which have no exact measure except by statutory regulation.

THE ENGLISH SYSTEMS—In Great Britain, in 1266, the 51st Act of the reign of Henry III declared

"that by the consent of the whole realm of England the measure of the King was made—that is to say, that an English silver penny called the sterling, round and without clipping, shall weigh *thirty-two grains of wheat*, well dried and gathered out of the middle of the ear; and twenty pence (pennyweights) do make an ounce and twelve ounces a pound, and eight pounds do make a gallon of wine, and eight wine gallons do make a bushel, which is the eighth of a quarter."

The 16-ounce pound (*avoirdupois pound*), undoubtedly of Roman origin, was introduced at the time of the first civilization of the British island. However, according to Gray, the word *haberdepois* was first used in English laws in 1303. A statute of Edward I (1304 AD) states "that every *pound* of money or of *medicines* is of *twenty shillings weight*, but the pound of all other things is *twenty-five shillings weight*. The *ounce* of *medicines* consists of *twenty pence*, and the *pound* contains *twelve* ounces [the Troy Pound], but in other things the pound contains *fifteen* ounces, in both cases the ounce weighing twenty pence."

These laws unfold the theory of the ancient weights and measures of Great Britain, and reveal the standards (ie, a natural object, grains of wheat). A difference existed then between the Troy and the avoirdupois pound, but the weights now in use are $\frac{1}{16}$ heavier than those of Edward I, due to the change subsequently made in the value of the coin by the sovereign. In addition, the true pennyweight standard was lost, and, in the next revision of the weights and measures, the present troy and avoirdupois standards were adopted.

The *troy weight* is of still earlier origin. The great fairs of the 8th and 9th centuries were held at several French cities, including Troyes, the gathering place of traders from all countries. Coins frequently were mutilated, so they were sold by weight, and the standard weight of Troyes for selling coin was adopted for precious metals and medicines in all parts of Europe. The troy ounce and the avoirdupois ounce originally were intended to have the same weight, but after the revision it was found that the avoirdupois ounce was lighter by 42½ gr (grains) than the troy ounce. The subsequent adoption of troy weight by the London College of Physicians in 1618, on the recommendation of Sir Theodore Turquet de la Mayerne who compiled their first pharmacopoeia, has entailed upon all apothecaries who are governed by British customs to this day the very great inconvenience of buying and selling medicines by one system of weights (the *avoirdupois*) and compounding them by another (the *apothecary* or *troy*).

In the next century efforts were made toward reforming the standards, and in 1736 the Royal Society began the work that ended in the preparation, by Mr. Bird under the direction of the House of Commons, of the standard *yard* and standard *pound* troy in 1760. Copies of these were prepared and no intentional deviation has been made since.

The growing popularity of the French metric system—and the desirability of securing a standard that could be recovered easily in case of loss or destruction, and that should be commensurable with a simple unit—prompted steps in England to secure these advantages in 1816. The labors of English scientists led to the adoption of the *imperial* measures and standards, which were legalized January 1, 1826; imperial standards, are now in use in Great Britain, thus introducing another element of confusion into an already complicated subject. In this system the *yard* is equivalent to 36 inches, and its length was determined by comparison with a pendulum beating seconds of mean time, in a vacuum, at the temperature of 62°F at the level of the sea in the latitude of London, a length that was found to be 39.1393 inches. The *pound troy* (containing 5760 gr) was determined by comparison with a given measure of distilled water under specified conditions. Thus, a cubic inch of distilled water was weighed with brass weights in air at 62°F, the barometer at 30 inches, and it weighed 252.458 gr. The standard for measures of capacity in Great Britain (either dry or liquid) is the *imperial gallon*, which contains 10 lb avoir (each 7000 gr) of distilled water weighed in air at 62°F, the barometer standing at 30 inches. The *bushel* contains eight such gallons.

Washington, in his first annual message to Congress, January 1790, recommended the establishment of uniformity in currency, weights, and measures. Action was taken with reference to the currency and recommendations were made by Jefferson, then the Secretary of State, for the adoption of either the currently used English systems or a decimal system. However,

nothing was accomplished until 1819 to 1820, when efforts again were made in the US to secure uniformity in the standards that were in use by the several states. Finally, after a lengthy investigation, on June 14, 1836, the Secretary of the Treasury was directed by Congress to furnish each state in the Union with a complete set of the revised standards, and thus the *troy pound* (5760 gr), the *avoirdupois pound* (7000 gr), and the *yard* (36 inches) are all identical with the British standards. However, the US *gallon* is quite different; the old wine gallon of 231 inch³—containing 58,372.2 gr of distilled water at its maximum density, weighed in air at 62°F, the barometer standing at 30 inches—was retained. The bushel contained 77.274 lb of water under the same conditions, thus making the dry quart about 16% greater in volume than the liquid quart.

In 1864 the use of the metric measures was legalized in Great Britain, but was not made compulsory, and in 1866 the US followed the same course. By the US law of July 28, 1866, all lengths, areas, and cubic measures are derived from the international meter equivalent to 39.37 inches. Since 1893 the US Office of Standard Weights and Measures has been authorized to derive the yard from the meter: one yard equals 3600/3937 m, and the customary weights are referred to the kilogram by an Executive order approved April 5, 1893. Capacities were to be based on the equivalent; dm³ equals one liter, the decimeter being equal to 3.937 inches. The gallon still remains at 231 inch³ and the bushel contains 2150.42 inch³. This makes the liquid quart equal to 0.946 liter and the dry quart equal to 1.1013 liter, whereas the imperial quart is 1.1359 liter. The customary weights are derived from the international kilogram, based on the value that one avoir lb equals 453.5924277 g and that 5760/7000 avoir lb equals one troy lb.

Avoirdupois weight is used in general in the US for commercial purposes, including the buying and selling of drugs on a large scale and occasionally on prescription orders.

THE METRIC SYSTEM—The idea of adopting a scientific standard for the basis of metrology that could be reverified accurately was suggested by a number of individuals after the Renaissance. Jean Picard, the 17th-century French astronomer, proposed to take as a unit the length of a pendulum beating one sec of time at sea level, at latitude 45°.

In 1783, the English inventor James Watt first suggested the application of decimal notation, and the commensurability of weight, length, and volume. The French National Assembly in 1790 appointed a committee to decide the preferability of the pendulum standard or a terrestrial measure of some kind as a basis for the new system. The committee reported in 1791 in favor of the latter, and commissions were appointed to measure an arc of meridian and to perfect the details of the commensurability of the units and of nomenclature. However, certain inaccuracies were inherent in the early standards, so they do not bear to each other the intended exact relationships. The present accepted standards are defined in publications of the National Institute of Standards and Technology (NIST).

In its original conception, the meter was the fundamental unit of the metric system, and all units of length and capacity were to be derived directly from the meter, which was intended to be equal to one ten-millionth of the earth's quadrant. Furthermore, it originally was planned that the unit of mass, the kilogram, should be identical with the mass of a cubic decimeter of water at its maximum density. At present, however, the units of length and mass are defined independently of these conceptions.

For all practical purposes, calibration of length standards in industry and scientific laboratories is accomplished by comparison with the material standard of length: the distance between two engraved lines on a platinum-iridium bar, *The International Prototype Meter*, which is kept at the International Bureau of Weights and Measures.

The *kilogram* is defined independently as the mass of a definite platinum-iridium standard, the *International Prototype Kilogram*, which also is kept at the International Bureau of Weights and Measures. The *liter* is defined as the volume of a kilogram of water, at standard atmospheric pressure, and at the temperature of its maximum density, approximately 4°C. The *meter* is thus the fundamental unit on which are based all metric standards and measurements of length and area and of volumes derived from linear measurements.

Of basic scientific interest is that on October 14, 1960, the 11th General Conference on Weights and Measures, meeting in Paris, adopted a new international definition for the standard of length: the meter is now defined as the length equal to 1,650,763.73 wavelengths of the orange-red light of the krypton-86 isotope. This standard will be used in actual measurements only when extreme accuracy is needed.

The kilogram is the fundamental unit on which are based all metric standards of mass. The liter is a secondary or derived unit of capacity or volume. The liter is larger by about 27 ppm (parts per million) than the cube of the tenth of the meter (the cubic decimeter): one liter = 1.000027 dm^3.

The conversion tables in this publication that involve the relative length of the yard and meter are based upon the relation: one m = 39.37 inch, contained in the act of Congress of 1866. From this relation it follows that one inch = 25.40005 mm (nearly).

In recent years engineering and industrial interests the world over have urged the adoption of the simpler relation, one inch = 25.4 mm exactly, which differs from the preceding value by only five ppm. This simpler relation has not as yet been adopted officially by either Great Britain or the US but is in wide industrial use.

In the US, the abbreviation *cc* (for cubic centimeter) still persists in general use and is taken as synonymous for the more correct milliliter. The US Pharmacopeia (USP) IX and National Formulary (NF) IV adopted the term *milliliter* with its abbreviated form *mil*, but it proved so unpopular in practice that the following pharmacopeial convention directed the return to the older term cubic centimeter (cc). However, in 1955, USP XV and NF X once again adopted the term milliliter with the abbreviation mL.

National jealousies and the natural antipathy to changing established customs interfered greatly with the adoption of the metric system during the early part of the 19th century. At present the metric system is in use in every major country of the world. In the US and Great Britain it is legalized for reference to and definition of other standards, and it is in exclusive use by nearly all scientists and by increasing segments of industry and the public. In the US the metric system was legalized in 1866, but not made compulsory; in the same year the international prototype meter and kilogram were adopted as fundamental standards. The US silver coinage was based upon the metric system, the half dollar being exactly 12.5 g and the quarter and the dime being of the proportionate weights.

As corporations became more international, the need for a universal standard increased. Since 1875 there has been established and maintained an International Bureau of Weights and Measures, with headquarters at Paris. This Bureau is managed by an international committee that enjoys universal representation. One objective of the committee is to make and provide prototypes of the meter and kilogram for the subscribing nations; approximately 40 such copies have been prepared.

The US prototype standards of both the meter and the kilogram mass, constructed of a platinum-iridium alloy, were brought from Paris in 1890 and are now in the custody of the NIST in Washington, DC. They have been reproduced and distributed by our own government to the various states having bureaus needing such replicas. The original US prototype meter was taken back to Paris in 1957 for reverification and was found to have altered only 3 parts in 100,000,000 after 67 years of use. Thus, there was no demonstrable change within the limits of experimental error.

Adoption of the krypton-86 wavelength of light definition for the meter gives the different countries the means to check their prototype meter bars without returning them to Paris at periodic intervals for comparison with the international meter bar.

Orthography and Reading

ORTHOGRAPHY—There are two methods of orthography of the metric units in use. In the original French, the units are spelled met*re*, lit*re*, and gram*me*; in the method proposed by the American Metric Bureau, the units are spelled met*er*, lit*er*, and gram. For three decades after the original adoption of the metric system, the USP and NF adopted met*er* and lit*er*, but used the French gram*me*. Now these official compendia use the spelling *gram*.

READING—Some difficulty usually is experienced by those unfamiliar with the metric system in reading the quantities. In the linear measures in pharmacy, centimeters and millimeters are used almost exclusively; thus, 0.05 m would not be read five hundredths of a meter, but rather five centimeters (5 cm); if the millimeter column contains a unit, as in 0.055 m, it is read 55 millimeters (55 mm) in preference to fifty-five thousandths of a meter.

Fractions of a millimeter must be read decimally, as 0.0555 m, fifty-five and five-tenths millimeter (55.5 mm). In measures of capacity, cubic centimeters (cc) or milliliters (mL) are used exclusively for quantities of less than a liter. The terms half-liter, quarter-liter, 100 milliliters, and one milliliter are denoted by 500 mL, 250 mL, 100 mL, and one mL.

In weight, when the quantity is relatively large and in commercial transactions, the *kilogram* is abbreviated to *kilo*. When less than a *kilogram* and not less than a *gram*, the quantity is read with the gram for the unit. Thus, 2000 g would be read either as 2000 grams or as 2 kilos, and 543 g would be read 543 grams; 2543 g is sometimes read 2 kilos and 543 grams, although 2543 grams usually is preferred.

For quantities below the *gram*, decigram and centigram usually are not used, but rather *milligram* has been regarded as the most convenient unit. With the increase in the use of extremely small doses of very potent drugs and the wide application of more delicate analytical procedures, the term *microgram* (mcg, µg, or γ), for thousandths of a milligram, is used frequently to designate quantities up to 999 µg (less than 1.000 mg).

Both the metric and English systems of weights and measures are in use in the US. Even though the metric system nearly has replaced the English system, the pharmacist must have a practical knowledge of both.

WEIGHTS

The Metric System

The USP of 1890 adopted the metric system of weights and measures to the exclusion of all others except for equivalent dosage statements, and the British Pharmacopoeia of 1914 did likewise. In 1944 the Council on Pharmacy and Chemistry of the American Medical Association adopted the metric system exclusively. The advantages of the metric or decimal system, and its simplicity, brevity, and adaptability to everyday needs are now conceded universally.

FRACTIONAL AND MULTIPLE PREFIXES—In many experimental procedures, including some in the pharmaceutical sciences, very small (and occasionally very large) quantities of weight, length, volume, time, or radioactivity are measured. To avoid the use of numbers with many zeros in such cases, the NIST recognizes prefixes to be used to express fractions or multiples of the International System of Units (SI), which was established in 1960 by the General Conference on Weights and Measures (see the foregoing discussion). The recognized prefixes, which in use are adjoined to an appropriate unit (as, for example, in such quantities as nanogram, picomole, microcurie, microsecond, or megavolt) are defined in Table 11-1.

Table 11-2 lists some metric weights. The prefixes, which indicate multiples, are of Greek derivation: deka, 10; hecto, 100; kilo, 1000. Fractions of the units are expressed by Latin prefixes: deci, 1/10; centi, 1/100; milli, 1/1000.

Table 11-1. Prefixes for Fractions and Multiples of SI Units

FRACTION	PREFIX	SYMBOL	MULTIPLE	PREFIX	SYMBOL
10^{-1}	deci	d	10	deka	da
10^{-2}	centi	c	10^2	hecto	h
10^{-3}	milli	m	10^3	kilo	k
10^{-6}	micro	μ	10^6	mega	M
10^{-9}	nano	n	10^9	giga	G
10^{-12}	pica	p	10^{12}	tera	T
10^{-15}	femto	f	10^{15}	peta	P
10^{-18}	atto	a	10^{18}	exa	E

Only a few of the most convenient denominations are employed in practical work. Whole numbers from one to 1000 usually are expressed in terms of grams, while the kilogram is used as the unit for larger quantities. Quantities between one milligram and one gram usually are referred to in terms of milligrams; microgram (μg or mcg) is used in quantitative analysis, biological studies, and for minute dosage statements.

The English Systems

In the US, both the avoirdupois and apothecary systems of weight measurement sometimes are used in handling medicines. It must be emphasized *that pharmacists may buy their drugs by avoirdupois weight*. These two systems differ:

1 pound avoirdupois = 7000 gr and is abbreviated lb.
1 pound apothecary = 5760 gr and is abbreviated ℔.
1 ounce avoirdupois = 437.5 gr and is abbreviated oz.
1 ounce apothecary = 480 gr and is abbreviated ℥.

The *grain* avoirdupois is exactly the same as the *grain* apothecary. The apothecary pound is therefore 1240 gr *lighter* than the avoirdupois pound, and the apothecary ounce is therefore 42.5 gr *heavier* than the avoirdupois ounce.

The abbreviations of the denominations of apothecary weight are represented by the signs ounce, ℥; dram, ℈; scruple, ℈; and grain, gr. These long have been in use but possibly may be mistaken for one another in rapid or careless writing. The abbreviations or signs of avoirdupois weight differ from those of apothecary weight, and care should be used not to confound them; they are lb (sometimes written #), pound: oz, ounce: gr, grain. Tables 11-3, 11-4, and 11-5 show three English systems of weight.

Jewelers evaluate precious stones with troy weight, which is very similar to apothecary weight. The apothecary and troy grain, ounce, and pound are identical, but the ounces are subdivided differently. The *carat*, used by jewelers, is equal to 3.168 troy grains or four carat grains. When used to express the fineness of gold, one carat signifies 1/24 part. A 14-carat ring is 14/24 pure gold.

As indicated in the footnote to Table 11-6, a number of special metric system units are used in various pharmacopeial and nonofficial descriptions, tests, and assays of drugs and other substances to express linear measurements of very small dimension. These units and their symbols or abbreviations are listed in Table 11-7, together with their equivalents in terms of the other metric units and the inch.

Table 11-2. Metric Weight

1 microgram	μg	=	0.000001	g
1 milligram	mg	=	0.001	g
1 centigram	cg	=	0.01	g
1 decigram	dg	=	0.1	g
1 gram	g	=	1	g
1 dekagram	dag	=	10	g
1 hectogram	hg	=	100	g
1 kilogram	kg	=	1000	g

Note: The abbreviation μg or mcg is used for microgram in pharmacy, rather than gamma (γ) as in biology.

Table 11-3. Avoirdupois Weight

POUNDS	OUNCES	GRAINS
1 =	16 =	7000
	1 =	437.5

Note: 2000 lb = 1 ton, and 2240 lb = 1 long ton.

Table 11-4. Apothecary Weight

POUNDS	OUNCES	DRAMS	SCRUPLES	GRAINS
1 =	12 =	96 =	288 =	5760
	1 =	8 =	24 =	480
		1 =	3 =	60
			1 =	20

Table 11-5. Troy Weight

POUNDS	OUNCES	PENNYWEIGHTS	GRAINS
1 =	12 =	240 =	5760
	1 =	20 =	480
		1 =	24

Table 11-6. Metric Linear Measure

1 nanometer	(nm)	= 0.000000001 m (0.001 μm: 10^{-9} m: 10 Å)
1 micrometer	(μm)	= 0.000001 m (0.001 mm: 10^{-6} m: 10,000 Å)
1 millimeter	(mm)	= 0.001 m
1 centimeter	(cm)	= 0.01 m
1 decimeter	(dm)	= 0.1 m
1 meter	(m)	= 1 m
1 dekameter	(dam)	= 10 m
1 hectometer	(hm)	= 100 m
1 kilometer	(km)	= 1000 m

Although the meter (m) is observed to be the initial unit, it is seldom necessary to use it in pharmaceutical practice, and the same holds true for a number of the above measures. The micrometer (μm), millimeter (mm), and centimeter (cm) are employed in the description of many official drugs. Measurements pertaining to spectrometric and colorimetric tests and assays of many official drugs are recorded in micrometers (μm) or reciprocal centimeters (cm^{-1}) for infrared and in nanometers (nm) for ultraviolet and visible wavelengths of light, respectively.

Table 11-7. Equivalent Linear Measurements

UNIT	INCHES	MM	μM	NM	Å
1 inch	1	25.4	25,400	2.54×10^7	2.54×10^8
1 mm (millimeter)	0.0394	1	1000	10^6	10^7
1 μm (micrometer)	3.94×10^{-5}	10^{-3}	1	1000	10,000
1 nm (nanometer)	3.94×10^{-8}	10^{-6}	10^{-3}	1	10
1 Å (angstrom unit)	3.94×10^{-9}	10^{-7}	10^{-4}	0.1	1

MEASURES

Systems

Two systems of linear measure are used in the US: English and metric. Two systems of liquid measure are used: apothecary (also called the wine measure or US liquid measure) and metric. The units of the English system of linear measure (inch, foot, yard, and mile) are well-known, and needn't be described here. The units of the metric systems of linear and liquid measure, and of the apothecary (wine, US liquid) system of liquid measure, with their respective equivalents, are given in Tables 11-7, 11-8, and 11-9.

Pharmacists who fill Canadian or British prescriptions should also be familiar with the substantially different British imperial liquid measure system; the units, with their equivalents, are given in Table 11-10.

The following facts concerning the US system of liquid measure (see Table 11-9) should be noted:

1. The apothecary fluidounce (f ℥) of distilled water weighs 455 gr at 25°C.
2. The apothecary pint contains 16 f ℥.
3. The US gallon contains 128 f ℥ or 231 inch³. One gallon of distilled water weighs 8.337 avoir lb at 62°F. The US pint therefore weighs 1.04 avoir lb and the pound of distilled water measures only 0.96 pt. *One pound does not measure one pt.*

The following facts concerning the imperial system (see Table 11-10) should be noted:

1. The imperial fluidounce of distilled water weighs 437.5 gr at 15.6°C (60°F). It therefore weighs one avoir oz.
2. The imperial pint contains 20 f ℥.
3. The imperial gallon contains 160 f ℥. One gal of distilled water weighs 10 avoir lb; 16 f ℥ in this system therefore weighs one avoir lb.

From the above, one can deduce the following:

1. The US fluidounce and minim are larger than the imperial fluidounce and minim (℧). One US minim or fluidounce equals 1.04 imperial minims or fluidounces.
2. The imperial pint and gallon are much larger than the US pint and gallon.

It is, therefore, inaccurate to use measuring devices calibrated in the US system in measuring quantities directed in English prescriptions when the imperial measure is intended. Conversely, devices calibrated in the imperial system should not be used to measure quantities directed in US prescriptions when the US measure is intended. For example, Canadian pharmacists using American graduated cylinders should calculate percentage solutions on the basis of 454.6 gr of distilled water to the fluidounce. This is one more argument in favor of adoption internationally by all pharmacists of the metric system of weights and measures.

Table 11-8. Metric Liquid Measure

1 microliter	(µL)	=	0.000001	L
1 milliliter	(mL)	=	0.001	L
1 centiliter	(cL)	=	0.01	L
1 deciliter	(dL)	=	0.1	L
1 liter	(L)	=	1	L
1 dekaliter	(daL)	=	10	L
1 hectoliter	(hL)	=	100	L
1 kiloliter	(kL)	=	1000	L

Note: The standard of capacity is the *liter,* which is the volume of one kg of distilled water at its maximum density (approx 4°C). Microliters (µL) are used to measure volumes of solutions used in chromatographic procedures for the separation and quantitative determination of some official drugs.

Table 11-9. Apothecary or Wine Measure (US)

GALLON	PINTS	FLUIDOUNCES	FLUIDRAMS	MINIMS
1	8	128	1024	61,440
	1	16	128	7,680
		1	8	480
			1	60

THE RELATIONSHIPS OF WEIGHTS AND MEASURES

When the systems of weights and measures in use in the US are examined, the lack of close relation between the different units is appreciated at once. Nevertheless, if the following points are used carefully, many pharmaceutical problems will be greatly simplified.

1. Pharmacists may weigh themselves, buy merchandise, sell over the counter, and calculate postage, etc., using avoirdupois weight, which contains *437.5 gr in one oz.*
2. Pharmacists may compound formulas by apothecary weight, which contains *480 gr in one ℥.*
3. One apothecary fluidounce of water weighs *455 gr* at 25°C. Since 480 ℧ weigh 455 gr, one m weighs 455/480 = 0.95 gr.
   1 ℧ does *not* weigh one gr.
   1 f ℥ does *not* weigh one ℥.

Practical Equivalents

Tables of weights and measures and a table of practical equivalents should be kept in a conspicuous and convenient place in the prescription department, and the following equivalents, which are given with practical accuracy, should be committed to memory. Other equivalents may be calculated from these.

Linear Measure
1 meter = **39.4 inches**
1 inch = 2.54 cm = **25.4 mm**
1 micrometer = **1/1000 mm** = 10^{-6} m = 1/25,400 inch
Liquid Measure
1 milliliter = **16.2 m**
1 fluidounce = **29.6 mL**
1 pint = **473 mL**
1 gallon = **3790 mL**
Weight
1 kilogram = **2.20 lb avoir**
1 pound avoir = **454 g**
1 ounce avoir = **28.4 g**
1 ounce apothecary = **31.1 g**
1 pound apothecary = **373 g**
1 gram = **15.4 gr**
1 grain = **64.8 mg**

The USP *Table of Metric Doses with Approximate Apothecary Equivalents* is reproduced in the Appendix, along with information concerning its permissible uses.

Approximate Measures

In apportioning doses for a patient, the practitioner usually is compelled to order the liquid medicine to be administered in

Table 11-10. Imperial Measure (British)

GALLON	PINTS	FLUIDOUNCES	FLUIDRAMS	MINIMS
1	8	160	1280	76,800
	1	20	160	9,600
		1	8	480
			1	60

certain quantities that have been established by custom, and estimated as:

HOUSEHOLD MEASUREMENT	APOTHECARY NOTATION	METRIC VOLUME
1 tumblerful	f ℥ viii	240 mL
1 teacupful	f ℥ iv	120 mL
1 wineglassful	f ℥ ii	60 mL
2 tablespoonfuls	f ℥ i	30 mL
1 tablespoonful	f ʒ iii or ℥ ss	15 mL
1 dessertspoonful	f ʒ ii	8 mL
1 teaspoonful	f ʒ i	5 mL
½ teaspoonful	f ʒ ss	2.5 mL

Note: one drop is often considered to be one minim, but this is incorrect, as drops are variable.

In almost all cases, careful tests have found that modern teacups, tablespoons, dessertspoons, and teaspoons to average 25% greater capacity than the theoretical quantities just given. The physician and the pharmacist therefore should recommend the use of accurately graduated medicine droppers, teaspoons, and calibrated measuring devices, which may be procured at a small cost (Fig 11-1).

Approximate Dose Equivalents

For many years the apothecaries' system of weights and measures was used widely by physicians and pharmacists when considering the doses of medicinal substances, and it was customary

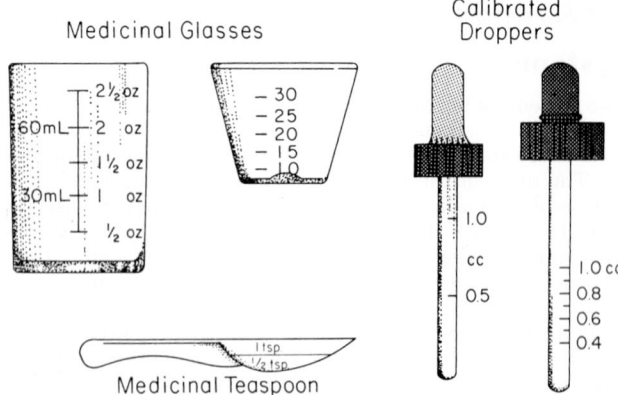

Figure 11-1.

to translate these apothecary doses into relatively exact amounts when the metric equivalents were mentioned. Today, however, doses are established primarily in the metric system without considering the relation of these metric figures to the corresponding quantities in any other system of weights and measures.

It should be emphasized that exact alternative formulas in the avoirdupois system of weights and measures are not obtained by using approximate equivalents but, for the purpose of compounding, should be calculated with the use of practical equivalents.

WEIGHING AND MEASURING

Having studied the several systems of weights and measures, students may now learn to apply their knowledge to the *weighing* and *measuring* of pharmaceuticals. The former process requires the use of the *balance*, or, for manufacturing purposes, *scales*, and the latter process requires the use of the *measure*, the *graduate,* and the *pipet.* The successful performance of many of the operations in pharmacy depends on a thorough knowledge of the principles of the balance and a correct understanding of its care and use; because weighing is nearly always the preliminary step in any compounding, it will be discussed first.

There is a relativity of accuracy in weighing (or measuring) that must not be overlooked, as illustrated by the following graded list: coal, salt, sugar, epsom salt, penicillin G, morphine, digoxin, vitamin B_{12}, and radium. One of the most important things for the pharmacist to learn is the degree of tolerance or error permissible in weighing or measuring any particular ingredient. Obviously, the final item on the list, radium, must be measured with much greater precision and accuracy than coal, the first item.

The empiric weighing and measuring methods of the kitchen, embodied in such concepts as a handful, a pinch, or "sweeten to suit your taste," have no place in pharmacy. Accurate work can be accomplished only by means of suitable apparatus.

WEIGHING

In pharmacy, weighing usually refers to ascertaining a definite weight of material to be used in compounding a prescription or manufacturing a dosage form.

The *balance* may be defined as an instrument for determining the relative weights of substances. It should be *selected correctly* for the specific task at hand, *used skillfully, protected from damage,* and *checked periodically*, if accurate results are to be obtained. Of even greater importance is its *construction.* Standards for balances are given by the NIST.[1]

Construction of the Balance

For systematic consideration pharmaceutical balances may be classified as follows: single-beam (equal-arm or unequal arm), compound lever, torsion and electronic.

SINGLE-BEAM EQUAL-ARM BALANCES—The principle on which single-beam equal-arm balances (or scales) operate is clearly evident in the construction of the classical two-pan analytical balance. This type has a metallic lever or beam, divided into two equal arms at the center by a knife-edge, on which it is supported. At exactly equal distances from this point of support, and situated in the same plane, are placed the end knife-edges; these suspend the pans, which carry the substances to be weighed. A properly constructed balance of this type should meet the following requirements:

1. *When the beam is in a horizontal position, the center of gravity should be slightly below the point of support, or central knife-edge, and perpendicular to it.*
   The relative sensitivity of the balance depends on the fulfillment of this principle, which may be illustrated roughly by forcing a pin through the center of a circular piece of pasteboard. If the edge of the pasteboard is touched slightly, it does not oscillate at all, but rather revolves around the center to a degree corresponding to the impulse given it. In this position it illustrates neutral equilibrium. If the pin is removed and inserted at a very short distance above the center, and the edge of the pasteboard touched as before, it will oscillate slowly, corresponding to a very sensitive beam, the point of support being slightly above the center of gravity as in the balance. If the pin is removed again and inserted far above the center, and the same impulse imparted to the edge, it will oscillate quickly, illustrating stable equilibrium characteristic of a beam that comes to rest quickly and is not particularly sensitive. Unstable equilibrium may be illustrated by balancing the disc so that the point of support is below the center. The slightest touch then causes it to reverse its position completely and finally come to rest with the center of gravity below the point of support.
2. *The end knife-edges must be exactly equal distances from the central knife-edge; they all must be in the same plane and the edges absolutely parallel to each other.*

It is very apparent that the conditions of a good prescription balance cannot be satisfied if there is inequality in the length of the arms of the beam. The distance from the central knife-edge to the one on the left must be exactly the same as the distance from the central knife-edge to the one on the right, otherwise unequal weights would be required to establish equilibrium. If the central knife-edge is placed either above or below a line drawn so that it connects the end knife-edges, the loading of the pans either will cause the beam to cease oscillating or diminish the sensitivity in proportion to the load. If the knife-edges are not parallel, the weight of a body will not be constant upon every part of the pan, but will be greater if placed near the edge on one side, and correspondingly less at a point directly opposite.

3. *The beam should be inflexible, but as light in weight as possible, and the knife-edges in fine balances should bear upon agate plates.* The rigidity of the beam is necessary because any serious deflection caused by a loading of the pans would lower the end knife-edges and thus accuracy in weighing would be impossible. The beam should not be heavier than necessary because the sensitiveness of the balance thereby would be lessened; to diminish friction, which constantly increases with the age and use of a balance, the bearings of the knife-edges should be agate plates, which are polished flat pieces of the very hard mineral called agate.

A single-beam equal-arm balance with the rider beam graduated to 28 g in increments of 0.2 g, and to 1 oz in increments of 0.01 oz, is shown in Figure 11-2.

UNEQUAL-ARM BALANCES—The unequal-arm balance is the type is preferred for laboratory work when large amounts are to be weighed (Fig 11-3). The lever principle on which these scales are constructed is based on the law of physics that at equilibrium the force applied at one end of the lever multiplied by the length of the arm (distance from the fulcrum to the point where the force is applied) must be equal to the product of the force acting at the opposite end of the lever and the length of the other arm. The inequality in the length of the arms of this beam permits the convenient use of movable weights upon the graduated longer arm of the beam, thus dispensing with the use of small weights, which are liable to be lost. This scale is of great advantage in laboratory or manufacturing work because it is particularly adapted for weighing liquids; a sliding tare is set on one beam for the weight of the container, and other sliding weights can be adjusted to the weight of liquid desired. These are available with the beams graduated either in the avoirdupois or metric system.

COMPOUND-LEVER BALANCES—The principle of the compound lever was first applied in the construction of balances by Robervahl of Paris, in about 1660 AD. It was skillfully adapted for both prescription balances and the general counter and platform scales. The principal objection to this type of scale, when compared with single-beam balances, consists in the multiplicity of points of contact and suspension, thus necessarily in-

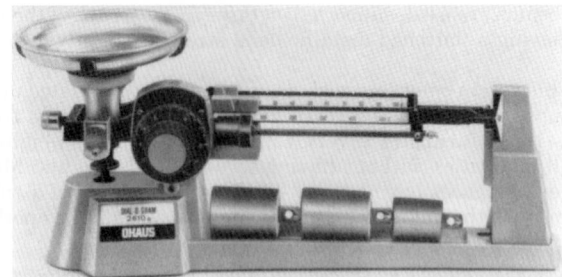

Figure 11-3. Manufacturing laboratory scale and weights (courtesy, Ohaus).

creasing friction and the liability to disarrangement; however, their general convenience has made them popular.

TORSION BALANCES—A simple illustration of the principle of torsion is afforded by tying a stout piece of cord to a firm support and inserting a lead pencil in the middle of the cord between the strands, at right angles to it. If the free end of the cord is stretched tightly, resistance is offered to any effort to turn the lead pencil over; if the pencil is released, it at once flies back to its original position. *Torsion* is the term applied to this method of twisting. The principle of supporting the beam of a balance on a tightly stretched wire, with the view of doing away with knife-edges and diminishing friction, occupied the attention of inventors for years.

In 1882 Prof. Roeder and Dr. Springer contrived an ingenious torsion balance that gave promise of valuable results. Two illustrations of this original balance were shown on page 54 of the first edition of *Remington's Practice of Pharmacy* in 1885. Improvements have increased its efficiency greatly. The most important difficulty in applying the principle of torsion resistance was overcome by placing a weight just above the center of gravity (Fig 11-4). Torsional resistance tends to keep the beam in a horizontal position, while the elevation of a weight above the center of gravity, by its tendency to produce unstable equilibrium, exercises an opposite effect—the beam is inclined to be top heavy and, therefore, to tip on either side. If now the weight is made adjustable by mounting it upon a perpendicular screw so that it can be raised or lowered, it is possible to arrange these opposite forces so that one exactly neutralizes the other. In this manner sensitivity is obtained.

The torsion principle has been applied to prescription balances, as well as analytical balances and scales designed to carry heavier loads. In the torsion prescription balance

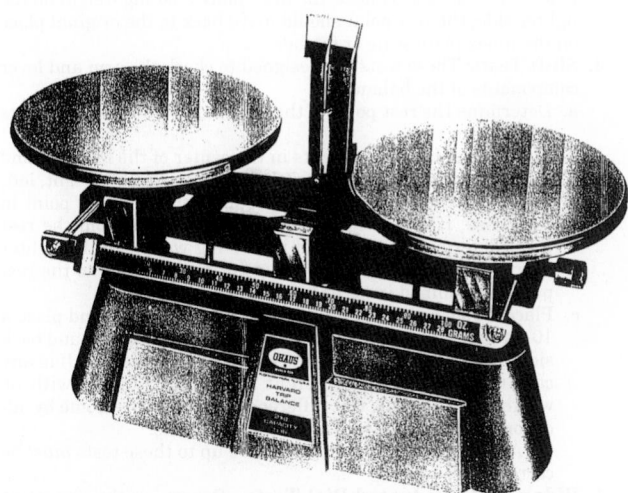

Figure 11-2. Single-beam equal-arm balance (courtesy, Ohaus).

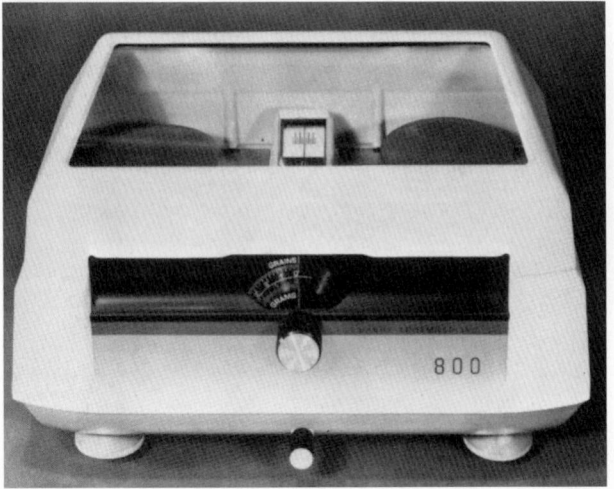

Figure 11-4. Troemner/800 prescription balance (courtesy, Troemner).

two beams are used, supported on three frames, each of the latter having a flattened metallic band stretched tightly over its edge.

The torsion balance, which has a rider beam graduated upon the upper edge from 1/8 to 15 gr and on its lower edge from 0.01–1.0 g, furnishes a very convenient means of weighing small quantities without having to use small weights. Most modern balances have a direct-reading dial instead of a rider beam, with the metric scale on the upper scale and the apothecary scale on the lower.

The prescription balance may be placed upon a base containing a drawer that can be used for holding weights or powder papers.

ELECTRONIC BALANCES—Electronic balances are single pan balances with digital or direct-reading features (Fig 11-5). Taring a weighing paper, weigh boat, or beakers is done automatically with the push of a button or lever without the need of external balancing weights. These balances are much more sensitive than the traditional prescription balance, are easier and quicker to use, but are usually more expensive than a torsion balance.

Prescription Balances

The most common type of prescription balance uses the taut-wire frame or torsion principle (see Fig 11-4). Such balances, manufactured to meet the requirements of the NIST Class III balances, have a maximum maintenance sensitivity of six mg with no load and with full load (ie, addition of the 6 mg weight to one pan causes the indicator or the rest point to be shifted not less than one division on the index plate). The Class III balance is used to weigh quantities up to 60 g, depending on the stated capacity and subject to the physical limit of the amount of the material that can be placed on the pan. Electronic balances typically have a sensitivity less than 10 mg (easily meeting standards for a Class III balance) and can weigh small quantities of drug more accurately than a torsion balance. All prescription departments must have a Class III balance.

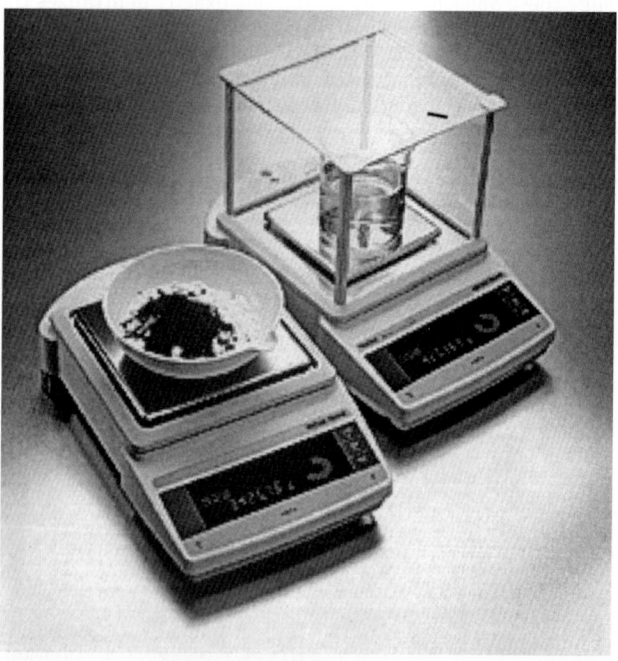

Figure 11-5. Electronic single pan balance.

REQUIREMENTS—A prescription balance should meet the following general requirements:

1. It should be constructed so as to support its full capacity without developing undue stresses, and should not be thrown out of adjustment by repeated weighings of the capacity load. (The capacity of the balance will be seen on the metal plate attached to it.) If the capacity is not stated, it is assumed to be at least 15 g (1/2 oz). The Class III balances usually have a capacity of 60 g (2 oz).
2. The removable pans of a torsion prescription balance should be of equal weight. If the pans show any difference in weight, they should be adjusted by leveling the balance or using small pieces of paper. Pans with any appreciable corrosion or wear should be refinished or replaced.
3. A prescription balance should have a leveling device, usually leveling feet or screws, so that the balance can be adjusted to a level position. A balance that does not have these is not entitled to be designated as a prescription balance.
4. The balance that has a rider or graduated dial should have, at the end of the graduation, a stop that halts the rider or dial at the zero reading. The reading edge of the rider should be parallel to the graduations on the beam.
5. The indicator points, when there are two on the balance, should be sharp, and their ends should not be separated by more than one mm (0.04 inch) when the scale is in balance. The distance from the face of the index plate to the indicator pointer or pointers should be small (1 mm or less) to protect the operator against making errors resulting from parallax, because it is unlikely that the eye of the operator will be exactly in line with the indicator and the division on the index plate. The indicating elements as well as the lever system of the balance should be protected against drafts. The balance should have a lid that allows a weighing to be made when the lid is closed.
6. A torsion prescription balance must have a mechanical means for arresting the oscillation of the mechanism.

TESTING—Certain tests may be used to satisfy the user regarding the construction and character of a torsion balance when its origin, history, or condition is in doubt. Additional tests are carried out by the NIST, manufacturers, and local and state testing agencies.

A Class III torsion prescription balance meets the following basic tests. Use a set of *test weights* and keep the rider or graduated dial at zero unless directed to change its position.

1. **Sensitivity Requirement:** Level the balance, determine the rest point, place a 10-mg weight on one of the empty pans, and again determine the rest point. Repeat the operation with a 10-mg weight in the center of each pan. The rest point is shifted not less than one division of the index plate each time the 10-mg weight is added. The sensitivity requirement for an electronic balance is supplied by the manufacturer.
2. **Arm Ratio Test:** This test is designed to check the equality of length of both arms of the balance. Determine the rest point of the balance with no weight on the pans. Place 30 g of test weights in the center of each pan and determine the rest point. If the second rest point is not the same as the first, place a 20-mg weight on the lighter side; the rest point should move back to the original place on the index plate scale or farther.
3. **Shift Tests:** These tests are designed to check the arm and lever components of the balance.
   a. Determine the rest point of the indicator without any weights on the pans.
   b. Place one of the 10-g weights in the center of the left pan, and place the other 10-g weight successively toward the right, left, front, and back side of the right pan, noting the rest point in each case. If in any case the rest point differs from the rest point determined in (*a*), add the 10-mg weight to the lighter side; this should cause the rest point to shift back to the rest point determined in (*a*) or farther.
   c. Place a 10-g weight in the center of the right pan, and place a 10-g weight successively toward the right, left, front, and back sides of the left pan, noting the rest point in each case. If in any case the rest point is different from that obtained with no weights on the pans, this difference should be overcome by addition of the 10-mg weight to the lighter side.
      A balance that does not measure up to these tests *must* be corrected.
4. **Rider- and Graduated-Dial Tests**—Determine the rest point for the balance with no weight on the pans. Now place on the left

pan the 500-mg test weight and move the rider to the 500-mg point on the beam. Now determine the rest point. If it is different from the zero rest point, add a 10-mg weight to the lighter side. This should bring the rest point back to its original position or farther. Repeat this test, using the 1-g test weight and moving the rider or graduated dial to the 1-g division. If the rest point is different it should be brought back at least to the zero rest point position by the addition of 10 mg to the lighter pan. If the balance does not meet this test, the graduated beam or the rider must be corrected. For balances equipped with a dial scale, the dial must be corrected.

PROTECTION—The necessity for protecting the delicate mechanism of a balance is overlooked frequently, notwithstanding the possibility of having a precision apparatus irretrievably ruined by lack of care in using or cleaning it or in protecting it while at rest. The position chosen for the balance or scales should be on a level and firm counter, desk, or table, where it will be subjected to little risk of damage from dampness, dust, or corrosive vapors and where the knife-edges will not be liable to become dulled by jarring or other vibrations.

In the analytical class of balances, protection is afforded by enclosing them in glass cases having sash doors in the front, sides, or back. They are protected against damage from vibration by a lever for elevating or locking the beam, so that the knife-edges are not in contact with any surface when not in use. To prevent damage from jarring while the balance is in use, from a weight falling on the pan, or other accident, the finest balances are provided with pan supports, which break the fall and serve the additional purpose of quickly arresting the beam, thus saving time while weighing.

In using a prescription balance, neither the weights nor the substance that is to be weighed should be placed on the balance pans while the beam is free to oscillate. The desired weight should be placed upon one pan (usually the one on the right-hand side) and an amount of the substance to be weighed, approximately the desired weight, upon the opposite pan. The beam should be released by means of the lever, and if the substance is in excess, the beam should be locked and a small portion removed and the beam again released and the oscillations observed. This procedure should be repeated until the correct amount is obtained. In case of a deficiency of the substance to be weighed, the reverse procedure is followed until the correct amount is obtained. With practice this can be done very deftly and very quickly and the sensitivity of the balance retained for years.

Substances that react with metals, such as iodine, and those that are adhesive, such as the extracts, should not be weighed directly upon the pans, but rather upon counterpoised watch crystals, or upon glazed paper, care being taken to balance the papers before weighing the substance. In cleaning the balances, great care should be exercised; polishing powders should be used sparingly, as a portion is very apt to find its way into crevices and elude detection until an attempt is made to adjust the balances, when the increased weight of one of the sides of the beam leads to its discovery. Frequent cleaning with soft leather generally is sufficient to keep a balance in good order, but once neglect makes it necessary to use more active measures, some simple polishing powder for the metal work, soapsuds for the nickel plate, and simple brushing for the lacquered brass are all that is necessary.

As the pans are subjected to more wear and tear than any other part of the balance, it is economical to use *solid* rather than *plated* pans because constant friction wears off the plating and the additional cost for replating soon absorbs the difference in price. Equipped in this way, and with agate bearings, a prescription balance is durable and really inexpensive because it will remain fully equal to the most exacting demands for a long time.

Weights Used in Pharmacy

The weights used by the pharmacist are very important, and care in their selection and examination is necessary. False economy must be avoided, as the use of cheap, inaccurate weights ultimately leads to serious consequences. Official inspectors have found pharmacies using prescription weights that were so worn that the characters on their faces had disappeared; also, weights have been found with bits of hardened extract and dirt almost entirely obscuring their characters. An unused set of standard weights should be kept on hand so that at least once a year the weights in daily use can be tested and adjusted or rejected if necessary. The standard weights should be used also when the balance is tested. The set should contain the following weights in a well-fitted box with forceps: one 50-g, two 20-g, one 10-g, one 5-g, two 2-g, one 1-g, one 500-mg, two 200-mg, one 100-mg, one 50-mg, two 20-mg, and one 10-mg, all adjusted to NIST tolerances for analytical or Class P weights.

METRIC WEIGHTS—For weighing larger quantities, japanned iron metric weights are available. They are preferably hexagonal, to distinguish them from the round avoirdupois weights. Sets of brass weights, usually in the range of 10 g to 1000 g, fitted into holes of appropriate size in a block of plastic (*block weights*), are especially convenient for many weighing operations. For prescription compounding, accurate sets of weights ranging from 10 mg to 50 g are available.

For analytical purposes, metric weights are used exclusively; usually, the highest weight is 100 g, the lowest 1 mg. The weights from one g upward are of finely lacquered brass or of nonmagnetic stainless steel or rhodium-plated bronze. The smaller weights are made of squares of platinum or aluminum foil, with one edge turned up to permit them to be handled easily with the forceps. Fractions of a milligram are weighed by means of the rider on the graduated beam of the balance.

In analytical work and in using the Class III balance in prescription work, the weights should never be handled with the fingers but always with the forceps, which accompany an accurate set of weights. In the more expensive sets of weights the forceps are tipped with bone, ivory, or plastic to prevent the wearing away of the weights during handling. With proper care the accuracy of a fine set of weights may be maintained for years.

COMMON AVOIRDUPOIS WEIGHTS—Avoirdupois weights usually are made of iron, and they are flat and circular and japanned to prevent rusting. These weights form a pyramidal pile, and range from ½ oz to 4 lb; if found to be incorrect, they may be adjusted by adding to or diminishing the amount of lead that is hammered into a depression in the base of each weight. They sometimes are made of brass in this form, and sometimes of zinc (the latter, however, are brittle and unserviceable). For general use in the pharmacy, the cylindrical weights, known technically as block weights, are preferable. The advantages of block weights are that the gaps left by missing weights are readily noticeable, and the greater part of the surface of the weight is protected from the action of corrosive vapors when the weights are not in use.

APOTHECARY WEIGHTS—Apothecary weights may be obtained either as *block weights* or in the less-desirable *flat* forms. The round, flat, brass *dram* weights, which have the denomination stamped on their faces in raised characters, still are used but should be replaced. With flat weights, the denomination is often only faintly stamped on the face and thus is liable to be obliterated by constant use or by corrosive contact.

Undoubtedly, the best grain weights are the aluminum wire weights. The wire weights are less susceptible to corrosive action than are the brass weights. Also, the wire weights are more easily and quickly distinguished from one another than are other weight forms, so there is less likelihood of dangerous mistakes: the number of sides in the wire weights at once gives the denomination (Fig 11-6).

Aluminum grain weights, which are cut out of aluminum plates, are also less liable to be corroded. They usually can be more accurately adjusted than brass weights. The corners of the aluminum weights are clipped, and each weight usually is pressed into a curved form so that it may be picked up easily (Fig 11-7).

The need for apothecary weights in modern practice is decreasing. Apothecary weights can easily be converted to the corresponding metric weights, which are easier to use and less

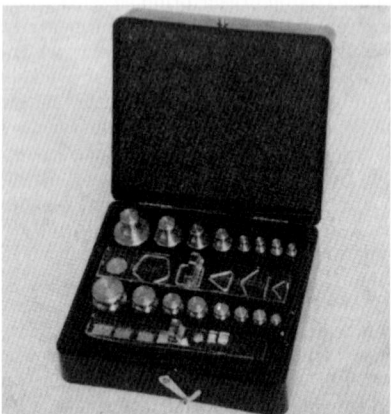

Figure 11-6. Metric and Apothecary weight set (courtesy, Troemner).

prone to error. In addition, electronic balances do not use external weights. Typically, an electronic balance can display weights in several systems as the discretion of the operator.

Minimum Weighable Quantity

All of the balances described must be used within a degree of error that can be tolerated in prescription compounding and in pharmaceutical manufacturing. The USP allows a maximum error of 5% in a single weighing operation. Since the sensitivity requirement of a balance represents the absolute error in using that balance, the percent error will depend on the amount of drug weighed and will increase as the amount of drug decreases.

The Minimum Weighable Quantity (MWQ) with no more than 5% error can be calculated for any balance knowing the sensitivity requirement (SR) (ie, the absolute error) from the following:

$$MWQ = SR \frac{100\%}{5\%}$$

Examples

1. Calculate the MWQ with no more than a 5% error for a balance with a sensitivity requirement of 10 mg.

$$MWQ = 10 \text{ mg} \frac{100\%}{5\%} = 200 \text{ mg}$$

2. Calculate the MWQ with no more than a 3% error for a balance with a sensitivity requirement of 2.5 mg.

$$MWQ = 2.5 \text{ mg} \frac{100\%}{3\%} = 83.3 \text{ mg}$$

MEASURING

In pharmacy, *measuring* usually refers to the exact determination of a definite volume of liquid. Many types of apparatus are

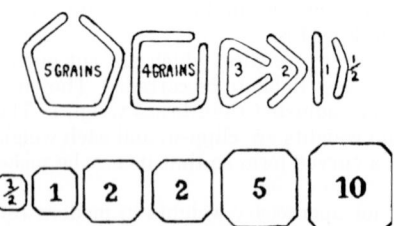

Figure 11-7. Aluminum wire and aluminum grain weights.

used in this operation, depending on the kind and quantity of liquid to be measured and the degree of accuracy required. (The NIST has requirements for graduates.[1])

Large Quantities

Glass measures are preferred for measuring liquids. Although glass measures are subject to breakage, they can indicate volume more accurately because of the transparency of glass.

THE MENISCUS—When an aqueous or alcoholic liquid is poured into a graduate, surface forces cause its surface to become concave—the portion in contact with the vessel is drawn upward. This phenomenon is known as the formation of a *meniscus* (Fig 11-8), and in determining the volume of a liquid *the reading must be made at the bottom of this meniscus.* This regulation has been established by the NIST, and all glass measuring vessels are graduated on this basis. Liquids with large contact angles, such as mercury, form an *inverted meniscus,* and the reading then is made at the top of the curved surface.

PROCEDURE—Pharmaceutical manufacturers package liquid preparations in glass or plastic containers equipped with a plastic screw-cap. These containers serve as a stock bottle from which liquids may be poured directly into a graduate. The procedure for pouring liquid from screw-capped containers is as follows:

1. Remove the cap and place it on the counter while the transfer of liquid is made.
2. While holding the graduate in the left hand, grasp the original container with the label in such a position that any excess of liquid will not soil the label if it should run down the side of the bottle.
3. Raise the graduate and hold it so that the graduation point to be read is on a level with the eye, and measure the liquid. (The extension of the graduating mark into a circle that passes entirely around the graduate is an improvement that obviates the necessity of placing the graduate upon a level place, as the corresponding mark upon the opposite side may be seen through the glass and the graduate easily leveled even when held in the hand.)
4. Replace the cap, and return the bottle to the counter or shelf.
5. Pour the liquid into the bottle or mortar for dispensing or compounding.

METALLIC MEASURES—Metallic measures are nearly cylindrical in shape, but are slightly wider at the bottom. These are generally used for measuring liquids when the quantity is over a pint. A set usually consists of five (gallon, half-gallon, quart, pint, and half-pint) of these measures. Measures made of tinned iron, or of the enameled sheet iron called agateware, are greatly inferior to those made of *tinned copper* or *stainless steel;* tinned-iron measures soon become rusty, and particles of enameling can chip off, leaving the exposed iron to contaminate the measured liquids.

The initial cost of copper or stainless-steel measures is greater than tinned iron, but they are far more durable. Care

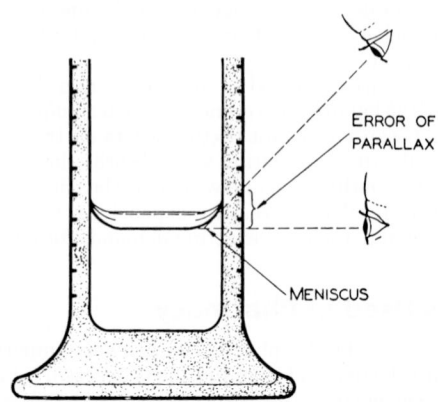

Figure 11-8. Error of measurement due to parallax.

must be taken to protect them from blows that will cause dents as these may be serious enough to detract from their accuracy. Cylindrical metric measures, usually made of monel metal or stainless steel and having a diameter just half their height, are available in various sizes. Such containers are relatively expensive, but their resistance to corrosion and wear is a tremendous advantage. Copper, of course, should not be used where it is likely to catalyze oxidation.

GRADUATED GLASS MEASURES—Graduated glass measures nearly always are used for quantities of 500 mL or one pt or less. There are of two forms, *conical* and *cylindrical* (Fig 11-9, 11-10). The conical graduate is suitable for some measurements because of the greater ease with which it can be handled, but cylindrical measures are more accurate because of their uniform and smaller average diameter. In a graduated cylinder, the error in volume caused by a deviation of ±1 mm in reading the meniscus remains constant along the height of the uniform column; the same deviation causes a progressively larger error in a conical graduate because the diameter, and thus the volume of the 1-mm column, increases along its vertical axis. It is safe to assume that practically all good-grade modern graduates comply with the NIST requirements for internal diameters at stated volumes.

A study has indicated that, to improve accuracy, the lower portions of graduates should not be used, and therefore should not be marked.[2] A composite tabulation (Table 11-11) shows the calculated and the assigned blank portions of graduates. The elimination of the lower markings on graduates was suggested, and in 1955 the NIST specifications for graduates used this principle.[1] The NIST Handbook states, "A graduate shall have an initial interval that is not subdivided, equal to not less than one-fifth and not more than one-fourth of the capacity of the graduate." For accurate measurement of volumes less than 1.5 mL, a graduated pipet or a graduated dropper could be used.

EFFECT OF LIQUID AND CONTAINER—It is difficult to measure accurately when pouring from a completely filled bottle because of the uneven flow of the liquid. After the first portion of the liquid is removed, the shape of the bottle does not influence the ease of pouring to any appreciable extent unless the neck is extremely narrow.

Viscous liquids pour slowly, but their accurate measurement is not difficult. Experiments showed that when glycerin is poured into a graduate without letting the liquid run down the inside surface, the precision of measurement can be very high. Naturally, the chance of hitting the inner surface is greater with smaller than with larger graduates. The increase in possible deviation then is caused by the slow movement of the viscous liquid to the desired mark.

Viscous liquids introduce another factor: drainage time. Graduates are calibrated to contain or deliver indicated volumes within specified limits. Aqueous, alcoholic, and hydroalcoholic liquids can be drained from a graduate in 30 seconds so completely that the delivered and contained volumes are fairly close. When 25 mL of glycerin was measured in the same cleaned and dried cylinders, the received volume measured 23.7 mL af-

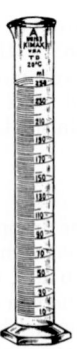

Figure 11-10. Glass cylindrical graduate (courtesy, Kimble Glass).

ter the same time period. Silicone-treated glassware, which now is used frequently, drains completely in a few seconds.

The viscosity factor might be altered when another liquid is to be mixed with the glycerin by measuring and mixing both liquids in a suitable graduate.

Small Quantities

For measuring smaller quantities of liquids, graduated glass tubes of small diameter should be used. The narrower bore permits greater distances between the graduations on the apparatus, thus allowing greater accuracy in making the reading. For example, with a buret the pharmaceutical chemist can estimate volumes to the nearest 1/100 mL.

Pipets and similar apparatus are more accurate and convenient than very small graduates. The graduations on very small graduates are necessarily in the very small, lowest portion of a comparatively tall measure. To measure 1 mL of a volatile oil in a graduate, the surface that the oil must traverse when this measure is inverted is so great that probably 20% of the oil will be left adhering to the measure. In liquid preparations in which the smaller liquid is miscible with the larger quantity of diluting liquid, the graduate may be rinsed and this loss recovered, but inconveniences are largely overcome and greater accuracy secured by using a pipet.

In administering small quantities of liquids, the very convenient *drop* is almost always used. It should be emphasized that one *drop is not equivalent to 1* ℳ and that *60 drops are not equivalent to one f ℥.* This impression doubtlessly arose because 60 ordinary drops of *water* are about equal to one f ℥, but the volume of a drop of fluid depends on many factors, including density, temperature, viscosity, surface tension, and the size and nature of the orifice from which it is dropped. Thick, viscous liquids, such as the mucilages and the syrups, necessarily produce large drops because the drop adheres to the surface of the glass as long as its weight does not overcome its power of adhesion, whereas chloroform, a mobile liquid that has very little adhesion to the dropping surface, produces very small drops. The greater the surface tension, the larger the

Table 11-11. Unmarked (Unreliable) Portions of Graduates

| CAPACITY OF GRADUATE (mL) | CALCULATED BLANKS (1951) | | NIST BLANKS (mL) |
	2.5%[a] ALLOWED (mL)	5%[a] ALLOWED (mL)	
5	3.0	1.5	1
10	4.4	2.2	2
25	11.8	5.9	5
50	15.8	7.9	10
100	20.9	10.5	20
250	36.3	18.2	50
500	66.5	33.2	100
1000	—	—	200

[a] Calculations by Goldstein and Mattocks[2] based on deviation of ±1 mm from graduation mark and allowable errors of 2.5% and 5%.

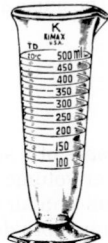

Figure 11-9. Glass conical graduate (courtesy, Kimble Glass).

drop, and the greater the extent of surface to which the drop adheres, the larger, proportionally, the drop.

A *normal or standard drop measure* was recommended by the Brussels Conference of 1902 for international adoption. This dropper is recognized in the USP.

MEDICINE DROPPER[3]

The Pharmacopeial medicine dropper consists of a tube made of glass or other suitable transparent material that generally is fitted with a collapsible bulb and, while varying in capacity, is constricted at the delivery end to a round opening having an external diameter of about 3 mm. The dropper, when held vertically, delivers water in drops each of which weighs between 45 mg and 55 mg.

When drops are specified on a prescription, the usual custom has been to employ an *eyedropper,* but now the standard dropper should be supplied. When accuracy is required, it is particularly important to use a specially calibrated dropper for administering potent medicines. The volume error incurred in measuring any liquid by means of a calibrated dropper should not exceed 15%, under normal conditions.[3]

TEASPOON

For household purposes, an American Standard Teaspoon has been established by the American National Standards Institute as containing 4.93 ± 0.24 mL. In view of the almost universal practice of employing teaspoons ordinarily available in the household for the administration of medicine, the teaspoon may be regarded as representing 5 mL and is so accepted by the USP.

It must be kept in mind that the actual volume delivered by a teaspoon of any given liquid is related to the latter's viscosity and surface tension, among other influencing factors.

THE HUMAN FACTOR—The *human factor of carefulness* is of paramount importance in every pharmaceutical operation in which accuracy is essential. Accurate measurement of liquids requires accurate equipment, careful manipulation, good vision, and a steady hand.

DENSITY AND SPECIFIC GRAVITY

Several terms are used to express the mass (weight) of equal volumes of different substances.

Absolute density is the ratio of the mass of an object, determined in or referred to a vacuum, at a specified temperature, to the volume of the object at the same temperature. This relationship is expressed mathematically as:

$$\text{Absolute Density} = \frac{\text{Mass in grams (in a vacuum)}}{\text{Volume in millimeters}}$$

Apparent density differs from absolute density only in that the mass of the object is determined in air; the mass is influenced by the difference in the buoyant effect of air on the object being weighed, and on the standard masses (weights) used for comparison. If the object and masses are made of the same material, or have the same density, there will be no difference in the buoyant effect, and the apparent density will be identical with the absolute density.

Relative density is an expression sometimes employed to indicate the mass of 1 mL (not cc, which is very slightly different) of a standard substance, such as water, at a specified temperature, relative to water at 4°C taken as unity. Thus, at 4°C the relative density of water is 1.0000, whereas its absolute density at the same temperature is 0.999973. Water attains its maximum absolute density of 0.999973 at 3.98°C. To convert a relative density of water to absolute density, the former should be multiplied by 0.999973.

Specific gravity may be defined as the ratio of the mass of a substance to the mass of an equal volume of another substance taken as the standard. For gases, the standard may be hydrogen or air; for liquids and solids, it is water.

From what has been stated, it is obvious that in a determination of specific gravity there will be, in general, a difference in the result if the masses (weights) are determined in air or in vacuum. If the masses are determined in, or referred to, a vacuum, the result is a *true specific gravity* (sometimes called *absolute specific gravity*); if the masses are determined in air, the calculated result is an *apparent specific gravity.* The difference between these specific gravities is, as a rule, very small.

A very important variable in specific gravity determinations is temperature, and this is doubly important because both the temperature of the substance under examination and the temperature of the standard may be different. The temperatures are commonly shown as a ratio, with the temperature of the water always being indicated in the denominator. The common practice with regard to the determination of specific gravity is that defined by the USP: "Unless otherwise stated, the specific gravity basis is 25°/25°, ie, the ratio of the weight of a substance in air at 25° to that of an equal volume of water at the same temperature."

But it is not always convenient, or desirable, to determine the weight of both the substance and the water at 25°, or even to determine the weight of the substance at the same temperature as that at which the water is weighed. Thus, the substance may be weighed at 25° and compared with the weight of an equal volume of water at 4°, in which case the specific gravity is reported as being on a 25°/4° basis. In the case of theobroma oil, which is solid at 25°, the specific gravity is determined on a 100°/25° basis; for alcohol, it is determined on a 15.56°/15.56° basis because many years ago the US government adopted 60°F (15.56°C) as the temperature at which alcoholometric measurements are to be made for government control of alcoholic liquids.

It is apparent that a completely informative statement of specific gravity must indicate the temperature of the substance under examination, as well as that of the equal volume of water. Furthermore, it should be stated whether the determinations of mass (weight) were made on an *in-vacuum* or *in-air* basis; the latter case, the material of construction of the weights also should be indicated (as the buoyant effect of air on weights depends on their volume).

Calculations

The principle underlying the determination of the specific gravity of either a liquid or a solid is the same: to find the ratio of the mass (weight) of the substance to that of an equal volume of water. This may be expressed by a simple relationship:

$$\text{Specific gravity} = \frac{W_s}{W_w}$$

where W_s is the weight of the substance, and W_w the weight of an equal volume of water.

DENSITY

Density is defined as the mass of a substance per unit volume. It has the units of mass over volume. *Specific gravity* is the ratio of the weight of a substance in air to that of an equal volume of water. In the metric system both density and specific gravity may be numerically equal, although the density figure has units. In the English system, density and specific gravity are not numerically equal; for example, the density of water is 62.4 lb/ft^3 and the specific gravity is 1. This shows the convenience of the metric system. The equations for calculating density, weight, and volume are

$$\text{Density} = \frac{\text{Weight}}{\text{Volume}}$$

$$\text{Weight} = \text{Density} \times \text{Volume}$$

$$\text{Volume} = \frac{\text{Weight}}{\text{Density}}$$

Given any two variables, the third one can be calculated.

Examples

1. A pharmacist weighs out 2 kg of glycerin (density, 1.25 g/mL). What is the volume of the glycerin?

$$\text{Volume} = \frac{2000 \text{ g}}{1.25 \text{ g/mL}} = 1600 \text{ mL}$$

2. What is the weight of 60 mL of oil whose density is 0.9624 g/mL?

$$\text{Weight} = 60 \text{ mL} \times 0.9624 \text{ g / mL} = 57.7 \text{ g}$$

3. Calculate the weight of 30 mL of sulfuric acid (density, 1.8 g/mL).

$$\text{Weight} = 30 \text{ mL} \times 1.8 \text{ g / mL} = 54 \text{ g}$$

4. If a prescription order requires 25 g of concentrated hydrochloric acid (density, 1.18 g/mL), what volume should the pharmacist measure?

$$\text{Volume} = \frac{25 \text{ g}}{1.18 \text{ g/mL}} = 21.2 \text{ mL}$$

Problems (Answers on page 125)

1. What is the weight in grams of one L of alcohol (density, 0.816 g/mL)?
2. What is the volume (mL) of one lb (avoir) of glycerin (density, 1.25 g/mL)?
3. What is the volume (mL) of 65 g of an acid whose density is 1.2 g/mL?

PHARMACEUTICAL CALCULATIONS

Pharmaceutical dispensing and compounding calculations use simple arithmetic. The errors that may arise often are due to carelessness, as in improper placing of decimal points, incorrect conversion from one system of measurement to another, or uncertainty over the system of measurement to be used. Before proceeding with any calculation, it is imperative that the problem presented (in a prescription, chart order, formula, etc) be read carefully, that the information given and required be identified, and that the procedure to be used in the calculation be selected.

Before students read this part of the chapter and attempt to solve the problems, the information in the preceding part of this chapter must be understood thoroughly. Often, several steps are necessary to solve problems. Shortcuts should not be taken unless one is certain they are proper. Many problems can be solved by more than one procedure, such as by ratio and proportion or by dimensional analysis. If students find a procedure that is more logical to them and gives the correct answer, it should be used. Thus, the solutions to sample problems used here generally should be considered suggestions, rather than the only way to solve a given type of problem.

Mathematical Principles

A few mathematical principles (eg, common decimal fractions, exponents, powers and roots, significant figures, and logarithms) will be reviewed, as these are areas where students often become careless or have forgotten skills. Following this, various types of practical pharmaceutical problems that the pharmacist may be required to solve are discussed and solutions are given. Where practical, rules for solving these problems are given. No attempt is made to elaborate on any mathematical theory.

The problems generally consist of determining the quantity or quantities of material(s) required to compound prescriptions properly and make products used to aid the compounding of prescriptions. The materials used to compound prescription orders may be pure or mixtures of substances in varying strengths. The strengths of mixtures may be denoted in different ways. Conversions may be necessary between systems of varying strengths or between different measuring systems. At the end of each section, sample problems are given for the student to solve, the answers to which appear on page 125.

Because of the decreasing importance of the apothecary system, the metric system is emphasized here. Chemicals and preparations most likely will be purchased using the avoirdupois or metric systems. Prescription orders are filled in the system indicated on the order, usually the apothecary or metric systems.

The student should become familiar with the terminology used in writing prescription orders, such as Latin words and abbreviations used in giving directions to the pharmacist and patient. The prescriber occasionally may use Roman numerals instead of Arabic numerals, so students must be familiar with these (even if the practice is declining).

SIGNIFICANT FIGURES

Weighing and measuring can be carried out with only a certain maximum degree of accuracy; the result always is approximate due to the many sources of error such as temperature, limitations of the instruments employed, personal factors, and so on. Pharmacists must achieve the greatest accuracy possible with their equipment, but it would be erroneous to claim that they have weighed 1 mg of a solid on a Class III prescription balance, which has a sensitivity requirement of 10 mg, or that they have measured 76.32 mL of a liquid in a 100-mL graduate, which can be read only to 1 mL. When quantities are written, the numbers should contain only those digits that are *significant* within the precision of the instrument.

Significant figures are digits that have practical meaning. In some instances zeros are significant; in other instances they merely indicate the order of magnitude of the other digits by locating the decimal point. For example, in the measurement 473 mL all the digits are significant, but in the measurement 4730 mL the zero may or may not be significant. In the weight 0.0316 g the zeros are not significant but only locate the decimal point. In any result the last significant figure is only approximate, but all preceding figures are accurate.

When 473 mL is recorded, it is understood that the measurement had been made within ± 0.5 mL or somewhere between 472.5 and 473.5 mL. The student should stop to consider the full implications of this specifically that the measurement is subject to a maximum error of:

$$\frac{0.5}{473} \times 100 = (\text{approx}) \ 0.1\% \text{ or } 1 \text{ part in } 1000$$

A zero in a quantity such as 473.0 mL is a significant figure and implies that the measurement has been made within the limits 472.95 mL and 473.05 mL or with a possible error of:

$$\frac{0.05}{473} \times 100 = (\text{approx}) \ 0.01\% \ \text{or} \ 1 \ \text{part in} \ 10,000$$

Thus, 473 is correct to the nearest mL, and 473.0 is correct to the nearest 0.1 mL.

Rules

1. *When adding or subtracting, retain in the sum or remainder no more decimal places than the least number entering into the calculations.* For example,

11.5 g	11.50 g
2.65 g	2.65 g
3.49 g	3.49 g
17.64 g	17.64 g

Answer: 17.6 g *Answer:* 17.64 g

In the first column 11.5 g was weighed to 0.1 g or with an accuracy of ±0.05 g. Although the other two weighings were made with an accuracy of ±0.005 g, the sum can be expressed properly only to one decimal place.

In the second column 11.50 g was weighed to the nearest 0.01 g or with an accuracy of ±0.005 g. Since all weighings were made with this degree of accuracy, the sum may be stated as in the example, 17.64 g.

Retain all figures possible until all the calculations are completed and then retain only the significant figures for the answer. Additions or subtractions involving both large and small quantities, each expressed with maximum significance, are often useless. For example, if one were to add 1.2 and 0.041 g, the physical sum would be 1.2 g, regardless of the fact that the two numbers add numerically to 1.241. To express the physical sum as 1.241 g would convey an erroneous degree of accuracy with which the quantity was known.

2. *When multiplying or dividing, retain in the answer no more significant figures than the least number entering into the calculation.* The meaning of this rule may be illustrated by the use of equivalents during conversions from one measuring system to another. Table 11-12 gives different equivalent values and the number of significant figures to which the answer is correct. Always use an equivalent that will give the desired degree of accuracy. Repeated multiplication of an approximation increases the error progressively; therefore, retain all figures during calculations and drop insignificant figures as the final step.

FRACTIONS

Common Fractions

An example of a common fraction is 3/8. It is read as "three-eighths" and indicates three parts divided by eight parts of the same thing. The units with both numbers must be the same. Pharmacists measure 3/8 of a fluidounce into a graduate, they measure 3 fluidrams, out of 8 fluidrams (a fluidounce contains 8 fluidrams).

The following principles should be applied when using common fractions:

1. The value of a fraction is not altered by multiplying or dividing both numerator and denominator by the same number.

2. Multiplying the numerator or dividing the denominator by a number, multiplies the fraction by that number.
3. Dividing the numerator or multiplying the denominator by a number divides the fraction by that number.
4. To add or subtract fractions, form fractions with the *lowest common denominator*, perform the arithmetical operation, and reduce to the lowest common denominator.
5. To multiply fractions, multiply all numbers above the line to form the new numerator and multiply all numbers below the line to form the new denominator. Cancel if possible to simplify and reduce to the lowest common denominator.
6. To divide by a fraction, multiply by the reciprocal of the fraction.

Decimal Fractions

Fractions with the power of 10 as the denominator are known as *decimal fractions* and are written by omitting the denominator and inserting a decimal point in the numerator as many places from the last number on the right as there are ciphers of 10 in the denominator.

The following principles should be applied when using decimal fractions:

1. When adding or subtracting decimals, align the decimal points under each other.
2. When multiplying decimals, proceed as with whole numbers, then place the decimal point in the product as many places from the first number on the right as the sum of the decimal places in the multiplier and the multiplicand.
3. When dividing by a decimal fraction, move the decimal point to the right, in both divisor and dividend, as many places as it is to the left in the divisor to form a whole number in the divisor; proceed as with whole numbers. The decimal point in the quotient should be placed immediately above the decimal point in the dividend.
4. When converting a common fraction into a decimal fraction, divide the numerator by the denominator and place the decimal point in the correct place.
5. When converting a decimal fraction into a common fraction, place the entire number, as the numerator, over the power of 10 containing the same number of ciphers of 10 as there are decimal places. Cancel, if possible, to simplify.

EXPONENTS, POWERS, AND ROOTS

In the expression $2^4 = 16$, the following names are given to the terms: 16 is called the *power* of the *base 2* and 4 is the *exponent* of the power. If the exponent is 1, it usually is omitted. The following laws should be recalled:

1. The product of two or more powers of the same base is equal to that base with an exponent equal to the sum of the exponents of the powers; eg, $2^5 \times 2^3 = 2^8$.
2. The quotient of two powers of the same base is equal to that base with an exponent equal to the exponent of the dividend minus the exponent of the divisor; eg, $2^8 \div 2^3 = 2^5$.
3. The power of a power is found by multiplying the exponents; eg, $(2^8)^3 = 2^{24}$.
4. The power of a product equals the product of the powers of the factors; eg, $(2 \times 3 \times 4)^2 = 2^2 \times 3^2 \times 4^2$.
5. The power of a fraction equals the power of the numerator divided by the power of the denominator; eg,

$$\left(\frac{2}{3}\right)^2 = \frac{2^2}{3^2}$$

The root of a power is found by dividing the exponent of the power by the index of the root; eg,

$$\sqrt[3]{3^6} = 3^{\frac{6}{3}} = 3^2$$

Any number other than 0 with an exponent 0 equals 1; eg, $2^0 = 1$. A number with a negative exponent equals one divided by the number with a positive exponent equal in numerical value to the negative exponent; for example,

$$2^{-4} = \frac{1}{2^4}$$

Table 11-12.

WEIGHT(G)		EQUIVALENT WEIGHT (GR/G)		EQUIVALENT WEIGHT (GR)	SIGNIFICANT FIGURES
4.522	×	15.432	=	69.78	4
4.522	×	15.43	=	69.77	4
4.522	×	15.4	=	69.6	3
4.522	×	15	=	68	2

Logarithms

Logarithms (logs) were invented to facilitate the solution of involved and lengthy problems. Many calculations that are difficult by ordinary arithmetical processes are performed rapidly and easily with the aid of logs; the advent of modern calculators and computer spreadsheet programs has made this use of logs obsolete. Logs still appear, however, in many chemical and pharmacokinetic equations.

The log of a number is the exponent of the power to which a given base must be raised in order to equal that number.

$$Y = a^x$$

$$\log_a Y = x$$

John Napier, of Scotland, who discovered logs over three centuries ago, used the Natural Log Number, 2.71828+, as the base. Henry Briggs, using Napier's discovery a few years later, introduced 10 as the base, which is the most convenient for practical purposes. Napier's system is called natural logs, and Briggs' system is called common logs. In this latter system the natural numbers are regarded as powers of the base 10 and the corresponding exponents are the logs; eg,

$$6 = 10^{0.7782}$$

$$\log_{10} 6 = 0.7782$$

For natural logs,

$$6 = e^{1.792}$$

$$\ln_e 6 = 1.792$$

LAWS AND RULES

The following laws, governing the use of logs, are based on the laws of exponents, and hence hold for any log system.

1. The log of a product equals the *sum* of the log of the component numbers; for example, for 25×2:

   $$\log(25 \times 2) = \log 25 + \log 2 = 1.3979 + 0.3010 = 1.6989$$

2. The log of a quotient equals the log of the numerator minus the log of the denominator; for example, for $25 \div 2$:

   $$\log(25/2) = \log 25 - \log 2 = \log 10^{1.3979} - \log 10^{0.3010}$$
   $$= 1.3979 - 0.3010 = 1.0969$$

3. The log of a power of a number equals the log of the number multiplied by the exponent of the power; for example, for $(25)^{12}$:

   $$\log(25)^{12} = 12 \log 25 = 12 \times 1.3979 = 16.7748$$

4. The log of a root of a number equals the log of the number divided by the index of the root; for example, for $\sqrt{25}$

   $$\log \sqrt{25} = \log 25^{1/2} = \frac{\log 25}{2} = \frac{1.3979}{2} = 0.6990$$

5. The log of a negative power of a number equals the reciprocal of the number multiplied by the exponent of the power; for example, $(5)^{-2}$:

   $$\log(5)^{-2} = -2 \log 5 = -2 \times 0.6990 = -1.398$$

The Log of a Number

The logarithm of a number can be easily obtained from a calculator or computer spreadsheet program.

1. Find the logarithm of 273.

   $$\log 273 = 2.4362$$
   $$\ln 273 = 5.6095$$

2. Find the logarithm of 0.08206.

   $$\log 0.08206 = -1.08587$$
   $$\ln 0.08206 = -2.5003$$

The Antilog of a Number

To find the number corresponding to a given log (or antilog), the reverse procedure of that discussed above is employed (ie, the appropriate numerical base is raised to the exponent expressed by the logarithm).

1. Find the number corresponding to the antilog 3.8357.

   $$\log X = 3.8357$$
   $$X = 10^{3.8357} = 6850$$

2. Find the number corresponding to the natural log 0.4351.

   $$\ln X = 0.4351$$
   $$X = e^{0.4351} = 2.71828^{0.4351} = 1.5451$$

3. Using the Henderson-Hasselbalch equation for an acidic substance, find the ratio of ionized to un-ionized drug at a pH of 3.0. The pK_a of the drug is 7.4.

   $$pH = pK_a + \log \frac{[\text{Salt}]}{[\text{Acid}]}$$

   $$\log \frac{[\text{Salt}]}{[\text{Acid}]} = pH - pK_a$$

   $$\log \frac{[\text{Salt}]}{[\text{Acid}]} = 3.0 - 7.4 = -4.4$$

   $$\frac{[\text{Salt}]}{[\text{Acid}]} = 10^{-4.4} = 3.98 \times 10^{-5}$$

Pharmaceutical Problems

The student who knows algebra, has studied the previous sections of this chapter, and recognizes the Roman numerals and Latin abbreviations used on prescription orders (for directions to the pharmacist and patient by the prescriber) should have sufficient knowledge to solve the routine problems encountered in a pharmacy. The various symbols and abbreviations and their meanings must be well understood. Explanation of practical problems, representative of those faced in practice, are presented below. Practice problems follow each section and the answers to these problems are found at the end of this chapter (page 125).

To solve each problem properly, the following procedure is suggested:

1. Analyze the problem carefully so that all data are clearly fixed in the mind; determine what is given and what is asked.
2. Select the most direct method of solving the problem. Not all problems can be solved properly in one step. Look up doses, equivalents, and abbreviations when you are not sure.
3. Prove or check the result.

Many problems encountered in pharmacy still utilize the apothecary and avoirdupois systems; however, solving these problems in contemporary practice is based on converting these systems into metric units prior to solving the problem mathematically. This approach will be followed in this text. Methods for the mathematical manipulation of apothecary and avoirdupois units and direct problem solving in these systems can be found in previous editions of *Remington*.

ADDITION

Review weighing and measuring systems discussed earlier in this chapter.

Rules

1. Add like quantities. Using the metric system, if the quantities are not alike, change them to a common unit.
2. When adding decimals, keep the decimal points directly under each other.
3. When adding fractions, reduce to the lowest common denominator (LCD), add the resulting numerators, and reduce the fraction, if possible, by canceling.

Examples

1. Add 3 kg, 33 g, and 433 mg.
   Convert to a common unit. The gram is convenient because it is the unit of weight.

$$3 \text{ Kg} \times \frac{1000 \text{ g}}{\text{Kg}} = 3000 \text{ g}$$

$$33 \text{ g} = 33 \text{ g}$$

$$433 \text{ mg} \times \frac{1 \text{ g}}{1000 \text{ mg}} = 0.433 \text{ g}$$

Answer = 3033.433 g

Problems

1. Add 25 mg, 25 g, 210 mg, 2 kg, 1.75 g, 215 mg, 454 g, and 30 mg.
2. The following quantities of a drug were removed from a container: 31 g, 225 g, 855.6 g, and 45.4 g. What is the total weight removed from the container?

SUBTRACTION

Rules

1. Subtract only like quantities. If the quantities are not alike, change to a common unit.
2. Treat common and decimal fractions as indicated in the section on addition.

Examples

1. Subtract 285 mL from 1 L. Convert to a common unit.

$$\begin{array}{r} 1000 \text{ mL} \\ -\ 285 \text{ mL} \\ \hline 715 \text{ mL} \end{array}$$

Answer: 715 mL

Problems

1. How much is left in a 5 L container after the removal of 895 mL?
2. A pharmacist buys 5 g of a potent drug and at different times dispenses 0.2 g, 0.85 g, 90 mg, and 150 mg on prescription orders. How much of the drug remains?

MULTIPLICATION

Rules

1. The product has the same denomination as the multiplicand.
2. If the multiplicand is composed of different denominations in the metric system, form a common unit before multiplying and reduce the product to measurable units.
3. Multiply fractions and decimals as in any arithmetic problem, and reduce fractional quantities to measurable or weighable units.

Examples

1. What will be the total weight of the ingredients in a prescription order for 25 units, each unit containing 0.4 g of Solid F, 0.01 g of

Solid G, and 5 mg of Solid H? First, convert to a common unit such as grams.

0.4 g + 0.01 g + 0.005 g = 0.415 g total weight of one unit

0.415 g/unit × 25 units = 10.375 g total weight of all units

2. Multiply 22.4 mL by 2.65.

$$\begin{array}{r} 22.4 \text{ mL} \\ \times\ 2.65 \\ \hline 59.36 \text{ mL} \end{array}$$

Problems

1. Multiply 48.5 mL by 3.24.
2. A certain preparation is to contain 0.0325 g of a chemical in each mL of solution. How much must be weighed out to make 5 L of the solution?
3. How much cod liver oil is necessary to make 2500 capsules, each containing 0.33 mL?
4. How many mg are used to make 1500 units, each of which contains 250 µg of a drug?

DIVISION

Rules

1. The quotient always has the same denomination as the dividend.
2. If the dividend is composed of different denominations, form a common unit in the metric system before dividing and reduce the quotient to weighable or measurable quantities.
3. Treat fractions, and decimals as explained in the multiplication section.

Examples

1. Divide 3 L by 25.

$$\frac{3 \text{L}}{25} = 0.120 \text{ L or } 120 \text{ mL}$$

Problems

1. How many 65 mg capsules can be made from 50 g of a drug?
3. The dose of a drug is 0.1 mg. How many doses are contained in 15 mg of the drug?
5. How many 325 mg capsules of a drug can be filled from a 454 g amount?

CONVERSION

As long as the student knows the interrelationships of the various units within the different weighing and measuring systems (eg, 20 gr = 1 Э, 3 Э = 1 ʒ; 1000 mg = 1 g), there are only three conversions necessary to memorize in order to convert between the apoth, avoir, and metric systems. These are

$$1 \text{ gr (avoir)} = 1 \text{ gr (apoth)}$$

$$1 \text{ gr} = 64.8 \text{ mg}$$

$$1 \text{ f ʒ} = 29.6 \text{ mL}$$

Learn them!

With these three conversions the student is able to derive all other necessary conversions.

Apothecary Conversions

Various equalities within the apothecary system may be calculated.

1. The number of grains in a dram, grains in a pound, and so on may be calculated using the following steps.

$$\frac{20 \text{ gr}}{Э} \times \frac{3 Э}{ʒ} = \frac{60 \text{ gr}}{ʒ}$$

$$\frac{60 \text{ gr}}{ʒ} \times \frac{8 ʒ}{ℨ} \times \frac{12 ℨ}{\text{lb}} = \frac{5760 \text{ gr}}{\text{lb}}$$

Cancel the units. If they do not cancel properly, something has been omitted.

2. Convert 1 ℥ (apoth) to weighable quantities in the avoir system

$$1 \text{ gr (apoth)} = 1 \text{ gr (avoir)}$$

Since 1 gr (apoth) = 1 gr (avoir), the number of grains in one system equals the number of grains in the other system; e.g., 480 gr (apoth) = 480 gr (avoir).

$$\frac{20 \text{ gr}}{\Theta} \times \frac{3 \, \Theta}{\Im} \times \frac{8 \, \Im}{\Im} = \frac{480 \text{ gr}}{\Im} \text{ (apoth)}$$

$$480 \text{ gr (apoth)} = 480 \text{ gr (avoir)}$$

$$437.5 \text{ gr} = 1 \text{ oz avoir}$$

$$\begin{array}{r} 480 \ \ \text{gr} \\ - \ 437.5 \ \text{gr} \\ \hline 42.5 \ \text{gr} \end{array}$$

Answer: 1 ℥ (apoth) = 1 oz, 42.5 gr (avoir).

3. Conversions in the metric system are made in the same manner. Convert 1 g to mg.

$$1 \text{ g} \times \frac{1000 \text{ mg}}{\text{g}} = 1000 \text{ mg}$$

Convert 1 g to kg.

$$1 \text{ g} \times \frac{1 \text{ kg}}{1000 \text{ g}} = 0.001 \text{ kg}$$

The same procedure is valid for volume measurements in the metric system.

4. Conversions between the apothecary and metric weight systems can be based on the conversion factor; 15.4 gr = 1 g, which may be restated as 15.4 gr/g or 1 g/15.4 gr.

a. How many mg equal 1 gr?

$$\frac{1 \text{ g}}{15.4 \text{ gr}} = 0.0648 \text{ g / gr} = 64.8 \text{ mg / gr or } 64.8 \text{ mg} = 1 \text{ gr}$$

b. How many grams are in 1 ℥?

$$\frac{1 \text{ g}}{15.4 \text{ gr}} \times \frac{480 \text{ gr}}{\Im} = \frac{311 \text{ g}}{\Im}$$

c. How many grams are in 1 oz (avoir)? *Remember*: 1 gr (apoth) = 1 gr (avoir).

$$\frac{1.000 \text{ g}}{15.4 \text{ gr}} \times \frac{437.5 \text{ gr}}{\text{oz}} = \frac{28.4 \text{ gr}}{\text{oz}}$$

d. Other weight conversions are then found in a similar manner.

5. Conversions between the apothecary and metric measuring systems can be based on the conversion factor; 1 f℥ = 29.6 mL, which may be restated as 1 f℥/29.6 mL or 29.6 mL/f℥.
a. How many ♏ are in 1 mL?

$$\frac{480 \, ♏}{\text{f}\Im} \times \frac{1 \text{ f}\Im}{29.6 \text{ mL}} = \frac{16.2 \, ♏}{\text{mL}}$$

Rules

1. The USP states that for prescription compounding one uses practical equivalents, defined as exact equivalents rounded to three (3) significant figures.
2. To calculate quantities required in pharmaceutical formulas, the USP directs the use of practical equivalents.
3. In converting doses the USP uses approximate equivalents. Use USP tables wherever possible.

Examples

1. Convert 1 pt, 4 f℥ into mL.
First, convert into f℥.

$$\frac{16 \text{ f}\Im}{\text{pint}} \times 1 \text{ pint} + 4 \text{ f}\Im = 20 \text{ f}\Im$$

Second, convert f℥ to mL.

$$20 \text{ f}\Im \times \frac{29.6 \text{ mL}}{\text{f}\Im} = 592 \text{ mL}$$

Answer: 1 pt, 4 f℥ = 592 mL.

2. What is the weight of 1200 g in the apothecary system?

$$1200 \text{ g} \times \frac{15.4 \text{ gr}}{\text{g}} = 18,480 \text{ gr}$$

Or:

$$1200 \text{ g} \times \frac{1 \text{ lb}}{373 \text{ g}} = 3.22 \text{ lb}$$

3. Convert 1 pound (apoth) into grams.

$$\frac{1 \text{ g}}{15.4 \text{ gr}} \times \frac{480 \text{ gr}}{\Im} \times \frac{12 \, \Im}{\text{lb}} \times 1 \, \cancel{\text{lb}} = 374 \text{ g}$$

4. Convert 25 gr to grams.

$$25 \text{ gr} \times \frac{1 \text{ g}}{15.4 \text{ gr}} = 1.62 \text{ g}$$

5. Convert 50 grams to grains.

$$50 \text{ g} \times \frac{15.4 \text{ gr}}{\text{g}} = 770 \text{ gr}$$

Problems

1. Convert:
   a. 6.50 grains into milligrams.
   b. 3/10 grain into milligrams.
   c. 3 ½ apoth ounces into grams.
   d. 2 ℥ into mg.
   e. 3 ½ avoir ounces into grams.
   f. 1 lb avoir into grams.
2. Convert:
   a. 550 g into weighable quantities in the avoir system.
   b. 450 mg into grains.
   c. 550 g into weighable quantities in the apoth system.
   d. 100 μg into grains.
   e. 1 kg into lb (avoir).
3. Convert the following doses into metric weights:
   a. 1/100 gr.
   b. 1/320 gr.
   c. 1/6 gr.
   d. 5 gr.
   e. 20 gr.
4. Convert:
   a. 200 m into mL.
   b. 3 f℥ into mL.
   c. 8 f℥ into mL.
   d. 1 pt into mL.
   e. 5 ♏ into mL.
   f. 0.1 mg into gr.
   g. 5 mg into gr.
5. Answer the following questions.
   a. How many gr are in 1 ℥?
   b. How many drams are in 1 ℥?
   c. How many grains are in 1 oz (avoir)?
   d. How many gr are in 1/2 lb (apoth)?
   e. Convert 250 gr to weighable quantities in the apothecary system.

HOUSEHOLD EQUIVALENTS

Common household equivalents are found on page 104. These are used to interpret the prescriber's instructions to the patient. The teaspoonful usually is indicated by the symbol f℥ or 5 mL, although 1 f℥ does not equal 5 mL. The problem of "the teaspoonful" has been discussed by Morrell and Ordway[4] and by Madlon-Kay and Mosch[5]. For practical purposes, a teaspoonful is equal to 5 mL, and 1 f℥ in the directions to the patient on the prescription means 1 teaspoonful.

For purposes of solving most compounding and dispensing problems, the exact equivalents rounded to three significant places should be used.

DOSAGE CALCULATIONS

Over the past years various rules for calculating infants' and children's dosages have been devised. All of them give only approximate dosages because they erroneously assume that the child is a small adult; some of them are still used because as yet no absolute method of calculating an infant or child's dose has been found. Children are sometimes more susceptible than adults to certain drugs. Doses for infants and children, where they are known, may be found in the USP Drug Information, the *Pediatric Dosage Handbook* published by APhA, and textbooks on pediatrics.[6–8] Doses should not be calculated when it is possible to obtain the actual infant or child's dose.

Rules for Approximate Doses for Infants and Children

1. *Young's Rule* (for children 2 years old and older)

$$\frac{\text{Age (years)}}{\text{Age (years)} + 12} \times \text{Adult dose} = \text{Child's dose (approx)}$$

2. *Clark's Rule*

$$\frac{\text{Weight (lb)}}{150} \times \text{Adult dose} = \text{Child's dose (approx)}$$

3. *Fried's Rule* (for infants up to 2 years old)

$$\frac{\text{Age (months)}}{150} \times \text{Adult dose} = \text{Child's dose (approx)}$$

4. *The Square Meter Surface Area Method* relates the surface area of individuals to dose. It is thought that this is a more realistic way of relating dosages.

$$\frac{\text{Body surface area of child}}{\text{Body surface area of adult}} \times \text{Adult dose} = \frac{\text{Child's dose}}{\text{(approx)}}$$

The average body surface area for an adult has been given as 1.73 square meters (m²); hence,

$$\frac{\text{Body surface area of child (m}^2)}{1.73 \text{ m}^2} \times \text{Adult dose} = \frac{\text{Child's dose}}{\text{(approx)}}$$

Calculating Doses for Individuals—of any age or size

Many drugs have doses stated as the amount of *drug/m² body surface area* and may be calculated as follows:

$$\frac{\text{Dose of drug}}{\text{m}^2 \text{ body surface area}} \times \text{Body surface area (m}^2) = \text{Dose}$$

Many physiological functions are proportional to body surface area, such as metabolic rate and kidney function.

Drug doses are often stated in *mg/kg body weight* and may be calculated as follows:

$$\frac{\text{Dose of drug}}{\text{kg body weight}} \times \text{Body weight (kg)} = \text{Dose}$$

This is the most common way of determining children's doses.

Drug doses also may be stated in *units,* as with vitamins A and D, penicillin, and hormones. This means that a certain quantity of biological activity of that drug is called 1 unit. When the term unit is used in connection with a drug, the calculations involved are the same as those for more familiar weight or volume notations. The USP often standardizes the unit for such drugs, so the expression "USP Units" is used. This means the units are calculated based on a USP assay procedure and reference standard.

Examples

1. The adult dose of a drug is 325 mg. What is the dose for a 3-year-old child?
   Use Young's Rule:

$$\text{Child's dose (approx)} \frac{3}{3 + 12} \times 325 \text{ mg} = 65 \text{ mg}$$

2. What is the dose for a 40 lb child if the average adult dose of the medicament is 10 mg?
   Use Clark's Rule:

$$\text{Child's dose (approx)} = \frac{40}{150} \times 10 \text{ mg} = 2.67 \text{ mg}$$

3. What is the dose for an 8-month-old infant if the average adult dose of a drug is 250 mg?
   Use Fried's Rule:

$$\text{Infant's dose (approx)} = \frac{8}{150} \times 250 \text{ mg} = 13.3 \text{ mg}$$

4. If the average adult dose of a drug is 50 mg, what is the dose for a child who has a body surface area equal to 0.57 m²?

$$\text{Child's dose (approx)} = \frac{0.57}{1.73} \times 50 \text{ mg} = 16.5 \text{ mg}$$

Problems

1. What is the dose of a drug for a 9-month-old infant if the average adult dose is 25 mg?
2. What is the dose of a drug for a 6-year-old child if the average adult dose is 98 mg?
3. What is the dose of a drug for a child who weighs 28 lb if the average adult dose is 100 mg?
4. What is the dose of a drug for an individual who has a 1.21 m² body surface area? The average adult dose is 400,000 units.
5. What is the dose of a medicament for a child that weighs 66 lb if the dose is stated as 2.5 mg/kg body weight?
6. What is the dose of a drug for an average adult patient if the dose of the drug is 45 mg/m²?

PROBLEM-SOLVING METHODOLOGY

The problem-solving method illustrated in solving pharmaceutical problems is *dimensional analysis* (which is based on *ratio and proportion*). Dimensional analysis is widely used in many scientific disciplines and offers a consistent way to solve problems. Dimensional analysis also overcomes many difficulties students and pharmacy practitioners have in problem interpretation and provides a well-defined, consistent starting point in the solution of pharmaceutical problems.

DIMENSIONAL ANALYSIS

The basis for dimensional analysis is the formation of relationships between quantities, multiplication and canceling units until only the units of the desired answer remain.

As an example, if 100 g of a drug cost $1.80, how much will 25 g cost?

Begin by collecting all of the information in the problem and identify all relationships with units and labels. In this problem, we know the following:

$$\frac{\$1.80}{100 \text{ g drug}}, 25 \text{ g drug}$$

Identify the units you want for the answer.

$$= \$$$

Identify a relationship from the problem that contains the unit(s) desired for the answer, forming the skeleton of the process.

$$\frac{\$1.80}{100 \text{ g drug}} \times ? = \$$$

Complete the process by using terms from the problem (or equivalents) necessary to cancel out units until only the unit(s) of the answer remain on the left side.

$$\frac{\$1.80}{100 \text{ g drug}} \times 25 \text{ g drug} = \$$$

Solve mathematically.

$$\text{Answer} = \$0.45$$

Dimensional analysis can be used to solve most pharmaceutical problems, regardless of complexity, using a consistent procedure:

1. Collect all the information and relationships in the problem complete with units and labels.
2. Identify the unit(s) and label of the answer.
3. Select a starting point corresponding to the unit(s) and label of the answer in the numerator.
4. Complete the process using relationships in the problem and known conversions to cancel units.
5. Solve the problem mathematically.

More complex problems use the same basic procedure; eg, if 100 g of a drug cost $1.80, what would be the cost of the drug to prepare 4 f℥ of a solution containing 5 g of the drug per teaspoonful?

Step 1: Collect all information and relationships:

$$\frac{\$1.80}{100 \text{ g drug}}, \frac{5 \text{ g drug}}{1 \text{ tsp}}, 4 \text{ f℥}$$

Step 2:

$$= \$$$

Step 3:

$$\frac{\$1.80}{100 \text{ g drug}} \times ? = \$$$

Step 4:

$$\frac{\$1.80}{100 \text{ g drug}} \times \frac{5 \text{ g drug}}{1 \text{ tsp}} \times \frac{1 \text{ tsp}}{5 \text{ mL}} \times \frac{29.6 \text{ mL}}{1 \text{ f℥}} \times 4 \text{ f℥} = \$$$

(The 3rd and 4th terms are known definitions and equivalents needed to cancel units.)

Step 5:

$$\text{Answer} = \$0.53$$

With practice, steps 2 through 4 can be written in one operation.

Examples

1. Determine the amount of each ingredient contained in one dose of the following prescription.
℞	Solid A	300 mg
	Solid B	150 mg
	Solid C	200 mg

   M ft capsules, D.T.D. No 12.

   The directions to the pharmacist are to mix and make 12 capsules each containing in the three solids in the amounts indicated. Thus, the dose of each ingredient is as stated in the prescription.
2. How much of each ingredient is contained in one dose of the following prescription?
℞	Solid E	7.2 g
	Solid F	0.24 g
	Solid G	1.2 g

   M div capsules, No 24.

In this prescription the prescriber requests that 24 capsules be made from the three ingredients. The amounts of the ingredients requested are considerable, and drugs usually do not have doses of 7.2 g or 1.2 g, so division of the amounts by the number of doses (24) is required. The pharmacist should check a textbook or compendium to confirm the average adult dose.

$$\text{Drug E: } \frac{7.2 \text{ g}}{24 \text{ capsules}} \times 1 \text{ capsule} = 0.300 \text{ g}$$

$$\text{Drug F: } \frac{0.24 \text{ g}}{24 \text{ capsules}} \times 1 \text{ capsule} = 0.010 \text{ g}$$

$$\text{Drug G: } \frac{1.2 \text{ g}}{24 \text{ capsules}} \times 1 \text{ capsule} = 0.050 \text{ g}$$

3. A prescription calls for 10 units of a drug to be taken 3 times a day. How much will the patient have taken after 7 days?

$$\frac{10 \text{ units}}{\text{dose}} \times \frac{3 \text{ doses}}{\text{day}} \times 7 \text{ days} = 210 \text{ units}$$

4. If 250 units of an antibiotic weigh 1 mg, how many units are in the 15 mg?

$$\frac{250 \text{ units}}{\text{mg}} \times 15 \text{ mg} = 3750 \text{ units}$$

5. If the dose of a drug is 0.5 mg/kg of body weight/24 hours, how many grams will a 33-lb infant receive per 24 hours and per week?

$$\frac{1 \text{ g}}{1000 \text{ mg}} \times \frac{0.5 \text{ mg}}{\text{kg} \times 24 \text{ hours}} \times \frac{1 \text{ kg}}{2.2 \text{ lb}}$$

$$\times 33 \text{ lb} \times 24 \text{ hours} = 0.00750 \text{ g}$$

$$\frac{0.00750 \text{ g}}{\text{day}} \times \frac{7 \text{ days}}{\text{week}} \times 1 \text{ week} = 0.0525 \text{ g}$$

6. A patient is to receive 260 μg of a drug 4 times a day for 14 days. How many 1/250-gr tablets must be dispensed?

$$\frac{1 \text{ tablet}}{\frac{1}{250} \text{ gr}} \times \frac{1 \text{ gr}}{64.8 \text{ mg}} \times \frac{1 \text{ mg}}{1000 \text{ μg}} \times \frac{260 \text{ μg}}{\text{dose}} \times \frac{4 \text{ doses}}{\text{day}}$$

$$\times 14 \text{ days} = 56.2 \text{ tablets} = 57 \text{ tablets}$$

7. An antibiotic is available as an injection containing 10 mg antibiotic/mL. How many mL are needed for an infant weighing 8 kg, the dose being 1.4 mg/kg of body weight?

$$\frac{1 \text{ mL}}{10 \text{ mg}} \times \frac{1.4 \text{ mg}}{\text{kg}} \times 8 \text{ kg} = 1.12 \text{ mL}$$

8. A preparation for coughs contains 1.5 g of an expectorant per 100 mL. How many gr of the expectorant are there in a teaspoonful?

$$1 \text{ tsp} = 5 \text{ mL}$$

$$\frac{15.4 \text{ gr}}{1 \text{ g}} \times \frac{1.5 \text{ g}}{100 \text{ mL}} \times \frac{5 \text{ mL}}{1 \text{ tsp}} \times 1 \text{ tsp} = 1.16 \text{ gr}$$

Problems

1. Calculate the dose for each ingredient in the following prescription.
℞	Chemical J	10 mg
	Chemical K	50 mg
	Chemical L	300 mg

   M ft capsules, D.T.D. No 14.
2. Calculate the dose of each ingredient in the following prescription.
℞	Drug Q	10.5 g
	Drug R	6.3 g

   M div 21 doses.

3. An 8 f℥ prescription contains 6 f℈ of a tincture. If 1 teaspoonful 4 times a day is prescribed, how much tincture does the patient take per dose and how much is taken daily?
4. How many 0.3-mL doses are contained in 15 mL of a solution?
5. If 1 mg of a hormone equals 22.5 units, how many mg are required to obtain 1 unit?
6. If a bottle contains 80 units of a drug/mL, how many mL must the patient take to get a 60-unit dose? If the bottle contains 10 mL total volume of the drug solution, how many days' supply will patients have if they use 60 units a day?
7. A 10-mL ampule contains a 2.5% solution of a drug. How many mL are needed to give a dose of 150 mg?
8. The dose of an antibiotic is 75 mg for a child. How much of a flavored suspension containing 125 mg antibiotic/5 mL must be given to the child per dose?
9. How many mg of a drug are there in each teaspoonful of a syrup that contains 0.5% of the drug?

REDUCING AND ENLARGING FORMULAS

Determine the total weight or volume of ingredients and convert, if necessary, to the system of the quantities desired. The quantities in the original and new formulas will have the same ratio.

Examples

1. The formula for a syrup is

Drug M	140 g
Sucrose	450 g
Purified Water qs	1000 mL

a. Find the quantities required for 100 mL.

$$\text{Drug M: } \frac{140 \text{ g}}{1000 \text{ mL}} \times 100 \text{ mL} = 14.0 \text{ g}$$

$$\text{Sucrose: } \frac{450 \text{ g}}{1000 \text{ mL}} \times 100 \text{ mL} = 45.0 \text{ g}$$

Purified Water: to make 100 mL

b. What quantities are required to compound 60 mL of the syrup?

$$\text{Drug M: } \frac{140 \text{ g}}{1000 \text{ mL}} \times 60 \text{ mL} = 8.40 \text{ g}$$

$$\text{Sucrose: } \frac{450 \text{ g}}{1000 \text{ mL}} \times 60 \text{ mL} = 27.0 \text{ g}$$

Purified Water: to make 60 mL

2. Calculate the amounts needed for 100 g of antiseptic powder as follows:

℞		
	Solid A	2 g
	Solid B	1 g
	Solid C	7 g
	Solid D	25 g
	Solid E	115 g
		150 g

$$\text{Factor} = \frac{100 \text{ g}}{150 \text{ g}} = 0.667$$

Solid A: 2 g × 0.667 = 1.33 g

Solid B: 1 g × 0.667 = 0.667 g

Solid C: 7 g × 0.667 = 4.67 g

Solid D: 25 g × 0.667 = 16.7 g

Solid E: 115 g × 0.667 = 76.7 g

3. Prescriptions, where the instruction to the pharmacist calls for making a certain number of doses of an ingredient or mixture of several ingredients, are a type of formula enlargement. The expression usually used is DTD, which means let such doses be given. Occasionally the prescriber will not use this expression, but inspection of amounts of the ingredients indicates that this is what is desired. For example,

℞		
	Solid H	50 mg
	Solid K	150 mg
	Liquid N	0.2 mL
	M ft capsules, D.T.D. No 24.	

The pharmacist checked the individual doses of the ingredients and found them to be slightly below the average adult dose, confirming that the prescriber wanted the quantities listed to be multiplied by 24.

$$\text{Solid H: } \frac{50 \text{ mg}}{\text{capsule}} \times 24 \text{ capsules} = 1200 \text{ mg or } 1.2 \text{ g}$$

$$\text{Solid K: } \frac{150 \text{ mg}}{\text{capsule}} \times 24 \text{ capsules} = 3600 \text{ mg or } 3.6 \text{ g}$$

$$\text{Liquid N: } \frac{0.2 \text{ mL}}{\text{capsule}} \times 24 \text{ capsules} = 4.8 \text{ mL}$$

Problems

1. The formula for a liquid preparation is

Liquid C	35 mL
Solid B	9 g
Liquid R	2.5 mL
Liquid P	20 mL
Purified Water, sufficient to make	100 mL

Calculate the quantities of the ingredients to make 2.5 L.
2. The formula for an ointment is

℞		
	Solid G	1
	Liquid D	30
	Solid M	3
	Ointment base, sufficient to make	100

Calculate quantities of the ingredients for 2 lb (apoth).
3. How much of each of the three solids and how much purified water are needed to properly compound the following prescription order?

℞		
	Solid N	0.1 mg
	Solid Q	2.5 mg
	Solid R	150.0 mg
	Purified Water, qs	5 mL
	M ft solution, D.T.D. No 48.	

4. How much of each ingredient is required to compound 90 mL of the following product?

Solid S	7.5 g
Solid T	25 g
Oil C	350 mL
Alcohol	250 mL
Purified Water, qs	1000 mL

PERCENTAGE

Percent, written as %, means per hundred. Fifteen percent is written 15% and means 15/100, 0.15, or 15 parts in a total of 100 parts. Percent is a type of ratio and has units of parts per 100 parts. Thus, 10% of 1500 tablets is 10/100 × 1500 tablets = 150 tablets.

To change percent to a fraction, the percent number becomes the numerator and 100 is the denominator. To change a fraction to percent, put the fraction in a form having 100 as its denominator; multiply by 100 so that the numerator becomes the percent.

$$\frac{1}{2} = \frac{50}{100}; \frac{50}{100} \times 100 = 50\%$$

$$\frac{1}{8} = \frac{12.5}{100}; \frac{12.5}{100} \times 100 = 12.5\%$$

Calculations involving percentages are encountered continually by pharmacists. They must be familiar not only with the arithmetical principles, but also with certain compendial interpretations of the different type percentages involving solutions and mixtures.

The USP states

Percentage concentrations of solutions are expressed as follows:

Percent weight in weight—(w/w) expresses the number of g of a constituent in 100 g of product.

Percent weight in volume—(w/v) expresses the number of g of a constituent in 100 mL of product, and is used regardless of whether water or another liquid is the solvent.

Percent volume in volume—(v/v) expresses the number of mL of a constituent in 100 mL of product.

The term *percent* used without qualification means, for mixtures of solids, percent weight in weight; for solutions or suspensions of solids in liquids, percent weight in volume; for solutions of liquids in liquids, percent volume in volume; and for solutions of gases in liquids, percent weight in volume. For example, a one percent solution is prepared by dissolving one g of a solid or one mL of a liquid in sufficient of the solvent to make 100 mL of the solution.

Ratio Strength

Ratio strength is another manner of expressing concentration. Such phrases as "1 in 10" are understood to mean that one part of a substance is to be diluted with a diluent to make 10 parts of the finished product. For example, a 1:10 solution means 1 mL of a liquid or one g of a solid dissolved in sufficient solvent to make 10 mL of solution. Ratio strength can be converted to percent by:

$$\frac{1 \text{ g substance}}{10 \text{ mL solution}} \times 100 \text{ mL solution} = 10 \text{ g substance}$$

$$\frac{10 \text{ g substance}}{100 \text{ mL solution}} = 10\%$$

The expression "parts per thousand" (eg, 1:5000) always means parts weight in volume when dealing with solutions of solids in liquids and is similar to the above expression. A 1:5000 solution means 1 g of solute in sufficient solvent to make 5000 mL of solution. This can be converted to percent by

$$\frac{1 \text{ g substance}}{5000 \text{ mL solution}} \times 100 \text{ mL solution} = 0.02 \text{ g substance}$$

$$\frac{0.02 \text{ g substance}}{100 \text{ mL solution}} = 0.02\%$$

The expression "trituration" has two different meanings in pharmacy. One refers to the process of particle-size reduction, commonly by grinding or rubbing in a mortar with the aid of a pestle. The other meaning refers to a dilution of a potent powdered drug with a suitable powdered diluent in a definite proportion by weight. It is the second meaning that is used in this chapter.

When pharmacists refer to a "1 in 10 trituration" they mean a mixture of solids composed of 1 g of drug plus sufficient diluent (another solid) to make 10 g of mixture or *dilution*. In this case the "1 in 10 trituration" is actually a solid dilution of a drug with an inert solid. The strength of a trituration may also be stated as percent *w/w*. Thus, the term trituration has come to mean a solid dilution of a potent drug with a chemically and physiologically inert solid.

The meanings implied by the USP statements in the section on percentage are illustrated below with a few examples of the three types of percentages.

Weight-in-Volume Percentages

This is the type of percent problem most often encountered on prescriptions. The volume occupied by the solute and the volume of the solvent are *not* known because sufficient solvent is added to make a given or known final volume.

EXAMPLES

1. Prepare 1 f℥ of a 10% solution.
   Since this is a solution of a solid in a liquid, this is a *w/v* solution.

$$\frac{10 \text{ g drug}}{100 \text{ mL soln}} \times \frac{29.6 \text{ mL}}{1 \text{ f℥}} \times 1 \text{ f℥} = 2.96 \text{ g drug}$$

   2.96 g is dissolved in sufficient purified water to make 29.6 mL of solution.

2. How much of a drug is required to compound 4 f℥ of a 3% solution in alcohol?

$$\frac{3 \text{ g drug}}{100 \text{ mL soln}} \times \frac{29.6 \text{ mL}}{1 \text{ f℥}} \times 4 \text{ f℥} = 3.55 \text{ g drug}$$

3. How much 0.9% solution of sodium chloride can be made from ½ ℥ of NaCl?

$$\frac{100 \text{ mL soln}}{0.9 \text{ g NaCl}} \times \frac{31.1 \text{ g}}{1 \text{ ℥}} \times 0.5 \text{ ℥} = 1730 \text{ mL soln}$$

4. How many grams of a drug are required to make 120 mL of a 25% solution?

$$\frac{25 \text{ g drug}}{100 \text{ mL soln}} \times 120 \text{ mL} = 30 \text{ g drug}$$

5. How would you prepare 480 mL of a 1 in 750 solution of an antiseptic?
   Remember: percent *w/v* is indicated.
   1 in 750 means 1 g of the antiseptic dissolved in sufficient solvent to make 750 mL solution.

$$\frac{1 \text{ g drug}}{750 \text{ mL soln}} \times 480 \text{ mL} = 0.64 \text{ g drug}$$

   Dissolve 0.64 g of antiseptic in sufficient solvent to make 480 mL solution.

6. How much of a substance is needed to prepare 1 L of a 1:10,000 solution?
   The ratio 1:10,000 means 1 g of a substance in 10,000 mL of solution.

$$\frac{1 \text{ g substance}}{10,000 \text{ mL soln}} \times \frac{1000 \text{ mL}}{1 \text{ L}} \times 1 \text{ L} = 0.1 \text{ g substance}$$

7. How would you prepare 120 mL of 0.25% solution of neomycin sulfate? The source of neomycin sulfate is a solution which contains 1 g neomycin sulfate/10 mL.

$$\frac{10 \text{ mL stock soln}}{1 \text{ g drug}} \times \frac{0.25 \text{ g drug}}{100 \text{ mL soln}} \times 120 \text{ mL soln} =$$

$$= 3 \text{ mL stock soln}$$

   Add sufficient purified water to 3 mL of stock solution to make 120 mL.

Problems

1. How would you make 3 f℥ of a 12.5% solution?
2. How many liters of a 4% solution can be made from 4℥ of a solid?
3. How many liters of an 8% solution can be made from 500 g of a solid?
4. How many grams of a drug are needed to make 4 L of a 1 in 500 solution?

Weight-in-Weight Percentages

Density must be considered in some of these problems. If a weight-in-weight solution is requested on a prescription, both the solute and solvent must be weighed, or the solute and the solvent may be measured if their densities are taken into consideration in determining the volumes. Since the solutions are made to a given weight, a given volume is not always obtainable.

EXAMPLES

1. What weights of solute and solvent are required to make 2 ʒ of a 3% w/w solution of a drug in 90% alcohol?

$$\frac{3 \text{ g solute}}{100 \text{ g soln}} \times \frac{31.1 \text{ g soln}}{1\,ʒ \text{ soln}} \times 2\,ʒ \text{ soln} = 1.87 \text{ g solute}$$

$$\frac{31.1 \text{ g soln}}{1\,ʒ \text{ soln}} \times 2\,ʒ \text{ soln} = 62.2 \text{ g soln}$$

$$62.2 \text{ g soln} - 1.87 \text{ g solute} = 60.3 \text{ g solvent}$$

2. The solubility of boric acid is 1 g in 18 mL of water at 25°C. What is the percentage strength, w/w, of a saturated solution?
1 g of boric acid + 18 mL of water make a saturated solution, 18 mL of water weighs 18 g; hence, the weight of solution is 19 g. The amount of boric acid present is 1 g in 19 g of solution; therefore, the following relationship can be set up:

$$\frac{1 \text{ g drug}}{19 \text{ g soln}} \times 100 \text{ g soln} = 5.26 \text{ g drug}$$

$$\frac{5.26 \text{ g drug}}{100 \text{ g soln}} = 5.26\%$$

3. How many grams of a chemical are needed to prepare 200 g of a 10% w/w solution?
10% w/w means 10 g of solute in 100 g total solution. The following relationship may be set up:

$$\frac{10 \text{ g solute}}{100 \text{ g soln}} \times 200 \text{ g soln} = 20 \text{ g solute}$$

4. How would one make a 2% w/w solution of a drug in 240 mL of alcohol? The density of alcohol is 0.816 g/mL.
   a. First, convert 240 mL to weight. Remember: alcohol is the solvent and it has a density different from that of water.

$$\frac{0.816 \text{ g alcohol}}{1 \text{ mL alcohol}} \times 240 \text{ mL alcohol} = 195.8 \text{ g } (196 \text{ g}) \text{ alcohol}$$

   b. 2% w/w means 2 g solute in 100 g solution. In this problem the final weight of solution is not known; 240 mL (196 g) of alcohol represents the solvent only. The solvent is 98% w/w of the total solution, so the following relationship may be set up:

$$\frac{2 \text{ g solute}}{98 \text{ g alcohol}} \times 196 \text{ g alcohol} = 4.00 \text{ g solute}$$

   c. Dissolve 4.00 g of the drug in 240 mL alcohol. The resulting solution will be 2% w/w and have a volume slightly larger than 240 mL because of the volume displacement of the drug.

5. How much of a 5% w/w solution can be made from 28.4 g of a chemical?

$$\frac{100 \text{ g soln}}{5 \text{ g chemical}} \times 28.4 \text{ g chemical} = 568 \text{ g soln}$$

6. How many mL of a 70% w/w solution having a density of 1.2 g/mL will be needed to prepare 600 mL of a 10% w/v solution?
   a. Drug needed

$$\frac{10 \text{ g drug}}{100 \text{ mL soln (10\%)}} \times 600 \text{ mL soln (10\%)} = 60 \text{ g drug}$$

   b. Weight of 70% solution needed

$$\frac{100 \text{ g soln (70\%)}}{70 \text{ g drug}} \times 60 \text{ g drug} = 85.7 \text{ g soln (70\%)}$$

   c. Volume of 70% solution needed.

$$\frac{1 \text{ mL soln (70\%)}}{1.2 \text{ g soln (70\%)}} \times 85.7 \text{ g soln (70\%)} = 71.4 \text{ mL soln (70\%)}$$

Compounding problems involving solid preparations (such as mixtures of powder) and semisolid preparations (such as ointments, creams, and suppositories) are also percent w/w. The following is an example of this.

1. How much drug is required to make 2 ʒ of a 10% ointment?

$$\frac{10 \text{ g drug}}{100 \text{ g oint}} \times \frac{31.1 \text{ g oint}}{1\,ʒ \text{ oint}} \times 2\,ʒ \text{ oint} = 6.22 \text{ g drug}$$

The same procedure could be used for such mixtures as powders and suppository masses. Instead of using units in the various measuring systems, quantities can be indicated "by parts." The term "parts" then can mean any unit in any measuring system, as long as the units are kept constant.

2. How many grams of each of the following three ingredients are required to make 30 g of the product?

    ℞   Solid A   0.5 part
          Powder B   3.0 parts
          Powder C, qs 30.0 parts

Since the product is a mixture of powders, percent w/w is indicated. In the above prescription order the total product is 30 parts because Powder C is used to "qs" or "make up to" 30 parts. Therefore, 0.5 g of Powder A and 3.0 g of Powder B are needed.

$$30 \text{ g total} - 0.5 \text{ g powder A} - 3.0 \text{ g powder B}$$
$$= 26.5 \text{ g powder C}$$

3. How much of each of the following ingredients is needed to make 60 g of the ointment?

    ℞   Solid D   3.0 parts
          Solid E   6.0 parts
          Ointment Base Q 30.0 parts
                        39.0 parts total

$$\frac{3.0 \text{ g solid D}}{39.0 \text{ g oint}} \times 60 \text{ g oint} = 4.62 \text{ g solid D}$$

$$\frac{6.0 \text{ g solid E}}{39.0 \text{ g oint}} \times 60 \text{ g oint} = 9.23 \text{ g solid E}$$

$$\frac{30.0 \text{ g base Q}}{39.0 \text{ g oint}} \times 60 \text{ g oint} = 46.2 \text{ g base Q}$$

4. What is the percent strength of a salt solution obtained by diluting 100 g of a 5% solution to 200 g?
Assign the 5% solution as soln 1
Assign the final solution as soln 2

$$\frac{5 \text{ g salt}}{100 \text{ g soln 1}} \times \frac{100 \text{ g soln 1}}{200 \text{ g soln 2}} \times 100 \text{ g soln 2} = 2.5 \text{ salt}$$

$$\frac{2.5 \text{ g salt}}{100 \text{ g soln 2}} = 2.5\% \text{ w/w}$$

Problems

1. How much of the drug and solvent are needed to compound the following prescription?

    ℞   Compound A   6% w/w
          Solvent, qs   4 ʒ

2. How many grams of solute are needed to prepare 240 g of a 12% w/w solution?
3. How many kg of a 20% w/w solution can be made from 1 kg of the solute?
4. How would you prepare, using 120 mL of glycerin (density, 1.25 g/mL), a solution that is 3% w/w with respect to a drug?

5. How much of each substance is needed to prepare a total of 24 g of the following suppository mass?

Compound K	0.3 g
Solid H	0.15 g
Suppository base, qs	2.0 g

6. How would one prepare 500 mL of a 15% *w/w* aqueous solution?
7. How much of each of the ingredients is required to make 1 kg of the following mixture?

Powder P	1 part
Powder Q	8 parts
Powder R	12 parts
Powder S	15 parts
Total	36 parts

8. How much of each ingredient is required to prepare the following ointment?

℞	Coal Tar Solution	10%
	Hydrophilic Ointment, qs	30 g

Volume-in-Volume Percentages

A direct calculation of percentage from the total volume is made. Volumes, unlike weights, may not be additive. However, this does not present a problem because the final solution is made up to the desired volume with the diluent.

Examples

1. How many minims of a liquid are needed to make 6 f℥ of a hand lotion containing 0.5% *v/v* of the liquid?

$$\frac{16.2 \; \text{℩ liq}}{1 \; \text{mL liq}} \times \frac{0.5 \; \text{mL liq}}{100 \; \text{mL lotion}} \times \frac{29.6 \; \text{mL lotion}}{1 \; \text{f℥ lotion}}$$
$$\times \; 6 \; \text{f℥ lotion} = 14.4 \; \text{℩ liq}$$

Add sufficient lotion to 14.4 m of the liquid to make 6 f℥ of the product.

2. How much 90% alcohol is required to compound 500 mL of a 10% alcohol mixture?

$$\frac{100 \; \text{mL (90%)}}{90 \; \text{mL alcohol}} \times \frac{10 \; \text{mL alcohol}}{100 \; \text{mL (10%)}} \times 500 \; \text{ml (10%)}$$
$$= 55.5 \; \text{mL (90%)}$$

Problems

1. How many minims of a liquid are needed to make 4 f℥ of a 12.5% *v/v* solution?
2. What volume of 50% *v/v* alcohol could be prepared from 1 L of 95% *v/v* alcohol?
3. What is the percentage strength, weight in weight, of a liquid made by dissolving 16 g of a salt in 30 mL of water?
4. How much drug will be required to prepare 1 f℥ of a 2.5% solution?
5. What is the percentage, weight in weight, of sugar in a syrup made by dissolving 5 kg of sugar in 8 kg of water?
6. How many grams of a drug are required to prepare 120 mL of a 12.5% aqueous solution?
7. How much drug is needed to compound a liter of a 1:2500 aqueous solution?
8. A solution contains 37% of active ingredient. How much of this solution is needed to prepare 480 mL of an aqueous solution containing 2.5% of the active ingredient?
9. How much of a drug is required to make 2 qt of a 1:1200 solution?

STOCK SOLUTIONS

To facilitate the dispensing of certain soluble substances, the pharmacist frequently prepares or purchases solutions of high concentration. Portions of these concentrated solutions are diluted to give required solutions of lesser strength. These concentrated solutions are known as *stock solutions*. This procedure is satisfactory if the substances are stable in solution or if the solutions are to be used before they decompose.

In the case of potent substances, a properly prepared stock solution permits the pharmacist to obtain accurately a quantity of solid that might otherwise be difficult to weigh. In the case of frequently prescribed salt solutions, a stock solution readily provides the required amount of salt without the necessity of weighing and dissolving it every time.

Stock solutions may be of various concentrations depending on the requirements for use. The stock solutions should be labeled properly and fractional parts needed to make various strengths also may be listed as a further convenience.

There is a type of compounding and dispensing problem that involves the concept of stock solutions. This involves the patient diluting a dose from the prescription order to a given volume to obtain a solution of desired concentration.

For example, how many grams of a salt are required to make 90 mL of a stock solution, 5 mL of which makes a 1:3000 solution when diluted to 500 mL?

Assign the stock solution as Soln 1
Assign the final dilution as Soln 2

$$\frac{1 \; \text{g salt}}{3000 \; \text{mL soln 2}} \times \frac{500 \; \text{mL soln 2}}{5 \; \text{mL soln 1}} \times 90 \; \text{ml soln 1} = 3.0 \; \text{g salt}$$

Problems

1. How much of a drug is needed to compound 120 mL of a prescription order such that when 1 teaspoonful of the solution is diluted to 1 qt, a 1:750 solution results?
2. How many grams of a drug are needed to make 240 mL of a solution of such strength that when 5 mL is diluted to 2 qt, a 1:2500 solution results?
3. An ampule of solution of an anti-inflammatory drug contains 4 mg of drug/mL. What volume of the solution is needed to prepare a liter of solution that contains 2 μg of the drug/mL?

PARTS PER MILLION

An expression that is occasionally used in compounding prescriptions is *parts per million* (ppm). This is another way of expressing concentration, particularly concentrations of very dilute preparations. A 1% solution may be expressed as 1 part/100; a 0.1% solution is 0.1 parts/100 or 1 part/1000. A one ppm solution contains 1 part of solute/1 million parts of solution; 5 ppm is 5 parts solute/1 million parts solution, and so on. Remember that the two parts must have the same units, except in the metric system where one g = one mL of water.

Sodium fluoride is a drug that may be prescribed by a dentist as a preventative for tooth decay in children. It is used only in very dilute solutions due to the drug's toxicity and because only minute quantities are needed. For example, how much sodium fluoride would be needed to prepare the following prescription?

℞	Sod Fluoride, qs
	Purified water, qs 60 mL
	Make soln such that when 1 f℥ is diluted to 1 glassful of water a 2 ppm soln results.
	Sig: 1 f℥ in a glassful of water a day.

The mathematics to solve this compounding problem are easy once the steps for calculating the answer are outlined. This problem should be worked "backward."

a. The amount of NaF needed is not known.
b. One glassful of water has a volume of 240 mL. The concentration of NaF in 240 mL is 2 ppm.
c. The NaF solution poured into the glass came from a teaspoonful dose (1 f℥), which is equal to 5 mL.
d. The 5-mL dose came from the prescription order bottle containing a NaF solution.

$$\frac{2 \; \text{g NaF}}{1,000,000 \; \text{mL dilution}} \times \frac{240 \; \text{mL dilution}}{5 \; \text{mL ℞}} \times 60 \; \text{mL ℞}$$
$$= 0.00576 \; \text{g NaF}$$

The pharmacist would weigh out 5.76 mg (actually, one would weigh out a larger quantity and take an aliquot part) and qs to 60 mL.

Another variation of this problem is the prescriber requesting the concentration in terms of fluoride ion (F^-). In this case the atomic weight of F^- and molecular weight of NaF are used in the calculation. If the request called for 2 ppm fluoride, the initial calculations would be the same as above, and an additional step would be added at the end. The 5.76 mg would now represent the weight of fluoride ion needed. This must be converted to weight of NaF. The molecular weight of NaF is 42 and the atomic weight of fluorine is 19. The following proportion can be set up.

$$5.76 \text{ mg fluoride} \times \frac{42 \text{ mg NaF}}{19 \text{ mg fluoride}} = 12.7 \text{ mg NaF}$$

Problems

1. How many mg of NaF are needed in the following prescription?

    ℞   Sodium Fluoride
                Purified water, qs to 90 mL
                M ft solution such that when 1 f℥ is diluted to 1 glassful of water a 3 ppm NaF soln results.

DILUTION AND CONCENTRATION

Stock solutions can be diluted to make a product that has a lower concentration; also mixtures of powders or semisolids (eg, ointments) can be diluted to give a product of lower concentration of the drug(s). The diluent is an inert solid or semisolid or base that does not contain any active ingredients.

Mixtures also may be concentrated by adding pure drug or mixing with a product containing a higher concentration of the drug. For example, how much of a diluent must be added to 50 g of a 10% ointment to make it a 5% ointment?

1. How many grams of active ingredient are in 50 g of 10% ointment?

$$\frac{10 \text{ g drug}}{100 \text{ g oint (10\%)}} \times 50 \text{ g oint (10\%)} = 5 \text{ g drug}$$

2. How many grams of a 5% ointment can be made from 5 g of active ingredient?

$$\frac{100 \text{ g oint (5\%)}}{5 \text{ g drug}} \times 5 \text{ g drug} = 100 \text{ g oint (5\%)}$$

3. How many grams of base must be added to the 50 g of the original 10% ointment?

$$100 \text{ g oint (5\%)} - 50 \text{ g oint (10\%)} = 50 \text{ g base}$$

The term *trituration* was used previously to mean a dilute powder mixture of a drug. It is often necessary to dilute this mixture further to obtain the required amount of drug.

1. How much of a 1 in 10 trituration of a potent drug contains 200 mg of the drug?
   A 1 in 10 trituration means 1 g of drug in 10 g of mixture or 1 g of drug plus 9 g diluent. *Remember*: mixtures of solids are percent *w/w*.

$$\frac{10 \text{ g trituration}}{1 \text{ g drug}} \times \frac{1 \text{ g drug}}{1000 \text{ mg drug}} \times 200 \text{ mg drug}$$
$$= 2 \text{ g trituration}$$

2. How much diluent must be added to 10 g of a 1:100 trituration to make a mixture that contains 1 mg of drug in each 10 g of the final mixture?
   a. Determine the amount of drug in 10 g of trituration.

$$\frac{1 \text{ g drug}}{100 \text{ g trituration}} \times 10 \text{ g trituration} = 0.1 \text{ g drug}$$

b. Determine the amount of mixture that can be made from 0.1 g (100 mg) of drug.

$$\frac{10 \text{ g mixture}}{1 \text{ mg drug}} \times \frac{1000 \text{ mg drug}}{1 \text{ g drug}} \times 0.1 \text{ g drug}$$
$$= 1000 \text{ g mixture}$$

c. Determine the amount of diluent needed.

$$1000 \text{ g mixture} - 10 \text{ g trituration} = 990 \text{ g diluent}$$

Problems

1. The following prescription order was received in a pharmacy. If the only ℞ cream available is a 10% concentration, how much of the 10% cream and how much diluent are required to compound the prescription?
    ℞   ℞ Cream 3% . . . . 30 g
2. How many grams of a 1:100 trituration contain 100 μg of the active ingredient?
3. How many grams of a 1:1000 dilution can be made from 1 g of a 1:25 trituration?

MIXING DIFFERENT STRENGTHS

Rules

1. The sum of the products obtained by multiplying a series of quantities by their respective concentrations equals the product obtained by multiplying a concentration by the sum of the quantities. For example, the sum of the products—obtained by multiplying the individual weights or volumes of a series of preparations by the concentration of a given ingredient contained in each preparation—is equal to the product obtained by multiplying the total weight of the series of preparations by the percentage of the given ingredient resulting from a homogeneous mixture of the same series of preparations.
2. When mixing products of varying strengths, the units and type of percent (*w/w, w/v, v/v*) must be kept constant.

Examples

1. What is the percent of alcohol in a mixture made by mixing 5 L of 25%, 1 L of 50%, and 1 L of 95% alcohol?
   a. Determine the total amount of alcohol in the three solutions and the total amount of solution (1 L = 1000 mL). Assume additivity of volumes on mixing.

$$\frac{25 \text{ mL alcohol}}{100 \text{ mL (25\%)}} \times 5000 \text{ mL (25\%)} = 1250 \text{ mL alcohol}$$

$$\frac{50 \text{ mL alcohol}}{100 \text{ mL (50\%)}} \times 1000 \text{ mL (50\%)} = 500 \text{ mL alcohol}$$

$$\frac{95 \text{ mL alcool}}{100 \text{ mL (95\%)}} \times 1000 \text{ mL (95\%)} = 950 \text{ mL alcohol}$$

b. Determine the percent of alcohol in the mixture. There is a total of 2700 mL of alcohol in 7000 mL of total solution.

$$\frac{2700 \text{ mL alcohol}}{7000 \text{ mL mixture}} \times 100 \text{ mL mixture} = 38.6 \text{ mL alcohol}$$

$$\frac{38.6 \text{ mL alcohol}}{100 \text{ mL mixture}} = 38.5\%$$

2. What is the strength of a mixture obtained by mixing 50 g of a 5%, 100 g of a 7.5% and 40 g of a 10% ointment?

$$\frac{5 \text{ g drug}}{100 \text{ g oint (5\%)}} \times 50 \text{ g oint (5\%)} = 2.5 \text{ g drug}$$

$$\frac{7.5 \text{ g drug}}{100 \text{ g oint (7.5\%)}} \times 100 \text{ g oint (7.5\%)} = 7.5 \text{ g drug}$$

$$\frac{10 \text{ g drug}}{100 \text{ g oint (10\%)}} \times 40 \text{ g oint (10\%)} = 4.0 \text{ g drug}$$

There is a total of 14.0 g of active ingredient in 190 g of total mixture.

$$\frac{14.0 \text{ g drug}}{190 \text{ g mixture}} \times 100 \text{ g mixture} = 7.37 \text{ g drug}$$

$$\frac{7.37 \text{ g drug}}{100 \text{ g mixture}} = 7.37\%$$

Problems

1. What percent of a drug is contained in a mixture of powder consisting of 0.5 kg, containing 0.038% of a drug, and 10 kg, containing 0.043% of a drug?
2. What is the strength of a mixture produced by combining the following lots of alcohol: 2 L of 95%, 2 L of 50%, and 7 L of 60%?
3. What is the percent of drug content in the following mixture: 2 kg of 3%, 300 g of 2.5%, and 500 g of 4.2% resin?

ALLIGATION ALTERNATE

Alligation is a rapid method of calculation that is useful to the pharmacist. The name is derived from the Latin *alligatio*, meaning the act of attaching, and it refers to lines drawn during calculation to bind quantities together. This method is used to find the proportions in which substances of different strengths or concentrations must be mixed to yield a mixture of desired strength or concentration. When the proportion is found, a calculation may be performed to find the exact amounts of the substances required.

Rules

1. Line up the concentrations of all the starting materials in a vertical column in order of concentration, traditionally from high to low. Pure drugs are defined as being 100%; solvents or vehicles are designated as 0%.
2. Place the concentration of the desired product in a second column such that it is bracketed by concentrations of starting materials. With two starting materials, the desired product simply falls between the two.
3. Cross subtract the two columns to give a parts formula that can be used to calculate specific amounts of each starting material.

Examples and Procedure

1. In what proportion must a preparation containing 10% of drug be mixed with one containing 15% of drug to produce a mixture of 12% drug strength?
Applying the above rules gives:

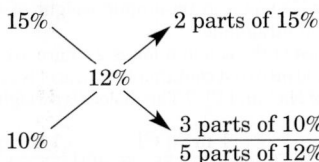

The concentrations of the starting material are lined up in the first column in decreasing or increasing order and the desired percent or concentration is placed in the center column. The third column is obtained by cross-subtracting as indicated by the arrows and gives a parts formula for mixing the two starting materials. Thus, mixing 2 parts of 15% drug preparation with 3 parts of 10% drug preparation will produce 5 parts of a drug mixture of the desired 12% strength.

2. In what proportion must 30% alcohol and 95% alcohol be mixed to make 500 mL of 50% alcohol? Set up the problem in the following manner:

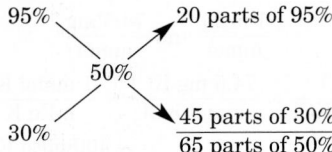

In a total of 65 parts, 20 parts of 95% alcohol + 45 parts of 30% alcohol are needed. Since the total is proportional to 500 mL, the following can be calculated:

$$\frac{20 \text{ parts (mL) } 95\%}{65 \text{ parts (mL) } 50\%} \times 500 \text{ (mL) } 50\% = 154 \text{ mL } 95\%$$

$$\frac{45 \text{ parts (mL) } 30\%}{65 \text{ parts (mL) } 50\%} \times 500 \text{ mL } 50\% = 346 \text{ mL } 30\%$$

Since volumes are not additive, sufficient water may be needed to make 500 mL.

3. How many grams of an ointment containing 0.18% of active ingredient must be mixed with 50 grams of an ointment containing 0.14% of active ingredient to make a product containing 0.15% of active ingredient?

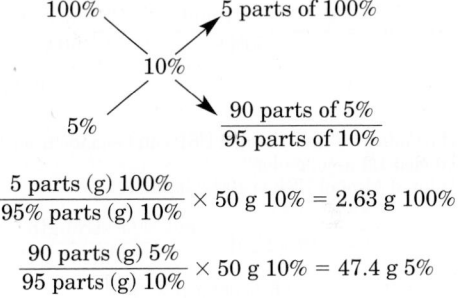

$$\frac{0.01 \text{ parts (g) } 0.18\%}{0.03 \text{ parts (g) } 0.14\%} \times 50 \text{ g } 0.14\% = 16.6 \text{ g } 0.18\%$$

4. Occasionally, it is necessary for a pharmacist to increase the strength of a product. For example, a prescription calls for 50 g of a 10% ointment. The pharmacist only has a 5% ointment and the pure ingredient available. How much of the 5% ointment and the pure ingredient are needed to compound the prescription?

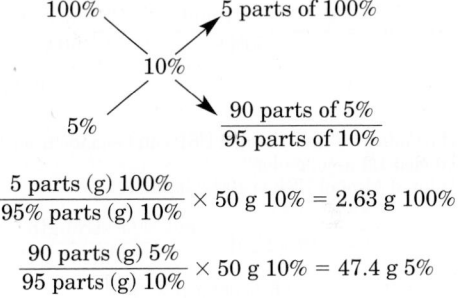

100%   5 parts of 100%

10%

5%   90 parts of 5%
            95 parts of 10%

$$\frac{5 \text{ parts (g) } 100\%}{95\% \text{ parts (g) } 10\%} \times 50 \text{ g } 10\% = 2.63 \text{ g } 100\%$$

$$\frac{90 \text{ parts (g) } 5\%}{95 \text{ parts (g) } 10\%} \times 50 \text{ g } 10\% = 47.4 \text{ g } 5\%$$

Problems

1. How much ointment containing 12% drug and how much ointment containing 16% drug must be used to make 1 kg of a product containing 12.5% drug?
2. In what proportion should 50% alcohol and purified water be mixed to make a 35% alcohol solution? (The purified water is 0% alcohol.)
Note: This problem may be solved by a method other than alligation as was shown above.
3. How many grams of 28% *w/w* ammonia water should be added to 500 g of 5% *w/w* ammonia water to produce a 10% *w/w* ammonia concentration?
4. How many mL of 20% dextrose in water and how many mL of 50% dextrose in water are needed to make 1 L of 35% dextrose in water?

PROOF SPIRIT

For tax purposes, the US government calculates the strength of pure or absolute alcohol (herein referred to as C_2H_5OH) by means of *proof degrees*. This means that 100 proof spirit contains 50% (by volume) or 42.49% (by weight) of C_2H_5OH, and its specific gravity is 0.93426 at 60°F. Thus, 2 proof degrees equals 1% (by volume) of C_2H_5OH. One proof gallon is one gal of 50% (by volume) of C_2H_5OH at 15.56°C (60°F). In other words, a proof gallon is a gallon that contains 1/2 gal of C_2H_5OH. A proof gallon is 100 proof.

The term *10 degrees under proof* (10° up) signifies that 100 volumes of the spirit contains 90 volumes of proof spirit plus 10 volumes of water, and *30 degrees over proof* (30° op) indicates that 100 volumes diluted with water yields 130 volumes of proof spirit. To prepare proof spirit, 50 volumes of C_2H_5OH are mixed with 53.71 volumes of water to allow for the contraction that occurs to yield 100 volumes of product.

The terms *proof strength, proof gallon,* and *proof spirit* are used so that the tax is levied only on the actual quantity of C_2H_5OH contained in any mixture. Therefore, it is sometimes necessary for the pharmacist to convert alcohol purchased to proof strength to compute tax refunds or convert proof strengths to percent for compounding purposes.

A quantity of solution that contains 1/2 gal of C_2H_5OH is said to contain one proof gal. Proof gallons may be calculated by the following two equations:

$$\text{Proof gal} = \frac{\text{gal} \times \text{v/v strength}}{50\% \text{ v/v}}$$

$$\text{Proof gal} = \frac{\text{gal} \times \text{proof strength}}{100 \text{ proof}}$$

The second equation is the same as the first because proof strength is always twice the % *v/v* strength. With these equations, given any two variables the third can be calculated.

Examples

1. What is the taxable alcohol in 1 pt of Alcohol USP?

$$1 \text{ pt} = \frac{1}{8} \text{ gal } (8 \text{ pt} = 1 \text{ gal})$$

Alcohol USP is 95% *v/v*; therefore,

$$\text{proof gal} = \frac{\text{gal} \times \% \text{ strength}}{50\%} = \frac{1/8 \text{ gal} \times 95\%}{50\%}$$

$$= 0.2375 \text{ proof gal}$$

2. How much Diluted Alcohol USP can be made from 1 qt of alcohol labeled 1/2 proof gallon?
   Diluted Alcohol USP is 49% *v/v*; therefore,

$$\text{Proof gal} = \frac{\text{gal} \times \% \text{ strength}}{50\%}$$

$$\text{gal} = \frac{0.5 \text{ proof gal} \times 50\%}{49\%} = 0.510 \text{ gal}$$

Problems

1. How many proof gallons are there in 1 qt of a preparation that is labeled 75% *v/v* alcohol?
2. How many proof gallons are there in a pint of an elixir that contains 14% alcohol?
3. How much Diluted Alcohol USP can be made from 1 gal of 190 proof alcohol?

SATURATED SOLUTIONS

Occasionally, it is necessary for a pharmacist to make saturated solutions. Solubility in the USP/NF is expressed as the number of milliliters of a solvent that will dissolve one g of a solid; for example, one g dissolves in 0.5 mL of water. In other words, if one g of a solid is dissolved in 0.5 mL of water, a saturated solution results. An example will illustrate this.

How much of a drug is needed to make 120 mL of a saturated solution if one g of the drug dissolves in 7.5 mL of water?

Calculate the amount of drug that can be dissolved in 120 mL water.

$$\frac{1 \text{ g drug}}{7.5 \text{ mL water}} \times 120 \text{ mL water} = 16 \text{ g drug}$$

When 16 g of the drug are dissolved in 120 mL of water, a saturated solution results that has a volume greater than 120 mL

because the solid will take up a certain volume. Only 120 mL would be dispensed.

What is the % *w/w* of the above solution?

$$120 \text{ g (mL) water} + 16 \text{ g drug} = 136 \text{ g solution}$$

$$\frac{16 \text{ g drug}}{136 \text{ g solution}} \times 100 \text{ g solution} = 11.8 \text{ g drug}$$

$$\frac{11.8 \text{ g drug}}{100 \text{ g solution}} = 11.8\% \text{ w/w}$$

Problems

1. What is the solubility of a chemical if a saturated aqueous solution is 0.5% *w/w*?
2. How many grams are needed to make 500 mL of a saturated solution if 1 g of the solute is soluble in 14 mL of solvent?

MILLIEQUIVALENTS

The quantities of electrolytes administered to patients are usually expressed by the term *milliequivalents* (mEq). The reason that weight units (mg, g) are not used is because the electrical activity of the ions, which in this instance is important, may be best expressed as mEq. (See Chapter 17 for additional discussion on electrolytic equilibria.)

A mEq is 1/1000 of an *equivalent* (Eq). An Eq is the weight of a substance that combines with or replaces one gram-atomic weight (g-at wt) of hydrogen. In pharmacy the terms equivalent and equivalent weight (Eq wt) have been used interchangeably. For problem solving it is convenient to identify the molar weight in terms of mg per mmol and the number of mEq per mmol as follows:

$$\text{Molecular weight} = \frac{\text{g}}{\text{mole}} = \frac{\text{mg}}{\text{mmol}}$$

$$\frac{\text{mEq}}{\text{mol}} = \text{valence}$$

For example, KCl has a molecular weight of 74.5; the above parameters would be 74.5 mg/mmol and one mEq/mmol.

Water of hydration contributes to the molecular weight (mol wt) of a compound but *not* to the valence, and the total mol wt is used to calculate mEq.

Examples

1. Calcium (Ca^{2+}) has a gram-atomic weight of 40.08. Determine the number of mEq/mmol.
   As the valence of the calcium ion is 2, there are 2 mEq/mmol.
2. A solution (100 mL) that contains 409.5 mg of NaCl/100 mL has how many mEq of Na^+ and Cl^-? The molecular weight of NaCl is 58.5.

$$\text{There is } \frac{1 \text{ mEq Cl}^-}{\text{mmol NaCl}} \text{ and } \frac{1 \text{ mEq Na}^+}{\text{mmol NaCl}}$$

$$\frac{1 \text{ mEq Cl}^-}{\text{mmol NaCl}} \times \frac{1 \text{ mmol NaCl}}{58.5 \text{ mg NaCl}} \times \frac{409.5 \text{ mg NaCl}}{100} \text{ mL}$$

$$\times 100 \text{ mL} = 7.0 \text{ mEq Cl}^-$$

Since NaCl is a 1:1 electrolyte, the solution contains 7.0 mEq of Cl^- and 7.0 mEq of Na^+.

3. A prescription order calls for a 500 mL solution of potassium chloride to be made so that it will contain 400 mEq of K^+. How many grams of KCl (mol wt: 74.5) are needed?

$$\frac{1 \text{ mEq}}{\text{mmol}} \text{ and } \frac{74.5 \text{ mg}}{\text{mmol}}$$

$$\frac{1 \text{ g KCl}}{1000 \text{ mg KCl}} \times \frac{74.5 \text{ mg KCl}}{\text{mmol KCl}} \times \frac{1 \text{ mmol KCl}}{\text{mEq K}^+}$$

$$\times 400 \text{ mEq K}^+ = 29.8 \text{ g KCl}$$

4. How many mEq of K^+ are in a 250-mg tablet of potassium phenoxymethyl penicillin (mol wt: 388.5; valence: 1)?

$$\frac{1 \text{ mEq } K^+}{\text{mmol Pen}} \text{ and } \frac{388.5 \text{ mg Pen}}{\text{mmol Pen}}$$

$$\frac{1 \text{ mEq } K^+}{\text{mmol Pen}} \times \frac{1 \text{ mmol Pen}}{388.5 \text{ mg Pen}} \times \frac{250 \text{ mg Pen}}{\text{Tab}}$$
$$\times 1 \text{ Tab} = 0.644 \text{ mEq } K^+$$

5. How many mEq of Mg are there in 10 mL of a 50% Magnesium Sulfate Injection? The mol wt of $MgSO_4 \cdot 7H_2O$ is 246.

$$\frac{2 \text{ mEq } Mg^{2+}}{\text{mmol drug}} \text{ and } \frac{246 \text{ mg drug}}{\text{mmol drug}}$$

$$\frac{2 \text{ mEq } Mg^{2+}}{\text{mmol drug}} \times \frac{1 \text{ mmol drug}}{246 \text{ mg drug}} \times \frac{1000 \text{ mg drug}}{\text{g drug}} \times \frac{50 \text{ g drug}}{100 \text{ mL}}$$
$$\times 10 \text{ mL} = 40.7 \text{ mEq } Mg^{2+}$$

6. A vial of Sodium Chloride Injection contains 3 mEq/mL. What is the percentage strength of this solution? The mol wt of NaCl is 58.5.

$$\frac{1 \text{ mEq}}{\text{mmol}} \text{ and } \frac{58.5 \text{ mg}}{\text{mmol}}$$

$$\frac{1 \text{ g}}{1000 \text{ mg}} \times \frac{58.5 \text{ mg}}{\text{mmol}} \times \frac{1 \text{ mmol}}{1 \text{ mEq}} \times \frac{3 \text{ mEq}}{\text{mL}} \times 100 \text{ mL} = 17.6 \text{ g}$$

$$\frac{17.6 \text{ g}}{100 \text{ mL}} = 17.6\%$$

Problems

1. What is the mEq wt of ferrous ion (Fe^{2+}) which has a atomic weight of 55.85 g?
2. What is the mEq wt of sodium phosphate ($Na_2HPO_4 \cdot 7H_2O$)?
3. How many mEq of Na^+ are in 60 mL of a 5% solution of sodium saccharin (mol wt: 241 g; valence: 1)?
4. How many mEq of Ca^{2+} are there in a 600-mg calcium lactate pentahydrate (mol wt: 308.30 g) tablet?
5. How many mEq of sodium are there in a 5 gr sodium bicarbonate tablet? The mol wt of $NaHCO_3$ is 84 and the valence is 1.
6. How many mEq of Na are there in 500 mL of 1/2 normal saline solution? Normal saline solution contains 9 g NaCl/L; mol wt NaCl is 58.5.
7. How much KCl is needed to make a pint of syrup that contains 10 mEq of K^+ in each tablespoonful? The mol wt of KCl is 74.5.

TEMPERATURE

Rules

The relationship of Centigrade (C) and Fahrenheit (F) degrees is:

$$9 \, (°C) = 5 \, (°F) - 160$$

Where °C is the number of degrees Centigrade, and °F is the number of degrees Fahrenheit.

Examples

1. Convert 77°F into °C.

$$9 \, (°C) = 5 \, (77) - 160$$

$$°C = \frac{385 - 160}{9} = 25°C$$

2. Convert 10°C into °F.

$$9 \, (10) = 5 \, (°F) - 160$$

$$°F = \frac{90 + 160}{5} = 50°F$$

Problems

Convert
  a. 30°C into °F
  b. 100°C into °F
  c. 37°C into °F
  d. 120°F into °C

REFERENCES

1. *Specifications, Tolerances, and Other Technical Requirements for Weighing and Measuring Devices.* NBS Handbook 44. Washington DC:US Department of Commerce, NBS, USGPO, 1989.
2. Goldstein SW, Mattocks AM. *Professional Equilibrium and Compounding Accuracy* (pamphlet). Washington DC: APhA, 1967.
3. USP XXVI, 2003.
4. Morrell CA, Ordway EM. *Drug Std* 1954; 22:216.
5. Madlon-Kay DF, Mosch FS. *J Family Pract* 2000; 49(8):741.
6. Shirkey HC. Dosage (posology). In Shirkey HC, ed. *Pediatric Therapy*, 5th ed. St Louis: Mosby, 1975, p 19.
7. Benitz WE, Tatro DS. *The Pediatric Drug Handbook*, 3rd ed. St Louis: Mosby, 1995.
8. Nelson JD. *Pocketbook of Pediatric Antimicrobial Therapy*, 4th ed. Dallas: Jodane, 1981.

ANSWERS TO PROBLEMS

DENSITY

1. 816 g
2. 363 mL
3. 54.2 mL

ADDITION

1. 2480 g or 2.48 kg
2. 1160 g or 1.16 kg

SUBTRACTION

1. 4100 mL or 4.11 L
2. 3.71 g

MULTIPLICATION

1. 157 mL
2. 163 g
3. 825 mL
4. 375 mg

DIVISION

1. 769 capsules + 15 mg remainder
2. 150 doses
3. 1396 capsules + 300 mg remainder

CONVERSIONS

1.
  a. 422 mg
  b. 19.4 mg
  c. 109 g
  d. 7780 mg
  e. 99.4 g
  f. 454 g
2.
  a. 1 lb, 3 oz, 173 gr
  b. 6.94 gr
  c. 1 ℔, 5 ʒ, 5 ʒ, 26 gr
  d. 0.00154 gr
  e. 2.2 lb
3.
  a. 0.648 mg
  b. 0.203 mg

c. 10.8 mg
d. 0.325 or 0.324 g
e. 1.299 or 1.296 g

4.
a. 12.3 mL
b. 11.1 mL
c. 237 mL
d. 473 mL
e. 0.309 mL
f. 0.00154 gr
g. 0.0772 gr

5.
a. 480 gr
b. 8 ℨ
c. 437 1/2 gr
d. 2880 gr
e. 4 ℨ, 10 gr

DOSAGE CALCULATION

1. 1.5 mg
2. 32.7 mg
3. 18.7 mg
4. 280,000 units
5. 75 mg
6. 77.9 mg

PROBLEM-SOLVING METHODOLOGY

1. D.T.D. No. 14 means dispense 14 such doses. Assuming the doses have been checked, they are for chemicals J, K, and L (10 mg, 50 mg, and 300 mg, respectively).
2. Drug Q: 0.5 g
   Drug R: 0.3 g
3. 0.469 mL/dose; 1.88 mL/day
4. 50 doses
5. 0.0444 mg
6. 0.75 mL contains 60 units: 13 1/3-day supply.
7. 6 mL
8. 3 mL
9. 25 mg

REDUCING AND ENLARGING

1. Liquid C 875 mL
   Solid B 225 g
   Liquid R 62.5 mL
   Liquid P 500 mL
2. Solid G 7.46 g
   Liquid D 224 g
   Solid M 22.4 g
   Base 492 g
3. Solid N 4.8 mg
   Solid Q 120 mg
   Solid R 7.2 g
   Add sufficient purified water to make 240 mL solution.
4. Solid S 0.675 g
   Solid T 2.25 g
   Oil C 31.5 mL
   Alcohol 22.5 mL

PERCENTAGE

w/v Solutions
1. Dissolve 11.1 g in sufficient solvent to make 3 f℥.
2. 2.84 L
3. 6.25 L
4. 8 g

w/w Products
1. Compound A 7.46 g
   Solvent 117 g
2. 28.8 g
3. 5 kg
4. Dissolve 4.64 g of drug in 120 mL (150 g) of glycerin.
5. Compound K 3.6 g
   Solid H 1.8 g
   Base 18.6 g
6. Dissolve 88.2 g of the solute in 500 mL of purified water. Dispense 500 mL

7. Powder P 27.8 g
   Powder Q 222 g
   Powder R 333 g
   Powder S 416 g
8. 3 g of coal tar solution; 27 g of hydrophilic ointment

PERCENT

(v/v, w/v, and w/w)
1. 240 ℔
2. 1900 mL
3. 34.8% *w/w*
4. 0.740 gr
5. 38.5% *w/w*
6. 15 g
7. 0.4 g
8. 32.4 mL of a 37% solution
9. 1.58 g

STOCK SOLUTIONS

1. 30.3 g
2. 36.3 g
3. 0.5 mL

PARTS PER MILLION

1. 13 mg

DILUTION AND CONCENTRATION

1. 9 g of 10% cream and 21 g of diluent (base)
2. 0.01 g
3. 40 g

MIXING PRODUCTS OF DIFFERENT STRENGTHS

1. 0.0428%
2. 64.5%
3. 3.16%

ALLIGATION ALTERNATE

1. 875 g of 12% ointment and 125 g of 16% ointment
2. 35 parts of 50% alcohol and 15 parts of purified water
3. 139 g of 28% ammonia water
4. 500 mL each of the 20% and 50% solutions are needed

PROOF SPIRIT

1. 0.375 proof gal
2. 0.035 proof gal
3. 1.94 gal

SATURATED SOLUTIONS

1. 1 g in 199 mL
2. 35.7 g of solute—dispense 500 mL

MILLIEQUIVALENTS

1. 27.9 mg/mEq
2. 134 mg/mEq
3. 12.5 mEq
4. 3.89 mEq
5. 3.86 mEq Na
6. 38.5 mEq Na
7. 23.5 g

TEMPERATURE

1.
a. 86°F
b. 212°F
c. 98.6°F
d. 48.9°C1.

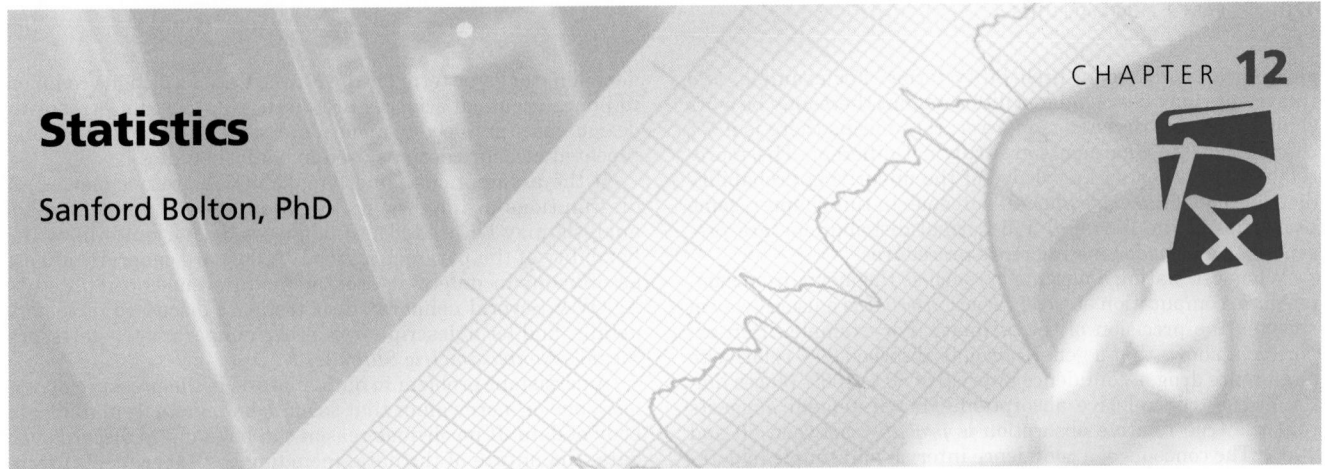

CHAPTER 12

Statistics

Sanford Bolton, PhD

Statistical methods are an integral part of the development, evaluation, and marketing of drug products. In this chapter, elementary definitions and some common statistical applications to problems of pharmaceutical interest will be presented and discussed.

Statistics is often thought of as a collection of numbers and averages, such as vital statistics, baseball statistics, or statistics derived from the census. Indeed, this is an important aspect of statistical thinking, and such collections of data and counting do play a role in pharmacy and medicine, such as in marketing or disease-incidence data. However, here more emphasis will be placed on the use of statistics in presenting, analyzing, and interpreting data that are often, but not necessarily always, derived from planned experiments.

OVERVIEW AND INTRODUCTION

Although the material in this chapter is elementary for the most part, those readers who have had little or no exposure to statistical methods may be overwhelmed by the large amount of information presented in a relatively small space. This introduction presents an overview of the chapter so that the student can get a feeling for what is contained here. Many illustrations are interspersed in the didactic discussion to show the applications in a practical way.

The first part of the chapter deals with *introductory definitions and methods*. An understanding of this material is essential if one wishes to use elementary techniques intelligently, or if one wishes to pursue more advanced topics. Definitions include statistical jargon, design of scientific experiments (both laboratory and clinical experiments), the concept of sampling (including methods of obtaining samples for experiments), and the concept and definition of probability distributions. These concepts lay the foundation for the understanding of practical applications of statistics to scientific research. Although not complete, an understanding of this introductory material should allow the student to feel confident about applying elementary methods to real data.

Some words of caution are necessary here. Real examples often have twists that are not obvious to the initiate, which make them different from simple textbook examples. At the beginning, students should try to seek advice from more experienced persons, preferably a statistician, to make sure that they are using the techniques in a proper manner.

For those with some background in statistics, the initial portion of the chapter should serve as a quick review and an introduction to the material that follows. The elementary definitions include the usual measures of central tendency and spread, such as the mean, median, standard deviation, variance, coefficient of variation, and range. The nature of *variation* and its basis for statistical thinking is discussed, as without variation, statistical reasoning would be unnecessary. Statistical approaches take the experimental variability (often referred to as *error*) into account during the analysis.

Statistical "proof" is different from mathematical proofs. In statistics, one is never sure of an answer or a decision. The decision has a given probability of being correct. Discrete and continuous variables are defined and discussed. Discrete variables include binomial measurements, which may have a "yes or no" outcome (eg, accept or reject). Continuous variables can have any number of outcomes and include typical measurements (eg, weight or assay).

Definitions of a population and a sample are presented; these are very important concepts in statistical reasoning. Definitions and examples of bias, precision, and accuracy are introduced. Examples are used to illustrate the fact that data may be precise but not accurate and vice versa.

The analysis of any data set depends on the *experimental design*, the detailed experimental procedure. A description of some common designs and the manner in which data may be collected are presented in this chapter. The integrity of data from any experiment is only as good as the design and the care that was taken to implement the design. Each experiment is different. Design and sampling considerations are different for questionnaire surveys, censuses (complete sampling), and laboratory or clinical experiments. Good experimental design should result in optimality, increased precision, and lack of bias. The *random selection* of objects to be included in an experiment and/or assigned to treatments is of vital importance in pharmaceutical and clinical research. In particular, controlled clinical studies should be designed as double-blind studies if at all possible. A *controlled study* is a designed study that includes a placebo or a positive control (eg, a known active drug).

Statistical inference and estimation are cornerstones of statistical applications in pharmaceutical research. Statistical inference results from the formulation and testing of a hypothesis, the *null hypothesis*. In this procedure, a hypothesis is formulated with regard to the true, but unknown, values of parameters of the data distribution that is investigated in an experiment. For example, the average potency of a commercial batch of tablets may be of interest, or the mean blood pressure reduction of a new drug compared to an effective marketed product may be assessed. The experimental outcome is observed and analyzed. Using statistical procedures that usually are based on the normal probability distribution, an inference based on probability is drawn as to whether the proposed hypothesis is true; eg, "Is the true average potency equal to 100 mg?" or "Are the two comparative drugs equally efficacious?"

Again, these inferences are not proofs. Two treatments may be declared to be equal, but only with a given degree of assurance expressed in probability terms. For example, two treatments may be considered different, but there may be a 5% chance that this decision is in error; that means there is a 5% chance that the treatments are truly not different. These procedures are based on knowledge of the underlying probability distribution of the experimental outcome. In this chapter, some properties of the binomial and normal distributions are presented as a basis for the inference procedures.

When estimating a parameter, such as the mean, from sample data, computation of a *confidence interval* is a useful way of showing the precision of the estimate. For example, if an experiment shows that a generic drug is absorbed 90% relative to a reference drug, a confidence interval of 80 to 100% places limits on the true relative absorption. This statement suggests that the true relative absorption is *probably* between 80 and 100%. The concepts of a confidence interval and simple hypothesis testing are discussed following the presentation of the properties of the normal and binomial distributions.

The *t test* is a common and well-known test that is used to make statistical decisions. This test is used to determine significance when comparing average results from two groups or treatments (a two-sample *t* test), or when comparing an average result to some hypothetical value (a one-sample *t* test). In the latter case, an example would be the comparison of the average dissolution time to some given compendial standard value. The *null hypothesis* is the hypothesis that is tested, and the *alternative hypothesis* is the hypothesis accepted if the null hypothesis is rejected. The test is deemed significant if the null hypothesis is rejected at a given probability level, the *alpha error* or *level of significance*. Thus, the alpha error is the probability of mistakenly rejecting the null hypothesis, usually taken as 5%. This, and other important concepts relating to statistical inference are presented in more detail in another part of the chapter.

The *t* test is appropriate for normally distributed variables. For dichotomous experimental outcomes following the binomial distribution, other statistical methods may be used. With sufficiently large samples, a *chi-square* test may be appropriate to compare the proportion of responders in two groups. A discussion of these tests is included following the examples of use of the *t* test.

The *F distribution* is introduced as used in a test to compare the variances of two independent samples. The more common use of the *F* test is in *analysis of variance* (ANOVA). The comparison of two means using the *t* test is the most elementary of comparisons. In more complicated experiments where more than two groups are being compared, and where the experimental design is complicated and includes many factors, the *t* test cannot be used. In these cases ANOVA is indicated.

A good deal of this chapter is devoted to ANOVA applications. Briefly, *ANOVA* is a method of separating the variance due to factors imposed on the experiment. For example, in a crossover design, subjects are treated on two occasions, Period I and Period II. If the results in one period tend to be higher than in the other, but the treatment differences are not affected, the variance due to period differences may be substantial without affecting the treatment comparison. By separating the variance due to period differences from the variation in the experiment, the residual error that is used to test treatment differences is smaller. This results in a more sensitive experiment—differences are detected more easily. If period differences exist and are not taken into account, the variance becomes part of the residual error, which is inflated, resulting in a less sensitive test.

Because of the more complex structure of experimental designs that are analyzed using ANOVA, several problems arise that need special attention. Procedures based on multiple comparisons have been devised to compare means in a pairwise fashion when more than two means are compared and it is not obvious how to identify significant effects. Also, in complex designs, the choice of the proper error term for an effect is not always obvious; ie, different effects may not all have the same

denominator error term for the *F* test. Various designs common to pharmaceutical sciences are discussed, including crossover designs used in bioequivalence and some clinical studies, and repeated measure designs used in clinical studies.

If the assumptions underlying ANOVA are not met, eg, if distributions are highly skewed, *nonparametric* methods of analysis may be used. These analyses do not quite have the flexibility of the parametric ANOVA, but are generally almost as efficient in detecting treatment differences compared to ANOVA. Several nonparametric tests are discussed. For more details, and for a description of other nonparametric tests, see Siegal's *Nonparametric Statistics*.[1]

A persistent problem in data analysis is the presence of *outliers*, one or more values that seem to be remote from the main body of data. If no obvious reason can be found to discard such data, the nature of the data, including the experimental technique and the history of such experiments, should be investigated carefully. If this investigation reveals no cause for the presence of the outlier(s), a statistical test may be applied to determine if the data can be discarded. If such procedures are applied, a report should include a description of what was done. Some people recommend performing the analysis with and without the outlier. In any event, before discarding an outlier, one should evaluate the consequences of this action.

The remainder of the chapter considers some specialized topics of interest to pharmaceutical scientists. An understanding of basic statistics is necessary to apply this material. Basic *Shewhart and Fraction Defective Control Charts* are discussed with examples. Often, Shewhart charts do not work for pharmaceutical processes where the material is heterogeneous (eg, solid dosage forms) or the manufacturing equipment is variable from batch to batch. In these cases, other approaches may give a satisfactory analysis.[8]

Regression analysis, a process familiar to most scientists, concerns the fitting of data to linear models, ie, to models that are linear in the parameters. In particular, the fitting of straight lines is common to many different fields of scientific research. The process of least-squares fitting and the statistical properties of the slope and intercept are discussed, with applications to stability, dose-response relationships, calibration plots, kinetics, and so on. In particular, an analysis of stability data to predict shelf life is presented in some detail. This analysis includes hypothesis tests for the slope and intercept, as well as confidence limits for the line.

Regression is used when one of the variables (X) is measured with little or no error, and the other variable (Y) is measured with error. *Correlation* is related to linear regression. This analysis may be appropriate when both variables are subject to error, and an estimate of the degree of their association is desired. A correlation coefficient is calculated, which can have values between +1 and −1. A correlation coefficient of 0 suggests that the variables are not correlated. Care should be exercised in the interpretation of correlation coefficients. A value of the correlation coefficient close to 1 does not prove that the variables have a linear relationship.

The chapter concludes with a discussion of *transformations*, which are useful when data distributions do not conform to that assumed for the statistical analysis. In particular, a transformation may help to normalize data that are not normal (eg, skewed). The most common transformation is the logarithmic transformation, which will equalize variances for data that have a relatively constant relative standard deviation, $S/\overline{X}$.

This chapter covers a wide variety of material in a small space. Although the concepts here should provide a basic understanding, much effort is needed to understand and apply statistics in the real world. The chapter bibliography should help students in this endeavor.

VARIABILITY AND VARIABLES—The prime reason for the need of statistical approaches to the analysis of real-life data is the inherent variability present in experimental data, in particular, in biological material and laboratory processes. Variability has the same meaning in statistics as it does in everyday usage. In its statistical sense, *variability* implies a lack of exact predictability of an experimental outcome. For example, although 50% of prescriptions are written for generic warfarin tablets, it cannot be predicted with certainty that a new prescription written by Dr Jones will be for the generic product. Conversely, the chance that the new prescription will be for the generic product is 1/2 or 0.50.

In statistical terms, variability commonly is called *error*. Measurement error does not mean that a mistake was made, but rather that the measurement yields inherently variable results.

A *variable,* simply put in statistical jargon, is a measurement that exhibits variability. Practically all measurements in scientific research and data collection are variable. Variables can be divided conveniently into two classes, discrete and continuous.

Discrete data have a countable number of possible outcomes. The number of animals that die when 12 animals are given 10 mg/kg of an experimental drug in an LD50 experiment, or the number of bottles missing a label in a packaging run of tablets, or the proportion of patients with a successful outcome in a clinical study, are examples of discrete variables. In the former case, the number of animals that could die in the experiment could be 0, 1, 2, 3, 4, 5, 6, 7, 8, 9, 10, 11, or 12. There are 13 possible outcomes. The number of dead animals is a discrete variable. Similarly, the number of bottles without labels is an integer that can vary between 0 and N, where N is the number of bottles in the run.

A *continuous* variable is one in which there are an unlimited (infinite) number of possible outcomes in some interval. The weight of a tablet may be any value between 180 and 220 mg, for example. The only limitation on the weight measurement is the accuracy and precision of the weighing device. Blood pressure measurement is a continuous variable. Although the actual measurement may appear to be limited to some countable number of outcomes—integers between 0 and 300, for example—this is due only to the approximate nature of the measuring instrument, the sphygmomanometer. With a more sophisticated device, one could expect a systolic blood pressure to be any value such as 160.629837465 torr. This exaggerated example is meant only to illustrate that the number of decimal places is limited only by the precision of the measuring device. To make this concept clearer, Table 12-1 gives further examples of discrete and continuous data encountered in pharmaceutical science.

SAMPLES AND POPULATIONS—Many experiments have as an objective the definition or comparison of two or more groups of data. For example, one may wish to compare the efficacy of two antihypertensive agents, or a new antipsychotic drug versus a placebo. Or it may be desired to estimate the average

Table 12-1. Examples of Discrete and Continuous Data

Measurement of LD$_{50}$—Although the number of animals dead at each of a series of doses is a discrete variable, the measurement of LD$_{50}$ is a continuous variable. For example, the LD$_{50}$ could take on any value between 1 and 100 mg, limited perhaps only by the precision of the analytical computations.

Preference Tests—If 100 consumers are asked for their preference for one of two products, the number who prefer one of the products is discrete.

Defects in Quality Control—The number of defects observed in a sample of 200 capsules sampled for quality control is a discrete variable.

Dissolution Test—The average time for 50% dissolution obtained from 12 tablets is a continuous variable. The 50% dissolution time is interpolated from the data. The dissolution time of the 12 tablets can have any number of possible outcomes of the average dissolution, limited only by the sensitivity of the measuring instruments, ie, the measurement of time and amount of drug dissolved.

drug content and variability of a batch of tablets. In virtually all such experiments, it is not realistic to observe all possible experimental units. In fact, sometimes the entire population of conceivable observations cannot be identified completely. The potential experimental material for a clinical study comparing an antipsychotic drug to a placebo would include not only patients but also persons with the disease who are not yet diagnosed. All of these people are the population or universe. Clearly, one would not perform an experiment that included the entire population for many reasons:

- All of these people could not be identified.
- The time or money to conduct such a huge experiment is not available.
- To include so many people in such an experiment could be dangerous or unethical.

It is not necessary to run such a large experiment to arrive at a fair conclusion regarding the efficacy of the drug. In fact, in most cases, the test consists of a relatively small *sample* taken from a relatively large *population*.

Another more concrete example is the process of sampling in quality control. It may be of interest to estimate the proportion of defective tablets or the average drug content and uniformity of tablets in a production batch. Certainly in the latter case every tablet in the batch would not be examined because the test is destructive, ie, the tablet is destroyed during the analysis for drug content. Rather, a sample of 20 tablets would be chosen to estimate the average drug content of the more than 1 million tablets in the batch.

Thus, in typical experiments in the pharmaceutical sciences, a small sample from the population is examined in order to make inferences about the large population.

THE AVERAGE OR MEAN—Suppose that a sample of n objects is taken from a population or universe in order to estimate some characteristic of the population, such as the average reduction of blood pressure after drug treatment, the average age of consumers purchasing an over-the-counter (OTC) acne product, or the average dissolution rate of drug from a tablet. The sample of n determinations can be designated by

$$x_1, x_2, x_3, \ldots, x_n$$

The sample mean, $\bar{x}$, is calculated as

$$\bar{x} = \frac{x_1 + x_2 + x_3 + \cdots x_n}{n} = \sum x_i/n$$

where i goes from 1 to n.

The *sample mean,* $\bar{x}$, estimates the *actual* or *true population mean,* designated as the Greek letter mu (μ). That is, the sample mean would not be expected to exactly equal the population mean μ in any given experiment, but should equal the population mean on the average. Figure 12-1 illustrates this idea.

Example 1—The weights, in mg, of nine tablets are

201	204	200
203	202	207
209	206	207

The average, $\bar{x}$, is $\sum x_i/n = 1839/9 = 204.33$ mg.

The *average* is a measure of the center of a set of data. Another measure of central tendency is the median. The *median* divides the data set in half; that is half of the data is below the median and half is above. For a sample with an odd number of observations, the median is the middle number—the ($n + 1$)/2 data point—after the data has been listed in order of magnitude.

200, 201, 202, 203, 204, 206, 207, 207, 209

For the tablet weights in this example, the median is 204 mg, the 5th, (9+1)/2, ordered value.

For an even number of data points, the median is the average of the two middle values after the data have been ordered.

MEASURES OF VARIATION—The mean alone is not sufficient to describe a set of data. When describing data, in

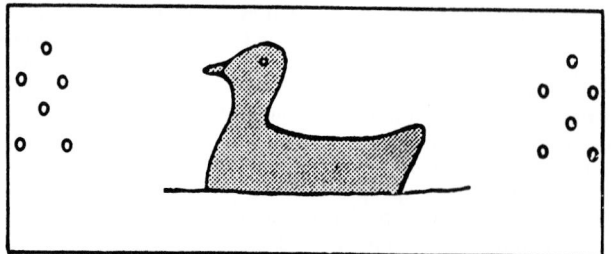

Figure 12-1. *On an average the duck was dead.* A hunter fired both barrels of a shotgun at a duck. The first hit 2 feet in front, the second hit 2 feet behind, and on an average the duck was dead. What the hunter really wanted was meat on the table. In duck hunting one wants to keep trying until a single shot hits the mark. But in estimating purity by a chemical test the best estimate is usually the average.

addition to the mean or average value, some measure of the variability or spread of the data should be calculated and reported. Two sets of data may have the same mean or average, but may have different distributions.

Example 2—The data in Example 1 have a mean of 204.33 mg. These data are reproduced below.

201	204	200
203	202	207
209	206	207

The following data set also has a mean of 204.33.

151	154	150
153	202	257
259	256	257

Clearly, the second set of data is spread out more, ie, it is more variable than the first set. The difference between the largest and smallest value in a data set is known as the *range*. For the first data set, the range is $209 - 200 = 9$. In the second data set, the range is $259 - 150 = 109$.

The standard deviation is a more common way of expressing the variability of data. The *standard deviation* of a sample of n values, designated as S or SD, is calculated as

$$S = \mathrm{SD} = \sqrt{\Sigma(x_i - \overline{x})^2/(n - 1)}$$

The standard deviation of the numbers 1, 3, 5, 9, and 12 is

$$\sqrt{\Sigma(x_i - \overline{x})^2/(n - 1)}$$
$$= \sqrt{[(1 - 6)^2 + (3 - 6)^2 + (5 - 6)^2 + (9 - 6)^2 + (12 - 6)^2]/4}$$
$$= \sqrt{80/4} = \sqrt{20} = 4.47$$

Exercise 1—Calculate the SD of the two sets of data in Example 2 above.

Answer: 3.08 and 52.65, respectively.

A shortcut formula for computing the SD is

$$\sqrt{[\Sigma\, x_i^2 - (\Sigma\, x_i)^2/n]/(n - 1)}$$

For the numbers 1, 3, 5, 7, 9, and 12, the computation is

$$\sqrt{[1^2 + 3^2 + 5^2 + 9^2 + 12^2 - 30^2/5]/4} = \sqrt{20} = 4.47$$

The sample SD calculated as shown above is an estimate of the *population SD*, designated as the Greek letter sigma (σ). As with the mean, the population SD is usually unknown. One can obtain an estimate of σ from the sample SD.

The SD measures the spread of a data set, but it is more difficult to interpret than the range. When the normal distribution is introduced, the SD will have a more tangible interpretation. For the moment, it can be said that the larger the spread of numbers in a data set, the larger the SD and vice versa.

The *coefficient of variation* or *relative standard deviation* (RSD) is defined as $\mathrm{SD}/\overline{x}$. This manner of expressing variability is useful when the SD is proportional to the magnitude of the measurement. This relationship often is seen in physical and biological measurements. For example, the analysis of large amounts of material often will have larger variability than the analysis of small quantities.

A very important concept in statistics is the *standard error of the mean,* designated as $s_{\overline{x}}$. Intuitively, one would expect that means of n observations would be less variable than the single, individual observations. The individual observations vary from extremes on the low side (below the average) to high values (above the average). When the means of 10 observations are taken, for example, the means will tend to be closer to the true average, μ, than the individual values. This can be better understood by visualizing the averaging effect of the mean, averaging extreme values with the other observations. In fact, the smaller variability of means can be proved mathematically; the SD of means of size n is equal to

$$s_{\overline{x}} = s/\sqrt{n}$$

For example, if the SD of individual values is 10, the standard error of means of size 25 is $10/\sqrt{25} = 2$. Thus, the means of size 25 are considerably less variable than the individual data points.

An examination of the equation for the standard error of the mean reveals that means constructed from very large sample sizes will be very stable, ie, nonvariable. If individual measurements are very variable, and a precise estimate of the mean is desired, this can be attained by making observations on a large number of samples. Of course, this is more easily said than done. Time and expense usually are limiting factors in data gathering and observation. However, it is true that the more observations, the more precise is the estimate of the mean (as well as estimates of other parameters such as the SD).

FREQUENCY DISTRIBUTIONS—A *frequency distribution* of a data set can be constructed by counting the number of data points falling into a series of intervals (usually of equal size). The frequency distribution and its corresponding graph, a *histogram* or *bar chart,* show the distribution of the data, its central value (eg, mean or median) and variability (eg, SD or range). Example 3 shows the weights of 50 weanling rats to be used in an experiment.

Example 3—The weights of 50 rats at weaning were as follows:

30g	47g	37g	29g	38g
32	42	32	30	34
34	32	33	37	36
39	33	45	40	35
43	41	35	32	41
36	27	28	35	30
38	28	41	37	34
41	36	32	30	37
31	31	35	28	25
26	49	34	34	33

Table 12-2 is a frequency distribution with 13 intervals derived from the data given in Example 3. A rule of thumb is to use 8 to 20 intervals, depending on the quantity and spread of the data. The histogram or bar chart of these data is shown in Figure 12-2.

BIAS, PRECISION, AND ACCURACY—*Precision* refers to the reproducibility of a series of measurements. If the values are very close to each other, the measurements are said to be precise. *Accuracy* refers to the closeness of measurements to the true value. For example, if a tablet contains exactly 200 mg of drug, and three analyses show a drug content of 205, 205, and 206 mg, it might be concluded that the analysis is precise, but not accurate. *Bias* refers to a systematic difference from the true value. Figure 12-3 illustrates these concepts.

The three assays observed above seem to be biased on the high side, ie, errors in the assay procedure result in too-high

Table 12-2. Frequency Distribution of Rat Weights

WEIGHT GROUP	FREQUENCY	WEIGHT GROUP	FREQUENCY
24–25 g	1	38–39	3
26–27	2	40–41	5
28–29	4	42–43	2
30–31	6	44–45	1
32–33	8	46–47	1
34–35	9	48–49	1
36–37	7		

values. Figure 12-3 shows that "precise" data need not be accurate. In fact, there need not be any relationship or correlation between the qualities of precision and accuracy. Note that biased data cannot be accurate but can be precise.

In addition to the concept of bias in the area of experimental measurements, it appears also in the field of experimental design. Bias can be introduced into an experiment, not because of an error in an experimental measurement, but because of poor judgment. For example, consider an experiment where the efficacy of oral and sublingual nitroglycerin are to be compared by administering both products to 20 patients on two different occasions and measuring the time to incidence of an angina attack in a treadmill test. Each of 20 patients will receive both the oral and buccal forms. If each patient receives the buccal drug on Monday and the oral drug on the following Sunday, a bias may be observed in the experimental results even if the measurements are not biased. This could be due to either the day of the week when the test was given (gloomy Monday versus a holiday weekend day) or an order effect where there is a different effect depending on which drug is given first. For example, there may be psychological factors causing the response to drug taken first to be systematically better (or worse) than that taken second, or the weather may be such as to cause more positive results on the first occasion. In the latter case, differences between the two dosage forms would be exaggerated (biased) in favor of the drug administered first, the buccal drug. To obviate this potential bias, we would give ten of the patients the oral drug first (Monday) and the buccal drug second (Sunday). The other ten patients would receive the products in opposite order. Perhaps, an improvement in this design would be to test the drugs on the same day of the week, eg, Monday.

DESIGN OF EXPERIMENTS AND COLLECTION OF DATA

The application of statistics in the analysis of data is optimal when the data are collected in a planned or designed manner.

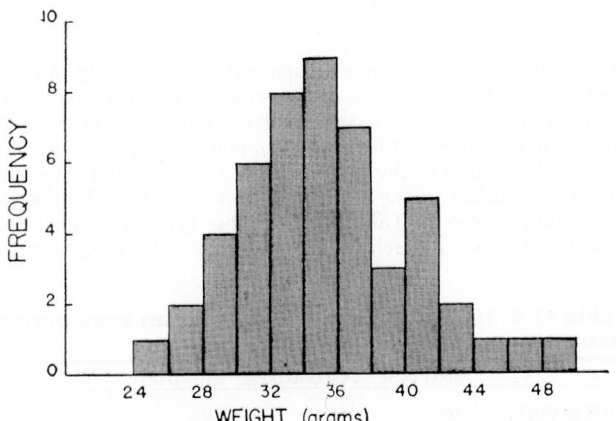

Figure 12-2. Bar chart showing frequency distribution of weights of 50 weanling rats (data in Example 3).

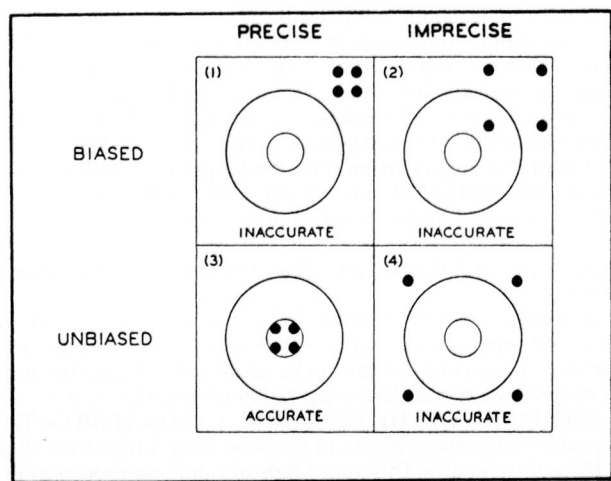

Figure 12-3. Diagram illustrating bias, precision, and accuracy. The shots on targets 1 and 2 are biased; in both cases the shots cluster away from the bull's-eye. The clusters on targets 3 and 4 both are unbiased; the center of each cluster is on the bull's-eye. The shots on targets 1 and 3 are precise; both sets are bunched together. The shots on targets 2 and 4 are scattered widely, hence imprecise. Only the shots on target 3 are accurate—precise and unbiased (courtesy, Lilly).

If data are analyzed after the fact (retrospective analysis), great care should be taken to examine the data for possible bias. For example, prescription-volume data gathered for the years 1970 to 1980 may be available only from cities with populations greater than 500,000 or from cities in the Western States. Clearly, conclusions from such data should not be applied indiscriminately to the entire country. Also, the information may have been gathered on a voluntary basis; without knowledge of the characteristics of those who did and did not supply the information, the conclusions could be tainted.

The manner in which data are collected is connected to the planning and design of experiments. In the collection of data, a small sample generally is taken from a large population or universe. Sometimes a sample is taken inadvertently when the original intention was to obtain data from the population. For example, when a questionnaire is sent to every pharmacist in the state, there always will be some people who do not respond to the questionnaire, and anything less than 100% response constitutes a sample. A variety of examples of sampling methods is illustrated below.

SAMPLING BY QUESTIONNAIRE—Suppose that questionnaires on the sales of certain drugs were sent to all pharmacists in a state and only 50% were returned. In this type of survey, the results tabulated from such a sample probably would be biased because those who did not return the questionnaire would not be represented in the sample.

It has been shown that persons who respond may have different characteristics from those who do not respond. In this hypothetical example, perhaps unanswered questionnaires were represented largely by pharmacists who had large drug sales and were too busy to answer. In another community, a pharmacist may have little or no sales of the drugs, resulting in a nonresponse. The reason for each unanswered questionnaire is unknown. These unreturned questionnaires cause a bias, the direction and magnitude of which is unknown.

Other potential errors in this type of response that may introduce bias include the way in which the question is asked, the order in which questions are asked, and the psychological interaction between the interviewer and respondent. Questionnaire and survey techniques that can be employed to reduce or eliminate bias in the sample of responses have been proposed by mathematical statisticians.[2]

For example, public opinion polls use certain statistical sampling techniques that not only reduce bias but also optimize the information gathered. The Census Bureau has information about the percentages of men, women, and children in the US in various income and nationality groups, in addition to many other detailed categorizations. A sample may be designed to contain the same proportion of particular group(s) as that in the population. Instead of mailing questionnaires, interviewers may be recruited and assigned quotas of the types of people to interview. The interviewers fill out the questionnaires for each respondent during the interview, ensuring a complete response.

It is not possible to elaborate fully on the various methods of sampling here. One should be aware of problems in sampling, and that a sampling design can be used that will give the limits of error of the resulting compilation for any given cost.[2]

SAMPLING IN THE CHEMICAL LABORATORY—The procedure for gathering data in the laboratory differs from that of the questionnaire. Different kinds of sampling processes include the sampling of material to be assayed chemically or physically, sampling of analytical reagents and instruments when multiple instruments are available, and sampling of analysts, the chemists who will perform the assay.

By way of illustration, several samples may be taken from a large lot of digitalis leaves for the chemical determination of acid-insoluble ash, or drug may be analyzed in samples taken from a blend. For the sample to be representative of the lot, the samples should be taken from different parts of the lot to ensure that every part of the lot is represented. Determinations from five samples taken from the same part of a lot (eg, the top of a container) probably will have values closer together than five samples taken from different parts of the lot (eg, the top, top-middle, middle, low-middle, and bottom of a container). Despite the good precision, the former five samples may give a biased estimate of the average value for the lot. The more heterogeneous the lot, the more effort should be expended in being sure that every part of the lot is represented by a sample. It might be that the granulation having the most drug is in the bottom of the lot; samples all taken from the top would give too low an estimate of average drug content of the lot in this example.

Another aspect of sampling in a chemical determination is the sampling of the chemists who perform the chemical analysis. If a single chemist makes several determinations on portions taken from the same sample of thoroughly mixed material, one expects the results to be more precise than if several chemists made these determinations. Probably the true reproducibility of a method can be indicated only in terms of how closely an analyst at one laboratory can check an analyst at another laboratory on exactly the same material. Thus, due to slight differences in technique, one chemist always might obtain higher results than another chemist. Thus, the technique of chemists will have an effect on the results and the reproducibility of the method.

SAMPLING IN BIOLOGICAL AND CLINICAL EXPERIMENTS—A typical animal experiment might involve determining the temperature response of rabbits to pyrogens. The results of such an experiment constitute a sample of all possible results that could be obtained from the population of all possible rabbits, laboratories, and technicians. Using different rabbits, laboratories, and technicians will give different results, all contributing to the variability or error in the experiment. The differences between results from two or more laboratories are usually greater than differences between results obtained by two or more technicians in the same laboratory.

Concurrent conditions—such as season of the year, temperature, and humidity—sometimes can contribute to the experimental variability. In biological experiments, differences between animals are relatively large, so experiments repeated in the same laboratory with different animals but under otherwise identical conditions will give different results. The use of statistical procedures gives an estimate of the amount of variation to be expected due to animal differences. The same can be said of clinical studies where more than one clinical site is needed to produce reliable, unbiased results.

Appropriate statistical designs and procedures will eliminate or account for potential bias in experiments. This point

Table 12-3. A Short Table of Random Numbers

39	61	09	51	68	81	26	30	52	20	61	41	25
89	35	48	61	72	10	84	34	10	44	72	94	77
37	98	37	56	40	30	70	31	75	03	68	32	15
20	55	68	05	53	73	60	28	96	48	91	81	18

may be illustrated by an extreme example, an illustration of what not to do. A technician wishes to compare two drugs as to their effects on the growth of rats. Thirty rats from a single cage are used; the first 15 rats caught are put on Drug 1 and the last 15 caught are put on Drug 2. The first 15 rats caught are less lively than the last 15, and because they are less lively they very likely differ in size and temperament from the last 15 rats. Thus, the results were biased from the very beginning, and one drug was favored merely because of the method of choosing the animals used for each drug.

Obviously, some method entirely free from subjective influences (unconscious or conscious) should be used. A table of random numbers[3] or computer-generated random numbers commonly is used to assign animals or patients to treatments. Table 12-3 is a short table of random numbers.

Example 4 (The use of the random number table)—Suppose that 10 patients are to be assigned to two treatment groups, five in each group. Table 12-3 can be used to assign patients randomly to groups. Patients first are numbered from 1 to 10. One way of assigning treatments to patients is to read across Table 12-3, and the first five distinct numbers will be assigned to the first treatment. The remaining patients are assigned to the second treatment. A zero will correspond to patient number 10. The first five numbers are 3, 9, 6, 1, and 0. (Note that if a number repeats itself, we skip the number and proceed to the next one.) Therefore, patients numbered 3, 9, 6, 1, and 10 are assigned to the first treatment. If 100 patients are to be assigned to the two treatments, two-digit numbers would be used: reading across, the 50 patients assigned to the first group would be numbered 39, 61, 9, 51, and so on.

There are many ways of using random numbers to ensure randomness in statistical experiments. The number of ways is limited only by the ingenuity of the experimenter. For example, random assignment could be accomplished by assigning patients to Group 1 or 2 as they enter the study, according to the appearance of an odd or even number in the random-number table.

In a biological assay, it often is advantageous to design a dosage schedule to take advantage of the reduced within-animal variation compared to between-animal variation. Because more than one dose may be given to a single animal, the order of dosing also must be designed to account for possible trends in response to consecutive doses caused by changes in the animal with time or due to site of application. This can be illustrated by an epinephrine assay (see *Remington's Practice of Pharmacy,* 14th ed, page 633), where a single dog is given 16 consecutive doses, the order of which is determined by a Latin square design, illustrated by

A	D	B	C
D	C	A	B
B	A	C	D
C	B	D	A

Note that in a Latin square each letter occurs only once in each row and each column of the square. A Latin square design was applied to an assay involving two levels of doses of the standard (high and low doses, s_H and s_L, respectively), and two levels of doses of the unknown (u_H and u_L), where the four doses correspond to the letters, A, B, C and D . The dosage schedule is given in Table 12-4. In this type of design each dose occurs once in each order of administration (eg, each of

Table 12-4. Typical Dosage Schedule for an Epinephrine Assay Using a Latin Square Design

	FIRST DOSE	SECOND DOSE	THIRD DOSE	FOURTH DOSE
First group	u_L	s_H	u_H	s_L
Second group	s_H	s_L	u_L	u_H
Third group	u_H	u_L	s_L	s_H
Fourth group	s_L	u_H	s_H	u_L

the four preparations are represented once in each group). In such an assay equal doses of epinephrine elicit a smaller and smaller rise in blood pressure with each succeeding dose. Therefore, order is important.

In all biological experimentation the design should be planned so that differences in treatment do not coincide with factors that could influence the outcome such as differences in age, weight, sex, dates of administration, and so forth. This is known as *confounding* in statistical jargon. For example, if males are given a control treatment and females are given a comparative active treatment, the differences between treatments are said to be confounded by sex. That is, it cannot be determined if the outcomes observed are due to treatment, sex, or a combination of these factors.

Animals or patients should be assigned to doses or treatments at random, taking advantage of the availability of optimal experimental designs. Fisher[4] has written an excellent book on planning or designing experiments, which explains fully the various types of designs mentioned here. Cochran and Cox[5] detail useful experimental designs and provide complete directions for the analysis of data using these designs. Another book by Cox[6] is less mathematically oriented and comprehended more easily.

DESIGN AND CONDUCT OF CLINICAL TRIALS—

Proof of the efficacy and safety of new drugs or treatments requires testing in human subjects. This is best achieved by carrying out *controlled clinical trials*. The use of a placebo treatment or an established treatment as a *control*, a basis of comparison, usually is necessary. Thus, the effects of treatment with those of a concurrently tested control or placebo are compared. The trial includes an adequate number of patients to allow a reliable projection of the results to future patients. Theoretically, the results cannot be projected beyond the types of severity of disease or the ages and sex of the patients included in the trial, although in practice this is not always the case.

The distribution of variables such as age, sex, differences in diagnosis, and initial severity of disease among treatments may be controlled by *stratification*. Usually patients are assigned to treatments at random, and allowances are made for the effects of the variables by using suitable statistical methods. A restricted randomization procedure is useful if it is desired to insure that about an equal number of patients enter the trial on each treatment. Table 12-5 illustrates a completely randomized design in which 15 patients are allocated at random, five to each of three treatments.

Note that the individual patients in each triad (the groups of three) are assigned randomly to one of the three treatments. Here the randomization is restricted in that each set of three patients when entered must be assigned to Treatments A, B and C. The patients are assigned to Treatments as they enter the trial. The first patient (#1) gets Treatment B. This scheme prevents runs in the randomization where a long consecutive number of patients are assigned to the same treatment. Another example is shown in Table 12-6 for a simple crossover design in which the individual patients take both Treatments consecutively, and are assigned randomly to one of two treatment order groups.

The latter design may be more efficient than a completely randomized design because each patient acts as his or her own control, thus eliminating patient-to-patient variability in the statistical analysis. However, this advantage may be offset if drug carryover effects are present, or if the severity of the dis-

Table 12-6. Crossover Design

GROUP	PATIENT	PERIOD 1	PERIOD 2
I	1 4 5 7 10	A	B
II	2 3 6 8 9	B	A

ease wanes in the second period to the point where treatment differences no longer can be demonstrated.

To be certain that the random allocation is followed strictly and to remove subjective bias on the part of both the patient and the clinical investigator in assessing the effects of the treatments, the clinical trial should be carried out blind. A *double-blind trial* is one in which neither the patient nor the investigator is made aware of the nature of treatment administered.

To ensure that the study remains blinded, all treatments must be packaged as identical-appearing dosage forms. This may require a great deal of ingenuity on the part of the packaging pharmacist, especially with respect to the taste of orally administered liquid products, the color and shape of tablets, and so on. In some cases, the characteristic side effects of the drugs make it difficult to keep a study blind. In these situations, one must rely more heavily on objective measures of response, and less on subjective measures. However, the *placebo effect* may also result in changes in so-called *objective* measure of response.

Federal regulations require that drugs shipped to clinical investigators must be labeled properly with the name of the drug. To keep the study blind, one suggested procedure is to use a two-part tear-off label.

One part is glued to the container and reveals only the patient's study number, the period number, and directions for taking the drug; the tear-off part shows the identity of the drug. The name of the drug is overlaid with a water-washable or erasable ink so as not to reveal the identity of the drug to the investigator. This portion of the label is torn off and stapled to the back of the clinical form. The investigator is instructed to break the code for an individual patient, if necessary, by washing off or erasing the overlaid ink.

Laboratory determinations in clinical studies usually include such measures as complete blood count, liver function tests, and analyses on urine and stool specimens. The occurrence of adverse effects may be recorded as ascertained by inquiry or as volunteered by the patient. It is informative also to determine the severity as well as the frequency of occurrence of adverse effects, and whether the investigator feels the effects were drug related.

Generally, it is more difficult to evaluate clinical data than laboratory animal data. Some of the contributing factors are

- The failure of patients to take the medication as directed and to report for examination at stated intervals.
- Patients' use of ancillary or concomitant medications.
- Incomplete data that may result from patients dropping out of the study for various reasons.

These factors are more prevalent among outpatients than among hospitalized patients. A trial secretary or Clinical Research Associate (CRA) can be of great help in assuring the completeness and accuracy of clinical forms.

Table 12-5. Allocation of Patients in Randomized Design

A	B	C	A	B	C
3	1	2	12	10	11
6	5	4	14	13	15
8	9	7			

THE BINOMIAL AND NORMAL PROBABILITY DISTRIBUTIONS

Statistical conclusions are based on *probability*. The process of *statistical inference* first considers an assumption about the distribution of the population data. If the observed data from the sample collected do not conform reasonably to the assumed distribution, the results are viewed as *significant,* ie, the sample data show significant differences from the assumed distribution. For example, it may be assumed or hypothesized that an antibiotic will cure 80% of the patients treated. If three of six patients are cured with the drug, this is the question: What is the probability that three or fewer of six patients treated will be cured if the probability of a single patient being cured is 80%? If this calculated probability is small, the probability of a cure is probably not 80%, but rather some lesser value.

To compute these probabilities, the properties of the assumed probability distribution must be known. Two important and often-used distributions in statistical theory are the binomial and normal distributions, which are examples of a discrete and continuous probability distribution, respectively. The experiment discussed in the preceding paragraph that related to the cure of patients treated with an antibiotic is an example of one application of the binomial distribution.

THE BINOMIAL DISTRIBUTION—The binomial distribution is applicable to data where one of two mutually exclusive and independent outcomes are possible as a result of a single observation or experimental trial. A patient may be cured or not cured. Only one of these two mutually exclusive events can occur at the time of observation. *Independence,* in this context, means that the probability of a cure for any given patient is 80%, regardless of the experimental outcome of the other patients in the study.

The problem to be solved is to compute the probability that three (or less) of six patients will be cured if the probability of a cure for an individual patient is 0.8, or 80%. The general solution to this problem uses the binomial distribution. If two independent and mutually exclusive outcomes are possible as the result of an experimental trial, the probability of x outcomes of one kind (arbitrarily called *successes*) in n binomial trials (n patients in this example) is

$$P(x) = \binom{n}{x} p^x q^{n-x}$$

where $P(x)$ is the probability of exactly x successes and n is the number of binomial trials.

$$\binom{n}{x} \text{ is } \frac{n!}{(x!)(n-x)!}$$

(! means factorial.   For example $5! = 5 \times 4 \times 3 \times 2 \times 1$.
$0! = 1$ by definition.)
p = probability of success
$q = 1 - p$ = probability of a failure
(note that $p + q = 1$)

Now it is possible to calculate the probability of exactly three successes (cures) in six trials (patients) if $P = 0.8$; ie, the probability of a success or cure is 0.8.

$$P(3) = \binom{6}{3} 0.8^3 0.2^3$$

$$= \frac{6 \times 5 \times 4 \times 3 \times 2 \times 1}{(3 \times 2 \times 1)(3 \times 2 \times 1)} \times 0.512 \times 0.008$$

$$= 20 \times 0.512 \times 0.008 = 0.082$$

Thus, the probability of exactly three cures in six patients is 0.082. This is interpreted to mean that the chance of observing exactly three successes in six binomial trials with $P = 0.8$ is approximately 8 in 100.

There are seven possible outcomes for the treatment of six patients as shown in Table 12-7, an example of a binomial probability distribution defined by $n = 6$ and $P = 0.8$. It lists all the possible outcomes, with the probability of each outcome. The sum of all the probabilities is equal to 1. This distribution is shown graphically in Figure 12-4. A knowledge of this distribu-

Table 12-7. Binomial Distribution for $n = 6$ and $P = 0.8$

NUMBER OF SUCCESSES	PROBABILITY OF OUTCOME	NUMBER OF SUCCESSES	PROBABILITY OF OUTCOME
0	0.0000026	4	0.24576
1	0.001536	5	0.39322
2	0.01536	6	0.262144
3	0.08192		

tion allows a decision to be made as to whether three or fewer cures in six patients is a probable outcome for patients treated with a drug that has a cure rate of 80%. The probability of observing three or less successes (0, 1, 2, or 3 successes) is $0.08192 + 0.01536 + 0.001536 + 0.0000026 = 0.0988$, or about 1/10. Is this sufficient evidence to say that the true probability of a cure for the drug is less than 0.8? This question will be discussed in more detail in the section on *Statistical Inference.*

Table 12-8 lists individual probabilities for $P = 0.2, 0.5,$ and 0.8, for N equal to 6 to 10, inclusive. For probabilities not listed in this table, the student should consult tables of binomial probability distribution[7] or use one of the statistical software packages listed at the end of this chapter.

Exercise 2—Calculate the probability of four successes in six trials for $P = 0.8$.

Answer: 0.246.

The mean of the binomial distribution can be expressed in two equivalent ways. In terms of probability (or proportions), the mean is equal to P, the probability of success. In terms of the number of successes in n trials, the mean is NP. Thus, for the binomial distribution with $P = 0.8$ and $N = 100$, the mean is $P = 0.8$ or $NP = 80$. That is, if 100 patients were treated with the antibiotic that has a cure rate of 80%, one could expect to see 80% or 80 patients cured of 100 treated <u>on the average</u>. The standard deviation of a binomial distribution is $\sqrt{pq}$ or $\sqrt{npq}$, depending on whether one is looking at P or NP, respectively. The standard deviation of the proportion of patients cured of 100 treated in the above example is

$$\sqrt{pq/n} = \sqrt{0.8 \times 0.2/100} = 0.04$$

The standard deviation of the number cured is

$$\sqrt{npq} = \sqrt{100 \times 0.2 \times 0.8} = 4$$

This can be interpreted as follows. If 100 patients are treated, it may be expected that 80 are cured on the average, but in any given experiment one probably would not see exactly 80 cured. The number cured will vary around 80, the mean, with a standard deviation equal to 4.

THE NORMAL DISTRIBUTION—The normal distribution can be considered as the underlying foundation of statistical theory and its applications. It is a continuous probability distribution with values ranging from $-\infty$ to $+\infty$. Each of the infinite number of different normal distributions is defined by its mean and standard deviation. The mean can be any positive or negative value, but the standard deviation must be a positive

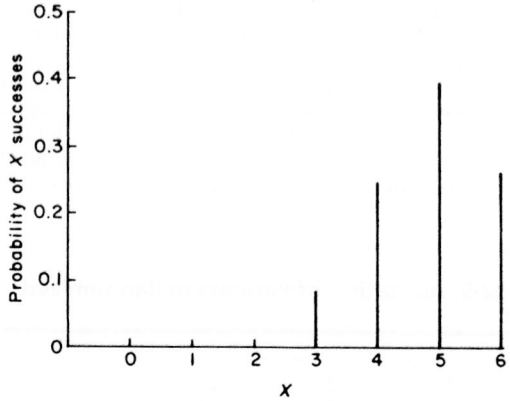

Figure 12-4. Binomial distribution for $n = 6$ and $P = 0.8$.

Table 12-8. Short Table of Binomial Probabilities

	P = 0.2										
	Probability of x successes in n trials										
x	0	1	2	3	4	5	6	7	8	9	10
n											
6	0.262	0.393	0.246	0.082	0.015	0.002					
7	0.210	0.367	0.275	0.115	0.029	0.004					
8	0.168	0.336	0.294	0.147	0.046	0.009	0.001				
9	0.134	0.302	0.302	0.176	0.066	0.017	0.003				
10	0.107	0.268	0.302	0.201	0.088	0.026	0.006	0.001			

	P = 0.5										
	Probability of x successes in n trials										
x	0	1	2	3	4	5	6	7	8	9	10
n											
6	0.016	0.094	0.234	0.313	0.234	0.094	0.016				
7	0.008	0.055	0.164	0.273	0.273	0.164	0.055	0.008			
8	0.004	0.031	0.109	0.219	0.273	0.219	0.109	0.031	0.004		
9	0.002	0.018	0.070	0.164	0.246	0.246	0.164	0.070	0.018	0.002	
10	0.001	0.010	0.044	0.117	0.205	0.246	0.205	0.117	0.044	0.010	0.001

	P = 0.8										
	Probability of x successes in n trials										
x	0	1	2	3	4	5	6	7	8	9	10
n											
6		0.002	0.015	0.082	0.246	0.393	0.262				
7			0.004	0.029	0.115	0.275	0.367	0.210			
8			0.001	0.009	0.046	0.147	0.294	0.336	0.168		
9				0.003	0.017	0.066	0.176	0.302	0.302	0.134	
10				0.001	0.006	0.026	0.088	0.201	0.302	0.268	0.107

value. Figure 12-5 shows two normal probability curves. The normal distribution is characterized by the symmetry about its mean; most of the data cluster around the mean. There are fewer values as the deviation is farther from the mean. The normal distribution is a theoretical probability distribution, not exactly observed in practical situations. However, much data approximate the normal distribution closely enough to make its application useful.

The Central Limit Theorem (CLT) is perhaps the most powerful theorem in statistics. It supports the pervasive use and importance of the normal distribution in statistical analyses. In simple terms, the CLT states that averages or means approach normality as n, the sample size, increases, no matter what the distribution of the individual variables. For data that are close to normal, means from even a small sample size will be approximately normal. For data that have distributions far from normal, larger sample sizes will be needed for the averages to be close to normal. The concept of the CLT is illustrated by the following example.[8]

The outcome of a disease after treatment can be (1) death = 1, (2) not cured but continue treatment = 2, and (3) cured = 3. The probabilities of these three outcomes are 0.1, 0.3, and 0.6, respectively. This distribution is shown in Figure 12-6. This is a discrete distribution (three possible outcomes in a single trial), and it clearly is not normal. Figure 12.7 shows the distribution of means of size 20 ($n = 20$). The means are obtained by treating 20 patients, assigning outcomes of 1, 2, or 3, according to the previous definition, and computing the mean. The distribution shown in Figure 12-7 was constructed from a computer simulation representing outcomes that can be expected in realistic situations. Note that the averages cluster almost symmetrically around 2.5 (the mean), and are beginning to look like a normal distribution. One also should note the small variability of the mean results, most values ranging between approximately 2.2 to 2.7. A single outcome varies from 1 to 3.

The CLT allows the use of statistical methods that assume an underlying normal distribution of the data when dealing with averages of data that do not come from a normal distribution.

COMPUTING PROBABILITIES FROM THE NORMAL DISTRIBUTION—The area under the normal curve is 1 and area represents probability. The probability of observing a single value from a continuous distribution such as the normal is 0. However, one can calculate the probability of observing values in any interval x_1, x_2—designated as $P(x_1 \leq x \leq x_2)$—by computing the area under the curve in that interval. Table 12-9 is a short compilation of cumulative probabilities from the standard normal curve (Fig 12-8) that has a mean of 0 and a standard deviation of 1. Table 12-9 shows the probability of

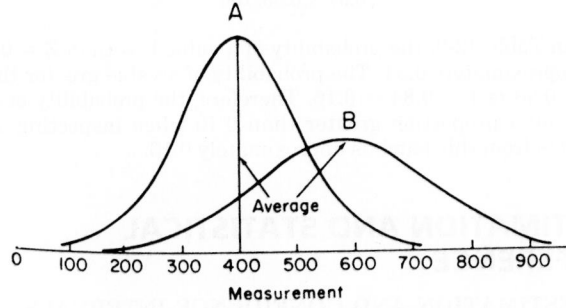

Figure 12-5. Normal probability curves.

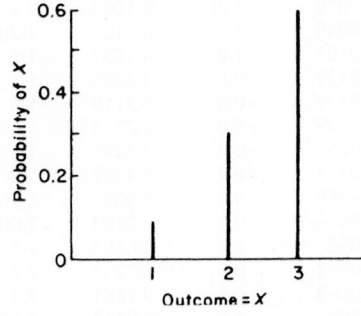

Figure 12-6. Probability distribution of outcomes after drug treatments.

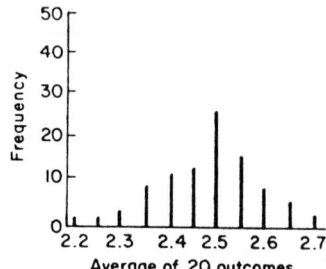

Figure 12-7. Simulation of distribution in Figure 12-6 with average of sample size of 20.

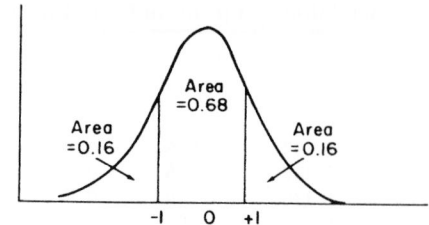

Figure 12-8. Standard normal distribution.

observing a value less than or equal to Z. For example, the probability of observing a value less than or equal to -1 from the standard normal distribution is 0.16. The symmetry of the normal curve indicates that the probability of a value being greater than or equal to $+1$ is also 0.16. Since the total area under the normal curve is 1 and area represents probability, the area less than or equal to $Z = +1$ is $1 - 0.16 = 0.84$. This relationship is illustrated in Figure 12-8. In general, to calculate the area in any interval, Z_1, Z_2, look up the cumulative areas corresponding to Z_1 and Z_2. The difference of the two areas is the area between Z_1 and Z_2, or the probability of observing a value in that interval.

Exercise 3—Calculate the probability of a value falling between -1.96 and $+1.28$ for the standard normal curve.

Answer: The area corresponding to $Z = -1.96$ is 0.025. The area corresponding to $+1.28$ is 0.90. The difference is 0.875. Thus, the probability of observing a value between -1.96 and $+1.28$ is 0.875.

Since there are an infinite number of normal distributions (defined by their means and standard deviations) a reasonable question is, How would one calculate probabilities from a normal distribution that is different from the standard normal distribution? Fortunately, there is a simple transformation that converts data from any normal distribution into the standard normal distribution; Table 12-9 can then be used to compute the probabilities.

The Z transformation is

$$\frac{x - \mu}{\sigma} = Z$$

Example 5—What is the probability that a tablet will weigh between 185 and 210 mg if tablet weights have an approximately normal distribution with mean 200 mg and a standard deviation of 10? Using the Z transformation,

$$(185 - 200)/10 = -1.5$$

$$(210 - 200)/10 = +1.0$$

The cumulative areas corresponding to $Z = -1.5$ and $Z = 1.0$ are found from Table 12-9. These areas are 0.07 and 0.84, respectively. Therefore, the probability of finding a tablet weighing between 185 and 210 mg is $0.84 - 0.07 = 0.77$. Note carefully that the transformation is equivalent to finding a value that is between -1.5 and $+1.0$ standard deviations from the mean (ie, 185 is -15 mg from the mean, which is equal to -1.5 standard deviation units).

What is the probability that a tablet will weigh less than 180.4 or more than 219.6 mg? The Z transformation results in the values -1.96 and $+1.96$. The student can verify that 95% of the values are found in this interval.

Several Z values appear frequently when testing for statistical significance:

- 68% of the values are within ± 1 standard deviation of the mean value.
- 80% of the values are within ± 1.28 standard deviations of the mean value.
- 90% of the values are within ± 1.65 standard deviations of the mean value.
- 95% of the values are within ± 1.96 standard deviations of the mean value.
- 99% of the values are within ± 2.58 standard deviations of the mean value.

NORMAL APPROXIMATION TO THE BINOMIAL DISTRIBUTION—The CLT can be applied to the binomial distribution if n, the number of binomial trials, is sufficiently large. As a general rule, if both np_0 and nq_0 are equal to or greater than 5 (p_0 is the true probability of success), the normal approximation can be used. For binomial distributions with p_0 close to 0.5, the approximation is good for values of np_0 and nq_0 smaller than 5. Under these conditions, $(p - p_0)/\sqrt{p_0 q_0/n}$ is approximately normally distributed with mean 0 and standard deviation 1 (the standard normal distribution). This transformation allows easy calculation of binomial probabilities. The approximation is improved if $1/(2n)$ is subtracted from the absolute value of the numerator. This is known as the *Yates continuity correction*.

Example 6—When inspecting 100 tablets for quality, what is the probability of observing a proportion of defective tablets equal to or greater than 0.10, if the true proportion defective is 0.07? Using the continuity correction,

$$Z = \frac{|0.10 - 0.07| - 1/200}{\sqrt{0.07 \times 0.93/100}} = 0.98$$

From Table 12-9, the probability of a value less than $Z = 0.98$ is approximately 0.84. The probability of a value greater than $Z = 0.98$ is $1 - 0.84 = 0.16$. Therefore, the probability of observing a proportion greater than 0.10 when inspecting 100 tablets from this batch is approximately 0.16.

ESTIMATION AND STATISTICAL INFERENCE

ESTIMATION AND CONFIDENCE INTERVALS—After gathering data from, for example, a survey or an experiment, it is often of interest to estimate the mean value or aver-

Table 12-9. Short Table of Areas for the Standard Normal Distribution (Area for Values Less Than Z)

Z	AREA	Z	AREA	Z	AREA
-3	0.0013	-1.28	0.1003	1.2	0.8849
-2.58	0.0049	-1.2	0.1151	1.28	0.8997
-2.3	0.0107	-1.0	0.1587	1.4	0.9192
-2.2	0.0139	-0.84	0.2005	1.5	0.9332
-2.1	0.0179	-0.8	0.2119	1.6	0.9452
-2.0	0.0228	-0.6	0.2743	1.645	0.950
-1.96	0.025	-0.4	0.3446	1.8	0.9641
-1.9	0.0287	-0.2	0.4207	1.9	0.9713
-1.8	0.0359	0.0	0.500	1.96	0.975
-1.7	0.0446	0.2	0.5793	2.00	0.9772
-1.645	0.050	0.4	0.6554	2.1	0.9821
-1.6	0.0548	0.6	0.7257	2.2	0.9861
-1.5	0.0668	0.8	0.7881	2.3	0.9893
-1.4	0.808	1.0	0.8413	2.58	0.9951
				3.00	0.9987

age of the population. As has been noted, the sample average, $\bar{x}$, is not exactly equal to the population average, μ, but in a well-designed and implemented experiment, $\bar{x}$ should be an unbiased estimate of the true mean. Thus, the best estimate of the true, but unknown, population average is the sample mean $\bar{x}$.

However, the mean of the sample gives no idea of the precision of this average. If the average assay of 10 tablets is 100 mg, it is not known how close this value is to the unknown true value. It would be important to have some estimate of the reliability of the result. *Confidence intervals*, or confidence limits, give an interval that may encompass the mean with a known probability. That is, a 95% confidence interval of 97 to 103 mg means that one would give 19 to 1 odds that the true mean is in this interval. It cannot be said for certain that the true mean is in the interval, but if the experiment were repeated many times and a 95% confidence interval constructed each time, then 19 of 20 such intervals would contain the true mean. For any given experiment, there is no way to tell if the true mean is in the interval, but it is known that the chances are 95% that the true mean is in the interval.

In statistical inference, no statements can be made with assurity. Statistical proofs are not like mathematical proofs. Statistical conclusions are couched in terms of probability. A statement such as "The means are significantly different," means that it is believed that the means are different but there is a chance, albeit a small one, that the conclusion is incorrect. However, the probability of making the wrong decision is known.

Symmetric confidence limits are computed as

$$\bar{x} \pm Z\,(\sigma_{\bar{x}})$$

where Z is an appropriate constant, depending on the probability statement (degree of confidence) associated with the confidence interval. For a normally distributed variable with standard deviation σ known, the value of Z is obtained from Table 12-9. For example, to obtain a 95% confidence interval, ± 1.96 standard deviations covers 95% of the area. For a 90% confidence interval, $Z = 1.65$; for a 99% confidence interval, $Z = 2.58$. Note that if the standard deviation is unknown but estimated from the sample data, the value of Z for normally distributed variables is replaced by t, obtained from the t distribution, which will be introduced in the next section.

Example 7—A drug shows an average blood pressure reduction of 9.8 torr when tested on 100 patients. The standard deviation is known to be 8 torr. A 95% confidence interval for the mean blood pressure reduction is

$$9.8 \pm 1.96 \times 8/\sqrt{100} = 9.8 \pm 1.57$$

A 99% confidence interval is

$$9.8 \pm 2.58 \times 8/\sqrt{100} = 9.8 \pm 2.06$$

Note that if the interval has a higher probability of containing the true mean, the confidence interval is wider.

Example 8—A survey of 1000 pharmacists showed that 30% have more than 15 yr of experience and 70% have less than 15 yr of experience. A 95% confidence interval on the proportion of pharmacists with more than 15 yr of experience is

$$p \pm 1.96\,\sqrt{pq/n} = 0.3 \pm 1.96\,\sqrt{0.3 \times 0.7/1000}$$
$$= 0.3 \pm 0.028$$

This means that the true proportion is between 0.272 and 0.328 with 95% probability.

On rare occasions, a *one-sided* or an *unsymmetrical* confidence interval may be appropriate. One use of a one-sided interval is described under linear regression as applied to stability prediction.

STATISTICAL INFERENCE AND THE *T* DISTRIBUTION—Statistics are used most often as a decision-making tool. The familiar phrase "the difference is statistically significant" results from the application of statistical inference to experimental data. The procedure allows a probability statement to be made about comparative data. Statements made using

this approach cannot be made with absolute certainty. Because experimental results generally come from sample data, one never can be sure of the exact properties of population data. However, decisions can be made with a known probability of error.

Example 9—Consider the estimation of the tablet potency of a batch of tablets based on an assay of 10 individual randomly selected tablets. The assay values (mg) are

$$
\begin{array}{ccccc}
98.6 & 99.3 & 97.9 & 100.3 & 99.6 \\
98.0 & 100.1 & 97.5 & 98.4 & 99.1
\end{array}
$$

The average is 98.88 mg and the standard deviation is 0.954. In this example, an estimate of the mean and standard deviation is obtained from a sample of size 10.

When the standard deviation is unknown but an estimate is available from a relatively small sample, the t distribution is used to describe the distribution of the means. The t distribution may be defined as the distribution of

$$\frac{\bar{x} - \mu}{\text{SD}/\sqrt{n}} = t$$

The t values show a symmetrical distribution centered at 0; ie, the mean is 0. The t distribution is spread out more than the standard normal distribution. Some commonly used points from the t distribution are shown in Table 12-10. The t distribution is defined by degrees of freedom (DF), which in Example 9 is $n - 1$. Note that when the DF are large (ie, n is very large), the values in the t table approach the corresponding values from the standard normal-curve table (see Table 12-9). For example, the value below which 97.5% of the area is found is 1.96 when the DF are infinite in the t table.

When the SD is unknown, values from the t table are used to construct confidence intervals in exactly the same manner as was done using Table 12-9. Table 12-10 shows t values that cut off areas of the t distribution in one tail or symmetrically in both tails of the distribution. For example, the two-tailed 5% points cut off 2.5% of the area in each tail. For DF = 9, t values below -2.262 and greater than $+2.262$ comprise 5% of the area. Conversely, it can be said that the probability of finding a t value between -2.262 and $+2.262$ is 95% for DF = 9.

Table 12-10 gives values for one-tailed probabilities for $P = 0.5\%$ and 2.5%. These values correspond to the two-tailed probabilities of 0.01 (1%) and 0.05 (5%). For example, for 9 DF, the probability of finding a t value greater than $+2.262$ (or -2.262) is 2.5%. Examples throughout the remainder of this chapter should make the use of the t table clear. In the current example of tablet assays, a 95% confidence interval can be constructed using the t distribution. The mean is 98.88 and the sample SD is 0.954. The t value for 95% of the area for 9 DF is 2.262. The 95% confidence interval is

$$98.88 \pm 2.262 \times 0.954/\sqrt{10} = 98.88 \pm 0.68$$
$$= 98.20 \text{ to } 99.56$$

This can be interpreted to mean that the probability is 95% that the true mean of the batch lies between 98.20 and 99.56 mg.

Are you surprised by the narrow limits of the interval based on only 10 tablets? The reason for the tight limits is the small standard deviation. Note that this does not guarantee that the true mean, μ, lies in this interval. As has been emphasized before, statistical statements and conclusions are probabilistic in nature.

T TEST—In addition to estimating the mean assay of a batch of 10 tablets, the 10 assay values were obtained to perform a statistical test comparing the average result to that expected based on the labeled potency of 100 mg. If every one of the 3,000,000 tablets in this batch were assayed, the average potency would be known. The random sample of 10 is representative of the entire batch, but it is extremely unlikely that the sample average exactly will equal the batch average. The question to be asked is, in view of the variability of the 10

Table 12-10. The *t* Table

Distribution of t Giving Both the Two-Sided or Two-Tailed Probability and the One-Sided or One-Tailed Probability According to Degrees of Freedom

DF	ONE TAIL							
	$P = 0.4$	$P = 0.3$	$P = 0.2$	$P = 0.1$	$P = 0.05$	$P = 0.025$	$P = 0.01$	$P = 0.005$
	TWO TAILS							
	$P = 0.8$	$P = 0.6$	$P = 0.4$	$P = 0.2$	$P = 0.1$	$P = 0.05$	$P = 0.02$	$P = 0.01$
1	0.325	0.727	1.376	3.078	6.314	12.706	31.821	63.657
2	0.289	0.617	1.061	1.886	2.920	4.303	6.965	9.925
3	0.277	0.584	0.978	1.638	2.353	3.182	4.541	5.841
4	0.271	0.569	0.941	1.533	2.132	2.776	3.747	4.604
5	0.267	0.559	0.920	1.476	2.015	2.571	3.365	4.032
6	0.265	0.553	0.906	1.440	1.943	2.447	3.143	3.707
7	0.263	0.549	0.896	1.415	1.895	2.365	2.998	3.499
8	0.262	0.546	0.889	1.397	1.860	2.306	2.896	3.355
9	0.261	0.543	0.883	1.383	1.833	2.262	2.821	3.250
10	0.260	0.542	0.879	1.372	1.812	2.228	2.764	3.169
11	0.260	0.540	0.876	1.363	1.796	2.201	2.718	3.106
12	0.259	0.539	0.873	1.356	1.782	2.179	2.681	3.055
13	0.259	0.538	0.870	1.350	1.771	2.160	2.650	3.012
14	0.258	0.537	0.868	1.345	1.761	2.145	2.624	2.977
15	0.258	0.536	0.866	1.341	1.753	2.131	2.602	2.947
16	0.258	0.535	0.865	1.337	1.746	2.120	2.583	2.921
17	0.257	0.534	0.863	1.333	1.740	2.110	2.567	2.898
18	0.257	0.534	0.862	1.330	1.734	2.101	2.552	2.878
19	0.257	0.533	0.861	1.328	1.729	2.093	2.539	2.861
20	0.257	0.533	0.860	1.325	1.725	2.086	2.528	2.845
21	0.257	0.532	0.859	1.323	1.721	2.080	2.518	2.831
22	0.256	0.532	0.858	1.321	1.717	2.074	2.508	2.819
23	0.256	0.532	0.858	1.319	1.714	2.069	2.500	2.807
24	0.256	0.531	0.857	1.318	1.711	2.064	2.492	2.797
25	0.256	0.531	0.856	1.316	1.708	2.060	2.485	2.787
26	0.256	0.531	0.856	1.315	1.706	2.056	2.479	2.779
27	0.256	0.531	0.855	1.314	1.703	2.052	2.473	2.771
28	0.256	0.530	0.855	1.313	1.701	2.048	2.467	2.763
29	0.256	0.530	0.854	1.311	1.699	2.045	2.462	2.756
30	0.256	0.530	0.854	1.310	1.697	2.042	2.457	2.750
40	0.255	0.529	0.851	1.303	1.684	2.021	2.423	2.704
60	0.254	0.527	0.848	1.296	1.671	2.000	2.390	2.660
120	0.254	0.526	0.845	1.289	1.658	1.980	2.358	2.617
∞	0.253	0.524	0.842	1.282	1.645	1.960	2.326	2.576

assays and the average result, can it be ascertained that these 10 tablets came from a population with an average of 100 mg? The solution to this question, an example of statistical inference, is obtained using a simple *t* test. This *t* test consists of the following steps, which can be considered typical in many designed experiments.

Construct a Null Hypothesis—A null hypothesis is an assumption about the parameter under investigation, which is the mean value in this example. The null hypothesis is a statement that assumes that the parameter is equal to some value, usually a null value. That is, the hypothetical value is considered to represent a situation of no change. How to construct the null hypothesis is not always obvious, but a few examples should make this concept clearer.

For the tablet assays, no change means that the population average, μ, is equal to the labeled potency, 100 mg. The null hypothesis is of the following form

$$H_o : \mu = 100 \text{ mg}$$

The statistical test allows a decision to be made: the sample of tablets are or are not representative of a population with mean 100 mg.

Construct an Alternative Hypothesis—An alternative hypothesis makes an assumption about alternative values of the parameter, usually encompassing complementary values. Thus, if H_0 is $\mu = 100$ mg, an alternative could include all values greater than or less than 100 mg. This is a two-sided alternative represented as $H_a : \mu \neq 100$ mg. In some cases, a one-sided alternative may be suitable. This may be expressed as $H_a : \mu > 100$ mg or $H_a : \mu < 100$ mg.

The process of statistical inference will result in one of two possible decisions: either accept or reject the null hypothesis. *Rejection* means the alternative is accepted. For a two-sided alternative, it is anticipated in advance that if the null hypothesis is not true, that the true average

could be either greater or smaller than the hypothetical or assumed value. A one-sided alternative is viable if the alternative only can take on either a lower or higher value than the hypothetical value, or only higher (or lower) values are of interest.

It is not clear always which alternative (one- or two-sided) is correct or appropriate for any given situation. Usually, two-sided alternatives must be considered because, in most situations, smaller and larger values of the parameter are possible and relevant. Some situations where one-sided alternatives may be best will be discussed.

Choose the Level of Significance—The level of significance also is known as the *alpha level* (α) or *error of the first kind*. This is the basis of the well-known statement (eg, the difference is significant at the 5% level). The α error is set in advance and has the following meaning. The level of significance or α error is the probability of erroneously stating that the difference between the observed value of the parameter (the mean in this example) and the hypothetical value is real or significant.

The α error commonly is chosen as 5%, although this is not obligatory. A more conservative approach would be to choose a level of 1%. This would mean that an error of the first kind, ie, erroneously declaring a difference, is only 1%. It will be seen that a larger difference is needed for significance if the α error is made smaller. That is, it is more difficult to find a significant difference.

Beta Error and Power—Usually, only the α error is chosen in advance of the experiment. However, it should be understood that there is a second kind of error that should be considered when making statistical decisions. This error, the *beta error* (β), is the probability of declaring no difference between the observed sample value and hypothesized value of the parameter when, in fact, a difference of size delta (δ) exists. The α level, β error, and sample size are related. Sample-size determination, an important topic, is discussed in most elementary statistics books.[8,9] When it is declared that differences are (or are not) significant, only the α level is considered, and not the β error.

Choose a Sample—The choice of a proper sample and the size of the sample are very important considerations in statistical experimentation and experimental design. The number of objects to be included in the sample is a consequence of the α and β errors. The manner in which samples are chosen will dictate the statistical analysis.

In this simple example, the choice of experimental units (tablets to be analyzed) appears to be uncomplicated. However, further thought reveals many alternatives. Ten tablets are to be chosen from 3,000,000. Some possible sampling schemes include (1) take the first 10 tablets from the batch, (2) take the last 10 tablets, (3) take tablets at regular intervals during the run and select 10 of these tablets at random, or (4) take 10 tablets at random from the entire batch. A random sample is one in which each object has an equal probability of being chosen (see under Sampling for more detail). Random samples will assure a valid statistical analysis.

Random sampling can be visualized as a kind of lottery device, in which all of the tablets are mixed and one selected. In many cases, random sampling is not convenient, or the design can be improved by using variations of random sampling schemes. Although the statistical analysis in the present example assumes a random sample, it would not be convenient to implement this procedure for a batch of 3,000,000 tablets. Scheme 3, above, is a more realistic sampling scheme; although it is not truly random, one can proceed as though it were random for this example. In this case, a sample size of 10 tablets is chosen, not for statistical reasons, but because this number has been written into the quality-control procedure. A better procedure would be to base the number of samples on the α and β levels.[8]

Determine Whether the Test Should Be One- or Two-Sided—In this example, a two-sided test is chosen because the observed average potency could be either lower or higher than the hypothetical value of 100 mg. That is, there is no reason to believe, based on the manufacturing process, that the observed value should deviate on one side rather than the other of the labeled potency.

Make Observations and Construct a *t* Test—Having gathered the tablets and performed the assays, the value of t is computed. This allows one to make the decision, significant or not significant. For a two-sided test, the t value is computed as

$$t_{n-1} = \frac{|\overline{x} - \mu|}{SD/\sqrt{n}}$$

where μ is the hypothetical mean defined by the null hypothesis. In this example, t is

$$t_{n-1} = \frac{|\overline{x} - \mu|}{SD/\sqrt{n}} = \frac{|98.88 - 100|}{0.954/\sqrt{10}} = 3.71$$

The t value then is compared to the t values in Table 12-10 at the specified α level with $n - 1$ DF. For a two-sided test, the absolute value of t is noted, because either small or large values of the difference $(\overline{x} - \mu)$ will lead to significance. If the observed value of t is equal to or greater than the value in the table, the difference between the observed and hypothetical values of the parameter, the mean in this example, is declared to be statistically significant. The value of t for a two-sided test at the 5% level for 9 DF is 2.262, the same value used for the 95% confidence interval. This is no coincidence, as will be shown below. Since the observed absolute value of t (3.71) is larger than the value in Table 12-10 (2.262), significance is declared. The true potency is apt not to be 100 mg, but rather some lower value, based on the observed value of 98.88.

An examination of the equation for t reveals that large differences between the observed and hypothetical mean coupled with a small SD of the mean lead to large values of t. This makes sense, from an intuitive point of view, as large differences with small variability suggest that the difference is real. Also, one should note that had the test showed a nonsignificant difference, it cannot be said with any assurance that the mean of the batch is 100 mg. In fact, it seems extremely unlikely that this should be true. The data simply do not provide sufficient evidence to show that the mean is different from 100 mg. In this case, the confidence interval would give a region in which the mean probably lies.

If the above test had been performed at the 1% level, it still might have been concluded that the mean of the batch was not 100 mg. The value of t at the 1% level with 9 DF from Table 12-10 is 3.25. As 3.71 is greater than 3.25, one would declare significance. A test significant at the 1% level gives greater assurance that the true mean differs from 100 mg, compared to a test significant at the 5% level.

There is a relationship between the two-sided t test and the confidence interval. For example, if the 95% confidence interval does not cover the hypothetical value defined by H_0, the test will show significance and vice versa. This suggests that the true mean is different from the hypothetical mean. In the example discussed above, the 95% confidence interval was calculated as 98.2 to 99.56, which does not cover the hypothetical value 100. Therefore, it may be concluded correctly that the t test will show a significant result at the 5% level. Had the confidence interval included 100, the t test would not be significant.

The example described above is known as a one-sample t test. In this test, the experimental design consists of determining the mean value of a random sample from a single population and comparing the mean to some hypothetical value. Thus, it may be of interest to compare the mean tail-flick value of an analgesic compound in rats to some value that represents activity based on previous experience, or to compare the average assay result of 10 tablets to the labeled amount or to a previously accumulated average, as may be available from quality-control records.

TWO INDEPENDENT SAMPLE *T* TEST—A common design in research involves the comparison of two treatments applied to two independent groups. For example, in a clinical study, a drug is compared to a placebo using 20 patients for the drug treatment and 20 different patients for the placebo treatment. Or the dissolution of tablets prepared by a marketed formulation is compared to the dissolution of tablets prepared from an experimental formulation. Note that this design differs from the one-sample test in that averages are obtained from two groups for purposes of comparison, whereas in the one-sample test, the average of a single group is compared to some hypothetical value.

Three key assumptions are necessary for the two independent sample t test to be valid: (1) each of the two groups are distributed normally, (2) each of the two groups are distributed with the same variance, and (3) the two samples are independent.

The independence assumption is very important. Independent samples mean that the results for any single individual do not influence the results of any other individual. In the case of a clinical trial, independence would mean that the treatment effect for one patient does not influence the result of a treatment for other patients. If one patient discussed the results of his or her medication with another patient in the study, their results would not be independent. If treatments are applied to more than one rat in a cage, their results would not be independent. In the latter case, competition for food and other animal interactions might favor the stronger animal and influence the treatment effect.

Equality of variance also is an important assumption. If the variances are reasonably close, the test should be conducted as usual. As a general rule, if the variances do not differ by more than a factor of four, no special procedure is needed. If the variances differ widely, a modified procedure should be used (the Behrens-Fisher test[10]). The normality assumption is less critical. The CLT results in approximate normality of means of nonnormal variables.

This statistical design consists of randomly dividing n objects into two groups of size n_1 and n_2. Treatment 1 is applied to the first group (n_1) and Treatment 2 is applied to the second group (n_2). Optimal treatment allocation in this design is to have an equal number of experimental units $(n/2)$ in each group if the primary objective is to compare the means of the two groups. However, if n_1 is not equal to n_2, the data are analyzed easily, and not much is lost if the two samples are close in size. In animal and human experiments, samples often are lost due to patient dropouts and animal deaths. An experiment that is carried out according to this plan sometimes is called a *parallel design*—two separate groups are treated in parallel.

The test is similar to the one-sample test. In a typical experiment to compare the mean results of the two samples, the null hypothesis is

$$H_o : \mu_1 = \mu_2$$

A two-sided alternative has an alternative hypothesis:

$$H_a : \mu_1 \neq \mu_2$$

Once the α level (usually 0.05) is specified and data are obtained, a t test is performed. This allows a decision to be made about the equality of the underlying population averages. As in the one-sample case, a value of t is computed as

$$= \frac{\text{Difference}}{\text{Standard error of difference}}$$

For calculation purposes,

$$t = \frac{\overline{x}_1 - \overline{x}_2}{s} \sqrt{\frac{n_1 n_2}{n_1 + n_2}}$$

where

$\overline{x}_1$ = mean of first sample of n_1 observations.
$\overline{x}_2$ = mean of second sample of n_2 observations.

and

$$s^2 = \frac{\sum x_{1i}^2 - (\sum x_{1i})^2/n_1 + \sum x_{2i}^2 - (\sum x_{2i})^2/n_2}{n_1 + n_2 - 2}$$

where

$\sum x^2_{1i}$ is the sum of squares of observations in first sample.
$\sum x_{1i}$ is the sum of observations in first sample.
$\sum x^2_{2i}$ is the sum of squares of observations in second sample.
$\sum x_{2i}$ is the sum of observations in second sample.
s^2 is the pooled variance of the two samples.

Example 10—Suppose one sample of four and one sample of five are taken, respectively, from each of two lots of amobarbital capsules and the amount of amobarbital is determined in each capsule. It is desired to determine if there is a significant difference between the two samples.

$$H_o{:}\mu_1 = \mu_2$$

where μ_1 and μ_2 represent the true averages of the two lots of capsules. This is a two-sided test at the 5% level.

Sample 1	Sample 2
10.1	9.8
13.6	9.6
12.5	11.4
11.4	9.1
$\sum x_{1i} = \overline{47.6}$	$\sum x_{2i} = \overline{50.0}$
$\sum x_{1i}^2 = 573.18$	$\sum x_{2i}^2 = 502.98$
$\overline{x}_1 = 11.90$	$\overline{x}_2 = 10.00$
$n_1 = 4$	$n_2 = 5$

$$s^2 = \frac{573.18 - (47.6)^2/4 + 502.98 - (50.0)^2/5}{4 + 5 - 2}$$

$$= \frac{573.18 - 566.44 + 502.98 - 500.00}{7} = \frac{9.72}{7} = 1.3886$$

$$s = 1.18$$

$$t = \frac{\overline{x}_1 - \overline{x}_2}{s} \sqrt{\frac{n_1 n_2}{n_1 + n_2}}$$

$$= \frac{11.90 - 10.00}{1.18} \sqrt{\frac{4(5)}{4 + 5}}$$

$$= 1.61(1.49) = 2.40$$

The degrees of freedom involved in the pooled standard deviation are 7, DF = $(n_1 - 1) + (n_2 - 1)$. In the t table (see Table 12-10), for $P = 0.05$ and DF = 7 (two tails) the value of t given is 2.365. The value of t calculated is greater than this. Therefore, since the probability of these two samples being drawn from the same population is less than 0.05, we conclude that they were drawn from different populations. (This conclusion may be wrong 5 times in 100.)It can be stated that there is a statistically significant difference between the two samples.

The examples illustrated so far have used a two-sided test. A one-sided test may be used when the difference can only occur in one direction or when only one direction is relevant.

Example 11—A drug is formulated to be dissolved more rapidly by substituting lactose for part of the lipoidal lubricant in the regular-release product. The formulator is convinced that this formulation change only could increase the rate of drug dissolution. A one-sided test at the 5% level is proposed when comparing the drug dissolution from the two

products. The time to 50% dissolution for six tablets of each product (minutes) is

Original product: 25, 22, 29, 30, 26, 24
Modified product: 18, 23, 24, 22, 19, 16

For this test, H_0 and H_a are defined as

$$H_o{:}\mu_1 = \mu_2$$
$$H_a{:}\mu_1 > \mu_2$$

where μ_1 is the 50% dissolution time for the original product.

If the test indicates rejection of the null hypothesis, it must be concluded that the new formulation has a faster dissolution time. If the test shows a nonsignificant difference, it is concluded that the data is insufficient to show that the new formulation reduces the dissolution time. Note that if the data show a longer dissolution time for the new formulation, a test would not be performed, but it would be concluded that the new formulation did not decrease the dissolution time. The average results and standard deviation for the two sets of data are

$$\overline{x}_1 = 26 \quad \overline{x}_2 = 20.33$$
$$\text{SD}_1 = 3.033 \quad \text{SD}_2 = 3.141$$
$$t = \frac{|26 - 19.17|}{3.087/\sqrt{3}} = 3.18$$

Note that the pooled standard deviation is equal to

$$\sqrt{\frac{\text{SD}_1^2 + \text{SD}_2^2}{2}}$$

when the sample sizes are equal in the two groups.

For a one-sided test, refer to one tail of the t distribution. For 10 degrees of freedom $(6 + 6 - 2)$, the t value, leaving 5% of the area in the upper tail, is 1.812 (see Table 12-10). Therefore, it is concluded that the new formulation causes faster dissolution of the drug. Note that it is easier to get significance with a one-sided test. Had the test been two-sided, the t would have had to exceed 2.228 at the 5% level for significance, according to Table 12-10.

PAIRED T TEST—In many situations, the scientist is interested in comparing the means of two experimental treatments using a paired-sample design. This differs from the independent two-sample design in that each of two different treatments may be applied to a single group of experimental units (eg, patients). In a bioavailability study, a generic drug is compared to a standard drug in each of 20 patients. A new analytical method is compared to a previously used method by comparing assay results on different concentrations of the same material divided into two parts.

The paired design has certain advantages over the two independent sample or parallel groups design. It has been noted that significance is determined by the ratio of the difference of the averages divided by the standard error. This ratio can be increased by reducing the standard error. One way is to increase the sample size. Another way of increasing the value of t is to reduce the variability.

In a two independent sample test, the variability is a result of the differences among different experimental units (differences among patients' responses to a drug, for example). In the paired test, the variability results from differences within experimental units. The within-individual variability should be less than the between-individual variability. (Theoretically, the measured between-individual variation includes the within-variation; therefore, the between-variation is larger than the within-variation.) Therefore, the paired-sample design has the advantage of reduced variability.

The paired-sample test also needs less experimental material. In a two independent sample design, comparing the response to two drugs, one might use 24 patients in each of two groups. In a paired design, each patient receives both drugs, on two different occasions if necessary. Thus, there is the need to recruit 24 patients rather than 48. For example, when testing a skin preparation, the products could be applied randomly to each arm of the 24 patients.

The paired design can be used only when there is a natural or easy way of pairing the experimental units. When comparing the dissolution of two different formulations, there seems to be no obvious way of pairing the tablets from the two different formulations, as is the case of applying two treatments to the same individual. In animal experiments, litter mates may be paired. Pairing implies that the paired units are more alike than are two different units. In clinical studies, test units may be paired or matched on the basis of certain characteristics such as sex, age, or severity of disease. Then each subject in the pair is assigned to one of the experimental treatments.

A disadvantage of the paired design is that if treatments cannot be applied concurrently, as may be the case where two drugs administered orally are to be compared, the time to complete the experiment can be extended. In the case of clinical studies, this may be an important detriment because time usually is of the essence. Also, as these studies are prolonged, the chances of patient dropouts increase, and time can influence the progress of the disease.

In the paired design, a missing value means that the single unpaired datum is of no value. In this design, each experimental unit (eg, each patient) essentially acts as its own control. That is, the comparison is made within each experimental unit. If one of the two paired values is missing, a comparison cannot be made.

Another potential disadvantage is that a *carryover effect* may be present. This means that effects from one treatment may affect the results of the other. For example, in a bioavailability study, if the first drug administered is not eliminated completely before the second drug is given, blood levels of the second drug will be contaminated. Or, in a clinical study, the first drug administered may modify the disease condition so that the effect of the second drug is not comparable directly with that of the first drug.

In any event, there are many situations where the advantages of the paired-sample design strongly suggest its use. For computational purposes, the formula is

$$t = \frac{\overline{d}}{s} \sqrt{n}$$

where

$\overline{d}$ = mean of the differences, $x_1 - x_2$, of the n pairs of observations

$$s^2 = \frac{\sum d_i^2 - (\sum d_i)^2/n}{n-1}$$

where

$\sum d_i^2$ = the sum-of-squares of the n differences
$\sum d_i$ = the sum of the n differences
n = the number of differences or pairs of observations

Example 12—The duration of loss of the righting reflex (minutes) was measured in 16 mice following treatment with a barbiturate. The drug was administered in the morning and the afternoon on two different occasions; the order of giving the morning or the afternoon dose was randomized in each mouse. It was desired to test the null hypothesis that the duration of loss of the righting reflex is the same in the morning and the afternoon (Table 12-11).

$$s^2 = \frac{354 - (40)^2/16}{16-1} = \frac{354 - 100}{15} = 16.9333$$

$$s = 4.11$$

$$t = \frac{\overline{d}}{s} \sqrt{n} = \frac{2.5}{4.11} \sqrt{16} = \frac{2.5(4)}{4.11} = 2.43$$

$$DF = n - 1 = 16 - 1 = 15$$

In the t table (see Table 12-10), for $P = 0.05$ and DF = 15 (two tails) the value of t is 2.131. The value of t calculated is greater than this. Therefore, as the probability of the morning and afternoon values being the same is less than 0.05, we conclude that they are different. Apparently, the duration of loss of the

Table 12-11. Loss of Righting Reflex on 16 Mice

MOUSE NO	AM x_1	PM x_2	DIFFERENCE $D = x_1 - x_2$
1	75	73	2
2	86	89	−3
3	93	89	4
4	87	79	8
5	91	95	−4
6	87	81	6
7	76	77	−1
8	83	89	−6
9	87	82	5
10	95	91	4
11	91	87	4
12	86	86	0
13	83	78	5
14	76	69	7
15	82	78	4
16	93	88	5

$\sum d_i = 40$
$\sum d_i^2 = 354$
$\overline{d} = 2.5$
$n = 16$

righting reflex in mice tested on the barbiturate in the morning was longer than when tested in the afternoon.

Note the similarity of the one-sample t test and the paired t test. The test is identical after differences between pairs have been calculated in the paired test. The null hypothesis in the paired test almost always is of the form $H_0{:}\delta = 0$, where δ is the hypothesized difference of the true means. It is hypothesized that the mean results of the two treatments are identical.

TESTS FOR PROPORTIONS—The t test is applicable for continuous data that is distributed normally. Much of the data that is seen in pharmaceutical experiments is dichotomous. That is, answers to a questionnaire regarding filling a prescription for a specified drug may be yes or no, or a bottle of tablets may be acceptable or not acceptable, or a patient may be cured or not cured. Tests similar to the t test may be constructed for binomial data. The principle is to compute proportions that are probable, based on the sample proportion. If the probable proportions do not include the hypothetical proportion, the null hypothesis is rejected.

For large sample sizes (n is large), such computations can be tedious and difficult. Therefore, the normal approximation to the binomial is used whenever possible. Fortunately, in most practical cases, the normal approximation is applicable. When comparing proportions from two independent samples when the normal approximation is clearly not applicable, the Fisher Exact test can be used.[8] (Statistical software programs can compute exact probabilities.) In general, use the rule that np and nq should be equal to or greater than 5 in order to use the normal approximation. In practice, this rule may be relaxed somewhat. When in doubt, a professional statistician should be consulted.

Simple statistical tests for proportions are analogous to the t tests. For a one-sample test, where the hypothetical value defined by H_0 is P_0, the ratio

$$Z = \frac{p - P_o}{\sqrt{P_o Q_o / n}}$$

may be computed, where p is the observed proportion and n is the number of binomial trials, the sample size.

The calculated value of Z is compared to the standard normal distribution, rather than the t distribution. Refer to Table 12-9 or to the last line in the t table, Table 12-10. For a two-sided test at the 5% level, the test statistic, Z, must exceed 1.96 for the difference to be considered significant.

Example 13—A one-sample test for proportions. A questionnaire was sent to pharmacists asking which of two cold medications the pharmacist would recommend to customers. A statistical test was proposed to decide which product was most recommended. The null hypothesis was that the two products, A and B, were recommended equally: $H_0: p_A = p_B = 0.50$. The test is two-sided at the 5% level. Two-hundred and fifty (250) pharmacists responded; Product A was recommended 145 times, and Product B was recommended 105 times.

The scientist conducting the experiment had sent out 400 questionnaires and was rightfully concerned about the nonresponders. However, she decided that there was no reason to suspect a bias because of the lack of 100% response and proceeded to analyze the data. The observed proportion of successes (A is a success) is 145/250 = 0.58 (or the observed proportion could be 0.42 as well). The absolute value of the numerator of the Z statistic will be the same for $p = 0.42$ or $p = 0.58$.

$$Z = \frac{|0.58 - 0.50|}{\sqrt{0.5 \times 0.5/250}} = 2.53$$

Since 2.53 exceeds the tabled value for α of 5% (1.96), it is concluded that Product A is the more recommended product. The normal approximation is improved if $1/(2n)$ is subtracted from the absolute value of the numerator, although the effect of the continuity correction is more evident for small sample sizes. In the present example, the corrected value of Z is 2.47. A 95% confidence interval for the proportion recommending Product A also was reported.

$$0.58 \pm 1.96 \sqrt{0.58 \times 0.42/250} = 0.519 \text{ to } 0.641$$

Exercise 4—Compute Z, with and without the continuity correction, if 141 of 250 pharmacists recommended Product A. Determine whether the result is significant by using a two-sided test at the 5% level.

CHI-SQUARE TEST—To test for differences of two proportions from two independent samples, the chi-square test is used. Chi-square (χ^2) is a probability distribution derived from the sum of squares of normal variables. The chi-square distribution is not symmetrical and can have only positive values. Table 12-12[3] is a short table of chi-square probabilities. This table is used in the same way as the normal and t tables: first compute a chi-square statistic and if the value exceeds the tabled value, a significant effect is declared.

Chi-square is calculated as

$$\chi^2 = \sum \frac{(\text{Observed frequency} - \text{Expected frequency})^2}{\text{Expected frequency}}$$

Example 14—In tossing a coin, 50% tails and 50% heads are expected. Suppose a coin is tossed 40 times and 25 heads and 15 tails are obtained, whereas 20 heads and 20 tails are expected. Is the coin biased or weighted in some way?

$$\chi^2 = \frac{(25 - 20)^2}{20} + \frac{(15 - 20)^2}{20} = 2.5$$

The degrees of freedom (DF) associated with χ^2 are one less than the number of categories. Here $\chi^2 = 2.5$ with 1 DF. The greater the disagreement between expected and observed, the larger will be χ^2. See Table 12-12 for probabilities of getting this value or larger. For 1 DF the probability of getting a value larger than 2.5 is somewhere between $P =$

Table 12-13. Survival Rates in Swine Dysentery

TREATMENT	SURVIVED	DIED	TOTAL
Drug	$a = 25$	$b = 14$	$a + b = 39$
Controls	$c = 21$	$d = 22$	$c + d = 43$
Totals	$a + c = 46$	$b + d = 36$	$N = 82$

0.20 and $P = 0.10$. To say that there is a statistically significant departure from the expected values, χ^2 would have to be larger than 3.84, which is the value for $P = 0.05$ at 1 DF. A value of χ^2 larger than 6.64 for 1 DF would indicate a statistically highly significant ($P < 0.01$) departure of the observed from the expected values.

The chi-square test commonly is used for comparing two percentages in a 2×2 or fourfold contingency table (Table 12-13).

Example 15—Table 12-13 gives the survival rates for drug-treated and control pigs with swine dysentery. The survival rates for the drug-treated and control pigs are $p_D = 25/39 = 64\%$ and $p_C = 21/43 = 49\%$, respectively. To test the null hypothesis that there is no difference in the survival rates of drug-treated and control pigs, χ^2 is calculated:

$$\chi^2 = \frac{(\text{Observed frequency} - \text{Expectancy frequency})^2}{\text{Expected frequency}}$$

The expected values in each of the four cells can be obtained by multiplying the column total by the row total and dividing this result by the grand total. The expected value for Cell a is $46 \times 39/82 = 21.9$. The expected frequencies for Cells b, c, and d are 17.1, 24.1, and 18.9, respectively. Note that the sum of the expected frequencies across any row or column equal the totals for the row or column. For example, the expected frequencies for b and d are 17.1 and 18.9, which sums to 36, the total number who died. The calculation of chi-square is

$$\frac{(25 - 21.9)^2}{21.9} + \frac{(14 - 17.1)^2}{17.1} + \frac{(21 - 24.1)^2}{24.1} + \frac{(22 - 18.9)^2}{18.9} = 1.91$$

The DF associated with an $R \times C$ contingency table $= (R - 1)(C - 1)$, so that for a 2×2 contingency table we have 1 DF. Table 12-12 shows that for 1 DF the probability of getting a value of χ^2 larger than the calculated value 1.91 is greater than $P = 0.10$. Since P is not equal to or less than 0.05, we conclude that there is insufficient evidence to indicate that the survival rates for the drug-treated and control pigs are different.

The chi-square test for comparing two correlated percentages for paired data takes a somewhat different form.

Example 16—Two different types of penicillin were given to each of 22 patients in random order, on successive occasions, and the presence or absence of a detectable blood level was determined (Table 12-14). The percentage of patients with detectable blood levels for the two forms of penicillin are $p_I = 16/22 = 73\%$ and $p_{II} = 8/22 = 36\%$. To test the null hypothesis that there is no difference in the percentage of patients with detectable blood levels for the two forms of penicillin, we calculate

$$\chi^2 = \frac{(|b - c| - 1)^2}{b + c} = \frac{(|10 - 2| - 1)^2}{10 + 2} = \frac{49}{12} = 4.08$$

In Table 12-13 for $P = 0.05$ and DF $= 1$, the value of χ^2 given is 3.84. The value of χ^2 calculated is greater than this. Therefore, as the probability of the percentages for Type I and Type II penicillin being the same is less than 0.05, we conclude that they are different.

Note that this test compares the number of patients who are positive on one test and negative on the other.

The chi-square distribution is an approximation of the discrete distribution represented by the fourfold table. The approximation can be improved by applying a *correction factor* for the Observed − Expected values. If the absolute difference is an exact integer (eg, 4.0), subtract 0.5 from the absolute difference; 4.0 would become 3.5. If the absolute difference has a decimal between 0.5 and 0 (eg, 3.8), change the decimal to 0.5; 3.8 would

Table 12-12. The Chi-Square Table[a]
Probability

DF	$P = 0.20$	$P = 0.10$	$P = 0.05$	$P = 0.01$
1	1.64	2.71	3.84	6.64
2	3.22	4.61	5.99	9.21
3	4.64	6.25	7.82	11.34
4	5.99	7.78	9.49	13.28
5	7.29	9.24	11.07	15.09
6	8.56	10.64	12.59	16.81
7	9.80	12.02	14.07	18.48
8	11.03	13.36	15.51	20.09
9	12.24	14.68	16.92	21.67
10	13.44	15.99	18.31	23.21
20	25.04	28.41	31.41	37.57
30	36.25	40.26	43.77	50.89

[a] Adapted from Fisher RA, Yates F. *Statistical Tables for Biological, Agriculture and Medical Research.* New York: Hafner, 1963.

Table 12-14. Data for Example 16

		TYPE II		
		+	−	Totals
Type I	+	$a = 6$	$b = 10$	16
	−	$c = 2$	$d = 4$	6
Totals		8	14	22

become 3.5. If the decimal is between 0 and 0.5, reduce the absolute difference to its integer value; 4.1 would become 4. In Example 15, the absolute difference of Observed − Expected would be reduced to 3.0. The corrected chi-square would be 1.79.

Exercise 5—Calculate the corrected chi-square for Example 15.

Answer: 1.79.

THE F DISTRIBUTION AND TESTS OF SIGNIFICANCE—The t distribution is suitable for a statistical test comparing two means. The F distribution is used to compare two variances, F being defined by the ratio of the variances, with $n_1 - 1$ DF in the numerator and $n_2 - 1$ DF in the denominator of the ratio

$$F_{n_1-1,n_2-1} = s_1^2/s_2^2$$

Similar to the chi-square distribution, the F distribution consists of only positive values and is a skewed distribution. The ratio of two variances is compared to values in the F table (Table 12-15[11]) with the appropriate DF in the numerator and denominator to test for statistical significance. If the calculated ratio exceeds the value in the table at a given α level, the variances differ at the α level of significance. The following two examples describe the use of the F test for comparing variances for independent and dependent samples.

Example 17 shows a test to compare the variances of two independent samples using the F test. Example 18 shows the test for comparing variances in related or paired samples, which uses the t statistic to determine significance. To compare the variances of samples from two independent populations, the calculation is

$$F = s_1^2/s_2^2 \text{ with } s_1^2 > s_2^2$$

where

$$s_1^2 = \frac{\sum x_{1i}^2 - (\sum x_{1i})^2/n_1}{n_1 - 1} = \text{larger variance}$$

$$s_2^2 = \frac{\sum x_{2i}^2 - (\sum x_{2i})^2/n_2}{n_2 - 1} = \text{smaller variance}$$

To test for significance, the F ratio is referred to the F table (see Table 12-15) with $f_1 = n_1 - 1$ and $f_2 = n_2 - 1$ DF. The null hypothesis that the two variances are the same is rejected at the $2P$ level of significance.

Example 17—Two treatments showed the results in Table 12-16. Entering Table 12-15 with $f_1 = 6$ and $f_2 = 5$ DF, we find that the tabulated values of F are 4.95 and 6.98 for $P = 2 (0.05) = 0.10$ and $P = 2 (0.025) = 0.05$, respectively. Thus, the probability of getting a value of F larger than the calculated value 5.75 is between $P = 0.05$ and $P = 0.10$. Since P is not equal to or less than 0.05, we conclude that there is insufficient evidence to indicate that the two variances are different.

If it is desired to compare the variances from paired data, the F test described above would be inappropriate. Instead, proceed as exemplified below.

Table 12-15. The F Table
10%, 5%, 2.5%, and 1% Points for the Distribution of F

T_2	P	1	2	3	4	5	6	7	8	9	10	20	30	40	60	120	∞
								f_1 DEGREES OF FREEDOM (FOR GREATER MEAN SQUARE)									
5	0.10	4.06	3.78	3.62	3.52	3.45	3.40	3.37	3.34	3.32	3.30	3.21	3.17	3.16	3.14	3.12	3.10
	0.05	6.61	5.79	5.41	5.19	5.05	4.95	4.88	4.82	4.77	4.74	4.56	4.50	4.46	4.43	4.40	4.36
	0.025	10.01	8.43	7.76	7.39	7.15	6.98	6.76	6.68	6.68	6.62	6.33	6.23	6.18	6.12	6.07	6.02
	0.01	16.26	13.27	12.06	11.39	10.97	10.67	10.45	10.27	10.15	10.05	9.55	9.38	9.29	9.20	9.11	9.02
10	0.10	3.28	2.92	2.73	2.61	2.52	2.46	2.41	2.38	2.35	2.32	2.20	2.16	2.13	2.11	2.08	2.06
	0.05	4.96	4.10	3.71	3.48	3.33	3.22	3.14	3.07	3.02	2.98	2.77	2.70	2.66	2.62	2.58	2.54
	0.025	6.94	5.46	4.83	4.47	4.24	4.07	3.95	3.85	3.78	3.72	3.42	3.31	3.26	3.20	3.14	3.08
	0.01	10.04	7.56	6.55	5.99	5.64	5.39	5.21	5.06	4.95	4.85	4.41	4.25	4.17	4.08	4.00	3.91
15	0.10	3.07	2.70	2.49	2.36	2.27	2.21	2.16	2.12	2.09	2.06	1.92	1.87	1.85	1.82	1.79	1.76
	0.05	4.54	3.68	3.29	3.06	2.90	2.79	2.71	2.64	2.59	2.54	2.33	2.25	2.20	2.16	2.11	2.07
	0.025	6.20	4.76	4.15	3.80	3.58	3.41	3.29	3.20	3.12	3.06	2.76	2.64	2.58	2.52	2.46	2.40
	0.01	8.68	6.36	5.42	4.89	4.56	4.32	4.14	4.00	3.89	3.80	3.36	3.20	3.12	3.05	2.96	2.87
20	0.10	2.97	2.59	2.38	2.25	2.16	2.09	2.04	2.00	1.96	1.94	1.79	1.74	1.71	1.68	1.64	1.61
	0.05	4.35	3.49	3.10	2.87	2.71	2.60	2.51	2.45	2.39	2.35	2.12	2.04	1.99	1.95	1.90	1.84
	0.025	5.87	4.46	3.86	3.51	3.29	3.13	3.01	2.91	2.84	2.77	2.46	2.35	2.29	2.22	2.16	2.09
	0.01	8.10	5.85	4.94	4.43	4.10	3.87	3.71	3.56	3.45	3.37	2.94	2.77	2.69	2.61	2.52	2.42
25	0.10	2.92	2.53	2.32	2.18	2.09	2.02	1.97	1.93	1.89	1.87	1.72	1.66	1.63	1.59	1.56	1.52
	0.05	4.24	3.39	2.99	2.76	2.60	2.49	2.40	2.34	2.28	2.24	2.01	1.92	1.87	1.82	1.77	1.71
	0.025	5.69	4.29	3.69	3.35	3.13	2.97	2.85	2.75	2.68	2.61	2.30	2.18	2.12	2.05	1.98	1.91
	0.01	7.77	5.57	4.68	4.18	3.86	3.63	3.46	3.32	3.21	3.13	2.70	2.54	2.45	2.36	2.27	2.17
30	0.10	2.88	2.49	2.28	2.14	2.05	1.98	1.93	1.88	1.85	1.82	1.67	1.61	1.57	1.54	1.50	1.46
	0.05	4.17	3.32	2.92	2.69	2.53	2.42	2.33	2.27	2.21	2.16	1.93	1.84	1.79	1.74	1.68	1.62
	0.025	5.57	4.18	3.59	3.25	3.03	2.87	2.75	2.65	2.57	2.51	2.20	2.07	2.01	1.94	1.87	1.79
	0.01	7.56	5.39	4.51	4.02	3.70	3.47	3.30	3.17	3.06	2.98	2.55	2.38	2.29	2.21	2.11	2.01
40	0.10	2.84	2.44	2.23	2.09	2.00	1.93	1.87	1.83	1.79	1.76	1.61	1.54	1.51	1.47	1.42	1.38
	0.05	4.08	3.23	2.84	2.61	2.45	2.34	2.25	2.18	2.12	2.08	1.84	1.74	1.69	1.64	1.58	1.51
	0.025	5.42	4.05	3.46	3.13	2.90	2.74	2.62	2.53	2.45	2.39	2.07	1.94	1.88	1.80	1.72	1.64
	0.01	7.31	5.18	4.31	3.83	3.51	3.29	3.12	2.99	2.88	2.80	2.37	2.20	2.11	2.02	1.92	1.81
60	0.10	2.79	2.39	2.18	2.04	1.95	1.87	1.82	1.77	1.74	1.71	1.54	1.48	1.44	1.40	1.35	1.29
	0.05	4.00	3.15	2.76	2.53	2.37	2.25	2.17	2.10	2.04	1.99	1.75	1.65	1.59	1.53	1.47	1.39
	0.025	5.29	3.93	3.34	3.01	2.79	2.63	2.51	2.41	2.33	2.27	1.94	1.82	1.74	1.67	1.58	1.48
	0.01	7.08	4.98	4.13	3.65	3.34	3.12	2.95	2.82	2.72	2.63	2.20	2.03	1.93	1.84	1.73	1.60
120	0.10	2.75	2.35	2.13	1.99	1.90	1.82	1.77	1.72	1.68	1.65	1.48	1.41	1.37	1.32	1.26	1.19
	0.05	3.92	3.07	2.68	2.45	2.29	2.18	2.09	2.02	1.96	1.91	1.66	1.55	1.50	1.43	1.35	1.25
	0.025	5.15	3.80	3.23	2.89	2.67	2.52	2.39	2.30	2.22	2.16	1.82	1.69	1.61	1.53	1.43	1.31
	0.01	6.85	4.79	3.95	3.48	3.17	2.96	2.79	2.66	2.56	2.47	2.03	1.86	1.76	1.66	1.53	1.38
∞	0.10	2.71	2.30	2.08	1.94	1.85	1.77	1.72	1.67	1.63	1.60	1.42	1.34	1.30	1.24	1.17	1.00
	0.05	3.84	3.00	2.60	2.37	2.21	2.10	2.01	1.94	1.88	1.83	1.57	1.46	1.39	1.32	1.22	1.00
	0.025	5.02	3.69	3.12	2.79	2.57	2.41	2.29	2.19	2.11	2.05	1.71	1.57	1.48	1.39	1.27	1.00
	0.01	6.64	4.60	3.78	3.32	3.02	2.80	2.64	2.51	2.41	2.32	1.87	1.69	1.59	1.47	1.32	1.00

Adapted from Snedecor GW, Cochran WG. *Statistical Methods*, 7th ed. Ames: Iowa State University Press, 1980.

Table 12-16. Data for Example 17

	A	B
	6	15
	4	4
	3	10
	7	10
	6	5
	4	11
		9
Σx_i	30	64
Σx_i^2	162	668
n_i	6	7
s_i^2	2.40	13.81
f_i	5	6

$$F = s_1^2/s_2^2 = 13.81/2.40 = 5.75$$
$$f_1 = n_1 - 1 = 7 - 1 = 6$$
$$f_2 = n_2 - 1 = 6 - 1 = 5$$

Example 18—A characteristic was measured before and after aging for each of 10 items (Table 12-17). Has the variability changed with aging?

$$\Sigma\,x_B^2 = 2,393.81 \qquad \Sigma\,x_A^2 = 2,252.72$$

$$\Sigma\,x_B x_A = 2,298.92$$

$$[x_B]^2 = 2,393.81 - (148.5)^2/10$$

$$= 188.59$$

$$[x_A^2] = 2,252.72 - (147.2)^2/10$$

$$= 85.94$$

$$[x_B x_A] = 2.298.92 - (148.5)(147.2)/10$$

$$= 113.00$$

$$t = \frac{(|x_B^2| - [x_A^2])\sqrt{n-2}}{2\sqrt{[x_B^2][x_A^2] - [x_B x_A]^2}} = \frac{(188.59 - 85.94)\sqrt{8}}{2\sqrt{(188.59)(85.94) - (113.00)^2}} = 2.476$$

$$DF = n - 2 = 10 - 2 = 8$$

In the t table (see Table 12-10), for $P = 0.05$ and DF = 8 (two tails), the value of t given is 2.306. The value of t calculated is greater than this. Therefore, because the probability of the variance before and after aging being the same is less than 0.05 it is concluded that they are different. Apparently, the variability decreased after aging.

The F distribution is used most often for the comparison of more than two means through the analysis of variance, and is equivalent to the t test if used to compare two means.

ANALYSIS OF VARIANCE (ANOVA) AND EXPERIMENTAL DESIGN—There is almost always more than one way to conduct an experiment to achieve a given objective. It was seen that when comparing the means of two treatment groups, two independent groups or a paired design could be used. For example, in a clinical study, two treatments could be applied to two separate and independent groups of patients, or each patient could take both treatments.

In the paired experiment, a further refinement could be added with regard to treatment order. For example, if drugs cannot be administered concurrently, the order of drug administration can be balanced. Half of the patients receive Drug A at the first administration and the other half receive A on the second administration. The patients who receive A on the first occasion will receive B on the second occasion and vice versa. This is known as a *crossover design*.

An alternative design is to assign each patient an order of administration randomly. In the latter case, it is likely that a balanced allocation would not be achieved, as in the crossover design. In fact, there is always a possibility, albeit a small one, that all patients will receive one and the same treatment first and the other treatment second, a situation that intentionally is avoided in the crossover design.

When more than two treatments are to be used in an experiment, a variety of designs are possible. In these cases, one design usually will be optimal, depending on the nature of the experiment, the treatments, and the experimental units or subjects. A common feature of most good designs is *symmetry*. That is not to say that all good designs are symmetrical. In some special cases, an asymmetrical design may be optimal, but this is not the usual circumstance.

The most simple analysis of variance design is known as a *one-way analysis of variance* (one-way ANOVA) or completely randomized design. This is the ANOVA analogy of the two independent sample t test. In the ANOVA design, there is interest in comparing the means of two or more treatment groups. As has been noted before, in the jargon of clinical trials this design often is one of a class known as parallel-groups designs.

In the following description, an example from clinical trials will be used. However, one should understand that tablets, bottles, or consumers could be substituted for patients and the process is the same: n patients are available for the experiment with t treatments. For example, 150 patients are to be assigned to three treatment groups, one placebo and two actives. The n patients are assigned randomly to the three groups (see the discussion on random assignment). The optimal assignment in the examples discussed in this chapter will result in equal numbers in each group, n/t units per group. Note that n is chosen to be divisible by t. If there are three treatments and $n = 150$, we randomly would assign 50 units per treatment. A loss of observations will not invalidate the analysis, as is also true in the two independent groups t test. Observations are made, and the null hypothesis that all t-means are equal is tested by an ANOVA procedure.

The ANOVA separates the total sum-of-squares, $\Sigma(x_i - \bar{x})^2$, into parts determined by the experimental structure. For the one-way ANOVA, the sum-of-squares consists of the between (among) and within sum-of-squares. The between sum-of-squares (BSS) represents differences among treatments, large values indicating large treatment differences (eg, if the treatment means are identical, the BSS will be 0 on the average). The within sum-of-squares (WSS) represents differences within treatments, or error; ie, the differences among objects (subjects in clinical studies) within a treatment is a measure of the variability of the observations.

An ANOVA table is prepared consisting of source of variation, degrees of freedom, sums-of-squares, and mean square. In the one-way ANOVA, the sources consist of the between, within, and total terms. The sum-of-squares divided by the DF is known as the mean square, between mean square (BMS) and within mean square (WMS) in the one-way ANOVA (Table 12-18).

For a one-way ANOVA, the DF for treatments is $t - 1$. The DF for error (within treatments) is $n - t$, where n is the total number of observations. The total sum-of-squares (SS) is exactly the sum of the between and within sums of squares. The error mean square (WMS) corresponds to the variance for the test, and in the case of two treatments, corresponds to the pooled variance in the t test.

Table 12-17. Measurement Before and After Aging

ITEM NO	BEFORE AGING	AFTER AGING
1	8.3	9.3
2	8.4	10.9
3	14.9	13.2
4	12.2	12.8
5	12.5	16.0
6	15.0	15.2
7	17.1	16.8
8	19.2	16.2
9	22.0	17.9
10	18.9	18.9
	$\Sigma x_B = 148.5$	$\Sigma x_A = 147.2$

Table 12-18. ANOVA for Example 19

SOURCE OF VARIATION	DEGREES OF FREEDOM	SUMS-OF-SQUARES	MEAN SQUARES	F RATIO
ANALYSIS OF VARIANCE				
Between regimens	$t - 1 = 9$	160.54	17.81	8.22
Within regimens	$\Sigma (n_i - 1)^a = 20$	43.33	$s^2 = 2.17$	
Total	$N - 1 = 29$	203.87		

$^a \Sigma(n_i - 1) = N - t.$

The ratio BMS/WMS has an F distribution under the null hypothesis, with $(t - 1)$ DF in the numerator and $(N - t)$ DF in the denominator. If the ratio exceeds the appropriate F value found in the table, then at least two of the treatments tested are significantly different. The computations consist of simple arithmetic, summing individual values and their squares. The following numerical example illustrates the computations and should clarify these concepts. Although it always is useful to practice some calculations, computer programs are available that should be used for most practical situations.

Example 19—Groups of three subjects each were given one of 10 food regimens and showed the weight gains (lb) in Table 12-19. These are unpaired data, and this type of study is referred to as a completely randomized experiment. There are only two sources of variation; the variation between regimens and the variation within regimens, as indicated in Table 12-18. The sums-of-squares are obtained as

$$\text{Total SS} = \Sigma x^2 - (\Sigma x)^2/N = 934 - (148)^2/30 = 203.87$$

$$\text{Between regimens SS} = \frac{(\Sigma x_1)^2}{n_1} + \frac{(\Sigma x_2)^2}{n_2} + \cdots + \frac{(\Sigma x_{10})^2}{n_{10}} - \frac{(\Sigma x)^2}{N}$$

$$= \frac{(7)^2}{3} + \frac{(3)^2}{3} + \cdots + \frac{(16)^2}{3} - \frac{(148)^2}{30}$$

$$= 160.54$$

$$\text{Within regimens SS} = 203.87 - 160.54 = 43.33$$

The mean squares are obtained by dividing the sums-of-squares by their corresponding DF. The mean square within regimens, s^2, is the pooled variance for the 10 samples. Since this is the only variance that can be identified as random sampling error (the mean square between regimens has in addition a component due to the variability among regimens), it becomes the denominator in the F ratio, so that

$$F = \frac{\text{mean square between regimens}}{\text{mean square within regimens}} = \frac{17.81}{2.17} = 8.22$$

To test for significance, the F ratio is referred to the F table (see Table 12-15) with $f_1 = t - 1 = 9$ and $f_2 = \Sigma(n_i - 1) = 20$ DF. We find that the calculated value 8.22 is larger than the tabulated value 3.45 for $P = 0.01$. Therefore, as the probability of these 10 samples being drawn from the same population is less than 0.05 (actually, it is less than 0.01), it is concluded that they are not all the same (ie, not all the means are equal).

MULTIPLE COMPARISONS IN ANOVA—If the F test is significant and more than two treatments are included in the experiment ($t > 2$), it may not be obvious immediately which

treatments are different. Some or all of the treatments may be different. Various multiple-comparison procedures have been proposed to solve this problem. It is not always apparent when a particular procedure is best, given the variety of procedures available. Several of these tests are described here, with discussion of their application. The general procedure is to list the ranked means from lowest to highest and underline the means that are not statistically significantly different from each other. Sometimes brackets or parentheses are used instead of an underline. The procedure is carried out by calculating a 5% allowance, which is defined as the critical difference between means which allows one to reject the null hypothesis ($\mu_i = \mu_j$) and accept the alternative hypothesis ($\mu_i \neq \mu_j$) for any two sample means $\bar{x}_i$ and $\bar{x}_j$ at $P = 0.05$. To calculate the 5% allowance the following data is required.

s^2 = pooled variance from the analysis of variance.
DF = degrees of freedom for the pooled variance from the analysis of variance.
n_i, n_j = the number of observations from which the means $\bar{x}_i$ and $\bar{x}_j$ were determined, respectively.
t = a critical value at $P = 0.05$ which depends upon the DF and the degree of conservatism desired as exemplified by the multiple comparison procedures described below.

Least Significant Difference Procedure—For this procedure

$$5\% \text{ allowance} = t \sqrt{s^2(1/n_i + 1/n_j)}$$

where t is the value of t from Table 12-10 (two tails). This is the least conservative procedure, and assures that the probability that any one comparison is judged to be significant by chance alone is 5%. However, the probability of one or more comparisons being judged significant would be greater than 5%. Applied to the results of Example 19,

$$s^2 = 2.17$$
$$n_i, n_j = 3,3$$
$$DF = 20$$

and $t = 2.086$ from Table 12-10 for 20 DF and $P = 0.05$ (two tails).

$$5\% \text{ allowance} = t \sqrt{s^2(1/n_i + 1/n_j)} = 2.086 \sqrt{2.17(1/3 + 1/3)} = 2.51$$

Thus, any two means differing by 2.51 or more are judged to be different.

Ranked Means

B	A, C	I	J	F, G	D, H	E
1.0	2.3	5.0	5.3	5.7	6.3	9.3

or, (BAC) $(IJFGDH)$ (E).

Any two means underscored by the same line (or included in the same parentheses) do not differ statistically at $P = 0.05$.

Any two means not underscored by the same line (or not included in the same parentheses) are statistically significantly different at $P \leq 0.05$.

Table 12-19. Weight Gains in Ten Food Regimens

	A	B	C	D	E	F	G	H	I	J	(t = 10 REGIMENS)
FOOD REGIMEN											
	2	1	2	4	9	3	6	7	4	4	
	3	2	4	8	8	8	5	6	4	6	
	2	0	1	7	11	6	6	6	7	6	
											Sums
Σx_i	7	3	7	19	28	17	17	19	15	16	$\Sigma x = 148$
Σx_i^2	17	5	21	129	266	109	97	121	81	88	$\Sigma x^2 = 934$
n_i	3	3	3	3	3	3	3	3	3	3	$N = 30$
$n_i - 1$	2	2	2	2	2	2	2	2	2	2	$\Sigma (n_i - 1) = 20$
$\bar{x}_i$	2.3	1.0	2.3	6.3	9.3	5.7	5.7	6.3	5.0	5.3	

Table 12-20. The Q Table
Upper 5% Points, Q, in the Studentized Range

DF	\(k\) (NUMBER OF TREATMENTS)																		
	2	3	4	5	6	7	8	9	10	11	12	13	14	15	16	17	18	19	20
10	3.15	3.88	4.33	4.66	4.91	5.12	5.30	5.46	5.60	5.72	5.83	5.93	6.03	6.12	6.20	6.27	6.34	6.41	6.47
11	3.11	3.82	4.26	4.58	4.82	5.03	5.20	5.35	5.49	5.61	5.71	5.81	5.90	5.98	6.06	6.14	6.20	6.27	6.33
12	3.08	3.77	4.20	4.51	4.75	4.95	5.12	5.27	5.40	5.51	5.61	5.71	5.80	5.88	5.95	6.02	6.09	6.15	6.21
13	3.06	3.73	4.15	4.46	4.69	4.88	5.05	5.19	5.32	5.43	5.53	5.63	5.71	5.79	5.86	5.93	6.00	6.06	6.11
14	3.03	3.70	4.11	4.41	4.64	4.83	4.99	5.13	5.25	5.36	5.46	5.56	5.64	5.72	5.79	5.86	5.92	5.98	6.03
15	3.01	3.67	4.08	4.37	4.59	4.78	4.94	5.08	5.20	5.31	5.40	5.49	5.57	5.65	5.72	5.79	5.85	5.91	5.96
16	3.00	3.65	4.05	4.34	4.56	4.74	4.90	5.03	5.15	5.26	5.35	5.44	5.52	5.59	5.66	5.73	5.79	5.84	5.90
17	2.98	3.62	4.02	4.31	4.52	4.70	4.86	4.99	5.11	5.21	5.31	5.39	5.47	5.55	5.61	5.68	5.74	5.79	5.84
18	2.97	3.61	4.00	4.28	4.49	4.67	4.83	4.96	5.07	5.17	5.27	5.35	5.43	5.50	5.57	5.63	5.69	5.74	5.79
19	2.96	3.59	3.98	4.26	4.47	4.64	4.79	4.92	5.04	5.14	5.23	5.32	5.39	5.46	5.53	5.59	5.65	5.70	5.75
20	2.95	3.58	3.96	4.24	4.45	4.62	4.77	4.90	5.01	5.11	5.20	5.28	5.36	5.43	5.50	5.56	5.61	5.66	5.71
24	2.92	3.53	3.90	4.17	4.37	4.54	4.68	4.81	4.92	5.01	5.10	5.18	5.25	5.32	5.38	5.44	5.50	5.55	5.59
30	2.89	3.48	3.84	4.11	4.30	4.46	4.60	4.72	4.83	4.92	5.00	5.08	5.15	5.21	5.27	5.33	5.38	5.43	5.48
40	2.86	3.44	3.79	4.04	4.23	4.39	4.52	4.63	4.74	4.82	4.90	4.98	5.05	5.11	5.17	5.22	5.27	5.32	5.36
60	2.83	3.40	3.74	3.98	4.16	4.31	4.44	4.55	4.65	4.73	4.81	4.88	4.94	5.00	5.06	5.11	5.15	5.20	5.24
120	2.80	3.36	3.69	3.92	4.10	4.24	4.36	4.47	4.56	4.64	4.71	4.78	4.84	4.90	4.95	5.00	5.04	5.09	5.13
∞	2.77	3.32	3.63	3.86	4.03	4.17	4.29	4.39	4.47	4.55	4.62	4.68	4.74	4.80	4.84	4.89	4.93	4.97	5.01

Adapted from Snedecor GW, Cochran WG. *Statistical Methods,* 7th ed. Ames: Iowa State University Press, 1980.

Studentized Range Procedure—For this method

$$5\% \text{ allowance} = \frac{Q}{\sqrt{2}} \sqrt{s^2(1/n_i + 1/n_j)}$$

where Q is the Studentized Range value for k treatments from Table 12-20.[12] This is one of the more conservative procedures, and it ensures that the probability of one or more comparisons being judged significant by chance alone is 5%. Applied to the results of Example 19,

$Q = 5.01$ from Table 12-20

for $k = 10$ treatments, 20 *DF* and $P = 0.05$.

$$5\% \text{ allowance} = \frac{Q}{\sqrt{2}} \sqrt{s^2(1/n_i + 1/n_j)} = \frac{5.01}{\sqrt{2}} \sqrt{2.17(1/3 + 1/3)} = 4.26$$

Thus, any two means differing by 4.26 or more are judged to be different.

Ranked Means

B	A, C	I	J	F, G	D, H	E
1.0	2.3	5.0	5.3	5.7	6.3	9.3

or, (BACI) (ACIJFGDH) (JFGDHE).

Duncan's New Multiple Range Procedure—For this method:

$$5\% \text{ allowance} = \frac{t_k}{\sqrt{2}} \sqrt{s^2(1/n_i + 1/n_j)}$$

where t_k are values for 2, 3, . . ., k treatments obtained from Table 12-21.[13] The critical values will be $A_2, A_3, . . ., A_k$, depending upon how many means are included in the range of ranked means being compared. This is next to the least conservative procedure. Applied to the results of Example 19,

$$5\% \text{ allowance} = \frac{t_k}{\sqrt{2}} \sqrt{s^2(1/n_i + 1/n_j)} = \frac{t_k}{\sqrt{2}} \sqrt{2.17(1/3 + 1/3)}$$

Values of t_k from Table 12-21 for $k = 2$ to 10 treatments, 20 DF, and $P = 0.05$ give the allowances in Table 12-22. Thus, the critical difference between E and B is 2.89 because the range includes 10 means, the critical difference between E and H is 2.64 because the range includes three means, and so on.

Ranked Means

B	A, C	I	J	F, G	D, H	E
1.0	2.3	5.0	5.3	5.7	6.3	9.3

or, (BAC) (IJFGDH) (E).

Dunnett's Procedure—The three procedures previously described are appropriate when it is desired to compare all possible pairs of means. Dunnett[14] considered the problem when the objective of the study is to compare several treatments with a standard or control. In his method,

$$5\% \text{ allowance} = t_d \sqrt{s^2(1/n_i + 1/n_j)}$$

Table 12-21. The Multiple Range Table
Values of t_k *for Duncan's New Multiple Range Test at the 5% Level of Significance*

DF	\(k\) (NUMBER OF TREATMENTS)								
	2	3	4	5	6	8	10	14	20
10	3.15	3.30	3.37	3.43	3.46	3.47	3.47	3.47	3.48
12	3.08	3.23	3.33	3.36	3.40	3.44	3.46	3.46	3.48
14	3.03	3.18	3.27	3.33	3.37	3.41	3.44	3.46	3.47
16	3.00	3.15	3.23	3.30	3.34	3.39	3.43	3.45	3.47
18	2.97	3.12	3.21	3.27	3.32	3.37	3.41	3.45	3.47
20	2.95	3.10	3.18	3.25	3.30	3.36	3.40	3.44	3.47
24	2.92	3.07	3.15	3.22	3.28	3.34	3.38	3.44	3.47
30	2.89	3.04	3.12	3.20	3.25	3.32	3.37	3.43	3.47
60	2.83	2.98	3.08	3.14	3.20	3.28	3.33	3.40	3.47
100	2.80	2.95	3.05	3.12	3.18	3.26	3.32	3.40	3.47
∞	2.77	2.92	3.02	3.09	3.15	3.23	3.29	3.38	3.47

Adapted from Duncan DB. *Biometrics II* 1948; 1.

Table 12-22. Critical Values using Duncan's Test for Example 19

k	T_k	A_k	k	T_k	A_k
2	2.95	2.51	7	3.34	2.84
3	3.10	2.64	8	3.36	2.86
4	3.18	2.70	9	3.38	2.87
5	3.25	2.76	10	3.40	2.89
6	3.30	2.81			

where t_D is Dunnet's t_D value for k treatments (excluding the standard or control) obtained from Table 12-23.

Like the Studentized Range procedure, this is one of the most conservative procedures, and it ensures that the probability of one or more comparisons between treatments and a standard or control being judged significant by chance alone is 5%. The one-tail values (listed in tables for $P = 0.10$) are used when the objective of the study is to select only those treatments that have higher (or lower) means than the standard or control. The two-tail values (listed in the table for $P = 0.05$) are used when the objective of the study is to select those treatments that are either higher or lower than the standard or control. Of course, the decision to carry out a one-tailed or a two-tailed test must be made before the study begins.

In Example 19, suppose J is a standard regimen, and it is desired to determine which regimens show different weight gains from J. Here, $t_D = 3.07$ from Table 12-23 for $k = 9$ treatments, 20 DF, and $P = 0.05$ (two-tails).

$$5\% \text{ allowance} = t_D \sqrt{s^2(1/n_i + 1/n_j)} \doteq 3.07 \sqrt{2.17(1/3 + 1/3)} = 3.68$$

Thus, any regimen mean that differs from the mean for Regimen J by 3.68 or more is judged to be different from J.

Ranked Means

B	A, C	I	J	F, G	D, H	E
1.0	2.3	5.0	5.3	5.7	6.3	9.3

It would be concluded that B showed a statistically significant smaller weight gain than J, E showed a statistically significantly larger weight gain than J, and there was insufficient evidence to indicate that the other regimens were different from J.

In the same example, if Regimen A is a control group and we knew beforehand that all of the other regimens had to be at least as good as the control or better, it may be desired to select those regimens that are statistically significantly better. We would proceed as follows:

$t_D = 2.60$ from Table 12.23 for $k = 9$ treatments, 20 DF, and $P = 0.10$ (this corresponds to a one-tail $P = 0.05$)

$$5\% \text{ allowance} = t_D \sqrt{s^2(1/n_i + 1/n_j)} = 2.60 \sqrt{2.17(1/3 + 1/3)} = 3.12$$

Thus, any regimen mean that is larger than the mean for Regimen A by 3.12 or more is judged to be better than A.

Table 12-23. The t_D Table
Values of t_D for Dunnett's Procedure for Comparing Several Treatments With a Control at the 5% Level of Significance (Use P = 0.10 Values for a One-Tailed Test and P = 0.05 Values for a Two-Tailed Test.)

DF	P	2	3	4	5	6	7	8	9
10	0.10	2.15	2.34	2.47	2.56	2.64	2.70	2.76	2.81
	0.05	2.57	2.76	2.89	2.99	3.07	3.14	3.19	3.24
11	0.10	2.13	2.31	2.44	2.53	2.60	2.67	2.72	2.77
	0.05	2.53	2.72	2.84	2.94	3.02	3.08	3.14	3.19
12	0.10	2.11	2.29	2.41	2.50	2.58	2.64	2.69	2.74
	0.05	2.50	2.68	2.81	2.90	2.98	3.04	3.09	3.14
13	0.10	2.09	2.27	2.39	2.48	2.55	2.61	2.66	2.71
	0.05	2.48	2.65	2.78	2.87	2.94	3.00	3.06	3.10
14	0.10	2.08	2.25	2.37	2.46	2.53	2.59	2.64	2.69
	0.05	2.46	2.63	2.75	2.84	2.91	2.97	3.02	3.07
15	0.10	2.07	2.24	2.36	2.44	2.51	2.57	2.62	2.67
	0.05	2.44	2.61	2.73	2.82	2.89	2.95	3.00	3.04
16	0.10	2.06	2.23	2.34	2.43	2.50	2.56	2.61	2.65
	0.05	2.42	2.59	2.71	2.80	2.87	2.92	2.97	3.02
17	0.10	2.05	2.22	2.33	2.42	2.49	2.54	2.59	2.64
	0.05	2.41	2.58	2.69	2.78	2.85	2.90	2.95	3.00
18	0.10	2.04	2.21	2.32	2.41	2.48	2.53	2.58	2.62
	0.05	2.40	2.56	2.68	2.76	2.83	2.89	2.94	2.98
19	0.10	2.03	2.20	2.31	2.40	2.47	2.52	2.57	2.61
	0.05	2.39	2.55	2.66	2.75	2.81	2.87	2.92	2.96
20	0.10	2.03	2.19	2.30	2.39	2.46	2.51	2.56	2.60
	0.05	2.38	2.54	2.65	2.73	2.80	2.86	2.90	2.95
24	0.10	2.01	2.17	2.28	2.36	2.43	2.48	2.53	2.57
	0.05	2.35	2.51	2.61	2.70	2.76	2.81	2.86	2.90
30	0.10	1.99	2.15	2.25	2.33	2.40	2.45	2.50	2.54
	0.05	2.32	2.47	2.58	2.66	2.72	2.77	2.82	2.86
40	0.10	1.97	2.13	2.23	2.31	2.37	2.42	2.47	2.51
	0.05	2.29	2.44	2.54	2.62	2.68	2.73	2.77	2.81
60	0.10	1.95	2.10	2.21	2.28	2.35	2.39	2.44	2.48
	0.05	2.27	2.41	2.51	2.58	2.64	2.69	2.73	2.77
120	0.10	1.93	2.08	2.18	2.26	2.32	2.37	2.41	2.45
	0.05	2.24	2.38	2.47	2.55	2.60	2.65	2.69	2.73
∞	0.10	1.92	2.06	2.16	2.23	2.29	2.34	2.38	2.42
	0.05	2.21	2.35	2.44	2.51	2.57	2.61	2.65	2.69

k (NUMBER OF TREATMENTS, EXCLUDING THE CONTROL)

Adapted from Dunnett CW. *Am Stat Assoc J* 1955; 50: 1096.

Ranked Means

B	A, C	I	J	F, G	D, H	E
1.0	2.3	5.0	5.3	5.7	6.3	9.3

It can be concluded that F, G, D, H, and E showed a statistically significantly better weight gain than A, and that there is insufficient evidence to indicate that B, C, I, and J were any better than A.

OTHER ANOVA DESIGNS COMMON TO PHARMACEUTICAL PROBLEMS—A somewhat more complex design is the *two-way ANOVA*. This design is analogous to the paired t test, but consists of more than two treatments; ie, more than one treatment is applied to the same experimental unit (eg, patient) or related units (eg, litter mates, males between 50 and 60 yr, etc). This design has the same advantages and disadvantages as the paired t test described earlier in this chapter. The ANOVA table is similar to the one-way table, but includes some new terms. The between-treatments term has the same interpretation as that in the one-way analysis, representing differences between treatments. A new term, between rows, represents the variability of the units to which the treatments have been applied (eg, patients). Finally, the table contains an error term, sometimes referred to as row $\times$ treatment interaction (patient $\times$ drug in a clinical trial).

The treatment mean square is divided by the error mean square (EMS) to form an F ratio, for purposes of performing a statistical test. Some complications can exist in the interpretation of this table and the F ratios. The examples here consider treatments as including all treatments of interest, and rows as a random selection of experimental units taken from a large population of such units.

For example, to compare a placebo, a generic drug, and a standard drug (three treatments) use a random selection of patients as the experimental units, with each patient to take each of the three treatments. Another example is the comparison of five analytical methods (five treatments) where 10 analysts, selected at random, each perform assays with each method.

Example 20—Three variations of an acne preparation and a control are to be tested for skin irritation. The four products, A, B, C, and the control, each are applied to sites on the backs of eight patients. The assignment of the four products to the four sites on the patient is random; ie, a random assignment of treatments to the four sites on each patient is done for each patient, using a random-number table. The products are applied, and after 24 hr, the degree of irritation is determined by assessing irritation subjectively on a scale of 1 to 10. A value of 1 means no irritation and a value of 10 means extreme irritation. The results are shown in Table 12-24.

The computations are similar to those for the one-way ANOVA. The sum-of-squares for treatments is obtained as before. The sum-of-squares for patients is determined exactly as for treatments except the operation is across rows. This is the same as rotating the table 90° and treating the rows as columns in the table matrix. The EMS (expected sum of squares) is obtained by subtracting the row and column sum-of-squares from the total sum-of-squares. The student may wish to follow the computations for this example, in general, however, the use of a statistical computer program is encouraged, as it is much quicker and eliminates potential arithmetical errors.

$$\text{Total SS} = \Sigma\, x_i^2 - (\Sigma\, x_i)^2/n, \text{ where } (\Sigma\, x_i)^2/n = CT$$

$$= 992 - 170^2/32 = 88.875$$

$$\text{Between treatments SS} = [49^2 = 50^2 + 39^2 + 32^2]/8 - 170^2/32$$

$$= 27.625$$

$$\text{Between rabbits SS} = [21^2 + 14^2 + \ldots 20^2]/4 - CT\ 3705/4 - CT$$

$$= 23.125$$

$$\text{Error} = \text{Total SS} - \text{Between treatments SS}$$

$$- \text{Between rabbits SS} = 88.875 - 27.625$$

$$- 23.125 = 38.125$$

Table 12-25 shows the ANOVA. Since the F ratio for treatments (5.07) exceeds the tabled F value with 3 and 21 DF at the 5% level, it can be concluded that at least two of the treatments differ. Although one may apply one of the a posteriori tests discussed under one-way ANOVA, inspection of the results suggests that results for Treatments A and B are similar and both are greater in magnitude than Treatments C and the control.

CROSSOVER DESIGN—A design that is popular in experimental research is the crossover design. This is in the class of paired-sample or two-way designs in that all treatments are applied to each experimental unit. For example, in practically all human bioequivalence studies, each subject takes all of the treatments. That is, if a control marketed drug is to be compared to two new formulations, each subject takes all three products.

The difference between the crossover and the two-way design (also known as a randomized block design) is that in the two-way design, the order or placement of treatments are assigned randomly to each patient. In the crossover design, an additional constraint, *order* or *balance*, is imposed on the experiment. For example, in a bioequivalence study of three products, these are taken sequentially during three periods. In the crossover design, each product appears an equal number of times in each period.

Table 12-26 shows how three products, A, B, and C, may be assigned to nine subjects in a bioavailability study. Note that Treatments A, B, and C appear exactly three times in each period and that each subject takes all three products. The balancing of order of administration compensates for period effects. If any extraneous variables affect the outcome differently in one period compared to another, all treatments may be affected equally. This would result in a fair comparison of the different treatments. In a purely random assignment of treatments, it would be unlikely that treatments would be assigned in such a balanced order. In an unbalanced design, differences due to periods would not affect treatments equally, resulting in a potential bias and a larger experimental error—the experimental error would include the usual causes of variability plus variability due to period effects. Thus, the crossover design can be considered an improvement over the two-way design in that the error has been reduced and the experiment made more efficient.

Many such designs are available, but care should be exercised to apply the correct design to each experimental situation. The crossover design is related to the Latin square design. Several very good references are available on principles of experimental design. In particular, the book by Cox[6] is recommended

Table 12-24. Skin Irritation Test

RABBIT	TREATMENT A	B	C	CONTROL	Σx	Σx^2
1	7	5	5	4	21	115
2	4	3	5	2	14	54
3	8	9	7	6	30	230
4	8	6	4	5	23	141
5	7	7	4	2	20	118
6	6	7	5	4	22	126
7	5	6	4	5	20	102
8	4	7	5	4	20	106
Totals	49	50	39	32	170	992

Table 12-25. ANOVA for Data of Table 12-24

SOURCE OF VARIATION	ANALYSIS OF VARIANCE DF	SUMS-OF-SQUARES	MEAN SQUARE	F RATIO
Between treatments	3	27.625	9.208	5.07
Between rabbits	7	23.125	3.304	
Error	21	38.125	1.815	
Total	31	88.875		

Table 12-26. Example of Crossover Design

SUBJECT	PERIOD 1	PERIOD 2	PERIOD 3
1	B	C	A
2	A	C	B
3	B	A	C
4	C	B	A
5	A	B	C
6	C	A	B
7	B	A	C
8	C	B	A
9	A	C	B

Table 12-28. ANOVA for Bioavailability Study

SOURCE OF VARIATION	DF	ANALYSIS OF VARIANCE SUMS-OF-SQUARES	MEAN SQUARE	F RATIO
Between subjects	8	29,834.1	3729.3	
Between treatments	2	1,116.5	558.3	3.15
Order	2	264.3	132.1	0.75
Error	14	1,947.2	177.0	
Total	26	33,162.1		

because it is not overly technical and can be understood without resorting to too much mathematics.

Example 21—Three drug formulations were administered to nine subjects in a bioavailability study according to the crossover design illustrated in Table 12-26. The area under the blood level curves were computed for each dosing, and the results are shown in Table 12-27.

The ANOVA (Table 12-28) separates the total variance into four parts: subjects, period (order of administration), treatments, and error.

$$\Sigma\,x_i = 2992 \qquad \Sigma\,x_i^2 = 364{,}720$$

$$\text{Total SS} = \Sigma\,x_i^2 - (\Sigma\,x_i)^2/n = 33{,}162.1$$

$$\text{Subject SS} = \Sigma\,(\text{row}^2)/3 - (\Sigma\,x_i)^2/n = 29{,}834.1$$

$$\text{Treatment SS} = \Sigma\,(\text{treat. sum}^2)/9 - (\Sigma\,x_i)^2/n = 1116.5$$

$$\text{Order SS} = [\Sigma\,I^2 + \Sigma\,II^2 + \Sigma\,III^2]/9 - (\Sigma\,x_i)^2/n = 264.3$$

$$\text{Error SS} = \text{Total SS} - \text{Subject SS} - \text{Treatment SS} - \text{Order}$$

$$\text{SS} = 1947.2$$

Neither treatments nor order are significant (see Table 12-15). For 2 and 14 DF, an F value of 3.70 is needed for significance. Treatment C has a higher average result, but fails to reach significance in this study. In the early days of bioequivalence testing, bioequivalence studies were designed to have a power of 0.8 to detect a difference of 20% between treatments. This means that a sufficient number of subjects should be included in the study so that if a true difference of 20% or more exists between two treatments, there will be at least an 80% chance of finding a significant difference. This method of evaluating equivalence has been replaced by a more meaningful confidence interval approach.[8]

If the crossover design becomes unbalanced, due to dropouts, or other conditions, a computer analysis can be used (eg, SAS).

Another experimental design common in clinical trials is the repeated-measures design, often called a *split-plot design*. For example, two treatments are compared by making observations in two independent groups of patients over time. Although an equal number of patients in each group is desirable, it is not necessary for the data analysis. The observations are made at the same time periods in both groups. The example shows the basic design and ANOVA table. The details of the calculations are not shown. Usually, a software program is used to analyze and summarize the data. The details of the analysis are given in Bolton[8] and Winer.[15]

Example 22—A pilot study to compare the effects of an antihypertensive drug versus placebo was designed with four patients on drug and four on placebo. Blood pressure changes from baseline were measured for 6 weeks at biweekly intervals. The results are shown in Table 12-29.

The ANOVA is shown in Table 12-30. The terms of interest are Treatments and Treatment × Times. The former term measures differences of the overall average results of the two treatments. The error term for Treatments is the mean square for Patients. The Treatment × Times term compares the time trends for the two treatments. The error term for the Treatment × Times effect is Patient × Times (treatments). If the trends are parallel, this term will not be significant. Significance for this term indicates a lack of parallelism, suggesting that differences between treatments depend on the time of observation.

As with most experimental data, a graphic display is recommended. Figure 12-9 is a plot of the average results versus time. The significant difference between treatments ($P < 0.05$) is apparent from the plot and the ANOVA. The time trends of both treatments are similar, and can be explained by the experimental variability (Treatment × Times is not significant).

NONPARAMETRIC TESTS OF SIGNIFICANCE—The validity of the t test for comparing two means depends to some extent (especially for small samples) on the assumptions that the two populations sampled are distributed approximately normally and have essentially equal variances. A procedure for testing the equality of variances has been discussed previously. Statistical procedures that do not depend on the assumption of normality are called nonparametric tests. Three commonly used procedures are the Rank Sum test for unpaired data, and the Signed-Rank Sum and Sign tests for paired data.

Rank Sum Test of Significance—The rank sum test of significance is the nonparametric analog of the two-independent sample t test. The n_1 and n_2 observations are taken from two independent groups. After the n_1 and n_2 observations are arranged in order of size, the combined values are ranked from 1, for the lowest, to $(n_1 + n_2)$ for the highest, and the sum of the ranks T of the n_1 observations in the smaller sample is computed. Values that are tied are given average ranks. Also calculate $T' = n_1(n_1 + n_2 + 1) - T$, and enter Table 12-31[16] with n_1, n_2, and T or T', whichever is smaller. If the calculated T (or T') is equal to or less than the tabled value, the null hypothesis is rejected at the significance level P.

Example 23—Data were available on the duration of loss of the righting reflex (min) for 10 mice given a standard barbiturate and for 11 mice given a test barbiturate (Table 12-32). Entering Table 12-31 with

Table 12-27. Results of Bioavailability Study

SUBJECT	PERIOD 1	PERIOD 2	PERIOD 3	SUM
1	B = 107	C = 102	A = 99	308
2	A = 100	C = 106	B = 89	295
3	B = 98	A = 90	C = 128	316
4	C = 71	B = 54	A = 63	188
5	A = 92	B = 111	C = 107	310
6	C = 113	A = 115	B = 91	319
7	B = 169	A = 187	C = 195	551
8	C = 88	B = 95	A = 77	260
9	A = 122	C = 168	B = 155	445
Period sum	I: 960	II: 1028	III: 1004	2992
Treatment sum	A: 945	B: 969	C: 1078	
Treatment average	105	107.7	119.8	

Table 12-29. Reduction in Diastolic Blood Pressure from Baseline

PATIENT	DRUG WEEK 2	4	6	PATIENT	PLACEBO WEEK 2	4	6
1	10	8	12	2	10	8	12
3	8	6	14	5	6	2	10
4	12	14	8	6	4	0	2
7	10	10	14	8	0	4	10
Average	10.0	9.5	12.0		5.0	3.5	8.5

Table 12-30. ANOVA for Example 22

SOURCE	DF	SS	MS	F
Patients	6	109	18.2	
Treatments	1	140.2	140.2	7.7
Times	2	60.3	30.2	3.5
Treatment × times	2	6.3	3.2	0.4
Patient × times (treatments)	12	104	8.7	
Total	23	419.8		

$n_1 = 10$, $n_2 = 11$, and $T' = 69.5$, we find that the calculated T' value 69.5 is less than the tabulated value 73 for $P = 0.01$. Therefore, because the probability of the standard drug and test drug values being the same is less than 0.05 (actually, it is less than 0.01), it is concluded that they are different. This test compares the medians of the two-populations sampled. The median of an ordered set of observations is defined as the middlemost value for an odd number of observations, and as the average of the two middlemost values for an even number of observations. Thus, the median for the standard drug is $(130 + 148)/2 = 139$ and the median for the test drug is 103.

Signed-Rank Sum Test of Significance—The signed-rank sum test of significance is the nonparametric analog of the paired t test. The differences between the n paired values are ranked in order of absolute size from 1, for the lowest, to n, for the highest, ignoring zero differences. Tied values are assigned an average rank. After the differences are ranked, the signs of the differences are attached to the ranks, and the sum of the positive ranks and of the negative ranks are obtained. Enter Table 12-33 with n = the number of non-zero differences and the sum T of positive or negative ranks, whichever is smaller. When the calculated T is equal to or less than the tabled T, the null hypothesis is rejected at the significance level P.

Example 24—The procedure is illustrated for data given in Example 12 (Table 12-34). Entering Table 12-33 with $n = 15$ and $T = 22.5$, we find that the calculated T value 22.5 is less than the tabulated value 25 for $P = 0.05$. Therefore, because the probability of the morning and afternoon values being the same is less than 0.05, it is concluded that they are different.

Sign Test—The sign test also is used for paired data, but it is not as powerful as the signed-rank test; it is more difficult to find significant differences when they exist with the sign test. Count the number of positive differences (b) and the number of negative differences (c), ignoring zero differences, and calculate

$$\chi^2 = \frac{(|b - c| - 1)^2}{b + c}$$

where $|b - c|$ is the absolute (ie, positive) difference $b - c$.

This is referred to the chi-square table (see Table 12-12) with DF = 1, the test being essentially the same as the chi-square test illustrated in Example 16.

Example 25—The procedure is illustrated for the data given in Examples 12 and 24.

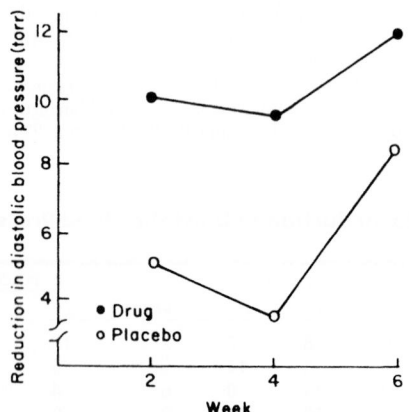

Figure 12-9. Plot of average results for Example 22.

$$b = \text{number of positive differences} = 11$$

$$c = \text{number of negative differences} = 4$$

$$\chi^2 = \frac{(|b - c| - 1)^2}{b + c} = \frac{(|11 - 4| - 1)^2}{11 + 4} = \frac{36}{15} = 2.40$$

Table 12-12 shows that for 1 DF the probability of getting a value of χ^2 larger than the calculated value 2.40 is between $P = 0.10$ and $P = 0.20$. Since P is not equal to or less than 0.05, it is concluded that there is insufficient evidence to indicate that the morning and afternoon values are different. This conclusion is not in agreement with that of the t test and the signed-rank test. The reason for this is that the statistical sign test considers only the sign of the difference and not the magnitude, and thus is a less-sensitive test in borderline situations such as this one.

REJECTION OF ABERRANT OBSERVATIONS—It is common practice among chemists and others working in the physical sciences to make observations in duplicate or triplicate. This is usually done for the purpose both of obtaining a more accurate result and also detecting mistakes in dilution, weighing, and so on. It is quite a common practice to reject the most extreme of the three results if it appears to disagree with the others.

Youden,[17,18] a chemist as well as a statistician, made a study of the problem of rejection of observations in an attempt to answer three questions:

1. If the extreme observation of triplicates is always rejected when only normal variation is present, how accurate is the result?
2. Is the average of the two closest observations as good an estimate as the average of all three?
3. By how much should the outlying observation of triplicates differ from the other two in order to be reasonably assured that this difference is due to a blunder rather than normal variation?

He found that rejection of the outlying observation resulted not only in the variation being greatly underestimated but the mean was biased.

If one wished to follow a simple rule of rejection[17,18] of observations in samples of three so as to reject not more than 5% of the extreme observations arising from normal variation, a rejection ratio of D/d greater than 20 would be required.

$$D/d = 20$$

where
D = difference between the most extreme observation and its closest neighbor
d = difference between two closest observations

In the USP there is an excellent chapter on the design and analysis of biological assays in which are included some tests for rejection of outlying observations. These and other tests can be applied to chemical, as well as, biological assays.[19] Two criteria are presented here, one for rejecting single suspect observations in one group and the other for rejecting a whole group of observations.

To use the first criterion, arrange the observations in the group in order of their magnitude and number them from 1 to n beginning with the supposedly erratic or outlying observation, thus

$$y_1, y_2, y_3, \ldots, y_n$$

where y_1 is the suspect observation. If there are 3 to 7 observations in the group, calculate

$$G_1 = \frac{y_2 - y_1}{y_n - y_1}$$

If there are 8 to 10 observations in the group, and the smallest value seems suspect, again arrange them in order from lowest to highest and calculate

$$G_2 = \frac{y_2 - y_1}{y_{n-1} - y_1}$$

Table 12-31. The Rank Sum Table
Values of T *or* T′, *Whichever Is Smaller, Significant at the 10%, 5%, and 1% Levels*

N_2	P	4	5	6	7	8	9	10	11	12	13	14	15	16	17	18	19	20
8	0.10	15	23	31	41	51												
	0.05	14	21	29	38	49												
	0.01	11	17	25	34	43												
9	0.10	16	24	33	43	54	66											
	0.05	14	22	31	40	51	62											
	0.01	11	18	26	35	45	56											
10	0.10	17	26	35	45	56	69	82										
	0.05	15	23	32	42	53	65	78										
	0.01	12	19	27	37	47	58	71										
11	0.10	18	27	37	47	59	72	86	100									
	0.05	16	24	34	44	55	68	81	96									
	0.01	12	20	28	38	49	61	73	87									
12	0.10	19	28	38	49	62	75	89	104	120								
	0.05	17	26	35	46	58	71	84	99	115								
	0.01	13	21	30	40	51	63	76	90	105								
13	0.10	20	30	40	52	64	78	92	108	125	142							
	0.05	18	27	37	48	60	73	88	103	119	136							
	0.01	14	22	31	41	53	65	79	93	109	125							
14	0.10	21	31	42	54	67	81	96	112	129	147	166						
	0.05	19	28	38	50	62	76	91	106	123	141	160						
	0.01	14	22	32	43	54	67	81	96	112	129	147						
15	0.10	22	33	44	56	69	84	99	116	133	152	171	192					
	0.05	20	29	40	52	65	79	94	110	127	145	164	184					
	0.01	15	23	33	44	56	69	84	99	115	133	151	171					
16	0.10	24	34	46	58	72	87	103	120	138	156	176	197	219				
	0.05	21	30	42	54	67	82	97	113	131	150	169	190	211				
	0.01	15	24	34	46	58	72	86	102	119	136	155	175	196				
17	0.10	25	35	47	61	75	90	106	123	142	161	182	203	225	249			
	0.05	21	32	43	56	70	84	100	117	135	154	174	195	217	240			
	0.01	16	25	36	47	60	74	89	105	122	140	159	180	201	223			
18	0.10	26	37	49	63	77	93	110	127	146	166	187	208	231	255	280		
	0.05	22	33	45	58	72	87	103	121	139	158	179	200	222	246	270		
	0.01	16	26	37	49	62	76	92	108	125	144	163	184	206	228	252		
19	0.10	27	38	51	65	80	96	113	131	150	171	192	214	237	262	287	313	
	0.05	23	34	46	60	74	90	107	124	143	163	182	205	228	252	277	303	
	0.01	17	27	38	50	64	78	94	111	129	147	168	189	210	234	258	283	
20	0.10	28	40	53	67	83	99	117	135	155	175	197	220	243	268	294	320	348
	0.05	24	35	48	62	77	93	110	128	147	167	188	210	234	258	283	309	337
	0.01	18	28	39	52	66	81	97	114	132	151	172	193	215	239	263	289	315

when $n_1 > 20$ and $n_2 > 20$, significance values are given to a good approximation by

$$n_1(n_1 + n_2 + 1)/2 - z \sqrt{n_1 n_2(n_1 + n_2 + 1)/12}$$

where z is 1.64 for the 10% level, 1.96 for the 5%, and 2.58 for the 1%.
The probability figures given are for a two-tailed test. For a one-tailed test, P is halved.

Adapted from Tate MW, Clelland RC. *Nonparametric and Shortcut Statistics.* Danville IL: Interstate Print, 1957.

Table 12-32. Data for Example 23

STANDARD DRUG	RANK	TEST DRUG	RANK
96	4.5	0	1
109	8	91	2
126	13	92	3
130	15	96	4.5
130	15	99	6
148	17	103	7
153	18	117	9
158	19	118	10
169	20	119	11
Died	21	120	12
		130	15
	$T = 150.5$		$n_2 = 11$
	$n_1 = 10$		

$$T' = n_1(n_1 + n_2 + 1) - T = 10(10 + 11 + 1) - 150.5 = 69.5$$

Table 12-33. The Signed-Rank Sum Table
Values of T *for Signed-Rank Test, Significant at the 10%, 5%, and 1% Levels*

	P					P		
n	0.10	0.05	0.01	n	0.10	0.05	0.01
5	0			18	47	40	27
6	2	0		19	53	46	32
7	3	2		20	60	52	37
8	5	3	0	21	67	58	43
9	8	5	1	22	75	65	49
10	10	8	3	23	83	73	55
11	14	10	5	24	91	81	61
12	17	13	7	25	100	89	68
13	21	17	9	26	110	97	75
14	25	21	12	27	120	106	83
15	30	25	16	28	130	116	91
16	35	29	19	29	141	126	100
17	41	34	23	30	152	136	109

Table 12-34. Signed Ranks from Example 24

DIFFERENCES	SIGNED-RANKS
2	2
−3	−3
4	6
8	15
−4	−6
6	12.5
−1	−1
−6	−12.5
5	10
4	6
4	6
0	ignore
5	10
7	14
4	6
5	10

Sum of positive ranks = 97.5
Sum of negative ranks = 22.5 = T
n = 15

If there are 11 to 13 observations, follow the same procedure, but use the statistic

$$G_1 = \frac{y_3 - y_1}{y_{n-1} - y_1}$$

If there are 14-25 observations, follow the same procedure, but use the statistic

$$G_4 = \frac{y_3 - y_1}{y_{n-2} - y_1}$$

If the largest value is open to suspicion as possibly being aberrant, arrange the observations in order from highest to lowest and number them, always labeling the suspect observation y_1.

If the calculated value of G_1, G_2, G_3, or G_4 is larger than the tabled value (which gives the probability of a value being so extreme as that observed), it can be assumed that the observation

Table 12-35. Criteria for Testing Extreme Value

STATISTIC	n, NUMBER OF OBSERVATIONS	CRITICAL VALUES
$G_1 = \dfrac{y_2 - y_1}{y_n - y_1}$	3	.988
	4	.889
	5	.780
	6	.698
	7	.637
$G_2 = \dfrac{y_2 - y_1}{y_{n-1} - y_1}$	8	.683
	9	.635
	10	.597
$G_3 = \dfrac{y_3 - y_1}{y_{n-2} - y_1}$	11	.679
	12	.642
	13	.615
$G_4 = \dfrac{y_3 - y_1}{y_{n-2} - y_1}$	14	.641
	15	.616
	16	.595
	17	.577
	18	.561
	19	.547
	20	.535
	21	.524
	22	.514
	23	.505
	24	.497
	25	.489

truly does not belong to the group and the observation is rejected. The values of G for a probability $P = 0.01$, that an outlier could occur at either end are shown in Table 12-35. This same criterion could be used for testing whether the largest or smallest average in a group of averages differs significantly from the remainder of the averages (Table 12-35).

Example 26—Suppose among the gains in weight of six rats after a feeding experiment, one weight was found to be much less than the other five. Can that observation be discarded? The six gains in weight are 36, 40, 38, 42, 20, and 39.

Rearrange these in order from smallest to largest and label $y_1, \ldots, y_6$, where $n = 6$.

$$
\begin{aligned}
y_1 &\quad 20 \\
y_2 &\quad 36 \\
y_3 &\quad 38 \\
y_4 &\quad 39 \\
y_5 &\quad 40 \\
y_6 &\quad 42
\end{aligned}
$$

$$G_1 = \frac{y_2 - y_1}{y_6 - y_1} = \frac{36 - 20}{42 - 20} = \frac{16}{22} = 0.727$$

Referring to the value of G_1 for $n = 6$ in the table, $G_1 = 0.698$ for $P = 0.01$. Since the calculated value of G_1 is larger than this value, reject the value of 20 and work with the remaining five values.

The second criterion for an aberrant observation as given in the USP compares the variation or range between various groups. It is a test for the homogeneity of the ranges (the range is again the highest value in a group minus the lowest value) and is for the purpose of locating outliers within one group of values. This method and its accompanying table are presented in considerable detail in the USP. The rejection of outliers using only statistical criteria is controversial. A knowledge of the characteristics or properties of the chemical or biological systems being studied should be used when making decisions to reject outlying data.

QUALITY CONTROL METHODS—A very short explanation is given here regarding the quality control methods that were developed primarily by Dr Walter Shewhart of the Bell Telephone Laboratories. A more complete explanation can be found in two short publications of the American Standards Association[20,21] and many texts, including Dixon and Massey.[22]

The quality control method for variables involves plotting the data as dots on a graph with the variable measured on the vertical axis and time (hours, days, etc) on the horizontal axis. The *control* is maintained by inserting on the chart the grand average and control limits that have been calculated from accumulated experience and drawn on the chart as parallel horizontal lines as shown in Figure 12-10. When all the dots fall within the limits, the results are said to be in a state of statistical control. When a dot falls outside the limits, a potential problem is indicated.

In a control chart, usually each dot is an average for a sample consisting of, say, four observations. The standard error of the average then is calculated for each group of four observations, and an average value for the standard error of the average is obtained. This is designated by $s_{\bar{x}}$. The grand average of all the averages plotted also is calculated and is labeled x. The *3-sigma*

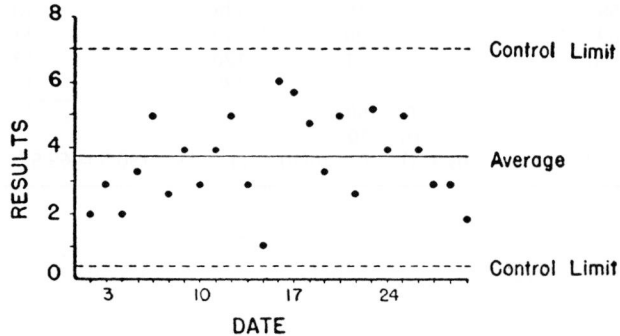

Figure 12-10. A typical quality control chart.

Table 12-36. Calculation of Standard Deviation from Range

SIZE OF SAMPLE (n)	AVERAGE NUMBER OF STANDARD DEVIATIONS IN THE AVERAGE RANGE (d)	SIZE OF SAMPLE (n)	AVERAGE NUMBER OF STANDARD DEVIATIONS IN THE AVERAGE RANGE (d)
2	1.128	7	2.704
3	1.693	8	2.847
4	2.059	9	2.970
5	2.326	10	3.078
6	2.534		

control limits used on the control chart can be obtained from

$$\text{Upper limit} = \bar{\bar{x}} + 3s_{\bar{x}}$$

$$\text{Lower limit} = \bar{\bar{x}} - 3s_{\bar{x}}$$

Thus, it can be seen that the control-chart technique is a graphic means of investigating whether the variation exhibited over a very short period of time is the same as the variation that occurs over a long period of time. If the two variations are identical and all of the plotted dots fall within the control limits, the experiments or processes that produced the data are said to be in a state of *statistical control*.

For many pharmaceutical processes, particularly heterogeneous processes, typical Shewhart control charts do not describe the process adequately. The process seems to not be in control. In these cases, alternative methods should be considered.[23] Control charts are a valuable tool for process validation.

It is possible to calculate the control limits by using the range in each group of four, instead of calculating the standard deviation. This is because, on the average, for samples of less than 10, the range and the standard deviation are related very closely. Given the number of observations in the sample, the standard deviation can be calculated by dividing the range by the appropriate figure given in Table 12-36 for the size of the sample, n. The factors for calculating 3-sigma limits from the range are given as Column A_2 in Table 12-37.

Control charts using 3-sigma limits can be obtained by the use of figures given in Table 12-37. The formulas are

$$\text{Upper limit for averages} = \bar{\bar{x}} + A_2\bar{R}$$

$$\text{Lower limit for averages} = \bar{\bar{x}} - A_2\bar{R}$$

$$\text{Upper limit for ranges} = D_4\bar{R}$$

$$\text{Lower limit for ranges} = D_3\bar{R}$$

$$\text{Where } \bar{R} = \text{average range}$$

These calculated limits are drawn on the charts as described above.

Example 27—A drug manufacturer keeps a record of the uniformity of the machine that is filling a given weight of a drug into ampuls. Samples of the finished product are taken at definite time intervals. The data are accumulated and arranged into groups of four ampuls according to the order in which they were taken from a filling machine. The av-

Table 12-37. Factors for 3-Sigma Limits[a]

SIZE OF SAMPLE (n)	FACTORS FOR $\bar{R}$ CHART		FACTOR FOR $\bar{X}$ CHART A_2
	D_3	D_4	
2	0	3.27	1.880
3	0	2.57	1.023
4	0	2.28	0.729
5	0	2.11	0.577
6	0	2.00	0.483
7	0.08	1.92	0.419
8	0.14	1.86	0.373
9	0.18	1.82	0.337
10	0.22	1.78	0.308

[a] This table contains data from the tables in Appendix 1 of Z1.3—1958.[20]

Table 12-38. Calculations for a Quality-Control Chart
On Averages and Ranges for Samples of 4 from a Filling Machine

TIME	AVERAGE (G)	RANGE (G)	TIME	AVERAGE (G)	RANGE (G)
Jan 6			Jan 7		
8 AM	38.1	1.5	8 AM	37.6	2.1
9 AM	37.6	2.1	9 AM	39.1	1.4
10 AM	38.3	1.1	10 AM	38.5	1.1
11 AM	36.5	2.4	11 AM	37.7	1.9
12 M	38.9	3.1	12 M	38.1	2.3
1 PM	37.8	2.8	1 PM	38.5	2.4
2 PM	38.5	1.7	2 PM	37.6	1.6
3 PM	39.4	1.6	3 PM	37.9	1.8
4 PM	36.4	2.5	4 PM	38.6	1.0

Grand average = $\bar{\bar{x}}$ = 38.1
Average range = $\bar{R}$ = 1.9
Control limits[a] for average = $\bar{\bar{x}} \pm A_2 \bar{R}$ = 38.1 ± 0.729(1.9)
Upper limit = 39.49
Lower limit = 36.71
Control limits[b] for range, are $D_3 \bar{R}$ and $D_4 \bar{R}$ or 0(1.9) and 2.28(1.9) which equal 0 and 4.33, respectively.

[a] A_2 is the factor for using the range to calculate 3-sigma limits for the average (ie, 3 times the standard error of the average). See Table 12-37 for $N = 4$.
[b] D_3 and D_4 are the factors for using the range to calculate 3-sigma limits for the range (ie, 3 times the standard error of the range). These values are taken from Table 12-37. In two instances the point plottings fell below the lower control limit, indicating a lower average fill than one might expect, ie, there is a lack of statistical control.

erage and the range are computed for each group of four as given in Table 12-38 according to the time the samples are taken. The resulting quality-control charts are shown in Figure 12-11.

CONTROL CHART FOR FRACTION DEFECTIVE—The control chart for fraction defective may be applied to results of an inspection that accepts or rejects individual items of a product. It is designed with the same objectives in mind as the $\bar{x}$ and $\bar{R}$ charts. Its most effective use is in the improvement of quality, although it also discloses the presence of assignable causes of variation. It provides management with an effective quality history. Fraction defective, p, may be defined as the ratio of the number of defective articles found in any inspection or series of inspections to the total number of articles actually inspected. This is expressed nearly always as a decimal fraction (Fig 12-12). The formula for the control limits on a fraction defective chart is

$$\bar{p} \pm 3 \sqrt{\frac{\bar{p}(1 - \bar{p})}{n}}$$

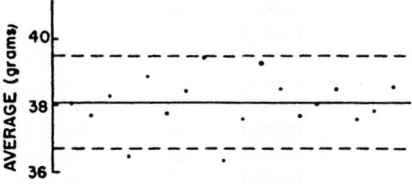

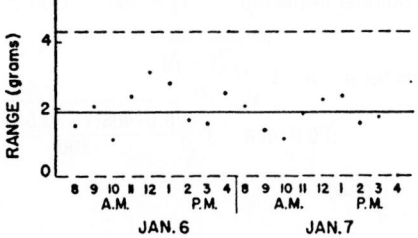

Figure 12-11. Quality control charts for data from Table 12-38.

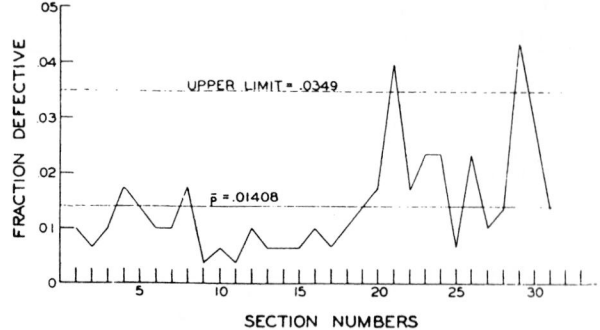

Figure 12-12. Control chart for fraction defective. (Courtesy Lilly)

Example 28—A department head in the capsule department of a pharmaceutical company keeps a record of the number of defective capsules found in sections of large lots of capsules (Table 12-39). Each section consists of approximately 19,000 capsules. In Table 12-39 and Figure 12-12, where points fall above the upper control limit, a greater number of defects are present than may be expected—there is a lack of statistical control. These sections are reinspected carefully and action is taken at the machine to correct the causes of bad quality.

The sample size, *n*, from each section is 300 capsules and typical data are shown in Table 12-39, plotted in Figure 12-12. Note that Sections 21 and 29 appear to be out of control. These sections were subjected to 100% reinspection. Approximately 4.5% of the capsules were defective and were removed.

ACCEPTANCE SAMPLING—Acceptance sampling has become one of the major fields of statistical quality control. It is used in many phases of manufacturing such as inspection of incoming materials, process inspection at various points in the manufacturing operations, and final inspection of the finished product. Sampling inspection usually is used in lieu of 100% inspection for several reasons:

1. The cost of 100% inspection is prohibitive.
2. 100% inspection is fatiguing and may result in the inspectors making errors.

3. The inspection operation may involve destructive testing.
4. A statistical sampling plan well applied may give better quality assurance than 100% inspection.

In sampling one must consider the laws of probability. The risk of rejecting good-quality material and the risk of accepting bad merchandise should be appraised. Sampling plans can be designed and applied in such a manner as to reduce these risks to a minimum and, over a period of time, give assurance of quality products.

The graph illustrating the performance of a sampling plan (ie, ability to discriminate between acceptable and unacceptable lots) is called an *operating characteristic curve* (OC curve). For any given quality of submitted material it is possible to determine the probability of acceptance.

Figure 12-13 is an example of an OC curve for the sampling plan described in Example 29. The government publication MIL-STD-105E[24] gives many different sampling plans with their corresponding OC curves. A plan that is appropriate for a product is chosen depending on lot size and seriousness of the defect.

Example 29—Example of a *statistical sampling plan*. A pharmaceutical manufacturer receives empty bottles of a particular size from a supplier in lots of 20,000 bottles each. The drug firm would like the producer to submit material that is not more than 1.0% defective most of the time, or specifically 95% of the time. See point *A*, Figure 12-13. However, the pharmaceutical firm has agreed to take one chance in 10 of accepting a lot that is 2.6% defective. See point *B*, Figure 12-13.

The acceptance sampling plan that complies with these specifications is as follows. Take a random sample of 540 bottles. Inspect the bottles for defectives. If zero to nine bottles are found defective, accept the lot; if 10 or more defectives are found, reject the lot. The operating characteristic curve for this plan is illustrated in Figure 12-13.[24]

One also can see that, using this sampling plan, submitted lots having 0.5% defective will be accepted about 99 times in 100 (probability of acceptance = 0.99) and thus rejected about one time in 100. Submitted lots having 1.75% defective will be accepted 50 times in 100 (probability of acceptance = 0.50) and rejected half the time.

STATISTICS OF THE STRAIGHT LINE—The use of straight lines to illustrate and define relationships or to help interpret data is common in research investigations. In phar-

Table 12-39. Data Collected from the Process in Example 28

SECTION NUMBER	NUMBER DEFECTIVES	FRACTION DEFECTIVE	SECTION NUMBER	NUMBER DEFECTIVES	FRACTION DEFECTIVE
1	3	0.01	17	2	0.0067
2	2	0.0067	18	3	0.01
3	3	0.01	19	4	0.0133
4	5	0.0167	20	5	0.0167
5	4	0.0133	21	12	0.04
6	3	0.01	22	5	0.0167
7	3	0.01	23	7	0.0233
8	5	0.0167	24	7	0.0233
9	1	0.0033	25	2	0.0067
10	2	0.0067	26	7	0.0233
11	1	0.0033	27	3	0.01
12	3	0.01	28	4	0.0133
13	2	0.0067	29	13	0.0433
14	2	0.0067	30	9	0.03
15	2	0.0067	31	4	0.0133
16	3	0.01			

$$\bar{p} = \frac{\text{Total number of defectives}}{\text{Total number inspected}} = \frac{131}{31 \times 300} = \frac{131}{9300} = 0.01408$$

Control limits for $\bar{p} = \bar{p} \pm 3 \sqrt{\frac{\bar{p}(1-\bar{p})}{n}}$

$$= 0.01408 \pm 3 \sqrt{\frac{0.01408(1-0.01408)}{300}}$$

Upper limit = 0.0349
Lower limit = 0

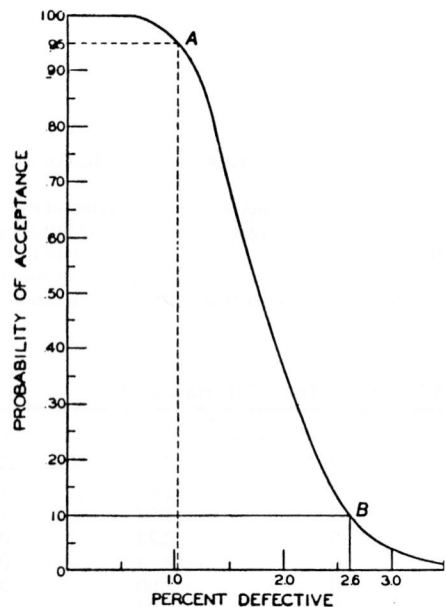

Figure 12-13. Operating characteristic curve. (From *Military Sampling Procedures and Tables for Inspection by Attributes*. MIL-STD-105E. Washington DC: USGPO, 1989.)

maceutical research, straight lines may be used for predictive purposes in stability studies, or to estimate future events such as sales figures in market research studies. Straight lines are found in many theoretical relationships in physical and biological chemistry. First-order and zero-order kinetics can be expressed in a linear fashion. Michaelis-Menten kinetics and the Arrhenius relationship can be transformed to a linear form. Dose-response curves often are linearized if the response is plotted versus log dose. In fact, it is almost always desirable to express a relationship in the form of a straight line, if at all possible.

Reasons for the desirability of straight-line relationships include the ease of extrapolation and interpolation as well as the simplification of the determination of the parameters of the line, the slope and the intercept. The straight line is defined by these two parameters and these often have biological and/or physical significance. Consider the example of a first-order kinetic relationship

$$C = C_0 e^{-kt}$$

where

C = concentration at time t
C_0 = concentration at time 0
k = first-order rate constant

This equation is not linear—a plot of C versus t will not result in a straight line. If the experimental data are gathered for C as a function of time, one usually is interested in defining the first-order relationship, in particular to evaluate the *constants* (sometimes called parameters) k and C_0. This is done most easily by linearizing the equation using a logarithmic (log) relationship. Using log to the base 10, the following linear relationship is obtained.

$$\log C = \log C_0 - kt/2.3$$

This has the form of a straight line. The general equation of a straight line can be expressed as

$$y = a + bx$$

where

y is the dependent variable.
a is the Y intercept (the value of y when $x = 0$).
b is the slope of the line.
x is the independent variable.

Figure 12-14 shows this linear relationship and calculation of the parameters.

The linearized first-order kinetic equation will show a straight line when log C is plotted versus time, with intercept log C_0 and slope $-k/2.3$. The linearized form makes it easy to obtain the values of C_0 and k. C_0 is the antilog of the intercept, log C_0, and $k = -2.3 \times$ slope.

One of the problems in estimating these values from real data is the variability; a plot does not clearly define a straight line. If variability is large, it may be very difficult to decide how to draw the line. Figure 12-15 shows real data from a pharma-

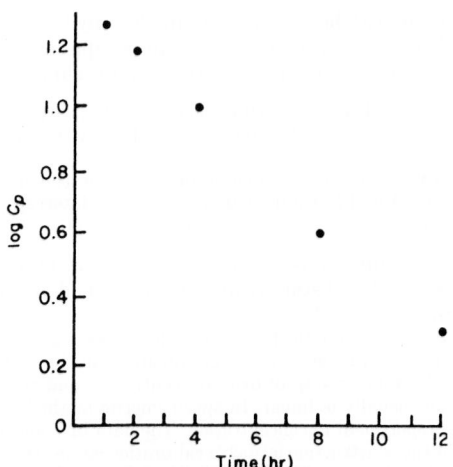

Figure 12-15. Drug plasma levels following an intravenous bolus dose of a drug.

cokinetic study where plasma drug concentrations are measured following an intravenous bolus injection of drug (a one-compartment model).

When confronted with a relationship that should be linear from a theoretical viewpoint but where the x,y values do not lie exactly on a single line, the lack of an exact fit will be considered to be due to variability (error) in y (the dependent variable). In most cases that are encountered, the x variable (the independent variable) tends to have little error relative to the y variable. For example, in a dose-response relationship, the drug is carefully prepared so that an almost unerring dose is administered. However, the response is unpredictable due to the biological variability of the natural material (eg, animals or bacteria). In a kinetic study, the x variable, time, can be measured with great accuracy. The dependent variable, concentration, is variable due to analytical error, for example. The best line for such variable data is called the least-squares (LS) line. This line is such that the sum of the squared deviations of each point from the line is minimized. That is, if the vertical distance from each point to the LS line is calculated, and the squares of these distances are summed, the LS line would minimize the sum-of-squares. Using methods of calculus, one easily can show that the slope and intercept of the LS line are as follows.[25]

$$b = \frac{\Sigma\, x_i y_i - \Sigma\, x_i \Sigma\, y_i / n}{\Sigma (x_i - \overline{x})^2}$$

$$a = \overline{y} - b\overline{x}$$

Example 30—Consider the data from Figure 12-15. See Table 12-40. The equation of the LS line is

$$\text{Log (Concentration)} = 1.345 - 0.0886\,(\text{Time})$$

$$k = -2.3(-0.0886) = 0.204$$

$$\therefore C = 22.1\, e^{-0.204t}$$

Table 12-40. Concentration vs Time for Example 30

Time (x)	1 hr	2 hr	4 hr	8 hr	12 hr
Concentration (μg/mL)	18	15	10	4	2
Log concentration	1.255	1.176	1.000	0.602	0.301

$$b = \frac{16.036 - 27(4.334)/5}{229 - 27^2/5} = -0.0886$$

$$a = 0.8669 + 0.0886\,(5.4) = 1.34534$$

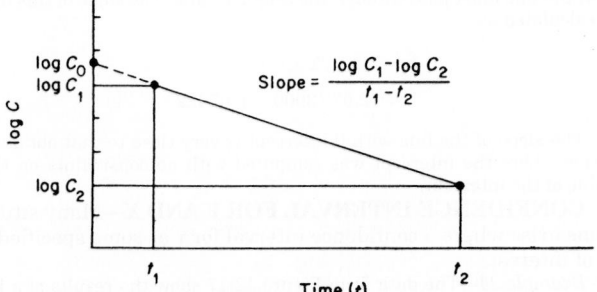

Figure 12-14. Plot of log C versus time.

This procedure can be used to fit a line for any two variables. If statistical inference procedures are to be applied to the line, certain assumptions about the data are necessary.

1. The x variable is measured without error. In practical situations, the error in x should be small compared to the error in the y variable.
2. The y variable is distributed normally with a true mean equal to $A + Bx$ (A and B are the true values of the intercept and slope) and with the same variance, σ^2, at all values of x.

With these assumptions, the confidence intervals for the line can be computed and statistical tests performed on the parameter estimates, a and b.

Example 31—In analytical procedures for drugs, a calibration curve often is constructed using known concentrations of the material to be analyzed. The relationship of drug concentration and the analytical measurement usually is linear. In spectrometric methods, absorption usually is proportional to concentration. The data in Table 12-41 were obtained for the construction of such a calibration curve. These data and the LS line are plotted in Figure 12-16. The LS slope, b, is

$$(72.67 - 2.421 \times 100/4)/500 = 0.02429$$

The LS intercept, a, is

$$0.60525 - 0.02429(25) = -0.002$$

The estimate of the variance of y, $s^2_{y.x}$ is

$$s^2_{y.x} = \frac{\Sigma\, y_i^2 - (\Sigma\, y_i)^2/n - b^2\{\Sigma\, x_i^2 - (\Sigma\, x_i)^2/n\}}{n-2}$$

$$= \frac{1.7607 - (2.421)^2/4 - 0.0249^2\{3000 - (100)^2/4\}}{2}$$

$$= [0.2954 - (0.02429)^2\{500\}]/2 = 0.000208$$

The value of the numerator is the sum-of-squares of the difference between the actual values of y and the value of y on the LS line, for each y. The divisor, $n-2$, is the number of data pairs minus 2, the DF. Thus, the estimate of the variance of y in this example has 2 DF. The reason that 2 is subtracted from the number of data points to obtain the DF is that two parameters are being estimated in the case of a straight line. In previous examples, such as the t test, only the mean is estimated for a treatment group, and DF = $n - 1$.

With an estimate of the variance, statistical procedures can be applied to these data if the assumptions, stated above, hold. Concentration is measured with little error, whereas the spectrometric readings, y, have error due to instrumental variability, sample processing, and handling (diluting, pipetting, etc), among other sources of variability. If it is assumed that the variance is the same at each concentration value and that the concentration values are distributed normally, the following statistical procedures can be used.

Confidence Limits and Test of the Slope—As in the statistical-hypothesis testing procedures described previously in this chapter, a test of the slope versus a hypothetical value can be performed. Also, confidence limits can be placed on the slope.

Example 32—Suppose that a value of 0.025 for the slope of the line is reported in an authoritative publication on this assay procedure. It is desired to determine if the slope in the experiment of Example 31 is different from 0.025 (ie, H_0:$B = 0.025$). The estimate of the variance of a slope is

$$s_b^2 = s^2_{y.x}/\Sigma(x_i - \bar{x})^2$$

The test is a two-sided t test with $n - 2$ DF of the following form:

$$t = \frac{|b - B|}{\sqrt{s_b^2}}$$

$$t = \frac{|0.02429 - 0.025|}{\sqrt{0.000208/500}} = 1.10$$

Table 12-41. Absorbance vs Concentration

Concentration	10 mg/L	20 mg/L	30 mg/L	40 mg/L
Absorbance	0.241	0.492	0.710	0.978

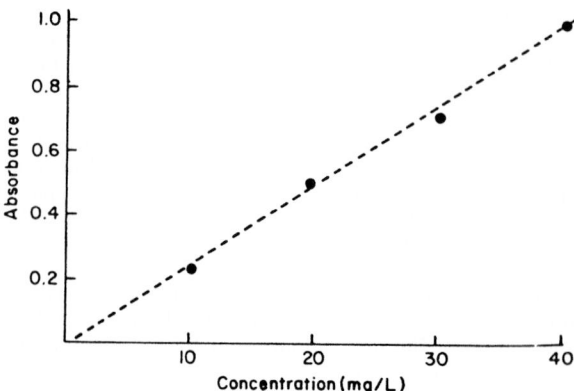

Figure 12-16. Beer's law plot.

Since t is less than the t value in the tables with 2 DF at the 5% level (see Table 12-10), it is concluded that the observed slope is not significantly different from 0.025. Note that a relatively large difference from 0.025 would be necessary to obtain significance because of the few DF in this test (the test is not very powerful). To increase the DF, more observations would be needed.

A confidence interval for the slope can be constructed in a manner similar to that described for means. A 95% confidence interval is

$$b \pm t\sqrt{s_b^2} = 0.02429 \pm 4.30\sqrt{0.000208/500}$$

$$= 0.00243 \pm 0.0028 = 0.0215 \text{ to } 0.0271$$

Confidence Limits and Test of the Intercept—Tests for the intercept and confidence limits are analogous to those presented immediately above for the slope. The variance estimate of the intercept is

$$S_a^2 = S^2_{y.x}[(1/n + \bar{x}^2/\Sigma(x_i - \bar{x})^2]$$

In Example 32, the calibration curve, a reasonable test would be to compare the intercept to zero. That is, one discovers whether zero concentration could correspond to a reading of zero. This would be a reasonable assumption if no interfering substances are present and if the optical density versus concentration relationship is a straight line from 0 to the highest concentration tested.

$$t = \frac{|-0.002 - 0|}{\sqrt{0.00028(1/4 + 625/500)}} = 0.1132$$

Since 0.1132 is less than the tabled value at the 5% level (see Table 12-10) with 2 DF, it is concluded that the intercept is not significantly different from zero.

A 95% confidence interval for the intercept is

$$-0.002 \pm 4.3\sqrt{0.00028(1/4 + 625/500)} = -0.002 \pm 0.082$$

These ideas as applied to analytical data are discussed in some detail by Youden.[26]

FITTING A LINE WITH AN INTERCEPT OF ZERO—

In some situations, it is desirable to force the LS line to have a y intercept equal to zero.

Example 33—In the Beer's Law line in Example 32, if it is known that there are no interfering substances and that the relationship is linear throughout the region of concentration being tested, the assumption that the line must pass through the origin is valid. The slope of this line is calculated as

$$b = \Sigma\, x_i y_i/\Sigma\, x_i^2$$

$$= 72.67/3000 = 0.02422$$

The slope of the line with 0 intercept is very close to that obtained above where the intercept was computed with no constraints on the value of the intercept.

CONFIDENCE INTERVAL FOR Y AND X—

Many situations arise where a confidence interval for y at some specified x is of interest.

Example 34—The data from Figure 12-17 show the results of a kinetic stability study, where drug content in tablets is measured as a function of time. The labeled content is 100 mg. The LS line was

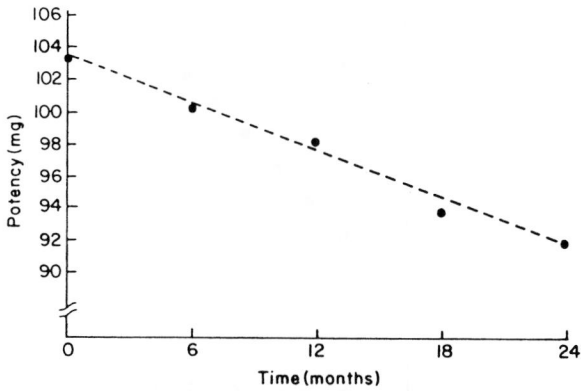

Figure 12-17. Tablet stability study.

calculated as $p = 103.3 - 0.483\,t$, where p is tablet potency and t is time. Note that the intercept is greater than 100 mg because a slight overage is built into the manufacturing process. The variance estimate, $S^2_{y,x}$, with 3 DF is equal to 0.367. In such stability studies, it often is of interest to predict the time for drug potency to reach 90% of the labeled amount in order to estimate shelf life or an expiration period. Substituting 90 for p (potency) and solving for time,

$$t = \frac{103.3 - 90}{0.483} = 27.54 \text{ months}$$

Therefore, the best estimate of the time to 90% potency is 27.54 months.

When establishing an expiration date, a conservative approach would take into account the error in the estimated values. A two-sided confidence interval can be constructed for the true value of y at a given x using

$$y \pm t \sqrt{S^2_{y,x}[1/n + (x - \overline{x})^2/\Sigma(x_i - \overline{x})^2]}$$

where y is a point on the LS line. The value of t (3 DF) for a two-sided 95% interval is 3.182. The width of the confidence interval depends on the value of x, being minimal when $x = \overline{x}$. The value of y when $x = \overline{x}$ is

$$y = 103.3 - 0.483(12) = 97.5$$

The 95% confidence interval when $x = \overline{x} = 12$ is

$$97.5 \pm 3.18 \sqrt{0.367[1/5 + 0/360]} = 96.64 - 98.36$$

Exercise 6—Calculate the 95% confidence interval for potency when $t = 24$ months.
Answer: 90.21 to 93.19.

Figure 12-18 shows 95% confidence intervals (confidence band) for the line calculated from the data of Figure 12-17. Note the hyperbolic shape, the interval being smallest at $\overline{x}$ and wider as x deviates more from its mean value. Using the lower line of the

confidence interval to compute the time to 90% potency yields a conservative estimate. In the example in Figure 12-18, a reasonable estimate of the expiration date would be 24.4 months. A one-sided interval (below the line) has been proposed as being more appropriate for stability data, as one usually is concerned with the loss of potency. For a 95% one-sided confidence interval, for 3 DF, the value of t from Table 12-10 is 2.353. Using this value of t to calculate the one-sided confidence interval, the one-sided confidence band shown in Figure 12-19 is obtained. For example, when $x = 12$ (months), the lower limit has the value 96.86 months.

With this approach, the expiration date would be set at 25.1 months (see Fig 12-19).

A confidence interval can be computed for x at a given value of y. This is sometimes known as inverse estimation. In the stability example, interest would be in computing a confidence interval for the time at which 90% of the potency remains. This time was estimated as 27.5 months. The formula for the confidence interval for x is more complex than that for y, but the computations are relatively simple.

$$\frac{(x - c^2\overline{x}) \pm t[s_{y,x}/b]\sqrt{(1 - c^2)/n + (x - \overline{x})^2/\Sigma(x_i - \overline{x})^2}}{1 - c^2}$$

where

$$c^2 = [t \cdot s]^2/[b^2\Sigma(x_i - \overline{x})^2]$$

Exercise 7—Use the above formula to show that a one-sided lower interval for x (time); 90% potency is 25.1.
Answer: This answer corresponds to the value of time taken from Figure 12-19.

COMPARISON OF THE SLOPES OF TWO LINES—A statistical test may be performed to compare the slopes of two lines, using a t test. The null hypothesis is

$$H_O{:}B_1 = B_2 \text{ or } B_1 - B_2 = 0$$

The t test compares the difference of the two slopes to the standard error of the difference. The variances of y for the two lines are assumed to be equal, and the estimates are pooled as in the two-sample t test

$$s^2 \text{ pooled} = \frac{s^2_{y,x}(n_1 - 2) + s^2_{y,x}(n_2 - 2)}{(n_1 + n_2 - 4)}$$

A two-sided t test with $(n_1 + n_2 - 4)$ DF is

$$t = \frac{|b_2 - b_1|}{\sqrt{s^2 \text{ pooled}(1/x_1^2 + 1/x_2^2)}}$$

where, x_1^2 and x_2^2 are $\Sigma(x_i - \overline{x})_1^2$ and $\Sigma(x_i - \overline{x})_2^2$, respectively.

Example 35—The line for the stability data depicted in Figure 12-17 has a slope of -0.483, with a variance estimate of 0.367 with 3 DF.

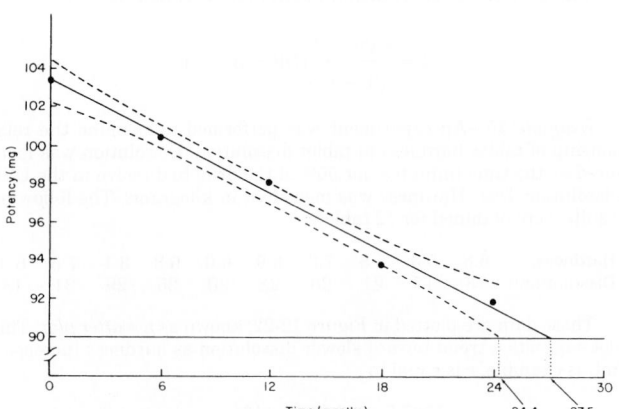

Figure 12-18. Two-sided confidence interval for stability data.

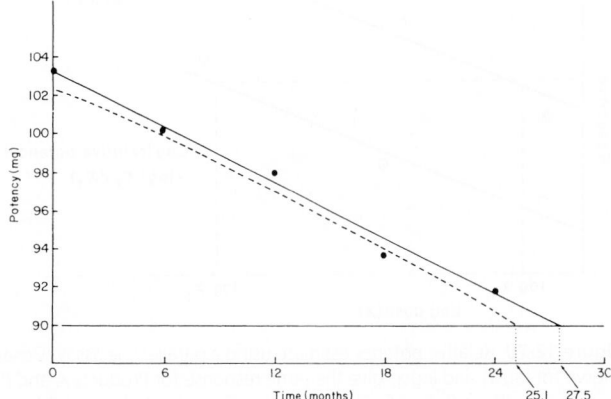

Figure 12-19. One-sided confidence interval for stability study.

The value of $\Sigma(x_i - \bar{x})^2$ is 360. Another formulation was prepared and tested for stability. Ten sampling times were used for the stability study, and the slope was determined to be -0.533. The variance estimate (8 DF) was 0.289, and $\Sigma(x_i - \bar{x})^2$ was equal to 2565. The test for equality of the slopes (rate of decomposition) is

$$t = \frac{|0.533 - 0.483|}{\sqrt{0.310(1/2565 + 1/500)}} = 1.84$$

Since 1.84 is less than the tabled t value for the 5% significance level with 11 DF, 2.20 (3 from one line and 8 from the other), it can be concluded that the slopes of the two lines are not significantly different.

In a biological assay, a common procedure is to determine the relative potency of two or more substances using the *parallel line assay*. In this procedure, the lines from a plot of response versus log dose are forced to be parallel and the distance between the lines is a measure of the relative potency. Before performing this procedure, a test is made to ensure that the lines are parallel. Nonparallel lines will cross, suggesting that at low doses one product gives a greater response, whereas at higher doses the other product gives the greater response. Figure 12-20[23] illustrates the principle of this assay. The computations are tedious, and the book by Finney[27] should be consulted for those who wish more detail on the statistical treatment of this and other biological assay methods.

CORRELATION—*Correlation* is related to, but should not be confused with, linear regression. It is a measure of the linear relationship between two variables but does not prove linearity. In fact, the usual formulas for determining the significance of the correlation assume that the variables already are related linearly. The question that is usually posed indirectly when testing the correlation is, can the value of one of the variables be used to predict the value of the second variable? This amounts to testing the slope of the line relating the variables versus 0. If the slope is significantly different from 0, then the variables have a *significant correlation*. Correlation is used when both variables are subject to error. If one variable is not subject to error (fixed), the linear regression approach to establish the relationship of the variables is more appropriate.

The measure of association is the correlation coefficient, r.

$$r = \frac{\Sigma x_i y_i - \Sigma x_i \Sigma y_i / n}{\sqrt{\Sigma(x_i - \bar{x})^2 \Sigma(y_i - \bar{y})^2}}$$

The correlation coefficient can vary between $+1$ and -1. A correlation coefficient of $+1$ would result if all points fall exactly on a single line with positive slope; this is a perfect positive correlation. Similarly, if all points fall on a line with negative slope, $r = -1$, a perfect negative correlation is observed. If $r = 0$, the variables are not correlated. These three cases are shown in Figure 12-21.

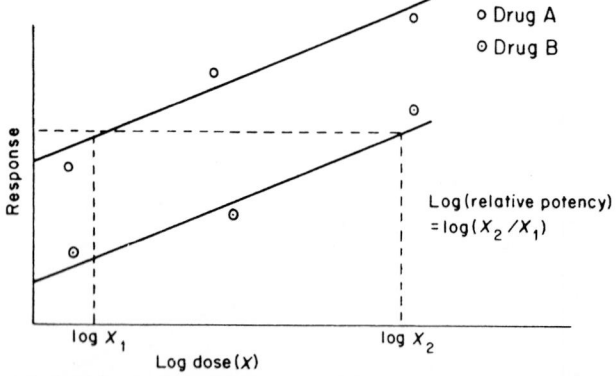

Figure 12-20. Relative potency estimate using a parallel line assay. Doses shown for log x_1 and log x_2 give the same response for Products A and B, respectively. (From Bolton S. *Pharmaceutical Statistics.* New York: Marcel Dekker, 1984, pp 416, 463.)

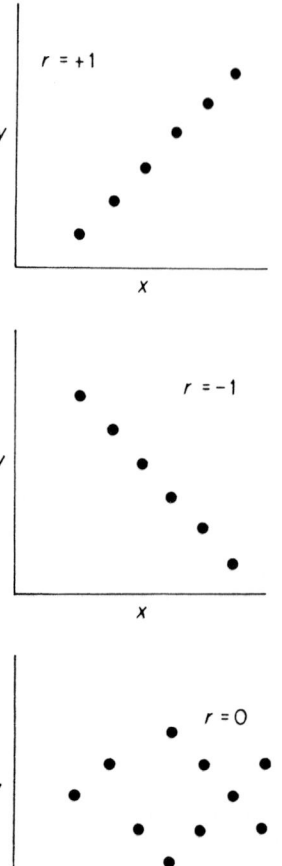

Figure 12-21. Correlation diagrams (scatter plots).

In real situations, these extreme results are seen rarely, but rather some intermediate value of r is observed. The statistical question of interest usually is concerned with the significance of the correlation—a test of r versus 0. One should appreciate, however, that the meaning of the correlation should be considered carefully. For example, if n, the number of data pairs, is large, correlation coefficients that are very small (practically insignificant) will be deemed statistically significant. Also, data that is not linear, but clearly related, may show small correlation coefficients.

Exercise 8—Compute the correlation between x and y for $x = -2, -1, 0, +1$ and $+2$, for the relationship $y = x^2$. *Answer: r = 0.*

The test of the correlation coefficient versus 0 is

$$t = \frac{r\sqrt{n-2}}{\sqrt{1 - r^2}} \quad (\text{DF} = n - 2)$$

Example 36—An experiment was performed to examine the relationship of tablet hardness to tablet dissolution. Dissolution was measured as the time (minutes) for 50% of the drug to dissolve in the USP Dissolution Test. Hardness was measured in kilograms. The following results were obtained for 12 tablets:

Hardness:	6.8	5.3	5.8	7.2	6.9	6.0	6.8	8.1	7.5	6.3
Dissolution:	18	17	21	26	28	20	25	29	31	18

These data are plotted in Figure 12-22, known as a *scatter plot*. This plot suggests a trend toward slower dissolution as hardness increases. In this example, r is equal to

$$\frac{1585.5 - 233(66.7/10)}{\sqrt{236.1 \cdot 6.321}} = 0.81$$

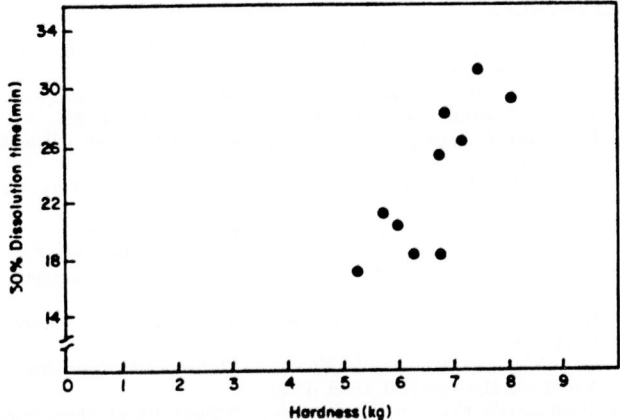

Figure 12-22. Scatter plot of hardness versus dissolution data (Example 36).

The test of the significance of the correlation coefficient shows $t = 3.94$ with 8 DF.

It is concluded that r is significantly different from 0, and hardness and dissolution are correlated ($P < 0.05$; see Table 12-10; $t = 2.228$ for significance at $P = 0.05$).

DATA TRANSFORMATIONS

Probabilities calculated from statistical analyses are based on assumptions underlying the nature of the data. The typical analyses presented in this chapter often assume normality of data and variance homogeneity. When dealing with means of a sufficiently large sample size, the assumption of normality is not critical. However, small sample sizes and a large deviation from normality can result in a significant violation of the normality assumption. When comparing samples from two or more groups, lack of homogeneity of variance (heteroscadiscity) is an important problem that can result in an unreliable analysis. One way of overcoming these problems is the use of *transformations*. Each data point is transformed, resulting in data that more closely fits the normality and variance homogeneity assumptions.[9]

The logarithmic, square root, and arcsine transformations will be presented here as examples of the more popular data transformations.

LOGARITHMIC (LOG) TRANSFORMATION—This transformation (log to the base 10 or log to the base e, ln, may be used) is most applicable for skewed data of the form illustrated in Figure 12-23. These data typically show a relatively constant coefficient of variation (CV). That is, the larger the value, the larger is the SD; the SD is proportional to the mean ($SD/\bar{x}$ is constant). This transformation is applicable to data that meet the above conditions and also are greater than 0; the log of 0 or a negative number is undefined.

This probably is the most common transformation for data in the pharmaceutical sciences. Many physical and biological measurements show larger variability as the size of the measurement increases. This is logical for many types of data. For example, the measurement of a large value such as the assay of a concentrated solution may be expected to show considerable variability about its mean (eg, 1000 mg/mL ± 50, a 5% variability). The assay of a dilute solution, 10 mg/mL, cannot show very large variation, particularly on the low side where zero (0) is the lower limit. If the CV were 5% (10 mg/ mL ± 0.5), a log transformation would be suitable. If the data are skewed (see Fig 12-23) and the CV is constant, a log transformation will tend to normalize the data distribution and equalize the variances.

When data are presented as ratios, a log transformation often is appropriate. Unless the data are extremely variable, the conclusions using the original or transformed data should be similar. The conclusions using the transformed data, however, will be more reliable if the transformation is appropriate.

Care should be taken that the log transformation does not help to improve one assumption while making another less valid. For data that are skewed but have constant variance, the normality assumption may improve while causing problems with the variance homogeneity assumption. Fortunately, the log transformation, when indicated, does not seem to cause such difficult and perplexing problems.

Example 37—The means of two treatment groups are to be compared where it is known that large values are associated with proportionally larger standard deviations. The measurements are 50% dissolution time in minutes (Table 12-42).

A two independent sample t test (two-sided) comparing the means shows

$$t = \frac{|43.17 - 61.17|}{19.11 \sqrt{1/3}} = 1.75$$

A log transformation results in the data in Table 12-43.

Neither test is significant at the 5% level but the log-transformed values in this example result in a test with a lower probability level.

Exercise 9—A bioequivalence study comparing two dosage forms, *A* and *B*, with six subjects in a paired design resulted in the following ratios of AUC_a/AUC_b:

$$1.27, 1.06, 0.90, 1.30, 1.15, 0.96$$

Calculate the mean, standard deviations and a 95% confidence interval for the data using the untransformed data and a log transformation. For the log transformation, calculate the antilogs for the lower and upper limit of the confidence interval. Repeat the calculations for the mean and standard deviation of the ratio of AUC_b/AUC_a. (Note that this is the reciprocal of the data presented above.) What can be said about the confidence intervals for the two kinds of ratios, *A/B* and *B/A*?

Answer:

Mean = 1.107; SD = 0.1627; CI = 1.107 ± 0.171. log transformation: Mean = 0.0400; SD = 0.0646; CI = 0.04 ± 0.0678

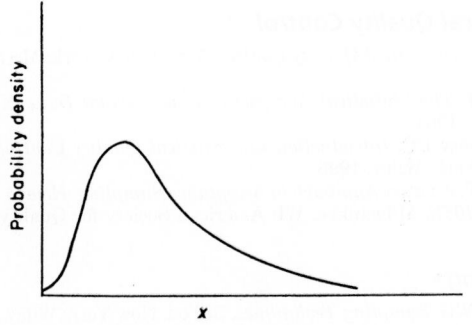

Figure 12-23. Example of a skewed distribution.

Table 12-42. 50% Dissolution Time for Two Formulations

	FORMULATION A	FORMULATION B
	27	65
	55	60
	33	98
	69	47
	36	57
	39	43
Mean	43.17	61.67
SD	15.75	19.59

Table 12-43. Log Transformation of Data of Table 12-42

	FORMULATION A	FORMULATION B
	1.431	1.813
	1.740	1.778
	1.519	1.991
	1.839	1.672
	1.556	1.756
	1.591	1.633
Mean	1.613	1.774
SD	0.150	0.126

$$t = \frac{1.613 - 1.774}{0.139 \sqrt{1/3}} = 2.01$$

CI = 0.938 − 1.282
Reciprocal: Mean = 0.92; SD = 0.1376
log transformation: Mean = −0.0400; SD = 0.0646

For bioequivalence data, a log transformation of AUC and C_{max} is currently recommended.

SQUARE-ROOT TRANSFORMATION—A square-root transformation is useful for data where the sample means are proportional or equal to the variances (s^2). The transformation will cause the data to have approximately homogeneous variance. This transformation may be used to replace the log transformation when the data consist of small numbers. If the numbers are less than 10 and zeros are present, $\sqrt{x+1}$ may be an appropriate transformation.[28] This transformation, like the log transformation, will tend to normalize distributions skewed to the right (distributions with a relative small number of very large values).

Exercise 10—Compute the mean and standard deviation of the following data before and after applying the square-root transformation ($\sqrt{x}$). Draw a histogram of the original and transformed values. Note the greater symmetry of the transformed data.

0, 11, 7, 3, 0, 15, 4, 2, 6, 9, 3, 0, 12, 5, 3, 6

Answer:

Original data:	$\bar{x} = 5.625$	SD = 4.272
Transformed data:	$\bar{x} = 2.00$	SD = 1.206

ARCSINE (INVERSE SINE) TRANSFORMATION—The arcsine (inverse sine) transformation is used for binomial data or data expressed as percentages or proportions. The transformation is arcsine $\sqrt{p}$, where p, the proportion or probability, is expressed as a decimal. The variance of a binomial proportion is pq/n, where p is the proportion of successes and q the proportion of failures in n binomial observations. If p varies in different treatment groups, the variance will vary. The arcsine transformation applied to the proportions tends to equalize the variances and normalize the data.[9] The variance of the transformed proportion is $821/n$ when the transformed data are in degrees. This transformation assumes that all proportions transformed have the same value of n. If n is approximately equal for the different groups, the transformation may still be used.

Example 38—Use a normal test to compare the proportion of rats who developed tumors in placebo-control and active-drug groups. In the placebo group, 15 of 100 animals developed tumors, whereas in the drug group, 22 of 100 developed tumors. The arcsines of $\sqrt{0.15}$ and $\sqrt{0.22}$ are 22.786 and 27.972, respectively. The normal test is

$$Z = \frac{|27.972 - 22.786|}{\sqrt{(821/100) + (821/100)}} = 1.28$$

The proportions are not significantly different.
Exercise 11—Calculate the value of chi-square for the test of these two proportions.
Answer: 1.625. Note that chi-square = Z^2 in this example.

REFERENCES

1. Siegal S. *Nonparametric Statistics.* New York: McGraw-Hill, 1956.
2. Kish L. *Survey Sampling.* New York: Wiley, 1995.
3. Fisher RA, Yates F. *Statistical Tables for Biological, Agriculture and Medical Research.* New York: Hafner, 1963, p 134 (Table 38).
4. Fisher RA. *The Design of Experiments,* 5th ed. Edinburgh: Oliver & Boyd, 1986.
5. Cochran WG, Cox GM. *Experimental Design,* 2nd ed. New York: Wiley, 1957.
6. Cox DR. *Planning of Experiments.* New York: Wiley, 1958.
7. United States Department of the Army. *Tables of the Binomial Probability Distribution.* Applied Mathematics Series No. 6 Washington, DC: USGPO, 1952.
8. Bolton S. *Pharmaceutical Statistics,* 3rd ed. New York: Marcel Dekker, 1997.
9. Dixon WJ, Massey FJ Jr. *Introduction to Statistical Analysis,* 3rd ed. New York: McGraw-Hill, 1969, p 324.
10. Snedecor GW, Cochran WG. *Statistical Methods,* 8th ed. Ames: Iowa State University Press, 1989, p 97.
11. Snedecor GW, Cochran WG. *Statistical Methods,* 7th ed. Ames: Iowa State University Press, 1980, p 476 (Table A14).
12. Snedecor GW, Cochran WG. *Statistical Methods,* 7th ed. Ames: Iowa State University Press, 1980, p 480 (Table A15).
13. Duncan DB. *Biometrics II* 1948; 1.
14. Dunnett CW. *Am Stat Assoc J* 1955; 50: 1096.
15. Winer BJ. *Statistical Principles in Experimental Design,* 2nd ed. New York: McGraw-Hill, 1971.
16. Tate MW, Clelland RC. *Nonparametric and Shortcut Statistics.* Danville IL: Interstate Print, 1957: p 137 (Table L).
17. Youden WJ. *Sci Monthly* 1953; 77: 143.
18. Youden WJ. *Natl Bur Std (US) Tech News Bull* 1949: 33 (July).
19. Dixon WJ, Massey FJ Jr. *Introduction to Statistical Analysis,* 3rd ed. New York: McGraw-Hill, 1969, p 328.
20. *Control Chart Method of Controlling Quality During Production (Std Z1.3).* New York: American Standards Association, 1958.
21. *Guide for Quality Control (Std Z1. 3).* New York: American Standards Association, 1958.
22. Dixon WJ, Massey FJ Jr. *Introduction to Statistical Analysis,* 3rd ed. New York: McGraw-Hill, 1969, p 142.
23. Bolton S. *Pharmaceutical Statistics.* New York: Marcel Dekker, 1984, pp 416, 463.
24. *Military Sampling Procedures and Tables for Inspection by Attributes.* MIL-STD-105E. Washington DC: USGPO, 1989.
25. Snedecor GW, Cochran WG. *Statistical Methods,* 8th ed. Ames: Iowa State University Press, 1989, p 151.
26. Youden WJ. *Statistical Methods for Chemists.* New York: Wiley, 1951.
27. Finney DJ. *Statistical Method in Biological Assay,* 4th ed. New York: Hafner, 1980.
28. Steel RGD, Torrie JH. *Principles and Procedures of Statistics.* New York: McGraw-Hill, 1960.

BIBLIOGRAPHY

Experimental Design

Cox DR. *Planning of Experiments.* New York: Wiley, 1992.
Fisher RA. *Statistical Methods for Research Workers,* 13th ed. Edinburgh: Oliver & Boyd, 1970.
Montgomery DC. *Design and Analysis of Experiments,* 4th ed. New York: Wiley, 1996.
Chow S-C, Liu J-P. *Statistical Design and Analysis in Pharmaceutical Science:* New York: Dekker, 1995.

Statistical Quality Control

Grant EL. *Statistical Quality Control,* 5th ed. New York: McGraw-Hill, 1980.
Mandel J. *The Statistical Analysis of Experimental Data.* New York: Dover, 1984.
Montgomery DC. *Introduction to Statistical Quality Control,* 3rd ed. New York: Wiley, 1996.
Weber RT. *An Easy Approach to Acceptance Sampling: How to Use MIL-STD-105E.* Milwaukee, WI: American Society for Quality Control, 1991.

Sampling

Cochran WG. *Sampling Techniques,* 3rd ed. New York: Wiley, 1997.
Deming WE. *Some Theory of Sampling.* New York: Wiley, 1984.

Yates F. *Sampling Methods for Censuses and Surveys.* New York: Hafner, 1981.

Biological Assay

Bliss CI. *The Statistics of Bioassay with Special Reference to the Vitamins.* New York: Academic Press, 1952.

Bliss CI. *Am Sci* 1957; 45: 449.

Finney DJ. *Statistical Method in Biological Assay,* 3rd ed. New York: Hafner, 1978.

Finney DJ. *Probit Analysis,* 4th ed. London, Cambridge University Press, 1980.

General

Bennett CA, Franklin NL. *Statistical Analysis in Chemistry and the Chemical Industry.* New York: Wiley, 1954.

Bolton S. *Pharmaceutical Statistics.* Third Edition, New York: Marcel Dekker, 1997

Brownlee KA. *Statistical Theory and Methods in Science and Engineering.* New York: Wiley, 1960.

Buncher CR, Tsay J. *Statistics in the Pharmaceutical Industry.* New York: Marcel Dekker, 1981.

Chow, Shein-Chung, Editor, Encyclopedia of Biopharmaceutical Statistics: New York: Marcel Dekker, 2000.

Davies OL. *The Design and Analysis of Industrial Experiments.* New York: Hafner, 1954.

Peace KE. *Biopharmaceutical Statistics for Drug Development.* New York: Marcel Dekker, 1988.

Snedecor GW, Cochran WG. *Statistical Methods,* 8th ed. Ames, Iowa State University Press, 1989.

Statistical Software Packages (Examples)

BMDP, Biomedical Computer Programs, University of California, Los Angeles, CA.

NCSS, NCSS Statistical Software, 329 North 1000 East, Kaysville, Utah 84037 (website: http://www.ncss.com, phone: 800-898-6109).

SAS, SAS Institute Inc, Cary, NC (website: http://www.sas.com/, e-mail: software@sas.com)

CHAPTER 13

Molecular Structure, Properties, and States of Matter

Eric J Lien, PhD

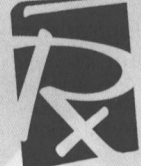

The many significant advances in the pharmaceutical sciences in recent years are in large part attributable to the accumulation of knowledge of the molecular structure and physicochemical properties of drugs, and to the correlation of this knowledge with that of the nature of biological reactions of drugs. This chapter discusses fundamental principles of atomic and molecular structure and certain physicochemical properties that are important in the pharmaceutical sciences, to aid in the understanding of drug action at the molecular level.

ATOMIC STRUCTURE

ATOMS AND ELEMENTARY PARTICLES—The atoms (from the Greek *atomos,* indivisible) were believed to be the minute, indivisible particles of which all material things were made. The search for the ultimate particle has been a continuous effort since the time of Democritus (about 460–370 BCE). Before the discovery of mesons and hyperons, the structure of matter was believed to be much simpler. The nucleus was thought to consist of protons and neutrons; and to form an atom, only electrons needed to be added in external shells. Therefore, protons, neutrons, and electrons were considered as the elementary particles. In theory, all the elements in the periodic table can be made by splitting neutrons into electrons and protons, and by combining these particles in proper ratios.

During the past three decades, nuclear physics progressively has probed atoms from their periphery to their center. The search for ultimate units of nuclear structure, by means of experiments consisting in large part of bombarding nuclei with high-energy particles, has revealed a spectrum of over 100 species, some of them unstable. Some of these particles are listed in Table 13-1. The proton is no longer considered an ultimate particle, but is believed to be made up of particles called *quarks* (from "three quarks for Muster Mark," in James Joyce's *Finnegans Wake*). One theory of quark structure of protons calls for nine kinds of quarks (along with antiquarks) and eight kinds of *gluons* (analogous to photons) to hold the quarks together. Whether these and other elementary particles are all composed of yet simpler elements remains to be investigated.[1]

In 1924, de Broglie raised the question that if light waves show corpuscular character, should not particles also show wave character? Now it generally is accepted that in the case of a photon there are two fundamental equations to be obeyed: $E = h\nu$ and $E = mc^2$, where E is the energy, h is Planck's constant, ν is the frequency and c is the speed of light. Combining both equations gives $h\nu = mc^2$ or $\lambda = c/\nu = h/mc = h/p$, where p is the momentum of the proton.

De Broglie proposed that a similar equation should govern the wavelength of the electron wave. It is interesting to note that x-ray diffraction is a good example of the use of the wave property of electromagnetic radiation.

Scattering of slow neutrons has been employed to provide information about the structure and dynamic properties of biological structures, for example, myoglobin and membranes.[2]

DALTON'S ATOMIC THEORY—In 1808, Dalton proposed his atomic theory on the basis of three generalizations: the Law of Conservation of Mass, the Law of Definite Proportions, and the Law of Multiple Proportions. The essential parts of the theory can be summarized as

1. All elements are composed of very small, discrete, indivisible particles called atoms.
2. All atoms of any one element are identical. Modern structural theory tells us that electronic differences between the atoms of an element may occur, but these differences arise as a consequence of electronic excitation. The lowest energy state of an atom is more appropriate for purposes of classification.
3. The atoms of no two elements are alike.
4. Atoms undergo no fundamental change during chemical reaction. There are subtle changes in the electronic character of atoms, although this does not change the identity of an atom.
5. Compounds are formed when atoms of two or more different elements combine to form a molecule.
6. In general, atoms combine in simple, integral ratios.

PERIODIC TABLE—The periodic classification of the elements is one of the most striking advances in generalizing many isolated facts; moreover, it contributes tremendously to the strength of the atomic theory and extends it to new sets of facts. The periodic table serves as an easily learned summary of almost limitless information about the chemical nature of the elements; it is of prime importance to students of pharmaceutical sciences as well as to students of chemistry.

After the publication of the independent researches of Mendeleyev and Meyer in 1869, the *periodic law* was well-established. The *periodic table* is an arrangement of the elements in accordance with the periodic law (see Periodic Chart of the Elements). The present arrangement is essentially the same as that of Mendeleyev, although there are now minor variations due to the incorporation of new elements and modern data. A few terms should be carried in mind for a thorough understanding of the table.

- *Atomic number (Z)* is the positive charge of the nucleus expressed as multiples of the electronic charge *e*.
- *Atomic weight* is the average weight expressed in atomic weight units of the natural atoms of an element existing as a mixture of isotopes in the same ratio as found in nature. An atomic weight unit, used in chemistry, is exactly 1/16 the average mass of the oxygen isotopes taken in the same ratio as they occur in nature. One atomic weight unit is equivalent to 1.000272 atomic mass units.
- An *isotope* is one of a group of nuclides of the same element (same Z), having the same number of protons in the nucleus but differing in the number of neutrons, resulting in different mass numbers.
- A *nuclide* is any one of the more than 1000 species of atoms and is characterized by the number of protons and neutrons in the nucleus.

Table 13-1. Subatomic Particles

GROUP	PARTICLES	RELATIVE MASS (ELECTRON = 1)	ELECTRIC CHARGE	MEAN LIFE-TIME (sec)
Heavy particles	α-Particle (He^{2+}, α)	7348	+2	Stable
	Triton (T, ^{3}H)	5451	+1	3.8×10^8
	Deuteron (D, d, ^{2}H)	3674	+1	Stable
	Neutron (n)	1837	0	7.2×10^2
	Proton (p, ^{1}H)	1837	+1	Stable
Hyperons	Λ° Particle	~2181	0	2.5×10^{-10}
	$\Sigma^\pm$ Particle	~2326	± 1	Σ^+ 0.8×10^{-10} Σ^- 1.6×10^{-10}
	$\Xi^\pm$ Particle	~2580	± 1	1.3×10^{-10}
Mesons	K meson (K$^\pm$)	966	± 1	1.2×10^{-8}
	K meson (K$^\circ$)	974	0	$10^{-9} - 10^{-10}$
	Pi meson ($\pi^\pm$)	273		2.6×10^{-8}
	Pi meson (π°)	264	0	1.9×10^{-16}
Leptons	Mu ($\mu^\pm$)	209 ± 2	± 1	2.2×10^{-6}
	Electrons (e$^-$, β^-)	1	-1	Stable
	Positron) (e$^+$, β^+)	1	+1	Stable
	Neutrino (ν)	0.01	0	Stable
	Photons (γ)	0	0	Stable

BOHR'S THEORY OF ATOMIC STRUCTURE—In 1913 Bohr proposed a theory of atomic structure for the interpretation of atomic spectra. His picture of the atom had the extranuclear electrons revolving around the nucleus in definite orbits. These orbits were assigned principal quantum numbers 1, 2, 3, . . ., n, counting outward from the nucleus.

When an electron absorbs a definite increment (quantum) of energy, it is promoted to an orbit of higher energy (excited state), and when it falls back to the original orbit, it emits radiation energy. The energy of the various levels in the atom can be related to the frequency of radiation that is emitted from or absorbed by the atom. This relationship is expressed by

$$\Delta E = E_2 - E_1 = h\nu \tag{1}$$

where ΔE is the difference of the energy in ergs between two levels, h is Planck's constant (6.624×10^{-27} erg sec) and ν is the frequency. Because the frequency is equivalent to the speed of light, c, divided by the wavelength, Equation 1 can be written as

$$\Delta E = hc/\lambda \tag{2}$$

When the electrons possess the lowest energy possible, the atom is said to be in its *ground state*.

The energy of an electron in an orbit is given by

$$E = \frac{-2\pi^2 Z^2 m e^4}{n^2 h^2} \tag{3}$$

where Z is the atomic number, m is the mass of the electron (9.1×10^{-28} g), e is the charge of the electron in electrostatic units (4.8×10^{-10} esu), n is the principal quantum number, and h is Planck's constant. One can calculate the radiation energy emitted when an electron falls from n_2 orbit to n_1 orbit by

$$E_2 - E_1 = \frac{2\pi^2 Z^2 m e^4}{h^2}\left(\frac{1}{n_1^2} - \frac{1}{n_2^2}\right) \tag{4}$$

When n_2 is ∞, Equation 4 gives the energy required for ionization; for example, the ionization potential of the hydrogen atom

can be calculated as

$$E_\infty - E_1 = \frac{2 \times (3.14)^2 \times (1)^2 \times 9.1 \times 10^{-28} \times (4.8 \times 10^{-10})^4}{(6.624 \times 10^{-27})^2}$$

$$\times \left(\frac{1}{(1)^2} - \frac{1}{(\infty)^2}\right)$$

$$= 2.18 \times 10^{-11} \text{ erg}$$

$$= \frac{2.18 \times 10^{-11} \text{ erg}}{1.60 \times 10^{-12} \text{ erg/electron volt (ev)}}$$

$$= 13.6 \text{ ev}$$

It is interesting to note that the quantum theory is founded on the principle that the energy of an atom or molecule does not change continuously but only by some definite whole number unit of energy referred to as a quantum.

MODERN MODEL OF ATOMIC STRUCTURE—After Bohr published his theory, there was a period of intense activity by theoreticians and experimental physicists. Based on mathematical principles and considerable experimental data, a more definite picture of atomic structure emerged. The modern interpretation of the atom is more elaborate than the original idea of Bohr. Four quantum numbers are used to describe the energy levels or orbitals of each electron.

The *principal quantum number, n,* is an approximate measure of the size of the electron cloud—that is, the order of magnitude of the potential energy. It has the values 1, 2, 3, . . ., 7, corresponding to the K, L, M, . . ., Q shells of electrons.

The *azimuthal quantum number, l,* is related to the shape of the electron cloud, indicating whether it is spherical, dumbbell-shaped, or of more complex geometry. It may have values of 0, 1, 2, . . ., $(n - 1)$, corresponding, respectively, to the terms s, p, d, or f used by spectroscopists; for example, a $4d$ electron would have an n number of 4 and an l value of 2.

The *magnetic quantum number, m_1,* is related to the orientation of the electron cloud in space. It has values of 0, ± 1, ± 2, . . ., $\pm l$. For a spherical cloud there is only one orientation. However, the dumbbell-shaped orbital, for example, could be oriented in three different directions corresponding to the x, y, and z axes of a set of Cartesian coordinates.

The *spin quantum number, s* (or m_s), gives the orientation of the magnetic component of an electron. There are only two discrete ways an electron can interact with an external magnetic field. Like a tiny magnet, it either can line up in the direction of the field or orient itself in the opposite direction. The electron's magnetic moment was at first pictured as being due to the rotation of the electron on its axis, and for this reason an electron was said to exhibit spin. The two spin quantum numbers, $s = +1/2$ and $s = -1/2$, were used to describe the two observable spin states.

Considerable progress has been made in the recent years in the application of quantum mechanical and molecular orbital theories in studying drug-receptor interactions and in correlating chemical structure with pharmacological activities of drugs (see Chapter 27).

ELECTRONIC CONFIGURATION OF THE ELEMENTS—Two rules are of extreme importance in explaining the building up of electronic shells of elements (Fig 13-1 and Table 13-2).

The *Pauli exclusion principle* states that an atom cannot exist in a state where two electrons in the same energy level or orbital have the same set of four quantum numbers. This is analogous to the principle in classical physics that no two bodies can be in the same place at the same time. Thus, two electrons in the K shell may have the same principal, azimuthal, and magnetic quantum numbers ($n = 1$, $l = 0$, $m_1 = 0$), but different spin quantum numbers ($s = +1/2$ and $s = -1/2$).

Hund's rule of maximum multiplicity states that when orbitals are of the same energy, electrons distribute themselves one to each orbital so as to maintain parallel spins; for example, oxygen, with an atomic number of eight, possesses eight elec-

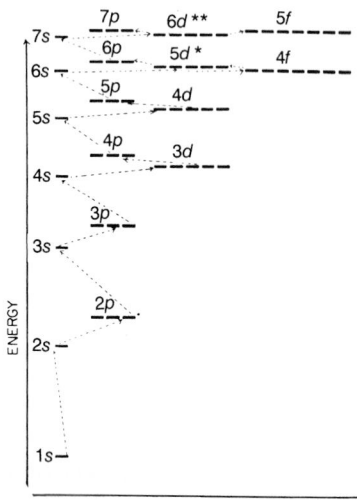

Figure 13-1. Atomic energy levels and the order of filling of orbitals: (*) a single $5d$ electron is added before the $4f$ orbitals can be filled; (**) one or more $6d$ electrons must be added before the $5f$ orbitals can be filled.

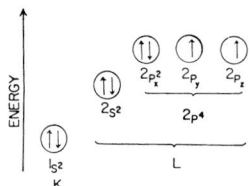

Figure 13-2. The electronic configuration of an oxygen atom.

trons. Two electrons are in the K shell ($1s^2$), and six are in the L shell. In the L shell, two electrons fill the $2s$ orbitals ($2s^2$) and the remaining four fill the $2p$ orbitals ($2p^4$).

According to Hund's rule, three electrons occupy $2p_x$, $2p_y$, and $2p_z$ orbitals and spin in the same direction (see the direction of the arrow in Fig 13-2); the fourth electron can pair up with any one of these three electrons (say $2p_x$). The electronic configuration for oxygen atom can be expressed as $1s^2\,2s^2\,2p_x^2\,2p_y\,2p_z$.

MOLECULAR STRUCTURE

A molecule is the smallest possible quantity of a substance. It is composed of two or more atoms, for example, N_2, O_2, $CHCl_3$, or H_2SO_4. There is a chemical bond between atoms when the forces acting between them are strong enough to give an aggregate with sufficient stability to make it convenient for the chemist to consider the aggregate as an independent molecular species. Different types of chemical bonds will be discussed in the following sections.

COVALENT BONDS—When two electrons of two atoms are paired and localized in the space between the two atoms, a *covalent bond* results. The paired electrons (with opposed spins) then will occupy the new molecular orbital encompassing the two atoms. It should be noted that the electron pair held jointly by two atoms is considered to do double duty by completing a stable electronic configuration for each atom.

For instance, in the case of methane, the carbon atom, with its two inner electrons and its outer shell of eight shared electrons, has assumed the stable 10-electron configuration of neon; and the hydrogen atoms have achieved the configuration of helium. Covalent and ionic bonds are found in both organic and inorganic chemistry.

THE UNIQUENESS OF CARBON

Since organic chemistry is concerned mainly with carbon and its compounds, closer attention is warranted to the kinds of bonds exhibited by the carbon atom.

Carbon (and, to a much lesser extent, boron and beryllium) is in a special class. Although only the twelfth most abundant element on earth, its compounds far outnumber those of the remainder of the periodic table combined. The exact number of existing carbon compounds is probably unknown, and the theoretical number is infinite. This uniqueness stems from the simple fact that carbon is capable of bonding with itself in many unusual modes.

Carbon-Carbon Bonds

Ordinarily, carbon is said to exhibit a valence of four. Thus, it can combine with four other monovalent atoms or groups or with four other carbon atoms in a linear or cyclic fashion, with or without branching, or any combination thereof.

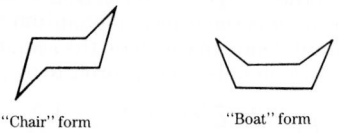

Also, carbon atoms can unite to each other or to other atoms such as nitrogen, oxygen, or sulfur by means of multiple bonds.

To compound the situation further, the structural diagrams just presented are not flat objects, but are three-dimensional. For example, a six-membered carbon ring may have several configurations, such as

"Chair" form   "Boat" form

This feature alone could essentially double the number of possible compounds of this type.

Table 13-2. Electronic Configurations of Some Elements in Their Ground States

n = SHELL		1	2		3			4		
l = SUBSHELL		K	L		M			N		
ATOMIC NO	ELEMENT	0 1S	0 2S	1 2P	0 3S	1 3P	2 3D	0 4S	1 4P	2 4D	3 4F
1	H	1								
2	He	2								
3	Li	2	1							
4	Be	2	2							
5	B	2	2	1						
6	C	2	2	2						
7	N	2	2	3						
8	O	2	2	4						
9	F	2	2	5						
10	Ne	2	2	6						
11	Na				1					
12	Mg				2					
13	Al				2	1				
14	Si	Neon core			2	2				
15	P				2	3				
16	S				2	4				
17	Cl				2	5				
18	Ar				2	6				

HYBRIDIZATION—What is so unusual about the constitution of the carbon atom that allows so many diverse compounds? Simply stated, the reason is *hybridization*, and a review of the electronic configuration of the atom is required to explain what hybridization is and how it is attained. The extra-nuclear configuration of an isolated carbon atom is $1s^2 2s^2 2p_x{}^1 2p_y{}^1 2p_z{}^0$, which means that there are two electrons in the $1s$ level, two in the $2s$ level, and two in the $2p$ level, but since the two $2p$ electrons reside in different subshells (p_x and p_y), they are unpaired. As only unpaired valence electrons are capable of bonding, it would be expected that carbon should exhibit a valence of two. However, in every instance (except for possibly carbon monoxide), carbon combines with four univalent atoms or groups.

Bond formation is a stabilizing (exothermic) process, and there is a tendency to form as many bonds as possible, even if the resulting molecular orbitals bear little resemblance to atomic orbitals that exist in the isolated or *ground* state of an atom. A carbon atom must be elevated or *excited* (energetically) to assume a valence state of four; to do this, four unpaired electrons must be created. This feat can be accomplished by promoting one electron from the $2s$ level to the vacant $2p_z$ level; thus, the resulting extranuclear electronic configuration becomes $1s^2 2s^1 2p_x{}^1 2p_y{}^1 2p_z{}^1$. More than enough energy is available during the process of bond formation to excite the $2s$ electron. Four unpaired electrons are now available for bonding purposes.

It might now be expected that carbon could form two different types of bonds, such as three bonds of a type using p orbitals ($2p_x$, $2p_y$, $2p_z$) and a fourth bond using the $2s$ orbital. But this is contrary to known fact—all four bonds are equivalent so far as bond energy and bond length are concerned.

The simplest two-dimensional picture of such a carbon atom, as noted in the diagram of the molecule dichloromethane, CH_2Cl_2, would be as in **A**.

$$\begin{array}{ccc} & Cl & \\ & | & \\ H\!-\!\!&C&\!\!-\!Cl \\ & | & \\ & H & \end{array} \qquad \begin{array}{ccc} & Cl & \\ & | & \\ H\!-\!\!&C&\!\!-\!H \\ & | & \\ & Cl & \end{array}$$

A   **B**

However, it readily can be observed that if the molecule were flat, it should exist in the two isomeric forms, **A** and **B**. As only one dichloromethane is known (and for other, more convincing, reasons) the structure as depicted is spatially incorrect. In 1874, LeBel and van't Hoff demonstrated, using the concept of *stereoisomerism*, that a carbon atom assumes a *tetrahedral* configuration. That is, each covalent bond is directed to a corner of a regular tetrahedron.

109.5°

To more clearly illustrate the three-dimensional aspect of this arrangement, the usual two-dimensional diagram is better shown by

$$\begin{array}{ccc} & X & \\ & | & \\ W\blacktriangleright\!\!&C&\!\!\blacktriangleleft Y \\ & \vdots & \\ & Z & \end{array} \qquad \begin{array}{ccc} & X & \\ & | & \\ Y\blacktriangleright\!\!&C&\!\!\blacktriangleleft W \\ & \vdots & \\ & Z & \end{array}$$

A   **B**

in which a solid line is understood to be in the plane of the paper, a broken line extends behind the plane, and solid arrowheads extend in front of the plane.

Study of the many kinds of three-dimensional organic models is very beneficial in the understanding of this concept. A cursory look at such models (or diagrams) indicates that **A** and **B** are not identical (not superimposable), but rather are in reality *isomers*. This situation, *stereoisomerism,* is a phenomenon that essentially doubles the number of possible compounds of this particular type.

Since the resultant bonds are comprised of one s and three p electrons, and neither are of the spherical s or linear p configuration but rather some combination thereof, they are said to be *hybridized*. This tetrahedral or sp^3 hybridization can be explained by the tendency for unshared electrons to get as far from each other as possible (the Pauli *exclusion* principle); for four bonds, the tetrahedral configuration satisfies this requirement. Covalent bonds, besides having characteristic bond length and energy, also are associated with direction in space.

Another peculiarity is associated with carbon-to-carbon bonding. In addition to the aforementioned tetrahedral, or sp^3, hybridization, two other possibilities are known to occur in the bonding of two carbon atoms: trigonal or sp^2, and linear (diagonal) or sp hybridization.

SIGMA (σ) AND PI (π) BONDS—Alkenes are examples of the sp^2 type of carbon-to-carbon bonding: the hybrid orbitals are directed toward the corners of an equilateral triangle. This permits the hybrid orbitals to be as far removed from each other as possible. An unhybridized p orbital also exists perpendicular to the plane of the sp^2 orbitals.

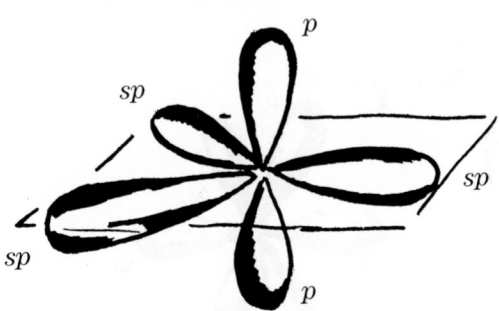

The union of two carbon atoms of this type produces a multiple bond involving two electron pairs (a double bond), as shown in the next set of figures. Overlap of the sp^2 orbitals forms a sigma (σ) bond and the p orbital overlap produces a pi (π) bond. A carbon-carbon double bond is not composed of two similar bonds, as might be interpreted from the usual notation of $C\!=\!C$ that is used. Rather, each bond is a distinct and separate entity and many physical and chemical properties confirm this feature.

All of the sigma bonds lie in the same plane, but the pi bonds project above and below the plane, as is evident from the previous diagram. As might be expected, because of the added "cementing" properties of the extra electrons, the carbon atoms of a multiple bond are held more closely. Thus the carbon-carbon bond distance for a double bond is 1.34 Å in ethylene, compared to 1.54 Å for the single carbon-carbon bond of ethane.

Another situation occurs due to the configuration of the sigma-pi double bond. Reference to the following illustration of the completed molecule shows that groups *a, b, c,* and *d* are in the same plane, and, by reversing the two substituent groups at either end of the molecule (as in **B** and **C**), an isomer is generated—a *geometric* isomer.

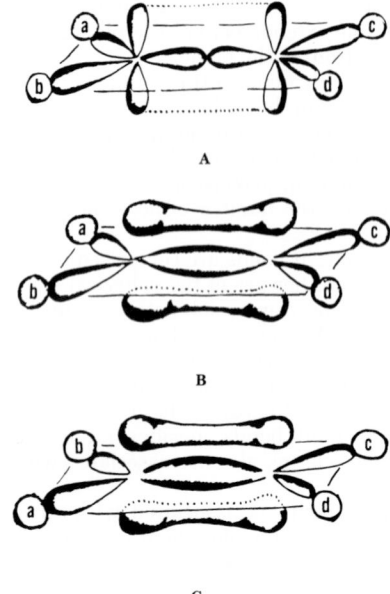

A

B

C

Again, this phenomenon leads to a doubling of the number of possible compounds of this particular type.

A third variety of hybridization that exists involves the coalition of one *s* and one *p* electron (*sp*). The resulting two *sp* orbitals produced are directed axially, 180° apart and 90° removed from the plane of the unhybridized *p* orbitals.

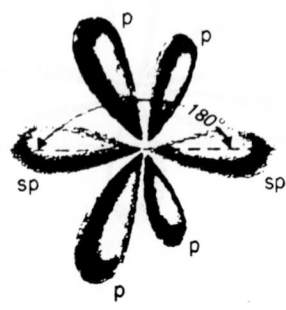

A combination of two carbon atoms exhibiting *sp* hybridization along the *sp* axis will yield carbon-carbon triple bonds.

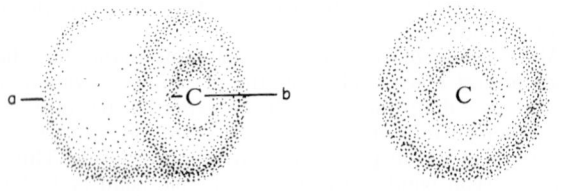

axial view

The *p* orbitals form a cylindrical sheath about the sigma bond. For a carbon-carbon triple bond the interatomic distance is smaller than a single or double bond, being 1.20 Å. Isomerism (geometric or stereoisomerism) is not possible with a triple bond as the substituents, **a** and **b**, are located axially.

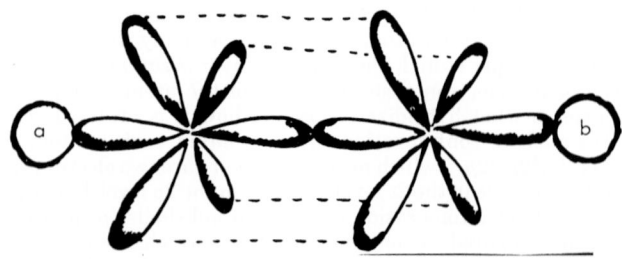

DELOCALIZATION AND RESONANCE—Benzene represents a large series of compounds exhibiting a kind of bonding that is perhaps as unique and different from the usual carbon-carbon bond types as is carbon from the rest of the periodic table. Although the six annular carbon atoms are bonded to each other via sp^2 orbitals (as with ethylene), the resultant molecule does not behave as an unsaturated compound. The compound is depicted as having a conjugate system of three double bonds (**B, C,** and **D**).

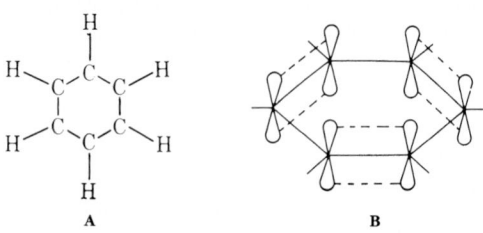

A   B

However, the benzene molecule does not behave chemically like a simple conjugated triene. Reactions normally occur by substitution of a hydrogen atom, rather than by the expected addition to the double bond. Also, two simple disubstitution products would be expected.

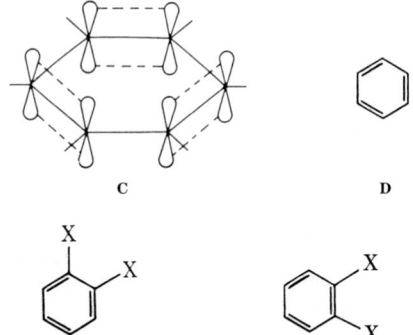

C   D

However, only one disubstitution product is known. Benzene, therefore, must exhibit an entirely different kind of bonding than those previously discussed. It is believed that the *p* orbitals, above and below the plane of the benzene ring, overlap in both directions and each electron can participate in several bonds. The ability of the π electrons to be active in joining several atoms results in stronger bonds and a more stable molecule. This phenomenon of *delocalization* of electrons results in a delocalization, or *resonance*, energy of stability.

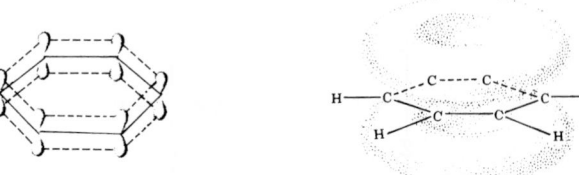

Due to the delocalization of the electrons only one type of bond exists and the classic alternate arrangement of single and double bonds between carbon atoms of the benzene molecule is misleading and incorrect. The carbon-carbon bond distance for benzene is 1.39 Å, lying between the single- and double-bond interatomic distance. The term *delocalization* better describes the resultant molecular orbital picture of benzene, as opposed to the concept of *resonance,* which may imply a rapid alternation between two or among several structural forms, which is totally incorrect.

Delocalization (resonance) stabilization is evidenced by many organic compounds that contain multiple bonds. Just as a lowering of energy results from the formation of molecular orbitals, whereby electrons are associated with two positive nuclei, a further lowering results if a molecular orbital is formed by using several nuclei. This extra energy-lowering increases the stability of a compound; the net energy difference derived from summing bond energies and that of the heat of combustion of the molecule is termed *resonance or delocalization energy.*

Several types of organic compounds, other than benzene, exhibit delocalization.

$$\left[R-C \underset{O}{\overset{O}{\lessgtr}} \right] \qquad CH_2{=\!=\!=}CH{=\!=\!=}CH{=\!=\!=}CH_2$$

Carboxylate ion   **1,3-Butadiene**

Delocalization accounts for the stability of *aromatic* compounds such as naphthalene, anthracene, pyridine, pyrimidine, thiophene, furan, etc. *Aromaticity* has become synonymous with the unusual stability and chemical behavior of benzene-like compounds. A quantum mechanical treatment of cyclic, conjugated systems indicates that aromaticity exists in those rings associated with $(4n + 2)$ π electrons, where n is an integer. Thus, rings having 6, 10, or 14π electrons may be aromatic (if they are planar), whereas those of 4, 8, or 12π electrons cannot be. The supporting mathematical theory is beyond the scope of this chapter, but chemical evidence easily suggests that compounds such as pyridine, thiophene, or furan do behave as benzene, while cyclooctatetraene—although a cyclic, conjugate system—behaves merely as a typical conjugated alkene and does not show the exceptional stability of an aromatic compound.

Carbon-Heteroatom Bonds

Practically all of the foregoing material pertains to the structure of a carbon-to-carbon or carbon-to-hydrogen bond. A majority of the compounds normally included in the area of organic chemistry also contain *heteroatoms* (atoms other than carbon and hydrogen), and the mode of bonding between carbon and the heteroatoms is of great importance. A rigorous treatment of this subject is beyond the limits of this chapter, but several general observations are in order.

Carbon forms a typical sigma bond with the univalent nonmetals (halogens) and with other electronegative polyvalent elements such as oxygen, nitrogen, sulfur, and phosphorus. Because of the differing electronegativities of the atoms on either side of the sigma bond, the bond is not entirely symmetrical and the slightly uneven distribution of bonding electrons causes an asymmetry leading to increased values of dipole moments with increased difference in electronegativities.

Multiple bonds also can exist between the polyvalent elements and carbon. Typical of this group is the carbonyl function ($=\!C\!=\!O$), an example of sp^2 hybridization. The carbon atom is joined to two other atoms and the oxygen atom by sigma bonds; the remaining p orbital of the carbon overlaps a p orbital of oxygen to form a typical pi bond. Thus, carbon and oxygen are joined by a double bond. Each of the three sigma bonds radiating from the carbon atom is at an angle of 120°, and the carbonyl portion and the two atoms to which it is attached lie in the same plane.

The electrons of the carbonyl double bond join two elements of quite different electronegativity, and hence are not shared equally, the electron cloud being pulled more strongly toward the electronegative oxygen atom. As the π electrons are of a lower energy than σ electrons, they are influenced more easily by the electronegative oxygen atom. This effect is much more pronounced with multiple bonds than for a single (sigma) bond and results in the occurrence of a permanent polarity. Therefore, aldehydes and ketones (which contain the carbonyl function) exhibit fairly large dipole moments (2.30–2.75 D) because of the polarity of the carbonyl group, as shown below. A lowercase delta (δ) indicates that a fractional charge of appropriate sign resides on the designated atoms.

$$
\begin{array}{c}
\delta^+ \quad \delta^- \\
R-C{=}O \\
| \\
R
\end{array}
$$

The structure of the carbonyl group largely determines the physical and chemical properties of aldehydes and ketones. Similar analogies can be drawn for carbon-to-sulfur and carbon-to-nitrogen multiple bonds.

Although carbon usually bonds to other elements by covalent-type linkages, several examples of ionic-type bonds are known (carbanion, R_3C^-; and carbonium ion or carbocation, R_3C^+), but these are very short lived and are primarily useful in explaining the *mechanisms* of various organic reactions via intermediates of transient existence.

Noncarbon Bonds

The magnitude of the number of organic compounds is not due solely to the intricacies shown in carbon-to-carbon and carbon-to-heteroatom bonds. The electronegative elements, especially nitrogen and oxygen, impart their individualities such that a carbon-to-oxygen or carbon-to-nitrogen bond can participate in new types of bonds not discussed previously. As an example, the *hydrogen bond* or *bridge* can cause intermolecular association which can lead to an apparent increase in molecular weight. The hydrogen bond also may be the reason for a drug binding to certain sites of activity. Formation of *chelates,* *clathrates,* coordination complexes, and so on also extends the number of compounds that would be possible if only classic types of bonding existed between elements. Chapter 14 deals in depth with the concepts mentioned in this paragraph.

Interatomic distances decrease appreciably to achieve the overlap needed to form pi bonds between atoms. The bond distance is characteristic of the atoms involved and the type of bond between them. Table 13-3 gives the bond energy and the bond distance for some covalent bonds.

Table 13-3. Covalent Bond Energy

BOND	BOND ENERGY, ΔH KCAL/MOL	BOND DISTANCE A
H—H	103.2[a]	0.74[c]
H—Cl	102.1[a]	1.27[c]
O—H	109.4[a]	0.96[b]
N—H	92.2[a]	1.01[b]
C—H	98.2[a]	1.09[b]
C—Cl	78.0[a]	1.77[b]
Cl—Cl	57.8[a]	1.99[c]
C—C	80.0[a]	1.54[b]
C=C	130.0[a]	1.33[b]
C≡C	193.0[a]	1.20[b]
C=O	152.0[b]	1.21[b]

[a]Data from Pitzer KS. *J Am Chem Soc* 1948; 70: 2140.
[b]Data from Fieser LF, Fieser M. *Introduction to Organic Chemistry.* Boston: DC Heath, 1957.
[c]Data from Pauling LC. *The Nature of the Chemical Bond,* 3rd ed. Ithaca, NY: Cornell University Press, 1960.

Table 13-4. Electronegativity Values for Some Elements

F	4.0	I	2.4	Be	1.5
O	3.5	P	2.1	Mg	1.2
N	3.0	H	2.1	Li	1.0
Cl	3.0	B	2.0	Ca	1.0
Br	2.8	Si	1.8	Na	0.9
S	2.5	Sn	1.7	K	0.8
C	2.5	Al	1.5	Cs	0.7

Adapted from Pauling LC. *The Nature of the Chemical Bond*, 3rd ed. Ithaca, NY: Cornell University Press, 1960, arranged in decreasing order.

POLAR BONDS: PARTIAL IONIC BOND AND IONIC BOND

BOND—There are many different types of partial ionic bonds between the two extremes of a covalent bond and an ionic bond. The tendency of a pair of atoms to form an ionic or a partial ionic bond is measured by the difference in their abilities to attract an electron, or in their *electronegativities*.

If a molecule acts as if it has a positive and negative pole (ie, has a partial separation of charge), it is called a *dipole*. A molecule with a dipolar bond is said to be *polar*, while an electrically symmetric molecule is designated as *nonpolar*.

The electronegativity values for some common elements are listed in Table 13-4. The relationship between electronegativity differences and the partial ionic character is shown in Table 13-5. It is interesting to point out that fluorine, the most electronegative of all elements, has not only unique chemical qualities but also important physiological properties. In very low doses fluorides can reduce the number of dental caries by well over 50%, while in excessive doses mottled enamel may result during the period of tooth formation. Lithium, a metal of very low electronegativity has been used in the treatment of manic depressive disorders; both the carbonate and citrate are the salt forms used clinically (see Chapters 24 and 82).

DIPOLE MOMENT—The process by which dipoles arise is known as *polarization*. The total polarization P can be written as

$$P = P_i + P_0 + P_a \tag{5}$$

The induced or electronic polarization, P_i, represents the shift of the electron cloud due to the influence of an electric field or an electromagnetic wave such as light. The induced molar polarization P_i can be determined from molar refraction measurements using the D-line of a sodium lamp, as the permanent dipole cannot follow an electromagnetic wave of such high frequency.

$$P_i = \frac{n_D^2 - 1}{n_D^2 + 2} \times \frac{M}{d} = MR \tag{6}$$

Equation 6 is known as the Lorentz-Lorenz equation, where n_D is the refractive index of the liquid measured with the D-line of a sodium lamp, M is the molecular weight, d is the density, and MR is the molar refraction (refractivity).

Table 13-5. The Difference in Electronegativities and Ionic Character of Some Chemical Bonds[a]

BOND	ELECTRONEGATIVITY DIFFERENCE, $X_a - Z_b$	PARTIAL IONIC CHARACTER, %
C—H	0.4	4
I—Br	0.4	4
I—Cl	0.6	9
O—H	1.4	30
C—F	1.5	44
Si—F	2.2	70
Be—F	2.5	79
K—F	3.2	92

Data from Pauling LC. *The Nature of the Chemical Bond*, 3rd ed. Ithaca, NY: Cornell University Press, 1960, arranged in increasing order.

Table 13-6. Atomic and Group Refractions for Sodium-D Light

ELEMENT	NA_D cc	ELEMENT	NA_D cc
C	2.42	N in	
H	1.10	Aliphatic oximes	3.93
O in OH	1.52	R—CONH$_2$	2.65
O in ester OR	1.64	R—CONHR'	2.27
O=	2.21	R—CONR'R"	2.71
F	1.22	NO$_2$ group in	
Cl	5.96	Alkyl nitrates	7.59
Br	8.86	Alkyl nitrites	7.44
I	13.90	Nitroparaffins	6.72
S in SH	7.69	Aromatic nitro compounds	7.30
S in RS	7.97		7.30
S in RCNS	7.91	Nitramines	7.51
S in RS	8.11	NO group in	
N in		Nitrites	5.92
Hydroxylamines	2.48	Nitrosamines	5.37
Hydrazines	2.47	Structural units	
RNH$_2$	2.32	Double bond	1.73
RNHR'	2.49	Triple bond	2.40
RNR'R"	2.84	3-membered ring	0.71
ArNH$_2$	3.21	4-membered ring	0.48
ArNHR	3.59	Oxirane	
ArNRR'	4.36	Terminal	2.02
R—C≡N	3.05	Nonterminal	1.85
Ar—C≡N	3.79	Conjugation—(see Ref 6)	

One also can calculate the induced molar polarization from the electron-group refractions given by Smyth, or from the Atomic Refractivities compiled by Fajans (see Fajans[8] and Table 13-6). For example, the molar refraction of methyl acetate,

$$CH_3\text{—}\overset{\displaystyle \underset{\|}{O}}{C}\text{—}O\text{—}CH_3$$

can be calculated as

$$Na_D$$

$$3 \times C = 3 \times 2.42 \quad = 7.26$$

$$6 \times H = 6 \times 1.10 \quad = 6.60$$

$$1 \times {=}O = 1 \times 2.21 \quad = 2.21$$

$$1 \times \text{—}O\text{—} = 1 \times 1.64 = 1.64$$

$$\text{Total} = 17.71$$

or

$$
\begin{aligned}
MR &= \frac{n_D^2 - 1}{n_D^2 + 2} \times \frac{M}{d} \\
&= \left[\frac{(1.3593)^2 - 1}{(1.3593)^2 + 2} \right] \times \left[\frac{74.08}{0.928} \right] \text{(at 20°)} \\
&= 17.57
\end{aligned}
$$

An apparent correlation between the activity of chloramphenicol analogs, as determined by microbial kinetics, and the group refraction of their aromatic substituents has been reported.[9]

In Equation 5, P_0 is the orientation polarization due to the permanent dipole and P_a is the atomic polarization, which may be neglected for practical purposes because it is only 5 to 10% of P_i. The orientation polarization, P_0, arises from the separation of charges due to the difference in electronegativities of the atoms.

Using an electromagnetic wave of much lower frequency than the frequency of light, such as a radio wave, one can measure the total polarization, as the permanent dipole as well as the electron cloud can follow the alternation of direction of the radio wave. In other words, one can calculate P from dielectric constant and molar volume (M/d) measurements.

$$P = \frac{\epsilon - 1}{\epsilon + 2} \times \frac{M}{d} \tag{7}$$

Combining Equations 5 through 7, Debye's equation (Eq 8) for a pure compound, and the Clausius-Mossotti equation (Eq 9), and neglecting P_a, gives Equation 10:

$$P = \frac{4}{3} \pi N_A \left(\alpha + \frac{\mu^2}{3kT} \right) \tag{8}$$

$$P_i = \frac{4}{3} \pi N_A \alpha \tag{9}$$

$$P_o = P - P_i = \frac{4}{3} \pi N_A \frac{\mu^2}{3kT} \tag{10}$$

where N_A is Avogadro's number, α is the induced polarizability (a measure of the ease of polarization by an electric field), μ is the dipole moment (esu · cm), k is the Boltzmann constant, and T is the absolute temperature. It should be noted that molar refraction is a molar property and induced polarizability is a molecular property.

Equation 8 can be written as

$$P = a + b/T \tag{11}$$

where $a = 4\pi N_A \alpha/3 = P_i$ and $b = 4\pi N_A \mu^2/9k$. Because Equation 11 is a linear equation, by plotting values of P at several temperatures (calculated from dielectric constant measurements) versus $1/T$, one can compute α and P_i from the intercept and the permanent dipole moment (μ) of the compound from the slope, b. This procedure usually is applied to gases.

For a pure liquid, one can obtain the total polarization, P, according to Equation 7 and the induced polarization, P_i, from refractive index and molar-volume measurements at a constant temperature (Eq 6). Regardless of the manner of obtaining P_i, the final equation for the calculation of the dipole moment, usually expressed in Debye units, is the same (Eq 12). One Debye unit (D) is equivalent to $10^{-18} \times$ esu · cm.

$$\mu = \sqrt{\frac{9kb}{4\pi N_A}} = 0.0128 \times 10^{-18} \sqrt{b}$$

$$= 0.0128 \times 10^{-18} \sqrt{(P - P_i)T} \text{ (esu · cm)}$$

$$= 0.0128 \sqrt{(P - P_i)T} \text{ (Debye units)} \tag{12}$$

There are other equations for calculating dipole moments from measured values of the dielectric constant, refractive index, and density of liquids. However, for pure liquids the results are not very satisfactory. The dipole moment of medicinal substances usually is measured in a nonpolar solvent (eg, benzene, cyclohexane, or heptane) or in a solvent with some polarity but without resultant moment (eg, dioxane).

It has been suggested that, to eliminate the inaccuracies that arise from treating the solvent in a different way than solutions, only the results of measurements on dilute solutions be used.

Correlations of biological activity with dipole moment have been reported for the insecticidal activity of chlorphenothane (DDT) isomers, the cholinesterase inhibitory activity of N-alkyl substituted amides, and the respiratory stimulation activity of cyclic ureas and cyclic thioureas. Investigations have shown that high dipole moment enhances central nervous system (CNS) stimulatory activity or toxicity, whereas low dipole moment favors anticonvulsant or CNS-depression activity. The use of dipole moment as a parameter in drug-receptor interaction and quantitative structure–activity relationship studies has been reviewed by Lien et al.[10–12]

When the electronegativities of the bonded atoms are quite different, a formal electron-pair bond can no longer exist. The bonding electron pair is now associated exclusively with the more electronegative atom, and an *anion* is formed. The atom that has lost its electron becomes positively charged, and a *cation* is formed.

COORDINATE COVALENT BONDS—A *coordinate covalent bond* is formed when only one atom donates both electrons; for example, the unshared electron pair on the nitrogen atom of an amine (a Lewis base) can serve to form such a bond with a proton or trimethyl boron (a Lewis acid).

Because the nitrogen suffers a loss of negative charge and the boron atom gains an equivalent negative charge, it is more realistic to depict the complex molecule as the *adduct*.

Amine oxides are other examples of coordinate covalent compounds.

Because oxygen is much more electronegative than boron (see Table 13-4), the ionic character of the N-oxide is more pronounced than that of the N—B bond. This is evidenced by the relatively high melting point, high solubility in water, and low solubility in nonpolar solvents of the amine oxides. One also can infer the polar character by a comparison of dipole moments: 6.2 D for KCl (ion pairs), 5.02 D for trimethylamine oxide, and 3.92 D for the trimethylamine-trimethylboron complex.

CHELATES—The term chelate (from the Greek *chela*, claw) describes this class of compounds appropriately. *Chelates* consist of a partial ring of atoms that close up by holding a given atom, usually a metal, in a molecular claw. The compounds capable of forming a ring structure with a metal are designated as *ligands* (see Chapter 14 for a thorough discussion of complex formation).

Cisplatin, a platinum coordination compound with the ammine groups at the *cis* position, has been used in the treatment of testicular and ovarian tumors in combination with other anticancer drugs (see Chapter 86).

Some biologically important compounds (eg, chlorophyll, hemoglobin, peroxidases, cytochromes, oxidases, ascorbic acid oxidase, tyrosinase, polyphenoloxidase, lactase, phosphatase, carboxylases, insulin, and cyanocobalamin) are naturally occurring chelates. Tetracyclines also are capable of forming chelates with metals. Chelating agents may be used for a number of purposes, such as sequestration of metals, stabilization of drug preparations vulnerable to oxidation in the presence of trace-metals, and the treatment of heavy metal poisoning.

MOLECULAR BONDS—Several classes of compounds contain *intermolecular coordinate covalent bonds* (eg, *sandwich* compounds, charge-transfer complexes, and the molecular-addition compounds). These types of bonds are referred to as *molecular bonds* for brevity.

METALLOCENES—In 1951 Kealy and Pauson accidentally discovered ferrocene by oxidizing cyclopentadienemagnesium bromide with anhydrous ferric chloride in ether solution. Ferrocene has aromatic character and is an unusually stable iron-containing orange product, formula $C_{10}H_{10}Fe$, that melts at 174° and boils at 249°; it is soluble in common organic solvents but insoluble in water. The generally accepted structure of ferrocene was first proposed by Woodward et al in 1952. X-ray and electron diffraction studies have shown that the iron is packed between two parallel cyclopentadienyl rings like a *sandwich* (**I**, below).

The solubility, volatility, and other properties of metallocenes are due to the covalent character of the molecular bonds. This indicates that each cyclopentadienyl ion donates an electron pair to the metal ion. Ferrocene is diamagnetic, hence the six $3d$ electrons of iron are paired up to make available two open $3d$ orbitals. A large number of metallocenes have been prepared and studied since the discovery of ferrocene.

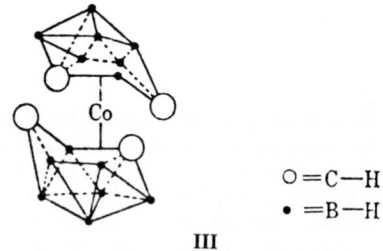

I
Ferrocene

• $= B—H$
○ $= C—H$
II
Structure of
$(\pi\text{-}C_5H_5)Fe(\pi(3)\text{-}1,2,\text{-}B_6C_2H_{11})$

○ $= C—H$
• $= B—H$

III

Several different aromatic rings (eg, indene, azulene, and benzene) also will form metallocenes. In many metallocenes, CO or NO molecules are found in place of one of the aromatic rings, and the metal may be Cr or Mn, as well as Fe. Metallocenes undergo most of the typical aromatic reactions.

It has been shown that daily oral administration of ferrocene produced hemosiderosis with an unusually high, dose-related accumulation of iron in dogs. A decrease in hemoglobin, packed-cell volume and erythrocyte count occurred within 4 weeks in dogs receiving 300 mg/kg of ferrocene. This and higher dosage resulted in cirrhosis, which was considered to be an effect of the hydrocarbon moiety.

There is a field of research that combines polyhedral carborane and transition metal chemistry. Several families of polyhedral species now are known in which a transition metal resides in the polyhedral surface (**II, III**).

CHARGE-TRANSFER COMPLEXES—Certain substances combine in a 1:1 molar ratio to form crystalline addition products. The molecular addition compound is held together by weak forces, such as van der Waals (dipole-dipole, dipole-induced dipole, induced dipole-induced dipole), ion-dipole, and even hydrogen bonds. Polynitroaromatic compounds, such as trinitrobenzene and picric acid, are well known for their ability to form charge-transfer complexes (pi complexes) (see Chapter 14).

Caffeine complexes with various drugs such as sodium benzoate, sodium salicylate, sulfonamides, barbiturates, and 5-chlorosalicylic acid.

AROMATIC SIGMA (σ) BOND COMPLEXES—Aromatic compounds react with $HCl \cdot AlCl_3$ or $HF \cdot BF_3$ to produce salts that ionize in highly polar nonaqueous solvents, for example, liquid hydrogen fluoride or sulfuric acid.

Using NMR spectrometry, Olah et al[13] detected the *p*-anisonium and the 2,4,6-trimethylphenonium ions produced by ionizing β-*p*-anisylethyl chloride and β-mesitylethyl chloride, respectively, in SbF_5—SO_2 at −70° to −60°.

Sigma complexes are molecular complexes resulting from the rupture of a sigma bond (eg, $H—AlCl_4$, $ArCH_2CH_2—Cl$); they also occur in Friedel–Crafts reactions. Because they are reactive toward water, no practical pharmaceutical uses have been made of these complexes. Refer to Chapter 14 for a more extensive treatment of complexation.

STEREOISOMERISM—Early in 1874 van't Hoff envisaged a double bond by joining two tetrahedrons at two corners and correctly predicted that unsymmetrically substituted derivatives of ethylene should exist in two stereochemical forms, or as a pair of *cis* and *trans* isomers.

cis   *trans*

As in the previous discussion of sigma and pi bonds, it was shown that in an alkene, rotation about the sigma bond is restricted by the overlap of *p* orbitals comprising the pi bond.

Stereoisomerism as a result of the rigid configuration about a double bond, or other rigid structure such as a ring, is known as *geometric isomerism*. It is interesting to note that in the case of the synthetic estrogens, the *cis* isomer of diethylstilbestrol is unstable and has less than one-tenth the activity of the *trans* isomer. One should note the structural similarity between *trans*-diethylstilbestrol and estradiol.

trans-Diethylstilbestrol   **Estradiol**

It has been reported that tamoxifen, a drug that structurally resembles *trans*-diethylstilbestrol, arrested or reduced breast tumor growth rate in 77% of patients given 20 mg of the drug orally twice a day. The compound is believed to block estrogen receptor sites.

Due to the presence of symmetry, the type of geometric isomerism occurring in substituted ethylenes usually is not associated with optical activity; some other site in the molecule ordinarily gives rise to optical isomerism.

Another type of geometric isomerism is found in ring compounds, the ring taking the place of the rigid double bond. For example, *trans*-2-phenylcyclopropylamine is more stable than the *cis* isomer and is a potent monoamine oxidase inhibitor.

trans-2-Phenylcyclo-
propylamine
(Tranylcypromine)

cis-2-Phenylcyclo-
propylamine

A substance that rotates the plane of polarized light is said to be *optically active*. *Optical rotation* may be considered as a consequence of the phenomenon of circular double refraction in which a beam of polarized rays is resolved into two circularly polarized rays, one turning clockwise and the other counterclockwise as the beam advances. In an optically active medium these rays have different velocities and on recombination they vibrate in a plane different from that of the incident ray. Refer to Chapter 35 for a more complete discussion.

The necessary and sufficient condition for a molecule to show optical activity is that the molecule should be asymmetric (ie, the molecule should not be superimposable with its mirror image); in other words, it should be *chiral* (from the Greek *cheir,* hand; thus, right- or left-handedness). Although many optically active compounds have asymmetric carbon atoms (carbon atoms bearing four different groups), not all compounds possessing asymmetric carbon atoms are optically active; for example, *meso*-tartaric acid has two asymmetric carbon atoms, but it is optically inactive due to the presence of a plane of symmetry within the molecule (*internal compensation*).

Optical isomerism due to restricted rotation (as with tetra-*ortho*-substituted biphenyls and dissymmetric polyphenyls) is well documented in Eliel's book (see the bibliography). Atoms other than carbon can serve as a center of asymmetry. For instance, optically active *N*-oxides, quaternary ammonium compounds, sulfonium and selenonium salts, and sulfoxides and sulfinic esters have been resolved. As living organisms are made of numerous chiral macromolecules, stereoselectivity commonly is observed for stereoisomers. Increasing emphasis is being placed on the use of the more active enantiomer (eutomer), instead of the racemic mixture (equal amounts of both eutomer and distomer) as the therapeutic agent (see Ariëns et al in the bibliography).

ENANTIOMERS—Molecules whose mirror images are nonsuperimposable are called *enantiomorphs, enantiomers,* or *optical antipodes*. Enantiomers have identical physicochemical properties in an optically inactive environment—they rotate the plane of polarized light to the same degree, but in opposite directions. The measurement of optical rotation is useful for the purpose of identifying and/or assaying an optically active

substance. The *specific rotation* is defined as

$$|\alpha|_D^t = \frac{\alpha}{l(g/v)}$$

where *D* is the D-line of sodium vapor lamp, *t* is the temperature, α is the observed rotation in degrees, *l* is the length of the cell in decimeters (1 dm = 10 cm) and *g*/*v* is the concentration in g/100 mL of solvent.

When equal amounts of *dextro* (+) and *levo* (−) isomers are mixed, a *racemic modification* arises. They are denoted as *d, l* (which no longer are used to designate direction of rotation of light) or ±. Racemic modifications are the products of most organic syntheses that involve a chiral center; they also may be obtained by racemization of a pure enantiomer. In a racemic modification the substance in bulk is not optically active, even though an individual molecule is optically active. The resultant rotation is zero as the concentration of the molecules that rotate light to the left is equal to those that rotate it to the right.

DIASTEREOISOMERS—Stereoisomers that are not mirror images of each other are called *diastereoisomers* or *diastereomers*. Diastereoisomerism exists when a given structural formula has at least two asymmetric atoms. Diastereoisomers should have different physicochemical properties like melting points, solubilities, and optical rotation.

(−) Erythrose   (+) Erythrose   (−) Threose   (+) Threose
I   **II**   **III**   **IV**

For one above example, compounds **I** and **II** or **III** and **IV** are enantiomers; compounds **I** and **III, I** and **IV, II** and **III** or **II** and **IV** are diastereomers.

ABSOLUTE CONFIGURATION—The designations (+), (−), *d,* and *l* refer to the rotation of plane polarized light by a molecule, but the actual three-dimensional arrangement in space of atoms in a chiral molecule may bear no relation to these descriptors. Even with the carbohydrates, the small capital D or L refers to the configuration of but a portion of a molecule relative to a reference compound, glyceraldehyde. Fortunately, the selection of the reference configurations for absolute and assumed configurations happened to coincide.

With the improvement of x-ray crystallographic techniques in the 1950s, it became possible to reveal the actual three-dimensional arrangement of atoms and the absolute configuration of (+)-tartaric acid was determined. This became a reference point to which other chiral molecules could be related, by chemical conversions, that previously had been demonstrated to retain or invert a configuration.

From these studies the *R* and *S*, or Cahn-Ingold-Prelog system (named after the chemists who devised the method), was developed. A series of *sequence rules* was promulgated, which is beyond the scope of this chapter. These rules accommodate geometric *cis* (*zusammen* or *Z*) and *trans* (*entgegen* or *E*) structures, as well as *R* (*rectus* or right) and *S* (*sinister* or left). The symbols *R* and *S* refer only to the right- or left-handedness of the chiral centers and not to the direction of rotation of polarized light.

OPTICAL ROTATORY DISPERSION (ORD)—*Optical rotatory dispersion* (ORD) involves the measurement of the angle of optical rotation of linearly polarized light at various wavelengths. Usually greater rotational angles are obtained at shorter wavelengths. The source of energy consists of a xenon arc and a monochromator to isolate the desired wavelength in the ultraviolet region. A photomultiplier and photometer are used to measure the intensity after the light has passed through the polarimeter.

As the wavelength of the polarized light is varied, the absolute value of rotation may increase continuously so that the plot of [α] versus λ is a plain curve (Line A, Fig 13-3). On the other hand, the rotation may change direction either from left to right or right to left, and show one or more maxima and minima.

The appearance of a maximum and a minimum in a plot of specific rotation versus wavelength is referred to as a *single Cotton effect* (Line B, Fig 13-3), whereas the appearance of several maximums and several minimums is referred to as a *multiple Cotton effect*. If, in approaching the region of the Cotton effect from long wavelengths, one passes first through a maximum and then through a minimum, the Cotton effect is called *positive*. If the minimum is reached first and then the maximum at shorter wavelength, it is called a *negative* Cotton effect.

The Cotton effect is due to the presence of an asymmetric center near a chromophoric group, such as =C=O, in the optically active molecule which has unequal absorption of right and left circularly polarized light. The concept of ORD is useful for the study of the stereochemistry of natural products, ketosteroids, and the analysis of randomly coiled and helical configurations of polypeptide chains.

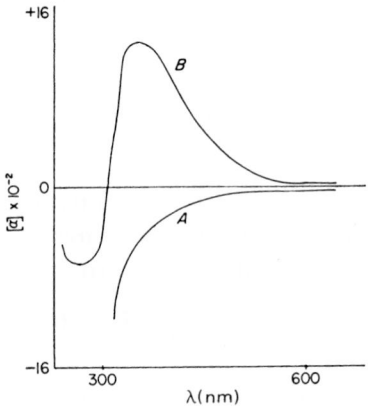

Figure 13-3. Rotatory dispersion curves: (*A*) levorotatory plain curve, (*B*) positive simple Cotton effect.

CIRCULAR DICHROISM (CD)—A *circular dichroic* curve is a plot of the molecular ellipticity [θ] versus the wavelength λ. The CD effect results from the fact that the right circularly polarized ray is *absorbed* differently from the left circularly polarized beam of light. The molecular ellipticity is defined as

$$[\theta] = 3300 \cdot \Delta\varepsilon, \Delta\varepsilon = \varepsilon_L - \varepsilon_R$$

where $\Delta\varepsilon$ is the differential dichroic absorption and ε_L and ε_R are the molar extinction coefficients for the left and right rays.

If in a dichrograph the oscillating crystal is oriented correctly, the plane-polarized beam of light passed through the instrument can be resolved into right and left components. These are passed through the optically active medium. When these unequally absorbed circular components are recombined in the region of electronic absorption, they give elliptically polarized light. Measurements involving CD have been used for studying drug–protein binding with 52 analgesic, sedative, and antidepressive drugs.[14] From this study it was suggested that a plane-ring system with high electron density (eg, benzodiazepine and dibenzazepine derivatives) appeared to be an essential factor for strong binding to human serum albumin.

CONFIGURATION AND CONFORMATION—The spatial arrangement of the groups about a central atom is referred to as the *configuration* of the atom. Three-dimensional models, their projections, or perspective drawings must be used to illustrate the difference between stereoisomers. The particular shape that a molecule assumes by free rotation about single bonds is referred to as its *conformation*.

An ethane molecule may have an infinite number of conformations because of rotation about the C—C bond; however, only a few conformations are possible that will make the molecular energy a minimum. The conformational preferences of some diastereoisomers have been determined from nuclear magnetic resonance (NMR) studies.

For a series of diastereoisomers involving a substituted phenylethyl skeleton, when the alkyl groups attached to each asymmetric center are small (eg, methyl), both *gauche*- and *trans*-conformers (rotamers)

have substantial populations because of the relatively low rotational barriers. Newman projection formulas are used for the illustrations, in which the molecules are viewed from front to back in the direction of the bond linking the asymmetric carbon atoms. In the following formulas, the center of the circle represents C-2 and the circle itself represents C-3 of 3-phenyl-2-butanol.

When the alkyl groups are bulky (eg, isopropyl), steric interactions cause these groups to prefer a *trans* orientation; the vicinal hydrogens are then *trans* in the *erythro* but *gauche* in the *threo* isomers.

For a more detailed discussion of potential-energy barriers in various systems, consult Eliel's book (see the bibliography).

The preferred conformation of serotonin has been calculated using molecular orbital theory. Complementary features of the serotonin receptor have been postulated, and the relationship of serotonin in its preferred conformation to the serotonin antagonist, lysergic acid diethylamide (LSD), has been presented as an explanation of LSD's antagonism.

INTERMOLECULAR BINDING FORCES

An understanding of intermolecular and intramolecular binding forces is very important in many different aspects of pharmaceutical sciences, such as in the manufacture of various preparations, in stability studies, and in the design of new drugs. A knowledge of these forces is not only essential for predicting some physicochemical properties of various dosage forms but also indispensable for the interpretation of drug action at the molecular level and for structure–activity correlations. Martin's classification[15] for various types of forces will be used in the following discussion.

REPULSIVE AND ATTRACTIVE FORCES—Intermolecular repulsive forces exist when two dipolar molecules are brought close together *head-to-head* or *tail-to-tail*, or when any two molecules are brought so close that their nonbonding electronic clouds interpenetrate. Otherwise, two molecules having opposite charges closer together than the like charges will attract each other. When the repulsive and the attractive forces are equal, the potential energy of the two molecules is a minimum and an equilibrium will be established. Similar forces may exist in the same molecule (intramolecular) as well as between different molecules. Only intermolecular forces will be discussed here.

VAN DER WAALS' FORCES—Due to electrostatic attraction, dipolar molecules tend to align themselves with neighboring molecules so that the negative pole of one molecule points towards the positive pole of the next, for example,

$$\overset{\leftarrow}{O=C}<\ldots\overset{\leftarrow}{NR_3}$$

This type of attraction is known as a *dipole–dipole* interaction and has a force of 1 to 7 kcal/mol. Dipole–dipole forces vary inversely as the fourth power of the distance between molecules, $F \propto (1/d^4)$.

The importance of the permanent dipole attractions in the stabilization of an α-helix has been pointed out. The electric dipoles in an α-helix add to one another along the direction of the axis. Two helices that wind in the same direction will, therefore, repel each other and two that wind in opposite directions will attract each other, as in DNA.

Permanent dipoles can induce a transient electric dipole in nonpolar molecules and produce *dipole-induced dipole*, or *Debye, forces*. These interactions involve an energy of about 1 to 3 kcal/mol.

When any two atoms belonging to different molecules are brought sufficiently close together, *induced dipole–induced dipole*, or *London, attractions* arise. In this case, the energy is about 0.5 to 1 kcal/mol. These forces originate from molecular internal vibrations. The temporary dipoles that this vibration creates in the constituent atoms induce dipoles in neighboring atoms of other molecules, and this process results in a net attraction. This type of force is responsible for the liquefaction of nonpolar gases. London forces vary inversely as the seventh power of the distance between molecules, $F \propto (1/d^7)$.

HYDROGEN BONDS—When a hydrogen atom holds two other atoms, a *hydrogen bond* (hydrogen bridge or H-bond) is formed. The two bonds attached to the same hydrogen cannot both be covalent bonds. The H-bond must be in part ionic. Indeed, the hydrogen bond usually is formed only between hydrogen and electronegative atoms. In addition, the atoms capable of forming H-bonds have at least one unshared electron pair.

Without hydrogen bonds this world would be much different, as water would boil at a temperature far below 0°. The surprisingly high boiling point of H_2O (100°), compared to H_2S (−60.7°) and H_2Se (−41.5°), can be attributed to the higher H-bonding ability of oxygen, which in turn is due to its smaller volume and higher electron density as compared to S and Se.

The most common atoms capable of forming H-bonds are F, O, N and, to a lesser degree, Cl and S. There also is some evidence that hydrogen attached to a triply-bound carbon (eg, HCN, HC≡CH, or $CHCl_3$) forms H-bonds. The strength of most H-bonds ranges from 1 to 7 kcal/mol.

H-BOND	BOND STRENGTH (kcal/mol)
F—H . . . F	7
O—H . . . O	4.5–7.6
O—H . . . N	4–7
C—H . . . π electrons	2–4
C—H . . . O	2–3
N—H . . . O	2–3
N—H . . . N	1.3

The strength of the H-bond depends on the solvent as well as the state. For instance, the H-bond strength of O—H . . . O for $(CH_3COOH)_2$ as a vapor is 7.64 kcal/mol, while that of $(CH_3COOH)_2$ in benzene is 4.85 kcal/mol. In water the H-bond has been estimated to have an energy of 4.5 kcal/mol; in ice, the bond strength is 6 kcal/mol. Hydrogen-bonding is responsible for the higher boiling point of a carboxylic acid compared with that of its ester. This is because in the free acid dimerization can occur by H-bonding, while this is impossible for an ester.

Hydrogen-bonding is also responsible for the high solubility of polyhydroxy compounds, such as sugars, in water. During the replication of DNA molecules, hydrogen bonds between base pairs are broken and rematched.

Various physical methods may be used to study H-bonding, such as molecular-weight determination, and infrared (IR) and NMR spectrometry.

ION-DIPOLE AND ION-INDUCED DIPOLE FORCES—Ion pairs in the solid state have bond strengths comparable to or even stronger than covalent bonds (100–200 versus 50–150 kcal/mol). However, in a biological system, due to hydration and the large amount of inorganic salts present for ion exchange, the bond strength would be weakened substantially to the neighborhood of 5 kcal/mol.

When an ionic bond is reinforced by the simultaneous presence of other forces, such as hydrogen-bonding, the bond becomes stronger (10 kcal/mol).

$$\begin{array}{ccc} H & & O \\ | & & \| \\ -N^{\oplus} & & {}^{\ominus}C- \\ | & & \\ H \quad H & \cdots\cdots & O \end{array}$$

An ion pair can attract a dipole or induce a dipole in a neighboring nonpolar molecule. The strength of an *ion-dipole* bond (eg, $R_4\overset{\oplus}{N}\ldots\overset{\leftarrow}{NR_3}$) is about 1 to 7 kcal/mol, and that of an *ion-induced* dipole (eg, $\overset{\oplus}{K}-\overset{\ominus}{I}\ldots I-I$) would be somewhat weaker.

HYDROPHOBIC INTERACTIONS—The association of nonpolar groups with each other in aqueous solution, arising because of the tendency of water molecules to exclude nonpolar molecules, is known as a *hydrophobic interaction,* or *hydrophobic bonding*. The word *hydrophobic* really is a misnomer, because it implies that the nonpolar molecule dislikes water—in fact, it is water that dislikes the nonpolar molecule.

The formation of hydrophobic bonds is favored because of an entropy effect. Before the formation of a hydrophobic bond, water molecules are arranged in an ordered fashion around exposed nonpolar groups. When hydrophobic interactions occur, the order is disrupted and results in a favorable entropy change, which is great enough to overcome the enthalpy for the interaction of the nonpolar groups; hence, the free energy is negative and the process is spontaneous. The strength of hydrophobic interactions has been reported to be 0.37 kcal/mol per CH_2 group.

A chain of 14 carbon atoms that binds with another nonpolar counterpart would have a bond strength of 5.2 kcal/mol. This bond, being stronger than an ionic bond or other weak forces in the biological system, then may dominate the mode of binding of a complicated drug molecule. The importance of hydrophobic interactions in stabilizing protein structure, drug-protein binding, transport, and storage of drugs and drug-receptor interaction has been noted in recent years. A summary of the different types of intermolecular forces and molecular recognition is given in Table 13-7.[10–12]

ADDITIVE PHYSICAL PROPERTIES

The division of physical properties into additive, constitutive, and colligative can be found in many textbooks. Additive physical properties depend on the number and kind of atoms in a

Table 13-7. Intermolecular Forces and Molecular Recognition

			Principles	
Like dissolves like (polar vs nonpolar)			II. Opposite charges attract each other (acids and bases; cations and I. anions)	
PROCESSES			FORCES INVOLVED (ALL INTERMOLECULAR FORCES ARE ELECTROSTATIC IN ORIGIN.)	
Non-Specific	Diffusion Dispersion Solution Mixing Phase transfer Passive absorption Excretion Non-chiral chromatographic separation		Non-stereospecific in general	Ionic, ion-dipole, ion-induced dipole Dipolar (dipole-dipole, Keesom forces; dipole-induced dipole, Debye forces; induced dipole-induced dipole, London forces) (*van der Waals'* forces) H-bonding Hydrophobic interactions
Self-Association	Crystallization Formation of 4° protein structure, DNA, RNA		All of the above, size, shape, complementarity, and group asymmetry are important	
Specific	Enzyme-substrate Drug-receptor Antigen-antibody DNA replication Transcription (DNA/RNA) Translation Active transport Facilitated transport Active secretion Chiral chromatographic separation		Stereospecific in general	All of the above Complementarity is involved Shape, group symmetry as well as size are important

molecule. Such additivity enables one to calculate many molecular values from a few fundamental constants. The best example is the calculation of molecular weights from atomic weights. The additive nature of molar refractions has been used for the calculation of induced polarization (see the discussion of dipole moment in Chapter 15).

MOLAR VOLUME—This term is self-explanatory. It is defined as the molecular weight divided by the density of a liquid (molar volume = MW/d). By using statistical analysis, it has been shown that the additivity of molar volume is better fulfilled at ordinary temperatures (20°) than at the boiling point of each individual substance. This is an interesting result, as from the *principle of corresponding states* it might be expected that additivity would hold better at the boiling point.

In the homologous series of nonbranched primary derivatives, the accuracy of a calculation of molar volume is relatively good. The deviations increase gradually with poly-substituted derivatives, 1,1-bis-derivatives, *ortho* derivatives, and branched isomers; nevertheless, the additivity scheme can serve as a first approximation.

PARTITION COEFFICIENTS AND THE Π CONSTANT—In the early theory of narcosis, lipid solubility was regarded as the most important factor for the inhibition of cell activity. At the beginning of the 20th century Meyer and Overton proposed that narcotic efficiency parallels the coefficient for the partition of a drug between oil and water. Although this theory cannot explain the mechanism of narcotic action, it does explain the role of transport to nerve tissues.

It is more logical to use partition coefficients than solubility in a single solvent for structure–activity correlations since, in a biological system, one is dealing with a heterogeneous system rather than a simple solution. Partition coefficients have been used in the study of drug absorption, distribution, metabolism, toxicity, and structure–activity correlation.

It has been shown that the partition coefficients for a given compound in two different solvent systems (eg, ether/water, octanol/water) are related as follows:

$$\log P_1 = a \log P_2 + b$$

where a and b are constants. This suggests that one can use the results from one set of solvents to predict results in a second set.

Hansch's group[16–20] systematically has extended the use of partition coefficients, measured from octanol/water, to serve as a measure of the ease of passage of organic molecules through various lipoprotein barriers and/or as a measure of the hydrophobic binding with protein (such as bovine serum albumin). From the partition coefficients of a variety of derivatives of the type X—C6H4OCH2COOH, X—C6H5, and C6H5(CH2)n—X, the substituent constants (π) for the aromatic and the aliphatic function (X) have been determined.

The π constant is defined as

$$\pi = \log P_X - \log P_H$$

where P_X is the partition coefficient of a derivative, and P_H is that of the parent compound. Although π varies continuously for a given function depending on its electronic environment, the variation generally is small; therefore, it is called *additive-constitutive*.

The application of $\log P$ and the additive-constitutive nature of constants for the correlation of biological activity with chemical structure has been illustrated in many cases. (See Chapter 28 for a discussion of the Hansch equation.) Table 13-8 lists the constants for some important functional groups.[16–18,21,22] One can calculate many $\log P$ values from a few constants. The method of calculation can be illustrated with diphenhydramine.

$\Sigma \pi = +4.26$ +0.30   −0.98   +0.50   −0.32

3.76 = calc log P
3.40 = obs log P

Heightened interest in the structures and properties of proteins as drugs or drug targets has been greatly stimulated by the recent developments of pharmacogenomics and proteomics. Of particular importance are the hydrophobic contribution con-

Table 13-8. π Constants for Some Functional Groups

FUNCTION X	AROMATIC SYSTEM[a]	ALIPHATIC SYSTEM
H—	0	0
F—	0.13	−0.17
Cl—	0.76	0.39
Br—	0.94	0.60
I—	1.15	1.00
CH_3—	0.50	0.50
$CH{\equiv}C$—		0.48
$CH_2{=}CH$—		0.70
C_2H_5—	1.00	1.00
$CH_2{=}CCH_3$		1.00
$\quad\mid$		
$CH_2{=}CHCH_2$—		1.20
$n\text{-}C_3H_7$—	1.50	1.50
$i\text{-}C_3H_7$—	1.30	1.30
$n\text{-}C_4H_9$—	2.00	2.00
$sec\text{-}C_4H_9$—	1.80	1.80
$t\text{-}C_4H_9$—	1.68	1.68
cyclo-C_3H_5—		1.21
cyclo-C_5H_9—	2.14	2.14
cyclo-C_6H_{11}—	2.51	2.51
Adamantyl	3.30	
C_6H_5—	2.13	2.13
—$(CH_2)_3$—	1.04	
—$(CH_2)_4$—	1.39	
—CF_3	1.07	
—CH_2OH	−1.03	−0.66
—CH_2COOH	−0.72	−0.76
—COOH	−0.32	−1.26
—COO⁻	−4.36	
—$CONH_2$	−1.49	−1.71
—$COOCH_3$	−0.01	−0.27
—$COCH_3$	−0.55	−0.71
—CN	−0.57	−0.84
—OH	−0.67	−1.16
—OCH_3	−0.02	−0.47
—OCH_2COOH	−0.86	
—$OCOCH_3$	−0.64	−0.91
$CH{=}NNHCONH_2$	−0.85	
$CH{=}NNHCSNH_2$	−0.27	
—O-β-glucose	−2.84	
—NH_2	−1.23	−1.19
—$N(CH_3)_2$	−0.18	−0.32
—NO	−0.12	
—NO_2	−0.28	−0.82
—$NHCOCH_3$	−0.97	
—$NHCOC_6H_5$	0.72	
—$N{=}NC_6H_5$	1.69	
—$NHCONH_2$	−1.01	
—$N(CH_3)_3$ $^+$	−5.96	
—SCH_3	0.62	
—SCF_3	1.58	
—SO_2CH_3	−1.26	
—SO_2CF_3	0.93	
—SF_5	1.50	
—SO_2NH_2	−1.82	

[a]Data from Hansch C, Anderson SM. *J Org Chem* 1967; 32:2583[16]; Hansch C, Anderson SM. *J Med Chem* 1967; 10:745[17]; Hansch C, et al. *J Med Chem* 1973; 16:1207[18]; Fujita T, et al. *J Am Chem Soc* 1964; 86:5175[21]; Iwasa J, et al. *J Med Chem* 1965; 8:150.[22]

[b]From X—C_6H_5 or X—$C_6H_4OCH_2COOH$ system. For different positions in the latter system slightly different values were reported in the original paper.[21] In cases where a strong interaction between two functions can occur (eg, in phenol or aniline series), different values should be used.

stants (faa) of different amino acids when they are incorporated into peptides or proteins. Table 13-9 summarizes the faa values of 21 common amino acids. The faa values range from −2.43 to + 1.47. This means when the most hydrophilic lysine is substituted with the most hydrophobic tryptophan, the logP in octanol/water is increased by 3.90 log units, and the partition coefficient P is increased by 7.94×10^3 fold.

X-RAY ANALYSES

In recent years the number of compounds of medicinal value that have been isolated from plant and animal sources and prepared by purely synthetic means has increased astronomically. In addition to the many compounds isolated, the more sophisticated isolation techniques now available have extended the capabilities of exploring biological molecules heretofore thought too complex to understand or investigate. The pharmaceutical chemist thus is faced with the task of identifying the chemical structure of a large number of complex materials in order to understand their biological functions.

For many of the compounds the chemist may rely on standard spectrometric methods (ie, IR, UV, NMR, and ORD), together with other chemical measurements, to elucidate molecular structure. Newer methods, especially mass spectrometry, have emerged as useful means of elucidating the structures of complex organic materials. In many instances these approaches have shortcomings, as they provide only fragmentary evidence about various portions of the molecule, which must be pieced together to get the picture of the whole compound (see also Chapter 34).

One of the most powerful of all techniques, when it is applicable, is that of x-ray crystallographic analysis. Using this method, the three-dimensional structure of a molecule can be determined without relying on any chemical information.

The maximum resolution that can be obtained through an ordinary light microscope under the most favorable conditions is about 2000 ÅÅ. This limitation is imposed primarily by the wavelength of the illumination. However, other forms of radiation capable of giving atomic resolution (1 ÅÅ or less) exist, namely electron beams, neutrons, and x-rays. Lenses have been constructed only for the first of these kinds of radiation, and at best they have a resolving power of about 6 ÅÅ. This resolution is insufficient to measure the distances between atoms. It is possible, however, to study the details of molecules without lenses, by means of diffraction experiments. Of the three types of radiation, x-rays have proved to be the most useful and fruitful for studying molecular structure.

Crystalline State

Atoms and molecules tend to organize themselves into their most favorable thermodynamic state, which under certain conditions results in their appearance as crystals. This form is characterized by a highly ordered arrangement of the molecules, associated with which is a three-dimensional periodicity. The repeating three-dimensional patterns, ideally depicted as *lattices*, are essential for x-ray structural analysis.

X-ray Diffraction

In 1912 von Laue and two of his students, Friedrich and Knipping, carried out an experiment with x-rays that opened the door to crystallographic structural analysis. They allowed a beam of nonhomogeneous x-rays to pass through a crystal of copper sulfate pentahydrate; they recorded, by means of photographic plates, the diffracted x-ray beam. A diagram of the experiment is shown in Figure 13-4.

The results showed that x-rays, which had been discovered by Roentgen less than two decades earlier, had wave characteristics (wavelength: approximately 1 Å). As a crystal is composed of a regular array of atoms with interatomic separations of the angstrom (Å) range, they were able to show that the diffraction pattern obtained on the plates was due to the crystal acting as a three-dimensional diffraction grating toward the x-rays.

This discovery led Bragg to make use of x-rays for the study of the internal structures of crystals. He considered that x-rays are reflected from planes of atoms within the crystal lattice. The reflections from a particular family of planes will occur

Table 13-9. The Hydrophobic Contribution Constants of Amino Acid Residues in Peptides and Proteins

AMINO ACID		HYDROPHOBIC CONTRIBUTION CONSTANT (faa) (measured in octanol/water, pH7)	COMMENTS
Lys (K)	⎫	− 2.43	Basic
Glu (E)	⎪	− 2.41	Acidic
Orn (O)	⎪	− 2.33	Basic
Asp (D)	⎬ Very Hydrophilic	− 2.32	Acidic
Arg (R)	⎪	− 1.86	Basic, guanadine group
Asn (N)	⎪	− 1.10	Monoamide group
Gln (Q)	⎭	− 1.09	Monoamide group
Ser (S)	⎫	− 0.78	Neutral, alcohol group
His (H)	⎪	− 0.54	Heterocyclic, imidazole
Gly (G)	⎪	− 0.51	Neutral
Thr (T)	⎬ Hydrophilic	− 0.50	Neutral alcohol group
Ala (A)	⎪	− 0.34	Neutral
Cys (C)	⎪	− 0.29	SH group
Pro (P)	⎭	− 0.18	Heterocyclic
Met (M)	⎫	0.43	Sulfur-containing
Val (V)	⎪	0.44	Neutral
Tyr (Y)	⎬ Hydrophobic	0.55	Aromatic, phenolic OH group
Ile (I)	⎪	0.87	Neutral
Leu (L)	⎭	0.97	Neutral
Phe (F)	⎫	1.23	Aromatic
Trp (W)	⎬ Very Hydrophobic	1.47	Heterocyclic, indole group

Adapted from Gao H, et al. *Pharma Res* 1995;12:1279 and Lien EJ, et al. Prog Drug Res 1997;48:9.

only at a particular angle of incidence and reflection. The essential condition for reflection is diagramed in Figure 13-5. In this figure the *crests* of the two incident waves will stay in phase if the thickened portion of the path (as shown in the diagram) of one wave is an integral multiple (n) of the wavelength (λ). The condition for reflection is given by the well-known Bragg equation:

$$\frac{\lambda}{2} = d_{nk,nk,nl} \sin \theta$$

The equation is satisfied only when $n = 1, 2, 3, \ldots$ If n is not a whole number, there will be destructive interference between the diffracted waves.

In any crystal there are an infinite number of families of planes that can be constructed. These planes usually are denoted by their Miller indices (hkl), as shown in Figure 13-6. These indices dictate the spacing between the planes (d_{hkl}) for a particular crystal. Because the highest value of θ that is theoretically possible to measure is 90° (reflected beam comes back along the incident beam's path), the number of planes (highest order) that one is capable of orienting in a diffracting position is limited by the wavelength of the radiation.

The planes that are accessible for a particular wavelength (x-ray) can be brought into a diffracting position by the proper orientation of the crystal relative to the collimated beam. In turn, many sets of planes can be recorded on a photographic plate by the movement of the crystal, when each of the planes will come into its diffracting position. In diffraction photographs, in which the crystal has been oscillated about an axis relative to the incident radiation, the various spots on the film arise from reflections from different planes; each spot can be indexed, according to the Miller indices of the respective plane, by its location on the film. The spacing between the various spots enables one to derive the distances and angles between the primitive translations—that is, the unit-cell dimensions.

In most cases little information can be gleaned from a knowledge of the unit-cell dimensions alone. To learn about the crystal and molecular structure, it is necessary to consider the intensities of the Bragg reflections.

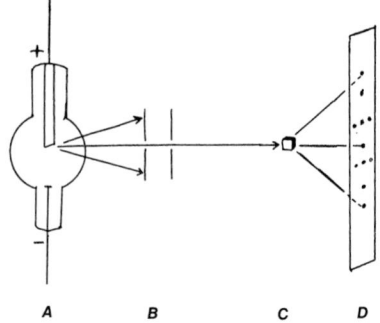

Figure 13-4. Diagram of Laue experiment:(*A*) x-ray tube, (*B*) lead slits, (*C*) crystal, (*D*) photographic plate.

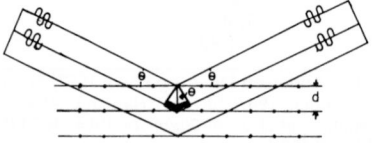

Figure 13-5. Bragg condition for reflection.

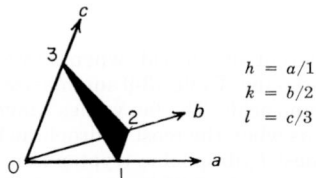

$h = a/1$
$k = b/2$
$l = c/3$

Figure 13-6. Crystal axes intercepted by a crystal plane.

Application of X-ray Diffraction

MOLECULAR WEIGHT—The measurement of the unit-cell parameters provides a means of accurately determining molecular weights of compounds. The density of a crystal can be obtained by means of flotation in mixtures of suitable liquids, the density of which may be altered by dilution until it matches that of the crystal.

The density (g/cm^3) is proportional to the molecular weight of the material in the unit cell.

The relationship is

$$\text{Mol wt} = \frac{Density \times V_{\text{cell}} \times N_a}{Z}$$

where N_a is Avogadro's number (6.023×10^{23}) and Z is the number of molecules in the unit cell. The unit-cell volume (V_{cell}) can be measured to a very high degree of accuracy. The number of molecules in the unit cell (Z) must be a whole number, with values of 1, 2, 4, and 8 being the most common among organic materials. When there is a high degree of solvation, it is necessary to approximate the amount of liquid bound by another means.

IDENTIFICATION OF MATERIALS—Every compound that is crystalline will give a characteristic x-ray diffraction pattern. These patterns can be very useful for identification purposes, and also for quantitative analysis of solid mixtures (see Chapter 34). They also have been used to a great extent by the pharmaceutical industry for the identification and classification of polymorphic and solvated forms of drugs. The *powder method*, in which the specimen is ground to a fine powder containing minute crystals oriented in every possible direction and a large number with their Bragg planes in correct orientation for reflection, is a valuable technique when quick comparisons of different forms are to be made and also when quantitative work is done. An example of such a comparison between the hydrated and anhydrous form of theophylline is shown in Figure 13-7.

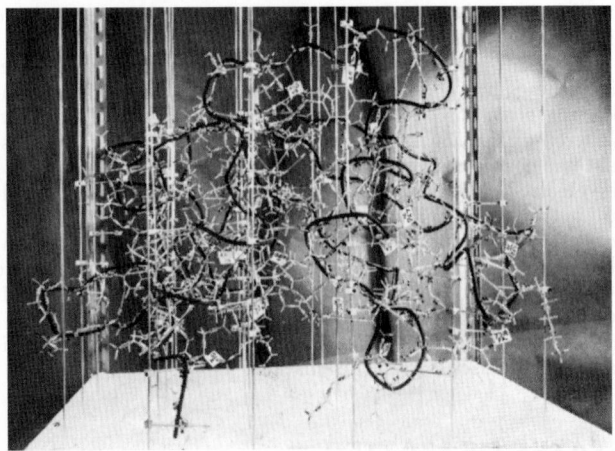

Figure 13-8. Model of bovine ribonuclease derived from x-ray data. The snakelike tube marks the backbone of the protein (courtesy, Dr G Kartha).

Extraction of quantitative information from diffraction patterns permits measurements of the physical and chemical stability of solid dosage forms. The kinetics of phase transformations are obtained easily by following the disappearance and/or appearance of various diffraction maxima corresponding to certain solid states as a function of time. One easily can visualize how this can be accomplished for theophylline hydrate by looking at the patterns in Figure 13-7.

STRUCTURE DETERMINATION—The body of substances of medicinal value whose structures were elucidated primarily by x-ray diffraction techniques is quite large. They range in molecular size from penicillin to vitamin B$_{12}$, and on up to the globular proteins. The structural determinations, in most instances, have played a major role in uncovering the secrets associated with the biological functions of the various molecules. A photograph of the ribonuclease molecule as determined by the x-ray studies of Kartha, Bello, and Harker is shown in Figure 13-8. This enzyme catalyzes the hydrolysis of phosphodiester bonds in RNA chains.

There also are large numbers of macromolecules of biological importance that do not form three-dimensional crystals in the usual sense, but will form fibers. The bundles of molecules in the fiber are aligned with respect to one another in a somewhat crystalline manner. These materials give x-ray diffraction patterns that have proved very useful in deriving molecular information. By fitting models to the x-ray pattern, many valuable biological polymers have had their secrets exposed. The two best examples are the α-helices of keratin and the double helix of deoxyribonucleic acid.

In recent years x-ray studies have been coupled with computer graphic and quantitative structure–activity relationship (QSAR) approaches in computer-assisted drug design (CADD) (see Chapter 28 for a more detailed discussion).

INTRAMOLECULAR BONDING AND CONFIGURATIONS—The precise determination of a crystal structure enables the bond lengths and angles between the various atoms to be determined accurately. This information is extremely valuable in the further understanding of how various chemical substituents influence the valence states and configurations of a molecule. With such knowledge, structure–activity relationships, which are of fundamental interest to the medicinal chemist, have much more depth. The observed bond orders also serve as experimental criteria by which theoretical models can be judged. It also is possible to compare quantum mechanical calculations relating drug interaction with actual observation.

Intramolecular steric effects, which tend to distort molecules, are unraveled easily by the scrutiny of their structures. It is possible to distinguish between repulsive and attractive effects of substituents. The torsional angles about var-

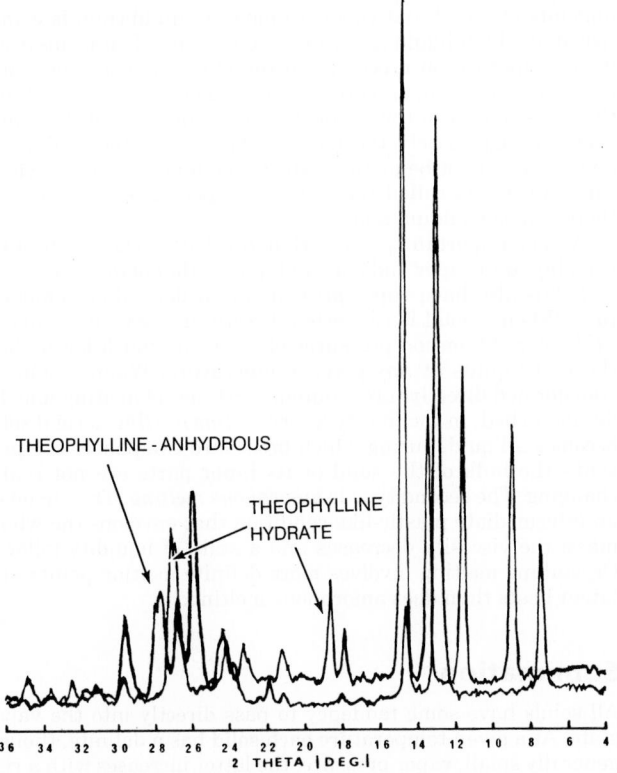

THEOPHYLLINE - ANHYDROUS

THEOPHYLLINE HYDRATE

36 34 32 30 28 26 24 22 20 18 16 14 12 10 8 6 4
2 THETA |DEG.|

Figure 13-7. A tracing of the powder-diffraction patterns of theophylline monohydrate and an anhydrous form.

ious bonds can be calculated from the atomic positions and are extremely helpful in correlating NMR data to structure.

In recent years the combination of x-ray and neutron-diffraction studies has enabled information on the bonding and nonbonding electrons within a molecule to be delineated clearly. Neutron-diffraction experiments enable atomic nuclei in a crystal to be positioned accurately; on the other hand, x-rays locate the electron clouds. Both types of data can be combined to calculate three-dimensional electron density maps with the inner-core electrons around each atom subtracted; this makes the unshared pairs and bonding electrons clearly visible. The atomic positions derived from neutron data are used for phases in calculating electron density maps with the x-ray data.

Refer to Chapter 34 for additional information on the physical methods discussed in this chapter.

STATES OF MATTER

The aim of this section is to discuss both generalities and specifics, most of which are not related explicitly to dosage forms, because the latter will be discussed in other chapters. Some of the principles should be useful to have in mind when dosage forms and their manufacture and processing are studied by the product-development pharmacist. It should be noted that due to the range of subjects covered by the section title it was necessary to take an eclectic approach in developing mostly qualitative discussions. The goal has been not to produce a difficult, in-depth section, but rather one that presents a mostly macroscopic overview of the significant states of matter.

Normally, matter exists in one of three states: solid, liquid, or gas. Although it is not pharmaceutically important, two other states of matter exist: the plasma state, in which matter exists as a hot gaseous cloud of atoms and electrons; and a more speculative state, possibly having only a momentary existence, is one which has characteristics of a superdense supermetal. The latter transient state is produced when material is subjected to very high pressures such as those used to make diamonds when compressing graphite.

To avoid the pitfalls of semantics, there is no need to call attention to other systems of classification, because for all practical purposes it is convenient to think only of the three most obvious states. These states are actually a continuum, with two common factors determining the position on the *scale of states*.

The first factor is the *intensity of intermolecular forces* of all kinds: solids have the strongest forces, and gases have the weakest. The other common factor is *temperature*. Obviously, as the temperature of a substance is raised, it tends to pass from a solid to a liquid to a gas. When the phrase "as temperature is increased" is used, it should be remembered that this is a relative phrase. Even at what is called room temperature, some of the effects of a temperature increase are present because room temperature is far above absolute zero.

SOLVATES AND HYDRATES—During the process of crystallization, some compounds have a tendency to trap a fixed molar ratio of solvent molecules in the crystalline (solid) state. These are called *solvates*. When water is used as the solvent, *hydrates* may be formed. Some recent pharmaceutical examples include gallium nitrate $(Ga(NO_3)_3 \cdot 9H_2O)$ and nafarelin acetate, where each decapeptide contains 1–2 molecules of acetic acid and 2–8 molecules of water.

As a point of historical interest, note that Lavoisier, the great "father of modern chemistry," thought of heat as a type of matter; the view even as late as the 18th century was that the three states of aggregation differ only with respect to how much heat they contain. Thus, although not all are satisfied with this phraseology, the term *enthalpy* (or *heat content*) is still used in thermodynamics.

Thinking further back to the ancient Greek philosophers and their original four elements (earth, air, fire, and water), note again the great significance attached to heat. Although the ancient philosophers' concepts of the nature of matter were not correct, they did recognize heat as an integral part of the scheme of things, and nothing could be truer. Heat, a vital form of energy, the mirror of molecular motion, is *the* form of energy of greatest importance to mankind.

As alluded to above, there is no clear line of demarcation between the states of matter, but the following arbitrary division may make the approach this section takes more coherent.

Changes of State

As a solid becomes a liquid and then a gas, heat is absorbed and the *enthalpy (heat content)* increases as the material passes through these phase changes. Thus, the enthalpy of a liquid is greater than that of its solid form, and the enthalpy of a gas is greater than that of its liquid form, because heat is absorbed when melting and vaporization occur. The *entropy* (a measure of the degree of total molecular randomness) also increases as materials go from solid to liquid to gas.

It is the balance of enthalpy, entropy, and temperature that determines if changes proceed spontaneously. Obviously, if systems tend to settle to states of lowest energy, it means that enthalpy and entropy considerations may counteract each other. Much of thermodynamics is concerned with explaining and quantitating the changes that systems undergo.

Latent heat is heat absorbed when a change of state takes place without a temperature change, as when ice turns to water at 0°. This example is one in which the heat required to produce the change of state is designated the *heat of fusion*. The counterpart, the *heat of vaporization*, is used when a change of state from liquid to gas is involved.

As molecules of a liquid in a closed, evacuated container continually leave the surface and go into the free space above it, some molecules return to the surface, depending on their concentration in the vapor. Ultimately, a condition of *equilibrium* is established, and the rate of escape equals the rate of return. The vapor then is saturated and the pressure is known as the *vapor pressure*.

Vapor pressure depends on the temperature, but not on the amounts of liquid and vapor, so long as equilibrium is established and both liquid and vapor are present. Heat is absorbed in the vaporization process, and therefore the vapor pressure increases with temperature. As the temperature is raised further, the density of the vapor increases, and that of the liquid decreases. Ultimately, the densities equal each other and liquid and vapor cannot be distinguished. The temperature at which this happens is called the *critical temperature*, and above it there can be no liquid phase.

A very important process that involves a change of state from liquid to vapor and back to liquid is that of *distillation*.

Solids also have vapor pressures that depend on temperature. When a solid is converted directly into gas, it is said to *sublime*. Sublimation pressures of solids are much lower than those of liquids at any given temperature. When a solid is transformed directly into a liquid, two types of melting may be distinguished. In the first type, *crystalline melting,* a rigid solid becomes a liquid, during which procedure two phases are present—the bulk of the solid or its inner parts are not really changing. The second type is *amorphous melting.* This involves an intermediate plastic-like condition that envelops the whole mass; the viscosity decreases and a state of liquidity follows. Crystalline melting involves more definite melting points and latent heats than does amorphous melting.

Sublimation

All solids have some tendency to pass directly into the vapor state. At a given temperature each solid has a definite, though generally small, vapor pressure; the latter increases with a rise in temperature. *Sublimation* is the term applied to the process of transforming a solid to vapor without intermediate passage through the liquid state. In pharmaceutical manufacturing the

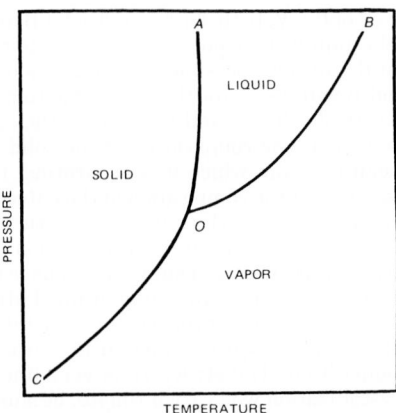

Figure 13-9. Phase diagram to illustrate the principle of sublimation.

process commonly includes also the condensation of the vapor back to the solid state.

A solid sublimes only when the pressure of its vapor is below that of the triple point for that substance. The *triple point* is the point, having a definite pressure and temperature, at which the solid, liquid, and vapor phases of a chemical entity are able to coexist indefinitely. If the pressure of vapor over the solid is above that of the triple point, the liquid phase will be produced before transformation to vapor can proceed.

Figure 13-9 depicts a phase diagram illustrating the principle involved. The line *OA* indicates the melting point of the solid form of a substance at various pressures; only along this line can both solid and liquid forms exist together in equilibrium. To the left only the solid form is stable; to the right only the liquid form remains permanently. The line *OB* shows the vapor pressure of the liquid form of the substance at various temperatures. It is called the *vapor-pressure curve* of the liquid and represents the conditions of temperature and vapor pressure for coexistence of liquid and vapor phases. Above this line only the liquid phase exists permanently; below it only vapor occurs. The line *OC* represents the vapor pressure of the solid at various temperatures. It is designated as the *sublimation curve* of the solid and represents the conditions of temperature and vapor pressure for the coexistence of solid and vapor phases. To the left of this line only solid can exist; to the right only the vapor form is stable. The intersection of the three lines, point *O*, is the triple point. It is apparent from the diagram that at pressures of vapor below that of the triple point it is possible to pass directly from the vapor to the solid state, and vice versa, simply by changing the temperature.

At pressures above the triple point the liquid phase must intervene in transformations between solid and vapor phases, in a closed system. Because the melting point of a solid commonly is taken at 1 atm (atmosphere) of pressure, it is evident that if the triple-point pressure is less than 1 atm, fusion of the solid form will occur on heating in a closed vessel. If, on the other hand, the triple-point pressure is greater than 1 atm, the solid form cannot be melted by heating at atmospheric pressure.

In a current of air, however, the conditions are somewhat different; some solids that melt when heated in a closed system now sublime appreciably even at ordinary temperatures, because the vapor pressure of the solid does not attain the triple-point pressure. Thus, camphor, naphthalene, *p*-dichlorobenzene, and iodine, all of which have a triple-point pressure below 1 atm, will vaporize in a current of air but melt when heated in a closed system.

Critical Point

The critical point is expressed as a certain value of temperature or pressure (or molar volume) above which or below which cer-

tain physical changes will not take place or certain states of being will not exist. At these points, some properties are constant and are referred to as the critical temperature, pressure, or volume. At the usual critical point, the properties of liquid and gas are identical and the phase diagram curve of *P* versus *T* ends. (Phase diagrams will be discussed later.) When a liquid changes to a vapor, increased disorder or randomness—and therefore increased entropy—results. At the critical temperature, the entropy of vaporization is zero, as is the enthalpy of vaporization, as the gas and liquid are indistinguishable.

Although the gas–liquid critical point is the one most discussed, others do occur. Each critical point marks the disappearance of a state. Note that most liquids behave similarly not only at their critical temperatures, but also at equal fractions of their critical temperatures. For example, the normal boiling points of many liquids are approximately equal fractions (about 60%) of their critical temperatures (in absolute temperature degrees).

Supercritical Fluid

Over the last decade, supercritical fluid chromatograph (SFC) and related unified chromatography techniques continue to grow, especially in food and natural products extractions and analysis.[25,26]

When the temperature and pressure of a liquid go beyond the critical points, a *supercritical fluid* may form. Under these stressed conditions, polar and nonpolar compounds are completely miscible. For example, dense fluid solvents, like supercritical CO_2 ($T_c = 31.1°$, $P_c = 73.8$ bar) and ethane ($T_c = 32.3°$, $P_c = 48.8$ bar) have been shown to offer advantages for the solubilization of amino acids. Other applications of supercritical fluids include chromatography of polar drugs and elimination of toxic wastes.[27,28]

Visualization of Changes of State

This section is to serve as an introduction to the following one on eutectics. When a pure substance cools and is transformed from a liquid to a solid, a graph (Fig 13-10) of decreasing temperature versus time is continuous. At the temperature at which solid crystallizes (ie, the *melting point*), the cooling curve becomes horizontal. The same is true at the *boiling point*—the temperature of a liquid at which the continuing application of heat no longer raises the temperature, but rather converts the liquid into vapor. It is the point where the vapor pressure of the liquid (or the sum of its components) equals that of the atmosphere above the liquid.

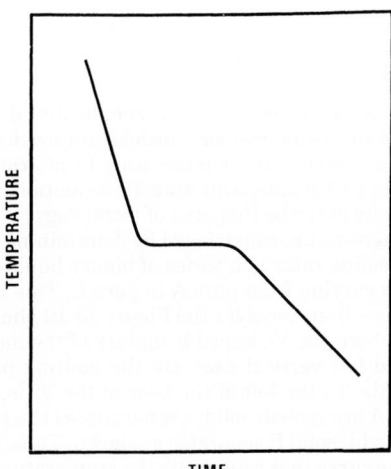

Figure 13-10. A single change of state as shown by a slowing of the cooling rate.

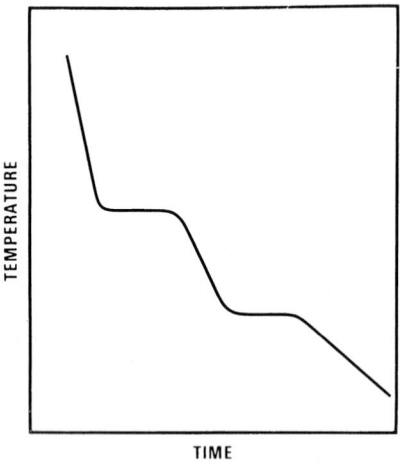

Figure 13-11. Two changes of state with resulting temporary decreases in cooling rate.

Increasing the pressure above the liquid or adding solutes raises the boiling point and *vice versa*. These plateaus observed at certain specific temperatures are due to the release of the heats of fusion or vaporization. Similarly, when solutions are cooled, the slope of the *cooling curve* (Fig 3-11) changes when one of the components starts to crystallize. Although a truly horizontal plateau may not be formed, as in the case of pure materials, the change in slope indicates precipitation of one of the components. If the same plateaus are formed when binary solutions of varied composition are cooled, it indicates that both components of the binary solution are coming out together. The temperature at which this occurs is the *eutectic temperature*, and the composition is generally called a *eutectic*.

Normally, cooling curves per se are converted to phase diagrams to facilitate visualization of the interrelationships as phase changes take place. If, instead of a minimum point or eutectic, a maximum point is observed, it may indicate that the components are reacting to form a solid compound that can exist in equilibrium with the melt over a range of compositions.

It is undoubtedly true that many unknown phase equilibria exist. Thus, when conditions are changed (eg, when a process is scaled up in a manufacturing process), different phase changes may take place and produce different final products. The pharmaceutical use of heterogeneous materials such as waxes and fats certainly provides ample opportunity for these changes to occur.

Eutectics

Although many very complex and complicated diagrams, including some three-dimensional models, are needed to characterize certain systems, most interesting to pharmacy are the diagrams (Fig 13-12) indicating eutectic formation. This section will only briefly describe this area of technology.

Phase diagrams are constructed by determining the melting points and cooling rates of a series of binary liquid solutions of compositions varying from pure A to pure B. This will be illustrated shortly—first, consider the Figure 13-12 phase diagram. The points where the V-shaped boundary of the melt intersect the right and left vertical axes are the melting points of the pure materials. To the left of the base of the V (ie, when solutions rich in A are cooled) solid A separates as the temperature falls; to the right, solid B separates as shown. Thus, the left arm of the V is the curve that represents the temperature conditions under which various liquid mixtures are in equilibrium with solid A, and the right arm of the V is that curve that shows which mixtures are in equilibrium with solid B.

At the point of the V, both solid A and solid B are in equilibrium with the liquid; this point, the lowest temperature at which any of the infinite possible combinations of liquid solutions of A and B will freeze (or the lowest melting point of any possible mixture of solids A and B) is called the *eutectic point*. Only at this point is the composition of the solid the same as that of the solution from which it is separating; this does *not* mean necessarily that the composition of the eutectic is a chemical compound of A and B. Thus, at the eutectic point, both A and B come out together in a constant proportion.

The eutectic composition is a simple two-phase mixture, but when made in situ it has a very fine-grained structure that could impart to it different properties (eg, solubility or gastrointestinal absorption rate), compared to a gross mixture of the same composition. The structure is very fine-grained because the crystallization was very intimate, because crystals of both phases were formed simultaneously. This is quite a different situation than one in which only one component is separating. It is important to remember that one can be only at one place on a phase diagram at any one time; that is, the diagram describes what a *particular* system is like at a certain temperature, which components are in the liquid and/or solid state, and the proportions of each.

The diagrams are constructed from information obtained on the cooling rates of binary solutions. Consider again a cooling curve analysis in which temperature versus time are plotted. The curves change slope to form plateaus when any solid phase separates; the plateaus tend to become more horizontal as absolute temperatures are lower because the intensity of radiation and conduction is lessened. A final plateau results when the whole liquid mass (or the last of it) solidifies. Thus, if a molten liquid having a composition lying *between,* for example, pure A and the eutectic were cooled, the following would be observed in a plot of temperature versus time (see Fig 13-11).

First, *T* drops with time; then solid A will come out of solution, release its heat of fusion, and thus slow the cooling rate to produce the first (upper) plateau. The temperature then starts to drop more sharply again as enough A comes out of solution, and the system changes composition until it contains only the eutectic composition.

When the eutectic composition is reached, the second solid (B) also coprecipitates, and the temperature remains constant (lower plateau) until all of A and B have solidified, after which, of course, the temperature will be able to drop further.

If the system being cooled started as the eutectic composition, only the lower break and plateau would be observed; that is, a pure material and a eutectic would have similarly shaped cooling diagrams.

Note then that a phase diagram can be constructed by studying a number of cooling curves made on a series of mixtures of known composition. To do this, the temperatures at which cool-

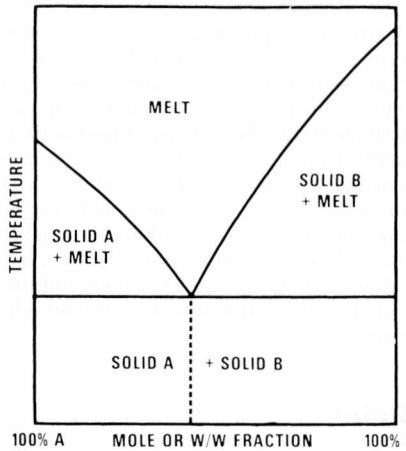

Figure 13-12. Simple phase diagram of system showing eutectic point.

ing-rate changes are plotted against each particular composition studied.

Note that Figure 13-12 is idealized in that no solid–solid solution of A and B is formed. If the two components are somewhat soluble in each other, the diagram would differ by having two thin solution areas along the left and right axes; such are partly in evidence in Figure 13-13.

Two pharmaceutical examples of eutectic formation are

1. A mixture of two common antipyretic-analgesic compounds: aspirin and acetaminophen. There always has been some "magic" associated with eutectic formation; indeed, as such a binary composition does melt at a lower temperature than other combinations, the eutectic probably does have weaker bonding forces, if any. And, being very fine grained, it dissolves more rapidly. It is known that many drug compounds form eutectics, and the aspirin-acetaminophen (APAP) eutectic (37% APAP by weight) does dissolve more quickly than a simple mixture of the two of the same composition. Because a formed eutectic is created under equilibrium conditions of intimate mixing as noted, the contact of the two compounds is much closer than that achievable by simply mixing the dry powders. The increase in dissolution rate obtained by using the eutectic may result in a greater speed of physiological absorption.

2. This example is illustrated in Figure 13-13. It was found that urea and acetaminophen formed a eutectic containing approximately 46% urea and 54% acetaminophen (by weight) which melted in the 110° to 115° range.

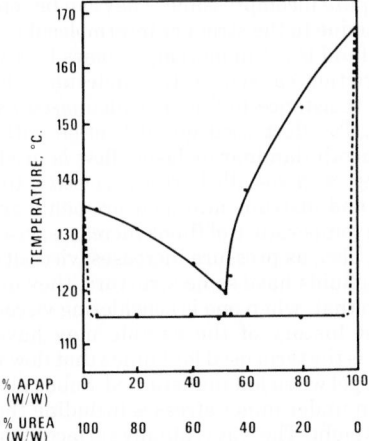

Figure 13-13. Phase diagram of the urea:acetaminophen (APAP) (46%:54%) eutectic melting in the 110 to 115° range. (From Goldberg AH, et al. J Pharm Sci 1966; 55:482.)

Gases

AEROSOLS—Gases are used directly in dosage forms in the field of aerosols. Although this subject, including the use of the so-called liquefied propellants, is covered elsewhere, note that pressure packs often use nitrogen, nitrous oxide, or carbon dioxide to expel the contents from their containers. The latter two gases are much more soluble in water, so some aeration (which may be desired) of the material discharged will take place.

Carbon dioxide is about six times as soluble in water as nitrogen, and nitrous oxide about four times as soluble as nitrogen. Thus, if it is desired to have some of the gas dissolved in the product, either nitrous oxide or carbon dioxide can be used. In organic solvents and in fatty materials, such as found in emulsions, nitrous oxide is somewhat more soluble than carbon dioxide. There is not a great deal of difference in solubility properties; however, the possibility exists that the pH-lowering effect of carbon dioxide as it forms carbonic acid may be just as undesirable, as it may cause precipitation of a carbonate in an alkaline product.

INHALERS—Inhalers are classified as being one of two types, surface or solution.

Surface-Type Inhaler—The volatile material resides on the surface of the pledget (cotton or other cellulosic material, usually). This represents a conventional adsorption situation; it is easy to appreciate the fact that the more surface area the pledget has, the greater the surface area of the material exposed to the airflow and the greater the opportunity for volatilization. Hence, a larger or more loosely packed pledget will cause a larger dose to emanate from an inhaler than will a smaller or tightly packed pledget.

It is convenient to make this type of inhaler if the volatile material itself is a liquid. The doses produced stay relatively high because the pledget charge is being depleted according to a zero-order scheme. This is reasonable because the volatile material has formed a multimolecular (as distinguished from a monomolecular) layer on the pledget surfaces. Thus, even though molecules are stripped off, the surface area—and hence the dose—remain essentially unchanged. However, as some areas of the pledget are denuded, the total exposed surface area of the volatile material decreases and so does the dose during successive uses.

Solution-Type Inhaler—The volatile material is dissolved in a suitable nonvolatile solvent, and this solution is placed on the pledget. The situation may be taken as an example of the operation of Raoult's and Henry's laws; that is, the vapor pressures of the components are proportional in some way to their concentrations. To keep the vapor-pressure contribution of the solvent low in order to enhance the vapor pressure of the solute, a solvent of very low vapor pressure is used as the vehicle.

In this inhaler type the exposed surface area of the material does not change as the inhaler is used; what does change is the concentration of the volatile material in the solvent. Thus, the dose gradually decreases according to a first-order scheme as the drug concentration decreases. Of course, the nature of the pledget and the inhaler body exert some effect here also, because if the airflow through the inhaler and the pledget does not permit volatilization of the material, insignificant, low doses will result.

If the drug is a volatile solid, the solution-type inhaler should be made because solids do not lend themselves to easy pledget-charging procedures even if a volatile solvent such as ether is used to deliver the material to the pledget during manufacturing.

Further amplification and clarification of the surface- and solution-type classification of inhalers might be achieved by considering the existing analogy to chromatographic systems. The surface-type inhaler corresponds to adsorption chromatography, with the material being adsorbed initially on a carrier and then desorbed by a passing stream of liquid or gas. The solution-type inhaler corresponds to partition chromatography, in which material in a solvent is supported by some medium, is partitioned between its original solvent and a passing stream of gas or liquid, and thus is removed.

Another point of significance concerns the relationship of the volatile active ingredient to the solvent. An increase in dose should result when the active ingredient is dissolved in solvents that cause it to deviate more positively from Raoult's law. Thus, the less the solute–solvent interaction and the greater the solute–solute interaction, the more pronounced will be the tendency toward volatilization of the solute. Using relative solubility as a gauge of such interaction, one would expect delivery of larger doses of a volatile solid from dibutyl phthalate (if the solute was less soluble in it) than from benzyl salicylate (if it was more soluble in it) at the same concentrations.

Although it might seem that the vapor pressure of the drug and additives would assume a position of primary importance, this does not appear to be the case. Vapor-pressure values represent an equilibrium situation, whereas what is involved in the inhaler situation is a process controlled by factors affecting rates of volatilization.

Although it is true that volatile materials usually have appreciable vapor pressures, it generally is not true that a compound with a vapor pressure value of twice that of another compound will volatilize twice as fast. Besides this fact, inhaler recovery times may be essentially zero and no equilibration time may be needed. Also, no decrease in dosage would be noted with the surface-type inhaler and no regular (ie, linear with concentration) decreases in dose would be noted with the solution-type inhaler if the vapor pressure was the controlling factor.

Unfortunately (from the standpoint of not having a more straightforward system to analyze), equilibrium and rate concepts are inextricably mixed in the present situation. This easily can lead to the basically incorrect tendency to try to predict kinetic data from thermodynamic values. However, because vaporization relatively is unencumbered with entropy and orientation factors, rates of volatilization often are qualitatively proportional to the equilibrium properties of the materials involved.

Equimolar quantities of the following compounds, allowed to evaporate at room temperature under the same conditions, will complete the evaporation process in this order: ether, acetone, chloroform, carbon tetrachloride, ethyl acetate, and water. This order corresponds both to the vapor pressures of the materials and their boiling points.

To further cloud the cause-and-effect relationship, the very magnitude of the numbers (the concentrations in mole fractions) is such that the partial vapor pressure of a volatile solid may increase proportionately with the mole fraction. Hence, although vapor-pressure concepts should not be neglected in inhaler development, it is the rates of volatilization that must be controlled or modified. For more information and experimental data on inhalers see Kennon and Gulesich.[30] Various drug-delivery systems for use with metered-dose inhalers (MDIs) are commercially available. They are intended for delivering oral aerosolized medication from MDIs to the lungs.

RELATIVE HUMIDITY—In the production of effervescent products, one of the most vital factors to be considered is the use of controlled-humidity conditions. It is well-known that the effective control of humidity is related closely to the success or failure of attempts to produce effervescent products.

It is useful to bring to light some of the facets of this area of technology. Two factors predominate when one views the situation: the effective concentration of water in the air and the temperature. In chemical reactions, particularly the kind involved here, the effect of temperature on an equilibrium condition is not very significant when compared to the influence manifested by concentration. Certainly, water of hydration, crystallization, or simple adsorption (which is tenaciously held at room temperature) does not disappear at temperatures under 100°F. What *is* effective and influential, however, in keeping and increasing such additional moisture on solids, is the *concentration* of water in the air.

The concept proposed here is that considerations based purely on relative humidity probably will be unfruitful. For purposes of illustration, Table 13-10 shows the amounts of water that are found under conditions encountered during the development of effervescent products. The following points may be drawn from this information. A 10% relative humidity (RH) at 36°F is equivalent to 25% RH at room temperature. Either of these conditions represents a fairly dry day, but certainly not a very dry day. Therefore, although heating the air surely lowers the RH, it probably does not lower the ability of the water in the air to cause trouble. Regardless of the temperature of the processing rooms, experience has shown that for water concentrations present at 72°F, the range of 10 to 15% RH should not be exceeded if minimum difficulties are desired.

Liquids

The liquid state may be considered an intermediate in the phase transitions from solid to gas. Liquids have neither the strong cohesive forces of solids nor the weak ones of gases. They are also intermediate in that they have neither the orderliness of a crystal nor the randomness of a gas. One then might consider a liquid a highly compressed gas or slightly released solid.

Due to the concept of molecular motion, there must be some free space in liquids. Also, if the motion is completely random, some spaces may be larger than others at a particular point in time. Thus, liquids may have holes, and this concept has explained phenomena such as the expansion of volume that materials undergo upon fusion (holes are created), diffusion in liquids, viscosity (movement of holes in the opposite direction of the viscous flow), and density decreases as temperature rises (the solubility of holes increases). It might be said that liquids are solutions of holes in material, whereas gases are solutions of matter in free space.

With respect to fluid mechanics, a fluid can be considered a material that cannot sustain shear forces when in static equilibrium. This is the factor distinguishing solids from fluids, the latter of which may be gases or liquids. This movement under the slightest stress sometimes is referred to as "no sideways friction." It can be seen in operation in the case where a sailor standing watch near the gangplank of a docked ship can step on a mooring rope and cause the ship to move toward the dock.

Liquids, just like gases, take the shape of their container, but only the lower part of it, as the liquid occupies a definite volume; gases, on the other hand, expand to fill their entire container. Intermolecular spaces are greater in a gas than in a liquid, thus they can be compressed. Relative to gases, both liquids and solids are quite incompressible. They can be considered already compressed due to the stronger intermolecular forces.

After a fluid is set in motion, it comes to rest because of the internal friction caused by the molecules sliding over each other; this resistance to flow is called *viscosity,* and it can be quantified. To effect good quantification with viscometers, a normal, smooth (laminar or layer) flow is needed. With excessive stirring, at a so-called *critical velocity,* the fluid becomes turbulent, and instrumental measurements are difficult to effect. As the temperature of fluids increases, viscosity decreases. In general, also, as pressure increases, viscosity increases.

Because fluids have some structure, they may change upon standing so that, when one is considering viscous behavior, the recent past history of the sample may have great effects. *Thixotropy* is the term used for liquids that flow freely if recently stirred, but gel when left undisturbed. Solids also flow, but more slowly, even under minor stresses including those produced by their own weight. The wavy, bumpy surface of tarred roads, particularly seen on hills, is a result of a flow phenomenon.

Of interest also is the *cluster* theory of liquids, the main concept being that localized order exists but does not extend to a great distance. One property explained by this visualization is that, as the temperature rises, the clusters disintegrate and viscosity decreases. Another is that transmitting momentum through a liquid is due not only to molecular movement, but also to the transmissions of elastic waves through the groups of semistationary clusters. It is possible that the cluster theory affords another way of looking at pharmaceutical complexes in solution.

Complexes

In addition to structure in solvents, it also is possible for solutes to create a structure of a sort within the solvent. Thus, it has been shown that benzocaine in water solution with caffeine exhibits a much-reduced rate of hydrolysis. In a somewhat similar vein, it also has been noted that different salts of the same compound (eg, hydrochloride versus nitrate) may exhibit different stability characteristics. Similarly, it has been shown that saccharin in certain chlorpromazine hydrochloride solutions enhances the light-stability of the drug. It appears that such changes are because the ionic environment may form a protective molecular overcoat or loose ionic atmosphere complex around the drug.

Table 13-10. Moisture Content (g/m³) Existing at the Conditions Noted

TEMPERATURE	RELATIVE HUMIDITY (%)			
	10	15	25	40
RT (22°C or 72°F)	1.9	2.9	4.8	7.7
Hot (36°C or 97°F)	4.1	6.2	10.3	16.5

Liquid Crystals

Lipids, when heated, usually do not pass directly from a crystalline to an isotropic structure, but rather assume intermediate liquid crystal phases. Of most interest pharmaceutically and physiologically is the concept that these structures are undoubtedly involved intimately in the structure, and hence in the function, of membranes and cells.

All biological systems are basically aqueous, and it is particularly in such systems that lyotropic mesomorphism (the formation of liquid-crystal phases in the presence of water) takes place; that is, the lipid phases undergo transformations involving crystal, liquid-crystal, and liquid forms. It is these changes that are mediators of the various physiological absorption, transport, storage, and excretory functions of cells. Many in vitro studies of biologically significant lipids have been performed in an attempt to elucidate the mechanisms of their interaction and behavioral properties in aqueous systems.

Liquid-crystals differ from solids and gases in that they have some freedom to move and to take on many different shapes while maintaining a high degree of order through quite long distances, relatively speaking. In the laboratory, liquid-crystals can be prepared from one component by heat treatment (thermotropic systems) or from one or more components by adding controlled amounts of water or other polar solvents (lyotropic mesomorphism). Note that the only molecules of significance here are asymmetric and have a definite long direction, so their tridimensional orientation is essential. This should be remembered throughout the discussion.

For present purposes, three types of liquid-crystal phases will be described briefly so that at least some appreciation for this particular state of matter may be gained. The phases generally are characterized as being nematic, smectic, or cholesteric.

Nematic Phase—Nematic molecules (Fig 13-14) are set in parallel arrangements and have restricted rotation about at least one axis. The molecules are parallel or nearly so. One might picture this as a long box filled with pencils with the latter being able to roll. Overall, the system might be considered to be thread- or cable-like. Another picture would be that of a group of logs going through a pipe. There is overlap of the pencils or logs somewhat, as there is with cars in an auto race.

Smectic Phase—The smectic or "two-dimensional" crystal (Fig 13-15) has its molecules arranged in layers with their long axes essentially normal (ie, at right angles) to the plane of the layers. Their centers of gravity are then mobile in two directions in their plane, and the molecules can rotate about one axis. Overall, one could consider the arrangement layer-like, with the degree of order just described in each layer.

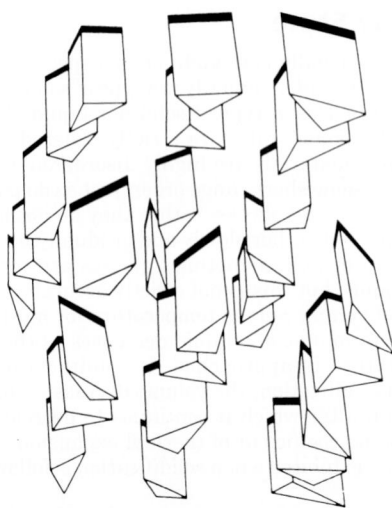

Figure 13-15. The smectic liquid–crystal phase. (Adapted from Fergason JL, Brown GH. *J Am Oil Chem Soc* 1968; 45:120.)

The smectic arrangement is similar to the nematic in that there is still essentially only one axis of rotation, except in this case there is no overlap. The logs go through the pipe as a member of a group—it would be like a series of drag races in which no one wins and all are tied. Each successive group, however, does not follow the same paths as the others; within any one group there may, or may not, be equal spacings sideways between the long axes. Note also that the thickness of the layers is about the same as the length of the molecules.

Cholesteric Phase—The cholesteric arrangement (Fig 13-16) is to some extent a combination of the nematic and smectic; the layers are nematic, but in addition certain layering formations that resemble the smectic phase are incorporated. In essence, the result is a helical, twisting repetition of the nematic phase that, corkscrew-like, slowly changes head direction (eg, the lead end of the pencil) as one proceeds to examine underlying layers of molecules. The cholesteric arrangement is, in toto, much thicker than a smectic layer.

All three structures are involved in building cells, and each type can (when viewed totally) form curved surfaces, membranes, or any other required micelle-like shapes. Some researchers have constructed cell models using these structures and have shown how the mechanics of many cellular functions can be visualized using the known properties of liquid crystals.

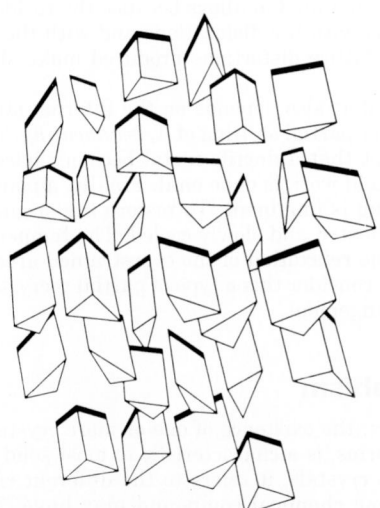

Figure 13-14. The nematic phase of a liquid crystal. (Adapted from Fergason JL, Brown GH. *J Am Oil Chem Soc* 1968; 45:120.)

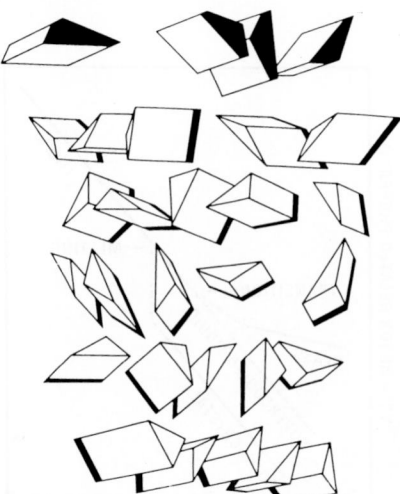

Figure 13-16. A 180° turn of the molecules in the cholesteric liquid–crystal phase. (Adapted from Fergason JL, Brown GH. *J Am Oil Chem Soc* 1968; 45:120.)

The Glassy State

Although glass usually is thought of as a specific, nonconducting, transparent solid, it actually is a type of solid matter. It can be considered neither a typical solid nor liquid. The atoms of most solid states generally are strictly ordered structurally, whereas glassy materials are highly disordered. Glasses may, however, have some short-range order, just as do polymers. Another characteristic of glasses is that they do not have specific melting points, but rather slowly and gradually become liquids when they are heated. Sometimes glasses are considered supercooled liquids, but this is not strictly accurate.

A graph of volume versus temperature for most substances shows that the volume of a liquid decreases as the crystallization temperature is approached. If solidification is accomplished by crystallization, the volume decreases sharply at the freezing point, after which it continues to decrease gradually depending on its coefficient of thermal expansion. This type of behavior is not exhibited when solidification is followed by glass formation.

The uniqueness of the glassy state is evident in its cooling curve. As indicated in Figure 13-17, as a glass-former is cooled, it does not suddenly undergo a large drop in volume (or density, or index of refraction) at any particular temperature or as it passes through the melting point, nor does its volume decrease as rapidly as that of a supercooled liquid, although it follows the curve of the latter initially during cooling. With supercooled liquids, the cooling curve is a simple continuation of the liquid curve itself, with no melting or transition points.

Atomically, the structure of the glassy state is marked by a random selection of polyhedral molecules considered to be linked together at their corners. Certain materials are easy to cast into a glassy state, others can be made glassy with great difficulty, and some seemingly not at all. At present there seems to be no specific theory to help predict this behavior. Materials that do form glasses appear, however, to have a very high viscosity at their melting point; this inhibits the formation of an ordered structure. In addition, non–glass-formers tend to exhibit large energy differences between the ordered form of the solid and the disordered liquid. Thus, the low-energy, ordered form of the solid tends to be developed. Obviously, the energetic tendencies here are balanced by entropy factors, which tend to favor states of minimum order.

Although the most well-known glass-formers are the metal oxides, many other materials can exist in the glassy state; even steel can be so cast if it is cooled very, very quickly. This technique produces glasses as the materials become solid before they have a chance to develop a crystalline structure. With regard to crystal formation, note that, in a crystallization process, when concentrated solutions of the material to be crystallized are cooled slowly, larger and more perfect crystals form.

Incomplete or imperfect crystallization, whether due to technique or to the nature of the material itself (eg, natural and synthetic high polymers), often causes the formation of crystallites, glasses, or liquid crystals. Crystallites have no recognizable regular crystal pattern; rather, they are, in a sense, incipient crystals. Many shapes and arrangements are possible such as globular, rows or clouds of globules, threads, cylinders, or rods.

Solids

The most significant physical property of the solid state is the high degree of order in which substances such as metals and minerals exist. The structure may be crystalline and lattice-like or noncrystalline, such as in plastic, glass, or gels, which are not lattice-like or only partly so. These latter materials do have much more order than liquids and gases. These materials also have, in varying degrees, some plastic and elastic properties, wherein some resistance to applied stresses exists, but when the stress reaches a certain intensity either slippage or fracture ensues.

Although different classifications exist, four major different types of bonds hold solids together; the strong bonds impart higher melting points to substances. In order of decreasing strength, the bond types are *metallic, ionic* (salts), *valence* (diamond), and *molecular* (many organic compounds). Thus, in some solids, the atoms or molecules or ions may be arranged in a regularly repeating pattern (crystalline state), whereas other solids are considered noncrystalline or amorphous if they do not have this characteristic of regularity. There is some blurring of the division, but in general, metals, minerals, rocks, and alloys are examples of the former class; glass, wood, ceramics, and plastics are examples of the latter.

Alloys are an example of a mixed solid having characteristics of regularity but being intermediate between the strictly crystalline and amorphous states. They are metal substances consisting of two or more elements, not counting the trace amounts of materials which make any element less than 100% pure. Alloys are solid solutions of one of two types. In the *interstitial* type, the smaller solute atoms occupy the interstices between the solvent atoms; the overall structure is quite like the parent or solvent metal. In the other type, *substitutional,* all atoms occupy (ie, contribute to building) a common lattice.

In general, alloys are stronger and harder than pure metals. This is probably because both dislocations in the crystalline lattice and the perfectly regular crystal structure of pure metals permit the planes of the crystals to slip over each other. These processes are inhibited in alloys because the resident or solute atoms interact with the dislocations and with the regular sections, so any lattice distortions produced make slipping more difficult.

A process that also depends on the internal structure, and possibilities for partial shifting of it, is *annealing.* This is based on the concept that a ductile metal becomes harder and less workable as cold work is done on it. Finally, a point is reached where cracking is imminent. To restore the original ductility, the metal is heated and slowly cooled. The temperatures used just permit the relaxation of the overstrained areas. A visualization might consider this a type of partial recrystallization or atomic rearrangement.

Polymorphism

Polymorphism, the existence of one or more crystalline and/or amorphous forms, is a characteristic of most solid substances. As applied to crystals, it refers to the different crystal structures the same chemical compound may have. The various forms also usually have different x-ray diffraction patterns, melting points, infrared spectra, and, most importantly from a pharmaceutical standpoint, different solubilities.

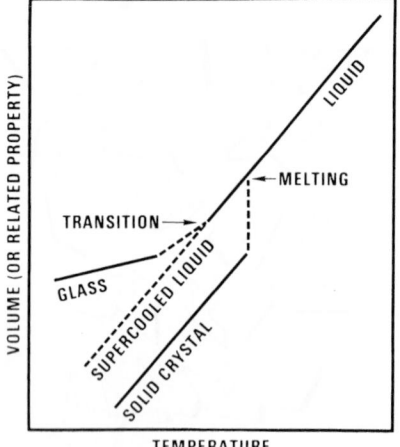

Figure 13-17. Composite cooling curve of liquids forming glass, supercooled liquid and solid-crystal states.

Particularly, in many cases in which dissolution in the gastrointestinal tract is the rate-limiting factor in absorption, differing solubilities may have a great effect, either good or bad. Different polymorphic forms are produced, depending on such factors as storage temperature, recrystallization solvent, and the rate of cooling (and, hence, the rate of crystallization) of the solvent. It appears that all organic materials exist in several polymorphic forms with the number of forms found depending on the effort spent searching.

In drugs, polymorphs of such diverse molecules from cortisone and prednisolone to aspirin have been found. As an example of the latter case, two different aspirin polymorphs form, depending on whether the material is crystallized from 95% alcohol or n-hexane. The two forms have different melting points, but, most importantly, the form produced from the hexane dissolves in water much more quickly. Toscani et al[32] have reported the stability hierarchy of three polymorphic forms of sulfanilamide.

REFERENCES

1. Feynman RP. *Science* 1974; 183:601.
2. Schoenborn BP. *Chem Eng News* 31, Jan 24, 1977.
3. Pitzer KS. *J Am Chem Soc* 1948; 70:2140.
4. Fieser LF, Fieser M. *Introduction to Organic Chemistry.* Boston: DC Heath, 1957, inside back cover.
5. Pauling LC. *The Nature of the Chemical Bond,* 3rd ed. Ithaca, NY: Cornell University Press, 1960, pp 225–226.
6. Pauling LC. *The Nature of the Chemical Bond,* 3rd ed. Ithaca, NY: Cornell University Press, 1960, p 93.
7. Pauling LC. *The Nature of the Chemical Bond,* 3rd ed. Ithaca, NY: Cornell University Press, 1960, Chap 3.
8. Fajans K. *Physical Methods of Organic Chemistry,* 2nd ed. Vol 1, Part II. New York: Wiley Interscience, 1949, p 1162.
9. Cammarata A. *J Med Chem* 1967; 10:525.
10. Lien EJ, et al. *J Pharm Sci* 1982; 71:641.
11. Lien EJ, et al. *J Pharm Sci* 1984; 73:553.
12. Lien EJ, et al. *Prog Drug Res* 1997; 48:9.
13. Olah GA, et al. *J Am Chem Soc* 1967; 89:711.
14. Sjoholm I, Szodin T. *Biochem Pharmacol* 1972; 21:3041.
15. Martin AN, et al. *Physical Pharmacy,* 3rd ed. Philadelphia: Lea & Febiger, 1983, 58–61.
16. Hansch C, Anderson SM. *J Org Chem* 1967; 32:2583.
17. Hansch C, Anderson SM. *J Med Chem* 1967; 10:745.
18. Hansch C, et al. *J Med Chem* 1973; 16:1207.
19. Hansch C, et al. *J Med Chem* 1977; 20:304.
20. Hansch C. *Farmaco Sci* 1968; 23:293.
21. Fujita T, et al. *J Am Chem Soc* 1964; 86:5175.
22. Iwasa J, et al. *J Med Chem* 1965; 8:150.
23. Gao H, et al. *Pharma Res* 1995; 12:1279.
24. Lien EJ, et al. *Prog Drug Res* 1997; 48:9.
25. Chester TL, et al. *Anal Chem* 2002; 74:2801.
26. Yang C, et al. *J Agr Food Chem* 2002; 50:846.
27. Lemert RM, et al. *J Phys Chem* 1990; 94:6021.
28. Crowther JB, Henion JD. *Anal Chem* 1985; 57:2711.
29. Goldberg AH, et al. *J Pharm Sci* 1966; 55:482.
30. Kennon L, Gulesich JJ. *J Pharm Sci* 1962; 51:278.
31. Fergason JL, Brown GH. *J Am Oil Chem Soc* 1968; 45:120.
32. Toscani S. *Pharm Res* 1996; 13:151.

BIBLIOGRAPHY

Ariëns EJ, et al. *Stereochemistry and Biological Activity of Drugs.* Boston: Blackwell, 1983.
Eliel EL. *Stereochemistry of Carbon Compounds.* New York: McGraw-Hill, 1962.
Hansch C, Leo A. Exploring QSAR. *Fundamentals and Applications in Chemistry and Biology.* Washington DC, ACS Professional Reference Book, 1995.
Hansch C, et al. Exploring QSAR. Hydrophobic, Electronic and Steric Constants, *ibid,* 1995.
Leo JA. *Chem Rev* 1993; 93: 1281.
Lien EJ. *SAR Side Effects and Drug Design.* New York: Dekker, 1987.

CHAPTER 14

Complex Formation

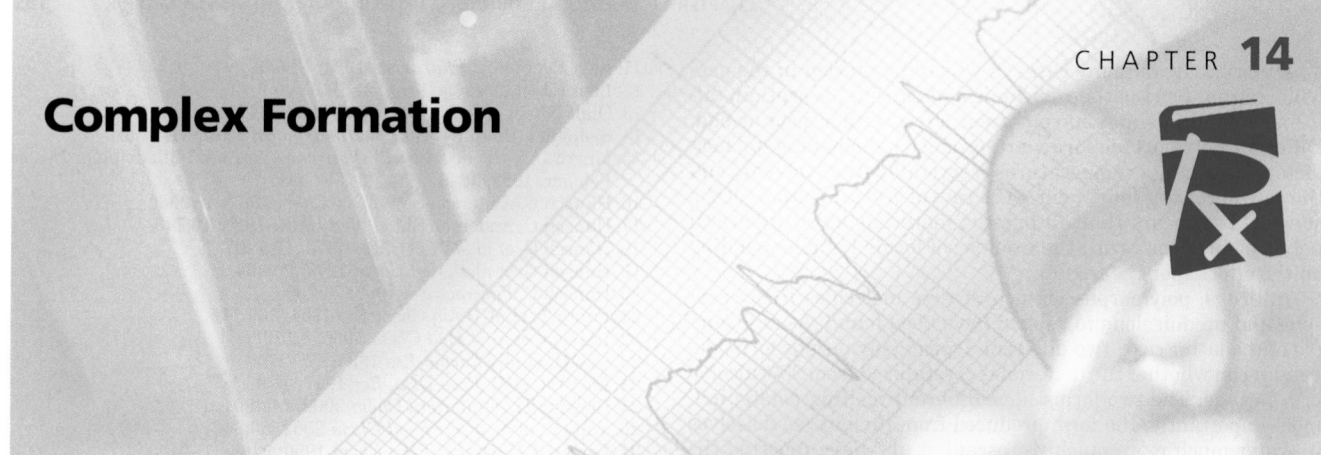

The word *complex* has many meanings in chemistry, so it is necessary at the outset to describe the types of systems that are included in this chapter. A complex is a species formed by the association of two or more interacting molecules or ions. To sharpen this concept the following definitions are provided:

- A *substrate, S,* is the interactant whose physical or chemical properties are observed experimentally.
- A *ligand, L,* is the second interactant whose concentration may be varied independently in an experimental study.
- A *complex* is a species of definite substrate-to-ligand stoichiometry that can be formed in an equilibrium process in solution, and also may exist in the solid state.

It is obvious that the complex must possess some properties that are different from those of its constituents; otherwise, there would be no evidence for its existence. Among the properties that may be altered upon complex formation are solubility, energy absorption, conductance, partitioning behavior, and chemical reactivity. It is by studying such properties of the substrate, as a function of ligand concentration, that complex formation may be recognized and described quantitatively. The terms *complex formation, complexation, binding,* and *association* are synonymous in the context of this chapter. Because complex formation is an equilibrium process, the methods of thermodynamics can be applied to describe it in the state of equilibrium. Moreover, the methods of chemical kinetics can be used to study the rate of approach to equilibrium. Finally, there may be interest in establishing the structure and properties of the complex.

These definitions are expressed succinctly in the following chemical equation for the formation of a complex S_mL_n.

$$mS + nL \rightleftharpoons S_mL_n$$

This shows that the distinction between substrate and ligand is arbitrary and is made solely for experimental convenience. The definition omits any consideration of the forces acting between substrate and ligand in the complex; thus, it is very general. Therefore, the phenomena of interest may be restricted further by specifying that complexes are not formed with classic covalent bonds.

TYPES OF COMPLEXES—The definition of a complex leads to a classification into two groups based on type of chemical bonding.

Coordination Complexes—These complexes are formed by coordinate bonds in which a pair of electrons is, in some degree, transferred from one interactant to the other. The most important examples are the metal-ion coordination complexes between metal ions and bases. Such complexes can be viewed as products of Lewis acid–base reactions. Proton acids then constitute a special case of this type.

Molecular Complexes—These species are formed by noncovalent interactions between the substrate and ligand. The noncovalent forces arise from electrostatic, induction and dispersion interactions, and they include, or give rise to, hydrogen-bonding, charge-transfer, and hydrophobic effects. Among the kinds of complex species that are included in this class are small molecule–small molecule complexes, small molecule–macromolecule species (eg, drug-protein and enzyme-substrate complexes), ion-pairs, dimers, and other self-associated species, inclusion complexes, intramolecular interactions (such as base–base interactions in the DNA helix), and clathrate complexes, in which the crystal structure of one interactant encloses molecules of the second interactant.

The following sections amplify these brief descriptions of coordination complexes and molecular complexes.

METAL-ION COORDINATION COMPLEXES

DESCRIPTIVE COORDINATION CHEMISTRY—Coordination complexes consist of a central metal ion (the substrate) bonded to an electron-pair donor (a base, the ligand). The ligand may be a conventional Brønsted base such as ammonia, an ion such as chloride ion, or even an aromatic compound. The complex may be neutral or charged. Coordination complexes also are called coordination compounds.

The number of bonds from the metal ion to the ligand (or ligands) is called the *coordination number* of the complex, and the maximum coordination number is evidently the largest possible number of such bonds. The maximum coordination number is determined by the electronic structure of the metal ion; numbers of 4 and 6 are most common, but other coordination numbers are possible. In solutions of Cu(II) in the presence of ammonia, these coordination complexes can form: $Cu(NH_3)^{2+}$, $Cu(NH_3)_2^{2+}$, $Cu(NH_3)_3^{2+}$, $Cu(NH_3)_4^{2+}$. The maximum coordination number of Cu(II) is 4.

A ligand, like ammonia, that has a single basic group capable of bonding to the metal ion is a *unidentate* ligand. A ligand having more than one accessible basic binding site is *multidentate*; for example, ethylenediamine, $H_2NCH_2CH_2NH_2$, is a bidentate ligand. If a metal ion binds to two or more sites on a multidentate ligand, a cyclic complex is formed necessarily; this cyclic complex is a *chelate*. Thus, ethylenediamine forms a chelate with Cu(II):

$$\begin{array}{c} NH_2 \quad H_2N \\ \diagdown \ Cu^{2+} \diagup \\ NH_2 \quad H_2N \end{array}$$

1

Table 14-1 shows several common multidentate ligands, and Table 14-2 lists abbreviations for some ligands. Thus, the complex shown in Structure **1** may be written $Cu(en)_2^{2+}$. Of course, this complex ion must be associated with an appropriate number of anions.

Table 14-1. Some Important Multidentate Ligands[a]

$H_2NCH_2CH_2NH_2$	Ethylenediamine
	2,2'-Bipyridine
	1,10-Phenanthroline
	8-Hydroxyquinoline (oxine)
	Dimethylglyoxime
	Ethylenediaminetetra-acetic acid

(structures shown)

CH₃C=NOH
CH₃C=NOH

$(HO_2CCH_2)_2NCH_2CH_2N(CH_2CO_2H)_2$

[a] Proton acid groups in these ligands are converted to basic groups upon the dissociation of the proton.

The nomenclature of coordination complexes is fairly complicated, and only the simplest features are reviewed here.[1]

1. If the complex is an ion, the cation is listed first, then the anion.
2. Ligands (names): neutral ligands are named as the molecule, except for H_2O (aquo) and NH_3 (ammine). Positive ligands end in -ium (eg, hydrazinium, $H_2NNH_3^+$) and negative ligands in -o (eg, acetato). Some exceptions are chloro, fluoro, cyano, oxo, and hydroxo (OH^-).
3. Ligands (order): the order is anionic, neutral, and cationic. There are subrules within these categories; for example, simple ions generally precede polyatomic ions, and organic ions appear last.
4. Complex names (endings): anionic complexes end in -ate or -ic (if named as the acid). Cationic or neutral complexes do not have characteristic endings.
5. Central atom or ion (oxidation state): given by a Roman numeral in parentheses; no sign is used for positive oxidation states, but a negative sign indicates a negative oxidation state.

Examples:

[Pt(en)(NH₃)₂ NO₂Cl]SO₄	Chloronitrodiammine ethylenediamine-platinum(IV) sulfate
NH₄[Cr(SCN)₄ (NH₃)₂]	Ammonium tetrathiocyanatodiammine-chromate (III)
[Co(en)₃]₂(SO₄)₃	Tris(ethylenediamine)cobalt(III) sulfate
K₄[Fe(CN)₆]	Potassium hexacyanoferrate(II)
K[CrOF₄]	Potassium oxotetrafluorochromate(V)

Not all coordination complexes can be formed simply by mixing the reactants in solution. It has been found convenient to classify coordination complexes as either *labile* or *inert* complexes:

A labile complex is one whose rates of formation and dissociation are faster than, or comparable to, the typical time of mixing of the reactant solutions. An inert complex is one whose formation and dissociation rates are slower than the typical time of mixing of the reactant solutions.

Table 14-2. Common Abbreviations of Some Ligands

LIGAND	ABBREVIATION
Pyridine	*py*
Thiourea	*tu*
Ethylenediamine	*en*
Glycine	*gly*
Oxalate	*ox*
2,4-Pentanedione (acetylacetone)	*acac*
1,10-Phenanthroline	*phen*
2,2'-Bipyridine	*bipy*
Ethylenediaminetetraacetate	*EDTA, Y*

Clearly, the classification of labile versus inert is arbitrary, but it has experimental utility because inert complexes can be investigated by conventional chemical techniques, as they may persist long enough to be studied as isolated species; however, labile complexes tend to dissociate upon perturbation of the chemical system. At a more fundamental level, the lability or inertness of a complex can be related to its electronic configuration.[2]

It is important to note that the labile or inert classification is a kinetic one and generally is distinct from a consideration of complex stability, which is a thermodynamic concept (to be treated subsequently). To express this distinction more concretely, consider the example of complex formation

$$S + L \underset{k_{-1}}{\overset{k_1}{\rightleftharpoons}} SL$$

where k_1 is the rate constant for association and k_{-1} is the dissociation rate constant. Then, approximately, if $(k_1[L] + k_{-1})$ is greater than the rate of mixing, the complex is labile. The stability of the complex, however, is described by the equilibrium constant for its formation, which is equal to the ratio k_1/k_{-1}.

Although labile complexes form and dissociate rapidly, even inert complexes can undergo reactions in which one or more ligands are replaced, thus forming a new complex. Such reactions are called substitution reactions, and because ligands are bases, these are nucleophilic substitutions. A nucleophile, or *nucleus-lover,* is an electron-rich species that reacts with an electrophilic site; nucleophilicity refers to reactivity, ie, kinetics. Basicity refers to equilibrium behavior. The following equation is a typical nucleophilic substitution reaction (a hydrolysis reaction) in which water is the nucleophile.

$$Co(NH_3)_5Cl^{2+} + H_2O \rightarrow Co(NH_3)_5(H_2O)^{3+} + Cl^-$$

ISOMERISM AND STEREOCHEMISTRY—From organic chemistry it is known that the geometry of bonding about the saturated carbon atom is that of a regular tetrahedron (the coordination number of carbon being 4). As a consequence, there is only one substance with the formula CA_2B_2, where C is carbon and A or B represent atoms or groups bonded to the carbon. For example, there is only one compound (methylene chloride) with the formula CH_2Cl_2.

It is otherwise with metal-ion coordination complexes having coordination number 4, for which it has been found that there may be two compounds of structure MA_2B_2, where M represents the metal ion. These two compounds are geometrical isomers, and their existence means that they have a square planar structure. For example, the two dichlorodiammineplatinum(II) isomers have these structures:

In the *cis* isomer, two like ligands are adjacent; in the *trans* isomer, they are opposite each other. The metal and the four ligand groups all lie in the same plane. Figure 14-1 shows alternative representations of the square planar complex structure. The demonstration of geometrical isomerism by chemical methods was based on the isolation of both isomers, which is possible if the complexes are inert.

There exists also the possibility of *cis* and *trans* isomerism in square planar complexes of the structure $M(AB)_2$, where AB is an unsymmetrical bidentate ligand, such as glycinate.

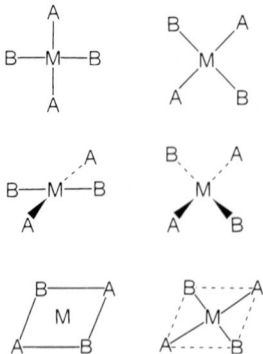

Figure 14-1. Equivalent representations of the square planar complex *trans*-MA$_2$B$_2$.

Most complexes of coordination number 4 have the square planar structure, but some are tetrahedral. Nearly all complexes with coordination number 6 are octahedral; ie, the coordinate bonds lie along the x, y, and z axes of a Cartesian coordinate system with the metal ion at the origin. This structure is consistent with the experimental observations that only two isomers can be isolated of each of the structures MA$_4$B$_2$ and MA$_3$B$_3$. The *cis* and *trans* isomers of the octahedral dichlorotetraamminecobalt(III) chloride have these structures:

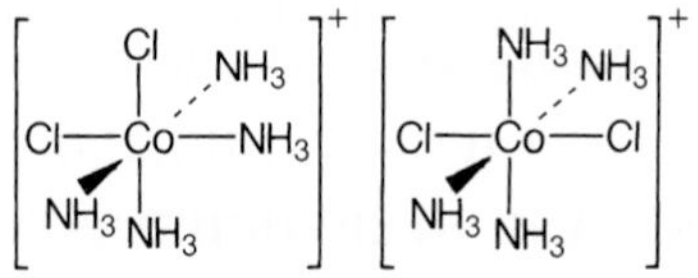

$$\left[\begin{array}{c}\text{Cl} \quad \text{NH}_3 \\ \text{Cl}-\text{Co}-\text{NH}_3 \\ \text{NH}_3 \text{ NH}_3\end{array}\right]^{+} \quad \left[\begin{array}{c}\text{NH}_3 \text{ NH}_3 \\ \text{Cl}-\text{Co}-\text{Cl} \\ \text{NH}_3 \text{ NH}_3\end{array}\right]^{+}$$

cis   *trans*

Figure 14-2 shows equivalent ways to draw an octahedral complex.

It should be noted that chloride in the above cobalt compounds plays two different roles; two chlorides are ligands, being coordinately bound to the cobalt, whereas the other chloride serves as a counterion to the complex cation.

Octahedral complexes can exhibit optical isomerism when two structures are related as nonsuperimposable mirror images. Such isomers are called *enantiomers*. The optical isomers of M(AA)$_3$, where AA is a symmetrical bidentate ligand, are shown in Figure 14-3, which also shows the specific example [Pt(*en*)$_3$]$^{4+}$.

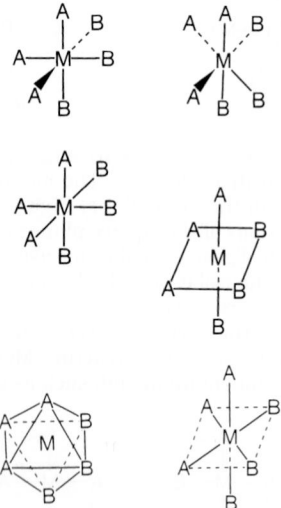

Figure 14-2. Equivalent representations of the octahedral complex *cis*-MA$_3$B$_3$.

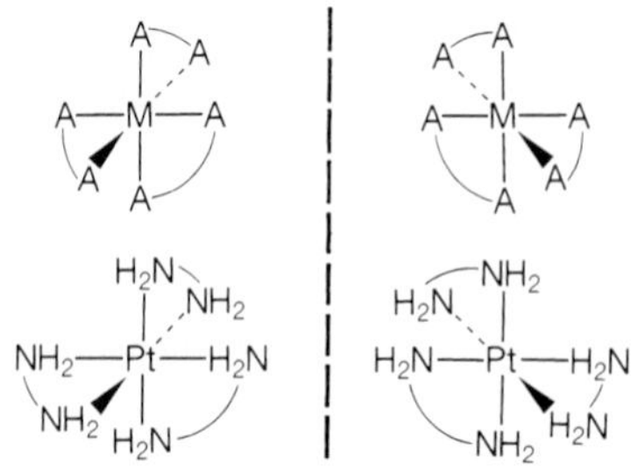

The existence of geometrical and optical isomers of coordination complexes has provided valuable insight into possible complex structures, as noted above; but, in addition, these isomers, when subjected to substitution reactions, have led to important inferences concerning the mechanisms of these reactions. For example, nucleophilic substitution reactions of square planar complexes are known to be bimolecular displacement processes, on the basis (in part) of complete retention of configuration; *cis* reactants yield *cis* products, and *trans* reactants yield *trans* products.[3] This rules out a dissociation (S$_N$1) mechanism. The reaction is believed to take place via a trigonal bipyramidal structure in which the metal-ion coordination number is increased as shown below.

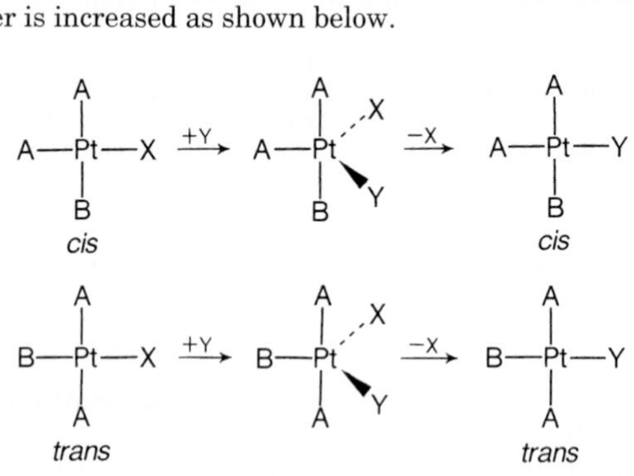

$$\begin{array}{ccc}
\text{A}-\text{Pt}-\text{X} & \xrightarrow{+\text{Y}} & \text{A}-\text{Pt} \cdots \text{X} \\
\text{B} & & \text{B} \quad \text{Y}
\end{array} \xrightarrow{-\text{X}} \text{A}-\text{Pt}-\text{Y}$$

cis   *cis*

trans   *trans*

THEORIES OF COORDINATE BONDING—A great range in complexing behavior is observed in the interactions of different metal ions with different ligands. A successful theory of coordinate bonding should be able to describe and predict the chemistry of coordination complexes given the identities of the metal ion and the ligand. Developments in this field have been concerned particularly with the transition elements, which may be defined as those elements having partly filled *d* or *f* shells in any of their common oxidation states[4]; with this definition, slightly more than half of the elements are transition elements. In addition, of course, some main group elements may form complexes.

A theory of coordinate complexing should be able to account for the coordination numbers of ions and the stereochemistry of their complexes. It should explain commonly observed regularities in complex stability, such as the *chelate effect:* the greater the number of sites of bonding of each ligand to the metal ion, the greater the complex stability. Another pattern is that of the complexes of certain divalent metal ions, whose stabilities vary in the order Mn < Fe < Co < Ni < Cu > Zn. The electronic absorption spectra (ie, the allowed electronic transitions) of complexes are a readily observed property that a theory should describe. Many metal coordination complexes absorb strongly in the visible region. Metal ions and their complexes also may have magnetic properties that can be accounted for theoretically. Substances having no unpaired electrons are diamagnetic, whereas those with unpaired electrons are paramagnetic,

Figure 14-3. Optical isomers of M(AA)$_3$ (top pair) and [Pt(*en*)$_3$]$^{4+}$ (bottom pair). Each enantiomer is a nonsuperimposable mirror image of the other as reflected in the central vertical plane.

and these properties easily are distinguished experimentally. Thus, a theory should be able to predict the number of unpaired electrons in the coordination complex.

Many theories have been developed, and they are essentially all different in concept. It is not possible here to treat any of them in detail, but their basic approaches will be outlined.

The *electrostatic* theory is completely classical (ie, nonquantum mechanical).[5] Ions are treated as spherical charges and molecules are treated as dipoles; the energy of a complex is calculated as a sum of charge–charge, charge–dipole, and charge-induced dipole terms and repulsive forces. Experimental values of dipole moments and intermolecular distances are employed in the calculations, which yield results for bond energies in remarkably good agreement with experimental values for many complexes. However, the theory necessarily is approximate, because it does not include quantum mechanical effects and it oversimplifies the structural differences among metal ions and ligands.

The *valence bond* theory of Pauling[6] is a quantum mechanical theory. A coordinate bond is formed when a pair of electrons on a ligand is donated to a vacant orbital on the metal ion. The coordination number is determined by the number of available orbitals, and the geometry of the complex is determined by the directional properties of the hybrid orbitals formed by combination of the atomic orbitals (the tetrahedral arrangement of hybrid sp^3 orbitals of carbon).

This theory has been quite successful in accounting for complex stereochemistry. It also can incorporate observations on magnetic type, as illustrated by the electronic configurations in Table 14-3.[7] From the vacant atomic orbitals of Fe^{2+} or Fe^{3+} there can be formed six equivalent hybrid orbitals of composition $3d^2 4s 4p^3$; thus, octahedral complexes are anticipated. Each ligand contributes two electrons to a hybrid orbital, resulting, in the case of $Fe(CN)_6^{4-}$, in a complex having no unpaired electrons and, therefore, diamagnetic; $Fe(CN)_6^{3-}$, on the other hand, possesses one unpaired electron, in agreement with experimental conclusions.

The valence bond theory is useful mainly in this qualitative pictorial way. In principle, bond energies can be calculated; in practice, this is extremely difficult.

As the coordinate bond has been treated thus far, it consists entirely of a pair of electrons donated by the ligand to a vacant metal orbital. Another type of donation is sometimes possible (as in the case of the two hexacyanato complexes shown in Table 14-3). If the ligand possesses vacant orbitals, the metal may contribute electrons from its d orbitals to vacant p or d orbitals on the ligand, thus producing a bond with double-bond character. This phenomenon is called *back-bonding*.

The *valence shell electron-pair repulsion* theory is a very simple approach to the prediction of complex geometry. This is based on the principle that the valence shell electrons of the metal are directed in space so as to minimize their total repulsive energy. Thus, if there were two electron pairs, they will distribute themselves on opposite sides of the central ion, and a linear complex will be formed. This theory is not able to calculate bond energies.

The *crystal field* theory has been very fruitful in the study of coordination complexes. (The word "crystal" in this context is a historical accident; the theory is applicable to complexes in so-

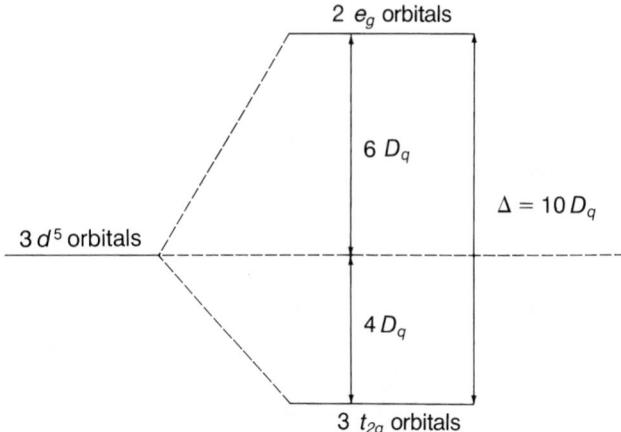

Figure 14-4. Energy-level diagram showing crystal-field splitting of the 5-fold degeneracy of metal-ion $3d$ orbitals in an octahedral complex.

lution as well as in the solid state.) The basis of the theory is seen readily with the example of an octahedral complex of a metal ion, such as iron. The five $3d$ orbitals are of equal energy (they are said to be 5-fold degenerate). According to crystal field theory, arranging the ligands colinear with d orbitals requires more energy (because of electron–electron repulsion) than does the approach of ligands between d orbitals. Two d orbitals (d_z and $d_{x^2-y^2}$) have lobes along the three Cartesian coordinates that define the geometry of the octahedral complex; thus, the electrical field of the ligands destabilizes (raises the energy of) these two orbitals. The other three orbitals (d_{xy}, d_{yz}, d_{xz}) are directed between the axes, so they are stabilized by the field of the ligands. Thus, the 5-fold degeneracy is split to produce two doubly degenerate orbitals (labeled e_g) and three triply degenerate orbitals (labeled t_{2g}), with no net energy change. This crystal-field splitting is shown in Figure 14-4. The total-energy difference Δ is conventionally labeled $10D_q$. It, therefore, follows that the e_g orbitals are destabilized by $6D_q$, and the t_{2g} orbitals are stabilized by $4D_q$.[8]

Now, the first orbitals to be filled upon formation of the complex will tend to be the lower energy t_{2g} orbitals, unless the stabilization is slight, in which case normal *Hund's rule* behavior will be observed, the electrons tending to remain unpaired. Thus, large splitting will lead to the formation of paired electrons (low-spin complexes), whereas small splitting will lead to more unpaired electrons (high-spin complexes).

A further subtlety can occur in which a distortion of the regular octahedral geometry takes place to lower the total energy of the system. This is known as the *Jahn-Teller effect*, with the result that for many octahedral complexes four of the ligands are coplanar with, and equidistant from, the metal ions; the other two ligands lie at a greater distance from the metal ion.

The crystal field theory has been developed in great detail, and many explanations and predictions have been achieved successfully. It especially is useful for explaining complex absorption spectra, and spectral measurements can be used to obtain values of the crystal field splitting, Δ.

The *molecular orbital* theory (which also is called the *ligand field* theory) is a quantum mechanical description in which molecular orbitals are constructed mathematically by the linear combination of atomic orbitals (MO-LCAO). The number of molecular orbitals (MOs) formed is equal to the number of atomic orbitals (AOs) taken, but the MOs are formed in pairs; one member of each pair is a symmetric, lower energy, bonding MO, and the other is an antisymmetric, higher energy, antibonding MO. The complex electronic configuration and energy are established by assigning electrons to the bonding MOs.

This concept is illustrated in Figure 14-5, shows a schematic MO diagram for an octahedral complex in which the ligand forms only single coordinate bonds (no back-bonding).[9] The

Table 14-3. Electronic Configurations of Some Iron Species According to Valence Bond Theory[a]

SPECIES	3D					4S	4P		
Fe^0	↑↓	↑	↑	↑	↑	↑↓	—	—	—
Fe^{2+}	↑↓	↑	↑	↑	↑	—	—	—	—
Fe^{3+}	↑	↑	↑	↑	↑	—	—	—	—
$Fe(CN)_6^{4-}$	↑↓	↑↓	↑↓	↑↓	↑↓	↑↓	↑↓	↑↓	↑↓
$Fe(CN)_6^{3-}$	↑↓	↑↓	↑	↑↓	↑↓	↑↓	↑↓	↑↓	↑↓

[a] Electrons in closed shells are not shown; thus, the electron configuration of Fe^0 is $1s^2 2s^2 2p^6 3s^2 3d^6 4s^2$.

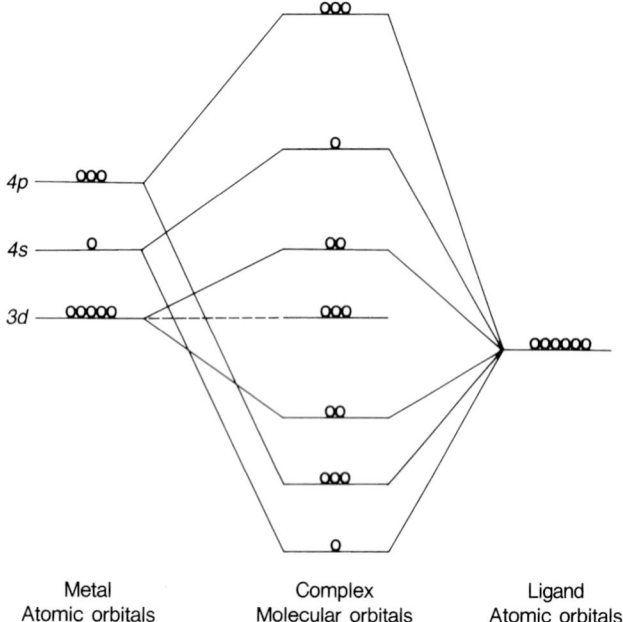

Figure 14-5. Schematic molecular orbital diagram for an octahedral complex. The vertical distance represents energy. Each circle denotes an orbital.

combination of AOs must take place according to certain quantum mechanical rules. For example, the metal s orbital combines with a ligand σ orbital to generate a bonding σ orbital and an antibonding σ^* orbital. The nine metal AOs combine with six ligand AOs to produce 15 MOs. The octahedral complex is formed by using the six bonding MOs (lowest energy MOs).

The MO theory is the most powerful of the theories of coordinate bonding, although quantitative calculations may be extremely difficult to make. Basolo and Pearson[10] have presented a comparison of the several theories.

Another view that has been found useful for its explanatory and predictive power is the *hard and soft acid–base* (HSAB) concept. A *hard acid* is defined as one in which the electron-pair acceptor atom is small in size, with high positive-charge density and low polarizability. A *soft acid* is large and polarizable. A hard base has high electronegativity and low polarizability, whereas a soft base is easily polarizable. Examples of these classes are listed in Table 14-4. Polarizability is a measure of the ease with which the electron cloud can be deformed under the influence of a field. Hardness and softness are related inversely.

The HSAB principle states that hard acids prefer to coordinate to hard bases and soft acids to soft bases. This empirical generalization can account qualitatively for much coordinate-complex chemistry. The HSAB concept has been extended by the introduction of a quantitative definition of hardness[11] as

$$\eta = \frac{(I - A)}{2}$$

where η is the hardness, I is the ionization potential (a measure of the ease with which an electron can be lost), and A is the electron affinity, which measures the ease with which an electron

Table 14-4. Examples of the Hard-Soft Classification of Lewis Acids and Bases

	ACIDS	BASES
Hard	H^+, Li^+, Na^+, K^+, Mg^{2+}, Ca^{2+}, Mn^{2+}, Al^{3+}	H_2O, OH^-, F^-, Cl^-, PO_4^{3-}, SO_4^{2-}, ClO_4^-, NO_3^-, NH_3
Soft	Cu^+, Ag^+, Au^+, HG_2^{2+}, Pd^{2+}, Pt^{2+}	I^-, SCN^-, CN^-

combines with the species. Pearson has related hardness to the MO theory and developed the quantitative aspects of HSAB theory.[11]

At the start of this chapter it was specified that complexes are not formed with covalent bonds, but in the case of coordination complexes it is seen that a coordinate bond may have extensive covalent character, even though both electrons are donated by one of the reactants. One of the goals of theory is to be able to calculate the fractions of ionic and covalent character of the coordinate bond. Very roughly, it may be expected that when the bond is between atoms that differ greatly in their electronegativities (propensities for attracting negative charge), the bond will be largely ionic, whereas if the atoms have similar electronegativities, the bond will be largely covalent.

MOLECULAR COMPLEXES

NONCOVALENT INTERMOLECULAR FORCES— Molecules in condensed systems (liquids and solids) experience mutual forces of attraction, which is why the systems are condensed. These forces are much weaker than those of "chemical" (ie, covalent) bonds, as shown by the ease with which they can be broken, such as by vaporization or dissolution. These are the noncovalent intermolecular forces.[12]

Two different kinds of solute molecules or ions are to be noted, labeled S (substrate) and L (ligand), in a solvent that is thought of conveniently (but somewhat artificially) as a homogeneous continuum; ie, for the present, neglect the molecular nature of the solvent. The intermolecular forces between S and L are of interest. The force of interaction F is related to the potential energy of interaction V by

$$F = -\frac{dV}{dr}$$

where r is the distance between the interacting species. It is conventional to express the intermolecular forces in terms of the corresponding energies. The most important noncovalent potential energy functions, as established by theoretical arguments, are listed in Table 14-5.

Table 14-5. Potential-Energy Functions for Noncovalent Interactions[a]

TYPE OF INTERACTION	POTENTIAL-ENERGY FUNCTION
Electrostatic	
Charge–charge	$+\dfrac{C_S C_L}{r}$
Charge–dipole	$-\dfrac{1}{3kT} \cdot \dfrac{C_S^2 \cdot \mu_L^2}{r^4}$
Dipole–dipole	$-\dfrac{2}{3kT} \cdot \dfrac{\mu_S^2 \cdot \mu_L^2}{r^6}$
Induction	
Charge-induced dipole	$-\dfrac{C_S^2 \cdot \alpha_L}{2r^4}$
Dipole-induced dipole	$-\dfrac{\mu_S^2 \cdot \alpha_L}{r^6}$
Dispersion	
Induced dipole–induced dipole	$-\dfrac{3}{4}\left[\dfrac{\varepsilon_S \cdot \varepsilon_L}{\varepsilon_S + \varepsilon_L}\right]\dfrac{\alpha_S \cdot \alpha_L}{r^6}$

[a] C is the charge on an ion, μ is permanent dipole moment, α is polarizability, r is intermolecular distance, ε is a specific energy term, T is absolute temperature, and k is Boltzmann's constant, where $k = R/N_A$.

The noncovalent forces are of three broad types:

- The *electrostatic* forces among ions and molecules possessing permanent dipole moments.
- The *induction* (or polarization) forces between an ion and a nonpolar molecule or a polar molecule and a nonpolar molecule.
- The *dispersion* (London) force, which operates between all molecules.

The *electrostatic* forces are the consequence of classical attraction and repulsion effects between charges. In the potential-energy terms in Table 14-5, the magnitudes of the charges are to be accompanied by their signs; a negative value for the energy is attractive, whereas a positive value is repulsive. Note that charges and dipole moments always appear as squared quantities.

The *induction* forces arise as a result of an ion or a polar molecule inducing a dipole in a neighboring molecule. Thus, their strength depends upon the ionic charge or the dipole moment of the inducing species and the polarizability (a measure of electron-cloud deformability) of the induced species.

The *dispersion* force is nonclassical in origin; ie, it is a quantum mechanical effect. At any moment the electronic distribution in one molecule, such as S, may result in the production of a dipole moment in S, even if it is a nonpolar molecule. This instantaneous dipole then can induce a dipole in L. The dispersion force, therefore, is general and acts among all molecules, both polar and nonpolar. (The term *van der Waals' force* sometimes is used to describe the dispersion force, but some authors use this term to include all noncovalent forces.)

It is important to notice that, for neutral molecules, the electrostatic, induction, and dispersion-energy terms all possess an intermolecular-distance dependence of r^{-6}. As two molecules approach each other they will experience a force of attraction that varies with distance as r^{-7}. They cannot continue to approach closely indefinitely because ultimately they experience repulsive forces as their electron clouds tend to repel each other, and at an even closer distance there is an internuclear repulsive force. The net force between molecules is a balance between the attractive and repulsive forces. This often is described by the potential-energy function below, which is called the Lennard-Jones 6-12 potential,

$$V = 4V_{min}\left[\left(\frac{r_0}{r}\right)^{12} - \left(\frac{r_0}{r}\right)^{6}\right] \quad (1)$$

where V_{min} is the value of V at the minimum in the "potential well," ie, where $r = r_{eq}$, the equilibrium intermolecular distance. This is the distance at which the attractive and repulsive forces are balanced. The term in r^{-12} is the repulsive term, that in r^{-6} is the attractive term, and r_0 is the value of r when $V = 0$. Figure 14-6 shows a plot of the Lennard-Jones 6-12 potential for a hypothetical system to illustrate the qualitative features of noncovalent interaction. Values of V_{min} are typically 5 kcal/mol, or less, which are much smaller than typical covalent bond energies.

Although Table 14-5 includes the most important noncovalent interactions, additional types of bonding often are invoked when describing complex formation. One of these is *hydrogen bonding*. The formation of a hydrogen bond (H-bond) between a proton-donor HA and a proton-acceptor B can be represented formally as

$$A - H + B \rightleftharpoons A - H \cdots B$$

The strength of the hydrogen bond is controlled, in part, by the acid strength of HA and the base strength of B, but the solvent also is very important. The A—H bond is mainly covalent in character, and the hydrogen bond H $\cdots$ B is predominantly electrostatic.[13] Structure **2** shows intermolecular hydrogen bonding in a dimer of acetic acid, and Structure **3** shows an intramolecular hydrogen bond of the salicylic acid anion.

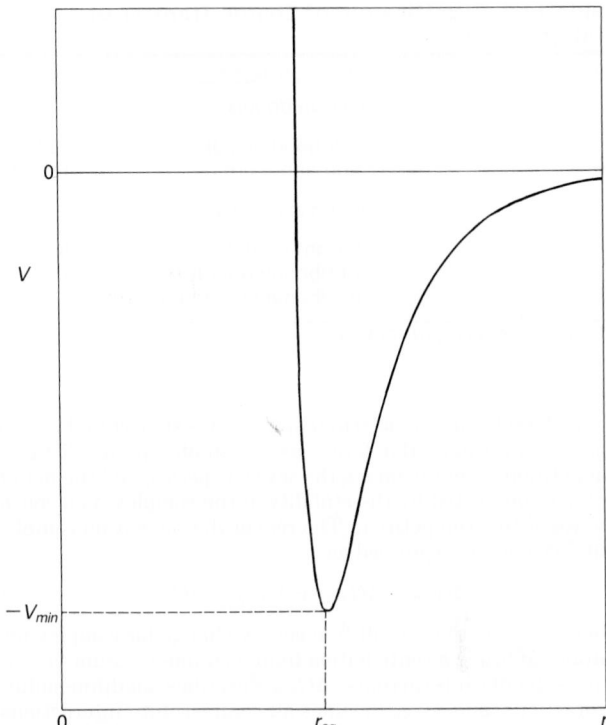

Figure 14-6. Potential-energy diagram according to Equation 1, the Lennard-Jones potential; r_{eq} is the equilibrium intermolecular distance, which minimizes the potential energy of the system.

Another type of bonding is *charge-transfer bonding*, which is a consequence of the transfer of an electron from a molecular orbital on an electron-donor molecule to an orbital on an electron-acceptor molecule. Because charge-transfer results in a change in electron configuration, it produces a change in the electronic energy levels and, therefore, in the ultraviolet-visible absorption spectra of the interacting molecules. The appearance of new absorption bands often is cited as evidence for charge-transfer bonding.

Since an electron transfer is involved in this type of bonding, the resulting bond may have some covalent character. In addition, the usual noncovalent forces of Table 14-4 also are present, and the contribution of the charge-transfer phenomenon to the overall stability of the complex depends upon the particular molecules involved. A classification of the types of electron donors and acceptors, with some examples, is given in Table 14-6.[16]

ROLE OF THE SOLVENT—The preceding discussion of intermolecular forces focused on the interactions between two molecules or ions that may be viewed as the substrate and the ligand in a complex-formation reaction. The solvent was ignored in this treatment, which strictly is applicable only in the vapor state. However, in this discussion, interest in complexes arises largely from their occurrence in solutions and solids, so the solvent must be introduced as a component of the system. Table 14-7 presents some useful groupings of solvents according to structure and chemical behavior.

Table 14-6. Classification of Charge-Transfer Donors and Acceptors

TYPE	ORBITAL INVOLVED	EXAMPLE
	Electron donors	
n	Nonbonding pair	$:NR_3$
$b\pi$	Bonding π orbital	Benzene
	Electron acceptors	
v	Vacant orbital	BCl_3
$a\pi$	Antibonding π orbital	TCNE[a]
$a\sigma$	Antibonding σ orbital	I_2

[a] Tetracyanoethylene, $(N\equiv C)_2C = C(C\equiv N)_2$.

As the solvent is a molecular species, it is subject to the same types of intermolecular forces as the solute species. Thus, a competition is set up among the several species, and the net effect, as manifested by the stability of the complex, is a consequence of this competition. The role of the solvent on complex stability may be expressed as

$$\Delta G_{net} = \Delta G_{MM} + \Delta G_{MS} + \Delta G_{SS} \qquad (2)$$

where ΔG_{net} is the overall free-energy change for complex formation, ΔG_{MM} is a contribution from medium–medium (ie, solvent–solvent) interactions, ΔG_{MS} describes medium–solute interactions, and ΔG_{SS} includes all solute–solute interactions. The value of ΔG_{SS} is determined by the substrate–ligand intermolecular interactions, but Equation 2 shows that the net stability of the complex also can be influenced by the solvent. The term ΔG_{MS} represents a solvation contribution, and its effect can be either stabilizing (if the complex is solvated more extensively than the reactants) or destabilizing (if the converse is applicable). The ΔG_{MM} term represents another way in which the solvent can influence complex stability.

Consider a nonpolar solvent, in which the *MM* interactions are weak (arising only from the dispersion force). In such a solvent the ΔG_{MS} term probably also will be small, and then the ΔG_{SS} term will make the major contribution to ΔG_{net}. If, on the other hand, the solvent is polar (such as water, in particular), the solvent–solvent interaction may be the predominant contributor to ΔG_{net}. The ΔG_{MM} term in water may be identified as the *hydrophobic effect*, which will be considered in more detail. There are two points of view from which the hydrophobic effect can be discussed.

One of these theories takes as its key feature the structure of water, ie, the intermolecular network of water molecules generated by their mutual hydrogen-bonding.[15] When a nonpolar solute dissolves in water, no H-bonds from water to the solute can form, so the water structure in the vicinity of the solute must be modified to compensate for the water–water H-bonds that were broken upon insertion of the solute into the water. The number of possible orientations of water molecules is decreased in the presence of the solute, so its dissolution is unfavorable entropically; this is why nonpolar compounds have low aqueous solubilities, according to this view.

When two such dissolved solute molecules come into contact, some of the *structured* water surrounding them must be released into the bulk medium, resulting in an increase in entropy, which (through its contribution to the ΔG_{MM} term) is the main driving force in the hydrophobic interaction of nonpolar molecules in water. Although this description is acceptable for nonpolar solutes, it must be modified for polar solutes, for which the main driving force may be either a favorable entropy change or a favorable enthalpy change.[16]

The second theory of the hydrophobic effect is the cavity model, which treats the solvent as a continuum. The surface tension γ of a solvent is a measure of its surface energy, and in water, whose surface tension is unusually high (72 dynes/cm), there is a strong driving force for the minimization of surface area. In order to dissolve a solute molecule in a solvent, a cavity must be created, and then the solute is inserted in the cavity. This can be thought of as "digging a hole in the solvent," and it takes an energy equal to the product of the surface area of the cavity (which is determined by the size of the solute molecule) and the surface tension of the solvent. Some of this energy cost may be offset by the subsequent interaction energy, through solvation, of the molecule with the solvent.

When two dissolved molecules unite to form a complex, the two cavities containing the separated species coalesce into a single cavity holding the complex. There is a net decrease in surface area (ΔA) in this process, and the product $\Delta A\gamma$ is the driving force for the complex formation. Figure 14-7 is a representation of this cavity model of the hydrophobic effect.

It now can be anticipated that if the hydrophobic effect makes a major contribution to the stability of a complex in water, the incorporation of an organic cosolvent into the medium (resulting in a lower surface tension) will decrease the stability of the complex. On the other hand, if the interest is in a complex (in a nonhydroxylic solvent) whose stability is derived largely from strong intermolecular substrate–ligand H-bonding, then incorporation of water or an alcohol will reduce the stability of the complex due to competition by the hydroxylic solvent.

Thus, it is seen that solvent effects on complex-formation can be varied and complicated, but that their study may offer insight into the nature of the intermolecular interactions responsible for the formation of the complex. A quantitative theory of solvent effects on complex formation has been developed.[17]

EXAMPLES OF MOLECULAR COMPLEXES—There is no systematic classification of molecular complexes, nor has a system of nomenclature been developed to describe complexes. Particular types may be classified in terms of the kinds of interactions involved in their formation, the kinds of interactants involved, or the kinds of complexes formed. Table 14-8 gives an outline of molecular complexes according to this classification.

Since molecular complexes are formed by noncovalent interactions, their bonding is localized less than that observed with covalent and coordinate bonds, which are highly directional. As a consequence, for many of these complexes it is not possible to indicate a specific complex structure. Hydrogen-bonded complexes are exceptions because of the requirements for the existence of the H-bond, and many H-bonded structures are known.

Studies by x-ray diffraction on crystalline complexes can reveal the mutual orientations of interactants in the solid state, but this knowledge does not indicate the nature or location of the noncovalent bonding directly. Theoretical calculations have

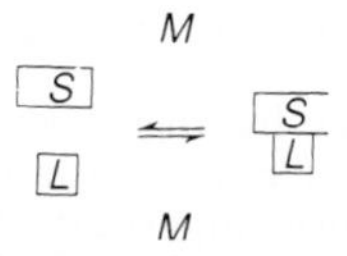

Table 14-7. Classification of Solvents

SOLVENT CLASS	EXAMPLES
Hydroxylic	Water, alcohols, glycols
H-bond donors	Water, alcohols, glycols, carboxylic acids, amides, imides, chloroform
H-bond acceptors	Amines, ethers, aldehydes, ketones
Dipolar aprotic[a]	Acetonitrile, dimethylsulfoxide, acetone, N,N-dimethylformamide
Nonpolar	Hydrocarbons, halogenated hydrocarbons

[a] These are solvents with large dipole moments and no readily donated proton.

Figure 14-7. Representation of complex formation between *S* and *L* (planar molecules viewed in cross section through the molecular planes) to form complex *SL*. The total surface area exposed to solvent *M* is less for the complex than for the separated species.

Table 14-8. Classification of Molecular Complexes

I. *Type of bonding or interaction*
   Charge-transfer
   Hydrogen-bonding
   Hydrophobic interaction
   Stacking interaction
II. *Type or structure of interactants*
   Small molecule–small molecule complex
   Small molecule–macromolecule binding
   Drug-protein binding
   Enzyme–substrate complex
   Drug–receptor complex
   Antigen–antibody complex
III. *Type or structure of complex*
   Self-associated aggregate
   Micelle
   Inclusion complex
   Clathrate

been helpful in suggesting how the substrate and ligand are positioned in the complex, and this approach is being used to design new drugs that can bind specifically to biological receptors.

Some examples of complexes, or of substrates and ligands that form complexes, will follow, using the outline in Table 14-8 as a guide.

Charge-transfer (CT) complexes, also called electron donor–acceptor (EDA) complexes, may be formed when one interactant can perform as the electron donor and the other as the electron acceptor. The appearance of a new electronic absorption band, not attributable to either the donor or the acceptor, often is taken as evidence for charge-transfer complexing. A classic example is provided by solutions of iodine in organic solvents. When I_2 is dissolved in aliphatic hydrocarbons or carbon tetrachloride, the solution has a violet color characteristic of iodine, but solutions in aromatic hydrocarbons, alcohols, or ethers are brown. It is inferred that, in these latter solvents, a complex is formed and, because of the color (spectral) change, charge-transfer is implicated. In solvents in which iodine forms a complex ("brown" solvents), the solvent is the electron donor and the iodine is the acceptor. Thus, from Table 14-6, the benzene–iodine complex may be described as a $b\pi$–$a\sigma$ CT complex, whereas the ethanol–iodine complex is an n–$a\sigma$ complex. Investigation of the benzene–bromine complex by X-ray crystallography shows that in the solid state the axis of the halogen molecule is perpendicular to the plane of the aromatic ring, as in Structure **4**. The structure of the complex in solution may, however, be different from this.

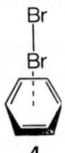

4

Referring to Table 14-8, it is noted that electron donors of the *n* type will be found among the amines, ethers, alcohols, and sulfides, whereas $b\pi$ donors include alkenes, alkynes, and aromatic hydrocarbons. Substitution on the donors by alkyl groups (which are electron-releasing) enhances their donor properties, unless the bulkiness of the substituent leads to steric hindrance. Hexamethylbenzene is a good electron donor. Lewis acids are electron acceptors, but among organic compounds the most important acceptors are unsaturated and aromatic compounds substituted with electron-withdrawing groups, exemplified by tetracyanoethylene, Structure **5**, picric acid, Structure **6**, and pyromellitic dianhydride, Structure **7**.

Structures **2** and **3** show hydrogen-bonding interactions. H-bonded complexes are observed readily in solvents that do not compete as H-bond donors or acceptors. The complex between phenol and pyridine in inert solvents is an H-bond complex. Perhaps the most famous hydrogen-bonded complexes are those of adenine-to-thymine and guanine-to- cytosine, which, as constituents of desoxynucleic acid, are responsible for the double-helix structure of the DNA molecule. Structure **8** shows the hydrogen bonds linking the cytosine of one polynucleotide strand to the guanine of a second strand.[18]

Any complex in aqueous solution may receive some portion of its stability from the hydrophobic effect, and for nonpolar interactants the hydrophobic contribution probably is the major one. According to the cavity model (see Fig 14-7), solvents other than water also can lead to complex formation via this surface-energy effect, although less effectively than in water because the surface tensions are lower; in solvents other than water this is called the *solvophobic effect*.

When two planar molecules undergo a primarily hydrophobic association, the total surface area of the complex exposed to the solvent can be minimized if the molecules are in plane-to-plane contact, as suggested in Fig 14-7. This plane-to-plane orientation is called a *stacking interaction*. The purine–pyrimidine H-bonded base pairs in DNA (Structure **8**) are planar assemblies that undergo stacking interactions with adjacent pairs.

Aside from the interactions specifically mentioned in Table 14-8, complex formation also can be the result of the several types of noncovalent interactions depicted in Table 14-5, and most complexes probably involve a combination of interactions.

The third class listed in Table 14-8 is not depicted so easily as is the second class. *Self-association* is a type of complexation in which a molecule forms complexes with others of its own species. If S represents a molecule capable of self-association, then S_2 is called its dimer, S_3 its trimer, S_4 its tetramer, and so on. Structure 2 shows a hydrogen-bonded dimer of acetic acid, which can exist in the vapor phase and in inert solvents. Benzene forms dimers in aqueous solution, as does caffeine; these planar molecules probably undergo hydrophobic stacking interactions in water.

A *micelle* is a special form of self-aggregated complex in which the interactant is a surfactant, a molecule possessing both a nonpolar and a polar portion. See Chapter 20 for an in-depth treatment of micelles.

Inclusion complexes are formed when a macrocyclic compound, possessing an intramolecular cavity of molecular dimensions, interacts with a small molecule that can enter the cavity. The macrocyclic molecule is called the *host,* the small, included molecule is the *guest,* and the inclusion process gives rise to *host–guest chemistry*. Both synthetic and naturally occurring

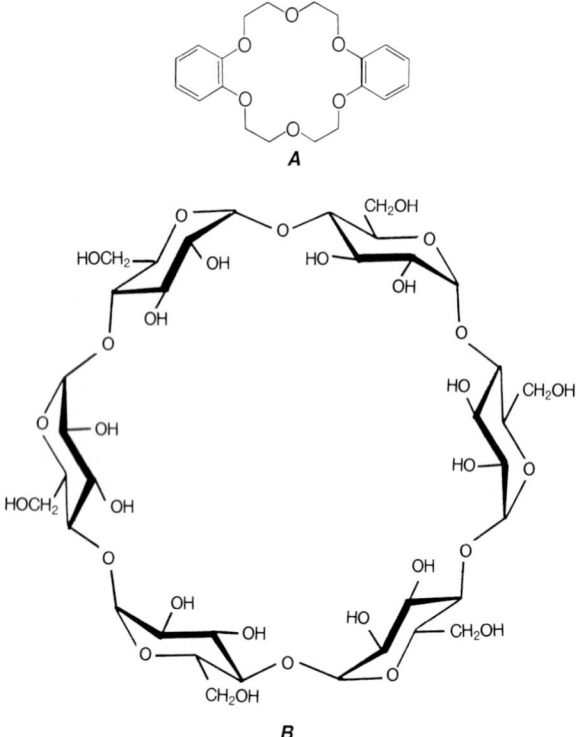

Figure 14-8. Structure of (*A*) dibenzo-18-crown-6 and (*B*) α-cyclodextrin.

macrocyclic hosts are known, and Figure 14-8*A* and *B* show an example of each. Crown ethers, such as the one shown in Figure 14-8*A*, present a nonpolar external molecular surface, but the interior of the cavity is relatively polar. As a consequence, polar guests such as ions can enter the cavity and, because their polarity now is masked by the surrounding host, exhibit unusual chemistry. For example, potassium permanganate, which is not soluble in nonpolar solvents, can be extracted into organic solvents from water in the presence of a crown ether.

The cyclodextrins are macrocyclic hosts that are formed by the action of certain bacterial enzymes on starch. They consist of α-D-glucose units joined with glycosidic (ether) linkages. The interior of the cavity is lined with these glycosidic bonds and, therefore, is relatively nonpolar (ie, relative to water), whereas the exterior of the molecule is quite polar because of the large number of hydroxy groups. The three commercially available cyclodextrins are called α-, β-, and γ-cyclodextrins (or, alternatively, cyclohexamylose, cycloheptaamylose, and cyclooctaamylose), and they consist of 6, 7, and 8 glucose units, respectively. The diameters of the cavities of the cyclodextrins are approximately 5 Å (for α), 6 to 7 Å (for β), or 8 to 9 Å (for γ). Thus, small guest molecules, or parts of molecules, may enter the host cavity to form inclusion complexes, whose stabilities are in part the result of the hydrophobic effect. Many properties of a guest molecule may be altered by inclusion in a cyclodextrin;[19] these include volatility, solubility, and chemical stability, so numerous practical applications have been suggested.[20] The stabilities of cyclodextrin complexes have been discussed.[21]

There is a special type of inclusion compound, called a *clathrate*, in which the host molecules form a crystal lattice containing spaces into which guest molecules can fit.[22] In cage clathrates, the cavity is a space completely surrounded by a network of host molecules. Some "gas" hydrates are examples; in these structures, a hydrogen-bonded network of water molecules, analogous to ice, encloses gaseous small molecules such as argon, methane, or nitrogen. The stoichiometry is not integral, but it can be explained on the basis of the hydrate crystal structure and size of the cages.[23]

Channel clathrates form when the host crystal contains continuous channels in which the guest can be included. Urea, $(H_2N)_2C{=}O$, forms channel clathrates with many long-chain molecules as the guests. Such clathrates have been used to isolate guest molecules from mixtures by crystallization in the clathrate form.

The literature on molecular complexes frequently now uses the term *molecular recognition*, which can be taken to mean a noncovalent interaction in which complementary features of the two interactants (exemplified by the hydrogen-bonding sites in Structure **8**) result in significant specificity in the complex-formation process.

COMPLEX STABILITY

Binding Constants and Stoichiometric Models

For the general complex-formation equilibrium

$$mS + nL \rightleftharpoons S_mL_n$$

the *overall binding constant*, β_{mn}, is defined

$$\beta_{mn} = \frac{[S_mL_n]}{[S]^m[L]^n} \tag{3}$$

where brackets denote molar concentrations. Actually, complexes probably form in a stepwise fashion by the coming together of two interactant species at a time. For example, the 1:2 complex SL_2 is formed in these two consecutive steps.

$$S + L \rightleftharpoons SL$$

$$SL + L \rightleftharpoons SL_2$$

Therefore, defining the stepwise binding constants as

$$K_{11} = \frac{[S]}{[S][L]} \tag{4}$$

$$K_{12} = \frac{[SL_2]}{[SL][L]} \tag{5}$$

Algebraic substitution shows that $\beta_{12} = K_{11}K_{12}$. Binding constants also are known as stability constants, formation constants, or association constants. The reciprocal quantity is a dissociation constant or an instability constant. These constants obviously depend on the identities of the substrate, S, and ligand, L; they also depend on the solvent and the temperature. Throughout most of this discussion the simplest example will be used, that of 1:1 complex formation, to illustrate concepts and methods, but in many situations it also may be necessary to consider the possibility of other stoichiometric ratios.[24]

The binding constant is an important measure of complex stability, and it is related to the standard free energy of complex formation by

$$\Delta G^0_{11} = -RT \ln K_{11} \tag{6}$$

where R is the gas constant and T is the absolute temperature. The standard free-energy change is related to the standard enthalpy change ΔH^0_{11} and the standard entropy change ΔS^0_{11} by

$$\Delta G^0_{11} = \Delta H^0_{11} - T\Delta S^0_{11} \tag{7}$$

ΔH^0_{11} can be determined from measurements of K_{11} at several temperatures. From

$$\log K_{11} = \frac{\Delta H^0_{11}}{2.303RT} + \text{constant} \tag{8}$$

a linear plot of $\log K_{11}$ against $1/T$ (a van't Hoff plot) yields ΔH^0_{11} from the slope. From Equation 7, ΔS^0_{11} then can be calculated.

Complex stability commonly is discussed in terms of K_{11}, log K_{11}, ΔG_{11}^0, or (less often) ΔH_{11}^0.

Before an experimentally measured binding constant can be accepted as a valid measure of complex stability, there must be a firm basis for believing that the stoichiometry has been identified correctly. This is achieved by formulating and then testing a hypothesis. This hypothesis is simply a statement or an equation giving the assumed stoichiometry; for example,

$$S + L \rightleftharpoons SL$$

which expresses the assumption of 1:1 stoichiometry. The test of this model consists of showing that K_{11} is a constant over all concentration ranges.

This procedure is oversimplified above, because it ignores nonideality effects that lead to differences between concentrations and activities. A more rigorous discussion is given elsewhere.[24]

This may be illustrated by building and testing a 1:1 model. The first step is to define K_{11} as in Equation 4. The second step is to write the material-balance relationship for the substrate.

$$S_t = [S] + [SL] \tag{9}$$

Here, S_t is the total substrate concentration. Also f_{11} is defined as the fraction of substrate in the complexed form.

$$f_{11} = [SL]/S_t \tag{10}$$

Algebraic combination of Equations 4, 9, and 10 yields

$$f_{11} = \frac{K_{11}[L]}{1 + K_{11}[L]} \tag{11}$$

Equation 11 is the *binding isotherm* for this model; it shows how f_{11} depends on the free-ligand concentration. The mathematical form of Equation 11 is very important in all 1:1 equilibria. The model is tested by measuring f_{11} (or some experimental variable that is proportional to f_{11}) and showing that it is quantitatively related to $[L]$ by Equation 11.

This procedure is of sufficient importance to be illustrated with a hypothetical example. Suppose $K_{11} = 10 \, M^{-1}$; by assigning reasonable values to $[L]$ the corresponding values of f_{11} can be calculated with Equation 11. The result is plotted in Figure 14-9. Several features are of interest. The binding isotherm is nonlinear; in fact, it is a rectangular hyperbola. At very low values of the free-ligand concentration the fraction bound rises sharply (the slope is relatively steep), but at high values of $[L]$ the curve flattens out and approaches the value $f_{11} = 1$, asymptotically. This change to a very small slope value at high $[L]$ is called a *saturation effect;* the physical interpretation is that in this region most of the substrate molecules are already bound (complexed) to ligand, so addition of more ligand cannot create additional complex as efficiently as at lower values of f_{11}. Notice, also, that when $f_{11} = \frac{1}{2}$, $[L] = 1/K_{11}$, as can be seen from

Equation 11. This condition is familiar in the context of acid–base chemistry, for at the condition of half-neutralization, $[H^+] = K_a$ or $pH = pK_a$, where K_a is defined to be a dissociation constant.

One way to test the assumed model against the experimental data is to perform a nonlinear least-squares regression analysis of f_{11} on $[L]$ according to Equation 11, observing the goodness of fit of the regression line to the data points. Another way is to rearrange Equation 11 into a linear form and plot the data accordingly. For example, Equation 11 is transformed easily to the "double-reciprocal" form

$$\frac{1}{f_{11}} = \frac{1}{K_{11}[L]} + 1 \tag{12}$$

This predicts that a plot of $1/f_{11}$ against $1/[L]$ will be linear if the model is valid. Other linear transformations also are possible, as shown below. Note that K_{11} can be evaluated from the slope of the double-reciprocal plot.

The *Michaelis-Menten equation* of enzyme kinetics has the same mathematical form as Equation 11, because it is based on the formation of a 1:1 enzyme-substrate complex. Another important example arises in the study of the binding of drugs to proteins. The simplest model of this process supposes that the protein possesses n identical, independent binding sites for drug L, each site having a site-binding constant of k. Mathematical treatment of this model leads to Equation 13 as the isotherm.

$$\bar{i} = \frac{nk[L]}{1 + k[L]} \tag{13}$$

where $\bar{i}$ is defined to be the average number of drug molecules bound per protein molecule at free-drug concentration $[L]$; $\bar{i}$ is defined by

$$\bar{i} = \frac{L_t - [L]}{S_t} \tag{14}$$

where L_t is the total drug concentration and S_t is the total protein concentration. The quotient $\bar{i}/n = \theta$ is called the degree of saturation.

Once again, in Equation 13, can be seen the characteristic hyperbolic dependence on ligand concentration. Drug–protein-binding often is analyzed with the aid of another linear transformation, Equation 15, according to which a plot of $\bar{i}/[L]$ against $\bar{i}$ will be linear.

$$\frac{\bar{i}}{[L]} = -k \cdot \bar{i} + n/k \tag{15}$$

From the slope and either intercept, the parameters n and k can be estimated. A plot according to Equation 15 is called a Scatchard plot. If the Scatchard plot is curved, evidently the simple model leading to Equation 13 is not valid.

Measurement of Complex Stability

If a property of the substrate is altered upon its complexation with a ligand, measurement of the property as a function of ligand concentration provides a means for estimating the binding constant. Many properties are suitable for this purpose. To demonstrate the method, a 1:1 complex formation will be used as a model, for just a few of these.

SPECTROMETRY—Suppose the absorption spectrum of the substrate is changed significantly upon binding. Figure 14-10 shows a typical example in which the ultraviolet spectrum of *p*-nitrophenol changes upon complexation with α- cyclodextrin. The presence of well-defined isosbestic points is consistent with the assumption of 1:1 stoichiometry. Selecting a wavelength at which a substantial change in absorption occurs and assuming that Beer's law is obeyed by all species, then, at total substrate concentration S_t in the absence of a ligand, the solution

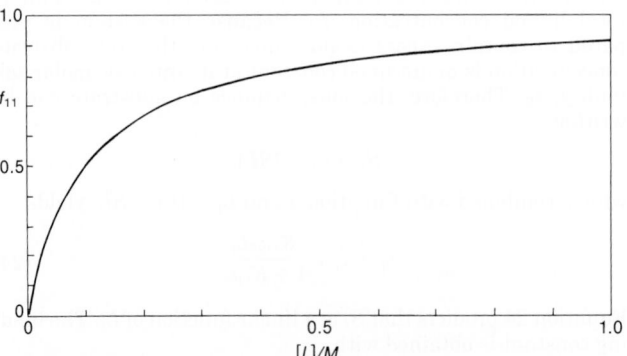

Figure 14-9. Plot of the 1:1 binding isotherm, Equation 11, with $K_{11} = 10 \, M^{-1}$.

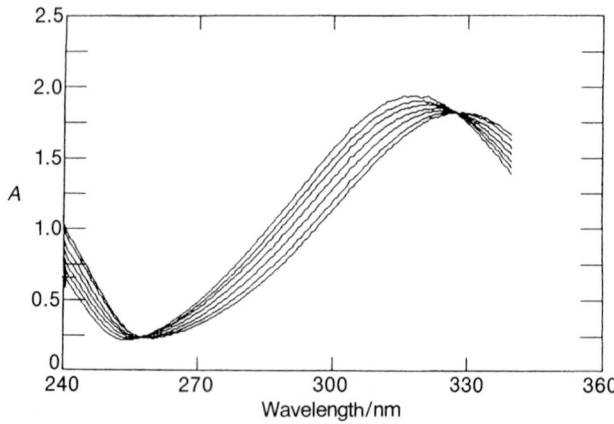

Figure 14-10. Ultraviolet absorption spectrum of *p*-nitrophenol in the presence of varying concentrations of α-cyclodextrin. The *p*-nitrophenol concentration is 1.99×10^{-4} M, and the cyclodextrin concentration ranges from zero (topmost spectrum) to 0.01 M.

absorbance is

$$A_0 = \varepsilon_S b S_t \qquad (16)$$

where b is the path length and ε_S is the molar absorptivity. In the presence of a ligand the absorbance is

$$A_L = \varepsilon_s b[S] + \varepsilon_L b[L] + \varepsilon_{11} b[SL] \qquad (17)$$

where ε_{11} is the absorptivity of the complex. Combining Equation 17 with the mass balances $S_t = [S] + [SL]$ and $L_t = [L] + [SL]$ gives

$$A_L = \varepsilon_S b S_t + \varepsilon_L b L_t + \Delta\varepsilon_{11} b[SL] \qquad (18)$$

where $\Delta\varepsilon_{11} = \varepsilon_{11} - \varepsilon_S - \varepsilon_L$. If the solution absorbance is measured against a reference solution containing the same total ligand concentration, L_t, the measured absorbance is

$$A = \varepsilon_S b S_t + \Delta\varepsilon_{11} b[SL] \qquad (19)$$

Equation 19 is combined with Equation 4 to give Equation 20, the binding isotherm, where $\Delta A = A - A_0$.

$$\frac{\Delta A}{b} = \frac{S_t K_{11} \Delta\varepsilon_{11}[L]}{1 + K_{11}[L]} \qquad (20)$$

Equation 20 is identical in form with Equation 11, and it can be analyzed in the same way. The two unknown parameters K_{11} and $\Delta\varepsilon_{11}$ are obtained from this analysis. From the data shown in Figure 14-10 the values $K_{11} = 256\,M^{-1}$ and $\Delta\varepsilon_{11} = -1726\,M^{-1}\,cm^{-1}$ (at 317 nm) were obtained.

There is a further matter to consider in this treatment of the data. Equation 20 is expressed in terms of free-ligand concentration $[L]$, but only the total ligand concentration L_t is known. From the relationship $L_t = [L] + [SL]$ is found

$$L_t = [L] + \frac{S_t K_{11}[L]}{1 + K_{11}[L]} \qquad (21)$$

The assumption that $[L] = L_t$, is used widely, but when this approximation is not justified, $[L]$ must be estimated with the aid of Equation 21. Methods have been devised to solve this problem.[25]

This spectrometric method is applicable in the ultraviolet, visible, and infrared regions. Nuclear magnetic resonance (NMR) spectrometry can be applied in a similar manner, but with NMR a change in the *chemical shift* is measured.

CHEMICAL REACTIVITY—If the rate of a chemical reaction (such as hydrolysis) undergone by the substrate is either increased or decreased by binding to the ligand, the stability constant can be measured. Consider this kinetic scheme:

$$S + R \xrightarrow{k_S} P$$

$$SL + R \xrightarrow{k_{11}} P$$

Here, R is a reagent that reacts with S and SL, but does not form complexes, P is the product of the reaction, and k_S, k_{11} are second-order rate constants. The mathematical development is similar to that in the spectrometric treatment, and the result is

$$\frac{k_S - k_S'}{k_S} = \frac{q_{11} K_{11}[L]}{1 + K_{11}[L]} \qquad (22)$$

where q_{11} is given by $q_{11} = 1 - k_{11}/k_S'$ and k_S' is the measured second-order rate constant in a solution having ligand concentration, $[L]$. If the reaction rate is decreased upon binding, then $k_s' < k_S$, and q_{11} will lie between 0 and 1. Equation 22 has the usual hyperbolic form, and is treated as described earlier for similar functions.

POTENTIOMETRY—If the activity of an ion is changed upon complex formation, it may be possible to make use of the measurement of electrical potential, E, according to the *Nernst equation:*

$$E = \text{constant} + \frac{RT}{nF} \ln a$$

where a is the ion activity, n is the number of electrons in the redox process, and F is the Faraday. Potentiometry is the most widely used method for the study of metal-ion coordination complexes, for which the activity of the metal ion, the ligand, or the hydrogen ion may be measured.[26]

Potentiometry also is applicable to structures that are weak acid–bases. If HA and A^- are the conjugate acid and base of such a substrate, with L being the ligand, two possible complexes can form:

$$HA + L \overset{K_{11a}}{\rightleftharpoons} HAL$$

$$A^- + L \overset{K_{11b}}{\rightleftharpoons} AL^-$$

The experiment consists of measuring the apparent acid dissociation constant K_a' of HA in the presence of the ligand. Mathematical treatment gives Equation 23 as the binding isotherm, where $'pK_a' = pK_a' - pK_a$, and pK_a is the value when $L_t = 0$.

$$\Delta pK_a' = \log\frac{(1 + K_{11a}[L])}{(1 + K_{11b}[L])} \qquad (23)$$

Thus, if $\Delta pK_a' \neq 0$, $K_{11a} \neq K_{11b}$; that is, the conjugate acid and base forms of the substrate have different affinities for the ligand. The sign of $\Delta pK_a'$ indicates which form of the substrate forms the stronger complex, and K_{11a} and K_{11b} can be evaluated from the dependence of $\Delta pK_a'$ on $[L]$.

SOLUBILITY—In this technique the total apparent solubility, S_t, of the substrate is measured as a function of total ligand concentration, L_t. Because the system is prepared to contain excess (solid) substrate, the free-substrate concentration is maintained constant at its intrinsic molar solubility, s_0. Therefore, the mass balance on substrate can be written

$$S_t = s_0 + [SL]$$

which, combined with Equation 4 and $L_t = [L] + SL$, yields

$$S_t = s_0 + \frac{K_{11} s_0 L_t}{1 + K_{11} s_0} \qquad (24)$$

Equation 24 predicts that S_t is a linear function of L_t. The binding constant is obtained with

$$K_{11} = \frac{\text{slope}}{s_0(1 - \text{slope})} \qquad (25)$$

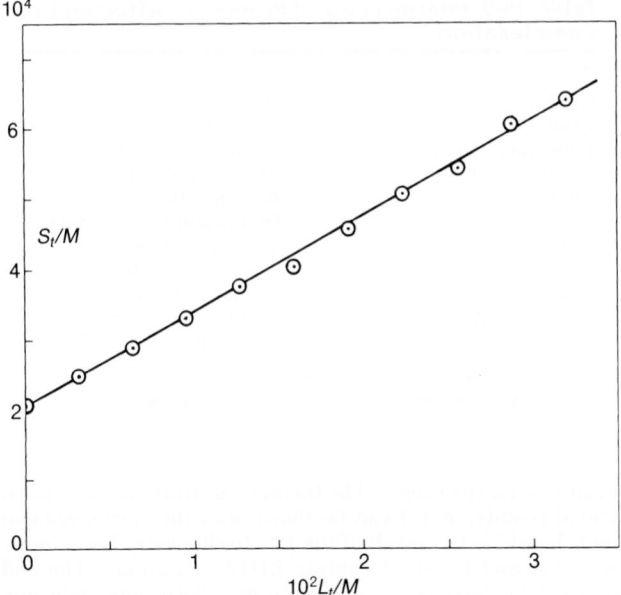

Figure 14-11. Solubility (S_t) of naphthalene as a function of concentration (L_t) of theophylline, in water at 25°.

Figure 14-11 is a plot according to Equation 24 for the system naphthalene (substrate)–theophylline (ligand). The equilibrium constant evaluated with Equation 25 is $K_{11} = 64\ M^{-1}$.

It will be noted that in the solubility method, the isotherm is linear, rather than hyperbolic. This is because [S] is held constant in this method, whereas in the methods discussed earlier, S_t is constant and [S] varies.

There are other methods that, like the solubility method, involve a distribution between two phases. The apparent partition coefficient of a solute between two immiscible solvents can be a measure of complex formation. Several chromatographic methods are based on a similar principle, the retention volume, or time, of a substrate being measured as a function of ligand concentration.

DIALYSIS—This is a technique applicable when one interactant, such as the substrate, is a very large molecule, and the other, the ligand, is a small molecule. Therefore, it is used widely to study the binding of drugs to proteins.

In dialysis, two compartments containing solvent are separated by a semipermeable membrane, ie, a membrane whose pores permit the free transport of the small ligand molecules but do not permit the passage of the large substrate molecule. In one compartment (No 1) this nondiffusible substrate is placed, and in the other (No 2) the diffusible ligand is placed. The system then is allowed to come to equilibrium.

At equilibrium the free-ligand concentration [L] is equal in the two compartments. The solutions in the two compartments are analyzed for their total ligand concentrations.

With the above designations of compartment numbers, we can write

$$(L_t)_1 = [L]_1 + [\text{bound } L]_1$$

$$(L_t)_2 = [L]_2$$

and the equilibrium condition is $[L]_1 = [L]_2$. Therefore, $\bar{\iota}$ can be calculated for compartment No 1 using Equation 14, because S_t, the total protein or macromolecule concentration, is known. The experiment is repeated at different ligand concentrations to obtain $\bar{\iota}$ as a function of [L]. The data then are analyzed in terms of the model equation.[25]

Factors Affecting Complex Stability

This is a large and poorly understood subject so any treatment must be cursory. Much of the earlier discussion on bonding and intermolecular forces is pertinent here.

Consider a general effect that operates in all systems having multiple equilibria. In the simplest example there exists a substrate, S, with n identical independent binding sites, so that complexes $SL, SL_2, SL_3, \ldots, SL_n$ may form, with corresponding binding constants $K_{11}, K_{12}, K_{13}, \ldots, K_{1n}$. Even though the binding sites are identical, it will be found that $K_{11} > K_{12} > K_{13}, \ldots, > K_{1n}$. This is a result of a *statistical effect*. The origin of the statistical effect can be demonstrated readily for the case $n = 2$. The formation of the 1:1 complex is favored over the formation of the 1:2 complex by a factor of 2, because there are two available sites for binding in reactant S, whereas there is only one available site in reactant SL. Moreover, dissociation of SL_2 is favored over dissociation of SL by a factor of 2 because SL_2 has twice as many ligands to surrender. The combination of these statistical factors leads to the result $K_{11} = 4K_{12}$, solely as a consequence of the statistical effect. This argument was generalized by Jones.[27]

Considering the stability of metal-ion coordination complexes, when successive complexes form, two additional factors may operate in addition to the statistical effect.

One of these is the *steric effect*, which is a result of the bulky nature of the ligand (relative to the H_2O that it replaces). As successive ligands are added to the metal ion, crowding inhibits the addition of the next ligand, resulting in a decrease in the value of the binding constants.

A second factor is the *electrostatic effect*, which plays a role when the central cation complexes with an anionic ligand. Then, as successive ligands approach the central ion they experience different fields, because the net charge on the central ion changes with the addition of each ligand.[26]

The *chelate effect* was mentioned earlier in this chapter. The formation of a cyclic complex upon binding of a metal ion to a multidentate ligand leads to greater complex stability than when the same metal ion complexes with an analogous unidentate ligand. Complex stability is favored especially by the formation of 5- and 6-membered rings. A multidentate ligand that is also a macrocycle (such as a crown ether) can form particularly strong complexes; this is called the *macrocyclic effect*.[28]

A useful approach in understanding complex stability is to seek correlations of stability with other properties of the interactants. For example, the *Irving-Williams order* of stability of complexes of divalent cations with a common ligand,

$$Mn^{2+} < Fe^{2+} < Co^{2+} < Ni^{2+} < Cu^{2+} < Zn^{2+}$$

can be correlated with the ionization potentials (corresponding to the last electron lost) of the ions. Similarly, for complexes of a common metal ion, with a series of structurally related ligands of measurable Brønsted basicity, the complex stabilities (expressed as the logarithms of the binding constants) often are correlated linearly with the pK_a values of the bases.[29] Bases of different structural classes (eg, aliphatic primary amines or substituted pyridines) usually give rise to different lines, showing that basicity is not the only controlling feature. The hard–soft acid–base concept described earlier provides additional insight into the effects that properties such as polarizability, electronegativity, ionization potential, electron affinity, and basicity can have in affecting complex stability.

In molecular complexes, it is useful to start with Equation 2, in which ΔG_{net} corresponds to ΔG_{11}^0 in Equation 6. The value of ΔG_{net} is determined by the three terms ΔG_{MM}, ΔG_{MS}, and ΔG_{SS}. If one of these terms greatly predominates over the others, then fairly simple correlations between ΔG_{11}^0 and a molecular property related to the dominant term might be expected. If, however, two or three terms contribute significantly to ΔG_{net}, they may combine in complicated ways, perhaps even opposing each other, so clear relationships may not be observed. Often the most fruitful experiments are those in which one interactant is held as a constant feature, and changes in the structure of the other interactant are made.

Table 14-5 provides some theoretical guidance. If solute–solute interactions of the dipole or induced-dipole type are important, one might anticipate correlations with interactant dipole moment or polarizability. In charge-transfer complexing, substituent effects that increase electron density in the donor or decrease it in the acceptor (Structures **5**, **6**, and **7** are examples of the latter type) may be expected to increase complex stability. Such effects have been observed.[30,31]

If the hydrophobic interaction makes an important contribution to complex stability, the incorporation of organic solvents will reduce the stability. According to the cavity theory of the hydrophobic effect, complex stability is related to the change in surface area upon complex formation, so it may be anticipated that, for such systems, complex stability is related to the size of the interactants. Such a dependence has been seen, but it is complicated by the presence of additional effects.[32] Another prediction of the cavity model is that, for a given complex, stability should be determined primarily by the solvent surface tension, and there is some experimental support for this prediction.[17,21,33]

COMPLEXES IN PHARMACY

APPLICATION TO DRUG DELIVERY—Some of the properties of a drug are so pertinent to dosage forms and drug delivery that it is reasonable to identify them as pharmaceutical or biopharmaceutical properties. Complex formation may affect these properties, sometimes to advantage and sometimes adversely. Many of these properties, with corresponding examples of drug complexes, are given in Table 14-9.[34]

A dosage form might be prepared either with the separate components S (the substrate or drug) and L (the ligand or complexing agent), or with the preformed solid complex.

In a solution dosage form the method of preparation makes no difference, because the complexation equilibrium immediately establishes the equilibrium composition. It must be remembered that the fraction of drug in the complexed form is given by Equation 11, so that the free-ligand concentration is a critical variable, and excess ligand may have to be added in order to "drive the equilibrium" in favor of the bound (complexed) form.

In a solid dosage form it may be preferable to incorporate the solid complex rather than a physical mixture of the drug and complexing agent. For many systems it has been shown that the complex provides faster dissolution and greater bioavailability than does the physical mixture. The processing characteristics (physical state, stability, flowability, etc) of the complex also may be better than those of the free drug.

Not all complexation is intentional or desirable, and some dosage-form *incompatibilities* may be the result of unwanted complexation reactions. For example, some widely used polyethers (Tweens, Carbowaxes, or PEGs) can form precipitates with H-bond donors such as phenols and carboxylic acids.

A substance used widely in liquid dosage forms as a complexer of metal ions is EDTA (ethylenediaminetetraacetic acid). The purpose of this application of complexation is to improve drug stability by inhibiting reactions (usually oxidations) that are catalyzed by metal ions, the complexed form of the metal ion being catalytically inactive. Citric acid (in the form of the citrate anion) also is used for this purpose.[35]

The cyclodextrins have been shown to have effects on all of the properties listed in Table 14-9, and many pharmaceutical applications have been proposed.[19,20,36,37]

COMPLEXES IN PHARMACEUTICAL ANALYSIS—The formation of metal-ion coordination complexes provides the basis of many analytical methods for the determination of metals. Titration of divalent and trivalent metal ions with a solution of EDTA is a standard procedure called complexometric or

Table 14-9. Pharmaceutical Properties Affected by Complexation

PROPERTY	EXAMPLE[a,b]
Physical state	Nitroglycerin-cyclodextrin
Volatility	Iodine-PVP
Solid-state stability	Vitamin A-cyclodextrin
Chemical stability	Benzocaine-caffeine
Solubility	Aspirin-caffeine
Dissolution rate	Phenobarbital-cyclodextrin
Partition coefficient	Benzoic acid-caffeine
Permeability	Prednisone-dialkylamides
Absorption rate	Salicylamide-caffeine
Bioavailability	Digoxin-cyclodextrin
Biological activity	Indomethacin-cyclodextrin

[a] Listed in order of drug-complexing agent.
[b] Citations of the original literature will be found in Ref 34.

chelatometric titration.[38] The theoretical titration curve is calculated readily, and it can be shown that the very large endpoint "break" is the result of the 1:1 stoichiometry between the metal ion and the multidentate EDTA tetraanion. The endpoint can be detected visually with metallochromic indicators or, potentiometrically, with ion-selective membrane electrodes.

Very low concentrations of metal ions can be determined spectrometrically by complexation with a ligand that produces a spectral change. If the complex absorbs in the visible region of the spectrum, this is called colorimetric analysis. Thousands of such methods have been developed.[39] Two examples are the determination of Fe(III) by complexation with 1,10-phenanthroline (see Table 14-1), and of Hg(II) by complexation with dithizone (diphenylthiocarbazone), $S=C(NHNHC_6H_5)_2$. Gravimetric analysis of metal ions can be accomplished via their precipitation as insoluble coordination complexes. For example, Ni(II) forms an insoluble square planar bis(dimethylglyoxime) complex, and many metal ions yield insoluble complexes with 8-hydroxyquinoline (see Table 14-1 for the structures of these ligands).

In some instances the analytical situation can be reversed to make the metal ion serve as the analytical reagent and the organic ligand as the sample. The *ferric hydroxamate* method for the detection and determination of carboxylic acid derivatives is a good example, in which a carboxylic acid derivative such as an ester, amide, or anhydride is reacted with hydroxylamine to form the corresponding hydroxamic acid.

$$R\overset{\overset{\textstyle O}{\|}}{-C}-X \ + \ NH_2OH \ \longrightarrow \ R\overset{\overset{\textstyle O}{\|}}{-C}-NHOH \ + \ HX$$

An excess of Fe(III) is added, and this forms a red-violet coordination complex with the hydroxamic acid; the concentration of the complex is determined spectrometrically.

Colorimetric analyses also can be based on molecular complex formation. Recall that charge-transfer complexation often is accompanied by the development of an intense charge-transfer absorption band, and this can be put to analytical use. For example, tertiary amines can be determined spectrometrically by complexation with tetracyanoethylene (Structure **5**).

Many complex formation reactions are used in conjunction with, or as the basis for, a separation, either by liquid–liquid extraction or chromatography. A classical method for amines, the *acid-dye method*, is based upon complex formation between an amine and a dye molecule. The complex is extracted from the aqueous phase in which it is formed into an organic solvent, where the dye concentration is measured spectrometrically.

The success of the method is based on the condition that only the complexed form of the dye is extractable, so each molecule of amine results in the complexation of one molecule of dye, and this is extracted into the organic phase, where its concentration is an indirect measure of the amount of amine. In order to ensure the nonextractability of the excess (uncomplexed) dye, a dye is used that is a neutral weak acid, and the aqueous pH is controlled at a level above the pK_a of the dye, thus converting it to its anionic form.[40] The principle can be reversed to determine acidic compounds with basic dyes.[41] In a similar way metal ions may be extracted into organic solvents upon complexation with hydrophobic ligands.

Chromatographic separations can make use of the same principle, most notably in a technique called *ion-pair chromatography*. In an application of great pharmaceutical importance, an amine sample in its cation form is complexed with a hydrophobic anion (eg, an alkyl sulfonate, RSO_3^-), and reverse-phase liquid chromatography is performed. The mobile phase is polar (often aqueous), and the stationary phase is nonpolar (eg, a C-18-bonded packing). Although the protonated amine has little affinity for the nonpolar stationary phase, its complex (called an *ion-pair*) with the hydrophobic counterion masks its polar nature, and the ion-pair can partition between the two chromatographic phases.

Several other forms of chromatography take advantage of complex formation between a sample solute and a molecular entity in the stationary phase to generate selective chromatographic retention behavior.

In *hydrophobic chromatography* the hydrophobic interaction provides the driving force for association.

Affinity chromatography is based on fairly specific interactions between the migrating solute and a ligand that is chemically bonded to the stationary phase. For example, an enzyme can be isolated by affinity chromatography on a column prepared with an inhibitor of the enzyme; formation of the enzyme-inhibitor complex on the column removes the enzyme from the sample mixture. In a similar way the very specific antigen–antibody interaction can be applied to isolate antibodies.

Another type of chromatography based on complex formation is *chiral chromatography,* used to separate optical isomers based on interactions between the isomers and a stationary phase that possesses chiral binding sites. For example, stationary phases have been prepared with covalently bound cyclodextrins, which are capable of effecting chiral separations.

PROTEIN-BINDING OF DRUGS—Systemically delivered drugs are made available to the tissues and organs of the body by means of the blood, which is a complicated mixture of substances, some of which are capable of forming complexes with drugs. Because it is widely accepted that the pharmacological response to a drug is determined by the concentration of the "free" (ie, unbound, uncomplexed) drug rather than the total drug concentration, drug-binding by constituents of the blood has important practical implications.

Of all the constituents of blood that might take part in complex formation, the most important and most studied is the protein serum albumin (HSA for human serum albumin, BSA for the closely related bovine serum albumin). The normal HSA concentration in the blood is remarkably high, being 3.5 to 4.5 g/100 mL, and the concentration can vary with age, exercise, stress, and disease.[42] It is a very soluble, very stable protein and consists of 585 amino acid residues, having a calculated molecular weight of 66,439 and a net charge of–15 units at pH 7. The amino acid sequence is known.[43]

Serum albumin is a strikingly indiscriminate complexing agent, having a significant affinity for very many compounds, including drugs. The molecule appears to be appreciably flexible and able to adapt its shape to fit the molecular shape of the ligand binding to it. There are multiple binding sites, but the number that are accessible appears to depend upon the particular ligand; moreover, not all the sites are equivalent.[42] The principal driving force for complexing is the hydrophobic interaction, and hydrophobic compounds, such as long-chain fatty acids (actually as their anions at physiological pH) are bound avidly to HSA. Typical site-binding constants are 10^4 to 10^8 M^{-1}. Certain metal ions also can bind to HSA, and the complex with Cu(II) is particularly stable.

Since the binding sites of HSA are evidently not all identical, the simple binding model exemplified by Equation 13 is not

applicable precisely, but this equation often forms the basis for discussions of the binding equilibria. Provided that this oversimplification is recognized, some useful insights can be gained. The symbolism is recast as follows: let P = protein, P_t = total protein concentration, D = drug (ligand), D_t = total drug concentration, and $[D]$ = free (unbound) drug concentration. Then $\bar{i} = (D_t - [D])/P_t$, is the average number of drug molecules bound per molecule of protein at free-drug concentration $[D]$. Equation 13 now is written

$$\bar{i} = \frac{nk[D]}{1 + k[D]} \tag{26}$$

In the context of drug-protein binding, workers often make use of the concepts *fraction of drug bound* (f_b) and *fraction of drug unbound* (f_u). Obviously, $f_b + f_u = 1$. One can write the definitions $f_u = [D]/D_t$ and $f_u = (D_t - [D])/D_t$. Algebraic combination of these expressions leads to

$$f_b = \frac{nkP_t}{1 + k[D] + nkP_t} \tag{27}$$

and

$$f_u = \frac{1 + k[D]}{1 + k[D] + nkP_t} \tag{28}$$

Equations 27 and 28 show that f_b and f_u depend upon the concentrations of both the protein and the drug. Clearly, however, when $k[D] << 1$ (ie, at very low free-drug concentrations), f_b and f_u essentially become independent of drug concentration, but this condition may not always hold in a therapeutic situation. Moreover, because f_b increases as P_t increases, changes in serum protein concentration as a result of physiological or pathological states may result in significant alterations in free-drug levels. Another implication is that for a strongly bound drug (high k) the protein-binding sites may become saturated with drug, so at higher doses a larger fraction of drug is in the free form.

There are several pharmacological or pharmacokinetic consequences of drug-protein binding.[44] Besides binding to proteins in the blood, drugs also may bind to constituents of the tissues in the organs perfused by the blood supply. If the binding ability of the blood (which may be roughly measured by the product nk) is greater than that of the tissues, the drug will tend to be retained in the blood, whereas tissue retention can occur for the opposite situation. Thus, the distribution of the drug can be affected by its binding characteristics.

The drug clearance also can be affected. If the extraction ratio for a tissue is high, the clearance is determined primarily by blood flow, and drug-protein binding has little effect on the clearance; if the extraction ratio is small, the clearance depends upon binding, and only the free drug is cleared.[44]

The pharmacokinetic parameters, volume of distribution, and elimination-rate constant may be dose-dependent if the protein can be saturated by the drug. A high loading dose may be appropriate in such a case to saturate the protein, followed by lower maintenance doses. It generally is advisable to perform experimental studies (eg, by dialysis) that allow free-drug concentration, as well as total-drug concentration, to be determined. Such studies can detect nonlinear dependencies of $[D]$ on D_t (ie, nonconstancy of f_b and f_u) and, therefore, can be helpful in developing dosage regimens to optimize therapeutic response and minimize undesirable side effects.

COMPLEXES IN THERAPEUTICS—Complexes occur widely in biological systems, so the application of complex formation processes in therapy is a reasonable approach to drug design. Among the most obvious and important biological manifestations of complexation are many metal-ion coordination complexes, whose study in this context constitutes a large part of bioinorganic chemistry. Examples of these complexes, with the metals involved, are hemoglobin (iron), cytochrome (iron), carboxypeptidase A (zinc), carbonic anhydrase (zinc), superoxide dismutase (zinc and copper), vitamin B_{12} (cobalt), chlorophyll (magnesium), and urease (nickel). Molecular complexation in biological systems also occurs, as noted earlier for DNA base-pairing and stacking interactions. The folding of proteins is a consequence of intramolecular noncovalent interactions. Charge-transfer interactions may play a role in physiological processes, and some membrane-transport processes may involve inclusion phenomena.

Numerous antimicrobial and antineoplastic agents are believed to exert their action by means of complex formation with DNA base-pairs. These drug molecules are large planar aromatic compounds, and they can be inserted between the planar base-pair assemblies in the DNA double helix; this type of inserted molecular interaction is called *intercalation*. Intercalating drugs include ethidium, quinacrine, proflavine, daunorubicin, adriamycin, and actinomycin D.[45]

The structure of *cis*-dichlorodiammineplatinum(II) (cisplatin, Structure **9**) is unusual for a drug.

9

This antineoplastic drug is a square planar complex of Pt(II). Its biological activity probably arises from the *cis* geometry.

Many toxic effects of excessive metal-ion concentrations can be treated by agents that form strong coordination complexes, via chelation, thus aiding the excretion of the metal. Among the metals whose toxicity can be treated by *chelation therapy* are iron, lead, copper, cobalt, nickel, mercury, and zinc. The standard chelating agents for this purpose are the monocalcium disodium salt of EDTA, dimercaprol (BAL, Structure **10**), and D-penicillamine (Structure **11**).

Iron poisoning is treated with the chelator, deferoxamine, Structure **12**.

12

REFERENCES

1. Basolo F, Pearson RG. *Mechanisms of Inorganic Reactions*, 2nd ed. New York: Wiley, 1967, Chap 1.
2. Basolo F, Pearson RG. *Mechanisms of Inorganic Reactions*, 2nd ed. New York: Wiley, 1967, p 141.
3. Basolo F, Pearson RG. *Mechanisms of Inorganic Reactions*, 2nd ed. New York: Wiley, 1967, p 375.
4. Cotton FA, Wilkinson G. *Advanced Inorganic Chemistry*, 4th ed. New York: Wiley-Interscience, 1980, p 619.
5. Basolo F, Pearson RG. *Mechanisms of Inorganic Reactions*, 2nd ed. New York: Wiley, 1967, p 60.
6. Pauling L. *The Nature of the Chemical Bond*, 3rd ed. Ithaca, NY: Cornell University Press, 1960, Chap 5.
7. Jones MM. *Elementary Coordination Chemistry*. Englewood Cliffs, NJ: Prentice-Hall, 1964, p 133.
8. Jones MM. *Elementary Coordination Chemistry*. Englewood Cliffs, NJ: Prentice-Hall, 1964, p 144.
9. Hanzlik RP. *Inorganic Aspects of Biological and Organic Chemistry*. New York: Academic Press, 1976, p 97.
10. Basolo, Pearson, *Mechanisms of Inorganic Reactions*, p 104.
11. Pearson RG. *J Chem Educ* 1987; 64: 561.
12. Israelachvili JN. *Intermolecular and Surface Forces*. New York: Academic Press, 1985, Chap 2.
13. Israelachvili JN. *Intermolecular and Surface Forces*. New York: Academic Press, 1985, p 98.
14. Mulliken RS, Person WB. *Molecular Complexes*. New York: Wiley-Interscience, 1969, Chap 1.
15. Tanford C. *The Hydrophobic Effect*, 2nd ed. New York: Wiley-Interscience, 1980.
16. Jencks WP. *Catalysis in Chemistry and Enzymology*. New York: McGraw-Hill, 1969, p 417.
17. Connors KA, Mulski MJ, Paulson A. *J Org Chem* 1992; 57: 1794.
18. Watson JD. *Molecular Biology of the Gene*, 2nd ed. New York: WA Benjamin, 1970, p 132.
19. Szejtli J. *Cyclodextrins and Their Inclusion Complexes*. Budapest: Akademiai Kiado, 1982.
20. Duchene D, ed. *Cyclodextrins and Their Industrial Uses*. Paris: Editions de Santé, 1987.
21. Connors KA. *Chem Rev* 1997; 97: 1325.
22. Hagan M. *Clathrate Inclusion Compounds*. New York: Reinhold, 1962.
23. Tsoucaris G. In: Duchene D, ed. *Cyclodextrins and Their Industrial Uses*. Paris: Editions de Santé, 1981, Chap 1.
24. Connors KA. *Binding Constants: The Measurement of Molecular Complex Stability*. New York: Wiley-Interscience, 1987.
25. Connors KA. *Binding Constants: The Measurement of Molecular Complex Stability*. New York: Wiley-Interscience, Chap 2.
26. Hartley FR, Burgess C, Alcock RM. *Solution Equilibria*. Chichester: Ellis Horwood/Halsted Press, 1980.
27. Jones MM. *Elementary Coordination Chemistry*. Englewood Cliffs, NJ: Prentice-Hall, 1964, p 333.
28. Cotton FA, Wilkinson G. *Advanced Inorganic Chemistry*, 4th ed. New York: Wiley-Interscience, 1980, p 73.
29. Hanzlik RP. *Inorganic Aspects of Biological and Organic Chemistry*. New York: Academic Press, 1976, p 118.
30. Andrews LJ, Keefer RM. *Molecular Complexes in Organic Chemistry*. San Francisco: Holden-Day, 1964, Chap 4.
31. Gur'yanova EN, Gol'dshtein IP, Romm IP. *Donor-Acceptor Bond*. New York: Wiley, 1975, Chap 5.
32. Cohen JL, Connors KA. *J Pharm Sci* 1970; 59:1271.
33. Connors KA, Sun S. *J Am Chem Soc* 1971; 93:7239.
34. Connors KA. *Pharm Mfg* 1985; 2(9):23.
35. Connors KA, Amidon GL, Stella VJ. *Chemical Stability of Pharmaceuticals*, 2nd ed. New York: Wiley-Interscience, 1987, p 100.
36. Pitha J, Szente L, Szejtli J. In: Bruck SD, ed. *Controlled Drug Delivery*, Vol I. Boca Raton, FL: CRC Press, 1983, Chap 5.
37. Duchene D, Vaution C, Glomot F. *Drug Develop Ind Pharm* 1986; 12:2193.
38. Connors KA. *A Textbook of Pharmaceutical Analysis*, 3rd ed. New York: Wiley-Interscience, 1982, Chap 4.
39. Sandell EB. *Colorimetric Determination of Traces of Metals*, 3rd ed. New York: Interscience, 1959.
40. Higuchi T, Bodin JI. In: Higuchi T, Brochmann-Hansen E, eds. *Pharmaceutical Analysis*. New York: Interscience, 1961.
41. Pesez M, Bartos J. *Colorimetric and Fluorometric Analysis of Organic Compounds and Drugs*. New York: Dekker, 1974, p 139.
42. Bridges JW, Wilson AGE. *Prog Drug Metab* 1978; 1:193.
43. Peters T Jr. *Adv Protein Chem* 1985; 37:161.
44. Tillement J-P, et al. *Adv Drug Res* 1984; 13:59.
45. Wilson WD, Jones RL. *Adv Pharmacol Chemother* 1981; 18:177.

ACKNOWLEDGMENTS—Kenneth A. Connors, PhD is acknowledged for his efforts in previous editions of this work.

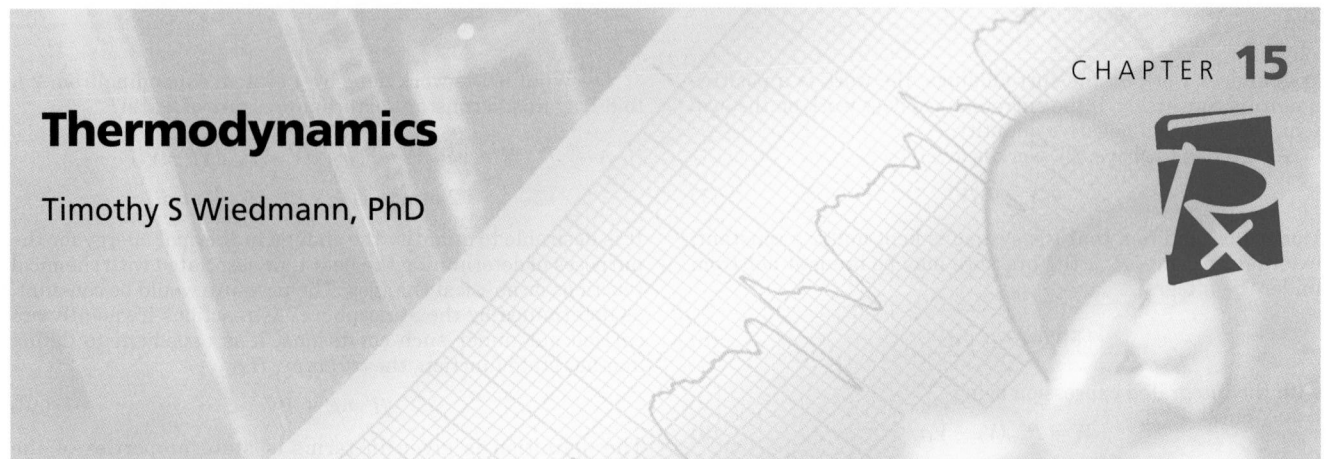

Thermodynamics

Timothy S Wiedmann, PhD

Thermodynamics rests upon three basic laws that took over 500 years to establish. Although quantum mechanics has defined the limits of its scope, the concepts laid out in this chapter have remained unchanged for over a century. The reader is therefore encouraged to appreciate not only the many years of effort spent in defining the laws of thermodynamics but also the likely fact that the contents will be relevant for a lifetime of applications.

The approach will involve the development of concepts within the framework of very specific examples, as the great value of thermodynamics lies in its general applicability. Simple examples will be used to introduce the concepts that form the basis of a thermodynamic description.

A *system* is that part of the universe under consideration and, as such, is separated from the *surroundings* or, equivalently, the rest of the universe. The focus of the analysis will center on how the properties of a system are altered through an interaction with the surroundings. The interaction occurs at the boundary that separates the system from the surroundings.

When a sufficient number of properties of the system have been specified as fixed values, then the system is at equilibrium. Certain systems at equilibrium have a simple equation that provides a relationship among the values of the properties. For example, a system containing an ideal gas has the properties of pressure, P, volume, V, number of mols, n and temperature (K), T related by

$$PV = nRT \tag{1}$$

where R is the gas law constant. Such a relationship is referred to as an *equation of state* because it specifies the relationship among the properties of a system in a definite state. Furthermore, if the system is at equilibrium, only three of the above values for the properties need to be specified, as the fourth may be calculated from the equation of state.

THE FIRST LAW

The first law of thermodynamics is a statement of the principle of conservation of energy; energy may neither be created nor be destroyed. It is mathematically written as

$$dE = \delta q - \delta W \tag{2}$$

where dE is the differential change in the internal energy, δq is the differential change in the absorbed heat, and δW is the differential change in the expended work.

The change in internal energy of a system in going from state A to state B is given by

$$\Delta E = \int_A^B dE \tag{3}$$

From this equation, it is observed that the internal energy is a state function since d represents an exact differential.

The implication is that the change in the internal energy depends only on the initial and final state and does not depend on how the change in state was achieved. Because the change in energy does not depend on the path, there is no net change in the energy for any system that undergoes a cyclic change. The expression is

$$\oint dE = 0 \tag{4}$$

This fact will be useful when a system undergoing a cyclic change is considered, as will be encountered with the discussion of a heat engine. And, finally, the equation provides only a relation for the change in the internal energy and does not provide an absolute value of the internal energy of the system in a particular state.

In the first law, the change in internal energy is related to heat flow and work done. The concepts of work and heat now will be defined precisely, thereby providing the framework for the use of the first law, as well as the other laws. In contrast to the internal energy, the differential change in heat and work are inexact differentials. This means that neither the heat nor the work are state functions of the system; thus, the integral of the differential depends on the path taken. To elaborate on this point, consider the change in going from state A to state B. The heat and work are given as

$$q = \int_A^B \delta q \ and \ W = \int_A^B \delta W \tag{5}$$

which will depend on what path was taken in going from state A to state B. The work and heat may be determined only if more information is provided concerning how the change in the state of the system was achieved.

WORK—The concept of *work* in thermodynamics may be expressed as a product of an *intensity factor* and a *capacity factor*; for example, mechanical work is given as

$$\delta W = Fdl \tag{6}$$

where the differential quantity of work done, δW, is the product of the force, F (intensity factor), and a differential distance, dl (capacity factor). Other types of work include *gravitational* (gravitational potential and mass), *electrical* (potential difference and quantity of electricity or charge), *surface increase* (surface tension and area) and, most important for our purposes, *volume expansion* or PV work (pressure and volume).

Some peculiarities of the work are that it appears only at the boundary and thus may be thought of as flowing into or out of the system. Work may be generated only through a change in the state of the system, and it is an algebraic quantity that may be positive or negative. The convention chosen is that if the system does work on the surroundings, the work is a positive quantity; conversely, if the surroundings does work on the system, the work is a negative quantity.

As alluded to above, PV work is given by

$$\delta W = PdV \tag{7}$$

Under the condition that the system is kept under a constant, external pressure, P_{ext}, the pressure may be brought out from under the integral

$$\delta W = P_{ext} \int dV \tag{8}$$

with the integrated expression being

$$W = P_{ext}(V_f - V_i) \tag{9}$$

where V_f and V_i are the final and initial volumes of the system. Therefore, it becomes clear that if the system expands ($V_f > V_i$) against a constant external pressure, the system does work on the surroundings, and $W > 0$. In dealing with PV work, a distinction concerning the nature of the boundary is made. The boundary can be rigid and not allow PV work or it may be movable, thereby permitting changes in the volume of the system. If there is no heat flow into or out of the system, $\delta q = 0$, the change in the internal energy may be calculated from the work,

$$\int dE = -W \tag{10}$$

or

$$\Delta E = -P_{ext}(V_f - V_i) \tag{11}$$

which indicates that, with the expansion of a system against a constant pressure and without heat flow, there is a decrease in the internal energy of the system. This convention agrees with intuition: work is done by the system at the expense of its internal energy.

HEAT—The other quantity appearing in the first law is *heat*. It shares many properties with work. Specifically, it also appears at the boundary and only with a change in the state of the system. By definition, heat flow into the system, which is taken to be a positive quantity, results in an increase in the internal energy of the system. For a system where there is no work done, $\delta W = 0$, the change in internal energy is given by

$$\int dE = \int \delta q \tag{12}$$

$$\Delta E = q \tag{13}$$

Thus, q often is referred to as a transfer of thermal energy.

Boundaries are classified as either *diathermal*, thereby allowing free exchange of heat, or conversely, *adiabatic*, where no heat flow is allowed. As an example, consider the change in internal energy for a system where only PV work is possible. The first law is written

$$\int dE = \int \delta q - \int PdV \tag{14}$$

where $\int PdV$ has been substituted for the work term.

Further, stipulating that the boundary be rigid, or $dV = 0$, the change in the internal energy is equal to the heat flow, or equivalently

$$\Delta E = q_v \tag{15}$$

where the subscript v has been added to the heat term to reflect the constraint of constant volume. Thus, adding a quantity of heat to the system increases the internal energy.

Q—What is the change in the internal energy and heat for a system that does 1.0 kcal of work on the surroundings? Assume a closed system where there is no exchange of matter across the boundary.

A—The adiabatic boundary prevents the transfer of heat, $q = 0$ and $\Delta E = 0 - 1.0$ or $\Delta E = -1.0$ kcal.

Q—What is the work done by a system expanding from 2 L to 8 L against a constant external pressure of 2 atm?

$$A— \qquad W = \int PdV = P_{ext} \int dV = P_{ext}(V_f - V_i)$$
$$= 2 \text{ atm } (8 \text{ L} - 2 \text{ L}) = 12 \text{ L atm.}$$

It is desirable to quantify the change in thermal energy for the purposes of determining the heat flow associated with chemical reactions or physical changes. The pressure would be constant, as determined by the atmosphere. As reactions frequently are carried out under such conditions, it is expedient to define another state function, the *enthalpy, H*.

$$H \equiv E + PV \tag{16}$$

The definition is given in terms of state properties of the system; however, to determine the change in the system, the differential is taken, resulting in

$$dH = dE + d(PV) \tag{17}$$

Expansion of the latter term yields

$$dH = dE + PdV + VdP \tag{18}$$

but because the pressure is constant, $VdP = 0$, the change in enthalpy becomes

$$dH = dE + PdV \tag{19}$$

However, from the first law the change in energy of systems restricted to PV work is

$$dE = \delta q_p - PdV \tag{20}$$

where δq_p is the heat absorbed under constant pressure. Combining the latter two equations reveals

$$dH = \delta q_p \tag{21}$$

or with integration

$$\Delta H = q_p \tag{22}$$

which implies that the enthalpy is no more than the heat absorbed by the system under the condition of constant pressure.

The heat capacity at constant pressure may be defined as

$$C_p \equiv (dq_p/dT) \tag{23}$$

or assuming the heat capacity is constant over the range of ΔT, given as

$$\int dq_p = \int C_p dT \tag{24}$$

and the integrated form

$$q_p = C_p \Delta T = \Delta H \tag{25}$$

Thus, knowing the heat capacity, the change in enthalpy of the system with a change in temperature may be determined.

In an analogous fashion, the heat capacity at constant volume may be defined as

$$C_v \equiv dq_v/dT \tag{26}$$

with the integrated form being

$$q_v = C_v \Delta T \tag{27}$$

assuming the heat capacity is constant over the range of ΔT.

Before proceeding to the application of these concepts to specific problems, the two types of processes involved with a change in the state of the system require elaboration. A process is *reversible* if, and only if, the difference between the driving and opposing force is infinitesimal; a process is *irreversible* if the forces are not infinitesimally different. The important point is that if a system is displaced from equilibrium by some vanishing small force, equilibrium may be restored by application of an equal force in the opposite direction. That is, the restoring force applied is equal in magnitude but is in the reverse direction of the force originally applied. The process then is said to be reversible. Any process that occurs in a different manner is irreversible, and the original state of the system may not be restored without some change in the surroundings. Because vanishing small forces cannot be achieved experimentally, all real processes are irreversible, although a reversible process can be approximated closely. Nevertheless, reversibility is an important concept to establish the maximum value of work associated with a process. If a specific transformation occurs that produces work, carrying out the process reversibly yields the maximum work that can be obtained. The actual process is carried out irreversibly and thereby must yield less work.

Q—Suppose a system containing 1 mole of an ideal gas at 300 K undergoes a reversible, isothermal compression from 4 to 2 liters. What are the values of ΔE, q, W, ΔH and the final pressure if, from the kinetic molecular theory, the internal energy of an ideal gas is known to be a function solely of the temperature?

A—Although $W = \int P dV$ is correct, the expression no longer may be integrated directly, because the pressure is not constant. However, the equation of state for an ideal gas provides the pressure in terms of the volume, that is, $P = nRT/V$; thus, upon substitution

$$\int \delta W = \int nRT dV/V$$

and with integration

$$W = nRT \ln (V_f / V_i)$$

$$= (1 \text{ mol})(0.082 \text{ L atm/mol K})(300 \text{ K}) \ln (2/4) = -17.1 \text{ L atm}$$

For all isothermal processes involving ideal gases, $\Delta E = 0$. Using this fact, the heat flow out of the system is

$$\Delta E = 0 = q - W$$

or

$$q = W = -17.1 \text{ L atm}$$

The change in enthalpy is found from the relationship

$$\Delta H = \Delta E + \Delta(PV)$$

and, noting that $\Delta(PV) = P_f V_f - P_i V_i = nRT - nRT = 0$, and from above, $\Delta E = 0$, thus, $\Delta H = 0$.

For the final part of the problem, calculation of the final pressure may be accomplished, again, by using the equation of state

$$P_f = nRT/V_f = (1 \text{ mol})(0.082 \text{ L atm/mol K})(300 \text{ K})/(2)$$

$$= 12.3 \text{ atm}$$

HEAT OF REACTION—The subject that deals with heat effects, associated with chemical reactions and certain physical processes, is known as *thermochemistry*. The heat of reaction is an important measure in chemical reactions. Consider the following reaction, which represents both a mass and energy balanced equation,

$$H_2(g, 1 \text{ atm}) + 1/2 O_2(g, 1 \text{ atm}) = H_2O(1)$$

$$\Delta H_{298} = -68,300 \text{ cal}$$

where ΔH_{298} is defined as the heat of reaction. This quantity specifies the change in enthalpy of the above reaction as written at the specified temperature of 298 K. The implication is that when a mole of H_2 combines with 1/2 mol of O_2 at 298 K, 68,300 cal of heat are released in this exothermic reaction, and the enthalpy of the system is reduced by the same value. Alternatively, a reaction is endothermic if heat is absorbed by the system from the surroundings, which would result in an increase in enthalpy of the system. Because this is a balanced energy equation, the reverse reaction of the breakdown of liquid

water into the respective components of H_2 and O_2 is an endothermic process requiring 68,300 cal of heat. The choice of the temperature of 298 K is arbitrary, although by convention it is taken as typical room temperature of 25°. It is important to note that, in general, the enthalpy change would be different if the reaction were carried out at another temperature.

The thermodynamic concept of the enthalpy change of the system may be extended to include coupled reactions. Because the enthalpy is a state function, only the difference between the initial and final state is important for determining the change in enthalpy for the entire process. This is simply Hess's law, which states that the enthalpy change of a reaction is the same, whether it occurs in one or several steps. Therefore, energy equations may be manipulated algebraically just like the corresponding mass balanced equations.

Consider the following two equations:

$$C(s) + O_2(g) = CO_2(g) \qquad \Delta H = -94,052 \text{ cal}$$

$$CO(g) + 1/2 O_2(g) = CO_2(g) \qquad \Delta H = -67,636 \text{ cal}$$

From these equations, the enthalpy change associated with the reaction

$$C(s) + O_2(g) = CO(g) + 1/2 O_2$$

may be calculated as

$$\Delta H = (-94,052) - (-67,636 \text{ cal}) = -26,416 \text{ cal}$$

HEAT OF REACTION AS A FUNCTION OF TEMPERATURE—At this point the information presented is useful if every reaction was carried out under standard conditions of 298 K and 1 atm pressure; however, most reactions are not. Nevertheless, the heat of the reaction may be calculated at any other temperature by the temperature dependence of the heat capacity.

Consider the problem of the heat of reaction for the freezing of water at $-10°$ (263 K). One should note that a simple phase change may be treated in a manner analogous to a chemical reaction for the purposes of calculating the enthalpy change.

The approach to the problem is to calculate the enthalpy change associated with the temperature change of the reactant (water) from 0° to $-10°$ and the product (ice) from $-10°$ to 0°, and then use the value for the enthalpy change at the melting point. The following schematic illustrates the approach and also provides insight into the concept of path independence of state functions.

$$H_2O\ (l, -10°)\ -?\ \rightarrow H_2O\ (s, -10°)$$
$$|\qquad\qquad\qquad \uparrow$$
$$\Delta H_I \qquad\qquad \Delta H_{III}$$
$$\downarrow\qquad\qquad\qquad |$$
$$H_2O\ (l, 0°)\ -\Delta H_{II} \rightarrow H_2O\ (s, 0°)$$

Specifically, the molar enthalpy for the reaction at $-10°$ is given by

$$\Delta H(-10°) = \Delta H_I + \Delta H_{II} + \Delta H_{III} \qquad (28)$$

with

$$\Delta H_I = \int c_p(H_2O, 1) dT = c_p(1)\Delta T$$

$$\Delta H_I = (8.7)(263 - 273) = \underline{-87 \text{ cal/mol}}$$

$$\Delta H_{II} = \underline{-1436 \text{ cal/mol}} \text{ (found in tables)}$$

$$\Delta H_{III} = \int c_p(H_2O, s) dT = c_p(s)\Delta T$$

$$\Delta H_{III} = (18)(273 - 263) = \underline{180 \text{ cal/mol}}$$

Thus, the enthalpy for the conversion of water to ice at $-10°$ is given by the sum or

$$\Delta H(-10°) = -87 - 1436 + 180 = \underline{-1343 \text{ cal/mol}}$$

As shown, the direction around the circle dictates the limits of integration (final less initial), thus care must be taken not to confuse them. The heat capacity was assumed to be independent of temperature, which in this case is reasonable for such a small temperature change (10°). However, in general, heat capacity is a function of temperature, which will not present severe difficulties if the functional relationship is known. In this case the temperature dependence may be substituted into the equation and then integrated with the appropriate limits. For example, the molar heat capacity of oxygen over the range of 300 to 1500 K has been determined experimentally and is approximated closely by

$$c_p = 6.0954 + 3.2533 \times 10^{-3}T - 10.171 \times 10^{-7}T^2 \quad (29)$$

The change in the molar heat of formation for oxygen from temperature T_1 to T_2 would then be given by

$$\int dH = \int (6.0954 + 3.2533 \times 10^{-3}T \\ - 10.171 \times 10^{-7}T^2)dT \quad (30)$$

$$\Delta H = [6.0954(T_2 - T_1) + (1/2)(3.2533 \times 10^{-3}) \\ [T_2{}^2 - T_1{}^2] + (1/3)(-10.171 \times 10^{-7})(T_2{}^3 - T_1{}^3) \quad (31)$$

HEAT OF SOLUTION—When a compound is dissolved in a solvent, the resulting enthalpy change of the system is referred to as the *heat of solution*. The heat evolved or absorbed reflects the energy required to disrupt the cohesive forces of the solid and the energy generated from interaction of the solute molecules with solvent molecules. There are two ways of expressing the enthalpy change per mol of material dissolved: the integral and differential heats of solution. The two conventions arise from the dependency of the heat of solution on the amount of solvent used to dissolve the solute. Thus, the *integral heat of solution* describes the enthalpy change when 1 mol of solute is dissolved to yield a specified concentration, perhaps a 1 molar solution, whereas the *differential heat of solution* provides a value of the enthalpy change when the amount of solute dissolved is negligible.

One way of understanding the difference between these representations, and also a way of remembering, is as follows:

- The integral heat of solution gives the enthalpy change for a discrete or integral change in concentration of the solution.
- The differential heat of solution provides the enthalpy change for an infinitesimally or differential (dC) change in concentration.

Q—If the differential heat of solution of two polymorphic forms of a drug were measured in water at standard temperature and pressure (STP) and form A had a larger heat than form B, which is more stable at STP?

A—More energy is required to dissolve form A; therefore, it must be the more stable polymorph at STP.

ENTROPY AND THE SECOND LAW

Although the first law provides the framework for calculating the change in energy associated with chemical reactions or physical changes in state, there is insufficient information to allow prediction of the likelihood of whether the change will occur. Consider a system composed of two parts that are at different temperatures, T_1 and T_2, separated by an impermeable, adiabatic partition. When the partition is removed, heat will flow from the part at a higher temperature to the part at a lower temperature. According to the first law, the energy of the whole system, the sum of parts one and two, has not changed.

Intuitively it is known that the above change will occur regardless of the fact that the first law does not provide a method of predicting the occurrence. Such changes are described as *spontaneous*, for the obvious reason that they occur without additional stimulation. It should be noted that this spontaneous change involved an increase in the disorder or, if

you will, the randomness of the system. Thus, the system initially was separated into two parts at different temperatures, but after thermal contact, a uniform temperature was reached. The *entropy*, *S*, is the function that provides a quantitative description of the randomness or disorder of the system and is fundamental for predicting the spontaneity of chemical reactions and physical changes. The entropy is a state function that depends only on the initial and final state of the system.

The definition of the entropy change is given by the seemingly surprising form

$$dS = \delta q_{rev}/T \quad (32)$$

where the subscript *rev* denotes that the heat flow occurs in a reversible manner. By carrying out the integration, the change in entropy for a reversible, isothermal change from state 1 to state 2 is given by

$$\Delta S = \int \delta q_{rev}/T = q_{rev}/T \quad (33)$$

With the introduction of entropy, the second law may be stated as follows:

For any spontaneous process in an isolated system, there is an increase in the value of entropy. Alternatively, the first and second laws may be combined with the classic thermodynamic statement, "the energy of the universe is constant; the entropy is increasing."

CARNOT CYCLE—Before giving specific examples for the calculation of the entropy, it is instructive to provide the background leading to the above definition. The concepts of heat and work have been developed already and thus can be used to show the origin of the entropy function. By permitting the flow of heat into a system, work may be done by the system. The hypothetical instrument that is capable of converting heat to work is referred to as a *heat engine* (Fig 15-1). The second law dictates that not all of the heat may be converted into work, even if all changes occur in a reversible manner. In fact, the maximum work, W_{max}, that may be obtained is specified by the heat flow into the system and the temperature difference over which the heat engine is operating; that is,

$$W_{max} = q_1(T_1 - T_2)/T_1 \quad (34)$$

where $T_1 > T_2$.

In 1824 Carnot established this equation, which perhaps may be understood best by introducing the *Carnot cycle*. Consider the system, as shown in Fig 15-1, containing an ideal

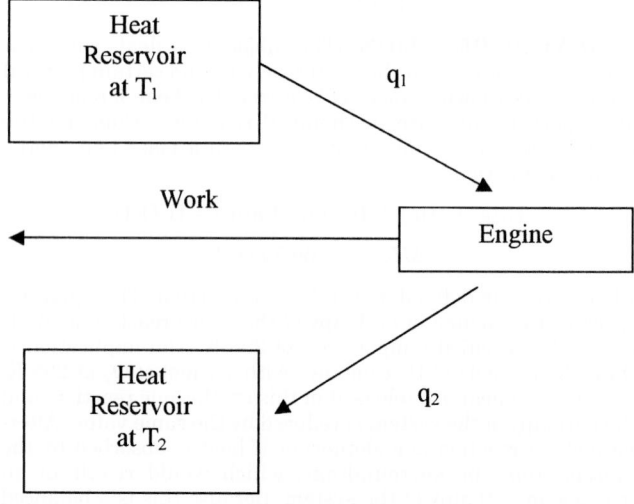

Figure 15-1. A schematic of one possible heat engine.

gas that can perform PV work due to its connections with two heat reservoirs. A *heat reservoir* is a system that has a constant temperature throughout, and the temperature is not affected by the transfer of heat into or out of the reservoir. Take a starting point at some pressure and volume and let the system undergo a cyclic, reversible change involving three other points on a pressure and volume diagram as shown in Figure 15-2. The first step is an isothermal expansion; the second is an adiabatic expansion; the third is an isothermal compression; and finally, the forth is an adiabatic compression. The proof of Equation 32 is provided by calculating the heat and work for each step and noting that not all of the heat energy may be converted into work.

As this is a cyclic change, the total energy change in one complete cycle, ΔE_{tot}, is zero. The change in energy, along with the heat and work with each step, may be determined using the first law. For the first step of the cycle, consisting of an isothermal expansion, the energy is given as

$$\Delta E_1 = q_1 - W_1 \tag{35}$$

Since the energy change for an isothermal process involving an ideal gas is zero, the heat is equal to the work:

$$q_1 = W_1 = \int P dV \tag{36}$$

Substituting for the pressure, to allow integration between the limits of the initial and final volumes, V_1 and V_2:

$$q_1 = \int nRT dV/V \tag{37}$$

$$q_1 = nRT \ln (V_2/V_1) \tag{36}$$

The second step is an adiabatic expansion. The heat flow is zero, and thus,

$$\Delta E_2 = -W_2 \tag{38}$$

The energy change may be obtained from the definition of the heat capacity at constant volume, or mathematically,

$$\int C_v \, dT = -W_2 \tag{39}$$

which is equal to the following, for an ideal gas.

$$C_v(T_2 - T_1) = -W_2 \tag{40}$$

The third step is an isothermal compression, which is essentially the reverse of the first step, with the volume limits altered accordingly:

$$q_3 = nRT \ln (V_4/V_3) \tag{41}$$

The final step is an adiabatic compression, which is dealt with in a manner similar to the second step by noting that $q_4 = 0$, yielding

$$C_v(T_1 - T_2) = -W_4 \tag{42}$$

Summing up the results for each individual step to obtain the total work for the cycle, W_{tot},

$$W_{tot} = nRT \ln (V_2/V_1) - C_v(T_2 - T_1) + nRT \ln (V_4/V_3) - C_v(T_1 - T_2) \tag{43}$$

which may be simplified by canceling terms, yielding

$$W_{tot} = nRT_1 \ln (V_2/V_1) + nRT_2 \ln (V_4/V_3) \tag{44}$$

The heat flow into the system occurs with the first step, thus

$$q_1 = nRT_1 \ln (V_2/V_1) \tag{45}$$

The efficiency of an engine, ε, is given by the amount of work extracted divided by the heat flow into the system,

$$\varepsilon = W_{tot}/q_1 \tag{46}$$

where $W_{tot} = W_{max}$ for reversible changes or, equivalently,

$$\varepsilon = [nRT_1 \ln (V_2/V_1) + nRT_2 \ln (V_4/V_3)]/[nRT_1 \ln (V_2/V_1)] \tag{47}$$

Although it is not obvious, it may be shown that $V_3/V_4 = V_2/V_1$, thus

$$\varepsilon = (T_1 - T_2)/T_1 \tag{48}$$

The efficiency is proportional to the difference in temperature between the heat reservoirs. In addition, there is no work done unless there is a difference in temperature between the heat reservoirs. Finally, 100% efficiency is obtained only when $T_2 \rightarrow 0$, which as will be noted from the third law, is impossible.

The above analysis elucidates the connection between entropy and heat flow. The second law provides the quantitative limit on the amount of work that can be done with a cyclic operation performed in a reversible manner. This result has the powerful implication that it is impossible to construct a perpetual motion machine. The latter is a hypothetical device that once set into motion continues to interconvert work and heat without exhausting its finite source of energy. No machine is 100% efficient; therefore, there can be no perpetual motion machine!

ENTROPY CHANGES FOR REVERSIBLE AND IRREVERSIBLE PROCESSES—Given the above background, the entropy changes associated with several reversible processes may be determined. Consider the melting of ice at the melting point under 1 atm pressure where $\Delta H_{fus} = 1436$ cal/mol (heat of fusion). The entropy of fusion, ΔS_{fus}, is given by

$$\int dS = \int \delta q/T \tag{49}$$

which may be determined from $\int \delta q = q_p = \Delta H$, because the pressure is constant and the temperature is the melting point. Thus,

$$\int dS = \Delta H_{fus}/T_m \tag{50}$$

$$\Delta S = 1436/273 = 5.275 \text{ cal/mol K}$$

The positive change in entropy also confirms intuition concerning such an event; liquids are in a state of more disorder than solids, thus the entropy also is greater in the liquid state.

Q—What is the entropy change for a reversible, adiabatic expansion of an ideal gas?

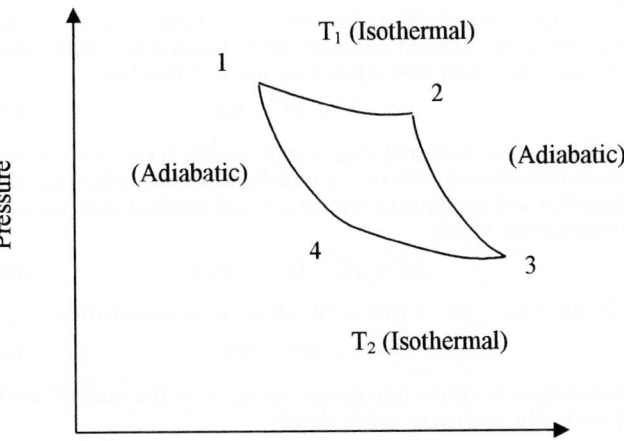

Figure 15-2. The four steps involved in the completion of the Carnot cycle, indicating the relationship among the pressure, volume, and temperature.

A—As $q = 0$ for an adiabatic change, $\Delta S = 0$.

Q—What is the relationship for the entropy change of a reversible expansion of an ideal gas, given that the pressure (isobaric condition) and heat capacity are constant over the range of T_1 to T_2?

A—Although $\Delta S = \int \delta q/T$, T is no longer a constant and, therefore, may not be taken outside the integral. However, note that

$$\Delta S = \int dH/T = \int (C_p/T)dT \tag{51}$$

$$\Delta S = C_p \ln (T_2/T_1) \tag{52}$$

The discussion, thus far, has been limited to reversible processes that are strictly impossible to achieve in the laboratory (even though such a process may be approximated very closely). The question is, what is the entropy change for an irreversible change? Here the entropy change is given by

$$dS > \delta q_{irr}/T \tag{53}$$

Thus, all real processes may be written as

$$dS \geq \delta q/T \tag{54}$$

This concept may be extended to determine the condition of spontaneity. Consider a system that is transformed irreversibly from state 1 to state 2 and then reversibly from state 2 back to state 1. The overall change is given by

$$\int_{State\ 1}^{State\ 2} \delta q_{irr}/T + \int_{State\ 1}^{State\ 2} + \delta q_{rev}/T < 0 \tag{55}$$

$$\int_{State\ 1}^{State\ 2} \delta q_{irr}/T + \int_{State\ 1}^{State\ 2} dS < 0 \tag{56}$$

which may be rearranged, with changing the limits of integration, to yield

$$\int_{State\ 1}^{State\ 2} \delta q_{irr}/T < \int_{State\ 1}^{State\ 2} dS \tag{57}$$

or, equivalently, for infinitesimal changes

$$\delta q_{irr}/T < dS \tag{58}$$

This is known as the *Clausius inequality*. For isolated systems, where boundaries do not permit the passage of energy or matter, $\delta q_{irr} = 0$, the result is given

$$dS > 0 \tag{59}$$

That is, for every spontaneous change in an isolated system there is an increase in the entropy.

The second law may be generalized in another way. The total entropy for any process is given by the sum of the entropy of the system and the surroundings; that is,

$$dS_{tot} = dS_{sys} + dS_{surr} \tag{60}$$

For reversible processes, the entropy change in a system is the negative of the entropy change produced in the surroundings. The total entropy, therefore, is zero. For irreversible processes the total entropy, system plus surroundings, increases. The mathematical statement of this relationship is

$$\sum \Delta S_{tot} = 0 \text{ reversible process} \tag{61}$$

$$\sum \Delta S_{tot} > 0 \text{ irreversible process} \tag{62}$$

THE THIRD LAW

The third law of thermodynamics simply defines the zero point of the entropy scale. The entropy of a pure, perfectly crystalline substance is zero at absolute zero. Intuitively, at the lowest possible temperature a system that has perfect three-dimensional order should have no entropy. The defining of a zero for the entropy is unlike the other state functions introduced previously. Thus, the value of the entropy, S, of a system in any state, in principle, may be calculated.

What would be the entropy of a crystalline solid at 150 K, S_{150}? This may be calculated as

$$\Delta S = S_{150} - S_0 \tag{63}$$

$$\Delta S = \int (c_p/T)dT - 0 \tag{64}$$

or

$$\Delta S = S_{150} \tag{65}$$

If the heat capacity over the range of 0 to 150 K is known, the value of the entropy may be calculated.

Free Energy

The concept of *free energy* is probably the most useful aspect of thermodynamics. The criteria for determining the spontaneity of a chemical reaction or phase change were presented above; however, it involved carrying out the change in an isolated system. One can imagine how inconvenient and often impossible it would be to apply such a constraint to the laboratory setting. For this sake, additional state functions have been defined to allow prediction of the spontaneity of a change in state. The rationale for the development of other functions was to allow maximum flexibility in their application. The two functions introduced are *Helmholtz free energy, A*, and *Gibbs free energy, G*. The functions for predicting spontaneity are

1. Isolated system: $dS > 0$
2. Isothermal and isochoric system: $dA < 0$
3. Isothermal and isobaric: $dG < 0$
4. Constant volume and entropy: $dE < 0$

Helmholtz free energy is defined as

$$A \equiv E - TS \tag{66}$$

Helmholtz free energy is the energy available to do pressure–volume work for reversible isothermal processes; a decrease in the Helmholtz free energy is equal to the capacity of the system to do work. An alternative view is that, for systems at constant volume and temperature, a change in state is spontaneous if, and only if, there is a decrease in the Helmholtz free energy. Thus, with the introduction of ΔA, the spontaneity of changes occurring at constant volume and temperature may be predicted.

As most reactions carried out in the laboratory are under conditions of constant pressure and temperature, Gibbs free energy is the most useful function and is defined as

$$G \equiv E + PV - TS \tag{67}$$

which can be converted into a more usable form by an analogous method used with the Helmholtz function. Taking the differential and applying the constraints of constant pressure and temperature yields

$$dG = dE + PdV - TdS \tag{68}$$

but $dE = \delta q - \delta W = TdS - \delta W$; thus, upon substitution,

$$-dG = \delta W - PdV \tag{69}$$

A decrease in Gibbs free energy is equal to the non-PV work done by the system or, equivalently,

$$dG = -\delta W_{(non-PV)} \tag{70}$$

which also provides the conditions of a spontaneous change under the constraints of constant temperature and pressure. A direct application of the relationship between Gibbs free energy and non-PV work is used in potentiometry.

These relationships for predicting spontaneity often are expressed in a differential form, which presents the state functions in a concise manner as well as facilitating their use to specific problems. The four differential equations are

$$dE = TdS - PdV \tag{71}$$

$$dH = TdS + VdP \tag{72}$$

$$dA = -SdT - PdV \tag{73}$$

$$dG = -SdT + VdP \tag{74}$$

These expressions represent the four fundamental equations of thermodynamics, which in reality are four ways of looking at one fundamental equation describing the conditions of spontaneity.

Q—One mol of liquid water is vaporized reversibly at 100° and 1 atm pressure. The molar heat of vaporization is 9.725 kcal/mol; what are q_p, ΔH, ΔE, ΔA, ΔG, and ΔS?

A—The value of q_p actually is given in the question, as the heat required to vaporize 1 mol of liquid is the definition of the molar heat of vaporization; thus, $q_p = 9.725$ kcal. Recognizing that the pressure is constant, $\Delta H = q_p = 9.725$ kcal. To calculate ΔE, the work first must be determined. The work is given by

$$W = \int PdV = P\Delta V \tag{75}$$

$$W = P(V_g - V_1) \tag{76}$$

However, the volume of the gas, V_g, is much larger than the volume of the liquid, V_1, which implies that the work is given by

$$W \approx PV_g \tag{77}$$

Assuming the gas is ideal, the work is

$$W = nRT = (1 \text{ mol})(1.987 \text{ cal/mol K})(373 \text{ K}) = 741 \text{ cal}$$

From the above, ΔE may be calculated from

$$\Delta E = q - w = 9725 - 741 = 8984 \text{ cal}$$

The change in entropy is a straightforward calculation, once the enthalpy is known:

$$\Delta S = \Delta H / T_m = 9725/373 = 26 \text{ cal/K}$$

Helmholtz free energy is given by

$$\Delta A = \Delta E - T\Delta S = 8984 - (373)(26.0) = -741 \text{ cal}$$

which also may have been obtained by recognizing that

$$\Delta A = -W_{\text{rev}} = -741 \text{ cal}$$

Finally, the change in Gibbs free energy is determined from

$$\Delta G = \Delta E + P\Delta V - T\Delta S = 8984 + 741 - (373)(26.0) = 0 \text{ cal}$$

which, too, may have been obtained by recognizing the absence of non-PV work.

STANDARD MOLAR GIBBS FREE ENERGY—The fundamental equation for Gibbs free energy has been given as

$$dG = -SdT + VdP \tag{78}$$

Consider the change in free energy with pressure at constant temperature. One may begin by defining a standard free energy, $G°(T)$, which corresponds to the free energy of the ideal gas under a pressure of 1 atm. Because the temperature is constant, the change in free energy is given by

$$\int dG = \int VdP \tag{79}$$

between the limits of 1 atm and the pressure, P. For an ideal gas, the volume is a strong function of pressure; thus, with substitution, and after integration, the result is

$$G(T, P) - G°(T) = \int (nRT/P)dP \tag{80}$$

Simplifying yields

$$G = G° + nRT \ln P \tag{81}$$

Dividing through by the number of mols gives

$$G/n = G°/n + RT \ln P \tag{82}$$

Molar free energy, G/n, is encountered so frequently it is given a special symbol, μ, and Equation 82 is written as

$$\mu = \mu° + RT \ln P \tag{83}$$

The molar free energy also is referred to as the *chemical potential.*

NONIDEALITY—Equation 83 describes the molar free energy of an ideal gas, but for real gases the molar free energy is not related directly to the pressure. Thus, a function, the *fugacity, f*, has been introduced, which provides the same functional form of equation for a real gas:

$$\mu = \mu° + RT \ln f \tag{84}$$

The fugacity is related to the pressure by the following equation, which is provided without derivation:

$$\ln f = \ln P + (1/nRT) \int (V - V_{\text{id}})dP \tag{85}$$

where V_{id} represents the volume of an ideal gas. This equation may be justified by considering the assumptions of an ideal gas, which are that the molecules are point particles without volume, and no intermolecular attractive or repulsive forces. Both of these effects have a direct impact on the measured volume; thus, the fugacity may be considered as a function that corrects for inaccuracies of these assumptions. Clearly, the fugacity approaches the pressure as the real volume approaches the ideal volume.

A similar approach is applied when dealing with mixtures. Consider the molar free energy of a mixture of gases. From Raoult's law, the partial pressure, P_i, of a gas is given by

$$P_i = x_i P \tag{86}$$

where x_i is the mol fraction of the ith component and P is the total pressure. Molar free energy is

$$\mu = \mu°(T) + RT(\ln P + \ln x_i) \tag{87}$$

For the purposes of evaluating mixtures, it generally is more convenient to define a new standard state, $\mu°(T, P)$, which consists simply of the pure gas at 1 atm, thereby yielding

$$\mu_i = \mu°_i(pure) (T, P) + RT \ln x_I \tag{88}$$

In fact, this equation is applicable not only to the gas state but any ideal state of aggregation. This becomes more apparent by letting the mole fraction go to unity (that is, a pure substance), whence the logarithmic term goes to zero and the molar free energy is equal to the standard-state molar free energy.

For solutions, there is a corresponding term that describes the departure for an ideal mixture, the *activity, a*. Equation 88 is applicable only for ideal mixtures. However, with the introduction of the activity, a, the above expression may be written as follows, which is general for all mixtures:

$$\mu_i = \mu°_i(T, P) + RT \ln a_I \tag{89}$$

For solutions, $\mu°_i (T, P)$ is the molar free energy of the liquid in the pure state.

Equilibria

Equilibrium is related intimately to spontaneity, thus the functions above used to predict the spontaneity also may be used for establishing conditions of equilibrium. In essence, if no spontaneous change is predicted, the system is at equilibrium.

Consider the following chemical reaction for an ideal gas:

$$aA \leftrightarrow bB$$

For this reaction, the equilibrium constant is written as

$$K = P_B{}^b / P_A{}^a \qquad (90)$$

Let the molar free energy of each component for the condition of equilibrium be defined as G_A and G_B, and as G_A' and G_B' for the nonequilibrium state. The changes in free energy at equilibrium and in a nonequilibrium state are given as

$$\Delta G = bG_B - aG_A \qquad (91)$$

$$\Delta G' = bG'_B - aG'_A \qquad (92)$$

The change in free energy between these two states is given by the difference between the changes in free energy; that is,

$$\Delta G' - \Delta G = b(G'_B - G_B) - a(G'_A - G_A) \qquad (93)$$

The difference between G'_B and G_B may be calculated for an ideal gas with the use of the fundamental equation given above:

$$dG = VdP - SdT \qquad (94)$$

which is related, under the condition of constant temperature, as

$$dG = VdP \qquad (95)$$

$$\Delta G = \int VdP \qquad (96)$$

$$\Delta G = \int (nRT/P)dP \qquad (97)$$

After integration between limits of the two states, it yields

$$\Delta G = nRT \ln (P'_B/P_B) \qquad (98)$$

Substituting into Equation 93, to find the overall change in ΔG:

$$\Delta G' - \Delta G = bRT \ln (P'_B/P_B) - aRT \ln (P'_A/P_A) \qquad (99)$$

The quantity under the logarithm is given a special definition because it may be generalized to other cases not involving ideal gases; thus, the reaction quotient is defined as

$$Q = [B']^b/[A']^a \qquad (100)$$

where including the equilibrium constant yields

$$\Delta G' - \Delta G = RT \ln Q - RT \ln K \qquad (101)$$

Under conditions of both constant pressure and temperature, dG and $\Delta G = 0$; thus,

$$\Delta G' = RT \ln Q - RT \ln K \qquad (102)$$

In a similar fashion to the standard enthalpies of formation of specific compounds, a standard Gibbs free energy, $\Delta G°$, for the above reaction, may be defined as the free energy associated with the conversion of a mols of reactants to b mols of products when the pressure and temperature are held constant, or $\Delta G' = \Delta G°$ and $\ln Q = 0$. The concentrations (or in this example, the pressures) are equal to unity, thus

$$\Delta G° = -RT \ln K \qquad (103)$$

This equation is of great importance because it provides the energy per mole of any chemical reaction, provided the equilibrium constant is known under standard conditions. Alternatively, the equilibrium constant may be calculated if the free energy is known. The universal applicability of thermodynamics also is displayed. Although it was derived for an ideal gas, it is equally applicable to reactions conducted in solution or even in the solid state.

TEMPERATURE DEPENDENCE OF THE EQUILIBRIUM CONSTANT—A related aspect is the question of the temperature dependence of the equilibrium constant or, from a different perspective, the temperature dependence of the change in free energy. Using the fundamental equations, it can

be shown that Gibbs free energy is related to the following state functions:

$$\Delta G° = \Delta H° - T\Delta S° \qquad (104)$$

The determination of the temperature dependence is obtained through the Gibbs–Helmholtz equation, which is derived as follows. First, both sides are divided by the temperature:

$$\Delta G°/T = \Delta H°/T - \Delta S° \qquad (105)$$

then, the derivative with respect to temperature is taken:

$$\partial(\Delta G°/T)/\partial T = \partial(\Delta H°/T)/\partial T \qquad (106)$$

$$\partial(\Delta G°/T)/\partial T = -\Delta H°/T^2 \qquad (107)$$

This is referred to as the *Gibbs–Helmholtz equation,* which provides the relationship between the change in Gibbs free energy with temperature and the enthalpy change. However, the standard free-energy change also is related to the equilibrium constant, which, in general, also is temperature dependent, as

$$\partial(\Delta G°/T)\partial T = -\partial(R \ln K)\partial T \qquad (108)$$

Combining Equations 105 and 107 yields

$$-\partial(R \ln K)/\partial T = -\Delta H°/T^2 \qquad (109)$$

which may be rearranged and integrated over the limits of T_1 and T_2, assuming that $\Delta H°$ is not a function of temperature, which is a reasonable approximation for a small temperature range:

$$\int \partial(\ln K) = -\int (\Delta H°/RT^2 \partial T) \qquad (110)$$

Thus, the temperature dependence of the equilibrium constant is given as

$$\ln [K_2/K_1] = \Delta H°/R[(1/T_1) - (1/T_2)] \qquad (111)$$

where K_1 and K_2 are the equilibrium constants at temperature T_1 and T_2, respectively. This is known as the *van't Hoff equation;* this equation is extremely important because of its wide applicability, to not only equilibrium constants of chemical reactions, but also other phenomena such as solubility, complexation, dissociation, and vapor pressure.

Q—If the equilibrium constant is 13.6 at STP, at what temperature will it be 20 if the standard enthalpy for the reaction is 8.3 kcal/mol?

A—Using the following equation:

$$(-R/\Delta H°) \ln (K_2/K_1) + 1/T_1 = 1/T_2$$

$$1/T_2 = (-1.987/8300) \ln (20/13.6) + 1/298$$

$$T_2 = 3.26 \times 10^{-3} = 306 \text{ K} = \underline{33°}$$

CLAPEYRON EQUATION—A special case of the van't Hoff equation is known as the *Clapeyron equation.* The interesting feature is that the free-energy change with temperature, in connection with phase changes, is approached in a different manner, with the same result. Consider a liquid in equilibrium with a vapor, such that the free energy associated with each phase, liquid and vapor, may be written from the fundamental equations as

$$dG_l = -S_l dT + V_l dP \qquad (112)$$

$$dG_v = -S_v dT + V_v dP \qquad (113)$$

However, because the phases are in equilibrium, $dG_l = dG_v$, or equating the above relationships,

$$-S_l dT + V_l dP = -S_v dT + V_v dP \qquad (114)$$

these can be rearranged to yield

$$(S_v - S_l)dT = (V_v - V_l)dP \qquad (115)$$

or with separation of the differential with the incremental changes to give

$$dP/dT = (S_v - S_l)/(V_v - V_l) \qquad (116)$$

or equivalent

$$dP/dT = \Delta S/\Delta V \quad (117)$$

The interesting aspect of this equation is that the derivative, dP/dT, is related to the discontinuous changes that occur with a phase change. Although this relation was derived for a liquid–vapor equilibrium, it is general and may be applied to any phase change.

The relationship may be manipulated further by recalling that $\Delta S = \Delta H/T$, where T is the temperature at the point of equilibrium. Thus, by substitution, the following is obtained:

$$dP/dT = \Delta H/T\Delta V \quad (118)$$

An approximation may be made, as before, by noting that $\Delta V = V_v - V_1 \approx V_v$, which for 1 mol of an ideal gas is $V_v = RT/P$ and affords

$$dP/dT = P\Delta H/RT^2 \quad (119)$$

The expression may be rearranged, thereby providing a means for measuring the change in enthalpy and entropy:

$$dP/P = (\Delta H/RT^2)dT \quad (120)$$

This is known as the *Clausius–Clapeyron equation*. Assuming ΔH is constant over the small temperature range between T_2 and T_1, this expression may be integrated yielding

$$\ln(P_2/P_1) = (\Delta H/R)[(1/T_1) - (1/T_2)] \quad (121)$$

Q—If the equilibrium constant is 1.3×10^{-2} at 25° and 1.7×10^{-1} at 150°, what are $\Delta H°$, $\Delta G°$, and $\Delta S°$?

A—The temperature of 25° is taken as the standard temperature; Gibbs free energy is given by

$$\Delta G° = -RT \ln K(298) = -(1.987)(298) \ln (1.2 \times 10^{-2})$$

$$= 2.62 \text{ kcal/mol}$$

The standard enthalpy change may be calculated from the temperature dependence as follows:

$$\Delta H° = R \ln [K(423)/K(298)]/[(1/T_1) - (1/T_2)] = 5.15 \text{ kcal/mol}$$

Finally, $\Delta S°$ may be calculated, knowing the free energy and enthalpy changes, from

$$\Delta S° = -(1/T)(\Delta G° - \Delta H°) = -(1/298)(2620 - 5150)$$

$$= 8.48 \text{ eu (entropy units)}$$

Q—Justify the following expression of the temperature dependence of the vapor pressure of a liquified gas:

$$\ln P = -\Delta H_{vap}/RT + C$$

where C is a constant.

A—Taking the indefinite integral of Equation 120,

$$\int dP/P = \int (\Delta H_{vap}/RT^2)dT$$

the result is obtained directly:

$$\ln P = (-\Delta H_{vap}/RT) + C$$

Solubility and Partitioning Behavior

Consider a system consisting of solid drug in equilibrium with a saturated solution. The molar free energy of the solute is the same everywhere, thereby permitting the following

$$\mu_{2,solution}(T,P,a_2) = \mu_{2,solid}(T,P) \quad (122)$$

from which

$$\mu°_{2,liquid}(T,P) + RT\ln a = \mu_{2,solid}(T,P) \quad (123)$$

where $\mu°_{2,liquid}$ is the chemical potential of the pure liquid solute. Solving for the activity of the pure liquid solute yields

$$\ln a_2 = [\mu_{2,solid}(T,P) - \mu°_{2,liquid}(T,P)]/RT \quad (124)$$

The relationship between activity and solubility is given as follows:

$$a_2 = \gamma_2 X_2 \quad (125)$$

where γ_2 is the activity coefficient of the solute in water. From this analysis, the mole fraction solubility is seen to depend only on the chemical potential of the solute. Thus, the ideal solubility of a drug is the same in every solvent. Furthermore, the difference in solubility observed between solvents is related to the nonideality of the solute, which is quantitatively determined by the activity coefficient.

The cause of nonideality arises from intermolecular interactions, which may be favorable leading to high solubility and a low activity coefficient. Alternatively, the interactions may be unfavorable, which lead to low solubility and high activity coefficient. For this reason, the activity coefficient quantitatively describes the escaping tendency of the solute from the solution.

In an analogous manner, the activity coefficients may be related to the partition coefficient. Consider a solute distributed between two immiscible solvents, A and B. At equilibrium, the chemical potential of the solute is the same in each phase, thus

$$\mu_{2A} = \mu_{2B} \quad (126)$$

and

$$\mu_2° + RT\ln a_A = \mu_2° + RT\ln a_B \quad (127)$$

The standard state for the solute in both solvents A and B, $\mu_2°$, must be the same since it is based on the pure liquid solute, the activities must be equal.

$$a_A = a_B \quad (128)$$

The partition coefficient is defined in terms of the mole fractions of infinitely dilute solutions,

$$P_{o/w} = (X_o)\infty/(X_w)\infty = \gamma_w/\gamma_o \quad (129)$$

where the activities of the solute in each phase have been cancelled. Noteworthy, in using this system of standard states is that for ideal oil and water solutions of solutes, the partition coefficient is unity, since the activity coefficients, γ_o and γ_w, are equal to one.

These two concepts have been combined by Yalkowski and his coworkers to predict the aqueous solubility of drugs. They proposed the following:

$$\ln(X_{2w}) = \ln(X_{2oct}) - \ln(P_{o/w}) \quad (130)$$

where X_{2w} is the mole fraction in water, $P_{o/w}$ is the octanol/water partition coefficient, and X_{2oct} is the mole fraction solubility of the solute in octanol. From above, the Po/w is given by the ratio of the activity coefficients, γ_w/γ_o. However, the drug in octanol generally forms an ideal solution, i.e. $\gamma_o = 1$. As such, the octanol/water partition coefficient is a measure of the activity coefficient of the drug in water. Finally, the mole fraction of the solute in an ideal solution of octanol may be determined from the heat of fusion and the melting point. The resulting predictive equation for the water solubility, which has yielded highly correlated data, is:

$$\ln X_2 = -(\Delta H_{fus}/R)(1/T - 1/T_m) - \ln P^x_{o/w} \quad (131)$$

The melting point and heat of fusion may be readily measured, and the partition coefficient can be estimated by group contribution methods. Thus, a conceptually elegant foundation has been developed into a practically useful scheme to estimate the water solubility of drugs from the thermal properties and the octanol/water partition coefficient of drugs.

PROTEIN BINDING—As a final example of equilibria, the protein-binding of drugs should be mentioned. Consider the case where a protein has a single binding site for a drug. A mass-balanced equation may be written as

$$[P] + [D] = [PD] \quad (132)$$

where $[P]$ is the concentration of unbound protein, $[D]$ is the concentration of unbound drug, and $[PD]$ is the concentration of the drug–protein complex. The equilibrium constant may be written for this reaction as

$$K_a = [PD]/[P][D] \tag{133}$$

where K_a is the association constant. Assuming ideality, the standard free energy for the above equilibrium may be immediately identified as

$$\Delta G° = -RT \ln (K_a) \tag{134}$$

This concept often is taken a step farther in order to characterize the nature of the binding site of the drug. This has application in structure–activity relationships used for predicting pharmacological activity.

Suppose the association constants of two structurally related drugs, K'_a and K''_a, were determined experimentally. The standard free energy of each association is given as $\Delta G°'$ and $\Delta G°''$. The effect of the change in the chemical structure on the energetics of the association then can be calculated from the association constants as

$$\Delta \Delta G° = \Delta G°'' - \Delta G°' = RT \ln (K'_a/K'_a) \tag{135}$$

where $\Delta \Delta G°$ is the standard free–energy change of protein-binding associated with the specific chemical modification.

Q—At room temperature and a protein concentration of 2 μM, the fraction of penicillin G and penicillin V bound was found to be 0.65 and 0.80, respectively. Calculate the change in the standard free energy of binding associated with the replacement of the benzyl group in penicillin G by the phenoxy moiety in penicillin V.

A—The fraction bound may be related to the equilibrium constant by assuming there is only one binding site on each protein molecule. The fraction of drug bound, F, is defined as

$$F = [DP]/([D] + [DP]) \tag{136}$$

and since the concentration of the drug–protein complex is given by

$$[PD] = K_a[P][D] \tag{137}$$

this may be substituted into the above equation yielding

$$F = K_a[P][D]/([D] + K_a[P][D]) \tag{138}$$

After canceling terms and solving for K_a, the desired expression is obtained:

$$K_a = F/[P](1 - F) \tag{139}$$

The association constants for each drug then are calculated:

$$K_a(G) = (0.65)/[2 \ \mu M](1 - 0.65) = 0.93 \ \mu M^{-1}$$

$$K_a(V) = (0.80)/[2 \ \mu M](1 - 0.80) = 2.0 \ \mu M^{-1}$$

From the association constants, the change in standard free energy associated with replacing the benzyl group with a phenoxy moiety is

$$\Delta \Delta G° = \Delta G°(V) - \Delta G°(G) = RT \ln (0.93/2.0)$$

$$\Delta \Delta G° - \underline{453 \ \text{cal/mol K}}$$

The change in the standard free energy is negative, in agreement with the concept that binding of the phenoxy group is more favorable than the benzyl group.

BIBLIOGRAPHY

Introductory

Alberty RA, Silbey RJ. *Physical Chemistry A Basic Theory and Methods,* 2nd ed. New York: Wiley, 1996.
Connors KA. *Thermodynamics of Pharmaceutical Systems, An Introduction for Students of Pharmacy.* New York: Wiley Interscience, 2002.
Levine IN. *Physical Chemistry,* 4th ed. New York: McGraw-Hill, 1995.
Reiss H. *Methods of Thermodynamics.* New York: Dover, 1997.

Comprehensive

Glasstone S. *Thermodynamics for Chemists,* New York: Van Nostrand, 1946.
Lewis GN, Randall M. *Thermodynamics.* Revised by Pitzer KS, Brewer L. New York: McGraw-Hill, 1961.
Kondepudi DK, Prigogine I. *Modern Thermodynamics: From Heat Engines to Dissipative Structures.* New York: Wiley, 1996.

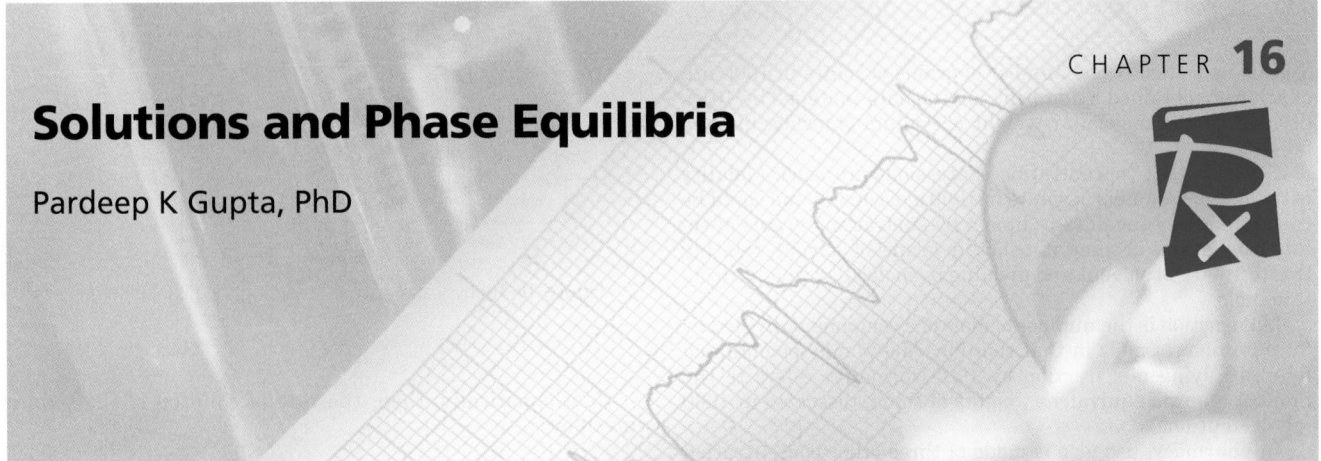

CHAPTER 16

Solutions and Phase Equilibria

Pardeep K Gupta, PhD

SOLUTIONS AND SOLUBILITY

A solution is a chemically and physically homogeneous mixture of two or more substances. The term *solution* generally denotes a homogeneous mixture that is liquid, even though it is possible to have homogeneous mixtures that are solid or gaseous. Thus, it is possible to have solutions of solids in liquids, liquids in liquids, gases in liquids, gases in gases, and solids in solids. The first three of these are most important in pharmacy, and ensuing discussions will be concerned primarily with them.

In pharmacy different kinds of liquid dosage forms are used and all consist of the dispersion of some substance or substances in a liquid phase. Depending on the size of the dispersed particle, they are classified as *true solutions, colloidal solutions,* or *disperse systems*. If sugar is dissolved in water, it is supposed that the ultimate sugar particle is of molecular dimensions and that a true solution is formed. On the other hand, if very fine sand is mixed with water, a suspension of comparatively large particles, each consisting of many molecules, is obtained. Between these two extremes lie colloidal solutions, the dispersed particles of which are larger than those of true solutions but smaller than the particles present in suspensions. In this chapter only true solutions will be discussed.

It is possible to classify broadly all solutions as one of two types. In the first type, although there may be lesser or greater interaction between the dispersed substance (the solute) and the dispersing medium (the solvent), the solution phase contains the same chemical entity as found in the solid phase; thus, upon removal of the solvent, the solute is recovered unchanged. One example would be sugar dissolved in water where, in the presence of sugar in excess of its solubility, there is an equilibrium between sugar molecules in the solid phase with sugar molecules in the solution phase. A second example would be dissolving silver chloride in water. Admittedly, the solubility of this salt in water is low, but it is finite. In this case the solvent contains silver and chloride ions and the solid phase contains the same material. The removal of the solvent yields initial solute.

In the second type the solvent contains a compound that is different from the one in the solid phase. The difference between the compound in the solid phase and solution is due generally to some chemical reaction that has occurred in the solvent. An example would be dissolving aspirin in an aqueous solvent containing some basic material capable of reacting with the acid aspirin. Now the species in solution would not only be undissociated aspirin, but aspirin also as its anion, whereas the species in the solid phase is aspirin in only its undissociated acid form. In this situation, if the solvent were removed, part of the substance obtained (the salt of aspirin) would be different from what was present initially in the solid.

Solutions of Solids in Liquids

REVERSIBLE SOLUBILITY WITHOUT CHEMICAL REACTION—From a pharmaceutical standpoint, solutions of solids in liquids, with or without accompanying chemical reaction in the solvent, are of the greatest importance, and many quantitative data on the behavior and properties of such solutions are available. This discussion will be concerned with definitions of solubility, with the rate at which substances go into solution, and with temperature and other factors that control solubility.

SOLUBILITY—When an excess of a solid is brought into contact with a liquid, molecules of the former are removed from its surface until equilibrium is established between the molecules leaving the solid and those returning to it. The resulting solution is said to be saturated at the temperature of the experiment, and the extent to which the solute dissolves is referred to as its *solubility*. The extent of solubility of different substances varies from almost imperceptible amounts to relatively large quantities, but for any given solute the solubility has a constant value at a given constant temperature.

Under certain conditions it is possible to prepare a solution containing a larger amount of solute than is necessary to form a saturated solution. This may occur when a solution is saturated at one temperature, the excess of solid solute is then removed, and the solution cooled. The solute present in solution, even though it may be less soluble at the lower temperature, does not always separate from the solution and there is produced a supersaturated solution. Such solutions, formed by sodium thiosulfate or potassium acetate, for example, may be made to deposit their excess of solute by vigorous shaking, scratching the side of the vessel in contact with the solution, or introducing into the solution a small crystal of the solute.

METHODS OF EXPRESSING SOLUBILITY—When quantitative data are available, solubilities may be expressed in many ways. For example, the solubility of sodium chloride in water at 25° may be stated as

1. 1 g of sodium chloride dissolves in 2.786 mL of water. (An approximation of this method is used by the USP.)
2. 35.89 g of sodium chloride dissolves in 100 mL of water.
3. 100 mL of a saturated solution of sodium chloride in water contains 31.71 g of solute.
4. 100 g of a saturated solution of sodium chloride in water contains 26.47 g of solute.
5. 1 L of a saturated solution of sodium chloride in water contains 5.425 mols of solute. This also may be stated as a saturated solution of sodium chloride in water is 5.425 molar with respect to the solute.

In order to calculate item 3 above from items 1 or 2, it is necessary to know the density of the solution, in this case 1.198 g/mL.

To calculate item 5, the number of grams of solute in 1000 mL of solution (obtained by multiplying the data in item 3 by 10) is divided by the molecular weight of sodium chloride, namely 58.45.

Several other concentration expressions are used. Molality is the number of mols of solute in 1000 g of solvent and could be calculated from the data in item 4 by subtracting grams of solute from grams of solution to obtain grams of solvent, relating this to 1000 g of solvent and dividing by molecular weight to obtain mols.

Mol fraction is the number of mols of a component divided by total number of mols in that solution. Mol % may be obtained by multiplying mol fraction by 100. Normality refers to the number of gram equivalent weights of solute dissolved in 1000 mL of solution.

In pharmacy, use also is made of three other concentration expressions. Percent by weight (% *w/w*) is the number of grams of solute per 100 g of solution and is exemplified by item 4 above. Percent weight in volume (% *w/v*) is the number of grams of solute per 100 mL of solution and is exemplified by item 3 above. Percent by volume (% *v/v*) is the number of milliliters of solute in 100 mL of solution, referring to solutions of liquids in liquids. The USP indicates that the term *percent,* when unqualified, means percent weight in volume for solutions of solids in liquids and percent by volume for solutions of liquids in liquids.

In pharmacopeial texts, when it has not been possible, or in some instances not desirable, to indicate exact solubility, a descriptive term is used. Table 16-1 indicates the meaning of such terms.

RATE OF SOLUTION—It is possible to define quantitatively the rate at which a solute goes into solution. The simplest treatment is based on a model depicted in Figure 16-1. A solid particle dispersed in a solvent is surrounded by a thin layer of solvent having a finite thickness, *l,* in centimeters. The layer is an integral part of the solid, and thus is referred to characteristically as the *stagnant layer.* This means that, regardless of how fast the bulk solution is stirred, the stagnant layer remains a part of the surface of the solid, moving wherever the particles moves. The thickness of this layer may get smaller as the stirring of the bulk solution increases, but it is important to recognize that this layer will always have a finite thickness however small it may get.

Using Fick's First Law of Diffusion, the rate of solution of the solid can be explained, in the simplest case, as the rate at which a dissolved solute particle diffuses through the stagnant layer to the bulk solution. The driving force behind the movement of the solute molecule through the stagnant layer is the difference in concentration that exists between the concentration of the solute, C_1, in the stagnant layer at the surface of the solid and its concentration, C_2, on the farthest side of the stagnant layer. The greater this difference in concentration ($C_1 - C_2$), the faster the rate of dissolution.

According to Fick's Law, the rate of solution also is directly proportional to surface area of the solid, *A* in cm², exposed to solvent and inversely proportional to the length of the path through which the dissolved solute molecule must diffuse.

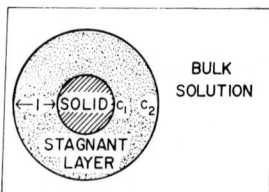

Figure 16-1. Physical model representing the dissolution process.

Mathematically, then, the rate of solution of the solid is given by

$$\text{Rate of solution} = \frac{DA}{l}(C_1 - C_2) \tag{1}$$

where *D* is a proportionality constant called the *diffusion coefficient* in cm²/sec. In measuring the rate of solution experimentally, the concentration C_2 is maintained at a low value compared to C_1 and hence is considered to have a negligible effect on the rate. Furthermore, C_1 most often is the saturation solubility of the solute. Hence Equation 1 is simplified to

$$\text{Rate of solution} = \frac{DA}{l}(\text{saturation solubility}) \tag{2}$$

Equation 2 quantitatively explains many of the phenomena commonly observed that affect the rate at which materials dissolve.

1. Small particles go into solution faster than large particles. For a given mass of solute, as the particle size becomes smaller, the surface area per unit of mass of solid increases; Equation 2 shows that as area increases, the rate must increase proportionately. Hence, if a pharmacist wishes to increase the rate of solution of a drug, its particle size should be decreased.
2. Stirring a solution increases the rate at which a solid dissolves. This is because the thickness of the stagnant layer depends on how fast the bulk solution is stirred; as stirring rate increases, the length of the diffusional path decreases. Because the rate of solution is proportional inversely to the length of the diffusional path, the faster the solution is stirred, the faster the solute will go into solution.
3. The more soluble the solute, the faster is its rate of solution. Again, Equation 2 predicts that the larger the saturation solubility, the faster the rate.
4. With a viscous liquid the rate of solution is decreased. This is because the diffusion coefficient is proportional inversely to the viscosity of the medium; the more viscous the solvent, the slower the rate of solution.

HEAT OF SOLUTION AND TEMPERATURE DEPENDENCY—Turning from the kinetic aspects of dissolution, this discussion will be concerned with the situation where there is thermodynamic equilibrium between solute in its solid phase and the solute in solution. (It is assumed that there is an amount of solid material in excess of the amount that can go into solution; hence, a solid phase is always present.) As defined earlier, the concentration of solute in solution at equilibrium is the saturation solubility of the substance.

When a solid (Solute *A*) dissolves in some solvent, two steps may be considered as occurring: the solid absorbs energy to become a liquid, then the liquid dissolves.

$$A_{(\text{solid})} \rightleftharpoons A_{(\text{liquid})} \rightleftharpoons A_{(\text{solution})}$$

For the overall dissolution, the equilibrium existing between solute molecules in the solid and solute molecules in solution may be treated as an equilibrium. Thus, for Solute A in equilibrium with its solution,

$$A_{(\text{solid})} \rightleftharpoons A_{(\text{solution})}$$

Using the Law of Mass Action, an equilibrium constant for this system can be defined, just as any equilibrium constant may be written as

Table 16-1. Descriptive Terms for Solubility

DESCRIPTIVE TERMS	PARTS OF SOLVENT FOR 1 PART OF SOLUTE
Very soluble	Less than 1
Freely soluble	From 1 to 10
Soluble	From 10 to 30
Sparingly soluble	From 30 to 100
Slightly soluble	From 100 to 1000
Very slightly soluble	From 1000 to 10,000
Practically insoluble, or insoluble	More than 10,000

$$K_{eq} = \frac{a_{(solution)}}{a_{(solid)}}$$

where a denotes the activity of the solute in each phase. Because the activity of a solid is defined as unity,

$$K_{eq} = a_{(solution)}$$

Because the activity of a compound in dilute solution is approximated by its concentration, and because this concentration is the saturation solubility, K_S, the van't Hoff equation (for a more complete treatment, see Martin et al[1]) may be used, which defines the relationship between an equilibrium constant (here, solubility) and absolute temperature.

$$\frac{d \log K_S}{dT} = \frac{\Delta H}{2.3RT^2} \qquad (3)$$

where $d \log K_S/dT$ is the change of $\log K_S$ with a unit change of absolute temperature, T; ΔH is a constant that, in this situation, is the heat of solution for the overall process (solid $\rightleftharpoons$ liquid $\rightleftharpoons$ solution); and R is the gas constant, 1.99 cal/mol/deg. Equation 3, a differential, may be solved to give

$$\log K_S = -\frac{\Delta H}{2.3RT} + J \qquad (4)$$

where J is a constant. A more useful form of this equation is

$$\log \frac{K_{S,T_2}}{K_{S,T_1}} = \frac{\Delta H(T_2 - T_1)}{2.3RT_1 T_2} \qquad (5)$$

where K_{S,T_1}, is the saturation solubility at absolute temperature T_1, and K_{S,T_2} is the solubility at temperature T_2. Through the use of Equation 5, if ΔH and the solubility at one temperature are known, the solubility at any other temperature can be calculated.

EFFECT OF TEMPERATURE—As is evident from Equation 4, the solubility of a solid in a liquid depends on the temperature. In the process of solution, if heat is absorbed (as evidenced by a reduction in temperature), ΔH is by convention positive and the solubility of the solute will increase with increasing temperature. Such is the case for most salts, as is shown in Figure 16-2 in which the solubility of the solute is plotted as the ordinate and the temperature as the abscissa, and the line joining the experimental points represents the solubility curve for that solute.

If a solute gives off heat during the process of solution (as evidenced by an increase in temperature), by convention ΔH is negative and solubility decreases with an increase in temperature. This is the case with calcium hydroxide and, at higher temperatures, with calcium sulfate. (Because of the slight solubility of these substances, their solubility curves are not included.) When heat is neither absorbed nor given off, the solubility is not affected by variation of temperature as is nearly the case with sodium chloride.

Solubility curves usually are continuous as long as the chemical composition of the solid phase in contact with the solution remains unchanged, but if there is a transition of the solid phase from one form to another, a break will be found in the curve. Such is the case with $Na_2SO_4 \cdot 10H_2O$, which dissolves with absorption of heat up to a temperature of 32.4°, at which point there is a transition of the solid phase to anhydrous sodium sulfate, Na_2SO_4, which dissolves with evolution of heat. This change is evidenced by increased solubility of the hydrated salt up to 32.4°, but above this temperature the solubility decreases.

These temperature effects are what would be predicted from Equation 4. When the heat of solution is negative, signifying that energy is released during dissolution, the relation between $\log K_S$ and $1/T$ is typified in Figure 16-3 (Curve A), where as $1/T$ increases, $\log K_S$ increases. It can be seen that with increasing temperature (T itself actually increases proceeding left in Fig 16-3A), there is a decrease in solubility. On the other hand, when the heat of solution is positive—that is, when heat is absorbed in the solution process—the relation between $\log K_S$ and $1/T$ is typified in Figure 16-3B. Hence, as temperature increases ($1/T$ decreases), the solubility increases.

EFFECT OF SALTS—The solubility of a nonelectrolyte in water either is decreased or increased generally by the addition of an electrolyte; it is only rarely that the solubility is not altered. When the solubility of a nonelectrolyte is decreased, the effect is referred to as *salting-out*; if it is increased, it is described as *salting-in*. Inorganic electrolytes commonly decrease solubility, though there are some exceptions to the generalization.

Salting-out occurs because the ions of the added electrolyte interact with water molecules, and thus, in a sense, reduce the amount of water available for dissolution of the nonelectrolyte. (Refer to the section on *Thermodynamics of the Solution Process* for another view.) The greater the degree of hydration of the ions, the more the solubility of the nonelectrolyte is decreased. If, for example, one compares the effect of equivalent amounts of lithium chloride, sodium chloride, potassium chloride, rubidium chloride, and cesium chloride (all of which belong to the family of alkali metals and are of the same valence type),

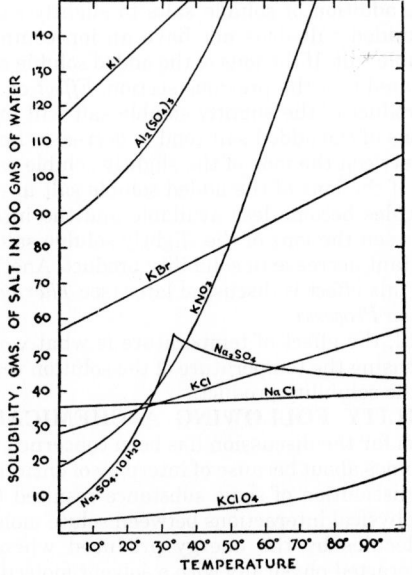

Figure 16-2. Effect of heat on solubility.

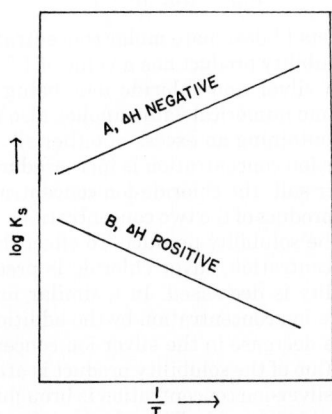

Figure 16-3. Typified relationship between the logarithm of the saturation solubility and the reciprocal of the absolute temperature.

lithium chloride decreases the solubility of a nonelectrolyte to the greatest extent and the salting-out effect decreases in the order given.

This is also the order of the degree of hydration of the cations; lithium ion—being the smallest ion and, therefore, having the greatest density of positive charge per unit of surface area (see Chapter 13 under *Electronegativity Values*)—is the most extensively hydrated of the cations, whereas cesium ion is hydrated the least. Salting-out is encountered frequently in pharmaceutical operations.

Salting-in commonly occurs when either the salts of various organic acids or organic-substituted ammonium salts are added to aqueous solutions of nonelectrolytes. In the first case, the solubilizing effect is associated with the anion; in the second, it is associated with the cation. In both cases the solubility increases as the concentration of added salt is increased. The solubility increase may be relatively great, sometimes amounting to several times the solubility of the nonelectrolyte in water.

SOLUBILITY OF SOLUTES CONTAINING TWO OR MORE SPECIES—In cases where the solute phase consists of two or more species (as in an ionizable inorganic salt), when the solute goes into solution, the solution phase often contains each of these species as discrete entities. For some such substance, *AB*, the following relationship for the solution process may be written.

$$AB_{(solid)} \rightleftarrows A_{(solution)} + B_{(solution)}$$

As there is an equilibrium between the solute and saturated solution phases, the Law of Mass Action defines an equilibrium constant, K_{eq}

$$K_{eq} = \frac{a_{A(solution)} \cdot a_{B(solution)}}{a_{AB(solid)}} \quad (6)$$

where $a_{A(solution)}$, $a_{B(solution)}$, and $a_{AB(solid)}$ are the activities of *A* and *B* in solution and of *AB* in the solid phase. Recall from the earlier discussion that the activity of a solid is defined as unity, and that in a very dilute solution (eg, for a slightly soluble salt) concentrations may be substituted for activities. Equation 6 then becomes

$$K_{eq} = C_A C_B$$

where C_A and C_B are the concentrations of *A* and *B* in solution. In this situation K_{eq} has a special name, the *solubility product*, K_{SP}. Thus,

$$K_{SP} = C_A C_B \quad (7)$$

This equation will hold true theoretically only for slightly soluble salts.

As an example of this type of solution, consider the solubility of silver chloride,

$$K_{SP} = [Ag^+][Cl^-]$$

where the brackets [ ] designate molar concentrations.

At 25° the solubility product has a value of 1.56×10^{-10}, the concentration of silver and chloride ions being expressed in mol/liter. The same numerical value applies also to solutions of silver chloride containing an excess of either silver or chloride ions. If the silver-ion concentration is increased by the addition of a soluble silver salt, the chloride-ion concentration must decrease until the product of the two concentrations again is equal numerically to the solubility product. To effect the decrease in chloride-ion concentration, silver chloride is precipitated, and hence its solubility is decreased. In a similar manner, an increase in chloride-ion concentration by the addition of a soluble chloride effects a decrease in the silver-ion concentration until the numerical value of the solubility product is attained. Again, this decrease in silver-ion concentration is brought about by the precipitation of silver chloride. This phenomenon of decrease in solubility due to the presence of one of the ions in solution is known as the *common-ion effect*.

The solubility of silver chloride in a saturated aqueous solution of the salt may be calculated by assuming that the concentration of silver ion is the same as the concentration of chloride ion, both expressed in mol/liter, and that the concentration of dissolved silver chloride is numerically the same as each silver chloride molecule gives rise to one silver ion and one chloride ion, because

$$[\text{dissolved AgCl}] = [Ag^+] = [Cl^-]$$

the solubility of AgCl is equal to $\sqrt{1.56 \times 10^{-10}}$, which is 1.25×10^{-5} mol/liter. Multiplying this by the molecular weight of silver chloride (143), we obtain a solubility of approximately 1.8 mg/liter.

For a salt of the type $PbCl_2$ the solubility product expression takes the form

$$[Pb^{2+}][Cl^-]^2 = K_{SP}$$

while for As_2S_3 it would be

$$[As^{3+}]^2[S^{2-}]^3 = K_{SP}$$

because from the Law of Mass Action

$$PbCl_{2(solid)} \rightleftarrows Pb^{2+}_{(solution)} + 2Cl^-_{(solution)}$$

and

$$As_2S_{3(solid)} \rightarrow 2As^{3+}_{(solution)} + 3S^{2-}_{(solution)}$$

For further details of methods of using solubility-product calculations, see textbooks on qualitative or quantitative analyses or physical chemistry.

Recall that the solubility-product principle is valid for aqueous solutions of slightly soluble salts, provided that the concentration of added salt is not too great. Where the concentrations are high, deviations from the theory occur and these have been explained by assuming that in such solutions the nature of the solvent has been changed. Frequently, deviations also may occur as the result of the formation of complexes between the two salts. An example of increased solubility, by virtue of complex-ion formation, is seen in the effect of solutions of soluble iodides on mercuric iodide. According to the solubility-product principle, it might be expected that soluble iodides would decrease the solubility of mercuric iodide, but because of the formation of the more soluble complex salt K_2HgI_4, which dissociates as

$$K_2HgI_4 \rightarrow 2K^+ + (HgI_4)^{2-}$$

the iodide ion no longer functions as a common ion.

It is possible to formulate some general rules regarding the effect of the addition of soluble salts to slightly soluble salts where the added salt does not have an ion common to the slightly soluble salt. If the ions of the added soluble salt are not highly hydrated (see the previous section, *Effect of Salts*), the solubility product of the slightly soluble salt will increase because the ions of the added salt tend to decrease the interionic attraction between the ions of the slightly soluble salt. On the other hand, if the ions of the added soluble salt are hydrated, water molecules become less available and the interionic attraction between the ions of the slightly soluble salt increases with a resultant decrease in solubility product. Another way of considering this effect is discussed later (see *Thermodynamics of the Solution Process*).

In general, the effect of temperature is what would be expected: increasing the temperature of the solution results in an increase of the solubility product.

SOLUBILITY FOLLOWING A CHEMICAL REACTION—Thus far the discussion has been concerned with solubility that comes about because of interplay of entirely physical forces. The dissolution of some substance resulted from overcoming the physical interactions between solute molecules and solvent molecules by the energy produced when a solute molecule interacted physically with a solvent molecule. The solution process, however, can be facilitated also by a chemical reaction. Almost always the chemical enhancement of solubility in aqueous systems is due to the formation of a salt following an acid–base reaction.

An alkaloidal base, or any other nitrogenous base of relatively high molecular weight, generally is slightly soluble in water, but if the pH of the medium is reduced by addition of acid, the solubility of the base is considerably increased as the pH continues to be reduced. The reason for this increase in solubility is that the base is converted to a salt, which is relatively soluble in water. Conversely, the solubility of a salt of an alkaloid or other nitrogenous base is reduced as pH is increased by addition of alkali.

The solubility of slightly soluble acid substances is, on the other hand, increased as the pH is increased by addition of alkali, the reason again being that a salt, relatively soluble in water, is formed. Examples of acid substances whose solubility is thus increased are aspirin, theophylline and the penicillins, cephalosporins, and barbiturates. Conversely, the solubility of salts of the same substances is decreased as the pH decreases.

Among some inorganic compounds a somewhat similar behavior is observed. Tribasic calcium phosphate, $Ca_3(PO_4)_2$, for example, is almost insoluble in water, but if an acid is added its solubility increases rapidly with a decrease in pH. This is because hydrogen ions have such a strong affinity for phosphate ions forming nonionized phosphoric acid that the calcium phosphate is dissolved in order to release phosphate ions. Or, stated in another way, the solubilization is an example of a reaction in which a strong acid (the source of the hydrogen ions) displaces a weak acid.

In all of these examples solubilization occurs as the result of an interaction of the solute with an acid or a base, and thus the species in solution is not the same as the undissolved solute. Compounds that do not react with either acids or bases are slightly, or not at all, influenced in their aqueous solubility by variations of pH. Such effects if observed are generally due to ionic *salt effects.*

It is possible to analyze quantitatively the solubility following an acid–base reaction by considering it as a two-step process. The first example is an organic acid, designated as *HA,* that is relatively insoluble in water. Its two-step dissolution can be represented as

$$HA_{(solid)} \leftrightarrows HA_{(solution)}$$

followed by

$$HA_{(solution)} \leftrightarrows H^+_{(solution)} + A^-_{(solution)}$$

The equilibrium constant for the first step is the solubility of $HA(K_S = [HA]_{solution})$, just as was developed earlier when no chemical reaction took place, and the equilibrium constant for the second step is the dissociation constant of the acid is

$$K_a = \frac{[H^+][A^-]}{[HA]}$$

Since the total amount of compound *in solution* is the sum of nonionized and ionized forms of the acid, the total solubility may be designated as $S_{t(HA)}$, or

$$S_{t(HA)} = [HA] + [A^-] = [HA] + K_a \frac{[HA]}{[H^+]} \tag{8}$$

and because $K_S = [HA]$, Equation 8 becomes

$$S_{t(HA)} = K_S\left(1 + \frac{K_a}{[H^+]}\right) \tag{9}$$

Equation 9 is very useful because it equates the total solubility of an acid drug with the hydrogen-ion concentration of the solvent. If the water solubility, K_S, and the dissociation constant, K_a, are known, the total solubility of the acid can be calculated at various hydrogen-ion concentrations.

Equation 9 demonstrates quantitatively how the total solubility of the acid increases as the hydrogen-ion concentration decreases (ie, as the pH increases).

It is possible to develop an equation similar to Equation 9 for the solubility of a basic drug *B,* such as a relatively insoluble nitrogenous base (eg, an alkaloid), at various hydrogen-ion concentrations. The solubility of the base in water may be represented in two steps as

$$B_{(solid)} \rightleftarrows B_{(solution)}$$

$$B_{(solution)} \rightleftarrows BH^+_{(solution)} + OH^-_{(solution)}$$

Again, if K_S is the solubility of the free base in water and K_b is its dissociation constant,

$$K_b = \frac{[BH^+][OH^-]}{[B]}$$

the total solubility of the base in water $S_{t(B)}$ is given by

$$S_{t(B)} = [B] + [BH^+] = [B] + \frac{K_b[B]}{[OH^-]} = K_S\left(1 + \frac{K_b}{[OH^-]}\right) \tag{10}$$

It is convenient to rewrite Equation 10 in terms of hydrogen-ion concentration by making use of the dissociation constant for water

$$K_W = [H^+][OH^-] = 1 \times 10^{-14}$$

Equation 10 then becomes

$$S_{t(B)} = K_S\left(1 + \frac{K_b}{K_W/[H^+]}\right) = K_S\left(1 + \frac{K_b[H^+]}{K_W}\right) \tag{11}$$

Equation 11 quantitatively shows how the total solubility of the base increases as the hydrogen-ion concentration of the solvent increases. If K_S and K_b are known, it is possible to calculate the total solubility of a basic drug at various hydrogen-ion concentrations using this equation.

Equations 9 and 11 have assumed that the salt formed following a chemical reaction is infinitely soluble. This, of course, is not an acceptable assumption, as suggested and demonstrated by Kramer and Flynn.[2] Rather, for an acidic or basic drug there should be a pH at which maximum solubility occurs where this solubility remains the sum of the solution concentrations of the free and salt forms of the drug at that pH. Using a basic drug *B* as the example, this would mean that a solution of *B*, at pH values greater than the pH of maximum solubility, would be saturated with free-base form but not with the salt form, and the use of Equation 11 would be valid for the prediction of solubility. On the other hand, at pH values less than the pH of maximum solubility, the solution would be saturated with salt form and Equation 11 is no longer really valid. Because in this situation the total solubility of the base, $S_{t(B)}$, is

$$S_{t(B)} = [B] + [BH^+]_s$$

where the subscript *s* designates a solution saturated with salt, the correct equation to use at pH values less than the pH maximum would be

$$S_{t(B)} = [BH^+]_s\left(1 + \frac{[OH^-]}{K_b}\right) = [BH^+]_s\left(1 + \frac{K_W}{K_b[H^+]}\right) \tag{12}$$

A relationship similar to Equation 12 likewise can be developed for an acidic drug at a pH greater than its pH of maximum solubility.

EFFECTING SOLUTION OF SOLIDS IN THE PRESCRIPTION LABORATORY—The method usually employed by the pharmacist when soluble compounds are to be dissolved in water in compounding a prescription requires the use of the mortar and pestle. The ordinary practice is to crush the substance into fragments in the mortar with the pestle and pour the solvent on it, meanwhile stirring with the pestle until solution is effected. If definite quantities are used and the whole of the solvent is required to dissolve the given weight of the salt, only a portion of the solvent should be added first, and, when this is saturated, the solution is poured off and a fresh portion of solvent added. This operation is repeated until the solid is dissolved entirely and all the portions combined. Other methods of affecting solution are to shake the solid with the liquid in a bottle or flask or to apply heat to the substances in a suitable vessel.

Substances vary greatly in the rate at which they dissolve; some are capable of producing a saturated solution quickly, others require several hours to attain saturation.

With hygroscopic substances like pepsin, silver protein compounds, and some others, the best method of effecting solution in water is to place the substance directly upon the surface of the water and then stir vigorously with a glass rod. If the ordinary procedure, such as using a mortar and pestle, is employed with these substances, gummy lumps form that are exceedingly difficult to dissolve.

The *solubility* of chemicals and the *miscibility* of liquids are important physical factors for the pharmacist to know, as they often have a bearing on intelligently and properly filling prescriptions. For the information of the pharmacist, the USP provides tabular data indicating the degree of solubility or miscibility of many official substances.

DETERMINATION OF SOLUBILITY—For the pharmacist and pharmaceutical chemist, the question of solubility is of paramount importance. Not only is it necessary to know solubilities when preparing and dispensing medicines, but such information is also necessary to effect separation of substances in qualitative and quantitative analysis. Furthermore, the accurate determination of the solubility of a substance is one of the best methods for determining its purity.

The details of the determination of the solubility are affected markedly by the physical and chemical characteristics of the solute and solvent and also by the temperature at which the solubility is to be determined. Accordingly, it is not possible to describe a universally applicable method, but in general the following rules must be observed in solubility determinations.

1. The purity of both the dissolved substance and the solvent is essential, because impurities in either affect the solubility.
2. A constancy of temperature must be maintained accurately during the course of the determination.
3. Complete saturation must be attained.
4. Accurate analysis of the saturated solution and correct expression of the results are imperative.

Consideration should be given also to the varying rates of dissolution of different compounds and to the marked effect of the degrees of fineness of the particles on the time required for the saturation of the solution.

THE PHASE RULE AND PHASE-SOLUBILITY ANALYSIS—Phase-solubility analysis is a useful and accurate method for the determination of the purity of a substance. It involves the application of precise solubility methods to the principle that constancy of solubility, in the same manner as constancy of melting point, indicates that a material is pure or free from foreign admixture. It is important to recognize that the technique can be used to obtain the exact solubility of the pure substance without the necessity of the experimental material itself being pure.

The method is based on the thermodynamic principles of heterogeneous equilibria that are among the soundest of theoretical concepts of chemistry. Thus, it does not depend on any assumptions regarding kinetics or structure of matter, but is applicable to all species of molecules, and is sufficiently sensitive to distinguish between optical isomers. The requirements for an analysis are simple, as the equipment needed is basic to most laboratories and the quantities of substances required are small.

The standard solubility method consists of five steps:

1. Mixing, in separate systems, increasing amounts of a substance with measured amounts of a solvent.

2. Establishment of equilibrium for each system at identical constant temperature and pressure.
3. Separation of the solid phase from the solutions.
4. Determination of the concentration of the material dissolved in the various solutions.
5. Plotting the concentration of the dissolved material of interest per unit of solvent (*y*-axis, or solution concentration) against the mass of total material per unit of solvent (*x*-axis or system concentration).

The solubility method has been established on the sound theoretical principles of the Gibbs phase rule: $F = C - P + 2$, which relates C, the number of components; F, the degrees of freedom (pressure, temperature, and concentration); and P, the number of phases for a heterogeneous equilibrium.

Solubility analyses are carried out at constant temperature and pressure, so a pure solid in solution would show only one degree of freedom, because only one phase is present at concentrations below saturation. This is represented by section AB in Figure 16-4. For a pure solid in a saturated solution at equilibrium (Fig 16-4, BC), two phases are present, solid and solution; there is no variation in concentration, and thus, at constant temperature and pressure, no degrees of freedom.

The curve ABC of Figure 16-4 represents the type of solubility diagram obtained for: (1) a pure material, (2) equal amounts of two or more materials having identical solubilities, or (3) a mixture of two or more materials present in the unique ratio of their solubilities. These latter two cases are rare and often may be detected by a change in solvent system.

Line segment BC of Figure 16-4 indicates purity because it has no slope. If, however, this section does exhibit a slope, its numerical value indicates the fraction of impurity present. Line segment BC, extrapolated to the *y*-axis at D, is the actual solubility of the pure substance.

A representative type of solubility curve, which is obtained when a substance contains one impurity, is illustrated in Figure 16-5. Here, at B the solution becomes saturated with one component. From B to C there are two phases present: a solution saturated with Component I (usually the major component) containing also some Component II (usually the minor component), and a solid phase of Component I. The one degree of freedom revealed by the slope of the line segment BC is the concentration of Component II, which is the impurity (usually the minor component). A mixture of d and l isomers could have

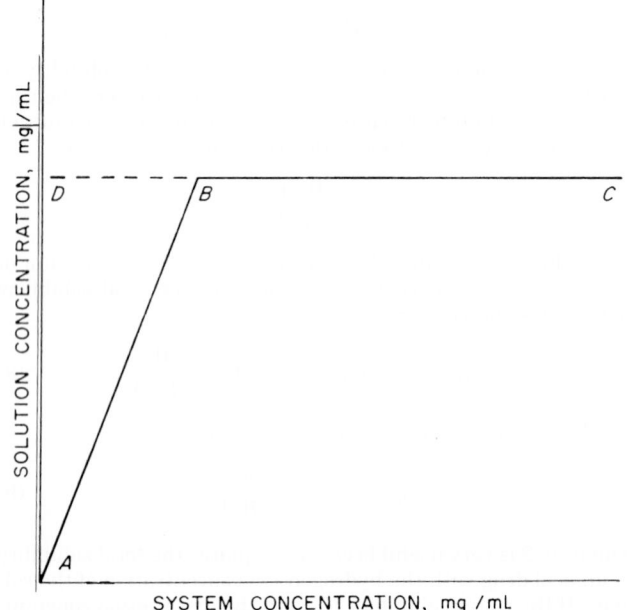

Figure 16-4. Phase-solubility diagram for a pure substance.

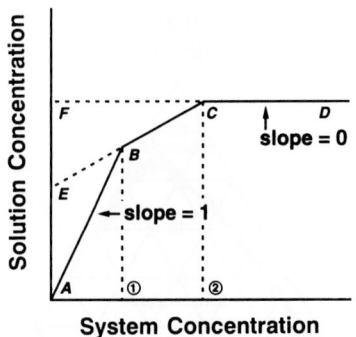

Figure 16-5. Type of solubility curve obtained when a substance contains one impurity.

such a curve, as would any simple mixtures in which the solubilities are independent of each other.

The section *CD* indicates that the solvent is saturated with both components of the two-component mixture. Here, three phases are present: a solution saturated with both components and the two solid phases. No variation of concentration is possible; hence, no degree of freedom is possible (indicated by the lack of slope of section *CD*). The distance *AE* on the ordinate represents the solubility of the major component, and the distance *EF* represents the solubility of the minor component.

The equilibration process is time consuming, requiring as long as 3 weeks in certain cases, but this is offset by the fact that all of the sample can be recovered after a determination. This adds to the general usefulness of the method, particularly in cases where the substance is expensive or difficult to obtain. A use for the method other than the determination of purity or of solubility is to obtain especially pure samples by recovering the solid residues at system concentration, corresponding to points on section *BC* in Figure 16-5. Thus, the method is useful not only as a quantitative analytical tool, but also for purification.

Solutions of Liquids in Liquids

BINARY SYSTEMS—The following types of liquid-pairs may be recognized as binary systems.

1. Those that are soluble completely in each other in all proportions. Examples: alcohol and water, glycerin and water, alcohol and glycerin.
2. Those that are soluble in each other in definite proportions. Examples: phenol and water, ether and water, nicotine and water.
3. Those that are imperceptibly soluble in each other in any proportion. Examples: castor oil and water, liquid petrolatum and water.

The mutual solubility of liquid pairs of Type 2 has been studied extensively and found to show interesting regularities. If a series of tubes containing varying, but known, percentages of phenol and water are heated (or cooled, if necessary) just to the point of formation of a homogeneous solution, and the temperatures at such points is noted, upon plotting the results a curve is obtained similar to that in Figure 16-6. On this graph the area inside the curve represents the region where mixtures of phenol and water will separate into two layers, while in the region outside of the curve homogeneous solutions will be obtained. The maximum temperature on this curve is called the *critical solution temperature,* that is, the temperature above which a homogeneous solution occurs regardless of the composition of the mixture. For phenol and water the critical solution temperature occurs at a composition of 34.5% phenol in water.

Temperature versus composition curves, as depicted in Figure 16-6, provide much useful information in the preparation of homogeneous mixtures of substances showing mutual-solubility behavior. At room temperature (here assumed to be 25°), by drawing a line parallel to the abscissa at 25°, we find that we actually can prepare two sets of homogeneous solutions, one containing from 0% to about 7.5% phenol and the other containing phenol from 72% to about 95% (its limit of solubility). At compositions between 7.5% and 72% phenol at 25° two liquid layers or phases will separate. In sample tubes containing a concentration of phenol in this two-layer region at 25° one layer always will be phenol-rich and always contain 72% phenol while the other layer will be water-rich and always contain 7.5% phenol. These values are obtained by interpolation of the two points of intersection of the line drawn at 25° with the experimental curve.

As it may be deduced, at other temperatures, the composition of the two layers in the two-layer region is determined by the points of intersection of the curve with a line (called the *tie line*) drawn parallel to the abscissa at that temperature. The relative amounts of the two layers or phases, phenol-rich and water-rich in this example, will depend on the concentration of phenol added. As expected, the proportion of phenol-rich layer relative to the water-rich layer increases as the concentration of phenol added increases. For example, at 20% phenol in water at 25°, there would be more of the water-rich layer than of the phenol-rich layer, whereas at 50% phenol in water there would be more of the phenol-rich layer. The relative portion of each layer may be calculated from such tie lines at any temperature and compositions as well as the amount of phenol present in each of the two phases. To determine how these calculations are made and for further discussion of this topic the student should consult Martin et al.[1]

A simple and practical advantage in the use of phase diagrams is pointed Martin et al.[1] Based on diagrams such as Figure 16-6, they point out that the most concentrated stock solution of phenol that should perhaps be used by pharmacists is one containing 76% *w/w* phenol in water (equivalent to 80% *w/v*). At room temperature this mixture is a homogeneous solution and will remain homogeneous to around 3.5°, at which temperature freezing occurs. It should be noted that Liquefied Phenol USP contains 90% *w/w* phenol and freezes at 17°. This means that if the storage area in the pharmacy falls to about 63°F, the preparation will freeze, resulting in a stock solution no longer convenient to use.

In the case of phenol and water, the mutual solubility increases with an increase in temperature and the critical solu-

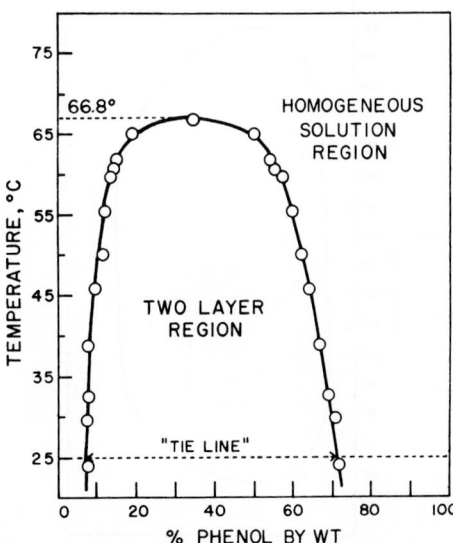

Figure 16-6. Phenol–water solubility. (From Campbell AN, Campbell AJR. *J Am Chem Soc* 1937; 59:2481.)

tion temperature occurs at a relatively high point. In a certain number of cases, however, the mutual solubility increases with decrease in temperature and the critical solution temperature occurs at a relatively low value. Most of the substances that show lower critical solution temperatures are amines as, for example, triethylamine with water.

In addition to pairs of liquids that show *either* upper or lower critical solution temperatures, there are other pairs that show *both* upper and lower critical solution temperatures and the mutual solubility curve is of the closed type. An example of this type of liquid pair is found in the case of nicotine and water (Fig 16-7). Mixtures of nicotine and water represented by points within the curve will separate into two layers, but mixtures represented by points outside of the curve are perfectly miscible with each other.

In a discussion of solutions of liquids in liquids it is evident that the distinction between the terms solute and solvent loses its significance. For example, in a solution of water and glycerin, which shall be considered to be the soluble and which the solvent? Again, when two liquids are only partially soluble in each other, the distinction between solute and solvent might be reversed easily. In such cases the term solvent usually is given to the constituent present in larger quantity.

TERNARY SYSTEMS—The addition of a third liquid to a binary liquid system to produce a ternary or three-component system can result in several possible combinations.

If the third liquid is soluble in only one of the two original liquids or if its solubility in the two original liquids is markedly different, the mutual solubility of the original pair will be decreased. An upper critical solution temperature will be elevated and a lower critical solution temperature lowered. On the other hand, the addition of a liquid having roughly the same solubility in both components of the original pair will result in an increase in their mutual solubility. An upper critical solution temperature then will be lowered and a lower critical solution temperature elevated.

An equilateral-triangle graph may be used to represent ternary systems. In this type of graph, each side of the triangle represents 0% of one of the components and the apex opposite that side represents 100% of that component. This is illustrated using a particularly common ternary system involving two solvents that are completely miscible and a third that is miscible with only one of the two. In Figure 16-8, water and alcohol are the miscible solvents and castor oil is the third solvent that is soluble in alcohol but not in water. Such diagrams could be ap-

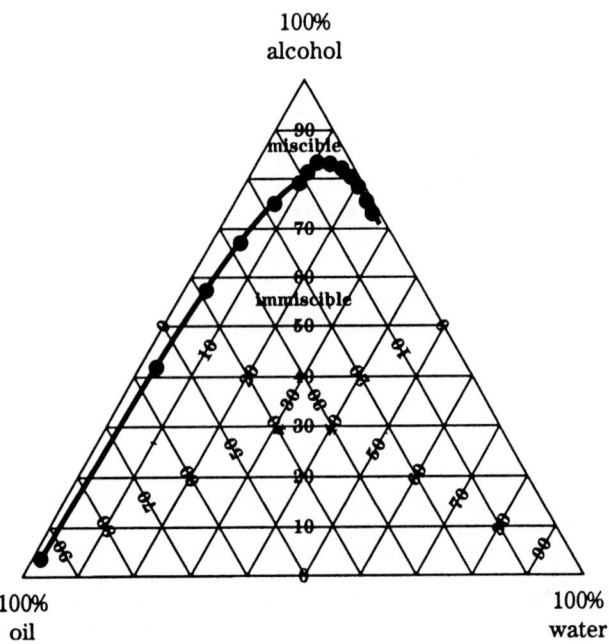

Figure 16-8. Phase diagram at constant temperature for a ternary system: two liquids completely miscible in one another with a third liquid soluble in only one of the two. (Data from Loran MR, Guth EP. *J APhA Sci Ed* 1951; 40:465.)

plied, for example, to surfactant/oil/water systems, flavor/water/alcohol systems, drug/propellant mixture systems, drug/water/propylene glycol systems or any other such system you might think of that would fit into this category.

The data in Figure 16-8 were obtained by determining the amount of water needed to just cloud solutions of oil in alcohol at different concentrations and at room temperature. The percentage of each solvent just clouding the system was then calculated and plotted as shown in the figure. For example, a cloudy solution developed at a mixture of about 67% alcohol, 27% oil, and 6% water. Note that the percentages of the three components must always equal 100%. In the region labeled *miscible*, any combination of the three components will result in a solution. The pharmacist can pick any combination in this region for reasons of taste, safety, stability, or cost. Figure 16-8 is constructed for room temperature; any other temperature would have its own phase diagram. Including temperature as a variable would create a three-dimensional relationship with ternary diagrams such as Figure 16-8 stacked in the *x–y* plane as a function of temperature on the *z*-axis.

Other possibilities exist in ternary liquid systems—for example, those in which two components are completely miscible and the third is partially miscible with each, and that in which all combinations of two of the three components are only partially miscible.

Solutions of Gases in Liquids

Nearly all gases are more or less soluble in liquids. One has but to recall the solubility of carbon dioxide, hydrogen sulfide, or air in water as common examples.

The amount of gas dissolved in a liquid in general follows *Henry's law,* which states that the weight of gas dissolved by a given amount of a liquid at a given temperature is proportional to its pressure. Thus, if the pressure is doubled, twice as much gas will dissolve as at the initial pressure. The extent to which a gas is dissolved in a liquid, at a given temperature, may be expressed in terms of the solubility coefficient, which is the volume of gas measured under the conditions of the experiment

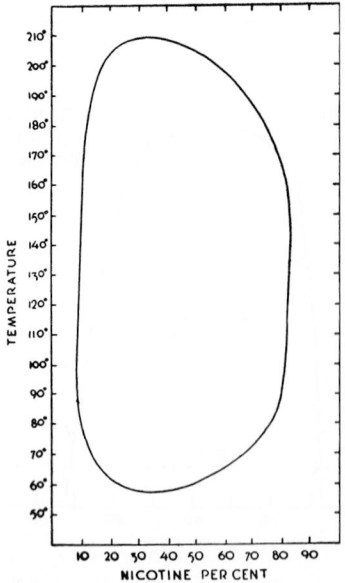

Figure 16-7. Nicotine–water solubility.

that is absorbed by one volume of the liquid. The degree of solubility also is expressed sometimes in terms of the *absorption coefficient,* which is the volume of gas, reduced to standard conditions, dissolved by one volume of liquid under a pressure of one atmosphere.

Although Henry's law expresses fairly accurately the solubility of slightly soluble gases, it deviates considerably in the case of very soluble gases such as hydrogen chloride and ammonia. Such deviations most frequently are due to chemical interaction of solute and solvent.

The solubility of gases in liquids decreases with a rise in temperature and, in general, also when salts are added to the solvent, the latter effect being referred to as the *salting-out* of the gas.

Solutions of gases potentially are dangerous when exposed to warm temperatures because of the liberation and expansion of the dissolved gas, which may cause the container to burst. Bottles containing such solutions (eg, strong ammonia solution) should be cooled before opening, if practical, and the stopper should be covered with a cloth before attempting its removal.

Solutions of Solids in Solids

Various mixtures of one solid in another are being considered in the pharmaceutical sciences primarily as a means to increase bioavailability. For example, melts of solid mixtures of drugs with excipients and eutectic mixtures are being investigated (see Chapter 13). It is possible to have a true solution of one solid in another to give rise to a continuum of one solid dispersed in another as depicted in Figure 16-9. Such a system is referred to as a *continuous* dispersion; it is very rarely found. To achieve this would mean that two materials would have to be of similar size, structure, and interaction energy so that they might enter and occupy a mutual crystalline structure at the molecular level. Hence, such solid solutions may occur only among racemic mixtures of chiral compounds. If it were possible to form a solid solution of a drug in a water-soluble excipient, bioavailability could increase dramatically because the drug would transfer into water as individual molecules.

There are three types of continuous dispersions depicted in Figure 16-9: [1] shows an *ideal* dispersion of constant melting point, while [2] and [3] (*nonideal* solutions) show dispersions having a maximum or minimum, respectively. Each of the latter dispersions show an upper or *liquidus line* and a lower or *solidus line* that might be viewed as representing the direction (cooling or heating) used to arrive at the temperature of melting or solidification in each mixture. The composition of the liquid and solid phases in the region between the two lines can be quantified in a way that is related to the tie-line treatment for phenol-water systems, although more complicated.

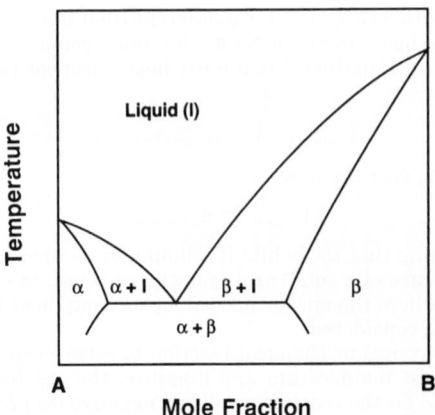

Figure 16-10. Phase diagram for a discontinuous solid solution for Solid *A* and Solid *B*: true solid solutions α and β are separated by a eutectic phase. (Adapted from Grant DJW, Abougela IKA. *Analytical Proceedings: Proceedings of the Analytical Division of the Royal Society of Chemistry.* Dec 1992.)

More common are the *discontinuous* solid dispersions illustrated in Figure 16-10 where two true solid solutions α and β are separated by a eutectic phase. Such a system is found for urea/acetaminophen; which exists as solid solutions in very small regions at very high urea concentration and very high acetaminophen concentration.

At this point it is worthwhile to briefly consider solid complexes. The interaction of a drug with an excipient to form a new solid phase through strong hydrogen-bond formation can give a solid phase that is not precisely a solid solution, but nonetheless potentially important in its effects on bioavailability—both in a positive and negative sense. The phase diagram in Figure 16-11 was obtained by fusing and cooling mixtures of griseofulvin (G) and phenobarbitone (P). When a complex is stable up to its melting point, the liquidus curve shows a peak referred to as a *congruent melting point.* Two congruently melting complexes, PG_3 and P_3G (at $x = 0.25$ and 0.75 in Fig 16-11), are found for the griseofulvin-phenobarbital system.

Thermodynamics of the Solution Process

In this discussion of the thermodynamics of the solution process, the solute is assumed to be in the liquid state, hence, the

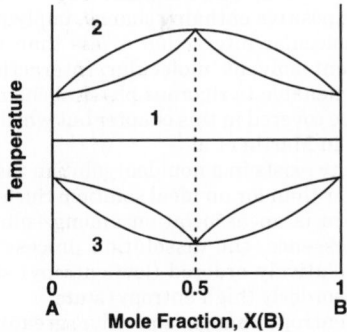

Figure 16-9. Phase diagram for a continuous solution of a Solid *A* in a Solid *B* (or of *B* in *A*: [1] is an ideal solution, [2] and [3], nonideal solutions. (Data from Duddu S. PhD thesis. University of Minnesota, 1993.)

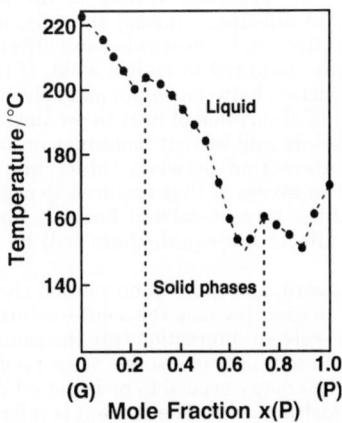

Figure 16-11. Temperature–concentration relationship for fused mixtures of griseofulvin (G) and phenobarbital (P). (Adapted from Grant DJW, Abougela IKA. *Analytical Proceedings: Proceedings of the Analytical Division of the Royal Society of Chemistry.* Dec 1992.)

heat of solution ($\Delta H'$) is a term different from that in Equation 3 (ΔH). The heat of solution for a solid solute going into solution as defined in Equation 3 is the net heat effect for the overall dissolution

$$A_{(solid)} \rightleftarrows A_{(liquid)} \rightleftarrows A_{(solution)}$$

Considering only the process,

$$A_{(liquid)} \rightleftarrows A_{(solution)}$$

and assuming that the solute is a liquid (or a super-cooled liquid in the case of a solid) at a temperature close to room temperature, where the energy needed for melting (heat of fusion) is not being considered.

For a physical or chemical reaction to occur spontaneously at a constant temperature and pressure, the net free-energy change, ΔG, for the reaction should be negative (see *Thermodynamics*, Chapter 15). Furthermore, it is known that the free-energy change depends on heat-related enthalpy ($\Delta H'$) and order-related entropy (ΔS) factors as seen in

$$\Delta G = \Delta H' - T\Delta S \qquad (13)$$

where T is the temperature. Recall also that the relation between free energy and the equilibrium constant, K, for a reaction is given by

$$\Delta G = -1 \, RT \ln K \qquad (14)$$

Equations 13 and 14 certainly apply to the solution of a drug. Because the solubility is, in reality, an equilibrium constant, Equation 14 indicates that the greater the negative value of ΔG, the greater the solubility.

The interplay of these two factors, $\Delta H'$ and ΔS in Equation 13, determines the free-energy change, and hence whether dissolution of a drug will occur spontaneously. Thus, if in the solution process $\Delta H'$ is negative and ΔS positive, dissolution is favored because ΔG will be negative.

As the heat of solution is quite significant in the dissolution process one must look at its origin. (For an excellent and more complete discussion of the interactions and driving forces underlying the dissolution process, see Higuchi.[6]) The mechanism of solubility involves severing of the bonds that hold together the ions or molecules of a solute, the separation of molecules of solvent to create a space in the solvent into which the solute can be fitted and the ultimate response of solute and solvent to whatever forces of interaction may exist between them. In order to sever the bonds between molecules or ions of solute in the liquid state, energy must be supplied, as is the case also when molecules of solvent are to be separated. If heat is the source of energy it is apparent that both processes require the absorption of heat.

Solute–solvent interaction, on the other hand, generally is accompanied by the evolution of heat as the process occurs spontaneously. In effecting solution there is, accordingly, a heat-absorbing effect and a heat-releasing effect to be considered beyond those required to melt a solid. If there is no, or very little, interaction between solute and solvent, the only effect will be that of absorption of heat to produce the necessary separations of solute and solvent molecules or ions. If there is a significant interaction between solute and solvent, the amount of heat in excess of that required to overcome the solute–solute and the solvent–solvent forces is liberated. If the opposing heat effects are equal, there will be no change of temperature.

When $\Delta H'$ is zero, and there is no volume change, an *ideal solution* is said to exist because the solute–solute, solvent–solvent, and solute–solvent interactions are the same. For such an ideal solution, the solubility of a solid can be predicted from its heat of fusion (the energy needed to melt the solid) at temperatures below its melting point. The student is referred to Martin et al[1] to see how this calculation is made.

When the heat of solution has a positive (energy absorbed) or negative (energy liberated) value, the solution is said to be a *nonideal solution*. A negative heat of solution favors solubility while a positive heat works against dissolution.

The magnitude of the various attractive forces involved between solute, solvent, and solute–solvent molecules may vary greatly and thus could lead to varying degrees of positive or negative enthalpy changes in the solution process. The reason for this is that the molecular structure of the various solutes and solvents determining the interactions can themselves vary greatly. For a discussion of these effects, see Martin et al.[1]

The solute–solute interaction that must be overcome can vary from the strong ion–ion interaction (as in a salt), to the weaker dipole–dipole interaction (as in nearly all organic medicinals that are not salts), to the weakest induced dipole–induced dipole interaction (as with naphthalene).

The attractive forces in the solvent that must be overcome are, most frequently, the dipole–dipole interaction (as found in water or acetone) and the induced dipole–induced dipole interaction (as in liquid petrolatum).

The energy-releasing solute–solvent interactions that must be taken into account may be one of four types. In decreasing energy of interaction these are ion–dipole interactions (eg, a sodium ion interacting with water), dipole–dipole interactions (eg, an organic acid dissolved in water), dipole–induced dipole interaction, to be discussed later (eg, an organic acid dissolved in carbon tetrachloride) and induced dipole–induced dipole interactions (eg, naphthalene dissolved in benzene).

Since the energy-releasing solute–solvent interaction should approximate the energy needed to overcome the solute–solute and solvent–solvent interactions, it should be apparent why it is not possible to dissolve a salt like sodium chloride in benzene. The interaction between the ions and benzene does not supply enough energy to overcome the interaction between the ions in the solute and therefore gives rise to a positive heat of solution. On the other hand, the interaction of sodium and chloride ions with water molecules does provide an amount of energy approximating the energy needed to separate the ions in the solute and the molecules in the solvent.

Consideration must next be given to entropy effects in dissolution processes. Entropy is an indicator of the disorder or randomness of a system. The more positive the entropy change (ΔS) is, the greater the degree of randomness or disorder of the reaction system and the more favorably disposed is the reaction. Unlike $\Delta H'$, the entropy change (an entropy of mixing) in an ideal solution, is not zero, but has some positive value as there is an increase in the disorderliness or entropy of the system upon dissolution. Thus, in an ideal solution with $\Delta H'$ zero and ΔS positive, ΔG would have a negative value and the process would therefore be spontaneous.

In a nonideal solution, on the other hand, where $\Delta H'$ is not zero, ΔS can be equal to, greater than, or less than the entropy of mixing found for the ideal solution. A nonideal solution with an entropy of mixing equal to that of the ideal solution is called a *regular solution*. These solutions usually occur with nonpolar or weakly polar solutes and solvents. Such solutions are accompanied by a positive enthalpy change, implying that the solute–solvent molecular interaction is less than the solute–solute and solvent–solvent molecular interactions. Regular solutions are amenable to rigorous physical chemical analysis, which will not be covered in this chapter but which can be found in outline form in Martin et al.[1]

The possibility exists in a nonideal solution that the entropy change is greater than for an ideal solution. Such a solution occurs when there is an association among solute or solvent molecules. In essence, the dissolution process occurs when starting at a relatively ordered (low entropy) state and progressing to a disorderly (high entropy) state.

The overall entropy change is positive, greater than that of the ideal case, and favorable to dissolution. As may be expected, the enthalpy change in such a solution is positive because association in a solute or solvent must be overcome. The facilitated solubility of citric acid (an unsymmetrical molecule), as compared to inositol (a symmetrical molecule), may be explained on the basis of such a favorable entropy change.[6]

The solubility of citric acid is greater than that of inositol, yet on the basis of their heats of solution, inositol should be more soluble. One may regard this phenomenon in another way. The reason for the higher solubility of citric acid is that, although there is no hindrance in the transfer of a citric acid molecule as it goes from the solute to the solution phase, when the structurally unsymmetrical citric acid attempts to return to the solute phase from solution, it must assume an orientation that will allow ready interaction with polar groups already oriented. If it does not have the required orientation, it will not return readily to the solute, but rather will remain in solution, thus bringing about a solubility larger than expected on the basis of heat of solution.

On the other hand, the structurally symmetrical inositol, as it leaves the solution phase, can interact with the solute phase without requiring a definite orientation; all orientations are equivalent. Hence, inositol can enter the solute phase without hindrance, and therefore no facilitation of its solubility is observed. In general, unsymmetrical molecules tend to be more soluble than symmetrical molecules.

Another type of nonideal solution occurs when there is an entropy change less than that expected of an ideal solution.

Such nonideal behavior can occur with polar solutes and solvents. In a nonideal solution of this type there is significant interaction between solute and solvent. As may be expected, the enthalpy change ($\Delta H'$) in such a solution is negative and favors dissolution, but this effect is tempered by the unfavorable entropy change occurring at the same time. The reason for the lower-than-ideal entropy change can be visualized where the equilibrium system is more orderly and has a lower entropy than that expected for an ideal solution. The overall entropy change of solution thus would be less and not favorable to dissolution.

One may rationalize the lower-than-expected solubility of lithium fluoride on the basis of this phenomenon. Compared with other alkali halides, it has a solubility lower than would be expected based solely on enthalpy changes. Because of the small size of ions in this salt there may be considerable ordering of water molecules in the solution. This effect must, of course, lead to a lowered entropy and an unfavorable effect on solubility. The effect of soluble salts on the solubility of nonelectrolytes may be considered as a result of an unfavorable entropy effect (see *Solubility of Solute Containing Two or More Species,* above).

PHARMACEUTICAL SOLVENTS

The discussion will focus now on solvents available to pharmacists and on the properties of these solvents. Pharmacists must obtain an understanding of the possible differences in solubility of a given solute in various solvents because they are often called on to select a solvent that will dissolve the solute. A knowledge of the properties of solvents will allow the intelligent selection of suitable solvents.

On the basis of the forces of interaction occurring in solvents one may broadly classify solvents as one of three types:

1. *Polar solvents*—those made up of strong dipolar molecules having hydrogen bonding (water or hydrogen peroxide).
2. *Semipolar solvents*—those also made up of strong dipolar molecules but that do not form hydrogen bonds (acetone or pentyl alcohol).
3. *Nonpolar solvents*—those made up of molecules having a small or no dipolar character (benzene, vegetable oil, or mineral oil).

Naturally, there are many solvents that may fit into more than one of these broad classes; for example, chloroform is a weak dipolar compound but generally is considered nonpolar in char-

acter, and glycerin could be considered a polar or semipolar solvent even though it is capable of forming hydrogen bonds.

Solvent Types

WATER—Water is a unique solvent. Besides being a highly associated liquid, giving rise to its high boiling point, it has another very important property, a high dielectric constant. The *dielectric constant* (ε) indicates the effect that a substance has, when it acts as a medium, on the ease with which two oppositely charged ions may be separated. The ease of solubilizing salts in solvents like water and glycerin can be explained on the basis of their high dielectric constant. Also, in general, the more polar the solvent, the greater its dielectric constant.

An important concept has been introduced to pharmaceutical systems: pharmacists frequently are concerned with dissolving relatively nonpolar drugs in aqueous or mixed polar aqueous solvents.[11] To understand what may be happening in such cases, factors concerned with the entropic effects arising from interactions originating with the nonpolar solutes must be considered. Previously it had been noted that the favorable entropic effect on dissolution was due to the disruption of associations occurring among solute or solvent molecules. Now consider the effects on solubility due to solute interactions in the solution phase—because the solutes under discussion are relatively nonpolar, the interactions are of the London Force type or a *hydrophobic association.*

This hydrophobic association in aqueous solutions may cause significant structuring of water with a resultant ordered or low-entropy system that is unfavorable to solution. Therefore, the solution of an essentially nonpolar molecular in water is not a favorable process. It should be stressed that this is due to not only an unfavorable enthalpy change but also an unfavorable entropy change generated by water structuring.

Such an unfavorable entropy change, known as the *hydrophobic effect,* is quite significant in the solution process. As an example of this effect, the aqueous solubility of a series of alkyl *p*-aminobenzoates shows a 10-million-fold decrease in solubility in going from the 1-carbon analog to the 12-carbon analog. These findings demonstrate clearly the considerable effect that hydrophobic associations can have.

ALCOHOLS—*Ethanol,* as a solvent, is next in importance to water. An advantage of ethanol is that growth of microorganisms does not occur in solutions containing alcohol in a reasonable concentration.

Resins, volatile oils, alkaloids, glycosides, etc are dissolved by alcohol, but many therapeutically inert principles, such as gums, albumin, and starch, are insoluble, which makes it more useful as a *selective* solvent. Mixtures of water and alcohol, in proportions varying to suit specific cases, are used extensively. They are often referred to as *hydroalcoholic solvents.*

Glycerin is an excellent solvent, although its range is not as extensive as that of water or alcohol. In higher concentrations it has preservative action. It dissolves the fixed alkalies, a large number of salts, vegetable acids, pepsin, tannin, and some active principles of plants, but it also dissolves gums, soluble carbohydrates, and starch. It also is of special value as a simple solvent (as in phenol glycerite), or where the major portion of the glycerin simply is added as a preservative and stabilizer of solutions that have been prepared with other solvents (see *Glycerines,* Chapter 41).

Propylene glycol, which has been used widely as a substitute for glycerin, is miscible with water, acetone, or chloroform in all proportions. It is soluble in ether and will dissolve many essential oils but is immiscible with fixed oils. It is claimed to be as effective as ethyl alcohol in its power of inhibiting mold growth and fermentation.

Isopropyl alcohol possesses solvent properties similar to those of ethyl alcohol and is used instead of the latter in a number of pharmaceutical manufacturing operations. It has the advantage in that the commonly available product contains not over 1% of water, whereas ethyl alcohol contains about 5% water, often a disadvantage. Isopropyl alcohol is employed in some liniment and lotion formulations. It cannot be taken internally.

General Properties—Low-molecule-weight and polyhydroxy alcohol forms associated structures through hydrogen bonds just as in water. When the carbon-atom content of an alcohol rises above five, generally only monomers then are present in the pure solvent. Although alcohols have high dielectric constants compared to other types of solvents, they are small compared to water. As has been discussed, the solubility of salts in a solvent should be paralleled by its dielectric constant. That is, as the dielectric constant of a series of solvents increases, the probability of dissolving a salt in the solvent increases. This behavior is observed for the alcohols. Table 16-2, taken from Higuchi,[6] shows how the solubility of salts follows the dielectric constant of the alcohols.

As mentioned earlier, absolute alcohol rarely is used pharmaceutically. However, hydroalcoholic mixtures such as elixirs and spirits frequently are encountered. A very useful generalization is that the dielectric properties of a mixed solvent, such as water and alcohol, can be approximated as the weighted average of the properties of the pure components. Thus, a mixture of 60% alcohol (by weight) in water should have a dielectric constant approximated by

$$\varepsilon_{(mixture)} = 0.6(\varepsilon_{(alcohol)}) + 0.4(\varepsilon_{(water)})$$

$$\varepsilon_{(mixture)} = 0.6(25) + 0.4(80) = 47$$

The dielectric constant of 60% alcohol in water is found experimentally to be 43, which is in close agreement with that just calculated. The dielectric constant of glycerin is 46, close to the 60% alcohol mixture. One would therefore expect a salt like sodium chloride to have about the same solubility in glycerin as in 60% alcohol. The solubility of sodium chloride in glycerin is 8.3 g/100 g of solvent and in 60% alcohol about 6.3 g/100 g of solvent. This agreement would be even closer if comparisons were made on a volume rather than weight basis. At least qualitatively it can be said that the solubility of a salt in a solvent or a mixed solvent closely follows the dielectric constant of the medium, or conversely that the polarity of mixed solvents is paralleled by their dielectric constant, based on salt solubility.

Although the dielectric constant is useful in interpreting the effect of mixed solvents on salt solubility, it cannot be applied properly to the effect of mixed solvents on the solubility of nonelectrolytes. It was seen earlier that unfavorable entropic effects can occur upon dissolution of relatively nonpolar nonelectrolytes in water. Such an effect due to hydrophobic association considerably affects solubility. Yalkowsky[11] studied the ability of cosolvent systems to increase the solubility of nonelectrolytes in polar solvents where the cosolvent system essentially brings about a reduction in structuring of solvent. Thus, by increasing, in a positive sense, the entropy of solution by using cosolvents,

it was possible to increase the solubility of the nonpolar molecule. Using as an example the solubility of alkyl *p*-aminobenzoates in propylene glycol-water systems, Yalkowsky reported that it is possible to increase the solubility of the nonelectrolyte by several orders of magnitude by increasing the fraction of propylene glycol in the aqueous system.[8] Sometimes, it is found that, as a good first approximation, the logarithm of the solubility is related linearly to the fraction of propylene glycol added by

$$\log S_f = \log S_{f=0} + \varepsilon f$$

where S_f is the solubility in the mixed aqueous system containing the volume fraction f of nonaqueous cosolvent, $S_{f=0}$ is the solubility in water, and ε is a constant (not dielectric constant) characteristic of the system under study. Specifically, when a 50% solution of prolyene glycol in water is used, there is a 1000-fold increase in solubility of dodecyl *p*-aminobenzoate, in comparison to pure water.

Another empirical equation sometimes used to estimate solubility of a poorly water-soluble substance in a mixed-solvent system is written as

$$\log S_t = \log S_w \times f_w + \log S_1 \times f_1 + \dots$$

where S_t is the total solubility, S_w and S_1 are solubilities in pure water and cosolvent 1, respectively, and f_w and f_1 are the fractions of water and cosolvent 1, respectively.

In a series of studies, Martin et al[9] have made attempts to predict solubility in mixed solvent systems through an extension of the *regular solution* theory. The equations are logarithmic in nature and can reduce in form to the equations of Yalkowsky.[8]

ACETONE AND RELATED SEMIPOLAR MATERIALS—Even though acetone has a very high dipole moment (2.8×10^{-18} esu), as a pure solvent it does not form associated structures. This is evidenced by its low boiling point (57°) in comparison with the boiling point of the lower molecular weight water (100°) and ethanol (79°). The reason why it does not associate is because the positive charge in its dipole does not reside in a hydrogen atom, precluding the possibility of its forming a hydrogen bond. However, if some substance that is capable of forming hydrogen bonds, such as water or alcohol, is added to acetone, a very strong interaction through hydrogen bonding will occur (see *Mechanism of Solvent Action*, below). Some substances that are semipolar and similar to acetone are aldehydes, low-molecular-weight esters, other ketones, and nitro-containing compounds.

NONPOLAR SOLVENTS—The nonpolar class of solvents includes fixed oils such as vegetable oil, and petroleum either (ligroin), carbon tetrachloride, benzene, and chloroform. On a relative basis there is a wide range of polarity among these solvents; for example, benzene has no dipole moment whereas that of chloroform is 1.05×10^{-18} esu.

It should be emphasized that when a solvent (such as chloroform) has highly electronegative halogen atoms attached to a carbon atom that also contains at least one hydrogen atom, such a solvent will be capable of forming strong hydrogen bonds with solutes which are polar in character. Thus, through the formation of hydrogen bonds such solvents will dissolve polar solutes. For example, it is possible to dissolve alkaloids in chloroform.

Mechanism of Solvent Action

A solvent may function in one or more ways. When an ionic salt is dissolved (eg, by water), the process of solution involves separation of the cations and anions of the salt with attendant orientation of molecules of the solvent about the ions. Such orientation of solvent molecules about the ions of the solute—a process called *solvation* (*hydration*, if the solvent is water)—is possible only when the solvent is highly polar, whereby the dipoles of the solvent are attracted to and held by the ions of the

Table 16-2. Solubilities of Potassium Iodide and Sodium Chloride in Several Alcohols and Acetone[a]

SOLVENT	g KI/100 g SOLVENT	g NACL/100 g SOLVENT
Water	148	35.9
Glycerin	…	8.3 (20°)
Propylene glycol	50	7.1 (30°)
Methanol	17	1.4
Acetone	2.9	…
Ethanol	1.88	0.065
1-Propanol	0.44	0.0124
2-Propanol	0.18	0.003
1-Butanol	0.2	0.005
1-Pentanol	0.089	0.0018

[a] All measurements are at 25° unless otherwise indicated.
Data from Duddu S. PhD thesis. University of Minnesota, 1993.

solute. The solvent also must possess the ability to keep the solvated, charged ions apart with minimal energy.

A polar liquid such as water may exhibit solvent action also by virtue of its ability to break a covalent bond in the solute and bring about ionization of the latter. For example, hydrogen chloride dissolves in water and functions as an acid as a result of

$$HCl + H_2O \rightarrow H_3O^+ + Cl^-$$

The ions formed by this preliminary reaction of breaking the covalent bond are subsequently maintained in solution by the same mechanism as ionic salts.

Still another mechanism by which a polar liquid may act as a solvent is that involved when the solvent and solute are capable of being coupled through hydrogen-bond formation.

The solubility of the low-molecular-weight alcohols in water, for example, is attributed to the ability of the alcohol molecules to become part of a water–alcohol association complex.

$$\begin{array}{cccc} H & R & H & R \\ | & | & | & | \\ H-O----H-O----H-O----H-O \end{array}$$

As the molecular weight of the alcohol increases, it becomes progressively less polar and less able to compete with water molecules for a place in the lattice-like arrangement formed through hydrogen bonding; high-molecular-weight alcohols are, therefore, poorly soluble or insoluble in water. When the number of carbon atoms in a normal alcohol reaches five, its solubility in water is reduced materially.

When the number of hydroxyl groups in the alcohol is increased, its solubility in water generally is increased greatly; it is principally, if not entirely, for this reason that such high-molecular-weight compounds as sugars, gums, and many glycosides, and synthetic compounds such as the polyethylene glycols, are very soluble in water.

The solubility of ethers, aldehydes, ketones, acids, and anhydrides in water and in other polar solvents also is attributable largely to the formation of an association complex between solute and solvent by means of the hydrogen bond. The molecules of ethers, aldehydes, and ketones, unlike those of alcohols, are not associated themselves, because of the absence of a hydrogen atom that is capable of forming the characteristic hydrogen bond. Notwithstanding, these substances are more or less polar because of the presence of a strongly electronegative oxygen atom, which is capable of association with water through hydrogen-bond formation.

Acetone, for example, dissolves in water, in all likelihood principally because of the following type of association:

$$\begin{array}{c} H \\ | \\ (CH_3)_2CO + H_2O \rightarrow (CH_3)_2CO \cdots H-O \end{array}$$

The maximum number of carbon atoms that may be present per molecule possessing a hydrogen-bondable group, while still retaining water solubility, is approximately the same as for the alcohols.

Although nitrogen is less electronegative than oxygen, and thus tends to form weaker hydrogen bonds, amines are at least as soluble as alcohols containing an equivalent chain length. The reason for this is that alcohols form two hydrogen bonds with a net interaction of 12 kcal/mol. Primary amines can form three hydrogen bonds; two amine protons are shared with the oxygens of two water molecules, and the nitrogen accepts one water proton. The net interaction for the primary amine is between 12 and 13 kcal/mol; hence, it shows an equal or greater solubility compared with corresponding alcohols.

The solvent action of nonpolar liquids involves a somewhat different mechanism. Because they are unable to form dipoles with which to overcome the attractions between ions of an ionic salt, or to break a covalent bond to produce an ionic compound or form association complexes with a solute, nonpolar liquids

are incapable of dissolving polar compounds. They only can dissolve, in general, other nonpolar substances in which the bonds between molecules are weak. The forces involved usually are of the induced dipole–induced dipole type. Such is the case when one hydrocarbon is dissolved in another, or an oil or a fat is dissolved in petroleum ether.

Sometimes it is observed that a polar substance, such as alcohol, will dissolve in a nonpolar liquid, such as benzene. This apparent exception to the preceding generalization may be explained by the assumption that the alcohol molecule induces a temporary dipole in the benzene molecule which forms an association complex with the solvent molecules. A binding force of this kind is referred to as a *permanent dipole–induced dipole force*.

SOME USEFUL GENERALIZATIONS—The preceding discussion indicates that enough is known about the mechanism of solubility to be able to formulate some generalizations concerning this important physical property of substances. Because of the greater importance of organic substances in the field of medicinal chemistry, certain of the more useful generalizations about organic chemicals are presented here in summary form. However, it should be remembered that the phenomenon of solubility usually involves several variables, and there may be exceptions to general rules.

One general maxim that holds true in most instances is, the greater the structural similarity between solute and solvent, the greater the solubility. As often stated to the student, *like dissolves like*. Thus, phenol is almost insoluble in petroleum ether but is very soluble in glycerin.

Organic compounds containing polar groups capable of forming hydrogen bonds with water are soluble in water, provided that the molecular weight of the compound is not too great. It is demonstrated easily that the polar groups OH, CHO, COH, CHOH, CH_2OH, COOH, NO_2, CO, NH_2, and SO_3H tend to increase the solubility of an organic compound in water. On the other hand, nonpolar or very weak polar groups, such as the various hydrocarbon radicals, reduce solubility; the greater the number of carbon atoms in the radical, the greater the decrease in solubility. Introduction of halogen atoms into a molecule in general tends to decrease solubility because of an increased molecular weight without a proportionate increase in polarity.

The greater the number of polar groups contained per molecule, the greater the solubility of a compound, provided that the size of the rest of the molecule is not altered; thus, pyrogallol is much more soluble in water than phenol. The *relative positions* of the groups in the molecule also influence solubility; thus, in water, resorcinol (*m*-dihydroxybenzene) is more soluble than catechol (*o*-dihydroxybenzene), and the latter is more soluble than hydroquinone (*p*-dihydroxybenzene).

Polymers and compounds of high molecular weight can be poorly soluble.

High melting points frequently are indicative of low solubility for organic compounds. One reason for high melting points

Table 16-3. Demonstration of Solubility Rules

CHEMICAL COMPOUND	SOLUBILITY[a]
Aniline, $C_6H_5NH_2$	28.6
Benzene, C_6H_6	1430.0
Benzoic acid, C_6H_5COOH	275.0
Benzyl alcohol $C_6H_5CH_2OH$	25.0
1-Butanol, C_4H_9OH	12.0
t-Butyl alcohol, $(CH_3)_3COH$	Miscible
Carbon tetrachloride, CCl_4	2000.0
Chloroform, $CHCl_3$	200.0
Fumaric acid (*trans*-butenedioic acid)	150.0
Hydroquinone, $C_6H_4(OH)_2$	14.0
Maleic acid, *cis*-butenedioic acid	5.0
Phenol, C_6H_5OH	15.0
Pyrocatechol, $C_6H_4(OH)_2$	2.3
Pyrogallol, $C_6H_3(OH)_3$	1.7
Resorcinol, $C_6H_4(OH)_2$	0.9

[a] The number of mL of water required to dissolve 1 g of solute.

is the association of molecules, and this cohesive force tends to prevent dispersion of the solute in the solvent.

The *cis* form of an isomer is more soluble than the *trans* form (Table 16-3).

Solvation, which is evidence of the existence of a strong attractive force between solute and solvent, enhances the solubility of the solute, provided there is not a marked ordering of the solvent molecules in the solution phase.

Acids, especially strong acids, usually produce water-soluble salts when reacted with nitrogen-containing organic bases.

COLLIGATIVE PROPERTIES OF SOLUTIONS

Up to this point our concern has been with dissolving a solute in a solvent. Once the dissolution has been brought about, naturally the solution has a number of properties that are different from that of the pure solvent. Of very great importance are the colligative properties that a solution possesses.

The *colligative properties* of a solution are those that depend on the number of solute particles in solution, irrespective of whether these are molecules or ions, large or small. Ideally, the effect of a solute particle of one species is considered to be the same as that of an entirely different kind of particle, at least in dilute solution. Practically, there may be differences that may become substantial as the concentration of the solution is increased.

The colligative properties that will be considered are

1. Osmotic pressure.
2. Vapor-pressure lowering.
3. Boiling-point elevation.
4. Freezing-point depression.

Of these four, all of which are related, osmotic pressure has the greatest direct importance in the pharmaceutical sciences. It is the property that largely determines the physiological acceptability of a variety of solutions used for therapeutic purposes.

Osmotic-Pressure Elevation

OSMOSIS—The phenomenon of osmosis is based on the fact that substances tend to move or diffuse from regions of higher concentration to regions of lower concentration. When a solution is separated from the solvent by means of a membrane that is permeable to the solvent but not to the solute (such a membrane is referred to as a *semipermeable* membrane), it is possible to demonstrate visibly the diffusion of solvent into the concentrated solution, as volume changes will occur. In a similar manner, if two solutions of different concentration are separated by a membrane, the solvent will move from the solution of lower solute concentration to the solution of higher solute concentration. This diffusion of solvent through a membrane is called *osmosis.*

There is a difference between the activity or escaping tendency of the water molecules found in the solvent and salt solution separated by the semipermeable membrane. Because *activity,* which is related to water concentration, is higher on the pure solvent side, water moves from solvent to solution in order to equalize *escaping-tendency* differences. The difference in escaping-tendency gives rise to what is referred to as the *osmotic pressure* of the solution, which might be visualized as follows. A semipermeable membrane is placed over the end of a tube and a small amount of salt solution placed over the membrane in the tube. The tube then is immersed in a trough of pure water so that the upper level of the salt solution initially is at the same level as the water in the trough. With time, solvent molecules will move from solvent into the tube. The height of the solution will rise until the *hydrostatic pressure* exerted by the column of solution is equal to the *osmotic pressure.*

OSMOTIC PRESSURE OF NONELECTROLYTES—Quantitative studies using solutions of varying concentration of a solute that does not ionize have demonstrated that osmotic pressure is proportional to the concentration of the solute; that is, twice the concentration of a given nonelectrolyte will produce twice the osmotic pressure in a given solvent. (This is not strictly true in solutions of fairly high solute concentration, but does hold quite well for dilute solutions.)

Furthermore, the osmotic pressures of solutions of different nonelectrolytes are proportional to the number of molecules in each solution. Stated in another manner, the osmotic pressures of two nonelectrolyte solutions of the same molal concentration are identical. Thus, a solution containing 34.2 g of sucrose (mol wt 342) in 1000 g of water has the same osmotic pressure as a solution containing 18.0 g of anhydrous dextrose (mol wt 180) in 1000 g of water. These solutions are said to be *iso-osmotic* (*isosmotic*) with each other because they have identical osmotic pressures.

OSMOTIC PRESSURE OF ELECTROLYTES—In discussing the generalizations concerning the osmotic pressure of solutions of nonelectrolytes it was stated that the osmotic pressures of two solutions of the same molal concentration are identical. This generalization, however, cannot be made for solutions of electrolytes—acids, alkalies, and salts (see Chapter 17).

For example, sodium chloride is assumed to ionize as

$$NaCl \rightarrow Na^+ + Cl^-$$

It is evident that each molecule of sodium chloride that ionizes produces two ions; if sodium chloride is completely ionized, there will be twice as many particles as would be the case if it were not ionized at all. Furthermore, if each ion has the same effect on osmotic pressure as a molecule, it might be expected that the osmotic pressure of the solution would be twice that of a solution containing the same molal concentration of nonionizing substance.

For solutions that yield more than two ions—for example,

$$K_2SO_4 \rightarrow 2K^+ + SO_4^{2-}$$

$$FeCl_3 \rightarrow Fe^{3+} + 3Cl^-$$

it is expected that the complete dissociation of the molecules would give rise to osmotic pressures that are three and four times, respectively, the pressure of solutions containing an equivalent quantity of a nonionized solute. Accordingly, the equation $PV = nRT$, which may be employed to calculate the osmotic pressure of a dilute solution of a nonelectrolyte, also may be applied to dilute solutions of electrolytes if it is changed to $PV = inRT$, where the value of i approaches the number of ions produced by the ionization of the stronger electrolytes cited in the preceding examples. For weak electrolytes i represents the total number of particles, ions, and molecules together in the solution, divided by the number of molecules that would be present if the solute did not ionize. The experimental evidence indicates that at least in dilute solutions the osmotic pressures approach the predicted values. It should be emphasized, however, that in more concentrated solutions of electrolytes the deviations from this simple theory are considerable, due to interionic attraction, solvation, and other factors.

BIOLOGICAL ASPECTS OF OSMOTIC PRESSURE—Osmotic pressure experiments were made as early as 1884 by the Dutch botanist Hugo de Vries in his study of *plasmolysis,* the term applied to the contraction of the contents of plant cells placed in solutions of comparatively high osmotic pressure. The phenomenon is caused by the osmosis of water out of the cell through the practically semipermeable membrane surrounding the protoplasm. If suitable cells (eg, the epidermal cells of the leaf of *Tradescanta discolor*) are placed in a solution of higher osmotic pressure than that of the cell contents, water flows out of the cell, causing the contents to draw away from the cell wall. On the other hand, if the cells are placed in solutions of lower osmotic pressure, water enters the cell, producing an expansion that is limited by the rigid cell wall. By immersing cells in a series of solutions of varying solute concentration, a solution may be found in which plasmolysis is barely detectable or absent. The osmotic pressure of such a solution is then the same, or very nearly the same, as that of the cell contents, and it is then said that the solution is *isotonic* with the cell contents. Solutions of greater concentration than this are said to be *hypertonic,* and solutions of lower concentration are called *hypotonic.*

Red blood cells, or erythrocytes, have been studied similarly by immersion into solutions of varying concentration of different solutes.[10] When introduced into water or into sodium chloride solutions containing less than 0.90 g of solute per 100 mL, human erythrocytes swell, and often burst, because of the diffusion of water into the cell and the fact that the cell wall is not sufficiently strong to resist the pressure. This phenomenon is referred to as *hemolysis.* If the cells are placed in solutions containing more than 0.90 g of sodium chloride per 100 mL, they lose water and shrink. By immersing the cells in a solution containing exactly 0.90 g of sodium chloride in 100 mL, no change in the size of the cells is observed; because in this solution the cells maintain their *tone,* the solution is said to be *isotonic* with human erythrocytes. For the reasons indicated it is desirable that solutions to be injected into the blood should be made isotonic with erythrocytes. The manner in which this may be done is described in Chapter 18.

DISTINCTION BETWEEN ISO-OSMOTIC (ISOSMOTIC) AND ISOTONIC—The terms *isosmotic* and *isotonic* are not to be considered as equivalent, although a solution often may be described as being both isosmotic and isotonic. If a plant or animal cell is in contact with a solution that has the same osmotic pressure as the cell contents, there will be no net gain or loss of water by either solution provided the cell membrane is impermeable to all the solutes present. As the volume of the cell contents remains unchanged, the *tone,* or normal state, of the cell is maintained, and the solution in contact with the cell may be described not only as being isosmotic with the solution in the cell, but also as being isotonic with it. If, however, one or more of the solutes in contact with the membrane can pass through the latter, it is evident that the volume of the cell contents will change, thus altering the tone of the cell; in this case the two solutions may be isosmotic, yet not be isotonic.

Vapor-Pressure Lowering

When a nonvolatile solute is dissolved in a liquid solvent the vapor pressure of the solvent is lowered. This easily can be described qualitatively by visualizing solvent molecules on the surface of the solvent, which normally could escape into the vapor, being replaced by solute molecules which have little if any vapor pressure of their own. For ideal solutions of nonelectrolytes the vapor pressure of the solution follows Raoult's law

$$P_A = X_A P_A^0 \qquad (15)$$

where P_A is the vapor pressure of the solution, P_A^0 is the vapor pressure of the pure solvent, and X_A is the mol fraction of solvent. This relationship states that the vapor pressure of the solution is proportional to the number of molecules of solvent in the solution. Rearranging Equation 15 gives

$$\frac{P_A^0 - P_A}{P_A^0} = (1 - X_A)X_B \qquad (16)$$

where X_B is the mole fraction of the solute. This equation states that the lowering of vapor pressure in the solution relative to the vapor pressure of the pure solvent—called simply the *relative vapor-pressure lowering*—is equal to the mol fraction of the solute. The *absolute lowering* of vapor pressure of the solution is defined by

$$P_A^0 - P_A = X_B P_A^0 \qquad (17)$$

Example Calculate the lowering of vapor pressure and the vapor pressure at 20°, of a solution containing 50 g of anhydrous dextrose (mol wt 180.16) in 1000 g of water (mol wt 18.02). The vapor pressure of water at 20°, in absence of air, is 17.535 mm.

First calculate the lowering of vapor pressure, using Equation 17 in which X_B is the mol fraction of dextrose, defined by

$$X_B = \frac{n_B}{n_A + n_B}$$

where n_A is the number of mols of solvent and n_B is the number of mols of solute. Substituting numerical values

$$n_B = \frac{50}{180.2} = 0.278$$

$$n_A = \frac{1000}{18.02} = 55.5$$

$$X_B = \frac{0.278}{55.5 + 0.278} = 0.00498$$

the lowering of vapor pressure is

$$P_A^0 - P_A = 0.00498 \times 17.535$$

$$= 0.0873 \text{ mm}$$

The vapor pressure of the solution is

$$P_A = 17.535 - 0.0873$$

$$= 17.448 \text{ mm}$$

Boiling-Point Elevation

In consequence of the fact that the vapor pressure of any solution of a nonvolatile solute is less than that of the solvent, the *boiling point* of the solution—the temperature at which the vapor pressure is equal to the applied pressure (commonly 760 mm)—must be higher than that of the solvent. This is clearly evident in Figure 16-12.

Freezing-Point Depression

The *freezing point of a solvent* is defined as the temperature at which the solid and liquid forms of the solvent coexist in equilibrium at a fixed external pressure, commonly 1 atmosphere (1 atm = 760 mm [torr] of mercury). At this temperature the solid and liquid forms of the solvent must have the same vapor

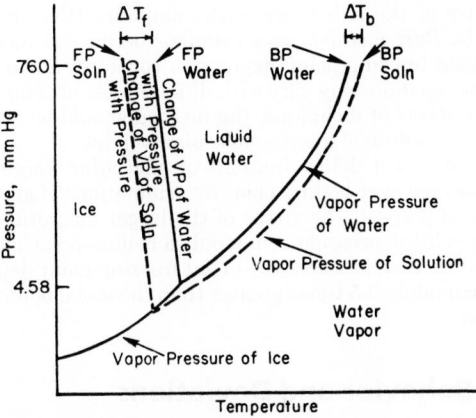

Figure 16-12. Vapor-pressure–temperature diagram for water and an aqueous solution, illustrating elevation of boiling point and lowering of freezing point of the latter.

pressure, for if this were not so, the form having the higher vapor pressure would change into that having the lower vapor pressure.

The *freezing point of a solution* is the temperature at which the solid form of the pure solvent coexists in equilibrium with the solution at a fixed external pressure, again commonly 1 atm. Because the vapor pressure of a solution is lower than that of its solvent, it is obvious that solid solvent and solution cannot coexist at the same temperature as solid solvent and liquid solvent; only at some lower temperature, where solid solvent and solution do have the same vapor pressure, is equilibrium established. A schematic pressure-temperature diagram for water and an aqueous solution, not drawn to scale and exaggerated for the purpose of more effective illustration, shows the equilibrium conditions involved in both freezing-point depression and boiling-point elevation (see Fig 16-12).

The freezing-point lowering of a solution may be quantitatively predicted for ideal solutions, or dilute solutions that obey Raoult's law, by mathematical operations similar to (though somewhat more complex than) those used in deriving the boiling-point elevation constant. The equation for the freezing-point lowering, ΔT_f, is

$$\Delta T_f = \frac{RT_0^2 M_A m}{1000 \Delta H_{fus}} = K_f m \tag{18}$$

where

$$K_f = \frac{RT_0^2 M_A}{1000 \Delta H_{fus}} \tag{19}$$

The value of K_f for water, which freezes at 273.1°K and has a heat of fusion of 79.7 cal/g, is

$$K_f = \frac{1.987 \times 273.1^2 \times 18.02}{1000 \times 18.02 \times 79.7} = 1.86° \tag{20}$$

The molal freezing-point depression constant is not intended to represent the freezing-point depression for a 1-molal solution, which is too concentrated for the premise of ideal behavior to be applicable. In dilute solutions the freezing-point depression, calculated to a 1-molal basis, approaches the theoretical value—the more dilute the solution, the better the agreement between experiment and theory.

To calculate the molecular weight of the solute, the freezing point of a dilute solution of a nonelectrolyte solute may be used (as was the boiling point). The applicable equation is

$$M_B = \frac{K_f 1000 w_B}{w_A \Delta T_f} \tag{21}$$

The molecular weight of organic substances soluble in molten camphor may be determined by observing the freezing point of a mixture of the substance with camphor. This procedure, called the *Rast method*, uses camphor because it has a very large molal freezing-point–depression constant, about 40. Because the *constant* may vary with different lots of camphor and with variations of technique, the method should be standardized using a solute of known molecular weight.

Freezing-point determinations of molecular weights have the advantage over boiling-point determinations of greater accuracy and precision by virtue of the larger magnitude of the freezing-point depression compared to boiling-point elevation. Thus, in the case of water the molal freezing-point depression is approximately 3.5 times greater than the molal boiling-point elevation.

Ideal Behavior and Deviations

In setting out to derive mathematical expressions for colligative properties, such phrases as for *ideal solutions* or for *dilute solutions* were used to indicate the limitations of the expressions. Samuel Glasstone defines an ideal solution as "one which obeys Raoult's law over the whole range of concentration and at all temperatures" and gives as specific characteristics of such solutions their formation only from constituents that mix in the liquid state without heat change and without volume change. These characteristics reflect the fact that addition of a solute to a solvent produces no change in the forces between molecules of the solvent. Thus, the molecules have the same escaping-tendency in the solution as in the pure solvent and the vapor pressure above the solution is proportional to the ratio of the number of solvent molecules in the surface of the solution to the number of the solvent molecules in the surface of the solvent—which is the basis for Raoult's law.

Any change in intermolecular forces produced by mixing the components of a solution may result in deviation from ideality; such a deviation may be expected particularly in solutions containing both a polar and a nonpolar substance. Solutions of electrolytes, except at high dilution, are especially prone to depart from ideal behavior, even though allowance is made for the additional particles that result from ionization. When solute and solvent combine to form solvates, the escaping-tendency of the solvent may be reduced in consequence of the reduction in the number of free molecules of solvent; thus, a negative deviation from Raoult's law is introduced. On the other hand, the escaping-tendency of the solvent in a solution of nonvolatile solute may be increased, because the cohesive forces between molecules of solvent are reduced by the solute; this results in a positive deviation from Raoult's law. Chapter 17 considers deviations from ideality in more detail.

Although few solutions exhibit ideal behavior over a wide range of concentration, most solutions behave ideally at least in high dilution, where deviations from Raoult's law are negligible.

COLLIGATIVE PROPERTIES OF ELECTROLYTE SOLUTIONS (See Chapter 17)—Earlier in this chapter attention was directed to the increased osmotic pressure observed in solutions of electrolytes, the enhanced effect being attributed to the presence of ions, each of which acts, in general, in the same way as a molecule in developing osmotic pressure. Similar magnification of vapor-pressure lowering, boiling-point elevation, and freezing-point depression occurs in solutions of electrolytes. Thus, at a given constant temperature the abnormal effect of an electrolyte on osmotic pressure is paralleled by abnormal lowering of vapor pressure; the other colligative properties are (subject to variation of effect with temperature) comparably intensified. In general, the magnitude of each colligative property is proportional to the total number of particles (molecules and/or ions) in solution.

While in *very* dilute solutions the osmotic pressure, vapor-pressure lowering, boiling-point increase, and freezing-point depression of solutions of electrolytes would approach values two, three, and four times greater for NaCl, Na_2SO_4, and Na_3PO_4 than in solutions of the same molality of a nonelectrolyte, two other effects are observed as the concentration of electrolyte is increased. The first effect results in less than 2-, 3-, or 4-fold intensification of a colligative property. This reduction is ascribed to interionic attraction between the positively and negatively charged ions. Consequently, the ions are not completely dissociated from each other and do not exert their full effect in lowering vapor pressure, etc. This deviation generally increases with increasing concentration of electrolyte. The second effect intensifies the colligative properties and is attributed to the attraction of ions for solvent molecules, which holds the solvent in solution and reduces its escaping-tendency, with consequent enhancement of the vapor-pressure lowering. Solvation also may reduce interionic attraction and thereby further lower the vapor pressure.

These factors (and possibly others) combine to effect a progressive reduction in the molal values of colligative properties as the concentration of electrolyte is increased 0.5 to 1.0 molal, beyond which the molal quantities either increase (sometimes quite abruptly) or remain almost constant.

Activity and Activity Coefficient

Various mathematical expressions are employed to relate properties of chemical systems (equilibrium constants, colligative properties, pH, etc) to the stoichiometric concentration of one or more molecular, atomic, or ionic species. In deriving such expressions it is either stated or implied that they are valid only so long as intermolecular, interatomic, and/or interionic forces may be ignored or remain constant, under which restriction the system may be expected to behave ideally. But intermolecular, interatomic and/or interionic forces do exist, and not only do they change as a result of chemical reaction, but they also change with variation in the concentration or pressure of the molecules, atoms, or ions under observation. In consequence, mathematical expressions involving stoichiometric concentrations or pressures generally have limited applicability. The conventional concentration terms provide a count of molecules, atoms, or ions per unit volume, but afford no indication of the physical or chemical activity of the species measured, and it is this activity that determines the physical and chemical properties of the system.

In recognition of this, GN Lewis introduced both the quantitative concept and methods for evaluation of activity as a true measure of the physical or chemical activity of molecular, atomic, or ionic species, whether in the state of gas, liquid, or solid, or whether present as a single species or in a mixture. *Activity* may be considered loosely as a corrected concentration or pressure that takes into account not only the stoichiometric concentration or pressure but also any intermolecular attractions, repulsions, or interactions between solute and solvent in solution, association, and ionization. Thus, activity measures the net effectiveness of a chemical species.

Because only relative values of activity may be determined, a *standard state* must be chosen for quantitative comparisons to be made. Indeed, because activity measurements are needed for many different types of systems, several standard states must be selected. Because this discussion is concerned mainly with solutions, the standard state for the solvent is pure solvent, while for the solute it is a hypothetical solution with free energy corresponding to unit molality under conditions of ideal behavior of the solution. The relationship of activity to concentration is measured in terms of an activity coefficient, which is discussed in Chapter 17.

Practical Applications of Colligative Properties

One of the most important pharmaceutical applications of colligative properties is in the preparation of isotonic intravenous and isotonic lacrimal solutions, the details of which are discussed in Chapter 18.

Other applications of the colligative properties are found in experimental physiology. One such application is in the immersion of tissues in salt solutions, which are isotonic with the fluids of the tissue, in order to prevent changes or injuries that may arise from osmosis.

The colligative properties of solutions also may be used in determining the molecular weight of solutes, or in the case of electrolytes, the extent of ionization. The method of determining molecular weight depends on the fact that each of the colligative properties is altered by a constant value when a definite number of molecules of solute is added to a solvent (see Chapter 17). For example, in dilute solutions the freezing point of water is lowered at the rate of 1.855 for each mol of a nonelectrolyte dissolved in 1000 g of water.

The boiling-point elevation may be used similarly for determining molecular weights. The boiling point of water is raised at the rate of 0.52° for each mol of solute dissolved in 1000 g of water; the corresponding values for benzene, carbon tetrachloride, and phenol are 2.57°, 4.88°, and 3.60°, respectively. The

observing vapor-pressure lowering and osmotic pressure likewise may be used to calculate molecular weights.

To determine the extent to which an electrolyte is ionized, it is necessary to know its molecular weight, as determined by some other method, and then to measure one of the four colligative properties. The deviation of the results from similar values for nonelectrolytes then is used in calculating the extent of ionization.

Quantitative Treatment of Solubility

The focus of discussion so far has been on the qualitative aspects of solubility. It is, however, important to understand some quantitative relationships that can help pharmaceutical scientists predict the solubility of new-drug entities in various solvents and allow them to choose the best solvent system for a given drug. The observation that structurally similar chemical entities have better solubility in each other is based on the fact that cohesive forces operating in such molecules are of the same order of magnitude. One measure of these cohesive forces is a quantity known as internal pressure (P_i). It is given by[1]

$$P_i = \left(\frac{\Delta H_v - RT}{V} \right) \qquad (22)$$

where ΔH_v is the heat of vaporization of a substance and V is its molar volume at temperature T. Since Equation 22 contains ΔH_v, which depends on the amount of energy required to break intermolecular (cohesive) bonds, P_i is a measure of cohesive forces among the molecules. This value is high in polar substances; for example, water has a P_i value of 550 cal/mL. Therefore, drugs with high internal pressure show higher solubility in water. The term P_i usually is reserved for solubility of liquids in liquids.

For a quantitative estimate of solubility of solids in liquids, it is assumed that in an ideal solution the heat of solution is equal to the heat of fusion (heat required to melt one mol of solid to liquid without changing its temperature). As ideal solubility does not depend on the nature of solvent, it can be expressed by[11]

$$-\log X_2^i = \frac{\Delta H_f}{2.303R} \left(\frac{T_0 - T}{T_0 T} \right) \qquad (23)$$

where X_2^i is the mol fraction solubility in an ideal solution, ΔH_f is the molar heat of fusion of solute, T_0 is the melting point of solute, and T is the solution temperature such that $T < T_0$.

In a nonideal solution, the mol fraction solubility (X) has to be replaced by thermodynamic activity (a) of the solute. This activity can be expressed in terms of mol fraction solubility as

$$a_2 = X_2 \gamma_2 \qquad (24)$$

in which γ_2 is a proportionality constant called the *activity coefficient*. The value of γ_2 in ideal solution is equal to its maximum value of 1. By taking the log of the above equation and substituting in Equation 23, one obtains the equation of nonideal solubility as

$$-\log X_2 = \frac{\Delta H_f}{2.303R} \left(\frac{T_0 - T}{T_0 T} \right) + \log \gamma_2 \qquad (25)$$

It can be seen that when $\gamma_2 = 1$, $\log \gamma_2$ is zero and the equation reduces to the ideal solubility equation.

In general, ideal solutions are rare. Solutions of nonpolar solutes in nonpolar solvents usually come close to being ideal. However, solutions involving polar solutes or solvents almost always show significant deviation from ideality. The value of γ_2 is hard to determine, and varies with concentration of solution. It can be, however, estimated by

$$\log \delta_2 = [(w_{11})^{1/2} - (w_{22})^{1/2}]^2 \frac{V_2 \Phi_1^2}{2.303RT} \qquad (26)$$

where w_{11} is the amount of work involved in separating solvent molecules to create space for a solute molecule, w_{22} is the work involved in breaking a solute molecule from its bulk, V_2 is the molar volume of solute at temperature T, Φ_1 is the volume fraction of the solvent, and R is the gas constant. The terms w_{11} and w_{22} are a measure of the internal energy or cohesive forces of the solvent and solute, respectively. It can be seen from Equation 26 that deviation from ideality is high if values of w_{11} and w_{22} are different from each other, or the molar volume of the solute is high. The w terms are also known as the *solubility parameters,* denoted as δ. Thus the equation of nonideal solubility can be written as

$$-\log X_2 = \frac{\Delta H_f}{2.303R}\left(\frac{T_0 - T}{T_0 T}\right) + \frac{V_2 \Phi_1^2}{2.303RT}(\delta_1 - \delta_2)^2 \quad (27)$$

The following observations can be made from Equation 27.

1. For dilute solutions Φ_1 is approximately equal to 1 and thus may be disregarded in estimating solubility in dilute solutions
2. The closer the values of δ_1 and δ_2, the greater the solubility for a given pair of solute and solvent. In fact, when $\delta_1 = \delta_2$, the equation reduces to the equation for ideal solution, in which case the solubility is at its maximum value and depends only on molar heat of fusion of the solute.
3. Solutions of larger solute molecules (high value of V_2) show higher deviation from ideality. It is not surprising therefore that solutions of polymers and other high-molecular-weight compounds show a very different behavior than ideal solution (see *Solutions of Polymers,* below).

The solubility parameters can be measured using property of the material that involves molecular or cohesive interactions. These include the molar heat of vaporization, surface tension, internal pressure, and several others. One method suggested by Hilderbrand et al[12] is to use the expression for internal pressure to estimate the value of solubility parameter as follows.

$$\delta = \left(\frac{\Delta H_v - RT}{V}\right)^{1/2} \quad (28)$$

The meanings of the symbols are the same as defined earlier.

The values of solubility parameters are available in several references for many commonly used drugs. As intermolecular forces are composed of many kinds of forces, including polar and nonpolar forces, the individual contribution of these forces can be included in quantitative estimate of solubility parameter. Hilderbrand and Scott[13] suggested Equation 29 for this purpose.

$$\delta^2 = \delta_D^2 + \delta_P^2 + \delta_H^2 \quad (29)$$

where δ_D is the partial solubility parameter arising from nonpolar interactions, δ_p is the partial solubility parameter from polar interactions, and δ_H is the partial solubility parameter from the hydrogen-bonding tendency among the molecules. The value of δ_D is fairly constant for all types of molecules, polar as well as nonpolar, because nonpolar forces operate in all of these molecules. This value ranges from 7 to 10 cal/cc. Because δ_p is due to polar forces, which are essentially absent in nonpolar compounds, its value range is broader, 0 to 13 cal/cc. The value of δ_H, on the other hand, has the highest contribution where present and has a range of 0 to 25 cal/cc Therefore, for nonpolar compounds such as linear hydrocarbons, the total value of δ is comprised entirely of δ_D, and is close to about 7. For this reason most hydrocarbons show a similar behavior of solubility. In the nonhydrogen-bonding compounds that are relatively polar, δ_p has significant contribution.

Solutions of Polymers

Solubility behavior of polymers is usually significantly different from that of small molecules. Although there is no well-defined value of molecular weight cutoff point between polymers and regular molecules, polymer solutions included in the discussion here will focus on molecules whose size approaches the colloidal range.

Depending upon the manner in which the monomers are connected to each other, polymers can be of several types. From the solubility standpoint, however, the nature of the monomers is of great significance. In general, the solubility behavior of homopolymers (consisting of monomers repeated N times) mimics the solubility behavior of the monomers. This implies that the homopolymers consisting of relatively hydrophobic monomers will be poorly soluble in water. Examples of such polymers include polystyrene and polyamines.

However, if the hydrophobic monomers form parts of the block polymers (consisting of blocks of one repeating monomer unit followed by a block of different monomer) or heteropolymers (several monomers attached in random manner), their contribution to solubility may not be as negative as one would expect from their structure. This is because polymers are long molecules and generally have the flexibility to fold themselves in a manner that allows their hydrophobic areas to be folded away from water, much the way amphiphiles aggregate to form a hydrophobic core. This arrangement allows the hydrophilic monomers to stay in contact with water, thereby allowing substantial solubility. Examples of such polymers include proteins (which may contain hydrophobic amino acid residues).

Many of the so-called *biological polymers* consist of monomers that carry a net negative or positive charge at near neutral pH. These are known as *polyelectrolytes,* and they are generally very soluble in water. Their solubility is driven by the electrostatic interactions between water and the charged monomers. Examples of such polymers include DNA, proteins, certain derivatized cellulose polymers, and carrageenans. Such polymers are of significant importance in pharmaceutical dosage forms as thickeners, additives, stabilizers, and controlled-release matrices.

Many biological polymers exist as random coil structures in aqueous solution. If the structure is treated as an approximate sphere, then its radius, known as the *radius of gyration (R_g)*, is a function of its molecular weight. In polymers of very high molecular weight (typically 100 kd or higher) this radius may be so large that the polymer in solution behaves like a particle, approaching the size of the colloidal range. The volume of this particle is given by[14]

$$V_{coil} = \frac{4}{3}\pi R_g^3 \quad (30)$$

where V_{coil} is the volume of a single polymer chain and R_g is the radius of gyration. When the value of this volume is large, the system no longer behaves as a dilute solution even when the molar concentration is small, and polymer-polymer interactions are significant. Depending on the polymer molecular weight, significant overlapping between the polymer chains may occur at concentration as low as 0.1%.[14] At higher concentration, the swollen polymer and free solvent may occupy comparable volumes in the solution.

Unlike in regular solutions, the solubility of polymers is driven primarily by the entropic changes. Upon mixing a polymer with a solvent, which is generally water in pharmaceutical solutions, two different kinds of entropic effects occur. One is the increase in entropy due to mixing of two molecular species. This effect is small in a dilute solution. The second effect is that the entropy of the polymer configuration increases due to swelling of the molecules and also due to greater flexibility in solution. Based on these entropic changes, Flory[15,16] derived Equation 31 to describe the overall entropic change (ΔS_{mix}) in a polymer solution.

$$\Delta S_{mix} = -R\left(n_s \ln \Phi_s + n_p \ln \Phi_p\right) \quad (31)$$

where n_s and n_p are the number of molecules of solvent and polymer, respectively, and Φ_s and Φ_p represent their volume fraction, respectively. The free-energy change (ΔG_{mix}) in the process of solubility can be written as

$$\Delta G_{mix} = RT\left(n_s \ln \Phi_s + n_p \ln \Phi_p\right) + \left(n_s + N_p n_p\right) w \Phi_p \Phi_s \quad (32)$$

The first term on the right side of Equation 32 is the entropy of mixing, and the second term is the enthalpy of mixing. N_p in the second term is the degree of polymerization, and w is the effective molar interaction parameter (effectively, w is the square of the difference between solubility parameters of the polymer and solvent, multiplied by Avogadro's number). It is clear from the above equation that the value of ΔG_{mix} and therefore the polymer solubility are driven primarily by the volume fraction of the polymer in solution.

METHODS TO INCREASE SOLUBILITY OF POORLY SOLUBLE DRUGS

A large number of promising drug candidates do not make it to the market due to poor bioavailability, due primarily to their poor solubility in aqueous medium. Recently, several strategies have been used to improve solubility profile of these drugs. The strategies used to improve drug solubility include the following.

1. Use of buffers
2. Use of cosolvents
3. Surfactants
4. Complexation
5. Solid dispersions

USE OF BUFFERS—The idea behind use of buffers to improve solubility is to create and maintain pH conditions in a system that cause the drug to be in its ionized state. As discussed previously in this chapter, ionized fraction of a drug is much more soluble in water due to its increased polarity relative to the un-ionized fraction. Buffers can also help in reducing the likelihood of drug precipitation when drug solution is diluted in an aqueous medium. Consistent with the principles of solubility changes with pH, acidic drugs are formulated under relative basic conditions, while the opposite is true for the basic drugs. Some examples of drugs that are formulated with buffer systems are Amikacin sulfate (pH 3.5–5.5, citrate buffer) and Midazolam hydrochloride (pH 3).[17–19] The drugs that make good candidates for use of pH variation or buffers are the ones that have the ability to ionize within a pH range of 2–8.

USE OF COSOLVENTS—A common way to increase drug solubility is through the use of a water miscible organic solvent. This strategy is based on the fact that poor solubility of drugs in water results due to great difference in polarity of the two components, water being of very high polarity, and the drug having low polarity. Addition of a cosolvent with a polarity value of less than that of water reduces the difference between polarity of the drug and water-cosolvent system, thereby improving solubility. Commonly used cosolvents for this purpose are the hydrogen bonding organic solvents such as ethyl alcohol, propylene glycol and glycerin.

The polarity scale of solvents is defined by a property known as dielectric constant. This value for water is 80, and for ethyl alcohol, propylene glycol and glycerin, it is 24,032 and 42, respectively. Most poorly soluble drugs have dielectric constant values of less than 20. Examples of some parenteral solution that contain cosolvents include Chlordiazepoxide (25% propylene glycol), Diazepam (10% ethyl alcohol and 40% propylene glycol), and digoxin (10% ethyl alcohol and 40% propylene glycol). Non-polar and non-ionizable drugs are good candidates for cosolvent systems.[17–19]

SURFACTANTS—Surfactants are molecules with well defined polar and non-polar regions that allow them to aggregate in solution to form micelles. Non-polar drugs can partition into these micelles and be solubilized. Depending on the nature of the polar area, surfactants can be non-ionic (eg, polyethylene glycol), anionic (eg, sodium dodecyl sulfate), cationic (eg, trialkylammonium) and Zwitterionic (eg, glycine and proteins). Among these, the most commonly used ones are the anionic and non-ionic surfactants. Since the process of solubilization occurs

due to presence of micelles, generally high concentrations of surfactants are needed to significantly improve drug solubility. One example of surfactant based solution is Taxol (paclitaxel), an anti-cancer drug that is solubilized in 50% solution of Cremophor. Other examples include Valrubicin in 50% Cremophor, and Cyclosporin in 65% Cremophor.[17–19]

COMPLEXATION—Complexation is the association between two or more molecules to form a noncovalent based complex that has higher solubility than the drug itself. From solubility standpoint, complexes can be put into two categories, stacking complexes and inclusion complexes. Stacking complexation is driven by association of nonpolar areas of the drug and complexing agent. This results in exclusion of the nonpolar areas from contact with water, thereby reducing total energy of the system. This aggregation is favored by large planar nonpolar regions on the molecules. Stacking can be homogeneous or mixed, but results in a clear solution.

Inclusion complexes are formed by insertion of drug molecule into a cavity formed by the complexing agent. In this arrangement, nonpolar area of the drug molecule is excluded from water due to its insertion in the complexing agent. One requirement for the complexing agent in such systems is that it has nonpolar core and polar exterior. The most commonly used inclusion complexing molecules are cyclodextrins. The cyclic oligomers of glucose are relatively soluble in water and have cavities large enough to accept nonpolar portions of many drug molecules. Cyclodextrins can consist of 6, 7, or 8 sugar residues and are classified as α, β, and γ, respectively. Due to geometric considerations, steroid molecules lend themselves very well for inclusion into cyclodextrin complexes.

SOLID DISPERSIONS—Solid dispersion refers to the dispersion of one or more active ingredients in an inert carrier or matrix at solid state prepared by the melting (fusion), solvent or the melting-solvent method. It has also been defined as the product formed by converting a fluid drug-carrier combination to the solid state. The term co precipitate or co evaporate has also been used frequently when a solid dispersion is prepared by solvent method.

Classification of Solid Dispersions—Solid dispersions can be classified as follows:

Simple eutectic mixtures
Solid solutions
Glass solutions of suspensions
Compound or complex formation between the drug and the carriers
Amorphous precipitations of drug in crystalline carrier

Simple Eutectic Mixtures—A simple eutectic mixture consists of two compounds that are completely miscible in the liquid state but only to a very limited extent in the solid state. A eutectic mixture of a sparingly water-soluble drug and a highly water-soluble carrier may be regarded thermodynamically as an intimately blended physical mixture of its two crystalline component. These components are assumed to crystallize simultaneously in very small particulate sizes. The increase in specific surface area therefore, is mainly responsible for the increased rate of dissolution of a poorly water-soluble drug.

Differential thermal analysis (DTA) of binary mixtures normally exhibits two endotherms, but a binary mixture of eutectic composition usually exhibits a single major endotherm. In the case of a simple Eutectic system, the thaw points of binary mixtures of varying compositions are equal to the eutectic temperature of the system.

Solid Solutions—Solid solution consists of a solid solute dissolved in a solid solvent. The particle size in solid solution is reduced to molecular level. Successful solubilization of Itraconazole has been achieved using solid solution techniques. Solid solutions of lower drug concentrations generally give faster dissolution rate, and drug dissolution improves considerably with an increase in molecular weight of a water-soluble polymer such as polyethylene glycol.

Glass Solutions of Suspensions—A glass solution is a homogeneous system in which a glassy or a vitreous form of the carrier solubilizes drug molecules. PVP has been used as a carrier in several formulations. In its matrix PVP dissolved an organic solvents undergoes a transition to a glassy state upon evaporation of the solvent.

Compound or Complex Formation Between the Drug and the Carriers—This system is characterized by complexation of two components in a binary system during solid dispersion preparation. The availability of a drug from the complex is dependent on the solubility, dissociation constant, and the intrinsic absorption rate of the complex. α, β, and γ CD in combination with polyethylene glycol (PEG) 6000 have been used to formulate such systems.

Amorphous Precipitation—Amorphous precipitation occurs when the drug precipitates as an amorphous form in the inert career. The high-energy state of the drug in this system generally produces much greater dissolution rates than the corresponding crystalline forms of the drug.

REFERENCES

1. Martin AN et al. *Physical Pharmacy: Physical Chemical Principles in Pharmaceutical Sciences*. Philadelphia: Lea & Febiger, 1993, pp 212–237.
2. Kramer SF, Flynn GL. *J Pharm Sci* 1972; 61:1896.
3. Campbell AN, Campbell AJR. *J Am Chem Soc* 1937; 59:2481.
4. Loran MR, Guth EP. *J APhA Sci Ed* 1951; 40:465.
5. Grant DJW, Abougela IKA. *Analytical Proceedings: Proceedings of the Analytical Division of the Royal Society of Chemistry*. Dec 1992, p 545.
6. Higuchi T. In: Lyman R, ed. *Pharmaceutical Compounding and Dispensing*. Philadelphia: Lippincott, 1949, p 159.
7. Duddu S. PhD thesis. University of Minnesota, 1993.
8. Yallowsky SH. *Techniques of Solubilization of Drugs*. New York: Dekker, 1981, p 91.
9. Martin A et al. *J Pharm Sci* 1982; 71: 849.
10. Setnikar I, Temelcou O. *J APhA Sci Ed* 1959; 48:628.
11. Hilderbrand JH, Wood SE. *J Chem Phys* 1933; 1:817.
12. Hilderbrand JH et al. *Regular and Related Solutions*. New York: Van Nostrand Reinhold, 1970, pp 22–23.
13. Hilderbrand JH, Scott RL. *Solubility of Nonelectrolytes*. New York: Dover, 1964, Chap 23.
14. Evans DF, Wennerstrom H. *The Colloidal Domain—Where Physics, Chemistry, Biology, and Technology Meet*. New York: VCH Publishers, 1994, pp 289–303.
15. Flory PJ. *Principles of Polymer Chemistry*. Ithaca, NY: Cornell University Press, 1953.
16. Flory PJ. *Statistical Mechanics of Chain Molecules*. New York: Interscience, 1969.
17. Strickley RG. *PDA J Pharm Sci Technol* 1999; 53:324.
18. Strickley RG. *PDA J Pharm Sci Technol* 2000; 54:69.
19. Strickley RG. *PDA J Pharm Sci Technol* 2000; 54:152.

CHAPTER 17

Ionic Solutions and Electrolytic Equilibria

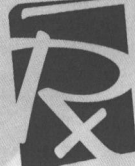

ELECTROLYTES

In a preceding chapter, attention was directed to the colligative properties of nonelectrolytes, or substances whose aqueous solutions do not conduct electricity. Substances whose aqueous solutions conduct electricity are known as *electrolytes* and are typified by inorganic acids, bases, and salts. In addition to the property of electrical conductivity, solutions of electrolytes exhibit anomalous colligative properties.

COLLIGATIVE PROPERTIES

In general, for nonelectrolytes, a given colligative property of two equimolal solutions will be identical. This generalization, however, cannot be made for solutions of electrolytes.

Van't Hoff pointed out that the osmotic pressure of a solution of an electrolyte is considerably greater than the osmotic pressure of a solution of a nonelectrolyte of the same molal concentration. This anomaly remained unexplained until 1887 when Arrhenius proposed a hypothesis that forms the basis for our modern theories of electrolyte solutions.

This theory postulated that when electrolytes are dissolved in water they split up into charged particles known as *ions*. Each of these ions carries one or more electrical charges, with the total charge on the positive ions (*cations*) being equal to the total charge on the negative ions (*anions*). Thus, although a solution may contain charged particles, it remains neutral. The increased osmotic pressure of such solutions is due to the increased number of particles formed in the process of ionization. For example, sodium chloride is assumed to dissociate as

$$Na^+Cl^- \xrightarrow{\text{H}_2\text{O}} Na^+ + Cl^-$$

It is evident that each molecule of sodium chloride that is dissociated produces two ions, and if dissociation is complete, there will be twice as many particles as would be the case if it were not dissociated at all. Furthermore, if each ion has the same effect on osmotic pressure as a molecule, it might be expected that the osmotic pressure of the solution would be twice that of a solution containing the same molal concentration of a nonionizing solute.

Osmotic-pressure data indicate that, in very dilute solutions of salts that yield two ions, the pressure is very nearly double that of solutions of equimolal concentrations of nonelectrolytes. Similar magnification of vapor-pressure lowering, boiling-point elevation, and freezing-point depression occurs in dilute solutions of electrolytes.

Van't Hoff defined a factor, i, as the ratio of the colligative effect produced by a concentration, m, of electrolyte, divided by the effect observed for the same concentration of nonelectrolyte, or

$$i = \frac{\pi}{(\pi)_0} = \frac{\Delta P}{(\Delta P)_0} = \frac{\Delta T_b}{(\Delta T_b)_0} = \frac{\Delta T_f}{(\Delta T_f)_0} \qquad (1)$$

in which π, ΔP, ΔT_b, ΔT_f refer to the osmotic pressure, vapor-pressure lowering, boiling-point elevation, and freezing-point depression, respectively, of the electrolyte. The terms $(\pi)_0$ and so on refer to the nonelectrolyte of the same concentration. In general, with strong electrolytes (those assumed to be 100% ionized), the van't Hoff factor is equal to the number of ions produced when the electrolyte goes into solution (2 for NaCl and $MgSO_4$, 3 for $CaCl_2$ and Na_2SO_4, 4 for $FeCl_3$ and Na_3PO_4, etc).

In *very* dilute solutions the osmotic pressure, vapor-pressure lowering, boiling-point elevation, and freezing-point depression of solutions of electrolytes approach values two, three, four, or more times greater (depending on the type of strong electrolyte) than in solutions of the same molality of nonelectrolyte, thus confirming the hypothesis that an ion has the same primary effect as a molecule on colligative properties. It bears repeating, however, that two other effects are observed as the concentration of electrolyte is increased.

The first effect results in less than 2-, 3-, or 4-fold intensification of a colligative property. This reduction is ascribed to interionic attraction between the positive and negatively charged ions, in consequence of which the ions are not dissociated completely from each other and do not exert their full effect on vapor pressure and other colligative properties. This deviation generally increases with increasing concentration of electrolyte.

The second effect intensifies the colligative properties and is attributed to the attraction of ions for solvent molecules (called *solvation*, or, if water is the solvent, *hydration*), which holds the solvent in solution and reduces its escaping tendency, with a consequent enhancement of the vapor-pressure lowering. Solvation also reduces interionic attraction and, thereby, further lowers the vapor pressure.

CONDUCTIVITY

The ability of metals to conduct an electric current results from the mobility of electrons in the metals. This type of conductivity is called *metallic conductance*. On the other hand, various chemical compounds—notably acids, bases, and salts—conduct electricity by virtue of ions present or formed, rather than by electrons. This is called *electrolytic conductance,* and the conducting compounds are electrolytes. Although the fact that certain electrolytes conduct electricity in the molten state is important, their behavior when dissolved in a solvent, particularly in water, is of greater concern in pharmaceutical science.

The electrical conductivity (or conductance) of a solution of an electrolyte is merely the reciprocal of the resistance of the solution. Therefore, to measure conductivity is actually to measure electrical resistance, commonly with a *Wheatstone bridge apparatus,* and then to *calculate* the conductivity. Figure 17-1 is a representation of the component parts of the apparatus.

The solution to be measured is placed in a glass or quartz cell having two inert electrodes, commonly made of platinum or gold and coated with spongy platinum to absorb gases, across which passes an alternating current generated by an oscillator at a frequency of about 1000 Hz. The reason for using alternating current is to reverse the electrolysis that occurs during flow of current that would cause polarization of the electrodes and lead to abnormal results. The size of the electrodes and their distance apart may be varied to reduce very high resistance or increase very low resistance to increase the accuracy and precision of measurement. Thus, solutions of high conductance (low resistance) are measured in cells having small electrodes relatively far apart, whereas solutions of low conductance (high resistance) are measured in cells with large electrodes placed close to each other.

Electrolytic resistance, like metallic resistance, varies directly with the length of the conducting medium and inversely with its cross-sectional area. The known resistance required for the circuit is provided by a resistance box containing calibrated coils. Balancing of the bridge may be achieved by sliding a contact over a wire of uniform resistance until no (or minimum) current flows through the circuit, as detected either visually with a cathode-ray oscilloscope or audibly with earphones.

The resistance, in ohms, is calculated by the simple procedure used in the Wheatstone bridge method. The reciprocal of the resistance is the conductivity, the units of which are *reciprocal ohms* (also called *mho*). As the numerical value of the conductivity will vary with the dimensions of the conductance cell, the value must be calculated as *specific conductance, L,* which is the conductance in a cell having electrodes of 1-cm^2 cross-sectional area and 1 cm apart. If the dimensions of the cell used in the experiment were known, calculating the specific conductance would be possible. Nevertheless, this information actually is not required, because calibrating a cell by measuring in it the conductivity of a standard solution of known specific conductance is possible—and much more convenient—and then calculating a *cell constant.* Because this constant is a function

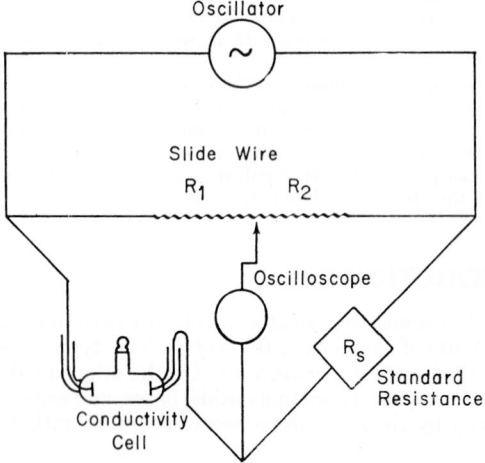

Figure 17-1. Alternating current Wheatstone bridge for measuring conductivity.

Table 17-1. Equivalent Conductances^a at 25°

G-EQ/L	HCL	HOAC	NACL	KCL	NAI	KI	NAOAC
Inf dil	426.1	390.6^a	126.5	149.9	126.9	150.3	91.0
0.0005	422.7	67.7	124.5	147.8	125.4	—	89.2
0.0010	421.4	49.2	123.7	146.9	124.3	—	88.5
0.0050	415.8	22.9	120.6	143.5	121.3	144.4	85.7
0.0100	412.0	16.3	118.5	141.3	119.2	142.2	83.8
0.0200	407.2	11.6	115.8	138.3	116.7	139.5	81.2
0.0500	399.1	7.4	111.1	133.4	112.8	135.0	76.9
0.1000	391.3	5.2	106.7	129.0	108.8	131.1	72.8

^{a} The equivalent conductance at infinite dilution for acetic acid, a weak electrolyte, is obtained by adding the equivalent conductances of hydrochloric acid and sodium acetate and subtracting that of sodium chloride.

only of the dimensions of the cell, it can be used to convert all measurements in that cell to specific conductivity. Solutions of known concentration of pure potassium chloride are used as standard solutions for this purpose.

EQUIVALENT CONDUCTANCE—In studying the variation of conductance of electrolytes with dilution it is essential to make allowance for dilution so that the comparison of conductances may be made for identical amounts of solute. This may be achieved by expressing conductance measurements in terms of *equivalent conductance,* Λ, which is obtained by multiplying the specific conductance, L, by the volume in milliliters, V_e, of a solution containing 1 g-eq of solute. Thus,

$$\Lambda = LV_e = \frac{1000L}{C} \qquad (2)$$

where C is the concentration of electrolyte in the solution in g-eq/L, that is, the normality of the solution. For example, the equivalent conductance of 0.01 N potassium chloride solution, which has a specific conductance of 0.001413 mho/cm, may be calculated in either of the following ways:

$$\Lambda = 0.001413 \times 100,000 = 141.3 \text{ mho cm}^2/\text{eq}$$

or

$$\Lambda = \frac{1000 \times 0.001413}{0.01} = 141.3$$

STRONG AND WEAK ELECTROLYTES—Electrolytes are classified broadly as *strong electrolytes* and *weak electrolytes.* The former category includes solutions of strong acids, strong bases, and most salts; the latter includes weak acids and bases, primarily organic acids, amines, and a few salts. The usual criterion for distinguishing between strong and weak electrolytes is the extent of *ionization.* An electrolyte existing entirely or very largely as ions is considered a strong electrolyte, while one that is a mixture of some molecular species along with ions derived from it is a weak electrolyte. For the purposes of this discussion, classification of electrolytes as strong or weak will be based on certain conductance characteristics exhibited in aqueous solution.

The equivalent conductances of some electrolytes, at different concentrations, are given in Table 17-1 and for certain of these electrolytes again in Figure 17-2, where the equivalent conductance is plotted against the square root of concentration. By plotting the data in this manner a linear relationship is observed for strong electrolytes, while a steeply rising curve is noted for weak electrolytes; this difference is a characteristic that distinguishes strong and weak electrolytes. The interpretation of the steep rise in the equivalent conductance of weak electrolytes is that the degree of ionization increases with dilution, becoming complete at infinite dilution.

Interionic interference effects generally have a minor role in the conductivity of weak electrolytes. With strong electrolytes, which are usually completely ionized, the increase in equivalent conductance results not from increased ionization but from

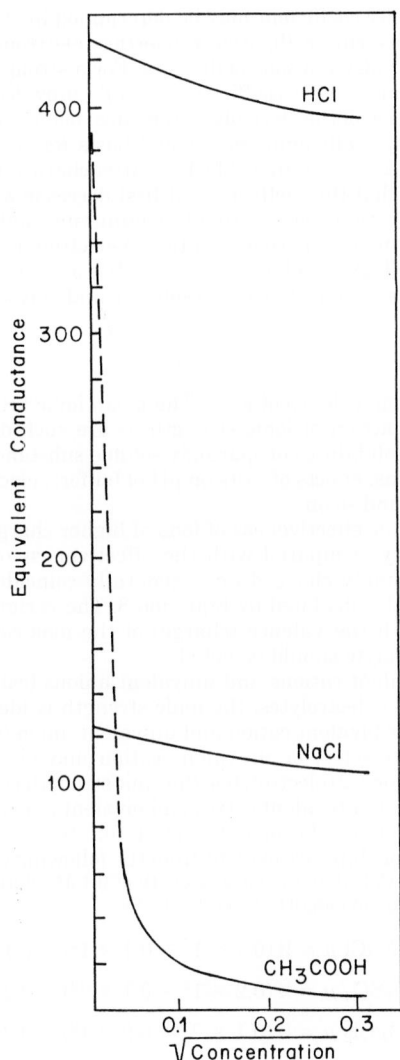

Figure 17-2. Variation of equivalent conductance with square root of concentration.

diminished ionic interference as the solution is diluted, in consequence of which ions have greater freedom of mobility (ie, increased conductance).

The value of the equivalent conductance extrapolated to infinite dilution (zero concentration), designated by the symbol Λ_0, has special significance. It represents the equivalent conductance of the completely ionized electrolyte when the ions are so far apart that there is no interference with their migration due to interionic interactions. It has been shown, by Kohlrausch, that the equivalent conductance of an electrolyte at infinite dilution is the sum of the equivalent conductances of its component ions at infinite dilution, expressed symbolically as

$$\Lambda_0 = l_0(\text{cation}) + l_0(\text{anion}) \qquad (3)$$

The significance of Kohlrausch's law is that each ion, at infinite dilution, has a characteristic value of conductance that is independent of the conductance of the oppositely charged ion with which it is associated. Thus, if the equivalent conductances of various ions are known, the conductance of any electrolyte may be calculated simply by adding the appropriate ionic conductances.

As the fraction of current carried by cations (*transference number* of the cations) and by anions (*transference number* of

anions) in an electrolyte may be determined readily by experiment, ionic conductances are known. Table 17-2 gives the equivalent ionic conductances at infinite dilution of some cations and anions. It is not necessary to have this information to calculate the equivalent conductance of an electrolyte, for Kohlrausch's law permits the latter to be calculated by adding and subtracting values of Λ_0 for appropriate electrolytes. For example, the value of Λ_0 for acetic acid may be calculated as

$$\Lambda_0(\text{CH}_3\text{COOH}) = \Lambda_0(\text{HCl}) + \Lambda_0(\text{CH}_3\text{COONa}) - \Lambda_0(\text{NaCl})$$

which is equivalent to

$$l_0(\text{H}^+) + l_0(\text{CH}_3\text{COO}^-) = l_0(\text{H}^+) + l_0(\text{Cl}^-) + (l0(\text{Na}^+)$$
$$+ l_0(\text{CH}_3\text{COO}^-) - l_0(\text{Na}^+) - l_0(\text{Cl}^-)$$

This method is especially useful for calculating for weak electrolytes such as acetic acid. As evident from Figure 17-2, the Λ_0 value for acetic acid cannot be determined accurately by extrapolation because of the steep rise of conductance in dilute solutions. For strong electrolytes, on the other hand, the extrapolation can be made very accurately. Thus, in the example above, the values of for HCl, CH$_3$COONa, and NaCl are determined easily by extrapolation as the substances are strong electrolytes. Substitution of these extrapolated values, as given in Table 17-2, yields a value of 390.6 for the value of Λ_0 for CH$_3$COOH.

IONIZATION OF WEAK ELECTROLYTES—When Arrhenius introduced his theory of ionization he proposed that the degree of ionization, α, of an electrolyte is measured by the ratio

$$\alpha = \Lambda/\Lambda_0 \qquad (4)$$

where Λ is the equivalent conductance of the electrolyte at any specified concentration of solution and Λ_0 is the equivalent conductance at infinite dilution. As strong electrolytes were then not recognized as being 100% ionized, and interionic interference effects had not been evaluated, he believed the equation to be applicable to both strong and weak electrolytes. It now is known that the apparent variation of ionization of strong electrolytes arises from a change in the mobility of ions at different concentrations, rather than from varying ionization, so the equation is not applicable to strong electrolytes. It does provide, however, a generally acceptable approximation of the degree of ionization of weak electrolytes, for which deviations resulting from neglect of activity coefficients and of some change of ionic mobilities with concentration are, for most purposes, negligible. The following example illustrates the use of the equation to calculate the degree of ionization of a typical weak electrolyte.

Example—Calculate the degree of ionization of 1×10^{-3} N acetic acid, the equivalent conductance of which is 48.15 mho cm^2/eq. The equivalent conductance at infinite dilution is 390.6 mho cm^2/eq.

$$\alpha = \frac{48.15}{390.6} = 0.12$$

$$\% \text{ ionization} = 100\alpha = 12\%$$

Table 17-2. Equivalent Ionic Conductivities at Infinite Dilution, at 25°

CATIONS	l_0	ANIONS	l_0
H$^+$	349.8	OH$^-$	198.0
Li$^+$	38.7	Cl$^-$	76.3
Na$^+$	50.1	Br$^-$	78.4
K$^+$	73.5	I$^-$	76.8
NH$_4^+$	61.9	AcO$^-$	40.9
½Ca^{2+}	59.5	½SO$_4^{2-}$	79.8
½Mg^{2+}	53.0		

The degree of dissociation also can be calculated using the van't Hoff factor, i, and

$$\alpha = \frac{i - 1}{v - 1} \qquad (5)$$

where v is the number of ions into which the electrolyte dissociates.

Example—A 1.0×10^{-3} N solution of acetic acid has a van't Hoff factor equal to 1.12. Calculate the degree of dissociation of the acid at this concentration.

$$\alpha = \frac{i - 1}{v - 1} = \frac{1.12 - 1}{2 - 1} = 0.12$$

This result agrees with that obtained using equivalent conductance and Equation 4.

MODERN THEORIES

The Arrhenius theory explains why solutions of electrolytes conduct electricity, and why they exhibit enhanced colligative properties. The theory is satisfactory for solutions of weak electrolytes. Several deficiencies, however, do exist when it is applied to solutions of strong electrolytes. It does not explain the failure of strong electrolytes to follow the law of mass action as applied to ionization; discrepancies exist between the degree of ionization calculated from the van't Hoff factor and the conductivity ratio for strong electrolyte solutions having concentrations greater than about 0.5 M.

These deficiencies can be explained by the following observations

1. In the molten state, strong electrolytes are excellent conductors of electricity. This suggests that these materials are already ionized in the crystalline state. Further support for this is given by x-ray studies of crystals, which indicate that the units comprising the basic lattice structure of strong electrolytes are ions.
2. Arrhenius neglected the fact that ions in solution, being oppositely charged, tend to associate through electrostatic attraction. In solutions of weak electrolytes, the number of ions is not large and it is not surprising that electrostatic attractions do not cause appreciable deviations from theory. In dilute solutions, in which strong electrolytes are assumed to be 100% ionized, the number of ions is large, and interionic attractions become major factors in determining the chemical properties of these solutions. These effects should, and do, become more pronounced as the concentration of electrolyte or the valence of the ions is increased.

It is not surprising, therefore, that the Arrhenius theory of partial ionization involving the law of mass action and neglecting ionic charge does not hold for solutions of strong electrolytes. Neutral molecules of strong electrolytes, if they do exist in solution, must arise from interionic attraction rather than from incomplete ionization.

ACTIVITY AND ACTIVITY COEFFICIENTS—Due to increased electrostatic attractions as a solution becomes more concentrated, the concentration of an ion becomes less efficient as a measure of its net effectiveness. A more efficient measure of the physical or chemical effectiveness of an ion is known as its *activity*, which is a measure of the concentration of an ion related to its concentration at a universally adopted reference-standard state. The relationship between the activity and the concentration of an ion can be expressed as

$$a = m\gamma \qquad (6)$$

where m is the molal concentration, γ is the activity coefficient, and a is the activity. The activity also can be expressed in terms of molar concentration, c, as

$$a = fc \qquad (7)$$

where f is the activity coefficient on a molar scale. In dilute solutions (below 0.01 M) the two activity coefficients are identical, for all practical purposes.

The activity coefficient may be determined in various ways, such as measuring colligative properties, electromotive force, solubility, or distribution coefficients. For a strong electrolyte, the mean ionic activity coefficient, $\gamma_\pm$ or $f_\pm$, provides a measure of the deviation of the electrolyte from ideal behavior. The mean ionic activity coefficients on a molal basis for several strong electrolytes are given in Table 17-2. It is characteristic of the electrolytes that the coefficients at first decrease with increasing concentration, pass through a minimum and finally increase with increasing concentration of electrolyte.

IONIC STRENGTH—Ionic strength is a measure of the intensity of the electrical field in a solution and may be expressed as

$$\mu = \frac{1}{2} \Sigma c_i z_i^2 \qquad (8)$$

where z_i is the valence of ion i. The mean ionic activity coefficient is a function of ionic strength as are such diverse phenomena as solubilities of sparingly soluble substances, rates of ionic reactions, effects of salts on pH of buffers, electrophoresis of proteins, and so on.

The greater effectiveness of ions of higher charge on a specific property, compared with the effectiveness of the same number of singly charged ions, generally coincides with the ionic strength calculated by Equation 8. The variation of ionic strength with the valence (charge) of the ions comprising a strong electrolyte should be noted.

For univalent cations and univalent anions (called *uniunivalent* or 1-1) electrolytes, the ionic strength is identical with molarity. For bivalent cation and univalent anion (*biunivalent* or 2-1) electrolytes, or univalent cation and bivalent anion (*unibivalent* or 1-2) electrolytes, the ionic strength is three times the molarity. For bivalent cation and bivalent anion (*bibivalent* or 2-2) electrolytes, the ionic strength is four times the molarity. These relationships are evident from the following example.

Example—Calculate the ionic strength of 0.1 M solutions of NaCl, Na_2SO_4, $MgCl_2$, and $MgSO_4$, respectively, for

$$NaCl \quad \mu = \frac{1}{2}(0.1 \times 1^2 + 0.1 \times 1^2) = 0.1$$

$$Na_2SO_4 \quad \mu = \frac{1}{2}(0.2 \times 1^2 + 0.1 \times 2^2) = 0.3$$

$$MgCl_2 \quad \mu = \frac{1}{2}(0.1 \times 2^2 + 0.2 \times 1^2) = 0.3$$

$$MgSO_4 \quad \mu = \frac{1}{2}(0.1 \times 2^2 + 0.1 \times 2^2) = 0.4$$

The ionic strength of a solution containing more than one electrolyte is the sum of the ionic strengths of the individual salts comprising the solution. For example, the ionic strength of a solution containing NaCl, Na_2SO_4, $MgCl_2$, and $MgSO_4$, each at a concentration of 0.1 M, is 1.1.

DEBYE–HUCKEL THEORY—The *Debye–Huckel equations*, which are applicable only to very dilute solutions (about 0.02 μ), may be extended to somewhat more concentrated solutions (about 0.1 μ) in the simplified form

$$\log f_i = \frac{-0.51 z_i^2 \sqrt{\mu}}{1 + \sqrt{\mu}} \qquad (9)$$

The mean ionic activity coefficient for aqueous solutions of electrolytes at 25° can be expressed as

$$\log f_\pm = \frac{-0.51 z_+ z_- \sqrt{\mu}}{1 + \sqrt{\mu}} \qquad (10)$$

in which z_+ is the valence of the cation and z_- is the valence of the anion. When the ionic strength of the solution becomes high (approximately 0.3 to 0.5), these equations become inadequate and a linear term in μ is added. This is illustrated for the mean ionic activity coefficient,

$$\log f_\pm = \frac{-0.51 z_+ z_- \sqrt{\mu}}{1 + \sqrt{\mu}} + K_s \mu \qquad (11)$$

Table 17-3. Values of Some Salting-Out Constants for Various Barbiturates at 25°

BARBITURATE	KCL	KBR	NACL	NABR
Amobarbital	0.168	0.095	0.212	0.143
Aprobarbital	0.136	0.062	0.184	0.120
Barbital	0.092	0.042	0.136	0.088
Phenobarbital	0.092	0.034	0.132	0.078
Vinbarbital	0.125	0.036	0.143	0.096

in which K_s is a *salting-out* constant chosen empirically for each salt. This equation is valid for solutions with ionic strength up to approximately 1.

SALTING-OUT EFFECT—The aqueous solubility of a slightly soluble organic substance generally is affected markedly by the addition of an electrolyte. This effect is particularly noticeable when the electrolyte concentration reaches $0.5\ M$ or higher. If the aqueous solution of the organic substance has a dielectric constant lower than that of pure water, its solubility is decreased and the substance is *salted-out*. The use of high concentrations of electrolytes, such as ammonium sulfate or sodium sulfate, for the separation of proteins by differential precipitation is perhaps the most striking example of this effect. The aqueous solutions of a few substances such as hydrocyanic acid, glycine, and cystine have a higher dielectric constant than that of pure water, and these substances are *salted-in*. These phenomena can be expressed empirically as

$$\log S = \log S_0 \pm K_s m \qquad (12)$$

in which S_0 represents the solubility of the organic substance in pure water and S is the solubility in the electrolyte solution. The slope of the straight line obtained by plotting $\log S$ versus m is positive for salting-in and negative for salting-out. In terms of ionic strength this equation becomes

$$\log S = \log S_0 \pm K'_s\, \mu \qquad (13)$$

where $K'_s = K_s$ for univalent salts, $K'_s = K_s/3$ for unibivalent salts, and $K'_s = K_s/4$ for bivalent salts. The salting-out constant depends on the temperature as well as the nature of both the organic substance and the electrolyte. The effect of the electrolyte and the organic substance can be seen in Table 17-3. In all instances, if the anion is constant, the sodium cation has a greater salting-out effect than the potassium cation, probably due to the higher charge density of the former. Although the reasoning is less clear, it appears that, for a constant cation, chloride anion has a greater effect than bromide anion upon the salting-out phenomenon.

ACIDS AND BASES

Arrhenius defined an acid as a substance that yields hydrogen ions in aqueous solution and a base as a substance that yields hydroxyl ions in aqueous solution. Except for the fact that hydrogen ions neutralize hydroxyl ions to form water, no complementary relationship between acids and bases (eg, that between oxidants and reductants) is evident in Arrhenius' definitions for these substances; rather, their oppositeness of character is emphasized. Moreover, no account is taken of the behavior of acids and bases in nonaqueous solvents. Also, although acidity is associated with so elementary a particle as the proton (hydrogen ion), basicity is attributed to so relatively complex an association of atoms as the hydroxyl ion. It would seem that a simpler concept of a base could be devised.

PROTON CONCEPT—In pondering the objections to Arrhenius' definitions, Brønsted and Bjerrum in Denmark and Lowry in England developed, and in 1923 announced, a more satisfactory, and more general, theory of acids and bases. According to this theory, an acid is a substance capable of yielding a proton (hydrogen ion), whereas a base is a substance capable of accepting a proton. This complementary relationship may be expressed by

$$\underset{\text{acid}}{A} \rightleftharpoons H^+ + \underset{\text{base}}{B}$$

The pair of substances thus related through mutual ability to gain or lose a proton is called a conjugate acid–base pair. Specific examples of such pairs are

Acid		**Base**
HCl	$\rightleftharpoons H^+ +$	Cl^-
CH_3COOH	$\rightleftharpoons H^+ +$	CH_3COO^-
NH_4^+	$\rightleftharpoons H^+ +$	NH_3
HCO_3^-	$\rightleftharpoons H^+ +$	CO_3^{2-}
$H_2PO_4^-$	$\rightleftharpoons H^+ +$	HPO_4^{2-}
H_2O	$\rightleftharpoons H^+ +$	OH^-
H_3O^+	$\rightleftharpoons H^+ +$	H_2O
$Al(H_2O)_6^{3+}$	$\rightleftharpoons H^+ +$	$Al(H_2O)_5OH^{2+}$

It is apparent that not only molecules, but also cations and anions, may function as acids or bases.

The complementary nature of the acid–base pairs listed is reminiscent of the complementary relationship of pairs of oxidants and reductants where, however, the ability to gain or lose one or more electrons—rather than protons—is the distinguishing characteristic.

Oxidant		**Reductant**
Fe^{3+}	$+\ e^- \rightleftharpoons$	Fe^{2+}
Na^+	$+\ e^- \rightleftharpoons$	Na
$\frac{1}{2}I_2$	$+\ e^- \rightleftharpoons$	I^-

However, these examples of acid–base pairs and oxidant–reductant pairs represent reactions that are possible in principle only. Ordinarily acids will not release free protons any more than reductants will release free electrons. That is, protons and electrons, respectively, can be transferred only from one substance (an ion, atom, or molecule) to another. Thus, it is a fundamental fact of chemistry that oxidation of one substance will occur only if reduction of another substance occurs simultaneously. Stated in another way, electrons will be released from the reductant (oxidation) only if an oxidant capable of accepting electrons (reduction) is present. For this reason oxidation–reduction reactions must involve two conjugate oxidant-reductant pairs of substances:

$$\text{oxidant}_1 + \text{reductant}_2 \rightleftharpoons \text{reductant}_1 + \text{oxidant}_2$$

where Subscript 1 represents one conjugate oxidant–reductant pair and Subscript 2 represents the other.

Similarly, an acid will not release a proton unless a base capable of accepting it is present simultaneously. This means that any actual manifestation of acid–base behavior must involve interaction between two sets of conjugate acid–base pairs, represented as

$$\underset{\text{acid}_1}{A_1} + \underset{\text{base}_2}{B_2} \rightleftharpoons \underset{\text{base}_1}{B_1} + \underset{\text{acid}_2}{A_2}$$

In such a reaction, which is called *protolysis* or a *protolytic reaction*, A_1 and B_1 constitute one conjugate acid–base pair, and A_2 and B_2 the other; the proton given up by A_1 (which thereby becomes B_1) is transferred to B_2 (which becomes A_2).

When an acid, such as hydrochloric, is dissolved in water, a *protolytic reaction* occurs.

$$\underset{\text{acid}_1}{HCl} + \underset{\text{base}_2}{H_2O} \rightleftharpoons \underset{\text{base}_1}{Cl^-} + \underset{\text{acid}_2}{H_3O^+}$$

The ionic species H_3O^+, called *hydronium* or *oxonium* ion, always is formed when an acid is dissolved in water. Often, for purposes of convenience, this is written simply as H^+ and is called hydrogen ion, although the "bare" ion practically is nonexistent in solution.

When a base (eg, ammonia) is dissolved in water, the reaction of protolysis is

$$\underset{\text{base}_1}{NH_3} + \underset{\text{acid}_2}{H_2O} \rightleftharpoons \underset{\text{acid}_1}{NH_4^+} + \underset{\text{base}_2}{OH^-}$$

The proton theory of acid–base function makes the concept of hydrolysis superfluous. When, for example, sodium acetate is dissolved in water, this acid–base interaction occurs

$$\underset{\text{base}_1}{CH_3COO^-} + \underset{\text{acid}_2}{H_2O} \rightleftharpoons \underset{\text{acid}_1}{CH_3COOH} + \underset{\text{base}_2}{OH^-}$$

In an aqueous solution of ammonium chloride the reaction is

$$\underset{\text{acid}_1}{NH_4^+} + \underset{\text{base}_2}{H_2O} \rightleftharpoons \underset{\text{base}_1}{NH_3} + \underset{\text{acid}_2}{H_3O^+}$$

Transfer of protons (protolysis) is not limited to dissimilar conjugate acid–base pairs. In the preceding examples H_2O sometimes behaves as an acid and at other times as a base. Such an amphoteric substance is called, in Brønsted's terminology, an *amphiprotic substance.*

ELECTRON-PAIR CONCEPT—The proton concept of acids and bases provides a more general definition for these substances, but it does not indicate the basic reason for proton transfer, nor does it explain how such substances as sulfur trioxide, boron trichloride, stannic chloride, or carbon dioxide—none of which is capable of donating a proton—can behave as acids. Both deficiencies of the proton theory are avoided in the more inclusive definition of acids and bases proposed by Lewis in 1923. In 1916 he proposed that sharing of a pair of electrons by two atoms established a bond (covalent) between the atoms; therefore, an acid is a substance capable of sharing a pair of electrons made available by another substance called a base, thereby forming a *coordinate covalent bond*. The base is the substance that donates a share in its electron pair to the acid.

The following equation illustrates how Lewis' definitions explain the transfer of a proton (hydrogen ion) to ammonia to form ammonium ion.

$$H^+ + \:\overset{\displaystyle H}{\underset{\displaystyle H}{:N:H}} \rightarrow \left[\overset{\displaystyle H}{\underset{\displaystyle H}{H:N:H}}\right]^+$$

The reaction of boron trichloride, which according to the Lewis theory is an acid, with ammonia is similar, for the boron lacks an electron pair if it is to attain a stable octet configuration, while ammonia has a pair of electrons that may be shared, thus,

$$\overset{\displaystyle Cl}{\underset{\displaystyle Cl}{Cl:B}} + \:\overset{\displaystyle H}{\underset{\displaystyle H}{:N:H}} \rightarrow \overset{\displaystyle Cl\ H}{\underset{\displaystyle Cl\ H}{Cl:B:N:H}}$$

LEVELING EFFECT OF A SOLVENT—When the strong acids such as $HClO_4$, H_2SO_4, HCl, or HNO_3 are dissolved in water, the solutions—if they are of identical normality and are not too concentrated—all have about the same hydrogen-ion concentration, indicating the acids to be of about the same strength. The reason for this is that each one of the acids undergoes practically complete protolysis in water.

$$\underset{\text{acid}_1}{HCl} + \underset{\text{base}_2}{H_2O} \rightarrow \underset{\text{base}_1}{Cl^-} + \underset{\text{acid}_2}{H_3O^+}$$

This phenomenon, called the *leveling effect of water,* occurs whenever the added acid is stronger than the hydronium ion. Such a reaction manifests the tendency of proton-transfer reactions to proceed spontaneously in the direction of forming a weaker acid or weaker base.

Since the strongest acid that can exist in an amphiprotic solvent is the conjugate acid form of the solvent, any stronger acid will undergo protolysis to the weaker solvent acid. $HClO_4$, H_2SO_4, HCl, or HNO_3 are all stronger acids than the

hydronium ion, so they are converted in water to the hydronium ion.

When the strong bases sodium hydride, sodium amide, or sodium ethoxide are dissolved in water, each reacts with water to form sodium hydroxide. These reactions illustrate the leveling effect of water on bases. Because the hydroxide ion is the strongest base that can exist in water, any base stronger than the hydroxide ion undergoes protolysis to hydroxide.

Intrinsic differences in the acidity of acids become evident if they are dissolved in a relatively poor proton acceptor such as anhydrous acetic acid. Perchloric acid ($HClO_4$), a strong acid, undergoes practically complete reaction with acetic acid to produce the *acetonium* ion (acid₂):

$$\underset{\substack{\text{acid}_1 \\ \text{(strong)}}}{HClO_4} + \underset{\substack{\text{base}_2 \\ \text{(strong)}}}{CH_3COOH} \rightarrow \underset{\substack{\text{base}_1 \\ \text{(weak)}}}{ClO_4^-} + \underset{\substack{\text{acid}_2 \\ \text{(weak)}}}{CH_3COOH_2^+}$$

but sulfuric acid and hydrochloric acid behave as weak acids. It is because perchloric acid is a very strong acid when dissolved in glacial acetic acid that it has found many important applications in analytical chemistry as a titrant for a variety of substances that behave as bases in acetic acid. Because of its ability to differentiate the acidity of various acids, it is called a *differentiating solvent for acids*; this property results from its relatively weak proton-acceptor tendency. A solvent that differentiates basicity of different bases must have a weak proton-donor tendency; it is called a *differentiating solvent for bases*. Liquid ammonia is typical of solvents in this category.

Solvents that have both weak proton-donor and proton-acceptor tendencies are called *aprotic solvents* and may serve as differentiating solvents for both acids and bases; they have little if any action on solutes and serve mainly as inert dispersion media for the solutes. Useful aprotic solvents are benzene, toluene, or hexane.

IONIZATION OF ACIDS AND BASES—Acids and bases commonly are classified as strong or weak acids and strong or weak bases depending on whether they are ionized extensively or slightly in aqueous solutions. If, for example, 1 N aqueous solutions of hydrochloric acid and acetic acid are compared, it is found that the former is a better conductor of electricity, reacts much more readily with metals, catalyzes certain reactions more efficiently, and possesses a more acid taste than the latter. Both solutions, however, will neutralize identical amounts of alkali. A similar comparison of 1 N solutions of sodium hydroxide and ammonia reveals the former to be more *active* than the latter, although both solutions will neutralize identical quantities of acid.

The differences in the properties of the two acids is attributed to differences in the concentration of hydrogen (more accurately hydronium) ion, the hydrochloric acid being ionized to a greater extent and thus containing a higher concentration of hydrogen ion than acetic acid. Similarly, most of the differences between the sodium hydroxide and ammonia solutions are attributed to the higher hydroxyl-ion concentration in the former.

The ionization of incompletely ionized acids may be considered a reversible reaction of the type

$$HA \rightleftharpoons H^+ + A^-$$

where HA is the molecular acid and A^- is its anion. An equilibrium expression based on the law of mass action may be applied to the reaction

$$K_a = \frac{[H^+][A^-]}{[HA]} \tag{14}$$

where K_a is the ionization or dissociation constant, and the brackets signify concentration. For any given acid in any specified solvent and at any constant temperature, K_a remains relatively constant as the concentration of acid is varied, provided the acid is weakly ionized. With increasingly stronger acids, however, progressively larger deviations occur.

Although the strength of an acid commonly is measured in terms of the ionization or dissociation constant defined in Equation 14, the process of ionization probably is never as simple as shown above. A proton simply will not detach itself from one molecule unless it is accepted simultaneously by another molecule. When an acid is dissolved in water, the latter acts as a base, accepting a proton (Brønsted's definition of a base) by donating a share in a pair of electrons (Lewis' definition of a base). This reaction may be written as

$$HA \ + \ H_2O \ \rightleftharpoons \ A^- \ + \ H_3O^+$$
$$\textbf{acid}_1 \quad \textbf{base}_2 \quad \textbf{base}_1 \quad \textbf{acid}_2$$

Application of the law of mass action to this reaction gives

$$K = \frac{[H_3O^+][A^-]}{[HA][H_2O]} \tag{15}$$

Because $[H_2O]$ is a constant, this equation may be written

$$K_a = \frac{[H_3O^+][A^-]}{[HA]} \tag{16}$$

This equation is identical with Equation 14 because $[H_3O^+]$ is numerically equal to $[H^+]$.

Acids that are capable of donating more than one proton are termed *polyprotic*. The ionization of a polyprotic acid occurs in stages and can be illustrated by considering the equilibria involved in the ionization of phosphoric acid:

$$H_3PO_4 + H_2O \rightleftharpoons H_2PO_4^- + H_3O^+$$
$$H_2PO_4^- + H_2O \rightleftharpoons HPO_4^{2-} + H_3O^+$$
$$HPO_4^{2-} + H_2O \rightleftharpoons PO_4^{3-} + H_3O^+$$

Application of the law of mass action to this series of reactions gives

$$K_1 = \frac{[H_2PO_4^-][H_3O^+]}{[H_3PO_4]} \tag{17}$$

$$K_2 = \frac{[HPO_4^{2-}][H_3O^+]}{[H_2PO_4^{-1}]} \tag{18}$$

$$K_3 = \frac{[PO_4^{3-}][H_3O^+]}{[HPO_4^{2-}]} \tag{19}$$

If the three expressions for the ionization constants are multiplied together, an overall ionization, K, can be obtained

$$K = K_1K_2K_3 = \frac{[PO_4^{3-}][H_3O^+]^3}{[H_3PO_4]} \tag{20}$$

Each of the successive ionizations is suppressed by the hydronium ion formed from preceding stages according to Le Chatelier's principle. The successive dissociation constants always decrease in value, as successive protons must be removed from species that always are charged more negatively. This can be seen from the data in Table 17-4, in which K_1 for phosphoric acid is approximately 100,000 times greater than K_2, which is in turn approximately 100,000 times greater than K_3. Although successive dissociation constants are always smaller, the difference is not always as great as it is for phosphoric acid. Tartaric acid, for example, has $K_1 = 9.12 \times 10^{-4}$ and $K_2 = 4.27 \times 10^{-5}$.

Ionization of a base can be illustrated by using the specific substance NH_3 for an example. According to Brønsted and Lewis, when the base NH_3 is dissolved in water, the latter acts as an acid, donating a proton to NH_3, which accepts it by offering a share in a pair of electrons on the nitrogen atom. This reaction is written

$$NH_3 + H_2O \rightleftharpoons NH_4^+ + OH^-$$
$$\textbf{base} \quad \textbf{acid}$$

Table 17-4. Dissociation Constants in Water at 25°

SUBSTANCE		K
Weak acids		
Acetic		1.75×10^{-3}
Acetylsalicylic		3.27×10^{-4}
Barbital		1.23×10^{-8}
Barbituric		1.05×10^{-4}
Benzoic		6.30×10^{-5}
Benzyl penicillin		1.74×10^{-3}
Boric	K_1	5.8×10^{-10}
Caffeine		1×10^{-14}
Carbonic	K_1	4.31×10^{-7}
	K_2	4.7×10^{-11}
Citric (1H$_2$O)	K_1	7.0×10^{-4}
	K_2	1.8×10^{-5}
	K_3	4.0×10^{-7}
Dichloroacetic		5×10^{-2}
Ethylenediaminetetra-acetic acid (EDTA)	K_1	1×10^{-2}
	K_2	2.14×10^{-3}
	K_3	6.92×10^{-7}
	K_4	5.5×10^{-11}
Formic		1.77×10^{-4}
Glycerophosphoric	K_1	3.4×10^{-2}
	K_2	6.4×10^{-7}
Glycine	K_1	4.5×10^{-3}
	K_2	1.7×10^{-10}
Lactic		1.39×10^{-4}
Mandelic		4.29×10^{-4}
Monochloroacetic		1.4×10^{-3}
Oxalic (2H$_2$O)	K_1	5.5×10^{-2}
	K_2	5.3×10^{-5}
Phenobarbital		3.9×10^{-8}
Phenol		1×10^{-10}
Phosphoric	K_1	7.5×10^{-3}
	K_2	6.2×10^{-8}
	K_3	2.1×10^{-13}
Picric		4.2×10^{-1}
Propionic		1.34×10^{-5}
Saccharin		2.5×10^{-2}
Salicylic		1.06×10^{-3}
Succinic	K_1	6.4×10^{-5}
	K_2	2.3×10^{-6}
Sulfadiazine		3.3×10^{-7}
Sulfamerazine		8.7×10^{-8}
Sulfapyridine		3.6×10^{-9}
Sulfathiazole		7.6×10^{-8}
Tartaric	K_1	9.6×10^{-4}
	K_2	4.4×10^{-5}
Trichloroacetic		1.3×10^{-1}
Weak bases		
Acetanilide		4.1×10^{-14} (40°)
Ammonia		1.74×10^{-5}
Apomorphine		1.0×10^{-7}
Atropine		4.5×10^{-5}
Benzocaine		6.0×10^{-12}
Caffeine		4.1×10^{-14} (40°)
Cocaine		2.6×10^{-6}
Codeine		9×10^{-7}
Ephedrine		2.3×10^{-5}
Morphine		7.4×10^{-7}
Papaverine		8×10^{-9}
Physostigmine	K_1	7.6×10^{-7}
	K_2	5.7×10^{-13}
Pilocarpine	K_1	7×10^{-8}
	K_2	2×10^{-13}
Procaine		7×10^{-6}
Pyridine		1.4×10^{-9}
Quinine	K_1	1.0×10^{-6}
	K_2	1.3×10^{-10}
Reserpine		4×10^{-8}
Strychnine	K_1	1×10^{-6}
	K_2	2×10^{-12}
Theobromine		4.8×10^{-14} (40°)
Thiourea		1.1×10^{-15}
Urea		1.5×10^{-14}

The equilibrium expression for this reaction is

$$K = \frac{[NH_4^+][OH^-]}{[NH_3][H_2O]} \quad (21)$$

With $[H_2O]$ constant, this expression may be written

$$K_b = \frac{[NH_4^+][OH^-]}{[NH_3]} \quad (22)$$

IONIZATION OF WATER—Although it is a poor conductor of electricity, pure water does ionize through a process known as *autoprotolysis*, in the following manner:

$$2H_2O \rightleftharpoons H_3O^+ + OH^-$$

Application of the law of mass action to this reaction gives

$$K = \frac{[H_3O^+][OH^-]}{[H_2O]^2} \quad (23)$$

where K is the equilibrium constant for the reaction. Because the concentration of H_2O (molecular water) is very much greater than either the hydronium-ion or hydroxyl-ion concentrations, it can be considered to be constant and can be combined with K to give a new constant, K_w, known as the *ion product* of water, and Equation 23 becomes

$$K_w = [H_3O^+][OH^-] \quad (24)$$

The numerical value of K_w varies with temperature; at 25° it is approximately equal to 1×10^{-14}.

Since the autoprotolysis of pure water yields one hydronium ion for each hydroxyl ion produced, $[H_3O^+]$ equal to $[OH^-]$. At 25° each has a value of 1×10^{-7} mol/L ($1 \times 10^{-7} \times 1 \times 10^{-7} = K_w = 1 \times 10^{-14}$). A solution in which $[H_3O^+]$ is equal to $[OH^-]$ is termed a *neutral* solution.

If an acid is added to water, the hydronium-ion concentration will be increased and the equilibrium between hydronium and hydroxyl ions will be disturbed *momentarily*. To restore equilibrium, some of the hydroxyl ions, originally present in the water, will combine with a *part* of the added hydronium ions to form nonionized water molecules, until the product of the concentrations of the two ions has been reduced to 10^{-14}. When equilibrium again is restored, the concentrations of the two ions no longer will be equal. If, for example, the hydronium-ion concentration is 1×10^{-3} N when equilibrium is established, the concentration of hydroxyl ion will be 1×10^{-11} (the product of the two concentrations being equal to 10^{-14}). As $[H_3O^+]$ is much greater than $[OH^-]$, the solution is said to be *acid* or *acidic*.

In a similar manner, the addition of an alkali to pure water momentarily disturbs the equilibrium between hydronium and hydroxyl ions. To restore equilibrium, some of the hydronium ions originally present in the water will combine with part of the added hydroxyl ions to form nonionized water molecules. The process continues until the product of the hydronium and hydroxyl ion concentrations again is equal to 10^{-14}. Assuming that the final hydroxyl-ion concentration is 1×10^{-4} N, the concentration of hydronium ion in the solution will be 1×10^{-10}. Because $[OH^-]$ is much greater than $[H_3O^+]$, the solution is said to be *basic* or *alkaline*.

RELATIONSHIP OF K_A AND $_{KB}$—A particularly interesting and useful relationship between the strength of an acid and its conjugate base, or a base and its conjugate acid, exists. For illustration, consider the strength of the base NH_3 and its conjugate acid NH_4^+ in water. The behavior of NH_3 as a base is expressed by

$$NH_3 + H_2O \rightleftharpoons NH_4^+ + OH^-$$

for which the equilibrium, as formulated earlier, is

$$K_b = \frac{[NH_4^+][OH^-]}{[NH_3]} \quad (25)$$

The behavior of NH_4^+ as an acid is represented by

$$NH_4^+ + H_2O \rightleftharpoons NH_3 + H_3O^+$$

The equilibrium constant for this is

$$K_a = \frac{[NH_3][H_3O^+]}{[NH_4^+]} \quad (26)$$

Multiplying Equations 25 and 26

$$K_a K_b = \frac{[NH_3][H_3O^+][NH_4^+][OH^-]}{[NH_4^+][NH_3]} \quad (27)$$

It is obvious that

$$K_w = K_a K_b \quad (28)$$

where K_w is the ion product of water as defined in Equation 24.

The utility of this relationship, which is a general one for any conjugate acid−base pair, is evident from the following deductions: (1) The strength of an acid may be expressed in terms either of the K_a or the K_b of its conjugate base, or *vice versa*; (2) the K_a of an acid may be calculated if the K_b of its conjugate base is known, or *vice versa*; and (3) the stronger an acid is, the weaker its conjugate base, or *vice versa*.

Bases that are capable of interacting with more than one proton are termed *polyacidic*, and can be illustrated by

$$PO_4^{3-} + H_2O \rightleftharpoons HPO_4^{2-} + OH^-$$

$$HPO_4^{2-} + H_2O \rightleftharpoons H_2PO_4^- + OH^-$$

$$H_2PO_4^- + H_2O \rightleftharpoons H_3PO_4 + OH^-$$

Applying the law of mass action to this series of reactions, and using the concepts outlined in Equations 25 to 28, the relationship between the various K_a and K_b values for phosphoric acid are

$$K_w = K_{a1} \times K_{b3} = K_{a2} \times K_{b2} = K_{a3} \times K_{b1} \quad (29)$$

where K_{a1}, K_{a2}, and K_{a3} refer to the equilibria given by Equations 17, 18, and 19, respectively; K_{b1}, K_{b2}, and K_{b3} refer to the reaction of PO_4^{3-}, HPO_4^{2-}, and $H_2PO_4^-$, respectively, with water.

ELECTRONEGATIVITY AND DISSOCIATION CONSTANTS—Table 17-4 gives the dissociation constants of several weak acids and weak bases, in water, at 25°. Strong acids and strong bases do not obey the law of mass action, so dissociation constants cannot be formulated for these strong electrolytes.

Table 17-4 shows that great variations occur in the strength of weak acids and weak bases. The effect of various substituents on the strength of acids and bases depends on the electronegativity of the substituent atom or radical. For example, the substitution of one chlorine atom into the molecule of acetic acid increases the degree of ionization of the acid. Substitution of two chlorine atoms further increases the degree of ionization, and introduction of three chlorine atoms produces a still stronger acid. Acetic acid ionizes primarily because the oxygen atom adjacent to the hydrogen atom of the carboxyl group has a stronger affinity for electrons than the hydrogen atom. Thus, when acetic acid is dissolved in water, the polar molecules of the water have a stronger affinity for the hydrogen of acetic acid than the hydrogen atoms of water. The acetic acid ionizes as a consequence of this difference in affinities.

When an atom of chlorine is introduced into the acetic acid molecule, forming $ClCH_2COOH$, the electrons in the molecule are attracted very strongly to the chlorine because of its relatively high electronegativity; the bond between the hydrogen and the oxygen in the carboxyl group is thereby weakened, and the degree of ionization increased. Introduction of two or three chlorine atoms weakens the bond further and increases the strength of the acid. On the other hand, substitution of chlorine into the molecule of ammonia reduces the strength of the base because of its decreased affinity for the hydrogen ion.

IONIC STRENGTH AND DISSOCIATION CONSTANTS—Most solutions of pharmaceutical interest are in a concentration range such that the ionic strength of the solution may have a marked effect on ionic equilibria and observed dissociation constants. One method of correcting dissociation constants for solutions with an ionic strength up to about 0.3 is to calculate an apparent dissociation constant, pK_a', as

$$pK_a' = pK_a + \frac{0.51\,(2Z-1)\,\sqrt{\mu}}{1+\sqrt{\mu}} \tag{30}$$

in which pK_a is the tabulated thermodynamic dissociation constant, Z is the charge on the acid, and μ is the ionic strength.

Example—Calculate pK_2' for succinic acid at an ionic strength of 0.1. Assume that pK_2 is 5.63. The charge on the acid species is -1.

$$pK_2' = 5.63\,\frac{0.51\,(-2-1)\,\sqrt{0.1}}{1+\sqrt{0.1}}$$

$$= 5.63 - 0.37 = 5.26$$

DETERMINATION OF DISSOCIATION CONSTANTS—Although the dissociation constant of a weak acid or base can be obtained in a wide variety of ways including conductivity measurements, absorption spectrometry and partition coefficients, the most widely used method is potentiometric pH measurement (see *Potentiometry*). The simplest method involving potentiometric pH measurement is based on the measurement of the hydronium-ion concentration of a solution containing equimolar concentrations of the acid and a strong-base salt of the acid. The principle of this method is evident from an inspection of Equation 16; when equimolar concentrations of HA (the acid) and A^- (the salt) are present, the dissociation constant, K_a, numerically is equal to the hydronium-ion concentration (also, the pK_a of the acid is equal to the pH of the solution). Although this method is simple and rapid, the dissociation constant obtained is not sufficiently accurate for many purposes.

To obtain the dissociation constant of a weak acid with a high degree of accuracy and precision, a dilute solution of the acid (about 10^{-3} to $10^{-4}\,M$) is titrated with a strong base, and the pH of the solution taken after each addition of base. The resulting data can be handled in a wide variety of ways, perhaps the best of which is the method proposed by Benet and Goyan.[1] The proton balance equation for a weak acid, HA, being titrated with a strong base such as KOH, would be

$$[K^+] + [H_3O^+] = [OH^-] + [A^-] \tag{31}$$

in which $[K^+]$ is the concentration of the base added. Equation 31 can be rearranged to give

$$Z = [A^-] = [K^+] + [H_3O^+] - [OH^-] \tag{32}$$

When a weak monoprotic acid is added to water, it can exist in the unionized form, HA, and in the ionized form, A^-. After equilibrium is established, the sum of the concentrations of both species must be equal to C_a, the stoichiometric (added) concentration of acid, or

$$C_a = [HA] + [A^-] = [HA] + Z \tag{33}$$

The term [HA] can be replaced using Equation 16 to give

$$C_a = \frac{[H_3O^+]Z}{K_a} + Z \tag{34}$$

which can be rearranged to

$$Z = C_a - \frac{Z[H_3O^+]}{K_a} \tag{35}$$

According to Equation 35, if Z, which is obtained from the experimental data using Equation 32, is plotted versus the terms $Z[H_3O^+]$, a straight line results with a slope equal to $1/K_a$, and an intercept equal to C_a. In addition to obtaining an accurate estimate for the dissociation constant, the stoichiometric concentration of the substance being titrated is also obtained. This is of importance when the substance being titrated cannot be purified, or has an unknown degree of solvation. Similar equations can be developed for obtaining the dissociation constant for a weak base.[1]

The dissociation constants for diprotic acids can be obtained by defining P as the average number of protons dissociated per mole of acid, or

$$P = Z/C_a \tag{36}$$

and

$$\frac{[H_3O^+]^2P}{(2-P)} = K_1K_2 + \frac{K_1[H_3O^+](1-P)}{(2-P)} \tag{37}$$

A plot of Equation 37 should yield a straight line with a slope equal to K_1 and an intercept of K_1K_2. Dividing the intercept by the slope yields K_2.

MICRO DISSOCIATION CONSTANTS—The dissociation constants for polyprotic acids, as determined by potentiometric titration, are known generally as *macro,* or *titration, constants*. As it is known that carboxyl groups are stronger acids than protonated amino groups, there is no difficulty in assigning K_1 and K_2, as determined by Equation 37, to the carboxyl and amino groups, respectively, of a substance such as glycine hydrochloride.

In other chemicals or drugs such as phenylpropanolamine, in which the two acidic groups are the phenolic and the protonated amino group, the assignment of dissociation constants is more difficult. This is because, in general, both groups have dissociation constants of equal magnitude. Thus, there will be two ways of losing the first proton and two ways of losing the second, resulting in four possible species in solution. This can be illustrated using the convention of assigning a plus ($+$) to a positively charged group, a 0 to an uncharged group, and a minus ($-$) to a negatively charged group. Thus, $+0$ would represent the fully protonated phenylpropanolamine, $+-$ the dipolar ion, 00 the uncharged molecule, and $0-$, the anion. The total ionization scheme, therefore, can be written

$$+0 \underset{k_2}{\overset{k_1}{\rightleftharpoons}} \begin{matrix} +- \\ \\ 00 \end{matrix} \underset{k_4}{\overset{k_3}{\rightleftharpoons}} 0-$$

The micro constants are related to the macro constants as

$$K_1 = k_1 + k_2 \tag{38}$$

$$K_1K_2 = k_1k_3 = k_2k_4 \tag{39}$$

It can be seen from Equation 38 that unless k_1 or k_2 is very much smaller than the other, the observed macro constant is a composite of the two and cannot be assigned to one or the other acidic group in a nonambiguous way.

Methods for determining k_1 are given by Riegelman et al[2] and Niebergall et al.[3] Once k_1, K_1, and K_2 have been determined, all of the other micro constants can be obtained from Equations 38 and 39.

pH

The numerical values of hydronium-ion concentration may vary enormously; for a normal solution of a strong acid the value is nearly 1, while for a normal solution of a strong base it is approximately 1×10^{-14}; there is a variation of 100,000,000,000,000 between these two limits. Because of the inconvenience of dealing with such large numbers, in 1909 Sørenson proposed that hydronium-ion concentration be expressed in terms of the logarithm (log) of its reciprocal. To this value he assigned the symbol pH. Mathematically it is written

$$pH = \log \frac{1}{[H_3O^+]} \tag{40}$$

Since the logarithm of 1 is zero, the equation also may be written

$$pH = -\log [H_3O^+] \tag{41}$$

from which it is evident that pH also may be defined as the negative logarithm of the hydronium-ion concentration. In general, this type of notation is used to indicate the negative logarithm of the term that is preceded by the p, which gives rise to the following

$$pOH = -\log [OH^-] \tag{42}$$

$$pK = -\log K \tag{43}$$

Thus, taking logarithms of Equations 28 and 24 gives

$$pK_a + pK_b = pK_w \tag{44}$$

$$pH + pOH = pK_w \tag{45}$$

The relationship of pH to hydronium-ion and hydroxyl-ion concentrations may be seen in Table 17-5.

The following examples illustrate the conversion from exponential to p notation.

1. Calculate the pH corresponding to a hydronium-ion concentration of 1×10^{-4} g-ion/L.

   Solution:

   $$pH = \log \frac{1}{1 \times 10^{-4}}$$

   $$= \log 10,000 \text{ or } \log (1 \times 10^{+4})$$

   $$\log (1 \times 10^{+4}) = +4$$

   $$pH = 4$$

Table 17-5. Hydronium-Ion and Hydroxyl-Ion Concentrations

	PH	NORMALITY IN TERMS OF HYDRONIUM ION	NORMALITY IN TERMS OF HYDROXYL ION
	0	1	10^{-14}
	1	10^{-1}	10^{-13}
	2	10^{-2}	10^{-12}
Increasing	3	10^{-3}	10^{-11}
acidity	4	10^{-4}	10^{-10}
	5	10^{-5}	10^{-9}
	6	10^{-6}	10^{-8}
Neutral point	7	10^{-7}	10^{-7}
	8	10^{-8}	10^{-6}
	9	10^{-9}	10^{-5}
	10	10^{-10}	10^{-4}
	11	10^{-11}	10^{-3}
Increasing	12	10^{-12}	10^{-2}
alkalinity	13	10^{-13}	10^{-1}
	14	10^{-14}	1

2. Calculate the pH corresponding to a hydronium ion-concentration of 0.000036 N (or g-ion/L). (*Note:* This more frequently is written as a number multiplied by a power of 10, thus, 3.6×10^{-5} for 0.000036.)

Solution:

$$pH = \log \frac{1}{3.6 \times 10^{-5}}$$

$$= \log 28,000 \text{ or } \log (2.8 \times 10^{+4})$$

$$\log (2.8 \times 10^{+4}) = \log 2.8 + 10^{+4}$$

$$\log 2.8 = +0.44$$

$$\log 10^{+4} = +4.00$$

$$pH = 4.44$$

This problem also may be solved as follows:

$$pH = -\log (3.6 \times 10^{-5})$$

$$\log 3.6 = +0.56$$

$$\log 10^{-5} = -5.00$$

$$= -4.44 = \log (3.6 \times 10^{-5})$$

$$pH = -(-4.44) = +4.44 = 4.44$$

The following examples illustrate the conversion of p notation to exponential notation.

1. Calculate the hydronium-ion concentration corresponding to a pH of 4.44.

   Solution:

   $$pH = \log \frac{1}{[H_3O^+]}$$

   $$4.44 = \log \frac{1}{[H_3O^+]}$$

   $$\frac{1}{[H_3O^+]} = \text{antilog of } 4.44 = 28,000 \text{ (rounded off)}$$

   $$[H_3O^+] = \frac{1}{28,000} = 0.000036 \text{ or } 3.6 \times 10^{-5}$$

This calculation also may be made as

$$+4.44 = -\log [H_3O^+]$$

or

$$-4.44 = +\log [H_3O^+]$$

In finding the antilog of -4.44 it should be kept in mind that the *mantissa* (the number to the right of the decimal point) of a log to the base 10 (the common or Briggsian logarithm base) is *always positive* but that the characteristic (the number to the left of the decimal point) may be *positive or negative*. As the entire log -4.44 is negative, it is obvious that one cannot look up the antilog of -0.44. However, the number -4.44 also may be written $(-5.00 + 0.56)$, or as more often written, $\overline{5}.56$; the bar across the characteristic indicates that it alone is negative, while the rest of the number is positive. Looking up the antilog of 0.56 it is found to be 3.6; as the antilog of -5.00 is 10^{-5}, it follows that the hydronium-ion concentration must be 3.6×10^{-5} mols/L.

2. Calculate the hydronium-ion concentration corresponding to a pH of 10.17.

   Solution:

   $$10.17 = -\log[H_3O^+]$$

   $$-10.17 = \log[H_3O^+]$$

   $$-10.17 = (-11.00 + 0.83) = \overline{11}.83$$

The antilog of 0.83 = 6.8.
The antilog of $-11.00 = 10^{-11}$
The hydronium-ion concentration is therefore 6.8×10^{-11} mol/L.

In the section *Ionization of Water*, it was shown that the hydronium-ion concentration of pure water, at 25°, is 1×10^{-7} N, corresponding to a pH of 7.

This figure, therefore, is designated as the neutral point, and all values below a pH of 7 represent acidity—the smaller the number, the greater the acidity. Values above 7 represent alkalinity—the larger the number, the greater the alkalinity. The pH scale usually runs from 0 to 14, but mathematically there is no reason why negative numbers or numbers above 14 should not be used. In practice, however, such values are never encountered because solutions that might be expected to have such values are too concentrated to be ionized extensively or the interionic attraction is so great as to materially reduce ionic activity.

The pH of the purest water obtainable, so-called 'conductivity water', is 7 when the measurement is made carefully under conditions to exclude carbon dioxide and prevent errors inherent in the measuring technique (such as acidity or alkalinity of the indicator). Upon agitating this water in the presence of carbon dioxide in the atmosphere (equilibrium water), the value drops rapidly to 5.7. This is the pH of nearly all distilled water that has been exposed to the atmosphere for even a short time and often is called 'equilibrium' water.

It should be emphasized strongly that the generalizations stated concerning neutrality, acidity, and alkalinity hold exactly only when (1) the solvent is water, (2) the temperature is 25°, and (3) there are no other factors to cause deviation from the simply formulated equilibria underlying the definition of pH given in the preceding discussion.

SPECIES CONCENTRATION

When a weak acid, H_nA is added to water, $n + 1$ species, including the un-ionized acid, can exist. After equilibrium is established, the sum of the concentrations of all species must be equal to C_a, the stoichiometric (added) concentration of acid. Thus, for a triprotic acid H_3A,

$$C_a = [H_3A] + [H_2A^-] + [HA^{2-}] + [A_3^-] \tag{46}$$

In addition, the concentrations of all acidic and basic species in solution vary with pH, and can be represented solely in terms of equilibrium constants and the hydronium-ion concentration. These relationships may be expressed as

$$[H_nA] = [H_3O^+]^n C_a / D \tag{47}$$

$$[H_{n-j}A^{-j}] = [H_3O^+]^{n-j} K_1, \ldots, K_j C_a / D \tag{48}$$

in which n represents the total number of dissociable hydrogens in the parent acid, j is the number of protons dissociated, C_a is the stoichiometric concentration of acid, and K represents the acid dissociation constants. The term D is a power series in $[H_3O^+]$ and K, starting with $[H_3O^+]$ raised to the nth power. The last term is the product of all the dissociation constants. The intermediate terms can be generated from the last term by substituting $[H_3O^+]$ for K_n to obtain the next-to-last term, then substituting $[H_3O^+]$ for K_{n-1} to obtain the next term, and onward until the first term is reached. The following examples show the denominator, D, to be used for various types of acids:

$$H_3A: D = [H_3O^+]^3 + K_1[H_3O^+]^2 + K_1K_2[H_3O^+] + K_1K_2K_3 \tag{49}$$

$$H_2A: D = [H_3O^+]^2 + K_1[H_3O^+] + K_1K_2 \tag{50}$$

$$HA: D = [H_3O^+] + K_a \tag{51}$$

The numerator in all instances is C_a multiplied by the term from the denominator that has $[H_3O^+]$ raised to the $n - j$ power. Thus, for diprotic acids such as carbonic, succinic, tartaric, and so on,

$$[H_2A] = \frac{[H_3O^+]^2 C_a}{[H_3O^+]^2 + K_1[H_3O^+] + K_1K_2} \tag{52}$$

$$[HA^-] = \frac{K_1[H_3O^+]C_a}{[H_3O^+]^2 + K_1[H_3O^+] + K_1K_2} \tag{53}$$

$$[A^{2-}] = \frac{K_1K_2C_a}{[H_3O^+]^2 + K_1[H_3O^+] + K_1K_2} \tag{54}$$

Example—Calculate the concentrations of all succinic acid species in a 1.0×10^{-3} M solution of succinic acid at pH 6. Assume that $K_1 = 6.4 \times 10^{-5}$ and $K_2 = 2.3 \times 10^{-6}$.

Equations 52–54 have the same denominator, D, which can be calculated as

$$\begin{aligned}
D &= [H_3O^+]^2 + K_1[H_3O^+] + K_1K_2 \\
&= 1.0 \times 10^{-12} + 6.4 \times 10^{-5} \times 1.0 \times 10^{-6} + 6.4 \\
&\quad \times 10^{-5} \times 2.3 \times 10^{-6} \\
&= 1.0 \times 10^{-12} + 6.4 \times 10^{-11} + 14.7 \times 10^{-11} \\
&= 21.2 \times 10^{-11}
\end{aligned}$$

Therefore,

$$[H_2A] = \frac{[H_3O^+]^2 C_a}{D}$$

$$= \frac{1.0 \times 10^{-12} \times 1.0 \times 10^{-3}}{21.2 \times 10^{-11}} = 4.7 \times 10^{-6} M$$

$$[HA^-] = \frac{K_1[H_3O^+]C_a}{D}$$

$$= \frac{6.4 \times 10^{-11} \times 1.0 \times 10^{-3}}{21.2 \times 10^{-11}} = 3.0 \times 10^{-4} M$$

$$[A^{2-}] = \frac{K_1K_2C_a}{D}$$

$$= \frac{14.7 \times 10^{-11} \times 1.0 \times 10^{-3}}{21.2 \times 10^{-11}} = 6.9 \times 10^{-4} M$$

PROTON-BALANCE EQUATION

In the Brønsted–Lowry system, the total number of protons released by acidic species must equal the total number of protons consumed by basic species. This results in a very useful relationship known as the *proton-balance equation* (PBE), in which the sum of the concentration terms for species that form by proton consumption is equated to the sum of the concentration terms for species that are formed by the release of protons. The PBE forms the basis of a unified approach to pH calculations, as it is an exact accounting of all proton transfers occurring in solution.

When HCl is added to water, for example, it dissociates yielding one Cl^- for each proton released. Thus, Cl^- is a species formed by the release of a proton. In the same solution, and actually in all aqueous solutions

$$2H_2O \rightleftharpoons H_3O^+ + OH^-$$

where H_3O^+ is formed by proton consumption and OH^- is formed by proton release. Thus, the PBE is

$$[H_3O^+] = [OH^-] + [Cl^-] \tag{55}$$

In general, the PBE can be formed in the following manner:

1. Start with the species added to water.
2. Place all species that can form when protons are released on the right side of the equation.
3. Place all species that can form when protons are consumed on the left side of the equation.
4. Multiply the concentration of each species by the number of photons gained or lost to form that species.
5. Add $[H_3O^+]$ the left side of the equation and $[OH^-]$ to the right side of the equation. These result from the interaction of two molecules of water as shown above.

Example—When H_3PO_4 is added to water, the species $H_2PO_4^-$ forms with the release of one proton; HPO_4^{2-} forms with the release of two protons; and PO_4^{3-} forms with the release of three protons, which gives the following PBE:

$$[H_3O^+] = [OH^-] + [H_2PO_4^-] + 2[HPO_4^{2-}] + 3[PO_4^{3-}] \quad (56)$$

Example—When Na_2HPO_4 is added to water, it dissociates into two Na^+ and one HPO_4^{2-}. The sodium ion is neglected in the PBE because it is not formed from the release or consumption of protons. The species HPO_4^{2-}, however, may react with water to give $H_2PO_4^-$ with the consumption of one proton, H_3PO_4 with the consumption of two protons, and PO_4^{3-} with the release of one proton to give the following PBE:

$$[H_3O^+] + [H_2PO_4^-] + 2[H_3PO_4] = [OH^-] + [PO_4^{3-}] \quad (57)$$

CALCULATIONS

The pH of solutions of acids, bases, and salts may be calculated using the concepts presented in the preceding sections.

Strong Acids or Bases

When a strong acid such as HCl is added to water, the following reactions occur:

$$HCl + H_2O \rightarrow H_3O^+ + Cl^-$$

$$2H_2O \rightleftharpoons H_3O^+ + OH^-$$

The PBE for this system would be

$$[H_3O^+] = [OH^-] + [Cl^-] \quad (58)$$

In most instances ($C_a > 4.5 \times 10^{-7} M$) the $[OH^-]$ would be negligible compared to the Cl^- and the equation simplifies to

$$[H_3O^+] = [Cl^-] = C_a \quad (59)$$

Thus, the hydronium-ion concentration of a solution of a strong acid would be equal to the stoichiometric concentration of the acid. This would be anticipated, because strong acids generally are assumed to be 100% ionized.

The pH of a 0.005 M solution of HCl therefore is calculated as

$$pH = -\log 0.005 = 2.30$$

In a similar manner the hydroxyl-ion concentration for a solution of a strong base such as NaOH would be

$$[OH^-] = [Na^+] = C_b \quad (60)$$

and the pH of a 0.005 M solution of NaOH would be

$$pOH = -\log 0.005 = 2.30$$

$$pH = pK_w - pOH = 14.00 - 2.30 = 11.70$$

Weak Acids or Bases

If a weak acid, HA, is added to water, it will equilibrate with its conjugate base, A^-, as

$$HA + H_2O \rightleftharpoons H_3O^+ + A^-$$

Accounting for the ionization of water gives the following PBE for this system:

$$[H_3O^+] = [OH^-] + [A^-] \quad (61)$$

The concentration of A^- as a function of hydronium-ion concentration can be obtained as shown previously to give

$$[H_3O^+] = [OH^-] + \frac{K_a C_a}{[H_3O^+] + K_a} \quad (62)$$

Algebraic simplification yields

$$[H_3O^+] = K_a \frac{(C_a - [H_3O^+] + [OH^-])}{([H_3O^+] - [OH^-])} \quad (63)$$

In most instances for solutions of weak acids, $[H_3O^+] \gg [OH^-]$, and the equation simplifies to give

$$[H_3O^+]^2 + K_a[H_3O^+] - K_aC_a = 0 \quad (64)$$

This is a quadratic equation* that yields

$$[H_3O^+] = \frac{-K_a + \sqrt{K_a^2 + 4K_aC_a}}{2} \quad (65)$$

since $[H_3O^+]$ can never be negative. Furthermore, if $[H_3O^+]$ is less than 5% of C_a, Equation 64 is simplified further to give

$$[H_3O^+] = \sqrt{K_aC_a} \quad (66)$$

It generally is preferable to use the simplest equation to calculate $[H_3O^+]$. However, when $[H_3O^+]$ is calculated, it must be compared to C_a in order to determine whether the assumption $C_a \gg [H_3O^+]$ is valid. If the assumption is not valid, the quadratic equation should be used.

Example—Calculate the pH of a $5.00 \times 10^{-5} M$ solution of a weak acid having a $K_a = 1.90 \times 10^{-5}$.

$$[H_3O^+] = \sqrt{K_aC_a}$$
$$= \sqrt{1.90 \times 10^{-5} \times 5.00 \times 10^{-5}}$$
$$= 3.08 \times 10^{-5} M$$

As C_a [($5.00 \times 10^{-5} M$)] is not much greater than $[H_3O^+]$, the quadratic equation (Equation 65) should be used.

$$[H_3O^+ = \frac{-1.90 \times 10^{-5} + \sqrt{(1.90 \times 10^{-5})^2 + 4(5.00 \times 10^{-5})}}{2}$$
$$= 7.06 \times 10^{-3}$$
$$pH = -\log (7.06 \times 10^{-3}) = 2.15$$

Note that the assumption $[H_3O^+] \gg [OH^-]$ is valid. The hydronium-ion concentration calculated from Equation 66 has a relative error of about 100% when compared to the correct value obtained from Equation 65.

When a salt obtained from a strong acid and a weak base—such as ammonium chloride, morphine sulfate, or pilocarpine hydrochloride—is dissolved in water, it dissociates as

$$BH^+X^- \xrightarrow{H_2O} BH^+ + X^-$$

in which BH^+ is the protonated form of the base B, and X^- is the anion of a strong acid. Because X^- is the anion of a strong acid, it is too weak a base to undergo any further reaction with water. The protonated base, however, can act as a weak acid to give

$$BH^+ + H_2O \rightleftharpoons B + H_3O^+$$

Thus, Equations 65 and 66 are valid, with C_a being equal to the concentration of the salt in solution. If K_a for the protonated base is not available, it can be obtained by dividing K_b for the base B, into K_w.

Example—Calculate the pH of a 0.026 M solution of ammonium chloride. Assume that K_b for ammonia is 1.74×10^{-5} and K_w is 1.00×10^{-14}.

---

* The general solution to a quadratic equation of the form

$$aX^2 + bX + c = 0 \quad \text{is} \quad X = \frac{-b \pm \sqrt{b^2 - 4ac}}{2a}$$

$$K_a = \frac{K_w}{K_b} = \frac{1.00 \times 10^{-14}}{1.74 \times 10^{-5}} = 5.75 \times 10^{-10}$$

$$[H_3O^+] = \sqrt{K_a C_a}$$

$$= \sqrt{5.75 \times 10^{-10} \times 2.6 \times 10^{-2}}$$

$$= 3.87 \times 10^{-6} \, M$$

$$pH = -\log(3.87 \times 10^{-6}) = 5.41$$

As C_a is much greater than $[H_3O^+]$ and $[H_3O^+]$ is much greater than $[OH^-]$, the assumptions are valid and the value calculated for pH is sufficiently accurate.

Weak Bases

When a weak base, B, is dissolved in water it ionizes to give the conjugate acid as

$$B + H_2O \rightleftharpoons BH^+ + OH^-$$

The PBE for this system is

$$[BH^+] + [H_3O^+] = [OH^-] \tag{67}$$

Substituting $[BH^+]$ as a function of hydronium-ion concentration and simplifying, in the same manner as shown for a weak acid, gives

$$[OH^-] = K_b \frac{(C_b - [OH^-] + [H_3O^+])}{([OH^-] - [H_3O^+])} \tag{68}$$

If $[OH^-] \gg [H_3O^+]$, as is true generally, then

$$[OH^-]^2 = K_b[OH^-] - K_b C_b = 0 \tag{69}$$

which is a quadratic with the following solution:

$$[OH^-] = \frac{-K_b + \sqrt{K_b^2 + 4K_b C_b}}{2} \tag{70}$$

If $C_b \gg [OH^-]$, the quadratic equation simplifies to

$$[OH^-] = \sqrt{K_b C_b} \tag{71}$$

Once $[OH^-]$ is calculated, it can be converted to pOH, which can be subtracted from pK_w to give pH.

Example—Calculate the pH of a $4.50 \times 10^{-2} \, M$ solution of a weak base having $K_b = 2.00 \times 10^{-4}$. Assume that $K_w = 1.00 \times 10^{-14}$.

$$[OH^-] = \sqrt{K_b C_b}$$

$$= \sqrt{2.00 \times 10^{-4} \times 4.50 \times 10^{-2}}$$

$$= \sqrt{9.00 \times 10^{-6}} = 3.00 \times 10^{-3} \, M$$

Both assumptions are valid.

$$pOH = -\log 3.00 \times 10^{-3} = 2.52$$

$$pH = 14.00 - 2.52 = 11.48$$

When salts obtained from strong bases and weak acids (eg, sodium acetate, sodium sulfathiazole, or sodium benzoate) are dissolved in water, they dissociate as

$$Na^+ A^- \xrightarrow{H_2O} Na^+ + A^-$$

in which A^- is the conjugate base of the weak acid, HA. The Na^+ undergoes no further reaction with water. The A^-, however, acts as a weak base to give

$$A^- + H_2O \rightleftharpoons HA + OH^-$$

Thus, Equations 70 and 71 are valid, with C_b being equal to the concentration of the salt in solution. The value for K_b can be obtained by dividing K_a for the conjugate acid, HA, into K_w.

Example—Calculate the pH of a $0.05 \, M$ solution of sodium acetate. Assume that K_a for acetic acid $= 1.75 \times 10^{-5}$ and $K_w = 1.00 \times 10^{-14}$.

$$K_b = \frac{K_w}{K_a} = \frac{1.00 \times 10^{-14}}{1.75 \times 10^{-5}}$$

$$= 5.71 \times 10^{-10}$$

$$OH^- = \sqrt{K_b C_b} = \sqrt{5.71 \times 10^{-10} \times 5.0 \times 10^{-2}}$$

$$= 5.34 \times 10^{-6} \, M$$

Both assumptions are valid:

$$pOH = -\log(5.34 \times 10^{-6}) = 5.27$$

$$pH = 14.00 - 5.27 = 8.73$$

Ampholytes

Substances such as $NaHCO_3$ and NaH_2PO_4 are termed *ampholytes* and are capable of functioning both as acids and bases. When an ampholyte of the type NaHA is dissolved in water, the following series of reactions can occur:

$$Na^+HA^- \xrightarrow{H_2O} Na^+ + HA^-$$

$$HA^- + H_2O \rightleftharpoons A^{2-} + H_3O^+$$

$$HA^- + H_2O \rightleftharpoons H_2A + OH^-$$

$$2H_2O \rightleftharpoons H_3O^+ + OH^-$$

The total PBE for the system is

$$[H_3O^+] + [H_2A] = [OH^-] + [A^{2-}] \tag{72}$$

Substituting both $[H_2A]$ and $[A^{2-}]$ as a function of $[H_3O^+]$ (see Equations 52 and 54), yields

$$[H_3O^+] + \frac{[H_3O^+]^2 C_s}{[H_3O^+]^2 + K_1[H_3O^+] + K_1 K_2}$$

$$= \frac{K_u}{[H_3O^+]} + \frac{K_1 K_2 C_s}{[H_3O^+]^2 + K_1[H_3O^+] + K_1 K_2} \tag{73}$$

This gives a fourth-order equation in $[H_3O^+]$, which can be simplified using certain judicious assumptions to

$$[H_3O^+] = \sqrt{\frac{K_1 K_2 C_s}{K_1 + C_s}} \tag{74}$$

In most instances, $C_s \gg K_1$, and the equation further simplifies to

$$[H_3O^+] = \sqrt{K_1 K_2} \tag{75}$$

and $[H_3O^+]$ becomes independent of the concentration of the salt. A special property of ampholytes is that the concentration of the species HA^- is maximum at the pH corresponding to Equation 75.

When the simplest amino acid salt, glycine hydrochloride, is dissolved in water, it acts as a diprotic acid and ionizes as

$$^+NH_3CH_2COOH + H_2O \rightleftharpoons {}^+NH_3CH_2COO^- + H_3O^+$$

$$^+NH_3CH_2COO^- + H_2O \rightleftharpoons NH_2CH_2COO^- + H_3O^+$$

The form, $^+NH_3CH_2COO^-$, is an ampholyte because it also can act as a weak base:

$$^+NH_3CH_2COO^- + H_2O \rightleftharpoons {}^+NH_3CH_2COOH + OH^-$$

This type of substance, which carries both a charged acidic and a charged basic moiety on the same molecule is termed a *zwitterion*. Because the two charges balance each other, the molecule acts essentially as a neutral molecule. The pH at which the zwitterion concentration is maximum is known as the *isoelectric point*, which can be calculated from Equation 75.

On the acid side of the isoelectric point, amino acids and proteins are cationic and incompatible with anionic materials such as the naturally occurring gums used as suspending and/or emulsifying agents. On the alkaline side of the isoelectric point, amino acids and proteins are anionic and incompatible with cationic materials such as benzalkonium chloride.

Salts of Weak Acids and Weak Bases

When a salt such as ammonium acetate (which is derived from a weak acid and a weak base) is dissolved in water, it undergoes the following reactions:

$$BH^+A^- \xrightarrow{H_2O} BH^+ + A^-$$

$$BH^+ + H_2O \rightleftharpoons B + H_3O^+$$

$$A^- + H_2O \rightleftharpoons HA + OH^-$$

The total PBE for this system is

$$[H_3O^+] + [HA] = [OH^-] + [B] \tag{76}$$

Replacing [HA] and [B] as a function of $[H_3O^+]$, gives

$$[H_3O^+] + \frac{[H_3O^+]C_s}{[H_3O^+] + K_a} = [OH^-] + \frac{K_a'C_s}{[H_3O^+] + K_a'} \tag{77}$$

in which C_s is the concentration of salt, K_a is the ionization constant of the conjugate acid formed from the reaction between A^- and water, and K_a' is the ionization constant for the protonated base, BH^+. In general, $[H_3O^+]$, $[OH^-]$, K_a, and K_a' usually are smaller than C_s and the equation simplifies to

$$[H_3O^+] = \sqrt{K_a K_a'} \tag{78}$$

Example—Calculate the pH of a 0.01 M solution of ammonium acetate. The ammonium ion has a K_a equal to 5.75×10^{-10}, which represents K_a' in Equation 78. Acetic acid has a K_a of 1.75×10^{-5}, which represents K_a in Equation 78:

$$[H_3O^+] = \sqrt{1.75 \times 10^{-5} \times 5.75 \times 10^{-10}}$$

$$= 1.00 \times 10^{-7}$$

$$pH = -\log(1.00 \times 10^{-7}) = 7.00$$

All of the assumptions are valid.

Buffers

The terms *buffer, buffer solution,* and *buffered solution,* when used with reference to hydrogen-ion concentration or pH, refer to the ability of a system, particularly an aqueous solution, to resist a change of pH on adding acid or alkali, or on dilution with a solvent.

If an acid or base is added to water, the pH of the latter is changed markedly, for water has no ability to resist change of pH; it is completely devoid of buffer action. Even a very weak acid such as carbon dioxide changes the pH of water, decreasing it from 7 to 5.7 when the small concentration of carbon dioxide present in air is equilibrated with pure water. This extreme susceptibility of distilled water to a change of pH upon adding very small amounts of acid or base is often of great concern in pharmaceutical operations. Solutions of neutral salts, such as sodium chloride, similarly lack ability to resist change of pH on adding acid or base; such solutions are called *unbuffered.*

Characteristic of *buffered solutions,* which undergo small changes of pH on addition of acid or base, is the presence either of a weak acid and a salt of the weak acid, or a weak base and a salt of the weak base. An example of the former system is acetic acid and sodium acetate; and of the latter, ammonium hydroxide and ammonium chloride. From the proton concept of acids and bases discussed earlier, it is apparent that such buffer action involves a conjugate acid–base pair in the solution. It will be recalled that acetate ion is the conjugate base of acetic acid, and that ammonium ion is the conjugate acid of am-

monia (the principal constituent of what commonly is called ammonium hydroxide).

The mechanism of action of the acetic acid–sodium acetate buffer pair is that the acid, which exists largely in molecular (nonionized) form, combines with hydroxyl ion that may be added to form acetate ion and water; thus,

$$CH_3COOH + OH^- \rightarrow CH_3COO^- + H_2O$$

The acetate ion, which is a base, combines with the hydrogen (more exactly hydronium) ion that may be added to form essentially nonionized acetic acid and water, represented as

$$CH_3COO^- + H_3O^+ \rightarrow CH_3COOH + H_2O$$

As will be illustrated later by an example, the change of pH is slight as long as the amount of hydronium or hydroxyl ion added does not exceed the capacity of the buffer system to neutralize it.

The ammonia–ammonium chloride pair functions as a buffer because the ammonia combines with hydronium ion that may be added to form ammonium ion and water; thus,

$$NH_3 + H_3O^+ \rightarrow NH_4^+ + H_2O$$

Ammonium ion, which is an acid, combines with added hydroxyl ion to form ammonia and water, as

$$NH_4^+ + OH^- \rightarrow NH_3 + H_2O$$

Again, the change of pH is slight if the amount of added hydronium or hydroxyl ion is not in excess of the capacity of the system to neutralize it.

Besides these two general types of buffers, a third appears to exist. This is the buffer system composed of two salts, as monobasic potassium phosphate, KH_2PO_4, and dibasic potassium phosphate, K_2HPO_4. This is not, however, a new type of buffer; it is actually a weak-acid/conjugate-base buffer in which an ion, $H_2PO_4^-$, serves as the weak acid, and HPO_4^{2-} is its conjugate base. When hydroxyl ion is added to this buffer the following reaction takes place:

$$H_2PO_4^- + OH^- \rightarrow HPO_4^{2-} + H_2O$$

and when hydronium ion is added,

$$HPO_4^{2-} + H_3O^+ \rightarrow H_2PO_4^- + H_2O$$

It is apparent that the mechanism of action of this type of buffer is essentially the same as that of the weak-acid/conjugate-base buffer composed of acetic acid and sodium acetate.

CALCULATIONS—A buffer system composed of a conjugate acid–base pair, NaA–HA (such as sodium acetate and acetic acid), would have a PBE of

$$H_3O^+ + [HA] = [OH^-] + [A^-] \tag{79}$$

Replacing [HA] and $[A^-]$ as a function of hydronium-ion concentration gives

$$[H_3O^+] + \frac{[H_3O^+]C_b}{[H_3O^+] + K_a} = [OH^-] + \frac{K_a C_a}{[H_3O^+] + K_a} \tag{80}$$

where C_b is the concentration of the salt, NaA, and C_a is the concentration of the weak acid, HA. This equation can be rearranged to give

$$[H_3O^+] = K_a \frac{(C_a - [H_3O^+] + [OH^-])}{(C_b + [H_3O^+] - [OH^-])} \tag{81}$$

In general, both C_a and C_b are much greater than $[H_3O^+]$, which is in turn much greater than $[OH^-]$ and the equation simplifies to

$$[H_3O^+] = \frac{K_a C_a}{C_b} \tag{82}$$

or, expressed in terms of pH, as

$$pH = pK_a + \log \frac{C_b}{C_a} \qquad (83)$$

This equation generally is called the *Henderson–Hasselbalch equation*. It applies to all buffer systems formed from a single conjugate acid–base pair, regardless of the nature of the salts. For example, it applies equally well to the following buffer systems: ammonia–ammonium chloride, monosodium phosphate–disodium phosphate, and phenobarbital–sodium phenobarbital. In the ammonia–ammonium chloride system, ammonia is obviously the base and the ammonium ion is the acid (C_a equal to the concentration of the salt). In the phosphate system, monosodium phosphate is the acid and disodium phosphate is the base. For the phenobarbital buffer system, phenobarbital is the acid and the phenobarbital anion is the base (C_b equal to the concentration of sodium phenobarbital).

As an example of the application of this equation, the pH of a buffer solution containing acetic acid and sodium acetate, each in 0.1 *M* concentration, may be calculated. The K_a of acetic acid, as defined above, is 1.8×10^{-5}, at 25°.

Solution:
First, the pK_a of acetic acid is calculated:

$$pK_a = -\log K_a = -\log 1.8 \times 10^{-5}$$

$$= -\log 1.8 - \log 10^{-5}$$

$$= -0.26 - (-5) = +4.74$$

Substituting this value into Equation 83:

$$pH = \log \frac{0.1}{0.1} + 4.74 = +4.74$$

The Henderson-Hasselbalch equation predicts that any solutions containing the same molar concentration of acetic acid as of sodium acetate will have the same pH. Thus, a solution of 0.01 *M* concentration of each will have the same pH, 4.74, as one of 0.1 *M* concentration of each component. Actually, there will be some difference in the pH of the solutions, for the *activity coefficient* of the components varies with concentration. For most practical purposes, however, the approximate values of pH calculated by the equation are satisfactory. It should be pointed out that the buffer of higher concentration of each component will have a much greater capacity for neutralizing added acid or base and this point will be discussed further in the discussion of buffer capacity.

The Henderson-Hasselbalch equation is useful also for calculating the ratio of molar concentrations of a buffer system required to produce a solution of specific pH. As an example, suppose that an acetic acid–sodium acetate buffer of pH 4.5 must be prepared. What ratio of the buffer components should be used?

Solution:
Rearranging Equation 83, which is used to calculate the pH of weak acid–salt type buffers, gives

$$\log \frac{[\text{base}]}{[\text{acid}]} = pH - pK_a$$

$$= 4.5 - 4.76 = -0.24 = (9.76 - 10)$$

$$\frac{[\text{base}]}{[\text{acid}]} = \text{antilog of } (9.76 - 10) = 0.575$$

The interpretation of this result is that the *proportion* of sodium acetate to acetic acid should be 0.575 mol of the former to 1 mol of the latter to produce a pH of 4.5. A solution containing 0.0575 mol of sodium acetate and 0.1 mol of acetic acid per liter would meet this requirement, as would also one containing 0.00575 mol of sodium acetate and 0.01 mol of acetic acid per liter. The actual concentration selected would depend chiefly on the desired buffer capacity.

BUFFER CAPACITY—The ability of a buffer solution to resist changes in pH upon addition of acid or alkali may be measured in terms of *buffer capacity*. In the preceding discussion of buffers, it has been seen that, in a general way, the concentra-

tion of acid in a weak-acid/conjugate-base buffer determines the capacity to "neutralize" added base, while the concentration of salt of the weak acid determines the capacity to neutralize added acid. Similarly, in a weak-base/conjugate-acid buffer the concentration of the weak base establishes the buffer capacity toward added acid, while the concentration of the conjugate acid of the weak base determines the capacity toward added base. When the buffer is equimolar in the concentrations of weak acid and conjugate base, or of weak base and conjugate acid, it has equal buffer capacity toward added strong acid or strong base.

Van Slyke, the biochemist, introduced a quantitative expression for evaluating buffer capacity. This may be defined as the amount, in gram-equivalents (g-eq) per liter, of strong acid or strong base required to be added to a solution to change its pH by 1 unit; a solution has a buffer capacity of 1 when 1 L requires 1 g-eq of strong base or acid to change the pH 1 unit. (In practice, considerably smaller increments are measured, expressed as the ratio of acid or base added to the change of pH produced.) From this definition it is apparent that the smaller the pH change in a solution caused by the addition of a specified quantity of acid or alkali, the greater the buffer capacity of the solution.

The following examples illustrate certain basic principles and calculations concerning buffer action and buffer capacity.

Example 1—What is the change of pH on adding 0.01 mol of NaOH to 1 L of 0.10 *M* acetic acid?
(a) Calculate the pH of a 0.10 molar solution of acetic acid:

$$[\text{H}_3\text{O}^+] = \sqrt{K_a C_a} = \sqrt{1.75 \times 10^{-4} \times 1.0 \times 10^{-1}} = 4.18 \times 10^{-3}$$

$$pH = -\log 4.18 \times 10^{-3} = 2.38$$

(b) On adding 0.01 mol of NaOH to a liter of this solution, 0.01 mol of acetic acid is converted to 0.01 mol of sodium acetate, thereby decreasing Ca to 0.09 *M*, and $C_b = 1.0 \times 10^{-2}$ *M*. Using the Henderson-Hasselbach equation gives

$$pH = 4.76 + \log \frac{0.01}{0.09} = 4.76 - 0.95 = 3.81$$

The pH change is, therefore, 1.43 unit. The buffer capacity as defined above is calculated to be

$$\frac{\text{mols of NaOH added}}{\text{change in pH}} = 0.011$$

Example 2—What is the change of pH on adding 0.1 mol of NaOH to 1 L of buffer solution 0.1 *M* in acetic acid and 0.1 *M* in sodium acetate?
(a) The pH of the buffer solution before adding NaOH is

$$pH = \log \frac{[\text{base}]}{[\text{acid}]} + pK_a$$

$$= \log \frac{0.1}{0.1} + 4.76 = 4.76$$

(b) On adding 0.01 mol of NaOH per liter to this buffer solution, 0.01 mol of acetic acid is converted to 0.01 mol of sodium acetate, thereby decreasing the concentration of acid to 0.09 *M* and increasing the concentration of base to 0.11 *M*. The pH is calculated as

$$pH = \log \frac{0.11}{0.09} + 4.76$$

$$= 0.087 + 4.76 = 4.85$$

The change of pH in this case is only 0.09 unit, about 1/10 the change in the preceding example. The buffer capacity is calculated as

$$\frac{\text{mols of NaOH added}}{\text{change of pH}} = \frac{0.01}{0.09} = 0.11$$

Thus, the buffer capacity of the acetic acid–sodium acetate buffer solution is approximately 10 times that of the acetic acid solution.

As is in part evident from these examples, and may be further evidenced by calculations of pH changes in other systems, the degree of buffer action and, therefore, the buffer capacity, depend on the kind and concentration of the buffer components, the pH region involved and the kind of acid or alkali added.

STRONG ACIDS AND BASES AS "BUFFERS"—In the foregoing discussion, buffer action was attributed to systems of (1) weak acids and their conjugate bases, (2) weak bases and their conjugate acids, and (3) certain acid–base pairs that can function in the manner either of system 1 or 2.

The ability to resist change in pH on adding acid or alkali is possessed also by relatively concentrated solutions of strong acids and strong bases. If to 1 L of pure water having a pH of 7 is added 1 mL of 0.01 *M* hydrochloric acid, the pH is reduced to about 5. If the same volume of the acid is added to 1 L of 0.001 *M* hydrochloric acid, which has a pH of about 3, the hydronium-ion concentration is increased only about 1% and the pH is reduced hardly at all. The nature of this buffer action is quite different from that of the true buffer solutions. The very simple explanation is that when 1 mL of 0.01 *M* HCl, which represents 0.00001 g-eq of hydronium ions, is added to the 0.0000001 g-eq of hydronium ions in 1 L of pure water, the hydronium-ion concentration is increased 100-fold (equivalent to two pH units), but when the same amount is added to the 0.001 g-eq of hydronium ions in 1 L of 0.001 *M* HCl, the increase is only 1/100 the concentration already present. Similarly, if 1 mL of 0.01 *M* NaOH is added to 1 L of pure water, the pH is increased to 9, while if the same volume is added to 1 L of 0.001 molar NaOH, the pH is increased almost immeasurably.

In general, solutions of strong acids of pH 3 or less, and solutions of strong bases of pH 11 or more, exhibit this kind of buffer action by virtue of the relatively high concentration of hydronium or hydroxyl ions present. The USP includes among its Standard Buffer Solutions a series of hydrochloric acid buffers, covering the pH range 1.2 to 2.2, which also contain potassium chloride. The salt does not participate in the buffering mechanism, as is the case with salts of weak acids; instead, it serves as a nonreactive constituent required to maintain the proper electrolyte environment of the solutions.

DETERMINATION OF pH

Colorimetry

A relatively simple and inexpensive method for determining the approximate pH of a solution depends on the fact that some conjugate acid–base pairs (indicators) possess one color in the acid form and another color in the base form. Assume that the acid form of a particular indicator is red, and the base form is yellow. The color of a solution of this indicator will range from red when it is sufficiently acid, to yellow when it is sufficiently alkaline.

In the intermediate pH range (the transition interval) the color will be a blend of red and yellow depending upon the ratio of the base to the acid form. In general, although there are slight differences between indicators, color changes apparent to the eye cannot be discerned when the ratio of base to acid form, or acid to base form exceeds 10:1. The use of Equation 83 indicates that the transition range of most indicators is equal to the pK_a of the indicator $\pm$ 1 pH unit, or a useful range of approximately two pH units. Standard indicator solutions can be made at known pH values within the transition range of the indicator, and the pH of an unknown solution can be determined by adding the indicator to it and comparing the resulting color with the standard solutions.

Another method for using these indicators is to apply them to thin strips of filter paper. A drop of the unknown solution is placed on a piece of the indicator paper and the resulting color is compared to a color chart supplied with the indicator paper. These papers are available in a wide variety of pH ranges.

Potentiometry

Electrometric methods for the determination of pH are based on the fact that the difference of electrical potential between two suitable electrodes dipping into a solution containing hydronium ions depends on the concentration (or activity) of the latter. The development of a potential difference is not a specific property of hydronium ions. A solution of any ion will develop a potential proportional to the concentration of that ion if a suitable pair of electrodes is placed in the solution.

The relationship between the potential difference and concentration of an ion in equilibrium with the electrodes may be derived as follows. When a metal is immersed into a solution of one of its salts, there is a tendency for the metal to go into solution in the form of ions. This tendency is known as the *solution pressure* of the metal and is comparable to the tendency of sugar molecules (eg, to dissolve in water). The metallic ions in solution tend, on the other hand, to become discharged by forming atoms, this effect being proportional to the *osmotic pressure* of the ions.

For an atom of a metal to go into solution as a positive ion, electrons, equal in number to the charge on the ion, must be left behind on the metal electrode with the result that the latter becomes negatively charged. The positively charged ions in solution, however, may become discharged as atoms by taking up electrons from the metal electrode. Depending on which effect predominates, the electrical charge on the electrode will be either positive or negative and may be expressed quantitatively by the following equation proposed by Nernst in 1889:

$$E = \frac{RT}{\text{n}F} \ln \frac{p}{P} \qquad (84)$$

where E is the potential difference or electromotive force, R is the gas constant (8.316 joules), T is the absolute temperature, n is the valence of the ion, F is the Faraday of electricity (96,500 coulombs), p is the osmotic pressure of the ions, and P is the solution pressure of the metal.

Inasmuch as it is impossible to measure the potential difference between one electrode and a solution with any degree of certainty, it is customary to use two electrodes and to measure the potential difference between them. If two electrodes, both of the same metal, are immersed in separate solutions containing ions of that metal—at osmotic pressure p_1 and p_2, respectively—and are connected by means of a tube containing a nonreacting salt solution (a so-called *salt bridge*), the potential developed across the two electrodes will be equal to the difference between the potential differences of the individual electrodes; thus,

$$E = E_1 - E_2 = \frac{RT}{nF} \ln \frac{p_1}{P_1} - \frac{RT}{nF} \ln \frac{p_2}{P_2} \qquad (85)$$

As both electrodes are of the same metal, $P_1 = P_2$ and the equation may be simplified to

$$E = \frac{RT}{nF} \ln p_1 - \frac{RT}{nF} \ln p_2 = \frac{RT}{nF} \ln \frac{p_1}{p_2} \qquad (86)$$

In place of osmotic pressures it is permissible, for dilute solutions, to substitute the concentrations c_1 and c_2 that were found (see Chapter 16), to be proportional to p_1 and p_2. The equation then becomes

$$E = \frac{RT}{nF} \ln \frac{c_1}{c_2} \qquad (87)$$

If either c_1 or c_2 is known, it is obvious that the value of the other may be found if the potential difference, E, of this cell can be measured.

For the determination of hydronium-ion concentration or pH, an electrode at which an equilibrium between hydrogen gas and hydronium ion can be established must be used in place of metallic electrodes. Such an electrode may be made by electrolytically coating a strip of platinum, or other noble metal, with platinum black and saturating the latter with pure hydrogen gas. This device functions as a *hydrogen electrode*. Two such electrodes may be assembled as shown in Figure 17-3.

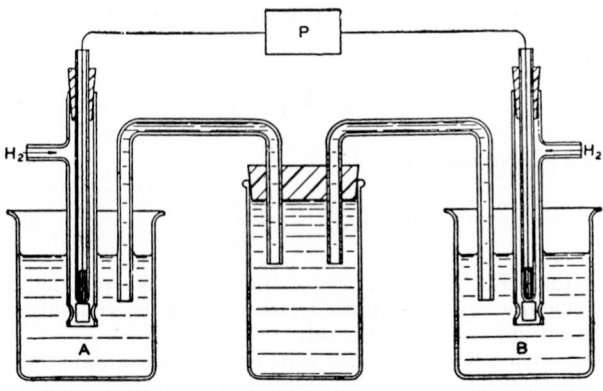

Figure 17-3. Hydrogen-ion concentration chain.

In this diagram one electrode dips into Solution A, containing a known hydronium-ion concentration, and the other electrode dips into Solution B, containing an unknown hydronium-ion concentration. The two electrodes and solutions, sometimes called *half-cells*, then are connected by a bridge of neutral salt solution, which has no significant effect on the solutions it connects. The potential difference across the two electrodes is measured by means of a potentiometer, P. If the concentration, c_1, of hydronium ion in Solution A is $1 N$, Equation 87 simplifies to

$$E = \frac{RT}{nF} \ln \frac{1}{c_2} \qquad (88)$$

or in terms of Briggsian logarithms

$$E = 2.303 \frac{RT}{nF} \log_{10} \frac{1}{c_2} \qquad (89)$$

If for $\log_{10} 1/c_2$ there is substituted its equivalent pH, the equation becomes

$$E = 2.303 \frac{RT}{nF} \text{pH} \qquad (90)$$

and finally by substituting numerical values for R, n, T, and F, and assuming the temperature to be 20°, the following simple relationship is derived:

$$E = 0.0581 \text{ pH} \quad \text{or} \quad \text{pH} = \frac{E}{0.0581} \qquad (91)$$

The hydrogen electrode dipping into a solution of known hydronium-ion concentration, called the *reference electrode,* may be replaced by a calomel electrode, one type of which is shown in Figure 17-4. The elements of a calomel electrode are mercury and calomel in an aqueous solution of potassium chloride. The potential of this electrode is constant, regardless of the hydronium-ion concentration of the solution into which it dips. The potential depends on the equilibrium that is set up between mercury and mercurous ions from the calomel, but the concentration of the latter is governed, according to the solubility-product principle, by the concentration of chloride ions, which are derived mainly from the potassium chloride in the solution. Therefore, the potential of this electrode varies with the concentration of potassium chloride in the electrolyte.

Because the calomel electrode always indicates voltages that are higher, by a constant value, than those obtained when the normal hydrogen electrode chain shown in Figure 17-3 is used, it is necessary to subtract the potential due to the calomel electrode itself from the observed voltage. As the magnitude of this voltage depends on the concentration of potassium chloride in the calomel-electrode electrolyte, it is necessary to know the concentration of the former. For most purposes a saturated potassium chloride solution is used that

produces potential difference of 0.2488 V. Accordingly, before using Equation 86 for the calculation of pH from the voltage of a cell made up of a calomel and a hydrogen electrode dipping into the solution to be tested, 0.2488 V must be subtracted from the observed potential difference. Expressed mathematically, Equation 92 is used for calculating pH from the potential difference of such a cell.

$$\text{pH} = \frac{E - 0.2488}{0.0581} \qquad (92)$$

In measuring the potential difference between the electrodes, it is imperative that very little current be drawn from the cell, for with current flowing the voltage changes, owing to polarization effects at the electrode. Because of this it is not possible to make accurate measurements with a voltmeter that requires appreciable current to operate it. In its place a potentiometer is used that does not draw a current from the cell being measured.

There are many limitations to the use of the hydrogen electrode:

- It cannot be used in solutions containing strong oxidants such as ferric iron, dichromates, nitric acid, peroxide, or chlorine or reductants such as sulfurous acid and hydrogen sulfide.
- It is affected by the presence of organic compounds that are reduced fairly easily.
- It cannot be used successfully in solutions containing cations that fall below hydrogen in the electrochemical series.
- Erratic results are obtained in the measurement of unbuffered solutions unless special precautions are taken.
- It is troublesome to prepare and maintain.

As other electrodes more convenient to use now are available, the hydrogen electrode today is used rarely. Nevertheless, it is the ultimate standard for pH measurements.

To avoid some of the difficulties with the hydrogen electrode, the *quinhydrone* electrode was introduced and was popular for a long time, particularly for measurements of acid solutions. The unusual feature of this electrode is that it consists of a piece of gold or platinum wire or foil dipping into the solution to be tested, in which has been dissolved a small quantity of quinhydrone. A calomel electrode may be used for reference, just as in determinations with the hydrogen electrode.

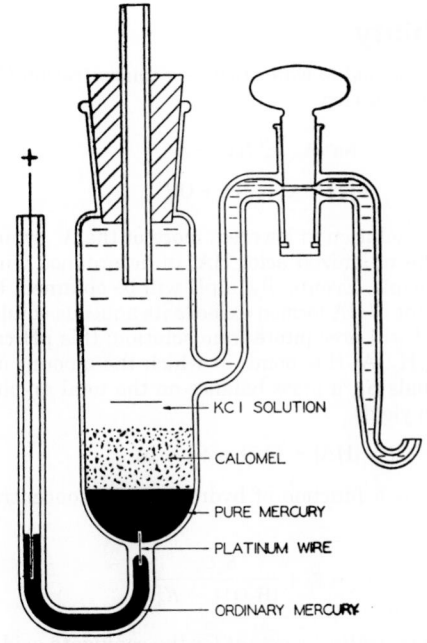

Figure 17-4. Calomel electrode.

Quinhydrone consists of an equimolecular mixture of quinone and hydroquinone; the relationship between these substances and hydrogen-ion concentration is

Quinone + 2 Hydrogen ions + 2 Electrons ⇌ Hydroquinone

In a solution containing hydrogen ions the potential of the quinhydrone electrode is related logarithmically to hydronium-ion concentration if the ratio of the hydroquinone concentration to that of quinone is constant and practically equal to 1. This ratio is maintained in an acid solution containing an excess of quinhydrone, and measurements may be made quickly and accurately; however, quinhydrone cannot be used in solutions more alkaline than pH 8.

An electrode that, because of its simplicity of operation and freedom from contamination or change of the solution being tested, has replaced both the hydrogen and quinhydrone electrodes is the *glass electrode*. It functions because when a thin membrane of a special composition of glass separates two solutions of different pH, a potential difference develops across the membrane that depends on the pH of both solutions. If the pH of one of the solutions is known, the other may be calculated from the potential difference.

In practice, the glass electrode usually consists of a bulb of the special glass fused to the end of a tube of ordinary glass. Inside the bulb is placed a solution of known pH, in contact with an internal silver–silver chloride or other electrode. This glass electrode and another reference electrode are immersed in the solution to be tested and the potential difference is measured. A potentiometer providing electronic amplification of the small current produced is employed. The modern instruments available permit reading the pH directly and provide also for compensation of variations due to temperature in the range of 0° to 50° and to the small but variable asymmetry potential inherent in the glass electrode.

PHARMACEUTICAL SIGNIFICANCE

In the broad realm of knowledge concerning the preparation and action of drugs few, if any, variables are so important as pH. For the purpose of this presentation, four principal types of pH-dependence of drug systems will be discussed: solubility, stability, activity, and absorption.

Drug Solubility

If a salt, NaA, is added to water to give a concentration C_s, the following reactions occur:

$$Na^+ A^- \xrightarrow{H_2O} Na^+ + A^-$$

$$A^- + H_2O \rightleftharpoons HA + OH^-$$

If the pH of the solution is lowered, more of the A^- would be converted to the unionized acid, HA, in accordance with Le Chatelier's principle. Eventually, a pH will be obtained, below which the amount of HA formed exceeds its aqueous solubility, S_0, and the acid will precipitate from solution; this pH can be designated as pH_p. At this point, at which the amount of HA formed just equals S_0, a mass balance on the total amount of drug in solution yields

$$C_s = [HA] + [A^-] = S_0 + [A^-] \tag{93}$$

Replacing $[A^-]$ as a function of hydronium-ion concentration gives

$$C_s = S_0 + \frac{K_a C_s}{[H_3O^+]_p + K_a} \tag{94}$$

where K_a is the ionization constant for the conjugate acid, HA, and $[H_3O^+]_p$ refers to the hydronium-ion concentration above

which precipitation will occur. This equation can be rearranged to give

$$[H_3O^+]_p = K_a \frac{S_0}{C_s - S_0} \tag{95}$$

Taking logarithms gives

$$pH_p = pK_a + \log \frac{C_s - S_0}{S_0} \tag{96}$$

Thus, the pH below which precipitation occurs is a function of the amount of salt added initially, the pK_a and the solubility of the free acid formed from the salt.

The analogous equation for salts of weak bases and strong acids (such as pilocarpine hydrochloride, cocaine hydrochloride, or codeine phosphate) would be

$$pH_p = pK_a + \log \frac{S_0}{C_s - S_0} \tag{97}$$

in which pK_a refers to the protonated form of the weak base.

Example—Below what pH will free phenobarbital begin to precipitate from a solution initially containing 1.3 g of sodium phenobarbital/100 mL at 25°? The molar solubility of phenobarbital is 0.0050 and its pK_a is 7.41. The molecular weight of sodium phenobarbital is 254.

The molar concentration of salt initially added is

$$C_s = \frac{g/L}{mol\ wt} = \frac{13}{254} = 0.051\ M$$

$$pH_p = 7.41 + \log \frac{0.051 - 0.005}{0.005}$$

$$= 7.41 + 0.96 = 8.37$$

Example—Above what pH will free cocaine begin to precipitate from a solution initially containing 0.0294 mol of cocaine hydrochloride per liter? The pKb of cocaine is 5.59, and its molar solubility is 5.60×10^{-3}.

$$pK_a = pK_w - pK_b = 14.00 - 5.59 = 8.41$$

$$pH_p = 8.41 + \log \frac{0.0056}{0.0294 - 0.0056}$$

$$= 8.41 + (-0.63) = 7.78$$

Drug Stability

One of the most diversified and fruitful areas of study is the investigation of the effect of hydrogen-ion concentration on the stability or, in more general terms, the reactivity of pharmaceutical systems. The evidence for enhanced stability of systems when these are maintained within a narrow range of pH, as well as of progressively decreasing stability as the pH departs from the optimum range, is abundant. Stability (or instability) of a system may result from gain or loss of a proton (hydrogen ion) by a substrate molecule—often accompanied by an electronic rearrangement—that reduces (or increases) the reactivity of the molecule. *Instability* results when the substance desired to remain unchanged is converted to one or more other, unwanted, substances. In aqueous solution, instability may arise through the catalytic effect of acids or bases—the former by transferring a proton to the substrate molecule, the latter by accepting a proton.

Specific illustrations of the effect of hydrogen-ion concentration on the stability of medicinals are myriad; only a few will be given here, these being chosen to show the importance of pH adjustment of solutions that require sterilization.

Morphine solutions are not decomposed during a 60-min exposure at a temperature of 100° if the pH is less than 5.5; neutral and alkaline solutions, however, are highly unstable. Minimum hydrolytic decomposition of solutions of cocaine occurs in the range of pH of 2 to 5; in one study a solution of cocaine hydrochloride, initially at a pH of 5.7, remained stable during 2 months (although the pH dropped to 4.2 in this time), while another solution buffered to about pH 6 underwent approximately 30% hydrolysis in the same time. Similarly, solutions of procaine hydrochloride containing some hydrochloric acid showed no appreciable decomposition; when dissolved in water alone, 5% of the procaine hydrochloride hydrolyzed, whereas when buffered to pH 6.5, from 19 to 35% underwent decomposition by hydrolysis. Solutions of thiamine hydrochloride may be sterilized by autoclaving without appreciable decomposition if the pH is below 5; above this, thiamine hydrochloride is unstable.

The stability of many disperse systems, and especially of certain emulsions, is often pH dependent. Information concerning specific emulsion systems, and the effect of pH upon them, may be found in Chapter 21.

Drug Activity

Drugs that are weak acids or weak bases—and hence may exist in ionized or nonionized form (or a mixture of both)—may be *active* in one form but not in the other; often such drugs have an optimum pH range for maximum activity. Thus, mandelic acid, benzoic acid, or salicylic acid have pronounced antibacterial activity in nonionized form but have practically no such activity in ionized form. Accordingly, these substances require an acid environment to function effectively as antibacterial agents. For example, sodium benzoate is effective as a reservative in 4% concentration at pH 7, in 0.06 to 0.1% concentration at pH 3.5 to 4, and in 0.02 to 0.03% concentration at pH 2.3 to 2.4. Other antibacterial agents are active principally, if not entirely, in cationic form. Included in this category are the acridines and quaternary ammonium compounds.

Drug Absorption

The degree of ionization and lipoid solubility of a drug are two important factors that determine the rate of *absorption* of drugs from the gastrointestinal tract, and indeed their passage through cellular membranes generally. Drugs that are weak organic acids or bases, and that in nonionized form are soluble in lipids, apparently are absorbed through cellular membranes by virtue of the lipoidal nature of the membranes. Completely ionized drugs, on the other hand, are absorbed poorly, if at all. Rates of absorption of a variety of drugs are related to their ionization constants and in many cases may be predicted quantitatively on the basis of this relationship. Thus, not only the degree of the acidic or basic character of a drug, but also consequently the pH of the physiological medium (eg, gastric or intestinal fluid, plasma, cerebrospinal fluid) in which a drug is dissolved or dispersed—because this pH determines the extent to which the drug will be converted to ionic or nonionic form—become important parameters of drug absorption. Further information on drug absorption is given in Chapter 58.

REFERENCES

1. Benet LZ, Goyan JE. *J Pharm Sci* 1965; 54:1179.
2. Riegelman S et al. *J Pharm Sci* 1962; 51:129.
3. Niebergall PJ et al. *J Pharm Sci* 1972; 61:232.

BIBLIOGRAPHY

Conway BE. *Ionic Hydration in Chemistry and Biophysics.* Amsterdam: Elsevier, 1980.
Denbigh K. *The Principles of Chemical Equilibrium*, 4th ed. London: Cambridge University Press, 1981.
Freiser H, Fernando Q. *Ionic Equilibria in Analytical Chemistry.* New York: Wiley, 1966.
Harned HS, Owen BB. *The Physical Chemistry of Electrolytic Solutions.* New York, Reinhold, 1958.

ACKNOWLEDGMENTS—Paul J Niebergall, PhD is acknowledged for his efforts in previous editions of this work.

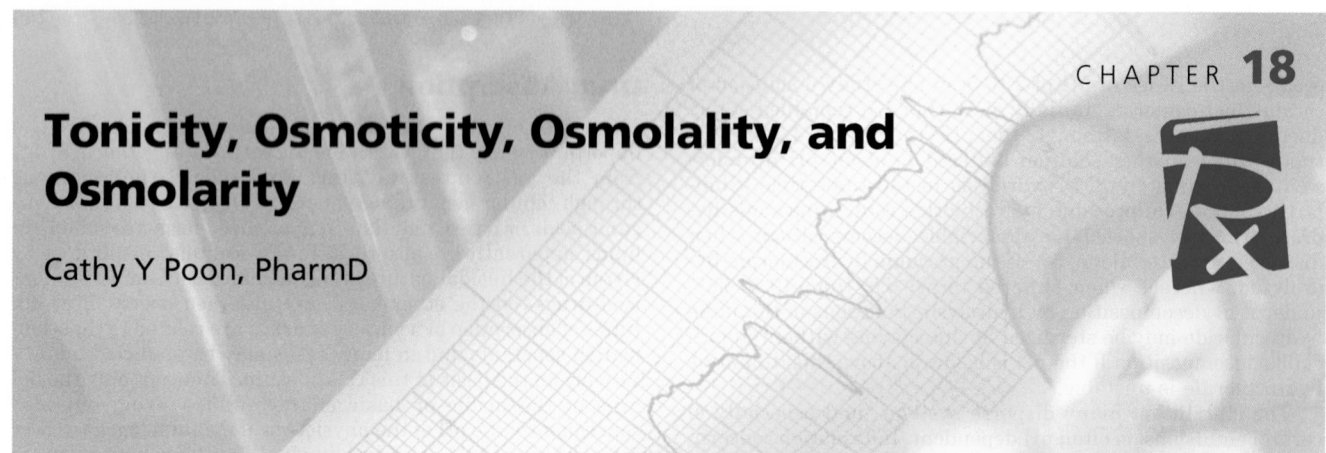

CHAPTER **18**

Tonicity, Osmoticity, Osmolality, and Osmolarity

Cathy Y Poon, PharmD

BASIC DEFINITIONS

If a solution is placed in contact with a membrane that is permeable to molecules of the solvent, but not to molecules of the solute, the movement of solvent through the membrane is called *osmosis.* Such a membrane often is called *semi-permeable.* As the several types of membranes of the body vary in their permeability, it is well to note that they are *selectively* permeable. Most normal living-cell membranes maintain various solute concentration gradients. A selectively permeable membrane may be defined either as one that does not permit free, unhampered diffusion of all the solutes present, or as one that maintains at least one solute concentration gradient across itself. Osmosis, then, is the diffusion of water through a membrane that maintains at least one solute concentration gradient across itself.

Assume that Solution A is on one side of the membrane, and Solution B of the same solute but of a higher concentration is on the other side; the solvent will tend to pass into the more concentrated solution until equilibrium has been established. The pressure required to prevent this movement is the osmotic pressure. It is defined as the excess pressure, or pressure greater than that above the pure solvent, that must be applied to Solution B to prevent passage of solvent through a perfect semipermeable membrane from A to B. The concentration of a solution with respect to effect on osmotic pressure is related to the number of particles (unionized molecules, ions, macromolecules, aggregates) of solute(s) in solution and thus is affected by the degree of ionization or aggregation of the solute. See Chapter 16 for review of colligative properties of solutions.

Body fluids, including blood and lacrimal fluid, normally have an osmotic pressure that often is described as corresponding to that of a 0.9% solution of sodium chloride. The body also attempts to keep the osmotic pressure of the contents of the gastrointestinal (GI) tract at about this level, but there the normal range is much wider than that of most body fluids. The 0.9% sodium chloride solution is said to be *iso-osmotic* with physiological fluids. In medicine, the term *isotonic,* meaning equal tone, is commonly used interchangeably with iso-osmotic. However, terms such as isotonic and tonicity should be used *only* with reference to a physiological fluid. Iso-osmotic actually is a physical term that compares the osmotic pressure (or another colligative property, such as freezing-point depression) of two liquids, neither of which may be a physiological fluid, or which may be a physiological fluid only under certain circumstances. For example, a solution of boric acid that is iso-osmotic with both blood and lacrimal fluid is isotonic only with the lacrimal fluid. This solution causes hemolysis of red blood cells because molecules of boric acid pass freely through the erythrocyte membrane regardless of concentration. Thus, isotonicity infers a sense of physiological compatibility where iso-osmoticity need not. As another example, a *chemically de-*
fined elemental diet or enteral nutritional fluid can be iso-osmotic with the contents of the GI tract, but would not be considered a physiological fluid, or suitable for parenteral use.

A solution is isotonic with a living cell if there is no net gain or loss of water by the cell, or other change in the cell, when it is in contact with that solution. Physiological solutions with an osmotic pressure lower than that of body fluids, or of 0.9% sodium chloride solution, are referred to commonly as being *hypotonic.* Physiological solutions having a greater osmotic pressure are termed *hypertonic.*

Such qualitative terms are of limited value, and it has become necessary to state osmotic properties in quantitative terms. To do so, a term must be used that will represent all the particles that may be present in a given system. The term used is *osmol:* the weight, in grams, of a solute, existing in a solution as molecules (and/or ions, macromolecules, aggregates, etc), which is osmotically equivalent to a mole of an ideally behaving nonelectrolyte. Thus, the osmol weight of a nonelectrolyte, in a dilute solution, generally is equal to its gram molecular weight. A *milliosmol,* abbreviated mOsm, is the weight stated in milligrams.

If one extrapolates this concept of relating an osmol and a mole of a nonelectrolyte as being equivalent, then one also may define an osmol in the following ways. It is the amount of solute that will provide 1 Avogadro's number (6.02×10^{23}) of particles in solution and it is the amount of solute that, on dissolution in 1 kg of water, will result in an osmotic pressure increase of 17,000 torr at 0° or 19,300 torr at 37°. One mOsmol is 1/1000 of an osmol. For example, 1 mol of anhydrous dextrose is equal to 180 g. One osmol of this nonelectrolyte is also 180 grams. One mOsmol would be 180 mg. Thus, 180 mg of this solute dissolved in 1 kg of water will produce an increase in osmotic pressure of 19.3 torr at body temperature.

For a solution of an electrolyte such as sodium chloride, one molecule of sodium chloride represents one sodium and one chloride ion. Hence, 1 mol will represent 2 osmol of sodium chloride theoretically. Accordingly, 1 osmol NaCl = 58.5 g/2 or 29.25 g. This quantity represents the sum total of 6.02×10^{23} ions as the total number of particles. Ideal solutions infer very dilute solutions or infinite dilution.

However, as the concentration is increased, other factors enter. With strong electrolytes, interionic attraction causes a decrease in their effect on colligative properties. In addition, and in opposition, for all solutes, including nonelectrolytes, solvation and possibly other factors operate to intensify their colligative effect. Therefore, it is very difficult and often impossible to predict accurately the osmoticity of a solution. It may be possible to do so for a dilute solution of a single pure and well-characterized solute, but not for most parenteral and enteral medicinal and/or nutritional fluids; experimental determination likely is required.

THERAPEUTIC CONSIDERATIONS

It generally is accepted that osmotic effects have a major place in the maintenance of homeostasis (the state of equilibrium in the living body with respect to various functions and to the chemical composition of the fluids and tissues, eg, temperature, heart rate, blood pressure, water content, or blood sugar). To a great extent these effects occur within or between cells and tissues where they cannot be measured. One of the most troublesome problems in clinical medicine is the maintenance of adequate body fluids and proper balance between extracellular and intracellular fluid volumes in seriously ill patients. It should be kept in mind, however, that fluid and electrolyte abnormalities are not diseases, but are the manifestations of disease.

The physiological mechanisms that control water intake and output appear to respond primarily to serum osmoticity. Renal regulation of output is influenced by variation in rate of release of pituitary antidiuretic hormone (ADH) and other factors in response to changes in serum osmoticity. Osmotic changes also serve as a stimulus to moderate thirst. This mechanism is sufficiently sensitive to limit variations in osmoticity in the normal individual to less than about 1%. Body fluid continually oscillates within this narrow range. An increase of plasma osmoticity of 1% will stimulate ADH release, result in reduction of urine flow, and, at the same time, stimulate thirst that results in increased water intake. Both the increased renal reabsorption of water (without solute) stimulated by circulating ADH and the increased water intake tend to lower serum osmoticity.

The transfer of water through the cell membrane occurs so rapidly that any lack of osmotic equilibrium between the two fluid compartments in any given tissue usually is corrected within a few seconds and, at most, within a minute or so. However, this rapid transfer of water does not mean that complete equilibration occurs between the extracellular and intracellular compartments throughout the entire body within this same short period of time. The reason is that fluid usually enters the body through the gut and then must be transported by the circulatory system to all tissues before complete equilibration can occur. In the normal person it may require 30 to 60 min to achieve reasonably good equilibration throughout the body after drinking water. Osmoticity is the property that largely determines the physiological acceptability of a variety of solutions used for therapeutic and nutritional purposes.

Pharmaceutical and therapeutic consideration of osmotic effects has been, to a great extent, directed toward the side effects of ophthalmic and parenteral medicinals due to abnormal osmoticity, and either to formulating to avoid the side effects or to finding methods of administration to minimize them. More recently this consideration has been extended to total (central) parenteral nutrition, to enteral hyperalimentation ("tube" feeding), and to concentrated-fluid infant formulas.[1] Also, in recent years, the importance of osmometry of serum and urine in the diagnosis of many pathological conditions has been recognized.

There are a number of examples of the direct therapeutic effect of osmotic action, such as the *intravenous* (IV) use of mannitol as a diuretic that is filtered at the glomeruli and thus increases the osmotic pressure of tubular urine. Water must then be reabsorbed against a higher osmotic gradient than otherwise, so reabsorption is slower and diuresis is observed. The same fundamental principle applies to the IV administration of 30% urea used to affect intracranial pressure in the control of cerebral edema. Peritoneal dialysis fluids tend to be somewhat hyperosmotic to withdraw water and nitrogenous metabolites. Two to 5% sodium chloride solutions or dispersions in an oleaginous base (Muro, *Bausch & Lomb*) and a 40% glucose ointment are used topically for corneal edema. Ophthalgan (*Wyeth-Ayerst*) is ophthalmic glycerin employed for its osmotic effect to clear edematous cornea to facilitate an ophthalmoscopic or gonioscopic examination. Glycerin solutions in 50% concentration Osmoglyn (*Alcon*) and isosorbide solution Ismotic (*Alcon*) are oral osmotic agents for reducing intraocular pressure.

The osmotic principle also applies to plasma extenders such as polyvinylpyrrolidone and to saline laxatives such as magnesium sulfate, magnesium citrate solution, magnesium hydroxide (via gastric neutralization), sodium sulfate, sodium phosphate, and sodium biphosphate oral solution, and enema (*Fleet*).

An interesting osmotic laxative that is a nonelectrolyte is a lactulose solution. Lactulose is a nonabsorbable disaccharide that is colon-specific, wherein colonic bacteria degrade some of the disaccharide to lactic and other simple organic acids. These, in toto, lead to an osmotic effect and laxation. An extension of this therapy is illustrated by Cephulac (*Marion Merrell Dow*) solution, which uses the acidification of the colon via lactulose degradation to serve as a trap for ammonia migrating from the blood to the colon. The conversion of ammonia of blood to the ammonium ion in the colon ultimately is coupled with the osmotic effect and laxation, thus expelling undesirable levels of blood ammonia. This product is employed to prevent and treat frontal systemic encephalopathy.

Osmotic laxation is observed with the oral or rectal use of glycerin and sorbitol. Epsom salt has been used in baths and compresses to reduce edema associated with sprains. Another approach is the indirect application of the osmotic effect in therapy via osmotic pump drug delivery systems.[2]

OSMOLALITY AND OSMOLARITY

It is necessary to use several additional terms to define expressions of concentration in reflecting the osmoticity of solutions. The terms include *osmolality,* the expression of osmolal concentration, and *osmolarity,* the expression of osmolar concentration.

OSMOLALITY—A solution has an osmolal concentration of one when it contains 1 osmol of solute/kg of water. A solution has an osmolality of *n* when it contains *n* osmol/kg of water. Osmolal solutions, like their counterpart molal solutions, reflect a weight-to-weight relationship between the solute and the solvent. Because an osmol of any nonelectrolyte is equivalent to 1 mol of that compound, then a 1 osmolal solution is synonymous to a 1 molal solution for a typical nonelectrolyte.

With a typical electrolyte like sodium chloride, 1 osmol is approximately 0.5 mol of sodium chloride. Thus, it follows that a 1 osmolal solution of sodium chloride essentially is equivalent to a 0.5 molal solution. Recall that a 1 osmolal solution of dextrose or sodium chloride each will contain the same particle concentration. In the dextrose solution there will be 6.02×10^{23} molecules/kg of water and in the sodium chloride solution one will have 6.02×10^{23} total ions/kg of water, one-half of which are Na^+ ions and the other half Cl^- ions.

As in molal solutions, osmolal solutions usually are employed where quantitative precision is required, as in the measurement of physical and chemical properties of solutions (ie, colligative properties). The advantage of the w/w relationship is that the concentration of the system is not influenced by temperature.

OSMOLARITY—The relationship observed between molality and osmolality is shared similarly between molarity and osmolarity. A solution has an osmolar concentration of 1 when it contains 1 osmol of solute per liter of solution. Likewise, a solution has an osmolarity of *n* when it contains *n* osmols/L of solution. Osmolar solutions, unlike osmolal solution, reflect a weight in volume relationship between the solute and final solution. A 1 molar and 1 osmolar solution would be identical for nonelectrolytes. For sodium chloride a 1 osmolar solution would contain 1 osmol of sodium chloride per liter which approximates a 0.5 molar solution. The advantage of employing osmolar concentrations over osmolal concentrations is the ability to relate a specific number of osmols or milliosmols to a volume, such as a liter or milliliter. Thus, the osmolar concept is simpler and more practical. Volumes of solution, rather than weights of solution, are more practical in the delivery of liquid dosage forms.

Many health professionals do not have a clear understanding of the difference between osmolality and osmolarity. In fact, the terms have been used interchangeably. A 1 osmolar solution of a solute always will be more concentrated than a 1 osmolal solution. With dilute solutions the difference may be acceptably small. For example, a 0.9% w/v solution of sodium chloride in water contains 9 g of sodium chloride/L of solution, equivalent to 0.308 osmolar; or 9 g of sodium chloride/996.5 g of water, equivalent to 0.309 osmolal, less than a 1% error. For concentrated solutions the percent difference between osmolarity and osmolality is much greater and may be highly significant; 3.5% for 5% w/v dextrose solution and 25% for 25% w/v dextrose solution. One should be alerted to the sizable errors that may occur with concentrated solutions or fluids, such as those employed in total parenteral nutrition, enteral hyperalimentation, and oral nutritional fluids for infants.

Reference has been made to the terms hypertonic and hypotonic. Analogous terms are hyperosmotic and hypo-osmotic. Assuming normal serum osmolality to be 285 mOsmol/kg, as serum osmolality increases due to water deficit, the following signs and symptoms usually are found to accumulate progressively at approximately these values: 294 to 298—thirst (if the patient is alert and communicative); 299 to 313—dry mucous membranes; 314 to 329—weakness, doughy skin; above 330—disorientation, postural hypotension, severe weakness, fainting, CNS changes, stupor, and coma. As serum osmolality decreases due to water excess the following may occur: 275 to 261—headache; 262 to 251—drowsiness, weakness; 250 to 233—disorientation, cramps; below 233—seizures, stupor, and coma.

As indicated previously, the mechanisms of the body actively combat such major changes by limiting the variation in osmolality for normal individuals to less than about 1% (approximately in the range 282–288 mOsmol/kg, based on the above assumption).

The value given for normal serum osmolality above was described as an assumption because of the variety of values found in the literature. Serum osmolality often is stated loosely to be about 300 mOsmol/L. Various references report 280 to 295 mOsmol/L, 275 to 300 mOsmol/L, 290 mOsmol/L, 306 mOsmol/L, and 275 to 295 mOsmol/kg.

In recent years, much attention has been directed at determining osmoticity of total parenteral nutrition solutions, enteral formulas, and parenteral and enteral medications.[3–5] Hyperosmoticity of parenteral and enteral formulas and medications serves as an indicator for potential risks, including thrombophlebitis, pain at injection site, diarrhea, and abdominal cramping. However, the terms osmolality and osmolarity often have been used interchangeably and caused much confusion for practitioners. Often, when the term osmolarity is used, one cannot discern whether this simply is incorrect terminology, or if osmolarity actually has been calculated from osmolality.

Another current practice that can cause confusion is the use of the terms *normal* or *physiological* for isotonic sodium chloride solution (0.9%). The solution surely is iso-osmotic. However, as to being physiological, the concentration of ions are each of 154 mEq/L whereas serum contains about 140 mEq of sodium and about 103 mEq of chloride.

The range of mOsmol values found for serum raises the question as to what really is meant by the terms hypotonic and hypertonic for medicinal and nutritional fluids. One can find the statement that fluids with an osmolality of 50 mOsmol or more above normal are hypertonic; and, if they are 50 mOsmol or more below normal, they are hypotonic. One also can find the statement that peripheral infusions should not have an osmolarity exceeding 700 to 800 mOsmol/L.[6] Examples of osmol concentrations of solutions used in peripheral infusions are (D5W) 5% dextrose solution, 252 mOsmol/L; (D10W) 10% dextrose solution, 505 mOsmol/L; and Lactated Ringer's 5% Dextrose, 525 mOsmol/L. When a fluid is hypertonic, undesirable effects often can be decreased by using relatively slow rates of infusion, and/or relatively short periods of infusion. For example, 25%

dextrose solution (D25W)—4.25% Amino Acids is a representative of a highly osmotic hyperalimentation solution. It has been stated that when osmolal loading is needed, a maximum safe tolerance for a normally hydrated subject would be an approximate increase of 25 mOsmol/kg of water over 4 hours.[7]

COMPUTATION OF OSMOLARITY

Several methods are used to obtain numerical values of osmolarity. The osmolar concentration, sometimes referred to as the *theoretical osmolarity,* is calculated from the w/v concentration using the following equation:

$$\frac{g}{L} \times \frac{mols}{g} \times \frac{osmol}{mol} \times \frac{1000\ mOsmol}{osmol} = \frac{mOsmol}{L} \tag{1}$$

The number of osmol/mol is equal to 1 for nonelectrolytes and is equal to the number of ions per molecule for strong electrolytes.

This calculation omits consideration of factors such as solvation and interionic forces. By this method of calculation, 0.9% sodium chloride has an osmolar concentration of 308 mOsmol/L and a concentration of 154 mOsmol/L in either sodium or chloride ion.

Two other methods compute osmolarity from values of osmolality. The determination of osmolality will be discussed later. One method has a strong theoretical basis of physical-chemical principles[8] using values of the partial molal volume(s) of the solute(s). A 0.9% sodium chloride solution, found experimentally to have an osmolality of 286 mOsmol/kg, was calculated to have an osmolarity of 280 mOsmol/L, rather different from the value of 308 mOsmol/L calculated as above. The method, using partial molal volumes, is relatively rigorous, but many systems appear to be too complex and/or too poorly defined to be dealt with by this method.

The other method is based on calculating the weight of water from the solution density and concentration

$$\frac{g\ water}{mL\ solution} = \frac{g\ solution}{mL\ solution} - \frac{g\ solute}{mL\ solution}$$

then

$$osmolarity\left(\frac{mOsmol}{L\ solution}\right)$$
$$= osmolality\left(\frac{mOsmol}{1000\ g\ water}\right) \times \frac{g\ water}{mL\ solution}$$

The experimental value for the osmolality of 0.9% sodium chloride solution was 292.7 mOsmol/kg; the value computed for osmolarity was 291.4 mOsmol/L. This method uses easily obtained values of density of the solution and of its solute content and can be used with all systems. For example, the osmolality of a nutritional product was determined by the freezing-point depression method to be 625 mOsmol/kg[10]; its osmolarity was calculated as $625 \times 0.839 = 524$ mOsmol/L.

Monographs in the USP for solutions provide IV replenishment of fluid, nutrients, or electrolytes, and for osmotic diuretics such as Mannitol Injection, require the osmolar concentration be stated on the label in osmol/L; however, when the contents are less than 100 mL, or when the label states the article is not for direct injection but is to be diluted before use, the label alternatively may state the total osmolar concentration in mOsmol/mL.

An example of the use of the first method described above is the computation of the approximate osmolar concentration (*theoretical osmolarity*) of a Lactated Ringer's 5% Dextrose Solution (*Abbott*), which is labeled to contain, per liter, dextrose (hydrous) 50 g, sodium chloride 6 g, potassium chloride 300 mg, calcium chloride 200 mg, and sodium lactate 3.1 g. Also stated is that the total osmolar concentration of the solution is approximately 524 mOsmol/L in part contributed by 130 mEq of Na^+, 109 mEq of Cl^-, 4 mEq of K^+, 3 mEq of Ca^{2+}, and 28 mEq of lactate ion.

The derivation of the osmolar concentrations from the stated composition of the solution may be verified by calculations using Equation 1.

Dextrose

$$\frac{50 \text{ g}}{\text{L}} \times \frac{1 \text{ mol}}{198 \text{ g}} \times \frac{1 \text{ osmol}}{\text{mol}} \times \frac{1000 \text{ mOsmol}}{\text{Osmol}} = 252 \text{ mOsmol/L}$$

Sodium Chloride

$$\frac{6 \text{g}}{\text{L}} \times \frac{1 \text{ mol}}{58.4 \text{ g}} \times \frac{2 \text{ osmol}}{\text{mol}} \times \frac{1000 \text{ mOsmol}}{\text{osmol}}$$

$$= 205 \frac{\text{mOsmol}}{\text{L}} \begin{cases} (102.7 \text{ mOsmol Na}^+) \\ (102.7 \text{ mOsmol Cl}^-) \end{cases}$$

Potassium Chloride

$$\frac{0.3 \text{ g}}{\text{L}} \times \frac{1 \text{ mol}}{74.6 \text{ g}} \times \frac{2 \text{ osmol}}{\text{mol}} \times \frac{1000 \text{ mOsmol}}{\text{osmol}}$$

$$= \frac{8.04 \text{ mOsmol}}{\text{L}} \begin{cases} (4.02 \text{ mOsmol K}^+) \\ (4.02 \text{ mOsmol Cl}^-) \end{cases}$$

Calcium Chloride

$$\frac{0.2 \text{ g}}{\text{L}} \times \frac{1 \text{ mol}}{111 \text{ g}} \times \frac{3 \text{ osmol}}{\text{mol}} \times \frac{1000 \text{ mOsmol}}{\text{osmol}}$$

$$= \frac{5.41 \text{ mOsmol}}{\text{L}} \begin{cases} (1.80 \text{ mOsmol Ca}^{2+}) \\ (3.61 \text{ mOsmol Cl}^-) \end{cases}$$

Sodium Lactate

$$\frac{3.1 \text{ g}}{\text{L}} \times \frac{1 \text{ mol}}{112 \text{ g}} \times \frac{2 \text{ osmol}}{\text{mol}} \times \frac{1000 \text{ mOsmol}}{\text{osmol}}$$

$$= \frac{55.4 \text{ mOsmol}}{\text{L}} \begin{cases} (27.7 \text{ mOsmol Na}^+) \\ (27.7 \text{ mOsmol lactate}) \end{cases}$$

The total osmolar concentration of the five solutes in the solution is 526, in good agreement with the labeled total osmolar concentration of approximately 524 mOsmol/L.

The mOsmol of sodium in 1 L of the solution is the sum of the mOsmol of the ion from sodium chloride and sodium lactate: 102 + 27.6 = 129.6 mOsmol. Chloride ions come from the sodium chloride, potassium chloride, and calcium chloride, the total osmolar concentration being 102 + 4.02 + 3.61 = 109.6 mOsmol. The mOsmol values of potassium, calcium, and lactate are calculated to be 4.02, 1.80, and 27.6, respectively.

The osmolarity of a mixture of complex composition, such as an enteral hyperalimentation fluid, cannot be calculated with any acceptable degree of certainty; therefore, the *osmolality* of such preparations should be determined experimentally.

OSMOMETRY AND THE CLINICAL LABORATORY

Serum and urine osmometry may assist in the diagnosis of certain fluid and electrolyte problems. However, osmometry values have little meaning unless the clinical situation is known. Osmometry is used in renal dialysis as a check on the electrolyte composition of the fluid. In the clinical laboratory, as stated above, the term *osmolality* is used generally, but usually is reported as mOsmol/L. It may seem unnecessary to mention that osmolality depends not only on the number of solute particles, but also on the quantity of water in which they are dissolved. However, it may help one to understand the statement that the normal range of urine osmolality is 50 to 1400 mOsmol/L, and for a random specimen is 500 to 800 mOsmol/L.

Serum Osmoticity

Sodium is by far the principal solute involved in serum osmoticity. Therefore, abnormal serum osmoticity is most likely to be associated with conditions that cause abnormal sodium concentration and/or abnormal water volume.

Thus, hyperosmotic serum is likely to be caused by an increase in serum sodium and/or loss of water. It may be associated with diabetes insipidus, hypercalcemia, diuresis during severe hyperglycemia, or with early recovery from renal shutdown. Alcohol ingestion is said to be the most common cause of the hyperosmotic state and of coexisting coma and the hyperosmotic state. An example of hyperosmoticity is a comatose diabetic with a serum osmoticity of 365 mOsmol/L.

In a somewhat analogous fashion, hypo-osmotic serum is likely to be due to decrease in serum sodium and/or excess of water. It may be associated with the postoperative state (especially with excessive water replacement therapy), treatment with diuretic drugs and low-salt diet (as with patients with heart failure, cirrhosis, etc), adrenal disease (eg, Addison's disease, adrenogenital syndrome), or SIADH (syndrome of inappropriate ADH secretion). There are many diseases that cause ADH to be released inappropriately (ie, in spite of serum osmoticity and volume having been normal initially). These include oat-cell carcinoma of the lung, bronchogenic carcinoma, congestive heart failure, inflammatory pulmonary lesions, porphyria, severe hypothyroidism, or cerebral disease (such as tumor, trauma, infection, and vascular abnormalities). It also may be found with some patients with excessive diuretic use. Serum and urine osmoticity are measured when SIADH is suspected. In SIADH there is hypo-osmoticity of the blood in association with a relative hyperosmoticity of urine. The usual cause is a malfunction of the normal osmotic response of osmoreceptors, an excess of exogenous vasopressin, or a production of a vasopressin-like hormone that is not under the regular control of serum osmoticity. The diagnosis is made by simultaneous measurement of urine and serum osmolality. The serum osmolality will be lower than normal and much lower than the urine osmolality, indicating inappropriate secretion of a concentrated urine in the presence of a dilute serum.

Cardiac, renal, and hepatic disease characteristically reduce the sodium/osmolality ratio, this being partially attributed to the effects of increased blood sugar, urea, or unknown metabolic products. Patients in shock may develop disproportionately elevated measured osmolality compared to calculated osmolality, which points toward the presence of circulating metabolic products.

There are several approximate methods for estimating serum osmolality from clinical laboratory values for sodium ion. They may be of considerable value in an emergency situation.

1. Serum osmolality may be estimated from

$$\text{mOsmol} = (1.86 \times \text{sodium}) + \frac{\text{blood sugar}}{18} + \frac{\text{BUN}}{2.8} + 5$$

(Na in mEq/L, blood sugar and BUN in mg/100 mL).

2. A quick approximation is

$$\text{mOsmol} = 2 \text{ Na} + \frac{\text{BS}}{20} + \frac{\text{BUN}}{3}$$

3. The osmolality is usually, *but not always*, very close to two times the sodium reading plus 10.

Urine Osmoticity

The two main functions of the kidney are glomerular filtration and tubular reabsorption. Clinically, tubular function is measured best by tests that determine the ability of the tubules to concentrate and dilute the urine. Tests of urinary dilution are not as sensitive in the detection of disease, as are tests of urinary concentration. As concentration of urine occurs in the renal medulla (interstitial fluids, loops of Henle, capillaries of the medulla, and collecting tubules), the disease processes that disturb the function or structure of the medulla produce early impairment of the concentrating power of the kidney.

Such diseases include acute tubular necrosis, obstructive uropathy, pyelonephritis, papillary necrosis, medullary cysts, hypokalemic and hypercalcemic nephropathy, and sickle cell disease.

Measurement of urine osmolality is an accurate test for the diluting and concentrating ability of the kidneys. In the absence of ADH, the daily urinary output is likely to be 6 to 8 liters or more. The normal urine osmolality depends on the clinical setting; normally, with maximum ADH stimulation, it can be as much as 1200 mOsmol/kg, and with maximum ADH suppression as little as 50 mOsmol/kg. Simultaneous determination of serum and urine osmolality often is valuable in assessing the distal tubular response to circulating ADH. For example, if the patient's serum is hyperosmolal, or in the upper limits of normal ranges, and the patient's urine osmolality measured at the same time is much lower, a decreased responsiveness of the distal tubules to circulating ADH is suggested.

Measurement of urine osmolality during water restriction is an accurate, sensitive test of decreased renal function. For example, under the conditions of one test, normal osmolality would be greater than 800 mOsmol/kg. With severe impairment the value would be less than 400 mOsmol/kg. Knowledge of urine osmolality may point to a problem even though other tests are normal (eg, the Fishberg concentration test, blood urea nitrogen, PSP excretion, creatinine clearance, or IV pyelogram). Knowledge of its value may be useful especially in diabetes mellitus, essential hypertension, and silent pyelonephritis. The urine/serum osmolality ratio should be calculated and should be equal to or greater than 3.

UNDESIRABLE EFFECTS OF ABNORMAL OSMOTICITY

OPHTHALMIC MEDICATION—It is generally accepted that ophthalmic preparations intended for instillation into the cul-de-sac of the eye should, if possible, be approximately isotonic to avoid irritation (see Chapter 43). It also has been stated that the abnormal tonicity of contact lens solutions can cause the lens to adhere to the eye and/or cause burning or dryness and photophobia.

PARENTERAL MEDICATION—Osmoticity is of great importance in parenteral injections, its effects depending on such factors as the degree of deviation from tonicity, the concentration, the location of the injection, the volume injected, the speed of the injection, and the rapidity of dilution and diffusion, etc. When formulating parenterals, solutions otherwise hypotonic usually have their tonicity adjusted by the addition of dextrose or sodium chloride. Hypertonic parenteral drug solutions cannot be adjusted. Hypotonic and hypertonic solutions usually are administered slowly in small volumes, or into a large vein such as the subclavian, where dilution and distribution occur rapidly. Solutions that differ from the serum in tonicity generally cause tissue irritation, pain on injection, and electrolyte shifts, the effect depending on the degree of deviation from tonicity:

Excessive infusion of *hypotonic* fluids may cause swelling of red blood cells, hemolysis, and water invasion of the body's cells in general. When this is beyond the body's tolerance for water, water intoxication results, with convulsions and edema, such as pulmonary edema.

Excessive infusion of *isotonic* fluids can cause an increase in extracellular fluid volume, which can result in circulatory overload.

Excessive infusion of *hypertonic* fluids leads to a wide variety of complications. For example, the sequence of events when the body is presented with a large IV load of hypertonic fluid, rich in dextrose, is as follows: hyperglycemia, glycosuria and intracellular dehydration, osmotic diuresis, loss of water and electrolytes, dehydration, and coma.

One cause of osmotic diuresis is the infusion of dextrose at a rate faster than the ability of the patient to metabolize it (as

greater than perhaps 400–500 mg/kg per hour for an adult on total parenteral nutrition). A heavy load of unmetabolizable dextrose increases the osmoticity of blood and acts as a diuretic; the increased solute load requires more fluid for excretion, 10 to 20 mL of water being required to excrete each gram of dextrose. Solutions such as those for total parenteral nutrition should be administered by means of a metered constant-infusion apparatus over a lengthy period (usually more than 24 hr) to avoid sudden hyperosmotic dextrose loads. Such solutions may cause osmotic diuresis; if this occurs, water balance is likely to become negative because of the increased urinary volume, and electrolyte depletion may occur because of excretion of sodium and potassium secondary to the osmotic diuresis. If such diuresis is marked, body weight falls abruptly and signs of dehydration appear. Urine should be monitored for signs of osmotic diuresis, such as glycosuria and increased urine volume.

If the IV injection rate of hypertonic solution is too rapid, there may be catastrophic effects on the circulatory and respiratory systems. Blood pressure may fall to dangerous levels, cardiac irregularities or arrest may ensue, respiration may become shallow and irregular, and there may be heart failure and pulmonary edema. Probably the precipitating factor is a bolus of concentrated solute suddenly reaching the myocardium and the chemoreceptors in the aortic arch and carotid sinus.[7]

Abrupt changes in serum osmoticity can lead to cerebral hemorrhage. It has been shown experimentally that rapid infusions of therapeutic doses of hypertonic saline with osmotic loads produce a sudden rise in cerebrospinal fluid (CSF) pressure and venous pressure (VP) followed by a precipitous fall in CSF pressure. This particularly may be conducive to intracranial hemorrhage, as the rapid infusion produces an increase in plasma volume and venous pressure at the same time the CSF pressure is falling. During the CSF pressure rise, there is a drop in hemoglobin and hematocrit, reflecting a marked increase in blood volume.

Hyperosmotic medications, such as sodium bicarbonate (osmolarity of 1560 at 1 mEq/mL), which are administered intravenously, should be diluted prior to use and should be injected slowly to allow dilution by the circulating blood. Rapid *push* injections may cause a significant increase in blood osmoticity.[8]

As to other possibilities, there may be crenation of red blood cells and general cellular dehydration. Hypertonic dextrose or saline infused through a peripheral vein with small blood volume may traumatize the vein and cause thrombophlebitis. Infiltration can cause trauma and necrosis of tissues. Safety, therefore, demands that all IV injections, especially highly osmotic solutions, be performed slowly, usually being given preferably over a period not less than that required for a complete circulation of the blood, for example, 1 min. The exact danger point varies with the state of the patient, the concentration of the solution, the nature of the solute, and the rate of administration.

Hyperosmotic solutions also should not be discontinued suddenly. In dogs, marked increase in levels of intracranial pressure occur when hyperglycemia produced by dextrose infusions is reversed suddenly by stopping the infusion and administering saline. It also has been shown that the CSF pressure in humans rises during treatment of diabetic ketoacidosis in association with a fall in the plasma concentration of dextrose and a fall in plasma osmolality. These observations may be explained by the different rates of decline in dextrose content of the brain and of plasma. The concentration of dextrose in the brain may fall more slowly than in the plasma, causing a shift of fluid from the extracellular fluid space to the intracellular compartment of the CNS, resulting in increased intracranial pressure.

Clinical Applications

Although there are many issues with abnormal osmoticity, most pharmacists are concerned with preventable adverse effects such as thrombophlebitis and pain at the injection site. The understanding of these potential risks from hyperosmotic parenteral medications has fine-tuned IV administration techniques. The site of administration—peripheral versus central venous catheter—plays a significant role in determining the final concentration of parenteral medications infused IV. Attention should be directed toward establishing the optimal osmolarity of IV administered parenteral medications via the peripheral venous route that will result in the least adverse effects.

Since the introduction of parenteral nutrition support, hyperosmoticity of these nutrition solutions remains a concern. The commonly accepted osmolarity of less than 900 mOsmol/L has been quoted for safe peripheral administration of parenteral nutrition solutions.[11,12] All attempts should be made to prepare solutions with osmoticity close to that of serum osmoticity or no greater than 900 mOsmol/L. This can be achieved by carefully selecting the diluent for dilution and determining the final concentration of the parenteral medication. Dextrose 5% in Water for Injection and Sodium Chloride 0.9% have been used routinely as diluents. When comparing the two diluents, parenteral medications diluted with Dextrose 5% in Water for Injection have a lower osmolarity than do solutions diluted with Sodium Chloride 0.9% at the same final concentration.

Several studies have been conducted to determine optimal final concentration of commonly used parenteral medications.[3–5] The published final concentrations for most parenteral medications are recommended for peripheral as well as central venous catheter IV administration for patients with no special needs, such as fluid restriction. In the event that fluid restriction is required or the recommended final concentration is not achievable, the parenteral medication should be administered via a central venous catheter, where immediate dilution and distribution is achieved rapidly. This will minimize potential for the phlebitis and pain at the injection site.

Osmoticity issues associated with parenteral medications are also applicable to *total parenteral nutrition* (TPN) solutions, especially via peripheral venous administration. Peripheral parenteral nutrition support remains an integral part of therapeutic options for hospitalized patients. The peripheral route of administration often is preferred for patients who require short-term therapy or supplemental nutrition support.

In clinical practice, however, many institutions use the macronutrient dextrose as the sole determinant for the safety of peripheral parenteral nutrition administration. For example, the approximate osmolarity of dextrose is 50 mOsmol/% of dextrose. Thus, a 10% dextrose solution equals 500 mOsmol/L. It is assumed that with *normal* protein and micronutrient requirements, the final osmolarity is estimated to be approximately 900 mOsmol/L. Therefore, guidelines for most institutions recommend any parenteral nutrition solution with a dextrose concentration less than or equal to 10% is safe for peripheral administration, irrespective of other components. Conversely, a parenteral nutrition solution with a final dextrose concentration greater than 10% should not be administered peripherally and should be considered for central venous catheter administration. Although this method appears to be practical and provides quick decision-making ability, it ignores the contributions of the other components, restricts its validity to adult parenteral nutrition solutions with *normal* protein and micronutrient requirements, and does not address neonatal and pediatric parenteral nutrition solutions. Because of the different fluid and nutrient requirements of neonates and pediatric patients, the final concentration of dextrose and amino acids is generally greater to provide the calories and protein requirements in a smaller volume of liquid. For example, protein requirements of neonates are much higher compared with adult requirements, 3 g/kg/day versus 1 g/k/day. Thus, the final percentage of amino acid in neonatal parenteral nutrition solution is generally higher. Coupled with an approximate osmolarity of amino acid equal to 100 mOsmol/%, amino acids may

contribute equally to the final osmolarity of a parenteral nutrition solution. Therefore, components other than dextrose cannot be ignored.

Currently, most institutions use automated compounding systems to prepare parenteral nutrition solutions. These systems often are computerized and include programs that will calculate the osmolarity of the final parenteral nutrition solution. This has helped clinicians determine the safety of parenteral nutrition solutions with various macro- and micronutrient combinations, thereby accounting for all components of parenteral nutrition solutions.

OSMOTICITY AND ENTERAL HYPERALIMENTATION

Some aspects of nutrition are discussed briefly here because of the potential major side effects due to abnormal osmoticity of nutritional fluids, and because there exists increasing dialogue on nutrition among pharmacists, dietitians, nurses, and physicians. The professional organization ASPEN (The American Society for Parenteral and Enteral Nutrition), for example, has a membership open to all of the above health practitioners. Pharmacists should be able to discuss these matters with other health professionals in terms of nutrition as well as medicine.

Osmoticity has been of special importance in the IV infusion of large volumes of highly concentrated nutritional solutions. Their hyperosmoticity has been a major factor in the requirement that they be injected centrally into a large volume of rapidly moving blood, instead of using peripheral infusion. Use of such solutions and knowledge of their value have led, more recently, to the use of similar formulations administered, not parenterally, but by instillation into some part of the GI tract, orally, by nasogastric tube, via feeding gastrostomy, or by needle-catheter jejunostomy. This method has given excellent total nutrition, for a period of time, to many patients and obviously avoids some of the problems associated with injections.

Enteral nutritional formulas can be modular, allowing individual supplementation of protein, carbohydrate, or fat. Other formulas are called *defined formula diets* and contain protein, carbohydrate, fat, minerals, and vitamins. These nutritionally complete formulations can be monomeric (or oligomeric), based on amino acids, short peptides, and simple carbohydrates, or can be polymeric, based on complex protein and carbohydrates.

These diets are necessarily relatively high in osmoticity because their smaller molecules result in more particles per gram than in normal foods. An example is a fluid consisting of L-amino acids, dextrose oligosaccharides, vitamins (including fat-soluble vitamins), fat as a highly purified safflower oil or soybean oil, electrolytes, trace minerals, and water. As it contains fat, that component is not in solution and therefore should have no direct effect on osmoticity. However, the potential for interactions can cause some significant changes in total particle concentration and indirectly affect the osmoticity.[13]

Although it is easily digested, dextrose contributes more particles than most other carbohydrate sources such as starch, and is more likely to cause osmotic diarrhea, especially with bolus feeding. Osmoticity is improved (decreased) by replacing dextrose with dextrose oligosaccharides (carbohydrates that yield on hydrolysis 2 to 10 monosaccharides). Flavoring also increases the osmoticity of a product, different flavors causing varying increases.

Commercial diets are packaged as fluids or as powders for reconstitution. Reconstitution is usually with water. These products are categorized on caloric density, (calories/mL), protein content, or osmolality (mOsm/kg of H_2O). Parenteral nutritional products, on the other hand, are labeled in terms of osmolarity (mOsm/L).

The enteric route for hyperalimentation frequently is overlooked in many diseases or post-trauma states, if the patient is not readily responsive to traditional oral feedings. Poor appetite, chronic nausea, general apathy, and a degree of somnolence or sedation are common concomitants of serious disease. This frequently prevents adequate oral alimentation and results in progressive energy and nutrient deficits. Often, supplementary feedings of a highly nutritious formula are taken poorly or refused entirely. However, the digestive and absorptive capabilities of the GI tract are frequently intact and, when challenged with appropriate nutrient fluids, can be used effectively. By using an intact GI tract for proper alimentation, the major problems of sepsis and metabolic derangement that relate to IV hyperalimentation largely are obviated, and adequate nutritional support is simplified greatly. Because of this increased safety and ease of administration, the enteric route for hyperalimentation should be used whenever possible.[14]

When certain foods are ingested in large amounts or as concentrated fluids, their osmotic characteristics can cause an upset in the normal water balance within the body. For a given weight of solute the osmolality of the solution is inversely proportional to the size of the particles. Nutritional components can be listed in an approximate order of decreasing osmotic effect per gram, as[15]

1. Electrolytes such as sodium chloride
2. Relatively small organic molecules such as dextrose (glucose) and amino acids
3. Dextrose oligosaccharides
4. Starches
5. Proteins
6. Fats (as fats are not water soluble, they have no osmotic effect)

Thus, in foods, high proportions of electrolytes, amino acids, and simple sugars have the greatest effect on osmolality and, as a result, on tolerance. The approximate osmolality of a few common foods and beverages is

	mOsmol/kg
Whole milk	295
Tomato juice	595
Orange juice	935
Ice cream	1150

When nutrition of high osmoticity is ingested, large amounts of water will transfer to the stomach and intestines from the fluid surrounding those organs in an attempt to lower the osmoticity. The higher the osmoticity, the larger the amount of water required; a large amount of water in the GI tract can cause distention, cramps, nausea, vomiting, hypermotility, and shock. The food may move through the tract too rapidly for the water to be reabsorbed, and result in diarrhea; severe diarrhea can cause dehydration. The hyperosmotic enteral effects have been observed by the administration of undiluted hypertonic oral medication.[16–17] Table I from this work lists average osmolality values of some commercially available drug solutions and suspensions. Thus, there is some analogy to the effect of hyperosmotic IV infusions.

Hyperosmotic feedings may result in mucosal damage in the GI tract. Rats given hyperosmotic feeding showed transient decrease in disaccharidase activity, and an increase in alkaline phosphatase activity. They also showed morphological alterations in the microvilli of the small intestines. After a period of severe gastroenteritis, the bowel may be unusually susceptible to highly osmotic formulas, and their use may increase the frequency of diarrhea. Infant formulas that are hyperosmotic may affect preterm infants adversely during the early neonatal period, and they may produce or predispose neonates to necrotizing enterocolitis when the formulas delivered to the jejunum through a nasogastric tube. The body attempts to keep the osmoticity of the contents of the stomach and intestines at approximately the same level as that of the fluid surrounding them. As a fluid of lower osmoticity requires the transfer of less water to dilute it, it should be tolerated better than one of higher osmoticity.

As to tolerance, there is a great variation from one individual to another in sensitivity to the osmoticity of foods. The majority of patients receiving nutritional formulas, either orally or by tube, are able to tolerate feedings with a wide range of osmoticities when the formulas are administered slowly and when adequate additional fluids are given. However, certain patients are more likely to develop symptoms of intolerance when receiving fluids of high osmoticity. These include debilitated patients, patients with GI disorders, pre- and postoperative patients, gastrostomy- and jejunostomy-fed patients, and patients whose GI tracts have not been challenged for an extended period of time. Thus, osmoticity always should be considered in the selection of the formula for each individual patient.

With all products, additional fluid intake may be indicated for individuals with certain clinical conditions. Frequent feedings of small volume or a continual instillation (pumped) may be of benefit initially in establishing tolerance to a formula. For other than iso-osmotic formulas, feedings of reduced concentration (osmolality less than 400 mOsmol/kg) also may be helpful initially if tolerance problems arise in sensitive individuals. Concentration and size of feeding then can be increased gradually to normal as tolerance is established.

A common disturbance of intake encountered in elderly individuals relates to excess solid intake rather than to reduced water intake. For example, an elderly victim of a cerebral vascular accident who is being fed by nasogastric tube may be given a formula whose solute load requires a greatly increased water intake. Thus, tube feeding containing 120 g of protein and 10 g of salt will result in the excretion of more than 1000 mOsmol of solute. This requires the obligatory excretion of a volume of urine between 1200 and 1500 mL when the kidneys are capable of normal concentration ability. As elderly individuals often have significant impairment in renal function, water loss as urine may exceed 2000 to 2500 mL per day. Such an individual would require 3 to 4 liters of water per day simply to meet the increased demand created by this high solute intake. Failure of the physician to provide such a patient with the increased water intake needed will result in a progressive water deficit that rapidly may become critical. The importance of knowing the complete composition of the tube feeding formulas used for incapacitated patients cannot be overemphasized.

OSMOLALITY DETERMINATION

The need for experimental determination of osmolality has been established. In regard to this there are four properties of solutions that depend only on the number of *particles* in the solution. They are *osmotic-pressure elevation, boiling-point elevation, vapor-pressure depression,* and *freezing-point depression.* These are called *colligative properties,* and if one of them is known, the others can be calculated from its value. Osmotic-pressure elevation is the most difficult to measure satisfactorily. The boiling-point elevation may be determined, but the values are rather sensitive to changes in barometric pressure. Also, for an aqueous solution the molal boiling point elevation is considerably less than the freezing-point depression. Thus, it is less accurate than the freezing-point method. Determinations of vapor-pressure lowering are quite easy, rapid, and convenient. A vapor pressure osmometer with a precision of <2 mOsmol/kg is reported by Dickerson et al.[16] Another commonly used method is that of freezing-point depression, which can be determined quite readily with a fair degree of accuracy (see *Freezing-Point Depression* in Chapter 16). It should be noted that the data in Appendix A can be converted readily to vapor-pressure lowering if desired.

The results of investigations by Lund et al[18] indicate that the freezing point of normal, healthy human blood is −0.52°. Inasmuch as water is the medium in which the various constituents of blood are either suspended or dissolved in this method, it is assumed that *any aqueous solution* freezing at −0.52° is *isotonic with blood.* Now it is rare that a simple aqueous solution of the therapeutic agent to be injected parenterally has a freezing point of −0.52°, and to obtain this freezing point it is necessary either to add some other therapeutically inactive solute if the solution is hypotonic (freezing point above −0.52°) or to dilute the solution if it is hypertonic (freezing point below −0.52°). The usual practice is to add either sodium chloride or dextrose to adjust hypotonic parenteral solutions to isotonicity. Certain solutes, including ammonium chloride, boric acid, urea, glycerin, and propylene glycol, cause hemolysis even when they are present in a concentration that is iso-osmotic, and such solutions obviously are not isotonic. See Appendix A.

In a similar manner solutions intended for ophthalmic use may be adjusted to have a freezing point identical to that of lacrimal fluid, namely −0.52°. Ophthalmic solutions with higher freezing points usually are made isotonic by the addition of boric acid or sodium chloride.

In laboratories where the necessary equipment is available, the method usually followed for adjusting hypotonic solutions is to determine the freezing-point depression produced by the ingredients of a given prescription or formula, and then to add a quantity of a suitable inert solute calculated to lower the freezing point to −0.52°, whether the solution is for parenteral injection or ophthalmic application. A final determination of the freezing-point depression may be made to verify the accuracy of the calculation. If the solution is hypertonic, it must be diluted if an isotonic solution is to be prepared, but it must be remembered that some solutions cannot be diluted without impairing their therapeutic activity. For example, solutions to be used for treating varicose veins require a high concentration of the active ingredient (solute) to make the solution effective. Dilution to isotonic concentration is not indicated in such cases.

FREEZING-POINT CALCULATIONS

As explained in the preceding section, freezing-point data often may be employed in solving problems of isotonicity adjustment. Obviously, the utility of such data is limited to those solutions where the solute does not penetrate the membrane of the tissue (eg, red blood cells) with which it is in contact. In such cases, Appendix A, which gives the freezing-point depression of solutions of different concentrations of various substances, provides information essential for solving the problem.

For most substances listed in the table, the concentration of an isotonic solution (one that has a freezing point of −0.52°) is given. If this is not listed in the table, it may be determined with sufficient accuracy by simple proportion using, as the basis for calculation, the figure that most nearly produces an isotonic solution. Actually the depression of the freezing point of a solution of an electrolyte is not absolutely proportional to the concentration but varies according to dilution; for example, a solution containing 1 g of procaine hydrochloride in 100 mL has a freezing-point depression of 0.12°, whereas a solution containing 3 g of the same salt in 100 mL has a freezing-point depression of 0.33°, *not* 0.36° (3 × 0.12°). Because the adjustment to isotonicity need not be absolutely exact, approximations may be made. Nevertheless, adjustments to isotonicity should be as exact as practicable.

EFFECT OF SOLVENTS—Besides water, certain other solvents frequently are employed in nose drops, eardrops, and other preparations to be used in various parts of the body. Liquids such as glycerin, propylene glycol, or alcohol may compose part of the solvent. In solving isotonicity adjustment problems for such solutions, it should be kept in mind that these solvent components contribute to the freezing-point depression but they may or may not have an effect on the *tone* of the tissue to which they are applied; thus, an *iso-osmotic* solution may not be *isotonic.* In such cases, it is apparent that the utility of the methods described above—or for that matter, of any other method of evaluating *tonicity*—is questionable.

TONICITY TESTING BY OBSERVING ERYTHROCYTE CHANGES

Observation of the behavior of human erythrocytes when suspended in a solution is the ultimate and direct procedure for determining whether the solution is isotonic, hypotonic, or hypertonic. If hemolysis or marked change in the appearance of the erythrocytes occurs, the solution is not isotonic with the cells. If the cells retain their normal characteristics, the solution is isotonic.

Hemolysis may occur when the osmotic pressure of the fluid in the erythrocytes is greater than that of the solution in which the cells are suspended, but the specific chemical reactivity of the solute in the solution often is far more important in producing hemolysis than is the osmotic effect. There is no certain evidence that any single mechanism of action causes hemolysis. The process appears to involve such factors as pH, lipid solubility, molecular and ionic sizes of solute particles, and possibly inhibition of cholinesterase in cell membranes and denaturing action on plasma membrane protein.

Some investigators test the tonicity of injectable solutions by observing variations of red blood cell volume produced by these solutions. This method appears to be more sensitive to small differences in tonicity than those based on observation of a hemolytic effect. Much useful information concerning the effect of various solutes on erythrocytes has been obtained by this procedure.

METHODS OF ADJUSTING TONICITY

There are several methods for adjusting the tonicity of an aqueous solution, provided, of course, that the solution is hypotonic when the drug and additives are dissolved. The most prominent of these methods are the freezing-point depression method, the sodium chloride equivalent method, and the isotonic solution V-value method. The first two of these methods can be used with a three-step problem-solving process based on sodium chloride.

1. Identify a reference solution and the associated tonicity parameter.
2. Determine the contribution of the drug(s) and additive(s) to the total tonicity.
3. Determine the amount of sodium chloride needed by subtracting the contribution of the actual solution from the reference solution.

The result of the third step also indicates whether the actual solution is hypotonic, isotonic, or hypertonic. If the actual solution contributes less to the total tonicity than the reference solution, then the actual solution is hypotonic. If, however, the actual solution contributes a greater amount to tonicity than the reference solution, the actual solution is hypertonic and can be adjusted to isotonicity only by dilution. This may not be possible on therapeutic grounds.

The amount of sodium chloride resulting in the third step also can be converted into an amount of other materials, such as dextrose, to render the actual solution isotonic.

FREEZING-POINT–DEPRESSION METHOD—The freezing-point method makes use of a *D value* (found in Appendix A) which has the units of degree centigrade/(*x*% drug). For example, in Appendix A, dexamethasone sodium phosphate has *D* values of 0.050°/(0.5% drug), 0.180°/(2.0% drug), 0.52°/(6.75% drug), etc. It is apparent that the *D* value is nearly proportional to concentration. If a *D* value is needed for a concentration of drug not listed in Appendix A, a *D* value can be calculated from the appendix by direct proportion, using a *D* value closest to the concentration of drug in the actual solution.

The reference solution for the freezing-point-depression method is 0.9% sodium chloride, which has a freezing-point depression of $\Delta T_f = 0.52°$. Using the three steps described above, the dexamethasone sodium phosphate solution in Example 1 can be rendered isotonic as follows:

EXAMPLE 1

Dexamethasone Sodium Phosphate	0.1%
Purified Water qs	30 mL

Mft Isotonic Solution
Step 1—Reference solution: 0.9% sodium chloride.

$$\Delta T_f = 0.52°$$

$$D = 0.050°/0.5\% \text{ (dexamethasone sodium phosphate)}$$

Step 2—Contribution of drug.

$$\frac{0.050°}{0.5\% \text{ drug}} \times 0.1\% \text{ drug} = 0.010°$$

Step 3—Reference solution − Actual solution.

$$0.52° - 0.01° = 0.51°$$

Sodium chloride needed.

$$\frac{0.9\% \text{ NaCl}}{0.52°} \times 0.51° = 0.883\% \text{ NaCl}$$

$$\frac{0.883 \text{ g NaCl}}{100 \text{ mL}} \times 30 \text{ mL} = 0.265 \text{ g NaCl}$$

The above solution could be made isotonic with any appropriate material other than sodium chloride by using the D value for that material. For example, to make the solution isotonic with dextrose with a D value, $D = 0.091°/1\%$;

$$\frac{1\% \text{ Dextrose}}{0.091°} \times 0.51° = 5.60\% \text{ Dextrose}$$

$$\frac{5.60 \text{ g Dextrose}}{100 \text{ mL}} \times 30 \text{ mL} = 1.68 \text{ g Dextrose}$$

EXAMPLE 2

Naphazoline HCl (N.HCl)	0.02%
Zinc Sulfate	0.25%
Purified Water qs	30 mL

Mft Isotonic solution
Step 1—Reference solution: 0.9% sodium chloride.

$$\Delta T_f = 0.52°$$

$$D = 0.14°/1\% \text{ (naphazoline HCl)}$$

$$D = 0.086°/1\% \text{ (zinc sulfate)}$$

Step 2—Contribution of drugs.

$$\frac{0.14°}{1\% \text{ N.HCl}} \times 0.02\% \text{ N.HCl} = 0.003°$$

$$\frac{0.086°}{1\% \text{ ZnSO}_4} \times 0.25\% \text{ ZnSO}_4 = 0.022°$$

$$0.003° + 0.022° = 0.025°$$

Step 3—Reference solution − actual solution.

$$0.52° - 0.025° = 0.495°$$

Sodium chloride needed.

$$\frac{0.9\% \text{ NaCl}}{0.52°} \times 0.495° = 0.857\% \text{ NaCl}$$

$$\frac{0.857 \text{ g NaCl}}{100 \text{ mL}} \times 30 \text{ mL} = 0.257 \text{ g NaCl}$$

The above solution could be made isotonic with any appropriate material other than sodium chloride by using the D value for that material.

For example, to make the solution isotonic with dextrose with a D value, $D = 0.091°/1\%$;

$$\frac{1\% \text{ Dextrose}}{0.091°} \times 0.495° = 5.44\% \text{ Dextrose}$$

$$\frac{5.44 \text{ g Dextrose}}{100 \text{ mL}} \times 30 \text{ mL} = 1.63 \text{ g Dextrose}$$

SODIUM CHLORIDE EQUIVALENT METHOD—A sodium chloride equivalent, E *value*, is defined as the weight of sodium chloride that will produce the same osmotic effect as 1 g of the drug. For example, in Appendix A, dexamethasone sodium phosphate has an E value of 0.18 g NaCl/g drug at 0.5% drug concentration, 0.17 g NaCl/g drug at 1% drug concentration and a value of 0.16 g NaCl/g drug at 2% drug. This slight variation in the sodium chloride equivalent with concentration is due to changes in interionic attraction at different concentration of drug; the E value is not directly proportional to concentration as was the freezing-point-depression.

The reference solution for the sodium chloride equivalent method is 0.9% sodium chloride as it was for the freezing-point-depression method.

The dexamethasone sodium phosphate solution in Example 1 can be rendered isotonic using the sodium chloride equivalent method as follows:

EXAMPLE 1

Dexamethasone Sodium Phosphate	0.1%
Purified Water qs	30 mL

Mft Isotonic Solution
Step 1—Reference solution: 0.9% sodium chloride.

$$\frac{0.9 \text{ g NaCl}}{100 \text{ mL}} \times 30 \text{ mL} = 0.270 \text{ g NaCl}$$

$$E = 0.18 \text{ g NaCl/g drug}$$

Step 2—Contribution of drug.

$$\frac{0.18 \text{ g NaCl}}{1 \text{ g drug}} \times \frac{0.1 \text{ g drug}}{100 \text{ mL}} \times 30 \text{ mL} = 0.0054 \text{ g NaCl}$$

Step 3—Reference solution − Actual solution.

$$0.270 \text{ g NaCl} - 0.0054 \text{ g NaCl} = 0.265 \text{ g NaCl}$$

The above solution can be made isotonic with a material other than sodium chloride, such as dextrose, by using the E value of that material. For example, to make the solution isotonic with dextrose, $E = 0.16$ g NaCl/g dextrose, the amount of sodium chloride needed in Step 3, can be converted to dextrose as follows:

$$\frac{1 \text{ g Dextrose}}{0.16 \text{ g NaCl}} \times 0.265 \text{ g NaCl} = 1.66 \text{ g Dextrose}$$

EXAMPLE 2

Naphazoline HCl (N.HCl)	0.02%
Zinc Sulfate	0.25%
Purified Water qs	30 mL

Mft Isotonic Solution
Step 1—Reference solution: 0.9% sodium chloride.

$$\frac{0.9 \text{ g NaCl}}{100 \text{ mL}} \times 30 \text{ mL} = 0.270 \text{ g NaCl}$$

$$E = 0.27 \text{ g NaCl/g N.HCl}$$

$$E = 0.15 \text{ g NaCl/g ZnSO}_4$$

Step 2—Contribution of drugs.

$$\frac{0.27 \text{ g NaCl}}{1 \text{ g N.HCl}} \times \frac{0.02 \text{ g N.HCl}}{100 \text{ mL}} \times 30 \text{ mL} = 0.002 \text{ g NaCl}$$

$$\frac{0.15 \text{ g NaCl}}{1 \text{ g ZnSO}_4} \times \frac{0.25 \text{ g ZnSO}_4}{100 \text{ mL}} \times 30 \text{ mL} = 0.011 \text{ g NaCl}$$

$$0.002 \text{ g NaCl} + 0.011 \text{ g NaCl} = 0.013 \text{ g NaCl}$$

Step 3—Reference solution − actual solution.

$$0.270 \text{ g NaCl} - 0.013 \text{ g NaCl} = 0.257 \text{ g NaCl}$$

The above solution can be made isotonic with a material other than sodium chloride, such as dextrose, by using the E value of that material. For example, to make the solution isotonic with dextrose, $E = 0.16$ g NaCl/g dextrose, the amount of sodium chloride needed in Step 3 can be converted to dextrose as follows:

$$\frac{1 \text{ g Dextrose}}{0.16 \text{ g NaCl}} \times 0.257 \text{ g NaCl} = 1.61 \text{ g Dextrose}$$

ISOTONIC SOLUTION *V* VALUES—The *V value* of a drug is the volume of water to be added to a specified weight of drug (0.3 g or 1.0 g, depending on the table used) to prepare an isotonic solution. Appendix B gives such values for some commonly used drugs. The reason for providing data for 0.3 g of drug is for convenience in preparing 30 mL (approximately 1 fluidounce) of solution, a commonly prescribed volume. The basic principle underlying the use of V values is to prepare an isotonic solution of the prescribed drug and then dilute this solution to final volume with a suitable isotonic vehicle.

The two solutions in the previous examples can be prepared as follows using the *V*-value method:

EXAMPLE 1

Dexamethasone Sodium Phosphate	0.1%
Purified Water qs	30 mL

Mft Isotonic Solution
Step 1—The V value for dexamethasone sodium phosphate can be calculated from the sodium chloride equivalent, E, as outlined in the footnote in Appendix B.

$$\frac{100 \text{ mL Soln}}{0.9 \text{ g NaCl}} \times \frac{0.17 \text{ g NaCl}}{1 \text{ g drug}} \times 0.3 \text{ g drug} = 5.67 \text{ mL Soln}$$

for a dilute solution:

$$5.67 \text{ mL Soln} \cong 5.67 \text{ mL H}_2\text{O there } V$$

$$= (5.67 \text{ mL H}_2\text{O})/(0.3 \text{ g drug})$$

Step 2—Amount of drug needed.

$$\frac{0.1 \text{ g drug}}{100 \text{ mL}} \times 30 \text{ mL} = 0.030 \text{ g drug}$$

Volume of water needed to prepare an isotonic solution.

$$\frac{5.67 \text{ mL H}_2\text{O}}{0.3 \text{ g drug}} \times 0.030 \text{ g drug} = 0.57 \text{ mL H}_2\text{O}$$

Step 3—To prepare the solution, dissolve 0.030 g of drug in 0.57 mL water, and qs to volume with a suitable isotonic vehicle such as 0.9% sodium chloride solution, 5.51% dextrose, or an isotonic phosphate buffer.

EXAMPLE 2

Naphazoline HCl (N.HCl)	0.02%
Zinc Sulfate	0.25%
Purified Water qs	30 mL

Mft Isotonic Solution
Step 1—The V value for naphazoline HCl can be calculated from the sodium chloride equivalent, E, as outlined in the footnote in Appendix B; the V value for zinc sulfate is taken directly from Appendix B.

$$\frac{100 \text{ mL Soln}}{0.9 \text{ g NaCl}} \times \frac{0.27 \text{ g NaCl}}{1 \text{ g N.HCl}} \times 0.3 \text{ g N.HCl} = 9.00 \text{ mL Soln}$$

for a dilute solution:

$$9.00 \text{ mL Soln} \cong 9.00 \text{ mL H}_2\text{O there V}$$

$$= (9.00 \text{ mL H}_2\text{O})/(0.3 \text{ g N.HCl})$$

$$V = 5.00 \text{ mL H}_2\text{O}/0.3 \text{ g ZnSO}_4$$

Step 2—Amount of drugs needed.

$$\frac{0.02 \text{ g N.HCl}}{100 \text{ mL}} \times 30 \text{ mL} = 0.006 \text{ g N.HCl}$$

$$\frac{0.25 \text{ g ZnSO}_4}{100 \text{ mL}} \times 30 \text{ mL} = 0.075 \text{ g ZnSO}_4$$

Volume of water needed to prepare an isotonic solution.

$$\frac{9.00 \text{ mL H}_2\text{O}}{0.3 \text{ g N.HCl}} \times 0.006 \text{ g drug} = 0.18 \text{ mL H}_2\text{O}$$

$$\frac{5.00 \text{ mL H}_2\text{O}}{0.3 \text{ g ZnSO}_4} \times 0.075 \text{ g ZnSO}_4 = 1.25 \text{ mL H}_2\text{O}$$

Step 3—To prepare the solution, dissolve 0.006 g of naphazoline HCl and 0.075 g zinc sulfate in 1.43 mL water, and qs to volume with a suitable isotonic vehicle such as 0.9% sodium chloride solution, 5.51% dextrose, or an isotonic phosphate buffer.

REFERENCES

1. Kaminski MV. *Surg Gynecol Obstet* 1976; 143:12.
2. Theeuwes F. *J Pharm Sci* 1975; 64:1987.
3. Wermeling DP et al. *Am J Hosp Pharm* 1985; 1739:42.
4. Crane VS. *Drug Intell Clin Pharm* 1987; 21: 830.
5. Santeiro ML et al. *Am J Hosp Pharm* 1990; 47:1359.
6. McDuffee L. *IL Council Hosp Pharm Drug Inf Newsl* 1978; 8 (Oct–Nov).
7. Zenk K, Huxtable RF. *Hosp Pharm* 1978; 13:577.
8. Streng WH et al. *J Pharm Sci* 1978; 67:384.
9. Murty BSR et al. *Am J Hosp Pharm* 1976; 33:546.
10. Bray AJ. Personal communication. Evansville, IN: Mead Johnson Nutritional Division, 1978.
11. Payne-James JJ et al. *J Parenter Enter Nutr* 1993; 17:468.
12. Miller SJ. *Hosp Pharm* 1991; 26:796.
13. Andrassy RJ et al. *Surgery* 1977; 82:205.
14. Dobbie RP, Hoffmeister JA. *Surg Gynecol Obstet* 1976; 143:273.
15. *Osmolality*. Minneapolis: Doyle Pharmaceutical, 1978.
16. Dickerson RN, Melnik G. *Am J Hosp Pharm* 1988; 45:832.
17. Holtz L, Milton J, Sturek JK. *J Parenter Enter Nutr* 1987; 11:183.
18. Lund CG et al. *The Preparation of Solutions Iso-osmotic with Blood, Tears, and Tissue.* Copenhagen: Danish Pharmacopoeial Commission, Einar Munksgaard, 1947.
19. Hammarlund ER *et al. J Pharm Sci* 1965; 54:160.
20. Hammarlund ER, Pedersen-Bjergaard K. *J APhA Sci Ed* 1958; 47:107.
21. Hammarlund ER, Pedersen-Bjergaard K. *J Pharm Sci* 1961; 50:24.
22. Hammarlund ER, Van Pevenage GL. *J Pharm Sci* 1966; 55:1448.
23. Sapp C et al. *J Pharm Sci* 1975; 64:1884.
24. *British Pharmaceutical Codex.* London: Pharmaceutical Press, 1973.
25. Fassett WE et al. *J Pharm Sci* 1969; 58:1540.
26. Kagan DG, Kinsey VE. *Arch Ophthalmol* 1942; 27:696.

BIBLIOGRAPHY

Alberty RA, Daniels F. *Physical Chemistry,* 7th ed. New York: Wiley, 1987.
Cowan G, Scheetz W, eds. *Intravenous Hyperalimentation.* Philadelphia: Lea & Febiger, 1972.
Garb S. *Laboratory Tests in Common Use,* 6th ed. New York: Springer, 1976.
Hall WE. *Am J Pharm Ed* 1970; 34:204.
Harvey AM, Johns RJ, Owens AH, et al. *The Principles and Practice of Medicine,* 18th ed. New York: Appleton Century Crofts, 1972.
Martin AN, Swarbrick J, Cammarata A. *Physical Pharmacy,* 4th ed. Philadelphia: Lea & Febiger, 1993.
Plumer AL. *Principles and Practice of Intravenous Therapy,* 4th ed. Boston: Little, Brown, 1987.
Ravel R. *Clinical Laboratory Medicine,* 5th ed. St Louis: Mosby, 1988.
Shizgal HM. *Ann Rev Med* 1991; 42:549.
Tilkian SM, Conover MH. *Clinical Implications of Laboratory Tests,* 4th ed. St Louis: Mosby, 1987.
Turco S, King RE. *Sterile Dosage Forms,* 3rd ed. Philadelphia: Lea & Febiger, 1987.
Wallach J. *Interpretation of Diagnostic Tests,* 4th ed. Boston: Little, Brown, 1986.

Appendix A Sodium Chloride Equivalents, Freezing-Point Depressions, and Hemolytic Effects of Certain Medicinals in Aqueous Solution

	0.5%		1%		2%		3%		5%		ISO-OSMOTIC CONCENTRATION[a]				
	E	D	E	D	E	D	E	D	E	D	%	E	D	H	pH
Acetrizoate methylglucamine	0.09		0.08		0.08		0.08		0.08	12.12	0.07			0	7.1
Acetrizoate sodium	0.10	0.027	0.10	0.055	0.10	0.109	0.10	0.163	0.10	0.273	9.64	0.09	0.52	0	6.9[†]
Acetylcysteine	0.20	0.055	0.20	0.113	0.20	0.227	0.20	0.341			4.58	0.20	0.52	100*	2.0
Adrenaline HCl											4.24			68	4.5
Alphaprodine HCl	0.19	0.053	0.19	0.105	0.18	0.212	0.18	0.315			4.98	0.18	0.52	100	5.3
Alum (potassium)			0.18				0.15		0.15		6.35		0.14	24*	3.4
Amantadine HCl	0.31	0.090	0.31	0.180	0.31	0.354					2.95	0.31	0.52	91	5.7
Aminoacetic acid	0.42	0.119	0.41	0.235	0.41	0.470					2.20	0.41	0.52	0*	6.2
Aminohippuric acid	0.13	0.035	0.13	0.075											
Aminophylline				0.098[c]											
Ammonium carbonate	0.70	0.202	0.70	0.405							1.29	0.70	0.52	97	7.7
Ammonium chloride			1.12								0.8	1.12	0.52	93	5.0
Ammonium lactate	0.33	0.093	0.33	0.185	0.33	0.370					2.76	0.33	0.52	98	5.9
Ammonium nitrate	0.69	0.200	0.69	0.400							1.30	0.69	0.52	91	5.3
Ammonium phosphate, dibasic	0.58	0.165	0.55	0.315							1.76	0.51	0.52	0	7.9
Ammonium sulfate	0.55	0.158	0.55	0.315							1.68	0.54	0.52	0	5.3
Amobarbital sodium			0.25	0.143[c]			0.25				3.6	0.25	0.52	0	9.3
d-Amphetamine HCl											2.64			98	5.7
Amphetamine phosphate			0.34	0.20			0.27	0.47			3.47	0.26	0.52	0	4.5
Amphetamine sulfate			0.22	0.129[c]			0.21	0.36			4.23	0.21	0.52	0	5.9
Amprotropine phosphate											5.90			0	4.2
Amylcaine HCl			0.22				0.19				4.98	0.18		100	5.6
Anileridine HCl	0.19	0.052	0.19	0.104	0.19	0.212	0.18	0.316	0.18	0.509	5.13	0.18	0.52	12	2.6
Antazoline phosphate											6.05			90	4.0
Antimony potassium tartrate			0.18				0.13		0.10						
Antipyrine			0.17	0.10			0.14	0.24	0.14	0.40	6.81	0.13	0.52	100	6.1
Apomorphine HCl			0.14	0.080[c]											
Arginine glutamate	0.17	0.048	0.17	0.097	0.17	0.195	0.17	0.292	0.17	0.487	5.37	0.17	0.52	0	6.9
Ascorbic acid				0.105[c]							5.05	0.52[b]		100*	2.2
Atropine methylbromide			0.14				0.13		0.13		7.03	0.13			
Atropine methylnitrate											6.52			0	5.2
Atropine sulfate			0.13	0.075			0.11	0.19	0.11	0.32	8.85	0.10	0.52	0	5.0
Bacitracin			0.05	0.03			0.04	0.07	0.04	0.12					
Barbital sodium			0.30	0.171[c]			0.29	0.50			3.12	0.29	0.52	0	9.8
Benzalkonium chloride			0.16				0.14		0.13						
Benztropine mesylate	0.26	0.073	0.21	0.115	0.15	0.170	0.12	0.203	0.09	0.242					
Benzyl alcohol			0.17	0.09[c]			0.15								
Bethanechol chloride	0.50	0.140	0.39	0.225	0.32	0.368	0.30	0.512			3.05	0.30		0	6.0
Bismuth potassium tartrate			0.09				0.06		0.05						
Bismuth sodium tartrate			0.13				0.12		0.11		8.91	0.10		0	6.1
Boric acid	0.50	0.288[c]									1.9	0.47	0.52	100	4.6
Brompheniramine maleate	0.10	0.026	0.09	0.050	0.08	0.084									
Bupivacaine HCl	0.17	0.048	0.17	0.096	0.17	0.193	0.17	0.290	0.17	0.484	5.38	0.17	0.52	83	6.8
Butabarbital sodium	0.27	0.078	0.27	0.155	0.27	0.313	0.27	0.470			3.33	0.27	0.52	0	6.8
Butacaine sulfate			0.20	0.12			0.13	0.23	0.10	0.29					
Caffeine and sodium benzoate			0.26	0.15			0.23	0.40			3.92	0.23	0.52	0	7.0
Caffeine and sodium salicylate			0.12	0.12			0.17	0.295	0.16	0.46	5.77	0.16	0.52	0	6.8
Calcium aminosalicylate											4.80			0	6.0
Calcium chloride			0.51	0.298[c]							1.70	0.53	0.52	0	5.6
Calcium chloride (6 H$_2$O)			0.35	0.20							2.5	0.36	0.52	0	5.7
Calcium chloride, anhydrous			0.68	0.39							1.3	0.69	0.52	0	5.6
Calcium disodium edetate	0.21	0.061	0.21	0.120	0.21	0.240	0.20	0.357			4.50	0.20	0.52	0	6.1
Calcium gluconate			0.16	0.091[c]			0.14	0.24							
Calcium lactate			0.23	0.13			0.12	0.36			4.5	0.20	0.52	0	6.7
Calcium lactobionate	0.08	0.022	0.08	0.043	0.08	0.085	0.07	0.126	0.07	0.197					
Calcium levulinate			0.27	0.16			0.25	0.43			3.58			0	7.2
Calcium pantothenate											5.50			0	7.4
Camphor			0.12[d]												
Capreomycin sulfate	0.04	0.011	0.04	0.020	0.04	0.042	0.04	0.063	0.04	0.106					
Carbachol				0.205[c]							2.82			0	5.9
Carbenicillin sodium	0.20	0.059	0.20	0.118	0.20	0.236	0.20	0.355			4.40	0.20	0.52	0	6.6
Carboxymethylcellulose sodium	0.03	0.007	0.03	0.017	0.145										
Cephaloridine	0.09	0.023	0.07	0.041	0.06	0.074	0.06	0.106	0.05						
Chloramine-T											4.10			100*	9.1
Chloramphenicol				0.06[d]											
Chloramphenicol sodium succinate	0.14	0.038	0.14	0.078	0.14	0.154	0.13	0.230	0.13	0.382	6.83	0.13	0.52	partial	6.1
Chlordiazepoxide HCl	0.24	0.068	0.22	0.125	0.19	0.220	0.18	0.315	0.17	0.487	5.50	0.16	0.52	66	2.7
Chlorobutanol (hydrated)			0.24	0.14											
Chloroprocaine HCl	0.20	0.054	0.20	0.108	0.18	0.210									
Chloroquine phosphate	0.14	0.039	0.14	0.082	0.14	0.162	0.14	0.242	0.13	0.379	7.15	0.13	0.52	0	4.3
Chloroquine sulfate	0.10	0.028	0.09	0.050	0.08	0.090	0.07	0.127	0.07	0.195					
Chlorpheniramine maleate	0.17	0.048	0.15	0.085	0.14	0.165	0.13	0.220	0.09	0.265					
Chlortetracycline HCl	0.10	0.030	0.10	0.061	0.10	0.121									
Chlortetracycline sulfate			0.13	0.08			0.10	0.17							

Appendix A Continued

	0.5%		1%		2%		3%		5%		ISO-OSMOTIC CONCENTRATION[a]				
	E	D	E	D	E	D	E	D	E	D	%	E	D	H	pH
Citric acid			0.18	0.10			0.17	0.295	0.16	0.46	5.52	0.16	0.52	100*	1.8
Clindamycin phosphate	0.08	0.022	0.08	0.046	0.08	0.095	0.08	0.144	0.08	0.242	10.73	0.08	0.52	58*	6.8
Cocaine HCl			0.16	0.090[c]			0.15	0.26	0.14	0.40	6.33	0.14	0.52	47	4.4
Codeine phosphate			0.14	0.080[c]			0.13	0.23	0.13	0.38	7.29	0.12	0.52	0	4.4
Colistimethate sodium	0.15	0.045	0.15	0.085	0.15	0.170	0.15	0.253	0.14	0.411	6.73	0.13	0.52	0	7.6
Cupric sulfate			0.18	0.100[c]			0.15		0.14		6.85	0.13		trace*	3.9
Cyclizine HCl	0.20	0.060													
Cyclophosphamide	0.10	0.031	0.10	0.061	0.10	0.125					8.92	0.10	0.52	0	8.0
Cytarabine	0.11	0.034	0.11	0.066	0.11	0.134	0.11	0.198	0.11	0.317					
Deferoxamine mesylate	0.09	0.023	0.09	0.047	0.09	−0.093	0.09	0.142	0.09	0.241					
Demecarium bromide	0.14	0.038	0.12	0.069	0.10	0.108	0.08	0.139	0.07	0.192					
Dexamethasone sodium phosphate	0.18	0.050	0.17	0.095	0.16	0.180	0.15	0.260	0.14	0.410	6.75	0.13	0.52	0	8.9
Dextroamphetamine HCl	0.34	0.097	0.34	0.196	0.34	0.392					2.64	0.34	0.52		
Dextroamphetamine phosphate			0.25	0.14			0.25	0.44			3.62	0.25	0.52	0	4.7
Dextroamphetamine sulfate	0.24	0.069	0.23	0.134	0.22	0.259	0.22	0.380			4.16	0.22	0.52	0	5.9
Dextrose			0.16	0.091[c]			0.16	0.28	0.16	0.46	5.51	0.16	0.52	0	5.9
Dextrose (anhydrous)			0.18	0.101[c]			0.18	0.31			5.05	0.18	0.52	0	6.0
Diatrizoate sodium	0.10	0.025	0.09	0.049	0.09	0.098	0.09	0.149	0.09	0.248	10.55	0.09	0.52	0	7.9
Dibucaine HCl				0.074[c]											
Dicloxacillin sodium (1 H2O)	0.10	0.030	0.10	0.061	0.10	0.122	0.10	0.182							
Diethanolamine	0.31	0.089	0.31	0.177	0.31	0.358					2.90	0.31	0.52	100	11.3
Dihydrostreptomycin sulfate			0.06	0.03			0.05	0.09	0.05	0.14	19.4	0.05	0.52	0	6.1
Dimethpyrindene maleate	0.13	0.039	0.12	0.070	0.11	0.120									
Dimethyl sulfoxide	0.42	0.122	0.42	0.245	0.42	0.480					2.16	0.42	0.52	100	7.6
Diperodon HCl	0.15	0.045	0.14	0.079	0.13	0.141					5.70			88*	5.5
Diphenhydramine HCl				0.161[c]											
Diphenidol HCl	0.16	0.045	0.16	0.09	0.16	0.180									
Doxapram HCl	0.12	0.035	0.12	0.070	0.12	0.140	0.12	0.210							
Doxycycline hyclate	0.12	0.035	0.12	0.072	0.12	0.134	0.11	0.186	0.09	0.264					
Dyphylline	0.10	0.025	0.10	0.052	0.09	0.104	0.09	0.155	0.08	0.245					
Echothiophate iodide	0.16	0.045	0.16	0.090	0.16	0.179					4.44	0.20	0.52	0	4.7
Edetate disodium	0.24	0.070	0.23	0.132	0.22	0.248	0.21	0.360			3.31	0.27	0.52	0	8.0
Edetate trisodium monohydrate	0.29	0.079	0.29	0.158	0.28	0.316	0.27	0.472							
Emetine HCl				0.058[c]			0.17		0.29			0.17			
Ephedrine HCl			0.30	0.165[c]			0.28				3.2	0.28		96	5.9
Ephedrine sulfate			0.23	0.13			0.20	0.35			4.54	0.20	0.52	0	5.7
Epinephrine bitartrate			0.18	0.104			0.16	0.28	0.16	0.462	5.7	0.16	0.52	100*	3.4
Epinephrine hydrochloride			0.29	0.16[b]			0.26				3.47	0.26			
Ergonovine maleate				0.089[c]											
Erythromycin lactobionate	0.08	0.020	0.07	0.040	0.07	0.078	0.07	0.115	0.06	0.187					
Ethyl alcohol											1.39			100	6.0
Ethylenediamine											2.08			100*	11.4
Ethylmorphine HCl			0.16	0.253[c]			0.15	0.26	0.15	0.43	6.18	0.15	0.52	38	4.7
Eucatropine HCl				0.088[c]											
Ferric ammonium citrate (green)				0.11[d]							6.83			0	5.2
Floxuridine	0.14	0.040	0.13	0.076	0.13	0.147	0.12	0.213	0.12	0.335	8.47	0.12	0.52	3*	4.5
Fluorescein sodium			0.31	0.181[c]			0.27	0.47			3.34	0.27	0.52	0	8.7
Fluphenazine 2-HCl	0.14	0.041	0.14	0.082	0.12	0.145	0.09	0.155							
d-Fructose											5.05			0*	5.9
Furtrethonium iodide	0.24	0.070	0.24	0.133	0.22	0.250	0.21	0.360			4.44	0.20	0.52	0	5.4
Galactose											4.92			0	5.9
Gentamicin sulfate	0.05	0.015	0.05	0.030	0.05	0.060	0.05	0.093	0.05	0.153					
D-Glucuronic acid											5.02			48*	1.6
Glycerin				0.203[c]							2.6			100	5.9
Glycopyrrolate	0.15	0.042	0.15	0.084	0.15	0.166	0.14	0.242	0.13	0.381	7.22	0.12	0.52	92*	4.0
Gold sodium thiomalate	0.10	0.032	0.10	0.061	0.10	0.111	0.09	0.159	0.09	0.250					
Hetacillin potassium	0.17	0.048	0.17	0.095	0.17	0.190	0.17	0.284	0.17	0.474	5.50	0.17	0.52	0	6.3
Hexafluorenium bromide	0.12	0.033	0.11	0.065											
Hexamethonium tartrate	0.16	0.045	0.16	0.089	0.16	0.181	0.16	0.271	0.16	0.456	5.68	0.16	0.52		
Hexamethylene sodium acetaminosalicylate	0.18	0.049	0.18	0.099	0.17	0.199	0.17	0.297	0.16	0.485	5.48	0.16	0.52	0*	4.0
Hexobarbital sodium				0.15[c]							4.30			100	4.8
Hexylcaine HCl											2.24	0.40	0.52	79*	3.7
Histamine 2HCl	0.40	0.115	0.40	0.233	0.40	0.466					4.10	0			4.6
Histamine phosphate				0.149[c]							3.45			40	3.9
Histidine HCl															
Holocaine HCl			0.20	0.12							5.67	0.16	0.52	92	5.0
Homatropine hydrobromide			0.17	0.097[c]			0.16	0.28	0.16	0.46					
Homatropine methylbromide			0.19	0.11			0.15	0.26	0.13	0.38	3.69			0	4.9
4-Homosulfanilamide HCl															
Hyaluronidase	0.01	0.004	0.01	0.007	0.01	0.013	0.01	0.020	0.01	0.033	6.39			64	5.6
Hydromorphone HCl															

Appendix A Continued

	0.5%		1%		2%		3%		5%		ISO-OSMOTIC CONCENTRATION[a]				
	E	D	E	D	E	D	E	D	E	D	%	E	D	H	pH
Hydroxyamphetamine HBr				0.15[d]											
8-Hydroxyquinoline sulfate											3.71			92	5.0
Hydroxystilbamidine isethionate	0.20	0.060	0.16	0.090	0.12	0.137	0.10	0.170	0.07	0.216	9.75			59*	2.5
Hyoscyamine hydrobromide															
Imipramine HCl	0.20	0.058	0.20	0.110	0.13	0.143					6.53			68	5.9
Indigotindisulfonate sodium	0.30	0.085	0.30	0.172											
Intracaine HCl															
Iodophthalein sodium				0.07[c]							4.97			85	5.0
Isometheptene mucate	0.18	0.048	0.18	0.095	0.18	0.196	0.18	0.302			9.58			100	9.4
Isoproterenol sulfate	0.14	0.039	0.14	0.078	0.14	0.156	0.14	0.234	0.14	0.389	4.95	0.18	0.52	0	6.2
Kanamycin sulfate	0.08	0.021	0.07	0.041	0.07	0.083	0.07	0.125	0.07	0.210	6.65	0.14	0.52	trace	4.5
Lactic acid				0.239[c]							2.30			100*	2.1
Lactose			0.07	0.040[c]			0.08		0.09		9.75	0.09		0*	5.8
Levallorphan tartrate	0.13	0.036	0.13	0.073	0.13	0.143	0.12	0.210	0.12	0.329	9.40	0.10	0.52	59*	6.9
Levorphanol tartrate	0.12	0.033	0.12	0.067	0.12	0.136	0.12	0.203							
Lidocaine HCl				0.13[c]							4.42			85	4.3
Lircomycin HCl	0.16	0.045	0.16	0.090	0.15	0.170	0.14	0.247	0.14	0.400	6.60	0.14	0.52	0	4.5
Lobeline HCl				0.09[b]											
Lyapolate sodium	0.10	0.025	0.09	0.051	0.09	0.103	0.09	0.157	0.09	0.263	9.96	0.09	0.52	0	6.5[†]
Magnesium chloride				0.45							2.02	0.45		0	6.3
Magnesium sulfate			0.17	0.094[c]			0.15	0.26	0.15	0.43	6.3	0.14	0.52	0	6.2
Magnesium sulfate, anhydrous	0.34	0.093	0.32	0.184	0.30	0.345	0.29	0.495			3.18	0.28	0.52	0	7.0
Mannitol				0.098[c]						5.07			0*		6.2
Maphenide HCl		0.27	0.075	0.27	0.153	0.27	0.303	0.26	0.448						
Menadiol sodium diphosphate											3.55	0.25	0.52		
Menadione sodium bisulfite											4.36			0	8.2
Menthol				0.12[d]							5.07			0	5.3
Meperidine HCl				0.125[c]											
Mepivacaine HCl	0.21	0.060	0.21	0.116	0.20	0.230	0.20	0.342			4.80			98	5.0
Merbromin				0.08[b]							4.60	0.20	0.52	45	4.5
Mercuric cyanide			0.15				0.14		0.13						
Mersalyl				0.06[b]											
Mesoridazine besylate	0.10	0.024	0.07	0.040	0.05	0.058	0.04	0.071	0.03	0.087					
Metaraminol bitartrate	0.20	0.060	0.20	0.112	0.19	0.210	0.18	0.308	0.17	0.505	5.17	0.17	0.52	59	3.8
Methacholine chloride				0.184[c]							3.21			0	4.5
Methadone HCl				0.101[c]							8.59			100*	5.0
Methamphetamine HCl				0.213[c]							2.75			97	5.9
Methdilazine HCl	0.12	0.035	0.10	0.056	0.08	0.080	0.06	0.093	0.04	0.112					
Methenamine			0.23				0.24				3.68	0.25		100	8.4
Methiodal sodium	0.24	0.068	0.24	0.136	0.24	0.274	0.24	0.410			3.81	0.24	0.52	0	5.9
Methitural sodium	0.26	0.074	0.25	0.142	0.24	0.275	0.23	0.407			3.85	0.23	0.52	78	9.8
Methocarbamol	0.10	0.030	0.10	0.060											
Methotrimeprazine HCl	0.12	0.034	0.10	0.060	0.07	0.077	0.06	0.094	0.04	0.125					
Methoxyphenamine HCl	0.26	0.075	0.26	0.150	0.26	0.300	0.26	0.450			3.47	0.26	0.52	96	5.4
p-Methylaminoethanolphenol tartrate	0.18	0.048	0.17	0.095	0.16	0.190	0.16	0.282	0.16	0.453	5.83	0.16	0.52	0	6.2
Methyldopate HCl	0.21	0.063	0.21	0.122	0.21	0.244	0.21	0.365							
Methylergonovine maleate	0.10	0.028	0.10	0.056							4.28	0.21	0.52	partial	3.0
N-Methylglucamine	0.20	0.057	0.20	0.111	0.18	0.214	0.18	0.315	0.18	0.517	5.02	0.18	0.52	4	11.3
Methylphenidate HCl	0.22	0.065	0.22	0.127	0.22	0.258	0.22	0.388			4.07	0.22	0.52	66	4.3
Methylprednisolone Na succinate	0.10	0.025	0.09	0.051	0.09	0.102	0.08	0.143	0.07	0.200					
Minocycline HCl	0.10	0.030	0.10	0.058	0.09	0.107	0.08	0.146							
Monoethanolamine	0.53	0.154	0.53	0.306							1.70	0.53	0.52	100	11.4
Morphine HCl			0.15	0.086[c]			0.14								
Morphine sulfate			0.14	0.079[c]			0.11	0.19	0.09	0.26					
Nalorphine HCl	0.24	0.070	0.21	0.121	0.18	0.210	0.17	0.288	0.15	0.434	6.36	0.14	0.52	63	4.1
Naloxone HCl	0.14	0.042	0.14	0.083	0.14	0.158	0.13	0.230	0.13	0.367	8.07	0.11	0.52	35	5.2
Naphazoline HCl			0.27	0.14[d]			0.24				3.99	0.22		100	5.3
Neoarsphenamine			0.11	0.063[c]			0.09	0.16	0.08	0.232	2.32		17		7.8
Neomycin sulfate			0.22	0.127[c]			0.19								
Neostigmine bromide			0.20	0.115[c]			0.18		0.17		4.98	0.17		0	4.6
Neostigmine methylsulfate			0.26	0.148[c]			0.21	0.36			5.22	0.17			
Nicotinamide			0.25	0.144[c]							4.49	0.20	0.52	100	7.0
Nicotinic acid				0.100[c]							5.94			100	6.9
Nikethamide	0.12	0.033	0.10	0.057	0.07	0.073									
Novobiocin sodium	0.08	0.017	0.08	0.038	0.08	0.084	0.08	0.129	0.08	0.255	10.82	0.08	0.52	0	5.0
Oleandomycin phosphate	0.13	0.037	0.13	0.074	0.13	0.144	0.12	0.204	0.10	0.285					
Orphenadrine citrate											.67			trace*	2.3
Oxophenarsine HCl	0.22	0.063	0.22	0.124	0.20	0.232	0.19	0.335			4.92	0.18	0.52	86	5.7
Oxymetazoline HCl	0.24	0.068	0.21	0.113	0.16	0.182	0.14	0.236	0.11	0.315					
Oxyquinoline sulfate	0.20	0.053	0.18	0.100	0.17	0.193	0.17	0.283	0.16	0.468	5.60	0.16	0.52	92	6.8
d-Pantothenyl alcohol			0.10	0.061[c]											
Papaverine HCl	0.25	0.071	0.25	0.142	0.25	0.288	0.25	0.430			3.65	0.25	0.52	97	5.3
Paraldehyde	0.30	0.083	0.29	0.165	0.29	0.327	0.28	0.491			3.18	0.28	0.52	91	3.8
Pargyline HCl															

Appendix A Continued

	0.5%		1%		2%		3%		5%		ISO-OSMOTIC CONCENTRATION[a]				
	E	D	E	D	E	D	E	D	E	D	%	E	D	H	pH
Penicillin G, potassium			0.18	0.102[c]			0.17	0.29	0.16	0.46	5.48	0.16	0.52	0	6.2
Penicillin G, procaine				0.06[d]											
Penicillin G, sodium			0.18	0.100[c]			0.16	0.28	0.16	0.46	5.90			18	5.2
Pentazocine lactate	0.15	0.042	0.15	0.085	0.15	0.169	0.15	0.253	0.15	0.420					
Pentobarbital sodium				0.145[c]							4.07			0	9.9
Pentolinium tartrate											5.95			55*	3.4
Phenacaine HCl				0.09[d]											
Pheniramine maleate				0.09[d]											
Phenobarbital sodium			0.24	0.135[c]			0.23	0.40			3.95	0.23	0.52	0	9.2
Phenol	0.35	0.20									2.8	0.32	0.52	0*	5.6
Phentolamine mesylate	0.18	0.052	0.17	0.096	0.16	0.173	0.14	0.244	0.13	0.364	8.23	0.11	0.52	83	3.5
Phenylephrine HCl			0.32	0.184[c]			0.30				3.0	0.30		0	4.5
Phenylephrine tartrate											5.90			58*	5.4
Phenylethyl alcohol	0.25	0.070	0.25	0.141	0.25	0.283									
Phenylpropanolamine HCl			0.38	0.219[c]							2.6	0.35		95	5.3
Physostigmine salicylate			0.16	0.090[c]											
Physostigmine sulfate				0.074[c]											
Pilocarpine HCl			0.24	0.138[c]			0.22	0.38			4.08	0.22	0.52	89	4.0
Pilocarpine nitrate			0.23	0.132[c]			0.20	0.35			4.84	0.20	0.52	88	3.9
Piperocaine HCl				0.12[d]							5.22			65	5.7
Polyethylene glycol 300	0.12	0.034	0.12	0.069	0.12	0.141	0.12	0.216	0.13	0.378	6.73	0.13	0.52	53	3.8
Polyethylene glycol 400	0.08	0.022	0.08	0.047	0.09	0.098	0.09	0.153	0.09	0.272	8.50	0.11	0.52	0	4.4
Polyethylene glycol 1500	0.06	0.015	0.06	0.036	0.07	0.078	0.07	0.120	0.07	0.215	10.00	0.09	0.52	4	4.1
Polyethylene glycol 1540	0.02	0.005	0.02	0.012	0.02	0.028	0.03	0.047	0.03	0.094					
Polyethylene glycol 4000	0.02	0.004	0.02	0.008	0.02	0.020	0.02	0.033	0.02	0.067					
Polymyxin B sulfate			0.09	0.052			0.06	0.10	0.04	0.12					
Polysorbate 80	0.02	0.005	0.02	0.010	0.02	0.020	0.02	0.032	0.02	0.055					
Polyvinyl alcohol (99% hydrol)	0.02	0.004	0.02	0.008	0.02	0.020	0.02	0.035	0.03	0.075					
Polyvinylpyrrolidone	0.01	0.003	0.01	0.006	0.01	0.010	0.01	0.017	0.01	0.035					
Potassium acetate	0.59	0.172	0.59	0.342							1.53	0.59	0.52	0	7.6
Potassium chlorate											1.88			0	6.9
Potassium chloride			0.76	0.439[c]							1.19	0.76	0.52	0	5.9
Potassium iodide			0.34	0.196[c]							2.59	0.34	0.52	0	7.0
Potassium nitrate			0.56	0.324[c]							1.62	0.56	0	5.9	
Potassium phosphate			0.46	0.27							2.08	0.43	0.52	0	8.4
Potassium phosphate, monobasic			0.44	0.25							2.18	0.41	0.52	0	4.4
Potassium sulfate			0.44								2.11	0.43	0	6.6	
Pralidoxime chloride	0.32	0.092	0.32	0.183	0.32	0.364					2.87	0.32	0.52	0	4.6
Prilocaine HCl	0.22	0.062	0.22	0.125	0.22	0.250	0.22	0.375			4.18	0.22	0.52	45	4.6
Procainamide HCl			0.22	0.13			0.19	0.33	0.17	0.49					
Procaine HCl			0.21	0.122[c]			0.19	0.33	0.18		5.05	0.18	0.52	91	5.6
Prochlorperazine edisylate	0.08	0.020	0.06	0.033	0.05	0.048	0.03	0.056	0.02	0.065					
Promazine HCl	0.18	0.050	0.13	0.077	0.09	0.102	0.07	0.112	0.05	0.137					
Proparacaine HCl	0.16	0.044	0.15	0.086	0.15	0.169	0.14	0.247	0.13	0.380	7.46	0.12	0.52		
Propiomazine HCl	0.18	0.050	0.15	0.084	0.12	0.133	0.10	0.165	0.08	0.215					
Propoxycaine HCl											6.40			16	5.3
Propylene glycol											2.00			100	5.5
Pyrathiazine HCl	0.22	0.065	0.17	0.095	0.11	0.123	0.08	0.140	0.06	0.170					
Pyridostigmine bromide	0.22	0.062	0.22	0.125	0.22	0.250	0.22	0.377			4.13	0.22	0.52	0	7.2
Pyridoxine HCl											3.05			31*	3.2
Quinacrine methanesulfonate				0.06[c]											
Quinine bisulfate			0.09	0.05			0.09	0.16							
Quinine dihydrochloride			0.23	0.130[c]			0.19	0.33	0.18		5.07	0.18	0.52	trace*	2.5
Quinine hydrochloride			0.14	0.077[c]			0.11	0.19							
Quinine and urea HCl			0.23	0.13			0.21	0.36			4.5	0.20	0.52	64	2.9
Resorcinol		0.161[c]									3.30			96	5.0
Rolitetracycline	0.11	0.032	0.11	0.064	0.10	0.113	0.09	0.158	0.07	0.204					
Rose Bengal	0.08	0.020	0.07	0.040	0.07	0.083	0.07	0.124	0.07	0.198	14.9	0.06	0.52		
Rose Bengal B	0.08	0.022	0.08	0.044	0.08	0.087	0.08	0.131	0.08	0.218					
Scopolamine HBr			0.12	0.07			0.12	0.21	0.12	0.35	7.85	0.11	0.52	8	4.8
Scopolamine methylnitrate			0.16				0.14		0.13	6.95	0.13	0	6.0		
Secobarbital sodium			0.24	0.14			0.23	0.40			3.9	0.23	0.52	trace	9.8
Silver nitrate			0.33	0.190[c]							2.74	0.33	0.52	0*	5.0
Silver protein, mild			0.17	0.10			0.17	0.29	0.16	0.46	5.51	0.16	0.52	0	9.0
Silver protein, strong				0.06[d]											
Sodium acetate			0.46	0.267							2.0	0.45	0.52		
Sodium acetazolamide	0.24	0.068	0.23	0.135	0.23	0.271	0.23	0.406			3.85	0.23	0.52		
Sodium aminosalicylate				0.170[c]							3.27			0	7.3
Sodium ampicillin	0.16	0.045	0.16	0.090	0.16	0.181	0.16	0.072	0.16	0.451	5.78	0.16	0.52	0	8.5
Sodium ascorbate											3.00			0	6.9
Sodium benzoate			0.40	0.230[c]							2.25	0.40	0.52	0	7.5
Sodium bicarbonate			0.65	0.375							1.39	0.65	0.52	0	8.3
Sodium biphosphate (H_2O)			0.40	0.23							2.45	0.37	0.52	0	4.1
Sodium biphosphate (2 H_2O)			0.36								2.77	0.32		0	4.0
Sodium bismuth thioglycollate	0.20	0.055	0.19	0.107	0.18	0.208	0.18	0.303	0.17	0.493	5.29			0	8.3
Sodium bisulfite			0.61	0.35							1.5	0.61	0.52	0*	3.0

Appendix A Continued

	0.5%		1%		2%		3%		5%		ISO-OSMOTIC CONCENTRATION[a]				
	E	D	E	D	E	D	E	D	E	D	%	E	D	H	pH
Sodium borate			0.42	0.241[c]							2.6	0.35	0.52	0	9.2
Sodium bromide											1.60			0	6.1
Sodium cacodylate			0.32				0.28				3.3	0.27		0	8.0
Sodium carbonate, monohydrated			0.60	0.346							1.56	0.58	0.52	100	11.1
Sodium cephalothin	0.18	0.050	0.17	0.095	0.16	0.179	0.15	0.259	0.14	0.400	6.80	0.13	0.52	partial	8.5
Sodium chloride			1.00	0.576[c]			1.00	1.73	1.00	2.88	0.9	1.00	0.52	0	6.7
Sodium citrate			0.31	0.178[c]			0.30	0.52			3.02	0.30		0	7.8
Sodium colistimethate	0.16	0.045	0.15	0.087	0.14	0.161	0.14	0.235	0.13	0.383	6.85	0.13	0.52	0	8.4
Sodium hypophosphite											1.60			0	7.3
Sodium iodide			0.39	0.222[c]							2.37	0.38	0.52	0	6.9
Sodium iodohippurate											5.92			0	7.3
Sodium lactate											1.72			0	6.5
Sodium lauryl sulfate	0.10	0.029	0.08	0.046	0.07	0.068	0.05	0.086							
Sodium mercaptomerin											5.30			0	8.4
Sodium metabisulfite			0.67	0.386[c]							1.38	0.65	0.52	5*	4.5
Sodium methicillin	0.18	0.050	0.18	0.099	0.17	0.192	0.16	0.281	0.15	0.445	6.00	0.15	0.52	0	5.8
Sodium nafcillin	0.14	0.039	0.14	0.078	0.14	0.158	0.13	0.219	0.10	0.285					
Sodium nitrate			0.68								1.36	0.66		0	6.0
Sodium nitrite			0.84	0.480[c]							1.08	0.83		0*	8.5
Sodium oxacillin	0.18	0.050	0.17	0.095	0.16	0.177	0.15	0.257	0.14	0.408	6.64	0.14	0.52	0	6.0
Sodium phenylbutazone	0.19	0.054	0.18	0.104	0.17	0.202	0.17	0.298	0.17	0.488	5.34	0.17	0.52		
Sodium phosphate			0.29	0.168			0.27	0.47			3.33	0.27	0.52	0	9.2
Sodium phosphate, dibasic (2 H$_2$O)			0.42	0.24							2.23	0.40	0.52	0	9.2
Sodium phosphate, dibasic (12 H$_2$O)			0.22				0.21				4.45	0.20		0	9.2
Sodium propionate			0.61	0.35							1.47	0.61	0.52	0	7.8
Sodium salicylate			0.36	0.210[c]							2.53	0.36	0.52	0	6.7
Sodium succinate	0.32	0.092	0.32	0.184	0.31	0.361					2.90	0.31	0.52	0	8.5
Sodium sulfate, anhydrous			0.58	0.34							1.61	0.56	0.52	0	6.2
Sodium sulfite, exsiccated			0.65	0.38							1.45			0	9.6
Sodium sulfobromophthalein	0.07	0.019	0.06	0.034	0.05	0.060	0.05	0.084	0.04	0.123					
Sodium tartrate	0.33	0.098	0.33	0.193	0.33	0.385					2.72	0.33	0.52	0	7.3
Sodium thiosulfate			0.31	0.181[c]							2.98	0.30	0.52	0	7.4
Sodium warfarin	0.18	0.049	0.17	0.095	0.16	0.181	0.15	0.264	0.15	0.430	6.10	0.15	0.52	0	8.1
Sorbitol (½ H$_2$O)											5.48			0	5.9
Sparteine sulfate	0.10	0.030	0.10	0.056	0.10	0.111	0.10	0.167	0.10	0.277	9.46	0.10	0.52	19*	3.5
Spectinomycin HCl	0.16	0.045	0.16	0.092	0.16	0.185	0.16	0.280	0.16	0.460	5.66	0.16	0.52	3	4.4
Streptomycin HCl			0.17	0.10[c]			0.16	0.16							
Streptomycin sulfate			0.07	0.036[c]			0.06	0.10	0.06	0.17					
Sucrose			0.08	0.047[c]			0.09	0.16	0.09	0.26	9.25	0.10	0.52	0	6.4
Sulfacetamide sodium			0.23	0.132[c]			0.23	0.40			3.85	0.23	0.52	0	8.7
Sulfadiazine sodium			0.24	0.14			0.24	0.38			4.24	0.21	0.52	0	9.5
Sulfamerazine sodium			0.23	0.13			0.21	0.36			4.53	0.20	0.52	0	9.8
Sulfapyridine sodium			0.23	0.13			0.21	0.36			4.55	0.20	0.52	5	10.4
Sulfathiazole sodium			0.22	0.13			0.20	0.35			4.82	0.19	0.52	0	9.9
Tartaric acid				0.143[c]							3.90			75*	1.7
Tetracaine HCl			0.18	0.109[c]			0.15	0.26	0.12	0.35					
Tetracycline HCl			0.14	0.081[c]	0.10										
Tetrahydrozoline HCl											4.10			60*	6.7
Theophylline				0.02[b]											
Theophylline sodium glycinate											2.94			0	8.9
Thiamine HCl				0.139[c]							4.24			87*	3.0
Thiethylperazine maleate	0.10	0.030	0.09	0.050	0.08	0.089	0.07	0.119	0.05	0.153					
Thiopental sodium				0.155[c]							3.50			74	10.3
Thiopropazate diHCl	0.20	0.053	0.16	0.090	0.12	0.137	0.10	0.170	0.08	0.222					
Thioridazine HCl	0.06	0.015	0.05	0.025	0.04	0.042	0.03	0.055	0.03	0.075					
Thiotepa	0.16	0.045	0.16	0.090	0.16	0.182	0.16	0.278	0.16	0.460	5.67	0.16	0.52	10*	8.2
Tridihexethyl chloride	0.16	0.047	0.16	0.096	0.16	0.191	0.16	0.280	0.16	0.463	5.62	0.16	0.52	97	5.4
Triethanolamine	0.20	0.058	0.21	0.121	0.22	0.252	0.22	0.383			4.05	0.22	0.52	100	10.7
Trifluoperazine 2HCl	0.18	0.052	0.18	0.100	0.13	0.144									
Triflupromazine HCl	0.10	0.031	0.09	0.051	0.05	0.061	0.04	0.073	0.03	0.092					
Trimeprazine tartrate	0.10	0.023	0.06	0.035	0.04	0.045	0.03	0.052	0.02	0.061					
Trimethadione	0.23	0.069	0.23	0.133	0.22	0.257	0.22	0.378			4.22	0.21	0.52	100	6.0
Trimethobenzamide HCl	0.12	0.033	0.10	0.062	0.10	0.108	0.09	0.153	0.08	0.232					
Tripelennamine HCl				0.13[d]							5.50			100	6.3
Tromethamine	0.26	0.074	0.26	0.150	0.26	0.300	0.26	0.450			3.45	0.26	0.52	0	10.2
Tropicamide	0.10	0.030	0.09	0.050											
Trypan blue	0.26	0.075	0.26	0.150											
...arsamide				0.11[c]											
...arine chloride				0.076[c]											
			0.59	0.34							1.63	0.55	0.52	100	6.6
				0.18[b]							2.93			100	6.3
	0.12	0.035	0.12	0.069	0.12	0.138	0.12	0.208	0.12	0.333	8.18	0.11	0.52	0*	6.1
	0.16	0.044	0.15	0.085	0.15	0.168	0.14	0.238	0.11	0.324					
	0.06	0.015	0.05	0.028	0.04	0.049	0.04	0.066	0.04	0.098					

Appendix A Continued

	0.5%		1%		2%		3%		5%		ISO-OSMOTIC CONCENTRATION[a]				
	E	D	E	D	E	D	E	D	E	D	%	E	D	H	pH
Viomycin sulfate			0.08	0.05			0.07	0.12	0.07	0.20					
Xylometazoline HCl	0.22	0.065	0.21	0.121	0.20	0.232	0.20	0.342			4.68	0.19	0.52	88	5.0
Zinc phenolsulfonate											5.40			0*	5.4
Zinc sulfate			0.15	0.086[c]			0.13	0.23	0.12	0.35	7.65	0.12	0.52		

[a] The unmarked values were taken from Hammarlund et al[19–22] and Sapp et al.[23]
[b] Adapted from Lund et al.[17]
[c] Adapted from *British Pharmaceutical Codex.*[24]
[d] Obtained from several sources.
[e] E, sodium chloride equivalents; D, freezing-point depression, °C; H, hemolysis, %, at the concentration that is iso-osmotic with 0.9% NaCl, based on freezing-point determination or equivalent test; pH, approximate pH of solution studied for hemolytic action; *, change in appearance of erythrocytes and/or solution[23–25]; †, pH determined after addition of blood.
Note: See also Budavari S, ed, *Merck Index,* 11th ed, Rahway, NJ: Merck, 1988: pp MISC 79–103.

Appendix B Isotonic Solution *V*—Values[26, a,b]

DRUG (0.3 g)	WATER NEEDED FOR ISOTONICITY (mL)	DRUG (0.3 g)	WATER NEEDED FOR ISOTONICITY (mL)	DRUG (0.3 g)	WATER NEEDED FOR ISOTONICITY (mL)
Alcohol	21.7	Epinephrine hydrochloride	9.7	Silver nitrate	11.0
Ammonium chloride	37.3	Ethylmorphine hydrochloride	5.3	Silver protein, mild	5.7
Amobarbital sodium	8.3	Fluorescein sodium	10.3	Sodium acetate	15.3
Amphetamine phosphate	11.3	Glycerin	11.7	Sodium bicarbonate	21.7
Amphetamine sulfate	7.3	Holocaine hydrochloride	6.7	Sodium biphosphate, anhydrous	15.3
Antipyrine	5.7	Homatropine hydrobromide	5.7		
Apomorphine hydrochloride	4.7	Homatropine methylbromide	6.3	Sodium biphosphate	13.3
Ascorbic acid	6.0	Hyoscyamine sulfate	4.7	Sodium bisulfite	20.3
Atropine methylbromide	4.7	Neomycin sulfate	3.7	Sodium borate	14.0
Atropine sulfate	4.3	Oxytetracycline hydrochloride	4.3	Sodium iodide	13.0
Bacitracin	1.7	Penicillin G, potassium	6.0	Sodium metabisulfite	22.3
Barbital sodium	10.0	Penicillin G, sodium	6.0	Sodium nitrate	22.7
Bismuth potassium tartrate	3.0	Pentobarbital sodium	8.3	Sodium phosphate	9.7
Boric acid	16.7	Phenobarbital sodium	8.0	Sodium propionate	20.3
Butacaine sulfate	6.7	Physostigmine salicylate	5.3	Sodium sulfite, exsiccated	21.7
Caffeine and sodium benzoate	8.7	Pilocarpine hydrochloride	8.0	Sodium thiosulfate	10.3
Calcium chloride	17.0	Pilocarpine nitrate	7.7	Streptomycin sulfate	2.3
Calcium chloride (6 H₂O)	11.7	Piperocaine hydrochloride	7.0	Sulfacetamide sodium	7.7
Chlorobutanol (hydrated)	8.0	Polymyxin B sulfate	3.0	Sulfadiazine sodium	8.0
Chlortetracycline sulfate	4.3	Potassium chloride	25.3	Sulfamerazine sodium	7.7
Cocaine hydrochloride	5.3	Potassium nitrate	18.7	Sulfapyridine sodium	7.7
Cupric sulfate	6.0	Potassium phosphate, monobasic	14.7	Sulfathiazole sodium	7.3
Dextrose, anhydrous	6.0			Tetracaine hydrochloride	6.0
Dibucaine hydrochloride	4.3	Procainamide hydrochloride	7.3	Tetracycline hydrochloride	4.7
Dihydrostreptomycin sulfate	2.0	Procaine hydrochloride	7.0	Viomycin sulfate	2.7
Ephedrine hydrochloride	10.0	Scopolamine hydrobromide	4.0	Zinc chloride	20.3
Ephedrine sulfate	7.7	Scopolamine methylnitrate	5.3	Zinc sulfate	5.0
Epinephrine bitartrate	6.0	Secobarbital sodium	8.0		

[a] This table of *Isotonic Solution Values* shows volumes in mL of water to be added to 300 mg of the specified drug in sterile water to produce an isotonic solution. The addition of an isotonic vehicle (commonly referred to as diluting solution) to make 30 mL yields a 1% solution. Solutions prepared as directed above are iso-osmotic with 0.9% sodium chloride solution but may not be isotonic with blood (see Appendix A for hemolysis data).
[b] The *V* values for drugs that do not appear in Appendix B but are listed in Appendix A can be calculated from the sodium chloride equivalent for 1% drug. *Example*—Calculate the *V* value for anileridine HCl (Appendix A defines *E* = 0.19).

$$\frac{100 \text{ mL Soln}}{0.9 \text{ NaCl}} \times \frac{0.19 \text{ g naCl}}{1 \text{ g drug}} \times 0.3 \text{ g drug} = 6.33 \text{ mL Soln}$$

for dilute solution

6.33 mL soln ≅ 6.33 mL water ∴ *V* = 6.33 mL water/0.3 g drug.

CHAPTER 19

Chemical Kinetics

Rodney J Wigent, PhD

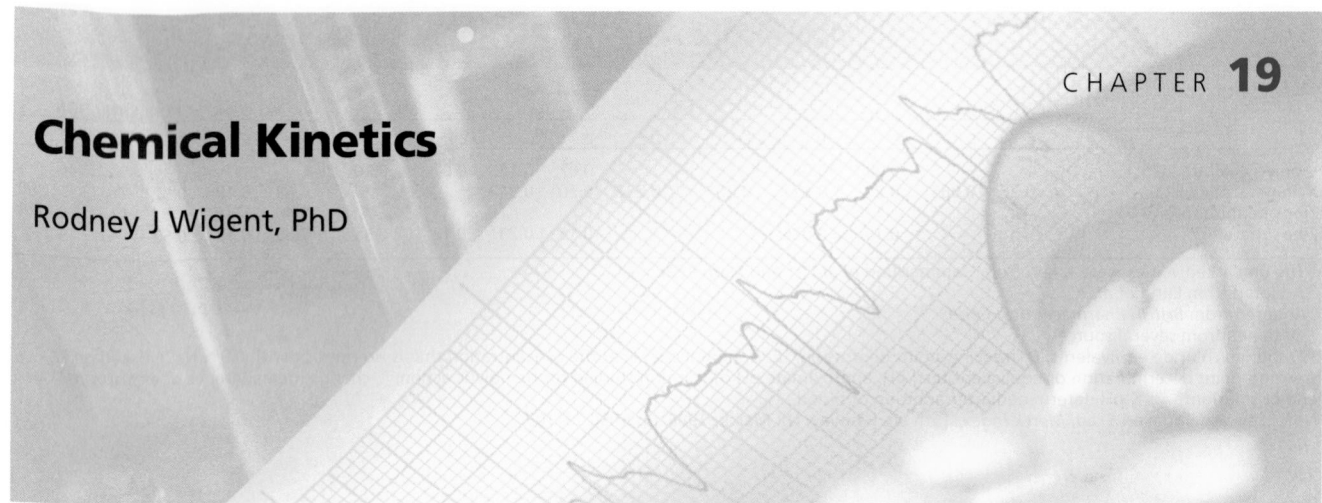

Thermodynamic parameters, such as ΔG, ΔE, ΔH, and ΔS, are state functions that only depend on the initial and final states of a chemical process—reactants and products—and are independent of the pathway taken to get to the final state from the initial state. *Chemical kinetics* is the discipline that is concerned with the mechanism by which a chemical process gets to its final state from its initial state and the rate in which this reaction proceeds. Therefore, chemical kinetics involves the study of rate of chemical change and the way in which this rate is influenced by the conditions of the concentration of reactants, products, and other chemical species that may be present, and by factors such as solvent, pressure, and temperature. From these studies, one or more mechanisms involving a series of elementary processes may be postulated to explain how the reactants are converted to products during a chemical process. Applied to pharmaceutics, such information permits a rational approach to the stabilization of drug products, and prediction of shelf life and optimum storage conditions.

This chapter is intended as a general introduction to this subject. A comprehensive review of experimental approaches and interpretation of data can be found in several texts, such as the books by House, Epenson and Houston, and the compilation of information relative to kinetic studies on pharmaceuticals by Garrett.[1]

REACTION RATE

The rate of a reaction is the velocity with which a reactant or reactants undergoes a chemical change. Experimentally, the rate of a reaction must be determined by directly or indirectly following the change in the concentration of the reactants or products as a function of time. When there is more than one reactant, such changes need to be normalized according to the stoichiometry of the reaction. For a reaction of the type

$$aA + bB + \ldots \rightarrow cC + dD + \ldots$$

where the uppercase letters represent chemical species and the lowercase letters represent stoichiometric coefficients, the rate in which reactants go to products can be determined by following the rate of the disappearance of the reactants as a function [of tim]e

$$\text{Rate} = -\frac{1}{a}\frac{d[A]}{dt} = -\frac{1}{b}\frac{d[B]}{dt} \qquad (1)$$

The brackets denote concentration (usually molar concentration unless otherwise indicated) and d represents the derivative function. The negative sign signifies that the concentration of the reactants is decreasing, as the rate must always be positive as long as the reaction is progressing from reactants to products.

The rate at which a reaction proceeds for the reaction type shown above also can be determined by following the appearance of the products as a function of time:

$$\text{Rate} = +\frac{1}{c}\frac{d[C]}{dt} = +\frac{1}{d}\frac{d[D]}{dt} \qquad (2)$$

where the positive signs indicate that the concentrations of the products are increasing. Note that these two expressions for rate are only for the type of reaction where the reactants go irreversibly to products, without going through any intermediates.

If $[A]_0$, $[B]_0$, $[C]_0$, and $[D]_0$ represent the initial concentration (ie, $t = 0$) of each of the reactants and products, at some time t (ie, $t = t$), the concentration of A decreases by aX (ie, $[A]_t = [A]_0 - aX$) and the concentration of B decreases by bX (ie, $[B]_t = [B]_0 - bX$).

Similarly, the concentrations of the products C and D increase by cX and dX, respectively (ie, $[C]_t = [C]_0 + cX$ and $[D]_t = [D]_0 + dX$). Thus, upon normalization, the rate expressed in Equations 1 and 2 reduces to Equation 3.

$$\text{Rate} = +\frac{dX}{dt} \qquad (3)$$

The *law of mass action* relates these experimentally determined rates to the concentration of all of the reacting species. This law states that, at a given temperature, the rate of the reaction is at each instant proportional to the product of the concentration of each of the reacting species raised to a power equal to the number of molecules of each species participating in the process. Accordingly, the law of mass action applied to the above reaction gives the following rate equation,

$$\text{Rate} = k[A]^n[B]^m \ldots \qquad (4)$$

where the proportionality constant k (referred to as the *specific rate constant* or as the *rate constant*) should be independent of the concentrations of all chemical species. The exponents n and m are known as the *order of the reaction* with respect to the components A and B, respectively; their sum represents the overall order of the reaction.

It is important to note that for a *net equation,* which is the sum of two or more elementary equations, there is no requirement that the order of the reaction with respect to a chemical species be identical to its stoichiometric coefficient in the net equation. Further, a proper rate equation should only consist of chemical species that are either reactants or products and should not contain any chemical species that are an intermediate during a chemical reaction.

It should be noted that unless the stoichiometric coefficient of the reactant or product that is being followed to determine the rate of the reaction is *unity* (one), the rate of the reaction is not equivalent to the change in the concentration of the chemical species with respect to time. For the case where there is only one chemical reactant, which has a stoichiometric coefficient that is greater than one, authors of articles and textbooks on kinetics often base the reaction rate only on the disappearance of the reactant without accounting for the stoichiometry. When this occurs, the resulting rate constant will be greater than the true rate constant by a factor equal to the stoichiometric coefficient. Thus, care must be taken to determine how the rates of reactions were determined when comparing rate constants of a reaction.

FIRST-ORDER REACTIONS

When the rate of a reaction is proportional to the first power of the concentration of a reactant, the rate equation is given by

$$\frac{dX}{dt} = k[A]_t = k([A]_0 - aX) \tag{5}$$

where a represents the stoichiometric coefficient for reactant A. For the case where $a = 1$, rearrangement of Equation 5 gives

$$\int \frac{dX}{([A]_0 - X)} = k \int dt \tag{6}$$

When Equation 6 is integrated over the limits of $t = 0$ (at which $X = 0$) to $t = t$ (at which $X = X$), the following first-order integrated rate equation is obtained:

$$[A]_t = [A]_0 e^{-kt} \tag{7}$$

Figure 19-1 shows a typical plot where reactant A exponentially decays to products according to Equation 7. The rate of the reaction—that is, the negative value of the tangent of this curve at any time—decreases with time as the concentration of the reactant decreases. Equation 7 can be linearized by rearrangement to give Equation 8.

$$\ln [A]_t = -kt + \ln [A]_0 \tag{8}$$

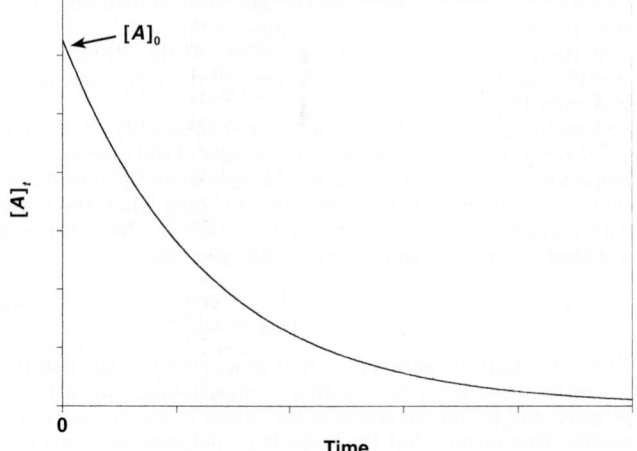

Figure 19-1. Plot of concentration of A versus time for a first-order reaction.

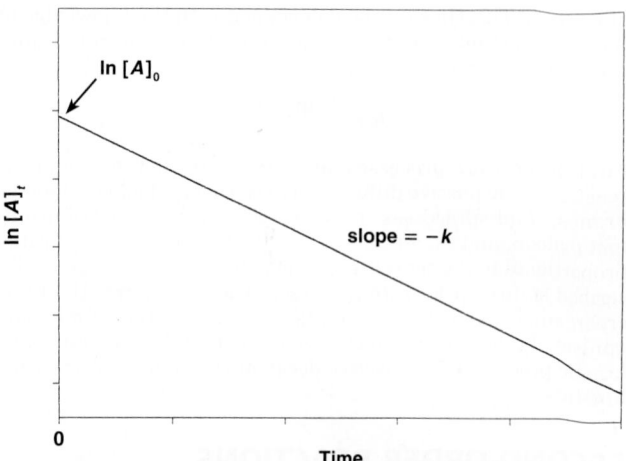

Figure 19-2. Plot of natural logarithm of the concentration of A versus time for a first-order reaction.

Equation 8 suggests that a plot of the natural logarithm of the concentration of the reactant as a function of time should give a linear plot with a slope equal to $-k$ and a y-intercept equal to the natural logarithm of the initial concentration of the reactant (Fig 19-2). Commonly a plot of the common logarithm of the concentration versus time is found in the literature for first-order reactions. In this case, according to Equation 9, the slope of this line would be equal to $-k/2.303$, and the y-intercept would be equal to the common logarithm of the initial concentration of the reactant.

$$\log [A]_t = -\frac{kt}{2.303} + \log [A]_0 \tag{9}$$

The rate constant, k, for a first-order reaction has a unit of reciprocal time (eg, s^1).

Sometimes it may be necessary to determine the rate constant k from only two concentrations of the reactant, $[A]_1$ and $[A]_2$, obtained at two different times, t_1 and t_2, in which case Equation 10 may be used.

$$k = \frac{1}{(t_2 - t_1)} \ln \frac{[A]_1}{[A]_2} \tag{10}$$

Another useful method for determining k is the fractional-life method, of which the half-life method is the most common. The *half-life method* involves measuring the time ($t = t_{1/2}$) that it takes for half of the initial concentration of the reactant to undergo reaction: $[A]_t = [A]_0/2$. Substituting these values into Equation 7 and rearranging to solve for k yields

$$k = \frac{\ln 2}{t_{1/2}} \tag{11}$$

It is apparent from Equation 11 that the half-life period for first-order reactions is constant and independent of the amount of reactant present. Thus, half of the initial concentration of the reactant undergoes reaction during the first half-life period, leaving 50% of the original concentration unreacted. During the second half-life period, which is identical to the time as the first half-life period for a first-order reaction, half of the remaining reactant reacts, leaving 25% of the initial concentration of the reactant unreacted. Similarly, after the third half-life period, 12.5% of the initial reactant would remain. After 10 first-order, half-life periods, only 0.098% of the original reactant remains unreacted. For precise studies, the rate of disappearance of a reactant should be followed over two or three half-life periods.

In some drug stability studies, it is necessary to determin the time that it takes for the loss of 10% of the drug, leav 90% of the original drug concentration; that is, $[A]_t = 0.9$

at $t = t_{0.90}$. This time can be determined with the knowledge of the rate constant by substituting these expressions into Equation 7 and rearranging to yield

$$t_{0.90} = \frac{\ln 0.90}{k} \qquad (12)$$

First-order rate processes are not restricted to chemical reactions. The passive diffusion of drugs across biological membranes, and processes of drug absorption, distribution, metabolism, and excretion often can be shown to occur at rates proportional to the concentration of a drug, and thus can be described as first-order rate processes. The rate of growth of microorganisms and the rate of killing or inactivation of microorganisms by heat or chemical agents usually follow first-order kinetic processes. Radioactive decay always follows first-order kinetics.

SECOND-ORDER REACTIONS

There are two forms of second-order reactions. For the first case, it is assumed that the rate of reaction is proportional to the concentration of reactant A raised to the power of 2—that is, the reaction is second order with respect to A, in which case the rate equation takes the form

$$\frac{dX}{dt} = [A]_t^2 = ([A]_0 - aX)^2 \qquad (13)$$

where a represents the stoichiometric coefficient of the reactant in the net equation. For the case where the stoichiometric coefficient of reactant A is 2, Equation 13 can be rearranged to give

$$\int \frac{dX}{([A]_0 - 2X)^2} = k \int dt \qquad (14)$$

When Equation 14 is integrated over the limits of $t = 0$ (at which $X = 0$) to $t = t$ (at which $X = X$), the following second-order integrated rate equation is obtained.

$$\frac{1}{[A]_t} = 2kt + \frac{1}{[A]_0} \qquad (15)$$

It should be noted that since the stoichiometry was taken into account in this derivation, the stoichiometric coefficient, 2, has been incorporated into Equation 15. If the rate of reaction was determined solely on the disappearance of reactant A without considering the stoichiometry, then the rate constant for this reaction would be twice as large as the true rate constant. This occurs quite frequently in the literature, so the reader should be aware of this situation.

The decomposition of hydrogen iodide is a second-order reaction; in the gaseous state, hydrogen iodide forms hydrogen gas and molecular iodine according to the reaction

$$2HI \rightarrow H_2 + I_2$$

The integrated rate expression for this reaction follows the form given by Equation 15.

Equation 15 suggests that, for a second-order reaction, if the reciprocal of the concentration of reactant A is plotted as a function of time, the slope of the line is equal to the rate constant k, and the y-intercept is the reciprocal of the initial concentration of A (Fig 19-3). Rearranging Equation 15 and solving for k yields

$$k = \frac{1}{t} \frac{[A]_0 - [A]_t}{[A]_0 [A]_t} \qquad (16)$$

The rate constant for second-order reactions has units of reciprocal concentration and seconds (eg, $M^{-1}s^{-1}$).

The second type of a second-order reaction occurs if the rate of reaction is proportional to the product of the concentration of both reactants, each raised to the power of 1, that is, first order with respect to both reactants. Equation 17 shows such a reaction.

$$= [A]_t[B]_t = ([A]_0 - aX)([B]_0 - bX) \qquad (17)$$

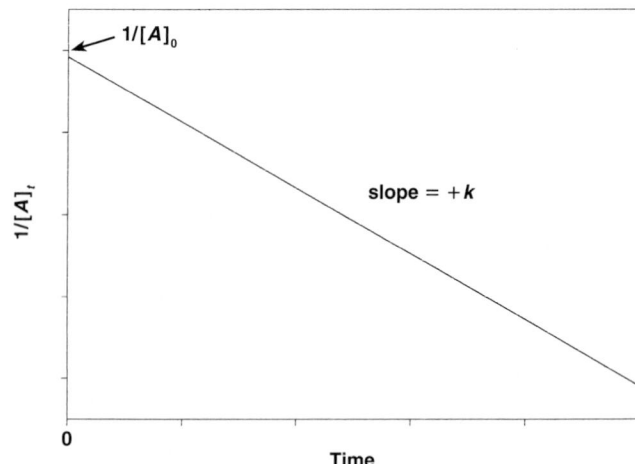

Figure 19-3. Plot of the reciprocal of the concentration of A versus time for a second-order reaction.

The stoichiometric coefficients of the reactants A and B are represented by a and b. For the case where a and b both equal 1, Equation 17 can be arranged to give the following:

$$\int \frac{dX}{([A]_0 - X)([B]_0 - X)} = k \int dt \qquad (18)$$

When Equation 18 is integrated over the limits of $t = 0$ (at which $X = 0$) to $t = t$ (at which $X = X$), the following second-order integrated rate equation is obtained:

$$\ln \frac{[A]_t}{[B]_t} = ([A]_0 - [B]_0)kt + \ln \frac{[A]_0}{[B]_0} \qquad (19)$$

This suggests that if the left side of Equation 19 is plotted against time, the slope of the line would be equal to $([A]_0 - [B]_0)k$ and the y-intercept is equal to the natural logarithm of the ratio of the initial concentrations of reactants A and B. Equation 19 does not apply if the initial concentration of the two reactants are equal; in this case, Equation 18 reduces to Equation 14 and the integrated rate equation for this system reduces to Equation 15.

An example of a second-order reaction in which two reactants are involved is the saponification of an ester, such as ethyl acetate, in alkaline solution:

$$CH_3COOC_2H_5 + OH^{-1} \rightarrow CH_3COO^{-1} + C_2H_5OH$$

The course of this reaction may be followed by determining, by titration at specified times, the concentration of hydroxide ions remaining unreacted during the course of the reaction. This information and the initial concentrations of the ethyl acetate and hydroxide can be used to determine the rate constant in Equation 19.

Fractional-life methods can be applied readily to second-order reactions for the case when the order of the reaction with respect to one reactant is 2, or for the case when the initial concentrations of each of two reactants are equal when the order with respect to each reactant is 1. For example, the half-life of a second-order reaction is given by Equation 20.

$$t_{1/2} = \frac{1}{k[A]_0} \qquad (20)$$

Unlike the half-life period for a first-order reaction, the half-life period for a second-order reaction is not constant, but rather is proportional to the reciprocal of the initial concentration of reactant. This means that the half-life period increases as a second-order reaction proceeds with time; thus, it takes twice as long to deplete a second-order reactant from 50 to 25% as it did to deplete the reactant from 100 to 50%.

THIRD-ORDER REACTIONS

Except for in the solution phase, third-order reactions are rare, as they require a simultaneous three-body collision of chemical species. There are a number of ways in which third-order reaction can occur—from a combination of three different chemical entities, for which the order of the reaction with respect to each of these is 1, to the simplest case in which three identical substances react, for which the order of the reaction with respect to that species is three. For the latter case, assuming the stoichiometric coefficient of the single reacting entity A is 3, then the rearranged rate equation is given by Equation 21.

$$\int \frac{dX}{([A]_0 - 3X)^2} = k \int dt \qquad (21)$$

Upon integration of Equation 21 over the limits of $t = 0$ (at which $X = 0$) to $t = t$ (at which $X = X$), the following third-order integrated rate equation is obtained.

$$\frac{1}{[A]_t^2} = 6kt + \frac{1}{[A]_0^2} \qquad (22)$$

Again, it should be noted, that if the stoichiometry was not taken into account and the *rate* was only determined by the rate of disappearance of reactant A, then Equation 22 would have 2 for the coefficient of kt instead of 6 and the value for the rate constant would be three times the value of the rate constant in Equation 22.

The equation for the half-life period for the case of Equation 22 is given by

$$t_{1/2} = \frac{1}{2k[A]_0^2} \qquad (23)$$

Another type of a third-order reaction occurs when the rate of the reaction is proportional to the product of the concentrations of two reactants, one raised to the power of 1 and the other raised to the power of 2; it is first order with respect to one reactant and second order with respect to the other reactant. Equation 24 shows the rate equation for such a reaction.

$$\frac{dX}{dt} = [A]_t^2 [B]_t = ([A]_0 - aX)^2([B]_0 - bX) \qquad (24)$$

If the stoichiometric coefficients, a and b, are both equal to 1, then Equation 24 can be rearranged and integrated over the limits of $t = 0$ (at which $X = 0$) to $t = t$ (at which $X = X$). The rate constant from this resulting equation is given by

$$k = \frac{1}{t} \frac{1}{[B]_0 - [A]_0} \frac{[A]_0 - [A]_t}{[A]_0 [A]_t} + \frac{1}{([B]_0 - [A]_0)^2} \ln \frac{[A]_t[B]_0}{[B]_t[A]_0} \qquad (25)$$

However, if the stoichiometric coefficients are $a = 2$ and $b = 1$, then when Equation 24 is rearranged and integrated over the limits of $t = 0$ (at which $X = 0$) to $t = t$ (at which $X = X$), the rate constant is determined by Equation 26.

$$k = \frac{1}{t} \frac{1}{2[B]_0 - [A]_0} \frac{[A]_0 - [A]_t}{[A]_0[A]_t} + \frac{1}{(2[B]_0 - [A]_0)^2} \ln \frac{[A]_t[B]_0}{[B]_t[A]_0} \qquad (26)$$

The rate constant for third-order reactions has units of reciprocal of the square of concentration per second (eg, $M^{-2}s^{-1}$).

Because of the rigors of the mathematics, when a third-order reaction is suspected, experimental conditions are often chosen so as to simplify the calculations. For example, for the third-order reaction in which the stoichiometric coefficients of the two reacting species are $a = 2$ and $b = 1$, such as that which led to the development of Equation 26, if the experimental conditions are set such that $[A]_0 = 2[B]_0$, it will lead to a much simpler integrated rate equation.

PSEUDO-ORDER REACTIONS

For some reactions, the rate of the reaction may be independent of the concentration of one or more of the reacting species over a wide range of concentrations. This may occur under these conditions:

1. One or more of the reactants enters into the rate equation in great excess compared to the others.
2. One of the reactants is a catalyst.
3. One or more of the reactants is constantly replenished during the course of a reaction.

If this happens, the constant concentration term(s) in the rate equation is combined with the rate constant to give an *apparent rate constant*. For example, if the concentration of A in Equation 4 remains constant, then Equation 4 can be rewritten as

$$\text{Rate} = (k[A]^n)[B]^m \ldots = k_{app}[B]^m \ldots \qquad (27)$$

where the apparent rate constant, k_{app} (sometimes referred to as the *pseudo-order rate constant*) now depends on the concentration of A raised to its power, n. Unfortunately, no information about n, the order of reaction with respect to A, can be determined from a single experiment. Rather, to gain an understanding of n, multiple experiments must be performed where the concentration of A is varied. A plot of the natural logarithm of k_{app} versus the natural logarithm of the concentration of A will give a slope that is equal to n.

In 1850, Wilhelmy performed the first quantitative kinetics study by following the rate of hydrolysis (inversion) of sucrose to glucose and fructose, according to the reaction

$$\underset{\text{sucrose}}{C_{12}H_{22}O_{11}} + \underset{\text{water}}{H_2O} \rightarrow \underset{\text{glucose}}{C_6H_{12}O_6} + \underset{\text{fructose}}{C_6H_{12}O_6}$$

Wilhelmy found that this reaction followed the rate equation

$$-\frac{d[C_{12}H_{22}O_{11}]}{dt} = k_{app}[C_{12}H_{22}O_{11}] \qquad (28)$$

which, upon rearrangement and integration, gives Equation 29.

$$\ln[C_{12}H_{22}O_{11}]_t = -k_{app}t + \ln[C_{12}H_{22}O_{11}]_0 \qquad (29)$$

This reaction is now known to be a second-order reaction, as it is first order with respect to both sucrose and water. As for most typical aqueous solutions, the molar concentration of water (approximately 55.5 mol of water per liter) greatly exceeds the concentration of the solute sucrose. Therefore, even at moderate concentrations of sucrose, there is only a minor change in the molar concentration of water and the concentration of the solvent is practically constant over the course of the reaction. This allows the concentration of water to be incorporated into the apparent rate constant and the reaction appears to be first order.

As another example, if component A reacts in aqueous solution to go to product B, according to the first-order rate equation given by Equation 5 and the stoichiometric coefficient a is 1 (unity), then the concentration of A as a function of time should follow the exponential form of the integrated rate equation given by Equation 7. However, if this reaction occurs in a saturated solution of A (ie, $[A]_{sat}$) in the presence of excess solid A, and if the rate of converting solid A to aqueous A is greater than the rate of reaction in solution, then the rate of disappearance of A is given by

$$\frac{dX}{dt} = k[A]_{sat} = k_{app} \qquad (30)$$

If Equation 30 is rearranged and integrated between the limits of $t = 0$ (at which $X = 0$) to $t = t$ (at which $X = X$) and defining $[B]_t = X$, the following zero-order rate equation is obtained,

$$[B]_t = k_{app}t \qquad (31)$$

which shows that as long as the solution remains saturated with A, the formation of B will occur at a constant rate. As a example, if a compound for which decomposition in solution first order is present in excess of its maximum solubility (a pension), the concentration of the reactant in solution will be invariant so long as there is excess solid reactant present. The kinetics of such a system would then follow Equation 30.

First- and second-order reactions are by far the most common types of rate processes encountered regarding drug stability. If a reaction is of higher order than first order, it often is convenient to adjust experimental conditions so that the concentrations of all but one of the reactants remain constant throughout the experiment. If, for example, the concentration of hydroxide ion in the saponification of an ester is in great excess of the concentration of ester, or if a buffer system is employed to control hydroxide-ion concentration, then the concentration of hydroxide ion essentially is invariant throughout the course of the experiment. The observed rate of the reaction, therefore, depends only on the changing concentration of the ester, and the reaction is said to be *pseudo first-order*. The apparent first-order rate constant, k_{app}, thus obtained is $k[OH^{-1}]$ and, of course, is different for each hydroxide-ion concentration. The actual rate constant, k, can be obtained easily by dividing the experimentally determined apparent first-order rate constant, $k[OH^{-1}]$, by the concentration of hydroxide ion maintained throughout the study.

In the study of complex reactions, it is often desirable to use this approach of maintaining the concentration of all but one of the reactants constant to facilitate determing the dependency of the reaction rate on each of the reactants in turn.

MORE COMPLEX REACTIONS

Many chemical reactions do not follow the simple reaction kinetics listed above, but rather they often consist of two or more elementary processes that may lead to more complicated rate equations. For example, comparison of experimental measurements of the rate of the disappearance of the reactants and the appearance of the products may indicate that the reactants must be forming one or more intermediates before proceeding to form the products. Often chemical reactions proceed reversibly to form products before an equilibrium is established. There are many cases were the reactants simultaneously proceed through different mechanisms to form two or more products. These situations can lead to negative or noninteger orders of reactions with respect to reactants and products within the rate equation. Quite often, a series of experiments must be performed in which certain conditions are controlled in order to establish the order of the reaction of individual species involved in the chemical reaction before an overall rate equation can be established. The next several sections will look as some of the more common complex reactions.

Reversible Reactions

Many reactions are known to be reversible where the reactants go to form products but the products will reversibly revert back to reactants. The simplest example of this is in the case where reactant A follows a first-order kinetic process with a forward rate constant, k_f, to produce product B.

$$k_f$$
$$A \rightarrow B$$

However, product B then follows a first-order rate process with a reverse rate constant, k_r, to reform reactant A.

$$k_r$$
$$B \rightarrow A$$

during the course of this reaction, reactant A is being 〔 〕ly depleted and formed, the rate at which reactant 〔 〕lated to the forward and reverse rates ac-〔 〕s 32 and 33:

$$\frac{d[A]}{dt} = \frac{d[A]_{forward}}{dt} - \frac{d[A]_{reverse}}{dt} \quad (32)$$

$$-\frac{d[A]_t}{dt} = k_f[A]_t - k_r[B]_t \quad (33)$$

If the initial concentration of B is zero, then at time $t = 0$ (initially) the rate equation is given solely by the forward rate equation. As the reaction proceeds, the reverse rate equation begins to contribute more and more substantially to the overall rate equation. Finally, a point will be reached at which the rate of the forward reaction is equal to the rate of reverse reaction and the overall rate is equal to 0. This is defined as a *dynamic equilibrium* and the concentration equilibrium constant, K_c, given by Equation 34, is equal to the ratio of the forward and reverse rate constants, where

$$K_c = \frac{[B]_{eq}}{[A]_{eq}} = \frac{k_f}{k_r} \quad (34)$$

$[B]_{eq}$ and $[A]_{eq}$ are the equilibrium concentrations of the product and reactant, respectively.

The rate equation expressed in Equation 33 can be rewritten to give

$$\frac{dX}{dt} = k_f([A]_0 - X) - k_r X \quad (35)$$

Rearrangement and integration of Equation 35 between the limits of $t = 0$ (at which $X = 0$) to $t = t$ (at which $X = X$) and defining $[B]_t = X$, the following expression for the concentration of A as a function of time is obtained:

$$[A]_t = \frac{k_f[A]_0 \exp[-(k_f + k_f)t] + k_r[A]_0}{(k_f + k_r)} \quad (36)$$

Simultaneous Reactions

Another very common reaction is when the reaction of one or more reactants lead to the formation of multiple products through different mechanistic pathways, each with characteristic rates:

$$k_1$$
$$A \rightarrow B$$

and

$$k_2$$
$$A \rightarrow C$$

For the case in which both reaction pathways are first order, then the rate of disappearance of reactant A is then given by Equation 37.

$$-\frac{d[A]_t}{dt} = k_1[A]_t + k_2[A]_t = (k_1 + k_2)[A]_t \quad (37)$$

Rearrangement and integration of Equation 37 gives

$$[A]_t = [A]_0 \exp[-(k_1 + k_2)t] \quad (38)$$

Since the rate of formation of product B is given by

$$\frac{d[B]}{dt} = k_1[A]_t \quad (39)$$

then, assuming that the initial concentration of B is 0, rearranging and integrating, and substituting Equation 38 into Equation 39 yields the following expression for the concentration of B as a function of time:

$$[B]_t = \frac{k_1[A]_0}{k_1 + k_2}(1 - \exp[-(k_1 + k_2)t]) \quad (40)$$

Using similar arguments, the concentration of C as a function of time is given by Equation 41.

$$[C]_t = \frac{k_2[A]_0}{k_1 + k_2}(1 - \exp[-(k_1 + k_2)t]) \quad (41)$$

It is of particular interest to note that if Equation 40 is divided by Equation 41, the ratio of the concentration of the products at any time is given by the ratio of the rate constants.

$$\frac{[B]_t}{[C]_t} = \frac{k_1}{k_2} \tag{42}$$

An example of this type of simultaneous reaction is the reaction of phenol with nitric acid to form both ortho- and para-nitrophenol through two simultaneous first-order reaction pathways. The relative concentrations of these two products is found to be given by Equation 42.

It is clear that if a kinetic experiment was performed without any a priori knowledge that the reaction is a simultaneous reaction, there is a danger that only the disappearance of a reactant or the appearance of only one of the products may lead to a faulty conclusion of the reaction mechanism. Care must be taken to attempt to identify and account for all of the chemical species in a chemical reaction to ensure that a proper rate mechanism is obtained.

Consecutive Reactions

One of the more common complex reactions is when a reactant decays through a series of consecutive reactions, forming one or more intermediates before forming a product. A simple case of a consecutive reaction is when reactant A proceeds through a first-order process to intermediate B which then decays to product C through another first-order process.

$$k_1 \quad k_2$$
$$A \rightarrow B \rightarrow C$$

For cases such as this, it is often convenient to consider the situation in which the initial concentrations of B and C are 0 and the sum of the concentrations of A, B, and C at any time is equal to the initial concentration of the reactant A. In this case, the rate of disappearance of A is given by Equation 43 and the rate of appearance of product C is given by Equation 44.

$$-\frac{d[A]_t}{dt} = k_1[A]_t \tag{43}$$

$$\frac{d[C]_t}{dt} = k_2[B]_t \tag{44}$$

The derivative of the concentration of the intermediate B with respect to time consists of the rate of formation of B from the product A and the disappearance of B as it proceeds to product C, as shown by

$$\frac{d[B]_t}{dt} = k_1[A]_t - k_2[B]_t \tag{45}$$

Upon integration and rearrangement of Equation 43, the concentration of reactant A as a function of time can be expressed by

$$[A]_t = [A]_0 \exp(-k_1 t) \tag{46}$$

It should be noted that Equations 44 and 45 are not considered to be valid rate equations because, by convention, the concentration of an intermediate may not appear in a final rate equation. Therefore, an expression for the concentration of B as a function of time in terms of only the reactant or product must be developed. Substituting Equation 46 into Equation 45 and rearranging and integrating yields the following expression for the concentration of B as a function of time.

$$[B]_t = \frac{k_1[A]_0}{k_2 - k_1} (\exp[-k_1 t] - \exp[-k_2 t]) \tag{47}$$

Equation 47 can be substituted into Equations 44 and 45 to give appropriate rate expressions. Then Equation 45 can be rear-

ranged and integrated to give an expression for the concentration of C as a function of time.

$$[C]_t = \frac{[A]_0}{k_2 - k_1} (k_2 - k_2 \exp[-k_1 t]) - (k_1 - k_1 \exp[-k_2 t]) \tag{48}$$

EFFECTS ON REACTION RATE

Temperature

The application of heat to increase the rate of a chemical reaction is a common laboratory procedure. The rate of most solvolytic reactions of pharmaceuticals is increased roughly 2- to 3-fold by a 10° increase near room temperature. In 1889 Arrhenius noted that the variation with temperature of the rate constant of chemical reactions could be expressed by

$$k = A \exp[-E_a/RT] \tag{49}$$

where, according to collision theory, E_a is the Arrhenius activation energy (ie, the difference between the average energy of reactive molecules and the minimum energy required for reactants to proceed to products); $\exp[-E_a/RT]$ is the Boltzmann factor, which represents the fraction of molecules having energies greater than or equal to E_a; the pre-exponential term A is a constant called the frequency factor; R is the gas constant (8.314 joule/mol-K or 1.987 cal/mol-K); and T is the absolute temperature. The Arrhenius equation can be expressed in a linear form according to Equation 50.

$$\ln k = \frac{E_a}{R}\frac{1}{T} + \ln A \tag{50}$$

Equations 49 and 50 are valid so long as the reaction mechanism does not change over the temperature range studied; a plot of the natural logarithm of the rate constant versus the reciprocal of the absolute temperature in which the rate constants are determined gives a negative slope that is equivalent to $-E_a/R$ (Fig 19-4). If a nonlinear plot is obtained, a thermally induced change in the reaction mechanism probably has occurred.

Differentiation of Equation 50 with respect to temperature, and then integrating between the limits of k_2 and k_1 at temperatures between T_2 and T_1 yields

$$\ln \frac{k_2}{k_1} = \frac{E_a}{R}\frac{T_2 - T_1}{T_2 T_1} \tag{51}$$

This equation allows E_a to be calculated for a reaction when the rate constants are known at two temperatures, or the rate con-

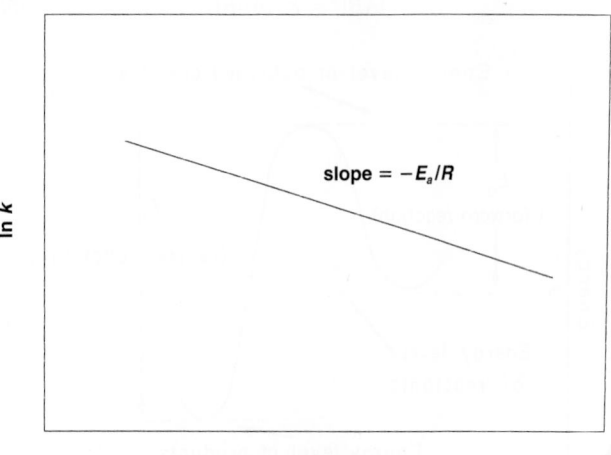

Figure 19-4. Variation of the rate constant with reciprocal absolute temperature, illustrating the Arrhenius equation.

stant at one temperature to be calculated if E_a and the rate constant at another temperature are known.

Most solvolytic reactions of pharmaceuticals exhibit activation energies in the range of 8 to 20 kcal/mol. Using Equation 50 and the appropriate activation energy, one readily can calculate that a reaction having an activation energy of 8 kcal/mol would show an approximately 1.5-fold increase in k for a temperature increase from 25° to 35°; a reaction having an activation energy of 20 kcal/mol would show a 3-fold increase in k for a similar temperature increase.

When two molecules undergo chemical interaction, it is reasonable to suppose that they first must collide and then, if conditions are right, undergo a rearrangement of certain electrons to form the bonds characteristic of the new molecules. However, not all collisions can cause a chemical change, or else chemical reactions would occur with great rapidity because collision frequencies are very high. While molecules or atoms must first collide if a reaction is to occur, the colliding molecules may not have an energy greater than or equal to the activation energy sufficient to overcome the mutual repulsion of the interacting molecules and enable them to approach close enough to each other to effect certain bond ruptures and/or establish new bonds characteristic of the products. The greater this energy requirement, the smaller the proportion of colliding molecules that will have the necessary energy, and the slower the reaction. In the Arrhenius equation, A is a factor related to frequency of collisions, and $\exp[-E_a/RT]$ is the probability that at temperature T a collision will occur with sufficient energy to provide a successful collision. The concept of energy of activation, in relationship to the energy of the reactants and of the products, is illustrated in Figure 19-5.

Eyring, in his transition state theory, proposed that reactants must proceed through an activated complex before proceeding to reactants. This is demonstrated by the reaction

$$K^* \qquad k'$$
$$\text{A+B} \Leftrightarrow [AB]^* \to \text{products}$$

where the reactants are considered to be in a rapid equilibrium with the activated complex or transition state, represented by $[AB]^*$, which then decays to products by a first-order process, according to the rate equation

$$\text{Rate} = k'[AB]^* \qquad (52)$$

However, as Equation 52 contains the concentration of the activated complex, an intermediate, it is not a valid rate equation and an expression in terms which include only the reactants or products must be substituted for this expression. Because the activated complex is in equilibrium with the reactants, the concentration of the activated complex can be given by

$$[AB]^* = K^*[A][B] \qquad (53)$$

where K^* is the equilibrium constant. Substituting Equation 53 into Equation 52 yields

$$\text{Rate} = K^*k'[A][B] = k[A][B] \qquad (54)$$

where k is equal to K^*k' and Equation 54 is a proper rate equation. Eyring was able to show that the rate constant, k', of any reaction is given by the expression

$$k' = \frac{RT}{N_a h} K^* \qquad (55)$$

where R is equal to 8.314 ergs/mol-K, N_a is Avogadro's number, and h is Planck's constant, which is equal to 6.625×10^{-27} erg-sec. K^* can be related to the thermodynamic parameters ΔG^*, ΔH^*, and ΔS^* through the equation

$$K^* = e^{-\Delta G^*/RT} = e^{(T\Delta S^* - \Delta H^*)/RT} \qquad (56)$$

If Equation 56 is substituted into Equation 55, after it has been divided by the absolute temperature, the following linear equation is obtained.

$$\ln \frac{k'}{T} = \ln \frac{R}{N_a h} + \frac{\Delta S^*}{R} - \frac{\Delta H^*}{R}\frac{1}{T} \qquad (57)$$

Thus, the thermodynamics of the formation of the activated complex can be determined from a plot of the natural logarithm of the ratio of the rate constant to absolute temperature versus the reciprocal absolute temperature.

CATALYSIS

In catalytic reactions, a molecule, called a catalyst, interacts with a reactant in a series of elementary processes in such a fashion as to lower the activation energy barrier (ie, E_a in Fig 19-5) of an uncatalyzed reaction. This change in mechanism causes the catalyzed reaction to run faster without changing the relative energy levels of either the reactants or products. During a catalytic reaction, the catalyst reacts with a reactant to form an intermediate that undergoes additional reaction(s) to form the product and the original catalytic molecule. Thus, while the catalyst is both consumed and produced in several elementary processes, there is no net change in the concentration of the catalyst during a catalyzed reaction but there is usually a substantial change in the rate in which the reaction occurs.

While there are several types of catalysis, such as homogeneous and heterogeneous catalysis, autocatalysis, etc., only a few general examples will be discussed here. Additional information about catalysis can be found in some of the references cited in the attached bibliography.

Specific Acid and Specific Base Catalysis

The terms *specific acid catalysis* and *specific base catalysis* refer to catalysis by the hydronium or hydrogen ion, and by the hydroxide ion, respectively. For example, if the rate of hydrolysis of an ester, such as ethyl acetate, is studied at a constant pH in a strongly buffered solution, the rate of disappearance of intact ester will be an apparent first-order reaction. If the reaction is studied in solutions buffered at several different pH values in a sufficiently acid pH region, a different apparent first-order rate constant will be observed for each pH value. The observed rate actually depends on the concentration of both the ester and hydrogen ion and, therefore, is a second-order reaction that appears to be a pseudo first-order reaction at the constant hydrogen-ion concentration in the buffer. Therefore, the observed first-order rate constant, k_{obs}, is proportional to the hydrogen ion concentration of the buffer system as shown by Equation 58.

$$k_{obs} = k_{acid}[H^+] \qquad (58)$$

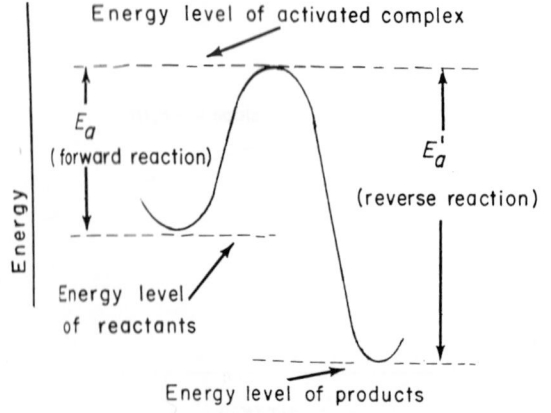

Energy level of activated complex

E_a (forward reaction)

E_a' (reverse reaction)

Energy level of reactants

Energy level of products

...on between activation energy and energy levels of re- and activated complex.

Taking the logarithm of Equation 58 yields

$$\log k_{\mathrm{obs}} = \log k_{\mathrm{acid}} + \log[\mathrm{H}^+] \qquad (59)$$

which upon applying the definition of pH yields

$$\log k_{\mathrm{obs}} = \log k_{\mathrm{acid}} - \mathrm{pH} \qquad (60)$$

Equation 60 suggests that a plot of $\log k_{\mathrm{obs}}$ versus pH will be linear with a slope of -1 and a y-intercept of $\log k_{\mathrm{acid}}$.

Similarly, if the same hydrolysis reaction is studied in buffered solutions at several pH values in a sufficiently alkaline region of the pH scale, the observed apparent first-order rate constants will be found to vary with hydroxide-ion concentration:

$$k_{\mathrm{obs}} = k_{\mathrm{base}}\,[\mathrm{OH}^-] \qquad (61)$$

and

$$\log k_{\mathrm{obs}} = \log k_{\mathrm{base}} + \log\,[\mathrm{OH}^-] \qquad (62)$$

However, the hydroxide ion concentration is related to the hydrogen ion concentration through the ionization constant of water, K_w, and Equation 60 becomes

$$\log k_{\mathrm{obs}} = \log k_{\mathrm{base}} + \log K_w + \mathrm{pH} \qquad (63)$$

Therefore, a plot of $\log k_{\mathrm{obs}}$ versus pH in a heavily buffered alkaline solution would yield a straight line with a slope of $+1$ and a y-intercept equal to $\log k_{\mathrm{base}} + \log K_w$.

Because of the equilibrium that exists between hydroxide and hydronium ions in aqueous solutions, each of these ions exists at all values of pH and the observed rate constant is actually given by the sum of Equations 58 and 61.

$$k_{\mathrm{obs}} = k_{\mathrm{acid}}\,[\mathrm{H}^+] + k_{\mathrm{base}}\,[\mathrm{OH}^-] \qquad (64)$$

The complete logarithm k_{obs} versus pH profile would be similar to that illustrated in Figure 19-6 for the hydrogen ion and hydroxide ion (specific acid and specific base) catalyzed hydrolysis of the ester atropine.[2] At relatively low values of pH the acid-catalyzed hydrolysis predominates; at relatively high values of pH the base-catalyzed hydrolysis predominates. The pH at which the minimum rate of hydrolysis is observed is a function of the relative magnitude of the specific rate constants k_{acid} and k_{base}. In the atropine example, the minimum rate of hydrolysis is at pH of 3.7, which indi-

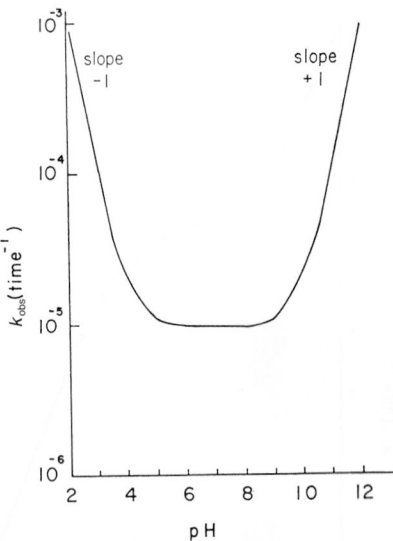

Figure 19-7. Apparent first-order rate of decomposition as a function of pH for a hypothetical case where $k_{\mathrm{H}^+} = k_{\mathrm{OH}^-} = 0.1$, $k_{\mathrm{H_2O}} = 1 \times 10^{-5}$. The uncatalyzed reaction predominates in the pH region 5 to 9.

cates that $k_{\mathrm{base}} > k_{\mathrm{acid}}$. If k_{base} equals k_{acid}, then, at 25°, the expected minimum rate of the reaction would be expected to occur at pH 7.

A reaction may be catalyzed not only by hydrogen ion and hydroxide ion, but also by other Brönsted acids or bases such as the solvent water. This is referred to as general acid/base catalysis. In this case, the observed rate constant is given by

$$k_{\mathrm{obs}} = k_{\mathrm{water}} + k_{\mathrm{acid}}\,[\mathrm{H}^+] + k_{\mathrm{base}}\,[\mathrm{OH}^-] \qquad (65)$$

where k_{water} is a pseudo-order rate constant that has the concentration of water, which is in large excess, incorporated into it. Figure 19-7 shows how a plot of the logarithm k_{obs} versus pH might appear in such a case. The flat region, where the rate of reaction apparently is not pH dependent, is the region where the solvent is much more important as a catalyst than either the hydrogen or hydroxide ions.

For compounds that are weak acids or weak bases, which can therefore exist in both ionized and nonionized species, the pH rate profiles become even more complex. Often, both the ionized and nonionized species are subject to decomposition and catalysis by hydrogen and hydroxide ion; but each of these species may react at a different rates. For example, the hydrolysis of the weakly basic drug procaine can be represented by[1]

$$-d[Pr]_{\mathrm{total}}/dt = k_1[OH^-][Pr] + k_2[OH^-][PrH^+] \qquad (66)$$

where Pr is the nonionized procaine molecule and PrH^+ is the protonated form. The concentration of each species can be related to the total procaine concentration by the relationships

$$[Pr] = \frac{[OH^-]}{K_b + [OH^-]} \cdot [Pr]_{total} \qquad (67)$$

and

$$[PrH^+] = \frac{K_b}{K_b + [OH^-]} \cdot [Pr]_{total} \qquad (68)$$

where K_b is the classical dissociation constant for the weak base procaine. The complete rate expression for procaine hydrolysis is given by Equation 69.

$$-\frac{d[Pr]_{total}}{dt} = \left[\frac{k_1[OH^-]^2}{K_b + [OH^-]} + \frac{k_2[OH^-]K_b}{K_b + [OH^-]} \right][Pr]_{total} \qquad (69)$$

The pH dependency of procaine hydrolysis is illustrated graphically in Figure 19-8[3] by a plot of logarithm k_{obs} versus pOH the pH region 7 to 13.

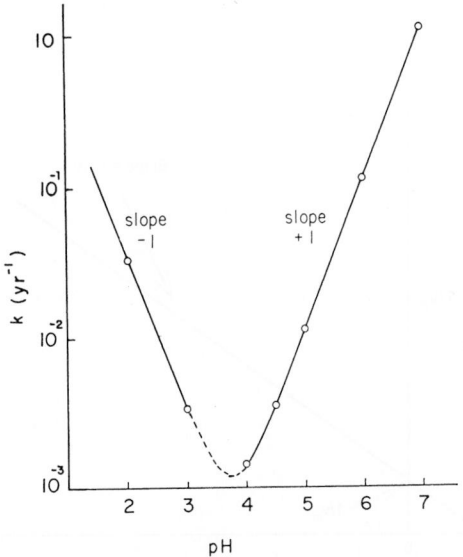

Figure 19-6. Apparent first-order rate of hydrolysis of atropine as a function of pH at 30°. The reaction is an illustration of specific hydrogen and hydroxide-ion catalysis. (From Kondritzer AA, Zvirblis P. *J APhA Sci Ed* 1957; 46: 531.)

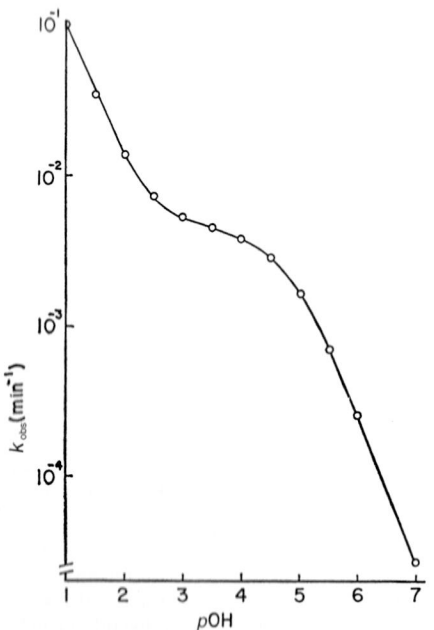

Figure 19-8. Apparent first-order rate of hydrolysis of procaine as a function of hydroxide-ion concentration at 40°. (From Higuchi T, Lachman L. *J APhA Sci Ed* 1955; 44: 52.)

General Acid or Base Catalysis

Acid or base catalysis is not restricted to the effect of hydrogen or hydroxide ion. Undissociated acids and bases often can be demonstrated to produce a catalytic effect, and in some instances metal ions and various anions can serve as catalysts. Mutarotation of glucose in acetate buffer is catalyzed by hydrogen ion, hydroxide ion, acetate ion, and undissociated acetic acid. Also, the rate of barbiturate hydrolysis in ammonia buffers is increased by increasing buffer concentration at constant pH as a result of catalysis by NH_3. Hydrolysis of the amide function of chloramphenicol exhibits, in addition to solvent and specific acid–base catalysis, general acid–base catalysis in phosphate and citrate buffers. General acid–base catalysis is to be anticipated if there is evidence of a significant solvent catalysis, as illustrated in the pH-rate profile of Figure 19-7.

Enzyme Catalysis

In biological systems, catalytic molecules, called enzymes (E), reversibly bind to a substrate (S) to form an intermediate (X) which then decomposes to give a product (P) and the original enzyme.

$$E + S \underset{k_r}{\overset{k_f}{\Longleftrightarrow}} X$$

and

$$X \overset{k_2}{\rightarrow} P + E$$

The rate of this reaction, v, will be given by $d[P]/dt = k_2[X]$. However, this is an improper rate equation as X is an intermediate. Michaelis and Menten used a steady state approximation (that sometime during the reaction the time rate of intermediate will be zero) to calculate the con-

$$[X] = \frac{k_f[E]_0[S]_0}{k_f[S]_0 + k_r + k_2} \tag{70}$$

Upon substitution of Equation 70 into the rate equation, the initial rate, v_0, (ie, The rate at time equal to zero) is given by Equation 71.

$$v_0 = \frac{k_f k_2 [E]_0}{k_f + \dfrac{k_r + k_2}{[S]_0}} = \frac{v_m}{1 + \dfrac{K_m}{[S]_0}} \tag{71}$$

where K_m, the Michaelis-Menten constant, is equal to $(k_r+k_2)/k_1$ and v_m, the maximum initial velocity of the reaction, is equal to $k_2 [E]_0$. The rate constant k_2 is often referred to as the turnover number which represents the number of molecules of product P created per second per mole of enzyme.

Equation 70 does not lend it self well to analysis as plots of v_0 vs. $[S]_0$ only asymptotically approachs the maximum velocity, $[S]_0$. Rearrangement of Equation 71 into Equation 72, known as the Lineweaver-Burk Equation, lends itself more readily to analysis as shown in Figure 19-9.

$$\frac{1}{v_0} = \frac{1}{v_m} + \frac{K_m}{v_m[S]_0} \tag{72}$$

An important area of study in enzyme kinetics is enzyme inhibition. There are two basic mechanisms in which an inhibitor, I, can inhibit and enzyme-catalyzed reaction. Competitive inhibition occurs when the inhibitor competes with the substrate, S, for the active binding site on the enzyme and blocks the catalytic action of the enzyme. In such a case, the formation of the enzyme-inhibitor complex is assumed to be in rapid equilibrium with the enzyme and inhibitor.

$$E + I \Leftrightarrow EI$$

Equation 73 shows the resulting Lineweaver-Burk Equation for the case of a competitive inhibitor.

$$\frac{1}{v_0} = \frac{1}{v_m} + \left[1 + \frac{[I]}{K_I}\right] \frac{K_m}{v_m[S]_0} \tag{73}$$

K_I is the dissociation constant for the enzyme-inhibitor complex, $[E][I]/[EI]$. Figure 19-10 shows a typical Lineweaver-Burk graph for competitive inhibition. Each plot represents a different concentration of the competitive inhibitor. Note that all three plots intersect at the same point on the y-axis indicating that the reactions all have the same maximum velocity. However, since they do not intersect at the same point on the x-axis then they have different Michaelis-Menten constants, K_m.

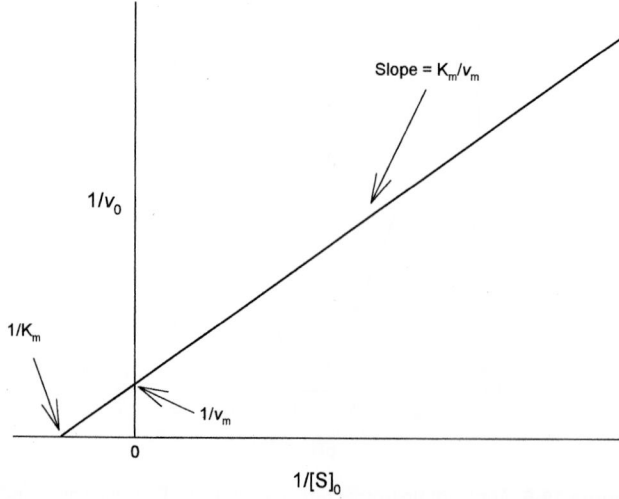

Figure 19-9. Lineweaver-Burk plot of modified Michaelis-Menten equation (Equation 72).

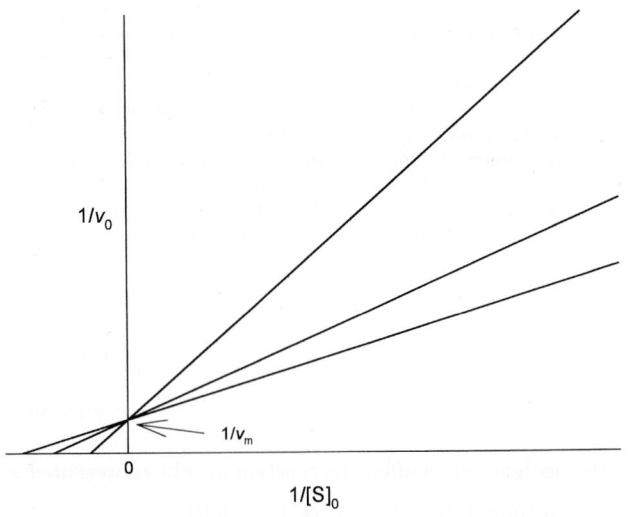

Figure 19-10. Lineweaver-Burk plot for competitive enzyme inhibition (Equation 73).

The other type of enzyme inhibition is noncompetitive inhibition. In this case the inhibitor does not bind to the active site of the enzyme but rather binds to another part of the enzyme or to the enzyme-substrate complex, X.

$$E + I \Leftrightarrow EI$$

and

$$X + I \Leftrightarrow XI$$

In this case, the equilibrium constant, K_I, is given by both [E][I]/[EI] and [X][I]/[XI]. The resulting Lineweaver-Burk equation is given by Equation 74.

$$\frac{1}{v_0} = \left[\frac{1}{v_m} + \frac{K_m}{v_m[S]_0}\right]\left[1 + \frac{[I]}{K_I}\right] \qquad (74)$$

Figure 19-11 shows a typical Lineweaver-Burk graph for noncompetitive inhibition. Each plot represents a different concentration of the competitive inhibitor. Note that all three plots intersect at the same point on the x-axis indicating that the reactions all have the same Michaelis-Menten constant, K_m.

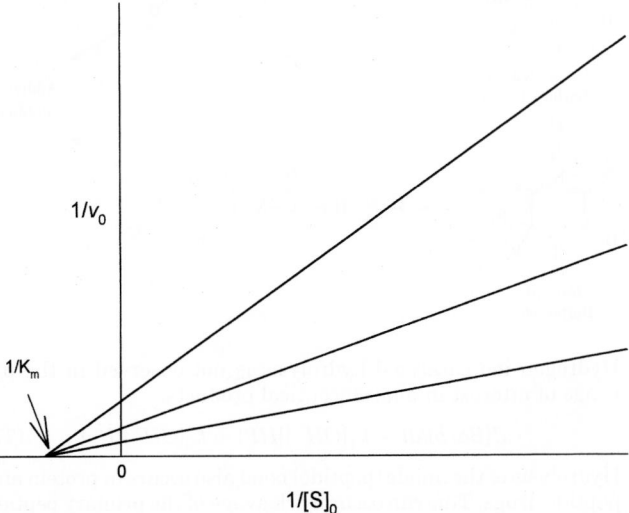

Figure 19-11. Lineweaver-Burk plot for noncompetitive enzyme inhibition (Equation 74).

However, since the plots do not intersect at the same point on the y-axis, then the reactions have different maximum velocities.

OTHER EFFECTS

Ionic Strength

In general, the effects of increasing concentrations of electrolytes on reaction rate can be predicted by consideration of the influence of ionic strength on interionic attraction. The Debye–Hückel equation may be used to demonstrate that increased ionic strength would be expected to decrease the rate of reaction between oppositely charged ions, and increase the rate of reaction between similarly charged ions. Thus, the hydrogen ion catalyzed hydrolysis of sulfate esters is inhibited by increasing electrolyte concentration.

$$\overset{H^+}{ROSO_3^- + H_2O \rightarrow ROH + HSO_4^-}$$

Reactions between ions and dipolar molecules, and reactions between neutral molecules generally are less sensitive to ionic strength effects than are reactions between ionic compounds. However, reactions that result in formation of oppositely charged ions as products may exhibit considerable increase in rate with increasing ionic strength.

Dielectric Constant of Solvent

Reactions involving ions of opposite charge are accelerated by solvents with low dielectric constants. For example, the rate of hydrogen ion-catalyzed hydrolysis of sulfate esters is much greater in low dielectric constant solvents, such as methylene chloride, than in water. Reaction between similarly charged species is favored by high dielectric constant solvents. Reaction between neutral molecules, which produce a highly polar transition state, such as the reaction of triethylamine with ethyl iodide to produce a quaternary ammonium salt, also will be enhanced by high dielectric constant solvents.

Hydrolysis (Solvolysis)

Hydrolysis of esters, such as procaine, aspirin, or atropine, represents one of the more common types of drug instability. *Ester hydrolysis* is either hydrogen- or hydroxide-ion catalyzed, although the catalysis that is important from the viewpoint of drug-product stability depends upon the specific compound and the pH of the solution. Amides generally are more stable than esters but are subject to catalysis by hydrogen and hydroxide ions, and often by general acids and bases. Some examples of the kinds of functional groups subject to hydrolytic cleavage

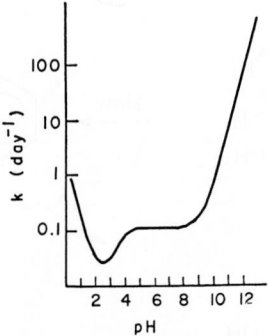

Figure 19-12. Apparent first-order rate of hydrolysis of aspirin as a function of pH at 17. (From Edwards LJ. *Trans Faraday Soc* 1950; 46: 7⁻

and species shown to be catalysts for the reactions are presented below.

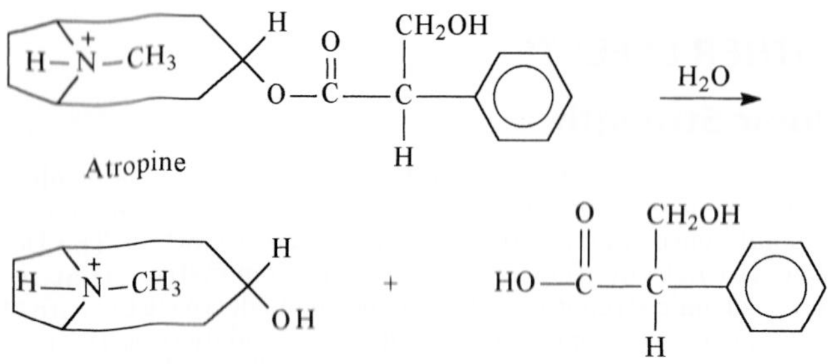

Atropine

Hydrolysis of the ester function of atropine is typical of ester hydrolysis in that only catalysis by the hydrogen or hydroxide ions are important. Figure 19-6 illustrates a pH-rate profile which might be considered typical for such a reaction. Below pH 3, the principal reaction is hydrogen-ion catalyzed hydrolysis of the protonated form of atropine. Above pH 5, the principal reaction is hydroxide ion catalyzed hydrolysis of the same species. Maximum stability at 30° is at pH 3.7.

Hydrolytic cleavage of aspirin to salicylic acid and acetic acid was studied by Edwards.[4]

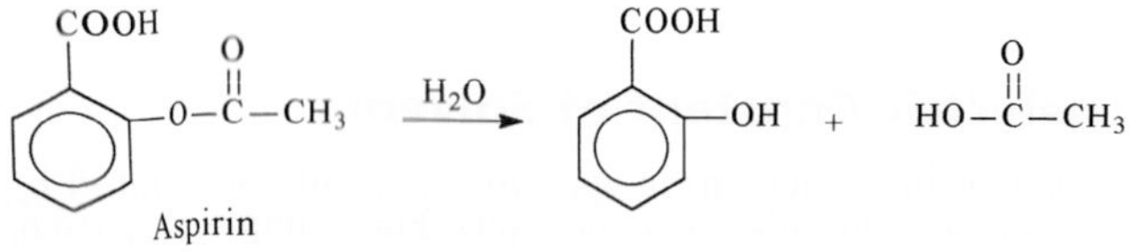

Aspirin

Edwards obtained the interesting pH-rate profile reproduced in Figure 19-12. The unusual pH-rate profile obtained for aspirin was attributed to a reaction of the form

$$-d[Aspirin]_{total}/dt = k_1[H^+][HA] + k_2[H^+][A^-]$$
$$+ k_3[OH^-][A^-] + k_0[A^-] \qquad (75)$$

where [HA] represents undissociated aspirin and [A⁻] represents aspirin anion. The pH-independent anion hydrolysis indicated for the pH region 5 to 9 has been attributed to intramolecular catalysis by orthocarboxylate anion, rather than to general acid–base catalysis by water. It is principally this intramolecular catalysis that is responsible for the high instability of aqueous solutions of aspirin in the pharmaceutically useful pH range. Fersht and Kirby[5] represented the intramolecular carboxylate ion reaction as a general base catalysis of attack by a water molecule. For nucleophiles such as ethanol, the terminal hydroxyl of polyethylene glycol (PEG) and the lysine ε-amino function in serum albumin also can participate in this reaction in the same manner as water. Thus, from aspirin in ethanol solution, ethyl acetate appears as a product; in polyethylene glycol, a polyethylene

glycol acetate is formed; and in a solution containing serum albumin (both *in vitro* and *in vivo*) aspirin produces an acetylated serum albumin. Whitworth et al.[6] reasoned that an aspirin solution prepared in a PEG solvent containing no free hydroxyl groups would provide an aspirin solution of improved stability. They used acetylated PEG 400 as a solvent for aspirin and demonstrated that in such a solvent less than 1% aspirin loss occurred after 30 days at 45°.

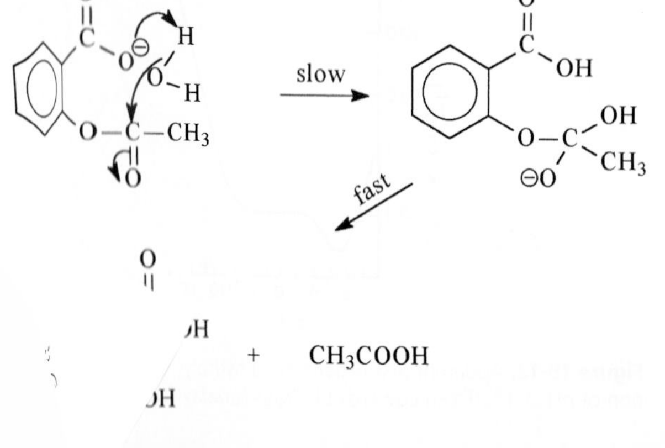

Chloramphenicol decomposition below pH 7 proceeds primarily through hydrolytic cleavage of the amide function.

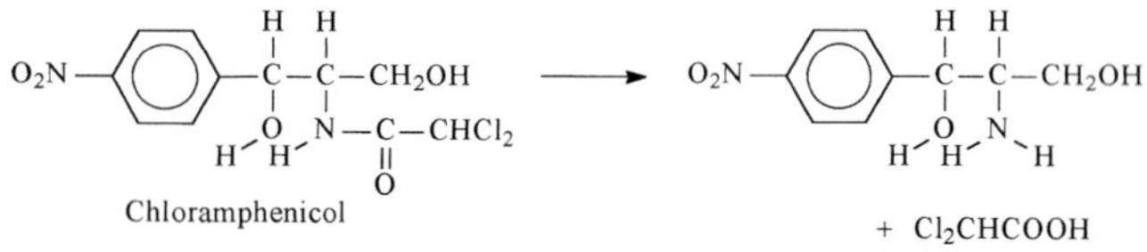

Chloramphenicol

In the presence of a buffer, the reaction may be represented as

$$-d[Camp]/dt = (k_0 + k_1[H^+] + k_2[OH^-]$$
$$+ k_{HB}[HB] + k_B[B])[Camp] \qquad (76)$$

In addition to hydrogen and hydroxide-ion catalysis there is an uncatalyzed (or water) reaction, and there may be general acid–base catalysis, represented above by the buffer species HB and B. In general, the rate of hydroxide-ion-catalyzed hydrolysis of amides is greater than rate of hydronium-ion-catalyzed hydrolysis.

Amides generally are much more stable than esters. Penicillins and cephalosporins are important exceptions to this rule because the amide bond is part of a strained four-membered ring (ie, a β-lactam). The decomposition of these compounds in aqueous solution is catalyzed by hydrogen ion, solvent, hydroxide ion, sugars, and many buffer species. Maximum stability occurs at about pH 7, but β-lactam antibiotics are too unstable to be formulated as solutions. For example, a buffered aqueous solution of penicillin G under refrigeration has a useful life of only about 1 week. Formation of the penicillanic acid by water-catalyzed rearrangement in acidic and neutral solutions is thought to be the first step in the degradation process.[7]

Barbiturate hydrolysis involves hydroxide-ion attack on both the undissociated acid, HP, and the ionized species, P⁻.

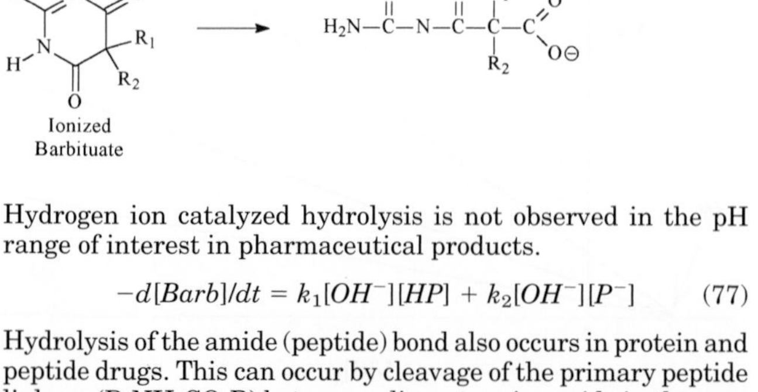

Unionized Barbituate

Ionized Barbituate

Additional Products

Hydrogen ion catalyzed hydrolysis is not observed in the pH range of interest in pharmaceutical products.

$$-d[Barb]/dt = k_1[OH^-][HP] + k_2[OH^-][P^-] \qquad (77)$$

Hydrolysis of the amide (peptide) bond also occurs in protein and peptide drugs. This can occur by cleavage of the primary peptide linkage (R-NH-CO-R) between adjacent amino acids in the peptide chain. Hydrolysis of the free side-chain amide groups of asparagine and glutamine (deamidation) is another degradation pathway for proteins. Insulin and recombinant human growth hormone undergo deamidation in solution.

Racemization

Many drugs are chiral and racemization is a common mechanism of degradation resulting in loss of biological activity. In proteins, a mixture of the D and L enantiomers is formed by base-catalyzed reaction of the natural L configuration. Acid-catalyzed racemization of epinephrine or base-catalyzed racemization of pilocarpine result in a loss of pharmacological activity.

Penicillin G

Benzylpenicilloic Acid

Benzylpenicillanic Acid

Oxidation

Compounds such as phenols, aromatic amines, aldehydes, ethers, and unsaturated aliphatic compounds are subject to oxidation upon exposure to air or oxidizing chemicals. Epinephrine, ascorbic acid, phenothiazines, and vitamin A are examples of important pharmaceutical products that are oxidized readily. Proteins can undergo oxidative degradation by oxidation of methionine, a thioether, to its corresponding sulfoxide. Oxidation of the carbon–carbon double bonds in unsaturated fatty acids (eg, oleic acid) results in the fats and oils tasting rancid.

Of particular concern are oxidations that occur when solutions are exposed to atmospheric oxygen. Such reactions, termed *autoxidation* or *self-oxidation,* are complex reactions that proceed via a free-radical mechanism. A free radical is a highly unstable (highly reactive) species containing an unpaired electron. Autoxidation reactions are autocatalytic in that free-radical reactions generate additional free radicals, causing a chain reaction.

A technique used to protect pharmaceuticals susceptible to autoxidation is to include in the formulation agents that will react readily with free radicals, but that will terminate the chain propagation either by forming relatively stable, resonance-stabilized free radicals or by forming products that do not include additional free radicals.

Photochemical Decomposition

Numerous dyes and drugs are subject to photochemical decomposition. Light-catalyzed oxidations and reductions of photoexcited species are common and are often mechanistically complex reactions involving free-radical intermediates. Pharmaceuticals such as riboflavin, nifedipine, and the phenothiazines are examples of common drugs that are extremely light sensitive.

Interaction Between Components

Because drugs are often combined in solution with buffers, antioxidants, flavoring agents, antimicrobial preservatives, and other drugs, potential interaction between the components of a formulation must be considered in pharmaceutical formulation

development. Some obvious interactions, such as the possibility of the reaction of a drug having a primary amino function with an aldehyde such as vanillin to produce a Schiff base, can be predicted; however, a number of interesting, less well-recognized reactions have been encountered.

In addition to buffer species acting as general acid–base catalysts, as previously indicated, some buffer species undergo specific interactions with drug molecules to form new chemical compounds. The formation of amides in aqueous solution from amines such as benzocaine and buffers such as citric acid has been observed.

The aromatic function of procaine reacts with glucose to form procaine *N*-glycoside; also, phenylethylamine reacts with dehydroacetic acid to form a Schiff base-type compound. Catechols have been shown to catalyze penicillin hydrolysis.

It has been demonstrated that bisulfite, an agent commonly employed to protect epinephrine against oxidative decomposition, is capable of inducing epinephrine degradation through attack on the chiral side chain.

Although a solution of folic acid alone is stable to light, a combination of riboflavin and folic acid showed a rapid loss of folic acid through formation of a coupled oxidation–reduction system in which riboflavin was photoreduced, with folic acid being used as a reducing substrate and being itself irreversibly oxidized. In the dark and in the presence of oxygen, the riboflavin was regenerated, and when the solution was again irradiated, the cycle was repeated with further destruction of folic acid. In this case, the riboflavin acts as a photosensitizer in this reaction and would cause the decomposition not only of folic acid, but also of ascorbic acid or any other easily oxidized substrate.

The presence of micellar surfactants and certain high-molecular- weight polymers commonly employed in pharmaceuticals also have been shown to lead to decreased drug stability in some cases. Both nonionic and anionic surfactants, as well as polymers such as polyvinylpyrrolidone, accelerate the photodecomposition of riboflavin in aqueous solution. Nonionic surfactants also are capable of increasing the rate of hydrolysis of sulfate esters which may be incorporated in or on the micellar surface.

Physical Instability

The introduction of an increasing number of drugs derived from developments in biotechnology necessitates greater awareness of instability occurring as a result of loss of drug activity through structural changes unrelated to disruption of covalent bonds. Protein-based drugs may lose activity as a result of a change in superstructure (secondary, tertiary, quaternary) that is independent of chemical modification. Superstructure changes, which may alter protein drug activity, include denaturation (unfolding), aggregation, surface adsorption, and precipitation. Treatments with potential for inducing such changes include temperature changes, pH extremes, and agitation or foaming resulting from shaking. High shear encountered in manufacturing or in drug delivery systems also may denature protein drugs. Detection of instability of a physical nature generally requires one or more biological assays, or physical assay methods that are sensitive to the critical superstructure change.

DRUG STABILIZATION

Some drug decomposition reactions, such as photolytic and oxidative reactions, are relatively easy to avoid by protecting the components from light (photodecomposition) or exclusion oxygen and by use of chain-terminating reagents or free-radi scavengers to minimize free-radical-mediated reactions. S ysis reactions, however, cannot be stopped by such procedures, but several techniques may be employed to retard reactions sufficiently to permit the formulation of a suitable drug product. The following approaches may be useful in attempts to retard solvolytic reactions.

Selection of Optimum pH, Buffer, and Solvent

Consideration of the mechanism of the reaction and the way in which the reaction rate is influenced by pH, buffer species, and solvent permits the selection of the optimum conditions for drug stability. Often, however, ideal conditions for maximum stability may be unacceptable from the viewpoint of pharmaceutically acceptable formulation or therapeutic efficacy; thus, it may be necessary to prepare a formulation with conditions less than optimum for drug stability. If a suitable compromise between conditions for maximum stability and conditions for a pharmaceutically acceptable formulation cannot be achieved, techniques such as those described below may be useful in retarding solvolysis reactions.

Specific Complexing Agents

The technique of stabilization by forming complexes in solution was introduced by Higuchi and Lachman,[8] who demonstrated that the rate of hydrolysis of the ester function of benzocaine was retarded significantly in the presence of caffeine, a reagent with which the benzocaine formed a soluble complex. It was demonstrated further that, in these systems, the complexed drug did not hydrolyze at all, and that the observed rate of hydrolysis could be ascribed to the concentration of the free or uncomplexed drug that was in equilibrium with the drug complex.

Boric acid chelation of the catechol function of epinephrine stabilizes epinephrine against attack by bisulfite and sulfite. The complex of povidone (polyvinylpyrrolidone) and iodine has been used for many years as a topical antiseptic because of its higher iodine concentration, slow release of iodine from the complex, and lower toxicity.

Surfactants

It has been demonstrated that the incorporation of benzocaine into surfactant micelles could retard significantly the rate of ester hydrolysis. Nonionic and anionic surfactants retarded the hydroxide-ion-catalyzed hydrolysis, but cationic surfactants somewhat increased the rate of hydroxide-ion-catalyzed hydrolysis. Similar observations have been reported for a number of drugs that are sufficiently lipophilic to be solubilized by surfactant micelles.

Suspensions

If the solubility of a labile drug is reduced and the drug is prepared in a suspension form, the rate at which the drug degrades will be related only to the concentration of dissolved drug rather than to the total concentration of drug in the product. Thus it has been demonstrated that penicillin G procaine suspensions degraded at a rate proportional to the low concentration of penicillin in solution. Because the penicillin in solution was in equilibrium with excess solid penicillin G procaine, the ⌐nicillin concentration in solution was constant and the observed order of reaction was apparently zero order.

temperature usually will retard solvolytic in the frozen state generally is an effective ᵤing degradative reactions. Several antibiotics

are sold as frozen solutions in flexible plastic bags. An exception is sodium ampicillin dissolved in 5% dextrose solution, which showed approximately 10% decomposition after 4 hr of storage at 5° and more than 13% loss after storage for the same period in the frozen state at $-20°$.

Stability Testing of Pharmaceutical Products

If a product is to be marketed, it must be stable over relatively long storage times at room temperature or at the actual temperature at which it will be shipped and stored prior to its ultimate use. Thus, the rate of degradation may have to be studied over an undesirably long period of time in order to determine the product's stability under normal storage conditions.

To avoid this undesirable delay in evaluating possible formulations, the manufacturer attempts to predict stability under conditions of room temperature or actual storage conditions by using data for the rate of decomposition obtained at several elevated temperatures. This is accomplished using an Arrhenius plot to predict, from high-temperature data, the rate of product breakdown to be expected at actual lower temperature storage conditions.

Prediction based on data obtained at elevated temperatures generally is satisfactory for solution dosage forms. Success is more uncertain when nonhomogeneous products are involved. Suspensions of drugs may not provide linear Arrhenius plots because often there is the possibility that the solid phase, which exists at elevated temperature, may not be the same solid phase that exists at room temperature. Such differences in the solubility of the several solid phases may invalidate the usual Arrhenius plots. These difficulties should be anticipated when polymorphic crystal forms or several different solvates are known to exist for a specific solute. Also, when solid dosage forms (eg, tablets) are subjected to high temperatures, changes in the quantity of moisture in the product may greatly influence the stability of the product.

Arrhenius plots also suffer limitations when applied to reactions that have relatively low activation energies and, therefore, are not accelerated greatly by an increase in temperature. Where usually it is desirable to determine drug stability by analyzing samples for the amount of intact drug remaining—in instances where there is very little drug decomposition and particularly when it is not convenient to accelerate the reaction by increasing temperature—it sometimes is advantageous to determine initial reaction rates from the determination of the amount of reaction product formed.

Using modern methods of analysis, such as high-performance liquid chromatography (HPLC), it is often possible to measure the rate of formation of a degradation product. By using this technique, very small amounts of degradation (less than 1% loss of parent compound) can be detected, resulting in a more sensitive indication of product stability than can be obtained by analyzing potency.

Since manufacturers are interested primarily in the time required to produce just a few-percent breakdown in their product, it is not uncommon to employ terminology such as $t_{0.90}$ or $t_{0.95}$, which is the time required for the drug to decompose to 90 or 95%, respectively, of original potency.

An Arrhenius-type plot, analogous to that illustrated in Figure 19-4, can be obtained by plotting the logarithm of the time required for the specified fractional decomposition versus the reciprocal of absolute temperature. The time required for the product to decrease in potency to 90% of original potency at room temperature then can be obtained directly from the plot.

REFERENCES

1. Garrett ER. In: Bean HS, et al, eds. *Advances in Pharmaceutical Sciences*, vol 2. New York: Academic Press, 1967, Chap 2.
2. Kondritzer AA, Zvirblis P. *J APhA Sci Ed* 1957; 46: 531.

3. Higuchi T, et al. *J APhA Sci Ed* 1950; 39: 405.
4. Edwards LJ. *Trans Faraday Soc* 1950; 46: 723.
5. Fersht AR, Kirby AJ. *J Am Chem Soc* 1967; 89: 4857.
6. Whitworth CA, et al. *J Pharm Sci* 1973; 62: 1184.
7. Yamana T, et al. *J Pharm Sci* 1977; 66: 861.
8. Higuchi T, Lachman L. *J APhA Sci Ed* 1955; 44: 52.

BIBLIOGRAPHY

Carstensen JT. *Drug Stability, Principles and Practices*. New York: Dekker, 1990.

Connors KA, et al. *Chemical Stability of Pharmaceuticals*, 2nd ed. New York: Wiley, 1986.
Espenson JH. *Chemical Kinetics and Reaction Mechanisms*, 2nd ed. New York: McGraw-Hill, 1995.
Fung HL. In: Banker GS, Rhodes CT, eds. *Modern Pharmaceutics*, 2nd ed. New York: Dekker, 1990, Chap 6.
House JE. *Principles of Chemical Kinetics*. Dubuque, IA: WC Brown, 1997.
Houston, PL. Chemical Kinetics and Reaction Dynamics, Boston: McGraw-Hill, Inc., 2001.
Lachman L, DeLuca P, Akers M. In: Lachman L, et al, eds. *The Theory and Practice of Industrial Pharmacy*, 3rd ed. Philadelphia: Lea & Febiger, 1986, Chap 6.

CHAPTER 20

Interfacial Phenomena

Paul M Bummer, PhD

Very often it is desirable or necessary in the development of pharmaceutical dosage forms to produce multiphasic dispersions by mixing together two or more ingredients that are not mutually miscible and capable of forming homogeneous solutions. Examples of such dispersions include:

Suspensions (solid in liquid)
Emulsions (liquid in liquid)
Foams (vapor in liquids)

Because these systems are not homogeneous and thermodynamically stable, over time they will show some tendency to separate on standing to produce the minimum possible surface area of contact between phases. Thus, suspended particles agglomerate and sediment, emulsified droplets cream and coalesce, and the bubbles dispersed in foams collapse to produce unstable and nonuniform dosage forms. One way to prevent or slow down this natural tendency for further phase separation is to add materials that can accumulate at the interface to provide some type of energy barrier to aggregation and coalescence. Such materials are said to exhibit *surface activity* or to act as *surface-active agents.*

In this chapter the fundamental physical chemical properties of molecules situated at interfaces will be discussed so that the reader can gain a better understanding of how problems involving interfaces can be resolved in designing pharmaceutical dosage forms by the use of surface-active agents.

INTERFACIAL FORCES AND ENERGETICS

In the bulk portion of each phase, molecules are attracted to each other equally in all directions, such that no resultant forces are acting on any one molecule. The strength of these forces determines whether a substance exists as a vapor, liquid, or solid at a particular temperature and pressure.

At the boundary between phases, however, molecules are acted upon unequally because they are in contact with other molecules exhibiting different forces of attraction. For example, the primary intermolecular forces in water are due to hydrogen bonds, whereas those responsible for intermolecular bonding in hydrocarbon liquids, such as mineral oil, are due to London dispersion forces.

Thus, molecules situated at the interface experience interaction forces dissimilar to those experienced in each bulk phase. In liquid systems such unbalanced forces can be satisfied by spontaneous movement of molecules from the interface into the bulk phase. This leaves fewer molecules per unit area at the surface (greater intermolecular distance) and reduces the actual area between dissimilar molecules.

Any attempt to reverse this process by increasing the area of contact between phases—that is, bringing more molecules into the interface—causes the interface to resist expansion and behave as though it is under a tension everywhere in a tangential direction. The force of this tension per unit length of interface generally is called the *interfacial tension,* except when dealing with the air–liquid interface, where the terms *surface* and *surface tension* are used.

To illustrate the presence of a tension in the interface, consider an experiment where a circular metal frame, with a looped piece of thread loosely tied to it, is dipped into a liquid. When the frame is removed and exposed to the air, a film of liquid will be stretched entirely across the circular frame, as when one uses such a frame to blow soap bubbles. Under these conditions (Fig 20-1A), the thread will remain collapsed. If a heated needle is used to puncture and remove the liquid film from within the loop (Fig 20-1B), the loop will stretch spontaneously into a circular shape.

The result of this experiment demonstrates the spontaneous reduction of interfacial contact between air and the liquid remaining; indeed, it illustrates that a tension causing the loop to remain extended exists parallel to the interface. The circular shape of the loop indicates that the tension in the plane of the interface exists at right angles or normal to every part of the looped thread. The total force on the entire loop divided by the circumference of the circle, therefore, represents the tension per unit distance of surface, or the surface tension.

Just as work is required to extend a spring under tension, work should be required to reverse the process seen in Figure 20-1A and B, thus bringing more molecules to the interface. This may be seen quantitatively by considering an experiment where tension and work may be measured directly. Assume that we have a rectangular wire with one movable side (Fig 20-2). Assume further that by dipping this wire into a liquid, a film of liquid will form within the frame when it is removed and exposed to the air. As seen earlier in Figure 20-1, when it comes in contact with air, the liquid surface will tend to contract with a force, F, as molecules leave the surface for the bulk. To keep the movable side in equilibrium, an equal force must be applied to oppose this tension in the surface. The surface tension, γ, of the liquid may be defined as $F/2l$, where $2l$ is the distance of surface over which F is operating. The factor 2 arises out of considering two surfaces, top and bottom. Upon expansion of the surface by a very small distance, Δx, the work done (W) is

$$W = F\Delta x \qquad (1)$$

and therefore,

$$W = \gamma 2l \Delta x \qquad (2)$$

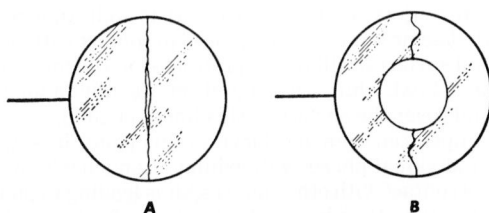

Figure 20-1. A circular wire frame with a loop of thread loosely tied to it: (*A*) a liquid film on the wire frame with a loop in it; (*B*) the film inside the loop is broken. (From Semat H. *Fundamentals of Physics,* 3rd ed. New York: Holt Reinhart Winston, 1957.)

Since

$$\Delta A = 2l\Delta x \tag{3}$$

where ΔA is the change in area due to the expansion of the surface, it may be concluded that

$$W = \gamma\Delta A \tag{4}$$

Thus, the work required to create a unit area of surface, known as the *surface free energy / unit area,* is equivalent to the surface tension of a liquid system—the greater the area of interfacial contact between phases, the greater the free-energy increase for the total system. Because a prime requisite for equilibrium is that the free energy of a system be at a minimum, it is not surprising to observe that phases in contact tend to reduce area of contact spontaneously.

Liquids, being mobile, may assume spherical shapes (smallest interfacial area for a given volume), as when ejected from an orifice into air or when dispersed into another immiscible liquid. If a large number of drops are formed, further reduction in area can occur by having the drops coalesce, as when a foam collapses or when the liquid phases making up an emulsion separate.

In the centigrade-gram-second (cgs) system, surface tension is expressed in units of dynes per centimeter (dyne/cm), while surface free energy is expressed in erg/cm². As an erg is a dyne-cm, both sets of units are equivalent. In the SI (international units) system, surface tension is expressed in mN/m and surface free energy in mJ/m².

Values for the surface tension of a variety of liquids are given in Table 20-1, and interfacial tension values for various liquids against water are given in Table 20-2. Other combinations of immiscible phases could be given, but most heterogeneous systems encountered in pharmacy usually contain water. Values for these tensions are expressed for a particular temperature. Because an increased temperature increases the thermal energy of molecules, the work required to bring molecules to the interface should be less, and thus the surface and interfacial tension will be reduced. For example, the surface tension of water is 76.5 dynes/cm at 0° and 63.5 dynes/cm at 75°.

As would be expected from the discussion so far, the relative values for surface tension should reflect the nature of intermolecular forces present, hence the relatively large values for

Table 20-1. Surface Tension of Various Liquids at 20°

SUBSTANCE	SURFACE TENSION (dyne/cm)
Mercury	476
Water	72.8
Glycerin	63.4
Oleic acid	32.5
Benzene	28.9
Chloroform	27.1
Carbon tetrachloride	26.8
1-Octanol	26.5
Hexadecane	27.4
Dodecane	25.4
Decane	23.9
Octane	21.8
Heptane	19.7
Hexane	18.0
Perfluoroheptane	11.0
Nitrogen (at 75 K)	9.4

mercury (metallic bonds) and water (hydrogen bonds), and the lower values for benzene, chloroform, carbon tetrachloride, and the *n*-alkanes.

Benzene, with π electrons, exhibits a higher surface tension than the alkanes of comparable molecular weight, but increasing the molecular weight of the alkanes (and hence intermolecular attraction) increases their surface tension closer to that of benzene. The lower values for the more nonpolar substances, perfluoroheptane and liquid nitrogen, demonstrate this point even more strongly.

Values of interfacial tension should reflect the differences in chemical structure of the two phases involved—the greater the tendency to interact, the less the interfacial tension. The 20-dyne/cm difference between air–water tension and that at the octane–water interface reflects the small but significant interaction between octane molecules and water molecules at the interface. This is seen also in Table 20-2 by comparing the values for octane and octanol, oleic acid and the alkanes, or chloroform and carbon tetrachloride. In each case the presence of chemical groups capable of hydrogen bonding with water markedly reduces the interfacial tension, presumably by satisfying the unbalanced forces at the interface. These observations strongly suggest that molecules at an interface arrange themselves or orient so as to minimize differences between bulk phases.

That this phenomenon occurs even at the air–liquid interface is seen when one notes the relatively low surface-tension values of very different chemical structures such as the *n*-alkanes, octanol, oleic acid, benzene, and chloroform. Presumably, in each case the similar nonpolar groups are oriented toward the air with any polar groups oriented away toward the bulk phase. This tendency for molecules to orient at an interface is a basic factor in interfacial phenomena and will be discussed more fully in succeeding sections.

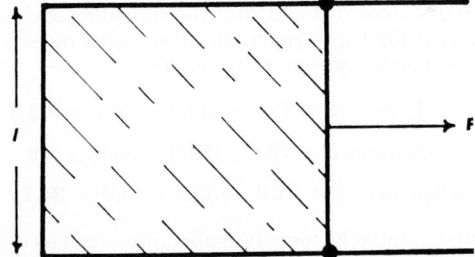

Figure 20-2. A movable wire frame containing a film of liquid being expanded with a force, *F.*

Table 20-2. Interfacial Tension of Various Liquids Against Water at 20°

SUBSTANCE	INTERFACIAL TENSION (dyne/cm)
Decane	52.3
Octane	51.7
Hexane	50.8
Carbon tetrachloride	45.0
Chloroform	32.8
Benzene	35.0
Mercury	428
Oleic acid	15.6
1-Octanol	8.51

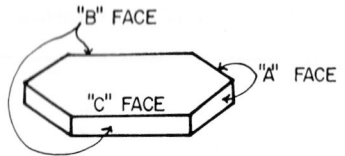

Figure 20-3. Adipic acid crystal showing various faces. (From Michaels AS. *J Phys Chem* 1961; 65: 1730.)

Solid substances such as metals, metal oxides, silicates, and salts, all containing polar groups exposed at their surface, may be classified as *high-energy solids,* whereas nonpolar solids such as carbon, sulfur, glyceryl tristearate, polyethylene, and polytetrafluoroethylene (Teflon) may be classified as *low-energy solids.* It is of interest to measure the surface free energy of solids; however, the lack of mobility of molecules at the surface of solids prevents the observation and direct measurement of a surface tension. It is possible to measure the work required to create new solid surface by cleaving a crystal and measuring the work involved. However, this work not only represents free energy due to exposed groups but also takes into account the mechanical energy associated with crystal fracture (ie, plastic and elastic deformation and strain energies due to crystal structure and imperfections in that structure).

Also contributing to the complexity of a solid surface is the heterogeneous behavior as a result of the exposure of different crystal faces, each having a different surface free energy/unit area. For example, adipic acid, $HOOC(CH_2)_4COOH$, crystallizes from water as thin hexagonal plates with three different faces, as shown in Figure 20-3. Each unit cell of such a crystal contains adipic acid molecules oriented such that the hexagonal planes (faces) contain exposed carboxyl groups, while the sides and edges (A and B faces) represent the side view of the carboxyl and alkyl groups and thus are quite nonpolar. Indeed, interactions involving these different faces reflect the differing surface free energies.[2]

Other complexities of solid surfaces include roughness and porosity.[3] Even in the absence of chemical contamination, such as that occurring during recrystallization, surface energy changes in a solid can be induced by unit operations such as milling, resulting in an altered pattern of drug dissolution.[4,5] In view of all these potential complications that are difficult to quantify, surface free energy values for solids, when reported, should be regarded as average values, often dependent on the method used and not necessarily the same for other samples of the same substance.

Table 20-3 lists some average values of γ_{sv} for a variety of solids, ranging in polarity from Teflon to copper, obtained by various indirect techniques.

ADHESIONAL AND COHESIONAL FORCES

Of prime importance to those dealing with heterogeneous systems is the question of how two phases will behave when brought in contact with each other. It is well known, for instance, that some liquids, when placed in contact with other liquid or solid surfaces, will remain retracted in the form of a drop (known as a *lens*), while other liquids may exhibit a tendency to spread and cover the surface of this liquid or solid.

Based upon concepts developed to this point, it is apparent that the individual phases will exhibit a tendency to minimize the area of contact with other phases, thus leading to phase separation. On the other hand, the tendency for interaction between molecules at the new interface will offset this to some extent and give rise to the spontaneous spreading of one substance over the other.

In essence, therefore, phase affinity is increased as the forces of attraction between different phases (*adhesional forces*) become greater than the forces of attraction between molecules of the same phase (*cohesional forces*). If these adhesional forces become great enough, miscibility will occur and the interface will disappear. The present discussion is concerned only with systems of limited phase affinity, where an interface still exists.

A convenient approach used to express these forces quantitatively is work of adhesion and work of cohesion. The *work of adhesion,* W_a, is defined as the free energy/cm^2 required to separate two phases at their boundary and is equal but opposite in sign to the free energy/cm^2 released when the interface is formed. In an analogous manner the *work of cohesion* for a pure substance, W_c, is the work/cm^2 required to produce two new surfaces, as when separating different phases, but now both surfaces contain the same molecules. This is equal and opposite in sign to the free energy/cm^2 released when the same two pure liquid surfaces are brought together and eliminated.

By convention, when the work of adhesion between two substances, A and B, exceeds the work of cohesion for one substance (eg, B), spontaneous spreading of B over the surface of A should occur with a net loss of free energy equal to the difference between W_a and W_c. If W_c exceeds W_a, no spontaneous spreading of B over A can occur. The difference between W_a and W_c is known as the *spreading coefficient, S.* Only when S is positive will spreading occur.

The values for W_a and W_c (and hence S) may be expressed in terms of surface and interfacial tensions, when one considers that upon separation of two phases, A and B, γ_{AB} ergs of interfacial free energy/cm^2 (interfacial tension) are lost, but that γ_A and γ_B erg/cm^2 of energy (surface tensions of A and B) are gained; upon separation of bulk-phase molecules in an analogous manner, $2\gamma_A$ or $2\gamma_B$ erg/cm^2 will be gained. Thus,

$$W_a = \gamma_A + \gamma_B - \gamma_{AB} \qquad (5)$$

and

$$W_c = 2\gamma_A \text{ or } 2\gamma_B \qquad (6)$$

for B spreading on the surface of A. Therefore,

$$S_B = \gamma_A + \gamma_B - \gamma_{AB} - 2\gamma_B \qquad (7)$$

or

$$S_B = \gamma_A - (\gamma_B + \gamma_{AB}) \qquad (8)$$

Using Equation 8 and the values of surface and interfacial tension given in Tables 20-1 and 20-2, the spreading coefficient can be calculated for three representative substances—decane, benzene, and oleic acid—on water at 20°.

$$\text{Decane: } S = 72.8 - (23.9 + 52.3) = -3.4$$

$$\text{Benzene: } S = 72.8 - (28.9 + 35.0) = 8.9$$

$$\text{Oleic Acid: } S = 72.8 - (32.5 + 15.6) = 24.7$$

As expected, relatively nonpolar substances such as decane exhibit negative values of spreading coefficient, whereas the more-polar materials yield positive values—the greater the polarity of the molecule, the more positive the value of S.

Table 20-3. Values of γ_{sv} for Solids of Varying Polarity

SOLID	Γ_{SV} (dyne/cm)
Teflon	19.0
Paraffin	25.5
Polyethylene	37.6
Polymethyl methacrylate	45.4
Nylon	50.8
~methacin	61.8
~lvin	62.2
~ne	68.7
~ride	155
	1300

The importance of the cohesive energy of the spreading liquid may be noted also by comparing the spreading coefficients for hexane on water and water on hexane.

$$S_{H/W} = 72.8 - (18.0 + 50.8) = 10.0$$

$$S_{W/H} = 18.0 - (72.8 + 50.8) = -105.6$$

Here, despite the fact that both liquids are the same, the high cohesion and air–liquid tension of water prevents spreading on the low-energy hexane surface, while the very low value for hexane allows spreading on the water surface. This also is seen when comparing the positive spreading coefficient of hexane to the negative value for decane on water.

To see whether spreading does or does not occur, a powder such as talc or charcoal can be sprinkled over the surface of water such that it floats; then, a drop of each liquid is placed on this surface. As predicted, decane will remain as an intact drop, while hexane, benzene, and oleic acid will spread out, as shown by the rapid movement of solid particles away from the point where the liquid drop was placed originally.

An apparent contradiction to these observations may be noted for hexane, benzene, and oleic acid when more of each substance is added: lenses now appear to form even though initial spreading occurred. Thus, in effect a substance does not appear to spread over itself.

It is now established that the spreading substance forms a monomolecular film that creates a new surface that has a lower surface free energy than pure water. This arises because of the apparent orientation of the molecules in such a film so that their most hydrophobic portion is oriented toward the spreading phase. It is the lack of affinity between this exposed portion of the spread molecules and the polar portion of the remaining molecules that prevents further spreading. This may be seen by calculating a final spreading coefficient where the new surface tension of water plus monomolecular film is used. For example, the presence of benzene reduces the surface tension of water to 62.2 dyne/cm so that the final spreading coefficient, is

$$S = 62.2 - (28.9 + 35.0) = -1.7$$

The lack of spreading exhibited by oleic acid should be reflected in an even more negative final spreading coefficient, as the very polar carboxyl groups should have very little affinity for the exposed alkyl chain of the oleic acid film. Spreading so as to form a second layer with polar groups exposed to the air also would seem very unlikely, thus leading to the formation of a lens.

WETTING PHENOMENA

In the experiment described above it was shown that talc or charcoal sprinkled onto the surface of water float despite the fact that their densities are much greater than that of water. In order for immersion of the solid to occur, the liquid must displace air and spread over the surface of the solid; when liquids cannot spread over a solid surface spontaneously, and, therefore, S, the spreading coefficient, is negative, we say that the solid is not wetted.

An important parameter reflecting the degree of wetting is the angle made by the liquid with the solid surface at the point of contact (Fig 20-4). By convention, when wetting is complete, the contact angle is 0°; in nonwetting situations it theoretically can increase to a value of 180°, where a spherical droplet makes contact with solid at only one point.

To express contact angle in terms of solid–liquid–air equilibria, one can balance forces parallel to the solid surface at the point of contact between all three phases (see Fig 20-4), as expressed in

$$\gamma_{SV} = \gamma_{SL} + \gamma_{LV} \cos \theta \qquad (9)$$

where γ_{SV}, γ_{SL}, and γ_{LV} represent the surface free energy/unit area of the solid–air, solid–liquid and liquid–air interfaces, re-

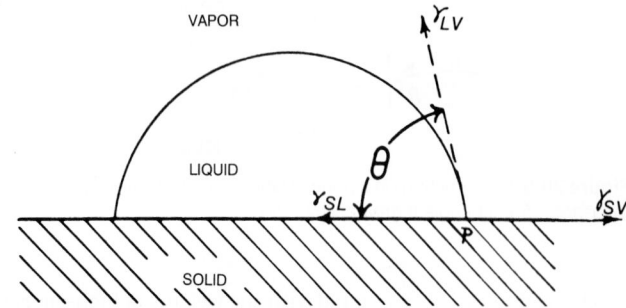

Figure 20-4. Forces acting on a nonwetting liquid drop exhibiting a contact angle of θ. (From Zisman WA. *Adv Chem Ser* 1964; 43: 1.)

spectively. Although difficult to use quantitatively because of uncertainties with γ_{SV} and γ_{SL} measurements, conceptually the equation, known as the Young equation, is useful because it shows that the loss of free energy due to elimination of the air–solid interface by wetting is offset by the increased solid–liquid and liquid–air area of contact as the drop spreads out.

The $\gamma_{LV} \cos \theta$ term arises as the horizontal vectorial component of the force acting along the surface of the drop, as represented by γ_{LV}. Factors tending to reduce γ_{LV} and γ_{SL}, therefore, will favor wetting, while the greater the value of γ_{SV}, the greater the chance for wetting to occur. This is seen in Table 20-4 for the wetting of a low-energy surface, paraffin (hydrocarbon), and a higher energy surface, nylon (polyhexamethylene adipamide). Here, the lower the surface tension of a liquid, the smaller the contact angle on a given solid, and the more polar the solid, the smaller the contact angle with the same liquid.

With Equation 9 in mind and looking at Figure 20-5, it is now possible to understand how the forces acting at the solid–liquid–air interface can cause a dense nonwetted solid to float if γ_{SL} and γ_{LV} are large enough relative to γ_{SV}.

The significance of reducing γ_{LV} was first developed empirically by Zisman[6] when he plotted cos θ versus the surface tension of a series of liquids and found that a linear relationship, dependent on the solid, often was obtained. When such plots are extrapolated to cos θ equal to 1, or 0° contact angle, a value of surface tension required to just cause complete wetting is obtained. Doing this for a number of solids, it was shown that this surface tension (known as the critical surface tension, γ_c) parallels expected solid surface energy γ_{SV}—the lower γ_c, the more nonpolar the surface.

Table 20-5 indicates some of these γ_c values for different surface groups, indicating such a trend. Thus, water with a surface tension of about 72 dyne/cm will not wet polyethylene ($\gamma_c = 31$ dyne/cm) but heptane, with a surface tension of about 20 dyne/cm, will. Likewise, Teflon (polytetrafluoroethylene) ($\gamma_c = 19$) is not wetted by heptane but is wetted by perfluoroheptane with a surface tension of 11 dyne/cm.

Table 20-4. Contact Angle on Paraffin and Nylon for Various Liquids of Differing Surface Tension

SUBSTANCE	SURFACE TENSION (dyne/cm)	CONTACT ANGLE (°)	
		PARAFFIN	NYLON
Water	72.8	105	70
Glycerin	63.4	96	60
Formamide	58.2	91	50
Methylene iodide	50.8	66	41
α-Bromonaphthalene	44.6	47	16
tert-Butylnaphthalene	33.7	38	spreads
Benzene	28.9	24	spreads
Dodecane	25.4	17	spreads
Decane	23.9	7	spreads
Nonane	22.9	spreads	spreads

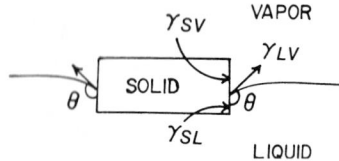

Figure 20-5. Forces acting on a nonwettable solid at the air+liquid+solid interface: contact angle θ greater than 90°.

One complication associated with the wetting of high-energy surfaces is the lack of wetting after the initial formation of a monomolecular film caused by the spreading substance. As in the case of oleic acid spreading on the surface of water, the remaining liquid retracts because of the low-energy surface produced by the oriented film. This phenomenon, often called *autophobic behavior,* is an important factor in many systems of pharmaceutical interest because many solids expected to be wetted easily by water may be rendered hydrophobic if other molecules dissolved in the water can form these monomolecular films at the solid surface.

CAPILLARITY

Because water shows a strong tendency to spread out over a polar surface such as clean glass (contact angle equal to 0°), one would expect to observe a meniscus forming when water is contained in a glass vessel such as a pipet or buret. This behavior is accentuated dramatically if a fine-bore capillary tube is placed into the liquid (Fig 20-6). Not only will the wetting of the glass produce a more highly curved meniscus, but the level of the liquid in the tube will be appreciably higher than the level of the water in the beaker.

The spontaneous movement of a liquid into a capillary or narrow tube due to surface forces is defined as *capillarity* and is responsible for a number of important processes involving the penetration of liquids into porous solids. In contrast to water in contact with glass, if the same capillary is placed into mercury (contact angle on glass: 130°), not only will the meniscus be inverted (Fig 20-7), but the level of the mercury in the capillary will be lower than in the beaker. In this case one does not expect mercury or other *nonwetting* liquids to penetrate pores easily unless external forces are applied.

To examine more closely the factors giving rise to the phenomenon of capillarity, consider the case of a liquid that rises to a height, h, above the bulk liquid in a capillary having a radius, r. As shown in Figure 20-6, if the contact angle of water on glass is 0, a force, F, will act upward and vertically

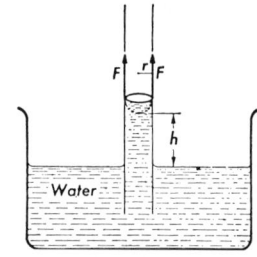

Figure 20-6. Capillary rise for a liquid exhibiting 0° contact angle. (From Semat H. *Fundamentals of Physics,* 3rd ed. New York: Holt Reinhart Winston, 1957.)

along the circle of liquid–glass contact. Based upon the definition of surface tension, this force will be equal to the surface tension, γ, multiplied by the circumference of the circle, $2\pi r$. Thus,

$$F = \gamma 2\pi r \qquad (10)$$

This force upward must support the column of water, and because the mass, m, of the column is equal to the density, d, multiplied by the volume of the column, $\pi r^2 h$, the force W opposing the movement upward will be

$$W = mg = \pi r^2 dgh \qquad (11)$$

where g is the gravity constant.

Equating the two forces at equilibrium gives

$$\pi r^2 dgh = \gamma 2\pi r \qquad (12)$$

so that

$$h = \frac{2\gamma}{rdg} \qquad (13)$$

Thus, the greater the surface tension and the finer the capillary radius, the greater the rise of liquid in the capillary.

If the contact angle of liquid is not 0 (Fig 20-8), the same relationship may be developed, except the vertical component of F which opposes the weight of the column is $F \cos \theta$ and, therefore

$$h = \frac{2\gamma \cos \theta}{rdg} \qquad (14)$$

This indicates the very important fact that if θ is less than 90°, but greater than 0°, the value of h will decrease with increasing contact angle until at 90° (cos θ = 0°), h = 0. Above 90°, values of h will be negative, as indicated in Figure 20-7 for mercury. Thus, based on these equations it may be concluded that capillarity will occur spontaneously in a cylindrical pore even if the contact angle is greater than 0°, but it will not occur at all if the contact angle becomes 90° or more. In solids with irregularly shaped pores the relationships between parameters in Equation 14 will be the same, but they will be more difficult to quantitate because of nonuniform changes in pore radius throughout the porous structure.

Table 20-5. Critical Surface Tensions of Various Polymeric Solids

POLYMERIC SOLID	Γ_C (dyne/cm AT 20°C)
Polymethacrylic ester of φ′-octanol	10.6
Polyhexafluoropropylene	16.2
Polytetrafluoroethylene	19
Polytrifluoroethylene	22
Poly(vinylidene fluoride)	25
Poly(vinyl fluoride)	28
Polyethylene	31
...lytrifluorochloroethylene	31
...vrene	33
...′ alcohol)	37
...methacrylate)	39
...le)	39
...ride)	40
...phthalate)	43
...ene adipamide)	46

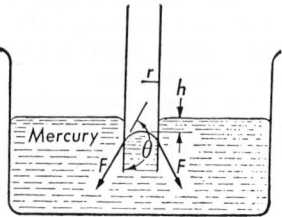

Figure 20-7. Capillary fall for a liquid exhibiting a contact angle, θ, that is greater than 90°. (From Semat H. *Fundamentals of Physics,* 3rd ed. New York: Holt Reinhart Winston, 1957.)

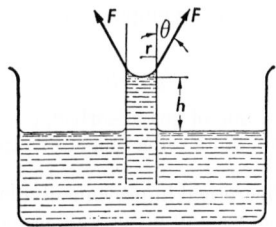

Figure 20-8. Capillary rise for a liquid exhibiting a contact angle, θ, that is greater than 0° but less than 90°. (From Semat H. *Fundamentals of Physics,* 3rd ed. New York: Holt Reinhart Winston, 1957.)

PRESSURE DIFFERENCES ACROSS CURVED SURFACES

From the preceding discussion of capillarity another important concept follows. In order for the liquid in a capillary to rise spontaneously it must develop a higher pressure than the lower level of the liquid in the beaker. However, because the system is open to the atmosphere, both surfaces are in equilibrium with the atmospheric pressure. To be raised above the level of liquid in the beaker and produce a hydrostatic pressure equal to hgd, the pressure just below the liquid meniscus, in the capillary, P_1, must be less than that just below the flat liquid surface, P_0, by hgd, and therefore

$$P_0 - P_1 = hgd \qquad (15)$$

Because, according to Equation 14,

$$h = \frac{2\gamma \cos \theta}{rgd}$$

then

$$P_0 - P_1 = \frac{2\gamma \cos \theta}{r} \qquad (16)$$

For a contact angle of 0°, where the radius of the capillary is the radius of the hemisphere making up the meniscus,

$$P_0 - P_1 = \frac{2\gamma}{r} \qquad (17)$$

The consequences of this relationship (known as the Laplace equation) are important for any curved surface when r becomes very small and γ is relatively significant. For example, a spherical droplet of air formed in a bulk liquid and having a radius r will have a greater pressure on the inner concave surface than on the convex side, as expressed in Equation 17. Direct measurement of the pressure difference, $(P_0 - P_1)$, for an air bubble of known radius allows the determination of the surface tension of either a pure liquid or a solution of surface active substance. Both static (constant radius) and dynamic (radius changing in a cyclic fashion as a function of time) measurements have been employed. The latter treatment, known as the pulsating bubble method, has been very useful in the study of some of the biophysical properties and associated disease states of pulmonary surfactant, a mixture of surface active materials lining the small airways of the mammalian lung.[7] One of the less appreciated advantages of this method for measuring surface tension is the need for only a very small sample size, typically on the order of 50 µL.

Another direct consequence of what Equation 17 expresses is the fact that very small droplets of liquid, having highly curved surfaces, will exhibit a higher vapor pressure, VP, than observed are over a flat surface of the same liquid at VP'. Equation 18, called the *Kelvin equation,* expresses the ratio of VP/VP' to droplet radius r, and surface tension γ:

$$\log \frac{P}{P'} = \frac{2\gamma M}{2.303 RT\rho r} \qquad (18)$$

where M is the molecular weight, R is the gas constant in erg/mol/degree, T is temperature, and ρ is the density in g/cm³. Values for the ratio of vapor pressures are given in Table 20-6 for water droplets of varying size. Such ratios indicate why it is possible for very fine water droplets in clouds to remain uncondensed despite their close proximity to one another.

This same behavior may be seen when measuring the solubility of very fine solid particles, as both vapor pressure and solubility are measures of the escaping tendency of molecules from a surface. Indeed, the equilibrium solubility of extremely small particles has been shown to be greater than the usual value noted for coarser particles; the greater the surface energy and smaller the particles, the greater this effect.

ADSORPTION

Vapor Adsorption on Solid Surfaces

It was suggested earlier that a high surface or interfacial free energy may exist at a solid surface if the unbalanced forces at the surface and the area of exposed groups are quite great.

Substances such as metals, metal oxides, silicates, and salts—all containing exposed polar groups—may be classified as high-energy or hydrophilic solids; nonpolar solids such as carbon, sulfur, polyethylene, or Teflon (polytetrafluoroethylene) may be classified as low-energy or hydrophobic solids (see Table 20-3). Whereas liquids satisfy their unbalanced surface forces by changes in shape, pure solids (which exhibit negligible surface mobility) must rely on reaction with molecules either in the vapor state or in a solution that comes in contact with the solid surface to accomplish this.

Vapor adsorption is the simplest model demonstrating how solids reduce their surface free energy in this manner. Depending on the chemical nature of the adsorbent (solid) and the adsorbate (vapor), the strength of interaction between the two species may vary from strong specific chemical bonding to interactions produced by the weaker, more nonspecific London dispersion forces. Ordinarily, these latter forces are those responsible for the condensation of relatively nonpolar substances such as N_2, O_2, CO_2, or hydrocarbons.

When chemical reaction occurs, the process is called *chemisorption;* when dispersion forces predominate, the term *physisorption* is used. Physisorption occurs at temperatures approaching the liquefaction temperature of the vapor; for chemisorption, temperatures depend on the particular reaction involved. Water-vapor adsorption to various polar solids can occur at room temperature through hydrogen-bonding, with binding energies intermediate to physisorption and chemisorption.

To study the adsorption of vapors onto solid surfaces, one must measure the amount of gas adsorbed/unit area or unit mass of solid, at different pressures of gas. Because such studies usually are conducted at constant temperature, plots of volume adsorbed versus pressure are known as *adsorption isotherms.* If the physical or chemical adsorption process is

Table 20-6. Ratio of Observed Vapor Pressure (*P*) to Expected Vapor Pressure (*P'*) of Water at 25°C With Varying Droplet Size

P/P'	DROPLET SIZE (µm)
1.001	1
1.01	0.1
1.1	0.01
2.0	0.005
3.0	0.001
4.2	0.00065
5.2	0.00060

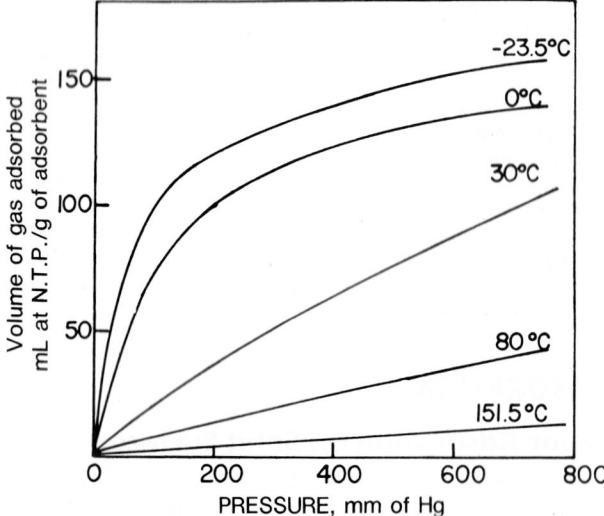

Figure 20-9. Adsorption isotherms for ammonia on charcoal. (From Titoff Z. *Z Phys Chem Leipzig* 1910; 74: 641.)

monomolecular, the adsorption isotherm should appear similar to those shown in Figure 20-9. Adsorption significantly increases with increasing pressure, followed by a leveling off, which is due either to a saturation of available specific chemical groups, as in chemisorption, or to the entire available surface being covered by physically adsorbed molecules. Adsorption reduction with increasing temperature occurs because the adsorption process is exothermic. In the case of physical adsorption at low temperatures after adsorption levels off, often a marked increase in adsorption occurs, presumably due to multilayered adsorption. In this case vapor molecules essentially condense upon themselves as the liquefaction pressure of the vapor is approached. Figure 20-10 illustrates one type of isotherm generally seen with multilayered physisorption.

To have a quantitative understanding of the adsorption process and to be able to compare different systems, two factors must be evaluated. It is important to know the capacity of the solid or the maximum amount of adsorption under a given set of conditions and the affinity of a given substance for the solid surface—how readily does it adsorb for a given amount of pressure? In effect, the second term is the equilibrium constant for the process. For many systems vapor-adsorption data may fit a

very general, but somewhat empirical equation, the Freundlich equation:

$$V_a = kp^n \tag{19}$$

where V_a is the volume of gas adsorbed, p is the gas pressure, and k and n are constants reflecting adsorption affinity and capacity.

A significant theoretical improvement along these lines was the theory of *monomolecular adsorption* proposed by Langmuir. He postulated that for adsorption to occur a solid must contain uniform adsorption sites, each capable of holding a single gas molecule. Molecules colliding with the surface may bounce off elastically or they may remain in contact for a period of time. It is this contact over a period of time that Langmuir termed *adsorption*.

Two major assumptions were made in deriving the adsorption equation:

1. Only those molecules striking an empty site can be adsorbed; hence, only monomolecular adsorption occurs.
2. The forces of interaction between adsorbed molecules are negligible and, therefore, the probability of a molecule adsorbing onto or desorbing from any site is independent of the surrounding sites.

With these assumptions and applying the kinetic theory of gases, it can be shown that

$$V_a = (V_m k'p)/(1 + k'p) \tag{20}$$

where V_m is the volume of gas covering all of the adsorption sites with a single layer of molecules and k' is a constant that reflects the affinity of the gas for the solid.

A test of fit to this equation can be made by expressing it in linear form.

$$\frac{p}{V_a} = \frac{1}{V_m k'} + \frac{p}{V_m} \tag{21}$$

The value of k' is, in effect, the equilibrium constant and may be used to compare affinities of different substances for the solid surface. The value of V_m is valuable because it indicates the maximum number of sites available for adsorption. In the case of physisorption the maximum number of sites is actually the total surface area of the solid; therefore, the value of V_m can be used to estimate surface area if the volume and area/molecule of vapor are known.

Since physisorption most often involves some multilayered adsorption, an equation based on the Langmuir equation, the B.E.T. equation, normally is used to determine V_m and solid surface areas. Equation 22 is the B.E.T. equation:

$$V_a = \frac{V_m cp}{(p_0 - p)[1 + (C - 1)(p/p_0)]} \tag{22}$$

where c is a constant and p_0 is the vapor pressure of the adsorbing substance.[9] Experimentally, the most widely used vapor for this purpose is nitrogen, which adsorbs nonspecifically on most solids near its boiling point at $-195°$ and appears to occupy about 16 Å^2/molecule on a solid surface.

Adsorption from Solution

By far one of the most important aspects of interfacial phenomena encountered in pharmaceutical systems is the tendency for substances dissolved in a liquid to adsorb to various interfaces. Adsorption from solution is generally more complex than that from the vapor state because of the influence of the solvent and any other solutes dissolved in the solvent. Although such adsorption generally is limited to one or two molecular layers at most, the presence of other molecules often makes the interpretation of adsorption mechanisms much more difficult than for chemisorption or physisorption of a vapor. Because monomolecular adsorption from solution is so widespread at all interfaces, we will first discuss the nature of monomolecular films and then return to a discussion of adsorption from solution.

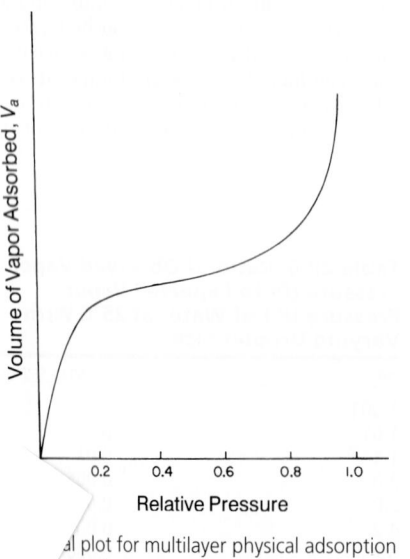

...al plot for multilayer physical adsorption
...lid surface.

Insoluble Monomolecular Films

It was suggested above that molecules exhibiting a tendency to spread out at an interface might be expected to orient so as to reduce the interfacial free energy produced by the presence of the interface. Direct evidence for molecular orientation has been obtained from studies dealing with the spreading on water of insoluble polar substances containing long hydrocarbon chains, such as fatty acids.

In the late 19th century Pockels and Rayleigh showed that a very small amount of olive or castor oil, when placed on the surface of water, spreads out, as discussed above. If the amount of material was less than could physically cover the entire surface, only a slight reduction in the surface tension of water was noted. However, if the surface was compressed between barriers, as shown in Figure 20-11, the surface tension was reduced considerably.

Devaux extended the use of this technique by dissolving small amounts of solid in volatile solvents and dropping the solution onto a water surface. After assisting the water-insoluble molecules to spread, the solvent evaporated, leaving a surface film containing a known amount of solute.

Compression and measurement of surface tension indicated that a maximum reduction of surface was reached when the number of molecules/unit area was reduced to a value corresponding to complete coverage of the surface. This suggested that a monomolecular film forms and that surface tension is reduced upon compression because contact between air and water is reduced by the presence of the film molecules. Beyond the point of closest packing, the film apparently collapses very much as a layer of corks floating on water would be disrupted when laterally compressed beyond the point of initial physical contact.

Using a refined quantitative technique based on these studies, Langmuir[11] spread films of pure fatty acids, alcohols, and esters on the surface of water. Comparing a series of saturated fatty acids, differing only in chain length, he found that the area/molecule at collapse was independent of chain length, corresponding to the cross-sectional area of a molecule oriented in a vertical position (see Fig 20-11). He further concluded that this molecular orientation involved association of the polar carboxyl group with the water phase and the nonpolar alkyl chain out toward the vapor phase.

In addition to the evidence for molecular orientation, Langmuir's work with surface films revealed that each substance exhibits film properties which reflect the interactions between molecules in the surface film. This is seen best by plotting the difference in surface tension of the clean surface γ_0, and that of the surface covered with the film γ, versus the area/molecule A produced by film compression (total area/the number of molecules). The difference in surface tension is called the surface pressure, π, and thus

$$\pi = \gamma_0 - \gamma \qquad (23)$$

Figure 20-12 depicts such a plot for a typical fatty acid monomolecular film. At areas greater than 50Å^2/molecule the molecules are far apart and do not cover enough surface to reduce the surface tension of the clean surface to any extent and thus the lack of appreciable surface pressure. Because the molecules in the film are quite free to move laterally in the sur-

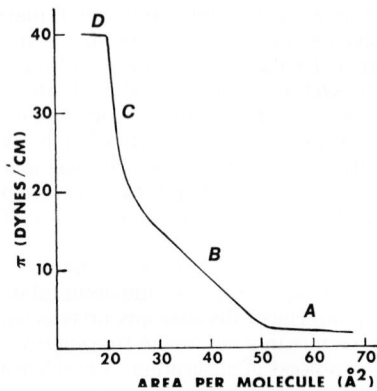

Figure 20-12. A surface pressure–area curve for an insoluble monomolecular film: Region *A*, gaseous film; Region *B*, liquid film; Region *C*, solid film; Region *D*, film collapse.

face, they are said to be in a two-dimensional *gaseous* or *vapor* state.

As the intermolecular distance is reduced upon compression, the surface pressure rises because the air–water surface is being covered to a greater extent. The rate of change in π with A, however, will depend on the extent of interaction between film molecules—the greater the rate of change, the more "condensed" the state of the film.

In Figure 20-12, from 50 to 30 Å^2/molecule, the curve shows a steady increase in π, representative of a two-dimensional "liquid" film, where the molecules become more restricted in their freedom of movement because of interactions. Below 30 Å^2/molecule, the increase in π occurs over a narrow range of A, characteristic of closest packing and a two-dimensional "solid" film.

Any factor tending to increase polarity or bulkiness of the molecule—such as increased charge, number of polar groups, reduction in chain length, or the introduction of aromatic rings, side chains, and double bonds—should reduce molecular interactions. On the other hand, the longer the alkyl chain and the less bulky the polar group, the closer the molecules can approach and the stronger the extent of interaction in the film.

Soluble Films and Adsorption from Solution

If a fatty acid exhibits highly gaseous film behavior on an aqueous surface, a relatively small change in π with A over a considerable range of compression should be expected. Indeed, for short-chain compounds such as lauric acid (12 carbons) or decanoic acid, not only is the change in π small with decreasing A, but at a point just before the expected closest packing area, the surface pressure becomes constant without any collapse.

If lauric acid is converted to the laurate ion, or if a shorter chain acid such as octanoic acid is used, spreading on water and compression of the surface produces no increase in π. These results illustrate that the more polar the molecule (hence, the more *gaseous* the film), the higher the area/molecule where a constant surface pressure occurs. This behavior may be explained by assuming that polar molecules form monomolecular films when spread on water but that, upon compression, they are caused to enter the aqueous bulk solution rather than to remain as an intact insoluble film. The constant surface pressure with increased compression arises because a constant number of molecules/unit area remain at the surface in equilibrium with dissolved molecules. The extent of such behavior will be greater for substances exhibiting weaker intermolecular interaction and greater water solubility.

Starting from the other direction, it can be shown that short-chain acids and alcohols (when dissolved in water) duce the surface tension of water, thus producing a su

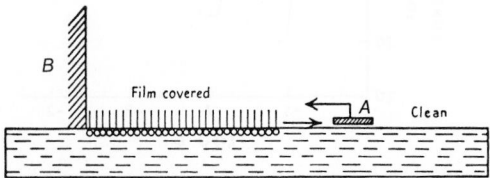

Figure 20-11. Insoluble monomolecular film compressed between a fixed barrier *B*, and a movable barrier *A*. (Osipow LI. *Surface Chemistry: Theory and Applications*. New York: Reinhold, 1962.)

pressure, just as with insoluble films (see Equation 23). That dissolved molecules are accumulating at the interface in the form of a monomolecular film is suggested from the similarity in behavior to systems where lightly soluble molecules are spread on the surface. For example, compressing the surface of a solution containing "surface-active" molecules has no effect on the initial surface pressure, whereas increasing bulk-solution concentration tends to increase surface pressure, presumably by shifting the equilibrium between surface and bulk molecules.

At this point one may ask, why should water-soluble molecules leave an aqueous phase and accumulate or *adsorb* at an air–solution interface? Because any process will occur spontaneously if it results in a net loss in free energy, such must be the case for the process of adsorption. A number of factors will produce such a favorable change in free energy:

- The presence of the oriented monomolecular film reduces the surface free energy of the air–water interface.
- The hydrophobic group on the molecule is in a lower state of energy at the interface, where it no longer is as surrounded by water molecules, than when it is in the bulk-solution phase.
- Increased interaction between film molecules also will contribute to this process.

A further reduction in free energy occurs upon adsorption because of the gain in entropy associated with a change in water structure. Water molecules, in the presence of dissolved alkyl chains are more highly organized or *ice-like* than they are as a pure bulk phase; hence, the entropy of such structured water is lower than that of bulk water.

The process of adsorption requires that the ice-like structure *melt* as the chains go to the interface, and thus an increase in the entropy of water occurs. The adsorption of molecules dissolved in oil can occur but it is not influenced by water structure changes, and hence, only the first factors mentioned are important here.

It is very rare that significant adsorption can occur at the hydrocarbon–air interface as little loss in free energy comes about by bringing hydrocarbon chains with polar groups attached to this interface. On the other hand, at oil–water interfaces, the polar portions of the molecule can interact with water at the interface, leading to significant adsorption.

Thus, whereas water-soluble fatty acid salts are adsorbed from water to air–water and oil–water interfaces, their undissociated counterparts, the free fatty acids, which are water insoluble, form insoluble films at the air–water interface, are not adsorbed from oil solution to an oil–air interface, but show significant adsorption at the oil–water interface when dissolved in oil.

From this discussion it is possible also to conclude that adsorption from aqueous solution requires a lower solute concentration to obtain the same level of adsorption if the hydrophobic chain length is increased or if the polar portion of the molecule is less hydrophilic. On the other hand, adsorption from nonpolar solvents is favored when the solute is quite polar.

Because soluble or adsorbed films cannot be compressed, there is no simple, direct way to estimate the number of molecules/unit area coming to the surface under a given set of conditions. For relatively simple systems it is possible to estimate this value by application of the Gibbs equation, which relates surface concentration to the surface-tension change produced at different solute activities. The derivation of this equation is beyond the scope of this discussion, but it arises from a classical thermodynamic treatment of the change in free ˘gy when molecules concentrate at the boundary between ˘ses. The equation may be expressed as

$$\Gamma = -\frac{a}{RT}\frac{d\gamma}{da} \tag{24}$$

s of solute adsorbed/unit area, R is the gas bsolute temperature and $d\gamma$ is the change in th a change in solute activity, da, at activity a.

For dilute solutions of nonelectrolytes, or for electrolytes when the Debye–Hückel equation for activity coefficient is applicable, the value of a may be replaced by solute concentration, c. Because the term dc/c is equal to $d \ln c$, the Gibbs equation is often written as

$$\Gamma = -\frac{1}{RT}\frac{d\gamma}{d \ln c} \tag{25}$$

In this way the slope of a plot of γ versus $\ln c$ multiplied by $1/RT$ should give Γ at a particular value of c.

Figure 20-13 depicts typical plots for a series of water-soluble surface-active agents differing only in the alkyl chain length. A greater reduction of surface tension occurs at lower concentrations for longer chain-length compounds. In addition, there are greater slopes with increasing concentration, indicating more adsorption (Equation 25), and an abrupt leveling of surface tension at higher concentrations. This latter behavior reflects the self-association of surface-active agent to form micelles which exhibit no further tendency to reduce surface tension. The topic of micelles will be discussed later in Chapter 21.

If one plots the values of surface concentration, Γ versus concentration c, for substances adsorbing to the vapor–liquid and liquid–liquid interfaces, using data such as those given in Figure 20-13, one generally obtains an adsorption isotherm shaped like those in Figure 20-9 for vapor adsorption. Indeed, it can be shown that the Langmuir equation (Equation 20) can be fitted to such data when written in the form

$$\Gamma = \frac{\Gamma_{\max}k'c}{1 + k'c} \tag{26}$$

where $\Gamma_{\max}$ is the maximum surface concentration attained with increasing concentration and k' is related to k in Equation 20. Combining Equations 24 and 26 leads to a widely used relationship between surface-tension change Π (see Equation 23), and solute concentration c, known as the Syszkowski equation.

$$\Pi = \Gamma_{\max}RT \ln (1 + k'c) \tag{27}$$

Mixed Films

It would seem reasonable to expect that the properties of a surface film could be varied greatly if a mixture of surface-active agents were in the film. As an example, consider that a mixture of short- and long-chain fatty acids would be expected to show a degree of *condensation* varying from the gaseous state when the short-chain substance is used in high amount to a highly condensed state when the longer chain substance predomi-

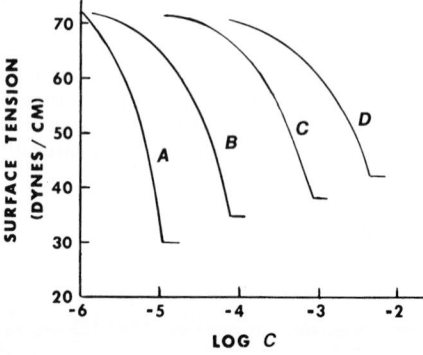

Figure 20-13. The effect of increasing chain length on the surface activity of a surfactant at the air–aqueous solution interface (each curve differs from the preceding or succeeding by two methylene groups with A, the longest chain, and D, the shortest).

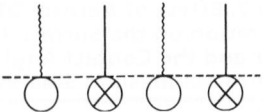

Figure 20-14. A mixed monomolecular film. ≧, a long-chain ion; o, a long-chain nonionic compound.

nates. Thus, each component in such a case would operate independently by bringing a proportional amount of film behavior to the system.

More often, the ingredients of a surface film do not behave independently, but rather interact to produce a new surface film. An obvious example would be the combination of organic amines and acids which are charged oppositely and would be expected to interact strongly. In addition to such polar-group interactions, chain–chain interactions strongly favor mixed condensed films. An important example of such a case occurs when a long-chain alcohol is introduced along with an ionized long-chain substance. Together the molecules form a highly condensed film despite the presence of a high number of like charges. Presumably this occurs as seen in Figure 20-14, by arranging the molecules so that ionic groups alternate with alcohol groups; however, if chain–chain interactions are not strong, the ionic species often will be displaced by the more nonpolar unionized species and will "desorb" into the bulk solution.

On the other hand, sometimes the more soluble surface-active agent produces surface pressures in excess of the collapse pressure of the insoluble film and displaces it from the surface. This is an important concept because it is the underlying principle behind cell lysis by surface-active agents and some drugs, and behind the important process of detergency.

Adsorption from Solution on to Solid Surfaces

Adsorption to solid surfaces from solution may occur if the dissolved molecules and the solid surface have chemical groups capable of interacting. Nonspecific adsorption also will occur if the solute is surface active and if the surface area of the solid is high. This latter case would be the same as occurs at the vapor–liquid and liquid–liquid interfaces. As with adsorption to liquid interfaces, adsorption to solid surfaces from solution generally leads to a monomolecular layer, often described by the Langmuir equation in the form:

$$x/M = [(x/M)mk^*c]/(1 + k^*c) \qquad (28)$$

where x is the amount of adsorbed solute, M is the total weight of solid, x/M is the amount of solute adsorbed per unit weight of solid at concentration c, k^* is a constant, and $(x/M)m$ is the amount of solute per unit weight covering the surface with a complete monolayer. However, as Giles[12] has pointed out, the variety of combinations of solutes and solids, and hence the variety of possible mechanisms of adsorption, can lead to a number of more complex isotherms. In particular, adsorption of surfactants and polymers, of great importance in a number of pharmaceutical systems, still is not understood well on a fundamental level, and may in some situations even be multilayered.

Adsorption from solution may be measured by separating solid and solution and either estimating the amount of adsorbate adhering to the solid or the loss in concentration of adsorbate from solution. In view of the possibility of solvent adsorption, the latter approach really only gives an apparent adsorption. For example, if solvent adsorption is great enough, it is possible to end up with an increased concentration of solute after contact with the solid; here, the term *negative adsorption* is used.

Solvent not only influences adsorption by competing for the surface, but as discussed in connection with adsorption at liquid surfaces, the solvent will determine the escaping tendency of a solute; for example, the more polar the molecule, the less the ad-

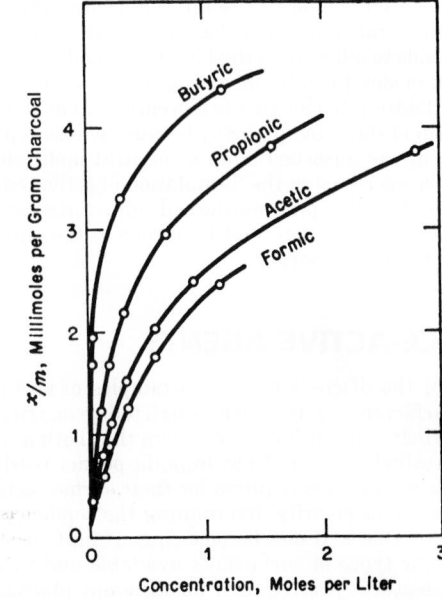

Figure 20-15. The relation between adsorption and molecular weight of fatty acids. (From Weiser HB. *A Textbook of Colloid Chemistry*. New York: Elsevier, 1949.)

sorption that occurs from water. This is seen in Figure 20-15, where adsorption of various fatty acids from water onto charcoal increases with increasing alkyl chain length or nonpolarity. It is difficult to predict these effects, but, in general, the more chemically unlike the solute and solvent and the more alike the solid surface groups and solute, the greater the extent of adsorption. Another factor that must be kept in mind is that charged solid surfaces, such as polyelectrolytes, will strongly adsorb oppositely charged solutes. This is similar to the strong specific binding seen in gas chemisorption, and it is characterized by significant monolayer adsorption at very low concentrations of solute. See Figure 20-16 for an example of such adsorption.

Adsorption onto activated charcoal has been shown to be extremely useful in the emergency treatment of acute overdosage of a variety of drugs taken by the oral route.[15] Overall effectiveness of commercially available activated-charcoal suspen-

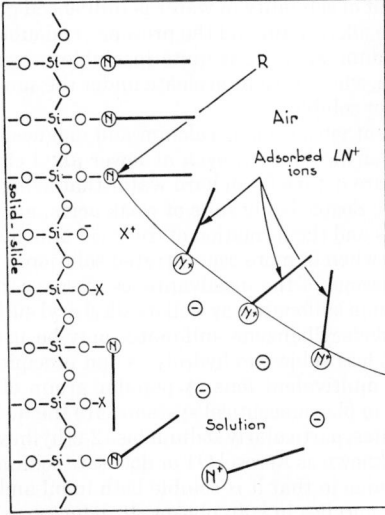

Figure 20-16. The adsorption of a cationic surfactant, LN⁺, onto a negatively charged silica or glass surface, exposing a hydrophobic surface the solid is exposed to air. (From Ter-Minassian-Saraga L. *Adv Chem* 1964; 43: 232.)

sions as an antidote in oral poisonings appears to be directly related to the total charcoal surface area.[16] Drug adsorption to charcoal tends to follow both the Langmuir model as well as the Freundlich model. In addition, a drug that is un-ionized at gastric pH will adsorb to charcoal to a greater extent than will the ionized form of the drug, probably because of less repulsive interactions in the adsorbed state of neutral molecules. Great care must be exercised in the formulation of activated-charcoal suspensions because pharmaceutical adjuvants employed in suspensions have the potential to adsorb to the charcoal and block sites for drug adsorption.

SURFACE-ACTIVE AGENTS

Throughout the discussion so far, examples of surface-active agents (surfactants) have been restricted primarily to fatty acids and their salts. It has been shown that both a hydrophobic portion (alkyl chain) and a hydrophilic portion (carboxyl and carboxylate groups) are required for their surface activity, the relative degree of polarity determining the tendency to accumulate at interfaces. It now becomes important to look at some of the specific types of surfactants available and to see what structural features are required for different pharmaceutical applications.

The classification of surfactants is quite arbitrary, but one based on chemical structure appears best as a means of introducing the topic. It is generally convenient to categorize surfactants according to their polar portions because the nonpolar portion usually is made up of alkyl or aryl groups. The major polar groups found in most surfactants may be divided as follows: anionic, cationic, amphoteric, and nonionic. As shall be seen, the last group is the largest and most widely used for pharmaceutical systems, so that it will be emphasized in the discussion that follows.

Types

ANIONIC AGENTS—The most commonly used anionic surfactants are those containing carboxylate, sulfonate, and sulfate ions. Those containing carboxylate ions are known as soaps and generally are prepared by the saponification of natural fatty acid glycerides in alkaline solution. The most common cations associated with soaps are sodium, potassium, ammonium, and triethanolamine; the chain length of the fatty acids ranges from 12 to 18.

The extent of solubility in water is influenced greatly by the length of the alkyl chain and the presence of double bonds. For example, sodium stearate is quite insoluble in water at room temperature, whereas sodium oleate under the same conditions is quite water soluble.

Multivalent ions, such as calcium and magnesium, produce marked water insolubility, even at lower alkyl chain lengths; thus, soaps are not useful in hard water that is high in content of these ions. Soaps, being salts of weak acids, are subject also to hydrolysis and the formation of free acid plus hydroxide ion, particularly when in more concentrated solution.

To offset some of the disadvantages of soaps, a number of long alkyl chain sulfonates, as well as alkyl aryl sulfonates such as sodium dodecylbenzene sulfonate, may be used; the sulfonate ion is less subject to hydrolysis and precipitation in the presence of multivalent ions. A popular group of sulfonates, widely used in pharmaceutical systems, are the dialkyl sodium sulfosuccinates, particularly sodium bis-(2-ethylhexyl)sulfosuc- best known as Aerosol OT or docusate sodium. This compound is unique in that it is soluble both in oil and water, and forms micelles in both phases. It reduces surface and interfacial tension to low values and acts as an excellent wetting agent in the manufacture of solid dosage forms (Table 20-7).

Alkyl sulfates are available as surfactants, but the most popular member of this group is sodium lauryl sulfate, which is used widely as an emulsifier and solubilizer in pharmaceutical systems. Unlike the sulfonates, sulfates are susceptible to pH-dependent hydrolysis leading to the formation of the long-chain alcohol.

CATIONIC AGENTS—A number of long-chain cations, such as amine salts and quaternary ammonium salts, often are used as surface-active agents when dissolved in water; however, their use in pharmaceutical preparations is limited to that of antimicrobial preservation rather than as surfactants. This arises because the cations adsorb so readily at cell membrane structures in a nonspecific manner, leading to cell lysis (eg, hemolysis), as do anionics to a lesser extent. It is in this way that they act to destroy bacteria and fungi.

Since anionic and nonionic agents are not as effective as preservatives, one must conclude that the positive charge of these compounds is important; however, the extent of surface activity has been shown to determine the amount of material needed for a given amount of preservation. Quaternary ammonium salts are preferable to free amine salts as they are not subject to effect by pH in any way; however, the presence of organic anions such as dyes and natural polyelectrolytes is an important source of incompatibility and such a combination should be avoided.

AMPHOTERIC AGENTS—The major groups of molecules falling into the amphoteric category are those containing carboxylate or phosphate groups as the anion, and amino or quaternary ammonium groups as the cation. The former group is represented by various polypeptides, proteins, and the alkyl betaines; the latter group consists of natural phospholipids such as the lecithins and cephalins. In general, long-chain amphoterics, which exist in solution in zwitterionic form, are more surface active than are ionic surfactants having the same hydrophobic group, because in effect the oppositely charged ions are neutralized. However, when compared to nonionics, they appear somewhere between ionic and nonionic.

PROTEINS—Considering the rapidly growing importance of proteins as therapeutic agents, the unique surface characteristics of these biological macromolecules deserve some special attention. Therapeutic proteins have been shown to be extremely surface active, and they adsorb to clinically important surfaces such as glass bottles and syringes, sterile filters, and plastic IV bags and administration sets; the result is treatment failures. In general, proteins can adsorb to a whole variety of surfaces, both hydrophobic and hydrophilic. From the standpoint of the surface, protein adsorption appears to be maximized when the electrical charge of the surface is opposite that of the protein or when the surface is extremely hydrophobic. From the standpoint of the protein, the extent of adsorption depends on the molecular weight, the number of hydrophobic side chains, and the relative distribution of cationic and anionic side chains. The effect of ionic strength is usually to enhance adsorption by shielding adjacent proteins from repulsive electrical interactions. Adsorption is also maximized when the pH of

Table 20-7. Effect of Aerosol OT Concentration on the Surface Tension of Water and the Contact Angle of Water with Magnesium Stearate

CONCENTRATION (M 3 106)	Γ_{SV}	θ (°)
1.0	60.1	120
3.0	49.8	113
5.0	45.1	104
8.0	40.6	89
10.0	38.6	80
12.0	37.9	71
15.0	35.0	63
20.0	32.4	54
25.0	29.5	50

the protein solution is equal to the pI (isoelectric point) of the molecule, again due to minimized electrical repulsion.

When different proteins compete for adsorption sites on a single surface, the effect of molecular weight becomes most striking. Early in the adsorption process the protein with the smaller molecular weight, which can diffuse to the surface more rapidly, initially occupies the interface. After some time, it is found that the larger molecular weight protein has displaced the smaller protein since the larger molecule has more possible interaction points with the surface and thus greater total energy of interaction.

The most important consequence of therapeutic protein adsorption is the loss of bioactivity, the reasons for which include loss of therapeutic agent by irreversible adsorption to the surface, possible structural changes in the protein induced by the interface, and surface-associated aggregation and precipitation of the protein. Each of these consequences is related to the structure adopted by the protein in the interfacial region. The native three-dimensional structure of a protein in solution is the result of a complex balance between attractive and repulsive forces. Surface can easily disrupt the balance of forces in proteins residing in the interfacial region and cause the molecule to undergo a change, unfolding from the native to the extended configuration. As it is unlikely that the extended configuration will refold back to the native state upon release from the interface, the protein is considered to be denatured. Like other polymers, the unfolding of the protein at the interface is thought to minimize the contact of apolar amino acid side chains with water.

In addition, electrical interactions, both within the protein and between the protein and the surface, strongly modulate the configuration assumed at the interface. Motion of the interface, such as comes about during shaking of a solution, appears to accelerate the surface-associated denaturation. Some proteins appear to be rather vulnerable to surface-induced structural alterations, whereas others are very resistant. Algorithms for predicting those proteins most vulnerable to the structure-damaging effects of interfaces are not yet available. Empirical observations suggest that those proteins easily denatured in solution by elevated temperatures may also be most sensitive to interfacial denaturation.

The best defense against untoward effects on the structure of proteins induced by surfaces appears to be prevention of adsorption. Research in the field of biomaterials has shown that surfaces that are highly hydrophilic are less likely to serve as sites for protein adsorption. Steric hindrance of adsorption by bonding hydrophilic polymers, such as polyethylene oxide, to a surface also appears to be successful in minimizing adsorption. Formulations of proteins intended for parenteral administration frequently contain synthetic surfactants to preserve bioactivity. The specific molecular mechanism of protection is not understood and can involve specific blocking of adsorption to the interface or enhanced removal from the interface before protein unfolding can occur. In support of the former mechanism is the observation that surfactants most successful at protecting proteins from interfacial denaturation contain long polyethylene oxide chains capable of blocking access of the protein to the surface.

PHOSPHOLIPIDS—All lecithins contain the L-α-glycerophosphoylcholine skeleton esterified to two long-chain fatty acids (often oleic, palmitic, stearic, and linoleic). Typically, for pharmaceutical use, lecithins are derived from egg yolk or soybean. Although possessing a polar zwitterionic *head* group, the twin hydrocarbon *tails* result in a surfactant with very low water solubility in the monomer state. With the exception of the skin, phospholipids make up a vast majority of the lipid component of cell membranes throughout the body. As a result, the biocompatibility of lecithin is high, accounting for the increasing popularity of use in formulations intended for oral, topical, and intravenous use. Egg yolk lecithins are used extensively as the main emulsifying agent in the fat emulsions intended for intravenous use.

The ability of the lecithins to form a tough but flexible film between the oil and water phases is responsible for the excellent physical stability shown the IV fat emulsions. In aqueous media, phospholipids are capable of assembling into concentric bilayer structures known as liposomes. The therapeutic advantage of such a lipid assembly for drug delivery depends upon the encapsulation of the active ingredient either within the interior aqueous environment or within the hydrophobic region of the bilayer. Deposition of the liposome within the body appears to be dependent upon a number of factors, including the composition of the phospholipids employed in the bilayer and the diameter of the liposome.

The unique surface properties of phospholipids are critical to the function of the pulmonary system. Pulmonary surfactant is a mixture of phospholipids and other associated molecules secreted by type II pneumocytes. In the absence of pulmonary surfactant (as in a neonate born prematurely), the high surface energy of the pulmonary alveoli and airways can be diminished only by physical collapse of these structures and resulting elimination of the air–water interface. As a consequence of airway collapse, the lung fails to act as an organ of gas exchange. Pulmonary surfactant maintains the morphology and function of the alveoli and airways by markedly decreasing surface energy through decreasing the surface tension of the air–water interface.

The most prevalent component of pulmonary surfactant, dipalmitoylphosphatidylcholine (DPPC), is uniquely responsible for forming the very rigid surface film necessary to reduce the surface tension of the interface to a value near 0. Such an extreme reduction in surface tension is most critical during the process of exhalation of the lung where the air–water interfacial area is decreasing. Although DPPC does form the rigid film, in the absence of additives it is unable to respread over an expanding interface typical of a lung during the inhalation phase. An anionic phospholipid, phosphatidylglycerol, in conjunction with a surfactant-associated protein, SP-C, appears to aid in the respreading of DPPC and to maintain mechanical stability of the interface. A truly remarkable feature is that pulmonary surfactant is able to carry out the cycle of reducing surface tension to near 0 during exhalation and then reexpanding over the interface during inhalation at whatever rate is necessary by the respiratory pattern.

Commercially available pulmonary surfactant replacement preparations contain DPPC as the primary ingredient. Agents that aid in the respreading of DPPC may differ depending upon the source of the surface-active material.

NONIONIC AGENTS—The major class of compounds used in pharmaceutical systems are the nonionic surfactants, as their advantages with respect to compatibility, stability, and potential toxicity are quite significant. It is convenient to divide these compounds into those that are relatively water insoluble and those that are quite water soluble. The major types of compounds making up this first group are the long-chain fatty acids and their water-insoluble derivatives. These include:

- Fatty alcohols such as lauryl, cetyl (16 carbons), and stearyl alcohols
- Glyceryl esters such as the naturally occurring mono-, di-, and triglycerides
- Fatty acid esters of fatty alcohols and other alcohols such as propylene glycol, polyethylene glycol, sorbitan, sucrose, and cholesterol. Included also in this general class of nonionic water-insoluble compounds are the free steroidal alcohols such as cholesterol.

To increase the water solubility of these compounds and to form the second group of nonionic agents, polyoxyethylene groups are added through an ether linkage with one of their alcohol groups. The list of derivatives available is much too long to cover completely, but a few general categories will be given.

The most widely used compounds are the polyoxyethylene sorbitan fatty acid esters, found in pharmaceutical formulations that are to be used both internally and externally. Closely related compounds include polyoxyethylene glyceryl steroidal esters, as well as the comparable polyoxypropylene esters. It is also possible to have a direct ether linkage with the hydrophobic group, as with a polyoxyethylene–stearyl ether or a polyoxyethylene–alkyl phenol. These ethers offer advantages because, unlike the esters, they are quite resistant to acidic or alkaline hydrolysis.

Besides the classification of surfactants according to their polar portion, it is useful to have a method that categorizes them in a manner that reflects their interfacial activity and their ability to function as wetting agents, emulsifiers, and solubilizers. Variation in the relative polarity or nonpolarity of a surfactant significantly influences its interfacial behavior, so some measure of polarity or nonpolarity should be useful as a means of classification.

One such approach assigns a hydrophile–lipophile balance (HLB) number for each surfactant; although the method was developed by a commercial supplier of one group of surfactants, it has received widespread application.

The HLB value, as originally conceived for nonionic surfactants, is merely the percentage weight of the hydrophilic group divided by 5 in order to reduce the range of values. On a molar basis, therefore, a 100% hydrophilic molecule (polyethylene glycol) would have a value of 20. Thus, an increase in polyoxyethylene chain length increases polarity, and hence the HLB value; at constant polar chain length, an increase in alkyl chain length or number of fatty acid groups decreases polarity and the HLB value. One immediate advantage of this system is that to a first approximation one can compare any chemical type of surfactant to another type when both polar and nonpolar groups are different.

Values of HLB for nonionics are calculable on the basis of the proportion of polyoxyethylene chain present; however, to determine values for other types of surfactants, it is necessary to compare physical chemical properties reflecting polarity with those surfactants having known HLB values.

Relationships between HLB and phenomena such as water solubility, interfacial tension, and dielectric constant have been used. Those surfactants exhibiting values greater than 20 (eg, sodium lauryl sulfate) demonstrate hydrophilic behavior in excess of the polyoxyethylene groups alone. Refer to Chapter 22 for further information.

Acknowledgment—The author is grateful to Professor George Zografi for his continuing mentorship and support.

REFERENCES

1. Semat H. *Fundamentals of Physics*, 3rd ed. New York: Holt Rinehart Winston, 1957.
2. Michaels AS. *J Phys Chem* 1961; 65:1730.
3. Ring TA. *Powder Tech* 1991; 65:195.
4. Elamin AA, et al. *Int J Pharmaceut* 1994; 111:159.
5. Dirkson JA, Ring TA. *Chem Eng Sci* 1991; 46:2389.
6. Zisman WA. *Adv Chem Ser* 1964; 43:1.
7. Putz G, et al. *J Appl Physiol* 1994; 76:1425.
8. Titoff Z. *Z Phys Chem Leipzig* 1910; 74:641.
9. Brittain HG. *Physical Characterization of Pharmaceutical Solids*. New York: Dekker, 1995.
10. Osipow LI. *Surface Chemistry: Theory and Applications*. New York: Reinhold, 1962.
11. Langmuir I. *J Am Chem Soc* 1917; 39:1848.
12. Giles CH. In: EH Lucassen-Reynders, ed. *Anionic Surfactants*. New York: Dekker, 1981, Chap 4.
13. Weiser HB. *A Textbook of Colloid Chemistry*. New York: Elsevier, 1949.
14. Ter-Minassian-Saraga L. *Adv Chem Ser* 1964; 43:232.
15. Cooney DO. *Activated Charcoal in Medical Applications*, Dekker, New York, 1995.
16. Modi NB, et al. *Pharm Res* 1994; 11:318.

BIBLIOGRAPHY

Adamson AW. *Physical Chemistry of Surfaces*, 5th ed. New York: Wiley Interscience, 1990.
David JT, Rideal EK. *Interfacial Phenomena*, 2nd ed. New York: Academic Press, 1963.
Hiemenz PC. *Principles of Colloid and Surface Chemistry*, 2nd ed. New York: Dekker, 1986.
MacRitchie F. *Chemistry at Interfaces*. San Diego: Academic Press, 1990.
Shaw DJ. *Introduction to Colloid and Surface Chemistry*, 4th ed. London: Butterworths, 1992.

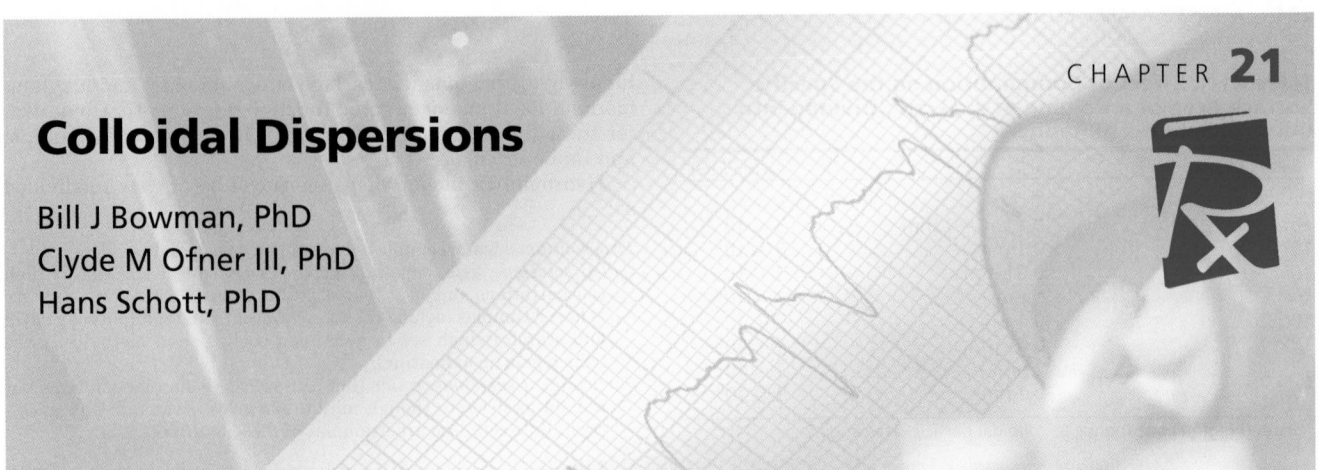

CHAPTER 21

Colloidal Dispersions

Bill J Bowman, PhD
Clyde M Ofner III, PhD
Hans Schott, PhD

The British chemist Thomas Graham applied the term "colloid" (derived from the Greek word for glue) *ca* 1850 to polypeptides such as albumin and gelatin; polysaccharides such as acacia, starch, and dextrin; and inorganic compounds such as gelatinous metal hydroxides and Prussian blue (ferric ferrocyanide). Contemporary colloid and surface chemistry deals with an unusually wide variety of industrial and biological systems. A few examples include catalysts, lubricants, adhesives, latexes for paints, rubbers and plastics, soaps and detergents, clays, ink, packaging films, cigarette smoke, liquid crystals, drug delivery systems, cell membranes, blood, mucous secretions, and aqueous humors.[1–3]

DEFINITIONS AND CLASSIFICATIONS

Colloidal Systems and Interfaces

Except for high molecular weight polymers, most soluble substances can be prepared as either low molecular weight solutions, colloidal dispersions, or coarse suspensions depending upon the choice of dispersion medium and dispersion technique.[4] Colloidal dispersions consist of at least two phases—one or more dispersed or internal phases, and a continuous or external phase called the *dispersion medium* or *vehicle*. Colloidal dispersions are distinguished from solutions and coarse dispersions by the particle size of the dispersed phase, not its composition. Colloidal dispersions contain one or more substances that have at least one dimension in the range of 1–10 nm at the lower end, and a few μm at the upper end (covering about three orders of magnitude). Thus blood, cell membranes, thinner nerve fibers, milk, rubber latex, fog, and beer foam are colloidal systems. Some materials, such as emulsions and suspensions of most organic drugs, are coarser than true colloidal systems but exhibit similar behavior. Even though serum albumin, acacia, and povidone form true or molecular solutions in water, the size of the individual solute molecules places such solutions in the colloidal range (particle size > 1 nm).[1–3,5–10]

Several features distinguish colloidal dispersions from coarse suspensions and emulsions. Colloidal particles are usually too small for visibility in a light microscope because at least one of their dimensions measures 1 μm or less. They are, however, often visible in an ultramicroscope and almost always in an electron microscope. Conversely, coarse suspended particles are usually visible to the naked eye and always in a light microscope. In addition, colloidal particles, as opposed to coarse particles, pass through ordinary filter paper but are retained by dialysis or ultrafiltration membranes. Also, unlike coarse particles, colloidal particles diffuse very slowly and undergo little or no sedimentation or creaming. Brownian motion maintains the dispersion of the colloidal internal phases.

An appreciable fraction of atoms, ions, or molecules of colloidal particles are located in the boundary layer between the particle and the dispersion medium. The boundary layer between a particle and air is commonly referred to as a *surface*; whereas, the boundary layer between a particle and a liquid or solid is commonly referred to as an *interface*. The ions/molecules within the particle and within the medium are surrounded on all side by similar ions/molecules and have balanced force fields; however, the ions/molecules at surfaces or interfaces are subjected to unbalanced forces of attraction. Consequently, a surface free energy component is added to the total free energy of colloidal particles and becomes important as the particles become smaller and a greater fraction of their atoms, ions, or molecules are located in the surface or interfacial region. As a result, the solubility of very fine solid particles and the vapor pressure of very small liquid droplets are greater than the corresponding values for coarse particles and drops of the same materials.

SPECIFIC SURFACE AREA—Decreasing particle size increases the surface-to-volume ratio, expressed as the *specific surface area* (A_{sp}). Specific surface area may expressed as the area (A, cm^2) per unit volume (V, cm^3) or per unit mass (M, gram). For a sphere, $A = 4\pi r^2$ and $V = 4/3\pi r^3$, then A_{sp} is:

$$A_{sp} = \frac{A}{V} = \frac{4\pi r^2}{4/3\pi r^3} = \frac{3}{r}\frac{cm^2}{cm^3} = \frac{3}{r}\ cm^{-1}$$

For density (d) of the material expressed as g/cm^3, the specific surface area is:

$$A_{sp} = \frac{A}{M} = \frac{A}{Vd} = \frac{4\pi r^2}{4/3\pi r^3 d} = \frac{3}{rd}\frac{cm^2}{g}$$

Table 21-1 illustrates the effect of comminution on the specific surface area of a material initially consisting of one sphere having a 1-cm radius. The specific surface area increases as the material is broken into a larger number of smaller and smaller spheres. Activated charcoal and kaolin are solid adsorbents having specific surface areas of about 6×10^6 cm^2/g and 10^4 cm^2/g, respectively. One gram of activated charcoal has a surface area equal to 1/6 acre because of its extensive porosity and internal voids.

Physical States of Dispersed and Continuous Phases

A useful classification of colloidal systems is based upon the state of matter of the dispersed phase and the dispersion medium (ie, whether they are solid, liquid, or gaseous).[2,7,8] Common examples and various combinations are shown in Table 21-2. The terms *sols* and *gels* are often applied to colloidal dispersions of a solid in a liquid or gaseous medium. *Sols* ten

Table 21-1. Effect of Comminution on the Specific Surface Area of a Volume of $4\pi/3$ cm³, Divided into Uniform Spheres of Radius R[a]

NUMBER OF SPHERES	R	A_{sp} (cm²/cm³)
1	1 cm	3
10^3	0.1 cm = 1 mm	3×10
10^6	0.1 mm	3×10^2
10^9	0.01 mm	3×10^3
10^{12}	1 μm	3×10^4
10^{15}	0.1 μm	3×10^5
10^{18}	0.01 μm	3×10^6
10^{21}	1 nm	3×10^7
10^{23}	0.1 nm	3×10^8

[a] Shaded region corresponds to colloidal particle-size range.

to have a lower viscosity and are fluid. If the solid particles form bridged structures possessing some mechanical strength, the system is then called a *gel*. Prefixes typically designate the dispersion medium. For example, hydrosol (or hydrogel), alcosol (or alcogel), and aerosol (or aerogel), designate water, alcohol, and air, respectively.

Interaction Between Dispersed Phases and Dispersion Mediums

Ostwald originated another useful classification of colloidal dispersions based on the affinity or interaction between the dispersed phase and the dispersion medium.[2,3,8] This classification refers mostly to solid-in-liquid dispersions. Colloidal dispersions are divided into the two broad categories, *lyophilic* and *lyophobic*. Some soluble, low molecular weight substances have molecules with both tendencies and associate in solution, forming a third category called *association colloids*.

LYOPHILIC DISPERSIONS

The system is said to be *lyophilic* (solvent-loving) if there is considerable attraction between the dispersed phase and the liquid vehicle (ie, extensive solvation). The system is said to be *hydrophilic* if the dispersion medium is water. Due to the presence of high concentrations of hydrophilic groups, solids such as bentonite, starch, gelatin, acacia, and povidone swell, disperse, or dissolve spontaneously in water to the greatest degree possible without breaking covalent bonds. Hydrophilic colloids often contain ionized groups that dissociate into

highly hydrated ions (eg, carboxylate, sulfonate, and alkylammonium ions) and/or organic functional groups that bind water through hydrogen bonding (eg, hydroxyl, carbonyl, amino, and imino groups).

Hydrophilic colloidal dispersions can be further subdivided as:

True solutions: water-soluble polymers (eg, acacia and povidone).
Gelled solutions, gels, or jellies: polymers present at sufficiently high concentrations and/or at temperatures where their water solubility is low. Examples include relatively concentrated solutions of gelatin and starch (which set to gels upon cooling) and methylcellulose (which gels upon heating).
Particulate dispersions: solids that do not form molecular solutions but remain as discrete though minute particles. Bentonite and microcrystalline cellulose are examples of these hydrosols.

Lipophilic or *oleophilic* substances have a strong affinity for oils. Oils are nonpolar liquids consisting mainly of hydrocarbons having few polar groups and low dielectric constants. Examples include mineral oil, benzene, carbon tetrachloride, vegetable oils (eg, cottonseed or peanut oil), and essential oils (eg, lemon or peppermint oil). Oleophilic colloidal dispersions include polymers such as polystyrene and unvulcanized or gum rubber dissolved in benzene, magnesium, or aluminum stearate dissolved or dispersed in cottonseed oil, and activated charcoal which forms sols or particulate dispersions in all oils.

LYOPHOBIC DISPERSIONS

The dispersion is said to be *lyophobic* (solvent-hating) when there is little attraction between the dispersed phase and the dispersion medium. *Hydrophobic* dispersions consist of particles that are only hydrated slightly or not at all because water molecules prefer to interact with one another instead of solvating the particles. Therefore, such particles do not disperse or dissolve spontaneously in water. Examples of materials that form hydrophobic dispersions include organic compounds consisting largely of hydrocarbon portions with few, if any, hydrophilic functional groups (eg, cholesterol and other steroids); some non-ionized inorganic substances (eg, sulfur); and oleophilic materials such as polystyrene or gum rubber, organic lipophilic drugs, paraffin wax, magnesium stearate, and cottonseed or soybean oils. Materials such as sulfur, silver chloride, and gold form hydrophobic dispersions without being lipophilic. There is no sharp dividing line between hydrophilic and hydrophobic dispersions. For example, gelatinous hydroxides of polyvalent metals (eg, aluminum and magnesium hydroxide) and clays (eg, bentonite and kaolin) possess some characteristics of both.[2,3,6,8] Common *lipophobic* dispersions include water-in-oil emulsions, which are essentially lyophobic dispersions in lipophilic vehicles.

Table 21-2. Classification of Colloidal Dispersions According to State of Matter

DISPERSE PHASE	DISPERSION MEDIUM (VEHICLE)		
	SOLID	LIQUID	GAS
SOLID	Zinc Oxide Paste USP, toothpaste (dicalcium phosphate or calcium carbonate with aqueous sodium carboxymethylcellulose binder), and pigmented plastics (titanium dioxide in polyethylene).	Sols: Bentonite Magma NF, Trisulfapyrimidines Oral Suspension USP, Alumina and Magnesia Oral Suspension USP, Tetracycline Oral Suspension USP, Betamethasone Valerate Lotion USP, and Prednisolone Acetate Ophthalmic Suspension USP.	Solid aerosols: Epinephrine Bitartrate Inhalation Aerosol USP, Isoproterenol Sulfate Inhalation Aerosol USP, smoke, and dust.
	Absorption bases (aqueous medium in Hydrophilic Petrolatum USP), emulsion bases Hydrophilic Ointment Lanolin USP), and butter foams (foamed plastics d rubbers) and pumice	Emulsions: Mineral Oil Emulsion USP, Benzyl Benzoate Lotion USP, and soybean oil in water for parenteral nutrition, milk, and mayonnaise. Foams, carbonated beverages, and effervescent salts in water.	Liquid aerosols: Metaproterenol Sulfate Inhalation Aerosol USP, Povidone-Iodine Topical Aerosol USP, mist, and fog. No colloidal dispersions.

ASSOCIATION COLLOIDS

Organic compounds that contain large hydrophobic moieties on the same molecule with strongly hydrophilic groups are said to be *amphiphilic*. The individual molecules are generally too small to be in the colloidal size range, but they tend to associate into larger aggregates when dissolved in water or oil. These compounds are designated *association colloids* because their aggregates are large enough to qualify as colloidal particles. Examples include surfactant molecules that associate into micelles above their critical micelle concentration (CMC) and phospholipids that associate into cellular membranes and liposomes, which have been used for drug delivery.

PROPERTIES OF COLLOIDAL DISPERSIONS

Particle Shape

Particle shape depends upon the chemical and physical nature of the dispersed phase and the method employed to prepare the dispersion *(preparation methods are described in later sections)*. Primary particles exist in a wide variety of shapes, and their aggregation produces an even wider variety of shapes and structures. Preparation methods such as mechanical comminution and precipitation generally produce randomly shaped particles unless the precipitating solids possess pronounced crystallization habits or the solids being ground possess strongly developed cleavage planes. For example, micronized particles of sulfonamides and other organic powders and precipitated aluminum hydroxide gels typically have irregular random shapes. An exception is bismuth subnitrate; hydrolyzing bismuth nitrate solutions with sodium carbonate precipitates lath-shaped particles. In addition, precipitated silver chloride particles show their cubic nature under the electron microscope. Lamellar or plate-like solids often preserve their lamellar shape during mechanical comminution because milling and micronization break up the stacks of thin plates, in addition to fragmenting plates in the lateral dimensions. In these materials, the molecular cohesion between layers is much weaker than the cohesion within layers. Examples of such materials include graphite, mica, and kaolin (Fig 21-1). In a like manner, macroscopic asbestos and cellulose fibers consist of bundles of microscopic and submicroscopic fibrils that have very small diameters. Mechanical comminution splits these bundles into their component fibrils as well as cutting them shorter. Figure 21-2 shows the individual, needle- or rod-shaped cellulose crystallites formed after breaking up the aggregated bundles of *microcrystalline cellulose*. These crystallites average 0.3 μm in length and 0.02 μm in width, which places them in the colloidal size range. Microcrystalline cellulose is a fibrous thickening agent and tablet additive made by the controlled hydrolysis of cellulose. Its manufacture is described in the 16–18th editions of this text, which also contain an electron micrograph of the porous, spongy, and compressible fibril bundle aggregates used in tableting.

Except in the special cases of clay and cellulose just mentioned, regular shaped particles are typically produced by condensation rather than disintegration methods. For example, *colloidal silicon dioxide* is a white powder consisting of submicroscopic spherical particles of rather uniform size (ie, narrow particle size distribution). It is manufactured by high-temperature, vapor-phase hydrolysis of silicon tetrachloride in an oxy-hydrogen flame (ie, a flame produced by burning hydrogen in a stream of oxygen). It is commonly referred to as fumed or pyrogenic silica because of this manufacturing process. Different grades are produced by different reaction conditions. Figure 21-3 shows the relatively large, single spherical particles of colloidal silicon dioxide. Their average diameter of 50 nm corresponds to the comparatively small specific surface area of 50 m²/g. Smaller spherical particles

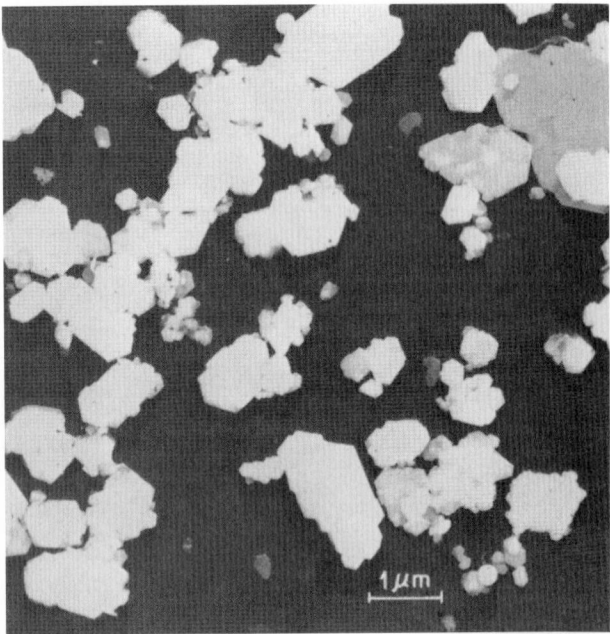

Figure 21-1. Transmission electron micrograph of a well-crystallized, fine-particle kaolin. Note hexagonal shape of the clay platelets (courtesy, John L. Brown, Engineering Experiment Station, Georgia Institute of Technology).

have a larger specific surface area. For example, the grade with the smallest average diameter, 5 nm, has a specific surface area of 380 m²/g. The finer-grade particles tend to sinter or grow together into chain-like aggregates resembling pearl necklaces during the manufacturing process (Fig 21-4). *Latexes* of polymers, such as latex-based paints, are aqueous dispersions prepared by emulsion polymerization. Their particles

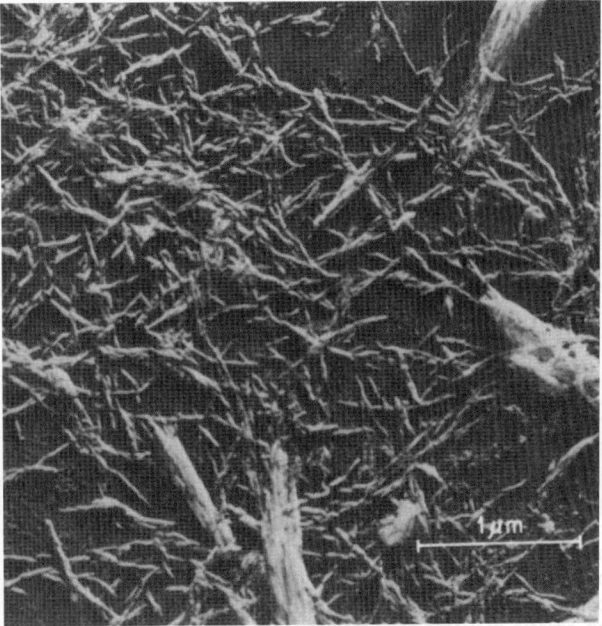

Figure 21-2. Transmission electron micrograph of Avicel RC-591 thickening grade microcrystalline cellulose. The needles are individual cellulose crystallites; some are aggregated into bundles (courtesy, FMC Corporation; Avicel is a registered trademark of FMC Corporation).

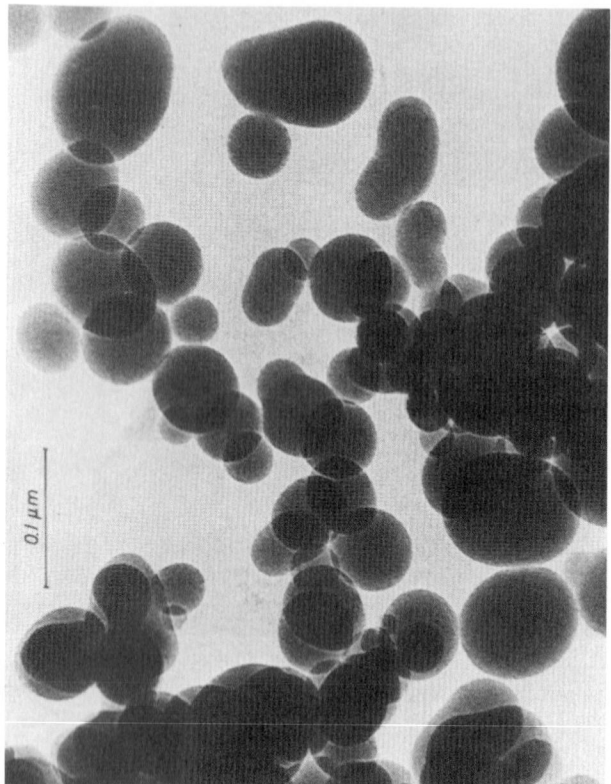

Figure 21-3. Transmission electron micrograph of Aerosil OX 50, ground and dusted on. The spheres are translucent to the electron beam, causing overlapping portions to be darker owing to an increased thickness (courtesy, Degussa AG of Hanau, Germany; Aerosil is a registered trademark of Degussa). The suffix 50 indicates the specific surface area in m²/g.

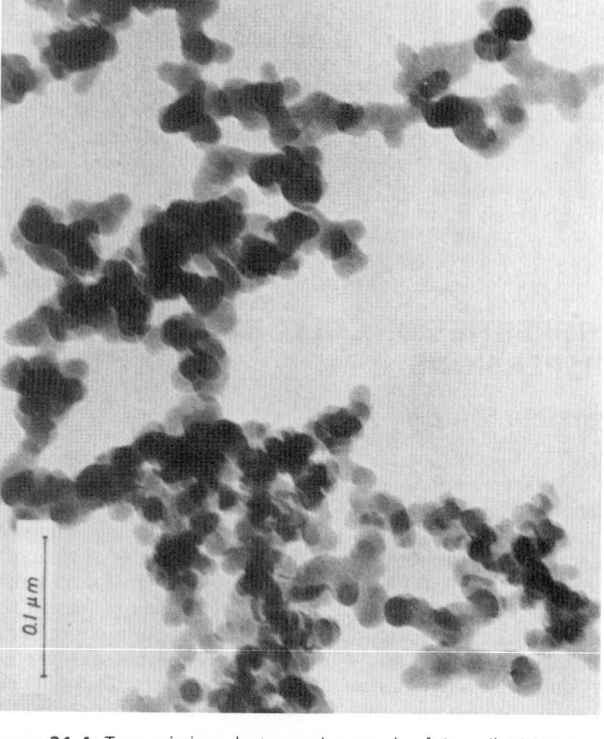

Figure 21-4. Transmission electron micrograph of Aerosil 130, ground and dusted on. The spheres are fused together into chain-like aggregates (courtesy, Degussa AG of Hanau, Germany; Aerosil is a registered trademark of Degussa). The suffix 130 indicates the specific surface area in m²/g.

are spherical because polymerization of the solubilized liquid monomers takes place inside spherical surfactant micelles. Some *clays* grow as plate-like particles possessing straight edges and hexagonal angles (eg, bentonite and kaolin) (Fig 21-1). Other clays have lath-shaped (nontronite) or rod-shaped particles (attapulgite).[11]

Emulsification produces spherical droplets to minimize the oil-water interfacial area. Cooling an emulsion below the melting point of the dispersed phase freezes the dispersed particles in a spherical shape. For instance, paraffin may be emulsified in 80°C water and then cooled to room temperature to produce a hydrosol containing spherical particles. Sols of viruses and globular proteins, which are hydrophilic, contain compact particles possessing definite geometric shapes. For example, the poliomyelitis virus is spherical, the tobacco mosaic virus is rod-shaped, and the serum albumins and globulins are prolate ellipsoids of revolution (football-shaped).

Diffusion and Sedimentation

The molecules of a gas or liquid are engaged in a perpetual and random thermal motion causing collisions with one another and with the container wall billions of times per second. Each collision changes the direction and the velocity of these molecules. The continuous motion of molecules of a dispersion randomly buffets any dissolved molecules and suspended particles. The random bombardment imparts movement called *Brownian motion* to solutes and phenomenon is named after the botanist Robert observed it under the microscope in an aqueous The Brownian motion of colloidal particles random movements of molecules in the liq-

uid or gaseous suspending medium and represents a three-dimensional random walk.

Suspended colloidal particles and solute molecules undergo both rotational and translational Brownian movements. For translational motion, Einstein derived the equation:

$$\bar{x} = \sqrt{2Dt}$$

where $\bar{x}$ is the mean displacement in the x-direction in time, t, and D is the *diffusion coefficient*. Einstein also showed that for spherical particles of radius, r, under conditions valid for Stokes' law and Einstein's law of viscosity:

$$D = \frac{RT}{6\pi\eta rN}$$

where R is the gas constant, T is the absolute temperature, N is Avogadro's number, and η is the viscosity of the suspending medium.

A common measure of the mobility of a dissolved molecule or suspended particle in a liquid medium is the diffusion coefficient. At room temperature, using units of cm²/sec, the value of sucrose in water is 4.7×10^{-6} and the value of serum albumin in water is 6.1×10^{-7}. Diffusion is a slow process on a macroscopic scale. Using the value of 1×10^{-7} cm²/sec, Brownian motion causes a particle to move in one direction an average distance of 1 cm in 58 days, 1 mm in 14 hours, or 1 μm in 0.05 seconds. As seen in the above equation, smaller molecules diffuse faster in a given medium. The radius of a sucrose molecule is smaller than that of a serum albumin molecule; the calculated values are 0.44 nm and 3.5 nm, respectively (assuming a spherical shape). Steroids have only slightly higher molecular weights than sucrose; however, their diffusion coefficients in petrolatum-based absorption bases are in the 10^{-10} to 10^{-8}

cm²/sec range. These much smaller diffusion coefficients are caused by the much higher vehicle viscosity. Passive diffusion (driven by a concentration gradient and carried out through Brownian motion) is important in the release of drugs from topical preparations and in the gastrointestinal absorption of drugs.

Brownian motion and convection currents maintain dissolved molecules and small colloidal particles in suspension indefinitely. This is true for all intrinsically stable systems when dissolution or dispersion occurs spontaneously and the corresponding free energy change is negative (see below). In metastable or diuturna dispersions, Brownian motion prevents sedimentation and may extend their life for years.

As particle size or r increases, Brownian motion decreases as seen by the $\bar{x}$ proportionality to $r^{-1/2}$. Larger particles have a greater tendency than smaller particles of the same material to settle to the bottom of the dispersion, provided the densities of the dispersed phase, d_P, and the liquid vehicle, d_L, are sufficiently different (sedimentation, when $d_P > d_L$). On the other hand, larger particles will rise to the top of the dispersion when $d_P < d_L$. This is known as creaming. The Stokes equation reflects the rate of *sedimentation/creaming*; it is expressed as:

$$h = \frac{2(d_P - d_L)r^2 g t}{9\eta}$$

where h is the height (or distance) that a spherical particle moves in time, t, and g is the acceleration of gravity. The equation illustrates that this rate is proportional to r^2. Consequently, as Brownian motion diminishes with increasing particle size, the tendency of particles to sediment or cream is increased. At a critical radius, the distance, h, that a particle settles/creams equals the mean displacement, $\bar{x}$, due to Brownian motion over the same time interval, t, and therefore, the two are equal.[12] Intravenous vegetable oil emulsions have little tendency to cream because their mean droplet size, ~0.2 μm, is smaller than the critical radius. In most pharmaceutical suspensions, sedimentation prevails.

Light Scattering

The optical properties of a medium are determined by its refractive index. Light will pass through the medium undeflected when the refractive index is uniform throughout. However, when there are discrete variations in the refractive index from the presence of particles or caused by small-scale density fluctuations, part of the passing light will be scattered in all directions. When a narrow beam of sunlight is admitted through a small hole into a darkened room, bright flashing points reveal the presence of the minute dust particles suspended in the air. A beam of light striking a particle polarizes the atoms and molecules of that particle and induces dipoles, which act as secondary sources and reemit weak light of the same wavelength as the incident light. This phenomenon is called *light scattering*. The scattered radiation propagates in all directions away from the particle. In a bright room, the light scattered by the dust particles is too weak to be noticeable.

Colloidal particles suspended in a liquid also scatter light. When an intense, narrowly defined beam of light is passed through a suspension, its path becomes visible because of the light scattered by the particles in the beam. This *Tyndall Beam* is characteristic of colloidal systems and becomes most visible when viewed against a dark background in a direction perpendicular to the incident beam. The magnitude of the turbidity or opalescence depends upon the nature, size, and concentration of the dispersed particles. For example, when clear mineral oil is dispersed in an equal volume of a clear, aqueous surfactant solution, the resultant emulsion is milky white and opaque due to light scattering. However, microemulsions containing emulsified droplets that are only about 40 nm in diameter (ie, much smaller than the wavelength of visible light) are transparent and clear to the naked eye.

The concentration of inorganic and organic colloidal dispersions and of bacterial suspensions can be measured by their Tyndall effect or turbidity. Turbidity, τ, is defined by an equation analogous to Beer's law for the absorption of light,[2,5–8] namely:

$$\tau = \frac{1}{l} \ln \frac{I_0}{I_t}$$

where I_0 and I_t are the intensities of the incident and transmitted light beams, and l is the length of the dispersion through which the light passes. The concentration of dispersed particles may be measured in two ways using turbidity. In *turbidimetry*, a spectrophotometer or photoelectric colorimeter is used to measure the intensity of the light transmitted in the incident direction. The theoretical and practical aspects of determining the particle size of suspensions by *turbidimetry* and the feasibility of estimating their particle-size distribution are discussed in two chapters by Kourti et al.[13] If the dispersion is less turbid, the intensity of light scattered at 90° to the incident beam is measured with a *nephelometer*. Both methods require careful standardization, using suspensions that contain known amounts of particles similar to those being studied. The turbidity of hydrophilic colloidal systems such as aqueous solutions of gums, proteins, and other polymers is far weaker than that of lyophobic dispersions. These solutions appear clear to the naked eye; however, their turbidity can be measured with a photoelectric cell/photomultiplier tube and used to determine the molecular weight of the solute.

The theory of light scattering was developed in detail by Lord Rayleigh. For white, nonabsorbing nonconductors or dielectrics like sulfur and insoluble organic compounds, the equation obtained for spherical particles whose radius is small compared to the wavelength of light (λ) is:[2,5–8]

$$I_s = I_0 \frac{4\pi^2 n_0^2 (n_1 - n_0)^2}{\lambda^4 d^2 c} (1 + \cos^2 \theta)$$

I_0 is the intensity of the unpolarized incident light; I_s is the intensity of light scattered in a direction making an angle, θ, with the incident beam and measured at a distance, d. The scattered light is largely polarized. The concentration, c, is expressed as the number of particles per unit volume. The refractive indices, n_1 and n_0, refer to the dispersion and the dispersion medium, respectively. Since the intensity of scattered light is inversely proportional to the fourth power of the wavelength, blue light (λ ≅ 450 nm) is scattered much more strongly than red light (λ ≅ 650 nm). Colloidal dispersions of colorless particles appear blue when the incident white light is viewed in scattered light (ie, in lateral directions such as 90° to the incident beam). Loss of the blue rays due to preferential scattering leaves the transmitted light yellow or red. Preferential scattering of blue radiation sideways accounts for the blue color of the sky, sea, cigarette smoke, and diluted milk and for the yellow-red color of the rising and setting sun viewed head-on.

The particles in pharmaceutical suspensions, emulsions, and lotions are generally larger than the wavelength of light, λ. When the particle size exceeds λ/20, destructive interference between the light scattered by different portions of the same particle lowers the intensity of the scattered light and changes its angular dependence. Rayleigh's theory was extended to large and strongly absorbing and conducting particles by Mie and to nonspherical particles by Gans.[1,2,5–8] It is possible to determine the average particle size and even the particle size distribution of colloidal dispersions and coarser suspensions by means of turbidity measurements using appropriate precautions in experimental techniques and interpretations.

DYNAMIC LIGHT SCATTERING—Light scattered by a moving particle undergoes a Doppler shift; its frequency increases slightly when the particle moves towards the photodetector and decreases slightly when it moves away. This shift is so small that it can only be detected by very intense, strictly monochromatic laser light. Because they are engaged in random Brownian motion, a set of colloidal particles scatters with a broadened frequency. Smaller particles diffuse faster than larger ones and therefore produce greater Doppler broadening. If the particles are spherical, monodisperse, and their concentration is so dilute that they neither attract nor repel one another, the frequency broadening can be used to estimate the particle diffusion coefficient, D. As noted above, the diffusion coefficient is inversely proportional to the particle radius. The measured radius is actually the hydrodynamic radius (r_H), which comprises the particle plus its attached water of hydration. The technique is called *dynamic* or *quasi-elastic light scattering*. The technique is also called *photon correlation spectroscopy* (PCS) because it counts and correlates the number of scattered photons over very short time intervals. For polydisperse spherical colloidal particles, it estimates the particle size distribution.[2,5,8,9] Particles that are asymmetric rather than spherical and/or extensively hydrated have a larger r_H and hence smaller D value than unsolvated spherical particles with the same dry volume. It is not possible to separate the effect of hydration upon r_H, and D from the effect of asymmetry by PCS alone; either hydration or particle shape must be determined by other means.[2,5,7–9]

In a related technique that uses a *fiber-optic Doppler anemometer* (FODA), a laser beam is carried into the interior of a colloidal dispersion via a fiber-optic cable. Particles in the small volume of dispersion around the immersed tip scatter light with the Doppler frequency shift back into the same fiber to the detector. This method is suitable for concentrated dispersions that are opaque to the laser beam and would have to be diluted extensively for conventional dynamic light scattering measurements[14] (see also the chapter by JC Thomas in reference 13).

Viscosity

Most lyophobic dispersions have viscosities only slightly greater than that of the liquid vehicle. This holds true even at comparatively high volume fractions of the disperse phase unless the particles form continuous network aggregates throughout the vehicle, in which case yield stresses are observed. By contrast, the apparent viscosities of lyophilic dispersions, especially of polymer solutions, are several orders of magnitude greater than the viscosity of the solvent or vehicle even at concentrations of only a few percent solids. Lyophilic dispersions are also generally much more pseudoplastic or shear-thinning than lyophobic dispersions.

Gel Formation

The flexible chains of dissolved polymers interpenetrate and entangle because of the constant Brownian motion of their segments. The chains constantly writhe and change their conformations. Each chain is encased in a sheath of solvent molecules that solvate its functional groups. For example, water molecules are hydrogen-bonded to the hydroxyl groups of polyvinyl alcohol, hydroxyl groups, and ether linkages of polysaccharides, ether linkages of polyethylene oxide or polyethylene glycol, amide groups of polypeptides and povidone, and carboxylate groups of anionic polyelectrolytes. This envelope of water of hydration prevents chain segments that are in close proximity from touching and attracting one another through interchain hydrogen bonds and van der Waals forces as they do in the solid state. The free solvent between the chains' solvation sheaths acts as a lubricant allowing the sol- chains to slip past one another when the solution flows. any factor that lowers the hydration of dissolved es will reduce or thin out the sheath of hydration nt chains. When hydration is low, contiguous t one another through secondary valence gen bonds and van der Waals forces, which d reversible cross-links between the chains at

their points of contact or entanglement, thus bringing about phase separation or precipitation. Hydrophobic bonding is an important contribution to the interchain attraction between polypeptide chains even in solution.

Most water-soluble polymers have a higher solubility in hot water than in cold water and tend to precipitate upon cooling because the sheaths of hydration surrounding adjacent chains become too sparse to prevent interchain attraction. Cooling dilute solutions tends to separate them into a solvent phase and a viscous liquid phase that contains practically the entire amount of polymer but still a large excess of solvent. This process is called *simple coacervation* and the polymer-rich liquid phase is referred to as a *coacervate*.[1,15] If the polymer solution is concentrated enough and/or the temperature is low enough, cooling causes the formation of a continuous network of precipitating chains attached to one another through weak crosslinks that consist of interchain hydrogen bonds and van der Waals forces at the points of mutual contact. Segments of regularly sequenced polymer chains will associate laterally into crystalline bundles or crystallites. However, irregular chain structures, such as those found in random copolymers, randomly substituted cellulose ethers and esters, and highly branched polymers like acacia, will prevent crystallization during precipitation from solution. In these cases, chain entanglements provide the sole temporary crosslinks. A network of associated polymer chains immobilizes the solvent, which may result in the separation of gelatinous precipitates or highly swollen flocs, and in the case of more concentrated polymer solutions, may even cause the solution to set to a gel.

The most important factors causing phase separation, precipitation, and gelation of polymer solutions are the chemical nature of the polymer and the solvent, temperature, polymer concentration, and polymer molecular weight. Lower temperatures, higher concentrations, and higher molecular weights promote *gelation* and produce stronger gels. For a typical *gelatin,* 10% solutions acquire yield values and begin to gel at about 25° C, 20% solutions gel at about 30° C, and 30% solutions gel at about 32° C. The gelation is reversible, and the gels liquefy when heated above these temperatures. Regardless of concentration, gelation is rarely observed above 34° C, and therefore, gelatin solutions do not gel at body temperature (ie, 37° C). Agar and pectic acid solutions set to gels at only a few percent of solids. Unlike most water-soluble polymers, methylcellulose, hydroxypropyl cellulose, and polyethylene oxide are more soluble in cold water than in hot water. Therefore, their solutions tend to gel upon heating (ie, *thermal gelation*) instead of cooling.

When dissolving powdered polymers in water, temporary gel formation often slows dissolution considerably. As water diffuses into loose clumps of the powder, their exterior frequently turns to a cohesive gel of solvated particles encasing the remaining dry powder. Such globs of gel dissolve very slowly because of their high viscosity and the low diffusion coefficients of the polymers. For large-scale dissolution, it is helpful to disperse the polymer powder in water at temperatures where the solubility of the polymer is lowest before it can agglomerate into lumps of gel. Most polymer powders, such as sodium carboxymethylcellulose, are dispersed with high shear in *cold* water before the particles can hydrate and swell into sticky gel grains that agglomerate into lumps. Once the powder is well dispersed, the mixture is heated with moderate shear to about 60°C for the quickest dissolution. Because methylcellulose hydrates more slowly in hot water, the powder is dispersed with high shear in 1/5 to 1/3 of the required amount of water heated to 80–90° C. Once the powder is finely dispersed, the remaining amount of water is added cold, or even as ice, and moderate stirring causes prompt dissolution. For maximum clarity, fullest hydration, and highest viscosity, the solution should be cooled to 0–10° C for about an hour. Alternatively, the polymer powder may be prewetted with a water-miscible organic solvent (eg, ethyl alcohol or propylene glycol) that does not swell the polymer. The solvent should be added in a proportion of 3–5 parts of solvent to one part of polymer. If other nonpolymeric, powdered adjuvants are to be incorporated into the solution, they are dry-blended with the polymer powder and should comprise only 1/4 or less of the blend for the best results.

Large increases in the concentration of polymer solutions may lead to precipitation and gelation. One way of effectively increasing the concentration of aqueous polymer solutions is to add inorganic salts. The salts will bind part of the water in the solution in order to become hydrated. Competition for water of hydration dehydrates the polymer molecules and precipitates them. This phenomenon is called *salting out* and may cause the polymer to separate as a concentrated, viscous liquid solution, a simple coacervate, or a solid gel. Because of its high solubility in water, ammonium sulfate is often used to precipitate and separate proteins from dilute solutions. However, salting out is reversible and subsequent addition of water redissolves the precipitated polymers and liquefies their gels.

HOFMEISTER OR LYOTROPIC SERIES—The effectiveness of electrolytes to cause salting out depends upon their extent of hydration. The *Hofmeister or lyotropic series* arranges ions in order of increasing hydration and increasing effectiveness in salting out hydrophilic colloids. The series for monovalent and divalent cations are

$$Cs^+ < Rb^+ < NH_4^+ < K^+ < Na^+ < Li^+$$

and

$$Ba^{2+} < Sr^{2+} < Ca^{2+} < Mg^{2+}$$

The Hofmeister series governs many colloidal phenomena, including the effect of salts upon the temperature of gelation, the swelling of aqueous gels, and the viscosity of hydrosols, and the permeability of membranes towards salts. The series is observed in many phenomena involving small atoms or ions and true solutions, including the ionization potential and electronegativity of metals; the heats of hydration of cations; the size of hydrated cations; the viscosity, surface tension, and infrared spectra of salt solutions; and the solubility of gases in salt solutions. This series also arranges cations in order of increasing ease in displacement from cation-exchange resins based on the smaller hydrated specie size (eg, K^+ displaces Na^+ and Li^+). Adsorption in the Stern layer of particles (see below) also illustrates the series. The lithium ion is more extensively hydrated, and therefore, Li^+ (aq), including the hydration shell, is larger than Cs^+ (aq). Due to its smaller size, the hydrated cesium ion can approach a negative particle's surface more closely than the hydrated lithium ion. Moreover, because of its greater electron cloud, the Cs^+ ion is more polarizable than the Li^+ ion. Therefore, the Cs^+ ion is more strongly adsorbed in the Stern layer.

For anions, in order of decreasing effectiveness in salting out, the lyotropic series is

$$F^- > citrate^{3-} > HPO_4^{2-} > tartrate^{2-} > SO_4^{2-} > acetate^- >$$

$$Cl^- > NO_3^- > ClO_3^- > Br^- > ClO_4^- > I^- > CNS^-$$

Iodides and thiocyanates, and to a lesser extent bromides and nitrates, actually tend to increase the solubility of polymers in water (ie, salt them in).[1,2,5–8] These large polarizable anions reduce the extent of hydrogen bonding among water molecules, and thereby, make more of the hydrogen-bonding capacity of water available to the solute. Most salts, except for nitrates, bromides, perchlorates, iodides, and thiocyanates, raise the temperature of precipitation or gelation of most hydrophilic colloidal solutions. Exceptions among hydrophilic colloids are methylcellulose, hydroxypropyl cellulose, and polyethylene oxide, whose gelation temperatures or gel melting points are lowered by salting out.

Most hydrophilic sols require electrolyte concentrations of 1 *M* or higher to induce precipitation or gelation. In addition, hydrophilic colloids disperse or dissolve spontaneously in water and their sols are intrinsically stable. Therefore, the polymer may be redissolved by removing the coagulating salt through dialysis or by adding more water. Whenever hydrophilic colloidal dispersions undergo irreversible precipitation or gelation, chemical reactions are involved. Neither dilution with water, heating, nor attempts to remove the gelling or precipitating agent by washing or dialysis will liquefy these gels.

Most of the hydrophilic and water-soluble polymers mentioned previously are only slightly soluble or insoluble in alcohol. Addition of alcohol to their aqueous solutions may cause precipitation or gelation because it lowers the dielectric constant of the medium and tends to dehydrate the hydrophilic solute. Alcohol also lowers the concentrations at which electrolytes salt out hydrophilic colloids. Therefore, alcohol is often referred to as a nonsolvent or precipitant. However, the addition of alcohol to an aqueous polymer solution may cause coacervation (ie, the separation of a concentrated viscous liquid phase) rather than precipitation or gel formation. Sucrose also competes for water of hydration with hydrophilic colloids and may cause phase separation. However, most hydrophilic sols tolerate substantially higher concentrations of sucrose than of electrolytes or alcohol. Lower viscosity grades of a given polymer are usually more resistant to the effects of electrolytes, alcohol, and sucrose than grades having higher viscosities and molecular weights.

The gelation temperature or gel point of gelatin is highest at its isoelectric point, where the attachment of adjacent chains through ionic bonds between carboxylate ions and alkylammonium, guanidinium, or imidazolium groups is most extensive. Since carboxyl groups are not ionized in strongly acidic media such as gastric juices, interchain ionic bonds are practically nonexistent in this environment and interchain attraction is limited to hydrogen bonds and van der Waals forces. Therefore, the combination of an acidic pH that is considerably below the isoelectric point and a temperature of 37° C completely prevents the gelation of gelatin solutions. Conversely, if a polymer owes its solubility to the ionization of these weakly acid groups, reducing the pH of its solution below 3 may lead to precipitation or gelation. This is observed with carboxylated polymers such as many gums, sodium carboxymethylcellulose, and carbomer. Adjusting the media to higher pH values returns the carboxyl groups to their ionized state and reverses the gelation or precipitation. However, gelation temperatures typically depend more upon temperature and concentration than pH.[16,17]

Hydrogen carboxymethylcellulose swells and disperses but does not dissolve in water. Only the sodium, potassium, ammonium, and triethanolammonium salts of carboxylated polymers are well soluble in water. In the case of carboxymethylcellulose, salts with heavy metal cations (eg, silver, copper, mercury, lead) and trivalent cations (eg, aluminum, chromic, ferric) are practically insoluble. Salts with divalent cations, especially of the alkaline earth metals, have borderline solubilities. Generally, higher degrees of substitution tend to increase the tolerance of carboxymethylcellulose toward salts.

When inorganic salts of heavy or trivalent cations are mixed with alkali metal salts of carboxylated polymers in solution, precipitation or gelation occurs due to metathesis. For instance, if a soluble copper salt is added to a solution of sodium carboxymethylcellulose, the double decomposition can be schematically written as:

$$R_1COO^-Na^+ + R_2COO^-Na^+ + CuSO_4 \rightarrow$$

R_1 and R_2 represent two carboxymethylcellulose chains, which are cross-linked by a chelated copper ion. Dissociation of the cupric carboxylate complex is negligible.

Electric Properties

ORIGIN OF ELECTRIC CHARGES—Particles can acquire charges from several sources. In *proteins,* one end group of the polypeptide chain and any aspartic and glutamic acid units contribute carboxylic acid groups, which are ionized into negatively charged carboxylate ions in neutral to alkaline media. The other chain end group and any lysine units contribute amino groups, while arginine units contribute guanidine groups, and histidine units contribute imidazole groups. The nitrogen atoms of these groups become protonated in neutral to acid media. These covalently attached anions and cations confer a negative and positive charge to the molecule, respectively. Therefore, proteins may be referred to as *polyelectrolytes* (polymeric electrolytes or salts). However, they are not the only organic polymers that contain ionic groups, and thus, many substances may be considered to be polyelectolytes. For example, natural polysaccharides of vegetable origin such as acacia, tragacanth, alginic acid, and pectin contain carboxylic acid groups, which are ionized in neutral to alkaline media. Agar and carrageenan, as well as the animal polysaccharides heparin and chondroitin sulfate, contain sulfate groups, which are strongly acidic and ionize even in acid media. Cellulosic polyelectrolytes include *sodium carboxymethylcellulose,* while synthetic carboxylated polymers include *carbomer,* a copolymer of acrylic acid.

Counterions are required for electroneutrality of the ionizing groups on polyelectrolytes. Counter-ions dissociate from ionogenic functional groups and can be replaced by other ions of like charge. For example, in neutral and alkaline media, Na^+, K^+, Ca^{2+}, and Mg^{2+} are among the counterions neutralizing the negative charges of the carboxylate groups, and if hydrochloric acid was used to make the medium acidic and to supply the protons, Cl^- is present to neutralize any of the cationic groups mentioned previously. These counterions are not an integral part of the protein particle but are located in its immediate vicinity. Alternatively, at a specific intermediate pH value (4.5–7 for most proteins), the carboxylate anions and the alkyllammonium, guanidinium, and imidazolium cations on the same molecule neutralize each other exactly. There is no need for counterions because the ionized functional groups are in exact balance. At this pH value, called the *isoelectric point,* the protein particle or molecule is neutral; its electrical charge is neither negative nor positive, but zero.[2,6,8]

Most inorganic particulate compounds are also charged. *Aluminum hydroxide,* $Al(OH)_3$, may be dissolved by acids and alkalis to form aluminum ions, Al^{3+}, and aluminate ions, $Al(OH)_4^-$, respectively. In neutral or weakly acid media (ie, acid concentrations too low to cause dissolution), an aluminum hydroxide particle has some positive charges attributed to Al^{3+} valences that have not been completely neutralized. The schematic below represents a portion of the surface of an aluminum hydroxide particle that has one such positive charge neutralized by a Cl^- counterion:

In weakly alkaline media (ie, base concentrations too low to transform the aluminum hydroxide particles completely into aluminate and dissolve them), the aluminum hydroxide particles bear some negative charges due to the presence of a few aluminate groups. The schematic below represents a portion of the surface of an aluminum hydroxide particle that has one such negative group neutralized by a Na^+ counterion:

At a pH of 8.5 to 9.1, there are neither $Al(OH)_2^+$ nor $Al(OH)_4^-$ ions on the particle surface but only neutral $Al(OH)_3$ molecules.[18,19] Therefore, the particles have no charge and do not need counterions for charge neutralization. This pH is considered to be the isoelectric point. In the case of inorganic particulate compounds such as aluminum hydroxide, it also is called the *zero point of charge.*

Bentonite clay is a lamellar aluminum silicate. Each lattice layer consists of a sheet of hydrated alumina sandwiched between two silica sheets. Isomorphous replacement of Al^{3+} by Mg^{2+} or of Si^{4+} by Al^{3+} confers net negative charges to the thin clay lamellas in the form of cation-exchange sites resembling silicate ions built into the lattice. The counterions producing electroneutrality are usually Na^+ (sodium bentonite) or Ca^{2+} (calcium bentonite).

Silver iodide sols can be prepared by the reaction:

$$AgNO_3 + NaI \rightarrow AgI(s) + NaNO_3$$

In the bulk of the silver iodide particles, there is a 1:1 stoichiometric ratio of Ag^+:I^- ions. If the above reaction is carried out with an excess of silver nitrate, there will be more Ag^+ ions than I^- ions in the surface layer of the particles. The particles will then be positively charged and the counterions surrounding them will be NO_3^-. If the reaction is carried out using an exact stoichiometric 1:1 ratio of silver nitrate to sodium iodide or with an excess sodium iodide, the surface of the particles will contain more I^- ions than Ag^+ ions.[6–8] The particles will then be negatively charged and the counterions surrounding them will be Na^+.

An additional mechanism through which particles acquire electric charges is by the adsorption of ions,[5,7,8,10] including ionic surfactants. This is discussed in more detail in a later section.

ELECTRIC DOUBLE LAYERS—As described previously, the surface layer of a silver iodide particle prepared using an excess of sodium iodide contains more I^- ions than Ag^+ ions; whereas, the bulk of the particle contains the two ions in an equimolar proportion. The aqueous solution in which such particles are suspended contains relatively high concentrations of Na^+ and NO_3^-, a lower concentration of I^-, and traces of H^+, OH^-, and Ag^+. The negatively charged particle surface attracts positive ions from the solution and repels negative ions. Therefore, the solution immediately surrounding the particle surface contains a much higher concentration of Na^+ (counterions) and a much lower concentration of NO_3^- ions than in the bulk solution. A number of Na^+ ions equal to the number of excess I^- ions in the surface (ie, the number of I^- ions in the surface layer minus the number of Ag^+ ions in the surface layer) and equivalent to the net negative surface charge of a particle are pulled towards its surface. These counterions tend to approach the particle surface as closely as their hydration spheres permit (Helmholtz double layer); however, thermal agitation of the water molecules tends to disperse them throughout the solution. Consequently, the layer of counterions surrounding the particle is spread out. The Na^+ ion concentration is highest in the immediate vicinity of the negative surface, where the ions form a compact layer called the Stern layer. The Na^+ ion concentration decreases with distance from the surface, throughout a diffuse layer called the Gouy-Chapman layer. Therefore, the sharply defined, negatively charged particle surface is surrounded by a cloud of Na^+ counterions required for electroneutrality. The combination of the two layers of oppositely charged ions constitutes an electric double layer, which is illustrated in the top part of Figure 21-5.

The electric potential of a plane is equal to the work required to bring a unit electric charge from infinity (in this case, from the bulk of the solution) to that plane against electrostatic forces. If the plane is the surface of a particle, the potential is called surface or ψ_0 potential, which measures the total potential of the double layer (Fig 21-5). This is the thermodynamic potential that operates in galvanic cells. Upon moving away from the particle surface towards the bulk solution in the direction of the horizontal axis, the potential drops rapidly across the Stern layer because the Na^+ ions in the immediate vicinity of the particle surface screen Na^+ ions that are farther removed in the diffuse part of the double layer from the effect of the negative surface charge. The decrease in potential across the Gouy-Chapman layer is more gradual. As the composition of the diffuse double layer gradually approaches that of the bulk liquid, where the anion concentration equals the cation concentration, the potential asymptotically approaches zero. In view of this indefinite end point, the thickness of the diffuse double layer (δ) is arbitrarily defined as the distance over which it takes the potential at the boundary between the Stern and Gouy-Chapman layers to drop to 0.37 *(equal to 1/e)* of its value (Fig 21-5).[1,2,4,6–10] The thickness of double layers usually ranges from 1 to 100 nm and decreases as the concentration of electrolytes in solution increases. This occurs more rapidly for higher valence counterions. The value of δ is approximately equal to the reciprocal of the Debye-Hückel theory parameter (κ).

The electrokinetic or ζ (zeta) potential has practical importance because it can be measured experimentally. In aqueous dispersions, organic particles containing polar functional groups, and even relatively hydrophobic inorganic particles, are surrounded by a layer of water of hydration, which is associated with the particles through ion-dipole and dipole-dipole interactions. When a particle moves, this shell of water, and all of the ions located inside it, moves along with the particle. Conversely, if water or an aqueous solution flows through a fixed bed of these solid particles, the hydration layer surrounding each particle remains attached to it. The electric potential at the plane of shear or slip separating the bound water from the free water is the ζ potential. It does not include the Stern layer and includes only the part of the Gouy-Chapman layer that lies outside the hydration shell (Fig 21-5).

STABILIZATION BY ELECTROSTATIC REPULSION—
When two uncharged hydrophobic particles are in close proximity, they attract each other by van der Waals secondary valences, mainly London dispersion forces. For individual atoms and molecules, these forces decrease with the seventh power of the distance between them. In the case of two particles, every atom of one particle attracts every atom of the other particle. Because the attractive forces are nearly additive, they decay much less rapidly with interparticle distance, approximately with the second or third power of the distance between them. Therefore, whenever two particles approach each other closely, the attractive forces take over and cause them to adhere. Coagulation occurs as the primary particles aggregate into increasingly larger secondary particles or flocs. If the dispersion consists of two kinds of particles, one having positive and the other negative charges, the electrostatic attraction between such oppositely charged particles is superimposed on the attraction by van der Waals forces and coagulation is accelerated. If the dispersion contains only one kind of particle with the same surface charge and charge density (the most common case) then electrostatic repulsion tends to prevent the particles from approaching closely enough to come within the effective range of each other's van der Waals attractive forces. This sta-

bilizes the dispersion against interparticle attachments or coagulation. The electrostatic repulsive energy has a range in the order of δ.

A quantitative theory of the interaction between lyophobic disperse particles was worked out independently by Derjaguin

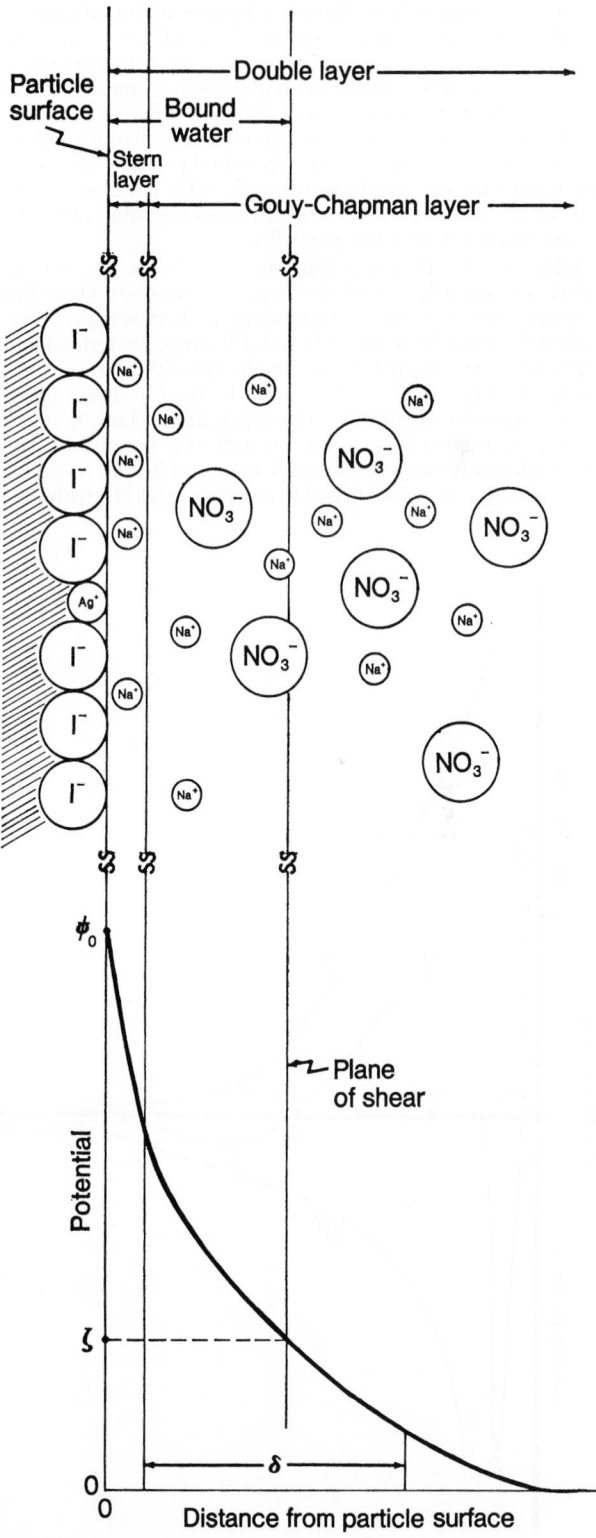

Figure 21-5. Electric double layer at the surface of a silver iodide particle (upper part) and the corresponding potentials (lower part). The distance from the particle surface, plotted on the horizontal axis, refers to both the upper and lower portions of the figure.

and Landau in the USSR and by Verwey and Overbeek in the Netherlands in the early 1940s.[1–3,5,7–9] Detailed calculations may be found in Chapter 21 of RPS-17. The so-called DLVO theory predicts and explains many, but not all, experimental data; its refinement to account for discrepancies is ongoing. The DLVO theory is summarized in Figure 21-6, where curve *WA* represents the van der Waals attractive energy, which decreases approximately by the second power of the interparticle distance, and curve *ER* represents the electrostatic repulsive energy, which decreases exponentially with interparticle distance. Because of the combination of these two opposing effects, attraction predominates at small and large distances; whereas repulsion may predominate at intermediate distances. Negative energy values indicate attraction and positive values indicate repulsion. The resultant curve *DPBAS*, obtained by algebraic addition of curves *WA* and *ER*, gives the total, net energy of interaction between two particles.

Interparticle attraction depends mainly upon the chemical nature and particle size of the dispersed material. Once these have been selected, the attractive energy between particles is fixed and cannot be readily altered. Electrostatic repulsion depends upon the ψ_0 potential, or the density of the surface charge, and upon the thickness of the double layer, both of which govern the magnitude of the ζ potential. Thus, dispersion stability correlates to some extent with this potential.[6] The ζ potential can be widely adjusted using additives, especially ionic surfactants, water-miscible solvents, and electrolytes. If the absolute value of the ζ potential is small, the resultant potential energy is negative and van der Waals forces of attraction predominate over electrostatic repulsion at all interparticle distances. Such sols coagulate rapidly.

The two identical particles, whose interaction is depicted in Figure 21-6, have a large (positive or negative) ζ potential, resulting in an appreciable positive or repulsive potential energy at intermediate distances. However, Brownian motion, convection currents, sedimentation, or stirring of the dispersion will eventually put them on a collision course. As the two particles approach each other, the two counterion atmospheres begin to interpenetrate or overlap at point A, corresponding to the distance, d_A. This produces a net repulsive (positive) energy because of the work involved in distorting the diffuse double layers and pushing water molecules and counterions aside. If the particles continue to approach each other, the repulsion between their surface charges increases the net potential energy of interaction to its maximum positive value at B, where most of the intervening water and counterions have been displaced. If the height of the potential energy barrier B exceeds the kinetic energy of the approaching particles, they will not come any closer to each other than the distance d_B and will then move away from each other. A net positive potential energy of about $25\,kT$ units usually suffices to keep them apart and renders the dispersion stable (k is the Boltzmann constant and T is absolute temperature). At $T = 298°K$, the required potential energy for stabilization corresponds to 1×10^{-12} erg or 1×10^{-5} J. The kinetic energy of a particle is of the order of kT.

On the other hand, if the kinetic energy of the approaching particles exceeds the potential energy barrier B, the particles will continue to approach each other past d_B, where the van der Waals forces of attraction become increasingly more important compared to the electrostatic repulsion. Therefore, the net potential energy of particle interaction decreases to zero and then becomes negative. This now pulls the particles closer together. When the particles touch, at a distance, d_P, the net energy has acquired a large negative value of P. This deep minimum in potential energy corresponds to a very stable situation in which the particles adhere. Since it is unlikely that enough kinetic energy can be supplied to the particles or that their ζ potential can be increased sufficiently to cause them to climb out of the potential energy well P, they are permanently attached to each other. When most or all of the primary particles agglomerate into secondary particles by this process, the sol coagulates. Any closer approach of the two particles than the touching distance d_P will cause a very rapid rise in potential energy along PD because the solid particles would interpenetrate each other and cause atomic orbitals to overlap (Born repulsion).

COAGULATION OF HYDROPHOBIC DISPERSIONS— The height of the potential energy barrier and the range over which the electrostatic repulsion is effective (or the thickness of the double layer) determine the stability of hydrophobic dispersions. Both factors are reduced by the addition of electrolytes. The transition between a coagulating and a stable sol is gradual and depends upon the time of observation. Therefore, standardized conditions must be used to classify a sol as either coagulated or coagulating, or stable (ie, fully dispersed).

To determine the coagulating concentration of a given electrolyte for a given sol, a series of test tubes is filled with equal portions of the sol. Identical volumes of electrolyte solutions having increasing concentrations are added to the test tubes with vigorous stirring. After a certain rest period (eg, 2 hours), the mixtures are agitated again. After an additional, shorter rest period (eg, 1/2 hour), they are inspected for signs of coagulation. The tubes are then classified into two group; one showing no signs of coagulation and the other showing at least some signs such as visible flocs. Alternatively, they can be classified into one group showing complete coagulation and another showing none or incomplete coagulation, such as some deflocculated colloid left in the supernatant. In either case, the separation between the two classes is quite sharp. The intermediate agitation breaks the weakest interparticle bonds and brings

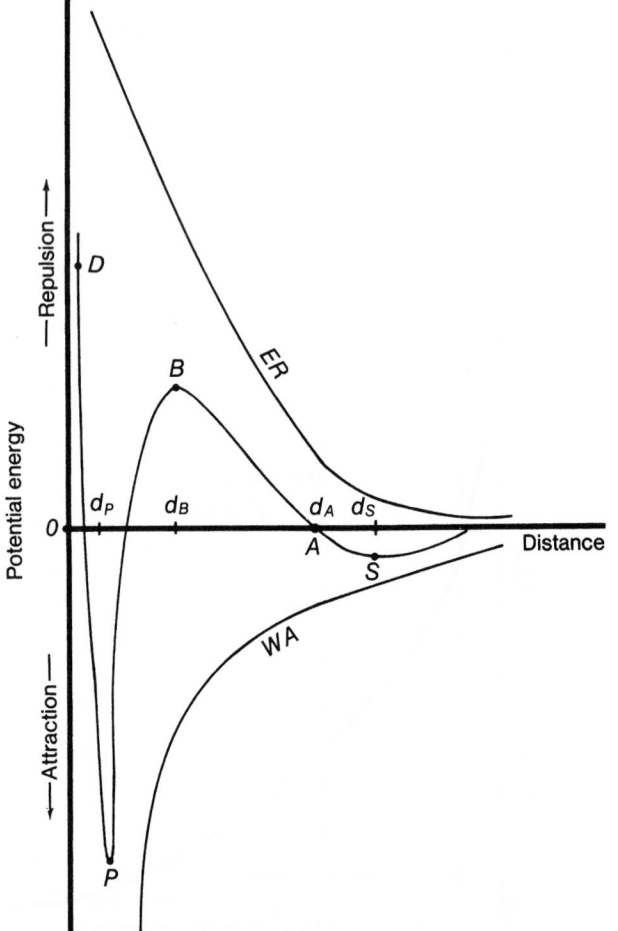

Figure 21-6. Curves representing the van der Waals energy of attraction (*WA*), the energy of electrostatic repulsion (*ER*), and the net energy of interaction (*DPBAS*) between two identical charged particles, as a function of the interparticle distance.

smaller particles into contact with larger ones, thus sharpening the distinction between coagulation and stability. After repeating the experiment with a narrower range of electrolyte concentrations, the coagulation value (c_{cv}) of the electrolyte (ie, the lowest concentration at which the electrolyte coagulates the sol) is established with good reproducibility.[2,6–8]

Typical c_{cv} values for a silver iodide sol prepared with an excess of iodide are listed in Table 21-3. The following conclusions can be drawn from the left half of Table 21-3:

1. The c_{cv} does not depend upon the valence of the anion. For example, nitrate and sulfate salts of the same metal have nearly identical c_{cv} values.

2. The differences between the c_{cv}'s of cations having the same valence are relatively minor. However, there is a slight but significant trend of decreasing c_{cv} with increasing atomic number in both the alkali and the alkaline earth metal groups. Arranging these cations in order of decreasing c_{cv} produces the Hofmeister or lyotropic series in decreasing size of hydrated specie. For monovalent cations, the lyotropic series is described above. The atomic weight of cesium is 19x greater than that of lithium, but the Cs+ ion in aqueous solution is less hydrated and therefore smaller than the hydrated Li+ ion. It is also more polarizable. Therefore, the Cs+ ion can approach the surface of a negatively charged particle suspended in water more closely and is more extensively adsorbed. This reduces its c_{cv} making cesium salts more effective coagulants than lithium salts for negatively charged hydrosols.

3. The coagulation values depend primarily upon the valence of the counterions, decreasing by one to two orders of magnitude for each unit increase in the valence of the counterions (Schulze-Hardy rule). According to the DLVO theory, the coagulation values vary inversely with the sixth power of the valence of the counterions. For mono-, di-, and trivalent counterions, they should be in the ratio:

$$\frac{1}{1^6} : \frac{1}{2^6} : \frac{1}{3^6} \text{ or } 100 : 1.6 : 0.14$$

The mean c_{cv} values for the mono-, di-, and trivalent counterions in Table 21-3 are 141, 2.45, and 0.068 *mmol/L*, respectively. This results in a ratio of 100:1.7:0.05, which is in satisfactory agreement with the DLVO theory.

The following conclusions can be drawn from the right half of Table 21-3:

4. The cations on the right side of Table 21-3 constitute obvious exceptions to the preceding conclusions. Ag^+ is a potential-determining counterion, those whose concentration determines the surface potential. When silver nitrate is added to the negatively charged silver iodide dispersion, some of its silver ions are incorporated into the negatively charged surface of the particles. This lowers the magnitude of the particle's surface charge by reducing the excess of I^- ions in the surface. Therefore, silver salts are exceptionally effective coagulating agents because they reduce the magnitude of both the ψ_0 potential and the ζ potential. Indifferent salts, which only reduce the ζ potential, require much higher salt concentrations for comparable reductions in this potential. The other potential-determining ion of silver iodide is the I^- ion. Alkali iodides have c_{cv} values higher than 141 mmol/L because they supply iodide ions that enter the surface layer of the silver iodide particles and increase its excess of I^- ions over Ag^+ ions, thereby making the ψ_0 potential more negative. Bromide and chloride ions act similarly but less effectively. The principal potential-determining ion for proteins is H^+ (and hence OH^-); those for aluminum hydroxide are OH^- (and hence H^+) and, Al^{3+} as well as Fe^{3+} and Cr^{3+}, which form mixed hydroxides with Al^{3+}.

5. The cationic surfactant and the alkaloidal salts (which also behave as cationic surfactants) on the right side of Table 21-3 constitute the second exception to the Schulze-Hardy rule. Surface-active compounds contain both hydrophilic and hydrophobic moieties within the same molecule. The dual nature of these compounds causes them to accumulate at interfaces. Dodecylammonium and alkaloidal cations are able to displace inorganic monovalent cations from the Stern layer of a negatively charged silver iodide particle. This occurs because they are not only attracted to the particle by electrostatic forces but also by van der Waals forces between their hydrocarbon moieties (ie, dodecyl chains in the case of the dodecylammonium ions) and the solid particle. Since they are strongly adsorbed from solution onto the particle surface and do not tend to dissociate from it, surface-active cations are very effective in reducing the negative ζ potential of silver iodide particles. Therefore, they have lower c_{cv} values than purely inorganic cations with the same valence.

6. Anionic surfactants, like those containing lauryl sulfate ions, also have a tendency to adsorb at solid-liquid interfaces. However, electrostatic repulsion between the negatively charged surface of the silver iodide particles, whose surface layer contains an excess of iodide ions, and the surface-active anions usually prevents adsorption from occurring below the critical micelle concentration. If adsorption does occur, it increases the density of the negative charges in the particle surface, and therefore, raises the ccv value of the anionic surfactant above the value corresponding to its valence.

The addition of water-miscible solvents such as alcohol, glycerin, propylene glycol, or polyethylene glycols to aqueous dispersions lowers the dielectric constant of the medium. This reduces the thickness of the double layer and, therefore, reduces the range over which electrostatic repulsion is effective, and lowers the size of the potential energy barrier. As a result, the addition of sufficient amounts of such solvents tends to coagulate aqueous dispersions. At lower concentrations, these solvents do not induce coagulation themselves, but make the dispersions more sensitive to coagulation by added electrolytes (ie, they lower the c_{cv} value).

Progressive addition of salts having counterions of high valence gradually reduces the ζ potential of colloidal particles to zero. Eventually, the sign of the ζ potential may be inverted, and its magnitude may then increase in the opposite direction. The ψ_0 and ζ potentials of aqueous sulfamerazine suspensions are negative above their isoelectric points, and those of bismuth subnitrate are positive. However, the addition of Al^{3+} to the former and of PO_4^{3-} to the latter in large enough amounts inverts the sign of their ζ potentials, while their ψ_0 potentials remain unchanged. Surface-active ions of opposite charge may also produce such charge inversions.

The superposition of the van der Waals attractive energy, with its long-range effectiveness, and the electrostatic repulsive energy, with its intermediate-range effectiveness, frequently produces a shallow minimum (designated S in Fig 21-6) in the resultant energy-distance curve at interparticle distances d_S that are several times greater than δ. If this minimum in potential energy is small compared to kT, Brownian motion prevents aggregation. For large particles, such as those of many pharmaceutical suspensions, and for particles that are large in one or two dimensions (eg, rods and plates), this *secondary minimum*

Table 21-3. Coagulation Values for Negative Silver Iodide Sol[a]

ELECTROLYTE	c_{cv} (mmol/L)	ELECTROLYTE	c_{cv} (mmol/L)
$LiNO_3$	165	$AgNO_3$	0.01
$NaNO_3$	140	$1/2(C_{12}H_{25}NH_3)_2SO_4$	0.07
$1/2(Na_2SO_4)$	141	Strychnine nitrate	1.7
KNO_3	136	$1/2$(Morphine sulfate)	2.5
$1/2(K_2SO_4)$	138		
$RbNO_3$	126		
Mean	**141**		
$Mg(NO_3)_2$	2.60	Quinine sulfate	0.7
$MgSO_4$	2.57		
$Ca(NO_3)_2$	2.40		
$Sr(NO_3)_2$	2.38		
$Ba(NO_3)_2$	2.26		
$Zn(NO_3)_2$	2.50		
$Pb(NO_3)_2$	2.43		
Mean	**2.45**		
$Al(NO_3)_3$	0.067		
$La(NO_3)_3$	0.069		
$Ce(NO_3)_3$	0.069		
Mean	**0.068**		

[a] Data from Kruyt HR. Colloid Science, vols I and II. Houston: Elsevier, 1949 and 1952 and unpublished data.

may be deep enough to trap them at distances d_S from each other. This requires a depth of several kT units. Such fairly long-range and weak energies of attraction produce loose aggregates or flocs that can be redispersed by agitation or by reducing the concentration of flocculating electrolytes.[1,2,5,7,8,10,20] This reversible aggregation process involving the secondary minimum is called *flocculation*. By contrast, aggregation in the deep primary minimum P is called *coagulation* and is irreversible.

ELECTROKINETIC PHENOMENA—When a dc electric field is applied to a dispersion, the particles move towards the electrode having a charge opposite to that on their surface. The counterions located inside their hydration shell are dragged along while the counterions in the diffuse double layer outside the plane of slip, in the free or mobile solvent, move toward the other electrode. This phenomenon is called *electrophoresis*. If the charged surface is immobile, as is the case with a packed bed of particles or a tube filled with water, application of an electric field causes the counterions in the free water to move towards the opposite electrode, dragging solvent with them. This flow of liquid is called *electroosmosis*, and the pressure produced by it is called *electroosmotic pressure*. Conversely, if the liquid is made to flow past charged surfaces by applying hydrostatic pressure, displacement of the counterions in the free water produces a potential difference between the two ends of the tube or bed called *streaming potential*. These three phenomena depend upon the relative motion of the charged surface and the diffuse double layer outside the plane of slip surrounding the surface. Actually, most of the diffuse double layer lies within the free solvent and, therefore, can move along the surface.[5-8, 21] All three electrokinetic phenomena measure the same ζ potential, which is the potential at the plane of slip.

Microelectrophoresis—The particles of pharmaceutical suspensions and emulsions, bacteria, erythrocytes and other isolated cells, latex particles, and many contaminant particles in pharmaceutical solutions are visible in a microscope. Therefore, their ζ potentials are conveniently measured by *microelectrophoresis*. A potential difference, E, applied between two electrodes that are dipped into a dispersion and separated by a distance, d, produces the potential gradient or field strength, E/d, expressed as V/cm. The average velocity, v, of the particles in response to the applied potential difference is determined using the eyepiece micrometer of a microscope and a stopwatch, and used to calculate the ζ potential by the Smoluchowski equation:

$$\xi = \left(\frac{4\pi\eta}{D}\right)\left(\frac{v}{E/d}\right) = \left(\frac{4\pi\eta}{D}\right)\mu$$

The electrophoretic mobility, μ, is equal to $v/(E/d)$ and is the velocity caused by a potential gradient of 1 V/cm. According to the Smoluchowski equation, particle size and shape do not affect the ζ potential. However, if the particle radius is smaller than or comparable to δ (in which case the particles cannot be detected in a microscope), a factor of 6 replaces the 4. The viscosity, η, and the dielectric constant, D, refer to the aqueous medium within the double layer and cannot be measured directly.[22] By using the values for water at 25°C, expressing the velocity in μm/sec and the electrophoretic mobility in (μm/sec)/(volts/cm), and converting into the appropriate units, the Smoluchowski equation is reduced to $\zeta = 12.9$ μ with ζ given as millivolts (mV). Zeta potentials as high as ± 180 mV have been reported.[1,6,21] If the particle surface has appreciable conductance, the absolute value of the ζ potential calculated by this equation may be too small.[2,7,21,22] Dispersions of hydrophobic particles having ζ potentials below ± 20–30 mV are frequently unstable and tend to coagulate.

The chief experimental precautions in microelectrophoresis measurements are:

1. Electroosmosis causes liquid to flow along the walls of the cell containing the dispersion. This in turn produces a return flow into the center of the cell. Therefore, the microscope must be focused on the stationary boundary between the two liquid layers that are flowing in opposite directions in order to measure the true velocity of the particles.

2. Following the motion of single particles in a microscopic field and measuring their velocity is only possible using very dilute dispersions. Therefore, many dispersions must be diluted before making such determinations. Since the ζ potential depends largely upon the nature, ionic strength, and pH of the suspending medium, dispersions should not be diluted with water but with solutions having compositions identical to their continuous phase (eg, with their own serum that has been separated by ultrafiltration or centrifugation).

When the particles cannot be individually observed using a microscope, other electrophoresis methods are employed.[6,8,21,23,24] In *moving boundary electrophoresis*, the movement of the boundary formed between a sol or solution and the pure dispersion medium in an electric field is studied. If the dispersed phase is colorless, the boundary is located by the refractive index gradient (Tiselius apparatus, frequently used with protein solutions). If several species of particles or solutes with different mobilities are present, each will form a boundary moving with a characteristic velocity. Unlike microelectrophoresis, this method permits the identification of different colloidal components in a mixture, the measurement of the electrophoretic mobility of each, and an estimation of the relative amounts present.

Capillary Electrophoresis—Capillary electrophoresis (CE)[25,26] is a widely used separation technique best suited for charged, water-soluble molecules having molecular weights ranging from those of amino acids and peptides to nucleic acids. CE has the following advantages: it provides fast and efficient separations, requires only minute amounts of sample, is applicable to a wide range of analytes, and (in contrast to HPLC) employs aqueous media rather than organic solvents.

Electrophoresis is carried out in horizontal capillaries of fused silica (which is transparent to ultraviolet) of 20 to 100 μm bore and 20 to 100 cm length. Both capillary ends are bent downward. Each end is immersed in a vial filled with a buffer solution that contains an electrode assembly. The electrodes are connected to an adjustable high-voltage dc power supply. As the dissolved analytes migrate past a detection window in the capillary, their concentrations are measured by ultraviolet absorption or by (often laser-induced) fluorescence. The silica capillaries are often coated externally with a very thin layer of polyimide to reduce their fragility. This plastic coating is burned off in the window area.

The capillary is filled with buffer solution, the sample is injected at one end, and a constant high potential difference E is applied, which produces a potential gradient or field strength in the range of 300 to 400 V/cm. If $E = 20,000$ V and the total capillary length $d_r = 57$ cm, then $E/d_r = 350$ V/cm. The velocity of migration, v, is the capillary length to the detector, d_L, divided by the migration time, t, of the analyte from the capillary injection end to the detection window. If $d_L = 50$ cm and $t = 10$ min $= 600$ sec, then $v = 50/600 = 0.083$ cm/sec. The electrophoretic mobility ($v/(E/d)$) is (0.083 cm/sec)/(350 V/cm) $= 2.4 \times 10^{-4}$ cm²/Vsec.

In addition to electrophoresis, electro-osmosis may play an important role in CE. The isoelectric point of hydrated silica is approximately 1.8. The weakly acidic silanol groups become increasingly ionized with increasing pH. Conditioning the capillary with a NaOH solution and then with the buffer ensures that its wall is charged uniformly with partially ionized silanol groups. These negatively charged sites attract cationic counterions from the buffer to form an electric double layer. When an electric potential is applied, the cations in the diffuse part of the double layer beyond the plane of shear (Fig 21-5) migrate toward the negative electrode, entraining water of hydration. Because of the small bore of the capillaries compared to the diffuse double layer thickness, the electro-osmotic flow (EOF) can be substantial. The EOF moves in a plug profile rather than the customary parabolic profile of laminar flow. At high pH, the EOF is strong because the silanol groups are extensively ionized. Amphoteric peptides are negatively charged and try to migrate toward the positive electrode or anode. This motion is often overwhelmed by a strong and opposite EOF, which drags them toward the negative electrode or cathode. These analytes move from the injection point in the anode compartment toward the cathode. The order of arrival at the detection window is: cationic analytes (whose electrophoretic migration toward the cathode is superimposed and accelerated by the EOF), nonionic analytes (which migrate exclusively by EOF), and anionic analytes (whose net migration velocity is that of the EOF minus their electrophoretic migration velocity toward the anode).

At low pH, the EOF is small and the peptides are positively charged. Their migration toward the cathode is then superimposed and accelerated by the EOF in the same direction. The direction of the EOF can be reversed by adding a cationic surfactant, such as cetyltrimethylammonium bromide, to the buffer. It will react and neutralize the silanol groups, and excess surfactant adsorbed on the silica will confer a positive charge to it. The Br^- counterions cause an EOF toward the anode. The EOF can be suppressed by coating the silica capillaries with a polymer or by using Teflon capillaries.

Unless the heat generated by the electric resistance of the buffer solution (Joule heating) is dissipated, it causes the temperature to increase with time and promotes temperature gradients across the capillary. This interferes with reproducibility and sharpness of the CE separations. The amount of heat generated is directly proportional to the square of the field strength (which is large) and to the conductivity of the buffer solution. While decreasing the voltage, using longer or smaller-bore capillaries and/or more dilute buffer solution would reduce the rate of heat generation; it would also increase the separation times.

Short separation times reduce the band broadening due to analyte diffusion, improving the resolution. Therefore, the capillary is cooled with a thermostatted liquid.

A variation of CE is micellar electrokinetic (capillary) chromatography (MEKC).[25, 26] The analytes are solubilized in micelles of an ionic surfactant, such as sodium dodecyl sulfate, which is added to the buffer solution at a concentration well above its critical micelle concentration of $8 \times 10^{-3} M$. MEKC is suited particularly to separate neutral analytes of limited water solubility, which are extensively partitioned into the micelles, but is also applicable to ionic analytes. Anionic analytes, being well soluble in water, either do not partition into the micelles or form mixed micelles with the anionic surfactant. Cationic analytes often form precipitates with anionic surfactants. Therefore, their separation by MEKC is best carried out with cationic surfactants.

The combination of a nonionic and an ionic surfactant produces mixed micelles. These have lower surface charge densities and larger sizes than the micelles of ionic surfactants, and hence they have lower electrophoretic mobilities. Thus, addition of a nonionic to an ionic surfactant narrows the migration time window, which is the difference between the migration times of the bulk solution in EOF and of the micelles, and often shortens the analysis time.

Analytes with molecular weights of 5000 or higher are not solubilized by micelles. Therefore, while they can be analyzed by CE, they cannot be analyzed by MEKC. Although anionic micelles tend to migrate toward the anode, a strong EOF in neutral or alkaline media will drag them toward the cathode, but with a velocity retarded by their own migration velocity. If a neutral analyte is partly solubilized in micelles and partly dissolved molecularly in the buffer solution, the latter portion has a shorter migration time because its velocity is that of the EOF.

Capillary gel electrophoresis[25,26] employs capillaries filled with a gel of cross-linked polyacrylamide, which suppresses EOF. Isotachophoresis and isoelectric focusing,[26] described in previous editions of this text, are other modalities of CE.

LYOPHILIC DISPERSIONS

Lyophilic dispersions consist either of polymers dissolved in a good solvent or of insoluble but extensively solvated particles dispersed in a liquid medium that has a high affinity or attraction for them. The free energy of dissolution or dispersion is $\Delta G_s = \Delta H_s - T \Delta S_s$, where ΔH_s and ΔS_s are the heat or enthalpy change, and the entropy change of dissolution or dispersion, respectively. For dissolution of polymers and dispersion of particulate solids to occur spontaneously, ΔG_s must be negative. Since both of these processes are exothermic (ie, occur with the evolution of heat), their ΔH_s is negative. Since the number of available conformations of the polymer chains increases considerably upon dissolution, and the number of positions and orientations of the solid particles increases considerably upon their dispersion in the liquid, their ΔS_s is positive (ie, there is an increase in randomness). The negative enthalpy change and the positive entropy change of dissolution/dispersion both contribute to making ΔG_s negative. Therefore, both types of colloidal systems are formed spontaneously when powders of solid polymers and particulate solids are brought into contact with the liquid dispersion medium. They are thermodynamically stable and reversible (ie, they are easily reconstituted after the dispersion medium has been removed). The van der Waals energies of attraction between dissolved macromolecules or between dispersed lyophilic solid particles are smaller than ΔG_s and are therefore insufficient to cause flocculation or coagulation of the dispersed phase. Furthermore, the solvation layers surrounding dissolved macromolecules and dispersed lyophilic particles form a physical barrier preventing their close approach.

Most liquid dispersed systems of pharmaceutical interest are aqueous. Therefore, most of the lyophilic colloidal systems discussed below consist of hydrophilic solids dissolved or dispersed in water. Most of the products mentioned below are official in the USP or NF, where more detailed descriptions may be found; they are also discussed in detail elsewhere in this text. Hydrophilic colloids can be divided into two classes (ie, soluble and particulate materials). Solutions of water-soluble polymers molecularly dissolved in water may be classified as colloidal dispersions because the individual molecules are in the colloidal particle size range: the diameter of a randomly coiled polymer chain commonly exceeds 10 nm. Particulate or corpuscular hydrophilic colloidal dispersions are formed by solids that swell and are peptized in water but whose primary particles do not dissolve or break down into individual molecules or ions.

Water-Soluble Polymers

Most of the hydrophilic colloidal systems used to prepare pharmaceutical dosage forms are molecular solutions of water-soluble, high molecular weight polymers. These polymers are either linear or slightly branched but not cross-linked. Water-soluble polymers may be divided into three classes according to their origin:

- *Natural polymers* include polysaccharides (acacia, agar, heparin sodium, pectin, sodium alginate, tragacanth, xanthan gum) and polypeptides (casein, gelatin, protamine sulfate). Of these, agar and gelatin are only soluble in hot water.
- *Cellulose derivatives* are produced by chemically modifying cellulose obtained from wood pulp or cotton to produce soluble polymers. *Cellulose* is an insoluble, linear polymer of glucose units in the ring or pyranose form joined by β-1,4 glucosidic linkages. Each glucose unit (except for the two at the terminal chain ends) contains a primary hydroxyl group on the No. 6 carbon and two secondary hydroxyls on the No. 2- and 3-carbons. Chemical modification of cellulose involves substitutions at these hydroxyl groups with the primary hydroxyl group being the most reactive. The extent of such reactions is expressed as *degree of substitution* (DS), the number of substituted hydroxyl groups per glucose residue. The highest value for DS is 3. Fractional values are most common because the DS is averaged over a multitude of glucose residues. A DS value of 0.6 indicates that some glucose repeat units are not substituted while others substituted once or even twice.

  Some soluble cellulose derivatives are listed below. Their DS values correspond to their respective pharmaceutical grades; the groups shown replace the hydrogen atoms of the cellulosic hydroxyls. Official derivatives include *methylcellulose* (DS = 1.65–1.93); (—O—CH$_3$) and *sodium carboxymethylcellulose* (DS = 0.60–1.00); (—O—CH$_2$COO$^-$Na$^+$). *Hydroxyethylcellulose* (DS $\cong$ 1.0); (—O—(CH$_2$CH$_2$O)$_n$H) and *hydroxypropylcellulose* (DS $\cong$ 2.5);

$$—O—(—CH—CH_2—O—)_nH$$
$$\overset{|}{CH_3}$$

  are manufactured by adding ethylene oxide and propylene oxide, respectively, to alkali-treated cellulose. The value of n is about 2.0 for hydroxyethylcellulose and not much greater than 1.0 for hydroxypropylcellulose. *Hydroxypropylmethylcellulose* is prepared by reacting alkali-treated cellulose first with methyl chloride to introduce methoxy groups (DS = 1.1–1.8) and then with propylene oxide to introduce propylene glycol ether groups (DS = 0.1–0.3). In general, the introduction of hydroxypropyl groups into cellulose slightly reduces its water solubility while promoting its solubility in polar organic solvents such as short-chain alcohols, glycols, and some ethers.

  The molecular weight of native cellulose is so high that soluble derivatives of approximately the same degree of polymerization would dissolve too slowly and their solutions would be excessively viscous even at concentrations of ≤1%. To overcome these difficulties, controlled degradation is used to break the cellulose chains into shorter segments. Commercial grades cellulose derivatives, such as sodium carboxymethylcellulose, come in various molecular weights or viscosity grades as well as with various degrees of substitution.

  Official cellulose derivatives that are insoluble in water but soluble in some organic solvents include *ethylcellulose* (DS = 2.2–2.7); (—OC$_2$H$_5$); *cellulose acetate phthalate* (DS = 1.70 for acetyl and 0.77 for phthalyl); *hydroxypropylmethylcellulose phthalate*; and *polyvinyl acetate phthalate*. *Collodion*, a 4.0% (w/v) solution of pyroxylin (cellulose dinitrate) in a mixture of 75% (v/v) ether and 25% (v/v) ethyl alcohol, is also a cellulose based, lyophilic colloidal system.

- *Water-soluble synthetic polymers* consist mostly of high molecular weight polyethylene glycols, or *polyethylene oxides*, and vinyl derivatives such as *polyvinyl alcohol, povidone* or polyvinylpyrrolidone, and *carbomer (Carbopol)*, a copolymer of acrylic acid.

A second classification of hydrophilic polymers is based upon their charge. *Nonionic* or uncharged polymers include methylcellulose, hydroxyethyl and hydroxypropyl cellulose, ethylcellulose, pyroxylin, polyethylene oxide, polyvinyl alcohol, and povidone. *Anionic* or negatively charged *polyelectrolytes* include carboxylated polymers (eg, acacia, alginic acid, pectin, tragacanth, xanthan gum, and carbomer) at pH values that result in the ionization of their carboxyl groups. Sodium alginate, sodium carboxymethylcellulose, and polypeptides (eg, sodium caseinate) at pH values above their isoelectric points are also anionic. Sulfuric acid is a stronger acidic group that exists as a monoester in agar and heparin and as a monoamide in heparin. *Cationic* or positively charged *polyelectrolytes* are rare. Examples include chitin, a polysaccharide found in the shells of beetles and crustaceans, and polypeptides at pH values below their isoelectric points. Protamines such as protamine sulfate are strongly basic due to their high arginine content and have isoelectric points around pH 12.

Particulate Hydrophilic Dispersions

The dispersed phase of these sols consists of solids that swell in water and spontaneously break up into particles having colloidal dimensions. The dispersed particles have high specific surface areas and are extensively hydrated. *Bentonite NF* is a hydrated aluminum silicate that crystallizes in a layer structure with individual lamellas 0.94 nm thick. Their top and bottom surfaces consist of sheets of oxygen ions from silica and an occasional sodium ion neutralizing a silicate ion-exchange site. The clay particles contain stacks of these lamellas. Water penetrates between these lamellas to hydrate the oxygen ions and causes extensive swelling. The bentonite particles in bentonite magma consist of single lamellas or packets of a few lamellas with intercalated water. Their specific surface area amounts to several hundred square meters per gram. *Kaolin USP* is also a hydrated aluminum silicate having a layer structure. In kaolin, hydrated alumina lattice layers alternate with silica layers. Therefore, one of the two external surfaces of a kaolin plate consists of a sheet of oxygen ions from silica whereas the other is a sheet of hydroxide ions from hydrated alumina. Both surfaces are well hydrated but water cannot penetrate into the individual lattice layers. Therefore, the particles do not swell in water or exfoliate into thin plates. As a result, kaolin plates dispersed in water are much thicker than those of bentonite, about 0.04 to 0.2 μm. *Magnesium Aluminum Silicate NF*, also known as Veegum®, is a clay similar to bentonite but contains magnesium; it is white whereas bentonite is gray. *Colloidal Activated Attapulgite USP* also consists of magnesium aluminum silicate. However, rather than having a lamellar habit like the other three clays, it crystallizes in the form of long needles approximately 20 nm in width.[27]

The following additional hydrophilic particles can also produce colloidal dispersions in water. *Titanium dioxide* is a white pigment with excellent covering power. *Colloidal silicon dioxide* consists of roughly spherical particles that are covered with siloxane and silanol groups. *Microcrystalline cellulose* is hydrophilic because of the hydroxyl and ether groups on the surface of the cellulose crystals. Gelatinous precipitates of hydrophilic compounds such as *aluminum hydroxide gel, aluminum phosphate gel,* and *magnesium hydroxide* consist of coarse flocs produced by agglomeration of the colloidal particles formed in the initial stages of precipitation.

LYOPHOBIC DISPERSIONS

Lyophobic dispersions are intrinsically unstable and irreversible because of the lack of attraction between the dispersed and continuous phases. Unlike lyophilic dispersions, their large surface free energy is not lowered by solvation, their dispersion process does not take place spontaneously, and they are not easily reconstituted. For lyophobic dispersions, ΔG_s is positive because of a positive (endothermic) ΔH_s term, which makes the reverse process (agglomeration) the spontaneous one. Aqueous dispersions of hydrophobic solids or liquids can be prepared by physical means that supply an appropriate amount of energy to the system. However, they are unstable. The van der Waals attractive forces between the particles are stronger than the solvation forces that promote particle dispersal, and therefore, the particles tend to aggregate. Most of the discussion of lyophobic dispersions deals with hydrosols consisting of hydrophobic solids or liquids dispersed in an aqueous media because water is the most widely used vehicle. Such hydrosols consist of aqueous dispersions of insoluble organic and inorganic compounds, which usually have low degrees of hydration. Organic compounds that are preponderantly hydrocarbon in nature and possess few hydrophilic or polar groups are hydrophobic, and therefore, insoluble in water.

Like all lyophobic dispersions, hydrophobic dispersions are intrinsically unstable. In their most thermodynamically stable state, the dispersed phase has coalesced into large crystals or drops, so that the specific surface area and surface free energy are minimized. Therefore, mechanical, chemical, or electrical energy must be supplied to break up the dispersed phase into smaller particles and overcome the resulting increase in surface free energy that occurs from the parallel increase in specific surface area.

Hydrophobic dispersions can be prepared by either dispersion methods (the reduction of coarse particles to colloidal dimensions through comminution or peptization) or condensation methods (the aggregation of small molecules or ions into particles having colloidal dimensions). Dispersion methods tend to produce sols that have wide particle size distributions. Conversely, condensation methods *may* produce essentially monodisperse sols provided specialized techniques are employed. Methods of purification to remove low molecular-weight, water-soluble impurities from hydrosols have been reviewed in the corresponding chapter of the previous *Remington* edition.

Preparation by Dispersion Methods

The first method, *mechanical disintegration* of solids and liquids into smaller particles before or during dispersion within a fluid vehicle, is frequently carried out by the input of mechanical energy via shear or attrition. Equipment such as colloid and ball mills, micronizers and, for emulsions, homogenizers is described elsewhere in this text and in Reference 27. Dry grinding with inert, water-soluble diluting agents also produces colloidal dispersions. For example, sulfur hydrosols may be prepared by triturating the powder with urea or lactose followed by shaking with water. Ultrasonic generators provide exceptionally high concentrations of energy. However, the successful dispersion of solids by means of ultrasonic waves can only be achieved with comparatively soft materials such as many organic compounds, sulfur, talcum, and graphite. In cases where fine emulsions are mandatory, such as soybean oil-in-water emulsions for intravenous feeding, emulsification by ultrasound waves is the method of choice.[27] The formation of aerosols is described elsewhere in this text.

Peptization is a second dispersion method used to prepare colloidal dispersions. The term is defined as the breaking up of aggregates (or secondary particles) into smaller aggregates (or primary particles) that are within the colloidal size range. Primary particles are those particles that are not formed from smaller ones. Peptization is synonymous with *deflocculation*. It can be brought about by the removal of flocculating agents, usually electrolytes, or by the addition of deflocculating or peptizing agents, usually surfactants, water-soluble polymers, or ions that adsorb onto the particle surface.[6,8] When powdered activated charcoal is added to water with stirring, the aggregated grains cannot be completely broken up and the resulting suspension is gray and translucent. The addition of

≤0.1% sodium lauryl sulfate or octoxynol 9 deflocculates the grains into finely dispersed particles and results in a deep black and opaque dispersion. Ferric or aluminum hydroxide that has been freshly precipitated with ammonia can be peptized with small amounts of acids which reduce the pH below the isoelectric points of the hydroxides. Even washing the gelatinous precipitate of $Al(OH)_3$ with water tends to peptize it. Therefore, in quantitative analyses, the precipitate is instead washed with dilute solutions of ammonium salts that act as flocculating agents.

Preparation by Condensation Methods

Sulfur is insoluble in water but somewhat soluble in alcohol. When an alcoholic solution of sulfur is mixed with water, a bluish-white colloidal dispersion results. In the absence of added stabilizing agents, the particles tend to agglomerate and precipitate upon standing. This technique of first dissolving a material in a water-miscible solvent such as alcohol or acetone and then producing a hydrosol by precipitation with water is applicable to many organic compounds. It has been used to prepare hydrosols of stearic acid, natural resins like mastic, and the so-called pseudo-latexes. Another less common physical condensation method is to introduce a current of sulfur vapor into water, which produces colloidal particles. Alternatively, the very fine powder produced by condensing sulfur vapor onto cold solid surfaces (sublimed sulfur or flowers of sulfur) can be dispersed in water by the addition of a suitable surfactant to produce a hydrosol.

Organic compounds that are weak bases, such as the alkaloids, are usually much more soluble at lower pH values, where they are ionized, than at higher pH values, where they exist as the free base. Therefore, increasing the pH of their aqueous solutions above their pKa may cause precipitation of the free base. Conversely, organic compounds that are weak acids, such as the barbiturates, are usually much more soluble at higher pH values, where they are ionized, than at lower pH values, where they exist as the free acid form. Therefore, lowering the pH of their aqueous solutions well below their pKa usually causes precipitation of the free acid. Depending upon the supersaturation (defined below) of the unionized bases or acids and the presence of stabilizing agents, the resultant dispersions may be within the colloidal range.

Chemical condensation methods include the reaction between hydrogen sulfide and sulfur dioxide (eg, by bubbling H_2S into an aqueous SO_2 solution):

$$2\,H_2S + SO_2 \rightarrow 3\,S + 2\,H_2O$$

The same reaction occurs when aqueous solutions containing sodium sulfide and sulfite are acidified with an excess of sulfuric or hydrochloric acid. Another reaction is the decomposition of sodium thiosulfate by sulfuric acid, using either very dilute or very concentrated solutions to obtain colloidally dispersed sulfur:

$$H_2SO_4 + 3\,Na_2S_2O_3 \rightarrow 4\,S + 3\,Na_2SO_4 + H_2O$$

Both reactions also produce pentathionic acid ($H_2S_5O_6$) as a by-product. The preferential adsorption of the pentathionate anion onto the surface of the sulfur particles confers a negative electric charge to the particles, thereby stabilizing the sol.[2,8,9] When powdered sulfur is boiled with a slurry of lime, it dissolves with the formation of calcium pentasulfide and thiosulfate. Subsequent acidification produces the colloidal "milk of sulfur," which upon washing and drying yields Precipitated Sulfur USP.

Sols of ferric, aluminum, chromic, stannic, and titanium hydroxides or hydrous oxides are produced by the hydrolysis of the corresponding chlorides or nitrates:

$$AlCl_3 + 3\,H_2O \rightleftharpoons Al(OH)_3 + 3\,HCl$$

Hydrolysis is promoted by boiling the solution and/or adding a base to neutralize the formed acid.[2]

Double decompositions that produce insoluble salts can also lead to colloidal dispersions. An example is silver chloride:

$$NaCl + AgNO_3 \rightarrow AgCl + NaNO_3$$

In addition, the reduction of gold, silver, copper, mercury, platinum, rhodium, and palladium salts with formaldehyde, hydrazine, hydroxylamine, hydroquinone, or stannous chloride forms hydrosols of the metals, which are strongly colored (eg, red or blue).[1,2,6,8]

KINETICS OF PARTICLE FORMATION—When the solubility of a compound in water is exceeded, its solution becomes supersaturated and the compound may precipitate or crystallize. The rate of precipitation, the resulting particle size (whether colloidal or coarse), and the particle size distribution (which can be narrow for mono- or homodispersed particles or broad for poly- or heterodispersed particles) depend upon two successive and largely independent processes. These are *nucleation* and *crystallization* (ie, growth of nuclei). When a solution of a salt or sucrose is supercooled or when a chemical reaction produces a salt in a concentration exceeding its solubility product, the separation of excess solid from the supersaturated solution is far from instantaneous. Clusters of ions or molecules called nuclei must exceed a critical size before they become stable and capable of growing into colloidal size crystals. These embryonic particles have much more surface for a given weight of material than larger and more stable crystals. Therefore, they have a higher surface free energy and greater solubility.

The occurrence of *nucleation* depends upon the *relative supersaturation*. If C is the actual concentration of the solute before crystallization and C_s is its solubility limit, then $C - C_s$ is the supersaturation and $(C - C_s)/C_s$ is the relative supersaturation. Von Weimarn recognized that the rate or velocity of nucleation (number of nuclei formed per liter per second) is proportional to the relative supersaturation. Nucleation seldom occurs at relative supersaturations below 3. However, this statement refers to homogeneous nucleation, where the nuclei have the same chemical composition as the crystallizing phase. If the solution contains solid impurities, such as dust particles in suspension, these may act as nuclei or centers of crystallization (heterogeneous nucleation).

Once nuclei have formed, *crystallization* begins. Nuclei grow by the aggregation of ions or molecules from solution. Crystallization continues until the supersaturation is relieved (i.e. until $C = C_s$) and may result in the formation of either colloidal or coarse particles. The rate of crystallization or growth of nuclei is proportional to the supersaturation:

$$\frac{dm}{dt} = \frac{A_{sp}D}{\delta}(C - C_s)$$

This equation is similar to the Noyes-Whitney equation that governs particle dissolution except that $C < C_s$ for the latter process, making dm/dt negative. In both equations, m is the mass of material crystallizing out in time t, D is the diffusion coefficient of the solute molecules or ions, δ is the length of the diffusion path or the thickness of the liquid layer adhering to the growing particles, and A_{sp} is their specific surface area. The presence of dissolved impurities may affect the rate of crystallization and even change the crystal habit, provided that these impurities are surface-active and become adsorbed onto the nuclei or growing crystals.[6] For instance, 0.005% polysorbate 80 or octoxynol 9 significantly retards the growth of methylprednisolone crystals in aqueous media.

Von Weimarn found that the particle size of the crystals depends strongly upon the concentration of the precipitating substance. At very low concentrations and slight relative supersaturation, diffusion is quite slow because the concentration gradient that drives the process is very small. Sufficient nuclei will usually form to relieve the slight supersaturation. However, crystal growth is limited by the small amount of excess dissolved material available to each particle and, therefore, the particles cannot grow beyond colloidal dimensions. This condition is represented by points A, D, and G of the schematic plot of von Weimarn (Fig 21-7). At intermediate concentrations, the extent of nucleation is somewhat greater and much more material is available for crystal growth. Therefore, coarse crystals form rather than colloidal particles. This condition is represented by points B, E, and H in Figure 21-7. At high concentrations, nuclei appear so quickly and in such large numbers that supersaturation is relieved before any appreciable diffusion can occur. The high viscosity of the medium also slows down the diffusion of excess dissolved ions or molecules, retarding crystal growth without substantially affecting the rate of nucleation. Therefore, a large number of very small particles results which, because of their proximity, tend to link and produce a translucent gel. This condition is represented by points C and F in Figure 21-7. Upon subsequent dilution with water, such gels usually yield colloidal dispersions. Thus, colloidal systems are usually produced at very low and high supersaturations.

Low solubility is a necessary condition for producing colloidal dispersions. If the solubility of the precipitate is increased, for instance by heating the dispersion, a new family of curves will result similar in shape to those shown in Figure 21-7 but are displaced to the right (towards higher concentrations) and upwards (towards larger particle sizes).[7,9,28,29] An additional phenomennon illustrated in Figure 21-7 is that aging increases particle size. Curves ABC, DEF, and GHI correspond to increasing time periods after mixing the reagents, namely, 10–30 minutes, several hours, and weeks to years, respectively. This gradual increase in the particle size of crystals in their mother liquor is a recrystallization process called *Ostwald ripening*. Very small particles have a higher solubility than large particles of the same substance due to their greater specific surface area and higher surface free energy. In a saturated solution containing precipitated particles with a wide range of particle sizes, the very smallest particles dissolve spontaneously and deposit onto the larger particles. The growth of the larger crystals at the expense of the very small ones occurs because this process lowers the free energy of the dispersion. Adding small amounts of surface-active compounds that adsorb at the particle surface slows down the process.

Increasing the solubility of the precipitate accelerates the spontaneous coarsening of colloidal dispersions upon aging. For instance, barium sulfate precipitated by mixing concentrated solutions of sodium sulfate and barium chloride is largely in the colloidal size range and passes through filter paper. The colloidal particles gradually grow in size by Ostwald ripening, forming large crystals that can be removed quantitatively by filtration. Heating the aqueous dispersion speeds recrystallization by increasing the solubility of barium sulfate in water.

Conversely, the addition of ethyl alcohol lowers the solubility of barium sulfate and slows Ostwald ripening, which allows the dispersion to remain in the colloidal state for years.

The relationship between particle size and solubility is given by the Ostwald-Freundlich or Kelvin equation which, for nonionic solutes, is[2,8,9]:

$$\ln \frac{S}{S_\infty} = \frac{2\gamma M}{rdRT}$$

where S and S_∞ are the solubility of colloidal particles having a radius r and the solubility of large, flat particles ($r = \infty$), respectively. For electrolytes, the mean ionic activity is included. The solid/solvent interfacial free energy, γ, can only be determined indirectly (for instance, by means of this equation). The ratio of the molecular weight of the solute to its density (M/d) equals its molar volume. Assuming $M = 500\ g/mol$, $d = 1.00\ g/mL$, and $\gamma = 30\ erg/cm^2$, and using the values of $8.314 \times 10^7\ erg/mol\text{-}K$ for the gas constant R and $298\ K$ for the absolute temperature T, dispersed particles having radii of 1×10^{-6} cm (10 nm), 1×10^{-5} cm (0.1 μm), 1×10^{-4} cm (1 μm), and 1×10^{-3} cm (10 μm) correspond to S/S_∞ ratios of 3.36, 1.13, 1.012, and 1.0012 respectively. Therefore, while particles having sizes at the lower end of the colloidal range are appreciably more soluble than coarser particles of the same compound, the solubility of finely ground drug or excipient powders (particle radii typically in the 1–10 μm range) is only increased by ≤1%.

Condensation methods generally produce polydisperse sols because nucleation continues while established nuclei grow. However, monodispersed colloidal sols may be prepared by precipitation using a technique that involves the formation of all nuclei in a single, brief burst. A sufficiently brief period of homogeneous nucleation relieves the supersaturation to such an extent that no new nuclei can subsequently form. Therefore, the nuclei created during the initial burst grow uniformly as the remaining excess of precipitating material diffuses and deposits onto them. The supersaturation never again reaches sufficiently high values for forming new nuclei because it is relieved by the continuous growth of the existing nuclei.[7,9,28,29] The controlled hydrolysis of salts of di- and trivalent cations in aqueous solutions at elevated temperatures has been used to produce colloidal dispersions of metal (hydrous) oxides having uniform sizes in a variety of well-defined shapes (eg, spheres or laths or cubes or discs). Complexation of the cations, concentration, and temperature control the rate of hydrolysis, and therefore, the chemical composition, crystallinity, shape, and size of the dispersed phase.[28,30]

Stabilization

It should be reiterated that hydrosols of hydrophobic substances are intrinsically unstable. While mechanical disintegration may break up the dispersed phase into colloidal particles, flocculation or coagulation causes the dispersed particles to become progressively coarser and fewer, ultimately resulting in the complete separation of a macroscopic phase. The reduction in surface area and in surface free energy accompanying flocculation or coagulation is small because irregular solid particles are rigid and only touch at a few points upon aggregation. However, these loose initial contacts may grow with time by sintering or recrystallization. Sintering is the "fusion" of primary particles into larger primary particles, which propagates from the initial small areas of contact. This recrystallization process is spontaneous because it decreases the specific surface area of the dispersed solid and the surface free energy of the dispersion. Sintering is analogous to Ostwald ripening, the recrystallization process that transfers solids from colloidal to coarse particles. Low solubility and the presence of adsorbed surface-active substances retard both processes.

If aqueous dispersions of hydrophobic solids are to resist reaggregation (ie, flocculation and coagulation), they must be

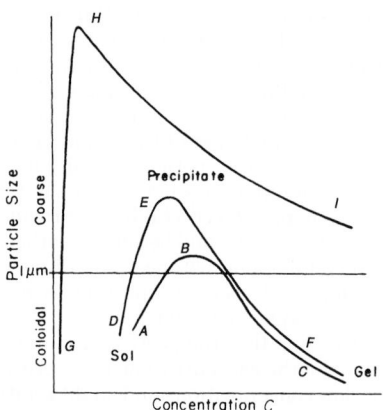

Figure 21-7. Effect of aging and concentration of the precipitating material upon particle size. Curves *ABC, DEF,* and *GHI* correspond to increasing aging. Both axes are on a logarithmic scale. Data from von Weimarn PP. In Alexander J, ed. *Colloid Chemistry*, vol I. New York: Chemical Catalog Co (Reinhold), 1926. See also *Chem Rev* 1926; 2:217 and Overbeek JThG. *Adv Colloid Interface Sci* 1982; 15:251.

stabilized during or shortly after the dispersion process. Stabilizing factors include the presence of electrical charges at the particle surface and the presence of adsorbed macromolecules or nonionic surfactants. The presence of positive or negative charges may result from the dissociation of the solid's ionogenic groups or the adsorption of ions such as ionic surfactants. These stabilizing factors do not alter the intrinsic thermodynamic instability of lyophobic dispersions, and therefore, ΔG_s remains positive and phase separation or aggregation is still energetically favored over dispersal. However, they establish kinetic barriers that delay the aggregation processes almost indefinitely; the dispersed particles cannot come together close enough for van der Waals attractive forces to produce coagulation.[5,6,8]

Stabilization may be provided by adsorbed surfactants. In a flocculated dispersion, groups of several particles are agglomerated into flocs. Frequently, the particles of a floc are in physical contact. When a surfactant is added to a flocculated sol, the dissolved surfactant molecules adsorb onto the surface of the particles. Surfactant molecules also tend to pry apart the flocs by wedging themselves in between the particle contact points. This action frees up additional surface area for surfactant adsorption. The breaking up of flocs or secondary particles is defined as deflocculation or peptization. Ophthalmic suspensions should be deflocculated because the large particle size of flocs causes irritation to the eye. Parenteral suspensions should also be deflocculated to prevent the larger particles from clogging hypodermic syringes, causing tissue irritation, or blocking capillary blood vessels. However, deflocculated suspensions tend to cake (ie, the sediment formed by gravitational settling is compact and may be hard to redisperse upon shaking). Caking in oral suspensions is prevented by controlled flocculation.

Surfactants tend to accumulate at interfaces because of their amphiphilic nature. This process is an *oriented physical adsorption*. Surfactant molecules arrange themselves at the interface between water and an organic solid or liquid of low polarity in such a way that the hydrocarbon chain is in contact with the surface of the solid particle or sticks inside the oil droplet while the polar head group is oriented towards the water phase. This orientation leaves the polar head group in contact with the water so that it can be hydrated and removes the surfactant's hydrophobic hydrocarbon chain from the bulk of the water, where it is unwelcome because it inferences with the hydrogen bonding between water molecules. Figure 21-8 shows that at a low surfactant concentration and at low surface coverage, the hydrocarbon chains of the adsorbed surfactant molecules lie flat against the solid surface. At higher surfactant concentrations, the surfactant molecules are adsorbed in an upright position to allow for the greatest number of molecules per unit surface area. In this position, the terminal methyl groups of the hydrocarbon tails are in contact with the hydrophobic particle surface and the hydrocarbon tails are in lateral contact with each other. London dispersion forces promote the attraction between both types of adjoining groups.

The adsorption of ionic surfactants increases the charge density and the ζ potential of the dispersed particles. These two parameters are low for water-insolubel organic substances. The increase in electrostatic repulsion between nonpolar particles due to the adsorption of surface-active ions stabilizes the dispersion against coagulation. This "charge stabilization" is described by the DLVO theory.

Most water-soluble nonionic surfactants are polyoxyethylated. Each molecule consists of a hydrophobic hydrocarbon chain combined with a hydrophilic polyethylene glycol chain (eg, $CH_3(CH_2)_{15}(OCH_2CH_2)_{10}OH$). Hydration of the ether groups and the terminal hydroxyl group renders the surfactant molecule water-soluble. It adsorbs at the interface between a hydrophobic solid and water, with the hydrocarbon moiety adhering to the solid surface and the polyethylene glycol moiety protruding into the water, where it is hydrated. Therefore, the particle surface is surrounded by a thin layer of hydrated polyethylene glycol chains. This hydrophilic shell forms a steric barrier that prevents close contact between particles and inhibits coagulation

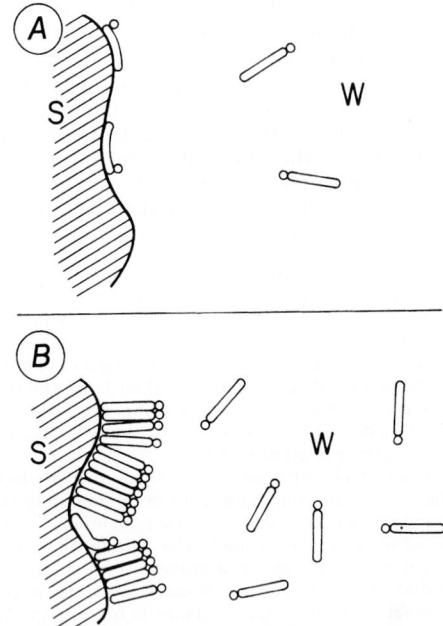

Figure 21-8. Schematic representation of the physical adsorption of surfactant molecules at a hydrophobic solid (S)/water (W) interface. Cylindrical portions and spheres represent the hydrocarbon chains and polar headgroups of the surfactant molecules, respectively. *A.* Low surfactant concentration/low surface coverage. *B.* Near critical micelle concentration/surface coverage near saturation.

("steric stabilization"). Nonionic surfactants also reduce the sensitivity of hydrophobic dispersions towards coagulation by salts (ie, they increase the coagulation values).[31]

The adsorption of water-soluble polymers provides a second mechanism for the stabilization of hydrophobic dispersions. Water-soluble polymers that have some hydrophobic groups may be surface active and adsorb at the interface between water and a hydrophobic organic solid because their hydrophobic groups limit their water solubility and render them amphiphilic. Such polymers also tend to accumulate at the air-water interface and, therefore, lower the surface tension of the aqueous phase. Conversely, polyelectrolytes that have a high concentration of ionic groups are excessively water-soluble, which reduces or eliminates their surface activity and tendency to adsorb at interfaces (eg, *sodium* carboxymethylcellulose). *Polyvinyl alcohol* is another polymer that does not adsorb extensively at interfaces due to a high concentration of hydroxyl groups, which makes it very water-soluble. Polyvinyl alcohol is manufactured by the hydrolysis of polyvinyl acetate, which is water-insoluble. Hydrolysis of ;85% of the acetyl groups produces a copolymer that is both water-soluble and surface-active. Other surface-active polymers include methylcellulose, hydroxypropyl cellulose, high-molecular-weight polyethylene glycols (polyethylene oxides), and proteins. The surface activity of proteins is due to the presence of hydrophobic groups at concentrations too low to cause insolubility in water. Proteins are denatured upon adsorption at air-water and solid-water interfaces.

As shown in Figure 21-9A, polymer molecules adsorb onto solid surfaces in the form of loops projecting into the aqueous phase rather than lying flat against the solid substrate. Only a small portion of an adsorbed polymer is in direct contact with the solid surface. However, because of its great chain length, there are enough of these contact points to anchor the adsorbed macromolecule firmly onto the surface. At sufficiently high concentrations, adsorbed polymers may form a layer surrounding the entire dispersed particles. This layer consists of the polymer chains as well as the water of hydration associated with them and any water mechanically trapped inside the chain loops. This sheath becomes an integral part of the particle surface and may prevent coagulation. The mechanisms by which adsorbed nonionic macromolecules prevent the coagulation of hydrophobic sols are the same ones operative in the stabilization of sols by nonionic surfactants. The hydrophilic polyethylene glycol moieties of the adsorbed surfactant molecules that protrude into the aqueous phase resemble the chain ends of the adsorbed macromolecules rather than their looped segments.

The following protective mechanisms are operative:

1. The layer of adsorbed polymer and enmeshed water surrounding the particles forms a *mechanical* or *steric barrier* ("*steric stabilization*") that prevents the particles from approaching each other closely enough for the interparticle attraction of London dispersion forces to produce coagulation. These forces are only effective over interparticle distances smaller than twice the thickness of the adsorbed polymer layer. These layers are somewhat elastic; they may be dented by a collision between two particles but tend to return to their original shape.

2. When two particles approach so closely that their adsorbed polymer layers overlap, the chain loops of the opposing layers compress and mix with or interpenetrate each other. The freedom of motion of the chain segments in the overlapped region becomes restricted, which produces a negative entropy change. Therefore, any reduction in interparticle distance, which is required for coagulation, results in a positive change in free energy. As a result, the reverse process of particle separation occurs spontaneously because disentangling the two opposing adsorbed polymer layers is more energetically favorable. The particles are thus prevented from coagulating by *entropic repulsion* through the mechanism of *entropic stabilization* of the sol. This mechanism predominates when the concentration of polymer in the adsorbed layer is low.

3. As the adsorbed polymer layers on two approaching particles overlap, the polymer concentration in the overlap region causes a local increase in osmotic pressure, which is relieved by an influx of water. This influx of water to dilute the polymer loops pushes the two particles apart, preventing coagulation.

4. If the adsorbed polymer has some ionic groups, stabilization by electrostatic repulsion or charge stabilization, as previously described, is an additional factor that prevents a close interparticle approach and coagulation.

5. The adsorption of water-soluble polymers changes the nature of the surface of hydrophobic particles to hydrophilic, resulting in an increased resistance to coagulation by salts.[32]

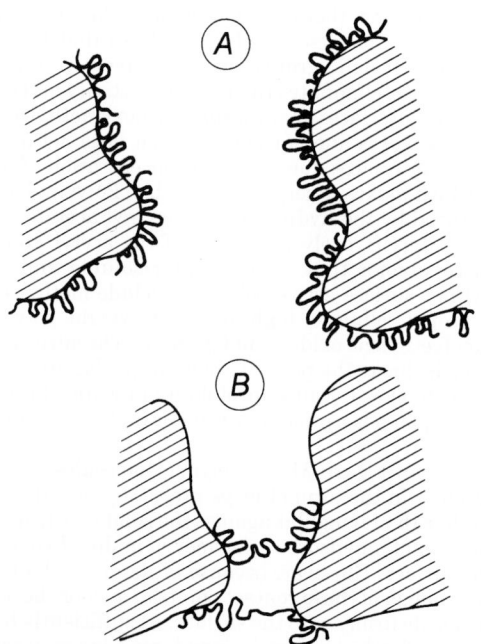

Figure 21-9. Protective action (*A*) and sensitization (*B*) of adsorbed polymer chains upon sols containing hydrophobic particles.

The water-soluble polymers whose adsorption stabilizes hydrophobic sols and protects them against coagulation are called *protective colloids*. *Gelatin* and *serum albumin* are the preferred protective colloids for stabilizing parenteral suspensions because of their biocompatibility. These two polymers, as well as casein (milk protein), dextrin (partially hydrolyzed starch), and vegetable gums like acacia and tragacanth are metabolized in the human body. Cellulose derivatives and most synthetic protective colloids such as *povidone* are not biotransformed. Because of this and their large molecular size, these polymers are not absorbed but excreted intact when administered in an oral dosage form.

Sensitization

Sensitization is the opposite of protective action (ie, a decrease in the stability of the hydrophobic sols). At concentrations well below those at which it exerts a protective action, a protective colloid may flocculate a sol in the absence of added salts and/or lower the coagulation values of the sol. In the case of nonionic polymers and of polyelectrolytes having charges of the same sign as the sol particles, flocculation results from the bridging mechanism illustrated in Figure 21-9*B*. At very low polymer concentrations, there are not nearly enough polymer molecules present to completely cover each sol particle. Since the particle surfaces are largely bare, a single macromolecule may be adsorbed onto two particles, thereby bridging the gap between them and pulling them close together. Flocs are formed when several particles become connected through polymer molecules that are adsorbed jointly onto two or possibly even three particles. Such flocculation usually occurs over a narrow range and at very low polymer concentrations. At higher concentrations, bridging is unlikely to occur because there is enough polymer to completely cover all of the particles and the adsorbed polymer stabilizes or peptizes the sol.[9,32]

If the polymer contains ionic groups of charge opposite to that of the sol particles, a limited amount of polymer adsorption neutralizes the charge of the particles and reduces their ζ potential to nearly zero. This eliminates stabilization by electrostatic repulsion. In addition, steric stabilization is ineffective because of the low surface coverage of the adsorbed polymer. Therefore, the sol either coagulates by itself or may be coagulated with a very small amount of sodium chloride. At higher polymer concentrations, where adsorption is more extensive, the charge on the particles is converted to the sign of the polyelectrolyte, which reactivates charge stabilization and adds steric stabilization. As a result, the coagulation value of the sol increases well above the original value. For example, partly hydrolyzed polyacrylamide containing about 20% of ammonium acrylate repeat units is an anionic polyelectrolyte. Addition of this polyacrylamide to aluminum hydroxide sols at a polymer concentration of 1:1,000,000 and a pH of 6–7, where the sols are positively charged and the polyelectrolyte is fully ionized, results in flocculation. At a polymer concentration of 1:10,000, the sols become negatively charged because extensive polymer adsorption introduces an excess of —COO⁻ groups over the =Al⁺ ions on the particle surface. This creation of negatively charged particles introduces electrostatic and steric stabilization, which makes the sols more stable against flocculation by salts than they were before the addition of the polyacrylamide.

Polymer B in Figure 21-10 illustrates this example. The curve in the lower plot indicates sensitization, with the coagulation value for sodium chloride lowered by as much as 60%. Zeta potential measurements may be used to distinguish between sensitization by bridging and sensitization by charge neutralization. The charge reversal caused by the adsorption of Polymer B is illustrated in the upper plot and indicates that charge neutralization is the cause of sensitization. If Polymer B had a ζ potential-polymer concentration plot similar to Polymer A, sensitization would be ascribed to bridging. The nonionic Polymer A in Figure 21-10 stabilizes the sol at all

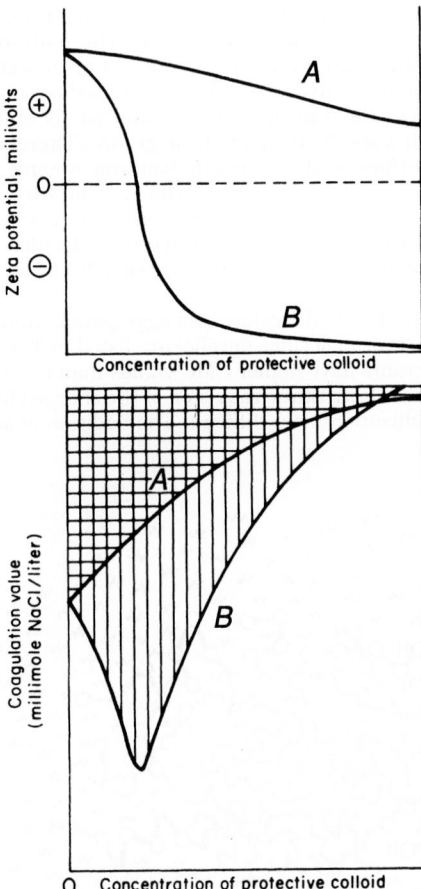

Figure 21-10. Protective action and sensitization: Polymer A exerts protective action at all concentrations, while Polymer B sensitizes at low concentrations and stabilizes at high concentrations. Horizontal and vertical hatching indicates region of flocculation for a sol treated with various concentrations of Polymers A and B, respectively. Clear region underneath indicates sol is deflocculated.

head groups but repels their hydrocarbon tails. Consequently, surfactants tend to concentrate and adsorb at air-water, oil-water, and solid-water interfaces. The surface tension of aqueous surfactant solutions decreases with increasing surfactant concentration up to a point, beyond which it remains nearly constant (Fig 21-11). Curves A and B in Figure 21-11 illustrate the surface tension (against air) and the interfacial tension (against oil) of an aqueous surfactant solution as a function of surfactant concentration. Surface-active impurities may cause a minimum in the surface tension (shown as a dotted curve) rather than a mere leveling off. Abrupt changes occur not only to the surface and interfacial properties but also to the surfactant solution's bulk properties such as equivalent conductivity (Curve D), co-ion and counterion activities in the case of ionic surfactants, colligative properties like osmotic pressure (Curve C), turbidity (but the increase is far too weak to be visible to the naked eye), refractive index, UV and NMR spectra, partial molar volume, relative viscosity, and the diffusion coefficients and solubility of water-insoluble, oil-soluble compounds (Curve E). All of these changes occur over a very narrow concentration range, which is shown as a crosshatched band and is referred to as the *critical micelle concentration* (CMC).

As the surfactant concentration in a liquid is increased, the amount of the surfactant adsorbed at the liquid-air and liquid-container interfaces increases and these interfaces become increasingly crowded. When the concentration is increased further, the surfactant molecules will continue to adsorb at these interfaces until tightly packed monolayers are formed and there is no longer any room for further surfactant adsorption. At this point, the surface and interfacial tensions reach their constant values,[33] and it would seem that the bulk solubility limit of the surfactant has been reached. However, if more surfactant is added to the solution, the excess surfactant molecules will begin to associate into small aggregates called *micelles* (at the CMC), while the concentration of nonassociated surfactant molecules remains nearly constant. Above the CMC, the concentration of micellar surfactant is equal to the total surfactant concentration minus the CMC. Diluting the surfactant solution to below the CMC causes the micelles to disperse or break up into single or nonassociated surfactant molecules.

concentrations. Neither sensitization by bridging nor by charge neutralization is observed. The reason that Polymer A slightly lowers the positive ζ potential of the sol is that the increasing amounts of adsorbed polymer chains gradually shift the plane of shear outward and away from the positively charged surface. If Polymer A were a cationic polyelectrolyte, the ζ potential-polymer concentration plot would gradually rise with an increase in polymer adsorption rather than drop.

Even water-soluble polymers which are too thoroughly hydrophilic to be adsorbed by hydrophobic sol particles can stabilize such sols. Their thickening action increases the viscosity of the sols. This slows down Brownian motion and sedimentation, giving the particles less opportunity to come in contact with each other and, therefore, decreasing flocculation.

ASSOCIATION COLLOIDS

Association colloids are formed by self-assembling enough small molecules to produce aggregates in the colloidal size range. This group of colloids includes surfactant micelles, microemulsions, and liposomes.

Formation of Surfactant Micelles

The dual or amphiphilic nature of surfactants or surface-active agents was discussed previously. Water attracts their polar

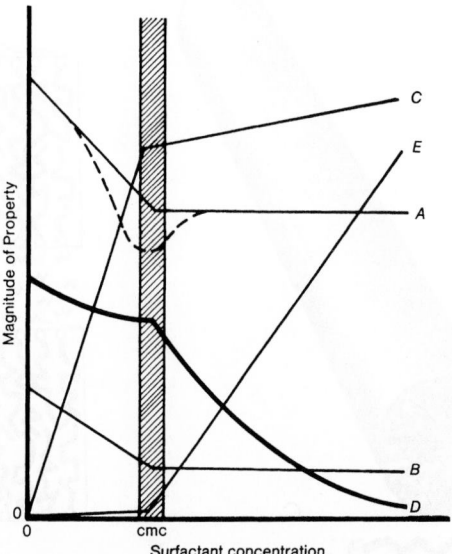

Figure 21-11. Effect of surfactant concentration and micelle formation on various properties of the aqueous solution of an ionic surfactant. *A:* Surface tension; *B:* interfacial tension; *C:* osmotic pressure; *D:* equivalent conductivity; *E:* solubility of a compound with very low solubility in pure water. (From Schott H, Martin AN. In Dittert LW, ed, *American Pharmacy*, 7th ed. Philadelphia: JB Lippincott, 1974.)

Micelles are not static aggregates; they dissociate, regroup and reassociate rapidly. The half-life of ionic surfactant micelles in the absence of additives is a small fraction of a second. Furthermore, there is a dynamic equilibrium (ie, an incessant exchange) between single surfactant molecules in solution, surfactant molecules adsorbed in monolayers at the interfaces, and surfactant molecules associated as micelles.

The shape of micelles in dilute aqueous surfactant solutions is approximately spherical (Fig 21-12A). The polar head groups of the surfactant molecules are arranged in an outer spherical shell while their hydrocarbon chains are oriented towards the center where they form a spherical core. These hydrocarbon chains are randomly coiled and entangled. The micellar interior has a nonpolar, liquid-like character resembling a liquid normal paraffin such as dodecane. In nonionic surfactant micelles, the polyoxyethylene moieties are oriented outwards and permeated by water while the hydrocarbon moieties form an "oil

droplet" core similar to ionic micelles (Fig 21-12B): this arrangement is energetically favorable. The hydrophilic head groups, located externally, are in contact with water and remain extensively hydrated. The hydrocarbon moieties are removed from the aqueous medium and partly shielded from contact with water by the polar head groups. Therefore, they no longer interfere with hydrogen bonding among the water molecules. This interference is the reason why surfactant molecules are pushed out of aqueous media towards interfaces. The hydrocarbon tails of the surfactant molecules, located in the micellar interior, attract one another by weak dispersion forces.[31,34–36]

Representative CMC values and aggregation numbers (number of surfactant molecules/micelle) are listed in Table 21-4.[36,37] Ionic surfactants have higher CMC values than nonionic surfactants because electrostatic repulsion of the charged head groups makes micellization more difficult. The addition of simple salts

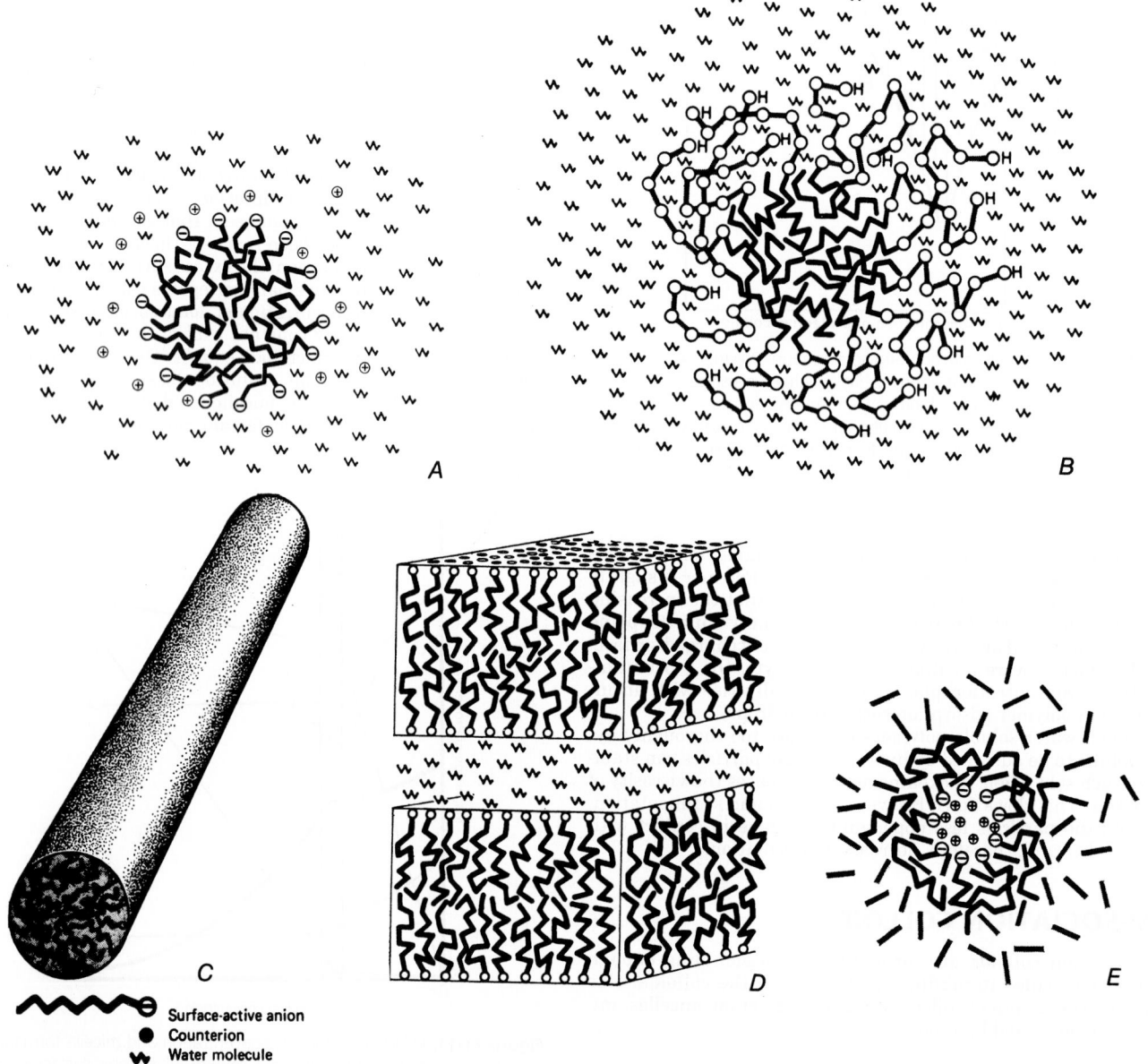

Surface-active anion
Counterion
Water molecule
Oil molecule

Figure 21-12. Different types of micelles. **A.** Spherical micelle of an anionic surfactant; **B.** spherical micelle of a nonionic surfactant; **C.** cylindrical micelle of an ionic surfactant; **D.** lamellar micelle of an ionic surfactant; **E.** reverse micelle of an anionic surfactant in oil. (From Schott H, Martin AN. In Dittert LW, ed, *American Pharmacy*, 7th ed. Philadelphia: JB Lippincott, 1974.)

Table 21-4. Critical Micelle Concentrations and Micellar Aggregation Numbers of Various Surfactants in Water at Room Temperature

STRUCTURE	NAME	CMC (mmol/L)	SURFACTANT MOLECULES/ MICELLE
n-$C_{11}H_{23}$COOK	Potassium laurate	24	50
n-$C_8H_{17}SO_3$Na	Sodium octane sulfonate	150	28
n-$C_{10}H_{21}SO_3$Na	Sodium decane sulfonate	40	40
n-$C_{12}H_{25}SO_3$Na	Sodium dodecane sulfonate	9	54
n-$C_{12}H_{25}OSO_3$Na	Sodium lauryl sulfate	8	62
n-$C_{12}H_{25}OSO_3$Na	Sodium lauryl sulfate[a]	1	96
	Docusate sodium	5	48
n-$C_{10}H_{21}N(CH_3)_3$Br	Decyltrimethylammonium bromide	63	36
n-$C_{12}H_{25}N(CH_3)_3$Br	Dodecyltrimethylammonium bromide	14	50
n-$C_{14}H_{29}N(CH_3)_3$Br	Tetradecyltrimethylammonium bromide	3	75
n-$C_{14}H_{29}N(CH_3)_3$Cl	Tetradecyltrimethylammonium chloride	3	64
n-$C_{12}H_{25}NH_3$Cl	Dodecylammonium chloride	13	55
n-$C_{12}H_{25}O(CH_2CH_2O)_8$H	Polyoxyl 8 dodecyl ether	0.13	132
n-$C_{12}H_{25}O(CH_2CH_2O)_8$H[b]	Polyoxyl 8 dodecyl ether	0.10	301
n-$C_{12}H_{25}O(CH_2CH_2O)_{12}$H	Polyoxyl 12 dodecyl ether	0.14	78
n-$C_{12}H_{25}O(CH_2CH_2O)_{12}$H[b]	Polyoxyl 12 dodecyl ether	0.091	116
p-$C_9H_{19}C_6H_4O(CH_2CH_2O)_{10}$H	Nonoxynol 10	0.07	276
p-$C_9H_{19}C_6H_4O(CH_2CH_2O)_{30}$H	Nonoxynol 30	0.24	44

[a] Interpolated for physiologic saline, 0.154 M NaCl.
[b] At 55° instead of 20°.

reduces these repulsive forces and, therefore, lowers the CMC values of ionic surfactants. Within any homologous surfactant series, the CMC decreases regularly with increasing hydrocarbon chain length and, therefore, with increasing surface activity of the surfactant. As is seen in Table 21-4, each additional methylene group decreases the CMC by approximately one-half. This is a consequence of Traube's rule, which states that, within a homologous series of surfactants, each additional methylene group decreases the molar concentration required to produce an equal lowering of the surface tension of water threefold. The addition of a methylene group reduces the CMC by a factor of antilog (1/3) = 2. The CMC of nonionic surfactants increases as the temperature decreases and as the percentage of polyoxyethylene increases.

The micelles of the surfactants listed in Table 21-4 are either spherical or ellipsoidal. They are rather small because their sizes were determined in relatively dilute solutions (containing only a few percent of surfactant) and mostly in pure water at room temperature. Their diameters are between 2 and 8 nm, which places them at the lower end of the colloidal size range. For this reason, surfactants are sometimes called *association colloids*. Adding salts increases the size of ionic micelles. Raising the temperature increases the size of nonionic micelles, especially if the temperatures are within 20° of their respective cloud points. These factors reduce the water solubility of ionic and nonionic surfactants, thereby rendering them more surface-active.

As micelles become larger, they also become more asymmetric. Their shape changes from spherical or ellipsoidal to cylindrical and eventually to lamellar. In cylindrical micelles, the polar head groups form the periphery and the hydrocarbon tails fill the interior of the cylinders (Fig 21-12C). In lamellar micelles, the surfactant molecules are arranged in parallel bimolecular sheets with a tail-to-tail orientation (ie, the hydrocarbon tails form the inner layer). Water is stratified between the sheets, thereby hydrating the external polar head groups (Fig 21-12D). In both types of micelles, the hydrocarbon tails are randomly coiled and in a liquid-like state.[12] In concentrated aqueous solutions containing 20% or more of surfactant, cylindrical micelles often line up parallel to each other and arrange themselves in hexagonal arrays. Likewise, lamellar micelles

are often packed parallel and equidistant from each other with the intervening water layers having a uniform thickness. These ordered solutions are liquid crystals or mesophases; they are birefringent and very viscous. Even though they are liquids, they have some of the properties of crystalline solids.[8,31,35,36]

Oil-soluble surfactants (eg, heavy metal soaps, docusate sodium, and nonionic surfactants with HLB values < 7) form aggregates when dissolved in organic liquids having low polarity such as hydrocarbons and chlorinated hydrocarbons. These micelles are inverted or turned inside out; their hydrocarbon tails are oriented outwards into the oil phase while their polar head groups are in the center of the micelle, where water can be solubilized (Fig 21-12E). Because the bulky head groups are in the center, the aggregation numbers for *reverse micelles* are small, usually between 3 and 20.[35,38]

Microemulsions

Microemulsions are liquid dispersions of water and oil that are made homogeneous, transparent, and stable by the addition of relatively large amounts of a surfactant and a cosurfactant.[10,39–41] *Oil* is defined as any liquid having low polarity and low miscibility with water (eg, toluene, cyclohexane, and mineral or vegetable oils). Microemulsions have intermediate properties between micelles containing solubilized oils and emulsions. Emulsions are lyophobic and unstable. Their preparation requires the input of considerable amounts of mechanical energy, which may be supplied by colloid mills, homogenizers, or ultrasonic generators. Conversely, microemulsions are on the borderline between lyophobic and lyophilic colloids. True microemulsions are thermodynamically stable and, therefore, form spontaneously when oil, water, surfactants, and cosurfactants are mixed together.[42]

Both emulsions and microemulsions may contain high volume fractions of the internal phase. For instance, some O/W systems contain 75% (v/v) of oil dispersed in 25% water, although lower volume fractions of the internal phase are more common.

Microemulsions droplet have a mean diameter range of approximately 6 to 100 nm and a narrow droplet size distribution. Since the droplet diameters are less than 1/4 of the wavelength of light (420 nm for violet and 660 nm for red light), microemulsions scatter little light. Therefore, they are transparent or at least translucent. By contrast, emulsions have broad droplet-size distributions and are generally opaque because the bulk of their droplets are greater than the wavelength of light and most oils have higher refractive indices than water.

Emulsions contan three components, namely, oil, water, and surfactant; whereas, microemulsions generally require a fourth component, a *cosurfactant.* Commonly used cosurfactants include linear alcohols of medium chain length that are sparingly miscible with water. The combination of surfactant and cosurfactant promote the generation of extensive interfaces through the spontaneous dispersion of oil in water, or vice-versa. The large interfacial area between the oil and water consists of a mixed interfacial film containing both surfactant and cosurfactant molecules. This film is called the "interphase" because it is thicker than the typical surfactant monolayers formed at the oil-water interfaces in emulsions. The interfacial tension at the oil-water interface in microemulsions approaches zero, which also contributes to their spontaneous formation. According to another viewpoint, microemulsions are regarded as micelles extensively swollen by large amounts of solubilized oil.

Micellar solutions, microemulsions, and emulsions can be of the O/W (oil-in-water) or W/O type. As mentioned previously, aqueous micellar solutions can solubilize oils in the hydrocarbon cores of the micelles. Conversely, oil-soluble surfactants like sorbitan monooleate and docusate sodium form reverse micelles in oils (Fig 21-12*E*) that are capable of solubilizing water in their polar centers. The solubilized oil in the former micelles and the solubilized water in the latter may in turn enhance the micellar solubilization of oil-soluble and water-soluble drugs, respectively.

Typical formulations for an O/W and a W/O microemulsion are shown in Table 21-5. The ratio of grams of surfactant to grams of solubilized or emulsified oil or water ranges from 2 to 20 for micellar solutions and 0.01 to 0.1 for emulsions. Microemulsions have intermediate values. For example, the ratios for the formulations in Table 21-5 are near unity. In industrial formulations, the ratios are closer to 0.1 to reduce costs. Microemulsions are used for a variety of applications including floor polishes, agricultural pesticides, tertiary petroleum recovery, and pharmaceutical delivery systems.

Liposomes

Liposomes are discussed by Crommelin and Schreier,[43] and by Rosoff.[44] They are spherical vesicles whose walls consist of hydrated bilayers of phospholipids. Phosphatidylcholines (lecithins), dispersed in excess water at temperatures where they are in a "fluid" or liquid-crystalline state, spontaneously form closed vesicles filled with trapped aqueous medium. Cooling the dispersion below the phase transition temperature of the lecithins orders the hydrocarbon chains of their fatty acids into a close—packed and more rigid structure (the gel state) and drastically lowers the permeability of solute molecules trapped inside the vesicles. The transition temperatures of dioleylphosphatidyl choline and dipalmityl phosphatidyl choline are $-15°$ and $41°$ C, respectively. Intercalating cholesterol molecules between adjacent lecithin molecules has a condensing effect on the bilayers, reducing their permeability considerably. The addition

of stearylamine confers a positive charge to liposomes and renders them impermeable towards cations. The incorporation of phosphatidic acids confers a negative charge and makes the liposomes permeable to cations. Anions generally diffuse rapidly through positive, negative, and neutral liposome membranes.

Liposomes are classified as unilamellar and multilamellar. The former are vesicles enclosed by a 6 to 7 nm thick single phospholipid bilayer. They range in size from 20 to 1000 nm (1 μm), depending on the method of preparation. Multilamellar liposomes consist of concentric phospholipid bilayers separated by aqueous layers of about 2.8 nm thickness. They have an onion-like structure with an aqueous core.

Methods of preparing liposomes include: subjecting aqueous lipid dispersions to high shear (including ultrasonication); forming their lipid films by solvent evaporation, followed by their hydration and dispersal in water; injecting solutions of lipids as water-immiscible (ether, petroleum ether) or water-miscible (alcohol) solvents into water. Vesicle formation is not restricted to lipids. Dioctadecyldimethylammonium chloride, dihexadecyl phosphate, and select nonionic surfactants also form vesicles, the latter called niosomes.

PHARMACEUTICAL APPLICATIONS

Colloidal materials are used for a variety of pharmaceutical applications including therapeutic and diagnostic agents, drug delivery systems, and pharmaceutical excipients. With the recent advances in biotechnology and protein engineering, many new drug substances are colloids including recombinant human insulin, interferons, interleukins, and monoclonal antibodies. Drug substances may also be prepared as colloidal sized particles to improve bioavailability or therapeutic activity (eg, colloidal sulfur).

Radioactive Colloids

Colloidal dispersions containing radioactive isotopes are being used as diagnostic and therapeutic agents in nuclear medicine.[45] *Colloid gold Au 198* is made by reducing a solution of gold (^{198}Au) chloride either by treatment with ascorbic acid or by heating with an alkaline glucose solution. Gelatin is added as a protective colloid. The particle size ranges from 5 to 50 nm with a mean of 30 nm, and the color of the sol is cherry-red in transmitted light. Violet or blue sols have excessively large particle sizes and should be discarded. Colloidal gold is used as a diagnostic and therapeutic aid and. The half-life of ^{198}Au is 2.7 days. *Technetium 99m sulfur colloid* is prepared by reducing sodium pertechnetate ^{99m}Tc with sodium thiosulfate. The product, a mixture of technetium sulfide and sulfur in the colloidal particle size range, is stabilized with gelatin. It is primarily used in liver, spleen, and bone scanning and has a half-life of 6.0 hours.

Crosslinked Polymers

When linear, water-soluble polymers are crosslinked, they swell in water but no longer dissolve. The crosslinks tie the macromolecular chains together by primary covalent bonds, transforming each particle into a single, giant molecule. The

Table 21-5. Microemulsion Formulations

COMPOUND	FUNCTION	CONTENT IN MICROEMULSIONS, %	
		O/W	W/O
Sodium lauryl sulfate	Surfactant	13	10
1-Pentanol	Cosurfactant	8	25
Xylene	Oil	8	50
Water		71	15

water-swollen grains of crosslinked polymers are permeable to low molecular weight solutes. Examples of crosslinked polyelectrolytes include the cation-exchange resin sodium polystyrenesulfonate copolymerized with divinylbenzene (used to reduce hyperkalemia by exchanging some of its Na^+ with $K^{+)}$ and the anion-exchange resins cholestyramine and colestipol hydrochloride (which reduce hypercholesterolemia by binding bile salt anions). Polycarbophil, a lightly crosslinked polymer of acrylic acid, only ionizes and swells in the nearly neutral small intestine, where it absorbs water and reduces the fluidity of diarrheal stool.

Colloidal Delivery Systems

Colloidal delivery systems include micelles, microemulsions, liposomes, parenteral emulsions, microspheres, nanoparticles, and drug-polymer conjugates.

MICELLES AND SOLUBILIZATION—Micelles have been used to solubilize poorly water-soluble compounds. For example, *Aquamephyton Injection* contains phytonadione (vitamin K_1) dissolved in the core of micelles of a polyoxyethylated fatty acid derivative. *Cernevit-12 for Infusion* consists of a mixture of fat-soluble vitamins (A, D, & E) solubilized by micelles, and water-soluble vitamins dissolved in water. As illustrated in Figure 21-12, the interior of surfactant micelles formed in an aqueous media consists of hydrocarbon tails in a liquid-like, disordered state. Therefore, the micelles resemble miniscule pools of liquid hydrocarbon surrounded by shells of polar head groups. Compounds that are poorly soluble in water but soluble in hydrocarbon solvents can be dissolved inside these micelles, and thereby brought homogeneously into the overall aqueous medium.

Being oleophilic, the solubilized molecules are primarily located in the hydrocarbon core of the micelles (Figure 21-13A). However, many water-insoluble drugs also contain polar functional groups such as hydroxyl, carbonyl, ether, amino, amide, and cyano groups. Upon solubilization, these hydrophilic groups are located among the polar headgroups of the surfactant in the periphery of the micelle in order to become hydrated (Figure 21-13B). For instance, when cholesterol or dodecanol is solubilized by sodium lauryl sulfate micelles, their hydroxyl groups penetrate between the sulfate ions and are even bound to them through hydrogen bonds, while their hydrocarbon portions are immersed among the dodecyl tails of the surfactant in the micelle core. Micelles of polyoxyethylated nonionic surfactants consist of an outer shell of hydrated polyethylene glycol moieties and a core of hydrocarbon moieties. Compounds like phenol, cresol, benzoic acid, salicylic acid, and esters of *p*-hydrobenzoic and *p*-aminobenzoic acids have some solubility in water and oils

but considerable solubility in liquids of intermediate polarity such as ethanol, propylene glycol, or aqueous solutions of polyethylene glycols. When solubilized by nonionic micelles, these compounds are located in the outer hydrated polyethylene glycol shell as shown in Figure 21-13C. Since these compounds have hydroxyl or amino groups, they frequently form complexes with the ether oxygens of the surfactant through hydrogen bonding.[31,34–36,38]

Micellar solubilization is generally nonspecific; any drug that is appreciably soluble in oils can be solubilized. Each compound has a solubilization limit, which depends upon temperature and the nature and concentration of the surfactant. There are two general categories of solubilizates. The first consists of comparatively large, asymmetrical and rigid molecules such as steroids and dyes that form crystalline solids. Because of a dissimilarity in structure, these compounds do not blend in with the normal paraffin tails that make up the micellar cores but remain as distinct solute molecules. They are sparingly solubilized by micelles with only a few molecules/micelle at saturation (Table 21-6). The number of carbon atoms in the micellar hydrocarbon core required to solubilize one molecule of a steroid or dye at saturation is of the same order of magnitude as the number of carbon atoms in bulk liquid dodecane or hexadecane required to dissolve one molecule of steroid or dye at saturation.

Since solubilization depends on the presence of micelles, it does not take place below the CMC. Therefore, such solubilization may be used to determine the CMC, particularly when the solubilizate is a dye or another compound easy to assay. Plotting the maximum amount of a water-insoluble dye solubilized by an aqueous surfactant, or the absorbance of its saturated solutions, versus the surfactant concentration produces a straight line that intersects the surfactant concentration axis at the CMC. Above the CMC, the amount of solubilized dye is directly proportional to the number of micelles, and therefore, proportional to the overall surfactant concentration. Below the CMC, no solubilization takes place. This is represented by Curve E in Figure 21-11.

The second category of compounds that may be solubilized is often liquid at room temperature and consist of relatively small, symmetrical and/or flexible molecules such as many constituents of essential oils. These molecules mix and freely blend in with the hydrocarbon portions of the surfactants in the core of the micelles and, therefore, become indistinguishable from them. Such compounds are extensively solubilized and in the process usually swell the micelles. They augment the volume of the hydrocarbon core and increase the number of surfactant molecules per micelle. Their solubilization frequently lowers the CMC.

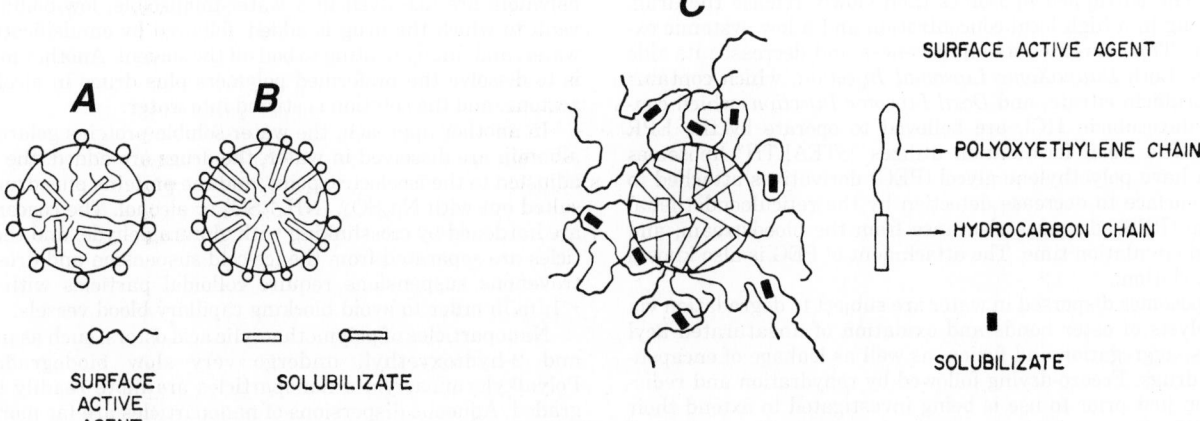

Figure 21-13. The locations of solubilizates in spherical micelles. **A.** Ionic surfactant (solubilized molecule has no hydrophilic groups); **B.** ionic surfactant (solubilized molecule has a hydrophilic group); **C.** nonionic surfactant (polar solubilizate). (From Shinoda K, Nakagawa T, Tamamushi B-I, Isemura T. *Colloidal Surfactants.* New York: Academic Press, 1963.)

Table 21-6. Micellar Solubilization Capacities of Different Surfactants for Estrone

SURFACTANT	CONCENTRATION RANGE (*M*)	TEMPERATURE (°C)	MOLES SURFACTANT/ MOLE SOLUBILIZED ESTRONE
Sodium laurate	0.025–0.23	40	91
Sodium oleate	0.002–0.35	40	53
Sodium lauryl sulfate	0.004–0.15	40	71
Sodium cholate	0.09–0.23	20	238
Sodium deoxycholate	0.007–0.36	20	476
Diamyl sodium sulfosuccinate	0.08–0.4	40	833
Dioctyl sodium sulfosuccinate	0.002–0.05	40	196
Tetradecyltrimethylammonium bromide	0.005–0.08	20	45
Hexadecylpyridinium chloride	0.001–0.1	20	32
Polysorbate 20	0.002–0.15	20	161
Polysorbate 60	0.0008–0.11	20	83

Data from Shinoda K, ed. *Solvent Properties of Surfactant Solutions.* New York: Dekker, 1967.

MICROEMULSIONS—O/W microemulsions are also formulated as aqueous vehicles for oil-soluble drugs to be administered by the percutaneous, oral, or parenteral routes. Oil-soluble drugs are incorporated into O/W emulsions by dissolving them in the oil phase before emulsification. Similarly, oil-soluble drugs are incorporated into microemulsions by prior dissolution within the oil phase. The advantage of microemulsions as dosage forms as compared to conventional emulsions is their smaller droplet size, which increases drug release, and their superior physical stability.

LIPOSOMES—Liposomes can be used as vehicles to deliver synthetic drugs, polypeptides, proteins, including enzymes and antibodies, and nucleic acids as well as recombinant DNA. Oil-soluble drugs are added to solutions of the lipid in organic solvents. Once the liposomes are formed, the drugs are solublilized by the hydrocarbon chains of the lipid bilayers. Water-soluble drugs are incorporated into the aqueous phase in which the liposomes are formed. The unencapsulated drug remaining in the external aqueous phase is then removed by dialysis, centrifugation, or ion exchange. *AmBisome Liposome for Injection* contains amphotericin B entrapped within a liposomal bilayer. Drugs have also been trapped within the inner, aqueous core of liposomes to protect them from enzymatic degradation as they circulate in the bloodstream.

An additional advantage of liposomes is their ability to target drugs to specific tissues in the body such as tumors. After IV administration, liposomes preferentially accumulate within tumors by what is known as the enhanced permeability and retention (EPR) effect because of their size. Tumor vasculature is typically more porous than most normal tissues of the body, which allows the permeation of colloidal sized materials. In addition, tumors typically lack significant lymphatic drainage, which results in the retention of these materials. The entrapped liposomes then slowly release the drug, resulting in a high local concentration and a low systemic exposure. This increases its effectiveness and decreases its side effects. Both *DaunoXome Lipsomal Injection*, which contains daunorubicin citrate, and *Doxil Lipsome Injection*, which contains doxorubicin HCl, are believed to operate by the EPR effect. The Doxil formulation utilizes "STEALTH" liposomes which have polyethylene glycol (PEG) derivatives attached to their surface to decrease detection by the reticuloendothelial system (RES), decrease clearance from the bloodstream, and extend circulation time. The attachment of PEG is also known as pegylation.

Liposomes dispersed in water are subject to degradation via hydrolysis of ester bonds and oxidation of unsaturated acyl chains, aggregation and fusion, as well as leakage of encapsulated drugs. Freeze-drying followed by rehydration and redispersion just prior to use is being investigated to extend their shelf life. The components of liposomes are similar to those of cell membranes. Therefore, they are nontoxic, biocompatible, and biodegradable. Liposomes have also been used as models to study the permeability of cell membranes.

MICROSPHERES—Microspheres are small, insoluble spherical particles consisting of a polymer matrix such as lactic/glycolic acid copolymer (PLGA).[46] Microspheres of gelatin or human serum albumin have been prepared in fairly narrow particle-size ranges from 10–20 nm through 45–55 μm. Drugs may be physically entrapped in the pores of the microspheres or chemically conjugated to the polymer matrix. Marketed drug products that utilize microspheres include *Lupron Depot for Suspension*, which is administered monthly by intramuscular injection and slowly releases leuprolide acetate, and *Nutropin Depot for Injectable Suspension*, which is administered 1–2× per month by subcutaneous injection and slowly releases somatropin of rDNA origin. In addition, microspheres have been labeled with a variety of β- and γ-emitting radionuclides such as ^{131}I, ^{99m}Tc, [113m]In, or [51]Cr. Such products have been used to scan the heart, brain, liver, urogenital and gastrointestinal tracts, and in pulmonary perfusion and inhalation studies.[45]

NANOPARTICLES—Nanoparticles are described in the chapter by Kreuter[42] as solid spherical polymeric particles ranging in size from 10 to 1000 nm (1 μm). The therapeutic agents are either adsorbed onto the nanoparticles, dissolved or dispersed throughout them, attached to their matrices by primary valences, trapped, or encapsulated. This definition of nanoparticles includes latexes, pseudolatexes, and even small microspheres, because it is not always easy to ascertain whether the particles consist of a solid, monolithic matrix or a shell, and whether the active ingredients are distributed throughout the particle or adsorbed onto its surface.

Polymeric nanoparticles are normally prepared in aqueous solutions of the drugs to be incorporated. Drugs having low water solubility may be solubilized by micelles. The most widely used technique is emulsion polymerization. It produces particles with controlled and fairly uniform sizes. Alternatively, preformed polymers are dissolved in a water-immiscible, low-boiling solvent, to which the drug is added, followed by emulsification in water, and finally heating to boil off the solvent. Another method is to dissolve the preformed polymers plus drugs in alcohol or acetone, and the solution is stirred into water.

In another approach, the water-soluble proteins gelatin and albumin are dissolved in water, the drugs are added, the pH is adjusted to the isoelectric point, and the proteins plus drugs are salted out with Na_2SO_4, $(NH_4)_2SO_4$ or alcohol. The coacervates are hardened by crosslinking with glutaraldehyde, and the particles are separated from the ice-cold suspension and dried. Intravenous suspensions require colloidal particles with sizes <1μm in order to avoid blocking capillary blood vessels.

Nanoparticles of polymethacrylic acid esters, such as methyl and 2-hydroxyethyl, undergo very slow biodegradation. Polyalkylcyanoacrylate nanoparticles are more readily biodegraded. Aqueous dispersions of nanoparticles are far more stable than those of liposomes. Moreover, they can be spray-dried or freeze-dried and reconstituted much more successfully. Any surfactants present in the dried powders aid redispersion of the nanoparticles in saline.

Like liposomes, intravenously injected nanoparticles are readily taken up by the RES phagocytic cells of the liver, spleen, and lungs. Also like liposomes, surface modification may extend the blood circulation time of nanoparticles or target them to specific tissues.

DRUG-POLYMER CONJUGATES—Polymers have also been used to produce soluble drug-polymer conjugates, which are formed by chemical reactions to produce covalent bonds between a drug and a polymeric molecule.[47] These polymer conjugates include synthetic polymers as well as biological polymers such as globular and fibrous proteins, antibodies and polysaccharides. For example, *Mylotarg for Injection* (gemtuzumab ozogamicin) consists of a conjugate between an IgG monoclonal antibody and calicheamicin, a chemotherapeutic agent. These conjugates are administered by IV infusion and the antibody targets the CD33 antigen found on the surface of leukemic blasts and immature normal cells of myelomonocytic lineage, but not on normal hematopoietic stem cells. The antibody-drug conjugate is believed to have a lysomotropic mechanism of action, ie, the antibody-antigen complex is internalized into the cell through endocytosis and entrapped within endosomal compartments. These endosomes merge with primary lysosomes to form secondary lysosomes, where the drug-antibody bonds are presumably broken by the acidic environment or cleaved by certain lysosomal enzymes. Once cleaved from the antibody, the drug is able to diffuse out of the lysosome and exert its pharmacological effect.

In-111 and Y-90 Zevalin consists of a conjugate between an ibritumoab antibody (a murine IgG) and either an indium-111 or yttrium-90 radioisotope. These conjugates are administered by IV infusion and attach to the CD20 antigen found on the surface of normal and malignant B-lymphocytes. However, the antibody-antigen complex is not internalized. The attachment of the antibody induces cell apoptosis and the close proximity of the radioisotope creates free radicals that damage nearby cells. *PEG-Intron Powder for Injection* also consists of a conjugate. In this case, interferon α-2b is conjugated with a PEG derivative. The conjugates are injected subcutaneously. The PEG derivative prevents detection by the RES and, therefore, decreases the clearance of interferon α-2b from the body.

The actively targeted conjugates described above may be contrasted to passively targeted macromolecular conjugates for solid tumor tissue. Passively targeted macromolecular conjugates have shown preferential accumulation in solid tumors because of the EPR effect. The preferential accumulation reduces systemic toxicity by reducing damage to non-cancerous organs. In addition, the EPR effect is more effective for macromolecules greater than 40 kDa but negligible for smaller molecules that are cleared more rapidly from the tumor interstitium.[48,49] These macromolecular conjugates have also demonstrated the potential to overcome drug resistance. The large conjugate can be taken up into cells by endocytosis, bypassing a drug resistance mechanism of deficient drug transport.[50] This uptake process may also avoid ATP-driven efflux pumps for the free drug[51] as well as block overexpression of these pumps.[52]

A doxorubicin-HPMA [N-(2-hydroxypropyl) methacrylamide] conjugate has been studied in phase I clinical trials. The maximum tolerated dose of this conjugate is several times higher than that of the free drug. This observation was ascribed to the EPR effect.[53] A methotrexate-albumin conjugate was investigated to overcome the short *in vivo* half-life and low tumor accumulation rates of the free drug in phase I and II clinical trials in Germany.[54,55] A camptothecin PEG conjugate has been evaluated in a phase II clinical trial.[56] Other macromolecular drug conjugates under investigation include ampoly(styrene-*co*-maleic acid-half-*n*-butylate)-conjugated neocarzinostatin,[57] dextran-mitomycin C,[58] and gelatin-methotrexate.[59]

Excipients

Most of the excipients, adjuvants or non-therapeutic ingredients of dosage forms listed below are monographs in the NF or USP.

Colloids are also used as pharmaceutical excipients for a variety of purposes including thickening agents. Colloidal thickening agents or viscosity builders belong to four chemical categories. *Semi-synthetic cellulose derivatives* include methylcellulose, carboxymethylcellulose sodium, hydroxypropyl methylcellulose, and hydroxypropyl cellulose. *Natural polymers* include acacia, tragacanth, xanthan gum, sodium alginate, and carrageenan. *Synthetic polymers* include carbomer, a co-polymer of acrylic acid; poloxamer, a block copolymer of ethylene oxide and propylene oxide; polyvinyl alcohol; and povidone (polyvinylpyrrolidone). *Particulate colloids* include bentonite, colloidal silicon dioxide, and microcrystalline cellulose. These viscosity builders may be used to decrease the dissolution rate of controlled release dosage forms, to decrease the sedimentation or creaming rates of dispersed systems, to improve the taste-masking abilities of liquid vehicles, and to provide consistency to ointments. Many of the water-soluble viscosity builders mentioned above are surface-active and are also used as emulsifying and suspending agents. Even particulate colloids are used to stabilize emulsions and suspensions.

Colloidal silicon dioxide is a white powder consisting of submicroscopic spherical particles of fairly uniform size in the range of 5–50 nm or higher. It is used to thicken liquid dosage forms and in tablets. The surface of colloidal silicon dioxide particles contains siloxane (Si-O-Si) and silanol (Si-OH) groups. When colloidal silicon dioxide powder is dispersed in nonpolar liquids, the particles tend to adhere to one another through hydrogen bonds between these surface groups. The spherical particles of finer grade colloidal silicon dioxide are linked together into short chain-like aggregates as shown in Figure 21-4. This creates loose three-dimensional networks that increase the viscosity of the liquid vehicles even at levels as low as a few percent. The hydrogen-bonded structures are torn apart by stirring but rebuilt while at rest, conferring a thixotropic nature to the thickened liquids.

Aerosol 200 is the grade most widely used as a pharmaceutical adjuvant. Its primary spheres, which are extensively sintered together, have an average diameter of 12 nm. At levels of 8 to 10%, it thickens liquids of low polarity such as vegetable and mineral oils to the consistency of ointments, imparting considerable yield values to them. Hydrogen-bonding liquids such as alcohols and water solvate the silica spheres, thereby reducing the hydrogen bonding between particles. Therefore, the higher silica levels of 12–18% or more are required to gel these solvents.

The grades that consist of relatively large and unattached spherical particles, such as those in Figure 21-3, are less efficient thickening agents because they lack the high specific surface area and asymmetry of the finer grades. The consistency of ointments thickened with colloidal silicon dioxide is not appreciably reduced at higher temperatures. Incorporation of colloidal silicon dioxide into ointments and pastes, such as those of zinc oxide, also reduces the syneresis or *bleeding* of the liquid vehicles.

Colloidal silicon dioxide is also used in dry dosage forms. The spherical particles are nonporous and have a density of 2.13 g/cm^3. However, the bulk density of their powder is a mere 0.05 g/cm^3. Because the powder is extremely light, it is frequently used to increase the fluffiness or bulk volume of powder formulations. In addition, the high porosity of colloidal silica enables it to absorb a variety of liquids from fluid fragrances to viscous tars, transforming them into free-flowing powders that can be incorporated into tablets or capsules. The porosity in colloidal silicon dioxide is due entirely to the enormous void space between the particles, which themselves are solid. When these ultrafine particles are incorporated at levels as low as 0.1–0.5% into a powder consisting of coarse particles or granules, they coat the surface of the granules and act as tiny ball bearings and spacers. This improves the flowability of the powder and eliminates caking, which is important in tableting. In addition, colloidal silicon dioxide is used to improve tablet disintegration. It is also used as a glidant and as a moisture absorber.

Microcrystalline cellulose is manufactured by controlled hydrolysis of purified native cellulose, which dissolves the amorphous matrix but leaves the crystallites intact. The needle or rod-shaped crystallites act as suspending agents in water, producing thixotropic structured vehicles. At concentrations of about 15%, the cellulose microcrystals gel water to an ointment consistency by swelling and producing a continuous network of rods that extends throughout the entire vehicle. Attraction between the elongated particles is presumably due to flocculation in the secondary minimum. Treatment of the microcrystalline mass with sodium carboxymethylcellulose facilitates its disintegration into primary needle-shaped particles and enhances their thickening action.

Gelatinous precipitates of inorganic hydrophilic compounds such as *aluminum hydroxide gel, aluminum phosphate gel,* and *magnesium hydroxide* consist of coarse flocs produced by the agglomeration of colloidal particles formed in the initial stage of precipitation. They possess large internal surface areas, which is one of the reasons why the first two are used as substrates for adsorbed vaccines and toxoids. *Alumina and magnesia oral suspensions*, a mixture of gelatinous precipitated aluminum and magnesium hydroxides, as well as aluminum hydroxide gel, are used as antacids.

Gelation is used to manufacture the following suppository bases: glycerinated gelatin suppositories; glycerin suppositories (in which glycerin is solidified with sodium stearate that crystallizes out as a network of needles upon cooling the hot solution); and polyethylene glycol suppositories (in which low molecular-weight liquid PEGs, such as PEG 400, are stiffened by high molecular-weight PEGs such as 3350 or 4000, which are waxy solids). A pharmaceutical application of gelation in a nonaqueous medium is the manufacture of *Plastibase* or *Jelene* (*Squibb*), which is prepared using 5% of a low-molecular-weight polyethylene and 95% of mineral oil. The polymer is soluble in mineral oil above 90°C, which is close to its melting point. When the solution is cooled below 90°C, the polymer precipitates and causes gelation. The mineral oil is immobilized in the network of entangled, adhering, insoluble polyethylene chains, which probably even associate into small crystalline regions. Unlike petrolatum, this gel can be heated to about 60°C without any substantial loss in consistency.

Crospovidone and croscarmellose sodium are crosslinked povidone and carboxymethylcellulose sodium, respectively. These crosslinked polymers swell rapidly and extensively in aqueous media and, therefore, are frequently used as tablet disintegrants. Starch performs the same function; its major constituent, amylopectin, is highly branched and insoluble in water but swells considerably. Because crosslinked hydrophilic polymers swell extensively without dissolution, they are also used as matrices for controlled-release dosage forms.

REFERENCES

1. Lyklema J. *Fundamentals of Interface and Colloid Science*, vols I–III. San Diego: Academic Press, 1993–2000.
2. Hunter RJ. *Foundations of Colloid Science*, vols I and II. Oxford: Clarendon Press, 1987 and 1991.
3. Everett DH. *Basic Principles of Colloid Science.*, London: Royal Soc Chem, 1988.
4. von Weimarn PP. In Alexander J, ed. *Colloid Chemistry*, vol I. New York: Chemical Catalog Co (Reinhold), 1926. See also *Chem Rev* 1926; 2:217.
5. Vold RD, Vold MJ. *Colloid and Interface Chemistry.* Reading, MA: Addison-Wesley, 1983.
6. Mysels KJ. *Introduction to Colloid Chemistry.* New York: Wiley-Interscience, 1959.
7. Shaw DJ. *Introduction to Colloid and Surface Chemistry*, 4th ed. Oxford: Butterworth-Heinemann, 1992.
8. Hiemenz PC, Rajagopalan R. *Principles of Colloid and Surface Chemistry*, 3rd ed. New York: Dekker, 1997.
9. Ross S, Morrison ID. *Colloidal Systems and Interfaces.* New York: Wiley, 1988.
10. Adamson AW. *Physical Chemistry of Surfaces*, 5th ed. New York: Wiley, 1990.
11. van Olphen H. *An Introduction to Clay Colloid Chemistry*, 2nd ed. New York: Wiley, 1977.
12. Schott H, Martin AN. In Dittert LW, ed, *American Pharmacy*, 7th ed. Philadelphia: JB Lippincott, 1974.
13. Provder T, ed. *Particle Size Distribution II Assessment and Characterization*, ACS Symposium Series 472, American Chemical Society, Washington, DC, 1991.
14. Ross DA, et al. *J Colloid Interface Sci* 1978; 64:533 and 1980; 76:478.
15. Morawetz H. *Macromolecules in Solution*, 2nd ed. New York: Wiley-Interscience, 1975.
16. Veis A. *The Macromolecular Chemistry of Gelatin.* New York: Academic, 1964.
17. Ward AG, Courts A, eds. *The Science and Technology of Gelatin*, Chap 6. New York: Academic Press, 1977.
18. Parks GA. *Chem Rev* 1965; 65:177.
19. Schott H. *J Pharm Sci* 1977; 66:1548.
20. Sonntag H, Strenge K. *Coagulation and Stability of Disperse Systems.* New York: Halstead, 1972.
21. Hunter RJ. *Zeta Potential in Colloid Science.* New York: Academic Press, 1981.
22. Davies JT, Rideal EK. *Interfacial Phenomena*, 2nd ed. New York: Academic Press, 1963.
23. Bier M, ed. *Electrophoresis*, vols I and II. New York: Academic, 1959 and 1967.
24. Shaw DJ. *Electrophoresis.* New York: Academic, 1969.
25. *Primer on Capillary Electrophoresis*, vols I–VII. Fullerton, CA: Beckman Instruments, 1993-1995.
26. Camilleri P. *Capillary Electrophoresis*, 2nd ed. Boca Raton, FL: CRC Press, 1998.
27. Lachman L, Lieberman HA, Kanig JL. *The Theory and Practice of Industrial Pharmacy*, 3rd ed. Philadelphia: Lea & Febiger, 1976.
28. Overbeek JThG. *Adv Colloid Interface Sci* 1982; 15:251.
29. LaMer VK, Dinegar RH. *J Am Chem Soc* 1950; 72:4847.
30. Matijevic E. *Acc Chem Res* 1981; 14:22 and *Ann Rev Mater Sci* 1985; 15:483.
31. Schick MJ, ed. *Nonionic Surfactants—Physical Chemistry.* New York: Dekker, 1987.
32. Vincent B. *Adv Colloid Interface Sci* 1974; 4:193.
33. Schott H. *J Pharm Sci* 1980; 69:852.
34. Shinoda K, Nakagawa T, Tamamushi B-I, Isemura T. *Colloidal Surfactants.* New York: Academic Press, 1963.
35. Attwood D, Florence AT. *Surfactant Systems.* London: Chapman & Hall, 1983.
36. Rosen MJ. *Surfactants and Interfacial Phenomena*, 2nd ed. New York: Wiley, 1989.
37. Mukerjee P, Mysels KJ. *Critical Micelle Concentrations of Aqueous Surfactant Systems*, NSRDS-NBS 36. Washington DC, Natl Bur Std, 1971.
38. Shinoda K, ed. *Solvent Properties of Surfactant Solutions.* New York: Dekker, 1967.
39. Bourrel M, Schechter RS. *Microemulsions and Related Systems.* New York: Dekker, 1988.
40. Solans C, Kunieda H, eds. *Industrial Applications of Microemulsions.* New York: Dekker, 1996.
41. Schott H. In: Gennaro AR, ed. *Remington: The Science and Practice of Pharmacy,* 19th ed, Chap 20. Easton: Mack, 1995.
42. Ruckenstein E. *Chem Phys Lett* 1978; 57:517 and *J Colloid Interface Sci* 1978; 66: 369.
43. Kreuter J, ed. *Colloidal Drug Delivery Systems.* New York: Dekker, 1994.
44. Rosoff M, ed. *Vesicles.* New York: Dekker, 1996.
45. Owunwanne A, Patel M, Sadek S. *The Handbook of Radiopharmaceuticals.* London: Chapman & Hall, 1995.
46. Burgess DJ, Hickey AJ. In Swarbrick J, Boylan JC, ed. *Encyclopedia of Pharmaceutical Technology*, 2nd ed. New York: Dekker, 2002.
47. Putnam D, Kopacek J. *Adv Polym Sci* 1995; 122:55.
48. Maeda H, Wu J, Sawa T, Matsumura Y, Hori K. *J Control Rel* 2000; 65:271.
49. Jang SH, Wientjes MG, Lu D, Au JL-S. *Pharm Res* 2003; 20:1337.
50. Ryser H J-P, Shen W-C. *Cancer* 1980; 45:1207.
51. Omelyanenka V, Gentry C, Kopeckova P, Kopecek J. *Inter J Cancer* 1998; 75:600.
52. Minko T, Kopeckova P, Kopecek J. *J Control Rel* 1999; 59:133.
53. Vasey PA, Kaye SB, Morrison R, et al. *Clin Cancer Res* 1999; 5:83.
54. Hartung G, Stehle G, Sinn H, et al. *Clin Cancer Res* 1999; 5:753.
55. Scheulen ME, Gatzemeier U, Pawel J, et al. *Annual Meeting of the American Association of Clinical Oncology (ASCO)*, Orlando, FL, May 2002, Abs. #1888.
56. Enzon, Inc. *Products under Development* (http://www.enzon.com/-develop.html), 2001.
57. Maeda H. *Adv Drug Deliv Rev* 2001; 46:169.
58. Mehvar R. *J Control Rel* 2000; 69:1.
59. Bowman B, Ofner III CM: *Pharm Res* 2000; 17:1309.

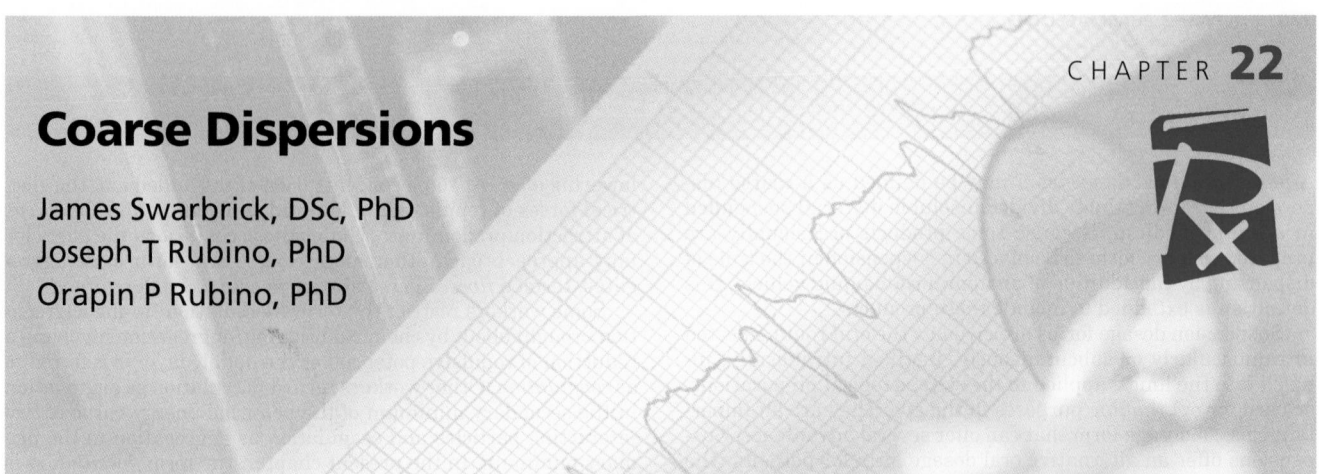

CHAPTER 22

Coarse Dispersions

James Swarbrick, DSc, PhD

Joseph T Rubino, PhD

Orapin P Rubino, PhD

This chapter includes the formation of suspensions and emulsions and the factors that influence their stability and performance as dosage forms. For the purpose of the present discussion, a dispersed system, or dispersion, will be regarded as a two-phase system in which one phase is distributed as particles or droplets in the second, or continuous, phase. In these systems, the dispersed phase frequently is referred to as the discontinuous or internal phase, and the continuous phase is called the external phase or dispersion medium. Discussion will be restricted to those solid–liquid and liquid–liquid dispersions that are of pharmaceutical significance, namely, suspensions and emulsions. However, more complicated phase systems (eg, a combination of liquid and liquid crystalline phases) can exist in emulsions. This situation will be discussed in the section dealing with emulsions.

All dispersions may be classified into three groups based on the size of the dispersed particles. Chapter 21 deals with one such group—colloidal dispersions—in which the size of the dispersed particles is in the range of approximately 1 nm to 0.5 μm. Molecular dispersions, the second group in this classification, are discussed in Chapter 20. The third group, consisting of *coarse dispersions* in which the particle size exceeds 0.5 μm, is the subject of this chapter. Knowledge of coarse dispersions is essential for the preparation of both pharmaceutical suspensions (solid–liquid dispersions) and emulsions (liquid–liquid dispersions).

THE DISPERSION STEP

The pharmaceutical formulator is concerned primarily with producing a smooth, uniform, easily flowing (pouring or spreading) suspension or emulsion in which dispersion of particles can be effected with minimum expenditure of energy.

In preparing suspensions, particle–particle attractive forces need to be overcome by the high shearing action of such devices as the colloid mill, or by use of surface-active agents. The latter greatly facilitate wetting of lyophobic powders and assist in the removal of surface air that shearing alone may not remove; thus, the clumping tendency of the particles is reduced. Moreover, lowering of the surface free energy by the adsorption of these agents directly reduces the thermodynamic driving force opposing dispersion of the particles.

In emulsification, shear rates are frequently necessary for dispersion of the internal phase into fine droplets. The shear forces are opposed by forces operating to resist distortion and subsequent breakup of the droplets. Again surface-active agents help greatly by lowering interfacial tension, which is the primary reversible component resisting droplet distortion. Surface-active agents also may play an important role in determining whether an oil-in-water (O/W) or a water-in-oil (W/O) emulsion preferentially survives the shearing action.

Once the process of dispersion begins there develops simultaneously a tendency for the system to revert to an energetically more stable state, manifested by flocculation, coalescence, sedimentation, crystal growth, and caking phenomena. If these physical changes are not inhibited or controlled, successful dispersions will not be achieved or will be lost during shelf-life.

INTERFACIAL PROPERTIES

Because suspensions and emulsions are dispersions of one phase within another, the process of dispersion creates a tremendous increase in interfacial area between the dispersed particles or droplets and the dispersion medium. When considering the interfacial properties of dispersed particles, two factors must be taken into account, regardless of whether the dispersed phase is solid or liquid. The first relates to an increase in the free energy of the surface as the particle size is reduced and the specific surface increased. The second deals with the presence of an electrical charge on the surface of the dispersed particles.

SURFACE FREE ENERGY—When solid and liquid materials are reduced in size, they tend to agglomerate or stick together. This clumping, which can occur either in an air or liquid medium, is an attempt by the particles to reduce the excess free energy of the system. The increase in surface free energy is related to the increase in surface area produced when the mean particle size is reduced. It may be expressed as

$$\Delta F = \gamma \Delta A \tag{1}$$

where ΔF is the increase in surface free energy in ergs, ΔA is the increase in surface area in cm^2, and γ is the interfacial tension in dyne/cm, between the dispersed particle or droplet and the dispersion medium. The smaller ΔF is, the more thermodynamically stable is the suspension of particles. A reduction in ΔF is effected often by the addition of a wetting agent (discussed in Chapter 20), which is adsorbed at the interface between the particle and the vehicle, thereby reducing the interfacial tension. This causes the particles to remain dispersed and settle relatively slowly. Unfortunately, in solid–liquid suspensions, the particles can form a hard cake at the bottom of the container when they eventually settle. Such a sediment, which can be extremely difficult to redisperse, can lead to dosing errors when the product is administered to the patient.

SURFACE POTENTIAL—As discussed in Chapter 20, both attractive and repulsive forces exist between particles in a liquid medium. The balance between these opposing forces determines whether two particles approaching each other actually make contact or are repulsed at a certain distance of separation. Although much of the theoretical work on electrical surface potentials has been carried out on lyophobic colloids, the theories developed in this area have been applied to suspensions and emulsions.

SUSPENSIONS

A *pharmaceutical suspension* may be defined as a coarse dispersion containing finely divided insoluble material suspended in a liquid medium. Because some products occasionally are prepared in a dry form to be placed in suspension at the time of dispensing by the addition of an appropriate liquid vehicle, this definition is extended to include these products.

Suspension dosage forms are given by the oral route, injected intramuscularly or subcutaneously, instilled intranasally, inhaled into the lungs, applied to the skin as topical preparations, or used for ophthalmic purposes in the eye. They are an important class of dosage form that can offer several advantages. Suspensions offer an alternative oral dosage form for patients who cannot swallow a tablet or capsule such as pediatric and geriatric patients. Oral antibiotics, analgesic and antipyretic drugs are commonly administered as suspensions to these groups of patients. Suspensions are often used to deliver pooly water-soluble drugs that cannot be formulated as a solution. In addition, drugs that have an unpleasant taste may preferably be formulated as a suspension to reduce interaction of drug with taste receptors in the mouth. Because suspended drug must undergo a dissolution step prior to crossing biological membranes, suspensions offer a way to provide sustained release of drug by parenteral, topical, and oral routes of administration

There are certain criteria that a well-formulated suspension should meet. The dispersed particles should be of such a size that they do not settle rapidly in the container. However, in the event that sedimentation does occur, the sediment must not form a hard cake. Rather, it should be capable of redispersion with a minimum of effort on the part of the patient. Finally, the product should be easy to pour, have a pleasant taste, and be resistant to microbial attack.

The three major concerns associated with suspensions are

1. Ensuring adequate dispersion of the particles in the vehicle.
2. Minimizing settling of the dispersed particles.
3. Preventing caking of these particles when a sediment forms.

Much of the following discussion will deal with the factors that influence these processes and the ways in which settling and caking can be minimized.

FLOCCULATION AND DEFLOCCULATION—Zeta potential, φ_z, is a measurable indication of the potential existing at the surface of a particle. When φ_z is relatively high (25 mV or more), the repulsive forces between two particles exceed the attractive London forces. Accordingly, the particles are dispersed and are said to be *deflocculated*. Even when brought close together by random motion or agitation, deflocculated particles resist collision due to their high surface potential.

The addition of a preferentially adsorbed ion whose charge is opposite in sign to that on the particle leads to a progressive lowering of φ_z. At some concentration of the added ion, the electrical forces of repulsion are lowered sufficiently and the forces of attraction predominate. Under these conditions the particles may approach each other more closely and form loose aggregates, termed *flocs*. Such a system is said to be *flocculated*.

Some workers restrict the term "flocculation" to the aggregation brought about by chemical bridging; aggregation involving a reduction of repulsive potential at the double layer is referred to as *coagulation*. Other workers regard flocculation as aggregation in the secondary minimum of the potential energy curve of two interacting particles and coagulation as aggregation in the primary minimum. In the present chapter, the term *flocculation* is used for all aggregation processes, irrespective of mechanism.

The continued addition of the flocculating agent can reverse the above process, if the zeta potential increases sufficiently in the opposite direction. Thus, the adsorption of anions onto positively charged, deflocculated particles in suspension will lead to flocculation. The addition of more anions eventually can generate a net negative charge on the particles. When this has achieved the required magnitude, deflocculation may occur again. The only difference from the starting system is that the net charge on the particles in their deflocculated state is negative rather than positive. Some of the major differences between suspensions of flocculated and deflocculated particles are presented in Table 22-1.

FLOCCULATION KINETICS—The rate at which flocculation occurs is a consideration in the stability of suspended dispersions. Whether flocculation is judged to be rapid or slow depends on the presence of a repulsive barrier between adjacent particles. In the absence of such a barrier, and for a monodispersed system, rapid flocculation occurs at a rate given by the Smoluchowski equation

$$\delta N/\delta t = -4\pi DRN^2 \qquad (2)$$

where $\delta N/\delta t$ is the disappearance rate of particles/mL, R is the distance between the centers of the two particles in contact, N is the number of particles per mL, and D is the diffusion coefficient. Under these conditions the rate is proportional to the square of the particle concentration. The presence or absence of an energy barrier is influenced strongly by the type and concentration of any electrolyte present. When an energy barrier does exist between adjacent particles, the flocculation rate likely will be much smaller than predicted by Equation 2.

SETTLING AND ITS CONTROL

To control the settling of dispersed material in suspension, the pharmacist must be aware of those physical factors that will af-

Table 22-1. Relative Properties of Flocculated and Deflocculated Particles in Suspension

DEFLOCCULATED	FLOCCULATED
1. Particles exist in suspension as separate entities.	1. Particles form loose aggregates.
2. Rate of sedimentation is slow, as each particle settles separately and particle size is minimal.	2. Rate of sedimentation is high, as particles settle as a floc, which is a collection of particles.
3. A sediment is formed slowly.	3. A sediment is formed rapidly.
4. The sediment eventually becomes very closely packed, due to weight of upper layers of sedimenting material. Repulsive forces between particles are overcome and a hard cake is formed that is difficult, if not impossible, to redisperse.	4. The sediment is packed loosely and possesses a scaffold-like structure. Particles do not bond tightly to each other, and a hard, dense cake does not form. The sediment is easy to redisperse, so as to reform the original suspension.
5. The suspension has a pleasing appearance, as the suspended material remains suspended for a relatively long time. The supernate also remains cloudy, even when settling is apparent.	5. The suspension is somewhat unsightly, due to rapid sedimentation and the presence of an obvious, clear supernatant region. This can be minimized if the volume of sediment is made large. Ideally, volume of sediment should encompass the volume of the suspension.

fect the rate of sedimentation of particles under ideal and non-ideal conditions. Also important are the various coefficients used to express the amount of flocculation in the system and the effect flocculation will have on the structure and volume of the sediment.

Sedimentation Rate

The rate at which particles in a suspension sediment is related to their size and density and the viscosity of the suspension medium. Brownian movement may exert a significant effect, as will the absence or presence of flocculation in the system.

STOKES' LAW—The velocity of sedimentation of a uniform collection of spherical particles is governed by *Stokes' law,* expressed as

$$v = \frac{2r^2(\rho_1 - \rho_2)g}{9\eta} \tag{3}$$

where v is the terminal velocity in cm/sec, r is the radius of the particles in cm, ρ_1 and ρ_2 are the densities (g/cm^3) of the dispersed phase and the dispersion medium, respectively, g is the acceleration due to gravity (980.7 cm/sec^2), and η is the Newtonian viscosity of the dispersion medium in poises (g/cm sec). Stokes' law holds only if the downward motion of the particles is not sufficiently rapid to cause turbulence. Micelles and small phospholipid vesicles do not settle unless they are subjected to centrifugation.

While conditions in a pharmaceutical suspension are not in strict accord with those laid down for Stokes' law, Equation 3 provides those factors that can be expected to influence the rate of settling. Thus, sedimentation velocity will be reduced by decreasing the particle size, provided that the particles are kept in a deflocculated state. The rate of sedimentation will be an inverse function of the viscosity of the dispersion medium.

However, too high a viscosity is undesirable, especially if the suspending medium is Newtonian rather than shear-thinning (see Chapter 23), because it then becomes difficult to redisperse material that has settled. It also may be inconvenient to remove a viscous suspension from its container. When the size of particles undergoing sedimentation is reduced to approximately 2 μm, random Brownian movement is observed and the rate of sedimentation departs markedly from the theoretical predictions of Stokes' law. The actual size at which Brownian movement becomes significant depends on the density of the particle as well as the viscosity of the dispersion medium.

EFFECT OF FLOCCULATION—In a deflocculated system containing a distribution of particle sizes, the larger particles naturally settle faster than the smaller particles. The very small particles remain suspended for a considerable length of time, with the result that no distinct boundary is formed between the supernatant and the sediment. Even when a sediment becomes discernible, the supernatant remains cloudy.

When the same system is flocculated (in a manner to be discussed later), two effects are immediately apparent. First, the flocs tend to fall together, so a distinct boundary between the sediment and the supernatant is readily observed; second, the supernatant is clear, showing that the very fine particles have been incorporated into the flocs. The initial rate of settling in flocculated systems is determined by the size of the flocs and the porosity of the aggregated mass. Under these circumstances it is perhaps better to use the term *subsidence,* rather than sedimentation.

Quantitative Expressions of Sedimentation and Flocculation

Frequently, the pharmacist needs to assess a formulation in terms of the amount of flocculation in the suspension and compare this with that found in other formulations. The two

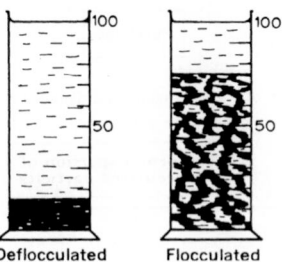

Figure 22-1. Sedimentation parameters of suspensions. Deflocculated suspension: $F\infty = 0.15$. Flocculated suspension: $F = 0.75$; $\beta = 5.0$.

parameters commonly used for this purpose are outlined below.

SEDIMENTATION VOLUME—The *sedimentation volume, F,* is the ratio of the equilibrium volume of the sediment, V_u, to the total volume of the suspension, V_0. Thus,

$$F = V_u/V_o \tag{4}$$

As the volume of suspension that appears occupied by the sediment increases, the value of F, which normally ranges from nearly 0 to 1, increases. In the system where $F = 0.75$, for example, 75% of the total volume in the container is apparently occupied by the loose, porous flocs forming the sediment. This is illustrated in Figure 22-1. When $F = 1$, no sediment is apparent even though the system is flocculated. This is the ideal suspension for, under these conditions, no sedimentation will occur. Caking also will be absent. Furthermore, the suspension is esthetically pleasing, there being no visible, clear supernatant.

DEGREE OF FLOCCULATION—A better parameter for comparing flocculated systems is the *degree of flocculation, β,* which relates the sedimentation volume of the flocculated suspension, F, to the sedimentation volume of the suspension when deflocculated, $F\infty$. It is expressed as

$$\beta = F/F_\infty \tag{5}$$

The degree of flocculation is, therefore, an expression of the increased sediment volume resulting from flocculation. If, for example, β has a value of 5.0 (see Fig 22-1), this means that the volume of sediment in the flocculated system is five times that in the deflocculated state. If a second flocculated formulation results in a value for β of say 6.5, this latter suspension obviously is preferred, if the aim is to produce as flocculated a product as possible. As the degree of flocculation in the system decreases, β approaches unity, the theoretical minimum value.

FORMULATION OF SUSPENSIONS

The formulation of a suspension possessing optimal physical stability depends on whether the particles in suspension are to be flocculated or to remain deflocculated. One approach involves use of a structured vehicle to keep deflocculated particles in suspension; a second depends on controlled flocculation as a means of preventing cake formation. A third, a combination of the two previous methods, results in a product with optimum stability. The various schemes are illustrated in Figure 22-2.

DISPERSION OF PARTICLES—The dispersion step has been discussed earlier in this chapter. Surface-active agents commonly are used as wetting agents; maximum efficiency is obtained when the HLB value lies within the range of 7 to 9. A concentrated solution of the wetting agent in the vehicle may be used to prepare a slurry of the powder; this is diluted with the required amount of vehicle. Alcohol and glycerin may be used sometimes in the initial stages to disperse the particles, thereby allowing the vehicle to penetrate the powder mass.

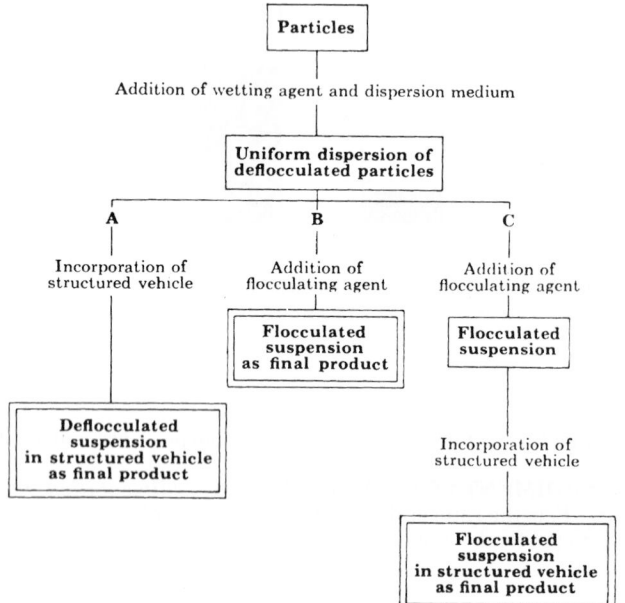

Figure 22-2. Alternative approaches to the formulation of suspensions.

Only the minimum amount of wetting agent should be used, compatible with producing an adequate dispersion of the particles. Excessive amounts may lead to foaming or impart an undesirable taste or odor to the product. Invariably, as a result of wetting, the dispersed particles in the vehicle are deflocculated.

STRUCTURED VEHICLES—*Structured vehicles* are generally aqueous solutions of polymeric materials, such as the hydrocolloids, that are usually negatively charged in aqueous solution. Typical examples are methylcellulose, carboxymethylcellulose, bentonite, and carbomer. The concentration employed will depend on the consistency desired for the suspension that, in turn, will relate to the size and density of the suspended particles. They function as viscosity-imparting suspending agents and, as such, reduce the rate of sedimentation of dispersed particles.

The rheological properties of suspending agents are considered elsewhere (Chapter 23). Ideally, these form pseudo-plastic or plastic systems that undergo shear-thinning. Some degree of thixotropy is also desirable. Non-Newtonian materials of this type are preferred over Newtonian systems because, if the particles eventually settle to the bottom of the container, their redispersion is facilitated by the vehicle thinning when shaken. When the shaking is discontinued, the vehicle regains its original consistency, and the redispersed particles are held suspended. This process of redispersion, facilitated by a shear-thinning vehicle, presupposes that the deflocculated particles have not yet formed a cake. If sedimentation and packing have proceeded to the point where considerable caking has occurred, redispersion is virtually impossible.

CONTROLLED FLOCCULATION—When using the controlled flocculation approach (see Fig 22-2*B* and *C*), the formulator takes the deflocculated, wetted dispersion of particles and attempts to bring about flocculation by the addition of a flocculating agent; most commonly, these are electrolytes, polymers, or surfactants. The aim is to *control* flocculation by adding that amount of flocculating agent that results in the maximum sedimentation volume.

FLOCCULATION USING ELECTROLYTES—*Electrolytes* are probably the most widely used flocculating agents. They act by reducing the electrical forces of repulsion between particles, thereby allowing the particles to form the loose flocs so characteristic of a flocculated suspension. As the ability of particles to come together and form a floc depends on their surface charge,

zeta potential measurements on the suspension, as an electrolyte is added, provide valuable information as to the extent of flocculation in the system.

This principle is illustrated by reference to the following example, taken from the work of Haines and Martin.[2] Particles of sulfamerazine in water bear a negative charge. The serial addition of a suitable electrolyte, such as aluminum chloride, causes a progressive reduction in the zeta potential of the particles. This is due to the preferential adsorption of the trivalent aluminum cation. Eventually, the zeta potential will reach zero and then become positive as the addition of $AlCl_3$ is continued.

If sedimentation studies are run simultaneously on suspensions containing the same range of $AlCl_3$ concentrations, a relationship is observed (Fig 22-3) between the sedimentation volume F, the presence or absence of caking, and the zeta potential of the particles. To obtain a flocculated, noncaking suspension with the maximum sedimentation volume, the zeta potential must be controlled so as to lie within a certain range (generally less than 25 mV). This is achieved by the judicious use of an electrolyte. A comparable situation is observed when a negative ion such as PO_4^{3-} is added to a suspension of positively charged particles such as bismuth subnitrate.

Work by Matthews and Rhodes[3–5] involving both experimental and theoretical studies has confirmed the formulation principles proposed by Martin and Haines. The suspensions used by Matthews and Rhodes contained 2.5% *w/v* of griseofulvin as a fine powder together with the anionic surfactant sodium dioxyethylated dodecyl sulfate (10^{-3} mcolar) as a wetting agent. Increasing concentrations of aluminum chloride were added and the sedimentation height (equivalent to the sedimentation volume, see Chapter 21) and the zeta potential recorded. Flocculation occurred when a concentration of 10^{-3} molar aluminum chloride was reached. At this point the zeta potential had fallen from -46.4 to -17.0 mV. Further reduction of the zeta potential, to -4.5 mV by use of 10^{-2} molar aluminum chloride did not increase sedimentation height, in agreement with the principles shown in Figure 22-3.

Matthews and Rhodes then went on to show, by computer analysis, that the DLVO theory (see Chapter 21) predicted the results obtained—namely, that the griseofulvin suspensions under investigation would remain deflocculated when the concentration of aluminum chloride was 10^{-4} molar or less. Only at concentrations in the range of 10^{-3} to 10^{-2} molar aluminum

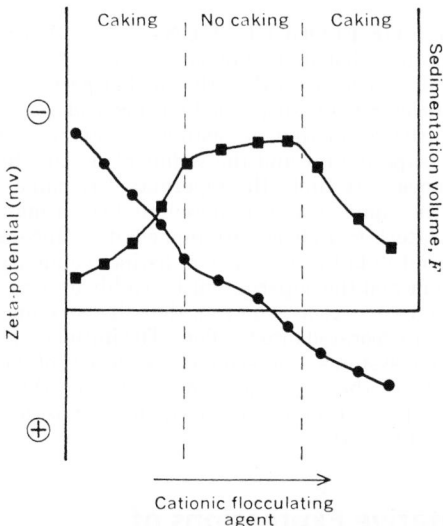

Figure 22-3. Typical relationship between caking, zeta potential, and sedimentation volume, as a positively charged flocculating agent is added to a suspension of negatively charged particles. ●: zeta potential. ■: sedimentation volume.

chloride did the theoretical plots show deep primary minima, indicative of flocculation. These occurred at a distance of separation between particles of approximately 50 Å, which led Matthews and Rhodes to conclude that coagulation had taken place in the primary minimum.

Schneider et al[6] have published details of a laboratory investigation (suitable for undergraduates) that combines calculations based on the DLVO theory carried out with an interactive computer program with actual sedimentation experiments performed on simple systems.

FLOCCULATION BY POLYMERS—*Polymers* can play an important role as flocculating agents in pharmaceutical suspensions. As such, polymers can have an advantage over ionic flocculating agents in that they are less sensitive to added electrolytes. This leads to a greater flexibility in the use of additives such as preservatives, flavoring, and coloring agents that might be needed for the formulation.

The effectiveness of a polymer as a stabilizing agent for suspensions primarily depends on the affinity of the polymer for the particle surface as well as the charge, size, and orientation of the polymer molecule in the continuous phase. Many pharmaceutically useful polymers contain polar functional groups that are separated by a hydrocarbon backbone. As a result of this structure, a polymer molecule may adsorb to particle surfaces while maintaining a degree of interaction with the solvent. As observed with ionic flocculating agents, polymers can produce both flocculated and deflocculated suspensions. It is believed that the primary mechanism by which polymers act as flocculants is due to the bridging of the polymer between the surfaces of different particles. The effect can be highly concentration dependent as illustrated in Figure 22-4. The effect has been interpreted as follows.

At very low concentrations of polymer, a large number of sites on the surface of the dispersed solid are available for adsorption of polymer. Bridging between particles occurs as a result of the simultaneous adsorption of a polymer molecule onto the surfaces of different particles. At very low polymer concentrations, the number of particle–particle bridges is relatively low. At somewhat higher concentrations of polymer, sufficient binding sites are still available on the particles, permitting additional interparticle attachments to form. It is these intermediate concentrations that result in optimum flocculation and sedimentation volume. At high concentrations of polymer, complete coverage of the particle surface with polymer occurs and insufficient binding sites remain on the particles to permit interparticle bridging. In this case, the degree of flocculation is low, but the close association of individual particles is inhibited by a phenomenon known as steric stabilization. In general, *steric stabilization* refers to the ability of adsorbed polymers to prevent close approach and cohesion of dispersed particles due to the fact that the mixing of polymers adsorbed at the particle surfaces is energetically unfavorable. Suspensions formulated with relatively high concentrations of polymer would be deflocculated and therefore tend to have small sedimentation volumes.

Flocculation using polymers may be influenced by the length of time and magnitude of mixing during the formulation process. In some cases, gentle mixing could result in a flocculated suspension; however, continued or more vigorous mixing could result in reorientation of the polymer at the particle surface with fewer interparticle bridges formed. The opposite phenomenon may also occur. Polymers are also frequently used to produce structured vehicles with relatively high viscosity. This effect may overshadow any effect on flocculation and is typically considered the most important use for pharmaceutical polymers in suspensions. Practical considerations in the formulation of suspensions using polymers have been presented by Scheer.[7]

The sedimentation volume achieved by addition of polymeric flocculating agents may or may not agree with DLVO theory. For example, Kellaway and Najib[8] found that sulfadimidine suspensions stabilized with the anionic polymer sodium carboxymethylcellulose obeyed the expected relationship between electrophoretic mobility, a measurement that is proportional to

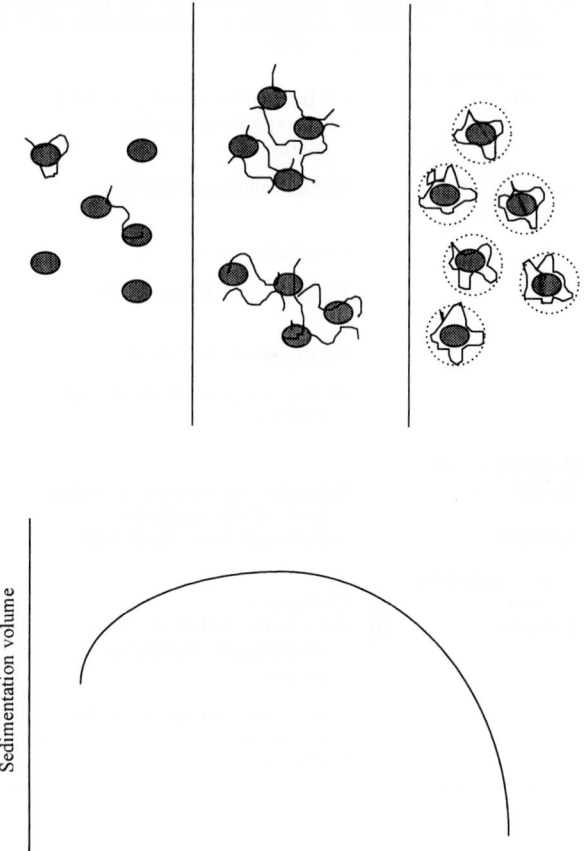

Figure 22-4. Flocculation by hydrophilic polymers. Optimal degree of flocculation and sedimentation volume occurs when a large number of interparticle bridges are formed. High concentrations of polymer result in a deflocculated suspension via steric repulsion.

zeta potential, and to sedimentation volume in agreement with Figure 22-3. However, stabilization of the suspension with the nonionic polymer polyvinylpyrrolidone (PVP) did not obey the expected relationship between electrophoretic mobility and sedimentation volume. At high concentrations of PVP, particles had a low zeta potential, but contrary to the predictions of Figure 22-3 a low sedimentation volume was observed. Although adsorption of the polymer reduced the charge at the plane of shear, flocculation did not occur. This is believed to be due to steric stabilization of the particles at high concentrations of PVP with few interparticle bonds resulting in a low degree of flocculation.

The conformation of the polymers in the continuous phase may also have an effect on the degree of flocculation. At concentrations where flocculation occurs, polymers that have a linear conformation in the continuous phase will generally be more effective flocculants than polymers that are coiled in the continuous phase.

In some situations, a combination of polymeric and ionic flocculating agents have been used. In general, the sensitivity of the dispersed solid to flocculation by added electrolyte is enhanced by the presence of the polymer.

Table 22-2 contains a list of suspending agents that have been used in the formulation of pharmaceutical suspensions. Many of these can serve dual functions as flocculating/stabilizing and viscosity enhancing agents.

FLOCCULATION USING DETERGENTS—Both ionic and nonionic *detergents* can be used to produce flocculation in suspensions. Ionic detergents can produce flocculation in a

Table 22-2. Suspending Agents Used in the Formulation of Pharmaceutical Suspensions

TYPE OF POLYMER	EXAMPLES	STRUCTURE	COMMERCIAL NAMES
Cellulose derivatives			
Anionic	Carboxymethylcellulose (CMC)	Cellulose ether	
	Microcrystalline cellulose blends	Crystalline cellulose + cellulose ether	Avicel
Nonionic	Methylcellulose (MC)	Cellulose ether	Methocel, Metocel, Tylopur, Culminol, Celocol, Walsroder
	Ethylcellulose (EC)		EC - Ethocel
	Hydroxyethylcellulose (HEC)		HEC - Natrasol, Cellocize, Bermocol, Tylose, Blanose
	Hydroxypropylcellulose (HPC)		HPC - Klucel, Lacrisert
	Hydroxypropylmethylcellulose (HPMC)		HPMC - Methocel, Methlose, Pharmacoat, Culminol, Tylose, Celocol
Natural polymers			
Anionic	Alginates, carageenan, xanthan gum, acacia, tragacanth	Polysaccharide	
Nonionic	Locust bean gum, guar gum	Polysaccharide	
Synthetic polymers			
Anionic	Carbomers	Crosslinked polyacrylate	Carbopol
Nonionic	Polyvinyl pyrrolidone (PVP), polyvinyl alcohol (PVA) poloxamer		Plasdone, Povidone, Kollidon
Clays	Magnesium aluminum silicate (Veegum), bentonite	Hydrated aluminum silicate	
	Hectorite	Magnesium hectorite	

manner that is similar to other electrolytes; they can reduce the zeta potential of the dispersed particles. Nonionic detergents have also been observed to reduce the zeta potential of dispersed particles. Both flocculation and deflocculation can occur. Relatively high concentrations of nonionic detergents can form a hydrated layer around particles that can lead to deflocculation via a mechanism that is similar to steric stabilization described for polymers. Alternatively, some liquid detergents can induce flocculation through the formation of liquid bridges between particles. High-molecular-weight detergents would be expected to behave similarly to polymers with regard to their action as a flocculant or stabilizer of suspensions.

FLOCCULATION IN STRUCTURED VEHICLES—The ideal formulation for a suspension would seem to be when flocculated particles are supported in a structured vehicle. As shown in Figure 22-2 (under *C*), the process involves dispersion of the particles and their subsequent flocculation. Finally, a lyophilic polymer is added to form the structured vehicle. In developing the formulation, care must be taken to ensure the absence of any incompatibility between the flocculating agent and the polymer used for the structured vehicle. A limitation is that virtually all the structured vehicles in common use are hydrophilic colloids and carry a negative charge. This means that an incompatibility arises if the charge on the particles is originally negative. Flocculation in this instance requires the addition of a positively charged flocculating agent or ion; in the presence of such a material, the negatively charged suspending agent may coagulate and lose its suspendability. This situation does not arise with particles that bear a positive charge, as the negative flocculating agent that the formulator must employ is compatible with the similarly charged suspending agent.

A method that can be used to circumvent incompatibilities between an anionic suspending agent and a cationic flocculating agent is to reverse the charge on the particle through the use of a positively charged surface active material such as gelatin. Adsorption of gelatin to the surface of a negatively charged particle can reverse the particle charge when the continuous phase is

adjusted to a relatively low pH. This may permit flocculation to be achieved with an anionic flocculating agent such as citrate ion or phosphate ion. Addition of these flocculating agents would be compatible with polymeric suspending agents that largely consist of molecules of anionic charge. Martin *et al*[9] have suggested that this effect can also be achieved using surface active amines, provided their toxicity does not prevent their use.

PARTICLE SIZE AND DISTRIBUTION—Particle size is an important consideration for the physical stability of a suspension. As predicted by Stokes' law, particles of small diameter tend to settle more slowly compared to larger particles; however, small particles will have an increased tendency to cake upon settling if they are not flocculated. In addition, particle–particle interactions can also have a significant effect on suspension stability. For suspensions with a relatively high percentage of solids, interparticle interactions may produce more viscous or thixotropic dispersions. Smaller particles will have a high surface area/weight ratio that favors interactions between the particles and may produce desirable rheological characteristics.

In addition to the effects on the physical properties of a suspension, particle size has important implications on the biopharmaceutical performance of the drug. Aqueous suspensions can effectively serve as a means to deliver poorly water-soluble drugs by the enteral, parenteral, and topical routes. For drugs whose solubility in water is low, the dissolution rate of the drug particles may be a primary factor that limits absorption of the drug. In these cases, the rate and extent of absorption of the drug may be enhanced through the use of small particles. Small particles dissolve faster than larger particles due to the increased surface area per unit weight of drug of the former. Lastly, the uniformity of dosing over the life of the product will be enhanced by ensuring that a relatively small particle size is achieved. This is especially true for suspensions whose individual doses are withdrawn from a larger container, such as suspensions for oral use. Additional information on the bioavailability of drug from suspensions is presented at the end of this chapter.

As most pharmaceutical powders are polydipserse rather than monodisperse, the distribution of particle sizes may also play an important role in the physical stability of a suspension. A relatively narrow distribution of particle sizes is desirable for good stability. A narrow particle size distribution provides a more uniform settling rate and allows for better predictability of suspension properties from batch to batch of finished suspension. In addition, the phenomenon of Ostwald ripening will be minimized when the distribution of particles is narrow. *Ostwald ripening* is the phenomenon in which larger particles grow in size due to the dissolution of smaller particles. This phenomenon could result in pharmaceutically unstable suspensions (caking) and alter the bioavailability of the product through an alteration in the dissolution rate. The use of an appropriate polymer with an affinity for the surface of the dispersed solid reduces or eliminates crystallization in suspensions that may occur due to Ostwald ripening or dissolution/crystallization phenomenon caused by temperature fluctuations. This effect occurs at concentrations of polymer that provide complete surface coverage of the particles. Thus, a hydrophilic colloid, such as a cellulose derivative, with high affinity for the particle surface is often added initially to the suspension formulation to provide a protective action.

In flocculated suspensions, a narrow distribution of particles also tends to result in floccules with a more opened structure. If a flocculated suspension is prepared using a powder with a wide distribution of particles, the floccules would consist of links between larger particles with small particles filling the voids created by the interparticle links between larger particles. This would create a floccule that is more dense compared to the more open structure that would be expected from a floccule composed of particles of more uniform size. The more opened floc structure is desirable, as it may exhibit thixotropic properties in addition to a large sedimentation volume.

NONAQUEOUS SUSPENSIONS—Although most pharmaceutical suspensions have a primarily aqueous continuous phase, formulation of a drug in a nonaqueous continuous phase is occasionally required. Suspension of a water-soluble drug in a nonaqueous vehicle may provide a means to prepare a liquid formulation of a drug that has poor long-term stability in aqueous solution. Dispersions of drugs in oleaginous vehicles can also provide a sustained release form of drug as observed with certain depot injections and topical products.

Aerosols represent another important class of nonaqueous suspensions. The physical stability of suspended drugs in nonaqueous propellents for aerosol products can have a significant impact on the uniformity of dose and operation of the aerosol system. Caking of the suspended particles can cause clogging of the various mechanical components of the aerosol system.

According to Coulomb's law, the force between two charges is inversely proportional to the dielectric constant of the medium between the charges:

$$f \propto \frac{q_1 q_2}{Dx} \qquad (6)$$

where f is the force between the particles, q_1 and q_2 are the charges on the particles, D is the dielectric constant, and x is the distance between the charges.

In general, most nonaqueous pharmaceutical liquids have a dielectric constant that is lower than water. This would result in a greater attraction between ions or particles of opposite charge and greater repulsion between ions or particles of similar charge.

The effect of a continuous phase of low dielectric constant can therefore affect a suspension formulation in different ways. The use of added electrolytes will be less useful due to their low degree of ionization and poor solubility in some nonaqueous media. In addition, the density of charges on the particle surfaces will be reduced, but repulsion between particles may be facilitated. The result is that controlled flocculation using electrolytes is difficult to achieve as with aqueous suspensions, and caking may occur upon settling. Thus, alternate means of producing pharmaceutically acceptable suspensions must be employed.

Nonionic surfactants of low HLB values can be used to improve the physical stability of the suspensions. Stearic and other aliphatic acids and stearate salts, particularly aluminum monostearate, have been used as suspending agents. These materials increase the viscosity of the oil and produce a structured medium that can hinder the settling of drug particles. Alternatively, thickening agents such as Avicel, colloidal silicon dioxide, and long-chain alcohols can be used to reduce the sedimentation rate in nonaqueous suspensions.

Few studies have been performed to predict formulation and physical stability of drugs in nonaqueous suspensions. Parsons *et al*[10] found that the suspension properties of a number of solids in a nonaqueous aerosol propellant depended on the surface properties of the solids. Solids that had relatively polar surfaces tended to aggregate to larger extents than solids with relatively nonpolar surfaces. The moisture content of the dispersed solid and continuous phase may also play an important role on the aggregation of the solid. Adsorbed moisture on the dispersed solid may help to create a liquid bridge between particles when dispersed in certain nonaqueous solvents. If carefully controlled, this could provide a means to obtain some degree of flocculation in certain nonaqueous vehicles. Examples are discussed by Hiestand.[1]

CHEMICAL STABILITY OF SUSPENSIONS—Particles that are completely insoluble in a liquid vehicle are unlikely to undergo most chemical reactions leading to degradation. However, most drugs in suspension have a finite solubility, even though this may be of the order of fractions of a microgram per milliliter. As a result, the material in solution may be susceptible to degradation. However, Tingstad *et al*[11] developed a simplified method for determining the stability of drugs in suspension. The approach is based on the assumptions that

1. Degradation takes place only in the solution and is first order.
2. The effect of temperature on drug solubility and reaction rate conforms with classical theory.
3. Dissolution is not rate-limiting on degradation.

PREPARATION OF SUSPENSIONS—The small-scale preparation of suspensions may be undertaken readily by the practicing pharmacist with the minimum of equipment. The initial dispersion of the particles is best carried out by trituration in a mortar, the wetting agent being added in small increments to the powder. Once the particles have been wetted adequately, the slurry may be transferred to the final container. The next step depends on whether the deflocculated particles are to be suspended in a structured vehicle, flocculated, or flocculated and then suspended. Regardless of which of the alternative procedures outlined in Figure 22-2 is employed, the various manipulations can be carried out easily in the bottle, especially if an aqueous solution of the suspending agent has been prepared beforehand.

For detailed discussion of the methods used in the large-scale production of suspensions, see the relevant section in Chapter 39.

EMULSIONS

An *emulsion* is a dispersed system containing at least two immiscible liquid phases. The majority of conventional emulsions in pharmaceutical use have dispersed particles ranging in diameter from 0.1 to 100 μm. As with suspensions, emulsions are thermodynamically unstable as a result of the excess free energy associated with the surface of the droplets. The dispersed droplets, therefore, strive to come together and reduce the surface area. In addition to this flocculation effect, also observed

icant in promoting stability by causing repulsion between approaching drops. This potential is likely to be greater when an ionized emulsifying agent is employed. Electrical potential has been shown to be a significant factor for maintaining the stability of intravenous fat emulsions that are stabilized with lecithin.

CONCENTRATION OF EMULSIFIER—The main objective of an emulsifying agent is to form a condensed film around the droplets of the dispersed phase. An inadequate concentration will do little to prevent coalescence. Increasing the emulsifier concentration above an optimum level achieves little in terms of increased stability. In practice the aim is to use the minimum amount consistent with producing a satisfactory emulsion.

It frequently helps to have some idea of the amount of emulsifier required to form a condensed film, one molecule thick, around each droplet. Suppose we wish to emulsify 50 g of an oil, density = 1.0, in 50 g of water. The desired particle diameter is 1 μm. Thus,

> Particle diameter = 1 μm = 1×10^{-4} cm
> Volume of particle = $(\pi d^3/6) = 0.524 \times 10^{-12}$ cm^3
> Total number of particles in 50 g = $(50/0.524 \times 10^{-12}) = 95.5 \times 10^{12}$
> Surface area of each particle = $\pi d^2 = 3.142 \times 10^{-8}$ cm^2
> Total surface area = $3.142 \times 10^{-8} \times 95.5 \times 10^{12} = 300 \times 10^4$ cm^2

If the area each molecule occupies at the oil–water interface is 30 Å^2 (30×10^{-16} cm^2), we require

$$\frac{300 \times 10^4}{30 \times 10^{16}} = 1 \times 10^{21} \text{ molecules}$$

A typical emulsifying agent might have a molecular weight of 1000. Thus, the required weight is

$$\frac{1000 \times 10^{21}}{6.023 \times 10^{23}} = 1.66 \text{ g}$$

To emulsify 10 g of oil would require 0.33 g of the emulsifying agent.

While the approach is an oversimplification of the problem, it does at least allow the formulator to make a reasonable estimate of the required concentration of emulsifier.

EMULSION RHEOLOGY—The emulsifying agent and other components of an emulsion can affect the rheologic behavior of an emulsion in several ways, as summarized in Table 22-3.[14] It should be borne in mind that the droplets of the internal phase are deformable under shear and that the adsorbed layer of emulsifier affects the interactions between adjacent droplets and also between a droplet and the continuous phase. The means by which the rheological behavior of emulsions can be controlled have been discussed by Rogers.[15]

Mechanism of Action

Emulsifying agents may be classified in accordance with the type of film they form at the interface between the two phases.

MONOMOLECULAR FILMS—Those surface-active agents that are capable of stabilizing an emulsion do so by forming a monolayer of adsorbed molecules or ions at the oil–water interface (Fig 22-6). In accordance with Gibbs' law (Chapter 20) the presence of an interfacial excess necessitates a reduction in interfacial tension. This results in a more stable emulsion because of a proportional reduction in the surface free energy. Of itself, this reduction is probably not the main factor promoting stability. More significant is the fact that the droplets are surrounded now by a coherent monolayer that prevents coalescence between approaching droplets. If the emulsifier forming the monolayer is ionized, the presence of strongly charged and mutually repelling droplets increases the stabil-

Table 22-3. Factors Influencing Emulsion Viscosity

1. Internal phase
   a. Volume concentration (φ); hydrodynamic interaction between globules; flocculation, leading to formation of globule aggregates.
   b. Viscosity (η_1); deformation of globules in shear.
   c. Globule size, and size distribution, technique used to prepare emulsion; interfacial tension between the two liquid phases: globule behavior in shear; interaction with continuous phase; globule interaction.
   d. Chemical constitution.
2. Continuous phase
   a. Viscosity (η_0), and other rheological properties.
   b. Chemical constitution, polarity, pH; potential energy of interaction between globules.
   c. Electrolyte concentration if polar medium.
3. Emulsifying agent
   a. Chemical constitution; potential energy of interaction between globules.
   b. Concentration, and solubility in internal and continuous phases; emulsion type; emulsion inversion; solubilization of liquid phases in micelles.
   c. Thickness of film adsorbed around globules, and its rheological properties, deformation of globules in shear; fluid circulation within globules.
   d. Electroviscous effect.
4. Additional stabilizing agents
   a. Pigments, hydrocolloids, hydrous oxides.
   b. Effect on rheological properties of liquid phases, and interfacial boundary region.

From Davies JT, Rideal EK. *Interfacial Phenomena*. New York: Academic Press, 1961, Chap 8.

ity of the system. With un-ionized, nonionic surface-active agents, the particles may still carry a charge; this arises from adsorption of a specific ion or ions from solution.

MULTIMOLECULAR FILMS—Hydrated lyophilic colloids form multimolecular films around droplets of dispersed oil (see Fig 22-6). The use of these agents has declined in recent years because of the large number of synthetic surface-active agents available that possess well-marked emulsifying properties. Although these hydrophilic colloids are adsorbed at an interface (and can be regarded therefore as surface active), they do not cause an appreciable lowering in surface tension. Rather, their efficiency depends on their ability to form strong coherent multimolecular films. These act as a coating around the droplets and render them highly resistant to coalescence, even in the absence of a well-developed surface potential. Furthermore, any hydrocolloid not adsorbed at the interface increases the viscosity of the continuous aqueous phase; this enhances emulsion stability.

SOLID PARTICLE FILMS—Small solid particles that are wetted to some degree by both aqueous and nonaqueous liquid phases act as emulsifying agents. If the particles are too hydrophilic, they remain in the aqueous phase; if too hydrophobic, they are dispersed completely in the oil phase. A second requirement is that the particles are small in relation to the droplets of the dispersed phase (see Fig 22-6).

Chemical Types

Emulsifying agents also may be classified in terms of their chemical structure; there is some correlation between this classification and that based on the mechanism of action. For example, the majority of emulsifiers forming monomolecular films are synthetic, organic materials. Most of the emulsifiers that form multimolecular films are obtained from natural sources and are organic. A third group is composed of solid particles, invariably inorganic, that form films composed of finely divided solid particles.

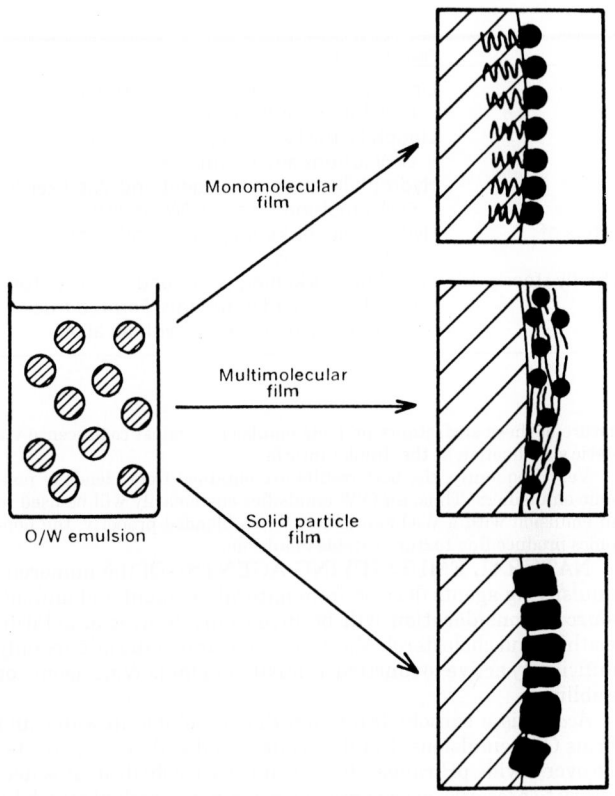

Monomolecular film

Multimolecular film

Solid particle film

O/W emulsion

Figure 22-6. Types of films formed by emulsifying agents at the oil–water interface. Orientations are shown for O/W emulsions. ▨: oil. □: water.

Accordingly, the classification, adopted divides emulsifying agents into *synthetic, natural,* and *finely dispersed solids* (Table 22-4). A fourth group, the *auxiliary materials* (Table 22-5) are weak emulsifiers. The list of agents is not meant to be exhaustive, but rather merely illustrates the various types available.

SYNTHETIC EMULSIFYING AGENTS—Synthetic emulsifying agents, a group of surface-active agents that act as emulsifiers, may be subdivided into anionic, cationic, and nonionic, depending on the charge possessed by the surfactant.

Anionics—In the anionic subgroup, the surfactant ion bears a negative charge. The potassium, sodium, and ammonium salts of lau-ric and oleic acid are soluble in water and are good O/W emulsifying agents. They do, however, have a disagreeable taste and are irritating to the gastrointestinal (GI) tract; this limits them to emulsions prepared for external use. Potassium laurate, a typical example, has the structure

$$CH_3(CH_2)_{10}COO^-K^+$$

Solutions of *alkali soaps* have a high pH; they start to precipitate out of solution below pH 10 because the un- ionized fatty acid is now formed, and this has a low aqueous solubility. Further, the free fatty acid is ineffective as an emulsifier, so emulsions formed from alkali soaps are not stable at pH values less than about 10.

The calcium, magnesium, and aluminum salts of fatty acids, often termed the *metallic soaps,* are water insoluble and result in W/O emulsions.

Another class of soaps are salts formed from a fatty acid and an organic amine such as triethanolamine. These O/W emulsifiers also are limited to external preparations, but their alkalinity is considerably less than that of the alkali soaps and they are active as emulsifiers down to around pH 8. These agents are less irritating than the alkali soaps.

Sulfated alcohols are neutralized sulfuric acid esters of such fatty alcohols as lauryl and cetyl alcohol. These compounds are an important group of pharmaceutical surfactants. They are used chiefly as wetting agents, although they do have some value as emulsifiers, particularly when used in conjunction with an auxiliary agent.

Sulfonates—Sulfonates are a class of compounds in which the sulfur atom is connected directly to the carbon atom, giving the general formula

$$CH_3(CH_2)_nCH_2SO_3^-Na^+$$

A frequently used compound is sodium lauryl sulfate. Sulfonates have a higher tolerance to calcium ions and do not hydrolyze as readily as the sulfates. A widely used surfactant of this type is dioctyl sodium sulfosuccinate.

Cationics—The surface activity in the cationic group resides in the positively charged cation. These compounds have marked bactericidal properties. This makes them desirable in emulsified anti-infective products such as skin lotions and creams. The pH of an emulsion prepared with a cationic emulsifier lies in the pH 4 to 6 ranges. Because this includes the normal pH of the skin, cationic emulsifiers are advantageous in this regard also.

Cationic agents are weak emulsifiers and generally are formulated with a stabilizing or auxiliary emulsifying agent such as cetostearyl alcohol. The only group of cationic agents used extensively as emulsifying agents are the quaternary ammonium compounds. An example is cetyltrimethyl-ammonium bromide.

$$CH_3(CH_2)_{14}CH_2N^+(CH_3)_3\ Br^-$$

Cationic emulsifiers should not be used in the same formulation with anionic emulsifiers because they will interact. The incompatibility

Table 22-4. Classification of Emulsifying Agents

TYPE	TYPE OF FILM		EXAMPLES

Synthetic (surface-active agents)	Monomolecular	*Anionic*
		Soaps
		  Potassium laurate
		  Triethanolamine stearate
		Sulfates
		  Sodium lauryl sulfate
		  Alkyl polyoxyethylene sulfates
		Sulfonates
		  Dioctyl sodium sulfosuccinate
			Cationic
			Quaternary ammonium compounds
			  Cetyltrimethyllammonium bromide
			  Lauryldimethylbenzylammonium chloride
			Nonionic
			Polyoxyethylene fatty alcohol ethers
			Sorbitan fatty acid esters
			Polyoxyethylene sorbitan fatty acid esters
			Polyoxyethylene polyoxypropylene block copolymers
			  (poloxamers)
			Lanolin alcohols and ethoxylated lalnolin alcohols

Natural	Multimolecular	*Hydrophilic colloids*
		  Acacia
		  Gelatin	

	Monomolecular	Lecithin Cholesterol	

Finely divided solids	Solid particle	*Colloidal clays*
		  Bentonite
		  Veegum
		Metallic hydroxides
		  Magnesium hydroxide	

Table 22-5. Auxiliary Emulsifying Agents

PRODUCT	SOURCE AND COMPOSITION	PRINCIPAL USE
Cetyl alcohol	Chiefly $C_{16}H_{33}OH$	Lipophilic thickening agent and stabilizer for O/W lotions and ointments
Glyceryl monosterate	$C_{17}H_{35}COOCH_2CHOHCH_2OH$	Lipophilic thickening agent and stabilizer for O/W lotions and ointments
Methylcellulose	Series of methyl ethers of cellulose	Hydrophilic thickening agent and stabilizer for O/W emulsions; weak O/W emulsifier
Sodium carboxymethylcellulose	Sodium salt of the carboxymethyl esters of cellulose	Hydrophilic thickening agent and stabilizer for O/W emulsions
Stearic acid	A mixture of solid acids from fats, chiefly stearic and palmitic	Lipophilic thickening agent and stabilizer for O/W lotions and ointments. Forms a true emulsifier when reacted with an alkali

may not be immediately apparent as a precipitate, but virtually all of the desired antibacterial activity will generally have been lost.

Nonionics—Nonionics, undissociated surfactants, find widespread use as emulsifying agents when they possess the proper balance of hydrophilic and lipophilic groups within the molecule. Their popularity is based on the fact that, unlike the anionic and cationic types, nonionic emulsifiers are not susceptible to pH changes and the presence of electrolytes. The number of nonionic agents available is legion; the most frequently used are the glyceryl esters, polyoxyethylene glycol esters and ethers, and the sorbitan fatty acid esters and their polyoxyethylene derivatives. More recently, the polyoxyethylene/polyoxypropylene block copolymers have become popular surfactants and emulsifying agents.

A glyceryl ester, such as glyceryl monostearate, is too lipophilic to serve as a good emulsifier; it is used widely as an auxiliary agent (see Table 22-5) and has the structure

$$CH_2OOCC_{17}H_{35}$$
$$|$$
$$CHOH$$
$$|$$
$$CH_2OH$$

Sorbitan fatty acid esters, such as sorbitan monopalmitate

[*R* is $(C_{15}H_{31})COO$]

are nonionic oil-soluble emulsifiers that promote W/O emulsions. The polyoxyethylene sorbitan fatty acid esters, such as polyoxyethylene sorbitan monopalmitate

[Sum of *w*, *x*, *y* and *z* is 20; *R* is $(C_{15}H_{31})COO$]

are hydrophilic water-soluble derivatives that favor O/W emulsions.

Polyoxyethylene glycol esters, such as the monostearate, $C_{17}H_{35}COO(CH_2OCH_2)_nH$, also are used widely.

Polyoxyethylene/polyoxypropylene block copolymers

$$HO(CH_2CH_2O)_a(CHCH_2O)_b(CH_2CH_2O)_cH$$
$$|$$
$$CH_3$$

also known as *poloxamers* consist of combined chains of oxyethylene with oxypropylene where the oxyethylene portion imparts hydrophilicity and the oxypropylene portion imparts lipophilicity. The molecules are synthesized as long segments of the hydrophilic portions combined with long segments of the hydrophobic portions, with each portion referred to as a *block*. This organization produces hydrophilic and hydrophobic domains that impart the surface active character to these agents. Poloxamers have been used in the formulation of intravenous emulsions and can impart structure to vehicles and interfacial films that can protect the dispersed phase against coalescence. The polymeric

nature of these surfactants protects emulsions against coalescence via steric stabilization at the droplet interface.

Very frequently, the best results are obtained from blends of nonionic emulsifiers. Thus, an O/W emulsifier customarily will be used in an emulsion with a W/O emulsifier. When blended properly, the nonionics produce fine-textured stable emulsions.

NATURAL EMULSIFYING AGENTS—Of the numerous emulsifying agents derived from natural (ie, plant and animal) sources, consideration will be given only to acacia, gelatin, lecithin, and cholesterol. Many other natural materials are only sufficiently active to function as auxiliary emulsifying agents or stabilizers.

Acacia is a carbohydrate gum that is soluble in water and forms O/W emulsions. Emulsions prepared with acacia are stable over a wide pH range. Because it is a carbohydrate it is necessary to preserve acacia emulsions against microbial attack by the use of a suitable preservative.

Gelatin, a protein, has been used for many years as an emulsifying agent. Gelatin can have two isoelectric points, depending on the method of preparation. So-called Type A gelatin, derived from an acid-treated precursor, has an isoelectric point of between pH 7 and 9. Type B gelatin, obtained from an alkali-treated precursor, has an isoelectric point of approximately pH 5. Type A gelatin acts best as an emulsifier around pH 3, where it is positively charged; on the other hand, Type B gelatin is best used around pH 8, where it is negatively charged. The question as to whether the gelatin is positively or negatively charged is fundamental to the stability of the emulsion when other charged emulsifying agents are present. To avoid an incompatibility, all emulsifying agents should carry the same sign. Thus, if gums (such as tragacanth, acacia, or agar) that are negatively charged are to be used with gelatin, then Type B material should be used at an alkaline pH. Under these conditions the gelatin is similarly negatively charged.

Lecithin is an emulsifier obtained from both plant (eg, soybean) and animal (eg, egg yolk) sources and is composed of various phosphatides. The primary component of most lecithins is phosphatidylcholine and the term "lecithin" is often used to describe purified samples of phosphatidylcholine. Frequently, lecithins that are used as emulsifiers also contain mixtures of phosphatides, including phosphatidylserine, phosphatidylinositol, phosphatidylethanolamine, and phosphatidic acid in addition to phosphatidylcholine. Although phosphatidylcholine is a zwitterionic compound, the presence of other phosphatides such as phosphatidylinositol and phosphatidic acid, as well as small quantities of lysophosphatides, result in an emulsifier that imparts a net negative charge to dispersed particles.

Lecithin can be an excellent emulsifier for naturally occurring oils such as soy, corn, or safflower. Highly stable O/W emulsions can be formed with these oils. Purified lecithins from soy or egg yolk are the principal emulsifiers for intravenous fat emulsions. Lecithin provides stable emulsions with droplet sizes of less than 1 μm in diameter. It is critical that a small, uniform particle size be maintained in these emulsions to eliminate the risks of fat embolism after intravenous injection. The excellent stability observed with these emulsions may be the result of the large negative zeta potential that results from the small quantity of charged lipids present in lecithin as well as the ability of the lecithin to form mesophases resembling liposomes. During manufacture of the emulsions, homogenization produces small droplets that are surrounded by concentric layers of phospholipids. The latter may form a protective layer that prevents coalescence of the droplets. As an emulsifier, lecithin produces the best results at a pH of around 8.

As with any natural product, the content of lecithins will vary from source to source and their emulsifying properties and toxicity may also vary. For highly critical applications, such as intravenous emulsions, the source and composition of the lecithin must be carefully controlled and monitored.

Cholesterol is a major constituent of wool alcohols, obtained by the saponification and fractionation of wool fat. It is cholesterol that gives wool fat its capacity to absorb water and form a W/O emulsion.

FINELY DISPERSED SOLIDS—Finely dispersed solids are emulsifiers that form particulate films around the dispersed droplets, producing emulsions that are coarse-grained but have considerable physical stability. It appears possible that any solid can act as an emulsifying agent of this type, provided it is reduced to a sufficiently fine powder. In practice, the group of compounds used most frequently are the colloidal clays.

Bentonite is a white to gray, odorless and tasteless powder that swells in the presence of water to form a translucent suspension with a pH of about 9. Depending on the sequence of mixing it is possible to prepare both O/W and W/O emulsions. When an O/W emulsion is desired, the bentonite is first dispersed in water and allowed to hydrate so as to form a magma. The oil phase is then added gradually with constant titration. Because the aqueous phase is always in excess, the O/W emulsion type is favored. To prepare a W/O emulsion, the bentonite is first dispersed in oil; the water is then added gradually.

Although *Veegum* is used as a solid particle emulsifying agent, it is employed most extensively as a stabilizer in cosmetic lotions and creams. Concentrations of less than 1% Veegum will stabilize an emulsion containing anionic or nonionic emulsifying agents.

AUXILIARY EMULSIFYING AGENTS—Auxiliary emulsifying agents include those compounds that are normally incapable themselves of forming stable emulsions. Their main value lies in their ability to function as thickening agents and thereby help stabilize the emulsion. Agents in common use are listed in Table 22-5. Auxiliary emulsifying agents that are amphiphilic in nature are, in some cases, capable of forming gel or liquid crystalline phases with the primary emulsifying agent when combined with water and oil. This type of behavior may help to stabilize emulsions due to an increased viscosity, as observed in topical creams. Alternatively, gel or liquid crystalline phases may prevent coalescence by reducing van der Waals forces between particles or by providing a physical barrier between approaching particles of the internal phase. This latter effect is thought to be an important function in phospholipid-stabilized emulsions that must maintain a low viscosity to permit administration via the intravenous route. Additional information is provided by Eccleston.[12]

Emulsifying Agents and Emulsion Type

For a molecule, ion, colloid, or particle to be active as an emulsifying agent, it must have some affinity for the interface between the dispersed phase and the dispersion medium. With the monolayer and multilayer films, the emulsifier is in solution, and therefore it must be soluble to some extent in one or both of the phases. At the same time it must not be overly soluble in either phase; otherwise, it will remain in the bulk of that phase and not be adsorbed at the interface. This balanced affinity for the two phases also must be evident with finely divided

Table 22-6. Relationship between HLB Range and Surfactant Application

HLB RANGE	USE
0–3	Antifoaming agents
4–6	W/O emulsifying agents
7–9	Wetting agents
8–18	O/W emulsifying agents
13–15	Detergents
10–18	Solubilizing agents

solid particles used as emulsifying agents. If their affinity, as evidenced by the degree to which they are wetted, is either predominantly hydrophilic or hydrophobic, they will not function as effective wetting agents.

The great majority of the work on the relation between emulsifier and emulsion type has been concerned with surface-active agents that form interfacial monolayers. Thus, the present discussion will concentrate on this class of agents.

HYDROPHILE–LIPOPHILE BALANCE—As the emulsifier becomes more hydrophilic, its solubility in water increases and the formation of an O/W emulsion is favored. Conversely, W/O emulsions are favored with the more lipophilic emulsifiers. This led to the concept that the type of emulsion is related to the balance between hydrophilic and lipophilic solution tendencies of the surface-active emulsifying agent.

Griffin[16] developed a scale based on the balance between these two opposing tendencies. This so-called *HLB scale* is a numerical scale, extending from 1 to approximately 50. The more hydrophilic surfactants have high HLB numbers (in excess of 10), whereas surfactants with HLB numbers from 1 to 10 are considered to be lipophilic. Surfactants with a proper balance in their hydrophilic and lipophilic affinities are effective emulsifying agents because they concentrate at the oil–water interface. The relationship between HLB values and the application of the surface-active agent is shown in Table 22-6. Some commonly used emulsifiers and their HLB numbers are listed in Table 22-7. The utility of the HLB system in rationalizing the choice of emulsifying agents when formulating an emulsion will be discussed in a later section.

RATE OF COALESCENCE AND EMULSION TYPE—Davies[13] indicated that the type of emulsion produced in systems prepared by shaking is controlled by the relative coalescence rates of oil droplets dispersed in the oil. Thus, when a

Table 22-7. Approximate HLB Values for a Number of Emulsifying Agents

GENERIC OR CHEMICAL NAME	HLB	WATER DISPERSIBILITY
Sorbitan trioleate	1.8	No dispersion
Sucrose distearate	3.0	
Propylene glycol monostearate	3.4	
Glycerol monostearate (non–self-emulsifying)	3.8	Poor dispersion
Propylene glycol monolaurate	4.5	
Sorbitan monostearate	4.7	
Glycerol monostearate (self-emulsifying)	5.5	
Sorbitan monolaurate	8.6	Milky dispersion
Polyoxyethylene-4-lauryl ether	9.5	
Polyethylene glycol 400 monostearate	11.6	Translucent to clear
Polyoxyethylene-4-sorbitan monolaurate	13.3	Clear solution
Sucrose stearate	14.5	
Polyoxyethylene-20-sorbitan monopalmitate	15.6	
Polyoxyethylene-40-stearate	16.9	
Sodium oleate	18.0	
Sodium lauryl sulfate	40.0	

mixture of oil and water is shaken together with an emulsifying agent, a multiple dispersion is produced initially that contains oil dispersed in water and water dispersed in oil (see Fig 22-5).The type of the final emulsion that results depends on whether the water or the oil droplets coalesce more rapidly. If the O/W coalescence rate (Rate 1) is much greater than W/O coalescence rate (Rate 2), a W/O emulsion is formed because the dispersed water droplets are more stable than the dispersed oil droplets. Conversely, if Rate 2 is significantly faster than Rate 1, the final emulsion is an O/W dispersion because the oil droplets are more stable.

According to Davies,[13] the rate at which oil globules coalesce when dispersed in water is given by the expression

$$\text{Rate 1} = C_1 e^{-W_1/RT} \qquad (8)$$

The term C_1 is a collision factor that is directly proportional to the phase volume of the oil relative to the water, and is an inverse function of the viscosity of the continuous phase (water). W_1 defines an energy barrier made up of several contributing factors that must be overcome before coalescence can take place. First, it depends on the electrical potential of the dispersed oil droplets, as this affects repulsion. Second, with an O/W emulsion, the hydrated layer surrounding the polar portion of emulsifying agent must be broken down before coalescence can occur. This hydrated layer is probably around 1 nm thick with a consistency of butter. Finally, the total energy barrier depends on the fraction of the interface covered by the emulsifying agent.

Equation 9 describes the rate of coalescence of water globules dispersed in oil:

$$\text{Rate 2} = C_2 e^{-W_2/RT} \qquad (9)$$

Here, the collision factor C_2 is a function of the water–oil phase volume ratio divided by the viscosity of the oil phase. The energy barrier W_2 is, as before, related to the fraction of the interface covered by the surface-active agent. Another contributing factor is the number of $-CH_2-$ groups in the emulsifying agent; the longer the alkyl chain of the emulsifier, the greater the gap that has to be bridged if one water droplet is to combine with a second drop.

Davies[13] showed that the HLB concept is related to the distribution characteristics of the emulsifying agent between the two immiscible phases. An emulsifier with an HLB of less than 7 will be preferentially soluble in the oil phase and will favor formation of a W/O emulsion. Surfactants with an HLB value in excess of 7 will be distributed in favor of the aqueous phase and will promote O/W emulsions.

PREPARATION OF EMULSIONS

Several factors must be taken into account in the successful preparation and formulation of emulsified products. Usually, the type of emulsion (ie, O/W or W/O) is specified; if not, it probably will be implied from the anticipated use of the product. The formulator's attention is focused primarily on the selection of the emulsifying agent, or agents, necessary to achieve a satisfactory product. No incompatibilities should occur between the various emulsifiers and the several components commonly present in pharmaceutical emulsions. Finally, the product should be prepared in such a way as not to prejudice the formulation.

Selection of Emulsifying Agents

The selection of the emulsifying agent or agents is of prime importance in the successful formulation of an emulsion. The pharmacist must ensure that, in addition to its emulsifying properties, the material chosen is nontoxic and that the taste, odor, and chemical stability are compatible with the product. Thus, an emulsifying agent that is entirely suitable for inclusion in a skin cream may be unacceptable in the formulation of an oral preparation due to its potential toxicity. This consideration is most important when formulating intravenous emulsions.

THE HLB SYSTEM—With the increasing number of available emulsifiers, particularly the nonionics, the selection of emulsifiers for a product was essentially a trial-and-error procedure. Fortunately, the work of Griffin[16,17] provided a logical means of selecting emulsifying agents. Griffin's method, based on the balance between the hydrophilic and lipophilic portions of the emulsifying agent, is now widely used and has come to be known as the HLB system. It is used most in the rational selection of combinations of nonionic emulsifiers, and we shall limit our discussion accordingly.

As shown in Table 22-6, if an O/W emulsion is required, the formulator should use emulsifiers with an HLB in the range of 8 to 18. Emulsifiers with HLB values in the range of 4 to 6 are given consideration when a W/O emulsion is desired. Some typical examples are given in Table 22-7.

Another factor is the presence or absence of any polarity in the material being emulsified, because this will affect the polarity required in the emulsifier. Again, as a result of extensive experimentation, Griffin evolved a series of "required HLB" values—that is, the HLB value required by a particular material if it is to be emulsified effectively. Some values for oils and related materials are contained in Table 22-8. Naturally, the required HLB value differs depending on whether the final emulsion is O/W or W/O.

Fundamental to the utility of the HLB concept is the fact that the HLB values are algebraically additive. Thus, by using a low HLB surfactant with one having a high HLB it is possible to prepare blends having HLB values intermediate between those of the two individual emulsifiers. The following formula serves as an example.

O/W Emulsion

Liquid petrolatum (Required HLB 10.5)	50 g
Emulsifying agents	5 g
Sorbitan monooleate (HLB 4.3)	
Polyoxyethylene 20 sorbitan monoleate (HLB 15.0)	
Water, qs	100 g

By simple algebra it can be shown that 4.5 parts by weight of sorbitan monooleate blended with 6.2 parts by weight of polyoxyethylene 20 sorbitan monooleate will result in a mixed emulsifying agent having the required HLB of 10.5. Because the formula calls for 5 g, the required weights are 2.1 and 2.9 g, respectively. The oil-soluble sorbitan monooleate is dissolved in the oil and heated to 75°; the water-soluble polyoxyethylene 20 sorbitan monooleate is added to the aqueous phase that is heated to 70°. At this point the oil phase is mixed with the aqueous phase and the whole is stirred continuously until cool.

The formulator is not restricted to these two agents to produce a blend with an HLB of 10.5. Table 22-9 shows the various proportions required, using other pairs of emulsifying agents,

Table 22-8. Required HLB Values for Some Common Emulsion Ingredients

SUBSTANCE	W/O	O/W
Acid, stearic	—	17.0
Alcohol, cetyl	—	13.0
Lanolin, anhydrous	8	15.0
Oil, cottonseed	—	7.5
Mineral oil, light	4	10–12.0
Mineral oil, heavy	4	10.5
Wax, beeswax	5	10–16.0
Microcrystalline	—	9.5
Paraffin	—	9.0

to form a blend of HLB 10.5. When carrying out preliminary investigations with a particular material to be emulsified, it is advisable to try several pairs of emulsifying agents. Based on an evaluation of the emulsions produced, it becomes possible to choose the best combination.

Occasionally, the required HLB of the oil may not be known, in which case it becomes necessary to determine this parameter. Various blends are prepared to give a wide range of HLB mixtures and emulsions are prepared in a standardized manner. The HLB of the blend used to emulsify the best product, selected on the basis of physical stability, is taken to be the required HLB of the oil. The experiment should be repeated using another combination of emulsifiers to confirm the value of the required HLB of the oil to within, say, ± 1 HLB unit.

There are methods for finding the HLB value of a new surface-active agent. Griffin[17] developed simple equations that can be used to obtain an estimate with certain compounds. It has been shown that the ability of a compound to spread at a surface is related to its HLB. In another approach a linear relation between HLB and the logarithm of the dielectric constant for a number of nonionic surfactants has been observed.

An interesting approach, developed by Davies,[13] is related to his studies on the relative rates of coalescence of O/W and W/O emulsions. According to Davies, hydrophilic groups on the surfactant molecule make a positive contribution to the HLB number, whereas lipophilic groups exert a negative effect. Davies calculated these contributions and termed them HLB Group Numbers (Table 22-10). Provided the molecular structure of the surfactant is known, one simply adds the various group numbers in accordance with the following formula:

$$HLB = \Sigma(\text{hydrophilic group numbers}) - m(\text{group number}/-CH_2-\text{group}) + 7$$

where m is the number of $-CH_2-$groups present in the surfactant. Poor agreement is found between the HLB values calculated by the use of group numbers and the HLB values obtained using the simple equations developed by Griffin. However, the student should realize that the absolute HLB values per se are of limited significance. The utility of the HLB approach (using values calculated by either Griffin's or Davies' equations) is to

1. Provide the formulator with an idea of the relative balance of hydrophilicity and lipophilicity in a particular surfactant.
2. Relate that surfactant's emulsifying and solubilizing properties to other surfactants. The formulator still needs to confirm experimentally that a particular formulation will produce a stable emulsion.

Later, Davies and Rideal[18] attempted to relate HLB to the C_{water}/C_{oil} partition coefficient and found good agreement for a series of sorbitan surfactants. Schott showed, however, that the method does not apply to polyoxyethylated octylphenol surfactants. Schott concluded that "so far, the search for a universal correlation between HLB and another property of the surfac-

Table 22-10. HLB Group Numbers

	GROUP NUMBER
Hydrophilic groups	
$-SO_4^-Na^+$	38.7
$-COO^-K^+$	21.1
$-COO^-Na^+$	19.1
N (tertiary amine)	9.4
Ester (sorbitan ring)	6.8
Ester (free)	2.4
$-COOH$	2.1
Hydroxyl (free)	1.9
$-O-$	1.3
Hydroxyl (sorbitan ring)	0.5
Lipophilic groups	
$-CH-$	
$-CH_2-$	
CH_3-	-0.475
$=CH-$	
Derived groups	
$-(CH_2-CH_2-O)-$	$+0.33$
$-(CH_2-CH_2-CH_2-O)-$	-0.15

From Wedderburn DL. In: *Advances in Pharmaceutical Sciences*, vol 1. London: Academic Press, 1964, p 195.

tant that could be determined more readily than HLB has not been successful."[19]

The HLB system gives no information as to the *amount* of emulsifier required. Having once determined the correct blend, the formulator must prepare another series of emulsions, all at the same HLB, but containing increasing concentrations of the emulsifier blend. Usually, the minimum concentration giving the desired degree of physical stability is chosen.

When varying the amounts of emulsifier in an emulsion it is useful to consider the use of a phase diagram to select the proper ratio of oil/water/surfactant. The use of the phase diagram to aid in the formulation of emulsions has been discussed by Swarbrick.[20] This approach can provide a systematic way to optimize an emulsion formulation and help to identify the existence of liquid crystalline phases that, when present in an emulsion formulation, can enhance the stability. Because liquid crystals exhibit birefringence, observation of prototype emulsions under polarized light microscopy can be a useful tool to identify combinations of water–oil and emulsifier that produce liquid crystals. It should be noted that liquid crystals are often formed when relatively high concentrations (eg, 20% or more) of surfactant are used in a formulation. The toxicity of the emulsifier for the intended use (eg, topical, oral, or parenteral) must be considered in addition to the physical characteristics.

MIXED EMULSIFYING AGENTS—Emulsifying agents are frequently used in combination because a better emulsion usually is obtained. This enhancement may be due to several reasons, one or more of which may be operative in any one system. Thus, the use of a blend or mixture of emulsifiers may

1. Produce the required hydrophile–lipophile balance in the emulsifier.
2. Enhance the stability and cohesiveness of the interfacial film.
3. Affect the consistency and feel of the product.

The first point has been considered in detail in the previous discussion of the HLB system.

With regard to the second point, Schulman and Cockbain in 1940 showed that combinations of certain amphiphiles formed stable films at the air–water interface. It was postulated that the complex formed by these two materials (one, oil-soluble; the other, water-soluble) at the air–water interface was also present at the O/W interface. This interfacial complex was held to be responsible for the improved stability. For example, sodium cetyl sulfate, a moderately good O/W emulsifier, and elaidyl alcohol or cholesterol, both stabilizers for W/O emulsions, show evidence of an interaction at the air–water interface. Furthermore, an O/W emulsion prepared with sodium cetyl sulfate and

Table 22-9. Nonionic Blends Having HLB Values of 10.5

SURFACTANT BLEND	HLB	REQUIRED AMOUNTS (%) TO GIVE HLB = 10.5
Sorbitan tristearate	2.1	34.4
Polyoxyethylene 20 sorbitan monostearate	14.9	65.6
Sorbitan monopalmitate	6.7	57.3
Polyoxyethylene 20 sorbitan monopalmitate	15.6	42.7
Sorbitan sesquioleate	3.7	48.5
Polyoxyethylene lauryl ether	16.9	51.5

elaidyl alcohol is much more stable than an emulsion prepared with sodium cetyl sulfate alone.

Elaidyl alcohol is the *trans* isomer. When oleyl alcohol, the *cis* isomer, is used with sodium cetyl sulfate, there is no evidence of complex formation at the air–water interface. Significantly, this combination does not produce a stable O/W emulsion either. Such a finding strongly suggests that a high degree of molecular alignment is necessary at the O/W interface to form a stable emulsion. This high degree of molecular alignment may be a prerequisite event for the formation of lamellar liquid crystalline or gel phases. As illustrated in Figure 22-7, the combination of certain long chain acids and alcohols with water can result in the formation of micelles and liquid crystals. It has also been observed that when liquid crystals or gels form in an emulsion, increased stability is generally observed. As discussed previously, gel or liquid crystalline phases can have an important effect in inhibiting coalescence in emulsions.

When using combinations of emulsifiers, care must be taken to ensure their compatibility, as charged emulsifying agents of opposite sign are likely to interact and coagulate when mixed.

STERIC STABILIZATION—Many useful nonionic surfactants consist of hydrophobic portions composed of fatty acids or other lipophilic organic compounds and hydrophilic portions composed of polyoxyethylene chains. When used to prepare O/W emulsions, the oxyethylene chains protrude into the aqueous side of the O/W interface while the hydrophobic portion of the emulsifier will be primarily located in the oil side. As in the case of suspensions, approaching oil droplets will be influenced by van der Waals attractive forces as well as repulsive forces. For an emulsion that is stabilized by a non-ionic surfactant, the repulsive forces consist of electrostatic and non-electrostatic forces. The electrostatic repulsive forces are similar to those discussed for suspensions and depend largely upon the zeta potential of the oil droplets.

Non-electrostatic forces may also arise from a phenomenon that is frequently described as *steric stabilization*. This effect has been explained as follows. First, as emulsion droplets approach, the adsorbed layers of surfactant on each droplet begin to mix. The hydrophilic oxyethylene chains behave as soluble polymers; as their concentration increases in the region of interfacial mixing, segments of the polymers from separate droplets compete for water molecules. This results in restricted movement of the polymer chains or a loss of entropy. Likewise, a positive heat of solution (enthalpy) may result from the mixing of the polymers in the interfaces. The loss of entropy and/or increase in enthalpy results in an increase in the free energy of mixing, meaning that spontaneous mixing in the interfacial region is not favorable. The particles will tend to separate in order to reverse the temporary increase in the free energy of mixing.

An additional effect that causes repulsion of the droplets may be a result of the increased osmotic pressure that results in the area of contact between the two emulsion droplets. The concentration of oxyethylene groups in the region of overlap between the two droplets increases, necessitating an influx of water into the region. This increase in osmotic pressure has the effect of forcing the droplets apart. Thus, in addition to their favorable effect of reducing interfacial tension, nonionic surfactants that possess long, hydrophilic chains provide additional emulsion stabilization via the energetically unfavorable result of mixing of polymer chains at the droplet–droplet interface.

Method of Preparation

Different methods are employed, depending on the type of emulsifying agent used and the scale of manufacture. Traditionally, the mortar and pestle was used for the small scale preparation of emulsions stabilized by the presence of such agents as acacia and tragacanth. However, the use of these agents has declined drastically in recent years; as a result, the use of the mortar and pestle has declined as well. (Refer to the 18th edition of this text, page 306, for details of the mortar and pestle method.)

An increasing number of emulsions are being formulated with synthetic emulsifying agents, especially of the nonionic type. The components in such a formulation are separated into those that are oil-soluble and those that are water-soluble. These are dissolved in their respective solvents by heating to about 70° to 75°. When solution is complete, the two phases are mixed and the product is stirred until cool. This method, which requires nothing more than two beakers, a thermometer, and a source of heat, is necessarily used in the preparation of emulsions containing waxes and other high-melting-point materials that must be melted before they can be dispersed in the emulsion. The relatively simple methodology involved in the use of synthetic surfactant-type emulsifiers is one factor that has led to their widespread use in emulsion preparation. This, in turn, has led to a decline in the use of the natural emulsifying agents.

With hand homogenizers, an initial rough emulsion is formed by trituration in a mortar or shaking in a bottle. The rough emulsion then is passed several times through the homogenizer. A reduction in particle size is achieved as the material is forced through a narrow aperture under pressure. A satisfactory product invariably results from the use of a hand homogenizer and overcomes any deficiencies in technique. Should the homogenizer fail to produce an adequate product, the formulation, rather than the technique, should be suspected.

For a discussion of the techniques and equipment used in the large-scale manufacture of emulsions, see Chapter 39.

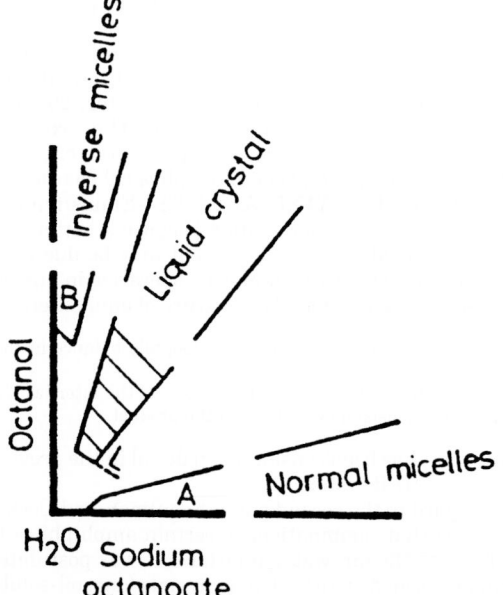

Figure 22-7. Phase diagram illustrating the formation of micellar and liquid crystalline phases in mixtures of a long-chain alcohol, long-chain acid, and water. Compositions that form the lamellar liquid crystalline phase can provide enhanced emulsion stability. (From Friberg S, Larson K. In: Brown GH, ed. *Advances in Liquid Crystals*, vol 2. New York: Academic Press, 1976, p 173.)

STABILITY OF EMULSIONS

Several criteria must be met in a well-formulated emulsion. Probably the most important and most readily apparent requirement is that the emulsion possess adequate physical stability; without this, any emulsion soon will revert back to two separate bulk phases. In addition, if the emulsified product is to have some antimicrobial activity (eg, a medicated lotion), care must be taken to ensure that the formulation possesses the required degree of activity. Frequently, a compound exhibits a lower antimicrobial activity in an emulsion than, say, in a solution. Generally, this is because of partitioning effects between the oil and water phases, which cause a lowering of the *effective* concentration of the active agent. Partitioning has also to be taken into account when considering preservatives to prevent microbiological spoilage of emulsions. Finally, the chemical stability of the various components of the emulsion should receive some attention, as such materials may be more prone to degradation in the emulsified state than when they exist as a bulk phase.

In the present discussion, detailed consideration will be limited to the question of physical stability. Reviews of this topic have been published by Garrett[21] and Kitchener and Mussellwhite.[22] For information on the effect that emulsification can have on the biologic activity and chemical stability of materials in emulsions, see Wedderburn,[23] Burt[24] and Swarbrick.[20]

The theories of emulsion stability have been discussed by Eccleston[25] in an attempt to understand the situation in both a simple O/W emulsion and complex commercial systems. A recent review by the same author[12] has discussed the stability of multiple phase emulsions and the role of bilayer gels and liquid crystalline phases on the physical stability of these systems.

The three major phenomena associated with physical stability are

1. The upward or downward movement of dispersed droplets relative to the continuous phase, termed *creaming* or *sedimentation*, respectively.
2. The *aggregation* and possible *coalescence* of the dispersed droplets to reform the separate, bulk phases.
3. *Inversion*, in which an O/W emulsion inverts to become a W/O emulsion and *vice versa*.

CREAMING AND SEDIMENTATION—*Creaming* is the upward movement of dispersed droplets relative to the continuous phase; *sedimentation*, the reverse process, is the downward movement of particles. In any emulsion one process or the other takes place, depending on the densities of the disperse and continuous phases. This is undesirable in a pharmaceutical product where homogeneity is essential for the administration of the correct and uniform dose. Furthermore, creaming, or sedimentation, brings the particles closer together and may facilitate the more serious problem of coalescence.

The rate at which a spherical droplet or particle sediments in a liquid is governed by Stokes' law (Equation 3). Other equations have been developed for bulk systems, but Stokes' equation is still useful because it points out the factors that influence the rate of sedimentation or creaming. These are the diameter of the suspended droplets, the viscosity of the suspending medium, and the difference in densities between the dispersed phase and the dispersion medium.

Usually, only the use of the first two factors is feasible in affecting creaming or sedimentation. Reduction of particle size contributes greatly toward overcoming or minimizing creaming, because the rate of movement is a square-root function of the particle diameter. There are, however, technical difficulties in reducing the diameter of droplets to below about 0.1 μm. The most frequently used approach is to raise the viscosity of the continuous phase, although this can be done only to the extent that the emulsion still can be removed readily from its container and spread or administered conveniently.

AGGREGATION AND COALESCENCE—Even though creaming and sedimentation are undesirable, they do not necessarily result in the breakdown of the emulsion, as the dispersed droplets retain their individuality. Furthermore, the droplets can be redispersed with mild agitation. More serious to the stability of an emulsion are the processes of aggregation and coalescence. In *aggregation* (flocculation) the dispersed droplets come together but do not fuse. *Coalescence*, the complete fusion of droplets, leads to a decrease in the number of droplets and the ultimate separation of the two immiscible phases. Aggregation precedes coalescence in emulsions; however, coalescence does not necessarily follow from aggregation. Aggregation is, to some extent, reversible. Although it is not as serious as coalescence, it will accelerate creaming or sedimentation, because the aggregate behaves as a single drop.

Aggregation is related to the electrical potential on the droplets, but coalescence depends on the structural properties of the interfacial film. As discussed previously, it has been recognized that combinations of emulsifiers produce more stable emulsions than a single emulsifier alone. One reason for this synergy, as suggested by Shulman and Cockbain, is that appropriate combinations of surfactants form densely packed complex films at the oil–water interface. Additional beneficial effects of mixed emulsifier films could result from an increase in viscosity of the interfacial emulsifier film. A viscous interfacial film could enhance emulsion stability because thinning of the film at the points of droplet to droplet contact would be inhibited. An additional explanation for the beneficial effect of mixed-film emulsifiers suggests that appropriate mixtures of surfactants provide a more elastic interfacial film. A more elastic interfacial film would resist rupture upon collision of emulsion droplets.

It has also been observed that when emulsifiers are combined in certain concentrations and proportions, liquid crystalline phases can be formed. The preparation of emulsions with surfactants that form liquid crystalline states can have greater stability against coalescence compared to emulsions that are formulated in the absence of liquid crystalline states. Friberg and Larson[26] have explained the enhanced stability of emulsions due to liquid crystals in terms of a reduced van der Waals attraction between emulsion droplets. Such an effect depends upon the formation of layers or lamellae around the emulsion droplets. Each layer of liquid crystal contributes to a further reduction in the van der Waals attractive force.

An additional effect of liquid crystals may be related to the high viscosity that often is observed upon their formation. Liquid crystals possess a viscosity that is on the order of 100-fold greater than most oil–water interfaces. The high viscosity may result in reduced rates of coalescence. A key factor that may be important for the stabilizing effect of liquid crystals is the location of the liquid crystalline phase in relation to the dispersed droplets. To effectively inhibit coalescence, the liquid crystals should concentrate at the interface between the droplet and the continuous phase. This may not occur with all oil–water–surfactant combinations.

Particle-size analysis can reveal the tendency of an emulsion to aggregate and coalesce long before any visible signs of instability are apparent. The methods available have been reviewed by Groves and Freshwater.[27]

INVERSION—An emulsion is said to *invert* when it changes from an O/W to a W/O emulsion, or *vice versa*. Inversion sometimes can be brought about by the addition of an electrolyte or by changing the phase-volume ratio. For example, an O/W emulsion having sodium stearate as the emulsifier can be inverted by the addition of calcium chloride, because the calcium stearate formed is a lipophilic emulsifier and favors the formation of a W/O product.

Inversion often can be seen when an emulsion, prepared by heating and mixing the two phases, is being cooled. This takes place presumably because of the temperature-dependent changes in the solubilities of the emulsifying agents. The phase inversion temperature (PIT) of nonionic surfactants has been shown by Shinoda and Kunieda[28] to be influenced by the HLB number of the surfactant—the higher the PIT value, the greater the resistance to inversion.

Apart from work on PIT values, little quantitative work has been carried out on the process of inversion; nevertheless, it would appear that the effect can be minimized by using the proper emulsifying agent in an adequate concentration. Wherever possible, the volume of the dispersed phase should not exceed 50% of the total volume of the emulsion.

BIOAVAILABILITY FROM COARSE DISPERSIONS

All dosage forms must be capable of releasing the drug in a known and consistent manner following administration to the patient. Both the rate and extent of release are important. Ideally, the extent of release should approach 100%, while the rate of release should reflect the desired properties of the dosage form. For example, with products designed to have a rapid onset of activity, the release of drug should be immediate. With a long-acting product, the release should take place over several hours or days, depending on the type of product used. The rate and extent of drug release should be reproducible from batch to batch of the product, and should not change during shelf-life.

The principles on which biopharmaceutics is based are dealt with in some detail in Chapters 57 to 59. Although most published work in this area has been concerned with the bioavailability of solid dosage forms administered by the oral route, the rate and extent of release from both suspensions and emulsions are also important and so must be considered in some detail.

BIOAVAILABILITY FROM SUSPENSIONS—Suspensions of a drug may be expected to demonstrate improved bioavailability compared to the same drug formulated as a tablet or capsule. This is because the suspension already contains discrete drug particles, whereas tablet dosage forms must invariably undergo disintegration in order to maximize the necessary dissolution process. Frequently, antacid suspensions are perceived as being more rapid in action and therefore more effective than an equivalent dose in the form of tablets. Bates et al[29] observed that a suspension of salicylamide was more rapidly bioavailable, at least during the first hour following administration, than two different tablet forms of the drug; this study was also able to demonstrate a correlation between the initial *in vitro* dissolution rates for the several dosage forms studied and the initial rates of *in vivo* absorption. A similar argument can be developed for hard gelatin capsules, where the shell must rupture or dissolve before drug particles are released and can begin the dissolution process. Such was observed by Antal et al[30] in a study of the bioavailability of several doxycycline products, including a suspension and hard gelatin capsules. Sansom et al[31] found that mean plasma phenytoin levels were higher after the administration of a suspension than when an equivalent dose was given as either tablets or capsules. It was suggested that this might have been due to the suspension having a smaller particle size.

In common with other products in which the drug is present in the form of solid particles, the rate of dissolution, and thus potentially the bioavailability of the drug in a suspension, can be affected by such factors as particle size and shape, surface characteristics, and polymorphism. Strum *et al*[32] conducted a comparative bioavailability study involving two commercial brands of sulfamethiazole suspension (Product A and Product B). Following administration of the products to 12 normal individuals and blood samples taken at predetermined times over a period of 10 hr, the Strum study found no statistically significant difference in the extent of drug absorption from the two suspensions. The absorption rate, however, differed, and from *in vitro* studies it was concluded that product A dissolved faster than Product B, and that the former contained more particles of smaller size than the latter, differences that may be responsible for the more rapid dissolution of particles in Product A. Product A also provided higher serum levels during *in vivo* tests 0.5 hr after administration. The results showed that the rate of absorption of sulfamethiazole from a suspension depended on the rate of dissolution of the suspended particles, which in turn was related to particle size. Previous studies[33,34] had shown the need to determine the dissolution rate of sus-

pensions to gain information as to the bioavailability of drugs from this type of dosage form.

The viscosity of the vehicle used to suspend the particles has been found to have an effect on the rate of absorption of nitrofurantoin but not the total bioavailability. Thus Soci and Parrott[35] were able to maintain a clinically acceptable urinary nitrofurantoin concentration for an additional 2 hr by increasing the viscosity of the vehicle.

BIOAVAILABILITY FROM EMULSIONS—There are indications that improved bioavailability may result when a poorly absorbed drug is formulated as an orally administered emulsion. However, little research appears to have been done to directly compare emulsions and other dosage forms such as suspensions, tablets, and capsules; thus, it is not possible to draw unequivocal conclusions as to advantages of emulsions. If a drug with low aqueous solubility can be formulated so as to be in solution in the oil phase of an emulsion, its bioavailability may be enhanced. It must be recognized, however, that the drug in such a system has several barriers to pass before it arrives at the mucosal surface of the GI tract.

For example, with an O/W emulsion, the drug must diffuse through the oil globule and then pass across the oil–water interface. This may be a difficult process, depending on the characteristics of the interfacial film formed by the emulsifying agent. In spite of this potential drawback, Wagner et al[36] found that indoxole, a nonsteroidal anti-inflammatory agent, was significantly more bioavailable in an O/W emulsion than in either a suspension or a hard gelatin capsule. Bates and Sequeira[37] found significant increases in maximum plasma levels and total bioavailability of micronized griseofulvin when formulated in a corn O/W emulsion. In this case, however, the enhanced effect was not due to emulsification of the drug in the oil phase *per se*, but more probably because of the linoleic and oleic acids present having a specific effect on GI motility.

REFERENCES

1. Hiestand EN. *J Pharm Sci* 1964; 53:1.
2. Haines BA, Martin A. *J Pharm Sci* 1961; 50:228, 753, 756.
3. Matthews BA, Rhodes CT. *J Pharm Pharmacol* 1968; 20(Suppl): 204S.
4. Matthews BA, Rhodes CT. *J Pharm Sci* 1968; 57:569.
5. Matthews BA, Rhodes CT. *J Pharm Sci* 1970; 59:521.
6. Schneider W et al. *Am J Pharm Ed* 1978; 42:280.
7. Scheer AJ. *Drug Cosmet Ind* 1981; (Apr):40.
8. Kellaway I.W, Najib NM. *Int J Pharm* 1981; 9:59.
9. Martin AN *et al. Physical Pharmacy*, 3rd ed. Philadelphia: Lea & Febiger, 1983, p 551.
10. Parsons GE et al. *Int J Pharm* 1992; 83:163.
11. Tingstad J et al. *J Pharm Sci* 1973; 62:1361.
12. Eccleston GM. In *Encyclopedia of Pharmaceutical Technology*, vol 5. New York: Dekker, 1992, p 137.
13. Davies JT. In: *Proceedings of the International Congress on Surface Activity*, 2nd ed. London: Butterworth/Academic, 1957, p 426.
14. Sherman P. In: *Emulsion Science*. New York: Academic Press, 1968, Chap 4.
15. Rogers JA. *Cosmet Toiletries* 1978; 93(7):29.
16. Griffin WC. *J Soc Cosmet Chem* 1949; 1:311.
17. Griffin WC. *J Soc Cosmet Chem* 1954; 5:249.
18. Davies JT, Rideal EK. *Interfacial Phenomena*. New York: Academic Press, 1961, Chap 8.
19. Schott J. *J Pharm Sci* 1971; 60:649.
20. Swarbrick J. *J Soc Cosmet Chem* 1968; 19:187.
21. Garrett ER. *J Pharm Sci* 1965; 60:1557.
22. Kitchener JA, Musselwhite PR. In: *Emulsion Science*. New York: Academic Press, 1968, Chap 2.
23. Wedderburn DL. In: *Advances in Pharmaceutical Sciences*, vol 1. London: Academic Press, 1964, p 195.
24. Burt BW. *J Soc Cosmet Chem* 1965; 16:465.
25. Eccleston GM. *Cosmet Toiletries* 1986; 101(11):73.

26. Friberg S, Larson K. In: Brown GH, ed. *Advances in Liquid Crystals*, vol 2. New York: Academic Press, 1976, p 173.
27. Groves MJ, Freshwater DC. *J Pharm Sci* 1968; 57:1273.
28. Shinoda K, Kunieda H. In: *Encyclopedia of Emulsion Technology*. New York: Dekker, 1983, Chap 5.
29. Bates TR et al. *J Pharm Sci* 1969; 58:1468.
30. Antal EJ et al. *J Pharm Sci* 1975; 64:2015.
31. Sansom LN et al. *Med J Aust* 1975; 2:593.
32. Strum JD et al. *J Pharm Sci* 1978; 67:1659.
33. Bates TR et al. *J Pharm Sci* 1973; 62:2057.
34. Howard SA et al. *J Pharm Sci* 1977; 66:557.
35. Soci MM, Parrott EL. *J Pharm Sci* 1980; 69:403.
36. Wagner JG et al. *Clin Pharmacol Ther* 1966; 7:610.
37. Bates TR, Sequeira JA. *J Pharm Sci* 1975; 64:793.

BIBLIOGRAPHY

Adamson AW. *Physical Chemistry of Surfaces*, 4th ed. New York: Wiley-Interscience, 1980.

Attwood D, Florence AT. In: *Surfactant Systems; Their Chemistry, Pharmacy and Biology*. London: Chapman & Hall, 1983, p 469.

Becher P. *Emulsions: Theory and Practice*, 2nd ed. New York: Reinhold, 1965.

Becher P. *Encyclopedia of Emulsion Technology*, vols 1–3. New York: Dekker, 1983–1988.

Davies JT, Rideal EK. *Interfacial Phenomena*. New York: Academic Press, 1963.

Eccleston GM. In: *Encyclopedia of Pharmaceutical Technology*, vol 5. New York: Dekker, 1992, p 137.

Hiemenz PC. *Principles of Colloidal and Surface Chemistry*, 2nd ed. New York: Dekker, 1986.

Matijevic E, ed. *Surface and Colloid Science*, vols 1–4. New York: Wiley, 1971.

Osipow LI. *Surface Chemistry*. New York: Reinhold, 1962.

Parfitt G. *Dispersion of Powders in Liquids*. New York: Applied Science, 1973.

Sherman P. *Emulsion Science*. New York: Academic Press, 1964.

Sherman P. *Rheology of Emulsions*. New York: Macmillan, 1963.

Vold RD, Vold MJ. *Colloid and Interface Chemistry*. Reading MA: Addison-Wesley, 1983.

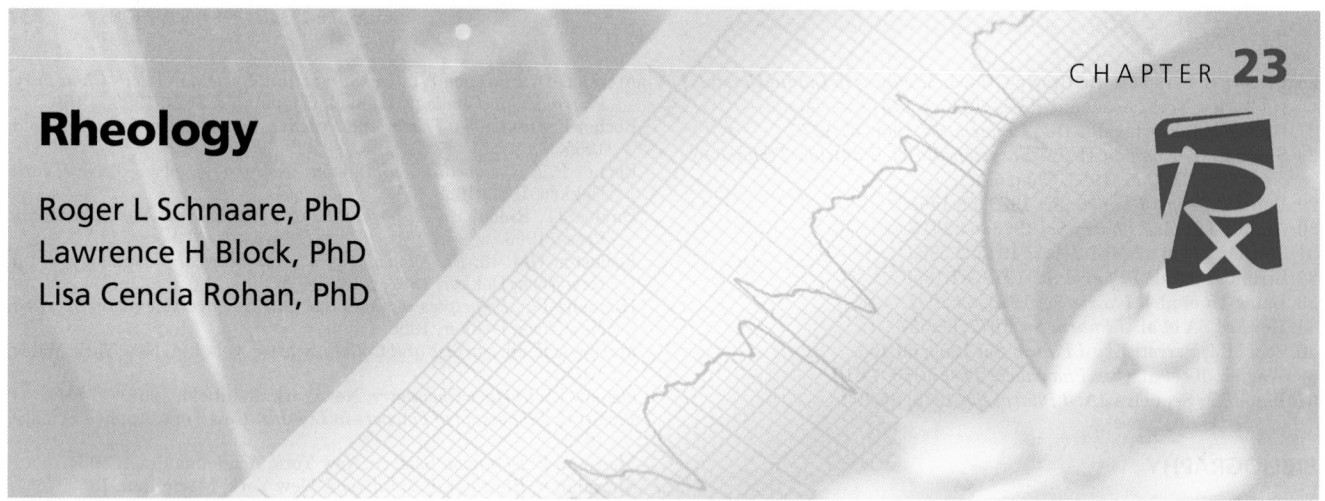

CHAPTER 23

Rheology

Roger L Schnaare, PhD

Lawrence H Block, PhD

Lisa Cencia Rohan, PhD

Rheology is the branch of physics that deals with deformation, including flow, of matter. Although this definition was proposed in 1929, the recognition of rheological phenomena dates back to antiquity.[1] The earliest application of rheology (*ca* 1600 BCE) is associated with the Egyptian Amenemhet who made a 7° correction to the drainage angle of a water clock in order to account for the temperature dependent variation in water flow during the course of a day. Archimedes's claim (*ca* 250 BCE)—"Give me but one firm spot on which to stand, and I will move the earth."—was based on the application of solid mechanics, the oldest branch of the physical sciences.[1]

Reiner[2] describes a simple mechanical experiment in which he lets three different materials—a pencil, a ball of plasticine, and a known mass of water—fall from some height onto the surface of a table. Newton's second law tells us that $F = m \cdot a$, where F is the force acting upon each of these materials of mass m, and a is the acceleration of the center of mass of each material. Since F is proportional to m, a is the same for each of these materials. Consequently, these three bodies fall towards the table in exactly the same manner. Their material differences do not become apparent until they reach the table top. At that point, the pencil rebounds somewhat, the plasticine stays put, and the water spreads over the tabletop and, on reaching the edge, flows off. These very different outcomes—which mechanics is unable to explain—are the focus of rheology.

The ubiquity of rheological phenomena in pharmacy is evident in the levigation or mixing of ointments on slabs, the use of a mortar and pestle to prepare suspensions and emulsions, the flow of emulsions through colloid mills and pumps, the use of roller mills for compacting powders or processing ointments, and the mechanical properties of glass or plastic containers and of rubber or polymeric closures. Squeezing ointments, creams, or toothpaste from a collapsible tube, spreading lotion on the skin, or spraying liquids from atomizers or aerosol cans all involve rheological phenomena. The fluidity of solutions to be injected by syringe or infused intravenously, the flexibility of tubing used in catheters, and the strength of sutures and ligatures are important rheological properties. Drug release from dosage forms and delivery systems is often controlled or modulated by the rheological properties of the formulation matrix. Although at a molecular level, diffusion is governed, in part, by the rheological behavior of the environment. Rheological principles govern the circulation of blood and lymph through capillaries and large vessels, the flow of mucus, the transit of the luminal contents through the gastrointestinal tract, the bending of bones, the stretching of cartilage, and the contraction of muscles.

The fundamentals of rheology are presented in the following section in the sequence that underscores their temporal recognition and application in pharmacy rather than their historic development in physics.

FUNDAMENTALS

The jargon of rheology can be problematic for the uninitiated. For example, as Scott Blair[3] notes, *stress* and *strain*, in everyday English, have virtually the same meaning. Rheologists, however, use the word *stress* to refer to a system of forces, whether applied in a *compressive*, *extensional*, or *shear* mode, and *strain*, to a change in size or shape.

Rheological principles stem from two fundamental laws derived in the late 17th century: Robert Hooke's law of elasticity (*ca* 1676) and Isaac Newton's law of flow (1687). The corresponding equations, which embody these laws, characterize Hookean and Newtonian materials, respectively. When a force is applied to a body, the two rheological extremes of behavior are the pure elastic deformation of a Hookean solid and the pure viscous flow of a Newtonian liquid. Pure (ideal) elasticity means that the body returns to its original form once the stress is removed, while pure (ideal) viscosity means that the liquid flows even under the smallest stress and does not return to its original shape or form once the stress is removed[4]. The resistance to deformation, or flow, is described by the modulus of elasticity or Young's modulus, E, for an elastic body undergoing extension, and by η, the coefficient of viscosity for a liquid.

Elastic deformation of solids is described by Hooke's law,

$$dl = \frac{\sigma}{E}, \qquad (1)$$

where dl is the elastic deformation or extension in length l caused by the application of stress σ. This is illustrated in Figure 23-1.

Viscous deformation, i.e. viscous flow, occurs in accordance with Newton's law,

$$\sigma = \eta\dot{\gamma} \qquad (2)$$

wherein the applied stress σ results in flow with a velocity gradient, $\dot{\gamma}$ or rate of shear. The proportionality constant η is termed *viscosity*, while its reciprocal is called *fluidity*. Viscosity has also been described as the *internal friction* in the fluid as it corresponds to the resistance of the fluid to the relative motion of adjacent layers of liquid. This is illustrated in Figure 23-2. Imagine a liquid contained between two very large, parallel plates as being divided into a stack of very thin, parallel layers much like a deck of cards, as shown in Figure 23-2. Shear is applied to the liquid by pulling or pushing the top plate with a constant force F per unit area A, ie F/A, or σ, while holding the bottom plate stationary. The top liquid layer, in contact with the moving plate, adheres to it and moves with the same velocity as the plate. The second layer, adjacent to the top one, is dragged

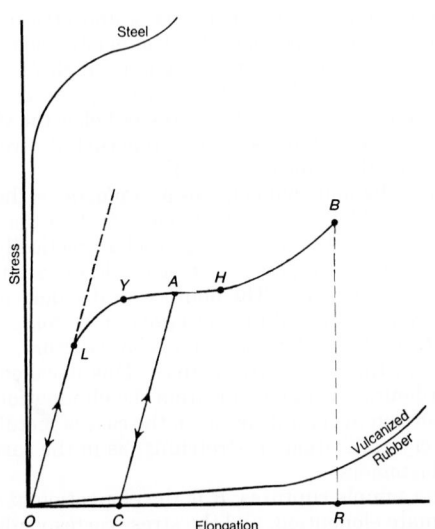

Figure 23-1. Elastic deformation in accordance with Hooke's Law.

Table 23-1. Approximate Shear Rates for Pharmaceutical Operations

OPERATION	RATE OF SHEAR, s^{-1}
Pouring from a bottle	50
Spreading lotion on skin	400–1000
Levigating ointment on slab with spatula	400–1000
Injecting through hypodermic syringe	4,000
Dispensing nasal spray from plastic squeeze bottle	20,000
Processing in colloid mill	10^5–10^6

shearing stress, τ, have been replaced by $\dot{\gamma}$ and σ, respectively, in accordance with more widely accepted nomenclature recommendations.[5,6]

Characteristic shear rates for pharmacy-related activities are listed in Table 23-1. Even for a given process, the shear rate can vary within wide limits, depending on the scale of the process and the processing rate. Thus, when a lotion is rubbed into the skin, if the hand (moving surface) slides across the skin (stationary surface) with a velocity $v = 45$ cm/s and if the thickness of the lotion film is $x = 0.05$ cm, then, according to Equation 3, the rate of shear is $\dot{\gamma} = (45$ cm/s$)/(0.05$ cm$) = 900$ s^{-1}. For a given force and a constant viscosity, the rate of shear is uniform throughout the layer of lotion.

The flow of liquids by parallel layers moving past each other and dragging adjacent layers along (as in Fig 23-2) is called *laminar* or *streamline flow*. At higher velocities and/or if the plates have rough surfaces, eddies or swirls develop whereby mass transfer occurs from one layer or lamina to another. Theoretically, this complex phenomenon—referred to as *turbulent flow*—may be described by a set of partial differential equations, known as the Navier-Stokes equations, which govern fluids in motion. However, explicit solutions of these nonlinear equations, originally derived in the 1840s on the basis of laws of conservation of mass, momentum, and energy, remain elusive.

From a historic rheological viewpoint, deformation of matter was first described in ideal terms. Precise differentiations were made among perfect, rigid *Euclidean* bodies (solids), ideal *Hookean* elastic solids, *Pascalian*, or inviscid, liquids, and *Newtonian* liquids. For ideal Euclidean solids, only mass (or density) is relevant; rigid bodies do not undergo deformation under stress. When stress is applied to an ideal Hookean elastic solid, the deformation induced is fully recovered when the stress is removed. Inviscid liquids exhibit no resistance to flow when stressed, whereas Newtonian liquids undergo flow at a rate that is proportional to the stress applied.

Unfortunately, most solids and fluids encountered in pharmacy do not exhibit ideal behavior consistent with the classical models that evolved with Hooke, Pascal, or Newton. By the 19th century, evidence for more complex, nonideal rheological behavior began to accumulate and the clear-cut dividing line between Hookean or elastic solids and Newtonian or viscous liquids became increasingly blurred. Some systems that behave as elastic solids when subjected to small stresses, or to moderate stresses of short duration, will undergo permanent deformation, resembling very viscous liquids, if the stresses are larger and/or applied for longer periods of time. For many materials, the temporal dependence of their rheological properties necessitates careful consideration of their handling prior to and during the process of rheological evaluation. Nonetheless, an understanding of ideal rheological behavior is necessary before deviations from ideality can be considered.

along by friction, but its velocity is reduced somewhat by the resistance of the layers beneath it. Each layer is pulled forward by the layer moving above it but is held back by the layer underneath it, over which it moves and which it drags along. The farther the liquid layers are from the moving plate, the smaller their velocities. The bottom layer adheres to the stationary plate and has zero velocity. Thus, the velocity of the liquid layers increases in the direction x perpendicular to the direction of flow y. The *shear strain* or deformation in shear, γ, is the displacement y divided by the height, x, of the sheared or deformed portion of the liquid, as shown in Figure 23-2. It equals the tangent of the displacement angle θ that, at low θ values, is approximately equal to θ expressed in radians: $\gamma = \dfrac{y}{x} = \tan\theta \cong \theta$.

In due time, all layers except the bottom one undergo infinite deformation. What distinguishes one liquid from another is the rate at which the deformation increases with time. This is called the *rate of* (deformation in) *shear*, $\dot{\gamma}$ or $d\gamma/dt$, the derivative of γ with respect to time, t. An equivalent definition for $\dot{\gamma}$ is the *velocity gradient,* ie, the rate at which the velocity, v, changes with the distance, x, perpendicular to the direction of flow:

$$\dot{\gamma} = \frac{d\gamma}{dt} = \frac{dv}{dx} \qquad (3)$$

The rate of shear or velocity gradient, $\dot{\gamma}$ indicates how fast the liquid flows when a shear stress is applied to it. Its unit according to both definitions is s^{-1}, since γ is dimensionless, velocity is expressed in m/sec, and x in m.

It should be noted that the symbols used in the past in the pharmaceutical literature for the rate of shear, D, and for the

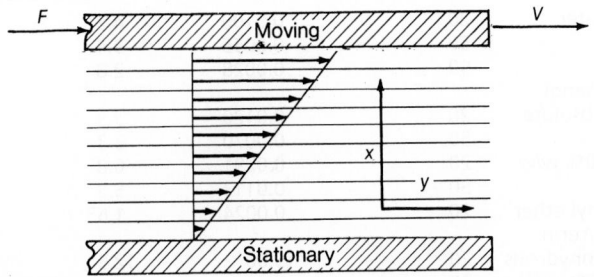

Figure 23-2. Laminar flow of a liquid contained between two parallel plates.

Elastic Solids

In the stretching or extension of an elastic solid, the deformation is said to be in tension. The deformation or strain of the stretched body, or its elongation, is the difference between its

Table 23-2. Values of Modulus of Elasticity[a] of Representative Solids of Pharmaceutical or Biomedical Interest

MATERIAL	YOUNG'S MODULUS (DYNES/CM^2)
Steel	2.2×10^{12}
Glass	6×10^{11}
Potassium chloride	2.3×10^{11}
Silk, viscose rayon	1.5×10^{11}
Microcrystalline cellulose	1.3×10^{11}
Polystyrene	3.4×10^{10}
Polyethylene (low density)	2.4×10^{9}
Rubber (vulcanized)	2×10^{7}
Tooth enamel	4.7×10^{11}
Bone	2.2×10^{11}
Tendon	1.3×10^{9}
Muscle	6×10^{6}
Soft tissue	7.5×10^{4}
Gelatin gels	
10% solids	2.4×10^{5}
20% solids	1.0×10^{6}
30% solids	1.5×10^{6}

[a]At room temperature.

length while under tension, l_s and its original length, l, which is equal to the length after the stress is released, expressed as a fraction of the original length, namely, $(l_s - l)/l$. Other modes of deformation are by bending or flexure, torsion, compression and shear.

For an ideal elastic solid, Hooke's law (Equation 1) states that the stress is directly proportional to the strain. This relationship is obeyed by real solids at moderate stresses and strains sustained for short periods of time. The *modulus of elasticity* or *Young's modulus, E,* is a measure of the stiffness, hardness, or resistance to elongation. There is also a modulus of shear or rigidity and a compression or bulk modulus. *Tensile compliance* is the reciprocal of Young's modulus, or the ratio of strain to stress.

In the CGS system, the units of stress are dynes/cm^2 or, since force = mass × acceleration, (g-cm/sec^2)/cm^2 = g/(cm sec^2). To convert dynes/cm^2 to the SI unit, Newton/m^2 or Pascal, divide by 10. Since strain is dimensionless, Young's modulus has the same dimensions as stress. Modulus values for a range of solids of pharmaceutical or biomedical interest are listed in Table 23-2.

Figure 23-3 shows representative stress-strain curves in tension, also called load-elongation curves. The cross-sectional area, A, of the solid becomes smaller as it is stretched. Therefore, to calculate the actual or true tensile stresses, the forces are divided by A_s, the cross-sectional area at each appropriate elongation. Stress-strain curves often are plotted with the strain or extension, the dependent variable, on the abscissa while consistency or flow curves (see below) usually are plotted with stress, the independent variable, on the abscissa. The practice followed here is to plot stress on the ordinate for both stress-strain and consistency curves, in order to make modulus and viscosity, respectively, the slopes of these curves.

The characteristic portions in the representative stress-strain curve *OLYAHB* in Figure 23-3 are as follows. Hooke's law of proportionality between stress and strain is obeyed throughout the linear portion *OL*. The elastic modulus of the solid is the slope of *OL* or the tangent of the angle *LOC*. The material behaves elastically up to the yield point *Y,* where the stress is called *yield stress*. When stresses below the yield stress are applied to the sample and then released, it stretches and contracts along the same curve *OLY*.

Beyond *Y,* the material behaves as a *plastic,* rather than as an elastic solid. Along the (nearly) horizontal portion *YAH,* the material is ductile; it flows or creeps under practically constant stress like a viscous liquid. If the stress is released at *A,* the sample retracts along *AC*. The nonrecoverable deformation *OC* is called *permanent set.* Many materials undergoing such "cold flow" are strengthened by some change in structure, causing an upturn *HB* in the stress-strain curve. This is called work (or strain) hardening. It may result from the elimination of flaws, from a reduction in crystal size as in the case of metals, or from reversible crystallization on stretching, as in the case of homo polymer elastomers.

At *B,* the sample ruptures; *R* is the elongation at the break or the ultimate elongation, and the stress corresponding to *B* is the ultimate strength or tensile strength. These values, as well as the load-elongation curve beyond *Y,* depend on the rate at which the sample is stretched.

The area *OLYAHBRCO* under the stress-strain curve is the energy or work required to break or rupture the material. It measures its toughness or brittleness. Glass is hard because of its high elastic modulus. Owing to the absence of a yield point and to a very low elongation to break, it is brittle as opposed to steel, which undergoes work hardening, has a high elongation to break, and is tough. Plastics are medium-hard or soft. Those that exhibit comparatively high elongations at break, like polyethylene but unlike polystyrene, are tough. Vulcanized rubbers are tough even though they are soft (low elastic modulus) because their elongation to break is very high, namely, 600–800%.

Newtonian Fluids

The viscosity of simple liquids, ie, pure liquids consisting of small molecules and solutions where solute and solvent are small molecules, depends only on composition, temperature, and pressure. It increases moderately with increasing pressure and markedly with decreasing temperature. For solutions of solid solutes, the viscosity usually increases with concentration. Simple liquids follow Newton's law (Equation 2) of direct proportionality between shear stress and rate of shear, so that their viscosity is independent of the shear stress or the rate of shear. Their flow behavior is thus referred to as *Newtonian*. Representative Newtonian viscosities are listed in Table 23-3.

Table 23-3. Newtonian Viscosities and Activation Energies for Viscous Flow[a]

MATERIAL	TEMPERATURE (°C)	VISCOSITY (POISE)	ACTIVATION ENERGY FOR VISCOUS FLOW (KCAL/MOLE)
Water	20	0.0100	4.2
	50	0.0055	3.4
	99	0.0028	2.8
Ethanol			
Absolute	20	0.0120	3.3
	50	0.0070	3.3
40% *w/w*	20	0.0291	6.8
	50	0.0113	5.3
Ethyl ether	20	0.0024	1.65
Glycerin			
Anhydrous	20	15.00	12.5
95% *w/w*	20	5.45	10.6

[a]At 1 atm pressure.

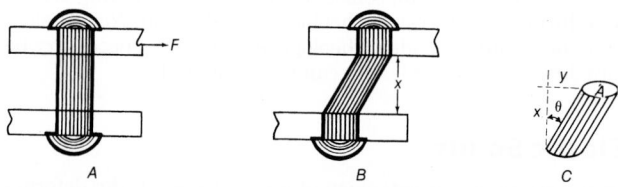

Figure 23-3. Stress-strain curves in tension. Loads or tensile stresses are corrected for actual cross-sectional areas.

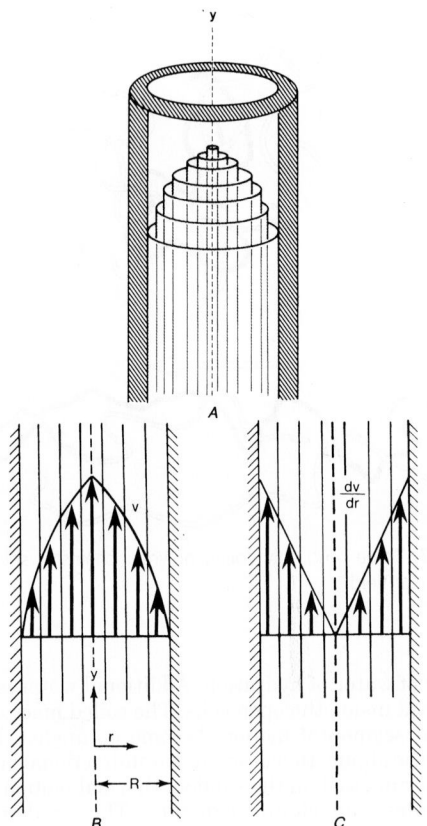

Figure 23-4. Laminar flow of a liquid through a cylindrical duct. **A.** Three-dimensional view of telescoping layers. **B.** Cross-section showing radial distribution of velocity. **C.** Cross-section showing radial distribution of velocity gradient.

Fluid flow through cylindrical pipes or capillaries is laminar, ie, Newtonian, at low velocities, for small tube radii, or for liquids of high viscosity. The liquid layers are very thin cylinders concentric with the duct[2]. During flow, they telescope past one another as shown in Figure 23-4A. The arrows in Figure 23-4B represent the velocity v of the individual cylindrical layers of radius r; v is maximal in the center of the tube and decreases in the radial direction, ie, in the direction r (previously x) perpendicular to the direction of flow y. The velocity is zero in the outermost liquid layer adjacent to and adhering to the wall, whose radius is equal to the inside radius of the tube R. In the center of the tube, where v is maximum, the velocity gradient $dv/dr = \dot{\gamma}$ is zero. This is shown in Figure 23-4C, where the arrows represent $\dot{\gamma}$ and the velocity gradient is maximum at the wall.

If V is the volume of liquid flowing through a cylindrical tube of radius R in time t, the volumetric flow rate is V/t, and the shear rate at the wall is

$$\dot{\gamma}_{\text{wall}} = \frac{4}{\pi R^3}\,(V/t) \qquad (4)$$

The shear stress is zero in the center of the tube and maximum at the wall:

$$\sigma_{\text{wall}} = \frac{R\Delta P}{2l} \qquad (5)$$

The liquid flows through the tube due to pressure, either caused by its own weight (hydrostatic) or produced by a pump. This pressure exceeds the innate viscous friction of the liquid and is converted into heat. The pressure drop, ΔP, along a length l of the tube is the difference between the pressure at the beginning and at the end of the tube.

As viscosity is shear stress divided by rate of shear, and as both vary in the x-direction perpendicular to the direction of

flow, both must be evaluated at the same location. Using the values at the wall of a cylindrical tube, dividing Equation 5 by Equation 4, and rearranging gives

$$\frac{V}{t} = \frac{R^4 \Delta P}{8 l \eta} \qquad (6)$$

This is Poiseuille's law, found experimentally by this French physician while studying the flow of liquids through capillary tubes representative of blood vessels. [The poise is also named in his honor.]

In the human body, the pumping action of the heart supplies the driving pressure for the flow of blood, which is the difference between the arterial and venous pressure. Digitalis glycosides increase the force of contraction of the heart muscle and make the heart a more efficient pump. This increases ΔP and, hence, the rate of flow of blood V/t. Vasodilator drugs like nitroglycerin or hydralazine hydrochloride increase the radius of blood vessels by relaxing the vascular smooth muscles. Since the flow rate varies with the fourth power of the radius of the blood vessel, a mere 5% increase in radius causes a 22% increase in the flow rate at constant blood pressure, because $(1.05)^4 = 1.22$.

Plots of shear stress (on the y-axis) as a function of the rate of shear (on the x-axis) are referred to as flow curves or rheograms. The rheograms of typical Newtonian liquids, like those of Figure 23-5, are straight lines going through the origin. Viscosity is the slope of such a line or the tangent of the angle it makes with the horizontal axis. Of the two liquids shown in Figure 23-5, A has a higher viscosity than B because $\alpha > \beta$, so that η_A $(= \tan \alpha) > \eta_B$ $(= \tan \beta$; $\eta_A = \sigma_2/\dot{\gamma}_2 = \sigma_1/\dot{\gamma}_1$ and $\eta_B = \sigma_1/\dot{\gamma}_3 = \sigma_3/\dot{\gamma}_2$. A given shear stress, σ_1, produces a greater rate of shear, $\dot{\gamma}_3$, in the more fluid Liquid B than $\dot{\gamma}_1$ in the more viscous Liquid A. Alternatively, to produce a given rate of shear, $\dot{\gamma}_2$, in the two liquids requires a higher shear stress, σ_2, for the more viscous Liquid A than σ_3 for the more fluid Liquid B.

In the CGS system, viscosity is defined as the tangential force per unit area, in dynes/cm^2, required to maintain a difference in velocity of 1 cm/s between two parallel layers of liquid 1 cm apart. Its unit is therefore dynes/cm^2-sec^{-1} or g/cm-s, which is called a *poise*. Because many common liquids including water have viscosities of the order of 1/100 of a poise, their viscosity is often expressed in *centipoise*. In the SI system, the unit of viscosity is Newton/m^2-s^{-1} or Pascal•s, which equals 10 poise. Typical Newtonian viscosities are listed in Table 23-3.

The variation of viscosity with temperature often is described by an *Arrhenius equation*:

$$\eta = Ae^{E_a/RT}$$
$$\text{or} \qquad\qquad (7)$$
$$\ln \eta = \ln A + \frac{E_a}{RT}$$

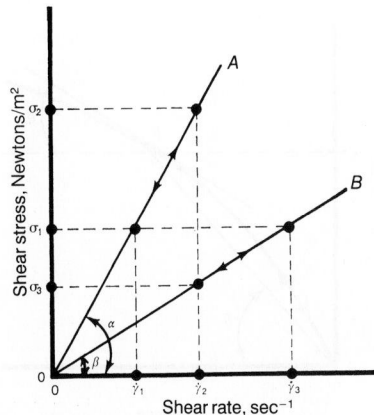

Figure 23-5. Rheograms or flow curves of two Newtonian liquids.

where A and E_a are constants, T is the absolute temperature and R is the molar gas constant. Values of E_a, the *activation energy* for viscous flow, are listed in Table 23-3. Large values of E_a indicate that the viscosity decreases substantially with rising temperature. According to Equation 7, plots of ln η as a function of the reciprocal of the absolute temperature should be straight lines with slopes of E_a / R. For associated, eg, hydrogen-bonded, liquids such plots are often somewhat curved.

According to Eyring's "*hole theory*," liquids contain vacancies or holes that are essential to flow. The activation energy is used largely to form these holes.[7] E_a is about 1/3 to 1/4 of the latent heat of vaporization for nonassociated liquids.

Non-Newtonian Fluids

Fluids that do not obey Newton's law (Equation 2) are described as *non-Newtonian fluids*. The rheological behavior of non-Newtonian fluids may be characterized either as time-*independent* or time-*dependent* non-Newtonian fluids.

TIME-INDEPENDENT NON-NEWTONIAN FLUIDS— *Shear-thinning fluids.* Many colloidal systems, especially polymer solutions and flocculated solid/liquid dispersions, become more fluid the faster they are stirred. This *shear-thinning* behavior is often referred to as *pseudoplasticity*, but the latter term is outdated and potentially misleading. Shear-thinning behavior is an example of non-Newtonian flow because the viscosity, at constant temperature and composition, is not constant as required by Newton's law of viscous flow (Equation 2), but decreases with increasing shear. As the increase in shear rate is greater than the increase in the corresponding shear stress, the flow curve of Figure 23-6 is concave toward the shear-rate axis.

There is an apparent viscosity for each value of shear rate or shear stress, which can be expressed in two different ways. At point P in Figure 23-6, the apparent viscosity can be taken as the slope of the secant to the flow curve at P, or tan θ, which is the viscosity of a Newtonian liquid whose flow curve passes through P. This is equal to the ratio $\sigma_P / \dot{\gamma}_p$. The second method defines the apparent viscosity as the slope of the tangent to the flow curve at P, ie, $d\sigma_P/d\dot{\gamma}_p = \tan \phi$. Since both θ and ϕ decrease with increasing shear stress or shear rate, so does the viscosity.

The shear-thinning behavior of polymer or macromolecule solutions arises from the alignment of neighboring macromolecules and the degree of their entanglement and concomitant immobilization of solvent. In aqueous solution, for example, the flexible, thread-like macromolecules are buffeted constantly by the surrounding water molecules in thermal agitation. This causes continuous random motion of chain segments by translation and by rotation around bonds between the atoms that make up the macromolecular backbone. These thermal fluctuations result in the formation of loose, roughly spherical coils that are permeated by water. The macromolecule chains are encased

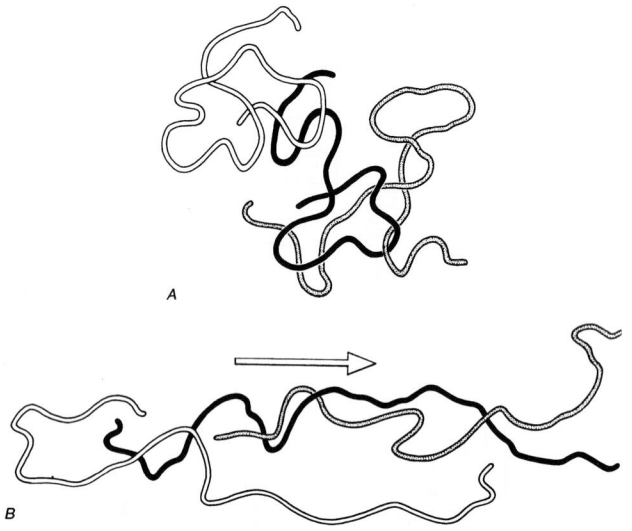

Figure 23-7. Three randomly coiled polymer chains in solution. **A.** At rest; **B.** In shear field.

in sheaths of water of hydration. Additional water is mechanically trapped inside the open coils. The coiled macromolecules, in constant segmental motion, become entangled (Figure 23-7A). Upon the application of shear, a unidirectional laminar motion is superimposed on the random thermal motion of the water molecules and chain segments. The randomly coiled, entangled macromolecules tend to disentangle themselves and to align themselves in the direction of flow, as shown in Figure 23-7B. The viscosity of the solution—its resistance to flow—depends on the size and shape of the flow units. The imposition of increasing shear in these systems enables the macromolecule "chains" to uncoil progressively and become streamlined or elongated, thereby offering less resistance to flow than the original, approximately spherical, shapes. At the same time, the amount of water trapped inside the coils and dragged along decreases. Furthermore, the chains become gradually more disentangled. Reduced entrapment of water and decreased entanglement of the macromolecules reduce the size of the flow unit, thereby reducing the viscosity. A further reduction in viscosity results from shear-induced uncoiling of the macromolecules. Thus, the apparent viscosity at a given rate of shear reflects the degree of randomization, coiling, entanglement, and alignment of the macromolecules, and the extent to which solvent molecules are associated with the macromolecules.

Dispersions of flocculated solid particles exhibit shear-thinning if the particle-particle bonds are too weak to withstand the applied shear stresses. Examples of weak interparticle bonds include weakly flocculated particles, in a secondary minimum, or electrostatically attracted lamellar clay platelets with positively charged edges and negatively charged faces that produce a "house-of-cards" structure in an aqueous suspension.

Shear progressively breaks up these aggregates at a rate that increases with increasing shear stress, releasing increasing amounts of trapped water. Brownian motion tends to rebuild the aggregates at a rate that is independent of shear. There is an average equilibrium size for the aggregates at each rate of shear that decreases with increasing shear, resulting in a decrease in the resistance to flow, or viscosity, as the shear increases.

At extremely low shear rates, well below 1 s^{-1}, the rate of disentanglement and alignment of polymer chains and the rate of breaking up of aggregates of particles under the influence of shear are negligible compared to the rate of entanglement and randomization of polymer chains and to the rate of aggregation of particles produced by Brownian motion, respectively. Hence, the flow units are neither noticeably deformed nor reduced in

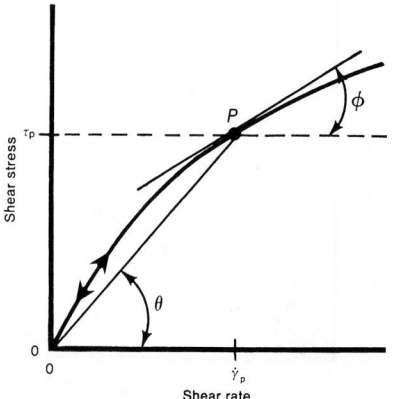

Figure 23-6. Flow curve of a shear-thinning liquid.

size by shear, and the systems exhibit Newtonian flow, with a constant and high viscosity designated as the *lower Newtonian* or *zero-shear viscosity,* η_0.

At very high shear rates, the dissolved polymer chains are wholly disentangled and well aligned in the direction of flow, and the aggregates of particles are broken up as far as possible. There is no residual structure left which can be broken up by further increments in shear rate: The viscosity levels off at a constant value called the *upper Newtonian viscosity,* η_∞. Turbulent flow and shear-induced rupture of polymer chains may set in before the upper Newtonian regime is reached. As can be seen in Figure 23-8, η_∞ is considerably lower than η_0. The value of the non-Newtonian viscosity observed at intermediate shear rates, including those encountered in most practical situations, depends on the amount of residual structure. It is, therefore, called *structural viscosity.*

Dilatancy—In contrast to shear-thinning, *shear-thickening* or *dilatancy*, ie an increase in viscosity with increasing shear, is rare. It is shown by concentrated dispersions of particles which do not tend to aggregate or stick together, provided the amount of liquid present is not much larger than that needed to fill the voids between the particles. Sediments of suspensions from which the supernatant liquid has been decanted are sometimes dilatant. When such a concentrated suspension is poured or stirred slowly, there is just enough liquid to lubricate the slipping of one particle past another, and the viscosity is low. When stirred fast, the particles get into each other's way, block each other and bunch up rather than slipping past each other. Large voids form between the unevenly clustered particles, and as the liquid seeps into these, the suspension appears dry—as if the suspended solids had expanded or become dilated. This phenomenon, which results in progressive viscosity increases, becomes more severe with increasing shear. When high shear is followed by low shear or rest, the particles that had been crowded together separate again, the interparticle void volume decreases, and the viscosity drops as the suspension appears wet again. Wet sand offers small resistance to slow flow or penetration, but stiffens and appears dry when deformed fast.

Among the few systems reported[8] to exhibit dilatant flow are suspensions of starch in water, aqueous glycerin or ethylene glycol containing about 40–50% *v/v* starch, and concentrated suspensions of inorganic pigments in water and in nonpolar liquids with enough surfactant added to deflocculate the disperse phase completely, eg, red iron oxide (12% *v/v* in water or 18% *v/v* in carbon tetrachloride), zinc oxide (30% *v/v* in water or 33% *v/v* in carbon tetrachloride), barium sulfate (39% *v/v* in water), and titanium dioxide (30–50% *v/v* in water).

Plasticity—Semisolids that do not flow at low shear stresses (exhibiting reversible deformation like elastic solids) but flow like liquids above their yield value (ie yield stress) are termed

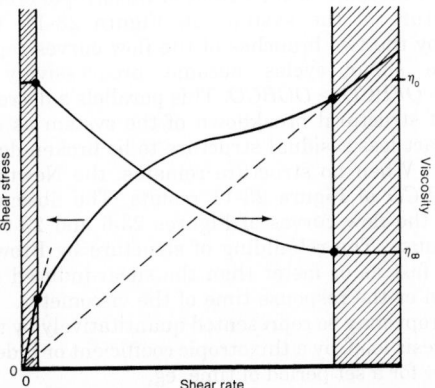

Figure 23-8. The three flow regions of a shear-thinning liquid. Shaded areas refer to lower (left) and upper (right) Newtonian regions; center area represent shear-thinning behavior.

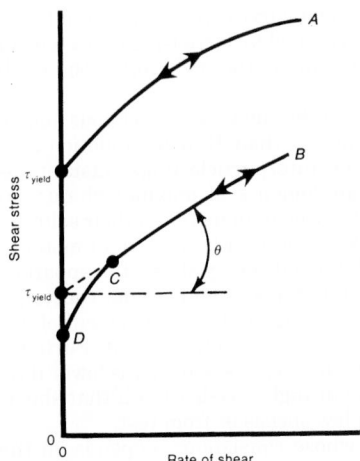

Figure 23-9. Flow curves of two plastic systems.

plastics or *Bingham bodies.* This type of rheological behavior is called *plasticity.* Plasticity is often exhibited by semisolids characterized as structured media, ie semisolids that have a *cross-linked* three-dimensional network of polymers, macromolecules, or particulates extending throughout the system.

Figure 23-9 shows the flow curves for two plastic systems. System *B* has a lower yield value than System *A* and Newtonian behavior at stresses above the yield value; $BC\sigma_{\text{yield}}$ is a straight line of inclination θ, so that the *plastic viscosity* of *B*, ie, its viscosity above the yield value, is the slope of this line or $\tan \theta$:

$$\eta_{\text{plastic}} = \frac{\sigma - \sigma_{\text{yield}}}{\dot{\gamma}}. \qquad (8)$$

This is equivalent to moving the origin of the flow curve from zero stress to the yield stress, and treating System *B* as a Newtonian liquid at stresses beyond. Semisolids with high yield values are described as "hard." When their plastic viscosity is high, they are described as "stiff."

Some Bingham bodies have flow curves that deviate from straight lines at stresses close to the yield stress, such as the portion *CD* in the flow curve of System *B*, where flow occurs even below the yield stress. This phenomenon is called *plug flow* because the material moves in chunks or as a plug rather than by laminar motion, often through slippage at the wall of the duct. In such cases, the yield value usually is obtained by extrapolating the linear portion *BC* to the stress axis.

System *A* is shear-thinning *above* its yield stress. This type of flow behavior is observed frequently with suspensions thickened with dissolved polymers, where the vehicle itself is shear-thinning.

TIME-DEPENDENT NON-NEWTONIAN FLUIDS—In the previous discussion, shear-thinning and plastic behavior was seen to arise from competition between the detachment of entanglement links among dissolved macromolecules or the rupturing of van der Waals links among dispersed particles by shear, and the reestablishment of such links by Brownian motion. The balance between breakdown and restoration of links shifts more and more toward breakdown as the shear increases. Reduction in interchain or interparticle links results in smaller flow units and lower apparent viscosity. It was assumed tacitly that the system adapts itself to changing shear "instantaneously," ie, so fast that by the time the instrumental conditions had been changed to higher or lower shear and readings then taken, the equilibrium between breakdown and restoration of links at the new shear already had been reached, producing flow units of the new average equilibrium size and the corresponding new apparent viscosity. Points representing pairs of $\dot{\gamma}$, σ values determined at increasing and at decreasing shear rates or shear stresses in Figures 23-5, 23-6, and 23-9 fall on the same single curves. It is immaterial whether a given shear rate was reached by increasing or decreasing the speed of the viscometer. This is the meaning of the double arrows on these curves.

Thixotropy—If the suspension is viscous and/or the particles are large and heavy, their Brownian motion is too slow to restore the broken interparticle links "instantaneously." Likewise, the entanglements of polymer chains are slow to be reestablished by Brownian motion if their solution is viscous. If the rate of link restoration by Brownian motion is lower than the rate of link breakdown by shear, the apparent viscosity decreases even while the system is under constant shear, as the size of the particle aggregates or the extent of macromolecular entanglement is progressively reduced. Furthermore, the apparent viscosity at a given shear rate is lower if the system was stirred recently at high speeds than if that shear rate was approached from low speeds or from rest.

Materials, whose consistency depends on the duration of shear as well as on the rate of shear, are said to be thixotropic or to exhibit *thixotropy*. Their apparent viscosity depends not only on temperature, composition, and rate of shear or shear stress, but on the previous shear history and time under shear.

The extreme behavior is an isothermal, reversible sol-gel transformation produced by rest and by shear, respectively. For example, an aqueous dispersion of 8% w/w sodium bentonite sets to a gel within an hour or two after preparation when undisturbed, but flows and can be poured within many minutes after it had been stirred above the yield value. After prolonged rest it reverts to a gel as the Brownian motion rebuilds the house-of-cards structure throughout the material.

Thixotropy in a shear-thinning liquid is shown in Figure 23-10. Starting with the system at rest (at the origin O) and gradually increasing the speed of the viscometer produces the "up" branch $ODAB$ of the flow curve. After the maximum shear rate $\dot{\gamma}_1$ and shear stress σ_3 corresponding to point B have been reached, the speed of the instrument is reduced. If there is not enough time for Brownian motion to regenerate completely, the structure torn down at the high speed, the liquid will be less viscous, and the "down" branch of the flow curve, $BCO,$ is lower than the "up" branch. Thus, the shear stress required to maintain the rate of shear $\dot{\gamma}_2$ has been reduced from σ_1 to σ_2, and the apparent viscosity has dropped from $\sigma_1/\dot{\gamma}_2$ to $\sigma_2/\dot{\gamma}_2$. This contrasts with the flow curve of Figure 23-6, where the "up" and "down" branches coincide.

When starting from rest, if the speed is not increased all the way up to $\dot{\gamma}_1$ but only to $\dot{\gamma}_2$ corresponding to point A in Figure 23-10 and then decreased, the "down" branch is AEO: Since the maximum speed is lower than previously, less struc-

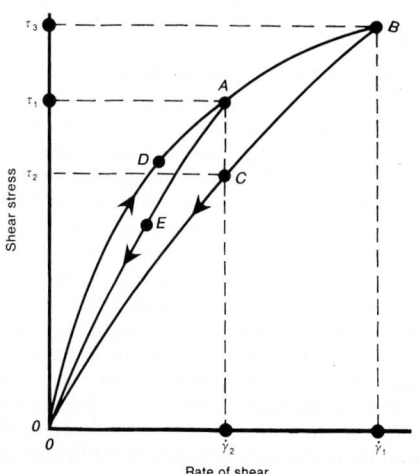

Figure 23-10. Flow curves of a shear thinning liquid exhibiting thixotropy.

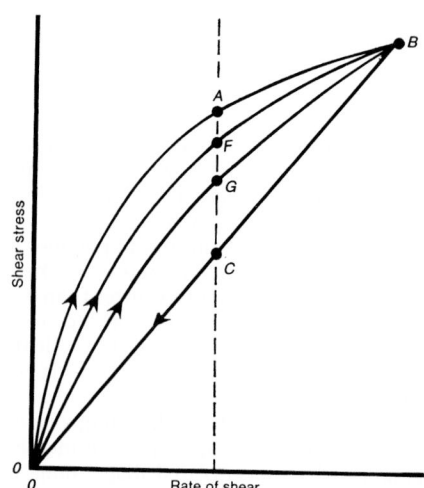

Figure 23-11. Flow curves representing successive shear cycles for a thixotropic, shear-thinning liquid.

ture is broken down and the apparent viscosity is not reduced by as much.

If the liquid in the instrument is kept at rest for a sufficient time period after it was subjected to the shear cycle *ODABCO*, Brownian motion rebuilds its structure, restoring its original high consistency. Starting from rest, the flow curve is again *ODABCO*. If no rest period is allowed and the shear cycle is repeated as soon as the "down" branch is completed, the next "up" branch is below *ODAB*, say, *OFB* in Figure 23-11. A third shear cycle following immediately after the second may give the "up" branch *OGB*. The "down" branch *BCO* may be curved as in Figure 23-10 or straight as in Figure 23-11. If the buildup of structure is very slow, there may be no structure left after the third shear cycle. In that case, the "up" branch coincides with the straight "down" branch *BCO* and the liquid has become Newtonian. This is only temporary because the flow curve reverts to *OABCO* of Figure 23-11 after a prolonged rest period.

Thixotropy frequently is superimposed on plastic flow behavior. The yield value may disappear after one or more shear cycles, as in curve C of Figure 23-12; it may be reduced as in curve B (sometimes called *false body* behavior), or it may remain unaltered as in curve A.

The difference between the *up* and *down* branches of a flow curve illustrates a common phenomenon called *hysteresis*. The area enclosed by the two branches (eg, areas *ODAEO* and *ODABCO* in Figure 23-10) or by the two branches and the stress axis (as in Figure 23-12 *B* and *C*) is called the *hysteresis loop*. Its size is a measure of the extent of thixotropic breakdown in the structure of the system. In Figure 23-11, the areas enclosed by the two branches of the flow curves representing successive shear cycles become progressively smaller: *OABCO > OFBCO > OGBCO*. This parallels a decrease in the amount of structural breakdown of the system as each cycle leaves intact less residual structure to be broken down in the next cycle. When no structure remains, the Newtonian flow curve *OCBCO* of Figure 23-11 results. The absence of hysteresis in the flow curves of Figures 23-6 and 23-9 is due to another cause: The rebuilding of structure by Brownian motion is as fast as or faster than the shear-induced structural breakdown or the response time of the viscometer.

Thixotropy may be represented quantitatively by the area of the hysteresis loop, by a thixotropic coefficient or index (*T.I.*) at a specific $\dot{\gamma}$ for a set period of time, eg,

$$TI = \frac{\sigma\,\big|_{\text{before shearing}}}{\sigma\,\big|_{\text{after shearing at }0.01\text{s}^{-1}}} \tag{9}$$

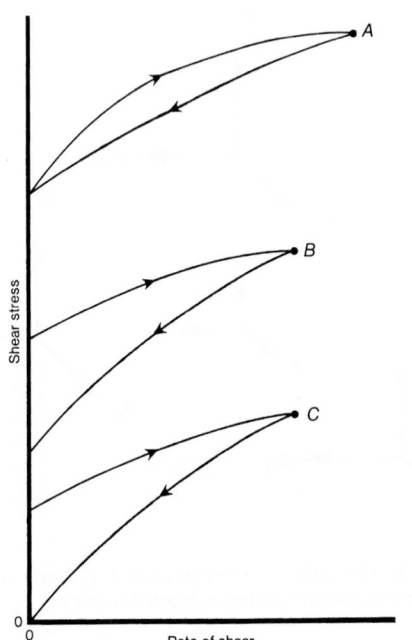

Figure 23-12. Flow curves of plastic systems exhibiting thixotropy (see text).

by shearing samples at various $\dot{\gamma}$ as a function of time and fitting all of the data to an equation of the form

$$\eta = A\dot{\gamma}^{B}t^{C} \qquad (10)$$

where *A* is a proportionality constant, and the exponents *B* and *C* are indices of shear-thinning and thixotropy, respectively. As B increases, the fluid becomes more shear-sensitive; as C increases, the fluid becomes more time-dependent.[9] A simple alternative method involves the measurement of the decay of shear stress or apparent viscosity as a function of time at a constant rate of shear. This method is illustrated in Figure 23-13. When a system is stirred at a constant shear rate, it eventually reaches constant or equilibrium values for shear stress and apparent viscosity. This is shown by the leveling off of the curve. Equilibration at a given shear rate may take half an hour or longer.

Thixotropy is particularly useful in the formulation of pharmaceutical suspensions and emulsions. These must be poured easily from containers, which implies low viscosity. Low viscosity, however, causes rapid settling of solid particles in suspensions and rapid creaming of emulsions. Solid particles that have settled out frequently stick together, producing a sediment difficult to redisperse ("caking" or "claying"). Creaming in emulsions is a first step towards coalescence. Thixotropy can be used to resolve this dilemma. A thixotropic agent such as sodium bentonite magma, other colloidal clays (magnesium bentonite, attapulgite), colloidal silicon dioxide, or microcrystalline cellulose is incorporated into the suspensions or emulsions to confer a high apparent viscosity or even a yield value. High viscosities retard sedimentation and creaming since, according to Stokes' law, the rate of sedimentation or creaming is inversely proportional to the viscosity of the medium. If the system possesses a yield value, sedimentation or creaming is prevented altogether since there is no flow below the yield stress, ie the apparent viscosity at low shear becomes infinite. When it is desired to pour some of the suspension or emulsion from its container, it is shaken well, at shear stresses considerably above the yield value. The agitation breaks down temporarily the thixotropic structure such as the house-of-cards scaffold of bentonite, reducing the yield value to zero and lowering the apparent viscosity. This makes for easy pouring. Back on the

shelf, the viscosity slowly increases again and the yield value is restored as Brownian motion rebuilds the house-of-cards structure of bentonite. This prevents sedimentation and caking of the suspended particles and creaming of the emulsion droplets; the disperse particles again become trapped in the plastic matrix. The optimum flow curve for such formulations is that of Figure 23-12*C*.

Rheopexy and Negative Thixotropy—Once the links among suspended particles or the entanglements among dissolved polymer chains have been broken by shear, their restoration by Brownian motion is slow if the suspensions or solutions are viscous. In such cases slow flow, gentle agitation, or moderate and rhythmic vibration may accelerate the rebuilding of the structure, ie, the restoration of the links between particles or macromolecules by Brownian motion. Low shear rates thus hasten the reappearance of high apparent viscosities or onset of gelation in thixotropic sols. In the case of sheared dispersions of bentonite, gentle vibration or rotation of the beaker speeds up the rebuilding of the house-of-cards structure. The material's recovery of some of its presheared viscosity at a faster rate when it is gently sheared, compared to when it is allowed to stand, is called *rheopexy*. Rheopexy is not to be confused with *negative thixotropy* (ie, anti-thixotropy), which is defined as a reversible time-dependent increase in viscosity at a particular shear rate as a result of shear-induced buildup of structure over time.

VISCOELASTICITY—Normal condensed matter is either solid or liquid. The molecules of an ideal solid are fixed in place while those of an ideal liquid are mobile. *Soft condensed matter* occupies a middle ground between the solid and liquid states as it typically possesses a structure that is on a substantially larger scale than atomic or molecular dimensions, ie the *mesoscopic* scale. [*Soft condensed matter*, *soft matter*, and *nanostructured systems* are, in effect, *colloids* or *colloidal dispersions* but the latter terms are being increasingly supplanted in the scientific literature by the former terms.] As a result, the *macroscopic* rheological behavior of soft condensed matter is determined by the structure and dynamics at the mesoscopic scale and is often described as *viscoelastic* in nature. When stressed, viscoelastic materials simultaneously exhibit some of the properties of elastic solids and some of the properties of viscous liquids: some deformation occurs instantaneously upon the application of stress and continues as long as the stress is applied. Upon removal of the stress, there is partial recovery of the original shape. In effect, viscoelastic systems are capable of storing part of the deformation energy elastically and reversibly. The relative proportions of elastic deformation and viscous flow are dependent upon the duration of time that stress is applied. In effect, the rheological characterization of viscoelastic materials depends, in part, on the experimental methodology employed. One useful parameter is the dimensionless *Deborah* number, N_{De}, defined by Reiner[10] as

$$N_{De} = \frac{\lambda}{t_{p}} \qquad (11)$$

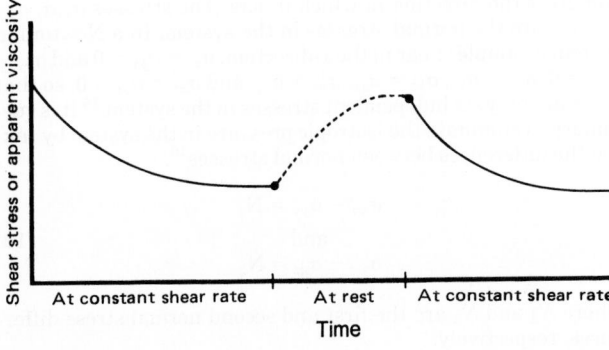

Figure 23-13. Time dependence of shear stress or of apparent viscosity of a thixotropic system.

where λ is the stress relaxation time (defined as the time required for the stress to decay to $1/e = 36.8\%$ of its initial value) and t_p is the process or observation time. When material is instantaneously deformed, the structure is perturbed as viscous flow occurs, and its microstructural elements, whether molecules or particles, are in a higher energy state. It takes some time for these molecules or particles to diffuse to a location where their energy state is equivalent to the pre-stress level.[11] The relaxation time for viscoelastic materials is of the same order of magnitude as the observation time ($N_{De} \approx 1$) while the relaxation time for a Newtonian fluid would be 0 (ie, relaxation time is instantaneous) and that for a Hookean solid would be ∞ (ie, no relaxation occurs). For nonideal materials, then, $N_{De} << 1$ are indicative of liquids and $N_{De} >> 1$, of solids.

Silicone putty (*Silly Putty*) is an example of a viscoelastic material. It has a comparatively short mean relaxation time (~ 1 s) at room temperature. It bounces, behaving like an elastic solid when the time of observation or of application of stress is short, but flows and shows little elasticity when slowly stretched. However, viscoelasticity is widespread even among liquids and plastic materials which seem to lack elasticity or stringiness to the touch, especially if they are tested at small deformations. Higher deformations or rates of shear approaching use conditions frequently rupture the elastic network in these materials, causing the loss of the elastic components of their rheological properties. For instance, fluid emulsions are often slightly viscoelastic at very low shear due to flocculation of the disperse droplets and interlinking of the flocs; they flow readily and lose all recovery properties under slightly higher shear.[12] Davis[13] determined the viscoelastic properties of oleaginous, emulsion, and absorption-type ointment bases by creep measurements. Radebaugh and Simonelli[14] evaluated the viscoelastic properties of powder-filled semisolids using starch dispersions in lanolin as their model. As gels, pastes, and polymer or macromolecule solutions often exhibit substantial viscoelasticity, this aspect of rheological behavior should not be ignored.

Unusual rheological phenomena associated with viscoelastic flow include the *Weissenberg effect*, in which fluid climbs up a shaft or impeller rotating in the fluid, and the *die swell effect*, wherein fluid exiting from a tube or capillary expands to two or more times the diameter of the tube. The Weissenberg effect is occasionally encountered in mixing operations while the die swell effect may be experienced during extrusion processes. Both phenomena result from the so-called *normal stress* effect in viscoelastic flow, ie the tendency of some viscoelastic fluids to flow in a direction normal to the direction of shear. Experimentally observable stresses normal to the direction of shear arise from fluid motion and the isotropic hydrostatic pressure in the system. In Newtonian fluids, the stresses generated by the flow act parallel to the direction of shear; Figure 23-14 presents a schematic view in x, y, and z coordinates of the stresses operating within a system subjected to shear.

The stresses in the system are denoted by σ_{xx}, σ_{xy}, σ_{xz}, σ_{yx}, σ_{yy}, σ_{yz}, σ_{zx}, σ_{zy}, and σ_{zz}, where the first subscript letter indicates the direction of the plane in which the shear stress lies and the second gives the direction in which it acts. The stresses $\sigma_{xx}\sigma$, σ_{yy}, and σ_{zz} are the normal stresses in the system. In a Newtonian system in simple shear in the x-direction, $\sigma_{xx} \sim \sigma_{yy} = 0$ and $\sigma_{yy} - \sigma_{zz} = 0$, $\sigma_{xy} = \sigma_{yx}$, $\sigma_{xz} = \sigma_{zx}$, $\sigma_{yz} = \sigma_{zy}$, and $\sigma_{xz} = \sigma_{yz} = 0$, so that there are only six independent stresses in the system.[15] It is customary to eliminate the isotropic pressure in the system by taking the differences between normal stresses[16]:

$$\sigma_{xx} - \sigma_{yy} = N_1$$
$$\text{and} \qquad (12)$$
$$\sigma_{yy} - \sigma_{zz} = N_2$$

where N_1 and N_2 are the first and second normal stress differences, respectively.

In effect, stresses normal to the direction of shear are different from those in the parallel direction. Fluids that exhibit no

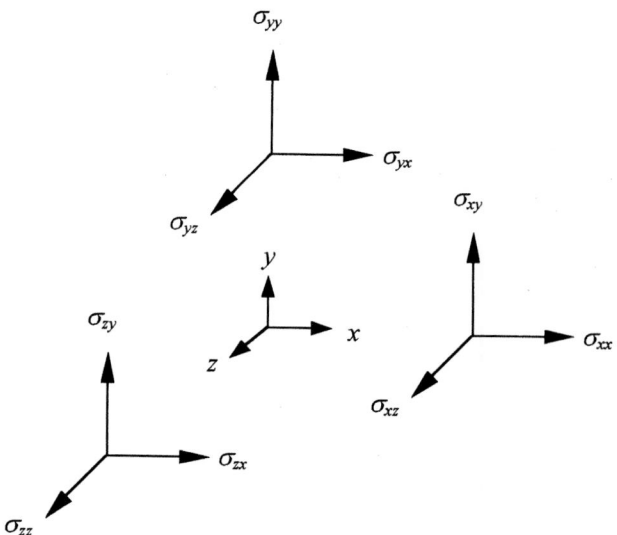

Figure 23-14. Schematic representation in x, y, and z coordinates of stresses operating within a system subjected to shear.

normal stress effects but only time-independent non-Newtonian viscous flow are sometimes characterized as *generalized Newtonian fluids*. However, when normal stress effects *are* evident, the fluids are viscoelastic in nature. Another indicator of viscoelasticity related to the Deborah number, N_{De}, is the dimensionless *Weissenberg* number, N_{Wi}, that characterizes the importance of elasticity in the flow by expressing the ratio of the first elastic normal stress difference to the shear stress:

$$N_{Wi} = \frac{N_1}{\sigma}. \qquad (13)$$

For Newtonian fluids, $N_{Wi} \equiv 0$; for viscoelastic fluids $N_{Wi} > 0$. In the course of addressing scale-up issues in biotechnology, Zlokarnik[17] has estimated N_{Wi} for various aqueous hydrocolloid solutions (carboxymethyl cellulose sodium, 1–2% w/v; xanthan gum, 0.05–0.2% w/v) used in cell culture studies; typical N_{Wi} values range from 1 to 10. In effect, the substantial viscoelastic nature of these systems must not be ignored if scale-up is to be successful.

In the realm of pharmaceutical solids, plasticity and viscoelasticity are observed during the course of tableting. This is not unexpected given the conditions of extreme stress used in the compaction of compressed tablets. The viscoelastic parameters of a number of drugs and excipients have been measured, under various conditions, during the stress-unloading phase of the tablet compaction cycle in a rotary tablet press.[18,19]

Rheological Models

LIQUIDS—Many liquids of pharmaceutical interest follow the empirical *power law* or *Ostwald-de Waele equation* over a wide range of shear rates, where

$$\dot{\gamma} = K\sigma^n$$
$$\text{or} \qquad (14)$$
$$\log \dot{\gamma} = \log K + n \log \sigma$$

In many references in the literature, the power law is given as $\sigma = k\dot{\gamma}^n$, so that values of $n > 1$ correspond to dilatant or shear thickening behavior and values of $n < 1$ to shear-thinning behavior. Of course, for Newtonian liquids $n = 1$.

For so-called *power-law liquids*, a plot of $\log \dot{\gamma}$ versus $\log \sigma$ yields a straight line of slope n. The power law equation has the advantage of representing flow behavior in terms of only two constants, K and n. On the other hand, it has the disadvantage of all power laws, namely, the dimensions of the intercept K

depend on the value of n, the specific shear rate at which K is evaluated, and the nature of the rheometer.[2]

For $n = 1$, $K = 1/\eta$, and Newton's law (Equation 2) results. Thus, the exponent, n, is an index of the deviation from Newtonian flow behavior. The more n differs from unity, the more non-Newtonian is the flow behavior, ie, the more substantial the viscosity decrease or increase with increasing shear. Among pharmaceutical liquids, the most commonly encountered deviants from time-independent Newtonian behavior are those described as *shear-thinning* fluids for which the power law exponent $n > 1$; less commonly encountered are *dilatant* fluids for which $n < 1$. Shear-thinning and dilatant liquids frequently follow this empirical *power law* or (Equation 8) over a wide range of shear rates.

OTHER EMPIRICAL EQUATIONS AND MODELS— Many empirical equations and models have been developed over the years in an effort to describe the flow behavior of non-Newtonian systems. One of the more successful relationships is the Herschel-Bulkley model,

$$\sigma = k\dot{\gamma}^n + \sigma_0 \qquad (15)$$

in which σ_0 is the yield stress and k is a consistency coefficient. For dilatant or shear thickening systems, $k > 0$, $1 < n < \infty$, and $\sigma_0 = 0$; for shear-thinning systems, $k > 0$, $0 < n < 1$, and $\sigma_0 = 0$; and, for Bingham plastics, $k > 0$, $n = 1$, and $\sigma_0 > 0$.

VISCOELASTIC MATERIALS— Viscoelastic behavior is often represented in terms of a mechanical model. Two of the basic elements used in such a model are a helical spring (which obeys Hooke's law and is characterized by a modulus E) and a dashpot (ie, a cylindrical container with a loosely fitting piston filled with a Newtonian liquid, characterized by its viscosity, η). When the deformation is in shear rather than in tension, Young's modulus E is replaced with the rigidity or shear modulus G. When a spring and a dashpot are connected in series, they form a Maxwell element (Figure 23-15A); when they are connected in parallel, they form a Voigt-Kelvin element (Figure 23-15B). Several Maxwell and/or Voigt-Kelvin elements can be combined in parallel and/or in series to represent the complex viscoelastic behavior of solutions and semisolids. A simple combination is Burgers' model, which consists of a Maxwell and a Voigt-Kelvin element in series (Figure 23-15C) and is characterized by two elastic moduli and two viscosities.

When a constant load or stress, σ_0, is applied to a Maxwell element, the elastic spring extends immediately to the recoverable strain or elongation, $\gamma_{el} = OA = \sigma_0/E$ (Figure 23-16A). The

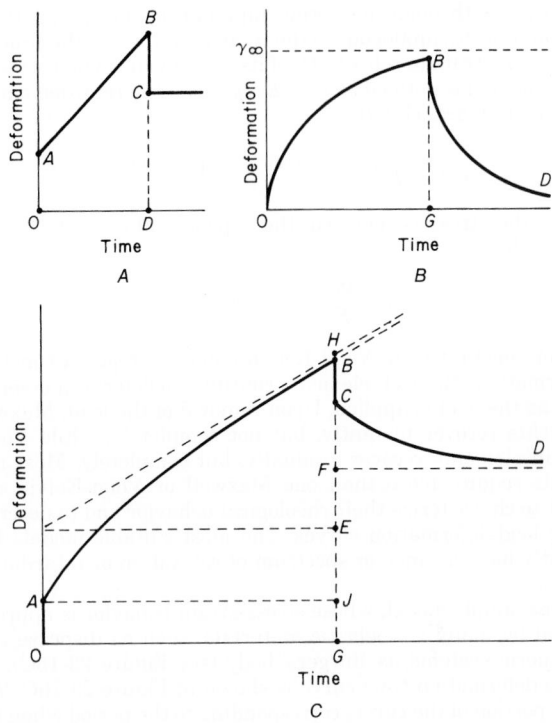

Figure 23-16. Deformation of three rheological models at constant applied stress. **A.** Maxwell element. **B.** Voigt-Kelvin element. **C.** Burgers' body.

piston in the dashpot pulls upwards gradually; this permanent deformation, γ_{vis}, is directly proportional to time, t. The two deformations are additive: $\gamma = \gamma_{el} + \gamma_{vis}$. At time D, $\gamma = BD = BC + CD = OA + CD$. When the stress is removed at time D (Point B), the spring retracts immediately and fully, and the specimen contracts from B to C by a length, $\gamma_{el} = BC = OA$. The permanent or nonrecoverable deformation, or creep, is $\gamma_{vis} = CD = \sigma_0 t/\eta$.

In plots like those of Figure 23-16, compliance (ie, strain per unit stress) often is used instead of strain. Compliance (eg, shear or tensile) is the reciprocal of modulus.

If the Maxwell element is stretched to a given deformation, γ_0, the stress required to maintain this deformation constant decreases gradually. As the piston of the dashpot is pulled gradually upwards and the dashpot extended, it increasingly relieves the stress on the spring, which gradually contracts. After a long time, as $\gamma \rightarrow \gamma_{vis}$, $\sigma \rightarrow 0$.

If the initial stress is σ_0 and the stress at time, t, is σ, the stress relaxation is

$$\sigma = \sigma_0 e^{-(Et/\eta)} = \sigma_0 e^{(-t/\theta)} \qquad (16)$$

The exponent Et/η is dimensionless and the ratio $\theta = \eta/E$, which has the dimension of time, is the relaxation time.

When a constant stress σ_0 is applied to a Voigt-Kelvin element (Figure 23-16B), the spring can stretch only as fast as the slow extension of the viscous dashpot permits. The greater the viscosity of the liquid in the dashpot, the greater is this retardation. The stress is shared by spring and dashpot, ie, $\sigma_0 = E\gamma + \eta\dot{\gamma}$. As σ_0 stretches the spring-dashpot assembly, the retarded elastic deformation of the specimen increases with time until, at $t = \infty$, the spring reaches the full extension corresponding to the applied stress: $\gamma_\infty = \sigma_0/E$. No additional deformation then takes place. When the stress is removed at time G, the specimen retracts fully to its original shape where $\gamma = 0$, because of the elasticity of the spring, but the motion is damped along the exponential curve BD, which is the mirror image of OB, because the plunger is pulled back only slowly to its origi-

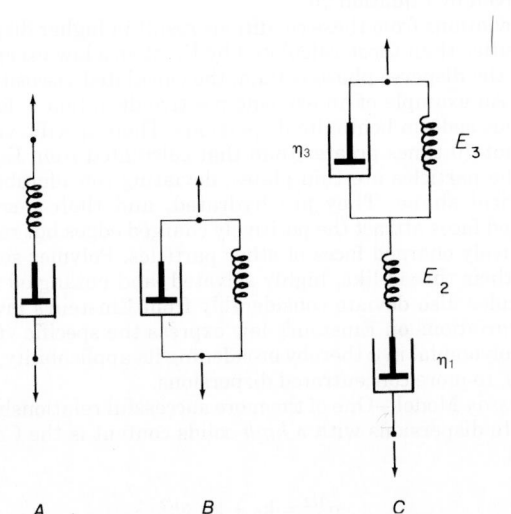

Figure 23-15. Elements of mechanical models for viscoelastic behavior. **A.** Maxwell element. **B.** Voigt-Kelvin element. **C.** Burgers' model. Arrows show applied force or load.

nal position through the viscous liquid in the dashpot. A retardation time, θ_d, analogous to the relaxation time, is the time required for strain to relax to $1/e$ of its initial value when stress is removed and is defined as $\theta_d = E/\eta$. Along the retarded elastic deformation branch OB

$$\gamma = \frac{\sigma_0}{E}(1 - e^{-t/\theta_d}) = \gamma_\infty(1 - e^{-t/\theta_d}) \tag{17}$$

When the stress is removed, the exponential curve CD is described by

$$\gamma = \frac{\sigma_0}{E} e^{-t/\theta_d} = \gamma_\infty e^{-t/\theta_d} \tag{18}$$

Under constant load, Voigt-Kelvin elements reach a constant deformation; Maxwell elements continue to deform in creep as long as the load is applied. Upon removal of the load, Maxwell elements recover instantly, but not completely, while Voigt-Kelvin elements recover gradually, but completely. Most materials require more than one Maxwell or Voigt-Kelvin element to characterize their rheological behavior and to describe their load-deformation curves. The most suitable models frequently have a range or spectrum of relaxation or retardation times.

One simple model, whose stress-strain behavior is approximated by many viscoelastic materials, such as disperse and polymeric systems, is Burgers' body (see Figure 23-15C). Its creep deformation-time curve is shown in Figure 23-16C. The OAB portion of the curve, corresponding to the period when the model is under a constant stress, σ_0, consists of two segments. When the load is applied, *spring* 2 stretches instantly and the specimen is elongated from O to A. On a molecular level, this corresponds to the elastic stretching of bonds between primary structural units, such as primary particles aggregated into flocs or crystallites in a semicrystalline polymer above its glass transition temperature. If the stress is removed at A, the specimen would recover its original structure completely.

The second segment, AB, results from the combination of the recoverable deformation of *spring* 3, retarded by *dashpot* 3 which is connected in parallel, and the non-recoverable creep of *dashpot* 1. The recoverable deformation predominates in the initial, strongly curved region of AB. In this region, interparticle bonds break and reform. The remainder of AB, which approaches a straight line, represents mainly the creep of *dashpot* 1. Here, some of the bonds that break are too slow to reform within the test period. The rupture of such interparticle bonds releases some structural units, which flow past one another to produce the permanent deformation.

At time G, the overall deformation is the sum of the instantaneous deformation of *spring* 2 (BC or AO or JG), of *spring* 3 damped by *dashpot* 3 (CF) and of *dashpot* 1 (HE). The first two deformations are completely recoverable; the third is not recovered at all.

$$\gamma = BG = JG + EJ + BE = \frac{\sigma_0}{E_2} + \frac{\sigma_0}{E_3}(1 - e^{-t/\theta_d}) + \frac{\sigma_0}{\eta_1}t \tag{19}$$

where the retardation time $\theta_d = \eta_3/E_3$.

The recovery, BCD, follows a pattern similar to the deformation. When the stress is removed at time G, *spring* 2 retracts instantly and the specimen contracts along $BC = OA$. The retraction of *spring* 3 is retarded by *dashpot* 3 along CD. The nonrecoverable part of the deformation, due to *dashpot* 1, is represented by $FG = HE$.

DISPERSE SYSTEMS—Many pharmaceutical preparations are dispersions of solids or liquids in liquid or semisolid vehicles, and their usefulness often depends on their flow properties. Few disperse systems are Newtonian. Most exhibit non-Newtonian flow behavior, some of it time-dependent, often in conjunction with elastic deformation.

Einstein's Law of Viscosity—This is the simplest equation derived to describe the flow behavior of dispersions. Unfortunately, it applies only to Newtonian and idealized systems.

$$\eta_{sp} = \frac{\eta_{12}}{\eta_1} - 1 = \frac{\eta_{12} - \eta_1}{\eta_1} = 2.5\phi \tag{20}$$

The Newtonian viscosities η_{12} and η_1 are those of the dispersion and of the liquid vehicle or solvent, respectively; η_{sp} represents the specific viscosity of the dispersion, ie, the increase in viscosity of the dispersion over that of the solvent, expressed as a multiple of the viscosity of the solvent; ϕ is the volume fraction of the disperse phase [Blood contains 45% v/v of red and 1% v/v of white cells; the corresponding ϕ values are 0.45 and 0.01.] The viscosity of a dispersion obeying Einstein's law depends only on the viscosity of the solvent and on the volume of solvent replaced by the disperse phase, not on the size of its particles.

Assumptions operative in Einstein's law of viscosity include negligible gravitational and inertial effects and the absence of turbulence. Particles of the dispersion are large compared to the solvent molecules (ie, the discontinuities between the solvent molecules are negligible compared to the size of the dispersed particles) but small compared to the dimensions of the viscometer (eg, gap between the coaxial cylinders or diameter of the capillary). The particles of the dispersion neither attract nor repel one another. [In reality, as most dispersions consist of particles of like charge, the viscosity of such dispersions increases due to interparticle electrostatic repulsion (the *electroviscous effect*). In aqueous dispersions, viscosity increases can be minimized by adding electrolytes.]

In addition, Einstein's law assumes that the solvent is continuous and that the particles are unsolvated, smooth, and rigid spheres (eg, glass beads, polymer latex particles, and many spores and fungi). However, emulsion droplets are deformable and the liquid inside them can circulate. This decreases the distortion of the flow pattern around the droplets and reduces the numerical constant in Equation 20 *below* 2.5. Rigid anisometric particles offer increased resistance to flow, raising the constant *above* 2.5. If the solvation layer of solvated spherical particles is included in ϕ, their dispersions may obey Equation 20. Examples of the latter are solutions of globular proteins at their isoelectric point, where their net electric charge is zero.

Furthermore, the "ideal" dispersions addressed by Einstein's law are considered to be so dilute that the distortion of the laminar streamlines of the solvent at the surface of one particle does not overlap and reinforce the distortions around its neighbors. However, at higher disperse phase concentrations, the perturbation of laminar flow produced by one particle reaches into the fields of other particles. This produces additional resistance to flow and increases η_{sp} and η_{12} above the values given by Equation 20.

Deviations from these conditions result in higher dispersion viscosities than those calculated by Einstein's law except that, when the disperse phase is fluid, the calculated viscosity is too high. An example of an extreme positive deviation is found in aqueous sodium bentonite dispersions. Their specific viscosity is about 70 times greater than that calculated from Equation 20. The particles are thin plates, deviating considerably from spherical shape. They are hydrated, and their negatively charged faces attract the positively charged edges but repel the negatively charged faces of other particles. Polymer solutions with their thread-like, highly solvated, and entangled macromolecules also deviate considerably from Einstein's law. Several variations on Einstein's law express the specific viscosity as a polynomial in ϕ thereby broadening its applicability, for example, to more concentrated dispersions.

Casson Model—One of the more successful relationships applied to dispersions with a *high* solids content is the Casson[20] model,

$$\sigma^{1/2} = k_0 + k_1 \dot{\gamma}^{1/2} \quad, \tag{21}$$

where k_0 and k_1 are constants which depend on the properties of the dispersion medium and the disperse phase. Although the

Casson equation has been used empirically in modeling the rheological properties of a wide range of concentrated dispersions, it was originally derived from basic principles with the assumption that the disperse phase behaved as rigid rods.

Computational Rheology

Empirical relationships aside, numerical methods for the characterization of non-Newtonian flow were developed in the 1960s, but it is only relatively recently that computational rheology has emerged to address previously intractable problems such as three-dimensional transient flows of polymeric liquids, non-isothermal non-Newtonian flows, or turbulent flow of generalized Newtonian and viscoelastic materials.[21] Computer software, in consort with modern rheometer design, has also facilitated the development of more complex models of deformation and flow under flow regimes ranging from the laminar to the turbulent, even encompassing the transitional flow regime in which flow is neither completely laminar or completely turbulent. In all likelihood, the net effect of these advances is to demystify rheological principles and allow the *a priori* estimation of the mechanical properties of the living and nonliving systems with which we contend.

BIORHEOLOGY

Biorheology is the study of deformation and flow in biological systems. Biological fluids are generally both elastic and viscous. Hence they are viscoelastic materials. Biological fluids are rheologically complex due to their multicomponent nature. The altering effects of disease compound the complexity of evaluating the rheology of physiological fluids. Several journals cover issues related to rheological characterization of biological fluids and tissues and the effect of disease and drugs on these properties. These include *Biorheology*, *Journal of Biomechanics*, and *Clinical Hemorheology and Microcirculation*. It is important to understand the rheological properties of biological materials for a greater understanding of their implications in both the healthy and diseased state. Rheological parameters of biological materials are also important in successful drug delivery to the body.

Hemorheology

The main function of blood is to act as a transport medium. It transports almost everything that is essential for the various organs of the body. Blood is composed of solid particles (red cells, white cells, and platelets) suspended in a fluid medium (plasma).[22] Early investigators conceptualized blood as a viscous fluid, assuming that the viscosity controls its flow properties.[23] However, blood is not a fluid in the ordinary sense; it is a fluidized suspension of elastic cells, which characterizes its rheological behavior. Blood is a non–Newtonian fluid with viscoelastic properties. At low shear rates, blood viscosity is higher because of the tendency of erythrocytes to aggregate. At high shear rates, which are typical for the arterial side and capillaries, blood viscosity is lower and constant because of erythrocyte deformation.[22,24,25] Comprehensive studies show that the shear dependence of the viscosity of blood may be attributed exclusively to the formation or disintegration of erythrocyte aggregation. The formation of aggregates is reversible and increases at decreasing shear rates.[26–28] The Casson equation has been suggested to describe mathematically the flow curve of blood.[28] In the circulation, the rheological behavior of blood is determined by the interactions of the erythrocyte cells with the vessel walls.[22,29] When blood is allowed to flow through capillary tubes of decreasing caliber, a second non-Newtonian characteristic is observed. Below a critical vessel caliber of 1mm, blood viscosity becomes dependent upon vessel radius. Viscosity drastically decreases when the vessel caliber is approximately

$12-15\mu m$. This phenomenon is known as the *Fahraeus-Lindqvist* or *Sigma Effect*.[29,30] Three possible contributory causes are:

1. The hematocrit value is lower for blood in capillaries. For instance, blood flowing through a capillary of $50\mu m$ diameter has only 70% of the red blood cells of blood flowing through large vessels.

2. Red blood cells are biconcave discs with an average diameter (d) of $7.5\mu m$. Their size is by no means negligible compared to the radius (R) of capillaries. This leads to a reduction in the apparent viscosity by a factor of $(1+d/R^2)$ according to the so-called *Sigma Effect*.[31]

3. The tubular pinch effect consists of an accumulation of red cells in an annular region located at a distance of about 60% of the tube radius from the tube axis during laminar flow of blood through cylindrical capillaries. Almost colorless plasma flows in the vicinity of the capillary wall. Blood flowing in the center of the tube is also deficient in red cells. This phenomenon commonly is observed when suspensions of spherical or asymmetric particles flow through ducts whose diameter is only a low multiple of the particle size.[31]

In the diameter range between $30\mu m$ and $300\mu m$ the effective blood viscosity can be predicted using the hematocrit reduction resulting from the *Fahraeus* effect.[29] The apparent viscosity can be determined in macro-viscometers.[29]

The flow properties of blood are determined by the hematocrit (Hct) value, plasma viscosity, red cell aggregation, and deformability.[22,29] The studies of blood viscosity factors present an important mechanism to better understand the pathways of cardiovascular disorders. It also allows utilization of blood viscosity tests in diagnostics, prognostic, and preventive medicine.[26] Elevated Hct levels have been associated with adverse cardiovascular outcomes including arteriosclerosis, coronary heart disease (CHD), angina pectoris, myocardial infarction, and CHD incidence.[32–34] Individuals who exercise regularly have been found to have reduced blood and plasma viscosity compared with nonexercisers.[33] On the other hand, after heavy exercise or during severe asthma attacks, serum mean lactate levels increase. In high concentrations, lactic acidosis produces erythrocyte swelling, increasing the Hct level and increasing whole-blood viscosity at high and low shear rates.[24]

Artificial Blood Substitutes (ABS) offer an alternative to blood transfusion. They have the ability to replace temporally the volume expansion and oxygen transport functions of transfused blood.[35–40] In the normal circulation system, vascular receptors have been calibrated to respond to a determined pressure and shear force exerted by normal blood. When ABS are introduced, new biorheological properties of the blood mixture can occur. Depending on the flow properties of the specific ABS, peripheral resistance of the circulatory system, and vascular receptor responses might be altered.[35] ABS can be divided in 3 classes: hemoglobin based products, perflurocarbon based products, and volume plasma expanders. Hemoglobin-based products include conjugates of hemoglobin with larger molecules (dextran or polyethyleneglycol), intramolecular cross-linked hemoglobins, polymerized hemoglobins, and liposome encapsulated hemoglobin.[37] Perfluorocarbon-based products have the ability to dissolve significant quantities of oxygen. Perfluorochemicals are immiscible with water, consequently must be emulsified before introduction to the bloodstream.[35–37] Due to the small size of the emulsion particles ($<0.2\mu m$ diameter), perfluorocarbon emulsions have the ability to perfuse into smaller capillaries where red blood cells are normally unable to perfuse due to their size limitation.[38] A study of a perfluorocarbon emulsions has shown that they exhibit non-Newtonian behavior.[35] Plasma expander products are non-oxygen carriers. Their purpose is to expand the blood volume after significant blood loss. The most common gelling agents used in these products are gelatin and starch. These products are viscous in nature. Rheological behavior studies of red blood cells when in contact with various polymeric plasma expanders are ongoing[36]

Lymph

The lymphatic system drains most regions of the body. Lymph is a clear to white viscous fluid. The chemical composition of lymph is very similar to that of plasma. Generally the composition of lymph differs from plasma in the concentration of its constituents. Lymph component concentration varies as a function of body region. The major components of lymph include proteins, enzymes, lipids, electrolytes, nonelectrolytes, iron and transferrin, and coagulation factors. A large number of white blood cells are present in the lymphatic fluid. The rheological properties of lymph are more complex than those of plasma. Very little information is available with regard to the rheological properties of lymph.

Mucus

Mucus is a weak viscoelastic gel.[41] It is a translucent or opaque, gel-like, stringy, slimy secretion. A mucus covering lines all the internal tracts of the body, the respiratory tract (nose, trachea, bronchi, and bronchioles), gastrointestinal tract, and female reproductive tract. It both lubricates and protects mucosal surfaces. More than 95% of mucus is water. The other components of mucus include glycoproteins or mucins (0.5–5%), inorganic salts (1%), proteins (0.5–1%), lipids, and mucopolysaccharides.[42] The primary component of mucus, the glycoproteins, are responsible for its gelling properties. The glycoproteins within mucus covalently bind to each other through disulfide bonds. Mucus secretions that reside in different locations of the body vary with respect to their rheological properties. This variability is required such that the physiological functions of the mucus secretions can be met. The rheological properties of mucus are a function of anatomical location, and the physiological and pathological state.[43] The rheology of mucus can be affected by ion content, hydration state, and pH.

The viscosity and elasticity of mucus can be altered using mucus thinning or mucus thickening agents. Di and Trivalent cations can thicken mucus in a concentration dependent manner. Reduction of mucus viscoelasticity by mucolytic agents which split mucus glycoproteins into smaller subunits such as N-acetylcysteine, dithiothretol, bromhexine, and erdosteine has been reported.[43] Acetylcysteine is one of the sulfhydryl mucolytics that disrupt disulfide bonds in mucus.[50,51] Changes in rheological properties can also be induced by other drug substances.

EYE—Mucus is primarily produced by goblet cells in the conjunctiva. The mucus is secreted onto the surface of the conjunctiva and the upper lid distributes the mucus in a thin film over the surface of the cornea.[44] The tear film is essential to provide a perfect optical surface for the eye. It is consisted of three distinct layers:

1. Mucus layer: present on top of the epithelial cells of the cornea. It is 10 to 100 times more viscous than the aqueous layer.[45]
2. Aqueous layer: present above the mucus layer. The lacrimal glands supply it.
3. Lipid or fatty layer: that covers the aqueous layer.[46]

The whole tear fluid is considered a non-Newtonian fluid, which means that the viscosity depends on the shear rate. The greater the shear rate, the lower the viscosity. The rationale of this is that the viscosity must be high enough to allow the tear film to maintain a continuous layer, covering the exposed area of the ocular surface.[47]

The *vitreous humor* is a clear gel, which occupies the posterior compartment of the eye, located between the *crystalline lens* and the *retina* and occupying about 80% of the volume of the eyeball. Normally, it is of a very consistent thickness, or viscosity, and is crystal clear. With age, the vitreous humor changes from a gel to a liquid. As it does so, the vitreous mass gradually shrinks and collapses, separating and falling away from the *retina*.[48] Certain pathological conditions result in changes in the viscosity of intraocular fluids.

MOUTH, NOSE, AND RESPIRATORY TRACT—

Mouth—Saliva is an exocrine secretion composed of water, bicarbonate, enzymes and mucoproteins.[25] It is produced predominantly by the salivary glands which include the parotid, submandibular, and sublingual glands. It is viscoelastic in nature. The viscosity of secretions from the parotid gland is less than the viscosity of secretions produced by the submadibular and sublingual glands. This is due to the lack of mucin in these secretions. Sublingual gland secretions contain a large amount of mucus making them very thick and viscous. In an adult the total amount of saliva produced daily is 500 to 1500 ml.[49]

Nose—Nasal secretions consist of a combination of glycoproteins, lipids, DNA, and ions in 95% water.[50] It is produced at a resting rate of 0.5 to 1mL of mucus/cm^2 mucosa over a period of 24h.[50] Mucins, a high molecular weight glycoproteins present in the nasal mucus, contain a large amount of sugar residues.[50] Due to this large amount of sugar and consequent polymerization of disulfide bonds, it is thought that mucins have a considerable influence on the rheological properties of mucus.[50–52]

Nasal mucus is thought to consist of a biphasic layer, which is a superficial gel layer that contains most of the glycoproteins overlying an aqueous layer in contact with cilia. Mucociliary transport depends on both ciliary activity and the rheological properties of nasal mucus. The nasal mucus traps and transports airbone particles and endogenous products.[50,52]

The mucus layer behaves as a non-Newtonian viscoelastic fluid. Studies have shown that the correlation between the mucociliary transport rate and the elastic modulus/dynamics viscosity change below and above the optimal viscoelasticity (close to 15 Pa/s).[50] Several methods have been developed to measure mucus viscosity including capillary viscometer (the simplest one),[53] coaxial cylinder sensor system,[54] magnetic microrheometer,[55] and controlled stress technique.[50]

Diseases and presence of drugs may alter the rheological properties of mucus. In chronic inflammation, there is a hypertrophy of the submucosal glands and an increase in the goblet cells, which results in an increase in the volume of mucus.[50] In chronic sinusitis, there is an increase in the submucosal cells, but the number of goblets cells are not significantly increased. In this case, the dynamic viscosity of the mucus was found to be 1.6 Pa/s.[50,52]

Respiratory Tract—The mucus present on the respiratory epithelium is produced by surface cells and submucosal glands. The various constituents of bronchial mucus provide a surface protective membrane. It is considered a membrane that moves. Bronchial mucus consists mainly of lipids and glycoconjugates.[56] Samples are generally difficult to analyze because are mixed with saliva and are not homogeneous. Consequently, the precise composition of bronchial mucus is not well elucidated.[56,57]

Sputum is defined as secretions from the lungs, bronchi, and trachea. Bronchial mucus samples can be collected from sputum or aspirated from fiberoptic bronchoscopy.[56] Sputum exhibits non-Newtonian rheological behavior.[57] The viscosity of sputum is influenced by the state of body hydration. Sputum produced overnight is more viscous than that produced during the day.[57]

Bronchial mucus has been shown to be shear thinning[57] Increases in bronchial mucus viscosity result in breathing difficulty. In chronic hypersecretory lung diseases, viscosity of bronchial mucus is increased. For example, lung epithelial mucus has increased viscosity in cystic fibrosis patients.[58] Patients with cystic fibrosis have a decrease in mucus water content and an increase in the DNA and total phospholipid content of mucus resulting in increase in viscosity and changes in the viscoelastic properties of the mucus.[50,54] In these cases, physiotherapies to change viscoelastic properties and improve mucus clearance have been used.[60–62]

The lung-lining layer is composed principally of phospholipids, the most prevalent being dipalmitoyl-phosphatidylcoline. This surfactant layer forms a film and spreads through the alveolar surface.[25] Evidences suggested that this lining material is continually replenished.[25] However, the rheological properties of this fluid have not been established.[63]

GASTROINTESTINAL TRACT—A water insoluble gel layer covers the mucosal surfaces of the stomach, duodenum, and colon. Gastric mucus is a non-Newtonian substance. Mucus secretions in the gastrointestinal tract have a viscoelastic gel structure. This gel structure is of a three-dimensional arrangement comprised of both entanglement and covalent and noncovalent association of mucin. The viscosity of this mucus is affected by pH. It has been shown that the viscosity of mucus in the stomach is greater at pH 2 than that at pH 7 with a maximum in viscosity being observed at pH 3–4.[64,65] In addition the viscoelastic properties can be modified by the presence of albumin which increases the viscosity of the gel.[66] Given that this mucus is viscoelastic in nature the stress contains both a storage modulus (G')(elastic component) as well as a loss modulus (G")(viscous component). Mucus gels from the stomach have been shown to have a storage modulus value which is greater than that of the loss modulus.[67] Tan δ values (the ratio of the loss modulus to the storage modulus) obtained for gastric mucus were found to be less than 0.4, characteristic of a viscoelastic gel.[67] The mucus in the gastrointestinal tract responds to pathological and physiological changes. Various drug molecules, stresses, and disease states can result in alterations in gastric mucus visocisty. The ulcerative processes that can occur in the stomach are a result of the weakening of the normal gastric mucosal barrier.

REPRODUCTIVE TRACT SECRETIONS—*Vaginal Fluid*—Vaginal fluid is made up of a vaginal transudate, secretions from Bartholin's and Skene's glands, exfoliated epithelial cells, residual urine, and fluids from the upper reproductive tract such as cervical mucus and fluid from the uterus and endometrial tubes.[68]

Cervical Mucus—The components of cervical mucus are mucus glycoproteins, plasma proteins, other proteins (eg, lactoferrin), enzymes, amino acids, cholesterol, lipids, and a range of inorganic ions.[69] Cervical mucus exhibits non-Newtonian viscosity and is a viscoelastic, highly hydrated substance. It is produced by secreting cells within the cervical canal or cervical os. Its primary functions are protection and transport. Mucus glycoproteins interact to form a gel. There have been two models proposed for the macromolecular arrangement of mucus glycoprotein. The first is Odeblad's model, which describes the arrangement of mucus as a micellar system with associated bound water molecules.[70,71] The second model proposed by Blandau and Lee suggests that in the high viscosity phase of mucus the glycoproteins within behave as a random coil structure without crosslinking.[72,72]

A number of factors have been shown to impact the viscoelastic properties of cervical mucus. The fucose/sialic acid ratio of cervical mucins present impacts the viscoelasticity. The viscoelasticity of cervical mucus may also be altered by serum albumin, which increases mucus viscosity. The gel structure of cervical mucus is susceptible to alteration by proteolytic enzymes.[73] In a study evaluating the nonlinear viscoelastic properties of cervical mucus conducted by Tam et al, the viscosity was shown to vary from 17 to 600 poise whereas values obtained for shear modulus ranged from 20 to 250 dynes/cm². The relaxation times for human cervical mucus ranged from 1 to 10 seconds.[74] The viscosity of cervical mucus is hormonally regulated. The viscosity changes of cervical mucus that occur during the menstrual cycle are also the result of variation in water content. At midcycle the amount of cervical mucus increases due to estrogen-induced increases in gel hydration. Cervical mucus becomes less viscoelastic at this point, thus the penetration of spermatozoa is facilitated.[75] The transfer of spermatozoa to the uterus is highly dependent on the rheological properties of the cervical mucus. The rheological properties of cervical mucus can be used to predict ovulation. The rheology of cervical mucus is not only altered by menstrual cycle stage but also varied by pathological state. It has been shown that bacterial vaginosis organisms degrade the protective mucus gel.[76]

Semen—Semen is a semi-gelatinous cellular suspension containing spermatozoa (the male gametes) and secretions from the male reproductive accessory glands. Temporal variations exist in the rheological properties of semen. The viscous component of post ejaculatory semen can be characterized by power law model.[77] Semen exhibits pseudoplastic behavior. The viscosity of normal semen at 230 s⁻¹ and 25° was found to be 4.3 ± 0.2 cp.[78]

Synovial Fluid

Fluids which lubricate and cushion the joints are known as synovial fluids. The structure of these fluids is quite complex. Synovia or synovial fluid is a clear liquid not only contained in joint cavities but also in bursae and tendon sheaths. Synovial fluid is a dialysate of blood plasma[79]and consists of electrolytes and proteins. An important component of synovial fluid is hyaluronic acid. This is the substance that is primarily responsible for this fluid's rheological properties. The consistency of synovial fluid is comparable to that of an egg white. This fluid is highly viscous and exhibits non-Newtonian behavior due primarily to the presence of hyaluronic acid. The fluid owes its viscoelastic behavior to the complex between hyaluronic acid and soluble proteins (mainly albumin). The storage modulus of healthy synovial fluid is high and decreases with age.[80]

Normal synovial fluid is a weak highly hydrated gel. Its zero shear viscosity ranges from 100 to 1000 poise. Synovial fluid is strongly pseudo plastic. At a shear rate of 100 sec⁻¹, the apparent viscosity is significantly smaller than the zero-shear viscosity. There are considerable variations between the rheological properties of normal synovial fluid from different human subjects.

The shear modulus (G) (analogous to the modulus of elasticity (E) when the deformation is in shear rather than in tension) of synovial fluid at low shear rates is surprisingly low. The combination of an extremely high zero-shear viscosity and an extremely low initial shear modulus renders their ratio, the relaxation time very long: [(126 to 300 poise)/(20 to 40 dynes/cm²)] ≅ 3 to 10 sec.

Increasing shear affects the modulus in two opposite ways. Progressive disentanglement of the long hyaluronic acid molecules with the attached protein side chains breaks up their network and tends to lower the modulus. However, as the shear rate increases, the relaxation time cannot keep pace with it. This results in incomplete relaxation, which causes the polymer chains to stiffen and tends to increase the modulus. Consequently, the shear modulus retains a nearly constant value, ranging from 20 to 40 dynes/cm² between 0 and 100 sec⁻¹, and increases moderately at higher shear rates. Because increasing shear rates lower the apparent viscosity of synovial fluid strongly but leave the shear modulus nearly unchanged, they shorten the relaxation time considerably.

The rheological properties of synovial fluid are well adapted to its functions. Its very high viscosity at low or zero shear, combined with its viscoelasticity, enable it to maintain the space or clearance between articular surfaces. Its lubricity is aided by its pronounced pseudoplasticity. When a joint moves rapidly and the motion-induced shear and pressure are high, the apparent viscosity is lowered substantially and the amount of energy dissipated as heat by viscous friction is reduced commensurately. However, the amount of energy stored elastically during the loading phase of a motion cycle is nearly the same as at rest because the elastic properties of synovial fluid (eg, the elastic component of the complex viscosity and the shear modulus) undergo only small changes with increasing shear. Therefore, the lubricating film of synovial fluid between articular surfaces is squeezed out only very slowly by pressure and protects the cartilage from wear.

Because motion-induced shear lowers the apparent viscosity of synovial fluid so strongly, while leaving its shear modulus nearly constant or somewhat higher, it shortens its relaxation times appreciably. Shorter relaxation times permit the stress-relaxation mechanisms to be carried to completion within each loading-unloading cycle during articular motion. Thus, synovial fluid can store energy elastically during each new loading phase without building up excessive peak stresses.

The rheological properties of synovial fluid are altered by disease. Although protein content in pathological synovial fluid is unaltered, joint diseases reduce the hyaluronic acid content of synovial fluid. The concentration of hyaluronic acid in normal synovial fluid ranges from 1.5 to 2.9 g/L. Hyaluronic acid concentration is reduced to levels of 1.1 to 1.4 g/L with meniscus lesions, 0.9 g/L in degenerative diseases, and to less than 0.5 g/L in inflammatory disease. This reduction in hyaluronic acid content impair the rheological/functional properties of synovial fluid. These alterations in rheological properties are not only contributable to decreased concentration of hyaluronic acid. In addition decreases in hyaluronic acid molecular weight in pathologic conditions alters synovial fluid rheological properties. Decreases in zero shear viscosity occur in diseased synovial fluid. Pathological synovial fluid is much less pseudoplastic than the normal fluid. Viscoelasticity is reduced considerably by inflammatory joint diseases. Assessment of synovial fluid rheological properties can be used as a promising diagnostic tool.

Cerebrospinal fluid

Cerebrospinal fluid is a clear fluid secreted by the choroids plexuses of the ventricles of the brain. It circulates in the space surrounding the spinal cord and brain. It serves to protect these areas from physical impact by providing a water cushion.[25] Cerebrospinal fluid is a newtonian fluid with a viscosity similar to water.[15] At 37° its viscosity lies in the range of 0.7 to 1 mPa.s.[81]

RHEOLOGICAL MEASUREMENTS

A wide variety of viscometers is available commercially; they vary in regards to range of shear, sample size, ease of operation, reproducibility, and cost. It is necessary to select an instrument which provides the information desired for a specific application. Information on selected suppliers along with web sites is listed in Table 23-4. This section outlines the basic aspects of some of the more frequently used types of viscometers (rheometers).

All of the equations routinely used with viscometers yield viscosities, shear rates, and shear stresses based on the assumption that the fluid is Newtonian. The viscosity, in particular, is an apparent viscosity defined as the ratio of shear stress to shear rate. For non-Newtonian fluids and in order to compare data from one viscometer to another, the pseudo-Newtonian data must be corrected for non-Newtonian behavior.

Table 23-5. Viscometer Parameters

TYPE OF VISCOMETER	x_γ	x_σ
Flow	Time of fluid flow	Fluid density
Rotary	Rotation speed of rotating element	Torque
Falling object	Velocity of falling object	Diameter of object

One very important potential problem is measuring the apparent viscosity of a material at a single rate of shear instead of covering a wide range of shear. A Newtonian, a pseudoplastic, a plastic, and a dilatant fluid may all have the same apparent viscosity if their flow curves have a common intersection point since apparent viscosity is defined as (shear stress)/(shear rate), whereas their flow curves may demonstrate very dissimilar behavior.

Measuring the apparent viscosity over a range of shear rates but maintaining the material for only short times at each shear rate also can give misleading results by missing thixotropic or time-dependent effects. The latter usually are detected by measuring the flow curve first at increasing shear rates and, after reaching the desired maximum value, at decreasing shear rates. An alternate technique is to keep the material at a constant shear rate for a given period of time and to observe the decay, if any, of the shear stress with time.

General Viscometer Types

There are three principal methods for measuring viscosity: (1) based on the rate of flow of a liquid through an orifice or a duct of simple geometry such as a capillary viscometer, (2) based on the resistance of a rotating element in contact with or immersed in the liquid such as a concentric cylinder viscometer, and (3) based on the velocity of an object rolling or falling through the liquid under the effect of gravity (or of an air bubble rising through the liquid) such as the falling or rolling sphere viscometer.

The apparent viscosity with any viscometer can be determined following calibration of the viscometer with a standard Newtonian oil:

$$\eta = K_\eta \, (x_\gamma, x_\sigma) \qquad (22)$$

where K_η is the viscometer constant for determining viscosity and x_γ and x_σ are experimental parameters related to shear rate and shear stress respectively. Alternately, shear rate and shear stress can be determined separately as follows:

$$\dot{\gamma} = K_\gamma \, x_\gamma \qquad (23)$$

and

$$\sigma = K_\sigma \, x_\sigma \qquad (24)$$

Table 23-4. Selected Viscometer Companies With Web Addresses

COMPANY	VISCOMETERS AND SERVICES	WEB ADDRESS
Brookfield Engineering	Broad Line Of Laboratory & Process Viscometers, Rheometers & Accessories For The Measurement & Control Of Viscosity	www.brookfieldengineering.com
Cannon Instrument Co.	Glass Capillary Viscometers, Automatic Viscometers, Rotational Viscometers, Special Purpose Viscometers, Viscosity Baths, Viscosity Standards	www.cannon-ins.com
Rheometric Scientific	A broad range of rheometers, controlled stress or controlled strain measurements.	www.rheosci.com
Thermo Haake	Rheometers & Viscometers Including Extension, Shear, Capillary, Rotation, Oscillation, Controlled Stress & Controlled Strain & Extrusion Capillary Rheometers	www.thermo.com
Reologica Instruments	Customized Research Rheometers, Accessories, & Measuring Systems	www.reologicainstruments.com
Gilson Company	Automatic, Brookfield, Saybolt, Kinematic, Absolute	www.globalgilson.com
Grace Instrument Co.	Extra High/Low Shear Viscometers, Rheometers	www.graceinstrument.com

where K_γ and K_σ are the viscometer constants for determining shear rate and shear stress respectively. K_γ and K_σ are related to K_η as follows:

$$K_\eta = \frac{K_\gamma}{K_\sigma} \qquad (25)$$

The experimental parameters x_γ and x_σ for the three basic types of viscometers are listed in Table 23-5.

CAPILLARY VISCOMETER—The glass capillary Cannon-Fenske, Ubbelohde, and Ostwald viscometers are the most popular instruments based on the first method. The duct is a cylindrical capillary, and the driving force causing the liquid to flow through it is its weight. Thus, ΔP in Poiseuille's law (Equation 6) is replaced by the hydrostatic pressure $h\rho g$ of a liquid column of height h and density ρ; g is the acceleration of gravity.

$$\eta = \left(\frac{\pi R^4 hg}{8L\,V}\right)\rho t \text{ or } \eta = K_\eta \rho t \qquad (26)$$

therefore:

$$K_\eta = \left(\frac{\pi R^4 hg}{8L\,V}\right) \qquad (27)$$

A standard volume of the liquid is transferred into the viscometer. Liquid is then drawn into the upper reservoir bulb of the instrument by suction (Figure 23-17). The efflux time, t, required for the liquid level to fall from the upper to the lower benchmark, emptying the upper reservoir, is measured with a stopwatch. The height, h, is the difference between the liquid levels in the two arms of the viscometer. The height, h, decreases as liquid flows through the capillary, but its time-averaged value is constant for a given viscometer containing a constant volume of liquid.

Calibration of the viscometer consists in determining the constant K_η experimentally with a liquid of known viscosity and density by measuring the efflux time t as described from Equation 26;

$$K_\eta = \frac{\eta}{\rho t} \qquad (28)$$

The viscosity for an unknown liquid is then determined from Equation (29);

$$\eta = K_\eta \rho t \qquad (29)$$

The liquid used to calibrate the viscometer should have approximately the same flow time t as the unknown, in order to

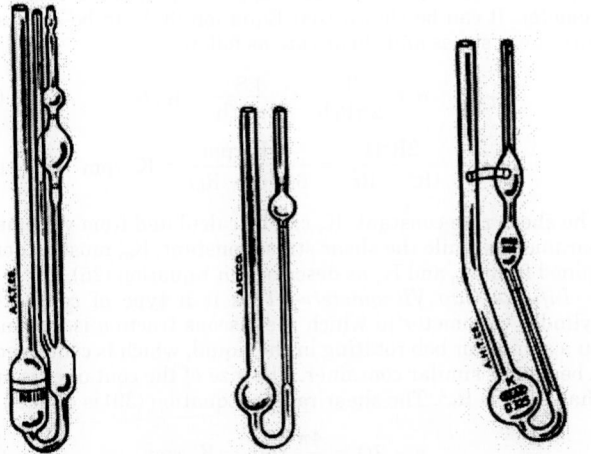

Figure 23-17. Capillary Viscometers: Ubbelohde, Ostwald, and Cannon-Fenske.

minimize two corrections when using Equation (8). The major portion of the potential energy represented by the hydrostatic pressure head is dissipated in overcoming the viscous resistance against flow in the capillary tube, ie, the friction of layer slipping past concentric layer. This portion is converted into heat. However, a small portion of the potential energy is required to accelerate the liquid as it enters the capillary from the reservoir (*kinetic energy correction*). Another small amount is used up in the streamlines converging from the broad reservoir into the narrow capillary and in spreading the streamlines upon issuing from the capillary (entrance or end effects, also called the *Couette correction*). These two corrections are included experimentally in the constant K_η.

It is not necessary to evaluate K_η if the viscosity of one liquid relative to a reference liquid is sufficient. It suffices to measure the flow time t_1 for the reference liquid of known viscosity η_1 and density ρ_1, and to compare it with the flow time t_2 for the liquid of density ρ_2 whose viscosity η_2 is to be determined. The equation

$$\eta_2 = \frac{t_2\rho_2}{t_1\rho_1}\,\eta_1 \qquad (30)$$

gives the unknown viscosity.

If the viscosity of the reference liquid is not known a relative viscosity, η_r, can be determined as defined in the following equation.

$$\eta_r = \frac{\eta_2}{\eta_1} = \frac{t_2\rho_2}{t_1\rho_1} \qquad (31)$$

If the density of the liquid is not known a kinematic viscosity can be determine which is defined as the absolute viscosity divided by the fluid density as:

$$\text{kinematic viscosity} = \frac{\eta}{\rho} = K_\eta t \qquad (32)$$

Kinematic viscosity has the units of stoke(s) or centistoke(s) and is not numerically or dimensionally equivalent to the viscosity in cps.

Shear rate and shear stress can be determined explicitly from Equations (23) and (24) as they apply to capillary viscometers. It can be shown that Equation (26) can be separated into shear stress and shear rate as follows:

$$\dot{\gamma} = \frac{4V L}{\pi R^3 t} = K_\gamma\,\frac{L}{t} \qquad (33)$$

and

$$\sigma = \frac{hgR}{2L}\,\rho = K_\sigma\rho \qquad (34)$$

It follows that K_γ, x_γ, K_σ, and x_σ in Equations (23) and (24) are defined as $4V/\pi R^3$, L/t, $hgR/2L$ and ρ, respectively.

It would appear that K_γ and K_σ in Equations (33) and (34) could be calculated directly since all of the parameters in their definition appear to be measurable. In reality the length of the capillary, L, cannot be measured precisely due to the corrections discussed above. Consequently, K_σ must be determined from calibration of the capillary viscometer with a Newtonian standard. This can be done conveniently by determining K_η experimentally, calculating K_γ directly from viscometer parameters, and then calculating K_σ from the relationship defined in Equation (25).

A range of shear rates and shear stresses can be obtained for a given liquid by using a series of glass capillary viscometers of different diameters since the usual glass capillary viscometer affords viscosity measurements at only one time-averaged value of shear rate. The efflux times should exceed 200 sec to minimize the kinetic energy correction and the possible error when starting and stopping the stopwatch. A range of shear rates can be obtained with a single capillary viscometer if external pressure is applied to force the liquid through the capillary. A variety of capillary extrusion viscometers operating under pressure are commercially available.

ROTATIONAL VISCOMETERS—These instruments depend on the fact that a solid rotating body immersed in a liquid is subjected to a retarding force due to the viscous drag, which is proportional to the viscosity of the liquid. The advantages of rotational viscometers are that the shear rate can be varied over a wide range of values, and that continuous measurements at a given shear rate or shear stress can be made for extended periods of time, affording measurements of the time-dependency as well as of the shear-dependency of the viscosity.

The entire liquid sample is in shear for as long as the rotational viscometer is being operated. Its temperature rises progressively as the energy used to overcome its viscous resistance is transformed into heat; the higher the viscosity, the greater the heat buildup. Since the viscosity of liquids depends strongly on temperature, accurate temperature control is essential. Rotational viscometers have arrangements for circulating water from a constant-temperature bath past the liquid sample, eg, around the cup. In capillary viscometers, only a small portion of the test liquid is sheared at any given moment, and the measurements are intermittent. Despite the minimal heat buildup, glass capillary viscometers are also usually operated in constant-temperature baths.

In the *MacMichael* type viscometer, the outer cup is rotated at a constant though adjustable speed. The torque on the bob is measured as the deflection or twist of the torsion wire from which the bob is suspended.

In the *Stormer* type viscometer, the cup is stationary and the bob or rotor is driven by weights suspended at the end of a pulley to which the shaft of the bob is connected. The shear stress is varied by applying different weights. The shear rate is measured by the speed of rotation of the bob; the number of revolutions per minute (rpm) is determined by means of a revolution counter connected to the shaft of the bob, and a stopwatch.

In most modern rotational viscometers, the cup likewise is fixed. The bob is rotated at a constant though adjustable speed that can be varied over a wide range of rpm or shear rates. The torque on the rotating bob required to maintain a constant speed of rotation against the viscous drag of the liquid is measured with a dynamometer consisting of a torsion spring interposed between the motor and the bob. The deflection or twist of the spring generates an electric signal by means of a potentiometer. The shear stress is read as the deflection of a needle on the torque scale. Modern rotational viscometers are interfaced with computers in order to simplify data collection and interpretation.

Coaxial-Cylinder Viscometer—The geometry of a coaxial-cylinder viscometer is shown in Figure 23-18. The viscosity is calculated by means of the *Margules* equation:

$$\eta = \frac{(R_c^2 - R_b^2)}{4\pi h R_b^2 R_c^2}\left(\frac{T}{\Omega}\right) = K_\eta'\left(\frac{T}{\Omega}\right) \tag{35}$$

where R_c and R_b are the radii of the cup and bob, respectively, h is the height of the bob immersed in the liquid, T the torque, and Ω the angular velocity of the bob in radians/sec.

The angular velocity of the bob is usually expressed in terms of rpm ($\Omega = (2\pi/60)$ rpm); torque is proportional to number of divisions, S, on the viscometer scale, ie, T = k S. These relationships are substituted into Equation (35) to give:

$$\eta = \frac{(R_c^2 - R_b^2)k}{120 h R_c^2 R_b^2}\left(\frac{S}{rpm}\right) = K_\eta\left(\frac{S}{rpm}\right) \tag{36}$$

The calibration factor K_η, can be determined experimentally for each combination of cup and bob by means of a viscosity standard.

Equation (36) was derived for two coaxial cylinders of infinite length. The *end effect* is the traction on both end surfaces of the bob if it is completely immersed in the liquid or on its bottom surface if it is only partly immersed. Thus, h in Equations (35) and (36) is an "effective" height of the bob. One way to cor-

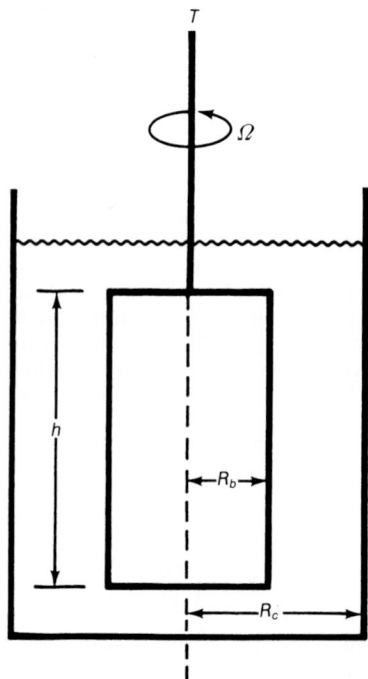

Figure 23-18. Geometry of a coaxial-cylinder (cup and bob) viscometer.

rect for the end effect is by adding an increment Δh to the height h of the bob to arrive at an effective height. For a partly immersed bob with a flat bottom, Δh is frequently of the order of 0.1h. The added height can be determined experimentally for each material by filling the annular gap to different depths of immersion of the bob. The ratio T/Ω is plotted against the height or depth of immersion h. The negative intercept of this usually straight line with the h axis represents Δh.

The end effect is more conveniently accounted for by calibrating the viscometer with a viscosity standard as was done with a capillary viscometer in Equation (26). However, since a rotational viscometer can be operated over a range of shear rates, the constant, K_η, is best determined from the slope of a plot of scale reading, S, vs. rpm as defined by a rearrangement of Equation (36);

$$S = \frac{\eta}{K_\eta} rpm \tag{37}$$

Shear rate and shear stress can be determined explicitly from Equations (23) and (24) as they apply to a coaxial-cylinder viscometer. It can be shown that Equation (35) can be separated into shear stress and shear rate as follows;

$$\sigma = \frac{T}{2\pi R_b^2 h} = \frac{kS}{2\pi R_b^2 h} = K_\sigma S \tag{38}$$

$$\dot\gamma = \frac{2R_c^2\Omega}{(R_c^2 - R_b^2)} = \frac{4\pi R_c^2 rpm}{60(R_c^2 - R_b^2)} = K_\gamma rpm \tag{39}$$

The shear rate constant, K_γ can be calculated from viscometer parameters while the shear stress constant, K_σ, must be determined from K_η and K_γ as described in Equation (25).

Infinite Gap Viscometers—This is a type of concentric-cylinder viscometer in which the viscous traction is measured on a spindle or bob rotating in the liquid, which is contained in a beaker or similar container. The size of the container is such that $R_c^2 \gg R_b^2$. The shear rate in Equation (39) is defined as:

$$\dot\gamma = 2\Omega = \frac{4\pi}{60} rpm = K_\gamma rpm \tag{40}$$

while the shear stress remains as defined in Equation (38).

The viscometer spindle can be inserted not only into beakers in the laboratory but also into kettles, reactors, and mixing tanks in the plant. Thus, the viscometer can be adapted for continuous in-line viscosity measurements. A guard can be mounted around the spindle to prevent it from being deflected laterally and thereby cause misalignment of the shaft. The guard also ensures that the condition, $R_c^2 >> R_b^2$, is maintained.

Cone-and-Plate Viscometers—These instruments consist of a rotating cone with a very obtuse angle and a stationary lower flat plate. The plate is raised until the apex of the cone just touches its surface. The liquid fills the narrow triangular gap between cone and plate (Figure 23-19). Its surface tension prevents it from spreading on the plate. The plate is maintained at a constant temperature by circulating water. The cone is driven at controlled speeds that can be varied continuously. The viscous drag on the rotating cone exerts a torque on a dynamometer that is proportional to the shear stress. The angle θ formed by cone and plate is usually less than 3°, and the average gap width is less than 2 mm. An added advantage of the instrument is that sample volumes smaller than 0.5 cm^3 can be used.

For small values of θ in radians, the viscosity is determined as:

$$\eta = \frac{3\theta}{2\pi R_b^2}\left(\frac{T}{\Omega}\right) = \frac{180\theta k}{4\pi R_b^2}\left(\frac{S}{rpm}\right) = K_\eta\left(\frac{S}{rpm}\right) \quad (41)$$

where k, S, T, and Ω are as defined previously and R_b is the maximum cone radius. Equation (41) can be expressed in terms of shear stress and shear rate as follows:

$$\sigma = \frac{3T}{2\pi R_b^2} = \frac{3k}{2\pi R_b^2}\, S = K_\sigma S \quad (42)$$

and

$$\dot{\gamma} = \frac{\Omega}{\theta} = \frac{2\pi}{60\theta}\, rpm = K_\gamma\, rpm \quad (43)$$

As with concentric-cylinder viscometers, K_η is determined by calibration with a viscosity standard, K_γ is calculated from viscometer parameters and K_σ is calculated from K_η and K_γ.

Parallel-Plate Viscometers—A parallel-plate or rotating-disk viscometer is similar to a cone and plate viscometer except that the rotating plate is parallel to the fixed plate. The equations are as follows where d is the distance between the plates:

$$\eta = \frac{d}{\pi R_b^4}\left(\frac{T}{\Omega}\right) = \frac{60dk}{2\pi^2 R_b^4}\left(\frac{S}{rpm}\right) = K_\eta\left(\frac{S}{rpm}\right) \quad (44)$$

$$\sigma = \frac{T}{2\pi R_b^3} = \frac{k}{2\pi R_b^3}\, S = K_\sigma S \quad (45)$$

$$\dot{\gamma} = \frac{R\Omega}{2d} = \frac{\pi R}{60d}\, rpm = K_\gamma\, rpm \quad (46)$$

The constants, K_η, K_σ and K_γ are determined as described above for the cone and plate viscometer.

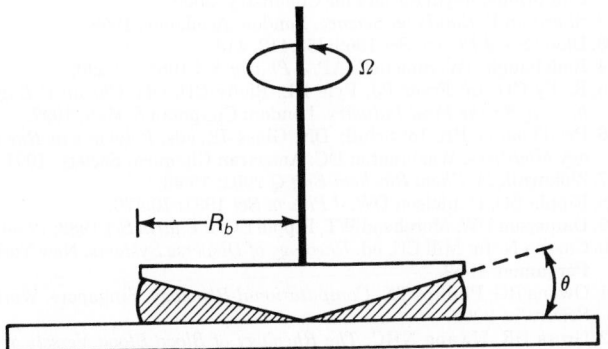

Figure 23-19. Geometry of a cone-and-plate viscometer.

FALLING BALL OR NEEDLE VISCOMETERS—With these instruments, viscosities are determined by measuring the velocity of a falling or rolling ball, a falling needle, or a rising air bubble in the liquid being studied. This method is best suited for Newtonian liquids because it measures viscosities at a single shear rate.

When a sphere of radius, R, and density, ρ_2, descends vertically through a liquid of density, ρ_1, the driving force is the effective weight of the sphere, ie, the weight of the sphere minus the weight of the liquid it displaces. It equals the volume of the sphere multiplied by the net density $\rho_2 - \rho_1$ and by the acceleration of gravity g, namely $(4\pi R^3/3)(\rho_2 - \rho_1)g$. The viscous resistance of the liquid is given by Stokes' law, namely, $6\pi\eta Rv$. When the sphere attains the terminal or constant velocity, v, (which occurs soon after it is dropped into the liquid column), the two opposing forces are equal, so that the viscosity is, in general, governed by Stokes' law:

$$\eta = \frac{2R^2(\rho_2 - \rho_1)\, g}{9v} \quad (47)$$

When deriving his law, Stokes assumed that the velocity of sedimentation was very low and that the liquid medium extended at an infinite distance from the ball. Among the factors requiring correction, therefore, is the proximity of the wall.

The viscosity can then be determined from the following:

$$\eta = \frac{2R^2 g}{9}\left(\frac{(\rho_2 - \rho_1)}{v}\right) = K_\eta\left(\frac{(\rho_2 - \rho_1)}{v}\right) \quad (48)$$

where v is the velocity in cm/sec of the falling, rolling, or rising object. Most viscometers of this type have a known distance marked on the instrument so that one merely measures the time for the object to move between the marks. Equation (48) then becomes:

$$\eta = \frac{2R^2 g}{L9}(\rho_2 - \rho_1)\, t = K_\eta(\rho_2 - \rho_1)\, t \quad (49)$$

where L is the distance between the two marks on the viscometer and t is the time for the object to travel between the marks. Calibration of the viscometer involves determining K_η using a viscosity standard for each ball or object.

Shear stress and shear rate can be determined from the following:

$$\sigma = \frac{Rg}{3}(\rho_2 - \rho_1) = K_\sigma(\rho_2 - \rho_1) \quad (50)$$

$$\dot{\gamma} = \frac{3L}{2R}\left(\frac{1}{t}\right) = K_\eta\left(\frac{1}{t}\right) \quad (51)$$

Instead of spheres, viscosities can be obtained from the velocity of sedimentation of cylindrical metal needles with hemispherical ends falling vertically through liquids contained in glass capillaries. The latter have much larger diameters than the needles and are closed at the bottom. To make measurements at different shear rates, hollow needles are used and their densities are varied with different inserts.[50]

For very viscous liquids, values of the Newtonian or the apparent viscosity at a single shear rate can be measured with a metal rod plunger immersed concentrically in a vertical cylindrical glass tube filled with the liquid. The tube is closed at the bottom and thermostatted. The diameter of the metal plunger is ≈68% of the inside diameter of the glass tube. The weight of the plunger forces the liquid upward through the narrow annular space between plunger and tube. The terminal or steady-state velocity of descent of the plunger is proportional to the viscosity of the liquid.

All of these instruments have guides to ensure that the probes descend along the vertical axis of the cylindrical containers.

Tensile And Torsion Testers/ Penetrometers—In the case of semisolids or very viscous liquids, a cone or needle attached to a holding rod is released and plunges vertically into the sample

Table 23-6. Non-Newtonian Correction Factors

VISCOMETER	CORRECTION FACTOR, f(n)
Capillary Viscometer	$f(n) = \dfrac{3n + 1}{4n}$
Cup-and-Bob Viscometer	$f(n) = 1 + K_1\left(\dfrac{1 - n}{n}\right) + K_2\left(\dfrac{1 - n}{n}\right)^2$
	Where: $K_1 = \dfrac{S^2 - 1}{2S^2}\left(1 + \dfrac{2}{3}\ln S\right)$
	$K_2 = \dfrac{S^2 - 1}{6S^2}\ln S$
	And $S = \dfrac{R_c}{R_b}$
Cup-and-Bob Viscometer − Infinite Gap	$f(n) = \dfrac{1}{n}$
Cone-and-Plate Viscometer	$f(n) = 1$
Parallel Plate Viscometer	$f(n) = \dfrac{3 + n}{4}$

under the influence of its own or added weight. The depth of penetration within a given time interval, eg, 10 sec, is used to rate the consistency of the material. The results cannot be translated into viscosity and yield values.

A modern variation of this principle is illustrated by the "Texture Analyzer" (www.texturetechnologies.com), which can provide a wide range of static and dynamic measurements of penetration and stress.

Comparison Between Instruments

When a material is to be studied over a wide range of shear rates, more than one viscometer may be used because each individual instrument may have too limited a range. When the flow curves are plotted as shear stress versus rate of shear, instruments of different dimensions and even based on different principles produce a single curve for a given material at a given temperature if the material is Newtonian. The shear rate and shear stress are measured at the surface of the bob in coaxial-cylinder viscometers, at the wall of the capillary in capillary viscometers and at the ball surface in a falling ball viscometer. When studying a material with two viscometers, it is advisable to use both instruments in the range of overlapping shear rates to ensure that the corresponding flow curves do indeed coincide. When flow curves are plotted in units other than shear stress and shear rate, such as torque units versus rpm, they depend on the geometry of the viscometer and are not directly comparable between viscometers.

In addition, all of the preceding discussion provides Newtonian parameters, even if the material being evaluated is non-Newtonian. In this case non-Newtonian corrections must be applied in order for flow curves from different viscometers to be comparable.

Non-Newtonian Corrections[83,84]

All of the preceding equations have been derived based on Newtonian behavior, which means that the shear rate is constant everywhere in the viscometer, ie, at the bob surface or at the cup surface in a cup-and-bob viscometer. This is not true for non-Newtonian fluids. Comparison of non-Newtonian fluids requires that viscosity data be corrected to a common reference point. The result is a correction to the shear rate term in reference to a fixed point in the viscometer, ie, the bob surface in a cup-and-bob viscometer and the wall in a capillary viscometer, and depends on both the viscometer and the fluid being tested.

In general, the correction takes for form:

$$\dot{\gamma}_{\text{corrected}} = \dot{\gamma}f(n) \qquad (52)$$

where f(n) is the correction factor and n is the slope of a log − log plot of shear stress vs. shear rate. For many non-Newtonian fluids of pharmaceutical interest, n is a constant. If the log − log plot is not linear, n must be determined numerically at each data point. Flow curves plotted as shear stress vs. corrected shear rates are then comparable between viscometers.

Correction factors for the most common viscometers are given as follows in Table 23-6.

REFERENCES

1. Doraiswamy E. *Rheology Bull* 2002; 71:1.
2. Reiner M. *Deformation, Strain, and Flow*, 2nd ed. New York: Interscience, 1960.
3. Scott Blair GW. *Elementary Rheology*, London: Academic Press, 1969, p 2.
4. Houwink R, de Decker HK eds. *Elasticity, Plasticity and Structure of Matter*, 3rd ed. London: Cambridge University Press, 1971.
5. Dealy JM. *J Rheol* 1995; 39:253.
6. Hackley VA, Ferraris CF. *Guide to Rheological Nomenclature: Measurements in Ceramic Particulate Systems.* NIST Special Publication 946, National Institute of Standards and Technology, Washington DC, 2001.
7. Ree T, Eyring H, in Eirich FR, ed, *Rheology*, vol. 2, New York: Academic Press, 1958.
8. Fisher EK, *Colloidal Dispersions.* New York: Wiley, 1950.
9. Braun DB, Rosen MR. *The Rheology Modifiers Handbook: Practical Use and Application.* New York: William Andrew, 1999.
10. Reiner M. *Physics Today* 1964; 17(1):62.
11. Goodwin JW, Hughes RW. *Rheology for Chemists: A Introduction.* Cambridge: Royal Society for Chemistry, 2000.
12. Sherman P. *Emulsion Science.* London: Academic, 1968.
13. Davis SS. *J Pharm Sci* 1969; l58:412, 418.
14. Radebaugh GW, Simonelli AP. *J Pharm Sci* 1984; 73:590.
15. Rielly CD. In: Fryer PJ, Pyle DL, Rielly CD, eds. *Chemical Engineering for the Food Industry.* London: Chapman & Hall, 1997.
16. Prud'homme RK. In: Schulz DN, Glass JE, eds. *Polymers as Rheology Modifiers.* Washington DC: American Chemical Society, 1991.
17. Zlokarnik M. *Chem Biochem Eng Q* 2001; 15:43.
18. Rippie EG, Danielson DW. *J Pharm Sci* 1981; 70:476.
19. Danielson DW, Morehead WT, Rippie EG. *J Pharm Sci* 1983; 72:342.
20. Casson N. In: Mill CC, ed. *Rheology of Disperse Systems.* New York: Pergamon, 1959.
21. Owens RG, Phillips TN. *Computational Rheology.* Singapore: World Scientific, 2002.
22. Gross DR, Hwang NHC. *The Rheology of Blood, Blood Vessels and Associated Tissues.* NATO Advanced Study Institute on Biorheology, 1980.

23. Lowe GDO. Nature and clinical importance of blood rheology. In: Lowe GDO, ed. *Clinical Blood Rheology*. Boca Raton, FL: CRC Press, 1988, pp 1–10.

24. Reinhart WH, et al. *J Crit Care* 2002; 17(1):68.

25. Patton HD, et al. Textbook of Physiology, vol 2, 21st ed. Philadelphia: WB Saunders, 1989.

26. Dintenfass L. Rheology of blood in diagnostic and preventive medicine. 1976.

27. Gomes N, et al. Shear stress modulates tumor cells adhesion to the endothelium. *Biorheology* 2003; 40:41.

28. Chmiel H, Walitza E. *On the Rheology of Blood and Synovial Fluids*. 1980.

29. Chien S, Dormandy J, Ernst E, et al. *Clinical Hemorheology*. 1987.

30. http://www.coheadquarters.com/PennLibr/MyPhysiology/index1.htm

31. Ruch TC, Patton HD. *Physiology and Biophysics*. Philadelphia: WB Saunders, 1965.

32. Brown DW, et al. *Am Heart J* 2001; 142:657.

33. Church TS, et al. *Am Heart J* 2002; 143:349.

34. Basaria S, et al. *Clin Endocrinol* 2002; 57:209.

35. Sushil S, Peach JP, Hitt DL, et al. *2001 Bioengineering Conference*, ASME 2001. BED, vol. 50.

36. Winslow RM. *Curr Opin Hematol* 2002; 9:146.

37. Winslow RM. *Annu Rev Med* 1999; 50:337.

38. Spahn DR. *Crit Care* 1999; 3(5):R93.

39. Lowe KC. *Blood Rev* 1999; 13:171.

40. Spahn DR. *Adv Drug Delivery Rev* 2000; 143–151.

41. Madsen F, et al. *J Controlled Release* 1998; 50:167.

42. Madsen F, Eberth K, Smart J. *Biomaterials* 1998; 19:1083.

43. Sanders NN, DeSmedt SE, Demeester J. *J Pharmaceut Sci* 2000; 89:835.

44. Lenaerts V, Gurny R. *Bioadhesive Drug Delivery Systems*. Boca Raton, FL: CRC Press, 1990.

45. Sharma A, et al. *Coll Surf B* 1999; 14:223.

46. Ehlers N. *Acta Ophthalmol* 1965; 81(suppl):3.

47. Tiffany JM. *Int Ophthalmol* 1991; 15:371.

48. *Anatomy, pathology, and physiology of the human eye.* http://www.tedmontgomery.com/the_eye/index.html

49. Hold K, de Boer D, Zuidema J, et al. *Int J Drug Testing*

50. Quraishi MS, Jones NS, Mason J. *Clin Otolaryngol* 1998; 23(5):403.

51. Rhee CS, et al. *Arch Otolaryngol Head Neck Surg* 1999; 125:101.

52. Majima Y, et al. *Am J Respir Crit Care Med* 1999; 160:421.

53. Alder KB, Wooten O, Dulfano MJ. *Arch Environ Health* 1993; 27:364.

54. Braga PC, et al. *Biorheology* 1992; 29:285.

55. King M. In: Braga PC, Allegra L, eds. *Methods in Bronchial Mucology*. New York: Raven, 1998, pp 73–83.

56. Reid LM, Bhaskar KR. In: *Mucus and Related Topics*. Symposia of the Society for Experimental Biology. 1989, pp 201–220.

57. Blair S. *An Introduction to Biorheology*. New York: Elsevier Scientific Publishing Company, 1974.

58. Sanders N, De Smedt C, Demeester J. *J Pharmaceut Sci* 2000; 89:835.

59. Shibuya Y, Wills PJ, Cole PJ. *Respirology* 2003; 8:181.

60. App EM, et al. *Chest* 1998; 114:171.

61. Del Donno M et al. The effect of inflammation on mucociliary clearance in asthma. *Chest*. 2000. 118, 1142–1149.

62. Mandelberg A, et al. *Chest* 2003; 123:481.

63. Labiris NR, Dolovich MB. *J Clin Pharmacol* 2003; 56:588.

64. Goddard AF, Spiller RC. *Alimentary Pharmacology and Therapeutics* 1996; 10:105.

65. Grubel P, Cave DR. *Alimentary Pharmacology and Therapeutics* 1998; 12:569.

66. List SJ, Findlay BP, Forstner GG, et al. *Biochem J* 1978; 175:565.

67. Chantler E, Ratcliffe NA. Gastrointestinal mucus gel rheology. In: *Mucus and Related Topics*. Society for Experimental Biology, 1989, pp 65–71.

68. Owen DH, Katz DF. *Contraception* 1999; 59:91.

69. Burruano BT, Schnaare RL, Malamud D. *Contraception* 2002; 66:137.

70. Odeblad E. In: Elstein M, Moghissi KS, Borth R, eds. *Cervical Mucus in Human Reproduction*. Copenhagen: Scriptor, pp 58–74.

71. Chantler EN, Elder JB, Elstein M. Structure and function of cervical mucus. In: *Mucus in Health and Disease*. New York: Plenum Press, 1982, pp 251–263.

72. Lee WI, Verdugo P, Blandau RJ, et al. Molecular arrangement of cervical mucus: a reevaluation based on laser light-scattering spectroscopy. *Gynecologic Investigation* 1977; 8(5–6):154.

73. Wolf DP, Blasco L, Khan MA, et al. *Fertility and Sterility* 1977; 28(1):41.

74. Tam PY, Datz DF, Berger SA. *Biorheology* 1980; 17:465.

75. Katz DF. *American Journal of Obstetrics & Gynecology* 1991; 165(6 Pt 2):1984.

76. Olmsted SS, Meyn LA, Rohan LC, et al. *Sexually Transmitted Diseases* 2003; 30(3):257.

77. Dunn PF, Picologlou BF. *Biorheology* 1977; 14:277.

78. Medeluk G, Gonzalez Flecha FL, Castello PR, et al: *Journal of Andrology*. 2000; 21:262.

79. Hlavacek M. *Biorheology* 2001; 38:319.

80. Rohn CL. *American Laboratory News* 2000 (June).

81. Bloomfield IG, et al. *Pediatr Neurosurg* 1998; 28(5):246.

82. www.brookfieldengineering.com

83. Steffe JF. *Rheological Methods in Food Process Engineering*, 2nd ed. East Lansing, MI: Freeman Press, 1992, www.egr.msu.edu/~steffe/freebook

84. Van Wazer JR, Lyons JW, Kim KY, et al. *Viscosity and Flow Measurement*. New York: Interscience Publishers, 1962.

PART **3**

Pharmaceutical Chemistry

Pardeep K Gupta, PhD
Associate Professor of Pharmaceutics
Director of BS Program in Pharmaceutical Sciences
University of the Sciences in Philadelphia
Philadelphia, PA

CHAPTER 24

Inorganic Pharmaceutical Chemistry

Clarence A Discher, PhD[†]

Thomas Medwick, PhD

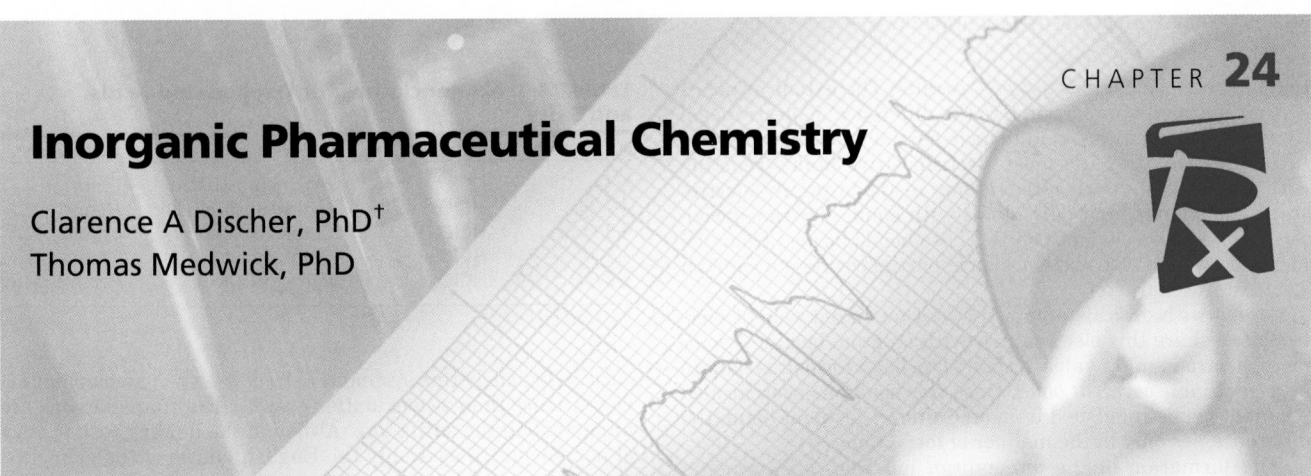

Inorganic chemicals have been used in pharmacy and medicine for many reasons, ranging from therapeutic agents to nutritional supplements to pharmaceutical necessities. In this chapter a review of some chemical principles and properties of elements is followed by a discussion of the wide variety of useful inorganic chemicals.

BASIS OF CHEMICAL REACTIONS

Although many subatomic particles have been identified, only the protons and neutrons of the nucleus of an atom and the extranuclear electrons will be considered here.

Each atom of an element is described uniquely by two pure numbers: its atomic number and its atomic weight. The atomic number gives the number of protons present in the nucleus and, therefore, its positive charge. Because the ground state atom must be neutral, this in turn defines the number of extranuclear electrons. The difference between the atomic number and the atomic weight of a given *isotope* of an element defines the number of neutrons in the nucleus. (Atomic weights in the tables are not whole numbers because they represent the weighted average of the atomic weights of all isotopes present.)

The electrons are arranged in major quantum groups (energy levels or orbitals) occupying the space about the nucleus. Each electron is assigned four quantum numbers:

The principle quantum number, n, describes the relative position of an energy level with respect to the other energy levels present.

The subquantum number, l, describes the different electron distributions possible for a given value of n.

The magnetic quantum number, m_l, is best described as the magnetic contribution to the angular momentum due to the movement of the electrons in space.

The magnetic spin quantum number, m_s, is the magnetic component contributed by the spin of the electron.

The permitted values for n are 1, 2, 3, . . . , for l are 0, 1, 2, . . . $(n-1)$, for m_l are $-1, . . . 0, . . . +1$, and for $m_s \pm 1/2$. Returning to the subquantum number l, when l is 0 the electrons occupying the suborbital are known as s electrons; when l is 1, they're known as p electrons; when l is 2, they're known as d electrons; and when l is 3, they're known as f electrons. Thus if 2 electrons occupy suborbital 0 of major quantum group 3, they are represented as $3s^2$.

In assigning electrons to the atom the Aufbau Principle is used. It is an application of quantum theory, Hund's rules, and the Pauli exclusion principle. Simply stated, a given entering electron must occupy the lowest unoccupied energy level of the

atom. In other words, each electron must have a unique set of quantum numbers.

As a result of the above process, all atoms, except hydrogen and the inert gases, have one or more completely occupied lower major quantum groups and have the suborbitals of their highest major quantum group only partially filled. The electrons of this outer, partially filled, energy level give each element its distinct chemical properties. These are the *valence electrons.*

Chemical reactions entail the removal of valence electrons, adding electrons to a partly filled valence shell, or sharing a pair of valence electrons between two atoms. Most atoms attempt to achieve a rare gas outer shell (ns^2 or ns^2np^6) by these processes. The energy required for the removal of the electron of least energy is known as the *first ionization potential*. It is unique for each element. The metals have low ionization potentials and, therefore, readily form cations. Nonmetals have high ionization potentials.

The attraction of a nucleus for electrons is termed its *electronegativity*. Metals have low electronegativities (they are electropositive), whereas nonmetals (especially the halogens) have high electronegativities. This allows the latter to attract additional electrons to form anions.

When atoms with widely differing electronegativities react, such as sodium, 0.93, and chlorine, 3.98, an electron transfer takes place. The one valence electron of sodium ($3s^1$) enters the incompletely filled ($3s^23p^5$) valence shell of the chlorine. Sodium now has an inert gas (Ne) electron structure with a +1 charge. The chlorine achieves the argon structure with a −1 charge. There is no formal electron-pair bond between the two entities. A crystal of sodium chloride consists of equal numbers of sodium and chloride ions held in place by the interaction of the spherically symmetrical positive cation field and the spherically symmetrical negative anion field. These ionic (electrostatic) compounds are characterized by high boiling and melting points and most are water soluble.

If two reacting atoms have similar electronegativities, such as two hydrogen atoms, a sharing of electrons takes place. One electron is donated to the bond from an incompletely filled suborbital of each atom. A covalent bond is formed by the overlap of the two atomic orbitals involved. With the formation of the bond a molecule results. The bonding electrons are no longer restricted to their atomic orbitals. They now are free to move in a molecular orbital between the two atoms in what is known as a σ molecular orbital.

When the electronegativities of the two atoms involved in the formation of a covalent bond are not identical the atom with the higher electronegativity tends to attract the electrons of the molecule more strongly than its partner. This leads to polariza-

[†]Deceased

tion of the molecule and a *dipole* results. The extent of polarization is directly proportional to the difference in electronegativities. Such bonds are said to have partial ionic character.

In practice, only the most electropositive atoms reacting with the most electronegative atoms result in purely electrostatic compounds, and only atoms with equal electronegativities form purely covalent bonds. Those bonds formed from elements between these extremes have partial covalent or partial electrostatic character.

Atoms with orbitals occupied by an unshared pair of electrons can share this electron pair with an atom lacking two or more electrons in its valence shell. The bond formed is said to be a *coordinate covalent bond.* Once this bond has been formed it cannot be distinguished from an ordinary covalent bond; the difference lies only in the manner of formation.

The formation of the ammonium ion from an ammonia molecule, which has an unshared electron pair, and a hydrogen ion, which has an empty *s* orbital, illustrates this type of reaction.

Covalent compounds have low melting and boiling points, and usually are insoluble in water. Solubility in water can be induced by introducing an acid or base group into the molecule. Reaction with base or acid will now give a soluble salt.

Other types of bonding exist. Those of interest are weakly bonded; the compounds formed decompose more readily than the electrostatic and covalent types. Hydrogen bonding (bridging) is quite common. Dipole–dipole bonding also is possible; very weak associations result.

Complexes are compounds or ions formed when an atom or cation *central unit* acts as a center about which anions or molecules, ligands, arrange themselves. The central unit is said to have a coordination number equal to the number of complexing ligands. The maximum number of ligands that can arrange themselves about the central unit is known as its *maximum coordination number* and is a function of the size of the central unit. Usual maximum coordination numbers are 2, 4, 6, or 8. The number of ligands that can coordinate with the central unit also is a function of ligand size. Thus, even though the maximum coordination number of aluminum is 6, only four of the relatively large chloride ions can be accommodated as ligands, for example, $[AlF_6]^{3-}$ versus $[AlCl_4]^{1-}$.

The bonding involved in the formation of complexes can be coordinate covalent or electrostatic. Bonds depending on permanent dipoles are also common, such as with hydrates.

NOMENCLATURE

The great advances in chemistry during the past several decades have made necessary constant revision of systems of nomenclature, designed to give precise information with respect to the composition of chemical compounds. Whereas oil of vitriol and lunar caustic at one time were useful names, today they must be looked upon as trivial.

CLASSICAL NOMENCLATURE—Prior to elucidation of the structure of coordination complexes, the naming of compounds was handled reasonably well by using nonnumerical prefixes and suffixes and Latin or Greek numerical prefixes. In general the main function of these prefixes and suffixes was to indicate the oxidation state of elements of variable valence, although some were intended to connote structural characteristics.

Systematic nomenclature must consider two problems; order of citation and stoichiometry. Order of citation is usually well defined; for salts and salt-like compounds the most electropositive element is named first, for example, sodium chloride. For nonmetals the International Union of Pure and Applied Chemistry (IUPAC) recommends the following order of citation: B, Si, C, Sb, As, P, N, H, Se, S, I, Br, Cl, O, F.

Cations with a single oxidation state simply are named as the element. If a cation has two oxidation states the suffix *-ous* is used to indicate the lower oxidation state; for example, mercurous; the suffix *-ic* indicates a higher oxidation state: mer-

Table 24-1. Nomenclature for Oxygenated Acids and Salts

CL OXID STATE	ACID FORMULA	ACID NAME	ANION NAME
−1	HCl	*Hydro*chloric acid	Chlor*ide*
+1	HClO	*Hypo*chlor*ous* acid	*Hypo*chlor*ite*
+3	HClO$_2$	Chlor*ous* acid	Chlor*ite*
+5	HClO$_3$	Chlor*ic* acid	Chlor*ate*
+7	HClO$_4$	*Per*chlor*ic* acid	*Per*chlor*ate*

curic. (Obviously this system breaks down when an element exists in more than two oxidation states.) The simple anions are named using the suffix *-ide.* Although the newer Stock system of nomenclature uses only the English names of the elements, classical nomenclature uses the stems of the Latin names in identifying the cations of copper, gold, tin, lead, and iron.

For the oxygenated anions a system of prefixes and suffixes was developed to indicate the oxidation state of the central atom. These are illustrated in Table 24-1 using the chlorine anions.

Sometimes one or more oxygen atoms of the anion are replaced by another element. The stem of the name of the substituting element is used as a prefix to the name for the fully oxygenated anion, for example, $Na_2S_2O_3$ is sodium thiosulfate, or Na_3AsS_4 is sodium thioarsenate (sodium tetrathioarsenate).

In addition to variable oxidation numbers, oxygenated acids (and their salts) present two other nomenclature problems: (1) a variation in the degree of hydration of the parent acid anhydride and (2) the naming of the different salts arising from partial neutralization of polyprotic acids. Table 24-2 shows the prefixes used for naming the phosphoric acids (P^{5+}).

For salts of diprotic acids, the salt resulting from neutralization of only one proton per acid molecule is named by using the prefix *bi-* or the words *hydrogen* or *acid* with the anion; for example, NaHCO$_3$ is sodium bicarbonate, acid carbonate, or hydrogen carbonate. The latter form is preferred. Several methods have been devised for the triprotic acids. These are shown in Table 24-3. Due to very strongly basic reaction of the solutions of Na$_3$PO$_4$ and other tertiary phosphates, the pharmacist must be alert, especially when using containers labeled sodium phosphate.

It is evident from Table 24-3 that the numerical Greek prefixes hemi-, mono-, sesqui-, di-, tri-, tetra-, penta-, hexa-, hepta-, octa-, ennea- (nona-), and deca- also are used in naming compounds. In fact there are compounds such as N$_2$O$_4$, dinitrogen tetraoxide, that must be named using numerical prefixes because modern systems of nomenclature are unable to identify them precisely.

STOCK NOMENCLATURE—Classical nomenclature is satisfactory for simpler compounds involving atoms with one or two oxidation states. It cannot indicate proper stoichiometry when atoms having three or more oxidation states are involved. The Stock system of nomenclature attempts to overcome the problem.

In the Stock system simple cations are named as the element followed by its oxidation state, expressed in Roman numerals enclosed in parentheses—for example, Fe^{2+} is iron(II), Fe^{3+} is iron(III), and Fe^{6+} is iron(VI). Simple anions use the suffix *-ide* as before. However, complex anions are named using the stem of the name of the central unit and the suffix *-ate* fol-

Table 24-2. Nomenclature for the Phosphoric Acids

WATER MOLECULES	RESULTANT ACID	NAME
H$_2$O + 1/2P$_2$O$_5$	HPO$_3$	*Meta*phosphoric acid *Pyro*phosphoric acid
2H$_2$O + P$_2$O$_5$	H$_4$P$_2$O$_7$	*Di*phosphoric acid
3H$_2$O + P$_2$O$_5$	H$_3$PO$_4$	*Ortho*phosphoric acid Phosphoric acid[a]
5H$_2$O + 3P$_2$O$_5$	H$_5$P$_3$O$_{10}$	*Tri*phosphoric acid

[a] The phosphoric acid of commerce and science is orthophosphoric acid.

Table 24-3. Nomenclature of the Phosphate Salts

FORMULA	NaH_2PO_4	Na_2HPO_4	Na_3PO_4
Preferred name	Sodium dihydrogen phosphate	Sodium monohydrogen phosphate	Sodium phosphate
Other names	Monobasic sodium phosphate	Dibasic sodium phosphate	Tribasic sodium phosphate
	Primary sodium phosphate	Secondary sodium phosphate	Tertiary sodium phosphate
USP 23	Monobasic sodium phosphate	Dibasic sodium phosphate	—

lowed by its oxidation state, in Roman numerals enclosed in parentheses. The ligand(s) involved are cited before the central unit of the complex. If two or more different ligands are present they are cited in alphabetical order, ignoring Greek prefixes. The number of each of the individual ligands involved is indicated by the use of Greek numerical prefixes. These latter rules also govern the citing of ligands associated with complex cations. The preferred nomenclature for common ligands is given in Table 24-4.

Stock names are not used for complex anions with well-established classical names. These include sulfate, sulfite, nitrate, nitrite, carbonate, phosphate, thiosulfate, cyanate, and thiocyanate.

EWENS-BASSETT SYSTEM—Sometimes it is advantageous to cite the charge on a complex ion rather than the oxidation state of the central unit. The Ewens-Bassett system gives the charge of the complex ion in Arabic numerals enclosed in parentheses, after the name. Other than this, the rules for naming a compound are similar to the Stock system. Thus, the common ferrocyanide ion, $[Fe(CN)_6]^{4-}$ becomes hexacyanoferrate(II) using Stock nomenclature, and hexacyanoferrate(−4) using the Ewens-Bassett system. Table 24-5 gives some examples of modern nomenclature.

A more thorough review of inorganic nomenclature may be found in Discher et al[1] or Huheey, Keiter, and Keiter.[2] A comprehensive report on the subject will be found in Report of the Commission on Nomenclature of Inorganic Chemistry, issued by IUPAC.[3]

THE PERIODIC TABLE AND FAMILIES OF ELEMENTS

The periodic table constitutes a valuable tool that systematizes the physical and chemical properties of the elements.

The utility of the periodic table lies in its ability to provide clues to the physical and chemical behavior of the elements and their compounds. Mendeleyev, the chemist who first arranged atoms systematically, could predict the existence and behavior of elements unknown during his time, such as ekasilicon, now known as germanium. A knowledge of periodic relationships enabled atomic scientists to postulate the properties of unknown post-uranic elements successfully so that

procedures could be designed for their recovery from atomic reaction products.

Based on periodic law, the periodic table arranges the elements into horizontal rows, with the same outermost, partly filled, major quantum groups, and into vertical columns that have elements with the same valence electron structures. As a result, in any given vertical group (*family*) the members exhibit similar behavior patterns. Differences are a matter of degree, depending upon atomic radius and the type of closed shell underlying the valence electron(s).

The preferred way of designating columns in the periodic table is controversial. In this chapter the vertical groups of the periodic table are identified by the Roman numerals I to VIII, except for the inert gases which are assigned as Group 0. Each group divides into two subfamilies, A and B. In this chapter the *typical elements* will be designated the A subgroup—thus, I-A is the alkali metals; the transition element members of the family will be designated the B subgroup. Group VIII is not divided into A and B subgroups. It consists of three triads of elements. The members of a given triad are remarkably similar in both physical and chemical properties, such as the first triad of cobalt, nickel, and iron.

Hydrogen ($1s^1$) and helium ($1s^2$) constitute the first row of the periodic table. Although helium clearly is the first member of Group 0, hydrogen customarily is placed at the head of both Group I-A, the alkalies, and Group VII-A, the halogens. Like the alkali metals, it exists as the monovalent cation H^+, but like the halogens, it also can exist as the monovalent anion H^-, the hydride ion.

Many of the vertical groups of the periodic table have common names. Those already identified are Group 0, the inert gases; Group I-A, the alkali metals; Group II-A, the alkaline earths; and Group VII-A, the halogens. Additional named groups are Group VI-A, the chalcogens; Group I-B, the coinage elements; and Group II-B, the volatile elements.

Those elements in which a d orbital is filled partially, starting at Group III-B and ending at Group II-B, are known as the *transition elements*. Horizontal similarities exist to a varying degree in the transition elements, especially in the lower oxidation states. As an example, the element palladium, to the left of silver, forms an insoluble chloride, $PdCl_2$, which is soluble in ammonia.

The lanthanides and actinides (inner transition elements) are fourteen member families in which f orbitals have 1 to 14 electrons. Each family has very strong horizontal similarities because the electrons in the partly filled external s, p, and d orbitals are identical for most.

Because the energy levels of the electrons in the d and f orbitals of the transition elements and the inner transition elements, respectively, differ only slightly, these elements give rise to colored compounds. The energy emitted when an excited electron falls to a vacant lower level within the d or f orbitals is that of radiation in the visible range of light.

Starting at the upper-right corner of the periodic table, as one proceeds down and to the left, the elements assume increasing metallic character; they become more basic, and less electronegative (more electropositive). The simple anions become less stable and the simple cations more stable. Thus, it may be said the nonmetals occupy the upper-right area of the periodic table and the metallic elements are found to the left and toward the bottom. The so-called *heavy metals* are found in the two bottom rows. Metallic elements, for the most part, are *protein precipitants,* the major exception being the alkali metals. Being pro-

Table 24-4. Nomenclature for Common Ligands

LIGAND	PREFERRED PREFIX	LIGAND	PREFERRED PREFIX
H_2O	Aqua	HS^-	Mercapto
NH_3	Ammine	S^{2-}	Thio (sulfo)[a] (sulfido)
CO	Carbonyl	S_2^{2-}	Disulfido
F^-	Fluoro	SO_3^{2-}	Sulfito
Cl^-	Chloro	SO_4^{2-}	Sulfato
Br^-	Bromo	$S_2O_3^{2-}$	Thiosulfato
I^-	Iodo	NO	Nitrosyl
O^{2-}	Oxo (oxy)	ONO^-	Nitrito
O_2^{2-}	Peroxo (peroxy)	NO_2^-	Nitro
OH^-	Hydroxo (hydroxy)	CN^-	Cyano
$C_2O_4^{2-}$	Oxalato	SCN^-	Thiocyanato
$NH_2CH_2CH_2NH_2$	Ethylenediamine, or *en*	NCS^-	Isothiocyanato

[a] Forms in parentheses are also used.

Table 24-5. Examples of Modern Nomenclature

FORMULA	CLASSIC NAME	STOCK NAME	EWENS-BASSETT[a]
$K_2[HgI_4]$	Potassium mercuric iodide	Potassium tetraiodomercurate (II)	(−2)
$[Ag(NH_3)_2]^+$	Silver ammonia ion	Diamminesilver (I) ion	(+1)
$Na_3[Au(S_2O_3)_2]$	Sodium gold thiosulfate	Sodium dithiosulfatoaurate (I)	(−3)
$[Fe(H_2O)_6]Cl_3$	Hydrated ferric chloride	Hexaaquairon (III) chloride	(+3)
$BiOCl$	Bismuthyl chloride	Bismuth (III) chloride oxide	c
$[Ni(CO)_4]$	Nickel carbonyl	Tetracarbonyl nickel (O)	c
$[(NH_3)_5CoO_2Co(NH_3)_5]^{4+}$	—	Decammine-μ-peroxodicobalt (III) ion[b]	(+4)
$Na_2[Fe(CN)_5(NO)] \cdot 2H_2O$	Sodium nitroprusside	Sodium pentacyanonitrosylferrate (III) dihydrate	(−2)

[a] This number, as shown, substitutes for the Roman numeral of the Stock name.
[b] This ion illustrates the use of μ to indicate a bridging structure, in this case the peroxo group.
[c] Not applicable.

tein precipitants, metals, especially heavy metals, are toxic. For example Ba, Tl, Pb, and Hg are violent poisons.

From the above it is obvious there must be an area in the periodic table where the elements are equally acidic and basic, that is, *amphoteric*. If a line is drawn diagonally through hydrogen and beryllium and through aluminum, germanium, antimony, and polonium, the elements on the line and some adjacent to it, are amphoteric. Thus, as a base, aluminum forms compounds such as aluminum chloride; as an acid, it forms sodium aluminate equally well.

In every *typical* element family the first member of the family can be quite unlike the other members. It more closely resembles the second member of the adjacent group to the right. These diagonally related elements are known as *diagonals* or *bridge* elements. They are

IA	IIA	IIIA	IVA	VA	VIA	VIIA
Li	Be	B	C	N	O	F
Na	Mg	Al	Si	P	S	Cl

Beryllium and aluminum constitute a bridge pair. Beryllium fluoride is water soluble (but poorly ionized), whereas the fluorides of magnesium and the other alkaline earths are sparingly soluble. Unlike magnesium and the alkaline earths, beryllium readily acts as the central ion of complexes, both in the solid state and in solution. Like aluminum, beryllium is amphoteric, gives rise to alums, catalyses the Friedel-Craft reaction, and so on.

Tables 24-6 to 24-17 will summarize some useful properties and facts concerning the groups of the periodic table. The sec-

ond and third row *triads* of Group VIII and the lanthanides and actinides are not included in these tables because they present no important applications in pharmacy and medicine.

The *orbital electrons* are important because they predict the possible oxidation states, the shielding of the nuclear charge, and the polarizability for each element. Those oxidation states that have been identified for each element also are listed.

The *atomic radius* and the *ionic radii* give an indication of the relative size of the members of a family. The negative ions of an element are always larger than the neutral atom; the positive ions are always smaller. Because of the increasing effective nuclear charge for a given element, cations of higher charge always are smaller than those with a lower charge. This is important because it gives an indication of the effective coordination number of cations and atoms as central units of complexes.

The *ionization potential* is a measure of the energy required to remove an electron by overcoming the attractive force of the nucleus. *Note:* This use of the word *potential* is improper; ionization potential is a measure of energy. It is related to atomic size; removal of the first electron from beryllium and barium requires 9.3 ev and 5.2 ev, respectively. Because the removal of one electron effectively increases the nuclear charge by one unit, the second ionization potential is about double that of the first, 18.2 ev and 9.95 ev for beryllium and barium, respectively.

Electronegativity, discussed previously, gives an indication of the type of bonding resulting when two atoms react. It gives an indication of the extent of polarization in covalent compounds. It also is used to determine the order of citation in the naming of binary compounds.

ELEMENTS OF GROUP 0

Because the inert gases were unknown at the time, Mendeleyev made no provision for them in his proposed atomic table. With their subsequent discovery Group 0 seemed the most appropriate designation. The group fits very nicely into Mendeleyev's arrangement. Its presence explains the extreme transition of properties in going from the very electronegative halogen family to the very electropositive alkali metal family. This shift in properties in going from halogen to inert gas to alkali metal is shown clearly by the change in the valence electron structures:

$$(n-1)s^2(n-1)p^5 \rightarrow (n-1)s^2(n-1)p^6 \rightarrow (n-1)s^2(n-1)p^6ns^1$$

All Group 0 elements except radon occur in the atmosphere. Helium also occurs in commercial quantities in certain natural gases in the southwestern US. Argon, neon, krypton, and xenon are produced from liquid air by fractional distillation. Helium is produced similarly from the natural gases named above. Radon is recovered from the natural decay products of radium.

The inert gases are monoatomic and are colorless, odorless gases under ordinary conditions of temperature and pressure. They vary widely in atomic mass and atomic volume. These dif-

ferences are reflected in the values of their physical constants (Table 24-6).

Each inert gas, except helium, is characterized by an outermost electron shell of the *inert gas* structure, ns^2np^6 (see Table 24-6). Helium has the $1s^2$ structure; the ns^2 structure is achieved in many stable cations, for example, Pb^{2+}. Because all electrons are paired, the chemical inertness of the group is predictable and is reflected in terms of peak ionization potentials and various other characteristics. However, under unusual reaction conditions, there is evidence of hydrate formation. Some relatively stable fluorides, such as XeF_2, XeF_4, and XeF_6, a crystalline sodium perxenate, and possibly a perkryptate, are known.

However, in comparison with other elements, those of Group 0 still are classed logically as chemically inert.

Helium, because of its low density and low solubility in blood is used to prepare synthetic airs.

Argon is relatively plentiful as it is a byproduct of the fractionation of liquid air for the production of oxygen and nitrogen. It is used as an inert atmosphere for industrial processes in

Table 24-6. The Elements of Group 0[a]

ELEMENT	HELIUM	NEON	ARGON	KRYPTON	XENON	RADON
Symbol	He	Ne	Ar	Kr	Xe	Rn
Atomic number	2	10	18	36	54	86
Atomic weight[b]	4.003	20.18	39.95	83.80	131.3	(222)[d]
Orbital electrons	$1s^2$	$[He]2s^2p^6$	$[Ne]3s^23p^6$	$[Ar]3d^{10}4s^24p^6$	$[Kr]4d^{10}5s^25p^6$	$[Xe]4f^{14}5d^{10}6s^26p^6$
Atomic radius (A)	1.80	1.60	1.92	2.00	2.20	2.29
Ionization potential,[c] ev	24.6	21.6	15.8	14.0	12.1	10.7
% by volume in air	5×10^{-4}	15×10^{-4}	0.94	11×10^{-5}	9×10^{-6}	—

[a] Physical data are from reference 4. Atomic and ionic radii are from Pauling[5] and modified by the work of Shannon and Prewitt.[6] See also reference 7.
[b] Given to four significant figures.
[c] First ionization potential, unless otherwise noted.
[d] Atomic weights in parenthesis are now known exactly.
Note: The above apply to Tables 24-6 to 24-17.

which nitrogen, the usual inert atmosphere, reacts with the materials present.

Krypton and xenon have been investigated for possible use as anesthetics. However, the sparsity of these elements in nature imposes severe limitations on such use. ^{133}Xe is used for diagnostic studies both by inhalation and intravenous injection.

Radon is used instead of radium in the treatment of certain types of cancer. Sealed tubes containing the gas are embedded in the tissues to be treated. Both radium and radon emit alpha particles in the first stage of their radioactive decay. Radon is a public health concern because it has been found in the basements of some private homes.

ELEMENTS OF GROUP I

The elements of Group I (Tables 24-7 and 24-8) are characterized by having only one valence electron, ns^1. The subgroups differ in that Group I-A has an underlying, stable, inert gas shell, $(n-1)s^2(n-1)p^6ns^1$, whereas in Group I-B this has been replaced by a completed d shell, $(n-1)d^{10}ns^1$.

These elements are strongly metallic, giving rise to cations, M^+. Because electrons can be removed from the underlying d shell, Group I-B elements can exhibit higher positive oxidation states, M^{2+} and M^{3+}.

the salts are neutral to strongly basic, depending on the strength of the anion as a Brønsted base. Most distinguishing properties of the salts and their solutions are due to the anion present, rather than the cation; if they are colored, the anion is responsible.

The cations hydrate in aqueous media; the degree of solvation decreases with increasing atomic number. In the crystalline state only lithium and sodium regularly form hydrates. Potassium and ammonium salts (below) rarely are hydrated; if hydrated, the water usually is associated with the anion.

Elements of Group I-A

Group I-A comprises the most reactive of all the metallic elements, and the activity increases with atomic number. The cations of these elements are stable chemically; the free elements are not found in nature. The single positive charge of the nucleus is screened effectively by the inert gas shell, thus these cations have little or no polarizing effect on anions and molecules and therefore do not form complexes.

The hydroxides give alkaline solutions, alkalinity increasing with atomic number. Alkali metal salts of common inorganic and organic acids are ionic, are usually colorless and, with few exceptions, are readily soluble in water. Aqueous solutions of

SODIUM AND POTASSIUM

Except for those properties due to mass and degree of hydration, sodium and potassium compounds are remarkably similar. Sodium salts are selected more frequently for use on a strictly economic basis. In addition, because of the lower atomic weight of sodium, there usually are more reactive units per gram when using sodium salts. (However, the greater hydration of the sodium versus the potassium salts may partially or entirely erase this latter advantage.)

Despite the foregoing factors, subtle differences often favor use of the potassium salt. Generally, a given potassium salt is more soluble in nonpolar solvents. Potassium salts generally are

Table 24-7. Elements of Group I-A

ELEMENT	HYDROGEN	LITHIUM	SODIUM	POTASSIUM	RUBIDIUM	CESIUM	FRANCIUM
Symbol	H	Li	Na	K	Rb	Cs	Fr
Atomic number	1	3	11	19	37	55	87
Atomic weight	1.008	6.94_1	22.99	39.10	85.47	132.91	(223)
Orbital electrons	$1s^1$	$[He]2s^1$	$[Ne]3s^1$	$[Ar]4s^1$	$[Kr]5s^1$	$[Xe]6s^1$	$[Rn]7s^1$
Oxidation states	$-1, +1$	$+1$	$+1$	$+1$	$+1$	$+1$	$+1$
Atomic radius (Å)	0.37	1.50	1.86	2.31	2.44	2.62	—
Ionic radius (Å)	1.36 (-1)[a]	0.60 $(+1)$	0.95 $(+1)$	1.33 $(+1)$	1.48 $(+1)$	1.69 $(+1)$	1.76 $(+1)$
Ionic (hydrated) radius (Å)	—	3.40	2.76	3.32	2.28	2.28	—
Ionization potential	13.527	5.39	5.14	4.34	4.18	3.89	—
Electronegativity,[b] ev	2.1	0.98	0.93	0.82	0.82	0.79	0.7
% of earth's crust	0.127	6.5×10^{-3}	2.8	2.6	3.1×10^{-2}	7×10^{-4}	—

[a] Hydride ion; figure in parenthesis is the oxidation state.
[b] Pauling scale.[5]

Table 24-8. The Elements of Groups I-B and II-B

ELEMENT	COPPER	SILVER	GOLD	ZINC	CADMIUM	MERCURY
Symbol	Cu	Ag	Au	Zn	Cd	Hg
Atomic number	29	47	79	30	48	80
Atomic weight	63.54	107.87	196.97	65.38	112.4	200.5_9
Orbital electrons	$[Ar]3d^{10}4s^1$	$[Kr]4d^{10}5s^1$	$[Xe]4f^{14}5d^{10}6s^1$	$[Ar]3d^{10}4s^2$	$[Kr]4d^{10}5s^2$	$[Xe]4f^{14}5d^{10}6s^2$
Oxidation states	+1, +2	+1, +2	+1, (+2), +3	+2	+2	+1, +2
Atomic radius (Å)	1.40	1.70	1.70	1.40	1.60	1.50
Ionic (crystal) radii (Å)	0.96 (+1)	1.26 (+1)	1.37 (+1)	—	—	1.27 (+1)
	0.72 (+2)	0.89 (+2)	0.99 (+3)	0.88 (+2)	1.09 (+2)	1.16 (+2)
Ionization potential, ev	7.724	7.574	9.223	6.92	8.99	10.42
Electronegativity	1.90	1.93	2.54	1.65	1.69	2.00
% of earth's crust	10^{-4}	10^{-8}	10^{-9}	1.3×10^{-2}	1.5×10^{-5}	ca 10^{-6}

less deliquescent than the corresponding sodium salt; for example, potassium permanganate is used rather than the deliquescent sodium permanganate. Finally, the living cell differentiates between the two cations; sodium is the cation of the extracellular fluids, whereas potassium is the cation of the intracellular fluids.

Sodium compounds are used widely in pharmacy and medicine. With a few exceptions, such as sodium chloride in electrolyte replenishers, the therapeutic activity is referable to the anionic component of the salt. Sodium is commonly the cation of choice to optimize the pharmaceutical utility of organic medicaments, as in methiodal sodium, phenobarbital sodium, or sodium citrate.

Because of the propensity of sodium ion to promote retention of water in the tissues, sodium salts are used with caution in the treatment of cardiac and renal conditions in which edema is a problem. Some drugs, such as hydrochlorothiazide, promote excretion of potassium ion to an extent requiring auxiliary dietary intake of potassium, usually as the chloride or gluconate. Potassium ion has a diuretic effect. The thiazides also cause the excretion of magnesium ion.

RUBIDIUM AND CESIUM

Rubidium and its cation are very similar in behavior to potassium. Neither rubidium nor cesium find application in pharmacy and medicine at this time.

LITHIUM

Being a bridge element, the behavior of the element lithium and its compounds often is decidedly different from that of the other members of the alkali family. At room temperature the free metal is much less reactive with water; on burning it forms the normal oxide rather than the peroxide. Lithium carbonates and phosphates are only slightly water-soluble. Its chloride is soluble in organic solvents. Lithium salts are highly hydrated. In all of these properties lithium resembles magnesium, and to some extent calcium, more closely than sodium.

Lithium has no normal physiological role. In its former therapeutic applications (eg, lithium bromide) the activity was inherent in the anion. However, because of the toxic character of the lithium ion, as revealed by use of lithium chloride in salt substitutes, continued use of these lithium compounds is not justified. Lithium Carbonate USP and Lithium Citrate USP have been found valuable in the treatment of hypomanic and manic states. However, these patients must be monitored carefully for blood lithium levels because of the toxicity of the cation.

AMMONIA AND AMMONIUM COMPOUNDS

Ammonia [NH_3] coordinates readily with a proton to form the ammonium ion [NH_4]$^+$. This ion displays many of the properties of the alkali metal ions. Its salts show a striking resemblance to

potassium and rubidium salts, with which they are commonly isomorphous. The relationship extends to solubilities, as evidenced by the general water solubility of ammonium salts of inorganic and organic acids, but the low water solubility of such salts as the bitartrate, chloroplatinate, and perchlorate.

However, there are important differences. *Ammonium hydroxide* (mainly a solution of ammonia molecules in water) is feebly basic. The equilibrium

$$NH_3 + H_2O \rightleftharpoons NH_4^+ + OH^-$$

lies strongly to the left unless the hydroxyl ion is removed by neutralization. Solutions of ammonium salts are acidic rather than basic.

Ammonium salts commonly used therapeutically include the carbonate, chloride, and bromide. The bromide is used as a central depressant. Both the chloride and carbonate are common ingredients in expectorant preparations.

In aqueous solution form, ammonia is used in pharmacy as a mild alkalizer. It often is preferred to the alkali bases because of its volatility, any excess being detected by its odor, and it is removed readily by heat. The ammonia in household use contains 10% NH_3 and is known as 16° ammonia (degrees Baumé, a concentration term).

Elements of Group I-B

The Group I-B elements have been known since antiquity. Because they occur in the free metallic state, are relatively easy to recover from their ores, and they are very malleable, they have been used throughout history to make decorative vessels and jewelry. They have been employed for centuries as a measure of monetary wealth and for the fabrication of coins, hence the family name *coinage metals*.

These elements and their compounds are strikingly different from those of Group I-A. Colored compounds are numerous. The hydroxides and many of the simple salts are insoluble in water. All readily act as the central unit of complexes. The soluble compounds of these elements are toxic. A summary of their important characteristics is given in Table 24-8.

COPPER

Of the monovalent compounds, copper(I) oxide, Cu_2O, and copper(I) chloride, Cu_2Cl_2, are used most frequently. Important copper(II) (cupric) salts are the oxide, CuO, and sulfate, $CuSO_4 \cdot 5H_2O$. Copper compounds are toxic.

Copper is an essential trace element. Small quantities enhance the physiological utilization of iron. It occurs in the respiratory pigment hemocyanin, in many enzymes, and is distributed widely in foods.

Copper compounds have been used in a variety of medicinal applications. Copper gluconate, cupric chloride dihydrate, and cupric sulfate pentahydrate are the officially cited copper compounds at this time. The radioactive ^{64}Cu isotope has been employed in mineral metabolism studies. Copper(II) sulfate is the basis for Fehling's and Benedict's Solutions, the classic test solutions for reducing sugars. Various copper compounds find commercial application as fungicides and insecticides, and they are particularly effective algaecides.

SILVER

With the exception of the nitrate and fluoride, the common salts of silver in the +1 oxidation state are insoluble or only slightly soluble in water. Many, including the oxide, react with and dissolve in ammonia water; the iodide and sulfide are important exceptions. Silver also forms a +2 series of salts. Silver has an oligodynamic action. Water distilled in contact with silver metal remains sterile over long periods of time.

Because of the ability of silver ion to precipitate protein and chloride in the affected tissue, silver compounds such as silver nitrate are employed to provide local germicidal action. Silver sulfadiazine is used topically as a germicide. Silver is released slowly from these *in situ* precipitates to give lasting germicidal action. Cosmetic problems can result because of discoloration due to the photosensitivity of silver ion.

Preparations containing silver or silver compounds in colloidal solution once were used widely as topical antiseptics; eg Mild Silver Protein, for which there is a renewed interest in ophthalmology. By increasing their concentration, silver ions may be used to bring about protein precipitation. To reduce brittleness, some silver chloride (5%) is formed in silver nitrate by adding hydrochloric acid or potassium chloride; the product, Toughened Silver Nitrate, is cast into sticks and used as a styptic.

The ready reducibility of silver ion to elemental silver gives rise to various instability problems and incompatibilities. Because silver compounds are light sensitive, they must be protected by the use of light-resistant containers. The soluble silver salts are toxic. However, the toxicity usually is limited, owing to local precipitation of adherent layers of silver protein and silver chloride.

GOLD

Two series of gold compounds exist: for example, AuCl, gold(I) chloride (aurous chloride); and $AuCl_3$, gold(III) chloride (auric chloride). Gold readily acts as the center for the formation of complexes, for example, $Na_3[Au(S_2O_3)_2]$, sodium dithiosulfatoaurate(I), sodium dithiosulfatoaurate(-3), gold sodium thiosulfate.

Chemically gold salts are characterized by instability to heat, light, and even very mild reducing agents. Simple gold(I) salts can undergo *autoxidation,* giving rise to finely divided metal and the corresponding gold(III) compound. The stability

of the gold ions is improved by complexation. This particularly is true if a sulfur linkage is available. Because of the ease of reduction, gold compounds must be handled with exceptional care and, if possible, dispensed separately.

At the present time, gold compounds are employed in the treatment of lupus erythematosus and rheumatoid arthritis. Aurothioglucose and gold sodium thiomalate are listed in the USP. Because these gold compounds are absorbed poorly when given orally, parenteral administration is required.

Dimercaprol (BAL) is used as an antidote if the patient shows signs of gold toxicity. Auranofin, [(2,3,4,6-tetra-*O*-acetyl-1-thio- β-d-glucopyranosato)(triethylphosphine)gold], is available in a tablet dosage form and is showing some success in the oral treatment of rheumatoid arthritis.

The radioactive isotope ^{198}Au is employed therapeutically in the treatment of certain malignancies.

Each element in Group II is characterized by the presence of two *s* electrons in the outermost orbital. Subgroup II-A elements have a $(n-1)s^2(n-1)p^6ns^2$ outer electron structure, except for the small beryllium atom whose structure is $1s^22s^2$. Subgroup II-B differs in that its underlying electron structure is the filled *d* orbital, $(n-1)d^{10}ns^2$.

Elements of Group II-A

Although Group II-A is called the *alkaline earth group,* there is some question whether magnesium, and especially beryllium, should be included under that title. Except for amphoteric beryllium, these elements are strictly metallic. Like the alkali metals, because of chemical reactivity, they do not occur free in nature. They function uniformly in the +2 oxidation state (Table 24-9).

The similarity existing between calcium, strontium, and barium is especially striking. Calcium, strontium, and barium react readily with water to form hydroxides with the simultaneous evolution of hydrogen. Magnesium reacts similarly but only at elevated temperatures. The hydroxides of beryllium and magnesium are insoluble in water; that of beryllium is amphoteric. Although less soluble than the alkali hydroxides, the hydroxides of calcium, strontium, and barium give strongly basic solutions. The carbonates, phosphates, sulfates, and fluorides are insoluble; they are important in analytical work.

Except for hydrate formation, the three heavier members of the family do not form complex ions. Magnesium forms a few crystalline complexes of the type K_2MgF_4.

BERYLLIUM

Being amphoteric, the element beryllium appears both as simple salts and berylates. The cation complexes readily, as in $[Be(H_2O)_4]^{2+}$ or $[Be(NH_3)_4]^{2+}$. As a *bridge element,* beryllium

Table 24-9. The Elements of Group II-A

ELEMENT	BERYLLIUM	MAGNESIUM	CALCIUM	STRONTIUM	BARIUM	RADIUM
Symbol	Be	Mg	Ca	Sr	Ba	Ra
Atomic number	4	12	20	38	56	88
Atomic weight	9.012	24.31	40.08	87.62	137.3	226.03
Orbital electrons	[He]$2s^2$	[Ne]$3s^2$	[Ar]$4s^2$	[Kr]$5s^2$	[Xe]$6s^2$	[Rn]$7s^2$
Oxidation states	+2	+2	+2	+2	+2	+2
Atomic radius (Å)	0.90	1.70	1.74	1.92	1.98	—
Ionic (crystal) radius (Å) (coordination number 6)	0.31 (+2)[a]	0.65 (+2)	0.99 (+2)	1.13 (+2)	1.35 (+2)	1.43 (+2)
Ionization potential, ev (II)[b]	9.3	7.6	6.1	5.7	5.2	5.252
	18.2	15.0	11.9	11.0	9.95	10.099
Electronegativity	1.57	1.31	1.00	0.95	0.89	0.9
% of earth's crust	6×10^{-4}	2.1	3.6	0.03	0.025	1.3×10^{-10}

[a] Coordination number 4.
[b] Second ionization potential.

resembles aluminum in its behavior. This similarity is so striking that many early workers considered beryllium a lighter member of the aluminum family before Mendeleyev correctly placed it in Group II. Although its ionic diameter is considerably greater than that of beryllium, the higher +3 charge on the aluminum ion results in a polarizing ability similar to that of beryllium. Both elements dissolve in caustic alkalis and both form a protective coating on their surface when placed in nitric acid. The halides of both elements have similar solubilities in organic solvents. Both elements act as Lewis acids and give rise to alums.

Beryllium metal and its compounds are extremely toxic when ingested, inhaled, or absorbed through the skin. None of its compounds are employed as therapeutic agents.

MAGNESIUM

Magnesium is a relatively abundant element that is chemically active. The cation, Mg^{2+}, is stable under all conditions ordinarily met in pharmaceutical practice. Magnesium compounds are employed for a variety of purposes in therapeutics. Many of its insoluble compounds are used as gastric antacids. The hydroxide and sulfate are used as cathartics, and the sulfate as an anticonvulsant. A concentrated solution of the sulfate often is used topically as a bath so that, by osmotic action of the concentrated sulfate solution, a local infection may be drawn to the surface of the skin and be expelled.

Toxic manifestations following magnesium administration are relatively rare; calcium gluconate given intravenously is an effective antidote. The stearate is employed as a lubricant in the preparation of compressed tablets. The artificial radioactive isotope ^{27}Mg, has been employed in research involving photosynthesis.

There is an increasing awareness of the critical importance of magnesium ions in human biochemistry. Because ion- specific electrode potentiometry now allows measurement of free, unbound magnesium ions, plasma concentrations may be measured and the concentration in the cytosol may be inferred. As the second most plentiful cation inside the cell and a natural calcium channel blocker, magnesium ions are important in many cardiovascular diseases. Successful absorption from the gastrointestinal tract appears to depend on the nature of the magnesium salt that is used.

CALCIUM

Calcium is a relatively reactive metal whose cation is stable. However, soluble calcium salts undergo metathesis with soluble borates, carbonates, citrates, oxalates, phosphates, sulfates, and tartrates to yield insoluble calcium compounds. These reactions often lead to pharmaceutical incompatibilities.

Calcium is indispensable to life. Calcium, and to a much lesser degree, magnesium, is the cation of hydroxyapatite, the major constituent (98%) of the bones and teeth. Calcium is essential to many physiological processes. Therapeutic categories represented by official calcium compounds include: antacids and calcium replenishers.

Calcium is frequently the cation of choice to carry therapeutically active anions, such as calcium aminosalicylate and calcium cyclobarbital. In some instances, this is referable to better physical characteristics of the calcium compound; in others, it is a deliberate attempt to avoid an unnecessary intake of sodium. The artificial radioactive ^{45}Ca isotope has been employed in studies involving mineral metabolism.

STRONTIUM

The behavior of the element strontium is very similar to calcium. Ingested, its distribution is similar to that of calcium. At this time it has no application in pharmacy or medicine. In the

past it has been used as the carrier cation for therapeutically active anions, as in strontium bromide.

BARIUM

Chemically, barium is the most active of Group II-A. Its cation is stable under all ordinary conditions. Barium hydroxide is soluble and is a strong base. Because of this, it often finds application in analytical and synthetic operations.

In sharp contrast to the lighter members of Group II-A all barium compounds that are soluble either in water or in dilute acid are poisonous. The most readily available antidote for barium ingestion is magnesium sulfate (Epsom Salt).

With the exception of barium sulfate, which finds use as a radiopaque, barium compounds are not employed as medicinal agents. Barium hydroxide lime is employed as a carbon dioxide absorber. Artificial radioactive isotopes of barium have been employed in pharmacokinetic investigations.

Elements of Group II-B

Because zinc, cadmium, and mercury (see Table 24-8) have comparatively low boiling points, 907°, 768°, and 357°, respectively; they are referred to frequently as the *volatile metals*. The common oxidation state is +2, but mercury also exists in the +1 state. This latter state is achieved by the formation of a covalent, two electron bond between two mercury atoms. Thus the mercury(I) ion (mercurous) is always written Hg_2^{2+}. The filled $(n-1)d^{10}$ orbital is stable in this family. Unlike Group I-B there are no oxidation states involving loss of a d electron. There is increasing covalent character in the salts of these elements; for example, fused zinc chloride conducts electric current whereas the mercury chlorides do not. These elements readily complex with most common ligands and concentrated solutions exhibit autocomplexation. Only zinc is sufficiently amphoteric to form a stable oxygen complex, ZnO_2^{2-}, the zincate ion.

ZINC

All soluble zinc salts show some degree of hydrolysis,

$$Zn^{2+} + 2H_2O \rightleftharpoons [Zn(OH)]^+ + H_3O^+$$

Thus, all zinc salts of weak Brønsted bases show an acid reaction.

Zinc has many therapeutic applications in the treatment of various external surfaces of the body and in wound healing, taste acuity, and various ophthalmic problems (eg, macular degeneration). Strong zinc sulfate solution is used as an emetic; its emetic action is so rapid that little or no zinc salt is absorbed. Zinc is present in all living organisms; it is distributed widely in foods. It is an essential trace element and an essential component of carbonic anhydrase and many other enzymes.

Zinc compounds soluble in water or in the gastric fluid, eg, ZnO, may be poisonous. There is a relatively wide margin of safety between the required intake and toxic intake. The most readily available antidote is sodium bicarbonate (baking soda).

Artificial radioactive isotopes of zinc have been employed in studies of mineral metabolism.

CADMIUM

Cadmium is truly intermediate in properties to zinc and mercury. Soluble cadmium compounds are astringent; $CdSO_4$ has been used both as a topical astringent and for eye infections. Cadmium sulfide has been introduced for the treatment of seborrheic dermatitis. In Japan, Itai-Itai disease is believed to be caused by drinking water contaminated with cadmium.

Table 24-10. The Elements of Group III-A

ELEMENT	BORON	ALUMINUM	GALLIUM	INDIUM	THALLIUM
Symbol	B	Al	Ga	In	Tl
Atomic number	5	13	31	49	81
Atomic weight	10.81	26.98	69.72	114.8	204.3_7
Orbital electrons	$[He]2s^22p^1$	$[Ne]3s^23p^1$	$[Ar]3d^{10}4s^24p^1$	$[Kr]4d^{10}5s^25p^1$	$[Xe]4f^{14}5d^{10}6s^26p^1$
Oxidation states	+3	(+1), +3	+1, +2, +3	+1, +3	+1, +3
Atomic radius (Å)	0.82	1.25	1.26	1.44	2.0
Ionic (crystal) radius (Å)	—	—	1.90 (+1)	1.90 (+1)	1.64 (+1)
(coordination number 6)	0.20 (+3)[a]	0.675 (+3)	0.76 (+3)	0.94 (+3)	1.03 (+3)
Ionization potential, ev	8.30	5.95	6.0	5.8	6.1
(II)[b]	25.15	18.82	20.4	18.8	20.3
(III)[b]	37.92	28.44	30.6	27.9	29.7
Electronegativity	2.04	1.61	1.81	1.78	1.62
% of earth's crust	3×10^{-4}	8.13	1.5×10^{-3}	10^{-5}	ca 10^{-4}

[a] Coordination number 4.
[b] Second and third ionization potential.

MERCURY

Mercury is a true metal. As indicated previously, it alone of the family has two series of salts. Mercury and its compounds are extremely toxic. Mercury metal, because of its low boiling point, has an appreciable vapor pressure even at room temperature.

All common mercury salts are poisonous. The best antidote for mercury poisoning, particularly the bichloride, is Sodium Formaldehyde Sulfoxylate NF. Egg albumen may be used in an emergency if the poisoning is discovered shortly after ingestion. The white of one egg should be administered for each 250 mg of mercuric chloride ingested. Emesis should be induced promptly thereafter. If mercury is spilled it should be recovered immediately. Mercury that falls into cracks and other difficult to clean places is removed best by covering with powdered sulfur, allowing several days for conversion to sulfide, then vacuuming.

In former years, metallic mercury was important therapeutically as a cathartic and parasiticide, but it has been replaced largely by more efficacious and less toxic medicaments. The FDA has now issued guidelines for the over-the-counter use of mercury compounds. The April 22, 1998 *Federal Register* contained an FDA announcement about OTC mercury compounds, a summary of which is given here.

"Since 1980, the FDA has instituted progressively restrictive rules on mercury-containing OTC drug products. Now in the absence of any components or data from manufacturers supporting the use of these products, FDA has declared all mercury-containing drugs for OTC products as 'not generally recognized as safe and effective' or 'misbranded.' Effective October 19, 1998, the new rule outlaws well-known products such as Mercurochrome (merbromin), calomel (mercurous chloride), and thimerosal for all OTC first-aid antiseptics, diaper rash products, and vaginal contraceptives."

Monographs for Ammoniated Mercury (ointment and ophthalmic ointment) and Nitromersol (and topical solution) are found in the USP.

The radioactive nuclides ^{197}Hg and ^{203}Hg are used in a diagnostic capacity.

ELEMENTS OF GROUP III

Group III of the periodic table includes some 36 elements which, on the basis of external electron structure, divide into the usual Group III-A (Table 24-10) with 5 elements, and Group III-B with 31 elements. Subgroup III-B further divides into the usual transition elements (Table 24-11), the *lanthanides* (14 elements) and *actinides* (14 elements). (See the Periodic Chart of the Elements in the back of this textbook.) The lanthanide cerium, as cerium(IV), is a widely used analytical reagent. Because the lanthanides and actinides have no applications in pharmacy, further discussion is unnecessary.

The members of this family are very reactive and do not appear in nature in the free state. They have no known biological role.

Table 24-11. Transition Elements

	GROUP III-B			GROUP IV-B		
ELEMENT	SCANDIUM	YTTRIUM	LANTHANUM	TITANIUM	ZIRCONIUM	HAFNIUM
Symbol	Sc	Y	La	Ti	Zr	Hf
Atomic number	21	39	57	22	40	72
Atomic weight	44.96	88.91	138.9	47.90	91.22	178.5
Orbital electrons	$[Ar]3d^14s^2$	$[Kr]4d^15s^2$	$[Xe]5d^16s^2$	$[Ar]3d^24s^2$	$[Kr]4d^25s^2$	$[Xe]4f^{14}5d^26s^2$
Oxidation states	3+	3+	3+	2+, 3+, 4+	2+, 4+	(2+), 4+
Atomic radius (Å)	1.51	1.8	1.87	1.36	1.45	1.44
Ionic radii (Å)	0.81 (3+)	0.93 (3+)	1.15 (3+)	1.00 (2+)	—	—
(coordination number 6)				0.75 (4+)	0.86 (4+)	0.85 (4+)
Ionization potential, ev	6.7	6.5	5.6	6.82	6.84	ca 5.5
Electronegativity	1.54	1.53	1.3	—	—	—
% of earth's crust	0.44	0.022	4.5×10^{-4}	0.629	0.028	—

Elements of Group III-A

In this family of elements an electron appears in the p orbital of the valence shell for the first time; each element has the structure ns^2np^1. Theoretically two oxidation states are possible. The first, $+1$, arises by the loss of the single p electron. The resulting helide structure, ns^2, has sufficient stability to give rise to stable ions such as Ga^+, In^+, and Tl^+. Aluminum has this oxidation state only at elevated temperatures and it is not evident with B, Sc, Y, La.

With the loss of all three valence electrons the $+3$ oxidation state appears in all the elements of the family. With increasing atomic number the $+3$ state becomes more electrovalent in character. Boron trichloride is a covalent compound, aluminum chloride is for practical purposes covalent, and gallium(III) chloride has some covalent character. Because a normal octet is not achieved in these compounds, an electron deficient structure results. As there are only three electron pairs in the valence shell the electron-pair repulsive forces are weaker, and the molecules become electron-pair acceptors.

Due to the weaker repulsive forces, these MX_3 molecules give rise to triangular structures with hybrid sp^2 orbitals. The metal occupies the center of the triangle. By accepting a fourth electron-pair the octet is completed and sp^3 hybrids form. The addends rearrange to give tetrahedral structures with the metal ion in the center of the tetrahedron.

Because the initial compounds, such as $AlCl_3$, are electron-pair deficient, they are Lewis acids. As such, they act as catalysts for the Friedel-Crafts synthesis.

Members of this family give rise to an interesting series of double salts, the *alums*. The common formula is $M^+_2 M^{3+}_2(SO_4)_4 \cdot 24H_2O$, where M^+ is a monovalent ion (eg, Na^+, K^+, Rb^+, NH_4^+, Tl^+) and M^{3+} is a trivalent ion (eg, Al^{3+}, Tl^{3+}, Cr^{3+}, or Fe^{3+}). The prototype of these double salts is alum, $K_2Al_2(SO_4)_4 \cdot 24H_2O$.

BORON

Boron appears only in the $+3$ oxidation state and is a nonmetal. Several oxyacids are known. Metaboric acid, $(HBO_2)_n$, and the metaborate ion do not exist as monomers. Orthoboric acid, $(H_3BO_3)_n$, exists as a hydrogen-bonded layered structure, which explains the flaky form in which it is available. Discrete H_3BO_3 molecules exist in the gaseous state and in solution. It is a weak acid, ionizing in solution.

$$H_3BO_3 + 2H_2O \rightleftharpoons H_3O^+ + [B(OH)_4]^-$$

The pH of a $0.1M$ solution is 5.3. In addition there is a tetraborate, available as borax, usually formulated as $Na_2B_4O_7 \cdot 10H_2O$. In water the tetraborate ion reacts as

$$[B_4O_5(OH)_4]^{2-} + 5H_2O \rightleftharpoons 2[B(OH)_3] + 2[B(OH)_4]^-$$

The strong alkalinity of solutions of all borates is due to the reaction

$$[B(OH)_4]^- \rightleftharpoons [B(OH)_3] + [OH]^-$$

Boric acid is soluble in polyhydroxy compounds such as glycerol. In anhydrous media esterification takes place to form *glyceroborate*. In aqueous media glyceroboric acid forms an acid that is valuable in the analytical determination of boric acid.

Since it is a bridge element, certain properties of boron resemble those of silicon, its diagonal neighbor in Group IV-A. The boron hydrides and boranes resemble the silanes. The borohydride ion, $[BH_4]^-$, is available commercially as the sodium salt, which is a valuable reducing agent.

Boron and its compounds are toxic, both by ingestion and by absorption through broken or inflamed skin. Numerous fatalities have occurred; especially depressing are infants deaths as a result of the use of dusting powders containing boric acid.

However, some dietary mineral formulas include boron in some form, such as amino acid chelate, because boron appears to be involved in bone metabolism.

Boric acid and the borates have no germicidal activity and, at best, are feebly bacteriostatic. On the basis of their toxicity and negligible antiseptic value the use of these compounds is unwarranted.

Boric acid in various dosage forms is employed as a topical anti-infective; in solution it is used as an eye wash. Sodium borate is bacteriostatic and is a frequent ingredient of cold creams, eye washes, and mouthwashes. Sodium perborate is an oxidizing type of local anti-infective. Various borate buffers are used in collyria. A common incompatibility in the use of these buffers is the precipitation of insoluble borates from neutral or alkaline buffers. All common metals, except the alkalies, precipitate as insoluble borates.

Boric Acid and Sodium Borate (borax) are cited in the NF.

ALUMINUM

Aluminum is the most abundant of the metals and the third most abundant element, being exceeded in natural occurrence only by oxygen and silicon. The metal and its hydroxide are amphoteric, but only those compounds in which it acts as a base are pharmaceutically important. As a result of its high charge, small diameter, and electron-pair deficiency, the aluminum (III) ion is incapable of independent existence in polar solvents. Due to the very high field strength surrounding this ion, complexation always takes place.

Many insoluble aluminum compounds find use as gastric antacids. Due to their astringency, soluble aluminum salts are used for various skin conditions and in antiperspirants and deodorants. Kaolin is used as an adsorbent and demulcent, and bentonite is useful as a suspending agent. In paste form, elemental aluminum is employed topically as a protective.

There is some concern about chronic aluminum toxicity and its effect on the brain, possibly manifesting itself in the elderly. The use of aluminum sulfate at very low levels in water purification and the presence of aluminum in baking powder is being questioned.

GALLIUM, INDIUM, AND THALLIUM

The remaining elements of Group III-A, gallium, indium, and thallium, are not of interest in pharmacy except for the use of their radioactive isotopes as diagnostic aids, ^{67}Ga, ^{111}In, ^{113}In, and ^{201}Tl.

Thallium compounds are among the most toxic and are absorbed from the intestine and through the skin from ointments and creams. Its action is somewhat similar to that of arsenic. Deaths have been recorded from a thallium cosmetic use. Thallium compounds have been used in insecticides, especially ant poisons. Thallium(I) is similar to potassium ion in that TlOH is a strong base and their salts are isomorphous. Thallium(III) is similar in behavior to aluminum(III) and gold(III).

Gallium is interesting because, except for mercury, it has the lowest melting point of the metals ($29.75°$). It also is unusual for its $+2$ oxidation state. Because this requires an odd electron it is difficult to explain why gallium(II) compounds are not paramagnetic. It has been postulated that equal numbers of gallium(I) and gallium(III) ions may exist in these compounds to give a formula $M^+[MX_4]^-$. Gallium(III) has properties very similar to iron(III). In fact, gallium (III) binds to transferrin, an iron transport protein, and appears to be useful in treating cancer-related hypercalcemia.

Indium is quite similar to both aluminum and gallium. It too, under very special conditions, exists as a divalent chloride.

Elements of Group III-B

Some properties of the Group III-B elements are given in Table 24-11. These three elements exhibit only the +3 oxidation state and are quite similar. The differences are mostly of degree, de-pendent on the increasing atomic radius. As scandium is the smallest, it has the greatest polarizing power and most readily forms complexes of the type K_3ScF_6. Yttrium has properties approximately midway between scandium and lanthanum. This gradation of properties is shown nicely with the three hydroxides: $Sc(OH)_3$ is a weak base, $Y(OH)_3$ is stronger, and $La(OH)_3$ is a very strong base.

ELEMENTS OF GROUP IV

The elements of this group are similar in that each has four valence electrons, two of which are s electrons. However, the remaining two valence electrons enter different orbitals to give the structure ns^2np^2 for Group IV-A and $(n-1)d^2ns^2$ for Group IV-B. Because of this there is a strong tendency for all members of the family except carbon and silicon to form *inert pair* ions. Except for the larger atoms, many of the compounds are covalent or predominantly covalent. All elements of the family show the +4 oxidation state. Important characteristics of these elements are found in Tables 24-11 and 24-12.

Elements of Group IV-A

Of the Group IV-A elements (Table 24-12), carbon and silicon usually are considered apart from germanium, tin, and lead because of their nonmetallic character and property of catenation. Boron, with which silicon forms a bridge element pair, is quite similar to silicon. The +2 oxidation state rarely is encountered in carbon and silicon. The bonding in carbon is covalent; corresponding silicon bonds have a somewhat greater electrovalent character. Simple carbon compounds are either linear (CO_2), planar triangular (CO_3^{2-}), or tetrahedral (CCl_4). Because the radius of the carbon atom is small, and it lacks d orbitals to expand its valence shell, carbon never increases its coordination number beyond four. Unlike carbon, because of its available d orbitals, silicon can achieve sp^3d^2 hybridization and appears in the octahedral configuration, SiF_6^{2-}, with a maximum coordination number of six. Similarly, germanium, tin, and lead have a maximum coordination number of six.

Carbon is exclusively nonmetallic. Metallic properties appear with silicon and germanium and become predominant in tin and lead. The oxides of carbon and silicon are acidic, whereas those of the other elements of the group are amphoteric. The characteristics such as electron configuration, atomic size, and electronegativity of the carbon atom combine to give the chemistry of carbon a uniqueness that is the basis for the classical division of the field of chemistry into inorganic and organic disciplines.

Silicon also is unique for the extensive range of complex, insoluble alumino-silicates it forms.

CARBON

Carbon appears widely distributed in nature, both in the free and combined states. The free element is produced in various forms, such as coke, lampblack, or charcoal. Activated charcoals are prepared from ligneous materials (sometimes pretreated with a dehydrating agent) by carbonization in the absence of air. This is followed by heat and/or chemical treatment to increase surface area and porosity. Activated charcoal is available in two forms: finely powdered (300 to 350 mesh) for use in liquid media; and coarse, hard, porous particles for gas absorption. The fine form is official in the USP, and is used as an adsorbent in the treatment of diarrhea.

Carbon dioxide usually is obtained as a byproduct from either the production of alcohol by fermentation or by recovery from the stack gases of power plants. Unlike carbon monoxide, its toxicity is not due to interaction with hemoglobin, but through suffocation. Carbon dioxide is an effective respiratory stimulant, cited in the USP.

Under appropriate conditions, carbon forms many binary compounds, such as cyanogen, carbon disulfide, carbon tetrachloride, and numerous carbides. Its important inorganic acids are carbonic, percarbonic (peroxocarbonic) and the pseudobinary hydrocyanic acid (HCN). All are weak acids and are available primarily in the form of salts.

Sodium bicarbonate and the slightly soluble carbonates or basic carbonates of calcium, magnesium, and aluminum find extensive use as gastric antacids. Potassium bicarbonate is used as a source of potassium ion in electrolyte replenishers. Bismuth subcarbonate is an astringent and protective. Ammonium carbonate is an effective reflex stimulant and expectorant.

Table 24-12. The Elements of Group IV-A

ELEMENT	CARBON	SILICON	GERMANIUM	TIN	LEAD
Symbol	C	Si	Ge	Sn	Pb
Atomic number	6	14	32	50	82
Atomic weight	12.01	28.08	72.5_9	118.6_9	207.2
Orbital electrons	$[He]2s^22p^2$	$[Ne]3s^23p^2$	$[Ar]3d^{10}4s^24p^2$	$[Kr]4d^{10}5s^25p^2$	$[Xe]4f^{14}5d^{10}6s^26p^2$
Oxidation states	4− to 4+	4− to 4+	2+, 4+	2+, 4+	2+, 4+
Atomic radius (Å)	0.77	1.17	1.22	1.41	1.54
Ionic (crystal) radii	2.60 (4−)	2.71 (4−)	0.87 (2+)	0.93 (2+)	1.20 (2+)
(coordination number 6)	0.30 (4+)[a]	0.54 (4+)	0.67 (4+)	0.83 (4+)	0.91 (4+)
Ionization potential, ev	11.264	8.149	8.09	7.30	7.38
Electronegativity	2.55	1.90	2.01	1.58	1.87
% of earth's crust	2.7×10^{-2}	27.7	7×10^4	6×10^{-4}	1×10^{-3}

[a] Coordination number 4.

SILICON

Next to oxygen, silicon is the most abundant element on earth. It does not appear free in nature. Silicon forms an inert oxide, silicon dioxide (silica), which occurs abundantly in nature in both amorphous and crystalline states such as sand, quartz, opal, or siliceous earths.

Siliceous earth (diatomaceous earth, Fuller's earth, Kieselguhr, Celite) and *infusorial earth* are the siliceous skeletal remains of diatoms and infusoria. The deposits are in the form of spicules, rods, and stars of silica. Because of their shapes, these materials act as excellent, inert, nonadsorbent filter aids. Because of their moderate hardness they are used as mild abrasives. Purified Siliceous Earth is official in the NF.

Synthetic amorphous silicas are manufactured by two methods. *Silica fume* is prepared by condensation of silica from its vapor phase. *Silica gel* is prepared by hydrolysis of inorganic or organic orthosilicates. Structurally, both forms may be considered condensation polymers of the silicic acids. They are available in various commercial grades, differing in such variables as particle size, degree of hydration, surface type (silanol and/or siloxane), porosity, and hardness. By selection of the product having the desired properties, amorphous silicas find employment as gas adsorbents, desiccants, carriers, fillers, thickeners, and abrasives. Colloidal Silicon Dioxide (fumed form) is official in the NF; Silicon Dioxide, a more general monograph title, replaces the title Silica Gel and now provides for both forms of SiO_2, silica gel and precipitated silica.

Silicosis, a lung condition resembling chronic tuberculosis, develops after long exposure (7 years or more) to *respirable dust* (silica particles 5 μm or less in mean diameter).

Silicon forms numerous silicic acids, such as metasilicic acid [H_2SiO_3], orthosilicic acid [H_4SiO_4], or disilicic acid [$H_6Si_2O_7$]. These and others occur in nature as silicates. Except for the alkali salts, silicates are insoluble in water or acids, but they are attacked readily by hydrofluoric acid, forming gaseous silicon tetrafluoride. The alkali silicates do not occur in nature, but rather are prepared by fusion of finely divided silica with the desired alkali base or carbonate.

The *insoluble* silicates have structural arrangements dominated by the large diffuse oxide ion. Because cations of high charge, such as Si^{4+} or Al^{3+}, are small and compact, they have only a secondary role in determining the structures. Physical properties such as density, hardness, and refractive index are determined almost completely by the *oxygen-packing* arrangement.

There are two *close-packed* oxide ion arrangements, cubic and hexagonal. In each, the oxygen arranges in identical layers; the difference arises from the placement of the layers with respect to one another. Two types of openings are possible between neighboring spheres. The smaller openings are occupied by small cations, such as Si^{4+}, resulting in a tetrahedral arrangement of four oxide ions around each cation. The larger openings between adjacent oxide ions are occupied by somewhat larger cations, such as Li^+, Mg^{2+}, or Fe^{3+}. Six oxide ions surround each cation in an octahedral arrangement. The aluminum ion, which is intermediate in size, can occupy either tetrahedral or octahedral spaces.

When cations too large to occupy either of the inter-oxide ion spaces, such as NH_4^+, Na^+, K^+, Ca^{2+}, are present, the oxide structure opens in one of two ways. Groups of the oxide ion layers separate to give an overall layered structure with the large cations forming a new layer between. The clays have this structure. Or the oxide ions may spread in a three-dimensional manner to give room-like cavities within the structure. The cavities are occupied by the large cations. Feldspars and zeolites have this latter structure.

A persistent problem preventing early workers from successfully elucidating silicate structures was their failure to recognize that ions of the ideal structure may be substituted to some extent by other ions of the same radius, irrespective of charge. This phenomenon, *isomorphous replacement,* is widespread among the silicates. Because of this, empirical formulas based on analytical data are meaningless. The illustrative formulas used in the following discussions are *ideal* formulas. Because of isomorphous replacement, the actual formula of a given silicate may differ somewhat from the ideal.

Before discussing specific insoluble silicates it must be said that all are chemically inert. The properties that distinguish them and determine their use are structural or related to surface phenomena.

Chain silicates are unidimensional arrangements of silicate tetrahedra sharing two oxygens per tetrahedron; in effect each chain is a macroanion. Because these chains consist of Si—O bonds having 50% covalent character, they are difficult to break. Electrical neutrality is maintained by placing a sufficient number of cations, usually K^+ and/or Ca^{2+}, between the chains. Electrostatic forces being weaker than covalent forces, these crystals cleave readily to give rise to the typical fibrous structure of asbestos, such as serpentine asbestos, $(HO)_6Mg_6(Si_4O_{11})\cdot H_2O$. These asbestos chains are useful as filter aids and as insulation. *Note:* Asbestosis is a pulmonary condition similar to silicosis.

Attapulgite, $Mg_5(Si_8O_{20})(OH)_2\cdot 8H_2O$, is a double-chain structure with rather large open spaces between the chains. These spaces are occupied by water molecules, which provide hydrogen bonding to hold the chains together. It has adsorptive properties similar to kaolin.

The layer silicates include talc (talcum, soapstone), the micas, the chlorites (no relationship to ClO_2^-) and the three clay minerals, the montmorillonites (bentonites), kaolins, (kaolinite) and the illites.

Talc, $Mg_3(OH)_2Si_4O_{10}$, is the softest mineral known. There are no cementing cations or molecules between silicate layers; they are held together by van der Waals forces. Consequently, the talc layers cleave easily to give the characteristic smooth, unctuous feel. Talc adheres readily to the skin, is chemically inert, and has very low adsorptive powers. It is used in dusting powders as a protective and lubricant, to prevent irritation due to friction. It also is used in medicated dusts and used widely in cosmetic applications. There are no problems in its use on intact skin, but talc must not be used on broken skin, wounds, or surgical incisions. This precludes its former use as a dusting powder and lubricant for surgical gloves.

Because of its inertness and nonadsorptive character, talc is a useful filter aid. Only particles which are passed by a No 80 sieve, but retained by a No 100 sieve, should be used. Finer particles suspend and are not removed easily by subsequent filtration. Talc is official in the USP.

In mica, $Al_2[(OH)_2(Si_3O_{10})]K$, and chlorite, $Mg_3[(OH)_2(Si_4O_{10})]$, negatively charged silicate layers are bound together by cations. Thus, these silicates cleave readily along the cation layer because the electrostatic forces are weaker than the covalent bonds within the silicate layer. Neither has pharmaceutical applications.

The clays—montmorillonite (Smectite), $Al_4[(OH)_4(Si_8O_{20})]\cdot 3_nH_2O$ and kaolinite, $[(OH)_6Al_4][(OH)_2(Si_4O_{10})]$—are layer structures built of alternating layers of aluminum oxide (hydrargillite) and silicate. The montmorillonites have higher $SiO_2:Al_2O_3$ ratios with much isomorphous replacement of aluminum. Magnesium never is present in the kaolins.

The distinguishing feature of the bentonite (montmorillonite) clays is the insertion of up to three distinct layers of hydrogen-bridged water molecules between the aluminosilicate layers. Not all water hydrogens are needed to bond the water molecules within their layer; the unused hydrogens bind the layers to each other and to the aluminosilicate layers. These water layers may be removed, one at a time, by heat. The thickness of the individual crystals decreases in steps as each water layer is removed. By treating with water, the water layers are restored, one at a time, with a return to the original thickness. This may be repeated indefinitely. Because of this phenomenon, bentonite clays are known as *swelling clays.*

The bentonites have gelling properties that make them useful suspending agents, as well as ion-exchange properties and detergent properties. Bentonite and Bentonite Magma are official in the NF, as is Purified Bentonite, a colloidal montmorillonite.

Kaolins are found always in the form of microcrystals of colloidal dimensions. The properties are somewhat similar to bentonite. They are used as clarifying agents and are good excipients for inorganic salts. They find employment as intestinal adsorbents and protectives. Externally they are used as dusting powders. Kaolin is official in the USP.

The *three-dimensional* or *lattice silicates* have been described previously. In the feldspars, $KAlSi_3O_8$, the most common rock, the large cations (eg, K^+) are trapped in enlarged cavities within the aluminosilicate network. On the other hand, in the zeolites, $CaAl_2Si_4O_{12} \cdot 6H_2O$, and in the synthetic *molecular sieves,* these cavities have connecting openings, or hallways, between one another and to the exterior of the crystal. Thus the cations (and water molecules) in these cavities are free to move about within the crystal and may be exchanged with external cations. These latter silicates are valuable as ion exchangers, desiccants, carriers for catalysts and for the separation of organic gases, as with ethylene from ethane. Certain forms of molecular sieves have been tried as antacids.

Pumice is a porous rock of volcanic origin, usually found in the vitreous state. Being a three dimensionally linked sodium aluminosilicate it is a hard, chemically inert, nonadsorptive material. In the powdered form it is used as a filter medium and dispersing agent. It is found in dental preparations as an abrasive.

Magnesium trisilicate is prepared by precipitation, using a soluble silicate and a soluble magnesium salt. Although it has an analytical composition approaching disilicate, it is actually a mixture of magnesium hydroxide, hydrated magnesium oxide, and silica gel. The insoluble magnesium compounds are responsible for the antacid action; the silica gel acts as a protective. Magnesium trisilicate also is employed as a suspending agent.

GLASS—*Glass* is a generic term used to identify vitreous silicate materials prepared by fusing a base, such as Na_2CO_3 and $CaCO_3$, with pure silica. On cooling, a clear vitreous mass results. There is no clearly defined melting point; a gradual softening takes place on heating as a result of the somewhat haphazard arrangement of the silicon–oxygen bonds.

Certain other cations may be included, such as manganese dioxide, to hide the blue-green color of the iron usually present in silica; borates, to reduce the coefficient of expansion; and potassium ion to give a brown and light-resistant glass.

Since the surface of the glass is an exposed oxide network, it can be reactive. On standing in contact with aqueous solutions, alkali will leach from it. This leaching is accelerated by heat, as occurs with sterilization. The surface of glass also has adsorbing powers, but this can be a problem only in extremely dilute solutions. The compendia usually specify the type of glass container to be used for certain materials and include tests for four types of glass.

SILANES AND SILOXANES—The close relationship between carbon and silicon has prompted much interest in the *organic chemistry of silicon*. The compounds involved are analogs of carbon compounds or compounds in which silicon functions in place of one or more of the carbon atoms. Simple silanes and their derivatives, such as silane $[SiH_4]$, silanol $[SiH_3OH]$, and disiloxane $[H_3SiOSiH_3]$, have been known for a long time. The present interest is in complex compounds that contain both carbon and silicon. The silicones (alkylsiloxanes), condensation polymers of various types of alkylsilanols, represent a field finding extensive commercial application. Simethicone USP, a polymeric dimethylsiloxane, is employed as an antifoaming agent. It has found use as an antiflatulent in gastric bloating and in postoperative gaseous distention in the gastrointestinal tract.

GERMANIUM

The properties of the element germanium are intermediate to those of silicon and tin. Germanium, found in bis-β-carboxyethyl germanium sesquioxide, is purported to have immune system enhancing and antitumor effects. Germanium also has remarkable electrical properties, which make it valuable in the manufacture of semiconductors and other microelectronic parts.

TIN

Tin forms compounds in both +2 and +4 oxidation states. The lower oxidation state is somewhat electrostatic but the higher state is largely covalent in character. Both oxides are amphoteric, giving rise to stannate(II) (stannite) $[SnO_2]^{2-}$, and stannate(IV) (stannate) $[SnO_3]^{2-}$ ions.

The only official compound is stannous fluoride tin(II) fluoride, applied topically as a dental prophylactic. Experimental evidence demonstrates the superiority of this fluoride over other soluble fluorides for this application. The ready susceptibility of tin(II) fluoride to oxidative and hydrolytic decomposition causes problems in the preparation and storage of suitable dosage forms. Various tin dioxide [tin(IV) oxide] preparations have been used externally for their germicidal effect, particularly against staphylococcal organisms that are often resistant to other germicides.

LEAD

Lead is the most metallic element of the group. However, some residual amphoteric character is present, particularly in the +4 oxidation state. At one time, lead compounds found employment in pharmacy and medicine, usually as astringents. However, because of its highly toxic nature as a *cumulative poison*, it is no longer used. It is absorbed readily in the intestinal tract and broken skin, and is deposited in the bone.

Elements of Group IV-B

Because of their minor importance, a detailed treatment of Group IV-B elements is unnecessary. Some important characteristics are given in Table 24-11. All members of the group occur in nature only in the combined state. The +2 and +4 oxidation states are common to all. All members of the group possess amphoteric properties and their cations readily form complexes.

TITANIUM

Titanium forms three oxides (TiO, Ti_2O_3, and TiO_2) and corresponding binary salts. The soluble salts of divalent and trivalent titanium are violet or red and are powerful reducing agents.

The most important compound is the dioxide, TiO_2, which is official in the USP. It is used as a solar-ray protective. As such, it is a popular ingredient in various lotions and creams for the prevention of sunburn. This action is the result of its high covering power as a white pigment, a consequence of its high refractive index.

ZIRCONIUM AND HAFNIUM

Hafnium occurs in small quantities in zirconium ores. As a consequence, unless highly purified, zirconium compounds include varying percentages of hafnium. Zirconium as the hydrous oxide or carbonate has been used as a lotion or cream for contact dermatitis. There are a number of basic aluminum–zirconium compounds used as antiperspirants. However, the prohibition against the use of zirconium in aerosols where inhalation is possible is still in effect.

Table 24-13. The Elements of Group V-A

ELEMENT	NITROGEN	PHOSPHOROUS	ARSENIC	ANTIMONY	BISMUTH
Symbol	N	P	As	Sb	Bi
Atomic number	7	15	33	51	83
Atomic weight	14.01	30.97	74.92	121.7_5	208.98
Orbital electrons	$[He]2s^22p^3$	$[Ne]3s^23p^3$	$[Ar]3d^{10}4s^24p^3$	$[Kr]4d^{10}5s^25p^3$	$[Xe]4f^{14}5d^{10}6s^26p^3$
Oxidation states	$3-, 1+, 3+, 5+$	$3-, 3+, 5+$	$3-, 3+, 5+$	$3-, 3+, 5+$	$3-, 3+, 5+$
Atomic radius (Å)	0.70	1.06	1.21	1.41	1.5
Ionic (crystal) radii (Å)	1.32 (3+)	0.58 (3+)	0.72 (3+)	0.90 (3+)	1.17 (3+)
(coordination number 6)	0.27 (5+)	0.52 (5+)	0.60 (5+)	0.74 (5+)	0.90 (5+)
Ionization potential, ev	14.48	11.10	10.5	8.5	8.0
Electronegativity	3.04	2.19	2.18	2.05	2.02
% of earth's crust	4.6×10^{-8}	0.12	5×10^{-4}	10^{-4}	2×10^{-5}

ELEMENTS OF GROUP V

The elements of this group have five valence electrons. Two of the electrons occupy s orbitals. The three remaining electrons are in different orbitals in the A and B subgroups, giving the structures ns^2np^3 and $(n-1)d^3ns^2$, respectively.

Elements of Group V-A

This group displays strikingly regular gradations in properties, ranging from exclusively nonmetallic nitrogen to almost exclusively metallic bismuth (Table 24-13). Oxidation states of +3 and +5 are common to all. Bismuth functions primarily in the +3 state. All members except bismuth also exist in a −3 oxidation state. Hydrides are of the covalent MH_3 type, characterized by an unshared electron pair. This allows these hydrides to form coordinate covalent bonds. The oxides of nitrogen and phosphorus are acidic. Those of arsenic and antimony are amphoteric, but are sufficiently acidic for the elements to be classified as nonmetals. The common oxide of bismuth, Bi_2O_3, is basic; the less-important pentoxide is acidic.

NITROGEN

Nitrogen occurs free in the atmosphere (78%) and combined in nitrates and organic compounds. It is a colorless, tasteless, and odorless inert gas. It is nonflammable and does not support combustion. Due to its stable triple-bond structure, the N_2 molecule shows little reactivity with other elements. The free nitrogen atom is very reactive.

The inertness of nitrogen is the result of the bonding existing in the molecule. There is a σ bond between the atoms and two π bonds, which fuse to form an electron cloud (doughnut) encasing the entire molecule. This electron cloud effectively prevents breaking of the σ bond for reaction with other elements. The cyanide ion and carbon monoxide have electron structures similar to that of the nitrogen molecule and also show an extraordinary stability.

Nitrogen is prepared primarily by the fractional distillation of liquid air. At the temperature of the electric arc it combines with oxygen forming nitrogen(V) oxide, which is converted into nitric acid. In the presence of catalysts and at great pressure and elevated temperature, it combines with hydrogen to form ammonia.

Unlike phosphorus and the other members of the family, nitrogen does not expand its coordination sphere beyond three. The nitric acid of chemistry is the meta acid. There is no ortho acid (hypothetically H_3NO_4). Nitrogen in the +5 state is too small to accommodate four oxygen atoms.

Therapeutically inactive, elemental Nitrogen NF is employed pharmaceutically as an inert atmosphere in ampules and other containers of substances that would be affected adversely by air. Nitrogen(I) Oxide (nitrous oxide) USP, is an inhalatory general anesthetic. Sodium Nitrite USP is used as an antidote to cyanide poisoning; it also is a vasodilator but is slower acting than the organic nitrite and nitrate esters commonly used for this purpose. The nitrate ion frequently is used as an anion for medicinally active cations, such as silver nitrate and thiamine mononitrate.

Very significant work has shown that the simple, paramagnetic molecule, nitric oxide, NO, is an important neurotransmitter produced by neurons and other cells, causing responses such as vasodilation by acting as a ligand for iron in a heme group with a resulting lowering of blood pressure. This knowledge rationalizes the action of drugs such as the organic nitrites and sodium nitroprusside.

Nitrite ion is toxic; it reacts with hemoglobin to form methemoglobin. Nitrites are also potentially dangerous because they can form N-nitroso derivatives of amines and amides, which may be carcinogenic. Nitrate ion is reducible to nitrite in the intestine and may cause methemoglobinemia. For the above reasons the use of nitrates and nitrites as food preservatives has been questioned.

PHOSPHORUS

Phosphorus exists in two common allotropic forms, yellow and red. Yellow phosphorus (white phosphorus) has a distinctive, disagreeable, ozone-like odor. On exposure to air, or when heated at about 50°, it ignites spontaneously. It is almost insoluble in water, but is soluble in chloroform, benzene, or carbon disulfide. It is poisonous, and on the skin it causes severe, slow to heal burns. Copper(II) sulfate is used as an antidote.

Red phosphorus is a brown to red amorphous powder. It is nonpoisonous and nonflammable in air, except at high temperatures. It is insoluble in any common solvent.

The use of inorganic phosphorus compounds in modern medicine is restricted primarily to the orthophosphates. Tribasic calcium, magnesium, and aluminum phosphates are used as gastric antacids, and the monobasic alkali phosphates are effective urinary acidifiers. Dibasic sodium phosphate is the active ingredient in various saline cathartics and enemas.

Phosphoric Acid NF, is used to form soluble salts of insoluble medicinal bases. The dihydrogen phosphate–monohydrogen phosphate system is a valuable buffer in physiological ranges. Hypophosphorous Acid NF is an antioxidant, used primarily with iodide and iron(II) salts. The radioactive isotope, ^{32}P, is employed therapeutically.

Table 24-14. Transition Elements

ELEMENT	GROUP V-B			GROUP VI-B		
	VANADIUM	NIOBIUM	TANTALUM	CHROMIUM	MOLYBDENUM	TUNGSTEN
Symbol	V	Nb	Ta	Cr	Mo	W
Atomic number	23	41	73	24	42	74
Atomic weight	50.94	92.91	180.95	52.00	95.94	183.8_5
Orbital electrons	$[Ar]3d^34s^2$	$[Kr]4d^45s^1$	$[Xe]4f^{14}5d^36s^2$	$[Ar]3d^54s^1$	$[Kr]4d^55s^1$	$[Xe]4f^{14}5d^46s^2$
Oxidation states	2+, 3+, 4+, 5+	2+, 3+, 4+, 5+	2+, 3+, 4+, 5+	2+, 3+, 4+, 6+	2+ . . . 6+	2+ . . . 6+
Atomic radius (Å)	1.22	1.34	1.34	1.18	1.30	1.30
Ionic (crystal) radii (Å) (coordination number 6)	0.40 (5+)	0.70 (5+)	0.73 (5+)	0.76 (3+) 0.58 (6+)	0.79 (4+) 0.73 (6+)	0.80 (4+) 0.74 (6+)
Ionization potential, ev	6.71	6.79	ca 6	6.77	7.38	7.98
Electronegativity	—	—	1.33	1.66	2.2	2.36
% of earth's crust	0.021	—	—	2×10^{-2}	ca 5×10^{-4}	ca 1.5×10^{-4}

Phosphorus is essential to plant and animal life. A complex basic calcium phosphate, called hydroxyapatite, constitutes the main inorganic component of bones and teeth. Dihydrogen phosphate and monohydrogen phosphate ions constitute the ion pair of one of the buffer systems of the blood and body fluids. The phosphate moiety has important roles in the metabolism of various organic materials, such as carbohydrates.

ARSENIC

Inorganic arsenic compounds rarely are employed in modern medicine. There no longer are official compounds; arsenic trioxide and potassium arsenite were the last; they were used as alteratives, tonics, and antileukemics. In the past, Potassium Arsenite Solution (Fowler's Solution) was used as an antileukemic agent. There is available an arsensic trioxide injection (1 mg/mL) that has been used to treat promyelocytic leukemia. The treatment must be carefully supervised owing to possible serious side effects that include ECG abnormalities. Sodium arsenate, (^{74}As), has been used as a diagnostic aid.

Arsenic compounds are poisonous. If they are still in the gastrointestinal tract, a freshly prepared mixture of iron(III) and magnesium hydroxides is administered orally as an antidote. If the arsenic has already been absorbed, dimercaprol by intramuscular injection is effective.

ANTIMONY

Antimony compounds have physiological reactions resembling those of arsenic. The compounds are potentially toxic. Except for Antimony Potassium Tartrate (antimonyl potassium tartrate, tartar emetic) USP, and for Antimony Sodium Tartrate USP, antimony compounds are no longer in common medical usage. Both antimony potassium and antimony sodium tartrates are used in the treatment of schistosomiasis, a parasitic disease involving flukes.

BISMUTH

With the exception of sodium bismuthate, [$NaBiO_3$] in which the bismuth functions anionically in the +5 oxidation state, the important bismuth compounds of commerce are the Bi^{3+} variety. The basic salts—bismuth subcarbonate, bismuth subgallate, and bismuth subnitrate—are employed for their astringent, mildly germicidal, and antacid properties.

Bismuth Subnitrate, Bismuth Subgallate, and Milk of Bismuth are official in the USP. Milk of Bismuth owes its antacid properties to the hydroxyl and carbonate ions present. Because of the adherent properties, it provides protective action. The small amount of dissolved bismuthyl ion present exerts a mild antiseptic effect. Colloidal bismuth subcitrate is used clinically in the treatment of peptic ulcer disease.

Hydrogen sulfide, from the breakdown of proteins in the gut, reacts with bismuthyl ion to form the insoluble, dark brown, bismuth(III) sulfide. As a result stools appear black. Soluble bismuth compounds are poisonous; intramuscular dimercaprol is an effective antidote.

Elements of Group V-B

Unlike previous transition elements, the valence electron structure of the Group V-B elements is not identical. Vanadium and tantalum have a $(n-1)d^3ns^2$ structure, whereas niobium has the structure $(n-1)d^4ns^1$ (Table 24-14). The difference has no apparent effect on their chemistry. In addition to the Group V oxidation states, +3 and +5, these elements also appear in a +2 and +4 oxidation state. The −3 oxidation state does not occur. There is a close similarity between niobium and tantalum. Tantalum, because of its size, has a maximum coordination number of eight and the compounds of these elements are colored.

The Group V-B elements are of little pharmaceutical importance; only tantalum metal is employed therapeutically. Because tantalum is unaffected by the body fluids, it is used in sheet form for the surgical repair of bones. Muscle tissue will attach itself to tantalum as though it were bone.

ELEMENTS OF GROUP VI

The members of Group VI have six valence electrons. Although theoretically a −2 oxidation state is possible for all, −2 and −1 appear only in the subgroup A elements. The common positive oxidation states are +4 and +6; +1 and +2 also exist.

Elements of Group VI-A

There is a very clear gradation of properties in the Group VI-A family (the chalcogens). Oxygen is nonmetallic in character

Table 24-15. The Elements of Group VI-A

ELEMENT	OXYGEN	SULFUR	SELENIUM	TELLURIUM	POLONIUM
Symbol	O	S	Se	Te	Po
Atomic number	8	16	34	52	84
Atomic weight	16.00	32.06	78.9_6	127.6	(209)
Orbital electrons	$[He]2s^22p^4$	$[Ne]3s^23p^4$	$[Ar]3d^{10}4s^24p^4$	$[Kr]4d^{10}5s^25p^4$	$[Xe]4f^{14}5d^{10}6s^26p^4$
Oxidation states	2−, 1−	2−, 2+, 6+	2−, 4+, 6+	2−, 4+, 6+	4+, 6+
Atomic radius (Å)	0.66	1.04	1.16	1.37	1.53
Ionic (crystal) radii (Å)					
(simple anion)	1.26 (2−)	1.70 (2−)	1.84 (2−)	2.07 (2−)	1.08 (4+)
(coordination number 6)	—	0.43 (6+)	0.56 (6+)	0.57 (6+)	0.81 (6+)
Ionization potential, ev	13.61	10.36	9.75	9.0	—
Electronegativity	3.44	2.58	2.55	2.1	2.0
% of earth's crust	46.6	0.052	10^{-7}	10^{-7}	10^{-14}

whereas polonium is metallic; the other members show both characteristics. Polonium is further distinguished by its natural radioactivity.

The sulfur–selenium–tellurium triad displays especially strong family relationships. Allotropic varieties of each element in the triad are numerous. Although there are quantitative differences, each functions generally in the −2, +4, and +6 oxidation states, forming many analogous compounds. Some of the more important characteristic properties of Group VI-A elements are presented in Table 24-15.

OXYGEN

In free form, oxygen constitutes about one-fifth of air, by weight. The primeval atmosphere of the earth probably had no oxygen. In combined form, it constitutes about seven-eighths, by weight, of water and important fractional parts of minerals such as $CaCO_3$ or Fe_2O_3. The industrial process for preparing oxygen is the fractional distillation of liquid air. When liquid air is allowed to evaporate under controlled conditions, the nitrogen and inert gases escape initially, followed by nearly pure oxygen.

The weighted atomic mass of the mixture of naturally occurring oxygen isotopes formerly was the standard for all chemical atomic weights. This standard has been replaced by the most abundant carbon isotope, ^{12}C. The isotopes of oxygen have been separated and introduced into specific molecules as tracer elements.

Oxygen USP is employed as a therapeutic gas in the treatment of conditions involving hypoxia. Ozone, O_3, an allotropic form of oxygen, is a powerful oxidizing agent. Ozonized air (air treated to convert some of its oxygen into ozone) is used in various disinfecting and bleaching operations.

Chemically, oxygen is very reactive, combining directly, under appropriate conditions, with all elements except mercury, silver, gold, and members of the platinum family. It is electronegative with respect to all elements except fluorine. The oxides of nonmetallic elements are acidic, while those of metals are basic. The oxides of many elements, such as antimony and tellurium, are amphoteric. In all, oxygen has the −2 oxidation number.

Hydrogen peroxide and the peroxides are a series of oxygen compounds in which oxygen has an oxidation number of −1. They are valuable oxidizing and reducing agents.

Hydrogen peroxide is prepared by the electrolysis of a concentrated solution of either sulfuric acid or ammonium sulfate. Persulfate, $[S_2O_8{}^{2-}]$, forms in the anode compartment. After electrolysis the analyte is reacted with water and the hydrogen peroxide formed is separated by distillation under reduced pressure.

Pure concentrated hydrogen peroxide is stable. However, commercial preparations must be stabilized; usually, a preservative is added such as acetanilid. Traces of mineral acid (eg, phosphoric acid) often are added, as the stability increases in acid medium.

Hydrogen peroxide is available as the 3, 6, 30, 70, and 90% solutions. Concentration also is expressed as volume strength, the volume of oxygen gas released from one volume of solution; ten volume is 3%. Hydrogen Peroxide Concentrate USP is the 30% solution. It is a powerful oxidant and must not be used on the skin. Hydrogen Peroxide Topical Solution USP is the 3% solution. It is a mild, fast acting, oxidizing germicide that will destroy most pathogenic bacteria. Hydrogen peroxide, 6%, is the only common bleach mild enough for use on hair.

Hydrogen peroxide is available as a solution in anhydrous glycerine (1.5%) and as urea peroxide, a stable crystalline 1:1 compound, usually in 4 to 10% solution in anhydrous glycerine. A monograph for Carbamide Peroxide is found in the USP, and the monograph for Carbamide Peroxide Topical Solution USP has a generic purity rubric statement. These preparations are preferable to hydrogen peroxide in treatment of oral and ear infections. Zinc peroxide and sodium perborate, a compound that has a hydrogen peroxide molecule in its hydration complement, have been listed in past compendia.

SULFUR

Sulfur is an element that exists in several allotropic forms. At room temperature α-sulfur (rhombic sulfur) is the stable form. At the equilibrium point, 96°, β-sulfur (monoclinic sulfur) becomes the stable form. Other allotropes exist. Commercial, Sublimed Sulfur USP and Precipitated Sulfur USP are α-sulfur. Precipitated sulfur has a smaller particle size than sublimed; therefore, it is more reactive.

As an ointment, precipitated sulfur is used as the scabicide. Sulfur ointments and lotions are used in dermatological applications as keratolytics. Elemental sulfur also has fungicidal action. Sublimed sulfur is used as a cathartic.

Sulfur appears in three series of compounds. The first, based on the −2 oxidation state, gives rise to hydrogen sulfide and the sulfides. The second and third series, based on +4 and +6 oxidation states, give rise to the two sulfur oxides and their acids and salts.

Hydrogen sulfide and soluble sulfides in solution react readily with suspended, finely divided sulfur to give rise to mixtures of polysulfides, $S_2{}^{2-}$, $S_3{}^{2-}$, $S_4{}^{2-}$, $S_5{}^{2-}$, usually written $S_n{}^{2-}$.

Sulfurated Potash consists largely of potassium polysulfides, sulfate, and thiosulfate. It is prepared by careful heating of a mixture of potassium carbonate and sublimed sulfur. The compound is very soluble in water, giving an alkaline reaction. The polysulfide component is soluble in ethanol. Sulfurated potash is used in the form of lotions, ointments, and aqueous solutions for the treatment of psoriasis and other chronic skin conditions and has parasiticidal activity.

Sulfurated potash must be stored in tightly sealed containers to prevent reaction with carbon dioxide and oxygen. It is incompatible with acid.

White Lotion USP is prepared by adding freshly prepared, filtered, sulfurated potash solution to zinc sulfate solution.

Table 24-16. The Elements of Group VII-A

ELEMENT	FLUORINE	CHLORINE	BROMINE	IODINE	ASTATINE
Symbol	F	Cl	Br	I	At
Atomic number	9	17	35	53	85
Atomic weight	19	35.45	79.90	126.90	(210)
Orbital electrons	$[He]2s^22p^5$	$[Ne]3s^23p^5$	$[Ar]3d^{10}4s^24p^5$	$[Kr]4d^{10}5s^25p^5$	$[Xe]4f^{14}5d^{10}6s^26p^5$
Oxidation states	1−	1−, 1+, 3+, 5+, 7+	1−, 1+, (3+), 5+	1−, 1+, (3+), 5+, 7+	—
Atomic radius (Å)	0.64	0.99	1.14	1.33	—
Ionic (crystal) radii (Å)					
(halide anion)	1.19	1.67	1.82	2.06	—
(coordination number 6)	0.022 (7+)	0.41 (7+)	0.53 (7+)	0.67 (7+)	0.76 (7+)
Ionization potential, ev	17.42	13.01	11.84	10.44	—
Electronegativity	3.98	3.16	2.96	2.66	2.2
% of earth's crust	8×10^{-2}	3×10^{-2}	1.6×10^{-4}	3×10^{-5}	—

The order of mixing is important. It is an astringent and protective.

Selenium Sulfide (and Lotion) USP is employed as a 2.5% suspension in the topical treatment of seborrheic dermatitis (dandruff). Care is essential to prevent introduction into the eyes or mouth. In addition, the hands must be cleansed thoroughly after using because selenium is toxic. Cadmium sulfide also is used in the treatment of seborrheic dermatitis. Although it is less irritating, it requires the same precautions as selenium sulfide.

Sulfur Dioxide NF usually is prepared industrially by burning sulfur. It is the acid anhydride of sulfurous acid and its salts, the sulfites. All are used in pharmaceutical practice as antioxidants and preservatives.

Attempts to crystallize sodium bisulfite yield, instead, normal sodium sulfite crystals. If the crystallization is carried out under a sulfur dioxide atmosphere crystals of the metabisulfite, $Na_2S_2O_5$, form. On dissolving metabisulfite in water, a solution of bisulfite results

$$S_2O_5{}^{2-} + H_2O \rightarrow 2HSO_3{}^-$$

Sodium Metabisulfite NF should be used when sodium bisulfite is specified. It is used as an antioxidant. A monograph for Potassium Metabisulfite is included in the NF.

Sodium Thiosulfate USP is prepared from the sulfite by reaction with sulfur. Because the sulfite ion has an unshared electron pair, and elemental sulfur lacks one electron pair for completion of a stable octet, a coordinate covalent bond forms easily, giving the thiosulfate ion. It is used as an antidote for cyanide poisoning. It is a valuable analytical reagent for the determination of iodine.

In the +6 oxidation state sulfur gives rise to sulfuric acid and the sulfates. Sulfuric acid is an important acid and is listed in the NF. Several sulfates are cited officially but with the exception of sodium sulfate (saline cathartic), all applications are ascribed more appropriately to the cation present, such as barium sulfate or bleomycin sulfate.

SELENIUM AND TELLURIUM

In general, selenium and tellurium compounds are analogous to those of sulfur. Observed differences are largely those to be expected in terms of relative atomic size and electronegativity.

Although selenium is toxic in large doses, it is an important trace element. It is absorbed very slowly through the skin. Toxicity usually is not a problem if it is applied to small areas of unbroken, unirritated skin. Prolonged contact with the skin results in contact dermatitis. The use of selenium sulfide, the only official compound, is described in the section on sulfides. Selenomethionine Se 75 Injection USP is used in the diagnosis of pancreatic tumors and growths.

Tellurium has no medicinal applications at this time.

Elements of Group VI-B

The Group VI-B elements are metallic in behavior. The lower oxidation state oxides are basic, whereas those of the higher oxidation states are acidic, giving rise to the chromates, molybdates, and tungstates. The cations of high oxidation numbers have a tendency to unite with oxygen to give stable -yl cations, such as CrO^{2+} chromyl. These elements show great similarity in behavior to their horizontal neighbors in Groups V-B and VII-B. Some properties are given in Table 24-14.

Chromium and molybdenum are essential trace elements. Monographs for Chromic Chloride (and Injection) and Ammonium Molybdate (and Injection) are found in the USP and Chromium Picolinate is listed in the NF. Chromium has a wide margin of safety between amounts usually ingested and those showing adverse effects. The radioactive isotope, ^{51}Cr, is employed as a biological tracer in certain hematological procedures. Their compounds are important in analytical pharmaceutical operations.

ELEMENTS OF GROUP VII

The elements of Group VII subdivide into Group VII-A (Table 24-16), members of which have an outer electron configuration ns^2np^5, and Group VII-B (Table 24-17) with the $(n-1)d^5ns^2$ valence electron configuration.

The halogens are nonmetallic in character; the transition elements of the family are metallic. Except for the higher oxidation states of +5 and especially +7, the elements of the subgroups and their compounds are quite dissimilar. The free halogens are colored, but almost all of their compounds are not.

Elements of Group VII-A

Examination of the valence electron structure of Group VII-A elements suggests −1, +1, +3, +5, and +7 as possible oxidation states. Fluorine, the most electronegative element, appears only as the simple fluoride ion (which readily acts as a ligand). Only chlorine forms compounds in all five oxidation states.

The halogen binary compounds may be ionic and/or covalent, depending on electronegativity differences. All halogens unite

None of the elements of the second triad have compounds of medicinal value, but platinum, a member of the third triad, is used in cancer chemotherapy as cisplatin, cis-diaminedichloroplatinum(II); monographs for Cisplatin and Cisplatin for Injection are found in the USP. Carboplatin, cis-diamine (1,1-cyclobutanedicarboxylato)platinum, is another compound used in cancer therapy.

Elements of the First Triad

The important oxidation states are +2, achieved by the loss of the two s electrons, and +3 in which an additional d electron is lost (see Table 24-17). The stability of the +2 oxidation state increases from iron to nickel. The free metals and the +2 cations are important reducing agents. The cations have a tendency to form both cationic and anionic complex ions of high stability.

IRON

Iron is distributed widely in nature. It functions in divalent and trivalent states to form iron(II) ferrous and iron(III) ferric compounds, respectively. Iron(II) compounds are usually green in the hydrated state and white in the anhydrous state. Iron(III) salts are usually yellow to brown in the hydrated state but vary in color when anhydrous. Aqueous solutions of iron(III) salts hydrolyze strongly to give acid solutions. Iron(II) salts undergo slight hydrolysis and are oxidized easily in solution. The behavior of the iron(III) ion is similar to that of aluminum(III).

Iron, in either oxidation state, readily forms soluble coordination complexes with ligands such as phosphate, citrate, tartrate, and amines. Iron does not precipitate from many of these complexes with the usual iron precipitants.

Iron is an essential trace element. It is the important element in the transportation of oxygen by hemoglobin. It functions in various cytochromes, which are essential oxidative enzymes of the body cells.

A study carried out in Finland has cast doubt on the advisability of the routine use of hematinics because men with higher levels of ferritin (an iron storage protein) were found to be more prone to heart attacks. Interpretation of the results included speculation about iron's ability to give rise to free radicals after reaction with oxygen. The caveat that persists is that ferritin levels must be measured and found to be low before an iron deficiency is pronounced requiring use of a hematinic. The use of hematinics without substantiated need is not advised.

Numerous iron(II) and iron(III) compounds, complexes, and solutions have been used as hematinics in the past. However, because of their greater gastrointestinal irritation and poor absorption, iron(III) compounds and their preparations are used rarely today. Ferrous Fumarate (Tablets and, together with Docusate Sodium, Extended Release Tablets), Ferrous Gluconate (Tablets, Capsules, and Elixir), Ferrous Sulfate (Oral Solution, Syrup, and Tablets) and Dried Ferrous Sulfate are official in the USP. Iron Dextran Injection, a colloidal iron(III) hydroxide with partially hydrolyzed dextran, and Iron Sorbitex Injection, a complex of iron with sorbitol and citric acid, are cited in the USP as injectable forms for patients with poor gastrointestinal tolerance or poor absorption of iron. Reduced iron formerly was used as a hematinic; it survives today in the fortification of foods such as flour.

Iron(III) compounds are astringent. Sodium nitroprusside USP, $Na_2[Fe(CN)_5(NO)] \cdot 2H_2O$, is a vasodilator. A monograph for Sterile Sodium Nitroprusside is provided in the USP.

COBALT

The important cobalt salts of commerce are those of cobalt(II). Most contain water of hydration and are red in color, but when rendered anhydrous they are blue. Because of this color change anhydrous cobalt(II) chloride is included in dehydrating agents for gases to indicate when they are spent.

There is evidence that the presence of traces of cobalt may catalyze the physiological utilization of iron. This has led to the introduction of medicinal specialty products containing iron in association with cobalt designed for use in the treatment of iron deficiency anemias. Cyanocobalamin (vitamin B_{12}) is the only cobalt compound officially cited. The radioactive isotopes, ^{57}Co and ^{60}Co, are used diagnostically and therapeutically.

NICKEL

The important nickel compounds are in the +2 oxidation state. There are no nickel compounds of medical importance.

WATER

Water is omnipresent. About 75% of the earth's surface is covered with liquid water. Land masses in polar regions are covered with thick sheets of ice. In vapor form, water is an important constituent of the earth's atmosphere. In combined form, water occurs abundantly in many minerals, such as gypsum ($CaSO_4 \cdot 2H_2O$). In addition, water occurs in all animal and vegetable tissues; it constitutes some 70% of the human body and over 90% of vegetables such as cucumbers and watermelons.

Together with ammonia and hydrogen fluoride, water is distinguished from other covalent hydrides by the strong hydrogen bonds existing between adjacent molecules. Despite the ability of fluoride ion to form stronger hydrogen bonds than oxide, hydrogen bonding reaches its peak in water because two protons are available per molecule. Hydrogen fluoride has only one available proton per molecule and ammonia has only one open site per molecule for hydrogen bonding.

Because of the extensive hydrogen bonding, the physical properties of water are unique among the other hydrides. Most obvious is the existence of water as a liquid under normal conditions. All other covalent hydrides are gases. The heat of fusion and melting point, heat of vaporization and boiling point, specific heat, surface tension, viscosity, and dielectric constant of water are all much higher in absolute value than those of other covalent hydrides. The world as we know it would be impossible without these unusual properties of water.

Water is a chemically stable compound. Even at 2000 K, less than 1% is dissociated into its elements. The K_w for water is only 10^{-14}. Despite this relative nonreactivity it acts as a solvent, especially for ionic compounds, as a ligand, as an acid or base, and as an oxidizing or reducing agent. In traces, water is frequently a catalyst. The acid–base properties are discussed later.

Because of its strong permanent dipole, water often acts as a ligand in complex substances. Almost all cations form one or more hydrates, divalent cations being more highly hydrated than the monovalent because of their stronger electrostatic fields. Having reduced field strengths because of their greater size, large cations (eg, cesium) do not hydrate. Many anions hydrate; for example, $CuSO_4 \cdot 5H_2O$ is actually $[Cu(H_2O)_4][SO_4 \cdot H_2O]$.

Water acts as a solvent for an unusual range of substances. This solvent action results from one or more of its properties: small size, strong permanent dipole, high dielectric constant, and availability of protons for hydrogen bonding.

NATURAL WATERS

Naturally occurring waters contain dissolved minerals indigenous to the region. Such waters are described variously as mineral waters, lithia waters, sulfur waters, and so on. Owners of springs or other sources of such waters often claim fanciful therapeutic effects but, in general, these claims have not been substantiated.

Natural waters contain varying amounts of suspended matter, such as clay, sand, microorganisms, and fragments of plants and animals. Commonly, they are a very dilute solution (parts per million or ppm) of calcium, magnesium, iron(III), sodium, and potassium ions, having bicarbonate, sulfate, and chloride as counterions.

The dissolved bicarbonate constitutes *temporary* hardness whereas sulfate and chloride constitute *permanent* hardness. In addition, natural water contains traces of dissolved atmospheric gases, ammonia, and metabolic decomposition products. Waters in inhabited areas often include dissolved minerals such as nitrate, phosphate, and organic compounds from homes, industry, and farms. Detergents and dissolved traces of insecticides and herbicides are proving especially troublesome. The Environmental Protection Agency (EPA) has water-quality criteria for a number of priority pollutants.

POTABLE WATER

Potable water is water that is *fit to drink.* Providing potable water is one of the most important functions of modern communities. The overall process involves the removal of insoluble matter through appropriate coagulating, settling, and filtering processes; destruction of pathogenic microorganisms by aeration, chlorination, or other methods; and improvement of palatability through aeration and filtration through charcoal.

Activated charcoal also removes some harmful trace impurities (eg, trihalomethanes) not removed or destroyed by previous operations. In regions where water is excessively hard, *softening* is effected by adding lime or ammonia to partially remove dissolved salts by precipitation as carbonates (Ca^{2+} and Mg^{2+}) and hydroxide [iron(III)]. To assure an adequate provision of the essential element fluorine, fluoridation is accomplished by adding sodium fluosilicate. Standards for potable water are issued by the EPA.

In emergencies water may be purified (rendered free of viable microorganisms) by boiling for 15 to 20 minutes, or by treatment with halazone or iodine.

PURIFIED WATER AND OTHER WATERS USED IN PHARMACY

Purified water is prepared by distillation, ion-exchange (deionized, demineralized), reverse osmosis, or other methods. Potable water, meeting EPA standards, is used in its preparation. The object is the removal of dissolved solids. Ion-exchange and reverse osmosis are particularly effective in removing electrolytes. Distillation is not effective in the removal of weak electrolytes and nonelectrolytes if they are volatile.

Purified water may be rendered sterile and pyrogen-free by repeated distillation.

Primarily because of its solvent powers and physiological inertness, water is an extremely important pharmaceutical agent. It is official in six different monographs: Purified Water, Sterile Purified Water, Water for Injection, Bacteriostatic Water for Injection, Sterile Water for Inhalation, Sterile Water for Injection, and Sterile Water for Irrigation. General Chapter <1231> in the USP is an excellent summary of the various waters and a guide to their use.

HEAVY WATER

The isotopes of hydrogen have been named deuterium (two neutrons) and tritium (three neutrons). The presence of three neutrons in tritium results in an unstable nucleus. However, like hydrogen, deuterium is stable and gives rise to deuterium oxide, D_2O. This compound occurs in ordinary water in a few parts per million. Because of its greater molecular weight, the physical properties of deuterium oxide differ from those of water (eg, bp 101.4°, sp gr 1.10).

Deuterium oxide has no known therapeutic role. It has been used as a research tool in biological and pharmacological investigations. Use of deuterium oxide for drinking purposes has caused retardation or stunted growth in experimental mammals. It is available commercially and finds use as a moderator in nuclear reactors and as a solvent in nuclear magnetic resonance studies.

ACIDS, BASES, AND BUFFERS

ACIDS AND BASES

Acid–base theories range from the limited, classic Arrhenius theory to the comprehensive theory of Lewis. In between are the Franklin solvent system of acids and bases and the Brønsted proton donor theory.

As the body functions with aqueous media and pharmaceuticals frequently are dispensed in aqueous solution, the Brønsted theory is convenient for use in pharmacy. A molecule or ion that can provide a proton (proton donor) is an *acid;* one that can accept a proton (proton acceptor) is a *base.* On accepting a proton, a base becomes an acid; on losing its proton, the acid becomes a base. An acid and its base are related by the presence or absence

of a proton, and are known as a *conjugate pair.* The transfer of a proton from the acid of one conjugate pair to the base of another conjugate pair is *neutralization.* Some conjugate pairs of pharmaceutical interest are given in Table 24-18. It is evident that acids and bases may be cations, neutral molecules, or anions. Some structures may be members of two different conjugate pairs, as an acid in one and as a base in the other.

A strong acid is an acid that loses its proton easily; a *weak acid* holds its proton tenaciously. The conjugate base of a strong acid is a *weak base,* whereas that of a weak acid is a *strong base.* In neutralization, the proton goes to the strongest of the bases present. The percent ionization and the ionization constant are measures of the strength of a given acid.

Acids and bases are used in pharmacy for analytical procedures, as buffer systems, and to dissolve insoluble medicinals. To accomplish the latter the insoluble compound must have a functional group capable of acting as a strong base or as an acid. Lidocaine Hydrochloride Injection USP and Niacin Injection USP are examples. The former is prepared by reacting lidocaine with hydrochloric acid; the diethylamino group is a stronger base than either the water molecule or the chloride ion. Lidocaine goes into solution as a cation. Niacin Injection is prepared by reacting niacin with either sodium carbonate or sodium hydroxide; the carboxyl group loses its proton to the carbonate or hydroxyl ion and the niacin goes into solution as an anion.

Table 24-18. Conjugate Acid–Base Pairs

ACID	BASE	ACID	BASE
H_2O	OH^-	H_2SO_4	HSO_4^-
H_3O^+	H_2O	HSO_4^-	SO_4^{2-}
NH_4^+	NH_3	H_3PO_4	$H_2PO_4^-$
RNH_3^+	RNH_2	$H_2PO_4^-$	HPO_4^{2-}
HCl	Cl^-	$[A](H_2O)_6]^{3+}$	$[A](H_2O)_5(OH)]^{2+}$
H_2CO_3	HCO_3^-	$[A](H_2O)_5(OH)]^{2+}$	$[A](H_2O)_4(OH)_2]^+$
HCO_3^-	CO_3^{2-}	$H_3BO_3 \cdot H_2O$	$[B(OH)_4]^-$

In neutralization, as above, the pharmacist must be cognizant of two requirements that are not important in ordinary chemical neutralizations. The counterion being introduced—chloride ion and sodium ion, respectively, in the above examples—must be compatible physiologically with the body fluids. Also, because strong acids or bases are being used, there can be no excess acid or base because of the corrosive nature of these reagents.

Acids and bases are also necessary for the preparation of effervescent mixtures, a medicinal dosage form sometimes used to render a medicinal more palatable for oral administration. Sodium bicarbonate is used as the carbon dioxide source. Solid acids such as citric acid, tartaric acid, or sodium dihydrogen phosphate are used, frequently in combination. Reaction rate is very important in these formulations. Sodium bicarbonate must have the correct particle size; if too fine, the reaction is too violent, and if too coarse, the reaction is too slow. To lower the activity of the acid, a normal salt of the acid is included in the mixture as a diluent.

Some acids and bases listed in the compendia at present are Calcium Hydroxide, Potassium Bicarbonate, Potassium Hydroxide, Sodium Bicarbonate, Sodium Carbonate, Sodium Hydroxide, Strong Ammonia Solution, Acetic Acid, Hydrochloric Acid and Diluted Hydrochloric Acid, Nitric Acid, Sulfuric Acid, Phosphoric Acid and Diluted Phosphoric Acid.

Stability and storage problems of these compounds must be considered. All strong bases are subject to reaction with carbon dioxide if proper closures are not maintained. Volatile compounds, such as ammonia and hydrogen chloride, must be sealed tightly at all times, as must hygroscopic compounds such as sodium hydroxide.

BUFFERS

Buffers are used to maintain the pH of a medicinal at an optimal value. A *buffer* is a solution of a weak acid and its conjugate base, the base being provided by one of its soluble salts.

PHYSIOLOGICAL CONTROL OF pH

Brønsted acids and bases have been used to maintain and adjust the pH of body fluids for many years. By far the greatest interest has been in development of gastric antacids. However, an adequate number of suitable reagents are available for systemic pH adjustments.

GASTRIC ANTACIDS

The present official magnesium antacids include Magnesium Hydroxide, Milk of Magnesia, Magnesia Tablets, Alumina and Magnesia Oral Suspension (and Tablets), Magnesium Carbonate, Magnesium Carbonate and Sodium Bicarbonate for Oral Suspension, Magnesium Oxide, Magnesium Phosphate, and Magnesium Trisilicate (and Tablets). The official aluminum antacids include Aluminum Hydroxide Gel, Dried Aluminum Hydroxide Gel (and Capsules and Tablets), Aluminum Phosphate Gel, Dihydroxyaluminum Aminoacetate (and Magma, and Capsules and Tablets), Dihydroxyaluminum Sodium Carbonate (and Tablets), Alumina, Magnesia, and Calcium Carbonate Oral Suspension (and Tablets), Alumina and Magnesium Trisilicate Oral Suspension (and Tablets), and the Alumina and Magnesia preparations already listed. The calcium antacids include Precipitated Calcium Carbonate (and Tablets), Calcium Carbonate and Magnesia Tablets, and Calcium and Magnesium Carbonates Tablets. Magaldrate, an aluminum magnesium hydroxide sulfate, is official, as is its Oral Suspension and Tablets. Miscellaneous official antacids include Milk of Bismuth, Sodium Bicarbonate, and Potassium Bicarbonate.

There are other gastric antacid dosage form monographs, some including simethicone, an antiflatulent, and they are

Magnesium Oxide Capsules (and Tablets); Basic Aluminum Carbonate Gel; Dried Basic Aluminum Carbonate Gel Capsules (and Tablets); Alumina and Magnesium Carbonate Oral Suspension (and Tablets); Alumina, Magnesium Carbonate, and Magnesium Oxide Tablets; Alumina, Magnesia, and Simethicone Oral Suspension (and Tablets); Calcium Carbonate Oral Suspension; and Magaldrate and Simethicone Oral Suspension (and Tablets). A monograph for Magnesium Hydroxide Paste, which contains about 31 g of magnesium hydroxide per 100 g, describes a suspension that is an intermediate in the manufacture of Milk of Magnesia and other suspensions of magnesium hydroxide.

SYSTEMIC ALKALIZERS AND ACIDIFIERS

Sodium Bicarbonate USP and Potassium Bicarbonate USP are used as systemic alkalizers. Because the bicarbonates are unstable to heat, chemical problems arise in the sterilization of bicarbonate solutions,

$$2HCO_3^- \rightleftharpoons CO_3^{2-} + CO_2 + H_2O$$

To depress the forward reaction the solution can be saturated with carbon dioxide. To prevent the loss of the gas, which would result in the permanent formation of the strong carbonate base, the ampules used must be sealed tightly before sterilization, and must be made of glass sufficiently strong to withstand the gas pressure developed during sterilization. On cooling the reverse reaction becomes dominant.

Ammonium Chloride USP, Monobasic Sodium Phosphate USP, and Calcium Chloride USP are employed as systemic acidifiers.

ELECTROLYTES AND ESSENTIAL TRACE ELEMENTS

The roles and behavior of inorganic elements in the electrolyte and essential trace elements categories are discussed elsewhere in this book, but it is instructive to review the physical and chemical properties that make possible their respective roles. Examination of orbital electron structures, ionic radii, oxidation states, etc, as given in Tables 24-7 through 24-17, can yield valuable clues to their behavior.

The transition elements have incompletely filled 18-electron outer shells and each can exist in several different oxidation

states. In most cases the shift between two electron states is relatively easy; for example,

$$Fe^{2+} \rightleftharpoons Fe^{3+} + e^-$$

As a result, the transition elements can act as electron sinks and are active in those systems involved in oxidation or reduction reactions.

On the other hand, an element such as zinc achieves a completely filled outer 18-electron shell on becoming zinc ion. In the 2+ oxidation state this shell becomes stable. Unlike the tightly held spherical 8-electron shell the 18-electron shell is *mushy* and deformed or polarized easily by external fields. In turn, it can cause polarization of other moieties. This ion is not found in redox systems, but rather in systems such as carbonic anhydrase, which aid in the splitting or forming of molecules.

Unlike the incompletely filled shells of the transition elements or the 18-electron shell of the zinc ion, 8-electron shell ions ordinarily are stable and are not deformed easily by external fields. Those 8-electron outer shell ions with a high charge (eg, calcium) have intense charge densities in the volume surrounding the ion. This results in strong interactions with the fields of other moieties to form strong permanent associations. However, an 8-electron shell effectively screens the single charge of ions such as sodium. They are, therefore, chemically inert with very weak interactions with other ions. This explains their simple roles in the body fluids as osmotic regulators, etc.

There are a number of monographs for parenteral infusions intended to supply electrolytes, water, and carbohydrates as nutrients. In addition to monographs in the USP for Ringer's and Dextrose Injection and Lactated Ringer's and Dextrose Injection (with Half-Strength and Modified variations), a series of monographs are found with the designation Multiple Electrolytes in each title; these monographs offer choices of cations from Na^+, K^+, Ca^{2+}, Mg^{2+}, and NH_4^+; of anions from chloride, acetate, citrate, lactate, gluconate, phosphate, and sulfate; plus a choice of carbohydrate nutrient from invert sugar and dextrose. These monographs indicate an awareness of the importance of inorganic cations (including magnesium) and anions and provide a variety of choices to allow treatment of patients on an individualized basis.

In addition to providing official standards for various infusions used as parenteral rehydration solutions or electrolyte replenishers, USP has a generic monograph for Oral Rehydration Salts, a dry mixture of sodium chloride, sodium bicarbonate (or sodium citrate), potassium chloride, and dextrose to be dissolved and used to treat chronic diarrhea.

In recent years there has been an increased awareness of the importance of minerals in the diet and of the value of mineral supplements. Generally, gluconates, like other organic salts, are less irritating to the gastrointestinal tract; thus, the following metal gluconates are found in the USP: Zinc, Sodium, Copper, Magnesium, and Manganese. The USP includes a monograph USP for Selenious Acid Injection, which can provide a source of selenium as a mineral supplement.

In a new USP section entitled Nutritional Supplements are monographs for Mineral Capsules and Mineral Tablets. The minerals present in these dosage forms are potassium, calcium, magnesium, phosphorous, zinc, iron, manganese, copper, molybdenum, fluorine, chromium, iodine, and selenium.

When it is necessary to administer trace elements parenterally, the monograph entitled *Trace Elements USP* describes a sterile solution that may be used to administer zinc, copper, chromium, manganese, selenium, iodine, and molybdenum.

TOPICAL AGENTS

OXIDIZING GERMICIDES

Hydrogen Peroxide, Sodium Hypochlorite, Iodine, and/or their various solutions are cited in the USP. Hypochlorous acid, the active moiety in sodium hypochlorite solution, owes its germicidal activity to both oxidizing and chlorinating activity.

PRECIPITATING GERMICIDES

Silver Nitrate, Silver Nitrate Ophthalmic Solution, and Toughened Silver Nitrate are listed in USP, as is Ammoniated Mercury. Zinc Acetate, Zinc Chloride, Zinc Sulfate, and Zinc Undecylenate also are official. Only two boron compounds are cited in NF: Boric Acid and Sodium Borate. The antimony compounds listed are Antimony Potassium Tartrate USP and Antimony Sodium Tartrate USP.

ASTRINGENTS

Aluminum ion in solution is an excellent local astringent over wide concentration ranges. It also is mildly antiseptic. Aluminum Chloride USP once was used in this application, but the high acidity of its solutions caused problems. The acidity results from ionization of the hexaaquo ion

$$[Al(H_2O)_6]^{3+} + H_2O \rightleftharpoons [Al(OH)(H_2O)_5]^{2+} + H_3O^+$$

and is about that of acetic acid. Today, the mixture of two compounds (aluminum hydroxychloride, aluminum chlorhydrate, aluminum chlorhydrol) obtained by partial neutralization of aluminum chloride is used.

$$[Al(H_2O)_6]^{3+} + OH^- \rightarrow [Al(OH)(H_2O)_5]^{2+} + H_2O$$

$$[Al(OH)(H_2O)_5]^{2+} + OH^- \rightarrow [Al(OH)_2(H_2O)_4]^+ + H_2O$$

The reaction is stopped before complete conversion to the dihydroxy hydrate. The resulting solution (or dried product) retains the excellent astringent (and deodorant) properties of the aluminum ion, but the pH of the solutions approximates neutrality (5 to 6).

Aluminum Subacetate Topical Solution USP is essentially a solution of the above ions prepared from aluminum sulfate using carbonate ion ($CaCO_3$) as the base. Aluminum Sulfate and Ammonium Alum and Potassium Alum are found in the USP and also are used as astringents. Alum may be either the potassium or ammonium form. It is shaped into a pencil form to be used as a styptic.

Iron(III) and aluminum ions are very similar. Iron(III) is astringent, and preparations of ferric salts for such use formerly were recognized. Although it is efficient in this capacity, its staining property is a major disadvantage. Lime water, a saturated solution of fresh calcium hydroxide, is used as a local astringent. Bismuth subnitrate and the other bismuth sub-salts are used as astringents and protectives.

PROTECTIVES

In order to possess good adhering properties, protectives must be in very finely powdered form. They also must be relatively inert, insoluble compounds. A wide range of compounds are suitable as protectives. They usually are used externally, but some applications involve the gastrointestinal tract. Some are slightly soluble (eg, ZnO) and give some astringent action; others (eg, kaolin) have adsorbent action.

Zinc Oxide, Calamine (and Calamine Lotion and Phenolated Calamine Lotion), and Zinc Stearate (all USP) are used for their protective and slightly astringent properties. Calamine is the calcined native zinc oxide ore. The iron oxide impurity gives calamine a flesh color that is cosmetically more appealing. Zinc stearate, a mixture of fatty acid zinc soaps, has an unctuous feel. White Lotion USP is used for its astringent and protective powers.

Magnesium trisilicate, basic aluminum carbonate, and chalk are used as protectives, as are the various insoluble bismuth sub-salts. Talc is used because of its smooth, unctuous feel. Kaolin and bentonite are used as they also have some absorptive properties; titanium dioxide is used as a solar screen.

INORGANIC PIGMENTS

The most important innocuous pigments are the iron oxides. They give colors throughout the visible spectrum. Three variables are involved: particle size, oxidation state, and degree of hydration.

MISCELLANEOUS INORGANIC APPLICATIONS

ARTIFICIAL ATMOSPHERES

Five gases are official: nitrogen, oxygen, helium, carbon dioxide, and nitrogen(I) oxide (nitrous oxide or laughing gas). Nitrogen is used as a diluent for oxygen and may be used as a protective atmosphere for easily oxidized medicinals.

Helium, because of its low density compared to nitrogen, is used to prepare a gaseous mixture composed of 20% oxygen and helium. This mixture is used to alleviate respiration difficulties. Because of the low solubility of helium in blood, the same mixture is used as an atmosphere for those performing under high atmospheric pressures (deep-sea divers, caisson workers). When ordinary air is used, rapid decompression causes bubbles of gaseous nitrogen to form in the blood; the resulting painful, and sometimes fatal, condition is known as the bends.

Oxygen is used when respiratory problems exist. Ordinarily, it is diluted with nitrogen or helium; 100% oxygen should not be used continuously. In hyperbaric oxygen therapy, oxygen is breathed inside a tank at up to 3 atm (atmospheres) of pressure. Although the amount of oxygen carried by the hemoglobin is little affected, the higher oxygen pressure increases the amount of dissolved oxygen in the plasma (Henry's law).

It is possible to produce oxygen that is medicinally useful on site, as in a hospital or nursing home, by the use of oxygen concentrators. There are two types of membranes that are used in the concentrators, permeable plastic membranes and molecular sieves. The monograph for Oxygen 93% USP sets standards for the oxygen produced by the molecular-sieve process.

Nitrogen(I) oxide usually requires 20 to 25% oxygen during administration. It is used for surgical operations of short duration. Xenon has a general anesthetic action but is too rare for use. Magnesium ion has anesthetic action; however, the anesthetic dose and the toxic dose of magnesium are too close for use as a general anesthetic. Magnesium Sulfate Injection USP is used as an anticonvulsant and central depressant.

CARBON DIOXIDE ABSORBERS

When, as in general anesthesia, a patient rebreathes air, dangerous levels of carbon dioxide build up. To prevent this *carbon dioxide absorbers* are used. Soda Lime NF is prepared by fusing calcium hydroxide with sodium hydroxide and/or potassium hydroxide with sufficient diatomaceous earth to yield a hard, nonfriable product. For Barium Hydroxide Lime USP, barium hydroxide is substituted for the alkali hydroxide. The particles formed must be large enough to allow free passage of air, but small enough to give a large surface area for absorption. The particles must be hard to prevent dust formation with handling. Entrainment of absorber dust in the breathed air could cause serious alkali burns in the respiratory tract. A colored indicator is included in the preparation to indicate when the carbon dioxide capacity is depleted.

RESPIRATORY STIMULANTS

Carbon dioxide is used as a respiratory stimulant, usually with 5 to 7% oxygen. Because it is the normal respiratory stimulant it is of no value where the respiratory center is already depressed. Carbon dioxide also is used as an inert gas in the headspace over medicinals in sealed containers.

Ammonium Carbonate NF is used as a respiratory stimulant. The name is a misnomer, as it is a mixture of ammonium bicarbonate and ammonium carbamate. At room temperature it decomposes to ammonia and carbon dioxide, two respiratory stimulants.

$$NH_4HCO_3 + NH_2CO_2NH_4 \rightarrow 3NH_3 + 2CO_2 + H_2O$$

The substance must be stored in tightly sealed containers.

Aromatic Ammonia Spirit USP is prepared from ammonium carbonate, strong ammonia solution, various aromatic oils, alcohol, and water. Light-resistant containers must be used.

EXPECTORANTS

Water vapor, an excellent expectorant, is currently considered the best. Ammonium chloride and carbonate, and ammonium and potassium iodides are used commonly as expectorants. Hydriodic acid syrup was official at one time. If the iodides are used in solution, they must be protected by an antioxidant such as sodium thiosulfate.

LAXATIVES, ENEMAS, AND IRRIGATION SOLUTIONS

Cathartics are divided into classes according to mode of action. With the exception of sulfur, the inorganic cathartics are saline (osmotic, bulk) laxatives. For laxative action one or both of the ions of the salt must not be absorbed, or be absorbed with difficulty. This sets up an osmotic imbalance in the intestinal tract that the body attempts to correct by secreting water into the intestine. The large volume of fluid in the intestine acts as a mechanical stimulus for peristalsis.

The commonly used salts of the monohydrogen phosphate, monohydrogen tartrate, tartrate, and citrate ions are absorbed slowly, but in laxative doses their osmotic action is rapid and effective. They are swept out of the intestinal tract before appreciable absorption can take place. Sulfate ion is relatively nonabsorbable and is used either as the magnesium or sodium salt (Epsom Salt and Glauber's Salt, respectively).

Insoluble laxatives, such as Milk of Magnesia, must be dissolved in the stomach before they can exert a laxative effect. The soluble magnesium sulfate and citrate of magnesia are used widely as laxatives. However, soluble magnesium salts frequently are not recommended as laxatives because of the danger of absorbing free magnesium ion. Dibasic Sodium Phosphate, Sodium Phosphates Oral Solution, Sodium Citrate and Citric Acid Oral Solution, Potassium Sodium Tartrate, Milk of Magnesia, and Sodium Sulfate are cited officially.

PEG 3350 and Electrolytes for Oral Solution USP (Polyethylene- glycol 3350, $NaHCO_3$, $NaCl$, Na_2SO_4 and KCl) is a dry mixture that is to be dissolved at the time of use and then consumed within a prescribed time in order to function as a cathartic and accomplish oral colonic lavage in preparation for a barium enema or a colonoscopic examination.

Sulfur, when ingested, has an irritant laxative effect. The element is thought to be reduced to hydrogen sulfide by reducing agents present in the intestinal fluid. Hydrogen sulfide is a mild intestinal irritant.

Sodium Phosphates Enema USP is a mixture of dibasic and monobasic sodium phosphates or dibasic sodium phosphate and phosphoric acid in water to give a pH of 5 to 5.8.

Some solutions are used for irrigating various parts of the body. For example, Citric Acid, Magnesium Oxide, and Sodium Carbonate Irrigation USP is defined as a sterile solution that, after the chemical reactions between citric acid and the other two compounds are completed and the resulting solution is sterilized, is suitable for use as a urinary bladder irrigant; its acidic pH is conducive to dissolving any bladder calculi in patients such as those using an indwelling catheter.

RADIOPAQUES AND IMAGING AGENTS

Radiopaque compounds are capable of interfering with the passage of x-rays. This interference is directly proportional to atomic number. The soft tissues of the body are composed of atoms of very low atomic number (1, 6, 7, 8, 15, and 16) that do not interfere sufficiently to be discerned. To make the soft tissues, the lumen of organs, and body channels show, high atomic number atoms must be used.

Because of the toxicity of these elements, the choices are limited. Only two, barium and iodine, atomic numbers 56 and 53, have proved useful. Barium Sulfate USP and Barium Sulfate for Suspension USP are used for studies of the intestinal tract. Iodine is incorporated into organic molecules designed to concentrate in the organ or cavity to be studied, such as Iopanoic Acid USP designed for visualization of the gall bladder. Each molecule of the acid has three iodine atoms.

The introduction and development of magnetic resonance imaging (MRI) as a means of getting images of parts of the body by noninvasive methods has made medical diagnoses simpler and more scientific. The use of gadolinium (element 64) in various complexes such as a cationic diethylenetriamine pentaacetic acid complex with a meglumine anion has dramatically facilitated the visualization of intracranial lesions by paramagnetic enhancement.

STRUCTURAL REPAIRS

Occasionally, temporary or permanent replacement of support structures is necessary. The materials used should be chemically inert and insoluble in the body fluids, they must be nontoxic, and they must have the strength to withstand any physical stress to which they are subjected. Tantalum has been used as a bone replacement for temporary braces of long bones, and to close openings in the skull. Silver has found similar applications. It reacts slightly with body fluids, but as insoluble silver chloride is the principal product, this is not a serious threat. Mercury amalgams of gold and silver are used for dental fillings

but this venerable use of mercury is being questioned because of possible chronic toxicity. Zinc-eugenol cement also is used for dental fillings.

Plaster of Paris is used for temporary support structures, especially for broken bones. The formula, $CaSO_4 \cdot 1/2H_2O$, suggests a hemihydrate, but there is experimental evidence indicating the existence of local gypsum ($CaSO_4 \cdot 2H_2O$) nuclei in anhydrous calcium sulfate.

Plaster of Paris also is used for taking dental impressions; because it expands slightly on setting, it fills all spaces completely to give a true surface replica.

EPILOGUE

Because of space considerations, many less important and older inorganic medicinals have been omitted. The chemistry given necessarily is abbreviated. For further details of basic chemistry and omitted uses and products see Discher et al.[1] For more thorough discussions of the etiology and treatment involving inorganic substances, see the appropriate chapters of this text or of Block et al.[8] For the chemistry and use of many products no longer in general use or entirely abandoned, refer to one of the older editions of Rogers, Soine, and Wilson.[9]

An excellent text by Rayner-Canham[10] considers the basic properties and descriptive aspects of many inorganic compounds and includes some biochemical and biological information. In addition, Emsley's excellent book[11] gives information about the presence of elements in humans and provides the background and history for the use of inorganic compounds for medicinal purposes.

REFERENCES

1. Discher CA, Medwick T, Bailey LC. *Modern Inorganic Pharmaceutical Chemistry,* 2nd ed. Prospect Heights, IL: Waveland Press, 1985.
2. Huheey HE, Keiter EA, Keiter RL. *Inorganic Chemistry: Principles of Structure and Reactivity,* 4th ed. New York: Harper Collins, 1993.
3. Leigh GJ, ed. *Nomenclature of Inorganic Chemistry, IUPAC,* 3rd ed. Oxford: Blackwell Science, 1990.
4. Bailar JC, ed. *Comprehensive Inorganic Chemistry.* New York: Pergamon, 1973.
5. Pauling L. *Nature of the Chemical Bond,* 3rd ed. Ithaca, NY: Cornell University Press, 1960.
6. Shannon RD, Prewitt CT. *Acta Crystallogr* 1969; B25: 925.
7. Lide DR, ed. *Handbook of Chemistry and Physics,* 71st ed. Boca Raton, FL: CRC Press, 1990.
8. Block JH, et al. *Inorganic Medicinal and Pharmaceutical Chemistry.* Philadelphia: Lea & Febiger, 1974.
9. Rogers CH, Soine TO, Wilson CO. *A Textbook of Inorganic Pharmaceutical Chemistry.* Philadelphia: Lea & Febiger, 1952.
10. Rayner-Canham G. *Descriptive Inorganic Chemistry.* New York: WH Freeman, 1996.
11. Emsley J. *Nature's Building Blocks.* New York: Oxford University Press, 2001.

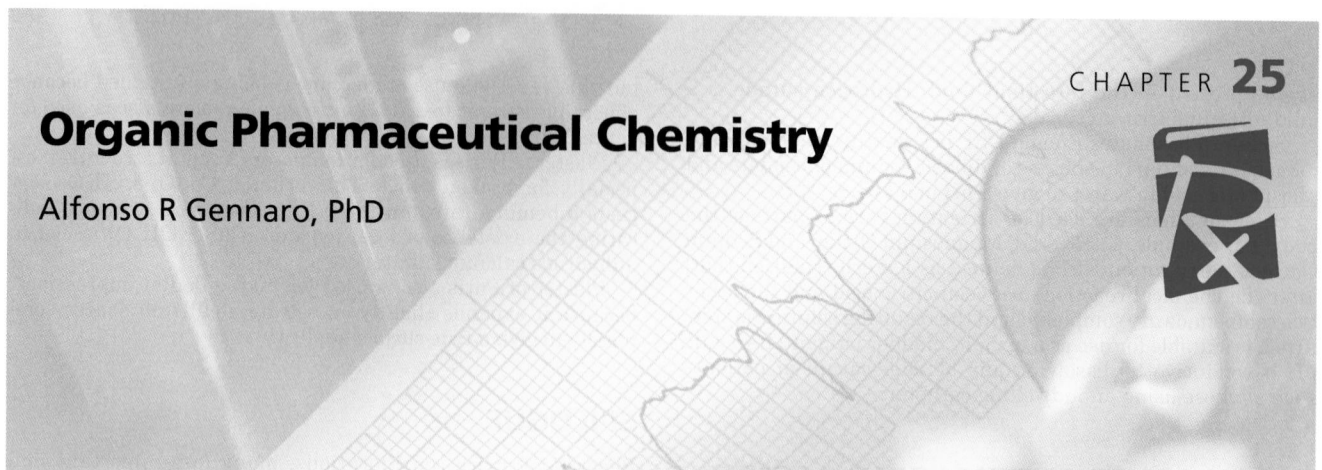

CHAPTER 25

Organic Pharmaceutical Chemistry

Alfonso R Gennaro, PhD

It is not the purpose of this chapter to provide a fundamental treatment of organic chemistry. Readers are expected to have pursued the usual basic courses in organic chemistry and be cognizant of the various advanced texts and other readily available works of reference. (See Bibliography) Accordingly, this chapter is restricted primarily to a listing of the more prominent structural types of organic compounds, a brief presentation of the various nomenclature systems and of the major chemical classes of official (USP/NF) pharmaceuticals, followed by a discussion on the identification of organic functional groups and the possible assignment of an approximate acidic, basic, or neutral value to these groups. A detailed treatment of the individual pharmaceuticals is provided at other locations in this book (refer to the index).

TYPES OF ORGANIC COMPOUNDS

A comprehensive understanding of organic chemistry would be extremely difficult were it not for the fact that the hundreds of thousands of known compounds fall conveniently into a very much smaller number of general types based on molecular structure. Similarities and differences among the physical and chemical properties of the diverse compounds thus become more apparent and understandable, and this is useful both in providing explanations for observed phenomena and in making predictions for possible applications of known compounds and compounds projected for synthesis.

Organic compounds may be classified in many ways, the desired intricacy of any particular scheme depending on the purpose of performing the classification. Thus, for one purpose it may suffice to construct a single, broad class of hydroxy compounds, while for other purposes it is desirable to subdivide this broad class into alcohols and phenols and perhaps even subdivide these further into subclasses of alcohols and phenols. It is appropriate here, for purposes of convenient reference, to list those types of compounds most commonly encountered in the systematic study of organic chemistry and to display their general (type) formulas. The types of compounds that are pertinent, especially to pharmacy, are treated in greater detail later in the chapter where examples of official drugs belonging to each class also are provided.

To enhance the utility of this chapter as a reference tool, the listing in Appendix A is alphabetical rather than by any chemical classification scheme. Prefatorily, the following explanatory notes are provided.

Unless otherwise specified, the formulas shown are for compounds containing only one of the particular functional groups involved. Formulas for compounds containing more than one of the same functional group can be derived easily.

Naturally occurring classes of compounds such as carbohydrates, proteins, alkaloids, glycosides, or lipids are not treated as types of compounds in this classification. A separate, more detailed presentation of these is provided in Chapter 26.

Although a few heterocyclic types such as imines (azacyclic), anhydrides of dibasic acids (oxacyclic), lactides (dioxacyclic) automatically enter into the listing, it will be observed that parent heterocycles in general (eg, thiophene, pyridine, dioxane) are not included. Heterocycles represented in official drugs are listed later in the chapter.

In type formulas, such as in Appendix A, the symbol R is employed conventionally to denote a hydrocarbon radical. Unless otherwise specified, it may be aliphatic, alicyclic, or aromatic, and its valence varies to satisfy the requirements of its attachment to the rest of the molecule. The degree of saturation in R does not enter into the scheme. When a formula contains more than one R, the radicals may be either identical or different. In a few instances it is possible, that even if two monovalent Rs are replaceable by a single divalent R, the same type of compound is retained, as with aliphatic ketones ($R_2C{=}O$) and cyclic ketones ($R{=}C{=}O$).

The type formulas assume a useful broader meaning if R, instead of being restricted to designate only a *hydrocarbon* radical, is permitted to (1) be a residue from a heterocycle and (2) carry substituent groups. The latter definition automatically extends the listing to embrace polyfunctional compounds, but it also introduces the complicating feature of the *order of precedence* of functional groups. This matter is discussed later in the chapter.

Unless otherwise specified, the symbol X stands for a member of the halogen family. In addition to the type formulas, one or more specific examples of each type of compound also are provided, showing how the formulas usually appear in somewhat condensed form and illustrating the manner in which the type names become parts of individual compound names. However, it should be remembered that, although correct, such names are not always the preferred names in modern nomenclature practice.

A linear formula with a horizontal line above the symbols indicates a ring structure; the line is a bond joining the two atoms at each end. For example, $\overline{CH_2CH_2CH_2CH_2COO}$ is δ-valerolactone. The oxygen atom on the right end is bonded to the carbon atom on the left end, forming a 6-membered ring.

The only formulas and structures that will be depicted will be those of pharmaceutical interest.

NOMENCLATURE OF ORGANIC COMPOUNDS

In the early decades of organic chemistry, newly discovered compounds commonly were provided with names which indicated either the source or some outstanding property of the compound. Thus, marsh gas, wood alcohol, salicylic acid, cadaverine, morphine, chlorophyll, and thousands of other similar names were invented. As more and more compounds were isolated or synthesized, it became apparent, however, that some systematic manner of naming organic compounds in terms of their structure would have to be devised. Early systems of nomenclature, while adequate for the period in which they were invented, soon required modification as the number of known compounds increased. The result has been that the system (or rather the combination of systems) now in use represents an evolution covering many decades.

That a truly effective system of nomenclature is bound to be very complex becomes obvious when one reflects that it must not only discriminate, unequivocally, among the many millions of compounds already known, but also must allow adequate provision for encompassing new compounds, which are being synthesized by the thousands each year. Fundamentally, therefore, such discrimination means that each specific name coined through the system must account for (1) the quantitative elementary composition (molecular formula) and (2) all of the structural features for one, and only one, specific compound.

The IUPAC and CAS Systems of Nomenclature

Of the various comprehensive systems which had been proposed, and used to a varying extent, the two most widely employed and most thoroughly updated through revision and enlargement are those devised by the International Union of Pure and Applied Chemistry (IUPAC) and the Chemical Abstracts Service (CAS). Each of these systems represents an implementation of the rules devised by the IUPAC Commission on the Reform of the Nomenclature of Organic Chemistry, which has been engaged actively and continuously in the subject for many decades.

The two systems are identical in many respects. The CAS system intentionally departs from that of IUPAC wherever such departure contributes to the main purpose of *Chemical Abstracts*—indexing the world's chemical literature. Recognizing the desirability to maintain compatibility between the two systems, however, CAS identifies each such departure and displays the alternative IUPAC treatment.

Because of the difficulty in converting many structural formulas into unique, descriptive names, CAS now assigns a *Registry Number* to every chemical compound (organic and inorganic). All editions of the USAN (see Chapter 27) and commencing with USP XIX and NF XIV, all monographs for pure chemical entities carry the CAS Registry Number, which uniquely identifies every compound. In the same editions of USP and NF, "New Chemical Abstracts Names" were assigned. Also, CAS has completely revised the older system (which parallels IUPAC rules) so that computer searches may be made using nomenclature fragments, rather than topological features, to locate molecular fragments as well as complete molecules.

It obviously is inappropriate and space-prohibitive to include in this text a discussion of the multiplicity of details in either of these two systems. Suffice it to state that, from a structural viewpoint, each system adequately must describe for each compound the following:

Composition and configuration of the carbon skeleton
Interruptions of the carbon skeleton by heteroatoms
State of hydrogenation of the skeleton
Presence and location of substituents, ie, atoms or groups of atoms
    (radicals) functioning in place of hydrogen
Features of stereoisomerism

The reader desirous of the details of the systems should consult the continuing series of reports issued by the IUPAC Commission on the Nomenclature of Organic Chemistry, and the CAS publication entitled *The Naming and Indexing of Chemical Compounds from Chemical Abstracts*. The latter, which first appeared as an introduction to the subject index of volume 56 of *Chemical Abstracts*, has undergone very extensive revision and enlargement. The introduction to the subject index of volume 66 provides a useful summary treatment. The publication of the American Chemical Society, *The Ring Index*, also offers a very detailed systematic presentation of closed-chain systems identified through the literature up to 1963.

Because of major changes in nomenclature and indexing procedures, mainly dictated by computerization of nomenclature and two-dimensional structures, each quinquennial index to *Chemical Abstracts* is accompanied by an index guide that allows the user to follow the transition between the old and new (or modified) nomenclature.

Three general features common to both systems deserve special comment, specifically the employment of trivial names, the order of precedence of functional groups, and permissive ambiguity.

TRIVIAL NAMES—A *trivial name* is one that does not describe a compound rigidly in terms of the absolute structure notations embodied in the system, but rather has earned worldwide recognition as being specific for that compound. Acetic acid (for ethanoic acid), purine (for 7*H*-imidazo[4,5-*d*]pyrimidine), and pregnane (for 10β,13β-dimethyl-17β-ethyl-9α,14α, 5β,8β-perhydrocyclopenta[*a*]phenanthrene) are common examples. Without allowing for the judicious employment of such trivial names, any scheme of nomenclature would be hopelessly complex and of little, if any, practical use. On the other hand, the wholesale, indiscriminate admission of trivial names to a system equally is disastrous.

Arriving at a satisfactory compromise between these two extremes obviously requires detailed deliberation, and the compromise position taken by IUPAC also has been adopted by CAS: trivial names admitted by IUPAC are also those admitted by CAS. However, with the advent of computer techniques, long or unwieldy names are handled with relative ease. Thus, trivial and systematic names are assuming equal importance, because a trivial-name index cannot be computer-searched to locate fragments of two-dimensional structures as these fragments are not evident in the name. But with long, systematic names, every portion of a parent molecule, substituent, functional group, and so on is apparent in the name and will yield to the computer search.

PRECEDENCE ORDER OF FUNCTIONAL GROUPS—An *order of precedence* (priority) for functional groups is necessary to manage polyfunctional compounds systematically. As a simple example, in the absence of a systematic method, the compound $NH_2CH_2CH_2CH_2OH$ could be named either as an aminopropanol or as a hydroxypropylamine. But in the order of precedence, hydroxyl is higher than amino and, because the system requires that only the function of highest priority shall be represented by the suffix part of the name, the systematic name becomes 3-amino-1-propanol. The order of precedence of functional groups is described clearly (see Table 1 of the introduction to the subject index of *Chemical Abstracts*, volume 66, or the *11th Collective Index*, volumes 96 to 105, Appendix IV, *Chemical Substance Index Names*) and is identical in both the IUPAC and CAS systems.

PERMISSIVE AMBIGUITY—*Ambiguity* (lack of complete structural specificity) is permitted to the extent that it reflects structural features of a compound that either are unknown or have not yet been incorporated into the system. Prohibition of such ambiguity would disallow the cataloging of a very significant percentage of known compounds, especially among those that involve features of stereoisomerism.

Compendial Nomenclature

The lack of adherence to the principles of systematic nomenclature, in both the commercial and academic worlds, has led to a multiplicity in the types of chemical names in actual use. It is not at all unusual to find a specific compound referred to by several different names, each of which is correct chemically. This, of course, creates a very confused state that, if it persists in the indexing literature, often renders searching via nomenclature extremely difficult, and frequently, impossible. It is for this reason that, wherever possible, *Chemical Abstracts* translates the nonsystematic nomenclature of the author into its CAS equivalent.

Recognizing the advantages of adhering to a standard system of nomenclature, the official compendia (USP/NF) elected to adopt names preferred by CAS. The principle of operation is simply that either the title or one of the subtitles of an official chemical must be the currently preferred CAS name. It is well to observe that the structural relationships established on the basis of the principal functional group automatically may hide relationships involving functional groups of lesser priority (eg, amphetamine is named as a derivative of phenethylamine, whereas hydroxyamphetamine becomes a derivative of phenol; similarly, sulfamerazine is named as a derivative of sulfanilamide, whereas phthalylsulfacetamide becomes a derivative of phthalanilic acid). Beginning with USP XIX and NF XIV each monograph carries the "new CAS name" along with the CAS preferred name currently in use. Also included is the Chemical Abstracts System *Registry Number,* which provides a unique identifier and simplifies locating a specific compound or drug in the literature, especially using a computer search.

Chemical Syllables

In addition to whatever numbers, numerical syllables, and individual Greek and English letters are required, systematic chemical names consist of a collection of syllables, each of which carry a chemical connotation of some sort. Many, such as chloro-, hydroxy-, and methyl-, clearly indicate specific elements or radicals.

Many others, such as andro- (from the Greek, "man"), tauro- (Latin, "bull"), neo- (Greek, "new"), or pseudo- or ψ (Greek, "false"), are of no chemical significance from a structural viewpoint, but often are very useful in forming the so-called trivial or common names for complex molecules such as androsterone, taurocholic acid, neoantergan, pseudoglobulin—the correct chemical names for these structures are often extremely cumbersome. Because of their lack of structural chemical significance, however, these will not be discussed further here.

The third group of these syllables consists of miscellaneous prefixes and suffixes and is of sufficient importance to warrant abbreviated treatment, because, like those of the first group, these have structural significance and often constitute a necessary part of systematic chemical names. A list of the more commonly encountered ones of this group is provided in Appendices B and C. Many of these have multiple meanings, and the definitions given herein represent the most common sense in which they are used in organic chemistry. Those shown in italics are used commonly in italicized form and/or enclosed in parentheses when used in organic nomenclature. It also must be remembered that the precise meanings shown here do not always apply to trivial names (eg, the meaning of -ene or of -ylene does not apply to acetylene; similarly, the meaning of -ol (alcohol) does not apply to benzol). Caution always must be exercised in attempting to attach significance to the various parts of such common names.

The systematic treatment of cyclic systems uses a generous miscellany of syllables with specific meanings; for listings and explanations, consult the *Ring Index* and Appendix E.

RADICALS AND GROUPS IN ORGANIC CHEMISTRY

Through the concept and use of radicals and groups, a logical and very helpful classification of the huge number of organic compounds is possible. Furthermore, knowledge of the chemical properties of commonly used individual radicals makes pos-

sible either a prediction or an explanation of the chemical properties of compounds because, in general, the chemical properties of a compound are completely or partially the combined properties of the radicals present in the molecule.

Several hundred different radicals have been recognized, named, and classified. A comprehensive list ordered by both names and formulas is published periodically as part of the *Collective Index* to *Chemical Abstracts,* as *Appendix IV,* in the *Chemical Substance Index Names* found in the index guide for volumes 96 to 105 of *Chemical Abstracts.*

For purposes of convenient reference, a list of radicals and groups frequently encountered in pharmaceutical chemistry is provided in Appendix D. Classification into chemical types has been sacrificed in favor of an alphabetical arrangement. Included in the list are many inorganic radicals that frequently are present in organic combination.

Chemical Notation Systems

The complexity and the cumbersome nature of modern organic chemical nomenclature have encouraged attempts to develop "shorthand expressions," variously referred to as notations, ciphers, codes, and alphamerics, which for certain purposes would be more convenient to use than the chemical names. Several systems have been proposed (eg, the NAS-NRC provided a comprehensive review of the history of the various systems), although none have fully survived. In general, they involved assigning chemical meanings to the characters usually available on, or readily adapted to, a standard typewriter or computer keyboard and devising rules for their use in constructing the notations. A recent addition to the nomenclature/notation foray is **SMILES**, an acronym for *S*implified *M*olecular *L*ine *E*ntry *S*pecification. This is a valence model of a structure, not a computer data structure, and is relatively simple to master. (A tutorial is available at http://www.daylight.com/.)

Final assessment of the overall utility of notations has yet to be made; they particularly are appealing because their brevity (compared with descriptive chemical nomenclature as illustrated in Table 25-1) greatly increases storage efficiency in printed indexes and computer memories and facilitates computerized searching. In addition, they automatically avoid the troublesome "trivial name feature" encountered in practical nomenclature. However, they are not pronounceable words and do not eliminate the need for descriptive chemical nomenclature in the written and spoken word.

Several of these notations have been found useful for retrieving compounds on a structural basis from specialized files of compounds stored in computers using the same notations. The extent to which techniques for accomplishing such retrieval may be applied usefully to a file comprising the universe of chemical compounds is the subject of considerable interest and study.

Special typewriters have been devised whereby structural formulas may be coded directly on punched tape and also stored in the memory of a computer in the form of a matrix (a connection table of atoms) that can be searched at any future time on an atom-by-atom basis. This technique permits retrieval of compounds on a highly intimate structural basis that need not involve either nomenclature or the above-mentioned notations. Auxiliary devices exist for regenerating the actual structural formulas of retrieved compounds either by actual printout or by display on a computer monitor screen.

Table 25-1. Illustrations of Notation Brevity

DESCRIPTIVE CAS NAME	SMILES NOTATION
1-Chloro-3-methylbutane	ClCCC(C)C
4-Aminobenzoic acid	Nc1ccc(C(=O)O)CCl
1-Naphthalenemethanol	OCc1c2ccccc2cc1

Organic Chemical Literature

The constantly accelerating rate of research and development during the past five decades has created severe literature problems, not only in the areas of basic chemistry but also in the other fields of science and technology where chemical information is primarily applied, rather than generated. The history of *Chemical Abstracts* (*CA*) illustrates the magnitude of this so-called "information explosion." Commencing in 1906, the Chemical Abstracts Service (CAS) required 32 years for *CA* to produce its first million abstracts (1938), but only 17 years for the second million (1955), 8 years for the third million (1963), 6 years for the fourth million (1969), 5 years for the fifth million (1974), and somewhat less than 5 years for the sixth million (1979). By late 1983 the seventh million was surpassed, and the 8-million mark was reached in early 1987. Over 10 million abstracts were published by the end of 1992. One prediction suggests 20 million abstracts will be achieved by the year 2005.

Currently, the volume of chemical literature is so great that many libraries simply do not have enough shelf space to accommodate bound volumes and have resorted to microfilming, microfiche or, more drastically, cancellation of hardcopy in favor of electronic journals. More important is the fact that selective retrieval of information from the hardcopy literature has become an extremely arduous task. As a consequence, various industrial, academic, and governmental institutions (several pharmaceutical firms actually pioneered the effort) have developed computerized systems of storage and retrieval of those kinds of chemical information pertinent to their specific interests.

Currently, *Chemical Abstracts* may be searched via *SciFinder* or *SciFinder Scholar* and information may be found at the website *www.info.cas.org*. This facility allows a very rapid and thorough search of CAS to date; the current information is available on computer even before the printed copy reaches the subscriber. The *Institute for Scientific Information* (ISI) in Philadelphia also has computerized its abstract journal, *Index Chemicus*, a text and substructure searchable database which has several million compounds in its registry, and is adding new compounds at a rate of about 200,000 per year (See *www.isinet.com*.) Computer programs are available to customers that provide the capability to search and retrieve compound data either on the basis of structural features, or properties, applications, and bibliographic information.

The huge and continuing flood of published literature also has taxed severely the abilities of abstracting services to keep current. The magnitude of the task is illustrated by the experience of CA, which shows that the approximate number of papers and patents abstracted annually increased from 50,000 in 1950 to 120,000 in 1959; 230,000 in 1968; 400,000 in 1973; over half a million in 1978; approached 750,000 in 1983; and exceeded 1 million in 1988. The lag between publication of original articles and that of their abstracts has been sufficiently severe to foster the production of various so-called "current awareness tools" and specialty publications such as *Index Chemicus* and *Current Contents of ISI* and *Chemical Titles, Chemical-Biological Activities* (CBAC), *Polymer Science and Technology* (POST), *Basic Journal Abstracts* (BJA), and *CA Condensates* of CAS; which also are computer-based publications.

ORGANIC PHARMACEUTICALS

The contrast between the drugs of today and those of yesterday is a dramatic one in several respects. A century ago, humans relied almost exclusively on nature to produce the organic drugs they needed, and the contributions of pharmacy were confined largely to the preparation of extracts, tinctures, or other dosage forms of the crude drugs, and to the isolation of active principles, especially alkaloids and glycosides.

Synthetic drugs began to appear at a noticeably accelerated rate in the 1920s, and this generally is attributed to the very large expansion of the American chemical industry fostered by World War I. Many observers view the advent of the sulfa drugs in the early 1930s as the beginning of the modern era of synthetics.

The great majority of new basic drugs are distinct organic chemical compounds. Most of these are products of synthetic organic chemistry, although some, such as taxol, ACTH, and many of the antibiotics, hormones, and anticancer drugs are products of natural origin. Even with drugs of the latter group, however, the chemist has played a very important role in devising processes to produce them economically, not only in the large quantities required, but also in a sufficient state of purity. He also has succeeded in the deliberate chemical alteration of these naturally occurring compounds and produced derivatives that are either more potent or superior in some other respect (eg, dehydrocholic acid, dihydroergotamine, fluorocorticosteroids, semisynthetic penicillins, methyltestosterone).

Such molecular modification of known pharmacodynamic compounds, both natural and synthetic, constitutes one of the main kinds of research effort in the field of chemotherapy. Although it is true that such effort frequently results in cluttering the market with drugs that may not be superior to those being imitated, nevertheless, a critical review of the results achieved over the past half century provides abundant evidence that the effort yields a gratifying percentage of new, highly beneficial drugs (see Chapter 28). Many of the new admissions to the official compendia are of such genesis.

Chemical and Pharmacological Classifications

During the early years of the modern era of synthetic organic pharmaceuticals, it was common to classify these new drugs on a chemical basis. This was logical, not only because they were fundamentally the products of chemical research but also because the sciences of pharmacology and biochemistry were still in their early stages of development. Indeed, the ever-increasing need for more precise knowledge concerning the efficacy and safety of new drugs has fostered, to a significant degree, the rapid growth of these sciences to their present impressive status, and will undoubtedly continue to do so in the future. The most comforting result is that these complementary efforts continuously are providing medical science with better tools and knowledge to the end that effective prevention and treatment of human physiological and psychological ills constantly are becoming more and more of a science and less and less of an art.

The guiding hypothesis underlying all efforts to classify organic pharmaceuticals on a chemical basis is simply that some correlation will exist between the chemistry of the compounds and their actions and uses as medicinal agents. Early efforts to discover useful correlations were based largely on gross structural considerations with particular emphasis on the presence and location of chemically active (functional) groups. In a more sophisticated form, such efforts continue today, and the net result has been the accumulation of a very large body of knowledge on the broad subject of drug action. This knowledge materially strengthens the belief that the pharmacodynamics of drugs ultimately will be explicable in terms of their chemical characteristics. It also points indisputably to the fact that a complete understanding of the mechanisms of drug action is far in the future and that it will involve much more information than presently can be visualized from structural formulas and molecular models. (Refer to Chapter 28, *Structure-Activity Relationships and Drug Design*.)

It has become clear that the pharmacological actions of drugs must be viewed as functions of the *total* molecules. For example, all barbituric acids contain the malonylurea fragment, but the relative actions of the different barbiturates vary widely with respect to quantitativeness, onset time, and duration, depending upon substituents at the 1, 3, and 5 positions (Chapter 80, *Sedative and Hypnotic Drugs*). The official sulfa drugs provide another example. The antibacterial portion common to all sulfas is the parent compound sulfanilamide, but chemical alterations at the N^1 and N^4 positions produce derivatives that differ importantly in their actions and chemotherapeutic applications.

Dependence of pharmacological activity on *total* molecular structure commonly is evident with drugs that are polyfunctional from a chemical viewpoint. The sulfa drugs provide a good example of this as elimination of either the amino or sulfonamido portions, or even a change in their relative positions, results in loss of bacteriostatic activity. Similarly, aspirin loses its analgetic action if either its carboxyl or acetoxy group is removed completely or if the relation of these groups is other than *ortho.*

Similar dependence is common in the area of stereochemistry. Thus, the *trans* form of diethylstilbestrol is estrogenically potent whereas the *cis* form is not. This is reminiscent of the α- and β-forms of estradiol, the latter being about ten times as potent as the former. As an example involving diastereoisomers, the widely different mydriatic and pressor potencies of ephedrine and pseudoephedrine might be cited. Similar differences in physiological activity also are commonly observed between enantiomorphs. Thus, the D- and L-ephedrines differ markedly in mydriatic and pressor potencies; the D- forms of the α-amino acids are vastly inferior to the L- forms as nutrients, and (−)-epinephrine is more than 20 times as potent a sympathomimetic agent as the (+)-form.

From the preceding discussion, it is clear that difficulties may be encountered whenever one attempts to classify organic drugs on a chemical basis and obtain a system that simultaneously separates these drugs on a pharmacological basis. As will be seen in subsequent parts of this text, drugs that fall into the same chemical category often display, collectively, quite a number of different actions. Conversely, drugs of widely different chemical characteristics frequently provide the same kind of action when used as medicinal agents. Since, from a practical viewpoint, these agents are important because of the actions they provide (irrespective of their chemical composition), in subsequent chapters of this text drug monographs are grouped and presented on a pharmacological basis.

HETEROCYCLES PRESENT IN OFFICIAL PHARMACEUTICALS

Many important biochemical compounds and drugs of natural origin contain heterocyclic ring structures. Numerous examples occur, among the carbohydrates, essential amino acids, vitamins, alkaloids, glycosides, and antibiotics. The presence of heterocyclic structures in such diverse types of compounds is indicative strongly of the profound effects such structures exert on physiological activity, and recognition of this is reflected abundantly in efforts to find useful synthetic drugs. Examples include researches leading to a wide variety of modern drugs such as chlordiazepoxide (tranquilizer), methazolamide (carbonic anhydrase inhibitor), guanethidine (antihypertensive), stanozolol (anabolic), dapsone (leprostatic), cyclophosphamide and thiotepa (antineoplastics), hydrochlorothiazide (diuretic and antihypertensive), imipramine (antidepressant), lucanthone (antischistosomal), and many others.

As is to be expected, this trend in research is reflected in the changing character of the contents of official drug compendia. Intensive research in diverse hetero areas continues to yield new medicinal agents, and Appendix E is designed to portray partially the spectrum of heterocycles presently represented in USP/NF drugs. The classification is patterned after that employed in the *Ring Index* and in *Chemical Abstracts.* The rings are presented in the order of increasing complexity. The boldface figures show the total number of atoms in the rings, and the number of boldface figures indicates the number of rings present in the systems. As an example, the notation 5, 6 indicates a system composed of two rings, one of which contains five atoms while the other one contains six atoms. The notations, such as $C_3NS\text{-}C_6$, portray the kind and number of atoms present in the ring or rings. Associated with each of these formulas are the

graphic formulas and *Ring Index* names[1] of the individual heterocycles and, in italics, one or more examples of official drugs (or the portions of them) containing these heterocycles.

Structures and numbering schemes[2] are according to the *Ring Index* and thus do not portray any inherent features of stereospecificity.[3] It will be observed that some of the names for the heterocycles are trivial (eg, pyrimidine, nortropane) while others are rigidly systematic. Trivial names are employed in the table wherever advisable; ie, wherever, through continued use, they have become recognized by chemists (as reflected by IUPAC adoption and *Chemical Abstracts* indexing) as denoting the structures to which they refer. In all other instances, systematic names must be used to distinguish between the heterocycle of interest and its isomeric forms. Presentation is exclusively on the basis of the *most complex ring "system"* containing the hetero atom or atoms; the term *"system"* meaning either a single ring or a combination of rings of the fused, bridged, or spiro types. For example, quinine is presented *only* as a quinoline derivative and *not* also as a pyridine derivative, even though quinoline also is a benzopyridine. Similarly, caffeine is presented only as a purine derivative and not as either a pyrimidine or an imidazole derivative, even though purine also is an imidazopyrimidine.

In a complete presentation of this type, drugs containing two or more *separate* hetero ring systems would appear under each of the systems; eg, quinine would emerge both as a quinoline and quinuclidine derivative. Wherever possible, only that portion of the official title is used that embraces the heterocycle; eg, thiamine is used instead of thiamine hydrochloride.

The final volume (IV) of the *Ring Index* was published in 1964 and index numbers are no longer assigned to ring structures by CAS. Identifiers for all compound types (including ring systems) have been organized into a *Parent Compound Handbook,* published by CAS, which consists of the following index categories.

Parent Name—This includes the names of all parent compounds and undefined natural products arranged in alphabetical order. Complex parent names are permuted so that root terms, buried in the names, may be located.

Parent Formula—Compounds are arranged according to the Hill system (carbon first, hydrogen second, with other elements following in alphabetic order), but omitting hydrogen atoms in the molecular formula. Ring systems are grouped in the same fashion as the *Ring Index* (see Appendix E) under the appropriate molecular formula.

Registry Number—These are arranged in ascending CAS registry number order with associated *Parent Compound Identifiers.*[4]

Stereoparent—This consists of CAS *Index Parents* whose names imply stereochemistry and whose structures are known. The arrangement is alphabetical with *CA* references for undefined or partially defined natural products.

---

[1] Heterocyclic structures often are synthesized actually or theoretically by relatively simple chemical operations such as condensation or dehydrogenation of aliphatic structures. Because of this, many authors prefer to name such compounds in a manner designed to disclose the relationship to the aliphatics, rather than employ *Ring Index* or *CAS* nomenclature, as is used in Appendix D

[2] Extreme caution must be exercised in interpreting position numbers (locants) as given the same compound by different texts, reference works or authors. The situation often exists in which two different numbering schemes, through long-continued usage, have become established firmly for a particular ring system. This leads to the use of different numbers as locants in an otherwise identical pair of names for the same compound. Also, authors frequently indulge in the reprehensible practice of inventing their own numbering schemes.

[3] The *Ring Index,* 2nd ed, Washington DC: American Chemical Society, 1960 and supplements. Also, for each annual, quinquennial and decennial Index to *Chemical Abstracts.*

[4] An identifier consists of a 5-letter code through which an entry may be found in the Parent Compound File. Each section of this file is assigned a range of identifiers bt which the type of parent may be recognized. The ranges are:

BBBBB to BPZZY	Cage parents
BQBBR to BZZZP	Acyclic stereo parents
CBBBC to DZZZR	Cyclic stereo parents
FBBBF to ZZZZK	Ring parents

Ring Analysis—This includes ring systems only, arranged by the classical *Ring Index* system and states the *CA* name and *Parent Compound Identifier*.

Ring Substructure—Rings are listed by; A *component ring formula* for each individual ring system listed in the *Ring Analysis Index,* arranged according to the Hill system, but not including hydrogen atoms. All entries are permuted to allow searching on any atom.

The *current CA index name* of a ring parent and cyclic stereoparent; a *Parent compound Identifier*.

ACIDS AND BASES

Organic pharmaceuticals are often complex molecules that have a variety of acidic and basic functional groups. The behavior of these groups in an aqueous environment will influence the activity of the drug, its transport through the body and its passage from one body compartment to another. There are two main theories of acids and bases, the *Brønsted* theory and the *Lewis* theory. According to the Brønsted theory an acid is a group that can donate a proton (a hydrogen ion), and a base is a group that can accept (bond to) a proton. Because a proton has no electrons, the base must be able to provide a pair of electrons to form a new bond. A Lewis acid is a group that can accept an electron pair and therefore must have an empty orbital. Groups that can donate an electron pair are termed *Lewis bases*. In this chapter the discussion will focus on Brønsted acids and bases. See also Chapter 17 *Ionic Solutions and Electrolytic Equilibria.*

Groups which function as acids must have a proton that can be removed in the presence of a base. In the laboratory extremely strong bases can be used in nonaqueous solvents to remove protons from alkyl groups and aromatic rings. Although such reactions are extremely important for drug synthesis, the concern of this chapter is with drugs in an aqueous environment. In water, the strongest base that can exist is hydroxide ion, OH^-, while the strongest acid is the hydrated proton or hydronium ion, H_3O^+. Although there are several exceptions, most hydrogen atoms bonded to carbon are not sufficiently acidic to be removed in aqueous solution. In general hydrogen atoms bonded to O, N, S, and sometimes P (in general, any electronegative atom) are potentially removable in aqueous solution. When an acid donates a proton, a new species called the *conjugate base* of the acid is formed.

$$CH_3COOH \xrightleftharpoons{K_a} CH_3COO^\ominus + H^\oplus$$
$$\text{acid} \qquad\qquad \text{conjugate base}$$

which has a charge one unit less than that of the acid from which it is derived. Thus, acetic acid, which is electrically neutral, dissociates to a proton and its conjugate base, acetate ion, which has a charge of −1. An equilibrium is established between the acid and its conjugate base. The equilibrium constant, which is known as the acid dissociation constant (K_a), is a property of the acid in question. Because K_a values generally are exponential numbers, it is convenient to use $-\log K_a$ which is referred to as the pK_a of the acid. In water, the pK_a scale runs from 0 to 14 with the lowest values corresponding to the strongest acids. Refer to Chapter 17 for a more extensive treatment of this concept.

Basic groups require a pair of electrons, which are used to bond with a proton. This electron pair can be either an unshared pair or a formal negative charge. Bases such as ammonia or amines bond with protons using the lone unshared pair of electrons on the nitrogen atom. Other bases, such as hydroxide, use the electron pair made available by dissociation of the cation, to bond with protons. When a neutral base accepts a proton its charge increases by one unit and a new species is formed, called the *conjugate acid* of the base.

$$:NH_3 + H^\oplus \xrightleftharpoons{K_b} NH_4^\oplus$$
$$\text{base} \qquad\qquad \text{conjugate acid}$$

Ammonium ion (+1 charge) is the conjugate acid of ammonia; water (0 charge) is the conjugate acid of hydroxide ion. The equilibrium constant for base dissociation is called the K_b of the base. In water, the pK_b scale extends from 0 to 14 with low values representing the strongest bases. There is a relationship between the pK_a of an acid and the pK_b of its conjugate base in water.

$$pK_a \text{ (acid)} + pK_b \text{ (conjugate base)} = 14$$

A similar relationship holds for bases and their conjugate acids.

$$pK_b(\text{base}) + pK_a(\text{conjugate acid}) = 14$$

Acids are in equilibrium with their conjugate base forms. One of these species will be charged and the equilibrium ratio, therefore, will determine the extent to which the molecule is ionized in solution. This has profound implications in medicinal chemistry because the extent of ionization of a drug in the body will affect its transport from one compartment to another. Examination of the expression for acid dissociation shows that the equilibrium constant

$$K_a = [A^-][H^+]/[HA]$$

Taking the logarithm of both sides of the equation gives

$$\log K_a = \log [A^-] + \log [H^+] - \log [HA]$$

Multiplying both sides of the equation by −1 gives

$$-\log K_a = -\log [A^-] - \log [H^+] + \log [HA]$$

Substitution of pK_a for $-\log K_a$ and pH for $-\log [H^+]$ gives

$$pK_a = pH + \log [HA]/[A^-]$$

This is known as the Henderson–Hasselbalch equation and gives the relationship between the pK_a of an acid[5] and the ratio of its acid form to conjugate base form at a given pH. *It is important to remember that while pK_a is a property of the molecule, pH is a property of the medium (solvent).* In this case (for electrically neutral acids) the ratio $[HA]/[A^-]$ is the ratio of [nonionized]/[ionized] species.

A more general form of the equation can be expressed as

$$pK_a = pH + \log [\text{acid form}]/[\text{conjugate base form}]$$

This is easy to remember because the *base* goes in the *basement*. For charged acids, such as conjugate acids of amines, the equation appears as

$$pK_a = pH + \log [BH^+]/[B]$$

Here, the ratio $[BH^+]/[B]$ equals the ratio of [ionized]/[nonionized] species.

The Henderson–Hasselbalch equation allows for calculation of the percent ionization of an acid at a given pH. This can be calculated as

$$\% \text{ ionization} = 100 [\text{ionized}]/[(\text{ionized} + \text{non-ionized})]$$

An example of a Henderson–Hasselbalch calculation using phenol as the acid at pH 7.

phenol   phenolate ion

[5]In medicinal chemistry only pK_a is recognized to eliminate confusion. Those compounds with a pK_a greater than pK_w are bases; the greater the pK_a, the stronger the base. Henceforth, only pK_a will be used.

pK_a (phenol) = 9.9

$9.9 = 7 + \log [PhOH]/[PhO^-]$

$2.9 = \log [PhOH]/[PhO^-]$

$794 = [PhOH]/[PhO^-]$

Thus, the ratio of phenol to phenolate ion (PhO^-) at pH 7 is 794:1, the compound is largely non-ionized. The percent ionization is calculated to be

$$\% \text{ ionization} = 100[1/(1 + 794)]$$

$$\% \text{ ionization} = 0.126\% \text{ at pH 7}$$

A second example is provided for the extent of ionization of aniline at pH 7. Aniline ($PhNH_2$) is a base with a pK_a of 4.6 for the anilinium ion ($PhNH_2^+$). Using the Henderson–Hasselbalch equation gives

$$4.6 = 7 + \log [PhNH_3^+]/[PhNH_2]$$

$$-2.4 = \log [PhNH_3^+]/[PhNH_2]$$

$$0.004 = [PhNH_3^+]/[PhNH_2]$$

The ratio of ionized to non-ionized aniline at pH 7 equals 1:251. The percent ionization at pH 7 is

$$\% \text{ ionization} = 100 [1/(1 + 251)]$$

$$\% \text{ ionization} = 0.4\% \text{ at pH 7}$$

Some compounds have several acidic or basic groups or a combination of acidic and basic groups. In these cases, the pK_a of the strongest acid is used for Henderson–Hasselbalch calculations because this is the group that will dissociate most readily. It also should be recognized that compounds that possess quaternary ammonium groups (N attached to four alkyl or aryl groups but not hydrogen) have a permanent +1 charge which is unaffected by the pH of the medium. Such compounds will *always* be 100% ionized and calculation of the extent of ionization of the molecule is unnecessary.

It was stated previously that in an aqueous environment hydrogen atoms attached to O, N, S, or P may be acidic and that an equilibrium is established between the acid form and its conjugate base. Groups that stabilize (lower the energy of) the conjugate base will drive the equilibrium farther to the right and thereby increase the strength of the acid. Such groups stabilize the conjugate base by providing a mechanism for the dispersal of any developing negative charge. Electronic effects from functional groups will therefore have an effect on the strength of nearby acidic and basic sites.

The electronic effects of functional groups can be divided into *field*, *inductive*, and *resonance* effects. The nature of these effects and how they are balanced, is the deciding factor for the type of electronic effect expressed by an individual functional group. *Field effects* are through-space effects on polarizability due to electronegativity differences.

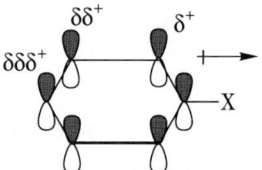

field effect

Polarizability is the ease of distortion of the electron cloud. Attachment of a highly electronegative atom to a system will draw electron density toward that atom, thereby rendering other portions of the molecule positively charged. Field effects tend to decrease with increasing distance. *Inductive effects* are the polarization of bonds as a result of electronegativity differences.

inductive effect

Thus an electronegative atom polarizes the bond attached to it by increasing the electron density in its vicinity. The opposite side of that bond acquires a degree of positive charge. This in turn polarizes the adjacent bond, and so on. These effects, which are transmitted through bonds, also decrease with distance from the electronegative atom.

Resonance effects involve the actual movement of electrons through a π-bond system. The π-bond system acts as a conductor of electrons, much as wires conduct the flow of electricity, which can be moved in either direction depending on the needs of the system. This is especially prominent in conjugated systems (those with alternating double and single bonds). The movement of electrons through a conjugated system allows for charges to be dispersed over several atoms (delocalization). This lowers the energy of the system relative to an isolated charge. In contrast to field and inductive effects, resonance effects decrease much more slowly with distance. Stabilization increases as the number of atoms over which the charge is dispersed increases. Resonance effects generally contribute more extensively to the overall electronic effect of a functional group than do field or inductive effects.

Among the functional groups which are classified as being electron-withdrawing are the carbonyl-based groups (aldehydes, ketones, esters, carboxylic acids, amides, etc), nitro, nitrile (cyano), sulfinyl, sulfonyl, halo, quaternary ammonium, trifluoromethyl, vinyl, ethynyl, and phenyl. The relative contributions of field, inductive, and resonance effects to the overall electronic effect of these functional groups is discussed below.

The carbonyl group (=C=O) is an integral part of a large number of functional groups such as ketones, carboxylic acids, amides, esters, and carbamates. Field and inductive effects within this bond system arise because of the electronegativity difference between oxygen and carbon. Electrons in both the σ- and π-bonds are polarized so that the greater density occurs near oxygen. The carbon atom acquires a partial positive charge which can attract excess electrons from neighboring groups. If a negative charge develops adjacent to a carbonyl group, that charge is stabilized not only by electrostatic effects, but also by resonance, which can delocalize the negative charge onto the carbonyl oxygen.

Another powerful electron-withdrawing group is the nitro group ($-NO_2$). Although this group is electrically neutral overall, the nitrogen always carries a positive charge that is balanced by a negative charge on one of the oxygen atoms. Two resonance structures can be drawn which distribute the negative charge over both oxygen atoms. The positively charged nitrogen can stabilize an adjacent negative charge by electrostatic attraction as well as by resonance.

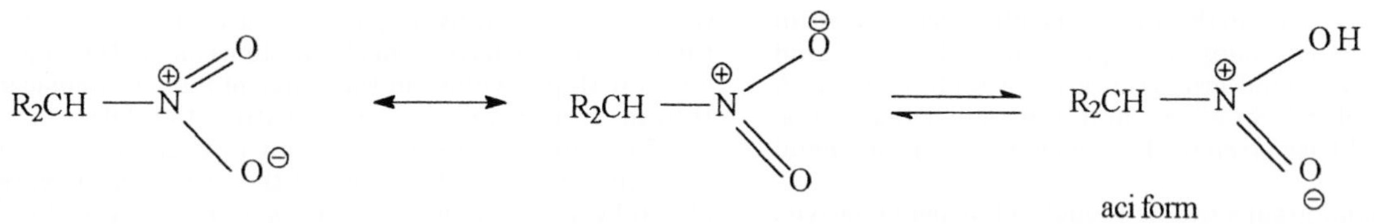

A nitrile possesses a carbon–nitrogen triple bond. The electronegativity difference between carbon and nitrogen results in carbon having a partial positive charge. The larger effect of this functional group however, comes from resonance stabilization of an adjacent negative charge onto the nitrogen.

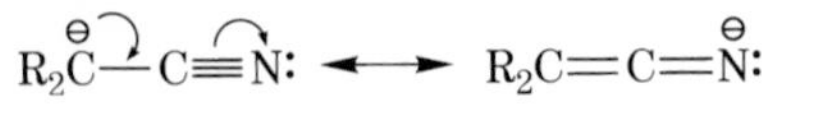

The difference between a sulfinyl and a sulfonyl group is that the former has one and the latter two S=O bonds. A major resonance form of the sulfinyl group has a S—O single bond with a formal positive charge on sulfur and a negative charge on oxygen. Sulfonyl has two such resonance structures. The preference for these structures over those with double bonds is a result of the relative inefficiency of p-orbital overlap due to the difference in size between sulfur and oxygen. Despite this, however, resonance stabilization of an adjacent negative charge does contribute to the electron-withdrawing capability of these functional groups.

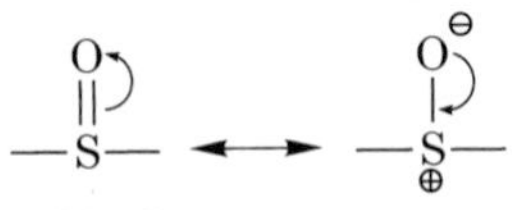

sulfinyl

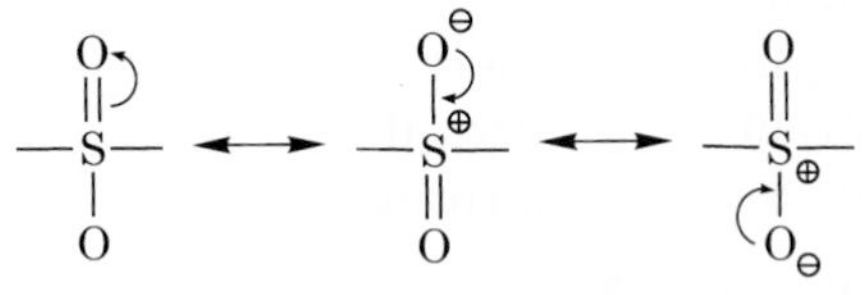

sulfonyl

The halides (F, Cl, Br, I) are much weaker electron withdrawing groups than might be expected. Fluorine, which is the most electronegative element, exerts strong field and inductive effects on an adjacent carbon atom. Additional electron density cannot be withdrawn by resonance because there are no available vacant orbitals. The lone-pair electrons on fluorine can however, be donated by resonance. As a result of this push–pull effect, the resonance and field (+ inductive) effects nearly cancel and fluorine usually exerts only a small electron-withdrawing effect.

electron-withdrawal by
field and inductive effects

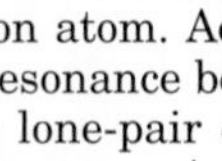

electron-donation by
resonance

Chlorine is less efficient at donating electrons by resonance because of its size relative to carbon. It does exert substantial field and inductive effects, and therefore behaves as an electron-withdrawing group. The electronegativity difference between carbon and bromine is small, and electron-donation by resonance is inefficient. As a result, bromine generally behaves as a weak electron-withdrawing group. Iodine is weaker still because of decreased field and inductive effects.

Functional groups such as quaternary ammonium and trifluoromethyl exert their electronic effects primarily through field and inductive effects. The quaternary ammonium group has a permanent positive charge on nitrogen, which stabilizes an adjacent negative charge electrostatically. Because there are no lone-pair electrons or vacant orbitals, resonance with this group is not possible. Direct resonance with a trifluoromethyl group does not occur. The three highly electronegative fluorine atoms exert multiple field and inductive effects on the carbon atom to which they are attached, which can then in turn stabilize an adjacent negative charge in a similar fashion.

Unsaturated groups such as phenyl, vinyl or ethynyl can function as electron withdrawing groups by delocalizing any excess electron density throughout the π-system.

Functional groups, which are classified as being electron donating, include alcohols, ethers, amines, and alkyl groups. Each of these will stabilize a developing positive charge and, when attached to basic atoms, tend to increase the association constant.

Alcohols and ethers have similar inductive effects to those present in carbonyl groups but experience decreased field effects due to the lack of a polarizable π-bond. Although carbonyl groups have the ability to delocalize excess electron density onto the oxygen, this is not possible for alcohols and ethers. Unshared electrons on the oxygen, however, can be delocalized by resonance to help stabilize a developing positive charge. In the process a new C=O bond is formed and the charge is delocalized onto oxygen. Although it is unfavorable to place a positive charge on an electronegative atom, this is compensated by the formation of a new bond. The predominance of resonance over field and inductive effects is observed by the fact that alcohols and ethers behave as electron-donating groups.

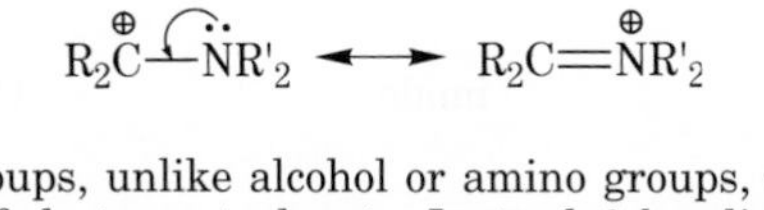

A similar situation exists for amino groups where the lone-pair electrons can be donated to form a C=N bond and thereby delocalize an adjacent positive charge onto the nitrogen. Because nitrogen is less electronegative than oxygen, it can better tolerate the charge. Amino groups are generally stronger electron donating substituents than either alcohols or ethers.

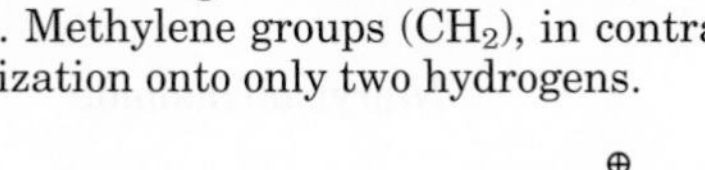

Alkyl groups, unlike alcohol or amino groups, do not have lone-pairs of electrons to donate. Instead, δ-bonding electrons, especially those from C—H bonds, can be donated in a process known as *hyperconjugation*, or *no-bond resonance*. Hyperconjugation allows an adjacent positive charge to be delocalized by resonance onto a proton. Such effects are greatest for methyl groups because the charge can be delocalized onto three different hydrogens. Methylene groups (CH_2), in contrast, allow for charge delocalization onto only two hydrogens.

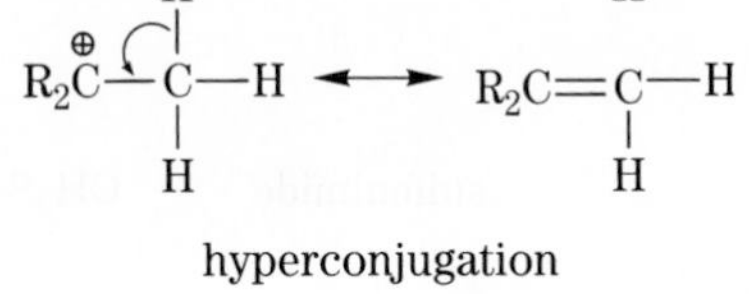

hyperconjugation

It has been observed that in the absence of other factors, certain electron-withdrawing groups affect pK_a values of oxygen- and nitrogen-based functional groups in a predictable manner. A knowledge of such effects allows first-order predictions to be made of acid and base strength for a wide range of functional groups.

Some functional groups can be thought of as being derived from water by replacement of one or both hydrogens. Alcohols, for example, can be derived from water by replacement of one hydrogen by an alkyl group. Replacement of hydrogen by an aryl group (aromatic ring) gives a phenol. If both hydrogens are replaced by alkyl or aryl groups, an ether is formed. Water and simple alcohols are neutral (pK_a 14) with respect to their acid–base properties. Ethers are neutral by virtue of the fact that they have no hydrogen to donate. In contrast, unsubstituted phenols behave as moderate to weak acids in aqueous solution with pK_a values in the range of 9 to 10. Replacement of H by an aryl group increases acid strength relative to water by 4 to 5 pK_a units. Substitution by an alkyl group however, has a negligible effect on pK_a. If one of the hydrogens of water is replaced by an acyl group (carbonyl), a carboxylic acid is formed. Such compounds typically have pK_a values in the range of 4 to 5. An acyl group therefore lowers the pK_a by 9 to 10 pK_a units. Substitution of a sulfonyl group for H increases acidity by 14 to 15 pK_a units. The resulting compounds, called sulfonic acids, are nearly as acidic as sulfuric acid in aqueous solution. A listing of the *approximate* pK_a values for a number of organic compounds is presented below.

ether	$H_3C—O—CH_3$	neutral	
alcohol	$H_3C—O—H$	neutral	
water	$H—O—H$	neutral	
phenol	$Ph—O—H$	pK_a 9–10	acid strength increases
carboxylic acid	$\overset{\overset{\displaystyle O}{\|}}{CH_3C}—O—H$	pK_a 4–5	
sulfonic acid	$\overset{\overset{\displaystyle O}{\|}}{\underset{\underset{\displaystyle O}{\|}}{CH_3S}}—O—H$	pK_a <1	↓
ammonia	$H—NH_2$	pK_a 5	
1° amine	$H_3C—NH_2$	pK_a 10	base strength decreases
2° amine	$H_3C—NH—CH_3$	pK_a 10	
arylamine	$Ph—NH_2$	pK_a 5	↓
diarylamine	$Ph—NH—Ph$	pK_a 1–2	base

base / acid

amide	$\overset{\overset{\displaystyle O}{\|}}{CH_3C}—NH_2$	neutral	
N-arylamide	$\overset{\overset{\displaystyle O}{\|}}{CH_3C}—NH—Ph$	pK_a 12–13	
imide	$\overset{\overset{\displaystyle O}{\|}}{CH_3C}—NH—\overset{\overset{\displaystyle O}{\|}}{C}CH_3$	pK_a 9	
sulfonamide	$\overset{\overset{\displaystyle O}{\|}}{\underset{\underset{\displaystyle O}{\|}}{CH_3S}}—NH_2$	pK_a 9	acid strength increases
N-arylsulfonamide	$\overset{\overset{\displaystyle O}{\|}}{\underset{\underset{\displaystyle O}{\|}}{CH_3S}}—NH—Ph$	pK_a 6–7	↓
sulfonimide	$\overset{\overset{\displaystyle O}{\|}}{\underset{\underset{\displaystyle O}{\|}}{CH_3S}}—NH—\overset{\overset{\displaystyle O}{\|}}{C}CH_3$	pK_a 4	

Electron-withdrawing substituents, when attached to a basic group, will decrease base strength by making it more difficult to donate lone-pair electrons for bonding with protons. Some nitrogen-containing functional groups can be thought of as being derived from ammonia by replacement of one, two, or three hydrogen atoms. Ammonia has a pK$_a$ of about 9 and behaves as a moderately strong base in aqueous solution. Primary, secondary and tertiary alkyl amines can be formed from ammonia by replacement of one, two or three hydrogens, respectively, by alkyl groups. Such compounds have approximately the same base strength as ammonia in aqueous solution, indicating that the alkyl groups have little effect on pK$_a$.

Replacement of one hydrogen of ammonia by an unsubstituted aryl group gives a very weak base with a pK$_a \approx 4$. A second aryl group further lowers the pK$_a$ to about 2. A single aryl substituent therefore has an effect (≈ 5 pK units), while a second such group displays an effect that is half again as great (2 to 3 pK units). The effect of a third group is not as easily quantified because of nonlinear effects such as steric hindrance.

Replacement of one of the ammonia hydrogen atoms by an acyl group gives an amide. Such compounds are virtually neutral in aqueous medium, suggesting that the acyl group decreased the pK$_a$ by 3 to 4 units, the same magnitude as it increased acid strength in the water model. The electron withdrawing carbonyl group restrains the lone pair electrons of the nitrogen atom to such an extent that it can no longer abstract protons.

Substitution of a second acyl group on ammonia gives an imide. Imides behave as acids in aqueous solution with pK$_a$ values of about 9. The second electron withdrawing group not only makes donation of lone pair of electrons difficult, but weakens the N—H bond to the point that dissociation can occur. The resulting conjugate base is stabilized by the two carbonyl groups. It is to be noted that the second acyl group had about half the effect (5 pK units) of the first. A sulfonyl group, when substituted for hydrogen on ammonia, gives a sulfonamide, which is acidic with a pK$_a$ of 9 to 10. A single sulfonyl group therefore alters the pK by 14 to 15 units.

Estimates of pK$_a$ values can be made for functional groups derived from the water and ammonia systems. The data seen in Table 25-2 are useful. When two different substituents are attached to nitrogen, the group having the larger effect is taken as the first group and that with the smaller effect as the second group. Thus, *N*-methylaniline is calculated to have a pK$_a$ of about 4 (using the first group value for the aryl substituent) and not pK$_a$ of 5 to 6, as would be obtained if the methyl group were taken for the first group. *It is important to realize however, these estimates exclude steric and other electronic effects and may vary from the actual (experimental) values by several pK units.*

Hybridization also can affect base strength as observed in the series amine, imine, nitrile where the hybridization of nitrogen changes from sp^3 to sp^2 to sp. Although amines function as moderately strong bases (pK$_a \approx 9$), imines are much weaker with pK$_a$ values near 4. Nitriles are essentially neutral (pK$_b \sim 1$). The effect of hybridization is to shorten the bond length and the general trend is that bond length decreases and electronegativity increases as the percent of s-character of the bond increases (25% for sp^3; 33% for sp^2; and 50% for sp). The shorter bond lengths and higher electronegativity associated with the nitrogen atom of nitriles results in the lone-pair being held much closer to nitrogen than it is for imines or amines. Since, basicity is a func-

tion of how readily the lone-pair is shared, it is reasonable that amines would be the most basic, and nitriles the weakest bases, within this series. Aromatic nitrogen atoms, such as found in pyridine and pyrimidine, are also sp^2 hybridized and are similar to imines with regard to their base-strength (pK$_a \approx 4$).

amine   imine   nitrile

pyridine   pyrimidine

Two functional groups that are common in pharmaceuticals are amidine and guanidine. Refer to Appendix A of this chapter for a listing of functional groups and names. These can be considered as amino derivatives of imines. Amidines, which have a single amino group attached to the imine carbon, are strong bases with pK$_a$ values near 11. Guanidines are even more basic (pK$_a \approx 13$) and have two amino groups attached to the imine carbon. The higher basicity of these functional groups as compared to imines is due to two factors: (1) the effect of the electron-donating amino nitrogen(s), which can increase electron density at the imino nitrogen by resonance, and (2) the conjugate acid form is stabilized by charge delocalization among each of the nitrogens again as a result of resonance. These effects are more pronounced for guanidines, which have an additional resonance structure available. In these functional groups it is the doubly-bound nitrogen that serves as the basic site. The single-bonded nitrogen is neutral due to the electron-withdrawing effect of the double bond and the lack of resonance stabilization for the conjugate acid form of this nitrogen. It is important to note, however, that if the amino nitrogen carries at least one hydrogen, tautomeric structures are possible in which either nitrogen can be bonded to hydrogen, with the other then becoming the basic site.

Tautomers are structures that differ in the placement of one small group or atom, usually hydrogen. In amidines, hydrogen can shift rapidly back and forth between the two nitrogen atoms (with the consequent relocation of a pair of electrons) unless structural features favor a particular tautomeric structure.

amidines   guanidines

tautomers

Table 25-2. pK Effect of Functional Groups as Substituents on H$_2$O and NH$_3$

FUNCTIONAL GROUP	EFFECT AS FIRST GROUP, PK UNITS	EFFECT AS SECOND GROUP, PK UNITS
H, Alkyl	0	0
Aryl, vinyl	4	2–3
Acyl	10	5
Sulfonyl	15	7–8

Another situation where tautomerization occurs involves protons on carbons adjacent to a carbonyl group. Ketones, for example, have two tautomeric structures known as the *keto* and *enol* forms. In the enol form, a hydrogen from an adjacent carbon migrates onto the carbonyl oxygen, with concomitant formation of a new C=C bond. The resulting hydroxyl group is acidic (when viewed as water with one hydrogen substituted by a vinyl group, a pK$_a$ of 9 would be predicted). For ordinary ketones however, the equilibrium constant heavily favors the keto form and in aqueous solution ketones behave as neutral compounds. If a second carbonyl group is attached to a carbon with at least one hydrogen the situation changes. In such compounds the equilibrium constant favors a much higher percentage of the enol tautomer due to stabilization by hydrogen bonding with the second carbonyl group. Such 1,3-dicarbonyl compounds behave as weak acids in aqueous solution.

SUMMARY

With the ability of the modern computer to manipulate millions of bits of data in a trice, the prediction of many physical and chemical constants for known and potential chemical entities, solely based on data available in a library of known information has really come to the fore. There exist programs that predict quite accurate values for pK$_a$, log P (octanol–water partition coefficient), fragmentation patterns for compounds in mass spectra, the interpretation of IR and NMR spectra, and so on, coupled with extensive databases of experimentally derived constants. (One such program may be viewed at http://www.acdlabs.com/.)

BIBLIOGRAPHY

Hart H, Craine LE, Hart DJ. *Organic Chemistry: A Short Course,* 11th ed. (With CD-ROM), New York: Houghton Mifflin College, 2002.
Morrison RT, Boyd RN. *Organic Chemistry,* 7th ed. Boston: Prentice-Hall, 2002. Also available on CD-ROM.
Survey of Chemical Notation Systems. Publication no 1150. Washington DC: National Academy of Science—National Research Council, 1964.
Chem Eng News 1955; 33: 2838.
Chem Eng News, Unique labels for compounds, 2002; 26: Nov
Solomons TWG. *Fundamentals of Organic Chemistry,* 6th ed. New York: Wiley, 1998.
Smith MB, March J. *Advanced Organic Chemistry,* 5th ed. New York; Wiley, 2000
Weininger J. *J Chem Inf Comput Sci* 1988; 28:31.
www.iupac.org/publications/ci/2002/2404/XML.html
www.iupac.org/projects/2000/2000-025-1-800.html

Appendix A Types of Organic Compounds

CLASS	EXAMPLES	CLASS	EXAMPLE
Acetals RC(H or R)(OR)$_2$ (*cf* Ketals)	CH$_3$CH(OCH$_3$)$_2$ acetaldehyde dimethyl acetal (1,1-dimethoxyethane)(CH$_3$)$_2$ C(OC$_2$H$_5$) acetone diethyl acetal (2,2-diethoxypropane)	Aldehydes RCHO Alkoxides (see *Alcoholates*) Alkylhalosilanes R(SiH$_2$)$_n$X *where one or more H's may be substituted by additional R's or X's*	CH$_3$CHO acetaldehyde CH$_3$SiH$_2$Cl methylchlorosilane
Acid Anhydrides 1. Of Monocarboxylic Acids RCOOCOR	(CH$_3$CO)$_2$O acetic (acid) anhydride	Alkylsilanes R(SiH$_2$)$_n$H *where one or more H's may be substituted by additional R's*	CH$_3$SiH$_3$ methylsilane C$_2$H$_5$SiH$_2$SiH$_2$C$_2$H$_5$ *sym*-diethyldisilane
2. Of Dicarboxylic Acids RCOOCO	CH$_2$CH$_2$COOCO succinic (acid) anhydride	Alkylsilanols Types here illustrated are limited to derivatives of silane; ie, (mono)-silane, SiH$_4$. There are similar derivatives of the di-, tri-, etc, silanes.	
Acid Halides (Acyl Halides) RCOX	CH$_3$COCl acetyl chloride		
Acids (Carboxylic) (other acids are listed under their characteristic names, eg, *Sulfonic Acids, Thio Acids,* etc)			RSiH$_2$OH RSiH(OH)$_2$ RSi(OH)$_3$ Alkylsilanols alkylsilanediols alkylsilanetriols R$_2$SiHOH R$_2$Si(OH)$_2$ dialkylsilanediols dialkylsilanols R$_3$SiOH trialkylsilanols
RCOOH Acyloins (α-Hydroxy Ketone) RCOCH(OH)R	CH$_3$COOH acetic acid CH$_3$COCH(OH)CH$_3$ acetoin C$_6$H$_5$COCH(OH)C$_6$H$_5$ benzoin	Alkylsiloxanes Various linear and cyclic types. (see *Silicones*). A common linear type consisting of condensation polymers of dialkylsilanediols is shown.	HO(SiR$_2$O)$_n$SiR$_2$OH
Alcoholates (Alkoxides) ROMetal *where R is aliphatic or alicyclic*	C$_2$H$_5$ONa sodium ethylate sodium ethoxide	Amides RCONH$_2$	CH$_3$CONH$_2$ acetamide
Alcohols ROH *where R is aliphatic or alicyclic*	C$_2$H$_5$OH ethyl alcohol (ethanol) CH$_2$(CH$_2$)$_4$CHOH cyclohexyl alcohol (cyclohexanol)	Amidines RC(=NH)NH$_2$	CH$_3$C(NH)NH$_2$ acetamidine

Appendix A　Continued

CLASS	EXAMPLES
Amines $RN(H \text{ or } R)(H \text{ or } R) RNH_2$ types = Amino Compounds	CH_3NH_2 methylamine $(C_2H_5)_2NH$ diethylamine $CH_3N(C_2H_5)C_3H_7$ methylethylpropylamine
Amino Acids $R(NH_2)COOH$	$CH_2(NH_2)COOH$ aminoacetic acid
Ammonium Derivatives $[RH_3N]^+X^-$ *where X = OH or a salt anion and any or all H's may be R's. If N is a ring member, specific "ium" nomenclature is employed to denote the heterocycle.*	$[(CH_3)_4N]^+I^-$ tetramethylammonium iodide $[(C_2H_5)_2N^+H_2]Cl^-$ diethylammonium chloride (diethylamine hydrochloride) $[CH{=}CHCH{=}CHCH{=}N^+{-}(CH_3)]Br^-$, 1-methyl pyridinium bromide
Anilides $RCONHR'$ *where NHR' is derived from aniline* *Note—If NHR' is derived from:* toluidine xylidine anisidine phenetidine	$CH_3CONHC_6H_5$ acetanilide Compounds are termed: toluidides xylidides anisidides phenetidides
Anils (Schiff bases) $RCH{=}NR$	$C_6H_5CH{=}NC_6H_5$ *N*-Benzylideneaniline
Azides (Acyl Azides) $RCON{=}N^+{=}N^-$	$CH_3CON{=}N^+{=}N^-$ acetyl azide
Azido Compounds $RN{=}N^+{=}N^-$	$C_2H_5N{=}N^+{=}N^-$ azidoethane
Azines $R_2C{=}NN{=}CR_2$	$(CH_3)_2C{=}NN{=}C(CH_3)_2$ acetone azine
Azo Compounds $RN{=}NR$	$C_6H_5N{=}NC_6H_5$ azobenzene
Azoxy Compounds $RN{=}N(O)R$	$C_6H_5N{=}N(O)C_6H_5$ azoxybenzene
Benzils (Aromatic α-Diketones) $RCOCOR$ *where R is aromatic*	p-$CH_3C_6H_4COCOC_6H_4CH_3$-p p,p'-dimethylbenzil
Benzoins (Aromatic α-Hydroxy Ketones) $RCH(OH)COR$ *where R is aromatic*	p-$CH_3C_6H_4CH(OH)CO$-$C_6H_4CH_3$-p p,p' dimethylbenzoin or p-toluoin
Betaines $R_3N^+(CH_2)_nCOO^-$	$(CH_3)_3N^+CH_2CH_2COO^-$ β-alanine, trimethylbetaine
Borates (see *Esters*) **Carbonates (see *Esters*)** **Carbylamines (see Isocyanides; Isonitriles)** RNC	C_6H_5NC phenyl { carbylamine, isocyanide or isonitrile
Cynates $ROCN$	C_6H_5OCN phenyl cyanate
Cyanides (see *Nitriles*) **Cyanohydrins** $RC(CN)(OH)(H \text{ or } R)$	$CH_3C(CN)(OH)CH_3$ acetone cyanohydrin

CLASS	EXAMPLE
Diazoamino Compounds (Triazene Derivatives) $RN{=}NNHR$	$C_6H_5N{=}NNHC_6H_5$ diazoaminobenzene or 1,3-diphenyltriazene
Diazo Compounds *Type A* $RNNX$ *where X = OH or a salt anion*	$C_6H_5N{=}NCl$ benzenediazochloride
Type B $RN{=}NOMetal$ (diazoates)	$C_6H_5N{=}NONa$ sodium benzenediazoate
Type C $C(H \text{ or } R)(H \text{ or } R)$-$={N^+}{=}N^-$	$CH_2{=}N^+{=}N^-$ diazomethane
Diazonium Compounds $RN_2^+X^-$ *where X = OH or a salt anion*	$[C_6H_5N_2{}^+]OH^-$ benzenediazonium hydroxide
Epoxy Compounds $CH_2(CH_2)_nCH_2O$ *where n = zero or greater and any or all H's may be R's*	$\overline{CH_2CH_2O}$ epoxyethane $CH_3\overline{CHCH_2CH(CH_3)O}$ 2,4-epoxypentane
Esters (of Carboxylic Acids) $RCOOR$	$CH_3COOC_2H_5$ ethyl acetate

Esters (of Inorganic Oxy Acids)

The listing here is intentionally limited to esters of the more important oxy acids of nitrogen, phosphorus, sulfur, boron, silicon, and carbon. In each instance, the type formula shown is for the ester which results from the replacement of all acidic H's by R's. Where more than one R is present, acid esters (ie, esters still containing one or more unreplaced H's) are possible.

Nitrates	$RONO_2$	$C_2H_5NO_3$, ethyl nitrate
Nitrites	$RONO$	C_2H_5ONO, ethyl nitrite
(Ortho)phosphates	$(RO)_3PO$	$(C_2H_5)_3PO_4$, (tri)ethyl phosphate
Metaphosphates	$ROPO_2$	$C_2H_5PO_3$, ethyl metaphosphate
Pyrophosphates	$(RO)_2PO{-}O{-}{-}PO(OR)_2$	$(C_2H_5)_4P_2O_7$, (tetra)ethyl pyrophosphate
(Ortho)phosphites	$P(OR)_3$	$(C_2H_5)_3PO_3$, (tri)ethyl phosphite
Hypophosphites *cf Phosphonic Acids*	$H_2P(O)(OR)$	$C_2H_5H_2PO_2$, ethyl hypophosphite
Sulfates	$(RO)_2SO_2$	$(C_2H_5)_2SO_4$, (di)ethyl sulfate
Sulfites	$(RO)_2SO$	$(C_2H_5)_2SO_3$, (di)ethyl sulfite
Orthoborates	$B(OR)_3$	$(C_2H_5)_3BO_3$, (tri)ethyl orthoborate
Metaborates	$ROBO$	$C_2H_5BO_2$, ethyl metaborate
Orthosilicates	$Si(OR)_4$	$(C_2H_5)_4SiO_4$, (tetra)ethyl orthosilicate
Metasilicates	$(RO)_2SiO$	$(C_2H_5)_2SiO_3$, (di)ethyl metasilicate
Orthocarbonates	$C(OR)_4$	$(C_2H_5)_4CO_4$, (tetra)ethyl orthocarbonate
Carbonates	$(RO)_2CO$	$(C_2H_5)_2CO_3$, (di)ethyl carbonate
Ethers ROR		$CH_3OC_2H_5$ ethyl methyl ether

Appendix A Continued

CLASS	EXAMPLES
Fluorophosphates (see *Phosphorofluoridates*)	
Glycerides $RCOOCH_2CH(OCOR)CH_2$- OCOR	$C_3H_5(C_2H_3O_2)$ or $(CH_3COO)_3$- C_3H_5 glyceryl triacetate or triacetin
Glycols $HOCH_2(CH_2)_nCH_2OH$ *where n = zero or greater*	$CH_2(OH)CH_2OH$ ethylene glycol $CH_2(OH)CH_2CH_2OH$ trimethylene glycol
Guanidino Compounds $NH_2(C{=}NH)NHR$	$NH_2(C{=}NH)NHC_2H_5$ 1-ethylguanidine
Haloalkylsilanes $XR(SiH_2)_nH$ *where one or more of the H's in R may be substituted by additional X's and one or more of silicon hydrogens may be substituted to additional RX groups*	$ClCH_2SiH_3$ (chloromethyl)silane
Halohydrins XCH_2CH_2OH *where either or both of the CH_2's may be CHR or CR_2*	$ClCH_2CH_2OH$ ethylene chlorohydrin
Hemiacetals RC(H or R)(OR)(OH)	$CH_3CH(OC_2H_5)OH$ acetaldehyde ethylhemiacetal (1-ethoxyethanol)
Hydrazides $RCONHNH_2$	$CH_3CONHNH_2$ acetic acid hydrazide
Hydrazines RN(H or R)N(H or R)- (H or R)	$C_6H_5NHNH_2$ phenylhydrazine
Hydrazones R_2(or RH)C${=}NNH_2$	$(CH_3)_2C{=}NNH_2$ acetone hydrazone $C_6H_5CH{=}NNH_2$ benzaldehyde hydrazone
Hydrocarbon Halides (Alkyl, Alkylene, Alkylidene, Alkenyl, Aryl, Arylene, etc Halides) RX_n *where n = valence of R*	CH_3Cl methyl chloride (chloromethane) $CH_2{=}CHBr$ vinyl bromide CH_3CHCl_2 ethylidene chloride C_6H_5I phenyl iodide (iodobenzene)
Hydroxamic Acids RC(=NOH)OH	$CH_3CH_2C(=NOH)OH$ propionohydroxamic acid
Hydroxy Acids RCH(OH)COOH	$CH_3CH(OH)COOH$ α-hydroxypropionic acid or lactic acid
Hypophosphites (see *Esters*)	
Imides (Carboximides) RCON(H or R)CO	$\overline{CH_2CH_2CONHCO}$ succinimide 1,2-ethanedicarboximide
Imidic Acids RC(NH)OH	$CH_3C(=NH)OH$ acetimidic acids
Imines R=NH	$\underline{CH_3CH_2}{=}NH$ ethylideneimine $\underline{CH_2CH_2NH}$ ethyleneimine
Iodonium Compounds $[R_2I]^+X^-$ *where X = ~~OH~~ or a salt anion*	$[(C_6H_5)_2I]^+Br^-$ diphenyliodonium bromide

CLASS	EXAMPLE
Iodoso Compounds RIO	C_6H_5IO iodosobenzene
Iodoxy Compounds RIO_2	$C_6H_5IO_2$ iodoxybenzene
Isocyanates RCNO	C_6H_5NCO phenyl isocyanate
Isocyanide Dichlorides (Imidocarbonyl Chlorides) $RN{=}CCl_2$	$C_2H_5NCCl_2$ ethyl isocyanide dichloride, ethylimido- carbonyl chloride
Isocyanides (see *Carbylamines*)	
Isonitriles (see *Carbylamines*)	
Isothiocyanates (Isosulfocyanates; Thiocarbimides; Mustard Oils) RNCS	CH_3NCS methyl isothiocyanate, etc
Ketals $R_2C(OR)_2$ (Commonly treated as *Acetals, qv* above)	$(CH_3)_2C(OC_2H_5)_2$ acetone diethylketal (2,2-diethoxypropane)
Ketenes RC(H or R)=C=O	$(CH_3)_2C{=}C{=}O$ dimethyl ketene
Keto Acids (monobasic) $H(CH_2)_nCO(CH_2)_nCOOH$ *where n = zero or greater and any or all H's may be R's. May also be polybasic.*	CH_3COCH_2COOH 3-oxobutyric acid or acetoacetic acid $HOOCCH_2COCOOH$ ketosuccinic acid or oxalacetic acid
Ketones RCOR *where R's are aliphatic or alicyclic. If one or both R's are aromatic, compounds are termed Phenones.*	$CH_3COC_2H_5$ ethyl methyl ketone or 2-butanone $C_6H_5COCH_3$ acetophenone
Lactams $\overline{CH_2(CH_2)_nCONH}$ *where n = 2 or more and any or all H's may be R's.*	$\overline{CH_2CH_2CH_2CH_2CONH}$ δ-valerolactam (2-piperidone)
Lactides $\overline{CH_2COOCH_2COO}$ *where any or all of the H's may be R's*	$CH_3\overline{CHCOOCH(CH_3)COO}$ 2-hydroxypropionic acid lactide "lactide"
Lactims as per lactams except $\overline{CH_2(CH_2)_nCONH}$ becomes $\overline{CH_2(CH_{2n}C(OH)}{=}N$	$\overline{CH_2CH_2CH_2CH_2C(OH)}{=}N$ δ-valerolactim
Lactones $\overline{CH_2(CH_2)_nCOO}$ *where n = 2 or more and any or all H's may be R's*	$\overline{CH_2CH_2CH_2CH_2COO}$ δ-valerolactone
Mercaptans (see *Thiols*)	
Mercaptides RSMetal	C_2H_5SNa sodium ethylmercaptide
Mercaptoles $R_2C(SR)_2$	$(CH_3)_2C(SC_2H_5)_2$ acetone diethylmercaptole
Morpholides $RCON\overline{(CH_2)_2OCH_2CH_2}$	$CH_3CON\overline{CH_2CH_2OCH_2CH_2}$ acetomorpholide (4-acetylmorpholine)
Nitrates (see *Esters*)	
Nitriles (Cyanides; Carbonitriles) RCN	CH_3CH_2CN propionitrile, ethyl cyanide

Appendix A Continued

CLASS	EXAMPLES	CLASS	EXAMPLE

Nitrites (see *Esters*)

Nitro Compounds
RNO$_2$

CH_3NO_2 nitromethane
$C_6H_5NO_2$ nitrobenzene

Nitroso Compounds
RNO

C_6H_5NO nitrosobenzene

Organometallic (Metallo-organic) Compounds
Note—Restricted here to compounds having a direct metal–carbon linkage.
Commonest types are:
MR$_V$ and R$_{(V-1)}$MX
where
  M = metal functioning with valence v
  R = *univalent*
    unsubstituted, or, substituted, hydrocarbon radical
  X = *univalent anion*

$(CH_3)_2Zn$ dimethylzinc
$(C_2H_5)_4Pb$
  tetraethyl lead

CH_3MgBr
  methylmagnesium bromide

$C_6H_5HgNO_3$ phenylmercuric nitrate; Ag_2C_2 silver acetylide

Osazones
[Bis(phenylhydrazones)]
(H or R)C(=NNHPh)-C(=NNHPh)(R or H)
where Ph = phenyl

$C_6H_5C(=NNHPh)C(=NNH-Ph)C_6H_5$
benzil osazone [Benzil bis(phenylhydrazone)]

Oximes
RC(H or R)=NOH

$CH_3CH=NOH$ acetaldoxime
$(CH_3)_2C=NOH$
  dimethylketoxime
  (acetone oxime)

Oxo Compounds (see *Aldehydes, Ketones, Quinones, Keto Acids*)

Ozonides

RCH-O-O-CH-R

$CH_3CHOOCHCH_3$
  2-butene ozonide

Peptides (Polypeptides)
NH$_2$(RCONH)$_n$RCOOH

$NH_2(CH_2CONH)_2CH_2COOH$
  glycine tripeptide
  glycylglycylglycine

Peroxides
ROO(R or H)

Peroxy Acids
RC(O)OOH

$C_2H_5OOC_2H_5$ ethyl peroxide

$CH_3C(O)OOH$ peroxyacetic acid

Phenolates (Phenoxides)
ROMetal
where R is aromatic

C_6H_5ONa
  sodium phenolate
  sodium phenoxide

Phenols
ROH
where R is aromatic

p-$CH_3C_6H_4OH$
  p-methylphenol (p-cresol)

Phenones (see *Ketones*)
Phenoxides (see *Phenolates*)
Phosphates (see *Esters*)
Phosphites (see *Esters*)
Phospho Compounds
RPO$_2$

$C_6H_5PO_2$ phosphobenzene

Phosphonic Acids
RPO(OH)$_2$

$CH_3PO(OH)_2$ methylphosphonic acid or methanephosphonic acid

Phosphorofluoridates (Fluoro-phosphates)
FPO(OR)$_2$

$FPO[OCH(CH_3)_2]_2$ diisopropyl phosphororfluoridate or diisopropyl fluorophosphate

Phosphorus Compounds (General)
In addition to the compounds in this listing, phosphorus forms a very large number of types of compounds containing direct linkages between the phosphorus atom and halogens, cyanogen, nitrogen, and sulfur. Many of these contain also phosphorus-oxygen linkages. For a comprehensive presentation of organic compounds containing phosphorus, see the report entitled *Organic Compounds Containing Phosphorus*, which is available from *Chemical Abstracts Service*.

Phthaleins, simplest type only
RC(R'OH)$_2$OCO
where R is o-phenylene, R' is p-phenylene and either or both may be substituted.

o-$C_6H_4C(p$-$C_6H_4OH)_2OCO$ phenolphthalein

Piperidides
RCON(CH$_2$)$_4$CH$_2$

$CH_3CONCH_2CH_2CH_2CH_2CH_2$ acetopiperidide (1-acetylpiperidine)

Quaternary Ammonium Compounds
[R$_4$N]$^+$X$^-$
where X = OH or a salt anion

$[(CH_3)_4N]^+Cl^-$
  tetramethylammonium chloride

Quinones
O=R=O
where R is a quinoid cycle

p-$O=C_6H_4=O$
  p-benzoquinone

Salts (Metal)

Formulas as for the acids except that the acidic H's are replaced by metal equivalent.

Semicarbazones
RC(H or R)=NNHCONH$_2$

$(CH_3)_2C=NNHCONH_2$ acetone semicarbazone

Silicates (see *Esters*)

Silicon Compounds (General)
Because of its position in Group IV of the Periodic Table, it is not surprising that silicon enters freely into organic-type chemical combinations. Like carbon, although to a much lesser extent, silicon forms stable chain compounds containing —SiSi— linkages. Compounds which contain hydrogen as the only other element are termed silanes: eg, SiH_4, silane (silicane, silicomethane); Si_2H_6, disilane (disilicoethane) and Si_3H_8, trisilane. Cyclosilanes, $SiH_2(SiH_2)_nSiH_2$ are also well-known. These silicon-hydrogen compounds are analogous to the alkanes and cycloalkanes in the carbon family of compounds. They form various types of derivatives: eg, SiH_3OH, H_2SiO, $HSiOOH$, $HOSiH_2SiH_2OH$, $SiHCl_3$, $H_2Si=NH$, $(SiH_3)_2NH$, etc. These structures are analogous to carbon compounds. Silicon also shows a strong tendency to form stable-chain compounds containing —SiOSi— linkages which are the siloxanes: eg, $H_3SiOSiH_3$, disiloxane, $H_3SiOSi-H_2OSiH_3$, trisiloxane; etc. Analogous compounds containing the imino group instead of oxygen, are also well-known. These are the silazanes: eg, $H_3SiNHSiH_3$, disilazane; $H_3SiNHSiH_2$—NH-SiH$_3$, trisilazane; etc.

It will be noted that none of the above types of compounds contain carbon and, in this sense, they are not organic compounds. However, the alkyl derivatives, which are very numerous, are organic in the same sense as alkyl derivatives of hydrogen compounds of other elements such as nitrogen and sulfur. Since

Appendix A Continued

CLASS	EXAMPLES	CLASS	EXAMPLE

the alkyl groups in the derivatives also may contain substituent functional groups, it readily is apparent that there are a great many types of organic silicon compounds. Only a few of the better known types are included in this listing.

Silylalkanols (Silicoalcohols)

Alcohols in which one (or more) of the CH hydrogens is replaced by silyl (SiH$_3$) or substituted silyl groups. In contrast to the silanols, compounds of this type contain hydroxyl in true organic combination. There are many subtypes.

(C$_2$H$_5$)$_3$SiCH$_2$CH$_2$OH
2-(triethylsilyl)ethanol

Sulfamic Acids

RNH(or R$_2$N)SO$_2$OH

CH$_3$NHSO$_2$OH methanesulfamic acid; (C$_2$H$_5$)$_2$NSO$_2$OH diethylsulfamic acid

Sulfates (see *Esters*)

Sulfenamides

RSNH$_2$

C$_6$H$_5$SNH$_2$ benzenesulfenamide

Sulfenic Acids

RSOH

C$_6$H$_5$SOH benzenesulfenic acid

Sulfenyl Halides

RSX

C$_6$H$_5$SCl benzenesulfenyl chloride

Sulfides (Thio Ethers)

RSR

(CH$_3$)$_2$S (di)methyl sulfide (di)methyl thioether

Sulfimides

RCONHSO$_2$

o-C$_6$H$_4$CONHSO$_2$
o-benzosulfimide (saccharin)

Sulfinamides

RSONH$_2$

C$_6$H$_5$SONH$_2$
benzenesulfinamide

Sulfinic Acids

RSOOH

C$_6$H$_5$SOOH benzenesulfinic acid

Sulfinyl Halides

RSOX

C$_6$H$_5$SOCl benzenesulfinyl chloride

Sulfites (see *Esters*)

Sulfonamides

RSO$_2$NH$_2$

C$_6$H$_5$SO$_2$NH$_2$
benzenesulfonamide

Sulfones

RSO$_2$R

(C$_2$H$_5$)$_2$SO$_2$ diethyl sulfone

Sulfonic Acids

RSO$_2$OH

C$_6$H$_5$SO$_2$OH benzenesulfonic acid

Sulfonium Compounds

[R$_3$S]$^+$X$^-$
where X is OH or a salt anion. If S is a ring member, specific "ium" nomenclature is employed to denote the heterocycle.

[(CH$_3$)$_3$S]$^+$I$^-$
trimethylsulfonium iodide

[$\overline{\text{CH}_2\text{CH}_2\text{CH}_2\text{CH}_2\text{CH}_2\text{S}}^+$-(C$_2H_5$)]PtCl$_6$$^-$
1-ethylhexahydrothia-pyrylium chloroplatinate

Sulfonyl Halides

RSO$_2$X

C$_6$H$_5$SO$_2$Cl benzenesulfonyl chloride

Sulfoxides

RSOR

(C$_2$H$_5$)$_2$SO diethyl sulfoxide

Sultams

Analogous to Lactams, *qv* with —SO$_2$— replacing —CO—

Sultones

Analogous to Lactones, *qv* with —SO$_2$— replacing —CO—

Thetins

R$_2$S$^+$CH$_2$COO$^-$

(CH$_3$)$_2$S$^+$CH$_2$COO$^-$
S,S-dimethylthetin

Thio Acids

1. Thiolic RCOSH

CH$_3$COSH thioloacetic acid ethanethiolic acid

2. Thionic RCSOH

CH$_3$CSOH thionoacetic acid ethanethionic acid

3. Thionothiolic RCSSH (Dithioic)

CH$_3$CSSH thionothioloacetic acid ethanedithioic acid

Thio Aldehydes

RCHS

CH$_2$CHS thioacetaldehyde

Thiocyanates (Sulfocyanates; Rhodanates)

RSCN

C$_6$H$_5$SCN phenyl thiocyanate, etc

Thio Ethers (see *Sulfides*)

Thiols (Mercaptans, Acid Sulfides, Hydrosulfides; Sulfhydryl Compounds)

RSH

C$_2$H$_5$SH ethanethiol
ethyl { mercaptan / acid sulfide / hydrosulfide

Thiones (Thio Ketones)

RCSR

CH$_3$CSCH$_3$ propanethione dimethyl thioketone

Thionium Compounds (see *Sulfonium Compounds*)

Thioureides-Ureides (*qv*) with the urea oxygen replaced by sulfur.

Ureides, simplest types only

acyclic RCONHCONH (H or COR)

CH$_3$CONHCONH$_2$ acetic acid ureide; acetylurea

cyclic $\underline{\text{RCONHCONHCO}}$

$\underline{\text{CH}_2}$CONHCONHCO malonic acid ureide (malonylurea); (barbituric acid)

Urethanes (Carbamate Estes)

NH$_2$COOR

NH$_2$COOC$_2$H$_5$ ethyl urethane (ethyl carbamate)

Appendix B Prefixes

ald- (or aldo-) — refers to *aldehyde,* as aldoxime and aldohexose

allo- — signifies a *close* (usually isomeric) *relationship,* as allocholesterol (coprostenol) is an isomer of cholesterol

anhydro- — denotes *abstraction of water,* as anhydrohydroxyprogesterone

anti- — equivalent to *trans, qv,* in certain geometric isomers, eg, *anti*-benzaldoxime

apo- — usually signifies *formation from the compound* whose name is attached, as apomorphine may be formed (produced) from morphine

ar- — abbreviation for *aromatic,* as aryl

as- — abbreviation for *asymmetric*

bis- — used instead of di-, meaning *two,* before complex expressions, as in bis(*m*-nitrophenyl)-

cis- — refers to that *geometric isomer* in which the two groups are on the *same* side of a plane produced through rigid bonding, preventing free rotation (eg, unsaturation, ring formation, etc)

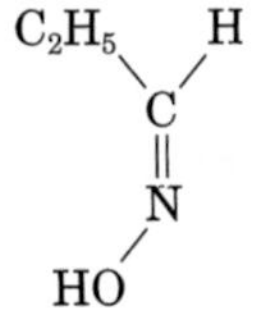

$$C_2H_5 \quad H$$
$$C$$
$$\parallel$$
$$N$$
$$HO$$

cyclo- — indicates a *cyclic* structure, as cyclopropane

d- — see *dextro-*

D- — signifies a *structural relationship* to D-glyceraldehyde without any reference to direction of optical rotation, as D-glucose

de- (or des-) — denotes *removal of something,* as hydrogen in dehydrocholic acid, and oxygen in desoxyephedrine

Δ (the capital Greek on, letter *delta*) — used to indicate, or focus attention

 — *double bonds,* as in Δ^2-butene [$CH_3CH{=}CHCH_3$]

dehydro- — see *de-*

desoxy- — see *de-*

dextro- [or *d-* or (+)-] — signifies *dextrorotatory* form, as *d*-glucose

dl- (or *d,l*-) — see *racemic*

E and Z — *E* (entgegen), *Z* (zusammen); descriptors used to distinguish stereoisomers differing in the spatial distribution of groups about a doubly-bonded atom pair. *E* signifies that the group of higher priority (by the Cahn-Ingold- Prelog sequence) on one of the atoms and the group of higher priority on the other atom are on opposite sides of the double bond. *Z* signifies that these higher priority groups are on the same side of the double bond. For further discussion, see *J Am Chem Soc 90:* 509, 1968. Examples:

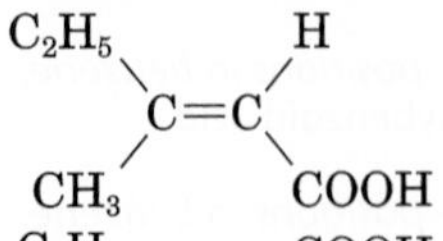

$$C_2H_5 \quad H$$
$$C{=}C$$
$$CH_3 \quad COOH$$

(*E*)-3-methyl-2-pentenoic acid

$$C_2H_5 \quad COOH$$
$$C{=}C$$
$$CH_3 \quad H$$

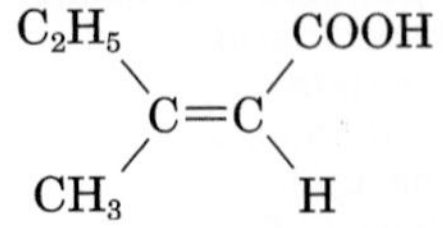

(*Z*)-3-methyl-2-pentenoic acid

epi- (or ep-) — connotes a *difference in steric configuration,* as epicholesterol is the 3α-hydroxy epimer of cholesterol; also used to signify a bridge, as in epichlorohydrin and 1,3-epoxybutane.

epoxy- — see *epi-*

gem- — refers to *two groups attached to the same carbon atom,* as the *gem*-dimethyl grouping in 2,2-dimethylpropane or camphor

hetero- — means *different,* or *not all the same,* as in heterocyclic

hom- (or homo-) — indicates a *homolog* of another compound, as homatropine

hydro- (or hydr-) — refers to *hydrogen,* as hexahydrobenzene and hydracrylic acid

hypo- — signifies a *lower state of oxidation* in relation to another compound, as hypoxanthine

i- — sometimes used instead of iso-

iso- (rarely, *i-*) — denotes an *isomer* of another compound, as isobutane and isopropyl alcohol

levo [or *l-* or (−)-] — signifies *levorotatory* form, as *l*-ephedrine

L- — signifies a *structural relationship* to L-glyceraldehyde without any reference to direction of optical rotation, as L-glucose

m- — see *meta-*

meso- — signifies *optical inactivity due to internal compensation,* as mesotartaric acid

meta- (or *m-*) — indicates the *1,3-positions* in benzene, as in *m*-dihydroxybenzene

n- — abbreviation for *normal,* as *n*-butyl alcohol

N — a locant, indicating substitution on a nitrogen atom, as in *N*-methylaniline

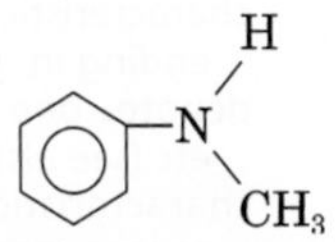

$$H$$
$$N$$
$$CH_3$$

nor- — indicates a *relationship, usually through alkylation or isomerization,* between the compound whose name carries the prefix and the compound whose name does not. Examples: ephedrine is an *N*-methylated norephedrine; camphane is a trimethylated norcamphane; and leucine (2-amino-4-methylpentanoic acid) is an isomer of the normal form represented by norleucine (2-aminohexanoic acid).

Appendix B Continued

o-	see *ortho-*
ortho- (or *o-*)	signifies the *1,2- positions in benzene,* as in *o*-hydroxybenzoid acid
p-	see *para-*
para- (or *p-*)	signifies the *1,4- positions in benzene,* as in *p*-aminobenzoic acid
per-	signifies *maximum state of substitution or addition,* as in perchloroethane, C_2Cl_6; perchloroethylene, $Cl_2C{=}CCl_2$; perhydrobenzene, C_6H_{12}. Sometimes used synonymously with peroxy, *qv*
poly-	indicates a *union of several* identical molecules or molecular fragments, as in polymers and polysaccharides
R and S	R (rectus), S (sinistere); notations used in the Cahn-Ingold-Prelog convention to describe configuration about a chiral center. The system utilizes a set of rules to establish a priority rating for the substituent groups around a center and the rating is then applied to the structure to describe the configuration. Unlike the D-L system, the convention does not involve comparisons with reference compounds. For further discussion, see *J Chem Ed 41 (Mar):* 116, 1964.
racemic [or dl- or (±)-	signifies *optical inactivity due to equimolecular mixture of* (+)- and (−)- *forms*
s-	see *sym-*
S and R	see *R* and *S*
sec-	abbreviation for *secondary,* as in *sec*-butyl alcohol and *sec*-amines
sub-	denotes a *basic salt,* as in aluminum subacetate

sym- (or *s-*)	abbreviation for *symmetrical,* as in *sym*- dichloroethane, $ClCH_2CH_2Cl$; specifically signifies the 1,3,5 positions in benzene, as in *sym*-trinitrobenzene
syn-	equivalent to *cis, qv,* in certain geometric isomers, eg, *syn*-benzaldoxime
t-see *tert-*	
tert- (or *t-*)	abbreviation for *tertiary,* as in *tert*-butyl alcohol and *tert*-amines
tetrakis-	used instead of tetra, meaning *four,* before complex expressions (see bis-)
trans- (or *anti*)	refers to that *geometric isomer* in which the two groups are on *opposite* sides of a planar bond (see *cis*)

tris-	used instead of tri-, meaning *three,* before complex expressions (see bis-)
uns-	see *unsym-*
unsym- (or *uns-*)	abbreviation for *unsymmetrical,* as in *unsym*- dichloroethane, CH_3CHCl_2; specifically signifies the 1,2,4 positions in benzene, as in *unsym*-trihydroxybenzene
v-	see *vic-*
vic- (or *v-* or *adj-* or *a-*)	signifies the *1,2,3 positions in benzene* as *vic*-trimethylbenzene
Z and E	see *E and Z*

Appendix C Suffixes

-al	indicates an *aldehyde,* as methanal, HCHO
-ane	indicates *saturated hydrocarbon or saturated heterocycle* as ethane, androstane or furane
-ase	characteristic ending for *enzymes,* as zymase, amylase, polypeptidase, etc
-ate	characteristic ending for *salts and esters of acids* ending in -ic, as acetate, phosphate, etc
-ene	denotes *one double bond,* as ethane, butadiene, etc (see also *-ylene*)
-ine	characteristic ending for various *basic nitrogen compounds such as amines or alkaloids,* as histamine, epinephrine, morphine, etc
-ite	characteristic ending for *salts and esters of acids* ending in -ous, as phosphite, nitrite, etc
-oic	refers to the *—COOH group,* as in ethanoic, benzoic, etc, acids
-ol	characteristic ending for *alcohols, phenols, naphthols, etc,* as in ethanol, cyclohexanol, etc
-one	indicates a *ketone,* as in propanone, acetophenone, etc
-osan	generic ending for *polysaccharides,* as pentosans, hexosanes, etc
-ose	characteristic *carbohydrate* ending, especially for *sugars,* as dextrose, sucrose, etc
-oside	generic ending for *glycosides,* as glucoside, rhamnoside, etc

-oyl	characteristic ending for *acyl* radicals, as ethanoyl (for acetyl), carbamoyl, etc
-yl	indicates a *group* or *radical,* especially a *univalent hydrocarbon radical,* as methyl, phenyl, etc
-ylene	signifies a *bivalent hydrocarbon radical* or *group* with the free bonds on *different* carbon atoms, as in ethylene [$—CH_2CH_2—$] and o-phenylene

; used also to indicate a *double bond* in olefin hydrocarbons, as in ethylene [$CH_2{=}CH_2$]

-ylidene	signifies a *bivalent hydrocarbon radical* or *group* with the free bonds on the *same* carbon atom, as in ethylidene [$CH_2CH{=}$] and benzylidene

-yne	denotes *one triple bond,* as in ethyne [$CH{\equiv}CH$], ethynyl [$CH{\equiv}C—$], etc

Appendix D Organic Groups and Radicals[a]

acetamido	CH₃CONH—

acetamido — CH_3CONH-

acetate — CH_3COO- or $C_2H_3O_2^-$

acetonyl — CH_3COCH_2-

acetoxy — see *acetate*

acetyl — CH_3CO-

acridinyl — $C_{13}H_8N-$ (5 isomers)

acyl — generic term signifying an acid minus its OH group or groups as *acetyl*, $CH_3\text{-}CO-$ or *carbonyl*, $=CO$

adipoyl — $-CO(CH_2)_4CO-$

alanyl — $CH_3CH(NH_2)CO-$

alkoxy — generic term signifying a radical consisting of an alkyl joined to oxygen as *methoxy*, CH_3O- and *ethoxy*, C_2H_5O-

alkyl — generic term signifying a saturated hydrocarbon radical with a valence of one as *methyl*, CH_3- or *ethyl*, C_2H_5-

alkylamino — generic term signifying RNH— wherein R is an *alkyl*

allyl — $CH_2=CHCH_2-$

amide (amido) — $-CONH_2$, see carbamoyl

amidino — $H_2NC(=NH)-$

amine (amino) — $-NH_2$

aminoacetate — H_2NCH_2COO-

aminobenzoate — $H_2NC_6H_4COO-$ (*o-*, *m-* and *p-* isomers)

n-amyl (amyl) — see *pentyl*

tert-amyl — see *tert-pentyl*

anilino — C_6H_5NH-

anthryl — $C_{14}H_9-$, from anthracene (3 isomers)

aryl — generic term signfying an aromatic hydrocarbon radical as; phenyl

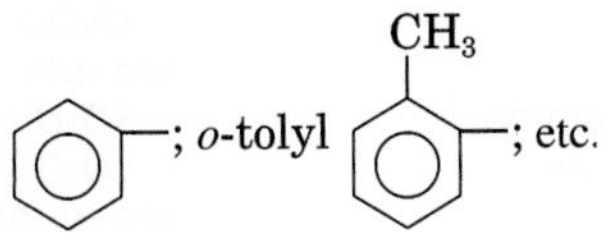

⬡ —; *o*-tolyl ⬡(CH₃) —; etc.

auro — $Au-$

azido — $-N=N^+=N^-$

azo — $-N=N-$

azoxy — $-N(O)=N-$

benzal — see *benzylidene*

benzamido — C_6H_5CONH-

benzenesulfonamido — $C_6H_5SO_2NH-$

benzenesulfonyl — $C_6H_5SO_2-$

benzhydryl — see *diphenylmethyl*

benzoate — C_6H_5COO- or $C_7H_5O_2^-$

benzoyl — C_6H_5CO-

benzoyloxy (benzoxy) — see *benzoate*

benzyl — $C_6H_5CH_2-$

benzylidene — $C_6H_5CH=$

biphenylyl — $C_6H_5C_6H_4-$ (3 isomers)

bisulfate — $HOSO_2O-$ or SO_4H^-

bisulfide — $-SH$; see *thiol*

bisulfite — $HOSOO-$ or SO_3H^-

borate (orthoborate) — $B(-O-)(-O-)(-O-)$ or BO_3^{3-}

bromo (bromide) — $Br-$

brosyl — *p*-bromobenzenesulfonyl

n-butyl (butyl) — $CH_3(CH_2)_3-$

sec-butyl — $CH_3CH_2CH(CH_3)-$

tert-butyl — $(CH_3)_3C-$

butyrate (butanoate) — $CH_3CH_2CH_2COO-$ or $C_4H_7O_2^-$

cacodyl — see *dimethylarsino*

carbamate (carbamoyloxy) — H_2NCOO-

carbamoyl — H_2NCO-, see *amide*

carbethoxy — see *ethoxycarbonyl*

carbomethoxy — see *methoxycarbonyl*

carbonyl — $=CO$

carboxyl (carboxy) — $-COOH$

cetyl — see *hexadecyl*

chloro (chloride) — $Cl-$

chloromercuri — $ClHg-$

cinnamoyl — $C_6H_5CH=CHCO-$

cinnamyl — $C_6H_5CH=CHCH_2-$

citrate — $-OOCCH_2C(OH)(COO-)CH_2COO-$ or $C_6H_5O_7^{3-}$

cresyl — $CH_3C_6H_4O-$ (3 isomers)

cyanato (cyanate) — $N\equiv C-O-$

cyan (cyanide) — $-CN$

cyclohexyl — $C_6H_{11}-$

cyclopentyl — C_5H_9-

cyclopropyl — C_3H_5-

n-decyl (decyl) — $CH_3(CH_2)_9-$ or $C_{10}H_{21}-$

dialkylamino — R_2N- wherein R's are *alkyls*

diazo — $-N(\equiv N)$

diazoamino — $-N=N-NH=$

diazonium — $N^+(\equiv N)-$

dimethylamino — $(CH_3)_2N-$

dimethylarsino — $(CH_3)_2As-$

diphenylmethyl — $(C_6H_5)_2CH-$

dodecyl — $CH_3(CH_2)_{11}-$

epoxy — $-O-$ oxygen united to two different atoms already united in some other way

ethenyl — see *vinyl*

ethoxy — C_2H_5O-

ethoxycarbonyl — C_2H_5OCO-

ethyl — C_2H_5-

ethylamino — C_2H_5NH-

ethylene — $-CH_2CH_2-$

ethylenedioxy — $-OCH_2CH_2O-$

ethylidene — $CH_3CH=$

ethylthio — CH_3CH_2S-

ethynyl — $HC\equiv C-$

fluoro (fluoride) — $F-$

fluorophosphate — see *phosphorofluoridate*

formamido — $HC(=O)NH-$

formate — $HCOO-$ or CHO_2^-

formyl — $-CHO$

furfuryl — $OCH=CHCH=CCH_2-$ (two isomers, but 1 used unqualified to refer specifically to the 2-form)

furfurylidene — $OCH=CHCH=CCH=$ (two isomers, but used unqualified to refer specifically to the 2-form)

furyl — C_4H_3O- (2 isomers)

glucosyl — $C_6H_{11}O_5-$

glyceryl — $-CH_2-CH-CH_2-$ or $C_3H_5\equiv$

glycinate — NH_2CH_2COO-

glycyl — NH_2CH_2CO-

guanidino — $H_2NC(=NH)NH-$

n-heptyl (heptyl) — $CH_3(CH_2)_6-$

hexadecyl — $CH_3(CH_2)_{15}-$

hexamethylene — $-CH_2(CH_2)_4CH_2-$

n-hexyl (hexyl) — $CH_3(CH_2)_5-$ or $C_6H_{13}-$

hydrazino — H_2NNH-

hydrazo — $-NHNH-$

hydroxy (hydroxyl) — $-OH$

hydroxyamino — $HONH-$

hydroxyimino — $HON=$

hydroxymethyl (methylol) — $HOCH_2-$

imide — $=NH$, as in succinimide (cyclic)

imino — $HN=$

indolyl — C_8H_6N- (several isomers)

iodo (iodide) — $I-$

isoamyl — see *isopentyl*

isobutyl — $(CH_3)_2CHCH_2-$

Appendix D **Continued**

isocyanato (isocyanate) $O{=}C{=}N{=}$

isocyano (isocyanide) $-NC$

isonitrile (isonitrilo)   see *isocyano*

isopentyl $(CH_3)_2CHCH_2CH_2-$

isopropoxy $(CH_3)_2CHO-$

isopropyl $(CH_3)_2CH-$

isothiocyano (isothiocyanato, isothiocyanate) $S{=}C{=}N-$ or NCS^-

keto   see *oxo*

lactate $CH_3CH(OH)COO-$ or $C_3H_5O_3^-$

malonyl $-COCH_2CO-$

mandelate $C_6H_5CH(OH)COO-$

menthyl $C_{10}H_{19}-$ (several isomers)

mercapto (mercaptan) $-SH$; see *thiol*

mercuri $-Hg-$

mesityl $2,4,6-(CH_3)_3C_6H_2-$

methenyl   see *methylidene*

methoxy CH_3O-

methoxycarbonyl CH_3OCO-

methoxyphenyl $CH_3OC_6H_4-$ *o-*, *m-* and *p-*isomers

methyl CH_3-

methylene $CH_2{=}$

methylenedioxy $-OCH_2O-$

methylidene $-CH_2-$

methylidyne $HC{\equiv}$

methylol   see *hydroxymethyl*

methylsulfonyl (methanesulfonyl) CH_3SO_2-

methylthio CH_3S-

morpholino $CH_2CH_2OCH_2CH_2N-$

naphthyl $C_{10}H_7-$ (from naphthalene; α and β isomers)

neopentyl $(CH_3)_3CCH_2-$

nitramino O_2NNH-

nitrate $-ONO_2$

nitrile   see *cyano*

nitrilo ${\equiv}N$

nitrite $-ONO$

nitro $-NO_2$

nitroso $-NO$

n-nonyl (nonyl) $CH_3(CH_2)_8-$

n-octyl (octyl) $CH_3(CH_2)_7-$

oleate $CH_3(CH_2)_7CH{=}CH(CH_2)_7COO-$ or $C_{18}H_{33}O_2{}^-$

oxalate (oxalato) $-OOCCOO-$ or $C_2O_4^{2-}$

oxalyl $-COCO-$

oxo $O{=}$

oxy $-O-$ as a connective

palmitate $CH_3(CH_2)_{14}COO-$ or $C_{16}H_{31}O_2^-$

n-pentyl (pentyl) $CH_3(CH_2)_3CH_2-$

tert-pentyl $CH_3CH_2C(CH_3)_2-$ (1,1-dimethylpropyl)

perchlorate O_3Cl-O- or $ClO_4{}^-$

perchloryl O_3Cl-

peroxy $-O-O-$

phenethyl $C_6H_5CH_2CH_2-$

phenoxy C_6H_5O-

phenyl C_6H_5-

phenylene $C_6H_4{=}$ (*o-*, *m-* and *p-*isomers)

phenylsulfonyl   see *benzenesulfonyl*

phosphate (orthophosphate) PO_4^{3-}

phosphino H_2P-

phospho $-PO_2$

phosphono $(HO)_2OP-$

phosphoro $-PP-$

phosphoroso $-PO$

phthalate $o-C_6H_4(COO-)_2$

phthaloyl $o-C_6H_4(CO-)_2$

picrate $2,4,6-(NO_2)_3C_6H_2O-$

picryl $2,4,6-(NO_2)_3C_6H_2-$

piperidino $CH_2CH_2CH_2CH_2CH_2N-$

piperidyl   2-, 3-, or $4-C_5H_{10}N-$

pivaloyl $(CH_3)_3CCO-$

propenyl $CH_3CH{=}CH-$

propionate (propanoate) CH_3CH_2COO- or $C_3H_5O_2-$

propionyl CH_3CH_2CO-

propoxy $CH_3CH_2CH_2O-$

n-propyl (propyl) $CH_3CH_2CH_2-$

propylene $CH_3-CH-CH_2-$

pyranyl C_5H_5O- (3 isomers)

pyrazolidinyl $C_3H_7N_2-$ (many isomers)

pyridyl C_5H_4N- (3 isomers)

pyrimidinyl (pyrimidyl) $C_4H_3N_2-$ (3 isomers)

quinolyl C_9H_6N- (7 isomers)

salicyl $o-C_6H_4(OH)CO-$

salicylate $o-C_6H_4(OH)COO-$ or $C_7H_5O_3^-$

silyl $-SiH_3$

stearate $CH_3(CH_2)_{16}COO-$ or $C_{18}H_{35}O_2^-$

stibo O_2Sb-

styryl $C_6H_5CH{=}CH-$

succinate $-OOCCH_2CH_2COO-$ or $C_4H_4O_4^{2-}$

succinoyl $-OCCH_2CH_2CO-$

sulfamoyl H_2NSO_2-

sulfanilamido $p-H_2NC_6H_4SO_2NH-$

sulfanilyl $p-H_2NC_6H_4SO_2-$

sulfate $-OSO_2O-$ or SO_4^{2-}

sulfhydryl   see *thiol*

sulfide $-S-$; characteristic of thioethers as (*di*)ethyl sulfide (ethyl thioether), $C_2H_5-S-C_2H_5$

sulfinyl $-SO-$

sulfite $-OSOO-$ or SO_3^{2-}

sulfo   see *sulfonic acid*

sulfonamido $-SO_2NH-$

sulfonate $-SO_2O-$

sulfone   see *sulfonyl*

sulfonic acid $-SO_2OH$

sulfonyl (sulfone) $-SO_2-$

sulfoxide   see *sulfinyl*

sulfuryl   see *sulfonyl*

tartrate $-OOCCH(OH)CH(OH)COO-$ or $C_4H_4O_6^{2-}$

tetradecyl $CH_3(CH_2)_{12}CH-$

tetramethylene $-CH_2(CH_2)_2CH_2-$

tetrazolyl $CHN_4{=}$ (isomers)

thenyl $C_4H_3SCH_2-$ (2 isomers)

thiazolyl C_3H_2NS- (3 isomers)

thienyl C_4H_3S- (2 isomers)

thio   see *sulfide*

thiocarbonyl ${=}CS$

thiocyano (thiocyanato, thiocyanate) $-SCN$

thiol (thiolo, mercapto) $-SH$

thionyl   see *sulfinyl*

toloxy (tolyloxy) $CH_3C_6H_4O-$ (*o-*, *m-* and *p-*isomers)

toluenesulfonyl $CH_3C_6H_4SO_2-$ (*o-*, *m-* and *p-*forms)

tolyl $CH_3C_6H_4-$ (*o-*, *m-* and *p-*isomers)

tosyl   = *tolylsulfonyl, qv*

trimethylene $-CH_2CH_2CH_2-$

trityl $(C_6H_5)_3C-$

ureido $H_2NCONH-$

valerate (pentanoate) $CH_3(CH_2)_3COO-$ or $C_5H_9O_2^-$

vinyl $CH_2{=}CH-$

xanthenyl (xanthyl) $C_{13}H_9O-$ (5 isomers)

xenyl   see *biphenylyl*

xylyl $(CH_3)_2C_6H_3-$ (6 isomers)

[a]Anionic radicals have slightly different names than given here when present as ligands. Examples: acetate versus acetato; nitrite versus nitrito; thiol versus thiolo.

Appendix E Heterocycles in Official Drugs

3 C₂N

Aziridine (11)[a]
Example: *Thiotepa*

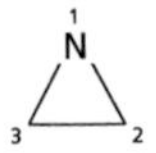

5 C₃OS

1,3-Oxathiole (133)
4,5-dihydro form
Example: *Nivirapine*

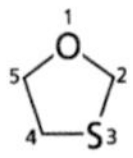

5 C₄N

1H-Tetrazole (61)
Examples: *cefamandole; Cefazolin.*

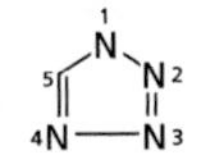

C₂N₂S

1,2,5-Thiadiazole (89)
Example: *Timolol.*

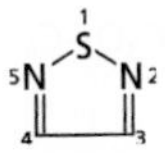

1,3,4-Thiadiazole (90)
Examples: *Acetazolamide; Cefazolin;
Sulfamethizole.*

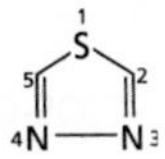

1,3,4-Thiadiazoline (90)
Example: *Methazolamide.*

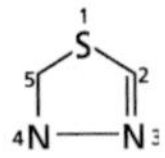

C₃NO

Oxazolidine (119)
Example: *Paramethadione*

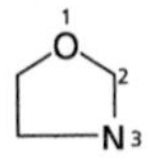

Isoxazole (118)
Examples: *Cloxacillin, Isocarboxazid;
Sulfisoxazole.*

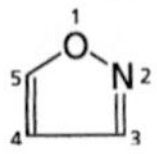

Isoxazolidine (118)
Example: *Cycloserine.*

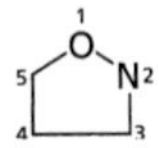

C₃NS

Thiazole (122)
Examples: *Thiabendazole; Thiamine.*

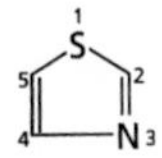

C₃N₂

Imidazole (127)
Examples: *Azathioprine; Histamine;
Pilocarpine.*

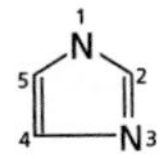

2-Imidazoline (127)
Example: *Phenytoin*

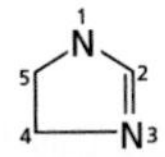

Imidazoline (127)
Example: *Nitrofurantoin*

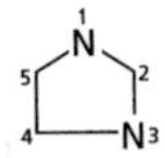

3-Pyrazoline (124)
Example: *Antipyrine.*

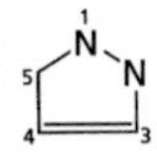

Pyrazolidine (124)
Examples: *Phenylbutazone; Sulfinpyrazone.*

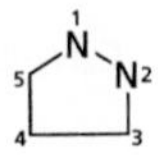

C₃O₂

1,3-Dioxolane (136)
Examples: *Ketoconazole; Propylene Carbonate.*

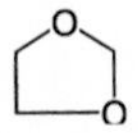

C₄N

Pyrrole (142)
Example: *Pyrvinium Pamoate.*

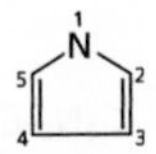

Pyrrolidine (142)
Example: *Methsuximide*

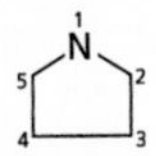

C₄O

Furan (145)
Example: *Nitrofurantoin*

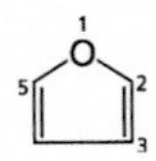

2,5-Dihydrofuran (145)
Examples: *Ascorbic Acid; Digitoxin.*

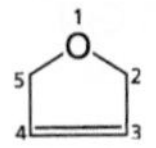

Tetrahydrofuran (145)
Examples: *Polysorbate; Sorbitan;
Streptomycin; Sucrose.*

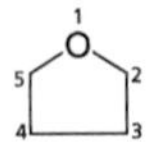

C₄S

Thiophene (149)
Example: *Cefoxitin*

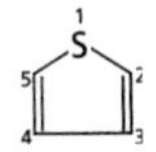

6 C₃NOP

Tetrahydro-2H-1,3,2-oxazaphosphorine
(7746)
Example: *Cyclophosphamide.*

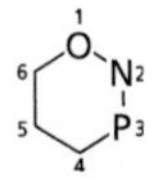

C₃O₃

s-Trioxane (222)
Example: *Paraldehyde.*

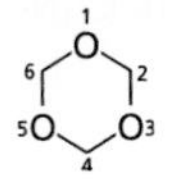

C₄NO

Morpholine (239)
Examples: *Pramoxine; Timolol.*

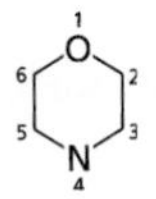

C₄N₂

Pyrimidine (249)
Example: *Pyrimethamine.*

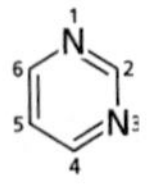

1,2,3,4-Tetrahydropyrimidine (249)
Example: *Propylthiouracil.*

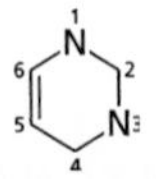

1,4,5,6-Tetrahydro form (249)
Example: *Oxyphencyclimine.*

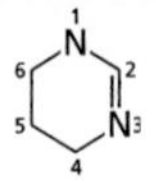

Hexahydropyrimidine (249)
Examples: *All barbituric and thiobarbituric
acids; Primidone.*

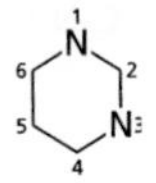

Pyrazine (250)
Example: *Amiloride.*

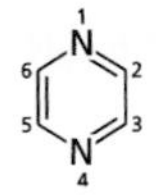

Piperazine: Hexahydropyrazine (250)
Example: *Prochlorperazine.*

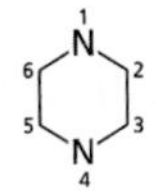

C₅N

Pyridine (277)
Examples: *Cetylpyridinium Chloride;
Niacinamide.*

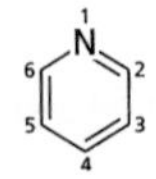

1,4-Dihydropyridine (4H-Pyridine) (277)
Example: *Propyliodone.*

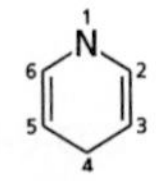

Piperidine; Hexahydropyridine (277)
Example: *Meperidine.*

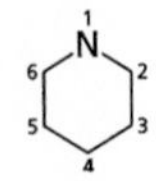

Tetrahydropyran (278)
Examples: *Lactose; Streptomycin.*

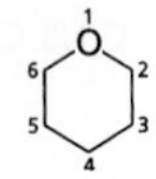

7 C₆N

Hexahydroazepine (355)
Example: *Tolazamide.*

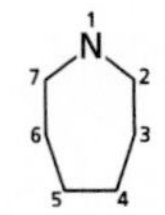

8 C_7N

Octahydroazocine (414)
Example: *Guanethidine*.

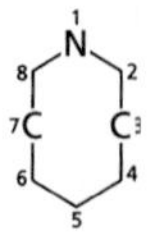

14 C_{13}O

Oxacyclotetradecane (534)
Example: *Erythromycin*.

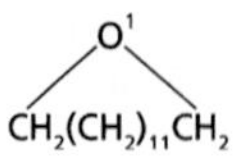

15 C_{13}NO

1-Oxa-6-azacyclopentadecane
Example: *Azithromycin*.

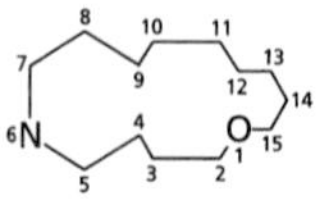

16 C_{11}N_5

1,4,7,10,13-Pentaazacyclo-
hexadecane
Example: *Capreomycin*.

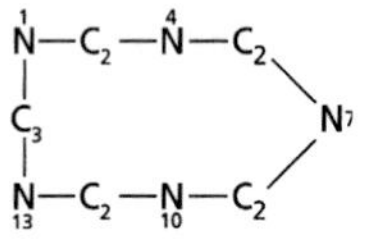

23 C_{16}N_2

1,4,7,10,13,16,19-
Heptaazacyclotricosane
(11705)
Examples: *Colistin;*
Colistimethate Sodium.

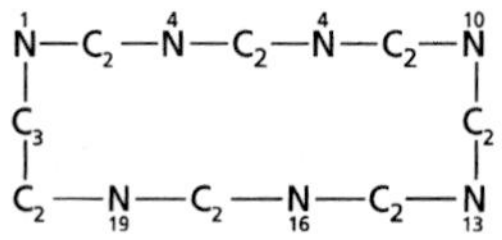

3,5 C_3-C_4N

3-Azabicyclo[3.1.0]hexane (690)
Example: *Trovafloxacin*

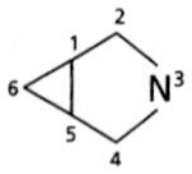

4,5 C_3N-C_3NO

4-Oxa-1-azabicyclo[3.2.0]heptane
Example: *Clavulanate Potassium.*

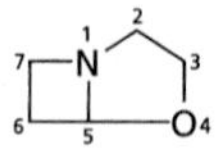

C_3N-C_3NS

4-Thia-1-azabicyclo[3.2.0]
heptane (774)
Example: *Penicillins.*

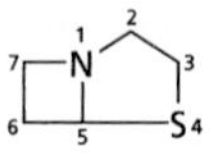

4,6 C_3N-C_5N

1-Azabicyclo [4.2.0] octane (810)
$\triangle^{2,3}$-form
Example: *Loracarbef*

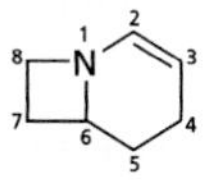

C_3N-C_4NS

5-Thia-1-azabicyclo[4.2.0]oct-2-ene
(11757)
Example: *Cefotaxin*

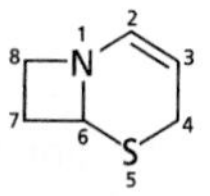

5,5 C_3N_2-C_4S

1H-Thieno[3,4-d]imidazole,
hexahydro form (945)
Example: *Biotin.*

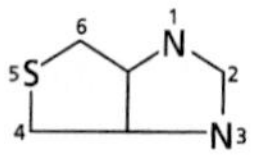

C_5O-C_5O

Furo[3,2-b]furan, hexahydro
form (996)
Example: *Isosorbide Dinitrate.*

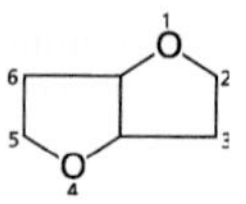

C_3NS-C_6

Benzothiazole (1152)
Example: *Ethoxzolamide.*

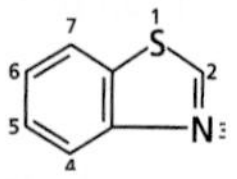

1,2-Benzisothiazole, 2,3-dihydro
form (1150)
Example: *Saccharin.*

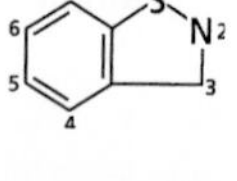

C_3N_2-C_4N_2

1H-Pyrazolo[3,4-d]pyrimidine (1174)
Example: *Allopurinol.*

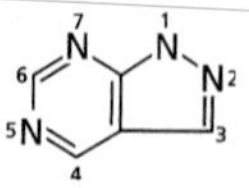

Purine[b] (1179)
Examples: *Caffeine; Dimenhydrinate.*

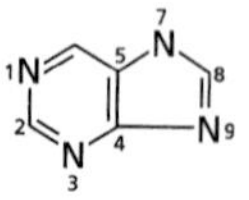

C_3N_2-C_6

Benzimidazole (1213)
Examples: *Cyanocobalamin;*
Droperidol; Thiabendazole.

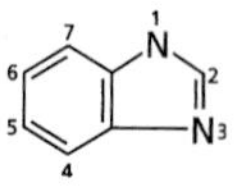

C_3O_2-C_6

1,4-Dioxaspiro[4.5]decane (1238)
Example: *Guanadrel.*

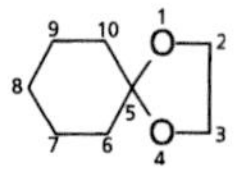

C_3OS-C_6

3H-2,1-Benzoxathiole (1222)
Example: *Phenolsulfonphthalein.*

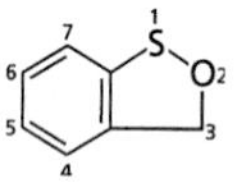

C_4N-C_5N

Nortropane (1281) or 8-azabicyclo-
[3.2.1]octane
Examples: *Atropine; Cocaine.*

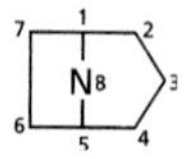

C_4NC_6

Indole (1286)
Example: *Indomethacin.*

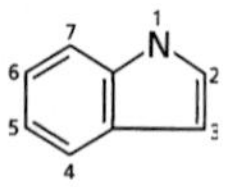

Indoline (1286)
Example: *Indigotindisulfonate*
Sodium.

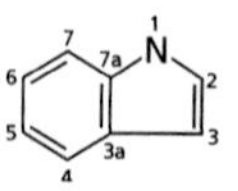

Isoindoline (1290)
Example: *Chlorthalidone.*

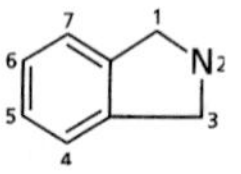

C_4O-C_5

Phthalan; (1,3-Dihydroisobenzofuran)
(1330)
Example: *Phenolphthalein.*

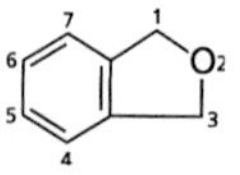

6,6 C_3N_25-C_6

2H-1,2,4-Benzothiadiazine (8074)
Example: *Chlorothiazide.*

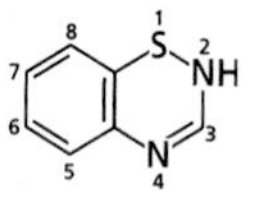

3,4-dihydro form (8074)
Examples: *Hydrochlorothiazide;*
Polythiazide.

C_4N_2-C_4N_2

Pyrimido[5,3-d]pyrimidine (1585)
Example: *Dipyridamole.*

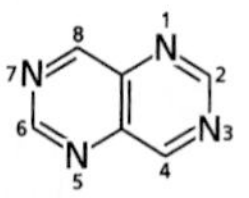

Pteridine (1587)
Example: *Methotrexate.*
1,4,5,6,7,8-hexahydro form.
Example: *Leucovorin.*

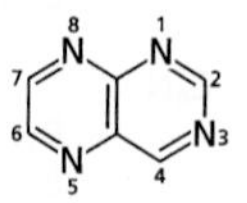

C_1N_2-C_6

Phthalazine (1628)
Example: *Hydralazine.*

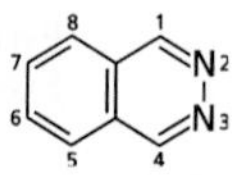

Quinazoline (1626)
Example: *Methaqualone.*

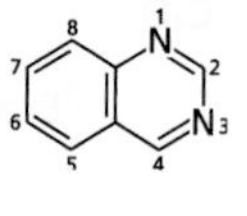

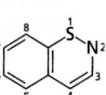

Appendix E Continued

C₄NS-C₆

2*H*-1,2-Benzothiazine (1577)
Example: *Piroxicam.*

C₅N-C₅N

1,8-Naphthyridine, 1,4-dihydro
form (1683)
Example: *Nalidixic Acid.*

Quinuclidine (1690)
Examples: Clidinium Bromide;
Quinine.

C₅N-C₅

Quinoline (1707)
Examples: *Chloroquine; Quinine.*

Isoquinoline (1708)
Example: *Papaverine.*
1,2,3,4-tetrahydro form
Example: *Emetine.*

C₅O-C₅

2*H*-1-Benzopyran (1727)
Examples: *Dicumarol; Warfarin.*

Chroman (Dihydrobenzopyran)
(1727)
Example: *Vitamin E*

6,7 C₆-C₅N₂

3*H*-1,4-Benzodiazepine (1829)
Example: *Chlordiazepoxide.*

2*H*-1,4-Benzodiazepine,
1,3-dihydro form (12067)
Examples: *Diazepam; Oxazepam.*

C₅-C₅NS

1,5-Benzothiazepine (1825)
1,2,3,4-Tetrahydro form
Example: *Dilitiazem*

6,36 C₅O-C₃₄O₂

14,39-Dioxabicyclo[33.3.1]
nonatriacontane
Example: *Amphotericin.*

3,5,6 C₂O-C₄N-C₅N

3-Oxa-9-azatricyclo[3.3.1.0²,⁴]
nonane (2072)
Examples: *Methscopolamine
Bromide; Scopolamine.*

3,6,24 C₂O-C₅O-C₂₂O₂

6,11,28-Trioxatricyclo[22.3.1.0⁵,⁷]
octacosane
Example: *Natamycin.*

5,5,5 C₃N₂-C₄S-C₄S

Imidazo[4,5-c]thieno[1,2-a]thiolium
or thieno[1′,2′:1,2]thieno[3,4-d]
imidazol-5-ium, decahydro
form (2215)
Example: *Trimethaphan Camsylate.*

5,5,6 C₃NO₂-C₄N-C₄N₂

8*H*-Oxazolo[3,2-a]pyrrolo[2,1-c]-
pyrazine, perhydro form (2319)
Example: *Ergotamine.*

C₃N₂-C₄N-C₆

3*H*-Imidazo[2,1-a]isoindole, 2,5-
dihydro form (2384)
Example: *Mazindol.*

C₄N-C₄N-C₆

Pyrrolo[2,3-b]indole, 1,2,3,3a,8,8a-
hexahydro form (2442)
Example: *Physostigmine.*

5,6,6 C₃O₂-C₄N₂-C₆

[1,3]-Dioxolo[4,5-g]cinnoline,
1,4-dihydro form (2806)
Example: *Cinoxacin.*

C₃O₂-C₅N-C₆

[1,3]-Dioxolo[4,5-g]isoquinoline,
5,6,7,8-tetrahydro form (2810)
Example: *Noscapine.*

C₄N-C₅-C₆

1*H*-Benz[e]indolium (2933)
Example: *Indocyanine Green.*

C₄O-C₅O-C₆

7*H*-Furo[3,2-g][1]benzopyran (2988)
Examples: *Methoxsalen; Trioxsalen.*

C₄O-C₆-C₆

Spiro[benzofuran-2(3H),1′-[2]-
cyclohexene] (3028)
Example: *Griseofulvin.*

5,6,7 C₂N₃-C₆-C₅N₂

4*H*-[1,2,4]Triazolo[4,3-a][1,4]
benzodiazepine
Examples: *Alprazolam, Triazolam.*

C₄S-C₆-C₅N₂

Thieno[2,3-b][1,5]benzodiazepine
Example: *Olanzapine*

6,6,6 C₃N₃-C₃N₃-C₃N₃

Hexamethylenetetramine (3237) or
1,3,5,7-Tetraazatricyclo [3.3.1³,⁷]
decane
Example: *Methenamine.*

C₄N₂-C₅N-C₆

4*H*-Pyrazino[2,1-a]isoquinoline,
1,2,3,6,7,11b-hexahydro form (10470)
Example: *Praziquantel.*

Appendix E Continued

C4NO-C6-C6
3H-Phenoxazine (3289)
Example: *Dactinomycin.*

C4NS-C6-C6
Phenothiazine (3314)
Examples: *Chlorpromazine;*
Prochlorperazine.

Phenazathionium (3315) or
Phenothiazin-5-ium
Example: *Methylene Blue.*

C4O2-C5O-C6
4H-Pyrano[2,3-b][1,4]benzodioxin,
decahydro form (12687)
Example: *Spectinomycin.*

C4N2-C4N2-C6
Benzo[g]pteridine, 2,3,4,
10-tetrahydroform (3340)
Example: *Riboflavin.*

C5N-C5N-C6
2H-Benzo[a]quinolizine, 1,3,4,6,7,-
11b-hexahydro form (3487)
Example: *Emetine.*

C5N-C6-C5
Acridine[b] (3523)
Examples: *Acrisorcin; Quinacrine.*

2,6-Methano-3-benzazocine,
1,2,3,4,5,6-hexahydro form (3535)
Example: *Pentazocine.*

C5O-C6-C6
Xanthene[b] (3571)
Example: *Propantheline.*

3H-Isoxanthene[b] (3569)
Examples: *Fluorescein Sodium;*
Rose Bengal Sodium.

6H-Dibenzo[b,d]pyran, 6a,7,8,
10a-tetrahydroform (3581)
Example: *Dronabinol.*

C5S-C5C5
Thioxanthene[b] (3607)
Example: *Thiothixene.*

6,6,7 C5N-C5N-C5N2
Dipyrido[3,2-b:2',3',e][1,4]diazepine
5,11-dihydro form
Example: *Nivirapine*

C5N-C6-C7
5H-Benzo[5,6]cyclohepta[1,2-b]-
pyridine 6,11-dihydro form
Example: *Azatadine.*

5H-Dibenz[b,f]azepine (3689)
Example: *Carbamazepine.*

10,11-dihydro form (3689)
Examples: *Desipramine; Imipramine.*

C6C6-C5NO
Dibenz[b,f][1,4]oxazepine (3697)
Example: *Loxapine*

C6C6-C6O
Dibenz[b,e]oxepine, 6,11-dihydro
form (3697)
Example: *Doxepin.*

3,5,5,6 C2N-C4N-C4N-C6
Azirino[2',3':3,4]pyrrolo[1,2-a]indole
(12848),1,1a,2,8,8a,8b-hexahydro
form
Example: *Mitomycin.*

5,6,6,6 C4N-C5N-C6-C6
Indolo[4,3-fg]quinoline,4,6,6a,7,8,9-
hexahydro form (4550)
Examples: *Ergonovine; Ergotamine.*

C5O-C6-C6-C6
Cyclopental[5,6]naphtho[1,2c]-
pyran, perhydro form (4760)
Example: *Oxandrolone.*

5,6,6,9 C4N-C5N-C6-C6N
10H-3,7-Methanoaza-
cycloundecino-
[5,4-b]indole,
1,2,4,5,6,7,8,9-
octahydro form (13276)
Examples: *Vinblastine; Vincristine.*

5,6,6,24 C4O-C6-C6-C22NO
2,7-(Epoxypentadecanimino)
naphtho[2,1-b]]furan
Example: *Rifampin.*

6,6,6,6 C5N-C6-C6-C5
4H-Dibenzo[de,fg]quinoline,
5,6,6a,7-
tetrahydro form (5171)
Example: *Apomorphine.*
2H-10,4a-Iminoethanophenan-
threne,[b] *cis*-1,3,4,9,10,10a-
hexahydro form
(5180)
Examples: *Dextromethorphan;*
Levorphanol.

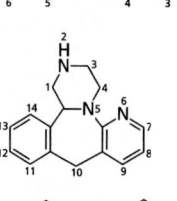

6,6,6,7 C4N2-C6-C6-C6N
Pyrazino[2,1-a]pyrido[2,3-c][2]-
benzazepine, 1,2,3,4,10,14b-
hexahydro form
Example: *Mirtizapine*

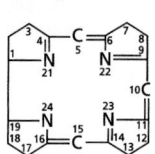

5,5,5,5,15 C4N-C4N-C4N-C4N-C11H4
Corrin[b] (5475)
Example: *Cyanocobalamin.*

Appendix E **Continued**

5,5,6,6,6 C₃NO-C₆-C₆-C₆-C₆

1*H*-Cyclopenta[7,8]phenanthro-
[3,2-*d*]-isoxazole, 2,3,3*a*,-
3*b*,4,5,10,10*a*,10*b*,11.12.12*a*-
dodecahydro form (11036)
Example: *Danazol.*

C₃N₂-C₅-C₆-C₆-C₆

8*H*-Cyclopenta[7,8]phenanthro-
[3,2-*c*]-pyrazole, 1,2,3,3*a*,3*b*,-
4,5,5*a*,6,7,10,10*a*,10*b*,11,12,-
12*a*-tetradecahydro form
(FKRBA)
Example: *Stanozolol.*

C₄N-C₄N-C₅N-C₆-C₆

1*H*-Indolizino[8,1-*cd*]
carbazole, 3a,4,5,5a,6,11,12,
13a-octahydro form (11605)
Examples: *Vinblastine; Vincristine.*

5,6,6,6,6 C₄N-C₅N-C₅N-C₆-C₆

Benz[*g*]indolo[2,3-*a*]quinolizine,
1,2,3,4,4a,5,7,13,13b,14,14a-
dodecahydro form (5784)
Example: *Reserpine.*

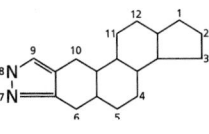

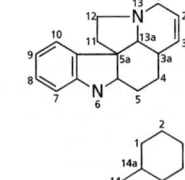

C₄O-C₅N-C₆-C₆-C₅

4*aH*-8,9*c*-Iminoethanophenan-
thro-[4,5-*bcd*]furan, 5922)
5,7a,8,9-tetrahydro form
Examples: *Codeine; Morphine;
Nalorphine.*
5,6,7,7a,8,9-hexahydro form
Examples: *Hydrocodone;
Hydromorphone.*

C₄O-C₅O-C₆-C₆-C₅

Spiro[phthalan-1,9'-xanthene] (5935)
or Spiro[isobenzofuran-1-(3*H*), 9']
9*H*]xanthene]
Example: *Fluorescein.*

6,6,6,6,6,6,18 C₅N-C₆-C₆-C₆-C₆-C₁₆-O₂

Octahydro form of
Ring Index No 7408.
Examples:
*Tubocurarine;
Metocurine.*

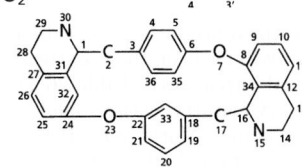

---

[a] Characters in parentheses are either the *Ring Index* number or the *Parent Compound Identifier.*
[b] Exception to the numbering rule.

Table 26-2. Current FDA Qualified Health Claims

PRODUCT	PERMITTED QUALIFIED CLAIM
Dietary supplement containing selenium	Some scientific evidence suggests that consumption of selenium may reduce the risk of certain forms of cancer or Some scientific evidence suggests that consumption of selenium may produce anticarcinogenic effects in the body
Dietary supplements containing vitamin E and/or vitamin C	Some scientific evidence suggests that consumption of antioxidant vitamins may reduce the risk of certain forms of cancer.
Whole or chopped almonds, hazelnuts, peanuts, pecans, some pine nuts, pistachio nuts, and walnuts	Scientific evidence suggests but does not prove that eating 1.5 ounces per day of most nuts [such as *name of specific nut*] as part of a diet low in saturated fat and cholesterol may reduce the risk of heart disease.
Dietary supplements containing the omega-3 long chain polyunsaturated fatty acids eicosapentaenoic acid (EPA) and/or docosahexaenoic acid (DHA)	Consumption of omega-3 fatty acids may reduce the risk of coronary heart disease.
Dietary supplements containing vitamin B6, B12, and/or folic acid	As part of a well-balanced diet that is low in saturated fat and cholesterol, folic acid, vitamin B6, and vitamin B12 may reduce the risk of vascular disease.
Dietary supplements containing soy-derived phosphatidylserine	Consumption of phosphatidylserine may reduce the risk of dementia in the elderly or Consumption of phosphatidylserine may reduce the risk of cognitive dysfunction in the elderly
Dietary supplements containing folic acid	0.8 mg folic acid in a dietary supplement is more effective in reducing the risk of neural tube defects than a lower amount in foods in common form.

pounds was both difficult and costly, especially for compounds present in very low concentrations. However, this has been made easier by continued advances in extraction, concentrating, and identifying processes. Since natural products already have a function in nature, and therefore, typically already display pharmacological activity, they are seen as improving the odds of synthesizing a good drug compared to starting with a completely new structure. Such compounds are proving to be very useful as starting points for combinatorial chemistry and the synthesis of lead drug compounds.

The remaining portion of this chapter will focus upon the active constituents of natural products such as foods and herbals and provides a discussion of the fundamental characteristics of the following, essentially chemical, classes of naturally occurring products:

Carbohydrates and Glycosides
Proteins, Peptides, and Amino Acids
Lipids (Fixed Oils and Fats, Waxes, Phospholipids, and Prostaglandins)
Sterols and Saponins
Alkaloids
Phenols
Volatile Oils, Resins, and Miscellaneous Isoprenoids

CARBOHYDRATES AND GLYCOSIDES

Composition and Structure

Carbohydrates consist of carbon, hydrogen, and oxygen and include numerous aliphatic polyhydric alcohols and their condensation products. The aliphatic polyhydric alcohols are frequently termed *monosaccharides* (sometimes simply *saccharides* or simple sugars) and have either the primary alcohol function oxidized to an aldehyde or the secondary alcohol function oxidized to a ketone. They have the empirical formula $(CH_2O)_n$, where $n \geq 2$ for aldehydes and ≥ 3 for ketones. Monosaccharides may be subclassified into *aldoses* and *ketoses* according to whether they contain an aldehyde or a ketone group and into *dioses, trioses, tetroses*, etc. according to the

number of carbon atoms they contain. For example, xylose may be considered an *aldopentose* (containing an aldehyde function and a total of five carbon atoms); similarly, fructose may be considered a *ketohexose* (containing a ketone function and a total of six carbon atoms).

The carbon skeleton of the common monosaccharides is unbranched and each carbon atom contains a hydroxy group except for the one containing the carbonyl oxygen that is combined in an *acetal* or *ketal* linkage. The total scheme for the aldoses and the ketoses is shown in Table 26-4 with the intermediate —CH(OH)— groups represented by horizontal lines drawn on the side to which the OH group is attached. Starting with the aldotrioses, the insertion of each —CH(OH)— group introduces a chiral center (asymmetric carbon atom), giving rise to an increasing number of stereoisomers. The enantiomorphs of each stereoisomeric pair are distinguished by the *configurational* notations D- and L-, referring respectively to whether the OH of the last inserted —CH(OH)— is on the right or left of the vertical axis when the formulas are drawn in the stick configuration as shown in Table 26-4. It is important to remember that the D- and L- notations have nothing to do with the direction of optical rotation and also that the actual demonstration of whether a given stereoisomer is D- or L- is a matter of extensive laboratory experimentation. It also should be noted that the prefixes D- and L- refer to the asymmetric carbon atom farthest removed from the carbonyl carbon atom. Two saccharides differing only in the configuration around the carbon atom adjacent to the carbonyl group are called *epimers* of each other. For example, D-glucose and D-mannose are epimers with respect to the second carbon atom.

Measurements of various characteristics, such as the propensity to function as reductants, the ability to form acetal derivatives, mutarotation, etc., have demonstrated conclusively that the open-chain formulas shown above do not represent the true structure of at least the higher monosaccharides such as the pentoses and hexoses. For example, in aqueous solution, many of the higher monosaccharides behave as if an additional chiral center is present. In reality, the structures are cyclic and may be looked upon as internal

Table 26-3. Popular Herbal Medicines—Their Bases and Source

HERBAL PRODUCT	SOURCE	ACTIVE INGREDIENT(S)	COMMON USES	COMMON SIDE EFFECTS	SUPPORTING EVIDENCE
Bilberry	*Vaccinium myrtillus*	Vitamins A & C, flavonoids, anthocyanin, and glucoquinine.	Improve eyesight, increase bloodflow, and treatment of diabetes	None known	Studies have indicated an improvement in eyesight, due mainly to the effects of vitamin A.
Black Cohosh	*Actaea racemosa* aka. *Cimicifuga racemosa*	Remifemin (brand name of standardized extract)	Menopausal symptoms, peripheral artery disease, and hypercholesterolemia	Overdose: nausea, dizziness, visual disturbances, nervous system abnormalities, increased perspiration and brachycardia. Large doses may induce miscarraige.	Studies have shown measurable effect on reproductive hormones. Studies have also shown that established breast tumor cell lines were not stimulated, leading scientists to consider Black Cohosh for studies as a substitute for hormone replacement therapy.
Cat's Claw	*Uncaria tormentosa*	Several alkaloids including: rhynchophylline, mytraphylline, gambirine, and hirsutine, also six quinovic acid glycosides	Inflammation, as an astringent, gastric ulcer, rheumatism, contraception, and cancer	Few to none.	Studies have verified; some anti-cancer claims, as well as some immunostimulant properties. The major effective ingredient, rhynchophylline may decrease blood pressure to the point of being hypotensive at certain doses.
Chamomile	*Matricaria recutita*	Bisabolol and flavanoids	Inflammation, GI spasms, and as a sedative	Persons allergic to the Compositae family may experience anything from contact dermatitis to anaphylaxis.	Anti-inflammatory and antipyretic claims are supported in animal models. Its main active ingredient, rhynchophylline, has also been shown to decrease blood pressure to the point of being hypotensive at certain doses.
Chaste Tree	*Vitex agnus-castus*	Monoterpene derivatives (limonene, 1,8-cineol, bornyl acetate, α- and β-pinene, sabinene), flavonoids (castican, orientin, isovitexin), and iridoid glycosides (agnuside, aucubin).	Menstrual irregularities, hormone imbalance, breast pain, uterine pain, and decreased sex drive in males	GI symptoms, rash, itching, headaches, and menstrual abnormalities can occur.	Progesterone/Estrogen balance was improved in studies. Its inhibition of prolactin release has also been supported, this can aid in the correction of luteal phase defects.
Cranberry	*Vaccinium macrocarpon*	Hippuric acid, although recent studies have suggested other alternatives.	Treatment, or prevention, of urinary tract infections	GI symptoms, such as diarrhea, can occur at very high doses.	Significant decrease in urinary pH has been observed in studies. However, treatment is still unproven as bacterial susceptibility and minimum effective dose were unclear.
Echinacea	*Echinacea augustifolia* (common); *E. purpuree* (commerce)	Isobutylamides	To decrease the length of cold or prevent its contraction	Those allergic to the daisy family should avoid due to immune response symptoms.	Some evidence points toward a shortening of duration for the common cold; however, prevention has been shown to be doubtful at best.
Evening Primrose	*Oenothera biennis*	Gamma-linolenic acid (GLA)	Breast disorders, PMS, breast pain, cardiovascular disease, rheumatiod arthritis, multiple sclerosis, atopic eczema, and other dermatologic disorders	None Known	Cholesterol—studies have shown that the active ingredient is successful in significantly lowering blood cholesterol; however, in the concentration found in primrose oil, such a decrease is substantially less, if any. Breast cancer—studies have indicated only a slight decrease in recurrence in those patients who have recovered from breast cancer. Premenstrual syndrome—studies have indicated a decrease in symptoms associated with primrose oil.

Table 26-3. Popular Herbal Medicines—Their Bases and Source (continued)

HERBAL PRODUCT	SOURCE	ACTIVE INGREDIENT(S)	COMMON USES	COMMON SIDE EFFECTS	SUPPORTING EVIDENCE
					Rheumatiod arthritis—studies have indicated a drop in NSAID usage among those taking primrose oil, suggesting some level of efficacy; however, disease modification has not been shown.
Feverfew	*Tanacetum parthenium*	Parthenolide	Fever, migraine prophylaxis, arthritis, manstrual pain, asthma, and dermatitis	Abrupt discontinuation can result in a withdrawal syndrome; increased heart rate has also been reported. Should not be used in children < 2 years old, or in pregnant or lactating women.	Severity and incidence of migraine headaches has been shown to be decreased in those taking feverfew.
Garlic	*Allium sativum*	Alliin[(+)-S-allyl-L-cysteine sulfoxide]	High blood sugar, hypercholesterolemia, and hyperlipidemia	None known	Garlic has been shown clinically to increase HDL, decrease LDL and total cholesterol. It has also been shown to have antioxidant properties and to decrease platelet aggregation.
Ginger	*Zingiber officinale*	Gingerols; shogaol	Prevent motion sickness, for cough, stomachache, and gallbladder disease.	In large amounts, CNS depression may occur. May affect cardiac function and anticoagulant activity.	Ginger has been shown to dramatically increase the amount of time needed to reach a state of motion sickness. It also decreases cardiac workload by increasing vasodilation. It has a strong antimicrobial effect.
Ginkgo	*Ginkgo biloba*	Flavonol and flavone glycosides (eg, of quescetin and kaempferol); rutin	Raynaud's disease, stress, tinnitis, dementia, cerebral insufficiency, anxiety, asthma, and circulation problems	Rare, but may include heart palpitations, dizziness, headache and dermatological reactions.	Ginkgo has been shown to increase cerebral blood flow and decrease cerebral deficiency. It has also been shown to decrease inflammatory response in the lungs reducing severity of asthma attacks. It also increases microcirculation and improvement in pathologic blood flow diseases has been observed.
Ginseng	*Panax quinque-folius*	Ginsenosides (triterpenoid saponin glycosides)	Decreased energy, cancer, immune support, and cardiovascular problems	Nervousness is the most common side effect; also some breast nodulation and vaginal bleeding have been reported.	An increase in CNS stimulatory and inhibitory effects has been observed in patients taking Ginseng. An increase in overall cognitive function has been established as well. However, no studies to date have linked ginseng and improved physical performance.
Goldenseal	*Hydrastis canadensis*	Isoquinolone alkaloids (hydrastine, canadine, and berberine)	Topical infections and as an anticatarrhal	Side effects are rare, but contraindicated in patients with hypertension or pregnancy. In very high doses, can cause nausea, anxiety and seizures.	Clinically, it has been shown to have modest antimicrobial activity, most effective topically.
Grape Seed	*Vitus vinifera*	Essential fatty acids and tocopherols	Nutritional supplement (fatty acid)	Hepatotoxicity in animal studies.	Clinically, it has been shown to have anti-enzyme properties resulting in a decrease in breakdown of compounds important for tissue structure, such as collagen, elastin, and hyaluronic acid.

(continues)

Table 26-3. Popular Herbal Medicines—Their Bases and Source *(continued)*

HERBAL PRODUCT	SOURCE	ACTIVE INGREDIENT(S)	COMMON USES	COMMON SIDE EFFECTS	SUPPORTING EVIDENCE
Green Tea	*Camellia sinensis*	Catechins and polyphenol components	Cancer, hyperlipidemia, prevention of dental carries, as an antimicrobial, antimutagenic, and an antioxidant	Caffeine in green tea may cause nervousness and increased heart rate, and should be avoided during pregnancy.	Clinically, it has been shown to decrease total cholesterol; however, triglycerides and HDL were unchanged. Also, antimicrobial activity has been shown especially against mouth flora. It also has been shown to inhibit the growth of some harmful GI pathogens, although the dose was 9 cups per day.
Hawthorn	*Crataegus laevigata*	Oligomeric procyanidins (epicatechin and flavonoids)	Hypertension, abnormal heart rate, artherosclerosis, angina pectoris, and as an antispasmodic and a sedative.	Hypotension and sedation can be experienced at high doses. May interfere with digoxin blood levels.	Studies have shown that hawthorn increases vasodilation and coronary artery flow, as well as to stabilize heart rate. It has also been shown to decrease lipid levels.
Horse Chestnut	*Aesculus hippo-castanum*	Aesculin	Edema, inflammation, and venous insufficiency	Use should be avoided due to classification as an unsafe herb by the FDA because of toxicity. Topical products containing this herb may also be carcinogenic.	Increased vascular resistance and tone has been indicated. A decrease in complaints and edema measures was shown in patients with peripheral edema. Anti-inflammatory properties have also been supported.
Kava Kava	*Piper methys ticum*	Kava lactones	Mild to moderate anxiety and as a sedative	Should not be used during pregnancy or by patients with depression. Use should be limited to 3 months to avoid habit-forming tendancies. Also, problems with vision and a condition similar to pellagra have been reported.	Studies have supported Kava's positive effect on patients with mild to moderate anxiety. It has also been demonstrated as an effective anticonvulsant. In addition, kava has an antithrombotic effect on platelet aggregation.
Licorice	*Glycyrrhiza uralensis*	Carbenoxalone	GI complaints	Lethargy and quadriplegia may result from long-term daily consumption.	Licorice has been shown to increase the lifespan of gastric epithelial cells. It has been demonstrated to be less effective than Cimetidine at treating gastric and duodenal ulcers.
Milk Thistle	*Silybum marianum*	Silymarins (flavano-lignanssilybin, isosilybin, dehy-drosilybin, silydianin, and silychristin)	Liver damage prophylaxis, antitoxin	Mild allergic reactions and mild GI symptoms.	Milk thistle has been shown to normalize liver enzymes; however, improvement in the evolution and mortality of cirrhosis is not supported.
Saw Palmetto	*Serenoa repens*	Probable active compounds are: phytosterols, fatty acids and their ethyl esters, and monoacylgly-cerides.	Symptoms associated with benign prostatic hyperplasia	Should be avoided during pregnancy, but no other side effects aside from mild GI symptoms.	Clinically, several symptoms associated with benign prostatic hyperplasia have been shown to decrease in those taking saw palmetto. It has not been shown to have any effect on prostate size or presence of prostate specific antigen in the blood.
St John's Wort	*Hypericum perforatum*	Hypericin, hyperforin, and related naptho-dianthrones	Depression and viral infection	Rare, but may include constipation, other GI symptoms, dry mouth, dizziness and photosensitivity. Mania and sexual disturbance occur even more rarely.	Clinical trials have shown that patients taking St. John's Wort have a significant decrease in serotonin reuptake as well as an increased dopamine function. Also, several viruses (influenza, herpes simplex 1 & 2 and some retroviruses) have susceptibility to this compound. St. John's Wort has also demonstrated potent antimicrobial activity.

Table 26-3. Popular Herbal Medicines—Their Bases and Source *(continued)*

HERBAL PRODUCT	SOURCE	ACTIVE INGREDIENT(S)	COMMON USES	COMMON SIDE EFFECTS	SUPPORTING EVIDENCE
Valerian	*Valeriana officinalis*	Valepotriates, valerenic acid, and valeranone	Restlessness and sleep disorders	Few to none.	Valerian has been demonstrated to improve sleep disorders very effectively. Also, antianxiety studies have indicated efficacy in treating those symptoms.

Data from DerMarderosian A, et al. *Guide to Popular Natural Products,* 2nd ed. St. Louis, MO: Facts and Comparisons, 2001; and *United States Pharmacopeia and National Formulary (USP 27–NF 22).* Rockville, MD: The United States Pharmacopeial Convention, Inc., 2003.

hemiacetals formed by condensation of the carbonyl oxygen atom and one of the alcoholic hydroxyls. Although such a reaction can involve any of the hydroxyl groups, theoretical considerations suggest that the γ- and δ-hydroxyl groups are situated more ideally to participate in the cyclization, thus giving rise to furanose (containing a furan ring) and pyranose (containing a pyran ring) structures. Experimental evidence indicates that the aldohexoses, in their normal monosaccharide states, exist largely in the more stable pyranose form. For example, the open-chain formula (**A**) for D-glucose gives way to the corresponding cyclic structures (**B**):

A **B**

α-form β-form

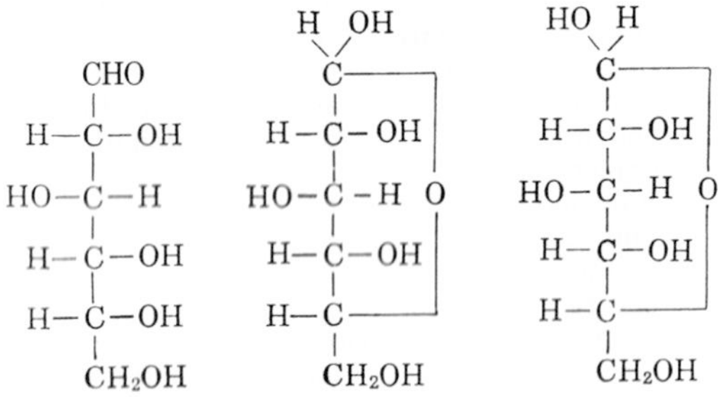

The two stereoisomeric forms of (**B**), conventionally distinguished by α- and β- nomenclature, arise because the cyclization automatically renders the former aldehyde carbon atom asymmetric. This isomerization occurs spontaneously in aqueous solution and causes the specific rotation to change until a final equilibrium value is reached. This process is termed *mutarotation.* Incidentally, both the α- and β-forms of D-glucose are well known with the commercial form (dextrose) being the α- variety. Isomeric forms of monosaccharides that differ from each other only in configuration of the chiral carbon atom derived from the carbonyl group are *anomers* and the newly formed asymmetric carbon atom is termed the *anomeric carbon.*

The two-dimensional representations of cyclic structures as in (**B**) have largely been superseded by the Haworth Projection models. In these models, the ring is usually represented as planar (although strict planarity is not implied), and the disposition of hydrogen atoms and substituents is portrayed by a vertical assignment upward or downward from the ring plane. Haworth structures for some selected hexoses are shown below, along with the conventional ring numbering. Note that the edge of the ring nearest the reader is represented by bold lines; thus, the plane of the ring is perpendicular to the page. For comparison, both the furanose and pyranose structures are shown for α-D-glucose.

α-D-Glucose (α-D-Glucopyranose)

α-D-Glucose (α-D-Glucofuranose)

β-D-Glucose (β-D-Glucopyranose)

α-D-Fructose (α-D-Fructopyranose)

α-D-Mannose (α-D-Mannopyranose)

α-D-Galactose (α-D-Galactopyranose)

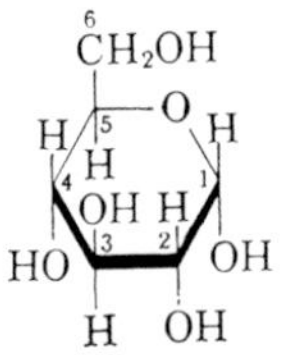

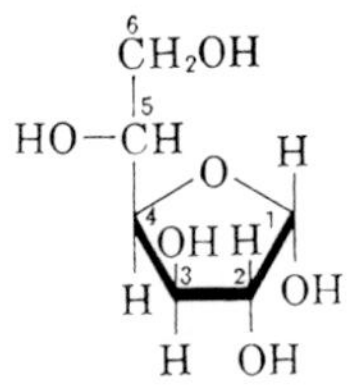

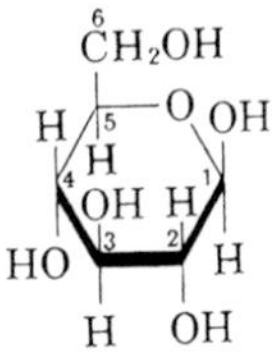

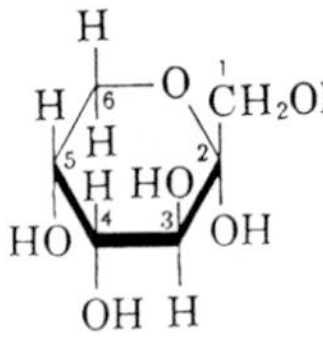

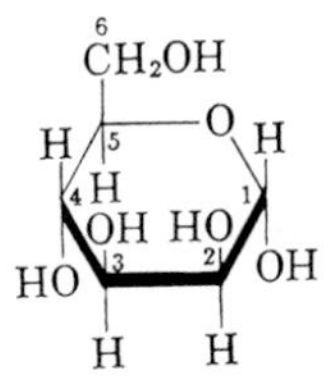

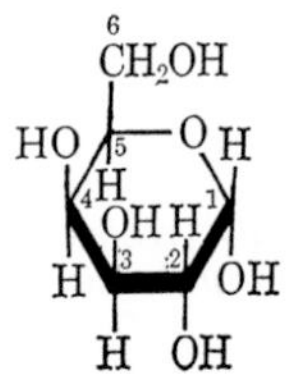

The Haworth projections are somewhat misleading, however, because they suggest that the five and six-member furanose and pyranose rings are planar, which is not the actual case. The pyranose rings exist in two conformations, the *chair* form and the *boat* form. The chair form of the pyranose ring, which is relatively rigid and much more stable than the boat form, predominates in aqueous solutions of hexoses. The substituent groups in the chair form are not equivalent geometrically or chemically; they fall into two classes, *axial* and *equatorial.* The equatorial hydroxyl groups of pyranoses are esterified more readily than axial groups.

Boat

Chair

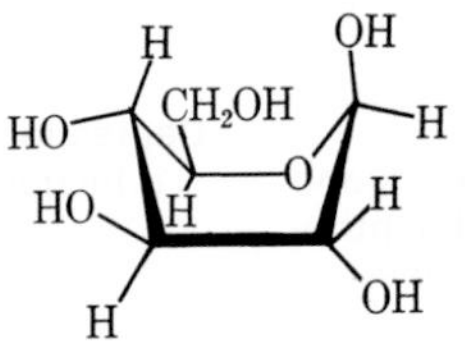

The condensation products of the monosaccharides, whose fundamental structural units are either aldoses or ketoses, are

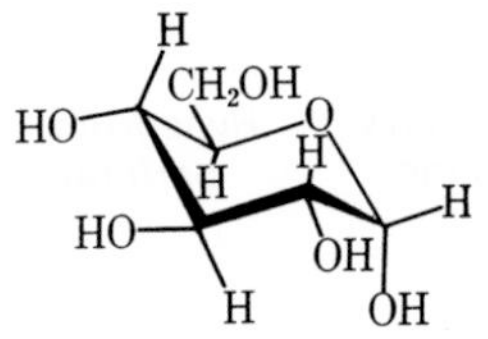

Table 26-4. Monosaccharides[a]

ALDOSES

DIOSE	TRIOSE	TETROSES	PENTOSES	HEXOSES
Glyceraldehyde (Parent molecule of the Aldoses)[c]	D-Glyceraldehyde	D-Erythrose	D-Ribose	D-Allose
				L-Talose
			L-Lyxose	D-Gulose
				L-Mannose
		L-Threose	D-Xylose	D-Glucose
				L-Idose
			L-Arabinose	D-Galactose
				L-Altrose
	L-Glyceraldehyde	D-Threose	D-Arabinose	D-Altrose
				L-Galactose
			L-Xylose	D-Idose
				L-Glucose
		L-Erythrose	D-Lyxose	D-Mannose
				L-Gulose
			L-Ribose	D-Talose
				L-Allose

KETOSES[b]

TRIOSE	TETROSES	PENTOSES	HEXOSES
Dihydroxyacetone (Parent molecule of the ketoses)[d]	D-Erythrulose	D-Ribulose	D-Psicose
			L-Tagatose
		L-Xyloketose	D-Sorbose
			L-Fructose
	L-Erythrulose	D-Xyloketose	D-Fructose
			L-Sorbose
		L-Ribulose	D-Tagatose
			L-Psicose

[a] Scheme is terminated with hexoses although some higher members are known.

[b] Scheme is limited to 2-ketohexoses. Other ketoses are not usually treated in carbohydrate chemistry.

[c] In all aldose representations, the vertical line stands for CH_2OH. Thus, for example, the representation for D-Glyceraldehyde actually portrays

$$
\begin{array}{c} CHO \\ H-C-OH \\ CH_2OH \end{array}
$$

; the representation for L-Threose actually portrays

$$
\begin{array}{c} CHO \\ H-C-OH \\ HO-C-H \\ CH_2OH \end{array}
$$

; etc.

[d] In all ketose representations, the symbol $\parallel O$ stands for $C=O$. Thus, for example, the representation for D-Erythrulose actually portrays

$$
\begin{array}{c} CH_2OH \\ C=O \\ H-C-OH \\ CH_2OH \end{array}
$$

the representation for L-Xyloketose actually portrays

$$
\begin{array}{c} CH_2OH \\ C=O \\ HO-C-H \\ CH_2OH \end{array}
$$

etc.

sometimes referred to as *saccharide anhydrides*. They are sub-classified into disaccharides, trisaccharides, etc. according to the number of monosaccharide units present. *Polysaccharides* contain many monosaccharide units joined in long linear or branched chains. Most polysaccharides contain recurring monosaccharide units of either a single or alternating type. The term *polysaccharide* may be used broadly to embrace all of the condensation products including the disaccharides or more restrictively excluding the disaccharides and sometimes the tri- and tetrasaccharides. In this case, the di- to decasaccharides may be grouped under the term *oligosaccharides* (from the Greek, *oligo, a few*).

The structures and systematic names of the four best-known disaccharides are shown below. The systematic bracketed names identify precisely the location of the oxygen bridge joining the two monosaccharide residues. Also note that, in the case of sucrose, the stable furan conformation is shown as being dominant for the fructose portion of the molecule.

Sucrose
[β-D-**Fructofuranosyl**-α-D-**glucopyranoside**]

Lactose (α-Lactose)
[4-(*O*-β-D-**Galactopyranosyl**)-α-D-**glucopyranoside**]

Maltose
[4-(*O*-α-D-**Glucopyranosyl**)-α-D-**glucopyranoside**]

Cellobiose
[4-(*O*-β-D-**Glucopyranosyl**)-β-D-**glucopyranoside**]

The naturally occurring polysaccharides (eg, the starches, cellulose, glycogen, and inulin) are formed primarily from pentoses and hexoses but vary considerably in size and structure. For example, inulin is a relatively small polymer composed of approximately 30 fructose (fructofuranose) units; whereas, cellulose is a relatively large polymer probably containing no less than 1000 glucopyranose units. In some polysaccharides, such as cellulose, evidence is strong that the polymers are purely linear; in others, such as starch and glycogen observed experimental data requires that considerable branching is present along the chain. Polysaccharides often are classified on the basis of their monomers; for example, pentosans are polymers of pentoses and hexosans are polymers of hexoses. Frequently, such classification is rendered more specific. For example, cellulose is a glucosan (the hexose unit is D-glucose) and inulin is a fructosan (the hexose unit is D-fructose). The complete systematic names of carbohydrates are considered cumbersome and consequently find little use in ordinary chemical practice. Recognizing this, both IUPAC and *Chemical Abstracts* admit the commonly used trivial names.

Physical and Chemical Properties

The common monosaccharides, namely the pentoses and hexoses, are white, crystalline solids that usually melt rather sharply but with simultaneous decomposition. They are readily soluble in water, much less soluble in methanol or ethanol, and relatively insoluble in ether. The common disaccharides, all hexoses, also display these characteristics. The soluble, lower molecular weight carbohydrates are also characterized by a sweet taste but their relative sweetness varies considerably. For example, lactose is only about ⅙, maltose about ⅓, and glucose about ¾ as sweet as sucrose. Fructose, on the other hand, is about 1.7 times sweeter than sucrose. The higher polysaccharides such as starch, cellulose, and inulin are amorphous, do not melt sharply, and are much less water-soluble; however, they typically have the capacity to absorb significant amounts of water and often form gels.

All carbohydrates are optically active, and their specific rotations serve as one means of differentiation. Many display the phenomenon of *mutarotation*, a continuing change in the value of the rotation until a final fixed value is attained. For example, a freshly prepared aqueous solution of α-D-glucose has an $[\alpha]_D^{20}$ of +113°, but gradually changes to a final value of +52°. It has been frequently demonstrated that such changes in rotation are due to structural shifts and that the final value is quantitatively characteristic of the components present in the equilibrium mixture. In the case of glucose, this ultimate equilibrium value is derived from an aqueous solution containing about ⅓ of the α-D-form ($[\alpha]_D^{20} = +112.2°$) and about 2/3 of the β-D-form ($[\alpha]_D^{20} = +18.7°$). The attainment of the equilibrium state is hastened by acid and especially base. However, hastening the action of the equilibrium should be done with very dilute solutions of acids or alkali such as ammonia. Concentrated acids will yield other compounds such as 5-hydroxymethylfurfural from D-glucose and high concentrations of alkali or strong alkali themselves cause D-glucose to form D-fructose and D-mannose through enediol structures in an equilibrium reaction.

The chemical properties of the carbohydrates are, in general, those expected based upon their structural features previously described. They display all the chemical reactions characteristic of alcohol and carbonyl groups. The aldehyde group of an aldose and the terminal hydroxyl group are each capable of being oxidized to the corresponding mono- or dicarboxylic acid. The carbonyl function can also undergo reduction to a primary or secondary alcohol. Both aldoses and ketoses exhibit the usual addition reactions typical of the carbonyl function. For identification purposes, the carbonyl and adjacent alcohol functions will form phenylhydrazine derivatives known as *osazones*, which give characteristic melting points and exhibit definite crystalline structures. It should be noted that glucose, fructose, and mannose yield the same osazone because the differences in structure and configuration about carbon atoms 1 and 2 are abolished. Also, reactions with copper or silver ions under proper conditions, in which the metal ion is reduced in valence and the carbohydrate is oxidized, are employed to distinguish *reducing* from *nonreducing* sugars (as is the strong acid/substituted furfural reaction described above). The hydroxyl groups can be esterified or etherified, a process often used to decrease the polarity and thus increase volatility for identification and separation purposes, especially in gas and liquid chromatography and mass spectrometry.

All polysaccharides can be hydrolyzed to the simple monosaccharides of which they are composed. Either chemical (boiling with dilute acid) or enzymatic procedures can be employed with the latter showing much more specificity. In some instances, it is possible to hydrolyze only α-linkages or even cleave at a specific monosaccharidic linkage within the polymer chain. Many microorganisms possess the ability to hydrolyze carbohydrates to simple alcohols, ketones, or acids, usually resulting in the production of carbon dioxide, by the process known as *fermentation*. Ethanol, acetic acid, citric acid, 2-butanone, and butyl alcohol are several of the products derived from sucrose by such a procedure. There are specific microorganisms used in quite efficient fermentation processes to transform l-sorbose, a glucose derivative, into ascorbic acid (vitamin C), which is actually the γ-lactone of a hexanoic acid having an enediol structure at carbon atoms 2 and 3.

Occurrence and Uses

Carbohydrates are the first products to arise from photosynthesis, and therefore, occur abundantly in nature. It has been estimated that more carbohydrate material occurs naturally than all other organic material combined. Although they are preponderantly important within the vegetable kingdom, carbohydrates also occur abundantly and have very important nutritional and biological roles in the animal world. Glucose and fructose are the only monosaccharides that occur in the free state to any important extent. They are present in the juices of many ripe fruits. Among the disaccharides, only sucrose (cane or beet sugar) and lactose (milk sugar) occur in important quantities. Prominent, naturally occurring, hexosan polysaccharides include cellulose (the primary structural material in the vegetable world), starch (the primary carbohydrate fuel reserve in the vegetable world; found primarily in seeds and underground roots in the form of granules or grains), and glycogen (the primary carbohydrate fuel reserve in the animal world; often dubbed as animal starch and found primarily in the liver). Pentosan polysaccharides occur abundantly in cereal straws and beans and yield the industrially important furfural upon suitable treatment with sulfuric acid.

Carbohydrate derivatives (chemical combinations with noncarbohydrate substances or slightly altered carbohydrates) occur plentifully in nature. The monosaccharide phosphate esters, D-ribose and α-deoxyribose, are pentose constituents of RNA and DNA, respectively. Other classes include the gums and mucilages (in which the terminal groups have been oxidized forming uronic acid), pectins, glycoproteins, and glycolipids (cerebrosides). Chitin, a condensation polymer of *N*-acetyl-D-glucosamine (which contains NH₂ instead of OH in the 2 position), comprises the skeletal material of crabs, lobsters, and insects of the arthropoda class. This same acetylglucosamine is also present in hyaluronic acid, an important constituent of connective tissue. Many bacteria have been shown to produce complex carbohydrate materials and some are known to have immunological importance. A special class of derivatives, the *glycosides*, is discussed in a following section.

Due to their sweet taste, the soluble low molecular weight carbohydrates are often used as sweeteners by the food and pharmaceutical industries. Fructose, due to its significantly sweet taste, may be used as a sweetener in smaller quantities than other sugars; and therefore, is often used as a substitute for sucrose to lower the caloric content of certain foods. For this reason, fructose is frequently used to manufacture candies for persons suffering from diabetes. Lactose is commonly used as diluent for the preparation of solid dosage forms such as tablets and capsules. The ability of many polysaccharides to absorb water is a physical property that has found numerous uses. For example, cotton fibers (primarily cellulose) are used for various types of surgical dressings, starch is used as dusting powder, pectin and carrageen (a mixture of polysaccharides from algae) are used as gelling agents, and dextran (α,1,6-glucan) is used as a blood plasma replacement and matrix for column chromatography. Polysaccharides are also commonly used as suspending agents, tablet binders and disintegrants, emulsifiers, and film formers in the preparation of various pharmaceutical dosage forms. In addition, several polysaccharides may be used as therapeutic agents. For example, psyllium, from plantago seed, is commonly used as a laxative; acacia gum is used in lozenges

as a demulcalent for cough, diarrhea, and throat problems; and the sodium salt of alginic acid, a polysaccharide from brown seaweed, is used for the treatment for GERD.

Glycosides

COMPOSITION AND STRUCTURE—*Glycosides* may be defined broadly as condensation products of saccharides with various kinds of organic hydroxy, and occasionally thiol compounds (usually noncarbohydrate in nature), with the added restriction that the OH of the hemiacetal portion of the carbohydrate must participate in the condensation. It is obvious that the polysaccharides also are encompassed in this broad definition. The nonsugar portion is termed an *aglycone* (or *aglycon*), or a *genin,* and a majority have cyclic structures. From a structural viewpoint, the glycosides may be looked upon as internal acetals. In modern terminology, the glycosides are usually classified according to their sugar moiety. For example, in glucosides, the sugar moiety is glucose; in fructosides, it is fructose; in galactosides, it is galactose, and so on (Table 26-5). The sugar in a large number of glycosides is D-glucose; therefore, in older literature, the term *glucoside* is used in a generic sense and is synonymous with the modern term *glycoside*. Classification according to the complexity of the sugar moiety is also employed frequently; for example, *monosides* are monosaccharide sugars, *biosides* are disaccharides, and *triosides* are trisaccharides. Classification on the basis of the aglycones, while feasible, is intricate because of the large variety of aglycones; however, with certain classes of glycosides (such as the cardiotonics) such subclassification is occasionally encountered in the literature.

Two series of stereoisomeric glycosides are known, the α- and β-glycosides. Taking the methyl-D-glucosides as a simple example, they are represented by:

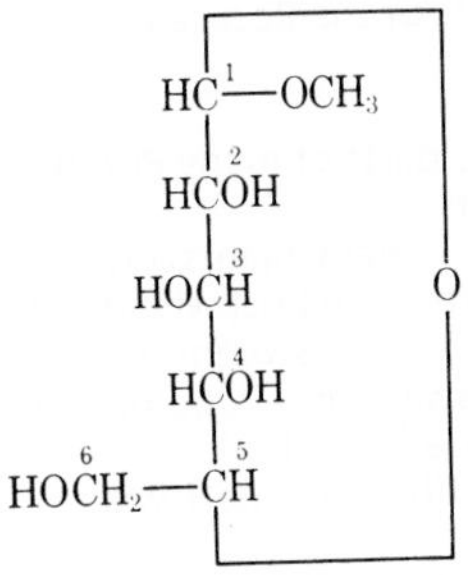

α-Methyl-D-glucoside 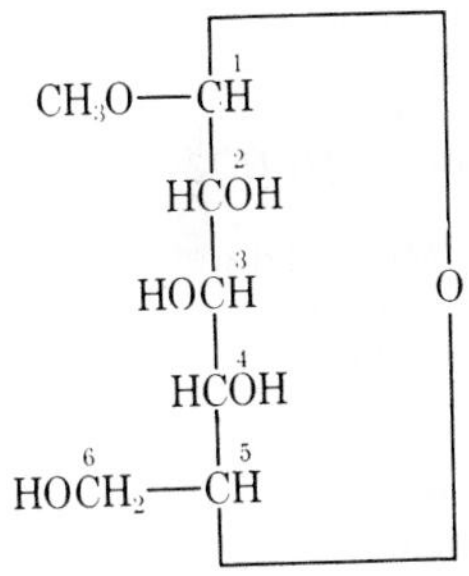   **β-Methyl-D-glucoside**

The glycosidic linkage is formed by dehydration involving a hydroxyl group of the aglycone (in the above example, methanol) and the hydroxyl group on the hemiacetal carbon of the sugar, thus forming an acetal type of structure. If the −OR (in the above example, −OCH₃) group is in the same steric sense as the CH₂OH group on C-5 (for D-family sugars), the glycoside configuration is designated as β-; if it is in the opposite steric sense, it is designated as α-. The great majority of naturally occurring glycosides are of the β- variety. For an illustration of how this relationship is reflected in the Haworth-type formulas, see amygdalin below, which is a typical β- glycoside, and therefore, the formula is written with the linking oxygen on the same plane as the CH₂OH group on C-5.

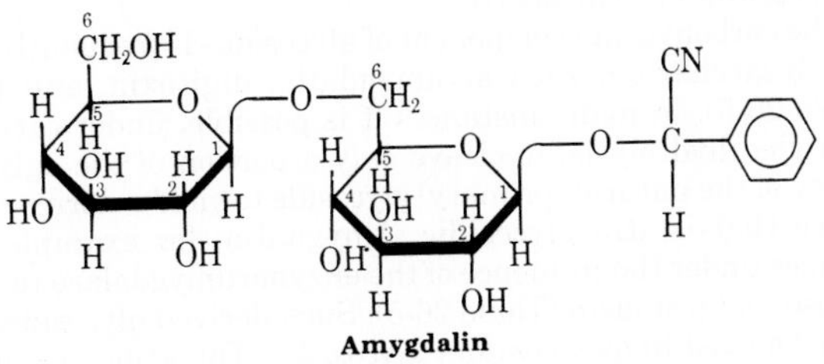

Amygdalin

Table 26-5. Selected Glycosides

NAME AND MOLECULAR FORMULA [a]	SOURCES [b]	AGLYCONE (GENIN)	SUGAR MOIETIES [c]
Amygdalin $C_{20}H_{27}NO_{11}$	Seeds of Amygdalaceae, Drupaceae, and Pomaceae; principally from almonds	D-Mandelonitrile → Benzaldehyde + HCN	Gentiobiose → 2 D-Glucose
Arbutin (Ursin) $C_{12}H_{16}O_7$	Leaves of plants of the Ericaceae and Rosaceae	Hydroquinone	D-Glucose
Coniferin (Abietin; Laricin) $C_{16}H_{22}O_8$	Plants of the Coniferae (ie, pine, spruce, and fir)	Coniferyl alcohol [4-Hydroxy-3-methoxycinnamyl alcohol]	D-Glucose
Cymarin $C_{30}H_{44}O_9$	Various species of Apocynum	Strophanthidin (a steroid) Cymarose	Cymarose (3-Methyl-digitoxose)
Daphnin $C_{15}H_{16}O_9$	Bark and flowers of varieties of Daphne	7,8-Dihydroxycoumarin	D-Glucose
Digitoxin $C_{41}H_{64}O_{13}$	Leaves of *Digitalis lanata* and *purpurea*	Digitoxigenin (a steroid)	3 Digitoxose (Digitoxose is a 2,6-bisdesoxy-aldohexose)
Digoxin $C_{41}H_{64}O_{14}$	Leaves of *Digitalis lanata* or *Digitalis orientalis*	Digoxigenin (12-Hydroxydigit-oxigenin) (a steroid)	3 Digitoxose
Frangulin $C_{21}H_{20}O_9$	Seeds and barks of various species of Rhamnus, especially alder buckthorn	4,5,7-Trihydroxy-2-methylanthraquinone	Rhamnose
Lanatoside A $C_{49}H_{76}O_{19}$	Leaves of *Digitalis lanata*	Digitoxigenin (a steroid)	2 Digitoxose + Acetyldigitoxose + D-Glucose
Lanatoside B $C_{49}H_{76}O_{20}$	Leaves of *Digitalis lanata*	Gitoxigenin (16-Hydroxy-digit-oxigenin - a steroid)	2 Digitoxose + Acetyldigitoxose + D-Glucose
Lanatoside C $C_{49}H_{76}O_{20}$	Leaves of *Digitalis lanata*	Digoxigenin (a steroid)	2 Digitoxose + Acetyldigitoxose + D-Glucose
Ouabain (G-Strophanthin) $C_{29}H_{44}O_{12}$	Seeds of *Strophanthus gratus* and varieties of Acokanthera	Ouabagenin (a steroid)	Rhamnose
Phlorizin (Phlorhizin; Phloridzin) $C_{21}H_{24}O_{10}$	Roots and leaves of various plants of the Rosaceae	Phloretin [β-(p-Hydroxyphenyl)-2,4,6-trihydroxypropiophenone]	D-Glucose
Prunasin $C_{14}H_{17}NO_6$	Various parts of many Prunus plants	D-Mandelonitrile → Benzaldehyde + HCN	D-Glucose
Rutin (Melin, Eldrin, and others) $C_{27}H_{30}O_{16}$	Occurs in many plants. Chief source is the buckwheat plant, *Fagopyrum esculentum*	Quercetin [3,3′,4′,5,7-Pentahydroxyflavone]	Rutinose → L-Rhamnose + D-Glucose
Salicin $C_{13}H_{18}O_7$	Various Salix and Populus plants, especially the bark	Saligenin [o-Hydroxybenzyl alcohol]	D-Glucose
Scillaren A $C_{36}H_{52}O_{13}$	Bulbs of *Urginea maritima*	Scillaridin A (a steroid)	Scillabiose → L-Rhamnose D-Glucose
Sinigrin (Potassium Myronate) $C_{10}H_{16}KNO_9S_2$	Seeds of *Brassica nigra, Brassica juncea*, and other plants of the Cruciferae	$CH_2{=}CHCH_2N{=}C(SH)OSO_3K →$ $CH_2{=}CHCH_2NCS + KHSO_4$	D-Glucose
K-Strophanthin-β $C_{36}H_{54}O_{14}$	Seeds of *Strophanthus kombé*	Strophanthidin (a steroid)	Strophanthobiose → Cymarose + D-Glucose

[a] Shown as the anhydrous forms. As isolated, many glycosides are hydrated.
[b] Typical and well known, but not exclusive.
[c] Produced upon complete hydrolysis unless otherwise indicated.

This compound, like all other glycosides, contains several asymmetric carbon atoms and is optically active. In this instance the aglycone is also optically active due to the asymmetric carbon to which the phenyl, nitrile, hydrogen, and gentiobiose residues are attached.

The carbohydrate component of glycosides is frequently a di- or polysaccharide, such as amygdalin, digitoxin, and rutin (Table 26-5). In many instances it is possible, under carefully controlled hydrolysis, to cleave only a portion of the aglycone moiety of the natural (primary) glycoside to yield a derived substance that is still glycosidic. Amygdalin, for example, hydrolyzes under the influence of the enzyme amygdalase to yield glucose and prunasin (Table 26-5). Such derived glycosides are often referred to as *secondary glycosides*. The same enzyme is often able to hydrolyze different glycosides, but the α- and β-stereoisomers of the same glycoside cannot usually be hydrolyzed by the same enzyme. For instance, *Emulsin* has been found to hydrolyze only β-glycosides; therefore, those glycosides that are attacked by emulsin, such as amygdalin, are regarded as β-glycosides. Maltase hydrolyzes only α-glycosides.

PHYSICAL AND CHEMICAL PROPERTIES—The greater portion of the known glycosides, when pure, are colorless or white, optically active, and soluble in alcohol or diluted alcohol. The aglycones of the majority of glycosides are cyclic structures, and therefore, many have aromatic properties. The most characteristic chemical property of the glycosides is their susceptibility to hydrolysis, whereby they yield their sugar and nonsugar moieties. There are no simple identifying tests for glycosides. It is through identification of the hydrolytic decomposition products that the composition of glycosides is commonly revealed. Methods for the detection of glycosides and for their quantitative determination involve the estimation of reducing sugars before and after hydrolysis by boiling with dilute acids or by the action of enzymes. Acid hydrolysis of glycosides is non-specific and occurs for both *alpha-* and *beta-*glycosidic linkages. On the other hand, enzymatic hydrolysis is often quite specific, as mentioned previously. It should be noted that there are two enzymes, namely emulsin of almond kernels and myrosin of black mustard seeds, each of which has the ability to hydrolyze a considerable number of different glycosides.

OCCURRENCE—Glycosides are distributed widely in the plant kingdom but rarely found in animals. Many fruits and other plant parts (ie, seeds, barks, and leaves) contain them. In addition, the pigments of flowers (anthocyanins) are of glycosidic character. Glycosides are extracted from the plant material by water, alcohol, or a mixture of the two. They occur in small amounts, and their isolation in a pure state is usually difficult and laborious. In addition, the enzymes responsible for hydrolyzing a particular glycoside frequently occur in the same plant along with the glycosides but usually in different cells. When the structure of the plant is destroyed by grinding or other means, the enzyme contacts the glycoside and soon exerts its hydrolytic action. Therefore, it is necessary to destroy any enzymes that are present before attempting to isolate glycosidal constituents. As a result, the processes used for glycoside production and purification vary according to the nature of the material and the glycoside. Many naturally occurring compounds not usually classed among the glycosides actually contain glycosidic linkages in their structures. Examples include gentamycin, amikacine, netilmicin, tobramycin, novobiocin, and streptomycin among the antibiotics, solanine and various other alkaloids (glucoalkaloids), and nucleosides (consist of a purine or pyrimidine base linked with D-ribose or D-2-deoxyribose). Certain glycosides will be covered in more detail within the following sections that pertain to their aglycone portion.

PROTEINS, PEPTIDES, AND AMINO ACIDS

Composition and Structure

Unlike carbohydrates, proteins vary widely in composition, not only from one species to another but also among the various tissues and cellular fluids within a given species. These differences in composition result in different physical and chemical properties that are reflected in the diverse biofunctions in which proteins participate. The intimate roles these compounds play in the fundamental processes of tissue formation, regeneration, and function makes this class of substances the primary component of all living matter, and hence, the term *protein* (from the Greek, *first*). All proteins contain carbon, hydrogen, oxygen, and nitrogen. Nitrogen constitutes approximately 16% of most proteins, which leads to the rough factor of 6.25 generally employed to convert the amount of protein nitrogen found by analysis to the amount of total protein. Other elements such as sulfur, phosphorus, iodine, copper, iron, and occasionally zinc may be present.

The fundamental structural units of proteins are α-amino acids, about 20 of which prominently participate in protein formation (Table 26-6). These building-block molecules contain at least one carboxyl group and one α-amino group, but differ in the structure of the remainder of the molecule. All except the simplest one, glycine, are capable of existing in both D- and L- configurations with respect to their α-carbon, but proteins contain only the L-enantiomers. The actual protein molecule consists of long-chain polymers that have resulted from condensation of the amino acids, thus producing amide or peptide linkages:

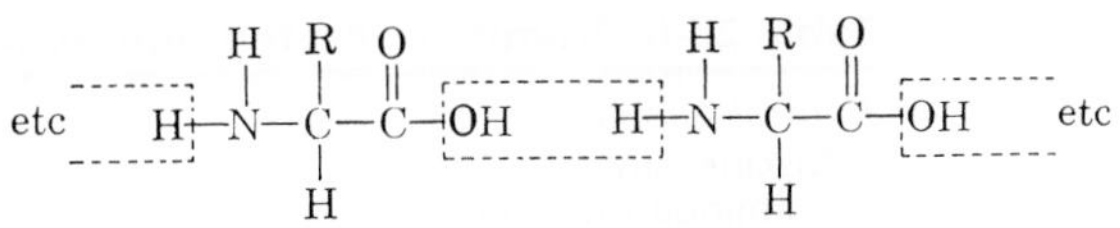

In addition to the 20 standard amino acids in Table 26-6, several others of relatively rare occurrence have been isolated from hydrolysates of some specialized types of proteins. All are derivatives of a standard amino acid. *Hydroxylysine*, the 5-hydroxy derivative of lysine, is present in collagen (as is *hydroxyproline*). *Desmosine* and *isodesmosine* occur in the fibrous protein *elastin*. As noted below, *desmosine* can be visualized as being formed from four lysine molecules with their side-chain moieties joined to form a substituted pyridine ring. Certain muscle proteins have been found to contain several ε-*N*-methylated analogs of *lysine* and *histidine*. β-*Alanine*, α-*aminobutyric acid, homocysteine, homoserine, citrulline, ornithine, canavinine, djenkolic acid,* and β-*cyanoalanine* are some naturally occurring amino acids that are not found in proteins. Some amino acids such as γ-*aminobutyric acid*, α-*aminoadipic acid, pipecolic acid,* and δ-*acetylornithine* exist only in the free state.

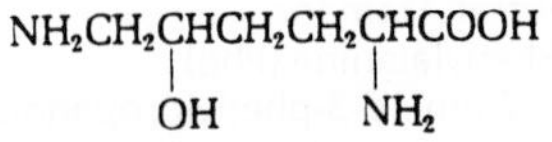

5-Hydroxylysine

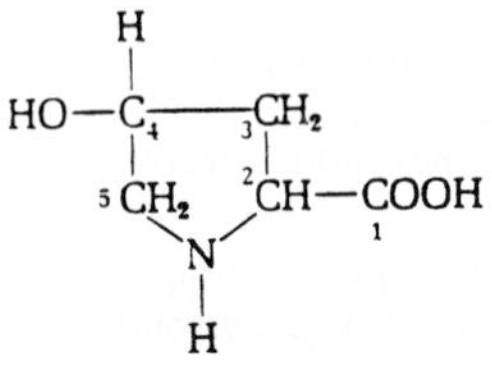

4-Hydroxyproline

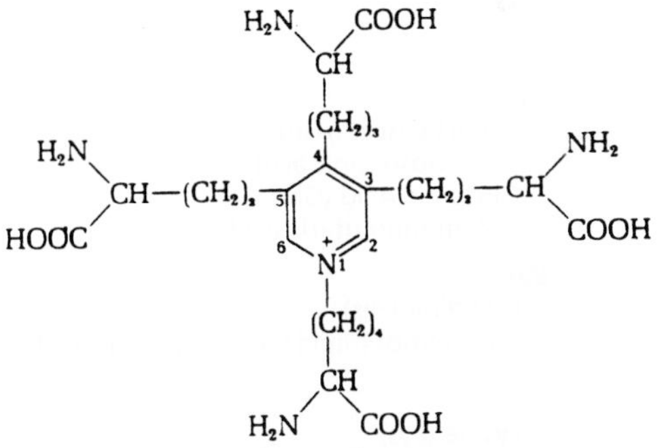

Desmosine

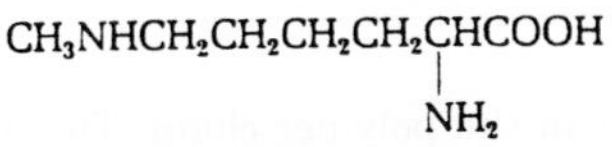

ε-N-Methyllysine

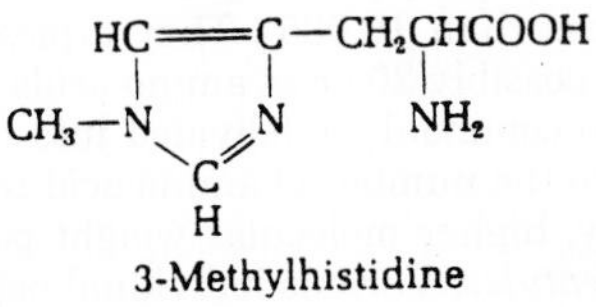

3-Methylhistidine

Proteins are macromolecules that differ from each other primarily in the number, type, and sequence of amino acid

Table 26-6. Prominent Protein Amino Acids

Neutral Aliphatic

Glycine (Gly)
  aminoacetic acid $CH_2(NH_2)COOH$

Alanine (Ala)
  2-aminopropanoic acid $CH_3CH(NH_2)COOH$

Serine (Ser)
  2-amino-3-hydroxypropanoic acid $CH_2(OH)CH(NH_2)COOH$

Threonine (Thr)
  2-amino-3-hydroxybutanoic acid $CH_3CH(OH)CH(NH_2)COOH$

Valine (Val)
  2-amino-3-methylbutanoic acid $CH_3CH(CH_3)CH(NH_2)COOH$

Leucine (Leu)
  2-amino-4-methylpentanoic acid $CH_3CH(CH_3)CH_2CH(NH_2)COOH$

Isoleucine (Ile)
  2-amino-3-methylpentanoic acid $CH_3CH_2CH(CH_3)CH(NH_2)COOH$

Neutral Thioaliphatic

Cysteine (CySH)
  2-amino-3-mercaptopropanoic acid $CH_2(SH)CH(NH_2)COOH$

Cystine (CyS-SCY)
  3,3'-dithiodi(2-aminopropanoic acid) $SCH_2CH(NH_2)COOH$

Methionine (Met)
  2-amino-4-(methylthio)butanoic acid $CH_2(SCH_3)CH_2CH(NH_2)COOH$

Neutral Aromatic

Phenylalanine (Phe)
  2-amino-3-phenylpropanoic acid

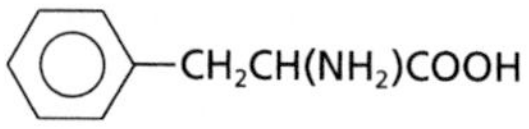

Tyrosine (Tyr)
  2-amino-3-(p-hydroxyphenyl) propanoic acid

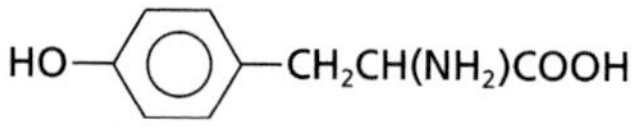

Neutral Heterocyclic

Proline (Pro)
  2-pyrrolidinecarboxylic acid

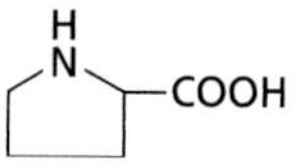

Hydroxyproline (Hyp)
  4-hydroxy-2-pyrrolidinecarboxylic acid

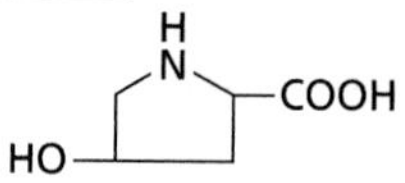

Tryptophan (Trp)
  α-aminoindole-3-propanoic acid

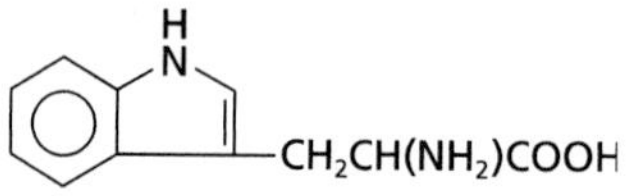

Acidic

Aspartic Acid (Asp)
  aminosuccinic acid $HOOCCH_2CH(NH_2)COOH$

Glutamic Acid (Glu)
  2-aminoglutaric acid $HOOCCH_2CH_2CH(NH_2)COOH$

Basic

Histidine (His)
  α-amino-4-imidazolepropanoic acid

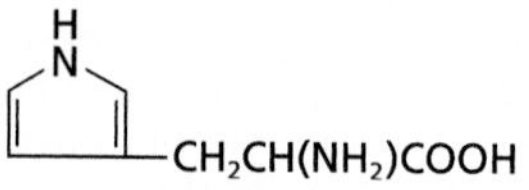

Lysine (Lys)
  2,6-diaminohexanoic acid $CH_2(NH_2)CH_2CH_2CH_2CH(NH_2)COOH$

Arginine (Arg)
  2-amino-5-guanidinopentanoic acid $NH_2C(=NH)NH-CH_2CH_2CH_2CH(NH_2)COOH$

residues present in the polymer chain. The number of amino acid molecules within proteins ranges from perhaps as few as 30 and up to tens of thousands. The term peptide is used in reference to very small hydrolytic fragments of proteins (generally having a MW less than 10,000). They typically contain anywhere from 2 to possibly 20 or so amino acids joined via amide linkages and are commonly subdivided into di-, tri-, etc, peptides according to the number of amino acid residues they contain. Collectively, higher molecular weight peptides are often termed as *polypeptides*. Various individual peptides have been isolated from protein hydrolysates or synthesized, such as oxytocin. With regard to classification or categorization, there is little distinction between peptides and polypeptides, except that the latter usually refers to compounds that carry a number

of amino acid residues but usually do not involve a distinct upper limit of residues. For example, the polypeptide hormone prolactin carries 199 residues. The simplest naturally occurring peptides are the dipeptide *penicillins* and *cephalosporins*. The MW of proteins may be determined by various methods, such as diffusion, sedimentation, viscosity, x-ray analysis, light-scattering, ultracentrifugation, electron microscopy, and gel permeation. MW values for common proteins range from about 10^4 to about 10^7; the value found for a given protein often varies depending upon the determination method used.

As for the elucidation of protein composition, two fundamental problems exist, the quantitative assay of the individual amino acids and the determination of the amino acid sequence in the chain. Each is a highly specialized field of endeavor and

Table 26-7. Amino Acid Composition of Selected Proteins[a]

	IUPAC ABBREVIATION	GELATINS	MILK: MIXED PROTEINS	CASEIN	SERUM ALBUMIN*	γ-GLOBULIN	HEMOGLOBLIN: HORSE	INSULIN	CLOSTRIDIUM BOTULINIUM TOXIN
Alanine	Ala	9.2	...	3.0	6.2	...	7.4	4.5	3.9
Arginine	Arg	8.8	4.2	4.1	6.0	4.8	3.7	3.1	4.6
Aspartic Acid	Asp	6.3	...	7.1	10.3	8.8	10.6	6.8	20.1
Cystine	Cys-Scy	0.1	1.0	0.3	6.5	3.1	1.0	12.5	0.8
Glutamic Acid	Glu	11.7	21.5	22.4	17.0	11.8	8.2	18.6	15.6
Glycine	Gly	30.5	2.3	2.7	2.0	4.2	5.6	4.3	1.4
Histisdine	His	0.7	2.8	3.1	4.0	2.5	8.7	4.9	1.0
Hydroxyproline	Hyp	14.5	...	0	0	0?	0?	0?	...
Isoleucine	Ile	1.9	7.5	6.1	3.0	2.7	0?	2.8	11.9
Leucine	Leu	3.2	11.0	9.2	12.0	9.3	15.2	13.2	10.3
Lysine	Lys	5.1	8.7	8.2	12.7	8.1	8.5	2.5	7.7
Methionine	Met	0.9	3.2	3.4	1.3	1.1	1.0	0	1.1
Phenylalanine	Phe	2.1	5.5	5.0	7.0	4.6	7.7	8.1	1.2
Proline	Pro	6.3	...	11.3	5.1	8.1	8.5	2.5	2.6
Serine	Ser	3.8	4.3	6.3	7.0	11.4	5.8	5.2	4.4
Threonine	Thr	2.2	4.7	4.9	7.1	8.4	4.4	2.1	8.5
Tyrosine	Tyr	0.7	6.0	6.3	5.5	6.8	3.0	13.0	13.5
Tryptophan	Trp	0	1.5	1.2	1.0	2.9	1.7	0	1.9
Valine	Val	2.1	7.0	7.2	6.0	9.7	9.0	7.8	5.3

[a] The data in this table were taken from a more comprehensive table by Hawk et al. *Practical Physiological Chemistry*, 13th ed. New York: Blakiston, 1954. All values are in g/100 g of protein except those marked * which are in g/16 g total nitrogen.

relies upon modern techniques such as selective adsorption (ion- exchange, paper, thin-layer, high-performance liquid, and gas-liquid chromatography), electrophoresis, countercurrent distribution, and isotope-dilution methods. The amino acid composition of various selected proteins is presented in Table 26-7.[18] In view of the diverse analytical methods employed, slight variations in reported values are expected and often encountered in the literature. With simple (nonconjugated) proteins, the total mass of the amino acids exceeds the mass of the source protein because of the water that becomes fixed during hydrolytic cleavage of the peptide linkages. The precise sequence of amino acid residues is now known for a considerable number of proteins, including insulin, ribonuclease, tobacco mosaic virus, and many of the hemoglobins, immunoglobulins, and other specialized proteins.

Protein structure is typically divided into four levels:

Primary—The amino acid sequence, as determined by sequencing techniques.
Secondary—The folding of polypeptide chains into coiled structures as determined by X-ray diffraction, optical rotatory dispersion, and electron photomicrography.
Tertiary—The arrangement of chains into specific layers and/or fibers.
Quaternary—The organization of many monomeric units, each displaying primary, secondary, and tertiary structure, associated to form a quaternary structure.

A fifth level is believed to consist of aggregates of different proteins, each composed of the four fundamental structural levels. These macromolecular complexes are believed to be involved in fatty acid synthesis and electron transport.

Physical and Chemical Properties

A satisfactory practical classification of proteins based solely upon either composition or structure has not been achieved, partly because of their wide diversity and partly because of incomplete knowledge. Classifications in terms of occurrence and function are encountered frequently in the literature but these are designed for special purposes and usually do not embrace all proteins. A classification based primarily upon physical and chemical properties such as solubility, coagulability, conjugation, denaturation, and hydrolysis characteristics and having some practical utility has evolved gradually over the years and is presented below.

Simple proteins are naturally occurring proteins that yield only α–amino acids or their derivatives upon hydrolysis. They may be of several types and include:

Albumins, which are soluble in water and coagulated by heat; examples include ovalbumin in egg white and serum albumin in blood.
Globulins, which are insoluble in water but soluble in dilute salt solutions and coagulable by heat; examples include serum globulin in blood.
Glutelins, which are insoluble in water or dilute salt solution but soluble in dilute acid and alkali; examples include glutenin in wheat.
Prolamines, which are insoluble in neutral solutions but soluble in 80% alcohol; examples include zein in corn and gliadin in wheat.
Albuminoids, which are dissolved only by boiling in strong acids; examples include keratins in hair and horny tissue, elastins in tendons and arteries, and collagens in skin and tendons.
Histones, which are basic in reaction, soluble in water but insoluble in dilute ammonia, and not easily heat-coagulable; examples include thymus histone and hemoglobin.
Protamines, which are strongly basic in reaction and soluble in water, dilute acid, and ammonia; examples include salmin and sturin in fish sperm. They precipitate many other proteins.

Conjugated proteins are proteins that are combined in nature with some nonprotein substance. They are classified according to the nature of the prosthetic (nonprotein) group. The classes, which are not mutually exclusive, include:

Phosphoproteins, which contain a phosphoric acid moiety as the prosthetic group; examples include casein in milk and ovovitellin in egg yolk.
Nucleoproteins, which contain a nucleic acid as the prosthetic group; examples include nuclein in cell nuclei.
Glycoproteins, which are simple proteins united to a carbohydrate group; examples include mucins in vitreous humor and saliva.
Chromoproteins, which contain a colored prosthetic group; examples include hemoglobin in blood and flavoproteins.
Lipoproteins, which contain lipid materials, such as sterols, fatty acids, or lecithin.
Metalloproteins, which contain a metal as the prosthetic group; examples include enzymes such as tyrosinase, arginase, and xanthine oxidase.

In general, pure proteins are relatively odorless and tasteless and have varying colors. Many proteins have been obtained in crystalline form, but unlike crystalline substances in general, this is not necessarily evidence of homogeneity as some have been further resolved into two or more components through chromatographic, electrophoretic, and other procedures. Upon heating, proteins decompose with or without simultaneous liquefaction and emit the characteristic odor of singed hair. In their normal biological environment, they are highly hydrated. Because proteins are polyelectrolyte macromolecules with multifunctional groups, they typically differ greatly in their physical properties such as solubilities in water, salt solutions, monohydric and polyhydric alcohols, and dilute acids and bases. Proteins often form colloidal solutions from which heat usually precipitates the protein in a coagulated form. Precipitation in an unaltered form is frequently accomplished, especially at their isoelectric point, by means of salt solutions such as sodium chloride and ammonium sulfate or by diluted ethanol. Dilution with acetonitrile is often sufficient to precipitate protein from extracted serum samples.

The exceptional vulnerability of proteins in general to chemical attack often requires careful control of reaction conditions; nevertheless, their chemical characteristics are quite in accord with those to be expected from the functional groups present. Peptides are readily soluble in water, noncoagulable by heat, and are not precipitated by saturation with ammonium sulfate. Precipitates are formed with amino acids on the addition of various reagents such as heavy metal salts, and certain acids such as picric, phosphotungstic, trichloroacetic, or sulfosalicylic acids.

In addition to the modern chromatographic, electrophoretic, and other procedures mentioned previously, the advent of post–column-derivatization techniques in which peptides and amino acids are made chromophoric by the use of such fluorescent derivatives as the fluorescamine derivative, the PTH amino acid derivatives, the derivative formed by reaction in the orthophthaldehyde method, and the *dansyl* and *dapsyl* derivatives makes it possible to determine the concentration of individual amino acids and small peptides in mixtures in the *nanomole* and *picomole* range. In addition, the hydrolysis of proteins yields amino acids that, upon treatment with *nitrous acid*, liberate nitrogen. This reaction along with other techniques forms the basis of Van Slyke's nitrogen distribution method, which has important uses in clinical chemistry. Amino acids and the free amino groups in proteins react with ninhydrin resulting in either yellow, pink, or violet color depending upon the amino acid. The presence of peptide linkages can be shown by means of the *Biuret* test. Numerous color tests are available for individual amino acids, including the *Ehrlich* and *Hopkins–Cole* tests for tryptophan, the *Sakaguchi* test for arginine, the *nitroprusside* test for cystine and cysteine, the *Millon* test for tyrosine, the *xanthoproteic* test for tyrosine and phenylalanine, the *Pauly diazo* test for histidine and tyrosine, and the *basic lead* test for the sulfur-containing acids.

Occurrence and Uses

Proteins are synthesized by the ribosomes in the cytoplasm and especially those associated with endoplasmic reticulum. Although proteins are present in all living matter, important differences in their distribution are clearly evident. In plants, for which the structural parts are essentially carbohydrate in nature, protein concentration is usually very much higher in the seed than in any of the other plant parts. No similar gross variation is observed in the animal world, but different tissues vary considerably in the approximate percentage of protein they contain (ie, skin—27%, skeletal muscle—21%, brain—11%, adipose tissue—5%).

Insoluble proteins are usually isolated simply by removing contaminating material by means of a suitable array of solvents. Débridement is often facilitated through the appropriate use of enzymes. Soluble proteins are usually obtained first as crude extracts in aqueous solutions and after subjecting the solution to dialysis to remove contaminating solutes, the protein is obtained either through precipitation by means of salt solutions or organic solvents or through lyophilization techniques. When

first isolated, proteins are frequently mixtures. Separation into individual components was formerly accomplished only by means of tedious fractional precipitation operations. Currently, it is achieved much more conveniently and completely through chromatographic procedures using ion-exchange resins or various cellulose derivatives and preparative HPLC.

In addition to their role in nutrition and as building blocks of proteins, the amino acids are precursors of many important biomolecules, including various hormones, vitamins, coenzymes, alkaloids, and porphyrins. The aromatic amino acids are particularly versatile as precursors for many alkaloids, such as morphine, codeine, and papaverine and a number of hormones such as the thyroid hormone, thyroxine; the plant hormone, indoleacetic acid; and an adrenal hormone, epinephrine.

Hormonal polypeptides are produced in the mammalian hypothalamus and are stored in the posterior pituitary. Examples include the partially cyclic octapeptides oxytocin, vasopressin, argitocin, argipressin, and lypressin. The polypeptides *ACTH (adrenocorticotropic hormone), lipotropin, prolactin,* and *somatotropin* also originate in the pituitary. The hypothalamus produces the polypeptide hormones or factors corticoliberin (CRF), gonadorelin (GnRH), protirelin (TRH), and somatotropin-releasing factor (GHF), which are transported to the anterior pituitary. Glutathione is a peptide hormone that is present in nearly all living cells. Other peptides (nonhormonal) in the hypothalamus network are neurotensin (anorexiant), a tridecapeptide, and substance P, an undecapeptide. The nerve tissue prevalent calcitonin gene-related peptide (CGRP) (37 residues) is 1000 times more potent than acetylcholine or substance P. Cyclic polypeptides such as bacitracin and polymixin from *Bacillus* sp. act as antibiotics, as do the penicillins and cephalosporins mentioned previously.

LIPIDS

Lipids, also known as *lipins* or *lipoids,* are fat or fat-like substances that occur widely in plants (mainly fruits and seeds) and animals (special deposits and in complex, active tissues such as the brain and liver). They contain only carbon, hydrogen, and oxygen atoms except for complex lipids such as phospholipids. Like the carbohydrates and proteins, the lipids constitute a very important group of organic substances from a physiological standpoint. However, unlike the carbohydrates and proteins, the lipids comprise a rather heterogeneous group of substances in terms of chemical composition. In general, lipids are hydrophobic in nature, which is very important to their physiological/pharmacological activities, and are soluble in solvents such as ether and chloroform and insoluble in water. They may be divided into the following classes according to their chemical structure:

Fixed Oils and Fats—Esters of glycerol and fatty acids. An example is olive oil. Fixed oils that are solid at ordinary temperatures are commonly called *fats*. An example is lard.

Waxes—Esters of high-molecular-weight, monohydric alcohols and high-molecular-weight fatty acids. An example is spermaceti.

Phospholipids (Phosphatides)—Esters consisting of glycerol in combination with fatty acids, phosphoric acid, and certain nitrogenous compounds. Pharmaceutically, the most important members of this group are the lecithins.

Prostaglandins—Essential fatty acids derived from prostanoic acid and having cyclic structures.

Fixed Oils and Fats

COMPOSITION AND STRUCTURE—*Fixed oils* and *fats* are mixtures of glyceryl esters of the higher-molecular-weight aliphatic acids, especially oleic, palmitic, and stearic acids. The natural fatty acids are nearly all straight-chain and contain an even number of carbon atoms (C_4 to C_{26}). The individual glyceryl esters themselves are frequently referred to as *glycerides*.

Mono-, di-, and triglycerides containing one, two, or three molecules of fatty acid esterified with one molecule of glycerol, respectively, have been prepared synthetically, but only the triglycerides occur commonly in nature. Three glycerides, *olein* (*glyceryl trioleate* [$C_3H_5(C_{18}H_{33}O_2)_3$]), *palmitin* (*glyceryl tripalmitate* [$C_3H_5(C_{16}H_{31}O_2)_3$]), and *stearin* (*glyceryl tristearate* [$C_3H_5(C_{18}H_{35}O_2)_3$]), are common to many fixed oils. Olein has a mono-unsaturated structure with the double bonds having a cis configuration. Palmitin and stearin have saturated structures.

The glycerides in a fixed oil may be simple or mixed. In *simple glycerides,* such as olein, palmitin, or stearin, all three fatty acid groups are identical. In the more frequently encountered *mixed glycerides,* more than one type of fatty acid is present. Because of the many possible combinations in the mixed glycerides, different fats having entirely different physical properties often show the same chemical analysis. The following formula illustrates a mixed glyceride:

$$C_{15}H_{31}COOCH_2 \quad \alpha'$$
$$C_{17}H_{35}COOCH \quad \beta$$
$$C_{17}H_{33}COOCH_2 \quad \alpha$$

α-Oleo-α',β-palmitostearin
(or 1-oleo-3-palmito-2-stearin)

PHYSICAL AND CHEMICAL PROPERTIES—Fixed oils and fats are rather distinctive in their physical properties. They are greasy to the touch and leave a permanent oily stain upon filter paper. They are all lighter than water and insoluble therein, but are soluble in ether, chloroform, and some other water-immiscible solvents. A few of them, such as castor oil, are soluble in alcohol. When purified, they are nearly colorless and have a bland odor and taste that has little distinctiveness. The yellow color of fats is usually due to the presence of carotene, which is one of the provitamins A. Glycerides of unsaturated fatty acids have lower melting points than those of saturated acids with the same number of carbon atoms. Although most vegetable oils are liquid at room temperature and most animal fats are solids, there are notable exceptions, such as cocoa butter (solid) and cod liver oil (liquid). The difference in consistency between fixed oils and fats is caused by the relative proportions of liquid and solid glyceryl esters that are present. Fixed oils contain a relatively high proportion of liquid glycerides (polyunsaturated glycerides), such as glyceryl oleate; whereas, fats are relatively rich in solid glycerides (mostly saturated), such as glyceryl stearate. For example, *olein* is a liquid at ordinary temperatures but *palmitin* is a solid (melting point, 60°C). *Stearin* melts at 71°C. When heated moderately, fats liquefy and oils become less viscous. Upon aging, fixed oils often develop a precipitate of stearin that will reliquefy on warming.

Olein and glyceryl esters of other unsaturated acids may be converted into stearin in the presence of a catalyst such as finely divided nickel by *hydrogenation.* Liquid oils such as cottonseed, corn, soybean, and peanut are transformed (hardened) by this process into solid fats for commercial use. The proprietary cooking fat, Crisco (*Procter & Gamble*), is a well-known example. Through partial hydrogenation, the consistency of such hardened oils may be widely varied. However, this process, used in making many margarine preparations, is a mixed blessing because it produces some *trans* unsaturated fats, which may have unwanted health effects.

Fixed oils are to be distinguished sharply from *volatile oils,* also known as *ethereal* or *essential oils.* From a composition viewpoint, the volatile oils differ from fixed oils in that they do not contain glyceryl esters. Physically, fixed oils are nonvolatile under ordinary conditions (hence the name *fixed* oils). Fixed oils may be classified into drying and nondrying oils. The *drying oils,* when exposed to the air, undergo oxidation and resinify forming a tough, hard film. Linseed oil is an example of this class, which find their greatest use in the manufacture of paints and varnishes. The *nondrying oils,* when exposed to the air, remain sticky to the touch for an indefinite period, and therefore, cannot be used in paints and varnishes. Olive oil and expressed almond oil are examples. The drying quality of fixed oils is caused by the presence of characteristic unsaturated fatty acids, such as linoleic and linolenic acids.

When heated strongly, fats undergo decomposition with the production of acrid, flammable vapors; when ignited, they burn with a sooty flame. The acridity of an overheated fixed oil or fat is largely due to the formation of *acrolein* (*propenal*). The property common to all fats and fixed oils is their propensity to undergo hydrolysis to yield glycerol and the fatty acids representative of the fat or oil. Uncatalyzed, the reaction proceeds very slowly; however, it is usually accelerated by employing high temperatures and pressures and by the presence of either acids or alkalies. If alkalies are employed, the liberated acids are converted automatically into their corresponding metallic salts. Because such salts ordinarily are referred to as soaps, the alkali-catalyzed hydrolysis of fats and fixed oils is known as *saponification.* Many naturally occurring enzymes also catalyze fat and fixed oil hydrolysis. Such enzymes are termed *lipases;* steapsin in human pancreatic juice is an important example.

The analytical factors of greatest importance in identifying fixed oils and in judging their quality are:

Iodine Value (the number of grams of iodine monochloride, expressed as iodine, absorbed by 100 g of sample under prescribed conditions) measures the degree of saturation. Iodine is taken up at the double bonds, and therefore, unsaturated oils, such as the drying oils, typically have higher iodine values.

Saponification Value (the number of milligrams of potassium hydroxide required to neutralize the free acids and saponify or hydrolyze the esters in 1 g of sample).

Acid Value (the number of milligrams of potassium hydroxide required to neutralize the free acids in 1 g of sample).

The refractive index, specific gravity, color, odor, and congealing point of fixed oils and fats are of little value in determining their purity or quality. Some oils, such as cottonseed and sesame, are identifiable using specific tests, but the identification of most fixed oils is only inferentially possible after taking many physical and chemical factors into account. Gas chromatography (the FAME methods) is a useful means by which the identification of fixed oils may be accomplished. There are many gas chromatographic methods that bring about the separation of free fatty acids or fatty acid methyl esters and the resulting chromatographic pattern may be used to identify the fixed oil. Near IR spectroscopy may also determine the degree of saturation because the value is directly related to HC=CH stretch bands at 2130 nm.

OCCURRENCE AND USES—Generally, the biosynthesis of fatty acids requires acyl-CoA or fatty acyl carrier protein (ACP). In plants, this occurs in the mitochondria and chloroplasts; in animals, this occurs in the cytoplasm. Of all the fatty acids, oleic, palmitic, and stearic are the most widely distributed. Stearic acid is mostly found in animal fats, but it is occasionally an important constituent in vegetable oils. Saturated fatty acids lower than C_{12} are found in the milk of mammals; however, butter fat contains all of the even-numbered fatty acids from C_4 to C_{18} as well as oleic acid. Olein is the predominating constituent in many vegetable oils and the more fluid animal oils. Palmitin predominates in palm and coconut oil and stearin predominates in many of the solid fats.

Most fixed oils and fats are obtained from the plant or animal tissues in which they occur by *expression* and can be fractionated to some extent into glycerides. Generally, the source material is first ground and subsequently submitted to hydraulic pressure. Heat may also be used when necessary. The oils obtained by the first expression are usually of the highest commercial value. For example, virgin olive oil results from the first pressings of olives. Olein is separated and purified by cold expression; the other constituents are retained due to their lack of fluidity at low temperatures. Stearin may be separated by expression under controlled temperature conditions that remove the olein and palmitin. Sometimes the expressed oil from plant tissues is of crude quality and requires subsequent purification, as in the case of cottonseed oil. Fixed oils and fats are frequently bleached by treatment with Fuller's earth or similar clays and subsequently filtered. Some oils used for technical purposes are obtained by extraction using *volatile solvents* rather than expression. Animal fats and oils are usually separated from tissues by a process known as *rendering,* which consists of heating the tissues until the fat melts and separates.

Fats and fixed oils contain certain unsaturated fatty acids that are essential to human nutrition. Their absence in the diet produces eczematous skin conditions and, in experimental animals, has resulted in scaly skin, emaciation, necrosis, and premature death. Evidence exists to support the view that fats (oils) such as safflower, corn, cottonseed, and soybean, which are rich in linoleic acid and other unsaturated acids, play an important role in the mobilization and utilization of serum cholesterol. It has been hypothesized that olive oil and canola oil (rapeseed) are even more effective in providing a favorable high-density lipoprotein/low-density lipoprotein (HDL/LDL) ratio. Combined with a controlled dietary fat intake, these oils can also ensure a favorable total serum cholesterol/HDL ratio. This is of particular interest in hypercholesterolemia, which is observed commonly in atherosclerosis. Peanut, almond, and sesame oils are used extensively as vehicles in the preparation of intramuscular injections. Theobroma oil found in cocoa butter is frequently used for the preparation of suppositories. Some derivatives of glycerides are soaps and related surface-active compounds, which are employed as detergents and germicides. A few oils are used medicinally. For example, castor oil is used as a cathartic, cod liver oil as an antirachitic, and olive oil as an emollient. Salts of several of the fatty acids are fungicidal, such as zinc undecylenate, which is prepared from the undecylenic acid in castor oil.

Waxes

Waxes, like fixed oils and fats, are esters of fatty acids. However, they differ in that the alcohol represented is *not* glycerol. In place of this trihydric alcohol is a sterol or one of the higher, even-numbered, monohydric alcohols from C_{16} to C_{36}. Therefore, they are typically solids and poorly water-soluble. In addition, unlike fats, which are primarily esters, waxes often contain significant amounts of free alcohols, sterols, and fatty acids (C_{24} to C_{36}); some of the waxes obtained from plants also contain paraffin hydrocarbons. The sterols and hydrocarbons presesnt in waxes are unsaponifiable. In addition, the esters are usually much more resistant to saponification than the glycerides of fats and fixed oils; they may only be saponified using alcoholic alkali. Therefore, waxes typically have high saponification values. Also, as a result of their free fatty acid content, they typically have high acid values. Conversely, iodine values are typically low. These characteristics have been exploited as a way to determine if waxes have been adulterated with fats. Waxes are frequently used to prepare pharmaceutical dosage forms. For example, wool fat is used as an emollient base for creams and ointments and beeswax and spermaceti are used to stiffen ointment preparations.

Phospholipids (Phosphatides)

CLASSIFICATION AND STRUCTURE—The *phospholipids* include all lipoidal constituents that contain phosphorus in their molecules and have been categorized as lecithins, cephalins, and sphingomyelins. Their chemical composition in all cases is revealed through quantitative measurement of the products resulting from hydrolysis under various conditions. They appear to be essential components of every plant and animal cell. The cis-double bond in the polyunsaturated fatty acids allows membrane lipids to remain mobile at relatively low temperatures. This is particularly critical for plants, which have no way of controlling their temperature. The only phospholipids having pharmaceutical applications are the lecithins.

When completely hydrolyzed, each lecithin molecule yields two molecules of fatty acid and one molecule each of glycerol, phosphoric acid, and a basic nitrogenous alcohol compound (usually choline). The fatty acids obtained from lecithins are usually oleic, palmitic, and stearic. The phosphoric acid may be attached to glycerol in either a α- or β-position forming *α-glycerophosphoric acid* or *β-glycerophosphoric acid*, respectively, and producing the corresponding series of lecithins known as α- and β-lecithins. The representations below are in the *zwitterion* (internal salt) form; the naturally occurring lecithins are of the α-variety. *Choline,* a very strong base, is a member of the vitamin B complex. It functions in the body to prevent accumulation of fat in the liver; also, as the acetylated derivative *acetylcholine,* it is released at parasympathetic nerve endings when these nerves are stimulated and thus controls the transmission of impulses across cholinergic synapses.

α-Lecithin   **β-Lecithin**

Choline

Acetylcholine

Lecithins oxidize readily and darken in color upon exposure to air. Commercially, lecithin is obtained by extraction processes. *Ovolecithin (vitellin)* from egg yolks, *vegilecithin* from soybeans, and purified lecithin from calves brains are used as emulsifiers, antioxidants, and stabilizers in foods and pharmaceutical preparations.

Prostaglandins

CLASSIFICATION AND STRUCTURE—The natural prostaglandins are unsaturated, hydroxylated fatty acids. They are derivatives of the parent compound, *prostanoic acid*, with nine principal groups or series of modifications being recognized, as listed in Table 26-8.

Prostanoic acid
5-Octylcyclopentaneheptanoic acid

The abbreviations in Table 26-8 often are shortened to the last letter, by dropping the PG prefix. A subscript following the ab-

Table 26-8. Prostaglandins

	SUBSTITUENTS					
ABBREVIATION	C=C	>C=O	—OH	—O—O—	—OOH	—O—
PGA$_1$	10,13E	9	15S	—	—	—
PGB$_1$	8(12), 13E	9	15S	—	—	—
PGC$_1$	11, 13E	9	15S	—	—	—
PGD$_1$	13E	11	9α, 15S	—	—	—
PGE$_1$	13E	9	11α, 15S	—	—	—
PGF$_1$	13E	—	9α, 11α, 15S	—	—	—
PGG$_1$	13E	—	—	9α, 11α	15S	—
PGH$_1$	13E	—	15S	9α, 11α	—	—
PGR	See PGA series	—	—	—	—	—
PGI$_2$	5Z, 13E	—	11α, 15S	—	—	6, 9α

breviation pertains to the prostaglandin depicted in Table 26-8 or the following modifications:

Subscript 3—Two additional double bonds, at C-5 (*Z*) and C-17 (*Z*)
Subscripts α *or* β—indicate the configuration at C-9 and the same designation used for the steroids is employed; α is *down* and β is *up*. At C-15 the Cahn–Prelog–Ingold convention defines the chirality and the *S* configuration (α or dotted line) is found in most natural substances.

Thus, the compound PGF$_{2\alpha}$, or simply, F$_{2\alpha}$ (dinoprost, prostin F$_2$ alpha) is:

PGF$_{2\alpha}$

The subscript 2 depicts a *trans* (E) configuration at C-13 and *cis* (Z) at C-5, alpha hydroxyl at C-9, and a *cis* (α) diol at C-9 and C-11.

Prostaglandins are formed from the 20-carbon straight-chain carboxylic acid arachidonic acid and closely related fatty acids such as dihomo-γ-linoleic acid. The enzymatic process using vesicular extracts from sheep or bulls yields mainly the E series. Employing lung homogenates as the enzyme source, F$_\alpha$ compounds have been formed by a similar process. It has been suggested that the biological activity of the prostaglandin molecule is associated with a right-handed chirality, best visualized as a right-handed wedge in which all the hydrophilic functional groups are oriented to one side and the hydrophobic groups to the other side of the molecule while both ends are hydrophilic.

OCCURRENCE—Prostaglandins are associated with most mammalian tissues and have also been established as components of some higher plants. They can be extracted from most animal tissues with human seminal fluid containing the highest concentration and the greatest number of prostaglandins (31). However, the total prostaglandin production in the adult human is only of the order of 1 to 2 mg/24 hours. Many prostaglandins are characterized by both their generally short lifetime and multiplicity of effects. Metabolism occurs by hydroxylation, oxidation, and/or degradation of the carboxylic acid chain. The prostaglandins are perhaps the most versatile, ubiquitous, and powerful substances found in humans. They are involved in platelet aggregation, blood pressure, gastrointestinal motility, gastric acid secretion and *cytoprotection,* relief of glaucoma, pain and inflammation, nerve conduction, fetal development, uterine contraction (abortifacients and induce labor), thermoregulation and fever production, food intake, vasodilation and vasoconstriction, bronchodilation and bronchoconstriction, topical vasodilation, baldness, and the movement of fluid and electrolytes across membranes.

During the early stages of prostaglandin development, pharmacological studies were the major consumer of the natural materials. The small amounts required were supplied fairly rapidly by biosynthesis. The need to find compounds that were more selective and more stable than the natural prostaglandins led to an overwhelming outburst of synthetic activity in the late 1960s that continues today.[19, 20] Currently, prostaglandins are on the market or are under clinical investigation for potential applications in treating fertility problems, as oxytocic agents, as bronchodilators, and in a variety of uses in animal husbandry. In addition, prostacyclin is used to prevent blood clotting in cardiopulmonary bypass operations and to protect the stomach mucosa against rebound ulceration during the use of nonsteroidal anti-inflammatory agents (NSAIDs) employed for arthritis.

It was thought for a long time that the mechanism of action of the prostaglandins in anti-ulcer therapy was the inhibition of gastric acid secretion. However, a recent study shows that the anti-ulcer effect may result from both antisecretory and cytoprotective properties of the prostaglandins. PGE$_1$ has been introduced for a rare but frequently life-saving application. In certain instances of congenital heart disease, the normal closure of the *ductus arteriosus* is undesirable until corrective surgery has guaranteed the passage of blood to the lungs. Such surgery is more likely to be successful if PGE$_1$ is infused into the blood of the infant to prevent closure of the ductus until after successful surgery. Although the general implication is that prostaglandins are too irritating to be used as potent ocular hypertensive agents for glaucoma by direct ocular application, some success has been obtained with latanoprost.[21] Table 26-9 shows the structures of some representative prostaglandin derivatives currently marketed and under investigation.

STEROLS AND SAPONINS

Sterols

The *sterols* are alcohols structurally related to the *steroids,* naturally occurring compounds obtained from plants and animals that contain the partly or completely hydrogenated 17*H*-cyclopenta[*a*]phenanthrene nucleus. Typical examples include the familiar cholesterol and ergosterol. In addition to the sterols, the naturally occurring steroids include various other substances, such as compounds of adrenal origin, certain alkaloids, antirachitic vitamins, bile acids, cardiac glycosides, saponins, sex hormones, and toad poisons. The general formula for the basic structure of these compounds may be represented below.

General steroid formula

Table 26-9. Structures of Representative Prostaglandins

NAME	FORMULA	OH	DOUBLE BONDS	R_1	R_2	OTHER
Alprostadil	$C_{20}H_{34}O_5$	11α, 15α	13—14	—OH	n-C_4H_9	9-oxo
Carboprost (Prostin/15 M) (Tromethamine salt)	$C_{21}H_{35}O_5$	9α, 11α, 15α	5—6 cis, 13—14	—OH	n-C_4H_9	15β-CH_3—
Cloprostenol Sodium	$C_{22}H_{28}ClNaO_6$	9α, 11α, 15α	5—6, 13—14	—OH	m-ClC_6H_4O	—
Dinoprost (Prostin F_2) (Tromethamine)	$C_{20}H_{34}O_5$	9α, 11α, 15α	5—6, 13—14	—OH	n-C_4H_9—	—
Dinoprostone (Prostin E_2)	$C_{20}H_{32}O_5$	9α, 15α	5— 6, 13—14	—OH	n-C_4H_9-	9-oxo
Enprostil	$C_{23}H_{28}O_6$	11α, 15α	4— 5—6 (allene)	—OCH_3	—O · C_6H_5	9-oxo
Epoprostenol Sodium (Prostacyclin)	$C_{20}H_{31}NaO_5$	11α, 15α	13— 14^a	—ONa	n-C_4H_9-	15β-CH_3
Latanoprost	$C_{26}H_{40}O_5$	9α, 11α, 15α	5—6 cis	$OCH(CH_3)_2$	$CH_2C_6H_5$	—
Misoprostil	$C_{22}H_{38}O_5$	11α, 16β	13—14	—OCH_3	n-C_4H_9	9-oxo, 16β-CH_3
Nocloprost	$C_{22}H_{37}ClO_4$	11α, 15α	5—6 cis, 13—14	—OH	n-C_4H_9	9β-Cl, 16-di-CH_3
Rioprostil	$C_{21}H_{38}O_4$	11α, 16β (1—OH)^b	13— 14	(footnote^b)	n-C_4H_9	9-oxo
Rosoprostol Sodium	$C_{18}H_{33}NaO_3$	9β	—	—ONa	-C_2H_5	—
Vapiprost HCl	$C_{30}H_{39}NO_4$	11β	4— 5	—OH	n-C_4H_9	(footnote^c)
Viprostol	$C_{23}H_{36}O_5$	11α, 16β	5—6 cis, 13—14	—OCH_3	n-C_4H_9	9-oxo, 16β-vinyl

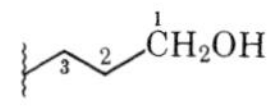

In actual conformation, however, the structure is not planar. The rings are lettered and numbered conventionally as indicated. Usually one or more rings are completely saturated and several centers of asymmetry are present. This, plus restricted rotations due to ring fusions, results in rather complex stereochemical relationships. In the naturally occurring compounds, substitutions in the rings occur most frequently on C-3, C-17, and C-11; C-18/C-19 may or may not be present (ie, CH_3). The direction in which a substituted group located at centers of asymmetry projects from the plane of the ring system is commonly indicated by the use of α- and β-. A α-substituent is viewed as projecting beneath the ring plane and is represented by a broken line; a β-substituent is viewed as projecting above the ring plane and is represented by a solid line.

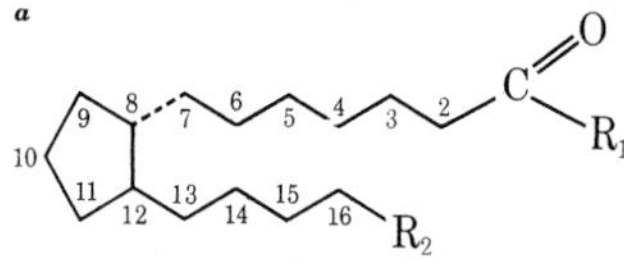

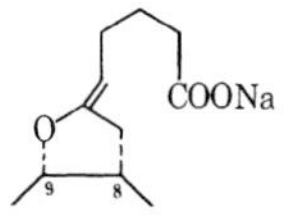

The prefixes *cis* and *trans* are often employed (but *not* in standardized nomenclature) to distinguish the α- and β- members of a pair of compounds that are otherwise stereochemically identical. However, this requires the selection of a substituting group to serve as a reference point in the steroid molecule; a *rule* frequently used is that the nearest angular (branching off at a ring fusion) methyl group is selected. For example, in the case of the sterols, the angular methyl group nearest to the 3-hydroxyl group is the one at C-10 and is represented as having the β-configuration. Thus, 3-β-hydroxycholestane becomes *cis*-3-hydroxycholestane and 3-α-hydroxycholestane becomes *trans*-3-hydroxycholestane. Most naturally occurring sterols have the 3-hydroxyl group in the β-, or *cis*-, position. The prefix *epi*- is often employed to specifically designate the corresponding epimers. In this case, the epimer contains the 3-hydroxyl group in the α- or trans- position; examples are epicholesterol and epicoprosterol.

Different investigators use slightly different methods of classifying the steroids. One method is to divide them into five classes according to the type of substituent group at carbon 17 (ie, group R):

Sterols—R is an aliphatic side chain. They contain one or more OH groups attached in an alicyclic linkage.

Sex Hormones—C-17 bears a ketonic or hydroxyl group and frequently carries a two-carbon side chain.
Cardiac Glycosides—R is a lactone ring. The glycosides also contain carbohydrates linked through oxygen in other parts of the molecule. Hydrolysis yields this carbohydrate and the *cardiac aglycone*.
Bile Acids—R is a five-carbon side chain terminating in a carboxylic acid group.
Sapogenins—R contains an oxacyclic (ethereal) ring system.

The parent hydrocarbon of natural sterols is cholestane, which exists in two forms depending on the configuration of the hydrogen atom at C-5. These are drawn below and labeled with their standard (IUPAC) names and, in parentheses, their trivial names:

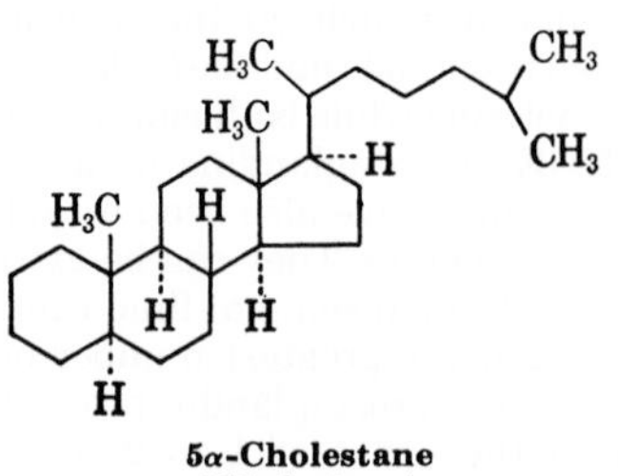

5α-Cholestane
(Cholestane)

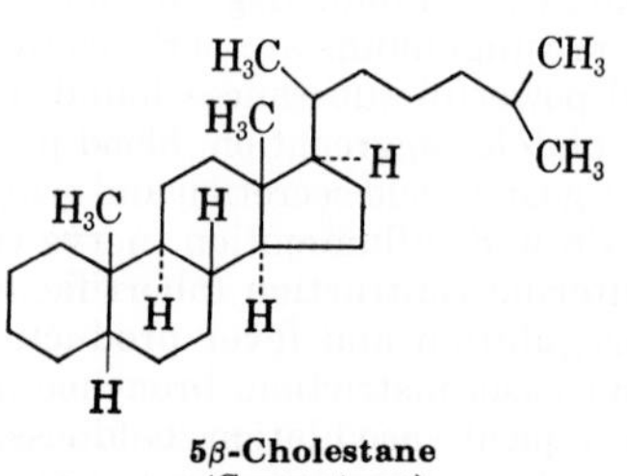

5β-Cholestane
(Coprostane)

As mentioned previously, the characteristic function of natural sterols is the 3-hydroxyl in the *beta-* orientation. Thus, 5α-cholestan-3β-ol and 5β-cholestan-3β-ol are looked upon as the parent sterols. Other sterols may be named as derivatives of them, although most have commonly accepted trivial names such as cholesterol, ergosterol, and stigmasterol. These parent sterols are shown below along with their various names. The two cholesterols are also illustrated. Note that in the cholest-5-enols, there is no H at C-5 and thus no α- or β- accompanies the numeral 5.

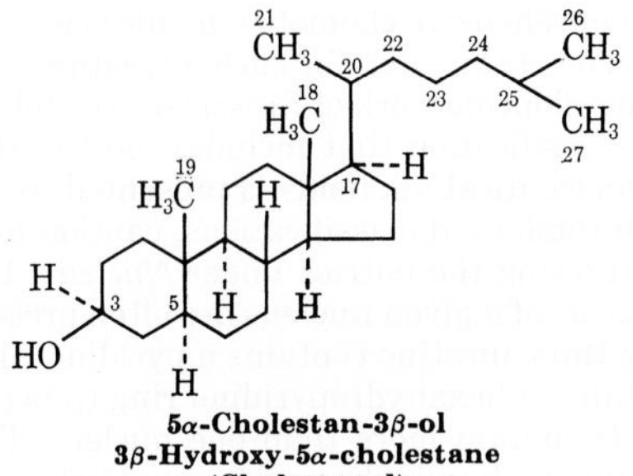

5α-Cholestan-3β-ol
3β-Hydroxy-5α-cholestane
(Cholestanol)

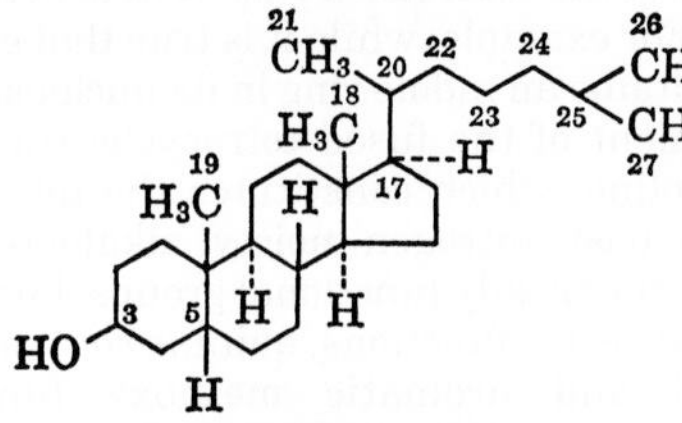

5β-Cholestan-3β-ol
3β-Hydroxy-5β-cholestane
(Coprostanol)

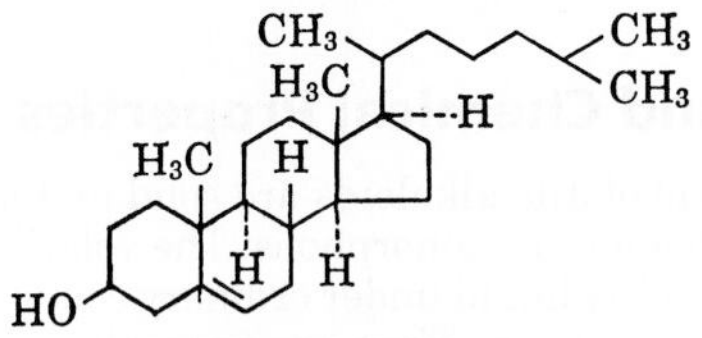

Cholest-5-en-3β-ol·
3β-Hydroxycholest-5-ene
(Cholesterol)

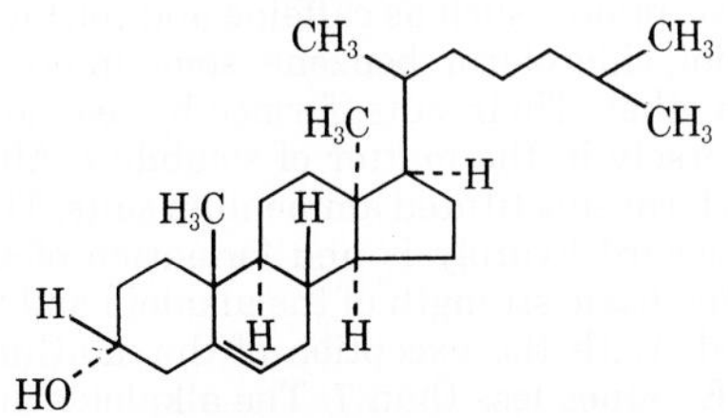

Cholest-5-en-3α-ol
3α-Hydroxycholest-5-ene
(Epicholesterol)

Several empirical color reactions have been developed for steroid identification. Most prominently cited are the Salkowski, Liebermann–Burchard, and Rosenheim reactions. For discussion of these, consult reference texts in biochemistry. Sterols occur abundantly in nature and often constitute a sizable fraction of the total unsaponifiable portion of lipoidal extractive matter from animal and vegetable tissue. The 3β-hydroxysteroids readily form sparingly soluble molecular complexes with the glycoside digitonin. These complexes are referred to as *digitonides,* and they find extensive application in various research operations involving isolation and characterization of the individual steroids.

Several sterols undergo intramolecular rearrangement under the influence of controlled ultraviolet radiation resulting in compounds that display antirachitic (vitamin D) activity. For example, ergosterol, a mycosterol occurring abundantly in yeast and ergot, is readily converted with good yield to ergocalciferol (vitamin D₂). The structure shown below emphasizes the locus of scission of the cyclic nucleus.

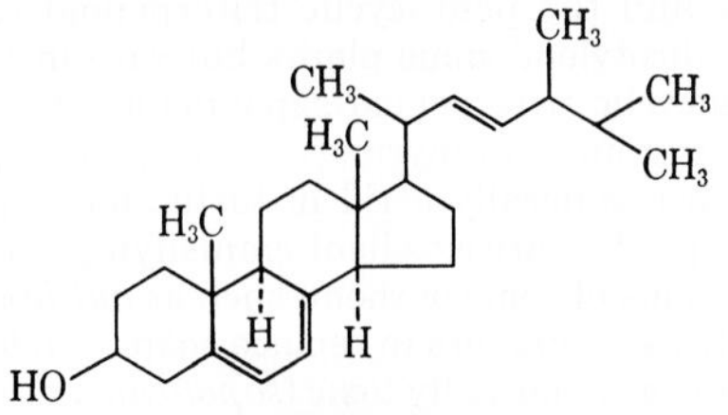

Ergosterol
5,7,22 E-Ergostatrien-3β-ol

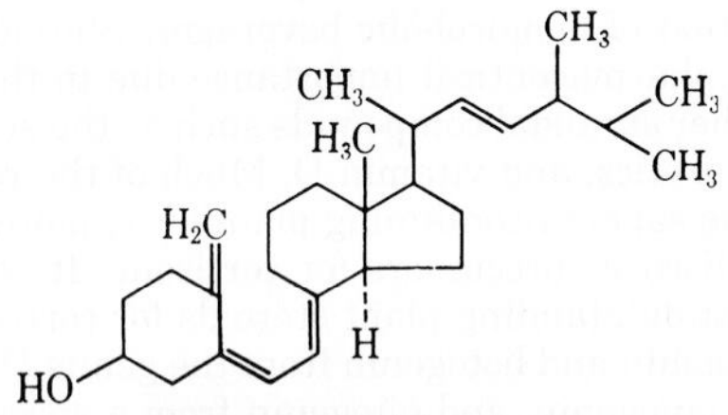

Ergocalciferol (vitamin D₂)
9,10-Seco-5Z,7E,10(19),22E-ergostatetraen-3β-ol

In a similar fashion, the natural vitamin D₃ metabolite, 1α,25-dihydroxycholecalciferol (calcitriol), is formed by ultraviolet conversion, hydrolysis, and heat isomerization from 1α,25-diacetoxy-7-dehydrocholesterol. Calcitriol (Rocaltrol, *Roche*) is used for the hypocalcemia associated with chronic renal dialysis.

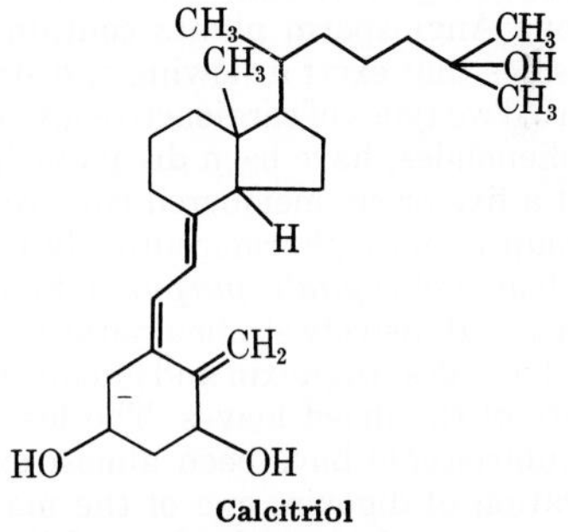

Calcitriol
(1α,2β,5Z,7E)-9,10-secocholesta-
5,7,10(19)-triene-1,3,25-triol

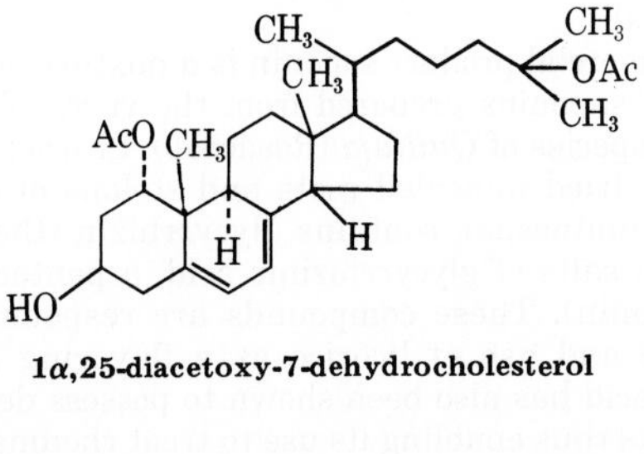

1α,25-diacetoxy-7-dehydrocholesterol

Saponins

The saponins are a group of amorphous, colloidal glycosides that are readily soluble in water and that produce froth when the aqueous solution is agitated. Two general types are well known, namely *steroid* (typically tetracyclic triterpenoids) as in digitonin, and *pentacyclic triterpenoids* as in aesculin. Both of these types have a glycosidic linkage at C-3 and are biosynthesized via mevalonic acid and isoprenoid units. Saponins have a high molecular weight and polarity with many conforming to the general formula $C_nH_{2n-8}O_{10}$. The aglycones, usually freed by acid-catalyzed hydrolysis, are termed *sapogenins*.[22] The saponins are distributed widely in the botanical kingdom with the steroidal type less distributed than the pentacyclic triterpenoid types. Steroidal saponins are found in both mono- and dicotyledons and the pentacyclic triterpenoid saponins are abundant in dicotylendonous plants but rare in monocotylendons.[23] Pentacyclic triterpenoid saponins are typically classified into three groups, α-amyrin, β-amyrin, and lupeol.

Saponins are generally acrid in taste and in powder form cause sneezing. They are excellent emulsifying agents, and the aqueous solutions of some of them, such as *quillaja* bark, were used formerly as detergents to replace soap. In addition, many of the saponins are markedly toxic (*sapotoxins*) and usually exert a powerful hemolytic action on red blood corpuscles. However, when taken orally they are comparatively harmless. For example, sarsaparilla is rich in saponins but is widely used in the preparation of nonalcoholic beverages. Steroidal saponins are of great pharmaceutical importance due to their relationship with other steroidal compounds such as the sex hormones, cortisone, diuretics, and vitamin D. Much of the research conducted on the saponin-containing plants was motivated by the attempt to discover precursors for cortisone. It would appear that the most outstanding plant steroids for cortisone production are diosgenin and botogenin from the genus *Dioscorea* and hecogenin, manogenin, and gitogenin from a species of *Agave*. In addition, some naturally occurring steroidal saponins are used therapeutically themselves. For example, the roots of *Panax ginseng* (Araliaceae) contain numerous steroidal and triterpenoid saponins classified as ginsenosides and panaxosides that are responsible for its therapeutic activity. Ginseng has gained popularity in the West in recent years for improvement in concentration and as an adaptogenic (resistance to stress and disease).

A very important group of steroidal glycosides, characterized by their physiological action, are the cardioactive glycosides. Numerous Angiosperm plants contain C23 and C24 sterodial glycosides that exert a slowing and strengthening effect on the heart. Two types of cardioactive glycosides, cardenolides and bufadienolides, have been distinguished based upon the presence of a five or six membered ring, respectively. The cardenolide group is most pharmaceutically important. Digitalis, the dried leaves of *Digitalis purpurea* (Scrophulariaceae), has been the most extensively studied natural source of cardenolide cardiac glycosides. Digitoxin and gitoxin are the main active components of the dried leaves. The leaves of *Digitalis lanata* (Scrophulariaceae) have been almost exclusively used for the preparation of digoxin, one of the most widely used drugs for the treatment of congestive heart failure. Cardiac glycosides similar to those of digitalis are also found in the oleander plant *(Nerium oleander)* and the lily of the valley (*Convallaria majalis)*.

The commercial product saponin is a mixture of pentacyclic triterpenoid saponins prepared from the yucca plant or from the bark of species of *Quillaja* (Rosaceae). Licorice, which consists of the dried unpeeled roots and stolons of *Glycyrrhiza glabra* (Leguminosae), contains glycyrrhizin (the potassium and calcium salts of glycyrrhizinic acid, a pentacyclic triterpenoid saponin). These compounds are responsible for the sweet taste and use of licorice as a flavoring agent. Glycyrrhizinic acid has also been shown to possess deoxycorticosterone effects thus enabling its use to treat rheumatoid arthritis, Addisons's disease, and various inflammatory conditions.[24]

ALKALOIDS

Composition and Structure

These basic compounds at first were called vegetable alkalies; later these were renamed *alkaloids,* meaning alkali-like. All al-
kaloids contain carbon, nitrogen, and generally oxygen (a typical exception is nicotine) but members of this group are classified as alkaloids based upon chemical properties of a basic nitrogen, which confers their alkali-properties. However, the group is very varied in regards to their physiological role, taxonomy, and biogenesis. In addition, there is no clear-cut distinction between alkaloids and naturally occurring complex amines because they typically contain one or more nitrogen atoms, usually wholly or partly in a hetercyclic ring. Therefore, alkaloids have been classified in a variety of ways such as botanical source, chemical structure, and pharmacological action. Any attempt at comprehensive chemotaxonomic classification is far beyond the scope of this text; for such a treatment, consult the continuing encyclopedic work of Brossi (see the bibliography).

A partial classification that includes most of the more important pharmaceutical alkaloids is presented in Table 26-10. As in all such condensed classifications, caution must be exercised in interpreting the entries under *Nucleus*. Different hydrogenated forms of a given nucleus are often present in different alkaloids; thus, nicotine contains a pyridine ring; whereas, piperine contains a hexahydropyridine ring (piperidine). Also, some alkaloids contain more than one nucleus. For example, quinine contains both quinoline and quinuclidine. In many instances, the nuclei shown in Table 26-10 are merely the best-known fragment of the total fused ring system actually present in the alkaloid. For example, while it is true that each of the ergot alkaloids contains an indole ring in its nucleus, the indole is actually a fragment of the fused tetracyclic ring system, indolo[4,3-*fg*]quinoline, which constitutes the total nucleus. In addition to their basic nitrogen moiety, alkaloids usually contain one or more chemically functional groups. For example, cocaine contains two ester functions, quinine contains both a secondary alcohol and aromatic methoxy functions, and ergonovine contains a substituted amide function. Some alkaloids such as solanine and tomatine actually occur as glycosides.

Physical and Chemical Properties

Most of the nonvolatile alkaloids are solid and mainly crystallizable, though a few are amorphous. The volatile ones, such as nicotine, are mainly liquid under ordinary conditions and these often contain no oxygen. They are generally white. However, berberine is yellow and sanguinarine, itself colorless, yields red salts. They are either insoluble or sparingly soluble in water, with a few exceptions, such as caffeine and colchicines, but soluble in alcohol, chloroform, benzene, some in ether, and a few in petroleum ether. Their salts, formed by reaction with acids, behave conversely in the matter of solubility. Alkaloids unite with acids to form substituted ammonium salts. The stability of these salts toward hydrolysis and formation of the free base varies with the basic strength of the alkaloid and the nature of the acid used. With the exception of the xanthine alkaloids, most have pK values less than 7. The alkaloids are freed from their salts by the addition of alkali. In the same manner, *alkaline salts* such as the *acetates, carbonates, citrates, benzoates, salicylates,* and *basic phosphates* of sodium, potassium, and ammonium will precipitate the free alkaloid or, in some instances, will convert it to a less-soluble salt. As a general rule, alkaloids are incompatible with *oxidizing agents,* some undergoing oxidation readily upon exposure to air. Various antioxidants such as sodium metabisulfite are effective in retarding this deterioration. Oxidation is more rapid in alkaline solution and buffers are commonly used to maintain a suitable pH to prevent degradation. The rate of hydrolysis of ester and glycosidic alkaloids is also pH dependent.

Various kinds of tests have been devised to identify known alkaloids. Their effective use, however, usually requires some relevant knowledge of the history of the sample under examination. In general, these tests involve combinations of two or more of the following: melting points of the alkaloid and at least one of its salts or other derivatives; specific rotation; solubility

Table 26-10. A Partial Classification of Alkaloids

NUCLEUS	PLANT GENERA	ALKALOIDS
Benzazulene	*Aconitum, Delphinium*	Aconitine, delphinine, delsoline
Diterpenoid	*Taxus*	Cephalomannine β-hydoxybaccatn, taiwanxan, taxagafine, taxine, taxol
Imidazole	*Pilocarpus*	Pilocarpine, pilocarpidine, pilosine, pseudopilocarpine, pseudojaborine, isopilocarpinea
Indole	*Peganum, Psilocybe, Stropharia, Evodia, Corynanthe, Claviceps, Physostigma, Strychnos, Rauwolfia*	Brucine, ergonovine, ergotamine, harmine, physostigmine, psilocybin, reserpine, strychnine, yohimbine
Isoquinoline	*Hydrastis, Papaver, Corydalis, Berberis, Chondodendron, Ipecacuanha, Sanguinaria*	Anhalonine, bebeerine, berberine, cephaeline, codeine, corydaline, cotarnine chloride, emetine, erythramine, erythroidine, hydrastine, menispermine, morphine, papaverine, sanguinarine, tubocurarine chloride
Phenylalkylamine	*Ephedra, Lophophora*	Ephedrine
Purine	*Guarana, Cola, Coffea, Thea, Theobroma*	Caffeine,[a] theobromine,[a] theophylline[a]
Pyridine	*Anabasis, Areca, Conium, Lobelia, Piper, Punica, Ricinus, Nicotiana*	Anabasine, aphylline, arecaidine, arecoline, coniine, guvacine, lobeline, nicotine, pelletierine, piperine, ricinine, trigonelline
Quinoline	*Cinchona, Cusparia*	Cinchonine, cinchonidine, cusparine, ethylhydrocupreine, quinacrine, quinine, quinidine
Quinolizine	*Anagyris, Laburnum, Lupinus, Sophora*	Anagyrine, cytisine, lupanine, lupinine, matrine, sparteine
Spirobenzylisoquinoline	*Fumaria, Corydalis*	Corpaine, fumaricine, fumariline, fumaritine, ochrobirine, ochrotensimine, ochrotensine, sibiracine
Steroidal[b]	*Solanum, Veratrum, Lycopersicon, Holarrhena, Schoenocaulon*	Cevadine, cevine, conessine, jervine, rubijervine, solanidine, solanine, tomatidine, veratramine, eratridine
Tropane	*Erythroxylon, Atropa, Datura, Hyoscyamus, Scopola*	Atropine, benzoylecgonine, cocaine, eucatropine, homatropine, hygrine, hyoscyamine, scopolamine

[a] Some authors do not classify these relatively feebly basic compounds as alkaloids.
[b] Various nuclei are represented in this group. In general, they have some resemblance to the steroid (cyclopentanophenanthrene) nucleus.

in various solvents; color producing reactions with specified reagents; and microscopic examination of the crystals obtained by the action of suitable precipitants under controlled conditions. Closely related alkaloids such as morphine and codeine do not differ sufficiently in their absorption of ultraviolet light to permit differentiation on the basis of their respective spectrograms. However, the infrared spectrum of an alkaloid is individual and identification can be made with certainty. Modern high-resolution NMR techniques make possible even more definitive identification.

Occurrence and Uses

The building blocks of the alkaloids are presumed to be amino acids and their metabolic degradation products. Formaldehyde sources (ie, glyoxylic and formic acids) are also available and biological processes of deamination, decarboxylation, and oxidation are operative. Various genera of 158 botanical families have yielded compounds with alkaloidal properties. A few are obtained from cryptogams (flowerless plants) but the majority are extracted from the phanerogams (flowering plants), most of them being from dicotyledons. Among the monocotyledons, some useful alkaloids are found in species of the Amaryllidaceae and Liliaceae families. Alkaloids are also found in some fungi (ie, lysergic acid derivatives), the skins of amphibians, and some mammals (ie, indole and isoquinoline).

Phytochemists estimate that less than 5% of the known flowering plants have been investigated for possible alkaloid content. Specific alkaloids of complex structures are ordinarily confined to specific plant families (ie, *hyoscyamine* in Solanaceae and *colchicine* in Liliaceae). However, the occurrence of ergot alkaloids in the fungus *Claviceps purpurea* and certain *Ipomoea* species (Convolvulaceae) is an exception, which may be attributed to either parallel or conversion evolution of certain complex biochemical pathways. In their native environment, alkaloids usually exist in the form of salts, frequently of the simple organic acids such as lactic, malic, tartaric, or citric. Unusual, often distinctive, acids are also en-

countered, such as quinic with cinchona alkaloids, and meconic with opium alkaloids.

Alkaloids may be recovered from their parent plant material by extraction. In a representative type of processing, the crude, milled plant material is moistened with an aqueous alkali such as sodium carbonate, sodium bicarbonate, or lime to liberate the alkaloids from their salts and percolated with benzene, ether, or some other suitable water-immiscible solvent. The solvent layer is extracted with dilute acid to convert the alkaloids into salts and to bring them into the aqueous phase. The free alkaloids are precipitated by the addition of alkali and separated by appropriate means. The specific operations involved are based upon the physical and chemical properties of the alkaloids sought. Purification is usually accomplished by the crystallization of the alkaloidal salts but distillation and other procedures may also be employed. In some cases, when the alkaloid content of a plant is low and large volumes of dilute aqueous solutions are obtained, it is advantageous to adsorb the alkaloids on ion-exchange resins. If the alkaloids adsorbed onto a resin differ sufficiently in basicity, it may be possible to effect at least a partial separation of the alkaloids during the course of the elution from the resin. An excellent example of the problems encountered and of some of the techniques employed in the separation of a complex mixture of alkaloids is provided by the review of researchers on the *Vinca* alkaloids.[25]

Most alkaloids are physiologically active, some being extremely poisonous, although typically harmless to plants. In the majority of instances, they are responsible for the pharmacological actions of the plants from which they are derived. Notwithstanding the many extremely valuable synthetic medicinal and antibiotic agents that have been added to the list of weapons against disease, the alkaloids still constitute an indispensable and most potent group of substances for the treatment and mitigation of functional disturbances and relief from suffering. It is for this reason that some of the larger pharmaceutical firms maintain continuing programs for the pharmacological screening of alkaloids, both new and old. For example, reserpine, much valued for its antihypertensive and psychotherapeutic actions, emerged from such a program in the 1950s, and an intensive effort with the *Vinca* (*Catharanthus*) alkaloids yielded some oncolytic drugs of value in the treatment of certain types of cancer. A number of naturally occurring alkaloids are made synthetically and there are also a number of synthetic drugs having an alkaloidal character.[25] Distinction should be made between *total synthesis,* in which the end product is the result of chemical processes that employ only materials that can be built up from the elements (carbon, hydrogen, oxygen, etc), and *partial synthesis* in which the end product is produced from a naturally occurring complex substance that is already closely related structurally to the desired end product (ie, the synthesis of ergonovine from lysergic acid).

Major Classes of Alkaloids

As mentioned previously, various alkaloidal classification systems have been employed. Each system has its advantages and disadvantages and more needs to be learned about the occurrence, composition, and physiological actions of the alkaloids before a comprehensive classification having maximum practical utility can be produced. We will classify the pharmaceutically relevant alkaloids based upon their biosynthesis from a particular amino acid derivative and discuss each of the following classes individually:

- Ornithine-derived alkaloids—The ornithine derivatives, proline and putrescine constitute the basic structures
- Phenylalanine-, tyrosine-, and dihydroxyphenylalanine-derived alkaloids
- Tryptophan-derived alkaloids
- Miscellaneous alkaloids—Not biosynthesized from amino acids or biosynthesis has not been fully established.

ORNITHINE-DERIVED ALKALOIDS

The **tropane alkaloids** will be considered in two groups: (1) atropine and related alkaloids and (2) cocaine. They are grouped together because all are derivatives of tropane. The alkaloids of the atropine group are closely related chemically (Table 26-11). Most of the natural alkaloids are esters of *mandelic acid* or *tropic acid* with *tropine* or *scopine*. Scopine is epoxytropine, the only difference being the 6,7-oxygen bridge. Esters of tropine are called *tropeines* (ie, tropine mandelate is mandelyltropeine). *Atropine* is a racemic variety of tropine tropate, *hyoscyamine* is the levorotatory enantiomorph of

Table 26-11. Atropine and Related Alkaloids and Derivatives

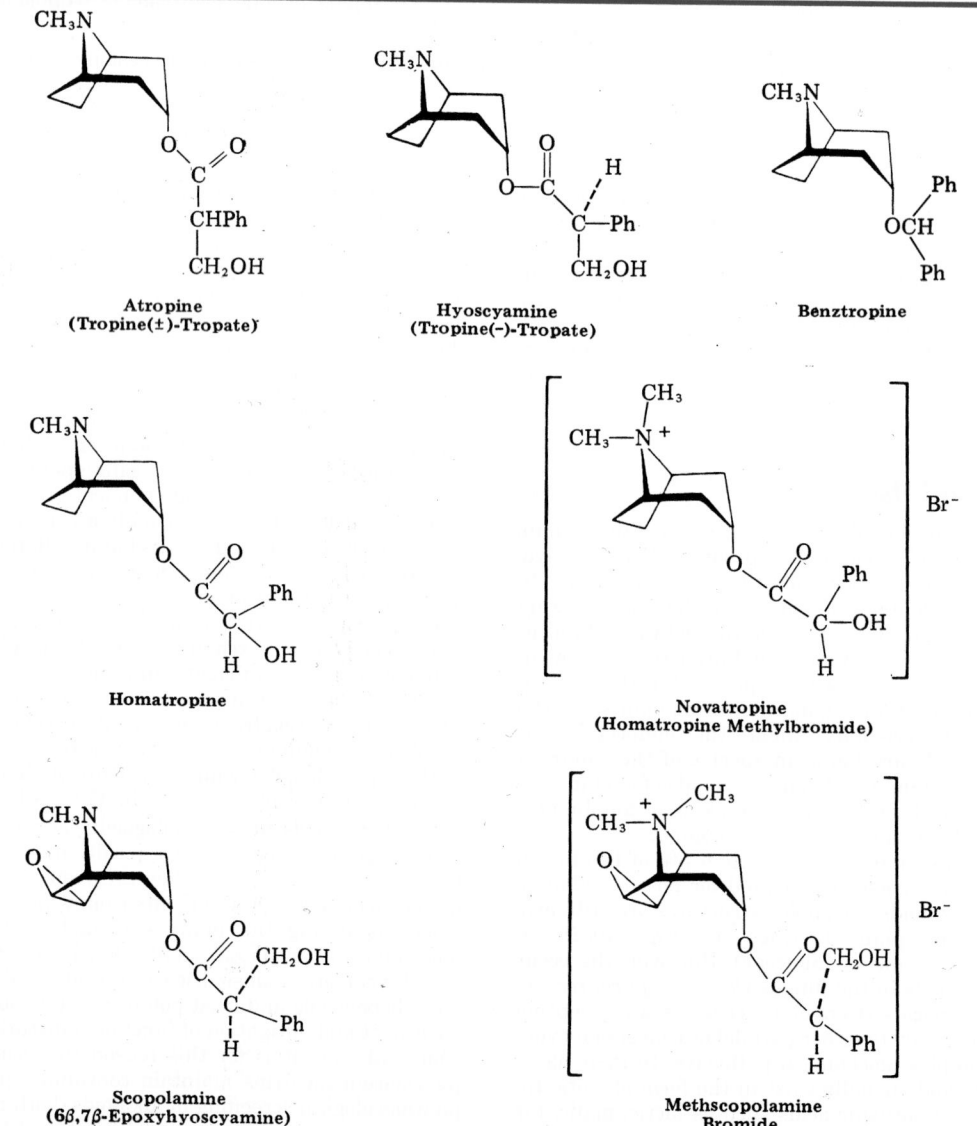

Atropine
(Tropine(±)-Tropate)

Hyoscyamine
(Tropine(−)-Tropate)

Benztropine

Homatropine

Novatropine
(Homatropine Methylbromide)

Scopolamine
(6β,7β-Epoxyhyoscyamine)

Methscopolamine
Bromide

tropine tropate, and *scopolamine* is scopine tropate. These esters may be hydrolyzed by heating in water.

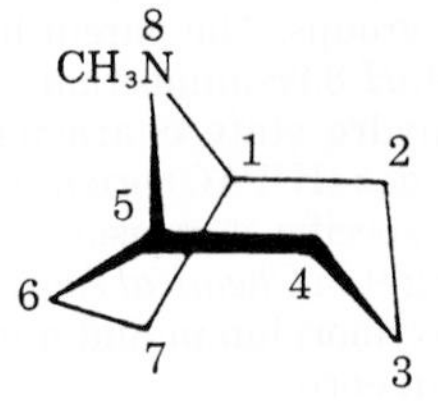

Tropane

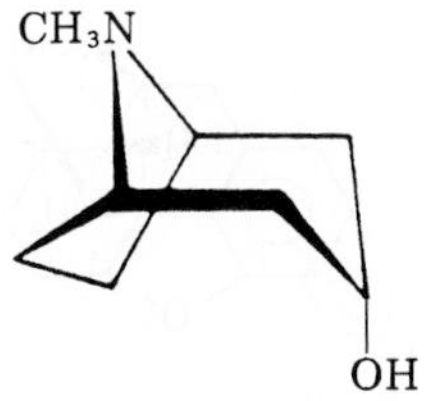

Tropine (*endo*-8-Methyl-8-azabicyclo[3.2.1]octane-3-ol)

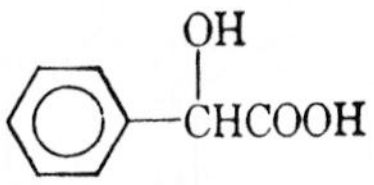

Mandelic Acid

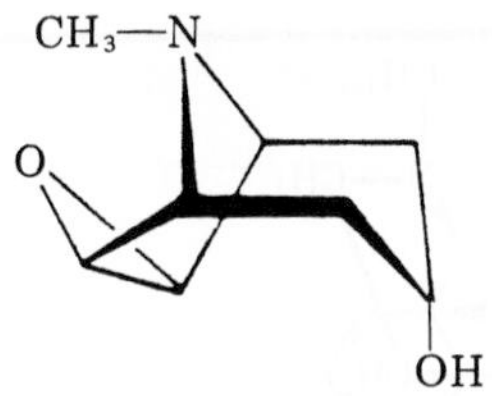

Scopine ([7(*S*)-(1α,2β,4β,5α,7β)]-9-Methyl-3-oxa-9-azatricyclo[3.3.1.0²,⁴]nonan-7-ol)

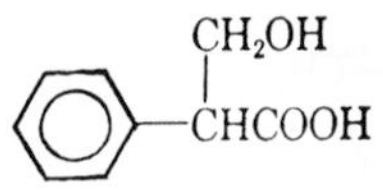

Tropic Acid

Eumydrine is also related closely; it is 8-methylatropinium nitrate, a quaternary ammonium salt. Homatropine is tropine mandelate and novatropine is 8-methylhomatropinium bromide. Benztropine is the benzhydryl ester of tropine (Table 26-11).

Atropa belladonna (nightshade), *Hyoscyamus niger* (henbane), and *Datura stramonium* (jimson weed) all yield mydri-

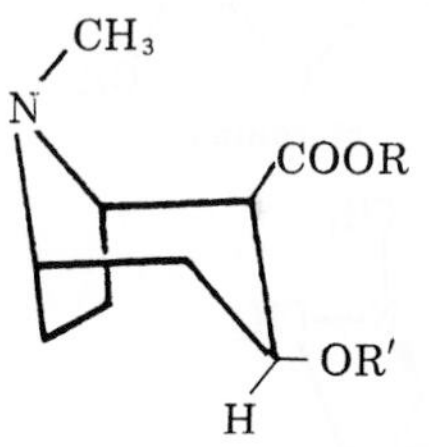

Table 26-12. Ecgonine Derivatives

R	R'	NAME OF DERIVATIVE
H	H	Ecgonine
CH_3	C_6H_5CO-(benzoyl)	Cocaine
H	CH_3	Methylecgonine
H	$C_6H_5CH=CHCO$-(cinnamoyl)	Cinnamoylecgonine
H	C_6H_5CO	Benzoylecgonine

atic alkaloids, characteristic of the Solanaceae family. There are also many other plants of this family that are being used largely in the manufacture of the various alkaloids. Atropine rarely occurs as such in any of the plants but is always the product of the racemization of the levo-isomeride hyoscyamine, which is converted into atropine by the action of weak alkalies. This racemization involves the conversion of the (−)-tropic acid moiety of hyoscyamine to (±)-tropic acid. The most characteristic physiological property of the Solanaceous alkaloids is their mydriatic effect (pupil dilation of the eye). This property is the basis for their most sensitive identification test. As little as one drop of a 1 in 25,000 solution will cause a distinct dilation of the pupil of a cat's eye. Atropine also simulates the CNS and causes a decrease in secretions; hyoscyamine does not stimulate the CNS and is used as a sedative for motion sickness.

The cocaine group of tropane alkaloids is distinguished chemically from the atropine group by the presence of an *exo*-carboxyl (or esterified carboxyl) at the 2-position and by the *exo*-configuration (instead of *endo*-) of the 3-ester function. Therefore, they become derivatives of ecgonine ([1R-(*exo,exo*)]-3-hydroxy-8-methyl-8-azabicyclo[3.2.1]octane-2-carboxylic acid) having the general structure:

Table 26-13. Classification of Opium Alkaloids

Benzylisoquinoline Group	Codamine [$C_{20}H_{25}NO_4$][a]	Narcototine [$C_{21}H_{21}NO_7$][e,c]
	Gnoscopine [$C_{22}H_{23}NO_7$][b,c]	l-Narcotine [$C_{22}H_{23}NO_7$][b,c]
	Laudanidine [$C_{20}H_{25}NO_4$][a]	Oxynarcotine [$C_{22}H_{23}NO_8$][b,c]
	dl-Laudanine [$C_{20}H_{25}NO_4$][a]	Papaverine [$C_{20}H_{21}NO_4$][e]
	Laudanosine [$C_{21}H_{27}NO_4$][a]	Xanthaline [$C_{20}H_{19}NO_5$][e]
	Narceine [$C_{23}H_{27}NO_8$][d]	
Phenanthrene Group	Codeine [$C_{18}H_{21}NO_3$][f]	Neopine [$C_{18}H_{21}NO_3$][g]
	Morphine [$C_{17}H_{19}NO_3$][f]	Thebaine [$C_{19}H_{21}NO_3$][h]
	ψ-Morphine [$(C_{17}H_{18}NO_3)_2$][f]	
Tetrahydroisoquinoline Group	Hydrocotarnine [$C_{12}H_{15}NO_3$][b]	
Quinoline Group	Aporeine [$C_{18}H_{17}NO_2$][i]	
Cryptopine Group	Cryptopine [$C_{21}H_{23}NO_5$][j]	Protopine [$C_{20}H_{19}NO_5$][h]
Alkaloids of Unknown Structure	Lanthopine [$C_{23}H_{25}NO_4$]	Papaveramine [$C_{21}H_{25}NO_6$]
	Meconidine [$C_{21}H_{23}NO_4$]	Rhoeadine $C_{21}H_{21}NO_6$]
Derivatives of Natural Alkaloids	Apomorphine[k]	Metopon (methyldihydromorphinone)
	Dionine (ethylmorphine)	Nalorphine (N-allylnormorphine)
	Heroin (diacetylmorphine)	Naloxone
	Hydrocodone (dihydrocodeinone)	Oxymorphone
	Hydromorphone (dihydromorphinone)	Oxycodone

[a] 1,2,3,4-tetrahydroisoquinoline; (1708).
[b] 5,6,7,8-tetrahydro-1,3-dioxolo[4,5-*g*]isoquinoline; (2810).
[c] 1,3-dihydroisobenzofuran (phthalan); (1330).
[d] 2,3-dihydrobenzofuran (coumaran); (1328).
[e] isoquinoline; (1708).
[f] 5,7a,8,9-tetrahydro-4a*H*-8,9c-iminoethanophenanthro[4,5-*bcd*]furan; (5922).
[g] 5,6,8,9-tetrahydro-4a*H*-8,9c-iminoethanophenanthro[4,5-*bcd*]furan; (5922).
[h] 8,9-dihydro-4a*H*-8,9c-iminoethanophenanthro[4,5-*bcd*]furan; (5922).
[i] 6,7,7a,8-tetrahydro-5*H*-benzo[*g*]-1,3-benzodioxolo[6,5,4-*de*]quinoline; (5846)
[j] 6,7,12,13,14,15-hexahydrobenzo[*e*]-1,3-dioxolo[4,5-*l*][2]benzazecine; (4874).
[k] 4*H*-dibenzo[*de, g*]quinoline; (5171).

Table 26-12 portrays the identities of R and R' for the common ecgonine derivatives. Alkaloids within this group are commonly found in cocoa leaves. They have local anesthetic properties but also have highly addictive properties, and, therefore, they are only used for ophthalmic, ear, nose, and throat surgery.

The **tobacco alkaloids** derived from ornithine are represented by nicotine, which consists of a pyridine moiety associated with a pyrrolidine ring. Nicotine is derived from the genus *Nicotiana* and is present in tobacco smoke and some insecticides. Nicotine has also been used in chewing gums, nasal sprays, and transdermal patches for smoking cessation.

PHENYLALANINE-, TYROSINE-, AND DIHYDROXYPHENYLALANINE-DERIVED ALKALOIDS

OPIUM ALKALOIDS—*Opium* is the latex obtained by incision of the unripe capsules of the opium poppy, *Papaver somniferum* (Papaveraceae). The many alkaloids obtained from the opium poppy are divided into the following chemical groups: *Benzylisoquinoline, Phenanthrene, Tetrahydroisoquinoline, Quinoline, Cryptopine, Alkaloids of Unknown Structure,* and *Derivatives of Natural Alkaloids* (Table 26-13). It will be observed that the pharmaceutically important alkaloids displayed in Table 26-14 derive from the so-called benzylisoquinoline (papaverine) and phenanthrene (morphine/codeine) groups. The parent heterocycle of the phenanthrene group is 4a*H*-8,9*c*-iminoethanophenanthro[4,5-*bcd*]furan. In the hexahydro state characteristic of codeine and morphine, its *Ring Index* (IUPAC) orientation and numbering are shown below. The specific stereoisomer present in these alkaloids is shown at the right in *Chemical Abstracts* format, which treats it as a 4,5α-epoxymorphinan and numbers it by the familiar Cahn–Robinson sequence.

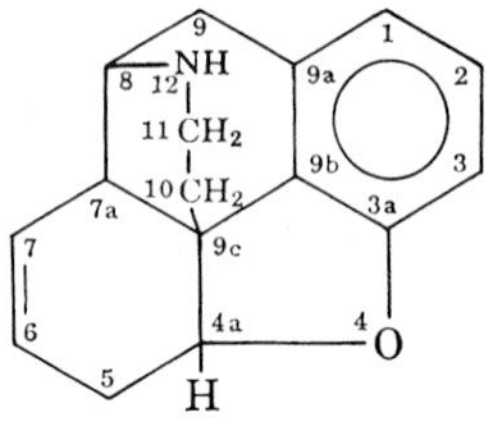

IUPAC 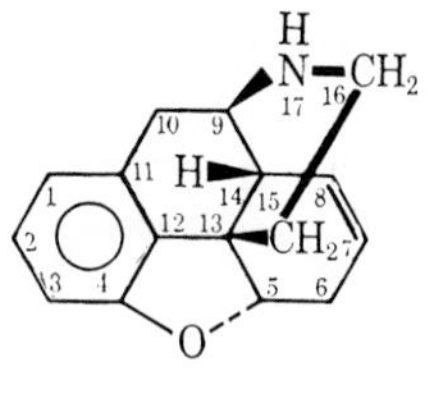   **Chemical Abstracts**

Table 26-14. Opium Alkaloids and Derivatives

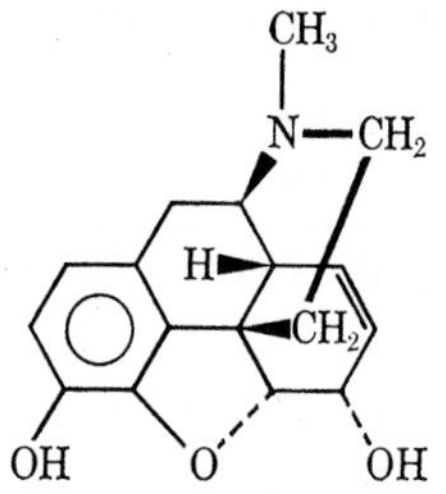

Morphine

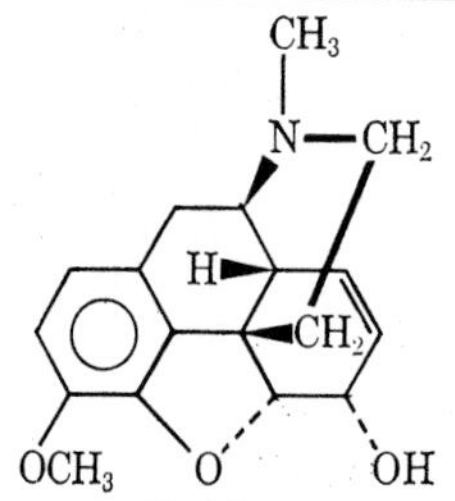

Codeine

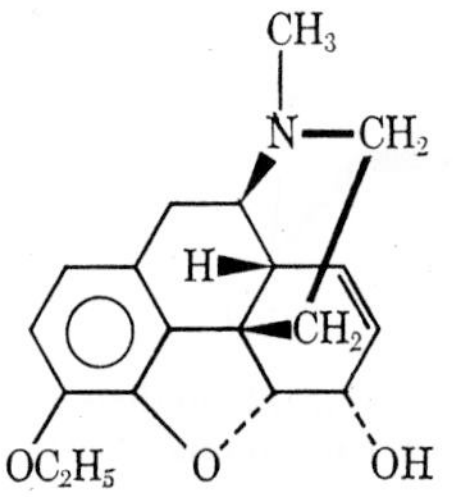

Ethylmorphine

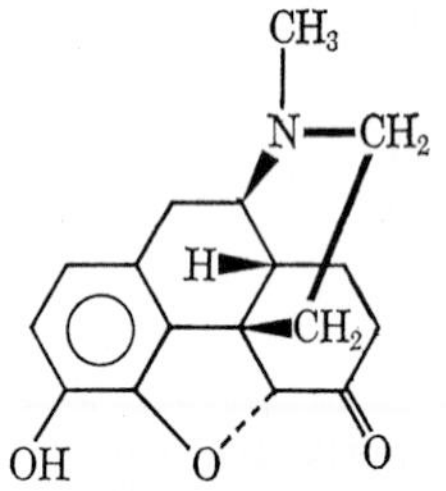

Hydromorphone

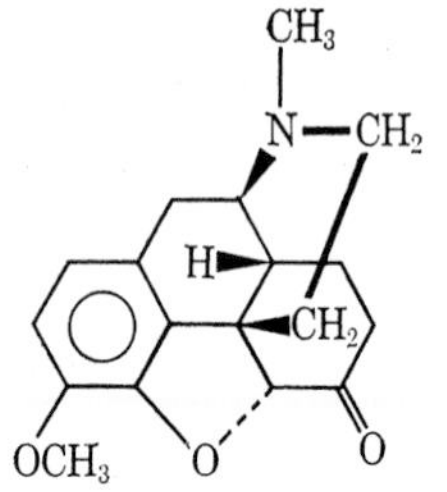

Hydrocodone

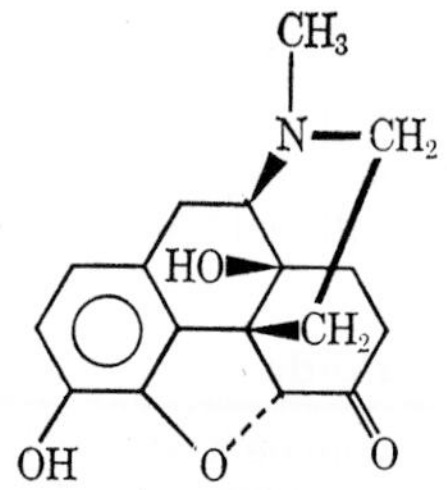

Oxymorphone

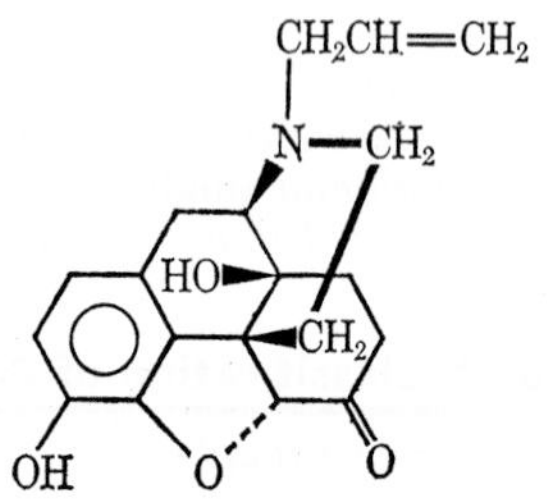

Naloxone

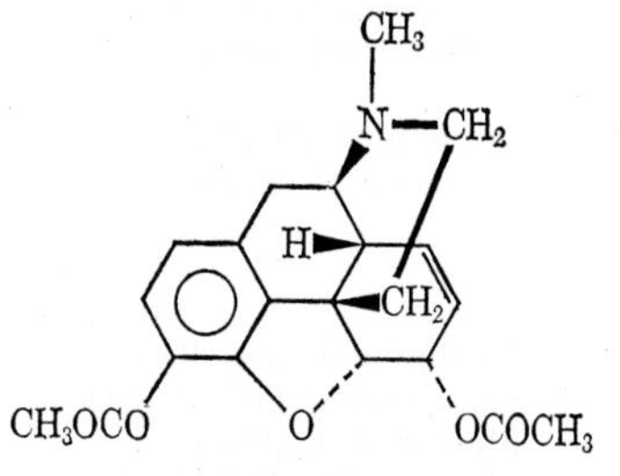

Heroin

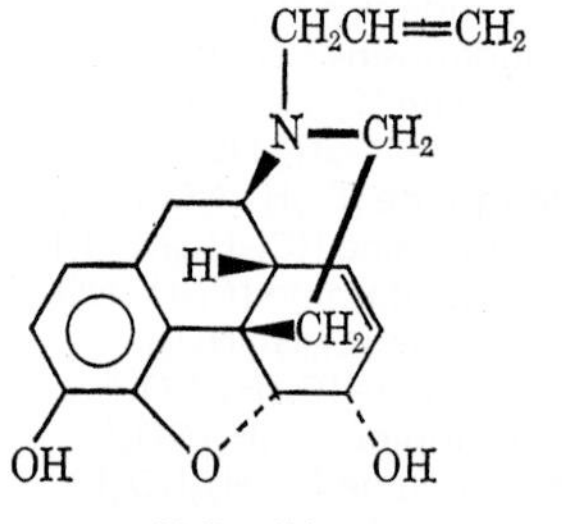

Nalorphine

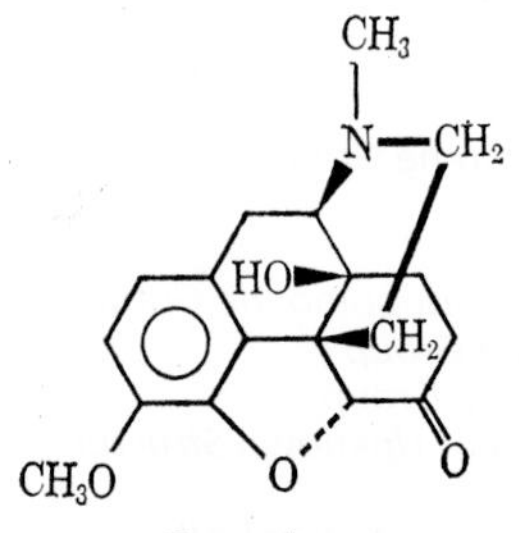

Oxycodone

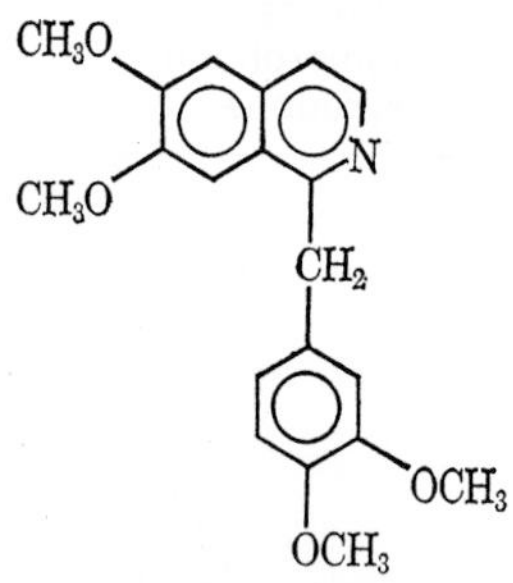

Papaverine

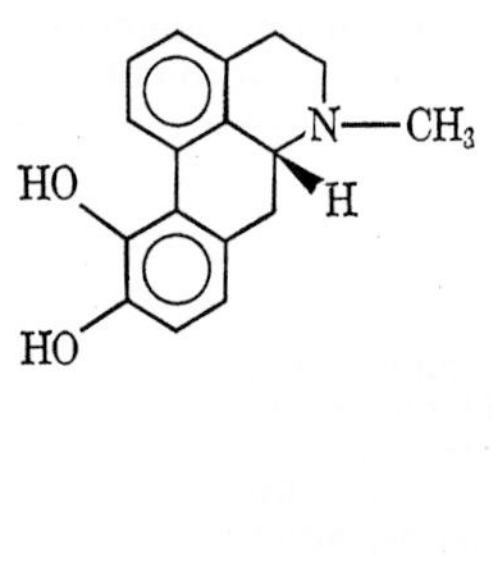

Apomorphine

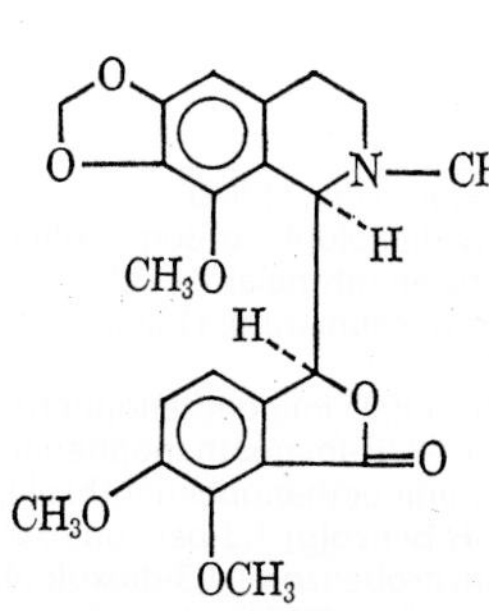

Noscapine (*l*-Narcotine)

Papaverine is a very weak base and slightly toxic. Morphine is a stronger base, alkaline to litmus, and highly toxic. Morphine and codeine have been used to treat pain, as hypnotics, and to treat diarrhea. Codeine has also been used as a cough suppressant.

Additional pharmaceutically relevant, phenylalanine-, tyrosine-, and dihydroxyphenylalanine-derived alkaloids include the following:

- Ephedrine and pseudoephedrine are derived from various species of *Ephedra* (Ma-huang) (Ephedraceae) and used for a variety of therapeutic actions including the relief of asthma.
- Colchicine is derived from the seed or corn of *Colchicum autumnale* (Liliaceae). It is an amorphous, yellowish-white solid that darkens upon exposure to light. It is a weak base that results in a yellow color when mixed with strong mineral acids. It is soluble in water, alcohol, and chloroform and slightly soluble in ether. It is used therapeutically to relieve gout.
- Emetine is derived from the root of *Cephaelis ipecacuanha* (Rubiaceae) and used as an expectorant and emetic.
- Tubocurarine is derived from *Chondrodendron tomentosum* (Menispermaceae) and used as a muscle relaxant. Such "curare" alkaloids are found in South American arrow poisons.

TRYPTOPHAN-DERIVED ALKALOIDS

Cinchona **Alkaloids**, such as the quinoline alkaloids (quinine and quinidine, a pair of diastereoisomers) and their 6-demethoxy derivatives (cinchonine and cinchonidine), are derived from the dried bark of the stem or root of various species of *Cinchona* (Rubiaceae). The structural formulas in Table 26-15 indicate the close relationships between the various members of this group of alkaloids. Examination of the formulas of these compounds shows that they all contain a *quinoline* ring attached through a hydroxymethylene group to a *quinuclidine* ring.

Quinuclidine   Quinoline

By altering the side chains attached to these rings and by esterifying and/or oxidizing the alcohol group, a large number of compounds have been produced and investigated.

Both *Quinine* and *quinidine* have a *methoxy* group attached to the quinoline ring and a *vinyl* group attached to the quinuclidine ring. Each has the same four chiral centers, but the diastereoisomerism involves only the configurations at the carbinol and 2-quinuclidine carbon atoms. *Cinchonine* and *cinchonidine* differ from these two alkaloids in that they do not have a methoxy group on the quinoline ring. Quinidine and cinchonine are dextrorotatory; whereas, quinine and cinchonidine are levorotatory. *Hydroquinine,* obtained from quinine by reduction with hydrogen and a catalyst, has the same structure as quinine except the vinyl group is reduced to an ethyl group. *Cupreine,* another naturally occurring *Cinchona* alkaloid, has an OH group in place of the methoxy group and *hydrocupreine* is cupreine with an ethyl group instead of a vinyl group. Therefore, quinine is the 6-methyl ether of cupreine and hydroquinine is the corresponding ether of hydrocupreine. Woodward and Doering first synthesized quinine in 1944 but the process is too costly for commercial use.

The salts of the alkaloids are typical amine salts. Since there are two nitrogen atoms present in the molecules of the *Cinchona* alkaloids, it is possible to form salts containing one or two equivalents of acid, such as mono- and dihydrochlorides. Quinine and its diastereoisomer, quinidine, are characterized

Table 26-15. Cinchona Alkaloids and Derivatives

Quinine   Quinidine   Cinchonine

Cinchonidine   Hydroquinine   Quinine Ethylcarbonate

Cupreine   Hydrocupreine   Ethylhydrocupreine

by the blue fluorescence of their solutions in dilute sulfuric or other oxyacids and by the *thalleioquin reaction*. The addition of two drops of bromine TS to 5 mL of a saturated solution of quinine or quinidine or a 1:1000 solution of their salts, followed by 1 mL of ammonia TS, produces an emerald green color due to the formation of thalleioquin. Quinine and quinidine are differentiated by their optical rotations and by their behavior toward alkali tartrate. In neutral or slightly acid solutions, quinine is precipitated by this reagent, but quinidine is not. On the other hand, quinidine, in moderately dilute solutions, is precipitated by soluble iodides but quinine is not affected. The same differences are exhibited by cinchonidine and its diastereoisomer, cinchonine; the former is levorotatory and, like quinine, is precipitated by alkali tartrates but cinchonine is dextrorotatory and unaffected by the reagent.

Other than quinine, quinidine, cinchonine, and cinchonidine, 18 other alkaloids have been isolated from cinchona barks. Some of these, such as cupreine, are found in only one kind of bark and some are doubtlessly split products (ie, not existing naturally in the bark but the result of the action of chemical agents upon them). The acids present are *quinic acid (hexahydro-1,3,4,5-tetrahydroxybenzoic acid), quinotannic acid,* and *quinovic acid (3β-hydroxyurs-12-ene-27,28-dioic acid)*. Also present are *α-quinovin* (a glycoside), *cinchona-red*, other coloring matter, and a volatile oil. The quinine and total alkaloid content is highest in the bark from the cultivated variety. Java bark, representing a highly cultivated plant, contains 7 to 10% of total alkaloids, of which about 70% is quinine. In the bark from the uncultivated plant, cinchonine and cinchonidine predominate.

Quinine was used as a treatment for malaria until the advent of synthetic anti-malarials during WWII. Quinidine also has anti-malarial properties and is used as a prophylaxis for cardiac arrhythmias and a treatment for arterial fibrillations. Java bark is infrequently used in the US but is employed elsewhere as a cheap substitute for quinine. It shares the *antimalarial*, *antipyretic*, and *analgetic* actions of quinine, but the alkaloidal salts are to be preferred to the galenical preparations. One of the principal difficulties in preserving its galenical preparations arises from the alteration and precipitation that the cinchotannic acid and its compounds undergo on storage. Glycerin has proved to be very useful by dissolving and holding these in solution, and hence it is present in nearly all of the preparations.

Ergot Alkaloids are derived from *Ergot*, a morbid growth formed when the fungus *Claviceps purpurea* develops on various plants of the *Gramineae* (grass) and *Cyperaceae* (sedge) families such as rye, wheat, oats, barley, and rice. If the infestation of the plant occurs naturally, the resulting ergot is called *natural* ergot; if the infestation is brought about artificially (ie, wholly or partly by human intervention), the resulting ergot is referred to as *cultivated* ergot. Ergots from different plants vary in composition, and therefore, they are not medicinally equivalent. It is for this reason that rye is stipulated as the source of official ergot. Ergot has yielded 12 different, well-defined alkaloids, each of which is an *N*-monosubstituted amide of either *normal* or *iso*lysergic acids. The substituting group on the amide nitrogen is commonly referred to as the *peptide moiety* of the alkaloid because it always contains one or more peptide (amide) linkages. In addition to alkaloids, ergot contains various carbohydrates, glycerides, sterols (ie, ergosterol and fungisterol), amino acids (ie, histidine, leucine, and tyrosine), amines (ie, histamine and tyramine), quaternary ammonium compounds (ie, choline and betaine), and coloring principles.

As mentioned, ergot alkaloids are all substituted amide derivatives of lysergic acid, which is shown below along with the official compounds and the important, but unofficial, diethylamide. It is the lysergic acid group that is their important medicinal constituent. Ergometrine, known in the US as ergonovine, produces an oxytocic effect (induces/assists with labor) and has been used as an analgesic for migraine headaches. Ergonovine, simpler by far than any of the other ergot alkaloids,

is commercially available both as the natural alkaloid and as a synthetic compound. It is soluble in water and dilute alcohol.

Lysergic Acid
(9,10-Didehydro-6-methylergoline-8β-carboxylic Acid)

Ergonovine (R = CH₃)
Methylergonovine (R = CH₂CH₃)

An understanding of the ergot alkaloids requires knowledge of the isomerism of lysergic acid, which exists in two diastereoisomeric forms depending on the spatial configuration of the carboxyl group relative to the 5β-hydrogen. In the *normal* lysergic acid (commonly called lysergic acid), this relative configuration is of the *cis* variety (carboxyl in β-configuration); in the *isolysergic acid*, it is of the *trans* type (carboxyl in α-configuration). *Chemical Abstracts* treats lysergic and isolysergic acid compounds as derivatives of ergoline, which is the 4,6,6aβ,7,8,9,10,10aα-octahydro form of indolo[4,3-*fg*]quinoline, *Ring Index* No 4550.

N,N-Diethyl-D-lysergamide, a compound of considerable interest, does not occur in nature. The physiologically active isomer is the (+)-enantiomorph of the *N,N*-diethylamide of normal lysergic acid and is commonly referred to as LSD-25 or simply LSD. Methods for its synthesis from lysergic acid have been developed. In normal subjects, LSD elicits a temporary combination of physiological and psychological effects that collectively mimic syndromes characteristic of psychotic states such as schizophrenia. LSD has been the subject of intense clinical investigation since the mid-1960s. There are no established therapeutic applications at present but it has found some application as a tool in psychopharmacology and in psychiatric diagnosis. Discovery of the psychotogenic activity of LSD has led to extensive research with various types of lysergic acid derivatives. It also has given rise to serious social problems.

N,N-**Diethyl-D-lysergamide (LSD)**

***Rauwolfia* Alkaloids,** such as reserpine, are obtained from several *Rauwolfia* species. Interest in the remarkable therapeutic properties of these powerful agents became so keen that reserpine alkaloid injections and tablets were admitted to the *USP XV* (by the 1959 supplement). Rescinnamine soon followed in *NF XI* in 1960 and syrosingopine gained *NF XII* recognition in 1965. Currently, only reserpine has official status. The general structure of these three alkaloids is shown below. *Chemi-*

cal Abstracts uses the familiar Barger-Scholz numbering. It will be observed that they are all esters of methyl reserpate with the only difference being in the identity of the acyl represented in the ester group at locus 18 of the heteronucleus. By the *Chemical Abstracts* system, methyl reserpate is the methyl ester of 18β-hydroxy-11,17-dimethoxy-3β,20α-yohimban-16β-carboxylic acid and yohimban is the 4aβ,13bα,14aα stereoisomer of the 1,2,3,4,4a,5,7,8, 13,13b,14,14a-dodecahydro form of *Ring Index* No 5874, benz[*g*]indolo[2,3-*a*]quinolizine. Reserpine and rescinnamine occur naturally; syrosingopine is synthetic.

Alkaloid	Acyl
Reserpine	**3,4,5-trimethoxybenzoyl**
Rescinnamine	**3,4,5-trimethoxycinnamoyl**
Syrosingopine	**carbethoxysyringoyl**

The genus *Rauwolfia,* natural order *Apocynaceae,* contains almost 50 species that grow in tropical and semitropical regions (India, Burma, Ceylon, Java, etc). The most extensively investigated species are *Rauwolfia serpentina* Benth, *R canescens* Linn, *R vomitoria* Afzel, and *R heterophylla* Roem. In ancient literature, mention is made of the use of *Rauwolfia* as a remedy for snakebites and scorpion stings, as a febrifuge, and as a cure for dysentery. The sedative action of the drug was also noted, for it was considered useful in *moon's disease* (lunacy), to induce sleep in children, and in hypochondria. Despite this long history, very few pharmacological and chemical studies were undertaken on *Rauwolfia* until the Indian investigators Bose and Sen reported successful clinical trials with the drug in 1941; the Indian chemists Siddiqui and Siddiqui isolated the first crystalline alkaloid from the plant in 1931. At present, at least 25 substances have been reported from *Reserpentina* alone, which, when assayed as directed, contains not less than 0.15% of reserpine-rescinnamine group alkaloids, calculated as reserpine. *Rauwolfia* preparations (known collectively as Rauwolfia) are available in the form of powdered whole root, extracts, selected alkaloidal fractions, the pure crystalline alkaloids *reserpine* and *rescinnamine,* and the synthetic *syrosingo pine.* The most prominent actions of its alkaloids are upon the cardiovascular and central nervous systems. They are widely employed as *antihypertensive agents* and as *adjuncts in psychotherapy.*

Vinca **Alkaloids**—During the late 1950s, pharmacological inquiries into the purported antihyperglycemic activity of principles contained in *Vinca rosae* Linn (Madagascan periwinkle of the Apocynaceae family) led to the initial discovery that two of the alkaloidal constituents, vincaleukoblastine (vinblastine) and leurocristine (vincristine), possessed certain demonstrable kinds of oncolytic (antitumor) activity. The overall result of these discoveries has been that the plant has been the subject, for several decades, of one of the most intensive phytochemical studies on record. Over 70 different alkaloids have been demonstrated to be present and more than half of these were recognized as new chemical compounds. The complete structure for most of the isolated compounds has been determined. An excellent review of the accomplishments during the first 7 years of intense research on the *Vinca* alkaloids is available.[25]

The therapeutic efficacy of vincaleukoblastine and leurocristine as antineoplastic agents has been established. The structures of these two closely related alkaloids are portrayed below. The four-ring heterosystem is a stereospecific hydrogenated form of 10*H*-3,7-methanoazacycloundecino[5,4-*b*]indole, *Ring Index* No 13276, and the five-ring system is a similar form of 1*H*-indolizino[8,1-*cd*]carbazole, *Ring Index* No 11065.

Vinblastine (vincaleukoblastine), R = CH₃
Vincristine (leurocristine), R = CHO
Vinglycinate, R = CH₃, R' = OCOCH₂N(CH₃)₂
Vindesine, R = CH₃, R' = OH, R'' = CONH₂

The costliness of vinblastine and vincristine provided increased interest in producing them synthetically. The five-ring indoline system is known to be available from other natural alkaloid sources. Vinglycinate and vindesine are additions wherein the structure has been modified synthetically.

An additional pharmaceutically relevant tryptophan-derived alkaloid is physostigmine, which is derived from calabor seeds, the dried ripe fruit of *Physostigma venenosum* (Leguminosae) and used to contract pupils and oppose the effect of mydriatics.

MISCELLANEOUS ALKALOIDS

The purine base alkaloids, better known as the **xanthine alkaloids,** have three medicinal important agents. They are secondary metabolites and are all methylated derivatives of 2,6-dioxypurine (xanthine). Three alkaloids, caffeine (1,3,7-trimethylxanthine), theophylline (1,3-dimethylxanthine), and theobromine (3,7-dimethylxanthine), comprise the bulk of this group. The structural relationships of the purine or xanthine alkaloids are portrayed in Table 26-16; purine is the parent molecule of each. The common practice of portraying the two-dimensional structure in box form is still primarily used. For example, the xanthine structure can be represented by:

Other bases closely related to purine are *hypoxanthine, adenine,* and *guanine,* all of which are found normally in animal tissues. The primary significance of the last two bases is the fact that they are constituents of nucleic acids and nucleoproteins that are found in cell nuclei and that hypoxanthine is produced in the body during the first stage of adenine oxidation. Subsequent oxidation yields *xanthine* and, finally, *uric acid.* In humans, the end product of protein metabolism is *urea.* In certain animals, the end product is *allantoin,* which is formed by further oxidation of uric acid. The two-dimensional structures of these compounds are illustrated in Table 26-16. The oxygen-containing compounds are depicted here in keto form but they often are shown in texts in enol form, as illustrated below with xanthine. The presence of oxygen in several of these structures also causes a slight alteration in the position of unsaturation because of the tautomerization that can occur. The enol forms often are named specifically to reflect the hydroxyl groups, such as purine-2,6,8-triol or 2,6,8- trioxypurine for uric acid.

Table 26-16. Xanthine Alkaloids

Xanthine
(3,7-Dihydro-1*H*-purine-2,6-dione)

Theophylline
(1,3-Dimethylxanthine)

Theobromine
(3,7-Dimethylxanthine)

Caffeine
(1,3,7-Trimethylxanthine)

1*H*-Purine

Adenine
(1*H*-Purin-6-amine)

Hypoxanthine
(1,7-Dihydro-6*H*-purine-6-one)

Guanine
(2-Amino-1,7-dihydro-6*H*-purine-6-one)

Uric Acid
(7,9-Dihydro-1*H*-purine-2,6,8(3*H*)-trione)

Allantoin
(2,5-Dioxo-4-imidazolidinyl)urea

The xanthines are very weak bases having a pK_b of approximately 13 to 14. They form readily hydrolysable salts with the stronger acids. By tautomeric shift of hydrogen from nitrogen to keto oxygen (enolization), a weakly acidic H (pK_a of about 9) is formed on the resulting OH group. Thus xanthine, along with various other oxopurines and their derivatives, forms salts with the stronger bases. Having no NH group to participate in enolization, caffeine is an exception.

keto structure   **enol structure**

The xanthines are characterized by the murexide reaction, which involves evaporating a nitric acid solution of the test sample to dryness and treating the residue with ammonia, whereupon a purplish-red color develops. The color is due to the formation of murexide, an ammonium salt of purpuric acid. Uric acid and various other purine derivatives also respond to this test.

Xanthine alkaloids are present in numerous plants including tea leaves obtained from *Thea sinensis* (Ternstroemiaceae), cocoa seeds/beans obtained from *Theobroma cacao* (Sterculiaceae), and coffee seeds/beans obtained from *Coffea arabica* and other *Coffea* species (Rubiaceae). A significant quantity of caffeine is present in tea and coffee and is responsible for their CNS stimulatory and diuretic effects. Theobromine has less CNS stimulatory and diuretic effects than caffeine. Theophylline is similar to caffeine except that is has a shorter and stronger diuretic effect and more significantly relaxes involuntary muscles.

The **imidazole alkaloid**, pilocarpine, is derived from various species of *Pilocarpus* (Rutaceae). It may be biosynthesized from histidine or threonine. It is an ophthalmic cholinergic drug used to contract the pupil and act as an antagonist to atropine. It also increases irrigation and decreases ocular pressure in the treatment of glaucoma.

PHENOLS

Phenols are very widespread in nature and are probably the largest group of secondary plant metabolites. They range from simple structures having a single aromatic ring to highly complex polymeric structures and often exist in glycosidic forms.

Phenols are biosynthesized through the shikimic acid pathway and may have aromatic rings derived through acetate condensation. They are frequently used as coloring agents, flavorings, aromatizers, and antioxidants. Phenols may be divided into several classes. Those of pharmaceutical importance are the simple phenolic compounds, tannins, anthraquinones, and flavonoids.

Simple phenolic compounds consist of a single phenolic ring and often possess alcholic, aldehydic, and carboxylic acid groups. Examples include vanillin, a phenolic aldehyde, and salicylic acid, a phenolic acid. Vanillin is found in the unripe fruits of varius species of *Vanilla* (Orchidaceae). It exists as the glycoside, glucovanillin, which yields vanillian and glucose upon hydrolysis. It has been used widely in both the food and perfume industries. Capsaicin (the vanillyl amide of isodecenoic acid) is found in the dried ripe fruit of different species of *Capsicum* (Solanaceae). It has been used internally for atonic dyspepsia and flatulence. Externally, it is frequently used as a counterirritant.

Tannins are more complex phenol compounds. They generally have molecular weights ranging from 1000 to 5000 and typically consist of a substantial number of phenolic groups (~1.5 per 100 MW), which are associated with an o-dihydroxy and o-trihydroxy orientation. Tannins having lower molecular weights are considered as pseudotannins. "True" tannins may be classified as hydrolysable, condensed, or complex. Hydrolysable tannins exist as glycosides with a glucose molecule and may be hydrolysed by acids or enzymes such as tannase. Their solutions turn blue with iron salts. Condensed tannins or proanthocyanidins have polymeric flavan-3-ol like structures. They are not associated with a sugar molecule, and therefore, are not readily hydrolyzed by acids or enzymes. Instead, they are usually precipitated as red insoluble compounds known as phlobaphenes. Complex tannins are formed from the joining of a hydrolysable and a condensed tannin.

Tannins are soluble in water, dilute bases, alcohol, glycerol, and acetone but generally sparingly soluble in other organic solvents. They occur widely in plants and are found in greatest quantity in dead or dying cells. Their inhibitory effects upon enzymes may contribute to the protective effects of bark. Tannins are also used commercially by the leather industry and have been used for dying and manufacturing ink. They have also been used therapeutically as a hemostatic agent and as antidiarrheals. Their ability to precipitate heavy metals, alkaloids, and glycosides has resulted in their use as antidotes in such poisonings. However, their use has recently been limited to topical astringents due to the discovery that tannic acid may cause severe necrosis of the liver.

Anthraquinones may exist in the free state or as glycosides with the sugar attached in various locations. The derivatives of anthraquinones may be di-, tri- (emodin), or tetrahydroxy (carminic acid) phenols. There may also be additional groups present such as methyl, hydroxymethyl (aloe-emodin), and carboxyl (carminic acid). Anthraquinones derivatives are often orange-red in color and soluble in hot water or dilute alcohol. This class also includes reduced derivatives of anthraquinones, the anthranols and anthrones, which are isomers and may exist in either form in solution. Anthrone is pale yellow, non-fluorescent, and insoluble in basic solutions; whereas, anthranol is brownish-yellow and strongly fluorescent in basic solutions. Anthranol derivatives are commonly found in aloes. Oxanthrones are intermediate products between anthraquinones and anthranols and may be converted to anthraquinones upon oxidation. They are found in cascara bark. Dianthrones are compounds formed by the combination of two like or unlike anthrone molecules resulting from mild oxidation. Two chiral centers are found in dianthrones, and therefore, a dianthrone consisting of two identical anthrone molecules may exist in two forms in addition to a *meso* form. Dianthrones are found in species of *Cassia, Rheum,* and *Rhamnus* with the sennidins (aglycones of sennosides) being the best-known examples. Anthraquinones and their derivatives generally have dyeing and purgative properties. The laxative action occurs only in the large intestine and, therefore, their therapeutic effect may take up to 6 hr to occur.

A variety of anthraquinone and anthrone derivatives have been isolated from senna pods, which consist of the dried, ripe fruits of *Cassia senna* and *Cassia angustifolia* (Leguminosae). Senna has been used for its purgative effects and remains to be a very important pharmaceutical laxative. Cascara bark is the dried bark of *Rhamnus purshianus* (Rhamnaceae) and contains a variety of anthracene derivatives present as both *O*- and *C*-glycosides. The primary glycosides are more active than the aloins whereas the free anthraquinones and dimers have less purgative activity. The cascarosides have a sweet and more pleasant taste than the aloins. Cascara is available as a liquid extract, elixir, or tablets and has a purgative active very similar to senna. Various types of anthraquinones and anthrones are found in the dried, underground parts of rhubarb, particularly *Rheum palmatum* and *R. officinale* (Polygonaceae), and are responsible for the purgative effects of these plants. Barbalion, the 10-glucopyranosyl glycosidic derivative of aloe-emodin-anthrone, is found in all commercial varieties of aloes, which are the solid residue obtained by evaporating the liquid that drains from the cut leaves of various species of *Aloe* (Liliaceae). This resin of aloes has been used for its purgative effects and should not be confused with "aloe vera," which is a mucilage found in the parenchymatous cells of the *Aloe vera* leaf. The red, dianthrone pigment, hypericin, is found in the dried, flowering, aerial parts of *Hypericum perforatum* (Guttiferae) or St. John's Wort. It has sedative and antiseptic properties. It also acts as a photosensitizer in mammals. Carminic acid is a *C*-glycoside anthraquinone derivative found in cochineal, which is a colorant derived from the dried female insects of *Dactylopius coccus*.

Flavonoids constitute the largest group of naturally occurring phenols and have been receiving much attention recently.[26] Flavonoids may exist in both the free and glycosidic state (typically the *O*-glycosoide form). They are formed from three acetate units and a phenylpropane unit and are distinguished by the state of oxygenation of the C3 unit. The dimeric forms, biflavonyls, are also well known. Flavonoids may be grouped into a number of classes such as flavones, flavonols, flavonones, xanthones, and isoflavones. Specific examples include hesperidin (the rhamnoglucoside of hesperetin or methyl eriodictyol) and rutin (the rhamnoglucoside of quercetin). The glycoside forms are typically soluble in water and alcohol but insoluble in organic solvents. Flavonoids dissolve in basic solutions resulting in a yellow color, which increases with pH and the number of hydroxyl groups but dis-

appears to a colorless solution upon the addition of acid. The flavones are most commonly found in the cell sap and young tissue of higher plants (particularly Polygonaceae, Rutaceae, Leguminosae, Unbelliferae, and Compositae) but are widely distributed in nature. Their therapeutic activity may result from their effect upon arachidonic acid metabolism.[27] They posses anti-inflammatory, anti-allergic, antithrombitic, and vasoprotective (decreased capillary fragility) effects. They also prevent tumor promotion and protect the gastric mucosa. Some flavonoids also have antibacterial and antifungal activity and flavonoligans such as silybin (a 1,4-dioxan produced from the oxidative combination of taxifolin and coniferyl alcohol and found in one of the milk-thistles, *Carduus marianus* (Compositae)) have anti-hepatoxic properties.

VOLATILE OILS, RESINS, AND MISCELLANEOUS ISOPRENOIDS

Composition and Structure

Volatile, or essential, oils differ from the other classes previously discussed in that they are complex mixtures of a variety of hydrocarbons and oxygenated compounds. In some countries they are called *olea aetherea*. In some instances they are called *essences*, a name that conflicts with our ordinary use of the word to designate an alcoholic solution of a volatile oil. The following groups of compounds occur in the volatile oils: hydrocarbons, alcohols, acids, esters, aldehydes, ketones, phenols and phenol ethers, lactones, and various nitrogen and sulfur organic compounds. In some cases, such as mustard oil and bitter almond oil, they are derived from glycosides. The hydrocarbons of chief importance are the *terpenes* ($C_{10}H_{16}$) and the *sesquiterpenes* ($C_{15}H_{24}$; literally, *one and one-half terpenes*). The terpenes have the formula C_nH_{2n-4} and typically occur in the following configurations:

- Three double bonds and no ring, such as *myrcene* (found in Myrcia Oil) and *ocimene* (found in the volatile oil from the leaves of *Ocimum gratissimum*)
- Two double bonds and one ring, such as *limonene* (widespread occurrence but especially in the citrus oils)
- One double bond and two rings, such as either α-*pinene* or β-*pinene* (the first of which is of very widespread occurrence; together, these two terpenes comprise at least 90% of the bulk of turpentine oil).

Terpenes

α-Pinene   **β-Pinene**

Limonene

Myrcene

The sesquiterpenes have the formula C_nH_{2n-6}, and therefore, occur in even more varied configurations. Sesquiterpenes are biosynthesized from farnesyl pyrophosphate and may have linear, monocyclic, or bicyclic structures.[28] They are secondary metabolites with some being formed as the result of some stress or injury to the plant. Although a number of these hydrocarbons have been isolated, many of their structures are not definitely known. Among those of known structure are *zingiberene* (from Ginger oil) and *bisabolene* (from Bisabol myrrh oil).

Hydrocarbons other than the terpene types are sometimes present. An example is the saturated hydrocarbon *n*-heptane (C_7H_{16}), which occurs in the volatile oil obtained from the oleoresin of *Pinus sabiniana* and *P jeffreyi* and from the fruits of *Pittosporum resiniferum* (the so-called *petroleum nut* of a tree growing in the Philippines). However, many of the essential oils owe their character and their value to constituents other than hydrocarbons. Among these are organic *acids* such as acetic, benzoic, cinnamic, and phenylacetic; *alcohols* such as benzyl alcohol, borneol, cinnamyl alcohol, citronellol, geraniol, linalool, menthol, phenylethyl alcohol, and terpineol; *aldehydes* such as anisaldehyde, cinnamaldehyde, benzaldehyde, citral, piperonal or heliotropin, salicylaldehyde, and vanillin; *ketones* such as carvone, camphor, thujone, and pulegone; *esters* such as bornyl acetate, methyl salicylate, benzyl benzoate, geranyl acetate, and linalyl acetate; *phenols* such as thymol, carvacrol, and chavicol; *phenol ethers* such as anethol, eugenol, and safrol; and many other more complex compounds such as coumarin and indole.

Alcohols

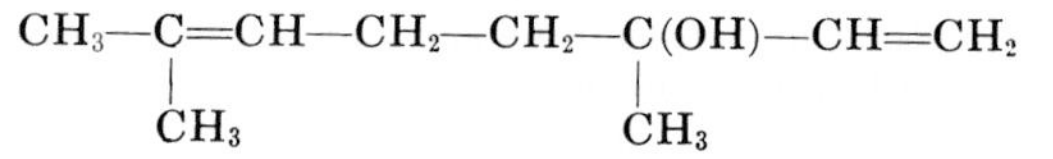

$CH_3-C=CH-CH_2-CH_2-C(OH)-CH=CH_2$
with CH_3 and CH_3 substituents
Linalool

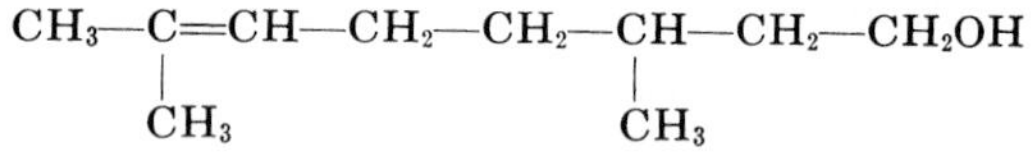

$CH_3-C=CH-CH_2-CH_2-CH-CH_2-CH_2OH$
with CH_3 and CH_3 substituents
Citronellol

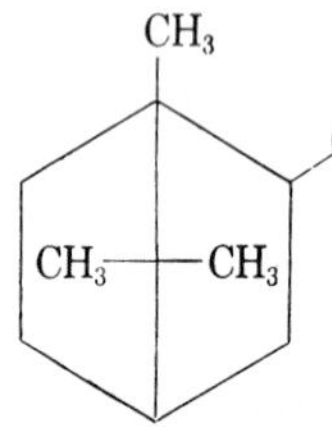

Borneol

Aldehydes

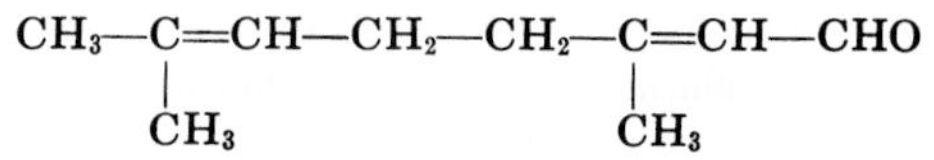

$CH_3-C=CH-CH_2-CH_2-C=CH-CHO$
with CH_3 and CH_3 substituents
Citral
(*cis*-**Neral**)
(*trans*-**Geranial**)

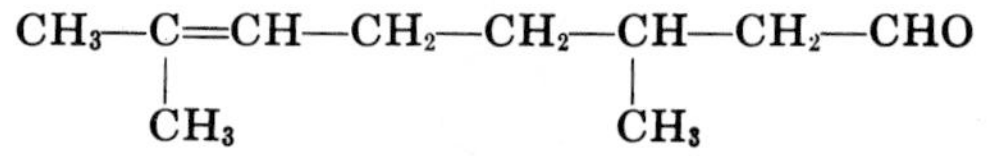

$CH_3-C=CH-CH_2-CH_2-CH-CH_2-CHO$
with CH_3 and CH_3 substituents
Citronellal

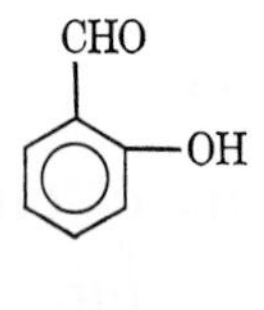

Salicylaldehyde 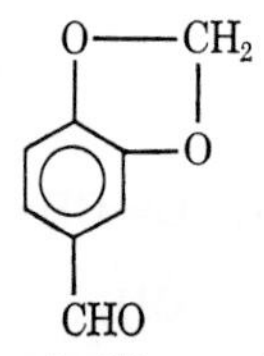   **Heliotropin (Piperonal)**

Ketones

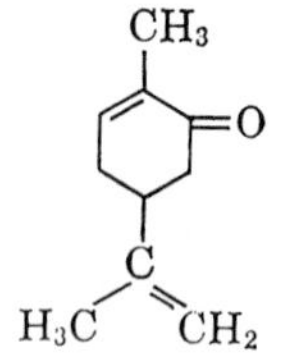

Carvone 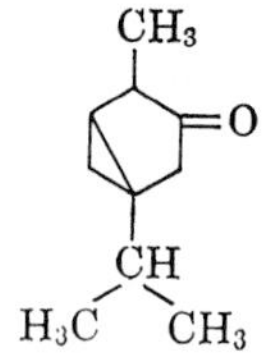   **Thujone** 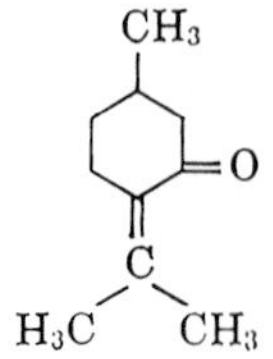   **Pulegone**

Phenols and Phenol Ethers

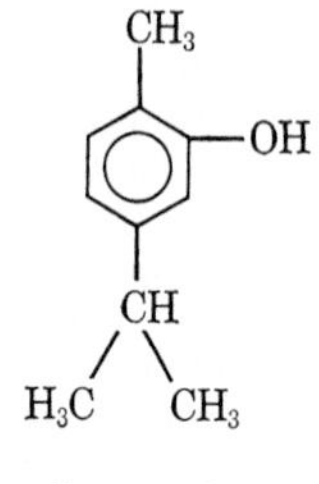

Carvacrol 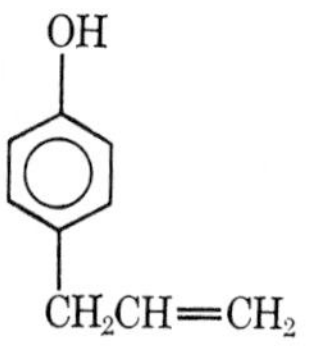   **Chavicol**

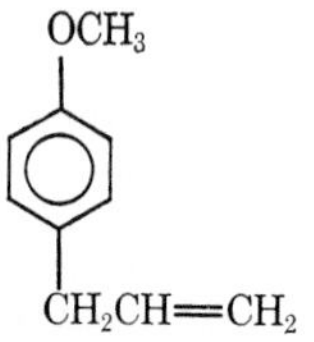

***O*-Methylchavicol** 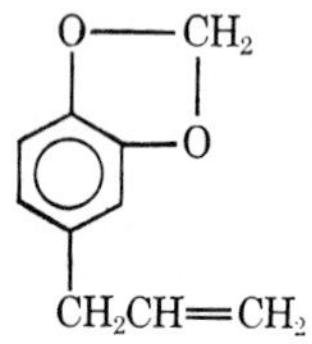   **Safrol**

Physical and Chemical Properties

The properties of volatile oils differ greatly from those of fixed oils. Most of the volatile oils are colorless when pure and fresh or can be made colorless by redistillation. Upon exposure to the air, they acquire various colors, becoming green, as in oil of wormwood; yellow, as in oil of peppermint; red, as in oil of origanum; and brown, as in oil of cinnamon. The blue color of oil of chamomile is an inherent property of the oil even when freshly distilled and is due to the highly unsaturated hydrocarbon *chamazulene* $(C_{15}H_{18})$. Their volatility results in their aromatic properties. The odors and tastes of volatile oils are determined by their oxygenated compound content, and therefore, they are extremely variable and their most characteristic feature. The odor of an oil is modified by exposure to the air. Oil of turpentine may be rectified by redistillation in an atmosphere of carbon dioxide, or *in vacuo*, so that it will be almost odorless or have an agreeable, fragrant odor. However, a very slight exposure to the air is sufficient to restore its well-known unpleasant odor. Other terpene-containing oils are quickly oxidized and the delicacy and fineness of their flavor and odor are seriously impaired. This is especially true of orange and lemon oils. Some volatile oils are sweet; others have a mild, pungent, hot, acrid, caustic, or burning taste.

The specific gravity of official volatile oils also varies (from 0.842 to 1.172) with the majority of them being lighter than water. Optical activity is used to determine the purity of many oils. Refractive index serves as a delicate test for both the identity and purity of oils. Because most volatile oils consist of complex mixtures of many types of compounds, their boiling point is of little significance. In general, the terpenes and sesquiterpenes are practically insoluble in water but soluble in alcohol, ether, chloroform, benzene, petroleum benzin, and the fixed and volatile oils. Even though water is a poor solvent for volatile oils, it acquires a decided odor and flavor when brought in contact with the oil in a finely divided state, as in the preparation of medicated waters. Alcohol, ether, chloroform, glacial acetic acid, petroleum ether, benzene, and many other organic solvents will dissolve volatile oils. Alcohol is a better solvent for oxygenated oils than for terpenes. Many official oils are required to meet specific solubility tests in 70%, 80%, or 95% alcohol. Volatile oils freely dissolve fixed oils, fats, resins, camphors, and usually sulfur and phosphorus.

Exposure to light and air impairs the quality and destroys the fragrance of volatile oils. Peroxides frequently develop in oils containing terpenes and, after extended exposure, the oils thicken and become resinified, or deposit crystalline compounds. The whitening of corks after insertion for a long time in bottles containing certain volatile oils is caused by the bleaching action of the peroxides that are gradually produced during the oils decomposition. This is only true for oils containing notable amounts of terpenes. Therefore, such volatile oils should be kept in well-filled, tightly stoppered, amber-colored bottles in a cool place. A suggestion has been made to replace the air in the original packages with nitrogen to prevent oxidation. Storage in metal cans causes pronounced deterioration in odor and the development of color. In some volatile oils, such as thyme, a separation into a solid and a liquid portion occurs upon standing in the cold. The solid portion is frequently known by the name *stearoptene* and the liquid portion is called *eleoptene*. Some stearoptenes are of commercial importance (eg, thymol, camphor, and menthol).

Occurrence and Uses

Volatile oils are found in various plant organs and tissues. They usually constitute the savory and odorous principles of the plants in which they exist and they either preexist in the tissues or are produced by the reaction of certain constituents when the tissues are brought into contact with water, which results in hydrolysis of their glycosides. Volatile oils are often associated with other substances such as resins and gums, and as mentioned previously, they typically resinify themselves upon exposure to air. They are generally obtained from plants by distillation with steam, distillation *per se* (or without the use of water), expression, and extraction. Volatile oils are sometimes actually formed through destructive distillation (ie, the oils of tar and amber). These are occasionally referred to as *pyrolea* or *empyreumatic oils*. Volatile oils are commonly used for flavoring and perfuming. Many volatile oils also have additional therapeutic effects. For example, camphor is used as an external rubefacient, clove and thyme have been used as antiseptics due to their high phenol content, caraway has been used as a carminative and antispasmodic, cinnamon oil has been used as a germicide, and ginger has been used as an anti-inflammatory, anti-platelet, anti-ulcer, antibacterial/fungal, and anti-emetic.

Resins

Resins are usually the oxidized terpenes of volatile oils and are more or less solid, amorphous products having a complex chemical nature. They typically consist of a mixture of acids, alcohols, esters, and phenols with inert compounds known as resenes. They should not be referred to as balsams, which contain a high amount of aromatic balsamic acids and consist primarily of fixed oils and waxes. Resins typically soften or melt upon heating and are insoluble in water but dissolve to different extents in alcohol, chloroform, and ether. As a result of their poor water solubility, they typically have little taste. Resins are typically found as normal physiological products in plant ducts and cavities but their yield increases upon injury. This further differentiates them from balsams, which are usually not formed until injury occurs making them of pathological origin. Resins are often associated with volatile oils and gums. For example, natural oleoresins, such as turpentine, consist of a mixture of volatile oils and resins, and gum resins are natural mixtures of gums and resins.

Podophyllum resin is derived from the dried rhizome and roots of *Podophyllum peltatum* (Berberidaceae) also know as May-apple or Wild Mandrake. Its chief active constituents are lignans, which are C18 compounds biosynthesized from the dimerization of two C6-C3 units, such as coniferyl alcohol, at the β-carbon of the side chains. The most important lignans present in this resin are β-peltatin and α-peltatin.[29] The resin also contains smaller amounts of the closely related 4′-demethylpodophyllotoxin. Podophyllum resin has cytotoxic activities and is used in the treatment of soft warts. Etoposide (4′-demethylepipodophyllotoxin ethylideneglucoside) is a lignan derivative obtained semisynthetically from podophyllotoxin and has been used in the treatment of small-cell lung cancer, testicular cancer, lymphomas, and leukemias.

Miscellaneous Isoprenoids

In addition to the isoprenoids mentioned previously, several others are of pharmaceutical importance. Valeranone is a sesquiterpene component of the volatile oil from valerian, which consists of the rhizome, stolons, and roots of *Valeriana officinalis* (Valerianaceae) and is responsible for the herbs sedative properties.[30] The sesquiterpene lactones, parthenolide and 3β-hydroxyparthenolide, are used to standardize feverfew, which is derived from various species of *Parthenium* (Compositae) and has been used for the treatment of fever, arthritis, migraine, and other disorders.[31] The leaves of *Ginkgo biloba* (Ginkgoaceae) contain several diterpene lactones (ginkgolides A, B, C, J, and M) that are platelet-activating factor antagonists. They have been characterized to consist of a tertiary butyl group and six 5-member rings. Carotenes are C_{40} tetraterpenoids often associated with chlorophyll and participate in photosynthesis. They may also be found in other plants organs. Carotenes are yellow or orange-red in color. For example, the carotenoids, lycopene and citraurin, are responsible for the color of red tomatoes and oranges, respectively. As a result, carotenes have been used extensively as colorants. They also possess vitamin A activity, which is a diterpenoid produced in animal livers by enzymatic hydrolysis of β-carotene. The taxane diterpenoid derivative, taxol, is derived from the bark of the pacific yew, *Taxus brevifolia*, (Taxaceae). Taxol consists of a four-membered oxetane ring and a complex ester side-chain. These structures provide taxol with its anti-cancer activity.

REFERENCES

1. Estes JW. Food as medicine. In: Kiple KF, Ornelas KC, eds. *The Cambridge World History of Food*. Cambridge: Cambridge University Press, 2000.
2. Lust JB. Herbs and history. In: *The Herb Book*. New York: Benedict Lust Publications, 1974, pp 3–9.
3. Simpson BB, Ogorzaly MC. Medicinal plants. In: Prancan KM, Barter PW, Luhrs M, eds. *Economic Botany: Plants in Our World*. New York: McGraw-Hill, 1995, pp 376–382.
4. El-Assal GS. *The Lancet* 1972; (Aug 5):272–274.
5. Der Marderosian A. Foods and "health foods" as drugs. In: *Encyclopedia of Pharmaceutical Technology, Vol. 6*. New York: Marcel Dekker, 1992, pp 251–274.
6. Kratz AM. *JAMA* 1998; 1:1.
7. Varro ET. *The Honest Herbal*, 3rd ed. New York: Haworth Press, 1993, pp xi–xvi.
8. Eisenberg DM, Kessler RC, Roster C, et al. *N Engl J Med* 1993; 328(4):246–252.
9. USP. *The Standard*. January/February 1998: 3.
10. Anonymous. *Journal of the American Dietetic Association* 1999; 99(10): 1278–1285.
11. Der Marderosian A. Foods and health foods as drugs. In: Schicher H, Phillipson JD, Loew D, eds. *Acta Horticulturae*. WOCMAP. 1993, pp 81–93.
12. DerMarderosian A, et al. *Guide to Popular Natural Products*, 2nd ed. St. Louis, MO: Facts and Comparisons, 2001.
13. *United States Pharmacopeia and National Formulary (USP 27–NF 22)*. Rockville, MD: The United States Pharmacopeial Convention, Inc., 2003.
14. Debromer D. *American Druggist* 1992; 205(5):34–40.

15. Kottke MK. *Drug Development and Industrial Pharmacy* 1998; 24(12):1177–1195.
16. Lipp FJ. *Alternative Therapies* 1996; 2(4):36–41.
17. Der Marderosian A. *New Ideas in Herbal Therapy.* New York: POW-ERx-PAK Communications, 1998
18. Hawk PB, et al. *Practical Physiological Chemistry,* 13th ed. New York: Blakiston, 1954.
19. Nelson NA, et al. *Chem Eng News* Aug 16, 1982: 30.
20. Newton RF, Roberts SM. *Tetrahedron* 1980; 36:2163.
21. Stjernschantz J, Bahram R. *Drugs of the Future* 1992; 17(8):691.
22. Patel AV, et al. *Fitoterapia* 1987; 58:67.
23. Mahato SB, et al. *Phytochemistry* 1988; 27:3037 and 1991; 30:1357.
24. Gibson. *Lloydia* 1978; 41:348.
25. Voboda GH, et al. *J Pharm Sci* 1962; 51:707.
26. Harborne JB, ed. *The Flavonoids: Advances in Research Since 1986.* London: Chapman and Hall, 1993.
27. Pathak D, et al. *Fitoterapia* 1991; 62:371.
28. Fraga,BM. *Nat Prod Rep* 1993; 10:397.
29. Jackson DE, Dewick PM. *Phytochemistry* 1984; 23:1147.
30. Houghton J. *Ethnopharmacol* 1988; 22:121.
31. Berry. *Pharm J* 1994; 253:806.

BIBLIOGRAPHY

Armstrong FB. *Biochemistry,* 3rd ed. New York: Oxford University Press, 1989.
Briggs MH, ed. *Advances in Steroid Biochemistry and Pharmacology.* New York: Academic Press, 1970.
Brossi A. *The Alkaloids*, vols 22, 38, 39. New York: Academic Press, 1983, 1990.
Crabbe P, ed. *Prostaglandin Research.* New York: Academic Press, 1977.
Cuthbert MF, ed. *The Prostaglandins: Pharmacologic and Therapeutic Advances.* Philadelphia: JB Lippincott, 1973.
Devlin TM. *Textbook of Biochemistry,* 3rd ed. New York: Wiley-Liss, 1992.
Drugs of the Future, vols 11–17. Barcelona, Spain: JR Prous, 1986–1992.
Evans WC. *Trease and Evans' Pharmacognosy,* 14th ed. London: WB Saunders, 1999.
Guenther E. *The Essential Oils,* 6 vols. New York: Van Nostrand, 1949–1952.
Gunstone F. *An Introduction to the Chemistry and Biochemistry of Fatty Acids and Their Glycerides,* 2nd ed. London: Chapman & Hall, 1968.
Hesse M. *Alkaloid Chemistry.* New York: Wiley-Interscience, 1981.
Honeyman J, Guthrie RD. *An Introduction to the Chemistry of Carbohydrates.* 3rd ed. Oxford: Clarendon, 1968.
Karim SSM, ed. *Prostaglandins: Chemical and Biochemical Aspects.* Baltimore: University Park Press, 1976.
Korolkovas A. *Essentials of Medical Chemistry,* 2nd ed. New York: Wiley, 1988.
Leach SJ, ed. *Physical Properties and Techniques of Protein Chemistry.* New York: Academic Press, (Part A) 1969, (Part B) 1970, (Part C) 1973.
Oesterling TO, et al. *J Pharm Sci* 1972; 61:1861.
Pelletier SW, ed. *Chemistry of the Alkaloids.* New York: Van Nostrand, 1970.
Putnam FW. *The Plasma Proteins,* 2nd ed, 3 vols. New York: Academic Press, 1975.
Rafauf R. *Handbook of Alkaloids and Alkaloid Containing Plants.* New York: Wiley, 1970.
Roberts SM, Newton RF. *Prostaglandins and Thromboxanes.* Boston: Butterworths, 1982.
Rosenfeld I. *Dr. Rosenfeld's Guide to Alternative Medicine.* New York: Fawcett Columbine, 1996.
Shamma M. *The Isoquinoline Alkaloids: Chemistry and Pharmacology.* New York: Academic Press, 1972.
Tyler VE. *Herbs of Choice.* New York: Haworth Press, 1994.
Tyler VE. *The Honest Herbal,* 3rd ed. New York: Haworth Press, 1983.
Wolff M. *Burger's Medicinal Chemistry and Drug Discovery,* 5th ed. vols 1, 4, 5. New York: Wiley, 1995, 1997.
Zubay G. *Biochemistry.* Reading, MA: Addison-Wesley, 1983.

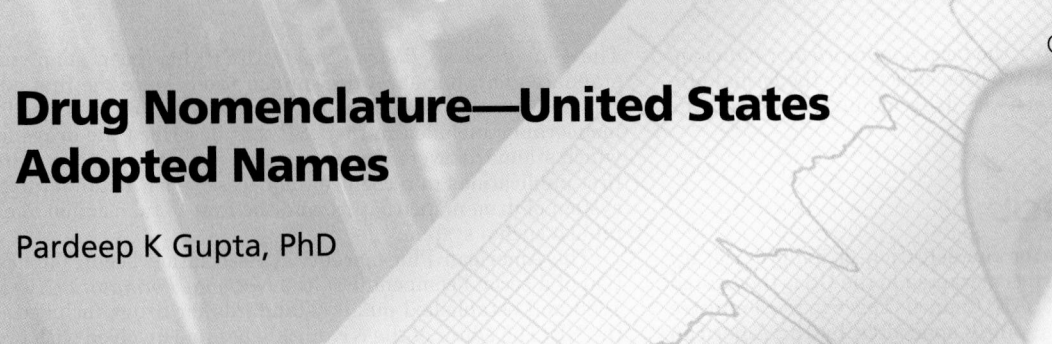

CHAPTER 27

Drug Nomenclature—United States Adopted Names

Pardeep K Gupta, PhD

Advances in the scientific disciplines continue to occur at such an accelerated rate that the processing of information has become a separate and distinct discipline in its own right. Precise and current terminology is an important tool of science, and nowhere is it more important than in medicine and pharmacy. Drug nomenclature, particularly, would become confusing, meaningless, and incomprehensible without a well-developed system of rules.

It is not unusual for each drug entity to be known by several chemical names, more than one code number, several trivial designations, a formally selected nonproprietary name, and one or more trademarks. Therefore, it is essential that a logical, well-defined nonproprietary nomenclature system is available to facilitate the exchange of drug information.

This chapter describes the mechanisms for creating nonproprietary drug names that are used in the US. It includes history, scope, function, and operation of the nomenclature system devised by the United States Adopted Names (USAN) Council. A brief introduction of the policies of the World Health Organization (WHO) International Nonproprietary Name (INN) program and its relationship to the USAN Council have been added.

DRUG NAME TYPES

The term *drug nomenclature* implies that drugs may have several types of names, each having its own function, and indeed this is the case. Although some names are scientifically precise, others may be ambiguous or misleading.

The first type of name, usually applied to compounds of known composition, is the *chemical name*. Among the several conventions that exist for creating chemical names, the most widely established is the American Chemical Society's Chemical Abstracts Services (CAS) Index naming system. Use of this system results in the creation of systematic (CAS Index) names for chemical entities that serve as a key to the chemical literature of the world. The CAS system is used by the USAN program.

For substances of plant or animal origin that cannot be classified as pure chemical compounds, scientific identification is given in terms of precise *biochemical, botanical, or zoological names*. Such designations are also scientifically exact, but like their chemical counterparts, they tend to be complex, unwieldy, and generally not useful to the physician, pharmacist, or other users of drug nomenclature.

Most developing drug materials while being investigated acquire a *code designation* as a convenient means of referring to the compound before it has been assigned either a nonproprietary name or a trademark. Such codes are generally a letter and number combination, eg, SC-40230 (bidisomide, *Searle*), Ro 4-3780 (isotretinoin, *Roche*), or RP 56976 (docetaxel, *Rhone-Poulenc*

Rorer). The letter(s) generally represent an abbreviation of the research laboratory name; the numbers are assigned by the firm in an arbitrary manner or following some internally created convention. Codes may be acronyms or letter combinations derived from portions of the chemical or common name (eg, AZT for azidothymidine or TPA for tissue plasminogen activator).

Code designations usually are considered as convenient "shop labels" and are meant to be discarded when a more appropriate name is selected. However, many of these codes appear in early scientific literature dealing with investigative work prior to the selection of a nonproprietary name. Frequently they are used in clinical studies in the absence of a nonproprietary name to identify the chemical entity. Code designations, therefore, must be considered a part of drug nomenclature, but they are not acceptable for general use. In themselves, these codes give no information about the compound they represent.

The use of acronyms instead of the proper nonproprietary names may also be dangerous because many contractions are extremely similar, such as DDI (didanosine) and DDC (zalcitabine). Similarly, AZT, is commonly used for the antiviral zidovudine (derived from *azidothymidine,* its shortened chemical name). However, AZT can just as readily represent the immunosuppressant azathioprine. Medication errors due to use of acronyms have been reported both by the Institute for Safe Medication Practices and the USP Medication Errors Reporting Program.

Trivial names occasionally are assigned to a new compound, usually by the researchers working on it. Nomenclature agencies strongly discourage the use of trivial names as generally they are coined haphazardly and are usually not suited for adoption as official nonproprietary names. Too frequently trivial names are confusingly similar to existing names, which may lead to confusing them with established nonproprietary names.

When a new drug has successfully survived the successive research stages and testing to the point where it appears it may become a marketable product, a *trademark* is developed by the manufacturer. Properly registered trademarks become the legal property of their owners and cannot be used freely in the public domain. Selected for their brevity and ease of recall, trademarks usually give little or no scientific information about the drug.

Each type of name described thus far aims to serve its specific purpose; however, none fulfill the need for a single, simple, informative designation available for unrestricted public use. The *nonproprietary name* is the only name intended to function in this capacity. The nonproprietary name often is referred to as the *generic name,* but this practice is inaccurate, as each nonproprietary name is specific for a given compound, even though it may possess a stem that is common to a related group of drugs.

Throughout this chapter, the term *nonproprietary name* applies to those names that have been selected by the formal process of negotiation between the drug manufacturer and the USAN Council.

THE USAN COUNCIL

The agency responsible for the selection of nonproprietary names for single-entity drugs marketed in the US is the United States Adopted Names (USAN) Council. This expert committee on drug nomenclature is jointly sponsored by the American Medical Association (AMA), the United States Pharmacopeial Convention Inc (USPC), and the American Pharmaceutical Association (APhA). All three agencies were involved in the selection of drug names for many years prior to the establishment of the USAN Council in the 1960s. The aim of USAN is the global standardization and unification of drug nomenclature and related rules to ensure that drug information is communicated accurately and unambiguously. The Council conducts its negotiation activity by correspondence. Twice a year, the Council convenes to discuss nomenclature policy, liaison activity, and new nomenclature strategies.

The USA Council Secretariat is located at the AMA headquarters in Chicago, Illinois. The agency works closely with the World Health Organization (WHO) International Nonproprietary Name (INN) Committee, and various national nomenclature groups. In addition, USAN program has liaison organizations all over the world. As of 2003, these organizations include the following:

The *United States Pharmacopeia* (USP) has been supplying standards for pharmaceutical preparations since the first edition appeared in 1820. Because there was a need for titles for monographs included in the USP that described the drugs for which standards were being prepared, the USP was one of the first publications to recognize the necessity for a standardized system of drug nomenclature and the first to take action to establish such a system.

The American Pharmaceutical Association began publication of a second compendium, the *National Formulary* (NF) in 1888 and established quality standards for drugs included in the NF. The editor of the NF quickly became involved with providing nonproprietary names for the monographs published in the NF.

In 1906, the US government legally recognized the significance of the work being done by the USP and the NF by declaring both publications *official* compendia. Since that time, monograph titles have had the status of official nonproprietary names.

As new pharmaceutical products increased in number, other organizations recognized the need for formally approved names while the drug entity was still in its investigational stages. The AMA Council on Pharmacy and Chemistry (CPC), later known as the Council on Drugs, was created in 1905 as an advisory body to the Board of Trustees to encourage rational drug use by physicians. In conjunction with screening and evaluating new remedies, the CPC initiated a nomenclature program to provide nonproprietary names for individual drugs available commercially under more than one trademark. This activity continued until the early 1940s when the Council on Drugs began to re-

Chemical Abstracts Service
2540 Olentangy River Road
PO Box 3012
Columbus, OH 43210-0012
Attn: Sabine P. Kuhn, PhD **WHO INN Committee Secretariat**
World Health Organization
1211 Avenue Appia
Geneva 27-Switzerland
Attn: Raffaella Balocco-Mattavelli, PhD

CHINA
The Deputy Chief
Drug Standard Division II Pharmacopeia Commission
Ministry of Health
Temple of Heaven
Beijing 100050
People's Republic of China

ITALY
DCE Commission - Denominazione
Communi Italiane
Director-General
Pharmaceutical Division
Ministero della Sanità
Viale della Civiltà Romana 7
1-00144 Roma

RUSSIA
Director
Pharmedinfo
Ministry of Health
PO Box 195
Moscow 103051, Russian Federation

UNITED KINGDOM
BAN - British Approved Names
The Secretary
British Pharmacopoeia Commission
Market Towers
1 Nine Elms Lane
London SW8 5NQ

BELGIUM
L'Inspecteur en chef-Directeur
Ministère de la Santé Publique et de l'EnvironementInspection
générale de la Pharmacie
Pharmacie Cité administrative de l'Etat
Cité administrative de l'Etat Quartier Vésale 333 B1010
Bruxelles

FRANCE
DCF Denominations
Communes Francaises Agence du Medicament
Agence du MedicamentDirection des Laboratoires
et des Controles
Unite Pharmacopee

JAPAN
JAN–Japanese Accepted Names
Japanese Ministry of Health and Welfare
New Drugs Division
Pharmaceuticals Affairs Bureau
1-2-2, Kasumigaseki, Chiyoda-ku
Tokyo 100

SPAIN
Ministerio de Sanidad Y Consumo
Direccion General de Farmacia
Centro Instit de Info de Medicamentos,
CINIME–Paseo del PrDO 18-20, Planta 15
28014 Madrid

quire a nonproprietary name for every active compound listed in all AMA publications.

The 1938 Food, Drug and Cosmetic (FD&C) Act stipulated that the *common or usual name* should be used as part of drug labeling to identify the drug entity. In the absence of such a name (or until a name attained such status), a chemical name was to be used.

The Drug Amendments of 1962 replaced the "common or usual" terminology with the more meaningful requirement that nonproprietary names must be "simple and useful." Also, for the first time, the Commissioner of the Food and Drug Administration (FDA) was given the authority to designate the official name if he determined that such action was necessary or desirable.

Despite the nomenclature activities of the AMA, USP, and APhA, large numbers of drug products did not become the subject of either the NF, the USP, or the Council on Drugs monographs and continued to be identified by their chemical names, trivial names, or trademarks selected by the manufacturers. As medicine and pharmacy advanced and drugs became more specific in their actions and structurally more complex, other nomenclature-related needs were recognized that made it apparent that each new drug needed a nonproprietary name selected early in its development. A systematic approach to assure drug name appropriateness and acceptability to AMA, USP, NF, and the drug manufacturer now became more obvious. Each new drug also needed a *global name*—one name used and accepted worldwide.

A significant step toward supplying this need was taken in June 1961, with the formation of the AMA-USP Nomenclature Committee. The names adopted by this committee were deemed acceptable as potential compendia monograph titles, and the acronym *USAN* (United States Adopted Name) was coined to designate names formally processed and approved by the Committee. The APhA participated in the program from its inception but did not become a full and official sponsor until January 1964, at which time the name of the committee was changed to the USAN Council.

The FDA and the USAN Council conducted an unofficial liaison until early 1967 when it was determined that a formal cooperative effort in the development of nonproprietary names would be more beneficial to both. In June 1967 an official agreement was signed between the sponsors of the USAN Council and the FDA that required the FDA to appoint annually one voting member to the Council. This contract stipulated that the FDA would accept as the "official or established" name any drug name the USAN Council adopted. In this agreement, the Commissioner of the FDA reserved the right to select the official name in those instances in which the USAN Council could not reach consensus. It should be noted that the designation of a name as an *official* or *established name* by the FDA did not follow automatically, but rather was accomplished by publication, subject to public comment, in the *Federal Register*. All parties upheld this agreement until it was modified 17 years later.

On November 26, 1984, the Commissioner of Food and Drugs and the Secretary of Health and Human Services published in the *Federal Register* an amendment to the FD&C Act that stated in part that

> "the Food and Drug Administration agrees with 'Guiding Principles for Coining US Adopted Names for Drugs', published in USAN and the USP Dictionary of Drug Names . . . [, and that] the established name . . . will ordinarily be either the compendial name of the drug or, if there is no compendial name, the common or usual name of the drug. Interested persons, in the absence of the designation of an official name, may rely on the USAN listed in USAN and the USP Dictionary of Drug Names as being the established name in accordance with the Federal Food, Drug, and Cosmetic Act."

Today, the USAN Council is comprised of five members: one member is appointed by each of the three sponsoring organizations, one is a liaison member from the FDA, and one is a member-at-large who must be approved by the three sponsoring organizations. Council members are nominated by their sponsoring organization annually. Every year their nomination must be approved by the boards of trustees of the other sponsoring organizations, who also approve the nominees for the FDA liaison and the member-at-large positions. Council members may serve for up to 10 consecutive years. The council members for 2003 are:

Daniel L Boring, PhD (FDA)
Everett Flanigan, PhD (USP)
William M Heller, PhD (Member-at-Large)
John E Kasik, MD, PhD (AMA)
Anthony Palmieri, III, PhD, (APhA)

At an early stage in the development of the USAN Council, it was anticipated that occasional disagreements might arise between the Council and a manufacturer over the selection of a particular nonproprietary name. In the majority of such cases, the Council and the firm can, in time, work out an acceptable compromise; however, in rare instances, an impasse may develop that needs adjudication by someone not directly involved with the USAN Council or the drug manufacturer. The USAN Review Board was established as the final arbitrator of nomenclature disputes when normal procedures have failed. Each sponsoring organization nominates two members to the Review Board annually; nominations must be approved annually by the Boards of Trustees of the other sponsoring organizations. No term limits have been placed on member's participation on the Review Board. Members of the Review Board for 2003 are

Donald R. Bennett, MD, PhD (AMA), (*Chair*)
Jordan Cohen, PhD (USP)
Stuart Feldman, PhD (APhA)
Alice Jean Matuszak, PhD (APhA)
Lauren A. Woods, MD, PhD (AMA)
Gary L. Yingling, JD (USP)
Joseph G. Valentino, JD, USP, *serves as the Review Board Secretary*

The USAN Review Board secretariat is supported by the USP. Joseph G Valentino, JD, serves the Board as Secretary. At the time of any appeal to the Board, representatives of the drug firm involved in the specific case can participate in the deliberations, but they have no voting privileges. The Secretary of the USAN Council becomes the spokesperson for the Council. The determination of the USAN Review Board is final and not subject to appeal.

PROCEDURE FOR OBTAINING A USAN

The negotiation of a USAN originates with a drug manufacturer, a licensee of that firm, or its legal representative. On rare occasions, a formal request for a nonproprietary name will be initiated by an individual who has developed a substance of potential therapeutic usefulness to the point where there is a distinct possibility of the compound being marketed in the US. Occasionally, the initiative for the development of a USAN is assumed by the FDA or the USP. The criteria set by the Council for initiating the negotiation process states that the drug must have progressed in its development to the point where clinical studies have been started. At that time an Investigational New Drug (IND) application must have been approved by the FDA.

The USAN application form was standardized in the early 1970s. Currently, each nomenclature request must be submitted on this form and accompanied by detailed chemical, pharmacological, and manufacturing information and reprints of clinical studies or other published information. Use of this form facilitates handling data and ensures that pertinent items have not been omitted. Requests for USAN are expected to conform to the established Guiding Principles for the Selection of Nonproprietary Names for Drugs and to be reasonably free from conflicts with other names, including both trademarks and nonproprietary names. Forms can be obtained by writing to USAN Secretariat at the AMA Headquarters, 515 N State Street, Chicago, IL 60610, or by photocopying the forms appearing in the current edition of the *USAN Handbook*.

A description of how a proposed name eventually becomes an adopted USAN will illustrate the process. Assume that a submission for a new single-entity drug has been received by the USAN Secretariat. Under ideal circumstances, inspection of the submitted material indicates that timing of the negotiation is correct relative to clinical investigation, information supplied is properly entered on the USAN submission form, and adequately substantiated by CAS information and scientific data, and that the suggested names include the proper stem for the class of compounds being considered. The negotiator assigned to the USAN application will begin processing the submission without delay. Obviously, if information is missing or incomplete, valuable time will be lost contacting the applicant for the needed data.

The initial step undertaken by the USAN staff coordinator is a review of the chemical information including the chemical name, structural and molecular formulas, and the molecular weight listed on the application. The coordinator verifies the accuracy of the CA Index name and Registry number against the CAS Registry File database. The chemical information then is forwarded to the USAN Council's chemical consultant for assignment of the IUPAC name and an expert review of the structural and molecular formulas as listed by the firm.

The main work on the submission involves a detailed check of the suggested names for conflicts with other names; verification of the assignment of the proper stem based on a study of the new compound relative to similar compounds, pharmacological action, therapeutic indication, formal ballot polling of the Council for an informed opinion on the suitability of the suggested names; publication of the names under consideration on the USAN Web site (www.ama-assn.org/go/usan), and the *USP Pharmacopeial Forum* to allow other manufacturers the opportunity to examine all suggested names for possible conflict; and communication with the submitting firm to obtain its approval of a tentatively adopted name or the reaction to counterproposals from the Council. Verifying chemical structure and support for therapeutic indication/method of action requires utilization of the CAS Registry File, Prouse Trilogy, STN database, Medlines, MedScape and other pertinent databases. In addition, the USAN and USP Dictionary of Names, the WHO INN list, Merck Index, and Martindale may be used to verify that the proposed name is not in conflict with an existing nonproprietary or trade name.

Selecting even a tentatively adopted USAN often requires considerable negotiation between the Council and the applicant. The Council conducts its negotiation activities by correspondence. *It is important to note that generally a name will not achieve the first level of tentative adoption until it has been found unanimously acceptable to all members of the USAN Council and to the submitting firm.*

Once a tentatively adopted USAN has been selected, the USAN Secretariat forwards this name and appropriate background information to the WHO INN Committee Secretariat located in Geneva, Switzerland. Names under review by the USAN Council are forwarded to nomenclature agencies of several countries. Input from other countries helps avoid selection of a USAN that has an unacceptable and unintended negative or pejorative connotation in another language. The INN Committee undertakes an evaluative procedure not unlike that conducted by the USAN Council, and this process takes approximately five months, but may extend longer. A formal negotiation is initiated to accept the tentative USAN or to consider an INN counterproposal if there is a problem with use of the original name in other countries. *Only when it becomes apparent that the tentative name is acceptable to the USAN Council, the submitting manufacturer, and, in most cases, the INN Committee will it be formally adopted as a USAN.* Therefore, a USAN will be as-

signed in the shortest possible time if the principals involved can reach agreement with minimal negotiations.

USAN adoptions are scheduled for the last Wednesday of each month. A Letter of Adoption and a Nomenclature Statement formally notifies the applicant that the negotiation process has been completed and that a USAN has been issued for the compound.

After the applicant has reviewed the Nomenclature Statement, the USAN is submitted for publication in the journal *Clinical Pharmacology and Therapeutics* (New Names column), and the *Pharmacopeial Forum* (Nomenclature Column), and posted in the "What's New" section of the USAN Web site. Reprints of "New Names" column are distributed to the drug manufacturers, libraries, and pharmaceutical press representatives.

USAN Nomenclature Statements are published for each definable chemical substance and is identified by two chemical names: the first name is the Chemical Abstracts (CA) Index name; the second is a systematic name developed in accordance with rules devised by the International Union of Pure and Applied Chemistry (IUPAC). Occasionally, a third chemical name may be added, one that has become firmly established through extensive use. In conjunction with use of CA nomenclature, a CAS Registry number is included in the published entry. Structural and molecular formulas and the molecular weight are listed where applicable. The manufacturer supplies the intended therapeutic classification. The name of the manufacturer, brand name, manufacturer code designation, and trivial name formerly used are included to further identify the new USAN. Reprints of the monthly "New Names" column are available on request from the USAN Council Secretariat.

After reviewing the complex USAN negotiation process, one can appreciate that the time required to approve a USAN varies considerably depending on a number of factors. The time between submission of an application and adoption of a USAN averages about 8 months and ranges from 4 to 26 months. A significant portion of this time, about five months or longer, may be required for processing by WHO. The time required may be appreciably shorter when adopting a USAN for a compound that already has INN status (ie, a compound already marketed outside the United States) or when the name does not have to be considered by the INN Committee (EG, contact lens plastics, surgical sutures). The negotiation time is shortest when the name being suggested is for a new salt or ester of a compound that already has an adopted USAN (ie, for a USAN modified). Such names are routinely processed by the USAN Secretariat and adopted following completion of review of chemical information. Such negotiations may take only 3 to 4 months.

The process chart for the process of approval can be found in Chart 27-1.

LIAISON RELATIONSHIP WITH THE US FOOD AND DRUG ADMINISTRATION

The FDA and the USAN Council conducted an unofficial liaison until early 1967 when it was determined that a formal cooperative effort in the development of nonproprietary names would be more beneficial to both. In June 1967, an official agreement was signed between the sponsors of the USAN Council and the FDA to appoint annually one voting member to the Council. This contract stipulated that the FDA would accept as the "official or established" name any drug name the USAN Council adopted. In this agreement, the Commissioner of the FDA reserved the right to select the official name in those instances in which the USAN Council could not reach consensus. It should be noted that the designation of a name as an "official or established" name by the FDA did not follow automatically but was accomplished by publication, subject to public comment, in the *Federal Register*. All parties upheld this agreement until it was modified 17 years later.

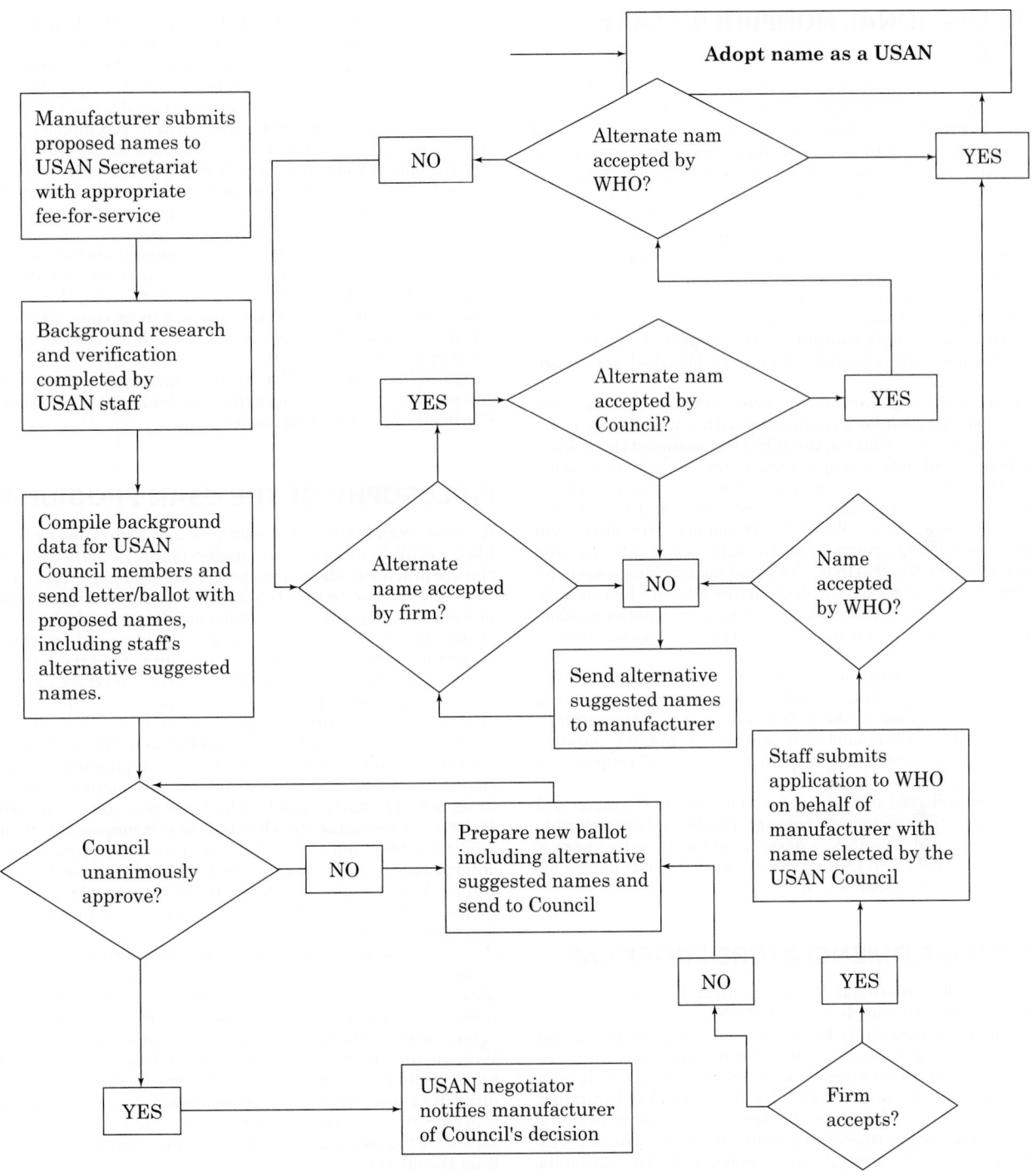

Chart 27-1. Process Chart for Approval Process.

On November 26, 1984, the Commissioner of Food and Drugs and the Secretary of Health and Human Services published in the *Federal Register* an amendment to the FD&C Act that stated in part that " . . . the Food and Drug Administration agrees with *"Guiding Principles for Coining US Adopted Names for Drugs,"* published in *USAN and the USP Dictionary of Drug Names* . . . "and that . . . the established name . . . will ordinarily be either the compendia name of the drug or, if there is no compendia name, the common or usual name of the drug. Interested persons, in the absence of the designation of an official name, may rely on the USAN listed in *USAN and the USP Dictionary of Drug Names* as being the established name in accordance with the Federal Food, Drug, and Cosmetic Act."

The FDA also plays a role when a manufacturer seeks to register a trademark (proprietary name) for a drug entity that has been assigned a USAN. Within the Center for Drug Evaluation and Research (CDER) of the FDA, the Labeling and Nomenclature Committee (LNC) provides recommendations on the acceptability of proposed proprietary names. One of the criteria for rejection is use of USAN syllables or stems in the proposed trademark.

INTERNATIONAL NONPROPRIETARY NAMES

The USAN Council functions primarily to serve the health professions in the US. However, at a time when drug manufacturers market their products in many countries and medical and pharmaceutical literature is widely translated around the world, the need for cooperation in nomenclature activities among the major drug-producing countries clearly is evident.

In addition to the USAN Council, nomenclature agencies exist in Great Britain, France, Italy, Japan, Spain, the Nordic countries, and Switzerland. These agencies function at varying levels of authority and work with their pharmaceutical industries to select appropriate nonproprietary names for drugs marketed within their borders. These agencies maintain liaisons with each other and coordinate the approval of identical nomenclature rules and the selection of identical nonproprietary names.

To prevent the confusion that arises when several nonproprietary names used for a single drug, either in the same country or in different countries, the WHO has assumed the responsibility for coordinating drug nomenclature at the international level. Through its Committee on Nonproprietary Names, whose members are drawn from representatives of the national nomenclature agencies, WHO has developed procedures and formulated guiding principles for the selection of International Nonproprietary Names (INN). National nomenclature agencies usually act as agents for the drug manufacturers by referring mutually selected designations (usually *prior* to national adoption) to the WHO with a request that these names be selected as INN.

A drug manufacturer located in a country without a nomenclature agency is permitted to make a direct submission for a nonproprietary name to the INN Committee or, alternatively, to an established nomenclature agency in another country, preferably a country in which the pharmaceutical preparation is likely to be marketed.

INN are selected for substances that can be characterized unequivocally by a chemical name or formula, and exceptions to this rule are rare. The INN is designated for the active part of the molecule only. The INN program does not select names for mixtures or herbal substances.

THE WHO NOMENCLATURE PROGRAM

In 1915 the International Pharmaceutical Federation established a Committee on International Nomenclature and assigned it the responsibility for identifying each pharmaceutical substance by a globally available and unique nonproprietary name. The WHO Constitution in 1946 relegated the duty of drug nomenclature to the WHO. By 1953, the WHO initiated the selection and publication of International Nonproprietary Names (INN) for pharmaceutical substances. The present INN program is administered by the Secretariat (Dr. Raffaella Balocco-Matavelli) located in Geneva, Switzerland. Nonproprietary names are selected biannually by members of the WHO Expert Advisory Panel on the International Pharmacopoeia and Pharmaceutical Preparations, Nomenclature Section. This advisory panel is comprised of representatives from national nomenclature groups (ie, the USAN Council Secretary, the British Approved Names (BAN) Committee Secretary, the French, Japanese, and Spanish nomenclature Secretariats, and representatives from Nigeria, Tunisia, and Poland. The process of INN selection is similar to that utilized to select a USAN. After the manufacturer submits an application, review and objections periods are followed by selection of the INN. Details of the process are explained below.

Under its charter, the WHO is empowered simply to *recommend* specific actions or procedures to its Members States. The WHO INN Committee initially publishes in *WHO Drug Information* the selected names as "proposed International Nonpro-

prietary Names (pINN)." From the date of publication, 4 months are allowed for member states or other interested parties to submit comments or objections to any proposal. An objection generally reflects a belief that the proposal is confusingly close to (ie, conflicts with) a name already in use. If no objection is received, the proposed INN will attain the status of recommended INN. Subsequently, WHO will publish the name as a "recommended International Nonproprietary Name (rINN)." The WHO publishes lists of rINN on a biannual basis. Many member states then recognize the rINN as the sole or preferred nonproprietary name for use in their respective countries.

A cumulative list of INN and the guidelines for coining an INN (*INN for Pharmaceutical Substances*) can be obtained from the World Health Organization in Geneva, Switzerland. The INN Cumulative List now contains more than 7000 names for drug entities. The INN Committee adds 120 to 150 new designations each year.

Guidelines on the Use of International Nonproprietary Names (INN) for Pharmaceutical Substances is available, on CD-ROM, for public distribution.

PHILOSOPHY OF THE USAN PROGRAM

A closer examination of nonproprietary names for drugs will likely result in an inaccurate understanding of present nomenclature practices. Many drug names for products on the market were coined prior to the creation of systematized nomenclature procedures, principles, and drug classifications. Indeed, many of the older names demonstrate the obvious need for selection of useful, simple, and appropriate nonproprietary names for drugs. Existing names, therefore, reflect a mixture of old and new nomenclature practices and philosophies. In many instances, poor naming of drugs was due to the now discarded practice of condensing the full chemical name into a chemically oriented nonproprietary name, eg, (1) amphetamine was assigned to the parent central stimulant, and methamphetamine to its methyl analog; and (2) the large perazine antipsychotic series—butaperazine, prochlorperazine [Compazine], trifluoperazine [Stelazine]—have very close names, represented by chlorpromazine [Thorazine] and triflupromazine [Vesprin]. Names for each new member in the perazine or promazine series were devised by adding a structure-based prefix, such as *but-* (butyl group), *prochlor-* (*propyl-* and *chloro-*), *trifluo-* (*trifluoro-*) to the base name *-perazine*. At the time this practice came into being, the chemistry of most drugs was not too complex, nor were there that many drugs on the market. The nomenclature confusion was lessened because each of these agents was marketed under a short, memorable trademark. With advancing chemical complexity of drug entities, however, nonproprietary names so derived became increasingly long and difficult to spell, pronounce, or remember. Using the above presented *perazine* series as an example, one can see that it becomes increasingly more difficult to distinguish one *perazine* from the others.

In addition to the problems caused by the complexity of the word itself, chemically derived names have been criticized because they fail to provide useful information to anyone but a scientist involved in drug development.

Nonproprietary nomenclature is intended primarily for physicians, pharmacists, and those in related health professions. A physician is not concerned with the sometimes subtle structural manipulation of molecules that produce a potential new drug. His or her primary concern is to understand the drug's pharmacological and therapeutic properties. Therefore, it must be emphasized again that nonproprietary names should be coined in such a way as to be most useful to the health professionals who are their primary users.

A well-coined nonproprietary name should be distinctive. How many hundreds of drug names begin with the familiar letters *di-*, *tri-*, *meth-*, *chlor-*, *oxy-*, or *phen-*? Repetitious use of chemical prefixes leads to similar, look-alike, and sound-alike names, so this practice has now been discarded. By abandoning strict adherence to chemical antecedents, names can be made not only simpler but also unique.

To assign meaningful nonproprietary names to new drug compounds, it is necessary to indicate through the name any relationship that exists between the new entity and established drugs. Conversely, inappropriate names suggesting nonexistent relationships are misleading and must be avoided. The USAN Council has used standardized prefixes, infixes, or suffixes in nonproprietary names to classify and relate new chemical entities to existing drug families. These standardized syllables collectively are called *stems*, and they can emphasize a special chemical nucleus, a pharmacological property, or a combination of both these attributes.

Chemically derived stems
cef- (cephalosporins)
 *cef*otetan, *cef*metazole, *cef*ixime
-nab- (can*nab*inols)
 dro*nab*inol, ti*nab*inol
-conazoles (antifungal imidazoles)
 keto*conazole*, flu*conazole*, cis*conazole*
Pharmacologically derived stems
-stat- (enzyme inhibitors)
 alre*stat*in, lova*stat*in
-vir- (antivirals)
 aciclo*vir*, riba*vir*in, *vir*oxime
-astine (antihistaminics)
 acriv*astine*, temel*astine*, zep*astine*
Combination Stems
-olol (propranolol-type beta-blockers)
 tim*olol*, aten*olol*
-profen (ibuprofen-type anti-inflammatory/analgesic agents)
 ibu*profen*, flurbi*profen*
-tecan (camptothecine antineoplastics)
 topo*tecan*, irino*tecan*

The USAN recommended list of stems (see Appendix A) is revised and updated regularly to keep pace with the changing chemical and pharmacological nature of new drugs.

Again, a random survey of names for drugs currently in use will show a mixture of "old" and "new" nomenclature practices. In fact, such a survey, presented below, should illustrate effectively the principles behind the newer nomenclature approach.

Figure 27-1 presents a pair of compounds named many years ago, meprobamate and carisoprodol, that are related both chemically and pharmacologically; despite these similarities, the drugs have dissimilar names.

The opposite situation is illustrated in Figure 27-2; the relationship between fluorometholone and oxymetholone is limited to the classification of both agents as steroids: fluorometholone is an anti-inflammatory corticosteroid, and oxymetholone is an anabolic 17α-alkylated testosterone derivative used as an erythropoietic. This class of compounds, however, is so large and so diverse that the common ring nucleus alone is hardly sufficient to warrant the use of a common stem (-*metholone*).

The steroids are, in fact, typical of several large groups of compounds that (within each group) exhibit somewhat similar chemical and pharmacological properties. Because of diversity within the group, however, it is desirable to establish subseries of names based on the nature of the substituent groups and on the placement of such substituents. In recent years the USAN

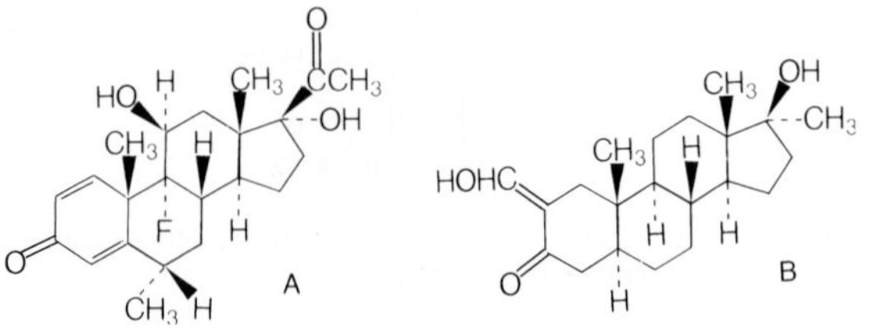

Figure 27-2. Illustrative of poor practice in nomenclature are the compounds fluorometholone (A) and oxymetholone (B). The compounds are not as closely related as the names suggest.

Council increasingly has developed this principle, which is typified by the examples in Figure 27-3.

Figure 27-3 depicts a basic glucocorticoid structure (glucocorticoids, in themselves, being a division of the broader category of steroids) in which the R groups indicate the positions at which the principal differences in the subseries occur. There is no common suffix for the entire glucocorticoid series, but the suffixes -*olone*, -*sone*, and -*onide* are indicative of this series and are used in the stems of the various subseries.

A more recent example of stem subdivision is represented by the various subgroups formed based on the stem *vir*: the *vir* stem represents drugs exhibiting antiviral properties, which was further subdivided to form the subclassification -*amivir* for antivirals capable of inhibiting the enzyme neuraminidase, -*ciclovir* for acyclovir-type antivirals, -*virsen* for antisense antivirals, -*navir* for antiviral HIV protease inhibitors, plus other lesser known subclasses of antivirals.

The use of common stems to indicate particular classes of drugs is reexamined constantly by the USAN Council. The development of nomenclature for the tetracycline series of drugs (Fig 27-4) demonstrates the review and revision processes by which the Council's principles are assessed to ensure their validity in the light of current nomenclature requirements. The first drugs in this series were chlortetracycline and oxytetracycline, both of which can be converted chemically to the parent compound, tetracycline. Further research led to still another variant, demethylchlortetracycline, which, in keeping with the standard practice of the time, was named in strict accordance

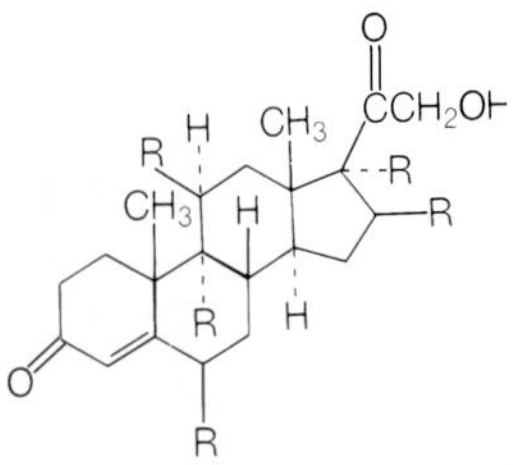

Figure 27-3. The R groups indicate the position on the glucocorticoid nucleus where the principal modifications occur. Such changes give rise to various structurally defined subseries differentiated by means of the following stems:

-olone

	-cinolone	triamcinolone fluocinolone
	-cortolone	fluocortolone clocortolone
-sone		
	-sone	cloticasone ticabesone
	-met(h)asone	dexamethasone mometasone
-onide (16,17-acetal)		
	-cinonide	amcinonide fluocinonide

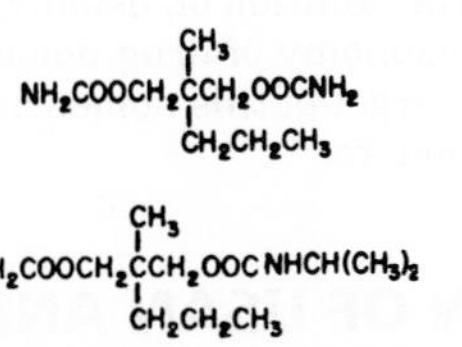

Figure 27-1. Meprobamate (*top*) and carisoprodol (*bottom*) are closely related chemically and pharmacologically; the assigned names, however, do not indicate this relationship.

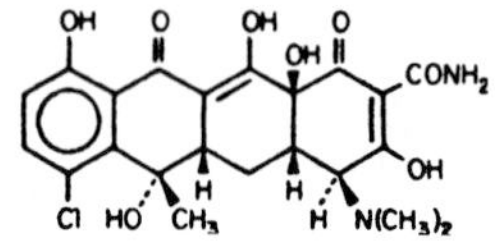

Figure 27-4. Chlortetracycline. Other names in this series include rolitetracycline, meclocycline, and amicycline.

with its chemical derivation to represent the desmethyl variant of chlortetracycline. The next member of this series to require a nonproprietary name was characterized by a distinctive pyrrolidine group and, following traditional patterns, the name might have become pyrrolidinotetracycline. Instead, the first step was taken toward simplifying names in this series by shortening the prefix, and the resulting name became rolitetracycline. The logical next step taken by the USAN Council members was to drop the syllables *tetra* from the suffixes of newer nonproprietary names for drugs in this group, thus yielding simpler and more useful designations. Examples of such designations are amicycline, sancycline, and doxycycline; the series stem became *-cycline*.

Although it is a very difficult thing to do for several valid reasons, occasionally the need and the opportunity arise to go back and change the poorly coined name of a well-established drug. Such was the case with demethylchlortetracycline. The name of this compound, which is commercially available as the hydrochloride salt, was changed to demeclocycline hydrochloride.

Captopril and the subsequently named angiotensin-converting enzyme inhibitors (enalapril, spirapril, quinapril, etc) were assigned names using the *pril* stem derived from *proline,* a common structural feature present in members of this series (Fig 27-5). The second member, enalapril, a tripeptide derivative, is a substituted alanylethyl ester. Later, when the di-acid form of enalapril was made available, the *pril* stem was modified to *prilat* (eg, enalaprilat) to accommodate this structural change from the ethyl ester to the acid.

The *stat* stem has been used to identify various enzyme inhibitors. As the series developed, it became apparent that subdivision was needed to group chemically related agents inhibiting a specific enzyme. Two very prominent subgroups in this series are (1) *-vastatin* HMG-CoA reductase inhibitors (mevastatin, lovastatin, simvastatin, pravastatin), and (2) *-restat-* for the aldose-reductase inhibitors (alrestatin, tolrestat) as seen in Figure 27-6.

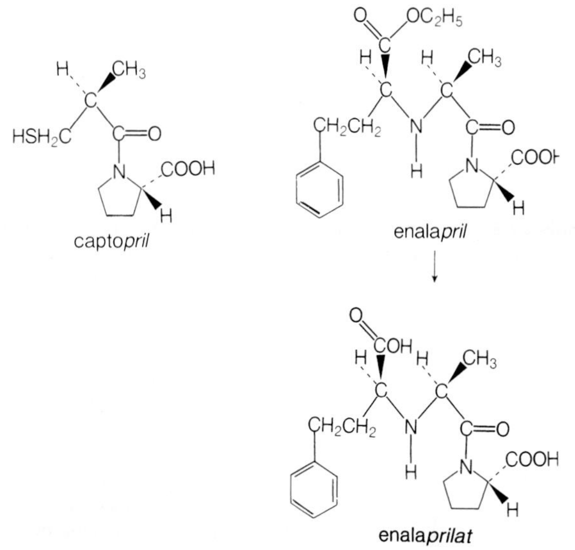

Figure 27-5. The *pril* series of related angiotensin-converting enzyme inhibitors. Hydrolysis of the ethyl ester of enalapril produced the modification from *pril* to *prilat*.

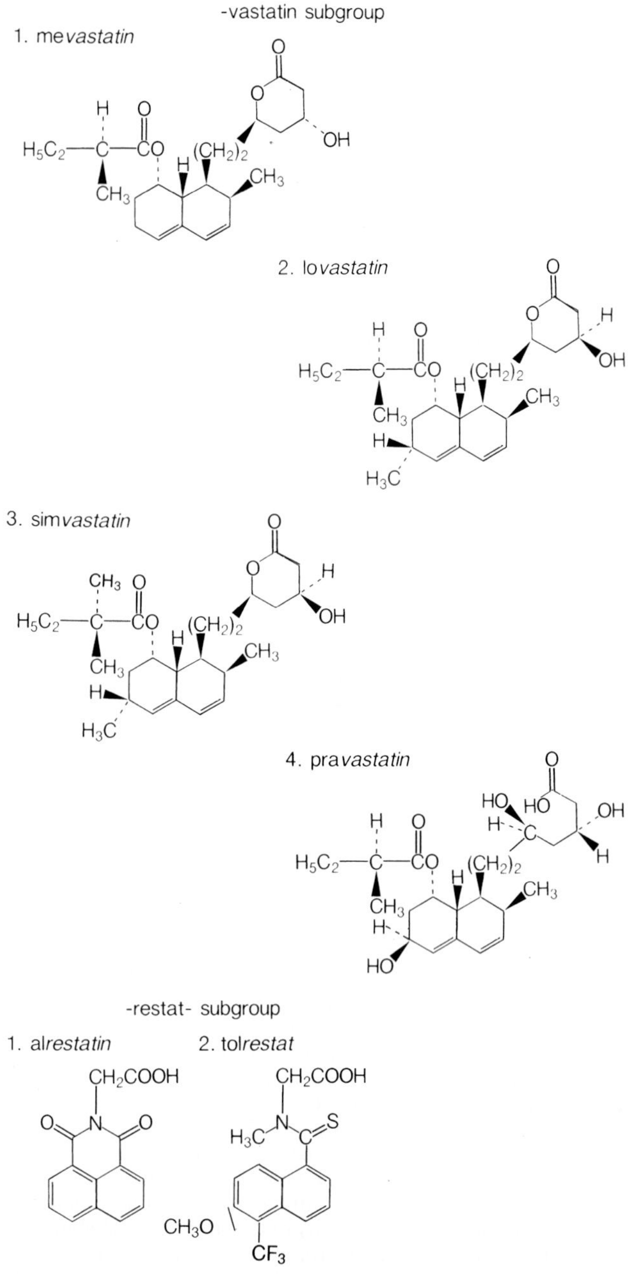

Figure 27-6. The *-vastatin* and *-restat* subgroups within the large stat (enzyme inhibitors) series.

These examples illustrate the USAN Council's developed policy of coining meaningful nonproprietary names. Its aim is to select short, unique names that are informative and useful to the primary health providers, the medical and related health professionals. These examples also illustrate the Council's policy of establishing classifications of stems based on chemical and/or pharmacological similarities and of subdividing stem classifications by the addition of, usually, structurally based infixes to create a taxonomy of drug nomenclature useful to the intended primary target of this nomenclature system, the various health practitioners.

PROTECTION OF USAN AND INN

After adoption of a USAN, the entry is submitted for publication in the "New Names" column in the journal of *Clinical Pharmacology and Therapeutics* and is transmitted to the USP for publication in the annually released *USP Dictionary of USAN and International Drug Names*. The 35th edition of the USP dictionary contained 8713 nonproprietary drug name entries, with more than 4115 trademarks.

With the growing number of USAN/INN and brand names, the possibility of conflicts between nonproprietary names, between trademarks, and between trademarks and nonproprietary names has increased significantly. A frequent source of conflict in the latter category is the practice of *piggybacking* on the USAN/INN or the incorporation of a nomenclature stem in the trademark. If trademark registration is obtained for names containing an officially reserved stem, this may diminish the freedom of the USAN and the INN programs in the selection of further nonproprietary names in the same series of substances.

To inhibit this practice at the WHO INN level, the issue of piggybacking and incorporation of the official stems into trademarks was taken up in a resolution of the World Health Assembly WHA46.19. Based on recommendations made by the WHO Expert Committee on the use of Essential Drugs, resolution WHA46.19 on Nonproprietary Names for pharmaceutical substances was adopted in May 1993, during the 46th World Health Assembly.

WHA resolution WAH46.19 was discussed by the USAN Council, and on January 22, 1996, the USAN Council approved the following statement as part of its nomenclature policy.

Co-Existence of Nonproprietary Names and Trademarks

In devising the Guiding Principles for coining USAN for drugs, the program originators included a rule stating that a USAN "should be free from conflict with other nonproprietary names and with established trademarks and should be neither confusing nor misleading." Through its various name-screening procedures, the Council Staff attempts to comply with this requirement. Unfortunately, the same kind of protection is not afforded to nonproprietary names by many drug manufacturers. The USAN Council, WHO INN Committee, and other nomenclature committees have actively discouraged the undesirable practices of devising trademarks from the nonproprietary names or incorporating into trademarks the *stems* used by the nomenclature committees to create new nonproprietary names.

USAN Statement on WHA Resolution 46.19

As the designated drug nomenclature agency of the US, the USAN Council is responsible for the selection of simple and useful nonproprietary names for drugs and such related substances as pharmaceutic aids, contact lens plastics, surgical materials, diagnostic agents, carriers, and excipients. The USAN Council cooperates and works with the WHO in devising nonproprietary names for drugs, in standardizing drug nomenclature, and in establishing rules governing the classification of new substances.

In 1993, the WHO Executive Board placed Resolution WHA46.19 before the World Health Assembly (WHA) seeking to encourage the WHO member states to intensify their efforts to discourage manufacturers from devising trademarks derived from recommended International Nonproprietary Names (rINN) and from including INN stems in trademarks. Resolution WHA46.19 was adopted by the 46th WHA on May 12, 1993. Resolution WHA46.19 was discussed by the USAN Council on January 28, 1994. The USAN Council agreed in principle with the resolution statements and supported the premises stated in the resolution.

The expression of general support for WHA Resolution 46.19, although in keeping with the historical support by the USAN Council for harmonization of global drug nomenclature policies, has led to a misapprehension of USAN Council views in some US-based and multinational pharmaceutical corporations and associations. A statement of the USAN Council's views is provided below.

WHO Resolution WHA46.19: Nonproprietary Names for Pharmaceutical Substances

The Forty-sixth World Health Assembly Requests Member States:

"... to enact rules or regulations, as necessary, to ensure that international nonproprietary names (or the equivalent nationally approved generic names) used in labeling and advertising of pharmaceutical products are always displayed prominently."

The principle that the USAN should be prominently displayed is not an issue in the US, as this has been required by the FD&C Act for more than three decades. Section 502(E) requires, for labeling, that

"[t]he established name ... is printed prominently and in type at least half as large as that used thereon for any proprietary name or

designation for such drug ... to encourage manufacturers to rely on their corporate name and the international nonproprietary names, rather than on trademarks, to promote and market multisource products introduced after patent expiration."

The USAN Council also recognizes that trademarks constitute intellectual property for their holders. USAN Council encourages manufacturers of multisource prescription drug products, other than those who obtained the original NDA approvals, to rely on the USAN and their corporate names in marketing such products instead of creating additional trademarks. Nevertheless, USAN Council recognizes that the use of trademarks is common and valuable in marketing over-the-counter drug products and is often useful in special cases with prescription drug products. Such special cases may arise when, for example, (1) there are differences in bioavailability between a drug product marketed by an innovator firm and a later version introduced by the same or another firm, and (2) drug products, containing the same drug substance but with different uses, are introduced "to develop policy guidelines on the use and protection of international nonproprietary names, and to discourage the use of names derived from INNs, and particularly names including established INN stems as trade-marks." The USAN Council discourages the use in trademarks of substantial portions of USAN and established USAN stems. This practice is an infringement on USAN and an impediment to the work of USAN Council in establishing new USAN in a class of drugs. It should be noted that USAN Council attempts to avoid establishing USAN that are in conflict with US and foreign trademarks as well as other nonproprietary names of drugs. Furthermore, the USAN Council is cognizant of the US FD&C Act, Section 508(A), which states, in part, "[I]n no event ... shall the secretary establish an official name so as to infringe a valid trademark."

Conclusion

The USAN Council was established to serve the health professions in the US by

1. Selecting simple, informative, and unique nonproprietary names for drugs.
2. Establishing a logical nomenclature classification based on pharmacological and/or chemical relationships.
3. Formulating nomenclature rules for selecting appropriate nonproprietary names for drugs.

The USAN Council, other national nomenclature groups, and the WHO Nomenclature Committee aim for global standardization and unification of drug nomenclature and related rules to ensure that drug information is communicated accurately and unambiguously.

GUIDING PRINCIPLES FOR COINING UNITED STATES ADOPTED NAMES FOR DRUGS

By definition, nonproprietary names are not subject to proprietary trademark rights, but exist entirely in the public domain. This feature distinguishes them from the trademarked names that have been registered for private use. A USAN is a nonproprietary name selected by the USAN according to principles developed to ensure safety, consistency, and logic in the choice of names. These principles take into account practical considerations, such as the existence of trademarks and the fact that the intended uses of substances for which names are being selected may change. These guidelines are and must be sufficiently flexible to be revised if this is considered to be desirable and/or necessary.

General Rules

1. A nonproprietary name should be useful primarily to health practitioners, especially physicians, dentists, pharmacists, nurses, educators, and veterinarians.
   a. The primary criterion for judging usefulness is suitability, including safety for use in the routine processes of prescribing, ordering, dispensing, and administering drugs throughout the United States.
   b. The second criterion is suitability for use in educational programs for students in medically oriented professions and for use in scientific and lay publications.
   c. The third criterion is suitability for use internationally for drug identification, for the exchange of information and translation into different languages.

2. Attributes that contribute to usefulness are simplicity (brevity and ease of pronunciation), euphony, and ready recognition and recall.
   a. The name for the active moiety of a drug should be a single word, preferably with no more than four syllables.
   b. The name for the active moiety may be modified by a single term, preferably with no more than four syllables, to show a chemical modification, such as salt or ester formation (eg, cortisone acetate from cortisone, cefamandole sodium from cefamandole, erythromycin acistrate from erythromycin).
   c. Only under compelling circumstances is a name with more than one modifying term acceptable (eg, pharmaceuticals containing radioactive isotopes, the different classes of interferons).
   d. Acronyms, initials, and condensed words may be acceptable in otherwise appropriate terminology.
3. A name should reflect characteristics and relationships that will be of practical value to the users.
   a. A common, simple word element (a "stem") should be incorporated in the names of all members of a group of related drugs when pertinent, common characteristics can be identified (eg, similarity of pharmacological action). When pharmacological similarity is found in drugs of distinctly different chemical nature, stems should differ (eg, the antipsychotics, promazine and haloperidol; the nonsteroidal anti-inflammatory agents [NSAID], ibuprofen, etodolac, and isoxicam).
   b. Distinctive terminology should be used for specific drugs or groups (eg, insulin I 131, dextran 40, interferon alfa-2a and interferon alfa-n1; licryfilcon A and licryfilcon B; epoetin alfa and epoetin beta).
4. A name should be free from conflict with other nonproprietary names and with established trademarks and should be neither confusing nor misleading.
   a. Prefixes that imply "better," "newer," or "more effective," or evoke the name of the manufacturer, dosage form, duration of action or rate of drug release should not be used.
   b. Prefixes that refer to an anatomical connotation or medical condition are not acceptable.
   c. Prefixes that indicate a chemical element or compound (Ca, Ni, and Stannous) are not acceptable.
5. Preference should be given to names of established usage provided they conform to these guiding principles and are determined to be free from conflict with existing nonproprietary names and trademarks.
6. Identical negotiations submitted by two or more manufacturers will be conducted in accordance with the Council's practice of maintaining confidentiality. The applicants involved will not be notified of the multiple sources of the submission. However, the name selected by the USAN Council will need to be accepted by each manufacturer involved in the negotiation process.
7. A request for a USAN should be made after the drug manufacturer or sponsor has submitted an Investigational New Drug (IND) application to the Food and Drug Administration (FDA) to obtain permission to initiate studies on humans.
8. Deferred Negotiations:
   a. The USAN Council Secretariat will defer an ongoing negotiation for 6 months plus one additional 3-month extension upon receipt of a written request from the manufacturer. If the USAN Council has selected a name candidate and recommended this name to the manufacturer, the maximum deferral is one 6-month period.
   b. The negotiation will be canceled after the maximum 9-month deferral has lapsed.
   c. If the negotiation is to be reopened at a later time, it will receive a new USAN file number and will be treated as a new application. The manufacturer will be expected to submit a new USAN negotiation form, update the background information, and submit the appropriate user's fee.

Specific Rules

1. Because of the international exchange of drug information, specific guidelines have been formulated to ensure appropriate translation of nonproprietary names into other languages. The following rules of preferred spelling should be used when coining USAN designations:
   a. the letter "f" should be used instead of "ph"
   b. the letter "t" should be used instead of "th"
   c. the letter "e" should be used instead of "ae" or "oe"
   d. the letter "i" should be used instead of "y"
   e. the letter "h" should be avoided
   f. the letter "k" should be avoided.
   g. the letter "j" should be avoided.
   h. the letter "w" should be avoided.
   i. "ar", "rac", "lev", "dex", or "es" are reserved for stereochemical configurations

2. Additionally, these letter combinations are restricted until further notice. Please avoid the following prefixes:
   a. the beginning letter "z"
   b. the beginning letter combination of "me"
   c. the beginning letter combination of "str"
   d. chemical connotations such as, "ben", "bu", "cat", "cel", "fen", "flu", "piro"
   e. Chemical symbols unless present in the compound, "al", "ba", "ca", "li", "ni"

In order to facilitate the development of names that will be accepted on an international level please note:

A. The following letter combinations pose pronunciation problems in several languages:

   -ch-
   -rs-
   -xn-

B. The letter sequence "-m" and "-n" followed by consonants may be regarded as difficult.
   1) "m" before a consonant other than "p", "n", or "b"
   2) -nb-, and -np- should be avoided
C. The letter sequence "-vr" should be avoided.
D. In addition, it should be kept in mind that there is, in some languages, no distinction between:

   "b" and "v" or "p"
   "l" and "r"
   before "e" and "i": "z" and "g"

3. Isolated letters, numbers, or hyphenations are restricted to those groups of substances for which such usage fulfills a clearly demonstrable purpose (eg, interferon alfa-2b, paflufocon A, technetium Tc 99m siboroxime).
4. Group relationships in a name preferably should be indicated by use of syllables or stems; conversely, use of the stem for other than the appropriate group should be avoided. When multiple stems are available, the stem conveying the most information should be used.
5. Esters, salts, chelates, and complexes ordinarily require a two-word name to indicate the inactive as well as the active portion.
6. The preferred order for the name of an inorganic salt is cation-anion (eg, sodium bromide). The same order is preferred for well-known salts of simple organic acids (eg, sodium lactate, magnesium citrate, potassium acetate). However, for more complex organic compounds, the pharmacologically active portion should be identified first (eg, oxacillin sodium, ibuprofen piconol, dexibuprofen lysine).
7. A name for a salt or ester generally should be derived from the name of the pharmacologically active moiety or corresponding acid (eg, sodium acetate or ethyl acetate, derived from acetic acid). When a nonacid suffix is used, as in the penicillin series, a salt should be named without modification of the parent acid name (eg, oxacillin sodium, derived from oxacillin). Names for different salts or esters of the same active moiety should differ only in the name of the inactive portion; exceptions are permissible when the salt and ester forms possess pharmacologic activity.
8. A name for the salt form of the pharmacologically active moiety is specific to the number of molecules used to react with the active moiety (eg, balsalazide *di*sodium, gusperimus *tri*hydrochloride). If only one molecule is used to react with the active moiety, the designation for the salt name is used without reference to the mono- prefix (eg, besipirdine hydrochloride, afovirsen hydrochloride). [This rule was formulated and approved in January 1993; different requirements were applied prior to this date.]
9. A name for a quaternary ammonium substance should designate the cation and anion separately (eg, octonium bromide, not octonine methylbromide). The name assigned to the cation must contain the *-ium* suffix stem.
10. A name for a complex of two or more components should list the name of the principal active ingredient followed by a coined designation for the second component ending with an "-ex\'\'" suffix to indicate "complex\'\' " (eg, bisacodyl tann*ex*, doxycycline fosfa*tex*). Complexes formed from sulfonated diethenylbenzene-ethenylbenzene copolymers and an active ingredient should list the name of the principal active ingredient followed by "polistirex\'\' " (eg, chlorpheniramine *polistirex*, codeine *polistirex*).
11. A name for a drug containing a radioactive atom should list, in the order given: (1) the name of the drug containing the radioactive atom, (2) the element symbol, (3) the isotope number, and (4) the name of the carrier agent, if any (eg, rose bengal sodium I 131, cyanocobalamin Co 60, potassium bromide Br 82, technetium Tc

99m butilfenin, technetium Tc 99m medronate, indium In 111 oxyquinoline, indium In 111 satumomab pendetide).

12. A name for a substance generally should not indicate the state of hydration, the morphology, or the mode of preparation. Reference to the water of hydration is retained in the chemical information (chemical names, formulas, weight) but is excluded from the nonproprietary name. The degree of hydration becomes a part of the chemical entity identified by the USAN.

13. Under the terms of the Orphan Drug Act of 1983, the development and marketing of drug products that are of limited commercial application but that are potentially useful in relatively rare disease conditions are encouraged. The selection of a name for an orphan drug may be based on special considerations. Therefore, when the name for an orphan drug appears to follow a more chemically oriented terminology style than is customary for drug nomenclature generally, this is not to be regarded as a basis or a precedent for a future selection of a USAN.

14. A name coined for a new chemical entity routinely does not specify the stereoisomeric form of the molecule in the nonproprietary name. If the stereochemical configuration has been determined, this information is presented in the chemical name(s) and is reflected in the structural formula. A USAN can, therefore, identify the racemic mixture (eg, carnitine, ibuprofen, tetramisole), the levo isomer (eg, remoxipride, quadazocine), or the dextro form (eg, butopamine). Subsequently, if a name is needed for a different enantiomer or for the racemic form, the following prefixes should be added to the existing name:

 a. For the racemate, the rac-/race- prefix is used (eg, racemethionine, racepinephrine, ractopamine).
 b. For the levorotatory form, the "(S)" isomer, the lev-/levo- prefix is used (eg, levocarnitine, levamisole, levcromakalim, levdobutamine).
 c. For the levo rotatory form but for the "(R)" isomer, ["R(-)"-isomer], the "ar-" prefix is added to the base name.
 d. For the dextrorotatory form, the "(R)" isomer, the dex-/dextro- prefix is used (eg, dexamisole, dexibuprofen, dextroamphetamine, dexverapamil, dexrazoxane, dexfosfoserine, dexniguldipine).
 e. For the dextro rotatory form but for the "(S)" isomer ["S(+)"- isomer], the "es-" prefix is added to the base name.

15. Official names have been selected for a number of radicals and adducts used to form salts or esters of the pharmacologically active moiety. In a majority of cases, these names represent contractions of the chemical name assigned to the radical or adduct. In four specific cases, the official name identifies a multicomponent adduct:

 • *acistrate* identifies the 2'-acetate (ester) and octadecanoate (salt) (eg, erythromycin acistrate).
 • *probutate* identifies the double ester 1-oxobutoxy and 1-oxopropoxy (eg, hydrocortisone probutate).
 • *estolate* identifies the double salt propanoate and dodecyl sulfate (eg, erythromycin estolate).
 • *hyclate* identifies the monohydrochloride salt, hemiethanolate, hemihydrate combination (eg, doxyclin hyclate).

The complete list of official names for radicals is presented under Appendix B.

Specific Nomenclature Rules for Contact-Lens Materials

The USAN Council began its involvement in the area of polymer nomenclature in 1971 and formulated the first nomenclature rules for assigning nonproprietary names to contact lens materials in 1972. Based on then-available polymer technology and input from the Food and Drug Administration, lens polymers were divided into the *filcon* (hydrophilic) and the *focon* (hydrophobic) series.

The following nomenclature rules, approved by the USAN Council in 1994, represent several expansions and revisions of the initial guidelines:

General Rules

For nomenclature purposes, contact lens materials are divided into hydrophilic and hydrophobic groups, depending on their water content. The hydrophilic lens materials with water content equal to or more than 10% by weight at ambient temperature are assigned "filcon" names. "Focon" names are assigned to hydrophobic lens materials with water content less than 10%.

In addition to water content, nomenclature for contact lens materials depends primarily on the polymeric composition, ie, the repeating monomer units comprising the lens material. These repeating units include linear monomers, and crosslinking entrapped color additives or ultraviolet absorbers are excluded in establishing the polymeric composition of the contact lens material for nomenclature purposes.

The first member of a series is assigned a unique nonproprietary name containing the proper *-filcon* or *-focon* suffix stem. A separate capital letter "A" is added after each parent designation. Subsequent designations for polymers consisting of identical monomers receive the same parent name but a different appended letter (B, C, D, etc). These letters are needed to differentiate between polymers of identical monomeric units but with different ratios of units that have different physiochemical properties, as determined by water content, oxygen permeability [Dk] value, specific gravity, refractive index, surface charge, wetting angle, elasticity, and toughness of the lens.

A contact lens material having the same repeating monomeric units as a named substance but made by a different manufacturing process (eg, lathe-cut versus cast-molded) is not required to obtain a new USAN if the lens material has the same water content and oxygen permeability as the initially named polymer.

The addition of a surface treatment to an existing lens material that has been assigned a USAN does not require a new USAN.

 a. A new USAN will not be assigned to contact lens materials containing chemically bound or physically entrapped color additives. The USAN Council defers to FDA labeling rules to identify color additives used to make tinted lenses.
 b. A new USAN will not be assigned to contact lens materials containing either chemically bound or physically entrapped ultraviolet absorbers. The USAN Council defers to the Food and Drug Administration labeling rules to identify UV absorber used to make these lenses.

A revision of the guiding principles regarding the publication timeframe of USAN for contact lens materials, was approved by the USAN Council at their February, 10, 2003, meeting. Therefore, information on USAN for contact lens materials, will not be published until the manufacturer files a Premarket Approval Application (PMA) with the FDA's Center for Devices.

Contact lens materials are not assigned nonproprietary names by the World Health Organization International Nonproprietary Names Committee. Names for contact lens polymers have USAN status only.

Specific Nomenclature Rules for Biological Products

The USAN Council has been involved in coining names for various biological products: the insulins, interferons, interleukins, growth hormones, colony-stimulating factors, cytokines, and monoclonal antibodies. With increasing development of highly purified biological extracts and recombinant materials, the Council expects to have an increasingly greater role in developing nomenclature rules for these agents.

Listed below are specific guidelines created by the USAN Council, in conjunction with the FDA, the US FDA Center for Biologics Evaluation and Research (CBER), and the WHO INN Committee.

Interferons—The following multi-tiered style for creating nonproprietary names for new interferons was adopted by the USAN Council:

1. The word *interferon* is the first element in the name. Interferon is defined as the class name for a family of species-specific proteins (or glycoproteins) that are produced according to information encoded by species of interferon genes, and exert complex antineoplastic, antiviral, and immunomodulating effects. The three main forms of interferon used in therapy are interferon alfa (formerly leukocyte or lymphoblastoid interferon), interferon beta (formerly fibroblast interferon), and interferon gamma (formerly immune interferon).

2. The appropriate Greek letter (spelled out) is the second word of the name: alfa, beta, gamma.

3. An appropriate Arabic numeral and letter are appended to the Greek letter by a hyphen (no space) to delineate subcategories. The numbers conform to the recommendation of the Interferon Nomenclature Committee. The lowercase letter is assigned by the drug nomenclature agencies to differentiate one manufacturer's interferon from another's. Examples of pure interferon substances are

interferon alfa-2a
interferon alfa-2b
interferon beta-1a
interferon beta-1b
interferon gamma-1a

4. For mixtures of naturally occurring interferons, the lowercase letter *n* precedes the number. Examples of names of mixtures of interferons obtained from a natural source, whether the exact percentage of a mixture is known or not, are

interferon alfa-n1
interferon alfa-n2

Interleukins—The suffix *-leukin* is used in naming interleukin 2 (IL-2) type substances, eg,

aldesleukin
celmoleukin
teceleukin

Somatotropins—The following guidelines have been developed for somatotropin analogs:

1. The *som-* prefix is used for growth hormone derivative, eg,

somatropin for human growth hormone
somatrem for methionyl human growth hormone

2. The *som-* prefix and the *-bove* suffix are required for bovine somatotropin derivatives, eg,

somidobove
sometribove
somagrebove

3. The *som-* prefix and the *-por* suffix are required for porcine somatotropin derivatives, eg,

somalapor
somenopor
sometripor
somfasepor

Colony-Stimulating Factors—The following guidelines have been selected for recombinant colony-stimulating factors:

1. The suffix *-grastim* is used for granulocyte colony-stimulating factors (G-CSF), eg,

lenograstim
filgrastim

2. The suffix *-gramostim* is used for granulocyte macrophage colony-stimulating factors (GM-CSF), eg,

molgramostim
regramostim
sargramostim

3. The suffix *-mostim* is used for macrophage colony-stimulating factors (M-CSF), eg,

mirimostim

4. The suffix *-plestim* is used for interleukin 3 (IL-3) factors classified as pleiotropic colony-stimulating factors, eg,

muplestim
daniplestim

Erythropoietins—The word *epoetin* is used for recombinant human erythropoietin, followed by the appropriate Greek letter (spelled out). The word *epoetin* describes erythropoietin preparations that have an amino acid sequence identical to the endogenous cytokine; the words *alfa, beta, gamma* are added to designate the preparations that differ in the composition and the nature of the carbohydrate moieties. Erythropoietins assigned USAN are

epoetin alfa
epoetin beta
epoetin gamma

Monoclonal Antibodies—The following guidelines have been devised for monoclonal antibodies:

1. The suffix *-mab* is used for monoclonal antibodies and fragments.
2. Identification of the animal source of the product is an important safety factor based on the number of products that may cause source-specific antibodies to develop in patients. The following letters were approved as product source identifiers: *u* = human, *e* = hamster, *o* = mouse, *i* = primate, *a* = rat, *xi* = chimera, and *zu* = humanized. These identifiers are used as infixes preceding the *-mab* suffix stem, eg,

-umab (human)
-omab (mouse)
-ximab (chimera)
-zumab (humanized)

3. The general disease state subclass must be incorporated into the name by use of a code syllable. The following disease state subclasses were approved based on products currently before the Council. Additional subclasses will be added as necessary.

Disease or Target Class

Viral	*-vir-*
Bacterial	*-bac-*
Immune (immunomodulator)	*-lim-*
Tumors	
colon	*-col-*
melanoma	*-mel-*
mammary	*-mar-*
gonad	
testis	*-got-*
ovary	*-gov-*
prostate	*-pr(o)-*
miscellaneous	*-tum-*
Cardiovascular	*-cir-*

4. In order to create a unique name, a distinct, compatible syllable should be selected as the starting prefix.
5. Sequence of stems—the order for the key elements is as follows:
   a. Infix representing the target disease state, the source of the product.
   b. The monoclonal root *-mab* used as a suffix (eg, bi*ciromab*, satu*momab*, neb*acumab*, se*virumab*, and tu*virumab*).
   c. When combining a target or disease infix stem with the source stem for chimeric (*xi*) or humanized (*zu*) monoclonal antibody, the last consonant of the target/disease specific syllable is dropped, eg,

targe	source	*-mab* stem	USAN
-cir-	*-xi-*	*-mab*	abci*ximab*
-lim-	*-zu-*	*-mab*	dacli*zumab*

These modifications were deemed necessary to facilitate pronunciation of the resultant designation.

6. If the product is radiolabeled or conjugated to another chemical such as a toxin, identification of this conjugate is accomplished by use of a separate, second word or other acceptable chemical designation. For monoclonals conjugated to a toxin, the *-tox* stem must be included as part of the name selected for the toxin (eg, in zolimomab aritox, the designation aritox was selected for ricin A-chain). For radiolabeled products, the word order is: name of the isotope, element symbol, isotope number, and name of the monoclonal antibody, eg, technetium Tc 99m biciromab, indium In 111 altumomab pentetate.
7. A separate, distinct name must be assigned to any linker/chelator used to conjugate the monoclonal antibody to a toxin, isotope, or for pegylated monoclonal antibodies, eg, telimomab aritox, indium In 111 satumomab, pendetide, and enlimomab pegol. For the USAN Council to initiate the selection of a name for a monoclonal antibody or fragment, the nomenclature application must provide the following relevant information:
   1. The immunoglobulin class and subclass and the type of associated light chain. Identity of the fragment of the immunoglobulin used (if applicable).
   2. Identity of the fragment of the immunoglobulin used (if applicable).
   3. Species source from which the coding region for the immunoglobulin originated and specific, complete origin of all parts of chimeric, humanized, or semi-synthetic immunoglobulins.
   4. The antigen specificity of the immunoglobulin, including its source.
   5. The clone designation (specify if vector or vector-cell combination).
   6. For conjugated monoclonal antibodies, the identity of any linkers, chelators, toxins, and/or isotopes present in the product.
   7. Identity of other modifications to the antibody, eg, reduction of disulfide bonds, glycosylation or deglycosylation, amino acid modification, or substitution.

BIBLIOGRAPHY

Guidelines on the Use of International Nonproprietary Names (INNs) for Pharmaceutical Substances. Geneva, Switzerland: WHO, 1998.

International Nonproprietary Names (INN) for Pharmaceutical Substances (Cummulative List No 9). Geneva, Switzerland: WHO, 1996.

SAN Handbook 4. Chicago: AMA, 1995.

Trademark Bulletin. Washington, DC: PhRMA, published monthly.

USAN Council: New Names. *J Clin Pharmacol Therap,* published monthly.

USP Dictionary of USAN and International Drug Names 1998. Rockville, MD: USPC.

Appendix A Stems Used by the USAN Council

STEM	DEFINITION	EXAMPLES
-abine	(see -arabine, -citabine)	
-ac	anti-inflammatory agents (acetic acid derivatives)	bromfen**ac**
		dexpemedol**ac**
-acetam	(see -racetam)	
-actide	synthetic corticotropins	ser**actide**
-adol or	analgesics (mixed opiate receptor agonists/antagonists)	taz**adol**ene
-adol-		spir**adol**ene
		levonantr**adol**
-adox	antibacterials (quinoline dioxide derivatives)	carb**adox**
-afenone	antiarrhythmics (propafenone derivatives)	alpra**fenone**
		dipra**fenone**x
-afil	PDE5 inhibitors	tadal**afil**
-aj-	antiarrhythmics (ajmaline derivatives)	lor**aj**mine
-aldrate	antacid aluminum salts	mag**aldrate**
-algron	alpha$_1$-adrenoreceptor agonists	dabuz**algron**
-alol	combined alpha and beta blockers	labet**alol**
		medrox**alol**
-amivir	(see -vir)	
-andr-	androgens	n**andr**olone
-anib	angiogenesis inhibitors	semax**anib**
-anserin	serotonin 5-HT$_2$ receptor antagonists	alt**anserin**
		trop**anserin**
		adat**anserin**
-antel	anthelmintics (undefined group)	carb**antel**
-arabine	antineoplastics (arabinofuranosyl derivatives)	faz**arabine**
		flud**arabine**
aril-, -aril, -aril-	antiviral (arildone derivatives)	plecon**aril**
		arildone
		fos**aril**ate
-arit	antirheumatics (lobenzarit type)	lobenz**arit**
		clobuz**arit**
-arol	anticoagulants (dicumarol type)	dicum**arol**
-arot-	arotinoids	et**arot**ene
		sum**arot**ene
		taz**arot**ene
-arotene	arotinoid derivatives	bex**arotene**
		lin**arotene**
		taz**arotene**
arte-	antimalarials (artemisin derivatives)	**arte**flene
-ase	enzymes	alglucer**ase**
		dorn**ase** alfa
	subgroups:	
-dismase	superoxide dismutase activity (exception: orgotein)	su**dismase**
-teplase	tissue-type plasminogen activators	al**teplase**
		du**teplase**
		sil**teplase**
-uplase	urokinase-type plasminogen activators	sar**uplase**
		nasar**uplase**
-ast	antiasthmatics/antiallergics	
	(not acting primarily as antihistamines; leukotriene biosynthesis inhibitors)	
subgroups:		
-lukast	leukotriene receptor antagonists	cina**lukast**
		pobi**lukast**
-milast	type IV phosphodiesterase inhibitors	picla**milast**
-trodast	thromboxane A$_2$ receptor antagonists	sera**trodast**
-zolast	benzoxazole derivatives	ecla**zolast**
		onta**zolast**
-(a)tadine	tircyclic histaminic-H1 receptor antagonists, loratadine derivatives	deslor**atadine**
		rup**atadine**
		soman**tadine**
-astine	antihistaminics (histamine-H$_1$ receptor antagonists)	eb**astine**
-atadine	tricyclic antiasthmatics	olop**atadine**
		lor**atadine**
-azenil	benzodiazepine receptor agonists/antagonists	bret**azenil**
		flum**azenil**
-azepam	antianxiety agents (diazepam type)	lor**azepam**

Appendix A Continued

STEM	DEFINITION	EXAMPLES
-azepide	cholecystokinin receptor antagonists	dev**azepide**
-azocine	narcotic antagonists/agonists (6,7-benzomorphan derivatives)	quad**azocine**
		ket**azocine**
-azoline	antihistamines/local vasoconstrictors (antazoline type)	ant**azoline**
-azosin	antihypertensives (prazosin type)	dox**azosin**
-bactam	beta-lactamase inhibitors	sul**bactam**
-bamate	tranquilizers/antiepileptics (propanediol and pentanediol groups)	mepro**bamate** fel**bamate**
-barb or	barbituric acid derivatives	pheno**barb**ital
-barb-		seco**barb**ital
		etero**barb**
-begron	beta 3 adrenoreceptor agonist	tali**begron**
-bendazole	anthelmintics (tibendazole type)	cam**bendazole**
-bersat	anticonvulsants; antimigraine (benzoylamino-benzpyran derivatives)	cara**bersat** tidem**bersat**
bol- or	anabolic steroids	**bol**andiol
-bol-		mi**bol**erone
-bufen	non-steroidal anti-inflammatory agents, fenbufen derivatives	indo**bufen**
-bulin	antineoplastics (mitotic inhibitors; tubulin binders)	mivo**bulin**
-butan	antiseptics (dapabutan type)	dapa**butan**
		lopo**butan**
-butazone	anti-inflammatory analgesics (phenylbutazone type)	mofe**butazone**
-caine	local anesthetics	dibu**caine**
calci- or	vitamin D analogues	**calci**potriene
-calci-		ta**calci**tol
-camra	antivirals (intracellular adhesion molecules, icam-1 derivatives**)**	trema**camra**
-camsule	camphorsulfonic acid derivatives used as UVA sunscreens	e**camsule**
-casan	caspase (interleukin–1b) converting enzyme inhibitors	pralna**casan**
-castat	(see -**stat)**	
-carbef	antibiotics (carbacephem derivatives)	lora**carbef**
-cavir	(see -vir)	
cef-	cephalosporins	**cef**azolin
-cept	receptors	al**vircept**
subgroups:		
-facept	lymphocyte function-associated with antigen 3 (LFA) receptor	ale**facept**
-farcept	interferon receptors	pi**farcept**
-lefacept	lymphocyte function-associated antigen 3	ale**facept**
-nercept	tumor necrosis factor receptors	le**nercept**
-vircept	antiviral receptors	al**vircept**
-cet	receptors (small molecule)	
subgroup:		
-calcet	calcium	te**calcet**
-cetrapib	cholesterol ester transfer protein inhibitors	tor**cetrapib**
-cic	hepatoprotectives (timonacic type)	limazo**cic**
-ciclovir	(see vir-)	
-cidib	cyclin dependent kinase inhibitor	alvo**cidib**
-cidin	natural antibiotics (undefined group)	grami**cidin**
-ciguat	guanaline cyclase activator	ata**ciguat**, atri**ciguat**
-cillin	penicillins	ampi**cillin**
-citabine	antivirals (nucleosides)	gem**citabine** fia**citabine** zal**citabine**
-clidine	muscarinic agonists (various indications)	veda**clidine** talsa**clidine**
-clone	hypnotics/tranquilizers (zopiclone type)	pago**clone**
-cog	blood coagulation factors	
subgroups:		
-eptacog	blood coagulation factor VII	**eptacog** alfa (activated)
-nonacog	blood coagulation factor IX	**nonacog** alfa
-octocog	blood coagulation factor VIII	mor**octocog**-alfa **octocog** alfa
-cogin	blood coagulation cascade inhibitor	tifa**cogin**
-conazole	systemic antifungals (miconazole type)	flu**conazole** oxi**conazole**
-cort-	cortisone derivatives	hydro**cort**isone

Appendix A **Continued**

STEM	DEFINITION	EXAMPLES
-coxib	cyclooxygenase-2 inhibitors	cele**coxib** pare**coxib** valde**coxib**
-cridar	(see -dar)	
-crinat	diuretics (ethacrynic acid derivatives)	bro**crinat**
-crine	acridine derivatives	amsa**crine** quina**crine**
-cromil	antiallergics (cromoglicic acid derivatives)	nedo**cromil**
-curium (also -curonium)	neuromuscular blocking agents (quaternary ammonium compounds)	atra**curium** al**curonium** pipe**curonium**
-cycline	antibiotics (tetracycline derivatives)	mino**cycline**
-dan	positive inotropic agents (pimobendan type)	prinoxo**dan** indoli**dan**
-dapsone	antimycobacterials (diaminodiphenylsulfone derivatives)	ace**dapsone**
-dar	multidrug resistance inhibitors	
subgroups:		
-cridar	acridine carboxamide derivatives	ela**cridar**
-icodar	pipecolic acid derivatives	bir**icodar**
-quidar	quinoline derivatives	lami**quidar** zozu**quidar**
-spodar	ciclosporin D derivatives	val**spodar**
-denoson	selective A_1 adenosine receptor subtype agonists	teca**denoson**, bino**denoson**
-dermin	(see -ermin)	
dil-, -dil- or -dil	vasodilators (undefined group)	foste**dil**
-dipine	phenylpyridine vasodilators (nifedipine type)	daro**dipine** felo**dipine**
-dismase	(see -ase)	
-distim	(see -stim)	
-ditan	antimigraine (5-HT$_1$ receptor agonists)	alni**ditan**
-dopa	dopamine receptor agonists	levo**dopa**
-dralazine	antihypertensives (hydrazine-phthalazines)	hy**dralazine** en**dralazine**
-dronate	calcium metabolism regulators	eti**dronate** tilu**dronate**
-dutant	(see -tant)	
-ectedin	ecteinascodin derivatives	mon**ectedin**
-ectin	antiparasitics (ivermectin type)	dorame**ctin** moxide**ctin**
-elestat	(see -stat)	
-elvakin	(see -kin)	
-emcinal	erythromycin derivatives lacking antibiotic activity	mit**emcinal**
-entan	endothelin receptor antagonists	bos**entan**
-eptacog	(see -cog)	
-eptakin	(see -kin)	
-erg-	ergot alkaloid derivatives	p**erg**olide
-eridine	analgesics (meperidine type)	anil**eridine**
-ermin	growth factors	
subgroups:		
-bermin	vascular endothelial growth factors	tel**bermin**
-dermin	epidermal growth factors	muro**dermin**
-fermin	fibroblast growth factors	erso**fermin**
-nermin	tumor necrosis factors	so**nermin** taso**nermin**
-plermin	platelet derived growth factors	beca**plermin**
-sermin	insulin-like growth factors	meca**sermin**
-termin	transforming growth factors	ce**termin**
subgroup:		
-otermin	bone morphogenetic proteins	dib**otermin** alfa
estr- or -estr-	estrogens	**estr**one fen**estr**el
-estrant	estrogen antagonists	fulv**estrant**
-etanide	diuretics (piretanide type)	bum**etanide**
-exakin	(see -kin)	
-ezolid	oxazolidinone antibacterials	epere**zolid** line**zolid**
-farnib	farnesykltransferase inhibitor	tipi**farnib**

Appendix A Continued

STEM	DEFINITION	EXAMPLES
-fenamate	"fenamic acid" ester or salt derivatives	eto**fenamate**
-fenamic acid	anti-inflammatory agents (anthranilic acid derivatives)	flu**fenamic acid**
-fenin	diagnostic aids ((phenylcarbamoyl)methyl iminodiacetic acid derivatives)	arclo**fenin**
-fenine	analgesics (fenamic acid subgroup)	flocta**fenine**
-fentanil	narcotic analgesics (fentanyl derivatives)	al**fentanil**
		mir**fentanil**
		bri**fentanil**
-fentrine	phosphodiesterase inhibitor	puma**fentrine**
-fermin	(see -ermin)	
-fiban	fibrinogen receptor antagonists (glycoprotein II$_b$/III$_a$ receptor antagonists)	lami**fiban**
		tiro**fiban**
-fibatide	(see -tide)	
-fibrate	antihyperlipidemics (clofibrate type)	beza**fibrate**
-filcon	hydrophilic contact lens materials	alpha**filcon** A
		xylo**filcon** A
		mipa**filcon** A
-fingol	sphingosine derivatives	cede**fingol**
		sa**fingol**
-flapon	5-lipoxygenase-activating protein (FLAP) inhibitors	qui**flapon**
-flurane	general inhalation anesthetics (halogenated alkane derivatives)	en**flurane**
-focon	hydrophobic contact lens materials	tri**focon** A
		pasi**focon** B
		sata**focon** A
-formin	hypoglycemics (phenformin type)	bu**formin**
-fradil	calcium channel blockers acting as vasodilators	mibe**fradil**
-fulven	antineoplastic, acylfulven derivatives	virido**fulven**
-fungin	antifungal antibiotics (undefined group)	kala**fungin**
-fylline	theophylline derivatives	enpro**fylline**
		bami**fylline**
		cipam**fylline**
-gab-	gabamimetics	fen**gab**ine
gado-	gadolinium derivatives (principally for diagnostic use)	**gado**diamide
		gadoteridol
		gadobenate
-gapil	neuronal apoptosis	omi**gapil**
-gapit	neuronal apoptosis	omi**gapit**
-ganan	antimicrobial, bactericidal permeability increasing polypeptide	ise**ganan**
		pexi**ganan**
-gatran	thrombin inhibitors (argatroban type)	efe**gatran**
-gest-	progestins	me**gest**rol
-giline	MAO inhibitors, type B	sele**giline**
-gillin	antibiotics (*Aspergillus* strains)	mito**gillin**
gli-	hypoglycemic agents (glipizide type)	**gli**flumide
-gliptin	antidiabetics, didpeptidyl aminopeptidase-IV inhibitors	vilda**gliptin**
-glitazar	antidiabetics, PPAR agonists (not thiazolidene derivatives)	far**glitazar**
-glitazone	antidiabetics (thiazolidene derivatives)	en**glitazone**
		pio**glitazone**
		tro**glitazone**
-glumide	CCK antagonists, antiulcer, anxiolytic agent	ami**glumide**
		itri**glumide**
-golix	GnRH receptor antagonists (nonpeptide)	rupu**golix**
-gosivir	(see -vir)	
-gramostim	(see -stim)	
-grastim	(see -stim)	
-grel- or	platelet antiaggregants (primarily thromboxane synthetase inhibitors)	itazi**grel**
-grel		dimeta**grel**
		fure**grel**ate
guan-	antihypertensives (guanidine derivatives)	**guan**octine
-ibat	ileal bile acid transport inhibitor	barix**ibat**
-icam	anti-inflammatory agents (isoxicam type)	enol**icam**
		tenox**icam**
-icodar	(see -dar)	
-ifen(e)	antiestrogens of the clomifene and tamoxifen groups	nitrom**ifene**
		ralox**ifene**
		drolox**ifene**
-ilide	class III antiarrhythmic agents	ibut**ilide**
		risot**ilide**
		dofet**ilide**

Appendix A Continued

STEM	DEFINITION	EXAMPLES
-imepodib -imex	inosine monophosphate dehydrogenase inhibitors immunostimulants	mer*imepodib* forfen*imex* roquin*imex* uben*imex*
-imib-	acycloA:cholesterol acetyltransferase (ACAT) enzyme inhibitors	eldac*imib*e lec*imib*ide oct*imib*ate
-imod	immunomodulators	ivar*imod* pidot*imod*

subgroup:
    -mapimod
    -imus
	
	mitogen-activated protein (MAP) kinase inhibitors
	immunosuppressives
		
		dor*mapimod*
		tacrol*imus*
		napir*imus*
		gusper*imus*
		sirol*imus*

io- -irudin -isant -isomide -ium (also -onium)	iodine-containing contrast media anticoagulants (hirudin type) histamine H3 receptor antagonists antiarrhythmics (disopyramide derivatives) quaternary ammonium derivatives	*io*damide des*irudin* cipral*isant* bid*isomide* clidin*ium* disiqu*onium* polixet*onium*
-kacin	antibiotics obtained from *Streptomyces* *kanamyceticus* (related to kanamycin)	ami*kacin*
-kalant	potassium channel antagonists	almo*kalant* teri*kalant*
-kalim	potassium channel agonists	croma*kalim* apri*kalim*
-kalner	opener of large conductance calcium-activated (map-k) K+ channels	flindo*kalner*
-kef-	enkephalin agonists (various indications)	met*keph*amide caso*kef*amide
-kin	interleukin type substances	

subgroups:
    -decakin
    -dodekin
    -elvekin
    -eptakin
    -exakin
    -leukin
	
	interleukin-10 analogues and derivatives
	interleukin-12 analogues and derivatives
	interleukin 11 analogues and derivatives
	interleukin 7 analogues and derivatives
	interleukin 6 analogues and derivatives
	interleukin 2 analogues and derivatives
		
		ilo*decakin*
		edo*dekin* alfa
		opr*elvekin*
		
		at*exakin* alfa
		tece*leukin*
		aldes*leukin*

-nakin	interleukin 1 analogues and derivatives	

subgroups:
    -onakin
    -benakin
    -nonakin
    -octakin
    -penkin
    -trakin
    -kinra
	
	1-α analogues and derivatives
	1-β analogues and derivatives
	interleukin 9 analogues and derivatives
	interleukin 8 analogues and derivatives
	interleukin 5 analogues and derivatives
	interleukin 4 analogues and derivatives
	interleukin receptor antagonists
		
		pit*onakin*
		mobe*nakin*
		
		em*octakin*
		
		bine*trakin*

subgroups: -nakinra -kiren	 interleukin 1 (IL-1) receptor antagonists renin inhibitors	 a*nakinra* dite*kiren* terla*kiren* zan*kiren*
-lazad -leptin -leukin -lipim -lubant	lipid peroxidation inhibitors leptin derivatives (see -kin) lipoprotein lipase activators leukotriene receptor antagonists (treatment of inflammatory skin disorders)	tiri*lazad* metre*leptin* ibro*lipim* tico*lubant*
-lukast -lutamide	(see -ast) antiandrogens	 bica*lutamide* f*lutamide*
-lutril	neutral endopeptidase inhibitors possessing additional endothelin	dag*lutril*
-mab	monoclonal antibodies	imciro*mab* abcixi*mab* capro*mab* daclixi*mab*

Appendix A Continued

STEM	DEFINITION	EXAMPLES
		detumo**mab**
		enlimo**mab**
-mantadine or	antivirals/antiparkinsonians	ri**mantadine**
-mantine	(adamantane derivatives)	dopa**mantine**
-mastat	(see -stat)	
-meline	cholinergic agonists (arecoline derivatives	xano**meline**
	used in treatment of Alzheimer's disease)	
-mer	polymers	cadexo**mer**
		carbeti**mer**
-mesine	sigma receptor ligands	ig**mesine**
		pana**mesine**
-mestane	antineoplastics (aromatase inhibitors)	plo**mestane**
-metacin	anti-inflammatory agents (indomethacin type)	zido**metacin**
-micin	antibiotics (*Micromonospora* strains)	madura**micin**
		genta**micin**
-monam	monobactam antibiotics	gloxi**monam**
		oxi**monam**
		tige**monam**
-morelin	(see -relin)	
-moren	non-peptidic growth hormone secretagogues	ibuta**moren**
-mostim	(see -stim)	
-motine	antivirals (quinoline derivatives)	fa**motine**
-moxin	monoamine oxidase inhibitors	ben**moxin**
	(hydrazine derivatives)	do**moxin**
-mustine	antineoplastics (chloroethylamine derivatives)	car**mustine**
-mycin	antibiotics (*Streptomyces* strains)	linco**mycin**
nab- or	cannabinol derivatives	**nab**azenil
-nab-		dro**nab**inol
-nakin	(see -kin)	
nal-	narcotic agonists/antagonists (normorphine type)	**nal**mefene
-navir	(see vir-)	
-nercept	(see -cept)	
-nermin	(see -ermin)	
-nertant	neurotensin receptor antagonists	remi**nertant**
-netant	(see -tant)	
-neurin	neurotensin receptor antagonists; neurotropins	abri**neurin**
-nicline	nicotinic acetylcholine receptor agonists	alti**nicline**
-nidap	nonsteroidal anti-inflammatory agents (tenidap type)	ilo**nidap**
		te**nidap**
-nidazole	antiprotozoal substances (metronidazole type)	ti**nidazole**
nifur-	5-nitrofuran derivatives	**nifur**atel
		nifuratrone
-nixin	anti-inflammatory agents (anilinonicotinic acid derivatives)	clo**nixin**
-nonacog	(see -cog)	
-nonakin	(see -kin)	
-octacog	(see -cog)	
-octakin	(see -kin)	
-olol	beta-blockers (propranolol type)	tim**olol**
		aten**olol**
-olone	steroids (*not* prednisolone derivatives)	minax**olone**
-onide	topical steroids (acetal derivatives)	amcin**onide**
-opilone	epothilone	fil**opilone**
-orex	anorexiants	flud**orex**
-orphan	narcotic antagonists/agonists	
dextro-	(morphinan derivatives)	meth**orphan**
		dextr**orphan**
-osuran	urotensin receptor antagonists	pal**osuran**
-otermin	bone morphogenetic proteins	dib**otermin** alfa
-otilate	hepatoprotectants, di-isopropyl-1,3-dithiol-malonate derivatives	miv**otilate**
-oxacin	antibacterials (quinolone derivatives)	difl**oxacin**
		ciprofl**oxacin**
-oxan	alpha-adrenoceptor antagonists (benzodioxane derivatives)	imil**oxan**
-oxanide	antiparasitics (salicylanilide derivatives)	brom**oxanide**
-oxef	antibiotics (oxacefalosporanic acid derivatives)	flom**oxef**
-oxetine	antidepressants (fluoxetine type)	dap**oxetine**
		sepr**oxetine**
-pafant	platelet-activating factor antagonists	a**pafant**
		daco**pafant**
		tulo**pafant**
		lexi**pafant**
-pamide	diuretics (sulfamoylbenzoic acid derivatives)	ali**pamide**

Appendix A Continued

STEM	DEFINITION	EXAMPLES
-pamil	coronary vasodilators (verapamil type)	tia**pamil**
-pamine	dopaminergics (butopamine type)	foso**pamine**
		ibo**pamine**
-panel	AMPA receptor antagonists	fana**panel**
		irum**panel**
		talam**panel**
-parcil	antithrombotics	beci**parcil**
		ili**parcil**
-parcin	glycopeptide antibiotics	avo**parcin**
-parin	heparin derivatives and low molecular weight (or depolymerized) heparins	he**parin**
		tinza**parin**
		dalte**parin**
-parinux	antithrombotyic indirect selective synthetic factor Xa inhibitors	fonda**parinux**
-paroid	antithrombotics (heparinoid type)	dana**paroid**
		sul**paroid**
peg-	PEGylated compounds	**peg**caristim
		pegnartograstim
		pegvisomant
-penem	antibacterial antibiotics (carbapenem derivatives)	imi**penem**
-penkin	(see -kin)	
perflu-	blood substitutes and/or diagnostics (perfluorochemicals)	**perflu**bron
		perflunafene
-peridol	antipsychotics (haloperidol type)	halo**peridol**
-peridone	antipsychotics (risperidone type)	ris**peridone**
		ilo**peridone**
		oca**peridone**
-perone	antianxiety agents/neuroleptics (4'-fluoro-4-piperidinobutyrophenone derivatives)	duo**perone**
-pezil	acetylcholinesterase inhibitors used in the treatment of Alzheimer's disease	ico**pezil**
		done**pezil**
-pidem	hypnotics/sedatives (zolpidem type)	zol**pidem**
		al**pidem**
-pirdine	cognition enhancers	lino**pirdine**
		besi**pirdine**
		sibo**pirdine**
-pirox	antimycotics (pyridone derivatives)	ciclo**pirox**
-pitant	(see -tant)	
-plact	platelet factor 4 analogs and derivatives	iro**plact**
-pladib	phospholipase A2 inhibitors	eco**pladib**
		vares**pladib**
-planin	antibacterials (*Actinoplanes* strains)	mide**planin**
		ramo**planin**
		teico**planin**
-platin	antineoplastics (platinum derivatives)	cis**platin**
-plermin	(see -ermin)	
-plestim	(see -stim)	
-plon	non-benzodiazepine anxiolytics, sedatives, hypnotics	ocina**plon**
		zale**plon**
-poetin	erythropoietins	e**poetin** alfa
		e**poetin** beta
-porfin	benzoporphyrin derivatives	verte**porfin**
		temo**porfin**
-pramine	antidepressants (imipramine type)	lofe**pramine**
-prazan	acid pump inhibitors, not dependent on acid activation	omida**prazan**
-prazole	antiulcer agents (benzimidazole derivatives)	ome**prazole**
		disu**prazole**
subgroup:		
-maprazole	acid pump inhibitors	pu**maprazole**
pred-, -pred- or -pred	prednisone and prednisolone derivatives	**pred**nicarbate
		clo**pred**nol
		oxiso**pred**
-pressin	vasoconstrictors (vasopressin derivatives)	desmo**pressin**
-pride	sulpiride derivatives	remoxi**pride**
		zaco**pride**
-pril	antihypertensives (ACE inhibitors)	enala**pril**
		temoca**pril**
		spira**pril**
-prilat	antihypertensives (ACE inhibitors) (diacid analogs of the -pril entity)	enala**prilat**
		spira**prilat**
-prinim	nootropic agents, purine derivatives	lete**prinim**

Appendix A Continued

STEM	DEFINITION	EXAMPLES
-tirelin	(see -relin)	
-tirome	antihyperlidaemic, thyromimetic derivatives	ani**tirome**
		axi**tirome**
-tocin	oxytocin derivatives	oxy**tocin**
-toin	antiepileptics (hydantoin derivatives)	albu**toin**
-tox(a)-	toxins	ur**toxa**zumab
-traposin	aP2 inhibitors	sel**traposin**
-trexate	antimetabolites (folic acid derivatives)	metho**trexate**
-trexed	antineoplastic thymidylate synthase inhibitors	peme**trexed**
		rali**trexed**
		nola**trexed**
-tricin	antibiotics (polyene derivatives)	mepar**tricin**
-triptan	antimigraine agents (5-HT$_1$ receptor agonists)	nara**triptan**
		oxi**triptan**
		suma**triptan**
-triptyline	antidepressants (dibenzo[a,d]cycloheptane derivatives)	ami**triptyline**
-troban	antithrombotics (thromboxane A$_2$ receptor antagonists)	dal**troban**
		sulo**troban**
-trodast	(see -ast)	
-troline	antipsychotics (dopamine D$_2$ antagonists)	carvo**troline**
		gevo**troline**
trop- or	atropine derivatives	benz**trop**ine
-trop-		
-uplase	(see -ase)	
-uracil	uracil derivatives used as thyroid antagonists and as antineoplastics	fluoro**uracil**
-uridine	antivirals; antineoplastics (uridine derivatives)	idox**uridine**
-vaptan	vasopressin receptor antagonists	coni**vaptan**
		relco**vaptan**
-vastatin	(see -stat)	
-verine	spasmolytic agents (papaverine type)	mebe**verine**
vin- or	vinca alkaloids	**vin**epidine
-vin-		apo**vin**camine
vir-, -vir-	antiviral substances (undefined group)	ganciclo**vir**
or -vir		en**vir**adine
		viroxime
		al**vir**cept
		dela**vir**dine
subgroups:		
-amivir	neuraminidase inhibitors	zan**amivir**
-cavir	carbocyclic nucleosides	lobu**cavir**
-cyclovir/	antivirals (acyclovir type)	des**ciclovir**
-ciclovir		fam**ciclovir**
		pen**ciclovir**
-gosivir	glucosidase inhibitor	cel**gosivir**
-navir	HIV protease inhibitors (saquinavir type)	droxi**navir**
		indi**navir**
		rito**navir**
-virdine	antivirals (non-nucleoside reverse transcriptase inhibitors; pyridine derivatives)	ate**virdine**
		dele**virdine**
-virenz	antivirals (non-nucleoside reverse transcriptase inhibitors; benzoxazinone derivatives)	efa**virenz**
-virsen	antivirals (antisense)	afo**virsen**
		fomi**virsen**
		treco**virsen**
-vircept	(see -cept)	
-virdine	(see vir)	
-virenz	(see vir)	
-vudine	antineoplastics; antivirals (zidovudine group) (exception: edoxudine)	sta**vudine**
		lami**vudine**
		alo**vudine**
-xaban	antithrombotic; factor X inhibitor	tami**xaban**
-xanox	antiallergic respiratory tract drugs (xanoxic acid derivatives)	ti**xanox**
-(x)antrone	antineoplastics, mitoxantrone derivatives aza-anthracenedione class of antitumor agents	pi**xantrone**
-zolamide	carbonic anhydrase inhibitors	brin**zolamide**
		dor**zolamide**
		se**zolamide**
-zolast	(see -ast)	
-zomib	proteozome inhibitors	borte**zomib**

Appendix A Continued

The following USAN stems have received official approval by the USAN Council at the July 14, 2003 USAN Council meeting:

STEM	DEFINITION	EXAMPLES
-algron	alpha$_1$-adrenoreceptor agonists	dabuz*algron*
-casan	caspase (interleukin-1b) converting enzyme inhibitors	pralna*casan*
-gliptin	didpeptidyl aminopeptidase-IV inhibitors	vilda*gliptin*
-lutril	neutral endopeptidase inhibitors possessing additional endothelin	dag*lutril*
-imod	mitogen-activated protein (MAP) kinase inhibitors	dor*mapimod*
-mapimod		
-nertant	neurotensin receptor antagonists	remi*nertant*
-pladib	phospholipase A2 inhibitors	eco*pladib*
-punil	motochondrial benzodiazepine receptor (MBR) selective antagonists (purine derivatives)	ema*punil*
-proget	nonsteroidal ligand for the progesterone receptor	tana*proget*
-osuran	urotensin receptor antagonists	pal*osuran*
-otermin	bone morphogenetic proteins	dib*otermin* alfa
-tinib	tyrosine kinase inhibitors	caner*tinib*, ima*tinib*, mubri*tinib*

This list represents common stems for which chemical and/or pharmacologic parameters have been established. These stems and their definitions have been approved by the USAN Council and are recommended for use in coining new nonproprietary names for drugs that belong to an established series of related agents. The list is not exhaustive in that it does not include all stems used by the Council and other national or international nomenclature groups. It is the nature of the nomenclature process that new, potential stems are constantly being created and that definitions of older stems may need to be modified as new information becomes available.

Appendix B Contractions for Radicals and Adducts

CONTRACTION	CHEMICAL NAME AND GRAPHIC FORMULA
aceturate	*N*-acetylglycinate $CH_3CONHCH_2COO^-$
acistrate	2'-acetate (ester) and octadecanoate (salt) CH_3-CO- and $CH_3-(CH_2)_{16}-CO-$
axetil	1-acetoxyethyl CH_3COCH- with CH_3
besylate	benzenesulfonate ($-SO_3^-$)
camsylate	camphorsulfonate ($CH_2SO_3^-$)
caproate	hexanoate $CH_3(CH_2)_4COO^-$

CONTRACTION	CHEMICAL NAME AND GRAPHIC FORMULA
closylate	*p*-chlorobenzenesulfonate $Cl-\langle\rangle-SO_3^-$
cyclotate	4-methylbicyclo[2.2.2]oct-2-ene-1-carboxylate $CH_3-\langle\rangle-COO^-$
cypionate	cyclopentanepropionate $CH_2CH_2COO^-$
dapropate	*N*,*N*-dimethyl-β-alanine $H_3C-N(CH_3)-CO_2^-$
diolamine	diethanolamine $HN(CH_2CH_2OH)_2$
edamine	ethylenediamine $H_2N-CH_2CH_2-NH_2$

Appendix B Continued

CONTRACTION	CHEMICAL NAME AND GRAPHIC FORMULA	CONTRACTION	CHEMICAL NAME AND GRAPHIC FORMULA
edetate*	ethylenediaminetetraacetate	hyclate	monohydrochloride, hemiethanolate hemihydrate

edetate* — ethylenediaminetetraacetate

NaOOCCH₂   CH₂COONa

        NCH₂CH₂N

NaOOCCH₂   CH₂COONa

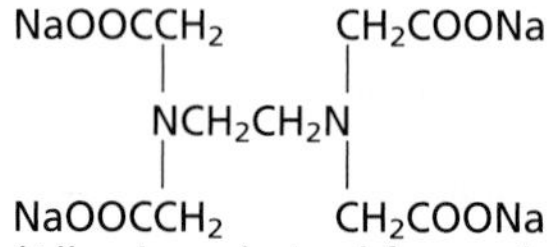

(All anions derived from edetic acid; edetate sodium is portrayed here.)

hyclate — monohydrochloride, hemiethanolate hemihydrate

$HCl \cdot \frac{1}{2}C_2H_5OH \cdot \frac{1}{2}H_2O$

isethionate — 2-hydroxyethanesulfonate

CH₂CH₂SO₃⁻

OH

edisylate — 1,2-ethanedisulfonate

CH₂SO₃⁻

CH₂SO₃⁻

meglumine — *N*-methylglucamine

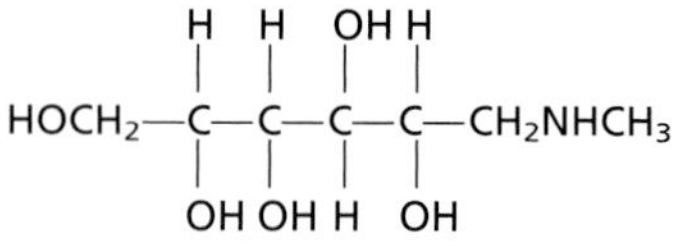

HOCH₂—C—C—C—C—CH₂NHCH₃ (with H, H, OH, H above and OH, OH, H, OH below)

enanthate — heptanoate

CH₃(CH₂)₅COO⁻

mesylate — methanesulfonate

CH₃SO₃⁻

epolamine — 1-pyrrolidineethanol

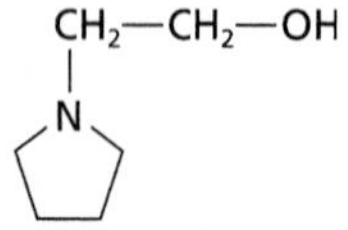

CH₂—CH₂—OH attached to N of pyrrolidine ring

mofetil — 2-(4-morpholinyl)ethyl

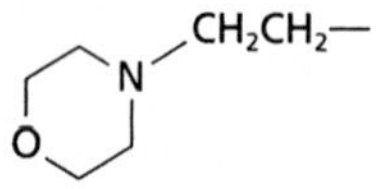

morpholine ring with N—CH₂CH₂—

erbumine — 2-methyl-2-propanamine

H₂NC(CH₃)₃

napsylate — 2-naphthalenesulfonate

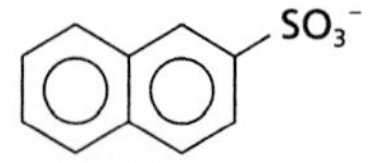

naphthalene ring with SO₃⁻

estolate — propanoate and dodecyl sulfate (salt)

CH₃CH₂COO—in ester linkage plus C₁₂H₂₃OSO₃⁻

esylate — ethanesulfonate

CH₃CH₂SO₃⁻

olamine — ethanolamine

H₂NCH₂CH₂OH

etabonate — (ethoxycarbonyl)oxy

O
||
CH₃CH₂OCO⁻

pamoate — 4,4'-methylenebis[3-hydroxy-2-naphthoate]

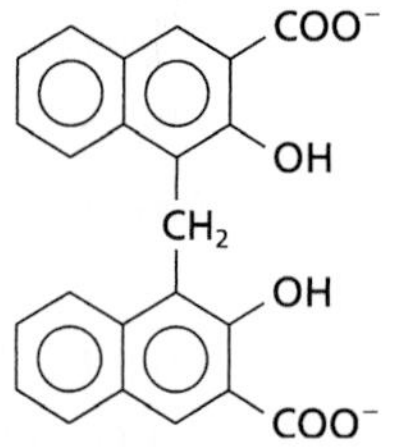

naphthalene rings with COO⁻, OH, CH₂, OH, COO⁻

fostedate — tetradecyl hydrogen phosphate

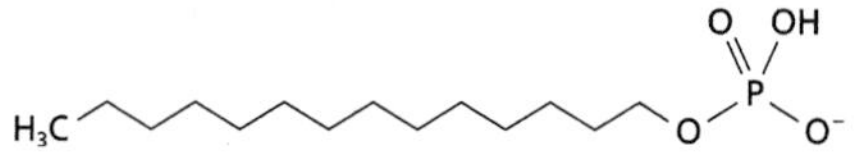

H₃C—(chain)—O—P(=O)(OH)—O⁻

gluceptate — glucoheptonate

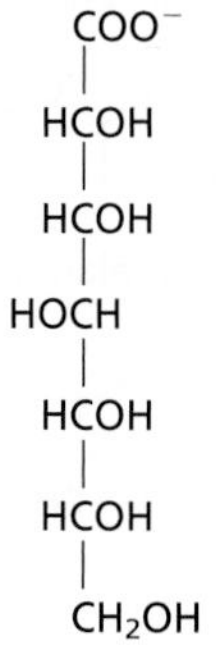

COO⁻

HCOH

HCOH

HOCH

HCOH

HCOH

CH₂OH

pendetide — N^6-[*N*-[2-[[2-[bis(carboxymethyl)-amino]ethyl](carboxymethyl)amino]-ethyl]-*N*-(carboxymethyl)glycyl]-N^2-(*N*-glycyl-L-tyrosyl-L-lysine-tyrosyl)

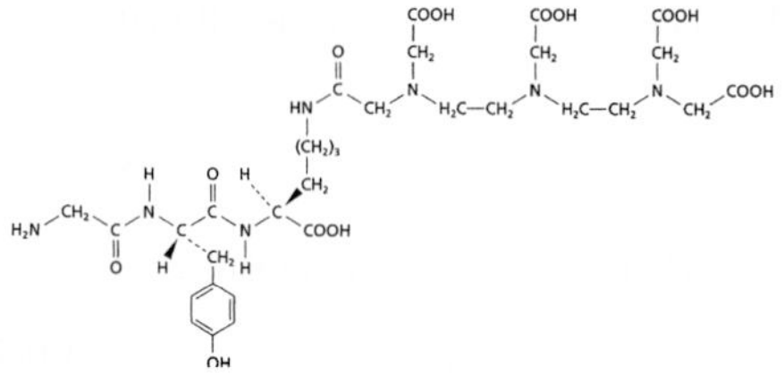

(complex structure)

hybenzate — *o*-(4-hydroxybenzoyl)benzoate

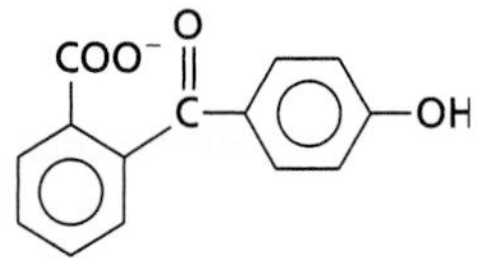

benzene ring with COO⁻ and C(=O)—benzene ring—OH

phenpropionate — 3-phenylpropionate

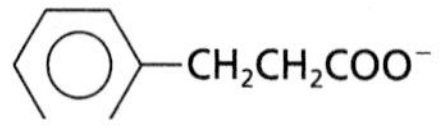

benzene ring—CH₂CH₂COO⁻

Appendix B Continued

CONTRACTION	CHEMICAL NAME AND GRAPHIC FORMULA	CONTRACTION	CHEMICAL NAME AND GRAPHIC FORMULA
pivalate	trimethylacetate 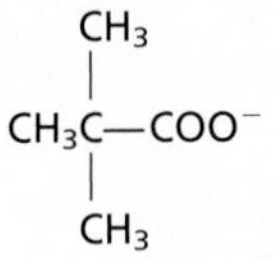	tebutate	*tertiary* butyl acetate 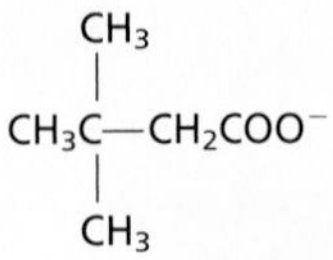

pivalate — trimethylacetate

$$CH_3C(CH_3)(CH_3)-COO^-$$

$$\begin{array}{c} CH_3 \\ | \\ CH_3C-COO^- \\ | \\ CH_3 \end{array}$$

tebutate — *tertiary* butyl acetate

$$\begin{array}{c} CH_3 \\ | \\ CH_3C-CH_2COO^- \\ | \\ CH_3 \end{array}$$

pivoxetil — 1-(2-methoxy-2-methyl-1-oxopropoxy)ethyl

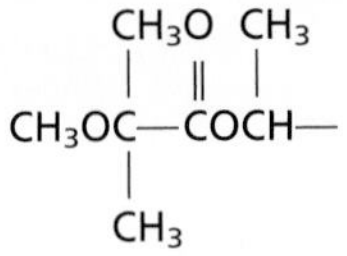

$$\begin{array}{c} CH_3O \quad CH_3 \\ | \quad \| \quad | \\ CH_3OC-COCH- \\ | \\ CH_3 \end{array}$$

tosylate — *p*-toluenesulfonate

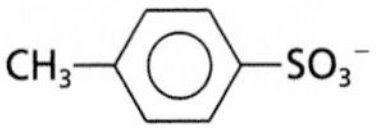

$$CH_3-\langle\bigcirc\rangle-SO_3^-$$

pivoxil — (2,2-dimethyl-1-oxopropoxy)methyl

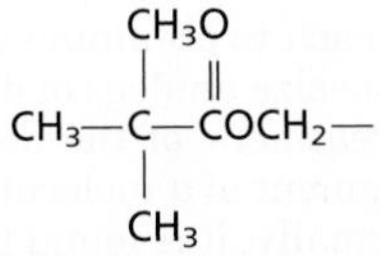

$$\begin{array}{c} CH_3O \\ | \quad \| \\ CH_3-C-COCH_2- \\ | \\ CH_3 \end{array}$$

triflutate — trifluoroacetate

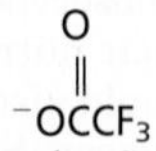

$$\begin{array}{c} O \\ \| \\ {}^-OCCF_3 \end{array}$$

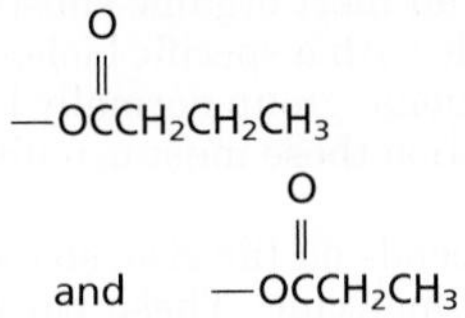

trolamine — triethanolamine

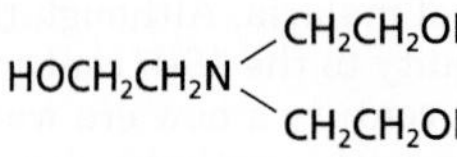

$$HOCH_2CH_2N\begin{array}{c} CH_2CH_2OH \\ \\ CH_2CH_2OH \end{array}$$

probutate — (1-oxobutoxy) (ester) and (1-oxopropoxy) (ester)

$$\begin{array}{c} O \\ \| \\ -OCCH_2CH_2CH_3 \end{array}$$

and

$$\begin{array}{c} O \\ \| \\ -OCCH_2CH_3 \end{array}$$

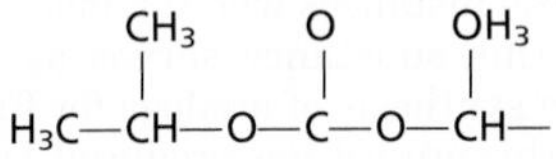

xinafoate — 1-hydroxy-2-naphthalenecarboxylate

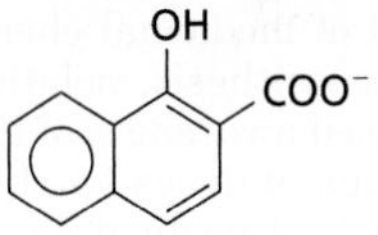

proxetil — 1-[(isopropoxycarbonyl)oxy]ethyl

$$\begin{array}{c} CH_3 \quad O \quad OH_3 \\ | \quad \| \quad | \\ H_3C-CH-O-C-O-CH- \end{array}$$

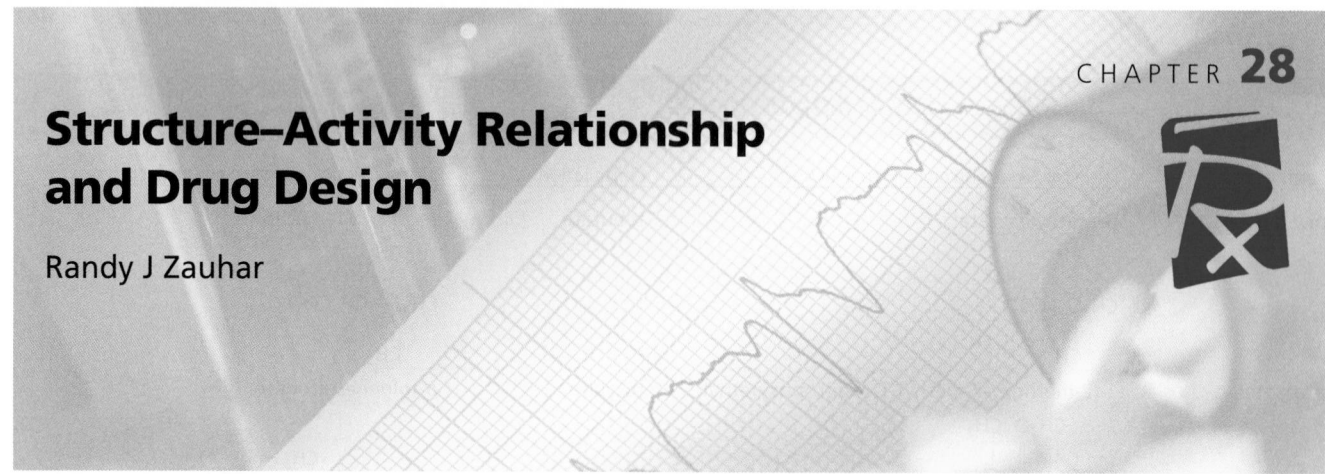

CHAPTER 28

Structure–Activity Relationship and Drug Design

Randy J Zauhar

For centuries humans have observed not only that natural substances could be used for their nutritional value and for treatment of diseases, but they could also bring about toxic or lethal effects. The Chinese Emperor Sheng Nang in 2735 BCE compiled a book of herbs and employed *Chang Shan* in the treatment of malaria. Although the majority of the drugs used from antiquity to the 19th century came from natural sources, in the past century a new era was brought about by treatment of diseases with synthetic drugs. Also, the modification of natural products, through various synthetic processes, has provided useful semisynthetic drugs.

The field of medicinal chemistry has evolved from an emphasis on the synthesis, isolation, and characterization of drugs to an increased awareness of the biochemistry of disease states and the design of drugs for the prevention of diseases. An important aspect of medicinal chemistry has been to establish a relationship between chemical structure and biological activity. An increased consideration in recent years has been to correlate the chemical structure with chemical reactivity or physical properties and these correlations can, in turn, be related to their therapeutic actions.

Although there has been a great deal of success in understanding the relationship between chemical structure and biological activity in a number of areas, especially for antibacterial drugs, there are still many human afflictions that require new and improved drugs. Cancer, viral infections, cardiovascular disease, and mental disease need new agents and approaches for treating and preventing these maladies. As more information is gained as to causative factors of different diseases, the move will be from the empirical approach to the rational design of new drugs. General principles of drug design have been and are continuing to be developed in medicinal chemistry.

In developing drugs with specific activities, several approaches are used. The effects of natural products or synthetic drugs are determined on various biological systems (or screens) to identify lead compounds with specific biological activities. Once the effect of the drug is known, the medicinal chemist and pharmacologist work together to improve the activity of a known active molecule or "lead molecule." This process normally goes through a synthesis—biological test—synthesis—biological test cycle until a drug with the desired activity is obtained. Today, the structure of receptors and function of enzymes, which may be involved in the pathogenesis of a disease, are understood better. These molecules, in turn, are used as targets for the design of drugs that act as agonists or antagonists of receptors or inhibitors of the enzymes. Thus, this information adds a new phase to the cycle, which is now drug design—synthesis—biological activity—drug design, and so on.

ANALOG APPROACH

The most frequent approach to obtaining drugs to treat a particular disease is to synthesize analogs of drugs that are known to be effective in the treatment of the disease. The *pharmacophore* is a chemical segment of a molecule that is responsible for biological action. Normally, it is found that the specific type of biological activity of a molecule depends on more than just one functional group. Consequently, the addition of a single functional group to an inert organic substance ordinarily does not imbue a molecule with a specific biological activity because more than one functional group normally is required for potent activity, and in addition these must usually be arranged with a specific geometry.

Drug activity depends on the size, shape, and degree of ionization of the drug molecule. These parameters are studied by making analogs or molecular modifications of a parent molecule. In those instances where a molecule has a known biological action, this substance serves as a prototype or lead molecule for the synthesis of analogs for further biological testing. In the past this process has produced a greater number of active analogs than just preparing and testing molecules obtained through a random process. In addition, structure–activity relationship studies often are used to determine the pharmacophore and also to obtain drugs with increased potency, greater selectivity, increased or decreased duration of action, low toxicity, and increased stability.

Finally, economics may be a prime reason for the search for analogs if a natural product is too difficult to obtain or if a synthetic molecule is too expensive to prepare in quantities needed for the manufacturing process.

Homologs

A *homologous series* refers to a series of analogs that differ in structure by a simple increment in the molecular formula. For example, these may be produced by sequential chemical change that includes increasing or decreasing the length of a carbon chain. A series of homologs of this type is used to provide insight into the relationship of biological activity and chemical changes that involve only the number of methylene groups. This type of determination has provided valuable information as to the importance of the partition coefficient and biological action. Often, the compounds with short, alkyl chains are low in activity; as the chain length is increased, the biological activity increases to an optimum point, and as more methylene groups are added, activity decreases. An interesting example of this phenomenon is the activity of the *n*-alkylresorcinols in which the optimum biological activity, as measured by phenol coefficients against *B typhosus*, is hexylresorcinol (**1**)

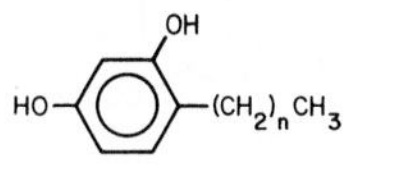

hexylresorcinol (n = 5)
1

with six carbon atoms ($n = 5$) in the side chain. If the alkyl chain is lengthened or decreased, a decrease in activity is observed relative to hexylresorcinol.

There are times in which changing the number of methylene groups may lead to a change in the type of biological activity rather than its intensity. For example, it is known that alkyltrimethylammonium analogs (**2**)

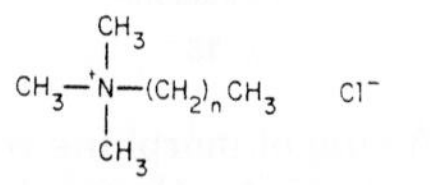

alkyltrimethylammonium
2

possess different types of activity depending on the length of the alkyl group.

If the alkyl group is up to six carbons ($n = 5$), as in 2, the compounds are muscarinic agonists. Thus, these compounds have activity similar to acetylcholine (**3**)

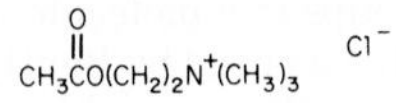

acetylcholine chloride
3

on muscarinic receptors. With seven carbons ($n = 6$) to eight ($n = 7$) carbons, these compounds are partial agonists; when the length is greater than nine carbons ($n = 8$), these compounds are muscarinic antagonists.

Molecular Fragmentation

The synthesis and biological evaluation of molecular fragments of a *lead* compound often is used in structure–activity studies. This process also may be called *molecular simplification, molecular dissociation,* or *disjunction.* Often, this process is used when the structure of a natural product is elucidated and possibly new biological action. When the natural product may be too difficult or expensive to obtain for drug use, the process of trial and error is used to determine which portion of the molecule is required for a desired biological activity. Several illustrations of the molecular fragmentation approach will be given in which the starting point is a natural product.

Cocaine (**4**),

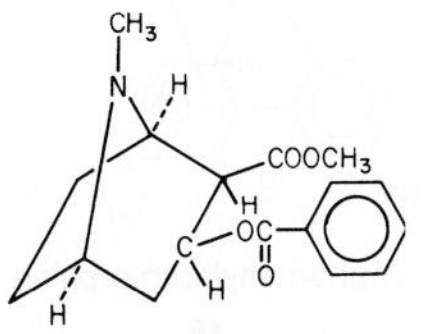

cocaine
4

an alkaloid obtained from *Erythroxylon coca*, has served as the prototype molecule for the development of a number of local

anesthetics. The carbomethoxy group of cocaine is not required for local anesthetic action, as can be seen with tropacocaine, which lacks this group (**5**).

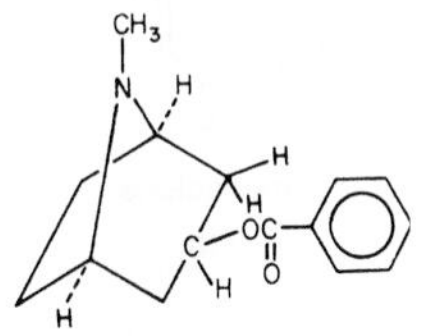

tropacocaine
5

The synthesis of β-eucaine (**6**)

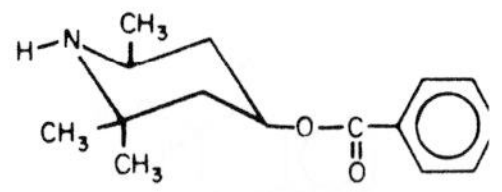

β-eucaine
6

and subsequent biological testing showed that a tropane ring system also was not a prerequisite for local anesthetic activity.

The synthesis of procaine (**7**)

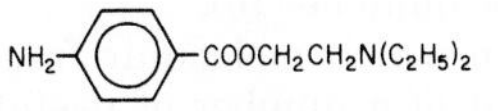

procaine
7

demonstrated that the critical part of the molecule required for activity was the hydrophilic amine segment attached to an intermediate chain, which in turn was attached to a lipophilic ester function. Many analogs of procaine have potent local anesthetic activity. The amine section of procaine can be removed to give benzocaine (**8**),

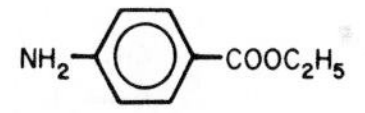

benzocaine
8

a substance known to possess local anesthetic activity. However, the mechanism of action of benzocaine in the production of local anesthesia is different from that of procaine. Therefore, one must be cautious in relating chemical changes to activity, particularly because the drug may retain activity but the mechanism by which the activity is produced may change.

Vitamin K_1 (**9**)

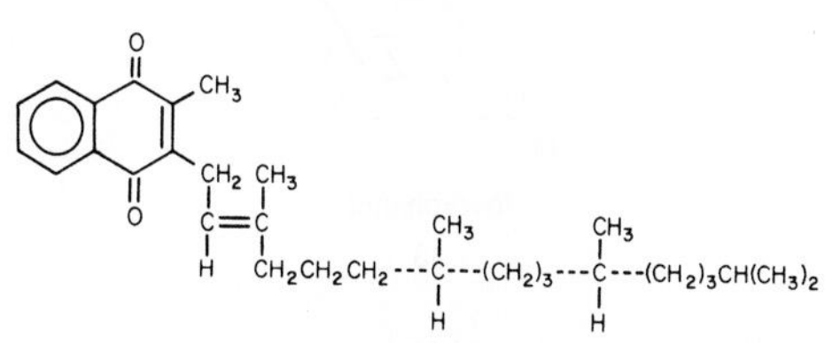

vitamin K₁
9

is a natural product (phytonadione) composed of a naphthoquinone bearing a 2-methyl group and a side-chain phytyl group at the 3 position. It is known that vitamin K is useful in preventing hemorrhage and attempts have been made to prepare drugs that were less complex but maintained vitamin K activity.

Menadione (**10**)

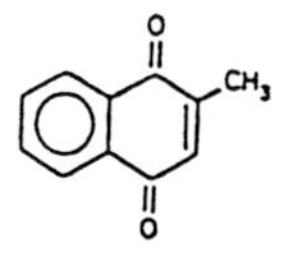

menadione

10

is a highly active, vitamin K–like drug that can be prepared by the oxidation of 1-methylnaphthalene with chromic acid. It is an analog of vitamin K that lacks the phytyl side chain at the 3 position. A bisulfite-addition product, menadione sodium bisulfite (**11**),

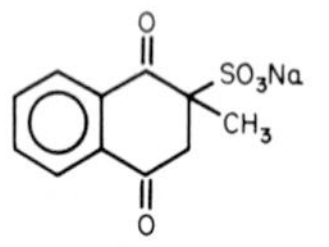

menadione sodium bisulfite

11

is available as a water-soluble anticoagulant. The substance is known to decompose under appropriate conditions to liberate menadione, the free quinone (**10**).

Another area in which molecular fragmentation has led to the development of a number of useful drugs is with the analgesics related to morphine. The structure of morphine was determined in 1925; subsequently, many analogs were prepared and examined for analgesic activity. In most instances new analogs were prepared with the goal of possibly separating the analgesic effects from the undesirable effects of dependence liability, nausea, constipation, and respiratory depression.

It can be seen that, through molecular fragmentation, one can reduce the number of ring systems from the pentacyclic, morphine (**12**)

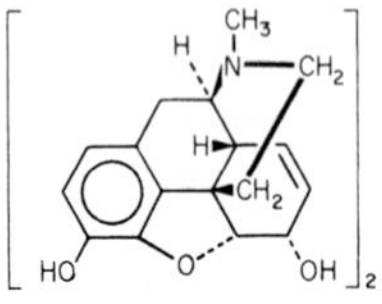

morphine

12

to a tetracyclic, levorphanol (**13**),

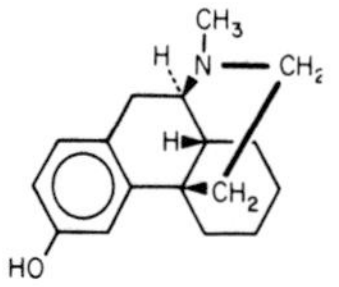

levorphanol

13

and a tricyclic, pentazocine (**14**),

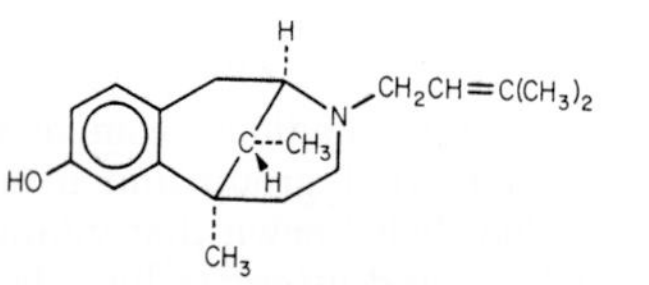

pentazocine

14

a bicyclic, meperidine (**15**);

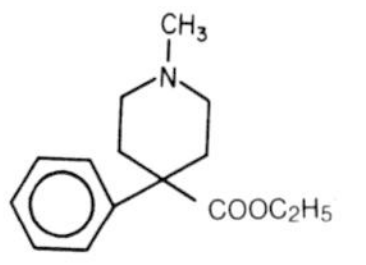

meperidine

15

and to (**16**), methadone,

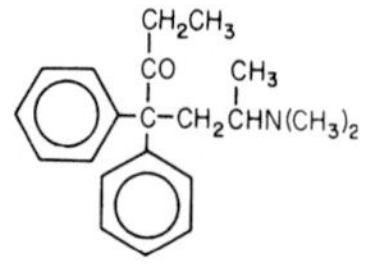

methadone

16

which has only the A ring of morphine remaining, but still retains potent analgesic activity. Certainly, the amine and aromatic ring play an important role in the production of analgesic activity. The intermediate carbon atoms between the amine and the phenyl ring do not have to be in a specific configuration for the molecule to possess analgesic activity.

Addition of Functional Groups

Another approach often used in structure–activity relationships is to add functional groups to a molecule with known biological activity. This approach was used by Bently and Hardy[1] to see if a molecule more complex than morphine could be synthesized that would interact with the analgesic receptor but, because of its complex structure, would not interact with the receptors that produced side effects. One of the analogs, etorphine (**17**),

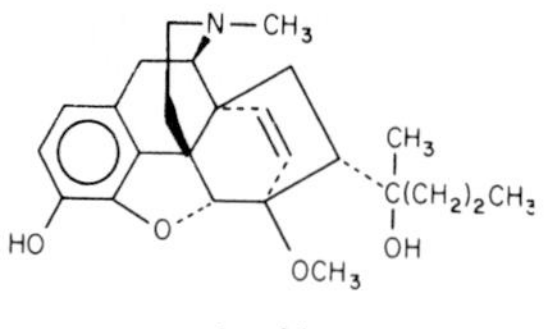

etorphine

17

is some 1000 times more potent than morphine and is used primarily in veterinary medicine to immobilize large animals. Of major importance is the fact that etorphine and related agents have enhanced potency, suggesting that etorphine may bind to an additional site that dramatically enhances the analgesic activity of morphine.

It also is known that replacement of the N-methyl group with the larger N-phenethyl group to give N-phenethylnormorphine (**18**)

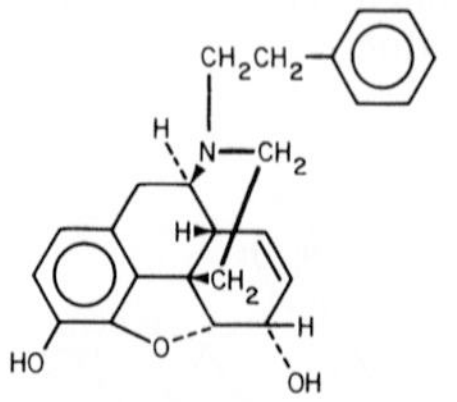

N-phenethylnormorphine

18

produces a compound six times as potent as morphine. An important observation is that not only may a quantitative change be brought about by modifying the N-methyl group of morphine but also a qualitative change in activity is observed if it is changed to an *N*-allyl group as shown in **19**,

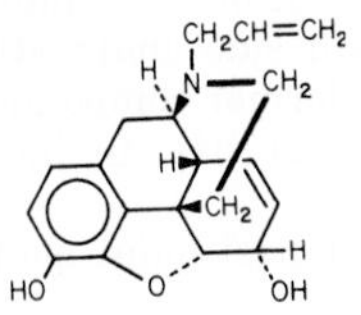

nalorphine

19

to produce *N*-allylnormorphine (nalorphine), a morphine antagonist. This finding has stimulated a great deal of study of structure–activity relationships with the *N*-substituents to find potent agonists, antagonists, and mixed agonist-antagonists of opioid receptors.

In other drug categories, it has been shown that tolazoline (**20**)

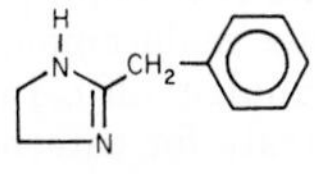

tolazoline

20

is an antagonist of α-adrenergic receptors, while the addition of another phenyl ring produces naphazoline (**21**),

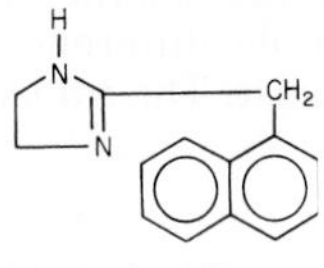

naphazoline

21

which is an α-adrenergic agonist. This is a rather unusual transformation of an antagonist into an agonist by the addition of a functional group.

Isosteric Replacements

The concept of *isosterism* or *bioisosterism* has been used for a number of years in the search for new drugs. This has been an extremely important approach in the design of antimetabolites. In 1919, Langmuir[2,3] first defined *isosteres* as those molecules or groups of atoms that have the same number and types of electrons. For example, N_2 and CO or N_3^- and NCO^- are examples of isosteres. These substances have similar physical properties. Later, Friedman[4] introduced the concept of *bioisosteres,* compounds that fit the broadest definitions for isosteres and have a similar type of biological activity. This concept included drugs with agonist or antagonist activity. When a substance is found that does possess promising therapeutic activity, the medicinal chemists will attempt to prepare closely related compounds with improved properties such as greater potency or fewer side effects. In the past, a considerable amount of intuition had been used by medicinal chemists in selecting bioisosteric replacements. The standard isosteric replacements are divided into five classes, as illustrated in Table 28-1.

A variety of nonclassic bioisosteric replacements also are known and include paired examples such as H and F, —CO_2H and —SO_3H and —CO— and —SO_2—.

Some of the examples of isosteric replacement that have provided useful drugs are a fluorine replacement of the hydrogen in uracil (**22**)

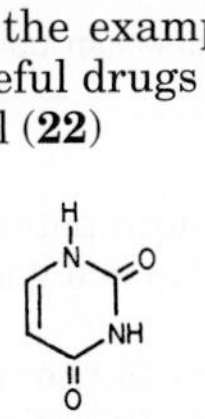

uracil	5-fluorouracil	hypoxanthine
22	**23**	**24**

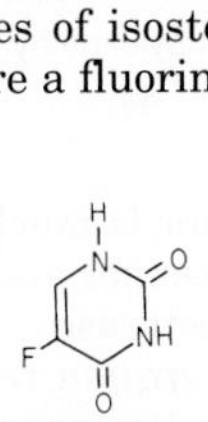

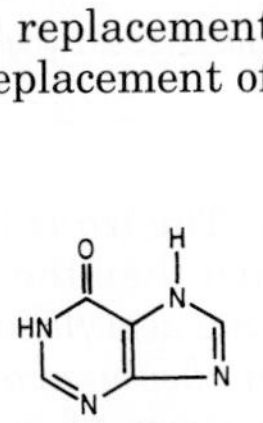

Table 28-1. Isosteric Replacements

CLASS 1 (MONOVALENT)	2 (DIVALENT)	3 (TRIVALENT)	4 (TETRAVALENT)	5 (RINGS)
F, Cl, Br, I	—O—	—N=	=C=	—CH=CH—
OH, SH	—S—	—P=	=Si=	—S—
NH_2, PH_2	—Se—	—As=	=N^+=	—O—
CH_3	—Tc—	—Sb=	=P=	—NH—
		=CH—	=As=	
			=Sb^+=	

to give 5-fluorouracil (**23**), a very useful anticancer drug; and the replacement of the carbonyl oxygen in hypoxanthine (**24**) to give 6- mercaptopurine (**25**),

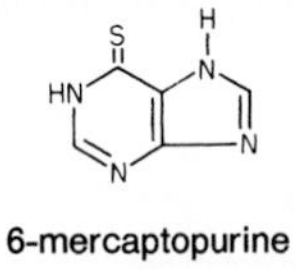

6-mercaptopurine	chlorpromazine
25	**26**

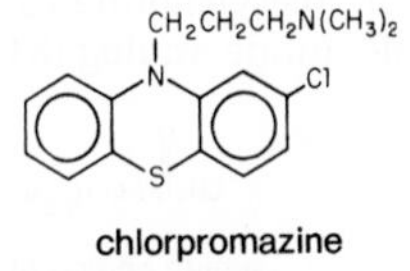

a potent antitumor antimetabolite. The replacement of oxygen by sulfur in chlorpromazine (**26**) to give the oxygen isostere (**27**)

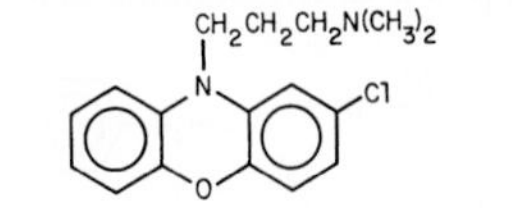

oxygen isostere of chlorpromazine

27

produced a compound with 1/10 the tranquilizing activity of the parent molecule.

The replacement of the ester function of procaine (**7**), a local anesthetic, with an amide function produced procainamide (**28**),

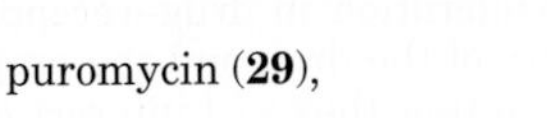

procainamide

28

which has found an important role in the treatment of cardiac arrhythmias. An important difference between the two drugs is that the amide function, which allows for similar biological activity, is more stable chemically, can be given orally, and is not affected by the esterases that catalyze the hydrolysis of procaine.

The antibiotic puromycin (**29**),

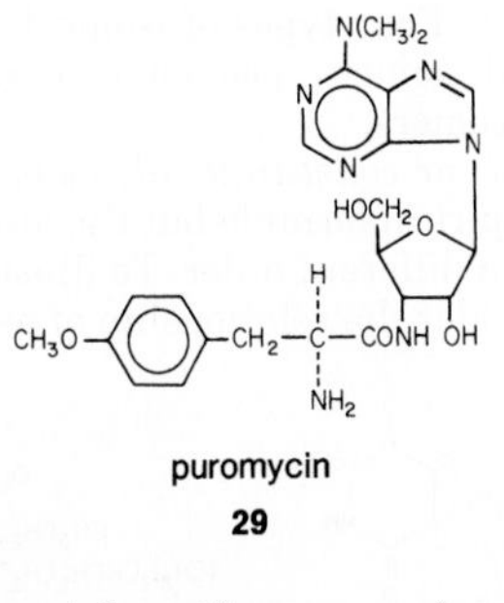

puromycin

29

which has antibacterial, antitumor, and antitrypanosomidal activity, inhibits protein synthesis by interfering with the utilization of transfer-RNA. Puromycin is the isosteric analog of the aminoacyl-*t*-RNA (**30**);

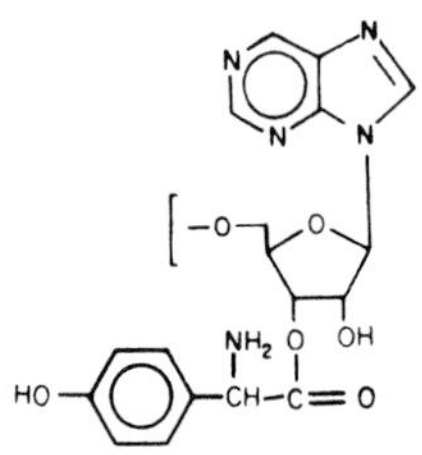

terminus of tyrosinyl-*t*-RNA
30

after puromycin is taken up, it blocks the subsequent protein synthesis.

The isosteric replacement of ester groups does not always produce compounds with significant biological activity, as the modification of acetylcholine ester (**3**) with an amide function resulted in the amide analog (**31**)

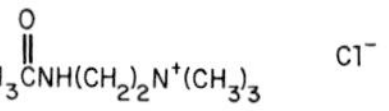

amide analog of acetylcholine
31

that does not show significant agonist or antagonist activity. One of the oldest nonclassic isosteric replacements that provided an important class of antibacterial agents was the replacement of carboxylic acid group of *p*-aminobenzoic acid (PABA, **32**)

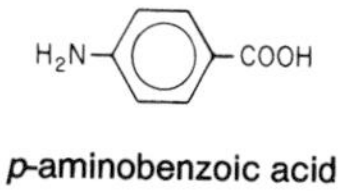

p-aminobenzoic acid	sulfanilamide
32	**33**

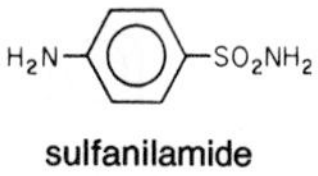

with a sulfonamide group to give sulfanilamide (**33**).

A final illustration of bioisosteric replacement in drug design is the replacement of the thiourea functional group of metiamide (**34**),

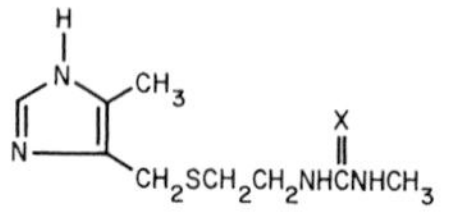

X = S, metiamide
34

X = NCN, cimetidine
35

a histamine H_2-blocker, with the cyanoguanidine group to produce the popular antiulcer drug cimetidine (**35**). This bioisosteric replacement overcame the granulocytopenia toxicity that had been observed with metiamide.

Stereochemistry

An important consideration in drug–receptor interactions is the stereochemistry of the drug and the proper positioning of functional groups so that they will interact optimally with an enzyme or receptor. Four types of isomeric drugs will be considered: positional isomers, geometrical isomers, optical isomers, and diastereomers.

With *positional*, or *constitutional*, *isomers* the compounds have the same empirical formula but the atoms of the molecule are rearranged in a different order. To illustrate positional isomers, one can consider the relationship of pentobarbital (**36**)

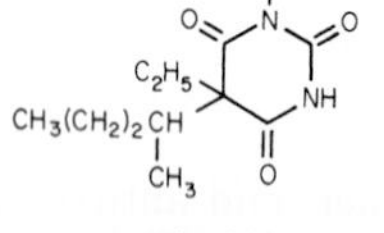

pentobarbital	amobarbital
36	**37**

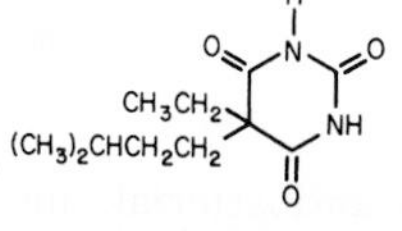

and amobarbital (**37**), both of which belong to the barbiturate family. These positional isomers differ only in the makeup of the 5-carbon side chain attached to the barbiturate ring system. The former compound has a short duration of action while the latter has an intermediate duration of action.

Another example of positional isomers is *N*-(*tert*-butyl)-norepinephrine (**38**)

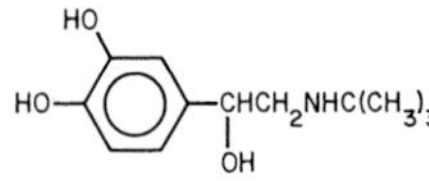

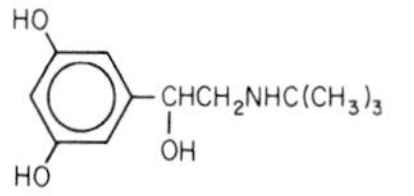

N-tertiary-butyl norepinephrine	terbutaline
38	**39**

and terbutaline (**39**). The resorcinol portion of 39 has served as a biologically effective replacement of the catechol group in 38. The resorcinol analog (**39**), in contrast to the catechol (**38**), is not a substrate for catechol-*O*-methyltransferase (COMT), an important metabolic enzyme; therefore, it has a longer duration of action. Terbutaline is a useful selective β_2-adrenergic stimulant for the treatment of bronchial asthma and related conditions, and it can be administered orally.

Geometrical isomers are another important set of molecules in which a possible difference in biological activity between isomers may exist. The *trans*, or *E*, isomer of triprolidine (**40**)

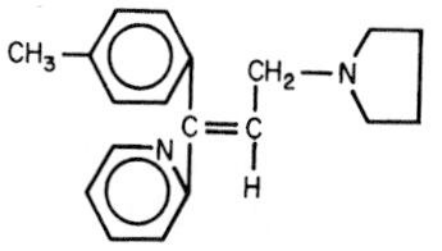

(*trans* or *E*-isomer) triprolidine	(*cis* or *Z*-isomer) triprolidine
40	**41**

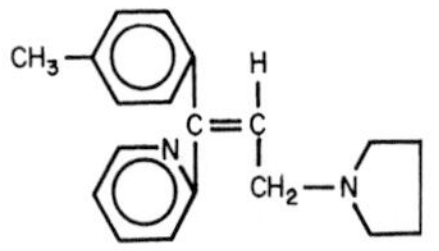

is over 1000 times as potent as the *cis*, or *Z*, isomer (**41**) as a H_1-histamine antagonist. Another example of a set of geometrical isomers is the *cis* and *trans*-2-acetoxycyclopropyltrimethyl ammonium iodides (**42** and **43**),

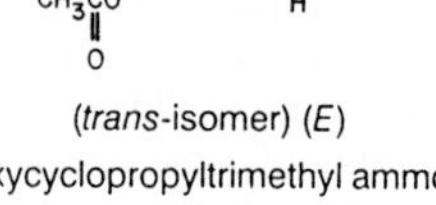

(*cis*-isomer) (*Z*)
cis-2-acetoxycyclopropyltrimethyl ammonium iodide
42

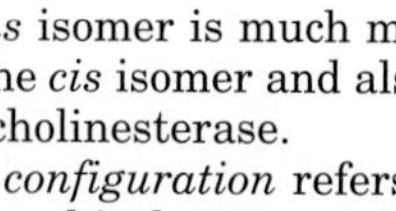

(*trans*-isomer) (*E*)
trans-2-acetoxycyclopropyltrimethyl ammonium iodide
43

respectively. The *trans* isomer is much more potent as a muscarinic agonist than the *cis* isomer and also is a good substrate for the enzyme acetylcholinesterase.

The term *absolute configuration* refers to the arrangement of atoms in space of a chiral compound. In a number of instances there is a distinct difference in biological activity of the *optical isomers* (enantiomers). For example, the $R(-)$

isomer of epinephrine (**44**)

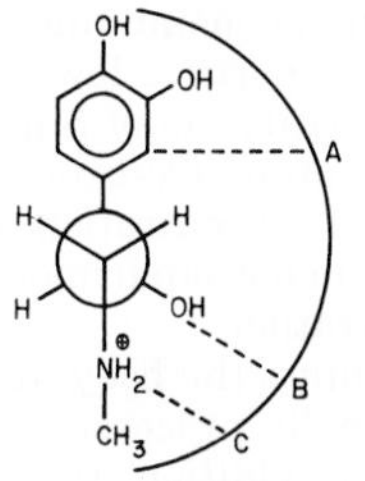

R (−) isomer
epinephrine
44

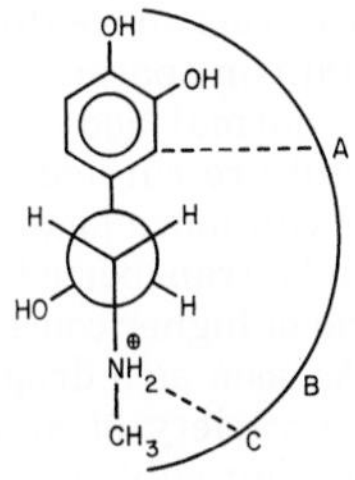

S (+) isomer
epinephrine
45

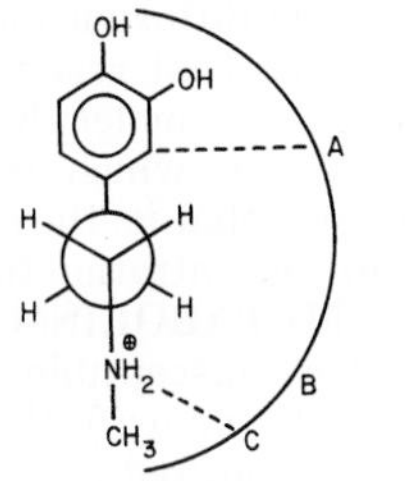

epinine
46

is more potent on both α- and β-adrenergic receptors than the S(+) isomer (**45**). The binding of the isomers of epinephrine and epinine (**46**) (the desoxy analog of epinephrine) is illustrated. The three points of binding on the receptor are the catechol binding site (*A*), hydroxy binding site (*B*), and anionic binding site (*C*).

According to the Easson–Stedman theory,[5] the relative order of activity of the isomers on adrenergic receptors are *R* > *S* ∼ deoxy. Only the *R* isomer can bind to all three sites, whereas both the *S* isomer and the deoxy isomer, which show similar activity, can bind only to two of the sites. Refer to Chapter 13 for a discussion of isomerism.

Although enantiomers have the same chemical and physical properties, except for the direction of rotation of polarized light, diastereomers have different physical properties. *Diastereomers* are compounds with two or more chiral centers. While 1*R*,2*S*(−)-ephedrine (**47**)

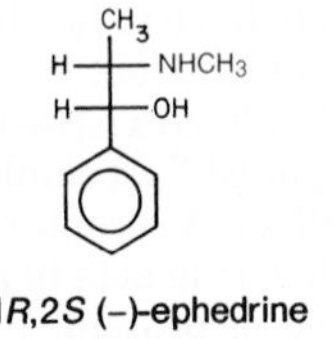

1R,2S (−)-ephedrine
47

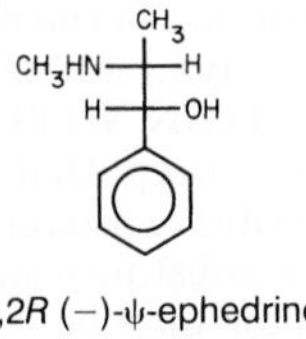

1R,2R (−)-ψ-ephedrine
48

has direct activity on both α- and β-adrenergic receptors, the 1*R*,2*R* (−)-Ψ-ephedrine (**48**) shows α-adrenergic blocking activity. Both diastereomers show indirect adrenergic activity.

An important strategy often used in drug design is to take a conformationally flexible molecule and to convert it into a conformationally rigid molecule in order to find the optimum conformation for binding to a drug receptor. This approach may be used to introduce selectivity for receptors, eliminate undesired side effects, and learn about the spatial relationships of functional groups for receptors.

Dopamine (**49A**)

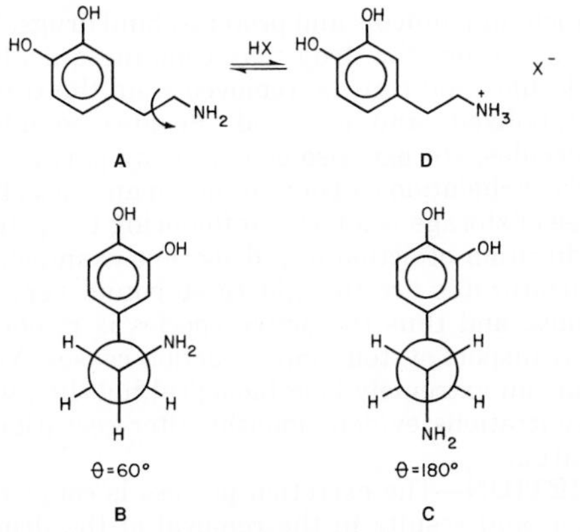

θ=60°
B

θ=180°
C

dopamine
49

can exist in an infinite number of conformations about the side-chain carbon–carbon bond. Two such conformations are illustrated [θ = 60° *gauche* and θ = 180° *trans* conformation (49B and C)].

Apomorphine (**50**)

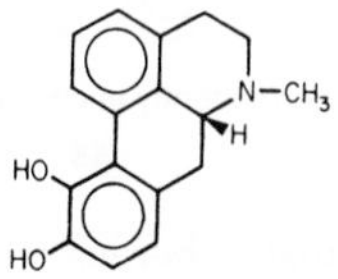

apomorphine
50

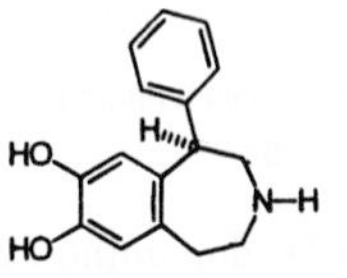

51

and 6,7-dihydroxy-2-aminotetralin (ADTN) (**52**)

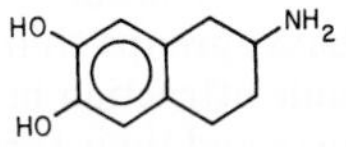

6,7-dihydroxy-2-aminotetralin (ADTN)
52

are two potent dopamine D_1 and D_2 agonists that exist in the *trans* conformation, whereas the selective D_1 agonist SKF 38393 (**51**) does not exist in a similar conformation. Apomorphine, a conformationally rigid molecule, can bind to both D_1 and D_2 dopamine receptors.

In other instances, a drug molecule may need conformational flexibility for proper binding to the receptor to produce biological activity in an induced-fit receptor model. Thus, conformational flexibility may in some instances be a prerequisite for drug agonist activity.

Ionization

Many of the substances used as drugs are weak acids or weak bases. Therefore, an important question is whether the charged or uncharged form of the drug binds to the receptor. Also of importance is the degree of ionization and the effect ionization may have upon absorption and distribution. In general, the ionization can be demonstrated as

$$[\text{Weak Acids}] \quad \underset{\text{(nonionized drug)}}{AH} \quad \rightleftharpoons \quad \underset{\text{(ionized drug)}}{A^- + H^+}$$

$$[\text{Weak Bases}] \quad \underset{\text{(ionized drug)}}{BH^+} \quad \rightleftharpoons \quad \underset{\text{(nonionized drug)}}{B + H^+}$$

It is very difficult to know which molecular form of the drug is active if the charged and uncharged forms are in equilibrium in physiological solution; for example, with dopamine the pK_a of the amine is ∼10. Thus, although most of the drug in solution is in the ionized form (49D), the un-ionized form of the drug molecule still may be the active form.

The quaternary salt of dopamine (**53**)

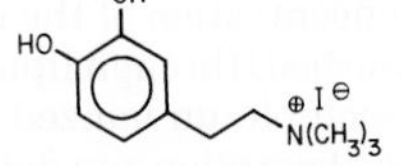

quaternary salt of dopamine
53

has been prepared and exhibits agonist activity on D_2-receptors, indicating that the ionized form of the drug is an active molecular species. However, it is almost impossible to determine if a primary, secondary, or tertiary amine is active as the un-ionized form of the drug because these amines are always in equilibrium under physiological conditions.

It has been shown that the permanently charged dimethylsulfonium analog (**54**)

dimethylsulfonium analog	permanently uncharged sulfide
54	**55**

is active as a D_2-dopamine agonist, whereas the permanently uncharged sulfide (**55**) is inactive as a D_2-dopamine agonist.[6] This suggests that the uncharged form of a dopamine agonist is unlikely to produce D_2-dopamine activity. It also has been found using this approach that both charged agonists and antagonists are responsible for binding to and activating dopamine D_2-receptors. This work, along with observations made using agents that interact with carboxyl groups that block dopaminergic receptors, indicates an ionic attraction between dopamine D_2-agonists and D_2-antagonists and their target receptor.

In order to improve on the pharmacological activity of a drug or to enhance metabolic stability, various replacements of acid and basic groups have been attempted. One of the bioisosteric replacements of an acid functional group often employed is that of the tetrazole group, which has a $pK_a \sim 4.9$. It was found that the tetrazole analog (**56**)

tetrazole analog of nicotinic acid	nicotinic acid
56	**57**

of nicotinic acid (**57**) was more active as an antihyperlipidemic than the parent molecule, nicotinic acid.

Drug Disposition

It should be recognized that a number of factors can affect the interaction of a drug with a receptor, including interatomic distances, shape, size, absolute configuration, rigidity, flexibility, and charge distribution. Some or all of these factors play a part in the consideration of drug design. Normally, by starting the drug-design process at the level of receptors or enzymes, the variables such as absorption, transportation, metabolism, and excretion are set aside temporarily in order to optimize affinity and potency. Regardless of how the medicinal chemist chooses to modify the structure, the process of developing a drug is very complex and the additional factors that must be considered in obtaining a useful drug will be discussed below.

ABSORPTION—Most drugs are administered orally and pass through the stomach, small intestine, and colon; they may be absorbed at any location. During their passage through the gastrointestinal (GI) tract, drugs will experience a range of pH changes starting at about 1.5 in the stomach and reaching as high as pH 8 in the colon. Additionally, drugs are subjected to a variety of enzymes and complexing agents, all of which tend to reduce the effective concentration of the compound.

For a drug to be absorbed (through lipid membranes), it must be present in the fat-soluble un-ionized form. The pK_a of the drug and the pH of the absorption site determine the ease of absorption. Acidic drugs (eg, aspirin) are absorbed best from the stomach, whereas basic compounds (eg, ephedrine) are absorbed preferentially in the small intestine. Permanently ionized molecules (eg, quaternary ammonium salts) lack lipid solubility and usually are absorbed poorly from any region of the GI tract.

TRANSPORT—The blood is the primary carrier of drugs throughout the body. Independent of the method of administration, the drug must pass through several membranes on its way to the active site. Solubility, degree of ionization, and other colligative properties all affect the transport process. Other factors that complicate the transport process include complexation or protein-binding. Most drugs move through a membrane by a simple diffusion mechanism (passive transport); a few compounds that resemble normal body substrates may bind to transport molecules and are carried via an *active-transport* process in which drugs can move against a concentration gradient—that is, they can be transported from a compartment of low concentration to one of higher concentration.

METABOLISM—As soon as a drug enters the body, it becomes susceptible to a variety of metabolic processes that usually *detoxify* the foreign substance. In addition, through oxidation, reduction, hydrolysis, esterification, or conjugation the drug usually is made more water soluble, to enhance its excretion from the body. However, there are instances when a drug metabolite actually may be the active compound, having activity similar to the original compound. Usually, after several biotransformations, the modified form is excreted.

The liver is the primary site of detoxification, but enzyme processes also may occur in the stomach, intestine, and other areas in the body. The metabolic reactions occurring in the liver traditionally are separated into two categories.

1. The drug undergoes what might be termed *functional-group changes,* such as ring or side-chain hydroxylation, nitrogroup reduction, aldehyde oxidation, dealkylation, or deamination.
2. The drug undergoes what is called *conjugation,* in which the metabolized compound combines with solubilizing groups such as glucuronic acid or glycine to form excretable conjugates.

Because drugs can undergo such a wide variety of chemical changes in the body, the specifics of which are unpredictable, the medicinal chemist must at least be aware of these metabolic processes. At some point in the development of a new drug, the molecular structure of the drug may have to be altered in order to change the way in which it is metabolized.

INTERACTION WITH ACTIVE SITES—Ehrlich[7] first introduced the concept that a drug must first combine with a *receptor* (active site) to produce an effect. A receptor is considered to be a cellular substance on which a drug acts to produce its effects. A receptor may be composed of protein, RNA, or DNA. Proteins are an important set of receptors, and drug action may be a consequence of the influence of a drug on an enzyme. Often, the drugs reserved for cancer and viral diseases interact with DNA.

An *enzyme system* is composed of a *coenzyme,* usually nonprotein in nature; an *apoenzyme* (the protein portion), which also may enjoin a nonprotein prosthetic group; and *cofactors,* often inorganic metallic ions and the substrate, which is acted upon by the enzyme. The *active site* on the enzyme may consist of an anionic, cationic, acidic, basic, and/or neutral sites. In addition, the physical shape of the site is such that the contour of the molecule that interacts with the receptor must have a proper shape to insure a *fit* on the receptor.

BINDING AND STORAGE—It is known that other substances, including mucins and proteins, bind drugs. If the binding force is strong, the drug may combine quickly with the macromolecules and thus be removed from the transport system, metabolized, and excreted. Besides complexation to macromolecules, storage also can occur by partitioning in the body lipids or chelation by bony tissue. In any case, the location and degree of storage is a factor influencing the potency, toxicity, and duration of action of a drug. For example, the short-acting barbiturates are thought to be bound very rapidly by body tissues, and thus the active species is removed quickly from the transport system and its action ceases. Yet suramin sodium has an extremely long biological half-life, with noticeable concentrations evident months after cessation of dosing with the drug.

EXCRETION—The excretion process is coupled closely to metabolism and results in the removal of the drug from the body. Elimination may occur via the kidney, liver, skin, lungs, or GI tract. The route of excretion used is determined largely by the drug; the volatile compounds (ether, alcohol) excrete via the lungs, poorly absorbed or insoluble substances through the GI tract with the feces, and very few through the skin. The main route of elimination is through the kidney. The biochemical aspects relating to the complexity of the biosystem that the drug must survive are intricate and little understood.

QUANTITATIVE STRUCTURE–ACTIVITY RELATIONSHIPS

A long-standing goal of workers in the area of quantitative structure–activity relationships (QSAR) has been the development of quantitative methods of determining the activities of a series of compounds. One of the earliest hypotheses that attempted to relate activity to a physicochemical parameter was the Meyer–Overton narcosis theory.[8] In 1901, both men working independently observed that, for general anesthetics, activity was related to the lipid/water partition coefficient; cyclopropane with a value of 65 was far more effective than nitrous oxide with a coefficient of 2.2.

In the field of theoretical chemistry, Hammett[9] was the first to demonstrate that the pKa values of substituted benzoic acids could be predicted as a function of the various substituents attached to the ring and their abilities to either donate or withdraw electrons from the carboxyl group. These results then were extended to other reactions and other series of compounds using the same substituent constants derived from the benzoic acid series. In the Hammet equation,

$$\log k/k_0 = p\sigma \tag{1}$$

where k is the rate constant for the reaction of a substituted aromatic compound, k_0 is the rate constant for the unsubstituted aromatic compound, p is the reaction constant, and σ is the substituent constant. Later work led to substituent constants in which the electronic effect is separated into inductive and resonance terms; in the Taft equation, a term E_s is defined as a measure of the steric requirements of a substituent.

In more recent times there have been numerous mathematical attempts to correlate molecular structure with drug activity. Many of these attempts were destined to fail because they grossly oversimplified what is now known as a very complex problem, even more so than *simple* chemical reactivity. Moderate success has been achieved within narrow limits of drug type, but a universal equation has yet to find expression.

One of the most successful investigators in this field is Hansch,[10] who derived a general equation based on linear free-energy considerations. Inherent in this equation is the ability to incorporate parameters that encompass the full range of known biological requirements for drug activity. Among these are terms for biological transport, drug/enzyme binding energies, substituent effects (both electronic and steric), and electron densities of possible active sites on the drug molecule.

The most general form of the Hansch equation usually is written

$$\log 1/C = -a(\log P)^2 + b \log P + p\sigma + c \tag{2}$$

Activity is expressed as $1/C$, where C is the concentration of a drug required to elicit a given response and P is the octanol/water partition coefficient, a measure of the hydrophobic bonding power of the drug. Its magnitude is indicative of the constant, p, which is characteristic of a given molecular type; and σ is the Hammett substituent constant, which is a measure of the electronic effect on the rate of reaction.

The equation also is expressed as

$$\log 1/C = -a\pi^2 + b\pi + p\sigma + c \tag{3}$$

where $\pi = \log P_x - \log P_H$. P_x is the partition coefficient of the substituted molecule, and P_H is the partition coefficient of the parent unsubstituted molecule. The particular benefit of the π term is the observation by Hansch that π values are additive and thus numerous partition coefficients can be calculated

without the necessity of synthesizing and measuring P_x of the actual compound. An example was the calculation of P_x values for a series of substituted benzeneboronic acids. The values of π were taken from the known series of substituted benzoic acids and, when added to the log P_H value for benzeneboronic acid, gave values of log P_x for the substituted boronic acids (**58**).

substituted boronic acid
58

When these values were used in a Hansch equation to predict drug penetration into brain tissue, excellent correlation with experimental values was obtained.

Another feature of Hansch's work is the use of the technique of regression analysis. In seeking structure–activity correlation it often is not necessary to include all of the defined parameters in the equation to obtain good results. In effect, what has been done is to fit the data to several forms of the equation using the method of least squares, to determine which equation is statistically the best. Thus, if good correlation can be obtained by including only π values, it is probable that the electronic effect of the substituent is not critical for drug activity in that series.

Postulates as to specific drug mechanisms thus can be made when activity dependence, or lack thereof, is found for a given parameter. Further expansions of the equation also permit mechanistic considerations to be formulated. The $p\sigma$ term (actually a log k term) can be expanded to include a steric parameter (E_s) or electron-density parameters for various parts of a molecule. Thus, if inclusion of a steric substituent constant leads to improved correlation, the steric requirements of the drug/enzyme interaction can be better understood. Several examples are given below for derived equations in which excellent correlation with experimental results is found when one or more parameters are omitted.

For the antibacterial effects on gram-negative bacteria of a series of diguanidines, the structures of which are shown in **59**,

diguanidines
59

substituted phenols
60

the equation

$$\log 1/C = -0.081\,\pi^2 + 1.483\pi - 1.578 \tag{4}$$

predicts quantitative activity very accurately. Substituent effects are neglected here because molecular modification involves only a change in the number of methylene groups.

For the antibacterial activity of substituted phenols of the structure indicated by 60, the equation

$$\log 1/C = 0.684 \log P - 0.921\sigma + 0.268 \tag{5}$$

fits the data best.

It would seem that substituents that donate electrons ($-\sigma$ values) would have the highest activity, but in the series studied, these compounds have relatively small values of log P, and this offsets much of the substituent effect. Thus, the most active compounds were those that had the best balance between partition coefficient and electronic effect.

For a series of phosphonate esters known cholinesterase inhibitors (**61**),

phosphonate esters
61

the equation that gave the best correlation was

$$\log K = -0.152\pi - 1.68\sigma + 4.053 E_s + 7.212 \qquad (6)$$

where K is the inhibition constant, σ is the substituent constant for aliphatic systems, and E_s is the Taft steric constant. Here is a series in which the steric effect of the substituents plays an important role. The bulkier groups cause a decrease in cholinesterase inhibition.

These are just a few of the many structure–activity correlations that Hansch has been able to formulate. A study of those equations of best-fit also can give an indication of how to modify a structure to affect biological activity. In a study of thyroxine derivatives, it was predicted (and substantiated) that the replacement of iodine by a *t*-butyl group should lead to a more active molecule. To date, the Hansch equation is one of the most ambitious attempts to explain drug activity in terms of structural variations.

To obtain a good statistical correlation in fitting data to an equation that should lead to the prediction of the most active compound in a series, the more compounds that are prepared, the better the results. At least five compounds should be prepared for each variable on the right side of the equation; and the greater the number of compounds synthesized, the more likely an optimum compound will be found.

Topliss[11] devised an operational scheme (**62**),

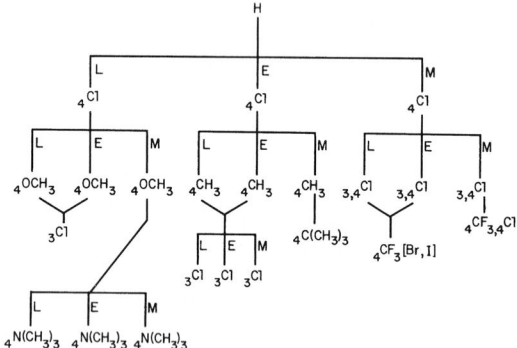

Topliss decision tree appraoch
62

which shows the beginning steps in this decision-tree approach) for the optimization of compounds using the substituent constants π and σ values used in the Hansch method. However, this approach avoids the mathematical and statistical requirements of the Hansch equation. For optimum aromatic substitution a *p*-chloro analog is prepared; if this is more (*M*) active than the parent, unsubstituted compound (*H*), a positive π and σ value is thought to be important, and the next type of substitution would be a 3,4-dichloro analog. If the *p*-chloro analog is less active (*L*), a 4-methoxy substituent would be the next compound to be prepared and tested; if equally (*E*) active, a 4-methyl substituent would be tried. Using this selection-grid approach, the optimum compound normally can be found with a fewer number of synthesized compounds than with the Hansch approach. A similar type of scheme has been devised by Topliss for side-chain substitutions.

In recent years, advances in computing power have made possible QSAR studies that do not rely solely on experimentally-derived parameters that describe substituent effects, but instead compute various descriptors (HOMO and LUMO energies, partial atomic charges, molecular dipole moment, polarizability) directly from the molecular wavefunction using both *ab initio* and semiempirical methods. For example, Olivero-Verbel and Pacheco-Londono[12] successfully modeled the cytotoxic and anti-HIV activity of 29 flavonoids using regression models based on descriptors such as atomic partial charges and total dipole moment computed using the Gaussian quantum-chemical package; Yao et al[13] constructed predictive models of the anti-cancer

activity of a series of indane nucleosides based on molecular surface area and the energy of the LUMO (lowest unoccupied molecular orbital); Clare and Supuran[14] built successful QSAR models for the activities of a series of 36 carbonic anhydrase inhibitors using as descriptors various quantities derived from *ab initio* quantum calculations, including partial atomic charges, components of molecular dipole moment projected along key chemical bonds, and molecular surface area.

Perhaps the most ambitious technique for directly correlating molecular structure with activity is CoMFA (Comparative Molecular Field Analysis). In this approach a three-dimensional grid is superimposed on a set of aligned molecules (usually a congeneric series, but not necessarily so), and electrostatic and steric potentials for the molecules are computed at each vertex of the grid. A multiple regression model is then constructed to relate experimental activities with the variations in the fields measured on the grid. The method can be used to create predictive models which have the added benefit of highlighting portions of the grid associated with large variations in activity (for example, regions where high positive electrostatic potential is correlated with high activity). It is possible to generate color-coded graphical displays that can serve as a guide in modifying molecules so as to realize increased activity. CoMFA has been successfully applied to a wide range of molecular targets, including HIV protease inhibitors,[15,16] androgenic compounds,[17] and opioids.[18]

MECHANISM-BASED DRUG DESIGN

Theories of drug design have evolved from the concept of drug-receptor interactions. In a viable biosystem, a variety of substrates are known to be metabolized through the intervention of enzyme systems. A large proportion of drugs are believed to act by altering the ability of the substrate to interact with the enzyme or receptor. Without attempting to be comprehensive, extensions of the drug-receptor concept that have some experimental verification will be discussed.

The theory of *metabolite antagonism,* or *antimetabolites,* is one that has gained credence. An antimetabolite can, through structural or functional group similarity, compete with a metabolite by blocking a site on an enzyme at which the metabolite ordinarily acts. This latter mechanism, *enzyme inhibition,* probably has been studied more than any other single mechanism. In its most recent version the theory postulates that there are sites of particular conformation on the surface of the enzyme. Spacing and chemical affinity are such that only a molecule having a shape that is the mirror image of the enzyme surface and has the correct chemical groups can interact with the enzyme.

The classic example of metabolite antagonism by a drug is sulfanilamide (**33**) and its derivatives. In work carried out by Woods,[19] sulfanilamide was shown to be antagonistic to *p*-aminobenzoic acid (PABA), a biological precursor of dihydrofolic acid. A fascinating feature of these studies was the demonstration that PABA would reverse the effect of sulfanilamide on a bacterial culture, an example of metabolite antagonism in reverse. Because the two compounds are isosteres, it is easy to see why they are mutually antagonistic.

Either the metabolite or its antagonist can attach itself to the critical area of the dihydrofolate synthetic enzyme surface. If the former occurs, PABA begins its transformation into dihydrofolic acid, but if the latter happens, the metabolic process ceases and, in the case of bacteria, multiplication is inhibited. The degree of inhibition depends on the relative concentrations of the substrate and the inhibitor. Selective toxicity is shown for bacteria because mammals do not need to synthesize dihydrofolic acid, but obtain it in their diets.

Another mode of drug action involves enzyme deactivation without actual competition. Here, the drug can react with the enzyme or even the enzyme-substrate complex and, in some manner, prevent the metabolism of the substrate. The nitrogen mustards, and other alkylating agents used for cancer chemotherapy, act in this fashion. These drugs are relatively nonspecific inhibitors that act by forming irreversible bonds with enzyme and nucleic acid molecules. In doing so they may not block necessarily a particular site, but rather many active sites; in this way, they inactivate enzymes and react with base residues of DNA, to form cross-links. Nitrogen mustards can prevent replication, and thus arrest cell division.

One of the recent advances in the treatment of hypertension came about through a better understanding of the mechanism of *angiotension*. The renin–angiotensin system (RAS) (**63**),

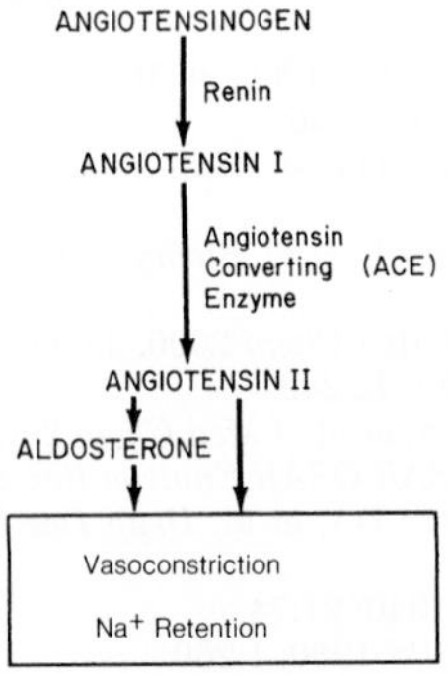

renin-angiotensin system
63

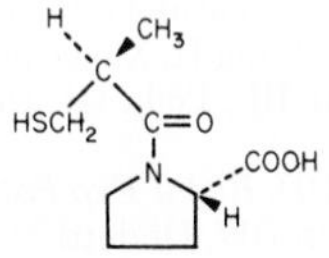

captopril
64

plays a key role in the maintenance of sodium and fluid volume, resulting in the regulation of blood pressure. The system is composed of two important enzymes: renin and angiotensin-converting enzyme (ACE). Renin converts angiotensinogen to the decapeptide angiotensin I; ACE acts upon angiotensin I to give the octapeptide angiotensin II, which is responsible for the peripheral effects leading to an elevation of blood pressure.

Although ACE was identified in the mid-1950s, it wasn't until 1977 that Cushman and Ondetti[20] reported a new drug, captopril (**64**), that competitively could inhibit ACE. This provided a major advance in the treatment of hypertension.

Based on the concepts learned from a knowledge of the binding points of captopril—that the mercapto group binds to Zn ion, the amide carbonyl to a hydrogen-bonding site, and the carboxylate to a positive center on the enzyme—new inhibitors have been synthesized. One of the most successful of these new analogs is enalaprilat (**65**),

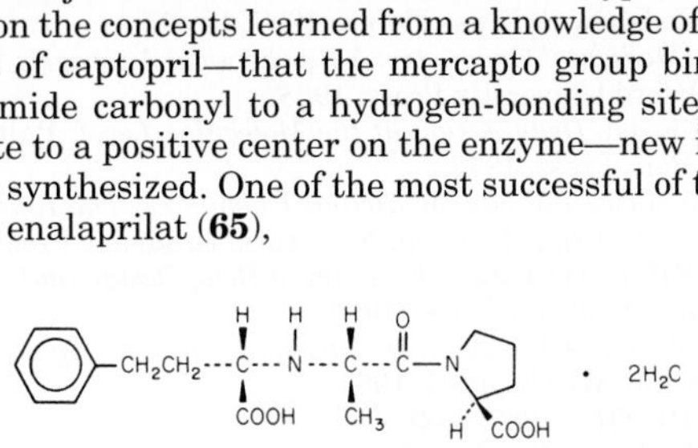

enalaprilat
65

which has the advantage of oral activity and lacks central effects. Modern approaches at preparing new drugs that will affect the RAS include inhibitors of renin and the preparation of angiotensin receptor antagonists.

Besides substrate analogs, the design of transition-state inhibitors also is an important approach to drug design. Transition-state analogs are intended to resemble the substrate in transition from substrate to products, and they should be stable substances. In designing this inhibitor, a very good understanding of the specific enzyme mechanism and the chemical nature of the transition state is needed. Another approach that is being used is to prepare k_{cat} or suicide-substrate inhibitors. In designing these types of inhibitors, the mechanism of the enzyme should be known; it is important to generate a reactive intermediate that, in turn, undergoes an irreversible reaction with the enzyme.

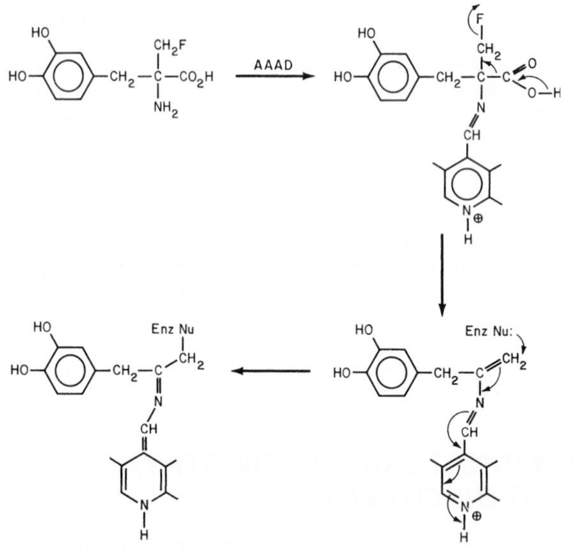

Figure 28-1.

Enzymes using pyridoxal phosphate have been used a great deal with this approach. An example is monofluoromethyl dihydroxyphenylalanine (Fig 28-1), which inhibits the enzyme aromatic amino acid decarboxylase (AAAD). The inhibition of the enzyme is shown with the cofactor in Figure 28-1. There are many examples of k_{cat} inhibitors, but at this time one of the most-used classes of drugs therapeutically are the propargylamine derivatives, which inhibit monoamine oxidase (MAO). The inhibitors form a covalent bond with the flavine portion of MAO.

COMPUTER USE IN DRUG DESIGN

One of the early uses of computer-assisted drug design (CADD)[21] was in the QSAR approaches of Hansch, as previously discussed. Other uses of the computer have been to apply computational chemistry to learn about the shape of molecules. In conformational studies, molecular mechanics and quantum mechanics calculations are carried out to provide insight as to the preferred conformations of a molecule. A variety of approaches are used to carry out such computations. Molecular mechanics calculations are fast, but require extensive lists of atom types and detailed sets of parameters, and will fail when confronted with novel chemical structures. On the other hand, high-level quantum calculations provide high accuracy and can be applied to any chemical structure, but are time-consuming and limited to relatively small compounds. Fast semiempirical quantum methods ranging from CNDO to PM3 fill an important gap, being applicable to a wide range of compounds and fast enough to be used with relatively large molecules. Although a preferred-conformation, low-energy form of a drug may be calculated using these concepts, this may not be the conformation required to produce drug activity.

Molecular modeling and molecular graphics have shown dramatic growth and are becoming an integral part of the drug-discovery process. *Molecular modeling* is the generation, manipulation, and representation of the three-dimensional form of molecules; *molecular graphics* refers to the use of computer graphics to represent the molecular structure. In the past, synthetic chemists have used molecular models, but computer modeling has enhanced the detailed display of molecular structures.

An important use of CADD is in the design of hypothetical drugs. For example, when the structure of an enzyme or receptor obtained through x-ray studies is known, one can begin to design hypothetical drugs that actually can be shown to interact with the active site. Computer programs such as GOLD[22] and UCSF DOCK[23] allow the positions, orientations, and conformations of putative drug molecules to be automatically optimized inside a receptor site, and their relative affinities to be predicted on the basis of binding energetics. A number of graphical rendering techniques can be used to highlight important interactions and features of interest, including the use of color and representations of molecular surfaces and volumes. This type of work, in combination with experimental methods such as x-ray, nuclear magnetic resonance (NMR), and infrared spectroscopy, should provide a powerful tool for the future design of drugs.

COMBINATORIAL CHEMISTRY AND DRUG DISCOVERY

The drug-discovery environment underwent a major evolution in the 1990s. These revolutionary changes are evident to those close to the drug-discovery process. The need for a more efficient and effective means of finding new drug molecules is one of a number of factors driving this new approach. Combinatorial chemistry has shown itself to be both effective and efficient in both drug-lead generation and the optimization of a new drug-lead molecule. An important part of this process is the introduction of new computing and chemical automation processes, along with the merging of the combinatorial chemistry with biology via high-throughput screening.

Two basic combinatorial processes are currently used.[24]

Parallel Synthesis This process was invented in the 1980s by H Mario Geysen. He used this approach initially to find the small segment of a protein that bound to antibodies. In parallel synthesis, reactions are carried out separately but simultaneously using different starting materials and reactants with such reactions yielding a single product. Thus, using an 8×12 array of reaction vessels and 20 different starting materials, one can obtain a library of 96 different compounds. Advances in robotics have allowed full automation of the routine chemistry involved. Pharmaceutical companies are expanding upon this process and are currently are generating thousands of new compounds every day.

Split and Mix Synthesis This method[24] was used in the late 1980s by Arpad Furka. The parallel synthesis affords a single product per reaction vessel, but a split and mix synthesis produces a mixture of compounds in each reaction vessel. This reduces the number of vessels needed per number of compounds, making it possible to prepare millions of compounds for a library. Split and mix synthesis has several complications compared to parallel synthesis; for example, it is difficult to keep track of the compounds in a given vessel. Furthermore, deconvolution of the mixture to identify the active component(s) of a mixture is also difficult and time-consuming.

The rate of discovery of new drugs has been accelerated greatly, almost beyond belief, by these new chemical technologies. Thus, combinatorial chemistry should increase cross-disciplinary research and already has started an exciting era in the discovery of new drugs.

REFERENCES

1. Bently KW, Hardy DG. *J Am Chem Soc* 1967; 89:3269.
2. Langmuir I. *J Am Chem Soc* 1919; 41: 868.
3. Langmuir I. *J Am Chem Soc* 1919; 41: 1543.
4. Friedman HL. National Academy of Sciences-National Research Council Publ No 206. Washington, DC: USGPO, 1951, p 295.
5. Patil PN, Miller DD, Trendelenberg U. *Pharmacol Rev* 1974; 26: 232.
6. Miller DD, et al. *TIPS* 1988; 9: 282.
7. Ehrlich P. *Lancet* 1913; 2: 445.
8. Doerge RF, ed. *Wilson and Gisvold's Textbook of Organic Medicinal Chemistry and Pharmaceutical Chemistry*, 8th ed. Philadelphia: Lippincott, 1982, p 15.
9. Hammett LP. *Physical Organic Chemistry.* New York: McGraw-Hill, 1940, p 184.
10. Hansch C, Fujita T. *J Am Chem Soc* 1964; 86:1616.
11. Topliss JG. *J Med Chem* 1972; 15:1006.
12. Olivero-Verbel J, Pacheco-Londono L. *J Chem Inf Comput Sci* 2002, 42:1241.
13. Yao S-W, Lopes VHC, Fernandez F, et al. *Bioorg & Med Chem* 2003; 11:4999.
14. Clare BW, Supuran CT. *Eur J Med Chem* 2000, 35:859.
15. Debnath AK. *J Med Chem* 1999, 42:249.
16. Nair AC, Jayatilleke P, Wang X, et al. *J Med Chem* 2002, 45:973.
17. Hong H, Fang H, Xie Q, et al. *SAR QSAR Environ Res* 2003, 14:373.
18. Podlogar BL, Poda GI, Demeter DA, et al. *Drug Des Discov* 2000, 17:34.
19. Woods DD. *Brit J Exp Pathol* 1940; 21:74.
20. Cushman DW, Ondetti MA. *TIPS* 1980; 1:260.
21. Hopfinger AJ. *J Med Chem* 1985; 28:1133.
22. Jones G, Willett P, Glen RC. *J Mol Biol* 1995, 245:43.
23. Oshiro CM, Kuntz ID. *J Comput-Aided Mol Design* 1995, 9:113.
24. Plunkett MJ, Ellman JA. *Sci Am* 1997; 276(4):69.

BIBLIOGRAPHY

Delgado JN, Remers WA, eds. *Wilson and Gisvold's Textbook of Organic Medicinal and Pharmaceutical Chemistry*, 9th ed. Philadelphia: Lippincott, 1991.
Foye WO. *Principles of Medicinal Chemistry*, 3rd ed. Philadelphia: Lea & Febiger, 1988.
Korolkovas A, Burckhalter JH. *Essentials of Medicinal Chemistry.* New York: Wiley Interscience, 1976.
Lien EJ. *SAR Side Effects and Drug Design.* New York: Dekker, 1987.
Martin YC. *Quantitative Drug Design.* New York: Dekker, 1978.
Natoff IL, Redshaw S. *Drugs Future* 1987; 12:475.
Nogrady T. *Medicinal Chemistry. A Biochemical Approach*, 2nd ed. New York: Oxford University Press, 1988.
Roberts GCK, ed. *Drug Action at the Molecular Level.* Baltimore: University Park Press, 1977.
Roberts SM, Price BJ, eds. *Medicinal Chemistry. The Role of Organic Chemistry in Drug Research.* New York: Academic Press, 1985.
Silverman RB. *The Organic Chemistry of Drug Design and Drug Action.* New York: Academic Press, 1992.
Smith HJ, Williams H, eds. *Introduction to the Principles of Drug Design.* Boston: Wright, PSG, 1983.
Vallotton MB. *TIPS* 1987; 8:69.
Williams M, Malick JB. *Drug Discovery and Development.* Clifton, NJ: Humana Press, 1987.
Wolff ME, ed. *The Basis of Medicinal Chemistry, Burger's Medicinal Chemistry*, 4th ed. New York: John Wiley. Part 1, 1980; Part 2, 1979; Part 3, 1981.

CHAPTER 29

Fundamentals of Medical Radionuclides

Jeffrey P Norenberg, MS, PharmD, BCNP, FASHP, FAPhA

William B Hladik III, MS, FASHP, FAPhA

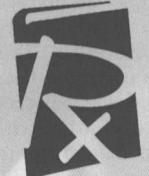

For years the alchemist sought the secret of *transmutation* without success. Today, this nuclear process—converting one element into another—is commonplace, but the knowledge of nuclear processes is of recent origin. It was not until 1896 that Becquerel observed the fogging of his photographic plates by a uranium salt. His observation aroused the curiosity of the Curies concerning the uranium ore, pitchblende, from which they isolated the elements polonium and radium. Research over the next few years by the Curies, Becquerel, Schmidt, Debierne, and others soon resulted in the discovery and isolation of still other new elements from uranium and thorium ores. These elements, too, were found to fog photographic plates.

It was known that the fogging of photographic plates was caused by some sort of radiation. By 1899 Rutherford concluded that this radiation was of two types, which he called *alpha* and *beta*. The next year Pierre Curie and Villard observed a third, very penetrating, type of radiation, which they called *gamma*.

The *theory of radioactive disintegration* was proposed by Rutherford and Soddy in 1903. They suggested that atoms of radioactive elements undergo spontaneous emission of alpha and beta particles with the formation of atoms of a new element. These deductions were amazing when one considers the status of atomic knowledge of that day.

The *electron*, later found to be physically identical with the beta particle, had been discovered by Thomson in 1897. In 1909 Rutherford and Royds identified the alpha particle as a helium nucleus; in 1911, data on alpha particle scattering provided the evidence needed for Rutherford to propose the *nuclear theory* of the atom, that the positive charge of an atom is concentrated in a centrally located *nucleus* rather than being interspersed with the negatively charged electrons.

Two years later, Bohr published his theory of atomic structure, based upon Rutherford's nuclear theory and the quantum theory of Planck. The same year (1913) Soddy proposed the name *isotope* (from the Greek, for "same place"). Aston had just separated two isotopes of neon by fractional diffusion in confirmation of Thomson's discovery of these two forms of neon in 1912.

Rutherford was the foremost nuclear scientist of his time. In 1919 it was he who first observed and identified *transmutation* of one element into another. It was achieved by bombarding nitrogen with alpha particles. In the process, the nitrogen was converted into an isotope of oxygen with a mass of 17. Rutherford died in 1937 believing that nuclear power would never be achieved. This was achieved only 5 years later when Fermi built the first nuclear reactor in Chicago.

Constructive research on the nucleus of the atom has resulted not only in the means to harness this tremendous power for the production of electricity and other forms of useful energy, but also has provided scientists with more than 2500 different species of atoms. These find innumerable applications in industry, medicine, pharmacy, agriculture, and other disciplines where the atom is used for the benefit of humanity.

The purpose of this chapter is to review some fundamental properties of radionuclides, including their nature and source, and methods for their detection and measurement. This basic information should facilitate a better understanding of how and when they can be applied to the disciplines of medicine and pharmacy.

APPLICATIONS OF RADIONUCLIDES IN MEDICINE AND PHARMACY

Radium has the distinction of being the first radionuclide used in medicine, employed as early as 1901. This nuclide was the most important medical radionuclide in use up to about 1946 when artificially produced radionuclides became available in quantity. Since that date, growth in the medical applications of radionuclides has been very rapid as their usefulness has become more and more apparent in medical diagnosis, therapy, and research and as greater numbers of physicians and other scientific personnel have been trained in their use. Current medical procedures employ more than 50 radionuclides in a wide variety of chemical and physical forms.

Other than for basic research, radionuclides are used in medicine and pharmacy in two different ways: as (1) sealed radiation sources or (2) radiopharmaceuticals.

As sealed radiation sources, their principal roles are in (1) therapy and (2) calibration of radiation detection instrumentation. For therapy, the choice of the radionuclide for a given application is governed largely by the properties of the radiation required for treatment; the type and energy of the radiation and range in tissues are prime considerations. For therapeutic applications, the radiation sources are either (1) externally beamed into cancerous tissue (teletherapy) or (2) implanted in the form of seeds, wires, or ribbons (or other physical forms) within, or in proximity to, cancerous tissue for specified periods of time (brachytherapy). For these purposes the chemical properties or chemical form of the radionuclide are relatively unimportant. Likewise, for calibration purposes, the nature of the radiation emitted is usually pertinent whereas the chemical properties are not.

A *radiopharmaceutical* is a preparation, intended for in vivo use, that contains a radionuclide in the form of a simple salt or a complex. It may exist as a solid, liquid, gas, or pseudogas. The chemical and physical identity and form of a radiopharmaceutical is very important because in each case, once administered, the radiopharmaceutical is intended to target certain tissues, binding sites, and/or biochemical pathways. Depending on its specific physicochemical and radiation properties, a radiopharmaceutical can be used for either diagnostic or therapeutic purposes, and in a few cases for both. For diagnostic applications, a radiopharmaceutical should not be pharmacologically active in that it should not produce a physiologic effect. It is administered in extremely small (tracer) quantities so that it does not alter the physiologic or pathophysiologic process which is being measured. The nature of the radiation emitted by a diagnostic radiopharmaceutical is important primarily for its ease of detection (ie, to obtain an image or other diagnostic data). On the other hand, for a therapeutic radiopharmaceutical, the type and energy of the radiation as well as its range in tissues are very important considerations, as was the case with sealed sources used for therapy. A radiopharmaceutical preparation designed for therapeutic purposes must contain enough radioactivity to produce the intended tissue effects.

The development, evaluation, preparation, testing, and clinical use of radiopharmaceuticals have led to the introduction of the specialty disciplines known as *nuclear medicine* and *nuclear pharmacy*. In the US alone, practitioners in these specialties are responsible for the care of approximately 40,000 to 50,000 patients each day on average.

RADIOACTIVITY AND RADIATION

Radioactivity is defined as the phenomenon by which one nuclide is spontaneously transformed into another nuclide with the emission of energy in the form of radiation. Therefore, a nuclide that undergoes a spontaneous nuclear reaction is said to be *radioactive*. Such elements are radioactive because the configuration of protons and neutrons in the nucleus produces an unstable structure. During the process of spontaneous transformation (*decay*) the ratio of neutrons to protons changes. After one or more decay processes, a stable nucleus is formed. Because of its special importance in nuclear pharmacy and nuclear medicine, radioactive decay is discussed in detail in a subsequent section. There are several types of radiation that may be emitted from radionuclides, each of which has found usefulness in some medical application.

RADIATION FROM RADIOACTIVE NUCLEI

Three types of radiation are emitted most frequently from radioactive nuclei: alpha, beta, and gamma.

Alpha particles, which constitute alpha radiation, are compound particles consisting of two protons and two neutrons. The alpha particle is identical with the helium nucleus—that is, a helium atom, less two orbital electrons. As an alpha particle loses energy, its velocity decreases. It then attracts electrons to its *K-shell* and becomes an ordinary helium atom. The range of alpha particles in air is about 5 cm; the range in tissue is less than 100 μm in tissue.

Beta radiation exists as two types because there are two kinds of electrons, the *negative electron* (or *negatron*), and the *positive electron* (or *positron*). The positron is identical with the negatron in all respects except for its charge of +1 instead of −1. The positron also is known as the *antiparticle* of the electron. When these electrons are emitted from radioactive nuclei, they are called *beta particles*. That is, the two particles β− and β+ are the same as e− and e+, respectively, except for their origin. Beta particles may have a range of over 3 m in air and up to about 1 mm in tissue (or more), depending on the specific energy of the beta particle.

Because alpha and beta particles release large amounts of energy over a short distance (*path*), they are locally destructive to tissue. As a result, radionuclides that emit these particles are useful as therapeutic agents if deposited internally or placed strategically in proximity to lesions (eg, therapeutic radiopharmaceuticals or sources for brachytherapy). To date, beta-emitting radionuclides have been used more commonly than alphaemitters in medicine, although several radiopharmaceuticals containing the latter are currently under investigation.

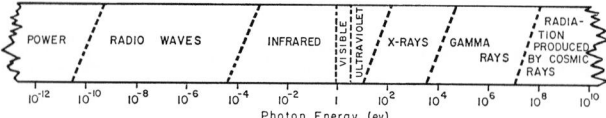

Figure 29-1. Electromagnetic spectrum.

Gamma radiation is different from alpha and beta radiation. Gamma radiation is electromagnetic, whereas alpha and beta radiation are particulate. Gamma rays are radiated as photons or quanta of energy at a velocity c of 3.0×10^{12} m/sec. They are often emitted as a result of *nuclear deexcitation*, which is required when nuclei produced in nuclear reactions are in an *excited state* rather than in the *ground state*. When excited, nucleons occupy high-energy quantum levels. They tend to lose excess energy, returning to the ground quantum state by *gamma ray emission*. Gamma radiation differs from X-rays, ultraviolet rays, and visible light only in wavelength (or frequency), as illustrated in Figure 29-1.

Gamma rays are the most penetrating of all types of radiation emitted by radionuclides (except neutrinos) and can pass easily through more than 25 cm of tissue or several centimeters of lead, again depending on the specific energy of the gamma ray. Radiotracers typically contain radionuclides that emit gamma rays. Gamma-emitting radionuclides are particularly useful for diagnostic radiopharmaceuticals; once the radiopharmaceutical has distributed within the body, the photons can penetrate the tissues and be detected externally using specially designed imaging equipment.

EXTRANUCLEAR RADIATION

There is a certain probability that, instead of emitting a gamma ray during nuclear deexcitation, the excited nucleus may transfer its excitation energy to an electron in an electron shell of its own atom. In this case, the electron is ejected from its shell provided that the excitation energy exceeds the electron binding energy. The ejected electron is called a *conversion* electron, and this entire process is referred to as *internal conversion*. When an electron is emitted from its electron shell, the vacancy will be filled with an electron from a more distant orbital shell. The energy difference between the two shells will be emitted as an x-ray. Because this process may result in multiple electron shell vacancies, a cascade effect may induce the emission of multiple x-rays.

Atomic deexcitation is a process that of necessity must follow any change in the identity of a nucleus. The daughter produced in a radioactive decay process is a different element. Orbital electrons find themselves in excited states and proceed to lose energy, either as *fluorescence* radiation or as *Auger electrons*, until a stable configuration is achieved.

Conversion electrons and Auger electrons are particulate radiation and thus are useful for therapeutic applications; x-rays are electromagnetic radiation, and hence are more applicable to radiotracer methodologies.

THE ATOM

To better understand the concepts of radioactivity and radiation, it is helpful to review selected properties of the atom.

ATOMIC STRUCTURE

A neutral atom consists of a positively charged nucleus (composed of protons and neutrons) with which orbital electrons are associated. The number of orbital electrons is equal to the number of protons in the nucleus, and the number of protons in the nucleus defines the *atomic number*, Z. The *neutron number*, N, is the number of neutrons in the nucleus, and the *mass number*, A, is equal to the sum of the protons and neutrons. Thus, $A = Z + N$.

The radius of an atom is approximately 10^{-10} m or 1 Å. The nucleus is roughly 1/100,000 the size of the atom. For example, the radius of the oxygen nucleus is about 3×10^{-15} m and that of the lead nucleus is about 7×10^{-15} m. To gain some appreciation of the smallness of the nucleus, let us suppose that the oxygen nucleus is magnified until it appears to be the size of a golf ball. The golf ball, similarly magnified, would appear to have a diameter of about 100 million miles, or roughly the distance from the earth to the sun.

Atoms are quite *empty*. The nucleus and orbital electrons occupy but a very small fraction of space in matter. Further, most of the mass of matter is concentrated in the nucleus, which has a density of 2.4×10^{14} g/mL. For example, 1 mL of the substance of which nuclei are made would weigh over 200 million tons. It is with this very unusual material of the nucleus that we are concerned in nuclear reactions and radioactivity.

NUCLIDES AND ISOTOPES

In 1912, Thomson developed an analytical process known as *positive ray analysis* by which he could measure the mass of particles such as atoms. When he attempted to determine the mass of the neon atom, two lines appeared on the screen of his apparatus, indicating two types of neon atoms having masses of 20 and 22, respectively. Using a process that would be the forerunner of mass spectrometry, Thomson demonstrated the existence of nuclei possessing the same number of protons (and, hence, of the same chemical element) but a different number of neutrons (and, hence, of different mass). Soddy later called these *isotopes*.

The atomic number, Z, of neon is 10. From the relationship $A = Z + N$, we can deduce that the difference between these two forms of neon lies in the number of neutrons, N, in the nucleus:

$$A = 20 = 10 + N \therefore N = 10$$
$$A = 22 = 10 + N \therefore N = 12$$

Today, at least eight isotopes of neon are known. These are illustrated in Figure 29-2.

Isotopes are species of nuclides that possess the same number of protons but a different number of neutrons. That is, isotopes are nuclides of the same chemical element and, therefore, have the same chemical properties but differ in mass. They also may differ in stability. Certain mass numbers may represent stable nuclei, whereas other mass numbers may represent radioactive nuclei. A *nuclide* is any one of the more than about 2500 known species of atoms characterized by the number of protons and the number of neutrons in the nucleus. Nuclides that have the same mass are called *isobars*. Nuclides which possess the same number of neutrons are called *isotones*. The nuclides illustrated in Figure 29-3—^{1}H, ^{2}H (deuterium), and ^{3}H (tritium)—are isotopes; ^{3}He and ^{4}He are isotopes also. On the

other hand, ^{3}H and ^{3}He are isobars, and ^{3}H and ^{4}He are isotones.

NUCLEAR NOTATION

In writing the symbol for a nuclide, the atomic number is written as a subscript preceding the symbol for the element, and the mass number is written as a superscript. Thus, the symbol $_7^{14}$N describes the nitrogen nucleus whose atomic number, Z, is 7 and whose mass, A, is 14.

$$_Z^A X_N$$

NUCLEAR EQUATIONS

A nuclear equation is a representation of a nuclear reaction. A nuclear reaction occurs when there is a change in the configuration of the nucleus of an atom. Nuclear reactions may occur spontaneously, as occurs during the decay of radionuclides; or they may be induced, as occurs during the production of artificial radionuclides. The nuclear equation expressing the first artificial transmutation observed by Rutherford is expressed by the notation:

$$_7^{14}N + _2^4He \rightarrow _1^1H + _8^{17}O$$

In this reaction, nitrogen of mass 14 is bombarded with a helium nucleus of mass 4 (ie, an alpha particle) to produce oxygen of mass 17 and a proton.

It will be noted that nuclear equations must balance. The sum of the masses on the left (14 + 4 = 18) must equal the sum of the masses on the right (1 + 17 = 18). Also, the sum of the atomic numbers on the left (7 + 2 = 9) must equal the sum of the atomic numbers on the right (1 + 8 = 9). This same nuclear reaction also may be represented by a *shorthand* notation:

$$^{14}N(\alpha, p)^{17}O$$

Target Nuclide (In, Out) Product Nuclide

RADIOACTIVE DECAY

STATISTICS

As stated previously, unstable nuclei that undergo a spontaneous nuclear reaction are said to be radioactive. If a single radioactive atom could be separated for observation, there would be no way to predict at which moment the decay of its nucleus would occur. If, however, a large number of similar radioactive atoms is considered, it becomes possible to predict how many will decay within a certain interval of time. This problem can be understood if a comparison is made to the similar situation existing with life insurance. Although the insuring company cannot predict when a particular policy holder will die, the fraction of a large group of policy holders who will die within a given time interval can be predicted. The larger the group considered, the more accurate the prediction. Such is the case with nuclei—the greater the number of nuclei considered, the more accurate the measurement of decay rate.

The need to recognize the influence of random decay upon analytical results is extremely important. When radioactivity is measured, the value μ, the true count, is required. Because radioactive decay is random, μ cannot be measured. It is expected that replicate measurements of count n_i of the same sample will give a range of values on either side of μ. The best estimate of μ is given by the average:

$$n = \sum_i n_i/N$$

where N is the number of replicate observations. The precision with which the decay rate can be measured is expressed by the standard deviation σ, which is a measure of the spread of data

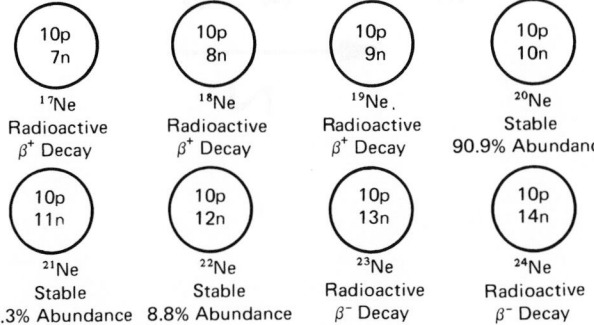

Figure 29-2. Isotopes of neon.

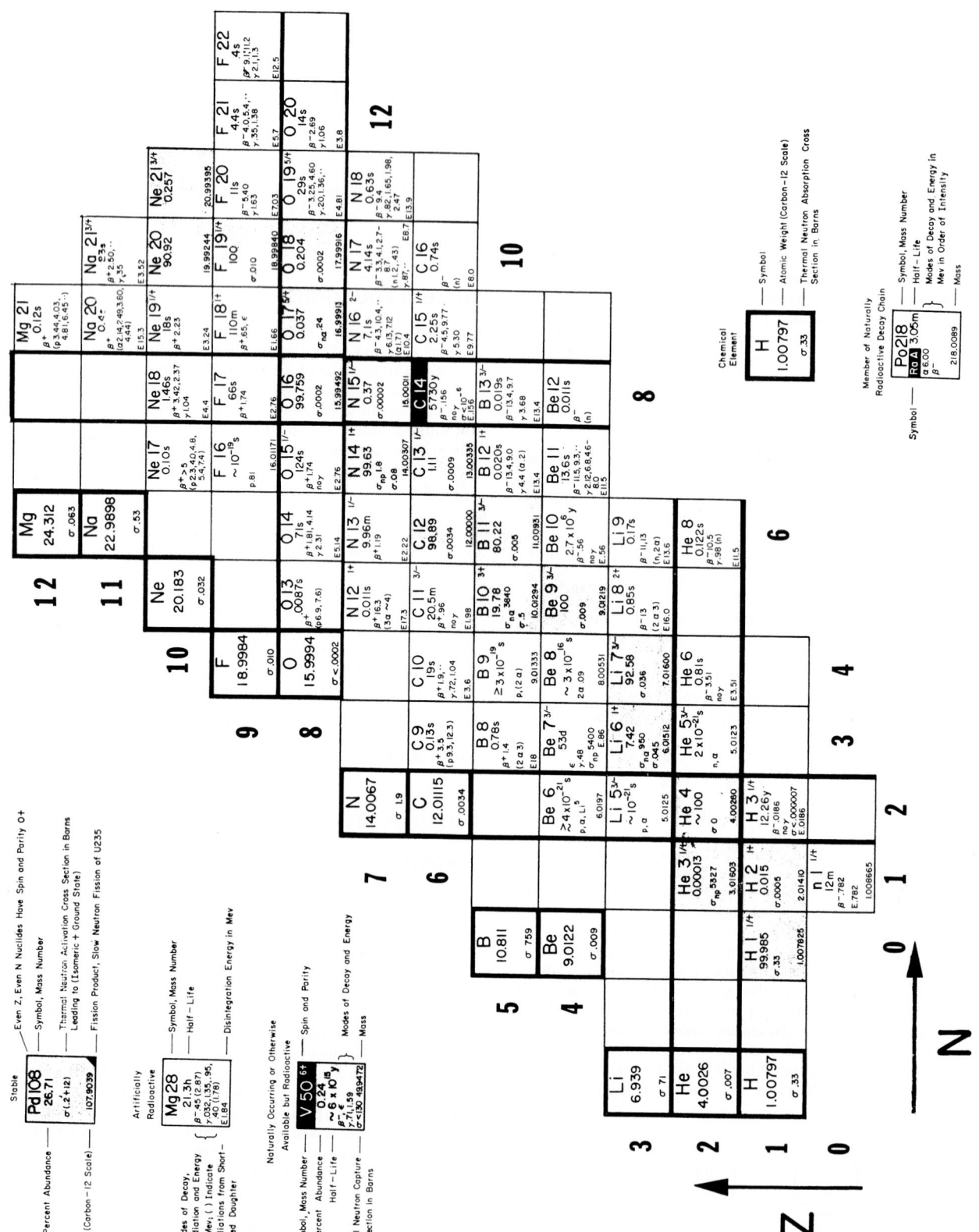

Figure 29-3. Chart of the nuclides—to mass number 21. Known nuclides now number about 2500 (courtesy, General Electric).

Table 29-1.

IF THE TOTAL NUMBER OF DECAYING ATOMS OBSERVED IS n THERE IS A 68% CHANCE THAT THE ERROR WILL BE LESS THAN $\sigma = \sqrt{n}$ OR A 68% CHANCE THAT THE OBSERVED VALUE IS IN ERROR BY NO MORE THAN 100 σ/n %

n	σ	100 σ/n%
50	7.07	14.14%
100	10.00	10.00%
500	22.36	4.47%
1000	31.62	3.16%
5000	70.71	1.41%
10000	100.00	1.00%
50000	223.60	0.44%

on either side of the mean. For radioactive decay, an estimate of σ is given by $\sqrt{n}$. There is a 68% chance that a particular measurement will fall within the range $n \pm \sigma$. About one-third of the observations result in values of n lying outside the range $n \pm \sigma$. The significance is illustrated by the statistical analysis in Table 29-1 and the normal probability curve depicted (refer to Chapter 12).

Assume that a radioactive sample is decaying at the rate of exactly 500 atoms per minute. If the number of decaying atoms during each of 100 different 1 minute intervals were measured, for 68 of these intervals the data would lie between $500 \pm \sqrt{500}$, or between 478 and 522. Data for the other 32% of the measurements will fall either below 478 or above 522, or greater than one standard deviation from the mean. Such variations, if truly of a statistical nature, should not be interpreted as indicating faulty equipment, faulty technique, or inaccurately calibrated samples. An increase in counting time to record a greater number of decay processes will result in an increase in counting accuracy.

When radionuclides are used in analytical procedures, the overall error in the measurement is due not only to random decay but also to instrument error, pipetting, weighing, and other procedural errors. The overall error can be estimated in terms of the sample standard deviation, s, where:

$$s = \sqrt{\frac{\sum_i (n_i - \bar{n})^2}{N - 1}}$$

If the only source of error is that due to random decay, the value of s should approach σ as N, the number of observations, approaches infinity.

KINETICS OF DECAY

Decay rate is the time rate at which atoms undergo radioactive disintegration. It is expressed by $-dN/dt$, where $-dN$ is the change in the number of atoms N, and dt is the change in the time t. The negative sign indicates merely that the number of atoms is decreasing in time. The rate of decay ($-dN/dt$) is proportional to the number of atoms N, present at any time t. Therefore, the rate of decay is expressed as:

$$-dN/dt = \lambda N$$

where λ is a proportionality constant usually called the *decay constant*. The decay of radioactive atoms, therefore, is a first-order reaction.

Integration of the equation above results in the useful relation:

$$\ln N_t/N_0 = -\lambda t$$

where N_0 is the number of atoms present at zero-time and N_t is the number of atoms present at time t. This relationship sometimes is used more conveniently in the exponential form, the "Common Radioactive Decay Equation":

$$N_t = N_0 e^{-\lambda t}$$

which is illustrated graphically in Figure 29-4.

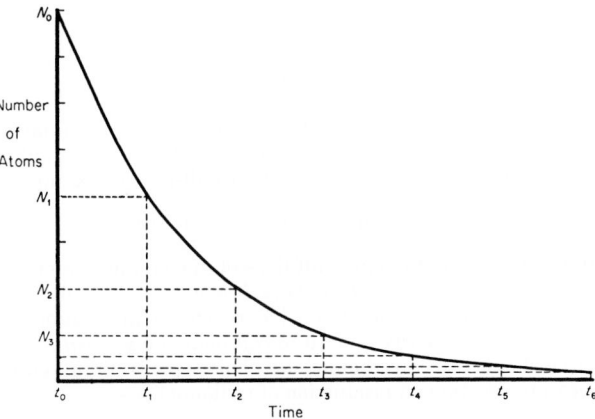

Figure 29-4. Energy-level diagram for the decay of phosphorus-32.

The rate of decay, $-dN/dt$, sometimes called the *activity*, is represented by the symbol A. Because the activity A is proportional to the number of atoms N, the following useful relationships also can be derived:

$$A = \lambda N$$

$$\ln A_t/A_0 = -\lambda t \quad \text{or} \quad A_t = A_0 e^{-\lambda t}$$

or

$$\ln A_t = \ln A_0 - \lambda t$$

The last relationship is shown in Figure 29-5.

The *absolute activity* usually is expressed as disintegrations per sec (*d/s* or *dps*) or disintegrations per minute (*d/m* or *dpm*). The *observed activity*, which is less than the absolute activity by a factor equal to the efficiency of the counting system, is expressed in counts per second (*c/s* or *cps*) or in counts per minute (*c/m* or *cpm*).

The *half-life* of a radioactive species is the time required for one-half of a given number of atoms to decay. The half-life, $t_{1/2}$, is related to the disintegration constant, λ, by

$$t_{1/2} = 0.693/\lambda$$

where $0.693 = \ln 2$.

Consecutive, *sequential*, or *series decay* results when a parent nuclide A decays to produce a radioactive *daughter* or *progeny* B, which, in turn, decays to C:

$$A \xrightarrow{\lambda_A} B \xrightarrow{\lambda_B} C$$

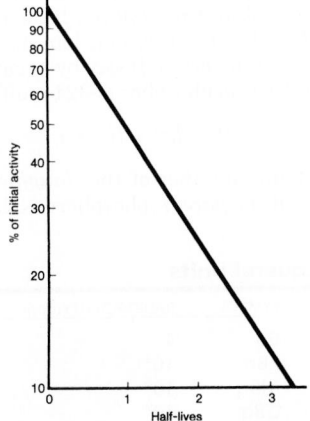

Figure 29-5. Radioactive decay curve.

If only atoms of A are present initially, the number of atoms of B present at time t is given by:

$$N_B = \lambda_A / \lambda_B - \lambda_A \, N_{Ao} \, (e^{-\lambda_A t} - e^{-\lambda_B t})$$

Of particular interest in nuclear medicine are combinations where the parent radionuclide has a relatively long half-life and the daughter radionuclide a short half-life, for example:

$$^{99}\text{Mo } 67 \text{ h} \rightarrow {}^{99m}\text{Tc } 6.0 \text{ h} \rightarrow {}^{99}\text{Tc}$$

After a time equal to many half-lives of the daughter, a state of *secular equilibrium* or *transient equilibrium* is achieved. At this time, *in-growth* of the daughter has reached a maximum. This process of series decay is used in *radionuclide generators* as a source of short-lived radionuclides. This topic is discussed further in the section on production of radionuclides.

UNITS OF RADIOACTIVITY

One gram of radium was selected as the unit of radioactivity and was called the *curie*. It has been extremely difficult to measure the absolute decay rate (dps) of a curie of radium, although the average of many measurements, using a variety of methods, is approximately 3.7×10^{10} dps. In view of these discrepancies, the International Radium Standards Commission has recommended the use of the arbitrary value of exactly 3.7×10^{10} until the third significant figure is agreed upon. Although originally defined in terms of radium, the curie has been used as a standard for the disintegration rate of any radionuclide. For example, 1 curie of carbon-14 means that amount of carbon-14 necessary to provide 3.7×10^{10} dps. Despite its continued use on a limited basis in the US, the curie has generally been replaced by the *becquerel,* Bq, named for Henri Becquerel, which is equal to an activity of one disintegrating atom per second (Table 29-2).

MODES OF RADIOACTIVE DECAY

When it is necessary to measure the absolute decay rate of a particular nuclear species, one must establish its mode of decay, or *decay scheme*, in order to determine the relationship of the number of particles or gamma rays emitted to the number of atoms actually undergoing decay. There are several important modes of decay.

Alpha decay is illustrated by the decay of polonium-210 to lead-206:

$$^{210}_{84}\text{Po} \rightarrow {}^{4}_{2}\text{He} + {}^{206}_{82}\text{Pb}$$

In this example, the nucleus of lead-206, which contains 82 protons and 124 neutrons, is stable and does not undergo further decay. The majority of nuclides that undergo alpha decay have atomic numbers greater than 82.

There are three types of *isobaric decay: negatron emission, positron emission,* and *electron capture.* If the ratio of neutrons to protons is too *high* for stability, a nucleus may decay by negatron emission (negatron decay). Decay by negatron emission is illustrated by the decay of phosphorus-32 to sulfur-32 (Fig 29-6):

$$^{32}_{15}\text{P} \rightarrow {}^{32}_{16}\text{S} + \beta^- + \nu$$

Note that the atomic number of the *daughter,* sulfur-32, is greater than that of the *parent,* phosphorus-32. In this process

Table 29-2. Becquerel Units

UNITS	SYMBOL	RADIOACTIVITY(dps)	CURIE EQUIVALENT
Becquerel	Bq	1	2.7×10^{-11} Ci
Kilobecquerel	kBq	10^3	2.7×10^{-8} Ci
Megabecquerel	MBq	10^6	2.7×10^{-5} Ci
Gigabecquerel	GBq	10^9	2.7×10^{-2} Ci
Terabecquerel	TBq	10^{12}	27 Ci

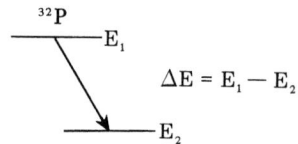

Figure 29-6. Energy level diagram.

a proton has been produced, but because a neutron has been consumed, there is no change in the mass number and thus the reaction is isobaric. This is explained by the *particle reaction:*

$$^1_0\text{n} \rightarrow {}^1_1\text{p} + \text{e}^- + \nu$$

which shows the decay of a neutron into a proton, a negative electron and a neutrino.

The beta particles emitted during the decay of a given radioactive species do not all possess the same energy but are emitted with a continuous energy distribution extending from zero to a specific maximum value, E_{max}. This posed an enigma for some time. The decay of phosphorus-32 of energy E_1 to sulfur-32 of energy E_2 should be associated with the release of energy equal to ΔE, where $\Delta E = E_1 - E_2$ (see Fig 29-6). A new particle, the *neutrino,* was postulated to explain the energy change not associated with the beta particle. Thus, the sum of the energies of the beta particle and its associated neutrino is equal to ΔE or E_{max} (Fig 29-7). Moreover, the average energy of a beta particle is equal to 1/3 E_{max}.

If the ratio of neutrons to protons is too *low* for stability, a nucleus may decay by *positron emission* (ie, *positron decay*):

$$^{11}_6\text{C} \rightarrow {}^{11}_5\text{B} + \beta^+ + \nu$$

In this instance the particle reaction that illustrates the change is:

$$^1_1\text{p} \rightarrow {}^1_0\text{n} + \text{e}^+ + \nu$$

Again, no change in mass number occurs (ie, the reaction is isobaric), since the decay of ^{11}C to ^{11}B is accompanied by the change of a proton into a neutron. The energies of the positrons extend from zero to E_{max} in a manner analogous to the energy distribution of negative beta particles because the neutrino is required to account for the balance of the energy.

An alternative to positron emission for increasing the neutron-to-proton ratio to a more stable condition is a process known as *electron capture.* In this process, an orbital electron is captured by the nucleus. An example is the decay of ^{201}Tl to ^{201}Hg:

$$^{201}_{81}\text{Tl} + \text{e}^- \text{ (K)} \rightarrow {}^{201}_{80}\text{Hg}$$

The corresponding particle reaction is:

$$\text{e}^- + {}^1_1\text{p} \rightarrow {}^1_0\text{n}$$

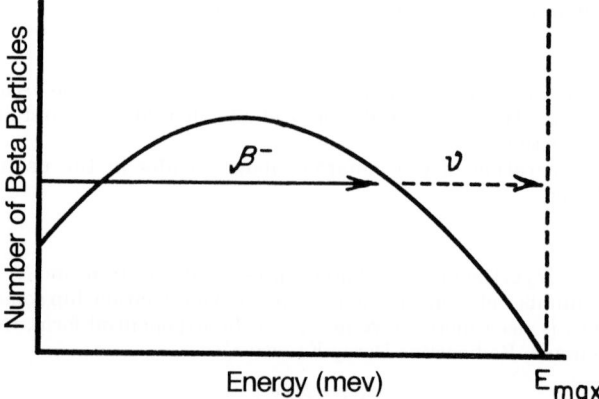

Figure 29-7. Typical beta spectrum.

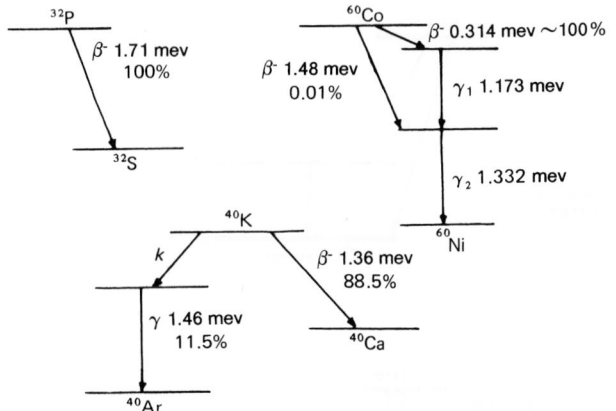

Figure 29-8. Modes of decay. Radioactive atoms may decay by any one of numerous processes. Negatron decay is shown by an arrow slanting to the right, electron or K-capture by an arrow slanting to the left and gamma emission by a vertical arrow.

Electron capture also has been called *K-capture* because the electron captured in the process is usually from the K shell. However, the electron may also come from the L or M shell.

The mode of decay is often represented by an energy-level diagram (Fig 29-8). Three different modes of decay are illustrated. The first is the simple beta decay of phosphorus-32. In this instance, each decaying atom of ^{32}P emits one beta particle. Thus, if the number of beta particles is measured, the number of decaying atoms also is known. The decay of an atom of cobalt-60 also results essentially in the emission of a single beta particle, but two gamma rays are also emitted. Thus, if the decay rate is measured by counting the number of beta particles emitted, a 1:1 ratio exists. If, on the other hand, the decay rate is determined from the number of gamma rays emitted, it must be remembered that the number of decaying atoms is equal to only one-half the number of gamma rays (neglecting a small correction for internal conversion). In the third example, the decay of ^{40}K results in the emission of beta particles in 88.5% of decay events. The other 11.5% of decay events are by electron capture. Thus, a microcurie of ^{40}K does not emit 3.7×10^4 beta particles per second, but only $0.885 \times 3.7 \times 10^4$ beta particles. Decay schemes for several radionuclides used in medicine are shown in Figure 29-9.

PRODUCTION OF RADIONUCLIDES

Most, if not all, radionuclides used in medicine and pharmacy are produced artificially. Table 29-3 is a compilation of medical radionuclides along with their physical properties. These radionuclides are produced by three general methods: (1) in a nuclear reactor as a fission by-product, (2) as the product of a neutron reaction—either by activation or transmutation, and (3) by use of a particle accelerator such as a cyclotron.

FISSION BY-PRODUCTS

Fission is a radioactive process in which a relatively heavy nucleus is divided into two new nuclei of nearly equal size with the simultaneous emission of two or three neutrons. Fission may be spontaneous, but normally the reaction is induced by bombardment of the parent nucleus with a neutron:

$$^{235}_{92}\text{U} + ^{1}_{0}\text{n} \rightarrow X + Y + 2.5\,\text{n}$$

where X and Y are fission products (new nuclei) with a Z value of between 30 and 65 and a sum of 92. Fission reactions may be self-sustaining. For each neutron consumed, an average of 2.5 new neutrons are produced that may initiate the fission of other nuclei. Such a reaction is called a *chain reaction*. If at least one

of the 2.5 neutrons produced is used to sustain the reaction, the reaction is said to be *critical*.

The following illustrates one of many combinations of fission reactions that are possible:

$$^{238}_{92}\text{U} + ^{1}_{0}\text{n} \rightarrow ^{131}_{50}\text{Sn} + ^{106}_{42}\text{Mo} + ^{1}_{0}\text{n} + ^{1}_{0}\text{n}$$

The ^{131}Sn and the ^{106}Mo are very radioactive and have very short half-lives. They immediately decay by a series of beta decay processes:

$$^{131}_{50}\text{Sn} \rightarrow ^{131}_{51}\text{Sb} \rightarrow ^{131}_{52}\text{Te} \rightarrow ^{131}_{53}\text{I}$$

$$^{106}_{46}\text{Mo} \rightarrow ^{106}_{43}\text{Tc} \rightarrow ^{106}_{44}\text{Ru} \rightarrow ^{106}_{45}\text{Rh}$$

Both ^{131}I and ^{106}Ru are available commercially as fission-produced radionuclides, although ^{106}Ru is not routinely used for medical applications.

Before use, the desired nuclide must be chemically separated from a large number of other fission-produced radionuclides. For many of the radionuclides produced by fission, separation of the desired nuclide from the mixture of fission products is too difficult or costly.

NEUTRON REACTIONS

Many radioactive nuclides used in radiopharmaceuticals are prepared by neutron activation (n, γ) or transmutation (n, p) reactions by placing a suitable target material in a nuclear reactor where it is bombarded by neutrons. By means of (n, γ) and (n, p) reactions, reactors produce radionuclides having a high neutron-to-proton ratio that typically decay by emission of a negatron. For example, radioactive phosphorus (^{32}P) can be prepared from stable phosphorus (^{31}P) by *neutron capture*:

$$^{31}_{15}\text{P} + ^{1}_{0}\text{n} \rightarrow ^{32}_{15}\text{P} + \gamma$$

The disadvantage of this method is that the radioactive phosphorus (^{32}P) is highly diluted with stable ^{31}P. Phosphorus-32 of low specific activity can be used for certain purposes, such as the investigation of phosphate fertilizers, but would be less useful for many biological and medical applications.

Radioactive phosphorus can be made by transmutation if high specific activities are required:

$$^{32}_{16}\text{S} + ^{1}_{0}\text{n} \rightarrow ^{32}_{15}\text{P} + ^{1}_{1}\text{p}$$

In this case, the radioactive phosphorus can be separated from the unreacted sulfur by chemical procedures. Where ^{32}P is made from ^{31}P, such chemical separations are not practical.

Transmutation is useful for the preparation of many radioactive nuclides, especially those of low atomic number. As the atomic number increases, (n, γ) reactions are favored over (n, p) reactions. For example, cobalt-60 is produced by the reaction ^{59}Co(n, γ)^{60}Co because the reaction ^{60}Ni(n, p)^{60}Co does not occur with sufficient frequency to make the process commercially feasible.

^{125}I($t_{1/2}$ = 60 d) is produced from ^{124}Xe:

$$^{124}\text{Xe(n, }\gamma)^{125}\text{Xe EC} \rightarrow ^{125}\text{I}$$

Secondary neutron capture results in the side reaction ^{125}I(n, γ)^{126}I. Because ^{126}I($t_{1/2}$ = 14 d) is an undesirable impurity in ^{125}I, it is removed through its own decay.

CYCLOTRON-PRODUCED RADIONUCLIDES

Certain radionuclides are cyclotron-produced. The cyclotron and similar *particle accelerators* can be used only with charged particles such as electrons, protons, alpha particles, or deuterons because the operation of such machines depends upon the interaction of magnetic and/or electrostatic fields with

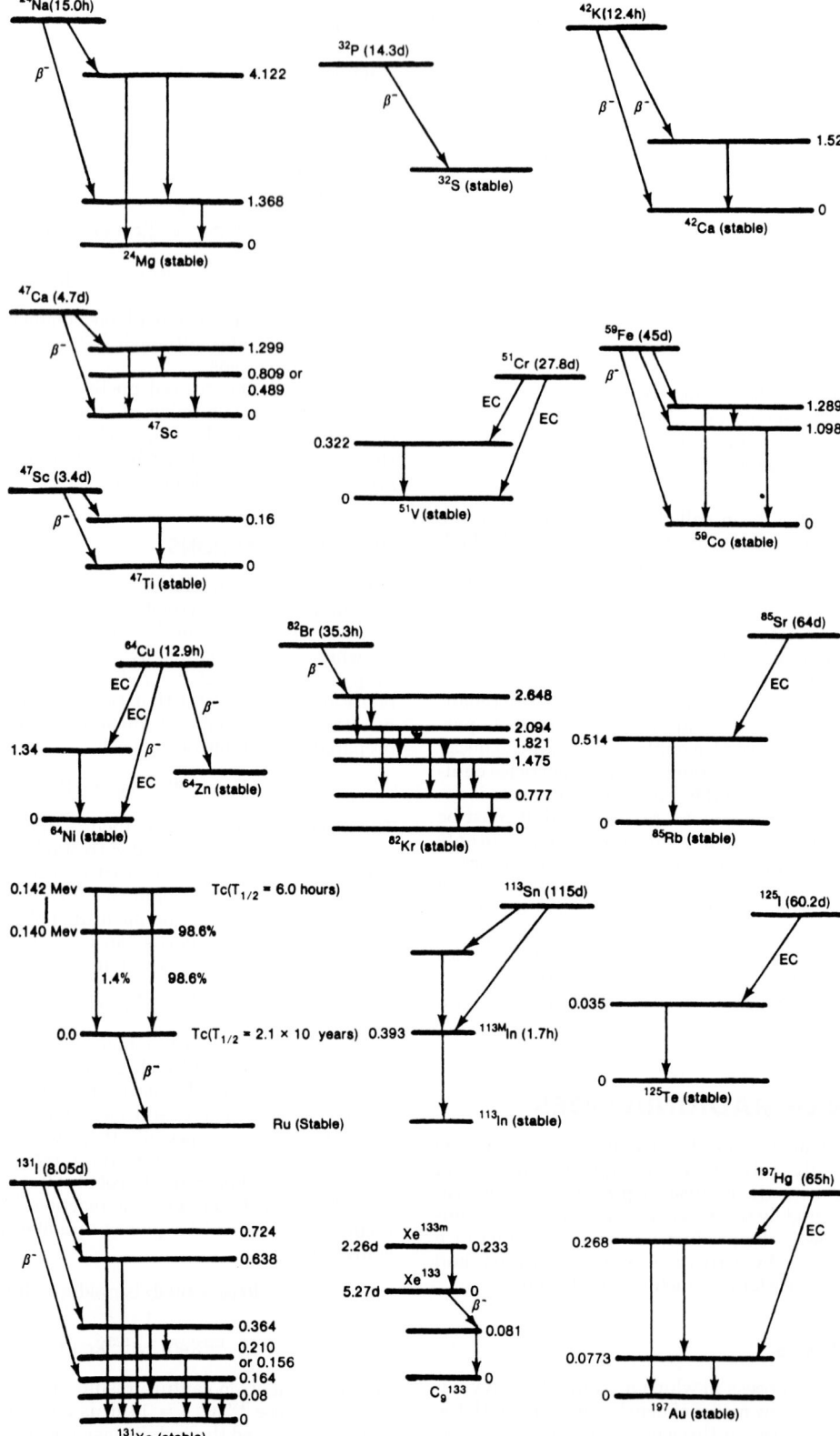

Figure 29-9. Decay schemes for nuclides commonly used in medicine.

Table 29-3. Physical Characteristics of Radionuclides Commonly Used in Medicine

NUCLIDE COMMON PRODUCTION	HALF-LIFE	DECAY MODE PRINCIPLE	EMISSIONS (MeV)	GAMMA RAY CONSTANT	R/mCi-HOUR AT 1 cm
^{11}C	^{14}N(p, α)^{11}C	20.4 minutes	β^+	0.97 β^+ (100%)	5.9
				0.511 γ (200%)	
^{13}N	^{16}O(p, α)^{13}N	10.0 minutes	β^+	1.2 β^+ (100%)	5.9
				0.511 γ (200%)	
^{14}C	^{14}N(n, p)^{14}C	5730 years	β^-	0.156 β^- (100%)	
^{15}O	^{14}N(d, n)^{15}O	2.05 months	β^+	1.74 β^+ (100%)	5.9
				0.511 γ (200%)	
^{18}F	^{18}O(p, n)^{18}F	110 minutes	β^+, EC	0.635 β^+ (97%)	5.7
				0.511 γ (194%)	
^{32}P	^{31}S(n, p)^{32}P	14.3 days	β^-	1.71 β^- (100%)	
^{51}Cr	^{50}Cr(n, γ)^{51}Cr	27.8 days	EC	0.320 γ (9%)	0.18
^{57}Co	^{56}Fe(p, γ)^{57}Co	271 days	EC	0.014 γ (9%)	0.57
				0.122 γ (86%)	
				0.136 γ (10%)	
^{60}Co	^{59}Co(n, γ)^{60}Co	5.27 years	β^-	0.31 β^- (99%)	13.2
				1.173 γ (100%)	
				1.332 γ (100%)	
^{67}Ga	^{68}Zn(p, 2n)^{67}Ga	78.3 hours	EC	0.093 γ (38%)	1.6
				0.184 γ (20%)	
				0.300 γ (16%)	
				0.394 γ (5%)	
^{68}Ga	^{68}Ge daughter	68.3 minutes	β^+, EC	1.9 β^+ (88%)	5.4
				0.511 γ (176%)	
^{81m}Kr	^{81}Rb daughter	13 seconds	IT	0.191 γ (66%)	1.6
^{82}Rb	^{82}Sr daughter	75 seconds	β^+, EC	3.15 β^+ (96%)	6.1
				0.511 γ (192%)	
^{89}Sr	^{88}Sr(n, γ)^{89}Sr	50.5 days	β^-	1.46 β^- (100%)	
^{90}Y	^{90}Sr daughter	64 hours	β^-	2.27 β^- (100%)	
^{99}Mo	fission	2.75 days	β^-	0.45 β^- (18%)	
				1.23 β^- (82%)	1.8
				0.181 γ (6%)	
				0.740 γ (13%)	
				0.778 γ (5%)	
^{99m}Tc	^{99}Mo daughter	6.02 hours	IT	0.140 γ (89%)	0.7
^{111}In	^{112}Cd(p, 2n)^{111}In	67.3 hours	EC	0.171 γ (90%)	3.2
				0.246 γ (94%)	
^{123}I	^{127}I(p, 5n)^{123}Xe daughter	13.2 hours	EC	0.159 γ (83%)	1.6
				0.027 $\times$ (71%)	
^{125}I	^{124}Xe(n, γ)^{125}Xe daughter	60.2 days	EC	0.036 γ (7%)	1.4
				0.027 $\times$ (110%)	
^{131}I	fission	8.04 days	β^-	0.61 β^- (90%)	2.2
				0.284 γ (6%)	
				0.364 γ (82%)	
				0.637 γ (7%)	
^{133}Xe	fission	5.25 days	β^-	0.35 β^- (100%)	0.5
				0.081 γ (36%)	
				0.031 $\times$ (39%)	
^{137}Cs	fission	30 years	β^-	0.51 β^- (94%)	3.3
				1.18 β^- (6%)	
				0.662 γ (84%)	
^{153}Sm	^{152}Sm(n, γ)^{153}Sm	46.3 hours	β^-	0.640 β^- (30%)	0.9
				0.710 β^- (50%)	
				0.810 β^- (20%)	
				0.103 γ (29%)	
^{186}Re	^{185}Re(n, γ)^{186}Re	3.72 days	β^-, EC	1.07 β^- (77%)	0.08
				0.93 β^- (23%)	
				0.137 γ (9%)	
^{201}Tl	^{203}Tl(p, 3n)^{201}Pb daughter	73 hours	EC	0.135 γ (3%)	0.47
				0.167 γ (10%)	
				0.070 $\times$ (74%)	
				0.080 $\times$ (20%)	

Data from Madsen MT, Ponto JA. *Medical Physics Handbook of Nuclear Medicine,* Madison, WI: Medical Physics, 1992; and individual product package inserts.

the charge (either + or −) of the particle undergoing acceleration. When the particles have been accelerated to a high velocity, even approaching the velocity of light and representing enormous energies, they are caused to strike a target containing the atoms to be bombarded. Sodium-22 is prepared in this way, by the interaction of high-velocity deuterons with magnesium. The nuclear equation is:

$$^{24}\text{Mg(d, }\alpha)^{22}\text{Na}$$

Cyclotrons produce neutron-deficient isotopes; that is, the neutron-to-proton ratio is low. These nuclides usually decay by positron emission or electron capture. Cyclotron-produced radionuclides are generally carrier-free because they are normally produced by transmutation.

The following reactions are typical for the cyclotron production of some medically useful nuclides:

$$^{10}\text{B(d, n)}^{11}\text{C}$$

$$^{11}\text{B(p, n)}^{11}\text{C}$$

$$^{11}\text{B(d, 2n)}^{11}\text{C}$$

$$^{14}\text{N(p, }\alpha)^{11}\text{C}$$

$$^{10}\text{B}(\alpha, \text{n})^{13}\text{N}$$

$$^{12}\text{C(d, n)}^{13}\text{N}$$

$$^{16}\text{O(p, }\alpha)^{13}\text{N}$$

$$^{14}\text{N(d, n)}^{15}\text{O}$$

$$^{15}\text{N(p, n)}^{15}\text{O}$$

$$^{16}\text{O(p, pn)}^{15}\text{O}$$

$$^{18}\text{O(p, n)}^{18}\text{F}$$

$$^{20}\text{Ne(d, }\alpha)^{18}\text{F}$$

$$^{70}\text{Zn(p, }\alpha)^{67}\text{Cu}$$

$$^{66}\text{Zn(d, n)}^{67}\text{Ga}$$

$$^{68}\text{Zn(p, 2n)}^{67}\text{Ga}$$

$$^{69}\text{Ga(p, 2n)}^{68}\text{Ge}$$

$$^{82}\text{Kr(p, 2n)}^{81}\text{Rb} \rightarrow {}^{81m}\text{Kr}$$

$$^{111}\text{Cd(p, n)}^{111}\text{In}$$

$$^{112}\text{Cd(p, 2n)}^{111}\text{In}$$

$$^{203}\text{Tl(p, 3n)}^{201}\text{Pb} \rightarrow {}^{201}\text{Tl}$$

Usually a nuclide can be made by more than one reaction. For example, ^{123}I can be prepared either directly or indirectly. Direct reactions include:

$$^{123}\text{Te(p, n)}^{123}\text{I}$$

$$^{121}\text{Sb(}^4\text{He, 2n)}^{123}\text{I}$$

$$^{122}\text{Te(d, n)}^{123}\text{I}$$

$$^{124}\text{Te(p, 2n)}^{123}\text{I}$$

Indirectly, the intermediate ^{123}Xe (or ^{123}Cs, which decays to ^{123}Xe) is prepared, which then decays to ^{123}I:

$$^{122}\text{Te(}^4\text{He, 3n)}^{123}\text{Xe} \rightarrow {}^{123}\text{I}$$

$$^{122}\text{Te(}^3\text{He, 2n)}^{123}\text{Xe} \rightarrow {}^{123}\text{I}$$

$$^{123}\text{Te(}^3\text{He, 3n)}^{123}\text{Xe} \rightarrow {}^{123}\text{I}$$

$$^{127}\text{I(p, 5n)}^{123}\text{Xe} \rightarrow {}^{123}\text{I}$$

$$^{124}\text{Xe(p, 2n)}^{123}\text{Cs} \rightarrow {}^{123}\text{Xe} \rightarrow {}^{123}\text{I}$$

RADIONUCLIDE GENERATORS

When clinical procedures require that a radionuclide be administered internally, it is advantageous to use a nuclide with a short half-life to minimize the radiation dose received by the patient. It is evident, however, that the shorter the half-life, the greater the problem of supply. One answer to this problem is the radionuclide generator, which uses the phenomenon of *sequential decay*. A radionuclide generator provides a mechanism for separating a clinically useful, short half-life daughter nuclide from a long-lived parent nuclide. Radioactive decay of the long-lived parent results in the production of a short-lived radioactive daughter nuclide that is *eluted* or *milked* from the generator by means of an appropriate eluant. Characteristics of a number of parent–daughter systems that have been used in radionuclide generators are found in Table 29-4.

The molybdenum-99/technetium-99m generator (Fig 29-10) consists of an alumina (Al_2O_3) column on which molybdenum-99 is adsorbed as ammonium molybdate. Radioactive decay of ^{99}Mo produces ^{99m}Tc, which is eluted from the column with 0.9% sodium chloride, USP. Upon elution, the ^{99m}Tc is in the form of sodium pertechnetate ($\text{Na}^{99m}\text{TcO}_4$). Elution repeated every 24 hours provides a satisfactory balance between concentration and quantity of eluted ^{99m}Tc. If a high activity of ^{99m}Tc is not required, the generator can be eluted more frequently. A typical elution curve for a ^{99}Mo/^{99m}Tc generator is shown in Figure 29-11. Normally the generator must be replaced about once a week due to the decay of ^{99}Mo.

RADIOLABELING OF COMPOUNDS TO PREPARE RADIOTRACERS AND RADIOPHARMACEUTICALS

RADIOLABELING METHODS

For medical and pharmaceutical purposes, some radionuclides can be used in their elemental or salt forms, and thus do not require extensive processing beyond their separation and purification following production. However, most radionuclides must be incorporated into some molecule or compound to form a useful radiotracer or radiopharmaceutical. There are several ways that radionuclides are incorporated into the final radiopharmaceutical, a process known as *radiolabeling*. Some of the more common methods of radiolabeling include the following.

Introduction of a Foreign Label—For example, ^{99m}Tc is not a natural part of any medically useful compound, and thus a method must be developed to chelate ^{99m}Tc to various compounds of interest.

Table 29-4. Selected Radionuclide Generators

PARENT ISOTOPE	HALF-LIFE	DAUGHTER ISOTOPE	HALF-LIFE	MODE OF DECAY
^{68}Ge	271 d	^{68}Ga	68 m	β^+
^{81}Rb	4.7 h	^{81m}Kr	13 s	I.T.
^{82}Sr	25 d	^{82}Rb	1.3 m	β^+
^{87}Y	80 h	^{87m}Sr	2.8 h	I.T.
^{90}Sr	28 y	^{90}Y	64 h	β
^{99}Mo	67 h	^{99m}Tc	6.0 h	I.T.
^{109}Cd	453 d	^{109m}Ag	39.2 s	I.T.
^{113}Sn	118 d	^{113m}In	1.7 h	I.T.
^{115}Cd	53.4 h	^{115m}In	4.5 h	I.T.
^{122}Xe	20 h	^{122}I	3.6 m	β^+
^{132}Te	3.2 d	^{132}I	2.3 h	β^-
^{137}Cs	30 y	^{137m}Ba	2.6 m	I.T.
^{144}Ce	285 d	^{144}Pr	17.3 m	β^-
^{178}W	21.5 d	^{178}Ta	9.4 m	β^+
^{191}Os	16 d	^{191m}Ir	4.9 s	I.T.
^{195m}Hg	41 h	^{195m}Au	30.6 s	I.T.
^{225}Ac	10 d	^{213}Bi	45.6 m	α, γ, β^-

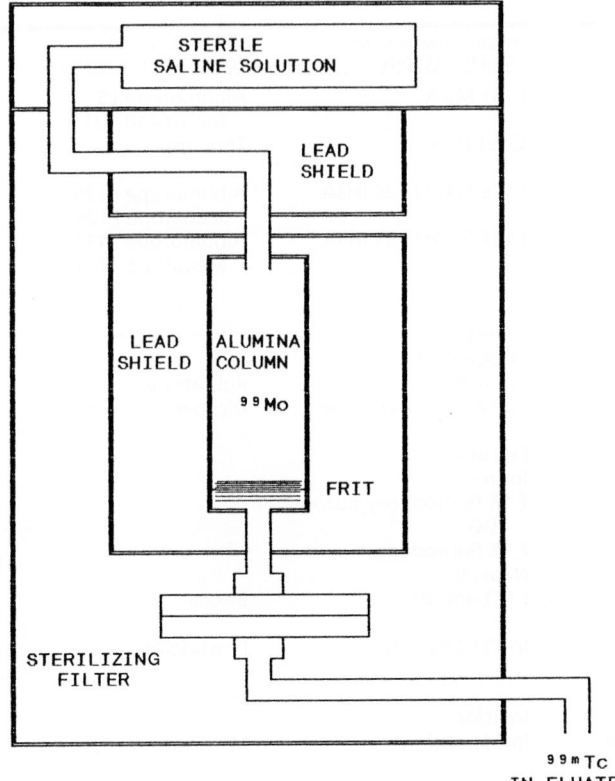

Figure 29-10. Schematic diagram of a radionuclide generator for the production of technetium-99m by elution from molybdenum-99 absorbed on an alumina column.

Isotope Exchange—This process occurs when a radioactive isotope is substituted for a stable atom of the same element that is already a natural part of the molecule. An example would be substituting ^{123}I for stable ^{127}I in some iodine containing molecule.

Labeling With Bifunctional Chelates—A *bifunctional chelate* is a molecule used to link another molecule with a radionuclide. An example would be linking ^{90}Y to a peptide without direct attachment to the peptide by using a compound such as 1,4,7,10-tetraazacyclododecane-1,4,7,10-tetraacetic acid (DOTA).

Biosynthesis—This reaction occurs when a radionuclide is incorporated into a molecule through some biosynthetic process. An example is when radioactive ^{57}Co is placed in the growth media of the bacteria that produces cyanocobalamin, vitamin B_{12}, as a metabolic by-product and yields radioactive vitamin B_{12} for use in the Schilling test.

DESIGN OF RADIOPHARMACEUTICALS

Not all radiopharmaceuticals use metal atoms as the radionuclide, but many do. When a molecule is radiolabeled with a metal atom, sometimes the metal atom does not change the biologic properties of the molecule into which it is incorporated; but sometimes it changes the biologic properties considerably. The result of the former instance is sometimes classified as a *metal-tagged* radiopharmaceutical, and the latter as a *metal essential* radiopharmaceutical. In the case of metal essential radiopharmaceuticals, the radioactive metal atom is absolutely essential in determining where that molecule will distribute in the body. Therefore, when designing a new radiopharmaceutical, one must be aware of how the addition of a metal atom (such as ^{99m}Tc) will affect the molecule in question.

In the design of radiopharmaceuticals, it is obviously important to select compounds that are likely to distribute to the organs or tissues of interest. As with nonradioactive drugs,

computer modeling can quite often be helpful. It is not always easy to match a radionuclide that has appropriate physical properties with a candidate compound for a particular diagnostic or therapeutic purpose. It is important to make sure that the chemistries are compatible and that the resulting molecule has the desired biodistribution pattern.

With radiodiagnostic agents, structure–distribution relationships (SDR) are used to design candidate molecules. The SDR are similar to using structure–activity relationships for designing pharmacologically active drugs. The goal of SDR are to optimize target site delivery of the candidate radiopharmaceutical. This involves predicting, investigating, and determining changes in the biokinetics of a candidate radiopharmaceutical by effecting small changes in its structure, such as through the addition of functional groups to the compound. The newly altered candidate is tested for its pharmacokinetic behavior and compared with the prototype. Eventually, the most effective radiopharmaceutical candidate is selected for animal and human testing.

TECHNETIUM RADIOPHARMACEUTICALS

Technetium 99m (^{99m}Tc) is the most commonly used metal atom in radiopharmaceuticals; over 75% of all radiopharmaceuticals include ^{99m}Tc as the radionuclide. Technetium-99m has desirable physical properties for imaging purposes. It has a 6-hour half-life and a 140 keV gamma photon that is emitted with high abundance and it lacks particulate alpha and beta emissions. It also has a versatile chemistry that allows it to be chelated with a variety of compounds (but certainly not all compounds).

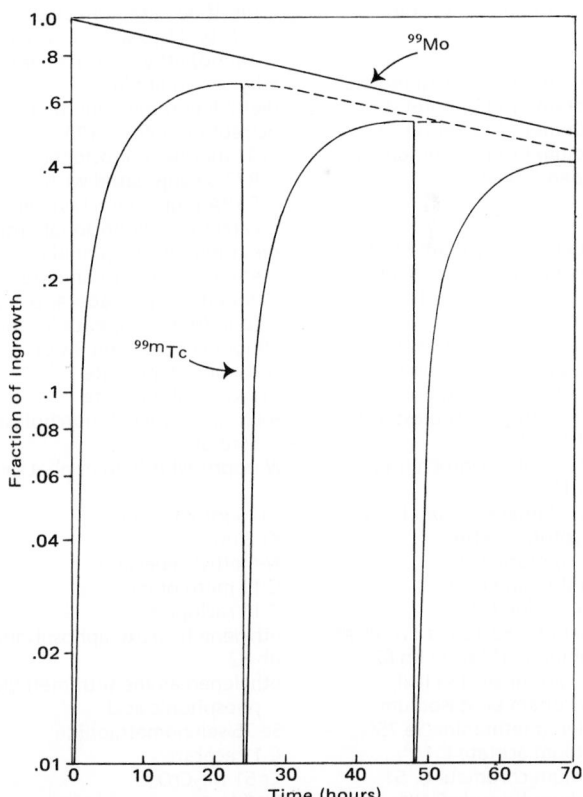

Figure 29-11. Elution curve. The lower solid lines show the theoretical activity of ^{99m}Tc in the generator as a result of ingrowth followed by elution of ^{99m}Tc at 24-hour intervals. If the generator were not eluted, ingrowth would follow the broken line and a transient equilibrium would be established. The upper solid line represents decrease in activity of ^{99}Mo, the parent nuclide, due to radioactive decay.

Table 29-5. Radiopharmaceutical Names

USAN/GENERIC NAME	LIGAND; COMMON CHEMICAL NAME	OTHER COMMON NAMES OR ABBREVIATIONS	COMMON TRADE NAMES
Albumin, aggregated iodinated I 131 serum[a]	macroaggregated albumin	I 131 MAA	Albumotope-LS; Macroscan-131
Albumin, chromated Cr 51 serum[a]		Cr 51 HSA	Tomatope
Albumin, iodinated I 125 serum	radio-iodinated serum albumin; iodinated human serum albumin	I 125 RISA; I 125 IHSA	Albumotope I 125; Jeanatope I 125
Albumin, iodinated I 131 serum	radio-iodinated serum albumin; iodinated human serum albumin	I 131 RISA; I 131 IHSA	Albumotope I 131; Megatope I 131
Ammonia N 13[a]	N 13 NH_3		
Carbon monoxide C 11[a]	C 11 CO		
Carbon C 14 urea	C 14 urea	PYtest	
Chromic phosphate P 32	P 32 colloid	Phosphocol	
Cyanocobalamin Co 57	vitamin B_{12}	Co 57 B_{12}	Rubratope
Cyanocobalamin Co 58/Co 57[b]	vitamin B_{12}/instrinsic factor	Co 58 B_{12}/Co 57 B_{12}-IF	Dicopac
Ferrous citrate Fe 59[a]	Fe 59 citrate	Ferrutope	
Fibrinogen I 125[a]	I 125 fibrinogen	Ibrin	
Fludeoxyglucose F 18[a]	2-fluoro-2-deoxy-D-glucose	F 18 fluorodeoxyglucose; FDG	
Fluorodopa F 18[a]	fluoro-levodopa	F 18 fluorodopa	
Gallium citrate Ga 67	Ga 67 citrate	Neoscan	
I 131 radiolabeled B1 monoclonal antibody[a]	iodinated IgG anti-B1 murine monoclonal antibody	I 131 anti-B1	Bexxar
Indium In 111 capromab pendetide	IgG 1 murine monoclonal 7E11-C5.3 conjugated with DTPA [antiprostate carcinoma monoclonal antibody]	In 111 CYT 356	ProstaScint
Indium In 111 chloride	In 111 Cl_3	Indiclor	
Indium In 111 imciromab pentetate[a]	IgG 2a murine monoclonal R11D10 Fab conjugated with DTPA [antimyosin monoclonal antibody]	In 111 antimyosin	Myoscint
Indium In 111 immune globulin intravenous pentetate[a]	immunoglobulin G (human polyclonal), disulfide with light chain, dimer, N,N-bis [2-[bis(carboxymethyl) amino]-ethyl] glycine conjugate	In 111 IgG	Macroscint
Indium In 111 oxyquinoline	8-hydroxyquinoline	In 111 oxine	
Indium In 111 pentetate	diethylenetriaminepentaacetic acid	In 111 DTPA	
Indium In 111 pentetreotide	octreotide-D-Phe-DTPA	In 111 octreotide	OctreoScan
Indium In 111 satumomab pendetide[a]	IgG1 murine monoclonal B72.3 conjugated with DTPA [anticolorectal/ovarian carcinoma monoclonal antibody]	In 111 CYT 099; CYT 103	OncoScint OR/OV
Iobenguane sulfate I 123[a]	meta-iodobenzylguanidine	I 123 MIBG	
Iobenguane sulfate I 131	meta-iodobenzylguanidine	I 131 MIBG	
Iocanlidic acid I 123[a]	iodobenzenepentadecanoic acid; (p-iodophenyl)pentadecanoic acid		
Iodocholesterol I 131[a]	19-iodocholest-5-en-3β-ol	I 131 iodocholesterol	
Iodohippurate sodium I 123[a]	ortho-iodohippurate	I 123 OIH	Nephroflow
Iodohippurate sodium I 131[a]	ortho-iodohippurate	I 131 OIH	Hippuran I 131; Hipputope
Iodomethylnorcholesterol I 131[a,b]	6-β-iodomethyl-19-norcholesto-5(10)en-3β-ol	NP 59	
Iofetamine hydrochloride I 123[a]	N-isopropyl-p-iodoamphetamine	I 123 IMP	Spectamine
Iothalamate sodium I 125	I 125 iothalamate	Glofil	
Krypton Kr 81m	Kr 81m		
Mesiperone C 11[a]	N-methylspiperone	C 11 NMSP	
Methionine C 11[a]	C 11 methionine		
Raclopride C 11[a]	C 11 raclopride		
Rhenium Re 186 etidronate[a]	ethylene hydroxydiphosphonate	Re 186 EHDP	
Rubidium chloride Rb 82	Rb 82	Cardiogen-82	
Samarium Sm 153 lexi-dronam pentasodium	ethylenediamine tetramethylene phosphonic acid	Sm 153 EDTMP	Quadramet
Selenomethionine Se 75[a]	Se 75 selenomethionine		
Sodium acetate C 11[a]	C 11 acetate		
Sodium chromate Cr 51	Cr 51 Na_2CrO_4	Chromitope	
Sodium fluoride F 18[a]	F 18 NaF		
Sodium iodide I 123	I 123 NaI		
Sodium iodide I 131	I 131 NaI	Iodotope	
Sodium pertechnetate Tc 99m	product from Mo-99/Tc-99m generator	Na^+ TcO_4^-	generators: Minitec; Technelite; Ultra-TechneKow
Sodium phosphate P 32	P 32 Na_3PO_4/Na_2HPO_4		
Stannic pentetate Sn 117[a,b]	tin (IV) diethylenetriaminepentaacetic acid	Sn 117 DTPA	

Table 29-5. Radiopharmaceutical Names (*continued*)

USAN/GENERIC NAME	LIGAND; COMMON CHEMICAL NAME	OTHER COMMON NAMES OR ABBREVIATIONS	COMMON TRADE NAMES
Strontium chloride Sr 89	Sr 89	Metastron	
Technetium Tc 99m albumin	Tc 99m HSA		
Technetium Tc 99m albumin aggregated	macroaggregated albumin	Tc 99m MAA	Pulmolite; Macrotec
Technetium Tc 99m albumin colloid[a]	Tc 99m AC	Microlite	
Technetium Tc 99m antimony trisulfide colloid[a]	Sb_2S_3	Tc 99m ASC	Lymph-Scan
Technetium Tc 99m apcitide	GP IIb/IIIa receptor peptide	Tc 99m P280	Accutech
Technetium Tc 99m arcitumomab	IgG murine monoclonal IMMU-4 Fab[anti-CEA monoclonal antibody fragment]	Tc 99m anti-CEA Fab	CEA-Scan
Technetium Tc 99m bectumomab[a]	IgG 2a murine monoclonal IMMU-LL2 Fab [anti-non-Hodgkin's lymphoma monoclonal antibody fragment]	Tc 99m IMMU-LL2	ImmuRaid-LL2
Technetium Tc 99m biciromab[a]	IgG murine monoclonal T2G1s Fab [antifibrin monoclonal antibody fragment]	Tc 99m antifibrin Fab	Fibroscint
Technetium Tc 99m bicisate	ethyl cysteinate dimer	Tc 99m ECD	Neurolite
Technetium Tc 99m depreotide			
Technetium Tc 99m disofenin	diisopropylacetanilidoiminodi-acetic acid	Tc 99m DISIDA	Hepatolite
Technetium Tc 99m etidronate[a]	ethylenehydroxydiphosphonate	Tc 99m EHDP	
Technetium Tc 99m exametazime	hexamethylpropyleneamineoxime	Tc 99m HMPAO	Ceretec
Technetium Tc 99m furifosmin[a]	ethylenebis(nitrilomethylidyne)bis (dihydrotetramethylfuranonato) bis(tris[methoxypropyl])-phosphine)	Tc 99m Q-12	TechneScan Q-12
Technetium Tc 99m gluceptate	glucoheptonate	Tc 99m GH; GHA	Glucoscan; TechneScan Gluceptate
Technetium Tc 99m lidofenin	dimethylacetanilidoimino diacetic acid	Tc 99m HIDA	TechneScan HIDA
Technetium Tc 99m mebrofenin	trimethylbromoacetanilidoimino-diacetic acid	Tc 99m BRIDA	Choletec
Technetium Tc 99m medronate	methylenediphosphonate	Tc 99m MDP	Osteolite; TechneScan MDP
Technetium Tc 99m mertiatide	mercaptoacetyltriglycine	Tc 99m MAG_3	TechneScan MAG3
Technetium Tc 99m nofetumomab merpentan	IgG murine monoclonal NR-LU-10 Fab [anti-small cell lung cancer mono-clonal antibody fragment]	Tc 99m NR-LU-10	Verluma
Technetium Tc 99m oxidronate	hydroxymethyldiphosphonate	Tc 99m HDP; HMDP	Osteoscan-HDP
Technetium Tc 99m pentetate	diethylenetriaminepentaacetic acid	Tc 99m DTPA	Techneplex
Technetium Tc 99m pyrophosphate		Tc 99m PYP	Phosphotec; Techne-Scan PYP
Technetium Tc 99m (pyro- and trimeta-) phosphates	Tc 99m PYP	Pyrolite	
Technetium Tc 99m red blood cells	Tc 99m RBC [in vitro]	UltraTag RBC	
Technetium Tc 99m sestamibi	hexakis(methoxyisobutyl)isonitrile	Tc 99m MIBI; hexamibi; RP 30A	Cardiolite; Miraluma
Technetium Tc 99m succimer	dimercaptosuccinic acid	Tc 99m DMSA	
Technetium Tc-99m sulesomab	IgG 1 murine monoclonal IMMU-MN3 Fab [anti-NCA-90 granulocyte cel antigen monoclonal antibody fragment]	Tc 99m IMMU-MN3	LeukoScan
Technetium Tc 99m sulfur colloid	Tc 99m SC	TechneColl; Tesuloid; TSC	
Technetium Tc 99m teboroxime[a]	boronic acid adduct of technetium dioxime; bis-cyclohexanedione dioxime methylborato-chlorotechnetium	SQ-30217; CDO-MEB; BATO	Cardiotec
Technetium Tc 99m tetrofosmin	1,2-bis[bis(2-ethoxyethyl)phos-phino] ethane	Tc 99m P53	Myoview
Thallous chloride Tl 201	Tl 201		
Water O 15[a]	O 15 H_2O		
Xenon Xe 127[a]	Xe 127		
Xenon Xe 133	Xe 133		

[a] Not commercially available (investigational, discontinued, or extemporaneously compounded).
[b] Official generic name not yet established.
Source: Table courtesy of James A Ponto.

Technetium-99m is derived from the decay of ^{99}Mo. Since ^{99}Mo is a decay product of ^{99m}Tc, it is chemically separated and used to make various ^{99m}Tc radiopharmaceuticals. This separation process occurs in what is known as a ^{99}Mo/^{99m}Tc radionuclide generator system, as was discussed in a previous section. The ^{99m}Tc is eluted from the generator in the form of sodium pertechnetate in the +7 oxidation state. As such, it is not very chemically reactive and will not bind to other compounds. The oxidation state of technetium must be reduced to a lower value in order to make it chemically reactive. This is typically done by using a reducing agent such as stannous ion.

Manufacturers develop compounds that can be labeled with ^{99m}Tc and used for imaging various organ systems or tissues. These compounds are frequently available in what are known as *reagent kits*. The reagent kits are vials containing the particular compound, usually in freeze-dried form, along with the stannous ion and any other necessary ingredients such as buffers or preservatives. The radioactive ^{99m}Tc, as pertechnetate, is added to the reagent kit vial and the stannous ion reduces the technetium, allowing it to chelate with the compound. Binding occurs through coordinate covalent bonds with certain moieties on the compound molecule, known as *ligands*. Some of the more common ligands that bind to technetium are —NH$_2$,

—NH$_3$$^+$, —CN, —SH, —COO—, —CO—, and —OH, among others. The radiolabeling of certain ^{99m}Tc radiopharmaceuticals involves the formation of an intermediate compound with a subsequent ligand exchange process (which usually requires a heating step) to form the final product.

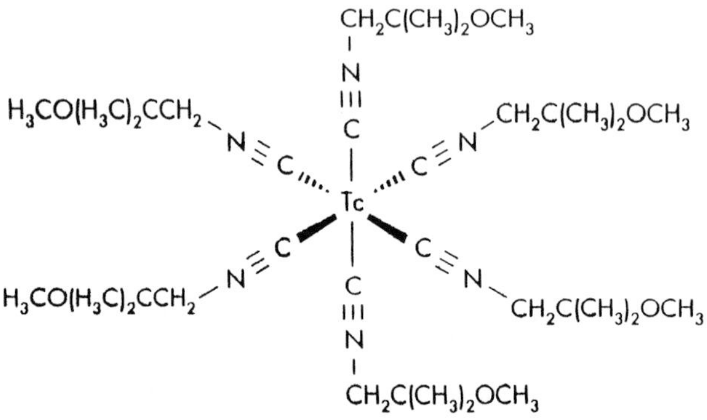

Technetium, in its various oxidation states, has a variety of coordination numbers. Compounds will complex with technetium in specific ways, depending on the oxidation state of technetium and the associated coordination number. Figure 29-12 illustrates how isonitrile molecules are complexed with ^{99m}Tc in the +1 oxidation state.

PREPARATION OF RADIOPHARMACEUTICALS

Some radiopharmaceuticals are prepared in their final form at the manufacturing site, whereas others are compounded at a nuclear pharmacy or nuclear medicine department. There are several levels of sophistication in compounding these agents, ranging from simple addition of radiopertechnetate to the reagent kit vial, to radiolabeling of autologous blood cells, custom radiolabeling of peptides and antibodies, and rapid *hot lab* chemistry compounding of short-lived positron-emitting radiopharmaceuticals. Different diagnostic and therapeutic needs require the use of different preparation techniques. Table 29-5 includes a list of radiopharmaceuticals currently in use.

Figure 29-12. Tc-hexakis-2-methoxyisobutylisonitrile (Tc-sestamibi).

BIBLIOGRAPHY

Baum S, et al. *Atlas of Nuclear Medicine,* New York: Appleton & Lange, 1993.

Merrick MV. *Essentials of Nuclear Medicine,* 2nd ed. New York: Springer-Verlag, 1997.

Emram AM. *New Trends in Radiopharmaceutical Synthesis and Quality Assurance and Regulatory Control.* Baltimore, 1991.

Sampson CB. *Textbook of Radiopharmacy Theory and Practice.* The Netherlands: Gordon and Breach, 1999.

Sorenson JA, et al. *Physics in Nuclear Medicine.* Philadelphia: WB Saunders, 1987.

Kowalsky RJ, et al. Radiopharmaceuticals in Nuclear Pharmacy and Nuclear Medicine. West Virginia: American Pharmaceutical Association, 2004.

PART 4

Pharmaceutical Testing, Analysis, and Control

Pardeep K Gupta, PhD

Associate Professor of Pharmaceutics

Director of BS Program in Pharmaceutical Sciences

University of the Sciences in Philadelphia

Philadelphia, PA

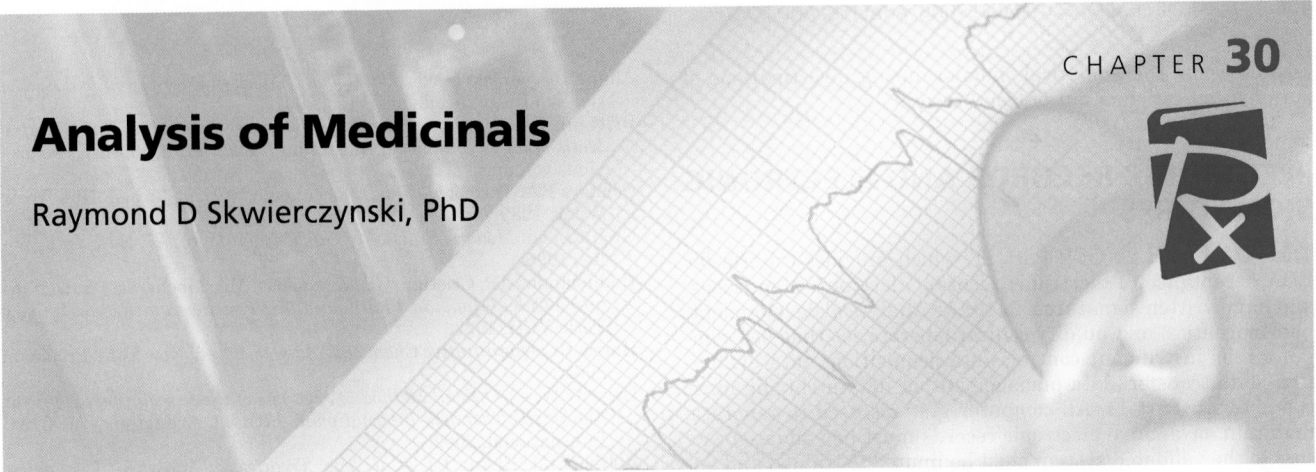

CHAPTER 30

Analysis of Medicinals

Raymond D Skwierczynski, PhD

From the time of the early apothecaries, who worked with meager equipment in small laboratories, pharmacists have made important contributions in the field of medicinal chemistry, both in discovering or isolating new therapeutic agents and in developing methods for standardizing and controlling medicinals. Today, such activity is rarely a function of the practicing pharmacist in the prescription laboratory or the industrial pharmacist in manufacturing laboratories. Rather, analytical chemists specializing in chromatographic, spectroscopic, and wet-chemical analyses perform this function. Some of the testing still involves classical titrimetric or gravimetric techniques. Other analytical techniques, such as two-dimensional nuclear magnetic resonance (NMR) spectroscopy and time-of-flight mass spectrometry (MS), are often performed by scientists with graduate and post-doctoral training in the methodology. But whether or not pharmacists may have occasion to conduct analyses, they at least should understand the basic principles involved in the standardization and control of the medicinal agents dispensed.

VALIDATION OF ANALYTICAL METHODS

The use of an analytical method is justified only after it has been found to be valid (has been *validated*). Both the Food and Drug Administration (FDA) and United States Pharmcopeia (USP) are vitally interested in formal assay method validation to be certain that methods are as they purport to be. In a section entitled *Validation of Compendial Methods*, the USP[1] describes analytical performance parameters that must be measured to validate an analytical procedure. Similar descriptions can be found in ICH Guidances.[2]

The degree to which a method is validated depends on the phase of development. All pharmaceutical companies have well-defined Standard Operating Procedures (SOPs) that state their validation requirements for different phases of development. Minimal validation is usually needed for preclinical, Phase I, and Phase II development. Typically the method's selectivity (ability to measure analyte in presence of any possible impurities, as in a stability-indicating assay), linearity (the concentration range over which concentration and response are related linearly), recovery (accuracy; the concentration of analyte measured relative to the concentration of analyte spiked into the sample), and repeatability (precision) are assessed. The stability of standard and sample solutions is also evaluated. Additional validation requirements are needed for methods used to support Phase III clinical studies, product registration, and clearance of drug substance and commercial drug product: limit of detection (concentration that gives the smallest perceptible response); limit of quantitation (lowest concentration measurable with good precision and accuracy); intra-laboratory reproducibility (different instruments, columns, analytical chemists within a laboratory); robustness (the capacity of a method to remain unaffected by small, but deliberate variations in method parameters); and reproducibility (method crossover between two laboratories). In the later stages of development, method validation is performed under a pre-approved validation protocol with defined procedure and acceptance criteria.

Compendial analytical methods usually do not require validation. Compendial microbial methods, however, may require validation as directed by individual company SOPs. Physical test methods, such as viscosity, pH, tablet hardness, melting point, require minimal or no validation prior to use.

INSTRUMENT QUALIFICATION

Instrumentation must be qualified prior to GMP use. An installation qualification (IQ) provides documented verification that all key aspects of a facility, utility system, or equipment installation adhere to appropriate codes, safety standards, approved design intentions, and that manufacturer's specifications for installation have been suitably considered. An operation qualification (OQ) provides documented verification that a facility, utility system, or equipment performs as intended throughout all anticipated established limits and tolerances. Performance qualification (PQ) provides documented verification that a facility, utility system, or equipment performs as intended under load conditions. Two documents are essential for any qualification: the qualification protocol and the qualification report. The qualification protocol describes the objectives, test procedures, and acceptance criteria. This document must be approved prior to execution of the qualification procedure. The qualification report summarizes the results of the qualification protocol versus the pre-determined acceptance criteria.

CALIBRATION, MAINTENANCE, AND USE

Instrumentation intended for GMP use must be calibrated to assure that equipment performs properly for the intended use. Calibration schedules are usually established so that instruments are calibrated on a monthly, quarterly, semi-annual, or annual basis. Between calibrations, company SOPs describe the frequency at which the instrument must be checked to assure that it is still working properly. For example, an analytical balance that is calibrated quarterly is usually checked on a weekly basis by weighing a NIST-traceable weight. Calibrations and calibration checks are recorded into a log book, as is preventative and corrective maintenance of instrumentation. Each sample analyzed is also logged. Detailed instrument records assist the analytical chemist during investigations of out-of-specification or out-of-trend results.

ELECTRONIC RECORDS AND ELECTRONIC SIGNATURES

The FDA issued 21 CFR Part 11, which provides criteria for FDA acceptance of electronic records, electronic signatures, and handwritten signatures, in 1997.[3] Analytical development, pharmaceutics, and quality control laboratories that use computers for instrument control, data acquisition, data evaluation, data transfer, data management, or data archiving must comply with Part 11. All computer systems used to generate, maintain, or archive electronic records must be validated. Access to the validated system must be limited to trained and authorized users; individual password-protected user accounts are required. Computer-generated, time-stamped audit trails that record the date and time of data acquisition, modification, or deletion by an authorized user are required. In addition, the integrity of original data files cannot be obscured. Standard Operating Procedures are required to manage and archive electronic files. Complete and accurate copies of the electronic records must be readily retrievable for agency inspection or review. Finally, policies that hold individuals responsible and accountable for actions initiated under their electronic signatures are required. An electronic signature is a computer data compilation of symbols that is executed, adopted, or authorized by an individual and is the legally binding equivalent of the individual's handwritten signature. In 2003, the FDA issued a new guidance[4] that limited the scope of Part 11 to apply only to records required by a predicate rule and when one or both or the following conditions apply: (1) Electronic records are used instead of paper; or (2) persons make printouts but still rely on the electronic records to perform regulated activities.[5]

ANALYTICAL BALANCES

The analytical balance is an indispensable requirement for any analytical procedure whether the method is a classic or stoichiometric analysis or a modern, instrumental method of a non-stoichiometric nature. If the determination of mass is not accurate and precise, the ultimate analytical result is unacceptable.

An analytical balance differs from a high-class prescription balance in the matter of sensitiveness. A satisfactory analytical balance is sensitive to the tenth of a milligram and should never be used for weighing a total load greater than that specified. The electronic analytical balance is of the null type, but the restoring torque is not applied by adding or removing weights but rather by varying a current applied to a coil in a magnetic field. The great advantage of the electromagnetic principle is the freedom from drift or change in sensitivity. The balances have a digital display, and tare-out capabilities, as well as internally programmed test and calibration routines. Some balances have small maximum capacity (about 0.1 to 1.0 g). Other electronic analytical balances using load cells are available with capacities of up to 200 g and a readability of $\pm$ 0.10 mg or $\pm$ 0.01 mg and have data outputs making them capable of incorporation into automated systems. Microbalances, which are useful when limited material is available, can be read to the nearest microgram.

SOURCES OF INFORMATION

The reference works needed in an analytical laboratory depend entirely upon the scope of work. For pharmaceutical testing of official substances, the USP-NF is, of course, given primary consideration. Other useful references are given below.

Ahuja S, Alsante, KM. *Handbook of Isolation and Characterization of Impurities in Pharmaceuticals.* Amsterdam: Academic Press, 2003.

Ahuja S, Scypinski S, eds. *Handbook of Modern Pharmaceutical Analysis.* San Diego: Academic Press, 2001.

Brittain, HG. *Profiles of Drug Substances, Excipients and Related Methodology,* Volume 31. Amsterdam: Elsevier, 2005. Also, see previous volumes.

Connors KA. *Textbook of Pharmaceutical Analysis,* 3rd ed. New York: Wiley, 1982.

Grob RL, ed. *Modern Practice of Gas Chromatography.* New York: Wiley, 1995.

Hadjiioannou TP, Cristian, GD, Koupparis, MA, Macheras, PE. *Quantitative Calculations in Pharmaceutical Practice and Research.* New York: VCH, 1993.

Harris DC. *Quantitative Chemical Analysis,* 6th ed. New York: Freeman, 2002.

Horwitz W, ed. *Official Method of Analysis of the Association of Official Analytical Chemists International,* 17th ed. Arlington, VA: AOAC International, 2002.

Kolthoff IM, Elving PJ, *et al.*, eds. *Treatise on Analytical Chemistry,* New York: Wiley, 1959–1993.

McLafferty FW, Turecek F. *Interpretation of Mass Spectra,* 4th ed. Sausalito, CA: University Science, 1993.

Miller JM, Crowther JB. *Analytical Chemistry in a GMP Environment,* New York: Wiley, 2000.

Munson JW, ed. *Pharmaceutical Analysis: Modern Methods,* New York: Dekker, part A, 1981; part B, 1984.

Ohannesian L, Streeter, AJ, eds. *Handbook of Pharmaceutical Analysis.,* New York: Dekker, 2001.

Reagent Chemicals, 9th ed. Washington, DC: American Chemical Society, 1999.

Rowe RC, Sheskey PJ, Weller PJ, ed. *Handbook of Pharmaceutical Excipients,* 4th ed. Washington, DC: American Pharmaceutical Association, 2003.

Sanders JKM, Hunter BK. *Modern NMR Spectroscopy: A Guide for Chemists,* 2nd ed. Oxford: Oxford University Press, 1993.

Schirmer RE. *Modern Methods of Pharmaceutical Analysis,* 2nd ed. Boca Raton, FL: CRC Press, 1991.

Skoog DA, Holler FJ, Nieman, TA *Priciples of Instrumental Analysis,* 5th ed. Philadelphia: Harcourt Brace, 1998.

Smith A, Heckelman P, O'Neill MJ, eds. *The Merck Index: An Encyclopedia of Chemicals, Drugs, and Biologicals,* 13th ed. Whitehouse Station, NJ: Merck & Co, 2001.

Snyder LR, Kirkland JJ, Glajch JL. *Practical HPLC Method Development,* 2nd Ed. New York: Wiley, 1997.

Swadesh JK. *HPLC Practical and Industrial Applications,* 2nd ed. Boca Raton, FL: CRC Press, 2001.

Watson JT. *Introduction to Mass Spectrometry,* 3rd ed. New York: Lippincott, Williams, and Wilkins, 1997.

Specialized Analytical Methods and Equipment

In the following section some important analytical methods used by pharmaceutical manufacturers are discussed. Practicing pharmacists do not, as a rule, require such sophisticated apparatus as is used for analysis, but they should at least be familiar with the types of analyses conducted with each instrument.

Some of the medicinal products are still being assayed by the time-honored procedures of gravimetric and titrimetric analysis, although here, too, the use of electronic balances and the recording titrator have improved these classic procedures considerably.

Familiar examples of analytical methods that are purely physical in their nature include those that involve the use of the microscope, the polarimeter, or the refractometer. The identity, relative purity, and crystallinity of many substances often are determined by microscopical examination. The polarimeter has long been recognized for its usefulness in assaying certain liquids, such as dextrose solutions, by determining their ability to bend or rotate the plane of polarized light. Polarimeters are available that measure the rotation of polarized light at wavelengths in addition to the D line of sodium (589 nm).

The determination of the moisture content in various substances involves several types of analytical measurement. These methods include drying in a desiccator or in a heated oven, either under ordinary atmospheric conditions or in vacuum under reduced pressure. A moisture balance, in which the sample pan is directly heated by an infrared lamp, eliminates removal of the sample from the balance. Other procedures involve distillation of vegetable drugs with toluene or with benzene, then noting the volume of water that separates in a graduated tube containing the distillate. A more specific and convenient procedure for determining water in many substances is the Karl Fischer titrimetric method. In this procedure, the water is quantitatively measured by titration under anhydrous conditions by the use of a reagent containing iodine, sulfur dioxide, pyridine, and methanol. The endpoint may be detected visually, or preferably by the use of the electrometric and automatic titration assembly. Some instruments use coulometric titration to generate the reagent at an electrode surface. Electrical methods for determining water are being applied now to a variety of industrial products, in some cases during continuous processing operations. These are based upon the principle that if a substance is placed between two condenser plates, the capacitance will vary with the dielectric constant of the medium between the plates. Because the dielectric constant of water is greater than that of other substances, the capacitance will vary with the amount of moisture present. Water content in granulations and solid-dosage forms can also be measured easily using near-infrared spectroscopy.

The determination and adjustment of pH or hydrogen ion concentration (activity) has become an important function in the control analysis of medicinal products. For a discussion of pH determination see Chapter 33. The use of microelectrodes allows pH to be measured in small volumes (0.5 mL) of solution.

Separation techniques, particularly chromatographic methods, are necessary and valuable in the analysis of pharmaceuticals. The partitioning of a solute between two immiscible solvents is used many times to isolate a drug from other components in a mixture. Open column chromatographic methods, once a mainstay in purification, have been replaced with preparative chromatographic techniques to isolate, purify, and often, concentrate drug, degradation product, or synthetic impurity from a dosage form matrix or a natural biological environment. Other separations such as solvent–solvent extraction, thin-layer chromatography, solid-phase extraction, or solid-phase micro-extraction may be required as a preparatory step when spectrometric analysis is to follow.

Gas chromatography (GC) and high-performance liquid chromatography (HPLC) represent two nonstoichiometric methods that have achieved very great popularity because of their capabilities. In GC, any compound, directly or with derivatization, can be analyzed if it has a perceptible vapor pressure and if a suitable column can be found. The use of various detectors adds another element of selectivity to the procedure. HPLC has been rapidly developing with the introduction of gradient pumping systems, integrated instrument control and data acquisition systems, a larger variety of columns, and sophisticated detectors. But the great attraction of chromatographic techniques to the industrial laboratory is the possibility of automation. The chromatographic procedure and instrumentation may be so designed that the method largely may be automated, involving automated sampling, separations, detection, recording, and finally, calculation and printing of results, leaving only the preparation of drug substance or of dosage form solutions to be done by the analytical chemist. Diode array detectors allow data acquisition over a range of analytical wavelengths. Mass spectrometric detectors can be used to obtain nominal masses of eluting substances or can be tuned to the mass of interest to quantify a substance that is not adequately separated from other substance or its matrix. Small-bore columns often afford shorter run times and conserve on solvent use. The subject of chromatography is discussed in Chapter 32.

Mass spectrometers and nuclear magnetic resonance (NMR) spectrometers are valuable instruments to identify new degradation products, extractables, leachables, and other impurities in drug substances and drug products. Organic and analytical chemists can often identify possible structures of an unknown molecule by re-constructing the molecule from its fragmentation pattern obtained from MS-MS analysis. The structures can be confirmed by two-dimensional proton and carbon-13 Fourier Transform NMR spectroscopy. High-frequency magnetic fields, complex pulse sequences, and innovative probes, like the cryoprobe, have greatly improved the sensitivity of NMR spectroscopy in recent years.

The modern spectrometer, which incorporates such features as microprocessor control and diode array detectors, has become an especially useful instrument for analysis, as it enables analytical chemists to seek the answers to their analytical problems with *eyes* that see not only in the visible range, but throughout the electromagnetic spectrum. The analytical possibilities in this direction can be understood more readily when one considers that the ultimate molecules and atoms that make up a material transmit, absorb, and scatter radiation according to their individual natures. Assay methods based upon absorption in the ultraviolet, infrared, and visible portions of the spectrum are used extensively. The principles underlying such determinations are discussed in Chapter 33. In some spectrometric analytical procedures, a colorless substance that must be analyzed is converted to a derivative having color, the intensity of the color being measured in a suitable spectrometer and compared with that developed by a known amount of a *reference standard* grade of the same substance.

Other widely used instruments which are quite suitable for routine colorimetric measurements are the colorimeter and the combination nephelocolorimeter, which is of considerable value in making quantitative turbidimetric measurements. High-through put robotic systems have added capability to analyze compounds synthesized using combinatorial methods. These systems require milligram quantities of drug and can analyze up to 96 compounds in a single sample plate. These systems have been interfaced to mass spectrometers for molecule identification and purification, X-ray diffractometers for salt selection and polymorph screening, and spectrophotometers and nephelometers for solubility and permeability measurements.

The fluorometer provides for measurement of fluorescence that may be present in the sample or that may be developed in the sample through derivatization. This method provides a means of evaluating the potency of many pharmaceutical products, as, for example, those containing thiamine hydrochloride. A solution in which the thiamine has been converted quantitatively into thiochrome is placed in the fluorometer where it is caused to fluoresce on exposure to light. This fluorescence intensity is compared with readings obtained on standard control samples prepared and observed under exactly the same conditions. This comparison serves as a basis on which the potency of the unknown vitamin sample can be calculated readily. At the opposite end of the electromagnetic spectrum are the infrared radiations. These are heat rays and their utilization marks another important contribution to analytical research. Infrared spectrometry involves placing the sample in a cell that is traversed by radiation from an infrared source. The transmitted radiation on passing into the spectrometer is dispersed into a spectrum by a prism of sodium chloride, or other salt, or by a diffraction grating. Fourier transform infrared spectrometers are available that can acquire an infrared spectrum very rapidly (see Chapter 33). An important application of infrared spectrometry in the USP is in the fingerprinting of organic compounds, by which means they may be identified. Pattern recognition techniques and the use of neural networks to compare spectra are very impressive.

The ability to detect and measure elements in a complex dosage-form system is very important because some elements such as the heavy metals, which may have been used in the synthesis, are toxic. The emission spectrograph is used for identification and for the quantitative measurement of many elements by providing photographic records of their emission spectra. These elements include most metals and some nonmetals, such as boron, silicon, and phosphorus. By determining the wavelengths of the lines, the various elements present in the sample may be determined by reference to wavelength tables. By the use of a densitometer, which measures the relative darkness of the lines, the quantitative evaluation is accomplished.

An emission technique that is largely solution based and is newer than emission spectroscopy is inductively coupled plasma optical emission spectrometry (ICP-OES). In this technique the sample solution is aspirated into an inductively-coupled plasma (argon gas), a medium whose temperature is about 10,000 K, a condition that results in atomization and excitation of even the most refractory elements (eg, sulfur). The results provide both qualitative and quantitative data in a rapid, efficient manner, identifying and measuring multiple elements from a single sample. The disadvantage of this technique is its high instrumental cost and its operating expense. The flame spectrometer serves a useful purpose in some industrial and hospital laboratories for making routine emission determinations, particularly of alkali metals and alkaline earth metals.

Electrochemical methods offer a level of selectivity that some spectroscopic analyses cannot provide. Ion-specific electrode potentiometry measures free-unbound species rather than the total amount of metal ion in a solution. The polarograph provides for rapid qualitative and quantitative analyses by automatic recording of current-voltage curves. In the operation of this instrument, reducible ions and organic compounds are reduced at the dropping mercury electrode, yielding polarograms that serve as records of the analysis. The polarogram establishes the identity of the substance by its half-wave potential, while the height of the step in the curve is taken as a direct measurement of concentration. Variations of polarography, such as differential pulse polarography, increase the sensitivity of quantitative analysis, whereas cyclic voltametry provides a means whereby the qualitative oxidation–reduction behavior of a species may be examined.

The nonstoichiometric methods used in drug analysis are discussed in Chapters 31, 32, and 34, and the stoichiometric analyses are treated in this chapter as they apply to specific drug substances and to specific dosage forms.

OFFICIAL PHYSICAL AND CHEMICAL ASSAYS

There appears to be a misconception on the part of some individuals concerning the assay procedures of the official compendia. A material may well fall within the assay limits stated in the individual monograph for a particular substance, and yet *not* be of suitable quality to conform to the complete specifications indicated for the compound, even though the assay is performed exactly as indicated in the official method. It is essential, then, to realize that even though a substance meets the purity specifications of an official monograph, as established by a chemical or physical assay procedure, it is *not* of USP quality unless it conforms to *all* of the specifications contained in the monograph for that material. Also, some official substances do not have an assay procedure, as such, listed in the monograph for the basic drug. A quantitative analytical method is not required in such cases because other specifications in the monograph serve to characterize the substance both quantitatively and qualitatively.

As dosage forms become more complex and active pharmaceutical ingredients become more potent, pharmaceutical companies may include additional testing or stricter acceptance criteria to ensure functionality of compendial excipients. For example, residual peroxide content of polyoxoether excipeints or of vehicles containing oxygen atoms may need to be monitored closely before the excipient is used to manufacture a drug that can easily oxidize. Another example is that lot-to-lot variation in polymers used in tablet coating may cause variation in dissolution behavior. Here the coating thickness may need to be adjusted during the manufacturing process in order to meet release-rate specification criteria.

In the following sections, various aspects of the official drug analyses are considered. The classic titrimetric and gravimetric methods are considered in some detail and, even though the subjects are treated in Chapters 32 and 33, some aspects of instrumental procedures are examined. Tables 30-3 and 30-4 contain the indicators and other reagents; some examples of the various classes of analyses are presented, together with an explanation of the chemical principles or other pertinent detail. A comprehensive tabulation of all official assays, which uses the classification outline of Appendix A, is found in Appendix B at the end of this chapter.

Because of the selectivity, specificity, and sensitivity that can be achieved by HPLC methods, there has been a definite tendency to choose HPLC procedures for the analysis of many drugs, as may be seen for USP-NF analyses in Appendix B. Chapter 32 presents a detailed consideration of HPLC.

THE PREPARATION OF SOLUTIONS

The preparation of a solution of a drug substance is vital to many methods of analysis. The nature of the system chosen to express the concentration of the solute is important, particularly in stoichiometric methods, because the nature of a chemical reaction is used to calculate the analytical result. The useful concentration systems, molarity, formality, molality, normality, and titer, are defined here.

Molarity = Mols of solute/liter = Millimols of solute/millimeter.
Formality = Number of formula weights/liter.
Formula Weight = Molecular weight in grams.
Molality = Mols of solute/1000 grams of solvent.

The most useful concentration system is normality, because the reaction capability of a reagent or an analyte is taken into account when solutions are prepared.

Normality = Number of equivalents/liter.
Equivalent = Grams of drug or reagent used/equivalent weight.
Milliequivalents = Grams of drug or reagent used/milliequivalent weight.
Equivalent Weight = Molecular weight in grams/n.
Milliequivalent Weight = Equivalent weight/1000.
n = number of reacting entities per reagent aggregate.

The number of reacting entities per reagent aggregate for acids is the number of accessible protons. For bases, it is the number of available basic anions or pairs of unshared electrons that can accept a proton. For oxidizing or reducing agents, it is the number of electrons that an aggregate can lose or gain in an electron transfer reaction as is seen from a half-reaction; for example, $MnO_4^- + 5\,e^- + 8\,H_3O^+ = Mn^{2+} + 12\,H_2O$. Textbooks that provide tables of standard oxidation or reduction potentials may be consulted for half reactions. The values of n for reagents are shown in Table 30-1.

A number of equations are useful when calculations in volumentric analysis are needed.

$$(\text{milliliters}_{\text{reagent}})(\text{normality}_{\text{reagent}}) = \frac{\text{grams}_{\text{analyte}}}{\text{milliequivalent weight}_{\text{analyte}}}$$

$$\frac{\text{grams}_{\text{analyte}}}{\text{grams}_{\text{sample}}} \times 100 = \%\ \text{analyte in sample}$$

Table 30-1. Reaction Capacity Values (n) for Selected Reagents

ACIDS	BASES	ELECTRON TRANSFER
HCl — 1	NaOH — 1	$KMnO_4$ — 5 (MnO_4^- — Mn^{2+})
H_2SO_4 — 2	$NH_3\text{-}H_2O$ — 1	I_2 — 2 (I_2 — $2I^-$)
H_3PO_4 — 2	$Ba\,(OH)_2$ — 2	$Na_2S_2O_3$ — 2 ($2S_2O_3^{2-}$ — $S_4O_6^{2-}$)
HOAc — 1	$CH_3CH_2NH_2$ — 1	$Na_2Cr_2O_7$ — 6 ($Cr_2O_7^{2-}$ — $2Cr^{3+}$)

The concept of titer is very useful because it allows a titrant to be labeled in terms of the analyte and simplifies calculations.

$$titer = \frac{\text{milligrams of analyte}}{\text{milliliter of titrant}}$$

For a titrant whose normality is 0.1000, the calculation is

(1.00) (0.1000) (milliequivalent weight of analyte) = titer

The USP-NF uses titer in titrimetric assays. Some examples are given in Table 30-2.

Titrimetric Assay Methods

The titrimetric assay procedure is the one most frequently encountered by the pharmaceutical chemist in the standardization of official products. Every titrimetric assay is based on the determination of the volume of a solution of known strength required to complete a chemical reaction with the substance being analyzed. Such a solution is called a *standard* or *volumetric solution* and is commonly referred to by the abbreviation *VS*.

Indicators for Determining Endpoints

It is imperative to avoid the error of using an insufficient amount of a volumetric solution, thus failing to complete a reaction; it is equally necessary to guard against overstepping a reaction by adding too much of the volumetric solution. To meet this situation, a group of chemicals known as *Indicators* is used. These are substances that show when the endpoint of a reaction has been reached, either by a change in color or by the formation of a precipitate.

INDICATOR SOLUTIONS

Solutions of indicators used for volumetric determinations are referred to as *Test Solutions* (TS), and those used for determination of hydrogen ion concentration are termed *pH indicators*.

Table 30-2. Titer Values for Selected Pharmaceuticals

ANALYTE	NATURE OF ANALYTICAL REACTION	n	TITRANT	TITER (1.00 mL =), mg
Ascorbic acid mw = 176.13	ET[a]	2	0.1N I$_2$	8.806
Chlorpromazine mw = 318.87	NAB[b]	1	0.1N HClO$_4$	31.89
Hydrogen peroxide concentrate mw = 34.01	ET	2	0.1N KMnO$_4$	1.701
Betaine hydrochloride mw = 153.61	NAB	1	0.1N HClO$_4$	15.36
Butabarbital mw = 224.26	P[c]	1	0.1N AgNO$_3$	22.43
Calcium acetate mw = 158.17	Complex[d]	1	0.05 N EDTA	7.909
Sodium hypochlorite solution mw = 74.44	ET	2	0.1 N Na$_2$S$_2$O$_3$	3.722
Sulfabenzamide mw = 276.32	NAB	1	0.1 N NaOMe	27.63
Zinc oxide mw = 81.39	AB[e]	2	1 N H$_2$SO$_4$	40.69

[a] ET indicates electron transfer.
[b] NAB indicates nonaqueous acid-base.
[c] P indicates precipitation.
[d] Complex indicates complex formation.
[e] AB indicates aqueous acid-base.

The indicators used for colorimetric pH determinations are either weakly acid or weakly basic. However, most indicators used for this purpose, such as the phthaleins and sulfonated phthaleins, behave like weak acids.

The usual concentration of the indicator solution is 0.05%. From 0.1 to 0.2 mL of the indicator solution is generally used for 10 mL of the liquid being examined.

Solutions of indicators of the basic type and of the phthaleins are prepared by dissolving them in alcohol. In preparing solutions of indicators containing an acid group, this group must first be neutralized with sodium hydroxide.

Unless otherwise stated each acid–base indicator solution is so adjusted that when 0.15 mL of the indicator solution is added to 25 mL of carbon dioxide-free water, 0.25 mL of 0.02 N acid or alkali, respectively, will develop the characteristic color changes.

The solutions should be kept in glass-stoppered bottles, and must be protected from light.

Indicators for Reactions Involving Neutralization

In the USP, indicators are used either to indicate the completion of a chemical reaction in volumetric analyses or to indicate the hydrogen ion concentration (pH) of solutions. Most of the indicators for acid–base titrations and for pH measurement are acidic. They contain a carboxyl, a sulfonic or a phenolic group. In many instances the same indicator is applicable either to acid–base titrations or to pH measurements, the difference being only in the preparation of the indicator solution. The following are the pH indicators of the Pharmacopeia; in each case Test Solutions (TS) of the following indicators are used.

Bromocresol Green (Bromocresol Blue: *Tetrabromo-m-cresolsulfonphthalein*)—Transition interval: from pH 4.0 to 5.4. Color change: from yellow to blue.

Bromocresol Purple (*Dibromo-o-cresolsulfonphthalein*)—Transition interval: from pH 5.2 to 6.8. Color change: from yellow to purple. This solution and the next two are satisfactory in the titration of weak bases.

Bromophenol Blue (*Tetrabromophenolsulfonphthalein*)—Transition interval: from pH 3.0 to 4.6. Color change: from yellow to blue.

Bromothymol Blue (*Dibromothymolsulfonphthalein*)—Transition interval: from pH 6.0 to 7.6. Color change: from yellow to blue.

Cresol Red (*o-Cresolsulfonphthalein*)—Transition interval: from pH 7.2 to 8.8. Color change: from yellow to red.

Cresol Red-Thymol Blue TS—Transition interval: from pH 7.7 to 9.1. Color change: from yellow to violet.

Malachite Green—The oxalate salt is used. Transition interval: from pH 0.0 to 2.0. Color change: from yellow to green.

Methyl Orange (*Helianthin or Tropaeolin D*)—The sodium salt of dimethylaminoazobenzenesulfonic acid or dimethylaminoazobenzene sodium sulfonate. Transition interval: from pH 3.2 to 4.4. Color change: from pink to yellow. Useful in the titration of weak bases.

Methyl Red (*Dimethylaminoazobenzene-o-carboxylic acid; o-carboxybenzeneazodimethylaniline*)—Transition interval: from pH 4.2 to 6.2. Color change: from red to yellow. Useful in the titration of weak bases.

Methyl Red-Methylene Blue TS—Transition interval: from pH 4.8 to 6.2. Color change: from red-violet to green.

Methyl Yellow (*p-Dimethylaminoazobenzene*)—Transition interval: from pH 2.9 to 4.0. Color change: from red to yellow.

Phenolphthalein—Use *Phenolphthalein* USP. Transition interval: from pH 8.0 to 10.0. Color change: from colorless to red. Useful in the titration of acids with strong bases.

Phenol Red—Use Phenolsulfonphthalein USP. Transition interval: from pH 6.8 to 8.2. Color change: from yellow to red.

Quinaldine Red (*5-Dimethylamino-2-styrylethylquinolinium iodide*)—Transition interval: pH 1.4 to 3.2. Color change: from colorless to red.

Thymol Blue (*Thymolsulfonphthalein*). Acid—Transition interval: from pH 1.2 to 2.8. Color change: from red to yellow. *Alkaline*—Transition interval: from pH 8.0 to 9.2. Color change: from yellow to blue.

Thymolphthalein—Transition interval: from pH 9.3 to 10.5. Color change: from colorless to blue.

Indicators for Reactions Involving Precipitation

Dichlorofluorescein TS.
Eosin Y (Sodium Tetrabromofluorescein) TS.
Ferric Ammonium Sulfate TS—8% in water. This indicator, well-known as *Ferric Alum*, generally is used when titrating with standard ammonium thiocyanate in the presence of silver nitrate. A red color of the ferric thiocyanate complex forms immediately when the silver thiocyanate has been completely precipitated.
Potassium Chromate TS—10% in water. This indicator gives a red precipitate of silver chromate in a neutral or slightly alkaline solution, after silver halides have been completely precipitated by titration with standard silver nitrate.
Sodium Alizarinsulfonate TS.
Tetrabromophenolphthalein TS.
Tetrabromophenolphthalein, Ethyl Ester TS.
Indicators for Nonaqueous Titrations
Azo-violet.
Crystal Violet (TS)—1% in glacial acetic acid.
Malachite Green—Use Malachite Green TS.
Methyl Red—Use Methyl Red TS.
Methyl Violet—Use Methyl Violet TS.
p-**Naphtholbenzein**—4-[α-(4-hydroxy-1-naphthyl)benzylidene]-1-(4*H*)[naphthalenone].
Phenol Red—Use Phenol Red TS.
Quinaldine Red—Use Quinaldine Red TS.
Thymol Blue—Use Thymol Blue TS.

Indicators for Complexometric Titrations

Diphenylamine TS.
Dithizone (*Diphenylthiocarbazone*) **TS.**
Eriochrome Black TS—0.05% aqueous solution (should be freshly prepared but can be stabilized).
Hydroxynaphthol Blue.
Murexide (*Acid Ammonium Purpurate*)
Used as a powder; usually mixed with an inert carrier (potassium sulfate) to facilitate handling.
Naphthol Green TS.
1-(2-Pyridylazo)-2-naphthol.

Indicators for Reactions Involving Changes in Valence

2,6-Dichloroquinone-chlorimide (*Dichlorophenolindophenol*)—Usually used as the sodium salt in a solution containing sodium bicarbonate to titrate ascorbic acid dosage forms. In oxidized form, it is blue in alkaline and rose-pink in acid solution; when reduced, it is colorless.
Dicyanobis(1,10-phenanthroline)iron II Dihydrate—An indicator that reacts similarly to ortho-phenanthroline.
Diphenylamine—Employed in titrations involving potassium dichromate as titrant. In reduced form it is colorless; in a reversible oxidation reaction it produces a brilliant violet diphenylbenzidine derivative.
Iodine—Free iodine serves as its own indicator in assays where it is liberated and determined volumetrically by titration with standard potassium iodate. The endpoint is the disappearance of the violet color of iodine in chloroform added to the mixture being titrated for the purpose of dissolving and concentrating the iodine.
Methyl Orange—Used as a test solution in titrations with potassium bromate; the color of this external indicator is discharged by excess titrant.
Nitrophenanthroline—An indicator that reacts similarly to *ortho*-phenanthroline.
***Ortho*-phenanthroline**—Used in 1.5% concentration in 1.5% ferrous sulfate solution as an indicator in titrations involving standard ceric sulfate solution. The color changes from red to pale green when the slightest excess of ceric sulfate is added to the oxidized solution.
Oxalic Acid VS—This standard solution generally is used without an indicator because most reactions in which it takes part depend on decolorization of potassium permanganate.
Potassium Permanganate VS—This highly colored solution is decolorized on being reduced, so a separate indicator is not required.
Potassium Thiocyanate—Used in conjunction with ferric chloride volumetric solution, a red compound is produced at the endpoint.

Starch Iodide Paste TS—Approximately 5% suspension of potato starch in 0.75% potassium iodide with zinc chloride preservative. May be used as an external indicator for titrations with sodium nitrite VS. Starch iodide paste test solution must show a definite blue streak when a glass rod, dipped in a mixture of 1 mL of 0.1 *M* sodium nitrite, 500 mL of water, and 10 mL of hydrochloric acid is streaked on a smear of the paste.
Starch-Potassium Iodide TS—0.5% KI in Starch TS. Must be freshly prepared.
Starch TS—A 0.5% suspension of arrowroot starch in water, freshly prepared. A blue color is produced by starch in the presence of free iodine.

INDICATOR PAPERS

Strong, white filter paper is treated with hydrochloric acid and washed with water until the washings no longer show an acid reaction to methyl red. It then is treated with ammonia TS and again washed with water, until the washings are no longer alkaline toward phenolphthalein. It then is dried thoroughly.

The dry paper is saturated with the proper strength indicator solution and carefully dried by suspending the paper in a room free from acid or alkali fumes.

The papers so prepared are kept in glass-stoppered bottles, and must be protected from light and moisture.

Lead Acetate Test Paper—Prepared from lead acetate TS.
Litmus Paper, Blue—Usually in the form of strips about 50 mm in length and 6 mm in width.
Litmus Paper, Red—Usually in the form of strips about 50 mm in length and 6 mm in width.
Mercuric Bromide Test Paper—Prepared from alcoholic mercuric bromide TS.
Phenolphthalein Paper—Prepared from a 0.1% solution of phenolphthalein in diluted alcohol.
Potassium Iodate-Starch Paper—Strips of white filter paper impregnated with a solution prepared by mixing a 5% solution of potassium iodate with an equal volume of freshly prepared starch TS.
Starch Iodate Paper—Strips of white filter paper impregnated with a mixture of equal volumes of starch TS and potassium iodate solution (1 in 20).
Starch Iodide Paper—Strips of white filter paper impregnated with a solution of 500 mg of potassium iodide in 100 mL of freshly prepared starch TS.
Turmeric Paper—Strips of white filter paper impregnated with turmeric solution prepared as directed in the USP.

Potentiometric Determination of Endpoints

The detection of the endpoint in titrimetric assays by use of colorimetric indicators may sometimes be difficult, especially if the solution being titrated is colored or turbid. In some instances, titration to the equivalence or true endpoint is essential, a requirement that is not met conveniently when an indicator is employed. In such cases the endpoint may be indicated potentiometrically, most commonly employing the millivolt scale of a pH meter. The potentiometric determination of endpoints depends on the fact that in most titrations the potential across two suitable electrodes immersed in the solution being titrated undergoes a sharp change at the true endpoint (equivalence point); this change corresponds to the point where an indicator undergoes marked change of color. In some titrations neither the change of color nor the change of potential is sharp at the endpoint, in which case titration to a predetermined voltage or voltage deflection is necessary. As it generally is more convenient to do this potentiometrically, rather than colorimetrically, this electrochemical method is employed. Suitable electrodes, such as a combination glass-calomel electrode, serve as a means of *detecting* the endpoint by sensing ionic activities.

It may be pointed out here that the change of other electrical properties, such as resistance or the amount of current flowing in a solution being titrated, may be used to indicate the endpoint in a titration. The general term *electrometric titrations* sometimes is applied to such titrations; specific titrations in this category are referred to as *amperometric, conductometric,* and *high-frequency titrations.*

Titrimetric Procedures

Table 30-3 contains the indicator abbreviations used in these sections. See Appendix A for explanation of abbreviations in parentheses appearing at the end of headings used throughout the rest of this chapter.

ACID–BASE REACTIONS

DIRECT OR RESIDUAL TITRATION OF AN ACID BY BASE (IA1A,IA2A)
In this category a free acid is titrated directly using the method indicated in the monograph to determine the endpoint.

Phosphoric Acid—Titrated in water with 1 *N* NaOH to a TP endpoint.

Boric Acid—The use of glycerin increases the acid strength of the boric acid by formation of a glycero-borate complex according to the equation given here.

$$H_3BO_3 \; + \; 2 \; H\!-\!\!\underset{\underset{CH_2OH}{|}}{\overset{\overset{CH_2OH}{|}}{C}}\!\!-\!\!OH \; = \; H_3O^{\oplus} \; + \; 2H_2O \; +$$

$$\left[\begin{array}{c} CH_2OH \qquad HOH_2C \\ H\!-\!C\!-\!O \qquad O\!-\!C\!-\!H \\ \quad \quad \;\; B \\ H_2C\!-\!O \qquad O\!-\!CH_2 \end{array} \right]^{\ominus}$$

Cellulose Acetate Phthalate—Phthalyl content.

Dibasic Sodium Phosphate—Treatment of the salt with hydrochloric acid forms phosphoric acid and the endpoint is determined potentiometrically from pH readings. Only one hydrogen of phosphoric acid is titrated in this procedure.

Oxyphenbutazone—Even though a phenol, it is sufficiently strong to be titrated directly.

Potassium Phosphate, Monobasic—See *Sodium Phosphate,* above.

Sodium Citrate and Citric Acid Oral Solution—For citric acid, titration to a phenolphthalein endpoint.

Sodium Phosphates Enema and Oral Solution—After the addition of a standard base, the solution is titrated potentiometrically, with standard acid, to two inflection points in the titration curve.

Sulfinpyrazone—The sulfonyl group (—SO₂—) makes the alpha-hydrogen sufficiently acid so that it may react with base.

Sulfur—Sulfur is oxidized to sulfuric acid by the *oxygen flask technique,* then titrated. In the *oxygen flask technique,* the sample is burned in a thick-walled iodine flask in an atmosphere of oxygen, in the presence of an absorbing solution (the nature of which depends on the sample being analyzed). After combustion the flask is shaken to absorb any gaseous product and treated as directed in the specific monograph.

TITRATION OF A LIBERATED ACID BY A BASE (IA1AI)
Cellulose, Oxidized—The sample is shaken with calcium acetate solution, to exchange calcium ion for hydrogen ion of the free carboxyl groups. The liberated hydrogen ion is then titrated with standard base.

Phenacemide (and Tablets)—The amide is hydrolyzed to phenylacetic acid, extracted with chloroform, evaporated, and the free acid titrated.

SØRENSEN FORMOL TITRATION (IA1AII)
Meprobamate (and Oral Suspension)—After hydrolysis of the ester.
Protein Hydrolysate Injection—For alpha-amino nitrogen.

In each case the free amino acid is treated with formaldehyde to form the methylimino or methylol derivative, reducing the basicity of the amino group so that the free carboxyl group may be titrated.

$$RCH(NH_2)COOH + HCHO = RCH(NHCH_2OH)COOH \; or$$
$$RCH(N\!\!=\!\!CH_2)COOH$$

RESIDUAL TITRATION OF EXCESS BASE AFTER INTERACTION WITH ACID (IA2B)
In this type of assay a measured excess of standard base is added to the prepared sample and the excess titrated with standard acid. Quite often a blank titration is performed, whereby the same volume of base, which was added to the sample, is titrated with standard acid. The difference in the volume of titrant used for the blank and sample is the volume of titrant equivalent to the sample.

Chloral Hydrate (and Capsules and Syrup)—The chloral-containing compounds are treated with excess standard sodium hydroxide which hydrolyzes the chloral to chloroform and sodium formate. Excess base is titrated with standard acid.

$$CCl_3CHO \cdot H_2O + NaOH = CHCl_3 + HCOONa + H_2O$$

With Chloral Hydrate Syrup a correction must be made for original acidity by a preliminary titration of the sample with base.

Ethyl Chloride—For ethyl chloride the halogen is hydrolyzed with excess standard alcoholic alkali and the excess titrated with acid.

Formaldehyde Solution—The formaldehyde is oxidized to formic acid with peroxide in the presence of excess standard base and the excess titrated.

Glutaral Concentrate—to a solution of hydroxylamine hydrochloride, neutralized to BpB with triethanolamine, a measured excess of triethanolamine is added, followed by the sample. The HCl liberated in the following reaction combines with triethanolamine and the excess is titrated with standard sulfuric acid. A blank is run on the reagents.

$$OHC(CH_2)_3CHO + 2NH_2OH \cdot HCl =$$
$$HON\!\!=\!\!CH(CH_2)_3CH\!\!=\!\!NOH + 2H_2O + 2HCl$$

Methenamine and Monobasic Sodium Phosphate Tablets—for sodium biphosphate.

All of the phosphates above are assayed by first precipitating ammonium phosphomolybdate from a dilute nitric acid solution of the sample:

$$AlPO_4 + 12(NH_4)_2MoO_4 + 24HNO_3 = (NH_4)_3PO_4 \cdot 12MoO_3 +$$
$$21NH_4NO_3 + Al(NO_3)_3 + 12H_2O$$

The precipitated yellow molybdate is filtered, washed free of adhering nitric acid, and dissolved in an excess of standard alkali:

$$(NH_4)_3PO_4 \cdot 12MoO_3 + 23NaOH = 11Na_2MoO_4$$

$$+ \; NaNH_4HPO_4 + (NH_4)_2MoO_4 + 11H_2O$$

Excess standard alkali then is titrated with standard acid.

DIRECT TITRATION OF BASE BY ACID (IA1B)
Oxtriphylline—For choline, using MeB.

Potassium Hydroxide—For potassium hydroxide using Phth and for potassium carbonate content using MeO.

Tromethamine (and for Injection)—For tromethamine using BcP.

TITRATION OF VOLATILE BASES AFTER DISTILLATION (IA2AI,IA1C)
Compounds in this category usually are hydrolyzed by boiling with strong alkali, and the ammonia or amines formed are distilled into excess standard acid or into a saturated boric acid solution. In either case, the excess standard acid is titrated with standard base, or the ammonia-boric acid complex titrated with acid; methyl red is the indicator for either method.

If the nitrogen content only is determined, the Kjeldahl procedure is used. The general procedure for the Kjeldahl method involves digestion of the sample with a mixture of sulfuric acid and potassium sulfate in the presence of a catalyst. Copper, selenium, or mercury salts have been used as catalysts. After conversion of the organic nitrogen to ammonia (ammonium ion in the acidic medium), alkali is added and the liberated ammonia is distilled and collected in standard sulfuric acid or in boric acid. Titration of the residual sulfuric acid or the ammonium ion in the boric acid solution allows calculation of the nitrogen content (IA1c).

Calcium Pantothenate—Nitrogen content by Kjeldahl method.
Glucagon—Nitrogen content by Kjeldahl method.
Ichthammol (and Ointment)—For ammonia; make alkaline and distill into excess standard acid.
Neostigmine Methylsulfate—Dimethylamine distilled.
Pyrazinamide—Amide hydrolyzed and ammonia distilled.

TITRATION OF METAL SALTS WITH ACID (IA1BI)
Caffeine and Sodium Benzoate Injection—The caffeine is extracted with chloroform, ether is added to the residual aqueous solution,

Table 30-3. Indicators, Color Developing Reagents, and Techniques[a]

AAP	4-Aminoantipyrine		MDB	Metadinitrobenzene
AAPF	4-Aminoantipyrine and potassium ferricyanide		MeB	Methylene blue
AC	Antimony trichloride		MeO	Methyl orange
ACBD	4-Amino-6-chloro-1,3-benzenedisulfonamide (diazotized)		MeP	Methyl purple, TS
ACT	Ammonium cobaltothiocyanate		MeR	Methyl red, TS
AMDB	Alkaline metadinitrobenzene		MeY	Methyl yellow (p-dimethylaminoazobenzene)
ANB	Alpha-nitroso-beta-naphthol (diazotized)		MP	Molybdophosphotungstate, TS
ANS	1,2,4-Aminonaphtholsulfonic acid		MRB	Methyl red—methylene blue, TS
AP	Alkaline picrate, TS		MV	Methyl violet, TS
AS	Ammonium molybdate and stannous chloride			
AT	Ammonium thiocyanate		Nb	Para-Naphtholbenzein
AV	Azoviolet		NiB	Nile blue hydrochloride
			Np	Nitrophenanthroline, TS
BcB	Bromocresol blue			
BcG	Bromocresol green		ON	Oxidized nitroprusside solution
BcP	Bromocresol purple		ONA	Ortho-Nitroaniline
BF	Basic fuchsin		Op	Ortho-Phenanthroline, TS
BM	Bratton-Marshall reagent; N-(1-naphthyl)ethylenediamine added to the diazotized solution		PAN	1-(2-Pyridylazo)-2-naphthol
BnF	Beta-Naphthoquinone sulfonate—formaldehyde		PBA	Para-Bromoaniline
BpB	Bromophenol blue		PC	Potassium chromate, TS
BPy	2,2'-Bipyridine		PDA	Para-Dimethylaminoazobenzene
BT	Blue tetrazolium		PDB	Para-Dimethylaminobenzaldehyde
BtB	Bromothymol blue		PdC	Palladium chloride
			PDS	Phenoldisulfonic acid
CAN	Ceric ammonium nitrate, TS		PH	Phenylhydrazine hydrochloride
C-S	Cyanogen bromide—sulfanilic acid		Phth	Phenolphthalein
CR	Cresol red, TS		Poten	Potentiometric determination of the endpoint
CRTB	Cresol red—thymol blue, TS		PR	Phenol red
CrV	Crystal violet, TS		PTB	Phenolphthalein—thymol blue
CTA	Chromotropic acid		PTC	Potassium thiocyanate
			PyA	Pyridine-acetic anhydride
DCF	Dichlorofluorescein			
DC	Diphenylcarbazone, TS		QR	Quinaldine red
DBP	Dicyanobis(1,10-phenanthroline)iron II dihydrate			
DBQ	2,6-Dibromoquinone chlorimide		R	Reinecke's salt
DcD	2,6-Dichloroquinone chlorimide			
DNP	2,4-Dinitrophenylhydrazine		SA	Sulfuric acid in methanol
DP	Diphenylamine, TS		SAF	Sodium acetate-potassium ferricyanide
DT	Dithizone		SAS	Sodium alizarinsulfonate, TS
			SD	Sudan IV
EBT	Eriochrome black T		SN	Sodium nitrite in acid solution
EY	Eosin Y, TS		SNF	Sodium nitroferricyanide, TS
			SaO	Safranin O
FAS	Ferric ammonium sulfate, TS		SPI	Starch-potassium iodide, TS, or paper or paste
FC	Ferric chloride, acid, TS		ST	Starch, TS
FCiT	Ferrocitrate reagent			
FCP	Folin-Ciocalteau-Phenol, TS		TB	Thymol blue
FEH	Ferric chloride and hydroxylamine		TBP	Tetrabromophenolphthalein, TS
FEN	Ferric nitrate		TBPE	Tetrabromophenolphthalein, ethyl ester, TS
FET	Ferrous tartrate reagent		TNP	Trinitrophenol (picric acid)
			TP	Thymolphthalein
HDA	Hexanitrodiphenylamine		TTC	Triphenyltetrazolium chloride
HNB	Hydroxynaphthol blue			
HQ	8-Hydroxyquinoline		UV	Ultraviolet radiation
IN	Isoniazid reagent		VS	Vanadyl sulfate
IP	Iron-phenol reagent			
MaG	Malachite green, TS		XyO	Xylenol orange

[a] These are coded in the last column of Appendix B. They usually are employed as solutions, and often are the official Test Solutions (TS).

and the mixture is titrated with acid, shaking vigorously. As free benzoic acid is liberated by titration with hydrochloric acid, it is immediately extracted into the ether phase. As the endpoint is exceeded, excess titrant causes the indicator (MeO) to change.

RESIDUAL TITRATION OF EXCESS ACID AFTER INTERACTION WITH BASE (IA2a)

For this category, a basic substance is treated with a measured excess of standard acid and the excess acid titrated with standard base.

Ammonia Spirit, Aromatic—For the total ammonia assay, the sample is boiled with excess standard acid and the excess titrated with sodium hydroxide. The ammonium carbonate is converted into an equivalent amount of sodium carbonate.

Magnesium Trisilicate—For magnesium oxide (MeO).

Zinc Undecylenate—Excess standard sulfuric acid is boiled with the salt, the liberated undecylenic acid is extracted with hexane, and the aqueous phase is titrated with standard base (MeO).

RESIDUAL TITRATION OF EXCESS ACID FOLLOWING LIBERATION OF A BASE BY A STRONGER BASE (IA2A)

Assays of this kind also are applied to extractions made of vegetable drugs containing alkaloidal principles and to the pharmaceutical preparations obtained from them.

All of the assays are based on the principle that relatively weak organic bases are displaced readily from their salts by a stronger base, such as sodium hydroxide, sodium carbonate, or ammonium hydroxide.

The last compound is more generally employed to liberate alkaloids from their salts. The liberated free bases are then extracted into an organic solvent (ether or chloroform) and the separated organic phase evaporated.

TITRATION OF CARBONATE RESIDUES FROM IGNITED SALTS (IA2AII)

In general the ignition of an alkali metal salt of a carboxylic acid forms sodium carbonate, carbon dioxide and water as exemplified by sodium citrate:

$$2Na_3C_6H_5O_7 + 9O_2 = 3Na_2CO_3 + 9CO_2 + 5H_2O$$

Excess standard acid is added to the ignition residue and the residue titrated with base. The volume of standard acid consumed is multiplied by the appropriate conversion factor to determine the amount of alkali salt in the sample taken.

Magnesium Citrate Oral Solution—For citric acid (Phth), after precipitation of calcium citrate and ignition of the filtered salt.

RESIDUAL TITRATION INVOLVING SAPONIFICATION OF AN ESTER (IA2bi)

In general, esters are determined by a saponification procedure of boiling the sample in excess standard alcoholic alkali, which acts as a mutual solvent. The excess alkali is determined with standard acid. A blank usually is run on the same volume of alkali used for the saponification procedure.

Oxandrolone—The ester is present in lactone form.

Peppermint Oil—For total menthol content. The free menthol first is acetylated with acetic anhydride to form the ester, menthyl acetate. After purification to remove excess acetic acid and water, the ester is subjected to the saponification procedure.

Polysorbates—Saponification value.

Polyvinyl Alcohol—Degree of hydrolysis.

Storax—Saponification value.

Tolu Balsam—Saponification value.

RESIDUAL TITRATION FOLLOWING AN ACYLATION REACTION (IA2aiii)

The general method involves the treatment of an alcohol with an acylating reagent, usually acetic anhydride or phthalic anhydride in pyridine. Any excess anhydride remaining after the esterification reaction is converted to the free acid with water, and the acid titrated with standard base. A blank usually is run employing all the reagents except the sample. The difference in titer between the blank and the sample is the volume of base equivalent to the alcohol content of the sample taken.

Polyethylene Glycol—For average molecular weight, using phthalic anhydride in pyridine.

RESIDUAL TITRATION FOLLOWING THE HYDROLYSIS OF ALKOXYL GROUPS (IA2bii)

A previously neutralized sample is saponified with excess standard base, and the excess is determined in the usual manner.

Pectin—For methoxyl groups (galacturonic acid).

PRECIPITATION REACTIONS

TITRATION OF LIBERATED NITRIC ACID (IB1E)

In assays of this type, silver nitrate reacts with the substance being assayed to form an insoluble silver derivative, simultaneously releasing an equivalent amount of nitric acid, which is titrated with standard alkali.

Oxtriphylline—For theophylline. The solution from the choline assay is treated with silver nitrate and the above method followed.

DIRECT TITRATION OF A THEOPHYLLINE–SILVER COMPLEX (IB1BI)

The theophylline–silver complex is separated by filtration, dissolved in nitric acid, and the liberated silver ion titrated with thiocyanate (FAS indicator).

Aminophylline—Some dosage forms, for theophylline.

RESIDUAL TITRATION OF A THEOPHYLLINE–SILVER COMPLEX (IB2ai)

The insoluble silver complex is precipitated from an ammoniacal solution of the sample by warming with excess standard silver nitrate. After filtration, the excess silver ion is determined in the filtrate by titration with thiocyanate (FAS indicator).

Dimenhydrinate—For 8-chlorotheophylline.

DIRECT TITRATION OF HALOGEN (IB1a)

These assays may involve the conversion of organic halogen to halide ion (if covalently bound) before titration. Silver nitrate is the titrant in all cases.

The following are titrated without previous treatment:

Anticoagulant Heparin Solution and Heparin Lock Flush Solution—For NaCl.

The following require hydrolysis with alkali:

Melphalan.

Methyclothiazide—Although two chlorine atoms occur in the molecule, only the benzylic halogen is sufficiently active to be hydrolyzed and then titrated with silver nitrate.

The following require refluxing with zinc and alkali to liberate the halogen:

Diatrizoate Meglumine (and Injection).

Diatrizoate Meglumine and Diatrizoate Sodium Injection—The assay gives both compounds and a correction is made for Diatrizoate Meglumine.

Diatrizoate Sodium (and Injection and Solution).

Diatrizoic Acid.

Iocetamic Acid (and Tablets).

Iodipamide.

Iodipamide Meglumine Injection.

Iopanoic Acid.

Iothalamate Meglumine Injection.

Iothalamate Meglumine and Iothalamate Sodium Injection.

Iothalamate Sodium Injection.

Iothalamic Acid.

Ipodate Calcium (and for Oral Suspension).

Ipodate Sodium (and Capsules).

RESIDUAL TITRATION OF HALOGEN (IB2aii)

Excess standard silver nitrate is added to a solution of the prepared sample containing ionic halogen. The excess silver nitrate is then titrated with standard ammonium thiocyanate. This method is known as the Volhard procedure. Nitrobenzene is added, in the titration involving silver chloride, to prevent its interaction with thiocyanate. Ferric Alum (FAS) is the usual indicator. Quite often the ionic halogen must be liberated from an organic compound.

Chlorobutanol—After hydrolysis with base.

Mannitol in Sodium Chloride Injection—For sodium chloride.

Sodium Chloride and Dextrose Tablets—For sodium chloride.

TITRATION WITH THIOCYANATE (IB1b)

Silver ion or mercury(II) ion is titrated with thiocyanate. With silver, insoluble silver thiocyanate is formed; with mercury(II) un-ionized mercuric thiocyanate is produced. Ferric alum (FAS) is the usual indicator.

Nitromersol (and Solution)—The sample is digested with sulfuric acid and peroxide, and oxidized with permanganate to form mercuric ion.

Phenylmercuric Acetate and Phenylmercuric Nitrate—Both are decomposed with formic acid to release mercury, which is scavenged with zinc metal and then dissolved in nitric acid.

TITRATION WITH THORIUM(IV) (IB1d)

Sodium Monofluorophosphate—The sample, acidified with sulfuric acid, is distilled and the fluoride-containing distillate is titrated with thorium nitrate solution, using sodium alizarinsulfonate indicator. Insoluble thorium tetrafluoride is formed in the acid solution, and when all the fluoride ion is precipitated the pink-red thorium salt of the indicator is produced.

REDOX REACTIONS

TITRATIONS INVOLVING DIRECT OXIDATION WITH CERIC SULFATE (IC1a)

Ceric sulfate is of value in titrating iron(II) salts in mixtures that contain excipients or diluents that have a reducing action on permanganate, but have no effect on ceric sulfate. The equation that applies is

$$2FeSO_4 + 2Ce(SO_4)_2 = Fe_2(SO_4)_3 + Ce_2(SO_4)_3$$

Ferrous Fumarate—Prior to titration with ceric sulfate, stannous chloride is added to ensure that all the iron is in the reduced state; excess tin is removed by precipitation with mercuric ion.

Homatropine Hydrobromide—Following hydrolysis with base, the mandelic acid thereby liberated is oxidized by the titrant.

Menadione—The quinone groups are reduced with zinc and acid to hydroquinone and then reoxidized with the titrant.

DIRECT TITRATION WITH POTASSIUM PERMANGANATE (IC1b)

The sample is oxidized directly by the permanganate titrant. No indicator is required, as a slight excess of permanganate imparts a distinct pink color indicating the endpoint.

Hydrogen Peroxide Concentrate (and Topical Solution).

TITRATION USING FERRIC ALUM AND PERMANGANATE (IC1bi)

In this reaction category an excess of ferric ammonium sulfate is added to the sample, which reduces the ferric iron to iron(II), and the latter is titrated with permanganate.

Titanium Dioxide—The sample is dissolved by heating with sulfuric acid and ammonium sulfate; the titanium(IV) is reduced to titanium(III) with zinc amalgam, and ferric alum is added to reoxidize the titanium with simultaneous formation of an equivalent amount of ferrous ion, which is titrated with permanganate.

RESIDUAL TITRATION USING OXALIC ACID AND PERMANGANATE (IC2e)

Potassium Permanganate—An excess of standard oxalic acid is reacted with a warm, acidified solution of the sample; the excess oxalic acid then is titrated with permanganate.

Sodium Nitrite—The nitrite first is oxidized to nitrate with an excess of standard permanganate and the unreacted permanganate is reduced with an excess of oxalic acid, which is titrated with more standard permanganate. The reason for using an excess of permanganate in the first step is to prevent loss of nitrous acid on acidifying the sodium nitrite; the addition of an excess of oxalic acid is to ensure reduction of permanganate to manganous ion rather than an intermediate of higher valence.

DICHLOROPHENOL-INDOPHENOL TITRATION (IC1c)

Ascorbic acid in Ascorbic Acid Injection may be oxidized quantitatively by titration with dichlorophenol-indophenol volumetric solution, which also serves as its own indicator. During the titration, the blue color of the dichlorophenol-indophenol solution is discharged by the reducing action of the ascorbic acid; when the endpoint is reached, a permanent reddish color is imparted by the slightest excess of titrant. The reaction is explained as

2,6-dichlorophenolindophenol
(blue in alkaline—
red in acid solution)

reduced indicator
(colorless)

SODIUM TETRAPHENYLBORON TITRATION (IE1)

Quaternary ammonium salts are capable of forming chloroform-soluble compounds with bromophenol blue as

bromophenol   quaternary   chloroform-
blue   salt   soluble product

The product is extracted from alkaline solutions into chloroform. Titration with sodium tetraphenylboron removes the quaternary salt from the product, discharging the color from the chloroform layer. In this assay, the quaternary salt and bromophenol blue, in a mixture of chloroform and water, are titrated with the sodium tetraphenylboron solution.

ASSAYS INVOLVING DIPHASIC AMINE-SURFACTANT TITRATION (IE2 AND 3)

Cetylpyridinium Chloride Lozenges—See *A*, below.
Docusate Calcium—See *B*, below (TBA).
Docusate Potassium—See *B*, below (TBA).
Docusate Sodium—See *B*, below (TBA).
Methylbenzethonium Chloride Dosage Forms—See *A*, below.
A.—In th—is type of assay, the amine salt is dissolved in chloroform, the indicator is added, and the mixture is shaken. The indicator dis-

solves in the organic phase. Titration of this two-phase system (with adequate shaking) with a surfactant solution, such as sodium lauryl sulfate, produces a water-soluble complex between amine and surfactant. As the endpoint is exceeded, the excess surfactant reacts with the basic dye (in the organic layer) and the indicator color changes from pale yellow to red (MeY), blue (BpB), or pink (SaO). Standardization of the titrant is effected using a pure sample of the substance being assayed as the standard.

B.—In this modification, the surfactant is the substance being assayed and is added to the chloroform-water–indicator mixture. The titration is now performed using a solution of a quaternary amine (cetalkonium chloride-CAC or tetrabutylammonium iodide-TBA) and the endpoint is reached when the color *disappears* from the chloroform layer.

DIRECT TITRATION WITH TITANIUM TRICHLORIDE (IC1f)

These titrations depend on the reduction of the colored sample and subsequent discharge of the color at the endpoint.

RESIDUAL TITRATION WITH TITANIUM TRICHLORIDE (IC2d)

The sample is heated with excess standard titanium trichloride, in an inert atmosphere. Excess reagent is determined by titration with ferric ammonium sulfate; as the indicator, thiocyanate ion gives a red endpoint.

TITRATION OF IODINE LIBERATED FROM POTASSIUM IODIDE (IC1lii)

Assays in this category involve addition of the substance being assayed to an acidified solution of potassium iodide as exemplified by the equation with cupric sulfate:

$$2CuSO_4 + 4KI = 2CuI + I_2 + 2K_2SO_4$$

The liberated iodine is titrated with thiosulfate; starch is employed as the indicator:

$$I_2 + 2Na_2S_2O_3 = 2NaI + Na_2S_4O_6$$

In many cases the sample requires an initial special treatment.

Ethiodized Oil Injection—See *A*, below.
Ethylcellulose—For ethoxyl, by the Zeisel alkoxy procedure.
Ferric Oxide—As for Ferrous Fumarate Tablets, replacing nitric acid with hydrochloric acid.
Ferrous Fumarate Tablets—The sample is decomposed with nitric and perchloric acids. Addition of KI to the iron(III) solution causes reduction of the iron and liberation of free iodine, which is titrated with thiosulfate.
Iodoquinol (and Tablets)—See *A*, below.
Iophendylate and Injection—Treatment with sodium biphenyl in toluene liberates iodide ion, which is extracted into dilute phosphoric acid. Addition of hypochlorite then liberates free iodine.
Methylcellulose Ophthalmic Solution and Oral Solution—Methoxyl; see *Ethylcellulose,* above.
Propyliodone (and dosage forms)—See *A*, below.
Selenium Sulfide (and Lotion)—After treatment with fuming nitric acid to form selenious acid. Potassium iodide then reduces the selenium, liberating iodine:

$$H_2SeO_3 + 4KI + 4H^+ = Se + 2I_2 + 4K^+ + 3H_2O$$

A.—Substances in this category are initially decomposed using the *Oxygen Flask Combustion Method,* and the sample is treated with bromine, as directed for *B*, below.

B.—The sample is fused with potassium carbonate, acidified, and oxidized with bromine to form iodate and bromide ions. The solution is boiled to expel bromine; phenol or formic acid is added to scavenge any remaining halogen; then KI is added and the iodate ion liberates free iodine, which is titrated.

TITRATIONS WITH POTASSIUM IODATE (IC1n)

When potassium iodate solution is titrated into an acidified solution of an alkali metal iodide, free iodine is liberated according to

$$5KI + KIO_3 + 6HCl = 6KCl + 3I_2 + 3H_2O$$

When this step of the reaction is complete, and if a sufficiently high concentration of hydrochloric acid is present, the liberated iodine is converted into iodine monochloride, as is shown by

$$KIO_3 + 2I_2 + 6HCl = KCl + 5ICl + 3H_2O$$

Combining both reactions,

$$KIO_3 + 2KI + 6HCl = 3KCl + 3ICl + 3H_2O$$

The endpoint of this titration is the disappearance of the iodine color from a few milliliters of chloroform, added to serve as an indicator.

Benzalkonium Chloride (and Solution)—Each equivalent of the quaternary chloride yields one equivalent of iodide ion, which is titrated according to the above reaction.

Hydralazine Hydrochloride Injection—The hydrazino group of hydralazine is oxidized by potassium iodate to nitrogen and is replaced by a hydroxyl group on the phthalazine ring in accordance with

Iodine Topical Solution—For sodium iodide; free iodine is first reduced by titration with arsenite.

Strong Iodine Solution—For potassium iodide; as for *Iodine Topical Solution.*

Iodine Tincture, Strong Iodine Tincture—For sodium iodide and potassium iodide; as for *Iodine Topical Solution.*

Stannous Fluoride—For tin(II); in HCl solution, KI is added and iodide is converted to iodine, which is titrated with iodate.

REACTION OF KI WITH EXCESS PERIODATE (IC1Liii)

Mannitol Injection—An acidified solution of the prepared sample is heated with periodate and acid, oxidizing the mannitol as

$$C_6H_{14}O_6 + 5HIO_4 = 2HCHO + 4HCOOH + 5HIO_3 + H_2O$$

The excess periodate and the iodate formed in the reaction react with KI to liberate iodine

$$HIO_3 + HIO_4 + 12HI = 7I_2 + 7H_2O$$

A blank is performed and the difference in the volumes of thiosulfate titrant is equivalent to the mannitol in the sample.

Mannitol in Sodium Chloride Injection—For Mannitol Injection, as above.

DIRECT TITRATION OF IODINE WITH THIOSULFATE (IC1l)

No preliminary preparation of the sample is necessary, as the iodine is present in the free state.

Povidone-Iodine—For available iodine.

RESIDUAL TITRATION OF IODINE FOLLOWING DICHROMATE PRECIPITATION (IC2ai)

These assays are based on the insolubility of the dichromate precipitated from an aqueous solution of the sample on the addition of excess standard potassium dichromate. After removal of the precipitate, the excess dichromate in the filtrate is determined by adding excess KI, which liberates free iodine and is titrated with thiosulfate.

$$Cr_2O_7{}^{2-} + 14H^+ + 6I^- = 3I_2 + 2Cr^{3+} + 7H_2O$$

RESIDUAL TITRATION OF EXCESS STANDARD IODINE (IC2a,f)

A sample of the assay material is oxidized or converted to a periodide or iodine substitution product with standard iodine, and the excess iodine is determined by titration with thiosulfate.

Phenelzine Sulfate—The hydrazine is oxidized by iodine as indicated by

$$C_6H_5CH_2NHNH_2 \cdot H_2SO_4 + 2I_2 + 5NaHCO_3 = C_6H_5CH_2I + 3NaI + Na_2SO_4 + 5CO_2 + 5H_2O + N_2$$

IODIMETRIC DETERMINATION OF PHENOLS (IC2a,c)

In these assays a bromophenol derivative is precipitated by adding a bromine (potassium bromate–potassium bromide) volumetric solution to a solution of the sample and acidifying to release free bromine, according to

$$5KBr + KBrO_3 + 6HCl = 6KCl + 3Br_2 + 3H_2O$$

The free bromine immediately reacts with the phenolic substance, as in the following equation using phenol as an example:

$$C_6H_5OH + 3Br_2 = C_6H_2Br_3OH + 3HBr$$

Potassium iodide then is added, and the excess bromine liberates free iodine:

$$2KI + Br_2 = 2KBr + I_2$$

It is titrated with thiosulfate. A blank is run on the same quantity of reagents, omitting the sample.

DIRECT TITRATION WITH STANDARD IODINE (IC1k)

The sample is titrated directly; starch TS is usually employed as the indicator.

Ascorbic Acid—A direct titration. If ascorbic acid is present in a multiple vitamin preparation, the dichlorophenol-indophenol procedure is employed.

Echothiophate Iodide (and for Ophthalmic Solution)—The ester first is hydrolyzed with pH 12 buffer to yield the free mercaptan, which then is oxidized, by titration with iodine, to the disulfide. Any free mercaptan in the original sample is corrected for by a preliminary titration. The following equations apply:

$$[(C_2H_5O)_2(PO)-S-CH_2CH_2N(CH_3)_3]^+I^- + H_2O$$
$$\text{Echothiophate}$$

$$= [HSCH_2CH_2N(CH_3)_3]^+I^- + (C_2H_5O)_2(PO)OH$$
$$2[HSCH_2CH_2N(CH_3)_3]^+I^- + I_2$$
$$\text{mercaptan}$$

$$= 2[-SCH_2CH_2N(CH_3)_3{}^+]I^- + 2HI$$

Sulfur Dioxide—On absorption in sodium hydroxide, bisulfite ion is produced and then titrated with iodine.

RESIDUAL TITRATION OF EXCESS THIOSULFATE WITH IODINE (IC2b)

Mechlorethamine Hydrochloride and Mechlorethamine Hydrochloride for Injection—Thiosulfate reacts with the active chlorine atoms according to

$$CH_3N(CH_2CH_2Cl)_2 \cdot HCl + NaHCO_3 + 2Na_2S_2O_3 = CH_3N(CH_2CH_2S_2O_3Na)_2 + 3NaCl + CO_2 + H_2O$$

DIRECT TITRATION OF IODINE WITH ARSENITE (IC1m)

Free or liberated iodine is titrated with a standard sodium arsenite solution.

Iodine Topical Solution—For iodine.

Iodine Solution, Strong—For free iodine.

Iodine Tincture and Strong Iodine Tincture—For free iodine.

DIRECT TITRATION WITH FERRIC CHLORIDE (IC1g)

Articles in this category are titrated with ferric chloride using thiocyanate indicator.

DIRECT TITRATION WITH STANDARD BROMINE (IC1h)

Thymol—A warm solution of the sample is titrated to produce a bromo-derivative, analogous to the determination of phenols. However, an excess is not employed, because methyl orange, whose color is bleached as the equivalence point is exceeded, is used as an indicator.

TITRATIONS INVOLVING SODIUM NITRITE SOLUTION (IC1J)

Most compounds in this group, being primary aromatic amines or derivatives that may be converted to such amines, are capable of undergoing quantitative diazotization of the amino group substituted on the aromatic ring, as illustrated by the following equation using *p*-aminobenzoic acid.

$$H_2NC_6H_4COOH + NaNO_2 + 2HCl = ClN_2C_6H_4COOH + NaCl + 2H_2O$$

The titration with sodium nitrite is performed potentiometrically in a solution containing crushed ice (to prevent decomposition of the diazonium salt), or until a drop of the titrated solution produces an immediate blue color with starch iodide paste used as an external indicator. Sulfonamides in which the reactive amino group is acylated must first be hydrolyzed to release the free amine form of the sulfonamide prior to diazotization.

Primaquine Phosphate (and Tablets)—This substance contains a secondary amino group and nitrosation rather than diazotization occurs, the =NH group being converted to =N—NO (*N*-nitroso).

Procaine and Tetracaine Hydrochlorides, Procaine and Tetracaine Hydrochlorides, and Levonordefrin Injection—For procaine and tetracaine, after removal as the thiocyanate.

COMPLEXATION REACTIONS

DIRECT WITH ETHYLENEDIAMINETETRAACETIC ACID (EDTA) (ID1a,IDib)

EDTA complexes with many polyvalent metals to form an undissociated chelate. A buffered solution of the sample is titrated with EDTA (as the disodium salt). The indicator used is a dye that forms a weak chelate with the analyte metal. At the endpoint the color changes when the indicator-metal complex can no longer exist.

Alumina and Magnesia Oral Suspension (and Tablets)—For magnesium hydroxide, using ammonium hydroxide and ammonium chloride buffer (EBT).

Calcium Pantothenate (and Tablets)—For calcium content.

Calcium Pantothenate, Racemic—For calcium content.

Edetate Calcium Disodium (and Injection)—Mercury(II) nitrate is the titrant.

Edetate Disodium (and Injection)—Primary standard calcium carbonate, after suitable preparation, is titrated with a solution of the *Assay Preparation*.

Edetic Acid—Calcium carbonate (primary standard) is titrated with a solution of the *Assay Preparation*.

Magaldrate (and Oral Suspension and Tablets)—For magnesium hydroxide.

Magnesia and Alumina Oral Suspension (and Tablets)—For magnesium hydroxide.

RESIDUAL TITRATION INVOLVING EDTA (ID2a)

To assay for aluminum, in many combinations containing both magnesium and aluminum a residual method is employed. Excess EDTA is added to a suitably buffered sample, and the excess determined by titration with standard zinc sulfate solution. By use of proper buffers and masking agents (weak complexing materials), it often is possible to determine mixtures of calcium and aluminum, calcium and magnesium, or zinc and aluminum without preliminary separation.

Alumina and Magnesia Oral Suspension (and Tablets)—For aluminum hydroxide (DT).

Aluminum Acetate Topical Solution—For aluminum oxide (DT).

Aluminum Subacetate Topical Solution—For aluminum oxide (DT).

Magaldrate (and Oral Suspension and Tablets)—For aluminum hydroxide (DT).

Magnesia and Alumina Oral Suspension (and Tablets)—For aluminum hydroxide (DT).

Acid–Base Reactions in Nonaqueous Solvents

Titrimetric methods employing nonaqueous solvents are used extensively for the assay of certain materials that cannot be titrated easily in aqueous systems. Water is a leveling solvent, and many weak acids or bases do not give a sufficiently sharp break in the titration curve to evidence a distinct endpoint. However, in a nonaqueous solvent such as glacial acetic acid, weak organic bases and their salts can be titrated with an acetic acid solution of perchloric acid. The strongest acid available in aqueous medium is the oxonium ion, H_3O^+, in acetic acid, but the proton of perchloric acid forms the acetacidium ion, $CH_3C(OH)_2^+$.

$$CH_3COOH + HClO_4 = CH_3C(OH)_2^+ + ClO_4^-$$

The reaction between acetacidium ion and an amine (a weak base) is illustrated by the following equation, forming the ammonium ion and acetic acid.

$$CH_3C(OH)_2^+ + RNH_2 = CH_3COOH + RNH_3^+$$

No difficulty is experienced in the titration of amine salts other than salts of halogen acids. In the latter case, mercury(II) acetate is added to form undissociated mercury(II) halide, thus preventing interference by the halogen acid, which would be liberated in its absence (Pifer–Wollish method).

Weak organic acids, such as carboxylic acids, phenols, barbiturates, sulfonamides, or enols, also may be titrated in nonaqueous medium using a strong base. These include the sodium or lithium salts of methanol or ethanol, and the reaction is of the ordinary neutralization type, as illustrated below for an organic acid with sodium ethoxide.

$$RCOOH + C_2H_5ONa = RCOONa + C_2H_5OH$$

In both types of titration, acid or base, the endpoint may be determined with indicators or potentiometrically as depicted in the accompanying chart (Table 30-4) taken from the USP.

TITRATION OF BASIC SUBSTANCES (IA1BII)

Dimenhydrinate—For diphenhydramine (poten).

Diphenoxylate Hydrochloride and Atropine Sulfate Oral Solution and Tablets—For diphenoxylate hydrochloride.

Mepivacaine Hydrochloride and Levonordefrin Injection—For mepivacaine.

Potassium Acetate—Titration of a salt of a carboxylic acid.

Potassium Sorbate—See Potassium Acetate.

Table 30-4. Systems for Nonaqueous Titrations

TYPE OF SOLVENT	ACIDIC (FOR TITRATION OF BASES AND THEIR SALTS)	RELATIVELY NEUTRAL (FOR DIFFERENTIAL TITRATION OF BASES)	BASIC (FOR TITRATION OF ACIDS)	RELATIVE NEUTRAL (FOR DIFFERENTIAL TITRATION OF ACIDS)
Solvent[a]	Glacial acetic acid	Acetonitrile	Dimethylformamide	Acetone
	Acetic anhydride	Alcohols	*n*-Butylamine	Acetonitrile
	Formic acid	Chloroform	Pyridine	Methyl ethyl ketone
	Propionic acid	Benzene	Ethylenediamine	Methyl isobutyl ketone
	Sulfuryl chloride	Chlorobenzene	Morpholine	*tert*-Butyl alcohol
		Ethyl acetate		
		Dioxane		
Indicator	Crystal violet	Methyl red	Thymol blue	Azo biolet
	Quinaldine red	Methyl orange	Thymolphthalein	Bromothymol blue
	p-Naphtholbenzein	*p*-Naphtholbenzein	Azo violet	*p*-Hydroxyazobenzene
	Alphazurine 2-G		*o*-Nitroaniline	Thymol blue
	Malachite green		*p*-Hydroxyazobenzene	
Electrodes	Glass-calomel	Glass-calomel	Antimony-calomel	Antimony-calomel
	Glass-silver-silver chloride	Calomel-silver-silver chloride	Antimony-glass	Glass-calomel
	Mercury-mercuric acetate		Antimony-antimony[b]	Glass-platinum[b]
			Platinum-Calomel	
			Glass-calomel	

[a] Relatively neutral solvents of low dielectric constant such as benzene, chloroform, or dioxane may be used in conjunction with any acidic or basic solvent to increase the sensitivity of the titration endpoints.
[b] In titrant.

TITRATION OF ACIDIC SUBSTANCES (IA1AIII)

A strong base is used to titrate very weak acids. Special precautions must be employed to exclude atmospheric carbon dioxide, which interferes with the titration. The titrants used frequently are indicated. Titrants employed are

1—Lithium methoxide solution.
2—Sodium methoxide solution.
3—Tetrabutylammonium hydroxide solution.
4—Tributylethylammonium hydroxide solution.

GRAVIMETRIC METHODS

In gravimetric methods of analysis, the assay results generally are obtained by determining either the weight of a substance in the sample, or the weight of some other substance derived from the sample, the equivalent weight of which serves as the basis for calculating the result. Separation of the substance ultimately weighed is accomplished frequently by purely physical methods. On the other hand, there are many instances in which it is necessary to use a chemical reaction to convert the substance to a corresponding amount of some other substance that can be separated, purified, and weighed. The various types of official gravimetric assays may be grouped conveniently into the following categories.

WEIGHING THE ACTIVE INGREDIENT AFTER SEPARATION (IIA)

The active principle is separated, dried and, weighed.

Caffeine and Sodium Benzoate Injection—For caffeine, after solution of the sodium benzoate in water.

Collodion—Pyroxylin is precipitated by water, dried, and weighed.

Estrone Injection—An elaborate purification procedure is involved whereby the estrone is converted to a water-soluble derivative using trimethylacethydrazide ammonium chloride (Girard's reagent for carbonyl compounds); the aqueous extract contains only ketonic material, as the reagent reacts only with carbonyl compounds. The aqueous extract then is decomposed with acid to regenerate estrone, which is extracted into chloroform; the solvent is removed and the residue weighed.

PRECIPITATION AND WEIGHING OF A DERIVATIVE OF THE ACTIVE INGREDIENT (IIB)

Anticoagulant Citrate Phosphate Dextrose Solution—For dextrose, a precipitate of Cu_2O, from reaction with Fehling's solution, is weighed.

Barium Sulfate—The sample is fused with sodium carbonate, forming barium carbonate, which is dissolved in acid; the barium is precipitated as the chromate, and is weighed.

Camphor Spirit—For camphor, as the 2,4-dinitrophenylhydrazone.

Ichthammol (and Ointment)—For total sulfur as barium sulfate after oxidation with nitric acid and perchlorate (see *Sulfur Ointment*).

Lanolin Alcohols—The cholesterol content is determined by precipitation as digitonide.

Magnesium Citrate Solution—For MgO as the 8-hydroxyquinolate.

Parachlorophenol, Camphorated—For *para*-chlorophenol: silver chloride is precipitated after release of chloride by oxidation with hot permanganate. For camphor: as the 2,4-dinitrophenylhydrazone.

Potash, Sulfurated—For sulfur by treatment with copper(II) sulfate to precipitate copper(II) sulfide, which is ignited to oxide and weighed.

Sorbitan Esters—The sample is saponified, the fatty acid is separated from the acidified aqueous solution, and it is weighed. The aqueous phase is concentrated and extracted with ethanol; the extract is concentrated to yield the *polyols*, which are weighed.

Sulfur Ointment—The sample is oxidized with nitric acid to convert sulfur to sulfate, which is precipitated and weighed as barium sulfate.

WEIGHING OF THE RESIDUE AFTER IGNITION OF THE SAMPLE (IIC)

Aluminum Monostearate—As aluminum oxide.

Silica Gel—See *Silicon Dioxide, Colloidal.*

Silicon Dioxide, Colloidal—Silica is determined by difference; the sample is weighed before and after treatment with hydrofluoric acid, which converts silica into the volatile silicon tetrafluoride. The difference in weight represents the silica content of the sample.

Zinc Oxide and Salicylic Acid Paste—For total zinc, as the oxide.

SPECTROMETRIC METHODS

Photometric analysis depends upon the measurement of the amount of light absorbed by a solution (*spectrophotometry*), a suspension (*turbidimetry*), the amount of light scattered by a suspension (*nephelometry*), or the intensity of the light emitted by an element when subjected to high temperatures (*flame photometry*). The measurement of light in the visible region (*colorimetry*) may be accomplished using a colorimeter or spectrometer or less accurately by visual comparison with color standards. See Chapter 33 for a more detailed treatment.

Radiant energy waves that are of importance to spectrophotometry range from 200 to 400 nm in the ultraviolet, from 400 to 750 nm in the visible range, and from 750 to 25,000 nm in the near infrared and infrared regions. The relatively large number of spectrometric assays that are described now in the official compendia testifies to the widespread development and general acceptance of the analytical methods that belong in this category.

VISIBLE ABSORPTION (COLORIMETRY) ASSAYS (IIIA)

If an absorption spectrometric analysis is specified in the USP-NF, a formula is provided to ensure accuracy in the calculation of the analytical result. In most cases, a numerical constant is found in the formula and may be deduced as follows. As Beer's Law holds for both the analyte (A) and standard (S) solutions, Equations 1 and 2 may be written

$$A_A = abc_A \ (1)$$

$$A_S = abc_S \ (2)$$

where A_A is the absorbance of the analyte solution whose concentration is C_A; A_S is the absorbance of the standard solution whose concentration is C_S; and a is the absorptivity of the drug substance, and b is the path length or cell thickness. If cells of the same thickness are used, Equation 1 may be divided by Equation 2 and the resulting expression solved for C_A to give

$$C_A = \frac{A_A}{A_S} C_S \qquad (3)$$

For a solution to have a proper concentration such that the absorbance may be in the range of the spectrometer, an initial analyte sample, large enough to minimize weighing errors, is chosen and the initial solution is then carried through a series of dilutions to produce the final desired solution concentration. The final analytical measurement should be related back to the original analyte sample, W_A, in milligrams; thus, Equation 4 may be written to indicate the total volume V_A in liters of solution of concentration, C_A in milligrams per liter, which would result if the entire quantity W_A were diluted directly.

$$W_A = V_A C_A \qquad (4)$$

Equation 4 may be solved for C_A and substituted into Equation 3 to yield Equation 5. Thus, the constant V_A is the numerical constant that is found in spectrometric analyses and represents the total volume of solution of concentration C_S that could be made from the entire initial analyte sample, W_A.

$$W_A = V_A \frac{A_A}{A_S} C_S \qquad (5)$$

It should be carefully noted that the spectrophotometric measurement allows the calculation of the mass of absorbing material, W_A. If the original sample is not pure drug substance but is a dilution, such as drug substance plus excipients, it should be clear that the percentage of the analyte in the sample taken, W_{sample}, is given by Equation 6.

$$\frac{W_A}{W_{sample}} \times 100$$

Under this heading are considered those assays that depend on the development of color or upon the color of the substance being assayed. The absorbances are measured accordingly at wavelengths that are within the visible range of the spectrum. These colorimetric assays generally consist of adding a reagent to the assay preparation or to the substance being tested, to produce a color that is compared with that of a standard preparation that has been prepared simultaneously and contains approximately an equal quantity of a reference standard. When the absorbance of a frequently assayed substance has been found to conform to Beer's law over a reasonable range of concentration, it is considered permissible to use a standard curve, prepared with the respective reference standard, for interpolation of the data obtained with the assay preparation.

In some instances characteristic colors are developed in *flame photometers* by subjecting an inorganic element or its compound in solution to an intensely hot flame. The intensity of the colors (radiations) is compared photometrically in a suitable spectrometer with standard solutions containing the same element.

The various models of available spectrometers are suitable for making these colorimetric measurements. Photoelectric colorimeters of the filter type, in which the light absorption is measured by sensitive photoelectric cells, also are used largely for making these determinations and several of these are commercially available.

DYE-COMPLEX METHOD (IIIA2)

Quaternary salts and many amines are capable of forming chloroform-soluble complexes with indicators, such as bromophenol blue. The usual procedure is to shake a mixture of the assay preparation, chloroform, and a buffer containing the indicator. The dye-complex partitions into the organic layer, which is separated and filtered to remove any adhering aqueous phase; the absorbance is then determined.

COLORIMETRY INVOLVING A CHROMOGENIC REAGENT (IIIA1,4)

When a three-digit number followed by a letter code is given, this indicates the analytical wavelength and color-developing reagent employed.

Anticoagulant Citrate Phosphate Dextrose Solution—For monobasic sodium phosphate; 660, ANS. For citrate; 425, PyA.

Carbachol Ophthalmic Solution—Hypochlorite is employed to form the *N*-chloroamide and this derivative with KI forms free iodine which reacts with starch TS, 590.

Mepivacaine Hydrochloride and Levonordefrin Injection—For levonordefrin; 530, FCiT.

Methenamine and Monobasic Sodium Phosphate Tablets—For methenamine; 570, CTA.

Norgestrel and Ethinyl Estradiol Tablets—For ethinyl estradiol; 536, H_2SO_4.

Procaine and Phenylephrine Hydrochlorides Injection—For phenylephrine; 500, AAP.

Procaine and Tetracaine Hydrochlorides and Levonordefrin Injection—For levonordefrin; 530, FCiT.

Propoxycaine and Procaine Hydrochlorides and Levonordefrin Injection—For levonordefrin; 530, FCiT.

Propoxycaine and Procaine Hydrochlorides and Norepinephrine Bitartrate Injection—For norepinephrine; 530, FCiT.

Propoxyphene Napsylate and Aspirin Tablets—For aspirin; 530, FEN.

Reserpine, Hydralazine Hydrochloride, and Hydrochlorothiazide Tablets—For reserpine; 390, SN. For hydralazine hydrochloride; 510, FAS-Op.

Terpin Hydrate and Dextromethorphan Hydrobromide Elixir—For dextromethorphan; 420, BcG.

SPECTROMETRIC ASSAYS IN THE ULTRAVIOLET (IIIB)

Spectrometric assays in which the absorbances are measured directly in the ultraviolet range are described in official monographs.

Applied to solutions, spectrometry is more specific than colorimetry because the absorption depends upon wavelength in a complicated manner that is generally characteristic of the chemical composition of the absorbing substance. Measurement of absorption at several wavelengths may permit identification of the solute as well as the determination of its concentration. Tests of this kind are made usually on solutions, rarely on pure liquids or solids.

Solvents used for dilution usually require special purification that is often exacting and different from the requirements for other uses. Some assays direct that blank runs be made on the solvent and reagents used to obtain a correction for their inherent absorbances.

REFERENCE STANDARDS

In practically all cases a *reference standard* is used in conjunction with the sample under assay. The standard preparation is prepared and observed in the same manner as the test specimen. The purpose of this specification is to avoid errors due to wavelength or slit-width variation among various spectrophotometers, as well as to avoid errors arising from differences in transmittance and placement of cells.

INFRARED ASSAYS (IIIC)

The quantitative estimation of compounds by infrared methods is quite similar to the techniques employed in the ultraviolet and visible regions. However, due to the difficulties involved in measuring the

absolute absorbance at a particular absorbance maximum, the *baseline* technique often is used. In this method a synthetic *baseline* is constructed between the minima at the sides of the absorption maximum, and a vertical line, intersecting the peak of the maximum, is erected perpendicular to the abscissa. The length of the vertical line, measured from the intersection of the synthetic baseline and the peak of the absorption maximum, is used as the absorbance in quantitative calculations, as illustrated in Figure 30-1. For a further discussion of the theory involved in infrared absorption, see Chapter 33.

ASSAYS INVOLVING FLAME PHOTOMETRY (IIID)

The *flame photometry method* deals with the emission of energy of a particular wavelength when a dilute solution of a metallic ion is sprayed into a colorless flame. The intensity of the emitted radiation is determined by a suitable spectrometer and compared to standards. Sodium, at 588 nm, and potassium, at 766 nm, are determined by this technique for the official substances indicated below.

Potassium Citrate and Citric Acid Oral Solution—For potassium.

Ringer's Injections and Irrigation—For potassium and sodium.

FLUOROMETRIC ASSAY METHODS (IIIE)

Riboflavin is assayed quantitatively by measuring its degree of fluorescence. Thiamine also is assayed by a fluorometric method, the principal difference from the riboflavin assay being that thiamine is oxidized first to thiochrome, the fluorescence of which is quantitatively measured in isobutyl alcohol solution. The intensity of fluorescence is measured at right angles to the incident monochromatic radiation in an instrument known as a fluorometer, or in certain spectrometers equipped with the required accessories. Quantitative evaluation of the fluorescence data is achieved through comparison with similar data obtained from solutions containing known amounts of the reference standard thiamine hydrochloride.

ATOMIC ABSORPTION ANALYSIS (IIIF)

Atomic absorption analysis is similar to flame photometry except that the photometer determines the decrease in intensity of a beam of energy passed through a flame into which the metallic ion under test is sprayed. The incident radiation is generated by a lamp, the cathode of which is fabricated from the same metal as the ions of the solution being assayed. See Chapter 33 for a detailed discussion.

NUCLEAR MAGNETIC RESONANCE METHODS (IIIG)

With NF XIV, a new spectrometric technique for the assay of organic pharmaceuticals was employed. Because this technique is an absorptive process, the area under the resonance peak is related to the concentration of that substance. The methods are similar to infrared or ultraviolet techniques, and an *internal standard* often is employed. See Chapter 33 for further discussion.

Amyl Nitrite (and Inhalant)—Benzyl benzoate internal standard.

POLAROGRAPHIC ANALYSIS (IVA1)

Quantitative polarographic methods of analysis are specified for several official substances. The *diffusion current* (i_d) is proportional to the concentration of the electroactive species under test, whereas the *half-wave potential* $(E_{1/2})$ is characteristic of the kind of electroactive species and is independent of concentration. In the official assay methods the diffusion current of a sample and a reference standard solution is measured under identical conditions, and the concentration of the sample is calculated from the ratio of the sample to reference standard diffusion currents. A review of the theory of polarography can be found in Chapter 33.

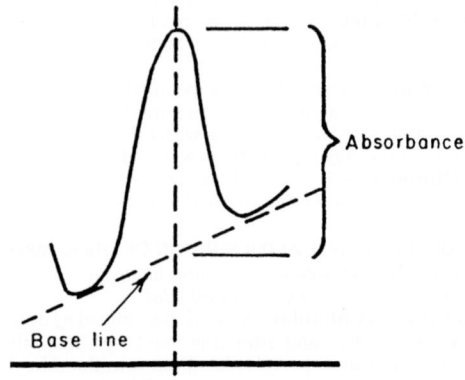

Figure 30-1. Illustration of baseline technique.

MISCELLANEOUS METHODS

GASOMETRIC ASSAY METHODS (VIA)

Gasometric methods of analysis depend on the measurement of the volume of a gas liberated under the conditions that are described in the assay, or of the decrease in volume of a gas when a suitable reagent is used to remove one of the gases present. These determinations usually are conducted in a gas buret or nitrometer, which is provided with a two-way stopcock and a two-way outlet and is properly connected with a balancing tube.

Carbon Dioxide—The sample is absorbed in 50% potassium hydroxide, and the volume of residual gas is measured.

Cyclopropane—The sample is absorbed by concentrated sulfuric acid, and the residual volume is measured.

Oxygen—The gas sample is exposed to the action of an ammoniacal copper solution, which reacts with oxygen. The residual volume is a measure of the impurities present.

ASSAYS INVOLVING VOLUMETRIC MEASUREMENTS (VIB)

Assays that depend on the separation and measurement of oily or aqueous immiscible layers are considered here. In general, these volumetric measurements are made possible as the result of processes that involve solvent separations, steam distillations, or chemical changes, in which an important constituent of the official substance (ie, volatile oil), such as an aldehyde, a ketone, or a phenol, is converted purposely to a water-soluble substance. In the latter case, the volume of residual oil is measured, and the assay result then is determined by difference.

Peppermint Spirit—For mixed oils; the oils are separated in a Babcock bottle after first mixing and centrifuging with kerosene and an acidified, saturated calcium chloride solution. A correction in the measured volume is made for the kerosene used.

ASSAYS DEPENDING ON MEASUREMENT OF OPTICAL ROTATION (VIC)

Many organic substances, or their solutions, have the property of rotating the plane of polarized light either to the right or to the left; this property is referred to as the optical activity or rotation of that substance. Measurement of this rotatory power serves as the basis for determining the purity, as well as the identity, of a number of official substances as the optical activity is a function of their chemical constitution, as well as their concentration. When the rotation is to the right, the dissolved substance is said to be dextrorotatory; whereas levorotatory substances are those that rotate the plane of polarized light to the left. The extent of observed rotation is measured and expressed in terms of degrees, and the instrument used in making these measurements is called a *polarimeter*.

The term *optical rotation* when used in the official monographs refers to *angular rotation,* and this represents the number of degrees a substance, or its solution, under specified conditions of wavelength of the polarized light, concentration, temperature, and length of the tube, will rotate the plane of polarization.

The *specific rotation,* [α], of a liquid is defined as the angular rotation in degrees through which the plane of polarization of polarized monochromatic light is rotated by passage through 1 decimeter (100 mm) of the liquid, calculated on the basis of a specific gravity of 1. In the case of solutions of an optically active substance, the specific rotation is calculated on the basis of a concentration of 1 g of solute in 1 mL of solution.

For calculating the specific rotatory power of an optically active liquid substance, or the solution of an optically active solid, the following formulas apply generally:

$$\text{For liquid substances, } [\alpha]_D^t = \frac{a}{ld}$$

$$\text{For solutions, } [\alpha]_D^t = \frac{100a}{lpd}$$

$$\text{or } [\alpha]_D^t = \frac{100a}{lc}$$

where

a = the observed rotation in degrees of the liquid at a temperature t, using a sodium light.

l = the length of the tube in decimeters.

d = the specific gravity of the liquid or solution at the temperature of observation.

p = the concentration of the solution expressed as the number of grams of active substance in 100 g of solution.

c = the concentration of the solution expressed as the number of grams of active substance in 100 mL of solution.

t = temperature of measurement.

D = D line of sodium (light source).

Anticoagulant Citrate Dextrose Solution—For dextrose.
Dextrose and Sodium Chloride Injection—For dextrose.
Diatrizoate Meglumine and Diatrizoate Sodium Injection—For diatrizoate meglumine.
Epinephrine Inhalation Solution, Sterile Oil Suspension, Nasal Solution—Rotation of the triacetyl derivative.
Epinephryl Borate Ophthalmic Solution—As for Epinephrine Nasal Solution.
Iothalamate Meglumine and Iothalamate Sodium Injection—For iothalamate meglumine.
Sodium Chloride and Dextrose Tablets—For dextrose.
Sterile Epinephrine Oil Suspension.

SPECIFIC GRAVITY (VID)

Many substances are mixtures of several compounds and can have varied composition. A simple assay procedure will not establish the purity or efficacy of such a material; therefore, they are characterized quite often by physical methods, one of which may be specific gravity.

ASSAYS INVOLVING MEASUREMENT OF RADIOACTIVITY (VIE)

In this type of assay, the radioactivity of a sample and of a calibrated radioactive standard are determined at the same time and under identical geometric conditions, as outlined in Chapter 29.

The radiochemical purity of many official radioactive substances is determined by first chromatographing the substance on a paper strip, then determining the radioactive distribution on the developed chromatogram.

ASSAYS OF ENZYME-CONTAINING SUBSTANCES (VIF)

The official enzymatic assays depend on the ability of enzymes to catalyze reactions of a certain type under the conditions that are described in the assay. These enzymes that bring about the conversion of starch into water-soluble sugars are known as diastatic enzymes. Other official enzyme-containing substances are those that digest proteins and peptides, changing them into peptones and eventually amino acids. These are called proteolytic enzymes. A third type of enzyme encountered in the official assays is the one that causes or prevents the coagulation of serum. In all of these assays the enzymatic activity of the sample is determined by comparison with that of a reference standard.

Chymotrypsin—A dilute hydrochloride solution of the sample is incubated with buffered *N*-acetyl-L-tyrosine ethyl ester in a spectrometer cell with the instrument set at 237 nm. The change in absorbance with respect to time is noted. One Chymotrypsin Unit is the activity causing a change in absorbance of 0.0075/min under the conditions of the assay.

Heparin Sodium (and Injection, Anticoagulant Heparin Solution, Heparin Calcium and Injection, and Lock Flush Solution)—The anticoagulant activity of heparin sodium is determined by its ability to inhibit the clotting of sheep plasma *in vitro*. Assay preparations are compared to a reference standard, and the calculation of potency is based on determinations of the extent of clotting which has occurred 1 hour after addition of heparin and calcium chloride to samples of citrated plasma.

Hyaluronidase Injection (and for Injection)—Hyaluronidase activity is assayed on the basis of the ability of preparations of the enzyme to decrease the turbidity of colloidal suspensions of a substrate consisting of potassium hyaluronate and protein *in vitro*. Assay preparations are compared to a reference standard, and the calculation of potency is based on measurements of the absorbance of solutions containing hyaluronidase, potassium hyaluronate, hydrolyzed gelatin, phosphate buffer, and serum.

Pancreatin (and for Capsules and Tablets)—The *starch digestive power* (amylase activity) is determined on a prepared sample by testing its quantitative ability to hydrolyze starch to the extent that no blue or reddish color develops upon the addition of iodine. The *casein digestive power* (protease activity) is determined by placing a suitably prepared casein solution in each of two tubes. To one tube is added a solution of Pancreatin and to the other tube is added a similar amount of Pancreatin Reference Standard. Both mixtures are diluted and incubated at 40°C for 1 hour. The addition of alcoholic acetic acid solution produces no more haze in the tube containing Pancreatin than in that containing the Reference Standard, indicating that the proteolytic activity of the former is at least as great as that of the latter. The *fat digestive power* (lipase activity) is determined on an olive oil substrate by titration of liberated fatty acid with base. The activity is determined from a standard curve in *mean acidity released* per minute.

Pancrelipase (and Capsules and Tablets)—The amylase activity is measured by hydrolysis of starch, after which the starch substrate is reacted with iodine. The lipase activity is determined by the digestion of olive oil and the concomitant production of acid. The protease activity is determined by the digestion of casein, after which the hydrolysis products are measured spectrophotometrically.

Protamine Sulfate (and Injection and for Injection)—The activity of Protamine Sulfate Injection is assayed on the basis of its ability to nullify the anticoagulant action of sodium heparin *in vitro*. Varying concentrations of sodium heparin are added to a series of test tubes containing uniform amounts of citrated sheep plasma, calcium chloride-thromboplastin solution, and Protamine Sulfate Injection. Calculation of potency is based on that amount of heparin sodium that results in a clotting time most nearly approaching the clotting time observed in the control tube.

Sutilains (and Ointment)—Using a casein substrate and a tyrosine reference standard, the amount of tyrosine cleared per unit time, measuring the absorbance at 275 nm, is related to the enzyme activity.

Trypsin, Crystallized (and for Inhalation Aerosol)—The method is similar to that used for *Chymotrypsin*; *N*-benzoyl-L-arginine ethyl ester hydrochloride is the substrate measured at a wavelength of 253 nm. One Trypsin Unit is the activity causing a change in absorbance of 0.003/min under the conditions of the assay.

PROXIMATE ASSAYS (VIG)

At one time the extensive use of vegetable drugs, extracts, and other galenicals in pharmacy required that the analyst be concerned with a great many *proximate assays*. Currently, more specific, well-defined medicinals, usually of synthetic origin, are in common use, so the proximate assay is required to a much lesser degree. By proximate assay is meant the determination of the amount of any organic constituent that may be present in any vegetable drug or plant to which its value or therapeutic activity is attributed. The separations depend mainly on the use of a variety of solvents selected after elaborate and painstaking research. Acid and alkali solutions, chloroform, ether, alcohol, or many other organic solvents play an important role in proximate assays.

Although largely associated with the alkaloidal content of vegetable drugs, proximate assays also include the determination of alcohol-soluble, ether-soluble, or water-soluble constituents of various drugs by solvent extraction.

ALKALOIDAL DRUG ASSAYS (VIG1)

Alkaloidal assays present the most important application of proximate assay methods with which the pharmaceutical chemist has to deal. Quantitative experiments necessarily must be done with great care, and in conducting proximate assays of alkaloidal drugs particular attention must be paid to all details. The alkaloidal substances to be separated are organic chemical compounds that are difficult to extract from the drug. They are present in comparatively small quantities and in many cases are easily destroyed by improper manipulation.

These assays are conducted largely through the use of immiscible solvents, such as chloroform, ether, or amyl alcohol, except where the properties of the alkaloid sought necessitate a special method, as for morphine in opium. Advantage is taken of the fact that the free alkaloids are practically insoluble in water (except colchicine, ephedrine, sparteine, nicotine, and a few others), whereas they are very soluble in one or more of the immiscible solvents such as chloroform or ether. The salts of the alkaloids behave in the reverse manner, being practically insoluble in the immiscible solvents and soluble in water. There are several exceptions, such as the salts of caffeine, theobromine, or colchicine; their bases are feebly basic, and the salts hydrolyze readily with the liberation of the free alkaloid.

Three general steps are required for the separation and estimation of alkaloids in vegetable drugs.

1. Extraction of the drug.
2. Subsequent separation and purification of the alkaloid.
3. Determination of the amount of alkaloid obtained, either by gravimetric or titrimetric means.

Extraction of the Crude Drug

After reduction to proper fineness by grinding, the drug may be *defatted* by extraction with petroleum benzin, or directly treated with a solvent to extract the active constituent. Depending on the alkaloid present, the drug is treated in one of the following methods:

1. Extraction with an organic solvent, after addition of ammonia to ensure the complete liberation of the basic alkaloid (belladonna and ipecac).
2. Extraction with water (morphine in opium).
3. Extraction with acidulated water, if the alkaloid is present as such or in the form of weakly combined organic salts.

The extraction procedure usually is accomplished by use of separatory funnels (separators) with mechanical agitation or in a Soxhlet extraction apparatus.

The assay processes for extracts, fluidextracts, tinctures, and powdered extracts of an alkaloidal drug are in general similar to those described for the crude drug. *Powdered and pilular extracts* usually are liquefied by the use of an appropriate solvent and then extracted directly. *Fluidextracts* often are diluted with water, and *tinctures* are concentrated to a small volume by means of a preliminary evaporation. After the mixture is made alkaline it is extracted, directly, with the most suitable solvent.

Automatic Extraction Apparatus—The need for an automatic extraction apparatus for use in the assay of alkaloidal galenicals prompted the design of an improved apparatus. The simple type is constructed easily, requires only a small amount of solvent and practically no attention, and gives a clear extraction in one operation.

In the simple type of apparatus (Fig 30-2) the same jacket, condenser, and boiling flask are used for light and heavy solvent. For light solvents, the funnel tube containing very small openings at its lower end is used in the jacket, as shown in *B*. For heavy solvents, as shown in *A*, the wide tube open at both ends is used.

The illustration shows the manner in which the extractors function. In both cases the extracting solvent is returned continuously to the boiling flask and reused. In *A*, the chloroform returns to the boiling flask under the bottom and around the inner jacket; in *B*, the nonaqueous layer is always on top and is returned by overflow.

Separation and Purification of the Alkaloid

The extract of the crude drug or galenical usually contains impurities that may interfere with the ultimate method of assay, especially in the case of extraction with immiscible solvents, whereby oils, tannins, and soluble coloring matter can obscure the endpoint in a titration or add to the weight of a gravimetric method. For these reasons, purification of the alkaloidal extract is accomplished by crystallization (as in the case of morphine in opium), removal of associated alkaloids by chemical methods, or by use of immiscible solvents. This latter method most often is employed and involves repeated extraction of the alkaloid from aqueous and organic solvent. For example, the original organic solvent extract containing the basic alkaloid is shaken with dilute acid, thus transferring the alkaloid to the aqueous layer due to the formation of the more polar acid salt. The aqueous acid layer then is made basic with ammonia (or a stronger base if required) and again extracted into an immiscible organic solvent as the free base. This process is repeated until the alkaloid is sufficiently pure for the final assay.

Estimation of the Alkaloid

Final determination of the alkaloid is accomplished either by a quantitative gravimetric or volumetric procedure, the latter being preferred. In the gravimetric method all, or a definite fraction (aliquot), of the solution containing the extract is evaporated to dryness in a tared

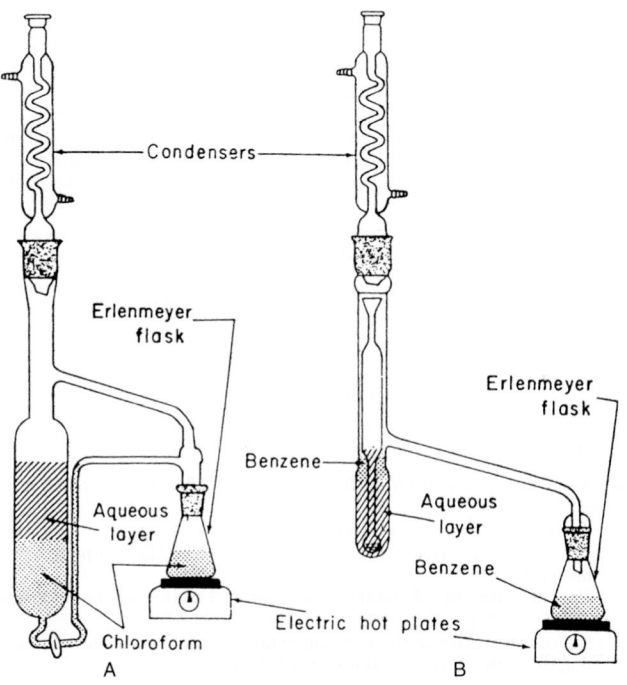

Figure 30-2. Automatic extraction apparatus for alkaloids.

container, the increase in weight of the container representing the weight (or some fraction thereof) of the alkaloid in the sample.

In the volumetric method the solvent is evaporated carefully to a small volume and an excess of standard acid plus a small amount of alcohol is added and the evaporation continued. The residual titration method is used, because the acid, by converting the alkaloid(s) to salt(s), prevents loss of some alkaloids that are fairly volatile in the form of the free base.

MISCELLANEOUS ASSAY METHODS OR FUNCTIONAL TESTS (VIK,M)

Barium Hydroxide Lime—The weight of carbon dioxide absorbed under specified conditions of rate of gas flow and time is determined.

Charcoal, Activated—The adsorptive power with respect to alkaloids (strychnine) and dyes (methylene blue) is determined by measuring the amount (if any) of unadsorbed material.

Mecamylamine Hydrochloride—Phase solubility analysis is applied to 50- to 250-mg portions of sample by equilibration with isopropyl alcohol and determination of the solution concentrations of the portions. From a plot of these concentrations versus the system concentrations, the purity of the sample may be calculated (see Chapter 16).

Soda Lime—See *Barium Hydroxide Lime,* above.

Sodium Alginate—The carbon dioxide, liberated when the sample is heated with hydrochloric acid in a special apparatus for alginates assay, is drawn into an excess of standard base and the excess titrated with acid (IA2b).

BIOLOGICAL ASSAYS (VIH)

Substances in this category may not need to be assayed by a chemical or physical method. If a biological assay is required, information concerning it may be found in Chapter 31. Some of these substances require batch certification by either the US Food and Drug Administration or the National Institutes of Health.

MULTIVITAMIN AND MULTIMINERAL DOSAGE FORMS (VIL)

The analysis of vitamins in a mixture of vitamins may be different from the procedures used when the individual vitamins or minerals are alone. The following methods are used in multivitamin and multimineral mixtures.

Vitamins

Vitamin A	HPLC; VB1a, 325 nm.
Vitamin D	HPLC; VB1a, 265 nm.
Vitamin E	HPLC; VB1b, 254 nm.
Vitamin K	HPLC; VB1b, 325 nm.
β-Carotene	Spectrometry; III A4, 452 nm.
Vitamin C	Titration; ICIK.
Biotin (1)	HPLC; VB1b, 200 nm.
Biotin (2)	Microbial; VIL.
Vitamin B$_{12}$ (1)	HPLC; VB1b, 280 nm.
Vitamin B$_{12}$ (2)	Microbial; VIL.
Folic Acid	HPLC; VB1b, 280 nm.
Calcium Pantothenate (1)	HPLC; VB1b, 210 nm.
Calcium Pantothenate (2)	Microbial; VIL.
Dexpanthenol or **Panthenol**	Microbial; VIL.
Niacin or **Niacinamide**	HPLC; VB1b, 280 nm.
Pyridoxine	HPLC; VB1b, 280 nm.
Riboflavin	HPLC; VB1b, 280 nm.
Thiamin	HPLC; VB1b, 280 nm.

Minerals

Metals—Atomic Absorption Spectroscopy, III F1, at λ given, in nanometers: Ca 422.7; Cr 357.9; Cu 324.7; Fe 248.3; Mg 285.2; Mn 279.5; Mo 313; K 766.5; Zn 213.8. Additional Mo: spectroscopy, III A4, 465 nm.

Nonmetals—F, potentiometry, IVB1; I, titration, IC10; P, spectroscopy, IIIA4, 650 nm; Se, (1) Atomic Absorption Spectroscopy, III, F1, 196 nm, (2) spectroscopy, III, B1, 380 nm, (3) fluorescene, III, E2, excitation 366 nm, emission 525 nm.

Dosage Forms

Minerals Capsules and Tablets
Trace Elements Injection
Oil-soluble Vitamin Capsules and Tablets
Water-soluble Vitamin Capsules and Tablets
Oil-and Water-soluble Vitamin Capsules and Tablets
Oil-and Water-soluble Vitamins with Minerals Capsules and Tablets
Water-soluble Vitamins with Minerals Capsules and Tablets

FIXED OILS AND WAXES (VII1)

The fixed oils (corn, cottonseed, olive) and waxes are composed largely of mixtures of fatty acid esters, and it is possible that each component has a relatively wide concentration limit without sacrificing the quality of the oil. It is for this reason that a single-substance assay is of little value; many parameters are necessary to stipulate the quality of the oil. Some of the many kinds of tests performed on the materials in this category include saponification value, acid number, acetyl value, iodine number, specific gravity, and melting range of fatty acids.

PENICILLIN CLASS ANTIBIOTIC ASSAYS (VIN2,3)

Penicillin G Determination

Penicillin G determination is a reversed-phase HPLC procedure that can measure the penicillin G content in an antibiotic drug substance by measuring responses of the major peaks in the chromatogram.

Iodometric Assay—Antibiotics

Treatment of penicillins with alkali or penicillinase causes the β-lactam to open, yielding a derivative with an acidic and an amine function (eg, penicillin yields penicilloic acid). The derivative consumes iodine, whereas the initial intact penicillin antibiotic does not. This behavior forms the basis for the iodometric assay.

Hydroxylamine (Hydroxamic Acid) Assay—Antibiotics

When penicillins are reacted with hydroxylamine, the β-lactam is opened and a hydroxamic acid derivative forms. The derivative reacts with iron III to produce a color whose intensity is used as a measure of the penicillins. This method is specific, because the β-lactam must be intact for the hydroxamic acid derivative to form. This assay has been automated.

MONOGRAPHS FOR COMPOUNDED PREPARATIONS

The USP has undertaken the development of monographs for compounded preparations. These compounded preparations represent those dosage forms that are not commercially available but for which there is a demonstrated need. The concept of a compliance assay has been introduced, and an assay is included in the monograph. The pharmacist who is compounding the preparation is not required to analyze the preparation; however, it is expected that the compounded preparation which results when the compounding directions are followed will meet the purity rubric requirements as determined by the compliance assay. The compliance assay is used in stability studies of the compounded preparation and provides the data from which a beyond-use date is specified in the monograph.

An example of a compounded preparation is Sodium Hypochlorite Topical Solution. The compliance assay is of the class IcIii and the beyond-use date is 7 days after that day on which the preparation was compounded. Cocaine and Tetracaine Hydrochlorides and Epinephrine Topical Solution, Hydralazine Hydrochloride Oral Solution, and Rifampin Oral Suspension are other compounded preparations whose monographs do not yet specify an assay, but each of which has a beyond-use date of 30 days. Other monographs will be added.

MONOGRAPHS FOR BOTANICALS AND NUTRITIONAL SUPPLEMENTS

The Revision Committee of the USP continues to provide monographs for botanicals and nutritional supplements. The list of monographs is growing with each supplement to the USP. The following is a partial list: Calcium with Vitamin D Tablets, Chamomile, Cranberry Liquid Preparation, Feverfew, Powdered Feverfew, Garlic, Powdered Garlic, Ginkgo, Oriental Ginseng, Powdered Oriental Ginseng, Milk Thistle, Powdered Milk Thistle, Saw Palmetto, Powdered Saw Palmetto, St John's Wort, Powdered St John's Wort, Valerian, Powdered Valerian, and Vitamins.

The approaches to qualitative and quantitative analysis in these botanical monographs are very similar. Thin-layer chromatography is used in all but one monograph (Cranberry Liquid Preparation) to identify plant principles. In some cases, characteristic color tests are used to supplement identification. For quantitative analysis, the quantity of a particular plant principle is determined by high-performance liquid chromatography (HPLC), using spectrophotometric detection in all but two cases. For Cranberry Liquid Preparation, there is an HPLC procedure that uses a refractive index detector to determine dextrose and fructose. In the monographs for Saw Palmetto and Powdered Saw Palmetto, gas chromatography (GC) is used to measure 11 methyl esters of fatty acids using flame ionization detection.

REFERENCES

1. United States Pharmacopeia 24/National Formulary 19 (USP24/NF19). Rockville, MD: United States Pharmacopeia Convention, 2002.
2. ICH Guidance for Industry Q2B Validation of Analytical Procedures: Methodology, November 1996.
3. FDA. Code of Federal Regulations, Title 21, Part 11 Electronic Records, Electronic Signatures–Final Rule. Federal Register, 1997; 62(54): 13429–13466.
4. FDA Guidance for Industry Q2B Part 11, Electronic Records, Electronic Signatures–Scope and Application, August 2003.
5. For a practical reference regarding Part 11 requirements, see Huber L, Winter, W. *BioPharm International*, February 2004 Supplement, S-4–S-9.

For the purpose of this chapter, the official chemical, physicochemical, and physical assay methods have been classified in an outline form. The first two classes are stoichiometric analyses; the next three are modern or nonstoichiometric analyses; the last class encompasses miscellaneous methods, including many older procedures and some more modern ones.

I. Titrimetric Methods
  A. Acid–Base Reactions
    1. Direct Titrations
      a. Titration of an acid by a base
        i. Titration of a liberated acid
        ii. Sørenson–Formol titration
        iii. Nonaqueous titration
      b. Titration of a base by an acid
        i. Titration of metal salts
        ii. Nonaqueous titration
        iii. Nonaqueous titration—Pifer–Wollish reagent
      c. Kjeldahl Determination
    2. Residual Titrations
      a. Titration of excess acid by a base
        i. After distillation of a volatile base
        ii. After addition to carbonate residues
        iii. After acylation reactions
        iv. Nonaqueous titration
      b. Titration of excess by an acid
        i. After saponification of an ester
        ii. After hydrolysis of an alkoxyl group
        iii. After distillation of a volatile base
  B. Precipitation Reactions
    1. Direct Titrations
      a. With silver nitrate
      b. With thiocyanate
        i. Of theophylline–silver compound
        ii. Of halogen
        iii. Of mercury
        iv. Of silver
      c. Of a halogen with mercuric ion
      d. Of a halogen with thorium (IV)
      e. Of liberated nitric acid
      f. Of thiol with mercuric ion
    2. Residual Titrations
      a. With thiocyanate
        i. Of theophylline–silver compound
        ii. Of silver
  C. Redox Reactions
    1. Direct Titrations
      a. Involving ceric sulfate or ceric ammonium nitrate
      b. Involving potassium permanganate
        i. Using ferric alum and potassium permanganate
      c. Involving dichlorophenol-indophenol
      d. Involving potassium dichromate
      e. Involving ferrous ammonium sulfate
      f. Involving titanium trichloride
      g. Involving ferric chloride
      h. Involving standard bromine
      i. Involving potassium ferricyanide
      j. Involving sodium nitrate
      k. With iodine
      l. Involving iodine and thiosulfate
        i. Iodimetric determination of phenols
        ii. Titration of iodine liberated from potassium iodide
        iii. Reaction of potassium iodide with excess periodate
      m. Of iodine with arsenite
      n. Involving potassium iodate
      o. With thiosulfate

    2. Residual Titrations
      a. Of excess standard iodine
        i. Titration of iodine following dichromate reaction
      b. Of excess thiosulfate with iodine
      c. Of generated iodine with thiosulfate
      d. Of residual titanium with iron (III)
      e. Of residual oxalic acid by potassium permanganate
      f. Of residual iodine by sodium thiosulfate
  D. Complexation Reactions
    1. Direct Titrations
      a. With EDTA
      b. With miscellaneous titrant
    2. Residual Titrations
      a. With EDTA
      b. With metal ion
  E. Large Anion Reagent and Large Cation Reagent Reactions
    1. Titrations with sodium tetraphenylboron
    2. Titration with sodium lauryl sulfate
    3. Titration with *tetra-n*-butyl ammonium iodide
    4. Titration with dioctyl sodium sulfosuccinate
II. Gravimetric Methods
  A. Weighing Drug after Separation
  B. Weighing a Derivative after Separation
  C. Weighing a Residue after Ignition
III. Spectrometric Methods
  A. Visible Absorption (Colorimetry)
    1. Steroid
    2. Dye–complex
    3. Direct
    4. Derivative formed
    5. Starch-iodine reaction
  B. Ultraviolet (UV) Absorption
    1. Direct
    2. Derivative formed
    3. Amphetamine
  C. Infrared (IR) Absorption
    1. Direct
    2. Derivative formed
  D. Flame Photometric Emission
  E. Fluorometric Emission
    1. Native fluorescence
    2. Fluorescent derivative formed
  F. Atomic Absorption (AA)
    1. Flame
    2. Furnace used
  G. Nuclear Magnetic Resonance (NMR) Absorption
    1. Absolute method
    2. Relative method
IV. Electrochemical Methods
  A. Voltammetry
    1. Polarography
    2. Differential pulse polarography
    3. Use of electrodes other than DME
  B. Potentiometry
    1. Ion-selective electrodes
V. Chromatographic Methods
  A. Gas Chromatography (GC)
    1. Direct assay
    2. Derivative formed

B. High-Performance Liquid Chromatography (HPLC)
   1. Direct assay
      a. Normal phase
      b. Reverse phase
   2. Derivative formed
      a. Normal phase
      b. Reverse phase
C. Thin-Layer Chromatography (TLC)
   1. Mobile phase
      a. Normal
      b. Reverse

VI. Miscellaneous Methods
A. Gasometric Assay
B. Assays Involving Liquid Volume Measurements
C. Assays Involving Optical Rotation
   1. Direct
   2. Derivative formed for assay

D. Assays Involving Specific Gravity
E. Assays of Radioactivity
F. Enzyme Assay
G. Proximate Assay
   1. Alkaloid assay
H. Biological Assay
I. Miscellaneous
   1. Fixed oils and waxes
J. Distillation
K. Functional Test
L. Vitamin Assays
M. Phase Solubility
N. Antibiotic Assays
   1. Microbial
   2. Iodometric
   3. Hydroxylamine
O. See individual components

This appendix presents a classification of the assay for the majority of official drugs taken from USP24–NF19. In column 1, the drug substance or dosage form is listed. Column 2 gives the assay category whose interpretation may be taken from Appendix A. Column 3 gives the analytical wavelength for spectrometric analyses (Class III) in nanometers for visible and ultraviolet regions and in micrometers for the infrared; it also gives the detector type that is used for chromatographic methods (Class V). For example, for GC methods, FID-P represents a flame ionization detector—temperature programmed mode, whereas TC-I means thermal conductivity detector—isothermal mode. For HPLC, UV-280 means UV detector used at 280 nm, RI indicates refractive index, and EC electrochemical detectors. Finally, column 4 lists the indicator employed in titration procedures or the internal standard, where used, for the chromatographic procedures and for the quantitative NMR analyses.

Appendix B. Assay Index of Official USP-NF Drugs

DRUG	ASSAY CATEGORY	ANALYTICAL WAVELENGTH AND/OR DETECTOR	INDICATOR OR INTERNAL STANDARD
Acebutolol Hydrochloride	VB1b	UV-254	
Acepromazine Maleate	VB1b	UV-280	
Injection	VB1b	UV-280	
Tablets	VB1b	UV-280	
Acetaminophen	IIIB1	244	
Capsules	VB1b	UV-243	
for Effervescent Oral Solution	VB1b	UV-243	
Oral Solution	VB1b	UV-243	
Oral Suspension	VB1b	UV-243	
Suppositories	VB1b	UV-243	
Tablets	VB1b	UV-243	
and Aspirin Tablets	VB1b	UV-280	benzoic acid
Aspirin and Caffeine Tablets	VB1b	UV-275	benzoic acid
and Codeine Phosphate Oral Solution	VB1b	UV-280	
and Codeine Phosphate Oral Suspension	VB1b	UV-220	
and Codeine Phosphate Capsules	VB1b	UV-280	
and Codeine Phosphate Tablets	VB1b	UV-280	
and Diphenhydramine Citrate Tablets	VB1b	UV-254, 265	guafenesin, xylometazoline
and Pseudoephedrine Tablets	VB1b	UV-214	
Capsules containing at least three of the following—acetaminophen, and salts of chlorpheniramine, Dextromethorphan, and Phenylpropanolamine	VB1b	UV-214, 280	
Oral Solution containing at least three of the following—acetaminophen, and salts of chlorpheniramine, Dextromethorphan, and Phenylpropanolamine	VB1b	UV-214, 280	
Tablets containing at least three of the following—acetaminophen, and salts of chlorpheniramine, Dextromethorphan, and Phenylpropanolamine	VB1b	UV-214, 280	
Capsules containing at least three of the following—acetaminophen, and salts of chlorpheniramine, Dextromethorphan, and Pseudoephedrine	VB1b	UV-214, 280	
Oral Powder containing at least three of the following—acetaminophen, and salts of chlorpheniramine, Dextromethorphan, and Pseudoephedrine	VB1b	UV-214, 280	
Oral Solutions containing at least three of the following—acetaminophen, and salts of chlorpheniramine, Dextromethorphan, and Pseudoephedrine	VB1b	UV-214, 280	
Tablets containing at least three of the following—acetaminophen, and salts of chlorpheniramine, Dextromethorphan, and Pseudoephedrine	VB1b	UV-214, 280	
Acetazolamide	IIC1		
Tablets	IVA1	7.38	
Acetazolamide for Injection	IIIB1	265	
Acetic Acid	IA1a		
Glacial	IA1a		
Irrigation	IA1a		
Otic Solution	IA1a		
Acetohexamide	IA1aiii		Phth
Tablets	IIIB1	247	Phth
Acetohydroxamic Acid	IIIA4	502	Phth
Tablets	IIIA4	502	Phth
Acetone	VA1	FID-P	TB
Acetylcholine Chloride for Ophthalmic Solution	IA2b		Phth
Acetylcysteine	VB1b	RI	(±)-phenylalanine
Solution	VB1b	UV-214	(±)-phenylalanine
and Isoproterenol Hydrochloride Inhalation Solution	VB1b	UV-214, 280	(±)-phenylalanine, acetaminophen
Acyclovir	VB1b	UV-254	
Capsules	VB1b	UV-254	
for Injection	VB1b	UV-254	
Ointment	VB1b	UV-254	
Oral Suspension	VB1b	UV-254	
Tablets	VB1b	UV-254	
Adenine	IAbii		Poten
Adenosine	IAbii		Poten
for Injection	VB1b	UV-254	
Air, Medical	VI		
Alanine	IA1bii		Poten

DRUG	ASSAY CATEGORY	ANALYTICAL WAVELENGTH AND/OR DETECTOR	INDICATOR OR INTERNAL STANDARD
Albendazole	IA1bii		
Oral Suspension	VB1b	UV-308	OB
Tablets	VB1b	UV-254	
Albuterol	IA1bii		
Tablets	IA1bii		CrV
Albuterol Sulfate	IA1bii		Nb
Alcohol Rubbing	IIIA2, IA2bi		OrB
Alcohol in Dextrose Injection	VIJ, VIC	410	Phth
Alfentanil Hydrochloride	IAbii		Nb
Injection	VB1b	UV-235	
Allopurinol	VB1b	UV-254	
Tablets	IIIB1	250	hypoxanthine
Allyl Isothiocyanate	IC11		FAS
Aloe	VIG		
Alprazlam	VB1a	UV-254	
Tablets	VB1a	UV-254	
Alprostadil	VB1b	UV-254	ethylparaben
Injection	VB1b	UV-254	ethylparaben
Alteplase	VIH		
for Injection	VIH		
Altretamine	VB1b	UV-227	
Capsules	VB1b	UV-227	
Alum	ID2a		DT
Ammonium	ID2a		DT
Potassium	ID2a		DT
Alumina and Magnesia Oral Suspension	ID2a, ID1a		DT, EBT
Tablets	ID2a, ID1a		DT, EBT
Alumina, Magnesia and Calcium Carbonate Oral	ID2a, ID1a, ID1a		DT, EBT, HNB
Suspension Tablets	ID2a, ID1a, ID1a		DT, EBT, HNB
Alumina, Magnesia, Calcium Carbonate, and Simethicone Tablets	ID2b, IIIF1, ID1a	285.2	dithizone
Alumina Magnesia and Simethicone Oral Suspension	IC2b, ID1a, IIIC1		DT, EBT
Tablets	IC2b, ID1a, IIIC1		DT, EBT
Alumina and Magnesium Carbonate Tablets	IIIF1		
Oral Suspension	IIIF1		
and Magnesium Oxide Tablets	ID1a, IIB, ID2a		DT
Alumina and Magnesium Trisilicate Oral Suspension	ID2a, ID1a		DT
Tablets	ID2a, IA2b		DT
Aluminum Acetate Topical Solution	ID2a		DT, Phth
Aluminum Chloride	ID1a		DT
Aluminum Chlorohydrate Solution	ID1a		DT
Aluminum Chlorohydrex Polyethylene Glycol	IC1a		DT

DRUG	ASSAY CATEGORY	ANALYTICAL WAVELENGTH AND/OR DETECTOR	INDICATOR OR INTERNAL STANDARD
Aluminum Chlorohydrex Propylene Glycol	IC1a		DT
Aluminum Dichlorohydrate	ID1a		DT
Solution	ID1a		DT
Polyethylene Glycol	ID1a		DT
Propylene Glycol	ID1a		DT
Aluminum Hydroxide Gel	ID2a		DT
Dried	ID2a		DT
Dried, Capsules	ID2a		DT
Dried Tablets	IIC		
Aluminum Monostearate	IA2b		Phth
Aluminum Phosphate Gel	ID1a		DT
Aluminum Sesquichlorohydrate	ID1a		DT
Solution	ID1a		DT
Polyethylene Glycol	ID1a		DT
Propylene Glycol			
Aluminum Subacetate Topical Solution	ID2a, IA2b		DT, Phth
Aluminum Sulfate	ID2a		DT
and Calcium Acetate Tablets for Topical Solution	ID1a		DT, EBT
Aluminum Zirconium Octachlorohydrate Solution			
Aluminum Zirconium Octachlorohydrex Gly Solution	ID1a		DT
Pentachlorohyrate Solution	ID1a		DT
Pentachlorohyrate Gly Solution	ID1a		DT
Tetrachlorohydrate Solution	ID1a		DT
Tetrachlorohydrex Gly Solution	ID1a		DT
Trichlorohydrate Solution	ID1a		DT
Trichlorohydrex Gly Solution	ID1a		DT
Amantadine Hydrochloride	IA1biii		Poten
Capsules	VA1	FID	naphthalene
Syrup	VA1	FID	naphthalene
Amcinonide	VB1b	UV-254	
Cream	VB1b	UV-254	
Ointment	VB1b	UV-254	dibutyl phthalate
Amikacin	VB2b	UV-340	
Amikacin Sulfate	VB2b	UV-340	
Sulfate Injection	VB2b	UV-340	
Amiloride Hydrochloride	IA1biii		CrV
Tablets	VB1b	UV-286	
and Hydrochlorothiazide Tablets	VB1b	UV-286	
Aminobenzoate Potassium	IC1j		Poten
Capsules	IIIB1	270	
for Oral Solution	IC1j		Poten
Tablets	IIIB1	270	

Appendix B. Assay Index of Official USP-NF Drugs

DRUG	ASSAY CATEGORY	ANALYTICAL WAVELENGTH AND/OR DETECTOR	INDICATOR OR INTERNAL STANDARD
Aminobenzoate Sodium	IC1j		Poten
Aminobenzoic Acid	IC1j		Poten
Gel	VB1b		salicylic acid
Topical Solution	IC1j		Poten
Aminocaproic Acid			
Injection	VB1b	UV-210	
Syrup	VB1b	UV-210	
Tablets	IA1bii		CrV
Aminoglutethimide	IA1bii		CrV
Tablets	VB1b	UV-240	
Aminohippurate Sodium Injection	VB1b	UV-240	
Aminohippuric Acid	IC1j		Poten
Aminophylline	IA1a		Poten
Delayed-release Tablets	VB1b	UV-254	
Enema	IB1bi		
Injection	IIIB1	270	
Oral Solution	VB1b	UV-254	
Suppositories	VB1b	UV-254	
Aminosalicylate Sodium	IB1bi		FAS
Tablets	IB1bi		FAS
Aminosalicylic Acid	VB1b	UV-254	sulfanilamide and acetaminophen
Tablets	VB1b	UV-254	sulfanilamide and acetaminophen
Amitraz	VA1	FID	Squalene
Concentrate for Dip	VA1	FID	Squalene
Amitriptyline Hydrochloride	IA1biii		CrV
Injection	VB1b	UV-254	
Tablets	IIIB1	265	
Strong Ammonia Solution	IA2a		MeR
Aromatic Ammonia Spirit	IA2a, IA1b		MeR, MeO
Ammonio Methacrylate Copolymer	IA1aiii		Poten
Ammonium Carbonate	IA2a		MeO
Ammonium Chloride	IB1a		EY
Injection	IA1c		FAS
Tablets, Delayed Release	IA1c		FAS
Ammonium Molybdate	IB		
Injection	IIF1		
Ammonium Phosphate	IA1b		Poten
Amobarbital Sodium	IIA		
for Injection	IIA		
Amodiaquine	IIIB1	342	
Amodiaquine Hydrochloride	IIIB1	342	
Tablets	IIIB1	342	
Amoxapine	IA1bii		CV
Tablets	VB1b	UV-254	
Amoxicillin	VB1b	UV-230	
Boluses	VB1b	UV-230	
Capsules	VB1b	UV-230	
Intramammary Infusion	VIN1		
for Oral Suspension	VB1b	UV-230	
for Injectable Suspension	VB1b	UV-230	SPI
Oral Suspension	VIN2		
Tablets	VB1b	UV-230	
and Clavulanate Potassium for Oral Suspension	VB1b	UV-220	
and Clavulanate Potassium Tablets	VB1b	UV-220	
Amphetamine Sulfate	IIIB3	257, 280	
Tablets	IIIB3	257, 280	
Amphotericin B	VIN1		
Cream	VIN1		
Injection	VIN1		
Lotion	VIN1		
Ointment	VIN1		
Ampicillin	VB1b	UV-254	SPI
Boluses	VIN2		
Capsules	VIN2		SPI
for Oral Suspension	VIN2		SPI
Soluble Powder	VIN2		SPI
for Injection	VB1b	UV-254	SPI
for Injectable Suspension	VIN2		
Sodium	VB1b	UV-230	
Sodium and Sulbactam Sodium	VB1b	UV-230	
and Probenecid for Oral Suspension	VIN2, IIIB1	257	SPI
Amprolium	VB1b	UV-254	
Oral Solution	VB1b	UV-254	
Soluble Powder	VB1b	UV-254	
Amrinone	IA1b		Poten
Injection	VB1b	UV-313	
Amyl Nitrite	IIIG1		
Inhalant	IIIG1		
Amylene Hydrate	VA1	TC-I	
Anileridine	IA1bii		benzyl benzoate
Injection	IIIA4	560	benzyl benzoate
Anileridine Hydrochloride	IA1biii		CrV
Tablets	IIIA4	560	CrV
Antazoline Phosphate	IA1bii		Poten
Anthralin	VB1a	UV-354	o-nitroaniline
Cream	VB1a	UV-354	o-nitroaniline
Ointment	VB1a	UV-354	o-nitroaniline
Anticoagulant Citrate Dextrose Solution	IIIA4, IA1a, IIB, VIC1	425, 660	Phth
Anticoagulant Citrate Phosphate Dextrose Solution	IIIA4, IA1a, IIB, VB1b, VIC1	425, 660	Phth
Adenine Solution	VB1b	UV-254	

DRUG	ASSAY CATEGORY	ANALYTICAL WAVELENGTH AND/OR DETECTOR	INDICATOR OR INTERNAL STANDARD
Anticoagulant Heparin Solution	VIF, IB1a		PC
Anticoagulant Sodium Citrate Solution	IA1bii		Poten
Antimony Potassium Tartrate	IC1k		ST
Antimony Sodium Tartrate	IC1k		ST
	IC11		ST
Antipyrine and Benzocaine Otic Solution	VB1b	UV-280	
Antipyrine, Benzocaine and Phenylephrine Hydrochloride Otic Solution	VB1b	UV-272	
Apomorphine Hydrochloride Tablets	IA1biii		CrV
	IA2a		MeR
Apraclonidine Hydrochloride Ophthalmic Solution	IAibii	UV-254	Poten
Arginine	VB1b		
Arginine Hydrochloride	IA1bii		
Injection	IA1biii		
Arsanilic Acid	IIIA4	520	
Ascorbic Acid	IC1b		
Injection	IC1k	UV-245	ST
Oral Solution	VB1b		
Tablets	IC1c		
	IC1c		
Ascorbyl Palmitate	IC1k		
Aspartame	IA1aiii		TB
	IA2b		Phth
Aspirin	VB1b	UV-254	
Boluses	IIIB1	280	
Capsules	VB1b	UV-280	
Delayed Release Capsules	VB1b	UV-280	
Delayed Release Tablets	VB1b	UV-280	
Effervescent Tablets for Oral Solution	ID1a		
Extended Release Tablets	VB1b	UV-280	
Suppositories	IIIB1	280	
Tablets	VB1b	UV-280	
Alumina and Magnesia Tablets	VB1b, ID2a	UV-280	phenacetin
Alumina and Magnesium Oxide Tablets	VB1b, ID2b, ID1a	UV-205	phenacetin dithizone, EBT
Caffeine and Dihydrocodeine Bitartraic Capsules	VB1b	UV-215	
Caffeine and Codeine Phosphate Tablets and Codeine Phosphate, Alumina and Magnesia Tablets	VB1b, ID2b, ID1c	UV-280	phenacetin phenacetin, DT, EBT
Astemizole	VB1b	UV-220	
Tablets	VB1b	UV-220	
Atenolol	VB1b	UV-226	
Injection	VB1b	UV-275	
Tablets	VB1b	UV-226	
and Chlorthalidone Tablets	VB1b	UV-275	
Atropine	IA1bii		CrV
Atropine Sulfate	IA1bii		Poten
Injection	VB1b	UV-218	
Ophthalmic Ointment	VA1	TC-I	homatropine hydrobromide

DRUG	ASSAY CATEGORY	ANALYTICAL WAVELENGTH AND/OR DETECTOR	INDICATOR OR INTERNAL STANDARD
Ophthalmic Solution	VA1	TC-I	homatropine hydrobromide
Tablets	VA1	TC-I	homatropine hydrobromide
Aurothioglucose Injectible Suspension	IIB		
	IIB		
Avobenzone	VA1	FID-P	
Azaperone Injection	VB1b	UV-243	
Azatadine Maleate	VB1b	UV-230	
Tablets	IA1bii	UV-254	CrV
Azathioprine	III1	283	
Tablets	IA1aiii		TB
Azathioprine Sodium for Injection	VB1b	UV-254	TB
Azithromycin	IVA1		
Capsules	VB1b	EC	
for Oral Suspension	VB1b	EC	
Aztreonam	VB1b	EC	
Injection	VB1b	UV-270	
for Injection	VB1b	UV-206	
Bacampicillin Hydrochloride for Oral Suspension	VB1b	UV-206	
Tablets	VIN2	UV-254	SPI
Bacitracin	VB1b	UV-254	
for Injection	None		
Ointment	None		
Ophthalmic Ointment	VIN1		
Soluble Methylene Disalicylate	None		
Soluble Powder	VN1		DT
and Polymyxin B Sulfates	VN1		DT
Topical Aerosol for Injection	VIN1		
Zinc	None		
Zinc Ointment	None		
Sterile Zinc	VIN1		
Zinc Soluble Powder	None		
Zinc and Polymyxin B Sulfate Ophthalmic Ointment	VIN1		
Zinc and Polymyxin B Sulfate Ointment	None		
Baclofen	IA1bii		
Tablets	VB1b		
Barium Hydroxide Lime	VIK	UV-265	Poten
Barium Sulfate	IIB		benzoic acid
Barium Sulfate Suspension for Suspension	IIB		
Beclomethasone Dipropionate	VB1b	UV-254	testosterone propionate
Belladonna Extract	VA1	TC-I	homatropine hydrobromide
Tablets	VA1	TC-I	homatropine hydrobromide

Appendix B. Assay Index of Official USP-NF Drugs

DRUG	ASSAY CATEGORY	ANALYTICAL WAVELENGTH AND/OR DETECTOR	INDICATOR OR INTERNAL STANDARD
Belladonna Leaf	VA1	TC-I	homatropine hydrobromide
Tincture	VA1	TC-I	homatropine hydrobromide
Bendroflumethiazide	IA1aiii		
Tablets	VB1b	UV-270	AV
Benoxinate Hydrochloride Ophthalmic Solution	IA1bii	308	Poten
Benzaldehyde	IIIB1		
Benzalkonium Chloride Solution	IA1ai		BpB
Benzethonium Chloride	IC1n		
Tincture	IC1n		
Topical Solution	IE1	BpB	BpB
Benzocaine	IIB		SPI
Cream	IE1		Poten
Gel	IC1j		Poten
Lozenges	IC1j		Poten
Ointment	VB1b	UV-294	Poten
Otic Solution	VB1b	UV-280	
Topical Aerosol	IC1j		
Topical Solution	IC1j		
and Menthol Topical Aerosol	IC1j		
Benzoic Acid and Salicylic Acid Ointment	VA1	FID	n-hexane
Benzoin	VB1b	UV-254	Phth
Benzonatate Capsules	VB1b	311, 275	Btb
Hydrous Benzoyl Peroxide	VIG	500	
Gel	IA2bi	UV-254	SPI
Lotion	IIIA4	UV-254	
Benztropine Mesylate Injection	IC11ii	UV-259	ethyl benzoate
Tablets	VB1b	UV-259	ethyl benzoate
Benzyl Alcohol	IA1a		MeR
Benzyl Benzoate	IA2bi		Phth
Lotion	IA2bi		Phth
Benzylpenicilloyl Polylysine Concentrate	IIIB2	282	Phth
Injection	IIIB2	282	

DRUG	ASSAY CATEGORY	ANALYTICAL WAVELENGTH AND/OR DETECTOR	INDICATOR OR INTERNAL STANDARD
Beta Carotene Capsules	IIIA3	455	
	IIIA4	452	
Betadex	VB1b	RI	CrV
Betaine Hydrochloride	IA1biii		
Betamethasone	VB1b	UV-240	propylparaben
Cream	VB1b	UV-240	propylparaben
Syrup	IIIA1	525	
Tablets	VB1b	UV-254	beclomethasone
Betamethasone Acetate	VB1b	UV-254	progesterone
Betamethasone Benzoate	VB1b	UV-254	betamethasone dipropionate
Gel	VB1b	UV-236	methyltestosterone
Betamethasone Dipropionate	VB1b	UV-254, 240	beclomethasone dipropionate
Topical Aerosol	VB1b	UV-254, 240	beclomethasone dipropionate
Cream	VB1b	UV-254, 240	beclomethasone dipropionate
Lotion	VB1b	UV-254, 240	beclomethasone dipropionate
Ointment	VB1b	UV-254, 240	beclomethasone dipropionate
Betamethasone Sodium Phosphate	VB1b	UV-254	beclomethasone dipropionate
Injection	VB1b	UV-254	beclomethasone dipropionate
and Betamethasone Acetate Suspension	VB1b	UV-254	butylparaben
and Betamethasone Acetate Injectable Suspension	VB1b	UV-254	methyltestosterone
Betamethasone Valerate	VB1b	UV-254	methyltestosterone
Cream	VB1b	UV-254	beclomethasone dipropionate
Lotion	VB1b	UV-254	beclomethasone dipropionate
Ointment	VB1b	UV-254	beclomethasone dipropionate
Betaxolol Hydrochloride Ophthalmic Solution	IA1bii	UV-280	Poten
Tablets	VB1b	UV-273	
Bethanechol Chloride	IA1biii		
Injection	IIB		
Tablets	IIIA4	590	CrV
Biotin	IA1b		
Biperiden	IA1bii		
Biperiden Hydrochloride Tablets	IA1biii		
Biperiden Lactate Injection	IIIA2	408	Phth
	IIIA2	408	CrV

DRUG	ASSAY CATEGORY	ANALYTICAL WAVELENGTH AND/OR DETECTOR	INDICATOR OR INTERNAL STANDARD
Butamben	IC1j	TC-I	SPI
Butane	VA1		
Butoconazole Nitrate	VB1b	UV-229	1-benzylimidazole
Nitrate Cream	VB1b	UV-225	CrV
Butorphanol Tartrate	IA1bii		
Injection	VB1b	UV-280	propylparaben
Butylated Hydroxyanisole	VA1	FID-I	4-tert-butylphenol
Butylparaben	IA2b		Poten
Caffeine	VB1b	UV-275	
and Sodium Benzoate Injection	IIA, IA1b		MeO
Calamine	IA2a		MeO
Calcifediol	VB1a	UV-254	testosterone
Capsules	VB1a	UV-254	testosterone
Calcium Acetate	ID1a		HNB
Tablets	ID1a		HNB
Calcium Ascorbate	ID1a		HNB
Calcium Carbonate	ID1a		HNB
Lozenges	IIF		
Tablets	ID1a		HNB
Oral Suspension	ID1a		HNB
and Magnesia Tablets	ID1a		HNB, EBT
and Magnesia and Simethicone Tablets	IIIF1		HNB
and Magnesium Carbonates Oral Suspension	ID1a	251.6, 422.7, 285.2	HNB, EBT
and Magnesium Carbonates Tablets	ID1a		HNB, EBT
Calcium with Vitamin D Tablets	VB1a	UV-265	
Calcium Chloride	ID1a		HNB
Calcium Citrate	ID1a		HNB
Calcium Glubionate Syrup	ID1a		HNB
Calcium Gluceptate	ID1a		HNB
Injection	ID1a		HNB
Calcium Gluconate	ID1a		HNB
Injection	ID1a		HNB
Tablets	ID1a		HNB
Calcium Hydroxide	IA1b		Phth
Topical Solution	ID1a		HNB
Calcium Lactate	ID1a		HNB
Tablets	ID1a		HNB
Calcium Lactobionate	ID1a		HNB
Calcium Levulinate	ID1a		HNB
Injection	ID1a		HNB
Calcium Pantothenate Tablets	VIII		
Dibasic Calcium Phosphate Tablets	ID1a		HNB
	ID1a		HNB
Tribasic Calcium Phosphate	ID1a		HNB
Calcium Saccharate	ID1a		HNB
Calcium Silicate	ID1a, IIC		HNB
Calcium Stearate	ID1a		HNB
Calcium Sulfate	ID1a		HNB
Calcium Undecylenate	IA2a		HNB
Camphor Spirit	iiB		MeO

DRUG	ASSAY CATEGORY	ANALYTICAL WAVELENGTH AND/OR DETECTOR	INDICATOR OR INTERNAL STANDARD
Bisacodyl	IA1bii		Nb
Rectal Suspension	VB1b	UV-254	
Suppositories	VB1b	UV-265	
Delayed Release Tablets	VB1b	UV-265	
Milk of Bismuth	IIC		
Bismuth Subcarbonate	D1a		XyO
Bismuth Subgallate	IIC		
Bismuth Subnitrate	ID1a		XyO
Bismuth Subsalicylate	ID1a, IIIA4	525	XyO
Bleomycin Sulfate	VIN1		
for Injection	VIN		
Boric Acid	IA1a		Phth
Bretylium Tosylate	IA1bii		CrV
Injection	VB1b	UV-220	
in Dextrose Injection	VB1B, IIC	UV-220	
Bromocriptine Mesylate	IA1bii		
Capsules	VB1b	UV-300	Poten
Tablets	VB1b	UV-300	
Bromodiphenhydramine Hydrochloride	IA1biii		CrV
Elixir	IA2a	262	MeR
Brompheniramine Maleate	IA1bii		CrV
Elixir	IA1bii		CrV
Injection	IIIB1	262	
Tablets	IIIB1	264	
and Pseudoephedrine Sulfate Syrup	VB1b	UV-254	naphazoline IIC1
Bumetanide	IA1a		PhR
Injection	VB1b	UV-254	ethylbenzaldehyde
Tablets	VB1b	UV-254	
Bupivacaine Hydrochloride and Epinephrine Injection	VB1b	UV-263, EC	dibutyl phthalate
Bupivacaine Hydrochloride in Dextrose Injection	IA1biii		CrV
Injection	VB1b	UV-263	dibutyl phthalate
	VB1b	UV-263	dibutyl phthalate
Buprenorphine Hydrochloride	IA1bii		CrV
Buspirone Hydrochloride	VB1b	UV-254	propylparaben
Tablets	VB1b	UV-254	
Busulfan	IA1ai		Phth
Tablets	IA1ai		Phth
Butabarbital	IIIB1	240	
Butabarbital Sodium	IIIB1	240	
Elixir	VA1	FID-I	secobarbital
Tablets	VA1	FID-I	secobarbital
Butalbital	VA1	FID-I	tetracosane
Acetaminophen, and Caffeine Capsules	VB1b	UV-254	
Acetaminophen, and Caffeine Tablets	VB1b	UV-216	phenacetin
Aspirin, and Caffeine Capsules	VB1b	UV-277, 210	
Aspirin Tablets	VB1b	UV-214	
Aspirin, and Caffeine Tablets	VB1b	UV-277, 210	
Aspirin, Caffeine, and Codeine Phosphate Capsules	VB1b	UV-277, 210	

Appendix B. Assay Index of Official USP-NF Drugs

DRUG	ASSAY CATEGORY	ANALYTICAL WAVELENGTH AND/OR DETECTOR	INDICATOR OR INTERNAL STANDARD
Capreomycin Sulfate for Injection	VIN		
Capsaicin	VIN		
Capsicum Oleoresin	VB1b	UV-281	
Captopril	VB1b	UV-280	
Tablets	IC1n		ST
and Hydrochlorothiazide Tablets	VB1b	UV-220	
Carbachol	VB1b	UV-210	
Intraocular Solution	IA1bii		CV
Ophthalmic Solution	IIIA5	590	
Carbachol	IIIA5	590	
Intraocular Solution	IA1biii		CrV
Ophthalmic Solution	IIIA5	590	
Carbamazepine	IIIA5	590	
Oral Suspension	VB1b	UV-230	
Tablets	VB1b	UV-254	
Carbamide Peroxide	IIIB1	285	
Topical Solution	IC2c		AM
Carbenicillin Disodium	IC1lii		ST
for Injection	VIN1		
Carbenicillin Indanyl Sodium	VIN1		
Tablets	VB1b	UV-210	
Carbidopa	VB1b	UV-210	
and Levodopa Tablets	VB1b	UV-280	
Carbinoxamine Maleate	VB1b	UV-280	
Tablets	IA1bii		CrV
Carbomer 934P	IA1bii		CrV
Carbon Dioxide	IA1a	RI	Poten
Carbon Monoxide C 11	VIA	RI	
Carboplatin	VIE	RI, UV-254	
Injection	VB1b	UV-230	
Carboxymethylcellulose Sodium	VB1b	UV-230	
Paste	IA1bii		Poten
Tablets	IA1bii		Poten
Carisoprodol	IA1bii		Poten
Tablets	IA2b		Phth
and Aspirin Tablets	VB1b	RI	
Aspirin and Codeine Phosphate Tablets	VB1b	RI	
Carrageenan	VB1b	RI, UV-254	
Carteolol Hydrochloride	None		
Ophthalmic Solution	VB1b	UV-252	
Tablets	VB1b	UV-252	
Casanthranol	VB1b	UV-252	
Cascara Sagrada Extract	IC1g, IIIA	515	
Cascara Sagrada	IIIA4	515	
Aromatic Fluidextract	IIIA4	515	
Tablets	IIA		
	IIIA4	515	
Castor Oil			
Aromatic	VA1	FID-I	bis(2-ethyl hexyl)-phthalate
Emulsion	VA1	FID-I	bis(2-ethyl hexyl)-phthalate
Cefaclor	VB1b	UV-265	
Capsules	VB1b	UV-265	
for Oral Suspension	VB1b	UV-265	
Cefadroxil	VB1b	UV-230	
Capsules	VB1b	UV-230	
for Oral Suspension	VB1b	UV-230	
Tablets	VB1b	UV-230	
Cefamandole Nafate	IVA2		
for Injection	IVA2		
Cefazolin Sodium	VB1b	UV-254	
Injection	VB1b	UV-254	
for Injection	VB1b	UV-254	
Cefixime	VB1b	UV-254	salicylic acid
for Oral Suspension	VB1b	UV-254	salicylic acid
Tablets	VB1b	UV-254	salicylic acid
Cefmenoxime for Injection	VB1b	UV-254	phthalimide
Hydrochloride	VB1b	UV-254	phthalimide
Cefmetazole	VB1b	UV-214	
Injection	VB1b	UV-214	
Cefmetazole Sodium	VB1b	UV-214	
for Injection	VB1b	UV-214	
Cefonicid Sodium	VB1b	UV-214	
for Injection	VB1b	UV-254	
Cefoperazone Sodium	VB1b	UV-254	
Injection	VB1b	UV-254	
for Injection	VB1b	UV-254	
Ceforanide	VB1b	UV-254	
for Injection	VB1b	UV-254	
Cefotaxime Sodium	VB1b	UV-235	
Injection	VB1b	UV-235	
for Injection	VB1b	UV-235	
Cefotiam Hydrochloride	VB1b	UV-254	
Injection	VB1b	UV-254	
for Injection	VB1b	UV-254	
Cefotetan	VB1b	UV-254	
Injection	VB1b	UV-254	
for Injection	VB1b	UV-254	
Cefotetan Disodium	VB1b	UV-254	
Cefoxitin	VB1b	UV-254	
Injection	VB1b	UV-254	
for Injection	VB1b	UV-254	
Cefpiramide for Injection	VIN3	480	
Cefprozil	VB1b	UV-254	
for Oral Suspension	VB1b	UV-280	
Tablets	VB1b	UV-280	

DRUG	ASSAY CATEGORY	AND/OR DETECTOR	ANALYTICAL WAVELENGTH INDICATOR OR INTERNAL STANDARD
Ceftazidime			
for Injection	VB1b	UV-254	
Injection	VB1b	UV-254	
Ceftizoxime Sodium	VB1b	UV-254	
Injection	VB1b	UV-254	salicylic acid
for Injection	VB1b	UV-254	salicylic acid
Ceftriaxone	VB1b	UV-254	salicylic acid
Injection	VB1b	UV-270	
for Injection	VB1b	UV-270	
Cefuroxime Injection	VB1b	UV-270	
for Injection	VB1b	UV-254	orcinol
Cefuroxime Axetil	VB1b	UV-254	orcinol
Tablets	VB1b	UV-278	acetanilide
Cefuroxime Sodium	VB1b	UV-278	acetanilide
Injection	VB1b	UV-254	orcinol
for Injection	VB1b	UV-254	orcinol
Microcrystalline Cellulose and Carboxymethyl-cellulose Sodium	IC1e	UV-254	orcinol
Oxidized Cellulose	IA1bii		Poten
Regenerated	IA1ai		
Powdered Cellulose	IA2b		
	IC1e		
Cephalexin	VB1b	UV-254	Phth
Capsules	VB1b	UV-254	Phth
for Oral Suspension	VB1b	UV-254	OP
Tablets	VB1b	UV-254	1-hydroxy-benzotriazole
Cephalexin Hydrochloride	VB1b	UV-254	1-hydroxy-benzotriazole
Cephalothin Sodium	VB1b	UV-254	1-hydroxy-benzotriazole
for Injection	VB1b	UV-254	1-hydroxy-benzotriazole
Injection	VB1b	UV-254	1-hydroxy-benzotriazole
Cephapirin Benzathine Intramammary Infusion	VIN	UV-254	
Cephapirin Sodium	VIN	UV-254	
for Injection	VB1b	UV-254	
Cephapirin Sodium Intramammary Infusion	VIN	UV-254	
Cephradine	VB1b	UV-254	
Capsules	VB1b	UV-254	
for Injection	VB1b	UV-254	
for Oral Suspension	VB1b	UV-254	
Tablets	VB1b	UV-254	
Cetostearyl Alcohol	VA1	FID-I	
Cetyl Alcohol	VA1	FID-I	
Cetylpyridinium Chloride	IE1	UV-254	BpB
Lozenges	IE2	UV-254	MeY
Topical Solution	IE1	UV-254	BpB
Activated Charcoal	VIK	UV-254	
Chloral Hydrate	IA2b		Phth
Capsules	IA2b		Phth
Syrup	IA2b		Phth
Chlorambucil	IA1a		Phth
Tablets	VB1b	UV-254	propylparaben

DRUG	ASSAY CATEGORY	WAVELENGTH AND/OR DETECTOR	ANALYTICAL INDICATOR OR INTERNAL STANDARD
Chloramphenicol	VB1b	UV-280	
Capsules	VB1b	UV-280	
Cream	VB1b	UV-280	
Injection	VIN1	UV-280	
Oral Solution	VB1b	UV-280	
Ophthalmic Ointment	VB1b	UV-280	
Ophthalmic Solution	VB1b	UV-280	
for Ophthalmic Solution	VB1b	UV-280	
Otic Solution	VB1b	UV-280	
Tablets	VB1b	UV-280	
and Hydrocortisone Acetate for Ophthalmic Suspension	VB1b	UV-280	
and Polymyxin B Sulfate Ophthalmic Ointment	VB1b	UV-280	
Polymyxin B Sulfate and Hydrocortisone Acetate Ophthalmic Ointment	VB1b	UV-280	
and Prednisolone Ophthalmic Ointment	VB1b	UV-280	
Chloramphenicol Palmitate	VB1b	UV-280	
Oral Suspension	VB1b	UV-280	
Chloramphenicol Sodium Succinate	IIIB1	276	
for Injection	VB1b	UV-275	sulfanilamide
Chlordiazepoxide	VB1b	UV-254	sulfanilamide
Tablets	VB1b	UV-254	sulfanilamide
and Amitriptyline Hydrochloride Tablets	VB1b	UV-254	sulfanilamide
Chlordiazepoxide Hydrochloride	VB1b	UV-254	sulfanilamide
Capsules	IIIB1	245	
for Injection	IA1bii		
and Clindinium Bromide Capsules	VB1b	UV-212	CrV
Chlorobutanol	IB2aii		
Chlorocresol	IC2f		
Chloroprocaine Hydrochloride	VB1b	UV-278	
Injection	VB1b	UV-278	
Chloroquine	IA1bii		
Chloroquine Hydrochloride	IIIB1	343	Poten
Injection	IIIB1	343	ST
Chloroquine Phosphate	IIIB1	343	CrV
Tablets	VB1b	UV-254	
Chlorothiazide	IIIB1	292	
Oral Suspension	VB1b	UV-254	
Tablets	IIIB1	292	
Chlorothiazide Sodium for Injection			
Chloroxylenol	VA1	FID-I	p-chlorophenol
Chlorpheniramine Maleate	IA1bii		CrV
Extended-release Capsules	VB1b	UV-261	
Injection	IIIB1	264	
Syrup	IIIB1	264	
Tablets	IIIB1	264	
and Pseudoephedrine Hydrochloride Oral Solution	VB1b	UV-261	

Appendix B. Assay Index of Official USP-NF Drugs

DRUG	ASSAY CATEGORY	ANALYTICAL WAVELENGTH AND/OR DETECTOR	INDICATOR OR INTERNAL STANDARD
Chlorpromazine	IA1bii		
Suppositories	IIIB1	254, 277	CrV
Chlorpromazine Hydrochloride	IA1bii		Poten
Injection	IIIB1	254, 277	
Oral Concentrate	IIIB1	277, 254	
Syrup	IIIB1	254, 277	
Tablets	IIIB1	254, 277	
Chlorpropamide	VB1b	UV-240	
Tablets	VB1b	UV-240	
Chlortetracycline Bisulfate and Sulfamethazine	VIN1		
Bisulfates Soluble Powder	VIN1, IC1j		
Chlortetracycline Hydrochloride	VIN1		
Ointment	VIN1		
Ophthalmic Ointment	VIN1		
Soluble Powder	VIN1		
Tablets	VIN1		
Chlorthalidone	VB1b	UV-254	2,7-naphthalenediol
Tablets	VB1b	UV-254	2,7-naphthalenediol
Chlorzoxazone	IIIB1	282	
Tablets	VB1b	UV-280	phenacetin
Cholecalciferol	VB1a	UV-254	
Solution	VB1b	UV-254	
Cholestyramine for Oral Suspension	IIIB2	318	
Sodium Chromate Cr51 Injection	IIIB1, VIE	370	
Chromic Chloride	IC1ii		
Injection	IIIF1	357.9	ST
Chymotrypsin	VIF		
for Ophthalmic Suspension	VIF		
Ciclopirox Olamine	IIIA4	440	
Cream	IIIA4	440	
Topical Suspension	IIIA4		
Cilastatin Sodium	IA1a		Poten
Cimetidine	VB1b	UV-220	
Tablets	VB1b	UV-220	
Injection	VB1b	UV-220	
in Sodium Chloride Injection	VB1b	UV-220	
Cimetidine Hydrochloride	VB1b	UV-220	
Cinoxacin	VB1b	UV-254	sulfanilic acid
Capsules	IIIB1	352	Phth
Cinoxate	IA2b		
Lotion	IIIB1	308	
Ciprofloxacin	VB1b	UV-278	
Injection	VB1b	UV-278	
Ophthalmic Solution	VB1b	UV-280	
Tablets	VB1b	UV-278	
Ciprofloxacin Hydrochloride	VB1b	UV-278	
Cisplatin	VB1b	UV-310	
for Injection	VB1b	UV-310	

DRUG	ASSAY CATEGORY	ANALYTICAL WAVELENGTH AND/OR DETECTOR	INDICATOR OR INTERNAL STANDARD
Citric Acid	IA1a		Phth
Magnesium Oxide and Sodium Carbonate Irrigation	VB1b, IIB, IIARI		
Clarithromycin	VB1b	UV-210	
for Oral Suspension	VB1b	UV-210	
Tablets	VB1b	UV-210	
Clavulanate Potassium	IA1bii	UV-220	Poten
Clemastine Fumarate Tablets	VB1b	UV-220	
Clidinium Bromide	IA1biii		Poten
Clindamycin Injection for Injection	VB1b	UV-210	
Clindamycin Hydrochloride	VB1b	UV-210	
Capsules	VB1b	UV-210	
Oral Solution	VB1b	UV-210	
Clindamycin Palmitate Hydrochloride	VA1	FID-I	cholesteryl benzoate
for Oral Solution	VA1	FID-I	cholesteryl benzoate
Clindamycin Phosphate	VB1b	UV-210	hydroxy acetophenone
Gel	VB1b	UV-210	
Injection	VA2	FID-I	hexacosane
for Injection	VA2	FID-I	hexacosane
Topical Solution	VB1b	UV-210	
Topical Suspension	VB1b	UV-210	
Vaginal Cream	VA1	FID-I	pyrene
Clioquinol	VA1	FID-I	pyrene
Cream	VA1	FID-I	pyrene
Ointment	IIIB1	267	
Compound Topical Powder and Hydrocortisone Cream	VA1, VB1b	FID, UV-254	pyrene
and Hydrocortisone Ointment	VA1, VB1b	FID, UV-254	pyrene
Clobetasole Propionate	VB1b	UV-240	beclomethasone dipropionate
Cream	VB1b	UV-240	beclomethasone dipropionate
Ointment	VB1b	UV-240	beclomethasone dipropionate
Topical Solution	VB1b	UV-240	beclomethasone dipropionate
Clocortolone Pivalate Cream	IIIA4	405	beclomethasone dipropionate
Clofazimine	IIIA4	390	
Capsules	IA1b		Poten
Clofibrate	IIIA1	491	
Capsules	IIIB1	226	
Clomiphene Citrate	IIIB1	226	
Tablets	VB1b	UV-233	
Clonazepam	VB1b	UV-233	
Tablets	VB1b	UV-254	
	VB1b	UV-254	

DRUG	ASSAY CATEGORY	ANALYTICAL WAVELENGTH AND/OR DETECTOR	INDICATOR OR INTERNAL STANDARD
Clonidine Hydrochloride	IA1bii		
Tablets	VB1b	UV-220	Poten
and Chlorthalidone Tablets	VB1b	UV-220	
Clorazepate Dipotassium	IA1bii		
Tablets	VB1b	UV-232	Poten
Clorsulon	VB1b	UV-254	
Clotrimazole	VB1b	UV-254	testosterone propionate
Cream	VB1b	UV-254	testosterone propionate
and Betamethasone Dipropionate Cream	VB1b	UV-254	progesterone
Lotion	VB1b	UV-254	testosterone
Lozenges	VB1b	UV-215	triphenylmethane
Topical Solution	VB1b	UV-254	testosterone propionate
Vaginal Tablets	VB1b	UV-254	testosterone propionate
Cloxacillin Benathine	VIN1		
Intramammary Infusion	VIN1	UV-225	
Cloxacillin Sodium	VB1b	UV-225	
Capsules	VB1b	UV-225	
for Oral Solution	VB1b		
Intramammary Infusion	VIN1		
Cyanocobalamin Co 57 Capsules	VIE		
Oral Solution	VIE		
Cocaine	IA1bii		CrV
Cocaine Hydrochloride	IA1biii		QR
Tablets for Topical Solution	IA2a		MeR
Cod Liver Oil	VIL		
Codeine	IA2a		Poten
Codeine Phosphate	IA1bii		MeR
Injection	IA1b		MeR
Codeine Sulfate	IA1bii		Poten
Tablets	IA2a		MeR
Colchicine	VB1b	UV-254	
Injection	VB1b	UV-254	
Tablets	VB1b	UV-254	
Colistimethate Sodium	VIN1		
for Injection	VIN1		
Colistin Sulfate	VIN1		
for Oral Suspension	VIN1		
and Neomycin Sulfate and Hydrocortisone Acetate Otic Suspension	VIN1, IIIA4	410	
Collodion	IIA		
Copper Gluconate	IC2f		ST
Corticotropin Injection	VIII		
for Injection	VIII		
Corticotropin Zinc Hydroxide Injectable Suspension	VIII		
Cortisone Acetate	VB1b	UV-254	methylparaben
Injectable Suspension	VB1b	UV-254	prednisone
Tablets	VB1b	UV-254	methylparaben
Creatinine	IA1c		
Cromolyn Sodium	IIIB1	326	
for Inhalation	IIIB1	326	
Inhalation Solution	IIIB1	326	
Nasal Solution	IIb1	326	
Crotamiton	IIIB1	242	
Cream	VB1b	UV-254	butyl benzoate
Cupric Chloride	IC1ii	324.8	ST
Injection	IIIF1		
Cupric Sulfate	IC1ii	324.8	ST
Injection	IIIF1		
Cyanocobalamin	IIIB1	361	
Injection	IIIB1	361	
Cyclizine Hydrochloride	IA1bii		Poten
Tablets	IIIB1	264	Poten
Cyclobenzaprine Hydrochloride	IA1bii		
Tablets	VB1b	UV-290	
Cyclomethicone	VA1	TC	
Cyclopentolate Hydrochloride	VB1b	UV-220	
Ophthalmic Solution	VB1b	UV-220	
Cyclophosphamide	VB1b	UV-195	ethylparaben
for Injection	VB1b	UV-195	ethylparaben
Tablets	VB1b	UV-195	ethylparaben
Cyclopropane	VIA		
Cycloserine	VIN1		
Capsules	VIN1		
Cyclosporine	VB1b	UV-210	
Capsules	VB1b	UV-210	
Injection	VB1b	UV-210	
Oral Solution	VB1b	UV-210	
Cyproheptadine Hydrochloride	IA1biii		CrV
Syrup	VB1b	UV-285	
Tablets	VB1b	UV-285	
Cysteine Hydrochloride	IC1ii		ST
Injection	IVA1		
Cytarabine	VB1b	UV-254	
for Injection	VB1b	UV-254	
Dacarbazine	IIIB1	323, 329	
for Injection	IIIB1	323	
Dactinomycin	VB1b	UV-254	
for Injection	VB1b	UV-254	
Danazol	IIIB1	285	
Capsules	VB1b	UV-270	
Dapsone	VB1a	UV-254	2-naphthalene-sulfonic acid
Tablets	VB1a	UV-254	2-naphthalene-sulfonic acid
Daunorubicin Hydrochloride	VB1b	UV-254	
for Injection	VB1b	UV-254	CrV
Decoquinate	IAbii	265	
Premix	IIIB1	485	
Deferoxamine Mesylate	IIIA4	485	
for Injection	IIIA4	485	

Appendix B. Assay Index of Official USP-NF Drugs

DRUG	ASSAY CATEGORY	ANALYTICAL WAVELENGTH AND/OR DETECTOR	INDICATOR OR INTERNAL STANDARD
Dehydrocholic Acid	IA1a		Phth
Tablets	IA1a		Phth
Demecarium Bromide			
Ophthalmic Solution	IA1bii		CrV
Demeclocycline	IIIB1	292	
Oral Suspension	VIN1		
Demeclocycline Hydrochloride	VIN1		
Capsules	VIN1		
Tablets	VIN1		
Denatonium Benzoate	IA1bii		CrV
Desflurane	VA1	FID	halothane
Desipramine Hydrochloride			
Tablets	IA1biii	255	Poten
Deslanoside	IIIB1		
Injection	IIIA1		FC
Desoximetasone	IIIA1		FC
Cream	VB1b	UV-254	ethylparaben
Gel	VB1b	UV-254	
Ointment	VB1b	UV-254	
Desoxycorticosterone Acetate	IIIA1	525	
Injection	IIIA1	525	
Pellets	IIIA1	525	
Desoxycorticosterone Pivalate	VB1b	UV-254	desoxycorticosterone
Injectable Suspension	VB1b	UV-254	desoxycorticosterone
Dexamethasone	IIIA1	525	
Topical Aerosol	VB1b	UV-254	
Elixir	IIIA1	525	
Gel	IIIA1	525	
Ophthalmic Suspension	VB1b	UV-254	
Oral Solution	VB1b	UV-254	
Tablets	VB1b	UV-254	
Dexamethasone Acetate	VB1b	UV-254	
Injectable Suspension	VB1b	UV-254	
Dexamethasone Sodium	VB1b	UV-254	CrV
Phosphate			
Inhalation Aerosol	IIIB1	239	
Cream	VB1b	UV-254	
Injection	VB1b	UV-254	
Ophthalmic Ointment	VB1b	UV-254	
Ophthalmic Solution	VB1b	UV-254	
Dexbrompheniramine Maleate	IA1bii	UV-254	CrV
and Pseudoephedrine Sulfate			
Oral Solution	VB1b		
Dexchlorpheniramine Maleate	IA1bii		CrV
Syrup	IIIB1	264	
Tablets	IIIB1	264	
Dexpanthenol	IA2aiv		CrV
Preparation	IA2aiv		CrV
Dextroamphetamine Sulfate	IA1bii		Poten
Capsules	VB1b	UV-254	
Elixir	IIIB1	257, 280	
Tablets	VB1b	UV-254	
Dextromethorphan	IA1bii		
Dextromethorphan Hydrobromide	VB1b	UV-280	
Syrup	VB1b	UV-280	
Dextrose Injection	VIC1		
and Sodium Chloride Injection	VIC1, IB1a		DCF
Diatrizoate Meglumine	IB1a		TBP
Capsules	IB1a		TBP
Tablets	IB1a		TBP
Injection	VIC1, IB1a		
and Diatrizoate Sodium			
Injection	IC1iii, IB1a		ST, TBP
and Diatrizoate Sodium			
Solution	IB1a		TBP
Diatrizoate Sodium	IB1a		TBP
Injection	IB1a		TBP
Solution	IB1a		TBP
Diatrizoic Acid	IA1bii		Poten
Diazepam	VB1b	UV-254	ethylparaben
Capsules	VB1b	UV-254	ethylparaben
Capsules, Extended-Release	VB1b	UV-254	tolualdehyde
Injection	VB1b	UV-254	ethylparaben
Tablets	VB1b	UV-254	hydrochlorothiazide
Diazoxide	VB1b	UV-254	hydrochlorothiazide
Capsules	VB1b	UV-254	hydrochlorothiazide
Injection	VB1b	UV-254	hydrochlorothiazide
Oral Suspension	IA1bii	UV-280	CrV
Dibucaine	IIIB1	247	
Cream	IIIB1	247	
Ointment	IA1biii	247	CrV
Dibucaine Hydrochloride	IIIB1		
Injection	VA1	FID-NI	
Dibutyl Sebacate	IAb, IC2a		
Dichloralphenazone	VA1	FID	ST
Dichlorodifluoromethane	VA1	FID	
Dichlorotetrafluoroethane	VB1b	UV-280	
Dichlorphenamide	IVA1		
Tablets	IA1bii		Poten
Diclofenac Sodium	IIIB1		
Delayed-release Tablets	VB1b	UV-254	
Dicloxacillin Sodium	VB1b	UV-225	
Capsules	VB1b	UV-225	
for Oral Suspension	VIN1		
Dicyclomine Hydrochloride	IA1biii		CrV
Capsules	VA1	FID	phenacetin
Injection	VA1	FID	phenacetin
Syrup	VA1	FID	phenacetin
Tablets	VA1	FID	phenacetin
Dienestrol	VB1b	UV-254	methyltestosterone
Cream	VB1b	UV-254	methyltestosterone
Diethanolamine	IA1b		BcG

DRUG	ASSAY CATEGORY	ANALYTICAL WAVELENGTH AND/OR DETECTOR	INDICATOR OR INTERNAL STANDARD
Diethylcarbamazine Citrate	IA1bii		Nb
Tablets	IA1bii		TB
Diethylphthalate	IA2b		Phth
Diethylpropion Hydrochloride	VB1b	UV-254	
Tablets	VB1b	UV-254	
Diethylstilbestrol	VB1b	UV-254	
Injection	IIIA4	418	
Tablets	VB1b	UV-254	
Diethylstilbestrol Diphosphate	IIIB1	241	
Injection	IIIB1	241	
Diethyltoluamide	IIIC1	14.1	
Topical Solution	IIIC1	14.1	
Diflorasone Diacetate	VB1b	UV-254	isoflupredone acetate
Cream	VB1b	UV-254	isoflupredone acetate
Ointment	VB1b	UV-254	isoflupredone acetate
Diflunisal	VB1b	UV-254	
Tablets	VB1b	UV-254	
Digitalis	VIH		
Powdered	VIH		
Capsules	VIH		
Tablets	VIH		
Digitoxin	VB1b	UV-218	
Injection	VB1b	UV-218	
Tablets	VB1b	UV-218	
Digoxin	VB1b	UV-218	
Elixir	VB1b	UV-218	
Injection	VB1b	UV-218	
Tablets	VB1b	UV-280	
Dihydrocodeine Bitartrate	IIIA4	585	
Dihydroergotamine Mesylate	IIIA4	585	
Injection	VIN1		
Dihydrostreptomycin Sulfate	VIN1		
Boluses	VIN1	UV-254	
Injection	VIN1	UV-254	
Dihydrotachysterol	VB1b	UV-254	
Capsules	VB1b	UV-254	
Oral Solution	VB1b	UV-254	
Tablets	VB1b	UV-254	
Dihydroxyacetone	IC1M		
Dihydroxyaluminum Aminoacetate	ID2a		ST
Magma	ID2a		DT
Dihydroxyaluminum Sodium Carbonate	ID2a		DT
Tablets	ID2a		DT
Diltiazem Hydrochloride	VB1b	UV-240	
Extended-release Capsules	VB1b	UV-240	
Tablets	VB1b	UV-240	
Dimenhydrinate	IA1bii, IB2aii		Poten, FAS
Injection	VB1b	UV-254	2-hydroxy benzyl alcohol
Syrup	VB1b	UV-254	2-hydroxy benzyl alcohol
Tablets	VB1b	UV-254	2-hydroxy benzyl alcohol

DRUG	ASSAY CATEGORY	ANALYTICAL WAVELENGTH AND/OR DETECTOR	INDICATOR OR INTERNAL STANDARD
Dimercaprol	IC1k		
Injection	IC1k		
Dimethicone	IIIC1		
Dimethyl Sulfoxide	None		
Gel	VA1	FID	dimethylformamide
Irrigation	VA1	FID-P	dimethylformamide
Topical Solution	VA1	FID	dimethylformamide
Dioxybenzone	IIIA3	325	
and Oxybenzone Cream	VC1b		
Diphenhydramine Citrate	IA1bii		Poten
Diphenhydramine Hydrochloride	VB1b	UV-254	
Capsules	VB1b	UV-254	
Elixir	VB1b	UV-254	
Injection	VB1b	UV-254	Poten
and Pseudoephedrine Capsules	VB1b	UV-254	Poten, homatropine hydrobromide
Diphenoxylate Hydrochloride	IA1biii	FID-I	
and Atropine Sulfate Oral Solution	IA1biii, VA1		
and Atropine Sulfate Tablets	VB1b	UV-206, 254	
Dipivefrin Hydrochloride	VB1b	UV-254	
Ophthalmic Solution	VB1b	UV-254	
Dipyridamole	IA1bii		Poten
Tablets	VB1b	UV-288	
Dirithromycin	VB1b	UV-205	
Delayed-Release Tablets	VB1b	UV-205	
Disopyramide Phosphate	IA1bii		Poten
Capsules	IIIB1	268	
Capsules, Extended-Release	IIIB2	261	
Disulfiram	VB1b	UV-250	
Tablets	VB1b	UV-250	
Dobutamine Hydrochloride	VB1b	UV-280	
Injection	VA2	FID-I	n-tricontance
for Injection	VB1b	UV-280	
Docusate Calcium	IE3		BpB
Capsules	IIIA2	545	
Docusate Potassium	IE3		BpB
Capsules	VB1b	RI	
Docusate Sodium	IE3	RI	BpB
Capsules	VB1b	UV-214	
Solution	VB1b	UV-214	
Syrup	IIIA2	650	
Tablets	VB1b	UV-210	
Dopamine Hydrochloride	IA1biii		Poten
Injection	VB1b	UV-280	
and Dextrose Injection	VB1b	UV-280, RI	
Doxapram Hydrochloride	IA1biii		CrV
Injection	VB1b	UV-225	diphenylhydramine
Doxepin Hydrochloride	VB1b	UV-254	
Capsules	VB1b	UV-254	
Oral Solution	IIIB1	292	
Doxorubicin Hydrochloride	VB1b	UV-254	2-naphthalene-sulfonic acid
Injection	VB1b	UV-280	2-naphthalene-sulfonic acid
for Injection	VB1b	UV-254	2-naphthalene-sulfonic acid

Appendix B. Assay Index of Official USP-NF Drugs

DRUG	ASSAY CATEGORY	ANALYTICAL WAVELENGTH AND/OR DETECTOR	INDICATOR OR INTERNAL STANDARD
Doxycycline	VB1b	UV-270	
Capsules	VB1b	UV-270	
for Injection	VB1b	UV-270	
for Oral Suspension	VB1b	UV-270	
Doxycycline Calcium Oral Suspension	VB1b	UV-270	
Doxycycline Hyclate	VB1b	UV-270	
Capsules	VB1b	UV-270	
Capsules, Delayed-Release	VB1b	UV-280	
for Injection	VB1b	UV-280	
Tablets	VB1b	UV-280	
Doxylamine Succinate	IA1bii		CrV
Syrup	IIIB1		
Tablets	VB1b	262	
Dronabinol	VB1b	UV-262	
Capsules	VB1b	UV-228	
Droperidol	IA1bii	UV-228	Nb
Injection	VB1b	UV-280	
Absorbable Dusting Powder	ID1a		EBT
Dyclonine Hydrochloride	VB1b	UV-254	
Gel	VB1b	UV-254	
Topical Solution	VB1b	UV-254	
Dydrogesterone	VB1b	UV-280	
Tablets	VB1b	UV-280	
Dyphylline	IA1bii		SD
Elixir	VB1b	UV-254	
Injection	VB1b	UV-254	
Tablets	VB1b	UV-254	
and Guaifenesin Elixir	VB1b	UV-230	
and Guaifenesin Tablets	VB1b	UV-230	
Echothiophate Iodide	IC1k		Poten
for Ophthalmic Solution	IC1k		Poten
Econazole Nitrate	IA1bii		Poten
Edetate Calcium Disodium	ID1b		DC
Injection	ID1b		DC
Edetate Disodium	ID1a		HNB
Injection	ID1a		HNB
Edetic Acid	ID1a		HNB
Edrophonium Chloride	IA1biii		CrV
Injection	IIIB1	273	
Multiple Electrolytes Injection Type 1	VIO		
Multiple Electrolytes Injection Type 2	VIO		
Multiple Electrolytes and Dextrose Injection Type 1	VIO		
Multiple Electrolytes and Dextrose Injection Type 2	VIO		
Multiple Electrolytes and Dextrose Injection Type 3	VIO		

DRUG	ASSAY CATEGORY	ANALYTICAL WAVELENGTH AND/OR DETECTOR	INDICATOR OR INTERNAL STANDARD
Multiple Electrolytes and Dextrose Injection Type 4	VIO		
Multiple Electrolytes and Invert Sugar Injection Type 1	VIO		
Multiple Electrolytes and Invert Sugar Injection Type 2	VIO		
Multiple Electrolytes and Invert Sugar Injection Type 3	VIO		
Trace Elements Injection	IIIF1, IC1lii, VB1b 213.8, 357.9, 279, ST	UV-226	
Emetine Hydrochloride	IA1bii		
Injection	IA2a		
Enalapril Maleate	VB1b	UV-210	CrV
Tablets	VB1b	UV-215	MeR
and Hydrochlorothiazide Tablets	VB1b	UV 215, 310	
Enalaprilat	VB1b	UV-210	
Enflurane	VA1	TC-P	
Ephedrine	IA2a		MeR
Ephedrine Hydrochloride	IA1biii		CrV
Ephedrine Sulfate	IA1bii		MeR
Capsules	IIIB2	242	
Injection	IA1bii	242	MeR
Nasal Solution	IIIB2	242	
Syrup	IIIB2	242	
Epinephrine	IA1bii		CrV
Inhalation Solution	VIC2		
Inhalation Aerosol	VIC2		
Injection	VB1b	UV-280	
Nasal Solution	VIC2		
Ophthalmic Solution	IIIB1	280	CrV
Epinephrine Bitartrate	IA1bii		
Inhalation Aerosol	IIIA4	530	
for Ophthalmic Solution	VIC2		
Ophthalmic Solution	VB1b	UV-280	
Epinephryl Borate Ophthalmic Solution	VIC2		
Epitetracycline Hydrochloride	VIN1	UV-280	phenol
Equilin	VB1b	UV-254	
Ergocalciferol	VB1a	UV-254	
Capsules	VB1a	UV-254	
Oral Solution	VIL		
Tablets	VB1b	UV-280	
Ergoloid Mesylates	VB1b	UV-280	
Capsules	VB1b	UV-280	m-chloroacetamilide
Oral Solution	VB1b	UV-280	papaverine HCl
Tablets	VB1b	UV-280	

DRUG	ASSAY CATEGORY	ANALYTICAL WAVELENGTH AND/OR DETECTOR	INDICATOR OR INTERNAL STANDARD
Ergonovine Maleate	IIIA4	550	
Injection	VB1b	UV-312	
Tablets	VB1b	UV-312	
Ergotamine Tartrate	IA1bii		CrV
Inhalation Aerosol	IIIA4	546	
Injection	IIIA4	545	
Tablets	VB1b	UV-254	ergonovine maleate
and Caffeine Suppositories	VB1b	UV-244, F-239	
and Caffeine Tablets	VB1b	UV-254, F-325	
Erythromycin	VB1b	UV-215	
Capsules, Delayed-Release	VIN1		
Intramammary Infusion	VIN1		
Injection	VIN1		
Ointment	VIN1		
Ophthalmic Ointment	VIN1		
Pledgets	VIN1		
Tablets	VIN1		
Tablets, Delayed-Release	VIN1		
Topical Gel	VIN1		
Topical Solution	VIN1		
Sterile Lactobionate	VIN1		
and Benzoyl Peroxide Topical Gel	VIN1, VB1b	UV-254	ethyl benzoate
Erythromycin Estolate	VIN1		
Capsules	VIN1		
Oral Suspension	VIN1		
Tablets	VIN1		
and Sulfisoxazole Acetyl Oral Suspension	VIN1, VB1b	UV-254	benzanilide
Erythromycin Ethylsuccinate	VIN1		
Injection	VIN1		
Sterile	VIN1		
Oral Suspension	VIN1		
for Oral Suspension	VIN1		
Tablets	VIN1		
and Sulfisoxazoleacetyl for Oral Suspension	VIN1, VB1b	UV-254	benzanilide
Sterile Erythromycin Gluceptate	VIN1		
Erythromycin Lactobionate for Injection	VIN1		
Sterile Erythromycin Lactobionate	VIN1		
Erythromycin Stearate	VIN1		
Tablets	VIN1		
Estradiol	VB1b	UV-205	ethylparaben
Pellets	VA2	FID-I	dotriacontane
Injectable Suspension	IIIA4	520	
Tablets	VB1b	UV-205	ethylparaben
Vaginal Cream	VB1b	UV-280	dydrogesterone
Estradiol Cypionate	VB1b	UV-280	testosterone benzoate
Injection	VB1b	UV-280	testosterone benzoate
Estradiol Valerate	VB1b	UV-280	testosterone benzoate
Injection	VB1b	UV-280	testosterone benzoate
Estriol	IIIB1	281	

DRUG	ASSAY CATEGORY	ANALYTICAL WAVELENGTH AND/OR DETECTOR	INDICATOR OR INTERNAL STANDARD
Conjugated Estrogens			
Tablets	VA2	FID-I	3-o-methylestrone
Esterified Estrogens	VA2	FID-I	testosterone
Tablets	IIIA4	635, 515	
Estrone	IIIA4	635, 515	
Injection	VB1b	UV-280	
Injectable Suspension	IIA		
Estropipate	VB1b	UV-268	p-nitroacetophenone
Tablets	VB1b	UV-213	p-nitroacetophenone
Vaginal Cream	VB1b	UV-213	p-nitroacetophenone
Ethacrynate Sodium for Injection	VB1b	UV-254	
Ethacrynic Acid	VB1b	UV-254	
Tablets	IVA1		
Ethambutol Hydrochloride	IA1biii		CrV
Tablets	IA1biii		CrV
Ethchlorvynol	VA1	TC-I	MRB
Capsules	IA1ai		
Ethinyl Estradiol	VB1b	UV-280	ethylparaben
Tablets	VB1b	UV-280	ethylparaben
Topical Gel	IC1ii		ST
Ethiodized Oil Injection	IIIB1	290	
Ethionamide	IIIB1	290	
Tablets	VB1b	UV-268	
Ethopabate	IA1aiii		AV
Ethosuximide	VB1b	UV-225	
Capsules	VB1b	UV-210	
Ethotoin	VB1b	UV-254	
Tablets	IA2b		ethylparaben
Ethyl Acetate	IA2b		Phth
Ethyl Chloride	None		Phth
Ethyl Oleate	IA1aiii		
Ethyl Vanillin	IC1ii		
Ethylcellulose	IC11		
Aqueous Dispersion	IA1b		TB
Ethylenediamine	IA2b		ST
Ethylparaben	VB1b	UV-200	
Ethynodiol Diacetate and Ethinyl Estradiol Tablets	VB1b	UV-210	BpB
and Mestranol Tablets	VB1b	UV-204	BtB
Etidronate Disodium	ID1b		
Tablets	ID1b		
Etodolac	IA1aiii		XyO
Tablets	VB1b	UV-274	XyO
Etoposide	VB1b	UV-254	Poten
Capsules	VB1b	UV-254	
Injection	VB1b	UV-254	
Eucalyptol	VA1	FID	
Eucatropine Hydrochloride Ophthalmic Solution	IA2a	242	MeR
Eugenol	IIIB2		
Famotidine	None		
Tablets	IAbii		Poten
Fenoprofen Calcium	VB1b	UV-272	
Capsules	VB1b	UV-272	
Tablets	VB1b	UV-272	

Appendix B. Assay Index of Official USP-NF Drugs

DRUG	ASSAY CATEGORY	ANALYTICAL WAVELENGTH AND/OR DETECTOR	INDICATOR OR INTERNAL STANDARD
Fentanyl Citrate			
Injection	IA1bii		Nb
Ferric Oxide	VB1b	UV-230	
Ferrous Fumarate	IIC		
Tablets	IC1a		Op
and Docusate Sodium	IC1ii		ST
Extended-release Tablets	IIIF1, VB1b	248.3, UV-214	
Ferrous Gluconate	IC1a		
Capsules	IIIA4	522	Op
Elixir	IC1a		
Tablets	IIIA4	522	Op
Ferrous Sulfate	IC1a		Op
Oral Solution	IC1a		Op
Syrup	IC1a		Op
Tablets	IC1a		Op
Dried	IC1a		Op
Flecainide Acetate	IA1aiii		
Tablets	VB1b	UV-254	Poten
Floxuridine	IA1a		
for Injection	IIIB1	268	Poten
Flucytosine	IA1bii		
Capsules	IIIB1	285	Poten
Injection	IIIA1	525	
Fludrocortisone Acetate	VB1b	UV-254	
Tablets	IIIA1	520	norethindrone
Flumethasone Pivalate	IIIB2	390	
Cream	VB1b	UV-254	
Flunisolide	VB1b	UV-254	norethindrone
Nasal Solution	VB1b	UV-254	
Flunixin Meglumine	IAbii		
Granules	IIIA3	283	
Injection	IIIA3	327	Poten
Paste	VB1b	UV-254	sodium benzoate
Fluocinolone Acetonide	VB1b	UV-254	norethindrone
Cream	VB1b	UV-254	norethindrone
Ointment	VB1b	UV-254	norethindrone
Topical Solution	VB1b	UV-254	norethindrone
Fluocinonide	VB1b	UV-254	norethindrone
Cream	VB1b	UV-254	
Gel	VB1b	UV-254	
Ointment	VB1b	UV-254	
Topical Solution	VB1b	UV-254	
Fluorescein	VA1	FID-P	
Injection	IIIE1	515	
Fluorescein Sodium	IIIE1	515	
Ophthalmic Strips	IIIE1	515	
and Benoxinate Hydrochloride Ophthalmic Solution	IIIE1, VB1b	515, UV-254	isopropyl alcohol
and Proparacaine Hydrochloride Ophthalmic Solution	IIIE1, VB1b	515, UV-270	
Fluorodopa F 18 Injection	VIE	UV-254	
Fluorometholone	VB1b	UV-254	
Cream	VB1b	UV-254	fluoxymesterone
Ophthalmic Suspension	VB1b	UV-254	
Fluorouracil	VB1b	UV-254	TB
Cream	VB1b	UV-254	
Injection	VB1b	UV-254	
Topical Solution	VB1b	UV-254	
Fluoxetine Hydrochloride	VB1b	UV-227	
Capsules	VB1b	UV-227	
Fluoxymesterone	VB1b	UV-254	methylprednisolone
Tablets	VB1b	UV-254	methylprednisolone
Fluphenazine Decanoate	IAbiii		CV
Injection	VB1b	UV-254	
Fluphenazine Enanthate	IA1bii	UV-254	CrV
Injection	IA1bii		CrV
Fluphenazine Hydrochloride	VB1b	UV-254	
Elixir	VB1b	UV-254	
Injection	IIIA4	485	
Oral Solution	IIIA4	485	
Tablets	VB1b	UV-254	
Flurandrenolide	VB1b	UV-240	prednisone
Lotion	VB1b	UV-240	testosterone
Tape	VB1b	UV-240	testosterone
Flurazepam Hydrochloride	IA1biii	UV-239	Poten
Capsules	VB1b	UV-239	
Flurbiprofen	IA1a	UV-254	Phth
Tablets	VB1b	UV-254	
Flurbiprofen Sodium	VB1b	UV-280	
Ophthalmic Solution	VB1b	UV-280	
Flutamide	VB1b	UV-240	
Capsules	VB1b	UV-254	testosterone
Folic Acid	VB1b	UV-280	
Injection	VIL		
Tablets	VIL		
Formaldehyde Solution	IA2b		BtB
Fructose	VIC1		
Injection	VIC1		
and Sodium Chloride Injection	VIC1, IB1a		
Basic Fuchsin	IC1f		DCF
Fumaric Acid	IA1a		
Furazolidone	IIIB1	367	
Oral Suspension	IIIB1	367	
Tablets	IIIB1	367	
Furosemide	IA1a		
Injection	VB1b	UV-254	Phth
Tablets	VB1b	UV-254	
Gadopentetate Dimeglumine	VB1b	UV-195	
Injection			

DRUG	ASSAY CATEGORY	ANALYTICAL WAVELENGTH AND/OR DETECTOR	INDICATOR OR INTERNAL STANDARD
Gallamine Triethiodide			
Injection	VB1b	UV-200	
Gallium Citrate Ga 67	VB1b	UV-200	
Injection	VIE		
Absorbent Gauze	None		
Petrolatum Gauze	None		
Gelatin	None		
Absorbable Film	None		
Absorbable Sponge	None		
Gemfibrozil			
Capsules	VB1b	UV-276	
Tablets	VB1b	UV-276	
Gentamicin Uterine Infusion	VIN1		
Gentamicin Sulfate	VIN1		
Cream	VIN1		
Injection	VIN1		
Ointment	VIN1		
Ophthalmic Ointment	VIN1		
Ophthalmic Solution	VIN1		
and Betamethasone Acetate			
Ophthalmic Solution	VB1b	UV-254	o-phenylphenol
and Betamethasone			
Valerate Ointment	VIN1, VB1b	UV-254	beclomethasone diproprionate
and Betamethasone			
Valerate Otic Solution	VIN1, VB1b	UV-254	beclomethasone diproprionate
and Betamethasone Valerate			
Topical Solution	VIN1, VB1b	UV-254	beclomethasone diproprionate
and Prednisolone Acetate			
Ophthalmic Suspension	VIN1, VB1b	UV-254	fluorometholone acetate
and Prednisolone Acetate			
Ophthalmic Ointment	VIN1, VB1b		
Gentian Violet	IC2d		FAS
Cream	IIIA3	435	FAS
Topical Solution	IC2d		
Pharmaceutical Glaze	IIA		
Glipizide	VB1b	UV-225	
Tablets	VB1b	UV-225	
Glucagon for Injection	VIH		
Gluconalactone	IA2bii		Phth
Glutaral Concentrate	IA2b		BpB
Glyburide	VB1b	UV-254	
Tablets	VB1b	UV-254	progesterone
Glycerin	IC1liii		ST
Ophthalmic Solution	IC1m		ST
Oral Solution	IC1m		ST
Suppositories	IC1m		
Glyceryl Behenate	None		
Glyceryl Monostearate	VA2	FID-I	hexadecyl hexadecanoate
Glycine	IA1bii		CrV
Irrigation	IA1a		Phth, TB
Glycopyrrolate	IA1biii		CrV
Injection	VB1b	UV-222	
Tablets	IIIA2	410	

DRUG	ASSAY CATEGORY	ANALYTICAL WAVELENGTH AND/OR DETECTOR	INDICATOR OR INTERNAL STANDARD
Gold Sodium Thiomalate	IIC		
Injection	IIC		
Gonadorelin Hydrochloride	VB1b, Ib1a	UV-220	Poten
Gonadorelin for Injection	VB1b	UV-220	
Chorionic Gonadotropin			
for Injection	VIH		
Gramicidin	VIH		
Griseofulvin	VIN1		
Capsules	VB1b	UV-254	3-phenylphenol
Oral Suspension	VB1b	UV-254	3-phenylphenol
Tablets	VB1b	UV-254	3-phenylphenol
Ultramicrosize Tablets	VB1b	UV-254	3-phenylphenol
Guaifenesin	VB1b	UV-276	3-phenylphenol
Capsules	VB1b	UV-276	
for Injection	IIIA1	276	
Syrup	VB1b	UV-276	benzoic acid
Tablets	VB1b	UV-276	hydrocodone bitartrate
and Codeine Phosphate Syrup	VA1	FID-I	benzoic acid, dextromethorphan HCl
and Pseudoephedrine			
Hydrochloride Capsules	VB1b	UV-263, 276	benzoic acid, dextromethorphan HCl
Pseudoephedrine Hydrochloride,			
and Dextromethorphan			
Hydrobromide Capsules	VB1b	UV-263, 276	
Guanabenz Acetate	IAbii		Poten
Tablets	VB1b	UV-254	ethylparaben
Guanadrel Sulfate	VB1b	RI	ethylparaben
Tablets	VB1b	Ri	
Guanethidine Monosulfate	IIIA4	500	
Tablets	IIIA4	412	butylparaben
Guanfacine Hydrochloride	VB1b	UV-220	
Tablets	VB1b	UV-220	
Halazone	IC1lii		ST
Tablets for Solution	IC1lii		ST
Halcinonide	IIIB1		
Cream	VB1b	239	progesterone
Ointment	VB1b	UV-254	butylparaben
Topical Solution	IA1bii	UV-254	progesterone
Haloperidol	IIIB1		
Injection	IIIB1	245	Nb
Oral Solution	VB1b	245	
Tablets	VA1	UV-254	
Helium	VIH, IB1a	TC-I	
Heparin Lock Flush Solution	VIH		PC
Heparin Calcium	VIH		
Injection	VIH		
Heparin Sodium	IA1a		
Injection	IIIB1		
Hexachlorophene	IIIB1		Poten
Cleansing Emulsion	IC2c	299	
Liquid Soap	VB1b	299	
Hexylresorcinol	IA1a	UV-280	ST
Lozenges	IIIA4		hexaphenone
Histamine Phosphate			
Injection	IA1a	460	TP
Tablets	IIIA4		

Appendix B. Assay Index of Official USP-NF Drugs

DRUG	ASSAY CATEGORY	ANALYTICAL WAVELENGTH AND/OR DETECTOR	INDICATOR OR INTERNAL STANDARD
Histidine Hydrobromide	IA1bii		
Homatropine Hydrobromide	IC1a		Poten
Ophthalmic Solution	IIIB2	242	Np
Homatropine Methylbromide	IA1biii		
Tablets	IIIA4	525	CrV
Homosalate	VA1	FID-P	
Hyaluronidase Injection	VIF		
for Injection	VIF		
Hydralazine Hydrochloride	VB1b	UV-230	
Injection	IC1n		
Tablets	VB1b	UV-230	
Hydrochloric Acid	IA1a		
Diluted	IA1a		
Hydrochlorothiazide	VB1b	UV-254	MeR
Tablets	VB1b	UV-254	MeR
Hydrocodone Bitartrate	VB1b	UV-280	
Tablets	IA1bii		
and Acetaminophen Tablets	VB1b	UV-280	Poten
Hydrocortisone	VB1b	UV-254	prednisone
Cream	VB1b	UV-254	
Enema	VB1b	UV-254	
Gel	VB1b	UV-254	acetaminophen
Lotion	VB1b	UV-254	
Ointment	VB1b	UV-254	
Injectable Suspension	IIIA1	525	
Tablets	VB1b	UV-254	prednisone
and Acetic Acid Otic Solution	VB1b, VA1	UV-254, FID-P	anisole
Hydrocortisone Acetate	VB1b	UV-254	
Cream	VB1b	UV-254	
Lotion	VB1b	UV-254	
Ointment	IIIA1	525	fluoxymesterone
Ophthalmic Ointment	IIIA1	525	fluoxymesterone
Ophthalmic Suspension	IIIA1	525	
Injectable Suspension	IIIA1	525	
Hydrocortisone Butyrate	VB1b	UV-254	
Cream	VB1b	UV-254	
Hydrocortisone Hemisuccinate	VB1b	UV-254	fluorometholone
Hydrocortisone Sodium Phosphate	IIIB2	239	
Hydrocortisone Sodium Succinate	IIIA4	410	
for Injection	IIIA1	525	
Hydrocortisone Valerate	VB1b	UV-254	fluorometholone
Cream	VB1b	UV-254	ethyl benzoate
Hydroflumethiazide	VB1b	UV-254	ethyl benzoate
Tablets	IIIB1	273	
Hydrogen Peroxide Concentrate	IIIB1	273	
Topical Solution	IC1b		
Hydromorphone Hydrochloride	IC1b		
Injection	IA1biii		CrV
Tablets	IIIA4	440	
	IIIA4	440	
Hydroquinone	IC1a		
Cream	IIIB1	293	DP
Topical Solution	VB1b	UV-280	
Hydroxocobalamin	VIE, IIIB2		
Injection	IIIB2	361	CrV
Hydroxyamphetamine	IA1biii	361	
Hydrobromide			
Ophthalmic Solution	IIB		
Hydroxychloroquine Sulfate	IIIB1	343	
Tablets	VB1b	UV-254	
Hydroxyprogesterone	IIIB1	240	
Caproate			
Injection	IIIB2	380	ST
Hydroxypropyl Cellulose	IC11	TC-I	toluene
Low-Substituted	VA2	TC-I	toluene
Ocular System	IIIa2	620	
Hydroxypropyl Methylcellulose	VA2	TC-I	toluene
Ophthalmic Solution	IIIA4	635	
Hydroxyurea	VB1b	UV-214	uracil
Capsules	VB1b	UV-214	uracil
Hydroxyzine Hydrochloride	IA1biii		Poten
Injection	VB1b	UV-254	
Syrup	VB1b	UV-232	
Tablets	VB1b	UV-232	
Hydroxyzine Pamoate	VB1b	UV-230	
Capsules	VB1b	UV-232	
Oral Suspension	VB1b	UV-232	
Hyoscyamine	IA1biii		
Tablets	VA1	TC-I	CrV
Hyoscyamine Hydrobromide	IA1biii		homatropine hydrobromide
Hyoscyamine Sulfate	IA1biii	TC-I	CrV
Elixir	VA1	TC-I	Poten / homatropine hydrobromide
Injection	VA1	TC-I	homatropine hydrobromide
Oral Solution	VA1	TC-I	homatropine hydrobromide
Tablets	VA1	TC-I	homatropine hydrobromide
Hypophosphorous Acid	IA1a		
Ibuprofen	VB1b	UV-254	homatropine hydrobromide
Oral Suspension	VB1b	UV-220	
Tablets	VB1b	UV-254	Phth
and Pseudoephedrine Hydrochloride Tablets	VB1b	UV-254	valerophenone
Ichthammol			valerophenone
Ointment	IA2a, IIB		butylparaben
Idarubicin Hydrochloride	IA2a		
for Injection	VB1b	UV-254	MeR
	VB1b	UV-254	MeR

DRUG	ASSAY CATEGORY	ANALYTICAL WAVELENGTH AND/OR DETECTOR	INDICATOR OR INTERNAL STANDARD
Idoxuridine	IA1aiii		
Ophthalmic Ointment	IIIB1	320, 283	TB
Ophthalmic Solution	IIIB1	320, 283	
Ifosfamide	VB1b	UV-195	ethylparaben
for Injection	VB1b	UV-195	ethylparaben
Imidurea	None		
Imipenem	VB1b	UV-300	
Imipenem and Cilastatin	VB1b	UV-254	
for Injection	VB1b	UV-254	
Imipenem and Cilastatin for Injectable Suspension	VB1b	UV-254	
Imipramine Hydrochloride	IA1biii		
Injection	IIIB1	250	CrV
Tablets	IIIB1	250	
Indapamide	VB1b	UV-254	p-chloro-acetanilide
Tablets	VB1b	UV-242	2-chloro-acetophenone
Indigotinsulfonate Sodium	IIIA3	610	
Injection	IIIA3	610	
Indium In 111 Chloride Solution	VIE		
Capromab Pendetide Injection	VIE		
Oxyquinoline Solution	VIE		
Pentetate Injection Solution	VIE		
Pentetreotide Injection	VIE		
Satumomab Pendetide Injection	VIE		
Indocyanine Green	IIIA3	785	
for Injection	IIIA3	785	
Indomethacin	VB1b	UV-254	
Capsules	IIIB1	318	
Capsules, Extended-Release	VB1b	UV-240	
Oral Suspension	VB1b	UV-240	
Suppositories	IIIB1	320	
Indomethacin Sodium	VB1b	UV-254	
for Injection	VB1b	UV-240	
Influenza Virus Vaccine	VIH		
Insulin	VB1b	UV-214	
Injection	VB1b	UV-214	
Human	VB1b	UV-214	
Human Injection	VB1b	UV-214	
Isophane Suspension	VB1b	UV-214	
Isophane Human Suspension	VB1b	UV-214	
Zinc Suspension	VB1b	UV-214	
Extended Zinc Suspension	VB1b	UV-214	
Prompt Zinc Suspension	VB1b	UV-214	
Human Zinc Suspension	VB1b	UV-214	
Extended Human Zinc Suspension	VB1b	UV-214	
Inulin	IIIA4	435	DCF
in Sodium Chloride Injection	IIIA4, IB1a	435	
Iobenguane I 123 Injection	VIE		
131 Injection	VIE		
Iodine	IC1I		ST
Topical Solution	IC1I		ST
Strong Solution	IC1I		ST
Tincture	IC1I		ST
Strong Tincture	IC1I		ST
Sodium Iodide I123 Capsules	VIE		
Solution	VIE		
Iodinated I125 Albumin Injection	VIE		
Iodinated I131 Albumin Injection	VIE		
Aggregated	VIE		
Iodohippurate Sodium I123 Injection	VIE		
Iodohippurate Sodium I131 Injection	VIE		
Rose Bengal Sodium I131 Injection	IIIA3, VIE	550	
Sodium Iodide I131 Capsules	VIE		
Solution	VIE		
Iodipamide	IB1a		TBPE
Meglumine Injection	IB1a		TBPE
Iodohippurate Sodium I123 Injection	VIE		
Iodoquinol	IC1Iii		ST
Tablets	IC1Iii		ST
Iohexol	IBk		TBPh
Injection	IBk		TBPh
Iopamidol	IA1b		Poten
Injection	IIb1	240	
Iopanoic Acid	IB1a		TBP
Tablets	IA1a		TB
Iophendylate	IC1Iii		ST
Injection	IC1Iii		ST
Iopromide	VB1b	UV-254	
Iothalamate Meglumine Injection	IB1a		Poten
Iothalamate Meglumine and Iothalamate Sodium Injection	VIC1, IB1a		Poten
Iothalamate Sodium Injection	IB1a		Poten
Iothalamic Acid	IB1a		Poten
Ioversol	IA2ai		Poten
Injection	IA2ai		Poten
Ioxaglate Meglumine and Ioxaglate Sodium Injection	VIC1		Poten
Ioxaglic Acid	IC1k		
Ioxilan	IB1a		Poten
Injection	VB1b	UV-245	TBP
Ipecac	VIG1, IIIB1	283, 350	MeR
Powdered	VIG1, IIIB1	283, 350	MeR
Syrup	VIG1, IIIB1	283, 350	MeR
Ipodate Sodium	IB1a		
Capsules	IB1a		
Iron Dextran Injection	IIIA4	510	EY
Iron Sorbitex Injection	IIIA4	510	EY
Isoamyl Methoxycinnamate	VA1	FID-P	
Isobutane	VA1	TC-I	
Isoetharine Hydrochloride	VB1b	UV-278	
Inhalation Solution	VB1b	UV-278	
Isoetharine Mesylate	VB1b	UV-254	
Inhalation Aerosol	VB1b	UV-254	
Isoflurane	VA1	TC-P	cyclohexanone
Isoflurophate	VA1	FID-I	cyclohexane
Ophthalmic Ointment	VA1	FID-I	
Isoleucine	IA1bii		Poten

Appendix B. Assay Index of Official USP-NF Drugs

DRUG	ASSAY CATEGORY	ANALYTICAL WAVELENGTH AND/OR DETECTOR	INDICATOR OR INTERNAL STANDARD
Isometheptene Mucate, Dichloralphenazone, and Acetaminophen Capsules	IC1lii, VB1b	UV-280	ST
Isoniazid			
Injection	IC1j		Poten
Syrup	IC1j		Poten
Tablets	IC1j		Poten
Isopropamide Iodide			
Tablets	VB1b	UV-254	CrV
Isopropyl Alcohol	IA1biii, IIIB1	280, 258	
Rubbing	VA1, VID	TC-I	
Isopropyl Myristate	VA1	FID-P	triethyleneglycol
Isopropyl Palmitate	VA1	FID-P	triethyleneglycol
Isoproterenol Hydrochloride	VB1b	UV-278	
Inhalation Aerosol	IIIA4	530	
Inhalation Solution	VB1b	UV-278	
Injection	VB1b	UV-280	
Tablets	VB1b	UV-280	
and Phenylephrine Bitartrate Inhalation Aerosol	IIIA4	495, 530	
Isoproterenol Sulfate	VB1b	UV-278	
Inhalation Aerosol	IIIA4	530	
Inhalation Solution	VB1b	UV-278	
Isosorbide Concentrate	VA1	TC-I	
Oral Solution	VA1	TC-I	
Isosorbide Dinitrate, Diluted	VB1b	UV-220	
Capsules, Extended-Release	VB1b	UV-220	nitroglycerin
Tablets	VB1b	UV-220	nitroglycerin
Tablets, Chewable	VB1b	UV-220	nitroglycerin
Tablets, Extended-Release	VB1b	UV-220	nitroglycerin
Tablets, Sublingual	VB1b	UV-220	nitroglycerin
Isotretinoin	IA1iii	UV-365	
Capsules	VB1a	269, 300	TB
Isoxuprine Hydrochloride	IIIB1	275	
Injection	IIIB1	275	
Tablets	IIIB1	UV-326	
Isradipine	VB1b		
Kanamycin	VIN1		
Capsules	VIN1		
Injection	VIN1		
Sulfate	VIN1		
Ketamine Hydrochloride	IA1biii		CrV
Injection	IIIB1	269	
Ketoconazole	IA1bii		Poten
Tablets	VB1b	UV-225	terconazole
Ketoprofen	VB1b	UV-215	
Ketorolac Tromethamine	VB1b	UV-313	
Injection	VB1b	UV-254	naproxen
Tablets	VB1b	UV-254	naproxen
Krypton Kr 81m	VIE		
Labetalol Hydrochloride	VB1b	UV-230	
Injection	VB1b	UV-254	
Tablets	VB1b	UV-230	Phth
Lactic Acid	IA2b		
Lactitol	VB1b	RI	
Lactulose Concentrate	VB1b	RI	
Solution	VIF		
Lanolin Alcohols	IIB		
Leucine	IA1bii	UV-254	
Leucovorin Calcium	VB1b		Poten
Injection	IIIB1	284	
Tablets	VB1b	UV-254	
Levamisole Hydrochloride	IA1a		
Tablets	VB1b	UV-215	Poten
Levmetamfetamine	IA1bii		
Levobunolol Hydrochloride	VB1b	UV-254	
Ophthalmic Solution	VB1b	UV-205	CrV
Levocarnitine	IA1bii	UV-225	
Injection	VB1b		
Oral Solution	VB1b		CrV
Levodopa	IA1bii	280	p-aminobenzoic acid
Capsules	VB1b	280	
Tablets	VB1b	241	Poten
Levonordefrin	IA1bii	UV-215	
Levonorgestrel and Ethinyl Estradiol Tablets	IIIB1		
Levorphanol Tartrate	IIIB1	UV-225	CrV
Injection	IA1bii	UV-225	
Tablets	IIIB1	UV-225	
Levothyroxin Sodium	VB1b	UV-254	MeR
Oral Powder	IA1bii	UV-254	MeR
Tablets	IA1bii	UV-246	MeR
Lidocaine	IA1bii	UV-254	
Topical Aerosol	VB1b		CrV
Ointment	VB1b		Poten
Oral Topical Solution	VB1b		CrV
Lidocaine Hydrochloride	IA1bii		
Injection	IA2a		
Jelly	IA1bii		
Topical Solution	VB1b	UV-254	
Topical Solution, Oral	IA2a		
and Dextrose Injection	VB1b	UV-254 EC	
and Epinephrine Injection	VB1b, VIC1	UV-261	norepinephrine bitartrate
and Epinephrine Bitartrate Injection	VB1b	UV-254, EC	norepinephrine bitartrate
Lime	ID1a	UV-261, EC	HNB

DRUG	ASSAY CATEGORY	ANALYTICAL WAVELENGTH AND/OR DETECTOR	INDICATOR OR INTERNAL STANDARD
Lincomycin Injection	VB1b	UV-210	
Lincomycin Hydrochloride	VB1b	UV-210	
Capsules	VB1b	UV-210	
Syrup	VB1b	UV-210	
Soluble Powder	IB2aii	UV-210	
Lindane			FAS
Cream	VA1	FID-I	methylene chloride
Lotion	VA1	FID-I	methylene chloride
Shampoo	VA1	FID-I	methylene chloride
Liothyronine Sodium	VB1b	UV-225	
Tablets	VB1b	UV-225	
Liotrix Tablets	VB1b	UV-225	
Lisinopril	VB1b	UV-210	
Tablets	VB1b	UV-215	
Lithium Carbonate	IA2a		MeO
Capsules	IIID	671	
Extended-release Tablets	IIIF1	671	
Tablets	IIID	671	
Lithium Citrate	IIID	671	
Syrup	IIID	671	
Lithium Hydroxide	IA1b		Phth
Loperamide Hydrochloride	IA1biii		Nb
Capsules	IIIA4	410	
Tablets	VB1b	UV-214	
Loracarbef	VB1b	UV-265	
Capsules	VB1b	UV-265	
for Oral Suspension	IA1biii	UV-265	
Lorazepam	VB1b	UV-240	
Injection	VB1b	UV-240	Poten
Oral Concentrate	VB1a	UV-240	
Tablets	VB1b	UV-240	
Lovastatin	VB1b	UV-238	
Tablets	VB1b	UV-238	
Loxapine Succinate	IA1bii	UV-254	Poten
Capsules	VB1b	UV-220	
Lypression Nasal Solution	IA1biii		
Lysine Acetate	IA1bii		Poten
Lysine Hydrochloride	IA1bii		Poten
Mafenide Acetate	IIIB1	267	
Cream	IIIB1	267	
Magaldrate	IA2a		Poten
Oral Suspension	IA2a		Poten
Tablets	IA2a		Poten
and Simethicone Tablets	IA2a, IIIC1		Poten
and Simethicone Oral Suspension	IA2a, IIIC1		Poten
Milk of Magnesia	ID1a		EBT
Magnesia Tablets	ID1a		EBT
Magnesium Aluminum Silicate	IIIF1	309, 285	MeO
Magnesium Carbonate	IA2a		EBT
and Citric Acid for Oral Solution	ID1a		EBT
and Sodium Bicarbonate for Oral Suspension	ID1a, IIIF1	589	EBT
Magnesium Chloride	ID1a		EBT
Magnesium Citrate	ID1a		EBT
Oral Solution	IA2a, IIB		Phth
for Oral Solution	ID1a		EBT
Magnesium Gluconate	ID1a		EBT
Tablets	ID1a		EBT
Magnesium Hydroxide	IA2a		MeR
Paste	ID1a		EBT
Magnesium Oxide	IA2a		MeO
Capsules	ID1a		EBT
Tablets	ID1a		EBT
Magnesium Phosphate	IA2b		Phth
Magnesium Salicylate	IIIB1	296	
Tablets	IIIB1	296	
Magnesium Silicate	IA2a, IIC		MeO
Magnesium Stearate	ID2a		EBT
Magnesium Sulfate	ID1a		EBT
Injection	ID1a		EBT
in Dextrose Injection	ID1a, VIC		
Magnesium Trisilicate	IA2a		MeO
Tablets	ID1a		EBT
Malathion	VB1b	UV-254	parathion
Lotion	VA1	FID-I	Phth
Malic Acid	IA1a		
Maltitol Solution	VB1b	RI	Poten
Mandelic Acid	IA1a		EBT
Manganese Chloride	ID1a		
Injection	IIIF1	279	
Manganese Gluconate	ID1a		EBT
Manganese Sulfate	ID1a		EBT
Injection	IIIF1	279	
Mannitol	VB1b	RI	
Injection	VB1b	RI	
in Sodium Chloride Injection	IC1iii		
Maprotiline Hydrochloride	IA1bii		ST, FAS
Tablets	VB1b	UV-272	Poten
Mazindol	IA1bii		
Tablets	VB1b	UV-254	CrV
Mebendazole	IA1bii		amitriptyline hydrochloride
Oral Suspension	IIIB1	247	Poten
Tablets	VB1b	UV-247	
Mebrofenin	IA1a		
Mecamylamine Hydrochloride	VIM		
Tablets	IA2a		TB
Mechlorethamine Hydrochloride for Injection	IC2b		
Meclizine Hydrochloride	IC2b		
Tablets	IA1biii		
Meclocycline Sulfosalicylate	VB1b	UV-340	MR
Cream	VB1b	UV-340	ST
Meclofenamate Sodium	VB1b	UV-340	ST
Capsules	IA1a		Poten
	IIIB1	336	Phth

Appendix B. Assay Index of Official USP-NF Drugs

DRUG	ASSAY CATEGORY	ANALYTICAL WAVELENGTH AND/OR DETECTOR	INDICATOR OR INTERNAL STANDARD
Medroxyprogesterone Acetate	VB1a	UV-254	progesterone
Injectable Suspension	VB1a	UV-254	progesterone
Tablets	VB1a	UV-254	progesterone
Mefenamic Acid	VB1b	UV-279	propylparaben
Capsules	VB1b	UV-279	propylparaben
Megestrol Acetate	VB1b	UV-280	MeR
Tablets	VB1b	UV-280	
Meglumine	IA1a		Poten
Melphalan	IB1a		Poten
Tablets	VB1b	UV-254	Poten
Menadiol Sodium Diphosphate	IC1a		
Injection	IC1a		
Tablets	IC1a		Op
Menadione	IC1a		
Injection	IIIA4	635	
Meningococcal Polysaccharide Vaccine			
Group A	None		
Group C	None		
Groups A and C Combined	None		
Menotropins	VIH		
for Injection	VIH		
Menthol Lozenges	VA1	FID	anethole
Menthyl Anthranilate	VA1	FID-P	
Meperidine Hydrochloride	VB1b	UV-230	
Injection	VB1b	UV-230	CrV
Syrup	IA1bii		
Tablets	VB1b	UV-230	
Mepivacaine Hydrochloride	IA1biii		CrV
Injection	IA1bii		MeR
and Levonordefrin Injection	IA1bii, IIIA4	530	MeR
Meprednisone	IIIB1	238	
Meprobamate	IA1aii		Phth
Oral Suspension	IA1aii		Phth
Tablets	VB1b		
Mercaptopurine	IA1aiii	UV-200	
Tablets	IIIB1		TB
Ammoniated Mercury	IA1bi	325	MeR
Mesalamine	VB1b	UV-254	
Extended-release Capsules	VB1b	UV-240	
Rectal Suspension	IA1bii	UV-254	sodium benzoate
Mesoridazine Besylate	IIIB1	262	
Injection	IIIB1	267	
Oral Solution	VB1b	UV-265	Poten
Tablets	IIIA4	547	
Mestranol	IC2c	UV-278	
Metacresol	VB1b	276	ST
Metaproterenol Sulfate	IIIB1	UV-278	
Inhalation Aerosol	VB1b		
Inhalation Solution	VB1b		
Syrup	VB1b	UV-278	
Tablets	VB1b	UV-278	
Metaraminol Bitartrate	IA1bii		CV
Injection	VB1b	UV-264	
Methacholine Chloride	IA1biii		
Methacrylic Acid Copolymer	IA1a		CrV
Dispersion	IA1A		Phth
Methacycline Hydrochloride	VIN1		Phth
Capsules	VIN1		
Oral Suspension	VIN1		
Methadone Hydrochloride	IA1biii		CrV
Injection	VA1	FID-I	procaine
Oral Concentrate	VB1b	UV-254	
Oral Solution	VB1b	UV-254	pyrilamine maleate
Tablets	VB1b	UV-254	
Methamphetamine Hydrochloride	VB1b	UV-254	
Tablets	VB1b	UV-254	
Methazolamide	VB1b	UV-257	
Tablets	VB1b	UV-265	
Methdilazine Hydrochloride	IIIB1	UV-252	MeR
Syrup	IIIA4	252, 275	
Tablets	IIIA4	460	
Methenamine	IA2a	460	
Elixir	IIIA4	570	
Tablets	IIIA4	570	
Methenamine Hippurate	IA1bii		Poten
Tablets	IA1a		TP
Methenamine Mandelate	IB1a		Poten
Delayed-release Tablets	IB1A		Poten
for Oral Solution	IB1a		Poten
Oral Suspension	IB1a		Poten
Tablets	IB1a		Poten
Methicillin for Injection	VB1b	UV-225	
Sodium	VB1b	UV-225	
Methimazole	IA1a		BtB
Tablets	IA1a		BtB
Methionine	IA1bii		Poten
Methocarbamol	IIIB1	274	
Injection	VB1b	UV-274	
Tablets	VB1b	UV-274	
Methohexital	IIIC1	5.93	caffeine
Sodium for Injection	VA1	FID-I	caffeine
Methotrexate	VB1b	UV-302	
Tablets	VB1b	UV-302	
Injection	IIIA4	UV-302	aprobarbital
for Injection	IA1bii	UV-302	
Methotrimeprazine			
Injection	VB1b	UV-254	CrV

DRUG	ASSAY CATEGORY	ANALYTICAL WAVELENGTH AND/OR DETECTOR	INDICATOR OR INTERNAL STANDARD
Methoxsalen	VB1b	UV-254	trioxsalen
Capsules	VB1b	UV-254	trioxsalen
Topical Solution	VB1b	UV-254	trioxsalen
Methoxyflurane	VA1	TC-I	
Methsuximide	IIIB1	247	
Capsules	IIIB1	UV-254	
Methyclothiazide	IB1a	268	EY
Tablets	IIIB1	FID-I	
Methyl Alcohol	VA1		
Methyl Salicylate	IA2b		Phth
Methyl Benzylidene Camphor	VA1	FID-P	
Methylbenzethonium Chloride	IC1n		
Lotion	IE4		SaO
Ointment	IE4		SaO
Topical Powder	IE4		SaO
Methylcellulose	VA2	TC-I	toluene
Ophthalmic Solution	IC1lii		ST
Oral Solution	IC1lii		ST
Tablets	IIA		
Methyldopa	IA1bii		CrV
Oral Suspension	VB1b	UV-280	
Tablets	IIIA4	520	
and Chlorothiazide Tablets	VB1b	UV-280	
and Hydrochlorothiazide Tablets	VB1b	UV-270	
Methyldopate Hydrochloride	VB1b	UV-280	
Injection	IIIB1	283	
Methylene Blue	IIIA3	663	
Injection	IIIA3	663	
Methylene Chloride	VA1	TC-I	
Methylergonovine Maleate	VB1b	FI	
Injection	VB1b	UV-240	
Tablets	VB1b	FI	
Methylparaben	IA2b		Poten
Methylparaben Sodium	IC2f		ST
Methylphenidate Hydrochloride	IA1bii		Nb
Tablets	VB1b	UV-210	
Tablets, Extended-Release	VB1b	UV-210	
Methylprednisolone	VB1b	UV-254	prednisone
Tablets	VB1b	UV-254	prednisone
Methylprednisolone Acetate	VB1b	UV-254	prednisone
Cream	IIIA1	525	
for Enema	VB1b	UV-254	prednisone
Injectable Suspension	VB1b	UV-254	prednisone
Methylprednisolone Hemisuccinate	VB1a	UV-254	fluorometholone
Methylprednisolone Sodium Succinate	IIIA1	525	
for Injection	VB1a	UV-254	fluorometholone
Methyltestosterone	VB1b	UV-241	
Capsules	IIIB1	241	
Tablets	IIIB1	241	
Methysergide Maleate	IA1bii		CrV
Tablets	VB1b	UV-318	
Metoclopramide Hydrochloride	IA1bii		Poten

DRUG	ASSAY CATEGORY	ANALYTICAL WAVELENGTH AND/OR DETECTOR	INDICATOR OR INTERNAL STANDARD
Metoclopramide Injection	VB1b	UV-215	
Oral Solution	VB1b	UV-215	
Tablets	VB1b	UV-215	
Metolazone	IIIB1	343	
Tablets	IIIB1	343	
Metoprolol Fumarate	IA1bii		Poten
Metoprolol Tartrate and Hydrochlorothiazide Tablets	VB1b	UV-254, 270	oxyprenolol, sulfanilamide
Metoprolol Tartrate	IA1bii		Poten
Injection	VB1b	UV-254	
Tablets	VB1b	UV-254	
Metronidazole	IA1bii		MaG
Gel	VB1b	UV-254	
Injection	VB1b	UV-320	
Tablets	IA1bii		Poten
Metyrapone	IIIB1	260	
Tablets	IIIA4	450	
Metyrosine	IA1bii		Poten
Capsules	IIIB1	274	
Mexiletine Hydrochloride	VB1b	UV-254	
Capsules	VB1b	UV-254	
Mezlocillin Sodium for Injection	VB1b	UV-210	
Mibolerone	VB1b	UV-210	
Oral Solution	VA1	FID-I	
Miconazole	IA1bii		
Injection	VB1b	UV-230	Nb
Miconazole Nitrate	IA1bii		Poten
Cream	VA1	FID-I	cholestane
Topical Powder	VA1	FID-I	cholestane
Vaginal Suppositories	VA1	FID-I	cholestane
Minerals Capsules	VIN1		
Minocycline Hydrochloride	VIL		
Capsules	VB1b	UV-280	medroxyprogesterone
for Injection	VB1b	UV-280	medroxyprogesterone
Oral Suspension	VB1b	UV-280	medroxyprogesterone
Tablets	VB1b	UV-280	
Minoxidil	VB1b	UV-254	
Tablets	VB1b	UV-254	
Topical Solution	VB1b	UV-254	
Mitomycin	VB1b	UV-365	
for Injection	VB1b	UV-365	
Mitotane	IIIB1	268	
Tablets	IIIB1	268	
Mitoxantrone Hydrochloride Injection	VB1b	UV-254	
Molindone Hydrochloride	VB1b	UV-254	butylparaben
Tablets	VB1b	UV-254	butylparaben
Mometasone Furoate	VB1b	UV-254	beclomethasone dipropionate
Cream	VB1b	UV-254	beclomethasone dipropionate
Ointment	VB1b	UV-254	beclomethasone dipropionate
Topical Solution	VB1b	UV-254	beclomethasone dipropionate

Appendix B. Assay Index of Official USP-NF Drugs

DRUG	ASSAY CATEGORY	ANALYTICAL WAVELENGTH AND/OR DETECTOR	INDICATOR OR INTERNAL STANDARD
Monensin	VB2b	520	
Granulated	VB2b	520	
Premix	VB2b	520	
Sodium	VB2b	520	
Mono- and Di-Glycerides	VA1	FID-I	hexadecyl hexadecanoate
Monoethanolamine	IA1b		BcG, MeR
Monosodium Glutamate	IA1bii		Poten
Monothioglycerol	IC1k		ST
Moricizine Hydrochloride	VB1b	UV-254	butamben
Tablets	VB1b	UV-254	butamben
Morphine Sulfate	VB1b	UV-284	
Injection	VB1b	UV-284	
Morrhuate Sodium Injection	IA2a		MeO
Mupirocin	VB1b	UV-229	
Ointment	VB1b	UV-229	
Nadolol	IA1bii		CrV
Tablets	VB1b	UV-220	
and Bendroflumethiazide Tablets	VB1b	UV-270	
Nafcillin Sodium	VB1b	UV-254	
Capsules	VIN1		
for Injection	VB1b	UV-254	
Injection	VB1b	UV-254	
for Oral Solution	VIN1		
Tablets	VIN1		
Naftifine Hydrochloride	VB1b	UV-270	
Cream	VB1b	UV-270	
Gel	VA1	FID	n-propyl alcohol
Nalidixic Acid	IA1aiii		TP
Oral Suspension	VB1b	UV-254	
Tablets	VB1b	UV-254	
Nalorphine Hydrochloride	IIIB1	285	
Injection	IIIB1	285	
Naloxone Hydrochloride	IA1biii	UV-229	MV
Injection	VB1b	UV-280	
Naltrexone Hydrochloride	VB1b	UV-280	
Tablets	VB1b	UV-238	
Nandrolone Decanoate	IIIB2	380	dimethyl phthalate
Injection	IIIA1		
Nandrolone Phenpropionate	IIIA4		
Injection	IA1biii		CrV
Naphazoline Hydrochloride	VB1b	UV-280	
Nasal Solution	VB1b	UV-285	
Ophthalmic Solution	IA1a	UV-254	Phth
Naproxen	VB1b	UV-254	ethylparaben
Oral Suspension	IA1bii		butyrophenone
Tablets	VB1b	UV-254	Nb
Naproxen Sodium			butyrophenone
Tablets	VB1b	UV-254	
Narasin Granular	VB2b	520	
Premix	VB2b	520	
Natamycin	VIN1		
Ophthalmic Suspension	VIN1		
Neomycin Sulfate	VIN		
Boluses	VIN1		
Cream	VIN1		
Ointment	VIN1		
Ophthalmic Ointment	VIN1		
Oral Solution	VIN1		
for Injection	VIN1		
Tablets	VIN1		
and Bacitracin Ointment	VIN1		
and Bacitracin Zinc Ointment	VIN1, IIIA1	525	
and Dexamethasone Sodium Phosphate Cream	VIN1, IIIA1	525	
and Dexamethasone Sodium Phosphate Ophthalmic Ointment	VIN1, VB1b	525, UV-254	fluoxymesterone
and Dexamethasone Sodium Phosphate Ophthalmic Solution	VIN1, VB1b	UV-238	
and Fluocinolone Acetonide Cream	VIN1, VB1b	UV-254	fluoxymesterone
and Fluorometholone Ointment	VIN1, VB1b	UV-240	
and Flurandrenolide Cream	VIN1, VB1b	UV-240	
and Flurandrenolide Ointment	VIN1, VB1b	UV-240	
and Flurandrenolide Lotion	VIN1, VB1b	UV-240	
and Gramicidin Ointment	VIN1		
and Hydrocortisone Cream	VIN1, VB1b	UV-254	
and Hydrocortisone Ointment	VIN1, VB1b	UV-254	
and Hydrocortisone Acetate Cream	VIN1, VB1b	UV-254	fluoxymesterone
and Hydrocortisone Acetate Ointment	VIN1, VB1b	UV-254	fluoxymesterone
and Hydrocortisone Acetate Lotion	VIN1, VB1b	UV-254	fluoxymesterone
and Hydrocortisone Acetate Ophthalmic Ointment	VIN1, VB1b	UV-254	fluoxymesterone
and Hydrocortisone Acetate Ophthalmic Suspension	VIN1, VB1b	UV-254	
and Methylprednisolone Acetate Cream	VIN1, IIIA1	525	
Neomycin and Polymyxin B Sulfates Solution for Irrigation	VIN1		
Cream	VIN1		
Ophthalmic Ointment	VIN1		
Ophthalmic Solution	VIN1		
and Bacitracin Ointment	VIN1		
and Bacitracin Ophthalmic Ointment	VIN1		
Bacitracin and Hydrocortisone Acetate Ointment	VIN1, VB1b	UV-254	fluoxymesterone

DRUG	ASSAY CATEGORY	ANALYTICAL WAVELENGTH AND/OR DETECTOR	INDICATOR OR INTERNAL STANDARD
Niacin	IIIB1	262	
Injection	IIIA4	450	
Tablets	VB1b	UV-262	
Niacinamide	VB1b	UV-254	
Injection	IIIA4	450	
Tablets	IIIA4	450	Poten
Nicotine	IA1bii	UV-260	
Transdermal System	VB1b	UV-254	
Nicotine Polacrilex	VB1b	UV-254	
Gum	VB1b	UV-235	
Nifedipine	VB1b	UV-235	
Capsules	VB1b	UV-235	
Nitric Acid	IA1a		MeR
Nitrofurantoin	VB1b	UV-254	theophylline
Capsules	VB1b	UV-254	theophylline
Oral Suspension	VB1b	UV-254	theophylline
Tablets	VB1b	UV-254	theophylline
Nitrofurazone	IIIB1	375	
Ointment	VB1b	UV-365	
Topical Solution	VB1b	UV-365	
Nitrogen	VA1	TC-I	
Nitrogen 97 Percent	VA1	TC-I	
Nitroglycerin Tablets	IIIA4	410, 600	
Diluted	VB1b	UV-220	pentaerythritol
tetranitrate	VB1b	UV-220	pentaerythritol
Injection			
tetranitrate	VB1b	UV-220	pentaerythritol
Ointment			
tetranitrate			
Nitromersol	IB1biii		FAS
Topical Solution	IB1biii		FAS
Nitrous Oxide	VA1	TC-I	
Nizatidine	VB1b	UV-254	
Capsules	VB1b	UV-230	
Nonoxynol 9	VB1b	UV-280	phenol
Norepinephrine Bitartrate	IA1biii		CrV
Injection	IIIB1	240	
Norethindrone	IIIB2	380	
Tablets	IIIB2, IIIE2	375, 556	
and Ethinyl Estradiol Tablets	VB1b	UV-200	
and Mestranol Tablets	IIIB1	240	
Norethindrone Acetate	IIIB1	240	
Tablets	VB1b	UV-220	valerophenone
Norethindrone Acetate and Ethinyl Estradiol Tablets	IIIB1	240	
Norethynodrel	IA1bii		
Norfloxacin	VB1b	UV-278	
Ophthalmic Solution	VB1b	UV-275	
Tablets	IIIB1	241	Poten
Norgestrel	IIIB2	380	
Tablets	IIIB1, IIIA4	241, 536	
and Ethinyl Estradiol Tablets	IA1biii		Poten
Nortriptyline Hydrochloride	VB1b	UV-239	
Capsules	IIIB1		
Oral Solution	IA1bii	239	CrV
Noscapine			

DRUG	ASSAY CATEGORY	ANALYTICAL WAVELENGTH AND/OR DETECTOR	INDICATOR OR INTERNAL STANDARD
Bacitracin and Hydrocortisone Acetate Ophthalmic Ointment and Bacitracin Zinc Ointment	VIN1, VB1b	UV-254	fluoxymesterone
and Bacitracin Zinc Ophthalmic Ointment	VIN1		
Bacitracin Zinc Ointment	VIN1		
Bacitracin Zinc Ophthalmic Ointment	VIN1, VB1b	UV-254	
Bacitracin Zinc and Hydrocortisone Ointment	VIN1, VB1b	UV-254	
Bacitracin Zinc and Hydrocortisone Ophthalmic Ointment	VIN1, VB1b	UV-254	
Bacitracin Zinc and Hydrocortisone Acetate Ophthalmic Ointment	VIN1, VB1b	UV-254	
Bacitracin Zinc and Hydrocortisone Ophthalmic Suspension	VIO		
Bacitracin Zinc and Lidocaine Ointment	VIO		
Bacitracin Zinc and Lidocaine Cream	VIN1, VB1b	UV-254	fluoxymesterone
and Dexamethasone Ophthalmic Ointment	VIN1, VB1b	UV-254	fluoxymesterone
and Dexamethasone Ophthalmic Suspension	VIN1, VB1b	UV-240	testosterone
and Flurandrenolide Lotion	VIN1		
and Gramicidin Cream	VIN1		
and Gramicidin Ophthalmic Solution	VIN1		
and Gramicidin and Hydrocortisone Acetate Cream	VIN1, VB1b	UV-254	fluoxymesterone
and Hydrocortisone Acetate Cream	VIN1, VB1b	UV-254	fluoxymesterone
and Hydrocortisone Ophthalmic Suspension	VIN1, VB1b	UV-254	
and Hydrocortisone Acetate Ophthalmic Suspension	VIN1, VB1b	UV-254	
and Lidocaine Cream	VIO		
and Prednisolone Acetate Ophthalmic Suspension	VIO		
and Hydrocortisone Otic Solution	VIN1, VB1b	UV-254	
and Hydrocortisone Otic Suspension	VIN1, VB1b	UV-254	
Bacitracin and Lidocaine Ointment	VIN1, VB1b	UV-230	
Neomycin Sulfate and Prednisolone Acetate Ophthalmic Suspension	VIN1, VB1b	UV-254	betamethasone
Neomycin Sulfate and Prednisolone Sodium Phosphate Ophthalmic Ointment	VIN1, IIIA1	525	
Neomycin Sulfate, Sulfacetamide Sodium and Prednisolone Acetate Ophthalmic Ointment	VIN1, IC1j, IIIA1	525	
Neomycin Sulfate and Triamcinolone Acetonide Cream	VIN1, VB1b	UV-254	fluoxymesterone
Neostigmine Bromide	VIN1, VB1b	UV-254	fluoxymesterone
Tablets	IA1bii		CV
Neostigmine Methylsulfate	IIIA4		
Injection	IA1c		MP
Netilmicin Sulfate	IIIA4		
Injection	VIN1		
	VIN1		

Appendix B. Assay Index of Official USP-NF Drugs

DRUG	ASSAY CATEGORY	ANALYTICAL WAVELENGTH AND/OR DETECTOR	INDICATOR OR INTERNAL STANDARD
Novobiocin Cream	VIN1		
Novobiocin Sodium	VIN1		
Intramammary Infusion	VIN1		
Nystatin	VIN1		
Cream	VIN1		
Lotion	VIN1		
Lozenges	VIN		
Ointment	VIN1		
Topical Powder	VIN1		
Oral Suspension	VIN1		
for Oral Suspension	VIN1		
Tablets	VIN1		
Vaginal Suppositories	VIN1		
Vaginal Tablets	VIN1		
and Neomycin Sulfate, Gramicidin, and Triamcinolone Acetonide Cream	VIO		
and Neomycin Sulfate, Gramicidin, and Triamcinolone Acetonide Ointment	VIO		
and Neomycin Sulfate, Thiostrepton, and Triamcinolone Acetonide Cream	VIO		
and Neomycin Sulfate, Thiostrepton, and Triamcinolone Acetonide Ointment	VIO		
and Triamcinolone Acetonide Cream	VIN1, VB1b	UV-254	fluoxymesterone
Ointment	VIN1, VB1b	UV-254	fluoxymesterone
Octocrylene	VA1	FID-P	
Octyldodecanol	VA1	FID-I	
Octyl Methoxycinnamate	VA1	FID-P	
Octyl Salicylalate	VA1	FID-P	
Ofloxacin	VA1bii		Poten
Ophthalmic Solution	VB1b	UV-294	
Oleovitamin A and D	VIL		
Capsules	VIL		
Omeprazole	VB1b	UV-280	
Ondansetron Hydrochloride	VB1b	UV-216	
Injection	VB1b	UV-216	
Opium	IIIB1	285	
Powdered	IIIB1	285	
Tincture	IIIB1	285	
Bland Lubricating Ophthalmic Ointment	None		
Orphenadrine Citrate	IA1bii		CrV
Injection	IIIA4	410	
Oxacillin Sodium	VB1b	UV-225	
Capsules	VB1b	UV-225	
for Injection	VB1b	UV-225	
Injection	VB1b	UV-225	
for Oral Solution	VB1b	UV-225	
Oxandrolone	IA2bi		Phth
Tablets	VA1	FID-I	n-octacosane
Oxazepam	IA1aiii	229	Poten
Capsules	IIIB1	229	
Tablets	IIIB1		
Oxfendazole	IA1bii		
Oral Suspension	VB1b	UV-254	
Oxprenol Hydrochloride	IA1bii		Poten
Extended-release Tablets	IIIB1	274, 300	
Tablets	IIIB1	274, 300	
Oxtriphylline	IB1e		MeB
Extended-release Tablets	VB1b	UV-275	
Oral Solution	VB1b	UV-275	
Tablets, Delayed Release	VB1b	UV-275	
Tablets	VB1b	UV-275	
Oxybenzone	IIIB1	285	
Oxybutynin Chloride	IAbii		CrV
Syrup	IIIA2	415	
Tablets	VB1b	UV-203	
Oxycodone and Acetaminophen	VB1b	UV-214	
Capsules	VB1b	UV-280	
Tablets	VB1b	UV-206	
Oxycodone Hydrochloride	VB1b	UV-280	
Oral Solution	IIIB1	281	
Tablets	VB1b	UV-300, 280	
and Aspirin Tablets	VB1b	UV-280	ethylparaben
Oxycodone Terephthlate	VIA		
Oxygen	VIA		
93 Percent	VB1b	UV-280	
Oxymetazoline Hydrochloride	VB1b	UV-280	
Nasal Solution	VB1b	UV-280	
Ophthalmic Solution	IIIB1	315	
Oxymetholone	IIIB1	315	
Tablets	IA1biii		
Oxymorphone Hydrochloride	IIIB1	282	MV
Injection	VB1b	UV-254	
Suppositories	IC2f		
Oxyquinoline Sulfate	VB1b	UV-254	procaine hydrochloride
Oxytetracycline	VB1b	UV-254	ST
Injection	VB1b	UV-254	
for Injection	VB1b	UV-254	
Tablets	VIN1		
and Nystatin Capsules	VIN1		
and Nystatin for Oral Suspension	VIN1		
Oxytetracycline Calcium	VIN1		
Oral Suspension	VIN1		
Oxytetracycline Hydrochloride	VIN1		
Capsules	VIN1		

DRUG	ASSAY CATEGORY	ANALYTICAL WAVELENGTH AND/OR DETECTOR	INDICATOR OR INTERNAL STANDARD
for Injection	VIN1		
Soluble Powder	VIN1		
and Hydrocortisone Ointment	VIN1, VB1b	UV-254	
and Hydrocortisone Acetate Ophthalmic Suspension	VIN1, VB1b	UV-254	
and Polymyxin B Sulfate Ointment	VIN1		
and Polymyxin B Sulfate Ophthalmic Ointment	VIN1		
and Polymyxin B Topical Powder	VIN1		
and Polymyxin B Vaginal Tablets	VIN1		
Oxytocin	VB1b	UV-220	
Injection	VB1b	UV-220	
Nasal Solution	VB1b	UV-220	
Oxytriphylline Tablets	VB1b	UV-275	
Padimate O	IA1bii		Poten
Lotion	VB1b, IA1b	UV-308	
Pamabrom	VIF	UV-280	caffeine, MeO
Pancreatin	VIF		
Tablets	VIF		
Pancrelipase	VIF		
Capsules	VIF		
Delayed-release Capsules	VIF		
Tablets	IA2aiv		CrV
Panthenol	VIF		
Papain	IA1biii		CrV
Tablets for Topical Solution	IIIB1		
Papaverine Hydrochloride	IIIB1	251	
Injection	IC2c	251	
Tablets	IIB, IIB		ST
Parachlorophenol	IIIB1		
Camphorated	IIIC1	242	
Paramethasone Acetate	IIIB1	6.04	
Tablets	VIN1	285	
Paregoric	VIN1		
Paromomycin Sulfate	IA2b, IA1a		
Capsules	VB1b		
Syrup	VB1b		
Pectin	VB1b		Phth
Penbutolol Sulfate	VB1b	UV-271	3,4-dimethyl-benzophenone
Tablets	VIO		
Penicillamine	VIN2	UV-270	
Capsules	VIN2	UV-210	
Tablets	VIN2	UV-210	
Penicillin G, Neomycin, Polymyxin B Sulfates, Hydrocortisone Acetate, and Hydrocortisone Sodium Succinnate Topical Suspension	VIN2	UV-210	
Penicillin G Benzathine	VIN2		SPI
Oral Suspension	VIN2		SPI
Injectable Suspension	VIN2		SPI
Tablets	VIN2		SPI
and Penicillin G Procaine Suspension	VIN2		SPI

DRUG	ASSAY CATEGORY	ANALYTICAL WAVELENGTH AND/OR DETECTOR	INDICATOR OR INTERNAL STANDARD
Penicillin G Potassium for Oral Solution	VB1b	UV-220	SPI
Injection	VIN2		
for Injection	VB1b	UV-225	SPI
Tablets	VB1b	UV-220	SPI
Penicillin G Procaine Intramammary Infusion	VIN2		
Injectable Suspension	VIN1		
for Injectable Suspension	VN2, VN1		SPI
and Dihydrostreptomycin Sulfate Intramammary Infusion	VIN2		
and Dihydrostreptomycin Sulfate Injectable Suspension	VIN1, VIN2		
Sulfate Injectable Suspension	VIN1, VIN2		
Dihydrostreptomycin Sulfate, Chlorpheniramine Maleate and Dexametasone Injectable Suspension	VIN2, VIN1, VA1, VB1b		brompheniramine, beclomethasone
Dihydrostreptomycin Sulfate and Prednisolone Injectable Suspension	VIN2, VIN1, VC1a		
and Prednisolone Suspension with Aluminum Stearate Suspension	VN2, VN1, IIIA2		525
Suspension	V1N2		SPI
Neomycin, Polymyxin B Sulfates and Hydrocortisone Acetate Topical Suspension	VIN1, VB1b	UV-254	fluoxymesterone
Novobiocin Sodium Intramammary Infusion	VIN1, VIN2		
Penicillin G Sodium for Injection	VB1b	UV-220	
for Injection	VB1b	UV-220	
Penicillin V for Oral Suspension	VIN2		
Tablets	VIN2		
Penicillin V Benzathine Oral Suspension	VIN2		
Penicillin V Potassium for Oral Solution	VIN2		
Tablets	VIN2		
Pentazocine	IA1bii	278, 296	CrV
Pentazocine Hydrochloride and Aspirin Tablets	IA1biii	UV-229	CrV
and Naloxone Tablets	IIIB1	278	
Pentazocine Lactate Injection	IIIB1		
Pentetic Acid	IC1		
Pentobarbital	IA1aiii		
Elixir	VA1	FID-I	Poten
Pentobarbital Sodium	IIIB1	240	
Capsules	VA1	FID-I	n-tricosane
Injection	IIA	FID	n-tricosane
Peppermint			
Oil	IA2bi		
Spirit	VIB		
Perflubron	VA1bii		
Perphenazine	IA1bii		
Injection	IIIA4	480	Phth
Oral Solution	VB1b	UV-254	
Syrup	IIIA4	480	
Tablets	IIIA4	480	
and Amitriptyline Hydrochloride Tablets	VB1b	UV-254	CrV

Appendix B. Assay Index of Official USP-NF Drugs

DRUG	ASSAY CATEGORY	ANALYTICAL WAVELENGTH AND/OR DETECTOR	INDICATOR OR INTERNAL STANDARD
Phenazopyridine Hydrochloride			
Tablets	IIIA3	390	
Phendimetrazine Tartrate	VB1b	UV-220	
Capsules	IA1bii		CrV
Tablets	VB1b	UV-256	salicylamide
Phenelzine Sulfate	VB1b	UV-256	salicylamide
Tablets	IC2f		ST
Pheniramine Maleate	VB2b	UV-254	
Phenmetrazine Hydrochloride	IA1bii		CrV
Tablets	IIIB1	256	
Phenobarbital	IIIB1	256	
Elixir	VB1b	UV-254	caffeine
Tablets	VB1b	UV-254	caffeine
Phenobarbital Sodium	VB1b	UV-254	caffeine
Injection	VB1b	UV-254	caffeine
for Injection	IIIB1	240	
Phenol	IC2c		ST
Liquefied	IC2c		ST
Phenoxybenzamine Hydrochloride	IA1aiii		Poten
Capsules	IIIB1	275	
Phensuximide	IIIB1	258	
Capsules	VB1b	UV-254	
Phentermine Hydrochloride	IA1biii		Poten
Capsules	VB1b	UV-254	
Tablets	VB1b	UV-254	
Phentolamine Mesylate	IA1aiii		
for Injection	IIIA4	410	
Phenylalanine	IA1bii		Poten
Phenylbenzimidazole Sulfonic Acid	IA1bi		phth
Phenylbutazone	VB1b	UV-254	desoxycorticosterone
Boluses	VB1b	UV-254	desoxycorticosterone
Injection	VB1b	UV-254	desoxycorticosterone
Tablets	VB1b	UV-254	desoxycorticosterone
Phenylephrine Hydrochloride	IC2c		ST
Injection	VB1b	UV-280	
Nasal Jelly	VB1b	UV-280	
Nasal Solution	VB1b	UV-280	
Ophthalmic Solution	VB1b	UV-280	
Phenylmercuric Acetate	IB1b		FAS
Phenylmercuric Nitrate	IB1b		FAS
Phenylpropanolamine Bitartrate	IA1bii		CrV
Phenylpropanolamine Hydrochloride	IA1biii		CrV
Capsules	VB1b	UV-254	theophylline
Capsules, Extended-Release	VB1b	UV-254	theophylline
Extended-release Tablets	VB1b	UV-254	theophylline
Oral Solution	VB1b	UV-254	theophylline
Tablets	VB1b	UV-254	theophylline
Phenytoin	IA1aiii	UV-229	AV
Oral Suspension	VB1b	UV-254	
Tablets	VB1b	UV-220	
Phenytoin Sodium			
Extended Capsules	VB1b	UV-254	
Injection	VB1b	UV-254	
Prompt Capsules	VB1b	UV-254	
Chromic Phosphate P32 Suspension	VIE		
Sodium Phosphate P32 Solution	VIE		
Phosphoric Acid	IA1a		TP
Diluted	IA1a		TP
Physostigmine	IA1bii		Poten
Physostigmine Salicylate	IA1bii		Poten
Injection	VB1b	UV-254	
Ophthalmic Solution	VB1b	UV-254	
Physostigmine Sulfate	IA1bii		Poten
Phytonadione	VB1a	UV-254	cholesteryl benzoate
Ophthalmic Ointment	VB1b	UV-254	Poten
Injection	VB1b	UV-254	
Tablets	VB1b	UV-215	
Pilocarpine	VB1b	UV-215	
Ocular System	VB1b	UV-220	
Pilocarpine Hydrochloride	VB1b	UV-220	
Ophthalmic Solution	VB1b	UV-220	
Pilocarpine Nitrate	VB1b	UV-220	
Ophthalmic Solution	VB1b	UV-220	
Pimozide	IA1bii	UV-280	3,4-dimethyl-benzophenone
Tablets	VB1b	UV-280	
Pindolol	VB1b	UV-219	
Tablets	VB1b	UV-254	nortriptyline
Piperacillin	VB1b	UV-220	
Piperacillin Sodium	VB1b	UV-220	
for Injection	VB1b	UV-220	
Piperazine	IA1bii		Poten
Piperazine Citrate	IA1bii		CrV
Syrup	IIB		
Tablets	IIB		
Piroxicam	VB1b	UV-254	
Capsules	VB1b	UV-254	
Plague Vaccine	None		
Plantago Seed	None		
Plasma Protein Fraction	None		
Platelet Concentrate	None		
Plicamycin	VB1b	UV-278	
for Injection	VB1b	UV-278	
Podophyllum	VIG		
Polacrilin Potassium	IIID	766	

DRUG	ASSAY CATEGORY	ANALYTICAL WAVELENGTH AND/OR DETECTOR	INDICATOR OR INTERNAL STANDARD
Poloxalene	IIIA2	630	
PEG 3350 and Electrolytes for Oral Solution	VB1b	RI	
Polymyxin B Sulfate	VIN1		
for Injection	VIN1		
and Bacitracin Zinc Topical Aerosol	VIN1		
and Bacitracin Zinc Topical Powder	VIN1		
and Hydrocortisone Otic Solution	VIN1, VB1b	UV-254	
Polyvinyl Acetate Phthalate	IIIB1	IIB	
Sulfurated Potash			
Potassium Acetate	IA1bii		CrV
Injection	IIIF1	766.5	
Potassium Benzoate	IA1bii		CrV
Potassium Bicarbonate	IA1b		MeR
Effervescent Tablets for Oral Solution	IIIF1	766.5	
and Potassium Chloride for Effervescent Oral Solution	IB2aii, IIIF1	766.5	FAS
and Potassium Chloride Effervescent Tablets for Oral Solution	IB2aii, IIIF1	766.5	FAS
Sodium Bicarbonate and Citric Acid Effervescent Tablets for Oral Solution	IIID, IA1a		Ph
Potassium Bitartrate	IA1a		Phth
Potassium Carbonate	IA1b		MeO
Potassium Chloride	IB1a		EY
Extended Release Capsules	IIIF1	766.5	
Extended Release Tablets	IIIF1	766.5	
for Injection Concentrate	IIIF1	766.5	
Oral Solution	IIIF1	766.5	
for Oral Solution	IIIF1	766.5	
in Dextrose Injection	VIC1, IB1a		DCF
in Dextrose and Sodium Chloride Injection	IIIF1, IB1a		DCF
in Lactated Ringer's and Dextrose Injection	IC1a, IIID, IB1a		
in Sodium Chloride Injection	IIIF1		lithiumnitrate
Potassium Bicarbonate and Potassium Citrate Effervescent Tablets for Oral Solution	VIO		
Potassium Citrate	IA1bii		CrV
and Citric Acid Oral Solution	IIID, IA1a	766	Poten, Phth
Extended-release Tablets	IIIA4	425	
Potassium Gluconate	IIIF1	766.5	
Elixir	IIIF1	766.5	
Tablets	IIIF1	766.5	
and Potassium Citrate Oral Solution	IIIF1		
and Ammonium Chloride Oral Solution	IIIF1, IVB1		
and Potassium Chloride Oral Solution	IIIF1, IVB1		
and Potassium Chloride for Oral Solution	IIIF1, IVB1		
Potassium Guaiacolsulfonate	IIIB1	279	

DRUG	ASSAY CATEGORY	ANALYTICAL WAVELENGTH AND/OR DETECTOR	INDICATOR OR INTERNAL STANDARD
Potassium Hydroxide	IA1b		Phth, MeO
Potassium Iodide	IB1a		Poten
Delayed-release Tablets	IB1a		Poten
Oral Solution	IB1a		Poten
Tablets	IB1a		Poten
Potassium Metabisulfite	IC2a		ST
Potassium Metaphosphate	IA2b		Phth
Potassium Nitrate	IA1a		Phth
Solution	IA1a		Phth
Potassium Permanganate	IC2e		
Monobasic Potassium Phosphate	IA1a		Poten
Dibasic Potassium Phosphate	IA2a		Poten
Potassium Phosphates Injection	IA1a, b		MeB
Potassium Sodium Tartrate	IA2aii		CrV
Potassium Sorbate	IA1bii		ST
Povidone-Iodine	IC11		Poten
Ointment	IC11		Poten
Topical Aerosol Solution	IC11		Poten
Topical Cleansing Solution	IC11		Poten
Topical Solution	IC11		
Pralidoxime Chloride	IIIB1	336	CrV
for Injection	IIIB1	336	
Pramoxine Hydrochloride	IA1biii		dibutyl phthlate
Cream	VB1b	UV-224	
Jelly	IIIB1	286	
Praziquantel	VB1b	UV-210	
Tablets	VB1b	UV-210	
Prazosin Hydrochloride	VB1b	UV-254	
Capsules	VB1b	UV-254	
Prednisolone	VB1b	UV-254	betamethasone
Cream	IIIA4	410	
Tablets	VB1b	UV-254	betamethasone
Syrup	VB1b	UV-254	betamethasone
Prednisolone Acetate	VB1b	UV-254	betamethasone
Ophthalmic Suspension	VB1b	UV-254	
Injectable Suspension	VB1b	UV-254	
Prednisolone Hemisuccinate	IIIB1	243	
Prednisolone Sodium Phosphate	IIIB1	241	
Injection	IIIB1	241	
Ophthalmic Solution	IIIB1	241	
Prednisolone Sodium Succinate for Injection	IIIA1	525	
Prednisolone Tebutate	VB1a	UV-254	
Injectable Suspension	IIIB1	254	
Prednisone	VB1a	UV-254	acetanilide
Oral Solution	VB1b	UV-254	
Injectable Suspension	VB1b	UV-254	
Syrup	VB1b	UV-254	
Tablets	VB1a	UV-254	acetanilide
Prilocaine Hydrochloride	IA1biii	UV-254	CrV
Injection and Epinephrine Injection	VB1b	UV-254, EC	
Primaquine Phosphate	IC1j		Poten
Tablets	IC1j		Poten

Appendix B. Assay Index of Official USP-NF Drugs

DRUG	ASSAY CATEGORY	ANALYTICAL WAVELENGTH AND/OR DETECTOR	INDICATOR OR INTERNAL STANDARD
Primidone	IIIB1	257	
Oral Suspension	VA1	FID-I	
Tablets	IIIB1	257	
Probenecid	VB1b	UV-254	
Tablets	IIIB1	257	
and Colchicine Tablets	IIIB1	244, 350	androsterone
Probucol	VB1b	UV-242	
Tablets	VB1b	UV-242	
Procainamide Hydrochloride	VB1b	UV-254	procaine hydrochloride
Capsules	VB1b	UV-254	procaine hydrochloride
Injection	VB1b	UV-254	procaine hydrochloride
Tablets	VB1b	UV-280	
Tablets, Extended-Release	VB1b	UV-280	
Procaine Hydrochloride	IC1j		Poten
Injection	IIIB1	280	
and Epinephrine Injection	IIIB1	280	
Tetracaine Hydrochloride	IC1j, IIIA4	530	SPI
and Levonordefrin			
Injection			
Procarbazine Hydrochloride	IA1a		Poten
Capsules	IVA1		
Prochlorperazine	IA1bii		
Oral Solution	VB1b	UV-254	
Suppositories	IIIB1	254, 278	CrV
Prochlorperazine Edisylate	IA1bii	CrV	
Injection	VB1b	UV-254	
Prochlorperazine Maleate	IA1bii		Poten
Tablets	VB1b	UV-254	trifluoperazine
Procyclidine Hydrochloride	IA1biii		Poten
Tablets	IIIA2	405	
Progesterone	VB1b	UV-254	methyltestosterone
Injection	VB1b	UV-254	methyltestosterone
Intrauterine Contraceptive	IIIB1	241	
System			
Injectable Suspension	VB1b	UV-254	methyltestosterone
Proline	IA1bii	CrV	
Promazine Hydrochloride	IIIB1	301	
Injection	IIIB1	301	
Oral Solution	IIIB1	301	
Syrup	IIIB1	301	
Tablets	IIIB1	301	
Promethazine Hydrochloride	IA1biii		CrV
Injection	IIIA4	470	
Suppositories	IIIA4	470	
Syrup	IIIB1	298	
Tablets	IIIA4	470	
Propafenone Hydrochloride	IA1b	TC-I	Poten
Propane	VA1		
Propantheline Bromide	IA1biii		Poten
Tablets	VB1b	UV-254	
Proparacaine Hydrochloride	IA1biii		CrV
Ophthalmic Solution	VB1b	UV-270	
Propionic Acid	IA1a		Phth
Propoxycaine Hydrochloride	IC1j		SPI
Procaine Hydrochloride and	IIIB1, IIIA4	272, 296, 530	
Levonordefrin Injection			
Procaine Hydrochloride and	IIIB1, IIIA4	272, 296, 530	
Norepinephrine Bitartrate			
Injection			
Propoxyphene Hydrochloride	IA1biii		CrV
Capsules	VB1b	UV-220	
and Acetaminophen Tablets	IIIB1, VA1	249, FID-I	n-tricosane
Aspirin and Caffeine	IIIA4, VA1	530, FID-I	n-tricosane
Capsules			
Propoxyphene Napsylate	IA1bii	FID-I	CrV
Oral Suspension	VA1	FID-I	n-tricosane
Tablets	VA1	UV-210, 245	n-tricosane
and Acetaminophen Tablets	VA1, IIIA4	FID-I, 530	n-tricosane
and Aspirin Tablets			
Propranol Hydrochloride	VB1b	UV-290	
Propranolol Hydrochloride	VB1b	UV-220	
Extended-release Capsules	VB1b	UV-290	
Injection	VB1b	UV-290	
Tablets	VB1b	UV-290	
and Hydrochlorothiazide	VB1b	UV-220	
Extended-release capsules			
and Hydrochlorothiazide	VB1b	UV-270	
Tablets			
Propyl Gallate	IIIB1	273	
Propylene Carbonate	IA1b		Phth
Propylene Glycol	VA1	TC-P	
Alginate	IA2bi		
Monostearate	IA2b		Phth
Propylhexedrine	IA1b		Phth
Inhalant	IA2a		MeR
Propylparaben	IA2b		MeR
Propylparaben Sodium	IC2f		BtB
Propylidone	IC1lii		ST
Injectable Oil Suspension	IC1lii		ST
Propylthiouracil	IA1ai		ST
Tablets	VB1b	UV-272	BtB
Protamine Sulfate	VIF		
Injection	VIF		
for Injection	VIF		
Protriptyline Hydrochloride	IA1biii	292	CrV
Tablets	IIIB1		
Pseudoephedrine	IA1biii		CrV
Hydrochloride			
Syrup	VB1b	UV-254	
Tablets	VB1b	UV-214	

DRUG	ASSAY CATEGORY	ANALYTICAL WAVELENGTH AND/OR DETECTOR	INDICATOR OR INTERNAL STANDARD
Pseudoephedrine Sulfate	IA1bii	UV-288	Poten
Pyrantel Pamoate	VB1b	UV-288	
Oral Suspension	VB1b		
Pyrazinamide	IA1c	UV-270	MeR
Tablets	VB1b		
Pyridostigmine Bromide	IA1biii		QR
Injection	IIIB1	269	
Syrup	IIIA2	415	
Tablets	VB1b	UV-270	
Pyridoxine Hydrochloride	VB1b	UV-280	p-hydroxybenzoic acid
Injection	IIIA4		
Tablets	IIIA4		
Pyrilamine Maleate	IA1bii		CrV
Tablets	IIIB1	312	
Pyrimethamine	IA1bii		QR
Tablets	IIIB1	273	
Pyrvinium Pamoate	IIIA3	505	
Oral Suspension	IIIA3	505	
Tablets	IIIA3	505	
Quazepam	IA1B	UV-254	Poten
Tablets	VB1b		ethylparaben
Quinidine Gluconate	IA1bii		Nb
Extended-release Tablets	VB1b	UV-235	
Injection	VB2b	UV-235	
Quinidine Sulfate	IA1biii		Nb
Capsules	VB2b	UV-235	
Tablets	VB2b	UV-235	
Tablets, Extended-Release	VB2b	UV-232	
Quinine Sulfate	IA1bii		Nb
Capsules	VB2b	UV-235	
Tablets	VB2b	UV-235	
Rabies Immune Globulin	None		
Vaccine	None		
Racepinephrine	IIIA4	530	
Inhalation Solution	VB1b	UV-280	
Hydrochloride	VB1b	UV-278	
Raclopride C 11 Injection	VIE		
Ranitidine Hydrochloride	VB1b	UV-230	
Injection	VB1b	UV-322	
Tablets	VB1b	UV-322	
Oral Solution	VB1b	UV-322	Poten
in Sodium Chloride Injection	VB1b, IB1a		
Rauwolfia Serpentia	IIIA4	390	
Powdered	IIIA4	390	
Tablets	IIIA4	390	
Rehydration Salts, Oral	VIC1, IIIF1, 121a		
Reserpine	VB1b	UV-268	
Elixir	IIIA4	390	
Injection	IIIA4	390	
Tablets	VB1b	UV-268	
and Chlorothiazide Tablets	IIIE2, IIIB1	292	

DRUG	ASSAY CATEGORY	ANALYTICAL WAVELENGTH AND/OR DETECTOR	INDICATOR OR INTERNAL STANDARD
Hydralazine Hydrochloride and Hydrochlorothiazide Tablets	IIIA4, IIIB1, IIIA4	390, 271, 510	
and Hydrochlorothiazide Tablets	IIIA4, IIIB1	500, 274	ST
Resorcinol	IC2c		ST, caffeine
and Sulfur Lotion	IC1k, VB1b	UV-280	
Ribavirin	VB1b	UV-207	
for Inhalation Solution	VB1b	UV-207	
Riboflavin	IIIE1	530	
Injection	IIIE1	530	
Tablets	IIIE1	530	
5'-Phosphate Sodium	IIIE1	530	
Rifabutin	VB1b	UV-254	
Capsules	VB1b	UV-254	
Rifampin	VB1b	UV-254	
Capsules	VB1b	UV-254	
for Injection	VB1b	UV-207	
Oral Suspension	None	None	Poten
and Isoniazid Capsules	VIN1, IC1h		
Rimexolone	VB1b	UV-242	
Ophthalmic Suspension	VB1b	UV-242	
Ringer's Injection	IIID, IB1a	766	DCF
Irrigation	IIID, IB1a	766	DCF
and Dextrose Injection	IIID, IB1a, VIC1	766	DCF
Lactated, Injection	IC1a, IIID, IB1a, VB1b	766, UV-210	HNB, DCF
Lactated and Dextrose Injection	IC1a, IIID, IB1a, VIC1	766	HNB, DCF
Half-strength Lactated and Dextrose Injection	IC1a, IIID, IB1a, VIC1	766	HNB, DCF
Modified Lactated and Dextrose Injection	IC1a, IIID, IB1a, VIC1	766	HNB, DCF
Ritodrine Hydrochloride	VB1b	UV-254	
Injection	VB1b	UV-275	
Tablets	VB1b	UV-275	
Roxarsone	VB1b	UV-280	
Rubidium Chloride Rb 82 Injection	VIE		
Saccharin	IA1a		Phth
Calcium	IA1ai		Phth
Saccharin Sodium	IA1ai		Phth
Oral Solution	VB1b		
Tablets	IIIB1	UV-257	
Salicylamide	IA1aiii	269	TB
Salicylic Acid	IA1a		Phth
Collodion	IA1a		BtB
Gel	IA1a		Phth
Plaster	IC2c		ST
Topical Foam	VB1b	UV-280	benzoic acid
Salsalate	VB1b	UV-263	
Capsules	VB1b	UV-263	
Tablets	VB1b		

Appendix B. Assay Index of Official USP-NF Drugs

DRUG	ASSAY CATEGORY	ANALYTICAL WAVELENGTH AND/OR DETECTOR	INDICATOR OR INTERNAL STANDARD
Sargramostim for Injection	VIE		
	VIE		
Scopolamine Hydrobromide	IA1bii		CrV
Injection	VA1	TC-I	homatropine hydrobromide
Ophthalmic Ointment	VA1	TC-I	homatropine hydrobromide
Ophthalmic Solution	VA1	TC-I	homatropine hydrobromide
Tablets	VA1	TC-I	homatropine hydrobromide
	IA1aiii		TB
Secobarbital Elixir	VA1	FID-I	butabarbital
Secobarbital Sodium	IIB		
Capsules	VA1	FID-I	butabarbital
Injection	IIIB1	260	
for Injection	IIB		
and Amobarbital Sodium Capsules	VA1	FID-I	aprobarbital
Selegiline Hydrochloride	VB1b	UV-205	
Tablets	VB1b	UV-205	
Selenious Acid	IC2c		
Injection	IIIF1		ST
Selenium Sulfide	IC1lii		ST
Lotion	IC1lii		ST
Selenomethionine	IA1bii		CrV
Sennosides A and B	IIIE2	505	
Tablets	IIIE2	505	
Serine	IA1bii		Poten
Silicon Dioxide	IIC		
Colloidal Silicon Dioxide	IIC		
Silver Nitrate	IB1b		FAS
Ophthalmic Solution	IB1b		FAS
Toughened	IB1b		FAS
Silver Sulfadiazine	VB1b	UV-254	
Cream	VB1b	UV-254	sulfamerazine
Simethicone	IIIC1	7.9	
Capsules	IIIC1	7.9	
Emulsion	IIIC1	7.9	
Oral Suspension	IIIC1	7.9	
Tablets	IIIC1	7.9	
Simvastatin	VB1b	UV-238	
Tablets	VB1b	UV-238	
Sincalide for Injection	VIH		
Sisomicin Sulfate	VIN1		
Injection	VIN1		
Soda Lime	VIK		
Sodium Acetate	IA1bii		Nb
C 11 Injection	VB1b, VIE	UV-210	
Injection	IIID	589	Nb
Solution	IA1bii		Phth
Sodium Alginate	IA2b		ST
Sodium Ascorbate	IC1k		

DRUG	ASSAY CATEGORY	ANALYTICAL WAVELENGTH AND/OR DETECTOR	INDICATOR OR INTERNAL STANDARD
Sodium Benzoate	IA1bii		CrV
Sodium Bicarbonate	IA1b		MeR
Injection	IA1b		MeR
Oral Powder	IA1b		MeO
Tablets	IA1b		MeR
Sodium Borate	IA1b		MeR
Sodium Carbonate	IA1b		MeR
Sodium Chloride	IB1a		DCF
Inhalation Solution	IB1a		DCF
Injection	IB1a		DCF
Bacteriostatic Injection	IB1a		DCF
Irrigation	IB1a		DCF
Ophthalmic Ointment	IB1a		DCF
Ophthalmic Solution	IB1a		DCF
Tablets	IB2aii		FAS
Tablets for Solution	IB2aii		FAS
Sodium Citrate and Dextrose Tablets	IB2aii, VIC1		FAS
and Citric Acid Oral Solution	IA1bii		Poten
Sodium Dehydroacetate	IIID, IA1a		Phth
Sodium Fluoride	IA1bii		Nb
Oral Solution	IVB1		
Tablets	IVB1		
and Acidulated Phosphate Topical Solution	IVB1		
and Phosphoric Acid Gel	IVB1		
and Phosphoric Acid Topical Solution	IVB1		
Sodium Formaldehyde Sulfoxylate	IC1k		ST
Sodium Gluconate	IA1bii		QR
Sodium Hydroxide	IA1b		Phth
Sodium Hypochlorite Solution	IC1lii		ST
Sodium Iodide	IC1n		
Sodium Lactate Injection	IA1bii		Poten
Solution	IA1bii		Poten
Sodium Lauryl Sulfate	None		
Sodium Metabisulfite	IC2a		ST
Sodium Monofluorophosphate	IB1d		SAS
Sodium Nitrite	IC2e		
Injection	IC2e		
Sodium Nitroprusside	IB1a		Poten
for Injection	VB1b	UV-210	
Monobasic Sodium Phosphate	IA1b		Phth
Dibasic Sodium Phosphate	IA2a		Poten
Sodium Phosphates Enema	IA1a		Poten
Injection	IA1a, b		Poten
Oral Solution	IA1a		Poten
Sodium Polystyrene Sulfonate Suspension	VB1b	RI	

DRUG	ASSAY CATEGORY	ANALYTICAL WAVELENGTH AND/OR DETECTOR	INDICATOR OR INTERNAL STANDARD
Sodium Propionate	IA1bii		CrV
Sodium Salicylate	IA1bii		CrV
Tablets	IA1b		BpB
Sodium Starch Glycolate	IA1bii		Poten
Sodium Stearate	VA2	FID-I	
Sodium Stearyl Fumarate	IA1a		QR
Sodium Sulfate	IIB		
Injection	IIB		
Sodium Thiosulfate	IC1k		ST
Injection	IC1k		ST
Sorbic Acid	IA1a		Phth
Sorbitan Monolaurate	IIA, IIA		
Sorbitan Monooleate	IIA, IIA		
Sorbitan Monopalmitate	IIA, IIA		
Sorbitan Monostearate	IIA, IIA		
Sorbitol	VB1b	RI	
Noncrystallizing Solution	VB1b	RI	
Solution	VB1b	RI	
Spectinomycin Hydrochloride	VA2	FID-I	triphenylantimony
for Injectable Suspension	VA2	FID-I	triphenylantimony
Spironolactone	VB1b	UV-254	
Tablets	VB1b	UV-254	
and Hydrochlorothiazide Tablets	IC1n, IVB1	UV-254	
Stannous Fluoride	IVB1	590	
Stanozolol	IA1bii		
Tablets	IIIB1	235	CrV
Stearic Acid	VA2	FID-I	
Purified	VA2	FID-I	
Stearyl Alcohol	VA1	FID-I	
Streptomycin Sulfate	VIN1	UV-214	
Injection	VIN1	UV-214	
for Injection	VIN1	UV-214	
Strontium Chloride Sr 89 Injection	IIIF1	UV-240	
Succinylcholine Chloride	VB1b	UV-230	
Injection	VB1b	UV-230	
for Injection	VB1b	RI	
Sucralfate	VB1b	RI	
Tablets	IA1aiii		
Sucrose Octaacetate	IA2b		Phth
Sufentanil Citrate	IAbii		NPB
Injection	VB1b	UV-240	
Compressible Sugar	VIC1		
Sugar, Inverted, Injection	IIB		
Sulbactam Sodium	VB1b	UV-230	TB
Sulconazole Nitrate	VB1b	UV-230	Poten
Sulfabenzamide	IA1aiii		Poten
Sulfacetamide	IC1j		
Sulfacetamide Sodium	IC1j		
Ophthalmic Ointment	VB1b	UV-254	
Ophthalmic Solution	VB1b	UV-254	
and Prednisolone Acetate Ophthalmic Ointment	VB1b	UV-254	norethindrone

DRUG	ASSAY CATEGORY	ANALYTICAL WAVELENGTH AND/OR DETECTOR	INDICATOR OR INTERNAL STANDARD
and Prednisolone Acetate Ophthalmic Suspension	VB1b	UV-254	
Sulfachlorpyridazine	VB1b	UV-265	
Sulfadiazine	VB1b	UV-254	
Tablets	VB1b	UV-214	
Silver Sulfadiazine	VB1b	UV-214	
Cream	IC1j		sulfamerazine
Sulfadiazine Sodium	IC1j		sulfamerazine
Injection	IC1j		Poten
Sulfadoxine	IC1j		Poten
and Pyrimethamine Tablets	VB1b	UV-254	phenacetin
Sulfamethazine	VB2b		Poten
Granulated		450	
Sulfamethizole	IC1j		Poten
Oral Suspension	IC1j		Poten
Tablets	IC1j		Poten
Sulfamethoxazole	IC1j		Poten
Oral Suspension	IC1j		Poten
Tablets	IC1j		Poten
and Trimethoprim for Injection	VB1b	UV-254	Poten
and Trimethoprim Oral Suspension	VB1b	UV-254	
and Trimethoprim Tablets	VB1b	UV-254	
Sulfapyridine	IC1j		Poten
Tablets	IC1j		
Sulfaquinoxaline	VB1b	UV-254	Poten
Oral Solution	VB1b	UV-254	Phth
Sulfasalazine	IIIB1	359	benzoic acid
Delayed-release Tablets	IIIB1	359	benzoic acid
Tablets	IIIB1	359	
Sulfathiazole	IC1j		TB
Sulfinpyrazone	IA1a		TB
Capsules	VB1b	UV-235	Poten
Tablets	IA1aiii	UV-235	Poten
Sulfisoxazole	IA1aiii		Phth
Tablets	IC1j		
Sulfisoxazole Acetyl	IC1j		
Oral Suspension	IA1a		Phth
Sulfur, Precipitated	IIB		
Ointment	IA1a		
Sulfur, Sublimed	IA1a		
Sulfur Dioxide	IC1k		Phth
Sulfuric Acid	IA1a		ST
Sulindac	IA1a		MeO
Tablets	VB1a	UV-332	Poten
Sulisobenzone	IA1a		
Suprofen	VB1b	UV-254	Poten
Ophthalmic Solution	VB1b	UV-254	
Tamoxifen Citrate	IA1bii		
Tablets	VB1b	UV-254	Poten
Technetium Tc 99m (All)	VIE		
Temazepam	VB1b	UV-220	
Capsules	VB1b	UV-254	benzophenone

Appendix B. Assay Index of Official USP-NF Drugs

DRUG	ASSAY CATEGORY	ANALYTICAL WAVELENGTH AND/OR DETECTOR	INDICATOR OR INTERNAL STANDARD
Terbutaline Sulfate	VB1b	UV-280	
Injection	VB1b	UV-280	
Inhalation Aerosol	VB1b	UV-280	
Tablets	VB1b	UV-280	
Terpin Hydrate	VA1	FID-I	biphenyl
Elixir	VA1	FID-I	biphenyl
and Codeine Elixir	VA1	FID-I	biphenyl, N-phenylcarbazole
Testolactone	IIIA4	415	
Tablets	IIIA4	415	
Testosterone	IIIB1	241	
Injectable Suspension	IIIB1	241	
Testosterone Cypionate	VA1	FID-I	cholesteryl caprylate
Injection	VA1	FID-I	cholesteryl caprylate
Testosterone Enanthate	IIIA4	380	
Injection	IIIA4	380	
Testosterone Propionate	IIIA4	380	
Injection	IIIA4	380	
Tetracaine	ICj	310	SPI
Ointment	IIIB1	310	
Ophthalmic Ointment	IIIB1	310	
and Menthol Ointment	VA1, IIIB1	FID-I, 310	1-decanol
Tetracaine Hydrochloride	ICj		Poten
Cream	IIIB1	310	
Injection	VB1b	UV-305	
Ophthalmic Solution	IIIB1	310	
Topical Solution	IIIB1	310	
for Injection	IIIB1	310	
in Dextrose Injection	VIC1	UV-280	
Tetracycline	VB1b		
Boluses	VIN1		
Oral Suspension	VB1b	UV-280	
Tetracycline Hydrochloride	VB1b	UV-280	
Capsules	VB1b	UV-280	
for Injection	VB1b	UV-280	
Ointment	VB1b	UV-280	
Ophthalmic Ointment	VIN1		
for Topical Solution	VIC1	UV-280	
Soluble Powder	VB1b		
Ophthalmic Suspension	VIN1		
Tablets	VB1b	UV-280	
Tetracycline Hydrochloride	VB1b	UV-280	
Capsules	VB1b	UV-280	
for Injection	VB1b	UV-280	
Ointment	VB1b	UV-280	
Ophthalmic Ointment	VIN1		
for Topical Solution	IIIB1	366	
Soluble Powder	VIN1		
Ophthalmic Suspension	VB1b	UV-280	
Tablets	VB1b	UV-280	
and Novobiocin Sodium Tablets	VIN1		
Novobiocin Sodium and	VIN1, VB1b	UV-254	betamethasone
Prednisol one Tablets	VIN1		
and Nystatin Capsules	IA1biii		
Tetrahydrozoline Hydrochloride	IIIA4	570	QR
Nasal Solution	VB1b	UV-280	
Ophthalmic Solution	VIE		
Thallous Chloride Tl 201 Injection			

DRUG	ASSAY CATEGORY	ANALYTICAL WAVELENGTH AND/OR DETECTOR	INDICATOR OR INTERNAL STANDARD
Theophylline	VB1b	UV-280	theobromine
Capsules	VB1b	UV-280	theobromine
Capsules, Extended Release	VB1b	UV-280	theobromine
in Dextrose Injection	VB1b, VIC1	UV-280	theobromine
Tablets	VB1b	UV-280	theobromine
Ephedrine Hydrochloride and	VB1b	UV-241	butabarbital sodium
Phenobarbital Tablets			
and Guaifenesin Capsules	VB1b	UV-280	caffeine
and Guaifenesin Oral Solution	VB1b	UV-280	theobromine
Theophylline Sodium Glycinate	VB1b	UV-280	theobromine
Elixir	IB2ai		FAS
Tablets	IA1biii		CrV
Thiabendazole	VB1b	UV-254	
Oral Suspension	VB1b	UV-254	
Tablets	VB1b	UV-232	
Thiacetarsamide	VB1b	UV-232	
Sodium Injection	VB1b	UV-254	
Thiamine Hydrochloride	VB1b	UV-254	methylbenzoate
Elixir	VB1b	UV-254	methylparaben
Injection	VB1b	UV-254	methylparaben
Tablets	IIIE2	365	
Thiamine Mononitrate	VB1b	UV-254	methylbenzoate
Elixir	VB1b	UV-254	methylparaben
Thiethylperazine Maleate	IA1bii		Poten
Suppositories	VB1b	UV-265	
Tablets	VB1b	UV-265	
Thimerosal	IIIF1	254	
Topical Aerosol	IIIF1	254	
Topical Solution	IIIF1	254	
Tincture	IIIF1	254	
Thioguanine	IIIB1	348	
Tablets	IIIB1	348	
Thiopental Sodium	IIIB1	304	
for Injection	IIIB1	304	
Thioridazine	IA1bii		Poten
Oral Suspension	IIIB1	265	
Thioridazine Hydrochloride	IA1bii		Poten
Oral Solution	IIIB1	265	
Tablets	VB1b	UV-265	
Thiostrepton	VB1b	UV-254	
Thiotepa	VB1b	UV-215	
for Injection	IIIC1	10.75	
Thiothixene	VB1b	UV-254	benzophenone
Capsules	VB1b	UV-254	
Thiothixene Hydrochloride	VB1b	UV-254	
Injection	VB1b	UV-254	
for Injection	VB1b	UV-254	
Oral Solution	VB1b	UV-254	
Threonine	IA1bii		Poten

DRUG	ASSAY CATEGORY	ANALYTICAL WAVELENGTH AND/OR DETECTOR	INDICATOR OR INTERNAL STANDARD
Thymol	IC1h		MeO
Thyroid	VB1b	UV-230	
Tablets	VB1b	UV-230	
Ticarcillin Disodium	VB1b	UV-220	
for Injection	VB1b	UV-220	
Ticarcillin Disodium and Clavulanic Acid Injection	VB1b	UV-220	
and Clavulanic Acid for Injection	VB1b	UV-220	
Ticarcillin Monosodium	VB1b	UV-220	CrV
Tiletamine Hydrochloride	IA1bii	FID	tetraphenylethylene
Tiletamine and Zolazepam for Injection	VA1	FID	
Tilmicosin	VB1b	UV-280	
Injection	VB1b	UV-280	
Timolol Maleate	IA1bii		Poten
Ophthalmic Solution	VB1b	UV-295	
Tablets	VB1b	UV-295	
and Hydrochlorothiazide Tablets	VB1b	UV-295	
Tioconazole	VB1b	UV-219	
Titanium Dioxide	IC1bi		
Tobramycin	VB2b	UV-365	
Injection	VIN1		
for Injection	VIN1		
Ophthalmic Ointment	VB2b	UV-365	
Ophthalmic Solution	VB2b	UV-365	
and Dexamethasone Ophthalmic Ointment	VB2b, VB1b	UV-365, 206	
and Dexamethasone Ophthalmic Suspension	VIN1, VB1b	UV-254	
and Fluorometholone Acetate Ophthalmic Suspension	VB2b	UV-365	
Tocainide Hydrochloride	IA1bii	UV-254	Poten
Tablets	VB1b	UV-254	
Tocopherols Excipient	VA1	FID-I	hexadecyl hexadecanoate
Tolazamide	VB1a	UV-254	tolbutamide
Tablets	VB1a	UV-254	tolbutamide
Tolazoline Hydrochloride	IA1biii		Poten
Injection	IIIA4	568	
Tolbutamide	VB1a	UV-254	tolazamide
Tablets	VB1a	UV-254	tolazamide
for Injection	VB1a	UV-254	tolazamide
Tolmetin Sodium	IA1bii		Poten
Capsules	VB1b	UV-254	
Tablets	VB1b	UV-254	
Tolnaftate	IIIB1	258	
Cream	VB1b	UV-254	progesterone
Gel	IIIB1	258	
Topical Aerosol Powder	IIIB1	258	
Topical Powder	VB1b	UV-254	progesterone
Topical Solution	IIIB1	258	
Trazodone Hydrochloride	VB1b	UV-254	butylparaben
Tablets	VB1b	UV-254	
Trenbolone Acetate	VB1b	UV-344	

DRUG	ASSAY CATEGORY	ANALYTICAL WAVELENGTH AND/OR DETECTOR	INDICATOR OR INTERNAL STANDARD
Tretinoin	IA1aiii		TB
Cream	VB1b	UV-365	
Gel	IIIB1	365	
Topical Solution	IIIB1	352	
Triacetin	IA2bi		Phth
Triamcinolone	VB1b	UV-254	hydrocortisone
Tablets	VB1b	UV-254	hydrocortisone
Triamcinolone Acetonide	VB1b	UV-254	fluoxymesterone
Topical Aerosol	VB1b	UV-254	fluoxymesterone
Cream	VB1b	UV-254	fluoxymesterone
Lotion	VB1b	UV-254	fluoxymesterone
Ointment	VB1b	UV-254	fluoxymesterone
Dental Paste	VB1b	UV-254	fluoxymesterone
Injectable Suspension	VB1b	UV-254	fluoxymesterone
Triamcinolone Diacetate	VB1b	UV-254	
Injectable Suspension	VB1b	UV-254	
Syrup	VB1b	UV-254	
Triamcinolone Hexacetonide	VB1b	UV-254	fluoxymesterone
Injectable Suspension	VB1b	UV-254	
Triamterene	IA1bii		Poten
Capsules	VB1b	UV-280	
and Hydrochlorothiazide Capsules	VB1b	UV-280	
and Hydrochlorothiazide Tablets	VB1b	UV-280	alprazolam
Triazolam	VB1b	UV-254	alprazolam
Tablets	VB1b	UV-254	Poten
Trichlorfon	IB1a		
Trichlormethiazide	VB1b	UV-254	methylparaben
Tablets	VB1b	UV-254	
Trichloromonofluoromethane	VA1	FID	
Tricitrates Oral Solution	IA1a, b, IIID	766	Phth
Triclosan	VA1	FID	
Trientine Hydrochloride	IAb		
Capsules	IIIA4	580	
Triethyl Citrate	IB2b		
Trifluoperazine Hydrochloride	IA1biii		Phth
Injection	IIIB1	255	CrV
Syrup	IIIB1	255	
Tablets	VB1b	UV-262	
Triflupromazine	IA1bii		
Oral Suspension	IIIB1	255	CrV
Triflupromazine Hydrochloride	IA1biii		
Injection	IIIB1	255	CrV
Tablets	IIIB1	255	
Trifluridine	VB1b	UV-254	
Trihexyphenidyl Hydrochloride	VB1b	UV-210	
Capsules, Extended-Release	VB1b	UV-210	
Elixir	VB1b	UV-210	
Tablets	VB1b	UV-210	
Trikates Oral Solution	IIIF1	766.5	
Trimeprazine Tartrate	VB1b	UV-254	
Syrup	VB1b	UV-254	
Tablets	VB1b	UV-254	

Appendix B. Assay Index of Official USP-NF Drugs

DRUG	ASSAY CATEGORY	ANALYTICAL WAVELENGTH AND/OR DETECTOR	INDICATOR OR INTERNAL STANDARD
Trimethobenzamide Hydrochloride	IA1biii		Poten
Capsules	IIIB1	258	
Injection	IIIB1	258	
Trimethoprim	IA1bii		Poten
Tablets	VB1b	UV-254	
Trimethoprim Sulfate	IA1bii		Poten
Trioxsalen	VB1b	UV-254	
Tablets	IIIB1	252	
Tripelenamine Hydrochloride	IIIB1	313	
Tablets	IA1biii		CrV
Triprolidine Hydrochloride	IA1biii		Poten
Syrup	VB1b	UV-254	
Tablets	VB1b	UV-254	
and Pseudoephedrine Hydrochloride Syrup	VB1b	UV-254	
and Pseudoephedrine Hydrochloride Tablets	VB1b	UV-254	
Trisulfapyrimidines Oral Suspension	VB1b	UV-254	
Tablets	VB1b	UV-254	
Trolamine Salicylate	IA1b		MeR
Troleandomycin	VIN1		
Capsules	VIN1		
Tromethamine	IA1b		BcP
for Injection	IA1b		BcP
Tropicamide	IA1bii		CrV
Ophthalmic Solution	IIIB1	253	
Crystallized Trypsin	VIF		
for Inhalation Aerosol	VIF		
Tryptophan	IA1bii		Poten
Tubocurarine Chloride	VB1b	UV-220	
Injection	VB1b	UV-220	
Tylosin	VIN		
Granulated	VIN		
Tyrosine	IA1bii		Poten
Tyrothricin	VIN1		
Undecylenic Acid	IA1a		
Compound Ointment	IIIF1, VA2	214, FID-I	Phth
Urea	IA1c		tridecanoic acid
Urea for Injection	IA1c		MRB
Ursodiol	VB1b	RI	MRB
Capsules	VB1b	RI	epiandrosterone
Valine	IA1bii		epiandrosterone
Valproic Acid	VA1	FID	Poten
Capsules	VA1	FID-I	nonanoic acid
Syrup	VA1	FID-I	biphenyl
Vancomycin	VIN1		biphenyl
Injection	VIN1		
Vancomycin Hydrochloride			
Capsules	VIN1		
for Injection	VIN1		
for Oral Solution	VIN1		
Sterile	VIN1		
Vanillin	IIIB1	308	
Varicella-Zoster Immune Globulin	None		
Vasopressin	VB1b	UV-220	
Injection	VB1b	UV-220	
Verapamil Hydrochloride	IA1biii		Poten
Extended-release Tablets	VB1b	UV-278	
Injection	VB1b	UV-278	
Tablets	VB1b	UV-278	
Vidarabine	VB1b	UV-262	
Ophthalmic Ointment	VB1b	UV-254	
Vinblastine Sulfate	VB1b	UV-262	
for Injection	VB1b	UV-262	
Vincristine Sulfate	VB1b	UV-297	
Injection	VB1b	UV-297	
for Injection	VB1b	UV-297	
Vitamin A	VIL		
Capsules	VIL		
Vitamin E	VA1	FID-I	hexadecyl hexadecanoate
Preparation	VA1	FID-I	hexadecyl hexadecanoate
Capsules	VA1	FID-I	hexadecyl hexadecanoate
Water-soluble Vitamins Capsules	VIL		
Water-soluble Vitamins Tablets	VIL		
Water-soluble Vitamins with Mineral Capsules	VIL		
Water-soluble Vitamins with Mineral Tablets	VIL		
Oil- and Water-soluble Vitamins Capsules	VIL		
Tablets	VIL		
with Mineral Capsules	VIL		
with Mineral Tablets	VIL		
Oil-soluble Vitamins Capsules	VIL		
Oil-soluble Vitamins Tablets	VIL		
Warfarin Sodium	VB1b	UV-280	propylparaben
for Injection	VB1b	UV-280	propylparaben
Xanthan Gum	IA2b	UV-280	propylparaben
Xenon Xe 127	VIE		
Xenon Xe 133	VIE		
Injection	VIE		Phth

DRUG	ASSAY CATEGORY	ANALYTICAL WAVELENGTH AND/OR DETECTOR	INDICATOR OR INTERNAL STANDARD
Xylazine	VB1b	UV-226	
Injection	VB1b	UV-254	
Xylazine Hydrochloride	VB1b	UV-254	
Xylitol	VA1		erithritol
Xylometazoline Hydrochloride Nasal Solution	IA1biii		Poten
Xylose	IIIA4	565	
	IIIA4	520	
Zalcitabine	VB1b	UV-270	
Tablets	VB1b	UV-280	
Zidovudine	VB1b	UV-265	
Capsules	VB1b	UV-265	
Injection	VB1b	UV-265	
Oral Solution	VB1b	UV-265	
Zinc Acetate	ID1a		EBT

DRUG	ASSAY CATEGORY	ANALYTICAL WAVELENGTH AND/OR DETECTOR	INDICATOR OR INTERNAL STANDARD
Zinc Carbonate	IA2a		MeO
Zinc Chloride	ID1a		EBT
Injection	IIIF1	213.8	
Zinc Gluconate	ID1a		EBT
Zinc Oxide	IA2a		MeO
Ointment	ID1a		EBT
Paste	IIC		
and Salicylic Acid Paste	IA1aiii		TB, PR
Zinc Stearate	ID1a		EBT
Zinc Sulfate	ID1a		EBT
Injection	IIIF1	213.8	
Ophthalmic Solution	ID1a		PAN
Zinc Undecylenate	IA2a		MeO
Zolazepam Hydrochloride	IA1bii		Poten

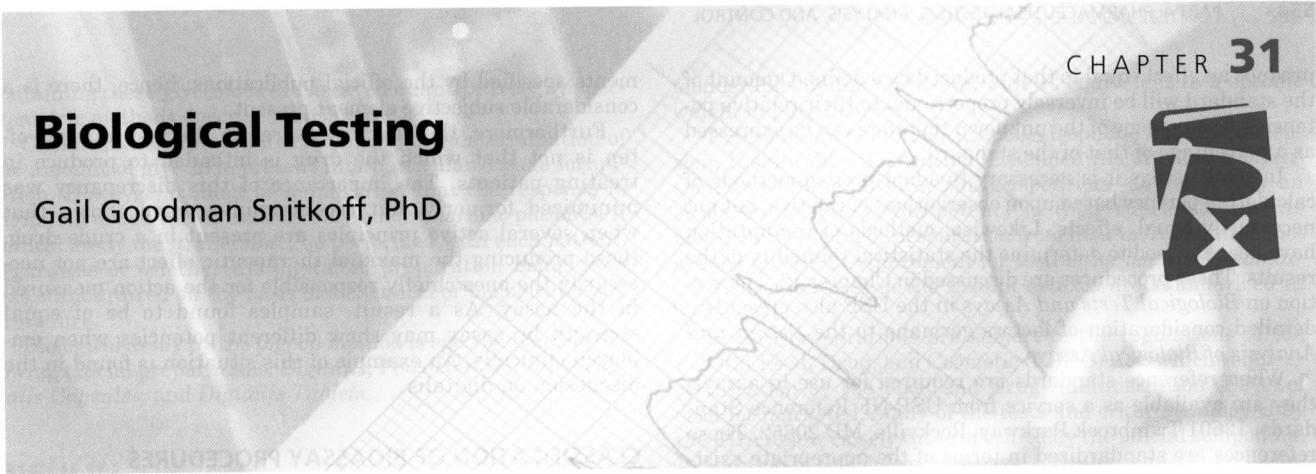

CHAPTER 31

Biological Testing

Gail Goodman Snitkoff, PhD

Biological testing includes the quantitative assay of drugs by biological methods as well as the application of qualitative biological tests. Such testing uses intact animals, animal preparations, isolated living tissues and cells, or microorganisms. In addition to drugs, biological tests are a requirement for plastics to be used as containers or closures for ophthalmic and parenteral preparations or to be used as implants, devices, or other related systems.

The practices of the USP are a good index of the state of biological testing. Currently there is a trend to use fewer animals in research and biological testing and to use alternatives such as cells and microorganisms in culture. This decrease in animal use can be observed in the decreased requirement for animal testing by the USP as documented in their monographs. Wherever possible, *in vitro* procedures should be used to complement or replace *in vivo* tests for evaluating the suitability of plastics.

The majority of currently available therapeutic agents are substances of known chemical composition that can be assayed by quantitative chemical or physical analyses. However, there are a limited number of useful drugs that cannot be assayed satisfactorily by chemical or physical means. Such drugs, which are primarily of natural origin, are assayed by biological methods. Biological standardization procedures generally are less precise, more time-consuming, and more expensive to conduct than are chemical assays; therefore, they generally are reserved for use:

1. If the chemical identity of the active principle has not been elucidated fully.
2. If no adequate chemical assay has been devised for the active principle, although its chemical structure has been established (eg, insulin).
3. If the drug is composed of a complex mixture of substances of varying structure and activity (eg, digitalis, posterior pituitary).
4. If purification of the crude drug, sufficient for the performance of a chemical assay, is not possible or practical (eg, the separation of vitamin D from certain irradiated oils).
5. If the chemical assay is not a valid indication of biological activity, due, for example, to lack of differentiation between active and inactive isomers.

There are several situations in which factors such as specificity, sensitivity, or practicality dictate the use of a biological rather than a chemical assay procedure.

A chemical assay quantitatively determines the amount of a specific compound or structural moiety present in a given sample. Once the concentration has been established an assumption is made relative to the biological activity of the sample. In contrast, a biological assay measures the actual biological activity of a given sample, which may represent the algebraic sum of the interaction of a number of chemical and physical-chemical factors. For example, the data obtained from a chemical assay will not provide information concerning the contribution to the net biological activity of trace amounts of substances that do not influence the chemical analysis. Such substances may produce qualitative variations in biological activity that may be responsible for unexpected side effects or toxic reactions. Furthermore, the enhancing or inhibiting influences of variations in the physical state of the active principle are not reflected in the results of a chemical assay. The safety, efficacy, and dependability of dosage of drugs are contingent upon standardization, and biological assays must be employed in some instances even though the chemical identities of the active principles in the preparation may be known.

ANIMAL TESTING

As animals are an important *unknown* factor in most biological assays, the need for their proper selection and adequate care is self-evident. Most laboratories seek a reliable source of animals that can supply their needs from colonies maintained for this purpose. In any one test it is desirable to use animals of only one strain. Usually bioassayists adopt a specified strain for all work of a particular type. This enables the bioassayist to gain experience concerning the expected normal variation. For some assays a specific sex must be employed (eg, estrogenic tests); in other assays either sex may be used, but the effect that sex may play in the response should not be overlooked. The male rat, for instance, has a faster growth rate than the female; therefore, indiscriminate use of both males and females in a rat growth test should be avoided. Differences in the response of the sexes may extend into other categories, such as response toward toxic materials. Animals used in these biological assays should always be handled according to the National Institutes of Health guidelines.[1]

BIOASSAY PROCEDURES

Bioassays are conducted by determining the amount of a preparation of unknown potency required to produce a definite effect on suitable test animals or organs under standard conditions.

REFERENCE STANDARDS

To minimize the source of error resulting from animal variation, standard reference preparations are used in certain bioassay procedures. The principle of the using a reference standard consists of successively testing the unknown and standard preparations on two groups of similar animals, or, in some cases (eg, epinephrine, posterior pituitary) on the same animal or organ. The amount of the unknown preparation required to

Table 31-1. Summary of Biological Assay Procedures

COMPENDIAL/ARTICLE	ACTIVITY ASSAYED	ANIMAL EMPLOYED	ROUTE OF ADMINISTRATION OF TEST MATERIAL	END POINT OF ASSAY	UNITAGE	ADDITIONAL BIOLOGICAL TESTS REQUIRED
Digitalis	Cardiac (cardiotonic) action	Pigeon	IV infusion	Cardiac arrest (death)	100 mg is equivalent to not less than 1 USP Digitalis Unit	—
Insulin injection	Hypoglycemic	Rabbit	SC injection	Reduction of blood glucose level	1 mL is equivalent to 40, 100, or 500 USP Insulin Units (potency not less than 95% and not more than 105% of that stated on the label)	Bacterial endotoxins
Insulin	Hypoglycemic	Rabbit	SC injection	Reduction of blood glucose level	Each mg has a biological potency of not less than 26.5 USP Insulin Units	Bacterial endotoxins
Insulin Human Insulin Human Injection	—	—	—	—	Biological potency (uses Insulin Assay, but rubric definition uses HPLC)	Bacterial endotoxins
Isophane Insulin Suspension	—	—	—	—	Biological Activity of the supernatant liquid (uses Insulin Assay, with modifications)	Bacterial endotoxins
Glucagon for injection	Hyperglycemic	Cat (injected IP with dextrose 16 hr prior to assay) Rat hepatocytes	IV injection	Elevation of blood glucose	—	Release of glucose
Oxytocin injection Oxytocin Nasal Solution	Contraction of isolated rat uterus	Rat	In vitro Water bath with addition of oxytocin	Magnitude of uterine contractions	1mg is equivalent to not less than 400 Oxytocin Units	Pressor activity—oxytocin injection must not contain excessive vasopressor activity as determined by elevation of arterial blood pressure following IV injection of the test sample in phenoxybenzamine pretreated rats
Vasopressin injection	Vasopressor	Rat (pretreated with phenoxybenzamine)	Intermittent IV injection	Elevation of arterial blood pressure	1mg is equivalent to not less than 300 Vasopressin Units	Oxytocic activity—vasopressin injection must not contain excessive oxytocic activity as determined by contraction of uterine smooth muscle isolated from the guinea pig
Posterior pituitary injection	Vasodepressor and vasopressor (Each mg of USP Posterior Pituitary Reference Standard represents 2.4 USP units of oxytocic activity and 2.1 USP units of vasopressor activity.)	Refer to assays for Oxytocin Injection and Vasopressin Injection	—	—	1 mL possesses USP Posterior Pituitary activity equivalent to not less than 85% and not more than 120% of the oxytocic activity and vasopressin activity stated on the label in USP Posterior Pituitary Units	—
Corticotropin injection Repository corticotropin injection Sterile corticotropin zinc hydroxide suspension						

Substance	Category	Animal	Method	Response	Requirement	Additional requirements
Corticotropin for Injection	Adrenal cortical stimulation	Hypophysectomized rat	SC injection	Reduction of ascorbic acid content of adrenal glands	—	Vasopressin activity—corticotropin injection must not contain excessive vasopressor activity as determined by elevation of arterial blood pressure following IV injection of the test sample in phenoxyben-amine-pretreated rats (this test is not required with Sterile Corticotropin Zinc Hydroxide Suspension)
Bacterial endotoxins Chorionic gonadotropin Chronic gonadotropin for injection	Gonad-stimulating	Female rat	SC injection daily for 3 days	Increase in weight of uterus	1 mg is equivalent to not less than 1500 USP Chorionic Gonadotropin Units	Estrogenic activity—chorionic gonadotropin must not contain excessive estrogenic activity as determined by cytological examination of vaginal smears taken from ovariectomized rats injected SC with the test sample
Bacterial endotoxins Acute toxicity (determined by minimal toxicity in mice injected IV with 1000 USP Chorionic Gonadotropin Units) Heparin sodium Heparin sodium injection Anticoagulant Heparin Solution Heparin Calcium Heparin Calcium Injection	Anticoagulant	Sheep	*In vitro* addition of heparin sodium to blood plasma	Inhibition of clot formation	1 mg is equivalent to not less than 140 USP Heparin Units when derived from intestinal mucosa or other tissues from domesticated foo animals.	Bacterial endotoxins
		—	—	—	—	
Heparin Lock Flush Solution Dihydroergotamine Mesylate, Heparin Sodium and Lidocaine Hydrochloride Injection Protamine sulfate Protamine sulfate injection Protamine sulfate for injection	Heparin neutralization	Sheep	*In vitro* addition of protamine sulfate to blood plasma containing known amounts of heparin sodium	Reduction of clotting time of heparinized plasma	1 mg neutralizes not less than 100 USP Units of heparin activity from lung tissue or not less than 100 USP Units of heparin derived from intestinal mucosa	Bacterial endotoxins
Cod liver oil	Antirachitic (vitamin D)	Rachitic rat	Oral feeding (one-half of total dose on day 1; one-half on day 3 or day 4)	Calcification of rachitic metaphysis of radius and tibia	1 g contains not less than 2.125 μg (85 USP Units) of vitamin D	1 g also contains not less than 255 μg (850 USP Units) of vitamin A (assayed by a spectrophotometric method)

of glucagon is determined by interpolation against a standard curve.

PARATHYROID

Parathyroid hormone is responsible for maintaining extracellular calcium ions at a constant concentration in the body. Porcine, bovine, and human parathyroid hormones are linear polypeptide chains of 84 amino acids with molecular weights of approximately 9500. Amino acids 1 to 27 of the *N*-terminal portion of the peptide are associated with biological activity.

The bioassay for Parathyroid Injection, which is found in USP XXI but is not included in the current USP (USP XXV), is based on measuring the increase in serum calcium in dogs. In this assay, the serum calcium levels are determined just prior to, and 16 to 18 hours after, the subcutaneous injection of the dose of Parathyroid Injection. Each mL of Parathyroid Injection possesses a potency of not less than 100 USP Parathyroid Units. One USP Parathyroid Unit represents 1/100th of the amount of Parathyroid Injection required to raise the calcium content of 100 mL of the blood serum of normal dogs, 1 mg within 16 to 18 hours after administration.

Parathyroid Injection is no longer available for clinical use. Parathyroid hormone was used extensively to raise plasma calcium levels in hypocalcemic patients. Presently, this is achieved more safely by the administration of calcium and/or vitamin D.

POSTERIOR PITUITARY, OXYTOCIN, AND VASOPRESSIN

Extracts of the posterior lobe of the neurohypophysis, when injected into responsive animals, may exert a variety of pharmacodynamic effects, including a rise in blood pressure, contraction of uterine smooth muscle (oxytocic effect), an increased renal tubular reabsorption of water (antidiuresis), and milk-ejection (galactokinesis) in the lactating mammary gland. Although there is no conclusive agreement on the number of different hormones elaborated by the neurohypophysis, two distinct active principles have been separated from extracts of this structure. These are *oxytocin,* which possesses primarily oxytocic and galactokinetic activities, and *vasopressin,* which exhibits predominantly pressor and antidiuretic activities. Both of these hormones are nonapeptides; the amino acid sequences of these fractions obtained from several animal species have been determined, and corresponding nonapeptide amides have been synthesized.

Posterior Pituitary Injection, which is prepared from the posterior lobe of the pituitary gland of domestic animals used for food by man, contains both oxytocic and vasopressor principles in varying amounts. Since oxytocin and vasopressin are available in purified form, Posterior Pituitary Injection, which represents a mixture of the active principles, is used relatively infrequently and is no longer included in the current edition of the USP (XXV).

The potency of Oxytocin Injection used to be determined by monitoring the decreases in blood pressure in an anesthetized chicken following intravenous administration of the Oxytocin Injection. Currently oxytocin activity is monitored by measuring the contraction of an isolated rat uterus. The contractile activity of the sample is compared to that of a reference standard. Oxytocin Nasal Solution, assayed by the same biological method as the Injection, is available for use as a lactational stimulant.

Currently, all commercially available preparations of oxytocin are prepared synthetically. Oxytocin Injection for intravenous or intramuscular administration contains not less than 400 USP oxytocin units per milligram. Oxytocin Injection is used to induce labor, control postpartum uterine bleeding, and treat incomplete abortion.

Vasopressin, also known as antidiuretic hormone, exerts antidiuretic activity and is a potent vasopressor. Vasopressin Injection is prepared synthetically or by extraction of the posterior lobe of the pituitary glands of domestic animals. The potency of Vasopressin Injection is determined by monitoring the elevations in blood pressure in a male rat following intravenous administration. Blood pressure elevations are monitored and compared to those obtained with a standard Vasopressin Injection, to determine potency of the assay sample relative to a USP Vasopressin Reference Standard. On a unit basis, the antidiuretic activity of Vasopressin is greater than or equal to 300 USP Vasopressin units per milligram.

Vasopressin Injection contains not less than 90% and not more than 110% of the USP Vasopressin Units stated on the label. Vasopressin Tannate is available commercially and used to prevent or control the symptoms and complications of diabetes insipidus caused by deficiency of endogenous antidiuretic hormone. All commercially available vasopression is prepared synthetically.

CORTICOTROPIN

Corticotropin (or ACTH, adrenocorticotropic hormone) is a polypeptide hormone that is synthesized and secreted by basophilic cells of the adenohypophysis. This hormone is a straight-chain polypeptide comprised of 39 amino acids. Corticotropin stimulates the release of cortisol, corticosterone, and aldosterone from the adrenal cortex. Stimulation of the median eminence of the hypothalamus causes the release of a polypeptide called corticotropin-releasing factor (CRF) into the circulatory system. CRF stimulates the release of corticotropin from the adenohypophysis. Endogenous corticosteroids influence the secretion of corticotropin through a negative feedback loop. Increased circulating levels of corticosteroids exert a negative influence on the adenohypophysis and decrease the secretion of corticotropin.

Corticotropin Injection is a sterile solution of the polypeptide hormone obtained from the pituitary glands of mammals used for food. It possesses the ability to stimulate the release of corticosteroids from the adrenal cortex. Corticotropin for Injection is the sterile, dry material of the polypeptide hormone and is made into a solution with suitable diluents, buffer, and an antimicrobial agent. Corticotropin Injection and Corticotropin for Injection can be administered by the subcutaneous, intramuscular or intravenous routes. Repository Corticotropin Injection is corticotropin in a solution of partially hydrolyzed gelatin and is intended for subcutaneous and intramuscular administration. Sterile Corticotropin Zinc Hydroxide Suspension is a suspension of corticotropin adsorbed on zinc hydroxide and is intended for intramuscular administration.

The Third International Standard for Corticotropin[2] has been adopted as the reference standard for corticotropin. In the biological assay[3] for corticotropin, rats are injected subcutaneously with specified diluted standard solutions and test solutions of corticotropin, 16 to 48 hours after the removal of the hypophysis. Three hours after the injections, the rats are anesthetized, and both adrenal glands of each rat are removed, and cleaned from adhering tissue, weighed and assayed for ascorbic acid content. The methodology involved in the preparation of the standard and test solutions, as well as the exact procedure of the bioassay, ascorbic acid determination and calculations are detailed in the USP. The bioassay for Corticotropin Injection and Corticotropin for Injection, labeled for intravenous administration, is identical to the procedure outlined above with the exception that the preparations are injected intravenously in the rats. For the bioassay of Sterile Corticotropin Zinc Hydroxide Suspension sufficient 0.1 *N* hydrochloric acid is added to the preparation for solubilization prior to being assayed in rats by the subcutaneous method.

Corticotropin Injection and Repository Corticotropin Injection also are assayed for vasopressin activity according to the procedure for Corticotropin Injection and the assay for Vasopressin Injection in the USP. Anesthetized rats are injected with a specified dose of USP Posterior Pituitary Reference Standard at 12- to 15-minute intervals and the blood pressure elevations are monitored and recorded. At the midpoint of the timed injections of the Reference Standard, specified dilutions of the Corticotropin Injection are injected into the rat and the blood pressure response is recorded. The blood pressure elevation observed with the Corticotropin Injection should not exceed the average elevation observed with the Reference Standard before and after the Corticotropin Injection.

CHORIONIC GONADOTROPIN

Chorionic gonadotropin is a gonad-stimulating principle, of placental origin, prepared from the urine of pregnant women. The biological activity of chorionic gonadotropin is essentially identical to that of the luteinizing hormone (interstitial cell-stimulating hormone) of the anterior pituitary. Chorionic gonadotropin is used in sequence with menotropins (human menopausal gonadotropins) in the treatment of infertility in women in whom anovulation is due to low or absent endogenous gonadotropins. Follicular growth and maturation are promoted by initial treatment with menotropins, followed by administration of chorionic gonadotropin to induce ovulation by simulating the normal preovulatory surge of luteinizing hormone.

Chorionic gonadotropin also is used in the treatment of cryptorchism in cases in which there is no apparent anatomical obstruction to descent of the testis. Combined therapy with this hormone and menotropins may promote spermatogenesis in patients with hypogonadotropic eunuchoidism. Diagnostically, chorionic gonadotropin is used to evaluate Leydig cell responsiveness.

Chorionic Gonadotropin for Injection is a sterile, dry mixture of chorionic gonadotropin with suitable diluents and buffers. Biological assay of the preparation is based on the increase in weight of the uterus excised from young female rats sacrificed 2 days after the last of three daily subcutaneous injections of dilutions of the test sample. The response is compared to that obtained in a series of animals similarly treated with USP Chorionic Gonadotropin Reference Standard. The uterotropic effects depend on elaboration of ovarian hormones in response to the gonad-stimulating activity of chorionic gonadotropin. Chorionic Gonadotropin for Injection is satisfactory if it contains not less than 80% and not more than 125% of the potency stated on the label.

It is also necessary to ascertain, biologically, that Chorionic Gonadotropin for Injection meets the requirements of the estrogenic activity test. This is accomplished by examination of vaginal smears taken from ovariectomized rats on each of three successive days following subcutaneous injection of 0.25 mL of chorionic gonadotropin test solution twice a day (morning and afternoon) for 2 days. The requirements of the test are met if the cellular elements in the smears consist of leukocytes and a few nucleated epithelial cells, but no cornified epithelial cells.

HEPARIN

Heparin consists of straight-chain mucopolysaccharides, called glycosaminoglycans, and has an average molecular weight of 15,000. The commercially available product consists of polymers of two alternating disaccharide units, namely, D-glucosamine-D-glucuronic acid and D-glucosamine-L-iduronic acid. It is an anticoagulant that prolongs the clotting time of blood and inhibits the formation of fibrin clots both *in vivo* and *in vitro*. It exerts its activity by forming a complex with antithrombin III to accelerate the inactivation of thrombin and to inhibit other coagulation proteases such as factor Xa, which is responsible for the conversion of prothrombin to thrombin.

The biological assay for heparin sodium consists of comparing the activity of the heparin sample and USP Heparin Sodium Reference Standard in preventing the clotting of citrated sheep plasma. The USP unit of heparin is the concentration of heparin that will inhibit 1.0 mL of citrated sheep plasma from clotting up to 1 hour after the addition of 0.2 mL of $CaCl_2$ solution (1:100). Because the potency of heparin varies from different preparations, heparin always should be expressed and prescribed in units, rather than by weight.

Heparin Sodium Injection USP is used in the prophylaxis and treatment of venous thrombosis and pulmonary embolism, in atrial fibrillation with embolization, and for the prevention of clotting in cardiac and arterial surgery. Commercially available preparations of Heparin Sodium Injection are obtained from bovine lung and porcine intestinal mucosa. Heparin Lock Flush Solution is prepared from porcine intestinal mucosa and is a sterile preparation of Heparin Sodium Injection containing sodium chloride in an amount to make it isotonic with blood. This preparation of heparin is used for clearing intermittent infusion sets. Heparin Calcium and Heparin Calcium for Injection are also available and are obtained from porcine intestinal mucosa.

PROTAMINE SULFATE

Protamine Sulfate is a mixture of simple proteins of low molecular weight that are rich in arginine. They are found in the sperm or mature testes of salmon and various other species of fish. Due to the high content of arginine, the protamines are strongly basic. In the absence of heparin, the intravenous administration of protamine exerts an anticoagulant effect through its interaction with platelets and fibrinogen. In the presence of heparin, protamine and heparin interact to form a stable salt that results in the loss of anticoagulant activity of both drugs.

The biological assay for protamine sulfate depends on the ability of protamine to neutralize the anticoagulant activity of heparin in citrated sheep plasma. In this assay, various amounts of heparin are added to plasma containing a constant concentration of protamine. A solution of calcium chloride containing thromboplastin is added to the above samples and the clotting times are monitored. A detailed description of this assay can be found in the USP. Each milligram of protamine sulfate, calculated on the dried basis, neutralizes not less than 100 USP Units of heparin activity derived from lung tissue or intestinal mucosa. Protamine Sulfate for Injection is a sterile mixture of protamine sulfate with one or more suitable, dry diluents. Protamine Sulfate Injection, a sterile isotonic solution of Protamine Sulfate, is used in the treatment of heparin overdosage.

VITAMINS

Chemical or spectrometric assay procedures are specified for all preparations of vitamin A, vitamin B_1 (thiamine), and vitamin D. A biological method for assaying vitamin D has been recently approved by the USP (4th Supplement, USP 23-NF 18). This assay measures the ability of vitamin D to stimulate calcification of the rachitic metaphysis in rats. Because calcification depends on adequate amounts of vitamin D, rats fed a diet deficient in vitamin D develop rickets; supplementation of the diet with adequate amounts of vitamin D results in recalcification of the bone. Briefly, the assay uses young rats (not older than 55 days) who have developed rickets on a *rachitogenic diet*. These rats are divided into groups and fed the rachitogenic diet that has been supplemented with either USP Cholecalciferol Reference Standard, unknowns, or no supplementation (control).

One half of the dose of vitamin D either as the USP Cholecalciferol Reference Standard or unknown is given to the rats on day 1 and day 3 (or 4) of the assay period. At the end of a fixed period (between 7 and 10 days) the rats are weighed and sacrificed. Any rats whose weight has decreased are removed from further analysis. The leg bones of the remaining rats are dissected out and assayed for amount of recalcification of the bones. The activity of the vitamin D may be determined by the amount of recalcification relative to the reference standards.

Additionally, a biological assay for determination of vitamin D activity of Cod Liver Oil, Nondestearinated Cod Liver Oil, Oleovitamin A and D, and descriptions of formerly official biological assay methods for vitamins A and B_1 will be found in the 13th edition of this text (*RPS*-13, pp 1600–1604).

SUMMARY TABLE

Major aspects of the biological assay procedures for several official articles are summarized in Table 31-1.

MICROBIAL ASSAYS

As previously noted in this chapter, *biological assay* refers to measurement of the relative potency or activity of compounds by determining the amount required to produce a specific, defined effect on a suitable test animal or organ under standard conditions. The experimental animals mentioned in specific test procedures described in the previous section include mice, rats, guinea pigs, rabbits, cats, dogs, and pigeons. As noted earlier, a biological assay may involve observations or measurements of effects obtained in any form of living matter, plant or animal. The term *microbial* (a contraction of microbiological) *assay* designates a type of biological assay, specifically, a biological assay performed with *microorganisms,* such as bacteria, yeasts, and molds.

In general, the principles involved in microbial assays are the same as those that apply to assays using higher forms of plant or animal life. One notable difference involves the relative size of the experimental population. In the bioassays described above, the response of each individual test animal is noted and the results are obtained when a series of animals are subjected to statistical analysis to calculate mean activity, standard error, and so on. In a typical microbial assay, each evaluation is performed with a culture of microorganisms, and the measurement represents the average response of an extremely large population of test organisms. In the case of most bioassays, a linear relationship exists between the *log dose* and the response, whereas in most microbial assays there is a linear relationship between the *dose* and the response (within certain limits). The importance of this relationship in the evaluation of microbial assays is considered in Chapter 12.

VITAMINS

Microbiological procedures are available for the assay of Calcium Pantothenate, Dexpanthenol, Niacin or Niacinamide, and Vitamin B_{12} activity of Cyanocobalamin Co 57 Solution and Capsules, and Cyanocobalamin Co 60 Solution and Capsules.

A fundamental requirement in a microbial assay for the activity of a vitamin or amino acid (factor) is the inability of the test organism to synthesize the factor being assayed. Furthermore, the test organism must require the factor being assayed for normal growth, and should be sensitive to very small amounts of the required factor. For these types of microbial assays, special media are prepared that are nutritionally complete in all respects except for the factor under study. Examples of these media may be found in the USP section <81>. Control tubes containing the suitable media inoculated with the test species exhibit no, or only minimal, growth. If the basic requirements specified above are satisfied, the growth response of the test organism is, within limits, proportional to the amount of factor added to the medium.

The extent of the growth response may be determined by turbidity or spectrometric measurement, or by titration of the acid produced as metabolic waste. The turbidity of the culture is proportional to the amount of microbial growth; the development of acidity also reflects quantitatively the growth response.

Sufficient levels of reference standard are included to enable construction of a dose response curve for each assay. The activity of the factor (or factor dilution) being tested is determined by interpolation from the standard curve.

Niacin or Niacinamide

The techniques and procedures used in the microbiological assay for niacin are common to many of the microbiological methods, and a description of the niacin method will serve to give the pattern generally employed.

THE MICROORGANISM

In the case of niacin, it has been clearly demonstrated that the assay organisms used metabolize only the forms of niacin that are available to the host in which they normally grow. The fact that some organisms are more limited than the host animal in their ability to use niacin derivatives serves as a basis for differentiating such compounds in biological materials. For example, in addition to the free niacin, *Lactobacillus plantarum* is able to use niacinamide, nicotinuric acid, cozymase, and niacinamide nucleoside.

Although a number of microorganisms require niacin for their metabolic processes and are unable to synthesize it for themselves, the acid-forming organism *L plantarum* is used most widely for assay purposes. It is nonpathogenic, easy to culture, and affected to only a limited degree by stimulatory or inhibitory substances normally found in foods or pharmaceutical preparations containing niacin. It may be grown on a simple stab-culture medium containing gelatin, yeast extract, and glucose, and is cultured for use in the assay tubes by direct transfer to the liquid medium consisting of the basic assay medium containing an optimum amount of added niacin.

One important advantage of microbiological procedures is that only a minute quantity of a vitamin is needed to give a measurable response. For example, the range of niacin added to the series of standard tubes is 0.05 to 0.50 µg/tube. Thus, the niacin content of extremely small amounts of biological materials may be measured readily. Modifications using microanalytical apparatus and a lower range of vitamin additions have been described for blood and tissue analysis.

THE TEST SOLUTION

The first step in the assay procedure is the preparation of the test solution of the material to be assayed. If the sample is a dry or semisolid material, the niacin is extracted by heating the sample in a measured volume of dilute H_2SO_4 in an autoclave for 30 minutes. Liquid preparations are autoclaved 30 minutes after addition of the H_2SO_4 to give a concentration of 1 N H_2SO_4. Although niacin is soluble in water, certain precursors, found particularly in cereals, are unavailable to the test organism unless hydrolyzed. Either acid or alkali is equally effective for the extraction but acid is preferred, owing to the possibility of hydrolysis of trigonelline in an alkaline solution. Preparation of the test solution is completed by neutralizing with strong NaOH solution, then diluting to a volume that contains 0.1 μg of niacin per milliliter. Further purification of the test solution is not ordinarily important, because *L plantarum* is relatively unaffected by substances that inhibit or stimulate other test organisms.

THE MEDIUM

The basic medium employed in a niacin assay is simple to prepare and, with properly treated casein hydrolysate, is otherwise nutritionally complete. Both dehydrated complete media and dehydrated casein hydrolysates are available commercially and appear to be entirely satisfactory for assay purposes. To prepare a medium suitable for assaying amino acids, the casein hydrolysate is replaced with an amino acid mixture, omitting only the amino acid being assayed.

Details of the microbial assay procedure for niacin (including preparation of standard niacin solution, spectrometric determination of cell density and calculation of the niacin content of the test samples) are given in the official compendium.

Calcium Pantothenate

In the assay of Calcium Pantothenate, stock complete media supplemented with casein hydrolysate and additional vitamins, as described in the USP, are prepared. Sets of tubes are supplemented with Calcium Pantothenate standards or test solutions. Inoculum of *L plantarium* are prepared in broth from agar slants. One drop of *L plantarium*–containing broth is used to inoculate 10 mL of the broth for test purposes. The amount of growth of the *L plantarium* culture is determined by measuring light transmittance in a spectrophotometer following 16 to 24 hours of incubation. A dose-response curve is drawn by plotting the transmittance for each level of the standard solution against the amount of Calcium Pantothenate in the respective tubes. The amount of Calcium Pantothenate contained in the test solution is determined by proper interpolation of the observed values with the standard curve.

Dexpanthenol

This assay is used to determine the amount of Dexpanthenol as an ingredient of multi-vitamin preparations or for identifying the amount of dextrorotary panthenol in a racemic mixture of dextro- and levo- panthenol.

Briefly, a modified panthenate medium is made and a set of tubes is supplemented with stock Dexpanthenol or unknown, 0.5mL of a standard stock culture of *Pedicoccus acidilactici* is added to 10mL of culture media and incubated for 16 hours. The cultures are then killed by heating and their turbidity is determined spectrophotometrically. A dose-response curve is plotted and the concentration of the unknown is determined by interpolating the unknown values with the standard curve.

Vitamin B$_{12}$ Activity

Determination of vitamin B$_{12}$ activity requires special treatment of the material to be assayed so that the vitamin is made available to the test organism, which is a culture of *Lactobacillus leichmannii*. The basic medium used is quite complex, prepared as a mixture in solution of a variety of essential nutrients. Measured amounts of the material to be assayed are added to one set of tubes containing this medium, and measured amounts of the Standard Cyanocobalamin Solution are added to a corresponding second set of tubes. The tubes are inoculated with a small amount of culture of the test organism and then incubated overnight. The extent of growth of the microorganisms is measured by determining light transmittance by means of a spectrometer. A concentration-response curve is drawn as described for Calcium Pantothenate, and the amount of vitamin B$_{12}$ contained in the test solution is determined by proper interpolation of the observed values on the standard curve.

ANTIBIOTICS

The term *antibiotic,* as used in the official compendia, designates a medicinal preparation containing a significant quantity of a chemical substance that is produced naturally by a microorganism, or artificially by synthesis, and that has the capacity to inhibit or destroy microorganisms in dilute solution. Under the terms of the Federal Food, Drug, and Cosmetic Act of 1938, batch certification for antibiotics, whether for human or veterinary use, was introduced in stages: 1945, penicillin; 1948, streptomycin; 1949, aureomycin, bacitracin, and chloramphenicol. In 1962, as part of the Kefauver-Harris Amendments, batch certification was applied to all antibiotics intended for human use. On 1982 the FDA issued regulations that exempted antibiotics from batch certification requirements so long as the articles complied with standards; however, Section 507 (Certification of Antibiotics) remains intact.

Standards of potency and purity for antibiotics are established by the FDA in the form of regulations published from time to time in the *Federal Register*. Because all recognized antibiotics are subject to the provisions of the regulations, these determine the official standards. The federal regulations governing all aspects of antibiotic testing are extremely detailed and are subject to periodic amendment; they should be consulted with regard to prescribed methods for the assay of individual antibiotics and their preparations.

In evaluation of the potency of antibiotic substances, the measured effect is inhibition of the growth of a suitable strain of microorganisms—that is, the prevention of the multiplication of the test organisms. The procedures employed in microbial assay of antibiotics may be divided into two broad classifications: the *Cylinder-Plate Method* and the *Turbidimetric Method.*

Cylinder-Plate Method

The Cylinder-Plate Assay of antibiotic potency is based on measurement of the diameter of zones of microbial growth inhibition surrounding cylinders containing various dilutions of test compound, which are placed on the surface of a solid nutrient medium previously inoculated with a culture of a suitable organism. Inhibition produced by the test compound is compared with that produced by known concentrations of a Reference Standard.

Turbidimetric Method

The Turbidimetric Assay of antibiotic potency is based on inhibition of microbial growth as indicated by measurement of the turbidity (transmittance) of suspensions of a suitable microorganism in a fluid medium to which have been added graded amounts of the test compound. Changes in transmittance produced by the test compound are compared with those produced by known concentrations of reference material.

Detailed descriptions of appropriate microbial assays for specific antibiotics (ie, cylinder-plate or turbidometric method) may be found in section <81> of USP 25-NF 20. This section also catalogs the test organisms to be used with each antibiotic.

BIOLOGICAL TESTS

In the context of *bioassay,* a biological test has as its objective the qualitative determination of a specific characteristic of a biological product or of the container in which it is supplied (eg, transfusion assemblies). These tests are designed to determine with a high degree of certainty the absence or presence of a type of activity (such as antibacterial activity or pressor activity), or quality (such as nonantigenicity or toxicity), or constituent (such as depressor substances or pyrogens). Animals are employed in some tests and microorganisms in others.

PYROGEN TEST

The USP pyrogen test requires healthy, mature rabbits to determine the absence or presence of pyrogens in products that can be tolerated by the rabbit. Three rabbits are used; each receives 10 mL of the test solution/kg by injection into an ear vein, completing the injection within 10 min. The rectal temperature is recorded at 1, 2, and 3 hr after the injection. The Decision Statements specify a limit on the temperature rise allowed for any one rabbit as 0.5° If a single rabbit has an increase in temperature 0.5° or greater then the test is expanded to include five additional rabbits (for a total of eight animals); after which the requirement for absence of pyrogen states that no more than three rabbits each exhibit a temperature rise of less than 0.5°, and the total temperature rise for all eight rabbits is 3.3° or less.

BACTERIAL ENDOTOXIN TEST

Since USP 21-NF 15, an alternative to the rabbit pyrogen test exists in the form of the Bacterial Endotoxin Test (BET). In this *in vitro* procedure, the aqueous extract of the circulating amebocytes of the horseshoe crab, *Limulus polyphemus,* called Limulus Amebocyte Lysate (LAL) is used because it causes the formation of a gel-clot if pyrogen (bacterial endotoxin) is present above a limiting concentration. Briefly, an aqueous sample is mixed with the LAL and incubated at 37°. The end point of the assay is determined spectrometrically by an increased turbidity due to gel formation or by the presence of a clot. This procedure requires a USP Reference Standard (defined potency of 10,000 USP Endotoxin Units per vial, endotoxin obtained from *Escherichia coli*) and provides a more sensitive detection of pyrogen (endotoxin) than does the rabbit test. Another advantage of the BET is that the presence of pyrogens may be detected in drugs that have definite physiological effects and for which the classic rabbit response could not be used.

The BET procedure has been widely adopted; for example, 216 monographs that used the rabbit pyrogen test now require the BET procedure instead. In 164 cases where the rabbit pyrogen test was unreliable, BET requirements are now found. BET is an ideal assay for ensuring that water used for pharmaceutical purposes is pyrogen free.

A discussion of pyrogens may be found in Chapter 40. This section discusses the nature, sources, and means of destruction of pyrogens. In addition, the testing for pyrogens is considered.

DEPRESSOR SUBSTANCES TEST

In the Depressor Substances Test, a female nonpregnant adult cat is anesthetized and the carotid or other suitable artery is exposed, separated from surrounding tissue, and monitored for continuous blood pressure. A femoral artery is exposed as a means to facilitate the intravenous injections of standard and test drugs. In this procedure, the depressor responses of the substance under test is compared to those responses elicited by several doses of a Standard Solution of Histamine. The substance under test is dissolved in a designated diluent to give the required concentration specified in the individual monograph. Refer to Biological Tests in the USP for the specific experimental steps required by the Depressor Substances Test.

BIOLOGICAL REACTIVITY TESTS, *IN VITRO* AND *IN VIVO*

In order to find suitable *in vitro* replacements for animal procedures, in 1985 the United States Pharmacopeial Convention established a standing group, the Subcommittee on *in Vitro* Toxicity, that has made impressive progress in gathering information about and in stimulating research into *in vitro* methods. The work of the Subcommittee has resulted in two proposed chapters, Biological Reactivity Tests *in Vitro,* and Biological Reactivity Tests *in Vivo.* Biological reactivity is the response of a biological system or the products of a biological system, such as cells from tissue culture, to an imposed stimulus.

In the Biological Reactivity Tests *in Vitro,* three tests called the *Agar Diffusion Test,* the *Direct Contact Test,* and the *Elution Test* are used to evaluate the suitability of elastomers and other polymers that are to have direct or indirect patient contact. The choice of test is dependent on the material, final product, and intended use.

Agar Diffusion and Direct Contact Tests

The Agar Diffusion Test is designed to assay elastomeric closures. In this assay, an agar layer protects tissue culture cells from contact with the material but allows diffusion of leachable chemicals from the polymers to reach the cells. To perform the test, monolayers of cultured cells are grown to 80% confluence in 60-mm diameter plates and the tissue culture media is replaced by media containing not more than 2% agar. After the agar has solidified, filter paper to which extracts from the polymers have been applied are placed on the agar.

The Direct Contact Test is designed for materials with a variety of shapes and also uses 80% confluent tissue culture cells. In the Direct Contact Test, the monolayers are incubated in direct contact with the samples. For both the Agar Diffusion and the Direct Contact Tests the cells are incubated with sample preparations or USP Negative Control Plastic RS or USP Positive Bioreaction Solid RS. After 24 hours of culture, the monolayer is examined microscopically and the observations made according to prescribed guidelines. The response is defined in terms of a series of Reactivity Grades.

Elution Test

The Elution Test evaluates the effects of extracts of polymeric materials on cultured cells. The materials are extracted into cell culture media (with or without serum supplementation) at either physiologic or nonphysiologic temperatures. When the monolayers are 80% confluent, the media is replaced with media containing the polymer extracts and the cells are incubated for an additional 48 hours at 37°. The evaluation once again is based on the microscopic appearance of the cells after incubation.

Systemic Injection Test

The Systemic Injection Test uses mice that receive an intravenous (IV) or intraperitoneal (IP) injection of a defined quantity of an extract of a plastic, after which the mice are observed just after the injection and then after 4, 24, 48, and 72 hours. The animal response from injection of the sample is compared with the animal response from injection of a blank (same quantity of the same extraction medium treated the same way). The sample passes the test only if the animals do not display biological reactivity significantly greater than that seen in the blank.

Intracutaneous Test

The Intracutaneous Test determines the local responses to the polymer extracts following intracutaneous injection into rabbits. The evaluation is based on erythema and eschar formation and on edema production and uses a defined response value to label the intensity of the biological reactivity. The difference between the sample and blank must be less than one for the test to be met.

Implantation Test

The Implantation Test is a procedure that evaluates the suitability of the polymeric materials intended for containers or container accessories for use in parenterals and for use in medical devices, implants, and other related systems that may come into direct contact with living tissue. This test uses adult rabbits into whose paravertebral musculature are implanted strips no smaller than 10×1 mm. The animals are maintained for at least 120 hours following implantation, after which they are sacrificed and the tissue around the implant examined grossly and microscopically for reactions to the implant. Reference standard material called USP Negative Control Plastic RS is provided to act as a control.

Safety Tests—Biologicals

The Safety Tests—Biologicals is a procedure used to determine the acceptability, in terms of safety, of biologicals and biotechnology derived products. A dose of 0.5 mL of a test solution containing the biological is injected IP into mice and guinea pigs, after which they are observed for 48 hours or 7 days, depending on the test.

Because biologicals derived from biotechnology may include contaminants from the cell lines as well as adventitious infectious agents, the Federal Government has drafted a number of *Points to Consider* for use in characterization of monoclonal antibodies and characterization of cell lines used to produce bio-

Table 31-2. Summary of Biological Test Procedures

COMPENDIAL ARTICLE	ACTIVITY ASSAYED	ANIMAL EMPLOYED	ROUTE OF ADMINISTRATION OF TEST MATERIAL	END POINT OF TEST PROCEDURE
Iron dextran injection	Absorption of iron compound	Rabbit	IM	No heavy black deposit of unabsorbed iron 7 days after injection
Diphtheria toxoid, tetanus toxoid and combinations with pertussis vaccine	Antigenicity	Guinea pig	SC	Not less than 80% survival (for at least 10 days) of immunized animals injected with test doses of toxin
Protein hydrolysate injection	Nutritional completeness	Rat	PO	Weight gain while maintained on test product and nitrogen-deficient diet
Isofluorophate ophthalmic ointment	Miotic	Rabbit	Ocular instillation	Pupil constriction
Insulin products	Lower blood sugar level	Rabbit	SC	Glucose analysis
Technetium	Tc99m–containing compounds	Distribution of radioactivity	Rats or mice IV	Residual radioactivity in specified tissues
Diphtheria toxoid, tetanus toxoid	Toxin poisoning	Guinea pig	SC	No symptoms of toxin poisoning within 21 days
Many articles	Pyrogen test or bacterial endotoxins test (BET)	Rabbits (Pyrogen)	IV (Pyrogen)	Rectal temperature increase not more than 0.6° (Pyrogen)
		LAL	*In vitro*	Increased turbidity by spectrophotometry or clot formation
Elastomeric closures, plastic containers, transfusion assemblies	Systemic toxicity of extract	Mouse	IP, IV	No toxic reaction within 72 hr
	Intracutaneous toxicity of extract	Rabbit	Intracutaneous	No significant irritation compared to blank
	Implantation toxicity of designated material	Rabbit	Aseptic implant	No significant encapsulation compared to blank
	Agar Diffusion, Direct Contact Elution Test	Tissue culture	*In vitro*	Minimal damage to monolayer cells
Biologics and biotechnology derived products	Toxicity	Mice Guinea pigs	IV, IP	Abnormal or untoward toxicity or death

Note: These tests are described in detail in the USP/NF and the Official Supplements.

logicals. The current approach is to focus on the production, identification, and characterization of the cells being used to produce the biological, the validation of the manufacturing process, and the testing of bulk and final product for safety. With regard to safety, the *Points to Consider* recommend testing for bacteria, fungi, and mycoplasma as well as tests for adventitious viruses including lymphocytic choriomeningitis virus, Epstein-Barr virus, cytomegalovirus and hepatitis B and C. If the cell lines being used are nonhuman lines, the recommendation includes assaying for viruses appropriate to the cell line. In addition, samples should be tested for retroviruses. Should viral contamination be found, the manufacturer should include steps to inactivate or remove the virus and these steps should be validated.

Medical devices labeled nonpyrogenic that make contact directly or indirectly with the cardiovascular system or other soft body tissue must meet the specifications for sterility, nonpyrogenicity, and safety as outlined under *Transfusion and Infusion Assemblies* in the USP. The pyrogen procedure uses the Bacterial Endotoxin Test (BET) using Limulus Amoebocyte Lysate (LAL) and, when appropriate, the rabbit pyrogen test. The mouse safety tests referred to before are used for extracts of the plastic.

Plastics for use in parental preparations, elastomeric closures for injections, and plastic containers for ophthalmics are subject to both *in vitro* and *in vivo* Biological Reactivity Tests. Plastic material from the three categories is tested for *in vitro* biological reactivity in the Agar Diffusion Test, Direct Contact Test, and Elution Test. Materials from plastics for use in parenteral preparations and elastomeric closures for injections that meet the *in vitro* tests are not required to undergo *in vivo* testing. Materials in the plastics for use in parenteral preparations category that do not meet the *in vitro* test requirements are subjected to the Systemic Injection, Intracutaneous, and Implantation Tests. Materials in the elastomeric closures for injections category that do not meet the *in vitro* test requirements are subjected to the Systemic Injection, Intracutaneous, and Pyrogen Tests. Materials intended for use in plastic containers for ophthalmics that do not meet the requirements of the *in vitro* tests are tested by the Systemic Injection and Intracutaneous Tests. Materials cannot be used for containers for ophthalmic preparations if they do not meet the requirements of the Systemic Injection and Intracutaneous Tests.

The USP search for alternatives to *in vivo* tests is an ongoing activity. Work is in progress for selective replacements for the Eye Irritation procedure: methods involving the irritation of the chorioallantoic membrane (from the chicken egg), the uptake of neutral red dye by living cell lyosomes, the total cell protein assay, and the rabbit corneal epithelial cell healing and other characteristics. Two bacterial tests are under study to determine their potential value, *v12*, the Bacterial Bioluminescence Test, a toxicity procedure applicable not only to extracts of plastics but also to solutions of bulk pharmaceuticals; and the bacterial colorimetric test, a procedure based on β- galactosidase measurement and with potential value in the determination of the biological reactivity of chemicals and extracts of plastics.

SUMMARY TABLE

An outline of compendial articles subject to identification, activity, or toxicity tests of a biological nature is presented in Table 31-2.

REFERENCES

1. *Guide for the Care and Use of Laboratory Animals.* NIH Publ No 86-23. Bethesda, MD: US Department of Health and Human Services, 1985.
2. Bangham DR, Mussett MV, Stack-Dunne MP. *Bull WHO* 1962; 27: 395.
3. Sayers MA, Sayers G, Woodbury LA. *Endocrinol* 1948; 42: 379.

GENERAL REFERENCE

USP 25/NF 20. Rockville, MD: USP Convention, 2002; and supplements.

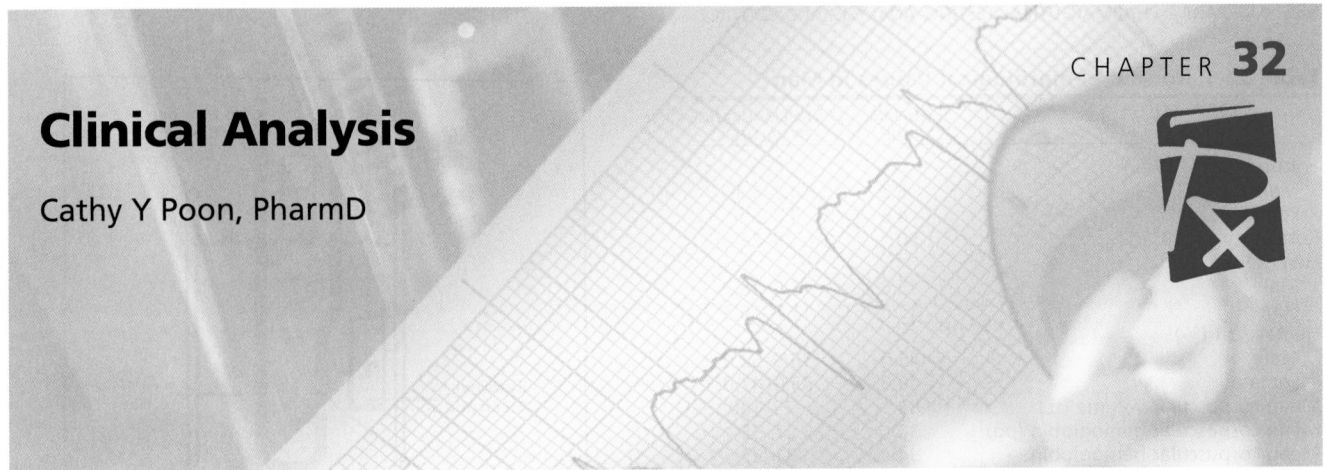

CHAPTER 32

Clinical Analysis

Cathy Y Poon, PharmD

The characterization and quantitation of the various components of blood, urine, and other body fluids are the primary functions of the clinical laboratory. The major divisions of clinical analysis are clinical biochemistry, hematology, blood-bank technology, histopathology, immunology, and microbiology. The accurate diagnosis of disease and determination of a potential therapeutic regimen frequently are based on the laboratory analysis of blood, urine, feces, gastric secretions, or cerebrospinal fluid. Modern medical practice is tending toward greater reliance on laboratory results as definitive measures of pathological or normal states.

Pharmacists should familiarize themselves with the basic principles involved in sample collection, analysis, and diagnostic significance of the various clinical parameters. Their role in community health necessitates comprehension of the methodology and diagnostic value of clinical laboratory procedures. The influence of various drugs and drug interactions on these parameters must be considered in both the clinical and drug-abuse situation.

HEMATOLOGY

The determination of the morphological, physiological, and biochemical properties of peripheral blood and the blood-forming organs (hematopoietic system) is a function of the hematology laboratory. The functional categories of hematology are (1) analysis of cellular elements, and specific biochemical and physiological parameters of peripheral blood and the hematopoietic system, (2) blood-coagulation analysis, and (3) blood-bank technology.

Peripheral blood is a biphasic liquid tissue system of cellular elements suspended in a liquid plasma phase. The cellular phase comprises about 45% of the blood volume and contains erythrocytes (red blood cells, RBC), leukocytes (white blood cells, WBC), and thrombocytes (platelets). The plasma phase is primarily water (90–92%) and protein (7%).

The hematological analysis of blood is concerned primarily with enumeration and differentiation of the various cellular elements. An analysis of the hematopoietic system (eg, bone marrow and lymphoid tissue) determines the status of blood-cell precursors in these tissues. Determinations of specific biochemical (hemoglobin) and physiological (blood or plasma volume) parameters are performed in a complete evaluation of the erythron system (blood and marrow RBC and their precursors). The normal hematological values in the adult are presented in Table 32-1.[1]

ERYTHROCYTES AND HEMOGLOBIN

The erythrocytic system is composed of the mature erythrocytes in peripheral blood and their precursors in bone marrow. The precursors of erythrocytes, as found in the erythropoietic system (red bone marrow), are classified as to the degree of nucleation and characteristics of cytoplasmic constituents. The sequence of erythrocyte formation in bone marrow—based on the gradual denucleation of the cell, generation of the chromatin structure, and changes in nucleolar structure and cytoplasmic constituents—is

pronormoblast → basophilic normoblast →
polychromatic normoblast → orthochromatic normoblast →
polychromatophilic erythrocyte → erythrocyte

The first four types are nucleated and normally are seen only in bone marrow. In normal erythrocyte formation these immature bone-marrow cells are designated as *normoblastic* or *normocytic*. In pernicious anemia and related conditions, they become abnormally large and are designated *megaloblastic* or *megalocytic*. In iron-deficiency anemia, these cells become abnormally small and are designated *microblastic* or *microcytic*, of the iron-deficiency type.

Normal blood contains 0.5% to 1.5% of circulating erythrocytes as reticulocytes. These cells contain a fine network of basophilic reticulum that is demonstrable on staining with a vital dye such as brilliant cresyl blue. The number of these cells in the blood is a measure of effective erythropoiesis. High-circulating reticulocyte values are an index of erythropoietic activity and are found in the first few days of life, after hemorrhage and after treatment of iron-deficiency or vitamin B_{12}-deficiency anemias.

The normal *erythrocyte* (normocyte) is a flexible, elastic, biconcave, enucleated structure with a mean diameter of 7.3 μm and a thickness near 2.2 μm. The chemical constituents of the red blood cell include water (63%), lipids (0.5%), glucose (0.8%), minerals (0.7%), nonhemoglobin protein (0.9%), methemoglobin (0.5%), and hemoglobin (33.6%). The primary function of the erythrocyte is transport of oxygen and carbon dioxide. The red cell membrane, a dynamic, semipermeable component of the cell, is associated with energy metabolism in the maintenance of the permeability characteristics of the cell to various cations (Na^+, K^+) and anions (Cl^-, HCO_3^-). The stroma of insoluble material that remains after red-cell disruption (hemolysis) constitutes 2% to 5% of the wet-cell weight; it is primarily protein (40–60%) and lipid (10–12%). The membrane includes stromatin (a fibrous or structural protein) and mucopolysaccharides associated with A, B, and O blood-group substances. The lipid fractions include phosphatides (lecithin, cephalin), cholesterol, cholesterol esters, neutral fats, cerebrosides, and sialic acid glycoproteins.

Erythrocytes may be enumerated by either visual or electronic procedures. In the visual procedures, a measured quantity of blood is diluted with a fluid, which is isotonic with blood and will prevent its coagulation. The diluted blood is then placed in a counting chamber (hemocytometer), and the num-

Table 32-1. Normal Hematological Values in Man

	NORMAL VALUE	NORMAL RANGE OF VALUES
Erythrocytes ($10^6/\mu L$)		
Male	5.2	4.2–6.1
Female	4.6	3.7–5.5
Reticulocytes ($10^3/\mu L$)	50	25–75
Hemoglobin (g/dL)		
Male	15.6	13.0–18.2
Female	13.6	11.0–16.3
Hematocrit (%)		
Male	45.0	36.5–52.0
Female	40.0	33.0–47.0
Mean corpuscular volume (fL)	88	75–100
Mean corpuscular hemoglobin (pg)	30	27–35
Mean corpuscular hemoglobin concentration (%)	34	31–37
Leukocytes ($10^3/\mu L$)	7.0	3.9–10.9
Leukocyte differential (%)		
Neutrophils	58	50–75
Bands	4	2–6
Eosinophils	2	1–5
Basophils	1	0–2
Lymphocytes	30	20–40
Monocytes	5	8–38
Platelets ($10^3/\mu L$)	300	150–450
Erythrocyte sedimentation rate (Westergren) (mm in 1 hr)		
Male	4	0–10
Female	10	0–20

From Simmons A. *Hematology—A Combined Theoretical and Technical Approach.* Philadelphia: WB Saunders, 1989, with permission from Elsevier.

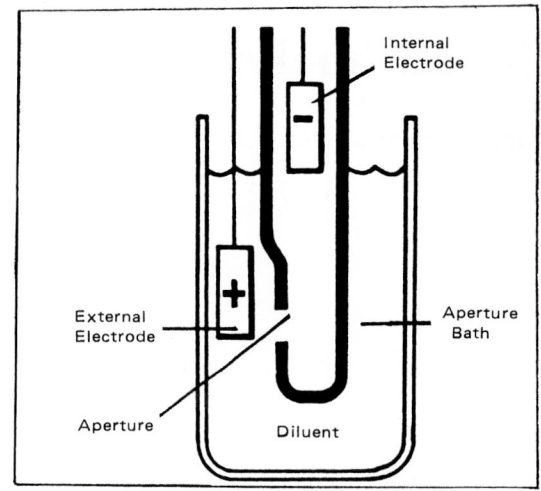

Figure 32-1. Coulter-counting cells by electronic impedance (courtesy, Beckman Coulter).

ber of cells in a circumscribed area is enumerated microscopically. Hayem's solution (sodium sulfate, 2.5 g; sodium chloride, 0.25 g; mercuric chloride, 0.25 g; distilled water, 100 mL), Toison's fluid (sodium sulfate, 8 g; sodium chloride, 1 g; methyl violet, 0.025 g; glycerin, 30 mL; distilled water, 180 mL) or 0.9% sodium chloride are used as diluting fluids. The overall error of this method is about 8%.

A greater degree of accuracy and reproducibility can be achieved by erythrocyte enumeration in an electronic counting apparatus, such as the Coulter Counter or various flow cytometric instruments. The Coulter method (Fig 32-1) determines the number and size of particles suspended in an electrically conductive liquid. The blood cells traverse a small aperture and displace their own volume in the diluent as to produce a change in resistance between the electrodes; the magnitude of the voltage pulse is proportional to cell volume, and the resultant pulses are then amplified, scaled, and automatically counted.

In instruments such as the Bayer ADVIA 120 (Fig 32-2), the principles of laser flow cytometry are used to count cells. Hydrodynamic focusing and laminar flow are combined in the system to count a large number of individual cells. Light focused by a laser diode is scattered by the cells as they pass through the flow channel. The scattered light is monitored by a photoelectric sensor and transfers the electrical pulses, which are processed by the systems circuitry. In addition to increased counting speed, the overall error of the electronic procedures is reduced to about 1%.

The *hematocrit value* is also a measure of the erythrocyte portion of blood. A sample of blood containing an anticoagulant

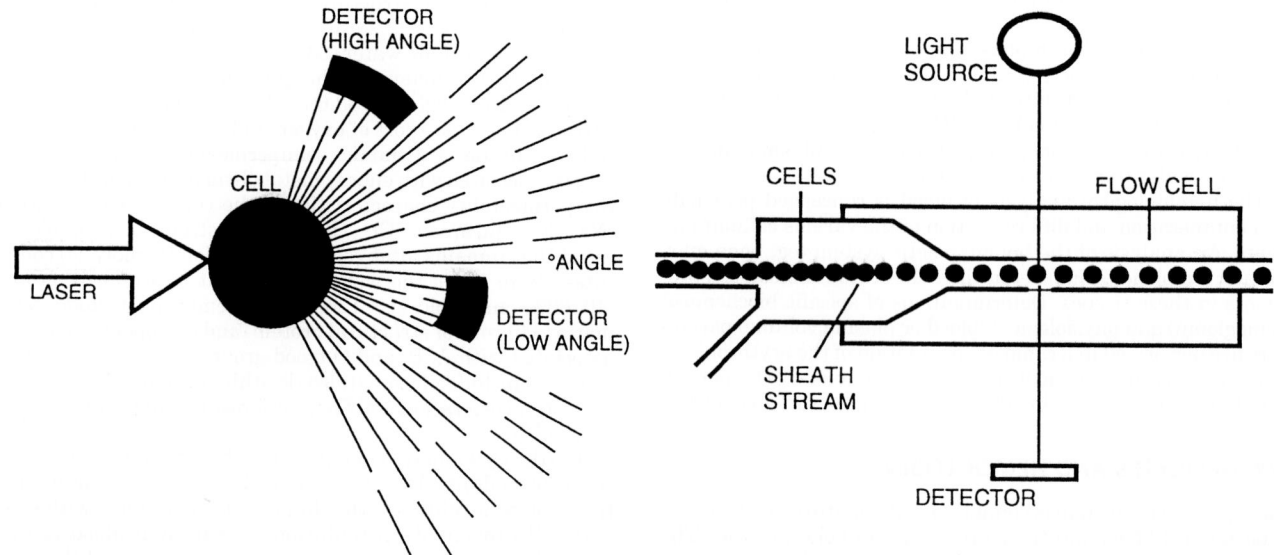

Figure 32-2. Sheath stream flow cell accomplishes hydrodynamic focusing, where cells pass single file through the detection area. Sensors detect high- and low-angle laser light-scatterer (courtesy, Bayer).

is placed in a graduated hematocrit capillary tube, centrifuged, and the volume ratio of packed red cells to total blood volume (hematocrit value) determined. The centrifuged sample appears as a red layer of packed erythrocytes over which is found an off-white layer of packed leukocytes and platelets, and a supernatant plasma phase. The hematocrit value is an index of both the number and size of the red cells.

Hemoglobin, a conjugated hemoprotein with an approximate molecular weight of 67,000 daltons, contains basic proteins, the globins, and ferroprotoporphyrin (heme). It is essentially a tetramer, consisting of four peptide chains, to each of which is bound a heme group. Heme, which constitutes about 4% of the weight of the molecule, consists of a divalent iron atom in the center of a pyrrole-porphyrin structure. Four distinct polypeptide chains (α, β, γ, δ) can be incorporated into hemoglobin. Normal adult hemoglobin is HbA = $\alpha_2^A\beta_2^A$. Fetal hemoglobin contains 2α and 2γ chains and is designated HbF = $\alpha_2^A\gamma_2^F$.

Differences in the structural sequences of amino acids in the peptide portion of the hemoglobin molecules are controlled genetically and are responsible for different types of hemoglobin. Based on the characteristic mobility of the hemoglobin, in an electric field (electrophoresis) on starch, paper, cellulose acetate, agar, or acrylamide gel media, many hemoglobin types have been recognized (see Chapter 33). Only types P, F, and A_1–A_4 are considered normal. Sickle-cell anemia and β- thalassemia are hemolytic anemias associated with abnormal hemoglobins (ie, Type S in sickle-cell anemia and abnormal production of the β chain in β-thalassemia). In homozygous *HbS disease,* sickling of the red cells is due to the low solubility of the abnormal hemoglobin in its reduced state, with the production of semicrystalline bodies (tactoids), which distort and elongate the cells. In the sickle-cell trait (heterozygous), the blood smear shows no sickle cells. In the homozygous condition, HbS accounts for nearly all of the hemoglobin with small amounts of HbF. In the heterozygous condition, HbS constitutes 50% or less of the hemoglobin, with the balance as HbA.

The detection of sickle-cell disease is performed by microscopic observation of the induction of red-cell sickling in the presence of a reducing agent such as sodium metabisulfite, or by quantitative determination of urea-dispersible turbidity induced by dithionite following reduction of HbS to deoxy-HbS in RBC lysates. The microscopic procedure will detect only homozygotes, whereas HbAS and HbS and its structural variant HbC-Harlem both are detected in the urea-dithionite technique. Commercial qualitative test kits are available for detecting sickle-cell trait and anemia by solubility determinations. All hemoglobins positive to the dithionite test must be electrophorized (cellulose acetate, citrate agar, or starch gel) to differentiate HbS from HbC and thalassemia traits. Drugs causing hemolysis in glucose 6-phosphate dehydrogenase (G6PD) deficiency include sulfones, nitrofurans, chloroquine, dimercaprol, nalidixic acid, and probenecid.

The *hemoglobin* concentration is measured spectrophotometrically after lysis of whole blood and conversion of hemoglobin to hematin, oxyhemoglobin, or cyanmethemoglobin. The addition of a strong base (NaOH) to pH 10 converts oxyhemoglobin, carboxyhemoglobin, and methemoglobin to hematin, which can be estimated photometrically. Weaker bases (Na_2CO_3 or NH_4OH) convert hemoglobin to oxyhemoglobin for analysis.

Total hemoglobin is measured also by conversion to cyanmethemoglobin using alkaline sodium cyanide–potassium ferricyanide reagent. Hemoglobin standards certified by the Clinical Standards Committee of the College of American Pathologists are used in these procedures, and all results are expressed as "grams hemoglobin per 100 mL (g/dL) blood."

In the normal state, the oxygen consumption of the RBC is low, and it is involved in the conversion of hemoglobin to oxidized (Fe^{3+}) methemoglobin (HbM), which cannot bind oxygen. The normal balance of HbM (<0.5%) is maintained by two en-

zyme systems: NADH and NADPH methemoglobin reductases. An inherited deficiency of the RBC enzyme, G6PD, will increase the rate of reduction of glutathione and methemoglobin, make the cell more vulnerable to oxidative attack, and result in susceptibility to drug-induced or immune-mediated nonspherocytic hemolytic anemia. G6PD deficiency is found predominantly in persons of Mediterranean descent, Southeast Asians, Africans, and American blacks. The enzyme can be quantitated spectrometrically or by fluoronephelometry by measuring the rate of reduction of nicotinamide adenine dinucleotide phosphate (NADP) in the presence of G6PD. Presumptive screening tests based on reduced glutathione (GSH) content of blood before and after incubation with acetylphenylhydrazine also are used.

Erythrocyte count, hemoglobin content, and hematocrit value are used to determine various blood indices in the diagnosis and treatment of anemia. These measurements are

$$Mean\ corpuscular\ volume\{MCV(fL)\} = \frac{Hematocrit\ (\%) \times 10}{Erythrocyte\ count\ (10^6/\mu L)}$$

$$Mean\ corpuscular\ hemoglobin\ \{MCH\ (pg)\}$$
$$= \frac{Hemoglobin\ (g/dL) \times 10}{Erythrocyte\ count\ (10^6/\mu L)}$$

$$Mean\ corpuscular\ hemoglobin\ concentration\ \{MCHC\ (\%)\}$$
$$= \frac{Hemoglobin\ (g/dL) \times 100}{Hematocrit\ (\%)}$$

Other parameters used to characterize red-cell variation include the red-cell distribution width (RDW). The RDW is calculated directly by the standard deviation and coefficient of variation from a red-cell size-distribution histogram. The difference in cell size may be used to monitor patients with pernicious or hemorrhagic anemia.

Anemias are classified as to red-cell volume and hemoglobin concentration. *Macrocytic* (large cell: MCV > 94), *normocytic* (normal cell: MCV, 82 to 92), or *microcytic* (small cell: MCV < 80) are the classifications according to cell volume. Cellular hemoglobin concentration categorizes the cells as to *hyperchromic* (MCHC > 38), *normochromic* (MCHC = 32 to 36), or *hypochromic* (MCHC < 30). Examples of anemias are

I. Hypochromic Microcytic—erythroid normoblastic anemia in bone marrow
   A. Iron Deficiency—low hemoglobin (Hbg) and RBC, low serum iron, high total iron binding capacity, absent hemosiderin
      1. Dietary—low iron intake
      2. Intestinal problems—decreased iron absorption
      3. Pregnancy, infants—increased iron requirements
      4. Iron loss—due to chronic hemorrhage, parasitic infections, GI tract lesions, excess menstrual bleeding
   B. Hereditary Sideroblastic—defect in the heme synthesis, an inability to utilize ingested iron
   C. Thalassemia—genetic abnormality that produces normal to increased HbgF and/or HbgA_2
II. Normochromic Normocytic
   A. Hemolytic—increased destruction of erythrocytes
      1. Autoimmune hemolytic
      2. Cold agglutinin hemolytic
      3. Mechanical destruction of RBCs
      4. Paroxysmal nocturnal hemoglobinuria
      5. Lymphomas and Hodgkin's disease
      6. Infections
   B. Hemoglobinopathies—abnormalities in structure of alpha or beta chains of hemoglobin molecule; normoblastic erythroid hyperplasia in bone marrow
      1. Sickle-cell
      2. Hemolysis
      3. Hemoglobin CC
   C. Acute Hemorrhage
   D. Other
      1. Aplastic Anemia, Leukemia, Malignancy
      2. Renal failure and drug-related anemias caused by chloramphenicol and antineoplastic drugs

III. Normochromic Macrocytic—due to deficiency of vitamin B_{12} or folate; bone marrow is hypercellular with increased erythroid precursors
1. Pernicious
2. Sideroblastic
3. Sprue—total iron-binding capacity is decreased; hemosiderin is increased in the bone marrow
4. Pregnancy

Determinations of the suspension stability of whole blood and erythrocyte fragility are useful adjuncts in the diagnosis of various diseases.

The *erythrocyte sedimentation rate* (ESR) is an estimate of the suspension stability of red blood cells in plasma; it is related to the number and size of the red cells and to the relative concentration of plasma proteins, especially fibrinogen and the α- and β-globulins. This test is performed by determining the rate of sedimentation of blood cells in a standard tube. Normal blood ESR is 0 to 15 mm/hr. Increases are an indication of active but obscure disease processes such as tuberculosis and ankylosing spondylitis. ESR is affected by anemia and does not respond linearly with changes in asymmetrical macromolecules such as fibrinogen and globins.

The *zeta sedimentation ratio* (ZSR) technique overcomes these disadvantages. It is based on a measure of the closeness with which RBC will approach each other after standardized cycles of dispersion and compaction.

The *erythrocyte fragility test* is based on resistance of cells to hemolysis in decreasing concentrations of hypotonic saline.

Increased osmotic fragility of the red cells is associated with various types of spherocytosis and acquired hemolytic anemia; increased resistance has been observed in thalassemia, sickle-cell anemia, and hypochromic anemia. The test can be performed manually by colorimetric estimation of hemoglobin released by hypotonic cell rupture or automatically in an instrument, which continually records the increase in light transmittance through a suspension of red cells in a continuously decreasing salt gradient during dialysis.

LEUKOCYTES

Mature *leukocytes* (white blood cells, WBC) in peripheral blood and their precursors in bone and lymphoid tissue comprise the leukocytic system. Various types of leukocytes are found in normal blood. Differentiation of the lymphocytic, monocytic, and granulocytic leukocyte types is based on cell size, color, chromatin structure, and cytoplasm constituents.

The primary function of leukocytes is the development of the various defense mechanisms and repair processes in inflammatory and immune-response mechanisms. The migration of leukocytes to the site of inflammation is associated with the release or activation of various biochemical substances (5-hydroxytryptamine, histamine, complement, immunoglobulins, prostaglandins, lysosomal enzymes). The tissue histiocyte or monocyte (macrophage) also can engulf and destroy foreign particles by the process of endocytosis and certain leukocyte types by phagocytosis.

The chemical composition of the leukocyte includes water (82%), nucleoprotein, phospholipids, and trace minerals. Enzyme content, glycogen, and histamine levels vary in the different types of white cells. Deficiency in enzymes associated with glycolytic metabolism (hexokinase) and increases in phosphomonoester hydrolases (alkaline phosphatase) have been observed in leukocytes of certain leukemia patients.

The precursors of granulocytic leukocytes are found in bone marrow and are classified according to the degree of cytoplasmic granulation, dye-affinity of the granules, and shape of the nucleus (Schilling, Arneth, or Cooke-Ponder Classification). As undifferentiated cells (myeloblasts) mature

promyelocyte → myelocyte → metamyelocyte →

band leukocyte → segmented leukocyte

metachromatic granules appear in the cytoplasm (granulocytes). All segmented leukocytes are motile, a requirement for participation in the inflammatory or phagocytic processes.

In the mature *basophilic* and *eosinophilic leukocytes*, these granules develop an affinity for a basic or acidic dye, respec-

tively; those cells containing granules that do not stain are called *neutrophils*. In peripheral blood, the mature granulocytic cells are designated *polymorphonuclear leukocytes: neutrophilic, eosinophilic,* or *basophilic.*

The other types of white cells normally observed in peripheral blood have no granules and are classified as to size and shape into the *monocyte* and *lymphocyte*, which are formed in lymphoid tissue. The small lymphocyte is thymic-derived and is found in the circulation and germinal centers of lymphoid tissue. The origin of the large lymphocyte is a gut-associated lymphoid stem cell that can further differentiate into the immunoglobulin-producing plasmacyte. The interaction of thymic (T) and bone-marrow (B) lymphocytes is the basis for the development and maintenance of humoral and cellular immune mechanisms.

Leukocytes are enumerated by procedures similar to those used for erythrocytes. In the visual procedures, the blood is diluted with a fluid (3% v/v acetic acid) that lyses the red cells, and the total leukocyte count is determined microscopically. Eosinophils also may be analyzed differentially with a diluting fluid that renders the red cells nonrefractile and invisible, and lyses the base-labile leukocytes, leaving the base-stable eosinophils intact. A suitable diluting fluid for this purpose is Pilot's Fluid (propylene glycol, 50 mL; distilled water, 40 mL; 1% phloxine, 10 mL; 10% sodium carbonate, 1 mL; and heparin sodium, 100 units). Electronic counting procedures are similar to those used for erythrocytes with the added advantages of speed, accuracy, and reproducibility.

The normal adult leukocyte value is 5000 to 10,000 cells μL^3. Values greater than 10,000 (*leukocytosis*) are encountered in the newborn infant, young children, leukemia, cancer, convulsive seizures of epilepsy, and after extreme exercise. Values of less than 5000 (*leukopenia*) are observed in certain microbial infections (eg, typhoid fever, measles, malaria, overwhelming septicemia), cirrhosis of the liver, pernicious anemia, radiation injury, and replacement of marrow by malignant tissue.

A *differential count of the leukocytes* provides information as to the relative numbers of each type. A thin film of blood is prepared on a microscope slide, stained with a polychromatic preparation such as the Leishman, Wright, or Giemsa stain, and analyzed microscopically. Wright's stain contains polychromed methylene blue and eosin dyes; the erythrocytes are stained pink; the nuclei of the leukocytes, purplish-blue; neutrophilic granules, violet-pink; eosinophilic granules, red; basophilic granules, blue; and platelets, blue.

The introduction of automated systems for differential white-cell counts has reduced the errors inherent with the subjective nature of the visual counting procedure. Differentiation of the various cell types can be made on the basis of cytochemistry and staining properties of enzymes specific for a single cell type. The granules of neutrophils and eosinophils are stained by action of their peroxidases on 4-chloro-1-naphthol to form a colored quinone in the presence of a peroxide and further differentiated by the optimum pH for peroxidase activity between these two cell types. The monocytic lipase is used as a specific marker by the reaction of basic fuchsin with α-naphthol liberated by lipase on α-naphthylbutyrate substrate. The lymphocytes are not stained in this procedure but are measured by electronic sizing.

Automated differential WBC counts also are obtained in systems that count large populations of cells by simultaneous measurement of two optical properties (axial light loss and/or narrow-angle scatter and/or multiple-wavelength fluorescence). Laser light also is used to differentiate cell size, granularity, and volume of cells. The collected light measured by forward versus right-angle scatter is converted to a histogram giving the percent of lymphocytes, monocytes, and granulocytes. Another type of system utilizes computer processing of two-dimensional images of the various cell types after staining, employing an automatic scanning microscope.

Polymorphonuclear neutrophilic leukocytes (neutrophils, "polys") normally comprise 62% (50–67%) of the total leukocyte count. These cells are irregular in shape (10–15 μm in diameter) and usually contain a multilobated nucleus with fine, lightly stained cytoplasmic granules. An immature or juvenile form of neutrophil, with a band-shaped nonsegmented nucleus constitutes 3% to 5% of peripheral blood leukocytes. Increases in the relative percentage of these cells (neutrophilia) are observed in acute microbial infections (eg, meningitis, smallpox, poliomyelitis), metabolic disorders (diabetic acidosis, gout), drug intoxication (digitalis, epinephrine), vaccination, coronary thrombosis, and malignant neoplasms.[2]

Polymorphonuclear eosinophilic leukocytes (eosinophils) normally comprise about 1% to 3% of total circulating white blood cells. In appearance they are similar to the neutrophil with the exception of large, red-stained cytoplasmic granules. Eosinophilia has been observed in certain skin diseases (psoriasis, eczema), parasitic infestations (pork round worm—trichinosis), certain hypersensitivity reactions, and in scarlet fever and pernicious anemia. Charcot-Leyden crystals, which are found in bronchial secretions from asthmatics, are derived from nucleoprotein-disintegration products of eosinophils.

Polymorphonuclear basophilic leukocytes (basophils) possess large cytoplasmic granules that stain a deep blue. These cells, which are primarily sources of blood heparin and histamine, constitute less than 1.0% of the leukocytes. Basophilic leukocytosis is seen in chronic myelocytic leukemia, hemolytic anemia, and Hodgkin's disease. Basophilic leukopenia occurs following radiation or therapy with glucocorticoids.

Lymphocytes have a cell diameter from 7 to 10 μm (small) to 10 to 18 μm (large). They have a round, or slightly indented, deeply stained nucleus and normally comprise 25% to 33% of the leukocytes. Lymphocytosis is seen in infectious mononucleosis, lymphocytic leukemia, rickets, and in most conditions associated with neutrophilic leukopenia (neutropenia).

Monocytes constitute 3% to 7% of the leukocytes. They are larger (12–20 μm) than the other leukocytes and possess an abundant, pale, bluish-violet-stained cytoplasm with a fine, reticulated chromatin structure in the nucleus. The monocytes (macrophages) phagocytize bacteria, parasitic protozoa, foreign particles, and even erythrocytes. Monocytosis is seen in certain microbial infections (tuberculosis, typhus, malaria), Hodgkin's disease and monocytic leukemia.

Drug therapy frequently causes neutrophil dysfunction, which can be characterized by a decreased number of mature neutrophils or a defect in cellular function resulting in the inability of the body to defend itself against infection. Drugs such as nitrogen mustard and chloramphenicol degenerate bone-marrow stem cells, and DNA synthesis is impaired by antimetabolites such as methotrexate and fluorouracil. Depolymerization of DNA is caused by procarbazine and alkylating agents. Mitosis is inhibited by colchicine and vinca alkaloids. The following outline lists drugs that cause granulocytopenia.[2]

Nonchemotherapeutic
rifampin
ristocetin
benzene
nitrous oxide
ethanol

Antithyroid
carbimazole
methimazole
thiouracil

Diuretics
acetazolamide
chlorthalidone
chlorothiazide
ethacrynic acid
hydrochlorothiazide
mercurials

Antihistamines
thenyldiamine
thenalidine
pyribenzamine

Phenothiazines
chlorpromazine
mepazine
methotrimeprazine
prochlorperazine
thioridizine

Antibiotics
chloramphenicol
carbenicillin
griseofulvin
isoniazid
novobiocin

Cardiovascular
diazoxide
procainamide
methyl dopa
quinidine
propranolol

As qualitative and quantitative changes in leukocytes in peripheral blood and their precursors in bone marrow and lymphatic tissue are associated with the various types of *leukemia*, this disease has been classified on the basis of the predominating type of leukocyte, ie, myelocytic (granulocytic), lymphocytic, monocytic, or plasmacytic. Leukemia may be either acute or chronic and involve the replacement of bone-marrow elements by malignant cells, infiltration of the reticuloendothelial system, anemia, thrombocytopenia, and hemorrhage. Leukemia usually is associated with an elevated WBC count and increase in the specific cell and its precursors in peripheral blood, but in certain instances there is an aleukemic blood picture with no evidence of leukocytosis. Leukocytes in acute leukemia are more immature ("blast"-type cells) than those encountered in the chronic type.

In many diseases of the hematopoietic system, it is necessary to examine the bone marrow to determine the rates of formation, maturation, and release of blood cells into the peripheral circulation. Using a puncture biopsy needle, samples of *bone marrow* may be obtained from the sternum, iliac crest, or proximal end of the tibia. Smears of marrow then are prepared, stained (Wright's stain or specialized histopathological procedure) and examined microscopically. The ratio of myeloid leukocyte to nucleated red cells in bone marrow, the presence of abnormal (*nonmyeloid*) cells, the number of platelet precursors (*megakaryocytes*), the signs of cell-maturation arrest, and the presence of focal lesions are important factors in the diagnosis of various disease states.

Systemic lupus erythematosus (SLE) is a disease characterized by numerous clinical and pathological manifestations associated with various organs. Although the disease chiefly affects the lymphatic system, the cardiac, renal, and articular systems also are involved. The diagnosis of this disease is based on the presence of an SLE-cell factor in the gamma-globulin fraction of blood in the diseased state. This factor dissolves the nuclei of leukocytes by depolymerization of deoxyribonucleic acid to form the SLE-body. If serum from patients with SLE is incubated with white cells, the "polys" will engulf the liberated SLE-body and form the typical SLE-cell with a characteristic progressive loss of nuclear detail. Drugs that cause SLE and produce a positive SLE-prep include hydralazine, procainamide, isoniazid, and phenytoin.

These antibodies to nucleoprotein also can be detected by immunologic techniques. In the double-antibody technique, the test serum containing antibodies to nuclear protein is incubated with a rat kidney slice (antigen). The second antibody is a fluorescein-labeled goat antihuman immunoglobulin (IgG) that binds to the human IgG, which is also bound to the antigen site in a positive test. The fluorescence is estimated by immunomicroscopy. Normal light-microscopy can be used if the goat-antihuman IgG is labeled with peroxidase.

THROMBOCYTES

The primary functions of *thrombocytes* (blood platelets) are the maintenance of hemostasis (arrest of blood flow from a vessel) and blood coagulation (clot formation). Platelets are oval to spherical in shape and have a mean diameter of 2 to 4 μm. They originate from an immature cell (megakaryocyte) in bone marrow; ranges of 140,000 to 450,000 μL have been reported in normal blood.

Adhesiveness, aggregation, and agglutination are the principal physical properties of platelets responsible for hemostasis and coagulation reactions. Chemically, they contain protein (60%), lipid (15%), and carbohydrate (8.5%). Their content of serotonin, epinephrine, and norepinephrine aids in promoting constriction at the site of injury. The release of "platelet thromboplastin," a cephalin-type phosphatide, and adenosine diphosphate (ADP) are important in blood coagulation.

Manual methods for the enumeration of blood platelets are notoriously imprecise due to the size and physical properties of the platelet. Indirect methods of analysis are based on the proportion of platelets to erythrocytes in a stained blood smear. Blood samples obtained directly from the fingertip puncture are diluted with an anticoagulant fluid that simultaneously will stain the platelets. The ratio of platelets to red cells then is determined microscopically, and the number calculated from the predetermined red-cell count (normal 3 to 8 platelets/100 RBC). In the direct procedures, a sample of blood is obtained by venipuncture, placed in a siliconized tube, diluted, and subsequently analyzed by counting the platelets in a microscopic counting chamber using conventional or phase-microscopy apparatus. Suitable diluting fluids are the Rees-Ecker Fluid (sodium citrate, 3.8 g; formaldehyde, 0.22 mL; brilliant cresyl blue, 0.05 g; water, qs 100 mL) or Brecker Fluid (1% ammonium oxalate). Automated procedures for platelet counting have increased the accuracy to ± 5% to 10%. Blood is collected in a special anticoagulant, diluted, and centrifuged at specified speeds to obtain a "platelet-rich" supernatant fluid, which then is counted in an automated counting apparatus similar to those used for RBC counting.

Methods for counting platelets in whole blood include electronic impedance instruments and laser-optical counters using hydrodynamic focusing.[3] These multiparameter hematology analyzers provide greater accuracy, precision, and increased rate of analysis performed on a small volume of blood. The automated instruments provide precise platelet measurements for monitoring chemotherapy-induced thrombocytopenia and transfusion therapy.

Persistent increases in platelet count (*thrombocythemia or piastrinemia*) have been observed in chronic myelocytic leukemia, polycythemia, megakaryocytic hyperplasia, and splenic atrophy. Acute or temporary increases in platelet values (*thrombocytosis*) are seen in trauma and asphyxiation.

Thrombocytopenia or a decrease in platelets to values less than 60,000/μL occurs in various purpuras or hemorrhagic states (idiopathic or symptomatic thrombocytopenic purpura). Inherited platelet defects include Glanzmann's thrombasthenia, which is characterized by prolonged bleeding time and poor clot retraction, whereas Bernard-Soulier Syndrome and Von Willebrand's disease demonstrates defective platelet adhesiveness. Defects in the release reaction include "Storage Pool Deficiency" and "Aspirin-like Syndrome."

A rare, inherited, structural, and functional platelet abnormality is the *grey-platelet syndrome,* characterized by large platelets lacking alpha granules and appearing grey on Wright's-stained peripheral blood smears. Patients have a history of bleeding, petechiae, easy bruising, and epistaxis. Diagnosis is confirmed by radioimmunoassay procedures to detect levels of platelet-specific alpha-granule proteins.

Leukemia, extensive burns, splenic disorders, and agents such as quinidine, sulfonamides, hydrochlorothiazide, diuretics, antiepileptics, and neuropharmacological agents have been implicated in the etiology of symptomatic thrombocytopenia. Decreases in platelet count also are accompanied by morphological changes in the size, shape, and cytoplasmic granulation of these cells and changes in adhesiveness and normal function in hemostasis and coagulation.

Studies on *platelet aggregation* have been of significant value in the study of platelet abnormalities and their role in disease states. The rate and extent of the aggregation and clotting response to adrenaline, ADP, collagen, and thrombin have been measured by observing changes in optical density of platelet-rich plasma on adding of these agents or other test substances. Low amounts of ADP give reversible aggregation, whereas a biphasic-aggregation pattern occurs with intermediate concentrations of ADP or with epinephrine. The second phase is the release of the platelets' endogenous ADP. High concentrations of ADP result in an irreversible aggregation. Aspirin acts as an inhibitor of the intrinsic-platelet ADP and the collagen reaction.

RETICULOCYTES

In normal peripheral blood 0.5% to 1.5% of the erythrocytes possess a fine reticulum in the cytoplasm. In blood smears prepared with Wright's, Giemsa, and other Romanowsky methods,

basophilic stippling of the erythrocytes occurs in lead poisoning (*plumbism*). This is not to be confused with the basophilic staining of the reticulocyte, which can only be seen when cells are stained by supravital procedures (mixture of dyes with wet blood prior to preparing of an air-dried blood smear). The observed granular filaments or reticulum of this immature erythrocyte are a result of endoplasmic coagulation by lipophilic dyes used in the supravital procedures. *Reticulocytes* can be enumerated manually by supravital staining of fresh blood with an anticoagulant-dye solution.

The usual method of expression is

$$\% \text{ Retics} = \frac{\text{No of reticulocytes}/1000 \text{ RBC}}{10}$$

The "corrected" reticulocyte count is calculated for a more meaningful clinical approach in the degree of anemia by expressing the percentage of reticulocytes per microliter of whole blood.

$$\begin{array}{c} \text{Corrected} \\ \text{reticulocyte} \\ \text{count} \end{array} = \begin{array}{c} \text{Reticulocyte} \\ \text{count} \end{array} \times \frac{\text{(Patient's hematocrit)}}{\text{(Normal hematocrit)}}$$

In indirect counting methods a thin film of the blood-dye mixture is prepared on a microscope slide, counterstained with Wright's stain, and the reticulocytes enumerated in proportion to a predetermined erythrocyte count. In direct procedures, reticulocytes are enumerated in wet films without counterstaining. Suitable dyes are brilliant cresyl blue, methylene blue, and Janus green. These methods are subject to a high counting error.

Flow cytometric analysis using RNA-staining fluorescent dyes has improved greatly the precision and accuracy of reticulocyte counts. Dedicated analyzers such as the Sysmex R-3000 Reticulocyte Analyzer (*TOA Medical Instruments*) examine hundreds of thousands of cells during a 45-sec counting cycle and can subclassify reticulocytes by age.

An increase in the number of reticulocytes is an index of accelerated hematopoiesis and is observed in acute hemorrhage or adequate therapeutic management of iron-deficiency or pernicious anemia. In cases of chronic blood loss or bone-marrow depression a decrease in reticulocytes is seen.

BLOOD-VOLUME AND ERYTHROPOIETIC MECHANISMS

The mean red-cell mass in normal males is 2095 ± 384 mL (30 mL/kg), the average plasma volume is 2766 ± 459 mL (40 mL/kg), and the total blood volume is 4861 ± 795 mL (70 mL/kg). The specific determination of *red-cell mass* is estimated accurately by tagging erythrocytes with ^{51}Cr *in vitro* or ^{59}Fe *in vivo*. These isotopes are incorporated into the β-polypeptide (Cr) or porphyrin (Fe) of hemoglobin in the RBC and subsequent isotope dilution in blood after injection of tagged erythrocytes is used for calculation of red-cell mass. In hemolytic anemia, there is also a decrease in the normal life span (108–120 days) of the erythrocyte as indicated by a decreased survival time of ^{51}Cr-tagged red cells in blood.

Plasma volume is estimated by measurement of hemodilution of intravenous-injected ^{125}I or ^{131}I human serum albumin. The activity of labeled albumin steadily decreases after injection due to the loss of albumin to the extravascular space. Estimates of zero-time radioactivity levels can be made by extrapolation of a typical first-order blood-level decay curve. Dyes (Evans Blue) and other isotopes are less satisfactory for accurate assessment of plasma volume. The total blood volume is equal to the red-cell mass and plasma volume.

Chronic expansion of the red-cell mass is seen in primary and secondary polycythemia associated with erythrocytosis due to hypoxia, tumors, and renal disease. In these conditions, there is an increased hemoglobin and hematocrit and absolute increase in red-cell mass. In relative polycythemia, the high hematocrit is due to contraction of the plasma volume. *Chronic expansion of the blood volume,* with a resultant decrease in hematocrit value, and in some cases a "hemodilution" anemia, is seen in cardiac failure, normal pregnancy, hepatic cirrhosis, splenomegaly, and arteriovenous fistula.

The metabolic defect in *pernicious anemia*, characterized by inadequate gastrointestinal absorption of vitamin B_{12}, is diagnosed readily by monitoring urinary radioactivity following oral administration of cyanocobalamin-[57]Co with and without intrinsic factor. The percent recovery of the isotope in normal patients is 3% to 25% and in pernicious anemia 0% to 2.5%.

Erythrocytes tagged with ^{51}Cr also are used in studying the effects of various compounds, such as the nonsteroidal anti-inflammatory drugs, on *gastrointestinal (GI) bleeding*. The patient's blood cells are tagged with ^{51}Cr and the agent under test is administered. If GI bleeding occurs, there is an increase in the ^{51}Cr content of fecal samples as a result of blood loss into the lumen of the GI tract.

Measurement of the absorption of radioactive iron (^{59}Fe), its tissue distribution (liver, spleen, precordium, sacral bone marrow), plasma elimination, and urinary excretion establish various *ferrokinetic parameters*. Iron is absorbed to the greatest extent as the ferrous salt in the upper small intestine. Absorption is decreased in iron overload, erythropoiesis, and various malignant, inflammatory, or infectious diseases. Iron is transported in plasma bound to transferrin, a specific iron-binding protein. Alterations in plasma iron and iron-binding capacity are seen in pregnancy, thalassemia major, and iron deficiency (hypochromic) anemia. Iron is stored in the liver, bone marrow, skeletal muscle, and spleen as ferritin and hemosiderin. The daily turnover of iron is about 35 mg, primarily from an "erythropoietic labile pool" in bone marrow.

Hemosiderosis is simply an increase in iron storage, whereas *hemochromatosis* denotes increased iron storage with associated tissue damage. Both of these states can result from oral or parenteral medicinal/transfusion iron overload. Iron excretion is limited and occurs by desquamation of iron-containing cells from the bowel, skin, and urinary tract. Iron-deficiency anemia is a symptom and not a disease. Treatment is based on evaluation of ferrokinetic parameters, correction of hemoglobin and tissue-iron deficiency, and recognition of the underlying cause (eg, chronic blood loss).

BLOOD COAGULATION

Hemostasis, the arrest of blood flow from a vessel, is regulated by extravascular (muscle, skin, and subcutaneous tissue), vascular (blood vessels), and intravascular (platelet-adhesion, clot-retraction, and blood-coagulation) mechanisms. The following discussion will be limited to those processes related to the blood-coagulation mechanism. When blood is allowed to clot, the free-flowing liquid is converted into a firm cell clot surrounded by serum. If an anticoagulant is added to blood, coagulation does not occur and the blood cells are suspended in a liquid phase—plasma. The clotting mechanism involves three stages: the formation of plasma *thromboplastin*, the conversion of *prothrombin* to *thrombin*, and the conversion of *fibrinogen* to *fibrin*.

The International Committee on Nomenclature of Blood Clotting Factors has numerically designated the blood-coagulation factors (Table 32-2). Fibrinogen and Factors V and VIII are absent in normal blood serum as a result of the clotting process. The absorption characteristics of certain blood-coagulation factors on calcium phosphate or barium sulfate are used in the differential analysis of specific factors. The interaction of coagulation factors may be initiated through either the intrinsic or extrinsic pathways. In the intrinsic system all the factors are present in the blood, while the extrinsic system is activated by the release of tissue thromboplastin. Figure 32-3 shows the activities of both pathways to form a stabilized fibrin clot.

In Stage 1 of the coagulation process, the contact of injured tissue with blood results in the activation of Factor XII, which reacts with calcium, plasma thromboplastin antecedent (PTA, Factor XI), plasma thromboplastin component (PTC, Factor IX), antihemophilic globulin (AHG, Factor VIII), and Factors III, V, and X to yield intrinsic or blood thromboplastin. This

Table 32-2. Blood-Coagulation Factors

FACTOR	SYNONYM
I	Fibrinogen
II	Prothrombin
III	Thromboplastin (tissue)
IV	Calcium
V	Labile factor, proaccelerin, Ac globulin
VI	Accelerin
VII	Stable factor, proconvertin, serum prothrombin conversion accelerator (SPCA)
VIII	Antihemophilic globulin (AHG)
IX	Christmas factor, plasma thromboplastin component (PTC)
X	Stuart-Prower factor
XI	Plasma thromboplastin antecedent (PTA)
XII	Hageman factor
XIII	Fibrin-stabilizing factor (FSF)

stage normally is completed in 3 to 5 min. Extrinsic or tissue thromboplastin is formed rapidly (<12 sec) in various tissues in the body such as lung and brain in the presence of calcium and Factors V, VII, and X.

In Stage 2, thromboplastin catalyzes the conversion of prothrombin to thrombin (8–15 sec) in the presence of Factors V, VII, X, and calcium.

In Stage 3, the thrombin rapidly converts fibrinogen into fibrin, which then forms a network of fibers that traps red cells and thus forms the blood clot.

Although the exact nature of the enzymatic sequences in the coagulation process is not clear, it is definitely a biological amplification process starting from the small reaction of tissue contact to rapid conversion of fibrinogen to fibrin.

Blood contains natural inhibitors of coagulation such as antithrombin, heparin, and antithromboplastin, which can prevent a particular reaction in the coagulation sequence. The dissolution of blood clots occurs by the action of the blood proteolytic enzyme—plasmin or fibrinolysin. Plasmin is formed

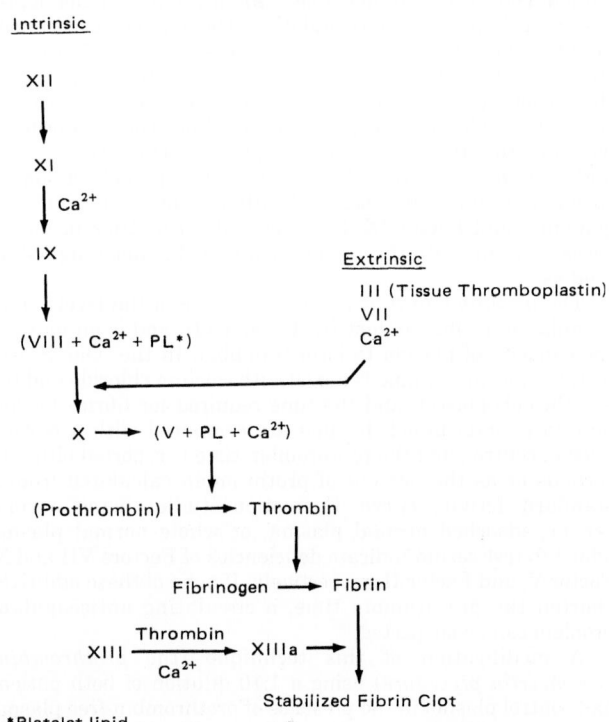

Figure 32-3. Blood coagulation process.

from its precursor, plasminogen, after activation by tissue and body fluids or substances of bacterial origin (streptokinase).

The routine tests performed in the coagulation laboratory are indices of vascular function (vascular phase and platelet adhesion) or intrinsic clotting mechanisms. Determinations of *bleeding time* and *capillary fragility* provide estimates of blood coagulation in the presence of platelets and tissue or vascular factors. In the Ivy method for determination of *capillary bleeding time,* a blood pressure cuff is placed on the forearm and inflated to 40 torr; a puncture wound is made and the time required for bleeding to stop is noted. *Bleeding time* is a screening test for disorders of platelet function or vascular defects but is usually normal in coagulation disorders. The test is useful in the differential diagnosis of Von Willebrand's disease (reduced factor VIII, with a normal bleeding time) from mild hemophilia. The normal bleeding time, as determined by this method, is 1 to 9 min. Dextran, pantothenyl alcohol and derivatives, penicillin G, nonsteroidal anti-inflammatory drugs, and streptokinase-streptodornase may cause a prolonged bleeding time. The Simplate 11 (*General Diagnostics*) is a standardized, disposable, spring-loaded bleeding-time device for platelet function testing. It uses two blades that are released automatically to produce two uniform incisions 6 mm long × 1 mm deep, making the procedure reliable and reproducible.

The *capillary fragility* or *tourniquet* test is based on the incidence of petechiae (small red marks) formation produced by an inflated blood pressure cuff over a 5-min period. Normally, a few tiny petechiae may appear. The most common cause of abnormalities in vascular-function and platelet-adhesion tests is thrombocytopenia.

An analysis of the *intrinsic coagulation mechanism* is concerned with the determination of the levels of the specific clotting factors in whole blood. In preliminary studies of a suspected hemorrhagic disorder, determinations of *coagulation time, clot retraction, platelet count, bleeding time,* and *capillary fragility* usually are performed.

In the Lee-White procedure, the coagulation time of whole blood is determined in regular or silicone tubes. Normal values are 8.5 to 15 min in glass and 19 to 60 min in silicone tubes. Anticoagulants and tetracyclines may cause increased times whereas corticosteroids and epinephrine cause decreased values. The siliconization of glassware prevents platelet aggregation, and thus delays coagulation. The samples used in the analysis of coagulation time are then inspected at 0.5, 1.0, 2.0, 4.0, and 24.0 hr after clotting to determine the time required for the various phases of clot retraction. The tubes also are observed for evidence of clot lysis or dissolution. The clot normally will start to retract in 30 min, completely retract within 24 hr and show no evidence of lysis over a 72-hr period. Prolonged coagulation times are associated with hemophilia, hypofibrinogenemia, and Factor IX deficiency. Abnormalities in any of these tests indicate the requirements for further coagulation studies.

The *prothrombin time test* is a measure of the levels of all coagulation factors, except III, IV, and VII, and is an index of the capacity of plasma to form thrombin. In the "One Stage" test, the plasma sample is mixed with calcium chloride and tissue thromboplastin, and the time required for fibrin-clot formation is determined. Results are compared with a normal plasma control, and the prothrombin time is reported either in seconds or as the percent of prothrombin calculated from a standard activity curve. Correction studies using normal serum, adsorbed normal plasma, or whole normal plasma added to test serum indicate deficiencies of Factors VII and X, Factor V, and Factor II, respectively. If none of these additives shorten the prothrombin time, a circulating anticoagulant problem can be suspected.

A modification of this technique (the *prothrombin-proconvertin procedure*) using a 1:10 dilution of both patient and control plasma in the presence of prothrombin-free plasma as a source of Factors I and V, is a more sensitive index of specific deficiencies in prothrombin, Factor VII, IX, and X.

Owren's *thrombotest,* as performed on whole blood, is sensitive to changes in both extravascular and intravascular clotting mechanisms, including Factor IX. The dosage of anticoagulant drugs, such as dicumarol, is adjusted in accordance with prothrombin-time determinations; patients are maintained usually within a therapeutic range of 20 to 40% of prothrombin activity (normal range, 80–130%). Reduced prothrombin levels, with prolonged prothrombin times, are observed in vitamin K deficiency, hemorrhagic disease of the newborn, excessive anticoagulant therapy, and liver and biliary disease. The interaction of other drugs with anticoagulants may cause increased prothrombin times. Drugs such as salicylates, phenylbutazone, oxyphenbutazone, indomethacin, and some sulfonamides increase the amount of active anticoagulant activity. Other drugs decrease the amount of vitamin K produced by gut bacteria, including chloramphenicol, kanamycin, neomycin, streptomycin, and the sulfonamides.

The *prothrombin consumption* test is an index of the efficiency of conversion of prothrombin to thrombin in the coagulation process. The blood sample is allowed to clot under standardized conditions and then the quantity of prothrombin complex removed in the serum is determined in the presence of extrinsic fibrinogen. At least 80% of the prothrombin is consumed normally. Reduced consumption of prothrombin (<80%) is observed in coagulation deficiencies (hemophilia) related to thromboplastin generation.

Other types of coagulation tests detect deficiencies in *thromboplastin generation mechanism.* The *thromboplastin generation time test* (TGT) provides a means of detecting specific deficiencies of Factors V, VIII, IX, X, XI, or XII. In the initial phase of this procedure, the clotting time of the patient's adsorbed plasma is determined in the presence of a standardized platelet factor reagent, calcium chloride, plasma substrate reagent (Factors I, II, and V), and the patient's serum. If the clotting time is abnormal (>16 sec), further tests are performed with the patient's plasma or serum. The adsorption of the plasma sample on barium sulfate removes Factors II, VII, IX, and X and facilitates differentiation of a Factor IX to X from V to VIII deficiency in the thromboplastin-generation mechanism. Thromboplastin generation is reduced in hemophilia and thrombocytopenia.

The *activated partial thromboplastin time* (PTT) *test* is based on the observation that hemophilic plasma has a normal clotting time in the presence of a complete thromboplastin (extrinsic-saline extract of brain tissue), as used in prothrombin determinations, but will give a markedly prolonged clotting time with an incomplete thromboplastin (cephalin). Cephalin is a thromboplastic, ether-soluble phospholipid factor with platelet-like activity. In this test, the clotting time of the patient's plasma is determined in the presence of calcium chloride and activated cephalin. This test is used primarily to detect deficiencies in Stage 1 of the coagulation mechanism and is rather sensitive to changes in Factors VIII and IX, as seen in classic hemophilia and Factor IX deficiency (Hemophilia B or Christmas disease).

In Stage 3 of the coagulation process, the presence of adequate levels of fibrinogen and thrombin is critical. *Fibrinogen levels* are analyzed semiquantitatively by determining the clotting time of a diluted plasma sample in the presence of extrinsic thromboplastin. This test is basically independent of prothrombin levels. Fibrinogen concentrations of 125 mg/dL or greater are adequate; deficiencies (hypofibrinogenemia) have been observed in liver disease, carcinomatosis, and in certain complications of pregnancy.

Increased levels of *fibrinogen degradation products* (FDP) have been demonstrated in serum due to primary activation of the fibrinolytic system (pathological fibrinolysis) or by secondary activation following increased blood clotting (disseminated intravascular coagulation). Fibrinogen (mol wt 3.4×10^5 daltons) is degraded sequentially to fragments X, Y, D, and E with molecular weights of 2.7, 1.65, 0.85, and 0.55×10^5 daltons, respectively. Fragments X and Y are more potent anticoagulants than fragments D and E and are responsible for hemorrhagic states in defibrination. Complexes between fibrin monomer, fragment X, and other FDP interfere with thromboplastin generation and platelet formation. FDP can be measured by immunological techniques involving latex agglutination of particles sensitized with specific antibodies to FDP or by a hemaglutination-inhibition test. The normal level of serum FDP is 4.9 ± 2.8 µg/mL. Increased levels are seen in acute myocardial infarction, menstruation, complications of pregnancy, hypoxic newborns, malignancy, and renal disease.

Deficiencies in the clotting mechanisms usually can be corrected partially and temporarily by transfusion of normal blood or plasma. When this fails, the presence of *circulating anticoagulants* (antithrombin, antithromboplastins, heparin) must be considered. Heparin acts indirectly by means of antithrombin III, which neutralizes several activated clotting factors (XIIa, activated Fletcher factor, XIa, IXa, Xa, IIa, and XIIIa). The pharmacological effect of an oral anticoagulant is the inhibition of blood clotting by interfering with vitamin K–dependent clotting factors II, VII, IX, and X. Circulating anticoagulants are detected by determining the effect of normal plasma on the clotting time (*recalcification time*) of the patient's oxalated plasma in the presence of calcium chloride. If the addition of the normal plasma does not shorten the prolonged recalcification time, a circulating anticoagulant state can be reported.

Because the end point of all coagulation tests is the conversion of fibrinogen to fibrin, it is vital that analysts rigidly standardize their concepts of fibrin formation in visual recording procedures. The use of mechanical instrumentation in the detection of clot formation has increased significantly the standardization, accuracy, and reproducibility of coagulation procedures. These instruments measure and record the process of fibrin formation via increased turbidity (coagulogram or photometric clot detection) or changes in electrical conductance in the reaction mixtures. As well as performing routine coagulation tests simultaneously or sequentially, updated systems can run Fibrinogen and Factor assays, achieving rapid throughput and accuracy. New performance features are available with many of the automated coagulation instruments. These include precise temperature regulation, digital displays, automatic dilutions of patient samples, and the ability to measure specific clotting factors using chromogenic substrates.

Hemophilia is a classic deficiency of AHG (Factor VIII), Christmas disease of PTC (Factor IX), and Hageman trait of Factor XII. Hereditary or acquired deficiencies of Factors II, V, VII, X, and XI also are associated with disease states. The process of blood coagulation, analysis of coagulation factors, and interpretation of results comprise a highly complex system. The coagulation laboratory and the physician function together in the diagnosis and treatment of coagulation-deficiency diseases.

BLOOD-BANK TECHNOLOGY

Blood-bank technology in the modern laboratory is part of the blood-transfusion service. As whole blood for transfusion and its components are biologically active therapeutic substances, a complete analysis of their chemical and biological characteristics is vital to the assurance of successful therapeutic effects. The transfusion service is responsible for

1. Receiving and examining of the donor.
2. Collecting, processing, and storing the blood.
3. Typing of recipient and donor for ABO and Rh blood-group factors.
4. Compatibility (cross-matching) testing before transfusion.
5. Issuing of blood for transfusion and extracorporeal circulation.
6. Evaluating transfusion complications.
7. Performance of special serological tests pertinent to blood groups and other factors.

In this section a discussion of pertinent factors related to the various phases of the transfusion service will be presented.

RECEIVING AND EXAMINING OF THE DONOR

A complete registry[4] of prospective donors should be maintained, with specific reference to age, sex, weight, address, occupation, and telephone number. Computerized blood banking has increased the efficiency of this service. Donors should preferably be between the ages of 21 and 60 and should weigh no less than 110 pounds. The donor may be rejected on the basis of previous or active incidence of certain microbial diseases (recurrent malaria, syphilis, infectious or homologous serum hepatitis, tuberculosis), bleeding abnormalities, convulsions, allergic syndromes, skin or heart diseases, diabetes, alcohol or drug addiction, pregnancy, cancer, recent immunization with live vaccine product, acquired immune deficiency syndrome (AIDS), or blood pressure abnormalities (acceptable blood pressure: between 100/50 and 200/100; pulse rate: 60 to 120/min). The screening of blood for exposure to human immunodeficiency virus (HIV) is crucial to reducing the risk of infection from transfusion. ELISA (enzyme-linked immunosorbent assay) screening tests for the detection of antibodies against HIV are available from manufacturers. More sensitive tests are available to detect viral DNA in body fluids.

A period of at least 8 weeks should have elapsed since blood was withdrawn and the blood hemoglobin level should be 12.5 to 13.5 g/dL or greater. Serum bilirubin and transaminase levels also should be evaluated in donors with previous incidence of jaundice.

COLLECTING, PROCESSING, AND STORING THE BLOOD

A tourniquet is applied to the arm of the donor to occlude the venous return, the skin area is sterilized, and the blood is collected by venipuncture (phlebotomy). NIH Formula A or B ACD (Acid-Citrate-Dextrose) or ACD-phosphate solutions are used as anticoagulants in the sterile blood-collecting containers. Evacuated containers may be of regular or silicone glass; collapsible plastic containers offer many advantages in donation, blood-banking, and transfusion procedures.

The preservation of the red cells in blood is improved by the complete removal of trapped air in the blood-collection apparatus, rapid cooling after collection, and storage at 4°. Properly collected whole blood is usually stable for 21 days at 1° to 6°. The deterioration of whole blood is related to increased cellular fragility (increased plasma K^+) and decreased glucose utilization. Blood that is used for correction of any bleeding tendency or clotting defect should be as fresh as possible. Leukocytes, platelets, and Factors V and VIII deteriorate in stored plasma or whole blood.

ABO BLOOD-GROUP CLASSIFICATION[5]

Human red cells can be classified into various groups or types on the basis of reactivity of certain blood factors (*agglutinogens*) located on the erythrocyte membrane. The Landsteiner system (Table 32-3) for the four blood groups is based on the presence or absence of either A or B agglutinogen on the cell surface (Group A, B, AB, or O, respectively).

Serum does not contain the antibody (*agglutinin*-IgM type) for the antigen present in an individual's own red cells, but does contain the isoagglutinin (eg, anti-B in blood group A) due to exposure, early in life, to bacterial and plant antigens similar in structure to the A-B antigens. The clumping or agglutination of the red cells by reaction of agglutinogen with agglutinin is used in blood-grouping techniques. In certain instances hemolysin antibodies, present in serum containing anti-A or anti-B agglutinins, cause the disruption of cells and release of hemoglobin (hemolysis).

Human blood cells are grouped by two separate reactions: cellular or "front" grouping and serum or *reverse* grouping. The blood group ordinarily is determined by testing an individual's red cells with standardized anti-A or anti-B serum (certified by the Bureau of Biologics, FDA). Confirmation of the blood group

Table 32-3. Blood-Group Systems

BLOOD GROUP	AGGLUTINOGEN IN CELL	AGGLUTININ IN SERUM	REACTION[a] WITH ANTI-A SERUM	REACTION[a] WITH ANTI-B SERUM	FREQUENCY (%) IN CAUCASIANS
A	A	Anti-B	+	−	41
B	B	Anti-A-A$_1$	−	+	10
AB	AB	None	+	+	4
O	None	Anti-A and B	−	−	45

[a] Agglutination.

(reverse typing) is accomplished by an analysis of an individual's agglutinin titer. In this procedure the individual's serum is heated at 56° for 10 min to destroy hemolysins, and then mixed with known Subgroup A$_1$ or B$_1$ human red (Rh-negative) cells in the agglutination test. These two tests should be in agreement prior to the release of blood for transfusion.

Although human blood cells of Group B react uniformly with Anti-B serum, Group A and AB cells show a wide range of reactivity with Anti-A or Anti-A$_1$B serum. Blood-group A may be further categorized into Subgroups A$_1$, A$_{int}$, A$_2$, A$_3$, A$_0$, and A$_x$ on the basis of the reaction with absorbed Anti-A, Anti-A$_1$-lectin, Anti-H-lectin, Anti-A$_{1,2}$, and Anti-AB serum and the presence of Anti-A$_1$ in the serum. Certain Group O individuals possess anti-H in their serum and are further subcategorized into the Bombay or O$_h$ phenotype. Tests for A, B, and H in saliva can establish the genotype of an individual, that is, A and H in saliva of blood-group A; B and H in B; H and O and A, B, H in AB. This is helpful in cases of poorly developed red-cell antigens or in the loss of cellular antigen in some patients with leukemia.

As the human blood cell contains many antigens with rather complex biochemical and immunochemical properties, the blood factors have been classified further into various subsystems. The Kell (K), Lutheran (Lu), Lewis (Le), Duffy (Fy), Kidd (Jk), MNS, Sutter (Js), Diego (Di), and P blood-factor systems are based on the detection of a specific antigen on or within the red cell by means of antibody (isohemagglutinin) reactions with specific antisera or panels of reagent red cells. Some of these factors (eg, Kidd, Kell, and Lewis) have been involved in transfusion reactions.

THE RH-HR SYSTEM AND ANTIHUMAN GLOBULIN TEST

The presence or absence of *Rh$_0$ antigen* in human blood is of prime importance in transfusion reactions, paternity disputes, and isosensitization phenomena. There are eight blood Rh phenotypes that are determined by their reaction with three specific serum agglutinins (Anti-Rh$_0$, Anti-rh′, and Anti-rh″): rh, rh′, rh″, rh′rh″, Rh$_0$, Rh′$_0$, RhO″, and Rh′$_0$Rh″$_0$. The rh groups do not contain the Rh$_0$ factor on the cell surface and are designated "Rh-negative." The terminology of the Wiener system (Rh, rh) is comparable to the Fisher-Race (CDE) as follows: rh′(C), Rh$_0$(D), rh″(E). The Rosenfeld system uses a numerical classification: Rh$_1$ = Rh$_0$.

The absence of the Rh antigen in about 15% of the population does not preclude the presence of other factors; the use of specific antisera (Anti-hr′ and Anti-hr″) has demonstrated the existence of the Hr factors (Hr$_0$, hr′, hr″). For example, the Rh-negative cell (rh″) possesses rh′hr′Hr$_0$ antigens. The antigen Rh$_0$(D) is the most potent immunogen of all the Rh antigens.

The Rh antibodies are either *saline agglutinins* (complete) or "blocking" antibodies (incomplete). The latter are of the IgG type. They are used in Rh testing procedures and are produced more commonly, and in higher titer, in the human isosensitization or autoantibody reactions. They will not agglutinate saline suspensions of normal Rh-positive red cells except in the presence of a high concentration of albumin, serum or conglutinin (AB serum with albumin) at a temperature of 35° to 37°.

In routine Rh testing procedures, a sample of blood (oxalated or heparinized) or a suspension of cells in serum or albumin is mixed with Anti-Rh$_0$ serum on a slide or in a tube at 37° to 47°. The presence of clumping indicates that the blood possesses Rh$_0$ antigen. Confirmation of an Rh-negative test may be performed by retesting with Anti-rh′Rh$_0$rh″ serum.

In Rh testing procedures, red cells from patients with acquired hemolytic anemia are partially coated with human autoantibody, and cells from erythroblastic infants are coated with maternal antibody globulins and may be clumped falsely by Rh typing serum containing a high protein concentration, or may appear to be Rh-positive in the saline-cell suspension test. Demonstration of anti-Rh$_0$(D) in an eluate from these antibody-coated cells can help to establish true Rh type.

Anti-Rh antibodies are not normally present in human serum; they may be acquired via isosensitization. The transfusion of Rh-positive blood to an Rh-negative recipient, or transfer of cells of Rh-positive fetus through the placental barrier to the Rh-negative mother, will result in formation of antibodies to Rh agglutinogens not present in the cells of the recipient or mother, respectively.

Hemolytic blood-transfusion reactions and hemolytic disease of the newborn (erythroblastosis fetalis) involve *isosensitization phenomena* usually related to the Rh$_0$ antigen. Hr and ABO antigens also can be responsible for hemolytic disease of the newborn. If an expectant mother is Rh-negative and the father is Rh-positive, the Rh genotype of the father should be determined. If the father is homozygous, the erythrocytes will contain a pair of Rh$_0$ factors and the offspring will inherit the Rh$_0$ factor; if he is heterozygous, one Rh$_0$ and one Hr$_0$ factor will be present and his offspring may or may not inherit the factor.

If the fetus is Rh-positive, the mother may be sensitized to the Rh antigen and in subsequent pregnancies the development of high titers of Anti-Rh$_0$ antibodies will result in hemolytic disease of the fetus. These antibodies enter the fetal circulation via the placental barrier, coat the red cells of the fetus, and cause excessive erythrocyte destruction, hyperbilirubinemia, and associated potential for brain damage, hydrops fetalis (edema), and congenital anemia of the newborn. This Rh disease can be avoided now by proper therapeutic use of Rh$_0$(D) Human Immune Globulin (Rh$_0$-GAM, *Ortho*) to prevent the postpartum formation of active antibodies in the Rh$_0$ (D)-negative, D^u-negative mother who has delivered an Rh$_0$(D)-positive or D^u-positive infant.

The *Coombs' antiglobulin test* is a method of detecting the blocking-type antibodies, globulins, and complement that are attached to red-cell antigens in isosensitization phenomena.

In the *direct* test procedure, a saline suspension of washed red cells is mixed with antihuman gamma globulin antiserum and agglutination is indicative of the combination of human antibody with antigen on the red cell, such as maternal incomplete isoantibody on infant's red cells in hemolytic disease of the newborn, autoimmune, drug-induced, alloantibody-induced hemolytic anemia, and after transfusion of incompatible red cells.

An *indirect* procedure is used to demonstrate the presence of blocking antibody in the serum of pregnant Rh-negative women and in transfusion reactions. In this procedure the patient's serum is incubated with a suspension of Group O Rh-positive red cells; the cells are washed and then antihuman globulin antiserum is added to detect the coating of the red cells with antibody globulin from the patient's serum by agglutination phenomena. If agglutination occurs in the first part of the procedure, a saline agglutinin is also present.

Anticomplement sera (anti-nongammaglobulin antiserum) are used to detect reactions involving anti-JK.

The Du allele is a clinically important variant of the Rh$_0$ factor and usually associated with rh′(C) and rh″(E). Individuals with this factor are considered Rh-positive; the red cells fail to react with anti-Rh$_0$ in the saline-tube method but react with incomplete anti-Rh$_0$(D) by other slide or tube techniques. Rh-negative donors should be tested for Du factor. If positive, their blood must only be given to Rh-positive recipients.

DRUG-RELATED PROBLEMS

Hematological abnormalities may be caused by the administration of drugs that can cause a positive direct antiglobulin test and immune hemolytic anemia, such as cephaloridine, cephalothin (*Keflin*), methyldopa (*Aldomet*), penicillin, L-dopa, quinidine, phenacetin, and insulin.

COMPATIBILITY TESTING

Cross-matching procedures are designed to detect incompatibilities in the blood of donors and recipient. The test is designed to prevent transfusion reaction and assure maximum benefit to the patient. Although erroneous ABO grouping usually will result in an incompatible cross match, no such protection exists in the Rh system. An incorrectly typed Rh-positive donor blood can result in primary immunization to $Rh_0(D)$ antigen if transfused to an Rh-negative recipient. For each transfusion, a *major* and *minor cross match* should be performed.

In the *major cross match* (1) a saline suspension of the donor's cells is mixed with the recipient's serum and (2) the donor's cells are suspended in recipient's serum or in serum with added albumin. The saline cross match is an additional check on the ABO typing and may detect incompatibilities caused by antibodies to M, N, S, P, and Lu subgroups. The high-protein or albumin cross-match can demonstrate antibodies in the Rh system. The presence of agglutination or hemolysis indicates incompatibility.

The *minor cross match* includes the donor's serum and the recipient's cells and is useful as a check of the ABO typing and an indication of the possibility of transfusion reactions caused by a rare antigen on the recipient's cells or uncommon antibodies directed against an antigen in the serum of the donor. The minor cross match has been replaced in many instances with screening of the donor's serum against a panel or pool of red cells of known antigenicity.

The *indirect antihuman globulin* procedure also must be performed with the recipient's serum and donor's cells with and without albumin (major side) and may be tested with the donor's serum and recipient's cells (minor side). The use of proteolytic enzymes (bromelain) enhances the agglutination of red cells by low-titer or weakly reacting Rh-Hr antibodies, probably by removing sialic acid residues on the RBC surface. The red cells used in the indirect Coombs' test are treated with the enzyme prior to absorption of antibodies and addition of antiglobulin reagent.

The usual cross-matching techniques involve (1) a room-temperature or 30° procedure, preferably with the addition of albumin, (2) a high-protein procedure, and (3) an antiglobulin procedure.

The presence of nonspecific *autoantibodies, cold agglutinins,* and *bacteriogenic agglutination* sometimes complicates the cross-matching procedure. If the recipient's serum reacts more strongly with his or her own cells than with the donor's, autoantibodies should be suspected. Cold agglutinins usually will agglutinate all blood, regardless of type, at low temperatures, but will not react at 37°. Agglutination as a result of bacterial contamination of blood is called panagglutination.

HEPATITIS TESTING

Post-transfusion hepatitis is associated with the transmission of virus-like particles referred to as *Australia* or *serum hepatitis antigen* or the *hepatitis-associated antigen* (HAA). All donor blood must be tested for the presence of HAA. Agar gel diffusion (AGD), counterelectrophoresis (CEP), complement fixation (CF), and rheophoresis procedures can be used.[6] The rheophore-sis procedure uses a modified gel-diffusion technique for the detection of HAA by precipitin-type reaction with HAA antibody. It offers the sensitivity of CEP and CF procedures with the simplicity of the AGD procedure. Other tests for HAA are based on radioimmunoassay (RIA) technique for detection of antigen by hemagglutination (HA) or HA-inhibition for the presence of HAA antibody. In the RIA technique, the donor's serum is added to a test tube coated with HAA antibody (solid RIA). If the serum contains HAA, it will bind to the antibody. ^{125}I-HAA is then added to the tube. If the antibody binding site is occupied previously with HAA from the donor's serum, ^{125}I-HAA will not bind and the determination of ^{125}I bound versus free is an index of HAA content of the donor's serum.

ISSUING OF BLOOD AND EVALUATING TRANSFUSION REACTIONS

Whole-blood, red-cell, or leukocyte suspensions, plasma, platelet-rich plasma, platelet concentrates, leukocyte-poor blood, AHF, factor IX complex, plasma protein fractions, and RhoGAM are products of the transfusion service.[7] Transfusion reactions are related to antibody phenomena or disease transmission. The hemolytic reaction resulting from the transfusion of incompatible cells is the most serious problem. The transfusion of microbially contaminated blood can result in a pyrogenic reaction or transmission of infectious diseases, such as malaria, syphilis, AIDS, or hepatitis. Allergic reactions (urticaria, asthmatic seizures), circulatory overload, embolic complications (blood clot, air emboli) also may be encountered. Leukocyte and platelet antibodies develop in repeat transfusions and in transplantation patients. The transfusion service is an integral unit in evaluating such complications.

TECHNIQUES OF ANALYSIS

This section will describe the principles of the procedures used in the analyses of various substances in blood, plasma, or urine. Examples of the significance of such tests in clinical diagnosis will be presented. For a complete description of the physiological and pharmacological aspects of these blood constituents, see the *Bibliography*.

INSTRUMENTATION

The development of instrumentation has accelerated progress in clinical chemistry. An excellent review of the principles and applications in clinical chemistry of automation, atomic-absorption spectroscopy, ultraviolet and visible spectrophotometry, fluorometry, phosphorimetry, infrared and Raman spectroscopy, microwave, and radiowave spectroscopy and nucleonics was prepared by Broughton and Dawson.[8] Quality-control techniques are a vital part of any clinical laboratory. Standard reference materials,[9,10] standardization of quantities and units,[11] and continual evaluation of precision and accuracy of various determinations[12] are incorporated into procedures of all reliable clinical laboratories. The manufacture of certified standards and reagents and the certification of clinical chemists and clinical laboratories are under the supervision of either the Food and Drug Administration (FDA), National Institutes of Heath (NIH), Pharmaceutical Manufacturers Association (PMA), American Association for Clinical Chemistry, the College of American Pathologists, and the National Committee for Clinical Laboratory Standards (NCCLS).

INTERACTION OF DRUGS WITH CLINICAL LABORATORY TESTS

Drugs may interfere with the interpretation of laboratory tests by three classes of mechanisms:

1. *Chemical or biochemical* interference due to reaction of a drug or its metabolite in biological fluids with test reagents in analytical procedures. Examples of Class 1 interference include false-positive urine glucose results due to the reducing properties of drugs or metabolites such as ascorbic acid, *p*-aminosalicylic acid, tetracycline, cephaloridine, and levodopa, which are excreted in urine. Spironolactone will result in an elevation of certain urinary ketosteroids through cross-reaction of the drug in the analytical procedure.
2. *Pharmacological* interference due to normal drug-induced alterations in various physiological parameters. Examples of Class 2 interference include the decrease in serum-potassium levels in patients receiving thiazide diuretics, the alteration in serum uric acid with probenecid, and the elevation in various plasma proteins and thyroid function tests with estrogen-progesterone combinations. Drug–drug interaction also can result in changes in these parameters. Guanethidine enhances the effect of the coumarin anticoagulants. Barbiturates induce hepatic microsomal enzyme synthesis and subsequently increase the metabolism and decrease the therapeutic effect of drugs, such as warfarin, even after these drugs are terminated.
3. *Toxicological* interference as a consequence of the toxicity of a drug. Examples of Class 3 interference include changes in liver- and kidney-function tests and hematological parameters (anemia, agranulocytosis, leukopenia) due to drug-induced toxicity and positive LE and ANA tests due to a "lupus-like" syndrome induced by hydralazine.

It is beyond the scope of this chapter to include a complete listing of drug interactions in laboratory tests. The reader is referred to an annual, readily available, computerized review of the effect of normal therapeutic drug doses, as well as overdoses, on clinical laboratory tests[13] and to other review articles.[14]

Blood

COLLECTION AND PREPARATION FOR CHEMICAL ANALYSIS

Using aseptic technique, a blood sample is obtained by venipuncture and usually drawn directly into evacuated glass tubes. The choice of anticoagulant, type of specimen, stability of test component, and use of preservatives depends on the type of analysis requested and the specific analytical procedure involved. If serum is desired, the blood sample is allowed to clot and the serum is separated by centrifugation. When whole blood or plasma is to be used in the analysis, an anticoagulant is added to the collecting tube.

The following concentrations of specific anticoagulants are used routinely per 10 mL blood: lithium, potassium, or sodium oxalate (15–25 mg), sodium citrate (40–60 mg), heparin sodium (2 mg), disodium or tripotassium ethylene-diaminetetraacetate (EDTA-Na$_2$, 10–30 mg), or ACD-Formula B solution (1.0 mL).

Heparin prevents blood coagulation by inhibiting the thrombin-catalyzed conversion of fibrinogen to fibrin. The other anticoagulants either precipitate blood calcium or convert ionized calcium into a nonionized (chelated) form that cannot function in the coagulation reaction. Heparin and EDTA do not alter the cellular elements of blood significantly. Sodium fluoride and thymol are used as preservatives or enzyme inhibitors to prevent the deterioration of various substances in the blood sample; for example,

glucose → lactic acid.

Preservatives and anticoagulants can interfere with some enzyme tests. Serum usually is used for these procedures.

The separation of plasma or serum, and chemical analysis, usually are performed as soon as possible after the collection of the sample. The addition of polystyrene granules to the blood sample prior to centrifugation facilitates the isolation of serum or plasma. Hemolysis interferes with analytical procedures for bilirubin, albumin, nonprotein nitrogens, pH, phosphorus, potassium, and various enzymes. The serum also should be observed for presence of lipemia. Changes in the ratio of CO$_2$, chloride, and electrolytes in cells and plasma, glycolytic conversion of glucose to lactic acid, hydrolysis of ester phosphate to free inorganic phosphate, bacterial conversion of urea to ammonia, and conversion of pyruvate to lactate are examples of changes that can occur in contaminated, improperly preserved, or unrefrigerated blood specimens.

The first stage in many of the classic manual chemical determinations is the removal of blood protein and preparation of *protein-free blood filtrate*. The protein is precipitated with tungstic acid, trichloroacetic acid, zinc hydroxide, or organic solvents, such as alcohol and acetone, and then filtered or centrifuged to remove the protein coagulum. Tungstic acid precipitation is performed by mixing 1 volume of blood or 2 volumes of plasma with 9 volumes of stabilized tungstic acid reagent. The filtrate obtained in this procedure should be in the pH range of 3.0 to 5.1 to assure the adequate removal of proteins (<2 mg/dL in filtrate).

The Somogyi filtrate is prepared by mixing 1 volume of blood with 5 volumes of water, 2 volumes of 5% zinc sulfate, and 2 volumes of 0.3 N barium hydroxide. The barium sulfate is precipitated and the zinc hydroxide formed in the reaction precipitates the blood proteins. Trichloroacetic acid (10%), in a ratio of 9:1 with blood, yields greater volumes of filtrate due to a more complete formation of protein agglomerates.

BLOOD GLUCOSE

Methods for determining blood glucose are based on the use of glucose as a reducing agent or on the enzymatic oxidation of glucose to gluconic acid. In the Folin-Wu technique, glucose is determined in a protein-free blood filtrate by reduction of alkaline cupric sulfate and subsequent reaction with phosphomolybdic or arsenomolybdic acid reagent to form a blue complex that can be estimated colorimetrically. The Nelson-Somogyi method uses a protein-free blood filtrate prepared with zinc hydroxide to remove most of the interfering reducing substances.

The presence of a terminal aldehyde in the glucose molecule is the basis of a colorimetric determination with phenolic hydroxyl reagents (phenol in aqueous methyl salicylate or phosphorylated 1,3-dihydroxybenzene) in the presence of strong sulfuric acid and heat. The *o*-toluidine procedure is a color reaction specific for hexoses—glucose, mannose, and galactose. Because aldohexoses other than glucose are normally present in very small concentrations, results obtained by this method approach the true value of glucose. *o*-Toluidine is condensed with glucose in glacial acetic acid to yield a green chromogen by forming an equilibrium mixture of a glycosylamine and Schiff base.

In the preceding techniques, interfering substances such as lactose, galactose, and glutathione are measured, and the value is reported in the nonspecific term "sugar." Enzymatic determination with glucose oxidase is the only test specific for blood glucose. Blood glucose is converted to gluconic acid and hydrogen peroxide by glucose oxidase; the peroxide is then estimated by iodimetric procedures or by oxidation of a chromogen (*o*-dianisidine or 2,2′-azino[diethylbenzothiazolinesulfonic acid]) in the presence of a peroxidase to form a colored product. Drugs that cause a slight increase in glucose values include ACTH, corticosteroids, D-thyroxine, diazoxide, epinephrine, estrogens, indomethacin, oral contraceptives, lithium carbonate, phenothiazines, phenytoin, thiabendazole, and diuretics. Drug interferences with *o*-toluidine methods, which cause a slight increase, include ascorbic acid, dextran, fructose, galactose, mannose, ribose, xylose, and bilirubin.

Another enzymatic procedure uses the hexokinase-catalyzed conversion of glucose to glucose 6-phosphate (G6P), and then to 6-phosphogluconate and nicotinamide-adenine-dinucleotide phosphate (NADPH) in the presence of NADP and G6P dehydrogenase. The NADPH thus formed is equivalent to the amount of glucose present and is estimated spectrometrically at 340 or 366 nm.

Normal fasting blood-sugar values for adults are 80 to 120 mg/dL; true glucose is 65 to 100 mg/dL. When the blood-sugar values exceed 120 (hyperglycemia), diabetes mellitus should be suspected and can be confirmed by evidence of diminished carbohydrate tolerance. The effect of ingested carbohydrate on blood sugar can be determined by the *glucose tolerance test;* 100 g of glucose (1.75 g/kg) in water or a flavored beverage is administered orally, and glucose determinations are performed on blood and urine samples at hourly intervals for 3 hr. Values above 160 at 1 hr and 110 at 2 hr in blood samples are abnormal. The renal threshold for glucose is 180 to 200 mg/dL of blood, and thus sugar should not appear in the urine of normal subjects in the tolerance test.

Hyperglycemia and decreased glucose tolerance are seen in diabetes mellitus (to 500 mg/dL) and hyperactivity of the adrenal, pituitary, and thyroid glands. *Hypoglycemia,* with a blood-sugar value of <60 mg/dL and increased glucose tolerance, is encountered in insulin overdose, glucagon deficiencies, and hypoactivity of various endocrine glands. Intravenous glucose tolerance studies are used to circumvent defective absorption of glucose in the GI tract, for example, in steatorrhea.

Monitoring hemoglobin A_{1c} is another way to follow patients with hyperglycemia. This is more specific for diagnosing diabetes but less sensitive than the glucose tolerance test.[15] Normally, hemoglobin A_{1c} accounts for 3% to 6% of the total hemoglobin, whereas in diabetics it is 6% to 12%. The concentration of Hgb A_{1c} in the blood reflects the patient's carbohydrate status over a period of time, providing a marker for hyperglycemia. *Pancreatic function tests* include studies on intravenous and oral glucose, glucagon, and tolbutamide tolerance. The beta cells of pancreatic islet tissue secrete insulin and the alpha cells secrete glucagon, a substance antagonistic to insulin and having a hyperglycemic effect induced by its glycogenolytic action. In *glucagon tolerance studies,* the effect of parenteral administration of glucagon on blood-sugar values is useful in the diagnosis of pancreatic and hepatic function. *Insulin and tolbutamide tolerance studies* are used in the diagnosis of endocrine disorders, differentiation of insulin-resistant diabetics, and determination of functional hypoglycemia and islet-cell tumors.

Galactosemia, the presence of galactose (>4.5 mg/dL) in blood, is usually due to an inborn error of galactose metabolism. Congenital deficiencies in galactokinase or galactose 1-phosphate uridyl transferase result in inadequate galactose metabolism with accumulation of galactose 1-phosphate in the liver. Oral administration of galactose in galactosemia leads to a decrease in blood glucose and an increase in concentrations of galactose in the urine and blood. Galactose is measured by estimation of NADH liberated in the conversion of galactose to galactonolactone in the presence of nicotinamide-adenine dinucleotide (NAD) and galactose dehydrogenase. Deficiencies in intestinal disaccharidases such as lactase will preclude efficient conversion of lactose to galactose and glucose, and oral administration of lactose will cause no increase in blood galactose and usually produce diarrhea. Galactose-loading studies are useful in the diagnosis of toxic or inflammatory conditions of the liver. In hepatic cirrhosis, there is a decrease in the galactose-metabolizing capacity of the liver due to the inhibition of hepatic diphosphogalactose-4-epimerase.

Lactic acid is a product of glucose metabolism; it is converted into pyruvic acid and NADH by lactate dehydrogenase (LDH) in the presence of NAD. Blood lactic acid is estimated by reaction with LDH to form pyruvate and NADH; the NADH level is determined spectrophotometrically at 340 nm and is a function of lactic acid concentration. It is elevated (>20 mg/dL) following exercise, anesthesia, and certain types of acidosis. The *blood lactate/pyruvate* ratio should be calculated to determine the presence of excess lactic acid in the blood in acidosis, thiamine deficiency, and decompensated heart disease.

Blood pyruvic acid is determined by the reverse procedure, that is, the conversion of pyruvate to lactate in the presence of LDH and NADH. Normal blood pyruvic acid ranges from 0.6 to 1.3 mg/dL by chemical methods and 0.3 to 0.7 mg/dL by enzymic procedures.

NONPROTEIN NITROGEN COMPOUNDS

Nonprotein nitrogen (NPN) compounds refer to all nitrogen-containing compounds in biological fluids exclusive of protein, including nitrogen from amino acids, low-molecular-weight peptides, urea, nucleotides, uric acid, creatinine, creatine, and ammonia. Blood NPN usually is determined by digesting a protein-free blood filtrate with sulfuric acid in the presence of a catalyst (SeO_2) to convert nitrogen to ammonium sulfate (Kjeldahl digestion); the excess acid is neutralized and ammonia determined by Nesslerization or reaction with alkaline hypochlorite.

The normal blood NPN is 25 to 45 mg/dL (48% urea N, 14% amino acid N, 4% creatine N, 1% creatinine N, 3% uric acid N, and 30% residual N). In renal damage, NPN is elevated to values ranging from 60 to 500 mg/dL (*azotemia*). As variations in NPN mainly reflect alterations in blood urea nitrogen (BUN), urea determinations are more sensitive and preferred as a guide to kidney function.

The primary pathway of nitrogen metabolism in man is the synthesis of urea from ammonia in the liver and then rapid renal excretion of urea. In renal disease (*nephritis*), the excretion of urea is diminished, and blood NPN and BUN are increased. In BUN procedures, *urea* is converted enzymatically to ammonia by urease; the ammonia then is determined by Nesslerization, reaction with phenol-alkaline hypochlorite, aeration into standard acid and subsequent titration or reaction with salicylate-nitroprusside reagent at pH 12 in the presence of alkaline dichloroisocyanurate to form a green chromogen that can be estimated colorimetrically. The ammonia also can be estimated by spectrophotometric determination of NAD produced in the conversion of ammonia and α-ketoglutarate to glutamate by NADH-L-glutamate dehydrogenase. Direct chemical determinations of urea are based on the reaction with 2,3-butanedione in an acid medium (Fearon reaction).

BUN (normal = 5–25 mg/dL) is increased in chronic and acute nephritis, metallic poisoning, and cardiac failure; reduced levels occur in rapid dehydration or following diuresis. In severe liver damage due to diminished urea formation, an increase in blood ammonia and decrease in BUN are observed. Urine urea output (6–17 g/day) is an index of *glomerular filtration rate* (GFR) *and kidney function.* Increased dietary protein and gastrointestinal hemorrhage will increase urine urea. Decreases in urea excretion involve either tubular reabsorption or secretion defects.

The *nitrogen balance* represents the balance between nitrogen input or produced (N_{in}) and nitrogen excreted (N_{out}); in normal individuals $N_{in} = N_{out}$. N_{out} is regulated by renal GFR; in renal disease GFR is decreased, $N_{in} > N_{out}$, and BUN is increased. The rate of urinary excretion of parenterally administered dyes (phenolsulfonphthalein), inulin sodium, *p*- aminohippurate, and mannitol are sensitive indices of GFR in *renal clearance studies.*

Creatine (methylguanidoacetic acid) and *creatinine* (creatine anhydride) are involved in the physiology of muscle contraction. Creatine phosphate is an intracellular source of high-energy phosphate bonds via the reaction of adenosine triphosphate (ATP) and creatine kinase. Creatinine is the waste product of creatine metabolism and is the normally excreted compound.

Serum creatinine is determined by reaction with alkaline picrate to form a red chromogen. These values usually represent 20% to 30% of noncreatinine-interfering substances. Absolute determinations can be made by the absorption of creatinine from protein-free blood filtrates on aluminum silicate prior to the final determination. Drugs causing nephrotoxicity result in a slight increase in creatinine, and those that interfere with color formation in the reaction include bromsulfophthalein (BSP), phenolsulfonphthalein (PSP), acetoacetate, ascorbic acid, levodopa, methyldopa, glucose, and fructose. Creatine is determined after hydrolytic conversion to creatinine with boiling, aqueous picric, or hydrochloric acid.

Renal clearance of endogenous creatinine is related to GFR and is normally 1 to 2 g/day (creatinine coefficient = 20–26 mg/kg/24 hours). Normal serum creatinine is 1 to 2 mg/dL; creatine 0.2 to 1.0 mg/dL. Higher values (5 mg/dL) indicate glomerular damage or cardiac insufficiency.

Uric acid is a catabolite of purine metabolism as derived from nucleic acids or nucleotide cofactors. Direct methods for determining uric acid involve the reaction with alkaline phosphotungstic acid to form a "tungsten blue," which is estimated colorimetrically. In another method, alcoholic NaOH is added to a protein-free filtrate to eliminate interfering reducing substances (ascorbic acid, glutathione) prior to the reduction of uric acid with acid copper chelate to form a cupric chromogen complex.

In indirect procedures, uric acid is hydrolyzed by the enzyme uricase; the decrease in absorbance at 290 to 293 nm is a function of the initial concentrations of uric acid. The normal blood value is 1.5 to 6.0 mg/dL. It is elevated in renal disease, gout due to increased metabolic pools of uric acid, and leukemia as a result of increased turnover of cellular nucleoprotein.

Amino acid determinations in blood are performed by conventional colorimetric ninhydrin techniques or reaction with alkaline β-naphthoquinone-4-sulfonate. Normal plasma values range from 3.9 to 7.8 mg/dL. A variety of metabolic disorders may be detected by analyzing for increased levels of specific amino acids in the urine or blood. Total urine amino acids are determined by formol titration; formaldehyde reacts with basic amino groups and thus permits subsequent titration of the acidic groups of the amino acids. Daily excretion of amino acid nitrogen ranges from 100 to 400 mg, constituting 1% to 2% of total urine nitrogen.

The identification and quantitation of specific amino acids in the blood and urine are accomplished by paper, thin-layer (TLC), column, and ion-exchange chromatographic and electrophoretic separation of electrolytically desalted blood or urine samples (see Chapter 33).

Abnormal amino acid metabolism (*aminoacidopathies*) usually results in the presence of abnormal quantities of specific amino acids in the urine (aminoaciduria). The aminoacidurias are divided into two main groups:

1. *Primary overflow aminoaciduria* in which blood amino acids are elevated phenylketonuria (PKU), maple syrup urine disease (MSUD), tyrosinosis, and alkaptonuria.
2. Aminoacidurias characterized by elevated amino acid urine levels with normal blood levels: *transport diseases* with a defect in the kidney tubule (eg, cystinuria), and "no-threshold" aminoaciduria in which the kidney has no mechanism for reabsorbing the amino acid involved (eg, homocystinuria).

PKU, a disease characterized by mental deficiency, is associated with the presence of phenylpyruvic acid in the urine and elevated serum phenylalanine levels due to a hereditary (autosomal recessive) deficiency of hepatic phenylalanine hydroxylase, which converts phenylalanine to tyrosine. The availability of treatment through dietary intake is predicated upon early detection. Many states have passed legislation for mass-screening for PKU in all infants. The Guthrie test is performed by placing filter paper discs impregnated with serum or blood on the surface of an agar culture medium containing β-(2-thienyl)alanine at a concentration sufficient to inhibit the growth of *Bacillus subtilis*. Phenylalanine will reverse this inhibition, and the Bacterial Inhibition Assay (BIA) is a direct measure of this amino acid. Serum phenylalanine determinations also can be performed by estimating the fluorescence of a complex with ninhydrin and copper in the presence of L-leucyl-L-alanine.

MSUD is characterized by the odor of the urine and is rapidly fatal to infants. It is associated with a deficiency in the oxidative decarboxylation of α-keto acids leading to an accumulation of both the keto and amino acids in the blood and urine (valine, leucine, isoleucine). TLC and BIA assays can be used to detect MSUD.

Alkaptonuria is a rare, hereditary disease in which homogentisic acid cannot be metabolized further due to a lack of homogentisic acid oxidase. This causes homogentisic acid-uria, ochronosis, and arthritis.

In *Hartnup disease*, indole and tryptophane appear in the urine due to defective renal and intestinal absorption of tryptophane. Tryptophane is an intermediary metabolite in the synthesis of *serotonin* (5-hydroxytryptamine) and 5-hydroxyindole acetic acid (HIAA). Excessive production of *serotonin* and the presence of its *HIAA metabolite* in the urine are associated with metastatic carcinoid tumors. HIAA is measured after removal of interfering keto acids with dinitrophenylhydrazine, extraction, and estimation with nitrosonaphthol reagent.

Routine screening tests for congenital metabolic defects and the substance under test in the newborn include PKU (phenylalanine), MSUD (leucine), tyrosinemia (tyrosine), homocystinuria (methionine), histidinemia (histidine), valinemia (valine), galactosemia (galactose or galactose uridyltransferase), orotic aciduria (orotidine-1-phosphate decarboxylase), arginosuccinuria (arginosuccinic lyase), hereditary angioneurotic edema (C¹-1-esterase inhibitor), and sickle-cell disease (hemoglobin S).

The analyses for these substances are based on BIA, metabolite bacterial inhibition assay (MIA), enzyme auxotroph bacterial assay (ENZ-Aux), fluorescent spot tests or TLC, and electrophoresis.

PROTEINS

The *plasma proteins* (albumins, globulins, and fibrinogen) are involved in nutrition, electrolyte and acid–base balance, transport mechanisms, coagulation, immunity, and enzymatic action. *Total plasma proteins* may be determined by Kjeldahl, Nesslerization, specific ion pair (bromcresol green dye plus albumin), or biuret procedures. The last technique is based on the reaction of —CONH— groups joined by carbon or nitrogen linkages in protein with alkaline copper sulfate to yield the biuret complex that can be estimated colorimetrically. Total protein also can be estimated by specific gravity, or refractometric or UV spectrometric methods. These methods are subject to large errors in the presence of a pathology involving increased glucose, lipid, urea, or abnormal protein concentrations.

The *albumin-globulin* (A/G) ratio is determined by the biuret method after precipitation of the globulins with a sodium sulfate–sulfite reagent. The normal range is 5.5 to 8.0 g/dL total protein with an A/G ratio of 1.4 to 2.4. Changes in total protein and A/G ratio occur in kidney and liver disease, hemorrhage, dehydration, rheumatoid arthritis, and multiple myeloma. Gastrointestinal albumin loss, as seen in GI bleeding, ulcerative colitis, sprue, and enteritis, can be detected by monitoring fecal radioactivity after intravenous injection of ^{51}Cr-human serum albumin.

The physiochemical properties of the plasma proteins—(mol wt 68,000 to 300,000 daltons) and isoelectric point (pH of minimum solubility and ionic neutrality)—provide the basis for the electrophoretic separation of plasma proteins (Fig 32-4). The plasma sample is spotted on a paper or cellulose acetate strip, or in a polyacrylamide gel (disc or gel electrophoresis) at pH 8.6. At this pH the proteins are electroanionic and, under the influence of electric current, will migrate to the anode at a rate dependent on their isoelectric point and, in the case of cellulose acetate or gel electrophoresis, their molecular size. The strips are then stained with a protein dye (bromophenol blue, Amido black, or Ponceau S), and the concentrations of the various proteins are estimated by densiometric scanning.

The normal ranges for the major proteins are (in g/dL): albumin 3.8 to 5.0; total globulin, 2.0 to 3.9; α_1-globulin, 0.1 to 0.5; α_2-globulin, 0.5 to 0.9; β-globulin; 0.5 to 1.2; γ-globulin, 0.7 to 1.6.

Ordinary electrophoresis does not identify the subgroups of *immunoglobulins*, IgA, IgM, IgG, and IgE. This is accomplished by immunoelectrophoresis, a process involving electrophoresis and immunodiffusion. The sample is electrophorized in an agar gel (zone electrophoresis) and then antiserum to the specific Ig or to total globulins is placed in a trough aligned parallel to the axis of the original electrophoresis. The serum proteins and

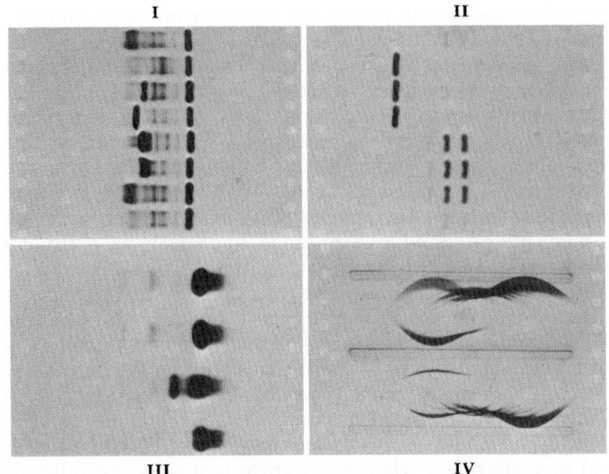

Figure 32-4. Electrophoretic separation of serum proteins (I), isoenzymes (II), hemoglobins (III), and immunoelectrophoresis of plasma protein (IV) (courtesy, Spinco).

antisera diffuse toward each other and form precipitin (antigen-antibody complex) lines. Ordinary cellulose acetate or gel electrophoresis will permit the recognition of diffuse, polyclonal elevation of serum immunoglobulins seen in chronic infections, isolated M-protein peaks of macroglobulinemia and multiple myeloma, and absent gamma component in a hypogammaglobulinemia or agammaglobulinemia. Immunoelectrophoresis will indicate specific Ig abnormalities or, by noting the presence of any displacement, bowing or broadening of the precipitin band will aid in the diagnosis of the paraimmunoglobulin monoclonal diseases such as multiple myeloma, macroglobulinemia, or chronic lymphatic leukemia.

Radial immunodiffusion is a simple process that also can be used for quantitation of IgA, IgM, and IgG.[16] It is performed by incorporating the antibody in an agar gel and then introducing the antigen or test sera into wells punched in the agar. The antigen diffuses radially out of the well into the surrounding gel media, and a visible precipitin line forms where the antigen and antibody have reacted. Quantitation of IgA, IgM, and IgG aids in the diagnosis and differentiation of collagen diseases, chronic infections, and liver disease. IgE is best quantitated by immunoelectrophoresis or RIA.

Nephelometric techniques detect immunological constituents by measuring the light-scattering properties of various antigen-antibody complexes in a test solution. The Hyland system measures the amount of laser-beam deflection at an angle by employing a photomultiplier tube that is sensitive in the red region of the spectrum. Results are calculated by an electronic-screening system and read in percent relative light-scatter on a digital readout. Automated electrophoresis instrumentation offers computer-controlled sample application, staining options, densitometry, and pattern interpretation for serum proteins and isoenzymes.

ENZYMES

Enzymes are proteins whose biological function is the catalysis of chemical reactions in living systems. Enzymes combine with the substances on which they act (substrates) to form an intermediate enzyme-substrate complex, which is then converted to a reaction product and liberated enzyme that continues its catalytic function. Enzymes are highly specific; a few exhibit absolute specificity and catalyze only one particular reaction, whereas others are specific for a particular type of chemical bond, functional group, or stereoisomeric structure.

Most serum enzymes of clinical significance are intracellular in origin and are elevated in hyperactivity disease, malignancy,

or injury to cardiac, hepatic, pancreatic, muscle, bone, and tissue. As the specific tissue involved will determine the type of enzyme that will be elevated, such determinations are valuable diagnostic tools in the differentiation of various pathological states.

Enzymes are named and classified according to the type of reaction that they catalyze and to their substrate specificities. Enzyme activity usually is expressed in International Units (IU) where 1 unit (U) is that amount of the enzyme that will catalyze the transformation of 1 μmole of substrate/min at a specific temperature, pH, and substrate-concentration conditions.

Transferases are enzymes that catalyze the transfer of amino or phosphate groups from one compound to another. Aspartate aminotransferase (AST) and alanine aminotransferase (ALT) are important in clinical diagnosis. These enzymes catalyze the transfer of the amino group from glutamic acid to keto acids (oxaloacetic or pyruvic) to form aspartic and α-ketoglutaric acids with AST (aspartate aminotransferase) and alanine and α-ketoglutaric acid with ALT (alanine aminotransferase).

Colorimetric methods are based on an estimation of the reaction products (oxaloacetic or pyruvic acid) with dinitrophenylhydrazine, or substrate (α-ketoglutaric acid) by coupling with 6-benzamido-4-methoxy-*m*-toluidinediazonium chloride.

Spectrometric methods are based on the reaction of the product pyruvate with lactic dehydrogenase and NADH, or of oxaloacetate with malic dehydrogenase and NADH. The rate of NADH utilization is measured by the decrease in absorbance at 340 or 360 nm and is directly proportional to transaminase activity.

Normal AST and ALT levels are < 40 U/L. AST is present in large amounts in liver, cardiac, and skeletal muscle, whereas ALT is found primarily in liver tissue. AST is elevated in myocardial infarction and Duchenne muscular dystrophy; AST and ALT are increased in liver disease, acute toxic or viral hepatitis, infectious mononucleosis, obstructive jaundice, and hepatic cirrhosis.

Creatine kinase (CK) is a transferase found in muscle and brain tissue. It catalyzes the transfer of phosphate groups from creatine phosphate to ADP to form ATP. Activated CK activity is measured by following the increase of ATP in the creatinine phosphate-ADP reaction in the presence of glutathione or cysteine thiol activators. The ATP can be measured by the fluorometric determination of light emitted by luciferinase conversion of luciferin to adenyl-oxyluciferin in the presence of ATP. Normal serum levels are < 50 U/L; it is elevated in myocardial infarction and Duchenne muscular dystrophy, but remains at normal levels in liver disease.

Ornithine transcarbamylase (OTC) in serum is the only enzyme of the urea cycle that has been used in the clinical investigation of liver disease. It catalyzes the conversion of ornithine to citrulline. The normal serum value is 0 to 0.4 U/L.

Oxidoreductases or *dehydrogenases* are enzymes that catalyze hydrogen transfer in cellular oxidation processes. *Lactic (LDH), α-hydroxybutyric (HBDH), malic (MDH), glutamic (GLDH), isocitric (ICDH), and sorbitol (SDH) dehydrogenases* are of diagnostic importance in myocardial and liver disease.

LDH catalyzes the reversible conversion of pyruvic to lactic acid in the presence of NADH. The activity may be estimated colorimetrically by forming the pyruvic acid hydrazone with 2,4-dinitrophenylhydrazine; spectrometric or fluorometric estimation of NADH in this reaction also is used to estimate enzyme activity. The normal serum LDH value is < 200 U/L (pyruvic → lactic) and < 50 U/L (lactate → pyruvate). LDH is increased to a much greater extent and for a more prolonged period than AST or CK in myocardial infarction; it also is increased to varying degrees in certain types of hepatic disease, disseminated malignancies, pernicious anemia, and muscular dystrophy.

Recent advances in protein chemistry and technical methodology have led to fractionation of enzymes, previously thought to be homogeneous, into heterogeneous moieties. These multiple-molecular forms of enzymes (*isoenzymes*) have similar substrate specificity but different biophysical properties. LDH,

MDH, CK, phosphatases, and leucine aminopeptidase exist in isoenzyme forms.

CK isoenzymes are important in the early detection of myocardial damage. Two CK molecular subunits, M and B, produce three isoenzymes: CK-MM found primarily in skeletal muscles, CK-MB in the myocardium, and CK-BB primarily from the brain. After acute myocardial infarction (MI), CK-MB appears in the serum in approximately 4 to 6 hr, reaches peak activity at 18 to 24 hr, and may disappear within 72 hr. Diagnostic testing of MI includes CK and LDH isoenzymes. Early detection of CK-MB allows the management of myocardial infarcts with agents such as streptokinase or tissue plasminogen activator (tPA). The methods of assessment include electrophoresis, column chromatography, and immunoinhibition.

Serum contains five LDH isoenzymes, each a tetramer composed of one or two monomers. LDH 1 and 2 are found in preponderance in heart, kidney, and RBC, whereas liver and skeletal muscle largely contain LDH 4 and 5. Intermediate forms prevail in lymphatic tissues and many malignancies. The fractionation of LDH isoenzymes is important in the differential diagnosis of cardiac, muscle, and liver disease. It can be accomplished with DEAE-cellulose chromatography, electrophoresis, sulfite, or urea inhibition of specific isoenzymes, thermal stability, and substrate-concentration requirements.

HBDH reduces α-ketobutyric acid to α-hydroxybutyric acid in the presence of NADH; estimation of the α-keto acid via hydrazone formation or NADH is the basis of activity measurements. The normal serum HBD level is <140 U/L; it is elevated in myocardial infarction. LDH 1 is high in HBDH activity. The ratio of total LDH/HBDH often is used in place of LDH isoenzyme determination. Ratios > 0.8 are seen in myocardial infarction and <0.6 in acute liver damage.

MDH and *SDH*, in the presence of NAD, catalyze the conversion of malate or sorbitol to oxaloacetate or fructose, respectively. They are of diagnostic value in MI (MDH > 48 U/L) and acute liver injury (SDH > 96 U/L).

ICDH oxidizes isocitrate, in the presence of NADP or NAD, to α-ketoglutarate; it is elevated (>5.0 U/L) in acute hepatitis.

Hydrolases are enzymes that catalyze the addition of the elements of water across the bond that is cleaved.

Amylases, lipases, phosphatases, 5'-nucleotidase, γ-glutamyl transferase, and *leucine aminopeptidase* are specific examples of clinically important hydrolases.

Salivary and pancreatic *amylases* hydrolyze the substrate starch to maltose and dextrins. Amylase activity can be measured by procedures based on the loss in certain properties of starch as it is hydrolyzed (*amyloclastic*), or by the generation of reducing substances (*saccharogenic*). The amyloclastic methods use the decrease in viscosity and turbidity of hydrolyzed water-soluble starch substrates, or the reaction of starch with iodine as the method of estimation. A newer procedure uses an improved substrate, ethylidene-G_7PNP, which prevents undesired hydrolysis of the substrate by α-glucosidase. This results in greater accuracy in amylase testing. Normal serum level using this methodology is ≤88 U/L; elevations are noted in acute pancreatitis, acute abdominal conditions (perforated peptic ulcer, common bile-duct obstruction), and salivary gland disease.

Lipases catalyze the conversion of triglycerides to glycerol and fatty acids. Classic clinical determination was based on the titrimetric analysis of fatty acids liberated from an emulsified olive oil substrate, a slow, tedious methodology requiring several hours of incubation. Modern methods are based on the hydrolysis by pancreatic lipase of 1,2-diglyceride to 2-monoglyceride and fatty acid. The 2-monoglyceride then is measured by coupled-enzyme reactions catalyzed by monoglyceride lipase, glycerol kinase, glycerolphosphate oxidase, and peroxidase. This assay is simple to perform and can be adapted easily to automated analyses. The measurement of serum lipase is used widely for the diagnosis of acute pancreatitis, in which a 10-fold increase above the upper reference limit (60 U/L) is sug-gestive of pancreatitis, pancreatic injury, or inflammation of organs contiguous to the pancreas.

Phosphatases catalyze the hydrolysis of orthophosphoric acid esters and are classified according to the pH of optimal activity into alkaline or acid phosphatases. Activity (alkaline, pH 8 to 10; acid, pH 4 to 6) is measured with phenyl phosphate, glycerophosphate, *p*-nitrophenyl phosphate, or thymolphthalein monophosphate substrates. With the latter two chromogenic substrates, the amount of *p*-nitrophenol or thymolphthalein liberated by phosphatase hydrolysis is estimated colorimetrically in an alkaline medium. With a glycerophosphate or phenyl phosphate substrate, the liberated phosphorus is determined by molybdenum blue formation with phosphomolybdic-phosphotungstic acids; phenol also may be estimated with 4-aminoantipyrine or Folin-Ciocalteau reagent.

Acid phosphatase activity may be differentiated by the use of inhibitors in the assay mixture; formaldehyde has no effect on acid phosphatase of prostatic origin, but it inhibits other acid phosphatases, whereas tartrate is a selective inhibitor of the prostatic enzyme. *Acid phosphatase* is of a primary diagnostic value in metastatic carcinoma of the prostate. Normal values for *alkaline phosphatase* activity depend on the substrate used; elevations in osteomalacia and in bone tumors depend on the degree of osteolytic or osteoblastic activity. The enzyme (isoenzyme) also is elevated in obstructive jaundice, and bone and liver disease.

The enzyme *5'-nucleotidase* is an alkaline phosphomonoesterase that hydrolyzes nucleotides with a phosphate radical attached to the 5'-position of the pentose (eg, adenosine monophosphate). The normal serum value is 17 U/L; it is elevated in hepatic disease.

Leucine aminopeptidase (LAP) is an exopeptidase that hydrolyzes the peptide bond adjacent to a free amino group. It liberates amino acids from the *N*-terminal group of proteins and polypeptides in which the free amino group is an L-leucine residue. Activity is determined by spectrophotometric estimation following hydrolysis of the amide bond of a leucin-amide substrate at 238 nm. Clinical estimations usually are performed on synthetic substrates, and as there is no correlation between cleavage of leucinamide and these substrates, the LAP-like activity is designated *leucine arylamidase*. A fluorometric determination of naphthylamine liberated from a leucyl-β-naphthylamide substrate or colorimetric determination of *p*-nitroaniline liberated from leucine-*p*-nitroanilide substrate also has been used. The normal value is 8 to 22 U/L; it is elevated in the last trimester of pregnancy, hepatobiliary disease, and pancreatic carcinoma.

Serum *γ-glutamyl transferase* (γGT) is increased in diseases of the liver, bile ducts, and pancreas. Together with alkaline phosphatase, LAP, and 5'-nucleotidase, γGT usually is tested in the group of cholestasis-indicating enzymes. The assay is based on the hydrolysis of γ-glutamyl-*p*-nitroanilide.

Serum lysozyme (muramidase) activity is increased in certain types of leukemia. Serum arginase, an enzyme that hydrolyzes arginine to ornithine and urea, and serum guanase are sensitive indicators of hepatic necrosis.

Lyases are enzymes which split C—C bonds without group transfer. *Aldolase* is a glycolic lyase that catalyzes the reversible splitting of fructose 1,6-diphosphate to form dihydroxyacetone phosphate and glyceraldehyde 3-phosphate. In the estimation of activity, the triose phosphate reaction products are hydrolyzed with alkali and the resultant trioses are reacted with 2,4-dinitrophenylhydrazine to form chromogenic hydrazones for colorimetric analysis. A spectrophotometric estimation is made by coupling the aldolase reaction products with a dehydrogenase acting on one of the triose phosphates and measuring concomitant changes in NADH. The normal value is < 8 U/L; it is elevated in muscular dystrophy, polymyositis, and acute hepatitis.

The significance of serum-enzyme changes in hepatitis is seen in Figure 32-5 and enzyme activity following myocardial infarction in Figure 32-6.

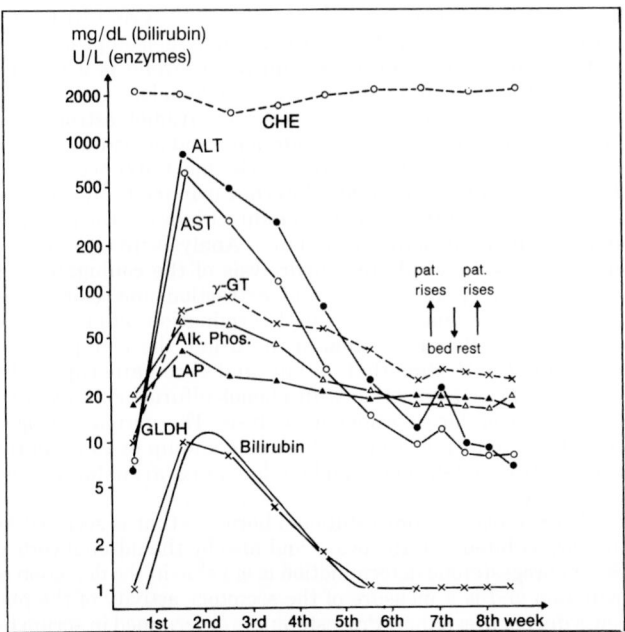

Figure 32-5. Typical course of alterations in serum enzyme activity in acute viral hepatitis. (Adapted from Schmidt E, Schmidt FW *Med Welt* 1970; 21:805.)

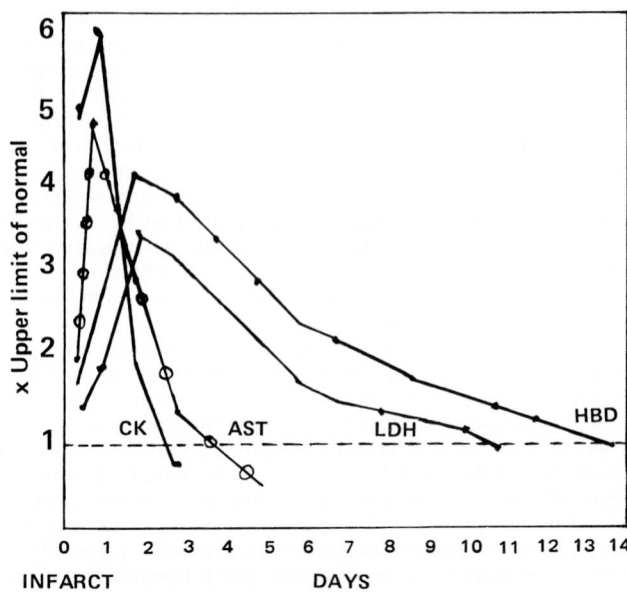

Figure 32-6. Serum enzymes following myocardial infarction, AST, CK, LDH, and HBD are compared.

LIPIDS

The major classes of blood lipids are *fatty acids, cholesterol, triglycerides, phospholipids,* and *lipoproteins.* Hyperlipidemia is not a single aberration, and there are a number of different hyperlipidemic states. Lipid-profile tests include measurements of cholesterol, triglyceride, phospholipids, and determination of lipoprotein phenotypes.

Cholesterol, a sterol molecule, is an essential substance in steroid-hormone synthesis by the adrenal cortex and bile acid production in the liver. It exists in blood as the free sterol and as cholesterol esters of fatty acids.

In the determination of *total cholesterol,* the serum is extracted with an alcohol–ether mixture and the cholesterol estimated colorimetrically after reaction with acetic anhydride–sulfuric acid reagent (Liebermann-Burchard reaction). The precipitation of free cholesterol with digitonin will differentiate free from esterified cholesterol. Chromatographic separation of cholesterol from its esters on alumina, silicic acid, or magnesium silicate columns with organic solvents also has been used.

Gas chromatographic procedures have resulted in the separation and quantitation of cholesterol, its metabolites, and precursors; this is a type of partition chromatography in which a volatilized sample is partitioned between a liquid stationary phase and a mobile gas phase. The normal-adult total-serum-cholesterol level is 150 to 270 mg/dL; it is increased in hyperlipidemia and specifically in hyper-β-lipoproteinemia, nephrosis, diabetes mellitus, and myxedema, and decreased in hyperthyroidism and hepatic disease. Free cholesterol comprises 20% to 40% and the ester fraction 60% to 80% of the total serum cholesterol.

Phospholipids are "compound" or "heterolipids" that contain phosphorus, a nitrogen base and a long-chain fatty acid. Lecithin (phosphatidylcholines) and cephalin (phosphatidylethanolamine or serine) are the principal plasma phospholipids, which normally comprise one-third of the total plasma lipids. They usually are bound to lipoproteins. These serum lipids are extracted into an alcohol–ether mixture, digested with sulfuric acid-hydrogen peroxide and the liberated phosphorus determined by colorimetric techniques. The normal lipid phosphorus is 6 to 11 mg/dL; about one-half is lecithin. The average ratio of cholesterol to lipid phosphorus when cholesterol is normal is 21. Phospholipid

changes usually are associated with cholesterol changes and are of interest in coronary artery and liver diseases and the hyperlipoproteinemias.

Sphingolipids differ from lecithin and cephalin. They are phosphate esters of sphingosine bound to choline or ethanolamine and primarily are found in brain tissue (eg, sphingomyelin, galactolipin). The *ratio of lecithin to sphingomyelin* (L/S) in amniotic fluid or resuscitated amniotic fluid from the oral cavity of the newborn is an accurate assessment of fetal maturity and the respiratory-distress syndrome. Changes in phospholipid biosynthesis during gestation reflect the aging of the fetal lung, as the L/S ratio normally increases.

Tay-Sachs disease is a lipid-storage disease in which the central nervous system degenerates because of the progressive intraneuronal accumulation of excess amounts of the sphingolipid ganglioside GM_2. The accumulation of GM_2 in Tay-Sachs disease has been shown to be caused by a lack of the enzyme hexosaminidase A. Therefore, the measurement of serum, WBC, or amniotic fluid *hexosaminidase A* is important in evaluating carriers and in diagnosing Tay-Sachs disease in the fetus.

Both hexosaminidase A (heat-labile) and hexosaminidase B (heat-stable) can catalyze the conversion of 4-methylumbelliferyl-*N*-acetylgalactosamine (a synthetic substrate) to *N*-acetylgalactosamine and 4-methylumbelliferone. The cleavage product, 4-methylumbelliferone, fluoresces under ultraviolet radiation, and the intensity of the fluorescence is a measure of the activity of the enzyme. In noncarriers, 50% to 75% of the total hexosaminidase activity is heat-labile (hexosaminidase A), and in carriers 20% to 45% of the total hexosaminidase activity is heat-labile.

The blood fatty acids occur in esterified (EFA) and nonesterified (NEFA) forms. *Triglyceride* determinations are of value in differentiating the hyperlipidemic states, that is, essential (diet-induced) hypertriglyceridemia from familial hypocholesterolemia with or without triglyceridemia. After the preliminary separation from phospholipids, triglycerides most often are determined in terms of their glycerol moiety. The glycerol released by saponification is oxidized to formaldehyde and the latter determined by fluorometric or colorimetric procedures. Triglycerides also can be determined by coupling the glycerol liberated from lipase/α-chymotrypsin treatment of serum with a glycerol kinase–pyruvate kinase–LDH system and spectrometric estimation of NADH. Normal triglyceride levels are 110 to 140 mg/dL. An increase in triglycerides will produce a milky appearance in serum (lipemic). EFA analyses are based also on the reaction of alkaline hydroxylamine with esters of fatty acids to form hydroxamic acids that produce a red color with ferric chloride.

Gas chromatographic procedures have been used to quantitate the various *fatty acids,* that is, palmitic, stearic, oleic, linoleic, and linolenic acids. Mono-, di-, and triglycerides also can be separated into classes and quantitated by column or thin-layer chromatography, and infrared spectrometry. The total fatty acids of plasma range from 200 to 450 mg/dL in the fasting state; they are derived from glycerides, cholesterol esters, and phospholipids.

All the lipids in plasma circulate in combination with protein. The free fatty acids are bound to albumin, and the lipids aggregate with other proteins to form *lipoproteins.* Electrophoresis and ultracentrifugation are the principal methods used to separate and identify lipoprotein families. *Chylomicrons* ($S_f > 400$), *pre-β-lipoproteins* (S_f 20–400), *β-lipoproteins* (S_f 0–20), and *α-lipoproteins* are the four major classes in order of increasing density and migration on cellulose acetate electrophoresis. Chylomicrons are representative primarily of dietary or exogenous triglycerides, pre-β-lipoproteins of endogenous glycerides, β-lipoproteins of cholesterol and its esters, and α-lipoproteins of cholesterol and phospholipids. Abnormal lipoproteins that may appear in plasma include floating β-lipoproteins, lipoprotein X, and complexes of normal lipoproteins with IgA and IgG myeloma proteins (autoimmune hyperlipoproteinemia). Age, sex, diet, fasting, posture changes, and trauma can alter the lipid profile.

The lipoprotein classes usually are separated by paper, agarose, or cellulose acetate electrophoresis. The strips are stained with fat-soluble dyes (Sudan Black or Oil Red O) and quantitated by densiometric scanning. Primary hyperlipoproteinemias are classified into normal and five abnormal types based on cholesterol and triglyceride levels and lipoprotein analysis. Hyperchylomicronemia (type I), hyper-β-lipoproteinemia (type II), broad β-band (type III), hyper-pre-β-lipoproteinemia (type IV), and hyper-pre-β-lipoproteinemia and chylomicronemia (type V) are the major classes. Carbohydrate and fat-tolerance studies, post-heparin lipase activity, and clinical symptomatology also are integrated into the diagnosis of the various subclasses. The presence or predisposition to coronary artery disease and other disease states is associated with the various types.[17]

STEROIDS AND OTHER HORMONES

The steroids possess a common structure, the perhydrocyclopentanophenanthrene nucleus, and include cholesterol, bile acids, androgens, and the adrenocortical, adrenomedullary, estrogenic, and progestational hormones.

Androsterone, dehydroepiandrosterone, etiocholan-3α-ol-17-one, 11-ketoandrosterone, 11-ketoetiocholanolone, 11β-hydroxyandrosterone, and 11β-hydroxyetiocholanolone are the principal *urinary 17-ketosteroids (17KS).* These androgenic hormones are derived from the adrenal and, in males, testicular function. The principal urinary steroid metabolites in this group of androgens are found both in the free form, and as conjugates of glucuronides, sulfates, or acetates. Their determination in urine involves the acid hydrolysis of the conjugates, extraction with organic solvent, reaction with alkaline *m*-dinitrobenzene (Zimmerman reaction), and colorimetric estimation of the chromogen. The individual 17KS can be separated by TLC prior to analysis to obtain further information on the individual steroids. The normal adult urine values are: male, 9 to 24 mg/day; female, 5 to 17 mg/day. Decreased excretion is seen in hypoactive disease of the pituitary, gonads, and adrenals. Increased excretion is seen in hyperplasia, cancer, or tumors of the adrenals.

Testosterone is the most potent androgen in blood. The measurement of urinary or serum testosterone is useful in distinguishing normal and hypogonadal males and in treating

hirsutism in the female. This hormone is determined by gas chromatography, competitive protein-binding, isotope dilution, or RIA procedures. Normal serum testosterone is 0.2 to 1.1 μg/dL in the male and <0.1 μg/dL in the female.

The natural *estrogenic hormones* are estradiol, estrone, and estriol, produced in the gonads, adrenals, and placenta. The relative amounts of the three estrogens rise and fall concomitantly during the menstrual cycle. Maternal urinary total-estrogen excretion, especially estriol, is an indirect index of the integrity and viability of the fetoplacental unit. Analysis involves acid or glucuronidase–arylsulfatase hydrolysis of the conjugates, removal of urinary glucose if present, extraction, and colorimetric or fluorometric analysis. In the determination, after acid hydrolysis and ether extraction of the urine, the estrogens are methylated with dimethyl sulfate and chromatographically separated prior to reaction with phenolsulfuric acid to yield a red chromogen for colorimetric analysis. The normal estrogen output is 4 to 60 μg/24 hr in the female and up to 25 μg in the male. Estrogen deficiency can be related to ovarian failure and pituitary deficiency.

Progesterone is a progestational hormone that is secreted by the corpus luteum of the ovary and also by the adrenal cortex. Serum progesterone determination is of value in the detection of ovulation and is a measure of the secretory activity of the placenta during pregnancy. Progesterone is determined in serum by RIA, double-isotope derivatization, gas-liquid chromatography, or competitive protein-binding techniques. Normal menstrual-cycle serum progesterone levels vary between 0 and 1.6 μg/dL.

Pregnanediol is the principal metabolite of progesterone. The urinary determination of pregnanediol excretion is an indirect index of progesterone levels but is subject to variation due to individual differences in hepatic metabolism of this hormone and is not representative of total endogenous progesterone production.

Adrenal cortex steroids include glucocorticoids, androgens, estrogens, progesterone, and mineralocorticoids. Glucocorticoids can be determined as plasma cortisol (plasma 17-OH corticosteroids), urinary-free (unconjugated cortisol), or total-urinary *17-OH corticosteroids.* The latter are determined in urine as *17-ketogenic steroids* (17KGS). The 17KS in urine are reduced with borohydride to alcohols; the 17-OH steroids are oxidized with sodium bismuthate or periodate to 17KS and quantitated by the alkaline dinitrobenzene method. The 17-OH steroids can be quantitated directly by the phenylhydrazine-sulfuric acid reaction after hydrolysis of glucuronide conjugates and chromatographic purification. The 17-OH steroid analysis only determines compounds with the dihydroxyacetone side chain, such as tetrahydrocortisol or tetrahydrocortisone; the 17KGS analysis includes the 17-OH-corticosteroids with the dihydroxyacetone side chain and the pregnanetriol type of compound. Normal 17KGS daily urinary excretion is 5 to 23 mg in the male and 3 to 15 mg in the female. They are reduced significantly in myxedema and adrenal or anterior pituitary insufficiency. Plasma cortisol usually is measured by fluorometric or gas chromatographic procedures.

Aldosterone is the most active member of the mineralocorticoid group. The determination of urinary aldosterone is of value in differentiating benign essential hypertension from primary aldosteronism (Conn's syndrome), which is caused by an adrenal adenoma and is accompanied by hypertension. A double-isotope derivatization technique is used. Urinary aldosterone is acetylated with ^{3}H-acetic anhydride; aldosterone-^{14}C-diacetate standard is added early in the procedure. The ^{3}H/^{14}C specific activity of the final product is measured after chromatographic purification and is a direct measurement of aldosterone. The normal aldosterone levels of about 10 μg/day are elevated in Conn's disease and usually are associated with low serum potassium, sodium retention, and low-concentration alkaline urine.

The anterior pituitary secretes three substances (*gonadotropins*) that regulate gonadal activity: *follicle-stimulating hormone (FSH), luteinizing hormone (LH)* or *interstitial cell hormone (ICSH),* and *luteotropin (LTH).* The gonadotropins are glycoproteins. Bioassay methods can be used to determine gonadotrophic activity. After fractionation and isolation, the urine extract is assayed in test animals as to the follicular growth of the ovaries in hypophysectomized animals or—increase in testicular, ovarian, or uterine weight in various–animal models. RIA techniques have been developed for these gonadotropins and represent the most sensitive and precise measurement method, although nonisotopic enzyme immunoassays (EIA) rapidly are becoming popular due to the increased costs of isotope disposal and their analytical performance equaling or surpassing RIA procedures.

Analysis of serum or urinary *placental lactogen (HPL)* and *chorionic gonadotropin (HCG),* a placental-derived protein hormone, is useful in the diagnosis of threatened abortion, hydatiform mole, and choriocarcinoma. HCG, pregnanediol, and progesterone as well as total and fractionated estrogens are useful in testing for pregnancy. HCG and HPL readily are measured by RIA or EIA, and low values are seen in threatened abortion and intrauterine fetal death.

The increase in HCG in the serum or urine of the pregnant female is the basis of a routine *pregnancy test.* Test components consist of an antigen in the form of HCG latex particles and an HCG antiserum. When antiserum is mixed with urine containing a detectable level of HCG, it is neutralized and no agglutination of latex-antigen particles occurs (*agglutination inhibition test*). The commercial application of the HCG assay gives laboratories a rapid, accurate pregnancy test by taking advantage of monoclonal antibody specificity and sensitivity. A monoclonal slide procedure on urine, Duoclon (*Organon Diagnostics*), uses two different monoclonal antibodies, one against HCG and one against the HCG$_B$ subunit for maximum specificity. Agglutination indicates a positive test with a sensitivity level of 500 miU HCG/mL, detecting pregnancy a few days after conception.

Human growth hormone and insulin are proteins that are of diagnostic value in growth-rate studies and diabetes. They are best quantitated by RIA.

Epinephrine and *norepinephrine* are biologically active catecholamines derived from the adrenal medulla and sympathetic nerve endings. Catecholamines are measured in the blood and urine after fractionation on alumina or ion-exchange columns, oxidation at pH 3.5 or 6, and subsequent fluorometric analysis. Urine catecholamines are increased to > 350 µg/24 hour in adrenal medullary tissue tumors (pheochromocytoma). The normal plasma level is 2.1 to 6.5 µg/L with about 80% as norepinephrine.

Vanillylmandelic acid (VMA) is the urine metabolite of these two catecholamines. Its quantity in urine reflects the endogenous secretion of catecholamines. VMA can be determined colorimetrically, after extraction of the urine with ethyl acetate, and diazotization with *p*-nitroaniline and ethanolamine in the presence of carbonate ion. VMA also can be measured spectrometrically following periodate oxidation to vanillin and solvent extraction. The normal output is 0 to 12 mg/24 hour.

Homovanillic acid (HVA) is not a metabolite of epinephrine or norepinephrine, but is produced from a common precursor, dopamine. Elevated HVA excretion is diagnostic in cases of neuroblastoma.

The biosynthesis of *serotonin* (5-hydroxytryptamine) and urinary excretion of its metabolite, 5-hydroxyindoleacetic acid (5-HIAA), are increased in argentaffine tumors. These have a very large capacity to metabolize tryptophane stores to serotonin. Urinary 5-HIAA increases from 1 to 7 mg/24 hr to as much as 1 g/24 hr in this type of tumor.

Bilirubin, a tetrapyrrole that is derived from senescent red-cell degradation, normally occurs in low concentration in the blood. In bile, it is present as the water-soluble conjugated acyldiglucuronide. In blood, bilirubin is bound tightly to plasma albumin. The reduction of bilirubin in the intestine yields urobilinogen, which is, in turn, oxidized to a brown pigment—urobilin.

Serum bilirubin is determined by coupling with diazotized sulfanilic acid to form azobilirubin for colorimetric analysis. The *direct* or *conjugated bilirubin* test is performed in aqueous media; the *indirect* or *free bilirubin* analysis is performed in methanol or caffeine-sodium benzoate solution. Normal values in serum are: direct, 0 to 0.3 mg/dL; total, 0 to 1.5 mg/dL.

Clinical jaundice is a yellowing of the tissues associated with hyperbilirubinemia; in hemolytic disease of the newborn due to Rh and ABO incompatibilities, indirect serum bilirubin is elevated, whereas acute hepatitis results in increases in the direct type.

ELECTROLYTES

The normal plasma electrolyte level is 154 mEq/L of cations and 154 mEq/L of anions. The osmotic effects of chloride, bicarbonate, sodium, and potassium are important in the maintenance of normal muscle contraction and water distribution between cells, plasma, and interstitial fluid.

Flame photometry, atomic-absorption spectrometry, neutron-activation analysis, x-ray fluorescence, ion-specific electrodes, and colorimetric techniques are used in the identification and determination of cations or anions in biological fluids. Advances in technology have developed multiphase systems capable of measuring not only sodium and potassium but also chloride, carbon dioxide, and calcium simultaneously.

Sodium and *potassium* serum concentrations are readily measured by flame photometry or highly sensitive and specific atomic-absorption spectrometry. The latter technique is similar to emission-flame photometry, except that it measures energy as it is absorbed by atoms rather than as it is emitted by atoms. Both techniques are based on the characteristic absorption or emission wavelengths of the cations. Ion-specific electrodes also are used for Na^+ and K^+ determinations, eliminating the use of a flame or combustible gas, and this can be performed on whole blood, plasma, or serum.

Chloride levels in serum or urine are determined by titration with acid mercuric nitrate solution in the presence of *s*-diphenylcarbazone indicator. They also may be determined potentiometrically with a silver–silver chloride pH electrode assembly. The normal serum values are 135 to 155 mEq Na/L, 3.9 to 5.6 mEq K/L, and 95 to 106 mEq Cl/L; urine levels are 150 to 197 mEq Na/day, 20 to 64 mEq K/day, and 180 to 270 mEq Cl/day.

Serum sodium, potassium, chloride, and *bicarbonate* determinations are useful indicators in adrenal cortical insufficiency, renal and cardiac failure, anuria, dehydration, alimentary tract diseases associated with diarrhea and vomiting, and increased renal electrolyte excretion (diuretic therapy).

The determination of excess *chloride* (>50 mEq/L) in the perspiration of patients with pancreatic *cystic fibrosis* is an accurate diagnostic tool. Perspiration is stimulated by placing the patient's hand in a plastic bag for 15 to 20 min or, preferably, by an iontophoresis technique in which pilocarpine nitrate ions are transported through small areas of the skin to produce local perspiration. The chloride content may be quantitated with silver nitrate–potassium chromate-impregnated papers or with ion-selective electrodes.

Bicarbonate, phosphates, sodium, potassium, and chloride concentrations are related to maintenance of acid–base balance in the body. The pH of the blood reflects the state of the acid–base balance and is related mathematically to HCO_3^- concentration and partial pressure of CO_2 ($_pCO_2$) in blood by the Henderson-Hasselbalch equation.

$$pH = 6.1 + \log \frac{[HCO_3^-]}{[H_2CO_3]} \tag{2}$$

Blood pH, as measured electrometrically, has a normal range of 7.36 to 7.40 for venous samples and 7.38 to 7.42 for arterial samples. The pCO$_2$ level in blood is determined by measuring the pH of the blood at three different pCO$_2$ concentrations—one native to the blood and the other two obtained by equilibration with gas mixtures of known pCO_2. Blood bicarbonate levels also may be determined by measuring the amount of acid neutralized by plasma or serum and pCO_2 calculated by Equation 2. The relationship between pCO_2 and carbonic acid concentration is

$$[H_2CO_3] = 0.03 \times pCO_2 \qquad (3)$$
$$\text{mM/L} \qquad\qquad \text{torr}$$

The role of oxygen and hemoglobin in respiration has been discussed previously. Measurements of blood pH and CO_2 content are used in differentiating respiratory acidosis (low pH, high CO_2) from metabolic acidosis (low pH, low CO_2).

Blood oxygen (pO_2) and *percent oxygen saturation* are measured by a polarographic method; the blood sample is placed in a chamber and separated from a combined platinum and silver–silver chloride electrode by a polypropylene membrane. By diffusion through the membrane, equilibrium is established between the pO_2 of the blood and a film of solution in contact with the electrode. A current, which is proportional to blood pO_2, is generated after the application of a polarizing voltage.

Calcium and *phosphorus* are important minerals in the processes of bone calcification, nerve irritability, muscle contraction, and blood coagulation. Calcium is present in plasma as an ultrafilterable (ionic and nonionic) form and a protein-bound fraction. Blood phosphorus consists of inorganic phosphorus, organic phosphate ester (G6P, ATP), and phospholipids.

Serum and urine calcium levels are determined routinely by titration with EDTA or EGTA using a fluorescent calcein or calcichrome indicator. Other methods are based on the colorimetric analysis of calcium–methylthymol blue complex in the presence of 8-quinolinol to prevent interference by magnesium. Bis-(o-hydroxyphenylimino)ethane forms a colored complex with calcium; in the presence of polyvinylpyrrolidone to inhibit phosphate interference, it is a sensitive and specific method for calcium. Total calcium is determined best by atomic-absorption spectrometry. As with all cations, calcium can be determined by emission- or absorption-flame photometry or ion-selective electrodes.

Inorganic phosphorus levels are determined by reaction with acid molybdate reagent to form phosphomolybdic acid which, in turn, is reduced with aminonaphtholsulfonic acid or *p*-dimethylaminophenol sulfate to give a blue complex which is estimated colorimetrically. Normal serum levels are 2.5 to 4.5 mg P/dL and 9 to 11 mg Ca/dL.

Calcium levels are decreased and phosphorus increased in hypoparathyroidism; an opposite effect is seen in hyperactivity of this gland. In rickets and osteomalacia, the concentrations of both elements are decreased. In establishing primary hyperparathyroidism and other causes of hypercalcemia, daily measurements for ionized calcium (Ca^{2+}) are replacing total Ca measurements using ISE technology.

Magnesium is an essential electrolyte that is a natural calcium channel blocker. This ion is involved with cardiac and vascular smooth muscle contraction. Hypomagnesemia may pose a risk to humans in terms of increased cardiovascular disease (such as cardiac arrhythmias and stroke), whereas hypermagnesemia may result in bradycardia, asystole, or respiratory insufficiency. A chemical analyzer (*Nova Biomedical*) is capable of measuring in 1 min Na, K, Ca, Mg, and the hematocrit in less than 200 μL of blood. Using an ion-specific electrode, the free, unbound magnesium ion activity is measured and may be related to intracellular levels of magnesium ions.

Copper, zinc, and iron are trace elements in blood. They are quantitated readily by flame photometric, colorimetric, or atomic-absorption techniques.

ORGAN FUNCTION TESTS

The analyses of various blood or urine constituents, determination of metabolic excretion rates of exogenous compounds or endogenous metabolites, and effect of exogenous stimuli on these parameters are used for evaluation of *in situ* activity and function of various organs. Organ function studies are performed in diseases associated with the liver, kidney, parathyroid, thyroid, pituitary gland, gastrointestinal tract, pancreas, adrenals, and gonads. The principles and significance of the analysis used in such evaluations have been described also in other sections of this chapter.

Tests for *hepatic function* are based on bilirubin metabolism and excretion, carbohydrate metabolism (galactose tolerance test), plasma-protein changes (cephalin flocculation test and A/G ratio), abnormal fat metabolism, detoxification mechanisms (hippuric acid synthesis), excretion of injected substances (BSP), prothrombin formation, and previously discussed enzyme levels.

Diseases of the liver are due to cellular alterations (hepatocellular) or obstructions to the flow of bile (obstructive jaundice). Hepatocellular liver disease can be chronic (postnecrotic cirrhosis, carcinoma) or acute (viral hepatitis, alcoholism, toxin- or chemical-induced).

The *cephalin flocculation* test is based on the flocculation of cephalin-emulsified cholesterol by γ-globulin. In normal serum an albumin-like protein will inhibit this reaction; in hepatic diseases, which produce abnormal γ-globulin or reduced albumin levels, the flocculation will occur.

The *detoxification mechanisms of the liver* can be evaluated by intravenous administration of sodium benzoate and estimation of the benzoic acid metabolite, hippuric acid, in the urine. In hepatoparenchymal disease, a reduced capacity of the liver to form hippuric acid by conjugation of glycine and benzoic acid is observed.

The ability of the liver to excrete an injected dye is determined in the *BSP test*; the serum is analyzed for dye concentration at a suitable time interval after intravenous administration of 2 to 5 mg BSP/kg. Radioiodinated (^{131}I) Rose Bengal Sodium dye also has been used in dye-excretion studies with isotopic estimation of urine dye levels.

Kidney function tests are based on the determination of blood nonprotein nitrogen (urea, uric acid, and creatinine), electrolytes, blood acid–base balance, routine urinalysis, and the clearance of administered compounds in the urine. Most *clearance studies* are performed with substances that are not resorbed or secreted by the renal tubules: inulin, mannitol, sodium *p*-aminohippurate, or ^{125}I-iothalamate sodium (sodium 5-acetamido-2,4,6-triiodo-*N*-methylisophthalamate). These are administered intravenously and the rate of urine clearance and glomerular filtration is estimated by analysis of the urine. The excretory capacity of the renal tubular epithelium can be determined by measuring the clearance rate of PSP. The dye is injected intravenously and the rate of its clearance in urine is determined. PSP is bound loosely to serum albumin and is removed rapidly from the blood by the renal tubules.

Sodium iodohippurate-(^{125}I), which is extracted almost completely from the blood on a single passage through the kidney, also has been used in renal function studies; a *renogram* or isotopic scan of both kidneys is performed. The test provides data on renal tubular secretion, renal vascular competence, and renal evacuation and is primarily useful as a comparison of individual kidney function. It is important to note that 50% of kidney function can be compromised without any significant change in the routine renal function parameters.

Thyroid function tests usually measure the circulating levels of the thyroid hormones, and not the end-organ effect. The thyroid gland converts inorganic iodide to *thyroxine (T_4)* and *triiodothyronine (T_3)*. T_3 and T_4 are stored in the colloid part of the gland as part of the thyroglobulin molecule. Hypothalamic *thyrotropin-releasing hormone (TRH)* mediates the release of the pituitary thyrotropin (*thyroid-stimulating hormone, TSH*). Excess levels of circulating T_4 depress, and low levels of T_4 increase, TSH release. TSH stimulates the proteolytic degradation of thyroglobulin to release T_4 and T_3, and increases organification of iodine. T_4 accounts for 90% of secreted thyroid hormones and exists in blood bound to *thyroxine-binding globulin (TBG)* or *thyroxine-binding prealbumin (TBPA)* or to albumin. T_3 is not protein-bound and has 5 to 10 times the biological potency of T_4 on a weight basis. Therefore, T_4 represents the major part of protein-bound iodine (PBI). The level of *free thyroxine (FT4)*, the active fraction in blood, is regulated by T_4 and T_3 release and the levels of binding proteins in blood and tissues.

The uptake of orally administered Na ^{131}I preparations by the thyroid gland can be estimated by isotopic scanning of the gland 24 hr after ^{131}I administration and is an index of glandular function (hyperactive, > 50% uptake; hypoactive, <15%).

PBI determinations are based on the precipitation of protein-bound thyroxine, removal of inorganic iodine by basic- or anion-exchange chromatography, alkaline incineration to convert thyroxine to inorganic iodide, and finally quantitation of iodide by reaction with arsenous acid and ceric ammonium sulfate. PBI is a good estimate of total circulating hormonal iodine. The normal range is 4 to 8 µg/dL serum.

T_4 can be determined by column chromatography in which it is separated and isolated by ion-exchange chromatography, and then analyzed colorimetrically. Nonisotope thyroid assays have been developed using fluorescence polarization methods for T_4 and free-thyroxin index. In the competitive protein-binding assay for T_4, serum T_4 competes with ^{125}I-T_4 for binding sites on a known amount of TBG. The ratio of bound to free ^{125}I is determined by adsorption of ^{125}I-T_4 not bound to TBG on an anion-exchange resin embedded in a polyurethane sponge or a porous dextran gel, and is a direct index of T_4 levels. The presence of mercurials, inorganic iodide, or iodinated radiographic compounds in serum interferes with the T_4 column and PBI procedures. The competitive-binding procedure is affected by the presence of highly protein-bound drugs or changes in TBG levels in serum. The normal range of serum T_4 is 2.9 to 6.4 µg/dL by column and 3.0 to 7.0 µg/dL by binding assay. T_4 and PBI are increased in hyperthyroidism and the early stages of hepatitis. T_4 and PBI are decreased in hypothyroidism and nephrosis.

FT4 also is determined in a competitive protein-binding assay in which ^{125}I-T_4 and serum are incubated, and then dialyzed to determine the percent dializable ^{125}I-T_4. FT4 analysis is used in suspected abnormalities in protein-binding globulins. T_4 binding capacity of serum TBG, albumin and prealbumin can be determined after electrophoretic separation of these proteins.

T_3 analysis is determined by the resin-uptake test. The uptake of ^{125}I-T_3 by a resin is determined in the presence of the test serum. In hyperthyroidism, the primary TBG-binding sites are saturated and ^{125}I-T_3 is taken up by the resin. The resin uptake is decreased in hypothyroidism, and most of ^{125}I-T_3 is bound to TBG in serum. A *free thyroxine index* can be obtained by multiplying T_3 (resin) × T_4 (competitive binding) × 0.01. This product deviates from normal in the same direction as T_3 and T_4 in hyper- and hypothyroidism. This product is stable during euthyroidism in spite of changes in binding proteins; for example, a euthyroid patient on phenytoin therapy will show a decreased TBG and T_4 and increased T_3, but (T_4 × T_3) is normal. The indication of hyper- or hypothyroidism in the presence of abnormal amounts of TBG is observed in the (T_4 × T_3) product.

The determination of *TSH* by RIA or EIA appears to be the most useful test in discriminating patients with primary hyperthyroidism from the euthyroidism or hypothyroidism secondary to pituitary disease. Serum TSH is increased in the primary disease state.

The *PBI conversion ratio* is an estimate of the rate of conversion of inorganic iodide to PBI. Radioiodide-(^{131}I) is administered to the subject; after 24 hr, a sample of blood is obtained and the ^{131}I to PB^{131}I is estimated by radiochromatographic procedures with ion-exchange resins (normal conversion, 13–42%).

Adrenocortical function is evaluated by estimation of serum or urinary 17-ketosteroids (17-KS) and 17-hydroxycorticosteroids (17-OH-CS) (androgen and corticosteroid metabolism), serum electrolytes (aldosterone metabolism), and blood adrenocorticotrophic hormone (ACTH) levels in the basal state, after stimulation with intramuscular or intravenous ACTH, or after adrenal inhibition with dexamethasone. In the normal individual, ACTH will increase plasma cortisol and urine 17-OH-CS, and dexamethasone will suppress plasma cortisol. Metapyrone, an inhibitor of 11β-hydroxylase, will cause selective secretion of compound S (11-deoxycortisol) by the adrenals in place of cortisol. Compound S will not inhibit the adrenal-pituitary feedback mechanism; the pituitary will secrete more ACTH and the adrenal will secrete more compound S. The determination of urinary 17-OH-CS or tetrahydro-compound S (THS) following metapyrone administration is a good index of the functional integrity of the pituitary-adrenal axis; patients with virilizing adrenal hyperplasia excrete excessive THS due to an 11β-hydroxylase defect.

Common clinical chemistry reference values are listed in Table 32-4.[18]

AUTOMATED ANALYSIS

The automation of analytical techniques used in blood and urine chemistry, hematology, blood typing, and immunology has increased the productivity and accuracy of the clinical laboratory.[19] *Computerization* of the automated analytical system also has increased the rapidity of reporting test results, reduced clerical error, and provided a unified and updated report of the laboratory tests for each patient.

In one of the first widely used multichannel chemistry analyzers, the SMA-6 (Sequential Multiple Analysis) Autoanalyzer (*Technicon*), a continuously operating, multiple-channel proportioning pump moved the samples, diluents, and reagent streams. Air bubbles segmented the flowing streams of samples and reagents, which then either flowed through dialyzers to remove interfering substances, and/or moved them directly into chambers preset at desired temperatures; they finally went into detection devices (colorimeters, fluorometers, flame photometers, spectrophotometers). A serum standard was run simultaneously with the samples. The results could be read directly from a recorder or were later coupled into a digital computer for numeric output. Sequential, multiple analyses in the SMA-12, a later model for 12-parameter analysis, was accomplished by distributing the sample to 12 different analytical streams, so that all 12 analyses were in progress at the same time. The *SMA-12 profile* usually determined calcium, inorganic phosphorus, glucose, BUN, uric acid, cholesterol, total protein, albumin, total bilirubin, alkaline phosphatase, LDH, and AST. SMA analyzers ushered in the era of automation in the clinical chemistry laboratory, spawning a high-technology industry that resulted ultimately in tremendous productivity gains, enhanced test accuracy and precision, and the ability to measure numerous constituents from microsamples in a very short time.

Typical high-throughput chemistry analyzers using standard *wet* reagent methodologies in combination with ion-specific electrodes (*ISE*) include the Synchron CX analyzers (*Beckman Coulter*), BM/Hitachi and the COBAS analyzers (*Roche Diagnostics*), and Dimension analyzers (*Dade Behring*). The non-ISE portions of these instruments basically are automated spectrometers, with robotic pipetting from on-board reagents to disposable or rewashed reaction cuvettes whose products are monitored continuously at one or more wavelengths. Stable calibration, sophisticated quality-control monitoring, off-hour preprogrammed maintenance, and self-diagnostics are regular features on these analyzers.

Vitros series analyzers (*Ortho Clinical Diagnostics*) have successfully implemented the use of "dry-slide" technology in which multilayered pads are impregnated with reagents, eliminating the need for extensive tubing and liquid reagent-handling components. Reaction end-products are measured using reflectance spectrometry in these analyzers, and analytical performance rivals or surpasses that of the more "conventional" instruments listed above.

Clinical chemistry technological innovations have enabled the laboratory to provide therapeutic drug-monitoring tests,

1.010 and 1.030 and is related to dietary habits of fluid and food ingestion and, secondarily, to the loss of fluid by other routes such as extensive sweating. The measurement of urine density or specific gravity is a part of "routine urinalysis," and as such provides information with regard to water and solids turnover in the body. The specific gravity information alone is not nearly so important as it may be in conjunction with other observations. Thus, if dehydration is suspected, a specific gravity in the midrange of 1.015 would cast doubt about dehydration unless there was a concurrent renal dysfunction.

The kidney possesses a remarkable ability to either form a concentrated urine or a very dilute urine ranging from a specific gravity of 1.001 to 1.032. This concentrating or diluting capacity is diminished in cases of a loss of renal function. In fact, one of the sensitive tests for measuring renal function involves the so-called dilution-concentration tests where fluid is administered or withheld, and the specific gravity of the urine is measured. With a serious loss of renal function, the kidney cannot excrete a urine in excess of 1.020 even with marked fluid restriction. In advanced renal disease the specific gravity of the urine may become "fixed" or constant in the range of 1.010 to 1.012, with all urine being of this specific gravity regardless of overhydration or dehydration.

Specific gravity is measured readily with a special hydrometer, called a urinometer. There is a correlation between the density of urine and its refractive index, and a special refractometer has been designed that gives readings in specific gravity units on a single drop of urine.

Certain abnormal constituents of urine, such as glucose or protein, when present in high concentrations, will cause significant increases in specific gravity. Certain x-ray contrast media, when excreted in the urine, also will cause marked increases in specific gravity.

Urine specific gravity is only an indirect index of solute concentration; that is, 1 mol of urea will produce a lower specific gravity than 1 mol of glucose. Osmolality is a direct measure of the molal concentration of solutes in solution regardless of their molecular weight; 1 mol of NaCl dissociates into 1 mol of chloride ion and 1 mol of sodium ion. Osmolality is determined in a direct-reading osmometer by comparing the freezing point of urine with that of a standard sodium chloride solution (see also Chapter 18).

The kidneys normally excrete 800 to 1400 mOsm/kg (an osmol is that weight of any substance when dissolved in water depresses the freezing point 1.86° of solutes/day). Humans concentrate urine and eliminate the daily solute load at a maximum volume of 1200 mOsm/kg water. Urine osmolality is an inverse function of urine volume in the normal catabolic state. Urine volume is regulated by the antidiuretic hormone (ADH) and sodium excretion by the hormone aldosterone. Increased osmolality of body fluids stimulates, and increased dilution inhibits, the release of ADH. The major determinant of body-fluid osmolality is sodium. Sodium conservation is mediated through the renin-angiotensin-aldosterone axis. Determinations of plasma and urine sodium, and osmolality and urinary volume, are of diagnostic value in Addison's disease, vasomotor nephropathy (acute tubular necrosis), inapparent volume depletion, incomplete urinary tract obstruction, and hepatorenal disease.

pH

Freshly voided urine usually has a slightly acid pH. The normal range is 5 to 8, and essentially this is also the abnormal pH range. The kidneys, by reason of excreting a urine of variable pH, provide a regulatory mechanism for the body to get rid of excess acid or alkaline waste products. Because the normal pH range and the abnormal pH range are comparable, the measurement of pH alone provides minimal information, but when used in conjunction with other information, it is a very useful urinary parameter. In conditions of acidosis, the urine is quite acid; in conditions of alkalosis, the urine pH is above 7. When metabolic or respiratory acidosis is suspected, an alkaline-urine pH result almost eliminates the possibility of acidosis. Conversely, if respiratory or metabolic alkalosis is suspected, the excretion of an acid urine indicates that alkalosis is likely not present.

Dip-and-read tests are used widely for pH testing; pH-meter measurements are used less commonly. In certain situations involving kidney stone susceptibility, it is quite important to maintain a narrow range of urinary pH. For example, in cystinuria an alkaline pH is maintained to keep the cystine solubilized and to avoid as much as possible the crystallization of cystine into renal calculi. The maintenance of urinary pH is also important for optimum results in certain types of drug therapy.

COLOR

Urine normally has a yellow color, mostly due to urochrome; the color varies from pale straw to dark amber. Darker specimens usually have a high specific gravity. Occasionally, either normal or abnormal urine may show a color different from yellow. Bilirubin may cause fresh urine to be dark in color. In addition, urine that is allowed to stand darkens because of the oxidation of urobilinogen to urobilin. Red, reddish-brown, or "smoky" urine usually is due to the presence of hemoglobin (hemoglobinuria), myoglobin (myoglobinuria), or red blood cells (hematuria). Porphyria is an uncommon cause of red coloration. Black urine can be caused by melanin, which may occur in the urine of patients with far-advanced malignant melanoma. An inborn error of metabolism, alkaptonuria, is characterized by the urinary excretion of homogentisic acid, which causes the urine to turn dark brown or black on standing. Many of the unusual colors occasionally found in urine are derived from exogenous sources, including both foods and drugs. Among these are the red color caused by beets, particularly in infants, the golden-yellow or orange-red color of metabolites of pyridium-like drugs or azo drugs, and the green or blue color from methylene blue.

ODOR

Normal, freshly voided urine has a faint aromatic and characteristic odor, which is more intense in concentrated specimens. If the urine is allowed to stand, the odor becomes strongly ammoniacal and unpleasant because of bacterial destruction of urea. Freshly voided urine having a foul odor indicates severe infection. A sweet, fruity odor may be due to ketones.

APPEARANCE

Freshly voided urine is usually clear. On standing, a precipitate may form that usually consists of amorphous urates if the urine is acid or calcium and magnesium phosphates if the urine is alkaline. The formation of a precipitate is more likely to occur if the urine is refrigerated. Most specimens will become clear again if they are warmed gently to room temperature. Large quantities of mucus, cells, leukocytes, or bacteria may cause cloudiness. Protein usually does not cause cloudiness.

PROTEIN

A small amount of protein is present in the urine obtained from healthy subjects, although the quantity is not sufficient to give a positive reaction with the tests commonly used for the recognition of protein in urine. The majority of the 25 to 50 mg of protein that is excreted daily is microprotein (low-molecular-weight polypeptide), with properties quite different than those of albumin and globulin, which are the principal proteins of the blood serum. Albumin and globulins do occur in the normal urine in minute concentrations.

Plasma proteins, hemoglobin, abnormal Bence-Jones protein, and proteins (nucleo-, phospho-, and glycoproteins) derived from leukocytes and mucus may be present in urine in nephritis, nephrosis, lesions of the urinary tract, GI dehydration, and renal congestion. Abnormal amounts of protein in the urine may be recognized by either precipitation or colorimetric tests. The precipitation depends on the heat coagulation of the protein or on the chemical precipitation of the protein. The most popular of the heat-precipitation tests is the heat- and-acetic acid test in which a tube of urine is heated to boiling after the addition of a drop or two of acetic acid. Sulfosalicylic acid is employed commonly in chemical precipitation tests; in this test, equal quantities of 3% sulfosalicylic acid and urine are mixed in a test tube, and the mixture is examined for turbidity indicative of precipitated protein.

Colorimetric tests for proteins involve *dip-and-read* type of systems and are based on the *protein error* of indicators. Certain indicators have a point of color change that is different in the presence of protein compared to the same system in the absence of protein. Thus, by buffering the indicator tetrabromophenol blue on this dip-stick at a specific pH, it is possible to have a yellow color in the absence of protein and a green or blue color in the presence of protein. This test, Albustix (*Bayer*), not only indicates the presence or absence of protein in the urine but also can be made to indicate the approximate amount of protein. Strongly alkaline or fermented urines will give false-positive results. The sensitivity of the colorimetric method is such that quantities of 10 to 20 mg of albumin/dL of urine can be recognized with confidence.

A positive test for protein in the urine may have any one of several meanings, and it is only when this information is related to other observations that it has optimum value. Proteinuria may be benign and appear following strenuous exercise or simply as a result of standing (orthostatic proteinuria). Protein frequently occurs in the urine during pregnancy and in some instances this is benign, but in other cases it indicates renal complications. Transient proteinuria may occur following severe infections, high fever, exposure to cold, and in congestive heart failure. Proteinuria may be an early and sensitive indicator of renal disease and may indicate an abnormality prior to other signs and symptoms of renal impairment in the glomerulus or tubules. In the majority of instances, there is no correlation between the amount of protein in the urine and the severity of the renal disease.

Patients with severe nephrosis may lose up to 25 g of protein/day. Such a marked loss of protein causes a decrease in plasma protein concentration with an accompanying edema. In both chronic and acute glomerulonephritis there is protein in the urine. Tumors of the kidney and renal infection usually will have an accompanying proteinuria. Bence-Jones protein is a unique protein that occurs in the urine of about 50% of patients with multiple myeloma. It has the unusual property of precipitating between 50° and 60° and dissolving at higher temperatures.

GLUCOSE (REDUCING SUBSTANCES)

Glucose normally occurs in urine in such low concentration that it escapes detection by the usual testing methods. The urine of untreated or poorly controlled diabetic patients characteristically contains easily detectable amounts of glucose. A positive test for glucose in urine usually suggests hyperglycemia and the diagnosis of diabetes mellitus; further studies, such as the glucose tolerance test to confirm the diagnosis, are indicated. Glucosuria also may occur when the renal tubules fail to reabsorb glucose normally, and glucose appears in the urine despite normal blood glucose levels, in contrast to true diabetes.

Glucose is the sugar almost always found in urine; however, lactose, galactose, levulose, sucrose, and pentoses may be encountered. These other sugars are identified by paper chromatography, selective fermentation, polarimetry, special chemical tests, or the formation of their osazones. Other reducing substances occur in urine and may cause falsely positive reducing reactions for glucose. Examples are ascorbic acid, glucuronides, many drugs, homogentisic acid, and the preservatives formalin and chloroform.

Benedict's test, the traditional test for glucose in urine, relies on the reduction of cupric ions in alkaline solution to reddish-orange insoluble cuprous oxide. The copper is reduced totally by large amounts of glucose and results in a brick-red sediment with no remaining blue color. Lesser concentrations form green to rust-colored solutions with some red sediment. A modification of this test, Clinitest (*Bayer*), is available in tablet form. The tablet contains copper sulfate, anhydrous sodium hydroxide, citric acid, and sodium carbonate. When added to dilute urine, the tablet dissolves and generates enough heat and effervescence to yield results comparable with the Benedict test.

A specific but extremely simple enzyme test for glucose is available—Tes-Tape (*Lilly*), Clinistix (*Bayer*), and Multistix (*Bayer*). Reagent strips are impregnated with glucose oxidase, peroxidase, and orthotolidine. When the stick is dipped into a solution of glucose, oxidation occurs and hydrogen peroxide is formed which oxidizes orthotolidine to a blue color. This test is more sensitive than Clinitest, but is not as reliable for estimating the concentration of glucose. The enzymatic test is specific and thus useful in determining whether a reducing substance is glucose. Diastix (*Bayer*) is a specific urine glucose test using glucose oxidase, which also indicates the quantity of glucose present.

KETONE BODIES

The ketone bodies acetone, acetoacetic acid, and beta-hydroxybutyric acid are present in the urine when fats are metabolized incompletely. Ketonuria is seen most commonly in poorly controlled diabetes and indicates ketonemia and diabetic acidosis. Other causes for ketonuria are starvation, fever, protracted vomiting, and Von Gierke's disease. Ketonuria also occurs following anesthesia. Acetoacetic acid and acetone produce a distinctive purple color when treated with a mixture of sodium nitroprusside, ammonium sulfate, and concentrated ammonium hydroxide. A similar reagent is available in tablet form (Acetest, *Bayer*). A drop of urine is placed on the tablet; if ketones are present, a lavender to deep-purple color develops in 30 sec. The color intensity indicates the concentration of ketones. The reagent strip Ketostix (*Bayer*), used as a dip-and-read test on urine or serum, contains the same reagents, which are available on Multistix (*Bayer*) and other multiple reagents as well. These tests will detect 5 to 10 mg acetoacetic acid/dL urine.

PHENYLPYRUVIC ACID

Phenylketonuria (PKU) is an inborn error of metabolism in which the normal conversion of phenylalanine to tyrosine in the body does not occur and there is a buildup of phenylalanine concentration in the blood. This metabolic disorder causes mental retardation. A portion of the phenylalanine is excreted by the kidneys into the urine and in the process is converted to phenylpyruvic acid (or phenylketone). If this genetic disorder is discovered soon after birth, it is possible to place the infant on a diet very low in phenylalanine-containing proteins and thus minimize the phenylalanine buildup in the body, averting the serious mental retardation that ordinarily is seen in the untreated PKU patient.

Recognition of PKU can be made by the use of a test for phenylpyruvic acid using a dip-and-read reagent composition containing ferric ions. This test, Phenistix (*Bayer*), can be used on urine from all newborn babies. A positive reaction gives a green color, whereas a normal infant's urine gives a pale-ivory or yellow color to the strip. PKU also can be recognized by employing a chemical or microbiological test for elevated phenylalanine in serum, as discussed under *Amino Acids*.

BILIRUBIN

Bilirubin is found in the urine of patients with hepatitis or obstructive jaundice but not in patients with hemolytic jaundice. Tests for bilirubin and urobilinogen combine to give excellent information in the differential diagnosis of jaundice. Tests for bilirubin are of two kinds: oxidation tests form a green color of biliverdin from bilirubin usually using ferric chloride as the oxidative reagent, and diazotization tests form colored compounds when bilirubin reacts with diazonium salts in a strongly acid medium. Most oxidation tests adsorb the bilirubin onto barium sulfate or similar material before the addition of Fouchet's reagent. The tablet test Ictotest (*Bayer*) is the most sensitive diazo test, and it uses an absorption mat to concentrate the bilirubin from 5 drops of urine. A reagent tablet is added to the moist spot on the mat and 2 drops of water are added to dissolve the effervescent reagent and wash some of it off the tablet onto the mat where the reaction takes place. A blue or purple color on the mat around the tablet in 30 sec indicates the presence of bilirubin. In addition, a dip-and-read test composition also based on the diazo reaction has been incorporated into the Bili-Labstix and Multistix (*Bayer*) multiple urinalysis reagent strips. It is less sensitive than the tablet test, but its convenience allows it to be used in routine urinalysis quite readily. An incidence of approximately 0.1% positives on health-screening population groups, 0.2% on clinic patients, and 0.9% on hospitalized patients has been reported.

UROBILINOGEN

Bilirubin in the bile is reduced to urobilinogen by bacteria in the lower intestine. A portion of the urobilinogen is reabsorbed from the intestine into the blood. A portion of this urobilinogen is excreted into the urine by the kidney, and the balance is re-excreted via the bile into the intestine. Although the quantity of urobilinogen in the urine is quite small, it is an important indicator of liver function and red-blood-cell catabolism.

If there is an obstruction to bile flow such as in obstructive jaundice, the amount of urobilinogen formed and reabsorbed into the blood and excreted in the urine is decreased. With impairment of liver function, the excretion of urobilinogen in the bile is decreased, the blood concentration increases, and there is a corresponding increase in urinary urobilinogen excretion. Actually, the increase in urinary urobilinogen is one of the most sensitive tests for impaired liver function, and this test may indicate an abnormality when all other tests of liver function remain unchanged from normal.

In hemolytic diseases in which there is an increased rate of hemoglobin breakdown, the amount of bilirubin formation is increased with a corresponding increase in urobilinogen formation and excretion in the urine. The concentration of urobilinogen in urine can be established by the use of a dip-and-read test that uses the interaction of urobilinogen and *p*-dimethylaminobenzaldehyde (Urobilistix, *Bayer*).

HEMATURIA, HEMOGLOBINURIA, AND MYOGLOBINURIA

Hematuria refers to a condition in which intact red blood cells appear in the urine. This condition is indicative of a specific defect in the microscopic functional unit (the nephron) of the kidney, or it may be indicative of bleeding in the kidney, the ureter, the bladder, or the urethra. In the female there may be variable numbers of red blood cells in the urine during menstruation.

Hemoglobinuria is a condition in which free hemoglobin is present in the urine without red blood cells. This may be caused by intravascular hemolysis as a result of a transfusion reaction or by poisoning or toxins. The free hemoglobin in the plasma is excreted by the kidney into the urine. In some situations actual total hemolysis of the red cells occurs after they have entered the urine. This occurs particularly with alkaline urines.

Myoglobin is the red respiratory pigment of muscle. This pigment is quite comparable to hemoglobin in its composition and chemical reactions. Myoglobin may be liberated from muscle cells in certain types of injury and, in such cases, will circulate in the plasma and be excreted in the urine. There are also certain genetic muscle disorders in which myoglobin is lost from the muscles and appears in the plasma and subsequently in the urine.

Chemical tests for red cells, free hemoglobin, and myoglobin are based on the peroxidase-like activity of hemoglobin or myoglobin. When a chromogen mixture such as orthotolidine and peroxide is exposed to this peroxidase activity, it will interact rapidly to generate an intense blue color. A dip-and-read solid state system is available called Hemastix (*Bayer*). This specific composition uses cumene hydroperoxide as the peroxide. The same dip-and-read test for occult blood is incorporated as a component part of multiple, urine dip-and-read tests such as Multistix (*Bayer*).

MICROSCOPIC EXAMINATION

Ordinarily, urine contains a number of formed elements or solid structures of microscopic dimensions. These are studied readily by centrifuging 10 to 15 mL of urine, pouring off the supernatant, and resuspending the sediment in the drop or so of urine that remains in the tube. This suspension of sediment is placed on a microscope slide and viewed with low-power magnification. Specific structures can be studied with higher magnification. The urinary sediments can be classified into unorganized (chemical substances) and organized (cells and casts) constituents.

In an alkaline urine, amorphous or crystalline ammonium-magnesium phosphates, calcium carbonate or oxalate crystals, and ammonium urate may occur normally. Amorphous or crystalline urates, uric acid, and calcium oxalates normally are seen in acid urines. The presence of tyrosine, leucine, or cystine crystals is associated with various diseases. Chemical crystals are identified by solubility in acid and/or alkali, colorimetric reactions, and crystalline structure.

The urine sediment ordinarily contains residues of epithelial cells, crystals, and an occasional red or white blood cell. Increased numbers of erythrocytes are seen when there is bleeding into the urinary tract. If the red cells are formed into a red-cell cast, it is suggestive that bleeding has occurred at the glomerular level. An increased number of leukocytes is suggestive of infection and inflammation of the kidney. Casts are microscopic concretions that have the form of a tubule; they have a matrix of precipitated protein and, depending on their appearance, may be identified as hyaline, granular, waxy, or red-cell casts. Renal-failure casts are larger and are associated with severe necrosis of the kidney.

Numerous crystals, mucus fibers, bacteria, yeast cells, spermatozoa, and parasites (such as *Trichomonas vaginalis*) may be identified in the urine sediment. The majority of these crystals do not have any unusual significance but in certain disorders may be indicative of crystal deposits in kidney tissue or predisposition to formation of calculi.

Tissue cells can be recognized in urine sediment. This provides an excellent means of detection and diagnosis of cancer of the lower urinary tract when the sediment is fixed in alcohol and stained by the Papanicolaou procedure. Exfoliative cytology of urine may be applied as a routine to all urology patients. In one large clinic, the number of positive cases found among urology patients was almost 5%, which is a much higher return of positive results than is obtained with routine staining of cervical smears.

BACTERIA

Freshly voided specimens of urine ordinarily contain a few microorganisms, which primarily represent bacteria picked up from the external genitalia. There are fewer contaminating organisms in a *clean-catch* specimen, which involves extensive washing of the external genitalia prior to collection of the specimen. A specimen collected at the midpoint of urination or a "midstream" specimen ordinarily has more organisms than a clean-catch specimen, but fewer than a so-called random specimen.

When there is an infection of the kidney or urinary tract, the number of organisms in the urine is increased markedly. Ordinarily, if the urine contains 100,000 or more organisms/mL, the result strongly suggests the presence of an active infection. Infection of the urinary tract with accompanying bacteriuria is relatively common in young girls and women. Quite often the condition is asymptomatic and is recognized only as a result of a study of the urine. If bacteriuria is not treated, it may lead to serious renal injury.

If there is a very large number of bacteria in the urine, the specimen actually may be turbid. This can be recognized by gross visual inspection of the urine. Bacteriuria also can be recognized by microscopic examination of the urine sediment, particularly if there is a large number of organisms present. The most widely employed procedure for recognizing bacteria involves plating a specimen of diluted urine on a culture plate, incubating it, and counting the number of colonies. A more convenient approach to this same measurement involves the use of a microscope slide coated with nutrient agar. Such a slide, when dipped in a urine specimen and then incubated, will indicate the presence or absence of bacteriuria and also the approximate count.

Methods to determine the presence of significant numbers of bacteria in urine samples have been developed and incorporated into various automated systems.[20] The Bac-T-Screen (*Marion*) system was a dispensing and filtering system used with a straining process to detect the presence of bacteria on special filter cards by noting the color change on the card. Analysis on the Abbott MS-2 was performed by photometric monitoring of bacterial growth, which changed the light transmitted in a broth culture over a period of time. A decrease in the light transmission due to turbidity or color identified a positive specimen.

The Lumac Biocounter M2010 measured bacterial ATP in urine by the bioluminescence produced in a luciferin-luciferase system. Once these rapid techniques were performed to determine which specimens had increased bacteria, further identification and sensitivity testing was performed. Chemical tests for the metabolic activity of bacteria have been used in studying bacteriuria. The most popular chemical test is that for nitrite. Ordinarily, all urine specimens contain nitrate, but do not contain nitrite. If *Escherichia coli* or certain other organisms are present in sufficient numbers, they will reduce the nitrate to nitrite.

A widely used advanced automated system, the VITEK System (*bioMérieux*) has a urine identification test card that can not only detect and enumerate bacteria from urine samples, but also selectively identify the organism or organisms present using nutritionally selective components and unique metabolic indicators.

CALCULI

Knowledge of the composition of renal and bladder calculi, or "stones," is essential in planning the therapeutic regimen for such diseases. Mixed calcium phosphate and oxalate stones usually occur over the entire urine pH range. Uric acid, cystine, and calcium hydrogen phosphate calculi generally are associated with acid urines, whereas magnesium ammonium phosphate calculi usually occur in alkaline urine. Hyperexcretion of one of the calculi components, pH, renal blockage, and the presence of foreign objects in the urinary tract are the most probable causal factors in the formation of renal calculi. Calcium oxalate stones are the most common type. The chemical content of the stones is established by routine qualitative analysis for calcium, magnesium, ammonium, phosphate, carbonate, oxalate, uric acid, and cystine. Subsequent confirmation by optical crystallography, x-ray diffraction, and infrared spectroscopy is also used in the characterization of the physical properties of the calculi.

Feces

Normal feces consist of undigested food remnants, products of digestion, bacteria, and secretions of the GI tract. *Macroscopic, chemical,* and *microscopic* determinations are performed rou-

tinely. The normal quantity of feces is about 200 g/day. The brown color is a result of the reduction of bilirubin to urobilinogen and then to uribilin (stercobilin); bilirubin is not normally present in feces, but porphyrins and biliverdin (a component of meconium) are excreted during the first days of life. Bilirubin can be detected by tests previously described for bile pigments.

Color changes in the stool can be the result of dietary intake or diagnostic for biliary obstruction and gastrointestinal bleeding.[21] Patients with steatorrhea and malabsorption may show a yellow bulky stool containing fat and gas. The feces is clay colored when bile is prevented from entering the gut. A red or black stool can occur when excessive doses of anticoagulants, phenylbutazone, or salicylates are taken, producing bleeding in the gastrointestinal tract. Substances that interfere with the coloration of the stool include antacids (whitish or speckling), bismuth salts (black), iron salts (black), pyridium (orange), senna (yellow to brown), and tetracyclines (red).

Fecal urobilinogen can be determined colorimetrically by reduction of urobilin to urobilinogen with alkaline ferrous sulfate, and then reaction with acidified p-dimethylaminobenzaldehyde (Ehrlich's reagent). It is increased from a normal range of 40 to 280 mg/day, to 400 to 1400 mg in hemolytic jaundice (dark brown stool), and is decreased in obstructive jaundice (clay-colored stool).

Porphyrins and *porphyrinogens* do not arise from hemoglobin catabolism, such as bilirubin, but are by-products of the synthesis of heme. Increases in fecal and urinary elimination of coproporphyrin, uroporphyrin, and protoporphyrin are valuable diagnostic aids in distinguishing the various hepatic and erythropoietic porphyrias. Fecal coproporphyrins (CP) and coproporphyrinogens (CPP) are determined after extraction, conversion of CPP to CP by iodine and triple-point spectrometric estimation at 380, 401, and 430 nm to correct for interfering substances (also see section on urinalysis).

Fecal occult blood is detected readily by the o-tolidine, benzidine, guaiac, or diphenylamine tests; this is valid only if the patient has been on a meat-free diet for 3 days. Guaiac and diphenylamine are preferred due to the carcinogenic potential of the other two chemicals.

The Seracult test kit (*Propper*) uses an impregnated guaiac paper slide for detecting occult blood, which is a useful screening test for colon cancer. Two slides are prepared each day for 3 days from different parts of the same stool while the patient is on a meat-free high-bulk diet. Interfering substances include aspirin, indomethacin, and corticosteroids because they can produce bleeding, and vitamin C, which interferes with the oxidation reaction of the test. If bleeding occurs high in the GI tract, the blood is digested and converted to acid hematin; 50 mL of blood in the feces will cause melena (black stool). Bleeding from the lower GI tract is apparent from red streaking of stools. Also, ^{51}Cr-tagged erythrocytes have been used to quantitate and locate the source of GI bleeding. The subject's red cells are mixed with an isotonic ^{51}Cr solution and then reinjected intravenously. If bleeding occurs, the ^{51}Cr-isotope content of the feces will be increased. Location of the hemorrhagic area also can be approximated by an isotopic scan of the abdominal area.

The presence of excessive quantities of *mucus* is usually indicative of dysentery, colitis, or other inflammatory processes in the intestinal mucosa. Strongly alkaline or acidic reaction in the feces is indicative of excessive quantities of protein or carbohydrate in the diet, respectively.

Quantitative determination of *fecal nitrogen* is useful in analysis of pancreatic function. In pancreatic disease, increases in fecal nitrogen will occur as a result of decreased secretion of pancreatic proteolytic enzymes. The normal individual will excrete 4% to 13% of ingested nitrogen in the feces; in chronic pancreatitis, 9% to 30% will be excreted. Fecal nitrogen can be determined by the Kjeldahl digestion procedure.

Fecal fat is present in the form of triglycerides of fatty acids (neutral fat), free fatty acids (FFA) and soaps. Fat determinations are based on the solubility of neutral fat and FFA in ether;

the soaps are insoluble in ether and have to be acid-hydrolyzed to their respective FFA prior to extraction. Neutral fat will liberate FFA only on alkaline hydrolysis. The FFA, isolated from the above fractionations, are then determined by titrimetric, colorimetric, or gas-chromatographic procedures.

Determinations of blood, urine, and fecal ^{125}I after oral administration of an iodinated glyceryl trioleate or ^{125}I-oleic acid preparation is an index of *pancreatic, biliary,* and *intestinal absorptive function* and correlates with *fecal fat excretion*. The bile must emulsify the ^{125}I-triglyceride prior to enzymatic hydrolysis by pancreatic lipase to yield FFA-^{125}I, which subsequently is absorbed and metabolized. An increased amount of ^{125}I in the feces is associated with pancreatic diseases (cystic fibrosis with achylia), obstructive jaundice, malabsorption disease (sprue, celiac disease), and steatorrhea. The latter entity can be differentiated as to a pancreatic lipase or intestinal absorptive defect. In the "absorptive disease," increased excretion of ^{125}I is seen after administration of ^{125}I-triolein or oleic acid. In the pancreatic defect, adequate absorption of ^{125}I oleic acid occurs but fecal ^{125}I is increased after the triolein meal.

A *microscopic examination* of emulsified feces includes analysis for the presence of crystals, food residues, body cells, bacteria, and parasites. Crystals of triple phosphate, calcium oxalate, fat and cholesterol, starch granules, vegetable fibers, and neutral fat globules are normally present. Octahedral needle-shaped crystals (Charcot-Leyden crystals) are present in parasitic infestation and mucous colitis. Excessive quantities of fat or starch are seen in malabsorption disease.

Adult, larval, or ova phases of parasites may be encountered in the feces. The most common parasitic infestations are caused by *cestodes* (tapeworms), *trematodes* (flukes), *nematodes* (roundworms), and *protozoa* (amoeba) (see the section on microbiology).

Toxicology

The determination of drug or chemical concentrations in biological fluids is an important aspect in diagnosing and treating the toxic syndrome induced by various agents in acute or chronic drug-abuse situations or in chemical poisoning.

Barbiturates, glutethimide, methaqualone, chlordiazepoxide, diazepam, diphenhydramine, ethchlorvynol, morphine, phenothiazines, and salicylates are encountered in drug-abuse situations. Preliminary screening of serum or urine samples for drug substances is accomplished through the use of homogeneous immunoassay techniques EMIT (enzyme-mediated immunologic technique) or FPIA (fluorescence polarization immunoassay), or less commonly by TLC. The analysis of serum or urine levels of intact drug or its metabolites usually is performed by extraction of the sample with an organic solvent, separation by gas-liquid (GLC), or high-performance liquid (HPLC) chromatography, and quantitation by spectrometric, fluorometric, or electrochemical techniques. The technique of GC-MS (gas chromatography–mass spectrometry) methodology has become the "gold standard" because of its great sensitivity and reliability. The interpretation of the serum- concentration data in relation to clinical significance and toxicology must not be limited to numbers.

In acute drug overdosage the time of drug ingestion, time of blood or urine sampling, and severity of clinical symptoms or time of death must be interpreted in reference to data on the absorption, tissue distribution, metabolism, and elimination of the drug and its metabolites. The specificity of the chemical assay as to interference from other drugs or metabolites of the parent drug must be considered. The use of GC-MS confirms the identity of specific drugs in biological matrices. The extent of absorption of many drug substances is not related directly to the dose when large amounts of a drug are ingested, in comparison to the therapeutic dose.

The tissue-distribution and metabolic rates can be affected by large drug overdoses in which renal or hepatic failure is encountered. The plasma-elimination rate also can be affected, and it is important to recognize the change in elimination kinetics and to be aware of the nature of plasma elimination as defined by a mono-, bi-, or polyexponential elimination curve. The drug overdose usually involves several drug substances and the chemical, metabolic, and pharmacological aspects of drug interaction must be considered.

The methodology for the analysis of drugs in biological fluids or tissues can be found in the books listed in the *Bibliography*. Classic analyses for serum *barbiturate* levels will be described in this section as a specific example of the analytical methodology.

Serum is extracted at pH 6.5 with chloroform; the chloroform extract is washed with pH 7 phosphate buffer and extracted with 0.45N NaOH. The UV spectrum of the alkaline aqueous layer is determined at pH 13 and 10.5. The UV spectra are characteristic and distinguish barbiturates, *N*-methylbarbituric acids, and thiobarbiturates. The barbiturates also can be detected by acidifying the alkaline layer, extracting with chloroform, and spotting this organic extract on a silica-gel TLC plate. Sequential spraying of the plate with $KMnO_4$, $HgSO_4$, and diphenylcarbazone will show R_f values and color reactions typical of the various barbiturates.

Blood barbiturates can be determined more accurately by a GLC procedure in which the retention times are used to identify the specific barbiturates. The degree of severity of clinical symptoms has been correlated with blood barbiturate levels. Comatose, areflexic signs are observed at 5.0 mg% amobarbital, 2.0 mg% pentobarbital, 8.0 mg% phenobarbital, and 1.5 mg% secobarbital.

Opiates, amphetamines, barbiturates, and methadone can be detected rapidly by "homogenous" immunoassay.[22] In this procedure, the addition of drug antibodies to a conjugate of drug and lysozyme results in the inhibition of lysozyme activity. The addition of free drug to this reaction mixture increases the enzyme activity in proportion to the amount of free drug added. The sensitivity of this type of assay is 0.1 μg/mL of amphetamine and barbiturates, 0.5 μg/mL of methadone, 0.3 μg/mL of opiates, and 1.0 μg/mL of benzoylecgonine, a cocaine metabolite. This assay is applicable to large drug-screening programs.

Electron-spin-labeling techniques also can be employed on large-scale drug-screening programs. In this procedure known amounts of drug antibodies are mixed with drug labeled with a stable nitroxide radical (spin-label) and with the specimen to be analyzed. Due to the competition for antibody between spin-labeled drug and drug in the specimen, the spin-labeled drug becomes detached from the antibody and can be detected by electron-spin resonance spectroscopy. This procedure is 1000 times more sensitive than TLC.

Blood-alcohol levels may be determined by aeration, distillation, gas chromatography, or specific enzymatic analysis with alcohol dehydrogenase. In the chemical techniques, the blood sample is either oxidized or distilled into a dichromate–sulfuric acid mixture; the excess dichromate is then determined by titration with potassium iodide or methyl orange–ferrous sulfate solutions or by colorimetric analysis. The gas chromatographic and enzyme procedures are specific for ethanol, whereas the chemical techniques are influenced by other volatile or oxidizable substances in the blood. The enzymatic method is based on the reaction of ethanol and NAD in the presence of alcohol dehydrogenase to form acetaldehyde and NADH; the acetaldehyde is removed with semicarbazide and the NADH formed in the reaction is estimated spectrophotometrically at 340 nm. Ethanol levels of >0.10% are indicative of intoxication and apparent psychomotor disturbance. Levels of 0.40% to 0.50% are associated with medullary and diencephalic disturbances such as tremors, coma, respiratory depression, peripheral collapse, and death.

Specific analysis of heavy metals is best performed by atomic absorption spectroscopy. Analyses for arsenic, beryllium, bismuth, copper, iron, lead, lithium, mercury, nickel, thallium, and zinc are encountered frequently in the toxicology laboratory. *Blood lead* is determined by forming a lead–dithiocarbamate chelate in the presence of ammonium pyrrolidinedithiocarbamate and extracting the chelate into methyl isobutyl ketone for subsequent atomic-absorption analysis. A lead concentration of > 60 µg/mL in children usually reflects significant absorption and accumulation of lead and is interpreted as an indicator of lead toxicity (plumbism).

Increased lead exposure will result in a decrease in *deltaaminolevulinic acid (ALA)* conversion to porphobilinogen by ALA-dehydrase in heme synthesis. ALA blood levels will increase to the point that ALA is excreted in the urine. Determination of urinary ALA is performed by removing urine porphobilinogen and urea by ion-exchange chromatography, reacting ALA with *p*-dimethylaminobenzaldehyde and determining the chromogen colorimetrically. Urinary ALA levels > 2.5 mg/dL are unacceptable in children and industrial lead workers. Urinary ALA levels are not as sensitive an indicator of lead toxicity as blood lead, but they can be used to monitor prophylactic treatment procedures.

Cholinesterase determinations are of value in the diagnosis of suspected cases of organophosphate or carbamate pesticide poisoning. Two types of cholinesterase are found in tissues. True cholinesterase is found in RBC and nerve tissue and exhibits a specificity for acetylcholine substrate. Pseudocholinesterase is found in plasma and has a greater affinity for hydrolyzing butyrylcholine and other esters. The organophosphate and carbamate insecticides inhibit both enzymes. The activity of the plasma enzyme is inhibited more rapidly than the RBC cholinesterase, and recovers more rapidly due to synthesis of new enzyme by the liver. The recovery of the erythrocyte enzyme is slow and is governed by red-cell turnover rate. Cholinesterase activity usually is determined spectrometrically using acetylthiocholine as the substrate. Cholinesterases split this substrate into acetic acid and thiocholine which reacts with 5,5'-dithiobis(2-nitrobenzoic acid) (Ellman's reagent) to form the yellow-colored 2-nitro-5-mercaptobenzoic acid. Increasing color intensity is directly proportional to cholinesterase activity. Expected values are 3167 to 6333 U/L (serum), 1667 to 5833 U/L (plasma), and 6000 to 9167 U/L in whole blood by this methodology.

Gastric Analysis

The chief constituents of gastric juice are hydrochloric acid, gastric proteases (pepsin and gastricsin), hematopoietic factor (intrinsic factor and vitamin B_{12} binders), gastric hormones, and mucosubstances (aminopolysaccharides, mucopolyuronides, mucoids, and mucoproteins). Tests for *gastric function*[23] usually are performed on gastric juice samples collected by direct intubation into the stomach. The fasting content (normal, <100 mL) of the stomach is removed and gastric secretion is collected in the basal state, or after stimulation by the oral administration of caffeine-benzoate or alcohol, or parenteral administration of histamine, insulin, or the hormone pentagastrin. Samples are collected by continuous aspiration and analyzed for acidity and gastric protease activity at various time intervals. The extent of recovery of total juice can be estimated by oral, nonabsorbable indicators (polyethylene glycol-^{14}C, phenol red and ^{125}I-HSA) instilled into the stomach prior to the aspiration. The recovery and specific concentration of these indicators in gastric juice is an index of gastric secretory volume, completeness of collection, and gastric emptying rate.

Gastric juice is a heterogeneous mixture of clear juice and flocculent, clear mucus. The *color* of the juice should be noted as to the appearance of blood, bile, and excessive quantities of mucus. The *acidity* can be determined by a simple pH measurement and conversion to mEq of H^+ or by titration of centrifuged gastric juice to pH 3.5, 4.5 and 7.4, the respective end points for free acid (HCl), protease activity, and physiological neutrality. The *basal acid output* is about 1 mEq/hour in normal subjects

and 2 to 4 mEq/hour in duodenal ulcer patients. The *peak acid output (PAO)* after histamine stimulation is 10 to 20 mEq/hour in normals and 40 to 50 mEq/hour in duodenal ulcer; PAO following pentagastric stimulation is similar to histamine. Gastric acid secretion is decreased in atrophic gastritis, gastric carcinoma, and certain types of gastric ulcer. Hypersecretion is seen in duodenal ulcer, Zollinger-Ellison (ZE) syndrome, and hyperparathyroidism.

In situ measurements of pH may be made with a *Heidelberg capsule apparatus*. In this technique the subject swallows a small pH-sensitive capsule (transmitter); radiowaves are transmitted from the capsule to a sensing device (receiver), and the signals are recorded as a function of pH. The normal pH of the stomach is 1.2 to 1.8.

The principal gastric proteases are *pepsin* and *gastricsin;* pepsinogen is a precursor that is converted to active pepsin by free HCl and by an autocatalytic process. *Total gastric protease activity* is determined on hemoglobin or radioiodinated human serum albumin (RISA) substrates at pH 1.8 to 3.1 (RISA-^{125}I); protease activity on hemoglobin will liberate tyrosine, which can be estimated spectrometrically at 280 nm. With RISA, liberated tyrosine-^{125}I, as estimated by isotopic procedures, is an index of proteolytic activity.

Pepsin activity can be distinguished from the total protease activity by estimation of the 3,5-diiodotyrosine liberated from *N*-acetyl-l-phenylalanyl-3,5-diiodotyrosine substrate at pH 2.1. Pepsin will react on this substrate; gastricsin will not. Normal gastric juice protease activity ranges from 200 to 1200 µg total protease activity/mL and 50 to 300 µg pepsin/mL. The presence of bile, blood, saliva, or excess mucus in the sample will decrease both acidity and gastric protease activity.

Gastrin, cholecystokinin, secretin, and *pancreozymin* are gastrointestinal hormones.[24] The role of gastrin and its interaction with other gastrointestinal hormones in the etiology and proliferation of ulcer disease is of recent interest. Accurate RIA techniques have been developed for gastrin and secretin-6-tyrosine due to the availability of a pure synthetic polypeptide. Biological assays based on the effect of these substances on gastric, pancreatic, and biliary secretion also have been used.

Gastrin is found in various species in two forms, G-I and G-II. The only difference is in sulfation of the 12-tyrosyl residue in G-II of the heptadecapeptide amides. Gastrin is found primarily in the gastrin-producing cells (G-cells) of the antral mucosa. The C-terminal tetrapeptide represents the biologically active part of the molecule. Gastrin infusion will stimulate secretion of gastric acid, pepsin, and intrinsic factor. It has a slight secretin-like effect and a powerful pancreozymin-like effect on pancreatic secretion. Gastrin also stimulates bile flow. The instillation of HCl into the stomach will inhibit gastrin release; protein and meal stimulation will increase serum gastrin.

The RIA of serum gastrin is of diagnostic value in the ZE syndrome, pernicious anemia, and duodenal ulcer. Basal serum gastrin levels in the normal individual are 20 to 30 µg/mL and increase about twofold after a protein meal stimulus.

Basal serum gastrin levels in duodenal ulcer are normal or slightly elevated, but increase four- to fivefold after a protein-meal stimulus. Basal serum gastrin levels are elevated in ZE to 500 to 4000 pg/mL due to the presence of a gastrin-producing tumor. The ZE patient is uniquely sensitive to intravenous calcium stimulation, which will increase both gastric acid secretion and serum gastrin in this syndrome. Basal serum gastrin levels also are elevated in gastric hyposecretion as seen in pernicious anemia and Type A gastritis and in chronic renal failure due to the decreased metabolic turnover of gastrin in the kidney.

The RIA of serum gastrin is based on the competition of gastrin in test sample with ^{125}I-gastrin for gastrin antibody binding sites. The antibodies used in this procedure are usually cospecific for G-I and G-II. However, they detect all forms of circulating gastrin: Big-Big Gastrin (G-39), Big Gastrin (mol wt 7000; G-33), gastrin heptadecapeptide (G-17, mol wt 2200), G-13 and G-8 (mini-gastrin). The Big components can be converted to gastrin by trypsin hydrolysis. The significance of changes in the ratio of the circulating gastrins is not known, but it has been suggested that G-39 and G-33 predominate in the basal state and cleave to G-17, which is the major serum form after a protein meal.

Other Body Fluids

Physical, chemical, and microscopic examination of cerebrospinal fluid, seminal fluid, synovial fluid, human milk, transudates, and exudates also are performed by the clinical laboratory. The principles of the various determinations are similar to those described for blood and urine.

MICROBIOLOGY

Clinical medical microbiology is a science concerned with the isolation and identification of disease-producing microorganisms: bacteria, fungi (including yeast), viruses, rickettsia, and parasites. The techniques employed in the isolation and identification of the suspect organisms involve the propagation on suitable primary culture media, selective isolation on special culture media, use of suitable living host material (mouse, embryonated egg, tissue culture, etc), determination of morphological and, where applicable, staining characteristics of the organism, and confirmation by biochemical and/or immunochemical analysis. Suitable animal inoculation, where applicable, may be employed to determine pathogenicity. Site, timing, technique (aseptic), instrumentation, and transportation of clinical specimens (blood, urine, feces, cerebrospinal fluid, etc) are prime variables involved in the final differentiation and confirmation process.

Rapid manual enzymatic and immunological test kits have been introduced to identify pathogens for cerebrospinal fluid analysis. The latex-agglutination test coats a specific antibody onto latex particles and when an antigen is present, the latex particles are visible.[25] In the coagglutination test, the specific antibody is bound to protein A on the surface of a staphylococcal cell and the presence of antigen produces agglutination.[25]

Staphylococcus aureus (*Micrococcus pyogenes* var *aureus*) is a Gram-positive coccus frequently found on normal human skin and mucous membranes and frequently associated with abscesses, septicemia, endocarditis, and osteomyelitis. Some strains elaborate an exotoxin capable of causing food poisoning. The primary isolation is on blood agar and in thioglycollate broth. With feces and other heavily contaminated specimens, phenylethyl alcohol agar and/or mannitol-salt agar should be inoculated to suppress growth of other bacteria. The identification of pathogenic staphylococci is based on colonial (pigmentation) and microscopic morphology (grape-like clusters), positive catalase production, positive coagulase production (staphylocoagulase-plasma clotting factor), and positive mannitol fermentation.

Streptococcus pyogenes is another Gram-positive coccus frequently associated with tonsillitis or pharyngitis, erysipelas, pyoderma, and endocarditis. Neopeptone agar containing 5% defibrinated sheep blood is preferred for primary isolation and to demonstrate characteristic hemolysin production by observing a zone of clear (beta) hemolysis around the colonies on blood agar. Streptococcal groups are identified by precipitin tests with group-specific antisera for A, B, C, D, F, and G. Streptex (*Diagnostic Product Corp.*) uses a latex agglutination system for identifying the Lancefield group of streptococci. Other groups usually are not associated with human clinical materials.

Legionella pneumophila identification includes specimen cultures on lung tissue or sterile body fluids (eg, pleural fluid or pericardial fluid). Direct fluorescent antibody method is a test for *L pneumophila*. Organisms are best seen in the acute stage of the disease. Because the antiserum is species-specific, polyvalent antisera are necessary for identification.

Neisseria gonorrhoeae is a Gram-negative diplococcus associated with the venereal disease gonorrhea. The identification is based on the primary isolation of the gonococcus from urethral exudates on chocolate agar or Thayer-Martin (TM) medium. The microscopic observation of Gram-negative intracellular diplococci resembling the gonococcus constitutes a presumptively positive diagnosis of gonorrhea. Confirmation of the oxidase enzyme activity of the gonococci is performed by a reaction with *p*-dimethylaminoaniline, which turns oxidase-positive colonies black. A positive oxidase test by Gram-negative diplococci isolated on TM medium constitutes a presumptively positive test for *N gonorrhoeae*. Final identification rests on typical sugar fermentation or specific (fluorescent antibody) staining.

Neisseria meningitidis is the primary cause of bacterial meningitis and septicemia. The primary isolation is based on culturing of a specimen (blood, spinal fluid, or nasopharyngeal secretions) on a Mueller-Hinton medium or chocolate agar containing a vancomycin-colistimethate-nystatin antibiotic mixture. The confirmation of the isolate by biochemical reactions (positive oxidase, positive catalase, etc) and serological agglutination with group-specific (A, B, and C) antiserum is used in the differentiation. Young cultures of groups A and C may show capsular swelling (Quellung reaction) in the presence of a specific antiserum.

The enteric bacilli (*Enterobacteriaceae*) are Gram-negative, nonsporulating rods associated with dysentery (*Shigella* spp) typhoid fever (*Salmonella typhi*), urinary tract and tissue infections (*Escherichia coli, Proteus* spp, and *Pseudomonas* spp), and pulmonary infections (*Klebsiella* spp). The primary isolation of enteric bacilli is on selective and differential infusion agar such as MacConkey and eosin-methylene blue (EMB), and enrichment media such as selenite broth and tetrathionate broth. The primary isolation of *Salmonella* spp is on Leifson's deoxycholate citrate agar (LDC) or *Salmonella-Shigella* agar (SS); if *Salmonella typhi* is suspected, brilliant green agar (BG) and bismuth sulfite agar (BS) may be used and would constitute a presumptively positive diagnosis of *S typhi*.

The confirmation and identification of enteric bacilli may be performed by serological tests and biochemical reactions: H_2S production (triple-sugar iron agar), indole production, acetylmethylcarbinol production, citrate utilization, urease, lysine, and arginine decarboxylase and phenylalanine deaminase activity. Enterotube (*Roche Diagnostics*) employs conventional media to perform 11 standard biochemical tests that can be inoculated simultaneously in one compartment tube, with a single bacterial colony. The serological identification of *Salmonella* and *Shigella* spp is based on the agglutination of antigens that fall into three categories: "K" capsular (*Klebsiella* spp and *Shigella* spp), "O" (*Salmonella* spp, *Arizona* spp, *E coli, Shigella* spp, etc), and "H" flagellar (*Salmonella* spp).

Other Gram-negative rods of medical importance are the hemophilic bacilli (*Bordetella pertussis*, whooping cough; and *Haemophilus influenzae,* bacterial meningitis), the hemorrhagic bacilli (*Pasteurella pestis*, bubonic plague; and *P tularensis*, tularemia), and pyrogenic bacillus (*Brucella melitensis*, undulant fever).

Spore-forming Gram-positive rods of medical importance belong to the genus *Clostridium*, which are associated with tetanus (*C tetani*), gas gangrene (*C perfringens* or *welchii*), and botulism (*C botulinum*). The isolation of these organisms requires anaerobic conditions. Once the strain to be identified is obtained in pure culture by single-colony selection, its morphological characteristics are noted; the strain then is grown in a variety of definitive media to determine catalase activity, hydrogen peroxide decomposition, and fermentation or hydrolysis of carbohydrates and organic acids. The analysis of fermentation products (gas chromatography) also is used for the identification of pathogenic anaerobic *Clostridia*. The major clostridial exotoxin type can be determined by typing with specific antitoxin sera. A Gram-positive, aerobic, sporeformer of medical importance is *Bacillus anthracis*, responsible for anthrax, a disease of animals that is transmissible to humans.

The mycobacteria are acid-fast bacilli associated with tuberculosis in man (*Mycobacterium tuberculosis*) and in cattle (*Mycobacterium bovis*), and leprosy (*Mycobacterium leprae*). Tubercle bacilli in man are isolated from sputum cultured on a tubed or bottled egg medium (Lowenstein-Jensen) following enzymatic digestion and concentration of the specimens. A provisional diagnosis of tuberculosis usually is made by demonstrating acid-fast bacilli microscopically, x-ray diagnosis, and a positive tuberculin skin test.

Other weakly and partially acid-fast bacilli of medical importance are members of the Actinomycetales, *Nocardia asteroides,* and *Nocardia brasiliensis*, which are responsible for severe pulmonary infections and cutaneous and subcutaneous abscesses.

Bacteriophages (phages) are a special group of viruses that are hosted by bacteria. Any given phage is highly host-specific and when in contact, lysis of the host occurs (phage-typing). They are used primarily as epidemiological tools in subtyping strains of *E coli*, staphylococci, or *Salmonella* spp that are presumed to be related epidemiologically. Phages also furnish ideal material for studying host-parasite relationships and virus multiplication.

The medically important fungal diseases include the superficial mycoses—fungal invasion is restricted to the outermost layers of the skin or to the hair shafts (such as *Microsporum audouini, Trichophyton* spp, *Epidermophyton floccosum*)—and the systemic pathogenic fungi (*Blastomyces dermatitidis, Coccidioides immitis, Histoplasma capsulatum, Candida albicans*). The diagnosis of the causative agent is based on the isolation of organisms on Sabouraud's dextrose agar or trypticase soy agar with or without cycloheximide and chloramphenicol to suppress the growth of saprophytic fungi and bacteria, macroscopic examination of morphological characteristics, and microscopic examination using potassium hydroxide (KOH) or lactophenol cotton-blue stain. Biochemical reactions usually are limited to *Candida* spp. Immunological reactions include skin tests, where applicable; agglutination tests, such as latex particle agglutination for histoplasmosis; and tube precipitin and complement-fixation tests.

An *antimicrobial susceptibility test* is a determination of the least amount of an antimicrobial chemotherapeutic agent that will inhibit the growth of a microorganism *in vitro,* using a tube-dilution method, agar cup, or disk-diffusion method. The test may function as an aid in the selection of a chemotherapeutic agent by the physician. Also, the concentration of antimicrobial agents in body fluids may be determined by biological assay with an organism of known susceptibility for the specific agent.

The laboratory diagnosis of *viral infections* is based upon

1. Examination of the infected tissues for pathognomonic changes or for the presence of viral material
2. Isolation and identification of the viral agent
3. Demonstration of a significant increase in antibody titer to a given virus during the course of the illness
4. Detection of viral antigens in lesions, using fluorescein-labeled antibodies
5. Electron microscopic examination of vesicular fluids or tissue extracts

Blood is used for serological tests but seldom for virus isolation. Acute and convalescent-phase blood specimens must be examined in parallel to determine whether antibodies have appeared or increased in titer during the course of the disease. Some examples of human viral infections are respiratory infections (Adenovirus group); diseases of the nervous system, such as polio and Coxsackie viruses of the picornavirus group; smallpox (poxvirus group); measles (paramyxovirus group); chicken pox (herpesvirus group); and influenza (myxovirus group).

Members of *Mycoplasmataceae* pleuropneumonia-like organisms (PPLO) are of a range of size similar to the larger viruses. They are highly pleomorphic because they lack a rigid cell wall, they can reproduce in cell-free media, and they do not revert to or from bacterial parental forms as the L-forms. Specimens (sputum, bronchial secretions, urinary sediment, etc) for the primary isolation of mycoplasmas (*Mycoplasma pneumoniae, M hominis,* etc) should be cultured on agar media containing peptone, serum, ascitic fluid, whole blood, or egg yolk. The species identification may be by growth inhibition on agar medium containing type-specific rabbit antisera. Antigenic variants or subspecies may be detected by immunodiffusion. Various PPLO are pathogenic, parasitic, or saprophytic. Mycoplasmas have a predilection for mucous membranes and are associated with primary atypical pneumonia and bronchitis.

Clinical parasitology is a science that is concerned with the parasitic protozoa (amoeba), the helminths (cestodes, tapeworms; trematodes, flukes; nematodes, roundworms), and the arthropods. The identification of protozoan ova is based on detailed microscopic morphology (nuclei and so on) using wet mounts (saline or iodine) or stained preparations (such as iron hematoxylin) obtained from fecal specimens (fresh or preserved with polyvinyl alcohol) that are concentrated by sedimentation, centrifugation, or flotation techniques. Trophozoite and/or cystic stages may be detected in fecal specimens associated with intestinal protozoa as in amebic dysentery caused by *Entamoeba histolytica.*

The commonly encountered helminths are *Necator americanus* (hookworm), *Trichuris trichiura* (whipworm), and *Enterobius vermicularis* (pinworm); they are identified by characteristic ova. Characterization of tapeworm segments (proglottids) or head (scolex) in a fecal specimen will differentiate *Taenia saginata* (beef tapeworm) from *Taenia solium* (pork tapeworm). Eggs of *T solium* and *T saginata* cannot be differentiated on a morphological basis.

Adult flukes oviposit a characteristic egg that may reach the urine, sputum, or feces. *Schistosoma japonicum* eggs have a small, indistinct spine; *S mansoni,* a distinct, large, lateral spine; and *S haematobium,* a distinct terminal spine.

Arthropoda is the largest of the animal phylum; arthropods are characterized by a segmented body, with the segments usually grouped in two or three distinct body regions; by a chitinous exoskeleton; several pairs of jointed appendages; and characteristic internal organs. Most arthropods can be preserved in 70% alcohol. They are of medical importance because they can infest humans and cause mechanical trauma or produce hypersensitivity from repeated exposure (eg, *Cimex lectularius,* the bedbug) or by toxin injection (eg, *Latrodectus mactans,* the black widow spider), by skin invasion (eg, *Sarcoptes scabiei,* the itch mite), and by transmitting disease (eg, *Anopheles* mosquitoes and malaria; fleas and *Yersinia pestis* or plague).

The serodiagnosis of parasitic diseases includes the following immunodiagnostic tests: complement-fixation (trichinosis), precipitin test (schistosomiasis), bentonite flocculation (ascariasis), hemagglutination (echinococcosis), latex agglutination (trichinosis), cholesterol flocculation (schistosomiasis), fluorescent antibody (malaria), and methylene blue dye test (toxoplasmosis).

IMMUNOCHEMISTRY

Clinical immunopathology[26] includes *general immunology* (immunofluorescence, immunodiffusion, immunoelectrophoresis, and agglutination tests), *radioimmunoassay* (RIA-hormones, vitamins, drugs, immunoglobulins), *tissue typing* (histocompatibility tests in organ transplants), *cellular immunology, cancer immunology,* and *immunohematology.* Examples of each of these disciplines are discussed in this section and other parts of this chapter.

The ELISA, *enzyme-linked immunosorbent assay,* detects antibodies by an indirect technique using enzyme-linked antibodies to label antigenic substances in tissue or body fluid. The antigen is attached to a solid matrix and reacts with a specimen that may contain a complementary antibody. The antihuman globulin, which is conjugated with the enzyme, is added and the antigen reacts with the bound antibody of the patient. By adding the substrate molecule the enzyme is detected. This analytical test system has been used to identify antibodies to viruses, parasites, bacterial products, and in quantitation of some drugs.

Antibody response is a complex process involving the lymphoid cell system response to foreign stimulus or antigen. Hematopoietic cells in the fetal yolk sac, liver, or marrow develop into lymphoid stem cells that, in turn, differentiate into T lymphocytes of thymic origin and B lymphocytes of bone-marrow origin. The T cells further differentiate into lymphoblasts, which are responsible for *cell-mediated cellular immunity* (graft-versus-host reaction, tissue transplant rejection, tuberculin skin testing, *delayed-type hypersensitivity*). B cells differentiate into plasma cells, which are responsible for humoral immunity, which is mediated by circulating serum immunoglobulins (*immediate-type hypersensitivity*).

Macrophages can cooperate in presentation of antigen to the T or B lymphoblasts. Cooperation between T and B cells, immunological memory, development of immune tolerance to antigens, and genetic control of the immune response are integral properties of the immune system and are related to development of immune deficiency and autoimmune disease.

The identification and determination of *immunoglobulins* (IgG, IgM, IgA) by radial immunodiffusion and immunoelectrophoresis were discussed in the section on proteins. *IgM* (γM) is the earliest antibody found in the primary immune response and falls rapidly after the onset of IgG antibody synthesis. *IgG* (γG) is the major class of antibody in both the primary and secondary immune response. IgG can cross the placenta to provide the early forms of antibody protection for the newborn. IgG and IgM can participate in the complement fixation reaction. *IgA* (γA) is found predominantly in saliva and secretions of the gastrointestinal and respiratory tracts. In contrast to IgM and IgG, only a small portion of total IgA is found in blood. IgA functions in protection against pathogens that enter the host through the respiratory or gastrointestinal tract. *IgD* (γD) is found in trace quantities in sera and its function is unknown. *IgE* (γE) is probably the most important antibody in acute hypersensitivity or allergic reactions. Reaction of mast cell- or basophil-bound IgE with antigen initiates the release of histamine, slow-reacting substance (SRS), serotonin, and bradykinin and the subsequent allergic response. IgE is best quantitated by RIA. Mean serum levels (mg/dL) in healthy adults are IgG 1200 ± 500, IgA 210 ± 140, IgM 140 ± 70, IgD 3, and IgE < 0.1.

Heterophile antibodies are agglutinins that are capable of reacting with antigens that are entirely unrelated to those that stimulate their production. These antibodies, which occur in the serum of patients with infectious mononucleosis or serum sickness, will agglutinate formalized horse erythrocytes. To distinguish the specific *heterophile agglutinins of infectious mononucleosis*, the serum sample is mixed with guinea-pig kidney tissue or beef erythrocyte stromata; the infectious mononucleosis antibody will be absorbed and inactivated by the beef cells but not by the kidney tissue, and subsequent agglutination of horse erythrocytes will occur only in the kidney-tissue system. This test is used to detect infectious mononucleosis even prior to clinical symptoms. The heterophile titer has no relation to the course or severity of the disease.

Two protein constituents of human plasma, *rheumatoid factor* (RF) and *C-reactive protein* (CRP) are of value in the differential diagnosis of rheumatoid diseases. CRP is a protein present in the serum of patients in the acute stages of bacterial and viral infections, collagen diseases, and other inflammatory processes. The presence of this antigen in serum is detected by agglutination of polystyrene latex particles sensitized with specific CRP antibody globulin. In the management of rheumatic fever, decreases in CRP blood levels are used to measure the effectiveness of therapy.

Rheumatoid arthritis is characterized by the presence of a reactive group of macroglobulins known as RF in blood and synovial fluid. RF is a protein of the IgM globulin fraction and is regarded as an autoantibody against antigenic determinants of IgG. Analysis of RF is based on agglutination procedures employing polystyrene latex particles coated with a layer of adsorbed human gamma globulin. The RF-antibody reaction causes a visible agglutination of the inert latex particles. CRP is not elevated in rheumatoid arthritis.

β-Hemolytic streptococci, the causative agent in rheumatic fever, produce streptolysin O and S, streptokinase, hyaluronidase, desoxyribonuclease, and NADase in the body. The growth of streptococci in tissue with elaboration of these proteins serves as the antigenic stimulus to evoke the production of specific antibodies (eg, *antistreptolysin-O, ASO*). The quantitation of the antibody titer to these enzymes is an index of the strength of the antigenic stimulus and the extent of the streptococcal infection. These antibodies can be detected by latex agglutination (ASO) or tests dependent on the inhibition of enzyme action by the antibody (anti-hyaluronidase inhibition of hyaluronic acid depolymerization by hyaluronidase).

The laboratory diagnosis of *syphilis* (treponemal disease) and the evaluation of a chemotherapeutic approach is based on serological tests. Demonstration of an antibody-like substance *reagin,* or of true antitreponemal antibody in the serum of infected individuals is accomplished by complement fixation or flocculation tests for reagin, or immunofluorescent techniques for treponemal antibody.

In the *complement fixation* tests (Kolmer CF), reagin reacts with a complex phosphatidic acid antigen (cardiolipin) and complement; the complement is bound and will not lyse hemolysin-sensitized red cells, which were added in the second phase of the test. In normal serum the reagin-cardiolipin complex is not formed, and the complement is free to react with hemolysin and lyse the erythrocytes.

Flocculation tests for determining syphilis use a cardiolipin-lecithin-cholesterol antigen that clumps in the presence of serum reagin occurring in nontreponemal diseases and syphilis (*Venereal Disease Research Laboratory, VDRL Test; rapid plasma reagin, RPR test*).

Treponemal antibody can be detected also by the reaction of the patient's serum with treponemal antigen and subsequent confirmation with fluorescein-labeled antihuman globulin as an indicator of primary antigen-antibody reaction (*fluorescent treponemal antibody, FTA test*). The patient's serum can be treated with an extract of treponemes prior to the FTA test to remove interfering antibodies and eliminate biological false-positives (FTA-Abs test). False-positives occur in related treponematosis such as yaws, pinta, and bejel. Increased reagin titers also occur in malaria, leprosy, infectious mononucleosis, chronic rheumatoid arthritis, or systemic lupus erythematosus and in patients on hydralazine therapy.

Febrile antibodies are present in the serum of patients with certain bacterial or rickettsial infections (spotted, typhus, or Q fever). In typhus the patient's serum contains a febrile antibody that will agglutinate a suspension of *Proteus OX-19* bacteria (Weil-Felix reaction). *Salmonella* O-H, *Pasteurella tularensis*, and *Brucella abortus* antigens are used in febrile antibody tests for diagnosis of typhoid or paratyphoid fever, tularemia, and brucellosis, respectively.

Toxoplasmosis is a major cause of birth defects. An expectant mother may become infected with oocysts in uncooked meat or from cat fur and may infect the fetus transplacentally. Toxoplasmosis testing is based on detecting serum antibody by a hemagglutination procedure. Red cells sensitized by exposure to toxoplasmosis antigen are agglutinated by the specific antibody.

Radioimmunoassay (RIA)[27] has been mentioned in various sections of this chapter as an analytical tool in the measurement of hormones, immunoglobulins, drugs, and steroids. The basic principle of RIA is

$$Ag^* + Ag + Ab \rightleftharpoons Ag^*Ab + AgAb + Ag^* + Ag$$

RIA is not to be confused with the *specific reactor assay,* which uses labeled antigen and nonantibody protein receptors for vitamin B_{12}, T^4, T^3, and cortisol assays.

All procedures are based on the observation that radiolabeled antigens (Ag*) compete with nonlabeled antigen (Ag) for binding sites on specific antibody (Ab) in the formation of antigen-antibody complexes (Ag*Ab, AgAb). When increasing amounts of Ag are added to the assay, the binding sites of Ab are saturated progressively and the antibody can bind less Ag*. Therefore, the ratio of bound to free Ag* (B/F) or percent Ag* bound is a direct index of the concentration of Ag in the assay.

The requirements for RIA are (1) preparation and characterization of Ag, (2) radiolabeling of Ag, (3) preparation of specific Ab, and (4) development of the assay system and methods to separate free (Ag, Ag*) from antibody bound (AgAb, Ag*Ab) antigen.

Antigens can be prepared from natural tissue sources or preferably synthesized. ^{3}H, ^{14}C, or ^{125}I-labeled antigens are used routinely in the assay. The biological and immunochemical activity of the antigen must not be altered in the tagging procedure, and the specific activity of Ag* must be extremely high so that tracer quantities can be used in the assay. Tritium labeling and iodination (^{125}I) produce the highest specific activity, but also increase susceptibility of Ag* to internal degradation and self-radiolysis, in contrast to ^{14}C. In many instances, the original antigen cannot be iodinated, but can be altered chemically in such a way as to retain full antigenic cross-reactivity in RIA; for example, cyclic adenosine monophosphate (cAMP) has no tyrosyl or histidyl residue for iodination; ^{125}I-succinylcyclic AMP-tyrosine methyl ester retains full cross-reactivity with antibodies to cAMP and is used in the assay.

Hormones, steroids, and drug substances are *haptens*. They do not produce the antibody response when injected by themselves, but will produce antibodies specific for the hapten when injected as a hapten-protein carrier conjugate. Gastrin (hapten) is coupled to albumin (protein-carrier) by treatment with carbodiimides (CCD), which couple functional carboxyl, amino, alcohol, phosphate, or thiol groups. Morphine must be converted to the 3-O-carboxymethyl derivative prior to CCD coupling with albumin to provide a functional coupling group in the hapten. The hapten-conjugate usually is emulsified in a mineral oil preparation of killed *Mycobacterium* (Complete Freund's Adjuvant) and injected intradermally in rabbits or guinea pigs on several occasions. The serum antibody must have both high specificity and affinity for the antigens.

The *assay system* contains Ag*, sample-containing endogenous Ag or a standard Ag and antibody, at specified pH (6.5 to 8.5). After incubation at 5° to 37° for anywhere from 1 hour to several days, free and antibody-bound antigen must be separated. This is accomplished by *double-antibody technique, solid-phase RIA, resin techniques,* or *salt or solvent precipitation.* In the double-antibody technique, antiglobulin (Ab′) serum is added to the assay system after incubation. Ab-Ag* and Ab-Ag complexes are antibody-globulin antigen complexes. The antiglobulin will react to form insoluble Ab′-Ab-Ag* and Ab′-Ab-Ag complexes, which can be removed by centrifugation. The free Ag*, Ag is in the supernate.

The solid phase RIA is performed by coating tubes with Ab; Ag and Ag* react, compete, and bind with Ab on the wall of the tube. Unreacted Ag and Ag* are separated by decanting and rinsing the tube. Ab also can be bound covalently with isothiocyanate to dextran gel particles. Ag and Ag* will compete and bind with Ab on particles. Bound antigen then can be separated from free antigen by centrifugation.

RIA has been applied to analysis of hormones (ACTH, angiotensin I and II, gastrin, HCG, FSH, GH, glucagon, HLH, HPL, insulin, thyroxine), steroid hormones (aldosterone, androstenedione, glucocorticoids, testosterone, estrones, progesterone), drug substances (digoxin, digitoxin, amphetamines, barbiturates, morphine, LSD, ouabain), endogenous substances (cAMP, cyclic GMP, prostaglandins, immunoglobulins, hepatitis antigen, carcinoembryonic antigen—CEA). Examples of the specific assays are discussed in other sections.

CEA and *α-1-fetoprotein* (AFP) are proteins found in fetal tissue. CEA analysis was first proposed as a specific test for the early detection of bowel cancer. Although the test does not have absolute specificity for this disease, it may prove of value as a diagnostic aid and therapy monitor. CEA can be detected by RIA. Serum levels > 2.5 ng CEA/mL are found in 60% to 70% of patients with adenocarcinoma of the colon; positive levels also are found in lower percentages in carcinomas of the pancreas, stomach, liver, breast, endometrium, ovary, kidney, and bronchus, as well as in other conditions such as gastrointestinal polyps, colitis, diverticulitis, and cirrhosis. CEA appears to be associated primarily with tumors of entodermally derived epithelial tissue. The similarity between CEA and cell-surface glycoproteins and sialic acids has stimulated considerable research interest in a new approach to cancer chemotherapy.

The study of *tissue-transplantation antigens* is an important factor in studies on tissue and organ transplants. ABO blood group antigens are involved in survival of skin and renal grafts. Because of the presence of natural occurring anti-A and B, avoidance of ABO incompatibility is important in clinical grafting. The *HL-A antigens* are found on tissue and on the white cells. There is one major histocompatibility locus, comprising a number of alleles or linked genes, on a single chromosome segment. Each allele controls four to five groups of major transplantation antigens. These HL-A isoantigens affect the survival of allogenic tissue grafts and organ transplants. HL-A antigens can be typed by a leukoagglutination method in which the patient's or donor's white cells are reacted with specific HL-A antisera. HL-A typing also can be performed by a cytotoxicity test in which lymphocytes are mixed with antisera and complement. The antibody can destroy the lymphocytes if a corresponding antigen is present on the cell surface.

REFERENCES

1. Simmons A. *Hematology—A Combined Theoretical and Technical Approach.* Philadelphia: WB Saunders, 1989, p 387.
2. Christensen RL, Triplett DA. *Lab Med* 1982; 13(11):666.
3. Bollinger P, Brailas CD, Drewinko B. *Lab Med* 1983; 14:492.
4. *Central File for Rare Donors.* Milwaukee: American Association of Blood Banks, nd.
5. Lockyer WJ. *Essentials of ABO-Rh Grouping and Compatibility Testing: Theoretical Aspects and Practical Applications.* Bristol, UK: Wright, 1982, p 56.
6. Berson S, Yalow R. *Gastroenterology* 1972; 62:1061.
7. *Federal Register* 37FR17419, Aug 26, 1972.
8. Broughton PMG, Dawson JB. *Adv Clin Chem* 1972; 15:288.
9. Solberg HE, Stamm D. *Clin Chim Acta* 1991; 202(1–2):S5.
10. Meinke W. *Anal Chem* 1971; 43:28A.
11. Vidall A, et al. *Clin Chim Acta* 1991; 202 (1–2):S23.
12. Fraser CG. *Arch Path Lab Med* 1992; 116(9):916.
13. Young DS. *Effects of Drugs on Clinical Laboratory Tests,* 4th ed. Washington, DC: AAAC Press, 1995.
14. Linnet K. *Clin Chem* 1988; 34(7):1379.
15. Peterson CM. *Diagn Med* 1980; 78(Jul/Aug):73.
16. *Radial Immunodiffusion and Immunoelectrophoreses for Qualitation and Quantitation of Immunoglobulins.* DHEW Publ HSM-72-8102. Washington DC: Department of Health, Education, and Welfare, 1972.
17. Warnick GR. *Scand J Clin Lab Invest* 1990; 198:9.
18. Statland BE. *Clinical Decision Levels for Lab Tests.* Oradell, NJ: Med Econ, 1983.
19. Godolphin W, et al. *Clin Chem* 1990; 36(9): 1551.
20. Szilagyi G, Aning V, Karmen A. *J Clin Lab Automation* 1983; 3:117.
21. Bradley GM. *Diagn Med* 1980; 63(Mar/Apr).
22. Rubenstein K, et al. *Biochem Biophys Res Comm* 1972; 47:846.
23. Baron J. *Scand J Gastroenterol* 1970; 5:9.
24. Sculkes A. *Aust NZ J Surg* 1990; 60(8):575.
25. Kuhn PJ. *Mod Lab Observer* 1983; 108(Sept).
26. Sell S. *Immunology, Immunopathology, and Immunity,* 4th ed. New York: Elsevier, 1987.
27. Patrono C, Peskar BA, eds. *Radioimmunoassay in Basic and Clinical Pharmacology.* New York: Springer-Verlag, 1987.

BIBLIOGRAPHY

Alois RM. *Principles of Immunology and Immunodiagnostics.* Philadelphia: Lea & Febiger, 1988.

Balows A, ed. *Manual of Clinical Microbiology,* 5th ed. Washington, DC: Am Soc Microbiol, 1991.

Beaver PC. *Clinical Parasitology,* 9th ed. Philadelphia: Lea & Febiger, 1984.

Beck WS, ed. *Hematology,* 5th ed. Cambridge: MIT Press, 1991.

Bick RL. *Disorders of Thrombis and Hemostasis: Clinical and Laboratory Practice.* Chicago: ASCP Press, 1992.

Brostoff J, et al. *Clinical Immunology.* New York: Gower Medical, 1991.

Chandrasoma P. *Concise Pathology.* Norwalk, CT: Appleton & Lange, 1991.

Coon JS, Weinstein RS. *Diagnostic Flow Cytometry.* Baltimore: Williams & Wilkins, 1991.

Dacie J, Lewis S. *Practical Hematology,* 5th ed. London: Churchill, 1984.

Davis FA. *Modern Blood Banking and Transfusion Practices.* Philadelphia: FA Davis, 1983.

Doucet LD. *Medical Technology Review.* Philadelphia: JB Lippincott, 1981.

Edwards PR, Ewing WH. *Identification of Enterobacteriaceae,* 4th ed. New York: Elsevier, 1986.

Faulkner W, et al. *Handbook Clinical Laboratory Data.* Cleveland: Chem Rubber, 1980.

Graff L. *A Handbook of Routine Urinalysis.* Philadelphia: JB Lippincott, 1983.

Hawcroft DM. *Diagnostic Enzymology.* London: Wiley, 1987.

Henry JB. *Clinical Diagnosis and Management by Laboratory Methods,* 19th ed. Philadelphia: WB Saunders, 1996.

Hicks JM, Young DS. *Directory of Rare Analyses.* Washington, DC: AACC Press, 1997.

Kaplan A, Szabo, LL. *Clinical Chemistry: Interpretation and Techniques,* 3rd ed. Philadelphia: Lea & Febiger, 1988.

Kaplan LA, Pesce AJ. *Clinical Chemistry,* 2nd ed. St Louis: Mosby, 1989.

Lamparczyk HK. *Analysis and Characterization of Steroids.* Boca Raton, FL: CRC Press, 1992.

Lee GR. *Wintrobe's Clinical Hematology,* 9th ed. Philadelphia: Lea & Febiger, 1993.

Lynch MJ. *Medical Laboratory Technology,* 4th ed. Philadelphia: WB Saunders, 1983.

Matsuda M, et al, eds. *Fibrinogen No 4: Current Basic and Clinical Aspects* (Proc, 1989 Workshop, Tokyo), New York: Elsevier, 1990.

Melamed MR, et al. *Flow Cytometry and Sorting,* 2nd ed. New York: Wiley-Liss, 1990.

Migle JB. *Laboratory Medicine-Hematology,* 6th ed. St Louis: Mosby, 1982.

Miller LE, et al. *Manual of Laboratory Immunology,* 2nd ed. Philadelphia: Lea & Febiger, 1991.

Moffat AC. *Isolation and Identification of Drugs,* 2nd ed. London: Pharmaceutical Press, 1986.

Narins RG, ed. *Diagnostic Techniques in Renal Disease.* New York: Churchill Livingstone, 1992.

Nyhan WL. *Abnormalities in Amino Acid Metabolism in Clinical Medicine.* Norwalk, CT: Appleton-Century-Crofts, 1984.

Patrono C, Peskar BA, eds. *Radioimmunoassay in Basic and Clinical Pharmacology.* New York: Springer-Verlag, 1987.

Sonnenwirth AC. *Gradwohl's Clinical Laboratory Methods and Diagnosis,* 8th ed. St Louis: Mosby, 1980.

Stahr HM, ed. *Analytical Methods in Toxicology.* New York: Wiley, 1991.

Stockley IH. *Drug Interactions,* 2nd ed. Oxford: Blackwell, 1991.

Tiwari JL, Terasaki PI, eds. *HLA and Disease Associations.* New York: Springer-Verlag, 1985.

Walker RH, ed. *Technical Manual.* Arlington, VA: American Association of Blood Banks, 1990.

Wentworth BB, ed. *Diagnostic Procedures for Mycotic and Parasitic Infections,* 7th ed. Washington, DC: American Public Health Association, 1988.

PERTINENT REFERENCE JOURNALS

Adv Clin Chem
Am J Clin Pathol
Am Clin Prod Rev
Am J Hosp Pharm
Am J Med Technol
Anal Chem
Biotechniques
Clin Chem
Clin Chim Acta
J Clin Lab Automation
J Lab Clin Med
Lab Med
Lab Notes Med Diag
Med Lab Obs
Med Lab Tech
Scand J Clin Lab Invest
Std Methods Clin Chem

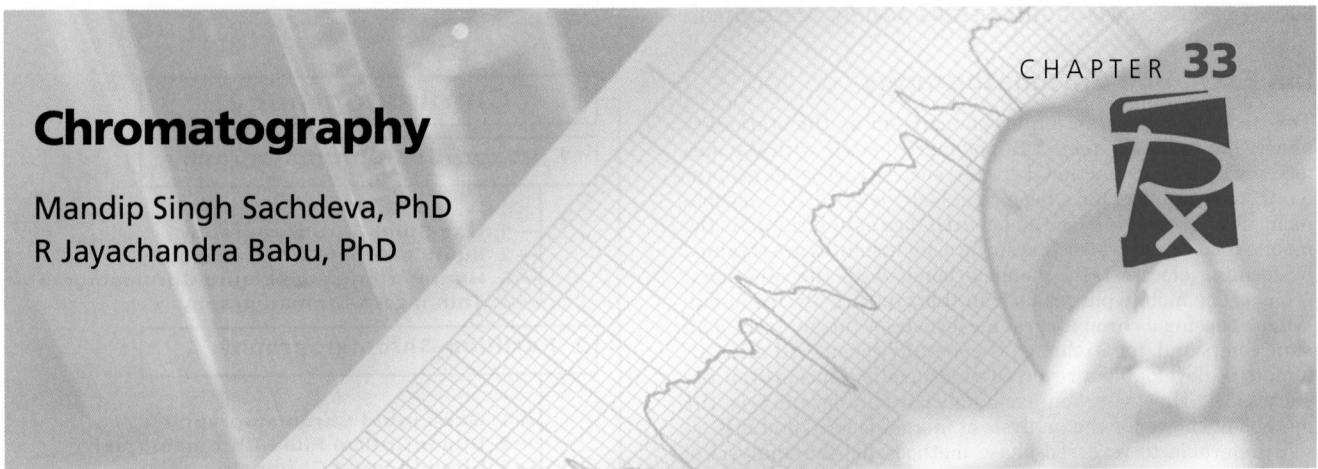

CHAPTER 33

Chromatography

Mandip Singh Sachdeva, PhD

R Jayachandra Babu, PhD

The term *"chromatography"* is derived from Greek, chroma meaning, *"color,"* and graphein meaning *"to write."* Mikhail Tswett (1906)[1] a Russian botanist used the technique to separate various plant pigments by passing solutions of them through glass columns packed with finely divided calcium carbonate. The separated species appeared as colored bands on the column and based on this phenomenon this process was called as chromatography. The chromatographic technique is now widely used for the separation, identification, and determination of the chemical components in complex mixture.

Chromatography according to USP can be defined as a procedure by which solutes are separated by a differential migration process in a system consisting of two or more phases, one of which moves continuously in a given direction and in which the individual substances exhibit different mobilities by reason of differences in adsorption, partition, solubility, vapor pressure, molecular size, or ionic charge density. The individual substances thus obtained can be identified or determined by analytical methods.[2] Thus, the term chromatography can be applied to a group of methods for separating molecular mixtures. One of the phases is a fixed bed of large surface area, whereas the other is a fluid that moves through or over the surface of the fixed phase. The components of the mixture must be of molecular dimensions, which require that they be in solution or in the vapor state. The relative affinity of the solutes for each of the phases must be reversible to ensure that mass transfer occurs during the chromatographic separation. The fixed phase is called the *stationary phase,* and the other is termed the *mobile phase.* The stationary phase may be a porous or finely divided solid or a liquid that has been coated in a thin layer on an inert supporting material. It is necessary that the stationary phase particles be as small and homogeneous as possible to provide a large surface area so that sorption and desorption of the solutes will occur frequently and efficiently. Depending on the type of chromatography employed, the mobile phase may be a pure liquid or a mixture of solutions (eg, buffers), or it may be a gas (pure or a homogeneous mixture).

Modern pharmaceutical formulations are complex mixtures including, in addition to one or more medicinally active ingredients, a number of inert materials such as diluents, disintegrants, colors, and flavors. To ensure quality and stability of the final product, the pharmaceutical scientist must be able to separate these mixtures into individual components prior to quantitative analysis. The complex nature of the polymers used in the manufacture of novel drug delivery systems makes the drug separation even more complicated. Moreover, comparison of the relative efficacy of different dosage forms of the same drug entity requires the analysis of the active ingredient in biological matrices such as blood, urine, and tissue.

Among the most powerful techniques available to the analyst for the resolution of these mixtures are a group of highly ef-

ficient methods collectively called *chromatography.* Because this technique is involved so intimately in all aspects of pharmaceutical research and development, the pharmacist or pharmaceutical scientist should possess a working knowledge of chromatographic principles and techniques. *Electrophoresis,* a separation technique especially useful for resolving mixtures of biological molecules, has some similarities to chromatography and is also discussed in this chapter.

CLASSIFICATION OF CHROMATOGRAPHIC METHODS

Chromatographic techniques can be classified into five types based on the type of equilibration process. These are (1) adsorption, (2) partition, (3) ion exchange, (4) pore penetration, and (5) affinity chromatography.

Adsorption Chromatography

The stationary phase is a solid on which the sample components are adsorbed. The mobile phase may be a liquid (*liquid-solid chromatography*) or a gas (*gas-solid chromatography*); the components distribute between the two phases through a combination of sorption and desorption processes. *Column chromatography* is a typical example of adsorption chromatography in which the solid stationary phase is packed in a tubular column, and the mobile phase is allowed to flow through the solid. *Thin-layer chromatography* is another example of sorption chromatography in which the stationary phase is a *plane,* in the form of a solid supported on an inert plate.

Partition Chromatography

The stationary phase is a liquid supported on an inert solid. Again, the mobile phase is a liquid (*liquid-liquid partition chromatography*) or a gas (*gas-liquid chromatography*). *Paper chromatography* is a type of partition chromatography in which the stationary phase is a layer of water adsorbed on a sheet of paper. In the normal mode of operations of liquid-liquid partition, a polar stationary phase (eg, water or methanol) is used with a nonpolar mobile phase (eg, hexane). This favors retention of polar compounds and elution of nonpolar compounds and is called *normal-phase chromatography.* If a nonpolar stationary phase is used along with a polar mobile phase, then nonpolar solutes are retained favoring elution of polar solutes. This is called *reversed-phase chromatography.*

Ion Exchange Chromatography

This technique uses an ion exchange resin as the stationary phase. Ion exchange resin is a polymeric matrix with the surface of which ionic functional groups, such as carboxylic acids or quaternary amines, have been chemically bonded. The mechanism of separation is based on ion exchange equilibrium. As the mobile phase passes over this surface, ionic solutes are retained by forming electrostatic chemical bonds with the functional groups. The mobile phases used in this type are always liquid. When choosing a chromatographic format for the analysis of an ionic compound, ion exchange is generally considered after attempts at developing a reversed-phase method has proven unsuccessful. However, ion-exchange chromatography is the method of choice for the analysis of inorganic ions, and it is often preferable to reversed-phase methods for the analysis of small organic ions.

Size Exclusion Chromatography

In this technique, the stationary phase is a polymeric substance containing numerous pores of molecular dimensions. The mobile phase containing analytes as solvated molecules are separated according to their size by their ability to penetrate a sieve-like structure (the stationary phase). Larger molecules that will not fit into the pores remain in the mobile phase and are not retained. This method is most suited to the separation of mixtures in which the solutes vary considerably in molecular size. The mobile phase in this type may be either liquid or gaseous. Size exclusion chromatography is used extensively for the preparative separations of macromolecules of biological origin as well as for the purification of synthetic-organic polymers.

Affinity Chromatography

This technique utilizes highly specific interactions between one kind of solute molecule and a second molecule covalently attached (*immobilized*) to the stationary phase. The immobilized molecule can be an *antibody* to a particular protein. When a crude mixture containing a large number of proteins is passed through the column, only the protein that reacts with the antibody is bound to the column. After washing all the other solutes off the column, the desired protein is dislodged from the antibody by changing the pH or ionic strength.

Capillary Electro-Chromatography (CEC)

Capillary electro-chromatography (CEC) can be defined as a liquid chromatographic method, in which the mobile phase is electro-osmotically driven through the chromatographic bed. The mobile phase in CEC has proven to be superior over other chromatographic methods in terms of its efficiency in separating ionic compounds and biomolecules.

The classifications given above for the various types of chromatographic processes can be deceptive in their simplicity. Except in isolated cases, pure adsorption or partition chromatography rarely occurs. In practice, separations frequently result from combination of adsorption and partitioning effects. The ultimate success of a chromatographic separation depends on the ability of analysts to recognize the limitations of the methods and adjust their experiments accordingly. The individual types of chromatographic techniques mentioned above are shown in Figure 33-1. The types of chromatography useful in qualitative and quantitative analysis that are employed in the USP assays and tests are Column, Gas, Paper, Thin-Layer, and High-Pressure or High-Performance Liquid Chromatography (HPLC). Paper and thin-layer chromatography are ordinarily more useful for purposes of identification because of their convenience and simplicity. Column chromatography offers a wide choice of stationary phases and is useful for the separation of individual compounds,

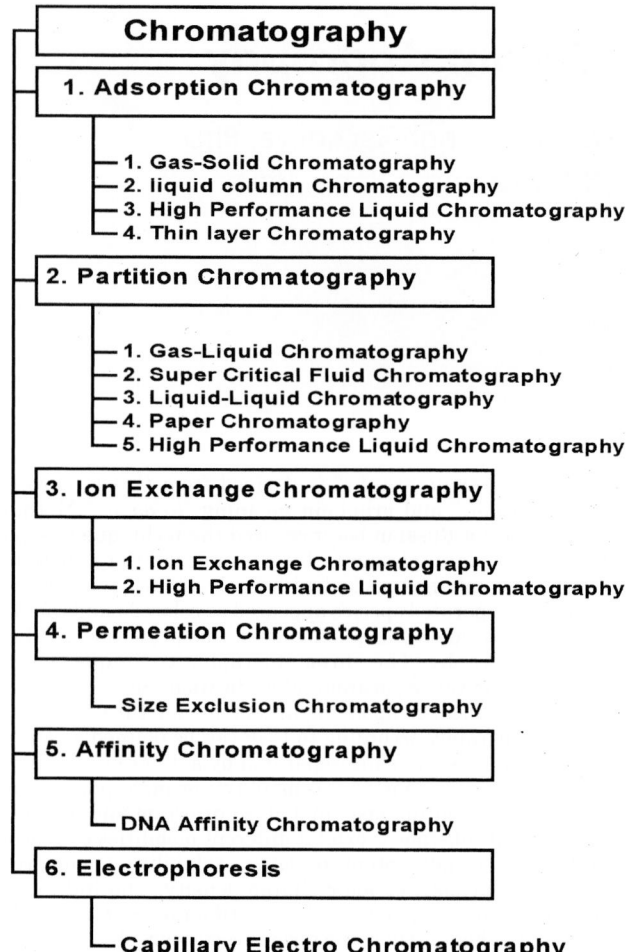

Figure 33-1. Classification of chromatographic techniques.

in quantity, from mixtures. Both GC and HPLC require elaborate apparatus and usually provide sophisticated methods to identify and quantify very small amounts of the material. A distinction needs to be made between *analytical* and *preparative-scale chromatography*. Analytical processes are used to identify and quantify tiny amounts of unknown materials. Preparative-scale chromatographic systems generally consist of a large cylindrical column within which the stationary material is packed. The mobile phase is invariably a liquid, and the stationary phase is either a solid, or a liquid supported by an adsorbent solid. Since the column is packed with stationary phase, liquid mobile phase must be forced through the column at a steady *pressure* for achieving the separation of the solutes of interest.

THE CHROMATOGRAPHIC PROCESS AND TECHNIQUES OF COLUMN DEVELOPMENT

To appreciate the theory and applications of chromatography, it is worthwhile to consider the events taking place in an ideal chromatograph. Conceptually, chromatography may be considered as being similar to the processes occurring in fractional distillation or sequential solvent extraction. In distillation, mixtures of liquids are separated by a series of steps involving vaporization and subsequent condensation. Each step involves an equilibrium between a vapor enriched in the more-volatile component and a liquid condensate of the same composition. Each single equilibration between the phases is termed a *theoretical plate,* and the length of the column required for one equilibration is called the *height equivalent to a theoretical plate (HETP).* The nomenclature has been adopted by chromatographers to describe the equivalent transfer of solute between the mobile and stationary phases.

In solvent extraction, a solute, commonly dissolved in an aqueous vehicle, is transferred partially in one step into an immiscible solvent. The amount of solute transferred is determined by its partition coefficient, which is the ratio of its concentration (in reality, activity) in the nonaqueous and aqueous phases, respectively. After the first step, the layers are separated, fresh solvent is brought in contact with the aqueous phase, and as a result, a new equilibrium based on the partition coefficient is established and more solute is transferred to the nonaqueous phase. Each of these extraction steps is equivalent to one theoretical plate and is analogous to the solute-transfer process occurring in a chromatographic system.

Chromatographic processes are classified according to the physical states of the mobile and stationary phases, that is, whether they are gaseous, liquid, or solid. Each of these techniques may be classified further depending on the method of mobile-phase development into *frontal analysis, displacement analysis,* and *elution analysis.*

FRONTAL ANALYSIS

In frontal analysis a large volume of a sample mixture is allowed to flow continuously through a chromatographic column. The most weakly retained component of the mixture emerges alone from the column first (Fig 33-2). After a period of time, during which the first component elutes continually at a constant rate, a sharp front appears indicating the appearance of the next most weakly retained compound. This now elutes as a mixture with the first component. The appearance of the next front indicates the emergence of the third most weakly retained compound in a mixture with the first two. This process continues until the effluent has the same composition as the sample being introduced into the column. After this point, no further separation can occur.

Because only the component that elutes first can be obtained in a pure state, frontal analysis never has been used extensively. However, research has indicated that it may be useful for the analysis of complex mixtures that cannot be resolved by other means. If the first derivative of the frontal chromatogram is taken, the resulting graph resembles exactly a normal elution pattern. The point of maximum height of the peak for each component corresponds to the inflection point of each rising front. The flat portions of the frontal chromatogram, being constant, give derivatives of zero and thus form the baseline. The computations of the derivatives can be done easily by a computer.

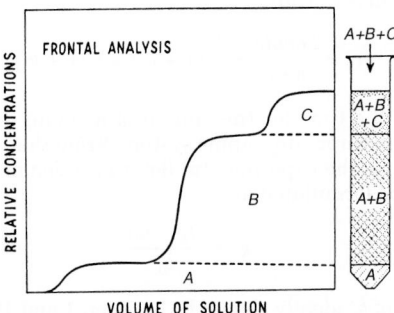

Figure 33-2. Frontal analysis for determining the number of components in a mixture. A solution containing a mixture of the Solutes *A*, *B*, and *C* is percolated through the adsorption column at the right. *A* is adsorbed least strongly and appears first in the effluent solution. This is followed by a mixture of *A* + *B* and finally *A* + *B* + *C*. The elution diagram illustrates the increasing concentration of solutes in the effluent.

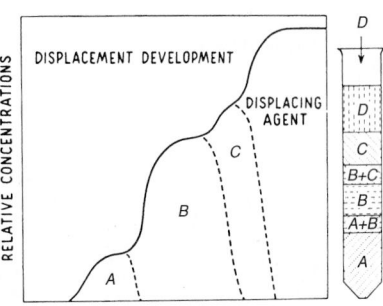

Figure 33-3. Displacement development for determining the number, nature and concentration of solutes. A sample containing Solutes *A* + *B* + *C* is applied to the top of an adsorption column. The chromatogram is developed with a solvent containing a displacing agent (*D*) that is adsorbed more strongly on the column than either *A*, *B*, or *C*.

DISPLACEMENT ANALYSIS

In displacement analysis, the sample mixture, dissolved in a small volume of solvent, is introduced onto the column as a narrow band at the top. The mobile phase, containing a *displacing agent,* then is allowed to pass through the column. The displacing agent is a substance that is retained more strongly by the stationary phase than any of the components of the sample mixture, and it, therefore, forces them off the surface of the stationary phase into the mobile phase.

As each of the displaced solutes move through the column in the mobile phase, it in turn acts as a displacing agent for less strongly retained compounds. The final result is that the solute that is bound least firmly is eluted first, followed in order by those more tightly bound and finally by the displacing agent. A displacement chromatogram is illustrated in Figure 33-3. The pattern is similar to that obtained with frontal analysis except that the trailing edge of each solute zone does not extend back through the length of the column.

Although displacement analysis is not used in quantitative studies, it has two potential advantages: it is possible to isolate in a pure state at least a portion of each of the compounds eluting from the column and in the course of the separation process the sample is concentrated, instead of being diluted as usually occurs in chromatographic analyses.

ELUTION ANALYSIS

Elution analysis is carried out by introducing the sample in as small a volume as possible onto the head of the column. The mobile phase then is allowed to flow through the system. The components with larger partition coefficients will be retarded in their passage through the system and will "elute" later. A typical elution chromatogram is shown in Figure 33-4.

The advantages of elution chromatography are that each component of a separated mixture can be isolated in a relatively pure state contaminated only by mobile phase and that the method can be used readily for quantitative analysis. If the composition of the mobile phase is not changed during the course of the development of the chromatogram, the technique is called *isocratic-elution analysis.*

A widely used modification of elution analysis, which is capable of overcoming the difficulties of long elution times and poor resolution of complex mixtures, is called *gradient-elution analysis.* In this adaptation two eluting solvents, one *weak* and one *strong,* are used to develop the chromatogram. The *weak* solvent has a lower affinity for the solutes, whereas the *strong* solvent has a higher affinity. The elution begins using only the weak solvent and, as the development progresses, the concen-

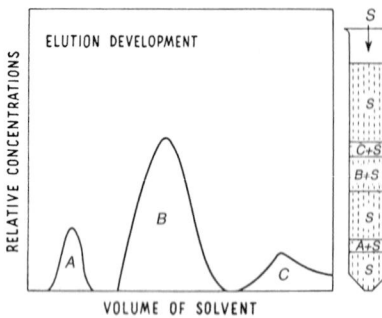

Figure 33-4. Elution development for separating components of a mixture. A sample containing Solutes $A + B + C$ is applied to the top of an absorption column, and the chromatogram developed by percolating pure solvent (S) through the column. The components separate as they pass down the column and are collected separately in the effluent.

tration of the strong solvent is increased gradually until the final mobile phase has a composition approaching that of the strong solvent. The mixing of the two solvents is done in a specially designed chamber at the top of the column. The result is that the composition and strength of the mobile phase change constantly during the analysis. Weakly retained solutes are eluted first by the weak solvent, and strongly retained solutes, which would not elute at all with the weak solvent or which would have undesirably long retention times, are eluted by the increasingly stronger mobile phase.

THEORY OF CHROMATOGRAPHY

Two theoretical approaches have been developed to describe the processes involved in the passage of solutes through a chromatographic system.

The *plate theory*, based on the work of Martin and Synge,[3] considers the chromatographic system as a series of discrete layers of theoretical plates. At each of these, equilibration of the solute between the mobile and stationary phases occurs. The movement of the solute is considered as a series of stepwise transfers from plate to plate.

The *rate theory*, discussed in the book by Giddings (see *Bibliography*), considers the dynamics of the solute particle as it passes through the void spaces between the stationary phase particles in the system as well as its kinetics as it is transferred to and from the stationary phase.

Aspects of both of these theories will be presented in the following discussion in order to exemplify the basic principles underlying the chromatographic process and introduce the experimental parameters necessary for the understanding and interpretation of chromatograms.

Chromatographic systems achieve their ability to separate mixtures of chemicals by selectively retarding the passage of some compounds through the stationary phase while permitting others to move more freely. Therefore, the chromatogram may be evaluated qualitatively, by determining the R_f, or *retardation factor*, for each of the eluted substances. The R_f is a measure of the fraction of its total elution time that any compound spends in the mobile phase. Because the solute particle proceeds down the column only when it is in the mobile phase, the R_f is related directly to the fraction of the total amount of solute that is in the mobile phase, and it can be expressed as

$$R_f = \frac{V_M C_M}{V_M C_M + V_S C_S} \tag{1}$$

where V_M is the volume of the mobile phase, and V_S is the effective volume of the stationary phase—the volume available for interaction with the solutes. The variables C_M and C_S indi-

cate the concentrations of the solute in the respective phases at any time. By dividing each term of the fraction by C_M, this can be simplified to

$$R_f = \frac{V_M}{V_M + K V_S} \tag{2}$$

where K, the partition coefficient, equals C_S/C_M, the ratio of the solute concentration in the stationary phase to that in the mobile phase and is an equilibrium constant that indicates the differential affinity of the solute for the two phases. It can be seen from this expression that a component with a large partition coefficient—one that is attracted strongly to the stationary phase—will have a small R_f and a long elution time because only a small fraction of its total mass will be in the mobile phase at any time. By dividing each term of the fraction by V_M, an alternate expression results

$$R_f = \frac{1}{1 + k'} \tag{3}$$

where the *capacity factor, $k' = KV_S/V_M$*. The capacity factor, which normally is constant for small samples, is a parameter that expresses the ability of a particular solute to interact with a chromatographic system. Because the volumes of the stationary and mobile phases are constant for any chromatographic experiment, k' is directly proportional to the partition coefficient. Therefore, the larger the value of k', the more the sample is retarded.

Both the retardation factor and the capacity factor may be used for qualitative identification of a solute or for developing strategies for improving separations. In terms of parameters easily obtainable from the chromatogram, the R_f is defined as the ratio of the distance from the origin traveled by the solute band to the distance traveled by the mobile phase in a particular time.

The R_f is used most conveniently in *complete chromatography,* such as paper and thin-layer chromatography, which occurs when the mobile phase is allowed to develop to a predetermined point in the system and then is stopped. Solutes then will have moved only a fraction of the distance traveled by the mobile phase. In *continuous chromatography,* as exemplified by the gas- and liquid-column techniques, mobile-phase development is permitted to continue indefinitely until the solutes elute from the end of the stationary phase. Measurement of the capacity factor, described below, is more useful in the latter cases.

The time that elapses from the start of the chromatogram to the elution maximum of the solute is called the *retention time, t_R,* a function of the length of the column and the rate of travel of the solute. The rate of travel is determined by

$$Rate = \mu\, R_f \tag{4}$$

where μ is the linear velocity of the mobile phase, usually expressed in cm/sec. Thus,

$$t_R = \frac{Length}{Rate} = \frac{L}{\mu}(1 + k') = t_0(1 + k') \tag{5}$$

where t_0 is the time for the elution of a solute that is not retained by the chromatographic system. From this, a convenient expression for the experimental determination of the capacity factor can be formulated as

$$k' = \frac{(t_R - t_0)}{t_0} \tag{6}$$

The values of k' ideally should be between 1 and 10; that is, solutes should be retained from 2 to 11 times as long as the unretained compound. Values of k' greater than 10 result in longer retention times and broad peaks, while values less than 1 lead to poor separation.

Another parameter used to describe the retardation of a solute is the *retention volume, V_R,* which is equal to the volume of mobile phase required to elute a compound from the system.

Therefore, the retention volume is equal to the product of the retention time and the flow rate of the mobile phase, $t_R F$, or $t_0(1 + k')F$. Because $t_0 F$ is equal to the volume of mobile phase in the system (V_M, or the *void volume*), the retention volume can be expressed as

$$V_R = V_M(1 + k') = V_M + K V_S \qquad (7)$$

Therefore, the retention volume of a solute depends on the relative volumes of the two phases and the partition coefficient. Because the phase volumes are identical for each solute in a mixture, the most important influence on retention arises from the partition coefficient. A large partition coefficient results in long retention since the solute spends more time in the stationary phase.

The retention time and retention volume frequently vary slightly from run to run due to small changes in operating parameters such as temperature and flow rate. To minimize the errors caused by these variations, retention time and/or volume frequently are measured with respect to another peak in the chromatogram, rather than from the origin. Because the peak of interest and the reference peak are affected similarly by the changes in experimental conditions, the retention measurements are more accurate. In these cases, the parameters are termed *relative retention time, RRT,* and *relative retention volume, RRV.*

The elution pattern of an ideal chromatographic peak is a curve whose shape is Gaussian. Thus, it can be described by parameters derived from the normal statistical distribution, ie, the standard deviation, σ, and the variance, σ^2. It can be seen clearly by reference to Figure 33-5 that the peak width at any point can be expressed as a multiple of the standard deviation. The inflection points are located at one standard deviation on either side of the mean at a level that is 60.7% of the overall height of the peak. The width at this point is therefore 2σ. If tangents to the peak are drawn through the inflection points and extended to the baseline, the width at the base, W_B, is 4σ. The width at one-half the height is 2.354σ (W_H).

Two further characteristics of the peak are the height and area. The area is equal to the integral of the equation representing the curve from the point where it leaves the baseline to the point where it returns and is proportional to the amount or concentration of the solute. The height is measured at the maximum and, therefore, corresponds to the greatest concentration in the zone. It is at the point of maximum height that retention times and volumes are measured.

Two parameters commonly used for estimating the effectiveness of a chromatographic system are N, the number of theoretical plates, and H, the height equivalent to a theoretical plate (HETP), which is defined as L/N, where L is the length of the column. Because the width and standard deviation of a peak can vary depending on experimental conditions, a better indicator of the sharpness of a peak is its *relative standard deviation* (RSD), σ/t_R. In practice, N is defined in terms of the re-

ciprocal of the RSD by the expression $N = (t_R/\sigma)^2$. Because it would be difficult to determine σ for each peak, the relationships given above ($W_B = 4\sigma$, $W_H = 2.354\sigma$) can be substituted to arrive at the equations

$$N = 16(t_R/W_B)^2 \text{ and } N = 5.545(t_R/W_H)^2 \qquad (8)$$

which are evaluated readily from the chromatogram. Although these are mathematically equivalent expressions, the former is used more frequently. However, the latter is useful particularly for nonideal peaks of unsymmetrical shape and possibly skewed or tailed, as the asymmetry is less pronounced at the half-height. At any particular retention time a system with a greater number of theoretical plates per unit length will produce a narrower peak and, therefore, will be capable of separating more complex mixtures.

Chromatographic systems are available in which N is 50,000/m or better. These values are established with selected test compounds, and the analyst should be aware that such levels would not be obtained with every sample. Because of intrinsic differences in the affinities of different compounds for the stationary phase, every solute will have a unique value for N in a particular system.

These procedures enable the chromatographer to derive from the experimental data a number of parameters, which characterize the retention behavior of individual compounds in a system. However, the greatest utility of chromatography lies in its ability to separate mixtures of solutes so that a number of individual substances may be quantitated or isolated in a pure state.

To develop strategies for accomplishing these objectives, consideration must be given to parameters that describe the interrelationships of both the retention- and peak-shape variables for more than one peak. The most significant of these parameters are *separation,* which is concerned with the relative positions of the band centers, and *resolution,* which describes the overlap of the leading and trailing edges of successive peaks. These are illustrated in Figure 33-6. In Figure 33-6A, a chromatogram with poor separation and resolution indicates the presence of two peaks, but is useful neither for quantitation nor for isolation of either substance. In Figure 33-6B, adequate separation has been achieved, but resolution remains poor because of overlap of the trailing edge of Peak 1 and the leading edge of Peak 2. In Figure 33-6C, the separation has remained constant while resolution has been optimized to lessen band overlap, resulting in an ideal chromatogram.

To achieve adequate separation of two adjacent peaks it is necessary to adjust the experimental variables so that the band centers or peak maxima elute at significantly different points on the chromatogram. This requires that the partition coefficients of the two solutes be sufficiently different so that one substance is retained more strongly than the other. Therefore, α, the *separation factor* or *selectivity factor,* may be defined as K_2/K_1, which is the ratio of the partition coefficient of the solute producing the second band to that of the solute producing the first. Because k', the capacity factor, is directly proportional to K, the separation factor also may be stated as the ratio of the respective k' values, k_2'/k_1'. From an experimental viewpoint, this is more useful, because k' can be determined more easily from peak retention parameters than K. Therefore, the separation factor usually is stated in terms of the *adjusted retention times* or *volumes* as

$$\alpha = \frac{(t_r)_2 - t_0}{(t_r)_1 - t_0} = \frac{(V_R)_2 - V_M}{(V_R)_1 - V_M} \qquad (9)$$

Because it is based on RRT and RRV, the separation factor also is termed the *relative retention.* In addition to being useful in optimizing chromatographic separation, α also has value in qualitative analysis by chromatography. If, under identical experimental conditions, an unknown compound has the same relative retention as a known substance, the identity of the

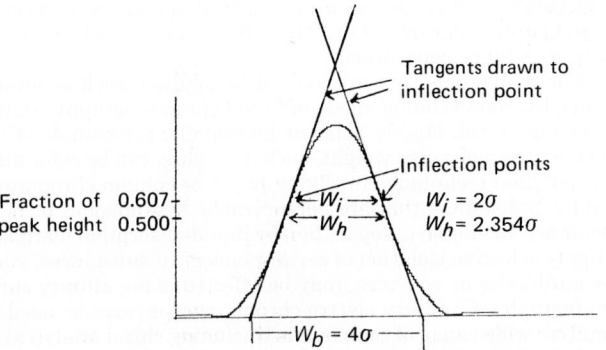

Fraction of 0.607
peak height 0.500

$W_i = 2\sigma$
$W_h = 2.354\sigma$
$W_b = 4\sigma$

Figure 33-5. Distribution characteristics of a typical Gaussian peak.

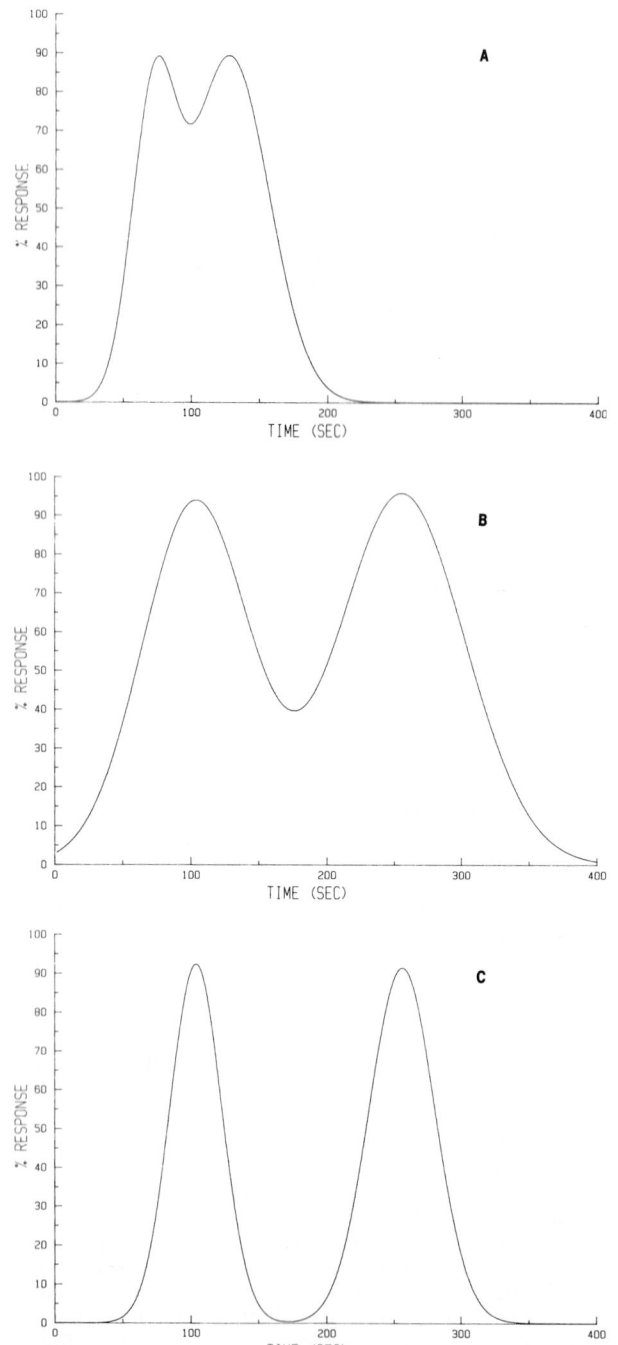

Figure 33-6. Effect of changes in separation and resolution on the elution pattern of adjacent peaks. **A.** The band centers are separated poorly and resolution is poor. **B.** Separation has been increased but band overlap remains, causing poor resolution. **C.** Peak separation is the same as in B, but overlap is reduced, giving good resolution.

unknown substance can be inferred. However, more positive identification, with greater confidence, requires that the same relative retention for the test sample be exhibited in two *different* chromatographic systems.

As shown in Figure 33-6B, it is possible to attain adequate separation of the peak maxima and yet fail to have a useful chromatogram because of overlap of the adjacent portions of the two peaks. In this case the partition coefficients of the two compounds are sufficiently different to effect separation, but the efficiency of the chromatographic system in terms of the

number of theoretical plates is low. For the purpose of comparison the *resolution* between two adjacent peaks can be defined as the distance between the band centers divided by the average peak width

$$R_S = \frac{2(t_{R2} - t_{R1})}{W_1 + W_2} \tag{10}$$

where the peak widths at the baseline are measured by drawing tangents through the inflection points and are, therefore, taken as four times the standard deviation. For two adjacent peaks of equal size, when $R_S = 1.00$ there will be a 4% contamination of each component by the other due to overlap. At $R_S = 1.25$ the overlap will be 2%, and at $R_S = 1.50$ it will be 0.3%. The calculation of resolution is useful especially when chromatography is being used to isolate pure compounds, as it gives the chromatographer an indication of where to start and end the collection of the peak to achieve the desired purity. An alternate equation that treats resolution in terms of easily measurable experimental parameters is

$$R_S = \left(\frac{N}{4}\right)\left(\frac{\alpha - 1}{\alpha}\right)\left(\frac{k'}{k' + 1}\right) \tag{11}$$

where N is the number of theoretical plates, α is the selectivity or separation factor, and k' is the capacity factor. Using this equation, the chromatographer can devise strategies for improving resolution by altering experimental conditions so as to affect one or all of N, α, or k' favorably. A more-detailed discussion of resolution, especially in those cases where the adjacent peaks are not equal in size and shape, can be found in the text by Snyder, Kirkland, and Glajch (see *Bibliography*).

TECHNIQUES OF CHROMATOGRAPHY

The five basic modes of chromatography—adsorption, partition, ion-exchange, size-exclusion, and affinity—can be applied to the analysis of pharmaceutical systems by a number of techniques that differ from each other according to the nature of the stationary and mobile phases and the apparatus used. Although it may be possible to analyze a sample using more than one of these methods, the choice of a particular technique depends on a number of factors, including the complexity of the sample, the chemical and physical properties of the compounds to be separated, the resolution required, the ease and speed of the technique and its ability to be automated, the availability and cost of the equipment, and the need to isolate the separated analytes.

If the materials are volatile and stable in the gas phase, GC may be the technique of choice because it is simple to perform, rapid, and capable of high resolution. If it is necessary to isolate eluted compounds in quantity, liquid- partition or thin-layer chromatography may be a more advantageous choice. Gas-chromatographic columns cannot handle large quantities of material and it is difficult to retrieve the eluants from the hot effluent gases. If the substances have a high molecular weight, such as proteins, triglycerides or polymers, liquid chromatography using the size-exclusion mode is necessary to achieve separation.

For compounds that are ionized in solution, such as amino acids, the ion-exchange mode of liquid chromatography particularly is useful. Highly polar or hydrophilic compounds of intermediate molecular weight, such as sugars, can be separated by partition techniques involving paper or column chromatography. Substances that are nonionizable, hydrophobic, or nonpolar are amenable to separation by liquid-adsorption methods. Highly selective isolation of certain biological substances, such as antibiotics or enzymes, may be effected using affinity chromatography. Capillary electro-chromatography can be used to analyze wide range of compounds (including chiral analytes) in biological fluids (eg, plasma, urine) in significantly shorter times than achieved by current GC and HPLC methods.

GAS CHROMATOGRAPHY

In 1941, in their paper on partition chromatography, which outlined the plate theory, Martin and Synge proposed the technique of gas chromatography (GC) with the following statement:

> "The mobile phase need not be a liquid but may be a vapor. Very refined separations of volatile substances should therefore be possible in a column in which a permanent gas is made to flow over gel impregnated with a non-volatile solvent in which the substances to be separated approximately obey Raoult's Law."[3]

In the subsequent 10 years, no one followed up on this suggestion, so Martin returned to it himself and with James developed the first separations using GC.[4] Once the validity and utility of the method had been demonstrated, other workers quickly adopted it, and GC became applied more rapidly and broadly to scientific research than any other analytical technique developed before that time. In GC, the sample is vaporized and injected onto chromatographic columns and then separated into many components. The elution is brought about by the flow of an inert gaseous mobile phase. In recent decade the development of gas chromatographic skill and its applications have been significant. Tens of thousands of papers have been published using GC as the analytical technique, and it is estimated that as many as 200,000 gas chromatographs are currently in use worldwide. The global market for GC instruments is estimated to be about $1 billion or over 30,000 instruments annually.[5]

Gas-chromatographic methodology is divided into two classes, depending only on the nature of the stationary phase as the mobile phase is always a gas. These are *gas–solid chromatography (GSC)*, in which the stationary phase is a solid adsorptive material and solute particles are removed from the mobile phase by electrostatic forces, and *gas–liquid chromatography (GLC)*, in which the stationary phase is a thin layer of liquid, coated, or bonded on the surface of an inert particle or on the walls of the column itself. In this method solute molecules are retained in the liquid phase based on their partition coefficients between it and the gaseous mobile phase.

Some of the advantages of GC are (a) fast analysis (typically in minutes); (b) efficient, providing high resolution; (c) sensitive, easy detecting ppm and often ppb; (d) non-destructive, making possible on-line coupling, eg, to mass spectrometer; (e) highly accurate quantitative analysis, typical RSDs of 1–5%; (f) requires small samples, typically μL; and (g) reliable and relatively simple and the technique is relatively inexpensive.

The disadvantages of GC include (a) it is limited to volatile samples; (b) not suitable for thermally labile samples; (c) fairly difficult for large, preparative samples; and (d) requires elaborate instrument such as mass spectroscopy, for confirmation of peak identity.[5]

Theory of Gas Chromatography

In the mid-1950s a group of Dutch chemical engineers began a study of the processes that caused band-broadening in chromatography. They derived an expression, commonly called the van Deemter equation, relating the height equivalent to a theoretical plate (HETP) to a number of experimental parameters, including the diameter of stationary phase particles, the diffusion coefficients of the solute in the stationary and mobile phases, and the flow rate of the mobile phase. For descriptive purposes the original, complicated equation frequently is given in the simplified form

$$\text{HETP} = A + B/\mu + C\mu \qquad (12)$$

where μ is the linear velocity, in cm/sec, of the mobile phase, and A, B, and C are coefficients that describe the various diffusion processes occurring in the chromatography that lead to band-broadening.

Coefficient A is called the *eddy diffusion* or *multiple-path coefficient* and is concerned with the different paths traveled by the molecules of a particular solute during their passage through the column. The particles of the stationary phase, whether irregularly or spherically shaped, are packed as tightly as possible, and the solute molecules must pass around them to proceed along the column. Because of the large number of possible paths, some molecules of the same kind will reach the end of the column before others. Faster molecules are found in the leading edge of the peak, and slower ones form the trailing edge. The net effect of this distribution is band-broadening. In a modern chromatographic column, which is packed with small, uniformly sized particles, the value of A is minimal and the contribution of this term to increasing the HETP is negligible. In a capillary GC column, which contains no solid particles, the value of A is zero.

Coefficient B in the van Deemter equation is termed the *coefficient of longitudinal diffusion*. Because the concentration of solute is lower at the edges of the band than in the center, a gradient exists and, during the travel of the band through the column, solute is diffusing continually through the mobile phase away from the center of the band. This phenomenon occurs at both the leading and trailing edges of the peak and contributes further to band-broadening. Because the equation predicts that the contribution to the HETP of this term is inversely proportional to the mobile phase velocity, the effect is more pronounced at low flow rates. Diffusion effects are more severe in GC than in liquid chromatography because diffusion coefficients are several orders of magnitude higher in a gas. The contribution of longitudinal diffusion to band-broadening can be lessened by the proper adjustment of flow rate and by increasing the viscosity of the mobile phase.

Coefficient C, the *coefficient of mass transfer,* is concerned with the transfer of the solute between the two phases. Because the mobile phase is moving rapidly, equilibrium between the two phases may not be attained. Therefore, some solute molecules in the mobile phase are not transferred to the stationary phase quickly enough, and, as a result, are carried ahead of the center of the band. Those in the stationary phase are retained too long and, hence, lag behind. In contrast to longitudinal diffusion, the contribution to the plate height of this term is directly proportional to flow rate; thus, to minimize the overall effect, a compromise in flow rate is necessary. Mass-transfer effects also may be lessened by using a very thin coating of stationary phase so that the area in contact with the mobile phase is maximized while diffusion deep into the stationary phase is reduced.

An efficient GC column will have several thousand theoretical plates, and capillary columns will have in excess of 10,000 theoretical plates. The HETP for a 1 m column with 10.000 theoretical plates would be 100 cm/10,000 plates = 0.01 cm/plate. In an HPLC, efficiency on the order of 400 theoretical plates per centimeter is typically achieved, and columns are 10 to 50 cm in length.

BASIC INSTRUMENTATION

The essential components of a gas chromatograph are the same whether the instrument is an inexpensive student-grade apparatus or a research instrument costing tens of thousands of dollars. The basic components are shown in the block diagram in Figure 33-7.

The *carrier gas,* which serves as the mobile phase, is supplied in steel tanks under high pressure. To reduce the pressure to a level compatible with the requirements of the instrument, a suitable two-stage diaphragm-controlled pressure regulator is fitted to the tank. The carrier gas, now at a pressure of approximately 40 to 80 psi, passes into a flow controller that allows the operator to adjust the flow rate to the desired operating level before the carrier gas moves into the instrument, which is contained within a thermostat controlled chamber capable of achieving temperatures ranging from less than ambient to as high as 400°.

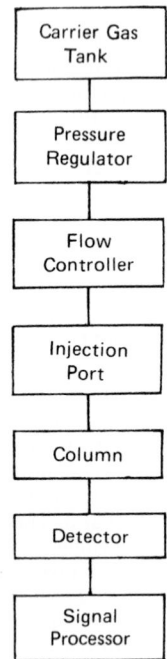

Figure 33-7. Block diagram of a gas chromatograph showing the essential components of the system.

The next component in the line of flow is the sample injection port. This is a small chamber, usually separately heated to a temperature slightly above that of the column, in which the analytical sample is made to vaporize rapidly before entering the column. The sample is introduced into the flowing gas stream through a self-sealing rubber or silicone *septum* using a microliter syringe. Injection of the sample solution may be done either manually or using and automatic injector, which gives more reproducible results. The sample may be injected into the chamber directly on the beginning of the column to minimize diffusion due to turbulence. Samples may be pure liquids, solids dissolved in liquid solvents, or gases. The gaseous mixture next enters the column, which is a tube, usually silica or stainless steel, 1 to 300 m long and with an internal diameter of 0.2 to 4.6 mm. The column may be straight, coiled, or U-shaped.

The interior of the column is filled with either a solid adsorbent material for GSC, or in the case of GLC, a liquid phase coated as a thin layer either directly on the walls or on a packing of small, inert solid particles. Based on their electrostatic attraction for the surface of the solid or their partition coefficients between the two fluids, the solutes are retained temporarily by the stationary phase. As the carrier gas continues to flow, the retained molecules diffuse back into the mobile phase.

At the end of the column, each of the separated solutes exists as a binary mixture with carrier gas and moves into the detector, which also may be heated to a level slightly higher than that of the column to prevent condensation of the solutes. The detector is a device that converts some physical property of the solute, such as thermal conductivity, ionizability, or electron-capturing ability, into an electrical signal that is proportional to the amount of solute in the carrier gas. This is amplified electronically and fed to a suitable signal processor that produces a record of the level of the signal versus time. The output also may be sent simultaneously to a computer for storage and calculation.

CARRIER GAS

The choice of the carrier gas is crucial to the success of the chromatography because it is the mobile phase. In theory any gas may be used, but for practical reasons such as inertness, purity, availability, and expense, usually helium or nitrogen and occasionally hydrogen, argon, or carbon dioxide are employed. The most prevalent carrier gas in the recent years is helium, and its usage is increased six-fold compared to 1970. One of the most important considerations is the purity of the gas, as a contaminated carrier gas will cause a drifting or elevated baseline or it may deposit its impurities on the column. Trace amounts of water can desorb other column contaminants and produce high detector background. Trace hydrocarbons in the carrier gas can cause a high background with most ionization detectors and thus limit their detectability. Water and trace hydrocarbons can be easily removed by installing a 5Å molecular sieve filter between the gas cylinder and the instrument. Drying tubes are commercially available, or they can be readily made by filling a 6-feet by 0.25″ column with GC grade 5Å molecular sieve. In either case, after two gas cylinders have been used, the sieve should be regenerated by heating to 300° C for 3 hours with a slow flow of dry nitrogen.[5] In addition, it is essential that the carrier gas be inert with respect to the sample components, the column-packing materials, and the components of the instrument. The viscosity also is important because low-viscosity gases such as hydrogen or helium allow higher flow rates to be maintained, whereas a gas with relatively high viscosity, such as nitrogen, may be useful in lessening longitudinal diffusion of the solutes and thereby reducing band-broadening.

STATIONARY PHASE

The interior of a GC column contains either an uncoated solid material for GSC or an inert *solid support* coated with a thin layer of *liquid phase* for GLC. The particles of the packing material are small (80- to 120-mesh) to minimize *void volume* (total volume of interstitial space between particles), while at the same time providing a large surface area for interaction with the solutes. Alternatively, in a column of capillary dimensions (<0.75 mm), the liquid phase may be coated directly on the wall.

In GSC the adsorbents most frequently used are activated charcoal, silica gel, alumina, or glass beads. For the analysis of low-molecular-weight compounds such as water or alcohols, molecular sieves may be used or columns may be chosen from a group of porous polymers made from styrene and divinylbenzene. These are manufactured in such a way that their porosity is controlled carefully, and their separation ability is achieved by a combination of adsorption and size exclusion.

For GLC, the most commonly used solid support material is diatomaceous earth, which is treated with acid and base to remove impurities and then calcined to activate the surface. Nonporous supports such as glass microbeads also have been used. The liquid phase is coated uniformly on the surface of the solid support usually at levels of 1% to 5% by weight. For the separation of compounds that are retained only slightly, amounts as high as 40% have been used. The liquid must be chemically stable, have a low vapor pressure at operating temperatures, and have specific solvent properties toward the compounds to be analyzed.

Today, there are in common use about 15 or 20 highly purified liquid phases that differ from each other in their overall polarity and specific selectivity for particular functional groups on the solute molecules. Most of these are based on silicone polymers with substituents such as phenyl, cyano, or trifluoropropyl introduced to affect polarity and selectivity. Methyl silicone and methyl phenyl silicone are the most commonly used liquid phases, and their use is increased from 28% in 1970 to 74% in 2000. Ethylene glycol polymers also are used frequently, mainly for the separation of polar compounds such as alcohols and amines, but the use of these compounds decreased by almost five times (32% in 1970 to 7% in 2000).[6] In the case of the nonpolar liquid phases, the elution of a mixture of solutes occurs usually in order of increasing molecular weight, as the larger the compound, the more nonpolar it likely is to be and the more strongly it will be retained. As the polarity of the liquid phase is increased, elution order will be based more on the relative polarities of the solutes, with the most polar substances being retained more strongly.

Several methods have been developed to facilitate the choice of the most-efficient stationary phase for a particular analysis. The Retention Index system of Kovats, a measure of the relative retention of a compound with respect to a series of *n*-alkanes, was formulated to catalog the relative polarities of the liquid phases. If the retention of the compound is determined on a polar and a nonpolar column, the difference in relative retention is a measure of the column polarity.

COLUMN DESIGN

Capillary Columns

Because of the relatively low viscosity of the mobile phase in GC, the contribution of solute diffusion to band-broadening can be substantial. In an effort to reduce the volume within which the solute can diffuse, narrow-diameter columns are used frequently. A small increase in efficiency has been achieved by using tubing with an inner diameter of about 1 mm. However, the greatest increase in efficiency has occurred with the use of *capillary columns*. The column diameter influences (i) broadening of chromatographic zones, (ii) column load quantity per column length unit, and (iii) the retention factor. The preferred column diameter in the capillary GC is 0.25 mm and 0.32 mm. Frequency of use of such columns in published literature is 73%. Researchers are interested in small diameter capillary columns, which are more compact and can be used in express-analysis and for the development of highly efficient columns.[6] The liquid phase is contained within these columns in either of two ways:

In more frequently used *wall-coated open tubular (WCOT)* columns the stationary phase is deposited as an extremely thin layer directly on the inner surface of the tube. This may be either as a film or, more frequently, by bonding it chemically to the wall of the capillary column. The latter is advantageous because it prevents *bleeding* or loss of the liquid phase due to its volatility at elevated temperatures.

In *support-coated open tubular (SCOT)* columns the inner surface of the tube is coated with a layer of inert support onto which the liquid is coated. Because of the irregularity of the support particles, the surface area of the SCOT column is larger, and therefore a more stationary phase is available to interact with the solutes. However, the mechanics of packing these columns are difficult, and they are not used as often as the WCOT type.

Because of its narrow diameter, the void volume in a capillary column is much lower than in the usual packed column and the ratio of V_S to V_M is high compared to a larger diameter column. In terms of plates per unit length, efficiencies four to five times greater than those of packed columns can be achieved by lessening eddy diffusion and increasing mass transfer (terms A and C in Equation 12). The absence of particles in the capillary decreases resistance to gas flow and permits the use of columns as long as 300 m. This results in much higher efficiencies, and columns of several hundred thousand theoretical plates are available.

The disadvantage of capillary columns is that they have low capacities due to the small volume of the stationary phase. Therefore, injection volumes must be very small (<0.1 μL) or injections must be made through a splitter that diverts more than 95% of the sample away from the column. The method also is not useful when it is desirable to collect the eluted solutes.

Packed Columns

Large-bore columns with inner diameters of 2.0 to 4.6 mm and packed with inert, solid particles coated with a thin layer of liquid phase also are used. They usually are made of stainless steel or glass and range in length from 1 to 3 m. They are attached at either end to the injection port and the detector, using compression fittings to achieve a gas-tight seal. Because the shape of the column has no effect on the chromatographic process, it is designed to conform to the dimensions of the oven. Shorter columns may be straight or U-shaped, but longer ones usually are coiled into a spiral.

For certain compounds, notably steroids, which are highly susceptible to degradation and molecular rearrangement on hot metal surfaces, glass columns are employed widely as their surfaces are relatively inert. The disadvantages of glass are that it is difficult to get a gas-tight seal at the injector and detector connections, and they are brittle enough to break under limited stress.

OPERATING CONDITIONS

Most chromatographic analyses are done in the *isothermal* mode in which the temperature of the instrument is maintained constant throughout the run. However, this method frequently is unsatisfactory for complex mixtures, when both volatile and comparatively nonvolatile solutes are present. If for these mixtures the column is operated at a high temperature, the low-boiling solutes will be eluted rapidly but not resolved while the less-volatile substances may be separated satisfactorily. At a lower operating temperature, all substances may be resolved, but the retention time for the less-volatile compounds will be excessively long and the peaks may be so broad as to be undetectable.

To obviate these problems, the technique of *temperature programming* may be used. In this method the temperature of the column is raised at a preset rate beginning at the time of injection of the sample. The programming rate may be constant during the run or, in more sophisticated instruments, periods of isothermal operation may be interspersed between temperature rises. The result of temperature programming is a chromatogram with evenly spaced peaks having good heights, resulting in an overall savings of time. The initial temperature should be chosen to minimize the retention time for the least-retained solute; the final temperature must be sufficient to elute the least-volatile compound in a reasonable time without exceeding the operating limits of the liquid phase.

DETECTORS

Detectors identify solutes as they exit the chromatographic column. As solutes are eluted from the GC column, they interact with the detector. The GC detector converts this interaction into an electrical signal that is sent to the data system. The magnitude of the signal is plotted versus time, and a chromatogram is generated. Gas chromatography detectors use one of several technology types to identify solutes as they exit the column.

Some of the commonly used methods include flame ionization, thermal conductivity, electron capture, nitrogen-phosphorous, flame photometric, and photo ionization type detectors as summarized in Table 33-1. These are grouped into two general classifications, *mass flow rate* detectors, which are sensitive to the rate of flow of the solute through the detector, and *concentration-sensitive* detectors, which respond to the concentration of solute in the mobile phase in the detector.[6,7]

The *Thermal Conductivity Detector (TCD)*, also called the *Hot Wire Detector (HWD)* or *katharometer*, is a concentration-sensitive detector and is used widely because it is a universal detector in that it responds to all solutes. In this device, a coil of fine wire, usually made of a tungsten–rhenium alloy, resides in a small chamber into which the column effluent flows. In practice most TCDs consist of a matched pair of wires, one of which is placed in the gas stream before it enters the column, while the other is at the end of the column. An electrical potential is placed across the wire filaments and they heat up due to their resistance.

Table 33-1. Summary of Commonly Used GC Detectors

NAME OF DETECTOR	TYPE	CARRIER GASES	SELECTIVITY	MINIMUM DETECTIBLE QUANTITY	OTHER CHARACTERISTICS
Flame ionization (FID)	Mass flow	Nitrogen or Helium	Organic compounds only	10^{-11}g (~50 ppb)	Excellent linearity and stability, Temperature limit −400°C
Thermal conductivity (TCD)	Concentration	Helium	Universal (all compounds)	10^{-9}g (~10 ppm)	Excellent linearity and good stability, Temperature limit −400°C
Electron capture (ECD)	Concentration	Make-up	Halides, nitrates, nitriles, peroxides, anhydrides, organometallics	10^{-9} to 10^{-12}g	Good linearity and fair stability
Nitrogen-phosphorus	Mass flow	Hydrogen and air	Nitrogen, phosphorus	10^{-12}g for P and 10^{-11}g for N_2	Very sensitive and highly specific
Flame photometric (FPD)	Mass flow	Hydrogen and air possibly oxygen	Sulphur, phosphorus, tin, boron, arsenic, germanium, selenium, chromium	10^{-7}g	Quenching or re-absorption of the light emitted by the selected species
Photo-ionization (PID)	Concentration	Make-up	Aliphatics, aromatics, ketones, esters, aldehydes, amines, heterocyclics, organ osulphurs, some organometallics	20^{-9}g	Good linearity and stability

Data from McNair HM, Miller JM. *Basic Gas Chromatography*. New York: John Wiley, 1997.

The resistance of the filament is a function of its temperature. When only carrier gas is flowing through the chamber, the filaments maintain a steady temperature, which is determined by the thermal conductivity of the gas; however, when a binary mixture of solute and carrier gas emerges from the column, the mixture has a different thermal conductivity and heat is conducted from the sample filament at a greater or lesser rate. This changes the resistance of the wire, and the change in resistance or current is a measure of the concentration of the solute in the detector.

The thermal conductivities of hydrogen and helium are as much as 10 times higher than those of most organic compounds, so even a small amount of solute will cause a large change in the output of the detector. Nitrogen, however, has conductivity close to that of most organic compounds, so sensitivity is lower with this carrier gas and, in fact, it is possible to obtain negative peaks. TCDs are simple, inexpensive, and nondestructive to the sample. They are relatively insensitive, however, compared to other detectors, and are generally not useful for analyses requiring detection of low levels of solutes such as drugs in biological fluids.

The *Flame Ionization Detector (FID)* is a mass flow detector and is the most frequently used detector in GC because it is highly sensitive, able to detect microgram quantities of solutes, and an almost universal detector. It responds well to most organic compounds but is insensitive to water and most inorganic substances. In this device, hydrogen and air or oxygen are introduced into the column effluent stream. The mixture is ignited and, as a result of the energy of the flame, electrons are stripped from the solutes and ions are formed. These charged particles migrate to a pair of oppositely charged collector electrodes in the chamber and cause a small electrical current to flow. The current, which is amplified to produce a useful signal, is proportional to the rate of flow of solute through the detector. In addition to their exceptional sensitivity, flame-ionization detectors are useful because of their large *linear dynamic range*. They will respond in a linear manner to amounts of solute that differ in concentration by several orders of magnitude.

Other highly sensitive detectors are available but their response is limited to compounds containing certain specific functional groups, such as nitrogen, phosphorus, or the halogens. This property of selectivity can be very useful, but even if the chromatographic separation is not optimal, an interfering solute will not be detected unless it contains the functional group for which the detector is specific. Thus, they impart a second level of selectivity to the procedure.

The *Electron Capture Detector (ECD)* is one of the most sensitive of detectors, being able to respond to nanogram, or even picogram, quantities of materials having functional groups that possess high electron affinity, such as the halogens or nitro groups. In this device, a radioactive source, usually ^{63}Ni, emits beta particles that interact with the carrier-gas molecules to form positive ions and electrons. These, in turn, migrate to oppositely charged electrodes in the detector chamber to produce a *standing current*. When a detectable solute elutes from the column, it is able to "capture" some portion of the electrons, thereby lowering the standing current. This decrease in the current is detected electronically and is proportional to the amount of solute.

The ECD is extremely sensitive to low levels of halogenated compounds such as pesticides. However, its linear response range is narrow, and it is very susceptible to permanent saturation if it is exposed to too high a concentration of a halogenated compound.

The *Thermionic Specific Detector (TSD)*, also called the *Nitrogen Phosphorus Detector (NPD)*, is a modified form of the FID that shows increased response to compounds containing nitrogen and phosphorus. It consists of a standard FID with an electrically heated bead of a solid alkali metal compound, such as rubidium silicate, suspended in the area above the flame assembly. In the presence of excess air, a plasma is formed in the area of the bead. This produces large numbers of ions from nitrogen- and phosphorus-containing compounds that are then detected at the collector electrodes, as in the FID. The mechanism of action is not understood fully, but its sensitivity for nitrogen- and phosphorus-containing compounds is 10^3 to 10^4 times greater than for other organic compounds. It, too, has important applications in pesticide-residue analysis.

Another modification of the FID, which has increased selectivity for sulfur and phosphorus containing compounds, is the *Flame Photometric Detector (FPD)*. The eluted compounds first are burned in the usual FID flame, from which the products of the pyrolysis then pass to another flame where sulfur and phosphorus atoms are excited to a higher energy state and subsequently detected by emission spectroscopy. The sensitivity of this device to sulfur and phosphorus is about 10^5 times greater than that for carbon compounds.

Probably the most sensitive and useful analyses can be made by combining a gas chromatograph with a mass spectrometer. Using a suitable separator to remove the carrier gas allows direct introduction of the solute into the ionization chamber of the *Mass Spectral Detector (MSD)* after it exits the column. This technique has the advantage of extremely high sensitivity (10^{-12} to 10^{-15} g) so that usually only one injection of the unknown is required. The GC-MS technique also is useful for quantitative analysis by using selective-ion monitoring.

There are a number of other detectors that are available for use in GC but are used less frequently because they do not offer significant advantages over the devices currently employed. These include detectors whose operating principles are based on coulometry, conductivity, or photoionization.

Some novel detector designs were reported during the past years including a chlorine-selective pulsed discharge emission detector (CI-PDED). This detector is based on reaction of krypton with chlorine and a unique detector design. A krypton ion produced in the krypton-doped helium pulsed discharge reacts with chlorinated compounds within the pulsed discharge to produce an excited species of KrCl* which emits at 221-222 nm[7].

SPECIAL TECHNIQUES

It is not unusual in the practice of GC to encounter samples that cannot be analyzed satisfactorily no matter what combination of mobile and stationary phases are used. For example, petroleum fractions contain tars and other high-boiling hydrocarbons that chromatograph with difficulty, if at all. In addition, many drugs that contain carboxylic acid or primary amine functional groups are volatile enough to chromatograph but will give badly tailed peaks due to nonideal interactions of the functional groups with the stationary phase. However, for research and quality-control purposes, the pharmaceutical and chemical industries require that these substances be analyzed; to overcome the problem posed by these compounds, special techniques such as *pyrolysis* and *derivatization* have been developed.

Pyrolysis GC is used frequently for the analysis of very high-molecular-weight compounds such as crude oil fractions, rubber vial closures, and packaging materials. In this technique, the high-molecular-weight substances are decomposed to lighter and more volatile compounds by controlled heating in a furnace, which may be external to the gas chromatograph or an integral part of the instrument. The resulting lighter compounds then will be chromatographed as usual, frequently using capillary columns.

Because the nature of the decomposition products rarely is known with any certainty, the chromatogram that is produced represents a "fingerprint" of the original sample. If the time and temperature of pyrolysis are controlled carefully, the method is reproducible and valuable for checking raw materials from different suppliers to determine if the source or the chemical composition has changed over a period of time.

A number of compounds, such as steroids, do not chromatograph well because they are not sufficiently volatile or they decompose at the higher temperatures needed for successful GC. Others, such as fatty acids, yield poorly shaped peaks. It frequently is possible to obviate these problems and obtain good chromatograms by forming derivatives of these substances. Many of the procedures used to produce derivatives in these cases are the same as those used in qualitative organic analysis, such as acylation of alcohols, formation of oximes and hydrazones of carbonyls, or esterification of fatty acids. However, for GC, a different class of derivatizing reagents called *silylating agents* has been used most often. These agents are intended to react with compounds containing labile protons such as alcohols, amines, carboxylic acids, or thiols to produce the corresponding ethers, silyl amines, esters, or thioethers. Because of the reduced polarity, the derivatives have greater volatility and stability than the original compounds. A number of derivatizing agents have been used, the most common of which are *N*-trimethylsilylimidazole (*TSIM*), *N,O*-bistrimethylsilyltrifluoroacetamide (*BSTFA*), and *N,O*-bistrimethylsilylacetamide (*BSA*). The by-products of the reactions are very volatile and elute very rapidly so they do not interfere with the chromatography.

Other than being useful as derivatizing agents, silylating compounds also are used to deactivate solid supports and the surfaces of glass columns. In these applications, they react readily with the silanol groups on the silica surface, thereby blocking polar sites that would interfere with the separation process.

QUALITATIVE ANALYSIS

Although GC is used primarily as a quantitative technique, it also is valuable in the qualitative analysis of unknown substances. This may be accomplished in either of two ways: by comparing the retention parameters of the unknown with known compounds, or by trapping the effluents as they leave the column and subjecting them to classic chemical or spectrometric identification procedures.

In terms of parameters derived from the chromatogram, the retention or relative retention times or their corresponding volumes are useful indicators of identity when compared with the same parameters for a known compound. The related variables, the capacity factor, k', and the separation factor, α, also may be used. If the unknown compound is suspected of being a member of a homologous series and sufficient known members of the series are available, plots of $\log t_R$ versus carbon number or $\log t_R$ on a polar column versus $\log t_R$ on a nonpolar column will give a straight line for homologs.

It also is possible to identify solutes after GC by collecting individual fractions as they elute from the column. This can be done manually or automatically using a fraction collector that is activated by the signal from the detector. In this manner the entire procedure can be automated and carried out unattended over an extended period of time to ensure that adequate amounts are collected for subsequent analysis.

QUANTITATIVE ANALYSIS

In addition to providing rapid and efficient separations of complex mixtures and qualitative information about the eluted substances, GC also can furnish the analyst with accurate and precise quantitative data.

The parameter that is proportional to the concentration of a compound in the GC effluent is the area under the elution peak, which is the integral of the elution curve from the point where it leaves the baseline to the point where it returns. Using computerized techniques, this integral can be determined exactly; however, a number of manual integration methods may be employed. These are based on the assumption that the shape of the peak is Gaussian; although they do not yield the true peak area, the results obtained are proportional to it and may be used with equal confidence. Some of the methods used for integration are

Triangulation—Tangents to the inflection points of the peak are drawn from the baseline to the point where they meet above the peak. The third side of the triangle is drawn along the baseline, and the area is determined by multiplying the base width by one-half the height. The resulting value is equal to 96% of the actual area of the Gaussian peak.

Height Times Width at Half-Height—The baseline portions of the chromatogram before and after the peak are joined with a straight line. The height is measured from this base and multiplied by the width at one-half height. The result is equal to 84% of the true area.

Height—If the conditions of temperature and flow rate are controlled rigorously, the peak height produced by a given quantity of solute will be constant from run to run. It therefore may be used directly as an estimate of the area.

Computer Integration—The computer, or integrator, converts the analog voltage produced by the detector into a digitized quantity and computes the results. This is by far the most precise method, as well as being applicable to peaks whose shape is not ideally Gaussian.

Once the relative areas of the peaks in the chromatogram have been determined, these data, which are proportional to the concentration of each of the species, must be used to determine exact concentrations. This is accomplished in one of three ways:

Area Normalization—The assumption is made that each substance in the injected mixture produces a separate peak in the chromatogram. The weight of the material in any peak is found by determining the ratio of its peak area to the sum of the total areas of all the peaks and multiplying this by the total weight of solute in the amount injected. This method is used infrequently because the initial assumption usually is not valid. It is, however, the standard default method on computerized integrators and is useful as a check on that reproducibility of repeated injections of the same sample.

External Standardization—A pure reference standard material corresponding to the substance to be determined is dissolved in a solvent at a known concentration. Exactly measured quantities of this solution (1, 2, 3, 4, and 5 μL) are injected successively. The areas of each of the peaks produced are plotted versus the mass of solute injected and a calibration curve is produced. Next, the unknown solution is injected, the area of the peak determined, and the concentration found by interpolation. This method is very accurate, but it is necessary that the analyst be skilled in the use of microliter syringes or that an automatic injector be used because the volumes injected must be known exactly. It also is assumed that instrument parameters remain constant for the period during which the samples are introduced, an assumption that is not always valid.

Internal Standardization—To obviate the difficulty of introducing precisely measured quantities into the GC, the internal standard method may be used. This procedure requires two standards: the *analytical standard*—a pure sample of the compound to be analyzed, and the other—an *internal standard*. This is normally a substance that elutes at a position near the substance being analyzed and is well resolved ($R_S > 1.25$), but that cannot be converted to the analyte under the conditions of the analysis. A series of solutions is prepared containing varying amounts of the analytical standard and constant amounts of the internal standard. These are chromatographed and a calibration curve is determined by plotting the ratio of the areas of the two peaks versus the ratios of their concentrations. The unknown then is dissolved in a suitable solvent, the same amount of internal standard is added, and the mixture is chromatographed. The ratio of the areas is calculated and, by interpolation on the calibration curve, the amount of the unknown determined. This method is the most frequently used technique for quantitative analysis by GC because it is not necessary to know the exact amount of solution injected. Usual practice is to prepare a solution of the internal standard in the solvent employed to dissolve reference standards or samples, thus ensuring unvarying ratios of standard or sample peak areas to that of the internal standard.

LIQUID CHROMATOGRAPHY

In 1906 Michael Tswett published a comprehensive paper on liquid chromatography in which he clearly explained the nature of the process and his appreciation of its potential. The method was not adopted widely until many years later. In 1941 Martin and Synge,[3] who had been unsuccessful in using countercurrent extraction for the separation of amino acids in wool samples, developed a liquid-chromatographic process in which they used a packed column containing water-saturated silica gel and a mobile phase of butanol-chloroform. They perfected the experimental techniques and explained the theoretical aspects of the procedure so thoroughly that they were awarded the Nobel Prize for this work in 1952.

Since that time, liquid chromatography has become one of the most versatile techniques available to the analyst because of its simplicity and capacity for high-resolution separations. Separations may be developed based on such diverse characteristics as the polarity of the solutes, their ionic nature, their molecular weight, their partitioning ability, or their ability to form affinity complexes.

The term liquid chromatography is used today to refer to those methods in which the separation takes place within a packed column. The packing material is the stationary phase and may be a solid with adsorptive or exclusion capabilities or an inert support coated with a liquid phase. A liquid mobile phase is used as the eluant. Although thin-layer chromatography and paper chromatography use a liquid mobile phase and a solid stationary phase, they differ in that the separations take place on a planar surface rather than in a column.

Liquid chromatography can be performed using either of two methods:

1. The classic procedure developed by Tswett, called *open-column chromatography*, in which the mobile phase is allowed to flow through the packed column under the influence of gravity or, at most, low pressure (eg, 50–100 psi).

2. The procedure in which the mobile phase is forced through the packed column under high pressure. The latter method is called *high-performance liquid chromatography* (HPLC) because of the extremely high efficiencies (as many as 50,000 plates/m) attainable, or *high-pressure liquid chromatography* because of the high pressures (1000–3000 psi) required. In HPLC, particle diameter is typically 10 μm or less and, as a result, columns are packed more tightly and develop high back pressures that necessitate pumping the mobile phase through the column.

Whether HPLC or open-column methods are used, the mode of separation depends primarily on the nature of the stationary phase. Five modes are available: adsorption, partition, ion-exchange, size-exclusion, or affinity. Each of these will be discussed in detail.

ADSORPTION CHROMATOGRAPHY

In the adsorption mode of liquid chromatography, as in gas–solid chromatography, solutes are retained as a result of the ability of the stationary phase to bond them temporarily to its active surface. The forces involved usually are relatively weak and effective only over short distances. These include van der Waals and London forces, dipole and induced-dipole interactions with polar groups on the active surface, charge-transfer forces, and hydrogen-bonding.

With this type of binding, termed *physical adsorption,* the energy required to break the bonds is small, and the mobile phase, through its ability to dissolve and displace the solutes effectively, can counteract these attractive forces. Therefore, an efficient chromatographic process can occur based on the competition between dissolution of the solute in the mobile phase and binding at the surface of the stationary phase. However, when stronger chemical bonds form between solutes and the adsorbent, as in the process of *chemisorption,* the mobile phase is not able to provide sufficient energy to desorb the solutes. In this case, equilibrium between the two phases is not reached, and solutes are adsorbed irreversibly or give unsatisfactory, tailed elution peaks.

Some of the most common of the large variety of substances that have been used as adsorbents are shown in Table 33-2. In addition to adsorptivity, surface area, particle size, and surface activity are of primary importance in determining the utility of a potential adsorbent. A large surface area is necessary to provide effective contact between the two phases and ensure frequent exchange of the solute. Although areas of 5 to 200 m²/g are quoted by suppliers of adsorbents, these values may be lower than the actual effective surface area, because the methods of measurement used do not account accurately for the porous nature of the adsorbent particles or the true shape of the solute molecules. Particle size is important, not only as an indicator of surface area, but also because it determines the resistance of the packed column to solvent flow. Although very small particles may provide a large area for solute interaction, they may pack so tightly that a reasonable flow rate cannot be achieved without using high-pressure techniques with a

Table 33-2. Adsorbents Used in Column Chromatography

Sucrose	(weakest)
Starch	
Inulin	
Talc	
Calcium carbonate	
Calcium phosphate	
Magnesia	
Silica gel	
Magnesium silicate	
Alumina	
Charcoal	(strongest)

Table 33-3. Characteristics of Solvents Used in Chromatography

SOLVENT	ELUOTROPIC VALUE, E⁰	DIELECTRIC CONSTANT	SOLUBILITY PARAMETER
Heptane	0.00	1.92	7.4
Hexane	0.01	1.88	7.3
Isooctane	0.01	1.94	7.0
Cyclohexane	0.04	2.02	8.2
Carbon tetrachloride	0.18	2.24	8.6
Toluene	0.29	2.38	8.9
Benzene	0.32	2.27	9.2
Ethyl ether	0.38	4.33	7.4
Chloroform	0.40	4.81	9.1
Methylene chloride	0.42	8.93	9.6
Tetrahydrofuran	0.45	7.58	9.1
Acetone	0.56	20.7	9.4
Dioxane	0.56	2.25	9.8
Ethyl acetate	0.58	6.02	8.6
Acetonitrile	0.65	37.50	11.8
Pyridine	0.71	12.30	10.4
l-Propanol	0.82	20.33	10.2
Ethanol	0.88	24.30	11.2
Methanol	0.95	32.70	12.9
Acetic acid	large	6.15	12.4
Water	large	78.54	21.0

consequent loss in sample capacity. Particles in the range of 75 to 150 μm in diameter are a useful compromise for open-column chromatography, providing a large surface area with good permeability. Surface activity refers to the energy of the active site of the adsorbent, and may vary depending on the nature of the substance and on the amount of water adsorbed. To provide a reproducible surface it is common practice to activate an adsorbent by heating it to expel most of the water and then to deactivate it to a desired level by exposure to a climate of known humidity, returning a known quantity of moisture to the adsorbent.

Among the commonly used adsorbents, silica gel and alumina have surfaces rich in hydroxyl groups and oxygen atoms, thus they interact strongly with polar solutes. Charcoal, activated at 1000° to make it nonreactive to polar compounds, has a very porous surface that slows down the adsorption–desorption process and makes it more prone to chemisorption. Separations on charcoal are based mainly on molecular weight, with larger compounds being retained more strongly. Magnesium silicate has an acid surface characteristic of the insoluble silicates and is similar to alumina in adsorptive properties.

Table 33-3 lists a number of the solvents most commonly used in liquid–solid chromatography cataloged in a standard order according to their relative energy of adsorption per unit surface area on alumina. A listing such as this is called an *eluotropic series,* and, although the relative energies of adsorption differ slightly on other surfaces, the choice of solvents usually is made according to this series. An exception to this is made in the case of charcoal; because of its tendency to adsorb nonpolar substances, the order of solvent strength is reversed.

The solvent used for a particular separation must be chosen with regard to the properties of the solutes as well as the stationary phase. For example, if a group of very polar compounds is to be separated using silica gel, the solvent must be polar enough to overcome the strong attraction between the solutes and the surface or very large retention times will result. If a mixture of less-polar solutes is to be analyzed, a weaker solvent must be used to permit a longer residence time on the column and more equilibrations between the phases. For a more detailed discussion of the methods used to correlate solute structure with retention time using adsorption chromatography the text by Snyder (see *Bibliography*) is recommended.

PARTITION CHROMATOGRAPHY

In this mode of liquid chromatography, mixtures of solutes are separated according to the relative tendencies of their components to partition between a mobile phase and a stationary phase consisting of a layer of liquid coated or bonded onto the surface of a solid support. The liquid is present as an extremely thin layer so that equilibration between the phases may be attained rapidly by minimizing the diffusion of the solutes into the stationary phase. The surface of the solid support frequently is treated (eg, by silylation) to eliminate adsorptive effects.

Although it has been used for many successful analyses, liquid–liquid partition chromatography was, until relatively recently, an inconvenient method to use experimentally. The liquid phase had to be coated onto the solid support by evaporation of a solution or by injecting it onto the column with the mobile phase flowing. In either case, it was difficult to obtain stationary phases that were stable and reproducible. In addition, the choice of mobile phase necessarily was restricted to those in which the liquid coating had limited solubility. For example, if a polyethylene glycol was to be used to provide a very polar stationary phase, a mobile phase of hexane or some other hydrocarbon of very low polarity had to be used. Even so, the liquid stationary phase would be stripped slowly but continually from the column, thereby changing the characteristics of the separation. To prevent stripping, either the mobile phase was saturated with the liquid phase material, or a precolumn containing a high concentration of the liquid phase coated on a solid support was inserted into the system before the analytical column. In either case, the nature of the mobile phase was changed and partition coefficients became less favorable.

Recently, the problems presented by unstable stationary phases have been solved by the development of *bonded-phase chromatography,* in which the liquid phase permanently is bonded chemically to the surface of the solid support. Silica gel, with its high surface population of hydroxyl groups, provides an excellent medium onto which various substances can be bonded using appropriately substituted silylating agents. For example, octadecyldimethylsilyl chloride reacts with silica gel to form a stable, nonpolar stationary phase called ODS (octadecylsilyl). Because of steric effects, not all of the hydroxyl groups of the silica gel are derivatized by the ODS reagent, so the remainder then are reacted with trimethylsilyl chloride in a process called *capping* (or *end-capping*) to reduce adsorption effects. Bonded phases are advantageous in that they can be made reproducibly from batch to batch and the surface does not change during the chromatographic process. They have the disadvantages of being expensive and effective only over the pH range within which the backbone of silica gel is stable, usually pH 2 to 7. Compared to the inconveniences of the former method, however, these disadvantages are not very restrictive, and the development of newer bonded phases using a polymeric support that is stable over a pH range of 1 to 13 promises to alleviate this problem.

Partition chromatography may be conducted in either of two ways: *normal* or *reversed phase.* In the normal phase mode, the stationary phase is a polar substance, such as polyethylene glycol or the untreated silica surface itself, and the mobile phase is nonpolar (eg, hexane). Under these circumstances polar compounds are retarded preferentially and nonpolar substances elute more quickly. In reversed-phase chromatography the stationary phase is nonpolar (eg, ODS) and the mobile phase is polar, usually a mixture of water, methanol, and/or acetonitrile. Nonpolar compounds are retained more strongly by this system, while polar solutes elute first. Reversed-phase separations are the most frequently used methods in HPLC.

Because of the efficiency and availability of reversed-phase materials, especially the ODS or C-18 type, attempts have been made to use them to separate mixtures of ionic compounds such as amino acids. Normally these compounds would not be retained in a reversed-phase packing, because they are too polar to partition appreciably onto the nonpolar stationary phase. Several techniques, all of which involve altering the mobile phase, have been developed to permit successful chromatography of ionic compounds using these stationary phases. These methods are called *ion-suppression chromatography, ion- pairing chromatography,* and *"soap" chromatography*.

Ion suppression is used for substances such as weak acids (pK_a >2) and weak bases (pK_a <8), which only are ionized partially at the neutral pH values characteristic of the usual mobile phases. For example, a carboxylic acid with pK_a = 5 will, at pH = 7, be present in both ionized and un-ionized forms with the anionic carboxylate predominating by a ratio of 100 to 1. To enhance the retention of the substance in a reversed-phase system, the pH of the mobile phase can be adjusted to a value low enough to suppress the ionization of the acid, for example, pH < 3. This causes the free acid to predominate and, as it is much less polar than the anion, it will be able to partition into the stationary phase.

For stronger acids or bases that remain ionized throughout the pH range (2–7) where silica is stable, ion-pairing chromatography is the technique of choice. In this method a reagent that dissociates to give ions opposite in charge to those of the solutes is added to the mobile phase. Although the mechanism of action has not been explained fully yet, the added ions may interact with the charged solutes in two ways.

First, they may combine directly with the charged solutes to form ion pairs that are nonpolar and will partition more readily into the stationary phase.

Alternatively, the nonpolar end of the ion-pairing reagent may itself partition into the stationary phase, leaving its polar end extending from the surface into the mobile phase, where it acts as an ion exchanger.

In either case, the retention of ionic solutes in the reversed phase materials is increased. Examples of ion-pairing reagents are heptanesulfonic acid, used for cationic species such as protonated amines, and tetra-*n*-butylammonium hydroxide, which pairs with anionic substances.

The third method, *soap chromatography*, is actually a form of ion-pairing in which the added reagent is a detergent or soap. Examples are sodium lauryl sulfate for cations and cetyltrimethylammonium chloride for anions. Soap chromatography is useful especially for the separation of proteins, because the soap not only neutralizes the charge on the molecule but also affects the conformation of the protein to allow it to interact more favorably with the stationary phase. The practical aspects of ion-pair chromatography are discussed in more detail by Gloor and Johnson.[8]

Another special technique that can be used with partition chromatography is *metal-ion complexation*. In this process, a small quantity of a metal ion, such as Ag^+, is added to the mobile phase in the chromatography of olefinic compounds. The ionic silver interacts with the double bonds, forming charge-transfer complexes and altering the partitioning behavior of the olefinic solute. This technique is useful for separating mixtures of compounds that differ in the extent and placement of the unsaturation.

Centrifugal partition chromatography (CPC) is a combination of countercurrent chromatography and partition chromatography where an automated liquid-liquid extraction process permitting hundreds of successive extractions taken place. The solute equilibrates between the stationary and mobile liquids by the phenomenon of partition. CPC is unique because no solid support is used for the stationary phase. Instead, the liquid stationary phase is retained in the column by a combination of centrifugal force, the special column geometry and the density difference between the two liquid phases.[9]

When a mixture of components is introduced into the mobile phase of the CPC column, it distributes according to the individual components' distribution coefficients while passing through the column. The centrifugal force field applied to the coiled columns promotes the retention of the stationary phase against a continuous flow of mobile phase. The mobile phase flow enables the two phases interact sufficiently for partition to occur.

CPC is used for many types of separations; racemic mixtures, natural products and amino acids are commonly separated on centrifugal partition columns. CPC is also utilized for enzymatic reaction. Some reviews have been published describing the basic principles of CPC and its applications.[10–12]

ION-EXCHANGE CHROMATOGRAPHY

Although ion-pairing techniques have proved useful in many cases for the separation of mixtures of ionic substances, the usual method for the analysis of these compounds is *ion- exchange chromatography*. This method provides a greater degree of selectivity due to the larger number of combinations of mobile and stationary phases that can be employed. It is especially useful for inorganic cations, amino acids, or similar groups of closely related compounds.

The stationary phase materials used to effect these separations are called *ion exchangers*, and they comprise a group of natural or synthetic organic or inorganic polymers that are capable of reversibly removing ions from a solution, while at the same time replacing them with ions of equivalent charge. At all times during this exchange process the principle of electro -neutrality must be obeyed both in the ion exchanger and the solution. An ion exchanger contains *fixed ions*, which are incorporated permanently into its insoluble skeleton, and loosely bound *counterions*, which are opposite in charge to the fixed ions and capable of being exchanged when charged species are adsorbed from solution. If the counterions are charged positively, the material is called a *cation exchanger*; if negative, it is an *anion exchanger*.

The inorganic polymers used in this type of chromatography are aluminosilicates, which have lattice, or cage-like, structures. Because of the preponderance of oxygen atoms in the polymer, it is charged negatively and the counterions, usually calcium or sodium, are positive. Therefore, they are cation exchangers. The naturally occurring members of this group are called *zeolites*, while the synthetic ones, which were developed to provide standardized structures with constant pore sizes, are called *molecular sieves*. Because of their low capacities for ion exchange, these inorganic substances are used primarily for the size separation of small molecules.

The most frequently used ion-exchange materials are organic copolymers made from styrene (vinylbenzene) and divinylbenzene (DVB). The styrene polymerizes to give long, twisted chains of carbon atoms, with a benzene ring at every other carbon. Divinylbenzene is added to cross-link these chains and give a three-dimensional bead-like structure. Commercially available ion-exchange resins are identified according to their percent cross-linking, as ×2, ×4, ×6, and so on, corresponding to the initial percentage of DVB in the reaction mixture.

Because the styrene–DVB copolymers have no intrinsic ion-exchanging properties of their own and act only as a skeleton, charged functional groups must be added. Reaction with chlorosulfonic acid places a sulfonic acid group on each of the nonlinked benzene rings, yielding a *strong cation exchanger*, that is, one in which the counterions can be removed easily from the fixed ions. If methacrylic acid is used in the polymerization in place of styrene, the resulting copolymer has carboxylic acid groups attached to the skeleton and functions as a *weak cation exchanger*, that is, one in which the counterions do not dissociate at low pH. *Strong anion-exchange* resins can be made from the same skeleton by introducing quaternary amine functional groups, while *weak anion exchangers* use polyamines as the ionizable groups.

Many other substances are used both as the skeletal components and the functional groups for ion exchange. Carbohydrate polymers, such as dextran and cellulose, when used as the insoluble matrix change the selectivity of a resin. For example, solute ions with attached polyaromatic groups, such as the anthraquinonesulfonic acids, do not chromatograph well on polystyrene-based ion exchangers, because they associate too strongly with the benzene rings of the resin. On a cellulose-based exchanger, however, separation is possible because the mechanism is limited entirely to the ion-exchange process. Silica gel also is used as a support matrix for preparing ion exchangers, especially in HPLC, where strength of the particle is important, as it must not be crushed by the high operating pressure of the system.

Other functional groups used frequently are diethylaminoethyl (DEAE) and triethylaminoethyl (TEAE), both of which are anion exchangers, and carboxymethyl (CM), which is used in cation-exchange resins. Attached to matrices of cellulose or dextran, these substances have been employed widely for the separation of proteins and peptides.

The mechanism of action in this mode of chromatography depends on the replacement of the counterions of the resin by the ionic species being separated. This can be illustrated by the procedure used for purifying water by passing it through a mixed-bed resin. Using sodium chloride as a typical contaminant, the mechanism is

(1) $RESIN—SO_3H + Na^+ = RESIN—SO_3Na + H^+$

(2) $RESIN—N(CH_3)_3OH + Cl^-$ (13)

       $= RESIN—N(CH_3)_3Cl + OH^-$

Water of the exceptionally high purity needed for making mobile phases for HPLC is prepared by an ion-exchange column, followed by passage through a charcoal adsorption column to remove nonionizable organic compounds and then microfiltrated to exclude particulate matter and bacteria.

For a mixture of solute ions that differ in charge, the more highly charged species are retained preferentially. Thus, on a sulfonic acid resin, aluminum is bound more strongly than calcium, and calcium more strongly than sodium. The binding of negatively charged species to strong anion exchange resins follows the same trend. Among substances of the same charge, retention is related to the size of the hydrated ions, with smaller ions being held more tightly. Because the smaller elements in the periodic table bind more molecules of water, their hydrated ions are larger; therefore, for the alkali metals the order of retention is $Cs^+ > Rb^+ > K^+ > Na^+ > Li^+$.

Another parameter that affects retention is the nature of the substituents attached to the charged portion of the solute species. Polystyrene resins exhibit preference for ions containing aromatic groups over aliphatic groups, because in addition to binding due to the electrostatic forces of ion exchange, the aromatic groups of the solute interact directly with the skeleton of the resin.

Ion-exchange chromatograms may be developed either by displacement or by elution methods. In the former case, an ion that is retained more strongly than any of the solute ions displaces them from the resin, and a continuous series of bands results (see Fig 33-3). In elution development, the eluting agent is an ion for which the resin has less selectivity than it has for the solute ions. Transfer of the solute ions to and from the resin depends on their exchange equilibria with the eluting ion. The resulting chromatogram consists of a series of separate Gaussian peaks, as in Figure 33-4.

Mobile phases used in ion-exchange chromatography are usually aqueous salt solutions that may be buffered to a desired pH or adjusted to a constant ionic strength. The choice of the mobile phase depends on knowledge of the selectivity of the resin for the solute ions and the influence of solution equilibria due to pH or complexation. Mixed aqueous-organic or organic solvents may be used if the stationary phase is not altered. Gradient elution is used for difficult separations.

Chromatofocusing, first described in 1978 by Sluyterman and Elgersma,[13] is a special method of ion-exchange chromatography that is of great utility in the separation of mixtures of proteins. In this case a buffer, adjusted to a specific pH, is added to an anion-exchange column previously adjusted to a different pH. As the buffers mix, a pH gradient is formed along the length of the column, ranging from the initial pH at the far end to that of the added buffer at the beginning. If the pH at the start of the column is lower than the isoelectric point of the protein to be analyzed, it will carry a positive charge and will not interact with the anion exchanger. Instead, it will migrate along the column to a point where the pH is just greater than the isoelectric point, at which time it will acquire a negative charge and bind to the resin. Thus, a group of proteins will arrange themselves on the column in order of their isoelectric points. As the pH gradient moves down the column, the proteins will migrate downward, so as to remain negatively charged, until each elutes from the column at its isoelectric point. The fractionation of complex mixtures of proteins is therefore possible using this method of separation.

SIZE-EXCLUSION CHROMATOGRAPHY

Size-exclusion chromatography (SEC), also called *gel filtration or molecular-sieve chromatography,* is an efficient technique used to separate groups of solutes based on their effective size in solution. The stationary phases used to attain these separations are polymers that have been cross-linked to yield an open network with numerous pores of consistent size. The degree of cross-linking is controlled carefully to yield a series of gels having different pore sizes and fractionation ranges. When a mobile phase containing a mixture of solutes of various sizes is passed through a column of these materials, molecules that are too large to fit within the pores are "excluded" and remain completely in the mobile phase. They are, therefore, eluted rapidly near the void volume. Molecules of smaller size are free to diffuse in and out of the pores so that, in effect, their path through the column is longer and they will elute later, as is depicted in Figure 33-8. The extent of retention depends on the size of the included molecules relative to the size of the pores. Thus, the smallest molecules will enter all of the pores, while molecules of intermediate size, because of the velocity of the mobile phase, will not have sufficient time to diffuse into all of the pores into which they would fit normally and, therefore, will be retained less effectively. The result is a chromatogram that consists of an initial peak containing all of the totally excluded substances, followed by a group of peaks representing all of the substances that have been retained partially and separated, and finally another single peak caused by all of the totally included solutes.

The stationary phases used in this mode of partition chromatography are of two types.

The *soft gels* are made usually from cross-linked carbohydrates, such as dextran (Sephadex), agarose (Sepharose), or polyacrylamide (Bio-Gel), the use of which was described first by Porath and Flodin.[14] These are very hydrophilic, and before the column can be packed, they must be mixed with the mobile phase until they have *imbibed* enough liquid to become swollen completely. Once the column has been packed, the composition of the mobile phase cannot be altered, because this would change the amount of imbibed solvent, resulting in shrinking of the bed, or in further swelling that may burst the column. These gels are used with mobile phases that are primarily aqueous, and the technique is called *gel filtration.* Because of the low structural strength of the soft gels they cannot be used under high pressure. Size-exclusion media made from silica gel with controlled pore sizes have been developed for HPLC; they do not deform under pressure and can be used with aqueous or nonaqueous mobile phases.

The *semirigid* or *rigid gels* consist of materials such as cross-linked polystyrene, controlled-porosity glass beads, or alkylated

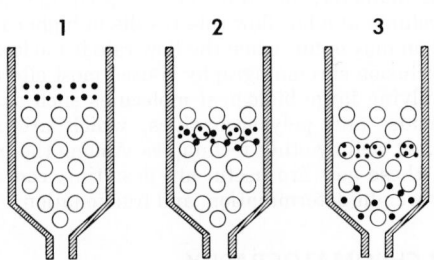

Figure 33-8. Size-exclusion chromatography. Small, soluble molecules (•) penetrate the pores of the gel (○) and are retarded. Macromolecules (●) are excluded from the gel matrix and elute first.

dextran. These can be used for the separation of organic-soluble polymers using nonaqueous mobile phases, such as chloroform, acetone, pyridine, or tetrahydrofuran. This technique is called *gel permeation,* and was described first in 1964 by Moore.[15]

Ideally, the only separation mechanism occurring in size-exclusion chromatography is that which depends on the diffusion of the solutes into and out of the pores. However, depending on the nature of the solute and the stationary phase, other retention mechanisms such as ion exchange, hydrophobic partitioning, or hydrogen-bonding may have an effect on certain solutes. These can result in long retention times, irreversible adsorption, or loss of activity in biological molecules. Such difficulties can be minimized by changing ionic strength or pH of the mobile phase to reduce charge effects, or by using additives such as detergents that modify the shape and charge of biological molecules.

Desalting is frequently necessary for the purification of biochemicals that have been separated from tissue using techniques involving buffers and precipitating reagents. In this procedure, a gel with a fairly low exclusion limit (ie, equivalent to a molecular weight of 1000–2000) is used. Because of the great differences in molecular weight between the biological molecules and the contaminating salts, short columns and high flow rates may be used. The macromolecules will be eluted in the void volume with little dilution, while the salts are retained on the column.

Concentration of dilute solutions of large molecules may be achieved with gels whose exclusion limit is less than the molecular weight of the substances involved. The solution is mixed with a small quantity of dry gel that will absorb 10 to 20 times its weight in water. Some salts and small molecules are taken up also, leaving the macromolecules in a solution of almost unchanged pH and ionic strength but significantly decreased volume.

Perhaps the greatest value of size-exclusion chromatography is for the fractionation and molecular-weight determination of macromolecules. It has been found that because the size of a molecule is approximately proportional to its molecular weight, M, the elution volume, V_E, can be expressed by

$$V_E = a + b \log M \qquad (14)$$

where a and b are constants dependent on the mobile and stationary phases. To determine the molecular weight of a substance, the system must be calibrated by using an extremely large molecule, such as blue dextran, to establish the void volume of the system, and a substance such as deuterium oxide or sucrose to determine the retention time for a totally included solute. A series of standard proteins or polymers then is used to calibrate the region between these limits. A typical calibration curve of V_E versus log M for a series of protein standards is shown in Figure 33-9. Once the elution volume of the unknown compound is determined, the molecular weight can be estimated by interpolation.

Packing of the column is very critical in SEC. The column dimensions range from 600 mm × 16 mm to 1000 mm × 50 mm, and the volume of the loaded sample should not exceed 5% of the column volume for preparative runs and 1% for analytical applications. The recommended flow rates, which depend on the column diameter, should not be increased. In general, running the column at a low flow rate results in higher resolution, but diffusion may occur, when the flow rate is too low.[16]

Size-exclusion chromatography is used most often in procedures involving large biological molecules such as proteins, nucleic acids, and polysaccharides, which are not chromatographed well by other techniques. Among the procedures for which these gels are useful are desalting, concentration, molecular-weight determination, and fractionation.

AFFINITY CHROMATOGRAPHY

In situations where very specific separations are desired, *affinity chromatography,* a highly specialized form of adsorption chromatography, may be employed. This technique makes use

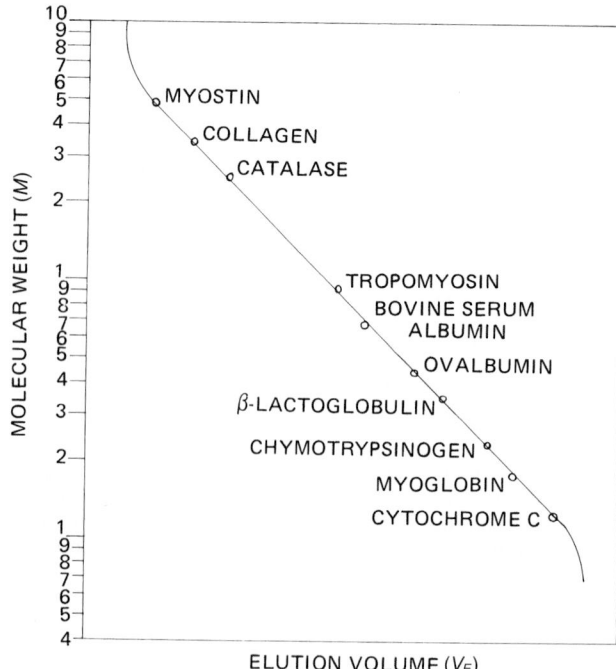

Figure 33-9. Typical size exclusion calibration curve of elution volume, V_E, versus log M for a series of protein standards.

of a specific ligand, which has been immobilized by being bound chemically to an insoluble matrix, to adsorb reversibly a single molecular species from a mixture of solutes. This method differs from other modes of chromatography already discussed in that, rather than attempting to separate a mixture of solutes for qualitative or quantitative analysis, it is concerned only with removing a single species from the mixture. It achieves its greatest utility as a highly specific purification technique for biological molecules.

Affinity chromatography owes its high degree of specificity to the nature of the binding forces between the ligand and the substance to be purified. Many biological molecules, as a result of their unique structure and conformation, form strong, noncovalent bonds to related compounds, as a drug would to a cellular receptor. The interactions between ligand and target molecule can be a result of electrostatic or hydrophobic interactions, Van der Waals' forces and/or hydrogen bonding. Examples of this are found in the association of enzymes with coenzymes, antigens with antibodies, lectins with carbohydrates, or polynucleotides with nucleic acids. If either member of the above-mentioned pairs is bonded permanently to a chromatographic matrix, it will be able to remove the other from solution without interacting significantly with any other solute in the mixture. Because the ligand-target molecule binding is reversible, a suitable mobile phase can be passed through the column to dissociate the pair and elute the purified substance.

The elution can be achieved by either specifically using a competitive ligand, or non-specifically, by changing the pH, ionic strength or polarity.[17] Some typical biological interactions, frequently used in affinity chromatography are (1) Enzyme - substrate analogue, inhibitor, cofactor; (2) Antibody - antigen, virus, cell; (3) Lectin - polysaccharide, glycoprotein, cell surface receptor, cell; (4) Nucleic acid - complementary base sequence, histones, nucleic acid polymerase, nucleic acid binding protein; (5) Hormone, vitamin - receptor, carrier protein; (6) Glutathione - glutathione-S-transferase or GST fusion proteins; 7) Metal ions - Poly (His) fusion proteins, native proteins with histidine, cysteine and/or tryptophan residues on their surfaces. Examples of the application of affinity chromatography are (1) Isolation of human immunoglobulins; (2) Purification of fusion proteins; (3) Proteins and peptides with exposed His, Cys, or Trp; (4) DNA binding proteins and coagulation factors.[17]

EXPERIMENTAL FACTORS AND INSTRUMENTATION

CLASSIC COLUMN CHROMATOGRAPHY

The experimental setup for performing this type of chromatography is relatively simple. The column into which the stationary phase is packed consists of a glass or Teflon tube, typically 10 to 50 mm in diameter and 5 to 100 cm in length, although much longer and wider columns have been used for difficult separations and preparative work. The bottom of the column is fitted with a stopcock or another type of flow restrictor to provide control over the flow rate of the mobile phase. The packing material is supported inside the column by means of a fritted glass disk or a piece of glass wool.

The packing may be introduced into the column either as a dry powder or as a slurry suspended in the mobile phase. In either case, it is essential that the bed be formed evenly with no air bubbles or channels to disrupt the flow of the mobile phase. If it is packed dry, the stationary phase is introduced in small quantities and allowed to settle with the aid of gentle tapping or vibrating on the outside of the column. If a slurry-packing technique is used, the stopcock is left open to allow the solvent to flow through the solid material and solvent is added, as necessary, to prevent the column from going dry while it is tapped to dispel air bubbles. When the bed has reached the desired height, the stopcock is closed and a layer of mobile phase left at the top of the bed. In slurry packing, positive pressure, vacuum, or a tamping rod may be used to ensure that the material is packed firmly.

The sample is placed on the top of the column in either of two ways. It may be mixed with a small portion of the stationary phase that then is packed as before or it may be dissolved in the mobile phase and deposited on the packing after the mobile phase has been allowed to run a slight distance into the stationary phase. More mobile phase then is added and the stopcock is opened to allow flow to begin. The chromatogram then may be developed by allowing the solvent to flow from a reservoir under the force of gravity or by introducing it under low pressure using a peristaltic pump. The effluent from the column is collected in fractions as a function of time or volume, and the eluates tested for the presence of the various solutes.

HIGH-PERFORMANCE LIQUID CHROMATOGRAPHY

Because of the relatively high pressures necessary to perform this type of chromatography, a more elaborate experimental setup is required. Figure 33-10 shows the block diagram of a complete HPLC apparatus. All of these components are not necessary to achieve successful analyses (see caption).

The *solvent reservoirs* are glass or stainless-steel containers capable of holding up to 1–2 liter of mobile phase, which may consist of pure organic solvents or aqueous solutions of salts or buffers. The substances used to prepare these mixtures should be of the highest purity available because contaminants eventually will be deposited on the column and disrupt the chromatography. The mobile phases are filtered to remove particulate matter that may clog the system, and they also are degassed using vacuum, sonication, or sparging with helium to eliminate outgassing in the pump or detector.

Because the particles that are used to pack HPLC columns are small enough (<50 μm) to prevent solvent flow by gravity, pumps that develop pressures up to 5000 psi are needed to force the mobile phase though the column. Two types are available: mechanical, which deliver at a constant flow rate, and pneumatic, which produce a constant pressure. Of the mechanical pumps, the most frequently used is the reciprocating piston type in which a motor-driven cam drives a sapphire plunger into a small liquid-end chamber to force out the solvent. Check valves control the flow of solvent into and out of the liquid end and prevent backflow. Because the flow pulses every time the plunger moves in and out, the pressure variations may cause an unstable baseline; thus, these pumps usually are equipped with a pulse-damping device. They may have two liquid chambers arranged in such a manner that, while one is filling, the other is delivering.

The pneumatic pumps may be either the gas-displacement type, which uses direct pressure from a highly compressed gas to force solvent out of a tube, or the pneumatic-amplifier type in which compressed gas at a lower pressure impinges on the large end of a piston to force the smaller end to deliver the liquid. The amplification of the original gas pressure is proportional to the ratio of the areas of the two ends of the piston. The pneumatic pumps have the advantage of pulseless operation.

If gradient analysis is necessary to achieve a particular separation, the most common way of forming the gradient is to include a second reservoir and pump and a *gradient controller*. This is an electronic device that synchronizes the operation of the two pumps to provide a mobile-phase mixture of the desired concentration. For example, if a 50–50 mixture of the solvents in the two reservoirs is desired at an overall flow rate of 1.0 mL/min, the controller will adjust the rate of delivery of each pump to 0.5 mL/min. The individual solvents then are combined in the *mixing chamber* and delivered to the chromatograph. The controllers are able to provide linear, convex, concave, or step gradients, thereby yielding a solvent mixture of constantly increasing strength to enable the resolution of complex mixtures.

In contrast to this high-pressure method of forming gradients, a low-pressure technique also is used frequently by some instrument suppliers. In this method, the mixing chamber is situated before a single pump. As many as four reservoirs are

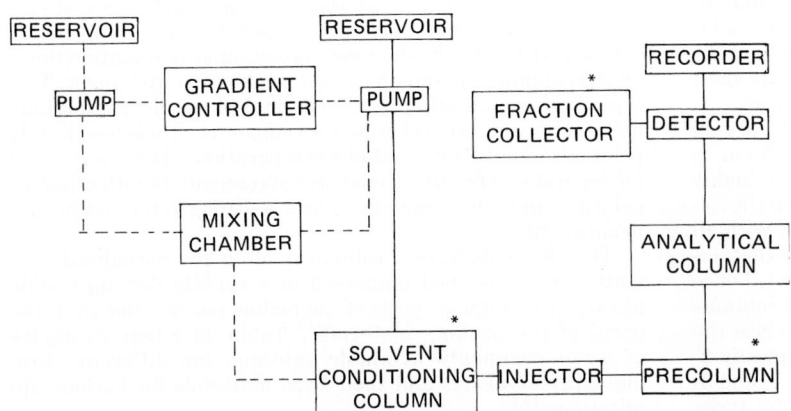

Figure 33-10. Block diagram of a complete HPLC. The items connected by dashed lines are necessary only for gradient elution. *These items are optional for both gradient and isocratic analysis.

connected to the mixing chamber, each reservoir having a remotely controlled valve. The gradient controller, either a separate device or a computer-resident software package, opens and closes the valves in the proper sequence so that the mixing chamber can generate mobile phase of the desired composition.

The next component, a *solvent-conditioning column,* is used only under special circumstances. Most HPLC column-packing materials are prepared from silica gel, which will dissolve slowly in solvents whose pH values are below 2 or above 7. This results in a shrinkage of the packing material, giving rise to void spaces in which separated solutes remix or are diluted, thereby leading to a loss of resolution. Therefore, to minimize this occurrence and to protect the expensive silica-based packing materials, a small column (5–10 cm) packed with HPLC-grade silica gel is inserted into the liquid stream after the pump but before the injector. The material in this column is dissolved preferentially, saturating the mobile phase and preserving the analytical column. Although there is some slight dissolution of the silica even in the pH range of 2 to 7, conditioning columns need not be used always and may be a disadvantage if fractions are collected with the object of recovering the solutes, as dissolved silica is difficult to remove from the solute.

The solute mixture is introduced into the chromatograph by means of a suitable *injection device.* Septum injectors are available, in which the sample solution is injected through a self-sealing rubber or Teflon disk using a microliter syringe. This may be done while the mobile phase is flowing or while it has been stopped temporarily. Although these devices are inexpensive and easy to use, it is difficult to achieve reproducible injections and automate their operation. Therefore, sample introduction is done mainly by using a rotary valve-and-loop injector. This consists of a stainless-steel and Teflon block that has been drilled to provide two alternate paths for solvent flow each selectable by a rotating valve. When the valve is in the "fill" position, the solvent flows through one path directly onto the column. In the other path there is a fixed-volume (10–1000 μL) loop of narrow-bore stainless-steel tubing, which is filled with the sample solution using a syringe or suction. When the valve is moved to the inject "position," the mobile phase path is diverted through the loop and washes its contents onto the column. The results obtained are very reproducible, and the injector can be automated by using a solenoid to change the valve position.

The next component in the instrument, called a *precolumn,* is optional and may be used for either of two reasons. When stationary phases consist of a thin layer of a liquid coated on a solid support, the liquid slowly dissolves in the mobile phase, causing a degradation of resolution. In this case, the precolumn will contain solid support coated with a higher percent of liquid phase than the analytical column to saturate the mobile phase and retard dissolution. Because most stationary phases used currently in HPLC are bonded permanently and not subject to dissolution, the precolumn is used mainly to protect the main column by trapping particulate matter and retaining substances, which would be irreversibly adsorbed on the analytical column. In this case it usually is called a *guard column.* The guard column is packed with a stationary phase identical to that in the main column, except that its particle size may be larger so that it will not restrict the flow. The larger material is relatively inexpensive and easy to pack so the contents of the guard column can be changed frequently. Because of its short length (2–10 cm), it usually does not affect the separation.

Most of the *analytical columns* used for HPLC are in straight lengths of stainless tubing, usually 5 to 25 cm in length, with an internal diameter of 2 to 4.6 mm, with highly polished interior walls. Compression end fittings attach the column to the HPLC apparatus. Stainless steel is useful with all organic and most aqueous buffers. However, chloride-containing buffers can slowly deteriorate the stainless steel, hence glass columns are recommended. Overall, stainless columns are used for most HPLC applications. Porous frits close the ends of column and retain the packing particles. Typically 2- and 0.5 μm- porosity stainless steel frits are used for 5- and 3-μm particles, respectively. Compression fitting column types

are available with the wide selection of different packing materials. Well-made columns of this type provide highest level of performance and reproducibility.

The column packing particles for HPLC support utilize silica or porous polymers. Three types of particles are available for HPLC separations: (1) *Totally porous microspheres*–these are most commonly used because of the favorable properties in terms of efficacy, sample loading, durability, convenience, and availability. These particles are generally available in 5 μm size and all types of HPLC methods are developed with these materials. (2) *Micropellicular particles*–these have a solid core (silica or polymer based) with a thin outer skin of interactive stationary phase usually in 1.5 to 2.5 μm size. These particles are very useful for fast separations of macromolecules and generate very sharp peaks. (3) *Perfusion particles*–These contain very large pores eg, 0.4 to 0.8 μm in the particles. At high flow rates, the solutes can enter and leave this pore structure through a combination of convective and diffusion processes. These are mainly used in the preparative separation of macromolecules.[18]

Particle size of HPLC column packing play very important role in the effective separations. Particle diameters of about 5 μm represent a good compromise in analytical columns in terms of column efficacy, back pressure, and durability. Smaller porous particles are available for faster separations. Pellicular particles as small as 1.5 μm are useful for extremely rapid separation of macromolecules such as proteins. A narrow particle size distribution of < ±50% from mean in all materials ensure stable, high efficacy packed beds with minimum pressure drop. On balance, columns of the 3- or 5- μm totally porous microspheres meet the requirements of most HPLC separations.

It is possible to coat, to graft or even to encapsulate the chromatographic support with another material called stationary phase or, since bonding is such a common procedure, the bonded phase. Stationary phases with aliphatic hydrocarbon chains and phenyl moieties are used for reversed phase chromatography; amines and diols are used for normal phase chromatography; unmodified or alkylated amines are used for cation exchange chromatography; sulfonates or carboxylates are used for cation exchange chromatography; and affinity ligands, such as protein A and heparin, are used for affinity chromatography. Other ligands, including bovine serum albumin are used in chiral chromatography.

The most popular bonded phases are C1, C4, C8, and C18. Silica based adsorbents modified with trimethylchlorosilane (C1) and buthyldimethylchlorosilane (C4) have a few applications in HPLC, mainly for protein separation or purification. These adsorbents show significant polar interactions, although they do not have specific interactions caused by acidic silanols. Octyl (C8) and octadecyl (C18) modified adsorbents are the most popular ones. Almost 80% of all HPLC separations have been developed with these adsorbents. Propylphenylsilane ligands attached to the silica gel show weak dipole-induced dipole interactions with polar analytes. Usually this type of bonded phase is used for group separations of complex mixtures. Amino-compounds show some specific interactions with phenyl-modified adsorbent. A cyano-modified surface is very slightly polar. Columns with this phase are useful for fast separations of mixtures consisting of very different components. These mixtures might show very broad range of retention times on the columns. Amino-phase is a weak anion-exchanger. This type of column is mainly used in normal-phase mode, especially for selective retention of aromatic compounds. Diols are slightly polar adsorbent for normal-phase separations. These are useful for separation of complex mixtures of compounds with different polarity, and which usually shows a strong retention on unmodified silica.

The chromatographic column is often conceptualized as a stationary phase bed immersed in a rapidly flowing mobile phase, with stagnant pools of the mobile phase situated in the pores of the packing material.[18] Table 33-4 lists examples of some commonly available columns for different chromatographic modes and their base materials for various applications.[19,20]

Table 33-4. Examples of Some Commonly Available HPLC Columns

TYPE OF COLUMN	BASE MATERIAL	APPLICATIONS	SUPPLIERS OF COLUMN
Reversed-phase	Highly aqueous type Silica, C18 functional group Particle size mostly 5 µm	For analysis of polar compounds, columns can beused under 100% aqueous conditions	Astec, Waters, ShiseidoNacalai, Tesque, Thermo Electron Alltech, Jones Chromatography, GL Sciences
Reversed-phase	Regular type, Silica, C18 functional group Particle size 3–10 µm, mostly 5 µm	For retaining polar compounds in a wide range of applications	Agilent, Higgins Analytical, Cohesive Techlologies Siseido, Dionex, ESA, Waters, Interchim
Reversed-phase	Regular type, Silica, Perfluorinated phenyl functional group, Particle size 5 µm	Recommended for analysis of isomers, available in analytical, microbore, capillary, and preparative sizes	ES Industries
Reversed-phase	Monolithic polymeric silica column with endcapped C8 phase, C8 functional group	High-speed analysis with low back-pressure	Merck
Reversed-phase	Base deactivated type, Silica base material, C8 functional group, Particle size 5 µm	High-speed analysis, available in analytical, microbore, and reparative sizes	Macherey-Nagel
Reversed-phase	High stability, polyamide base material, Polyamide functional group, Particle size 5 µm	Hydrophilic polymeric bead with pH 0–14 stability; can withstand high pressures and temperatures; recommended for protein separations	Zordi
Reversed-phase	Regular type, Silica, C12 functional group Particle size 4, 10 µm	pH 1.5–10 stability; recommended for tryptic digests and small peptides	Phenomenex
	Polymer type, PS-DVB base material, PS-DVB functional group, Particle size 5 µm	For separating peptides, nucleotides, and other small molecules and also LC–MS.	Amersham Biosciences
Reversed-phase	Polar end capped, high aqueous type, silica base material, C18 functional group Particle size 2, 4, 10 µm	Polar end capping enables use in 100% aqueous mobile phase; recommended for retaining nonpolar and highly polar compounds and for LC–MS applications	Phenomenex
Reversed phase	Methacrylate/Methacrylate	Small protein and polypeptide analysis	Alltech Associates
Superficially Porous reversed phase	Silica/C3, C8, C18	High-speed protein analysis	Agilent Technologies
Normal Phase	Highly purified silica / 3µm to 300 µm particles	Nonpolar compound analysis, High sample recovery	YMC Inc., Perkin-Elmer
Normal Phase	Diol stationary phase, 6–30nm pore size and 5–50 µm particle size.	Diol columns also provide better reproducibility when compared with bare silica columns.	YMC Inc.
Normal Phase	µBondapak-NH$_2$, amine bonded silica	Nonpolar compound analysis	Waters
Normal Phase	Alkyl cyano phase on silica	Nonpolar compound analysis	BTR Seperations
Hydrophilic interaction	Silica/	Polar pharmaceutical analysis	Waters
Hydrophobic interaction	Silica/Diol	Protein analysis, desalting	Nacalai Tesque
Hydrophilic interaction	Silica/Sulfonic and quaternary amine	Peptide analysis	SeQuant
Ion exchange, Cation type	Polymethyl methacrylate, Sulfopropyl functional group, Particle size 7 µm	For separating proteins and peptides	Tosoh Biosep
Ion exchange, Cation type	Silica, Sulfonic acid functional group, Particle size 5 µm	For LC–MS analyses and ion-exchange separations of proteins, peptides	Thermo Hypersil-Keystone
Ion exchange, Anion type	PS-DVB base material, Cryptand functional group, Particle size 5 µm	Ror separating mono- and polyvalent anions in a single run and for determining trace anions in concentrated acids	Dionex
Ion exchange, Cation type	PS–DVB–methacrylate, Carboxymethyl or Sulfoethyl functional group, Particle size 5 µm	For separating biomolecules at most pH values and at high flow rates	OraChrom
Chiral	Silica/Amylose tris (3, 5-dimethylphenyl carbamate)	For use on compounds, with aromatic, amide, carbamate, ester groups, alkyl amines, and compounds with multiple stereogenic sites.	Chiral Technologies

(continues)

Table 33-4. *(continued)*

TYPE OF COLUMN	BASE MATERIAL	APPLICATIONS	SUPPLIERS OF COLUMN
Chiral	Silica/Cellulose tris (3, 5-dimethylphenyl carbamate)	Particularly effective for beta blockers, compounds with similar functionality and steroids Examples: alprenolol, atenolol, flavanone, metoprodol, oxprenolol, pindolol, propranolol.	Chiral Technologies
Chiral	Silica/Vancomycin aglycon	General chiral compound analysis	Astec
Chiral	Acidic chiral compound analysis	Silica / Quinidine or Quinoline	Bischoff Chromatography
Turbo flow columns	Polymer or silica	Turbulent flow chromatography	Cohesive Technologies
Polymeric Biomolecules	Polymethacrylate PS–DVB / PS–DVB	Protein and peptide analysis DNA fragment analysis	Supelco Biochrom Labs
Trapping column	Silica, DVB / Various	Biological sample analysis	Optimize Technologies
Environmental	Silica / Proprietary	Polyaromatic hydrocarbon analysis	Restek
Protein column	PS–DVB / PS–DVB	Proteomic analysis	Polymer Laboratories
Capillary column	Silica / C18	Proteomic analysis, drug discovery, and LC–MS	SGE
Proteomics	Silica / C4, C8, C18	Protein, peptide, and tryptic digest analysis	Micro-Tech Scientific
Trapping column	Strong cation exchange	Biological sample analysis	Scivex/Upchurch Scientific
Turbulent flow column	Silica/Sulfonic acid	Turbulent flow chromatography	Cohesive Technologies
Affinity column	PS–DVB–methacrylate / Protein A	Antibody purification	OraChrom
Affinity column	Porous glass / Protein A, protein G	Antibody purification	Millipore
Ion exchange	PS–DVB / Sulfonic acid	Amino acid analysis	Pickering Laboratories
LC–MS	Silica / C18, strong cation exchange	Protein and proteomic analysis	New Objective

Data from Majors RE. *LCGC North America* 2003; 21:240; and Majors RE. *LCGC North America* 2002; 20:248.

DETECTORS FOR HPLC

Devices used for detection of analytes in column chromatography typically rely on differences in the physical or chemical properties of the eluent and the analyte. Alternatively the solvent may be evaporated to allow detection by mass spectrometry, flame ionization or other detection modes.[21, 22] Table 33-5 lists the different types of detectors used in HPLC instrumentation.

Table 33-5. Detectors Used in HPLC Instrumentation

Optical Detectors
  UV/Visible
  IR/Raman
  Optical Activity
  Evaporative Light Scattering
  Refractive Index
  Luminescent
  Fluorescence/Phosphorescence
  Chemiluminescence/Bioluminescence
Mass Spectrometry Detectors
  Time-of-Flight/MALDI
  Fourier Transform Ion Cyclotron Resonance
  Mass Spectrometry (FTICR-MS or FT-MS)
  Electrospray/Thermospray
Elemental Detectors
  Atomic Absorption/Emission
  Inductively Coupled Plasma (ICP)-Mass Spectrometry
  Microwave-Induced Plasma
Electrochemical Detectors
  Direct current amperometry (DCA)
  Conductivity
  Coulometry
  Polarography

The most frequently used instrument is an ultraviolet-visible spectrometer that has been fitted with a flow cell of very small volume (8 μL). The simplest of these are fixed at one wavelength, usually 254 nm, because most aromatic organic compounds absorb strongly at, or near, this wavelength and the low-pressure mercury lamps used as light sources have a strong emission line at this point. Fixed wavelength models are also available at 280 nm, where the aromatic amino acids of proteins and peptides absorb, or at 214 nm, where isolated double bonds such as the carbonyl group absorb. The fixed wavelength detectors have the advantages of low cost and high sensitivity, being able to detect some compounds at the low-nanogram range. Sensitivity sometimes can be increased by using a variable wavelength detector, as it can be set to the exact point of maximum absorptivity for the solute.

More elaborate models, called *photodiode array detectors*, also are available. These can scan the entire UV spectrum repeatedly during the elution of a peak to determine if more than one substance is co-eluting.

A much more sensitive, but less broadly applicable, detector is the fluorescence spectrometer. Sensitivities in the picogram range can be attained with those compounds that fluoresce naturally or can be made to do so by derivatization. The less expensive models of these instruments are filter fluorimeters whereas the more sensitive ones use a prism or grating to provide monochromatic excitation and emission radiation. A benefit of fluorescence detector versus UV detector is its ability to discriminate analyte from interference or background peaks.

The most generally applicable detector available for use in HPLC is the differential refractometer, which is capable of measuring refractive index changes of 10^{-4} to 10^{-5} RI units. The other detector that is similar in function to differential refractometer is called evaporative light scattering detector (ELS). Each of these detectors has a similar sensitivity for typical samples, allowing the analysis of compounds present on the range of 0.1 μg/ml and higher. These are so called *universal de-*

tectors as that give response to all sample components. Universal detectors are used primarily in two applications: (1) for detection of very low level compounds and (2) to provide a more representative analysis of unknown samples by means of area normalization. Although these detectors react to almost all organic and inorganic compounds, these are not as sensitive as spectrometers. In addition, changes in ambient temperature cause severe drift and it cannot be used with gradient elution because in both cases differences in the RI are attributable to the solvent and not the solution.

Detectors based on electrochemical measurements such as amperometry, coulometry, polarography, or photoconductivity are used for readily oxidizable or reducible compounds such as the catecholamines. With the development of separator interfaces that remove part or all of the mobile phase and the concurrent use of narrow-bore (≤2 mm) columns, spectrometric techniques such as mass spectrometry (LC-MS), and Fourier transform infrared (LC-FTIR) can be used as HPLC detectors. When a greater sensitivity is required than can be obtained from UV detection, the choice is usually fluorescence or an electrochemical detector. Electrochemical detection can be performed in either the oxidative or reductive mode, depending on the type of the analyte. Oxidative electrochemical detection is more commonly used because it is generally easier to (1) operate and run routine samples; (2) maintain the working electrode activity; and (3) avoid some of the preparative steps needed for routine reductive electrochemical detection. Reductive electrochemical methods also suffer from a poor signal / noise ratio due to reduction of dissolved oxygen in the solution.

DERIVATIZATION

Derivatization procedures are used with HPLC for a number of reasons:

- To allow chromatography of compounds that otherwise could not be detected by the instruments currently available, such as aliphatic amines, alcohols, and carboxylic acids.
- To improve resolution by adding a functional group that enhances the interaction of the solutes with the stationary phase, such as esterification of acids.
- To improve the sensitivity of the method, such as formation of fluorescent derivatives of amino acids.

Most of the derivatization reactions commonly used involve adding a substituted phenyl group to enhance detectability at 254 nm. These include the formation of *p*-bromophenacyl esters of alcohols, *p*-nitrobenzyl esters of carboxylic acids and *p*-nitrobenzyl oximes of carbonyls. Fluorescent derivatives (fluorescamine adducts of primary amines) are useful especially because they not only increase the sensitivity greatly, but they also allow selective detection of derivatizable compounds in the presence of coeluting substances that do not react with the reagent.

Derivatization may be done before the sample is introduced onto the column or after it has been eluted. Precolumn reactions provide a functional group, which may enhance the separation of the solutes as well as their detectability, for example, the formation of phthalaldehyde derivatives of amino acids.[23] Postcolumn derivatization allows the separation of the solutes based on their own functionalities but introduces a reagent into the column effluent before it reaches the detector in order to increase the sensitivity. Special items of equipment are available that have the capability of adding reagent, heating the reaction mixture, and providing a time delay to allow quantitative derivatization to occur before introducing the sample into the detector.

QUALITATIVE AND QUANTITATIVE ANALYSIS

The methods used for qualitative and quantitative analysis with HPLC are the same as those used with GC and the interested reader should consult that section for the relevant information.

RECENT DEVELOPMENTS IN HPLC

ION CHROMATOGRAPHY (IC)

Ion chromatography is a form of liquid chromatography that uses ion-exchange resins to separate atomic or molecular ions based on their interaction with the resin. This is a valuable technique for the analysis of inorganic and organic ions in trace amounts. Because there are other techniques, such as atomic absorption spectrometry, by which low levels of cations can be determined accurately, ion chromatography is most useful for the quantitation of anions. This method has a greatest utility for analysis of anions for which there are no other rapid analytical methods. It is also commonly used for cations and biochemical species such as amino acids and proteins.

The equipment usually consists of a resin or silica based low-capacity ion exchanger that permits the use of buffers of low ionic strength as eluants. This column is coupled to a conductivity detector. In those cases where the low signal generated by trace amounts of analytes is overwhelmed by the response due to the mobile-phase ions, a *suppressor column* may be used. This is a second ion-exchange column, which converts the ions of the mobile phase into molecular species of lower conductivity, thereby unmasking the analyte signal. The utility of ion chromatography has been demonstrated on samples as diverse as wastewater and biological fluids.

Ions in solution can be detected by measuring the conductivity of the solution. In ion chromatography, the mobile phase contains ions that create background conductivity, making it difficult to measure the conductivity due only to the analyte ions as they exit the column. This problem can be greatly reduced by selectively removing the mobile phase ions after the analytical column and before the detector. This is done by converting the mobile phase ions to a neutral form or removing them with an eluent suppressor, which consists of an ion-exchange column or membrane. For cation analysis, the mobile phase is often HCl or HNO_3, which can be neutralized by an eluent suppressor that supplies OH^-. The Cl^- or NO_3^- is either retained or removed by the suppressor column or membrane. The same principle holds good for anion analysis. The mobile phase is often NaOH or $NaHCO_3$, and the eluent suppressor supplies H^+ to neutralize the anion and retain or remove the Na^+.

SUPERCRITICAL FLUID CHROMATOGRAPHY

Supercritical fluid chromatography (SFC) is a relatively new chromatographic technique, having been commercially available in the recent years. As a result there is a large amount of research currently underway both in SFC method development and in hardware development. What differentiates SFC from other chromatographic techniques (GC and HPLC) is the use of a supercritical fluid as the mobile phase. This technique is based on the use as a mobile phase of a *supercritical fluid*, one held at or above its critical temperature, the point at which a gas cannot be liquefied no matter how high the pressure. The resulting liquid has density, viscosity, and diffusivity characteristics midway between its gaseous and liquid states. The lower density and viscosity, when compared to that of a liquid, allow faster separations than with ordinary HPLC, while the higher diffusion than that of a gas reduces longitudinal band-spreading.

The instrumentation employed is common to both HPLC and GC. Packed columns with reversed-phase bonded materials have been used as well as fused-silica open tubular capillary columns as long as 60 m. In addition to the usual HPLC detectors, the universal detectors used in GC such as the FID are also applicable. Solute retention may be influenced by gradient-programming of either the temperature or the pressure. The most commonly used mobile phase, carbon dioxide, has a critical temperature of 31° at 73 atmospheres and is an excellent solvent for many organic compounds as well as being inexpensive, nontoxic, and nonflammable.

Supercritical fluid chromatography has several main advantages over other conventional chromatographic techniques (GC and HPLC). Compared with HPLC, SFC provides rapid separations without the use of organic solvents. With the desire for environmentally conscious technology, the use of organic chemicals as used in HPLC could be reduced with the use of SFC. Because SFC generally uses carbon dioxide collected as a byproduct of other chemical reactions or is collected directly from the atmosphere, it contributes no new chemicals to the environment. In addition, SFC separations can be done faster than HPLC separations because the diffusion of solutes in supercritical fluids is about ten times greater than that in liquids (and about three times less than in gases). This result in a decrease in resistance to mass transfer in the column and allows for fast high resolution separations. Compared with GC, capillary SFC can provide high-resolution chromatography at much lower temperatures. This allows fast analysis of thermolabile compounds.

HYDROPHOBIC INTERACTION CHROMATOGRAPHY (HIC)

Separation and purification of active biological molecules such as proteins by normal reversed-phase techniques usually leads to denaturation and loss of activity due to the strong hydrophobic interactions with the supports or on account of the organic modifier (eg, acetonitrile or methanol) in the mobile phase. In HIC, supports are generally hydrophilic polymers, such as polyethylene glycol, onto which short hydrophobic ligands (eg, methyl, propyl, or butyl) have been bonded. Mobile phases are entirely aqueous with retention being controlled by the concentration of added salts such as ammonium sulfate or surfactants. High salt concentrations favor retention by increasing hydrophobic interactions with the column. Thus, the usual method of elution is gradient analysis with decreasing salt concentration. The weakness of the interaction with the stationary phase and the use of aqueous mobile phases enhance retention of biological activity.[24]

Hydrophobic interaction chromatography and reverse-phase chromatography (RPC) are closely related liquid chromatographic techniques. Both are based upon interactions between solvent-accessible non-polar groups (hydrophobic patches) on the surface of biomolecules and the hydrophobic ligands (alkyl or aryl groups) covalently attached to the gel matrix. The difference is that, adsorbents for RPC are more highly substituted with hydrophobic ligands than HIC adsorbents. The degree of substitution of HIC adsorbents is usually in the range of 10 to 50 mmoles/ml gel of C2–C8 alkyl or simple aryl ligands, compared with several hundred mmoles/ml gel of C4–C18 alkyl ligands usually used for RPC adsorbents. Consequently, protein binding to RPC adsorbents is usually very strong, which requires the use of non-polar solvents for their elution. RPC has found extensive applications in analytical and preparative separations of mainly peptides and low molecular weight proteins that are stable in aqueous-organic solvents. HIC is an alternative way of exploiting the hydrophobic properties of proteins, working in a more polar and less denaturing environment. Compared with RPC, the polarity of the complete system of HIC is increased by reducing the ligand density on the stationary phase and by adding salt to the mobile phase.[24]

Factors Affecting HIC

The main parameters to consider when selecting HIC media and optimizing separation processes on HIC media are:

1. Ligand type and degree of substitution: The type of immobilized ligand (alkyl or aryl) determines primarily the protein adsorption selectivity of the HIC adsorbent. In general, straight chain alkyl ligands show greater hydrophobic character than aryl ligands, which show mixed mode behavior where both aromatic and hydrophobic interactions are possible. It is also established that, at a constant degree of substitution, the protein binding capacities of HIC adsorbents increase with increased alkyl chain length.

The choice between alkyl or aryl ligands is empirical and must be established by screening experiments for each individual separation problem. The protein binding capacities of HIC adsorbents increase with increased degree of substitution of immobilized ligand and reach a plateau at a certain high degree of ligand substitution but the strength of the interaction increases. Solutes bound under such circumstances are difficult to elute due to multi-point attachment.

2. Type of base matrix: The two most widely used types of support are strongly hydrophilic carbohydrates (eg, cross-linked agarose, or synthetic copolymer materials). The selectivity of a copolymer support will not be exactly the same as for an agarose based support substituted with the same type of ligand.

3. Type and concentration of salt: The addition of various salts to the equilibration buffer and sample solution promotes ligand-protein interactions in HIC by salting out process. As the concentration of such salts is increased, the amount of proteins binding also increases almost linearly up to a specific salt concentration and continues to increase in an exponential manner at still higher concentrations.

4. pH: The effect of pH in HIC is not straightforward. In general, an increase in pH weakens hydrophobic interactions, probably as a result of increased titration of charged groups, thereby leading to an increase in the hydrophilicity of the proteins. On the other hand, a decrease in pH results in an apparent increase in hydrophobic interactions. Thus, proteins, which do not bind to a HIC adsorbent at neutral pH, bind at acidic pH

5. Effect of temperature: The binding of proteins to HIC adsorbents is entropy driven, which implies that the interaction increases with an increase in temperature. The Van der waals attraction forces, which operate in hydrophobic interactions, also increase with increase in temperature. However, an opposite effect was reported some times indicating that the role of temperature in HIC is of a complex nature. This apparent discrepancy is probably due to the differential effects exerted by temperature on the conformational state of different proteins and their solubilities in aqueous solutions. In practical terms, one should thus be aware that a downstream purification process developed at room temperature might not be reproduced in the cold room, or *vice versa*.

6. Additives: Low concentrations of water-miscible alcohols, detergents and aqueous solutions of chaotropic ("salting-in") salts result in a weakening of the protein-ligand interactions in HIC leading to the desorption of the bound solutes. The non-polar parts of alcohols and detergents compete effectively with the bound proteins for the adsorption sites on the HIC media resulting in the displacement of the latter. Chaotropic salts affect the ordered structure of water and/or that of the bound proteins. Although additives can be used in the elution buffer to affect selectivity during desorption, there is a risk that proteins could be denatured or inactivated by exposure to high concentrations of such chemicals. However, additives can be very effective in cleaning up HIC columns that have strongly hydrophobic proteins bound to the gel medium.

CHIRAL CHROMATOGRAPHY

Many medicinally useful agents occur naturally as members of a racemic pair of chiral isomers. Frequently, the medicinal activity resides in one of the isomers, while the other has no appreciable activity or is toxic. To reduce the chance of untoward effects in patients, it is desirable to separate the mixture into its constituent isomers. The enantiomers can also differ in absorption, distribution, protein binding, and affinity to the receptor.[25] In order to separate the mixture (*racemate, which is a 1: 1 mixture of isomers*) into discrete isomers, it is necessary to react the sample with a chiral compound to form two *diastereomers* or *diastereomeric* complexes. Diastereomers have different chemical and physical properties and can be resolved to individual isomers. The separation process involves the use of GC, supercritical fluid chromatography and HPLC, but HPLC is the most widely used of these methods.

Chiral seperation techniques can be classified as *indirect* and *direct* methods.[26] In the *indirect* separation technique, *chiral derivatizing agent* (CDA) is added to the mobile phase, which reacts with the isomers to form a mixture of two *diastereomers*. These have an additional chiral center, and their altered geometric structure permits separation (as they differ in physico-chemical properties) by conventional normal phase or reversed phase HPLC. These loosely bound complexes are adsorbed to the stationary phase with different affinities and thus are separated. This approach circumvents the need for expensive columns with chiral stationary phases and is more flexible. This technique needs high enantiomeric purity and stability of the CDA. Another disadvantage is that isolation of the pure isomers requires removal of the chiral reagent. Examples of CDAs include (1) 1-(9-fluorenyl)-ethylchloroformate and o-phtaldialdehyde in combination with chiral thiols; (2) (O,O0-R,R)-diacylated tartaric acid anhydrides; (3) (1R,2R)- or (1S,2S)-N-[(2-isothiocyanato)cyclohexyl]-3,5 dinitrobenzoylamide (DDITC); (4) 1-(6-Methoxy-2-naphthyl)ethyl isothiocyanate (NAP-IT) and 2-(6-methoxy-2-naphthyl)-1-propylchloroformate (NAP-C).[27]

In the *Direct method,* a chiral-separating reagent can be bonded (covalently or ionically or physically coated) to the stationary phase to form a *chiral stationary phase* (CSP). Silica or aminopropyl silica is commonly used as a starting support material, but particles of a polymeric chiral stationary phase are also available. The chiral isomers associate loosely with the bound reagent to form dissociable diastereomers with different retention times. Resolution of chiral isomers relies on the formation of transient diastereoisomers on the surface of the column packing. The compound that forms the most stable diastereoisomer will be most retained, whereas the opposite enantiomer will form a less stable diastereoisomer and will elute first. Majority of chiral separations reported in the literature are direct separations. Several hundreds of CSP columns are commercially available, although many of these columns are similar in structure and enantioselectivity.[28] Table 33-6 lists different types of CSP columns according to their chemistry and mechanism of chemical recognition. Some columns are better able to separate wide range of sample types. A very rough order of CSP universality is, protein type > carbohydrate type > Pirkle type > cyclodextrin type.[18] Some suggestions for the choice of CSP for different chemical categories are listed in Table 33-7.

MICROBORE CHROMATOGRAPHY

The microbore chromatography procedure, also known as microscale HPLC or *capillary HPLC*, combines extremely high efficiencies with speed and economy of operation. The columns used in this technique are narrow-bore (1 mm or less) fused-silica or glass-lined stainless steel. The tubes may be coated with liquid phase or packed (densely or loosely) with microparticulate stationary phases of the same types used in ordinary HPLC. Special equipment is necessary for operation in this mode, including pumps that can deliver accurate volumes at flow rates of 50 to 200 µL/min, injectors that introduce samples of less than 1 µL, and detector flow cells with volumes of as low as 45 µL.

Transferring standard HPLC methods to Microbore HPLC allows huge increase in sensitivity. Sensitivity of most HPLC detectors is concentration dependent. Thus, the sensitivity of standard HPLC column can be increased by a factor of 20 when 4mm i.d. columns (typical flow rate: 1ml/min) are replaced by 1mm i.d. columns (typical flow rate: 50µl/min). In addition, columns can be connected in series to achieve additive increases in efficiency, a procedure that is not possible with ordinary HPLC columns. Other advantages include significant savings in solvents, as flow rates lower than 50 µL/min are required, low operational costs and finally the possibility of direct coupling to a mass spectrometer (LC-MS). The major disadvantage is a result of the low solute capacity of the columns, which makes preparative work impractical.

Microscale HPLC columns can be hyphenated to infrared (IR) spectrometer or mass (MS) spectrometer for compound detection and characterization. Usage of microscale columns increases the mass sensitivity of a sample, IR and MS spectrometric techniques are hyphenated with microscale columns with great success.[31]

Increased mass sensitivity of micro-HPLC is significant in the analysis of biological samples. Microscale HPLC technique is successfully applied in the determination of bile acids in serum (detection levels, 0.13–0.28 pmole),[32] determination of dibutyl phthalate (DBP) in water (detection levels of tap water and commercially available purified water were 4.5 and 5.4 parts per billion, respectively),[33] determination of anti-oxidants in gasoline,[34] and determination of theophylline in serum and so on.

THE HIGH PERFORMANCE LIQUID CHROMATOGRAPHY METHOD DEVELOPMENT

High performance liquid chromatography is a widely used technique in the pharmaceutical and biopharmaceutical sectors. The HPLC method development essentially follows series of

Table 33-6. Different Types of CSP Columns for Chiral Chromatography

CSP TYPE	APPLICATION	MECHANISM OF CHIRAL SEPARATION
Pirkle type*	Beta blockers, Warfarin, Ibuprofen, and arylamides, aryl-epoxides aryl-sulphoxides	Hydrogen bonding, π-π interactions, dipole stacking
Cellulose/carbohydrate based	Small aliphatic and aromatic compounds, cyclopentenones, alkaloids, tropines, amines, beta blockers, beta lactams, dihydroxypryidines	Combination of attractive interactions and inclusion complexes
Protein based	Benzodiazepine, Warfarin and oxazepam, amines and acids, in general analytes with ionizable groups	Combination of hydrophobic and polar interactions
Cyclodextrin	The selectivity of a Cyclodextrin Phase is dependent on the size of the analyte. Alpha-cyclodextrin will include single Phenyl groups or Napthyl groups end-on. Beta-cyclodextrin will accept Napthyl groups and heavily substituted phenyl groups. Gamma-Cyclodextrin is useful for bulky steriod-type molecules	Inclusion complexation and hydrogen bonding
Ligand exchange type	Mainly for separation of alpha- amino acids	Coordination complexes with copper or other metals
Macrocyclic antibiotics+	All amino acids, amino acid derivatives such as methyl esters and peptides	π-π interactions, hydrogen bonding, inclusion complexation, ionic interactions and peptide binding.

* The columns within this group are mainly the result of the work of Bill Pirkle
+ The antibiotics immobilized with silica Rifamycin, Vancomycin and Ticoplanin to form CSPs.

Table 33-7. Suggested Columns for Different Compounds Types

CLASS OF COMPOUND	TYPE OF CSP TO USE	COLUMN TRADE NAME
Acids	Proteins, cellulose/Amylose, Pirkle	OVM, AGP, BSA, Chiralcel OD-OJ, Whelk-O-1
Amino Acids	Crown ether, ligand exchange, cyclodextrins, protein	CrownPak CR (+), 1-hydroxyproline, BSA, Cyclobond II
Amines	Proteins, cellulose/amylose, Pirkle, cyclodextrins	OVM, AGP, BSA, Chiralcel OD-OJ, CTA, DNBPG, naphthyl alanine, Whelk-O-1, Cyclobond II
Alcohols	Proteins, cellulose/ amylose, Pirkle, cyclodextrins	OVM, AGP, BSA, Chiralcel OB, OD-OJ, CTA, DNBPG, naphthyl alanine, Whelk-O-1, β-Cyclobond II
Esters	Pirkle, cellulose	DNBPG, Whelk-O-1, CTA
Sulfoxides	Pirkle, cellulose, protein	DNBPG, Whelk-O-1, Chiralcel OA, OB, BSA
Carbamates	Pirkle	DNBPG, Whelk-O-1
Ureas	Pirkle	DNBPG, Whelk-O-1
Crown ethers	Cyclodextrins	β-Cyclobond II
Metallocenes	Cyclodextrins	β-Cyclobond II
Thiols	Pirkle	DNBPG, β-GEM-1
Amino Acids	Pirkle	DNBPG, β-GEM-1
Succinamides	Pirkle	DNBPG, β-GEM-1
Hydantoins	Pirkle	DNBPG, β-GEM-1
Binaphthols	Pirkle	DNBPG, β-GEM-1
β-Lactams	Pirkle, cellulose	DNBPG, Whelk-O-1, Chiralcel OC, OF
Succinamides	Pirkle	DNBPG, β-GEM-1
Polycyclic aromatic hydrocarbons	Cyclodextrins	Cyclobond Ac
Cyclic drugs	Protein	BSA, AGP, OVM
Aromatic drugs	Protein	BSA, AGP, OVM
Lactones	Cellulose	Chiralcel OA, OB
Cyclic ketones	Pirkle, cellulose	Whelk-O-1, Chiralcel OA, OB
Alkaloids	Cellulose	Chiralcel OC, OD, OF, OG
Dihydropyridines	Cellulose	Chiralcel OC, OD, OG, OJ
NSAIDS	Pirkle, cellulose, protein	Whelk-O-1, Chiralcel OJ, AGP
Oxazolindones	Pirkle	DNBPG

From Snyder LR, Kirkland JJ, Glajch JL. *Practical HPLC Method Development*, 2nd ed. New York: John Wiley, 1997; 174. Copyright © 1997. Reprinted with permission of John Wiley & Sons, Inc.

steps as summarized in Figure 33-11.[29] In most cases, the desired separation can be achieved easily with only few experiments, and in other cases considerable number of experiments need to be performed. Before beginning a method development process for any given sample, the analyst needs to know several sample characteristics, eg, chemistry and physical properties of the sample, separation goal (whether qualitative or quantitative analysis), need for pretreatment of sample, detection method etc. The HPLC method development cannot be generalized, and there is no universal procedure that can be adopted for different types of samples. The development procedure varies according to the chemistry and nature of the analyte. The procedure given below gives more focus on analytes that follow reversed or normal phase separation.

Nature of the Sample and Defining Separation Goals

At the beginning of method development activity, information concerning the sample chemistry, composition, and properties has to be reviewed. These include sample solubility, number of compounds present in the sample, chemical structures, molecular weight of compounds, UV spectra, pKa of compounds and concentration range of compounds in the sample. Ideally, complete description of the sample is needed. For example, in a tablet containing the active and inactive ingredients, the goal of HPLC separation is primarily the assay of active drug. From the information on chemistry of the given sample, chromatographers can choose appropriate initial chromatographic conditions (ie, type of column and stationary phase needed, column dimensions, mobile phase composition, flow rate etc.). Many times the composition of many samples is not fully known at the beginning of HPLC method development (eg, samples containing impurities, degradation products, metabolites). In these cases, chromatographers follow an empirical procedure using a default column (mostly with reversed phase chromatographic conditions) and initial conditions as described under 'initial separation conditions'.

The chromatographer needs to define what is the goal of his analysis for the given sample . The chromatographic separation or analysis is carried out for one or more of the following reasons: (a) whether the goal is quantitative analysis of the active ingredient of the sample or qualitative detection of impurities in the given sample mixture, (b) number of samples to be analyzed at a given point of time (when a large number of samples must be processed at the same time, the run time can be decreased by decreasing column length and/or increasing the flow rate by compromising on the resolution of the samples), and (c) whether to resolve all the impurities or degradation products in a sample mixture; (many times it is essential to isolate all the impurities and degradation products from the active ingredient, but it may not be essential to resolve these impurities into individual components).

Sample Pretreatment and Need for Special Procedures

Sample preparation is an essential part of HPLC analysis intended to provide a homogeneous solution that is suitable for injection into the column. The sample should be prepared in such a way that it is relatively free from interferences and /or protect the column or equipment from damage. Furthermore, the sample solvent should be miscible in mobile phase without affecting the retention and resolution of the sample. Best results are often obtained when the composition of sample solvent is close to that of mobile phase since this minimizes base line upset and other problems. Some times it may be desirable to concentrate the analytes in the sample and / or derivatize them for improved detection or better separation.

Sample pretreatment includes large number of methodologies, as well as multiple operational steps and can therefore be a challenging part of HPLC method development. A sample pretreatment procedure should provide quantitative (>99%) recovery of analytes and involve minimum number of steps. The samples should be collected using a statistically validated process, stored in inert and tightly sealed containers. Several sample pretreatment processes are available for making the sample suitable for HPLC analysis. One or more of these methods are employed in the sample pretreatment.

(A) *Solid phase extraction:* Liquid is passed through solid phase, which selectively removes the analyte or interferences. Analyte can be eluted with a strong solvent and in some cases, interferences are retained and analytes are allowed to pass through solid phase. A wide variety of stationary phases is available for selective removal of desired inorganic, organic or biological analytes.

(B) *Liquid-liquid extraction:* Sample is partitioned between two immiscible phases, which are chosen to maximize differences in solubility.

(C) *Dilution:* Sample is diluted with a solvent compatible with HPLC mobile phase to avoid column overload or to be in linear range of detector.

(D) *Evaporation:* Liquid is removed by gentle heating at atmospheric pressure with flowing air or inert gas or vacuum. Rotary vacuum evaporator is commonly used and automated systems (eg, Turbovap) are also available.

(E) *Distillation:* Sample is heated to boiling point of solvent and volatile analytes are concentrated in vapor phase, condensed and collected.

(F) *Microdialysis:* A semi-permeable membrane is placed between two aqueous liquid phases, and sample solute transfer from one liquid to the other progresses based on differences in concentration. Sample enrichment techniques such as solid phase extraction are required to concentrate the dialysate. Microdialysis is used for examination of extracellular chemicals in living plant or animal tissue using molecular weight cut off membranes. Molecular weight cut-off membranes are used on-line with micro-LC columns. These membranes some times are used on-line to deproteinate samples prior to HPLC since large proteins cannot pass through membranes

(G) *Lyophilization:* Aqueous sample is frozen and water removed by sublimation under vacuum. For suspensions, filtration, centrifugation or sedimentation are carried out to remove particulate matter and the resultant solution is processed by one of the methods as described above. These are highly recommended to remove particulate matter and this prevents backpressure problems and preserves the column life.

Choosing Detector and Detector Settings

Before the first sample is injected during HPLC method development, we must be reasonably sure that the detection cell will sense all sample components of interest. In most cases, variable wavelength (spectrophotometric) or Photodiode-array (PDA) detectors are normally the choice because of their convenience and applicability for most samples. For many samples, good analytical results are obtained by careful selection of the detector wavelength. PDA detector permits simultaneous collection of chromatograms at different wavelengths during a single run, therefore providing more information on sample composition than is provided by a single wavelength run. The wavelength chosen for UV detection must provide acceptable absorbance by various analytes in the sample combined with acceptable light

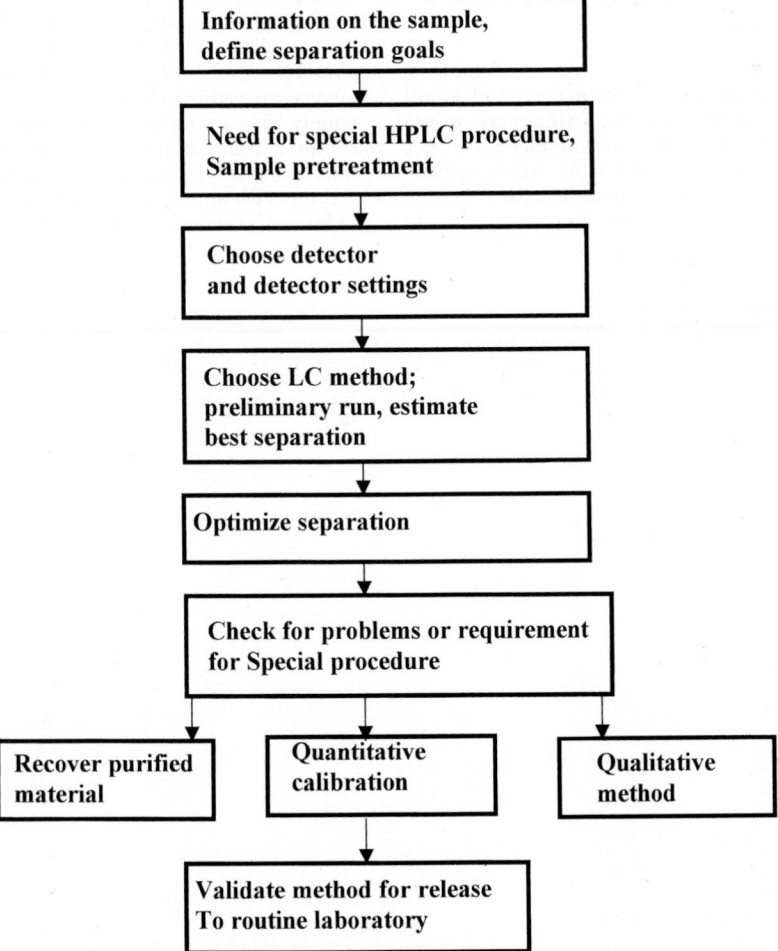

Figure 33-11. Steps in HPLC method development. From Snyder LR, Kirkland JJ, Glajch JL. *Practical HPLC Method Development*, 2nd ed. New York: John Wiley, 1997; 174. Copyright © 1997. Reprinted with permission of John Wiley & Sons, Inc.

transmittance by mobile phase. For some samples, it is also important to select a wavelength at which sample interferences have minimum absorption. For UV detection to provide adequate sensitivity for the analysis of major sample components, molar absorptivity (ε) must be greater than 10. For trace analysis, values greater than 100 (preferably >1000) are usually required for UV detection. The organic compounds for which UV detection is completely unsuitable are saturated hydrocarbons and their amino and nitrile derivatives. Saturated hydrocarbons substituted by ether (-O-), hydroxy (-OH), chloro (-Cl), carboxy (-COOH), or ester (-COOR) groups have marginal absorptivity and may require detection at low UV values (210–185 nm). Since many mobile phases and degradation products in the sample absorb strongly in this range, analysis in this region is somewhat restricted. Compound types other than those mentioned above generally have larger absorptivity values and can be detected at higher wavelengths (> 210 nm).

When the sample shows little or no UV response or analyte concentrations are too low for UV detection, other detectors such as electrochemical or fluorescence detector can be considered. Further, sample can be derivatized for enhanced detection. The use of mass spectrometer for HPLC detection (LC-MS) is becoming commonplace. A mass spectrometer can facilitate HPLC method development and avoid common problems by (1) identifying the components of individual peaks in the chromatogram, (2) distinguishing the analytes of interest from interfering substances, and (3) recognizing unexpected and overlapping interference peaks to avoid a premature finish to method development.

Choice of HPLC Method and Choosing Column and Initial Separation Conditions

HPLC analytes can be classified as *regular* or *special* samples. Regular samples are defined as typical mixtures of small molecules <1000 Da that can be separated using more-or-less standardized starting conditions.[29] Regular samples are either neutral or ionic. Ionic substances include acids, bases, organic salts (ionized strong acids or bases) or sometimes, the sample composition is completely unknown (ie, the sample could contain acids or bases). Initial separation of regular samples is achieved by *reversed phase* chromatography under standard column dimensions, solvent system and run conditions (Standard conditions include: 15 cm column length and 0.46 cm i.d., 5 μm particle size, C_{18} stationary phase, buffered acetonitrile mobile phase, pH 3.0, 1.5–2.0 ml/min flow rate, 35–45 °C column temperature and 25–50μl sample volume).[29] A gradient run is preferable to isocratic run to resolve the sample mixture. The initial gradient should be 5% to 100% acetonitrile in 60 min. This first gradient run can be used to decide (a) whether isocratic or gradient elution is recommended for analysis and b) if special reversed-phase conditions will be needed. Using these conditions, first exploratory run is carried out and then improved systematically. If the typical reversed-phase conditions provide insufficient sample retention, it suggests the use of either ion-pair or normal phase HPLC. In some cases, the sample may be strongly retained with 100% acetonitrile as mobile phase suggesting the use of non-aqueous reversed-phase chromatography or normal phase HPLC.

Special samples are usually separated with a different column and customized conditions. Examples of some special samples and their HPLC requirements are:

Inorganic ions isomers: Detection is primary problem; use ion chromatography.

Enantiomers: Require chiral conditions for separation as described in chiral chromatography.

Biological (proteins, peptides and oligonucleotides): Several factors make this kind 'special': These are molecular conformation, polar functionality and hydrophobicity. These are successfully resolved by ion pair or ion exchange chromatography.

Macromolecules: These may be separated by column packing with large pores (>>10-nm diameter) by size exclusion chromatography as described earlier.

The column is the heart of HPLC separation processes. The availability of stable HPLC column is essential in developing a rugged reproducible method. Commercial columns can differ widely among suppliers and even between supposedly identical columns from a single source. Such differences can have serious impact on developing the desired HPLC method. For selecting column with appropriate bonded phase, the first requirement is to know the chemistry of sample components. Molecular struc-

Table 33-8. Column Selection Chart

	PARTICLE SIZE (MICRONS)			COLUMN LENGTH (MM)			COLUMN INNER DIA (MM)			SURFACE AREA (M²/G)		PORE SIZE (Å)			CARBON LOAD (%)		
	3	5	10	30	150	300	2	4.6	22.5	200	300	60	100	300	30	10	20
What Do You Need? Default column#		*			*			*		*			*			*	
High efficiency	*																
High capacity											*	*					*
Low back pressure			*	*													
High resolution	*					*					*						*
High sample loadability									*		*	*					*
Capability to analyze samples with greater than 2000 molecular weights														*			
High stability																	
High sensitivity				*			*										
Fast analysis				*						*						*	
Low mobile-phase consumption				*			*										
Stability at pH extremes																	
Fast equilibration				*						*							

A default column is good for most applications.

Data from Young CS, Weigand R. *LCGC North America* 2002; 20:465.

Table 33-9. Effect of Column Dimensions and Particle Physical Characteristics on the Chromatographic Separations[30]

Column dimensions:

The column dimensions are the length and inner diameter of the packing bed.

Short: Short columns are 30–50 mm in length. They provide short run times and low back pressure.

Long: Long columns are 250–300 mm in length. They provide higher resolution and longer run times.

Narrow: Narrow-bore columns have inner diameters smaller than 2.1 mm. They provide higher detection sensitivity.

Wide: Wide-bore columns have 10–22 mm inner diameters. They enable the loading of large samples.

Particle shape:

Particles are either spherical or irregular.

Spherical particles have reduced backpressures and provide longer column life when used with viscous mobile phases such as 50:50 (v/v) methanol–water.

Irregular particles have higher surface areas and higher carbon loads, and they generally produce higher capacity factors for potentially greater resolution.

Particle size:

The particle diameter range is 1.5–20 μm.

Smaller particles offer higher efficiency. Choose 1.5 or 3 μm particles for resolving complex, multicomponent samples. Otherwise, choose 5- or 10-μm packings.

Surface area:

The surface area is the sum of particle outer surface and interior pore surface in square meters per gram.

High surface areas generally provide greater retention, capacity, and resolution for separating complex, multi component samples.

Pore size:

The pore size is the average size of the particles' pores or cavities. They range in value from 60 Å to 10,000 Å.

Larger pores allow larger solute molecules to be retained through maximum exposure to the surface area of the particles. Choose a pore size of 150 Å or less for samples with molecular weights less than 2000. Choose a pore size of 300 Å or greater for samples with molecular weights greater than 2000.

Bonding type:

The bonding type is the attachment mode of each bonded-phase strand to the base silica.

Monomeric: Monomeric phases have single-point attachments of bonded phase molecules. Monomeric bonding provides faster equilibration and higher column efficiency.

Polymeric: Polymeric phases have multiple-point attachments of bonded phase molecules. Polymeric bonding offers increased column stability, particularly when used with highly aqueous mobile phases. Polymeric bonding also enables columns to accept higher sample loading.

Carbon load:

The carbon load is the amount of bonded phase attached to the base material, expressed as the percentage of carbon.

High carbon loads generally offer greater resolution and longer run times for hydrophobic samples.

Low carbon loads shorten run times and often show different selectivity.

Endcapping:

Endcapping is the capping of exposed silanols with short hydrocarbon chains after the primary bonding step. Endcapping reduces peak tailing of polar solutes that interact excessively with the otherwise-exposed silanols. Nonendcapped packings provide a different selectivity than that of endcapped packings, especially for polar samples.

Data from Young CS, Weigand R. *LCGC North America* 2002; 20:465.

---

tures for all sample components should be known and two molecular structures that are the most similar need to be identified. Analyte retention occurs as the functional groups in question interact with the stationary and mobile phases and promote resolution of the pair by a process of differential migration. The intermolecular forces involved are Van der Waals interaction, dipole–dipole interaction, hydrogen bonding and π-π interactions. *C18, C8, and C4* are non-polar phases and retention for these phases is based upon Van der Waals interactions with hydrophobic compounds. Because the C8 phase has approximately 40% to 50% of the carbon loading of a C18 phase, its hydrophobicity and hence it's hydrophobic resolving power is less than that of a C18 phase. *Phenyl* phases also are nonpolar and retention for these phases is a mixed mechanism of hydrophobic and π-π interactions. The overall hydrophobic retention of a phenyl phase is similar to that of a C8 bonded phase but unique selectivity rests in its π-orbital interaction with analyte electron-deficient functional groups. *Cyano* phases have intermediate polarity. Retention is a mixed mechanism of hydrophobic, dipole–dipole, and π-π interactions. These phases are best used for analyzing polar organic compounds and they are versatile enough for use in both normal and reversed-phase modes. The *amino* phase is a polar phase that can be used in both normal and ion exchange modes. Retention is caused by dipole–dipole interactions or acid–base interactions. Amino phases commonly are used for carbohydrate analysis but they also can be used for analyzing both organic and inorganic ions.

The effect of column format and particle physical characteristics on the chromatographic separation is shown in Table 33-8.[30] The chart uses a default column as a starting point (first row). This profile represents an average analytical column that is good for most applications: 150 mm × 4.6 mm, 5-μm particles, 100-Å pore size, 200-m^2/g surface area, 10% carbon load, monomeric bonding, and spherical particles. To use the chart effectively, match the method goals with individual particle physical characteristics. Change only those physical parameters that are affected by specific method goals. For example, a goal of fast equilibration is best achieved by using a short 30 to 50 mm column with a silica surface area of 200 m^2/g. Assessing the most important method goals will lead to important decisions regarding the physical aspects of the column and conclude with the selection of an optimal column. Finally, recognize the optimum column as a possible compromise of method goals. For example, the optimum column for highest resolution of all sample components could sacrifice speed of analysis. This is because; resolution (Rs) is dependent in part upon the number of theoretical plates, which in turn is affected by column length and particle efficiencies. Table 33-9 describes the column and particle physical characteristics and how they affect chromatography. This gives the analyst information for deciding the column type and specifications of column that to be used for separation of given sample.

Optimizing Separation

The separation achieved in one or two runs usually will be less than adequate. After few additional trials, it may be tempting to accept a marginal separation, especially if no further improvement is observed. However experienced workers realize that a good separation requires more than minimal resolution of individual sample bands, particularly for a routine procedure used to analyze a number of samples. Specifically the experienced chromatographer will consider several aspects of separation summarized as follows[29]:

Resolution: Precise and rugged quantitative analysis requires that the base line resolution to be greater than 1.5.

Separation time: < 5 to 10 minutes is desirable for routine procedures.

Pressure: <2000 psi is desirable, <2500 psi is usually essential (new column assumed).

Peak height: Narrow peaks are desirable for large signal/noise ratios.

Solvent composition: Minimum mobile phase use per run is desirable.

The time required for separation of the given sample should be as short as possible. The run time goal should be compared with the 2-hour setup time typically required for HPLC procedure including mobile phase preparation, column installation, equilibration, base line achievement, replicate standards injected to confirm precision, reproducible retention, and acceptable separation. Thus, if only two or three samples are to be assayed at one time, a run time of 20 to 30 min is not excessive. When several samples are to be assayed, run times of 5 to 10 minutes is desirable.

Conditions for final HPLC method should be selected so that the operating pressure with a new column does not exceed 2500 psi and an upper pressure limit below 2000 psi is desirable. This is because during the life of a column, the backpressure may rise by a factor of as much as 2 due to gradual plugging of the column with particulate matter. Moreover, at a lower pressure, pumps, sample valves, and auto-samplers operate much better, seals last longer and columns tend to plug less thereby improving system reliability. For these reasons, a target pressure of less than 50% of the maximum capacity of the pump is desirable.

While changing the mobile phase, enough time must elapse for the column to come into equilibrium with the new mobile phase and temperature. Usually column equilibrium is achieved after passage of 10 to 20 column volumes of the new mobile phase through the column. However, this should be confirmed by carrying out a repeat experiment under similar conditions. When constant retention times are observed in two or three successive experiments, it can be assumed that column is equilibrated and the experiments are repeatable. Failure to ensure column equilibration and repeatable chromatograms can be a serious impediment to HPLC method development.

Check for Problems or Requirement for Special Procedure

Problems in the HPLC method development are mostly concerning with column and instrument usage and maintenance. Three most important kinds of problems in HPLC method development are: (1) variability in retention and resolution, (2) band tailing, and (3) short column lifetime.

Columns must maintain reproducible retention and resolution during use, otherwise the accuracy and precision of the method are compromised and new columns may be required frequently. Sometimes, a new column may give unsatisfactory separation. This means that the operating conditions must be modified to re-establish the required separation. The main reasons for variations in retention and resolution are: variation in support and bonding (from column-to-column), disturbance in the bed and loss of bonded phase (during column usage), changes in the instrument-to-instrument configuration and insufficient equilibration time between stationary and mobile phases. Problems associated with this kind of irreproducibility are usually solved by: (a) initially selecting a good column of less-acidic highly purified support (silica column) and maintaining the same stationary phase, particle size and column dimensions throughout the operation; (b) eliminating the chemical or silanol effects for silica based columns by using favorable mobile phase conditions (pH, buffer type and additives); (c) making sure that the column is properly equilibrated with the mobile phase; (d) using proper laboratory techniques that ensure day-to-day operation; (e) using retention mapping to provide corrective action when required; and (f) stocking columns, or establishing a continuing supply of the same column.

Tailing peaks cause inferior separations and reduced precision. Column plate numbers and band resolution are over estimated when tailing peaks are involved. Tailing peaks can also trail into a closely eluting following peak reducing the ability to quantitate each peak accurately. Peak asymmetry or band tailing can arise from several sources: Bad column, plugged frit, build-up of waste in column inlet, sample overload, wrong solvent for sample, extra-column effects, chemical or secondary retention (silanol) effects, inadequate buffering and contaminating heavy metals. During use, columns can develop severe band tailing usually due to void in the inlet of the column and/or a dirty partially plugged inlet frit. This can be eliminated by replacing the inlet frit of the column or reversing the direction of flow through the column. Purging the column with a strong solvent sometimes can eliminate the buildup in the column (eg, dichloromethane), methanol and ammonium hydroxide (96%, 4%, 0.1% respectively are often effective for reversed phase columns and methanol (100%) for normal phase columns).

Columns for normal phase chromatography are more stable (>1 year life, when used with clean samples) than are columns used for other HPLC procedures. Polymeric ion exchange columns display similar stability. On the other hand, silica based columns for reversed phase chromatography, ion pair and ion exchange chromatography are less rugged in the aqueous environments. Columns degrade for several reasons: (a) Partially blocked (plugged) frit or column bed; (b) adsorption of sample impurities; (c) initially poorly packed column; (d) mechanical or thermal shock creating voids; and (e) chemical attack on support or stationary phase. The increase in column backpressure, tailing bands, decrease in retention are some symptoms imminent to column 'death.'

Some steps for ensuring best column life-time and performance are to: (a) use well-packed columns; (b) minimize pressure surges to avoid mechanical and thermal shock; (c) use guard column and an in-line filter; (d) flush column frequently with strong solvent; (e) pretreat samples to minimize particulates; (f) use stable stationary phase (C_{18} is the best); (g) use organic buffers when operating at intermediate pH (pH 6.0–8.0); (h) use column temperatures of less than 40° C; (i) keep mobile phase pH between 3.0 and 8.0 for most silica based columns; (j) add 200 ppm sodium azide to aqueous mobile phases and buffers; and (k) for overnight and storage, purge out salt and buffers, leave the column in pure organic solvent (preferably acetonitrile).

Finally, quantitation and method validation are an important part of the method development process. The key components of a method validation study are: (a) accuracy and precision; (b) linearity; (c) range; (d) limit of detection and quantitation; (e) specificity; (f) ruggedness and robustness; (g) stability of samples and reagents; and (h) instruments and system suitability criteria. In addition, method documentation data from interlaboratory crossover studies and techniques for determining equivalent performance are to be studied.

THIN-LAYER CHROMATOGRAPHY

Thin-layer chromatography (TLC) is a method of analysis in which the stationary phase, a finely divided solid, is spread as a thin layer on a rigid supporting plate; and the mobile phase, a liquid, is allowed to migrate across the surface of the plate. It differs from the techniques previously discussed in that the separation does not take place in a closed column, but rather on a planar surface; and the mobile phase does not flow under the influence of gravity or high pressure, but is drawn across the plate by capillary action. Although separation efficiencies equivalent to those obtained with gas or high-pressure liquid chromatography cannot be obtained by this method, it has the advantages of speed, versatility, and simplicity.

A wide variety of stationary phases are available in size ranges suitable for use in TLC. Because the mechanism of this method is essentially the same as that of liquid-column chro-

Table 33-10. Stationary and Mobile Phases Used in TLC

TECHNIQUE	STATIONARY PHASES	MOBILE PHASES
Adsorption	Silica gel	Alumina
Charcoal	Nonpolar or polar organic solvents	
	Polyamide	Polar organics
Partition	Cellulose	
Silica gel	Mixed aqueous, organic solvents	
Reversed phase partition	ODS silica gel	
	Coated silica	
Acetylated cellulose	Mixed aqueous, polar solvents	
Ion exchange	Ion-exchange resins	
	DEAE- and CM-cellulose	
	Buffered aqueous solutions	
Size exclusion	Dextran gels	Aqueous buffers

matography, the only distinction being that the separation takes place on a flat surface, the same modes used in liquid chromatography—adsorption, partition, ion-exchange, and size-exclusion—are available for thin-layer separations. These processes are listed in Table 33-10, along with some of the more commonly used mobile and stationary phases.

Silica gel, the most frequently used stationary phase, is employed as such for adsorption TLC and modified for reversed-phase separations by coating with a thin layer of a nonpolar substance, such as silicone oil, or by binding a nonpolar functional group to it, such as octadecylsilyl (ODS). The surface of silica is acidic due to the presence of many silanol hydroxyl groups; therefore, it is best suited to the analysis of acidic compounds. It also is preferable for polar compounds such as amino acids and sugars. Alumina (aluminum oxide) has a basic surface and is chosen over silica gel for the separation of basic and weakly polar compounds.

Polyamide (nylon) is a long-chain polymer that, because it has many free amide and carboxyl groups on its surface, is an adsorbent with strong hydrogen-bonding abilities. It will readily bond phenols, carboxylic acids, quinones, and nitro compounds, all of which require polar solvents such as methanol and dimethylformamide to displace them. Less active and less frequently used sorbents are calcium phosphate, calcium carbonate, and diatomaceous earth. Cellulose, a polysaccharide, has numerous neutral hydroxyl groups on its surface and can adsorb water or polar solvents by hydrogen-bonding, making it useful for partition TLC.

To ensure that the stationary phase adheres firmly to the backing plate and does not flake off during the development, binders such as calcium sulfate (gypsum), starch, or carbomethylcellulose are added to the adsorbent.

The mobile phases in TLC are identical to those used in liquid chromatography, and can be chosen using the eluotropic series shown in Table 33-3. If possible, it is preferable to use a single solvent to develop the chromatogram rather than a multicomponent mixture, because solvents are adsorbed preferentially by the stationary phase, and as the mixture moves up the plate, the composition of the mobile phase is always changing. Compounds that travel a greater distance up the plate, therefore, will be exposed to a different mobile phase than those that are retained strongly. The solvents also should be volatile so they can be evaporated from the plate after the development is completed.

The selection of the optimum solvent or mixture for use as the mobile phase depends also on the nature of the solutes and stationary phase and largely is empirical. A useful procedure for initial trials is to run two separate plates, one using a very polar solvent (eg, ethanol), and the other employing a nonpolar

liquid (eg, hexane). After observing which type of mobile phase moves the solutes from the origin and determining their k' or R_f values, the solvent may be modified to increase selectivity and resolution in a number of ways. The polarity may be altered by adding other solvents chosen by consulting tables of strength or dielectric constant. Substances with functional groups similar to those of the solutes, such as ethers, alcohols, or carboxyls, may be added to increase the R_f value by promoting solubility in the mobile phase. Acids or bases (acetic acid or ammonia) may be added to affect the charges on the solutes to prevent tailing.

PREPARATION OF PLATES

Plates with dimensions of 20×20 cm are necessary to attain the greater efficiency required for more difficult separations. These are usually made of glass, but plastic, stainless steel, or aluminum backings also are used. The material must be cleaned scrupulously to prevent interaction of the solutes with contaminants on the backing.

To reduce band-broadening, the stationary phase should consist of small particles of uniform size so as to provide a large area for interaction and a small void volume. The particles are mixed with water or an organic solvent to form a slurry, a suitable binding agent is added, and fluorescent indicators such as zinc silicate may be included to aid in detection of the solutes after the development. The slurry is coated on the plates using a spreader, which will apply a uniform layer of adsorbent of desired thickness over the surface of entire plate and the plates are dried.

Instead of coating a plate with one sorbent, two different substances may be applied simultaneously so that the layer is made of a gradient mixture of both. For example, silica gel and alumina can be used to prepare a pH gradient across the width of the plates. This may yield separations that otherwise would be impossible.

The thickness of the layer of stationary phase is important to the success of the chromatography, as excessively thick layers allow the solutes to diffuse laterally and, as in liquid column chromatography, band-broadening results. Layers from 0.1 to 2.0 mm in depth are used most often, with thinner ones (250 μm) being most suitable for precise separations and thicker coatings for preparative work, due to their greater solute capacity.

SAMPLE APPLICATION AND DEVELOPMENT

After the plates have been dried and conditioned, if necessary, in a controlled humidity chamber, the samples, which may range from a few μg to mg dissolved in 10 to 1000 μL of a volatile solvent, are spotted usually with a capillary tube or a microliter syringe. Samples may be applied as spots or as thin streaks, but it is essential that all of the solvent be evaporated between repeated applications and the area of sample application be kept as small as possible, because the bands will broaden as they travel up the plate.

For ascending development of the thin-layer chromatogram, the plate is placed in a rectangular jar that contains developing solvent to a depth of about 0.5 cm. The atmosphere of the jar should be saturated completely with the mobile phase before development, a process usually performed by lining the jar with a piece of filter paper that has been wet with mobile phase. The plate then is removed from the tank, the mobile phase front is marked by scratching the surface, and the solvent is evaporated in an oven or, if the sample is heat labile, in the air. To increase resolution, the techniques of *multiple development* and *two-dimensional development* have been used.

In the *multiple development,* after the plate is dried, it is returned to the chamber and redeveloped in the same direction, using the same mobile phase. The process may be repeated as many times as is necessary to ensure effective separation.

In two-dimensional TLC, the sample is applied as a small spot in the lower left corner of the plate, about 2.5 cm from each edge. After the plate has been developed in the usual manner, it is dried, rotated 90° counterclockwise, and placed in another chamber with a different developing solvent. The separated spots produced by the first elution are now located at the origin of the second. This method is useful especially for complicated mixtures containing many components or groups of substances with different functionalities, because selectivity effects of the mobile phases can be exploited more efficiently using two solvents.

DETECTION METHODS

Once the chromatogram has been developed, the solute spots must be made visible in order to determine their R_f values. If the substances are highly colored (eg, dye pigments), there is no difficulty in visual detection. Most organic compounds do not absorb visible light and routinely ultraviolet (UV) light is used to examine the separation compounds to detect light emission. *Fluorescence quenching* is a particularly useful technique for detection of compounds that absorb at 254 nm.

The two most frequently employed nonspecific methods involve the use of iodine vapor and charring of organic compounds. Iodine associates with practically all organic compounds, especially with unsaturated or aromatic compounds forming charge-transfer complexes. In any case the solutes will become visible as brown spots. Charring is a very widely employed technique for the detection of carbon-containing compounds, because it is effective for almost all organic compounds. The process involves spraying the plate with sulfuric acid, usually as a 50% (v/v) mixture with methanol, and then heating it in an oven at 110° for 10 to 30 min. The organic compounds are destroyed by the acid and a dark deposit of carbon (charcoal) remains at the spot. Though this method is effective for most organic solutes, it is destructive and, hence, cannot be used if the compounds are to be removed from the plates.

The more specific methods of detection involve spraying the plates with reagents designed to react with specific functional groups to produce visible derivatives. These reactions may produce products of three types:

- Those that are detected directly in visible light (2,4-dinitrophenylhydrazones of carbonyls)
- Those that absorb UV and quench fluorescence (benzoate esters of alcohols)
- Those that fluoresce directly (phthalaldehyde derivatives of amino acids).

Some of the more common derivatizing reagents, and the classes of compounds with which they react, are shown in Table 33-11.

The incorporation of radioactive elements, such as ^{14}C or ^{3}H, into the solutes provides another convenient method of detection, because special instruments are available that will scan a TLC strip and produce a chart recording similar to that obtained in GC.

Table 33-11. Commonly Used Derivatizing Agents

COMPOUND CLASS	REAGENT	COLOR PRODUCED
General	Iodine vapor	Brown
General	Sulfuric acid (50%)	Black
Acids	Bromcresol green	Yellow
Aldehydes and ketones	2,4-Dinitrophenylhydrazine	Yellow-red
Amines and amino acids	Ninhydrin	Fluorescent
Alkaloids	Mercuric nitrate	Yellow to brown
Barbiturates	Diphenylcarbazone	Purple
Carbohydrates	Aniline phthalate	Gray-black
Lipids	Bromthymol blue	Light-green
Steroids	Antimony trichloride	Various

QUALITATIVE ANALYSIS

In thin-layer chromatography, qualitative correlations of unknown compounds with standards are accomplished primarily by comparing the R_f value, which is the distance from the origin to the point of maximum intensity in the spot divided by the total distance of solvent travel. This method is used with great success in monitoring drugs of abuse in the urine of addicts undergoing treatment.

QUANTITATIVE ANALYSIS

Quantitation may be performed either while the solute is still on the plate or after it has been removed. The solute can be isolated from the plate in a number of ways. The area of adsorbent containing the substance can be removed from the plate by scraping or by aspirating it into a Pasteur pipet. The compound then is eluted from the adsorbent using a suitable solvent, and the solid stationary phase is removed by centrifugation or filtration. The solute then may be identified or quantitated by the usual spectrometric or chromatographic methods.

In those cases in which the solute band cannot be seen except by chemical reaction, underivatized solute may be obtained by running portions of the same sample in adjacent lanes or a sample in one lane and a standard in the next. After development, the sample lane is masked with a piece of glass and the remainder of the plate is sprayed with developing reagent to determine the location of the desired spot. The other lane is uncovered and the adsorbent removed in the area adjacent to the visualized solute.

Since the bonding between the solutes and adsorbents is frequently quite strong, complete removal from the stationary phase often is not achieved. Therefore, quantitative analysis of the substance while it is still on the plate is more reliable. Manual methods, such as comparing the spot sizes and intensities between unknown and standard, using a template, or tracing the spot outline on paper and weighing it, have been used, but they are tedious and give high levels of variability.

An automated method called spectrodensitometry is much more convenient and is capable of yielding quantitation in the submicrogram range. In this method, the plate is placed on a movable stage that is driven by a motor so that the lane of Spectrodensitometric measurements may be made on substances that are colored or absorb UV, those that have been charred, those that quench fluorescence, and even on photographs or x-ray films. A more detailed discussion of the quantitative aspects of densitometry can be found in the paper by Touchstone.[35]

The applications of thin-layer chromatography include (a) detection of narcotic and stimulant drugs in a single sample using a combination of R_f value and the various colors produced by over-spraying with different reagents,[35] (b) identification and isolation of active chemicals from plants and crude extracts, (c) determination of glycerol in tobacco, (d) determination of aflatoxins in foodstuffs, (e) determination of selenium after derivatization with 2,3=diaminonaphthalene in water and serum, (f) determination of vitamin B_1 in Pharmaceutical Products, and (g) determination of essential oils in herbal drugs etc.

PAPER CHROMATOGRAPHY

Although successful paper-chromatographic separations of dyes, salts, and other substances had been reported as far back as the middle of the 19th century, the method was not used widely until 1944 when Consden and co-workers[36] rediscovered and developed it just as they had done for liquid-partition and GC. They not only optimized the experimental procedure but also developed the theory of the separation process and formulated equations to describe the factors influencing the technique. Their work led to an appreciation of the method and its subsequent widespread application.

The stationary phase consists of a sheet of filter paper; the tightly bound water is the actual stationary phase and as a mobile phase passes over the surface of the paper, the solutes distribute themselves between the bound layer of water and the mobile-phase solvent. Therefore, the mechanism that predominates is liquid–liquid or partition chromatography, although adsorption to the cellulose surface also may occur. Papers especially impregnated to permit ion-exchange and reversed-phase chromatography also are available.

STATIONARY PHASE

The paper used in this method is prepared especially from cotton fibers and highly purified so as to be about 99% alpha-cellulose, which consists of polymers of glucose with molecular weights above 50,000. The chains of cellulose are bound together by hydrogen bonds in two different types of cross-linking. About 6% of the weight of the cellulose consists of water molecules permanently bound to the sugar hydroxyl groups, while another 10% to 20%, depending on humidity, are held more loosely. Because of the potential variability of the water content of the paper, moisture must be controlled carefully in its manufacture, storage, and use to achieve reproducible results. Some of the more important chromatographic papers and their characteristics are shown in Table 33-12.

Another variable introduced in the manufacture of the paper concerns the orientation of the fibers in the direction of motion of the machines that form it. Because the mobile phase travels across the paper by capillary action, the physical orientation of the channels is important in determining the rate of movement and, as a result, the flow is greater in the direction of the fiber orientation (*grain*) and slower perpendicular to it. In addition, there is a distance effect resulting in a slower flow as the distance from the origin increases.

Modified cellulose papers with a higher carboxyl content or attached ion-exchange functional groups (diethylaminoethyl, DEAE; or carboxymethylcellulose, CM) are available for the separation of cations, amines, and amino acids. For hydrophobic substances, cellulose-ester papers or those impregnated with mineral oil or silicone oil are used with polar organic solvents. Glass-fiber paper (Whatman GF/A) has been used, the main advantage being that it is not affected by reagents that are too corrosive for cellulose.

MOBILE PHASE

The solvents used for paper-chromatographic analysis are similar to those employed in other forms of partition chromatography. However, because the surface of the paper binds solutes strongly, mobile phases tend to be more polar than those used in thin-layer chromatography. Mixtures of alcohols, such as butyl or isopropyl, and water commonly are employed with ammonia or acetic acid added to control the charge on the solutes and reduce tailing.

Many organic substances are insoluble in water but soluble in polar organic solvents. For these compounds, paper impregnated with 20% to 40% of formamide in ethanol is used. In most cases, chloroform (for hydrophilic substances), benzene (for substances of medium polarity), cyclohexane (for hydrophobic substances), or a mixture of these solvents is used as the mobile phase. The advantages of these solvents are good separating ability and relatively short developing times, ranging from 1 to 4 hr.

SAMPLE PREPARATION AND APPLICATION

Drugs frequently are applied to the paper in solution in volatile solvents, such as ethanol, acetone, or chloroform, in quantities of 0.1 to 1000 μg, depending on the sensitivity of the detection method and the purpose of the analysis. In the determination of pharmaceutical or biological materials in which test substances occur at low concentrations, an extraction step generally must be employed, because substances like proteins, lipids, and inorganic ions may have undesirable effects when present in large amounts and, therefore, must be removed before the sample is applied to the paper. To enhance separation and identification, it often is advantageous to chromatograph derivatives when the original compounds are volatile.

Samples are applied at an origin that is located approximately 7 to 9 cm from the upper edge of the paper for descending development, 3 to 5 cm from the lower edge in ascending development, and on a circle with a radius of 1 to 3 cm for radial development. The optimum size of the spot varies from 3 to 8 mm in diameter, and adjacent spots should be 2 to 3 cm apart. Samples are applied with capillary pipets or microliter syringes, using multiple applications for large sample volumes, and drying each spot between applications.

DEVELOPMENT OF THE CHROMATOGRAM

The development of a paper chromatogram takes place in a glass or glass-lined stainless steel chamber of a size commensurate with the dimensions of the paper. This may range from a test tube for a small strip to a large cabinet or jar able to contain papers almost 2 feet long. The chamber must be kept sealed and saturated with the mobile-phase solvents. If the mobile phase is a mixture (eg, butanol–water) the two reagents are saturated mutually by shaking in a separatory funnel; the layers are separated, and the butanol layer transferred to the mobile phase reservoir in the chamber. The aqueous layer then is poured into a second container and placed in the chamber; the chamber is sealed and the vapors of the two solvents are allowed to come to equilibrium. The paper is spotted and placed in the chamber, but not yet allowed to contact the mobile phase, and the cellulose is permitted to equilibrate with the vapors.

The chromatogram is developed by allowing the mobile phase to travel over the surface of the paper in one of a number of ways: *ascending, descending, radial, linear horizontal,* or *spiral.*

Once the solvent has reached a point near the end of the paper, the process is stopped by removing the sheet from the chamber and allowing the solvent to evaporate. The spots then are made visible by methods similar to those employed in TLC, with the exception of charring, which is not useful because of the cellulose paper.

Qualitative analysis also is accomplished in the same manner as in TLC. The R_f values are determined and compared with standards, as are the results of specific derivatization reactions. Areas of the paper containing the compound of interest may be cut out and treated with a solvent to elute the substances. In descending chromatography, spots may be eluted off

Table 33-12. Types and Properties of Common Chromatographic Papers

PAPER	THICKNESS (MM)	WATER ASCENT[A]	DEVELOPMENT TIME[B]	CHARACTERISTICS
Whatman				
No. 1	0.16	140–220	15–16	Standard paper
No. 3MM	0.31	140–180	11	Preparative
No. 4	0.19	70–100	9	Fast
No. 31ET	0.50	60–120	4	Very fast
No. 54	0.17	60–120	6	Washed, fast
Schleicher & Schuell				
2040a	0.18	90–140	7	Fast
2043b (MGI)	0.23	220–260	15	Standard paper
2045b (GI)	0.16	300–400	45	Slow
2071	0.67	274–290	23	Preparative

[a] Time in minutes for water to ascend 30 cm up the paper.
[b] In hours, for the system: L-butanol:acetic acid:water (4:1:5).

the paper and collected in small containers at the bottom of the chamber.

Quantitative analysis may be accomplished by comparing spot size and intensity with standards developed under identical conditions, by densitometry, or by subjecting the material to standard spectrometric methods after eluting it off the paper.

ELECTROPHORESIS

Electrophoresis is defined as the migration of charged molecules under the influence of an external electric field. Since its introduction in 1937 by Tiselius for the purification of proteins, it has been used widely, especially for the separation of complex mixtures of biological substances such as proteins, nucleic acids, and polysaccharides. The name *electrochromatography* has been used for this process because, in some cases, as in chromatography, a narrow zone of solute is applied to a support, and migration in the electric field is influenced by the adsorptive or steric exclusion properties of the support. Electrophoresis is discussed at this point because some of the techniques are similar to chromatographic techniques with which they are combined readily.

The migration of particles in an electrophoretic system depends on properties of the particles as well as the instrumental system. Based on Stokes' Law, the mobility of a particle, μ, may be calculated from

$$\mu = \frac{Q}{6\pi r n} \qquad (15)$$

where Q is the charge on the particle in esu, μ is in cm^2/volt-sec, r is the particle radius in cm, and n is the viscosity of the medium in poises.

For ions and peptides with a molecular weight of at least 5000 that do not obey Stokes' Law, Equation 16 is valid:

$$\mu = \frac{Q}{A\pi r^2 n} \qquad (16)$$

where A has a value that ranges from 4 to 6 and is related to the particle shape.

Solution conditions are important variables. The solution pH determines the nature of species. For example, an acidic pH would favor protonation of basic centers of a protein, resulting in a positively charged molecule, whereas an alkaline pH leads to loss of protons from the protein, producing a negatively charged molecule. It is not desirable to choose a pH such that the protein is at its isoelectric point and exists as the uncharged zwitterion, a species not mobile in the imposed electrical field.

Electrophoretic mobility decreases with the supporting electrolyte ionic strength. Generally, the ionic strengths employed in electrophoresis range from 0.01 to 0.10. The temperature of the solution is important because the solution viscosity varies with temperature and the mobility increases with temperature. Because heat is generated during the electrophoretic process, this must be provided for in apparatus design and in experimental conditions.

The phenomenon of electroendosmosis arises because the solution itself migrates in an electrical field. This migration, which results from surface charges on the apparatus walls, usually is increased when a gel is added to stabilize the electrolyte and prevent the mixing of separated zones because of thermal gradients or diffusion. The stabilizing media develop a negative charge that causes the electrolyte and all zones, even the neutral compounds, to be carried to the cathode. Electroendosmosis effects are large with agar gels but small with polyacrylamide gels.

When no stabilizing medium is present or when a very porous system is used, the separations of species is related to the charge-to-size ratios as is seen in Equation 15. If stabilizing media are present, interaction of the species undergoing separation with molecules of the media introduce another consideration into the process.

Electrophoresis commonly is performed using one of two techniques.

In *moving-boundary* or *free-boundary electrophoresis*, the apparatus consists of a U-shaped tube with provision for introducing the cathode and anode electrodes into each of the arms. The sample solution is introduced and each arm is filled carefully with a buffer solution. If the sample consists of compounds with different mobilities, their migration may be observed as several moving boundaries. This method yields information on isoelectric points and mobilities of the compounds but usually is not useful for the isolation of the components because complete separation rarely is achieved. Several problems are associated with the technique, including stabilization of ion boundaries, boundary anomalies, and the need for specialized equipment.

Zone electrophoresis makes use of a stabilizing medium to minimize the problems associated with free-boundary electrophoresis. Many types of stabilizing media are available including paper, starch gels or blocks, cellulose, and agar or polyacrylamide gels.

One of the simplest procedures in electrophoresis involves spotting a mixture of solutes in the middle of a paper strip, moistening the paper with some electrolyte, and placing it between two sheets of glass. The ends of the paper strip extending beyond the glass plates are immersed in beakers of the electrolyte. A potential of approximately 5 V/cm of paper length is placed on this system, from a direct-current source. Electrophoresis is allowed to continue for a period of several hours. Usually, sufficient movement occurs in that time to obtain good separations, but longer periods sometimes are required.

Many other supporting media have been used for electrophoretic separations. *Cellulose acetate* strips, which are used widely in clinical laboratories, produce excellent separations of 7 to 9 protein fractions in a few hours. This material is exceedingly fine and homogeneous, and little *tailing* is encountered due to negligible adsorption. It especially is useful for separating α_1-globulins from albumin and provides a good background for staining glycoproteins (see Chapter 32).

Electrophoresis in compact gels, which depends at least in part on size-exclusion effects to achieve separation, is used frequently for the separation of proteins and nucleic acids. Although starch gels have been used in this respect, agar and especially polyacrylamide gels are employed most often. The degree of cross-linking of the individual acrylamide polymer strands may be varied during the preparation to produce gels of different pore sizes. This allows the separation conditions to be varied according to the size of the solutes in the analysis mixture. The overall migration in these gels is a combination of movement under the influence of the electric field and size separation by the pores of the gel.

The most frequently used technique of *polyacrylamide gel electrophoresis* (*PAGE*) is the discontinuous buffer system developed by Laemmli[37]. In this procedure the sample is placed on a *stacking* gel with a low level of cross-linking and, therefore, a large pore size. During movement through this gel, the sample is concentrated into a narrow band and then deposited onto a *separating* gel that has a higher cross-linking and smaller pore size. The separation of the solutes occurs in this phase.

In a special modification of this technique used for the separation of proteins, a detergent, such as sodium dodecylsulfate (SDS), is introduced into the buffer. This interacts with the proteins to produce particles of consistent shape and uniform negative charge so that separation occurs according to size alone. This enables the simple determination of molecular weight because the migration distance is proportional to the logarithm of molecular weight, as in size-exclusion chromatography.

Various methods have been used for the detection of the sample bands on the *electrophoretograms*. They include reaction with specific reagents such as Comassie Blue for proteins or ethidium bromide for nucleic acids to form derivatives that are detectable spectrally, general reactions such as staining with silver, or autoradiography using included radioactive labels.

In a common method of detection known as *blotting,* the macromolecules either are transferred passively or electroeluted onto a suitable medium, such as nitrocellulose or a nylon membrane, following the electrophoretic separation. The membrane then is processed to detect the individual solutes. For nucleic acid separations, the membrane is developed using nucleotide probes of complementary sequence. These are known as Northern (for DNA) or Southern (for RNA) blots. Transferred proteins are detected with antibody probes in the technique of Western blotting.

Enzymatic and immunological methods also have been used to detect proteins following electrophoresis in gels. Immunochemical methods add an additional dimension to protein identification. Following electrophoresis in an agar gel backed with a microscope slide, an antibody is placed into a trough cut parallel to the direction of electrophoresis. The antibody and electrophoretically separated antigens diffuse toward each other resulting in precipitin arcs where antigen–antibody complexes form. This technique has been referred to as *immunoelectrophoresis.*

Polyacrylamide gels also have been used successfully for the fractionation of DNA and RNA. The technique yields separations that are superior to those obtained by zone centrifugation through sucrose density gradients; thus, the time of analysis is reduced greatly. Larger columns of starch, cellulose, or silica gel are suitable for preparative work, yielding highly purified fractions in sufficient quantity for chemical analysis.

A modification of one electrophoretic technique, called *isoelectric focusing,* rapidly is becoming an important tool for the separation of ampholytes, especially proteins. All proteins have an isoelectric point, pI, which is the pH value when the molecule has no net charge. When electrophoresis is run in a solution buffered at a constant pH, proteins having a net charge will migrate toward the opposite electrode so long as the current flows. The use of a pH gradient across the supporting medium causes each protein to migrate to an area of specific pH. Proteins are focused at the point in the gradient where they carry no net charge—the pI of the protein equals the pH of the gradient—thus resulting in sharp, well-defined protein bands.

Whereas separation by isoelectric focusing depends on the existence of a pH gradient in the system, the technique of *isotachophoresis* depends on the development of a potential gradient. A leading electrolyte (eg, chloride) with a higher mobility than the analytes, and a trailing electrolyte (eg, glycinate) with a lower mobility are used. The analytes are positioned between the electrolytes and, when the voltage is applied, they migrate in order of decreasing mobility. This establishes the potential gradient; from that point on, all the analytes move at the same speed. Isotachophoresis has been used for the separation of proteins as well as inorganic substances.

A technique that shares the attributes of both chromatography and electrophoresis is called *capillary electrophoresis* (CE). In this method, separation based on electrophoretic mobility takes place inside a capillary similar to those used in GC. The effective length of the capillary from the point of injection to the detector is commonly 25 to 50 cm, and the supporting electrolyte or "mobile phase" is usually a buffer, although a gel such as polyacrylamide may be used.

The apparatus used in this technique is very simple. The ends of the capillary are placed in buffer reservoirs, and these are established as anode and cathode by means of a DC power supply capable of delivering up to 30,000 V. At some point near the cathodic end of the capillary, a detector, usually an UV-visible spectrophotometer of the type used in HPLC, is placed so that a section of the capillary serves as its flow cell.

The sample is introduced at the anodic end, either by electromigration or positive pressure, and when potential is applied, net migration occurs in the direction of the cathode. Even substances with a net negative charge migrate in the direction of the cathode because of a phenomenon called the *electro-osmotic effect.* Because the capillary is made of silica, the surface contains many weakly acidic silanol groups. These dissociate in the presence of the buffer, leaving a negative charge at the surface and hydrated positive ions (H^+) in solution. When a potential is applied, the contents inside the capillary move toward the cathode, carrying along with them all of the analytes.

Neutral molecules move at the same speed as the electro-osmotic flow, while positively charged species move faster, their net speed being the sum of the electro-osmotic flow and their intrinsic electrophoretic mobility. Negatively charged molecules still move toward the cathode under the influence of the electro-osmotic flow, but they lag behind the other species. Within a group of similarly charged ions, separation is by electrophoresis.

The same modes as used in ordinary electrophoresis—zone, gel, isoelectric focusing, and isotachophoresis—are used in CE. However, none of these is successful in separating neutral molecules, a class exemplified by many pharmaceuticals. Although these substances will migrate under the influence of the electro-osmotic flow, they travel as a group and do not separate. Therefore, a mode called *micellar electrokinetic capillary chromatography* (MECC) is used in which a detergent, such as sodium dodecylsulfate (SDS), at a concentration above the critical micelle concentration, is included in the running buffer. As the resulting anionic micelles travel through the capillary, the neutral molecules partition in and out of the micelles selectively and separation is achieved.

Because the separation combines electrophoresis and chromatography, CE can achieve outstanding efficiencies even approaching 10^6 plates/m. However, sensitivity is lower than with chromatographic methods due to detection difficulties. The only detector in widespread use is the UV-visible spectrophotometer; however, because the optical path length across the capillary is on the order of 50 μm instead of the usual 1 cm, sensitivity to a particular compound is lowered by a factor of 200. However, research into improved systems, especially CE-MS, is actively continuing and applications in pharmaceutical analysis are increasing.[38]

REFERENCES

1. Tswett M. *Berichte der Deutschen botanischen Gesellschaft* 1906; 24:316.
2. *United States Pharmacopeia-National Formulary (USP26 NF21),* United States Pharmacopeial Convention; Rockville, MD, 2003: 2126.
3. Martin AJP, Synge RLM. *Biochem J* 1941; 35:1358.
4. Martin AJP, James AT. *Biochem J* 1952; 50:679.
5. McNair HM, Miller JM. *Basic Gas Chromatography.* New York: John Wiley, 1997.
6. Berezkin VG, Viktorova EN. *J Chromatogr A* 2003; 985:3.
7. Eiceman GA, Gardea-Torresdey J, Overton E, et al. *Anal Chem* 2002; 74:2771.
8. Gloor R, Johnson E. *J Chromatogr Sci* 1977; 15:413.
9. Marchal L, Legrand J, Foucault A. *Chem Res* 2003; 3:133.
10. van Buel MJ, van der Wielen LAM, Luyben KCAM. In: Foucault AP, ed. *Centrifugal Partition Chromatography, Chromatographic Science Series.* New York: Marcel Dekker,1994; 68.
11. Foucault AP. *J Chromatogr A* 2001; 906:365.
12. Den Hollander JL. *J Chromatogr B* 1998; 711:223.
13. Sluyterman LA, Elgersma O. *J Chromatogr Sci* 1978; 17:150.
14. Porath J, Flodin P. *Nature* 1959; 183:1657.
15. Moore JC. *J Polymer Sci (Gen Pap)* 1964; 2:835.
16. Barth HG, Boyes BE, Jackson C. *Anal Chem* 1994; 66:595R.
17. Amersham Biosciences Corp., *Affinity Chromatography, Principles and Methods,* Piscataway NJ: Amersham Biosciences Corp, 2002; 7.
18. Snyder LR, Kirkland JJ, Glajch JL. *Practical HPLC Method Development,* 2nd ed. New York: John Wiley, 1997; 174.
19. Majors RE. *LCGC North America* 2003; 21:240.
20. Majors RE. *LCGC North America* 2002; 20:248.
21. Snyder LR, Kirkland JJ, Glajch JL. *Practical HPLC Method Development,* 2nd ed. New York: John Wiley, 1997; 59.
22. LaCourse WR. *Anal Chem* 2002; 74:2813.
23. Jones BN, Paabo S, Stein S. *J Liq Chromatogr* 1981; 4:565.
24. Builder SE, Amersham Biosciences Corp. *Hydrophobic Interaction Chromatography: Principles and Methods.* Piscataway NJ: Amersham Biosciences Corp, 1993; 13.
25. Eichelbaum M, Gross AS. *Adv Drug Res* 1996; 28:1.
26. Haginaka J. *J Pharm Biomed Anal* 2002; 27:357.

27. Szymura-Oleksiak J, Bojarski J, Aboul-Enein HY. *Chirality* 2002; 14:417.
28. Schurig V. *J Chromatogr A* 2002; 965:315.
29. Snyder LR, Kirkland JJ, Glajch JL. *Practical HPLC Method Development*, 2nd ed. New York: John Wiley, 1997; 1.
30. Young CS, Weigand R. *LCGC North America* 2002; 20:465.
31. Jinno K, Tsuge S. In: Ishii D, ed. *Indroduction to Microscale High Performance Liquid Chromatography*. New York: VCH Publishers, 1988; 95.
32. Takeuchi T, Ishii D. *J High Resolut Chromatogr / Chromatogr Commun* 1983; 6:571.
33. Takeuchi T, Ishii D *J Chromatogr.* 1982; 253:41.
34. Ishi, D, Goto M, Takeuchi T. *J Chromatogr.* 1984; 291:398.
35. Touchstone JC, Levin SS, Murawec T. *Anal Chem* 1971; 43:858.
36. Consden R, Gordon AH, Martin AJP. *Biochem J* 1944; 38:224.
37. Laemmli UK. *Nature* 1970; 227:680.
38. Rabel SR, Stobaugh JF. *Pharm Res* 1993; 10:171.

BIBLIOGRAPHY

Cazes J, Scott RPW. *Chromatography theory.* New York: Marcel Dekker, 2002.

Deyl Z, ed. *Electrophoresis—A Survey of Techniques and Applications*, Vol 18. *Journal of Chromatography* Library. New York: Elsevier, 1979.

Dilts RV: *Analytical Chemistry.* New York: Van Nostrand, 1974.

Frei RW, Lawrence JF. *Chemical Derivatization in Analytical Chemistry*, vol 1, *Chromatography.* New York: Plenum, 1981.

Fries B, Sherma J. *Thin Layer Chromatography, Techniques and Applications*, 3rd ed. New York: Dekker, 1994.

Giddings JC. *Advances in Chromatography.* New York: Dekker, continuing series starting in 1965.

Giddings JC. *Dynamics of Chromatography*, Part 1. New York: Dekker, 1965.

Grob RL. *Modern Practice of Gas Chromatography*, 3rd ed. New York: Wiley, 1995.

Heftmann E. *Chromatography: Fundamentals and Applications of Chromatographic and Electrophoretic Method.* New York: Elsevier Science, 1983.

Satinder A. *Chromatography and Separation Science.* Boston: Academic Press, 2003.

Cserhati T. Esther F. *Chromatography in Environmental Protection.* Australia: Harwood Academic Publishers, 2001.

Cserhati T, Esther F. *Chromatography in Food Science and Technology.* Lancaster, PA: Technomic, 1999.

Kuksis A. *Chromatography of Lipids in Biomedical Research and Clinical Diagnosis.* New York: Elsevier Science, 1987.

Satinder A. *Chromatography of Pharmaceuticals: Natural, Synthetic, and Recombinant Product.* Washington: American Chemical Society, 1992.

Miller JM. Separation Methods in Chemical Analysis. New York: Wiley, 1975.

Reed E, ed. *Assay of Drugs and Other Trace Compounds in Biological Fluids*, vol 5, *Methodological Developments in Biochemistry.* Amsterdam: Elsevier, 1976.

Snyder LR, Kirkland JJ, Glajch JL. *Practical HPLC Method Development.* London: Wiley, 1997.

Snyder LR, Kirkland JJ. *Introduction to Modern Liquid Chromatography*, 2nd ed. New York: Wiley, 1979.

Snyder LR. *Principles of Adsorption Chromatography*, vol 3 of Giddings JC, Keller RA, eds. *Chromatographic Science Series.* New York: Dekker, 1968.

Touchstone J, Sherma J. *Techniques and Applications of Thin Layer Chromatography.* New York: Wiley, 1985.

Touchstone JC, Dobbins MF. *Practice of Thin Layer Chromatography*, 2nd ed. New York: Wiley, 1983.

Zweig G, Sherma J. *CRC Handbook of Chromatography.* Cleveland, OH: CRC Press, 1972.

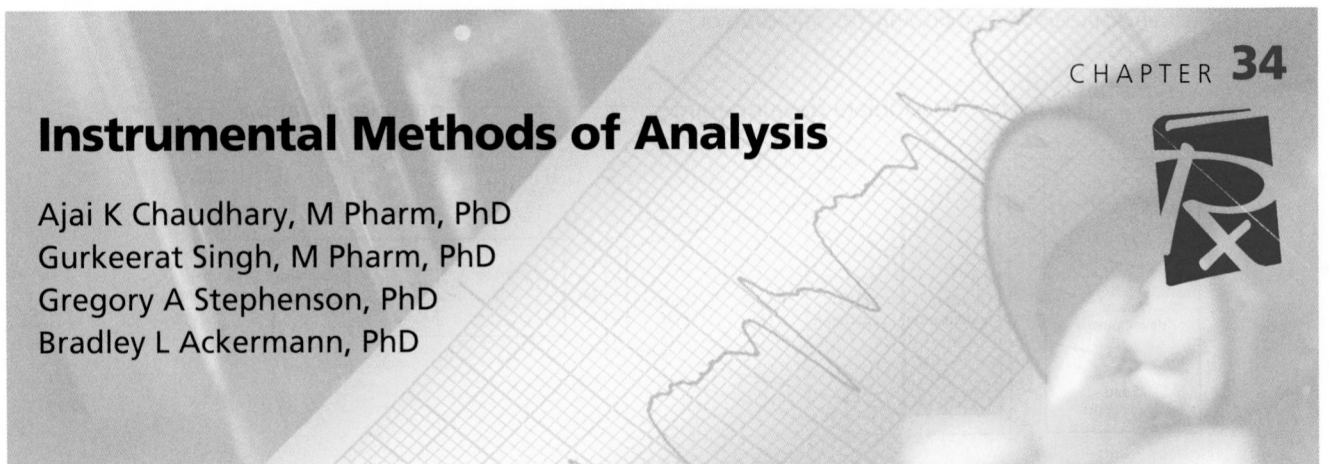

Instrumental Methods of Analysis

Ajai K Chaudhary, M Pharm, PhD

Gurkeerat Singh, M Pharm, PhD

Gregory A Stephenson, PhD

Bradley L Ackermann, PhD

CHAPTER **34**

Throughout the drug discovery and development phases, analysis and characterization of the new chemical entity, its metabolites, and its degradation products require deployment of a number of analytical techniques. This chapter describes the principles, instrumentation, and application of some of the major techniques used in these analyses.

Discovery Research is responsible for identifying new chemical entities that may be useful for treating a disease or disorder. The various phases of drug discovery and development are shown in Figure 34-1. There are three phases to Hypothesis Generation: Target Identification and Validation, Assay Development, and Lead Generation.

The first process in Hypothesis Generation is Target Identification/Validation. A target may be a site in the human body that is linked in some manner to a disease, such as a specific gene or process within the body. A target may also be outside the human body, such as viruses, bacteria, or parasites. The task at this point is to first identify potential target-disease linkages. The next step is to test the target-disease linkage hypothesis in order to validate them using biological tools. Assay Development is the next step in the Hypothesis Generation process. The goal of Assay Development is to develop screen(s), which will allow for the identification of a lead compound. This involves designing the screen(s), and actually screening compounds against it. Given a target, one can design a test or screen(s) to see if a given chemical compound will have the desired biological effect. Next, we must be able to test a large volume of chemicals against the screen(s). These chemical compounds may be naturally occurring or they may be chemically synthesized. The last process in the Hypothesis Generation and testing stage is Lead Generation. The goal of Lead Generation is to find a molecule that causes a specific biological response: "a hit". At this point the primary concern is to identify those chemicals that had some level of desired effect in the screen. These chemicals then become leads. These leads serve as the starting point for further synthesis using chemistry tools in the next step in the overall process—Lead Optimization.

The lead compounds identified from the Hypothesis Generation stage must be refined and optimized prior to continuation of research, so that the value of research expenses are maximized. This process is called Lead Optimization, the first stage in the Development phase. Optimization is accomplished through refinement of in-vitro and in-vivo testing, performing necessary toxicology and pharmacokinetic studies, developing scale-up processes for drug development, and providing assay, stability and ADME (Absorption, Distribution, Metabolism, Excretion) testing and studies.

First Human Dose (FHD) Preparation includes a variety of protocols and studies that intend to prepare a particular compound for administration to healthy human volunteers. During this pre-clinical development, the new drug substance (NDS) is synthesized, analytically characterized and formulated for initial toxicology studies. Toxicology studies are designed to evaluate the effect of the compound on animals to determine what levels of the compound can be safely administered to humans. During this period, drug disposition scientists study the absorption, distribution, metabolism, and excretion in animals to further determine what the likely disposition of the compound will be in humans. Initial studies in humans are called Phase Ia clinical trials. In these studies, compounds are given to volunteers in very low single doses, then gradually escalated to determine tolerance to the substance. Although most studies are conducted in healthy, male volunteers, some drugs may be initially given to patients. If single doses of the experimental therapy are well tolerated, multiple doses will be administered to determine if the drug accumulates in body tissues and to further define the likely therapeutic level. An important objective of early clinical studies is to identify a pharmacodynamic effect relevant to the therapeutic application to guide the selection of doses for the treatment of patients.

Phase Ib and II are the phases where a drug's safety and efficacy are evaluated. With the First Efficacy Dose [FED], clinical investigators begin to study the effect of the drug candidate in a few patients to determine if a therapeutic response is produced. If a response is seen, the correct dose and regimen for the drug will be determined in Phase II clinical trials, involving several hundred patients. Concurrent with clinical trials, the chemistry and manufacturing components prepare larger quantities of material to support future clinical trials and to provide material for long-term toxicology studies. Commercialization is the final, and undeniably the most expensive portion of the Drug Development process. The Phase III clinical involves hundreds or thousands of patients, to fully evaluate efficacy and safety.

Finally, after approval is obtained, the product is launched, and it is here that the product's utility is truly demonstrated. Physicians are educated about the mechanism of action and dosage form and regimen. Physicians closely monitor the marketplace for additional adverse reactions that may appear in large-scale deployment. Throughout the life of the product, a primary responsibility of product development and manufacturing is to continually improve manufacturing processes and develop alternative drug delivery forms to retain a strong, competitive market position. This is the goal of Global Optimization.

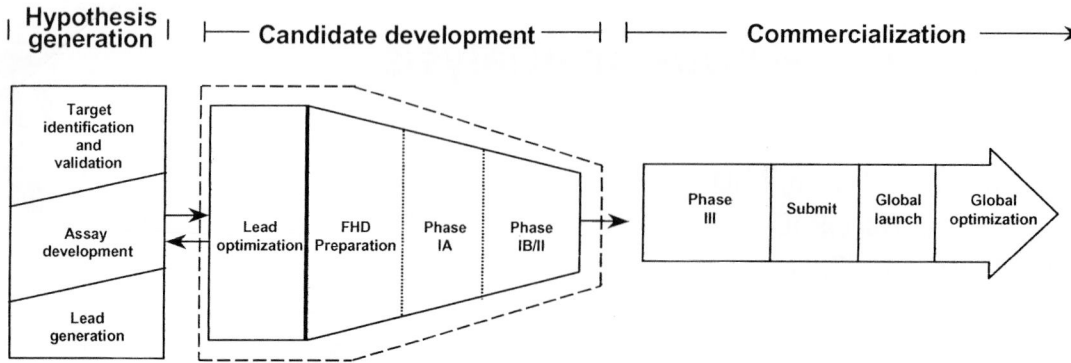

Figure 34-1. Drug development paradigm.

INSTRUMENTAL TECHNIQUES IN DRUG DISCOVERY AND DEVELOPMENT

Mass Spectrometry

Mass Spectrometry (MS) is an analytical spectroscopic tool primarily concerned with the separation of molecular (and atomic) species according to their mass. MS can be used in the analysis of many types of samples from elemental to large proteins and polymers. A mass spectrometer is an instrument that measures the masses of individual molecules that have been converted into ions, ie, molecules that have been electrically charged. The unit of mass is often referred to by chemists and biochemists as the Dalton (Da), and is defined as follows: 1 Da = (1/12) of the mass of a single atom of the isotope of carbon-12(^{12}C). This follows the accepted convention of defining the ^{12}C isotope as having exactly 12 mass units. A mass spectrometer measures the mass-to-charge ratio (m/z) of the ions formed from the molecules. The mass-to-charge ratio represents Daltons per fundamental unit of charge. In many cases, the ions encountered in mass spectrometry have just one charge (z = 1) so the m/z value is numerically equal to the molecular (ionic) mass in Da. Formation of gas phase samples ions is an essential prerequisite to the mass sorting and detection processes that occur in a mass spectrometer. Early mass spectrometers required a sample to be a gas, but due to recent developments, the applicability of mass spectrometry has been extended to include samples in liquid solutions or embedded in a solid matrix. The sample, which may be a solid, liquid, or vapor, enters the vacuum chamber through an inlet. Depending on the type of inlet and ionization techniques used, the sample may already exist as ions in solution, or it may be ionized in conjunction with its volatilization or by other methods in the ion source.

The gas phase ions are sorted in the mass analyzer according to their mass-to-charge (m/z) ratios and then collected by a detector. In the detector the ion flux is converted to a proportional electrical current. The data system records the magnitude of these electrical signals as a function of m/z and converts this information into a mass spectrum. A mass spectrum is a graph of ion intensity as a function of mass-to-charge ratio.

Some of the applications for mass spectrometry can be listed as follows:

- Accurate mass measurements can be used to match empirical formulae.
- Fragmentation fingerprints (specific to each compound) can be used to identify samples by comparison to fragment databases.
- Controlled fragmentation (through MS/MS and MS^n) can be used for structural elucidation of novel compounds.

- Common peaks observed in a spectrum can give useful information regarding functional groups.
- Relative isotope abundances are used to get information regarding the elements making up a compound.
- Complex mixtures can be analyzed via 'hyphenated' techniques such as GC-MS and HPLC-MS, thus negating the need for time-consuming sample purification.

MASS SPECTRA AND MOLECULAR STRUCTURE

With the low-energy electron beams in the order of 8 to 14 eV, it is possible to observe only the molecular ion (parent ion). Unlike other analytical methods, mass spectrometry gives an exact molecular weight. The mass spectrum of toluene shows a peak at $m/z = 92$ (m/z is the mass to charge ratio; for the parent ion this value also is the molecular weight), which is developed according to

$$\text{(toluene)} \xrightarrow{e} \left[\text{(toluene)} \right]^{+} + e \qquad (17)$$

With a high-energy electron beam, in the order of 70 eV, the parent ion disintegrates, due to the removal of several electrons, giving positively charged and uncharged fragments. Adopting the symbolism for the transfer of a single electron by a single-headed arrow, two typical examples for fragmentation can be given by

$$R\!\!\frown\!\!CH_2\!-\!NH_2 \longrightarrow R^{\cdot} + CH_2\!\!=\!\!\overset{+}{N}H_2$$

$$\begin{array}{c} \text{(benzoyl)}\!-\!\overset{\displaystyle C}{\underset{\displaystyle O}{\parallel}}\!-\!O\!-\!CH_2\!-\!CH_2\!-\!CH\!=\!CH_2 \\ \\ 77 \quad 105 \ 121 \quad 135 \quad 176 \end{array} \qquad (18)$$

The mass spectrum of a compound, therefore, is a display of masses of molecular fragments together with the mass of the parent ion versus the relative abundance of each species as depicted by the peak heights.

The graphic form of the mass spectrum of toluene and its tabular presentation are depicted in Figure 34-2. The most intense mass peak is referred to as the *base peak* and is assigned an arbitrary value of 100; the other peaks are normalized relative to the base peak. Because the ratio of fragment abundance for a given compound remains constant, a mass spectrum (like an IR spectrum) becomes a *fingerprint* for each molecule.

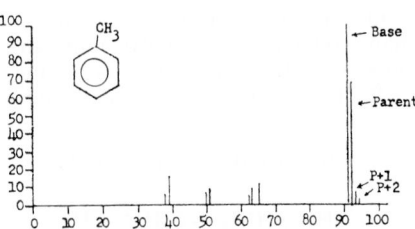

m/e	% of base peak		m/e	% of P
38	4.4		92 (P)	100
39	16		93 (P + 1)	7.37
45	3.9		94 (P + 2)	0.29
50	6.3			
51	9.1			
62	4.1			
63	8.6			
65	11			
91	100	(Base)		
92	68	(Parent)		
93	5.3	(P + 1)		
94	0.21	(P + 2)		

Figure 34-2. Relative abundance of various fragments shown in mass spectrum of toluene.

ISOTOPIC ABUNDANCE

The isotope abundance of atoms such as Cl, Br, S, and Si leads to the detection of these elements by mass spectrometry. For example, the ratio of ^{35}Cl to ^{37}Cl is 100 to 32.5.

For compounds of the general formula $C_wH_xN_yO_z$, contribution from the heavy isotopes can be calculated by

$$100 \frac{P+1}{P} = 1.11w + 0.015x + 0.37y + 0.037z \quad (1)$$

and

$$100 \frac{P+2}{P} = 0.002wx + 0.004wy + 0.006w(w-1) + 0.20z \quad (2)$$

where P is the monoisotopic peak (parent peak; equivalent to the nominal molecular weight value) and $P + 1$ and $P + 2$ are the monoisotopic mass number plus one and two mass numbers, respectively. The relative isotope abundance of the heavy isotopes of each element determines the height of the $P + 1$ and $P + 2$ peaks. By consulting special tables of abundance factors for the $P + 1$ and $P + 2$ peaks, it is possible to determine an exact molecular formula from mass spectral data.

The following example represents the use of isotopic contribution in structural elucidation.

A compound with a mass spectrum of $P = 110$ (100%), $P + 1 = 111$ (5.5%), and $P + 2 = 112$ (0.3%) could be sorted out of the following molecular formulas with the molecular weight of 110:

Formula	P + 1	P + 2
$C_3H_2N_4O$	4.84	0.30
$C_4H_2N_2O_2$	5.20	0.51
$C_4H_4N_3O$	5.57	0.33
$C_4H_6N_4$	5.94	0.15
$C_5H_2O_3$	5.55	0.73
$C_5H_4NO_2$	5.93	0.55

The data reveal that the molecular formula of the compound is $C_4H_4N_3O$.

Table 34-1. Isotopic Abundances of Some Common Elements

ELEMENT	P MASS	%	P+1 MASS	%	P+2 MASS	%
H	1	100	2	0.015		
C	12	100	13	1.1		
N	14	100	15	0.37		
O	16	100	17	0.04	18	0.2
F	19	100				
Si	28	100	29	5.1	30	3.4
P	31	100				
S	32	100	33	0.79	34	4.4
Cl	35	100			37	32.0
Br	79	100			81	97.3

The isotope abundance of atoms such as Cl, Br, S, and Si leads to the detection of these elements by mass spectrometry. For example, the ratio of ^{35}Cl to ^{37}Cl is 100 to 32.0. The isotopic abundance of some common elements is shown in Table 34-1. The higher isotopic abundance of halogens such as Cl or Br provides characteristic fingerprint to the mass spectrum of molecules containing these atoms. The mass spectrum of Cl_2 and Br_2 is shown in Figure 34-3.

This characteristic is further illustrated in mass spectrum of protonated molecular ions (MH^+) of the drug labetolol as shown in the Figure 34-4.

STRUCTURE ELUCIDATION BY FRAGMENTATION PATTERNS—The fragmentation patterns of a few representative chemical classes are illustrated below. More detailed information can be obtained by consulting reference books on mass spectrometry (see Bibliography).

Several empirical rules of molecular fragmentation are:

- Cyclic compounds show an intense parent peak and a peak at the mass number of the ring.
- Saturated cyclic compounds lose side chains at the α-carbon. The peaks resulting from the loss of two atoms from the ring is more intense than the peaks from the loss of one atom.
- In cyclic compounds containing a double bond next to the side chain, cleavage occurs at the bond β to the ring.
- In olefins, cleavage occurs β to the double bond.
- In compounds with heteroatoms, cleavage occurs at the bond β to the heteroatom.

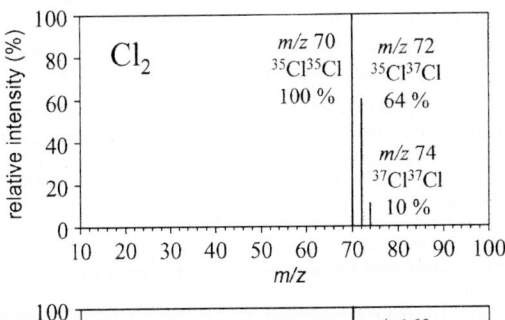

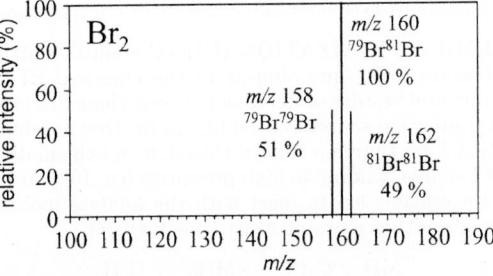

Figure 34-3. Mass spectrum of chlorine and bromine.

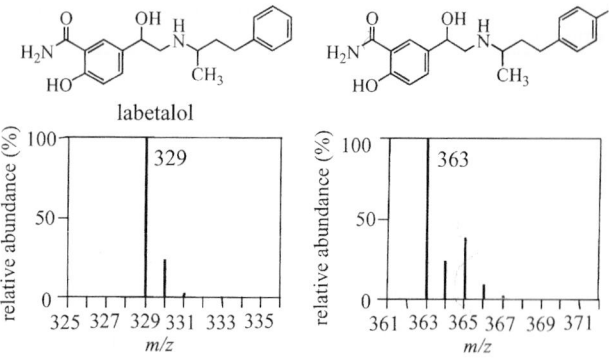

Figure 34-4. Mass spectrum: protonated molecular ions (MH+) of labetolol and its analog containing one chlorine atom.

- In hydrocarbon molecules, the ease of cleavage is in the following order: tertiary > secondary > primary. The positive charge remains on the branched fragment.
- In carbonyl containing compounds, cleavage occurs at this group, the positive charge remaining on the fragment containing the carbonyl function.

Molecular fragmentation may occur by one or a combination of the following processes: simple fission, simple rearrangement, complex fission, and complex rearrangement.

IONIZATION METHODS AND INSTRUMENTATION

The first step in producing the ions is the acquisition of energy by the molecules present in the sample. Some of the important methods of ionization are discussed below:

ELECTRON IMPACT (EI)—Electron impact ionization is the classical ionization technique in mass spectrometry. In the ion source ($10^{-7} - 10^{-5}$ mbar), the gaseous sample is bombarded with 70 eV electrons usually generated from a tungsten filament. Because the pressure is kept that low, ion-molecule reactions do not occur, eg, a $[M+H]^+$ signal due to proton transfer is not observed. The application of EI is restricted to thermally stable samples with low molecular masses (< ca. 2000 Da). Since the ion source temperature and the bombarding electron's energy are kept constant, the number and amount of fragments is constant for (almost) every mass spectrometer, too. Therefore, the number and amount of ionic fragments (*daughter ions*) and the amount of the M^+ is characteristic for each substance. Electron impact ionization has following characteristics:

- Can be used for GC/MS systems and direct inlet techniques.
- Produces "classical" compound spectra that are library searchable and/or interpretable.
- Useful for positive compound identification and/or structure elucidation.
- EI spectra are relatively easy to obtain.
- Comparatively rugged and sensitive ionization technique.
- Can be employed for analyzing air- and moisture-sensitive compounds.
- Analytes have to be vaporized - problems with thermal degradation.

CHEMICAL IONIZATION (CI)—Chemical Ionization is an ionization technique similar to the classical EI but the knowledge and results of ion-molecule reactions are exploited. In CI a similar ion source is used like in EI. One notable exception: The CI ion source is almost closed, ie, much smaller holes as the EI source, leading to high pressures (ca. 10^{-3} to 1 mbar). CI uses a reagent ion to react with the analyte molecules to form ions by either a proton or hydride transfer:

$$MH + C_2H_5^+ \rightarrow MH_2^+ + C_2H_4$$

$$MH + C_2H_5^+ \rightarrow M^+ + C_2H_6$$

The reagent ions are produced by introducing a large excess of methane (relative to the analyte) into an electron impact (EI) ion source. Electron collisions produce CH_4^+ and CH_3^+ which further react with methane to form CH_5^+ and $C_2H_5^+$:

$$CH_4^+ + CH_4 \rightarrow CH_5^+ + CH_3$$

$$CH_3^+ + CH_4 \rightarrow C_2H_5^+ + H_2$$

Sometimes other gases such as ammonia are also used as the reagent gas instead of methane.

Chemical ionization has following characteristics:

- Provides molecular weight information.
- Quantification is almost impossible without internal standards.
- CI can be used as ionization methods in GC/MS.

NEGATIVE-ION CHEMICAL IONIZATION (NCI)—Many important compounds of environmental or biological interest can produce negative ions under the right conditions. Negative ions can be produced by a number of processes. The electron energy is very low, and the specific energy required for electron capture depends on the molecular structure of the analyte. Benefits of NCI are efficient ionization, higher sensitivity and less fragmentation than positive-ion EI or CI. There is also a greater selectivity for certain environmentally or biologically important compounds. The limitations are that not all volatile compounds produce negative ions and a poor reproducibility of the measurements.

FAST-ATOM BOMBARDMENT (FAB)—In FAB a high-energy beam of netural atoms, typically Xe or Ar, strikes a solid sample causing desorption and ionization. It is used for large biological molecules that are difficult to get into the gas phase. The atomic beam is produced by accelerating ions from an ion source though a charge-exchange cell. The ions pick up an electron in collisions with neutral atoms to form a beam of high energy atoms. The FAB spectrum contains often only a few fragments and a signal for the pseudo molecular ion, eg, $[M+H]^+$, $[M+Na]^+$, adducts. This makes FAB useful for molecular weight determination. However, the low m/z region is crowded with signals resulting from the matrix. These matrix signals are not very reproducible. Therefore, spectra correction and interpretation is not easily accomplished.

MATRIX-ASSISTED LASER DESORPTION IONIZATION (MALDI)—MALDI is a method of vaporizing and ionizing large biological molecules such as proteins or DNA fragments. The biological molecules are dispersed in a solid matrix such as nicotinic or sinnapinic acid. A UV laser pulse ablates the matrix that carries some of the large molecules into the gas phase in an ionized form so they can be extracted into a mass spectrometer. MALDI allows determination of the molecular weight of molecules up to 500 kDa, routinely 5 to 100 kDa (polymers, biomolecules, complexes, enzymes), depending on the analyzer. The MALDI technique can be coupled with a time-of-flight analyzer (resolution and accuracy of the spectra are low but easy to handle and hence, most commonly used), quadrupole analyzer, ion traps or a fourier-transform mass spectrometer (expensive, difficult to handle, low dynamic range, but very accurate). Matrix-assisted laser desorption ionization has following characteristics:

- Soft ionization method provides molecular weight information.
- Suitable for analyzing very large bio- or synthetic polymers.
- Sensitivity depends strongly upon the analyte.
- Suitable for analyzing polar and even ionic compounds (e.g. metal complexes).
- Less fragmentation.
- Pulsed ionization technique, in contrast to EI, CI, FAB, ESI, and APCI.

ATMOSPHERIC PRESSURE IONIZATION (API)—API is used in conjunction with LC/MS techniques. The ions are formed at atmospheric pressure. It is a very soft ionization technique leading in formation of predominantly molecular ion with little or no fragmentation. There are two common types of atmospheric pressure ionization:

Electrospray Ionization (ESI)—The ESI source consists of a very fine needle and a series of skimmers. A sample solution is sprayed into the source chamber to form droplets. The droplets carry charge when the exit the capillary and as the solvent vaporizes the droplets disappear leaving highly charged analyte molecules. Electrospray ionization is the method of choice for proteins, oligonucleotides and metal complexes. However, the sample must be soluble in low boiling solvents (acetonitrile, MeOH, CH_3Cl, water. . .) and stable at very low concentrations, ie, 10^{-2}mol/l. The characteristics of ESI can be summarized as follows:

- Soft ionization method provides molecular weight information.
- Suitable for analyzing large bio- or synthetic polymers.
- Sensitivity depends strongly upon the analyte.
- Suitable for analyzing polar and even ionic compounds (e.g. metal complexes).
- Less fragmentation.
- Enables LC / MS coupling.

Atmospheric Pressure Chemical Ionization (APCI)— Atmospheric pressure chemical ionization is closely related to ESI. The ion source is similar to the ESI ion source. In addition to the electrohydrodynamic spraying process, a corona-discharge needle at the end of the metal capillary creates a plasma. In this plasma proton transfer reactions and to a small amount fragmentation can occur.

Depending on the solvents, only quasi-molecular ions like $[M + H]^+$, $[M + Na]^+$ and M^+. (In the case of aromatics), and/or fragments can be produced. Multiply charged molecules $[M + nH]^{n+}$, as in ESI, are not observed. The characteristics of APCI can be summarized as follows:

- Provides molecular weight information.
- Sensitivity depends strongly upon the analyte.
- Suitable for analyzing less polar compounds compared to ESI.
- Increased fragmentation compared to ESI.
- Enables coupling MS and LC with flow rate up to 1 ml/min.

INSTRUMENTATION

The typical instrumentation for mass spectrometry consists of the following components:

SAMPLE INLET—The sample introduction systems produce vapors from the samples or reduce the pressure of the gaseous samples. Sample inlets include batch inlet for gases, and direct heated probes for solid samples. Hyphenated interphases with on-line sample introduction techniques such as gas or liquid chromatographic systems and electrophoresis systems are used extensively.

ION SOURCE—All ion sources produce analyte ions and introduce a suitable ion beam into the analyzer. Various ionization techniques to produce these ions are discussed above.

MASS ANALYZER—The center of any mass spectrometer is the mass selective analyzer. The main function of a mass analyzer is to resolve ions of the same m/z from all other ions and to focus the individual ion beams of discrete mass onto a detector or into a second ionization chamber or into a collision cell. The mass analyzers in current use can be classified in to two distinct classes. The first set of analyzers accomplish ion separation in a linear, *in space*, mode. These analyzers are: quadrupole, magnetic and time-of-flight. The second set of analyzers accomplishes ion separation *in time*. These analyzers are: ion trap and ion cyclotron resonance (Fourier transform).

In the *quadrupole mass analyzer,* four electric poles (a quadrupole) replace the magnetic field application procedure. The ions entering from the top, travel with a constant velocity in a direction parallel to the poles (Z direction) and acquire stable oscillation in the X and Y directions. This usually is accomplished by applying a dc voltage as well as radio frequency (rf) to the poles. Only one m/z ratio can pass through the quadrupole mass analyzer and be detected for a given rf potential and rf frequency. Therefore, a very rapid sweep can be performed by varying the rf frequency while rf and dc potentials are constant or *vice versa*. An advantage of the quadrupole is

that it does not require focusing slits and this results in higher sensitivity, as the resolution is only a function of the number of cycles an ion spends in the field.

In *time of flight spectrometers,* the ions of different mass are given the same kinetic energy allowing them to acquire different velocities, and have a time of flight that depends only on their mass—the lighter the ions, the faster they can travel through the field-free region. Hence, the original beam of ions tends to separate into several layers of ions, depending on their mass that bombarded the cathode of the ion-detector sequentially, and their transit time is calculated. Because a complete mass spectrum can be repeated 20,000 times in 1 second, the *time of flight* instrument is extremely useful in kinetic studies of fast reactions.

ION DETECTOR—The ions in each ion beam of different m/z are "counted" at a collector tube. This yields an analog signal that is amplified to provide electron currents that are representative of the number of collected ions of a particular m/z value.

COMPUTER SYSTEM—Digitized electrical data from the ion collector is fed into a computer where it can be processed further and simultaneously matched with a host of possibly identical spectra stored in the computer. This allows rapid accumulation, manipulation, and interpretation of the mass spectra. Dedicated computers are an integral part of a mass spectrometer. These perform a variety of functions such as automatic tuning, mass calibration, processing data etc. The advancements in information technology have helped in making mass spectrometers more powerful in terms of data acquisition as well as data processing.

VACUUM SYSTEM—All mass spectrometers operate under high vacuum that helps in eliminating unwanted collisions among the ions and between ions and neutral molecules. High vacuum also helps in preventing gas discharge from high voltages used in certain ion detectors. High vacuum also minimizes background and cross contamination between successive samples particularly in hyphenated systems.

HPLC coupled with API (ESI and APCI) MS techniques is one of the most widely used MS techniques to answer the bioanalytical issues during drug development. The usefulness and versatility of this technique will be illustrated in following section.

The production of ions by evaporation of charged droplets obtained through spraying or bubbling, has been known about for centuries, but it was only fairly recently discovered that these ions may hold more than one charge. A model for ion formation in ESI, containing the commonly accepted themes, is described below:

Large charged droplets are produced by *pneumatic nebulization*; ie, the forcing of the analyte solution through a needle (Fig 34-5) at the end of which is applied a potential. The potential used is sufficiently high to disperse the emerging solution into a very fine spray of charged droplets all at the same polarity. The solvent evaporates away, shrinking the droplet size and increasing the charge concentration at the droplet's surface. Eventually, at the Rayleigh limit, Coulombic repulsion overcomes the droplet's surface tension and the droplet explodes. This *Coulombic explosion* forms a series of smaller, lower charged droplets. The process of shrinking followed by explosion is repeated until individually charged *naked* analyte ions are formed. The charges are statistically distributed among the analyte's available charge sites, leading to the possible formation of multiply charged ions under the correct conditions. Increasing the rate of solvent evaporation, by introducing a drying gas flow counter current to the sprayed ions increases the extent of multiple-charging. Decreasing the capillary diameter and lowering the analyte solution flow rate, ie, in nanospray ionization, will create ions with higher m/z ratios (ie, it is a softer ionization technique) than those produced by *conventional* ESI and are of much more use in the field of bioanalysis. A positive ion LC/ESI/MS spectrum of the drug ganciclovir (MW 255) is shown in Figure 34-6. A strong signal

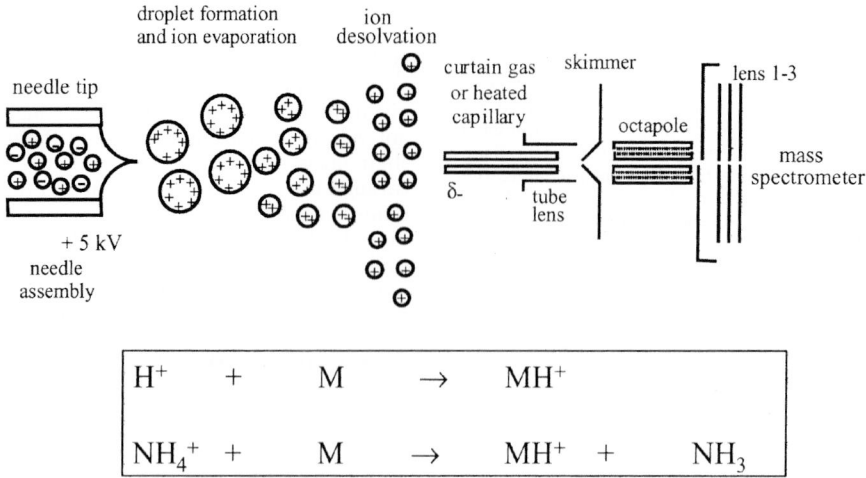

Figure 34-5. Positive electrospray ionization.

corresponding to protonated molecular [MH]$^+$ ion at m/z 256 is obtained. In negative ion LC/ESI/MS mode a strong signal corresponding to the loss of a proton [MH]$^-$ at m/z 254 is obtained.

TANDEM MASS SPECTROMETRY

Tandem mass spectrometry (MS/MS) is used to produce structural information about a compound by fragmenting specific sample ions inside the mass spectrometer and identifying the resulting fragment ions. This information can then be pieced together to generate structural information regarding the intact molecule. Tandem mass spectrometry also enables specific compounds to be detected in complex mixtures on account of their specific and characteristic fragmentation patterns.

A tandem mass spectrometer is a mass spectrometer that has more than one analyzer, in practice usually two. The two analysers are separated by a collision cell into which an inert gas (eg, argon, xenon) is admitted to collide with the selected sample ions and bring about their fragmentation. The analysers can be of the same or of different types, the most common combinations being:

quadrupole-quadrupole
magnetic sector–quadrupole
magnetic sector–magnetic sector
quadrupole–time-of-flight.

The basic modes of data acquisition for tandem mass spectrometry experiments are as follows:

PRODUCT OR DAUGHTER ION SCANNING—The first analyzer is used to select user-specified sample ions arising from a particular component; usually the molecular-related (ie, (M+H)$^+$ or (M-H)$^-$) ions. These chosen ions pass into the collision cell, are bombarded by the gas molecules which cause fragment ions to be formed, and these fragment ions are analyzed, ie, separated according to their mass to charge ratios, by the second analyser. All the fragment ions arise directly from the precursor ions specified in the experiment, and thus produce a fingerprint pattern specific to the compound under investigation. This type of experiment is particularly useful for providing structural information concerning small organic molecules. An example of product ion scanning is provided in Figure 34-7. ESI/MS analysis of the drug labetalol gives predominantly [MH]$^+$ ion at m/z 329. This ion upon collision-induced dissociation produces a series of fragment ions.

PRECURSOR OR PARENT ION SCANNING—The first analyser allows the transmission of all sample ions, while the second analyser is set to monitor specific fragment ions, which are generated by bombardment of the sample ions with the collision gas in the collision cell. This type of experiment is particularly useful for monitoring groups of compounds contained within a mixture, which fragment to produce common fragment ions, eg, aliphatic hydrocarbons in an oil sample, or glucuronide conjugates in urine.

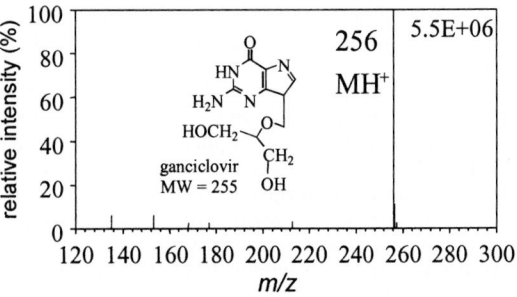

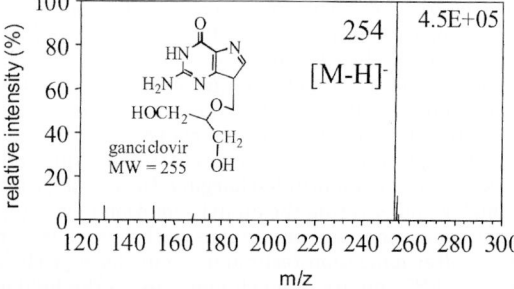

Figure 34-6. Positive (*upper panel*) and Negative (*lower panel*) LC/ESI/MS spectrum of ganciclovir.

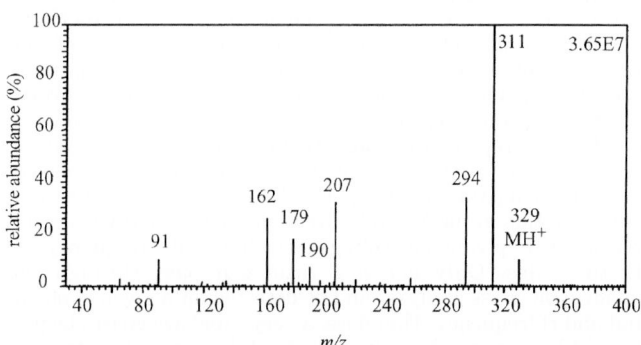

Figure 34-7. LC/ESI/MS/MS spectrum of labetelol.

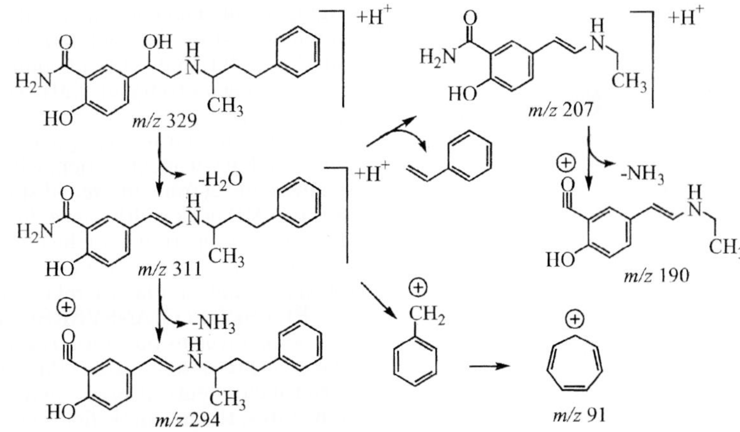

Figure 34-8. Product ions from labetelol.

CONSTANT NEUTRAL LOSS SCANNING—This involves both analysers scanning, or collecting data, across the whole m/z range, but the two are offset so that the second analyser allows only those ions, which differ by a certain number of mass units (equivalent to a neutral fragment) from the ions transmitted through the first analyser. This type of experiment could be used to monitor all of the carboxylic acids in a mixture. Carboxylic acids tend to fragment by losing a (neutral) molecule of carbon dioxide (CO_2), which is equivalent to a loss of 44 Da or atomic mass units. All ions pass through the first analyser into the collision cell. The ions detected from the collision cell are those from which 44 Da have been lost.

SELECTED/MULTIPLE REACTION MONITORING (SRM/MRM)—Both of the analysers are static in this case as user-selected specific ions are transmitted through the first analyzer and the second analyzer measures user-selected specific fragments arising from these ions. The compound under scrutiny must be known and have been well characterised previously before this type of experiment is undertaken. This methodology is used to confirm unambiguously the presence of a compound in a matrix, eg, drug testing with blood or urine samples. It is not only a highly specific method but also has very high sensitivity.

Nuclear Magnetic Resonance Spectroscopy

Nuclear magnetic resonance spectroscopy (NMR) is one of the most powerful tools used for the elucidating the structure of organic molecules. As with other forms of spectroscopy it involves the absorption of electromagnetic radiation, in this case in the radio frequency range (4–900 MHz). NMR is based on the fact that atomic nuclei have quantized spin states, which may be differentiated in the presence of a strong magnetic field. The application of energy in the form of a radio frequency, orthogonal to the applied magnetic field induces transitions between the allowed states resulting in the absorption of energy. The corresponding frequency of the absorbed energy depends, not only on the nuclei in question (eg, ^1H), but also depends on its electronic environment. Absorbed frequencies are therefore influenced by nature of chemical bonding, an attribute that ultimately leads to the use of NMR as a structural tool.

This section will deal primarily with proton (^1H) and carbon-13 (^{13}C) NMR, as these nuclei are the primary nuclei studied in organic chemistry. Following a brief discussion of NMR theory, sufficient background will be given to provide the reader with the fundamental knowledge of how NMR is used for structural elucidation. This discussion will include an examination of the major 2-D techniques used. The section will conclude with a brief overview of the instrumentation associated with FT-NMR along with a brief overview of important advances including

magic angle spinning (MAS) for the analysis of solids, the use of pulsed field gradients (PFG), and the evolution in probe technology for applications such as LC-NMR.

NMR THEORY

As early as 1924, Pauli suggested that certain atomic nuclei could have spin as well as a magnetic moment from rotation around their axes. He theorized that in the presence of an external magnetic field, nuclei could be split in to different energy levels. In other words, nuclei could align themselves either with or opposed to the magnetic field, much like the phenomenon observed with a bar magnet. Experimental verification of these theoretical concepts, however, did not occur until 1946 when Bloch at Stanford and Purcell at Harvard independently demonstrated that nuclei absorb electromagnetic radiation in the presence of a strong magnetic field. The two physicists shared the Nobel Prize in physics in 1952 for their work.

Quantum mechanics can be used to describe the properties of spinning nuclei. Specifically, the angular momentum of the spinning charge is expressed by the *spin quantum number*, I. The spin quantum number can adopt integer or half-integer values expressed in units of $h/2\pi$, where h is Plank's constant. As shown in Table 34-2, spin numbers vary for various nuclei depending on the relationship between the number of protons and neutrons in the nucleus.

Any nuclei of $I > 0$ placed in a magnetic field will assume a maximum number of orientations equal to $2I + 1$. Because $I = \frac{1}{2}$ for the proton, two orientations or spin states exist: aligned with field (low energy) and opposed to field (high energy). Pharmaceutical applications of NMR primarily focus on nuclei of $I = \frac{1}{2}$ (Table 2). As stated previously, two of these nuclei (^1H and ^{13}C) will be considered in the chapter.

The separation of the energy levels (spin states) is a function of the nuclear magnetic moment (μ), the external magnetic field (H_0) and the spin quantum number (I) according to equation 3.

$$E = \mu H_0 / I \qquad (3)$$

In the presence of a strong magnetic field, nuclei will precess about an axis parallel to the magnetic field. This process is depicted for a single nucleus in Figure 34-9.

Table 34-2. Spin Quantum Numbers for Various Nuclei

SUM OF PROTONS PLUS NEUTRONS	SPIN QUANTUM NUMBER (I)	EXAMPLES OF NUCLEI
Even	0	^{12}C, ^{16}O, ^{32}S
Odd	1/2	^1H, ^{13}C, ^{19}F, ^{31}P
Odd	3/2	^{127}I, ^{11}B, ^{79}Br
Even	1	^2H, ^{14}N

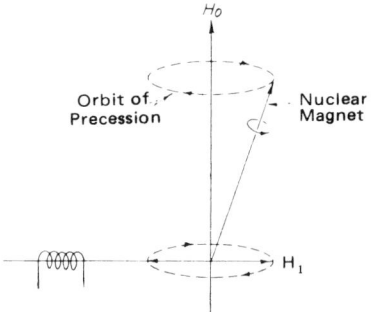

Figure 34-9. The spinning and precessing of a nuclear magnet in an external magnetic field.

The angular velocity of a precessing nucleus, ω_0, is related to the applied magnetic field according to:

$$\omega_0 = \gamma H_0 \qquad (4)$$

γ is the magnetogyric ratio (a constant for a given nucleus which is directly proportional to the magnetic moment). The greater the angular velocity, the greater the energy required to flip a nucleus from its low energy state (aligned with H_0) to its high energy state (opposed to H_0). During a NMR experiment, a sample is placed in a homogeneous magnetic field (H_0) and an external rf oscillator coil is used to introduce a second magnetic field orthogonal to H_0. When the applied rf frequency (ν) is equal to $\omega_0/2\pi$, a nuclei is able to absorb energy and flip to the excited state. As this occurs, a nucleus is said to be in "resonance" and the associated frequency is referred to as the resonance frequency. The energy absorbed in this transition induces a potential in a receiving coil placed orthogonal to both H_0 and the magnetic field of the oscillating coil. In older generation NMR instruments, referred to as continuous wave (CW), the applied frequency is held constant while H_0 is scanned. As different nuclei are consecutively brought into resonance, a voltage is induced proportional to the number of nuclei present in the sample. The NMR spectrum produced by this process is essentially a plot of applied frequency (ν) versus absorbed peak intensity. In this spectrum, peak intensity is expressed in arbitrary units; however, this signal reflects the concentration of the sample as well as the relative abundance of each type of magnetically distinct nucleus that exists in the molecule analyzed.

Fortunately, the resonance frequency of a particular nucleus (eg, ^1H) varies considerably according to its electromagnetic environment. Since this environment is strongly influenced by chemical structure, NMR is a powerful tool for the structural assignment of organic molecules. The specific correlation between resonance frequency and chemical structure is referred to by the term *chemical shift*. This concept will be discussed subsequently in more detail when we address the use of NMR for structure determination.

ABSORPTION AND RELAXATION

An interesting distinction about NMR compared to other forms of spectroscopy is that there are roughly equal populations among the higher and lower energy states. Actually, a slight excess of nuclei exists in the lower energy state. In the absence of an applied magnetic field the population of the two states is governed by a Boltzmann distribution. In most other forms of spectroscopy, the lowest energy state (ground state) is heavily populated relative to the excited states. For absorption of energy to occur, there must be an excess population in the lower state. However, because this excess in NMR is

slight, the phenomenon of signal saturation occurs readily as the lower state is depleted (ie, the two states achieve equal populations). This phenomenon also accounts for the relative insensitivity of NMR compared to other forms of spectroscopy.

The population in the upper state also depends on a phenomenon known as relaxation, which refers to any process that removes nuclei from an excited state. Relaxation is also important to NMR peak width, since the width of an absorption band is inversely proportional to the lifetime of the excited state. Two basic relaxation mechanisms are operative in NMR: spin-spin relaxation and spin-lattice relaxation.

SPIN-SPIN (TRANSVERSE) RELAXATION—Spin-spin relaxation involves the mutual exchange of energy between two proximal precessing nuclei. Basically, when two neighboring nuclei have identical precession rates, but exist in different spin states, the magnetic fields of each nucleus can interact to cause a mutual exchange in spin-states (low to high and high to low). Obviously, this type of relaxation does not help maintain an excess lower spin state population. It can, however, increase line broadening by decreasing the average lifetime of a nucleus in excited state.

SPIN-LATTICE (LONGITUDINAL) RELAXATION—Spin-Lattice relaxation involves the transfer of energy to lattice components (surrounding molecules) as nuclei return from the higher to a lower spin state. Energy dissipated to the lattice increases the vibrational, translational and rotational energy of adjacent nuclei. Because this process replenishes the lower state, it helps alleviate signal saturation. The extremely broad NMR signals observed for solids or viscous liquids are attributed in part to a limited facility for spin-lattice relaxation.

INTERPRETATION OF SPECTRA—To begin to understand how NMR is used for structural interpretation, it is important to introduce specific terms or concepts such as shielding, chemical shift, anisotropy and spin-spin coupling. Each of these terms will be described below in the context of proton NMR.

CHEMICAL SHIFT—The magnetic environment of any nucleus is influenced by circulating electrons, since electrons are capable of producing small magnetic fields. When these fields counteract the applied magnetic field (H_0), the nucleus is said to be shielded. A stronger magnetic field must therefore be applied to transition protons shielded by circulating electrons. As one might expect, shielding can be reduced by the presence of electron-withdrawing substituents, such as oxygen or halogens. Consequently, protons attached or adjacent to electronegative substituents require less magnetic field strength to achieve resonance and are said to be displaced downfield or deshielded.

Chemical shift is the term used to describe the unique magnetic field strength required to achieve resonance for any given proton. As discussed earlier, the required magnetic field for resonance (and thus chemical shift) is influenced by the electromagnetic environment of the proton. To correlate observed chemical shifts to chemical structure, it is important to define chemical shift in a manner that is independent of instrument or applied field strength. By convention, tetramethylsilane (TMS) is used as a reference in proton NMR and is assigned a chemical shift of zero. TMS was selected because its methyl protons are found well upfield from almost all known proton resonances owing to the electropositive nature of silicon (maximum shielding). Chemical shifts are defined by the following equation and are expressed in parts per million using the symbol δ.

$$\delta = (\nu_s - \nu_{TMS}/\nu_{rf}) \times 10^6 \qquad (5)$$

In equation (5), ν_s and ν_{TMS} are the field strengths (in Hz) for the sample and reference, respectively, while ν_{rf} refers to the frequency of the applied rf signal. Note, the reader should also be made aware of a second convention using the symbol τ (where $\tau = 10 - \delta$).

As δ (ppm) increases, the proton is said to be shifted downfield (a higher frequency/lower field required for resonance). For the purpose of illustration, the chemical shifts (ppm) for the methyl protons of the molecular series CH_3X are as follows: CH_3I (2.16), CH_3Br (2.68), CH_3Cl (3.05) and CH_3F (4.26). In this series the effect of electronegativity is clear as the most electronegative element fluorine creates the highest deshielding.

Chemical shifts are influenced by additional sources of magnetic fields correlated to chemical structure. Several cases involve the participation of π electrons. A classic illustration is the apparent anomaly in the chemical shift (δ) of acetylenic (2.35) and olefenic (4.60) protons. Since most methylenic protons have chemical shifts below 2 ppm, one might expect that the deshielding caused by the introduction of π electrons would result in higher deshielding for acetylene than ethylene. This phenomenon is explained by the illustration in Figure 34-10a and 34-10b where the magnetic field induced by the triple bond of acetylene acts in concert with H_0. This effect, referred to as *diamagentic anisotropy*, also accounts for the deshielding of the aromatic protons of the phenyl group (S 7–8 ppm) as well as the extreme deshielding observed for aldehyde protons (Fig 10b)

SPIN-SPIN COUPLING—Figure 34-11a depicts the NMR spectrum of ethanol. In this spectrum one might expect to observe three distinct peaks for CH_3, CH_2 and OH in the abundance of 3:2:1. Interestingly, this is not the case. Although three clusters of peaks are observed, two occur as multiplets. These multiplets are formed by a phenomenon called spin-spin coupling (often referred to as *splitting* or scalar coupling), which is caused by the influence of the spin states of neighboring protons transmitted through chemical bonds.

Figure 34-11b illustrates the probable nuclear arrangement of the —CH_2— and —CH_3 groups of ethanol. The spin coupling which leads to the observed multiplicity is sometimes called *3-bond* coupling since information about neighboring spin states is transmitted through three chemical bonds (ie, 2 C-H and 1 C-C). This means that the multiplicity observed in 1H-NMR spectra is due to the influence of protons on adjacent carbon atoms. The formula for spin-spin generated multiplicity is $2nI + 1$, where n is the number of equivalent nuclei of spin I. For ^1H and ^{13}C, this formula may be re-written as $n + 1$. In Figure 34-11a, the multiplet for the —CH_2— group is a quartet of peaks of the intensity ratio 1:3:3:1. The —CH_3 multiplet occurs as a triplet of intensity ratio 1:2:1. An explanation of this splitting pattern is shown in Figure 34-11b, which gives the possible combinations for parallel and antiparallel spin for —CH_3 (upper) and —CH_2- (lower). Note, this illustration is consistent with the n + 1 rule. In addition, the complete integration for the two multiplets gives a ratio of 3:2 as expected from the overall proton abundance of the two groups.

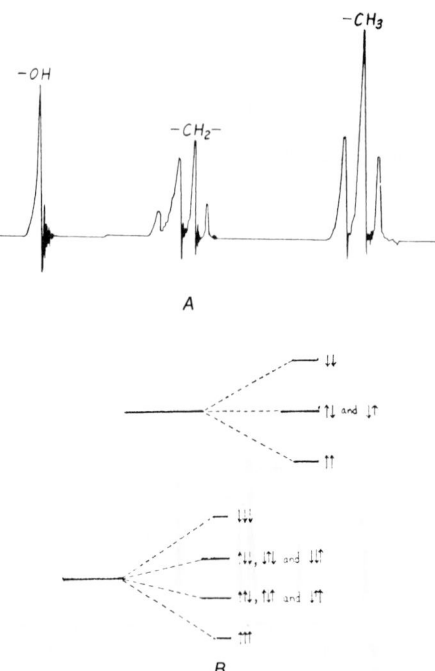

Figure 34-11. A. A high-resolution NMR spectrum of ethanol. **B.** Spin-spin splitting presentation of proximal CH_3 and CH_2.

Although spin-spin coupling adds complexity and reduces the sensitivity of NMR, it is an essential feature for organic structure elucidation because it allows the features in a NMR spectrum to be correlated to adjacent positions within a molecule. The distance between adjacent peaks within a multiplet is also diagnostic and is referred to as the scalar (through bond) coupling constant J. J values are on the order of a few Hz (rarely exceed 20 Hz). Coupling constants are generally denoted as J_{A-B}, where A and B refer to the corresponding positions on the molecule.

^{1}H-NMR SPECTRUM OF PROPRANOLOL—Several features of spectral interpretation are illustrated by the proton NMR spectrum of the common β-blocker, propranolol. Propranolol has 16 carbons as well as 21 hydrogens as labeled in Figure 34-12. Propranolol also has three heteroatoms, two of which have exchangeable hydrogens. Because this NMR spectrum was acquired in a deuterated solvent (CD_3OD), these active hydrogens were readily exchanged by deuterium and not observed in the NMR spectrum shown. Despite the use of deuterated solvents, the presence of the residual water in the sample is evident from the large water resonance at 4.83 ppm.

An illustration of spin-spin coupling is found in the three-carbon spin system defined by the isopropyl group. Figure 34-13a shows an expanded view of the multiplet centered at 3.49 ppm. This multiplet, which contains seven peaks, has a combined integration of 1.00 meaning that it represents a single proton. According to the n+1 rule, there must be a total of six protons on the neighboring carbon atoms, a situation that can only be explained by the methyl groups of the isopropyl moiety. Therefore, this peak is assigned to the methine proton of the isopropyl group (carbon 14).

The corresponding multiplet for the methyl groups (Fig 34-13b) is centered at 1.38 ppm and has a combined peak integration of 6. The expanded view of this multiplet reveals what appears to be a triplet, but is in reality an unresolved pair of doublets, each corresponding to one of the methyl groups. Because of the chiral center, these methyl groups are chemically nonequivalent and thus have slightly different chemical shifts. Each peak is split into a doublet by the methine proton.

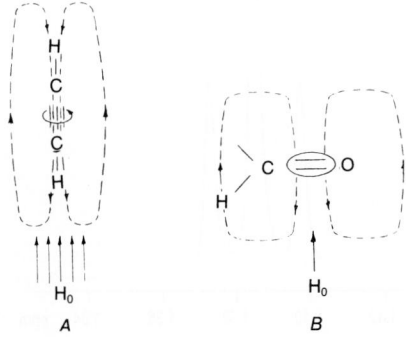

Figure 34-10. The electron-induced magnetic lines of force. **A.** Shielded acetylenic proton. **B.** Deshielded aldehyde proton.

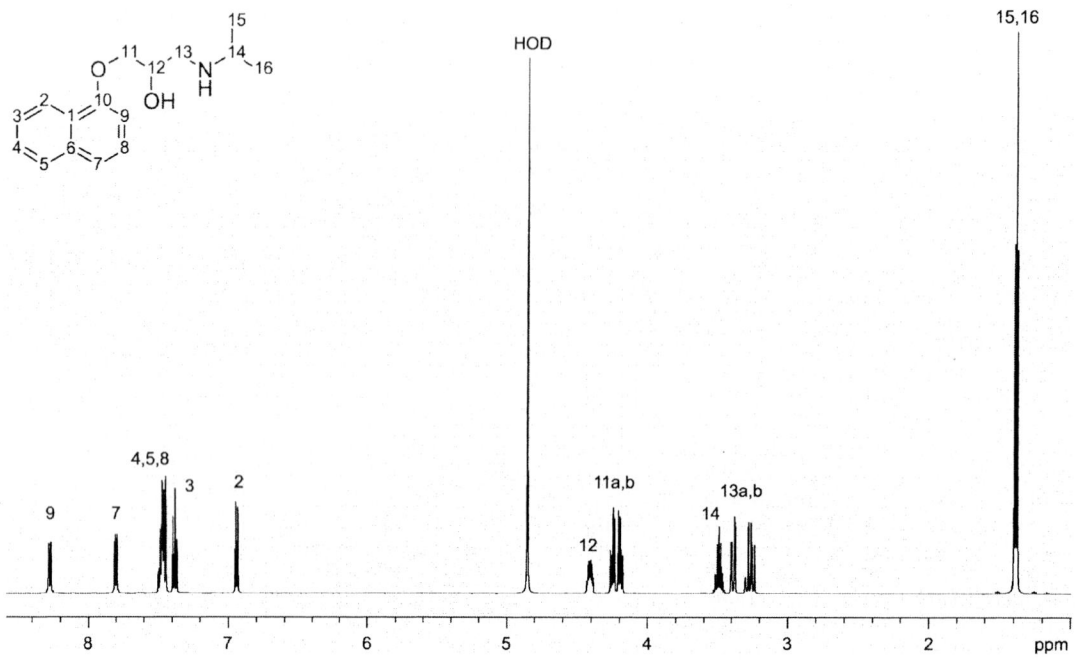

Figure 34-12. 1H-NMR spectrum of propranolol.

Table 34-3 provides a list of assignments for all 19 non-exchangeable protons in the ^{1}H-NMR spectrum of propranolol.

The assignments for propranolol were based on three pieces of information: chemical shift, peak integration and scalar coupling. Despite the complexity of the spectrum, the molecule can be broken down into 3 spin systems. The first system, corresponding to the isopropyl group, was already described. A second spin system is created by the interaction of the protons on carbons 11, 12, and 13. Multiplets for the protons on these carbons are centered at 4.22, 4.41 and 3.33, respectively. The proton on carbon 12 is readily identified since it is the most deshielded (attached to a primary alcohol) and has a peak integration of 1.00. In addition, this resonance exists as complex multiplet created from splitting by two adjacent methylene groups. One would predict that the protons on the methylene groups adjacent to carbon 12 would exist as doublets. This is true to a first approximation; however, additional splitting occurred resulting in the production of a doublet of doublets in each case (Fig 34-12). The proton pairs on carbons 11 and 13 are differentiated with the letters "A" and "B" in Table 34-3 indicating that they are not magneti-

cally equivalent. These sets of protons are said to be *diastereotropic*, a phenomenon introduced by the chiral site in propranolol. The assignments for the methylene protons on carbons 11 and 13 are consistent with predicted chemical shifts and peak integration across the complex doublets observed in each case.

The third system corresponds to the aromatic protons on the napthyl ring. Due to anisotropic effects the aromatic protons appear in the region from 6.5 to 8.5 ppm. Based on the information present in this region of the spectrum, it is possible to deduce the position of substitution on the napthyl ring. The reader is referred to Table 34-3 for a list of the assigned resonances in this region.

A technique frequently used in concert with ^{1}H-NMR is selective decoupling to identify the protons participating in a given spin system. Decoupling can be accomplished by irradiating the sample at the resonance frequency of one of the known protons. When this occurs, any peaks coupled to the proton in question automatically become decoupled causing any related multiplets collapse into a single peak. Historically, this process was repeated manually for each resonance, but for years has oc-

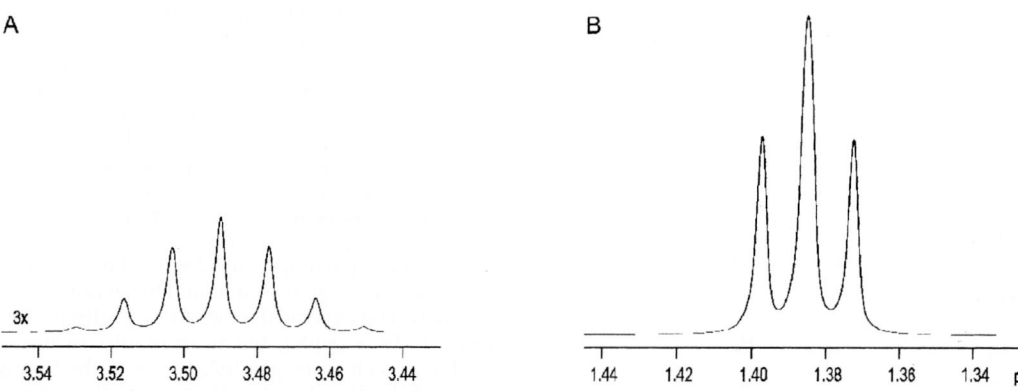

Figure 34-13. Expanded view of the muliplets related to the isopropyl moiety of propranolol. Figure 34-13a corresponds to the methine proton (carbon 14) and Figure 13b represents the methyl protons (carbons 14 and 15).

Table 34-3. Peak Assignments for the ¹H-NMR Spectrum of Propranolol

CHEMICAL SHIFT (PPM)	MULTIPLICITY	INTEGRATION (NO. OF PROTONS)	ASSIGNMENT (ATTACHED CARBON)
1.38	triplet (unresolved pair of doublets)	6	15, 16
3.26	doublet of doublets	1	13A
3.39	doublet of doublets	1	13B
3.49	septet	1	14
4.19	doublet of doublets	1	11A
4.25	doublet of doublets	1	11B
4.41	multiplet	1	12
4.83	singlet	n/a	residual water
6.94	doublet	1	2
7.38	triplet	1	3
7.47	multiplet	3	4, 5, 8
7.81	doublet	1	7
8.28	doublet	1	9

curred as an automated process using 2-D NMR pulse sequences. An illustration of this technique is provided in the subsequent discussion of 2-D methods.

NMR Instrumentation

HISTORICAL OVERVIEW

The use of NMR as a tool for organic structure elucidation is now almost fifty years old. Over this period a number of important advances in instrumentation have occurred. The use of NMR as a structural tool began in the 1950s when the notion of chemical shifts and the recognition of spin-spin coupling occurred. Advances during the 1960s included the application of Fourier transformation (FT), the use of signal averaging for improved sensitivity and the first utilization of the Nuclear Overhauser Effect (NOE) for structural determination. In the 1970s, NMR became a more widely adopted technique. It was during this decade that FT-NMR became a commercial reality along with the introduction of superconducting magnets and computer controlled instrumentation. The introduction of magic angle spinning for solids was also introduced. Many of the advances in the 1980s were related to the implementation of 2-D techniques as well as larger sized magnets to enable more complex structural elucidation, such as the analysis of peptides and proteins. These trends continued in the 1990s along with the routine implementation of pulsed field gradients, which have improved the overall data quality obtained by 2-D techniques. The 1990s also witnessed several advances in probe technology, including the introduction of a viable interface between HPLC and NMR. A high level overview of the important trends that have led to the capabilities associated with modern NMR appears in the remainder of this section. Greater detail may be obtained from the sources cited in the bibliography.

FT-NMR

One of the chief limitations of NMR is sensitivity. This is particularly true for ¹³C spectra which are about 6000-fold less intense that ¹H owing to a lower natural isotopic abundance and a weak magnetogyric ratio (γ). Although sensitivity issues still exist, NMR was revolutionized by the introduction of Fourier transform (FT) techniques. This technology has led to vastly improved sensitivity and has led to the introduction of 2-D NMR methods.

Prior to FT-NMR, data were acquired in a linear or scanned function. That is, the magnet was scanned over the range of desired chemical shift allowing nuclei to come into resonance in a consecutive fashion. In FT-NMR, data acquisition occurs in a multiplexed format, initiated by pulsing the sample with a 1–10

μsec pulse of radio frequency radiation encompassing multiple wavelengths (white noise). This step causes all protons to achieve resonance simultaneously. The induced voltage pattern detected from this process represents a complex time-domain signal known as the free induction decay (FID).

As depicted in Figure 34-14 the FID represents a complex pattern having a tapered shape. The fall-off in the FID signal is the result of spin-relaxation, whereas the complexity can be understood from the wealth of information encoded in a single FID transient. Obviously, the FID is of little use in its time-domain form. The act of Fourier transformation converts this time-domain signal into a frequency-domain pattern containing all information needed to reconstruct the complete NMR spectrum.

Typically, several FID transients are summed to produce a NMR spectrum. Signal averaging is commonly used to increase the signal-to-noise ratio in accordance with the Felgett advantage. With current technology, a complete ¹H NMR spectrum may be acquired using as little as 100 μg of material; however, low milligram quantities are typically used. For ¹³C NMR spectra, several milligrams are recommended and data are often acquired over several hours (eg, overnight acquisition).

2-D NMR SPECTROSCOPY

To mange the complexity of NMR spectra, two-dimensional methods were introduced.[1] The term 2-D NMR refers to the use of a variety of pulse sequences that allow a sample to be perturbed along two independent time domains. Using 2-D methods, NMR spectra are no longer linear; rather they express

1D ¹H

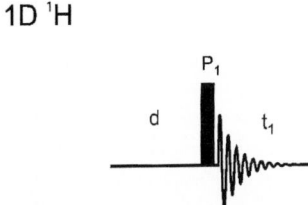

Figure 34-14. Pulse sequence for 1D 1H NMR data acquisition. The sample is irradiated with an rf-pulse (indicated as P1) containing multiple frequencies at an angle 90° with respect to the applied magnetic field. Following absorption of radiation, data acquisition occurs during the period shown as t1, to produce a time domain signal known as the free induction decay (FID). Fourier transformation is subsequently applied to derive frequencies corresponding to chemical shifts. The equilibration time between scans (inter scan delay) is depicted at the front of the sequence by the letter "d."

2D ^{1}H-^{1}H COSY

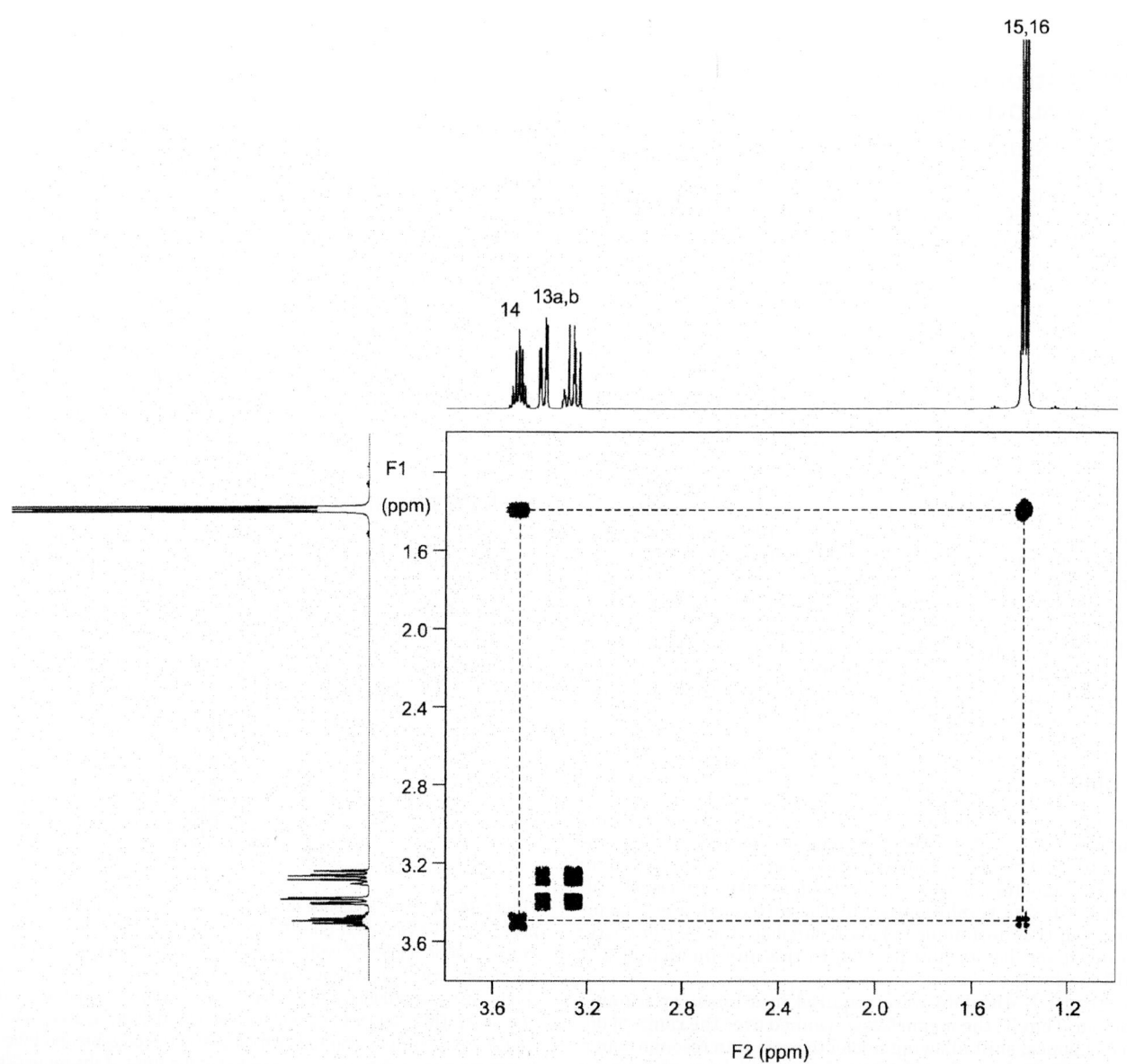

Figure 34-15. Pulse sequence for 2D 1H-1H NMR data acquisition by COSY. This sequence builds on the sequence 1D sequence shown in Figure 34-14 by inserting a second orthogonal rf-pulse (P2) prior to data acquisition, indicated as t2. To acquire a COSY spectrum, the evolution time between pulses P1 and P2 (t$_1$) is varied so that consecutive FIDs are acquired under different evolution times. This process ultimately yields a 2D contour map allowing scalar coupling interactions to be identified from cross-peaks in the 2D spectrum.

a matrix of all combinations of the two variables studied. Fourier transformation of each encoded time domain in the resulting FID yields a spectrum having two separate frequency axes. The 2-D spectrum is expressed in a plane defined by the two frequency axes with peak intensity displayed using a contour format.

The most widely used 2-D technique is named COSY, which stands for Correlation Spectroscopy. A generic pulse sequence for COSY appears in Figure 34-15. Comparison to the sequence in Figure 34-15 reveals the application of a second pulse along with the insertion of an additional time element shown in this Figure at t$_1$. In practical terms, COSY introduces a second decoupling dimension to a conventional ^{1}H-NMR allowing facile determination of all spin-systems present in a molecule.

Figure 34-16 displays the double quantum-filtered (DQF-COSY) spectrum of propranolol. The chemical shift region from 1 to 5 ppm is plotted orthogonally yielding a 2-D contour plot where the conventional 1-D ^{1}H-NMR spectrum is encoded along the diagonal of this plot. Peaks that fall off of the diagonal are referred to as "cross-peaks" because they allow two related portions of the NMR spectrum to be correlated. An ex-

Figure 34-16. Region of the double quantum filtered COSY 2-D NMR spectrum of propranolol. The dotted lines identify protons that are spin-coupled, as indicated by the presence of cross-peaks which fall off the central diagonal. The resonances indicated correspond to the isopropyl spin system.

Table 34-4. Commonly Used 2-D NMR Methods

EXPERIMENT	FULL NAME	NUCLEAR CORRELATION	INFORMATION
COSY	Correlation Spectroscopy	^{1}H-^{1}H Homonuclear	Assignment of spin systems and J$_{A-B}$ (scalar coupling constants)
NOESY	Nuclear Overhauser Enhancement Spectroscopy	^{1}H-^{1}H Homonuclear	Short range through space interactions (dipolar coupling)
HSQC	Heteronuclear Single Quantum Coherence	^{13}C-^{1}H Heteronuclear	An indirect method which allows gives carbon chemical shifts and single bondC-H connectivity
HMBC	Heteronuclear Multiple Bond Correlation	^{13}C-^{1}H Heteronuclear	Similar to HSQC, but gives information about C-H bond connectivity through as many as 4 bonds (long range).

ample illustrated in the Figure is the isopropyl spin-system discussed earlier. In this example the methine proton of carbon 14 (3.49 ppm) is shown to be spin-coupled to the methyl protons of carbons 15 and 16 by the perpendicular lines drawn on the spectrum connecting the resonances to the cross peak of interest. Application of the double quantum filtered variation of COSY has become quite popular since the cross peaks are split into finely divided multiplets providing information on the peak degeneracy produced by the associated spin-system. In addition, it is possible to derive coupling constants from the distance between adjacent peaks.

COSY is but one a several 2-D methods routinely used by NMR spectroscopists. Table 34-4 lists the most common 2-D methods and provides general information about their use. The techniques listed are classified as "homonuclear" meaning that common nuclei are involved or "heteronuclear" if the nuclei are different (eg, ^{1}H and ^{13}C). Heteronuclear methods are often "indirect" meaning the information is obtained indirectly about carbon atoms from their coupling to protons (improved sensitivity since ^{13}C not measured directly). The NOESY technique (based on the Nuclear Overhauser Effect) is particularly useful for distinguishing isomeric configurations since the signals involved arise from through space interactions (as opposed to through bond interactions).

PULSED FIELD GRADIENTS

In 1973 Lauterbur discovered that the use of linear gradients in applied magnetic field enable the determination of spatial position within the magnet.[2] This discovery ultimately led to the present day application of NMR for magnetic resonance imaging (MRI). In early 1990s, it was discovered that pulsed field gradients (PFG) could be used in conjunction with 2-D methods to improve overall data quality.[3]

Without going into detail, there are three basic benefits that have been derived through the application of PFGs. The first is that PFGs allow NMR spectra to be acquired without phase cycling. Phase cycling involves the acquisition of different types of data in alternate scans allowing the desired data to be combined from each scan. PFGs remove the considerable overhead associated with phase cycling resulting in faster data acquisition. The application of PFGs also leads to cleaner spectra by eliminating artifact peaks associated with phase cycling. Finally, PFGs help suppress the unwanted effects of solvent (eg, H$_2$O) in NMR spectra. Because of these advantages, PFGs have become the default mode for NMR data acquisition and are even used automate magnetic field "shimming" in the process NMR instrument optimization.

ADVANCES IN PROBE TECHNOLOGY

Magic Angle Spinning (MAS)–When NMR spectra are acquired for solids using standard methods, extremely broad peaks are produced caused by high proton dipolar and chemical shift anisotropy. These terms vanish when NMR spectra are ac-

quired for liquids and only the spin Hamiltonians for chemical shift and spin coupling contribute. The problem of line broadening in the NMR spectra of solids was largely overcome by the introduction of a technique known as magic angle spinning (MAS).[4] MAS requires a specialized NMR probe that spins the sample at a high rate (>5 kHz) while positioned at an angle of 54°44' relative to the applied magnetic field.

Microprobe Design–Conventional NMR probes use glass tubes (5 mm O.D.) for sample introduction. While various sample volumes may be used, the active volume (interacting with the rf-coil) represents a volume of 220 μL. Because NMR is a concentration-sensitive detector, increased sensitivity may be achieved by dissolving the sample in a reduced solvent volume and/or using a microprobe designed to maximize the sample presented to the rf-coil. Microprobes built for use with smaller tubes (1.0–3.0 mm O.D.) were introduced in the early 1990s for this purpose and may be used with volumes of < 100 μL in some cases.[5] It is important to note that for both conventional and microprobe designs, the solution in the tube must extend beyond the area eclipsed by the rf-coils as not to introduce sources of inhomogeneity. More recently, nanoprobes designs have been introduced (40 μL) in which the entire sample volume is presented to the rf-coil.[6] Because of the effects introduced at the liquid-air interface, nanoprobes must be used with MAS.

Flow Probes (LC-NMR)–An entirely new field of NMR spectroscopy has grown up around the use of NMR probes which incorporate a flow-through design.[7] Flow probes have a detector volume of 100–200 μL and permit sample introduction via flow injection analysis (FIA) or liquid chromatography (LC-NMR). FIA has proven useful for automating sample introduction for use with 96-well technology. LC-NMR offers the advantage of direct mixture analysis, avoiding the need for sample isolation. Although LC-NMR has been used with a number of applications,[8,9] a fundamental limitation of the technology results from the disparate time frames associated with HPLC and NMR data acquisition.

Very recently, a microflow NMR probe has been introduced having a volume of only 5 μl (2 μl active RF coil volume).[10] This design, constructed largely from fused silica capillary tubing, allows for the introduction of highly concentrated samples, reduces the consumption of deuterated solvents, and minimizes post-column band broadening during LC-NMR.

Cryoprobes–One of the most effective ways found to reduce the noise in NMR spectra is to reduce the temperature of the probe. Superconducting probes are now commercially available which use low temperature rf coils to reduce the overall noise level. In these experiments the coils are typically maintained at 20–25°K while the sample is left at room temperature. In most instances, a 4-fold reduction in noise can be expected using current technology.[11] It is important to note that an increase in signal-to-noise of 4-fold reduces the time needed for NMR acquisition by more than a factor of ten.

Magnet Size–Throughout the history of FT-NMR, superconducting magnets have steadily increased in size. At the time of this writing, the largest commercially available magnets are on the order of 900 MHz. In addition to providing greater spectral resolution, high field magnets allow data acquisition to proceed more rapidly since less time is required to achieve a usable resolving power. Despite the performance of such magnets, ultra high field instruments are not widely deployed in the field owing to their high cost. A more common magnet size used in the pharmaceutical industry today is 600 MHz.

SPECTROSCOPY

Continual advances in instrumental methods of analysis have helped to establish these techniques as the mainstream of the analytical laboratory. The conventional wet chemical methods are gradually playing a minor role in the analytical discipline. *Spectrometric methods,* instruments based on the absorption or emission of electromagnetic (EM) radiation as a result of its interaction with matter are described and their applications are explored. These include ultraviolet (UV), visible, infrared (IR), florescence, Raman and light scattering techniques.

A study of the theory and applications of spectrometric methods of analysis necessitates a brief understanding of electromagnetic (EM) theory. Maxwell first expressed the concept of the electromagnetic field in 1860. His equations theorized the existence of waves that travel through electromagnetic fields and whose properties are identical to those of light. The oscillation of an electron gives rise to EM radiation. As is illustrated in Figure 34-17, at each point in the direction of the beam, the electric field and magnetic field, represented by two vectors, are perpendicular to each other. The wavelength, λ, is defined as the distance between successive maxima or minima, and is expressed in nanometers (nm) or 10^{-9} meters, formerly known as Angstroms (Å), (one Å = 10^{-8} cm). The frequency in cycles per second (cps or Hz) is denoted by ν. The frequency is related to λ by $\nu = c/\lambda$, where c is the velocity of light in vacuum. The time required for the completion of one cycle is designated by τ, which is related to ν by $\tau = 1/\nu$. The reciprocal of wavelength, $1/\lambda$, is referred to as wave number, $\underline{\nu}$, expressed in reciprocal centimeters, cm^{-1}. The wave number is employed particularly in describing the position of peak maxima for IR spectra.

Planck, in 1900, formulated a concept of quantum restriction. He stated that oscillating atoms of a hot body can have only energies that are integral multiples of $h\nu$. In other words, the energy of an oscillator is discontinuous and any change in the energy can occur only by a jump between two energy states. Planck showed that the energy in a photon of light is related to wave frequency by the expression $E = h\nu = hc/\lambda$, where h is Planck's constant, 6.6256×10^{-27} ergs/sec. In 1903 Einstein conducted his experiments on the photoelectric effect of light. He concluded that electrons are emitted from the surface of a specific metal upon its illumination with light of a relatively low wavelength such as blue light.

Red light, irrespective of its intensity, fails to eject an electron from a similar metal. These findings by Michelson and Morley, Planck, Einstein, and others could not be explained by Maxwell's assigned wave properties. Considering these facts, a reliance on the dual nature of light, behaving both like a wave and a particle, seemed to be indispensable for resolving many physicochemical phenomena.

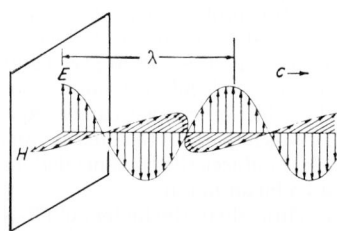

Figure 34-17. A plane-polarized electromagnetic radiation, *E,* electric vector, *H,* magnetic vector.

Molecular Interactions and EM Radiation

The presence of radiation of a particular frequency is necessary, but is not always sufficient, to induce a change in the energy level of a molecule. Quantum restrictions specify certain conditions for the interaction of radiation with a molecule. On many occasions energy is absorbed only if the radiation frequency corresponds to the components of the molecular frequency. This is referred to as resonance absorption.

The position of maximum absorption, λ_{max}, for a molecule in a particular region of the spectrum is a function of the total structure of the molecule with a transition energy corresponding to a given wavelength. The intensity of the absorption maximum, ϵ_{max}, is a function of the probability of EM radiation- molecule interaction and polarity of the excited state. At ground state (i.e. room temperature) a molecule is normally in its lowest energy state. The transition between E_1 and E_2, two energy states or levels of a molecule, occurs by the interaction of EM radiation with a molecule. The difference between E_1 and E_2 is designated by ΔE, whose frequency of radiation is expressed as $\Delta E = h\nu$ ergs.

Very high energies ($>10^8$ cm^{-1}) disturb and cause changes in the nucleus of the atom regardless of its environment. Lower energy however, causes a change in the electronic distribution around the nucleus.

Regions of the Spectrum

The whole range of EM radiations are divided arbitrarily into a number of regions. Interaction between a molecule and various kinds of EM radiation gives rise to a change in the electronic energy and/or kinetic energy of the molecule. In most cases, the energy absorbed is converted quickly to vibrational, rotational, and translational energy. However, in specific cases, emission occurs either immediately as in *fluorescence,* or after a short time as in *phosphorescence.* These specific changes in the energy of a molecule result in the generation of a characteristic spectrum that can be used for both structural elucidation and quantitative determination. Figure 34-18 depicts a wavelength and frequency scale for the different regions of the EM radiation spectrum.

A theoretical and practical description of various types of spectrometry of primary interest in the pharmaceutical industry is given in the following sections. The length of discussion of each topic is based on the extent of the applicability of the method in pharmaceutical analysis.

Absorption Spectrometry

Absorption spectrometry is the measurement of the selective absorption by atoms, molecules, or ions of electromagnetic radiation having a definite and narrow wavelength range, approximating monochromatic energy. Absorption spectrometry encompasses the wavelength regions; ultraviolet (200–380 nm), visible (380–780 nm), near infrared (780 nm to 2.5 μm) and infrared (2.5–40 μm). The region between 10 nm and 200 nm, known as the far UV or vacuum UV (as it requires the complete absence of air due to its interference), has minimal application in pharmaceutical analysis. Atomic absorption spectrometry involves the measurement of radiation absorbed by the unexcited atoms of a chemical substance that has been aspirated into a flame or other high-energy sources.

Theory

When electromagnetic radiation travels through a medium containing atoms, molecules, or ions, a number of events may take place.

- The intensity of the emergent energy may be identical to the intensity of the incident energy. This indicates that no absorption of radiation has occurred.

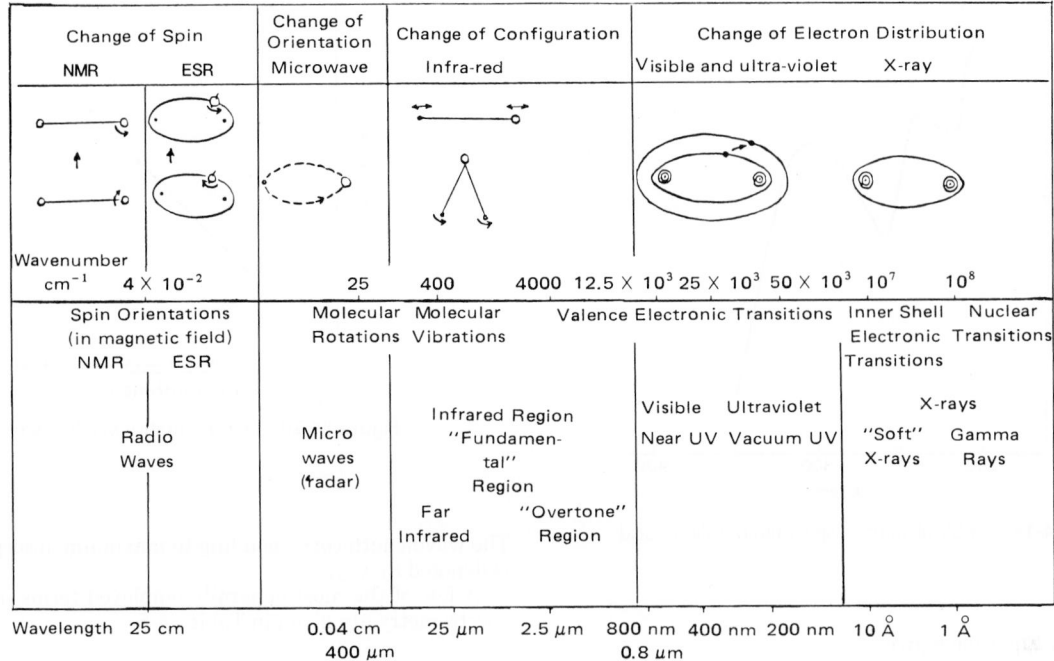

Figure 34-18. The electromagnetic spectrum.

- Reflection, refraction, and/or scattering may occur.
- The intensity of the emergent energy is less than that of the incident energy.

This latter condition indicates that some absorption has taken place (absorption spectrometry). As a result of this absorption, the species involved are activated from their lowest energy state (ground state) to higher energy states (excited states). For absorption to occur, the energy of the exciting radiation must match the quantified energy difference between the ground state and one of the excited states of the species. In atomic absorption, excitation occurs only through electronic transition. In visible and ultraviolet spectrometry, radiation energy can excite only the outermost or valence electrons. Accompanying the electronic excitation (E_e) is a change in vibrational energy (E_v) and rotational energy (E_r) of the molecule. For polyatomic molecules, vibrational and rotational transitions can occur in addition to electronic excitation. As a result, the molecular spectrum consists of closely spaced absorption bands instead of the sharp lines as in atomic absorption. Pure vibrational and some rotational transitions can be achieved by infrared radiation.

The duration of the excited state is brief (10^{-8} to 10^{-9} sec), its existence being terminated by any of several *relaxation* processes. The most common relaxation occurs with the production of heat, which may cause a slight increase in the temperature of the medium. Another form of relaxation results as the decomposition of the excited state into new species (photochemical reactions) according to

$$M + h\nu \rightarrow M^* \text{ (excited state)}$$

$$M^* \rightarrow M + \text{heat}$$

$$M^* \rightarrow M' \text{ (new species)}$$

Alternatively, relaxation may result in emission of radiation at specific wavelengths characteristic of the excited species (emission spectroscopy), or in emission of radiation at longer wavelengths than the incident beam, immediately (fluorescence) or after a short time (phosphorescence).

Ultraviolet and Visible Absorption Spectrometry

The UV and visible absorption bands are due to electronic transitions in the region of 200 nm to 780 nm. In case of organic molecules, the electronic transitions could be ascribed to σ, π, or n electron transition from the ground state to an excited state (σ^*, π^*, or n^*). Because the σ electron is involved firmly in the construction of a single bond, its transition requires much more energy (usually in far UV) than the n electron (nonbonding electrons) or less tightly bonded π electrons.

There are four types of absorption bands that occur due to the electronic transition of a molecule:

R-Bands: $n \rightarrow \pi^*$, in compounds with C=O or NO_2 groups $\epsilon_{max} < 100$

K-Bands: $\pi \rightarrow \pi^*$, in conjugated systems $\epsilon_{max} > 10,000$

B-Bands (benzenoid bands): due to aromatic and heteroaromatic systems, $\epsilon_{max} < 2000$

E-Bands (ethylenic bands): in aromatic systems, ϵ_{max} 2000 to 14,000

Beer's Law

If incident light with wavelength λ and intensity I_0 impinges on a solution with concentration c, and pathlength l of 1 cm, the radiant energy of the light decreases in an exponential fashion. Thus, if a given concentration of a substance absorbs 50% of the incident radiation, doubling the concentration will not absorb 100% but rather 75% of the light. The thickness of the sample or pathlength has a similar effect on the absorption. Mathematically, the radiation-concentration and radiation-pathlength relation can be expressed by

$$\frac{dI}{dc} = -k_1 I \text{ and } \frac{dI}{dl} = -k_2 I \tag{6}$$

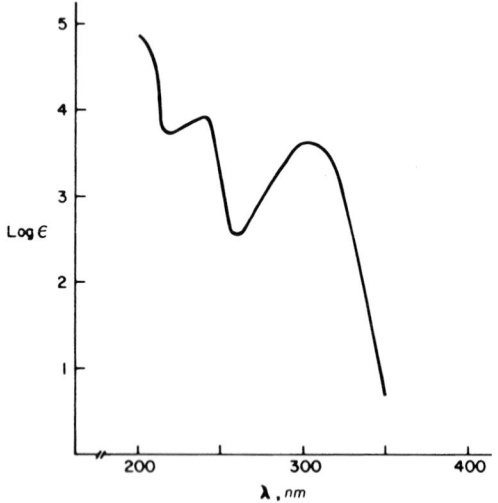

Figure 34-19. The UV absorption spectrum of salicylic acid.

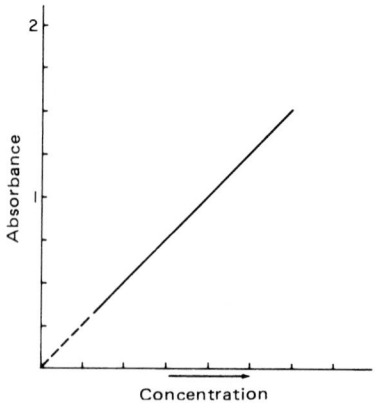

Figure 34-20. A representative Beer's law plot.

Integration of Equation 6 gives:

$$\int_I^{I_0} \frac{dI}{I} = -k_1 \int_0^c dc \text{ and } \int_I^{I_0} \frac{dI}{I} = -k_2 \int_0^l dl \qquad (7)$$

Evaluation of the integrals between limits, combining the two formulas, and incorporating the value 2.303 (for transforming the natural log into a log of base 10) in the constant provides the more familiar equation used in spectrometry,

$$\log (I_0/I) = \epsilon cl \qquad (8)$$

Where I_0 is the intensity of the incident energy, I is the intensity of the emergent energy, c is the concentration, l is the thickness of the medium (in cm), and ϵ is the molar absorptivity (formerly expressed as molar extinction coefficient) for concentration in mol/L.

If the concentration is expressed in g/L, absorptivity is designated by a instead of ϵ. The term $\log I_0/I$ or $\log (1/T)$ is referred to as absorbance, A (formerly stated as optical density or extinction); T is Transmittance or I/I_0. $E_{1cm}^{1\%}$, which is encountered less frequently in the literature, represents a concentration of 1% w/v and a 1-cm cell thickness and is used primarily in the investigation of those substances of unknown or undetermined molecular weight (usually impure natural products).

A typical UV absorption spectrum, shown in Figure 34-19, is the result of plotting wavelength (λ) versus absorptivity ($\log \epsilon$).

The wavelength corresponding to maximum absorptivity, ϵ_{max}, is denoted by λ_{max}.

A few of the most generally employed terms in absorption spectrometry are given in Table 34-5.

Quantitative Applications of UV and Visible Spectrophotometry

One of the major uses of UV and visible spectrometry is for quantitative analysis. An unknown concentration of a known compound, if it conforms to Beer's Law, can be determined by using Equation 8. A representative calibration curve, shown in Figure 34-20 is constructed by plotting absorbance (A) versus concentration.

For quantitative estimation, the samples for UV absorption can be examined in the form of a vapor or a solution. Both polar and nonpolar solvents can be employed to prepare an analytical sample. The cutoff point of a solvent, however, should be recognized as it renders the solvent useless at wavelengths below this value. This is the wavelength at which the absorbance of a solvent approaches unity, using water as a reference. The cutoff points for many solvents can be found in the literature and in solvent charts supplied by several suppliers of solvents.

An understanding of the limitations of Beer's law must be taken into consideration. Some of these are of such a fundamental nature that they constitute a real limitation of the law. The Beer's law during quantitative analysis does not take into consideration the effects of pH, temperature, wavelength, or solute–solvent and solute–solute interactions, such as association (intermolecular hydrogen bonding), dissociation, and chemical reaction. Because of these limitations, the law usually applies only to dilute solutions, where these interactions are insignificant. Another limitation to the Beer's law is the inability of most instruments to provide monochromatic radiation.

A simplified diagram of a UV-visible spectrometer is presented in Figure 34-21 and its major components are outlined in the Table 34-6.

Table 34-5. UV Terminologies

Chromophore	A moiety of molecule responsible for selective absorption of radiation in a given range
Auxochrome	A chemical group which does not give rise to an absorption band by itself, but upon being attached to a chromophore alters both the position and/or intensity of the peak
Bathochromic shift	A shift of the peak position (λmax) to a higher wavelength due to the effect of a substituent or solvent (red shift)
Hypsochromic shift	A shift in (λmax) to lower wavelength (blue shift)
Hyperchromic and Hypochromic shift	An increase and decrease in absorptivity

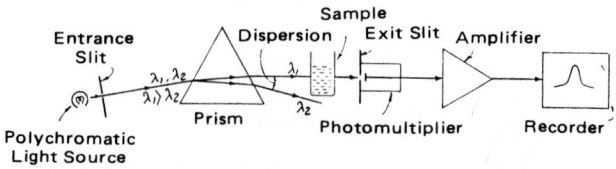

Figure 34-21. A classic UV-visible spectrometer (newer instruments use a grating instead of prisms).

Table 34-6. Comparative Characteristics of Spectroscopic Methods of Analysis

TECHNIQUE	WAVELENGTH (nm)	SOURCE	DETECTOR	SAMPLE	INFORMATION TYPE	APPLICATION
Absorption Spectrometry Ultraviolet/Far UV	200 to 380 nm	Hydrogen or deuterium lamp	Photomultiplier tube (photodiode array, Photon diode) and semiconductors (Charge transfer devices)	Vapor/solution	Little structural information but the presence of unsaturated sites in the molecule	Qualitative and quantitative analysis, confirmation analysis, multicomponent analysis, derivative spectrometry
Visible	380 to 780 nm	Tungsten lamp or deuterium arc lamp	Photomultiplier tube and semiconductors	Vapor/solution	Presence of unsaturated sites in the molecule	Quantitative analysis, confirmation analysis (purity control)
Infrared	2.5 to 40 μm	Nernst or globar unit	Thermocouple or bolometer	Gas, liquid or solid (NaCl, KBr, and CsBr pellets)	R-H vibrational mode	Characterization of molecules
Fourier transform Infrared (FT-IR)	2.5 to 40 μm	Zirconium oxide or rare earth oxides (Nernst Source), silicium carbide	Mercury cadmium telluride (MCT), deuterated triglycerine sulphate (DTGS) crystal or lithium tantalite (LiTaO$_3$)	Same as IR	Structural analysis	Qualitative powers of FT-IR coupled with separation technique as GC-FT-IR and LC-FT-IR
Diffuse Reflectance (Specular or diffuse or attenuated total reflection)	2 to 10 μm	Same as IR	Same as IR	Sample is diluted with KBr powder	Structural analysis	IR spectra of solid samples ie, drugs, pharmaceuticals, food products, soap powder, coal, clay, paper, painted surfaces, polymer foam, catalysts.
Infrared Microscopy Pattern Recognition Analysis	Same as IR UV and IR regions	Same as IR	Same as IR	Same as IR	Same as IR	Flaws and variations in bulk properties of matrices. Identification and differentiation of plastic materials used in Pharmaceutical packing
Hierarchical Cluster Analysis	UV and IR regions					
Emission Spectrometry		AC-, DC-, and AC spark				Qualitative detection of all metals and nonmetallic elements
Flame Photometry		No light source			Qualitative and quantitative analysis	Group IA and IIA metals (Quality control measurement of alkaline or alkaline earth metals)
Plasma Emission		No light source/ hollow cathode lamp				Elemental Analysis
Atomic absorption spectrometry		Discharge lamps (argon or neon)		Solution or in solid state	Qualitative/ quantitative analysis	
Fluorescence Spectrometry	Visible or UV range	Xenon arc lamp				PAH analysis in water, measurement of aflatoxins
Raman Spectrometry	4000 to 25 cm^{-1}	Helium/neon laser	Photomultiplier detector		Vibrational and rotational energy modification	Qualitative/quantitative analysis of inorganic, organic, and biological systems

In general, in single beam spectrometer the sample is placed in the compartment where it encounters monochromatic energy. In a double-beam instrument, this compartment contains a beam-chopping device or a beam-switching assembly that allows the beam to pass alternatively through the sample and reference cells (about 35 times/sec). This allows the sample-reference relationship to remain unaffected by slight changes in the source or optics of the instrument. The detector is usually a photomultiplier tube. The output from the detector is amplified and observed on a meter, a recorder or a cathode ray tube. Most next generation spectrometers are equipped for automatic and continuous recordings. Spectrometers employing the latest technology can be interfaced with a digital computer through an analog to digital converter for the direct determination of difference spectra of analytes as well as for the storage of reference spectra.

Modern Spectrometric Techniques

There has been significant progress in the use of holographic gratings and microprocessor control in the design of modern spectrometers. Recent models feature automatic control of all operating parameters such as wavelength selection and calibration, baseline correction, programmed scanning, first-, second-, third-, and fourth-derivative spectra, light-emitting diode (LED) readouts of absorbance or concentration in addition to screen monitoring and hard-copy printouts.

Also, due to the advent of stable microelectronics, in addition to the wide availability of microprocessor controlled and fully automated spectrometers, new interest is rising in all of the UV-visible absorption techniques that normally require substantial instrument control and data manipulation. These include simultaneous multicomponent analysis, reaction rate determinations, and dual-wavelength derivatives. Also, there is a significant increase in the use of *Difference Spectrometry* as a means for increasing sensitivity, improving detection limits, and decreasing noise as compared to conventional absorption spectrometry.

Other new high-sensitivity spectrometric techniques have gained wide attention recently, especially in trace analysis application and determination of solvent spectra. These new techniques include

- Laser-absorption intracavity techniques based on the dyelaser oscillating mechanism, which are capable of measuring absorbance's in the 5×10^{-6} range and are more suitable for aqueous systems.
- Wavelength modulation (peak-sensing) methods suitable for measuring two different samples simultaneously as well as double derivation of reflectivity, with a sensitivity of up to 1×10^{-7} g.
- Colorimetric methods for the measurement of energy absorbed by the solution using laser sources. These methods have a range of detection between 1×10^{-7} to 8×10^{-8} g and they include thermocouple colorimetry, photoacoustic colorimetry, and thermal lens techniques. Both photoacoustic and thermal lens methods suffer great loss of sensitivity in aqueous media.
- Photon-counting and diode-array detectors.

Diode-Array UV-Visible Spectrophotometry

Advances in technology have led to the development and implementation of photodiode detectors, which when placed in closely spaced linear arrays, offers rapid and accurate spectrum analysis. The primary advantage of linear-array detectors is that they permit the simultaneous analysis of an entire spectrum over a period of a few seconds. This is advantageous when performing kinetic studies involving rapidly changing events. A simplified diagram is presented in Figure 34-22.[12]

Diode-array detectors have an added advantage of increased wavelength resolution. Precision-matching of slit sizes to individual photodiodes and focusing the spectrum in a focal plane can enhance wavelength-resolving power to 1 to 2 nm.

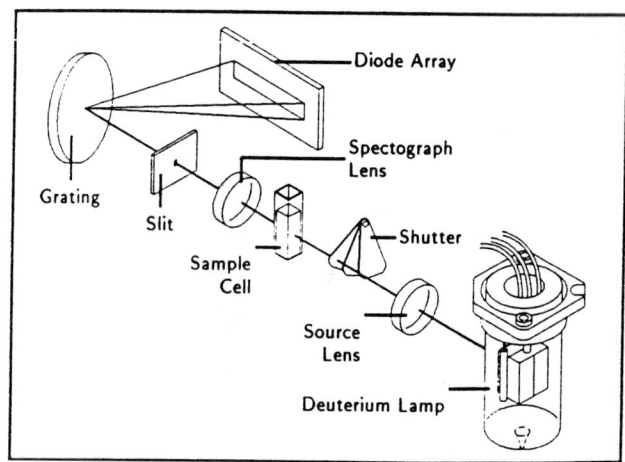

Figure 34-22. HP 8452A optical system with deuterium lamp.

Infrared Spectrometry (IR)

The range of EM radiation between 0.8 and 500 μm is referred to as infrared radiation. At present the IR spectrometer is one of the instruments most frequently employed in the characterization of organic molecules. Unlike the UV-visible spectral plots, the IR spectrum usually is represented with percent transmittance, rather than absorbance, as the ordinate (X-axis). Also, it is customary to use the unit of reciprocal centimeter (cm^{-1}) or the wave number for the abscissa (Y-axis) rather than the wavelength. This is because of the direct proportionality between the wave number and the energy as well as the frequency of the radiation; the frequency can, in turn, be related directly to molecular vibrational frequencies. An example of an IR spectrum is shown in Figure 34-23.[13] The most commonly used region of the IR spectrum in pharmaceutical chemistry is the region between 2.5 μm (4000 cm^{-1}) and 16 μm (625 cm^{-1}).

The near infrared region (NIR) or the overtone region refers to the segment from about 700 nm (12,500 cm^{-1}) to 2.5 μm (4000 cm^{-1}); the far infrared region (FIR) or the rotational region is between 400 and 20 cm^{-1}.

Theory

In order for IR radiation to be absorbed by a molecule, two criteria must be met: the molecule should possess a vibrational or rotational frequency identical to that of the impinging EM radiation, and a net change in the magnitude or direction of the dipole moment should occur as a result of radiation-molecule

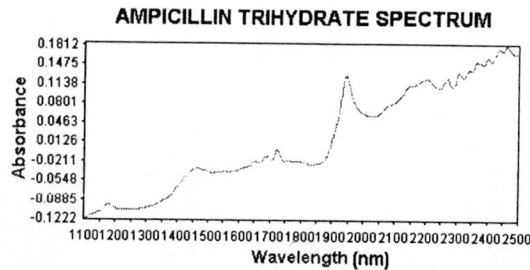

Figure 34-23. NIR diffuse reflectance spectrum of ampicillin trihydrate.

interaction. When IR radiation impinges upon a molecule at the suitable frequency, the vibration and/or rotation of the molecule is altered. If the frequency of the impinging EM radiation matches a natural vibrational frequency of the molecule, a net transfer of energy occurs that creates greater amplitude of vibration and, as a result, absorption of radiation occurs.

The longest wavelength (lowest energy) of IR radiation that induces a change in the vibratory motion of a molecule gives rise to an absorption band known as the *fundamental band*. There is only one fundamental band in a diatomic molecule, although multiples of the band frequency (ν), known as overtones, can occur as 2ν, 3ν, and so on.

Rotation of asymmetric molecules around their centers of mass results in a periodic dipole change that interacts with the incident EM radiation causing a higher frequency of the molecular rotation and absorption of radiation occurs. The energy required to cause a change in rotational levels only is very small (100 cm^{-1}) and comprises the far IR (FIR) region. Absorption by gases in this region appears as discrete, well-defined lines. However, because of the intramolecular collisions and interactions in liquids and solids, broadening of the absorption lines occurs and usually appears as a continuum. The FIR region, which experimentally is difficult to study, has limited application in pharmaceutical chemistry and thus will not be discussed further.

Because absorption of IR radiation alters both vibrational and rotational characteristics of a molecule, absorption bands are not defined lines but are bands that are centered upon one frequency. As the total kinetic energy is a combination of translational, rotational, and vibrational energies of a molecule (ie, $E_t = E_{tr} + E_r + E_v$), a polyatomic molecule consisting of n atoms will have 3n degrees of freedom of motion. The possible fundamental vibrational modes of a molecule can be calculated by subtracting 3 for translational energy and 3 for rotational energy (2, if the molecule is linear). This gives a total of 3n-6 possible vibrational modes. The theoretical number of fundamental absorption bands, however, is not observed due to such factors as weak absorptivity, coalescence of several closely located bands, and lack of required change in dipole moment. Because the 2 to 16 μm region normally employed for IR investigation covers both fundamental and *overtone* regions, the total number of absorption bands in an IR spectrum may greatly exceed the theoretical number.

The atomic stretching vibration can be approximated mechanically by Hooke's law, $F = -kx$, where F is the restoring force, k is the proportionality or the force constant (dyne/cm), and x is the displacement distance. For a diatomic molecule with atoms of masses m_1 and m_2, the frequency of fundamental vibration is expressed by

$$\nu = \frac{1}{2\pi} \sqrt{\frac{k}{\mu}} \tag{9}$$

or in terms of wave number by

$$\bar{\nu} = \frac{1}{2\pi c} \sqrt{\frac{k}{\mu}} \tag{10}$$

Where μ is known as the reduced mass, defined by

$$\mu = \frac{m_1 m_2}{m_1 + m_2} \tag{11}$$

Application of the equation for the C—H stretching frequency with $k = 5 \times 10^5$ dynes/cm, $m_1 = 19.8 \times 10^{-24}$ g, and $m_2 = 1.64 \times 10^{-24}$ g gives the value 3040 cm^{-1} (slightly higher than the observed value, 2950 cm^{-1}, which is caused by neglect of the environmental effect). The vibrational modes of a CH$_2$ group are depicted in Figure 34-24. It should be observed that more energy is required for the stretching vibration than for the bending vibration.

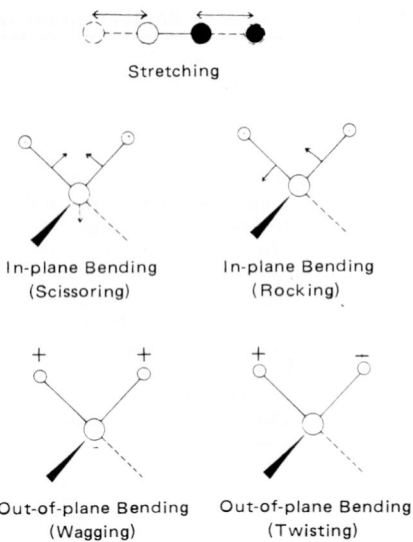

Figure 34-24. Types of molecular vibrations. Plus sign (+) indicates motion from plane of page toward reader, Minus sign (−) indicates motion from plane of page away from reader.[15]

The position of the absorption bands is determined by the symmetry of a molecule, the masses of atoms, the force constants of the chemical bonds, and the interaction of vibrations (Fermi interactions). Hydrogen bonding affects the position of the bands by shifting the frequency of the stretching vibration to a lower frequency and that of the bending vibration to a higher frequency.

Characterization of Molecules

There are two major applications of IR spectrometry in the characterization of various molecules: determination of the identity of a compound by means of spectral comparison with that of an authentic sample, and verification of the presence of functional groups in an unknown molecule. The latter aspect is quite important in the structural elucidation of synthetic organic compounds or substances isolated from natural sources.

The position of the absorption bands due to stretching and in-plane bending vibrations of the functional groups, such as C=O, C—H, N—H, O—H, are somewhat independent of the influence of the neighboring groups in the molecule. These bands usually occur at 4000 to 1300 cm^{-1}. The position of the bands below 1300 cm^{-1} is influenced markedly by neighboring groups in the molecule. The portion of the spectrum from 1300 to 400 cm^{-1} is referred to as the "fingerprint" region.

Extensive charts and tables of the characteristic group absorption frequencies for common organic functional groups can be found in many of the texts listed in the *Bibliography*. Several catalogs of reference spectra have been published, the most voluminous of which is that of the Sadtler Research Laboratories, currently in excess of 90,000 spectra.

The C—H stretching and bending vibrations occur at 3300 to 2800 cm^{-1}. Each type of hydrocarbon has its own characteristic band position; for example, saturated acyclic and cyclic hydrocarbons have stretching ν at 2960 to 2850 cm^{-1} and in-plane bending ν at 1470 to 1360 cm^{-1}; unsaturated olefinic C—H stretching at 3090 to 3000 cm^{-1} and unsaturated acetylenic C—H stretching ν at 3300 to 3270 cm^{-1}; aromatic C—H stretching ν at 3100 to 3000 cm^{-1} and the out-of-plane bending is at 900 to 650 cm^{-1}. The most characteristic band for aromatic compounds, however, is at 1610–1590 cm^{-1} (due to aromatic skeletal vibration). The characteristics of band frequencies are given in Table 34-7.

Table 34-7. Characteristics of Band Frequencies

O—H Vibration	Stretching at 3700 to 3350 cm^{-1}, depending on the extent of hydrogen bonding.
C—O Vibration	Stretching at 1280 to 1000 cm^{-1}, depending on whether it is an alcohol, phenol, ester, ether, etc.
C=O Vibration	Stretching at 1950 to 1640 cm^{-1}, These bands are quite intense and very conspicuous. Hydrogen bondings, field effect, and conjugation affect the position
N—H Vibration	Stretching at 3500 to 3300 cm^{-1}, hydrogen bonding at lower frequency. Bands for N$^+$H$_3$, N$^+$H$_2$, and N$^+$H occur at about 3200, 2700, and 2000 cm^{-1}, respectively.
C—N Vibration	Stretching of aliphatic compounds at 1210, aromatic at 1250 to 1350, C=N at 1680 to 1640, and for C≡N at 2250 cm^{-1}

Quantitative IR

IR spectrometry generally is employed for qualitative identification, with limited use in quantitative analysis. Because of the uniqueness of IR spectra, quantitative methods may not require prior separation of the analyte from excipients. The sensitivity of IR analysis, however, is poor, only 0.01 to 0.001 of the sensitivity of UV, and, therefore, it has only a few applications in quantitative analysis. The major components of IR spectrometer are illustrated in Figure 34-25. The most commonly used prism materials for dispersion of IR radiation are: 1) NaCl with a refractive index of 1.5442. This provides good dispersion at 2000 to 650 cm^{-1}, but poor dispersion beyond 2000 cm^{-1}; 2) KBr, with a refractive index of 1.53, disperses at 1600 to 370 cm^{-1}; and 3) CsBr, with a refractive index of 1.69, disperses at 1000 to 250 cm^{-1}. In recent years grating systems have been employed widely than the prism, primarily because of their high resolving power.

As seen in Figure 34-25, the source beam is reflected by mirrors to form the sample and reference beam. After passing through the sample and reference, the beams are chopped by a mirror that serves to focus each beam alternately onto the entrance slit of the monochromator. If the sample absorbs part of the radiation, the intensity of the two beams will be unequal.

This inequality results in the development of an out of balance signal in the detector. After amplification and rectification, the signal is relayed to a comb or wedge to drive the reference beam attenuator to reduce the intensity of the reference beam. As the difference between the two beams becomes zero,

the out of balance signal also becomes zero. The pen of a recorder, which is connected to the attenuator, will perform the function of plotting the absorption coordinates on a paper chart. The abscissa of the chart is a function of frequency, and the resulting tracing of percent transmission versus frequency is known as an IR spectrum.

Fourier Transform Infrared Spectrometry (FT-IR)

The wide availability of high-powered microcomputers at reasonable cost has helped popularize the applications of transform spectroscopy in general and Fourier transform in particular to several branches of spectrometry. These include IR, NMR, and MS. FT-IR, however, has been one of the first techniques developed; today, it is the instrumentation of preference over dispersive IR for handling ever smaller and more complex samples. Superior sensitivity and resolution, absolute wavelength accuracy, and higher precision of measurements are some of the reasons behind the rapid growth of FT-IR.

Basically, the technique is a coupling of a Michelson interferometer with a sensitive infrared detector. However, because of the enormous amount of data generated, a microcomputer is essential for data handling. In the Michelson interferometer, there is no monochromator and radiation of many frequencies passes through the sample. The source radiation is split between a fixed mirror and a movable one. The two reflected beams then are combined, either constructively or destructively, at the beam splitter, depending on the position of the movable mirror. As the path difference between the two beams is altered and, because only the nonabsorbed frequencies reach the detector, the signal pattern becomes the sample interferogram. For monochromatic radiation, the amplitude of the signal is a cosine function of the mirror position. For polychromatic radiation, the signal is a summation of all the constructive reinforcement or destructive interferences of each wavelength interacting with every other wavelength and results in a unique interferogram for each particular sample.

To handle the complex mathematical treatment needed for calculations, it was found that the cosine Fourier transform can relate the intensity of the interferogram as a function of the mirror travel, $I(x)$ (Eq 12) and the intensity of the frequency $I(v)$ (Eq 13) of the IR radiation:

$$I(x) = \int_{-\infty}^{\infty} I(v) \cos (2\pi v x)\, dv \qquad (12)$$

and after calculating (using a computer) the inverse transforms,

$$I(v) = \int_{-\infty}^{\infty} I(x) \cos(2\pi v x)\, dx \qquad (13)$$

by which the interferogram could be related back to the IR spectrum.

Modern FT-IR spectrometers provide full spectra that can be monitored continuously on a CRT screen while scanning. Standard software packages include spectral subtraction, baseline correction, integration, peak selection, multicomponent and factor analysis, quantitative analysis, and spectral library searching. The use of a new mercury cadmium telluride (MCT) detector, diffuse reflectance accessory, cylindrical interval reflection device, and transmission or reflectance microscopy are recent features that enhance the instrument's sensitivity and versatility.

Diffuse Reflectance

The diffuse reflectance technique has become very popular in recent years and is applicable to a wide range of solid samples. In this technique, IR radiation is focused on a sample and the

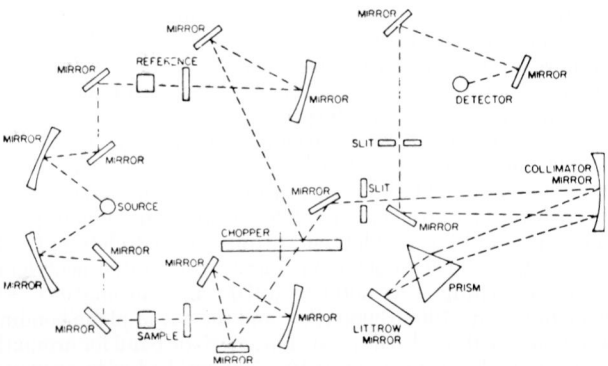

Figure 34-25. The optical system of a classic IR spectrometer (newer instruments use gratings instead of prisms).

reflected or scattered radiation is collected over a wide solid angle, hence the term *diffuse reflectance*. Sample handling is simple and straightforward. Extensive grinding or use of high pressure is not needed, which eliminates the risk of altering the sample structure. Some of the samples for which good IR spectra are obtained are drugs, pharmaceuticals, food products, soap powder, coal, clays, paper, painted surfaces, polymer foam, and catalysts. Many samples, such as inorganics, may be run in neat form. Dilution with KBr powder is often used to reduce the intensity of strong absorption bands.

Infrared Microscopy

Often the analyst is confronted with a sample that precludes exhaustive sample handling. At times these samples take the form of minute flaws or variations from the bulk properties of the matrix. Such samples arise from many sources: forensic, textile, packaging, polymers, films, coatings, paper, and electronic components, all of which can contain small discontinuous areas of questionable composition. When these imperfections arise, the analyst is asked to examine the spot or fragment so that its source in relation to the manufacturing process can be identified.

Infrared spectrometry is especially useful in these situations because it is nondestructive. In addition, the variety of sample-handling techniques available often permits a sample to be analyzed *in situ*. For those problems where it is impossible to extract the critical portion of the sample, this is especially important. Microsampling techniques are employed in IR to improve sensitivity or to restrict the field of view, and thus, eliminate gross background interference. Beam condensers and other magnification tools have been used for many years. Microscopes extend the utility of IR to samples of the order of 10 μm. Use of a microscope allows alignment of the small sample in the IR beam as well as focusing the energy.

Thermogravimetric analysis (TGA) coupled with FT-IR is a new way of monitoring the evolved gases generated during sample decomposition or volatilization caused by heating over time. Using TGA, identification of the components of the gases can be used to determine sample characteristics.

Advantages and Limitations of FT-IR

The speed and high sensitivity of FT-IR, which make it ideal for microanalysis, arise from two factors.

1. The use of what is known as the multiplex or the Fellgett advantage where a very high signal-to-noise ratio exists due to the fact that the sample; thus, the detector is affected by all frequencies at one time.
2. The radiation power throughput of the interferometer is significantly larger than for the dispersive instrument (about 40 times).

These advantages of FT-IR make it the technique of choice for coupling the qualitative power of IR to such separation techniques as gas and liquid chromatography (GC-FT-IR and LC-FT-IR).

Pattern Recognition Analysis

As the preceding sections of this chapter have shown, the spectra obtained in the UV and IR regions are very useful. This utility has been extended by the implementation of pattern recognition analysis. Subtle differences between data sets can be visualized easily, resulting in faster identifications and much quicker decisions. Two approaches, *Principal Component Analysis* (PCA, referred to previously in the near IR discussion), and *Hierarchical Cluster Analysis* (HCA) are mentioned here.

In PCA, new sets of variables or factors that are linear combinations of the original variables in the data set are calculated. The few dimensions in the new factor space that are needed to represent all of the significant information in the data are called principal components, whereas other factors represent noise components only. This view allows visualization of the natural clustering in the data, identifies outliers, and facilitates assignment of chemical or physical meaning to the data patterns that emerge.

The primary purpose of HCA is to present data in a manner that emphasizes the natural groupings in that data set. Distances between the samples (variables) in a data set are calculated and compared. When distances between samples are relatively small, the implication is that samples are similar. HCA results are presented in the form of a dendrogram; a tree-shaped distance map constructed using the sets of intersample distances. Dendrograms show clustering, and the branch lengths are proportional to the distances between the connecting clusters.

One of the activities that may benefit from the capabilities of pattern recognition analysis is the identification and differentiation of plastic materials used in pharmaceutical packaging. For a discussion of this very useful approach to data treatment, see the text by Massart, Vandefinste, and Deming in the Bibliography.

Emission Spectrometry, Flame Photometry, and Atomic Absorption

The study of atomic spectra is probably the most basic scientific phenomenon that has captured the curiosity and the imagination of physicists, astronomers, and chemists for centuries. The information gained from the intensive and unrelenting pursuit to establish its fundamental theories was a major factor behind the development of our modern physical and chemical sciences.

Theory

When gaseous ions or an aerosol form of metals and some nonmetallic elements are heated to a high temperature, the kinetic energy of the atoms or molecules is increased. Collisions occurring at such an elevated energy incur a high probability of transforming the kinetic energy into excitation energy. The electronically excited species are unstable, and if no chemical reaction occurs after 10^{-4} to 10^{-7} sec, the energy is lost by emission of EM radiation in the UV and visible region, with wavelengths that are characteristic of the species under investigation.

Commonly employed methods of excitation are flame, ac arc, dc arc, and ac spark. Flame provides low-energy excitation and is used for easily activated substances; it has been used more recently with great success in Inductively Coupled Plasmas (ICP) where a high temperature argon torch is used to excite most atoms. Electrical excitation by discharge also is very effective in volatilizing and exciting samples and a temperature range of 4000 to 8000K is attainable by this method. An ac spark provides excitation energies greater than the arc and is produced by application of a high voltage (10–50 kV) across the electrodes. Excitation also can be achieved with an optical ruby laser. The optical system of a typical emission spectrograph is shown in Figure 34-26. A diffraction grating can be used in place of a prism for radiation dispersion.

The major application of emission spectrometry is in the qualitative detection of all metals and most of the nonmetallic elements. Detection limits lie in the ppm or ppb range. Quantitative application, which used to be limited, has grown very rapidly lately, especially with the introduction of inductively coupled plasma techniques and laser sources. Currently, emission spectrometry provides an excellent rapid technique for the simultaneous or sequential quantitative determination of up to 30 elements.

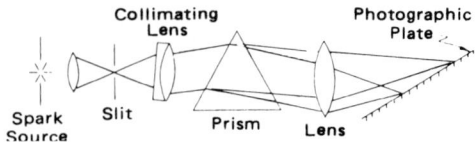

Figure 34-26. A simplified optical diagram of an emission spectrometer.

Flame Photometry (Flame Emission Spectrometry)

Flame photometry employs an emission-measuring device and uses a gas–air flame (1100°–1300°) for excitation. The detection is limited to group IA and IIA metals of the periodic table, which have a low-lying electronic level. Sodium is the most active in the series with a detection limit of 0.0002 ppm and beryllium is the least active with a detection limit of 25 ppm. The detection limit of a few elements is listed in Table 34-8.

Samples are dissolved in a solvent and introduced into the burner via an atomizer. Standard solutions used for analysis should be similar to the sample solution, as variables such as viscosity and temperature affect the nature of atomization, and thus the degree of excitation. In clinical laboratories the quantitative measurement of sodium, potassium, and calcium in biological samples is made by means of flame photometers.

Plasma Emission

Conventional atomization methods, such as combustion flame, furnaces, and electric arcs, are usually adequate for most of the traditional applications of atomic emission spectroscopy. These techniques, however, have several limitations, the most important of which are the instability of the atomization source, the possibility of chemical interaction such as metal oxide formation, the requirement of a relatively large size sample, low sensitivity, and finally, the inability to conduct simultaneous or sequential multielemental analyses. To overcome these limitations, new techniques called plasma emission spectroscopy have been developed.

Plasma is a partially ionized gas, usually a mixture of the sample vapor and a support gas. The plasma is generated electrically and once formed, a greater quantity of electric power can be transferred to it, raising its temperature to 9000K. Such a high temperature provides the analyst with a rich and stable source of atoms that act as a reservoir of free and highly excited atoms. The other advantages of plasma include a wide linear dynamic range, excellent sensitivity, high accuracy, and good precision. Also its suitability for simultaneous multielemental determinations at the ng/mL level has made it the method of choice for the analysis of trace constituents in samples of very limited volume.

Table 34-8. The Detection Limits of Some Elements Using Flame Photometry[a]

ELEMENT	WAVELENGTH (nm)	DETECTION LIMIT (ppm)
Barium	553.6	1.3000
Calcium	422.7	0.0030
Cesium	852.1	0.1000
Lithium	670.8	0.0020
Magnesium	285.2	0.2000
Potassium	766.5	0.0010
Sodium	589.3	0.0002

[a]Source: Courtesy Beckman.

Although there have been different types of plasma emission sources, the most popular sources that have gained wide application are the Direct-Current Argon Plasma and the Inductively Coupled Plasma.

Direct-Current Argon Plasma (DC Argon Plasma)

The main advantage of dc argon plasma is its excellent stability even in the presence of solvents, organics, and high acid or alkali concentrations. It usually consists of two carbon anodes, between which the plasma jet is formed, and a tungsten cathode. It requires about 1 kW of power and once ignited can be sustained by a low voltage. The plasma can sustain a temperature as high as 10,000K. Samples are introduced in an aerosol form, and their emission spectra are observed in a region isolated from the main plasma core, a procedure by which the sensitivity is enhanced greatly. Multielemental sequential analysis can be achieved easily with much lower detectable limits than with conventional flame emission.

The dc argon plasma also has a special advantage in the determination of trace amounts of arsenic and other nonmetallic elements. One limitation, however, is its unsuitability for automation, because the plasma supporting electrodes have to be replaced or reshaped after about 2 hours of operation.

Inductively Coupled Argon Plasma (ICP)

The main difference between inductively coupled argon plasma (ICP) and DC plasma is that the ICP derives its sustaining power by induction from a high frequency magnetic field. The pioneering work of Reed in the early 1960s laid the basis for ICP as an exciting new technique that can be used for the simultaneous determination of all of the periodic table elements with a lower limit of detectability in the ppb range.

ICP simply consists of a quartz tube (2.5 cm diameter) placed inside a coil that is connected to a high-frequency generator (4–50 MHz range) with output levels of 2.5 kW.[14] Because argon is a nonconductor, a seed of electrons (from a Tesla discharge coil) is first introduced before turning on the power. Argon is fed into the quartz tube and is ionized by the magnetic field produced by the induction coil. The seed electrons interact with the magnetic field and gain in intensity enough to ionize the gas flow and an eddy current, induced by the magnetic field, flows in circular closed paths around the discharge tube. After complete ionization, coned flame plasma is formed at the tip of the torch.

Because there is no electrode contact in ICP (as there is with dc plasma), the excitation and emission zones are separated from each other. This, besides the inert environment and the high temperature achieved, allows complete ionization of the sample with minimum chemical interference and a high signal-to-noise ratio of the sample's emission. These excellent conditions are the main reasons for the extreme sensitivity of ICP, typically in the ppb range.

Therefore, ICP offers the threefold potential of ultra-trace determinations on a multi-element basis, using a very small sample size (microliter or microgram level), in any type of matrix. ICP also is very amenable to complete automation and the simultaneous determinations of a vast array of both metals and metalloids.

Atomic Absorption Spectrometry (AA)

As early as 1860 Kirchhoff described the basic principles of atomic absorption (AA) spectra. It was not until 1955, however, that Walsh, Alkemade and Milatz demonstrated the theoretical background for its analytical applications. The simplicity of this technique makes it an attractive tool for the analysis of many elements. At present, many chemical and clinical laboratories use this method for the quantitative determination of most of the elements in multivitamin and mineral formulations, drugs, and biological fluids.

Theory

In AA spectrometry, the elements are transformed into the atomic vapor form by drawing an aerosol of the sample solution into an open flame. A fraction, or most of the freed atoms, are then excited by exposure to a suitable source of radiation. The radiation absorbed by the unexcited atoms is related to the sample concentration. In this sense, AA then could be envisaged as the inverse of emission spectrometry, where the radiation emitted by the thermally excited atoms is related to concentration. It should be emphasized that usually the fraction of atoms excited by heat (via a flame or an electric arc) is relatively small for most elements. Also the atomic absorption of any element is generally at its resonance line—that is, a narrow range of wavelengths, usually in the UV or visible region of the spectrum, corresponding to the electronic transition between the lowest excited state and the ground state.

FACTORS AFFECTING AA SPECTRA

Solvents—In general, an organic solvent enhances the absorption signal, and therefore, it may alter the absorption intensity.

Anions—These can bond strongly with metals and tend to reduce the signal intensity. EDTA chelation could eliminate such effect.

Metal Binding—Sometimes, the presence of one metal interferes with the signal of another. For example, either Si or Al interferes with a proper absorption signal of Sr if both are present in a solution. The signal can be improved by the addition of La, which preferentially binds the interfering metal.

Ionization—If a large quantity of the test element is ionized, a very weak absorption is observed. This is due to the ionic absorption occurring at wavelengths different from that of the atomic one. The condition can be improved by adding a large excess of easily ionized elements; for example, in the measurement of Ca, a large amount of sodium ion usually is added.

Emission from the flame itself is minimized by using a chopper between the lamp and the flame. As the amplifier is designed to amplify only an ac signal (that of the chopping frequency), the intensity of light from the hollow cathode tube can be observed and recorded. A reduction of intensity due to the presence of the sample in the flame then will be detected. The magnitude of the decrease in intensity is a function of the quantity of the sample in the flame.

It is desirable to dissolve the sample in an organic solvent and for higher sensitivity the strongest absorption line must be chosen. In general, the resonance line resulting from the lowest excited state is usually the line exhibiting the strongest absorption. The instruction manual of each instrument suggests the choice of the line and the sampling technique.

New Atomization Techniques in AA Spectrometry

While flame atomic absorption still is used widely for the routine determination of more than 60 elements with new records of detection limits, there has been a considerable interest in the use of other atomization techniques. These include the mercury cold vapor atomic absorption, hydride generation techniques especially for As and Se, and an electrothermal atomization method. Recent research has concentrated on the latter technique as a new powerful tool for the study of trace amounts of lead in different matrices.

Fluorescence Spectrometry (Fluorometry)

When certain chemical substances are excited electronically by the absorption of UV or visible radiation, they emit light at a longer wavelength. This phenomenon is called *luminescence* and depending on the lifespan of the excited species, two different processes could be distinguished. The first is fluorescence, where the luminescence stops within 10^{-8} to 10^{-4} sec after the source of excitation is removed, and the second is phosphorescence, where the luminescence continues for a slightly longer period of time ($\sim 10^{-4}$ to 10 sec).

Theory

Upon absorption of visible or UV radiation by a molecule (usually $\pi \rightarrow \pi^*$ transition), the electron from S_0 (singlet ground state) is promoted to S_1 or S_2 (singlet excited states). The excited species, may return to the ground state by dissipation of energy through collision or by vibrational relaxation of the excited state. The vibrationally relaxed species can return to the ground state with the emission of radiation with a wavelength longer than that which originally was absorbed. This radiation is referred to as fluorescence. Figure 34-27 illustrates different electron spin states.

There also is a nonradiative process in which the excited state gives off energy and proceeds to a lower energy (triplet) state T, by a decay process. A return from T to S_0 gives off a long-lived radiation, which is called phosphorescence. The absorption and emission of radiation is specific for a particular molecule. Figure 34-28 is an energy level diagram that summarizes the electronic processes.

In order for a molecule to fluoresce, an absorbing molecular structure is required. Fluorescence may be expected to occur generally with molecules containing a highly conjugated system. At least one electron-donating group such as NH_2 or OH should be a part of the conjugated system. Electron

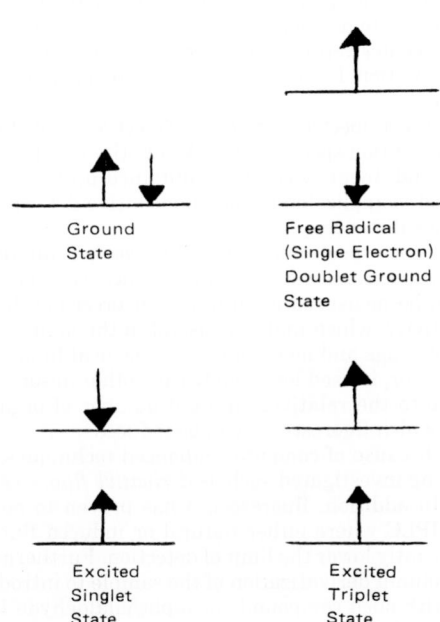

Figure 34-27. The different electron spin states.

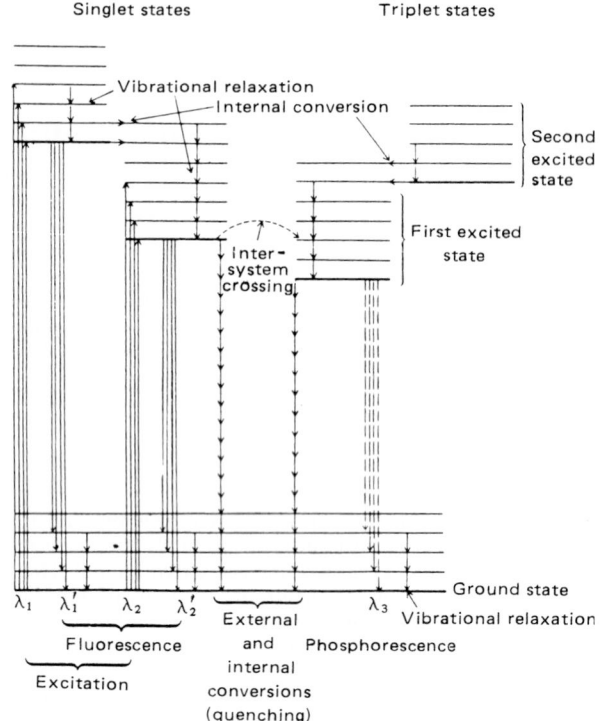

Figure 34-28. Energy level diagram for a photoluminescent system.[15]

Nonabsorptive Interaction of Matter with EM Radiation

The phenomenon of nonabsorptive interaction of matter with EM radiation is applied in such analytical procedures as light-scattering photometry, refractive index, and polarimetry. These interactions are not quantized, except for Raman spectroscopy, and therefore are considered to be nonspecific. However, each compound possesses its own characteristic interaction. The differentiation of stereoisomers with a polarimeter, the quantitative analysis of various substances with a refractometer, and the determination of the molecular weight of macromolecules by light scattering are examples of this type of instrumental analysis.

Light-Scattering Spectrometry

As in reflection and refraction, the scattering of radiation results when it passes through a transparent medium in which particles of a second phase are suspended. For EM radiation to be scattered by particles, two criteria should be met: the dimensions of particles should be equal to or smaller than the incident wavelengths, and the dispersing medium should have a refractive index different from that of the particles.

Particles of 0.1 to 1000 nm scatter EM in the UV and visible regions. If a beam of light is allowed to illuminate a colloidal suspension in a test tube, a pencil of light will be observed in the tube, due to the light-scattering phenomenon. This is known as the *Tyndall effect* and is an indication of the presence of suspended particles. The simplest kind of scattering is that observed by small, spherical and optically isotropic particles and is known as *Rayleigh scattering*.

Turbidimetry, nephelometry, and Raman spectrometry are analytical techniques based on the light scattering phenomenon. However, only Raman spectrometry will be discussed here.

Raman Spectrometry

In 1928 CV Raman, an Indian physicist, noted that under certain conditions, when an intense monochromatic light is scattered by molecules, the wavelength of a fraction of the scattered radiation is different from that of the incident beam. Figure 34-29 is a diagram of the various types of scattering of radiation. This shift (called the *Raman effect*) was found to be related to the chemical structure of the sample; therefore, it offered a new technique for structural elucidation and, in some cases, quantitative determination of several organic and inorganic compounds, in a way similar to IR spectroscopy.

Raman spectra, however, arise under certain conditions that are entirely different from IR. For example, molecules must undergo a change in their polarizability as they vibrate under quantum conditions, but are not required to have a dipole moment as in IR. Therefore, vibrations that are inactive in the infrared may be active in the Raman, such as homonuclear diatomic molecules. Also Raman spectra, unlike IR, can be used to study aqueous solutions.

The main limitation of Raman spectrometry, however, is that it is a weak effect, with low sensitivity and high vulnerability to much interference. Meticulous sample preparation is required, as any dust contamination would cause Tyndall scattering. Lately, laser sources, usually a helium-neon laser, have been employed to provide an intense, coherent, monochromatic beam, and this has improved the sensitivity significantly and raised new interest in the technique. Figure 34-30 is the Raman spectrum of carbon tetrachloride.

withdrawing groups such as COOH or NO_2 diminish, and in some cases prevent, fluorescence. Fluorescence is enhanced as the rigidity of the molecule increases, a reduction in the internal vibration of the molecule.

In case of dilute atomic vapors, resonance fluorescence occurs (at the same wavelength as the excitation), however, in more complex organic compounds in addition to the resonance radiation, emission of radiation at longer wavelength occurs (Stokes' shift).

The position and intensity of the fluorescence bands are affected by pH. The quantum yield, φ, of fluorescence is lower than unity due to a "quenching" process; that is, not all of the excited molecules return to the ground state by emitting fluorescence radiation. Energy may be lost by bond dissociation and deactivation.

Fluorescence spectrometry offers detection limits lower than those of absorption spectrometry. A quantity of 1.1 µg/L can be measured and linearity can be maintained up to 10,000 µg/L. The method is applicable in the quantitative determination of fluorescing substances.

Fluorescence spectrometry has the greatest inherent sensitivity of all spectrometric techniques. Concentrations as low as $10^{-7}M$ can be measured accurately and precisely. It also has high selectivity, which makes it useful in the analysis of trace amounts of drugs and metabolites in biological fluids. Fluorescence, however, is used less widely than other absorption techniques due to the relatively limited number of organic compounds in which fluorescence can be induced.

Lately, because of computer enhanced techniques, new areas are being investigated such as *derivative fluorescence spectrometry*. In addition, fluorescence has proven to be of great value in HPLC where either natural or induced fluorescence can significantly lower the limit of detection. Furthermore, pre- and post-column derivatization of the sample to introduce fluorescence with such compounds as *o*-phthalaldehyde is becoming increasingly common.

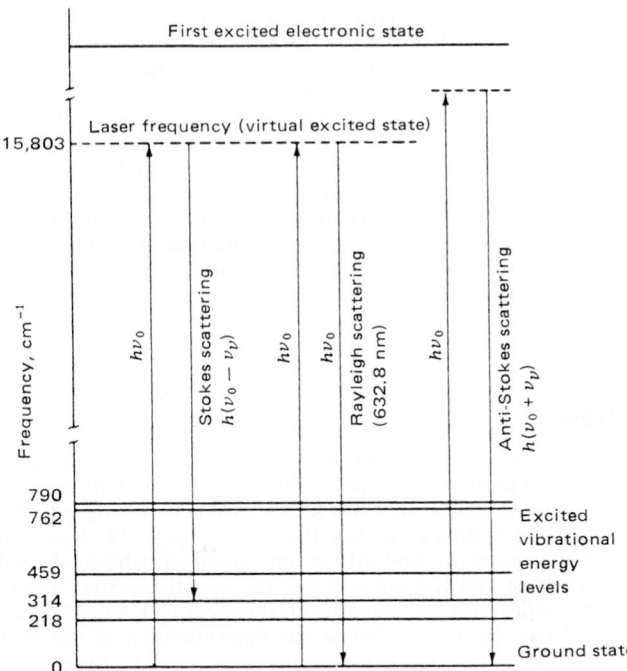

Figure 34-29. Energy interchange involved in Rayleigh and Raman scattering (CCl_4 molecule; source is a He-Ne Laser).[15]

Polarimetry

The fundamental principle of polarimetric analysis is based on the existence of optical activity in a substance, meaning the ability of a material to rotate plane-polarized light. Polarimetry is applicable to the determination of the molecular structure of substances that do not have a rotation–reflection symmetry axis. Determination of the sugar content of foodstuffs is an example of the quantitative application of polarimetry.

Modern polarimeters are capable of measuring optical rotation at more than just the traditional D-line of sodium. Some instruments measure optical rotation discretely at a number of different wavelengths. When the optical rotation is measured continuously as a function of wavelength, the technique known as *optical rotatory dispersion* (ORD) results. ORD has found some use in structural studies.

Solid-State Methods

Much must be accomplished in order to make an active pharmaceutical a viable product. The vast majority of pharmaceutical compounds are orally administered. The active molecule must be presented to the patient in a formulation in which the drug dissolves and is able to be absorbed through the small intestine. Furthermore, the drug must exist in a solid-state form that is sufficiently chemically and physically stable to produce the desired activity over a period of time, its shelf life, of typically two years or more. For this reason, solid-state chemistry and analytical methods play an important role in the development of the drug substance as both a bulk active pharmaceutical ingredient and as a formulated product.

Pharmaceuticals may exist in numerous solid forms having different physical properties. These forms include different salts of the pharmaceutical or neutral drug molecules. Each salt or neutral molecule may exist in number of physical states; it may exist in polymorphic forms, solvates and amorphous (non-crystalline) forms. As a consequence, a series of analytical techniques are employed that enable identification

of the existence of different forms, their characterization, and often quantification of mixtures of forms.[15–17] Ultimately one solid-state form is selected that provides the optimal physical properties. After the form is selected, analytical techniques are employed to ensure that the form that is in the final product is consistent with the form that was tested during clinical trials. Many of the spectroscopic techniques described previously, specifically solid-state NMR, FT-IR, and Raman spectroscopy are used for identification, by providing a fingerprint of the solid-state form. The differences in the spectra are due to perturbations of the molecular spectroscopy brought about by short-range molecular interactions such as differences in hydrogen bonding and conformation. Oftentimes the differences in the spectra are very subtle in spectroscopic methods. In contrast, x-ray diffraction patterns usually differ substantially from one crystalline form to another since diffraction probes the molecular organization within the three dimensional lattice, rather than perturbation of the molecular. Each technique has its own particular strength in solid-state characterization and as a consequence an integrated approach to characterization is recommended.[18]

Polarized Light Microscopy (PLM)

While it is not essential that molecules pack in an orderly crystalline environment, it is usually observed that drug substances do so. The crystalline environment provides a thermodynamically more favorable arrangement than does a disorderly "amorphous" form and has a higher, more efficient, density packing of molecules. As a direct result, crystalline arrangements of molecules typically give rise to more chemically stable drug substances, are less hygroscopic and give products that have better flow properties allowing for a more readily processed and formulated product. The simplest and most cost effective analytical technique used in pharmaceutical development is polarized light micrococpy (PLM).[19] For a fraction of the cost of other analytical techniques, PLM can be used to

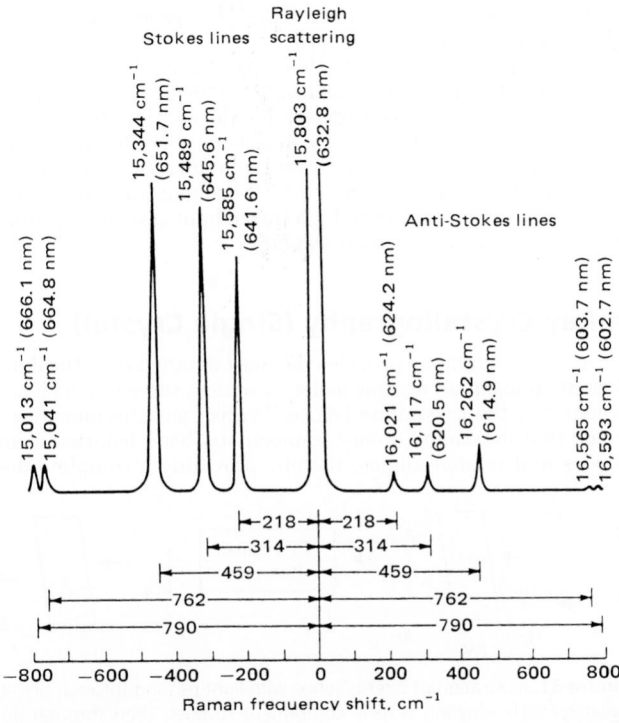

Figure 34-30. Raman spectrum of CCl_4 obtained with a He-Ne Laser.[15]

determine many physical properties of pharmaceutical compounds and plays a critical role in most laboratories due to its simplicity of use and the expediency with which information can be gained. Two important qualities that are instantly observed when one examines a solid are the presence of birefringence and the crystal habit or shape. The observation of birefringence under cross polarization indicates that the substance is crystalline, while crystal habit provides insight as to how well a material might process.

Theory

As was demonstrated earlier, molecules arranged in a crystal lattice are ordered and have a distinct orientation with respect to the facets of the crystal. Most organic molecular crystals crystallize in lower symmetry lattices; triclinic, monoclinic or orthorhombic lattices. Such lattices are termed anisotropic in that they possess more than one principal index of refraction and demonstrate the property known as double refraction. In double refraction, the light ray incident upon such a crystal is split into two components traveling at different velocities and in mutually perpendicular vibration directions. One can evaluate the crystalline quality of a sample by placing it between two polarizers and attempting to pass a beam of light through all three. Electromagnetic radiation can be represented as two vector components. As the ray passes through the first polarizer, only the fraction of the rays having vibrational direction parallel to the first polarizer, that is the vertical component, are transmitted to the crystalline sample. If the sample is an anisotropic crystalline solid, then this vertical component is again split into two components due to double refraction. As the rays strike the second, crossed polarizer, only the horizontal component is allowed to pass through to the eyepiece of the microscope, see Figure 34-31.

If the substance is isotropic, such as an amorphous solid, all of the light passing through the sample would remain unaltered (vertical) and would be removed by the second polarizer (PH).

The second rapidly assessed quality of a crystalline substances using microscopy is its external shape or "habit". Crystals that exhibit habits, where there is an elongated growth direction, can be problematic to develop due to poor flow properties and can significantly delay the speed with which a pharmaceutical can be developed.

The coupling of PLM with a hot stage can further extend the wealth of information that can be gained about a pharmaceutical solid.[20] It can be used to determine the melting characteristics and thermodynamic relationships between different crystal forms of a pharmaceutical. Polarized light microscopy can readily be automated using a precision X-Y sample stage and as result can easily be applied in high throughput crystal screening applications, as will be discussed later.

X-Ray Crystallography (Single Crystal)

X-ray crystallography provides the most detailed structural information about an organic molecule and its three dimensional packing in the crystalline lattice. Precise measurements are made that determine atomic connectivity, bond lengths, bond angles and torsion angles, thereby providing a complete de-

scription of the molecular conformation. X-ray crystallography is used to establish cis versus trans bond geometries and relative stereochemistry. It also enables one to establish absolute configurations of a molecule's chiral center(s) by relation to a known stereo-center of the molecule or by relation to a known stereo-center of a counter-ion forming a salt with the molecule. Even if a molecular structure contains only a single chiral center, its absolute stereochemistry can be established by the method of anomalous dispersion of a structure containing at least one heavy atom.[21] The greatest limitation of the technique is the requirement that material be isolated as a single crystal, having a smallest dimension on the order of 10 to 30 microns. Generally one skilled at crystallizations can meet this criterion in very short period of time.

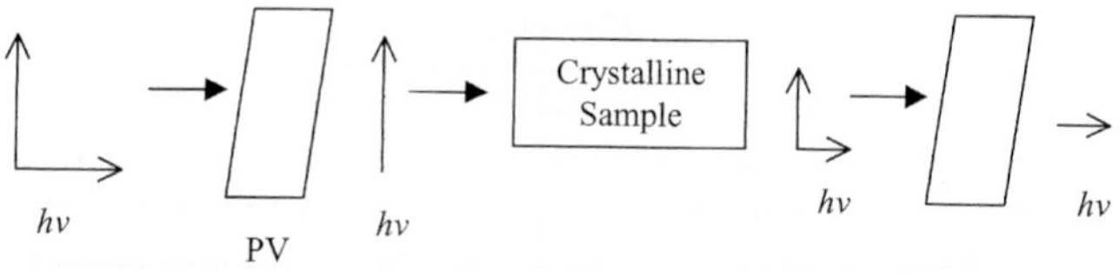

Theory

The precise internal order of crystals can be demonstrated when a crystal is used as a three-dimensional diffraction grating for radiation that has a comparable wavelength to the interatomic distances within the crystal. In 1912, Max von Laue suggested the first diffraction experiments be conducted by Friedrich and Knipping to test the hypothesis that X-rays are wavelike with wavelengths on the order of 1 Å.[22] The success of the experiment led to the determination of the first crystal structure, NaCl, that same year by W.L. Bragg.[23] A single crystal is composed of millions of regularly organized molecules in unit cells that are stacked upon one another in a space filling arrangement. The smallest repeating unit, the unit cell, can be described by six lattice parameters; three axial dimensions a, b, and c and three angles α, β and γ. (see Table 9). The volume of the unit cell can be described by the general relationship

$$V = abc \, (1 - \cos^2\alpha - \cos^2\beta - \cos^2\gamma + 2 \cos \alpha \cos \beta \cos \gamma)^{1/2}$$

Or may have parameters constrained due to the symmetry to one of seven crystal classes as described in Table 34-9.

A distribution of the primitive and centering operations of lattice points among the seven crystal classes result in 14 different Bravais lattices, where equivalent lattice points are related by translational symmetry alone. When rotation, mirror reflection, and inversion symmetry operations of the 32 unique point groups are applied to the 14 different Bravais lattices, 230 unique space groups are possible for the organization of molecules to fill three-dimensional space. After the lattice parameters are determined by indexing, inspection of systematic absences are used to determine the space group. Systematic absences in the diffraction pattern indicate the presence of symmetry elements that cause selective and predictable destructive interference to occur. Tabulation of the systematic absence relationships, along with the unit cell dimensions during space group determination is done by systematically considering each class of Bragg reflections. Once the space group is deduced, attempts are made to solve the structure. For small molecule structures, composed primarily of organic molecules, direct methods have become the dominant method for structure determination.[24] The crystal structure provides the atomic locations of all atoms in the unit cell of the crystal, as is illustrated in Figure 34-32. Molecular structure information is provided to the food and drug administration as a part of the proof of structure section of the new drug application (NDA), whereas the information about crystallographic packing and the physical properties of the solid are often provided in the control and manufacturing section of the NDA.

Cryocrystallography

Data sets are commonly collected at reduced temperature. This, in effect improves the certainty with which atoms can be located. This is because there is a large contribution of vibrational mo-

Figure 31. Illustration of birefringence with light passing through first a polarizer (PH) allowing verticle component to pass, then through an anisotropic crystalline solid followed by a polarizer (PH) that only allows the remaining horizontal component to pass to the eyepiece.

Table 34-9. Seven Crystal Systems, Their Unit-Cell Geometries, and Bravais Lattices

CRYSTAL SYSTEM	NO. OF INDEPENDENT PARAMETERS	PARAMETERS	LAUE SYMMETRY	LATTICE
Triclinic	6	$a \neq b \neq c; \alpha \neq \beta \neq \gamma$	$\bar{1}$	P
Monoclinic	4	$a \neq b \neq c; \alpha = \gamma = 90°; \beta \neq 90°$	2/m	P, C
Orthorhombic	3	$a \neq b \neq c; \alpha = \beta = \gamma = 90°$	mmm	P,C,I,F
Tetragonal	2	$a = b \neq c; \alpha = \beta = \gamma = 90°$	4/mmm	P,I
Rhombohedral	2	$a = b = c; \alpha = \beta = \gamma \neq 90°$	$\bar{3}$m	R
Hexagonal	2	$a = b \neq c; \alpha = \beta \neq \gamma$	6/mmm	P
Cubic	1	$a = b = c; \alpha = \beta = \gamma$	M3m	P,I,F

tion to the anisotropic displacement parameters describing the electron density surrounding the atoms of a molecule. While cryo-crystallography increases the quality of the structural determination, there are other benefits. A very high percentage of organic molecular crystals contain the solvent of recrystallization, where the solvent molecule in the crystal lattice is water (hydrate) or another solvent molecule. Many solvents used for crystallization of organic compounds are volatile and are readily lost from the crystal lattice due to desolvation at room temperature. Desolvation results in fracturing of the single crystal into thousands of smaller "desolvated" crystallites. Temperature reduction stabilizes the solvated structure and enables the crystal structure to be solved.[25]

X-Ray Powder Diffraction (XRPD)

In addition to determining whether a compound is crystalline or amorphous, the first instrumental technique applied is typically x-ray powder diffraction (XRPD). XRPD enables the direct determination of the presence of different crystalline forms of a compound. XRPD is often referred to as the gold standard for determination of the existence of drug polymorphism. A compound is termed to be polymorphic when it crystallizes with different molecular arrangements but identical chemical constituents.[26] If one were to dissolve samples containing two different polymorphs, the samples are no longer distinguishable, that is they will have identical solution NMR, mass spectra, solution-state IR or solution-state Raman spectra.[15] Polymorphs have different physical properties due to their different packing arrangements. The different arrangements are responsible for differences in solubility, rates of dissolution, and melting points. Just as graphite and diamond have identical chemical compositions but different physical properties, so too do different crystal forms of a drug substance.

X-ray powder diffraction can be used to determine the physical state of a drug and used as a quality control assay to ensure that the drug is present in the proper crystallographic form so as to ensure reproducible performance of the active pharmaceutical ingredient in the drug product, hence control of the manufacturing process.

Theory

In the powder method, crystals to be examined are reduced to a fine powder and placed in a beam of monochromatic x-rays. Each tiny crystal is oriented at random with respect to the incident beam. The crystal diffracts x-rays similar to a diffraction grating. The three-dimensional crystal functions like a series of plane gratings stacked one above the other, giving rise to diffraction of electromagnetic ray whose wavelength approximate the atomic spacing in the crystal lattice.[27] The wavelength of the x-rays, λ, is related to the angle of incidence, θ, and the interatomic distance, d, by the Bragg equation;

$$n\lambda = 2d \sin (\theta)$$

where n is the order of the diffraction, 1, 2, 3, and so on.

The analogy of planes in a crystal owe their existence to the repetition of molecules packed in the crystal lattice, since diffraction occurs as the result of the interaction of the radiation with the electrons of the atoms. The planes are separated by an interplanar spacing of atoms, d, commonly termed the d-spacing. Constructive interference occurs when the path difference that the two rays travel are an integral number of wavelengths before they constructively recombine. When the "Bragg condition" is fulfilled, a peak is detected that is representative of the interplanar spacing of the symmetry equivalent sets of Miller planes. Figure 34-33 provides an illustration of cones of diffraction that emanate from a powdered sample when a beam of x-rays strikes the crystalline sample. The position that the

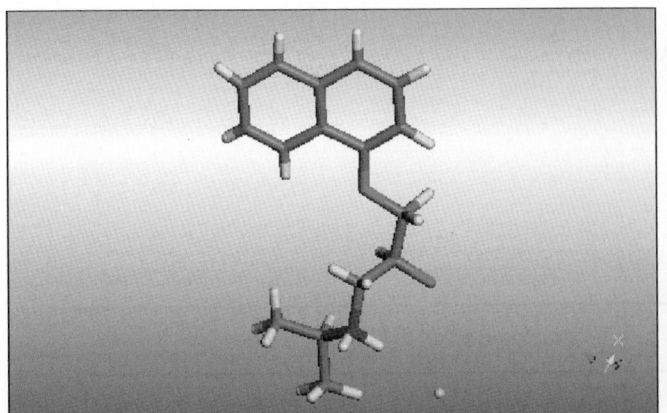
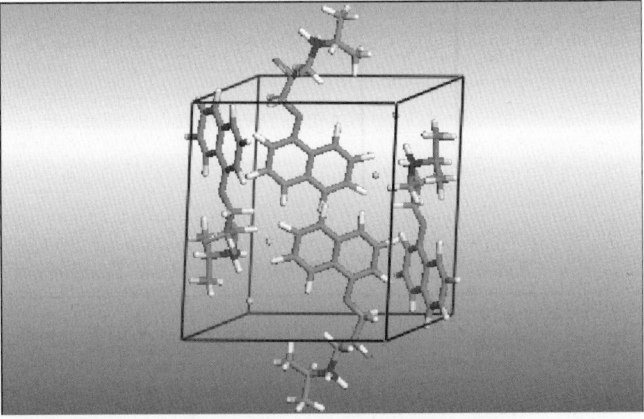

Figure 34-32. The 3-dimensional molecular structure of d,l-propranolol hydrochloride provides information about the molecular conformation and bonding whereas the its packing arrangement within the crystallographic unit cell is useful in understanding the physical properties of the crystalline form. See Color Plate 1.

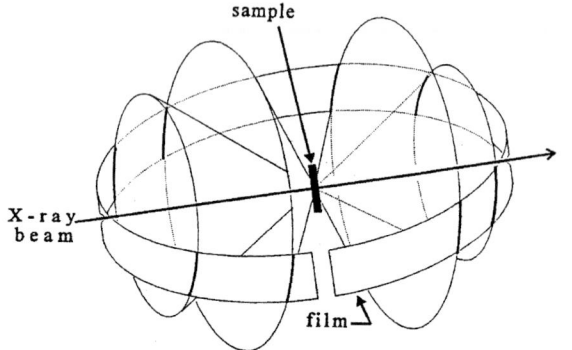

Figure 34-33. Cones of diffraction are produced by an x-ray beam striking a crystalline powder sample (reproduced with permission of Wiley-Interscience).[30]

Methodology

The x-ray diffractometer consists of an x-ray source that produces the x-rays, most commonly a sealed x-ray tube, a variety of optics that minimize divergence of the x-ray beam as it strikes the sample and travels toward the detector, see Figure 34-34.

In a typical powder diffraction experiment, the wavelength of radiation is constant. For the Bragg condition of diffraction to be satisfied, the angle of the diffracted beam that is detected must be the same as the angle of the incident x-ray beam. In the Bragg-Brentano geometry, this is accomplished by scanning the detector through an angle (2θ) while the sample is scanned through an angle (θ). An alternative approach requires movement of the heavier x-ray tube through an angle (θ) at the same rate as the detector is scanned through the angle (θ). Because of the historically more common (θ)-$2(\theta)$ geometry, powder patterns are usually depicted in a graph of intensity of diffraction (y-axis) versus the $2(\theta)$ angle of diffraction, see Figure 34-35.

Instrumentation

Many different detectors exist that can be applied to diffraction, varying in speed of data acquisition, sensitivity, and resolution. Similarly there are many different sources for generation of x-radiation, having different characteristic wavelength and intensity. Most commonly a copper $K\alpha$ radiation source is used, having a characteristic wavelength of 1.54056 Å. Scintillation or solid-state point detectors are used to detect the diffracted radiation. There are numerous potential experimental errors that occur in and x-ray diffraction experiment. The major factor influencing observed intensity is the lack of random orientation of crystallites in the powder sample, whereas the major error in

diffracted radiation intersects with the detector, in this case a piece of photographic film, is characteristic of the material.

The peak positions of the unit cell reflect its size and angular relations of the crystal system. The intensity detected is a function of the atoms that make up the crystal and their scattering factors, a function of the electron density surrounding the atoms comprising the sample, as well as the location of the atoms within the unit cell. As a consequence, the diffraction pattern provides a unique characterization of a crystalline substance representing both its crystallographic packing and its unit cell contents. Each substance scatters the beam in a particular diffraction pattern, producing a unique fingerprint for each crystal form.

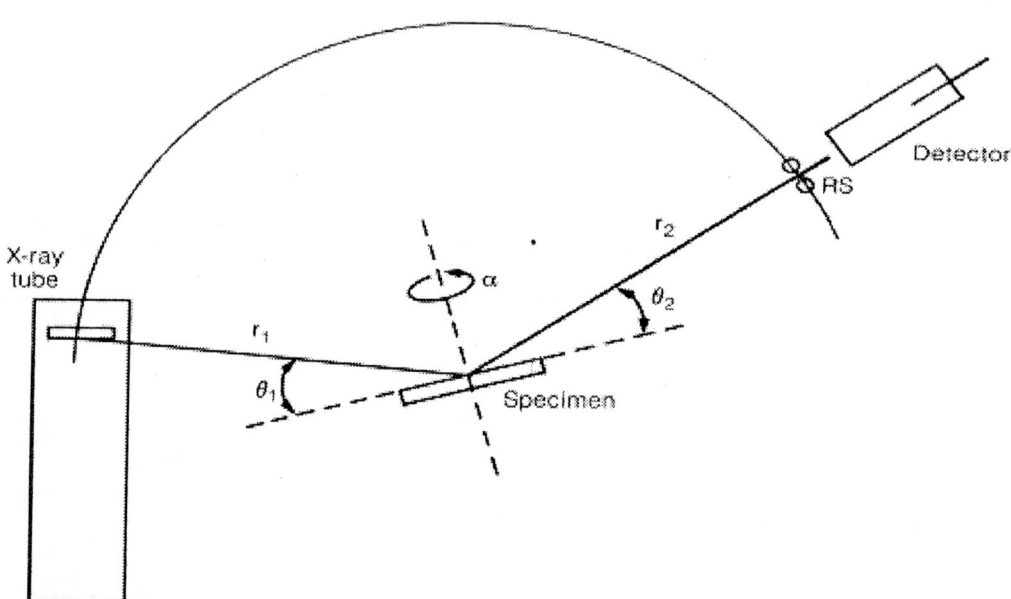

Type	Tube	Specimen	Receiving Slit	r_1	r_2
Bragg-Brentano $\theta:2\theta$	Fixed	Varies as θ *	Varies as 2θ	Fixed	$=r_1$
Bragg-Brentano $\theta:\theta$	Varies as θ	Fixed *	Varies as θ	Fixed	$=r_1$

Figure 34-34. Representation of the Bragg-Brentano geometry most commonly used the powder diffraction experiment uses a conventional x-ray tube source with a point detector (reproduced with permission Wiley-Interscience).[30]

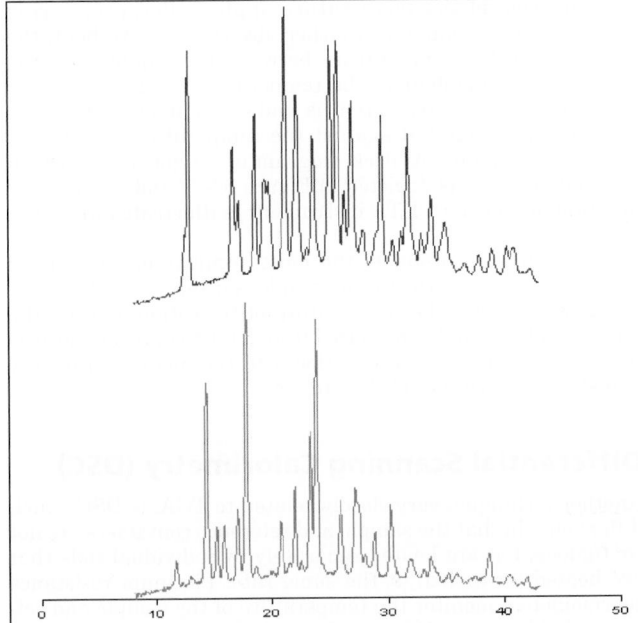

Figure 34-35. The x-ray powder diffraction patterns of two polymorphic forms of d,l-propranolol hydrochloride indicate differences in molecular arrangements within their different crystal lattices. See Color Plate 2.

angle of diffraction is due to sample displacement from the diffraction plane.[28–30] Using a properly aligned and calibrated instrument and appropriate sample preparation, these errors can be minimized.

Thermal Methods

Thermal analysis is a technique in which a physical property of a substance is monitored as a function of controlled temperature increase. Modern thermal analytical methods can measure weight loss on heating, melting points, heat and energy of tran-

sitions, and changes in form, in dimensions, or in the viscoelastic properties of the substance. They find wide applications in material characterization, purity determination of medicinal substances, study of relative heat stabilities and dynamic properties of new compounds, as well as in crystallography, chemical kinetics, and generation of phase diagrams.

Theory

Most thermodynamic events are accompanied by a loss of heat or require addition of heat from an external source to proceed. The event may be a phase transition, loss of a volatile component, or a chemical reaction. Each of these occurrences can be followed thermodynamically by noting either change of temperature of the sample under study or energy changes of the sample with respect to time. If the sample loses a volatile substance by evaporation, sublimation, or chemical conversion to a gas, it also is possible to follow the course of events by noting weight loss with respect to time, as the temperature of the sample is increased at a constant rate.

The general laws of thermodynamics, specifically those governing calorimetry, serve as the basis for understanding the theoretical concepts involved in the different thermal analytical methods of analysis. For equilibrium transitions, where $\Delta G = 0$ the heat of transition, ΔH_n is related to the entropy of transition ΔS_n by

$$\Delta S_n = \frac{\Delta H_n}{T_n} \qquad (14)$$

Modern instruments for thermal methods of analysis are based on these parameters: mass, temperature, and heat flow. Table 10 illustrates the use of these functions and typical data outputs.

Thermogravimetry (Thermogravimetric Analysis, TGA)

Thermogravimetric analysis (TGA), perhaps the simplest form of thermal analysis, uses a *thermobalance* as the analytical instrument. The apparatus may be no more than a

Table 34-10. Typical Curves Produced in Thermal Gravimetric Analysis (TGA), Differential Thermal Analysis (DTA) and Differential Scanning Calorimetry (DSC)

TECHNIQUE	PARAMETER MEASURED	INTRUMENT EMPLOYED	TYPICAL CURVE
Thermogravimetry	Mass	Thermobalance	
Differential thermal analysis (DTA)	$T_s - T_t (\Delta T)$	DTA apparatus	
Differential scanning calorimetry (DSC)	Heat flow, dH/dt	Calometer	

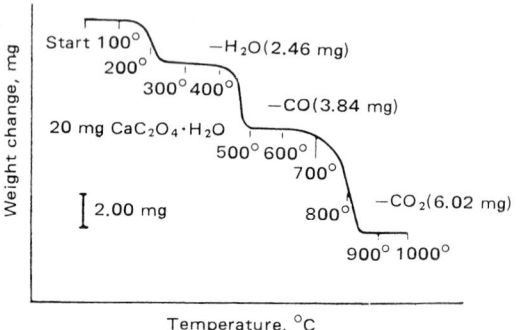

Figure 34-36. Thermogravimetric evaluation of calcium oxalate monohydrate, heating rate 6°/min.[19]

modified single pan analytical balance provided with a digital electronic output so that a plot of weight change (y-axis) can be made with respect to time or temperature. An infrared lamp may be the source of heat to irradiate the balance pan. Many modifications of such a device are used to determine the moisture content of tablet granulations, hydrated substances, and so on. Much more sophisticated instruments are also commercially available that include temperature programming and the use of a variety of beam, spring, cantilever, or torsion balances to determine changes in the weight of a sample. Because the atmosphere surrounding the heated sample may influence (retard or hasten) decomposition, provision often is made to control the atmosphere by addition of inert gases (nitrogen, helium) or reactive gases (oxygen, hydrogen, etc). The result of a thermogravimetric evaluation of calcium oxalate monohydrate may be seen in Figure 34-36.[31]

Recently several types of thermogravimetric devices have been coupled to a gas chromatograph, mass spectrometer, or FI-IR so that the effluent products of decomposition can thus be characterized.

A new development in TGA is the high-resolution technique.[32] The rate of heating of the sample is modified dynamically and continuously in response to changes in the sample decomposition so as to maximize weight change resolution. This technique allows use of very high heating rates while avoiding transition temperature overshoot, thereby optimizing time to complete a thermal analysis experiment.

Differential Thermal Analysis (DTA)

In differential thermal analysis (DTA), a sample and a thermally inert reference material are heated (or cooled) linearly with the aid of a programming device, and the temperature difference between the sample and the reference is measured

as a function of the temperature applied. Because, during transition, the sample may either absorb or evolve heat, the difference in the temperature between the sample and the standard is equivalent to the temperature of transition and can indicate if the transition is endothermic or exothermic. Usually, ΔT is plotted against the temperature, T, or as a function of time (t). A block diagram of a typical differential thermal analyzer is depicted in Figure 34-37 and a schematic diagram of a modern DTA instrument is illustrated in Figure 34-38.[33]

DTA data are probably the most accurate of all thermal techniques, because the thermocouple is inserted into the sample; however, only the temperature of transition and not the amount of heat can be measured from a DTA curve, as the area under the peak is not proportional to the amount of energy transferred into or out of the sample.

Differential Scanning Calorimetry (DSC)

Another technique, very closely related to TGA, is DSC which differs only in that the sample and reference containers are not contiguous, but are heated separately by individual coils that are heated (or cooled) at the same rate. Platinum resistance thermometers monitor the temperature of the sample and reference holders and electronically maintain the temperature of the two holders constant.

If a thermodynamic event occurs that is either endothermic or exothermic, the power requirements for the coils maintaining a constant temperature will differ. This power difference (ΔP) is plotted as a function of the temperature recorded by the programming device.

Unlike DTA, in DSC the amount of heat put into the system is exactly equivalent to the amount of heat absorbed or liberated during a specific transition (transition energy).

AUTOMATION OF INSTRUMENTAL METHODS

Beginning in the early 1990s, a well-chronicled trend occurred in the pharmaceutical industry involving the implementation of high throughput screening (HTS) methods for lead generation. Today HTS assays involving in vitro assays, such as ligand-receptor binding and enzyme inhibition are routinely performed using highly automated schemes capable of processing over 10,000 samples per day. When combined with other related trends, such as combinatorial chemistry, parallel synthesis, and systems biology, the demand for sample preparation and analysis has transformed the modern pharmaceutical laboratory into a highly automated workplace. Unfortunately, a full review of laboratory automation is beyond the scope of this communication. Instead, this section will highlight select examples of technologies or practices that have increased throughput for the major instrumental techniques introduced in this chapter.

Although laboratory automation will not be the primary focus of this section, it is appropriate to mention the significance

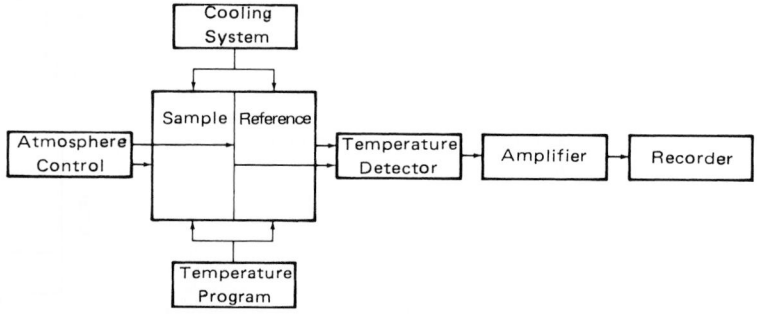

Figure 34-37. Block diagram of differential thermal analyzer.

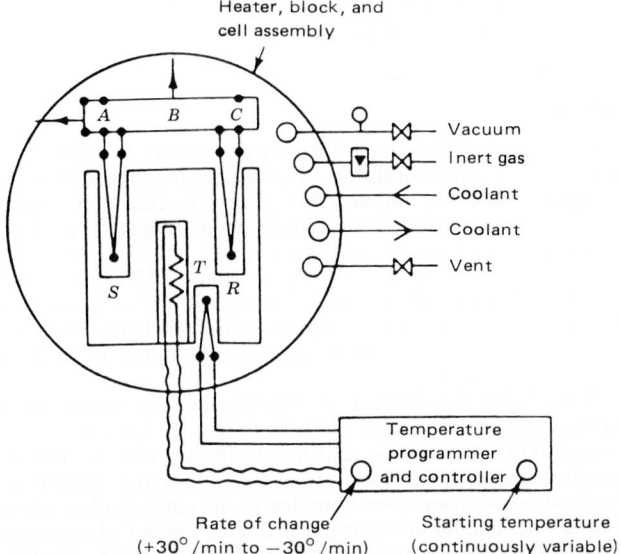

Heater, block, and
cell assembly

Vacuum

Inert gas

Coolant

Coolant

Vent

Temperature
programmer
and controller

Rate of change
($+30°$/min to $-30°$/min)

Starting temperature
(continuously variable)

Figure 34-38. Schematic diagram of the DuPont differential thermal analysis apparatus.[17]

of the microtiter plate, which has become the default format for sample handling. Originally, introduced as a format for ELISA (enzyme-linked immunosorbent assay), the microtiter plate consists of 96 wells arranged in a standard format of 8 rows of 12 wells. In addition to offering a convenient approach for processing high sample numbers (compared to individual tubes), the microtiter plate provides a standardized platform for automated liquid handling and keeps reagent costs to a minimum. Today, the capacity for sample preparation and analysis is often described in terms of "plates" referring to the 96-well microtiter plate. Larger capacity formats based on multiples of 96 have also become popular (ie, 384, 1536).

In contrast to the HTS methods involved in lead generation, most of the instrumental techniques discussed in this chapter involve serial detection and are thus not capable of extremely high throughput (a notable exception is the spectrophotometric plate reader, which allows direct detection in a 96-well format). Due to the serial format inherent to many forms of instrumental analysis, extensive focus has be given to technologies which automate either sample *preparation* and sample *analysis*. Each of these topics is addressed separately below.

Sample Preparation

For many forms of instrumental analysis sample preparation simply involves dissolution in an appropriate solvent at the desired concentration. A common example is structural confirmation of individual compounds or compound libraries by MS and/or NMR. For such applications, the compounds undergoing analysis exist either as neat solids or concentrated solutions (eg, DMSO stock solutions). Given that compounds are typically processed using automated methods for liquid handling, most analytical instruments are equipped with autosamplers which accommodate 96-well plates.

Bioanalysis

In contrast to the relatively limited sample preparation associated with routine applications of organic structural analysis, bioanalytical applications tend to require more extensive sample preparation. By definition, bioanalysis refers to quantitative analysis of a drug and or its metabolites in a biological matrix and is most often linked to the study ADME properties.

Matrices studied can either be of *in vitro* (eg, liver preparation, biological media or buffer) or *in vivo* (eg, plasma, urine, tissue homogenate) origin. Because of its ability to perform rapid, selective quantitation in complex matrices, LC/MS/MS has become the default tool used to investigate ADME properties. ADME applications may also be qualitative, such as profiling and structural identification of drug metabolites in biological matrices. Although similar sample preparations are used for qualitative and quantitative applications, the present discussion will be limited to quantitative bioanalysis.

Despite the power of LC/MS technology, bioanalysis requires some form of sample preparation to achieve acceptable sensitivity, precision and robust instrumental performance. Several review articles have been published on this subject.[34, 35] The method selected for sample preparation depends both on the complexity of the sample matrix and the required sensitivity. Sample throughput and costs are also important considerations. For most drug discovery applications simple desalting or protein precipitation (PP) is employed to maximize throughput. PP, typically used for plasma and tissue bioanalysis, can result from the simple addition of an organic solvent such as acetonitrile or methanol. Other procedures involving acid or salt ($ZnCl_2$) may also be used.

Assays that require greater sensitivity generally involve some form of sample extraction to clean up and concentrate the sample. The two most widely adopted formats are solid-phase extraction (SPE) and liquid-liquid extraction (LLE). In SPE, the biological sample is loaded onto a solid sorbent having an affinity for the analyte. The SPE cartridge is then washed to remove matrix components followed by subsequent elution of the analyte. LLE involves placing the sample into a mixture of two immiscible solvents. Differential partitioning of the analyte and matrix components serves as the basis for sample cleanup. Both methods afford greater selectivity than PP and may also be used to concentrate the sample. All three aforementioned sample preparation methods routinely employ 96-well format and frequently incorporate automated procedures for liquid handling.[36-38]

Historically, LC/MS/MS methods were applied to development applications, such as GLP toxicology or clinical sample analysis. Over the past five years the demand for drug discovery bioanalysis has dramatically increased due to the use of LC/MS/MS for exposure screening as well as the widespread implementation of *in vitro* screens to assess ADME properties. Common in vitro ADME screens include hepatic metabolic stability,[39] intestinal permeation,[40] blood brain barrier penetration,[41] protein binding[42] assessment of drug-drug interaction potential[43] and the investigation of specific drug transporters.[44] Using LC/MS/MS technology, Cole and co-workers cite the ability to perform 2000 samples per instrument per day for a variety of in vitro ADME screens.[45] Further reading on this topic is available from a number of published articles.[46]

As with *in vitro* applications, increased demand for *in vivo* sample analysis has also occurred. *In vivo* demand stems from the important need to quantify drug exposure in live-phase studies ranging from early exposure screening in pharmacology animals to large clinical trials in man. In these studies, the principal sample matrix is plasma, since the plasma concentration of a drug is used to derive pharmacokinetic or toxicokinetic parameters. One of the issues faced in discovery bioanalysis is the need to develop rapid methods to simultaneously quantify several analogs in a structural series, as opposed to a single clinical candidate. This challenge is significant when strategies such as sample pooling[47] or cassette dosing[48] are used to maximize the utilization of expensive LC/MS/MS instrumentation. To accommodate the need for simultaneous quantification, many analysts employ gradient elution techniques, often in conjunction with one of several methods available which allow sample preparation and analysis to occur on-line. Note, traditional bioanalytical sample preparation techniques occur off-line (ie, independent of sample analysis). Reported approaches to on-line sample cleanup include restricted access media,[49] turbulent flow liquid chromatography,[50] SPE[51] and immunoaffinity chromatography.[52] The common link to all of these approaches is the use of multiple columns, connected via multi-port HPLC valves, to derive an automated approach referred to as "column-switching." Under column-switching, a biological sample is loaded onto a dedicated extraction column that retains the target analyte while unwanted matrix components are washed to waste. After a defined period, the valve is switched to allow elution of the analyte onto a second column where chromatographic separation and detection are accomplished.

Perhaps the biggest difference regarding *in vivo* bioanalysis performed in drug discovery versus drug development is the sensitivity required. Discovery applications typically require quantification in the low ng/mL range, whereas development applications, such as the support of human clinical trials, often require quantification in the low pg/mL range. Nevertheless, a common thread is that LC/MS/MS is routinely used as the method of choice. Although many of the tools used for automation are common between discovery and development applications, the strategies used as well as the degree of regulatory oversight differ dramatically.

A final example of automated bioanalytical sample preparation is use of semi-automated systems for tissue preparation. Historically, tissue analysis is preceded by the homogenization of individual samples, a process that is both time and labor-intensive. Recently, a commercial instrument was introduced, which allows homogenization to be carried out in parallel by a series eight homogenization probes. The fully-automated system contains a platform, which accommodates 48 samples and has three wash stations to reduce inter-sample carry over. The demonstration of this system for bioanalysis of brain tissue samples has been recently published.[53]

Automated X-ray Diffraction

One of the most dramatic examples of automated spectroscopic sample preparation is in the field of x-ray diffraction (XRD). For years, XRD has been regarded as the definitive method for the determination of protein structure; however, the throughput of the technique has been limited by the ability to grow acceptable protein crystals. In addition to taking several days, protein crystallization still requires a significant degree of 'trail and error' as several permutations in conditions must be tested.

A major breakthrough occurred when it was discovered that viable protein crystallization can occur using small protein sample volumes ($< 1 \mu L$).[54] In addition to requiring less protein, such nano preparation methods reduce the time needed for crystallization by as much as 10-fold. Using automation, it is possible to test hundreds of crystallization methods per day using automated schemes. While several permutations of this technology exist,[55,56] most approaches employ a variation of a technique referred to as "hanging drop vapor diffusion".[56] This technology has been employed to direct the synthesis of compound libraries in the generation of more specific leads. Co-crystallization of lead compounds with the target protein is a secondary technique applied later during lead optimization.

Sample Analysis

Most forms of instrumental analysis provide the capability for unattended sample introduction, a process typically referred to as automated sample introduction or "autosampling." Moreover, sample introduction can either occur by direct means or through an on-line interface to one of several forms of chromatography. To date, chromatographic interfaces exist for following spectroscopic techniques: MS, UV, fluorescence, IR, NMR, and electrochemical. Obviously, a review of "hyphenated" chromatographic techniques is beyond the scope of this section. Instead, attention will be given to current trends in sample introduction associated with the major forms of spectroscopy.

NMR

Conventional NMR sample introduction occurs by inserting a narrow glass tube containing a liquid sample into the center of a superconducting magnet. For years, unattended sample analysis has occurred using robotic arms standard on all instruments which insert and retrieve the glass sample tubes from the magnet. As discussed previously, NMR flow probes have been introduced to permit coupling with HPLC. This same device is also used for flow injection analysis (FIA) providing another convenient means for automated, higher throughput sample analysis.[57]

NMR holds the distinction of being the first spectroscopic method to perform routine analysis in a mode known as "open access" (OA). Under OA, multiple users are able to perform standard analysis in a "walk-up" mode. In this environment, individual users place their samples in an autosampler, where they are queued for analysis in the order received. Many variations of OA exist, generally differing by the degree of instrumental control afforded to the walk up analyst. As one would expect, OA provides the most immediate turn around for sample analysis and works best when generalized analysis conditions can be employed. It is also important that the instrumentation be sufficiently robust to permit access by multiple users, often with limited training.

Mass Spectrometry

Routine application of MS in an OA environment did not occur until the introduction of the API-interface. The first reports of OA by MS occurred in 1994 and used APCI as the ionization mode.[58] ESI methods for OA have also been reported.[59] Both techniques are widely used in the pharmaceutical industry to support chemical synthesis. Although the most frequent format for OA sample introduction is FIA, it is important to note that OA by LC/MS is also a routine tool.[60]

Several approaches have been used to contend with the limitation imposed by the serial nature of MS detection. Using a novel redesign of a commercial autosampler, Morand and co-workers were able to perform FIA analysis in support of chemical synthesis at a rate of 3 seconds/injection (5 minutes/plate).[61] Several formats for ultra fast gradient elution have been employed with LC/MS[62] including the use of monolithic column formats.[63] For bioanalytical applications, full gradient elution routinely occurs with run times under 2 minutes. Staggered injections have also been used to increase LC/MS throughput.[64] This general methodology is applicable whenever analyte detection represents a finite part of the overall injection duty cycle.

Another approach taken is to combine multiple ESI sprayers with a single instrument. A commercial version of this methodology, referred to at MUX, employs a rotating cylinder containing an aperture to sequentially sample up to eight sprayers housed within a single API-MS interface.[65] Using the eight-sprayer format, each sprayer is sampled every 1.2 s allowing for multiple points to be acquired over a given chromatographic peak. MUX interfaces are used in conjunction with multi-injector autosamplers, where typically a gradient formed by a single HPLC system at elevated flow is prior to the autosampler to provide flow for multiple LC columns. Successful applications of this approach have been reported for both chemical synthesis support[66] and bioanalysis.[67]

An emerging trend in instrumental analysis is miniaturization. Often referred to as "lab-on-a chip," microfluidic applications, allowing sample analysis and detection to occur on a microchip, offer several advantages including reduced reagent costs and lower waste stream production. Current formats and applications for lab-on-a chip exist and have been

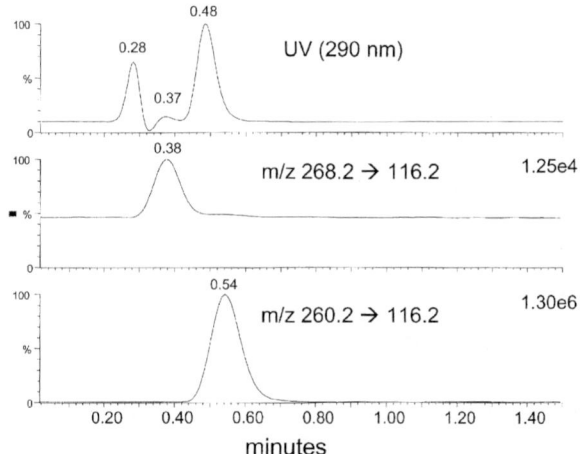

Figure 34-39. LC-UV-MS/MS anlysis of β-blocker drugs propanolol and metoprolol

reviewed.[68] The most common detection formats for microfluidics are spectrophotometric and include UV[69] and fluorescence.[70] Electrochemical detection has also been employed.[71] Recently, a silicon chip incorporating 100 individual ESI-MS nozzles was commercially introduced.[72] To date, this technology has been applied to a variety of applications including proteomics,[73] protein-ligand interactions[74] and bioanalysis.[75]

Application

Earlier in this chapter, the drug propranolol was introduced to illustrate the power of NMR for structural analysis. In the section that follows, further analysis of propranolol was conducted to provide additional examples of how common instrumental techniques are used for pharmaceutical analysis.

LC/M/MS Analysis of Propranolol

Due to its versatility, LC/MS has become one of the most widely used instrumental techniques for pharmaceutical analysis. LC/MS has the unique ability to extract structural information from complex mixtures with high sensitivity. Because of these attributes, LC/MS has been applied to several areas related to chemical synthesis. In early drug discovery, LC/MS is routinely used to confirm the structure of newly synthesized molecules and to obtain estimates of purity. Figure 34-39 displays data obtained from the LC-UV-MS/MS analysis of a binary mixture of two β-blockers, propranolol and metoprolol. In this example, LC/MS was conducted by reversed phase HPLC with on-line UV detection followed by positive ion electrospray ionization (ESI). Gradient elution was conducted using a mobile phase system consisting of methanol, water and formic acid at a flow rate of 0.25 ml/min. The column used was an Aquasil C18 (2.1 mm × 2 mm). In this example, the ratio of propranolol to metoprolol was 200:1.

The upper profile in Figure 34-39, which corresponds to the UV absorbance at 290 nm, contains three peaks at 0.28, 0.37 and 0.54 minutes. The two most highly retained peaks correspond to the metoprolol and propranolol, respectively, whereas the peak at 0.28 minutes represents the column void (ie, unretained material). The relative insensitivity of UV is apparent from the metoprolol peak, which was barely detected. The signal shown corresponds to approximately 0.625 ng injected on-column for metoprolol versus 125 ng for propranolol. The corresponding MS signals were acquired by tandem MS using SRM detection (see mass spectrometry section). The bottom profile, corresponding to metoprolol, indicates the superior sensitivity of MS detection. The results in Figure 34-39 reveal a slight shift in retention time between UV and MS. This delay is related to the transit time between detectors. The incorporation of spectroscopic detection on-line with MS is applied to several forms of pharmaceutical analysis including chemical synthesis, drug metabolism, natural product analysis, stability testing and impurity profiling.

As described in the section on mass spectrometry, SRM detection involves monitoring a compound-specific fragmentation transition, typically using a triple quadrupole mass spectrometer, for the purpose of enhancing detection. Because of the extraordinary selectivity conferred by this approach, SRM vastly improves the signal to noise for analytes detected in a complex matrix and is therefore routinely used for quantification of drugs and their metabolites in biomatrices (eg, plasma, tissue homogenate, urine). Figures 34-40 and 34-41 display the product ion mass spectra for propranolol and metoprolol, respectively. The structure of each molecule appears as an inset in the corresponding spectrum. In each case, the protonated molecule was selected by Q1 and induced to fragment by collisions with an argon target gas in the Q2. The data shown were obtained by scanning the third quadrupole (Q3) to transmit the product ions formed in Q2. As indicated in Figures 34-40 and 34-41, both drugs gave rise to a prominent fragment ion at m/z 116, formed by the loss of the corresponding phenol as a neutral molecule. This fragmentation transition was optimized and used to acquire the SRM data

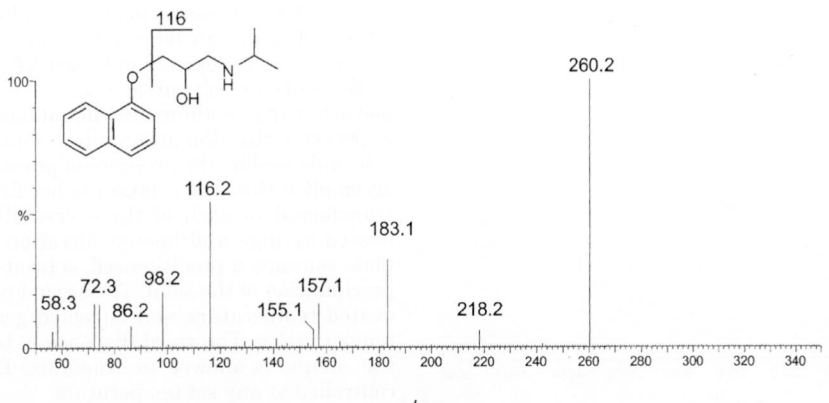

Figure 40. Product ion mass spectrum of propanolol

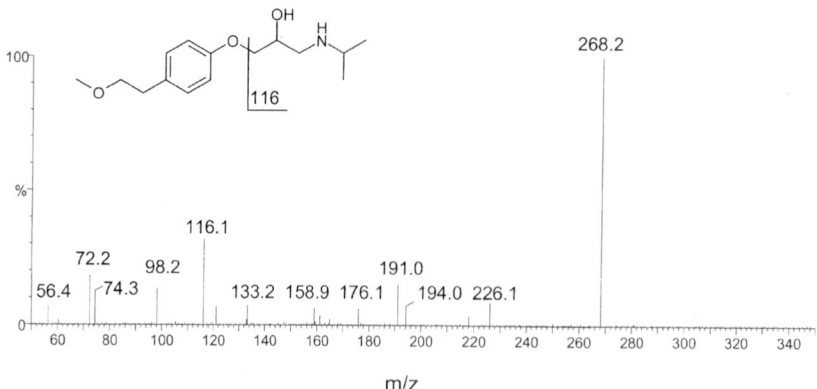

Figure 34-41. Product ion mass spectrum of metoprolol

presented in Figure 34-39. The corresponding SRM transitions used were as follows: propranolol (m/z 260.2 to 116.2) and metoprolol (*m/z* 268.2 to 116.2).

An illustration of how SRM detection is used for quantitative analysis is indicated by the calibration curve shown in Figure 34-42. To produce this curve, a series of neat propranolol standards were prepared and analyzed covering a range from 10 to 5000 ng/ml. All samples received a constant amount of metoprolol (25 ng/ml) acting as an internal standard. The calibration curve in Figure 34-42 plots the peak area ratio of propranolol to metoprolol versus propranolol concentration. Least squares linear regression analysis with 1/X weighting was used to fit a straight line through the data. The observed coefficient of determination (r^2) was 0.9978.

High Throughput Screening for Polymorphism of d, I-Propranolol Hydrochloride

At the very early stages of lead optimization, a vast number of molecules exist that demonstrate activity against target receptor sites. The number of molecules being evaluated and rate of attrition is high. In an effort to increase the rate that new compounds can be progressed from discovery to launch, a need has emerged to rapidly screen molecules for solid-state forms that posses acceptable biopharmaceutical and solid-state properties. The primary objective is to conduct meaningful toxicological studies on a solid form that can readily be developed and brought to market.

There are numerous counter-ions available for salt formation, particularly for actives containing basic moieties.[76] There are also numerous experimental variables that can result in successful crystallization. Three of the most common methods for crystallizing organic molecules are evaporation, precipitation by anti-solvent addition, and temperature reduction. The need for high throughput crystallization screening stems from the need to rapidly survey a large array of chemistries and crystallization variables in parallel. Critical to this end is the coupling of rapid experimental design with liquid and sample handling, followed by delivery of the isolated crystals in an arrayed format such that each individual sample can be characterized for desirable solid-state properties.

Central to the overall process is a database that provides the ability to track the chemistry and conditions and ability to rapidly analyze the data so that correlations can be made between the variables and crystallization outcomes.

Figure 34-43 provides the general strategy for crystallization screening of an active pharmaceutical. The same basic workflow design is used for salt formation or polymorph screening.

Design

The chemistry is designed such that a small amount of API is dispensed into individual wells and reacted with a stoichiometric amount of an acceptable counter ion. In the design, typically a 96 well plate is designed with the different counterions dispensed along a given column and different solvent or solvent combinations are dispensed along the rows, typically screening 12 counterions versus 8 different solvent combinations. In the case of a polymorphism, no counterion is dispensed. Each of the 96 wells has the same chemistry, but different solvent compositions. The design for crystallization screening of polymorphism screen is depicted in Figure 34-44.

Solvents or solvent mixtures for crystallization are dispensed, using an automated liquid handler. It is essential that every crystallization attempt be a unique experiment and that it be unbiased by the presence of preexisting nuclei. In order to accomplish this, the solution is hot filtered and the filtrate is transferred to each of three crystallization plates using a heated syringe and heated filtration assembly. One 96-well plate contains a predispensed, solvent-miscible antisolvent for precipitation of the solid. The second plate is maintained at elevated temperature and is cooled gradually to sub-ambient temperatures. The third dispense is to a 96-well plate where the sample is allowed to evaporate. Evaporation rate can be controlled at any set temperature.

An aliquot of sample is transferred initially to another 96-well plate to determine the solubility at elevated temperature

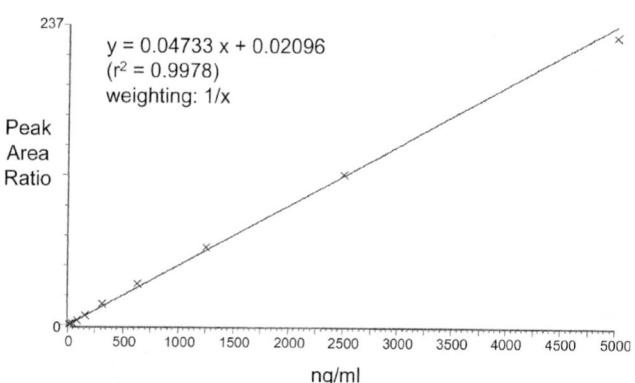

y = 0.04733 x + 0.02096
(r^2 = 0.9978)
weighting: 1/x

Figure 34-42. Standard curve for propanolol acquired by LC/MS/MS.

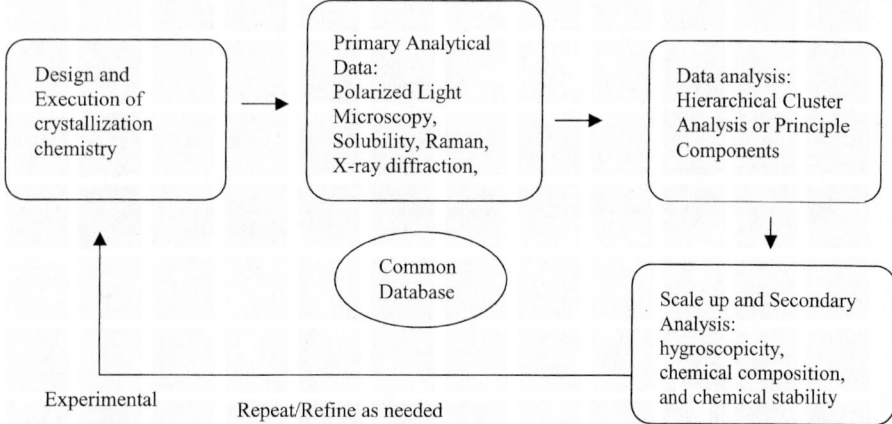

Figure 34-43. The design of the general workflow used for high throughput crystallization and solid-state characterization.

and another sample is transferred from the plate containing the sample that was cooled gradually, typically 55 and 10°C respectively. This sample is analyzed by HPLC or UV/VIS spectroscopy to provide an approximate measure of solubility. The solubility data can be useful in designing the next series of screening experiments.

Analysis of Experiments

One of the key elements working with small sample sizes is elimination of the transfer of the sample from one technique to another for analysis. Such transfers result in loss of sample. Central to the overall process is the ability for instrumentation to receive and examine samples in an arrayed, typically 96 well, format. The general procedure involves the use of a glass substrate on which the crystallization occurs. Birefringence assessment using polarized light microscopy and Raman microscopy and x-ray powder diffraction analysis is conducted directly on the glass substrate.

In the workflow for HTS crystal form we use polarized light microscopy to first assess whether or not a sample is crystalline and then use both x-ray powder diffraction and Raman microscopy to determine the number of forms present. The complementary methods for form assessment are used, since both techniques have advantages and disadvantages depending upon the particular sample. Figure 34-45 provides an illustration of the birefringence images and powder diffraction patterns from one of the three crystallization plates obtained in the HTS of d,l-propranolol hydrochloride, as can readily be seen there are at least two crystalline polymorphic forms. The plate layout, with each form is represented as a thumbnail whose color indicates its form, enables easy correlation of the crystallization outcome with the chemistry of the specific well.

After the different crystalline "hits" are identified, the chemistry information is used to try to validate the hits by scaling up the individual forms. Using the larger quantity of sample that is generated, other characterization tests are used to determine which form is best suited for further development. For crystalline salt forms, the stoichiometry of the salt is determined

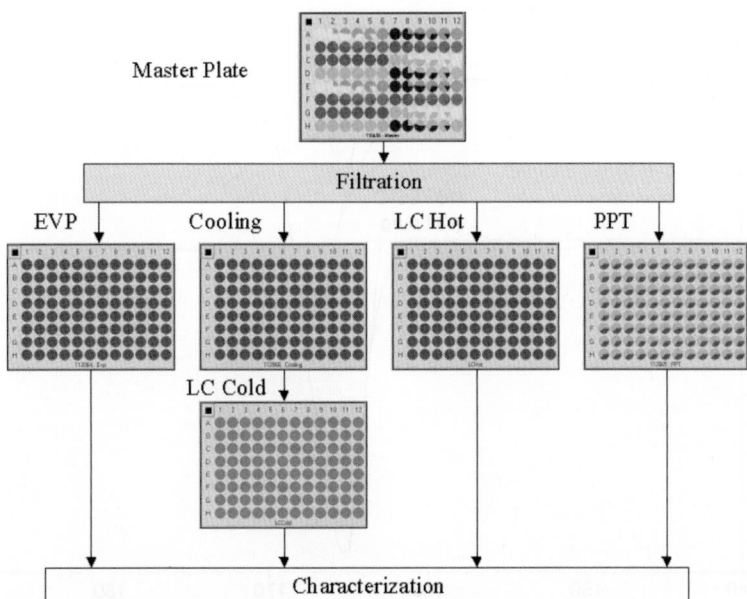

Figure 34-44. Design for the crystallization process for polymorphic form screening demonstrates hot filtration of the crystallization solution and its transfer to three crystallization plates and two plates for solubility determination. See Color Plate 3.

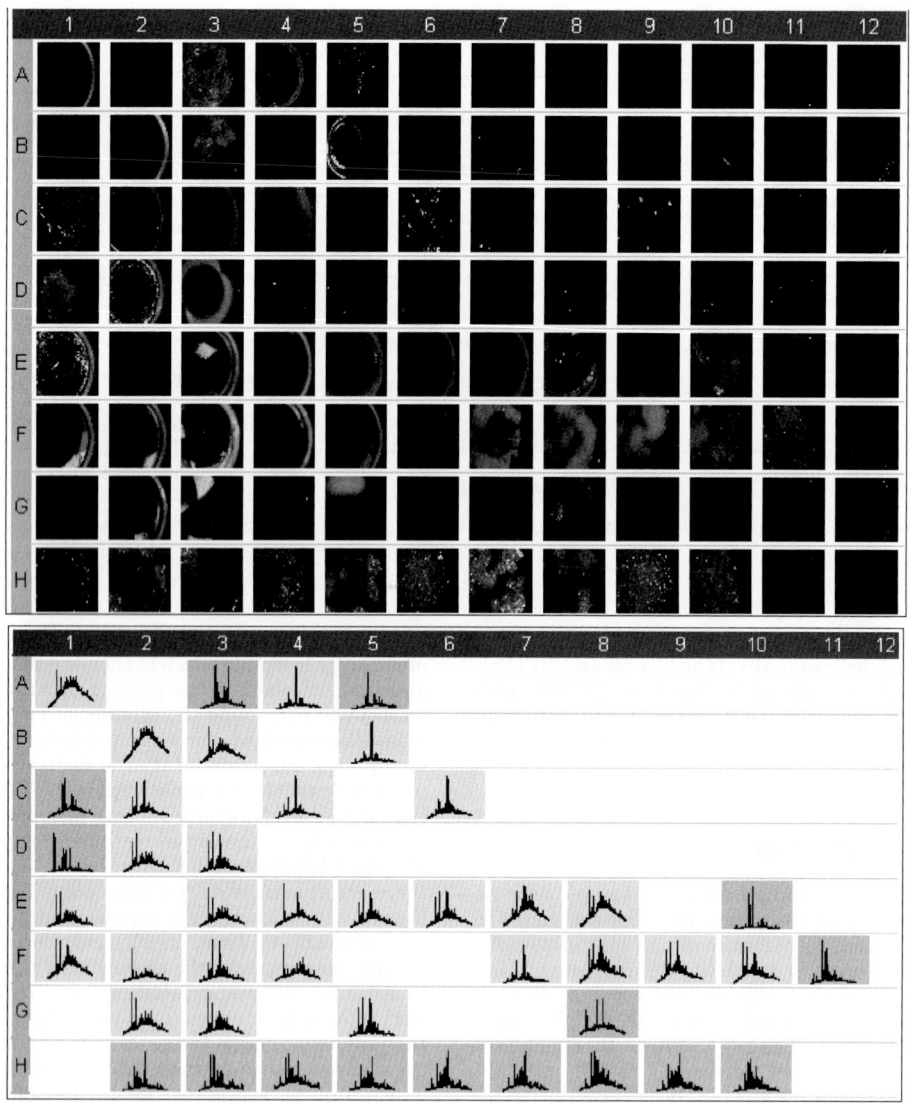

Figure 34-45. Birefringence images and powder diffraction patterns collected from the evaporative crystallization plate in the HTS of d,l-propranolol hydrochloride indicates two polymorphic crystal forms and their location within the 96-well plate, thus enabling correlation of crystallization chemistry with the crystal form obtained. See Color Plate 4.

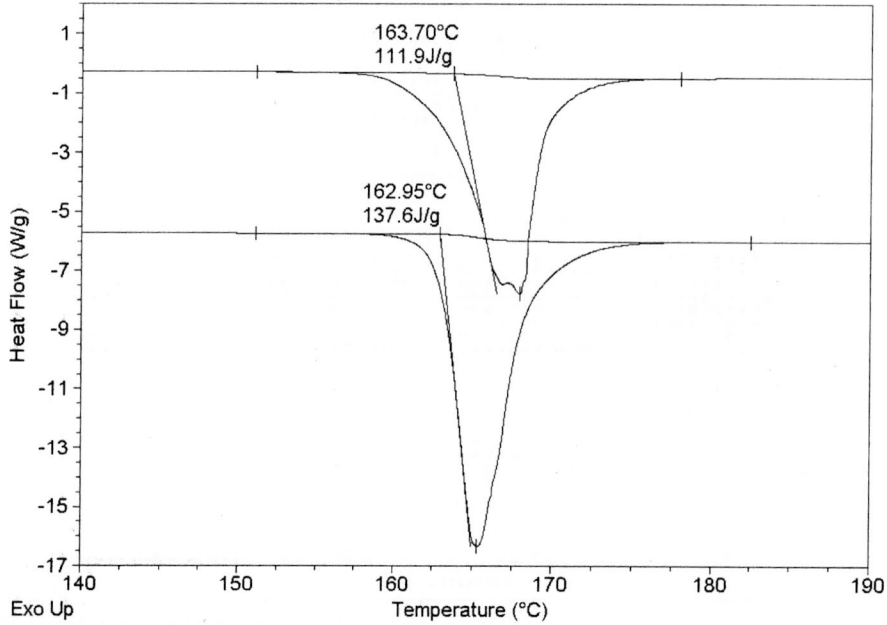

Figure 34-46. The DSC thermal curves of from two polymorphic forms of d,l-propranolol hydrochloride noting the onset temperature of melting and the enthalpy of fusion.

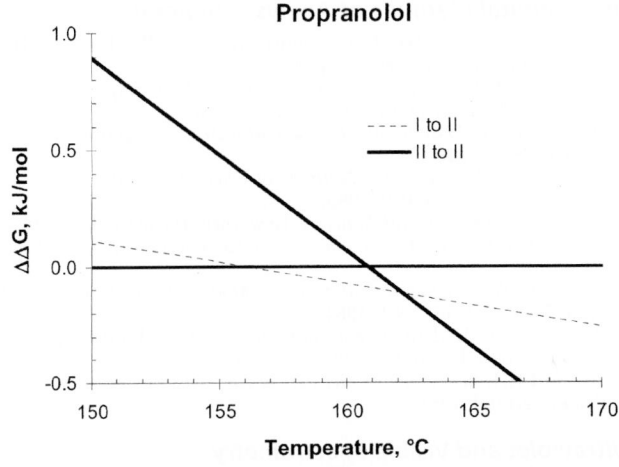

Figure 34-47. A temperature stability diagram of the two forms demonstrates that below 159°C the polymorphic form with the lower melting point is more stable whereas above the transition point, the higher melting polymorph is more stable.

using methods such as ^{13}C NMR or ion chromatography. The solid-state chemical stability of the forms is determined. The hygroscopic characteristics of the forms are assessed to ensure that the compound can be processed under normal ambient conditions. The thermodynamic relationship of polymorphic forms is determined so as to ensure that the most stable form under ambient temperature is produced. There is always a risk that a metastable form may eventually be unattainable during crystallization due to generation of a more stable. There have been numerous reports in which a metastable polymorphic form that was initially isolated could no longer be produced due to the appearance of a thermodynamically more stable form. On one occasion, the appearance of a more stable crystalline form of ritanovir, post product launch, resulted in a major product recall and an additional year of development due to the discovery of and the innovator's inability to isolate the crystalline form that was tested in clinical trials. One analytical method that is often used to determine crystal form stability is DSC. If the enthalpy of fusion of the higher melting form is greater than the lower melting form, then it is more stable at all temperatures between 0 K and its melting point and the polymorphs are related monotropically. If the difference in free energy versus temperature curves cross, then they are enantiotropically related and there is a temperature at which the lower melting polymorph is more stable than the higher melting polymorph, see Figure 34-46. In this trace it is evident that the higher melting polymorphic form has the lower enthalpy of fusion. The information indicates that the polymorphic forms of d,l-propranolol hydrochloride are enantiotropically related, with one melting at 162.95°C and the other at 163.7°C. That is the free energy of forms cross due primarily to differential changes in entropy with respect to change in temperature. A diagram of their stability versus temperature indicate that the transition temperature is 159°C, as is shown in Figure 34-47.

Acknowledgments

The authors gratefully acknowledge Jim Koers, MS, Scott Bradley, PhD, and Robert Behme (Eli Lilly and Company) for MS, NMR, and DSC data acquisition, respectively, related to propranolol. Scott is further acknowledged for helpful discussions related to NMR theory and practice.

The authors also express gratitude to Professor Ian Blair, PhD (University of Pennsylvania) for contributing material to the section on MS and for his continued mentorship.

REFERENCES

1. Freeman R, Morris GA. *Bull. Magn. Reson.* 1979; 1: 5.
2. Lauterbur PC. *Nature (London)* 1973; 242: 190.
3. Hurd, R.E. *J. Magn. Reson.* 1990; 87: 422.
4. Shaefer J, Stejskal EO. *J. Am. Chem. Soc.* 1976; 98: 1031.
5. Crouch RC, Martin GE. *J. Nat. Prod.* 1992; 55: 1343.
6. Keifer PA, Baltusis RDM, Tymiak AA, Shoolery JN. *J. Magn. Reson.* 1996; A 119: 65.
7. Albert K. *J. Chromatogr.* 1995; 703: 123.
8. Shockcor JP, Silver IS, Wurm RM, Sanderson PN, Farrant RD, Sweatman BC, Lindon JC. *Xenobiotica.* 1996; 26: 41.
9. Ehlhardt WJ, Woodland JM, Baughman TM, Vandenbranden M, Wrighton SA, Kroin JS, Norman BH, Maple SR. *Drug Metab Dispos.* 1998; 26: 42.
10. Olson DL, Norcross JA, O'Neil-Johnson M, Molitor PF, Detlefsen DJ, Wilson AG, Peck TL. *Anal Chem.* 2004; 76: 2966.
11. Logan TA, Murali N, Wang G, Jolivet C. *Magn. Reson. Chem.* 1999; 37, 512.
12. HP8452A *Diode-Array Spectrophotometer Handbook.* Palo Alto, CA: Hewlett Packard, 1990.
13. Skoog DA, Holler FJ, Nieman TA. *Principles of Instrumental Analysis, 5th Ed.* New York: WB Saunders, 1998.
14. Willard HH, Merritt LL, Dean JA, Settle PA. *Instrumental Methods of Analysis, 6th Ed.* New York: Van Nostrand, 1981.
15. Haleblian JK, McCrone W. *Journal of Pharmaceutical Sciences* 1969; 58: 911.
16. Byrn, SR, Pfeiffer RR, Stowell JG. *Solid-State Chemistry of Drugs,* 2nd ed. SSCI, Inc, West Lafayette IN, 1999.
17. Stephenson GA, Forbes RA, Reutzel-Edens SM. *Advanced Drug Delivery Reviews* 2001; 48: 67.
18. Yu L, Reutzel SM, Stephenson GA. *Pharmaceutical Science and Technology Today* 1998; 1: 118.
19. Bloss, FD. *An Introduction to the Methods of Optical Crystallography,* Saunders College Publishing, Marietta, OH, USA, 1961.
20. McCrone WC. *Fusion Methods in Chemical Microscopy,* Interscience Publishers, New York, USA, 1957.
21. Giacovazzo C, Monaco HL, Viterbo D, Scordari F, Gill G, Zanotti G, Catti M. *Fundamentals of Crystallography,* ED C. Giacovazzo. Oxford University Press. 165, 1992.
22. Friedrich W, Knipping P, Laue M. *Sitzb. Kais. Akad. Wiss.,* Munchen, 1912; 303: 22.
23. Bragg, WL. *Proc. Roy. Soc. London* 1913; (A) 89: 248.
24. Glusker JP, Lewis M, Rossi M. *Journal of Chemical Education* 1995; 72: A73.
25. Hope H. *Acta Crystallographica, Section B: Structural Science* 1998; B44: 22.
26. McCrone WC. *Physics and Chemistry of the Organic Solid State* 1965; 2: 725.
27. Bragg WL. *Proc. Roy. Soc. London* 1913; (A) 89: 248.
28. Klug HP, Alexander LE. *X-Ray Diffraction Procedures;* CAPLUS 716, 1954.
29. Cullity BD. *Elements of X-Ray Diffraction.* 2nd Ed., CAPLUS 555, 1978.
30. Jenkins R, Snyder R. eds. *Introduction to X-Ray Powder Diffractometry.* CAPLUS 544, 1996.
31. Strobel HA, Heineman WR. *Chemical Instrumentation: A Systematic Approach,* 3rd ed. New York: Wiley, 1989.
32. High Resolution Option Manual. New Castle, DE: Y/A Instruments, 1991.
33. Willard HH, Merritt LL, Dean JA, Settle PA. *Instrumental Methods of Analysis,* 6th ed. New York: Van Nostrand, 1981.
34. Ackermann BL, Berna MJ, Murphy AT. *Curr. Top. Med. Chem.* 2002; 2: 56.
35. Jemal M. *Biomed. Chromatogr.* 2000; 14: 422.
36. Allanson, JP, Biddlecombe RA, Jones AE, Pleasance S. *Rapid Commun. Mass Spectrom.* 1996; 10: 811.
37. Stenborner S, Henion J. *Anal. Chem.* 1999; 71: 2340.
38. Watt AP, Morrison D, Locker KL, Evans DG. *Anal. Chem.* 2000; 72: 979.
39. Di L, Kerns EH, Hong Y, Kleintop TA, McConnell OJ, Huryn DM. *J. Biomol. Screen* 2003; 8: 453.
40. Caldwell GW, Easlick SM, Gunnet J, Masucci JA, Demarest K. *J. Mass Spectrom.* 1998; 33: 607.
41. Chu I, Liu F, Soares A, Kumari P, Nomeir AA. *Rapid Commun. Mass Spectrom.* 2002; 16: 1501.
42. Fung EN, Chen YH, Lau YY. *J. Chromatogr. B. Analyt Technol Biomed Life Sci.* 2003; 795: 187.
43. Dierks EA, Stams KR, Lim HK, Cornelius G, Zhang H, Ball SE. *Drug Metab Dispos.* 2001; 29: 23.

44. Chen C, Hanson E, Watson JW, Lee JS. *Drug Metab Dispos.* 2003; 31: 312.
45. Janiszewski JS, Rogers KJ, Whalen KM, Cole MJ, Liston TE, Duchoslav E, Fouda HG. *Anal. Chem.* 2001; 73: 1495.
46. Kerns EH. *J. Pharm. Sci.* 2001; 1838.
47. Hop CECA, Wang Z, Chen Q, Kwei G. *J. Pharm. Sci.* 1998; 901.
48. Berman J, Halm K, Adkison K, Shaffer J. *J. Med. Chem.* 1997; 40: 3.
49. Needham SR, Cole MJ, Fouda HG. *J. Chromatogr. B.* 1998; 718: 87.
50. Ayrton J, Dear GJ, Leavens WJ, Mallett DN, Plumb RS. *Rapid Commun. Mass Spectrom.* 1997; 11: 1953.
51. Beaudry F, LeBlanc JYC, Coutu M, Brown N. *Rapid Commun. Mass Spectrom.* 1998; 12:1216.
52. Sen JW, Bergen HR 3rd, Heegaard NH. *Anal Chem.* 2003; 75: 1196.
53. Wang S, Mei H, Ng K, Workowski K, Astle T, Korfmacher W. *Proceedings of the 50th ASMS Conference on Mass Spectrometry and Allied Topics*, Orlando, FL, May 26–30, 2002.
54. Abola E, Kuhn P, Earnest T, Stevens RC. *Nat. Struct. Biol.* 2000; 7: 973.
55. Kuhn P, Wilson K, Patch MG, Stevens RC. *Curr. Opin. Chem. Biol.* 2002; 6:704.
56. Stout TJ, Foster PG, Matthews DJ. *Curr. Pharm. Des.* 2004; 10:1069.
57. Keifer PA. *Curr Opin Chem Biol.* 2003; 7: 388.
58. Taylor LCE, Johnson RL, Raso R. *J. Am Soc Mass Spectrom.* 1995; 6: 387.
59. Greaves J. *J Mass Spectrom.* 2002; 8: 777.
60. Mallis LM, Sarkahian AB, Kulishoff JM Jr, Watts WL Jr. *J Mass Spectrom.* 2001; 9: 889.
61. Morand KL, Burt TM, Regg BT, Chester TL. *Anal. Chem.* 2001; 73: 247.
62. Romanyshyn L, Tiller PR, Alvaro R, Pereira A, Hop CECA. *Rapid Commun. Mass Spectrom.* 2001; 15: 313.
63. Wu J-T, Zeng H, Deng Y, Unger SE. *Rapid Commun. Mass Spectrom.* 2001; 15: 1113.
64. King RC, Miller-Stein C, Magiera DJ, Brann J. *Rapid Commun. Mass Spectrom.* 2002; 16: 43.
65. Fang L, Cournoyer J, Demee M, Zhao J, Tokushige D, Yan B. *Rapid Commun Mass Spectrom.* 2002; 16: 1440.
66. Xu R, Wang T, Isbell J, Cai Z, Sykes C, Brailsford A, Kassel DB. *Anal Chem.* 2002; 74: 3055.
67. Yang L, Mann TD, Little D, Wu N, Clement RP, Rudewicz PJ. *Anal Chem.* 2001; 73: 1740.
68. Khandurina J, Guttman A. *J Chromatogr A.* 2002; 943: 159.
69. Weigl BH, Bardell RL, Cabrera CR. *Adv Drug Deliv Rev.* 2003; 55: 349.
70. Huikko K, Kostiainen R, Kotiaho T. *Eur J Pharm Sci.* 2003; 20: 149.
71. Jakeway SC, de Mello AJ, Russell EL. *Fresenius J Anal Chem.* 2000; 366: 525.
72. Schultz GA, Corso TN, Prosser SJ, Zhang S. *Anal. Chem.* 2000; 72: 4058.
73. Meng F, Du Y, Miller LM, Patrie SM, Robinson DE, Kelleher NL. *Anal. Chem.* 2004; 76: 2852.
74. Keetch CA, Hernanndez H, Sterling A, Baumert M, Allen MH, Robinson CV. *Anal Chem.* 2003; 75: 4937.
75. Dethy JM, Ackermann BL, Delatour C, Henion JD, Schultz GA. *Anal. Chem.* 2003; 75: 805.
76. *Handbook of Pharmaceutical Salts Properties, Selection, and Use* P. Heinrich Stahl, Camille G. Wermuth (Eds.) 2002.

BIBLIOGRAPHY

Mass Spectrometry

1. Busch KL, Glish GL, McLuckey SA. *Mass spectrometry/mass spectrometry,* VHC, New York, 1988.
2. Watson JT. *Introduction to Mass Spectrometry,* 3rd ed., Lippincott-raven, Philadelphia, 1997.
3. Willoughby R, Sheehan E, Mitrovich S. *A Global view of LC/MS,* Global View Publishing, Pittsburgh, 1998.
4. The American Society of Mass Spectrometry web page and associated links. (WWW.asms.org).
5. Murray KK. *J. Mass Spectrom.* 1999; 34: 1.

NMR

1. Skoog DA. *Principles of Instrumental Analysis.* Saunders College Publishing, Philadelphia, 1984
2. Lambert JB, Shurvell HF, Lightner DA, Cooks RG. *Organic Structural Spectroscopy.* Prentice Hall, Upper Saddle River, NJ, 1998.
3. Keifer PA. In ed. Jucker E. *In Progress in Drug Research,* Vol 55, Birkhauser Verlag, Basel, Switzerland, 2000.

Instrumental Methods of Analysis, General

1. Analytical Chemistry, Fundamental Reviews. Washington, DC: American Chemical Society, April 1982.
2. Borman SA. *Instrumentation in Analytical Chemistry, vol 2.* Washington, DC: American Chemical Society, 1982.
3. Christian GD, O'Reilly JE. *Instrumental Analysis,* 2nd ed. Boston: Allyn & Bacon, 1986.
4. Ewing GW. *Instrumental Methods of Chemical Analysis,* 5th Ed. New York, McGraw-Hill, 1985.
5. Mann CK. *Instrumental Analysis.* New York: Harper & Row, 1974.
6. Moore WJ. *Physical Chemistry,* 4th ed. Englewood Cliffs, NJ: Prentice-Hall, 1972.
7. Munson JW. *Pharmaceutical Analysis, Modern Methods,* Parts A, B. New York: Dekker, 1981, 1984.
8. Schirmer RE. *Modern Methods of Pharmaceutical Analysis,* 2nd Ed, vols 1, 2. Boca Raton, FL: CRC Press, 1991.
9. Willard HH. *Instrumental Methods of Analysis,* 6th Ed. New York: Van Nostrand, 1981.

Ultraviolet and Visible Spectrometry

1. *ASTM Index to Ultraviolet and Visible Spectra.* ASTM Tech Publ 357. Philadelphia: ASTM, 1963.
2. Braude EA. *Determination of Organic Structures by Physical Methods.* New York: Academic, 1955, pp 131–194.
3. Duncan ABF, Matsen FA. In: Weissberger A, ed. *Technique of Organic Chemistry,* vol 9, 2nd Ed. New York: Interscience, 1968–1970, p 581.
4. Harris TD. Anal Chem 1982; 54: 741A.
5. Hershenson HM. *Ultraviolet and Visible Absorption Spectra,* Index, 1930–1963, 6 vols. New York: Academic, 1966.
6. Jaffe HH, Orchin M. *Theory and Applications of Ultraviolet Spectroscopy.* New York: Wiley, 1962.
7. Lang L. ed. *Absorption Spectra in the Ultraviolet and Visible Region,* vols 1–17. New York: Academic, 1961–1973.
8. Montegu B, Langier A. *Fournier J. J Phys* [E] 1979; 12: 1153.
9. Organic Electronic Spectral Data, 1946–1967, vols 1–7. New York: Interscience, 1960–1971.
10. Scott AI. *Interpretation of the Ultraviolet Spectra of Natural Products.* New York: Pergamon, 1964.

Infrared Spectrometry

1. Bellamy LJ. *The Infrared Spectra of Complex Molecules,* 3rd Ed. New York: Wiley, 1975.
2. Colthup NB. *Introduction to Infrared and Raman Spectroscopy,* 3rd Ed. New York: Academic, 1990.
3. Dyer JR. *Organic Spectral Problems.* Englewood Cliffs, NJ: Prentice-Hall, 1972.
4. Griffiths PR, de Haseth JA. *Fourier Transform Infrared Spectrometry.* New York: Wiley, 1986.
5. Hershenson HM. *Infrared Absorption Spectra,* Index, 1947–1954, 2 vols. New York: Academic, 1965.
6. Hurley WJ. *J Chem Educ* 1966; 43: 236.
7. Lang L. ed. *Absorption Spectra in the Infrared Region,* vols 1, 2. London: Butterworths, 1974, 1976.
8. Low MJD. *J Chem Educ* 1970; 47: A163, A255, A415.
9. Fourier MA. *Hadamard and Hilbert Transforms in Chemistry.* New York: Plenum, 1982.
10. Martin AE. *Infrared Instrumentation and Techniques.* New York: Elsevier, 1966.
11. Massart DL, Vandefinste BGM, Deming SN. *Chemometrics: A Textbook.* New York: Elsevier, 1988.
12. Nyquist RA, Kegel RO. *Infrared Spectra of Inorganic Compounds.* New York: Academic, 1971.
13. *Catalog of Infrared Spectra.* Philadelphia: Sadtler Research Labs, nd.
14. Silverstein RM et al. *Spectrometric Identification of Organic Compounds,* 5th Ed. New York: Wiley, 1991.
15. Szymanski HA, Erickson RE. *Infrared Band Handbook,* rev Ed. New York: Plenum, 1970. Suppls 1 and 2 cover the 200 to 600 cm^{-1} region.
16. Vornhederand PF, Brabbs WJ. *Anal Chem* 1970; 42: 1454.

Emission Spectrometry, Flame Photometry, and Atomic Absorption Spectrometry

1. Ahrens LH, Taylor SR. *Spectrochemical Analysis,* 2nd ed. Reading, MA: Addison-Wesley, 1961.
2. Alkemade CTJ, Milatz JMW. *Appl Sci Res* 1955; B4: 289.
3. Alkemade CTJ, Milatz JMW. *J Opt Soc Am* 1955; 45: 583.
4. Brode WR. *Chemical Spectroscopy,* 2nd ed. New York: Wiley, 1943.
5. Dedina J, Rubeska I. *Spectrochim Acta B* 1980; 35B: 119.

6. Elwell WT, Gidley JAF. *Atomic Absorption Spectrophotometry*, 2nd rev Ed. New York: Pergamon, 1966.
7. Godden RG, Thomerson DR. *Analyst* 1980; 105: 1137.
8. Haswell SJ, ed. *Atomic Absorption Spectrometry*. New York: Elsevier, 1991.
9. Mavrodineanu R, ed. *Analytical Flame Spectroscopy*. Berlin: Springer-Verlag, 1971.
10. Meggers WF, et al. *Tables of Spectral-Line Intensities, parts 1, 2*. National Bureau of Standards (US) Monograph 32. Washington, DC: USGPO, 1961–1962. Revised edition: Corliess CH, 1967.
11. Pinta M. *Atomic Absorption Spectrometry*, vol 2. Application to Chemical Analysis, 2nd ed. Paris: Masson, 1980.
12. Reed TB. *J Appl Phys* 1961; 32: 821, 2534.
13. Reed TB. *Int Sci Technol*. June 1962; 142.
14. Styris DL, Kaye JH. *Spectrochim Acta B* 1981; 36B: 41.
15. Van Loon JC. *Analytical Atomic Absorption Spectroscopy, Selected Methods*. New York: Academic, 1980.
16. Walsh A. *Spectrochim Acta* 1955; 7: 108.
17. Willard H, et al. *Instrumental Methods of Analysis*, 6th Ed. New York: Van Nostrand, 1981.

Fluorescence and Phosphorescence Spectrometry

1. Guilbault GC. *Fluorescence: Theory, Instrumentation and Practice*. New York: Dekker, 1967.
2. Guilbault GC, ed. *Practical Fluorescence*. New York: Dekker, 1990.
3. Hercules DM, ed. *Fluorescence and Phosphorescence Analysis: Principles and Applications*. New York: Interscience, 1966.
4. Udenfriend S. *Fluorescence Assay in Biology and Medicine*. New York: Academic, 1962.

Light Scattering and Polarimetry

1. Crabbe P. *ORD and CD in Chemistry and Biochemistry*. New York: Academic, 1972.
2. Djerassi C. *Optical Rotatory Dispersion*. New York: McGraw-Hill, 1960.
3. Stacey K. *Light-Scattering in Physical Chemistry*. London: Butterworths, 1956.
4. Weissberger A, ed. *Physical Methods in Organic Chemistry*, vol 1, 3rd Ed, Part 2. New York: Interscience, 1960.

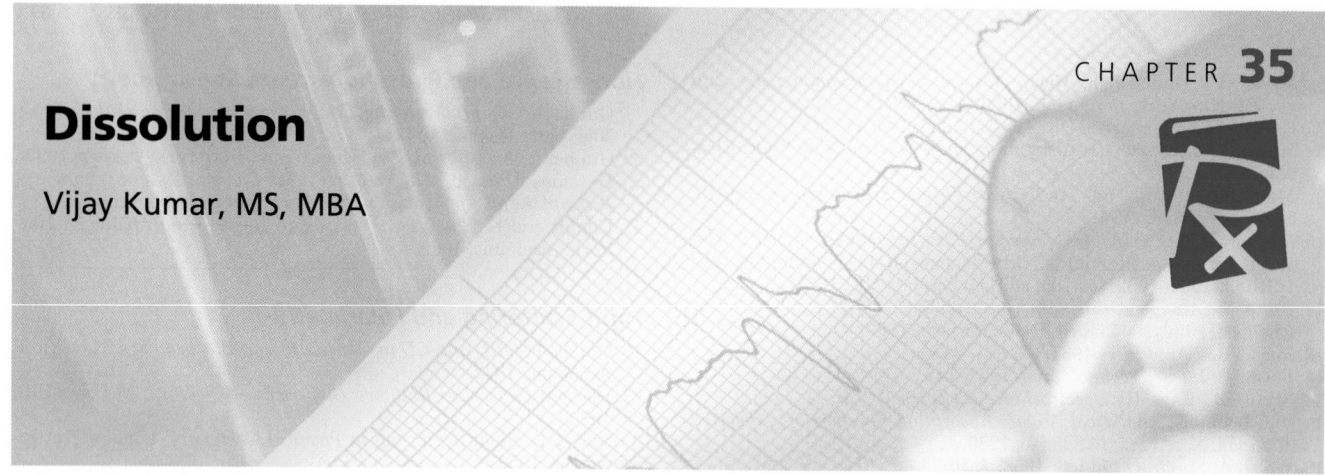

CHAPTER 35

Dissolution

Vijay Kumar, MS, MBA

Dissolution is the process by which a solid enters into solution. The earliest reference to dissolution is probably the 1897 article by Noyes and Whitney, titled as "The Rate of Solution of Solid Substances in Their Own Solution." The authors suggested that the rate of dissolution of solid substances is determined by the rate of diffusion of a very thin layer of saturated solution that forms instantaneously around the solid particle. They developed the mathematical relationship that correlates the dissolution rate to the solubility gradient of the solid. Their equation is still the basic formula upon which most of the modern mathematical treatments of the dissolution phenomenon revolve.

Interestingly, the work of Noyes and Whitney, together with the studies that followed in the early part of the 20th century, was primarily based on the physicochemical aspects of dissolution applied to chemical substances. The most prominent part of these investigations that deserve recognition are those of Nernst and Brunner in 1904 for their application of Fick's law of diffusion to the Noyes-Whitney equation, and those of Hixson and Crowell in 1931 for their development of famous "Cube Root Law" of dissolution.[1]

By the middle of the 20th century, emphasis started to shift to the examination of the effects of dissolution behavior of drugs on the biological activity of pharmaceutical dosage forms. One of the earliest studies with this purpose in mind was conducted by J Edwards in 1951 on aspirin tablets. He reported, "because of its poor solubility, the analgesic action of aspirin tablets would be controlled by its dissolution rate within the stomach and the intestine." No *in vivo* studies, however, were conducted by Edwards to support his postulate.

About 8 years later, Shenoy and colleagues proved the validity of Edward's suggestion of the *in vitro/in vivo* correlation by demonstrating a direct relationship between the bioavailability of amphetamine from sustained-release tablets and its *in vitro* dissolution rate. Other studies, especially those reported by Nelson, Levy, and others, confirmed beyond doubt the significant effect of the dissolution behavior of drugs on their pharmacological activities. Because of the importance of these findings, dissolution testing began to emerge as a dominant topic within both the pharmaceutical academia and the drug industry.

In the late 1960s dissolution testing became a mandatory requirement for several dosage forms. The role of dissolution in the absorption of drug products, however, still is far from being understood completely. In spite of the reported success of several *in vitro/in vivo* correlation studies, dissolution cannot be relied upon as a predictor of therapeutic efficiency. Rather, it is a qualitative tool that can provide valuable information about the biological availability of a drug as well as batch-to-batch consistency. Another area of difficulty is the fact that the accuracy and precision of the testing procedure is dependent, to a large extent, on the strict observance of so many subtle parameters and detailed operational controls.

In spite of these shortcomings, dissolution is considered today as one of the most important quality control procedure performed on pharmaceutical dosage forms. Whether or not it has been correlated with biological effectiveness, the standard dissolution test is a simple and inexpensive indicator of product's physical consistency. If one batch differs from the other in its dissolution characteristics, or if the dissolution profiles of the production batches show a consistent trend upwards or downwards, it sounds a sure warning that some factor in the raw material, formulation, or process is out of control.[1] Additionally, dissolution data seems to be a useful tool in the early stages of drug development and molecular manipulation. In the early stages of research, steps may be taken to optimize characteristics that will influence subsequent data concerning biological availability. Based on simple dissolution test, selection of a proper salt for a new drug can be done at early drug development stage.

Definition of Dissolution and Theoretical Concepts for the Release of the Drug from Dosage Forms

"Dissolution is defined as the process by which solid substances enters in solvent to yield a solution. Stated simply, dissolution is the process by which a solid substance dissolves. Fundamentally, it is controlled by the affinity between the solid substance and the solvent." The physical characteristics of the dosage form, the wettability of the dosage unit, the penetration ability of the dissolution medium, the swelling process, the disintegration and the deaggregation of the dosage forms are few of the factors that influence the dissolution characteristics of drugs. Wagner proposed a scheme depicted in Figure 35-1 for the processes involved in the dissolution of solid dosage forms.

This scheme was later modified to incorporate other factors that precede the dissolution process of solid dosage forms. Carstensen proposed a scheme incorporating the following sequence:

1. Initial mechanical lag
2. Wetting of the dosage form
3. Penetration of the dissolution medium into the dosage form
4. Disintegration
5. Deaggregation of the dosage form and dislodgement of the granules
6. Dissolution
7. Occlusion of some particles of the drug

Carstensen explained that the wetting of the solid dosage form surface controls the liquid access to the solid surface and, many times, is the limiting factor in the dissolution process. The speed of wetting directly depends on the surface tension at the interface (interfacial tension) and upon the contact angle, θ, between

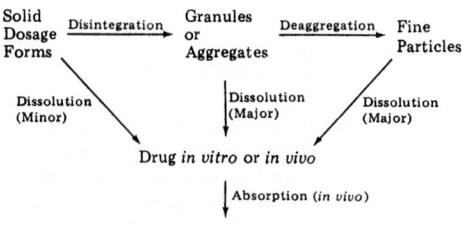

Figure 35-1. Dissolution process of solid dosage forms.

the solid surface and the liquid. Generally, a contact angle of more than 90° indicates poor wettability. Incorporation of a surfactant, either in the formulation or in the dissolution medium, lowers the contact angle and enhances dissolution. Also, the presence of air in the dissolution medium causes the air bubbles to be entrapped in the tablet pores and act as a barrier at the interface. For capsules, the gelatin shell is extremely hydrophilic, and therefore, no problems in wettability exist for the dosage itself (although it may exist for the powders inside).

After the solid dosage form disintegrates into granules or aggregates, penetration characteristics play a prime role in the deaggregation process. Hydrophobic lubricants, such as talc and magnesium stearate, commonly employed in tablet and capsule formulations, slow the penetration rate and, hence, the deaggregation process. A large pore size facilitates penetration, but if it is too large it may inhibit penetration by decreasing the internal strain caused by the swelling of the disintegrant.

After deaggregation and dislodgment occur, the drug particles become exposed to the dissolution medium and dissolution proceeds as previously discussed under Film Theory. Figure 35-2[2] graphically presents the model proposed by Carstensen.

It is apparent from Figure 35-2 that the rate of dissolution of the drug can become rate-limiting step before it appears in the blood. However, when the dosage form is placed into the gastrointestinal tract in solid form, there are two possibilities for the rate-limiting step. The solid must first dissolve, and the drug in solution must then pass through the gastrointestinal (GI) membrane. Freely water-soluble drugs will tend to dissolve rapidly, making the passive diffusion of the drug or the active transport of the drug rate-limiting step for absorption through the GI membrane. Conversely, the rate of absorption of poorly water-soluble drugs will be limited by the rate of dissolution of the undissolved drug or disintegration of dosage form.

The rate of dissolution of drug substance is determined by the rate at which solvent-solute forces of attraction overcome the cohesive forces present in the solid. This process is rate-limiting when the release of solute into solution is slow and the transport into the bulk solution is fast. In this case the dissolution is said to be interfacially controlled. Dissolution may also be diffusion controlled, where the solvent-solute interaction is fast compared to transport of solute into the bulk solution. In diffusion-controlled process, a stationary layer of solute adjacent to the solid/liquid interface is postulated and is commonly referred to as the diffusion layer. The saturation concentration of solute develops at the interface and decreases with distance across the diffusion layer.

MATHEMATICS OF DISSOLUTION

It has long being recognized that the release of the active drug from a drug product may be greatly influenced by the physicochemical properties of the drug as well as the dosage form.[3] The availability of the drug is usually determined by the rate of release of the drug from the physical system (dosage form). The release of the drug from its dosage form is usually determined by the rate at which it dissolves in the surrounding medium. The rate of dissolution of a chemical or drug from the solid state is defined as the amount of drug substance that goes into solution per unit time under standardized condition of liquid/solid interface, temperature, and solvent composition. In biopharmaceutics, rate of dissolution usually refers to the rate at which the drug dissolves from an intact dosage form or from fragments or particles from the dosage form during the test.[4]

The following section deals with the introductory concepts on mathematics of dissolution focusing primarily on intrinsic dissolution.

Intrinsic Dissolution

The rate of dissolution of a pure pharmaceutical active ingredient when conditions such as surface area, temperature, agitation or stirring speed, pH, ionic strength of the dissolution medium is kept constant is known as intrinsic dissolution rate. This parameter allows the screening of the drug candidates and aids in understanding their solution behavior under various biophysiological conditions.[5]

INTRINSIC DISSOLUTION RATE CONSTANTS—The rate at which a substance dissolves in a liquid to form a solution is governed by physical parameters such as the surface area of the substance at a given time during the process of dissolution, the shape of the substance, the characteristics of the solid/liquid interface, and the solubility of the substance in the liquid. Hence, dissolution can be considered a specific type of certain heterogeneous reaction which results in a mass transfer as a net effect between the escape and deposition of solute molecules at a solid surface. Mathematically, the process can be simply described as follows:

$$dM/dT = KA(C_s - C) \tag{1}$$

where, M is the mass of the substance remaining to be dissolved, A is the surface area exposed to the dissolution medium, C_s is the saturation concentration referred to as solubility in the dissolution medium, C is the amount dissolved or the concentration of the drug in solution at time t, K is the intrinsic dissolution rate constant or simply the dissolution rate constant.

The equation expresses the fact that when C is small, $C < 0.15C_s$, then K is proportional to C_s, since $(C_s - C)$ is large. If this applies, then to a good approximation we may write

$$dM/dT = KAC_s \tag{2}$$

Equation 2 is commonly referred to as a sink-condition equation, which implies that sink conditions exist during the process of dissolution. It must be noted, however, that A is a constant except initially, when only very small quantities of solute have dissolved and where there is an amount of solute far in excess of saturation.

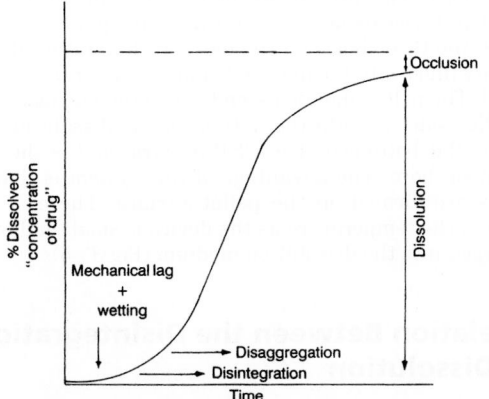

Figure 35-2. The S-shaped dissolution curve of solid dosage forms.

When the process of dissolution takes place under sink conditions, a stagnant film of liquid (dissolution medium) is adsorbed onto the solid, the thickness of this film being l cm. The liquid in the film that is in direct contact with the solid is saturated with drug in solution. The concentration of the drug in solution then drops as the distance from the dissolving solid surface increases. At the end of the film, l cm from the surface, the concentration in the film is the same as that in the bulk solution, C_b. The driving force behind the movement of solute molecules through the stagnant film is the concentration gradient that exists between the saturation concentration of the solute, C_s, in the stagnant layer at the surface of the solid and its concentration on the farthest side of the stagnant film, C_b. A schematic representation of dissolution as a physicochemical phenomenon is shown in Figure 35-3, the greater this difference in concentration, the faster the rate of dissolution.

Applying Fick's first law of diffusion to equation 2, the flux, J (defined as the rate of flow of material through 1 cm^2, ie,

$$J = \frac{dM/dT}{A}$$

can be expressed as

$$J = -D(\delta C/\delta x)$$

where D is the coefficient of diffusion; x is the distance as shown in the Figure 35-3. If the concentration gradient, $\delta C/\delta x$, is linear, if $C = C_s$ at the surface $(x = 0)$, and if $C = C_b$ (the bulk concentration at the interface between the bulk solution and the film, where $x = 1$), then

$$(\delta C/\delta x) = (C_b - C_s/l) \qquad (4)$$

Therefore,

$$\frac{1}{A}\frac{dM}{dT} = -D\frac{C_b - C_s}{l} = -K(C_s - C)$$

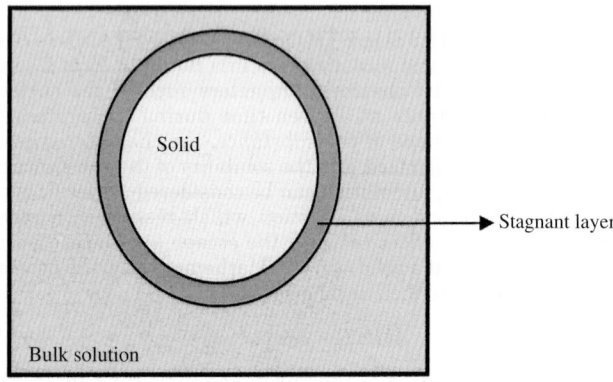

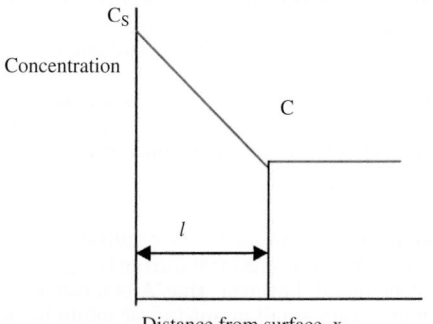

Figure 35-3. Physical model depicting a dissolution process.

Or simply

$$\frac{dM}{dT} = -KA(C_s - C)$$

If the agitation intensity of the system containing suspended particles is increased, the thickness of the film will decrease progressively. Hence k is a function of the test as well. Additionally, if the product of A (Cs 2 C) is maintained constant for many drug tested by the same test, the relative magnitude of k values will indicate the effective ease of dissolution. In practice, k also includes the dynamics of the shear rate between solid and the solvent, that is, the rate at which fresh solvent contacts the surface of the solid; highly complex processes, including diffusion rate through the boundary layers, depend upon this rate.

The shear rate depends upon a multitude of variables that must be controlled if the test is to be repeatable. Those variables include the flow pattern of solvent in the apparatus, turbulence, viscosity, surface tension, and dissolved gases, all of which are subject to uncontrolled input variables to the system, such as vibrations and system geometry. The theoretical basis for those inputs rests in the realm of chemical engineering's fluid flow and surface boundary theories, which are discussed elsewhere.[6]

The intrinsic dissolution rate has been used as a means to demonstrate the chemical purity and equivalency of the active pharmaceutical ingredient (API). The use of rotating disk system (USP Wood Apparatus), which is similar to USP procedure 1 is most common, though stationary disk systems, vertical diffusion cells, and enhancer cells can also be used to measure the intrinsic dissolution rates.[7]

Rotating Disk System (USP Wood Apparatus)

The apparatus consists of steel punch, a die, and a base plate. The base of the die has three threaded holes for the insertion of the screws and the attachment to the base plate. The material is placed in the die cavity, and the punch is inserted into the cavity and the material is compressed. The die is screwed onto the shaft holder, and the shaft holder is mounted on the stirring device. The shaft is a stainless steel rod with hollow die holder. Pellet and the die assembly are introduced all at once, when the dissolution drive mechanism is lowered. The dissolution is achieved by shear-like motion of the pellet in the dissolution medium. The dissolution vessel is standard curved bottom 1-L flask. Care should be taken that the air bubbles do not form on the surface of the pellet or else it will interfere with the dissolution rate (Fig 35-4).

Stationary Disk System

The apparatus consists of a steel punch, a die, and a base plate. The die base has three holes for the attachment of the base plate. The three fixed screws on the base plate are inserted through the three holes on the die. Punch is inserted into the die cavity filled with the material, and the material is then compressed. The pellet and die assembly can then be inserted with the pellet side up, into the bottom of the dissolution vessel, which is flat bottomed. The USP Apparatus 2 is the stirring mechanism here. The advantage of this system is that no air bubbles are formed on the pellet surface. There is also no change in the temperature as the device is small and is totally submerged into the dissolution medium (Fig 35-5).

Correlation Between the Disintegration and Dissolution

The close correlation between disintegration and dissolution has been studied by many investigators. Both processes exhibit

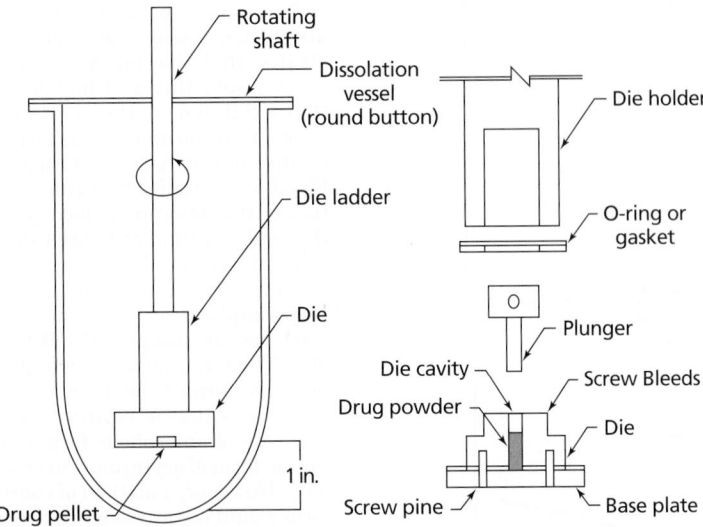

Figure 35-4. Rotating disk system (USP Wood apparatus).

"S"-shaped curves and a probit or a weibul function was suggested to explain the data. In general, however, disintegration has proved to be a poor indicator of bioavailability because of the turbulent agitation maintained during the test. Several other factors such as solubility, particle size, and crystalline structure, among others, have been found to affect the dissolution of the drug substance but have no relevance to disintegration.

Factors Affecting the Rate of Dissolution

The dissolution rate data can be meaningful only if the results of successive test on the same dosage form are consistent within reason. The dissolution test should yield reproducible result even when it is performed in different laboratories or with different personnel. To achieve high reproducibility, all variables that influence the test should be clearly understood and possibly controlled.

Factors affecting the dissolution rate of drugs from a dosage form include the following:

1. Factors related to the physicochemical properties of the drug
2. Factors related to drug product formulation
3. Effect of processing factors on the dissolution rate
4. Factors related to dissolution test parameters
5. Miscellaneous factors

FACTORS RELATED TO THE PHYSICOCHEMICAL PROPERTIES OF THE DRUG

EFFECT OF SOLUBILITY ON DISSOLUTION—The physicochemical properties of the drug substance play a prime role in controlling its dissolution from the dosage form. The modified Noyes and Whitney equation shows that the aqueous solubility of the drug is the major factor that determines its dissolution rate. Actually, some studies showed that drug-solubility data could be used as a rough predictor of the possibility of any future problems with bioavailability, a factor that should be taken into consideration in the formulation design.

EFFECT OF PARTICLE SIZE ON DISSOLUTION—According to Nernst- Brunner theory, the dissolution rate is directly proportional to the surface area of the drug. Since the surface area increases with the decreasing particle size, higher dissolution rates may be achieved through the reduction of the particle size. This effect has been highlighted by the superior dissolution rate observed after "micronization" of certain sparingly soluble drugs as opposed to the regularly milled form.

Several investigations have demonstrated an increased absorption rate for griseofulvin after micronization. Similar effects have been reported for chloramphenicol, tetracycline salts, sulfadiazine, and norethisterone acetate. In the case of chloramphenicol, it has been shown that formulations containing smaller particles (50–200 μm) were absorbed faster than formulations containing larger particles (400–800 μm). Figure 35-6 presents the effect of particle-size differences on the dissolution rate of phenacetin and phenobarbital.[8]

However, when employing this technique to enhance dissolution, it is important to recognize the fact that it is the effective surface area that has to be increased. The effective surface area is the surface area available to the dissolution fluid. If the drug is hydrophobic and the dissolution medium has poor wetting properties, reduction of particle size may lead to decreased effective surface area and hence a "slower" rate of dissolution.

Physical properties of the drug particles other than size also affect indirectly the effective surface area by modifying the shear rate of the fresh solvent that comes in contact with the solid. These properties include the particle shape and the density.

The mechanism by which the reduction in particle size improves dissolution is usually through the enhancement of the drug solubility. It is assumed that the drug solubility is independent of particle size. However, the drug solubility and the

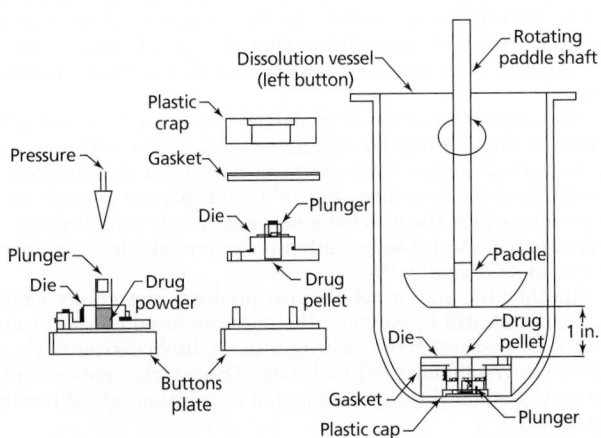

Figure 35-5. Stationary disk system (new apparatus).

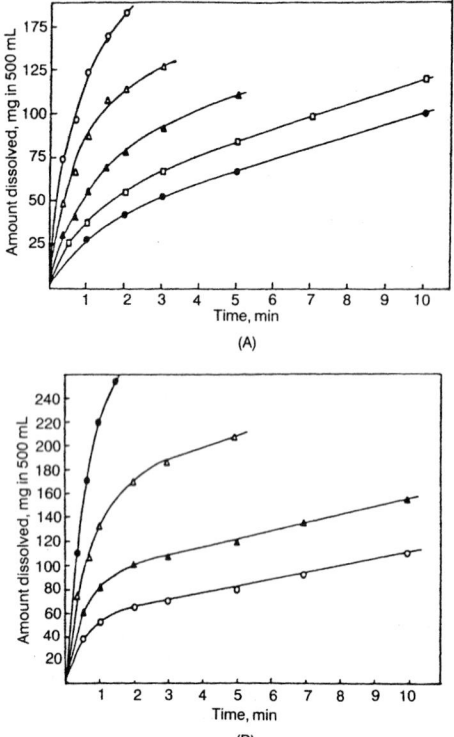

Figure 35-6. Effect of particle size on the dissolution rate of drugs from solid dosage forms.[3] **A.** Phenacetin: ○ particle size: 0.11–0.15 mm; △ particle size: 0.15–0.21 mm; ▲ particle size: 0.21–0.30 mm; □ particle size: 0.30–0.50 mm; ● particle size: 0.50–0.71 mm. **B.** Phenobarbital ● particle size: 0.07–0.15 mm; △ particle size: 0.15–0.25 mm; ▲ particle size: 0.25–0.42 mm; ○ particle size: 0.42–0.71 mm.

surface area can be correlated by the *Ostwald-Freundlich equation:*

$$\ln S = \frac{2M\gamma}{\rho RT}\frac{1}{r} = \frac{\alpha}{r}$$

where, M is the molecular weight, ρ is the density, γ is the interfacial tension or surface free energy of the solid, T is the temperature, R is the gas constant, r is the radius of the particle.

From the above equation

$$S = S_\infty \cdot e^{\frac{\alpha}{r}}$$

The equation shows that the solubility is inversely proportional to particle radius. Therefore, S could be viewed as the solubility of the microparticles and S_∞ as the solubility of the macro particles. However, it is obvious that the particle radius has to be reduced to a microlevel before it can effect a change in solubility.

This extreme reduction in particle size usually cannot be achieved through regular milling or even micronization procedures, and therefore other methods have been recommended. One of these involves formation of a *solid solution* or *molecular dispersion* where the molecules of the sparingly soluble drug either are dispersed interstitially in a water-soluble drug or replaced in its crystal lattice.

Another technique, which also produces extremely small particles but still larger than the ones produced by solid solution, is by dispersion of the drug into a soluble carrier such as polyvinylpyrrolidone (PVP) solution. These techniques usually are employed for the enhancement of dissolution rate of insoluble drugs.

EFFECT OF SOLID PHASE CHARACTERISTICS OF THE DRUG ON DISSOLUTION—Amorphicity and crystallinity, the two important solid-phase characteristics of drugs affect their dissolution profile. Numerous studies have demonstrated that the amorphous form of a drug usually exhibits greater solubility and higher dissolution rate as compared to that exhibited by the crystalline form. For example, it was shown that the amorphous form of novobiocin has a greater solubility and higher dissolution rate than the crystalline form. Blood-level studies confirmed such findings where administration of the amorphous form yielded about three to four times the concentration compared to the administration of the crystalline form. Similar differences were demonstrated for griseofulvin, phenobarbital, cortisone acetate, and chloramphenicol. Chloramphenicol palmitate is one example that exists in at least two polymorphs. The B form is apparently more bioavailable. The recommendation might be that manufacturers should use polymorph B for maximum absorption. One contradictory example is that of erythromycin esteolate, where the dissolution rate of amorphous form is markedly lower than the crystalline form of erythromycin esteolate, as exemplified by Figure 35-7. However, a method of controlling and determining crystal form would be necessary in the quality control process.[9]

EFFECT OF POLYMORPHISM ON DISSOLUTION—Polymorphic forms of drugs have been shown to influence changes in solubilizing characteristics and thus the dissolution rate of the drug in question. Numerous reports have shown that polymorphism and the state of hydration, solvation, and/or complexation markedly influence the dissolution characteristics of the drug. The drugs that exhibit influence on the dissolution behavior include tolbutamide, chloramphenicol, and others.

FACTORS RELATED TO DRUG PRODUCT FORMULATION

It has been shown that the dissolution rate of a pure drug can be altered significantly when mixed with various excipients during the manufacturing process of solid dosage forms. These excipients are added to satisfy certain pharmaceutical functions such as diluents (fillers), dyes, binders, granulating agents, disintegrants, and lubricants. Generically identical tablet and capsule products, manufactured by different pharmaceutical manufacturers, were found to exhibit significant differences in dissolution rates for their active ingredients. In certain cases, several studies showed that poor tablet and capsule formulations have been shown to cause a marked decrease in bioavailability and impairment of the clinical response. Such findings during the 1960s, especially in the case of digoxin and tolbutamide tablets, as well as chloramphenicol and tetracycline HCl (all lifesaving drugs), were the triggering factors that compelled the drug-regulatory agencies and compendial au-

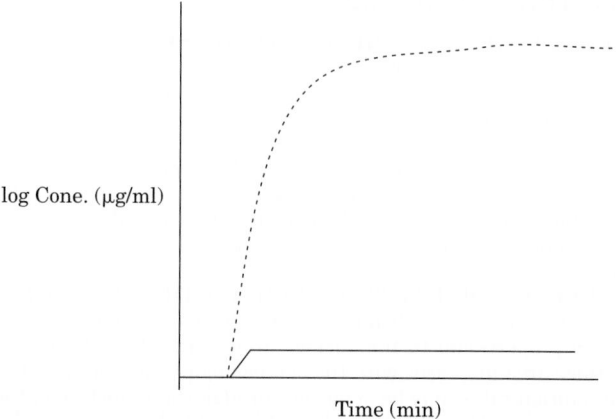

Figure 35-7. Dissolution performance of erythromycin estolate. (dotted line), Crystalline form; (solid line), Amorphous form.

thorities to institute the dissolution test as a legal requirement for most solid dosage forms.

EFFECT OF GRANULATING AGENTS AND BINDERS—Solvang and Finholt [10] have shown that Phenobarbital tablets granulated with gelatin solution provide faster dissolution rate in gastric fluid than those prepared using sodium carboxymethylcellulose or polyethylene glycol 6000 as a binder. This observation was attributed to the fact that gelatin imparts hydrophilic characteristics to the hydrophobic drug surface, whereas PEG 6000 forms complex with poor solubility, and sodium carboxymethylcellulose is converted to its less soluble acid form at low pH of the gastric fluid (Figure 35-8). Even gelatin obtained from various processes and origins has been shown to affect the dissolution rate of dosage forms.[11]

Various studies have been reported in the literature evaluating the effects of various granulating agents and binders on the dissolution rate of tablets.[12]

EFFECT OF DISINTEGRANTS AND DILUENTS—The type and amount of disintegrating agent employed in the formulation significantly controls the overall rate of dissolution of dosage form. Jaminet et al[11] employed several disintegrating agents in manufacturing of Phenobarbital tablets, including Primojel (sodium glycolate of potato starch), Nymcel (polymerized water-soluble brand of sodium carboxymethylcellulose), and Copagel (low viscosity grade of sodium carboxymethylcellulose). The effect on the dissolution rate of tablets by the addition of disintegrants before and after granulation was assessed. When added before granulation, Copagel gave tablets with a remarkably slow dissolution rate. However, when added after granulation, Copagel did not result in lowering the dissolution rate. Primojel was not found to be as effective, particularly on addition after granulation. Levy, in 1963, studied the effect of starch, the most commonly used diluent, on the rate of dissolution of salicylic acid tablets manufactured by the dry, double-compression process[13] (Fig 35-9). Increasing the starch content from 5% to 20% resulted in a dramatic increase in the dissolution rate (almost threefold). This was attributed to better and more thorough disintegration. Later, however, Finholt suggested that the hydrophobic drug crystals acquire a surface layer of fine starch particles that imparts a hydrophilic property to the granular formulation and thereby increases the effective surface area and hence the dissolution rate (see Fig 35-9).

EFFECT OF LUBRICANTS—The nature, quality, and quantity of lubricants added can affect the dissolution rate. The effect of various lubricants on dissolution rate of salicylic acid was studied and it was concluded that magnesium stearate, a hydrophobic lubricant, tends to retard the dissolution rate of salicylic acid tablets, whereas sodium lauryl sulfate enhances dissolution, due to its hydrophobic character combined with surface activity, which increases the microenvironment pH surrounding the weak acid and increases wetting and better solvent penetration into the tablets[14] (Fig 35-10) illustrates the effect of lubricants on the dissolution rate of tablets.

Effect of lubricants on the dissolution rate of drugs from dosage form would depend on properties of the granules, the lubricant itself, and the amount of lubricant used. If granules are hydrophilic and fast disintegrating, a water-soluble surface-active lubricant will have an insignificant effect on the dissolution. On the other hand, if the granules are hydrophobic, the surface-active lubricant will enhance dissolution. It was also found that hydrophobic lubricants, such as magnesium stearate, aluminum stearate, stearic acid, and talc, decrease the effective drug-solvent interfacial area by changing the surface characteristics of the tablets, which results in reducing its wettability, prolonging its disintegration time, and decreasing the area of the interface between the active ingredient and solvent.

FACTORS RELATED TO THE DISSOLUTION TEST PARAMETERS

METHOD OF GRANULATION—Wet granulation has been shown to improve the dissolution rates of poorly soluble drugs by imparting hydrophilic properties to the surface of the granules. Additionally the use of fillers and diluents such as starch, spray dried lactose, and microcrystalline cellulose tends to increase the hydrophilicity of the active ingredients and thus improve dissolution. Consequently, wet granulation

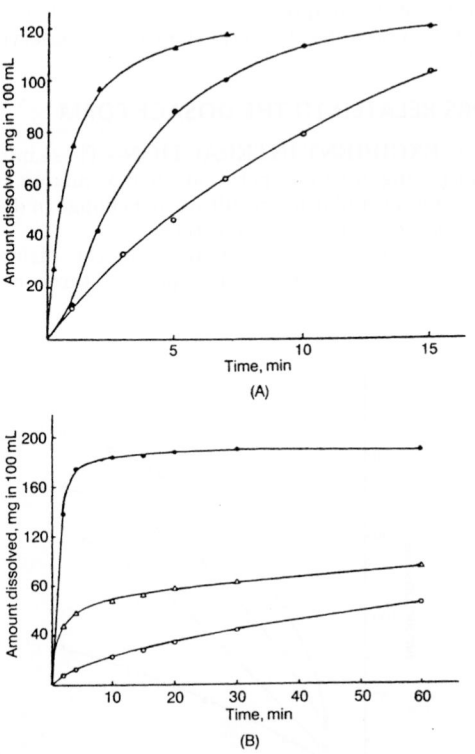

Figure 35-8. Effect of binders and granulating agents on dissolution rate of tablets.[5] **A.** Rate of dissolution of phenacetin from powder, granules, and tablets in diluted gastric juice (surface tension 42.7 dynes cm^{-1}, pH 1.85). O, phenacetin powder; ▲, phenacetin granules; ●, phenacetin tablets. **B.** Dissolution rate of phenobarbital tablets in diluted gastric juice (surface tension 39.4 dynes cm^{-1}, pH 1.50). ● Gelatin binder, <open triangle> CMC, <open circle> Polyethylene glycol 6000.

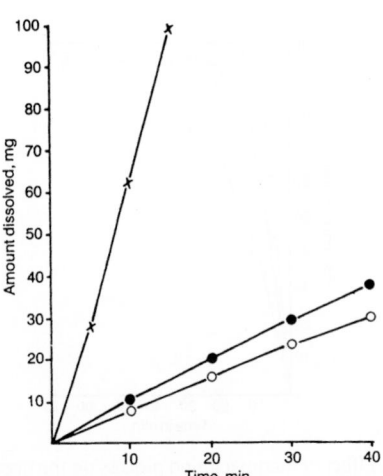

Figure 35-9. Effect of starch content on dissolution rate.[4] O, 5%; ●, 10%; ×, 20% starch in granules.

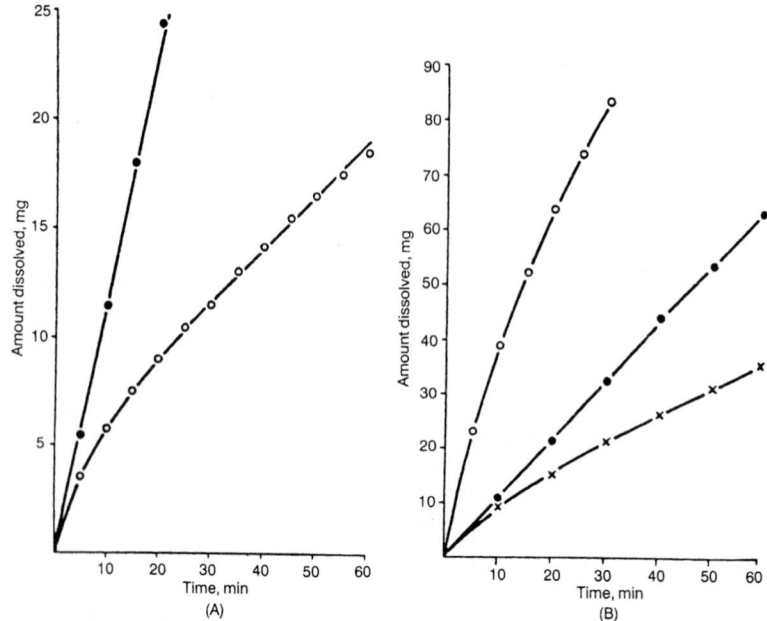

Figure 35-10. Effect of lubricant on the dissolution rate of tablets.[6] **A.** Effect of magnesium stearate on dissolution rate of salicylic acid from rotating discs made from fine salicylic acid powder. ○, 3% magnesium stearate; ●, no lubricant added. **B.** Effect of lubricant on dissolution rate of salicylic acid contained in compressed tablets (formula A). ×, 3% magnesium stearate; ●, no lubricant; ○, 3% sodium lauryl sulfate.

was considered superior to a dry or double-compression procedure. Figure 35-11 shows the effect of different granulation methods on the dissolution rate of tablets.[15]

It must be noted that with the advent of newer tableting machines and materials, it becomes more evident that the critical formulation and proper mixing sequence and time of adding the several ingredients are the main criteria that affect the dissolution characteristics of the tablets, not the method of granulation.

EFFECT OF COMPRESSION FORCE ON DISSOLUTION RATE—In his early studies of the physics of tablet compression, T Higuchi (1953), pointed out the influence of compression force employed in the tableting process on the apparent density, porosity, hardness, disintegration time, and average primary particle size of compressed tablets. There is always a competing relationship between the enhancing effect due to the increase in surface area through the crushing effect and the inhibiting effect due to the increase in particle bonding that causes an increase in density and hardness and, consequently, a decrease in solvent penetrability. The high compres-

sion may also inhibit the wettability of the tablet due to the formation of a firmer and more effective sealing layer by the lubricant under the high pressure and temperature that usually accompanies a strong compressive force[13] (Fig 35-12). The curve profile of the compressive force of the tablet versus dissolution rate can take one of several shapes, as is observed in Figure 35-13.[8]

FACTORS RELATED TO THE DOSAGE FORM

DRUG EXCIPIENT INTERACTION—These interactions can occur during any unit operation, such as mixing, blending, drying, and/or granulating, resulting in a change in dissolution pattern of the dosage form in question.

The effect of magnesium stearate on the disintegration time of tablets containing either potato starch or sodium

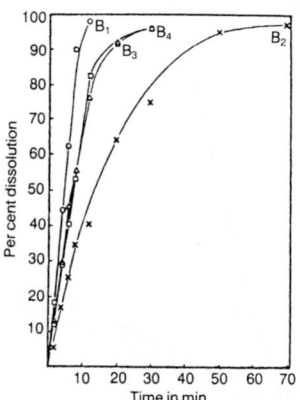

Figure 35-11. Effect of manufacturing process on the dissolution rate of tablets.[7] B_1, Direct compression with spray-dried lactose. B_2, Wet granulation with ethylcellulose and lactose. B_3, Acacia mucilage and lactose. B_4, Starch paste and lactose.

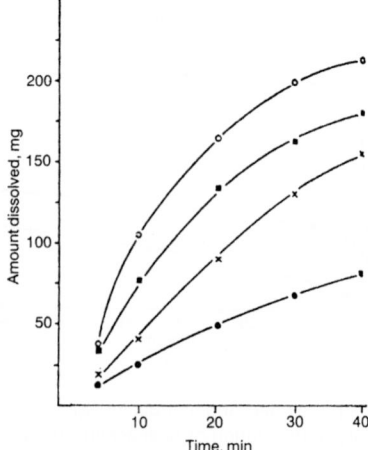

Figure 35-12. Effect of precompression pressure on the dissolution rate of salicylic acid contained in compressed tablets.[4] ●, 715 kg; ×, 1430 kg; □, 2860 kg; ○, 5730 kg pressure per cm.[2] (Average of five tablets each, formula D.)

starch glycolate was found to depend on the swelling characteristics of the disintegrants. These results were attributed to the formation of lubricant film during mixing, which resulted in an increase in disintegration time and thus delayed dissolution.[16]

It is essential that the formulator have a thorough understanding of these interactions so that the most appropriate excipients can be selected to enable the formulator to perform optimally. By minimizing, if not eliminating, these interactions, adverse effects on the performance of the final product can be avoided. It must also be noted that better process control is also possible with noninteracting drug-excipient interactions.

DEAGGREGATION—Deaggregation is often a prerequisite for dissolution. In such cases it can control dissolution. It was reported that two capsule formulations of sodium diphenylhydantoin showed significant deaggregation, dissolution, and thereby absorption rates. The formulation that deaggregated rapidly after the capsule shell was dissolved resulted in exposure of a larger surface area. This resulted in rapid dissolution at neutral pH but less rapid dissolution when both preparations were exposed to 0.1N hydrochloric acid. Aggregation of other formulation inhibited the conversion of most of its sodium salt to the free acid in acidic medium, whereas such conversion occurred readily with the rapidly disintegrating formulation. As a result, after neutralization of the medium, the latter dissolved and absorbed more readily and rapidly than did the former.

EFFECT OF TEST PARAMETERS ON THE DISSOLUTION RATE

ECCENTRICITY OF THE STIRRING DEVICE—USP 26/NF 21 specifies that the stirring shaft must rotate smoothly without significant wobble. Eccentricity can be measured with a machinist's indicator. It is measured in terms of total indicator reading (TIR), which determines the sum of the distance on both sides (180°C) of the axis of rotation.

GUIDING THE SHAFT—One must remember that the shaft of the stirring device extends about 6 in. beyond the chuck. An eccentricity of 0.005 in (0.11 mm) at a distance of 1 in (25 mm) from the chuck will be barely perceptible, but at 6 in it will amount to 0.30 in (0.75 mm), which is the maximum that can be tolerated.

The shaft mounting should not produce perfect concentricity but also allow for ease of vertical adjustment. That can best be obtained with a hollow drive shaft and chuck grip on the output with a guide on the other hand. They must be held to close concentricity tolerances with the axis of rotation of the drive tube. The further apart such guides, the better the probability of minimum wobble at the end of the shaft-provided the shaft is straight. The simple trigonometry is illustrated in the Figure 35-14.[1]

In the lower left view, the distance from the chuck to the basket is approximately 12 in (15 mm). If no guide bushing is used, any inherent eccentricity in the chuck is multiplied 12 times at the basket, which will certainly produce an eccentricity greatly exceeding the acceptable tolerances for eccentricity at the basket or paddle-if not when new, then after the chuck has been in use for a time.

In the lower right view, no guide bushing is used, but the shaft is supported at both the ends of the hollow shaft form A to A and the chuck is brought closer to the flask cover. The inherent eccentricity in the drive (A to A) can be held close at the factory, and the eccentricity of the basket cannot exceed it if the shaft is straight. In this case, the distance form A to A is about 6 in and matches the distance from the chuck head to the basket, also is about 6 in.

Even with a guide bushing, the system shown on the lower left is not recommended because the chuck may have a twist that is corrected by the bushing and that might cause a whip in the shaft with attendant vibration. These problems can be minimized by using a resilient grip in the chuck, such as a rubber "O" ring.

VIBRATION—Vibration is a common variable introduced into the dissolution system from myriad causes. It has the effect of changing the flow patterns of the liquid and of introducing unwanted energy to the dynamic system. Both effects may result in significant changes in the dissolution rates. The speeds of the rotational device selected by official compendium are 50 rpm or 100 rpm. Other speeds are specified for certain drugs. Precise speed control is best obtained with a synchronous motor that locks into the line frequency. Such motors are not only more rugged but are far more reliable. Periodic variations in rpm might result in possible disturbance in rotational devices, is commonly referred to as torsional vibration. Such vibration indicates a variation in the velocity of rotation for short periods of time-although the average velocity is well within ± 4% of the specified rate.

ALIGNMENT OF THE STIRRING ELEMENT—There are two important factors to be considered here. These are as follows:

Tilt—USP 26/NF 21 states that the axis of the stirring element shall not deviate more than 0.2 cm form the axis of the dissolution vessel, which defines centering of the stirring shaft to within ± 2 mm. It also constrains tilt. A series of tests suggest that tilt in excess of 1.5 (degrees) may increase dissolution rates using Method 2 from 2% to 25%,[17] which is still a significant variation. The user should be able to adjust his equipment to obtain alignment of the vertical spindles to within 1 (degrees) perpendicularly with the base of the drive to which the flasks are mounted. Such alignment cannot be ensured in the factory. Adjustments for perpendicularity must therefore be used in order to bring the equipment into alignment in its final position.[18]

Agitation Intensity—The degree of agitation, or the stirring conditions, is one of the most important variables to consider in dissolution. Given the background of various theories of dissolution, it is apparent that agitation conditions can markedly affect diffusion-controlled dissolution, because the thickness of the diffusion layer is

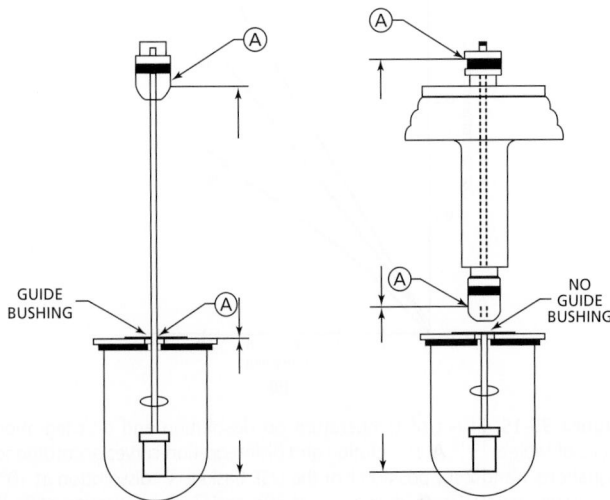

Figure 35-14. The rotating shaft should be supported at two places (A) to minimize wobble, shown by the two arrangements depicted.

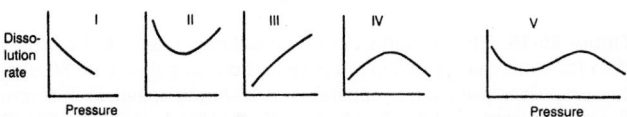

Figure 35-13. Different types of relations between compressional force of tablets and dissolution rate.

inversely proportional to agitation speed. Wurster and Taylor[19] employed the empirical relationship

$$K = a(N)^b \qquad (16)$$

where, N is the agitation rate, K the reaction (dissolution) rate, a and b are constants. For diffusion controlled processes, b = 1. Dissolution that is interfacial-reaction-rate-controlled will be independent of agitation intensity, and thus b = 0.

Agitation intensity within and between various *in vitro* dissolution testing devices can be varied by the dimensions and geometry of the dissolution vessel, volume of dissolution medium, and the degree of agitation or shaking. It is safe to predict that the two dosage forms having particles of differing sizes and densities will not experience identical dissolution system, even though the containers are being subjected to the same rate of rotation as of oscillation.

TEMPERATURE—Because drug solubility is temperature-dependent, careful temperature control during the dissolution process is very important and should be maintained within 0.5°. Generally, a temperature of 37° is always maintained during dissolution determinations. The effect of temperature variations of the dissolution medium depends mainly on the temperature/solubility curves of the drug and excipients in the formulation[20,21] (Fig 35-15).

For a dissolved molecule, the diffusion coefficient, D, depends on the temperature T according to the Stokes equation

$$D = kT/6\pi\eta r \qquad (17)$$

where k is the Boltzmann constant and $6\pi\eta r$ is the Stokes force for a spherical molecule (η is the viscosity in cgs or poise units, and r is the radius of the molecule).

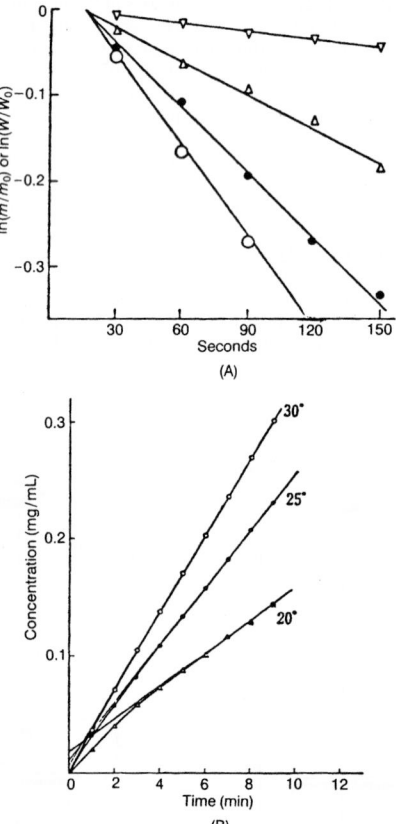

Figure 35-15. Effect of temperature on dissolution and disintegration rates of tablets.[15,16] **A.** Dissolution and disintegration curves according to Equations 1 and 2 for position II of the USP basket. ▽, dissolution at 10°; ○, dissolution at 20°; ●, dissolution at 30°; and ○, disintegration at 5°.[16] **B.** Dissolution of phenobarbital anhydrate at various temperatures (at 300 rpm).

DISSOLUTION MEDIUM

Selection of suitable fluid for dissolution testing depends largely on the solubility of the drug, as well as mere economics and practical reasons.

pH OF THE DISSOLUTION MEDIUM—Great emphasis and effort was first placed on simulating *in vivo* conditions, especially pH, surface tension, viscosity, and sink condition. Most of the early studies were conducted in 0.1N HCl or buffered solutions with a pH close to that of the gastric juice (pH ~ 1.2). The acidic solution tends to disintegrate the tablets slightly faster than water and thereby may enhance the dissolution rate by increasing the effective surface area. However, because of the corroding action of the acid on dissolution equipment, currently it is a general practice to use distilled water unless investigative studies show a specific need for the acidic solution to generate meaningful dissolution data. Another approach for avoiding the deleterious effects of hydrochloric acid is to replace it with acidic buffers, such as sodium acid phosphate, to maintain the required low pH.

SURFACE TENSION OF THE DISSOLUTION MEDIUM—Surface tension has been shown to have a significant effect on the dissolution rate of drugs and their release rate from solid dosage forms. Surfactants and wetting agents lower the contact angle and consequently improve penetration by the dissolution medium. Measurable enhancement in the dissolution rate of salicylic acid from an inert matrix was reported by Singh and co-workers when the contact angle, θ, was lowered from 92° (water) to 31° (using 0.01% dioctyl sodium sulfosuccinate)[22] (Fig 35-16). The surface tension also was correspondingly lowered from 60 to 31 dynes/cm. Similar findings were obtained in benzocaine studies when polysorbate 80 was used as the surface active agent[22] (see Fig 35-16).

Other studies conducted on conventional tablet formulations and capsules also showed significant enhancement in the dissolution rate of poorly soluble drugs when surfactants were added to the dissolution medium, even at a level below the critical micelle concentration, probably by reducing the interfacial

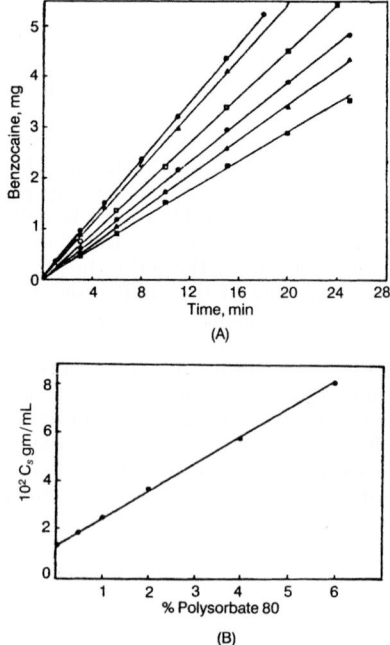

Figure 35-16. Effect of surfactants on dissolution rate.[17] **A.** Dissolution data for benzocaine in different concentrations of polysorbate 80 using the propeller-driven stirrer apparatus at a stirring speed of 150 rpm. Polysorbate conc: ○, 6%; △, 4%; □, 2%; ●, 1%; ▲, 0.5%; □, 0%. **B.** Solubilization data for benzocaine in different concentrations of polysorbate 80.

tension. Low levels of surfactants were recommended to be included in the dissolution medium as this seemed to give a better *in vivo* and *in vitro* correlation.

Finholt and Solvang compared the dissolution behavior of phenacetin and phenobarbital tablets in human gastric juice to that in dilute hydrochloric acid with and without various amounts of polysorbate 80 in the dissolution medium. The data showed that both pH and surface tension have significant influence on the dissolution kinetics of the drug studies. For example, they found that not only was the dissolution rate much faster in diluted gastric juice, but that it increased with decreasing particle size, whereas the opposite was the case when $0.1N$ HCl was used.

VISCOSITY OF THE DISSOLUTION MEDIUM—In case of diffusion-controlled dissolution processes, it would be expected that the dissolution rate decreases with an increase in viscosity. In the case of interfacial-controlled dissolution processes, however, viscosity should have little effect. The Stokes—Einstein equation describes diffusion coefficient, D, as a function of viscosity.

Braun and Parrott showed that the dissolution rate of benzoic acid is inversely proportional to the viscosity of the dissolution medium using various concentrations of sucrose and methylcellulose solutions[23] (Fig 35-17).

MISCELLANEOUS FACTORS

In addition to the factors discussed earlier, there are several other factors that can affect the dissolution characteristics of the drug product.

ADSORPTION—The adsorbent has an influence on the dissolution rate of a slightly soluble solid. It was also reported that the adsorbent is capable of increasing the dissolution rate observed in water under conditions of a decreased concentration gradient applying Nernst-Brunner film theory. Maximum dissolution rate can be obtained when a constant-concentration gradient is maintained. Adsorption isotherms can be employed

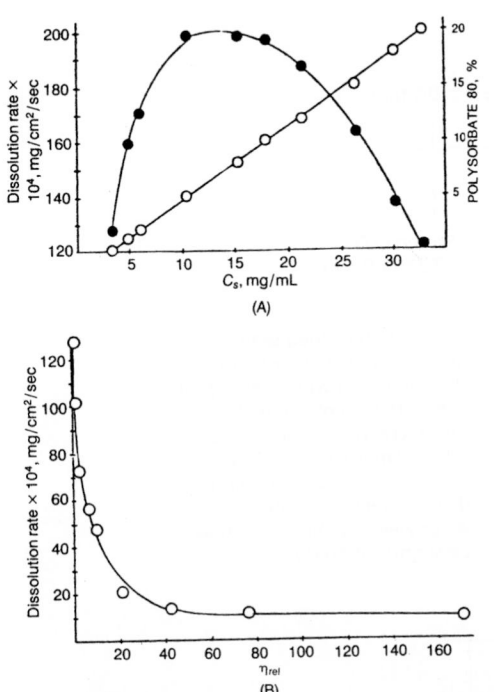

Figure 35-17. Effect of viscosity on dissolution rate.[18] **A.** Relationship of total solubility (C_s) of benzoic acid at 25° to dissolution rate and concentration of polysorbate 80. ●, rate; ○, concentration. **B.** Relationship of viscosity to dissolution rate of benzoic acid in aqueous methylcellulose solutions at 25°.

to calculate the approximate amount of adsorbent required to increase the slower dissolution rate.

SORPTION—The effect of water sorption on disintegration and dissolution properties, among other physical properties, of tablets containing microcrystalline cellulose was examined. It was concluded that water sorption from the atmosphere into the tablet containing microcrystalline cellulose is a very rapid first-order process, resulting in substantial changes in the physical properties. These changes are attributed to the breaking of the hydrogen bonds. The relative density of the tablets was found to decrease, resulting in increased disintegration time with increase in water sorption-rate constants. These changes were found to be irreversible.

HUMIDITY—In relation to the dissolution rate of a drug substance, humidity is usually associated with storage effects. Moisture has shown to influence the dissolution rate of many drugs from solid dosage forms. Environmental conditions to which dosage forms are exposed, moisture in particular, should be rigorously assessed if reproducible and reliable dissolution data are to be obtained. Additionally, humidity during the manufacture of the dosage forms should be carefully controlled to reproduce the quality of the product from batch to batch.

DETECTION ERRORS—Two most common variables leading to interlaboratory disagreement are the failure to use standards during analysis, and external vibration.[24] Extreme care must be exercised when laboratory methods are introduced into quality control to ensure that no part of the equipment interferes with sensitive determinations.

Despite the fundamental relationship between bioavailability and dissolution rate, the present evidence suggests that no single dissolution-rate test can be applied to all drugs. The possibility that a single test may be applied to drugs having similar physicochemical properties remains to be established. These observations are attributable, primarily, to the inability to assess and control the many variables affecting the dissolution process of a drug substance.

COMPENDIAL METHODS—When selecting apparatus for dissolution testing, routine quality control, new drug development, or complying with regulatory requirements, the analyst must follow the latest issue of compendia, including revisions. The modifications introduced in the dissolution testing methods during recent years are numerous that even revisions 2 or 3 years old may be outdated.

USP/NF Method 1 (Rotating Basket Method)—The USP/NF rotating basket method of dissolution testing essentially consists of a 1-in-diameter × 13/ 8-in-high stainless-steel 40-mesh wire basket rotated at a constant speed ranging between 25 and 150 rpm. It is immersed in 900 ml of dissolution medium in a vessel of 1000 ml capacity. The medium in the vessel is maintained at a constant temperature of 37 ± 0.5°C by means of a suitable water bath. The environment in which the apparatus is placed should not contribute significant motion, agitation, or vibration to the assembly. A fitted cover may be used to retard evaporation. The shaft is positioned so that its axis is not more than 2 mm at any point from the vertical axis of the vessel and rotates smoothly without any significant wobble (Fig 35-18).

The dosage unit is placed in a dry basket at the beginning of each test. Distance between inside bottom of the vessel and the basket is maintained at 25 ± 2 mm during the test.

In case of non-disintegrating dosage forms this apparatus is superior to Apparatus 2 since it constrains the dosage form in steady state fluid flow. This method may seem to be inferior for testing of dosage forms, which contain gums due to the clogging of screen matrix. In case of floating dosage forms this method performs well, but care should be taken that excipients do not clog the basket mesh.

USP/NF Method 2 (Rotating Paddle Method)—For all practical purposes the compendial specifications outlined for this method are identical to method 1 except that the paddle is substituted for the rotating basket.

The metallic or suitably inert, rigid blade and shaft comprise a single entity. The paddle and blade shaft may be coated with suitable inert coating. The dosage form is allowed to sink to the bottom of the vessel before rotation of the blade is started. This apparatus is frequently used for both disintegrating and non-disintegrating dosage form at 50 rpm. Other agitation speeds are acceptable with proper justification.

USP/NF permits variation in the paddle method involving the use of a helix of non-reactive material as a "sinker" for floating dosage forms. Anchoring accomplished by such a device has been severely studied (Fig 35-19).

USP/ NF Method 3 (Reciprocating Cylinder)—The assembly consists of a set of cylindrical, flat bottomed glass vessels; a set of glass reciprocating cylinders; stainless steel fittings (type 316 or equivalent) and screens that are made of suitable nonsorbing material and nonreactive material and that are designed to fit the top and bottoms of the reciprocating cylinders; and a motor and drive assembly to reciprocate the cylinders vertically inside the vessels and, if desired, index the reciprocating cylinders horizontally to a different row of vessels. The vessels are immersed in suitable water bath of any size that permits holding the temperature at 37 ± 0.5°C during the test. The components conform to the specifications as shown in the Figure 35-20 unless otherwise specified in the individual monograph.

One advantage of reciprocating cylinder is that gastrointestinal tract conditions can be easily simulated, as it is easy to make time dependent pH changes. This apparatus is most suitable for nondisintegrating (extended release) or delayed-release dosage (enteric coated) dosage forms.

USP Apparatus 4 (Flow-Through Cell)—The assembly consists of a reservoir and a pump for dissolution medium; a flow-through cell; a water bath that maintains dissolution medium at 37 ± 0.5°C. The pump forces the dissolution medium upwards through the flow-through cell. The pump has a delivery range between 240 and 960 ml/ hr, with the standard flow rates of 4, 8, and 16 ml/min. It must be volumetric to deliver constant flow independent of flow resistance in the filter device; the flow profile is sinusoidal with a pulsation of 120 ± 10 pulses per minute.

The components conform to the specifications as shown in the Figure 35-21 unless otherwise specified in the monograph.

The advantages of flow through cell apparatus most often cited are the ability to test drugs of very low aqueous solubility in the open loop mode and the ability to change the pH conveniently during the test. The disadvantage associated with it might be the operational difficulties of preparing large volumes of medium for operation in the open loop mode and the added time in the system set up and cleaning.

USP Apparatus 5 (Paddle Over Disk)—The Apparatus 2 is used, with the addition of a stainless steel disk assembly designed for holding the transdermal system at the bottom of the vessel. Temperature is maintained at 32 ± 0.5°C. A distance of 25 ± 2 mm between the paddle and blade and the surface of the disk assembly is maintained during the test. The vessel may be covered during the test to minimize evaporation. Disk assembly for holding the transdermal system is designed to minimize any 'dead' volume between the disk assembly and the bottom of the

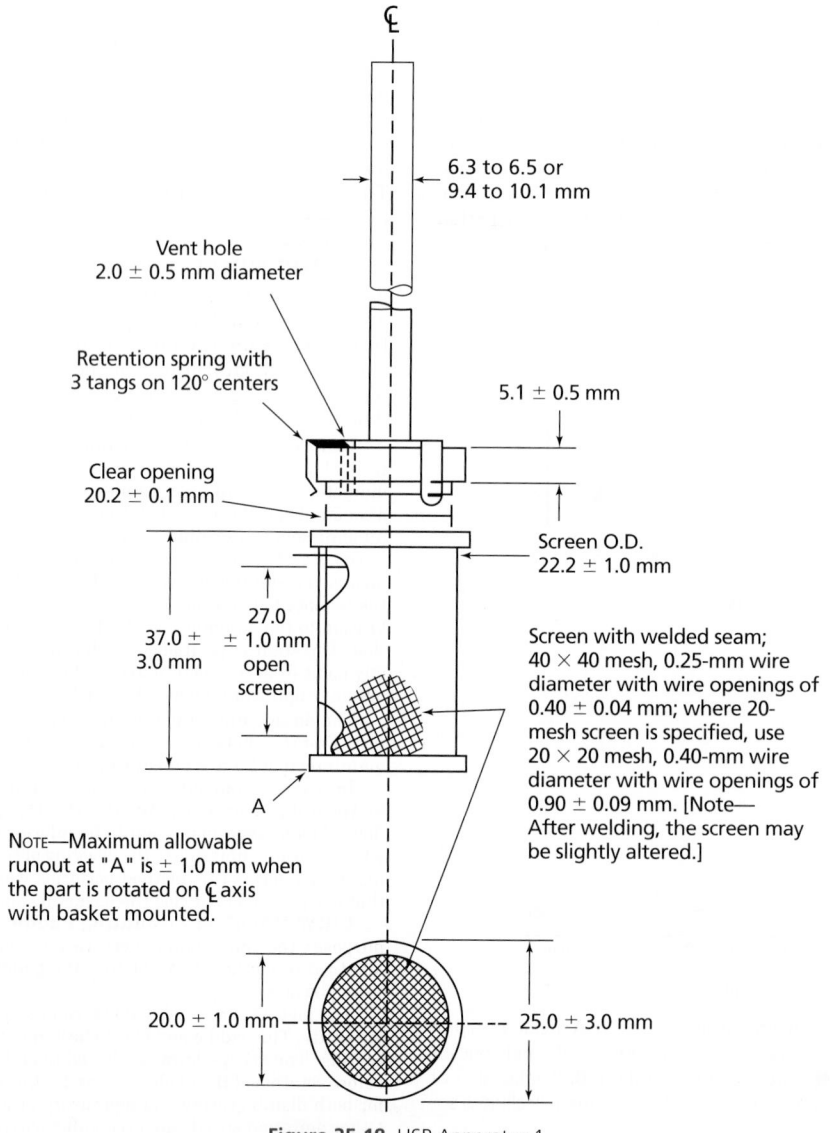

Figure 35-18. USP Apparatus 1.

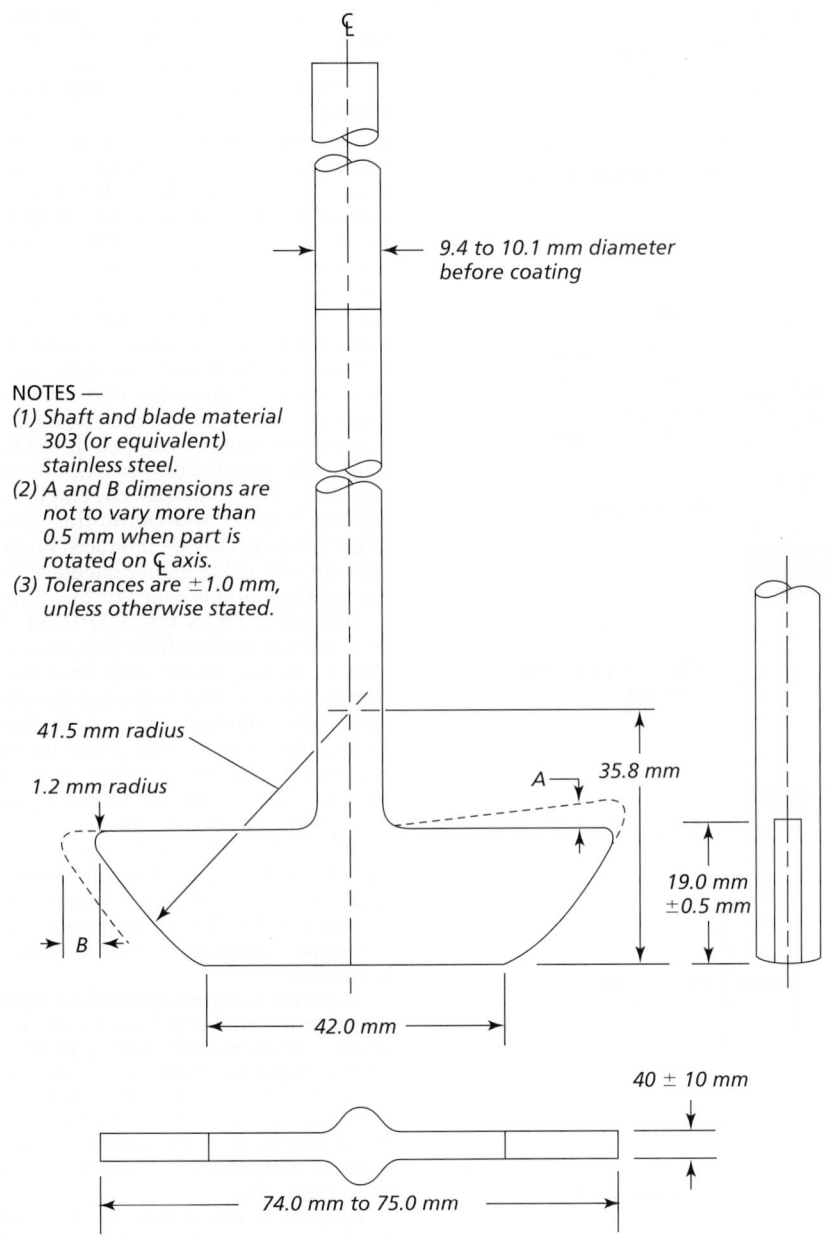

NOTES —
(1) *Shaft and blade material 303 (or equivalent) stainless steel.*
(2) *A and B dimensions are not to vary more than 0.5 mm when part is rotated on ₵ axis.*
(3) *Tolerances are ±1.0 mm, unless otherwise stated.*

9.4 to 10.1 mm diameter before coating

41.5 mm radius

1.2 mm radius

A

35.8 mm

19.0 mm ±0.5 mm

B

42.0 mm

40 ± 10 mm

74.0 mm to 75.0 mm

Figure 35-19. USP Apparatus 2.

vessel. Disk assembly holds the system flat and is positioned such that the release surface is parallel with the bottom of the paddle blade. For more specifications refer to Figure 35-22.

USP Apparatus 6 (Cylinder)—The vessel assembly used is same as Apparatus 1, except the basket and the shaft is replaced with a stainless steel cylinder stirring element and to maintain the temperature at $32 \pm 0.5°C$ during the test. The shaft and cylinder components of the stirring element are fabricated of stainless steel to the specifications as shown in Figure 35-23. The dosage units are placed on the cylinder at the beginning of each test. The distance between the inside of the vessel and the cylinder is maintained at 25 ± 2 mm during the test.

USP Apparatus 7 (Reciprocating Cylinder)—The assembly consists of a set of volumetrically calibrated or tared solution containers made of glass or other suitable inert material, a motor and drive assembly to reciprocate the system vertically and to index the system horizontally to a different row of vessels automatically if desired, and a set of suitable sample holders. For details on specifications refer to the Figure 35-24.

DISSOLUTION OF IMMEDIATE RELEASE SOLID ORAL DOSAGE FORMS—*In vitro* dissolution tests for immediate release solid oral dosage forms, such as tablets and capsules, are used to (I) assess the lot-to-lot quality of a drug product; (II) guide development of new formulations; (III) ensure continuing product quality and performance.

For the drug approval process, it is essential to have the current knowledge about solubility, permeability, dissolution, and pharmacokinetics of a drug product. Based on drug solubility and permeability, the following Biopharmaceutical Classification System (BCS) is recommended in the literature[25]:

Case 1: High solubility-High permeability drugs
Case 2: Low solubility- High permeability drugs
Case 3: High solubility- Low permeability drugs
Case 4: Low solubility-Low permeability drugs

This classification can be used as a basis for setting *in vitro* dissolution specifications and *in vivo—in vitro* correlation

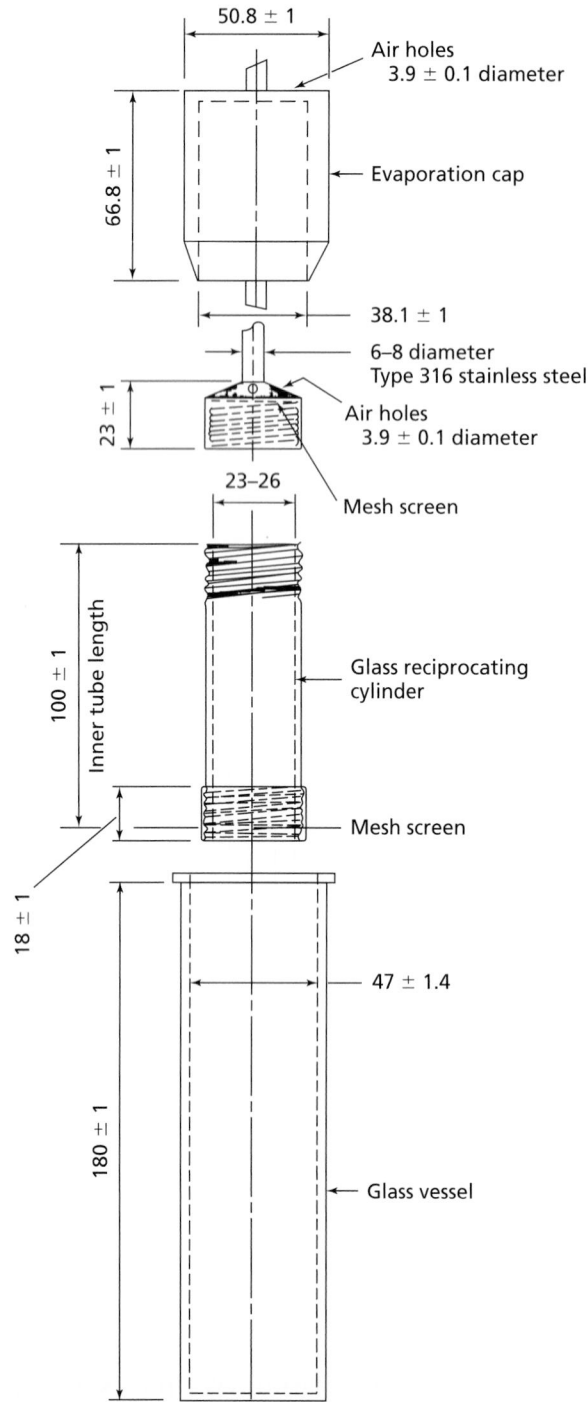

Figure 35-20. USP Apparatus 3. All measurements are expressed in mm unless noted otherwise.

relative rates of dissolution and intestinal transit. Drugs in low solubility, low permeability (Case 4) present significant problems for oral drug delivery.

DISSOLUTION OF ORALLY DISINTEGRATING TABLETS [26]—Orally disintegrating tablets (ODT) are solid dosage forms that disintegrate in the oral cavity leaving an easy to swallow residue. ODT in general have high porosity, low density, and low hardness. The time for disintegration for ODT is usually considered to be less than 1 minute. Development of dissolution methods for ODT is comparable to the approach taken for conventional tablets except when the tablets utilize taste masking. Media that can be used are 0.1 N hydrochloric acid, and pH 4.5 and 6.8 buffers. The most commonly used apparatus for running dissolution test for ODT is USP Apparatus 2 (Paddle method) with a paddle speed of 50 rpm. USP Apparatus 1 is less frequently used due to the physical properties of these tablets, as the tablet fragments or disintegrated tablet masses may become trapped in the basket yielding poorly reproducible dissolution profiles. Since dissolution for ODT is very fast, slower speeds are employed. In case of tablets exceeding 1 gram and containing relatively denser particles larger mounds may be produced on dissolution, which may be prevented by using higher paddle speeds. These two situations expand the suitable range to 25–75 rpm.

DISSOLUTION OF TOPICAL DOSAGE FORMS [27]— Drug-release studies from gels, creams, and ointments are becoming an important step both during the developmental stages of new formulations and as a routine quality control test for assuring the uniformity of the finished product. Also these studies often can provide useful information on some physicochemical parameters involved in the *in vivo* percutaneous absorption, such as the diffusion coefficient and the solubility of the drug in the specific vehicle used.

Although many investigators have conducted drug release-rate studies from topical dosage forms, it appears that no single apparatus or procedure has yet emerged as the most favored, or to be accepted widely as a quasi-standard for others in the field. According to FDA guidelines the most commonly used method is as follows:

In vitro dissolution method for topical dosage forms is based on an open chamber diffusion cell system such as a Franz cell system, fitted usually with a synthetic membrane. The test product is placed on the upper side of the membrane in the open donor chamber of the diffusion cell and a sampling fluid is placed on the other side of the membrane in a receptor cell. Diffusion of drug from the topical product to and across the membrane is monitored by assay of sequentially collected samples of the receptor fluid.

Aliquots removed from the receptor phase can be analyzed for drug content by high-pressure liquid chromatography (HPLC) or other analytical methodology.

DISSOLUTION OF SUSPENSIONS—Although most dissolution studies during the last two decades have concentrated on tablets and capsules, some studies have pointed to the importance of the dissolution characteristics of drugs administered in suspension. This hardly is surprising, as suspensions are similar to the disintegrated form of tablets and capsules; if dissolution has become a priority for these formulations; it is logical to extend its concept to suspensions. Indeed, several studies have shown that the absorption of several poorly soluble drugs administered in suspension formulations is dissolution rate—limited.

Such *in vivo/in vitro* correlation studies have confirmed the importance and the viability of dissolution rate determinations of suspensions as a discriminative test for rapid screening of new formulations and to control lot-to-lot variability within the same manufacturer and between different commercial manufacturers. In general, most of the dissolution apparatuses that have been described for tablets and capsules easily could be used for suspensions.

The USP Apparatus 2 (Paddle) has been used frequently at a rotation speed between 25 to 50 rpm. However, the rotating filter apparatus by Shah has gained wide acceptance for sus-

(IVIVC). The BCS suggests that for high solubility, high permeability (Case 1) drugs and in some cases for high solubility, low permeability (Case 3) drugs, 85% dissolution in 0.1N HCl in 15 minutes can ensure that the bioavailability is not limited by dissolution. In case of low solubility, high permeability drugs (Case 2), drug dissolution may be the rate-limiting step for drug absorption and an IVIVC may be expected. A dissolution profile in multiple media is recommended for drug products in this category. In case of high solubility, low permeability drugs (Case 3), permeability is the rate controlling step and a limited IVIVC may be possible, depending on the

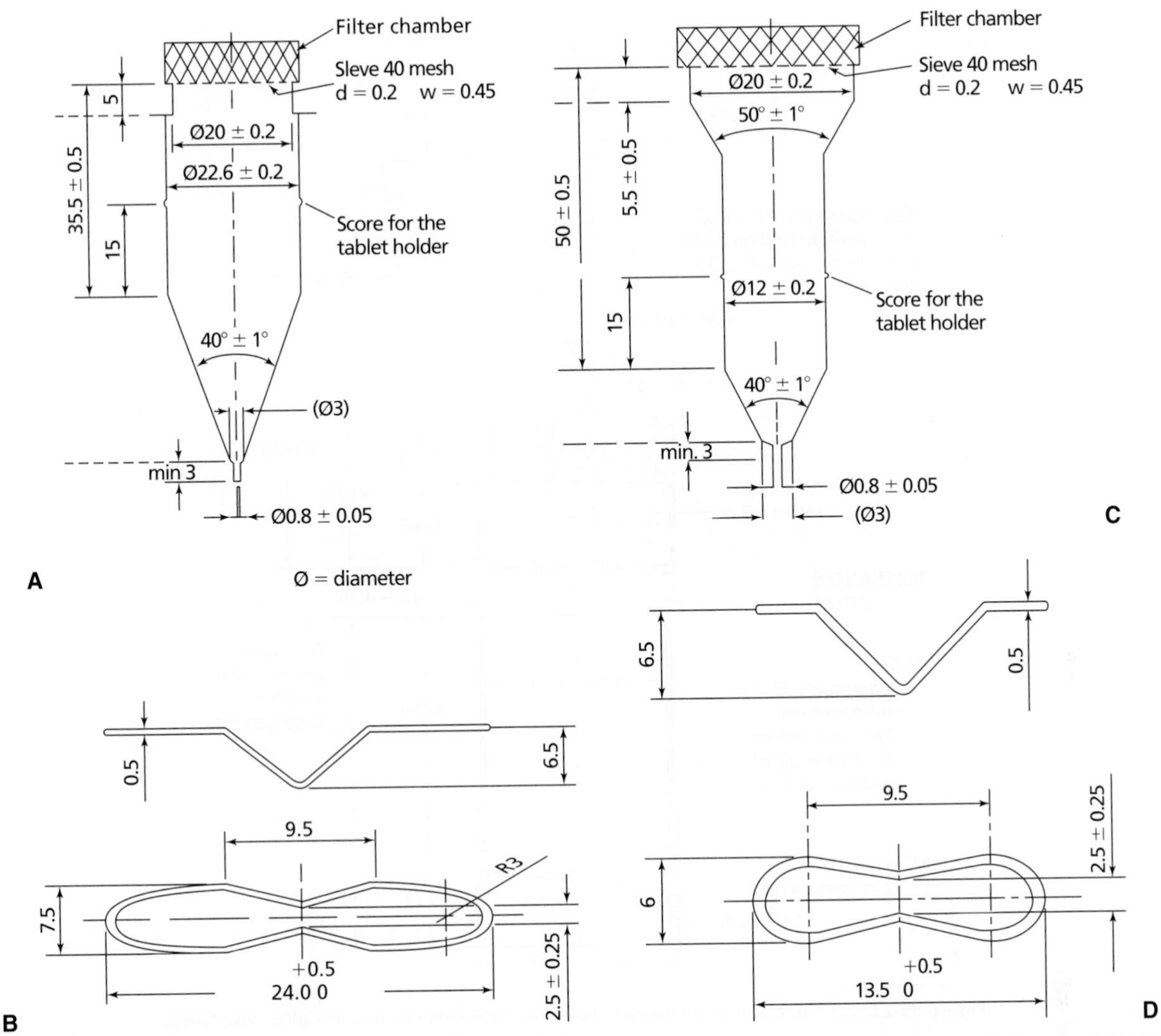

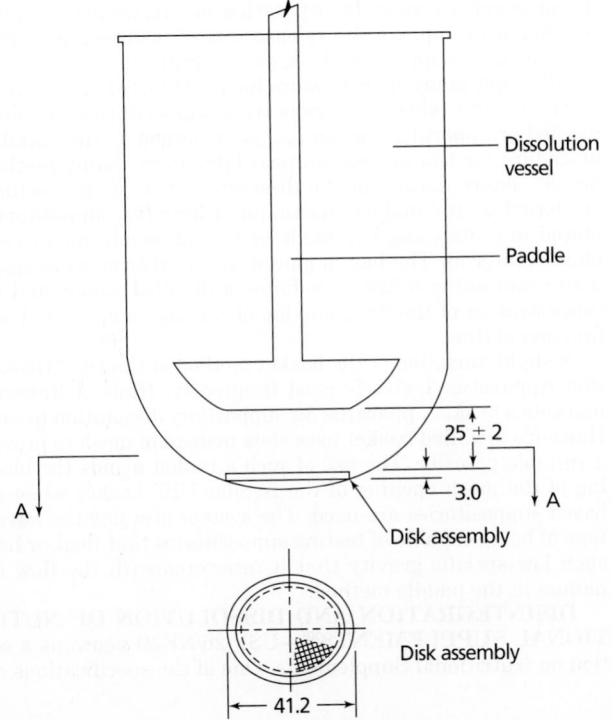

A. Large cell for tablets and capsules

Filter chamber

Sleve 40 mesh
d = 0.2   w = 0.45

Ø20 ± 0.2

Ø22.6 ± 0.2

Score for the
tablet holder

40° ± 1°

(Ø3)

min 3

Ø0.8 ± 0.05

35.5 ± 0.5

5

15

Ø = diameter

A

C. Small cell

Filter chamber

Sieve 40 mesh
d = 0.2   w = 0.45

Ø20 ± 0.2

50° ± 1°

Ø12 ± 0.2

Score for the
tablet holder

40° ± 1°

min. 3

Ø0.8 ± 0.05

(Ø3)

50 ± 0.5

5.5 ± 0.5

15

C

B. Tablet holder large cell

0.5

6.5

9.5

R3

7.5

24.0 +0.5 0

2.5 ± 0.25

B

D. Tablet holder small cell

6.5

0.5

9.5

2.5 ± 0.25

6

13.5 +0.5 0

D

Figure 35-21. USP Apparatus 4. **A.** Large cell for tablets and capsules. All measurements are expressed in mm unless noted otherwise. **B.** Tablet holder for the large cell. All measurements are expressed in mm unless noted otherwise. **C.** Small cell for tablets and capsules. All measurements are expressed in mm unless noted otherwise. **D.** Tablet holder for small cell. All measurements are expressed in mm unless noted otherwise.

Dissolution
vessel

Paddle

25 ± 2

3.0

A   A

Disk assembly

Disk assembly

41.2

Figure 35-22. USP Apparatus 5 (paddle over disk). All measurements are expressed in mm unless noted otherwise.

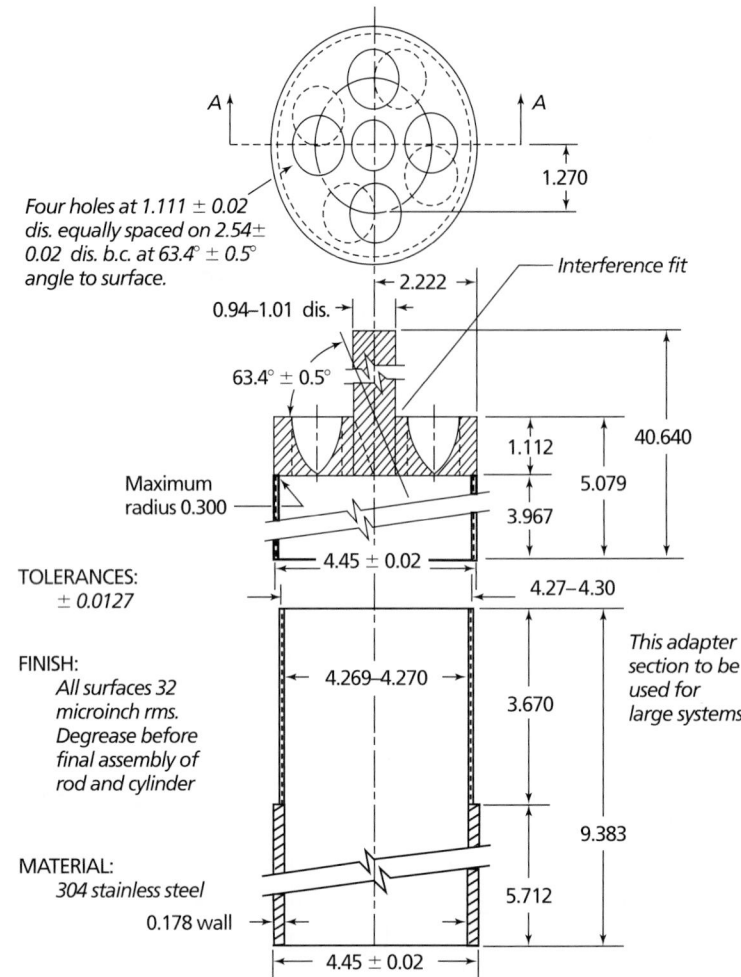

Four holes at 1.111 ± 0.02 dis. equally spaced on 2.54± 0.02 dis. b.c. at 63.4° ± 0.5° angle to surface.

Interference fit

0.94–1.01 dis.

63.4° ± 0.5°

2.222

1.270

Maximum radius 0.300

1.112

40.640

5.079

3.967

4.45 ± 0.02

4.27–4.30

TOLERANCES:
± 0.0127

FINISH:
All surfaces 32 microinch rms. Degrease before final assembly of rod and cylinder

4.269–4.270

This adapter section to be used for large systems

3.670

9.383

MATERIAL:
304 stainless steel

0.178 wall

5.712

4.45 ± 0.02

Figure 35-23. USP Apparatus 6. All measurements are expressed in cm unless otherwise noted.

pensions because it provides mild laminar liquid agitation, and it also functions as an *in situ* nonclogging filter. Sufficient volume of the dissolution medium should be used to maintain sink condition (about 900–1000 mL), and a temperature of 37° should be maintained.

DISSOLUTION OF SUPPOSITORIES—Although most of the early work on suppositories has been concerned with their physical characteristics, such as softening and liquefaction ranges, homogeneity, smoothness, and neutrality, several reports appeared in the early literature pointing to the direct correlation between their efficacy and the release characteristics of the active ingredients. It has been reported that fatty bases, such as the popular cocoa butter, tend to release hy-

drophobic drugs, which are highly soluble in the oily base, very slowly. Emulsification of the fatty base significantly improved the drug-release rate. Incorporation of surface-active agents was found to improve the release rate of water-soluble drugs from the fatty suppository base dramatically.

Although many investigators have conducted extensive research on the release of drugs from suppositories, no single method or apparatus design has yet emerged as the standard procedure for the pharmaceutical laboratory. Many methods for the determination of the dissolution rate of suppositories are based on the dialysis technique, where the suppository is placed in a dialyzing bag made of special membrane or cellophane material. The bag is placed in a beaker or wide-mouth bottle containing a known volume of distilled water, and the concentration of the drug outside of the bag is measured as a function of time.

A slight variation of the basket method of the USP Dissolution Apparatus 1 also is used frequently. Hanson Research markets a basket apparatus for suppository dissolution testing. Hanson's modified basket uses slots instead of mesh to provide a suitable porosity. The use of such a basket avoids the blocking of the mesh opening of the regular USP basket when oil-based suppositories are used. The system also has the advantage of being capable of testing suppositories that float or have such low specific gravity that it interferes with the flow dynamics in the paddle method.

DISINTEGRATION AND DISSOLUTION OF NUTRITIONAL SUPPLEMENTS[28]—USP 26/NF 21 contains a section on Nutritional Supplements. One of the specifications ap-

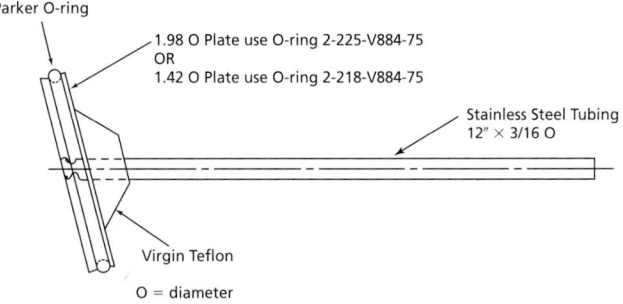

Parker O-ring

1.98 O Plate use O-ring 2-225-V884-75
OR
1.42 O Plate use O-ring 2-218-V884-75

Stainless Steel Tubing 12″ × 3/16 O

Virgin Teflon

O = diameter

Figure 35-24. USP Apparatus 7. Transdermal system holder-angled disk

pearing in the monographs for some of the supplement dosage forms is Disintegration and Dissolution, 2040. The dissolution procedures for the nutritional supplements use Apparatus 1 and Apparatus 2 and require measurement of one vitamin and folic acid (if applicable) and one mineral (if applicable). Oil-soluble vitamins are exempted from the dissolution requirement.

DISSOLUTION OF MODIFIED RELEASE DOSAGE FORMS[27]—

Extended Release—In addition to application/compendial release requirements, multipoint dissolution profiles should be obtained in three other media, for example, in water, 0.1N HCl, and USP buffer media at pH 4.5, and 6.8 for the drug product. Adequate sampling should be performed, for example, at 1, 2, and 4 hours and every 2 hours thereafter until either 80% of the drug from the drug product is released or an asymptote is reached. A surfactant may be used with appropriate justification.

Delayed Release—In addition to application/compendial release requirements, dissolution tests should be performed in 0.1 N HCl for 2 hours (acid stage) followed by testing in USP buffer media, in the range of pH 4.5-7.5 (buffer stage) under standard (application/compendial) test conditions and two additional agitation speeds using the application/compendial test apparatus (three additional test conditions). If the application/compendial test apparatus is the rotating basket method (Apparatus 1), a rotation speed of 50, 100, and 150 rpm may be used, and if the application/compendial test apparatus is the rotating paddle method (Apparatus 2), a rotation speed of 50, 75, and 100 rpm may be used. Multipoint dissolution profiles should be obtained during the buffer stage of testing. Adequate sampling should be performed, for example, at 15, 30, 45, 60, and 120 minutes (following the time from which the dosage form is placed in the buffer) until either 80% of the drug from the drug product is released or an asymptote is reached.

DISSOLUTION PROFILE COMPARISONS

In the presence of minor changes, single point dissolution tests have been employed in evaluating scale-up and post approval changes.[29] For major changes, a dissolution profile comparison performed under identical conditions for the product before and after the change is recommended. Dissolution profile comparison may be carried out using the model dependent or model independent methods. One such model independent approach has been explained in the following paragraph.

Model Independent Approach Using A Similarity Factor

This approach uses a difference factor (f_1) and a similarity factor (f_2) to compare the dissolution profiles. The difference factor (f_1) calculates the percent (%) difference the two curves at each time point and is a measurement of the relative error between the two curves:

$$f_1 = \left\{ \left[\sum_{t=1}^{n} |R_t - T_1| \right] / \left[\sum_{t=1}^{n} R_t \right] \right\} \cdot 100$$

Where n is the number of time points, R_t is the dissolution value of the reference batch (prechange) at time t, and T_t is the dissolution value of the test (postchange) batch at time t.

The similarity factor (f_2) is a logarithmic reciprocal square root transformation of the sum of squared error and is a measurement of the similarity in the percent (%) dissolution between the curves.

$$f_2 = 50 \cdot \log \left\{ \left[1 + \left(\frac{1}{n} \right) \sum_{t=1}^{n} |R_t - T_t|^2 \right]^{-0.5} \cdot 100 \right\}$$

In order to calculate the difference and similarity factor, first the dissolution profile should be done for 12 units each of the prechange and the postchange products. The difference factor (f_1) and similarity (f_2) can be calculated using the mean dissolution values from both curves at each time interval. For the curves to be considered similar, f_1 values should be close to 0,

and f_2 values close to 100. This model independent method is most suitable for dissolution profile comparison when three or four more dissolution time points are available.

Automation in Dissolution Testing

Due to the large amount of testing required in determining dissolution rate of drugs, automation of the process seemed almost a necessity and not simply a convenience to the analyst. Also, because of modular nature of the dissolution apparatus, automation can be accomplished easily in different ways and by various techniques.

At present, however, the setup of the apparatus, media preparation, and introduction of the dosage forms mostly are done manually. The rest of the process—including the withdrawal of samples, maintenance of a certain pH or of sink conditions, assay performance, and data acquisition and calculations—is in most cases fully automated. The automation process not only saves money, time, and effort on the part of the analyst, but more significantly it improves the overall reliability and enhances the reproducibility of testing procedures.

Several commercial companies have also introduced semi- and fully automated dissolution systems. Some of these are the Hanson Research Dissolution System (Northridge, CA; Dissoette and Dissograph apparatuses), Technicon (Tarrytown, NY; Sasdra apparatus), and Applied Analytical (Wilmington, NC).

Millipore's Waters Chromatography Division has introduced a fully automated dissolution system using a Waters pump, detector, and autosampler combined with a Hanson Research's dissolution bath and sample transfer system. Samples are analyzed by HPLC, which provides better specificity than ultraviolet (UV) methods of analysis.

Hewlett-Packard manufactures a fully automated dissolution-sampling and UV analysis system that can analyze samples from three dissolution baths. One such system is model 2100 C (Fig 35-25) dissolution test system.[30] The Model 2100C combines enhanced features with advanced communications to ensure reproducibility and control throughout the dissolution testing process. The operations are technician-friendly. Its convenient vessel layout simplifies manual or automatic sampling. It has built-in height adjustment and permanent centering which reduces operator errors. It also has chuckless spindles to reduce setup time. The precision control of variables provides most accurate and repeatable results. The unique water bath flow characteristics maintains vessel temperature to better than ± 0.1°C. It has versatile SystemLink™ for PC communication and printer output, and can be configured for use both with basket and paddles.

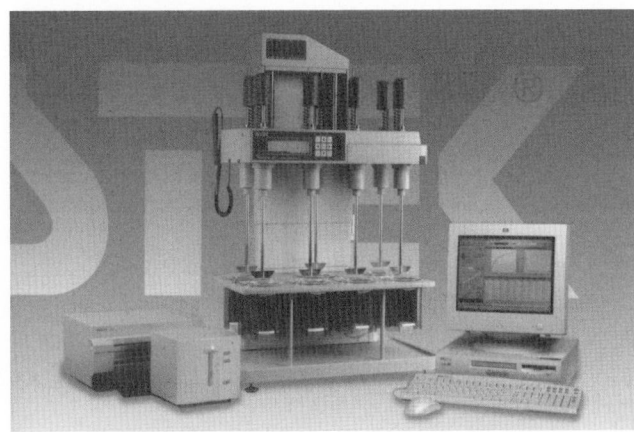

Figure 35-25. Distek dissolution system.

Validation of Dissolution Method

In general, the approach to validation of a dissolution method is similar to that of any other method. The following discussion briefly summarizes the approach to dissolution assay validation.[31]

LINEARITY, FILTER BIAS, AND RECOVERY STUDIES—The linearity of the detection method, the filter bias, and the recovery of drug from dissolution fluid containing placebo should be determined. System suitability tests for UV-Vis and chromatographic methods are also identified at this stage.

PRECISION AND RUGGEDNESS—Precision testing of the dissolution method should be performed on at least two lots of six tablets each on 2 days. The average of each run, as well as the standard and relative standard deviations, should be computed. Precision of the dissolution method is usually expressed as the standard deviation for a data set obtained on a single day.

EFFECT OF DISSOLVED GASES—Air dissolved in the media may form bubbles that in turn could coat the tablets or other dosage form. This is the most likely to happen as the medium is heated to test temperature (37°C). The coating can affect the drug release by altering the dissolution and disintegration or dissolution of the tablet. Accordingly, the effect of deaeration on the dissolution rate should be evaluated or deaerated medium should be specified in the procedure. Effective methods of deaeration include vacuum filtration, helium sparging, hot water placed under a vacuum with or without sonication, and the use of a commercially available medium dispensing device.[32]

AUTOMATION—Validation for automated systems is the same as for manual sampling. A simple experiment should be done in order to verify that the drug does not adsorb to the apparatus tubing and to quantify system carryover.

REFERENCES

1. Banakar UV. *Pharmaceutical Dissolution Testing*, 1st ed. New York: Marcel Dekker, 1991.
2. Carstensen TJ. *Dissolution—State of the Art 1982.* (Proc 2nd WI Update Conf) Madison, WI: Extension Services in Pharmacy, University of Wisconsin, 1982.
3. Morrison AB, Campbell JA. *J Pharm Sci* 1965; 54(1):1–8.
4. Wagner JG. *Biopharmaceutics and Relevant Pharmacokinetics*, 2nd ed. Hamilton: Drug Intelligence Publications, 1971, pp 190–196.
5. Abdou H. *Dissolution, Bioavailability and Bioequivalence.* Easton, PA: Mack, 1989, Chap 2.
6. Cox D, Douglas C, Furman W, et al. *Pharm Tech* 1978; 2(4):40–53.
7. Viegas TX, Curatella LVW, Brinker G. *Pharm Tech* 2001; 44–53.
8. Finholt P. In: Leeson LJ, Carstensen TJ, eds. *Dissolution Technology.* Washington, DC: APhA, 1974, p 108.
9. Aguiar AJ, Krc J, Kinkel AW, et al. *J Pharm Sci* 1967; 56(7):847–853.
10. Solvang S, Finholt P. *J Pharm Sci* 1970; 59(1): 49–52.
11. Jaminet F, Delattre L, Delporte JP. *Pharma Acta Helvetiae* 1969; 44(7):418–432.
12. Alam AS, Parrott EL. *J Pharm Sci* 1971; 60(2):263–266.
13. Levy G, et al. *J Pharm Sci* 1963; 52:1047.
14. Levy G, Gumtow RH. *J Pharm Sci* 1963; 52:1139.
15. Marlowe E, Shangraw R. *J Pharm Sci* 1967; 56:498.
16. Murthy KS, Samyn JC. *J Pharm Sci* 1977; 66(9):1215–1219.
17. Hanson W, Hanson R. *Pharm Tech* 1979; 3(3):42–50.
18. Thakker K, Naik N, Gray V, et al. *Pharm Forum* 1980; 6:177–185.
19. Wurster DE, Taylor PW. *J Pharm Sci* 1965; 54(5):670–676.
20. Nogami H. *Chem Pharm Bull* 1969; 17:499.
21. Carstensen TJ, et al. *J Pharm Sci* 1980; 69:291.
22. Singh P, et al. *J Pharm Sci* 1968; 57:959.
23. Braun R, Parrott E. *J Pharm Sci* 1972; 61:175.
24. Cartwright AC. *J Pharm Pharmacol* 1979; 31:434–440.
25. Amidon GL, Lennernas H, Shah VP, et al. *Pharm Res* 1995; 12:413–420.
26. Klancke J. *Dissolution Technologies* 2003; 10(2):6–8.
27. http://www.fda.gov/cder/guidance/1447fnl.pdf
28. US Pharmacopeia 26/ National Formulary 21
29. Moore JW, Flanner HH. *Pharm Tech* 1996; 20(6):64–74.
30. www.distek.com
31. Skug JW, et al. *Pharm Tech* 58, 1996.
32. Rohrs BR, Stelzer D J. *Dissolution Technologies* 1995; 2(2).

PART 5

Pharmaceutical Manufacturing

Linda Felton, PhD, BSPharm, RPh

Associate Professor of Pharmaceutics

University of New Mexico

College of Pharmacy

Albuquerque, NM

Although the purpose of using CCD is to bring about the separation of two or more substances, the basic principles of operation are best introduced by first considering the distribution pattern of a single solute in the two immiscible solvents.

1. Assume that the solute under consideration has a distribution coefficient of unity when distributed between chloroform and buffer solution and that there are no deviations from Nernst's law of distribution due to molecular association, dissociation, ionization, or chemical reactions.
2. Consider six containers such as 250-mL glass-stoppered Erlenmeyer flasks, each holding 50 mL of chloroform (lower phase) as shown in Figure 36-1 (Row A). Add to container No 0, 100 mg of solute under consideration dissolved in 50 mL of buffer solution, and shake until equilibrium has been established. Because equal volumes of solvent are used and the distribution coefficient of solute in these two solvents is unity, the solute at equilibrium will distribute itself in such a way that one-half is found in each of the upper and lower phases (Row B). Because 100 mg was originally present, 50 mg will be found in both layers of Container 0 (Row B).
3. Transfer the upper phase of Container 0 holding 50 mg of solute to Container 1 (Row B) and add fresh buffer solution to Container 0 (Row B). Shake both containers until equilibrium has been established. At equilibrium the quantity of solute in each phase of Containers 0 and 1 (Row C) will be 25 mg.
4. Transfer the upper phase of Container 1 (Row C) to Container 2 (Row C), and the upper phase of Container 0 (Row C) to Container 1. Add fresh buffer solution to Container 0 (Row C) and shake all three containers until equilibrium has been established. At equilibrium the quantity of solute (25 mg) in Container 2 (Row D) will have distributed itself so that one-half (12.5 mg) is in the upper phase and one-half (12.5 mg) is in the lower phase. Because 25 mg of solute was transferred to Container 1 from Container 0, 25 mg of solute will be present in each phase of Container 1 (Row D). The quantity (25 mg) of solute in Container 0 will distribute itself between the chloroform layer and freshly added buffer solution so that one-half (12.5 mg) will be present in each layer (Row D).

Continue this general procedure of transferring the upper phases of Containers 0, 1, and 2 to Containers 1, 2, and 3, respectively; then add fresh buffer to Container 0. Shake the four flasks until equilibrium is established. A distribution is obtained as shown in Row E. Continuing in a like manner will give a distribution as shown in Row F.

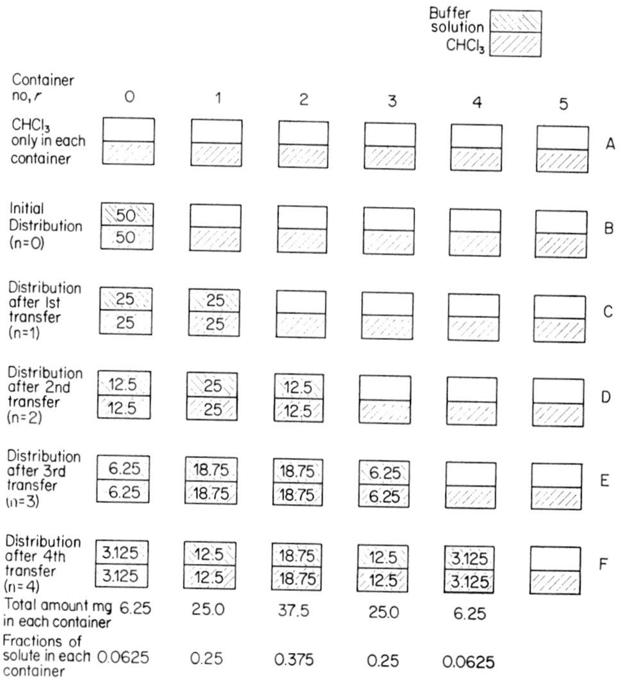

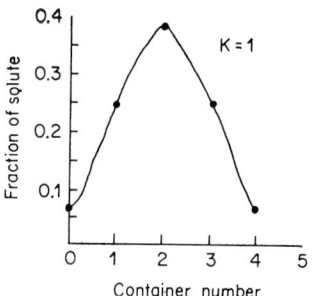

Figure 36-2. Distribution of solute after four transfers.

A plot of the fraction of solute in each container versus container number is shown in Figure 36-2. The significance of this curve is that the distribution of the solute shows a peak in which the maximum is located in a specific container and the location of the peak container is a function of the partition coefficient. Hence, it can be seen that two or more solutes with different K values can be separated effectively after the passage of a mixture through many tubes (usually 25 or more, depending upon K values) in a CCD apparatus.

Figure 36-2 illustrates the distribution of a solute after only four transfers. In actual practice between 8 and 2000 containers or tubes usually are used in multiple extractions of this kind. The tubes are connected in series in a train and are rocked simultaneously rather than individually to bring about distribution of solutes between the two phases. The device also permits the transfer of upper phases to the next tube in series, in one operation. A device of this type is called a countercurrent distribution apparatus.

To study the fraction of a given solute present in each tube r, after n number of transfers, it is convenient to use Equation 2,

$$f_{n,r} = \frac{n!}{r!(n-r)!}\left(\frac{1}{1+KR}\right)^n (KR)^r \qquad (2)$$

where K is defined as the partition coefficient and R is defined as the ratio of the volume of the upper phase to the volume of the lower phase, (V_u/V_l).

The use of Equation 2 is illustrated as follows: Calculate the fraction of solute in tubes no 0, 1, 2, 3, and 4 after four transfers are made in a CCD apparatus using equal volumes of upper and lower phases. The K value for the solute in the solvent system is assumed to be 1.0 in this example.

For Tube 3,

$$f_{4,3} = \frac{4!}{3!(4-3)!}\left(\frac{1}{1+1}\right)^4 (1)^3 = 0.25$$

By similar calculations the fraction of solutes in Tube 0, 1, 2, and 4 is found to equal

$$f_{4,0} = 0.0625; \ f_{4,1} = 0.25; \ f_{4,2} = 0.375; \ f_{4,4} = 0.0625$$

The distribution of solute using Equation 2 is shown in Figure 36-2.

When a large number of transfers (50) are made and K is near unity it is more convenient to use a Gaussian treatment[2] to calculate the fraction of solute in a particular tube. The appropriate equations are

$$y_x = \frac{1.00}{\sqrt{2\pi nKR/(KR+1)^2}} \exp\left\{-\left(\frac{x^2}{2nKR/(KR+1)^2}\right)\right\} \quad (3)$$

$$\tau_{max} = \frac{nKR}{KR+1} \qquad (4)$$

where y_x represents the fraction of solute with distribution coefficient K in the tube that is x distant from the peak tube; exp is the exponent of the base e, ex, exp2 = e^2; π = 3.14; K, R, and n are terms that have been defined previously and r_{max} represents the number of the tube containing the maximum amount of solute.

	Buffer solution				
	CHCl₃				

Container no, r	0	1	2	3	4	5	
CHCl₃ only in each container							A
Initial Distribution (n=0)	50 / 50						B
Distribution after 1st transfer (n=1)	25 / 25	25 / 25					C
Distribution after 2nd transfer (n=2)	12.5 / 12.5	25 / 25	12.5 / 12.5				D
Distribution after 3rd transfer (n=3)	6.25 / 6.25	18.75 / 18.75	18.75 / 18.75	6.25 / 6.25			E
Distribution after 4th transfer (n=4)	3.125 / 3.125	12.5 / 12.5	18.75 / 18.75	12.5 / 12.5	3.125 / 3.125		F
Total amount mg in each container	6.25	25.0	37.5	25.0	6.25		
Fractions of solute in each container	0.0625	0.25	0.375	0.25	0.0625		

Figure 36-1. Theoretical distribution of solute after varying numbers of transfer.

Distribution curves may be prepared from hypothetical data using Equations 3 and 4 or from a computer program using these equations. Figure 36-3 illustrates a series of curves for a solute in which $K = 1.0$ and $R = 1.0$ following 8, 32, and 128 transfers. It is interesting to observe that as the number of transfers increases, the amplitude of the curve decreases and the solute spreads through more and more tubes. At first thought, this would seem undesirable, but the significant point is that the fraction of vessels containing solute after 128 transfers is now much less than after 10 transfers.

Therefore, two solutes with different but similar K values can be separated in 128 transfers because each solute occupies a smaller fraction of total tubes. If this separation were attempted with 10 to 20 transfers, both solutes would occupy nearly all of the tubes and no separation would be obtained.

Figure 36-4 illustrates the distribution patterns obtained in a 16-transfer experiment for solutes having distribution coefficients that differ by one order of magnitude. Under no circumstances can a separation be obtained if the distribution coefficients of the solutes are equal.

The procedure of operation that has been considered thus far is known as the *fundamental procedure*. Here, the solute is distributed through a specified number of tubes and nothing is withdrawn from the system until the entire operation is completed. Then the tube contents are withdrawn and analyzed for the purpose of determining solute concentrations, or the solutes are withdrawn simply for the purpose of isolating them from a mixture.

Another procedure of operation that is of interest primarily due to its analogy to elution chromatography is known as *end withdrawal*. In this operation the fundamental procedure is followed for a predetermined number of transfers as previously described. Then the upper phase only of the last tube in the train is collected. All other upper phases are advanced to the next tube in succession and after equilibration the upper phase of the last tube, n, is again collected.

This process is continued until all upper phases have passed through n tubes containing lower phase. In elution chromatography the analogy is similar. However, fresh upper phase is added continuously to the first *tube* (called a *plate* in elution chromatography) until only upper phase is eluted from the column.

In summary, the degree of separation of two or more solutes using CCD depends upon the distribution coefficients of the solutes, nature and volume of the solvents used, and number of transfers taken.

CENTRIFUGATION

A large number of separations may be accomplished with the centrifuge. This apparatus consists essentially of a container in which a mixture of solid and liquid, or of two liquids, is rotated at high speeds so that the mixture is separated into its constituent parts by the action of centrifugal force. A solid or liquid, mixed with a liquid of lesser density, may be separated be-

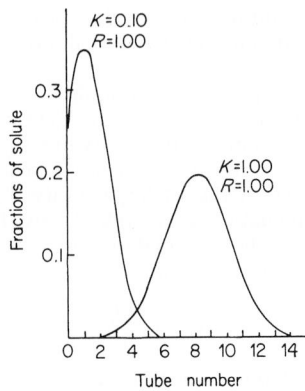

Figure 36-4. Distribution of two solutes with different K values.

cause the substance of higher specific gravity is thrown outward with greater force—it will be impelled to the bottom of the container, leaving a clear supernatant layer of pure liquid.

Centrifugation is useful particularly when separation by ordinary filtration is difficult, as in separating a highly viscous mixture. Separations may be accomplished more rapidly in a centrifuge than under the action of gravity. In addition, the degree of separation that is attainable may be greater because the forces available are of a far higher order of magnitude. The centrifuge has become a valuable analytical tool, particularly in biochemical and microbiological research. It has wide application in pharmaceutical laboratories and its use as a means of predicting emulsion stability has been suggested.

Two basic types of centrifuges are available: *sedimentation* and *filtration*. The *sedimentation type* of centrifuge depends on differences in the densities of the two or more phases comprising the mixture. This instrument is capable of separating both solid–liquid and liquid–liquid mixtures. *Filtration centrifuges*, however, are limited to the separation of solid–liquid mixtures only.

Sedimentation Centrifuges

The design of the bottle centrifuge and the disc centrifuge are based on the sedimentation principle (ie, separation by density difference).

BOTTLE CENTRIFUGE

The bottle centrifuge, which consists of a vertical spindle that rotates the containers in a horizontal plane, commonly is used to separate materials of different densities. Separation in a centrifugal field is brought about because denser particles in a mixture require greater forces to hold them in a circular path of a given radius than do lighter particles. Thus, the lighter particles are displaced toward the axis of the centrifuge by the heavier particles. During the centrifugation of blood, for example, a speed of 3000 rpm is required to separate blood corpuscles from serum. If the radius of the centrifuge is assumed to be 10 cm, the acceleration, a, acting on a particle can be approximated to be 10^6 cm/sec^2; or about 1000 times the acceleration due to gravity, g

$$a = 4\pi^2 N^2 r = \frac{4(3.14)^2(3000)^2(10)}{3600} = 10^6 \text{ cm/sec}^2$$

N = revolutions/sec; r = radius in cm

$$\frac{10^6 \text{ cm/sec}^2}{10^3 \text{ cm/sec}^2} = 100 \ (g)$$

10^3 cm/sec^2 = approximate acceleration due to gravity

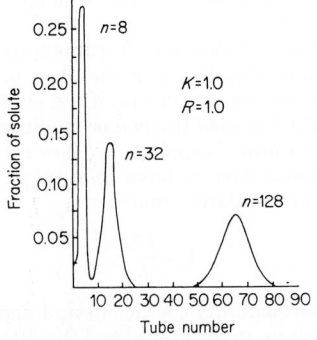

Figure 36-3. Distribution of solute after varying number of transfers.

Under these conditions, the blood corpuscles eventually migrate under the influence of centrifugal force to the tip of the centrifuge tube.

The separation of particles in a liquid medium also depends on the nature of the medium. A solid particle settling under the influence of acceleration due to gravity in a liquid phase accelerates until a constant terminal velocity is reached. The terminal velocity is known as the settling velocity of the particle and is described mathematically by Stokes' Law. It can be shown that Stokes' Law can be extended to those cases where settling takes place in a centrifugal field,

$$v_s = v_g \frac{\omega^2 r}{g} \qquad (5)$$

where v_s is the settling velocity of a particle in a centrifugal field, v_g is the settling velocity of a particle in a gravitational field (Stokes' Law), ω is the angular velocity of the particle in the settling zone, and r is the radius at which the settling velocity is determined.

Consider a solid particle at an initial position in a liquid medium and a distance r from the axis of rotation. Under these conditions,

$$v_s = dr/dt \qquad (6)$$

Substituting Equation 6 into Equation 5 gives

$$dr/dt = v_g \frac{\omega^2 r}{g} \qquad (7)$$

Rearranging and integrating between limits gives

$$\int_r^{rc} \frac{dr}{r} = \int_0^t v_g \frac{\omega^2 r}{g} dt \qquad (8)$$

$$\ln \frac{r_c}{r} = v_g \frac{\omega^2 t}{g} \qquad (9)$$

where r_c is the distance between the surface of the sedimented cake in the tip of the tube and the axis of rotation, and t is the time during which the particle is subjected to centrifugal acceleration while the particle travels the distance from r to r_c. Equation 9 shows that if centrifuging conditions for a given suspension are to be compared in different centrifuges, the speed, bottle size, centrifuge dimensions, and centrifuging time must be taken into consideration. Lavanchy and Keith[3] describe mathematical approaches that should be taken for this purpose.

ULTRACENTRIFUGE

When extremely fine solid matter must be separated from a liquid, such as in colloid or biological research, the ultracentrifuge is employed. In this instrument a relatively small rotor is operated at speeds exceeding 100,000 rpm and forces up to one million times gravity are exerted. High speeds are attained with air or oil turbines and bearings lubricated with a film of compressed air. Friction heat may be minimized by the use of high vacuum.

By placing the samples in specially constructed cells and spinning them in the ultracentrifuge, it is possible to separate the dispersed phase from the continuous phase rather rapidly. To aid the investigator, optical attachments may be employed to photograph the settling while the centrifuge is in operation.

Only small batches of material can be handled in these instruments during a single run. Ultracentrifuges are employed in the determination of particle size and molecular weight of polymeric and other high-molecular-weight materials such as proteins and nucleic acids by direct or indirect observation of the rate of separation of particles in solution or suspension.

Filtration Methods

The filtration centrifuge is restricted to the separation of solid–liquid mixtures. It is similar in principle to the sedimen-

tation type, but rather than containers it possesses a porous wall through which the liquid phase may pass but upon which the solid phase is retained. Analogous to filtration, this process requires consideration of the flow of liquid through the solid bed that accumulates on the porous plate.

FILTRATION

Filtration is the process of separating liquids from solids with the purpose of obtaining optically transparent liquids. This is accomplished by the intervention of a porous substance, called the *filter* or the *filtering medium*. The liquid that has passed through the filter is called the *filtrate*.

Mathematics of Filtration

In 1842 Poiseuille proposed a relationship for streamlined flow of liquids under pressure through capillaries. This equation in its simplified form is represented by

$$V = \frac{\pi \Delta p r^4}{8 L \eta}$$

where V = flow velocity, r = flow capillary radius, L = capillary length, η = viscosity of the fluid, and Δp = pressure differential at the two ends of the capillary.

The modified Poiseuille equation has been shown to be valid for liquid flow through sand, glass beads, and various porous media. It represents the foundation for all mathematical models of filtration that where developed subsequently. Of critical importance in this equation is the powerful effect of capillary radius; ie, by reducing it to 1/8 its size, the pressure differential must be increased more than 4000 times in order to obtain the same flow velocity, all other factors remaining constant.

On the basis of the Poiseuille formula, the Kozeny-Carman relationship was established. This may be expressed as

$$V = \left[\frac{e^3}{KS^2(1-e)^2} \right] \left[\frac{A \Delta p g}{\eta L} \right]$$

where A = cross-sectional area of porous bed (filter medium), e = porosity of bed, S = surface area of medium, K = constant, and the remaining symbols are the same as in the Poiseuille equation.

The Kozeny-Carman relationship, like Poiseuille's law states that the rate of flow is directly proportional to the pressure drop across the medium and to the area of the bed, and inversely proportional to the viscosity of the liquid and the thickness of the bed. To characterize the material composing the bed, two new quantities, e and S, are introduced, replacing capillary radius.

The use of a nondefinite constant K, rather than the definite constant in Poiseuille's equation, $\pi/8$, offers greater utility in the use of this equation in accounting for the geometry of the medium. The constant, K, generally ranges in value from 3 to 6. The Kozeny-Carman equation finds its greatest limitation in complex systems such as filter paper, but provides excellent correlation in filter beds composed of porous material.

In applying Poiseuille's law to filtration processes, one must recognize the capillaries found in the filter bed are highly irregular and nonuniform. Therefore, if the length of a capillary is taken as the thickness of the bed or medium and the correction factor for the radius is applied, the flow rate is more closely approximated. These factors have been taken into account in the formulation of the Darcy equation

$$V = \frac{k \Delta p}{L \eta}$$

where k is the permeability coefficient and depends on the nature of the precipitate to be filtered and the filter medium itself.

Computer-assisted design of microfiltration systems are underway.[4] This technique is used to design an optimum filtration system from actual filtration data, thereby predicting its performance with any given fluid.

In considering the nature of the precipitate, it is known that large particles are easier to filter than are small particles because of the tendency of the latter to enter into and occlude the pores of the bed, thus hindering the passage of the filtrate. In addition, the buildup of small particles on the filter tends to form a nonporous, densely packed bed that also resists passage of the filtrate.

Filtering Media

The filtering medium, whether a filter paper, synthetic fiber, or porous bed of glass, sand, or stone, is composed of countless channels that impart porosity to the medium. Almost without exception these channels or pores are nonuniform and possess a rather tortuous nature.

The mechanism of filtration basically involves a two-step process:

1. The filter medium itself resists the flow of solid material while permitting the passage of liquid.
2. During the course of the filtration the suspended, solid material builds up on the filter medium and thereby forms a *filter bed*, which acts as a second, and often more efficient, filter medium.

The ability of a filter medium to eliminate solid matter from a liquid is termed *retention*. It must be borne in mind that the filtration process must compromise retention with filtration rate, the speed at which the purified liquid (the filtrate) is recovered. To illustrate this point, it will be noted that a slab of marble will most effectively retain the solid material contained in a suspension; unfortunately, it would require a few centuries to collect the purified filtrate.

Both the retentive ability of a filter medium and filtration rate of a liquid through the medium depend on the porosity of the medium. Each factor, however, is influenced significantly by the viscosity of the liquid, the proportion of solid matter in the liquid, and the size, shape, and physical nature of the suspended solids.

The flow of a liquid through a filter bed follows the same basic rules that govern the flow of any liquid through a medium offering resistance. The *flow rate* through the medium will vary directly with the area of the medium, as well as the pressure drop or driving force across the bed.

$$\text{Rate of flow} \propto \frac{(\text{driving force})(\text{cross-sectional area})}{\text{resistance}}$$

The flow rate is retarded by the viscosity of the liquid being filtered and by any obstruction to flow. These obstructions include the resistance of the filter medium itself and the second filter bed or *filter cake* that builds up on the medium at a rate dependent on the solids content of the liquid. The resistance offered by the medium itself will not vary significantly during the filtration process. It depends on the thickness of the medium as well as its porosity. The resistance of the filter cake, on the other hand, is not constant and generally increases continuously during the operation. The resistance offered by the cake depends both on its thickness and physical nature. The thickness of the cake is dictated by the amount of filtrate passing through the filter and on the solids content of the liquid. The physical nature of the cake—whether it is loose, compacted, coarse, fine, granular, or gelatinous—determines whether or not it will readily allow the flow of liquid.

FILTER PAPER

Filter paper most frequently is employed in clarification processes required of the pharmacy practitioner. Only high-quality filter paper should be used to ensure maximum filtering efficiency. When possible the first few milliliters of filtrate should be discarded to eliminate (insofar as possible) contamination of the pharmaceutical product by free fibers associated with most filter paper. This is especially true in the preparation of ophthalmic solutions.

MEMBRANE FILTERS

Membrane filter media are produced from pure cellulose, cellulose derivatives, and polymeric materials. All have an extremely uniform micropore structure as well as an exceptionally smooth surface. The integral structure contains no fibers or particles that can work loose and contaminate a filtrate. This is a particular advantage in the filtration of ophthalmic solutions. The presence of these fibers is difficult to prevent when using many other filter media, including paper filters.

The efficiency of membrane filters is due to the uniform pore system that functions like a highly effective sieve. The pore size, of different types of these filters, ranges from 10 nm to 10 μm. All particles in liquids or gases that are larger than the pore of a given filter are retained on the surface. The thickness of these membrane filters ranges from 50 to 200 μm.

The pores that penetrate these filters pass directly through the entire thickness of the membrane, with a minimum of crosslinkage. Porosity or pore volume is estimated as 80% of the total fiber volume. The high porosity of these filters, coupled with the *straight-through* configuration of the pores, results in flow rates through membrane filters that are at least 40 times faster than flow rates through conventional filter media that possess the same particle size retention capabilities.

Major producers of these filters include the *Millipore Filter Corp*, Bedford, MA; *Gelman Instrument Corp*, Ann Arbor, MI; *Pall Corp*, Glen Cove, NY; *Nuclepore Corp*, Pleasanton, CA; and *Carl Schleicher & Schuell Co*, Keene, NH. The membrane filters are available as circular discs of varying diameter. Different types are available for use in the filtration of either aqueous or nonaqueous liquids. The discs generally are used in conjunction with specialized holders of either metal or glass composition. With small volumes (ie, less than 500 mL), solutions usually are filtered using vacuum techniques. Larger volumes require filtration under pressure provided by an inert gas such as nitrogen.

In addition to their obvious utility in routine filtration processes on both a laboratory and industrial scale, these filters have been used for a wide range of purposes, including chemical analysis, microbiological analysis, and bacterial filtration. The latter process provides an economical and rapid method for sterilizing heat-labile material (see Chapter 40).

OTHER FILTERING MEDIA

Many devices have been advanced to replace filter paper, which has many disadvantages, particularly for large-scale operations. A great many variations of filtering processes, each designed to fit the needs of special cases, are found in the modern pharmaceutical laboratory. The filter press, the centrifugal filter, the vacuum filter, sand-bed filter, charcoal filter, paper-pulp filter, and porous porcelain filter are all examples of specialized filtration methods. Each one of these possesses some advantageous quality, and it is the experience of the laboratory operators that guides them in their selection of appropriate filtering devices. Reference is made later in the text to many of these special-scale filters.

However, it would not be inappropriate to refer briefly to special filtering devices that may be useful in the prescription or research laboratory.

Cotton Filters—A small pledget of absorbent cotton, loosely inserted in the neck of a funnel, adequately serves to remove large particles of extraneous material from a clear liquid. Although this properly might be termed colation, the cotton also can be used to serve as a fairly efficient filter. It is sometimes necessary to return the liquid a number of times to secure perfect transparency. This should be remembered in filtering ophthalmic solutions through cotton, because small detached filaments are carried through on initial filtration.

Glass-Wool Filters—When solutions of highly reactive chemicals, such as strong acids, are to be filtered, filter paper cannot be used. In its place glass wool may be used just as one uses absorbent cotton for filtering. This material is resistant to ordinary chemical action, and when properly packed into the neck of a funnel it constitutes a very effective filtering medium.

Sintered-Glass Filters—These filters have as the filtering medium a flat or convex plate consisting of particles of Jena glass powdered and sifted to produce granules of uniform size that are molded together. The plates can be fused into a glass apparatus of any required shape (Fig 36-5). These filters vary in porosity, depending on the size of the granules used in the plate. They are very useful in the filtration of solutions such as those intended for parenteral injection. A vacuum attachment is necessary to facilitate the passage of the liquid through the filter plate (see Chapter 40).

Funnels

Funnels are conical-shaped utensils intended to facilitate the pouring of liquids into narrow-mouthed vessels. They also are used widely in pharmacy for supporting filter media. Funnels may be made of glass, polyethylene, metal, or any other material that serves a specific purpose. The community pharmacist will find the glass funnel to be quite adequate for all processes of clarification in prescription practice.

Most funnels used by the pharmacy practitioner are conical in shape and may be fluted, grooved, or ribbed for the purpose of facilitating the downward flow of the filtrate.

The *Büchner* type of funnel is used today largely in pharmaceutical laboratories. A piece of round filter paper is laid on the perforated porcelain diaphragm and the filtration conducted. This funnel is especially applicable to vacuum filtration (see the discussion, *Vacuum Filtration*).

FILTRATION OF VOLATILE LIQUIDS

It is evident that the ordinary methods of filtering liquids will not be practical for very volatile liquids because of the loss through evaporation, and the liability to explosion in the case of flammable volatile liquids. Funnels must be covered, the receiving vessel closed, and provision made for the escape of the confined air in the receiving vessel. The following method is quite useful. A rubber cover, perforated to admit a tube, is placed on top of the funnel; connection between the bottle and funnel is effected as shown in Figure 36-6.

AIDS TO FILTRATION

It has long been known that addition of an insoluble adsorbent powder to a liquid prior to its filtration greatly increases the

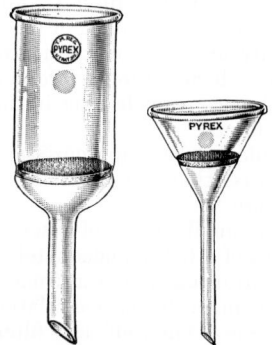

Figure 36-5. Sintered-glass filters.

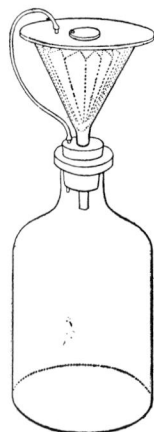

Figure 36-6. Filtration of volatile liquids.

efficiency of the process. Purified talc, siliceous earth (kieselguhr), clays, charcoal, paper pulp, chalk, magnesium carbonate, bentonite, silica gel, and others have been used for this purpose.

It must not be overlooked, however, that powdered substances employed for such purposes must be insoluble and inert, so not all of those in the foregoing list are applicable for general filtration.

Talc is nonadsorbent to materials in solution and is a chemically inert medium for filtering any liquid, provided it has been purified for this purpose and it is not the impalpably fine variety that will pass through the filter paper.

Kieselguhr is almost pure silica (SiO_2). It is as applicable as talc for general filtration purposes, with no danger of removing active constituents by adsorption.

Siliceous earths or clays, such as fuller's earth or kaolin in the hydrated form which is produced when they are brought into contact with aqueous liquids, are safe for general use only in filtering fixed oils. Liquids containing coloring matter or alkaloidal principles must not be filtered through these media, for adsorption of both color and alkaloids occurs and the filtrate is altered in comparison.

Charcoals, as a rule, possess adsorptive properties not only toward color but for many active constituents of medicinal preparations, such as alkaloids and glycosides. Consequently, charcoal should never be used as a filtering medium unless the removal of such constituents is desirable.

Chalk and *magnesium carbonate* readily react with acids and possess a finite solubility in water and aqueous fluids, with the production of alkalinity in the filtrate. This is particularly true of magnesium carbonate; the degree of alkalinity imparted to the filtrate is sufficiently great to cause precipitation of alkaloids. Either of these media, when added to an alkaloidal preparation prior to filtration, will precipitate and remove all of the alkaloidal constituents. Neither is suitable for general use.

RAPID FILTERING APPARATUS

Much attention has been given to methods for increasing the rapidity of filtration. This may be accomplished by applying pressure on the filter or by creating a vacuum in the receiving vessel.

VACUUM FILTRATION

One of the first practical efforts made to create a vacuum to aid filtration was by means of the Bunsen pump. Its action depends on the principle that a column of water descending through a tube from a height is capable of carrying with it the air contained in a lateral tube, if the latter is placed properly. This form of aspirator is practicable where water pressure is available.

Pumps Acting by Water Pressure—The various aspirator or vacuum pumps that operate under the influence of water pressure are all based on the same principle. The following are selected for illustration from the great variety in use. Figure 36-7 shows Chapman's vacuum pump. Valve *a* prevents the water from flowing into the bottle which carries the filter when the pressure of water ceases or is reduced.

On a larger scale, the vacuum for filtration is produced by one of the many types of vacuum pumps now available. The pump should be protected from vapors by placing a suitable vapor trap between the filter unit and the pump. The trap usually is cooled to very low temperatures by means of dry ice and acetone when very high vacuum is needed.

In assembling a filtering apparatus using the vacuum principle, it is necessary that there be no leaks in the connections from the filter to the aspirator. If filter paper is used in connection therewith, a plainly folded paper must be used and its tip must be protected against breakage by reinforcing it with a filter paper support or some other device. A Büchner filter also may be used, employing a specially strong filter paper.

In analytical work it is customary to use the Gooch crucible and flask (Fig 36-8) for rapid filtration. The flask, of especially thick glass, is provided with a side tube that is connected to a water aspirator pump. The perforated crucible bottom is converted into a filter bed of the required thickness by means of a filter mat placed over the perforations in the porcelain base.

FILTRATION UNDER PRESSURE

Figure 36-9 illustrates a sectional drawing of a plate-and-frame filter press. The material to be filtered enters the apparatus under pressure through a pipe at the bottom and is forced into one of the many chambers. A filter cloth is positioned on both sides of each chamber. As the material passes through the filtering cloth, solids remain behind in the chamber and the clear filtrate passes through and out of an opening located on top of the apparatus.

Rotary-drum vacuum filters are used widely in the pharmaceutical industry, especially in the preparation of antibiotics by the fermentation process. In this type of filtration a perforated drum, wrapped with a cloth or other suitable substance holding a filter medium, is immersed partially in a tank holding the material to be filtered (Fig 36-10).

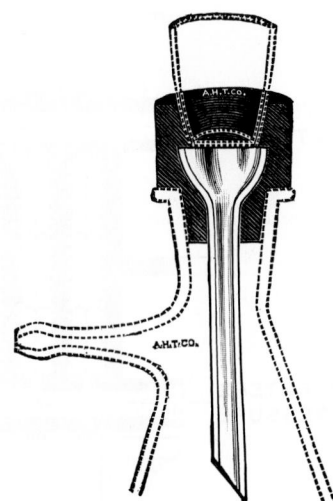

Figure 36-8. Gooch crucible arranged for vacuum filtration (courtesy, Thomas).

The drum is rotated through the slurry of material and a vacuum within the drum draws the material into and through the filter medium. During this step of the process, the filtrate is taken into the drum and collected, while the solid material remains deposited on the outer surface of the drum. This material is then removed by a scraper in the last step of the operating cycle, just before the rotating drum repeats another cycle.

CLARIFICATION AND DECOLORATION

Clarification

Clarification is the process by which finely divided solids and colloidal materials are separated from liquids without the use of filters. The process is employed to remove suspended oil from aqueous solutions, such as aromatic waters, and for the removal of undesirable solids that interfere with the transparency of such natural products as honey and fruit juices.

Clarification generally is resorted to when the contaminating material is finely subdivided, amorphous, or colloidal in nature and tends to plug a filtration medium rapidly. A number of methods are available to handle this difficult problem.

When the solids are not of a granular or free-filtering nature, it may be possible to improve the characteristics of the suspended solids. This may involve varying the temperature or pH of the medium. When a viscid liquid is heated, its viscosity and specific gravity are decreased and particles that are suspended in it will separate. Those particles that are more dense than the liquid will fall to the bottom, while those that are less dense will rise to the surface. In the latter case the minute bubbles of steam formed in the heating process become enveloped in the viscid particles, rise through their buoyancy, and a scum is formed that may be separated readily.

The dewaxing of oils at a reduced temperature offers a further example of the possibilities of contaminant modification. Oil that is chilled rapidly often produces an amorphous wax that will plug a straining medium. Slow chilling, on the other hand, produces a wax with a more crystalline nature, which has good filtration characteristics.

The simplest method of clarification, although not always feasible, is gravitational sedimentation. This method involves the least amount of labor and expense and is used frequently, particularly on a large scale, when haste is unnecessary. The deposit formed is called a *sediment* or *sludge*. These terms are not synonymous with *precipitate*. A sediment is solid matter separated merely by the action of gravity from a liquid in which it has been suspended. A precipitate, on the other hand,

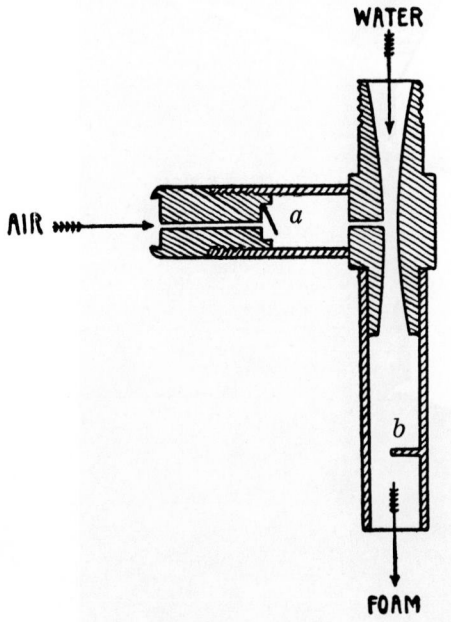

WATER

AIR ➤➤➤

a

b

FOAM

Figure 36-7. Chapman's pump.

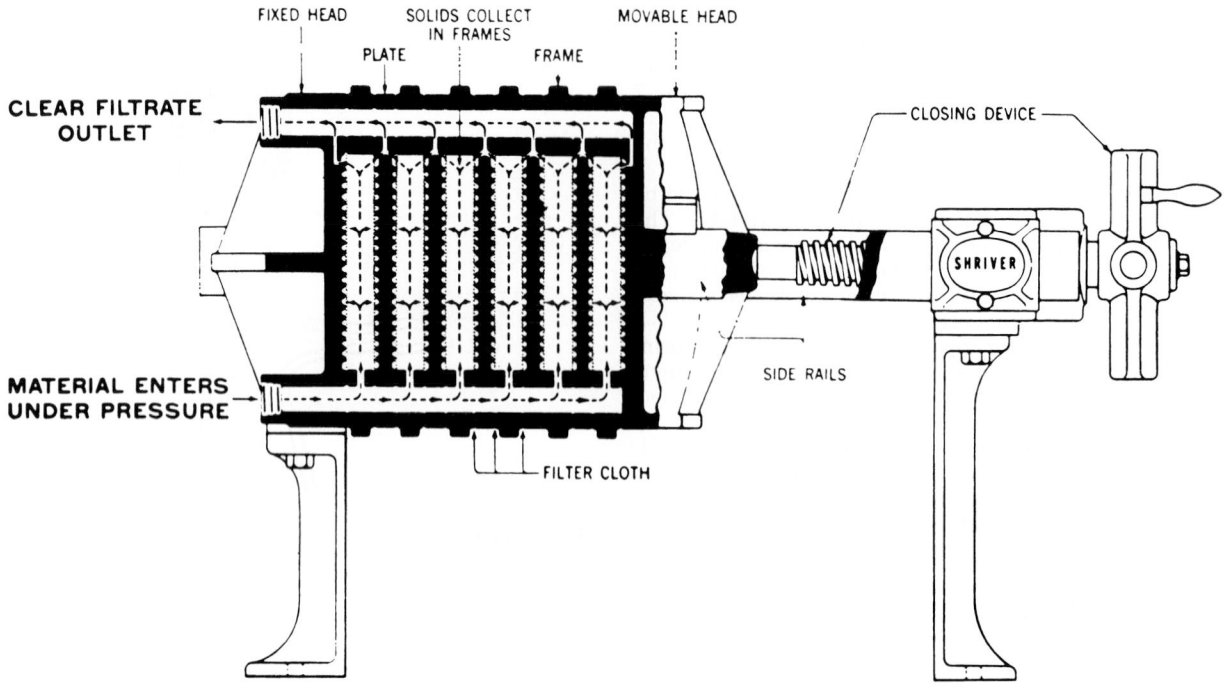

Figure 36-9. A plate-and-frame filter press (courtesy, Shriver).

is solid matter separated from a previously clear solution by physical or chemical change. Fixed oils usually are clarified by gravitational sedimentation. In vegetable oils the sediment consists principally of albuminous and gummy substances, cellular tissue, and water, all of which have been separated with the oil during the expression process.

The clarification process generally is carried out by adding a clarifying agent such as paper, pulp, talc, infusorial earth, as well as a number of other materials to the turbid liquid. These agents usually act to reduce turbidity by physical adsorption of the contaminating material, although a large number of specific, physical-chemical coagulants also are in use. After the addition of the clarifying agent, the mixture is agitated and the agents, along with the adsorbed impurities, are removed by filtration or any other suitable means. Albumin and gelatin are examples of clarifying agents obtained from natural sources.

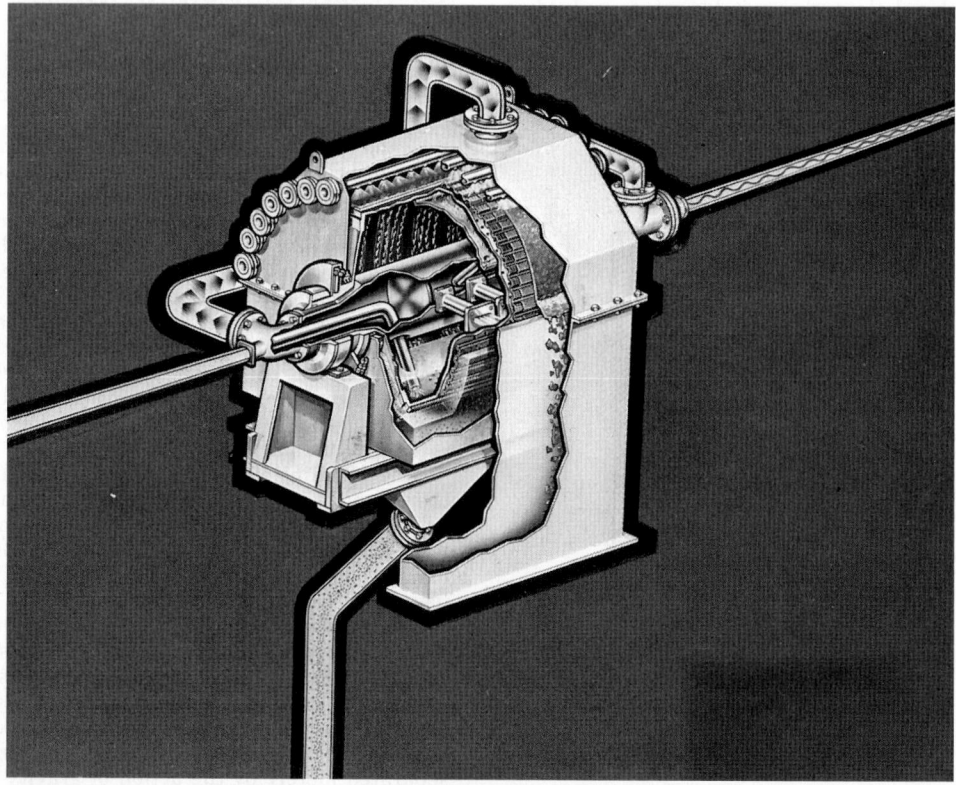

Figure 36-10. Rotary filter (courtesy, Bird Machine).

Substances of a synthetic nature, such as polyamines, also are used for this purpose.

Decoloration

Decoloration, or decolorization as it sometimes is called, is the process of depriving solutions of color by use of an appropriate adsorptive medium. In many respects it is closely related to the clarification process. Decoloration is used for removal of coloring matter from a number of raw materials, both natural and synthetic, and from many finished products. Animal charcoal (also called bone black), wood charcoal, or activated charcoal frequently are used as decolorizing agents. Clays such as bentonite, kaolin, and fuller's earth also are used for this purpose.

LOTION, DECANTATION, AND COLATION

Lotion

Lotion (displacement washing) is the process by which soluble impurities are removed from insoluble material by the addition of a suitable washing solvent. The wash liquid usually is separated from the purified solid by decantation or filtration. An expedient method of adding the washing solvent to the solid in a fine, controlled spray is by the use of wash bottles.

CONTINUOUS WASHING

The use of the wash bottle is limited to small operations. A simple method of automatically supplying the wash liquid in larger quantities is shown in Figure 36-11. This requires attention from the operator only at the beginning of the operation. The inverted bottle containing the washing solvent is furnished with a perforated stopper and a short glass tube. All that is necessary is to fill the bottle and adjust it over the funnel so that the end of the tube is at the height at which the level of liquid in the funnel is to be maintained. When the bottle is tilted slightly (if the tube selected is not too narrow in diameter), the liquid runs into the funnel until it rises to the orifice of the tube, whereupon the flow ceases. As the liquid gradually passes through the solid substance in the funnel, the level falls below the orifice, bubbles of air pass through the tube into the bottle, the liquid once more flows, and the operation continues until the upper bottle is empty. Many elaborate methods of continuous washing have been suggested, but the simple apparatus just described is quite satisfactory if a tube of proper diameter has been selected, one of such size that the force of capillary attraction will not be strong enough to prevent the passage of air.

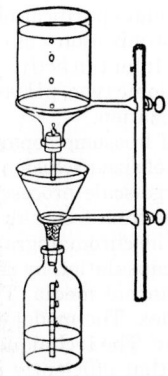

Figure 36-11. Continuous washing.

Decantation

The simplest method available for the separation of a solid from its soluble impurities is the technique of decantation. This method involves washing and subsequent agitation of the solid with an appropriate solvent, allowing the solid to settle and removing the supernatant solvent. These three steps are repeated as often as required to attain the desired purity of the solid. This method also is applicable to the simple separation of solids and liquids, such as after precipitation of a material from a mother liquor. Decantation provides an effective method for washing magmas and other gelatinous products.

Some degree of skill is required to decant liquids effectively. It is most convenient to decant from a lipped vessel that is not filled to capacity. In addition, the use of a stirring rod is suggested as a guide to steady the hand of the operator.

Colation

Colation or straining (from Latin *colare,* to strain) is the process of separating a solid from a fluid by pouring the mixture on a cloth or porous substance that will permit the fluid to pass through, but will retain the solid. This operation frequently is used for separating sediment or mechanical impurities of various kinds from liquids.

Colation should not be considered as a separate process but simply as a crude form of filtration, with larger pores in the straining medium than usually are employed for filtration.

The essential apparatus is a straining medium and a strainer support or frame. The straining medium is usually a cloth material such as flannel, muslin, wool, or cheesecloth. The material should be colorless and washed before use. Fabrics, particularly those of cotton, usually are treated or impregnated with a material called *sizing* to improve their appearance and quality for certain purposes; however, for use as a strainer, the fabric must be free of sizing because it causes contamination. Many different substances are used for sizing, some being soluble in cold water, others only in hot water. Thus, the proper method for their removal is to soak the fabric for a few hours in cold distilled water, rinse thoroughly; then cover with distilled water, boil for a few minutes, and rinse well in distilled water to remove the last traces of the gelatin, albumin, glue, or starch that may have been present in the sizing.

EXPRESSION

Expression is a process of *forcibly* separating liquids from solids. A number of mechanical principles have been recognized in the operation of expression, namely the use of the spiral twist press, the screw press, the roller press, the filter press, and the hydraulic press.

SPIRAL TWIST PRESS—The principle of this press is best and most practically illustrated in the usual process of manually expressing a substance contained in a cloth.

ROLLER PRESS—This is used for large-scale pressing of oily seeds, fatty substances, and so on. Care must be taken to apply the force gradually to the bag containing the material to be pressed, and not to use it on substances that will be corrosive to the rubber rollers.

HYDROSTATIC OR HYDRAULIC PRESS—Of the presses heretofore mentioned, each has some special advantage of use, but each also has some objectionable feature. The spiral twist is not powerful and its action is limited. The screw presses have friction with which to contend; the friction of a screw increases with the intensity of the pressure applied, and when a certain limit is reached all further force applied is wasted, and if continued may result in destruction of the press. The roller press is very limited in its action. Although the hydraulic press is expensive, after the first coat it is the most economical because the greatest power is obtained at the expense of the least labor. The principle of a hydraulic press is based on the fact that pressure exerted upon an enclosed liquid is transmitted equally in all directions. Tremendous pressures can be developed with hydraulic presses.

PRECIPITATION

Precipitation is the process of separating solid particles from a previously clear liquid—a solution—by physical or chemical changes. The separated solid is termed a *precipitate;* the cause of precipitation is the *precipitant;* and the liquid that remains in the vessel above the precipitate is called the supernatant liquid.

In pharmacy, precipitation may be useful for many purposes. It provides a convenient method of obtaining solid substances in the form of fine particles, such as the precipitation of calcium carbonate (precipitated chalk). White Lotion is an example of a preparation prepared by precipitation, in this case by mixing aqueous solutions of zinc sulfate and sulfurated potash to form an insoluble, finely divided zinc sulfide, free sulfur, and various polysulfides.

One of the most important uses of precipitation is in the purification of solids. The process as applied to purification is termed *recrystallization.* The impure solid usually is dissolved in a suitable solvent at elevated temperatures. On cooling, the bulk of the impurities remain solubilized while the purified solid product precipitates. This procedure is repeated as many times as necessary, using a number of solvents if required.

SEPARATION OF IMMISCIBLE LIQUIDS

The separation of liquids that are mutually soluble usually is effected by distillation, if one or both of the liquids are volatile. The separation of liquids that are immiscible is generally a simpler process.

Separations of this kind are necessary in analytical procedures, manufacturing operations, distillation of volatile oils, and accidental contaminations and admixtures, and are usually best made using a separatory funnel. When very small amounts of liquids are floating on the surface of another liquid, separation is accomplished most easily by using a pipet, medicine dropper, or glass syringe with an attached needle.

FLORENTINE RECEIVER

The separation of volatile oils from the water that accompanies them during steam distillation is a very important part of their manufacturing process. Where the volatile oil is lighter than water, the principle shown in Figure 36-12 may be used. The oil and water collect in the glass receiver during distillation, the oil floating on the top, while the water ascends the bent tube from the bottom; further addition of distillate causes the water to overflow from the side tube. The reverse action is produced in the receiver for light or heavy oils (Fig 36-13), in which either a lighter or a heavier fraction may be collected continuously.

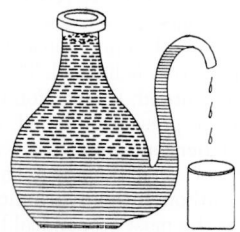

Figure 36-12. Florentine receiver.

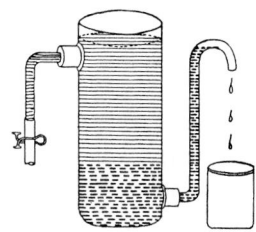

Figure 36-13. Receiver for light or heavy oils.

SPECIALIZED SEPARATION TECHNIQUES

Diffusion Phenomena

Diffusion is the spontaneous penetration of one substance into another under the potential of concentration gradient. Simply stated, material will tend to move from a region of higher concentration to one of lower concentration. The driving force or potential of such a process may be enhanced by the application of an electric field.

If the two regions of concentration noted are separated by a selective membrane, certain species will diffuse through the membrane, while other molecular species will be held back. When this selectivity is dictated by the porosity of the membrane, the process is termed *dialysis.* Dialysis is used principally for the separation of small molecules and ions contained in a mixture with colloidal material. The latter substances diffuse with difficulty or not at all. Materials such as gums, starch, albumin, and proteins fall into this colloidal, nondiffusible category.

The rate of diffusion across a semipermeable membrane is directly proportional to the concentration gradient between the two surfaces of the membrane and to the area of the membrane, but is inversely proportional to the membrane thickness. These factors are expressed in Fick's law of diffusion

$$\frac{dS}{dt} = \frac{kA(C_i - C_0)}{h}$$

where S is the amount of substance diffused at time t, k is a permeability constant, A is the membrane area, h is the membrane thickness, dS/dt is the diffusion rate, C_i is concentration on one side, and C_0 is concentration on the other side of the membrane.

Gel Filtration

The chromatography of cephalosporins in gel filtration chromatography has been demonstrated and shown to be important in the separation of high-molecular-weight impurities. The impurities frequently are associated with allergic responses in patients. This method has been demonstrated to serve as an excellent quality-control procedure for the impurities in cephalosporin preparations.[5]

Different types of Sephadex gels were used for separation. The study investigated various reagents necessary to perform the separation in an ultimate purification of the compound. The results indicated that optimization was capable of being done to separate the impurities from the active compound. The nature of the mobile phase, the ionic type, pH value, and molarity were important for the optimization.

A feasibility study of liposome separation that was undertaken to explore the use of size-exclusion chromatography, such as gel filtration of a large-scale process, demonstrated that it could separate liposomes from freeze-dried material in a chromosome preparation.[6] The chromatographic step was intended to improve the drug encapsulation by removing free (unincapsulated) drugs from external media. The selected stationary phase was G-50 Sephadex. The model drug used in the study was orciprenaline sulfate. The technique was able to produce a suitable size exclusion that efficiently removed the free drug from the liposome preparation.

In a study of liposomes loaded with calcitonin, it was necessary to observe the location of the protein to protect it from enzymatic digestion.[7] The analysis of the liposome produced from this protein was extracted using suitable gel separation of the liposome mixture to ensure the location of the protein within the system. It established the stability and the ultimate formation of the liposome product. This ensured the appropriate loading of the protein within the liposome product.

A process for purifying bovine pancreatic glucagon as a byproduct of insulin production was described.[8] The glucagon, containing supernatant from the alkaline crystalline crystallization of insulin, was precipitated using ammonium sulfate and isoelectric precipitation. The precipitate containing glucagon then was purified by ion-exchange chromatography on Q-Sepharose FF gel filtration on Sephadex G-25 and ion-exchange chromatography on S-Sepharose FF. Successful yields were obtained using this technique, which was successful because of the gel filtration procedure.

A report was presented on the characterization of adenosine receptors in porcine striatal membranes and their solubilization by detergent digitonin.[9] Once the drug was solubilized, the material was bound to sites after the removal of receptors from the lipid environment. Gel filtration on Superdex 200 accomplished the separation into appropriate molecular weights. Suitable purification was achieved by this means.

In another report of the use of gel filtration, the expression and purification of human gamma-glutamylcysteine synthetase were studied.[10] Specific proteins and polypeptides were isolated and their amounts characterized by the use of Superdex 200 along with ATP-affinity resins. Cyclosporin A has potential for wide clinical use, limited only by the very narrow therapeutic index.[11] Potentiation of its clinical efficacy is thus very desirable. Preliminary data had indicated that the mixture of cyclosporin A, with hyaluronate, could increase its efficiency. In this study, it was found that cyclosporin A could reduce the hypersensitivity in test animals when administered along with hyaluronate. To demonstrate the association of this mixture, gel filtration was required, which showed the protection of the molecule from being bound to red blood cells. This association would improve the clinical response and was proven only by the use of gel filtration.

Ultrafiltration

A new type of membrane coating has been developed for osmotic delivery that offers significant advantages over membrane coatings used in conventional osmotic tablets.[12] This coating has an asymmetric structure similar to the asymmetric membranes made for reverse osmosis membrane or ultrafiltration. The study demonstrated clearly how the porous membranes could work as a thin outer skin of a dosage form. The permeability of the coating to water can be controlled by the membrane structure, whose principles were derived from ultrafiltration principles. A porosimetric technique for verifying the integrity of virus-retentive membranes, which can be validated, has been studied.[13] This integrity test of filtration processes was specifically designed for and is useful for post-use membrane integrity testing.

Reverse Osmosis

As reverse osmosis (Fig 36-14) is used it is necessary to evaluate which new composite reverse osmosis membranes were developed with significant improved performance over commercially available conventional composite membranes. The ESPA membrane chemistry provides a high flux at low operating pressure while maintaining a very good salt and organic rejection. The membranes have been demonstrated to operate for several years. Appropriate transmission and field emission electron micrographs of the membrane demonstrated the struc-

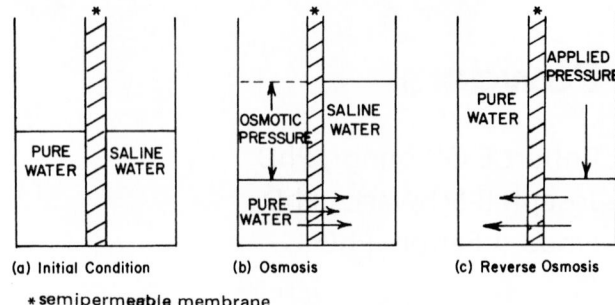

Figure 36-14. Principles of reverse osmosis.

ture of the membrane skin layer is the reason for the improved performance. This surface charge of the various membranes was demonstrated qualitatively using zeta-potential measurements. The newer membranes had a low surface charge and operated at a low pressure. In an effort to further improve the available reverse osmosis water-treatment membranes, other studies have been conducted over the past several years to evaluate specific ultra-low-pressure membranes. Very little information was available to the industry. It is possible to design membranes with 30% increase in productivity over conventional membranes. These improvements are particularly important to multistage systems for water purification. Recommendations have been made by many to improve the systems by using ultra-low-pressure membranes.

REFERENCES

1. Craig LC, Craig D. In Weissberger A. *Technique of Organic Chemistry,* vol 3, pt 1, 2nd ed. New York: Interscience, 1956, chap 2.
2. Rogers LB. In: Kolthoff IM, Elving PJ. *Treatise on Analytical Chemistry,* vol 2, pt 1. New York: Interscience, 1961, chap 22.
3. Lavanchy AC, Keith FW In: *Kirk-Othmer Encyclopedia of Chemical Technology,* vol 5, 3rd ed. NY: Interscience, 1991, p 194.
4. Weyand J. In: Shoemaker W. *What the Filterman Needs to Know about Filtration.* AIChE Symposium Series, no 171, vol 73. New York: American Institute of Chemical Engineers, 1977.
5. Changyin H, et al. *J Pharm Biomed Anal* 1994; 12:533.
6. Nemuri S, Rhodes C. *Pharm Acta Helv* 1994; 69:107.
7. Arien A, et al. *Pharm Res* 1995; 12:1289.
8. Andrade A, et al. *J Med Biol Res* 1997; 30:1421.
9. Costa B, et al. *Neurochem Int* 1998; 32:121.
10. Misra I, Griffith O. *Prot Express Purif* 1998; 13:268.
11. Gowland G. *Int J Immunother* 1998; 14:1.
12. Herbig S, et al. *J Contr Rel* 1995; 25:127.
13. Phillips M, Diheo A. *Biologicals* 1996; 24:243.

BIBLIOGRAPHY

Curling JM. *J Parenteral Sci Technol* 1982; 36:59.
Driscoll HT. *Filter Aids and Materials: Technology and Applications.* Park Ridge, NJ: Noyes Data Corp, 1977.
Hwang ST, Kammermeyer K. *Membranes in Separations,* vol 3. New York: Wiley Interscience, 1975.
Kolthoff IM, Elving PJ. *Treatise on Analytical Chemistry,* vol 5, pt 1. New York: Interscience, 1982.
Lachman L, et al. *The Theory and Practice of Industrial Pharmacy,* 3rd ed. Philadelphia: Lea & Febiger, 1986, chap 7.
Mink HP. *Application of a Multicomponent Membrane Transport Model to Reverse Osmosis Separation Processes.* ACS Symposium Series, no 281. Washington, DC: American Chemical Society, 1985.
Perry ES, Weissberger A. *Technique of Chemistry,* vol 12, 3rd ed. New York: Wiley Interscience, 1978.
Perry JH, et al. *Chemical Engineer's Handbook,* 6th ed. New York: McGraw-Hill, 1984.
Swarbrick J, Boylan J. *Encyclopedia of Pharmaceutical Technology.* New York: Dekker, 1990.
Townsend A. *Encyclopedia of Analytical Science.* New York: Academic, 1995.

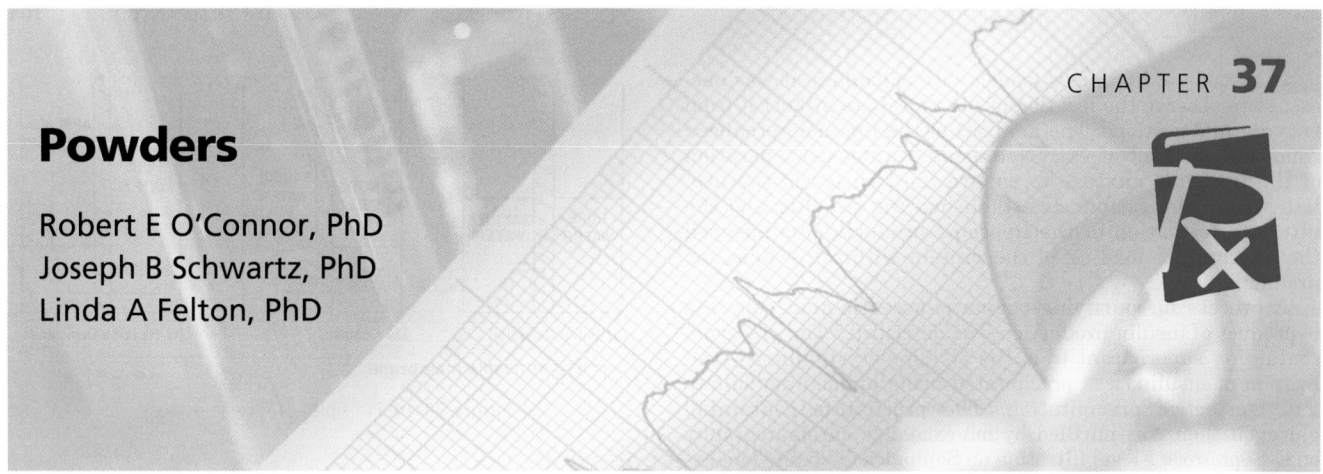

CHAPTER 37

Powders

Robert E O'Connor, PhD

Joseph B Schwartz, PhD

Linda A Felton, PhD

Powders are encountered in almost every aspect of pharmacy, both in industry and in practice. Drugs and other ingredients, when they occur in the solid state in the course of being processed into a dosage form, usually are in a more or less finely divided condition. Frequently, this is a powder whose state of subdivision is critical in determining its behavior both during processing and in the finished dosage form. Apart from their use in the manufacture of tablets, capsules, and suspensions, powders also occur as a pharmaceutical dosage form. Although the use of powders as a dosage form has declined, the properties and behavior of finely divided solid materials are of considerable importance in pharmacy. This chapter is intended to provide an introduction to the fundamentals of powder mechanics and the primary means of powder production and handling. The relationships of the principles of powder behavior to powders as dosage forms are discussed.

PRODUCTION METHODS

Molecular Aggregation

PRECIPITATION AND CRYSTALLIZATION

The precipitation and crystallization processes are fundamentally similar and depend on achieving three conditions in succession: a state of supersaturation (super cooling in the case of crystallization from a melt), formation of nuclei, and growth of crystals or amorphous particles.

Supersaturation can be achieved by evaporation of solvent from a solution, cooling of the solution if the solute has a positive heat of solution, production of additional solute as a result of a chemical reaction, or a change in the solvent medium by addition of various soluble secondary substances. In the absence of seed crystals, significant supersaturation is required to initiate the crystallization process through formation of nuclei. A nucleus is thought to consist of from 10 to a few hundred molecules having the spatial arrangement of the crystals that will be grown ultimately from them.

Such small particles are shown by the Kelvin equation to be more soluble than large crystals; therefore, they require supersaturation, relative to large crystals, for their formation and subsequent growth. It is a gross oversimplification to assume that, for a concentration gradient of a given value, the rate of crystallization is the negative of the rate of dissolution. The latter is generally somewhat greater.

Depending on the conditions of crystallization, it is possible to control or modify the nature of the crystals obtained. When polymorphs exist, careful temperature control and seeding with the desired crystal form are often necessary. The habit or shape of a given crystal form often highly depends on impurities in solution, pH, rate of stirring, rate of cooling, and the solvent. Very rapid rates of crystallization can result in impurities being included in the crystals by entrapment.

SPRAY-DRYING

Atomization of a solution of one or more solids via a nozzle, spinning disk, or other device, followed by evaporation of the solvent from the droplets is termed *spray-drying*. The nature of the powder that results is a function of several variables, including the initial solute concentration, size distribution of droplets produced, and rate of solvent removal. The weight of a given particle is determined by the volume of the droplet from which it was derived and by the solute concentration. The particles produced are aggregates of primary particles consisting of crystals and/or amorphous solids, depending on the rate and conditions of solvent removal. This approach to the powdered state provides the opportunity to incorporate multiple solid substances into individual particles at a fixed composition, independent of particle size, and avoiding difficulties that can arise in attempting to obtain a uniform mixture of several powdered ingredients by other procedures.

Particle-Size Reduction

Comminution in its broadest sense is the mechanical process of reducing the size of particles or aggregates. Thus, it embraces a wide variety of operations including cutting, chopping, crushing, grinding, milling, micronizing, and trituration, which depend primarily on the type of equipment employed. The selection of equipment in turn is determined by the characteristics of the material, the initial particle size and the degree of size reduction desired. For example, very large particles may require size reduction in stages simply because the equipment required to produce the final product will not accept the initial feed, as in crushing prior to grinding. In the case of vegetable and other fibrous material, size reduction generally must be, at least initially, accomplished by cutting or chopping.

Chemical substances used in pharmaceuticals, in contrast, generally need not be subjected to either crushing or cutting operations prior to reduction to the required particle size. However, these materials do differ considerably in melting point, brittleness, hardness, and moisture content, all of which affect the ease of particle-size reduction and dictate the choice of equipment. The heat generated in mechanical grinding, in particular, presents problems with materials that tend to liquefy or stick together and with the thermolabile products that may degrade unless the heat is dissipated by use of a flowing stream of water or air. The desired particle size, shape, and size distribution also must be considered in the selection of grinding or milling equipment. For example, attrition mills tend to produce spheroidal, more free-flowing particles than do impact-type mills, which yield more irregular-shaped particles.

FRACTURE MECHANICS

Reduction of particle size through fracture requires application of mechanical stress to the material to be crushed or ground. Materials respond to stress by yielding, with subsequent generation of strain. Depending on the time course of strain as a function of applied stresses, materials can be classified according to their behavior over a continuous spectrum ranging from brittle to plastic. In the case of a totally brittle substance, complete rebound would occur on release of applied stress at stresses up to the yield point, where fracture would occur. In contrast, a totally plastic material would not rebound nor would it fracture.

The vast majority of pharmaceutical solids lie somewhere between these extremes and thus possess both elastic and viscous properties. Linear and, to a lesser extent, nonlinear viscoelastic theory has been developed well to account for quantitatively and explain the simultaneous elastic and viscous deformations produced in solids by applied stresses.

The energy expended by comminution ultimately appears as surface energy associated with newly created particle surfaces, internal free energy associated with lattice changes, and as heat. Most of the energy expressed as heat is consumed in the viscoelastic deformation of particles, friction, and in imparting kinetic energy to particles. Energy is exchanged among these modes and some is, of course, effective in producing fracture. It has been estimated that 1% or less of the total mechanical energy used is associated with newly created surface or with crystal lattice imperfections.

Although the grinding process has been described mathematically, the theory of grinding has not been developed to the point where the actual performance of the grinding equipment can be predicted quantitatively. However, three fundamental laws have been advanced:

Kick's Law—The work required to reduce the size of a given quantity of material is constant for the same reduction ratio regardless of the original size of the initial material.

Rittinger's Law—The work used for particulate size reduction is directly proportional to the new surface produced.

Bond's Law—The work used to reduce the particle size is proportional to the square root of the diameter of the particles produced.

In general, however, these laws have been useful only in providing trends and qualitative information on the grinding process. Usually laboratory testing is required to evaluate the performance of particular equipment. A work index, developed from Bond's Law, is a useful way of comparing the efficiency of milling operations.[1] A grindability index, which has been developed for a number of materials, also can be used to evaluate mill performance.[2]

A number of other factors also must be considered in equipment selection. Abrasion or mill wear is an important factor in the grinding of hard materials, particularly in high-speed, close-clearance equipment (eg, hammer mills). In some instances mill wear may be so extensive as to lead to highly contaminated products and excessive maintenance costs that make the milling process uneconomical. Hardness of the material, which often is related to abrasiveness, also must be considered. This usually is measured on the Moh's scale. Qualitatively, materials from 1 to 3 are considered as soft and from 8 to 10 as hard. Friability (ease of fracture) and fibrousness can be of equal importance in mill selection. Fibrous materials, such as plant products, require a cutting or chopping action and usually cannot be reduced in size effectively by pressure or impact techniques. A moisture content above about 5% will in most instances also create a problem and can lead to agglomeration or even liquefaction of the milled material. Hydrates often will release their water of hydration under the influence of a high-temperature milling process and thus may require cooling or low-speed processing.

METHODS AND EQUIPMENT

When a narrow particle-size distribution with a minimum of fines is desired, closed-circuit milling is advantageous. This technique combines the milling equipment with some type of classifier (see *Particle-Size Measurement and Classification*). In the simplest arrangement, a screen is used to make the separation, and the oversize particles are returned to the mill on a continuous basis while the particles of the desired size pass through the screen and out of the grinding chamber. Overmilling, with its subsequent production of fines, thereby is minimized. Equipment also has been designed to combine the sieving and milling steps into a single operation (see *Centrifugal-Impact Mills and Sieves*).

To avoid contamination or deterioration, the equipment used for pharmaceuticals should be fabricated of materials that are chemically and mechanically compatible with the substance being processed. The equipment should be easy to disassemble for cleaning to prevent cross-contamination. Dust-free operation, durability, simplified construction, and operation and suitable feed and outlet capacities are additional considerations in equipment selection.

Although there is no rigid classification of large-scale comminution equipment, it generally is divided into three broad categories based on feed and product size:

1. *Coarse crushers* (eg, jaw, gyratory, roll, and impact crushers).
2. *Intermediate grinders* (eg, rotary cutters, disk, hammer, roller, and chaser mills).
3. *Fine grinding mills* (eg, ball, rod, hammer, colloid, and fluid-energy mills; high-speed mechanical screen and centrifugal classifier).

Machines in the first category are employed ordinarily where the size of the feed material is relatively large, ranging from 1½ to 60 inches in diameter. These are used most frequently in the mineral crushing industry and will not be considered further. The machines in the second category are used for feed materials of relatively small size and provide products that fall between 20- and 200-mesh. Those in the third category produce particles, most of which will pass through a 200-mesh sieve, although often the particle size of the products from fine grinding mills is well into the micron range.

The comminution effect of any given operation can be described mathematically in terms of a matrix whose elements represent the probabilities of transformation of the various-size particles in the feed material to the particle sizes present in the output. The numerical values of the elements in the transition matrix can be determined experimentally and the matrix serves to characterize the mill. Matrices of this type are frequently a function of feed rate and feed particle-size distribution but are useful in predicting mill behavior. Multiplication of the appropriate comminution matrix with the feed-size distribution line-matrix yields the predicted output-size distribution.

INTERMEDIATE AND FINE GRINDING MILLS

The various types of comminuting equipment in this class generally employ one of three basic actions or, more commonly, a combination of these actions.

1. *Attrition.* This involves breaking down of the material by a rubbing action between two surfaces. The procedure is particularly applicable to the grinding of fibrous materials where a tearing action is required to reduce the fibers to powder.
2. *Rolling.* This uses a heavy rolling member to crush and pulverize the material. Theoretically, only a rolling-crushing type of action is involved, but in actual practice some slight attrition takes place between the face of the roller and the bed of the mill.
3. *Impact.* This involves the operation of hammers (or bars) at high speeds. These strike the lumps of material and throw them against each other or against the walls of the containing chamber. The impact causes large particles to split apart, the action continuing until small particles of required size are produced. In some instances high-velocity air or centrifugal force may be used to generate high-impact velocities.

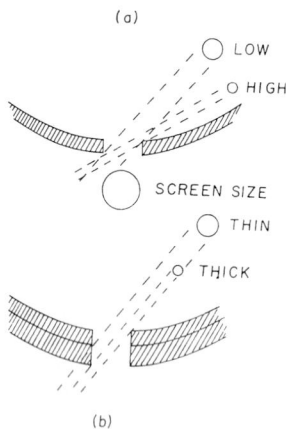

Figure 37-1. The influence of (**a**) mill speed and (**b**) screen thickness on particle size at a constant screen-opening size.[3]

Roller Mills—Roller mills in their basic form consist of two rollers revolving in the same direction at different rates of speed. This principle, which provides particle-size reduction mainly through compression (crushing) and shear, has been applied to the development of a wide variety of roller mills. Some use multiple smooth rollers or corrugated, ribbed, or sawtoothed rollers to provide a cutting action. Most allow adjustment of the gap between rollers to control the particle size of the product. The roller mill is quite versatile and can be used to crush a variety of materials.

An example of a pharmaceutical roller mill is the Crack-U-Lator, in which a series of ribbed rollers are adjusted to reduce sequentially the particle size of the product to produce the desired distribution. The design allows particles that are smaller than the gap between the rollers to pass to the next stage without unnecessary size reduction, thus reducing fines.

Hammer Mills—Hammer mills consist of a rotating shaft on which are mounted either rigid or swing hammers (beaters). This unit is enclosed with a chamber containing a grid or removable screen through which the material must pass. On the upper part is the feed hopper. As the material enters the chamber, the rapidly rotating hammers strike against it and break it into smaller fragments. These are swept downward against the screen where they undergo additional *hammering* action until they are reduced to a size small enough to pass through the openings and out. Oversize particles are hurled upward into the chamber where they also undergo further blows by the revolving hammers.

These mills operate at high speed and generally with controlled feed rate. Both impact and attrition provide the grinding action. Particle size is regulated by rotor speed, feed rate, type and number of hammers, clearance between hammers and chamber wall, and discharge openings. At a constant screen opening, the speed of the mill and the thickness of the screen will affect the particle size of the milled powder,[3] as shown in Figure 37-1. The higher the speed, the steeper the approach angle of the particle to the screen hole. Thus, for any screen size opening, the higher the blade speed, the smaller the particle obtained. Increasing the screen thickness will have a similar effect. In general flat-edged blades are most effective for pulverizing, while sharp-edged blades will act to chop or cut fibrous materials.

The FitzMill Comminutor (Fig 37-2) is an example of this type of mill. It can be used in either the hammer or knife-blade configuration and can be fitted with a wide range of screen sizes to fulfill a variety of milling specifications.

A wide range of particle sizes down to the micron size can be produced by these mills. The particle shape, however, is generally sharper and more irregular than that produced by compression methods. When very fine particles are desired, hammer mills can be operated in conjunction with an air classifier. Under such conditions a narrower particle-size distribution and lower grinding temperatures are obtained. Fine pulverizing of plastic material can be accomplished in these mills by embrittlement with liquid N_2 or CO_2 or by jacketing the grinding chamber.

Centrifugal-Impact Mills and Sieves—Centrifugal-impact mills and sieves are useful to minimize the production of fine particles, because their design combines sieving and milling into a single operation. The mill consists of a nonrotating bar or stator that is fixed within a rotating sieve basket. The particles that are smaller than the hole size of the sieve can pass through the mill without comminution; however, the particles or agglomerates larger than the hole size are directed by centrifugal force to impact with the stator. The sieve baskets also can be constructed to have a cutting edge that can aid in particle-size reduction without impact with the stator. The Quick Sieve (Fig 37-3), Turbo Sieve and CoMill are examples of this type of mill.

Cutter Mills—Cutter mills are useful in reducing the particle size of fibrous material and act by a combined cutting and shearing action. They consist of a horizontal rotor into which is set a series of knives or blades. This rotor turns within a housing, and into it are set stationary bed knives. The feed is from the top and a perforated plate or screen is set into the bottom of the housing through which the finished product is discharged. The particle size and shape is determined by the plate size, gap between rotor and bed knives, and size of the openings. A number of rotor styles are available to provide different particle shapes and sizes, though cutter mills are normally not designed to produce particles finer than 80- to 100-mesh.

Attrition Mills—Attrition mills make use of two stone or steel grinding plates, one or both of which revolve to provide grinding mainly through attrition. These mills are most suitable for friable or medium-hard, free-flowing material.

A double-runner attrition mill is an example of a mill that uses two rotating disks revolving in opposite directions. The particle-size reduction is controlled by varying the rotational speed of the disks, the space between the disks, and the size and number of ridges and indentations in the face of the disks. By appropriate combination with a classifier, particle sizes ranging from 10-mesh to 20 μm can be obtained by these attrition mills.

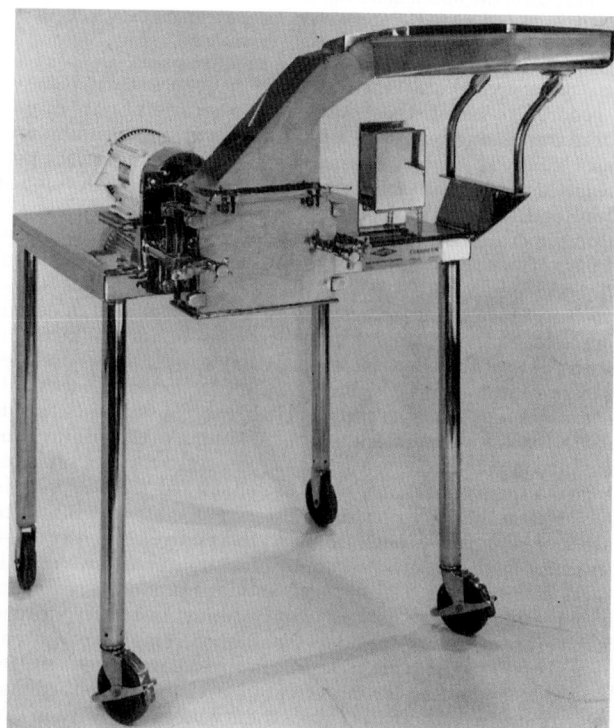

Figure 37-2. EZ-Clean FitzMill Comminutor (courtesy, Fitzpatrick).

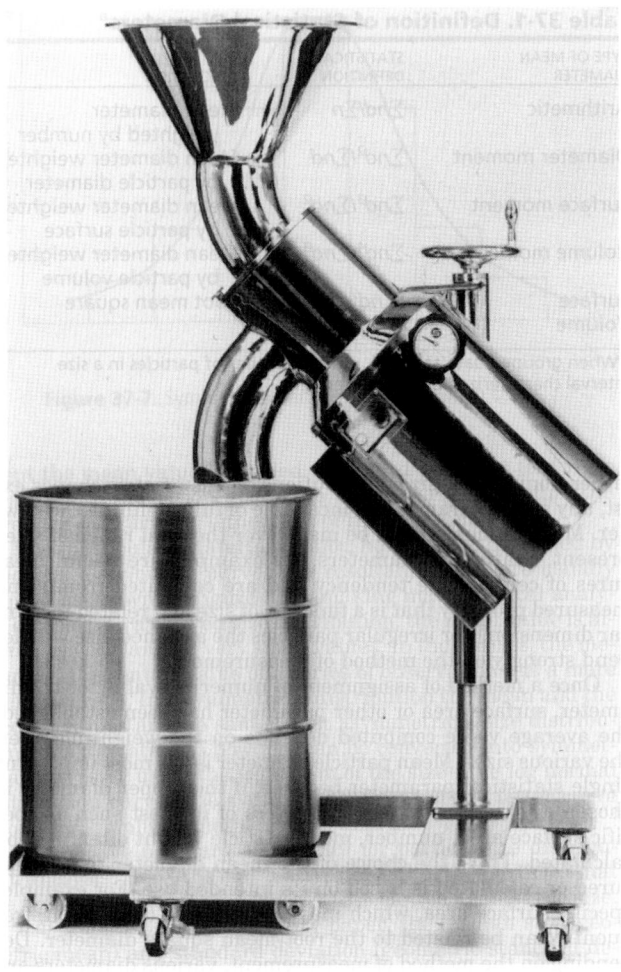

Figure 37-3. Quick Sieve (courtesy, Glatt Air).

Chaser Mills—Chaser mills are so called because two heavy granite stones, or chasers, mounted vertically like wheels and connected by a short horizontal shaft, are made to revolve or chase each other upon a granite base surrounded by a curb. Revolution of the chasers produces an upward current of air; this carries over the lighter particles, which fall outside the curb and subsequently are collected as a fine powder.

Pebble or Ball Mills—Pebble or ball mills, sometimes called *pot mills* or *jar mills,* are operated on the principle of attrition and impact. The grinding is effected by placing the substance in jars or cylindrical vessels that are lined with porcelain or a similar hard substance and containing *pebbles* or *balls* of flint, porcelain, steel, or stainless steel. These cylindrical vessels revolve horizontally on their long axis and the tumbling of the pebbles or balls over one another and against the sides of the cylinder produces pulverization with a minimum loss of material. Ball-milling is a relatively slow process and generally requires many hours to produce material of suitable fineness. To keep the grinding time within reasonable limits, coarse material (>10-mesh) should be preground before introduction into a ball mill. Figure 37-4 shows a sectional view of a single jar mill. *Rod mills* are a modification in which rods about 3 inches shorter than the length of the mill are used in place of balls. This results in a lower production of fines and a somewhat more granular product.

Vibrating Ball Mills—Vibrating ball mills, which also combine attrition and impact, consist of a mill shell containing a charge of balls similar to rotating ball mills. However, in this case the shell is vibrated at some suitable frequency, rather than rotated. These mills offer the advantage of being free of ro-

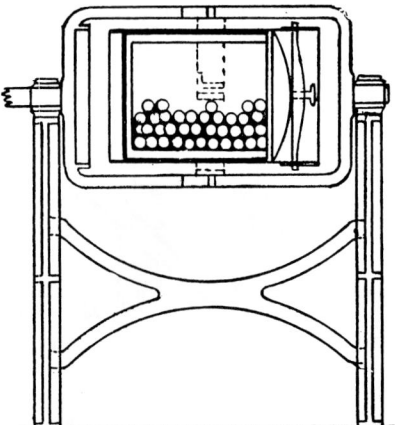

Figure 37-4. Single jar mill.

tating parts, and thus can be integrated readily into a particle classifying system or other ancillary equipment. Furthermore, there have been several studies that have demonstrated that the vibrating ball mill will grind at rates often as high as 20 to 30 times that of the conventional tumbling mill and offer a higher order of grinding rate and efficiency than other prevailing milling procedures.

Fluid-Energy Mills—Fluid-energy mills are used for pulverizing and classifying extremely small particles of many materials. The mills have no moving parts, grinding being achieved by subjecting the solid material to streams of high-velocity elastic fluids, usually air, steam, or an inert gas. The material to be pulverized is swept into violent turbulence by the sonic and supersonic velocity of the streams. The particles are accelerated to relatively high speeds; when they collide with each other, the impact causes violent fracture of the particles.

One type of fluid-energy mill is shown in Figure 37-5. The elastic grinding fluid is introduced through nozzles in the lower portion of the mill under pressures ranging from 25 to 300 psi. In this way, a rapidly circulating flow of gas is generated in the hollow, doughnut-shaped mill. A Venturi feeder introduces the coarse material into the mill and the particles enter into the jet stream of rapidly moving gas. The raw material is pulverized

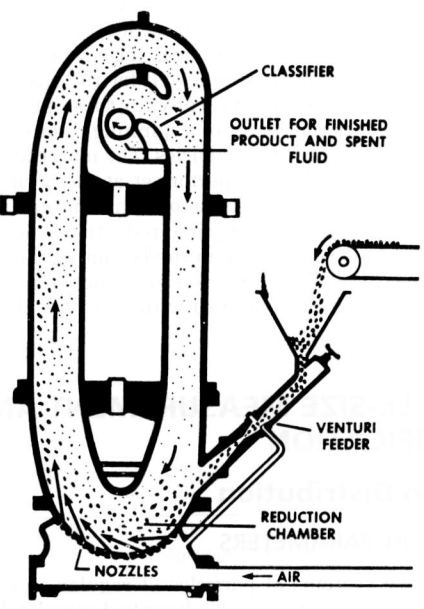

Figure 37-5. The Jet-O-Mizer fluid energy mill (courtesy, Fluid Energy).

light and to about 0.01 μm by the use of the ultramicroscope. The electron microscope finds its greatest usefulness in particle-size measurements in the range of 0.001 to 0.2 μm.

Although microscopic methods for particle size determination are time consuming, tedious, and generally require more skill than some of the other techniques, they offer a number of advantages. They supply information about particle shape and thickness that cannot be obtained by other methods and, in addition, supply a permanent record through use of photomicrographs.

A variety of semiautomated procedures have been developed to reduce the fatigue and tedium associated with manual counting of particles. These are represented by instruments such as the Imanco Quantimet 720 and the πMC System (*Millipore*), which scan the powder image in a manner similar to a TV scanner. The signal obtained is analyzed by a pulse-height analyzer and expressed as a particle-size distribution.

ADSORPTION OF GASES

Adsorption of a solute from solution or of a gas at low temperatures onto powdered material serves as a measure of the particle surface area, generally reported as specific surface (area/unit mass). Common adsorption techniques use the adsorption of nitrogen and krypton at low temperatures. The volume of the gas adsorbed by a powdered sample is determined as a function of gas pressure, and an appropriate plot is prepared. The point at which a monomolecular layer of adsorbate occurs is estimated from the discontinuity that shows in the curve. The specific surface area then can be calculated from knowledge of the volume of gas required to achieve this monolayer, and the area/molecule occupied by the gas, its molecular weight and density. Frequently, more complex expressions such as the Brunauer, Emmett, and Teller (BET) equation must be used to describe the surface adsorption of some materials and determine the volume of gas required to produce an adsorbed monolayer. The surface properties of a number of pharmaceuticals have been investigated by this technique.

PERMEABILITY

When a gas or liquid is allowed to flow through a powdered material, the resistance to this flow is a function of such factors as specific surface of the powder, area of the bed, pore space, pressure drop across the bed, and viscosity of the fluid. This resistance can be described and the specific surface calculated by the Kozeny–Carmen equation, which relates these factors. This method, although it does not provide a size distribution analysis, offers a rapid and convenient means of size estimation that is useful for some industrial operations.

Instruments that measure the rate of flow of a gas through a powder bed under controlled pressure differential are available commercially. The Sub-Sieve Sizer (*Fisher*) permits the reading of average particle size directly. The Blaine Permeameter (*Precision Scientific*) uses the principle of filling the void spaces in a powder with mercury and then weighing it. The void fraction is calculated from the known density of mercury at different temperatures.

The calculations involved in permeability techniques are often complicated and yield only an average size of particles. In measuring particles in the subsieve ranges, rather large deviations may be encountered. With larger mesh sizes, some good agreement is found between the results obtained by techniques employing permeability and microscopy, particularly if the powders are made up of spherical or near-spherical particles.

IMPACTION AND INERTIAL TECHNIQUES

The laws that govern the trajectories of particles in fluid streams are used in several methods of particle-size measure-

ment. Impaction devices are based on the dynamics of deposition of fine particles in a moving air stream when directed past obstacles of defined geometric form, or when forced from a jet device onto a plane surface.

The *cascade impactor,* described by Pilcher and co-workers,[4] forces particle laden air at a very high speed and fixed rate through a series of jets (each smaller than the preceding one) onto glass slides; impaction takes place in a series of stages. The velocities of the air stream and the particles suspended in it are increased as they advance through the impactor. As a result, the particles are classified by impaction on the different slides, with the larger particles on the top slides and the smaller ones on the downstream slides. Figure 37-10 illustrates the principle of the cascade impactor. The exact size of impacted particles on each slide subsequently must be determined. Size analyses may be obtained directly by theoretical treatment or prior calibration of the instrument.

Tillotson[5] described an instrument based on inertial principles similar to those of the cascade impactor. This instrument may be adapted for automatic readout of size distribution by means of light-scattering techniques and electronic counters. The method is claimed to provide complete particle-size distribution data in a few minutes.

AUTOMATIC PARTICLE SIZE COUNTERS

The principles of electronic and light sensing and light scattering techniques have been used to develop automated particle size counters that indirectly measure particle size.

Electrozone Sensing—The *Coulter Counter* determines the particle volume distribution of materials suspended in an electrolyte-containing solution. This instrument utilizes an electrical sensing zone and measures electrical pulses caused by the passage of particles through the zones. The instrument must be calibrated with monodispersed particles of known diameter. A table of size ranges of several methods

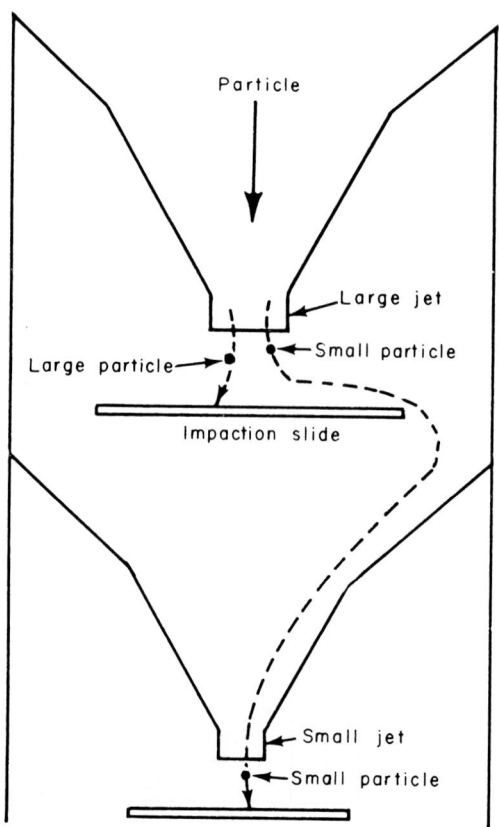

Figure 37-10. The principle of the cascade impactor.

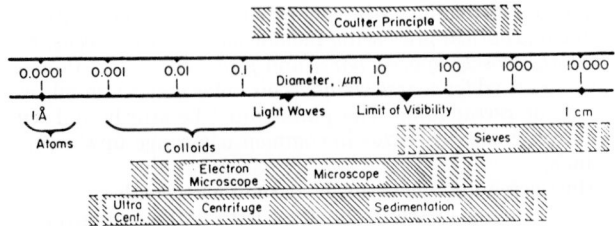

Figure 37-11. Size range of Coulter method compared with coverage of sieve, sedimentation, and microscopic methods, and overlap of electron microscope and centrifuge ranges (courtesy, Coulter).

compared with the Coulter principle is shown in Figure 37-11. Detection is limited by thermal and electrical noise and the ability to discriminate true signal pulses from background.

Photozone Sensing—The *HIAC Counter* measures the size distribution of particles suspended in either liquids or gases. The standard models will measure sizes from 2 to 2500 μm at pressures up to 3000 psi. Basically, in this instrument the particles pass a window, one by one. As each particle passes, depending on its size it interrupts some portion of a light beam. This causes an instantaneous reduction in the voltage from a photodetector that is proportional to the size of the particle. Several counting circuits with preset thresholds tally the particles by size.

Laser Diffraction—Laser diffraction or low angle laser light scattering has become one of the preferred methods for particle size characterization. The instrument consists of a laser light source (generally a He-Ne gas laser), a suitable detector such as a silicon photodiode, and a means of passing the sample through the laser beam. An ultrasonic probe may be used to improve particle dispersion. In this technique, particles are dispersed in a liquid or gaseous medium. The diffraction angle is inversely proportional to particle size. The instrument does not require calibration against a standard and dry powders may be measured directly by using pressure to pass the sample through the instrument. In addition, the method is nondestructive and samples can be recovered after testing. The latest instruments utilize the Mie theory of particle interaction with light and allow for accurate measurements over a large size range (typically 0.1 to 3000 μm)[6].

Size Classification

SIEVING

Sieving is one of the simplest and probably most frequently used methods for determining particle-size distribution. The technique basically involves size classification followed by the determination of the weight of each fraction.

In this technique, particles of a powder mass are placed on a screen made of uniform apertures. By the application of some type of motion to the screen, the particles smaller than the apertures are made to pass through. The sieve motion generally is either (1) horizontal, which tends to loosen the packing of the particles in contact with the screen surface, permitting the entrapped subsieve particles to pass through, or (2) vertical, which serves to agitate and mix the particles as well as to bring more of the subsieve particles to the screen surface.

One major difficulty associated with this method is the production of screens with uniform apertures, particularly in the very fine mesh sizes. As a result the practical lower limit for woven-wire mesh screens is about 43 μm (325-mesh). However, with the introduction of electroformed screens, sieves capable of analyzing particles in the 5-μm range are now available. In addition, "blinding" of the openings by oversized or irregular particles and inefficient presentation of the particles to the screen surface are problems associated with this technique. The use of horizontal and vertical screening motions, air jets, sudden periodic reversal of the sieve motion, and continuous cycling all have been used in an attempt to eliminate these problems.

For continuous operations, the screens are attached to mechanical or electromagnetic devices that supply the energy required to shake the particles through the openings in the screen and also to prevent accumulation of fines within the openings, as this tends to clog them and slow down the operation. The use

of an electromagnetic instead of mechanical drive provides a more gentle sieving action with a resultant decrease in sieve wear, blinding, and machine noise. Sieves may be used either in a sequence of sizes through which the material must pass or singly in the required size.

This apparatus is useful in obtaining size-analysis data under controlled conditions. The sample is placed in the top of the nest of standard sieves arranged in a descending order. The length of time and force of vibration to which the sample is subjected may be preset by variable time and voltage controls. The controlled vibration causes the powder particles to pass through the sieves, each fraction coming to rest in the sieve through which it cannot pass. For the purpose of analysis, the weight of each fraction is determined and the percentage calculated.

The Sonic Sifter (*Allen-Bradley* and *ATM*) is a laboratory sifter that uses sonic oscillation to classify particles. A mechanical pulse action is used to reduce blinding and agglomeration in the subsieve sizes. This combination of sonic and mechanical agitation permits dry sifting down to 5 μm. US Standard Sieves are available for this unit from 3 1/2- to 400-mesh and in precision electroformed mesh sizes from 150 to 5 μm.

Industrial-size mechanical sieves are varied in design and capacity, and include the gyratory, circular rotatory, vibrating, shaking, and revolving sifters. In gyratory sifters, the motion is in a single horizontal plane, but may vary from circular to reciprocal from the feed to the discharge end. The circular sifter also confines the screen motion to a horizontal plane, but in this case the total motion applied to the sieve is circular. The material enters the top of a gyratory sifter and spreads over the first sieve. Some of the finer particles drop through and are discharged into the *throughs* channel. The remaining powder moves to the next sieve in order, the process is repeated until complete separation is accomplished (Fig 37-12).

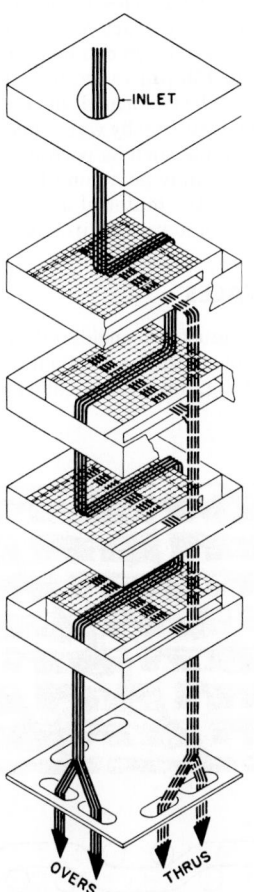

Figure 37-12. Gyratory sifter (courtesy, Sprout Waldron).

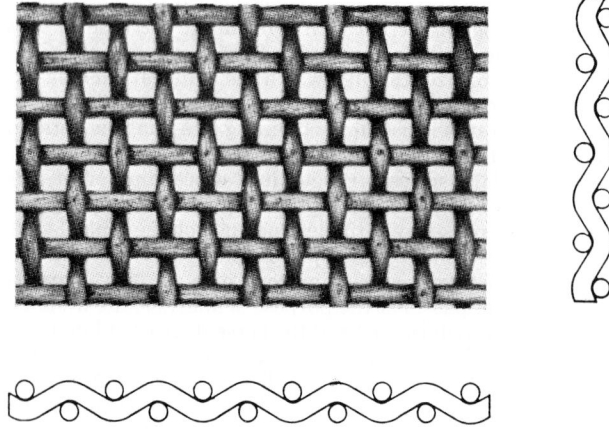

Figure 37-13. Plain weave screen.

In centrifugal screening, the material is pushed through a spinning vertical wire cloth cylinder. Sharp cuts in particle size can be obtained with this type of equipment. Downward air flow, instead of shaking and tapping, has been used to move the particles through the screen openings; alternating with a reverse air flow serves to prevent *blinding*, particularly with fine-mesh sieves.

WET SCREENING

The addition of water sometimes is employed to dissolve any unwanted binders, remove fines or surface contamination, and to reduce surface forces—particularly in micromesh sieves—that oppose the flow of particles through the sieve. Particles that tend to agglomerate or react with oxygen or moisture and thus cannot be dry-sieved often can be handled by wet-sieving. Particles in the 6- to 150-μm range have been classified with good precision using electroformed sieves. Some hydrophobic substances that resist wetting by water may be wet screened by the use of organic liquids such as petroleum ether, acetone, or alcohol. Wet screening may be accomplished by spraying both the screen surface and the material as it is fed onto the screen or by feeding a slurry of material directly onto the screen.

SCREENING SURFACES

A number of factors must be considered in selecting screening surfaces. Primary consideration is given to the size and shape of the aperture opening, the selection of which is determined by the particle size that is to be separated. Screens commonly used in pharmaceutical processing include *woven wire screens, bolting cloth, closely spaced bars,* and *punched plates*. Punched plates are used for coarse sizing; their holes may be round, oval, square, or rectangular. The plates must be sturdy and withstand rough service. Sizes in common use range upward from 1/4 inch.

Most screening, however, is accomplished with woven-wire screens ranging in size from those with 400 openings/inch to screens with 4-inch square openings or larger. There are numerous types of woven wire screens, including plain, twilled, and braided weave. An example of the plain and twilled weave is shown in Figures 37-13 and 37-14.

In the US, the two common standards are the *Tyler Standard* and *US Standard* sieves. In both these series the sieve number refers to the number of openings per linear inch. For most purposes, screens from the two series are interchangeable, though in a few instances the number designations are different. Because these numbers do not define the size of the openings, the Bureau of Standards has established specifications for *Standard Sieves,* as given in Table 37-2. These specifications also establish tolerances for the evenness of weaving, as irregularities from careless weaving might permit much larger particles to pass the sieve than would be indicated. The standard sieves used for pharmaceutical testing are of wire cloth.

SEDIMENTATION

The sedimentation method employs the settling of particles in a liquid of a relatively low density, under the influence of a gravitational or centrifugal field. In free settling (ie, no particle-particle interference), the particles are supported by hydraulic forces and their fall can be described by Stokes' law. However, in most real situations, particle–particle interference, nonuniformity, and turbulence are all present, resulting in more complex settling patterns. The Andreason pipet, which is based on sampling near the bottom of a glass sedimentation chamber, is perhaps the best known of the early instruments. With centrifugation, entrainment of particles in the currents produced by other particles also may interfere with fractionation.

Gravitational settling chambers often are used for large-scale separation of relatively coarse particles in the range of 100 μm. Centrifugal devices are useful for the separation of much smaller particles (5–10 μm).

Sedimentation balances are available that provide a means of directly weighing particles at selected time intervals as they fall in a liquid system. For continuous observations, automatic recording balances also are available. A commercially available instrument called a *Micromerograph* uses the principle of sedimentation in an air column. This instrument and others related

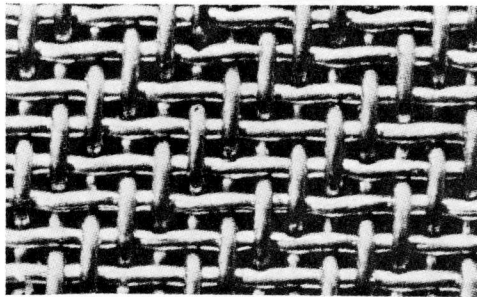

Figure 37-14. Twilled weave screen.

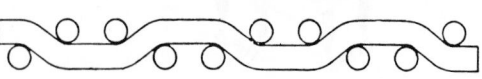

Table 37-2. Nominal Dimensions of Standard Sieves

| NO | SIEVE OPENING | | PERMISSIBLE VARIATION IN AVERAGE OPENING, % | PERMISSIBLE VARIATION IN MAXIMUM OPENING, % | WIRE DIAMETER, mm |
	mm	μm			
2	9.52	9520	±3	+5	2.11 to 2.59
4	4.76	4760	±3	+10	1.14 to 1.68
8	2.38	2380	±3	+10	0.74 to 1.10
10	2.00	2000	±3	+10	0.68 to 1.00
20	0.84	840	±5	+15	0.38 to 0.55
30	0.59	590	±5	+15	0.29 to 0.42
40	0.42	420	±5	+25	0.23 to 0.33
50	0.297	297	±5	+25	0.170 to 0.253
60	0.250	250	±5	+25	0.149 to 0.220
70	0.210	210	±5	+25	0.130 to 0.187
80	0.177	177	±6	+40	0.114 to 0.154
100	0.149	149	±6	+40	0.096 to 0.125
120	0.125	125	±6	+40	0.079 to 0.103
200	0.074	74	±7	+60	0.045 to 0.061

to it in principle offer more rapid determinations than those that use a liquid medium. There are, however, serious uncertainties in the method that must be taken into consideration. Deviations from Stokes' law and impaction of particles against the inner wall of the settling chamber are sources of possible error.

The Carey and Stairmand *photosedimentometer* photographs the tracks of particles as they fall in a dispersion medium. The size determination is derived from the length of the photographic track, which is an indication of the distance traveled by the particles, and the time of exposure of the photograph.

ELUTRIATION

In elutriation, the particles are suspended in a moving fluid, generally water or air. In vertical elutriation at any particular velocity of the fluid, particles of a given size will move upwards with the fluid, while larger particles will settle out under the influence of gravity. In horizontal elutriation a stream of suspended particles is passed over a settling chamber. Particles that leave the stream are collected in the bottom of the chamber. Normally, for all elutriation techniques, both undersize and oversize particles appear in each fraction and recycling is required if a clean cut is desired. By varying the fluid velocities stepwise, the sample may be separated into fractions. The amount in each fraction then can be determined and the size limits calculated by the use of the Stokes' equation or measured directly by microscopy. Air elutriation usually will give a sharper fractionation in a shorter time than will water elutriation.

Centrifugal elutriation is basically the same process, except in this case the fluid stream is caused to spin so as to impart a high centrifugal force to the suspended particles. The particles that are too large to follow the direction of flow separate out on the walls or bottom of the elutriator or cyclone. The finer particles escape with the discharge stream. Separation down to about 0.5 μm can be achieved with some centrifugal classifiers.

The DorrClone (*Dorr-Oliver*) (Fig 37-15) is an example of a centrifugal-type classifier. The feed enters tangentially into the upper section. Centrifugal forces in the vortex throw the coarser particles to the wall where they collect and then drop down and out of the unit. The fine particles move to the inner spiral of the vortex and are displaced upward and finally out of the top of the unit.

Inertial elutriators, which use an abrupt change in direction of the fluid stream to produce separation, are effective down to about 200-mesh. However, as with other elutriators, a clean cut usually cannot be obtained without recycling.

Felvation is a unique process that combines elutriation and sieving along with a varying fluid flow rate and a turbulent fluidized bed to achieve particle separation. The particles are fluidized within the felvation column. With a gradual increase of the fluid flow rate, the very fine particles are brought up to and then through a sieve surface set into the upper section of the column. These fines are filtered subsequently out of the fluid stream. A further increase in the fluid flow rate causes larger and larger particles to move through the sieve. The final stage is reached when particles just larger than the sieve aperture are elutriated up to the sieve.

Because of the way in which the particles are presented to the sieve, very little blinding of the openings occur. Furthermore, because the sieve need only serve as a go/no-go gauge and not as a supporting surface for the powder, a relatively small sieve surface is required. Thus, the more-uniform but more-expensive electroform sieves, even down to a 10-μm size, can be used in this process.

MISCELLANEOUS METHODS

Numerous other methods have been applied to particle size determination, including x-ray and electron diffraction, ultrasound, flotation, and electrostatic, magnetic, and dielectrophoretic methods. Newer techniques include photon

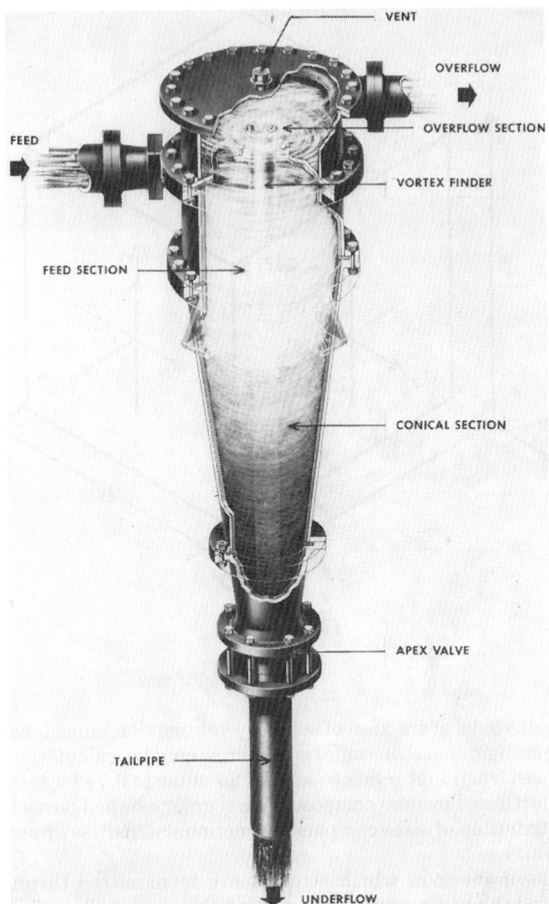

Figure 37-15. DorrClone, a hydrocentrifugal classifier (courtesy, Dorr-Oliver).

correlation spectroscopy, polarization intensity differential scattering, and fourier-transform infrared spectroscopy with diffuse reflectance. These techniques either are used principally as research tools or are industrial-scale methods of use outside the pharmaceutical industry. Detailed descriptions of their principles of operation and their applications can be found in the *Bibliography*.

SOLIDS HANDLING

Packing and Bulk Properties

BULK DENSITY; ANGLES OF REPOSE

Systems of particulate solids are the most complex physical systems encountered in pharmacy. No two particles in a powder are identical and the nature of momentum and energy exchange between particles defies description except in the most idealized and approximate terms. Bulk properties of powders are determined in part by the chemical and physical properties of their component solids and in part by the manner in which the various components interact. These interactions in turn frequently depend on the past history of the powder bed as well as on the ambient conditions.

The static properties of a particulate bed depend on particle–particle interactions and, in particular, on the way in which applied stresses are distributed through the bed. The number of contacts between particles and, hence, the average number of interparticulate contact points per particle increases as bed-packing increases. Packing may be expressed in terms of porosity,

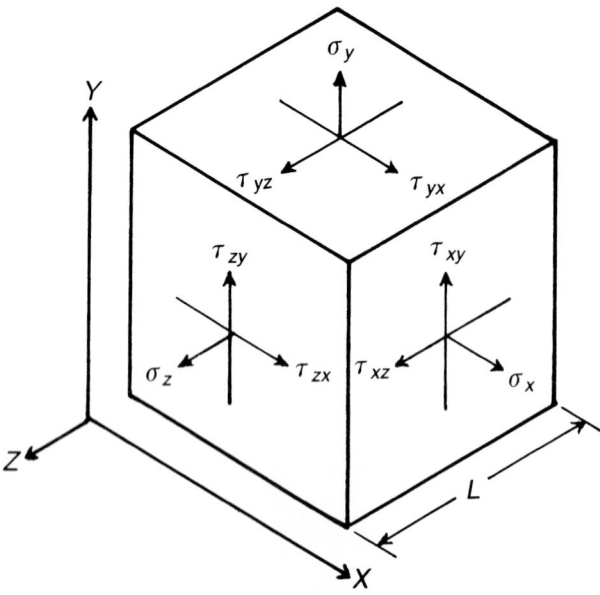

Figure 37-16.

percent voids, or fraction of solids by volume. Packings for regular arrangements of uniform spheres can be calculated and range in fractional solids from 0.53 for cubic to 0.74 for tetrahedral lattices. Powders composed of irregular-shaped particles in a distribution of sizes can pack to fractional densities approaching unity.

The manner in which stresses are transmitted through a bed and the bed's response to applied stress are reflected in the various angles of friction and repose. The most commonly used of these is the angle of repose, which may be determined experimentally by a number of methods, with slightly differing results. The typical method is to pour the powder in a conical heap on a level, flat surface and measure the included angle with the horizontal. Angles of repose range from 23° for smooth uniform glass beads to 64° for granular limestone. Cohesive materials frequently behave in an anomalous manner, yielding values in excess of 90°.

The angle of internal friction is a measure of internal stress distributions and is the angle at which an applied stress diverges as it passes through the bed. This angle together with the angle of slide are useful parameters in the design of storage/discharge bins. The latter angle is defined as the least slope at which a powder will slide down an inclined plane surface. Various other angles are in lesser use and will not be discussed here.

STATICS

Powders at rest experience stresses that vary with location throughout their volume and arise from pressures exerted by the container as well as from the weight of the bed above. Each point within the bed experiences both normal and shear stresses in general. Normal stresses may be either tensile or compressive. The powder bed will remain motionless and no flow will occur unless the normal and/or the shear strength is exceeded at some point within the bed. In general, the yield strengths, both normal and shear, are functions of the normal and shear stresses at the point of interest and depend upon the orientation of the axes of reference and the nature of the powder itself. It is apparent that to understand powder flow it is necessary to understand the conditions under which bed failure occurs and powder flow is initiated and sustained.

Consider the stresses that are applied to the faces of a small cube that is centered about a point chosen at random

within a powder bed. Normal stresses are designated σ_i, where the subscript indicates the axis normal to the face and shear stresses are designated τ_{ij}, where the first subscript indicates the face and the second indicates the direction of the applied force. If the cube has an edge length, L, which is not infinitesimal, and if a stress gradient exists within the region, the corresponding stresses on opposite faces of the cube will not be equal. However, if the cube is made progressively smaller, and as L approaches zero, the stress values will converge to those at the point of interest. These forces are illustrated in Figure 37-16. It can be seen from this diagram that the state of stress at a point can be described by nine stress components.

If the system is in static equilibrium, and is not being accelerated translationally or rotationally, the forces that otherwise would result in movement must be in balance and have the effect of canceling each other. For example, τ_{xy} must equal τ_{yx} if rotation about the z-axis is not to occur. In a similar manner, shear and normal stresses, which would lead to translational movement along any of the three axes, also must balance.

Because the directions of the mutually perpendicular axes in Figure 37-16 were chosen arbitrarily, any other orientation of the cube corresponding to another set of axes also must result in a balance of forces. However, the distribution of stress among normal and shear components will depend on the particular axes selected. Thus, the stress condition of a powder can be analyzed in terms of the dependence of the normal and shear stresses on the direction chosen for the reference axes. This can be done by a method of analysis devised by Mohr, and can be visualized using a Mohr circle diagram, which permits stresses at any given point within a powder bed to be graphically resolved into normal, σ, and shear, τ, stresses for any arbitrary choice of axes.

For simplicity, assume that stress in the z-direction is not a function of z and that stress gradients exist in the x and y directions only. Stresses then can be analyzed in the xy plane without reference to the z-axis. Figure 37-17 shows the relationship between stresses relative to two xy coordinate systems at an angle θ to each other. If the condition of stress in the powder remains constant and only the angle θ between the two sets of reference axes is allowed to change, the resolution of stress into normal and shear components will be different for each set of axes and will depend on θ. By means of

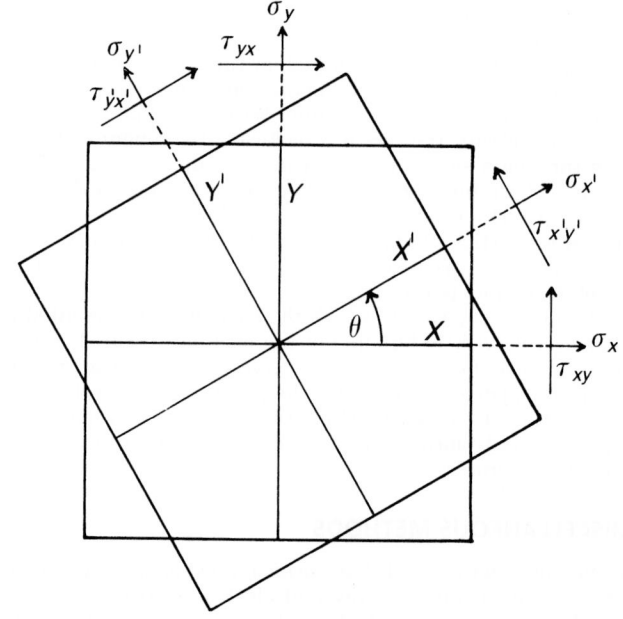

Figure 37-17.

trigonometry, the relationships between these two sets of stresses is shown to be

$$\sigma_{x'} = \frac{\sigma_x + \sigma_y}{2} + \frac{\sigma_x - \sigma_y}{2} \cos 2\theta + \tau_{xy} \sin 2\theta$$

$$\sigma_{y'} = \frac{\sigma_x + \sigma_y}{2} - \frac{\sigma_x - \sigma_y}{2} \cos 2\theta - \tau_{xy} \sin 2\theta$$

$$\tau_{x'y'} = -\frac{\sigma_x - \sigma_y}{2} \sin 2\theta - \tau_{xy} \cos 2\theta$$

These equations permit the calculation of σ and τ values for any desired set of axes if the values are known for any given set of axes. In particular, if σ is chosen properly, $\tau_{x'y'}$ can be made to vanish and normal stresses only will remain. The set of axes for which this is true are called the *principal axes* of stress and the corresponding σ's are called the *principal stresses*. All points within static beds of powders can be characterized by principal axes and stresses that will, in general, vary from point to point throughout the bed. The principal axes do not correspond necessarily to the orientation of the walls of the powder container.

These concepts can be extended to three dimensions. Thus, it is possible to find a set of three mutually perpendicular planes, on which there are no shear stresses acting, for each location within the powder. The normals to these planes are the principal axes. It also is possible to find a set of planes for which the shear stresses are a maximum and the normal stresses are equal. The associated axes are called the axes of maximum shear. These two sets of axes are important because they represent directions of bed failure were it to occur.

The relationships between stresses, as functions of θ, can be illustrated and determined graphically. Figure 37-18 is an example of a Mohr's circle diagram for stress. Such diagrams are based on the stress equations. This can be seen by comparing Figure 37-18 with the equations, noting the relationships of the stresses of θ. A Mohr diagram can be constructed for any point within the powder, permitting stresses to be resolved graphically into normal and shear components for any arbitrary choice of axes.

Steps in constructing a diagram are

1. Plot the center of the circle, p, on the σ axis at the average normal stress, $(\sigma_x + \sigma_y)/$
2. Plot point x and y with coordinates (σ_x, τ_{xy}) and (σ_y, τ_{xy}), respectively. Note that these three points lie on a diameter of the circle.
3. Draw a circle with its center at p and passing through points x and y.
4. Locate the $x'y'$ diameter using the angle 2θ.

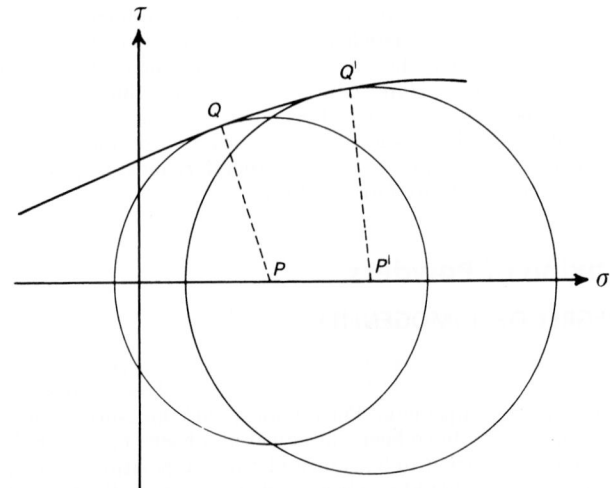

Figure 37-19.

The stress components corresponding to the new axes can be read off the graph. Both $\sigma_{x'}$ and $\sigma_{y'}$ are read off the same axes on the graph because both are normal stresses.

For the particular case in Figure 37-19, the principal axes lie at an angle of θ^* to the original axes. The axes of maximum shear stress lie at an angle of θ^- from the original axes because the xy line corresponding to maximum shear is perpendicular to the σ axis. Depending on the state of the powder, it is possible to have negative σ values, where the Mohr circle passes to the left of the τ axis.

The application of stress normal to a plane of shear influences the shear stress at which the powder fails. Because of this, a given powder will fail at various combinations of normal and shear stresses. These combinations can be expressed graphically by a line in the σ, τ plane that separates regions on the graph at which the powder either flows or is stable.

This is shown in Figure 37-19 for a typical powder. Various powders will display curves that uniquely define their failure characteristics. Each point on such a curve corresponds to a σ, τ combination at which failure occurs and can be analyzed by constructing a Mohr circle that passes through the point and is centered on the intersection of a line perpendicular to the point q and the σ axis. An example is shown in Figure 37-19.

BULK PROPERTIES

In addition to the angles of repose and friction that reflect bulk behavior, tensile and shear strength and dilatancy are of interest. Tensile strength is measured by forming a powder bed on a roughened and split plate. Half of the plate is laterally movable and the force necessary to rupture the bed by pulling the plate halves apart, minus sliding plate friction corrections, represents the bed tensile strength. Various methods of applying force to the movable plate are used, including tipping the plate from the horizontal and allowing it to react to gravity by rolling on steel balls.

Shear strength is determined from the force necessary to shear horizontally a bed of known cross-section. The Jenike shear cell is typical of those in use. It permits various loads to be applied normal to the plane of shear, whereby a shear failure locus can be determined. With the desired normal load applied, a steadily increasing shearing force is applied until failure occurs. These measurements are the basis for constructing powder-failure curves.

When packed powder beds are deformed, local expansion occurs along the failure planes, barring fracture of the particles themselves. This phenomenon is termed dilatancy and is a

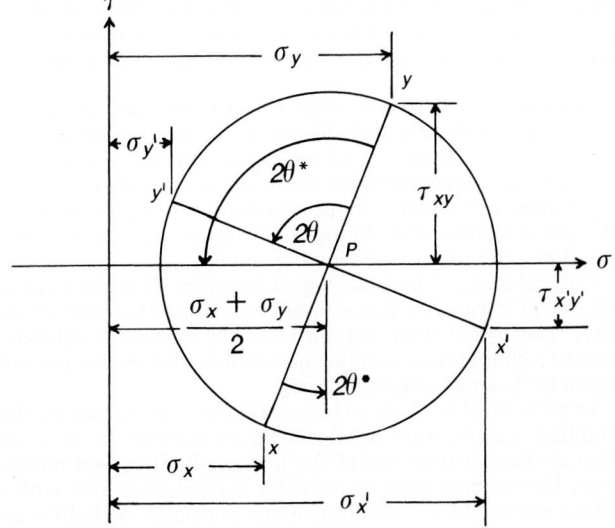

Figure 37-18.

direct consequence of the micromechanics of interparticulate movement. For one particle to move past another, it is necessary for it to move to the side in order to move forward when the particles are in an *interlocked* arrangement. Such arrangements predominate in packed beds with the consequence that the collective sideways movements in the failure zone produce bed expansion. Room for expansion therefore must be provided when packed beds are forced to flow.

Mixing of Powders

DEGREE OF HOMOGENEITY

Many mathematical expressions have been proposed and used to express the degree of homogeneity of powders composed of two or more components. For the most part, measures of mixture uniformity have been statistical and based on either the standard deviation or variance of the composition from its mean value. It should be recognized that these indices of mixing are scalar quantities and are incapable of uniquely describing the composition profile of a given powder bed. A practical definition of mixing uniformity should be selected to relate as closely as possible to the desired properties of the mix. The manner in which samples are taken (number, size, location of samples, and method of sampling) largely determines the validity and interpretation of the derived index[7].

The standard deviation is presented here as a representative index. It can be estimated solely from a set of n samples. If sample number i has composition x_i, and all samples are of uniform size, the sample standard deviation is defined in the usual way as

$$s = \sqrt{\sum_{i=1}^{n} (x_i - \overline{x})^2/(n - 1)}$$

where $\overline{x}$ is the mean composition estimated from the samples alone.

In sampling a bed, there should be assurance that the bed is sampled uniformly over its entirety. This can be done either by use of a *sampling thief* designed to probe the bed and collect samples at selected points or serially as the powder is discharged from the mixer.

The *scale of scrutiny* at which the powder is examined for uniformity is determined by the sample size. This should be chosen based on the ultimate use of the powder. For a tablet or capsule formulation, the appropriate sample size is that of the dosage form.

Two important concepts related to mixing uniformity have been described by Danckwerts as the scale and intensity of segregation. Assuming that zones having uniform but differing compositions exist in a powder bed, the scale of segregation is a function of the size of the zones. The intensity of segregation is, in turn, a function of the composition differences among zones. Generally, the process of mixing tends to reduce the intensity of segregation, whereas the scale of segregation passes through a minimum.

MECHANISMS OF MIXING AND SEGREGATION

Three primary mechanisms are responsible for mixing:

- Convective movement of relatively large portions of the bed.
- Shear failure, which primarily reduces the scale of segregation.
- Diffusive movement of individual particles.

Most efficient mixers operate to induce mixing by all three mechanisms. Thus, mixing can be considered to be a random shuffling-type operation involving both large and small particle groups and even individual particles. However, it should be noted that the use of random motion to achieve random distribution assumes that no other factors influence this distribution. This is rarely if ever the case in practice. Instead, a variety of properties of the powders being mixed influence this approach to complete randomness. Stickiness or slipperiness of particles must be considered, among other factors. As might be expected, the stickier the material, the less readily it mixes and demixes. Electrostatic forces on the particle surface also can produce marked effects on the mixing process, and in fact may produce sufficient particle-particle repulsion to make random mixing impossible.

By enabling particles to undergo movement relative to each other, mixers also provide the conditions necessary for segregation to occur. Any manipulation of a powder bed for purposes of conveying, discharging from a hopper, and so on provides the opportunity for segregation. Thus, many of the so-called mechanisms of segregation are actually conditions under which segregation can happen.

The segregation that occurs in free-flowing solids usually does so as a result of differences in particle size and, to a lesser extent, to differences in particle density and shape. The circumstances leading to segregation can be generalized from a fundamental physical standpoint. The necessary and sufficient conditions for segregation to occur are

1. Various mixture components exhibit mobilities for interparticulate movement that differ.
2. The mixture experiences either a field that exerts a directional motive force on the particles, or a gradient in a mechanism capable of inducing or modifying interparticulate movement.

The combination of these conditions results in asymmetric particle migrations and leads to segregation.

RATES OF MIXING AND SEGREGATION

Rate expressions analogous to those of chemical kinetics can be derived using any of the various indices of mixing as time-dependent variables. When this is done, it usually is found that mixing follows a first-order approach to an equilibrium state of mixedness. More recently, mixing has been described as a stochastic process (by means of stationary and nonstationary Markov chains) in which the probabilities of particle movement from place to place in the bed are determined. When applied to a mixer, this approach is capable of indicating zones of greater and lesser mixing intensity.

LARGE-SCALE MIXING EQUIPMENT

The ideal mixer should produce a complete blend rapidly with as gentle as possible a mixing action to avoid product damage. It should be cleaned and discharged easily, be dust-tight, and require low maintenance and low power consumption. All of these assets generally are not found in any single piece of equipment, thus requiring some compromise in the selection of a mixer.

Rotating-Shell Mixers—The drum-type, cubical-shaped, double-cone, and twin-shell blenders are all examples of this class of mixers. Drum-type blenders, with their axis of rotation horizontal to the center of the drum, are used quite commonly. These, however, suffer from poor crossflow along the axis. The addition of baffles or inclining the drum on its axis increases crossflow and improves the mixing action.

Cubical-and polyhedron-shaped blenders with the rotating axis set at various angles also are available. However, in the latter, because of their flat surfaces, the powder is subjected more to a sliding than a rolling action, a motion that is not conducive to the most efficient mixing.

Double-cone blenders, an important class of rotating-shell or tumbling mixers, were developed in an attempt to overcome some of the shortcomings of the previously discussed mixers. Here, the mixing pattern provides a good crossflow with a rolling rather than a sliding motion. Normally, no baffles are required, so cleaning is simplified. The twin-shell blender is another important tumbling-type blender. It combines the

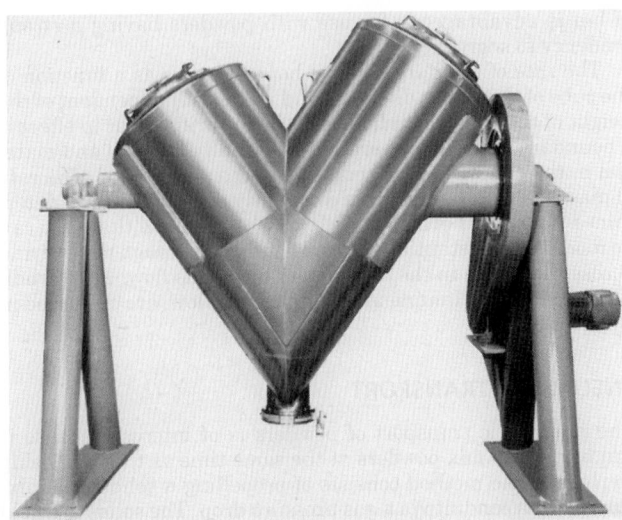

Figure 37-20. Cross-flow twin-shell blender (courtesy, Patterson-Kelley).

efficiency of the inclined drum-type with the intermixing that occurs when two such mixers combine their flow.

The Cross-Flow blender (*Patterson-Kelley*) (Fig 37-20) is an example of a twin-shell blender. The uneven length of each shell in this blender provides additional mixing action when the powder bed recombines during each revolution of the blender. The Zig-Zag blender, an extension of the twin-shell blender, provides efficient continuous precision blending.

Fixed-Shell Mixers—The ribbon mixer, one of the oldest mechanical solid–solid blending devices, exemplifies this type of mixer. It consists of a relatively long troughlike shell with a semicircular bottom. The shell is fitted with a shaft on which are mounted spiral ribbons, paddles, or helical screws, alone or in combination. These mixing blades produce a continuous cutting and shuffling of the charge by circulating the powder from end to end of the trough as well as rotationally. The shearing action that develops between the moving blade and the trough serves to break down powder agglomerates. However, ribbon mixers are not precision blenders; in addition, they suffer from the disadvantage of being more difficult to clean than the tumbler-type blenders and of having a higher power requirement.

Sigma-Blade and Planetary Paddle Mixers—Sigma-blade and planetary paddle mixers also are used for solid–solid blending, although most generally as a step prior to the introduction of liquids. Mixers with high-speed impeller blades set into the bottom of a vertical or cylindrical shell have been shown to be very efficient blenders. This type, in addition to its ability to produce precise blends, serves also to break down agglomerates rapidly. The mechanical heat buildup produced within the powder mix and the relatively high power requirement are often drawbacks to the use of this type of mixer; however; the shorter time interval necessary to achieve a satisfactory blend may offset these factors.

Vertical Impeller Mixers—Vertical impeller mixers, which have the advantage of requiring little floor space, employ a screw-type impeller that constantly overturns the batch (Fig 37-21). The fluidized mixer is a modification of the vertical impeller type. The impeller is replaced by a rapidly moving stream of air fed into the bottom of the shell. The body of the powder is fluidized, and mixing is accomplished by circulation and overtumbling in the bed (Fig 37-22). Generally, when precision solid–solid blending is required, the rotating twin-shell or the double-cone–type blenders are recommended.

Motionless Mixers—These are in-line continuous processing devices with no moving parts. They consist of a series of fixed flow-twisting or flow-splitting elements. The Blendex (*Ross & Son*), designed for blending of free-flowing solids, is constructed to operate in a vertical plane. Four pipes inter-

connect with successive tetrahedral chambers, the number of chambers needed depending on the quality of mix desired. The powders enter the mixer from overhead hoppers and free-fall through the mixer and are mixed by what is described as Interfacial Surface Generation. For two input streams entering this mixer the number of layers, L, emerging from each of the successive chambers, C, is $L = 2(4)^C$. Thus, for 10 chambers over 2 million layers are generated. This type provides efficient batch or continuous mixing for a wide variety of solids without particle-size reduction or heat generation with essentially no maintenance. Units are available to mix quantities ranging from 100 to 5000 lb/hour.

SMALL-SCALE MIXING EQUIPMENT

The pharmacist most generally employs the mortar and pestle for the small-scale mixing usually required for prescription compounding. However, spatulas and sieves also may be used on occasion. The mortar and pestle method combines comminution and mixing in a single operation. Thus, it is particularly useful where some degree of particle-size reduction as well as mixing is required, as in the case of mixtures of crystalline material.

The blending of powders with a spatula on a tile or paper, or spatulation, is used sometimes for small quantities of powders, often as an auxiliary blending technique or when the compaction produced by the mortar and pestle technique is

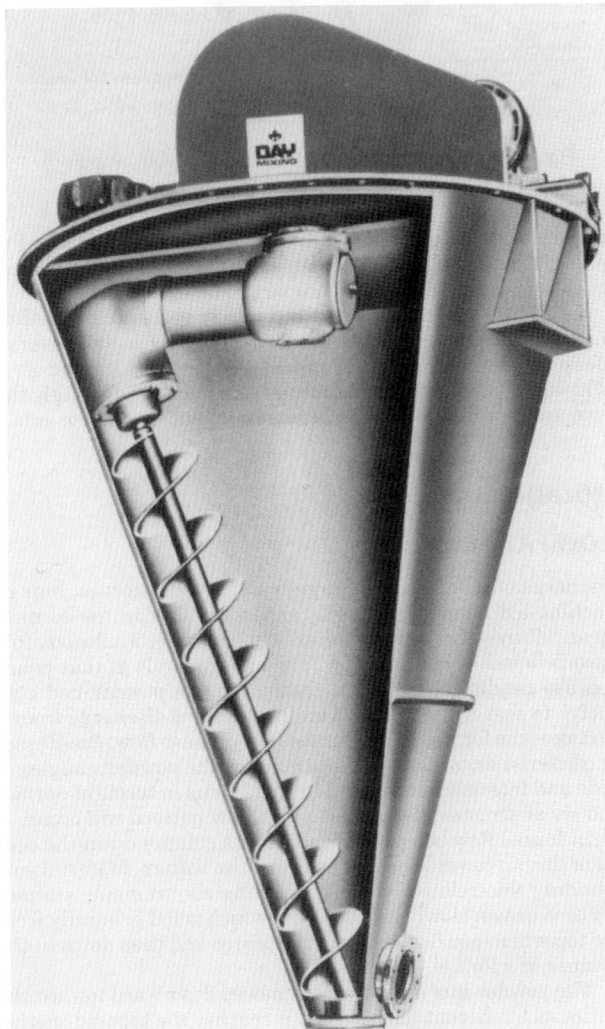

Figure 37-21. Cutaway view of the Mark II Mixer (courtesy, JH Day).

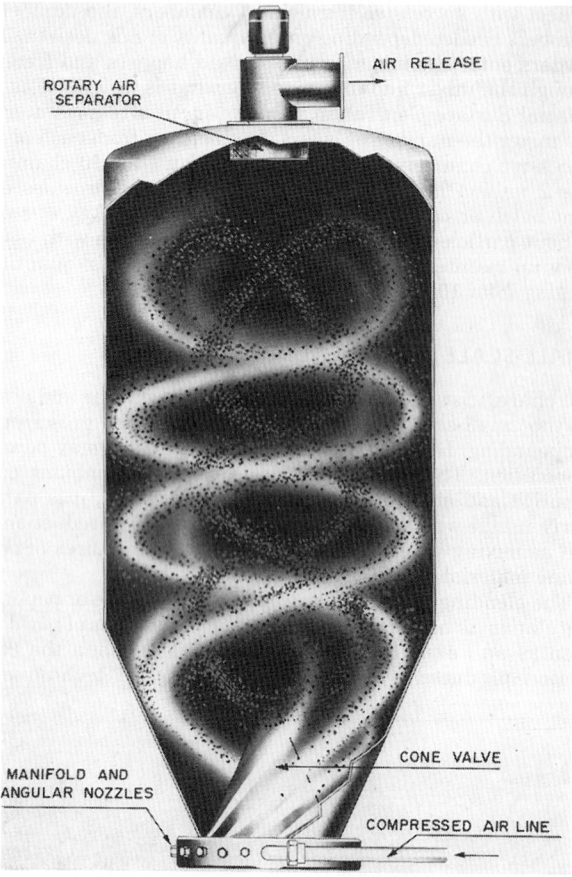

ROTARY AIR SEPARATOR

AIR RELEASE

MANIFOLD AND ANGULAR NOZZLES

CONE VALVE

COMPRESSED AIR LINE

Figure 37-22. Fluidized air mixer (courtesy, Sprout, Waldron).

undesirable. Spatulation is a relatively inefficient method of mixing, thus principles of geometric dilution must be employed. Spatulation is rarely used to prepare a finished dosage form.

Sieving usually is employed as a pre- or post-mixing method to reduce loosely held agglomerates and to increase the overall effectiveness of a blending process. When used alone as a solid–solid blending technique, several passes through the sieve are required to produce a reasonably homogeneous mix.

Storage and Flow

FLOW PATTERNS

Discharge of powders from large-scale mixers, storage, bins or machine-fed hoppers primarily generates flow in the form of shear failure—the powder behaves in a manner analogous to a viscous liquid in laminar flow. The analogy ends at that point, because conditions are then present in the powder bed conducive to segregation. The overall pattern of discharge from a bin takes the form of either funnel flow or mass flow. Bin-design characteristics, which take into account the powder's angles of slide and internal friction and its yield locus in terms of normal and shear stresses, determine which flow pattern will occur.

In funnel flow the powder moves in a column down the center of the bin toward the exit orifice at the bottom. Material surrounding this relatively rapidly moving core remains stationary or is drawn slowly into the core, which is fed primarily from the top where powder moves to the center and then down in the manner of a funnel.

The powder in a mass-flow bin moves downward toward the orifice as a coherent mass. When it reaches the tapered section of the bin leading to the orifice, it is compressed and flows in shear analogous to a plastic mass being compressed. This type

of bin is advantageous for use with powders having a strong tendency to segregate.

The rate of discharge from a hopper varies as a function of the cube of the orifice diameter and is nearly independent of the height of the bed. An arch forms over the orifice that in effect is a boundary between material in essentially free-fall and material in the closely packed condition of the powder bed. The rate of mass transport across this constantly renewed surface determines the rate of orifice flow. It has been shown that flow can be increased substantially if gas is pumped through the bed and across the orifice in the direction of the solids flow. Flow conditioners, an important means of improving flow, are discussed in Chapter 20.

PNEUMATIC TRANSPORT

The pneumatic transport of powders is of interest because it can be used to mix powders at the same time as they are being conveyed. The method consists of propelling a solids–gas mixture along a conduit via a gas pressure drop. The solids are held in suspension by the turbulence of the gas stream. At low-solids concentrations, where the particles are relatively small, the solids are dispersed uniformly over the pipe cross-section. However, at higher solids content or with larger particles, some stratification will occur in a horizontal pipe and solids will settle out if the pipe is overloaded.

Gas flow must be turbulent so as to suspend the solids; however, the solids behave as in laminar flow. Slippage between gas and solid occurs, particularly in vertical pipes; consequently, gas and solids flow rates are not in proportion to flow-stream composition. Further, smaller and less dense particles flow more rapidly than large and dense material and a chromatographic-like separation occurs. This is not a problem, however, once steady state is achieved. Because of the industrial importance of this process in many fields it has been investigated extensively and a number of useful theoretical and empirical expressions have been derived and may be used to predict conditions necessary for satisfactory pneumatic transport.

POWDERS AS A DOSAGE FORM

Historically, powders represent one of the oldest dosage forms. They are a natural outgrowth of the attempt to prepare crude drugs and other natural products in a more conveniently administered form. However, with declining use of crude drugs and increasing use of many highly potent compounds, powders as a dosage form have been replaced largely by capsules and tablets.

In certain situations, powders possess advantages and thus still represent a portion (although small) of the solid dosage forms currently being employed. These advantages are flexibility in compounding and relatively good chemical stability. The chief disadvantages of powders as a dosage form are they are time-consuming to prepare and they are not well suited for dispensing the many unpleasant-tasting, hygroscopic, or deliquescent drugs.

Bulk powders have another serious disadvantage when compared with divided and individually weighed powders: inaccuracy of dose. The dose is influenced by many factors, including size of measuring spoon, density of powder, humidity, degree of settling, fluffiness due to agitation, and personal judgment. Not only do patients measure varying amounts of powder when using the same spoon, but they often select one differing in size from that specified by their physician.

EXTEMPORANEOUS TECHNIQUES

In both the manufacturing and extemporaneous preparation of powders, the general techniques of weighing, measuring, sifting, and mixing, as described previously, are applied. However, the following procedures should receive special attention.

- Use of geometric dilution for the incorporation of small amounts of potent drugs.
- Reduction of particle size of all ingredients to the same range to prevent stratification of large and small particles.
- Sieving when necessary to achieve mixing or reduction of agglomerates, especially in the preparation of dusting powders or powders into which liquids have been incorporated.
- Heavy trituration, when applicable, to reduce the bulkiness of a powder.
- Protection against humidity, air oxidation, and loss of volatile ingredients.

Powders are prepared most commonly either as divided powders and bulk powders, which are mixed with water or other suitable material prior to administration, or as dusting powders, which are applied locally. They also may be prepared as dentifrices, products for reconstitution, insufflations, aerosols, and other miscellaneous products.

The manually operated procedures usually employed by the pharmacist today are *trituration, pulverization by intervention,* and *levigation.*

Trituration—This term refers to the process of reducing substances to fine particles by rubbing them in a mortar with a pestle. The term also designates the process whereby a mixture of fine powders is intimately mixed in a mortar. The circular mixing motion of the pestle on the powders contained in a mortar blends the powders and also breaks up their soft aggregates. By means of the application of pressure on the pestle, crushing or grinding also can be effected. When granular or crystalline materials are to be incorporated into a powdered product, these materials are comminuted individually and then blended together in the mortar.

Pulverization by Intervention—This is the process of reducing the state of subdivision of solids with the aid of an additional material that can be removed easily after the pulverization has been completed. This technique often is applied to substances that are gummy and tend to reagglomerate or that resist grinding. A prime example is camphor, which cannot be pulverized easily by trituration because of its gummy properties; however, on the addition of a small amount of alcohol or other volatile solvent, this compound can be reduced readily to a fine powder. Similarly, iodine crystals may be comminuted with the aid of a small quantity of ether. In both instances the solvent is permitted to evaporate and the powdered material is recovered.

Levigation—In this process a paste is first formed by the addition of a suitable nonsolvent to the solid material. Particle-size reduction then is accomplished by rubbing the paste in a mortar with a pestle or on an ointment slab using a spatula. Levigation generally is used by the pharmacist to incorporate solids into dermatological and ophthalmic ointments and suspensions.

THE MORTAR AND PESTLE

The mortar and pestle are the most frequently used utensils in small-scale comminution. Mortars made of various materials and in diverse shapes are available; although these often are used interchangeably, the different kinds of mortars have specific utility in preparing or grinding different materials.

Modern mortars and pestles are prepared usually from Wedgwood ware, porcelain, or glass. Although pharmacists often use different mortars interchangeably, each type has a preferential range of utility.

Glass mortars are designed primarily for use in preparing solutions and suspensions of chemical materials in a liquid. They also are suitable for preparing ointments which require the reduction of soft aggregates of powdered materials or the incorporation of relatively large amounts of liquid. Glass also has the advantage of being comparatively nonporous and of not staining easily and thus is particularly useful when substances such as flavoring oils or highly colored substances are used. Glass cannot be used for comminuting hard solids.

Wedgwood mortars are suited well for comminution of crystalline solids or for the reduction in particle size of most materials used in modern prescription practice. They are capable of adequately powdering most substances that are available only as crystals or hard lumps. However, Wedgwood is relatively porous and will stain quite easily. A Wedgwood mortar is available with a roughened interior, which aids in the comminution process but which requires meticulous care in washing because particles of the drugs may be trapped in the rough surface and cause contamination of materials subsequently comminuted in the mortar.

Porcelain mortars are very similar to Wedgwood, except that the exterior surface of the former is usually glazed and thus less porous. Porcelain mortars may be used for comminution of soft aggregates or crystals but more generally are used for blending powders of approximately uniform particle size.

Pestles are made of the same material as the mortar. Pestles for Wedgwood or porcelain mortars are available with hard rubber or wooden handles screwed into the head of the pestle. Also available are one-piece Wedgwood pestles. Pestles made entirely of porcelain are objectionable, because they are broken easily.

Pestles and mortars should not be interchanged. The efficiency of the grinding or mixing operation depends largely on a maximum contact between the surfaces of the head of the pestle and the interior of the mortar. The pestle should have as much bearing on the interior surface of the mortar as its size will permit. A pestle that does not *fit* the mortar will result in a waste of labor.

Divided Powders

Divided powders (*chartula* or *chartulae*) are dispensed in the form of individual doses and generally are dispensed in papers, properly folded. They also may be dispensed in metal foil, small heat-sealed plastic bags, or other containers.

DIVIDING POWDERS

After weighing, comminuting, and mixing the ingredients, the powders must be divided accurately into the prescribed number of doses. To achieve accuracy consistent with the other steps in the preparation, *each dose should be weighed individually* and transferred to a powder paper. Following completion of this step, the powder papers are folded.

FOLDING POWDERS

The operations of folding powder papers are illustrated in Figure 37-23. Care in making the several folds, and experience gained by repetition, are necessary to obtain uniformity when the powders finally are placed in the box for dispensing. Deviation from any of the three main folds will result in powders of varying height being formed, and variations in the folded ends likewise will be noticeable when the powders are placed side by side.

PACKAGING DIVIDED POWDERS

Specially manufactured paper and boxes are available for dispensing divided powders.

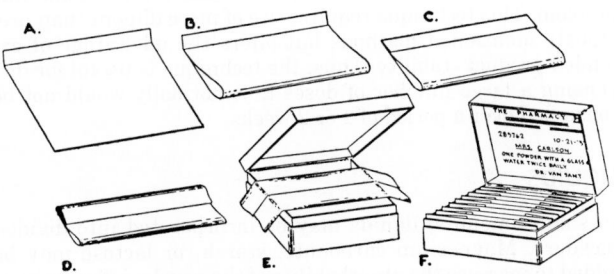

Figure 37-23. Folding powder papers.

Powder Papers—Four basic types of powder papers are available.

1. Vegetable parchment, a thin, semiopaque, moisture-resistant paper.
2. White bond, an opaque paper with no moisture-resistant properties.
3. Glassine, a glazed, transparent, moisture-resistant paper.
4. Waxed, a transparent waterproof paper.

Hygroscopic and volatile drugs can be protected best by using a waxed paper, double-wrapped with a bond paper to improve the appearance of the completed powder. Parchment and glassine papers offer limited protection for these drugs.

A variety of sizes of powder papers are available. The selection of the proper size depends on the bulk of each dose and the dimensions of the powder box required to hold the number of doses prescribed.

Powder Boxes—Various types of boxes are supplied in several sizes for dispensing divided powders. The hinged-shoulder box shown in Figure 37-23F is the most popular; these have the advantage of preventing the switching of lids with the directions for use when several boxes of the same size are in the same home. The prescription label may be pasted directly on top of the lid or inside the lid. In the latter case, the name of the pharmacy is lithographed on top of the lid.

SPECIAL PROBLEMS

The incorporation of volatile substances, eutectic mixtures, liquids, and hygroscopic or deliquescent substances into powders presents problems that require special treatment.

VOLATILE SUBSTANCES

The loss of camphor, menthol, and essential oils by volatilization when incorporated into powders may be prevented or retarded by use of heat-sealed plastic bags or by double wrapping with a waxed or glassine paper inside of a bond paper.

EUTECTIC MIXTURES

Liquids result from the combination of phenol, camphor, menthol, thymol, antipyrine, phenacetin, acetanilid, aspirin, salol, and related compounds at ordinary temperatures. These so-called eutectic mixtures may be incorporated into powders by addition of an inert diluent. Magnesium carbonate or light magnesium oxide are commonly used, effective diluents for this purpose, although kaolin, starch, bentonite, and other absorbents have been recommended. Silicic acid prevents eutexia with aspirin, phenyl salicylate, and other troublesome compounds; incorporation of about 20% silicic acid (particle size, 50 μm) prevented liquefaction even under the compression pressures required to form tablets.

In handling this problem, each eutectic compound should be mixed first with a portion of the diluent and gently blended together, preferably with a spatula on a sheet of paper. Generally, an amount of diluent equal to the eutectic compounds is sufficient to prevent liquefaction for about 2 weeks. Deliberate forcing of the formation of the liquid state, by direct trituration, followed by absorption of the moist mass, also will overcome this problem. This technique requires use of more diluent than previously mentioned methods but offers the advantage of extended product stability. Thus, the technique is useful for dispensing a large number of doses that normally would not be consumed over a period of 1 or 2 weeks.

LIQUIDS

In small amounts, liquids may be incorporated into divided powders. Magnesium carbonate, starch, or lactose may be added to increase the absorbability of the powders if necessary. When the liquid is a solvent for a nonvolatile heat-stable com-

pound, it may be evaporated gently on a water bath. Lactose may be added during the course of the evaporation to increase the rate of solvent loss by increasing the surface area. Some fluidextracts and tinctures may be treated in this manner, although the use of an equivalent amount of a powdered extract, when available, is a more desirable technique.

HYGROSCOPIC AND DELIQUESCENT SUBSTANCES

Substances that become moist because of affinity for moisture in the air may be prepared as divided powders by adding inert diluents. Double-wrapping is desirable for further protection. Extremely deliquescent compounds cannot be prepared satisfactorily as powders.

BULK POWDERS

Bulk powders may be classified as oral powders, dentifrices, douche powders, dusting powders, insufflations, and triturations.

ORAL POWDERS

Oral powders generally are supplied as *finely divided powders* or *effervescent granules*. The finely divided powders are intended to be suspended or dissolved in water or mixed with soft foods such as applesauce prior to administration. Antacids and laxative powders frequently are administered in this form.

Effervescent granules contain sodium bicarbonate and either citric acid, tartaric acid, or sodium biphosphate in addition to the active ingredients. On solution in water, carbon dioxide is released as a result of the acid–base reaction. The effervescence from the release of the carbon dioxide serves to mask the taste of salty or bitter medications.

Granulation generally is accomplished by producing a moist mass, forcing it through a coarse sieve and drying it in an oven. The moisture necessary for massing the materials is obtained readily by heating them sufficiently to drive off the water of hydration from the uneffloresced citric acid. The completed product must be dispensed in tightly closed glass containers to protect it against the humidity of the air.

Effervescent powders may be prepared also by adding small amounts of water to the dry salts to obtain a workable mass. The mass is dried and ground to yield the powder or granule. Care must be used in this procedure to ensure that the reaction that occurs in the presence of water does not proceed too far before it is stopped by the drying process. Should this happen, the effervescent properties of the product will be destroyed.

Other preparative techniques have been reported for effervescent powders such as a fluidized-bed procedure in which the powders are blended and then suspended in a stream of air in a Wurster chamber. Water is sprayed into the chamber, resulting in a slight reaction and an expansion of the particles to form granules ranging in size from 10- to 30-mesh. This approach apparently offers a number of advantages over the older techniques. The extent of reaction and particle size are controlled during the manufacture. A drying oven, trays, or even grinding devices are not required. Furthermore, the technique lends itself to a continuous as well as a batch operation.

The heat generated from the blending and mixing operation also has been used to mass the powders by causing the release of the water of hydration from the citric acid. The massed materials can be dried and sieved through a coarse sieve. This technique thus eliminates the need of an external heat source or a granulating solution.

DENTIFRICES

Dentifrices may be prepared in the form of a bulk powder, generally containing a soap or detergent, mild abrasive, and an anticariogenic agent.

DOUCHE POWDERS

Douche powders are completely soluble and are intended to be dissolved in water prior to use as antiseptics or cleansing agents for a body cavity. They most commonly are intended for vaginal use, although they may be formulated for nasal, otic, or ophthalmic use. Generally, because aromatic oils are included in these powders, they are passed through a No 40 or 60 sieve to eliminate agglomeration and ensure complete mixing. Dispensing in wide-mouth glass jars serves to protect against loss of volatile materials and permits easy access by the patient. Bulk-powder boxes may be used for dispensing douche powders, although glass containers are preferred because of the protection afforded by these containers against air and moisture.

DUSTING POWDERS

Dusting powders are locally applied nontoxic preparations that are intended to have no systemic action. They are applied to various parts of the body as lubricants, protectives, absorbents, antiseptics, antipruritics, antibromhidrosis agents, astringents, and antiperspirants. Dusting powders always should be dispensed in a very fine state of subdivision to enhance effectiveness and minimize irritation. When necessary, they may be micronized or passed through a No 80 or 100 sieve.

Extemporaneously prepared dusting powders should be dispensed in sifter-top packages. Commercial dusting powders are available in sifter-top containers or pressure aerosols. The latter, while generally more expensive than the other containers, offer the advantage of protection from air, moisture, and contamination, as well as convenience of application. Foot powders and talcum powders are currently available as pressure aerosols.

Although in most cases dusting powders are considered nontoxic, the absorption of boric acid through large areas of abraded skin has caused toxic reactions in infants. Accidental inhalation of zinc stearate powder has led to pulmonary inflammation of the lungs of infants. The pharmacist should be aware of the possible dangers when the patient uses these compounds as well as other externally applied products. See also Chapter 65.

INSUFFLATIONS

Insufflations are finely divided powders introduced into body cavities such as the ears, nose, throat, tooth sockets, and vagina. An insufflator (powder blower) usually is employed to administer these products. However, the difficulty in obtaining a uniform dose has restricted their general use.

Specialized equipment has been developed for the administration of micronized powders of relatively potent drugs. The Norisodrine Sulfate Aerohaler Cartridge (*Abbott*) is an example. In the use of this Aerohaler, inhalation by the patient causes a small ball to strike a cartridge containing the drug. The force of the ball shakes the proper amount of the powder free, permitting its inhalation. Another device, the Spinhaler turbo-inhaler (*Fisons*), is a propeller-driven device designed to deposit a mixture of lactose and micronized cromolyn sodium into the lung as an aid in the management of bronchial asthma.

Pressure aerosols also have been employed as a means of administering insufflations, especially for potent drugs. This method offers the advantage of excellent control of dose, through metered valves, as well as product protection.

TRITURATIONS

Triturations are dilutions of potent powdered drugs, prepared by intimately mixing them with a suitable diluent in a definite proportion by weight. They were at one time official as 1 to 10 dilutions. The pharmacist sometimes prepares triturations of poisonous substances such as atropine in a convenient concentration using lactose as the diluent, for use at the prescription counter. These medicinal substances are weighed more accurately and conveniently by using this method.

The correct procedure for preparing such triturations or any similar dilution of a potent powder medicament, to ensure uniform distribution of the latter, is

1. Reduce the drug to a moderately fine powder in a mortar.
2. Add about an equal amount of diluent and mix well by thorough trituration in the mortar.
3. Successively add portions of diluent, triturating after each addition, until the entire quantity of diluent has been incorporated.

Under no circumstance should the entire quantity of diluent be added at once to the drug that is to be diluted in the expectation that uniform dispersion of the latter will be more expeditiously achieved on brief trituration of the mixture.

REFERENCES

1. Parrott EL. In Lachman L, et al. *The Theory and Practice of Industrial Pharmacy,* 3rd ed. Philadelphia: Lea & Febiger, 1986, p 32.
2. Perry RH, et al. *Chemical Engineers' Handbook,* 7th ed. New York: McGraw-Hill, 1997: 8–8.
3. Byers JE, Peck GE. *Drug Dev Ind Pharm* 1990; 16(11): 1761–1779.
4. Pilcher JM, et al. *Proc Chem Spec Mfrs Assoc Ann Mtg* 1956; 66.
5. Tillotson D. *Aerosol Age* 1958; 3(5): 41.
6. Rawle A. *Adv. Colour Sci Tech* 2002; 5(1):1–12.
7. Muzzio FJ, et al. *Int J Pharm* 2003; 250:51–64.

BIBLIOGRAPHY

Alderborn G, Nystrom C., eds. *Pharmaceutical Powder Compaction Technology.* New York: Marcel Dekker, 1996.
Allen T. *Particle Size Measurement,* 5th ed. London: Chapman & Hall, 1997.
Brittain HG, ed. *Physical Characterization of Pharmaceutical Solids,* New York: Marcel Dekker, 1995.
Carstensen JT. *Advanced Pharmaceutical Solids,* New York: Marcel Dekker, 2000.
Hickey AJ and Ganderton D. *Pharmaceutical Process Engineering,* New York: Marcel Dekker, 2001.
Levin M, ed. Pharmaceutical Process Scale-Up, New York: Marcel Dekker, 2002.
Martin AN, et al. *Physical Pharmacy,* 4th ed. Philadelphia: Lea & Febiger, 1993.
Venables HJ, Wells JI. Powder Mixing, *Drug Dev Ind Pharm* 2001; 27(7): 599–612.

Property-Based Drug Design and Preformulation

Howard Y Ando, PhD

Galen W Radebaugh, PhD

The discovery and development of new chemical entities (NCEs) into stable, bioavailable, marketable drug products is a long, but rewarding process. Due to the tremendous cost of developing a NCE, and industry's need to enhance productivity, it is desirable to create NCEs that have suitable physical-chemical properties, rather than compensate for deficiencies solely by the formulation process. Hence, property-based design can enhance the likelihood a NCE will have the desired physical-chemical that will facilitate its ability to be developed into a stable, bioavailable dosage form. Even so, well-designed preformulation studies are necessary to fully characterize molecules during the discovery and development process so that NCEs have the appropriate properties, and there is an understanding of the deficiencies that must be overcome by the formulation process. This chapter provides guidance that will facilitate property-based design and the supporting preformulation studies necessary to direct formulation efforts to give NCEs the highest possibility of success.

EVOLUTION OF THE DRUG DISCOVERY PROCESS

The need for property-based design follows from the natural evolution of a research and development process that seeks to become more efficient. The growth and decline of markets and sectors is a natural process that applies to every life structure whether it is the universe, an individual, or a market sector. All have a sigmoidal curve with periods of vulnerability, growth, and decline. For the pharmaceutical new chemical entity (NCE) sector, this is shown in Figure 38-1 as NCE-1. Of course, the declining phase is of major concern and usually is seen only in retrospect. However, Charles Handy has pointed out that given enough foresight, organizations can renew themselves by changing their operational paradigm.[1] Ideally, they would initiate and build the basis for this change during the α phase (shown in Fig 38-1). If successful, they could then initiate the hypothetical second curve, labeled NCE-2 in Fig 38-1. What then are the causes for the aging of the NCE-1 cycle, and what will fuel the initiation and growth of the hypothetical NCE-2 cycle paradigm? The relevance of property-based design in this context is discussed below.

GROWTH CYCLE DETERMINANTS

NCE Paradigms

The first growth epoch for the pharmaceutical development was driven by the application of physical-chemical principles to the

design of dosage forms and delivery of NCEs. Physical chemistry provided scientists with a macroscopic, theoretical model, and as a young discipline, empirical experimentation predominated in the industrial design of dosage forms. Moreover, discovery and development phases occurred as separate and sequential phases. This was efficient and sufficient at the time, mainly because the targets were simpler. Evaluating the activity of new NCEs might involve bacterial cultures or perfused animal tissues. Testing for pharmacological activity in whole animals would then follow. Compounds that had poor development potential like limited aqueous solubility never showed any *in vivo* pharmacodynamic activity and were never advanced. In addition, indirect biomarkers were not needed because the physiological impact of an NCE could be readily measured and extrapolated from animals to humans (eg, blood pressure monitoring). However, new technological developments have caused the decline of this paradigm.

Advances in biotechnology fueled the second epoch starting in the 1980s because proteins could be synthesized from genetic information. Initially, bacteria and then mammalian cells were the source of these proteins. Such technology meant that these proteins could now be used as targets for discovery research. Individual receptors, enzymes, or transporters could now be synthesized in isolation from their parent tissue and could be used as surrogates for *in vivo* pharmacological activity. The banks of compounds that were accumulated during the first epoch, both in the academic and industrial setting, could now be screened for *in vitro* activity by high-speed robots.

The realization that a more integrated process of discovery was necessary became apparent only after a painful period. Early in this second epoch, a lot of energy was devoted to compounds that have been coined high affinity traps.[2] These are compounds that have very high *in vitro* activity but poor aqueous solubility. This occurred because of the needs of high throughput screening to automate the dispensing of compounds in a 96 well format. Because accurate and economical dispensing of powder is not possible, all reagents must be added as solutions. Liquid dispensing required a very general way to dissolve compounds. So the solution was to use small amounts of a very good, universal solvent, DMSO, that dissolved almost all organic compounds. The problem was that property-based factors like solubility and dissolution are not accounted for. Lipinski sounded the warning to the industry with his rule of five (RoF).[3] Subsequently, developmental scientists have put into place a number of high throughput physical property screens that could be used during the discovery phase; hence the realization of a need for property-based design. However, there are signs that this epoch may be reaching the end of its growth phase. DiMasi[4] has shown that the NCE-1 curve in Figure 38-1 for new INDs filings reached a plateau during the 1980s and has declined in the 1990s.

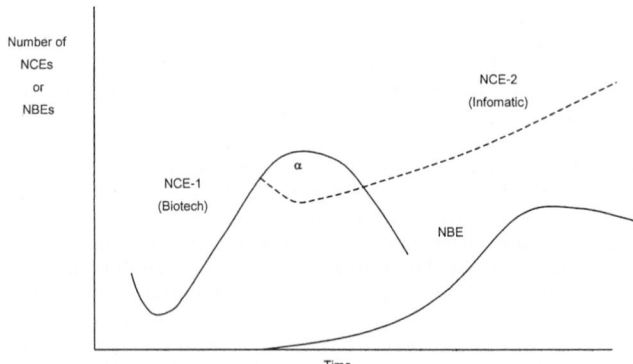

Figure 38-1. Charles Handy's sigmoidal growth curve. (From Handy C. The Age of Paradox. Cambridge, MA: Harvard Business School, 1995: 49-67. Copyright © 1995 by the Harvard Business School Publishing Corporation: all rights reserved.)

Because the biotechnology paradigm may now be reaching the limits of its efficiency, it is proposed that a new paradigm (Informatics) will begin to evolve, taking advantage of an increased molecular understanding of the crystalline state and advances in the computational sciences, especially machine learning. The α phase of Figure 38-1 may be upon us. This new paradigm, NCE-2, will be driven by both technological opportunities, especially infomatics, and pharmaco-economic constraints.

Pharmaco-Economic Constraints

COST—In a recent white paper by IBM consultants, it was pointed out that the innovative driving force for drug development is rapidly shifting from the manufacturers and physicians to consumers, which in many cases are managed care organizations (MCO). One of the most important imperatives of this new consumer is the control of rising health care cost. With their control of formularies, MCOs will exert considerable influence in the future on the direction and limits of innovation.[5]

REGULATORY AND SAFETY—At the same time, regulatory agencies are requiring electronic filing requirements that in the short term considerably increase cost, but in the long term have the potential to speed review. In addition, because our understanding of side effects has increased substantially during the biotechnology epoch, self-imposed industry and regulatory requirements for NCEs have become much more stringent. For example, safety screens are now available for certain types of potentially fatal arrhythmias (torsades de pointes syndrome) that have been found to be associated with drug binding to potassium channels in the heart's conduction fibers. Chromosomal genotoxicity screens are also available that can detect a drug's interference with normal mitotic spindle and microtubule complex formations, or DNA strand breakage.[6] All of these new insights increase what is expected for a new NCE before it can be introduced into the marketplace. How then can costs be reduced as NCE regulatory requirements increase?

RISK MINIMIZATION—DiMasi has shown that the clinical approval rates from more recent IND filings has improved.[7] Apparently, better preclinical screening has increases the success rate. Since filtering out poor clinical candidates during the preclinical screening stage should be much cheaper than having clinical candidates fail, highly efficient screening should be justified. On the other hand, even if current preclinical screening is efficient in increasing the clinical success rate, apparently it does not add to productivity as measured by the decline in IND filings in the 1990s.[6] The substantial improvements that are needed to reduce both cost and risk and to initiate the Informatic NCE-2 curve in Figure 38-1 will most likely need the simultaneous improvements of a number of infomatic-based at point α.

Such improvements would include computational (a) activity-based design, (b) safety-based design, and (c) property-based design. If all of these elements could be highly accurate and applied at very early stages of discovery, fewer resources would be expended on nonproductive activities. In addition, if the number of potential opportunities both from the number of targets due to genomic opportunities and from increased property-based design possibilities can be achieved, then higher productivity should result.

Cost Reduction by Learning Before Doing

A model for the cost saving of such a paradigm has been carried out in the chemical development arena, but the concepts should hold for the property-design area as well. Today, when discovery chemists find a compound that has promising activity, additional amounts need to be made for further testing. Here the speed at which a chemical can be manufactured is critical. Usually, any route that will make the compound the quickest to synthesize on a small scale is chosen. If however, the compound continues to show potential, it has to be scaled up for even further testing. In his study, Pisano found that the two most important elements for reducing cost of manufacturing chemicals are: (a) the optimal synthetic route, and (b) telescoping successive unit operations. Of these two elements, finding the optimal synthetic route is the most important. If the company can effectively utilize its past experience to make the route determination earlier, then costs are reduced most effectively. Figure 38-2 shows the savings of this *learning before doing*.[8] One can imagine sometime in the not too distant future discovery chemists making decisions on which compounds to move forward based on all of the discovery criteria previously discussed but also on chemical synthesis scalability and optimum route design. Not only would the speed for making NCEs benefit, but also the long-term cost and efficiency of the entire chemical development organization.

In summary, the development cost can in theory be drastically reduced if computational design of property, activity, and safety can be accomplished. Such savings have the potential to alter the pharmaceutical industry's focus on blockbuster NCEs to potentially smaller but still lucrative markets. Accomplishment of this goal would most likely initiate the NCE-2 curve of Figure 38-1. The biotechnology arena is a good model. In Figure 38-1, the new biologic entities (NBEs) are seen to be growing as the NCEs are shown to be flat or peaked.[4]

INTEGRATION OF DISCOVERY AND DEVELOPMENT

As discussed, the pharmaceutical industry has evolved from a sequential organization where problems were passed on from discovery to development (epoch 1) to one in which both drug activity and physical properties are considered very early in discovery (epoch 2). The RoF was one of the early movements to

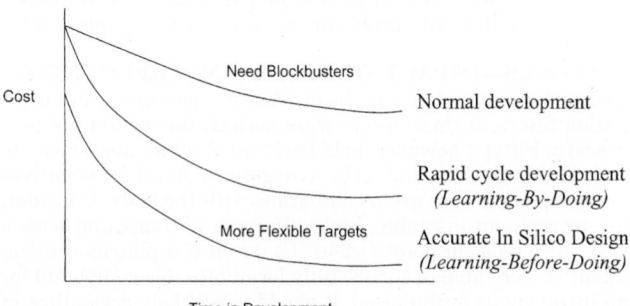

Figure 38-2. Cost savings by learning-before-doing.

foster integration of discovery and development. The ideal development of a NCE optimizes both "property-based" as well as "activity"-based design simultaneously. Continued improvements in efficiency will require that organizations be ready to adapt to new technologies and learnings. However, potential roadblocks to the integration of discovery and development efforts include high throughput (HT) decision-making, attrition, and the management of complexity.

HT Decision-Making

One of the attractive concepts for improving efficiency is that of successive screens. Currently, they come in two flavors, *in vitro* and computational to filter out poor drug candidates so resources are not wasted on unproductive activities.[9] The sequential paradigm

Discovery → Development

can now be replaced by the sequence

Discovery [design → synthesis] →
Selection [screen for activity → absorption → metabolism → toxicology] →
Development [formulation → animal pk testing → regulated toxicology → IND → initial clinical trials]

In essence, screens used in this manner are a way to simplify the complex process of discovering, selecting, and developing NCEs.

As efficient and useful as successive, hierarchical high throughput screens (HTSs) are for simplifying decision making, the question should be asked, "Have HTSs increased productivity?" As we alluded to under a previous section, productivity for IND filings (a measure of preclinical activity) has reached a plateau. This is most likely due to the use of successive filters in a decision-tree that then successively reduces future possibilities. If successive filters are employed, they could be prioritized so that earlier filters have higher quality. This would minimize the loss of potential opportunities.

Consider a situation of form selection in which scientists are trying to select the best molecule for development. In this multi-tiered approach, decision-making follows a progression of:

Hygroscopicity → thermal analysis & x-ray diffraction → accelerated solid-state stability

One impact of such decision-trees is that hygroscopic salts would rarely be developed (even if they have very advantageous bioavailability properties). If hygroscopicity were a property that prevented development, then any compound with this characteristic would be eliminated immediately. However, it is possible, with a good enough reason, to work with this situation.

Attrition

GAINS—Property-based screens have made tremendous gains over the last 5 years. This is due to the design of NCEs that have both activity and desirable physical properties such as solubility. These advances have been instrumental in reducing pharmacokinetic attrition during clinical trials.[7,10,11] On the other hand, more sophisticated technologies are needed to overcome low productivity problems associated with simple successive filters.

LOSSES—IMPACT OF FILTER IMPERFECTIONS—Reduced compound flow in the pipeline is a possible result of attrition filters. If these filters were perfect, this would not be a concern. Filters, however, hold back: (a) absolute negatives, (b) technical negatives, and (c) false negatives. Absolute negatives are compounds that are incompatible with the body. Consider, for example an insoluble, high affinity trap compound with a very high melting point (>240° C). Even if a pharmaceutical scientist were able to successfully formulate this compound for an intravenous formulation, it would most likely crystallize in the kidney. On the other hand, suppose water solubility was used as a filter. A technical negative that fails for adequate

water solubility, may still be biocompatible. A highly lipophilic compound with a melting point of 100° C would be a compound of this type. This compound may be deliverable by special formulations and has the potential to be a viable NCE from the property-design point of view. However, both of these compounds would be screened out if water solubility were used as an attrition filter. The final type of negative is a false negative in which the filter removes a perfectly viable compound.

To appreciate the impact of losing good compounds as false negatives and formulatable technical negatives, consider the following situation. Three filters A, B, and C are to be used in succession. To calculate their impact, assume that each has the following characteristics. Each will pass 50% of the positives correctly, will block correctly the 25% absolute negatives, but will also block 25% of compounds that are either false or technical negatives. For this battery of successive filters the throughput of positives is 12.5%. However, the correct throughput of positives and formulable compounds is 42%. Thus the pipeline possibilities were reduced unnecessarily by 236%. How many compounds are being filtered out that previously might have taken a considerable amount of time to develop but were developable? A key goal for property-design should be not to lose technical negatives that a company has the core competencies to develop rapidly.

PROPERTY-BASED DESIGN IN LEAD SELECTION

One of the keys for continuous improvement and moving into the Informatic α phase of Figure 38-1 is to make better use of existing data and to obtain higher quality data. In addition, the active participation of special groups that have domains of expertise is also needed. As we have seen, simple models can promote efficiency but more sophisticated refinements that take into account complexity are needed to increase productivity.

As an example, one area of extreme complexity is understanding disease. The biotechnology epoch of the 20th century that focused on a single gene–single protein approach just doesn't work well with multi-gene disorders such as cancer or Alzheimer's disease. In order to understand the basis for human genetic variability, the human genome project pooled and sequenced the genes and nucleotides of many individuals to establish a baseline. Single nucleotide deviations from this baseline are termed SNPs (single nucleotide polymorphisms). Although rare diseases can occur from SNPs (eg, sickle cell anemia and cystic fibrosis), the most common diseases (eg, diabetes and asthma) may encompass 20–50 SNPs and may involve 10 or more genes. Research efforts are now ongoing to establish blocks of SNPs that correlate with a given disease predisposition. If such correlations can be found, then drugs can be sought to prevent disease expression. The complexity of this undertaking will require a much more sophisticated approach to drug development. Understanding complexity in property-design will also expand possibilities.

Ideally, a property-based design strategy would be able to anticipate and predict the physical properties of a proposed molecule from structure alone. This would be coordinated with activity-based and safety-based strategies so that predictions would be made on this triad of design characteristics. Proposed molecules could then be evaluated from structure alone to see if they either had (a) the requisite properties, or (b) the potential to be further designed to have the requisite triad of design characteristics: activity, solubility, and safety. For this latter group, knowledge of functional groups that have the flexibility for being modified would have to be identified so that further predictions could be carried out on modified structures for triad characteristics. Property-base possibilities would include compounds that had:

a. Passive diffusion properties (solubility & membrane permeability)
b. Crystal packing disruptive potential for passive diffusion

c. Special vehicle delivery potential
d. Prodrug enhancement potential
e. Stability enhancement potential.

FORWARD-FOCUS VISION

Some of the terminologies that we have inherited from crisis situations like attrition and triage cast images of what is to be avoided and what choices have to be made with limited resources. While it is necessary to recognize these areas, a focus on them may inhibit forward thinking and new solutions to get where we want to go. The 'forward focus' model is an alternative way to think about producing more products that add shareholder value. The principles of the model are[12]:

(1) If we focus on obstacles, we expend time and energy on obstacles rather than on getting where we want to go.
(2) When we clearly focus on where we want to go, we do whatever we need to do to get there with minimal wasted energy.

Ironically, empirical evidence suggests that focusing on obstacles may attract what we want to avoid.[12] The forward-focus vision concentrates on the efficient utilization of resources to enable more NCEs to come to market faster, and with higher quality. Its advantage over an attrition-focus strategy is that more energy is expended using existing knowledge to enlarge property-space possibilities and on the development of novel approaches. It has been said that[13] "In the realm of possibility, we gain our knowledge by invention." We also invent rules, but these must be used with caution.

LIFECYCLE OF RULES—Rules are the compilations of knowledge that enable us to carry out business efficiently. Even the best rules, however, should be viewed in the context of a lifecycle. Changing circumstances or new knowledge can cause rules that were formulated in the past to become inappropriate. One of the most useful roles rules play is that they provide a reference for obtaining a more precise understanding of physical phenomena. Attrition also can be thought of in terms of a lifecycle and be made productive.

MAKING ATTRITION NON-PERISHABLE—While late clinical-stage attrition is very costly, the loss of resources involved in attrition of NCEs prior to Phase I clinical trials is even more costly. It is possible that more that 85% of pre-Phase I activity is taken up by compounds that never progress to clinical trials. While this is accepted as an inevitable part of the research and development process, a program for capturing the knowledge from all of these failed NCEs might very well enhance the efficiency of property-design.

ACCEPTANCE OF COMPLEXITY—Rules that capture the essence of complex phenomenon is one strategy for designing properties. Another approach is to accept that physical systems will be complex and that computational approaches may be needed to design systems that can accurately predict. Such systems can analyze more situations in more detail than an individual. One key element that enhances acceptance of such computational approaches is that the reasoning or scientific basis of the predictions be understandable. For continuous progress, phenomena need to be understood at the molecular level.

MOLECULAR PRINCIPLES

Grasping the structure of a subject is understanding it in a way that permits many other things to be related to it meaningfully. To learn structure, in short, is to learn how things are related.[14] Insight that will lead to improved property-based design will result from using a variety of molecular tools that will give scientists an understanding of the precise interactions that occur between molecules, whether they be interactions between molecules among themselves or between molecules with biological systems. The two types of molecular interactions that we will be focusing on in this section deal with interactions in (1) crystals and (2) membranes.

Crystalline interactions are of interest because they ultimately determine solubility, melting point, and dissolution of NCEs. If we can gain a molecular understanding of the intermolecular interactions that occur between the molecules in a crystal, then we can gain insight into how we can predict and design molecules that have the properties we desire from structure alone. This is the ultimate goal of property-based design. For simple crystals, containing only the same molecules (no solvents or salt counterions), we will use the term *cohesive* to characterize the type of intermolecular interactions of the same type of molecule.

Membrane interactions between an NCE and a biological membrane will be termed *adhesive*, because they are between different types of molecules. Adhesive interactions are those types of interactions that also occur between solvent molecules and the NCE when it is dissolved in the aqueous environment of the digestive tract. Solvent-solute interactions control the familiar like-dissolves-like concept. For example, lipid molecules dissolve in oil more than they do in water. We refer the reader to the work of Abraham[15] for extensive research into the solvation phenomena. In this discussion of molecular property-based design, we will begin to examine the types of cohesive interactions that can occur in a crystal which impact its solubility (or insolubility).

Crystalline Interactions

Molecules in a crystal organize themselves in a limited number of regular arrays, which are termed space groups. There are 230 possible crystalline space groups; however, because pharmaceutical molecules are complex and in general not symmetric, the number of actual space groups for drug-like molecules is only about 3. These are shown in Table 38-1. The impact of regular ordering of molecules in a crystal is that, for a given space group, rules can be stated that allow the entire crystal to be replicated through a sequential series of translation, reflection, inversion, and other analytical geometric operations. For example, the operation for the very common space group for drug-like molecules, P21/c, is shown in Figure 38-3. The fundamental unit that is replicated is the unit cell. This is obtained from single crystal x-ray diffraction evaluations of the NCE. This unit cell (sometimes termed the asymmetric unit) has information regarding the number of molecules in the asymmetric unit and the dimension and angles of the unit cell.

Ultimately, it is the molecular structure of the molecule that determines the space group and the number of molecules in the unit cell of a particular crystal. However, for a given molecule, the crystals that can form are not unique. Because molecules can assume different conformations, and because a variety of crystallization conditions can influence the crystal that forms, a variety of different polymorphic forms are possible (this will be discussed in detail in later sections). Polymorphic forms may have different physical properties, especially dissolution characteristics that could impact bioavailability and very often these different forms can interconvert. One objective of active pharmaceutical ingredient (API) design is to find the most stable crystalline form so that polymorphic changes do not occur once an NCE is formulated into a dosage form. It is the packing of the atoms in a given crystal that will be considered next and the forces that lead to insolubility.

CRYSTAL PACKING

Crystal packing is dominated by two opposing phenomena: (1) maximizing the number of hydrogen bonds (H-bonds) that can be formed for a given molecular structure, and (2) packing the atoms of the crystal as densely as possible (ie, close packing). Ultimately, molecular shape and the distribution of the H-bond donor and acceptor groups in a given molecule determine the most favored polymorphic form chosen by nature.

Table 38-1. Possible 3-Dimensional Crystalline Space Groups

CRYSTAL SYSTEM	NUMBER OF INDEPENDENT PARAMETERS	PARAMETERS	MATHEMATICAL ABUNDANCE	ORGANIC CRYSTAL ABUNDANCE
Triclinic	6	$a \neq b \neq c$; $\alpha \neq \beta \neq \gamma$	2	High ?
Monoclinic	4	$a \neq b \neq c$; $\alpha = \gamma$; >90	13	High $P2_1/c$
Orthorhombic	3	$a \neq b \neq c$; $\alpha = \beta = \gamma = 90$	59	Very Low $P2_12_12_1$
Tetragonal	2	$a = b = c$; $\alpha = \beta = \gamma = 90$	68	~0
Trigonal rhombohedra	2	$a = b = c$; $\alpha = = \gamma \neq 90$	6	~0
Trigonal hexagonal	2	$a = b = c$; $\alpha = = 90$; $\gamma = 120$	19	~0
Hexagonal	2	$a = b = c$; $\alpha = = 90$; $\gamma = 120$	27	~0
Cubic	1	$a = b = c$; $\alpha = \beta = \gamma = 90$	36	~0

H-bonds are non-covalent interactions that can occur within a given molecule (intramolecular) and between different molecules (intermolecular). Essentially they are electrostatic in nature and as such are long-ranging forces (force varies as $1/r^2$). Weak H-bonds usually have a higher multiplicity of interactions than strong H-bonds because they are more flexible, as illustrated Table 38-2. Intramolecular H-bonds form when the atoms in the molecule can be arranged such that a ring of covalently linked atoms (usually 6) is closed with 1 or more H-bond (Fig 38-4A). Intermolecular H-bonds form between different molecules of a crystal (Fig 38-4B–E).

High affinity traps with their associated insolubility and high melting points can be attributed to H-bonding networks and/or close packing. As a general rule, H-bonding network insolubility is associated with the number of H-bonds per molecule as well as the number of H-bond between molecules in a crystal. In Table 38-3, pairs of molecules are shown that have the same water solubilizing groups but differ in their H-bonding motifs. Figures 38-4B and C show molecules that form a dimer and a single chain, respectively. Each has 2 H-bonds per molecule but differ in the number of H-bonding neighbors. Similarly, Figures 38-4D and E show molecules that form single and double H-bonding chains, respectively. In this case, each molecule has the same number of H-bonding neighbors, but has a different number of H-bonds per molecule. For both pairs, Table 38-3 shows that increasing either the number of H-bonding neighbors or the number of H-bond per molecules reduces the effectiveness of the water-solu-

bilizing group. The negative influence of close packing on physical properties is most likely due to the introduction of van der Waals dispersion forces that vary as $1/r^6$. Zwitterion formation, conformationally restricted molecules, or high packing density molecules have the highest intrinsic insolubility potential.

Membrane Interactions and Permeability

THEORIES OF PASSIVE PERMEABILITY

The *water of desolvation* hypothesis, explored extensively by Burton and co-workers[16,17] states that the major barrier for passive permeability NCEs across cell membranes is the energy needed to remove bound water from the molecule so it can enter the hydrophobic portion of the lipid bilayer. Although both hydrophobic and hydrophilic NCEs would have some bound water associated with them in solution, the adhesive H-bonding between water and the polar groups of hydrophilic NCEs group would be much stronger and thus need to be broken before transport can take place. Strong supporting evidence for this concept has been found using the peptide bond as the polar moiety and has led to an experimental partitioning system, $P_{heptane/ethylene glycol}$, that appears to be more predictive of permeability than the widely accepted octanol/water partition coefficient.[16]

The *molecular rigidity hypothesis* posits that molecular weight itself is not a sufficient condition to impart reduced membrane permeability but may itself be a factor that is correlated with the number of rotatable bonds and polar surface

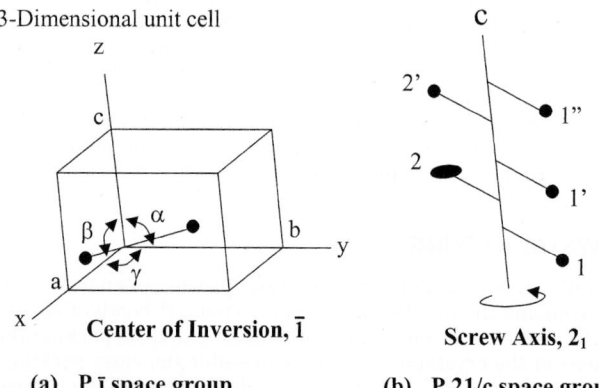

3-Dimensional unit cell

Center of Inversion, $\bar{1}$

(a) P $\bar{1}$ space group

Screw Axis, 2_1

(b) P $2_1/c$ space group

Figure 38-3. Repeat mechanism (space group rules).

Table 38-2. Comparison of Hydrogen

	BOND CHARACTERISTICS	
	WEAK	STRONG
Bond Character	Electrostatic Broad	Covalent Narrow
Bond Length	1.5 Å–3 Å	1.2 Å–1.5 Å
Directionality	160° ± 20°	~ 180°
Multiplicity	2,3,4 Centered A	2 Centered A
XH ---- A	XH	XH ---- A'
	A'	A''
2 Centered	3 Centered	4 Centered

area. If these two latter parameters are below certain values, then compounds that are sufficiently rigid and non-polar may be absorbed independent of molecular weight.[18] Some factors that can impart rigidity besides fused-ring systems are molecules that have intramolecular H-bonds that form a ring or cyclic peptides.

THEORIES OF ACTIVE PERMEABILITY

NUTRIENT UPTAKE MECHANISMS—The passive permeability limitations discussed above for polar or ionized molecules do not hold for a number of nutrients. Special site-specific transporter proteins are present in membranes that are used to bypass the lipophilic barrier of bilayer membranes.[19] Among these are transporters for peptides, amino acids, nucleoside and nucleobase, ascorbate, and a few other molecules such as glucose and urea. Application of the PEPT1 transporter to prodrug delivery will be discussed below.

XENOBIOTIC EFFLUX MECHANISMS—Membrane transporters belong to one the largest classes of proteins, termed ABC (ATP binding cassette) proteins that can transport against the concentration gradient of the substrate. The characteristics of these membrane proteins are: (a) 2 transmembrane domains [regions of the protein embedded in the membrane], and (b) 2 ABC units [which bind ATP].[20] Defects in ABC proteins are the cause of many human inherited diseases. In most studies, ABC proteins are the multidrug resistance proteins (MDR) that remove therapeutic agents from cells by an active efflux.

MDR1 (or Pgp1) is one of the most extensively studied ABC proteins. Its normal function is believed to protect cells and organisms from toxic substances.[21] There are 7 identified proteins that have been placed in the MDR family, all are organic anion transporters. MDR1, MDR2, and MDR3 have all been associated with multi-drug resistance.

PASSIVE-DIFFUSION DESIGN

One way to reduce conformational restriction is to open up a restricting ring. Alternatively, Figures 38-4 A, D & E discussed in a previous section shows that the substitution of a t-butyl group for a phenyl group dramatically increased solubility by

breaking up H-bonding so that each molecule only had 2 rather than 4 H-bonds per molecule. This was due to the bulkiness of the t-butyl group that prevented dimer formation.

PRODRUG DESIGN

Often NCEs have adequate biological activity but do not have the required physical properties to become a drug. For orally administered drugs, the compound needs to dissolve in the gastrointestinal tract and be absorbed by the intestinal membranes; for intravenous drugs, the compound must have adequate solubility in its dosing vehicle and in the blood so it can be delivered safely without causing embolisms. Prodrugs are one way to solve a number of safety and property-design problems and should be considered early in the design phase. Prodrugs are inactive analogs of biologically active compounds that can be converted into active compounds by the body's chemical processes. They are designed to have the critical properties that the parent compound lacks. Poor membrane permeability, poor solubility, and poor dissolution are problem areas that may be addressed by prodrugs. All three of these areas impact the passive absorption of drugs. Prodrug design has also been used to reduce toxicity.

Poor Membrane Permeability

One of the major roles of the outer limiting membranes of cells is to isolate it from its surroundings. Three factors that inhibit the passage of a drug molecule through biological membranes are: (a) charge, (b) water of hydration, and (c) molecular size. The importance of charge is related not only to the hydrophobic environment of the bilayers but also to the asymmetry of plasma membranes. Because these membranes are composed of two layers of phospholipids (a bilayer), the radius of curvature of micron-sized cells requires that phospholipids with small head groups be located in the inner leaflet of the bilayer to prevent excessive tension on the membrane.[22] The anionic phospholipid, phosphatidylserine (PS), resides almost exclusively in the inner leaflet due to an active process.[23] This negatively charged inner leaflet of the plasma membrane has

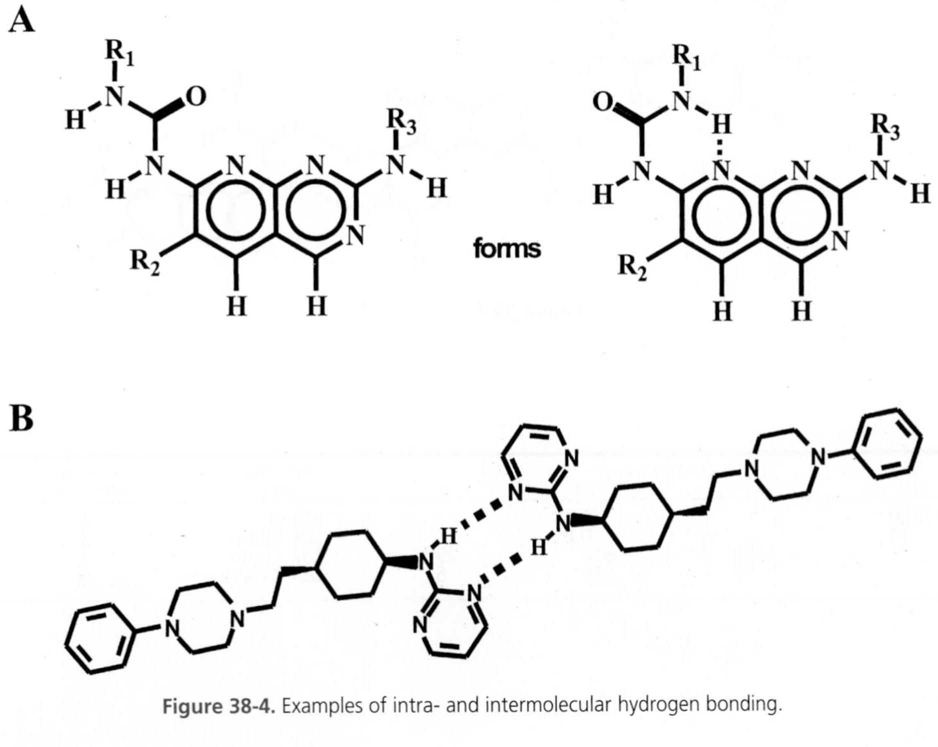

Figure 38-4. Examples of intra- and intermolecular hydrogen bonding.

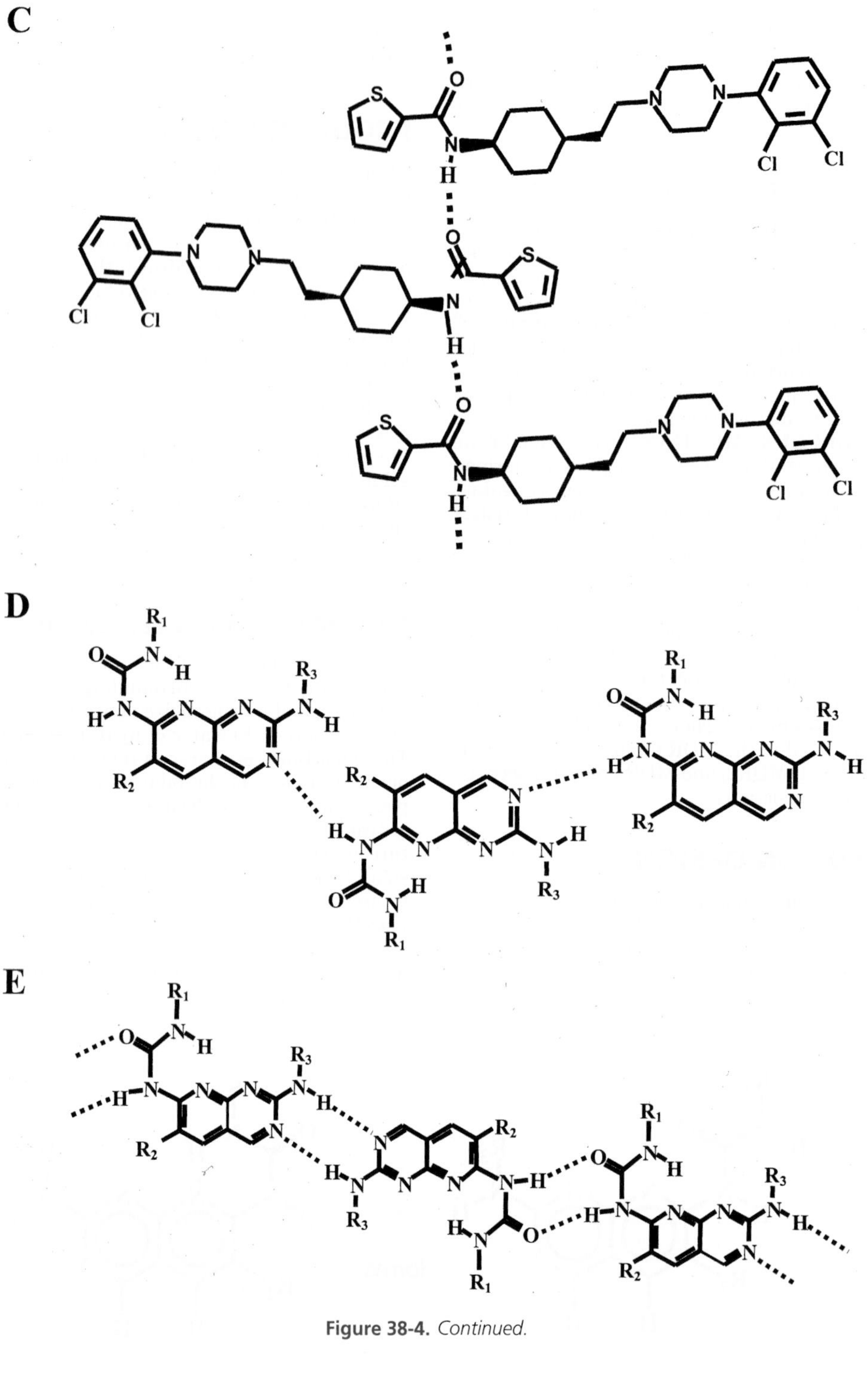

C

D

E

Figure 38-4. *Continued.*

Table 38-3.

pH	SOLUBILITY μg/mL				NETWORK TYPE	# H-BOND /MOLECULE	# H-BONDED NEIGHBORS
	1	5.6	7.3	13			
B	17600		8		Island	2	1
C	14		0.05		Sgl. Chain	2	2
D		1700	610	25	Sgl. Chain	2	2
E		16	10	6	Dbl. Chain	4	2

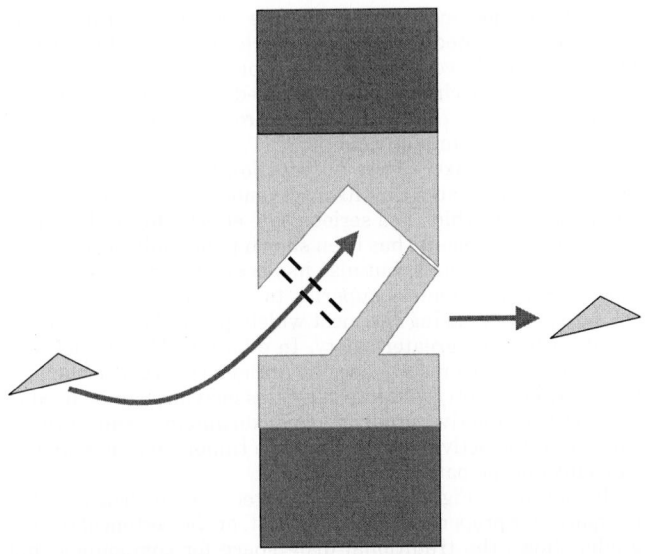

Figure 38-5. PepT1 cattle-gate mechanism.

been shown to control the tissue distribution of basic cationic drugs[24] and the permeability of the anthracycline base, doxorubicin, in a biphasic manner.[25] One might expect this inner leaflet would impact the absorption of anionic drugs. To circumvent these barriers to ionized and polar nutrients like peptides, amino acids, and nucleoside bases, cells developed a number of special transport proteins. Prodrug efforts are now ongoing to exploit these membrane transporters to enhance drug absorption.[26]

Use of Membrane Transporter Systems

Recently, some of the structural requirements of the plasma membrane peptide transporter, PEPT1, have been elucidated.[27-29] The binding requirements and the cattle-gate mechanism for PEPT1 are shown in Figure 38-5. Among the number of drugs reported to be transported by PEPT1 are ACE inhibitors (captopril, enalapril, lisinopril), penicillin, and cephalosporins (ceftibuten, cefadroxil). The advantage of this transporter is its high capacity (grams/meal). Successful prodrug strategies utilizing PEPT1 have been reported. The antiviral agent, Valtrex (valcyclovir-*GlaxoSmithKline*) is a prodrug of Zovirax (acyclovir). It has recently been observed that the H-bonding of the guanidine moiety of L-valaciclovir may enhance its PEPT1absorption.[30]

Reducing Ionization

Most Factor Xa inhibitors for preventing the activation of thrombin and blood clots have utilized a highly charged group, either a guanidine or an amidine group. These groups, however, limit the bioavailability of these compounds when used orally. One strategy to overcome this problem is to synthesize a prodrug which has a reduced charge for oral absorption but which can be converted in the systemic system to the active charged compound. Scientists at *Millennium* have recently designed a Factor Xa inhibitor that utilizes amidoximes as prodrugs for amindines.[31] These prodrugs showed good bioavailability but the conversion to the amidine was only 20%. Although the amidoxime prodrug approach apparently has been successful in masking charge for other chemical entities, in this situation, steric factors evidently retarded activation *in vivo*. This raises another concern with prodrugs: the potential toxicity of the intact prodrug moiety.

The pentamidines are very effective antimicrobial agents against a variety of pathogens and have been used to treat malaria and leishmaniasis. However, their use has been limited to systemic injections since a doubly charged drug is poorly absorbed. Exploration of amidoximes as prodrugs for amidines[32] has led to a new agent, DB 289, that has excellent bioavailability and is currently undergoing phase II clinical trials to treat *Pneumocystis carinii*, a fungal infection in infants that have immune deficiencies and in AIDS patients.[33] Studies with Caco-2 cell monolayers indicate that the greater permeability of the prodrug is due to its ability to transport passively across cell membranes by the transcellular route compared to the pericellular route of the parent compound.

Reducing Water of Hydration

In a previous section, the desolvation hypothesis was discussed in which the impact of strong H-bonds between NCE polar groups and water provides barriers for absorption (due to the need to remove this water before traversing the hydrophobic environment of bilayer acyl chains). Using prodrug strategies to make polar groups more lipophilic is one method to increase permeability and this has been accomplished for peptides by designing cyclic compounds that encourage intramolecular H-bonding and thus reduce water of hydration, make a more compact, rigid molecule, and minimize adhesive interactions with the membrane phospholipid head group.[34]

Size of Molecule

Although molecular weight has always been considered an important determinant of permeability, questions have recently arisen regarding the exact molecular property that determines a reduction of permeability with increasing molecular size as discussed in a previous section. We have discussed the hypothesis that increased molecular rigidity and a reduced polar surface area may enhance permeability. Results with cyclic peptides would seem to be consistent with this hypothesis as the Type I β-turn both reduces the polar surface area and enhances molecular rigidity. In addition, a molecule with more conformational flexibility would appear to present a larger size entity to the membrane.

POOR SOLUBILITY

Using prodrugs for solubility enhancement can take at least two different pathways: (a) increasing water solubility, and (b) disrupting crystal packing. The latter application has as much promise as the first, yet it is less obvious. The reader is referred to the previous discussion on crystal packing. Enhancing ionization with phosphate moieties has been used for both intravenous and oral applications. The intravenous is the earlier.

INCREASING IONIZATION—Fosphenytoin (Cerebyx-*Pfizer*) is an injectable, phosphate prodrug of phenytoin (Dilantin- *Pfizer*) for the treatment of epilepsy that is freely soluble and rapidly cleaved to phenytoin after injection (half-life 8–15 min). The aqueous solubility of the parent drug is 20–25µg/ml while the solubility of the prodrug is significantly greater (approximately 88,000µg/ml). Local toxicity (pain, burning, itching) that is associated with phenytoin administration due to its high pH formulation is greatly reduced since the more highly soluble prodrug can be formulated at physiological pHs.[35]

DISRUPTING CRYSTAL PACKING—Parecoxib sodium (Pharmacia) is a good example of using prodrugs to disrupt H-bonding and crystal packing as well as increasing pK_a to enhance solubility. For post-surgical pain management, a compound must not only be effective and have few side effects, but it must also be formulated so that a minimal injection volume is administered. Although valdecoxib (*Pharmacia*) possessed

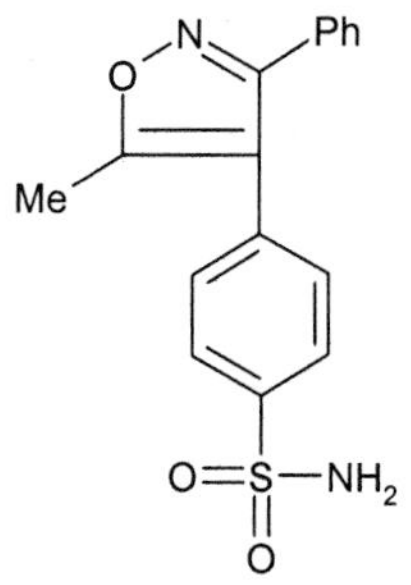

Parent: Valedcoxib
Solubility = 9 µg/mL

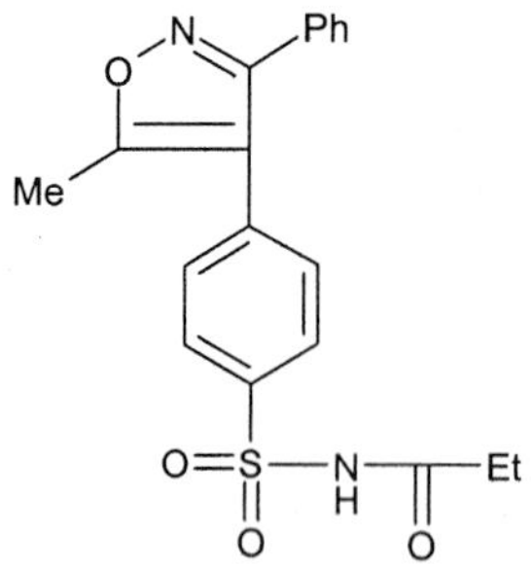

Prodrug: Parecoxib
Solubility = 44 µg/mL

Figure 38-6. Prodrug of valdecoxib increases solubility by decreasing H-bonding.

the required potency and safety profile, its solubility was insufficient for this application. Increased water solubility was imparted to the prodrug, parecoxib, by making a prodrug of valdecoxib (Fig 38-6).[36,37]

POOR DISSOLUTION

Prodrugs may be used to improve dissolution properties. For example, Fosamprevavir (Vertex - *GlaxoSmithKline*) is an oral prodrug of Amprenavir (Agenerase - Vertex - *GlaxoSmithKline*), an anti-viral for HIV infections. Although agenerase is approved for HIV treatment, its poor water solubility necessitated that the drug be formulated with large amounts of excipients for optimal dissolution and bioavailability. Typical clinical dosage routines included dosing at 1200 mg (8 capsules) twice or three times a day when plasma concentrations fell below therapeutic levels. The large number of capsules and the food and water restrictions associated with administration of this drug provide barriers to patient adherence with the prescribed therapeutic regimen. By synthesizing the highly soluble phosphate prodrug, fosamprevavir, it is anticipated that adequate drug levels can be achieved with out food or water restriction at 2-700 mg tablets twice daily.[38] Currently, fosamprevavir is completing Phase III clinical trials.

TOXICITY REDUCTION

Xeloda (capecitabine - *Roche*) is a prodrug of the anti-cancer drug 5FU.[39] The parent compound has a number of dose-limiting side effects including: myelo-suppression, intestinal toxicity, and reduction in bone marrow function. Capecitabine reduces the intensity of these side effects by utilizing intestinal,

liver and tumor enzymes to generate 5FU in the tumor cell. Camptosar (irinotecan HCl - *Pharmacia*) is a second line agent for advanced colorectal cancer. It is a prodrug of the natural alkaloid camptothecin[40] that is activated by carboxylesterase-2 when it occurs in the tumors. This prodrug greatly increases the solubility of camptothecin.

Taxol's (paclitaxel - *Bristol-Myers Squibb*) low aqueous solubility has necessitated that its intravenous formulation include Cremophor EL which has serious side effects. Recently, a prodrug, paclitaxel oleate, has been shown to not only be activated *in vitro* and in rabbits, but also has been shown to have pharmacokinetic parameters superior to paclitaxel.[41] This raises the possibility of using the most widely prescribed anti-cancer agent with much greater safety. In addition, *Merck* scientists have shown that prostate specific antigen (PSA), a serine protease with chymotrypsin-like activities enzyme, can be used to convert the inactive prodrugs of doxorubicin[42] and vinblactine[43] into the active agent within the tumor thereby reducing side effect of the parent drugs.

In summary, Figure 38-7 shows three types of drug possibility spaces for property-design. The first, at the bottom of the triangle, shows the traditional drug space for compounds that have adequate physical chemical properties and have been found by traditional discovery techniques. The second possibility space is shown in the middle section of the triangle. This space requires more active participation by the property designer to utilize all available tools when physical chemical problems arise. The techniques listed here for simplicity include special delivery systems (SDS) such as self-emulsifying drug delivery systems, prodrugs to break up crystal packing or to add water solubilizing or lipophilic groups, SDS for lipophilic prodrugs, and crystal packing disruptions designed to reduce H-bonding interactions and dense crystal packing. Technology will produce even more options for the future. Finally, there is the physiologically negative drug space or the region of high-affinity traps. These molecules usually have extremely high *in vitro* activity, but have been so over-designed for activity that they suffer from poor physical chemical properties. Sometimes these molecules can be delivered to the systemic system with clever formulations or drug delivery systems, but their poor physical properties ultimately reveal themselves when they crystallize out in the renal tubules of the kidney when solubilizing factors have diffused away from the drug molecules. The ability to anticipate the second possibility space and to avoid the negative-property space at the top of the triangle is a worthy goal for property-based design. This is the subject of the next section.

MACHINE LEARNING SYSTEMS

Artificial intelligence (AI) is a computational algorithm that would be called intelligent if a human exhibited it. One of AI's theses is that computers can simulate any effective procedure.

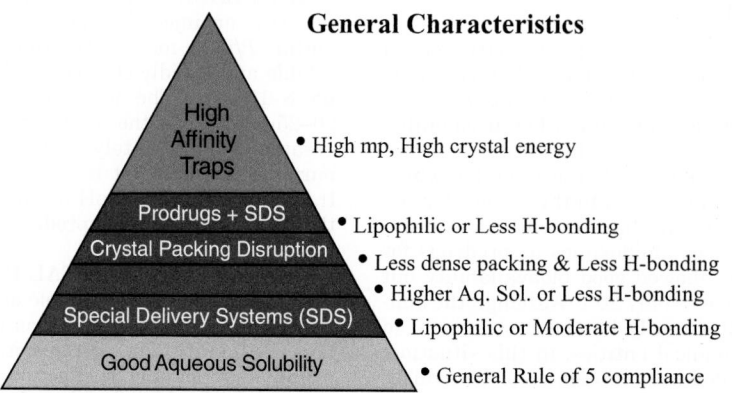

Figure 38-7. Possible and physiological-negative drug spaces. See Color Plate 5.

As John von Neumann once said: "Tell me what a machine cannot do, and I will always be able to make a machine that can do it!" Opponents of AI once defined intelligence as learning. Machine learning is AI's response to that challenge. In the following sections, *machine* will be used synonymously with a computational algorithm.

Machine learning is an area of AI that develops techniques that allow computers to, in some sense, "learn." If the pharmaceutical industry is to become more efficient and reduce cost, it must learn more efficiently. Since 90–95 % of the resources that are expended on NCE development are spent on compounds that will never advance, learning from this experience is an imperative. Machine learning may be the way the industry can reduce cost by learning before doing as we have shown in Figure 38-2. Activity-based design utilizing rapid machine learning techniques would efficiently use the results of high throughput screening to develop highly accurate pharmacophores. In addition, *in silico* activity screening and chemical route design technology would generate structures that are synthesizable, scalable, and match different aspects of these pharmacophores. Safety-based machines would accurately predict different features such as mutagenicity, clastogenicity, or QT-interval prolongation. And finally, property-based machines would be used to ensure that the design of such structures had the requisite physical properties so that traditional or specialized drug delivery could be accomplished. All of these activities would be carried out before a single molecule was synthesized. The impact on cost reduction of such a learning-before-doing paradigm also opens up new markets for NCEs.

Supervised learning is the most prevalent form of machine learning that is currently practiced. Because data in machine learning are termed examples, supervised machine learning is termed *learning by example*. In this type of learning, examples are presented to the machine, and after learning takes place, the machine is tested to see how well it can predict *unseen* examples. Just how accurately the machine can predict unlearned examples is termed the machine's *generalizability*. Example sets are usually subdivided into *training* and *test* sets to carry out the operations stated above. In general, the quality of a machine's future generalizability is highly dependent on how representative the training example set is of examples that are to be predicted in the future.

There are two main types of applications for machine learning, *regression* and *classification*. In regression, the goal is to predict an exact value of a physical property such as solubility or melting point. For classification, the training set is composed of both *positive* and *negative* examples. After training, the machine is asked to correctly separate unseen examples. Classification applications for machine learning are generally *binary* classification i.e. yes/no answers. For example, in the bioinformatics area, classification is used to predict whether a particular gene codes for a particular protein.

Unsupervised learning deals with learning the *structure* or *topology* of knowledge. Learning that fails to have an ability to grasp the general principles or the structure of a discipline will fall short of learning how things are related and how new information can be related in the future.[44] Learning 'without a teacher' is learning that *adapts* its behavior without being told (supervised learning) the appropriateness (reinforced learning) of an observation. However, by grasping the topology of the subject area, the learning machine will be more able to respond in an improved way in the future. Knowledge discovery and data mining are areas where this type of learning has immediate applications.

One of the major concerns in the machine learning community is the *opaqueness* of some of the algorithms. Humans, and especially physicians, distrust 'black boxes' even if they can be shown to be highly accurate. This concern has lead to new machines that are much more *transparent* in their reasoning. This leads to exciting collaborations between machines and domain experts, humans that are highly specialized in certain technical areas. *Expert systems* are *non-learning* computing systems in which the knowledge of the human domain expert is captured and stored as a set of rules in a knowledge base. A generic inference engine connects the user with the knowledge base so that the machine expert can respond to queries from the user. Machine learning systems, in distinction to expert systems, learn rules from data alone. This is potentially much more powerful since machines can examine data in larger quantities and more consistently than humans. If this process is transparent to humans, it provides a synergistic situation in which the domain expert and the machine can collaborate in solving new problems.

Property-design is based on the premise that all of the information that is needed to predict physical properties is contained in the molecular structure of the molecule alone. This means that the dependent variable (a physical property like solubility) must be computed from factors (independent variables) that are determined from the molecular structure only. The machine learning terminology for these independent variables is *features*; the molecular modeling term for these variables is *molecular descriptors*. There are many computational programs that can generate molecular features and a number of strategies for *feature selection*. The danger, however, is that users get caught up in 'group think' and become so dependent on software programs that innovative thinking is inhibited.

Several mathematical issues are associated with the algorithms of machine learning. The first is the functional relationship of the physical property with features. *Linear* relationships are the simplest type of functional dependence. The advantage of *linear regression analysis* is that humans can easily see and understand the relationships between what is being predicted and the features that are being used to predict (*transparency*). Visual inspection can be used to assess the quality of the prediction. Assuming that there is a linear dependence is both a strength and weakness of this type of analysis. On the one hand, linear system analysis is amenable to many different mathematical analytical methodologies, and, fortunately, many non-linear systems are linear over a narrow range of feature values. On the other hand, because most physical systems are non-linear over wider ranges, linear dependencies are accurate *locally* but often do not project to the same accuracy over wider ranges (ie, *globally*). Neural networks made the next advance in making predictions. They address the non-linear issue.

Artificial neural networks (ANN) are mathematical abstractions of a simple animal reasoning systems. These systems utilize a non-linear function, usually the hyperbolic tanh function, to model the relationship between the input features with respect to the output physical property. During the learning phase of ANNs, feature selection takes place on the training examples. Learning is a supervised reinforcement that focuses on minimizing error in the training set (empirical risk minimization). The features that have the strongest relationships to the dependent property are selected while taking into account multiple feature interactions. This learning process is often tedious and requires experienced personnel. More over, the complexity of the interactions or the dependence of the dependent property on the input features is hidden, i.e. the reasoning is *opaque*. Another issue with ANNs is that they are subject to *over fitting*. This is a phenomenon in which the ANN model is refined to such a degree that the training examples are very highly correlated to the dependent property but the model as a whole has very poor *generalalizability*. This is a result of learning being dependent on empirical risk minimization. Skilled usage of ANNs, however, can give us some of the most accurate machine learning predictions we have at the current time. In addition, one of the shortcomings of ANNs, a lack of memory, appears to have been addressed. ASNNs were designed with this defect in mind.

Associate neural networks (ASNN) address the issue of training set dependence and knowledge update[45,46] by combining ANN and K-nearest neighbor technology. With such machine learning technology, extensive and laborious training is carried out to generate ensembles of ANNs. The machine has the ability to determine the most appropriate ANN for a particular compound so that it can obtain the advantage of higher local accuracy while having a global span. In addition, it has the ability to learn new examples on-the-fly. This means that extensive training can be carried out on public databases while updating with respect to proprietary data is possible on an ongoing basis. Recent implementation of an ASNN for calculated LogP has shown 2–5-fold improvements using additional proprietary examples.[47] ASNNs partially address the local/global issue, but still suffer from being opaque. A newer machine learning paradigm has been introduced that addresses both of these issues, *support vector machines* (SVM).

SVMs are statistically constrained machines that were introduced in 1982 to explicitly address *generalizability*, *local/global*, and *linear/non-linear* issues.[48,49] In addition, some SVMs are *very transparent* and are very efficient in *feature selection*.[50] SVMs use mathematical functions, called kernels, that have a very special property: they can act as mediators that allow nonlinear data to be processed by linear algorithms. Their major strength is that they promote generalizability explicitly. In addition, SVMs are designed so that they converge on global optima only. They have been shown to give classification results superior to ANNs in the bioinfomatics area and some have regression capabilities. These machines use dual optimization routines that promote generalizability, global, non-linear, and feature efficient predictions, and are just being introduced into the chemoinfomatic arena.[51] In general, however, they are *opaque* techniques that require skill in parameter selection. One machine learning technique, however, excels in its transparency, *inductive logic programming* (ILP).

ACTIVE PHARMACEUTICAL INGREDIENT-BASED DESIGN AND PREFORMULATION

Once a NCE is selected for development, choosing the molecular form that will be the active pharmaceutical ingredient (API) is a critical milestone because all subsequent development will be affected by this decision. For preformulation, physical characterizations should be focused on making decisions that balance solid-state dissolution properties with material consistency under manufacturing and storage conditions. The advantages of having a rapidly dissolving amorphous state have to be balanced against the potential conversion of this state by time, moisture, and heat to a crystalline state that can be less soluble. Similarly, the increased solubility that often can occur with hydrochloride and sodium salts may have to be balanced with a potential for physical or chemical instability due to moisture and heat. These salts are attractive because they are simple to make and are relatively nontoxic. The salt selection process must project its considerations of the "best" properties to encompass dissolution, physical and chemical stability, toxicology, market-image formulations, large scale manufacturing, and product storage.

The following section will outline solid-state changes that might occur with varying moisture content, pH, and temperature. It will be illustrated that water (moisture) is one of the most important environmental factors that influences solid-state stability. The discussion will then focus on identifying the solid-state properties of an NCE that will make it a viable API. Ultimately, the best balance between absorption and material consistency is sought. Later, the discussion of engineering the solid state will explore why these requisite properties should be designed into NCEs from the earliest stages of discovery.

CHALLENGES TO THE SOLID STATE

Solids are a complex state of matter because intermolecular forces can arrange the molecules in a variety of different ways, each producing a different solid with potentially different physical properties. In this section, a symbolic nomenclature is introduced to specifically address changes that can occur in the solid state (Table 38-4). Application of this notation to the ef-

Table 38-4. List of Symbols

SYMBOL	MEANING
α	Amorphous solid state as left subscript designation
Σ	Surface of solid state as right subscript designation
δ	Defective region of solid state as left subscript designation
ρ	Density
I, II, III	Crystalline polymorphic forms of the solid state as left subscript designation
$+$	Positively charged, cationic species as superscript designation
$-$	Negatively charged, anionic species as superscript designation
0	Uncharged, free species as superscript designation
A	Active ingredient in the solid state
a	Dissolved form of the active ingredient
$_jA_\Sigma{}^i$	Surface of active ingredient of charge i and solid state j
B	Reactant of A in the solid state
b	Dissolved form of reactant
C_s	Saturation concentration
h	Monohydrate as left subscript designation
$0h$	Anhydrous as left subscript designation
nh	n-Hydrate as left subscript designation
$<h$	Reduced water content as left subscript designation
$>h$	Increased water content as left subscript designation
m	Mass
An^-	Negatively charged anionic counterion
i	Charge on the active ingredient as superscript designation
j	Solid state form of the active ingredient as left subscript designation
k_d	Dissolution rate constant
k_r	Recrystallization rate constant
P	Permeability
Cn^+	Positively charged cationic counterion
S_a	Surface area

fects of moisture, the major environmental factor influencing the solid state, will then be examined.

SOLID-STATE CHARACTER

In this chapter, $_jA_\Sigma{}^i$ is a notation that will be used to indicate solid-state changes. The A denotes the active drug entity. This may be a weak acid, a weak base, or a nonelectrolyte. When A dissolves, a denotes the presence of this entity in solution; thus, dissolution of the solid A in water to form a will be shown schematically as

$$A \xrightarrow{\text{H}_2\text{O}} \alpha \qquad (1)$$

The charge of A is denoted by the usual placement of a right superscript, i. The charge of A is assumed to be zero by default. For emphasis, a lack of charge may be shown explicitly as A^0. For a weak acid, A^0 represents the protonated form (in other notations this might be shown as HA). The ionized form of the weak acid, A^-, represents A^0 minus the weak acid proton. For a weak base, A^0 denotes the uncharged base that can be protonated to A^0H^+. Equations with A, shown with arrows, are not stoichiometric. Instead, they only show essential changes, so the focus can be placed on the relevant chemical, ionic, and solid-state alterations in the chemical entity. For example, in Equation 2, in which a chemical reaction changes the parent entity A into a different molecular solid B,

$$A \to B \qquad (2)$$

there is no attempt to show the specific details of the functional groups that were changed to bring about the formation of B. In a similar manner, consider a reversible acid–base reaction

$$A \underset{\longleftarrow}{\longrightarrow} A^i \qquad (3)$$

where i as a plus sign $(+)$ represents the cationic form, or a minus sign $(-)$ the anionic form, of A. The protonation or deprotonation of a weak basic or acidic group on A will simply be reflected in the charge change that occurs. The scheme is nonstoichiometric because counter ions and charge-balance considerations have not been included.

When a particular molecular organization or emphasis of the solid state is needed, it will be denoted with the left subscript j. A wide variety of different solid states, denoted by $_jA$, are possible. For example, amorphous solids that have randomly packed molecules are denoted as $_\alpha A$ in this chapter. Crystalline solids, on the other hand, have regular packing arrangements and are denoted in a number of ways. Two types of crystalline phases, polymorphs and solvates, are possible for a given molecule depending on the crystallization conditions.

Polymorphs are crystals that have the same molecule formula but have different crystal structures. The Roman numerals I, II, III, . . . are used to denote polymorphs; the most stable polymorph under ambient conditions is usually designated with Roman numeral I. This solid-state form of A will be denoted as $_IA$ in this chapter.

Solvates, on the other hand, are crystals in which a solvent is incorporated into the crystal structure (polymorphs of solvates could exist). The solvent may be highly bound in the crystal or it may be more loosely bound in channels within the crystal. To simplify this discussion, only water of solvation will be considered. Hydrated solids are denoted by $_{nh}A$, where n is a fraction or an integer. For example, $_{h/2}A$ denotes a hemihydrate while $_{3h}A$ denotes a trihydrate.

In some situations, it will be useful to emphasize that a particular chemical reaction or physical change is occurring on the surface of a particle. For these purposes, the right subscript Σ will be used to emphasize the surface of the solid state. It should be noted that the right superscript i, used for charge designation, and the left subscript j, used for solid-state designation, are only general placeholders for more specific instances that will be detailed below; on the other hand, the right subscript Σ specifically denotes the surface of a solid particle and not a more general entity. For most situations, the full notation will not be used.

In actual APIs, crystal defective regions A_δ are present. These were formed during large-scale synthesis and milling operations that reduced the API's particle size. In Figure 38-8, defective regions as well as crystalline and amorphous regions are shown diagrammatically.

WATER: A MAJOR ENVIRONMENTAL VARIABLE

The presence or absence of moisture is one of the most important environmental factors that can affect solid-state stability. The surface of an API particle can gain or lose water depending on the relative humidity (RH). Figure 38-8 shows how water vapor can form regions of dissolved drug on the surface of the API particle. The amorphous region would be expected to dissolve the fastest, and the crystalline region the slowest; that is, the rank order of dissolution would be $A_\alpha > A_\delta > {}_IA$. In the Figure 38-8 diagram, this is indicated by the font size of the saturated dissolved form of A, a_s, associated with each of these regions. This surface coating results in chemical and physical instability.

Chemical Instability: Water as a Molecular Mobilizer

In general, chemical reactivity is slow in solids because of the spacial separation of different reactive components. For example, if a small amount of an impurity that can act as a catalyst is distributed heterogeneously in an API or a dosage form, the overall rate of reaction is limited because the reaction only occurs in microenvironmental regions. However, in dosage forms, most APIs are usually in contact with moisture-bearing excipients and are stress-tested at elevated temperatures and humidity. The presence of an adsorbed layer of moisture increases the catalytic reactivity of the impurity because water, acting as a molecular mobilizer, can transport different chemical species laterally over the surface of the API.[52] Equation 4 shows a chain of reactions from A to a degradant B:

$$A \xrightarrow{[H_2O]_{vapor}} a \xrightarrow{[H_2O]_{vapor}\ catalytic\ impurity} b \xrightarrow{[H_2O]_{vapor}} B \qquad (4)$$

where b is the solubilized form of B. Moisture also induces solid-state changes in A. (Further discussion of moisture- induced chemical instability will be treated in the section *Hydrate Stability: Importance of the Critical Relative Humidity*.)

Microenvironmental pH: Moisture-Induced Sensitivity of Acid/Bases

Acid–base reactivity in the solid-state change will be enhanced by moisture. Equation 5 shows a moisture-induced change of an anionic salt to its free acid on the surface of a drug particle:

$$A_\Sigma^- \xrightarrow{[H_2O]_{vapor}} A_\Sigma^0 \qquad (5)$$

Conversely, Equation 6 shows a moisture-induced surface conversion of a cationic salt into its free base,

$$A_\Sigma^+ \xrightarrow{[H_2O]_{vapor}} A_\Sigma^0 \qquad (6)$$

where $A^+ = HA^+$. Because the amount of solid drug is large compared to the amount of moisture, Equations 5 and 6 have been diagramed as irreversible reactions. Such solid-state changes can alter the physical properties of the API. For example, if particles of the sodium salt of an insoluble acid form a surface coating of the free acid as in Equation 5, the dissolution rate of the surface will be retarded. Testing methods are needed during the salt selection stage to anticipate this type of solid-state change (see under *Salt Selection*).

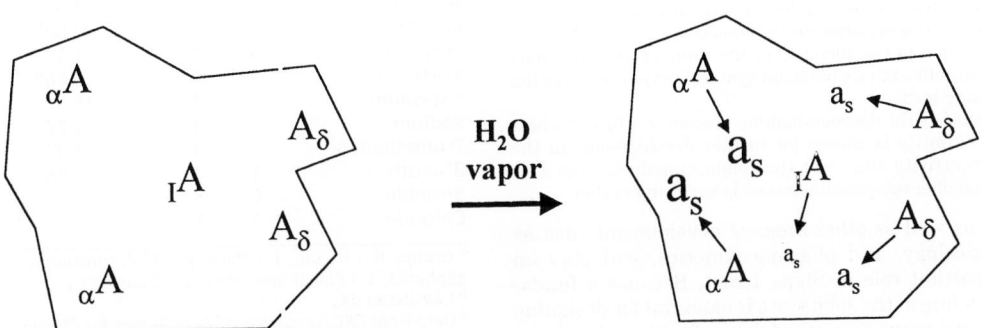

Figure 38-8. Surface of a milled API and dissolution of surface regions due to adsorbed moisture.

Solvent-Mediated Transformations of Polymorphs: Water as a Transporter

If two polymorphic forms can exist at a given temperature, the metastable polymorph will be more soluble (see *Salt Selection*). When this form is put in contact with water, the following solvent-mediated transformation can be promoted:

$$_{II}A \xrightarrow{H_2O} {}_1A \qquad (7)$$

Water, in the vapor phase, has also been shown to be capable of mediating transformations between amorphous and crystalline forms in both directions.[53]

$$_aA \underset{\leftarrow}{\xrightarrow{[H_2O]_{vapor}}} {}_1A \qquad (8)$$

Finally, transformations can occur that incorporate water into the crystal structure. Here, an anhydrous crystalline form is changed into the monohydrate,

$$_{II}A \xrightarrow{H_2O} {}_hA \qquad (9)$$

and a salt is transformed into a hemihydrate after passing through the amorphous form:

$$_{II}A^+ \xrightarrow{H_2O} {}_aA^+ \xrightarrow{H_2O} {}_{h/2}A^+ \qquad (10)$$

Equations 7 to 10 emphasize solid-state changes. It is likely that most of these transformations may occur only after dissolving and forming a or a species forming a^+.

DECISION-POINTS IN THE DISCOVERY AND DEVELOPMENT OF AN API

The term *active pharmaceutical ingredient* (API), also known as drug substance and bulk pharmaceutical chemical (BPC), highlights both a discovery and a development component. In this section, discovery Steps 1 to 4 will be introduced briefly. The focus will then shift to a detailed discussion of the developmental Steps 5 to 9. Using this background, the section Engineering in the Solid State will outline how early parallel integration of these activities can reduce the time from concept to market.

The term *expansion* is used when choices are being enlarged, and *selection* is used when choices are reduced by decision-making. Ultimately, the expansion and selection phases of discovery lead to a single choice, the best candidate for further development.

1. Library expansion refers to additions to a company's chemical library. Established pharmaceutical companies have amassed hundreds of thousands of compounds through previous discovery efforts. These collections are cataloged carefully and are used systematically in mass screens.
2. Series selection is a decision-making process in which the most active chemicals in the library are identified using a high-throughput biological assay. Typically, these assays are used to detect the ability of a small molecule to interact with a protein, in vitro. In the past, decisions regarding which leads will be pursued further were made based on activity, chemical diversity, patentability, and analog synthetic potential. Today, developmental potential increasingly is part of series selection decision-making.
3. Analog expansion is the increase in the number of compounds targeting a specific activity based on synthetic exploitation of the most promising leads.
4. *Analog selection* is the decision-making process in which the best new chemical entity is chosen for further development. In the past, *in vitro* activity alone was the dominating decision-maker; today, a blend of developmental issues is surfacing earlier.

Preformulation, as well as other areas of development such as metabolism, toxicology, and pharmacokinetics, will play an increasingly important role in Steps 1 to 4. Because a fundamental understanding of the solid state is essential for designing appropriate physical property methodologies for Steps 1 to 4, the remainder of this section will deal with how solid-state proper-

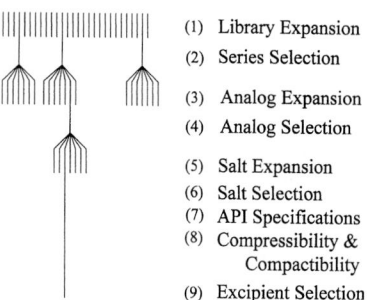

(1) Library Expansion
(2) Series Selection
(3) Analog Expansion
(4) Analog Selection
(5) Salt Expansion
(6) Salt Selection
(7) API Specifications
(8) Compressibility & Compactibility
(9) Excipient Selection

Figure 38-9. Typical API sequential decision-making: selection and expansion cycles.

ties affect absorption and consistency, the two major development issues for an API. Salt selection, which determines the character of $_jA^i$, is the first critical solid-state decision for preformulation in the developmental arena.

Salt Expansion: Exploring the Molecular Possibilities of A^I

The un-ionized (free) form of weak acids and bases, A^0, may not be the ideal molecular form for development. During the salt expansion Step 5 of Figure 38-9, salts are prepared to explore whether one of them would make a more suitable API. Salts are formed by reacting A^0 with an appropriate counter-acid or counter-base. In this discussion, HAn is used to represent a counter-acid that forms an anion An^-. Common counter-acids like HCl and maleic acid are listed in Table 38-5. Similarly, CnOH is used to represent a mineral base of counter cation Cn^+. Common mineral bases like NaOH and KOH are also shown in Table 38-5 along with organic counter-bases.

Table 38-5. Molecular Forms Marketed Worldwide Between 1983 and 1996

SALT FORM	FREQ.	GROUP^A	PK$_A$	CLOGP	MW
No salt form	390	0			
Hydrobromide	1	1	−8	0.45	80.91
Hydrochloride	102	1	−6.1	0.24	36.46
Sulfate	5	1	−3	−1.58	98.08
Nitrate	6	1	−1.44	2.09	63.01
Phosphate	2	1	2.15	−1.95	96.99
Glucuronate	1	1	3.22^b	−3.74	194.14
Acetate	8	1	4.76	−0.36	59.05
Maleate	3	2	1.92	−0.18	116.07
Fumarate	8	2	3.02	−0.18	116.07
Tartrate	1	2	3.03	−2.21	150.09
Citrate	1	2	3.13	−2.11	189.10
Succinate	2	2	4.21	−0.62	118.09
Mesylate	8	3	−1.20	−1.31	96.11
Acistrate	1	3	4.91^b	7.98	284.49
Besylate	2	4	−2.80^b	0.23	157.17
Tosylate	3	4	−1.34	0.88	171.20
Xinafoate	1	4	2.66^b	3.00	188.18
Potassium	1	1	16		39.10
Sodium	37	1	14.77		23.00
Tromethamine	2	1	8.07^c	−3.17	121.14
Bismuth	1	1	1.58		208.98
Bromide	6	5			79.90
Chloride	2	5			35.45

^{a} Groups: 0 = No salt, 1 = Polar, 2 = Multifunctional, 3 = Flexible aliphatics, 4 = Planar aromatics, 5 = Quaternary.
^{b} Calculated pK$_a$.
^{c} Data from *CRC Handbook of Basic Tables for Chemical Analysis*, page 469. From Serajuddin ATM, Sheen P, Augustine MA. To market, to market. In: Bristol J, ed. *Annu Rep Med Chem*. New York: Academic, 1983–1996.

When A^0 is a weak base, the salt, $(A^0H)^+ An^-$, is composed of the protonated form of the base, $(A^0H)^+$ and the ionized form of the counter-acid HAn, An^-. For salt formation, A^0 must be sufficiently basic to remove the proton from HAn (see *Salt-Forming Reactivity Potential*).

Salts have different physical properties than their free forms. Salt selection explores whether a particular salt might have properties that are more appropriate for an API than its parent form. Improving oral absorption by increasing the dissolution rate is often a goal of the salt expansion step. Salts generally dissolve faster in water than their free forms because dissolution is enhanced by the rapid hydration of the ionized salt species with water. Salts of weak bases generally lower the pH of water; salts of weak acids elevate it. For the salt of a weak base in water, the initial dissociation of the salt into the two ions, A^0H^+ and An^- is relatively complete. On the other hand, the deprotonation of A^0H^+ depends on the pK$_a$ of A^0, as shown by these reactions:

$$A^0H^+An^- \xrightleftharpoons{} A^0H^+ + An^- \text{ and } A^0H^+ \xrightleftharpoons[\text{high pK}_a]{\text{low pH}_a} A^0 + H^+ \quad (11)$$

It is the release of the H$^+$ in the second reaction by the salt that lowers the pH and increases the solubility (see *pH-Solubility Profiles*). Hydrochlorides are the most common salts of weak bases.

When A^0 is a weak acid, the salt that forms from a reaction with CnOH is A^-Cn^+ (A^- represents A^0 minus a proton). The most common salts for weak acids are the sodium salts.

Even though salts increase aqueous solubility, they only alter the pH of the solution so that more of the ionized form is present in solution. Salts do not change the ionizable character of the free form; this is an intrinsic property of the free acid or free base and their associated pK$_a$(s). pH-solubility profiles show the solubility relationship between salts and their free forms.

pH Solubility Profiles

For a weak base, a plot of solubility versus pH will show the highest solubility at low pH and the lowest solubility at high pH; for weak acids, the opposite is true. Such plots give a graphic view of the impact of ionization on solubility for an NCE. The pH range of the small intestine, where oral absorption generally occurs, is approximately 6.5 to 8. It is undesirable to have a compound totally charged or uncharged in this region. If it is entirely charged, there are no un-ionized species that can be transported across the GI membrane. If it is totally uncharged, there are no charged species to enhance solubility. For a monoprotic NCE, the pK$_a$ denotes the pH where the number of charged and uncharged species in solution are equal. On the ionized side of the pK$_a$, the solubility of the salt limits the maximum solubility. The solubility decline at very low pHs is due to activity and solubility-product effects.[54-56] On the un-ionized side, the solubility of A^0 (the intrinsic solubility) marks the lowest solubility. Salts promote a saturated solution to be formed at a pH that is on the ionized side of the pK$_a$. They cannot alter the pK$_a$ or the intrinsic solubility. Using these parameters, a qualitative pH-solubility profile can be constructed. Figure 38-10 shows pH-solubility profiles for different counter-acid salts.

The synthesis of salts depends on

1. A proton-exchange reactivity between A^0 and the counter-acid/base
2. A long-range order that permits crystal formation.

The discussion that follows will focus on forming salts from weak bases, because they comprise the majority of the new drug candidates. Weak acids would be treated analogously.

Salt-Forming Reactivity Potential

In order for a salt to form, both the weak base, A^0, and the counter-acid, HAn, must have sufficiently different pK$_a$ values such that a Brönsted-Lowry proton transfer from HAn to A^0 can take place. Table 38-5 gives potential counter-ions and their pK$_a$ values from a listing of all drugs approved worldwide from

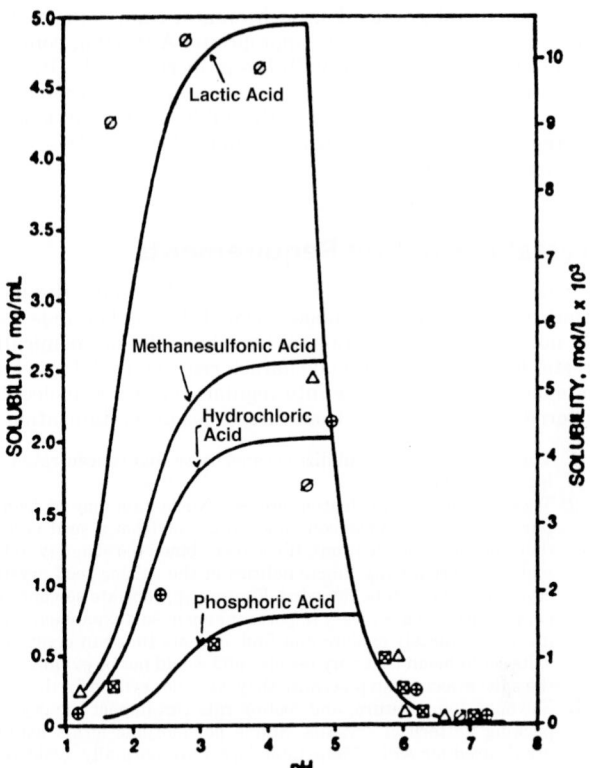

Figure 38-10. pH solubility profile of a weak base. (From Streng WH, et al. *J Pharm Sci* 1984;73:1679.)

1983 to 1996. An acid–base proton transfer should be possible as long as the pK$_a$ of HAn is less than that of the weak base A^0 (recall that the pK$_a$ of A^0 is referenced to its protonated form A^0H^+; see *Solid-State Character*). If ΔpK$_a$ is defined as

$$\Delta pK_a = pK_a \text{ (weak base)} - pK_a \text{ (H}An) \quad (12)$$

a salt-forming reaction should be possible as long as ΔpK$_a$ is positive. For example, a succinate salt (pK$_a$ 4.2) with doxylamine (pK$_a$ 4.4) is possible[57] where the ΔpK$_a$ is 0.2. Nevertheless, the greater the ΔpK$_a$, the greater the probability that a salt can be formed. Because the pK$_a$ values in Table 38-5 are calculated for an aqueous environment, this rule must be used only as a guide for salt-forming reactivity in organic solvents. In an organic solvent in which the dielectric constant is lower than water, the ionization equilibria would be shifted:

$$HAn \xrightarrow{\text{low dielectric solvents}} H^+ + An^- \quad (13)$$

$$AH^+ \xrightarrow{\text{low dielectric solvents}} H^+ + A^0 \quad (14)$$

For acridine bases, 50:50 ethanol:water weakens the aqueous pK$_a$ by 1.41 pH units. For the counter-acid, HAn, pK$_a$ weakening is greater than for the protonated base, A^0H^+, because of the greater solubility of HAn in the organic phase and the production of two charges upon ionization. The net effect of organic solvent weakening is to reduce the pK$_a$ difference between the counter-acid and the weak base. This lowers the salt-forming reactive potential. Therefore, in a given organic solvent, if salt formation fails to occur for a particular aqueous ΔpK$_a$, it is unlikely that salts can be formed in this organic solvent with a smaller aqueous ΔpK$_a$.

Varying Salt Properties Using Counter-Acid Groupings

For weak bases, salt-forming counter-acids can be used to alter an API's solubility, dissolution, hygroscopicity, stability, and processing.[57] Table 38-5 shows counter-acids organized into different functional groups. For each counter-acid, both the pK_a and the $\log P$ is given where appropriate. A starting point for salt expansion must begin with the properties of A^0. If, for a weak base, $\Delta pK_a = pK_{a\ A}^{\ 0} - pK_{a\ \text{counter-acid, }HAn} > 0$, then aqueous salts may be possible. Use of this table and the influence of different counter-acids are covered under *Decision-Tree, Goal-Oriented Approach*.

Crystal Formation Requirements

In general, crystalline solids, including salts, make the most promising APIs. The amorphous form of the solid state is usually not as stable as crystals, either physically or chemically. Crystal formation is a special characteristic of a solid in which the molecules self-organize into regular, repeating, molecular patterns. Solvents play at least three roles in crystallization.

1. They provide some solubilizing capacity so that concentrated solutions can be formed.
2. They promote the nucleation process. Nucleation may be from a pure solution (homogeneous nucleation) or from a seed crystal (heterogeneous nucleation). If a solvent binds too strongly to the molecular organizing functionalities of the salt or seed crystal, crystallization will be impeded. Finding appropriate solvents for crystal formation is a very important step in salt expansion. Failure to adequately explore and find solvents that can crystallize salts could mean that very usable salts would not be evaluated in the salt-selection step because they were not synthesized.
3. Solvents, temperature, and cooling rate can impact the crystal-packing pattern of crystals. Stable polymorphic forms usually are desired for APIs. Metastable forms are normally avoided in an API because they are prone to physical and chemical instability. Solvent conditions that promote metastable and stable crystal formations will be explored under *Metastable Polymorph Formation*.

SALT SELECTION: CHOOSING THE "BEST" API

Salt selection is the first important API decision from the development perspective. Once a salt is chosen, time-consuming and lengthy toxicological studies are initiated that would have to be repeated if the salt form is changed. This decision involves choosing a solid-state phase, $_jA$, which balances potentially conflicting needs: increasing absorption versus maintaining an API that is consistent and can be manufactured in a market-image dosage form (see *Compressibility and Compactibility*). Figure 38-11 shows some of the factors involved in this decision.

Permeability, solubility (C_S), and pK_a are intrinsic properties of A^0 that have been already determined in the analog selection phase (see Fig 38-9). The major dependent variables, absorption and consistency of the API, can be manipulated and balanced in salt selection. In the following sections, the impact of dissolution and particle size on absorption will be explored. In addition, the consistency of the API solid state under the influence of environmental destabilizing factors—such as exposure time (t), ultraviolet light (UV), pH, moisture (H_2O), temperature (T), and pharmaceutical processing operations like milling, compression, and compaction—will be considered.

Absorption Assessment

Oral absorption is generally viewed as two-step, sequential process:

$$A_{\text{solid}} \xrightleftharpoons[]{\text{dissolution}} a_{\text{GI tract}} \xrightleftharpoons[]{\text{permeation}} a_{\text{blood}} \qquad (15)$$

Either dissolution of solid drug, A_{solid}, after the dosage form disintegrates in the GI tract, or the permeation of the dissolved drug, $a_{\text{GI tract}}$, through the GI membrane could be the slowest process. The slower of these two steps determines the overall rate of absorption and is thus rate-limiting.

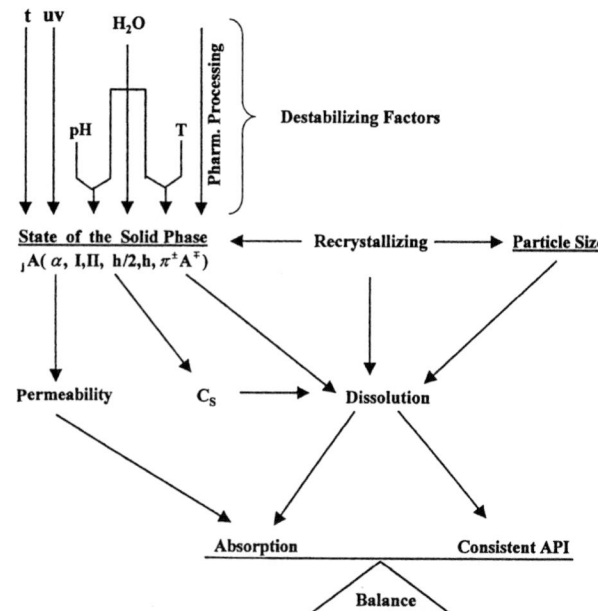

Figure 38-11. API salt selection decision: a balance between absorption and consistency.

Dissolution-limited absorption occurs when the rate of appearance in the GI tract by dissolution (a_{GI}) is slower than the rate of appearance in the systemic system (a_{blood}); *permeation-limited* absorption occurs when the a_{blood} appearance is the slowest process. The impact of these two rate processes on *in vitro–in vivo* (IVIV) correlations will be discussed in the section *Biopharmaceutical Classification of API*. Dissolution-limited absorption will now be considered.

The rate of dissolution of a particle is given by the Noyes–Whitney equation,

$$dA/dt = k_d S_a\ [C_s - C_{\text{bulk}}] \text{ (non-sink conditions)} \qquad (16)$$

where
A is the amount of drug dissolved.
dA/dt is the rate of dissolution (Q sometimes is used for this rate).
k_d is the intrinsic dissolution constant for the drug.
S_a is the total surface area of the dissolving particle.
C_S is the saturation solubility of the drug at the surface of the particle.
C_{bulk} is the concentration of the drug in the bulk solution.
Because the rate of dissolution depends on the concentration difference between C_S and C_{bulk}, the maximum rate of dissolution would occur if $C_{\text{bulk}} = 0$ (ie, if drug was removed from solution as fast as it dissolved). This would be analogous to a sink that could drain the water coming out of a water faucet as fast as it comes in so that the water level never built up. This analogy is the basis for referring to Equation 16 as nonsink conditions for dissolution, because drug does build up in the solution and the rate of dissolution is correspondingly reduced.

The expression for the maximum dissolution rate is found by setting C_{bulk} equal to 0[58]:

$$dA/dt = k_d S_a C_s \text{ (sink conditions)} \qquad (17)$$

This initial rate of the Noyes–Whitney equation is termed sink conditions for the dissolution rate.

PARTICLE-SIZE EFFECTS—For a spherical drug particle of radius r, amount m, and of density ρ, Equation 17 can be rewritten as:

$$dA/dt = (3k_d m/\rho)(1/r)C_s \qquad (18)$$

This expression emphasizes the inverse relationship between the dissolution rate, dA/dt, and the particle size r, assuming no dissolution rate-reducing factors are present such as adsorbed air bubbles or aggregated particles.

Smaller particles dissolve faster than larger particles. Thus milling, a pharmaceutical unit-operation, increases dissolution because the API particle size is reduced. On the other hand, when drug particles are suspended in an aqueous solution, particles can increase in size due to recrystallization growth[59]

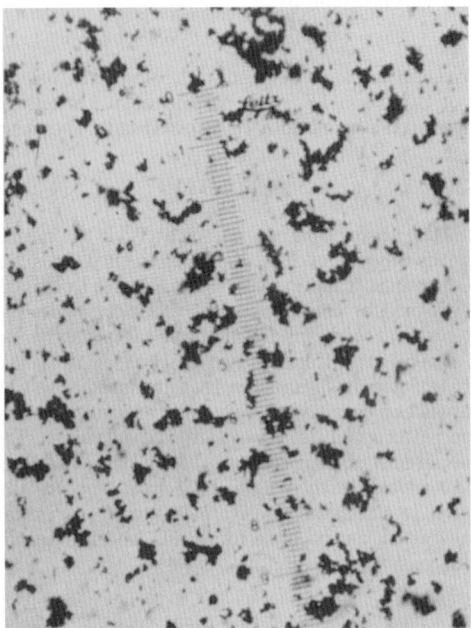

FORM I

INITIAL SUSPENSION

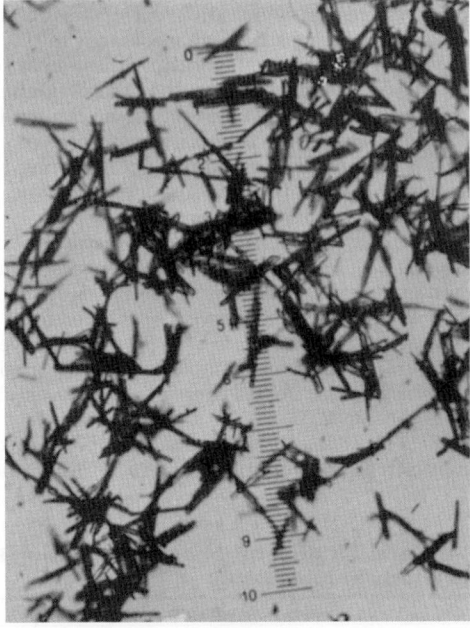

FORM I

SUSPENSION AFTER 6 HOURS.

Figure 38-12. Photomicrographs showing change in crystal size for a suspension of Form 1 of an experimental drug.

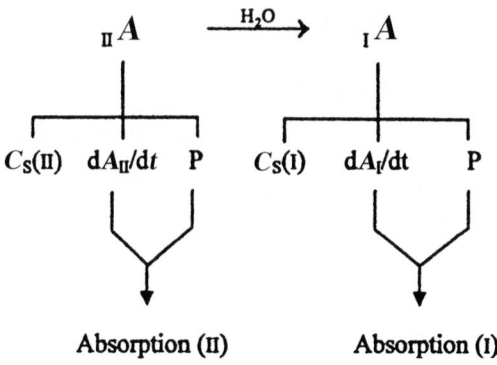

Figure 38-13. Absorption changes due to aqueous-phase transformations.

(Fig 38-12). Dosing such suspension orally would be expected to reduce absorption because of a reduction in the dissolution rate.

Reactive Media 1: Implications for Salts of Weak Acids and Weak Bases—When a drug reacts with gastric fluids, its dissolution deviates from Equation 17. For dissolution in 0.1 N HCl, acid–base reactivity is most important for salts of weak acids and for free bases. It has been found that the low pH environment of the stomach dissolves a salt of a weak acid 10 to 100 times faster than the weak acid itself.[60] On the other hand, it is the free base, and not its HCl salt, that dissolves faster in this same environment.[61] These deviations from Equation 17 have been shown to be due to differences between bulk-solution pHs and the pH at the surface of the drug particle. Thus, Equation 17 becomes

$$dA/dt = k_d S_a \, C_{s,h=0} \tag{19}$$

where $C_{S,h=0}$ is the saturation solubility at the surface of the API.

For weak acid salts, the surface pH has been calculated to be 6.2 to 6.5 for sodium salicylate (pK$_a$ 3.0) and 10.3 for sodium theophylline (pK$_a$ 8.4) in bulk solutions having pHs of 1.10 and 2.1, respectively. On the other hand, the weak base phenazopyridine (pK$_a$ 5.2) sees a surface pH of 3.3 to 3.6, while its HCl salt sees a surface pH of 1.2 for a bulk-solution pH of 1.10. If the solubility due to surface pH and not the pH of the bulk is considered, deviations from Equation 17 become understandable. For the HCl salt, the common-ion effect reduces its solubility from the maximum solubility of the pH-solubility profile at 3.45. Thus, the nonaggregated free base, in this situation, has a surface pH that is optimized to give the highest dissolution rate because it has the highest surface solubility.

Reactive Media 2: Implications for Anhydrates and Metastable Polymorphs—Aqueous-phase transformations are solid-state changes in which water acts as a mediator. During the transition from one form to another, dissolution behavior will reflect the switch from the dissolution rate of the initial solid state to that of the more stable state. Two types of aqueous-phase transformations were introduced in Equations 7 and 9: (1) a transformation from Polymorph II to Polymorph I and (2) a transformation from an anhydrous Form II to a hydrated form h.[62] In Figure 38-13, the transformation of Equation 7 is shown.

Because the permeability (P) of the dissolved drug is the same for the different crystalline forms, the impact on absorption will be due to differences in their solubilities (C_S) as defined in Equation 17 and thus will be reflected in the dissolution rates, dA_I/dt and dA_{II}/dt, being different.

When a solvent-mediated transformation like that shown in Equation 9 occurs, dissolution profiles become more complex. Figure 38-14 shows the biphasic dissolution characteristics for Equation 9. In this situation, an anhydrous substance, $_{0h}A$, becomes hydrated as it dissolves and forms a surface layer of $_hA$. It is this latter layer that controls subsequent dissolution. The concentration versus time plot for the net reaction is $_{0h}A$ (phase change). Note that initially the slope for $_{0h}A$ (phase change) approaches that of the very steep slope $_{0h}A$ (no phase change), and

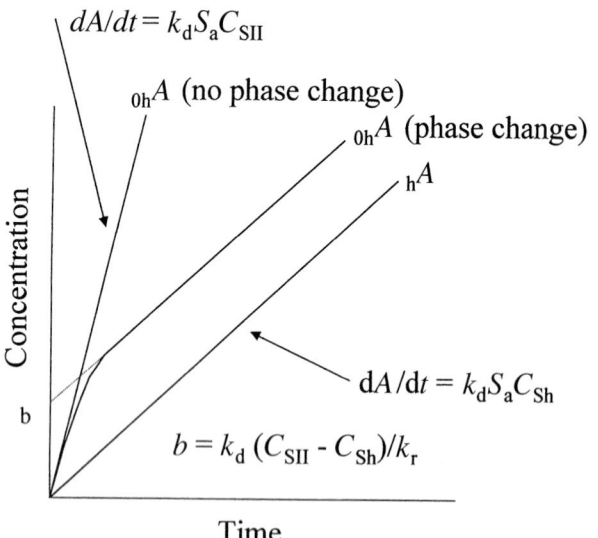

Figure 38-14. Biphasic dissolution of anhydrous to hydrous forms. (Data from Nogami H, Nagai T, Yotsuyanagi T. *Chem Pharm Bull* 1969;17:499.)

that the terminal slope approaches that of $_hA$ (no phase change), the hydrated form. Modifications of Equation 17 to take into account surface recrystallization of $_hA$ on $_{0h}A_\Sigma$ give the biphasic dissolution behavior,

$$dA/dt = k_d S_a \{C_{she}e^{-k_r{}^t} + C_{sh}[1 - e^{k_r{}^t}]$$ (20)

where k_r is the recrystallization rate constant for the second phase, k_d is the intrinsic dissolution constant, C_{SII} is the saturation concentration for the first phase, and C_{Sh} is the saturation concentration for the second hydrate phase.[63]

ENHANCED AND RETARDED DISSOLUTION DUE TO SINKS AND PLUGS

The increase in dissolution due to the particle-size reduction of an uncharged API, A^0, can be estimated from Equation 18. Equation 21 shows the resulting surface area increase, $\Sigma\uparrow$, and the corresponding dissolution enhancement.

$$A_\Sigma{}^0 \xrightarrow{\text{willing}} A_\Sigma{}^0\uparrow \xrightarrow{\text{faster}} a_S{}^0$$ (21)

This enhancement, however, is assumed to be under sink conditions and is driven by $C_S = a_S{}^0$ in Equation 17. If the concentration of drug does build up, dissolution is reduced by and is given by Equation 16. This slower dissolution is diagrammed in Equation 22 where $a_{\text{bulk}}{}^0\uparrow$ indicates the buildup of the drug in the bulk solution.

$$A^0 \xrightarrow{\text{slow}} a_{\text{bulk}}{}^0\uparrow$$ (22)

An ionizable drug, on the other hand, reduces $a_{\text{bulk}}{}^0$, which is indicated by $\downarrow$ in Equation 23 because it is rapidly converted to $a_{\text{bulk}}{}^+$, the ionized form. Thus, the ionized form ($a_{\text{bulk}}{}^+ = a_{\text{bulk}}{}^0\text{H}^+$) acts as a sink to remove $a_{\text{bulk}}{}^0$ and promotes the dissolution of A^0 by driving the reaction to the right:

$$A^0 \xrightarrow{\text{fast}} a_{\text{bulk}}{}^0\downarrow \xrightarrow{\text{very fast}} a_{\text{bulk}}{}^+ \quad (\text{sink})$$ (23)

Reduction of dissolution, on the other hand, can occur for an anhydrous API when the hydrated form recrystallizes on the surface as in Figure 38-14. This effect is the opposite of the sink concept, hence the term plugging. Equation 24 show the species involved in plugging. The subscript Σ emphasizes that this is a surface phenomenon.

$$_{0h}A_\Sigma \xrightarrow{\text{slow}} a_{\text{bulk}} \xrightarrow{\text{recrystallization}} {}_hA_\Sigma \xrightarrow{\text{slower}} a_{\text{bulk}}\downarrow \quad (\text{plug})$$ (24)

ACCEPTANCE CRITERIA GUIDANCE

A simple model to assess the impact of particle size on dissolution and absorption of a non-ionized drug considers the intestine as a single compartment.[63] If the number of particles of uniform size at time t is

$$N(t) = N_0 e^{-Qt/V}$$ (25)

where N_0 is the initial number of particles, Q is the flow rate out of the intestine, and V is the intestinal volume, then the surface area for spherical particles of uniform size, r, as a function of time can be given by

$$S_a = 4\pi r^2(t)N(t)$$ (26)

This expression can then be used in the non-sink dissolution expression of Equation 16, with certain assumptions including linear intestinal absorption, to approximate the fraction absorbed as

$$F \infty \frac{k_a X_d \hat{t}_r}{X_0}$$ (27)

where k_a is the absorption rate constant, X_0 is the administered dose, X_d is the amount of drug dissolved in the GI tract at $\hat{t}_r$, and $\hat{t}_r$ is the GI transit time. Further refinements to this model include accounting for polydispersed spherical powders and comparing cylindrical with spherical shape factors, with and without time-dependent diffusion layer thickness.

Finally, for poorly soluble drugs, simulated dose absorption studies have been carried out over different ranges of solubility, absorption rate constants, doses, and particle sizes. Table 38-6 shows the percent of drug absorbed for a drug that has a solubility of 10 μg/mL with a k_a of 0.01 min^{-1}. Note that, even though particle-size reduction from 100 to 10 μm increases the percent absorbed, as the dose increases, the impact of this reduction decreases dramatically.

Consistency Assessment

POLYMORPHIC STABILITY: IMPORTANCE OF THE TRANSITION POINT

Polymorphic systems, in which different crystalline forms of the same molecular composition can exist, vary in their ability to interconvert at different temperatures. The enantiotropic/monotropic classification is based on the observation that some systems can reversibly interconvert and some cannot. In enantiotropic systems, reversible interconversion between the different forms is possible. For monotropic polymorphic systems, interconversion is only possible in one direction, from a metastable form to a more stable form.

For enantiotropic systems, a critical temperature exists, the transition point, T_p, at which the rate of conversion from one form to another is equal. At temperatures below T_p, one form is more stable; at temperatures above T_p, another form is more stable (see the section *Solid-State Character*; the convention of designating Form I as the most stable polymorph breaks down for such systems because Form I cannot be the most stable form *both* above *and* below T_p).

Figure 38-15 shows a solubility versus temperature diagram for an enantiotropic polymorphic system.[64,65] For the enan-

Table 38-6. Reduced Absorption with Increasing Particle Size for a Poorly Soluble Drug

DOSE	PERCENT OF DOSE ABSORBED			
10 μm	25 μm	50 μm	100 μm	
1	91.3	66.9	38.5	17.5
10	70.0	50.0	30.7	15.4
100	9.0	8.7	8.0	6.3
250	3.6	3.6	3.4	3.1

Data from Johnson KC, Swindell AC. *Pharm Res* 1996; 13:1795.

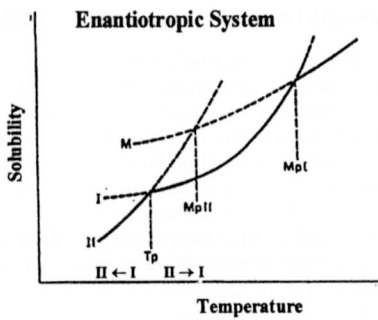
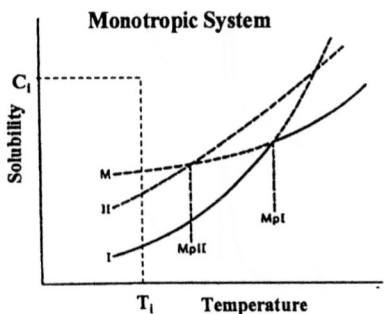

Figure 38-15. Thermal stability of polymorphic systems. (Data from Kuhnert-Bradnstatter M. *Thermomicroscopy in the Analysis of Pharmaceuticals.* New York: Pergamon, 1971; and Heleblian J, McCrone W. *J Pharm Sci* 1969;58:911.)

tiotropic system on the left, at constant pressure, there are three solubility versus temperature curves: Form II is the lowest, Form I is the next higher, and the melting curve is M. The critical temperature, T_p, occurs at the intersection of the Form II and I curves. At this point the solubilities of Form II and Form I are equal and the interconversion rate in any direction is zero.[65] Below the T_p, Form I interconverts to Form II; above the T_p, Form II converts to Form I. The melting point of Form I occurs at the intersection of the Form I curve and the melting curve M.

Because enantiotropic forms show a change in relative physical stability as temperature is changed, it is important to anticipate the impact of temperature on stability. An early warning sign that one is dealing with an enantiotropic system can be found by relating solubilities with thermal parameters. The higher melting Form I has a smaller heat of fusion. Equation 28 gives the relationship between the solubilities,

$$\ln\left[\frac{S_I(T)}{S_{II}(T)}\right] = \left[\frac{\Delta H_{II} - \Delta H_I}{RT}\right]\left[\frac{T_m - T}{T_m}\right] \qquad (28)$$

where S_I and S_{II} are the solubilities and ΔH_I and ΔH_{II} are the heats of fusion of Forms I and II, respectively.[66] The more stable form at a given temperature will have lower solubility at that temperature.

Enantiotropicity exists only when the transition point is below the melting point of Form I (see Fig 38-15). However, if a transition point is not found below the melting point of Form I, it does not mean that the system is monotropic.[65] The transition point, for example, could be below the lowest temperature studied.

For monotropic systems, interconversion is always from the metastable Form II to Form I. The solubility curve of Form II is always above that of Form I, and a transition point does not exist because a crystal cannot be heated above its melting point (see Fig 38-15). Oswald's Law of Stages dictates that if a system is supersaturated with respect to Form II at concentration C_i and T_i, the metastable Phase II will be the first solid phase that appears.[67] As Form II continues to crystallize, the supersaturation is reduced until it reaches its solubility. At this point, although there is no longer a driving force to crystallize more Form II, the solution continues to be supersaturated with respect to Form I. Thus, crystallization of Form I occurs at the expense of the dissolution of Form II.

POLYMORPHIC SOLUBILITY: DIFFERENCE BETWEEN EQUILIBRIUM AND DISSOLUTION-BASED SOLUBILITY

Assume Polymorphs I and II are possible for an NCE. Oswald's Law of Stages tells us that a supersaturated solution will first crystallize out as Form II and then ultimately Form I. Thus, the thermodynamic equilibrium solubility will be limited by the solubility of Form I. However, because the rate of nucleation of II and I is a function of a wide variety of variables, equilibrium solubility is not an especially useful parameter in estimating the impact of a polymorph form on the absorption of drug from a dosage form. A dissolution-based solubility definition is more useful in this regard. How might such a solubility be defined?

Because the metastable state Form II has a faster dissolution rate, $dA/dt_{II} > dA/dt_I$, where it is assumed that dissolution is carried out under sink conditions of Equation 17. Because $dA/dt = k_d S_a C_S$, we can conclude that $C_S(II) > C_S(I)$ if we assume that S_a and k_d are the same for both polymorphs. Thus, Equation 17 provides a working definition for the solubility differences between Polymorph II and Polymorph I, and it provides a method for measuring them from dissolution experiments. More precisely, it provides the solubility at the surface of the API, which is the solubility that is most relevant for dissolution (see the section *Reactive Media 1*).

POLYMORPH CHARACTERIZATION TECHNIQUES

At a given temperature, a fluid-phase transformation can cause a metastable polymorph to change into a more stable, less soluble polymorph. Using a hot-stage microscope, fluid-phase transformations as a function of temperature can be observed.[65] As the temperature is varied, the more soluble polymorph dissolves and the less soluble one grows. If a temperature can be found at which both polymorphs have the same solubility, then the system is enantiotropic, and the temperature is the transition point, T_p. Plots similar to Figure 38-15 can be constructed qualitatively in which the intersection is the measured transition point. These plots are important because they tell which form is most stable at low temperatures, and whether the system is enantiotropic.

Differential scanning calorimetry (DSC) is another characterization tool that is commonly used. It measures heat changes that occur when a solid undergoes phase transitions. Melting of a solid into a fluid, for example, requires an influx of heat into the crystal. Two techniques are useful for detecting polymorphic systems using DSC: scanning-rate variation and temperature cycling.

Scanning-rate variation has been shown to detect some reversible polymorphic systems. In Figure 38-16, crystallization of the more stable polymorph shows up as exothermic depressions as the scanning-rate increases.[68] Hot-stage microscopy can be used to confirm these thermal changes.

Temperature cycling using DSC also can be used to study the relative interconvertability of crystalline forms. A loss of the metastable, lower melting point polymorph of metoclopramide base was found after heating, cooling, and then reheating.[69] The more stable polymorph can often be observed as exotherms due to crystallization after heat–cool cycles.[70] In addition, storage of a metastable polymorph below the melting point of either polymorph can result in the formation of the more stable polymorph. For gepirone hydrochloride, this occurred after a heat treatment of 3 hours at 150° C.[68]

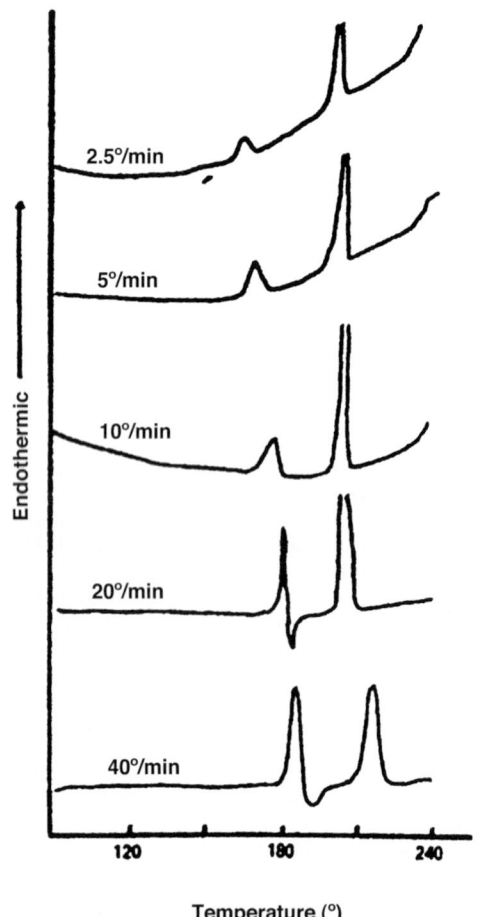

Figure 38-16. Detection of polymorphs by varying the DSC scanning rate.

Powder x-ray diffraction is the most powerful method for detecting polymorphs. Because different polymorphs have different crystal structures, the packing patterns of their atoms are different. Powder x-ray diffraction detects these packing differences as differences in diffraction patterns. Comparisons of diffraction scans between different polymorphs show characteristic differences that can be used for identification (fingerprinting) purposes.

Single-crystal x-ray diffraction is the most definitive characterization tool because the exact relative locations of atoms in the molecular crystal can be determined. However, most often, high-quality crystals for this type of analysis are not available from the bulk API (especially if the material was milled). Recrystallization of suitable crystals from saturated solutions may be possible. If the single-crystal x-ray diffraction problem can be solved, programs are now available that can convert single-crystal diffraction data to a powder x-ray diffraction pattern. This is necessary to ensure that the recrystallization process has not grown a new polymorph.

Solid-state nuclear magnetic resonance (NMR) is also a powerful technique for studying polymorphic systems. In this technique, a powder sample must be rotated at a special angle (the *magic angle*) with respect to the magnetic field so that preferential orientations of the powder particles are averaged. Microcalorimetry also has been used to characterize the thermodynamic properties of different polymorphs. Finally, diffuse reflectance infrared Fourier-transform spectroscopy recently has been used to quantify binary mixtures of polymorphs using the partial least-squares method for spectral analysis.[71]

METASTABLE POLYMORPH FORMATION

Exploring the potential that a given salt has for polymorph formation is a very important aspect of salt selection. It is important that the choice of the final molecular form be based on as much information as possible. Other factors being equal, a molecular entity that forms polymorphs is generally not as desirable as one that does not, because of the potential interconversion of polymorphs and a change in an API's dissolution. This could cause consistency problems both in the API and in the dosage forms. Special techniques are used to attempt to synthesize metastable polymorphs. Preparation of metastable polymorphs requires:

1. Supersaturating conditions for the metastable form, $_{II}A$.
2. Crystallization of the metastable state before the stable polymorph forms.
3. Stable conditions for the metastable polymorph so that conversion to the stable $_{I}A$ form is prevented.

These steps are shown in Figure 38-17.

For a monotropic system, the metastable state can only change to the stable state; for an enantiotropic system, the transition point is critical for interconversion. Therefore, the formation temperature should be as far above the transition point as practical.

The ideal solution conditions to prevent $_{II}A$ from converting to $_{I}A$ are such that the solution phase, a, should be highly supersaturated, of a small volume, and in a relatively poor solvent. Rapid cooling is the method of choice for maintaining supersaturation with respect to $_{II}A$. To help ensure that the rate of metastable crystallization is much greater than the rate of thermodynamic equilibration, small volumes and poor solvents for $_{I}A$ are used. The use of dry ice for rapid cooling with alcohol or acetone is common for these purposes. Once crystallization from the saturated solution phase, a, has occurred, it is important to filter and dry the precipitate as quickly as possible to prevent a fluid-phase transformation to the stable polymorph. Alternatively, if $_{I}A$ can be melted without degradation, complete melting and rapid cooling of the melt is an another method of forming metastable forms. This avoids two major problems of solution-phase metastable polymorph formation—filtration and drying, both of which can promote interconversion.

HYDRATE STABILITY: IMPORTANCE OF THE CRITICAL RELATIVE HUMIDITY

Relative humidity (RH) is the percentage of the maximum amount of moisture that air can hold. A substance is hygroscopic when it takes up this moisture from air. For a drug substance, the RH that is in equilibrium with a saturated aqueous solution of a solute is termed the critical relative humidity (CRH).[72] It is a key parameter that can influence the physical stability of solid-state hydrates. A number of studies have shown that the gain or loss of water from a hydrate can center on the CRH. Because water in organic crystals is never a passive entity (see *Hy-*

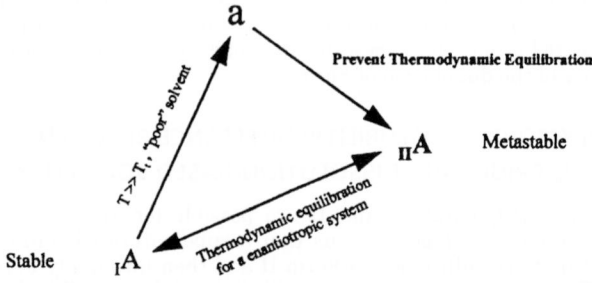

Figure 38-17. Formation of a metastable polymorph in a monotropic system.

drate Formation), solid-state changes in the crystal are very likely to follow.

For the tetrahydrate sodium salt of a tetrazolate derivative, a number of different solid-state forms are possible.[73]

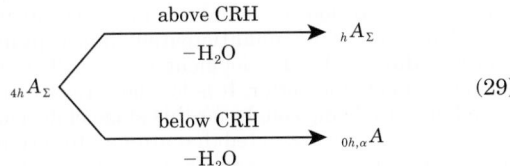

$$_{4h}A_\Sigma \begin{cases} \xrightarrow[\substack{\text{above CRH}\\ -H_2O}]{} {_hA_\Sigma} \\[2em] \xrightarrow[\substack{\text{below CRH}\\ -H_2O}]{} {_{0h,\alpha}A} \end{cases} \qquad (29)$$

The conversion of $_{4h}A$ to $_hA$ requires elevated temperature and a RH above the CRH. Water's plasticizing action in reducing the intermolecular H-bonding between adjacent molecules is believed to be the mechanism that facilitates the solid-state transformation to the more stable $_hA$ crystal form.[74] Similarly, elevation of both temperature and RH were required to convert the $_{0h}A$ form of paroxetine HCl to the $_{0.5h}A$ form.[75] Water also promoted a solid-state transformation of the αA form to the $_{0h}A$ form of a disodium leukotriene antagonist. The amorphous form initially picked up a small amount of water (2%) and then slowly released this water as the anhydrous form was formed. Conversely, the humidity-mediated conversion from $_{II}A$ to αA has been observed for another leukotriene antagonist.[76] Difficult hydrate situations have been dealt with by carefully defining the RH ranges of different species and setting specifications consistent with typical manufacturing environments.[77]

In general, hydrates that are more closely packed tend to be more physically stable with respect to moisture loss. The ideal solid state is one that is stable over a wide range of RH, such as the $_{0.5h}A$ form of paroxetine HCl.[75] For the sodium salt of the tetrazole derivative shown in Equations 29 and 30, the denser $_hA$ structure is physically more stable than the $_{4h}A$ structure. The latter loses four water molecules from crystal channels at a significantly lower temperature than the one water molecule of the $_hA$ form, which is integrated into the crystal structure in a more cohesive manner.[73] In the sections *H-Bonding Networks*, and *Hydrate Formation*, hydrate formation is discussed from a molecular point of view. Crystal formation involves two mutually opposing principles: (1) satisfying the molecule's intermolecular H-bonding needs and (2) packing the atoms in the crystal as closely as possible. Hemi- (h/2) and monohydrates (h) evidently satisfy both close packing and H-bonding needs more efficiently than hydrates that contain water in channels.

Hysteresis is a general term that is used when a material's response to a second exposure of a stress differs from a prior response. This has been observed in the moisture uptake of an API as a function of RH. A number of instruments are now available that can monitor a sample's weight as RH is cycled from 0% to 95%. The noncoincidence of the weight as the sample is back cycled from 95% to 0% indicates hysteresis. One explanation of this type of behavior is that surface-initiated changes occurred in the solid state below or above the sample's CRH. Dehydration of the surface below the CRH, as in Equation 29, with the formation of an amorphous coat of $_{0h,\alpha}A_\Sigma$ means that any subsequent water vapor will encounter a more hygroscopic surface than $_{4h}A_\Sigma$ and thus a different hydration kinetic behavior. On the other hand, conversion of $_{4h}A$ to $_hA$ above the CRH, as in Equation 30, will produce a different kinetic behavior upon rehydration. Thus, RH hysteresis may result from changes in both the kinetic and equilibrium behavior of the surface of the particle.

CHEMICAL STABILITY: COMMON DEGRADATION SEQUENCES—BELOW CRH

SORPTION/DESORPTION OF SURFACE WATER—If an anhydrous form of A is exposed to an RH below the CRH, water molecules will slowly adsorb onto the surface of the drug particle (denoted as $>0h$). Adsorption of up to a monolayer of water has been shown to provide partial protection from oxidation. Dehydrated foods, for example, are more stable when moisture coats reactive sites. For the anhydrous phenylbutazone, the oxidation rate has been shown to be lower below the CRH.[78] For a hydrate, however, the loss of surface water of hydration (denoted as h) at RHs below the CRH has been shown to increase reactivity. Equations 30 and 31 show both of these possibilities.

$$_{0h}A_\Sigma \xrightarrow[+H_2O]{\text{below CRH}} >_{>0h}A_\Sigma \quad \text{(partial oxidation protection)} \quad (30)$$

$$A \xrightarrow{\text{below CRH}} A \quad \text{(increase chemical reactivity)} \qquad (31)$$

FORMATION OF AN AMORPHOUS (A) SURFACE—A water enriched/depleted surface, $(>h/<h)$, is prone to further solid-state changes shown in Equations 32 and 33. For the water-enriched surface, a chemical reaction is shown in which the crystalline form of A $(j = I)$ reacts to form the product αB_Σ, which is amorphous. This type of surface hydrolysis at RHs below the CRH was shown to occur for meclofenoxate HCl decomposition[79] and for propantheline bromide hydrolysis.[80] For the latter, a lag time occurred that was attributed to the amount of time that was necessary to form a monolayer. For the water-depleted hydrate ($j = h$), the loss of water initiated the formation of an amorphous surface layer, αA_Σ. The consequences of these amorphous surfaces will now be explored.

$$_IA_\Sigma \xrightarrow{+H_2O} {_{I,>h}A_\Sigma} \to {_\alpha B_\Sigma} \qquad (32)$$

$$_{Ji}A_\Sigma \xrightarrow{-H_2O} {_{<h}A_\Sigma} \to {_\alpha A_\Sigma} \qquad (33)$$

TRANSFORMATION OF AMORPHOUS SURFACES—Because amorphous layers are more prone to be hygroscopic than crystalline solids, the chemical transformation of $_IA_\Sigma$ to αB_Σ in Equation 32 is significant because the latter can attract more water to the surface. Dissolution of αB_Σ shown in the first downward reaction of Equation 34 will then form a surface coated with b_Σ, as shown in Figure 38-8. The reaction of meclofenoxate HCl below the CRH to form amorphous dimethylaminoethanol HCl (see Eq 32) is a good example of this.[79] Next, the water adsorbed to the surface due to the dissolved form of B on the surface, b_Σ, promotes the dissolution of the surface of A, A_Σ, to form a surface coated also with a_Σ, the dissolved form of A on the surface, which then undergoes further decomposition to b_Σ. This is shown in the horizontal and final downward reactions of Equation 34.

$$\begin{array}{c} _\alpha B_\Sigma \\ \downarrow +H_2O \\ A_\Sigma \xrightarrow{b_t} a_\Sigma + b_\Sigma \\ \downarrow \\ b_\Sigma \end{array} \qquad (34)$$

In Equation 35, two possible solid-state changes for αA_Σ are shown. First, the reactive amorphous surface can undergo a degradation reaction to form C_Σ. Second, the surface can continue to lose water below the CRH so that the subsurface $_hA$ undergoes a solid phase transformation to a crystalline phase, $_IA$. The dehydration changes for cefixime trihydrate are examples of these reactions.[81] The partially dehydrated form of this compound was more unstable than the fully hydrated or the completely dehydrated crystalline forms.

$$_\alpha A_\Sigma \begin{cases} \xrightarrow{T} C_\Sigma \\[1em] \xrightarrow{-H_2O,\, T} {_IA_\Sigma} \end{cases} \qquad (35)$$

CHEMICAL STABILITY: COMMON DEGRADATION SEQUENCES—*ABOVE CRH*

When water is adsorbed to the surface of the particle above the CRH, the drug particle becomes coated with a dissolved drug layer, a_Σ, which is assumed to be saturated[52]:

$$A_\Sigma \xrightarrow{\text{excess H}_2\text{O}} a_\Sigma \qquad (36)$$

Degradation under these conditions is assumed to occur solely in the dissolved layer. This situation has been extensively discussed.[52] For the Maillard reaction, in which primary amines react with carbohydrates, adsorbed water initially increases the reaction rate to a maximum due to the enhancement of reactant mobility. Greater amounts of water then decrease the reaction rate due to dilution of the reactive species. Similarly, for free-radical auto-oxidation of unsaturated groups, reactivity increases above the CRH because of accelerated reactant mobility. Below the CRH, oxidation decreases due to the immobilization of hydrogen peroxides and trace metal catalysts and the protective effects of a monolayer of water that is insufficient to increase reactant mobility.

INFLUENCE OF SALT FORM ON HYGROSCOPICITY—Table 38-2 shows that the non-salt forms, including free bases, free acids, and nonelectrolytes, are the most popular molecular forms on the market. In general, these forms would be expected to be less hygroscopic than salt forms due to their un-ionized character. Although the sodium salt is the most popular weak acid form, this form has a tendency to be hygroscopic. Alternative salts that have proven useful in overcoming hygroscopicity are hydrogen sulfate[82] and tromethamine.[83,84]

Hygroscopic tendencies for weak bases might be overcome by using aromatic counter-ions. Aryl sulfonic acids were shown to provide moisture protection without decreasing dissolution for the sparingly soluble weak base, Xiobam.[85] The free-base form of this drug (pK_a 6.1) was hydrolyzed at 40°C/80% RH. On the other hand, one weak base (pK_a 3.67) was chosen for development because it was less reactive to moisture exposure than the HCl salt. The latter showed chemical instability with moisture and heat and was the only salt that could be formed.[86] Stronger bases like pelrinone (pK_a 4.71) can form stable and nonhygroscopic HCl salts.[87]

GRINDING IMPACT—Processing of solids can have a major impact on dissolution due to solid–solid phase changes. Grinding is one process that has been shown to cause changes in both polymorphs and hydrates. For the $_{III}A$ polymorph (Form C) of chloramphenicol palmitate,[88]

$$_{III}A \xrightarrow{\text{grinding}} {}_{II}A \xrightarrow{\text{more grinding}} {}_{I}A \qquad (37)$$

grinding causes a successive change to the $_{II}A$ polymorph (Form B) and finally to the $_{I}A$ polymorph (Form A).[89] Correspondingly, dissolution from the fastest to the slowest is in the order

$$_{\text{ground II}}A > {}_{\text{ground I}}A > {}_{II}A > {}_{I}A \qquad (38)$$

For hydrates, similar solid-state changes have been observed. When cefixime trihydrate is ground, a solid-phase transformation takes place:

$$_{3h}A \xrightarrow{\text{grinding}} {}_{\alpha,0h}A \qquad (39)$$

Water in this situation plays an essential role in crystal formation. Its removal causes a collapse of the crystal lattice.[90] Other pharmaceutical processing operations and their impact on crystals have been reviewed.[91]

SALT SELECTION DECISION-MAKING

The pressure to increase the productivity of the knowledge worker is readily apparent at the salt-selection stage. Because of increased productivity in discovery, the cascading impact on

development to choose rapidly the best molecular form is readily apparent; toxicological and bioavailability studies cannot proceed until the salt is chosen. Once these studies are initiated, it becomes very costly to change the molecular form because many of these biological studies would have to be repeated. More importantly, precious time and a competitive advantage will be lost. However, if an unanticipated, unacceptable property emerges during the development of an API, the sooner the change is made the better. It is for these reasons that efficient paradigms are being sought for this stage of development. Two approaches will be presented that attempt to optimize the probability of success with speed. Previous approaches were criticized for excessive characterization of poor candidates and for a lack of clear go/no-go decision-making.[92] As a practical consideration, it is essential that NCEs have high purity, and that salts be crystallized. In the following discussion, weak bases that are to be absorbed orally are used. Similar approaches can be developed for intravenous NCEs and for weak acids.

Multi-Tiered Selection Approach

One approach in which different critical parameters are used to filter a salt candidate's progression to the next stage has recently been proposed.[92] Crystalline salts are successively sorted by a three-tier system in the following way:

Tier 1. Hygroscopicity
Tier 2. Thermal analysis and x-ray diffraction
Tier 3. Accelerated solid-state stability

Tier 1 eliminates any form with excessive moisture sorption/desorption characteristics. Only the survivors progress to Tier 2. In this second tier, changes in crystal structure are examined under extremes of moisture conditions by using thermal analysis and powder x-ray diffraction to detect desolvation and aqueous-phase transformation problems. In addition, aqueous solubility is determined to address potential dissolution problems. The best candidates for formulation and manufacturing are considered here and survivors proceed onto Tier 3. In this third tier, accelerated thermal and photo-stability testing is carried out. This is considered to be the most time-consuming step so the limiting of candidates saves time and effort. Selected excipient compatibility testing may also occur at this stage. If Tier 2 eliminates all of the candidates, additional salts or free acid/bases are considered before reevaluating any salt that was dropped in an earlier tier.

Several comments can be made regarding this approach.

1. The HCl salt of ranitidine, due to its hygroscopicity,[93] probably would not have been a final candidate in the multi-tiered approach. Yet this is one of the most successful drugs ever marketed. This emphasizes a need for prioritizing the salt selection process so that as wide of a range of development issues are addressed as early as possible and that they all are put in perspective. If a hydrochloride salt has much better absorption properties than the free base but is hygroscopic, it would be very prudent for development to see if it can deal with this problem. Otherwise, bioavailability may be compromised by a single-minded emphasis on API consistency.
2. The free base is not considered in the multi-tiered approach unless all alternatives have failed despite its potentially favorable dissolution in gastric fluids and its sensitivity to particle size reduction with a reactive sink.

The decision-tree, goal-oriented approach discussed below addresses some of these issues.

Decision-Tree, Goal-Oriented Approach

An alternative approach to the multi-tiered go/no-go selection approach is one based on a decision-tree using statistical probabilities and functional grouping of counter-ions to seek prioritized physical properties. In Figure 38-18, prioritized problems are shown, absorption being the highest priority.

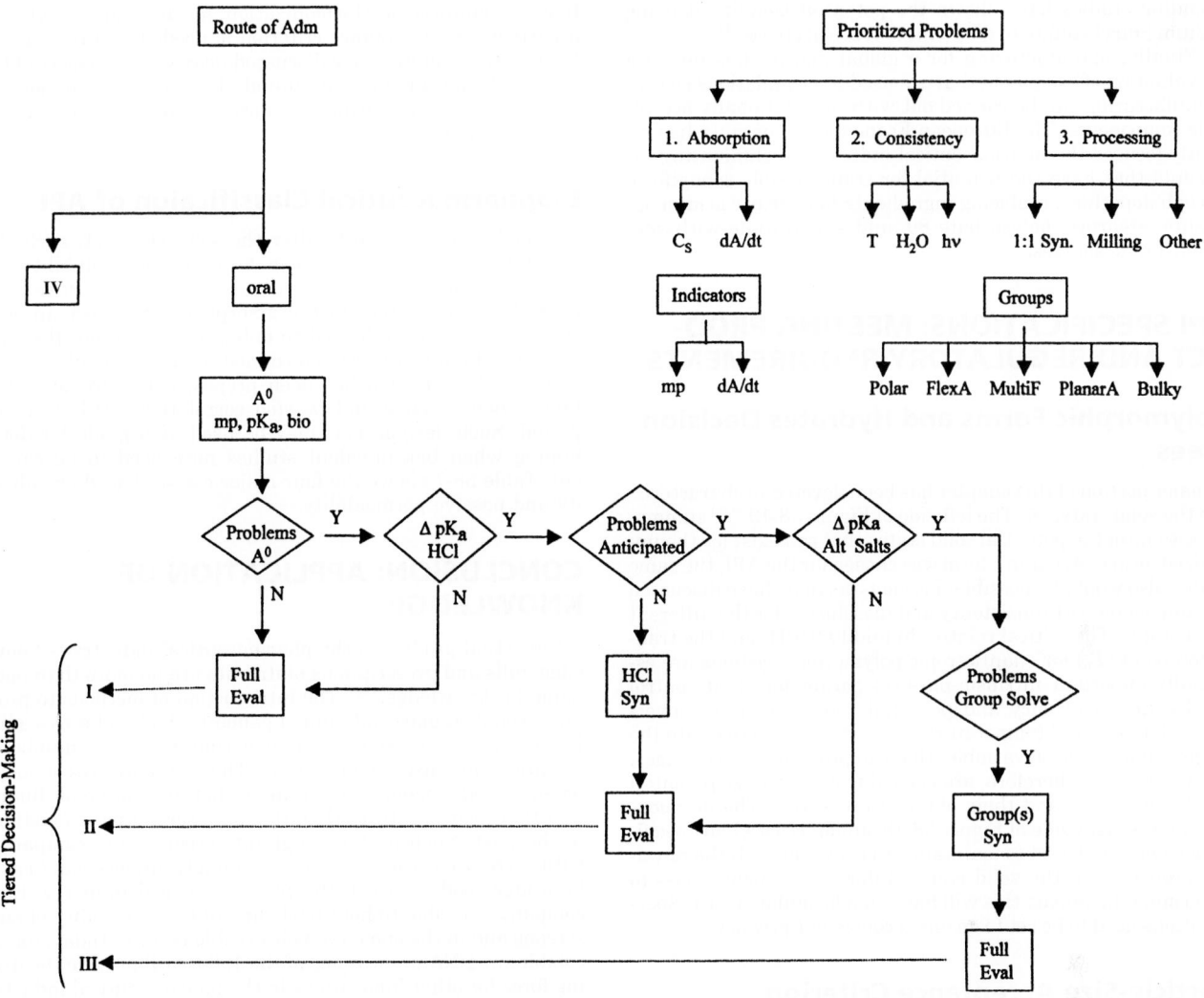

Figure 38-18. Absorption-dominated decision-tree.

The decision-tree considers the free base, the HCl salt, as well as other options. Although this approach uses statistical probabilities for molecular form consideration, ideally, a high-throughput, automated methodology would be available that could determine exhaustively which salts can form crystals and under which conditions. Feasible salts would then be synthesized and placed under accelerated stability and stressing conditions. This would allow for the maximum amount of exposure to the sample before a decision has to be made. Degradant evaluation need not be carried out on these stressed samples immediately; other issues may eliminate a particular candidate and make this unnecessary. However, evaluation for crystallinity should be carried out early to ensure that this does not impact physical or chemical stability. Physical property screens and absorption-dominated prioritization would then force a pharmaceutical evaluation to be made regarding the possibility of overcoming consistency and processing problems.[94] By using functional groupings (see Table 38-5), salt forms would be considered that could address specific problems.[57]

EXCIPIENT SELECTION: FORMULATION COMPATIBILITIES

Excipients serve many roles and are the backbone of a formulation. They may be needed to stabilize the API by providing an-

tioxidant, heavy-metal chelating, or light-protection properties. They also may be used to enhance bioavailability and to control the release from dosage forms. For solid dosage forms, they provide suitable properties for dispensing the API in accurate dosage units that have reproducible release properties. Diluents provide a flowable bulk, binders hold powders together, lubricants provide punch-releasing properties, and disintegrants help to disperse dosage forms in the GI tract. On the other hand, judicious choices must be made to prevent incompatibilities between the API and excipients.

Screens to detect drug-excipient incompatibilities recently have been developed using elevated temperature and added water to accelerate potential interactions in ternary and more complex powder blends.[95] Such methods have been shown to be capable of rapidly detecting chemical incompatibilities and giving good correlations with results using powder blends of drug and excipients at elevated temperatures and humidity.

Processing incompatibilities can be more difficult to troubleshoot than chemical incompatibilities. For example, tablet performance has been shown to vary for ketorolac tromethamine, depending upon the kind of starch that was used. Cornstarch showed a decreased disintegration time and dissolution rate as a function of blending time whereas pregelatinized starch showed no such dependency. The difference between these two excipients was attributed to the formation of drug/cornstarch agglomerates with magnesium stearate.[96]

Blending studies have shown the potential benefits of using sodium lauryl sulfate to offset these types of effects.[97]

Finally, manufacturing for a global market has forced a reevaluation of excipients that are used in formulations so that manufacturing can be carried out with internationally acceptable components. The European Economic Community has recently focused the pharmaceutical industry on eliminating excipients that have the potential for transmissible spongiform encephalopathies, replacing ingredients like stearic acid, magnesium stearate, polysorbate 80, and simethicone with vegetable grade sources.

API SPECIFICATIONS: MEETING PRODUCT AND REGULATORY REQUIREMENTS

Polymorphic Forms and Hydrates Decision Trees

A major portion of this chapter has been devoted to characterizing the solid state, $_jA$. The left side of Figure 38-19[98,99] summarizes some of the potential solid states that can exist for the unionized form of A; if a salt form was chosen for the API, the same states also would be possible. Previous sections have discussed the impact on API consistency and dissolution for the different solid states. The critical relative humidity (CRH) and the transition point (T_p) for enantiotropic polymorphic systems are especially important intrinsic physical parameters that control solid-state consistency and potential solid-state interconversion. Moisture and temperature, as we have discussed, are the major environmental variables that can promote these changes. Rapid methods, therefore, are needed to characterize potential solid-state forms and their physical properties. The decision-tree on the right side of Figure 38-19 summarizes when specifications need to be set to maintain API consistency. If the physical properties of the solid states differ, assessments need to determine the impact this will have on a formulated API. Specifications need to be set to ensure a consistent product.

Particle-Size Acceptance Criterion

Once the solid state, $_jA$, has been characterized, the potential impact of particle size on absorption can be assessed. Figure 38-20 shows a decision-tree approach, suggested by the International Committee on Harmonization, for determining whether a particle-size acceptance criterion is needed.[100] Previous sections in this chapter have discussed nearly every aspect of this tree. Although dissolution-limited absorption is a major concern, Figure 38-20 also includes dosage form issues such as content uniformity.

Biopharmaceutical Classificaion of API

Although it is possible to alter the solid state, $_jA$, such that dissolution and absorption can be enhanced, solubility and passive permeability are, in general, intrinsic properties of the NCE. Thus, even though the amorphous state, αA, in some situations can be stabilized to enhance dissolution, the equilibrium solubility will be determined by the least soluble solid state. A classification has been proposed to segregate situations when *in vitro* and *in vivo* correlations (IVIV) are expected. Such designations may be used as a guide for determining when bioequivalent studies may need to be carried out. Table 38-7 shows the four major classes based on solubility and passive permeability.

CONCLUSION: APPLICATION OF KNOWLEDGE

"The actual product of the pharmaceutical industry is knowledge; pills and prescriptions ointments are no more than packaging for knowledge."[101] The introduction of methods to probe and exploit human and animal genomics has had a cascading impact on the industry. These new concepts had a number of qualities that ensured adaptation. The systematic use of mechanism-based reagents was a tangibly better solution for finding new therapeutic entities than the more serendipitous methods of the past. Such high-throughput screens were compatible with increasing use of robotics whose advantages could easily be understood by all in the pharmaceutical industry. Each company was able to hold trial runs to test the utility of such screens and in the end obtain observable results. Today, the recombinant DNA innovations of the 1980s still provide the driving force for other innovations in the pharmaceutical industry: miniaturization, customizing, and artificial intelligence.

Miniaturization began in earnest with the micronization of the transistor concept onto silicone chips. In the pharmaceutical industry, mass screening, the demand for higher and higher

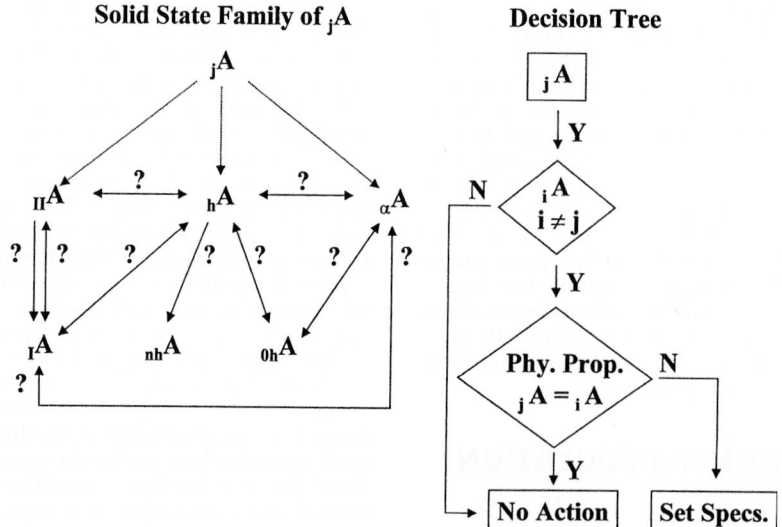

Figure 38-19. Solid-state forms and specification setting. (Data from Byrn S et al. *Pharm Res* 1995;9:84; and Byrn S et al. *Gold Sheet* 1996;30(6):1.)

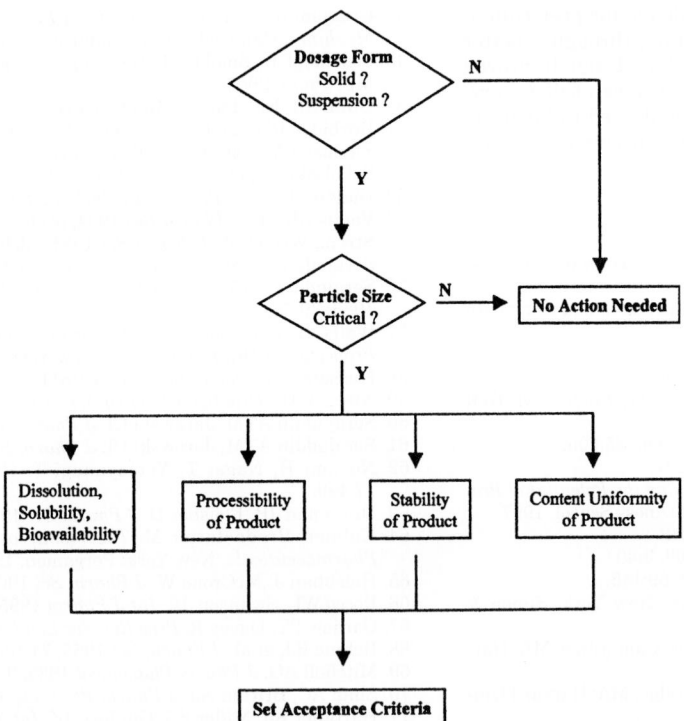

Figure 38-20. Decision-tree for drug substance particle-size distribution. (From Byrn S et al. Specifications for new drug substances and products: Chemical Substances, ICH4, Fourth International Conference on Harmonization. Brussels, July 1997.)

throughput, and the need to conserve chemical libraries have accelerated analytical and synthetic nanotechnology. This latter need is extremely important because chemical libraries are expendable resources that are not easily replaced. Old library entries were synthesized in gram quantities, and newer entries in milligrams. Conservation of this resource will require a combination of nanotechnology along with a host of regeneration technologies including combinatorial synthesis, high-throughput purification, and promotion of an increasingly diverse molecular library for mass screening. In addition, chromatographic columns, HPLCs, and electrophoresis on the nanoscale hold promise for extremely high resolution with extremely low material consumption. On this scale, area can efficiently be converted to a linear dimension. Thus a chip 10 × 10 mm can be converted easily to an electrophoretic path of 9.5 cm. The potential for massive parallel processing is evident when one considers the possibilities of 100 nanolaboratories on a single chip.

Customization at low cost also will be possible with new technology. DNA probes located on biochips will permit the individualization of a treatment course depending on a person's ability to metabolize a given drug. Such innovations likely will cause a cascading demand on development to individualize dosage forms. Finally, the rapid and parallel demands placed on preformulation will force more decisions to be made using artificial intelligence. High-throughput determinations of physical properties will result in high quality databases, which can in turn be systematically exploited by expert systems. Highly accurate predictions of solubility, permeability, and dissolution will be possible in the 21st century.

Although artificial intelligence is still in its infancy, the benefits of its applications can be appreciated from a consideration of the differences between knowledge and information. A chemical reaction database, for example, stores information on particular reactions. However, it cannot apply this information to new molecules. Expert systems, on the other hand, so codify knowledge that they can be applied to entirely new situations. Knowledge differs from information in that information is random and miscellaneous, and it tends to expand too rapidly and overwhelm us. Knowledge, on the other hand, requires that the structure of a subject be understood in a way that permits other things to be related to it in a meaningful way; it permits intuitive heuristic procedures to be developed to solve problems when no algorithms are available. Such applications of artificial intelligence, however, are still in the early-stage knowledge revolution, in which knowledge is applied to produce results. In the postcapitalist society, knowledge will be applied toward systematic innovation: "It will be applied systematically and purposefully to define what new knowledge is needed, whether it is feasible, and what has to be done to make knowledge more effective."

Knowledge and the productive application of knowledge are anticipated to be the sole factors that will drive the postcapitalist society into the 21st century. In the pharmaceutical industry, massive diffusion of innovations from discovery into de-

Table 38-7. *In Vitro/In Vivo* Correlation Expectations for Immediate-Release Products Based on Biopharmaceutics Class for Passive Absorption

CLASS	SOLUBILITY	PERMEABILITY	IVIV CORRELATION EXPECTATION
I	High	High	IVIV correlation if dissolution rate is slower than gastric emptying rate. Otherwise limited or no correlation.
II	Low	High	IVIV correlation expected if *in vitro* dissolution rate is similar to *in vivo* dissolution rate (unless dose is very high).
III	High	Low	Absorption (permeability) is rate-determining and limited or no IVIV correlation with dissolution rate.
IV	Low	Low	Limited or no IVIV correlation expected.

From Amidon GL, et al. *Pharm Res* 1995; 12:413.

velopment will pose an accelerating challenge for preformulation. To meet this challenge, preformulation, through a better understanding of the solid state, must seek to design improved characteristics into APIs at the earliest stages of discovery. This will be the edge that any company will need to facilitate the rapid movement of new therapeutics entries to marketplace. The patient is waiting!

REFERENCES

1. Handy C. *The Age of Paradox*. Cambridge, MA: Harvard Business School, 1995: 49–67.
2. Stella V. One of the many fine terms Dr. Stella has coined along with 'grease balls' and 'brick dust'.
3. Lipinski CA. *Adv Drug Del Rev* 1997; 23:3.
4. DiMasi JA. *Clin Pharmacol Ther* 2001; 69:286.
5. Arlington S, et al. *Pharma 2010: The Threshold of Innovation*. IBM Future Series, GS10-9439-00, 2000.
6. Kulling SE, Metzler M. *Food Chem Toxicol* 1996, 35:605.
7. DiMasi JA. *Clin Pharmacol Ther* 2001; 69:297.
8. Pisano GP. *The Development Factory–Unlocking the Potential of Process Innovation*. Cambridge, MA: Harvard Business School, 1997.
9. Sinko PJ. *Curr Opin Drug DiscDev* 1999; 2:42.
10. Caldwell GW. *Curr Opin Drug Disc Dev* 2000; 3:30.
11. Vankatesh S, Lipper RA. *J Pharm Sci* 2000; 89:145.
12. Oakley E, Krug D. *Enlightened Leadership*. New York: Simon & Schuster, 1994:76–93.
13. Zander RS, Zander B. *The Art of Possibilities*. Cambridge, MA: Harvard Business School, 2000.
14. Bruner JS. *The Process of Education*. Cambridge, MA: Harvard University Press, 1960:7.
15. Abraham MH, Le J. *J Pharm Sci* 1999; 88:868.
16. Goodwin JT, et al. *J Med Chem* 2001; 44:3721.
17. Goodwin JT, et al. *J Peptide Res* 1999; 53:355.
18. Veber DF, et al. *J Med Chem* 2002; 45:2615.
19. Anand BS, Dey S, Mitra AK. *Exp Opin Biol Ther* 2002; 2:607.
20. Klein I, Sarkadi B, Váradi A. *Biochem Biophy Acta* 1999; 1461:237.
21. Borst P, et al. *Biochem Biophy Acta* 1999; 1461:347.
22. Sheetz MP, Singer MJ. *Proc Nat Acad Sci* 1974; 71:4457.
23. Boon JM, Smith BD. *Med Res Rev* 2002; 22:251.
24. Yata N, et al. *Pharm Res* 1990; 7:1019.
25. Speelmans G, et al. *Biochem* 1994; 33:13761.
26. Anand BS, Dey S, Mitra AK. *Exp Opin Biol Ther* 2002; 2:607.
27. Bailey PD, et al. *Angew Chem Int Ed* 2000; 39:505.
28. Terada T, et al. *Pflugers Arch* 2000; 440:679.
29. Swaan PW, et al. *Receptor Channels* 1998; 6: 189.
30. Friedrichsen GM, et al. *Eur J Pharm Sci* 2002; 16:1.
31. Song Y, et al. *Bioorg Med Chem Lett* 2003; 13:297.
32. Hall JE, et al. *Antimicrob Agents Chemother* 1998; 42:666.
33. Zhou L, et al. *Pharm Res* 2002; 19:1689.
34. Gangwar S, et al. *Pharm Res* 1996; 13:1657.
35. Stella VJ. *Adv Drug Del Rev* 1996; 19:311.
36. Talley JJ, et al. *J Med Chem* 2000; 43:1661.
37. Talley JJ, et al. *J Med Chem* 2000; 43:775.
38. Corbett AH, Kashuba ADM. *Curr Opin Invest Drugs* 2002; 3:384.
39. Shimma N, et al. *Bioorg Med Chem* 2000; 8:1697.
40. Xu G, et al. *Clin Cancer Res* 2002; 8:2605.
41. Lundberg BB, et al. *J Controlled Release* 2003; 86:93.
42. Garsky VM, et al. *J Med Chem* 2002; 45:4706.
43. Brady SF, et al. *J Med Chem* 2001; 44:4216.
44. Bruner JS. *The Process of Education*. Cambridge, MA: Harvard University Press, Cambridge, 1960:7,17–32.
45. Tetko IV. *J Chem Inf Comput Sci* 2002; 42:717.
46. Tetko IV. *Neur Proc Lett* 2002; 16:187.
47. Tetko IV, Tanchuk VY. *J Chem Inf Comput Sci* 2002; 42:1136.
48. Cristianini N, Shawe-Taylor J. *An Introduction to Support Vector Machines*. Cambridge UK: Cambridge University Press, 2000.
49. Schölkopf B, Smola AJ. *Learning with Kernels*. Cambridge, MA: MIT Press, 2002.
50. Gunn SR, Kandola JS. *Machine Learning* 2002; 48:137.
51. Burbidge R, et al. *Comput Chem* 2001. 26:5.
52. Shalaev EY, Zografi G. *J Pharm Sci* 1996; 85:1137.
53. Sokoloski TD, et al. *Pharm Res* 1994; 11:S1.
52. Duddu SP, et al. *Pharm Res* 1994; 11: S1.
53. Vadas EB, et al. *Pharm Res* 1994; 8:148.
54. Streng WH, et al. *J Pharm Sci* 1984; 73:1679.
55. Serajuddin ATM, Mufson D. *Pharm Res* 1985; 2:65.
56. Serajuddin ATM, Sheen P, Augustine MA. *J Pharm Pharmacol* 1986; 39:587.
57. Wells JI. *Pharmaceutical Preformulation: The Physicochemical Properties of Drug Substances*. New York: Wiley, 1988:38.
58. Hussain A. *J Pharm Sci* 1972; 61:811.
59. Nielsen AE. *Croatica Chemica Acta* 1987; 60:531.
60. Serajuddin ATM, Jarowski CI. *J Pharm Sci* 1985; 74:148.
61. Serajuddin ATM, Jarowski CI. *J Pharm Sci* 1985; 74:142.
62. Nogami H, Nagai T, Yotsuyanagi T. *Chem Pharm Bull* 1969; 17:499.
63. Dressman JB, Fleisher D. *J Pharm Sci* 1986; 75:109.
64. Kuhnert-Bradnstatter M. *Thermomicroscopy in the Analysis of Pharmaceuticals*. New York: Pergamon, 1971:35–36.
65. Heleblian J, McCrone W. *J Pharm Sci* 1969; 58:911.
66. Rocco WL, Swanson JR. *Int J Pharm* 1995; 117:231.
67. Cardew PT, Davey R. *Proc Roy Soc Lond A* 1985; 398:415.
68. Behme RJ, et al. *J Pharm Sci* 1985; 74:1041.
69. Mitchell AG. *J Pharm Pharmacol* 1985; 37:601.
70. Shah AC, Britten NJ. *J Pharm Pharmacol* 1987; 39:736.
71. Hartauer KJ, Miller ES, Guillory JK. *Int J Pharm* 1992; 85:163.
72. Admirat P, Grenier JC. *J Rech Atmos* 1975; 9:97.
73. Kitamura S, et al. *Pharm Res* 1992; 9:138.
74. Tada T, et al. *J Pharm Sci* 1987; 76:S302.
75. Buxton PC, Lynch IR, Roe JM. *Int J Pharm* 1988; 42:135.
76. Vadas EB, Toma P, Zografi G. *Pharm Res* 1991; 8:148.
77. Morris KR, et al. *Int J Pharm* 1994; 108:195.
78. Yoshioka S, Shibazaki T, Uchiyama M. *J Pharmacobiodyn* 1986; 9:S6.
79. Yoshioka S, Shibazaki T, Ejima A. *Chem Pharm Bull* 1982; 30:3734.
80. Yoshioka S, Uchiyama M. *J Pharm Sci* 1986; 75:92.
81. Kitamura S, et al. *Int J Pharm* 1990; 59:217.
82. Gu L, et al. *Drug Devel Ind Pharm* 1987; 13:437.
83. Gu L, Strickley RG. *Pharm Res* 1987; 4:255.
84. Roseman TJ, Yalkowsky SH. *J Pharm Sci* 1973; 62:1680.
85. Walkling WD, et al. *Drug Dev Ind Pharm* 1983; 9:809.
86. Serajuddin ATM, et al. *J Pharm Sci* 1986; 75:492.
87. Hajdu J, Adams G, Lee H. *J Pharm Sci* 1988; 77:921.
88. Aguiar AJ. *J Pharm Sci* 1969; 58:963.
89. Kaneniwa N, Otsuka M. *Chem Pharm Bull* 1985; 33:1660.
90. Kitamura S, et al. *Int J Pharm* 1989; 56:125.
91. Grant DJW, York P. *Int J Pharm* 1986; 30:161.
92. Morris KR, et al. *Int J Pharm* 1994; 105:209.
93. Teraoka R, Otsuka M, Matsuda Y. *J Pharm Sci* 1993; 82:601.
94. Gould PL. *Int J Pharm* 1986; 33:201.
95. Serajuddin ATM, et al. *Pharm Res* 1991; 8(suppl):S103.
96. Chowhan ZT, Chi LH. *Pharm Technol* 1985; 9:84.
97. Wand LH, Chowhan ZT. *Int J Pharm* 1990; 60:61.
98. Byrn S, et al. *Pharm Res* 1995; 9:84.
99. Byrn S, et al. *Gold Sheet* 1996; 30(6):1.
100. Byrn S, et al. Fourth International Conference on Harmonization, Brussels, July 16, 1997.
101. Drucker P. *Post-Capitalist Society*. New York: Harper Business, 1993:182.

CHAPTER 39

Solutions, Emulsions, Suspensions, and Extracts

Michael M Crowley, PhD

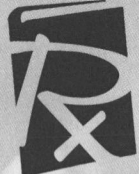

The dosage forms described in this chapter are prepared by employing pharmaceutically and therapeutically acceptable vehicles. The active ingredient(s) may be dissolved in aqueous media, organic solvent or combination of the two, by suspending the drug (if it is insoluble) in an appropriate medium, or by incorporating the medicinal agent into one of the phases of an oil and water emulsion. Such solutions, suspensions and emulsions are further defined in subsequent paragraphs but some, with similar properties and applications, are considered in greater detail elsewhere in *Remington*.

These dosage forms are useful for a number of reasons. They can be formulated for different routes of administration: orally, introduction into body cavities, or external application. The dose can easily be adjusted by dilution, making the oral liquid form ready to be administered to children or people unable to swallow tablets or capsules. Extracts eliminate the need to isolate the drug in pure form, allow several ingredients to be administered from a single source (eg, pancreatic extract), and permit the preliminary study of drugs from natural sources. Occasionally, solutions of drugs such as potassium chloride are used to minimize adverse effects in the gastrointestinal tract.

The preparation of these dosage forms involves several considerations on the part of the pharmacist, namely; purpose of the drug, internal or external use, solubility and concentration of the drug, selection of the liquid vehicle(s), physical and chemical stability of the drug and any excipients, preservation of the preparation, and use of appropriate excipients such as buffers, solubility enhancers, suspending agents, emulsifying agents, viscosity controlling agents, colors and flavors. Oral preparations require consideration be given to improving patient compliance by making an acceptable product; consequently, color, odor and taste must be considered. The viscosity of a product also must be considered so that it has the proper palatability for an oral preparation and has the appropriate suspending properties if it is an emulsion or suspension. The theory of solutions, which involves solubility, ionization, pH control through the use of buffers, and solubilization, is discussed in Chapters 16 (*Solutions and Phase Equilibria*) and 17 (*Ionic Solutions and Electrolyte Equilibria*). Because of the complexity of some manufactured products, compounding may be carried out with the aid of linear programming models to obtain the optimal product. Chapters 41 to 43 should be consulted for information on the preparation and characteristics of those liquid preparations that are intended for parenteral and ophthalmic use.

Much has been written about the biopharmaceutical properties of solid dosage forms. Many researchers begin their absorption studies of drugs administered in solution to assess the bioavailability relative to tablets and capsules. Absorption occurs when drugs are in a dissolved state, thus it is frequently observed that the bioavailability of oral dosage forms decreases in the following order: aqueous solution > aqueous suspension > tablet or capsule. Formulation may influence the bioavailability and pharmacokinetics of drugs in solution, including drug concentration, volume of liquid administered, pH, ionic strength, buffer capacity, surface tension, specific gravity, viscosity and excipients. Emulsions and suspensions are more complex systems; consequently, the bioavailability and pharmacokinetics of these systems may be affected by additional formulation factors such as surfactants, type of viscosity agent, particle size and particle-size distribution, polymorphism and solubility of drug in the oil phase.

Liquid preparations may be dispensed in one of three ways: (1) in its original container, (2) repackaging a bulk product at the time a prescription is presented by the patient or (3) compounding the solution, suspension, or emulsion in the dispensary. Compounding may involve nothing more than mixing marketed products in the manner indicated on the prescription or, in specific instances, may require the incorporation of active ingredients and excipients in a logical and pharmaceutically acceptable manner into aqueous or organic solvents that will form the bulk of the product.

The pharmacist, in the first instance, depends on the pharmaceutical manufacturer to produce a product that is safe, efficacious, elegant and stable until its expiration date when stored at conditions described on its label. Manufacturers guarantee efficacy of their products but, in some instances, consumer preference is variable. For example, cough syrups marketed by two different manufacturers may contain the same active ingredient(s), and the relative merits of the two products may appear interchangeable. In such instances the commercial advantage may be based on factors such as flavor, color, aroma, mouth feel and packaging.

SOLVENTS FOR LIQUID PHARMACEUTICAL PREPARATIONS

The pharmacist's knowledge of the physical and chemical characteristics of a given drug dictates the selection of the appropriate solvent for a particular formulation. In addition to solubility, solvent selection is also based on clarity, toxicity, viscosity, compatibility with excipients, chemical inertness, palatability, odor, color, and economy. In most cases, especially solutions for oral, ophthalmic or parenteral administration, water is the preferred solvent because it meets the majority of the above criteria better than other available solvents. Often, an auxiliary solvent is also employed to augment the solvent action of water or to contribute to a product's chemical or physical stability. Alcohol, glycerin, and propylene glycol have been frequently used for these purposes.

Solvents such as acetone, ethyl oxide, and isopropyl alcohol are too toxic for use in oral pharmaceutical preparations, but they are useful as solvents in organic chemistry and in the preparatory stages of drug development. For purposes such as this, certain solvents are officially recognized in the compendia. A number of fixed oils such as corn oil, cottonseed oil, peanut oil, and sesame oil serve useful solvent functions particularly in the preparation of oleaginous injections and are recognized in the compendia for this purpose.

WATER

The major ingredient in most of the dosage forms described herein is water. It is used both as a vehicle and as a solvent for the desired flavoring or medicinal ingredients. Its tastelessness, freedom from irritating qualities, and lack of pharmacological activity make it ideal for such purposes. There is, however, a tendency to assume that its purity is constant and that it can be stored, handled, and used with a minimum of care. Although it is true that municipal supplies must comply with Environmental Protection Agency (EPA) regulations (or comparable regulations in other countries), drinking water must be purified before it can be used in pharmaceuticals. Water quality can have a significant impact on the stability of pharmaceutical dosage forms.[1] In manufacturing environments, the design of purified water systems must meet standards outlined in the United States Pharmacopeia (USP) and be validated.[2–5]

Five of the eight solvent waters described in the USP are used in the preparation of parenterals, irrigations, or inhalations. *Purified Water* must be used for all other pharmaceutical operations, dosage forms, and, as needed, in all USP tests and assays. It must meet rigid specifications for chemical purity. Purified Water is water obtained by deionization, distillation, ion-exchange, reverse osmosis, filtration, or other suitable procedures. For parenteral administration, Water for Injection, Bacteriostatic Water for Injection, or Sterile Water for Injection must be used. Sterile water may be sterile at the time of production but may lose this characteristic if it is stored improperly.

The major impurities in water are calcium, iron, magnesium, manganese, silica, and sodium. The cations usually are combined with the bicarbonate, sulfate, or chloride anions. Hard waters are those that contain calcium and magnesium cations. Bicarbonates are the major impurity in alkaline waters. Deionization processes do not necessarily produce Purified Water that will comply with EPA requirements for drinking water. Resin columns retain phosphates and organic debris. Either alone or in combination, these substances can act as growth media for microorganisms. Observations have shown that deionized water containing 90 organisms / mL contained 10^6 organisms / mL after 24-hour storage. Ultraviolet radiant energy (240–280 nm), heat or filtration can be used to limit the growth of, kill, or remove microorganisms in water. The latter method employs membrane filters and can be used to remove bacteria from heat-labile materials.

The phenomenon of *osmosis* involves the passage of water from a dilute solution across a semi-permeable membrane to a more concentrated solution. Flow of water can be stopped by applying pressure to the concentrated solution equal to the osmotic pressure. The flow of water can be reversed by applying a pressure greater than the osmotic pressure. The process of reverse osmosis uses the latter principle; by applying pressure greater than the osmotic pressure to the concentrated solution (eg, tap water), pure water may be obtained. Organic molecules are rejected on the basis of a sieve mechanism related to their size and shape. Small organic molecules, with a

molecular weight smaller than approximately 200, will pass through the membrane material. Because there are few organic molecules with a molecular weight of less than 200 in the municipal water supply, reverse osmosis usually is sufficient for the removal of organic material. The pore sizes of the selectively permeable reverse-osmosis membranes are between 0.5 and 10 nm. Viruses and bacteria larger than 10 nm are rejected if no imperfections exist in the membrane. The membranes may and do develop openings that permit the passage of microorganisms. Because of the semi-static conditions, bacteria can grow both upstream and downstream of the membrane.

ALCOHOLS

Next to water, alcohol is the second most commonly used solvent in pharmacy for many organic compounds. When mixed with water, a hydroalcoholic mixture is formed capable of dissolving both alcohol-soluble and water-soluble substances, a feature especially useful for extraction and purification of active constituents from crude drugs and synthetic procedures. Alcohol, USP, is 94.9% to 96.0% by volume, at 15.56°C of C_2H_5OH and Dehydrated Alcohol, USP, contains not less than 99.5% C_2H_5OH by volume. Dehydrated alcohol is utilized when an essentially water-free alcohol is necessary. Alcohol is widely used for its miscibility with water and its ability to dissolve many water-insoluble ingredients including drug substances, flavors, and antimicrobial preservatives. Alcohol is used in liquid products as an antimicrobial preservative or in conjunction with parabens, benzoates, sorbates, and other agents. Diluted Alcohol, NF, is prepared by mixing equal volumes of Alcohol, USP, and Purified Water, USP. Due to contraction upon mixing, the final volume of such mixtures is not the sum of the individual volumes of the two components, but is generally about 3% less.

The United States Food and Drug Administration (FDA) has expressed concern about undesired pharmacologic and potential toxic effects of alcohol when ingested by children. For this reason, manufacturers of over-the-counter (OTC) oral drug products have been asked to restrict, if possible, the use of alcohol and include appropriate warnings in the labeling. For OTC oral products intended for children under 6 years of age, the recommended alcohol content limit is 0.5%; for products intended for children 6 to 12 years of age, the recommended limit is 5%; and for products recommended for children over 12 years of age and for adults, the recommended limit is 10%.

Rubbing Alcohol, USP must be manufactured in accordance with the requirements of the US Treasury Department, Bureau of Alcohol, Tobacco, and Firearms, Formula 23-H (8 parts by volume of acetone, 1.5 parts by volume of methyl isobutyl ketone, and 100 parts by volume of ethyl alcohol). It contains not less than 68.5% and not more than 71.5% by volume of dehydrated alcohol, the remainder consisting of water and the denaturants with or without color additives and perfume oils. Rubbing Alcohol contains in each 100 mL not less than 355 mg of sucrose octaacetate or not less than 1.40 mg of denatonium benzoate. The preparation may be colored with one or more color additives listed by the FDA for use in drugs and a suitable stabilizer may be added. The use of this denaturant mixture makes the separation of ethyl alcohol from the denaturants a virtually impossible task with ordinary distillation apparatus. This discourages the illegal removal and use of the alcoholic content of rubbing alcohol as a beverage. The product is volatile and extremely flammable and should be stored in tight containers remote from ignition sources. It is used externally as a soothing rub for bedridden patients, a germicide for instruments, and a skin cleanser prior to injection.

Isopropyl Rubbing Alcohol is about 70% by volume isopropyl alcohol, the remainder consisting of water with or without color additives, stabilizers, and perfume oils. It is used exclusively as a vehicle in topical products and applications. This preparation and a commercially available 91% isopropyl alcohol solution are commonly employed to disinfect needles and syringes for hypodermic injections of insulin and for disinfecting the skin.

Glycerin is a clear, syrupy liquid with a sweet taste and is miscible with water and alcohol. Glycerin is used in a wide variety of pharmaceutical formulations including oral, otic, ophthalmic, topical, and parenteral preparations. In topical pharmaceutical formulations and cosmetics, glycerin is used primarily for its humectant and emollient properties. In parenteral formulations, glycerin is used mainly as a solvent. In oral solutions, glycerin is used as a solvent, sweetening agent, antimicrobial preservative, and viscosity-increasing agent.

Propylene glycol has become widely used as a solvent, extractant, and preservative in a variety of liquid pharmaceutical formulations, including parenterals. Propylene glycol is a viscous liquid and is miscible with water and alcohol. It is a useful solvent with a wide range of applications and is often used in place of glycerin. As an antiseptic it is similar to ethanol, and against molds it is similar to glycerin and only slightly less effective than ethanol. Propylene glycol is also used as a carrier for emulsifiers and as a vehicle for flavors, as opposed to ethanol, due to its lack of volatility.

STABILITY CONSIDERATIONS

The stability of the active ingredient in the final product is a primary concern to the formulator. In general, drug substances are less stable in aqueous media than solid dosage forms, and it is important to properly stabilize and preserve solutions, suspensions, and emulsions that contain water. Acid–base reactions, acid or base catalysis, oxidation, and reduction can occur in these products. These reactions can arise from ingredient–ingredient interactions or container–product interactions. For pH sensitive compounds, any of these interactions may alter the pH and cause precipitation.

Vitamins, essential oils, and almost all fats and oils can be oxidized. Formulators usually use the word *auto-oxidation* when the ingredient(s) reacts with oxygen but without drastic external interference. Such reactions can be initiated by heat, light (including ultraviolet radiant energy), peroxides, or other labile compounds or heavy metals such as copper or iron. This initiation step results in the formation of a free radical that then reacts with oxygen. The free radical is regenerated and reacts with more oxygen (propagation). The reactions are terminated when the free radicals react with one another.

The effect of trace metals can be minimized by using chelating agents such as citric acid or EDTA. Antioxidants may retard or delay oxidation by rapidly reacting with free radicals as they are formed (quenching). Common antioxidants include propyl, octyl, and dodecyl esters of gallic acid, butylated hydroxyanisole (BHA), butylated hydroxytoluene (BHT), and the tocopherols or vitamin E. Connors and coworkers provide a detailed approach for the prevention of oxidative degradation of pharmaceuticals.[6] Common antioxidants and chelating agents used in pharmaceutical preparations are listed in Table 39-1.

The USP states that if a product must be repackaged, the container specified by the compendium must be used. For example, a suitable opaque plastic container should be used if a light-resistant container is specified. If a product is diluted, or where two products are mixed, the pharmacist should use his or her knowledge to guard against incompatibility and instability. Oral antibiotic preparations constituted into liquid form should never be mixed with other products. If the chemical stability of extemporaneously prepared liquid preparations is unknown, their use should be minimized and every care taken to ensure that product characteristics will not change during the time it must be used by the patient.

Because of the number of excipients and additives in these preparations, it is recommended all the ingredients be listed on the container to reduce the risks that confront hypersensitive patients when these products are administered. Finally, the pharmacist should inform the patient regarding the appropriate use of the product, the proper storage conditions, and the time after which it should be discarded.

PRESERVATIVES

In addition to stabilization of pharmaceutical preparations against chemical and physical degradation, liquid and semisolid preparations must be protected against microbial contamination. Nearly all products described in this chapter contain water and thus, with certain exceptions such as aqueous acids, will support microbial growth. Aqueous solutions, syrups, emulsions, and suspensions often provide excellent growth media for microorganisms such as molds, yeast, and bacteria (typically *Pseudomonas, E. coli, Salmonella,* and *Staphylococcus*).

Kurup and Wan describe many preparations that are not preserved adequately and are not able to resist microbial contamination.[7] Products such as ophthalmic and injectable preparations are sterilized by autoclaving (20 minutes at 15 pounds of pressure at 120°C followed by dry heat at 180°C for 1 hour) or filtration. However, many of them require the presence of an antimicrobial preservative to maintain aseptic conditions throughout their stated shelf life.[8] Certain hydroalcoholic and alcoholic preparations do not require addition of a chemical preservative if the alcohol content is sufficient to prevent microbial growth. In general, an alcohol content of 15% by weight in acid solutions and 18% by weight in alkaline solutions is sufficient to prevent microbial growth. Most alcohol containing preparations such as elixirs, spirits, and tinctures are self-preserving and will not require preservation. Indeed, the formulator should challenge any new preparation by procedures described in the General Tests and Assays, parts ⟨51⟩ and ⟨61⟩ of the USP and other methods reported in the literature.[9–12]

Table 39-1. Common Antioxidants and Chelating Agents Used in Liquid Pharmaceutical Dosage Forms

Antioxidants	Alpha tocopherol
	Ascorbic acid
	Acorbyl palmitate
	Butylated hydroxyanisole
	Butylated hydroxytoluene
	Monothioglycerol
	Potassium metabisulfite
	Propionic acid
	Propyl gallate
	Sodium ascorbate
	Sodium bisulfite
	Sodium metabisulfite
	Sodium sulfite
Chelating Agents	Citric acid monohydrate
	Disodium edetate
	Dipotassium edetate
	Edetic acid
	Fumaric acid
	Malic acid
	Phosphoric acid
	Sodium edetate
	Tartaric acid
	Trisodium edetate

When a preservative is required, its selection is based upon several considerations, in particular the site of use whether internal, external, or ophthalmic.[13] Several researchers have described various interactions that must be considered when preservatives are selected.[14,15] The major criteria that should be considered in selecting a preservative are as follows: It should be effective against a wide spectrum of microorganisms, stable for its shelf life, nontoxic, nonsensitizing, compatible with the ingredients in the dosage form, inexpensive, and relatively free of taste and odor.

The chosen preservative should be sufficiently stable and soluble to achieve adequate concentration to provide protection. This choice is more critical in two and three phase emulsion systems in which the preservative may be more soluble in the oil phase than in the aqueous phase.[12,16] The pH of the preparation must be considered to ensure that the preservative does not dissociate rendering it ineffective or degrade by acid or base catalyzed hydrolysis. The undissociated moiety or molecular form of a preservative possesses preservative capacity because the ionized form is unable to penetrate microorganisms. The preservative must be compatible with the formulation ingredients and the product container or closure. Finally, the preservative must not impact the safety or comfort of the patient when administered. For instance, preservatives used in ophthalmic preparations must be non-irritating. Chlorobutanol, benzalkonium chloride, and phenylmercuric nitrate are commonly used in these applications.

Although few microorganisms are viable below a pH of 3 or above pH 9, most aqueous pharmaceutical preparations are manufactured within the favorable pH range. Acidic preservatives such as benzoic acid, boric acid, and sorbic acid are less dissociated and more effective in acidic formulations. Similarly, alkaline preservatives are less effective in acidic or neutral conditions and more effective in alkaline formulations. The scientific literature is rife with examples of incompatibilities between preservatives and other pharmaceutical adjuncts.[17–19] Commonly used macromolecules including cellulose derivatives, polyethylene glycol and tragacanth gum have been reported to cause preservative failure due to binding and adsorption.[20,21]

The mode of action by which preservatives interfere with microbial growth, multiplication, and metabolism occurs through one of several mechanisms. Preservatives often alter cell membrane permeability causing leakage of cell constituents (partial lysis), complete lysis, and cytoplasmic leakage and / or coagulation of cytoplasmic constituents (protein precipitation). Other preservatives inhibit cellular metabolism by interference with enzyme systems or cell wall synthesis, oxidation of cellular constituents, or hydrolysis.

Preservatives commonly used in pharmaceutical products are listed in Table 39-2 with typical concentration levels. Preservatives may be grouped into a number of classes depending upon their molecular structure. These basic groups are discussed below.

Alcohols

Ethanol is useful as a preservative when it is used as a solvent; however, it does need a relatively high concentration, somewhat greater than 15%, to be effective. Too high a concentration may result in incompatibilities in suspension and emulsion systems. Propylene glycol also is used as a solvent in oral solutions and topical preparations, and it can function as a preservative in the range of 15% to 30%. It is not volatile like ethanol and is used frequently not only in solutions but also in suspensions and emulsions. Chlorobutanol and phenylethyl alcohol are other alcohols used in lower concentrations (about 1%) as preservatives.

Acids

Benzoic acid has a low solubility in water, about 0.34% at 25°C, but the apparent aqueous solubility of benzoic acid may be enhanced by the addition of citric acid or sodium acetate to the solution. The concentration range used for inhibitory action varies from 0.1% to 0.5%. Activity depends on the pH of the medium because only the undissociated acid has antimicrobial properties. Optimum activity occurs at pH values below 4.5; at values above pH 5, benzoic acid is almost inactive.[22] It has been reported that antimicrobial activity of benzoic acid is enhanced by the addition of the basic protein protamine.[23] Sorbic acid also has a low solubility in water, 0.3% at 30°C. Suitable concentrations for preservative action are in the range of 0.05 to 2%. Its preservative action is due to the nonionized form; consequently, it is only effective in acid media. The optimum antibacterial activity is obtained at pH 4.5, and practically no activity is observed above pH 6. Sorbic acid is subject to oxidation, particularly in the presence of light and in aqueous

Table 39-2. Common Preservatives Used in Liquid Pharmaceutical Dosage Forms and Their Typical Concentration Levels

ANTIMICROBIAL PRESERVATIVES	TYPICAL USAGE LEVEL (% W/W)	ANTIFUNGAL PRESERVATIVES	TYPICAL USAGE LEVEL (% W/W)
Benzalkonium Chloride	0.002–0.02%	Butyl Paraben	0.1–0.4%
Benzethonium Chloride	0.01–0.02%	Methyl Paraben	0.1–0.25%
Benzyl Alcohol	3.0%	Ethyl Paraben	0.1–0.25%
Bronopol	0.01–0.1%	Propyl Paraben	0.1–0.25%
Cetrimide	0.005%	Benzoic Acid	0.1–0.5%
Cetylpyridinium chloride	0.0005–0.0007%	Potassium sorbate	0.1–0.2%
Chlorhexidine	0.002–0.5%	Sodium Benzoate	0.1–0.2%
Chlorobutanol	0.5%	Sodium Propionate	5–10%
Chlorocresol	0.2%	Sorbic Acid	0.05–0.2%
Chloroxylenol	0.1–0.8%		
Cresol	0.15–0.3%		
Ethyl Alcohol	15–20%		
Glycerin	20–30%		
Hexetidine	0.1%		
Imidurea	0.03–0.5%		
Phenol	0.1–0.5%		
Phenoxyethanol	0.5–1.0%		
Phenylethyl Alcohol	0.25–0.5%		
Phenylmercuric Nitrate	0.002–0.01%		
Propylene Glycol	15–30%		
Thimerosal	0.1%		

solutions. Activity against bacteria can be variable because of its limited stability. Thus, sorbic acid is frequently used in combination with other antimicrobial preservatives or glycols in which synergistic effects occur.

Esters

Parabens are esters of *p*-hydroxybenzoic acid and include the methyl, ethyl, propyl, and butyl derivatives. The water solubility of the parabens decreases as the molecular weight increases from 0.25% for the methyl ester to 0.02% for the butyl ester. These compounds are used widely in pharmaceutical products, stable over a pH range of 4 to 8, and have a broad spectrum of antimicrobial activity, although they are most effective against yeasts and molds. Antimicrobial activity increases as the chain length of the alkyl moiety is increased, but aqueous solubility decreases; therefore, a mixture of parabens is frequently used to provide effective preservation. Preservative efficacy is also improved by the addition of propylene glycol (2–5%) or by using parabens in combination with other antimicrobial agents such as imidurea. Activity is reduced in the presence of nonionic surface active agents due to binding. In alkaline solutions, ionization takes place and this reduces their activity; in addition, hydrolytic decomposition of the ester group occurs with a loss of activity.

Quaternary Ammonium Compounds

Benzalkonium chloride is a mixture consisting principally of the homologs $C_{12}H_{25}$ and $C_{14}H_{29}$. This preservative is used at a relatively low concentration, 0.002% to 0.02%, depending on the nature of the pharmaceutical product. This class of compounds has an optimal activity over the pH range of 4 to 10 and is quite stable at room temperature. Because of the cationic nature of this type of preservative, it is incompatible with many anionic compounds such as surfactants and can bind to nonionic surfactants. It is used generally in preparations for external use or those solutions that come in contact with mucous membranes. In ophthalmic preparations, benzalkonium chloride is widely used at a concentration of 0.01–0.02% w/w. Often it is used in combination with other preservatives or excipients, particularly 0.1% w/v disodium edetate, to enhance its antimicrobial activity against strains of *Pseudomonas*. A concentration of 0.002–0.02% is used in nasal and otic formulations, sometimes in combination with 0.002–0.005% thimerosal. Benzalkonium chloride 0.01% w/v is also employed as a preservative in small-volume parenteral products.

Clearly, when the pharmacist dispenses or compounds liquid preparations, responsibility is assumed, along with the manufacturer, for the maintenance of product stability. General chapter ⟨1191⟩ of the USP describes stability considerations for dispensing, which should be studied in detail.[9] Stock should be rotated and replaced if expiration dates on the label so indicate. Products should be stored in the manner indicated on the manufacturer's label or in the compendium. Further, products should be checked for evidence of instability. With respect to solutions, elixirs, and syrups, major signs of instability are color change, precipitation, and evidence of microbial or chemical gas formation. Emulsions may cream, but if they break (ie, there is a separation of an oil phase) the product is considered unstable. Sedimentation and caking are primary indications of instability in suspensions. The presence of large particles may mean that excessive crystal growth has occurred (Ostwald Ripening). Additional details on these topics are provided in the pertinent sections of this chapter.

SOLUTIONS

A solution is a homogeneous mixture that is prepared by dissolving a solid, liquid, or gas in another liquid and represents a group of preparations in which the molecules of the solute or dissolved substance are dispersed among those of the solvent. Most solutions are unsaturated with the solute, in other words, the concentration of the solute in the solution is below its solubility limit. The strengths of pharmaceutical solutions are usually expressed in terms of % strength, although for very dilute preparations expressions of ratio strength are sometimes used. The term % when used without qualification (as with w/v, v/v, or w/w) means % weight-in-volume for solutions or suspensions of solids in liquids; % weight-in-volume for solutions of gases in liquids; % volume-in-volume for solutions of liquids in liquids; and weight-in-weight for mixtures of solids and semisolids.

Solutions also may be classified on the basis of physical or chemical properties, method of preparation, use, physical state, number of ingredients, and particle size. For the pharmacist, solutions are more defined by site of administration and composition than by physicochemical definitions. For instance, pharmaceutical solutions may be classified as an *oral solution*, *otic solution*, *ophthalmic solution*, or *topical solution*. These solutions may also be classified based upon their composition. *Syrups* are aqueous solutions containing a sugar; *elixirs* are sweetened hydroalcoholic (combinations of water and ethanol) solutions; *spirits* are solutions of aromatic materials if the solvent is alcoholic or *aromatic waters* if the solvent is aqueous. Depending on their method of preparation and concentration, *tinctures* or *fluid extracts* are solutions prepared by extracting active constituents from crude drugs.

Many pharmaceutical chemicals are only slowly soluble in a given solvent and require an extended time for complete dissolution. To increase the dissolution rate, a pharmacist may employ one or several techniques such as applying heat, reducing the particle size of the solute, utilizing of a solubilizing agent, or subjecting the ingredients to rigorous agitation. In most cases, solutes are more soluble in solvents at elevated temperatures than at room temperature or below due to the endothermic nature of the dissolution process. The pharmacist should ensure that the materials are heat stabile and non-volatile when using heat to facilitate the dissolution rate.

AQUEOUS SOLUTIONS

The narrower definition in this subsection limits the solvent to water and excludes those preparations that are sweet and/or viscid in character and nonaqueous solutions. This section includes those pharmaceutical forms that are designated as *Aromatic Waters, Aqueous Acids, Solutions, Douches, Enemas, Gargles, Mouthwashes, Juices, Nasal Solutions, Otic Solutions,* and *Irrigation Solutions*.

Aromatic Waters

The USP defines Aromatic Waters as clear, saturated aqueous solutions (unless otherwise specified) of volatile oils or other aromatic or volatile substances.[9] Their odors and tastes are similar, respectively, to those of the drugs or volatile substances from which they are prepared, and they are free from empyreumatic and other foreign odors. Aromatic waters may be prepared by distillation or solution of the aromatic substance, with or without the use of a dispersing agent. They are used principally as flavored or perfumed vehicles.

Peppermint Water USP and Stronger Rose Water USP are examples of aromatic waters. Concentrated waters, such as peppermint, dill, cinnamon, and caraway, may be prepared as follows:

Dissolve 20 mL of the volatile oil in 600 mL of 90% ethanol. Add sufficient purified water in successive small portions to produce 1000 mL. Shake vigorously after each addition. Add 50 g of sterilized purified talc, shake occasionally for several hours, and filter.

The aromatic water is prepared by diluting the concentrate with 39 times its volume of water.

The chemical composition of many of the volatile oils is known, and suitable synthetic substances may be used in preparing pharmaceuticals and cosmetics. Similarly, many synthetic aromatic substances have a characteristic odor; for example, geranyl phenyl acetate has a honey odor. Such substances, either alone or in combination, can be used in nonofficial preparations.

The principal difficulty experienced in compounding prescriptions containing aromatic waters is *salting out* certain ingredients such as very soluble salts. A replacement of part of the aromatic water with purified water is permissible when no other function is being served than that of a vehicle. Aromatic waters will deteriorate with time and should, therefore, be made in small quantities, protected from intense light and excessive heat, and stored in airtight, light-resistant containers.

Aqueous Acids

Inorganic acids and certain organic acids, although of minor significance as therapeutic agents, are of great importance in pharmaceutical manufacturing and analysis. This is especially true of acetic, hydrochloric, and nitric acids. Many of the more important inorganic acids are available commercially in the form of concentrated aqueous solutions. The percentage strength varies from one acid to another and depends on the solubility and stability of the solute in water and on the manufacturing process. Thus, Hydrochloric Acid contains from 36.5% to 38.0% by weight of HCl, whereas Nitric Acid contains from 69% to 71% by weight of HNO_3.

Because the strengths of these concentrated acids are stated in terms of percent by weight, it is essential that specific gravities also be provided if one is to be able to calculate conveniently the amount of absolute acid contained in a unit volume of the solution as purchased. The mathematical relationship involved is given by the equation $M = V \times S \times F$, where M is the mass in g of absolute acid contained in V mL of solution having a specific gravity S and a fractional percentage strength F.

As an example, Hydrochloric Acid containing 36.93% by weight of HCl has a specific gravity of 1.1875. Therefore, the amount of pure HCl supplied by 100 mL of this solution is given by:

$$M = 100 \times 1.1875 \times 0.3693 = 43.85 \text{ g HCl}$$

Although many of the reactions characteristic of acids offer opportunities for incompatibilities, only a few are of sufficient importance to require more than casual mention. Acids and acid salts decompose carbonates with liberation of carbon dioxide; in a closed container, sufficient pressure may be developed to produce an explosion. Inorganic acids react with salts of organic acids to produce the free organic acid and a salt of the inorganic acid. If insoluble, the organic acid will be precipitated. Thus, salicylic acid and benzoic acid are precipitated from solutions of salicylates and benzoates. Boric acid likewise is precipitated from concentrated solutions of borates. By a similar reaction, certain soluble organic compounds are converted into an insoluble form. Phenobarbital sodium, for example, is converted into phenobarbital that will precipitate in aqueous solution.

The ability of acids to combine with alkaloids and other organic compounds containing a basic nitrogen atom is used in preparing soluble salts of these substances. Certain solutions, syrups, elixirs, and other pharmaceutical preparations, may contain free acid, which causes these preparations to exhibit the incompatibilities characteristic of the acid. Acids also possess the incompatibilities of the anions that they contain and, in the case of organic acids, these are frequently of prime importance. These are discussed under the specific anions.

Diluted Acids

The diluted acids in the USP are aqueous solutions of acids of a suitable strength (usually 10% *w/v* but Diluted Acetic Acid is 6% *w/v*) for internal administration or for the manufacture of other preparations.

The strengths of the official undiluted acids are expressed as percentages in weight (*w/w*), whereas the strengths of the official diluted acids are expressed as percent in volume (*w/v*). It, therefore, becomes necessary to consider the specific gravities of the concentrated acids when calculating the volume required to make a given quantity of diluted acid. The following equation will give the number of milliliters required to make 1000 mL of diluted acid:

$$\frac{\text{Strength of diluted acid} \times 1,000}{\substack{\text{Strength of undiluted acid} \\ \times \text{ Specific gravity of undiluted acid}}}$$

Thus, if one wishes to make 1000 mL of Diluted Hydrochloric Acid USP (10% w/v) using Hydrochloric Acid that assays 37.5% HCl (sp gr 1.18), the amount required is

$$\frac{10 \times 1,000}{37.5 \times 1.18} = 226 \text{ mL}$$

Diluted Hydrochloric Acid, USP has been used in the treatment of achlorhydria. However, it may irritate the mucous membrane of the mouth and attack the enamel of the teeth. The usual dose is 2 to 4 mL, well-diluted with water. In the treatment of achlorhydria no attempt is made to administer more than a relief-producing dose.

Douches

A douche is an aqueous solution directed against a part or into a cavity of the body. It functions as a cleansing or antiseptic agent. An *eye douche*, used to remove foreign particles and discharges from the eyes, is directed gently at an oblique angle and allowed to run from the inner to the outer corner of the eye. *Pharyngeal douches* are used to prepare the interior of the throat for an operation and cleanse it in suppurative conditions. Similarly, there are *nasal douches* and *vaginal douches*. Douches usually are directed to the appropriate body part by using bulb syringes.

Douches are often dispensed in the form of a powder with directions for dissolving in a specified quantity of water (usually warm). However, tablets for preparing solutions are available (eg, Dobell's Solution Tablets) or the solution may be prepared by the pharmacist. If powders or tablets are supplied, they must be free from insoluble material in order to produce a clear solution. Tablets are produced by the usual processes but any lubricants or diluents used must be readily soluble in water. Boric acid may be used as a lubricant and sodium chloride normally is used as a diluent. Tablets deteriorate on exposure to moist air and should be stored in airtight containers.

Douches are not official as a class of preparations but several substances in the compendia frequently are employed as such in weak solutions. *Vaginal douches* are the most common type of douche and are used for cleansing the vagina and hygienic purposes. Liquid concentrates or powders, which may be prepared in bulk or as single-use packages, should be diluted or dissolved in the appropriate amount of warm water prior to use.

The ingredients used in vaginal douches include antimicrobial agents such as benzalkonium chloride, the parabens or chlorothymol, and anesthetics or antipruritics such as phenol or menthol. Astringents such as zinc sulfate or potassium alum, surface-active agents such as sodium lauryl sulfate, and chemicals to alter the pH such as sodium bicarbonate or citric acid also are used.

Enemas

A number of solutions are administered rectally for the local effects of the medication (eg, hydrocortisone) or for systemic absorption (eg, aminophylline). In the case of aminophylline, the rectal route of administration minimizes the undesirable gastrointestinal reactions associated with oral therapy.[24] Clinically effective blood levels of the agents are usually obtained within 30 minutes following rectal instillation. Corticosteroids are administered as retention enemas or continuous drip as adjunctive treatment of some patients with ulcerative colitis.

Enema preparations are rectal injections employed to evacuate the bowel (evacuation enemas), influence the general system by absorption, or to affect a local disease. The latter two are called retention enemas. They may possess anthelmintic, nutritive, sedative, or stimulating properties, or they may contain radiopaque substances for roentgenographic examination of the lower bowel.

Sodium chloride, sodium bicarbonate, sodium monohydrogen phosphate, sodium dihydrogen phosphate, glycerin, docusate potassium, and light mineral oil are used in enemas to evacuate the bowel. These substances may be used alone, in combination with each other, or in combination with irritants such as soap. Evacuation enemas usually are given at body temperature in quantities of 1 to 2 pt injected slowly with a syringe.

An official retention enema used for systemic purposes is aminophylline. Retention enemas are to be retained in the intestine and should not be used in larger quantities than 150 mL for an adult. Usually, the volume is considerably smaller, such as a few mL. *Microenema* is a term used to describe these small-volume preparations. Vehicles for retention microenemas have been formulated with small quantities of ethanol and propylene glycol, and no significant difference in irritation, as compared with water, was found. A number of other drugs such as valproic acid, indomethacin, and metronidazole have been formulated as microenemas for the purpose of absorption.

Gargles

Gargles are aqueous solutions frequently containing antiseptics, antibiotics, and/or anesthetics used for treating the pharynx and nasopharynx by forcing air from the lungs through the gargle that is held in the throat; subsequently, the gargle is expectorated. Many gargles must be diluted with water prior to use. Although mouthwashes are considered as a separate class of pharmaceuticals, many are used as gargles either as is, or diluted with water.

A gargle/mouthwash containing the antibiotic tyrothricin has been shown to provide levels of gramicidin, a component of tyrothricin, in saliva when used as a gargle rather than a mouthwash.[25] Higher saliva levels of gramicidin were obtained when a lozenge formulation was employed. Rapid relief of pharyngeal and oral pain was obtained when Cepacaine solution, which contains a topical anesthetic, was used as a gargle.[26]

Nystatin is administered in both powder and liquid form to treat oral fungal infections.[27] The medication is taken by placing one-half of the dose in each side of the mouth, swishing it around as long as possible, then gargling and swallowing. Hydrogen peroxide is a source of nascent oxygen and a weak topical antibacterial agent. Hydrogen peroxide topical solution has been used as a mouthwash or gargle in the treatment of pharyngitis or Vincent's stomatitis.[28,29] Hydrogen peroxide has also been applied in root canals of teeth or other dental pulp cavities. While used topically as a 1.5–3% solution for cleansing wounds, hydrogen peroxide is usually diluted with an equal volume of water for use as a mouthwash or gargle. Hydrogen peroxide gel is used topically as a 1.5% gel for cleansing minor wounds or irritations of the mouth or gums. A small amount of the gel is applied to the affected area, allowed to remain in place for at least 1 minute, and then expectorated; the gel may be used up to 4 times daily (after meals and at bedtime).

Mouthwashes

Mouthwashes are aqueous solutions often in concentrated form containing one or more active ingredients and excipients described below. They are used by swishing the liquid in the oral cavity. Mouthwashes can be used for two purposes, therapeutic and cosmetic. Therapeutic rinses or washes can be formulated to reduce plaque, gingivitis, dental caries, and stomatitis. Cosmetic mouthwashes may be formulated to reduce bad breath through the use of antimicrobial and/or flavoring agents.

Recent information indicates that mouthwashes are being used as a dosage form for a number of specific problems in the oral cavity; for example, mouthwashes containing a combination of antihistamines, hydrocortisone, nystatin, and tetracycline have been prepared from commercially available suspensions, powders, syrups, or solutions for the treatment of stomatitis, a painful side effect of cancer chemotherapy. Other drugs include allopurinol, also used for the treatment of stomatitis,[30] pilocarpine for xerostoma (dry mouth),[31] amphotericin B for oral candidiasis,[32] and chlorhexidine gluconate for plaque control.[33] Mouthwashes may be used for diagnostic purposes. For example, oral cancer and lesions are detected using toluidine blue mouth rinse.[34]

Commercial products (eg, Cepacol, Listerine, Micrin, or Scope) vary widely in composition. Tricca has described the excipients generally found in Mouthwashes as alcohols, surfactants, flavors, and coloring agents.[35] Alcohol is often present in the range of 10% to 20%. It enhances the flavor, provides sharpness to the taste, aids in masking the unpleasant taste of active ingredients, functions as a solubilizing agent for some flavoring agents, and may function as a preservative. Humectants such as glycerin and sorbitol may form 5% to 20% of the mouthwash. These agents increase the viscosity of the preparation and provide a certain *body* or *mouth feel* to the product. They enhance the sweetness of the product and, along with the ethanol, improve the preservative qualities of the product.

Surfactants of the nonionic class such as polyoxyethylene/polyoxypropylene block copolymers or polyoxyethylene derivatives of sorbitol fatty acid esters may be used. The concentration range is 0.1% to 0.5%. An anionic surfactant occasionally used is sodium lauryl sulfate. Surfactants are used because they aid in the solubilization of flavors and in the removal of debris by providing foaming action. Cationic surfactants such as cetylpyridinium chloride are used for their antimicrobial properties, but these tend to impart a bitter taste.

Flavors are used in conjunction with alcohol and humectants to overcome disagreeable tastes, at the same time flavors must be safe to use. The principle flavoring agents are peppermint, spearmint, cinnamon, wintergreen oils, menthol, or methyl salicylate. Other flavoring agents may be used singly or in combination. Finally, coloring agents also are used in these products.

Juices

A juice is prepared from fresh ripe fruit, is aqueous in character, and is used in making syrups that are employed as vehicles. The freshly expressed juice is preserved with benzoic acid and allowed to stand at room temperature for several days, until the pectins that naturally are present are destroyed by enzymatic action, as indicated by the filtered juice yielding a clear solution with alcohol. Pectins, if allowed to remain, would cause precipitation in the final syrup.

Cherry Juice and Tomato Juice are described in the USP. Artificial flavors now have replaced many of the natural fruit juices. Although they lack the flavor of the natural juice, they are more stable and easier to incorporate into the final pharmaceutical form. Commercial juices such as orange, apple, grape, and mixed vegetables have been used recently to prepare extemporaneous preparations of cholestyramine[36] and nizatidine.[37] Information on cranberry juice indicates that it may be effective in controlling some urinary tract infections and urolithiasis.[38]

Nasal Solutions

Nasal solutions are usually aqueous solutions designed to be administered to the nasal passages in drops or sprays. Other nasal preparations may be in the form of emulsions or suspensions. The adult nasal cavity has about a 20 mL capacity with a large surface area (about 180 cm^2) for drug absorption afforded by the microvilli present along the pseudo-stratified columnar epithelial cells of the nasal mucosa.[39] The nasal tissue is highly vascularized making it an attractive site for rapid and efficient systemic absorption. Another advantage of nasal delivery is that it avoids first-pass metabolism by the liver. For some peptides and small molecular compounds, intranasal bioavailability has been comparable to that of injections. However, bioavailability decreases as the molecular weight of a compound increases, and for proteins composed of more than 27 amino acids bioavailability may be low.[40] Various pharmaceutical techniques and functional excipients, such as surfactants, have been shown to be capable of enhancing the nasal absorption of large molecules.[41,42]

Many drugs are administered for their local sympathomimetic effects to reduce nasal congestion, such as Ephedrine Sulfate Nasal Solution, USP or Naphazoline Hydrochloride Nasal Solution, USP. A few other preparations, Lypressin Nasal Solution USP and Oxytocin Nasal Solution USP, are administered in spray form for their systemic effect for the treatment of diabetes insipidus and milk letdown prior to breast feeding, respectively. Examples of commercial products for nasal use are listed in Table 39-3.

Nasal solutions are formulated to be similar to nasal secretions with regard to toxicity, pH, and viscosity so that normal ciliary action is maintained. Thus, aqueous nasal solutions usually are isotonic and slightly buffered to maintain a pH of 5.5 to 6.5. In addition, antimicrobial preservatives, similar to those used in ophthalmic preparations, and appropriate drug stabilizers, if required, are included in the formulation.

Current studies indicate that nasal sprays are deposited mainly in the atrium and cleared slowly into the pharynx with the patient in an upright position. Drops spread more extensively

than the spray, and three drops cover most of the walls of the nasal cavity with the patient in a supine position and head tilted back and turned left and right.[43,44] It is suggested that drop delivery, with appropriate movement by the patient, leads to extensive coverage of the walls of the nasal cavity.

Most nasal solutions are packaged in dropper or spray bottles, usually containing 15 to 30 mL of medication. The formulator should ensure the product is stable in the containers and the pharmacist should keep the packages tightly closed during periods of nonuse. The patient should be advised that should the solution become discolored or contain precipitated matter, it must be discarded.

Otic Solutions

These solutions occasionally are referred to as ear or aural preparations. Other otic preparations include suspensions and ointments for topical application in the ear. Ear preparations are usually placed in the ear canal by drops or in small amounts for the removal of excessive cerumen (ear wax) or for the treatment of ear infections, inflammation, or pain.

The main classes of drugs used for topical administration to the ear include analgesics, such as benzocaine; antibiotics, such as neomycin; and anti-inflammatory agents, such as cortisone (Table 39-4). The USP preparations include Antipyrine and Benzocaine Otic Solution. The Neomycin and Polymyxin B Sulfates and Hydrocortisone Otic Solutions may contain appropriate buffers, solvents, and dispersants usually in an aqueous solution. The main solvents used in these preparations include glycerin or water. The viscous glycerin vehicle permits the drug to remain in the ear for a long time. Anhydrous glycerin, being hygroscopic, tends to remove moisture from surrounding tissues, thus reducing swelling. Viscous liquids such as glycerin or propylene glycol are used either alone or in combination with a surfactant to aid in the removal of cerumen (ear wax). To provide sufficient time for aqueous preparations to act, it is necessary for patients to remain on their side for a few minutes so the drops do not run out of the ear. Otic preparations are dispensed in a container that permits the administration of drops.

Irrigation Solutions

Irrigation solutions are sterile, non-pyrogenic solutions used to wash or bathe surgical incisions, wounds, or body tissues. Because they come in contact with exposed tissue, they must meet stringent USP requirements for sterility, total solids, and bacterial endotoxins. These products may be prepared by dissolving the active ingredient in Water for Injection. They are packaged in single-dose containers, preferably Type I or Type II glass, or suitable plastic containers, and then sterilized. A number of irrigations are described in the USP, including Acetic

Table 39-3. Examples of Commercial Nasal Preparations

PRODUCT NAME	MANUFACTURER	ACTIVE INGREDIENT	INDICATION
Atrovent Nasal Spray	Boehringer Ingelheim	Ipratropium bromide 0.06%	Seasonal or Allergic Rhinitis
Beconase AQ Nasal Spray	GlaxoSmithKline	Beclomethasone dipropionate, monohydrate 42 mcg	Seasonal or Allergic Rhinitis
Miacalcin	Novartis	Calcitonin-salmon, 2200 I.U. per mL	Postmenopausal osteoporosis
Nasalcrom Nasal Spray	Pharmacia	Cromolyn sodium 5.2 mg	Seasonal or Allergic Rhinitis
Nasarel Nasal Spray	IVAX	Flunisolide	Seasonal or perennial rhinitis
Nicotrol Nasal Spray	Pfizer	Nicotine 0.5 mg	Smoking Cessation
Neo-Synephrine	Bayer	Oxymetazoline hydrochloride 0.05%	Decongestion
Rhinocort Aqua Nasal Spray	Astra-Zeneca	Budesonide 32mcg	Seasonal or Allergic Rhinitis
Stadol Nasal Spray	Bristol-Myers Squibb	Butorphanol tartrate, 1 mg	Pain Relief, Migraines
Stimate Nasal Spray	Aventis	Desmopressin Acetate 1.5 mg/mL	Hemophilia A or von Willebrand disease
Synare Nasal Solution	Searle	Nafarelin acetate 2 mg/mL	Endometriosis
Tyzine	Bradley Pharmaceuticals	Tetrahydrozoline hydrochloride	Decongestion

Table 39-4. Examples of Commercial Otic Preparations

PRODUCT NAME	MANUFACTURER	ACTIVE INGREDIENT	INDICATION
Americaine-Otic	Celltech	Benzocaine	Local anesthetics
Cerumenex Ear Drops	Purdue	Triethanolamine polypeptide oleate-condensate	Removal of earwax
Chloromycetin Otic	Pfizer	Chloramphenicol	Antiinfective
Cipro HC Otic	Alcon	Ciprofloxacin hydrochloride and hydrocortisone	Acute otitis externa
Cortisporin	GlaxoSmithKline	Neomycin and Polymyxin B Sulfates and Hydrocortisone	Antibacterial and anti-inflammatory
Debrox Drops	GlaxoSmithKline	Carbamide peroxide	Removal of earwax
Floxin Otic	Daiichi	Ofloxacin	Antiinfective
Tympagesic	Savage	Antipyrine, Benzocaine, and Phenylephrine Hydrochloride	Topical anesthetic

Acid Irrigation for bladder irrigation, Dimethyl Sulfoxide Irrigation for relief of internal cystitis, Glycine Irrigation for transurethral prostatic resection, Ringer's Irrigation for general irrigation, Neomycin and Polymyxin B Sulfates Solution for Irrigation for infection, and Sodium Chloride Irrigation for washing wounds.

Extemporaneous formulations frequently are prepared using an isotonic solution of sodium chloride as the solvent. For example, cefazolin or gentamicin in 0.9% sodium chloride are used as anti-infective irrigations[45] and 5-fluororacil in 0.9% sodium chloride is employed for bladder irrigation.[46] Alum, either potassium or ammonium, in either sterile water or 0.9% sodium chloride for irrigation has been used for bladder hemorrhage. Amphotericin in sterile water has been used for the treatment of localized infections on the dermis, the bladder, and urinary tract.[47] All the extemporaneous preparations should meet the general requirements noted above for USP irrigations.

PREPARATION OF SOLUTIONS

The method of preparation for many solutions is given in the compendia. These procedures fall into three main categories: simple solutions, solution by chemical reaction, and solution by extraction.

Simple Solutions are prepared by dissolving the solute in most of the solvent, mixing until dissolved, then adding sufficient solvent to bring the solution up to the proper volume. The solvent may contain other ingredients that stabilize or solubilize the active ingredient. Calcium Hydroxide Topical Solution USP (Lime Water), Sodium Phosphates Oral Solution USP, and Strong Iodine Solution USP are examples.

Calcium Hydroxide Topical Solution USP contains, in each 100 mL, not less than 140 mg of $Ca(OH)_2$. The solution is prepared by agitating vigorously 3 g of calcium hydroxide with 1000 mL of cool, purified water. Excess calcium hydroxide is allowed to settle out and the clear, supernatant liquid dispensed. An increase in solvent temperature usually implies an increase in solute solubility. This rule does not apply, however, to the solubility of calcium hydroxide in water, which decreases with increasing temperature. The official solution is prepared at 25°C.

Solutions containing hydroxides react with the carbon dioxide in the atmosphere.

$$OH^- + CO_2 \rightarrow HCO_3^-$$

$$OH^- + HCO_3^- \rightarrow CO_3{}^{2-} + H_2O$$

Calcium Hydroxide Topical Solution, therefore, should be preserved in well-filled, tight containers, at a temperature not exceeding 25°C.

Strong Iodine Solution USP contains, in each 100 mL, 4.5 to 5.5 g of iodine, and 9.5 to 10.5 g of potassium iodide. It is prepared by dissolving 50 g of iodine in 100 mL of purified water

containing 100 g of potassium iodide. Sufficient purified water then is added to make 1000 mL of solution. One g of iodine dissolves in 2950 mL of water. However, solutions of iodides dissolve large quantities of iodine. Strong Iodine Solution is, therefore, a solution of polyiodides in excess iodide.

$$I^- + nI_2 \rightarrow I_{(2n+1)}{}^-$$

Doubly charged anions may be found also.

$$2I^- + nI_2 \rightarrow I_{(2n+2)}{}^{2-}$$

Strong Iodine Solution is used in the treatment of iodide deficiency disorders such as endemic goiter.

Several antibiotics (eg, cloxacillin sodium, nafcillin sodium, and vancomycin), because they are relatively unstable in aqueous solution, are prepared by manufacturers as dry powders or granules in combination with suitable buffers, colors, diluents, dispersants, flavors, and/or preservatives. These preparations, Cloxacillin Sodium for Oral Solution, Nafcillin for Oral Solution, and Vancomycin Hydrochloride for Oral Solution meet the requirements of the USP. Immediately prior to dispensing to the patient, the pharmacist adds the appropriate amount of water. The products are stable for up to 14 days when refrigerated.[48] This period usually provides sufficient time for the patient to complete the administration of all the medication.

Solutions by chemical reaction are prepared by reacting two or more solutes with each other in a suitable solvent. An example is Aluminum Subacetate Topical Solution USP. Aluminum sulfate (145 g) is dissolved in 600 mL of cold water. The solution is filtered, and precipitated calcium carbonate (70 g) is added, in several portions, with constant stirring. Acetic acid (160 mL) is added slowly and the mixture set aside for 24 hours. The product is filtered and the magma on the Buchner filter washed with cold water until the total filtrate measures 1,000 mL.

The solution contains pentaquohydroxo- and tetraquodihydroxoaluminum(III) acetates and sulfates dissolved in an aqueous medium saturated with calcium sulfate. The solution contains a small amount of acetic acid. It may be stabilized by the addition of not more than 0.9% boric acid. The reactions involved in the preparation of the solution are given below. The hexaquo aluminum cations first are converted to the nonirritating

$$[Al(H_2O)_5(OH)]^{2+} \text{ and } [Al(H_2O)_4(OH)_2]^+ \text{ cations.}$$

$$[Al(H_2O)_6]^{3+} + CO_3{}^{2-} \rightarrow [Al(H_2O)_5(OH)]^{2+} + HCO_3^-$$

$$[Al(H_2O)_6]^{3+} + HCO_3^- \rightarrow [Al(H_2O)_5(OH)]^{2+} + H_2O + CO_2$$

As the concentration of the hexaquo cations decreases, secondary reactions involving carbonate and bicarbonate occur.

$$[Al(H_2O)_5(OH)]^{2+} + CO_3{}^{2-} \rightarrow [Al(H_2O)_4(OH)_2]^+ + HCO_3^-$$

$$[Al(H_2O)_5(OH)]^{2+} + HCO_3^- \rightarrow [Al(H_2O)_4(OH)_2]^+ + H_2CO_3$$

The pH of the solution now favors the precipitation of dissolved calcium ions as the insoluble sulfate. Acetic acid now is added.

The bicarbonate that is formed in the final stages of the procedure is removed as carbon dioxide.

Aluminum Subacetate Topical Solution is used in the preparation of Aluminum Acetate Topical Solution USP (Burow's Solution). The latter solution contains 15 mL of glacial acetic acid, 545 mL of Aluminum Subacetate Topical Solution and sufficient water to make 1000 mL. It is defined as a solution of aluminum acetate in approximately 5%, by weight, of acetic acid in water. It may be stabilized by the addition of not more than 0.6% boric acid.

Often, drugs or pharmaceutical necessities of vegetable or animal origin often are extracted with water or with water containing other substances. Preparations of this type may be classified as solutions but, more often, are classified as extracts and are described at the end of this chapter.

SWEET AND OTHER VISCID AQUEOUS SOLUTIONS

Solutions that are sweet or viscid include syrups, honeys, mucilages, and jellies. All of these are viscous liquids or semisolids. The basic sweet or viscid substances giving body to these preparations are sugars, polyols, and / or polysaccharides.

Syrups

Syrups are concentrated, viscous, aqueous solutions of sugar or a sugar substitute with or without flavors and medical substances. When Purified Water alone is used in making the solution of sucrose, the preparation is known as *syrup*, or *simple syrup* if the sucrose concentration is 85%. Syrups are also used to apply sugar coatings to tablets, particularly those with disagreeable aromas or acrid taste. In addition to sucrose, certain other polyols, such as glycerin or sorbitol, may be added to retard crystallization of sucrose or to increase the solubility of added ingredients. Alcohol often is included as a preservative and also as a solvent for flavors; further resistance to microbial attack can be enhanced by incorporating antimicrobial agents. When the aqueous preparation contains some added medicinal substance, the syrup is called a *medicated syrup*. Flavored syrups are usually not medicated, but rather contain various aromatic or pleasantly flavored substances and are intended to be used as a vehicle or flavor for prescriptions, such as Acacia, Cherry, Cocoa, Orange, and Raspberry USP.

Flavored syrups offer unusual opportunities as vehicles in extemporaneous compounding and are accepted readily by both children and adults. Because they contain no, or very little, alcohol they are vehicles of choice for many of the drugs that are prescribed by pediatricians. Their lack of alcohol makes them superior solvents for water-soluble substances. However, sucrose-based medicines continuously administered to children apparently cause an increase in dental caries and gingivitis; consequently, alternate formulations of the drug either unsweetened or sweetened with noncariogenic substances should be considered. A knowledge of the sugar content of liquid medicines is useful for patients who are on a restricted calorie intake; a list has been prepared by Greenwood.[49]

As noted above, sucrose-based syrups may be substituted in whole or in part by other agents in the preparation of medicated syrups. A solution of sorbitol, or a mixture of polyols, such as sorbitol and glycerin, is commonly used. Sorbitol Solution, USP, which contains 64% by weight of the polyhydric alcohol sorbitol, is often used in sugar-free and children's preparations. However, reports of adverse reactions to sorbitol are largely due to its action as an osmotic laxative when ingested orally.[50] Ingestion of large quantities of sorbitol (> 20 g/day in adults) should therefore be avoided.

Syrups possess remarkable taste-masking properties for bitter or saline drugs. Syrups flavored with Glycyrrhizin, a triterpene glycoside extracted from licorice root, has been recommended for disguising the salty taste of bromides, iodides, and chlorides.[51] This has been attributed to its colloidal character and its double sweetness—the immediate sweetness of the sugar and the lingering sweetness of the glycyrrhizin. This syrup is also of value in masking bitterness in preparations containing the B complex vitamins. Acacia Syrup USP is of particular value as a vehicle for masking the disagreeable taste of many medicaments because of its colloidal character. Raspberry Syrup, USP is one of the most efficient flavoring agents and is especially useful in masking the taste of bitter drugs. Many factors, however, enter into the choice of a suitable flavoring agent. Literature reports are often contradictory and there appears to be no substitute for the taste panel when developing new formulations.[52]

It is important that the concentration of sucrose approach but not quite reach the saturation point. In dilute solutions sucrose provides an excellent nutrient for molds, yeasts, and other microorganisms. In concentrations of 65% by weight or more, the solution will retard the growth of such microorganisms. However, a saturated solution may lead to crystallization of a part of the sucrose under conditions of changing temperature. Several commercial medicated syrups are available for a variety of indications (Table 39-5).

Preparation of Syrups

Syrups are generally prepared using one of four techniques: solution with heat, solution by agitation, addition of sucrose to a liquid medication or flavored liquid, and percolation. The method of choice depends on the physical and chemical characteristics of the substances entering into the preparation. In many cases, syrups may be successfully prepared by more than one of the above methods, and the selection may simply be a matter of preference on the part of the pharmacist. Many of the compendial syrups do not have a designated method for preparation because most are commercially available and are not prepared extemporaneously by the pharmacist.

Solution with Heat is a suitable preparation method if the constituents are not volatile or degraded by heat, and when it is desirable to make the syrup rapidly. Purified water is heated to 80°–85°C, removed from its heat source, and sucrose is added with vigorous agitation. Then, other required heat-stable components are added to the hot syrup, the mixture is allowed to cool, and its volume is adjusted to the proper level by the addition of purified water. In instances in which heat labile agents or volatile substances, such as flavors and alcohol, are to be

Table 39-5. Examples of Commercial Medicated Syrups

PRODUCT NAME	MANUFACTURER	ACTIVE INGREDIENT & DOSE	INDICATION
Chlor-Trimeton	Schering-Plough	2 mg chlorpheniramine maleate / 5 mL	Allergic rhinitus
Children's Benadryl	Pfizer	12.5 mg diphenhydramine HCl / 5 mL	Allergic rhinitus
Demerol Syrup	Sanofi	50 mg meperidine HCl / 5 mL	Narcotic analgesic
Ditropan Syrup	Ortho-McNeil	5 mg Oxybutynin chloride / 5 mL	Overactive bladder
Dramamine	Pfizer	12.5 mg dimenhydrinate / 5 mL	Antiemitic
Phenergan Syrup	Wyeth-Ayerst	25 mg promethazine HCl / 5 mL	Antiemitic
Symmetrel Syrup	Endo	50 mg amantadine HCl / 5 mL	Antiviral

added, they are generally incorporated into the syrup after cooling to room temperature.

When heat is used in the preparation of syrups, there is almost certain to be an inversion of a slight portion of the sucrose. Sucrose, a disaccharide, may be hydrolyzed into monosaccharides, dextrose (glucose), and fructose (levulose). This hydrolytic reaction is referred to as *inversion*, and the combination of the two monosaccharide products is *invert sugar*. Sucrose solutions are dextrorotary, but as hydrolysis proceeds, the optical rotation decreases and becomes negative when the reaction is complete. The rate of inversion is increased greatly by the presence of acids; the hydrogen ion acts as a catalyst in this hydrolytic reaction. Invert sugar is more readily fermentable than sucrose and tends to be darker in color. Nevertheless, its two reducing sugars are of value in retarding the oxidation of other substances.

The fructose formed during inversion is sweeter than sucrose, and thus the resulting syrup is sweeter than the original syrup. The relative sweetness of fructose, sucrose, and dextrose is in the ratio of 173:100:74. Thus, invert sugar is $1/100 (173 + 74)1/2 = 1.23$ times as sweet as sucrose. Fructose is responsible for the darkening of syrup, as it is amber in color. If the syrup is significantly overheated, sucrose is carmelized and becomes darker. Excessive heating of syrups is undesirable because inversion occurs with an increased tendency to ferment. Syrups cannot be sterilized in an autoclave without some caramelization.

Agitation without Heat is used in cases in which heat would cause degradation or volatilize formulation constituents. On a small scale, sucrose and other formulation ingredients may be dissolved in purified water by placing the ingredients in a vessel of greater capacity than the volume of syrup to be prepared, allowing intense agitation without spillage. This process is more time-consuming than solution with heat, but the product has greater stability. Large glass-lined and stainless steel tanks equipped with mechanical mixers are employed in the large scale preparation of syrups.

Often, simple syrup or some other non-medicated syrup, rather than sucrose, is employed as the sweetening agent and vehicle. When solid agents are to be added to a syrup, it is best to dissolve them in a minimal amount of purified water and then incorporate the resulting solution into the syrup. When solid substances are added directly to syrups, they dissolve slowly because the viscous nature of the syrup does not permit the solid substance to distribute readily.

This method and that previously described are used for the preparation of a wide variety of preparations that are described popularly as syrups. Most cough syrups, for example, contain sucrose and one or more active ingredients. Many other active ingredients (eg, ephedrine sulfate, dicyclomine hydrochloride, chloral hydrate, or chlorpromazine hydrochloride) are marketed as syrups. Like cough syrups, these preparations are flavored, colored, and recommended in those instances where the patient cannot swallow the solid dosage form.

Addition of sucrose to a liquid medication or flavored liquid is often used with fluidextracts, tinctures. Syrups made in this way usually develop precipitates because alcohol is often an ingredient of the liquids thus used, and the resinous and oily substances solubilized by the alcohol precipitate when water is added. A modification of this process entails mixing the fluidextract or tincture with the water, allowing the mixture to stand to permit the separation of insoluble constituents, filtering, and then dissolving the sucrose in the filtrate. It is obvious that this procedure is not permissible when the precipitated ingredients are the valuable medicinal agents.

In the *percolation* method, either purified water or the source of the medicinal component is passed slowly through a bed of crystalline sucrose, thus dissolving it and forming a syrup. This latter method really involves two separate procedures: first the preparation of the extractive of the drug and then the preparation of the syrup. To be successful in using this process, technique is critical: (1) the percolator used should be

cylindrical or semicylindrical and cone-shaped as it nears the lower orifice; (2) a coarse granular sugar must be used, otherwise it will coalesce into a compact mass, which the liquid cannot permeate. The percolation method is applied on a commercial scale for the making of compendial syrups as well as those for confectionary use.

Ipecac syrup is prepared by percolation by adding glycerin and syrup to an extractive of powdered ipecac obtained by percolation. The drug ipecac consists of the dried rhizome and roots of *Cephaelis ipecacuanha* and contains the medicinally active alkaloids, emetine, cephaeline, and psychotrine. These alkaloids are extracted from the powdered ipecac by percolation with a hydroalcoholic solvent. The syrup is categorized as an emetic with a usual dose of 15 mL. This amount of syrup is commonly used in the management of poisoning in children when the evacuation of stomach contents is desirable. About 80% of children given this dose will vomit within a half hour. Bulimics have used ipecac to bring on attacks of vomiting in an attempt to lose more weight.[53] Pharmacists must be aware of this abuse and warn these individuals because one of the active ingredients is emetine. With chronic abuse of the syrup, emetine builds up toxic levels within body tissues and in 3 to 4 months can do irreversible damage to heart muscles resulting in symptoms mimicking a heart attack.

Syrups should be made in quantities that can be consumed within a few months, except in those cases where special facilities can be employed for their preservation; a low temperature is the best method. Concentration without super-saturation is also a condition favorable to preservation. The USP states that syrups may contain preservatives. Glycerin, methylparaben, benzoic acid, and sodium benzoate may be used to prevent bacterial and mold growth. Combinations of alkyl esters of *p*-hydroxybenzoic acid are effective inhibitors of yeasts that have been implicated in the contamination of commercial syrups. Syrups should be preserved in well-dried bottles, preferably those that have been sterilized. These bottles should not hold more than is likely to be required during 4 to 6 weeks and should be filled completely, carefully closed, and stored in a cool, dark place.

Some examples of syrup formulations are noted below:

Ferrous Sulfate Syrup

Ferrous Sulfate	40.0 g
Citric Acid	2.1 g
Peppermint Spirit	2 mL
Sucrose	825 g
Purified Water	to make 1000.0 mL

Dissolve the Ferrous Sulfate, Citric Acid, Peppermint Spirit, and 200 g of the Sucrose in 450 mL of Purified Water, and filter the solution until clear. Dissolve the remainder of the Sucrose in the clear filtrate, and add Purified Water to make 1000 mL. Mix, and filter, if necessary, through a pledget of cotton.

Amantadine Hydrochloride Syrup

Amantadine Hydrochloride	10.0 g
Citric Acid	2.1 g
Artifical Raspberry Flavor	2 mL
Methyl paraben	2 g
Propyl paraben	0.5 g
Sorbitol Solution	to make 1000 mL

Dissolve the amantadine hydrochloride, the Citric Acid, flavor and preservatives in the sorbitol solution.

Syrups are useful for preparing liquid oral dosage forms from not only the pure drug, as described above, but also injections, capsules, or tablets if the pure drug is not readily available. If the drug and all the excipients in the preparation, such as injectables or capsules, are water-soluble, a solution should result if a syrup is prepared. On the other hand, if the preparation to be used contains water-insoluble ingredients, as is usually the case with tablets and some capsules, a suspension will be formed. Several of these preparations have been described in the literature, in regard to their formulation, stability, and bioavailability. Some drugs that have been prepared from either the pure drug or an injectable form include midazolam, atropine, aminocaproic acid, terbutaline, procainamide, chloroquine, propranolol, and citrated caffeine.[54,55] If the appropriate salt of the drug is used, a solution will result.

When tablets are introduced to a syrup formulation, a suspension is often formed because there are water-insoluble ingredients used in tablet preparations. Examples of medicated syrups prepared from tablets are clonidine hydrochloride, cefuroxime axetil, famotidine, terbutaline sulfate, spironolactone, ranitidine, and rifampin.[56,57] The resulting suspensions should have a uniform distribution of particles so that a consistent dose is obtained. If the materials are not distributed uniformly, more appropriate suspending formulations should be considered, which are described later in the chapter. If pharmaceutical preparations contain a liquid that is insoluble in water, such as valproic acid or simethicone, to be incorporated into syrups, an emulsion will form and it will be difficult to prepare a uniform product.

Honeys

Honeys are thick liquid preparations somewhat allied to the syrups, differing in that honey, instead of syrup, is used as a base. They are unimportant as a class of preparations today, but at one time, before sugar was available and honey was the most common sweetening agent, they were used widely. Honey and sugar pastes are used to a small extent and have been discussed in the pharmaceutical literature for topical application for the treatment of certain types of ulcers and abscesses.[58]

Mucilages

Mucilages are thick, viscid, adhesive liquids, produced by dispersing gum in water, or by extracting the mucilaginous principles from vegetable substances with water. The mucilages all are prone to decomposition, showing appreciable decrease in viscosity on storage; they should never be made in quantities larger than can be used immediately, unless a preservative is added. Mucilages are used primarily to aid in suspending insoluble substances in liquids; their colloidal character and viscosity help prevent immediate sedimentation. Examples include sulfur in lotions, resin in mixtures, and oils in emulsions. Both tragacanth and acacia either are partially or completely insoluble in alcohol. Tragacanth is precipitated from solution by alcohol, but acacia, on the other hand, is soluble in diluted alcoholic solutions. A 60% solution of acacia may be prepared with 20% alcohol, and a 4% solution of acacia may be prepared even with 50% alcohol.

Recent research on mucilages includes the preparation of mucilage from plantain and the identification of its sugars, the preparation and suspending properties of cocoa gum, the preparation of glycerin ointments using flaxseed mucilage, and the consideration of various gums and mucilages obtained from several Indian plants for pharmaceutical purposes.

Several synthetic mucilage-like substances such as *polyvinyl alcohol, methylcellulose, carboxymethylcellulose,* and related substances are used at the appropriate concentration as mucilage substitutes, and emulsifying and suspending agents. Methylcellulose is used widely as a bulk laxative because it absorbs water and swells to a hydrogel in the intestine, in much the same manner as *psyllium* or *karaya* gum. Methylcellulose Oral Solution USP is a flavored solution of the agent. It may be prepared by adding slowly the methylcellulose to about one-third the amount of boiling water, with stirring, until it is thoroughly wetted. Cold water then should be added and the wetted material allowed to dissolve while stirring. The viscosity of the solution will depend upon the concentration and the specifications of the methylcellulose. The synthetic gums are non-glycogenetic and may be used in the preparation of diabetic syrups. Sodium carboxymethyl cellulose of a medium grade in water (0.25–1%) is generally suitable for preparing a suspending vehicle. Several formulas for such syrups, based on sodium carboxymethylcellulose, have been proposed.

Uniformly smooth mucilages sometimes are difficult to prepare because of the uneven wetting of the gums. In general, it is best to use fine gum particles and disperse them with agitation in a small quantity of 95% alcohol or in cold water (except for methylcellulose). The appropriate amount of water then can be added with constant stirring. A review of the chemistry and properties of acacia and other gums has been prepared.[59]

Jellies

Jellies are a class of gels in which the structural coherent matrix contains a high portion of liquid, usually water. They are similar to mucilages, in that they may be prepared from similar gums, but they differ from the latter in having a jelly-like consistency. A whole gum of the best quality, rather than a powdered gum, is desirable to obtain a clear preparation of uniform consistency. Although the specific thickening agent in the USP jellies is not indicated, reference usually is made in the monograph to a water-soluble, sterile, viscous base. These preparations also may be formulated with water from acacia, chondrus, gelatin, carboxymethylcellulose, hydroxyethylcellulose, and similar substances.

Jellies are used as lubricants for surgical gloves, catheters, and rectal thermometers. Lidocaine Hydrochloride Jelly USP is used as a topical anesthetic. Therapeutic vaginal jellies are available and certain jelly-like preparations are used for contraceptive purposes, which often contain surface-active agents to enhance the spermatocidal properties of the jelly. Aromatics, such as methyl salicylate and eucalyptol, often are added to give the preparation a desirable odor.

Jellies are prone to microbial contamination and therefore contain preservatives; for example, methyl *p*-hydroxybenzoate is used as a preservative in a base for medicated jellies. One base contains sodium alginate, glycerin, calcium gluconate, and water. The calcium ions cause a cross-linking with sodium alginate to form a gel of firmer consistency. A discussion of gels is provided later in the chapter.

NONAQUEOUS SOLUTIONS

It is difficult to evaluate fairly the importance of nonaqueous solvents in pharmaceutical processes. That they are important in the manufacture of pharmaceuticals is an understatement. However, pharmaceutical preparations, and, in particular, those intended for internal use, rarely contain more than minor quantities of the organic solvents that are common to the manufacturing or analytical operation. Products of commerce for internal use may contain solvents such as ethanol, glycerin,

propylene glycol, certain oils, and liquid paraffin. Preparations intended for external use may contain solvents in addition to those just mentioned, namely isopropyl alcohol, polyethylene glycols, various ethers, and certain esters.

Although the lines between aqueous and nonaqueous preparations tend to blur in those cases where the solvent is water-soluble, it is possible to categorize a number of products as nonaqueous. This section is, therefore, devoted to groups of nonaqueous solutions: the alcoholic or hydroalcoholic solutions (eg, elixirs and spirits), ethereal solutions (eg, collodions), glycerin solutions (eg, glycerins), oleaginous solutions (eg, liniments, oleovitamins, and toothache drops), inhalations, and inhalants.

Although the above list is limited, a wide variety of solvents are used in various pharmaceutical preparations. Solvents such as glycerol formal, dimethylacetamide, and glycerol dimethylketal have been suggested for some products produced by the industry. However, the toxicity of many of these solvents is not well established and, for this reason, careful clinical studies should be carried out on the formulated product before it is released to the marketplace. It is essential that the toxicity of solvents be tested appropriately and approved to avoid problems; for example, lives were lost in 1937 when diethylene glycol was used in an elixir of sulfanilamide. The result of this tragedy was the 1938 Federal Food, Drug, and Cosmetic Act, which required that products be tested for both safety and effectiveness.

COLLODIONS

Collodions are liquid preparations containing pyroxylin, a partially nitrated cellulose, in a mixture of ethyl ether and ethanol. They are applied to the skin by means of a soft brush or other suitable applicator and, when the ether and ethanol have evaporated, leave a film of pyroxylin on the surface. Salicylic Acid Collodion USP, contains 10% *w/v* of salicylic acid in Flexible Collodion USP and is used as a keratolytic agent in the treatment of corns and warts. Collodion USP and Flexible Collodion USP are water-repellent protectives for minor cuts, scratches, and chigger bites. Collodion is made flexible by the addition of castor oil and camphor. Collodion has been used to reduce or eliminate the side effects of fluorouracil treatment of solar keratoses.[60] Vehicles other than flexible collodion, such as a polyacrylic base, have been used to incorporate salicylic acid for the treatment of warts with less irritation.

ELIXIRS

Elixirs are clear, pleasantly flavored, sweetened hydroalcoholic liquids intended for oral use. The main ingredients in elixirs are ethanol and water but glycerin, sorbitol, propylene glycol, flavoring agents, preservatives, and syrups often are used in the preparation of the final product. The solvents are often used to increase the solubility of the drug substance in the dosage form. Elixirs are more fluid than syrups, due to the use of less viscous ingredients such as alcohol and the minimal use of viscosity-improving agents such as sucrose. They are used as flavors and vehicles such as Aromatic Elixir USP for drug substances; when such substances are incorporated into the specified solvents, they are classified as medicated elixirs, such as Dexamethasone Elixir USP and Phenobarbital Elixir USP.

The distinction between some of the medicated syrups and elixirs is not always clear. For example, Ephedrine Sulfate Syrup USP contains between 20 and 40 mL of alcohol in 1000 mL of product. Definitions are sometimes inconsistent and, in some instances, not too important with respect to the naming of the articles of commerce. To be designated as an elixir, however, the solution must contain alcohol. The alcoholic content will vary greatly, from elixirs containing only a small quantity to those that contain a considerable portion as a necessary aid to solubility. For example, Aromatic Elixir USP contains 21% to 23% alcohol; Compound Benzaldehyde Elixir USP, on the other hand, contains 3% to 5%.

Elixirs also may contain glycerin and syrup. These may be added to increase the solubility of the medicinal agent, for sweetening purposes, or to decrease the pharmacological effects of the alcohol. Some elixirs contain propylene glycol. Claims have been made for this solvent as a satisfactory substitute for both glycerin and alcohol.

Although alcohol is an excellent solvent for some drugs, it does accentuate the saline taste of bromides and similar salts. It often is desirable, therefore, to substitute some other solvent that is more effective in masking such tastes for part of the alcohol in the formula. In general, if taste is a consideration, the formulator is more prone to use a syrup rather than a hydroalcoholic vehicle.

Because only relatively small quantities of ingredients have to be dissolved, elixirs are more readily prepared and manufactured than syrups, which frequently contain considerable amounts of sugar. An elixir may contain both water- and alcohol-soluble ingredients. If such is the case, the following procedure is indicated:

> Dissolve the water-soluble ingredients in part of the water. Add and solubilize the sucrose in the aqueous solution. Prepare an alcoholic solution containing the other ingredients. Add the aqueous phase to the alcoholic solution, filter, and make to volume with water.

Sucrose increases viscosity and decreases the solubilizing properties of water and so must be added after the primary solution has been effected. A high alcoholic content is maintained during preparation by adding the aqueous phase to the alcoholic solution. Elixirs always should be brilliantly clear. They may be strained or filtered and, if necessary, subjected to the clarifying action of purified talc or siliceous earth.

Elixirs, and many other liquid preparations intended for internal use, such as the diabetic syrups thickened with sodium carboxymethylcellulose or similar substances, contain saccharin, aspartame, acesulfame potassium, and other sweeteners. Cyclamates and saccharin have been banned in some countries as ingredients in manufactured products. Much research has been done to find a safe synthetic substitute for sucrose.

Research concerning the preparation of a dry elixir has been conducted by Kim and co-workers.[61] Dry Elixirs containing a nonsteroidal anti-inflammatory drug and ethanol were encapsulated in a dextrin. The dissolution rate constant of the drug from the microcapsules usually increased considerably compared to the drug alone, possibly due to the cosolvent ethanol. It is suggested that this type of dosage form may be useful to improve the solubility, dissolution rate, and bioavailability of the drug.

Because elixirs contain alcohol, incompatibilities of this solvent are an important consideration during formulation. Alcohol precipitates tragacanth, acacia, and agar from aqueous solutions. Similarly, it will precipitate many inorganic salts from similar solutions. The implication here is that such substances should be absent from the aqueous phase or present in such concentrations that there is no danger of precipitation on standing.

If an aqueous solution is added to an elixir, a partial precipitation of alcohol soluble ingredients may occur. This is due to the reduced alcoholic content of the final preparation. Usually, however, the alcoholic content of the mixture is not sufficiently decreased to cause separation. As vehicles for tinctures and fluidextracts, the elixirs generally cause a separation of extractive matter from these products due to a reduction of the alcoholic content. Many of the incompatibilities between elixirs, and the substances combined with them, are due to the chemical characteristics of the elixir per se, or of the ingredients in the final preparation. Thus, certain elixirs are acid in reaction while others may be alkaline and will, therefore, behave accordingly.

Some example formulations of medicated elixirs are as follows:

Phenobarbital Elixir

Phenobarbital	4.00 g
Propylene Glycol	50 mL
Alcohol	200 mL
Sorbitol Solution	600 mL
Saccharin Sodium	5.0 g
Flavor	qs
Purified Water, to make	1000 mL

Theophylline Elixir

Theophylline	5.3 g
Citric Acid	10.0 g
Syrup	132.0 mL
Glycerin	50.0 mL
Sorbitol Solution	324.0 mL
Alcohol	200.00 mL
Flavor	q.s
Purified Water, to make	1000.0 mL

GLYCERINS

Glycerins or glycerites are solutions or mixtures of medicinal substances in not less than 50% by weight of glycerin. Most of the glycerins are extremely viscous and some are of a jelly-like consistency. Few of them are used extensively. Glycerin is a valuable pharmaceutical solvent forming permanent and concentrated solutions not otherwise obtainable. Glycerin is used as the sole solvent for the preparation of Antipyrine and Benzocaine Otic Solution USP. Glycerins are hygroscopic and should be stored in tightly closed containers.

INHALATIONS AND INHALANTS

Inhalation preparations are so used or designed that the drug is carried into the respiratory tree of the patient. The vapor or mist reaches the affected area and gives prompt relief from the symptoms of bronchial and nasal congestion. The USP defines Inhalations in the following way:

"Inhalations are drugs or solutions or suspensions of one or more drug substances administered to the nasal or oral respiratory route for local or systemic effect. Solutions of drug substances in sterile water for inhalation or in sodium chloride inhalation solution may be nebulized by the use of inert gases. Nebulizers are suitable for the administration of inhalation solutions only if they give droplets sufficiently fine and uniform in size so that the mist reaches the bronchioles. Nebulized solutions may be breathed directly from the nebulizer, or the nebulizer may be attached to a plastic face mask, tent or intermittent positive pressure breathing (IPPB) machine."

Another group of products, also known as metered-dose inhalers (MDIs) are propellant-driven drug suspensions or solutions in liquefied gas propellant (chlorofluorocarbons and hydrofluoroalkanes) with or without a cosolvent and are intended for delivering metered doses of the drug to the respiratory tract. An MDI contains multiple doses, often exceeding several hundred. The most common single-dose volumes delivered are from 25 to 100 µL (also expressed as mg) per actuation. Examples of MDIs containing drug solutions are Epinephrine Inhalation Aerosol, USP and Isoproterenol Hydrochloride and Phenylephrine Bitartrate Inhalation Aerosol, respectively. Both the solubility and stability of the drug in the propellant mixture must be investigated during formulation development. Ethanol is commonly used as a cosolvent hydrofluoroalkane propellants, and was reported to significantly increase the solubility of steroids.[62]

As stated in the USP, particle size is of major importance in the administration of this type of preparation. The various mechanical devices that are used in conjunction with inhalations are described in Chapter 50 (*Aerosols*). It has been reported that the optimum particle size for penetration into the pulmonary cavity is of the order of 0.5 to 7.0 µm.[63] Fine mists are produced by pressurized aerosols and hence possess basic advantages over the older nebulizers; in addition, metered aerosols deliver more uniform doses. A number of inhalations are described in the USP.

The USP defines "inhalants" as follows:

"A special class of inhalations termed "inhalants" consists of drugs or combinations of drugs that, by virtue of their high vapor pressure, can be carried by an air current into the nasal passage where they exert their effect. The container from which the inhalant is administered is known as an inhaler."

Amyl nitrate USP and Propylhexedrine Inhalant USP are two examples. Amyl nitrite is a clear, yellowish, volatile liquid that acts as a vasodilator when inhaled. The drug is prepared in sealed glass vials that are covered with a protective gauze cloth. Upon use, the glass vial is broken in the fingertips and the cloth soaks up the liquid which is then inhaled. The vials generally contain 0.3 mL of the drug substance. The effects of the drug are rapid and are used in the treatment of anginal pain.

Propylhexedrine is the active ingredient in the widely used Benzedrex Inhaler. Propylhexedrine is a liquid, vasoconstrictor agent that volatilizes slowly at room temperature. This quality enables it to be effectively used as an inhalant. The official inhalant consists of cylindrical rolls of suitable fibrous material impregnated with propylhexedrine, usually aromatized to mask its amine-like odor, and contained in a suitable inhaler. The vapor of the drug is inhaled into the nostrils when needed to relieve nasal congestion due to colds and hay fever. It may also be employed to relieve ear block and the pressure pain in air travelers. Each plastic tube of the commercial product contains 250 mg of propylhexedrine with aromatics. The containers should be tightly closed after each opening to prevent loss of the drug vapors.

LINIMENTS

Liniments are alcoholic or oil-based solutions or emulsions containing therapeutic agents intended for external application. These preparations may be liquids or semisolids that are rubbed onto the affected area; because of this, they were once called *embrocations*.

Liniments usually are applied with friction and rubbing of the skin, the oil or soap base providing for ease of application and massage. Alcoholic liniments are used generally for their rubefacient, counterirritant, mildly astringent, and penetrating effects. Such liniments penetrate the skin more readily than do those with an oil base. The oily liniments, therefore, are milder in their action but are more useful when massage is required. Depending on their ingredients, such liniments may function solely as protective coatings. Liniments should not be applied to skin that is bruised or broken.

Other liniments contain antipruritics, astringents, emollients, or analgesics and are classified on the basis of their active ingredient. Dermatologists prescribe products of this type but only those containing the rubefacients are advertised extensively and used by consumers for treating minor muscular aches and pains. It is essential that these applications be marked clearly "For External Use Only". Liniments containing a capsaicin are being investigated for treatment of pruritus.[64]

OLEOVITAMINS

Oleovitamins are fish liver oils diluted with edible vegetable oil or solutions of the indicated vitamins or vitamin concentrates (usually vitamin A and D) in fish liver oil. The definition is broad enough to include a wide variety of marketed products.

In oleovitamin A and D, USP, vitamin D may be present as ergocalciferol or cholecalciferol obtained by the activation of ergosterol or 7-dehydrocholesterol, or may be obtained from natural sources. Synthetic vitamin A, or a concentrate, may be used to prepare oleovitamin A. The starting material for the concentrate is fish liver oil, the active ingredient being isolated by molecular distillation or by a saponification and extraction procedure. These vitamins are unstable in the presence of rancid oils; therefore, these preparations should be stored in small, tight containers, preferably under vacuum or under an atmosphere of an inert gas, protected from light and air.

SPIRITS

Spirits, sometimes known as essences, are alcoholic or hydroalcoholic solutions of volatile substances. Like the aromatic waters, the active ingredient in the spirit may be a solid, liquid, or gas. The genealogical tree for this class of preparations begins with a distinguished pair of products, Brandy (*Spiritus Vini Vitis*) and Whisky (*Spiritus Frumenti*), and ends with a wide variety of products that comply with the definition given above. Physicians have debated the therapeutic value of the former products, and these are no longer compendial.

Generally, the alcohol concentration of spirits is rather high, usually over 60%. Because of the greater solubility of aromatic or volatile substances in alcohol than in water, spirits can contain a greater concentration of these materials than the corresponding aromatic waters. When mixed with water or with an aqueous preparation, the volatile substances present in spirits generally separate from solution and form a milky preparation. Salts may be precipitated from their aqueous solutions by the addition of spirits due to their lesser solubility in alcoholic liquids. Some spirits show incompatibilities characteristic of the ingredients they contain. For example, Aromatic Ammonia Spirit cannot be mixed with aqueous preparations containing alkaloids (eg, codeine phosphate). An acid–base reaction (ammonia-phosphate) occurs, and if the alcohol content of the final mixture is too low, codeine will precipitate. Spirits should be stored in tight, light-resistant containers and in a cool place. This tends to prevent evaporation and volatilization of either the alcohol or the active principle and to limit oxidative changes.

Spirits may be used pharmaceutically as flavoring agents and medicinally for the therapeutic value of the aromatic solute. As flavoring agents they are used to impart the flavor of their solute to other pharmaceutical preparations. For medicinal purposes, spirits may be taken orally, applied externally, or used by inhalation, depending upon the particular preparation. When taken orally, they are generally mixed with a portion of water to reduce the pungency of the spirit. Depending on the materials utilized, spirits may be prepared by simple solution, solution by maceration, or distillation. The spirits still listed in the USP/NF are aromatic ammonia spirit, camphor spirit, compound orange spirit, and peppermint spirit.

EMULSIONS

An emulsion is a two-phase system prepared by combining two immiscible liquids, in which small globules of one liquid are dispersed uniformly throughout the other liquid. The liquid that is dispersed into small droplets is called the dispersed, internal, or discontinuous phase. The other liquid is the dispersion medium, external phase, or continuous phase. Where oil is the dispersed phase and an aqueous solution is the continuous phase, the system is designated as an oil-in-water (O/W) emulsion. Conversely, where water or an aqueous solution is the dispersed phase and oil or oleaginous material is the continuous phase, the system is designated as a water-in-oil (W/O) emulsion. Emulsions may be employed orally, topically, or parenterally depending upon on the formulation ingredients and the intended application. Many pharmaceutical emulsions may not be classified as such because they are described by another pharmaceutical category more appropriately. For instance, certain lotions, liniments, creams, ointments, and commercial vitamin drops may be emulsions but may be preferentially referred to in these terms.

Emulsions possess a number of important advantages over other liquid forms:

- In an emulsion, poorly water-soluble drugs may be easily incorporated with improved dissolution rates and bioavailability.
- The unpleasant taste or odor of oils can be masked partially or wholly, by emulsification.
- The absorption rate and permeation of medicaments are can be controlled.
- Absorption may be enhanced by the diminished size of the internal phase.
- Formulation and technology for organ targeted delivery is available.
- Various particle sizes of the internal phase can be achieved by preparation technique, from micro emulsions (micron-sized particles) to nanoparticles.
- Water is an inexpensive diluent and a good solvent for the many drugs and flavors that are incorporated into an emulsion.

It is possible to prepare emulsions that are basically nonaqueous. For example, investigations of the emulsifying effects of anionic and cationic surfactants on the nonaqueous immiscible system, glycerin and olive oil, have shown that certain amines and three cationic agents produced stable emulsions. Although the USP definition is broad enough to encompass nonaqueous systems, emphasis is placed on those emulsions that contain water, as they are by far the most common in pharmacy.

When it is necessary to administer oils by the oral route, patient acceptance is enhanced when the oil is prepared in emulsion form. Thus, mineral oil (a laxative), valproic acid (an anticonvulsant), oil-soluble vitamins, vegetable oils, and preparations for enteral feeding are formulated frequently in an O/W emulsion form to enhance their palatability.

The bioavailability of oils for absorption may be enhanced when the oil is in the form of small droplets. Furthermore, the absorption of some drugs, such as griseofulvin may be enhanced when they are prepared in the form of an O/W emulsion.[65] Emulsion formulations of drugs such as erythromycin and physostigmine salicylate have been considered, in order to improve their stability.[66,67] Finally, the greatest use of emulsions is for topical preparations. Both O/W and W/O emulsions are used widely, depending upon the effect desired. Emulsion bases of the W/O type tend to be more occlusive and emollient than O/W emulsion bases, which tend to be removed more easily by water. The effects of viscosity, surface tension, solubility, particle size, complexation, and excipients on the bioavailability of emulsions have been reported.[68]

Although this section on emulsions focuses primarily on those for oral use and to a lesser degree those for topical application, it should be noted that there are a number of emulsions used parenterally that are described in specialized textbooks on this topic. For example, emulsions of the O/W type are used for intravenous feeding of lipid nutrients. These are used to provide a source of calories and essential fatty acids. These emulsions must meet exacting standards in regard to particle size, safety, and stability. Examples of commercial products include Diprivan Injectable Emulsion (*AstraZeneca*), EMLA Cream (*AstraZeneca*), Renova 0.02% Cream (*OrthoNeutrogena*), Bactroban Cream (*GlaxoSmithKline*), Cordran Lotion (*Watson*), Differin Cream (*Galderma*) and Renova 0.05% Cream (*OrthoNeutrogena*). Other specialized uses of emulsions include radiopaque emulsions that are used as diagnostic agents for x-ray examination.

THEORIES OF EMULSIFICATION

Several theories have been proposed to explain how emulsifying agents act in producing the multi-phase dispersion and in maintaining the stability of the resulting emulsion. Some of these theories apply to specific types of emulsifying agents and to certain conditions, such as pH of the system and the physicochemical nature and proportions of the internal and external phases). The most prevalent theories are the *surface-tension theory*, the *oriented-wedge theory*, and the *interfacial film theory*.

Liquids assume a shape to minimize their surface area, which is spherical for a small drop. In a spherical drop of liquid, there are attractive forces between the molecules, resisting distortion into a less spherical form. If two or more drops of the same liquid come into contact with one another, it is more thermodynamically favorable for them to coalesce, making a larger drop with a decreased surface area compared to the total surface area of the individual drops. The tendency of liquids to minimize their surface area can be measured quantitatively, and when the liquid is surrounded by air, the measurement is called the surface tension.

When a liquid is in contact with another liquid in which it is insoluble and immiscible, the force causing each liquid to resist breaking up into smaller particles is called interfacial tension. Surface active agents, or surfactants, are substances that reduce the resistance of a droplet to form smaller droplets. Surfactants are also called emulsifiers and wetting agents. According to the surface tension theory of emulsification, the use of surfactants results in a reduction in the interfacial tension of the two immiscible liquids, reducing the repellent force between the liquids and diminishing each liquid's attraction for its own molecules. Thus, surfactants enable large globules to break into smaller ones, and prevent small globules from coalescing into larger ones.

The oriented wedge theory proposes that the surfactant forms monomolecular layers around the droplets of the internal phase of the emulsion. The theory is based on the assumption that emulsifying agents orient themselves about and within a liquid relative to their solubility in that particular liquid. In a system containing two immiscible liquids, the emulsifying agent is preferentially soluble in one of the two liquids and becomes more embedded with that phase relative to the other. Many surfactants have a hydrophilic or water loving portion and a hydrophobic or water hating portion (but usually lipophilic or oil-loving), and the molecules will position or orient themselves in each phase. Depending upon the shape and size of the molecules, their solubility characteristics, and thus their orientation, the wedge shape theory proposes that emulsifiers will surround either oil globules or water globules.

Generally an emulsifying agent having a greater hydrophilic character than hydrophobic character will promote oil in water emulsions. On the other hand, water in oil emulsions result with the use of an emulsifyer that is more hydrophobic than hydrophilic. Putting it another way, the phase in which the emulsifying agent is more soluble will become the continuous or external phase of the emulsion. Although this theory does not represent a completely accurate depiction of the molecular arrangement of the emulsifier molecules, the concept that water soluble emulsifiers generally form oil in water emulsions is important.

The interfacial film theory proposes that the emulsifier forms an interface between the oil and water, surrounding the droplets of the internal phase as a thin layer of film adsorbed on the surface of the drops. The film prevents the contact and coalescing of the dispersed phase; the tougher and more pliable the film, the greater the stability of the emulsion. Naturally, the surfactant must be available to coat the entire surface of each drop of internal phase. Similar to the oriented wedge theory, the formation of an oil in water or a water in oil emulsion depends upon the degree of solubility of the emulsifier in the two phases, with water soluble agents encouraging oil in water emulsions and oil-soluble emulsifiers promoting water in oil emulsions.

In reality, none of the emulsion theories can individually explain the mechanism by which the many and varied emulsifiers promote emulsion formation and stability. It is more than likely that even within a given emulsion system, more than one of the theories of emulsification are applicable. For instance, reducing the interfacial tension is critical during initial formation of an emulsion, but the formation of a protective wedge of molecules or film of emulsifier is equally important for continued emulsion stability. Undoubtedly, many emulsifiers are capable of both tasks.

EMULSION FORMULATION INGREDIENTS

The first step in preparation of an emulsion is the selection of the emulsifier. The emulsifier must be compatible with the formulation ingredients and the active pharmaceutical ingredient. It should be stable, nontoxic, and promote emulsification to maintain the stability of the emulsion for the intended shelf life of the product. The selection of the oil phase for oral preparations depends upon the purpose of the product. For example, mineral oil is used as a laxative and corn oil is used for its nutrient properties. Vegetable oils can be used to dissolve or suspend pharmaceuticals such as oil-soluble vitamins.

Emulsions are thermodynamically unstable because of the large increase in surface energy that results from the combination of interfacial tension and large surface area of the dispersed phase and the different densities of the two phases. Thus, emulsions tend to cream—the less dense phase rises and the more dense phase falls in the container. Subsequently, the droplets can coalesce with a considerable reduction in surface free energy. Consequently, considerable research has been conducted on their preparation and stabilization. To prepare suitable emulsions that remain stable, a number of excipients are used in their preparation.

Emulsifiers often have a hydrophilic portion and a lipophilic portion with one or the other being more or less predominant. Griffin devised a method whereby emulsifying or surface-active agents may be categorized on the basis of their *hydrophilic-lipophilic balance or HLB value*. By this method, each agent is assigned an HLB value or number which is indicative of the substance's polarity, which may vary from 40 for sodium lauryl sulfate to 1 for oleic acid. Although the numbers have been assigned up to about 40, the usual range is between 1 and 20. Examples of HLB values for common emulsifiers used in pharmaceutical applications are listed in Table 39-6. HLB values have also been useful in describing the functional properties of materials. For example, HLB values from 1 to 3 typically exhibit anti foaming properties, values from 7 to 10 exhibit good wetting properties, values from 13 to 20 act as solubilizers, and values from 13 to 15 function as

Table 39-6. HLB Values of Common Emulsifiers Used in Pharmaceutical Systems

AGENT	HLB	CLASS
Oleic Acid	1.0	Anionic
Ethylene glycol distearate	1.5	Nonionic
Sorbitan tristearate (Span 65)	2.1	Nonionic
Glyceryl monooleate	3.3	Nonionic
Propylene glycol monostearate	3.4	Nonionic
Glyceryl monostearate	3.8	Nonionic
Sorbitan monooleate (Span 80)	4.3	Nonionic
Sorbitan monostearate (Span 60)	4.7	Nonionic
Diethylene glycol monolaurate	6.1	Nonionic
Sorbitan monopalmitate (Span 40)	6.7	Nonionic
Acacia	8.0	Anionic
Polyoxyethylene lauryl ether (Brij 30)	9.7	Nonionic
Polyoxyethylene monostearate (Myrj 45)	11.1	Nonionic
Triethanolamine oleate	12.0	Anionic
Polyoxyethylene sorbitan monostearate (Tween 60)	14.9	Nonionic
Polyoxyethylene sorbitan monooleate (Tween 80)	15.0	Nonionic
Polyoxyethylene sorbitan monolaurate (Tween 20)	16.7	Nonionic
Pluronic F 68	17.0	Nonionic
Sodium oleate	18.0	Anionic
Potassium oleate	20.0	Anionic
Cetrimonium Bromide	23.3	Cationic
Cetylpyridinium chloride	26.0	Cationic
Poloxamer 188	29.0	Nonionic
Sodium lauryl sulfate	40.0	Anionic

detergents. Oil in water emulsions typically have a weighted HLB value ranging from 8 to 16 while water in oil emulsions have weighted HLB values ranging from 3 to 8.

Materials that are highly polar or hydrophilic have been assigned higher numbers than materials that are less polar and more lipophilic. Generally, lipophilic surfactants have an HLB value from 0 to 10 and are known for their antifoaming, water in oil emulsifying or wetting properties. Hydrophilic surfactants have HLB values ranging from 10 to 20 and form oil in water emulsions. The HLB system also assigns values to oils and oil like substances. In using the HLB concept in the preparation of an emulsion, one selects emulsifying agents having the same or nearly the same HLB value as the oleaginous phase of the intended emulsion. When needed, two or more emulsifiers may be combined to achieve the proper HLB value.

The ionic nature of a surfactant is an important consideration when selecting a surfactant for an emulsion. Nonionic surfactants are effective over pH range 3 to 10; cationic surfactants are effective over pH range 3 to 7; and, anionic surfactants require a pH of greater than 8.[69]

Emulsifying agents may be divided into three classes: *natural emulsifying agents, finely divided solids,* and *synthetic emulsifying agents.*

1. **Natural Emulsifying Agents** are substances derived from vegetable sources and include acacia, tragacanth, alginates, chondrus, xanthan, and pectin. These materials form hydrophilic colloids when added to water and generally produce o/w emulsions. Although their surface activity is low, these materials achieve their emulsifying power by increasing the viscosity of the aqueous phase. Examples of emulsifying agents derived from animal sources include gelatin, egg yolk, casein, wool fat, cholesterol, wax, and lecithin. Because of the widely different chemical constitution of these compounds, they have a variety of uses, depending upon the specific compound, in both oral and topical preparations. All naturally occurring agents show variations in their emulsifying properties from batch to batch.
2. **Finely Divided Solids** are the colloidal clays: bentonite (aluminum silicate) and Veegum (magnesium aluminum silicate). These compounds are good emulsifiers and tend to be absorbed at the interface, increase the viscosity in the aqueous phase, and are often used in conjunction with a surfactant to prepare O/W emulsions. However, both O/W and W/O preparations can be prepared by adding the clay to the external phase. They are used frequently for external purposes such as a lotion or cream.
3. **Synthetic Emulsifying Agents** are very effective at lowering the interfacial tension between the oil and water phases because the molecules possess both hydrophilic and hydrophobic properties. These emulsifying agents are available in different ionic types: anionic, such as sodium dodecyl sulfate; cationic, such as benzalkonium chloride; nonionic, such as polyethylene glycol 400 monostearate; and ampholytic, such as long-chain amino acid derivatives. In addition to the emulsifying agents, *viscosity agents* are employed, namely the hydrophilic colloids such as naturally occurring gums, noted above, and partially synthetic polymers such as cellulose derivatives (eg, methylcellulose, hydroxypropylmethylcellulose, sodium carboxymethylcellulose) or a number of synthetic polymers that may be used, such as carbomer polymers. These materials are hydrophilic in nature and dissolve or disperse in water to give viscous solutions and function as emulsion stabilizers.

Other functional excipients are often utilized in emulsions. High molecular weight alcohols such as stearyl alcohol, cetyl alcohol, and glyceryl monostearate are employed primarily as thickening agents and stabilizers for o/w emulsions of certain lotions and ointments used externally. Cholesterol and cholesterol derivatives may also be employed in externally used emulsions and to promote w/o emulsions.

The aqueous phase of the emulsion favors the growth of microorganisms; because of this, a preservative usually is added to the product. Some of the preservatives that have been used include chlorocresol, chlorobutanol, mercurial preparations, salicylic acid, the esters of *p*-hydroxybenzoic acid, benzoic acid, sodium benzoate, or sorbic acid. The preservative should be selected with regard for the ultimate use of the preparation and possible incompatibilities between the preservative and the ingredients in the emulsion (eg, binding between the surfactant and the preservative). Low pH values of 5 to 6 and low concentrations of water are characteristics also likely to inhibit microbiological growth in emulsions.

Emulsions consist of an oil or lipid phase and an aqueous phase, thus the preservative may diffuse from the aqueous phase into the oil phase. It is in the aqueous phase that microorganisms tend to grow. As a result, water-soluble preservatives are more effective because the concentration of the unbound preservative in the aqueous phase assumes a great deal of importance in inhibiting the microbial growth. Esters of *p*-hydroxybenzoic acid appear to be the most satisfactory preservatives for emulsions.

Many mathematical models have been used to determine the availability of preservatives in emulsified systems. One model takes into account the O/W partition coefficient of the preservative, interaction of the preservative with the surfactant, interfacial tension and membrane permeability. However, because of the number of factors that reduce the effectiveness of the preservative, a final microbiological evaluation of the emulsion must be performed.

While emphasis concerning preservation of emulsions deals with the aqueous phase, microorganisms can reside also in the lipid phase. Consequently, it has been recommended that pairs of preservatives be used to ensure adequate concentration in both phases. Esters of *p*-hydroxybenzoic acid can be used to ensure appropriate concentrations in both phases because of their difference in oil and water solubilities.

The oxidative decomposition of certain excipients, the oil phase, and some pharmaceuticals is possible in emulsions, not only because of the usual amount of air dissolved in the liquid and the possible incorporation of air during the preparation of the product, but also the large interfacial area between the oil and water phase. The selection of the appropriate antioxidant briefly described at the beginning of the chapter depends on factors such as stability, compatibility with the ingredients of the emulsion, toxicity, effectiveness in emulsions, odor, taste, and distribution between the two phases.

PREPARATION OF EMULSIONS

After the purpose of the emulsions has been determined (eg, oral or topical use), the type of emulsions (O/W or W/O) and appropriate ingredients selected, and the theory of emulsification considered, then experimental formulations may be prepared. One method is suggested by Griffin[70]:

1. Group the ingredients on the basis of their solubilities in the aqueous and nonaqueous phases.
2. Determine the type of emulsion required and calculate an approximate HLB value.
3. Blend a low HLB emulsifier and a high HLB emulsifier to the calculated value. For experimental formulations, use a higher concentration of emulsifier (eg, 10% to 30% of the oil phase) than that required to produce a satisfactory product. Emulsifiers should, in general, be stable chemically, nontoxic, and suitably low in color, odor, and taste. The emulsifier is selected on the basis of these characteristics, as well as the type of equipment being used to blend the ingredients and the stability characteristics of the final product. Emulsions should not coalesce at room temperature, or when frozen and thawed repeatedly, or at elevated temperatures of up to 50°C. Mechanical energy input varies with the type of equipment used to prepare the emulsion. The more the energy input, the less the demand on the emulsifier. Both process and formulation variables can affect the stability of an emulsion.
4. Dissolve the oil-soluble ingredients and the emulsifiers in the oil. Heat, if necessary, to approximately 5° to 10°C over the melting point of the highest melting ingredient or to a maximum temperature of 70° to 80°C.
5. Dissolve the water-soluble ingredients (except acids and salts) in a sufficient quantity of water.
6. Heat the aqueous phase to a temperature that is 3° to 5°C higher than that of the oil phase.

emulsions of low viscosity ingredients and small volumes may be prepared using the appropriate equipment described below.

Agitators

Ordinary agitation or shaking may be used to prepare the emulsion. This method frequently is employed by the pharmacist, particularly in the emulsification of easily dispersed, low-viscosity oils. Under certain conditions, intermittent shaking is considerably more effective than ordinary continuous shaking. Continuous shaking tends to break up not only the phase to be dispersed but also the dispersion medium, thus impairing the ease of emulsification. Laboratory shaking devices may be used for small-scale production.

Mechanical Mixers

Emulsions may be prepared by using one of several mixers that are available. Propeller and impeller type mixers that have a propeller attached to a shaft driven by an electric motor are convenient and portable and can be used for both stirring and emulsification. This type operates best in mixtures that have low viscosity, that is, mixtures with a viscosity of glycerin or less. They are also useful for preparing emulsions. A turbine mixer has a number of blades that may be straight or curved, with or without a pitch, mounted on a shaft. The turbine tends to give a greater shear than propellers. The shear can be increased by using diffuser rings that are perforated and surround the turbine so that the liquid from the turbine must pass through holes. The turbines can be used for both low-viscosity mixtures and medium-viscosity liquids. The degree of stirring and shear by propeller or turbine mixers depends upon several factors, such as the speed of rotation, pattern of liquid flow, position in the container, and baffles in the container.

Production sized mixers include high-powered propeller, shaft stirrers immersed in a tank, or self-contained units with propeller and paddle systems. The latter usually are constructed so that the contents of the tank either may be heated or cooled during the production process. Baffles often are built into a tank to increase mixing efficiency. Examples of two production dispersion mixers are shown in Figures 39-1 and 39-2.

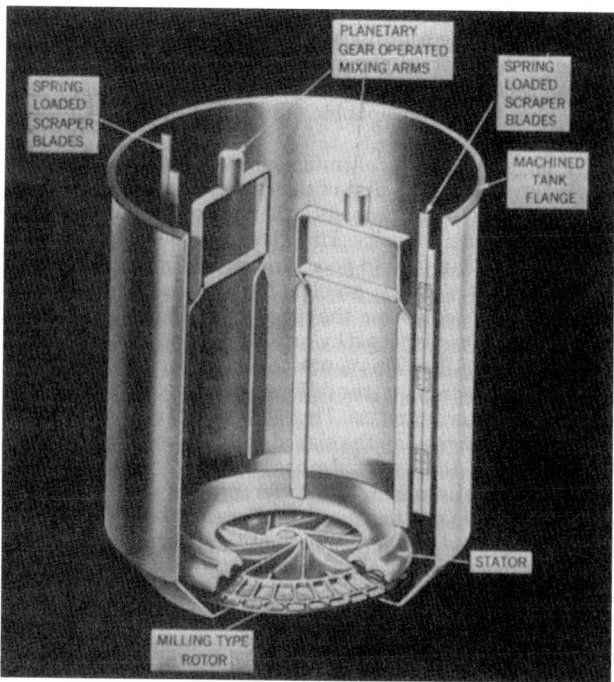

Figure 39-2. Standard paste-type dispersal mixer with cupped-rotor milling element and double-rotating mixing arm circulating element (courtesy, Abbe Eng).

Small electric mixers may be used to prepare emulsions at the prescription counter. They will save time and energy and produce satisfactory emulsions when the emulsifying agent is acacia or agar. The commercially available *Waring Blender* disperses efficiently by means of the shearing action of rapidly rotating blades. It transfers large amounts of energy and incorporates air into the emulsion. If an emulsion first is produced by using a blender of this type, the formulator must remember that the emulsion characteristics obtained in the laboratory will not necessarily be duplicated by the production-size equipment.

Colloid Mills

The principle of operation of the colloid mill is the passage of the mixed phases of an emulsion formula between a stator and a high-speed rotor revolving at speeds of 2,000 to 18,000 rpm. The clearance between the rotor and the stator is very small, but adjustable from 0.001 inches and up. The emulsion mixture, in passing between the rotor and stator, is subjected to a tremendous shearing action that effects a fine dispersion of uniform size. A colloid mill and various rotors are shown in Figures 39-3 and 39-4. The operating principle is the same for all, but each manufacturer incorporates specific features that result in changes in operating efficiency. The shearing forces applied in the colloid mill usually result in a temperature increase within the emulsion. It may be necessary, therefore, to use jacketed equipment to cool the emulsion during processing. Maa and Hsu have shown that droplet size of emulsions was mainly determined by shear force within the gap between the spinning rotor and stationary rotor.[81] Droplet size decreased with homogenization intensity and duration, increasing viscosity of the continuous phase, and with decreasing viscosity of the dispersed phase.

Colloid mills are used frequently for the comminution of solids and for the preparation of suspensions, especially suspensions containing solids that are not wetted by the dispersion medium, which are discussed later in this chapter.

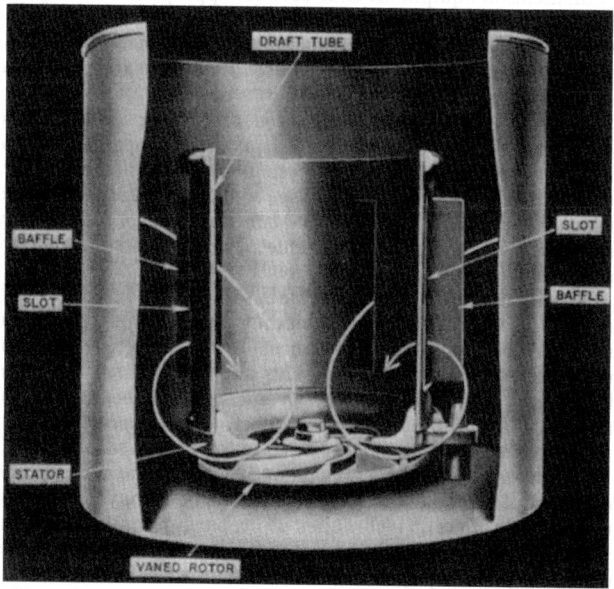

Figure 39-1. Standard slurry-type dispersal mixer with vaned-rotor mixing element and slotted draft-tube circulating element (courtesy, Abbe Eng).

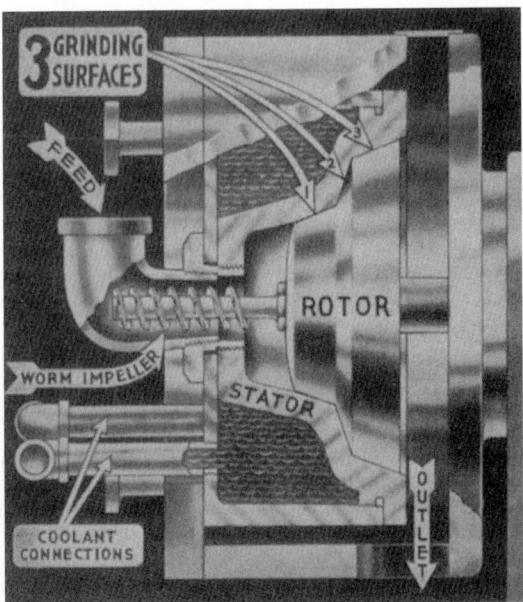

Figure 39-3. A cross section of a colloid mill (courtesy, Tri-Homo).

Homogenizers

Impeller types of equipment frequently produce a satisfactory emulsion; however, for further reduction in particle size, homogenizers may be employed.[82] Homogenizers may be used in one of two ways:

1. The ingredients in the emulsion are mixed and then passed through the homogenizer to produce the final product.
2. A coarse emulsion is prepared in some other way and then passed through a homogenizer for the purpose of decreasing the particle size and obtaining a greater degree of uniformity and stability.

The mixed phases or the coarse emulsion are subjected to homogenization and are passed between a finely ground valve and seat under high pressure. This, in effect, produces an atomization that is enhanced by the impact received by the atomized mixture as it strikes the surrounding metal surfaces. They operate at pressures of 1,000 to 5,000 psi and produce some of the finest dispersions obtainable in an emulsion.

Figure 39-5 shows the flow through the homogenizing valve, the heart of the high pressure, APV Gaulin homogenizer. The product enters the valve seat at high pressure, flows through the region between the valve and the seat at high velocity with

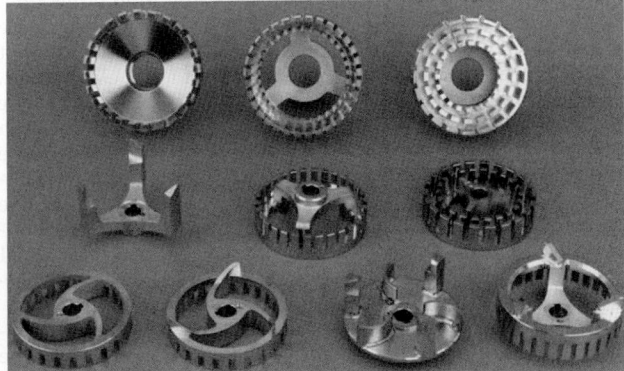

Figure 39-4. Types of rotors used in colloid mills. These may be smooth (for most emulsions), serrated (for ointments and very viscous products), or of vitrified stone (for the paints and pigment dispersions) (courtesy, Tri-Homo).

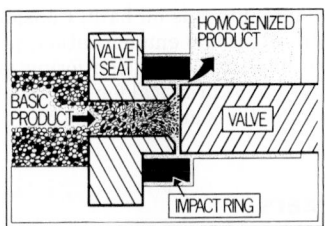

Figure 39-5. Material flow through a homogenizer (courtesy, APV Gaulin).

a rapid pressure drop, causing cavitation; subsequently, the mixture hits the impact ring causing further disruption and then is discharged as a homogenized product. It is postulated that circulation and turbulence are responsible mainly for the homogenization that takes place. Different valve assemblies, two-stage valve assemblies, and equipment with a wide range of capacities are available.

Two-stage homogenizers are constructed so that the emulsion, after treatment in the first valve system, is conducted directly to another where it receives a second treatment. A single homogenization may produce an emulsion that, although its particle size is small, has a tendency to clump or form clusters. Emulsions of this type exhibit increased creaming tendencies. This is corrected by passing the emulsion through the first stage of homogenization at a high pressure (eg, 3,000–5,000 psi) and then through the second stage at a greatly reduced pressure (eg, 1,000 psi). This breaks down any clusters formed in the first step.

For small-scale extemporaneous preparation of emulsions, the inexpensive hand-operated homogenizer is particularly useful. It is probably the most efficient emulsifying apparatus available to the prescription pharmacist. The two phases, previously mixed in a bottle, are hand-pumped through the apparatus. Recirculation of the emulsion through the apparatus will improve its quality.

A homogenizer does not incorporate air into the final product. Air may ruin an emulsion because the emulsifying agent is adsorbed preferentially at the air–water interface, followed by an irreversible precipitation termed *denaturization*. This is particularly prone to occur with protein emulsifying agents. Homogenization may spoil an emulsion if the concentration of the emulsifying agent in the formulation is less than that required to accommodate the increase in surface area produced by the process.

The temperature rise during homogenization is not very large. However, temperature does play an important role in the emulsification process. An increase in temperature will reduce the viscosity and, in certain instances, the interfacial tension between the oil and the water. There are, however, many instances, particularly in the manufacturing of cosmetic creams and ointments, where the ingredients will fail to emulsify properly if they are processed at too high a temperature. Emulsions of this type are processed first at an elevated temperature and then homogenized at a temperature not exceeding 40°C.

Homogenizers have been used most frequently with liquid emulsions, but now they may be used with suspensions, as the metal surfaces are formed from wear-resistant alloys that will resist the wear of solid particles contained in suspensions.

Ultrasonic Devices

The preparation of emulsions by the use of ultrasonic vibrations also is possible. An oscillator of high frequency (100–500 kHz) is connected to two electrodes between which is placed a piezoelectric quartz plate. The quartz plate and electrodes are immersed in an oil bath and, when the oscillator is operating, high-frequency waves flow through the fluid. Emulsification is accomplished by simply immersing a tube containing the emulsion ingredients into this oil bath. Considerable research has been done on ultrasonic emulsification, particularly with regard to the mechanism of emulsion formation. The method has not been proven to be practical for large-scale production of emulsions, but evaluations are underway.[83]

Microfluidizers

Microfluidizers have been used to produce very fine particles. The process subjects the emulsion to an extremely high velocity through micro-channels in to an interaction chamber; as a result, particles are subjected to shear, turbulence, impact, and cavitation. Two advantages of this type of equipment are lack of contamination in the final product and ease of production scale up.

LIPOSOMES

Liposomes have been one of the most extensively studied drug delivery systems.[84–87] Liposomes, meaning lipid body, may be broadly described as small vesicles of a bilayer of phospholipid encapsulating an aqueous space ranging from about 0.03 to 10 μm in diameter. Generally, the lipid membrane of a liposome consists of a bilayer-forming amphiphile, cholesterol, and a charge-generating molecule. The lipid membrane encloses a discrete aqueous compartment. This structure presents an overall hydrophilic membrane-like assembly, in which the apolar or lipophilic portion of the amphiphilic molecule points inward while the polar or hydrophilic portion points outward of the lamellar structure. These characteristics make liposomes useful as drug delivery systems. The enclosed vesicles can encapsulate water soluble drugs in the aqueous spaces or lipid soluble drugs in the membranes. Liposomes have been administered parenterally, topically, and by inhalation.

Liposomes offer several advantages as drug delivery systems: (1) they are biologically inert and completely biodegradable; (2) they can be prepared in various sizes, charge, compositions, and surface morphology; (3) liposomes can encapsulate both water-soluble and water-insoluble drugs, including enzymes, hormones, and antibiotics; (4) encapsulated drugs are less susceptible to degradation; (5) organ-targeted drug delivery is possible since the entrapped drug is delivered intact to various tissues and cells after the liposome is destroyed; and (6) other tissues and cells of the body are protected from the drug until it is released by the liposomes, thus decreasing the drug's toxicity. The primary disadvantage of liposomes is their rapid removal from the blood following intravenous administration by cells of the reticuloendothelial system, particularly by Kupfer cells in the liver. Drug release is slowed by phagocytes through endocytosis, fusion, surface adsorption, or lipid exchange.

Several different amphiphiles have been investigated to create liposomal structures (vesicles). Only the bilayer-forming lipid is the essential part of the lamellar structure, and the other components are to impart specific characteristics. For example, cholesterol adds rigidity to the vesicular structure rendering it less permeable. Phospholipids such as phosphatidyl choline (lecithin) were the first amphiphiles used to produce bilayer structures to mimic cell membranes.

Liposomes can be prepared into several morphologies, which have been classified according to the vesicular shape. *Multilamellar vesicles* (MLV) were first prepared by Bangham and have multiple bilayer structures surrounding a relatively small internal core, much like an onion.[88] *Oligolamellar vesicles* (OLV) have large central aqueous cores surrounded by 2 to 10 bilayers. *Unilamellar vesicles* (ULV) have a single bilayer structure surrounding an internal aqueous core. Unilamellar vesicles can be prepared in a variety sizes: small unilamellar vesicles (20–40 nm), medium unilamellar vesicles (40–80 nm), large unilamellar vesicles (10–1,000 nm), and giant unilamellar vesicles (> 1,000 nm).

Drug release in the blood following intravenous administration ranges from a few minutes to several hours depending upon the nature and composition of the lipids, surface properties, and size. In general, smaller unilamellar vesicles show much longer half-lives than multilamellar vesicles and large unilamellar vesicles. Negatively charged liposomes are cleared more rapidly from the circulation than neutral or positively charged liposomes. Circulation can be prolonged by blocking the reticuloendothelial system and allowing the liposomes to interact with vascular endothelial cells and blood cells. These "stealth liposomes" were developed by coating the liposomes with polymers such as polyethylene glycol, enabling liposomes to evade detection by the body's immune system.

Preparation of Liposomes

Liposomes have been prepared using a number of techniques including solvent evaporation, sonication, supercritical fluid techniques, spray drying, extrusion, and homogenization. A combination of these methods is often used, and the drug is added during the formation process. In this method, the lipid is dissolved in an organic solvent such as acetone or chloroform. The solvent is evaporated leaving a thin, lipid film on the walls of the container. An aqueous solution of the drug is added and placed in an ultrasonic bath. The sound waves displace the lipid from the container walls, and they self-assemble into spheres or cylinders entrapping the aqueous drug solution inside. If the drug is lipophilic, it is incorporated into the lipid phase and will reside within the lipophilic bilayers. Several advances have been made in liposome preparation to better control stability and size.

Liposomal products are now commercially available. Amphotec (distributed by *InterMune*, manufactured by *Ben Venue Laboratories*) is Amphotericin B Cholesteryl Sulfate Complex for Injection. It is a sterile, pyrogen-free, lyophilized powder for reconstitution and intravenous (IV) administration. Amphotec consists of a 1:1 (molar ratio) complex of amphotericin B and cholesteryl sulfate. Upon reconstitution, Amphotec forms a colloidal dispersion of microscopic disc-shaped particles. Each 50 mg single dose vial contains amphotericin B, 50 mg; disodium edetate dihydrate, 0.372 mg; lactose monohydrate, 950 mg; and hydrochloric acid, qs. Amphotec is indicated for the treatment of invasive aspergillosis in patients where renal impairment or unacceptable toxicity precludes the use of amphotericin B deoxycholate in effective doses and in aspergillosis patients where prior amphotericin B deoxycholate therapy has failed. The drug is reconstituted with Sterile Water for Injection by rapidly adding the water to the vial; it is shaken gently by hand, rotating the vial until all the solids have dissolved. The fluid may be opalescent or clear.[89] For infusion, it is further diluted in 5% dextrose injection. The product should not be reconstituted with any fluid other than Sterile Water for Injection; do not reconstitute with dextrose or sodium chloride solutions. Also, for further dilution, it should not be admixed with sodium chloride or electrolytes. Solutions containing benzyl alcohol or any other bacteriostatic agent should not be used as they may cause precipitation. An inline filter should not be used, and the infusion admixture should not be mixed with other drugs. If infused using a y-injection site or similar device, flush the line with 5% dextrose injection before and after infusion of Amphotec. After reconstitution, the drug should be refrigerated and used within 24 hours; do not freeze. If further diluted with 5% dextrose injection, it should be refrigerated and used within 24 hours.

Doxil (*Ortho Biotech*) is doxorubicin hydrochloride encapsulated in stealth liposomes for intravenous administration. The product is provided as a sterile, translucent, red liposomal dispersion in a 10 mL glass, single use vial. Each vial contains 20 mg of doxorubicin HCl at a concentration of 2 mg/mL and a pH of 6.5. The stealth liposome carriers are composed of N-(carbonyl-methoxypolyethylene glycol 2000) - 1,2–distearoyl–

sn–glycerol–3 - phosphoethanolamine sodium salt (MPEG-DSPE), 3.19 mg/mL; fully hydrogenated soy phosphatidylcholine (HSPC), 9.58 mg/mL; and cholesterol, 3.19 mg/mL. Each mL also contains ammonium sulfate, approximately 2 mg; histidine as a buffer; hydrochloric acid and/or sodium hydroxide for pH control; and sucrose to maintain isotonicity. Greater than 90% of the drug is encapsulated in the Stealth liposomes. The stealth liposomes are specially formulated to circulate in the body "undetected" by the mononuclear phagocyte system for a prolonged circulation time of about 55 hours. This is accomplished by pegylation, or binding methoxypolyethylene glycol on the surface of the liposomes. These liposomes are small, in the range of 100 nm in diameter. Doxil must be diluted in 250 mL of 5% dextrose injection prior to administration; once diluted it should be refrigerated and administered within 24 hours. It should not be mixed with any other diluent or any preservative-containing solution. It should not be used with in-line filters. The product is not a clear solution but a red, translucent liposomal dispersion. Unopened vials should be stored in a refrigerator but freezing should be avoided, even though short-term freezing (less than 1 month) does not appear to adversely affect the product.

SUSPENSIONS

The physical chemist defines the word "suspension" as a two-phase system consisting of an undissolved or immiscible material dispersed in a vehicle (solid, liquid, or gas). A variety of dosage forms fall within the scope of this definition, but emphasis is placed on solids dispersed in liquids. In more specific terms, the pharmaceutical scientist differentiates between such preparations as suspensions, mixtures, magmas, gels, and lotions. In these preparations, the substance distributed is referred to as the dispersed phase and the vehicle is termed the dispersing phase or dispersion medium. In a general sense, each of these preparations represents a suspension, but the state of subdivision of the insoluble solid varies from particles that settle gradually on standing to particles that are colloidal in nature.

The particles of the dispersed phase vary widely in size, from large, visible particles to colloidal dimensions, which fall between 1.0 nm and 0.5 μm in size. Course dispersions contain particles usually 10–50 μm in size, and include suspensions and emulsions. Fine dispersions contain particles of smaller size, usually 0.5–10 μm. Magmas and gels represent such fine dispersions. Particles in a coarse dispersion have a greater tendency to separate from the dispersion medium than do the particles of a fine dispersion. Most solids in a dispersion tend to settle to the bottom of the container because their density is higher than the dispersion medium.

Suspensions have a number of applications in pharmacy. They are used to supply drugs to the patient in liquid form. Many people have difficulty swallowing solid dosage forms; consequently a liquid preparation has an advantage for these people. In addition, the dose of a liquid form may be adjusted easily to meet the patient's requirements. Thus, if the drug is insoluble or poorly soluble, a suspension may be the most suitable dosage form. If a drug is unstable in an aqueous medium, a different form of the drug, such as an ester or insoluble salt that does not dissolve in water, may be used in the preparation of a suspension. Drugs, such as antibiotics, that are unstable in the presence of an aqueous vehicle for extended periods of time are most frequently supplied as dry powder mixtures for reconstitution at the time of dispensing. This type of preparation is designated in the USP by the title "for Oral Suspension." Suspensions that do not require reconstitution at the time of dispensing are simply designated as an "Oral Suspension." Examples of commercial products are presented in Table 39-7.

To improve the stability of an antibiotic such as ampicillin, formulations are made in such a way that the dispersion medium, water, is added upon dispensing to form a satisfactory suspension. Generally, the taste of pharmaceuticals can be improved if they are supplied in suspension form, rather than solutions; thus, chloramphenicol palmitate is used instead of the more soluble form, chloramphenicol. Another method to decrease the solubility of the drug is to replace part of the water with another appropriate liquid such as alcohol or glycerin. Insoluble drugs may be formulated as suspensions for topical use such as calamine lotion. Other preparations of suspensions, in addition to those noted above, include parenteral preparations (Chapter 41), ophthalmic preparations (Chapter 43), aerosol suspensions (Chapter 50), and medicated topicals (Chapter 44).

PHYSICAL CHARACTERISTICS OF SUSPENSIONS

Formulation of suspensions involves more than mixing a solid in a liquid. Knowledge of the behavior of particles in liquids, suspending agents, wetting agents, polymers, buffers, preservatives, flavors, and colors is required to produce an acceptable and satisfactory suspension. Suspensions should possess several basic chemical and physical properties. The dispersed phase should settle slowly, if at all, and be re-dispersed readily upon shaking. The solid particles should have a narrow particle size distribution, which does not cake on settling, and the viscosity should be such that the preparation pours easily. In addition, the product should have an elegant appearance, be resistant to microbial growth, and maintain its chemical stability.

Several factors influence the sedimentation rate of particles in a suspension. Stokes' law relates the diameter of the

Table 39-7. Examples of Commercial Suspensions

PRODUCT NAME	MANUFACTURER	ACTIVE INGREDIENT & DOSE	INDICATION
Carafate	Aventis	1 g sucralfate / 10 mL.	Antiulcer
Maalox	Novartis	225 mg aluminum hydroxide and 200 mg magnesium hydroxide / 5 mL	Antacid
Mepron	GlaxoSmithKline	750 mg atovaquone / 5 mL	Antiprotozoal
Mylanta Liquid	J&J-Merck	200 mg Aluminum Hydroxide, 200 mg Magnesium Hydroxide, and 20 mg simethicone / 5 mL	Antacid
Nystastin	Teva	100,000 units mycostatin / mL	Antifungal
Pepto-Bismol Liquid	Proctor & Gamble	262 mg bismuth subsalicyalte / 15 mL	Antidiarrheal
Pred-G ophthalmic suspension	Allegan	0.3% gentamicin and 1.0% prednisolone acetate	topical anti-inflammatory/ anti-infective
Viramune	Boehringer Ingelheim	50 mg of nevirapine / 5 mL	Antiviral

particles, the density of the particles and the medium, and the viscosity of the of the medium to the sedimentation rate:

$$\frac{dS}{dt} = \frac{d^2(\rho_p - \rho_M)g}{18\eta}$$

where

dS/dt is the sedimentation rate,
d is the diameter of the particles,
ρ_P is the density of the particles,
ρ_M is the density of the medium,
g is the gravitational constant,
η is the viscosity of the medium.

Stokes' equation was derived for an ideal situation with perfectly spherical particles in a very dilute suspension. It assumes the spherical particles settle without causing turbulence, without particle-to-particle collision, and without chemical or physical attraction or affinity for the dispersion medium. Obviously, the typical pharmaceutical suspension contains particles are irregularly shaped with a range of sizes, settling results in both turbulence and collision, and there is a reasonable affinity between the particles and suspension medium. However, the basic concepts of the equation offer an indication of the important variables for suspension of the particle and clues to formulation adjustments to decrease the rate of particle sedimentation.

Clearly, the sedimentation rate of large particles is greater than smaller particles, assuming all other factors remain constant. A slower rate of settling can be achieved by reducing particle size. Density also has a direct relationship with sedimentation rate: dense particles settle more rapidly than less dense particles. Most pharmaceutical suspensions are aqueous, and the density of the particles is generally greater than water; a desirable feature, since if they were less dense, they would float making a uniform product difficult to achieve.

The sedimentation rate is indirectly related to the medium viscosity, allowing the pharmaceutical scientist to manipulate settling by adjusting the viscosity of the medium. Settling is reduced by increasing the viscosity of the dispersion medium. One must keep in mind, a very high viscosity is not generally desirable, because it pours with difficulty and it is equally difficult to re-disperse. The viscosity characteristics of a suspension may be altered not only by the vehicle used, but also by the solids content. As the proportion of solid particles is increased in a suspension, so is the viscosity. In most cases, the physical stability of a pharmaceutical suspension is adjusted by the dispersed phase rather than through the dispersion medium. Generally, the dispersion medium supports the adjusted dispersed phase.

The most important consideration in formulation of suspensions is the size of the drug particles. In most pharmaceutical suspensions, the particle diameter is between 1 and 50 μm. The reduction in the particle size is beneficial to the stability of the suspension in that the rate of sedimentation is reduced as the particles are decreased in size. The reduction in particle size produces slow, more uniform rates of settling. However, reduction of the particle size to too great a degree of fineness should be avoided, since fine particles have a tendency to form a compact cake upon settling. The result may be that the cake resists breakup upon shaking and forms rigid aggregates of particles. Particle shape can also affect caking and product stability.[90]

Actions must be taken to prevent the agglomeration of particles into larger crystals or into masses, to avoid the formation of a cake. A common method to prevent rigid cohesion of small particles is through the intentional formation of a less rigid or loose aggregation of the particles by particle-to-particle bonding forces. An aggregation of this type is called a *floc* or *floccule*, in which particles form a lattice structure that resists complete settling and compaction. Flocs form a higher sediment volume than unflocculated particles, and the loose structure permits the aggregates to break up easily and redistribute with agitation. There are several methods of preparing flocculated suspensions, the choice depending on the drug and type of product desired. For example, clays such as bentonite are commonly used as flocculating agents in oral suspensions. The structure of bentonite and of other clays assists the suspension by helping to support the floc once formed. When clays are unsuitable, as in a parenteral suspension, a floc of the dispersed phase can be produced by an alteration in the pH of the preparation, generally to a region of low drug solubility. Electrolytes can also act as flocculating agents by reducing electrostatic interactions between the particles. Nonionic and ionic surfactants can also induce particle flocculation and increase the sedimentation volume.

Particle growth or *Ostwald ripening* is also a destabilizing process resulting from temperature fluctuations during storage. Temperature fluctuations may change particle size distribution and polymorphic form of a drug, if the solubility of the drug is temperature dependent. For example, if the temperature is raised, drug crystals may dissolve and form a supersaturated solution, which favor crystal growth on cooling. As the dissolved drug crystallizes out of solution, it will preferentially occur on the surface of a crystal in the suspension.

SUSPENSION INGREDIENTS

The external phase is usually water for oral preparations; however, other polar liquids such as glycerin or alcohol may be considered to control solubility, stability, and taste. The selection of the external phase is based upon taste, viscosity, density, and stability. Nonpolar liquids such as aliphatic hydrocarbons and fatty esters may be considered if the preparation is used for external purposes.

The main ingredients in a suspension are the drug and functional excipients that wet the drug, influence flocculation, control viscosity, adjust pH, and the external medium, usually water. In addition, flavoring, sweetening, and coloring agents and preservatives are employed. A *wetting agent* is a surfactant with an HLB value between 7 and 9. Surfactants with higher HLB values are recommended sometimes, such as polysorbates and poloxamers. They are employed at a low concentration (0.05–0.5%) to allow the displacement of air from hydrophobic material and permit the liquid, usually water, to surround the particles. If it is desirable to flocculate the particles, then flocculating agents are employed. Usually low concentrations, less than 1%, of electrolytes such as sodium or potassium chloride are employed to induce flocculation. Water-soluble salts possessing divalent or trivalent ions may be considered if the particles are highly charged.

Viscosity producing agents are generally polymers, including natural gums (acacia, xanthan) and cellulose derivatives, such as sodium carboxymethylcellulose and hydroxypropyl methylcellulose. These excipients are used at low concentrations to function as protective colloids, but at higher concentrations they function as viscosity increasing agents. At higher viscosity, the rate of settling of deflocculated particles is decreased providing additional stability to the flocculated suspension. The choice of an appropriate viscosity agent depends upon the use of the product (external or internal), processing equipment, and the duration of storage. Suspension preparations for internal use exhibiting good flow and suspending properties often contain sodium carboxymethylcellulose 2.5%, tragacanth 1.25%, or guar gum 0.5%. For external applications, Carbopol polymers have been successfully used. Other common viscosity-producing agents include acacia, methylcellulose, sodium alginate, or tragacanth.

Ideally, a suspension should be stable over a wide pH range. The chemical and / or physical stability of an active compound may occasionally require the pH of the medium to be maintained within a specified range. *Buffers* must be carefully considered so that they produce their intended effects without interference with other ingredients in the formulation. Buffers can influence the solubility of the active, preservative ionization and its activity, and ionic viscosity agents.

PREPARATION OF SUSPENSIONS

The preparation of suspensions involves several steps; the first is to obtain particles of the proper size, typically in the lower micrometer range. Oral preparations should not feel gritty, topical preparations should feel smooth to the touch, and injectables should not produce tissue irritation. Particle size and distribution also should be considered in terms of bioavailability, or from an in vitro perspective, the rate of release. Very small particles, less than 1 µm, will have a higher solubility than larger particles, but also have a faster *rate* of dissolution. Thus, particle size of the dispersed solid in a suspension can influence the rate of sedimentation, flocculation, solubility, dissolution rate, and ultimately, bioavailability.

Particle size reduction is generally accomplished by dry milling prior to the incorporation of the dispersed phase into the dispersion medium. *Milling* is the mechanical process of reducing particle size, which may be accomplished by a number of different types of machines. Hammer mills grind the powders by impact (Fig 39-6). Centrifugally rotating hammers or blades contact the particles and direct them against a screen, typically in the range of 4 to 325 mesh. The particles are forced through the screen, which regulates final particle size at the outlet of the milling chamber. The blade and screen act in conjunction to determine final product sizing, typically in the range of 10–50 µm.

Fluid energy or jet mills produce particles under 25 µm through violent turbulence in high velocity air (Fig 39-7). Compressed air forms a high speed, jet stream which passes the feed funnel and draws powders into grinding chamber. Pulverizing nozzles are installed around the grinding chamber and inject additional high-speed air into the grinding chamber in a rotational direction. The centrifugal air-flow accelerates particles and reduces particle size by particle to particle impaction and friction. The air-flow drives large particles toward the perimeter, but small particles move toward the center where they exit through the outlet.

A ball mill contains a number of steel or ceramic balls in a rotating drum. The balls reduce the particle size to a 20 to 200 mesh by both attrition and impact. Roller mills have two or more rollers that revolve at different speeds, and the particles are reduced to a mesh of 20 to 200 by means of compression and a shearing action. See Chapter 37 (Powders) for a more detailed discussion on particle size reduction of solids.

In the pharmacy, ceramic mortar and pestle are better for grinding and reducing particle size than glass. After reducing particle size, the drug powder is wetted thoroughly with a small

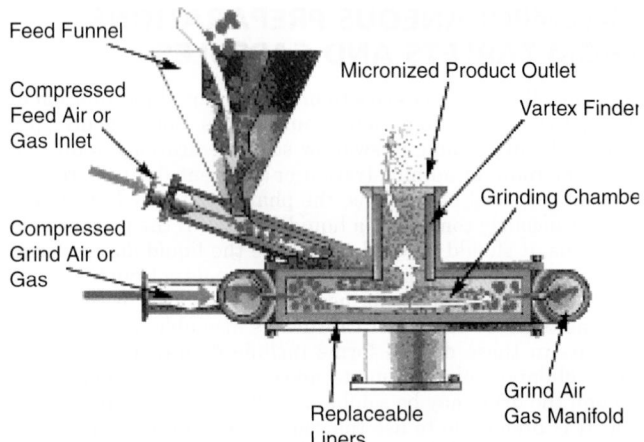

Figure 39-7. Schematic of particle size reduction in a fluid energy or jet mill (courtesy, Sturtevant Inc.).

quantity of water miscible solvent, such as glycerin or alcohol, which reduces the interfacial tension. The suspending agent in the aqueous medium is then added. Alternately, the suspending agent can be triturated with the drug particles using a small quantity of glycerin or alcohol and then brought up to volume with the diluent water and triturated to a smooth uniform product.

On a large scale, the fine drug particles are treated with a small portion of water that contains the wetting agent and allowed to stand for several hours to release entrapped air. At the same time, the suspending agent should be dissolved or dispersed in the main portion of the external phase and allowed to stand until complete hydration takes place. Subsequently, wetted drug particles should be added slowly to the main portion of the dissolved suspending agent. Other excipients such as electrolytes or buffers should be carefully introduced. The preservatives, flavoring agents, and coloring agents are added last. Finally, the formulation is processed with homogenizers, ultrasonic devices, or colloid mills to produce a uniform product.

A procedure for the preparation of Trisulfapyrimidines Oral Suspension is given below.

Trisulfapyrimidines Oral Suspension

Veegum	1.00 g
Syrup USP	90.60 g
Sodium Citrate	0.78 g
Sulfadiazine	2.54 g
Sulfamerazine	2.54 g
Sulfamethazine	2.54 g

Add the Veegum slowly and with continuous stirring to the syrup. Incorporate the sodium citrate into the Veegum–syrup mixture. Premix the sulfa drugs, add to the syrup, stir, and homogenize. Add sufficient 5% citric acid to adjust the pH of the product to 5.6. A preservative and a flavoring agent may be added to the product.

QUALITY CONSIDERATIONS

The quality of the suspension can be determined in a number of ways. Particle size, particle size distribution, and particle shape are often determined using photo microscopy or laser light diffraction techniques. Physical stability, the degree of settling, or flocculation may be determined using a device to measure the zeta potential. Viscosity may be determined by instruments such as the Brookfield viscometer or of the cone and plate configuration. Microbiological as well as stability testing according to ICH guidelines should be performed to determine the efficiency of the preservative and the appropriateness of the formulation with respect to time, temperature, and relative humidity.[91]

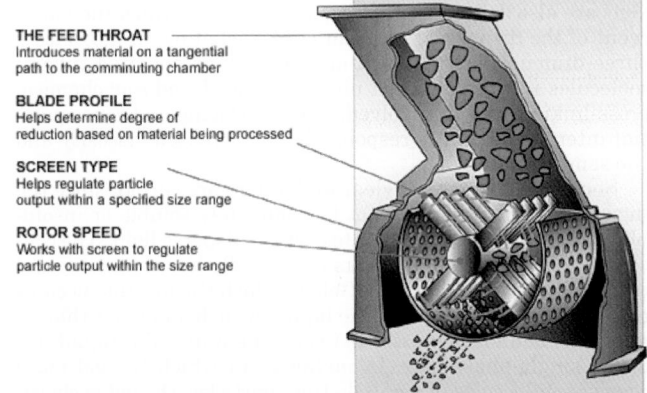

Figure 39-6. Material Flow through a Hammer Mill. Hammer mills operate by feeding material uniformly into a chamber in which a rotating blade assembly reduces the particles of the material by cutting or impacting them. The material discharges through a screen which regulates final particle size at the outlet of the milling chamber (courtesy, The Fitzpatrick Company).

EXTEMPORANEOUS PREPARATIONS FROM TABLETS AND CAPSULES

Occasionally, it is necessary to prepare a liquid formulation of a drug to meet certain patient requirements. Consequently, patients who are unable to swallow solid medications, require a different route of administration or different dosing strength present a special need. Thus, the pharmacist may have to extemporaneously compound a liquid product. If the pure drug is available, it should be used to prepare the liquid dosage form. If it is necessary to prepare a liquid dosage form from tablets or capsules, a suspension is formed if either the drug or one of the excipients in the tablets or capsules is insoluble. Insoluble excipients in these dosage forms include disintegrants, lubricants, glidants, colors, diluents, and coatings. Consequently, although the drug may be soluble in water, many excipients are not. It is preferable to use the contents of capsules, or tablets that are not coated. If coated, tablets with a water-soluble coat are preferred to those with functional enteric coatings and the like. In any case, the contents of the capsules or the tablets should be ground finely with a ceramic mortar and pestle and then wetted using alcohol or glycerin.

Preservatives may be included in the liquid formulation to enhance the stability. However, preservatives have been found to cause serious adverse effects in infants. Benzyl alcohol should be omitted from neonatal formulations because it can cause a gasping syndrome characterized by a deterioration of multiple organ systems and eventually death. Propylene glycol has also been implicated to cause seizures and stupor in some preterm infants. Thus, formulations for neonates should be purposely kept simple, and not compounded to supply more than just a few days of medicine

Finally, it may be desirable to use a hand homogenizer to prepare a more suitable product. Some drugs that have been formulated in this manner include clonidine hydrochloride and simple syrup,[92] cefuroxime axetil in an orange syrup vehicle,[93] and famotidine in cherry syrup.[94] Many other examples may be found in current hospital and community pharmacy journals such as the *American Journal of Hospital Pharmacy, Canadian Journal of Hospital Pharmacy, U.S. Pharmacist, International Journal of Pharmaceutical Compounding,* and *Drug Development and Industrial Pharmacy.* Frequently, stability data and, occasionally, bioavailability and/or taste data are provided.

To minimize stability problems of the extemporaneously prepared product, it should be placed in air-tight, light-resistant containers and stored in the refrigerator by the patient. Because it is a suspension, the patient should be counseled to shake it well prior to use and to be aware of any change that might indicate a stability problem with the formulation.

Tortorici reports an example of an extemporaneous suspension of cimetidine tablets that retained its potency at 40° over 14 days.[95] Twenty-four, 300 mg cimetidine tablets are compounded with 10 mL of glycerin and 120 mL of simple syrup. The tablets are triturated to a fine powder using a mortar, the mixture is levigated with the glycerin, and the simple syrup added. The suspension is mixed well, placed in a blender until smooth, and then refrigerated.

SUSTAINED RELEASE SUSPENSIONS

Sustained release suspensions represent a very specialized class of preparation. Sustained release, oral suspensions with morphine,[96] nonsteroidal anti-inflammatory agents,[97] and other drugs[98] have been described in the literature. However, limited commercial success has been achieved due to the difficulty in maintaining the stability. Formulation research for sustained release suspensions has focused on the similar technologies used in preparing sustained release tablets and capsules. *Celltech* licenses the Tussionex Pennkinetic system,

which uses a combination of ion exchange resin and particle coating.[99] This novel system exploits the likelihood of complexation between ionic drugs and ion-exchange resins, which are then coated with ethyl cellulose. When administered orally, the coated particles with encapsulated drug adsorbed onto the resin are slowly released by an ion exchange process.

Durect markets the SABER system for sustained release suspension applications. SABER uses a non-polymeric, non-water-soluble high-viscosity liquid carrier material (>5,000 cPs. at 37°C), such as sucrose acetate isobutyrate (SAIB), to provide controlled release of active ingredients.[100] The drug is mixed with a small amount of a pharmaceutically acceptable solvent to form a low viscosity solution or suspension, which is then mixed with the high viscosity carrier. The resulting suspension can be administered via injection, orally, or as an aerosol, forming an adhesive, biodegradable depot upon contact with tissues. After administration of the SABER formulation, the solvent diffuses away, leaving a viscous, adhesive matrix of the three components—SAIB, drug, and any additives. The release rate can be easily modified by the ratio of non-polymeric, non-water-soluble high-viscosity liquid carrier material present in the formulation. Extended systemic and local delivery for durations of 1 day to 3 months from a single injection has been demonstrated.

GELS AND MAGMAS

Gels are defined by the USP as:

> "...semisolid systems consisting of either suspensions made up of small inorganic particles or large organic molecules interpenetrated by a liquid. Where the gel mass consists of a network of small discrete particles, the gel is classified as a two-phase system. In a two-phase system, if the particle size of the dispersed phase is relatively large, the gel mass is sometimes referred to as a magma. Both gels and magmas may be thixotropic, forming semisolids on standing and becoming liquid on agitation.
>
> Single-phase gels consist of organic macromolecules uniformly distributed throughout a liquid in such a manner that no apparent boundaries exist between the dispersed macromolecules and the liquid. Single-phase gels may be made from synthetic macromolecules or from natural gums. The latter preparations are also called mucilages. Although these gels are commonly aqueous, alcohols and oils may be used as the continuous phase. For example, mineral oil can be combined with a polyethylene resin to form an oleaginous ointment base.
>
> Gels can be used to administer drugs topically or into body cavities."

Gels are also defined as semi-rigid systems in which the movement of the dispersing medium is restricted by an interlacing three-dimensional network of particles or solvated macromolecules in the dispersed phase. Physical and / or chemical cross-linking may be involved. The interlacing and consequential internal friction is responsible for increased viscosity and the semisolid state.

Some gel systems are clear and others are turbid, since the ingredients involved may not be completely soluble or insoluble, or they may form aggregates, which disperse light. The concentration of the gelling agents is generally less than 10%, and usually in 0.5 to 2.0% range. Gels in which the macromolecules are distributed throughout the liquid in such a manner that no apparent boundaries exist between them and the liquid are called single-phase gels. In instances in which the gel mass consists of floccules of small distinct particles, the gel is classified as a two-phase system and frequently called a magma or a milk. Gels and magmas are considered colloidal dispersions since they each contain particles of colloidal dimension.

Different types of colloidal dispersions have been given specific names. For instance, *sol* is a general term designating a dispersion of a solid substance in a liquid, a solid, or a gaseous dispersion medium. However, more often than not it is used to describe the solid liquid dispersion system. A prefix such as hydro- for water (*hydrosol*) or alco- for alcohol (*alcosol*) is used to specify the medium. Similarly, *aerosol* has similarly been developed to indicate a dispersion of a solid or a liquid in a gaseous phase.

The generally accepted size range for a substance "colloidal" is when particles fall between 1 nm and 0.5 μm. One difference between colloidal dispersions and true solutions is the larger particle size of the dispersed phase in colloidal systems. The optical properties of the two systems are also different. True solutions do not scatter light and therefore appear clear, but colloidal dispersions contain discrete particles scatter light.

Gelling Agents

Several compendial materials function as gelling agents, including acacia, alginic acid, bentonite, carbomer, carboxymethylcellulose sodium, cetostearyl alcohol, colloidal silicon dioxide, ethylcellulose, gelatin, guar gum, hydroxyethylcellulose, hydroxypropyl cellulose, hydroxypropyl methylcellulose, magnesium aluminum silicate, maltodextrin, methylcellulose, polyvinyl alcohol, povidone, propylene carbonate, propylene glycol alginate, sodium alginate, sodium starch glycolate, starch, tragacanth, and xanthan gum.

Alginic acid is refined from seaweed. It is a tasteless, practically odorless, white to off-white colored, fibrous powder. It is used in concentrations between 1% and 5% as a thickening agent, and swells in water to about 200 times its own weight without dissolving. Alginic acid can be cross-linked by addition of calcium salts, resulting in substantially higher viscosity. Sodium alginate produces a gel at concentrations up to 10%. Aqueous preparations are most stable between pH values of 4–10; below pH 3, alginic acid is precipitated. Sodium alginate gels for external use should be preserved.

Carbomer resins are high molecular weight, acrylic acid-based polymers. The pH of 0.5% and 1.0% aqueous dispersions are 2.7–3.5 and 2.5–3.0, respectively. There are many carbomer resins, with viscosity ranges available from 0 to 80,000 cPs., depending upon the pH to which it is neutralized. In addition to thickening, suspending, and emulsifying in both oral and topical formulations, carbomers are also used to provide sustained release properties in both the stomach and intestinal tract for commercial products. Alcohol is often added to carbomer gels to decrease their viscosity. Carbomer gel viscosity is also dependent upon the presence of electrolytes and the pH. Generally, a rubbery mass forms if greater than 3% electrolytes are added. Carbomer preparations are primarily used in aqueous systems, although other liquids can be used. In water, a single particle of carbomer will wet very rapidly but, like many other powders, carbomer polymers tend to form clumps of particles when haphazardly dispersed in polar solvents. Rapid dispersion of carbomers can be achieved by adding the powder very slowly into the vortex of the liquid that is very rapidly stirred. A neutralizer is added to thicken the gel after the carbomer is dispersed. Sodium hydroxide or potassium hydroxide can be used in carbomer dispersions containing less than 20% alcohol. Triethanolamine will neutralize carbomer resins containing up to 50% ethanol.

Carboxymethylcellulose (CMC) produces gels when used in concentrations of 4% to 6% of the medium viscosity grade. Glycerin may be added to prevent drying. Precipitation will occur at pH values less than 2, it is most stable at pH levels between 2 and 10, with maximum stability at pH 7 to 9. It is incompatible with ethanol. Sodium carboxymethylcellulose (NaCMC) is soluble in water and should be dispersed with high shear in cold water before the particles hydrate and swell. Once the powder is well dispersed, the solution is heated with moderate shear to about 60°C for fastest dissolution. These colloidal dispersions are sensitive to pH and the viscosity of the product decreases below pH 5 or above pH 10.

Tragacanth gum has been used to prepare gels that are stable at a pH range of 4–8. These gels must be preserved or sterilized by autoclaving. Tragacanth often lumps when added to water, thus, aqueous dispersions are prepared by adding the powder to rapidly mixed water. Also, lumps are also prevented by wetting the gum with ethanol, glycerin, or propylene glycol.

Colloidal silicon dioxide can be used to prepare transparent gels when used with other ingredients of similar refractive index. Colloidal silicon dioxide adsorbs large quantities of water without liquefying, and its viscosity is largely independent of temperature. Changes in pH affect the viscosity: it is most effective at pH values up to about 7.5. Colloidal silicon dioxide (fumed silica) will form a hydrophobic gel when combined with 1-dodecanol and n-dodecane. These are prepared by adding the silica to the vehicle and sonicating for about 1 minute to obtain a uniform dispersion, sealing, and storing at about 40°C overnight.

Gelatin gels are prepared by dispersing gelatin in hot water followed by cooling. Alternatively, gelatin can be wetted with an organic liquid such as ethyl alcohol or propylene glycol followed by the addition of the hot water and cooling. Magnesium aluminum silicate forms thixtropic gels at concentrations of about 10%. The material is inert and has few incompatibilities but is best used above pH 3.5. It may bind to some drugs and limit their availability.

Methylcellulose forms gels at concentrations up to about 5%. Since methylcellulose hydrates slowly in hot water, the powder is dispersed with high shear at 80–90°C in a portion of water. Once the powder is finely dispersed, the remaining water is added with moderate stirring. Alcohol or propylene glycol is often used to help wet the powders. High electrolyte concentrations will salt out the polymer, ultimately precipitating the polymer.

Poloxamer gels are made from selected forms of polyoxyethylene-polyoxypropylene copolymers in concentrations ranging from 15% to 50%. Poloxamers are white, waxy, free-flowing granules that are practically odorless and tasteless. Aqueous solutions of poloxamers are stable in the presence of acids, alkalis, and metal ions. Polyvinyl alcohol (PVA) is used at concentrations of about 2.5% in the preparation of various jellies, which dry rapidly when applied to the skin. Borax is a often used to gel PVA solutions. For best results, disperse PVA in cold water, followed by hot water. It is less soluble in the cold water.

Povidone, in the higher molecular weight forms, can be used to prepare gels in concentrations up to about 10%. It has the advantage of being compatible in solution with a wide range of inorganic salts, natural and synthetic resins, and other chemicals. It has also been used to increase the solubility of a number of poorly soluble drugs.

Two-Phase Gels

Two-phase gels containing bentonite may be used as a base for topical preparations such as plaster and ointment. Aluminum Hydroxide Gel, USP is an example of a two-phase gel. The USP states that "Aluminum Hydroxide Gel is a suspension of amorphous aluminum hydroxide in which there is a partial substitution of carbonate for hydroxide." The gel is usually prepared by the interaction of a soluble aluminum salt, such as a chloride or sulfate, with ammonia solution, sodium carbonate, or bicarbonate. The reactions that occur during the preparation are

$$3CO_3{}^{2-} + 3H_2O \rightarrow 3HCO_3{}^- + 3OH^-$$

$$[Al(H_2O)_6]^{3+} + 3OH^- \rightarrow [Al(H_2O)_3(OH)_3] + 3H_2O$$

$$2HCO_3{}^- \rightarrow CO_3{}^{2-} + H_2O + CO_2$$

The physical and chemical properties of the gel will be affected by the order of addition of reactants, pH of precipitation, temperature of precipitation, concentration of the reactants, the reactants used, and the conditions of aging of the precipitated gel.

Aluminum Hydroxide Gel is soluble in acidic (or very strongly basic) media. The mechanism in acidic media is

$$Aluminum\ Hydroxide\ Gel + 3H_2O \rightarrow [Al(H_2O)_3(OH)_3]^0$$

$$[Al(H_2O)_3(OH)_3]^0 + H_3O^+ \rightarrow [Al(H_2O)_4(OH)_2]^+ + H_2O$$

$$[Al(H_2O)_4(OH)_2]^+ + H_3O^+ \rightarrow [Al(H_2O)_5(OH)]^{2+} + H_2O$$

$$[Al(H_2O)_5(OH)]^{2+} + H_3O^+ \rightarrow [Al(H_2O)_6]^{3+} + H_2O$$

It is unlikely that the last reaction given proceeds to completion. Because the activity of the gel is controlled by its insolubility. Further, because a certain quantity of insoluble gel always is available, the neutralizing capability of the gel extends over a considerable period of time.

Aluminum hydroxide gels also may contain peppermint oil, glycerin, sorbitol, sucrose, saccharin, and various preservatives. Sorbitol improves the acid-consuming capacity by inhibiting a secondary polymerization that takes place on aging. In addition, polyols such as mannitol, sorbitol, and inositol have been shown to improve the stability of aluminum hydroxide and aluminum hydroxycarbonate gels.[101]

Single-Phase Gels

Single-phase gels are used more frequently in pharmacy for several reasons: semisolid state, high degree of clarity, ease of application, and ease of removal and use. The gels often provide a faster release of drug substance, independent of the water solubility of the drug, as compared to creams and ointments.

Some recent gel formulations include ophthalmic preparations of pilocarpine, carbachol, and betamethasone valerate; topical preparations for burn therapy, anti-inflammatory treatment, musculoskeletal disorders, and acne; peptic ulcer treatment with sucralfate gel; and bronchoscopy using lidocaine. Gels may be used as lubricants for catheters and bases for patch testing, and sodium chloride gels are used for electrocardiography.

Some gel formulation examples are provided below.

Methylcellulose and Carbomer Gel Base

Methylcellulose, 4000 cps	1.0 %
Carbomer 934	0.35 %
1 N Sodium hydroxide solution	qs to pH 7
Propylene glycol	16.7 %
Methyl paraben	0.015%
Purified water,	qs 100%

Disperse the methylcellulose in a portion of hot (80–90°C) water. Cool to room temperature, and disperse the Carbomer 934 in the gel using a bladed impeller. Adjust the pH of the dispersion to 7.0 by adding sufficient 1 N sodium hydroxide solution. Dissolve the methylparaben in the propylene glycol. Mix the methylcellulose, Carbopol 934 and propylene glycol fractions using caution to avoid incorporating air.

Sodium Alginate Gel Base

Sodium Alginate	10 g
Glycerin	10 g
Methyl Hydroxybenzoate	0.2 g
A soluble calcium salt (calcium gluconate)	0.5 g
Purified Water,	to make 100 mL

Place a portion of water in a beaker and add the glycerin and preservative. Stir this solution with a high speed mixer and add the sodium alginate. The calcium salt is added next, which increases the viscosity. Continue mixing until the preparation is homogeneous. The preparation should be stored in a tightly sealed wide mouth jar or tube.

Carbomer Gel

Carbomer 934	2 g
Triethanolamine	1.65 mL
Methyl Paraben	0.2 g

Propyl Paraben	0.05 g
Purified Water,	to make 100 mL

The parabens are dissolved in 95 mL of water with the aid of heat and allowed to cool. Carbomer 934 is added in small amounts to the solution using a high speed mixer until a smooth dispersion is obtained. The preparation is allowed to stand, permitting entrapped air to separate. Then the neutralizing agent, triethanolamine, is added very slowly to avoid entrapping air. Finally, the remaining water is then incorporated.

LOTIONS

Lotions are not defined specifically in the USP, but a broad definition describes them as either liquid or semi-liquid preparations that contain one or more active ingredients in an appropriate vehicle. Lotions may contain antimicrobial preservatives and other appropriate excipients such as stabilizers. Lotions are intended to be applied to the unbroken skin without friction. Lotions are usually suspensions of solids in an aqueous medium. Some lotions are, in fact, emulsions or solutions.

Even though lotions usually are applied without friction, the insoluble matter should be divided very finely. Particles approaching colloidal dimensions are more soothing to inflamed areas and effective in contact with infected surfaces. A wide variety of ingredients may be added to the preparation to produce better dispersions or to accentuate its cooling, soothing, drying, or protective properties. Bentonite is a good example of a suspending agent used in the preparation of lotions. Methylcellulose or sodium carboxymethylcellulose, for example, will localize and hold the active ingredient in contact with the affected site and at the same time be rinsed off easily with water. A formulation containing glycerin will keep the skin moist for a considerable period of time. The drying and cooling effect of a lotion may be accentuated by adding alcohol to the formula.

Dermatologists frequently prescribe lotions containing anesthetics, antipruritics, antiseptics, astringents, germicides, protectives, or screening agents, to be used in treating or preventing various types of skin diseases and dermatitis. Antihistamines, benzocaine, calamine, resorcin, steroids, sulfur, zinc oxide, betamethasone derivatives, salicylic acid, safflower oil, minoxidil, and zirconium oxide are ingredients common in lotions.

Lotions may be prepared by triturating the ingredients to a smooth paste and then adding the remaining liquid phase with trituration. High-speed mixers or colloid mills produce better dispersions and, therefore, are used in the preparation of larger quantities of lotion. Calamine Lotion USP is the classic example of this type of preparation and consists of finely powdered, insoluble solids held in more or less permanent suspension by the presence of suspending agents and/or surface-active agents. The formula and the method of preparation of Calamine Lotion, USP follows.

Calamine Lotion, USP

Calamine	80 g
Zinc Oxide	80 g
Glycerin	20 mL
Bentonite Magma	250 mL
Calcium Hydroxide Topical Solution	qs 1,000 mL

Dilute the bentonite magma with an equal volume of calcium hydroxide topical solution. Mix the powder intimately with the glycerin and about 100 mL of the diluted magma, triturating until a smooth, uniform paste is formed. Gradually incorporate the remainder of the diluted magma. Finally add enough calcium hydroxide topical solution to make 1000 mL, and shake well. If a more viscous consistency in the Lotion is desired, the quantity of bentonite magma may be increased to not more than 400 mL.

Many investigators have studied Calamine Lotion, and this has led to the publication of many formulations, each possessing certain advantages over the others, but none satisfying the collective needs of all dermatologists. Formulations containing hydrated microcrystalline cellulose and carboxymethylcellulose have a slower rate of sedimentation than the official preparation.

Although most lotions are prepared by trituration, some lotions are formed by chemical interaction in the liquid. White Lotion, USP is an example.

White Lotion

Zinc Sulfate	40 g
Sulfurated Potash	40 g
Purified Water,	qs 1,000 mL

Dissolve the zinc sulfate and the sulfurated potash separately, each in 450 mL of purified water, and filter each solution. Add slowly the sulfurated potash solution to the zinc sulfate solution with constant stirring. Then add the required amount of purified water, and mix.

Benzyl Benzoate Lotion USP is an example of a lotion that is also an emulsion. The formula and method of preparation are:

Benzyl Benzoate	250 mL
Triethanolamine	5 g
Oleic Acid	20 g
Purified Water	qs 1,000 mL

Mix the triethanolamine with the oleic acid, add the benzyl benzoate, and mix. Transfer the mixture to a suitable container of about 2000 mL capacity, add 250 mL of purified water, and shake the mixture thoroughly. Finally add the remaining purified water, and again shake thoroughly.

Triethanolamine forms a soap with the oleic acid and functions as the emulsifying agent to form a stable product. This type of emulsifying agent is almost neutral in water and gives a pH of about 8 and thus should not irritate the skin.

Certain lotions tend to separate or stratify on long standing, and they require a label directing that they be shaken well before each use. All lotions should be labeled "For External Use Only." Microorganisms may grow in certain lotions if no preservative is included. Care should be taken to avoid contaminating the lotion during preparation, even if a preservative is present.

Milk of Magnesia USP is a suspension of magnesium hydroxide containing approximately 80 mg of $Mg(OH)_2$ per milliliter. The specifications for double strength or triple strength are that these products should contain approximately 160 mg or 240 mg of $Mg(OH)_2$ per mL, respectively. It has an unpleasant, alkaline taste that can be masked with 0.1% citric acid (to reduce alkalinity) and 0.05% of a volatile oil or a blend of volatile oils. Magnesium hydroxide is prepared by the hydration of magnesium oxide.

For the most part, magmas are intended for internal use, although Bentonite Magma is used primarily as a suspending agent for insoluble substances for local application and occasionally for internal use. All magmas require a "Shake Well" label and "Avoid Freezing."

EXTRACTS

Extraction, as the term is used pharmaceutically, involves the separation of medicinally active portions of plant or animal tissues from the inactive or inert components by using selective solvents in standard extraction procedures. The products obtained from plants are relatively impure liquids, semisolids, or powders intended only for oral or external use. These include classes of preparations known as decoctions, infusions, fluidextracts, tinctures, pilular (semisolid) extracts, and powdered extracts. Such preparations popularly have been called galenicals, after Galen, the 2nd century Greek physician.

Extraction continues to be of considerable interest in order to obtain improved yields of drugs derived from plant and animal sources. For example, extraction of digitalis glycosides has been carried out using super critical carbon dioxide.[102] Other techniques include ultrasonics, rotary-film evaporators, hydrodistillation, liquid chromatography, multiple-solvent extraction, countercurrent extraction, and gravitation dynamics.

This discussion is concerned primarily with basic extraction procedures for crude drugs to obtain the therapeutically desirable portion and eliminate the inert material by treatment with a selective solvent, known as the menstruum. Extraction differs from solution in that the presence of insoluble matter is implied in the former process. The principal methods of extraction are maceration, percolation, digestion, infusion, and decoction. The quality of the finished product can be enhanced by standardizing primary extracts and carrying out analytical assays during production on the raw materials, intermediate products, and manufacturing procedures.

The processes of particular importance, insofar as the USP is concerned, are those of maceration and percolation, as described specifically for Belladonna Extract USP and Cascara Sagrada Extract USP. Most pharmacopeias refer to such processes for extraction of active principles from crude drugs. The USP provides general directions for both maceration and percolation under the heading of *Tinctures*.

Techniques of extraction continue to be investigated and applied to obtain higher yields of the active substance from natural sources. Some of these methods include the use of different grinding and shearing processes of plants, use of specific membranes for extraction, and different extraction procedures such as distillation, digestion, percolation, and microwaves.

MACERATION—In this process the solid ingredients are placed in a stoppered container with 750 mL of the prescribed solvent and allowed to stand for a period of at least 3 days in a warm place with frequent agitation, until soluble matter is dissolved. The mixture is filtered and, after most of the liquid has drained, the residue on the filter is washed with sufficient quantity of the prescribed solvent or solvent mixture; the filtrates are combined to produce 1000 mL.

PERCOLATION—The ground solids are mixed with the appropriate quantity of the prescribed solvent to make it evenly and uniformly damp. It is allowed to stand for 15 min, then transferred to a percolator and packed. Sufficient prescribed solvent is added to saturate the solids. The top is placed on the percolator, and when the liquid is about to drip from the apparatus, the lower opening is closed. The solids are allowed to macerate for 24 hours or for the specified time. If no assay is directed, the percolation is allowed to proceed slowly or at the specified rate gradually adding sufficient solvent to produce 1000 mL of solution. If an assay is required, only 950 mL of percolate are collected and mixed and a portion assayed as directed. The rest of the percolate is diluted with the solvent to produce a solution that conforms to the required standard and then mixed.

DIGESTION—This is a form of maceration in which gentle heat is used during the process of extraction. It is used when moderately elevated temperature is not objectionable and the solvent efficiency of the menstruum is increased thereby.

INFUSION—An infusion is a dilute solution of the readily soluble constituents of crude drugs. Fresh infusions are prepared by macerating the solids for a short period of time with either cold or boiling water. The USP has not included infusions for some time.

DECOCTION—This once popular process extracts watersoluble and heat stable constituents from crude drugs by boiling in water for 15 min, cooling, straining, and passing sufficient cold water through the drug to produce the required volume.

EXTRACTIVE PREPARATIONS

After a solution of the active constituents of a crude drug is obtained by maceration or percolation, it may be ready for use as a medicinal agent, as with certain tinctures or fluidextracts, or it may be processed further to produce a solid or semisolid extract.

Tinctures

Tinctures are defined in the USP as being alcoholic or hydroalcoholic solutions prepared from vegetable materials or from chemical substances, an example of the latter being Iodine Tincture. Traditionally, tinctures of potent vegetable drugs essentially represent the activity of 10 g of the drug in each 100 mL of tincture, the potency being adjusted following assay. Most other tinctures of vegetable drugs represent the extractive from 20 g of the drug in 100 mL of tincture.

The USP specifically describes two general processes for preparing tinctures, one by percolation and the other by maceration. Percolation includes a modification so that tinctures that require assay for adjustment to specified potency thus may be tested before dilution to final volume. Belladonna Tincture, USP is prepared in this manner. Compound Benzoin Tincture USP and Sweet Orange Peel Tincture, USP are prepared by the maceration procedure.

Fluidextracts

The USP defines fluidextracts as being liquid preparations of vegetable drugs, containing alcohol as a solvent or as a preservative, or both, so made that, unless otherwise specified in an individual monograph, each milliliter contains the therapeutic constituents of 1 g of the standard drug that it represents.

Extracts

Extracts are defined in the USP as concentrated preparations of vegetable or animal drugs obtained by removal of the active constituents of the respective drugs with suitable menstrua, evaporation of all or nearly all of the solvent, and adjustment of the residual masses or powders to the prescribed standards. There are three forms of extracts: semiliquids or liquids of syrupy consistency, plastic masses (known as *pilular* or *solid extracts*), and dry powders (known as *powdered extracts*). Extracts, as concentrated forms of the drugs from which they are prepared, are used in a variety of solid or semisolid dosage forms. The USP states that pilular extracts and powdered extracts of any one drug are interchangeable medicinally, but each has its own pharmaceutical advantages. Pilular extracts, so-called because they are of a consistency to be used in pill masses and made into pills, are also suited for use in ointments and suppositories. Powdered extracts are better suited for incorporation into a dry formulation, as in capsules, powders, or tablets. Semiliquid extracts, or extracts of a syrupy consistency, may be used in the manufacture of some pharmaceutical preparations.

Most extracts are prepared by extracting the drug by percolation. The percolate is concentrated, generally by distillation under reduced pressure. The use of heat is avoided where possible because of potential injurious effect on active constituents. Powdered extracts that are made from drugs that contain inactive oily or fatty matter may have to be defatted or prepared from defatted drug. Pure Glycyrrhiza Extract USP is an example of a pilular extract and Belladonna Extract USP is an example of a powdered extract.

BIBLIOGRAPHY

General

Nielloud F, Marti-Mestres G, eds. *Pharmaceutical emulsions and suspensions.* New York: Marcel Dekker, 2000.
Lieberman HA, Rieger MM, Banker GS, eds. *Pharmaceutical Dosage Forms. Volume 3: Disperse Systems,* 2nd ed. New York: Marcel Dekker, 1998.
Lachman L, Liebermann HA, Kanig J, eds. *The Theory and Practice of Industrial Pharmacy,* 3rd ed. Philadelphia: Lea & Febiger, 1986.

Solutions, Emulsions and Suspensions

Becher P. *Emulsions: Theory & Practice,* 3rd ed. New York: Oxford, 2001.
Becher P. *Encyclopedia of Emulsion Technology.* New York: Marcel Dekker, 1983.
Kreuter J. *Colloidal Drug Delivery Systems.* New York: Marcel Dekker, 1994.
Osborne DW, Amann AH. *Topical Drug Delivery Formulations.* New York: Marcel Dekker, 1990.
Yalkowsky SH. *Handbook of Aqueous Solubility Data.* Boca Raton: CRC Press, 2003.
Yalkowsky SH. *Techniques of Solubilization of Drugs.* New York: Marcel Dekker, 1981.

Equipment

Busse DJ. *Mfg Chem* 1990; 61:39.
Lagman B. *Drug Develop Ind Pharm* 1988; 14:2705.
Oldshue JY. *Fluid Mixing Technology.* New York: McGraw-Hill, 1983.

Excipient Properties

Kibbe AH, ed. *Handbook of Pharmaceutical Excipients,* 3rd ed. Washington, DC: American Pharmaceutical Association, 2000.
Reynolds JEF, ed. *Martindale, The Extra Pharmacopoeia,* 31st ed. London: Pharmaceutical Press, 1996.

REFERENCES

1. Wang J, Yang TY, Zhang JX. *Herald of Medicine* 2003; 22:642–643.
2. Schmidt-Nawrot J. *Pharm Ind* 2000; 62:464–469.
3. Eisinger HJ. *Pharm Ind* 2000; 62:469–473.
4. Pfafflin A. *Pharm Ind* 2000; 62:223.
5. Woiwode W, Huber S. *Pharm Ind* 2000; 62:377–381.
6. Connors KA, Amidon GL, Stella VJ. *Chemical Stability of Pharmaceuticals: A Handbook for Pharmacists,* 2nd ed. New York: Wiley-Interscience, 1986.
7. Kurup T, Wan L. *Pharm J* 1986; 37:761.
8. Novack GD, Evans R. *J Glaucoma* 2001; 10:483–486.
9. *United States Pharmacopeia 27 / National Formulary 22.* Rockville, MD: United States Pharmacopeial Convention, Inc., 2004.
10. Sutton SVW, Porter D. *J Pharm Sci Technol* 2002; 56:300–311.
11. Clesceri LS, Greenberg AE, Eaton AD, eds. *Standard Methods for Examination of Water and Wastewater,* 20th ed. Washington DC: American Public Health Association, 1998.
12. Moll F, Naeff REJ, Ehrhart EI, et al. *Pharm Ind* 1997; 59:258–264.
13. Coates D. *Manuf Chem Aerosol News* 1974; 45:19–20.
14. Steinberg DC. 1995; 110: 71–76.
15. Koch CS. *Parfuem Kosmet* 1994; 75:6–21.
16. Bruch CW. *Drug Cosmet Ind* 1976; 118:49–53; 161–162.
17. Ma MH, Lee T, Kwong E. *J Pharm Sci* 2002; 91:1715–1723.
18. Maa YF, Hsu CC. *Int J Pharm* 1996; 140:155–168.
19. Scalzo M, Orlandi C, Simonetti N, et al. *J Pharm Pharmacol* 1996; 48:1201–1205.
20. Coates D. *Manuf Chem Aerosol News* 1973; 44:34–37.
21. Coates D. *Manuf Chem Aerosol News* 1973; 44:41–42.
22. Hurwitz SJ, McCarthy TJ. *J Clin Pharm Ther* 1987; 12:107–115.
23. Boussard P, Devleeschouwer MJ, Dony J. *Int J Pharm* 1991; 72:51–55.
24. Gionchetti P, Venturi A, Rizzello F, et al. *Aliment Pharmacol Ther* 1997; 11:679–684.
25. Matula C, Nahler G, Kreuzig F. *Int J Clin Pharmacol Res* 1988; 8:259–261.
26. Breytenbach HS. *Curr Ther Res-Clin Exp* 1979; 26:640–643.
27. Allen LV. *US Pharmacist* 1990; 15:88–90.
28. Davis CC, Squier CA, Lilly GE. *J Periodont* 1998; 69:620–631.
29. Shibly O, Ciancio SG, Kazmierczak M, et al. *J Clin Dent* 1997; 8:145–149.

30. Hanawa T, Masuda N, Mohri K, et al. *Drug Dev Ind Pharm* 2004; 30:151–161.
31. Amerongen AVN, Veerman ECI. *Support Care Cancer* 2003; 11:226–231.
32. Ellis ME, Clink H, Ernst P, et al. *Eur J Clin Microbiol Infect Dis* 1994;13:3–11.
33. Ellepola ANB, Samaranayake LP. *Oral Dis* 2001; 7:11–17.
34. Joseph BK. *Med Princ Pract* 2002; 11:32–35.
35. Tricca RE. 1988; 142:32.
36. Jungnickel PW, Shaefer MS, Maloley PA, et al. *Ann Pharmacother* 1993; 27:700–703.
37. Abdel-Rahman SM, Johnson FK, Gauthier-Dubois G, et al. *J Clin Pharmacol* 2003; 43:148–153.
38. Krieger JN. *J Urol* 2002; 168:2351–2358.
39. Sarkar MA. *Pharm Res* 1992; 9:1–9.
40. Eppstein DA, Longenecker JP. 1988; 5:99–139.
41. Davis SS, Illum L. *Clin Pharmacokinet* 2003; 42:1107–1128.
42. Arnold J, Ahsan F, Meezan E, et al. *J Pharm Sci* 2002; 91:1707–1714.
43. Bateman ND, Whymark AD, Clifton NJ, et al. *Clin Otolaryngol* 2002; 27:327–330.
44. Tsikoudas A, Homer JJ. *Clin Otolaryngol* 2001; 26:294–297.
45. Adams WP, Conner CH, Barton FE, et al. *Plast Reconstr Surg* 2001; 107:1596–1601.
46. Connolly JG, Anderson C. *Can Med Assoc J* 1979; 121:318–320.
47. Abbas AAH, Felimban SK, Yousef AA, et al. *Med Pediatr Oncol* 2002; 39:139–140.
48. Mallet L, Sesin GP, Ericson J, et al. *N Engl J Med* 1982; 307:445.
49. Greenwood J. *Pharm J* 1989; 243:553–557.
50. Jain NK, Rosenberg DB, Ulahannan MJ, et al. *Am J Gastroenterol* 1985; 80:678–681.
51. Kim NC, Kinghorn AD. *Arch Pharm Res* 2002; 25:725–746.
52. Mitchell JC, Counselman FL. *Acad Emerg Med* 2003; 10:400–403.
53. Cooper C, Kilham H, Ryan M. *Med J Aust* 1998; 168:94–95.
54. Cote CJ, Cohen IT, Suresh S, et al. *Anesth Analg* 2002; 94:37–43.
55. Allen LV, Erickson MA. *Am J Health-Syst Pharm* 1998; 55:1915–1920.
56. Allen LV, Erickson MA. *Am J Health-Syst Pharm* 1998; 55:1804–1809.
57. Horner RK, Johnson CE. *Am J Hosp Pharm* 1991; 48:293–295.
58. Al-Waili NS. *Complement Ther Med* 2003; 11:226–234.
59. Nussinovitch A. *Water-Soluble Polymer Applications inFfoods.* Oxford: Blackwell Science, 2003.
60. Bedinghaus JM, Niedfeldt MW. *Am Fam Physician* 2001; 64:791–796.
61. Kim CK, Yoon YS, Kong JY. *Int J Pharm* 1995; 120:21–31.
62. Williams RO, Rogers TL, Liu J. *Drug Dev Ind Pharm* 1999; 25:1227–1234.
63. Smith KJ, Chan HK, Brown KF. *J Aerosol Med-Depos Clear Eff Lung* 1998; 11:231–245.
64. Weisshaar E, Dunker N, Gollnick H. *Neurosci Lett* 2003; 345:192–194.
65. Stozek T, Borysiewicz J. *Pharmazie* 1991; 46:39–41.
66. Park SJ, Kim SH. *J Colloid Interface Sci* 2004; 271:336–341.
67. Rubinstein A, Pathak YV, Kleinstern J, et al. *J Pharm Sci* 1991; 80:643–647.
68. Constantinides PP. *Pharm Res* 1995; 12:1561–1572.
69. Bhargava HN, Narurkar A, Lieb LM. *Pharm Tech* 1987; 11:46.
70. Griffin WC, Lynch MJ, Lathrop LB. *Drug Cosmet Ind* 1967; 101:41.
71. Nielloud F, Marti-Mestres G, eds. *Pharmaceutical Emulsions and Suspensions.* New York: Marcel Dekker, 2000.
72. Lachman L, Liebermann HA, Kanig J, eds. *The Theory and Practice of Industrial Pharmacy,* 3rd ed. Philadelphia: Lea & Febiger, 1986.
73. Binks BP. *Curr Opin Colloid Interface Sci* 2002; 7:21–41.
74. Florence AT, Whitehill D. *Int J Pharm* 1982; 11:277–308.
75. Okochi H, Nakano M. *Adv Drug Deliv Rev* 2000; 45:5–26.
76. Kassem MA, Safwat SM, Attia MA, et al. *STP Pharma Sci* 1995; 5:309–315.
77. Bourrel M, Schechter RS, eds. *Microemulsions and Related Systems: Formulation, Solvency, and Physical Properties.* New York: Marcel Dekker, 1988.
78. Rosano HL, Cavallo JL, Chang DL, et al. 1988; 39:201–209.
79. Lin TJ, Shen YF. *J Soc Cosmet Chem* 1984; 35:357–368.
80. Lin TJ. *J Soc Cosmet Chem* 1978; 29:117–125.
81. Maa YF, Hsu C. *J Control Release* 1996; 38:219–228.
82. Lieberman HA, Rieger MM, Banker GS, eds. *Pharmaceutical Dosage Forms. Volume 3: Disperse Systems,* 2nd ed. New York: Marcel Dekker, 1998.
83. Maa YF, Hsu CC. *Pharm Dev Technol* 1999; 4:233–240.
84. van Balen GP, Martinet CAM, Caron G, et al. *Med Res Rev* 2004; 24:299–324.
85. Derycke ASL, de Witte PAM. *Adv Drug Deliv Rev* 2004; 56:17–30.
86. Gregoriadis G, Florence AT, Patel HM, eds. *Liposomes in Drug Delivery.* Vol 2. Drug Targeting and Delivery. Langhorne, PA: Harwood Academic Publishers, 1993.
87. Lasic DD, Papahadjopoulos D, eds. *Medical Applications of Liposomes.* Amsterdam: Elsevier, 1998.
88. Bangham AD, Standish MM, Watkins JC. 1965; 13:238.
89. *Physicians' Desk Reference,* 58th ed. Montvale, NJ: Medical Economics, 2003.
90. Tsai SC, Botts D, Plouff J. *J Rheol* 1992; 36:1291–1305.
91. FDA. *Guidance for Industry. Stability Testing of Drug Substances and Drug Products.* Center for Drug Evaluation and Research (CDER). 1998; 1–114.
92. Levinson ML, Johnson CE. *Am J Hosp Pharm* 1992; 49:122–125.
93. Harris AM, Rauch AM. *Pediatr Infect Dis J* 1994; 13:838–838.
94. Echizen H, Ishizaki T. *Clin Pharmacokinet* 1991; 21:178–194.
95. Tortorici MP. *Am J Hosp Pharm* 1979; 36:22.
96. Morales ME, Lara VG, Calpena AC, et al. *J Control Release* 2004; 95:75–81.
97. Shah KP, Chafetz L. *Int J Pharm* 1994; 109:271–281.
98. Sjoqvist R, Graffner C, Ekman I, et al. *Pharm Res* 1993; 10:1020–1026.
99. Sheumaker JL. United States Patent #4,762,709. 1988.
100. Tipton AJ, Holl RJ. United States Patent #5,747,058. 1998.
101. Nail SL, White JL, Hem SL. *J Pharm Sci* 1976; 65:1195–1198.
102. Moore WN, Taylor LT. *J Nat Prod* 1996; 59:690–693.

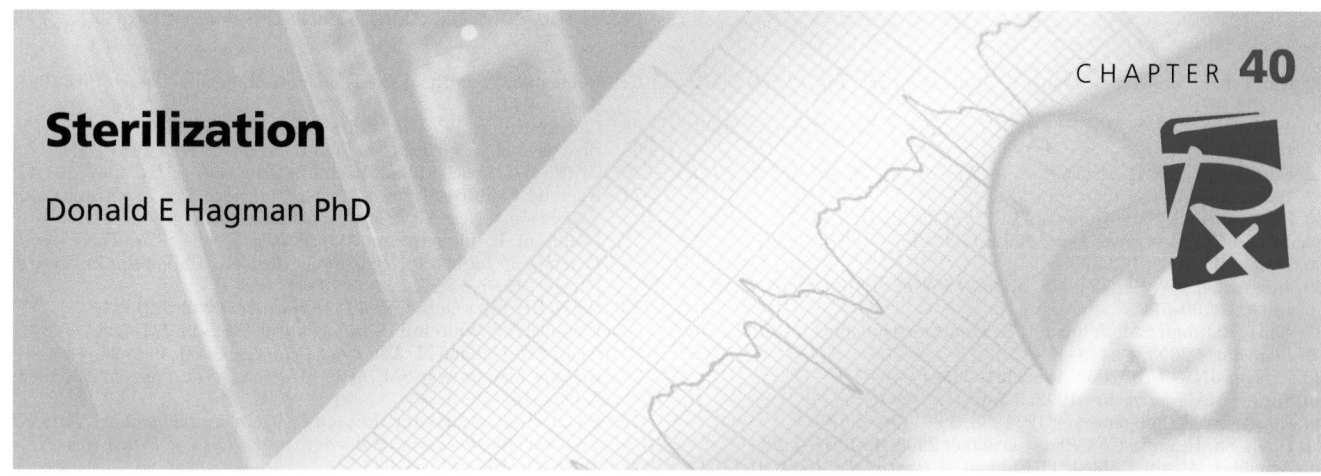

CHAPTER 40

Sterilization

Donald E Hagman PhD

Sterilization is an essential concept in the preparation of sterile pharmaceutical products. Its aim is to provide a product that is safe and eliminates the possibility of introducing infection.

Mergers and acquisitions of pharmaceutical companies create multinational organizations faced with complying with all of the regulatory agencies of the involved countries. To date there is no global regulatory agency that oversees the production of sterile pharmaceutical products. Multinational companies must be familiar with the regulations of all countries in which they operate and meet those regulations. Although it is not the intent of this chapter to delineate the sterilization standards for all countries, it is to provide a detailed description of the techniques used throughout the world to sterilize pharmaceutical products. There are many attempts to standardize practices throughout the multinational industry. These include the efforts of the International Council on Harmonization (ICH) and the issuance of various technical ISO standards and compendial efforts of the various countries like United States Pharmacopoeias (USP) to set some basic standards. Additionally, organizations like International Society for Pharmaceutical Engineering (ISPE) and Parenteral Drug Association (PDA) have issued various documents, which include all facets of the international regulatory requirements.

Sterilization is a process used to destroy or eliminate viable microorganisms that may be present in or on a particular product or package. The process requires an overall understanding and control of all parts of the preparation for use of a particular product. Those areas include the selection and acceptance of all materials used for the product and package, environment in which the product is prepared and used and the ultimate disposition of the remaining materials after use. Sterilization may be required for several steps of the process using any one or a combination of the techniques listed in this chapter.

The aim of a sterilization process is to destroy or eliminate microorganisms that are present on or in an object or preparation, to make sure that this has been achieved with an extremely high level of probability and to ensure that the object or preparation is free from infection hazards. The currently accepted performance target for a sterilization process is that it provide for a probability of finding a nonsterile unit of less than 1 in 1 million. That is, the process (including production, storage, and shipment) will provide a *Sterility Assurance Level* (SAL) equal to or better than 10^{-6}. This is achieved through the processing of products in validated equipment and systems. Thorough validation and periodic requalification is essential to meeting these sterility requirements.

The purpose of this chapter is to provide a basic understanding of the following sterilization methods currently being used in pharmaceutical technology and the equipment employed to carry out these methods:

Method	Equipment
Moist heat sterilization	Saturated steam autoclaves
	Superheated water autoclaves
	Air over steam autoclaves
Dry heat sterilization	Batch sterilizers
	Continuous tunnel sterilizers
Chemical *cold* sterilization	Ethylene oxide
	Vaporized hydrogen peroxide
	Hydrogen peroxide/steam
	Other gases
Radiation sterilization	Electromagnetic
	Particulate
Filtration	Membranes

DEFINITIONS

The following terms, relating to sterilization, should be understood by those carrying out sterilization processes or handling sterile products:

Antiseptic—A substance that arrests or prevents the growth of microorganisms by inhibiting their activity without necessarily destroying them.

Aseptic—Refers to areas and practices where the intent is to be sterile.

Aseptic Processing—Those operations performed between the sterilization of an object or preparation and the final sealing of its package. These operations are, by definition, carried out in the complete absence of microorganisms.

Bactericide—Any agent that destroys microorganisms.

Bacteriostat—Any agent that arrests or retards the growth of microorganisms.

Bioburden—The number of viable microorganisms present prior to sterilization; Usually expressed in colony-forming units of volume.

Disinfection—A process that decreases the probability of infection by destroying vegetative microorganisms, but not ordinarily bacterial spores. The term usually is applied to the use of chemical agents on inanimate objects.

Germicide—An agent that destroys microorganisms, but not necessarily bacterial spores.

Sanitization—A process that reduces the level of bioburden in or on a product or object to a safe level.

Sterile—The absolute absence of viable microorganisms. There is no degree or partiality.

Sterility Assurance Level (SAL)—An estimate of the effectiveness of a sterilization process. It usually is expressed in terms of the negative power of 10 (ie, 1 in 1 million = 10^{-6}).

Sterilization—A process by which all viable microorganisms are removed or destroyed, based on a probability function.

Terminal Sterilization—A process used to render products sterile to a preferred SAL.

Validation—The act of verifying that a procedure is capable of producing the intended result under prescribed circumstances and challenges to predefined specifications.

Viricide—An agent that will destroy viruses.

STERILITY AS A TOTAL SYSTEM

It is necessary to reiterate the concept already briefly addressed in the introduction. The task of the technology we are dealing with is to provide the product in sterile conditions to the end user. It is currently acknowledged that the quality of the product must be *built into* the process. This concept is particularly true when one of the essential qualities of the product is sterility.

Accordingly, the above-mentioned task is accomplished with a series of design, production, and distribution steps that can be summarized as activities for the selection and routine checking of the following items:

- Active constituents, additives, raw materials in general
- Water used both as solvent and as washing/rinsing agent
- Packaging suitable for the product and for the sterilization process that will be used
- Working environment and equipment
- Personnel

These procedures clearly have the purpose of providing the sterilization process with a product that has a minimum, definite, and consistent bioburden. There are also the following activities:

- Selection of the sterilization method that most suits the unit formed by the product and its packaging, and definition of the process variables for obtaining the intended SAL
- Selection of the machine that is most suitable for performing the selected method and of the utilities that this machine requires
- Qualification and validation of the machine and of the process
- Routine checking of the process
- Checking of the results of the sterilization process
- Proper storage of sterile goods and verification that their sterility is maintained with full reliability throughout the allowed storage period
- Delivering, opening, and using sterile goods without recontamination.

It also should be noted that, in December 2002, the US Food and Drug Administration (FDA) proposed new regulations for aseptic processing and terminal sterilization. The proposed rules as defined in their Concept Paper require that manufacturers of sterile products use validated and robust sterilization techniques wherever possible. The European Pharmacopeia and related pharmacopeias have modified their requirements in their rulings identified as Annex 1.

CONTAMINATION

Certain facts about microorganisms must be kept in mind when preparing sterile products. Some microbes (bacteria, molds, etc) multiply in the refrigerator, others at temperatures as high as 60°C. Microbes vary in their oxygen requirements from the strict anaerobes that cannot tolerate oxygen to aerobes that demand it. Slightly alkaline growth media will support the multiplication of many microorganisms while others flourish in acidic environments. Some microorganisms have the ability to use nitrogen and carbon dioxide from the air and thus can actually multiply in distilled water. In general, however, most pathogenic bacteria have rather selective cultural requirements, with optimum temperatures of 30° to 37°C and a pH of 7.0. Contaminating yeasts and molds can develop readily in glucose and other sugar solutions.

Actively growing microbes are, for the most part, vegetative forms with little resistance to heat and disinfectants. However, some forms of bacteria—among them the bacteria that cause anthrax, tetanus, and gas gangrene—have the ability to assume a spore state that is very resistant to heat as well as to many disinfectants. For this reason, an excellent measure of successful sterilization is whether the highly resistant spore forms of nonpathogenic bacteria have been killed.

The nature of expected contamination and the bioburden are important to pharmacists preparing materials to be sterilized. The raw materials they work with rarely will be sterile, and improper storage may increase the microbial content. Because the pharmacist seldom handles all raw materials in a sterile or protected environment, the environmental elements of the manufacturing area (air, surfaces, water, etc) can be expected to contribute to the contamination of a preparation. The container or packaging material may or may not be presterilized and thus may contribute to the total microbial load.

Understanding the nature of contaminants prior to sterilization and application of methods for minimizing such contamination is vital to preparing for successful pharmaceutical sterilization. Examples of such methods include:

- Maintenance of a hygienic laboratory
- Frequent disinfection of floors and surfaces
- Minimization of traffic in and out of the area
- Refrigerated storage of raw materials and preparations that support microbial growth
- Use of laminar airflow devices for certain critical operations
- Use of water that is of appropriate USP quality and is free of microbial contamination (It is preferable to use presterilized water to avoid any possible contamination.)

METHODS

General

The procedure to be used for sterilizing a drug, a pharmaceutical preparation, or a medical device is determined to a large extent by the nature of the product. It is important to remember that the same sterilization technique cannot be applied universally because the unique properties of some materials may result in their destruction or modification. Methods of inactivating microorganisms may be classified as either physical or chemical. Physical methods include moist heat, dry heat, and irradiation. Sterile filtration is another process, but it only removes, not inactivates, microorganisms. Chemical methods include the use of either gaseous or liquid sterilants. Guidelines for the use of many types of industrial and hospital sterilization are available.[1-10]

Each sterilization method can be evaluated using experimentally derived values representing the general inactivation rates of the process. For example, a death rate or survival curve for a standardized species can be diagramed for different sterilization conditions. This is done by plotting the logarithm of surviving organisms against time of exposure to the sterilization method. In most instances, these data show a linear relationship, typical of first-order kinetics, and suggest that a constant proportion of a contaminant population is inactivated in any given time interval. Based on such inactivation curves, it is possible to derive values that represent the general inactivation rates of the process. For example, based on such data, it has become common to derive a decimal reduction time or D value, which represents the time under a stated set of sterilization exposure conditions required to reduce a surviving microbial population by a factor of 90%.

D values, or other expressions of sterilization process rates, provide a means of establishing dependable sterilization cycles. Obviously, the initial microbial load on a product to be sterilized becomes an important consideration. Beyond this, however, kinetic data also can be used to provide a statistical basis for the success of sterilization cycles. A simple example will

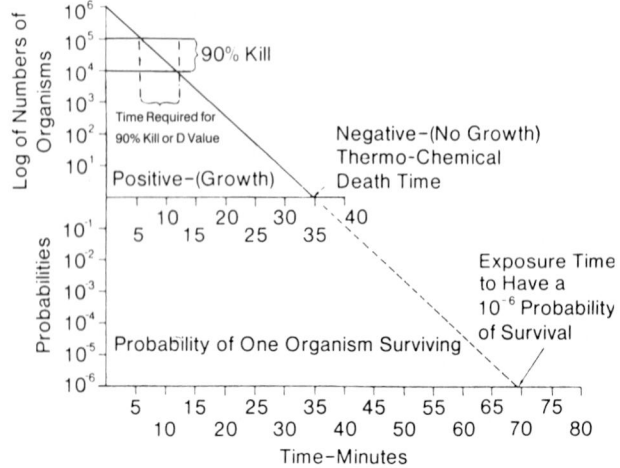

Figure 40-1. Sterilization model using D values.

suffice (Fig 40-1). When the initial microbial contamination level is assumed to be 10^6, and if the D value of the sterilization process is 7 minutes, complete kill is approached by application of 6 D values (42 minutes). However, at this point reliable sterilization would not be assured because a few abnormally resistant members of the population may remain. In this example, by extending the process to include an additional 6 D values, most of the remaining population is inactivated, reducing the probability of one organism surviving to one in 1 million.

Moist Heat

ESSENTIALS OF STEAM STERILIZATION KINETICS

Let us suppose a system contaminated by microorganisms (which we assume, for the sake of simplicity, to be pure and homogeneous) is immersed in pressurized saturated steam, at constant temperature; for example, it could be a vial containing an aqueous suspension of a certain spore-forming microorganism.

It has been shown experimentally that, under the above conditions, the reaction of thermal degradation of the microorganism obeys the laws of chemical reactions: the rate of reduction of the number of microorganisms present in the system in each moment is proportional to the actual number itself. The proportionality coefficient is typical of the species and conditions of the chosen microorganism.

Thus, the degradation reaction (the sterilization process) develops like a first-order chemical reaction in which the reaction rate is proportional, in each moment, only to the amount of microorganisms still to be inactivated. This seems to be obvious for dry sterilization, but less rigorous for steam sterilization, in which the water vapor molecules also seem to take part in the reaction. Actually, this bimolecular reaction is of the first order, as the steam is present in high excess during the entire reaction and its concentration may be regarded as constant.

The most frequently used mathematical expression of the above facts is

$$N = N_0 \, 10^{-t/D} \qquad (1)$$

where N_0 is the initial number of microorganisms, t is the elapsed exposure (equal to sterilization time), N is the number of microorganisms after the exposure time t, and D is the *decimal decay time,* defined as the time interval required, at a specified *constant* temperature, to reduce the microbial population being considered by 1/10 (ie, by one logarithmic value; eg, from 100% to 10% or from 10% to 1% of the initial value).

The D value is inversely proportional to the first-order reaction coefficient and is therefore typical of the species and condi-

tions of the chosen microorganism. Depending on the initial hypothesis of exposure at constant temperature, each D value always refers to a specified temperature.

Equation 1 allows one to draw a first very important conclusion: the time required to reduce the microorganism concentration to any preset value is the function of the initial concentration. The sterilization reaction is therefore neither an *all-or-nothing* process nor a *potential barrier* process as was once thought.

It also is evident immediately that the effect of sterilization at the same constant temperature will be very different depending on the D value of the contaminating microbial species (or on the largest D value in the usual case of mixed contamination). Figure 40-2 shows that the same reduction ratio for different species is achieved after exposure time proportional to the D value of each species. The graph derives only from Equation 1 and from the definition of D value. The basic hypothesis of the temperature being constant is thoroughly valid.

Sterility Is a Probable Effect of Exposure Time—Let us now consider what happens within a batch of units (vials, bottles, or others) with an initial constant unit contamination of 100 microorganisms equal to 10^2. If the D value at 121°C is assumed to be 1, after 1 min at 121°C, a reduction equal to 10^1 = 10 microorganisms is achieved; after another minute, only 10^0 = 1 microorganism is still surviving. After another minute, the surviving microbial population would be 10^{-1} = 1/10 microorganism. A contamination of 1/10 must not be understood to mean that each unit contains 1/10 of a microorganism, which is biologically meaningless (in this case the unit probably would be sterile) but that there is a probability of having 1/10 of the units still contaminated within the batch of sterilized units.

In fact, 3 min would be the necessary time to reduce the microbial population to a single surviving microorganism if the initial population were 10 times larger than the one at issue. This higher initial contamination could be regarded either as a 10 times larger number of microorganisms in the same unit, or as the initial contamination of a 10 times larger unit.

If the unit is not considered any longer as the single vial or bottle, but as the whole of all the items produced over a period of time, the initial number of microorganisms present in each item has to be multiplied times the number of items produced, and the exposure time to achieve the reduction to the same number of viable microorganisms left in the whole of the items produced, has to be increased correspondingly. The following example will be helpful to focus the matter.

A new sterile product in ampules has to be manufactured; the number of ampules to be produced over all the life period of the product is expected to be 10^{10}. The maximum number of contaminated ampules deemed to be acceptable is 10 = 1: this obviously means that the probability of having nonsterile ampules after sterilization must not exceed 10^{-10}. Let us also suppose that the microbial population within each ampule after the filling and the sealing does not exceed 10^3 microorganisms. These must be destroyed by means of moist heat-terminal sterilization at 121°C. The applicable D value is 1 min. The total number of microorganisms to be destroyed during the life of the product will be

$$10^{10+3} = 10^{13}$$

If this whole microbial population were exposed to moist heat at 121°C over a period of 13 min, it would be reduced to 10^{-13} times its initial number (ie, to $10^{13-13} = 10^0 = 1$. The exposure time of 13 min thus would be sufficient (under all the other above hypotheses) to prevent the total number of contaminated ampules from exceeding the value of 1.

From the point of view of each single ampule, 13 min of exposure would reduce the microbial population to the theoretical value of

$$10^{3-13} = 10^{-10}$$

To interpret this numeric value as the probability of still having one contaminated ampule in 10 billion sterilized ampules means that a single ampule will still be contaminated out of a whole lot of 10^{10}. This probability value is defined as PNSU (probability of nonsterile unit).

In recent times the PNSU as a sterility evaluation criterion is being replaced by the SAL. The name itself could generate some misunderstanding, because a level of assurance commonly is deemed to be good if high, but SAL seems to have been defined in such a way that its numerical value is the same as PNSU. This notwithstanding, it is sometimes calculated as the reciprocal value of PNSU. The SAP (sterility assurance probability) criterion has been proposed as well and SAP seems for the moment to have been granted the same definition of PNSU, even if it would be better understandable if its value approached unity after a satisfactory sterilization.

The above discussion and example lead to the conclusion that the optimum exposure time for a sterilization process must take into account not only the initial microbial population within the single item to be sterilized and the species and conditions of the contaminating microorganism, but also the total number of items expected to be sterilized over the life of the product.

Effect of Temperature Changes—All the above considerations have been developed under the basic assumption that the temperature is kept constant during the entire exposure time. It seems rather obvious that the D value will change as the temperature changes. If the D values experimentally obtained for a given microbial species are plotted on a semilogarithmic chart as the function of the temperature T, a path similar to Figure 40-3 is obtained.

In this case, it can be seen that D value is 1 min at 121°C (ie, the average value which very often is assumed to be acceptable in the absence of more exact experimental data). It also can be seen that D value varies by a factor of 10 if the temperature varies by 10°C.

The z value is defined as the temperature coefficient of microbial destruction, the number of degrees of temperature that causes a 10-fold variation of D (or, more generally, of the sterilization rate). The z values generally oscillate between 6 and 13 for steam sterilization in the range 100° to 130°C, and z value often is assumed to be equal to 10 in the absence of more precise experimental data.

The fact that D value varies by 10 times for a variation of 10°C when $z = 10$ must not lead to the false assumption that D varies by one time (ie, doubles) for an increase of 1°C. Obviously, this is not true. It is actually a matter of finding the number which yields 10 when raised to the tenth power. This number is 1.24. Therefore, a variation of 1°C entails a variation of D value of 24%. This is quite a significant number, which illustrates the dramatic effects that are generated when the sterilization temperature is also only a few degrees lower than the expected value, perhaps only in some areas of the sterilizer load.

It is also useful to remember that the effect of temperature variation decreases considerably as the temperature rises and drops to approximately 1/2 (or even less) for dry sterilization at approximately 200°C. Under these conditions the z value is about 20 instead of about 10. Therefore, the small temperature differences that can be so dramatic in steam sterilization have much less effect in dry sterilization.

The foregoing refers to average values because the actual D values and z values depend to a large extent on the medium that contains the microorganisms and on their history. At 121°C no microorganism has exactly D = 1 and $z = 10$. However, the combined use of these two parameters in calculating F_0 and PNSU provides ample margins of safety with regard to the microorganisms with which we deal commonly.

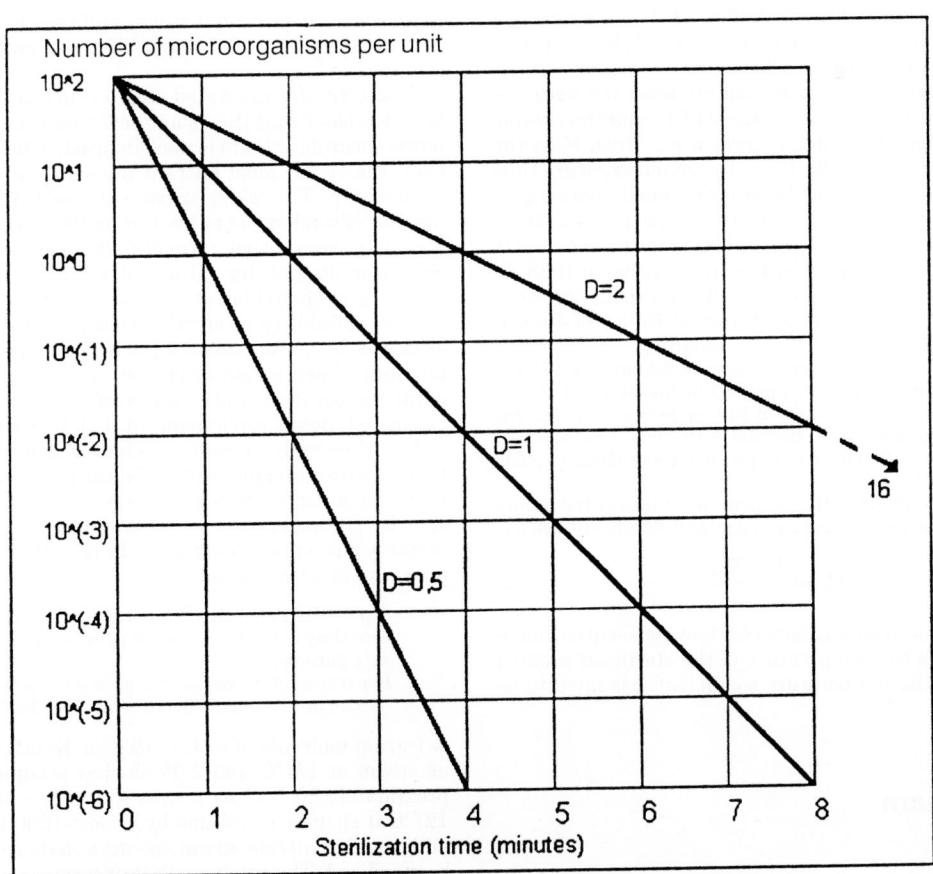

Figure 40-2. Effect of varying D values on sterilization rate (courtesy, Fedegari Autoclavi).

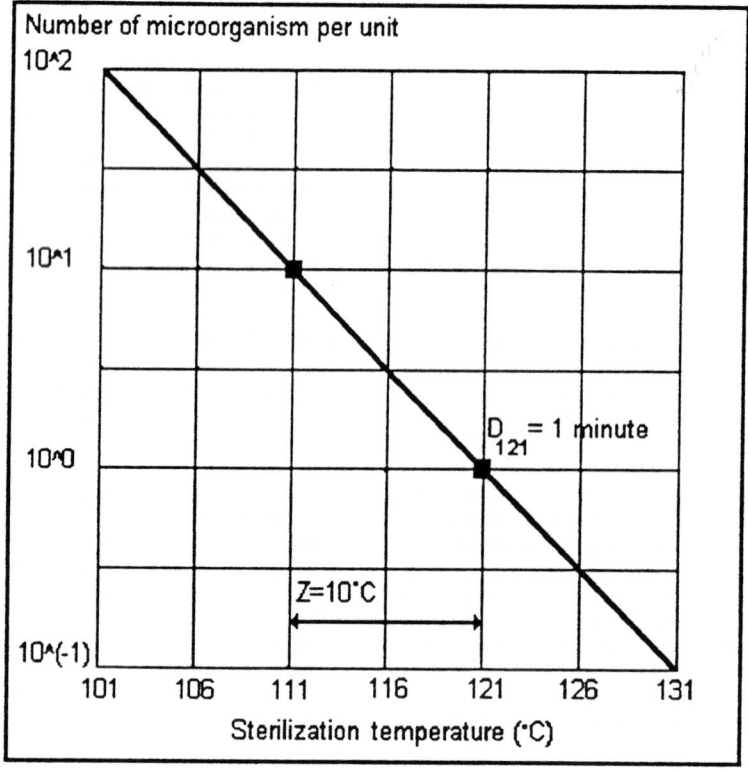

Figure 40-3. Effect of temperature on microbial destruction (courtesy, Fedegari Autoclavi).

F_0 or Equivalent Sterilization Time at 121°C—It is of the utmost interest to calculate the lethal effect of the exposure of a microbial population to a variable temperature, T, by relating it to an hypothetical sterilization performed at a constant temperature, T_0, for the time, t_0. If the constant reference temperature is assumed equal to 121.1°C (originally 250°F) and the z value equal to 10, the equivalent time is termed F_0. Thus, F_0 is the equivalent exposure time at 121.1°C of the actual exposure time at a variable temperature, calculated for an ideal microorganism with a temperature coefficient of destruction equal to 10.

First introduced in the *Laboratory Manual for Food Canners and Processors* by the National Canners Association in 1968, F_0 has become a common term in pharmaceutical production since the FDA used it extensively in the "Proposed Rules" of June 1, 1976 (21 CFR 212.3) with the following meaning:

F_0 means the equivalent amount of time, in minutes at 121.1°C (250°F), which has been delivered to a product by the sterilization process. For the calculation of it, a z value of 10°C or 18°F is assumed; the term z value means the slope of the thermal death time curve and may be expressed as the number of degrees required to bring about a 10-fold change in the death rate.

In practice, the knowledge of the temperature values as the continuous function of elapsing time is not available, and F_0 is calculated as

$$F_0 = \Delta t \; \Sigma \; 10^{\frac{T-121.1}{z}} \qquad (2)$$

where Δt is the time interval between two consecutive measurements of T, T is the temperature of the sterilized product at time t, and z is the temperature coefficient, assumed to be equal to 10.

Saturated Steam

PRINCIPLES

Sterilization with saturated steam is the method that provides the best combination of flexibility in operation, safe results and low plant and running costs. The sterilizing medium obviously is pressurized saturated steam and the typical operating temperature is 121°C (250°F), but higher or lower temperatures often are used.

The term *dry* saturated steam sometimes is used: it should be made clear that this is an *ideal* condition of steam, and that moist saturated steam is used in practice for sterilization. However, the steam must entrain the smallest possible amount of condensate. The *water vapor ratio* of the steam defines the amount of condensate entrained by 100 parts by weight of moist steam; a water vapor ratio of 0.95 means that 100 g of steam consist of 95 g of dry saturated steam plus 5 g of condensate which is, or should be, *at the same temperature as the steam*.

The reliability of sterilization performed with saturated steam is based on several particular characteristics of this medium. When steam condenses, it releases calories at a constant temperature and in a *considerable amount*: 1 kg of pure saturated steam condensing at 121°C (turning into water at 121°C, thus without cooling) releases as much as 525 kcal. The temperatures and pressures of saturated steam have a two-way correlation. Once the temperature of the steam is determined, so is its pressure, and *vice versa*. Saturated steam at 121°C inevitably has a pressure of 2.05 abs bar. This entails two very interesting practical possibilities:

1. A pure saturated steam autoclave can be controlled indifferently according to the temperature parameter or according to the pressure parameter.
2. Regardless of the parameter used for control, the second parameter can be used easily to cross-monitor the first one.

A 1 gram molecule of water (18 g, or 18 mL in the liquid state) as steam at 121°C and 2.05 abs bar occupies a volume of approximately 15 L. This means that when steam condenses at 121°C it shrinks in volume by almost 1000 times. Accordingly, additional available steam *spontaneously* reaches the object to be sterilized. The condensate that forms can be removed easily from the autoclave chamber by means of a condensate discharge or, with a more modern technique, by continuous and forced bleeding (as occurs for example in so-called *dynamic steam* sterilizers).

However, several other phenomena must be considered. To perform its microorganism inactivating action (coagulation of cellular proteins), the steam, or more generally the moist heat, must make contact with the microorganisms. This can occur directly or indirectly. For example, it occurs directly when the steam that is present in the autoclave chamber is in direct contact with a surgical instrument. It instead occurs indirectly when moist steam is generated (by heat exchange with the steam present in the chamber) inside a sealed ampule that contains an aqueous solution. However, it is evident that it is not possible to steam-sterilize the inside of an empty closed ampule or the contents of an ampule if they are constituted by an anhydrous oil-based solution.

The air that is initially present in the autoclave chamber and the *incondensables* that possibly are entrained by the steam (generally CO_2) have molecular weights, and thus densities, 1.5 to 2.0 times higher than steam (under equal temperature/pressure conditions). Therefore, the air must be eliminated initially from the chamber and the steam must not introduce incondensables in the chamber; otherwise, these tend to stratify in the lower portions of the chamber, creating intolerable temperature gradients.

When closed nondeformable containers that contain aqueous solutions are sterilized, the pressures inside them can reach values far above those of the chamber. All air has been removed from the chamber, which in fact only contains steam: accordingly, at 121°C the pressure is 2.05 abs bar. The container instead almost always has a head space that contains air (or other gases). During sterilization, the aqueous solution of the container produces a vapor pressure that is approximately equal to 2.05 abs bar, but this value is increased by the partial pressure of the air of the head space; assuming that its initial value is 1.0 bar, it will increase to approximately 1.3 bar due to heating.

Pressure increases also will occur due to the thermal expansion of the solution (which is not entirely compensated by the expansion of the glass of the container) and because any gases dissolved in the solution may leave it.

Generally, in the conditions described above the total pressure inside the container exceeds by approximately 1.4 bar the pressure in the chamber if the initial head space is, as usually occurs, 10 to 20% of the total volume of the container. This overpressure generally is well tolerated by glass ampules, even those of considerable capacity (20 to 30 mL). However, it becomes hazardous for glass containers fitted with rubber stoppers held in place by a seal (due to the risk of stopper lifting) and intolerable for deformable containers, such as rigid (and even flexible) plastic containers, prefilled syringes, or cans. In all these cases, it is necessary or convenient to use the *counterpressure* sterilization methods (described later).

SATURATED STEAM AUTOCLAVES

Materials—All autoclaves intended for the pharmaceutical industry are made of Class AISI 316 stainless steel, including valves and piping (Fig 40-4). Only the service elements arranged *downstream* of the autoclave (for example the vacuum pump or the condensate discharge) are accepted if they are made of other materials. The service elements *upstream* of the autoclave (eg, heat exchangers or water pumps) also must be made of stainless steel.

Silicone rubber or Teflon and derivatives thereof generally are used for the gaskets (of doors, valves, etc).

Structure—Saturated steam autoclaves generally have a quadrangular, or rarely cylindrical, chamber. The doors are generally quadrangular even if the structure is cylindrical; in this case, the doors are inscribed in the circumference. There may be one or two doors: when the autoclave leads to a sterile room, there are always two doors.

Two-door autoclaves often are used when this requirement does not occur but the need is nonetheless felt to separate the

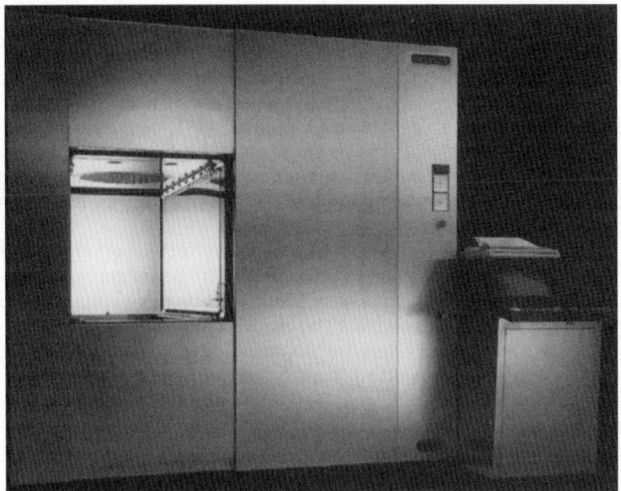

Figure 40-4. A modern computerized steam autoclave with horizontal sliding door (courtesy, Fedegari Autoclavi).

loading area, where products to be sterilized are placed, from the unloading area, where already sterilized products are placed. *This concept applies to all types of sterilizers.*

Doors may be of various kinds. The most common types are

- Hinged, manually operated, retained by radial locking bars, with a solid and fixed gasket
- Hinged, semiautomatically operated, retained by means of abutments in which the door engages automatically and with a movable gasket activated by compressed air
- Vertically or laterally sliding, with retention and gaskets as mentioned immediately above

Saturated steam autoclaves generally are jacketed. There is no room here to discuss the various kinds of jacket and their purposes. However, there are two ways to feed steam into the jacket and into the chamber:

Single Feed—the steam circulates first in the jacket and passes from the jacket into the chamber.
Separate Feed—usually the chamber is fed pure steam and the jacket is fed industrial steam.

Single-feed steam has some advantages in terms of control, but separate-feed steam is preferred because it provides better assurances of lack of microbiological and particle contamination.

MANAGEMENT SYSTEMS

The management systems used on currently manufactured autoclaves are programmable logic controllers (PLCs) or personal computers (PCs), or sometimes combinations of PLCs and PCs. This is also true for other kinds of autoclaves and sterilizers, which will be discussed later. However, a very large number of autoclaves controlled by electropneumatic systems are still in operation and still perform acceptable work. Naturally, the current control systems offer a kind of performance that was undreamed of earlier.

Pressure or temperature control (as mentioned previously, these parameters are interchangeable for a saturated steam autoclave) generally is performed with a proportional-integral-derivative method. Control by temperature is the generally accepted scheme because it is not influenced by trapped air. Sterilization can be time-managed or F_0-managed (with the F_0 being accumulated by heat probes enabled for this function), or time-managed with simultaneous calculation of F_0 for monitoring purposes.

Some management systems offer exceptional flexibility in composing programs and in setting parameters even to operators who have no knowledge of electronic programming. The information provided in real time (on same display device) is extremely detailed, as is the permanent information, which can be produced on paper or stored on various kinds of electronic medium.

PROCESS

Initial Removal of the Air from the Chamber—The main reason the air must be removed from the autoclave chamber has been pointed out above.

Loads often are made up of porous materials or materials packaged in sterilization paper or in plastic/paper bags, or contained in filter boxes. All these situations require reliable and rapid removal of the air from the load. The so-called *gravity* removal method is considered obsolete. Modern autoclaves have a water-ring vacuum pump that can produce a vacuum of approximately 70 residual mbar in the chamber. Accordingly, only about 10% of the air remains in the chamber. There are essentially two methods for completing air removal:

Pulsed Vacuum—Once the initial vacuum has been reached, the pump is stopped and steam is introduced in the chamber (up to approximately atmospheric pressure), then vacuum is produced again. Three or more of these vacuum/steam pulses are performed.

Dynamic Vacuum—Once the initial vacuum has been reached, the pump continues to run, but at the same time a 5- to 10-min injection of steam is performed (from the side of the chamber that lies opposite the vacuum drain).

Modern autoclaves are capable of performing either of these methods, chosen according to the load to be processed.

Heating-Sterilization—During heating phases, and much less during the sterilization phase, considerable amounts of condensate form in the chamber. Except for particular instances, this condensate must be removed from the chamber. There are basically two extraction methods:

• *A condensate trap located at the bottom of the chamber.* This is the simplest and cheapest method, but it causes significant pressure drops, and therefore temperature drops, inside the chamber due to the inertia of the condensate trap. Essentially, it discharges not only the condensate but also significant amounts of steam, which cause instantaneous expansion, and thus cooling, of the steam that remains in the chamber.

• *Dynamic steam.* This is the most reliable and elegant system, but is also more expensive. During the heating and sterilization phases, the vacuum pump is kept running and draws from the chamber all the condensate that forms in it through a low-capacity valve. A certain amount of steam is naturally aspirated continuously, and a dynamic condition of the steam is thus produced, hence the name of the method.

Autoclaves also are required to have a continuous steam bleed past the controlling sensor in the drain line.

Post-Sterilization Phases—These may be different according to the material to be sterilized and depending on the results to be obtained on the material itself. The most common solutions are listed below.

1. **Vacuum and Time-Controlled Vacuum Maintenance**—This method is used to dry and simultaneously cool loads of solid materials, both porous and nonporous. It is performed by restarting the vacuum pump until a preset value (eg, 100 mbar) is reached; the pump then is kept running for a preset time (eg, 20 min).

2. **Cooling by Circulating Cold Water in the Jacket**—This method is used to cool containers that are partially filled with solution (eg, culture media) and closed with sleeve (Bellco-type) stoppers. Naturally, with these loads Item 1 is not applicable, because the solution would boil, and Item 3 is dangerous due to possible contaminations. This method is performed by removing the steam present in the chamber through the introduction of compressed sterile air at a pressure that is equal to, or greater than, the sterilization pressure. Then, cold water is circulated in the jacket. The pressurized compressed air in the chamber has two purposes: (1) to prevent the solution from boiling and (2) to improve heat exchange between the load and the jacket.

3. **Cooling by Spraying Water on the Load**—This method generally is used for loads of filled and closed ampules and plastic intravenous containers. It is performed with deionized water (to avoid salt residues on the ampules) which is nebulized onto the load by means of a sparger provided in the ceiling of the chamber. Naturally the ampules, which preferably are arranged in an orderly fashion, must be contained in trays with a perforated bottom. Nebulization of the water causes a rapid condensation of the steam that produces a sudden pressure drop in the chamber, whereas the pressure inside the ampules still remains rather high because the solution cools rather slowly. Ampules of good quality (even large ones up to approximately 20 mL) tolerate this method adequately. Cooling stops when the solution inside the ampules has reached the temperature of 70° to 80°C. In this manner, the load, removed from the autoclave, still contains enough heat energy to dry spontaneously.

4. **Ampule Tightness with Fast Vacuum**—The pressure stress described in Item 3, above, is produced deliberately and increased by activating the vacuum pump as soon as the sterilization phase ends. The pressure in the chamber quickly drops to values that can reach 150 to 200 mbar (obviously this value can be controlled easily), whereas the pressure inside the closed ampules initially remains above 3.0 bar. The ΔP thus produced breaks ampules with *closed defects,* such as thinner regions, tensions in the glass, and closed cracks.

   Obviously, if the ampules have *open defects* (ie, holes at the tip or open cracks), the ΔP does not arise or is very small and thus the ampules rarely break. What happens instead is that the solution in the ampule boils and thus evaporates, reducing the volume of the solution. Unfortunately, this evaporation is very limited. Because it requires a considerable amount of energy, the solution cools very quickly and the boiling ends. One cannot rely on the transmission of heat from the adjacent ampules or from the jacket, because the chamber is evacuated. It is evident that in such conditions, solution in the liquid state leaks from the ampules; at least from the *open defects* that lie below the level of the solution. Accordingly, it may be convenient to load the ampules upside down (ie, with their tip pointing downward) if it is known that most defects occur at the tip or shoulder of the ampules. Naturally, the breakage of the ampules or the leakage of solution soils the load, which must therefore be washed and dried. With appropriate methods it usually is possible to achieve all this in the autoclave itself.

5. **Cooling as in Item 3, but with Air Counterpressure**—In many cases it is not possible or reasonable to subject the load, during cooling, to the pressure stress that arises with the method described in Item 3. In such cases, it is possible to remove the steam present in the chamber by replacing it with sterile compressed air at a pressure that is equal to, or higher than, the sterilization pressure. Only after this has occurred does the cooling water spray described in Item 3 begin. This method only prevents the load from suffering the pressure stress of the cooling phase, whereas the stress of the sterilization phase is unavoidable. Reference is made to the section on *Counterpressure Methods* below for an explanation of this phenomenon and for the autoclaves that allow to avoid it.

6. **Spontaneous Cooling**—In some particular cases it may be necessary to resort to this cooling method, which is the simplest but also obviously requires a very long time. Clearly, at the end of this cooling the autoclave will be in vacuum, and the longer the cooling the deeper the vacuum.

7. **Ampule Tightness Test with Dye Solution Penetration**—This test generally is performed with an aqueous solution of methylene blue. However, it is also possible to use other dyes. This test is effective only on *open defects* of ampules and is performed as follows:
   a. Vacuum in the chamber to approximately 100 to 150 mbar.
   b. The chamber is filled with the colored solution until the load is completely covered; the ampules must of course be contained in appropriate trays that do not allow them to escape, because they tend to float.
   c. During this filling operation, the chamber vacuum reached in Item 1 is maintained continuously by connecting the vacuum pump to the ceiling of the chamber.
   d. The colored solution is pressurized at 2 to 3 bar and is maintained in this condition for 30 to 60 min or more.
   e. The colored solution is discharged and recovered.
   f. The load is washed several times with spray water.
   g. The load is washed by flooding the chamber.
   h. The washing water is discharged.

There are alternatives to this method, such as electronic spark discharge inspection which detects leakage of liquid from the ampule by a decrease in resistance across electrodes placed across the ampule.

- The vacuum is not maintained continuously while the chamber is being filled with the colored solution.
- The vacuum is produced only after filling the chamber with the colored solution.
- The vacuum is not produced at all.

This test has in any case the following problems:

- It has been demonstrated extensively that with usual values for dye concentration, differential test pressure, and test time, tip holes with a diameter of less than 5 to 10 μm allow very small amounts of colored solution to enter. This prevents detection of the coloring of the ampules during subsequent checking.
- The preparation of sterile colored solution for each test entails very high costs.
- Recovery and reuse of the colored solution entails keeping it in conditions that prevent microbial proliferation (80°C) and subjecting it to sterilizing filtration prior to each test. All these procedures are expensive and complicated. In any case, the solution recovered from each test is contaminated chemically by the broken or defective tested ampules.
- Decolorization/destruction of the solution is very difficult, because methylene blue is very stable; however, good decolorization results have been achieved by using ozone. The use of amber glass ampules makes detection of the dye difficult.

STERILIZING THE AIR INTRODUCED IN THE CHAMBER

In the previous paragraphs we noted that it is often necessary to introduce air in the chamber, especially in post-sterilization phases. This air must be sterile, otherwise it may recontaminate the sterilized load and can, in any case, contaminate the sterile environment if the autoclave is of the two-door type connected to the sterile area.

The air generally is sterilized by filtration using a system that is part of the autoclave. It is thus necessary to

- Provide a filtration cartridge with sterilizing porosity
- Allow *in situ* sterilization of the assembled filtration system with an appropriate sterilization program of the autoclave itself
- Ensure that the filtration system and the line for connecting it to the autoclave maintain their sterility between one production sterilization program of the autoclave and the next
- Allow validation of all of the above described procedures

If one wishes to operate in perfect safety, the filtration system also should be subjected to an integrity test each time it is operated.

Counterpressure Methods

Autoclaves operating with counterpressure are defined as devices able to control, during sterilization, the pressure of the moist sterilizing medium independently of its temperature. Conventional pure saturated steam autoclaves do not belong to this category. The temperature of the pure saturated steam present in the chamber in fact automatically generates a specific pressure that cannot be modified without modifying the temperature as well. If the temperature of the steam is 121°C, its pressure is unavoidably 2.05 bar abs and *vice versa*, assuming no trapped air.

For many kinds of load it is necessary or convenient to use an autoclave operating with counterpressure. To understand this need, let us see what happens in a conventional autoclave during the sterilization of a rigid container partially filled with an aqueous solution and closed tight. For the sake of simplicity, let us assume that the container is filled with pure water.

A glass bottle is filled partially in standard conditions: 20°C and 1.013 bar; the bottle is closed with a rubber stopper and aluminum seal. In the head space there is a total pressure of 1.013 bar, which is actually the sum of two factors: a partial water-vapor pressure which corresponds to the vapor pressure of water at 20°C, ie, 0.025 bar, and a partial air pressure of 0.988 bar.

When the bottle is subjected to the sterilization phase at 121°C, these two factors change as follows:

	Initial Condition		Sterilization Condition
Partial water-vapor pressure	0.025	→	2.050 bar (1)
Partial air pressure	0.988	→	1.330 bar (2)
Total pressure in head space	1.013	→	3.380 bar abs

Value 1, 2.050 bar, is obviously the pressure of water vapor at 121°C and *corresponds to the pressure that occurs in the autoclave chamber*. Value 2, 1.330 bar, is a theoretical value that is calculated by applying the law of perfect gases to air:

$$0.988 \times \frac{121 + 273}{20 + 273} = 1.330$$

Therefore, the total pressure of 3.380 bar abs is also a theoretical value.

There are some reports that demonstrate that the *practical* value is slightly higher than the theoretical one and largely depends on the ratio between the head space and the volume of the filling solution. The practical pressure of the head volume is, on average, higher at 121°C by approximately 1.40 bar, with respect to the pressure in the chamber. This is caused by two mechanisms:

The thermal expansion of water is significantly greater than that of glass and increases very rapidly as the temperature rises. The specific volumes of water at the temperatures we are interested in are in fact

Temperature °C	Specific Volume mL/g
0	1.0002
4	1.0000 (maximum density)
20	1.0017
120	1.0606

In passing from 20° to 121°C, water increases its volume by approximately 6% according to the following ratio:

$$\frac{1.0606}{1.0017} = 1.058$$

This fact must be considered carefully by those who tend to reduce or eliminate the head space in containers and then are surprised to find that such containers explode or warp during sterilization. Solutions (especially if filtered under gas pressure) contain considerable amounts of dissolved gases that leave the liquid phase as the temperature rises.

The overpressure of approximately 1.40 bar that occurs in the bottle naturally generates a force of approximately 1.4 kg per cm^2 of internal surface of the bottle. A rubber stopper with a diameter of 24 mm is subjected to an expulsion force of approximately 6.3 kg.

These conditions therefore prevent or advise against the use of a pure saturated steam autoclave to sterilize solutions contained in a wide variety of containers. For example,

- Large-Volume Parenterals (LVP) in glass containers
- Small-Volume Parenterals (SVP) in glass vials with rubber stopper
- LVP or SVP in plastic containers (flexible, semirigid, or rigid plastic)
- Prefilled syringes
- Jars or similar containers with press-on or screw on closures
- Blisters containing various materials, such as disposable contact lenses

Two counterpressure methods currently in use are

- Superheated water spray method (water cascade process)
- Air overstream method (steam plus air method)

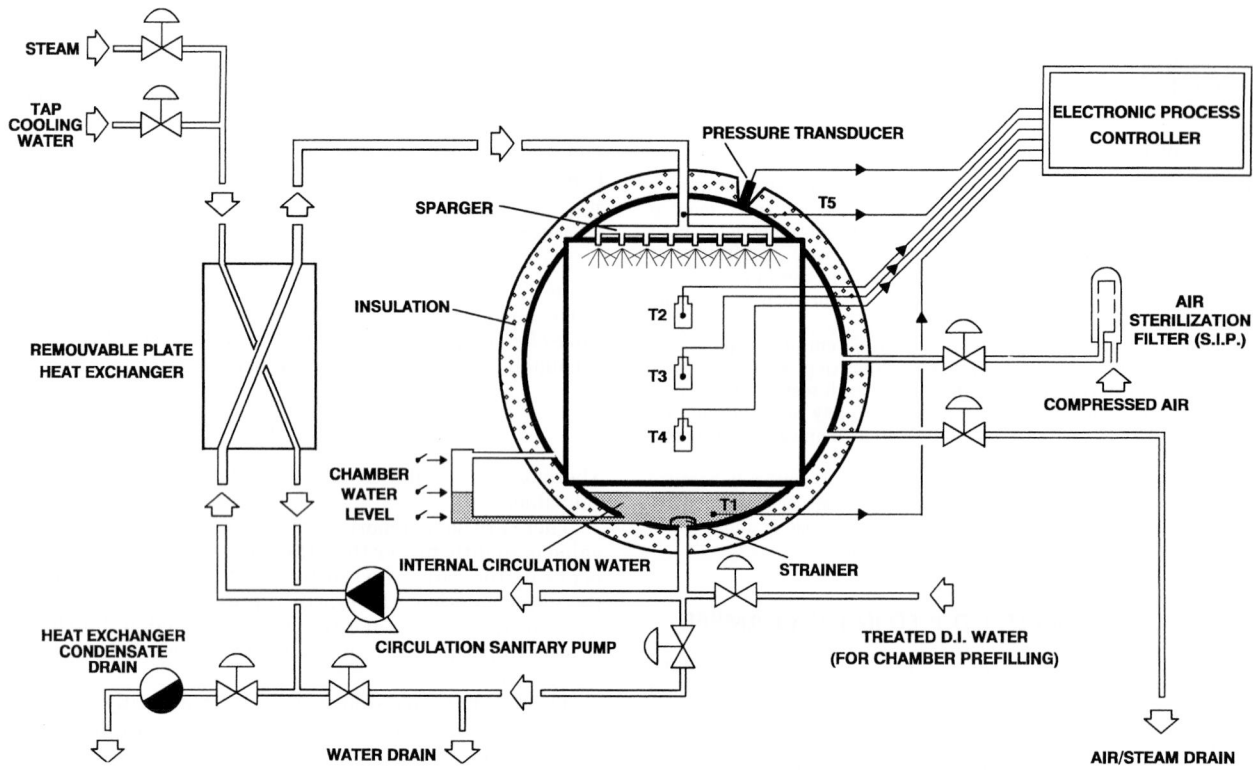

Figure 40-5. Superheated water-spray autoclave: simplified piping and instrumentation diagram (courtesy, Fedegari Autoclavi).

SUPERHEATED WATER SPRAY AUTOCLAVES

A typical functional diagram of this autoclave is shown in the Figure 40-5. Obviously, different solutions are also possible which, however, do not change the essence of the method. The chamber generally has a circular cross-section (with quadrangular door(s) inscribed in the circumference) and has a single wall.

At the beginning of the program, after the goods have been loaded, the lower circular sector is filled with purified water. The air contained in the chamber is *not* removed. The water, drawn by a sanitary-type pump, circulates in a heat exchanger (plate or other sanitary type), which is *indirectly* heated in countercurrent with industrial steam. The water returns then into the upper part of the chamber and is distributed to the load by a system of solid-cone spray nozzles. The uniform redistribution of the water on the lower layers of the load is ensured by appropriate perforated racks that support the load. Side spray bars sometimes are used, even if their actual usefulness is not demonstrated.

The heating of the circulation water, and therefore of the load, is gradual but quite fast; for example, the temperature of 121°C is reached in approximately 20 to 30 min *inside* 500-mL containers, mainly dependent on the solution and the material and shape of the containers.

The sterilization phase lasts 15 to 20 min, and temperature uniformity (in time and space) is excellent: it is well within the quite narrow limits required by FDA for LVP sterilization, ±0.5°C. This allows very small F_0 dispersions, and therefore minimum sterilization times.

The cooling phase is performed while the circulation water, now sterile, continues to circulate. However, cold tap water now flows in the plates of the exchanger, where steam was flowing earlier. In less than 15 min, the temperature *inside* the 500-mL containers drops to approximately 70°C, which is also the ideal temperature for obtaining a rapid and spontaneous drying of the load removed from the autoclave.

During all the phases of the process, an appropriate sterile air counterpressure is maintained inside the chamber to counterbalance the overpressure in the bottles. There are various methods for controlling this counterpressure in each phase. With computerized management, it is even possible to generate a total pressure (steam plus air) inside the chamber that is correlated, in each phase, to the average of the internal temperatures of two or more *witness* containers.

The load suffers no thermal or pressure shock and the differential pressure between containers and chamber can be eliminated or maintained in a direction convenient, in each phase, for the particular type of load. Even highly deformable products (semirigid plastic containers or plastic–aluminum blisters) or products that are particularly sensitive to differential pressures (eg, prefilled syringes) can be treated (from 60° to 127°C) without problems.

The autoclaves are obviously highly specialized machines, and as such they have some limitations in application:

- It is illogical to attempt to dry the load inside the autoclave by putting the chamber in vacuum or by circulating warm air.
- In the case of materials with concavities directed upward, these concavities will be filled with water at the end of the program: the most obvious solution is to load these materials upside down.
- When PVC bags are sterilized, the phenomenon of *blushing*—the whitening of the PVC due to water absorption—usually occurs. The intensity of this phenomenon and the time required for its disappearance depend on the type of PVC and of plasticizer employed. Blushing does not occur with rigid or semirigid plastic or with polylaminate plastics; it also is reduced considerably with PVC containing special plasticizers.

AIR OVER STEAM AUTOCLAVES

A typical functional diagram of this type of autoclave is shown in Figure 40-6. Alternatives are also possible in this case. The most important one is the use of horizontal fans placed on a side of the chamber. As in the previous case, the chamber has a cir-

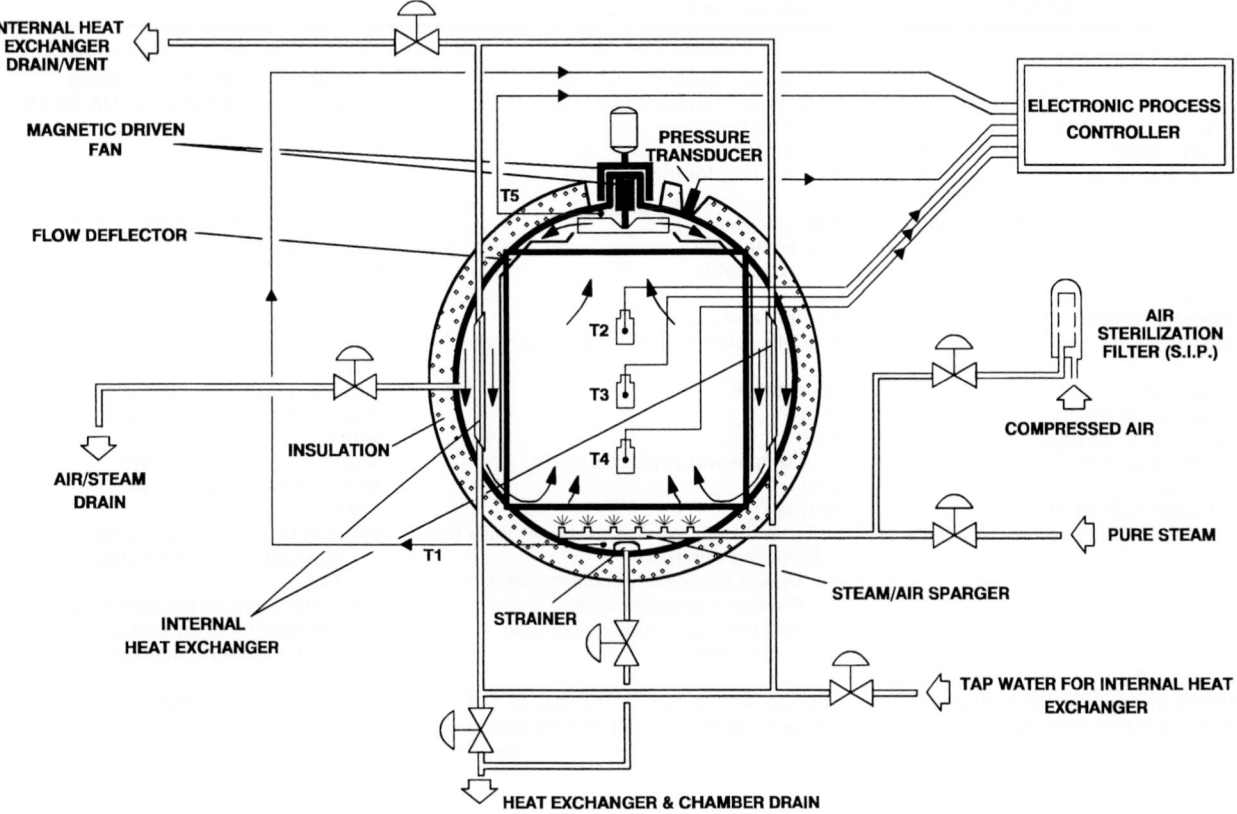

Figure 40-6. Air over steam autoclave: simplified piping and instrumentation diagram (courtesy, Fedegari Autoclavi).

cular cross-section (with a quadrangular door or doors inscribed in the circumference) and has a single wall.

There are two reasons for choosing a circular cross-section for autoclaves operating in counterpressure.

1. These autoclaves operate at significantly higher pressures than conventional pure saturated steam autoclaves, and generally are not put in vacuum. It is well known that a cylindrical structure withstands internal pressure much better than a quadrangular one.
2. The circular sectors of the chamber that are not occupied by the load are used to place elements required for the operation of these autoclaves.

The air is *not* removed initially from the chamber. The steam enters directly into the chamber through a sparger located in the chamber's lower portion. The partial air pressure of the mixture can be adjusted during the entire process, similarly to what occurs for the previously described superheated water spray autoclaves.

The fan(s) placed against the ceiling of the chamber and the flow deflectors have the purpose of homogenizing the steam plus air mixture that forms inside the chamber. The task of these fans is very important and demanding. In fact, for equal pressure and temperature conditions, the air is approximately 1.6 times denser than the steam (one only has to consider their respective molecular weights) and would tend to stratify on the bottom, producing intolerable temperature gradients.

The cooling phase consists of feeding air into the chamber (to condense and replace all the steam that is present) while maintaining the same sterilization pressure or possibly increasing it. Cold tap water then is fed into the heat exchangers, which are constituted by batteries of hollow plates located in the two circular sectors of the sides of the chamber (only one plate is shown in the diagram for the sake of simplicity). A tube heat ex-

changer can be used as an alternative. The load is thus cooled while constantly maintaining a controlled pressure inside the chamber.

However, this cooling comprises two solid-gas heat exchanges (plates → air; air → load) that, as is known, have a very poor efficiency. An attempt is made to improve this exchange by increasing the pressure of the air in the chamber (within the limits allowed by the product and the autoclave) so as to increase its density and therefore its heat-exchange capacity. The fans obviously continue to run during the cooling phase. Despite these refinements, the cooling phase is definitely longer than the same phase in superheated water spray autoclaves.

A critical mechanical aspect of these autoclaves is the tightness of the fan shaft. This aspect can be solved completely by using magnetic-drive fans.

With steam plus air mixture autoclaves, the blushing of PVC bags is less intense than with water spray autoclaves and generally affects essentially the regions where the bag rests on the supporting racks.

Table 40-1 compares the characteristics of the two kinds of counter pressure autoclaves.

Dry Heat Treatments

STERILIZATION AND DEPYROGENATION

Dry heat treatments have two targets: microorganisms and their by-products. The aim of sterilization is to destroy the ability of microorganisms to survive and multiply. Depyrogenation seeks to destroy the chemical activity of the by-products: pyrogens or endotoxins (these terms do not mean exactly the same thing, but we will consider them to be synonymous for the sake of simplicity).

Table 40-1. Counter Pressure Autoclave Comparison

CRITICAL COMPARISON	WATER SPRAY (WS) AUTOCLAVES	AIR OVER STEAM (AS) AUTOCLAVES
Temperature uniformity in time	Very good easily in $\pm 0.5°$ limits	Very good easily in $\pm 0.5°$ limits
Temperature uniformity in space	Very good requested by FDA for LVP	Very good requested by FDA for LVP
Total pressure uniformity in time	Very good	Very good
Counterpressure management flexibility	Excellent	Excellent
Consumption of high microbiological quality water	Yes, modest, for initial filling	No
Consumption of tap water for cooling	Yes, acceptable	Yes, approx. 3 times higher than WAS
Consumption of compressed air	Yes, acceptable	Yes, acceptblke
Consumption of industrial steam	Yes, acceptable	No
Consumption of ultraclean steam	No	Yes, acceptable
Condensate recovery	Possible and easy	Not possible
Cooling water recovery	Possible, recovered water is initially very hot	Possible, recovered water is initially very hot
Autoclave price	Acceptable	Approx. 1.1 times higher than WS
Total process duration	Short	Approx. 1.3 times higher than WS
Autoclave productivity/price	High	Approx. 70% of WS
Operation principle	Very simple and straightforward	More complicated than WS
Mechanical construction	Simple	More complicated than WS
Qualification/validation	Normal	Normal
Operating flexibility according to type of load	Suitable for any kind of container with the following remarks: • Upward concavities collect water • Product is unloaded wet • PVC bags can produce blushing phenomena	Suitable for any kind of container: • Upward concavities collect condensate only • Other kinds of container can be unloaded slightly damp • Blushing phenomena of PVC bags are limited
Possibility of combination with pure saturated steam processes	Strongly discouraged: It is complex and expensive and complicates validation	Very frequent, but moderately expensive

Both processes consist of an oxidation that is almost a combustion. However, the temperatures required to achieve depyrogenation are distinctly higher than those needed to obtain sterilization. We can summarize the situation as follows:

- If an effective dry heat depyrogenation is performed, sterilization generally is achieved *as well*.
- Effective dry heat sterilization can be performed even *without* achieving depyrogenation.
- If moist heat sterilization is performed, in normal operating conditions depyrogenation is *not* achieved.

The kinetics of dry heat treatments are not substantially different from those of moist heat sterilization. The values of the algorithms F_T and F_H (analogous to F_0) and those of the parameters D and z, however, are different not only from those of moist heat sterilization but also from each other. Furthermore, the two dry heat treatments are verified biologically with different biochallenges. Accordingly, the two dry heat treatments require different validation approaches.

The materials subjected to dry heat treatments naturally must be heat-stable: the most common are glass containers for parenterals. Elastomeric compounds generally are unable to tolerate these treatments.

The literature generally mentions the following operating conditions:

Sterilization: 160°C—120 to 180 min
                     170°C—90 to 120 min
                     180°C—45 to 60 min

Depyrogenation: 230°C—60 to 90 min
                     250°C—30 to 60 min

However, the current trend is toward using treatments at higher temperatures than those listed.

The sections that follow describe the most common types of equipment used to perform the above processes. If the load (bottles/vials/ampules made of glass or other materials) is wet when it is introduced, a large part of the energy required by the process is used initially to evaporate the water that wets the load, and the process accordingly takes more time. The equipment uses large amounts of air, which generally is recirculated partially and must be filtered in HEPA filters to have, in the critical regions of the equipment, the Class 100 environment. This is relatively easy to achieve in the sterilization phases (or regions) in which the *thermal situation* of the filters is stable. It is much less easy to achieve in the heating/cooling phases (or regions), because the changes in temperature entail expansions/contractions of the filters, with consequent release of particles.

DRY HEAT BATCH STERILIZERS

The forced-convection batch sterilizer is a type of dry heat unit widely used in the industry. It uses the principle of convective heat transfer to heat the load. Figure 40-7 is a schematic diagram of a modern unit. It shows a two-door sterilizer in which the unloading door leads to the sterile area. The two doors are, of course, parallel to the plane of the drawing and are hinged vertically.

The pressure inside the chamber must be controlled continuously so that it is slightly higher than the pressure in the loading area (nonsterile) and slightly lower than the pressure in the unloading area (sterile).

The unit is made entirely of stainless steel; particular care must be taken in selecting the insulating materials and in the methods for applying them. It is important also to avoid the forming of so-called *thermal bridges;* these allow dissipation, and thus excessive external temperatures of the sterilizer and *cold spots* in the chamber.

The main features shown in the sketch are:

1. Air-circulation fan
2. Water-cooled battery (for the cooling phase)
3. Circulation HEPA filters
4. Launch/recovery bulkheads
5. Trolley and load
6. Discharge duct
7. HEPA filter on the discharge duct to prevent back-flow contamination
8. Variable-speed fan for chamber pressurization (proportionally controlled)
9. Prefilter and HEPA filter on the chamber pressurization loop
10. Electric heater (proportionally controlled)

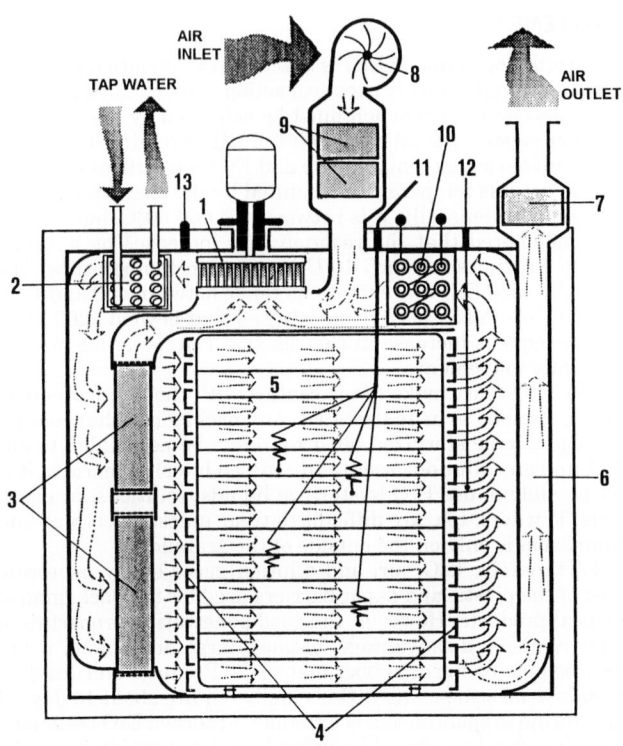

Figure 40-7. Dry heat batch sterilizer: simplified diagram (courtesy, Fedegari Autoclavi).

11. Four flexible Pt100 4-wire RTDs
12. Main control Pt100 4-wire RTD
13. Pressure transducer

DRY HEAT TUNNELS

The drying, sterilizing/depyrogenation, and cooling tunnel is the only continuous sterilizing apparatus widely used in the pharmaceutical industry (apart from filters). It basically consists of a horizontally rotating transport belt made of a stainless-steel mesh (some devices must be provided to confine the product on the transport belt without particulate generating friction), installed in a thermally insulated *tunnel* that directly connects an upstream cleaning machine to the downstream sterile area or to *isolated* devices.

Inside the tunnel, the product (most frequently glass vials) is dried; heat-treated either by radiant heat or, as more usual today, by hot air; and finally cooled. In both cases the internal part of the tunnel must be pressurized dynamically by ventilation at an intermediate pressure level between the downstream system and the loading room. From a process point of view, higher temperature and shorter exposure time are used than in batch sterilizers. During the last 10 years the practice has changed from 20 min at 280°C to 3 or 4 min at 300°C or more. Because a minimum safety margin is required for the duration of exposure, and glass of most types becomes more difficult to handle above 320°C and more fragile after such a treatment, it is likely that the trend toward higher temperature values has reached its practical limit.

In infrared (IR) radiant heat tunnels, heat is supplied by resistance-in-glass heaters located above and below the transport belt; prefiltered and HEPA-filtered air is fed into the cooling zone mainly for pressurizing and cooling. This air, a countercurrent slowly flowing through the entire tunnel, has also an important drying and preheating effect of the load in the infeed zone. Figure 40-8 schematically represents an IR

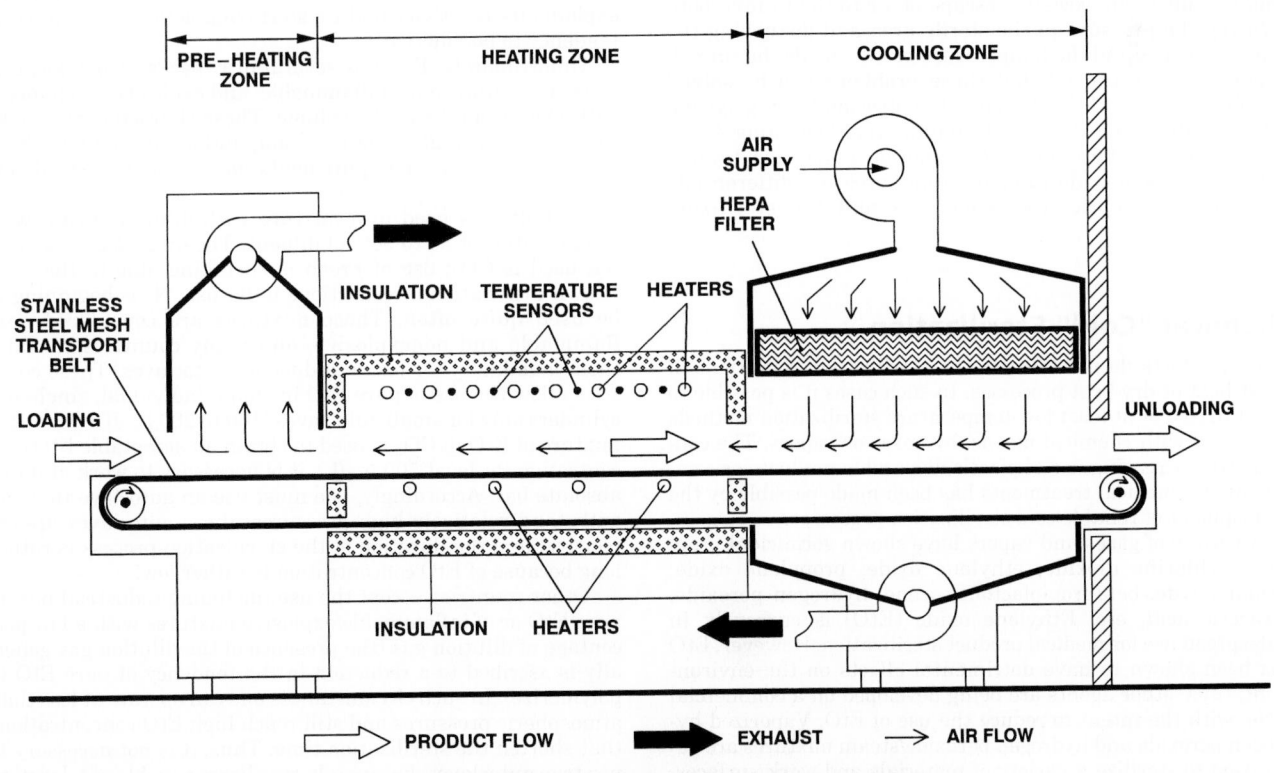

Figure 40-8. Dry heat tunnel: simplified diagram (courtesy, Fedegari Autoclavi).

tunnel: even if this type of apparatus is no longer widely used, the basic concepts have not been modified in the hot-air laminar flow tunnel, but airflow patterns are a little more complex.

Hot-air laminar flow (LF) tunnels do not radiate heat directly to the product, but rather heating is provided by circulation of hot filtered air forced onto the product. A circulation fan withdraws the air; it leaves the product through heating bars below the transport belt and is fed again to the inside of the tunnel through HEPA filters suitable for operating at high temperature. Airtightness of the coupling of HEPA filters with tunnel framework is of utmost importance from the point of view of particulate contamination. It must cope with the strong thermal expansion of different materials. Some makeup air is required in the heating zone, and the total number of installed fans may be as high as five or even six if an additional extraction below tunnel outfeed is required in case of high pressure in the sterile room.

Despite the complexity of its airflow, the LF tunnel has the main advantage of quicker heating and consequent shorter process time. This results in reduced size compared with the IR tunnel, because the belt speed cannot be reduced below a certain value. As the name itself declares, the air speed in the LF tunnel is kept around 0.5 m/sec (1.5 ft/sec), aiming to avoid particulate contamination.

The comparison between continuous tunnel and batch oven is favorable to the continuous tunnel from the point of view of handling the product. No batch work is needed after the unpacking of the components and loading of them into the cleaning machine until the final removal of the packaged product from the line after the filling and the following operations. This can be very important in the case of large-scale production.

The batch oven provides a much easier isolation of the sterile area. In the case of continuous tunnel, there must be a steady flow of air through the open connection from the sterile area to the tunnel. The pressure difference between the two systems must be such that the sterile area always is kept at a higher pressure level than the tunnel. Too big a difference would result in an excessive escape of air to the tunnel, both reducing the pressure in the sterile area and disturbing the laminar airflow and the temperature profile inside the tunnel. Experience has proved that these problems can be solved satisfactorily only if the design of the air-conditioning system of the sterile area is developed from the very beginning, keeping in mind the foreseen installation of a specified tunnel. Baffle systems also aid in maintaining pressure differentials between the aseptic-processing area and the sterilizing tunnel.

Chemical "Cold" Sterilization

Many products do not tolerate the sterilization conditions of moist-heat or dry heat processes. In such cases it is possible to resort to cold or at least low-temperature sterilization methods performed with chemical means, by gases or vapors. The continuously increasing use of plastic disposable products or components for medical treatments has been made possible by the development of reliable cold sterilization processes.

A variety of gases and vapors have shown germicidal properties: chlorine dioxide, ethylene oxide, propylene oxide, formaldehyde, betapropiolactone, ozone, hydrogen peroxide, peracetic acid, etc. Ethylene oxide (EtO) is currently in widespread use for medical product sterilization. However, EtO has been shown to have detrimental effects on the environment; thus, other agents are being developed on a commercial scale, with the intent to reduce the use of EtO. Vaporized hydrogen peroxide and hydrogen peroxide/steam mixtures are being used to sterilize a variety of materials and work surfaces. Chlorine dioxide recently has become available for these applications.

ETHYLENE OXIDE

The sterilizing action of EtO is based on an alkylation reaction: it is, accordingly, a truly chemical action rather than a physical one. This chemical reaction must be activated by the presence of water vapor (approximately 60% of RH or relative humidity) and is increased by temperature and EtO concentration.

The process temperature is limited by the characteristics of the product. Generally, it is between 40° and 60°C, but it must be remembered that the reaction rate increases by approximately 2.5 times for each 10°C increase in temperature. The normally used EtO concentrations range between 400 and 1200 mg/L. It has in fact been demonstrated that beyond 1200 mg/L the consequent increase in the reaction rate is no longer economically convenient.

The EtO must make *direct* contact with the microorganism for the microbe to be inactivated. Any packagings that contain the object to be sterilized must therefore be permeable to air, EtO, and any dilution gases (as discussed later). Generally, it is not possible to use EtO to sterilize liquids, solutions, or emulsions. Powders, too, are difficult to treat unless microbial contamination is only on the outside of the granules.

Fortunately, EtO, air, and dilution gases easily penetrate most of the plastic and paper barriers used for the packaging of medical products. However, the good penetrating properties of EtO are also a disadvantage, because large amounts of it are absorbed by plastic or rubber materials. Products sterilized on an industrial scale using EtO normally require about 14 days of quarantine to spontaneously eliminate absorbed EtO residuals. This time can be reduced by using forced desorption methods. Sterilized goods must be monitored for toxic EtO residual, ethylene glycol, and ethylene chlorhydrin breakdown products of EtO.

EtO in standard room conditions is a vapor (indeed, its boiling point is about 11°C at atmospheric pressure). It is colorless, heavier than air, and has an ether-like odor. Its formula is

$$CH_2 \text{---} CH_2$$
$$\underset{O}{\underline{\hspace{1.2cm}}}$$

The presence of the oxygen bridge, which can be opened easily, explains its reactivity and its sterilizing action, as well as its tendency to polymerize.

Unfortunately, EtO has several drawbacks: it is toxic, carcinogenic, teratogenic, inflammable, and explosive when mixed with more than 3% air by volume. These characteristics make the use of EtO highly controversial, and many countries have issued regulations or requirements for its use as a sterilizing agent.

EtO often is used in a mixture with dilution gases, with weight ratios of 85 to 90% of diluent. The diluent gas most often used is CO_2; use of Freon is shrinking, due to the well-known international restrictions to its use; N_2 is beginning to be used quite often. These mixtures are considered non-flammable and nonexplosive, and many countries consider them mandatory for use in industrial autoclaves. These countries allow the use of pure EtO in small, individual, single-use cylinders only for small autoclaves (100 to 200 L). If a 10 to 12% mixture of EtO in CO_2 is used to obtain an acceptable EtO concentration (at least 500 mg/L), it is necessary to work at 3 to 4 absolute bar. Accordingly, one must use an autoclave that can withstand relatively high pressures; these autoclaves are expensive, and the duration of the sterilization process is rather long because of EtO concentration is rather low.

Other countries accept the use (including industrial use) of pure EtO or of inflammable/explosive mixtures with a low percentage of dilution gas (the presence of the dilution gas generally is ascribed to a reduction in the tendency of pure EtO to polymerize). In such circumstances one can operate at less than atmospheric pressures and still reach high EtO concentrations that shorten the sterilization time. Thus, it is not necessary to use true autoclaves, but merely sterilizers capable of tolerating the very hard vacuum required for the initial elimination of the air from the chamber and from the load and for the final ex-

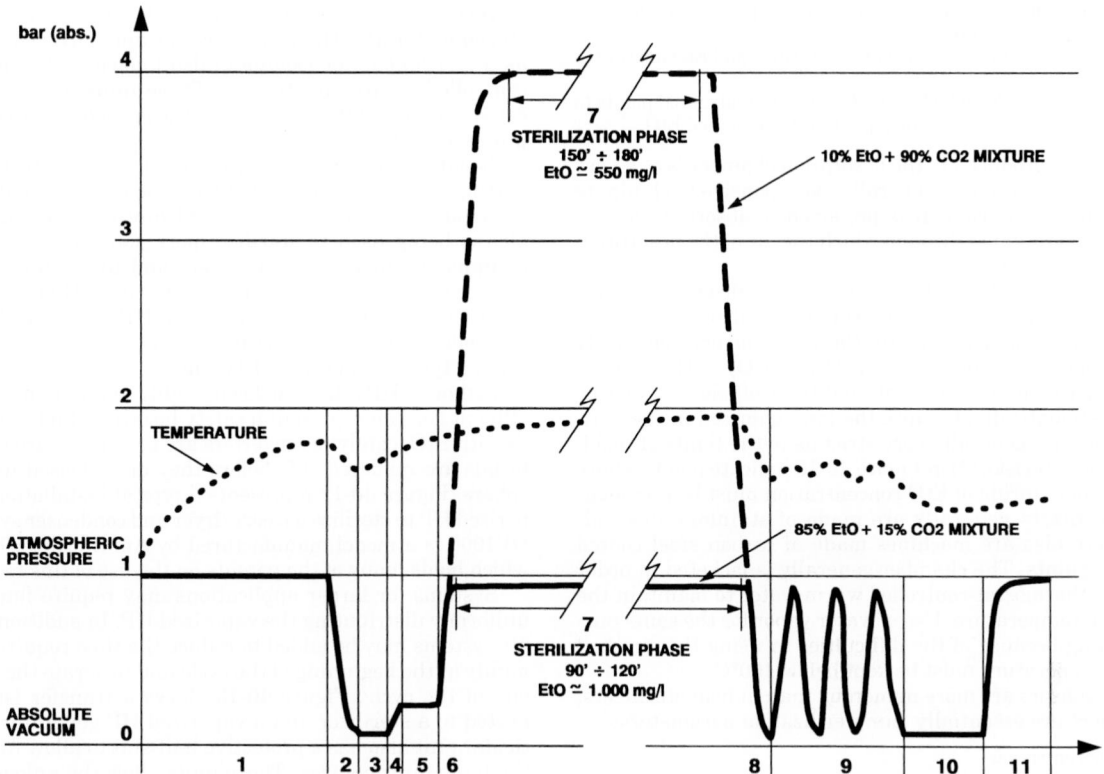

Figure 40-9. EtO sterilization pressure–time diagram: overpressure and subatmospheric pressure (courtesy, Fedegari Autoclavi).

traction of the EtO. Obviously, in these circumstances the use of plants constructed with explosion-proof criteria cannot be avoided.

The P/T/t diagrams of EtO sterilization are therefore different, depending on whether one or the other of the above described principles is used. A typical diagram of an overpressure sterilization with a mixture using 10% EtO and 90% CO_2 is shown in Figure 40-9. These are the steps:

1. Load and/or chamber heating
2. Vacuum
3. Vacuum hold for leak test
4. Humidification by steam injection
5. Penetration of humidity in the load
6. Loading of EtO mixture
7. Sterilization
8. EtO mixture evacuation
9. Air/vacuum pulses
10. Vacuum hold
11. Vacuum breaking

A typical diagram of a subatmospheric sterilization with a mixture using 85% EtO and 15% CO_2 is shown equally in Figure 40-9. One can see clearly that the phases are substantially the same as in Figure 40-8; the changes are the sterilization pressure, the EtO concentration, and therefore the duration of the sterilization phase.

In performing industrial sterilizations, which accordingly involve large loads, the load is heated and humidified before placing it in the sterilizer, in adequately conditioned rooms. Thus, the heating/humidification phases described above in the diagrams of Figures 40-8 and 40-9 are reduced drastically.

The layout of an industrial EtO sterilization plant is shown in Figure 40-10. This unit contains:

• The EtO or EtO-mixture cylinders
• The automatic devices that connect/disconnect the various cylinders to and from the sterilizer; disconnection of a cylinder (especially for mixture cylinders) often is controlled by its weight reduction, which must accordingly be checked individually

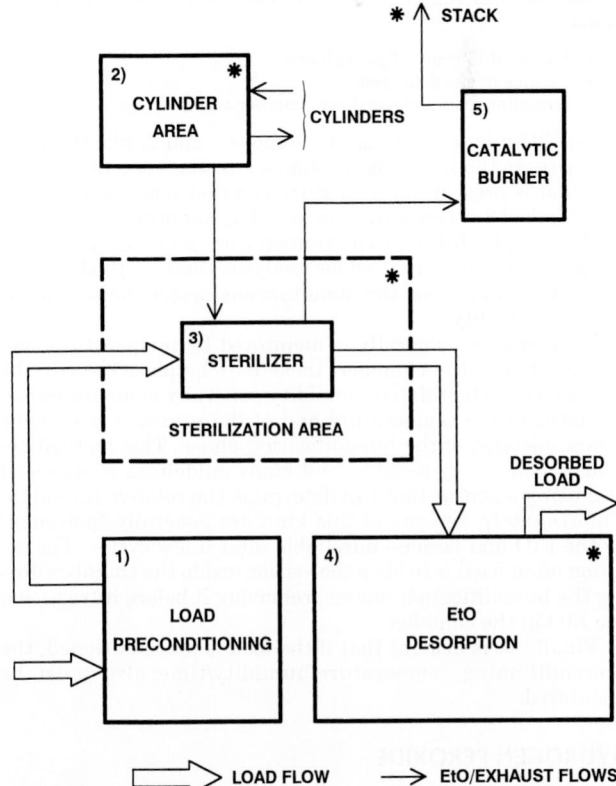

Figure 40-10. Flow diagram of an EtO sterilization industrial plant (courtesy, Fedegari Autoclavi).

- The heat exchanger that must provide the vaporization calories to the liquid EtO mixture
- The pressure reduction unit that brings the liquid EtO mixture to the vapor state
- Any cylinders of N_2, which is used in the most advanced plants to *wash,* after each process, the pipes that have carried EtO

The EtO that is produced in the desorption chamber is at a very low concentration and it is generally too expensive to eliminate it with a catalytic burner. It is preferred to absorb it on activated-charcoal columns through which the air of the desorption chamber is recirculated.

Obviously, the EtO discharged by the sterilizer (and possibly the EtO arriving from the desorption chamber) must not be discharged into the atmosphere. Catalytic burners generally are used today: they convert the EtO into $CO_2 + H_2O$. These burners must be highly efficient, and their efficiency must be checked systematically, because the laws enforced in the various countries are generally very strict as to the limits of residual EtO. The asterisks (*) in Figure 40-10 indicate points where continuous monitoring of EtO concentration must be provided.

EtO sterilizers generally are made of stainless steel, although there also are machines made of carbon steel coated with epoxy paints. The chamber generally is jacketed in order to circulate thermostat-controlled warm water to maintain the sterilization temperature. Use of water vapor for the same purpose is fading because of the difficulties in using this method when the temperature must be kept below 100°C.

Process sensors are more numerous than in heat sterilizers, because there are essentially four sterilization parameters:

- EtO concentration
- Temperature
- Humidity or relative humidity
- Time

The EtO concentration generally is monitored by the pressure rise that occurs in the chamber when the EtO mixture is introduced; a pressure transducer is therefore used as a sensor.

Many guidelines require, in addition to the pressure rise, a second monitoring method that can be chosen among the following:

1. Weight difference of gas cylinder
2. Volume of gas delivered
3. Sampling from the sterilizer chamber and analysis

When EtO mixtures are used, Methods 1 and 2, like the pressure rise method, assume confidence in the concentration of EtO that is present in the mixture and that reaches the sterilizer. Method 3 is certainly more reliable, but it also is more difficult to apply. Infrared spectrometry or gas chromatography methods generally are used for analysis; these methods can be continuous and allow the simultaneous determination of the relative humidity.

Temperature generally is monitored by temperature sensors located in the chamber; these may be placed inside the load as well. The relative humidity generally is monitored on the basis of the temperature and of the pressure rise of the steam injection of the humidification phase. This method obviously is not very reliable, and many guidelines recommend also using a sensor that can determine the relative humidity. Unfortunately, sensors of this kind are generally "poisoned" by the EtO and become unreliable after a few cycles. The solution often used is to keep the sensor inside the chamber during the humidification phases, removing it before introducing the EtO in the chamber.

Finally, it is evident that if the load is preconditioned, the preconditioning temperature/humidity/time also must be monitored.

HYDROGEN PEROXIDE

Hydrogen peroxide (HP), chemically H_2O_2, is normally a liquid at room temperature. However, it can be vaporized and the resultant gas is an effective sterilant for certain packaged materials and for equipment and enclosures used in processing sterile materials. The most frequent and successful use of HP as a sterilant is for *isolators* (also known as barriers, locally controlled environments, etc). These units are very sophisticated versions of their ancestors, the *glove boxes* used to isolate processes in the past.

Isolators now are used widely for sterility testing, transporting sterilized goods from moist and dry heat units to sterile areas or processing isolators, and processing of supplies. HP also is being used to sterilize more sophisticated processing equipment, such as freeze dryers and filling lines, and even may be used to sterilized small clean rooms. High humidity can inhibit the effectiveness of vaporized HP and must therefore be controlled during the exposure of the gas. Figure 40-11 represents a typical vaporized HP cycle.

Although HP is broken down readily to water and oxygen, the effluent gas can represent a safety hazard at higher levels. Just as with EtO, catalytic converters are used to ensure that all materials are rendered safe before they are released to the atmosphere. Figure 40-12 represents a typical installation using vaporized HP to sterilize a freeze dryer and condenser system. VHP DV1000 is a model manufactured by Am Sterilizer/Finn Aqua, which holds many of the patents on the use of this technology.

Systems for larger applications may require fans to aid in uniformly distributing the vaporized HP. In addition, auxiliary air systems may be added to reduce the time required to dehumidify at the beginning of the cycle and to aerate the load at the end of the cycle. Figure 40-13 shows a transfer isolator connected to a sterilizer and a vaporized HP generator. This particular unit also has a protective half-suit to allow full access to the large internal area. These units allow the unloading of the sterilizer directly into a sterilized isolator. The isolator excludes direct human intervention, which greatly reduces the potential for microbial contamination.

A typical freeze-dryer sterilization involves several vacuum *pulses* during which the temperature is brought to 40° to 60°C and the humidity is reduced (dry phase). A vacuum hold cycle is run to check for leaks and the temperature is reduced to about 25°C for the sterilization cycle. The sterilant is introduced and is monitored and controlled by weight using an electronic balance. Filtered air is pulsed with sterilant to push the vapors into any deadlegs and to compress the vapors, thus increasing the concentration. Finally, the vacuum is pulsed again to aerate the chamber, and the residual vapor is verified to be below acceptable levels before proceeding to the processing cycle.[11]

HYDROGEN PEROXIDE PLUS STEAM

For certain applications, one can combine moist heat and hydrogen peroxide methods. The combination can produce some effects that may be more desirable than either of the techniques run separately. Cycles can be as effective in shorter times and may improve the removal of residual peroxide. The system must be able to withstand exposure to steam at atmospheric pressure. The air-handling equipment can be moved outside the processing area, which simplifies the system and minimizes any mechanically generated particles, because the air, steam, and peroxide are introduced through the same type of HEPA filters used for laminar-flow hoods.[12,13]

The process area is raised to about 80°C by introducing dry heated air through the HEPA filters. The steam is introduced and surfaces are raised to about 100°C. During the steam cycle, hydrogen peroxide is introduced and is carried with the steam. When the cycle has been completed, the steam and peroxide are stopped and the dry heated air is started again. This aids in removal of residual condensate and helps break down the peroxide to water and oxygen. After sufficient heat has been introduced to dry and remove residuals, cool air is introduced to bring the unit to the desired operating temperature.

Because the hydrogen peroxide is mixed intimately with the steam, temperature can be used to monitor the progression of the cycle. However, the heated portions of the cycle must be

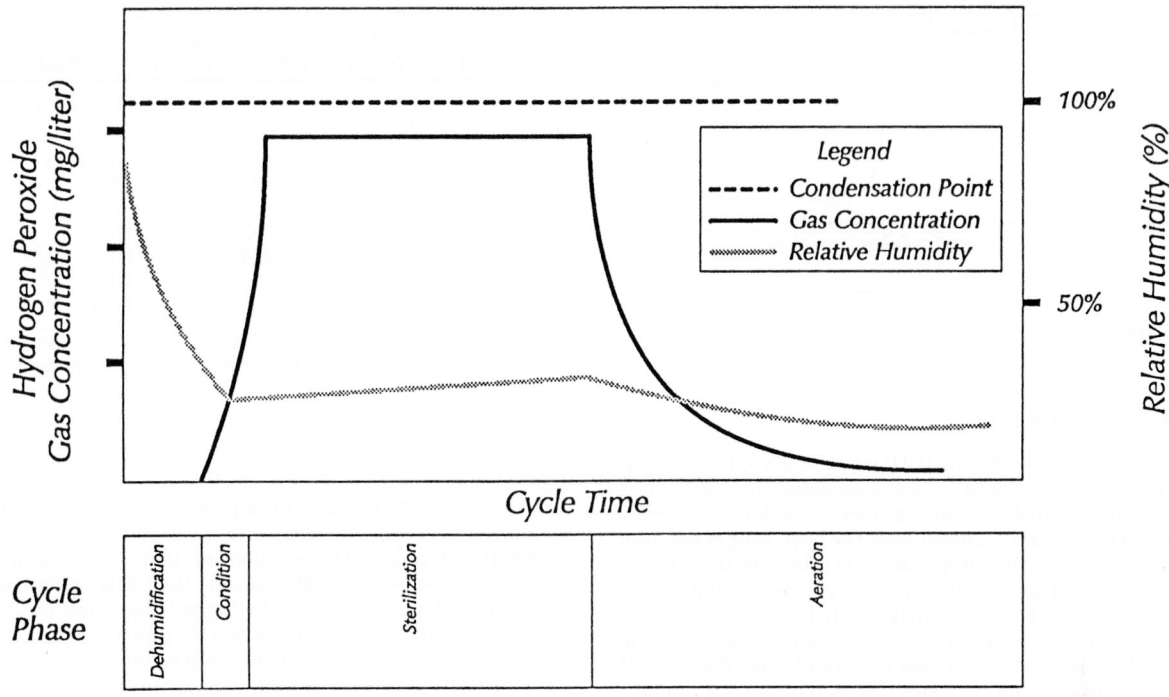

Figure 40-11. A typical vaporized HP cycle (courtesy, Am Sterilizer/Finn Aqua).

validated using biological indicators and residual peroxide measurements, to ensure their effectiveness in sterilizing and removing residuals to a safe level. Figure 40-14 diagrams a cycle using steam and hydrogen peroxide to sterilize as a filler in an isolator.

Figure 40-15 is included to show the synergistic effects of steam and hydrogen peroxide in some sterilization cycles. The challenge organism was *Bacillus stearothermophilus,* which typically is used to validate steam cycles. It should be noted that the kill rate was not only considerably faster, but was accomplished using atmospheric steam. This means that instead of 121°C the equipment was only subjected to 100°C and was exposed for 15 min less to achieve the same reduction in microorganism count.

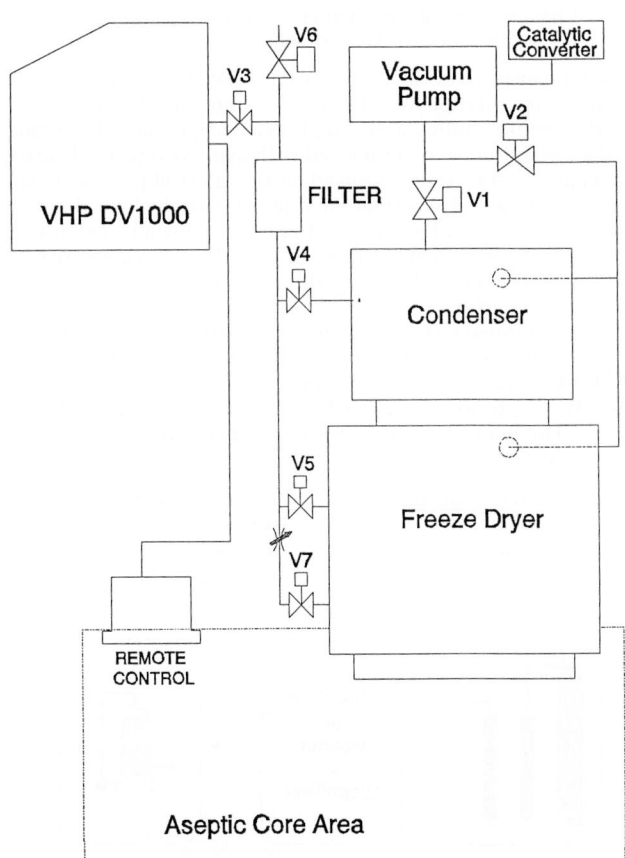

Figure 40-12. A typical installation using vaporized HP to sterilize a freeze dryer and condenser (courtesy, Am Sterilizer/Finn Aqua).

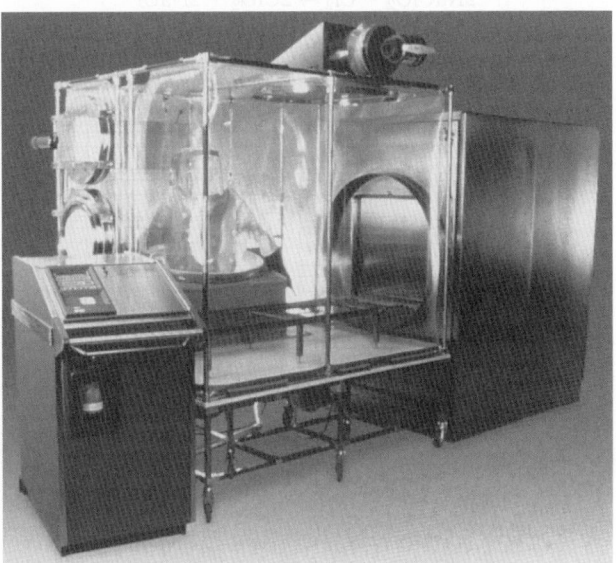

Figure 40-13. A transfer isolator connected to a sterilizer and a vaporized HP generator (courtesy, Am Sterilizer/Finn Aqua).

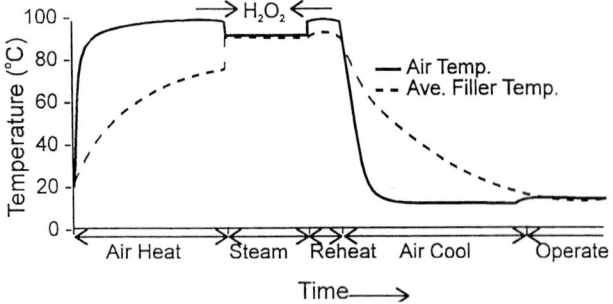

Figure 40-14. A steam/hydrogen peroxide cycle (courtesy, TL Systems and Despatch Industries).

CHLORINE DIOXIDE (CD)

The compound chlorine dioxide (CD) was discovered in 1811. It is a greenish-yellow gas with the common name euchlorine. It is a single electron transfer–oxidizing agent that has a chlorine-like odor. CD has been recognized since the beginning of the 20th century for its disinfecting properties. CD possesses the bactericidal, virucidal, and sporicidal properties of chlorine, but unlike chlorine, does not lead to the formation of trihalomethanes or react with ammonia to form chlorinated organic products (chloramines). These properties have led to the widespread use of CD in the treatment of drinking water. Despite numerous applications for CD in aqueous systems, only recently have the sterilizing properties of gaseous CD been demonstrated.

CD has been shown to have low toxicity in humans and is nonmutagenic and noncarcinogenic; it is not an ozone-depleting chemical. Used at comparatively low concentrations and at subatmospheric pressure, gaseous CD sterilization lacks many of the hazards associated with EtO, and it has been suggested as an attractive potential replacement.[14,15] Gaseous CD does not require expensive damage-limiting construction and is cost-competitive with EtO. Capability for spectrophotometric in-chamber measurement of gas concentration makes the process amenable for the validation of parametric release.

CD gas cannot be compressed and stored in high-pressure cylinders, but is generated upon demand using a column-based solid phase generation system. The chemical reaction used for CD generation is based upon the reaction of solid flaked sodium chlorite with dilute chlorine gas:

$$2NaClO_2 + Cl_2 \rightarrow 2ClO_2 + 2NaCl$$

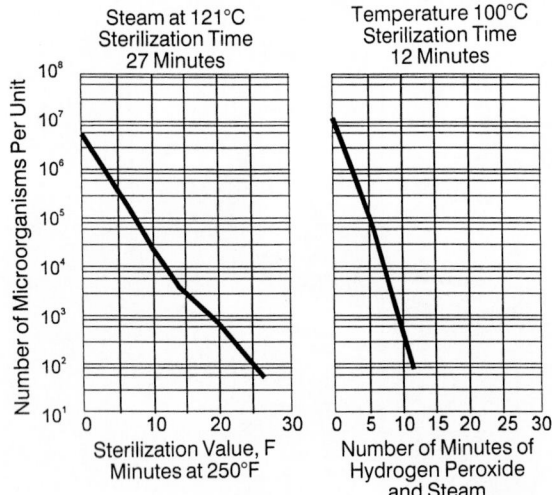

Figure 40-15. Comparison of steam under pressure with hydrogen peroxide/atmospheric steam mixture (courtesy, TL Systems and Despatch Industries).

Table 40-2. Effect of CD Gas Concentration on the Rate of Inactivation of 10^6 *B subtilis* Spores on Paper Strips Within a Load of Overwrapped Foil Suture Packages[a]

EXPOSURE PHASE TIME (min)	FRACTION NONSTERILE[b]		
	10 mg/L	20 mg/L	40 mg/L
0	NT	20/20	19/20
15	NT	19/20	1/20
30	20/20	4/20	0/20
60	9/60	0/60	0/20
90	3/20	NT	NT
180	0/20	NT	NT
240	0/20	0/20	NT

[a] The paper spore strips were placed next to the foil suture package and then overwrapped with Tyvek/Mylar. Sterilization exposures were performed at 30 to 32°.
[b] NT = not tested.

A block diagram for a CD gas sterilization system is shown in Figure 40-16. The output of the primary generation column is monitored spectrophotometrically, as is the gas concentration within the chamber. The scrubber system uses a sodium thiosulfate solution to chemically convert the CD to sodium sulfate. The scrubber system is highly efficient; therefore, the effluent released into the atmosphere is mainly process N_2 and air with the CD component reduced to low ppm levels. A typical gaseous CD sterilization process is quite similar to that used with EtO and has these steps:

1. Initial vacuum to remove air from the chamber and load.
2. Moisture conditioning at 70 to 85% relative humidity for 30 to 60 min.
3. CD gas injection: 10 to 30 mg/L.
4. Air or N_2 injection to attain a constant subatmospheric pressure, generally 80 kP$_a$.
5. CD gas exposure, generally 60 min.
6. Chamber and load aeration by evacuation and air replacement, tailored to load materials and density.

The temperature of the process in a sterilizer application is 30 to 32°C; for isolation systems, it is at ambient temperature.

Feasibility studies on the application of gaseous CD for medical sterilization were performed with over-wrapped foil suture packages.[16] The studies focused on the effect of gas concentration on the rate of inactivation of paper-strip biological indicators (BIs). The results of these studies are shown in Table 40-2. As with other gaseous sterilants, as the CD concentration increases, the time it takes to attain all sterile BIs becomes progressively shorter.

More detailed CD sterilization process development and validation studies were performed using polymethylmethacrylate (PMMA) intraocular lenses as the test system. A diagram of the sterilization process used for these studies is shown in Figure 40-17. The following results were obtained after 30 minutes of gas exposure at 30 mg/L (half cycle):

Packages/Load	Fraction Nonsterile
800	0/8, 0/8
1600	0/16, 0/16
25	0/25, 0/25

2% Cl$_2$ / 98% N$_2$
NaClO$_2$ Columns

Sterilizer or Isolator or Lyophilizer

Sodium thiosulfate "Scrubber"

Figure 40-16. Block diagram of a gaseous CD sterilization unit.

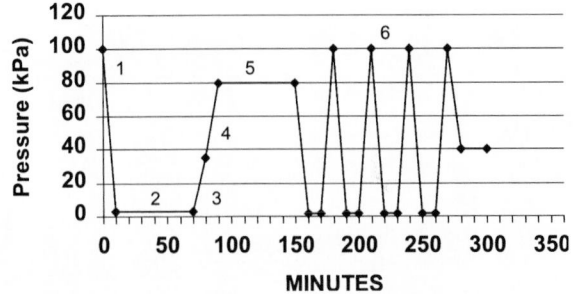

Figure 40-17. Pressure excursion diagram of a typical gaseous CD sterilization process. (1) Initial vacuum; (2) Moisture conditioning; (3) CD gas injection; (4) N_2 or air injection; (5) CD gas exposure phase; (6) aeration by evacuation and air replacement.

As can be seen, all of the *B. subtilis* BTs were sterilized and varying the load size had no discernible effect upon process lethality. CD also has been evaluated for the sterilization of blood oxygenators.[17]

CD also has great potential for the decontamination/sterilization of barrier-isolation systems. Initial studies on the efficacy of gaseous CD for the decontamination/sterilization of a sterility testing isolator used a gas concentration of 10 mg/L. This concentration yielded a relatively rapid process with a complete kill of 10^6 spores in approximately 15 min. The effect of gas concentration upon the observed D_{10} value with *B. subtilis* spores was determined at 10, 20, and 30 mg/L of CD:

mg/L CD	D Value in Seconds
10	45
20	16
30	7

As expected, the D_{10} value decreases with increasing CD concentration. These low D_{10} values yield very rapid decontamination/sterilization processes for barrier-isolation applications.

Very low residuals of CD are observed when examining product and packaging materials from medical devices or isolation technology systems. CD does not appear to have the *solvent-like* quality of EtO. Residual CD is generally less than 10 ppm following a 15-min exposure at 10 mg/L. Rapid aeration also is observed with levels often less than 1 ppm following 15 min of aeration. A typical aeration curve of CD from flexible-wall isolator PVC material is shown in Figure 40-18.

The impact of CD exposure on a number of polymeric materials and metals has been evaluated. Commonly used polymers such as ABS, nylon, PMMA, polyethylene, polypropylene, polystyrene, Teflon, and Viton appear highly compatible. Poly-

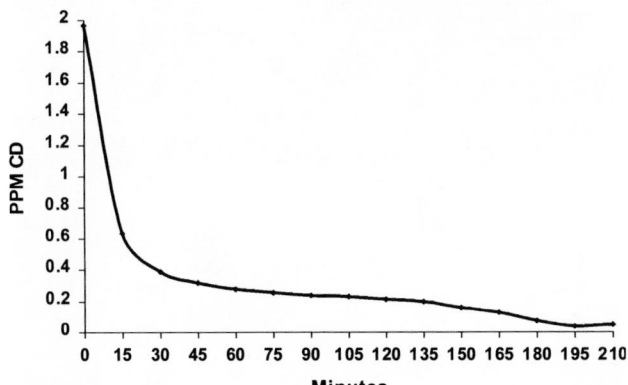

Figure 40-18. Aeration of CD from flexible-wall isolator PVC material; aqueous extraction from treated samples (10 mg/L, 15 min) followed by polarographic measurement of dissolved CD.

carbonates and polyurethanes, depending upon the particular formulation, may exhibit a loss in tensile properties and/or discoloration. Stainless steel is compatible with CD; uncoated copper and aluminum are affected.

OTHER GASES

Formaldehyde (HCHO) sometimes is used for sterilizing certain medical products. It is not in widespread use in the United States but as a gas or in combination with low-pressure steam, it is used in some European hospitals instead of ethylene oxide. Formaldehyde, a toxic chemical and a human carcinogen, is an alkylating agent and destroys microorganisms by alkylation of susceptible cell components.

Filtration

Filtration is the removal of particulate matter from a fluid stream. Sterilizing filtration is a process that removes, but does not destroy, microorganisms. Filtration, one of the oldest methods of sterilization, is the method of choice for solutions that are unstable to other types of sterilizing processes.

Pasteur, Chamberland, Seitz and Berkfeld filters have been used in the past to sterilize pharmaceutical products. These types of filters were composed of various materials such as sintered glass, porcelain, or fibrous materials (ie, asbestos or cellulose). The filtration mechanism of these depth filters is random adsorption or entrapment in the filter matrix. The disadvantages of these filters are low flow rates, difficulty in cleaning, and media migration into the filtrate. Fiber-releasing and asbestos filters now are prohibited by the FDA for the filtration of parenteral products.[18,19]

Over the past 35 years, membrane filters have become the method of choice for the sterilization of heat-labile sterile products. Membrane filters are thin, strong, and homogenous polymeric structures. Microorganisms, present in fluids, are removed by a process of physical sieving and are retained on or near the membrane surface. Membrane filters of 0.1 and 0.22-μm pore size are employed commonly as sterilizing filters.

When solutions are sterilized by filtration, the filters must be validated to ensure that all microorganisms will be removed under known conditions. Filter manufacturers normally validate sterilizing membrane filters using a protocol similar to the one developed by the Health Industry Manufacturers Association (HIMA).[20] In this procedure, *Pseudomonas diminuta* (ATTC 19146) is cultivated in saline lactose broth. Leahy and Sullivan[21] have shown that when *P. diminuta* is cultivated in this medium the cells are discrete and small (approximately 0.3 μm in diameter)—a range recommended for sterilizing filtration with 0.22-μm filters. Each cm^2 of the filter to be validated is challenged with 10^7 microorganisms at a differential pressure of 30 psig. The entire filtrate is collected and tested for viable microorganisms. The retention efficiency (log reduction value) of the membrane filter may be calculated using the procedure described in the HIMA protocol. Dawson and co-workers[22] have demonstrated that the probability of a nonsterile filtration with a properly validated membrane filter is approximately 10^{-6}. Another aspect in filter validation is adsorption of the product by the filter and extractables from the filter and housing.

Once the performance of the membrane filter has been validated, a nondestructive integrity test that has been correlated to the bacterial challenge test (the bubble point or diffusion test) can be used routinely prior to and after a sterilizing filtration to ensure that the membrane filter is integral.[23,24] Unique to membrane filtration is the condition that beyond a certain challenge level of microorganisms, the filter will clog. For a typical sterilizing filter this level is 10^9 organisms per cm^2. Initially, membrane filters were available only in disc configuration. Advances in membrane technology have provided filters in stacked-disc, pleated-cartridge and hollow fiber configurations. These advances have provided larger surface areas and higher

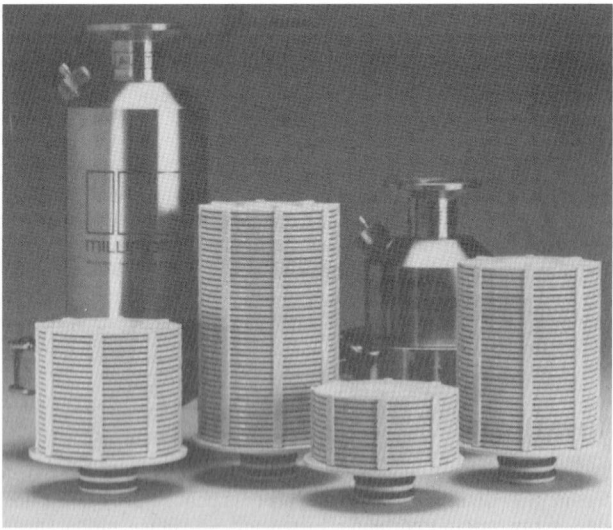

Figure 40-19. Stacked-disk membrane filters. This new technology allows filter manufacturers to supply filters with large surface area in relatively small packages (courtesy, Millipore); vaporized HP generator (courtesy, Am Sterilizer/Finn Aqua).

flow-rate capabilities. Figure 40-19 is an example of these larger surface area filters.

Membrane filters are manufactured from a variety of polymers, such as cellulosic esters (MCE), polyvinylidine fluoride (PVF), and polytetrafluoroethylene (PTFE). The type of fluid to be sterilized will dictate the polymer to be used. The listing below is intended to serve only as a guide for the selection of membrane filters for a particular application. The filter manufacturer should be consulted before making a final choice.

Fluid	Polymer
Aqueous	PVF, MCE
Oil	PVF, MCE
Organic solvents	PVF, PTFE
Aqueous, extreme pH	PVF
Gases	PVF, PTFE

Figure 40-20 is an example of a sterilizing filtration system commonly used in the pharmaceutical industry.

Positive pressure commonly is used in sterilizing filtrations. It has the following advantages over vacuum: it provides higher flow rates, integrity testing is easier, and it avoids a negative pressure on the downstream (sterile) side of the filtrate, thus precluding contamination. Membrane filters are sterilized readily by autoclaving, by *in-situ* steaming, or by using ethylene oxide.

In addition to their use in the pharmaceutical industry, membrane filters are used in many applications in the hospital pharmacy. The membrane filters commonly used in these applications are small disposable units. Examples of these are shown in Figures 40-21 and 40-22. Typical applications for membrane filters in hospital pharmacies include sterilization of intravenous (IV) admixtures and hyperalimentation solutions, sterilization of extemporaneously compounded preparations, sterility testing of admixtures, as well as in direct patient care (see Chapter 42).

Radiation Sterilization

The retail or hospital pharmacist probably has little opportunity to use radiation sterilization. However, they should be aware that many of the products sold in stores and used daily in hospitals are sterilized by this technology. Products such as contact lens solutions, bandages, baby bottle nipples, and teething rings (the kind containing water/gel) are a few exam-

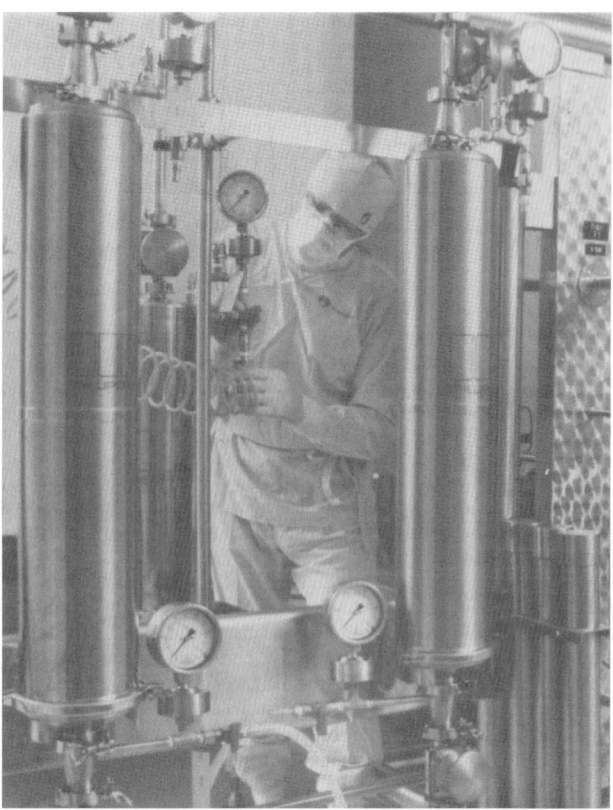

Figure 40-20. An example of a process filtration system in a pharmaceutical plant (courtesy, Millipore).

ples of the everyday type of product encountered in a pharmacy. Several drugs, including some anticancer drugs, also are terminally sterilized using gamma radiation.

The hospital pharmacist is likely to encounter the use of gamma or X-ray treatment of blood to eliminate white blood cells in host-versus-graft reactions following transplant surgery. The serum used for tissue cultures is frequently ster-

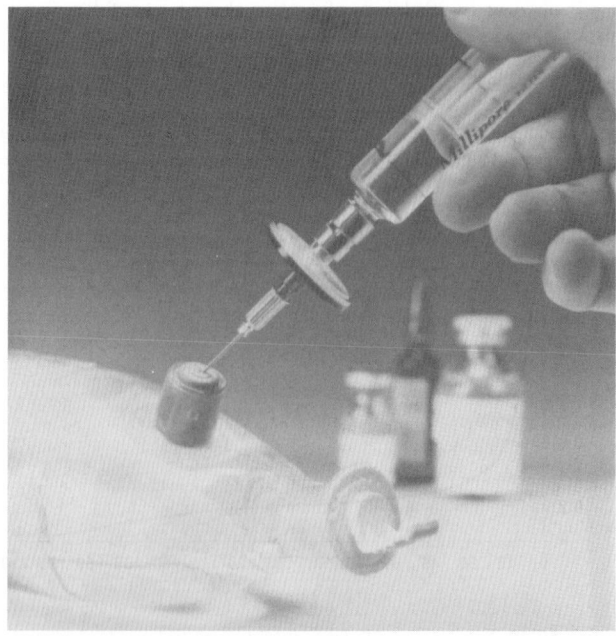

Figure 40-21. Intravenous additive filtration using a small disposable membrane filter (courtesy, Millipore).

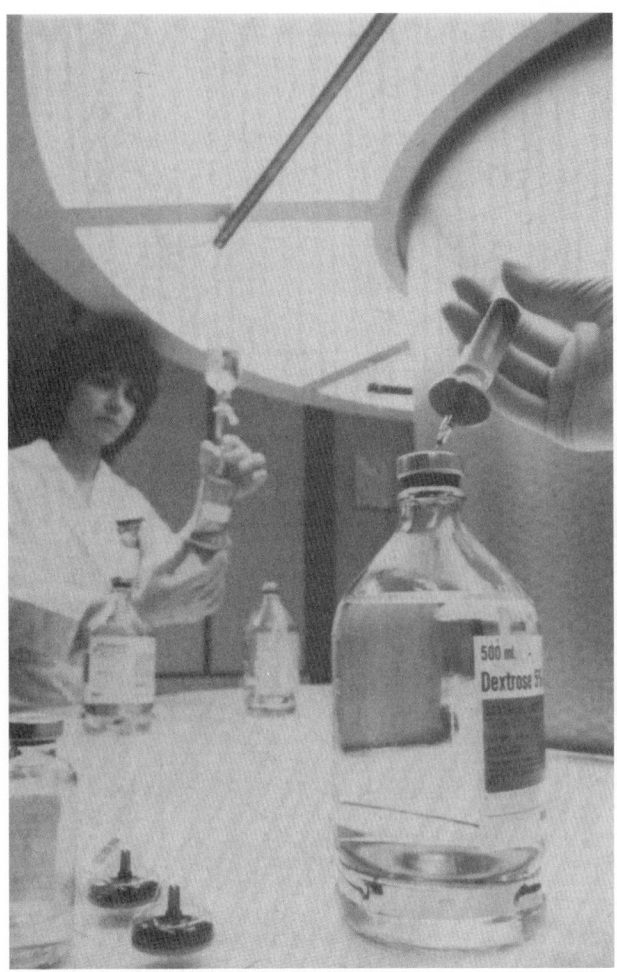

Figure 40-22. Intravenous additive filtration and sterility testing. Both procedures employ membrane filtration (courtesy, Millipore).

ilized with gamma radiation to eliminate viruses, virus-like particles, and mycoplasms.

The pharmaceutical industry historically has relied on steam, dry heat, ethylene oxide gas, filtration, and chemical processes to meet sanitization or microbial load reduction requirements. Sterilization by radiation may employ either electromagnetic radiation or particle radiation.

Electromagnetic radiation, composed of photons of energy, includes ultraviolet, gamma, X-, and cosmic radiation. Gamma radiation, emitted from radioactive materials such as Cobalt-60 or Cesium-137, is the most frequently used source of electromagnetic radiation. Of these two, only Cobalt-60 is used in the large industrial irradiator (Fig 40-23). Cesium-137 is used in blood irradiators.

Particulate or corpuscular radiation includes a formidable list of particles. The only one that currently is being employed for sterilization is the electron. These electrons are machine generated using the technique illustrated in Figure 40-24; Figures 40-25 and 40-26 illustrate two methods of presenting products to a commercial electron-beam sterilizer.

Radiation-processing technology, and its application in the manufacture of pharmaceuticals, is being investigated more actively now than at any other time. This renewed interest is in part due to the development of aseptic and barrier technology, as well as an overall improvement in the environment in which pharmaceuticals are manufactured.

In the past the use of a radiation dose of 25 kGy was required to ensure that all viable microbes had been inactivated, and that a SAL of 10^{-6} was achieved. This level of radiation

proved detrimental to many pharmaceuticals. With the advent of clean rooms, and aseptic and barrier technologies, the microbial environment has improved dramatically. No longer are spores or even the number of organisms as daunting. It is more appropriate now to determine the resistance of the bioburden to radioaction and to tailor the minimal sterilization dose to meet the most resistant strain of the bioburden. In this way many more drugs and other products are capable of being sterilized terminally. This provides an SAL of 10^{-6} or greater, depending upon the microorganism.

The increased use of radiation processing to sterilize medical devices has led to the development of more efficient and economical irradiation equipment and processes. It also has generated new scientific data. The positive experience of the medical-device industry should be a *signpost* for the pharmaceuticals industry.

Several pharmaceutical raw materials and finished products are being sanitized/sterilized successfully with gamma radiation. Although it is possible to use electron beam radiation, we are presently unaware of any pharmaceuticals being treated using this technology. This should not preclude others from investigating its potential. The superior penetrating ability of gamma radiation provides the edge for this technology in this application.

HOW RADIATION KILLS MICROORGANISMS

The principles of sterilization by irradiation have been known since the early 1940s. Basically, charged particles or electromagnetic radiation interact with matter to cause both ionization and excitation. Ionization results in the formation of ion pairs, comprised of ejected orbital electrons (negatively charged) and their counterparts (positively charged). Charged particles such as electrons interact directly with matter causing ionization, whereas electromagnetic radiation causes ionization through various mechanisms that result in the ejection of an orbital electron with a specific amount of energy transferred from the incident gamma ray. These ejected electrons then behave similarly to machine-generated electrons in ionization reactions. Thus, both particle and electromagnetic radiation are considered as ionizing radiation and differ from ultraviolet radiation in this respect.

Ionizing radiation kills or inactivates microorganisms through the interaction of the ion pairs or excitations altering the molecular structure or spatial configuration of *biologically active* macromolecules. In particular, those involved in cell replication are most critical. It can do this in two ways. The first is to deposit energy directly in a bond of the macromolecule. This can cause a rearrangement of its structure, altering or destroying its normal function. The second is to generate free radicals, primarily from the water contained within the cytoplasm. The free radicals thus generated react with the macromolecules to subvert their normal function. In either case the result is the loss of reproductive capability of the microorganism.

The number of microorganisms inactivated by a given radiation dose is a statistical phenomenon. It depends upon the sensitivity of the biologically active macromolecule(s) to alteration (denaturation), the number of alterations elicited within the cell and the ability of the cell to repair these alterations. Different microorganisms have different capabilities to withstand or repair such alterations. This sensitivity is referred to as the D_{10} value. The size of the microorganism, its state of hydration, and the presence or absence of radical scavengers affect the outcome of exposure to ionizing radiation.

The ability of gamma radiation to inactivate microorganisms has been well documented. New documentation relating to viruses or new strains/reclassifications of microorganisms is being added continually. The major benefit of using radiation sterilization as the terminal step in the manufacturing process, as opposed to autoclaving or dry heat methods, is the minimal product degradation usually observed with this technology.

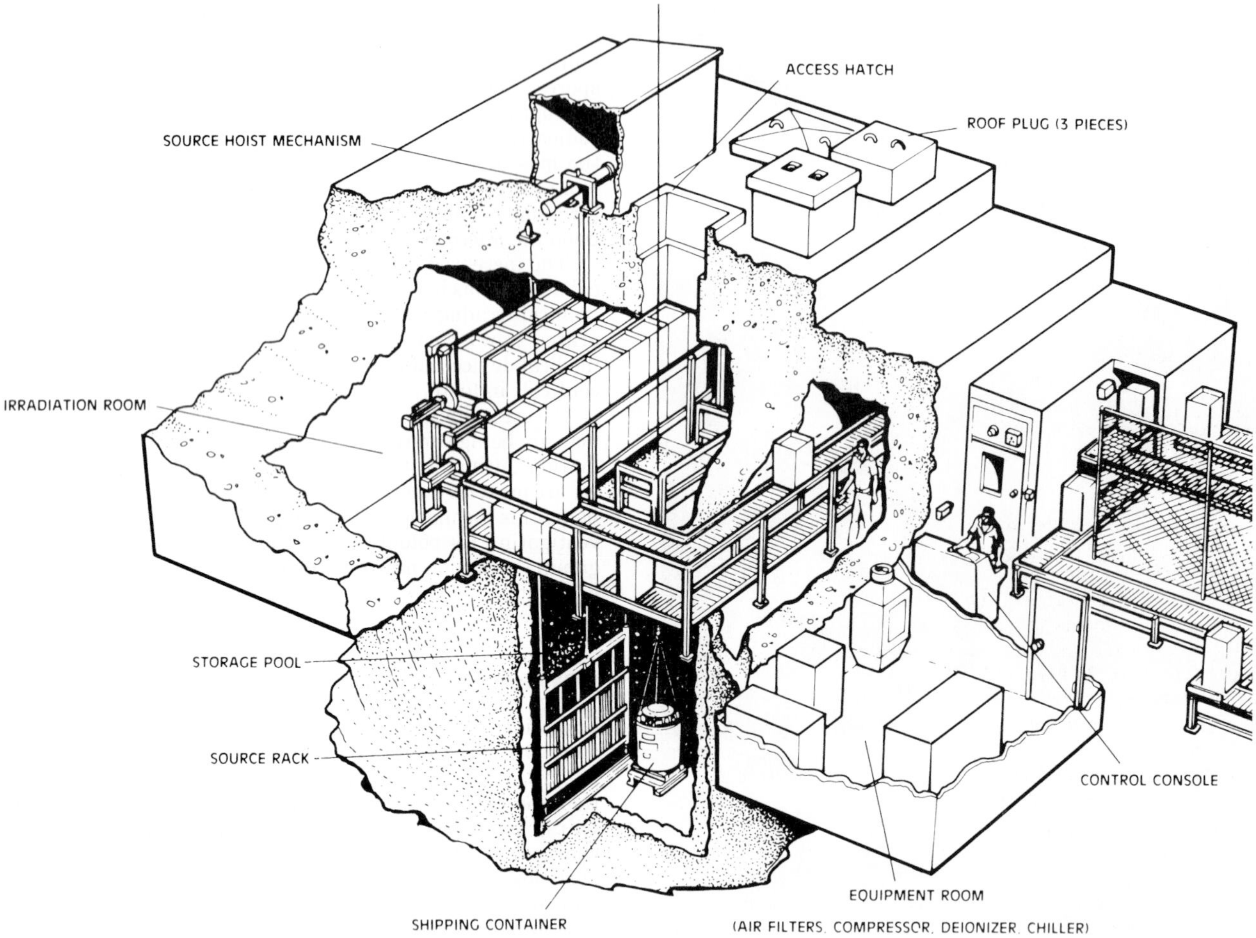

Figure 40-23. Tote box irradiator: automatic (courtesy, Nordion Intl).

The process has been in use in the medical device industry for over 25 years. Ample evidence as to its efficacy exists in scientific literature. Materials and processes have been developed to reduce the impact of radiation on the product. Some materials, such as Teflon and polypropylene, are severely degraded by radiation and must be avoided. It is the intent of this update to present some of the process developments that will facilitate the use of this technology for the terminal sterilization of pharmaceutical products. It also will assist those wishing to improve the microbial quality of raw materials entering the manufac-

turing process. Clean materials reduce the bioburden levels present in a clean room facility.

Sterilization by ionizing radiation requires consideration of the minimum and maximum doses (or the amount of radiation that is absorbed by the material), the energy level available (which along with the bulk density of the material will determine the depth of penetration), and the power output available (which determines the rate at which the dose can be applied).

The unit of absorbed dose is the Gray (Gy), where 1 Gy = 1 joule/kg, independent of the nature of the irradiated substance.

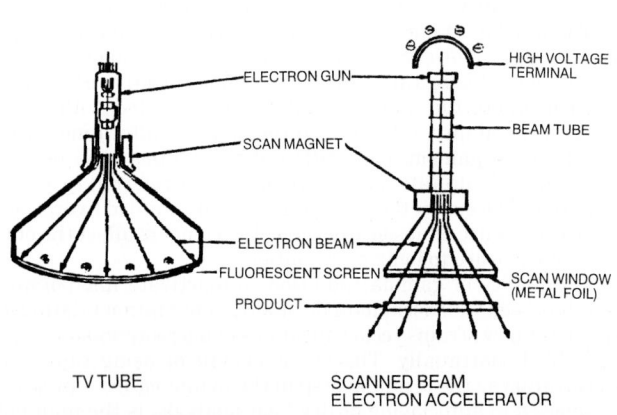

Figure 40-24. To produce an electron (courtesy, RDI).

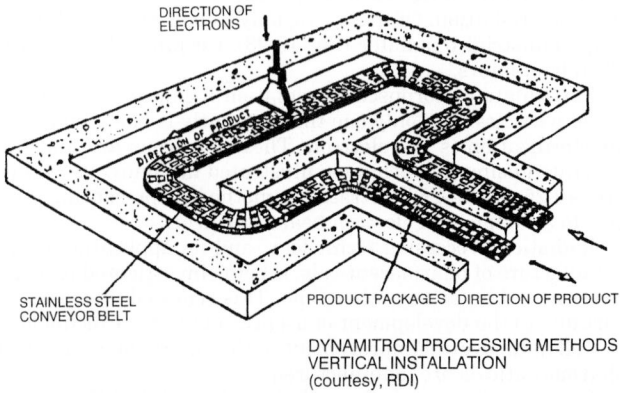

Figure 40-25. Dynamitron processing methods: vertical installation (courtesy, RDI).

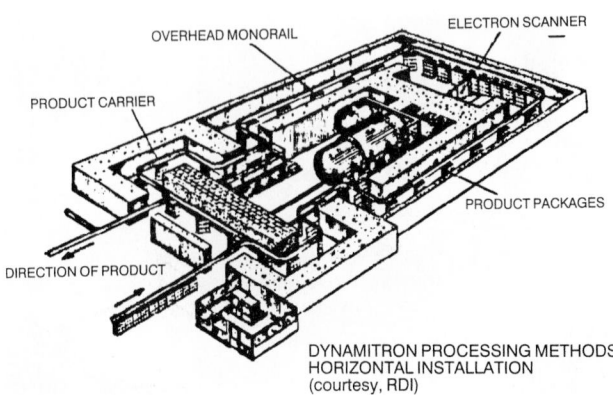

Figure 40-26. Dynamitron processing methods: horizontal installation (courtesy, RDI).

Sterilization doses, for convenience, are predominantly expressed in kilogray (kGy).

Many investigators have studied the relative resistance of microorganisms to sterilization by radiation. The consensus is that vegetative forms are most sensitive, followed by molds, yeasts, viruses and spore-formers. While historical practice has been to use 15 to 25 kGy, today the minimal sterilization dose is more closely tailored to the resistance of the bioburden. It is not unusual to use doses as low as 2 to 8 kGy. The use of the AAMI/ISO or EN standards is highly recommended.

Modern gamma sterilization facilities used by pharmaceutical and medical device companies generally hold up to 4 MCi of Cobalt-60. The largest facility holds 12 MCi. Figure 40-23 shows a schematic of a modern Cobalt-60 radiationsterilization facility.

Two types of electron accelerators are used in sterilization: alternating-current machines with ranges up to 50 kW of power and 5 to 12 meV of energy, and direct-current machines with ranges of 30 to 200 kW and 0.5 to 5 meV. These machines generate electrons at high voltage, accelerate the electrons, and project them into the product to be sterilized. The greater the machine power (kW), the more electrons can be generated per unit time. The higher the energy (meV), the greater the penetration capability of the electrons into the material to be sterilized.

Ultraviolet (UV) Radiation

Artificially produced UV radiation in the region of 253.7 nm has been used as a germicide for many years. Although UV radiation often is used in the pharmaceutical industry for the maintenance of aseptic areas and rooms, it is of limited value as a sterilizing agent.

Inactivation of microorganisms by UV radiation is principally a function of the radiant energy dose, which varies widely for different microorganisms. The primary mechanism of microbial inactivation is the creation of the thymidine dimers in DNA, which prevents replication. Vegetative bacteria are most susceptible, while bacterial spores appear to be 3 to 10 times as resistant to inactivation and fungal spores may be 100 to 1000 times more resistant. Bacterial spores on stainless-steel surfaces require approximately 800 μW min/cm^2 for inactivation. By comparison, the black spores of *Aspergillus niger* require an exposure of over 5000 μW min/cm^2. Even with an adequate dose, however, the requirements for proper application of germicidal UV radiation in most pharmaceutical situations are such as to discourage its use for *sterilization* purposes. On the other hand, as an ancillary germicidal agent, UV radiation can be useful.

When using UV radiation, it is very important that lamps be cleaned periodically with alcohol and tested for output: also its use requires that personnel be properly protected; eye protection is particularly important.

The principal disadvantage to the use of germicidal UV radiation is its limited penetration—its 253.7 nm wavelength is screened out by most materials, allowing clumps of organisms, and those protected by dust or debris, to escape the lethal action. The use of UV radiation as a sterilizing agent is not recommended unless the material to be irradiated is very clean and free of crevices that can protect microorganisms. Many organisms are capable of repairing the UV-induced DNA damage using photoreactivation (light repair) and dark repair.

PULSED LIGHT

Recently, high-intensity visible light has been developed to a level that allows it to be used for certain sterilization applications. The advantages include extremely short exposure times (eg, 2 to 3 pulses of a few seconds) and relative ease in shielding the operations to provide operator safety. It can be used for surface sterilization and certain terminal sterilization applications. This is limited to packaging materials that are transparent to the wavelengths used. It is applicable for certain plastic materials, but not for Type I glass. This technique requires additional study, but has been shown to be effective against all organisms studied thus far.

Aseptic Processing

Although not actually a sterilization process, aseptic processing is a technique frequently used in the compounding of prescriptions or commercial products that will not withstand sterilization but in which all of the ingredients are sterile. In such cases, sterility must be maintained by using sterile materials and a controlled working environment. All containers and apparatus used should be sterilized by one of the previously mentioned processes and such work should be conducted only by an operator fully versed in the control of contamination. The use of laminar-airflow devices or barrier technology for aseptic processing is essential.

With the availability of sterile bulk drugs and sterilized syringe parts from manufacturers, the purchase of several pieces of equipment permits pharmacies to produce filled sterile unit-dose syringes with minimum effort. The equipment needs have been described in a paper by Patel and associates.[25] Figure 40-27[25] illustrates this system.

PACKAGING

Following exposure of a product to a well-controlled sterilization treatment, the packaging material of the product is expected to maintain sterility until the time of use. Packaging must be durable, provide for permanent-seal integrity, and have pore sizes small enough to prevent entry of contaminants. Obviously, the packaging must be compatible with the method of sterilization.

The package design is important if the contents are to be removed without recontamination. Tearing of plastics or paper can be tempered by coatings, and sealed containers should be tested carefully to ensure retention of sterility at the time of use.

If sterile material passes through many hands, it is important to provide a tamperproof closure to indicate if the container has been opened inadvertently. These four features—compatibility with sterilization, proven storage protection, ease of opening, tamper-proofing—are highly desirable characteristics of medical packaging.

For hospitals and pharmacies, there are a wide variety of woven reusable materials or nonwoven disposable materials that provide acceptable sterile barriers and are offered by major packaging suppliers. These suppliers normally conduct extensive programs to ensure the ability of the material to maintain sterility. Both hospitals and industry have guidelines and accepted practices for sterile-product packaging.[5]

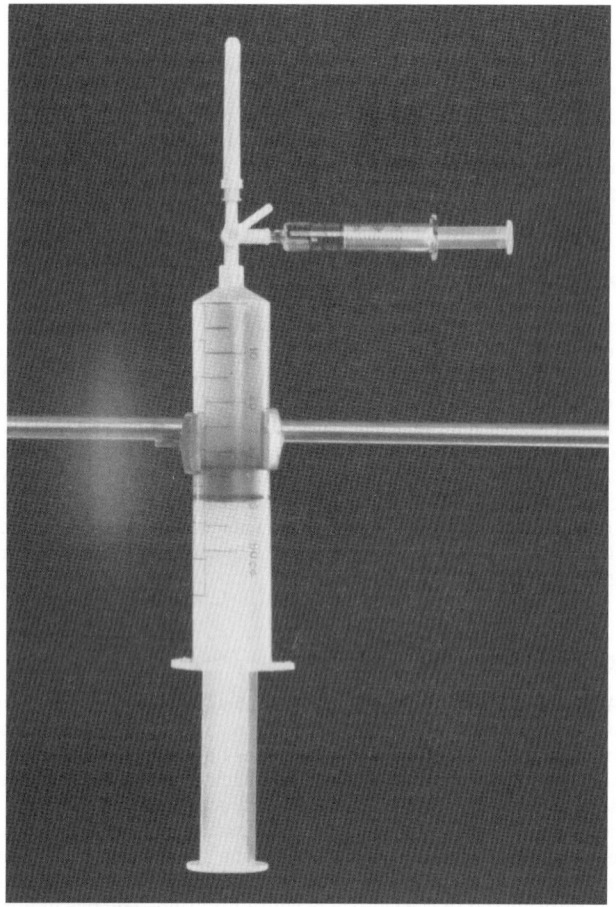

Figure 40-27. Unit-of-use system for sterile injectable medication.[19]

A review of the principles of sterile-material packaging by Powell[26] discusses the suitability of packaging materials for various sterilization methods, including resistance to bacteria, types of openings, strength of packaging, testing of packaging, and types of packaging. These topics also are discussed in Chapter 54.

UNIDIRECTIONAL AIRFLOW

Unidirectional airflow equipment is essential for proper performance of sterility tests and aseptic filling or assembling operations. These procedures require exact control over the working environment, but while many techniques and different types of equipment for performing these operations have been used over the years, unidirectional airflow devices are superior to all other environmental controls.

The unidirectional airflow procedure for producing very clean and dust-free areas was developed in 1961. In a unidirectional airflow device the entire body of air within a confined area moves with in one direction with uniform velocity along parallel flow lines. By employing prefilters and high-efficiency bacterial filters, the air delivered to the area essentially is sterile and sweeps all dust and airborne particles from the chamber through an open side. The velocity of the air used in such devices is generally 90 fpm ± 20%. Unidirectional airflow devices that deliver the clean air in a vertical, horizontal, or curvilinear fashion are available. The devices can be in the form of rooms, cabinets, or benches. For a comprehensive discussion of the biomedical application of unidirectional airflow the reader is referred to Runkle and Phillips.[27]

Each unidirectional airflow cabinet or bench should be located in a separate, small, clean room having a filtered air supply. The selection of the type of cabinet will depend on the oper-

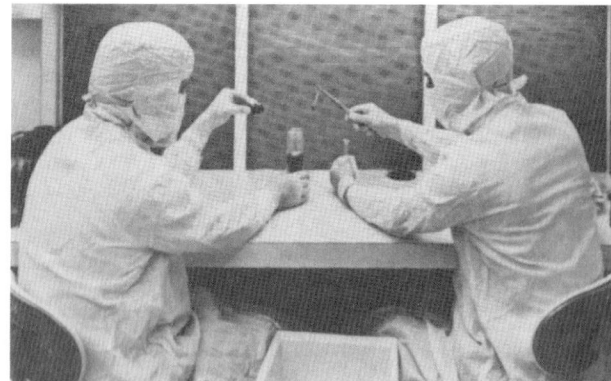

Figure 40-28. Sterility testing of plastic disposable syringes in a horizontal laminar-airflow bench (courtesy, Becton Dickinson & Co).

ation itself. For most sterility-testing operations, horizontal unidirectional airflow units appear to be superior to vertical-flow hoods because the air movement is less likely to wash organisms from the operator's hands or equipment into the sterility test media. Figure 40-28 shows the sterility testing of syringes in a horizontal unidirectional airflow hood. Figure 40-29 shows the design of a typical horizontal, unidirectional airflow hood.

The major disadvantage of the horizontal unidirectional airflow units is that any airborne particulate matter generated in the units is blown directly into the room and against the working personnel. In situations where infectious material is involved, or where one must prevent contamination of the environment with a powder or drug, the use of specifically designed vertical, recirculating unidirectional airflow units is recommended. Units are available that do an excellent job of providing both product and personnel protection. Such a unit is shown in Figure 40-30.

To achieve maximum benefit from unidirectional airflow, it is important first to realize that the filtered airflow does not itself remove microbial contamination from the surface of objects. Thus, to avoid product or test contamination, it is necessary to reduce the microbial load on the outside of materials used in sterility testing. Unidirectional flow will do an excellent job of maintaining the sterility of an article bathed in the airflow; however, to be accurate, the sterility-testing, or product-assembly procedure must create the least possible turbulence within the unit. Moreover, an awareness of the turbulent air patterns created by the operation is necessary to avoid performing critical operations in turbulent zones. To illustrate how effectively airborne particles are washed from an environment by laminar airflow, Figure 40-31 shows the distance that particles of various sizes will travel horizontally before falling 5 ft in a cross-flow of air moving at 50 fpm.

Unidirectional airflow clean benches should supply Class 100 air as defined in Federal Standard 209B.[28] They should be certified to this standard when installed and then tested periodically. An air velocimeter should be used at regular intervals to check the airflow rates across the face of the filter. Smoke tests are use-

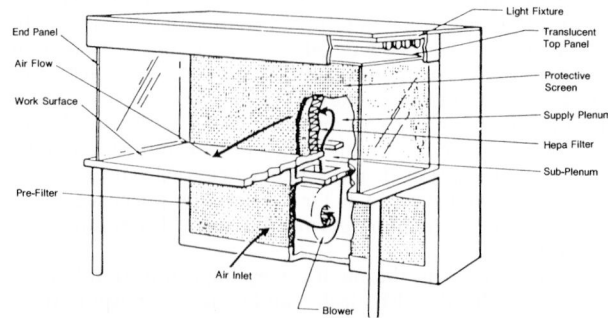

Figure 40-29. Horizontal laminar-airflow hood.

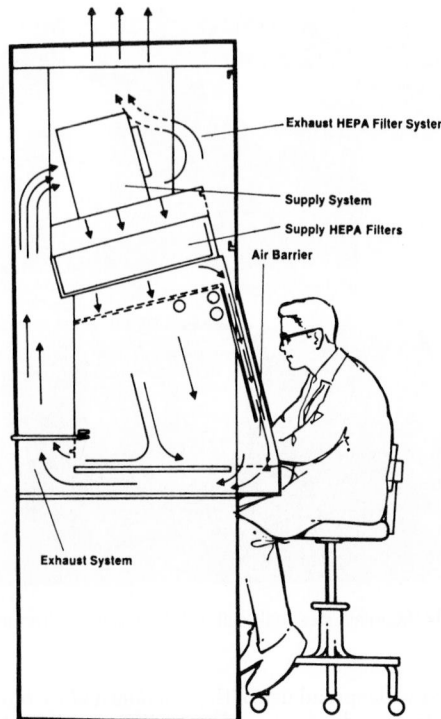

Figure 40-30. Sketch of a biological cabinet with vertical, recirculating laminar-airflow and HEPA-filtered exhaust. HEPA-filtered air is supplied to the work area at 90 fpm 20%. Airflow patterns in combination with a high-velocity curtain of air form a barrier at the front access opening that protects both the work and the worker from airborne contamination (courtesy, Bioquest).

ful in visualizing airflow patterns and a particle analyzer can be used to check the quality of the air. Filter efficiency testing determines the validity of the filter and its seal using a smoke (mean particulate diameter of 0.3 μm) and a light-scattering aerosol photometer. The smoke, at a concentration of 80 to 100 mg/L, is introduced to the plenum of the unit and the entire perimeter of the filter face is scanned with the photometer probe at a sampling rate of 1 ft³/min. A reading of 0.01% of the upstream smoke concentration is considered a leak.

In addition to the routine airflow measurements and filter-efficiency testing, biological testing should be done to monitor the effectiveness of laminar-airflow systems. Microbial air sampling and agar-settling plates are useful in monitoring these environments. Phillips evaluated horizontal laminar-flow hoods by tabulating the number of *false positives* appearing in sterility-test media over a period of time. These results (Table 40-3) showed very low numbers of *false positives*.

Table 40-3. False Positives Occuring in a Laminiar-Flow Hood[26]

PRODUCT	NO. OF UNITS STERILITY TESTED	NO. OF FALSE POSITIVES	% FALSE POSITIVES
Syringes	9793	2	0.02
Needles	4676	2	0.04
Misc	306	0	0

See Figure 40-29 for laminar-flow hood.

TESTING

After sterilization, there are several techniques for determining whether the particular lot of material is sterile. The only method for determining sterility with 100% assurance would be to run a total sterility test, that is, to test every item in the lot.

Representative probabilities are shown in Tables 40-4 and 40-5 to illustrate more specifically how low levels of contamination in treated lots of medical articles may escape detection by the usual sterility-test procedures. The data are calculated by binomial expansion, employing certain assumed values of percent contamination with large lot sizes (greater than 5000) and including standard assumptions with regard to the efficiency of recovery media and so on.

In Table 40-4 the probability data are calculated for lots with various degrees of assumed contamination when 10 random samples per lot are tested. For example, a lot that has one in each 1000 items contaminated (0.1% contamination) could be passed as satisfactory (by showing no positive samples from 10 tested) in 99 tests out of 100. Even at the 10% contamination level, contamination would be detected only two out of three times.

Table 40-5 shows the difficulty in attempting to improve the reliability of sterility tests by increasing sample size. For contamination levels as low as 0.1%, increasing the sample size from 10 to 100 has a relatively small effect in improving the probability of accepting lots. Even a sample size of 500 would result in erroneously accepting a lot 6 times out of 10. On the other hand, with a lot contaminated to the extent of 10%, by testing 100 samples the probability of acceptance of the lot would be reduced to a theoretical zero.

The information in Table 40-5 may be viewed in another way. If, for the probability values shown for each different sample size, the value that approximates the 95% confidence level ($P = 0.05$) is selected, it is clear that using 20 samples only will discriminate contamination levels of 15% or more. If the 20 tubes show no growth, the lot could, of course, be sterile but there would be no way of knowing this from the test. From such a test it could be stated only that it is unlikely that the lot would be contaminated at a level higher than 15%. It is clear from these data that product sterility testing is a poor method of validating sterilization procedures.

The USP provides two basic methods for sterility testing. One involves the direct introduction of product test samples into culture media; the second involves filtering test samples through membrane filters, washing the filters with fluids to remove inhibitory properties, and transferring the membrane

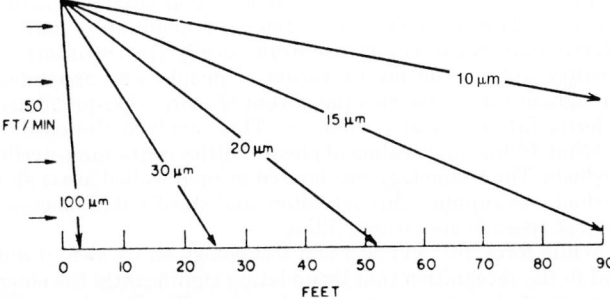

Figure 40-31. Distance traveled by particles settling from a height of 5 ft.

Table 40-4. Probabilities for Sterility Testing of Articles With Assumed Levels of Contamination

"TRUE" % CONTAMINATION	PROBABILITY OF DESIGNATED POSITIVES OUT OF 10 SAMPLES TESTED			
	0	2	5	10
0.1	0.990	(Total = 0.010)		
1.0	0.904	0.091		
5.0	0.599	0.315		
10.0	0.349	0.387	0.001	
30.0	0.028	0.121	0.103	
50.0	0.001	0.010	0.246	0.001

Table 40-5. Relationship of Probabilities of Acceptance of Lots of Varying Assumed Degrees of Contamination to Sample Size

NUMBER OF SAMPLES TESTED (n)	PROBABILITY OF NO POSITIVE GROWTH "TRUE" % CONTAMINATION OF LOT					
	0.1	1	5	10	15	20
10	0.99	0.91	0.60	0.35	0.20	0.11
20	0.98	0.82	0.36	0.12	0.04	0.01
50	0.95	0.61	0.08	0.007		
100	0.91	0.37	0.01	0.00		
300	0.74	0.05				
500	0.61	0.01				

aseptically to appropriate culture media. Test samples may be sterilized devices that simply are immersed aseptically into the appropriate culture-broth washings of the sterile object with sterile diluent, or dilutions of sterile materials. The USP recommends three aqueous diluting fluids for sterility tests while the Antibiotic Regulations list four; all are nontoxic to microorganisms. In the case of petrolatum-based drugs, a nonaqueous diluting fluid is required.

Many studies have been conducted to find the minimum number of culture media that will provide the greatest sensitivity in detecting contamination. Internationally recognized experts and bodies now recommend the use of two culture media: Soybean-Casein Digest Medium, incubated at 20° to 25°C, and Fluid Thioglycollate Medium, incubated at 30° to 35°C. The time of incubation specified usually is 7 days for the membrane filtration method and 7 to 14 days for the direct-inoculation method, depending on the method of sterilization. The requirements are described in detail in the USP.

The preferred method of verifying sterility is not by testing sterilized materials but by the use of biological indicators. This is not possible, however, when products are sterilized by filtration and filled aseptically into their final containers, as is the case with such important drugs as antibiotics, insulin, or hormones. The indicators generally are highly resistant bacterial spores present in greater numbers than the normal contamination of the product and with equal or greater resistance than normal microbial flora in the products being sterilized. Various properties of commercially available bacterial spores have been recommended for specific methods of sterilization based on unique resistance characteristics.

Commonly accepted species of bacteria used for biological indicators are shown in Table 40-6. Other species can be employed, probably without serious impact on the validity of sterility interpretation, so long as the prime requirements of greater numbers and higher resistance, compared to material contamination characteristics, are maintained.

Included with the materials being sterilized, biological indicators are imbedded on either paper or plastic strips or are inoculated directly onto the material being sterilized. Obviously, the indicator has greater validity in verifying sterility if it is located within product spaces that are the most difficult to sterilize. For example, in the case of a syringe, the location of a paper strip or inoculation of spores between the ribs of the plunger stopper is recommended.

The use of isolators (barrier technology) for processing materials is discussed in the section on advanced aseptic process-

Table 40-6. Species of Bacteria Used as Biological Indicators

METHOD OF STERILIZATION	BACTERIAL SPECIES
Moist heat	*B stearothermophilus*
Dry heat	*B subtilis*
Ethylene oxide	*B stearothermophilus*
Radiation	*B pumilus, B stearothermophilus, B subtilis*

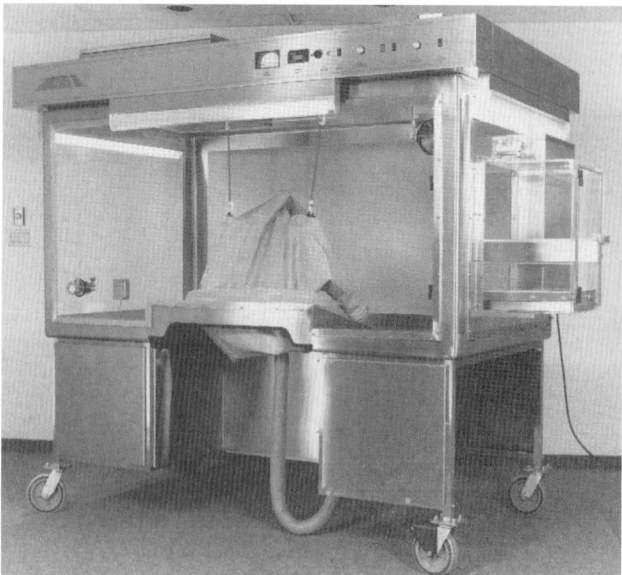

Figure 40-32. Stainless steel half-suit isolator (courtesy, Laminar Flow).

ing. The first widespread use of these modern *glove boxes* in the pharmaceutical industry was in sterility testing. As filling speeds became faster, batches became larger. This, coupled with more expensive drug substances, created the need to avoid false-positive sterility tests. Even with laminar-flow hoods becoming widely used, the large number of manipulations carried out by people, created a significant chance for contamination through the testing procedure.

Government standards for SAL basically eliminated the possibility to repeat sterility tests. This means that batches that fail for any reason cannot be released. They are only useful for investigation of potential contamination hazards. Industry in turn needed more assurance that the product was indeed not sterile and the test was valid. This led to the development of more sophisticated isolation units. Figure 40-32 shows a stainless-steel half-suit system that is typical of those used in sterility testing. The units can be *docked* to a sterilizer, which eliminates the possibility of contamination during transfer of materials to the test area. The units can be sterilized using vaporized hydrogen peroxide. The exterior of any test materials required to be transferred into the units also can be sterilized in this manner. Validation of these steps allows one to virtually eliminate false-positive test results. Most manufacturers have adopted this technique and have agreed to a policy of essentially no sterility retests. Only where obvious system breakdowns can be shown to have led to failures will a retest be considered.

ADVANCED ASEPTIC PROCESSING

Isolator technology also is being used with increasing frequency in the processing of sterile products and associated packaging materials. This is driven by the same need to minimize human intervention and thus increase dramatically the assurance of sterility (SAL). The minimization of people was expanded throughout the 1990s with the advent of more widespread use of form, fill, and seal technology. This involved the on-line molding, filling, and sealing of plastic bottles containing sterile products. The technology was housed in rigid walled areas and product was supplied through filters and sterilized in place, at the last possible area before filling.

While form, fill, and seal is a technology on its own, it did lead to the recognition that by updating significantly the older concepts of *glove boxes,* one could dramatically affect the sterility assurance of an aseptic process. People contribute the largest percentage of the contamination risk. By minimizing their interaction, the probability of nonsterility is greatly reduced.

Glove boxes were not designed to support modern (and especially more automated) operations. This may explain why they did not become popular as aseptic processing units. Usage began to expand only when the need for increased assurance drove designers to develop ergonomically designed isolators.

More recently, the manufacturers of high-speed processing equipment have begun to redesign their machinery in line with the principles of isolator units. Because the mechanics of these machines have been proved to be very reliable and require very little human intervention, the timing seems to be correct for such modifications. Isolator units are relatively inexpensive also. They have allowed for aseptic processing without the construction of large processing areas, sterile suites or gowning areas. The development of relatively safe sterilization methods, such as vaporized hydrogen peroxide (with or without atmospheric steam) also has allowed the technology to become more viable for widespread use. Prior to this, the use of toxic (and sometimes corrosive) materials was required. This limited their use to more sophisticated operators, who were able to afford the resources required to build and maintain facilities for their use.

TRAINING

It is desirable that personnel involved with sterilization or aseptic processing be instructed in the basic behavior of microorganisms. This would include the differentiation of vegetative, spore-forming, and slow-growing life forms such as molds and yeasts. This would allow those being trained in the operations to understand the reasons for many of the restrictions necessary to carry out these processes. It is imperative that each person involved in these operations be instructed in two main areas.

Safety is the first and foremost area of concentration for a training program. Each of the pieces of equipment and processes described above have unique hazards associated with them. The operators must be made to understand the dangers of steam under pressure and exposure to gaseous sterilants prior to their neutralization.

The equipment design and installation should undergo safety reviews prior to its general operation. This review for potential hazards must be done by highly trained individuals and should include computer control and piping systems. It is important that the equipment fail (should a failure occur) in a manner that is safe to the operators. Valves should fail in a way to vent pressure to some safe area and/or gases to a relatively safe, unoccupied site.

The second major area of training involves gowning for entry into the sterile areas and subsequent performance of aseptic operations. Personnel must be instructed in proper gowning techniques so that they do not contaminate the exterior of garments and gloves during the process. Gowning areas should be supplied with full-length mirrors so that personnel can verify that all areas of their body have been covered fully and properly prior to entering a sterile work area. Recent trends indicate that gowning training should be followed by personnel monitoring with contact plates containing growth media. This allows one to verify the effectiveness of the training and, should growth occur, one can use this growth as a training tool to emphasize the importance of careful attention to detail during the gowning process. Because these plates require incubation, one does not allow operators to enter the sterile area until the results of these tests have been collected and reviewed with the candidate.

Continuing with the above approach, those performing aseptic operations require additional training and subsequent verification. This principle of competency-based training (ie, verifying the capabilities of those being trained) is necessary to ensure that the operators have developed the skills to carry out these

vital operations while minimizing the risk of contamination. Again, it allows for constructive feedback to those who have not yet become fully accomplished in the techniques. It is prudent to reinforce these skills periodically through refresher sessions, and reverification of the skills. It has become standard practice to do unannounced spot-checks of the gloves and gowns of aseptic operators. This practice helps to maintain a level of vigilance, with regard to proper gowning and operating technique.

ACKNOWLEDGMENTS—Special thanks to the previous authors Barry Garfinkle and Martin Henley for writing such a good treatise on this subject. A thank you to the Cardinal-Health ElPaso, Texas facility for their review and comments on the radiation section.

REFERENCES

1. *Medical Device Sterilization Monographs* (Rep Nos 78-4.13 and 78-4.11). Washington, DC: Health Industry Manufacturers Association, 1978.
2. Block SS, ed. *Disinfection, Sterilization and Preservation,* 3rd ed. Philadelphia: Lea & Febiger, 1983.
3. *Steam Sterilization and Sterility Assurance, Good Hospital Practice* (AAMI Recommended Practice, ST.1-1980). Arlington VA: Assoc Adv Med Instrum, 1980.
4. *Guideline for Industrial Ethylene Oxide Sterilization of Medical Devices* (AAMI Recommended Practice, OPEO-87). Arlington, VA: Assoc Adv Med Instrum, 1987.
5. *In-Hospital Sterility Assurance—Current Perspectives, Aseptic Barrier Evaluation, Sterilizer Processing, Issues in Infection Control and Sterility Assurance* (AAMI Technol Assess Rep No 4-82). Arlington, VA: Assoc Adv Med Instrum, 1982.
6. *Hospital Steam Sterilizers* (Am Natl Std, ANSI/AAMI ST8-1982). Arlington, VA: Assoc Adv Med Instrum, 1983.
7. *Process Control Guidelines for Gamma Radiation Sterilization of Medical Devices* (AAMI Recommended Practice, RS-3/84). Arlington, VA: Assoc Adv Med Instrum, 1984.
8. *Performance Evaluation of Ethylene Oxide Sterilizers—Ethylene Oxide Test Packs, Good Hospital Practice* (AAMI Recommended Practice, EOTP-2.85). Arlington, VA: Assoc Adv Med Instrum, 1985.
9. *Biological Indicators for Saturated Steam Sterilization Processes in Health Care Facilities* (Am Natl Std, ANSI/AAMI ST 19-1985). Arlington, VA: Assoc Adv Med Instrum, 1986.
10. *Good Hospital Practice: Steam Sterilization Using the Unwrapped Method (Flash Sterilization)* (AAMI Recommended Practice, SSUM-9/85). Arlington, VA: Assoc Adv Med Instrum, 1986.
11. Johnson J. *Vaporized Hydrogen Peroxide Sterilization of Freeze Dryers.* ISPE Ann Meeting, Panama City, FL, 1993.
12. Lysfjord JP, et al. *The Potential For Use of Steam at Atmospheric Pressure to Decontaminate or Sterilize Parenteral Filling Lines Incorporating Barrier Isolation Technology.* Spring Mtg of the PDA, Philadelphia, 10 Mar 1993.
13. Edwards LM. *Pharm Eng* 1993; 13(2):50.
14. Rosenblatt, et al. *Use of Chlorine Dioxide Gas as a Chemosterilizing Agent,* US Pat 4,504,422 (Scopas Technol Corp), 1985.
15. Knapp JE, Rosenblatt DH, Rosenblatt AA. *Med Dev Diag Ind* 1986; 8:48.
16. Kowalski JB, Hollis RA, Roman CA. In: Pierce G, ed. *Developments in Industrial Microbiology,* vol 29. Amsterdam: Elsevier, 1988, p 239.
17. Jeng DK, Woodworth AG. *Artif Organs* 1990; 14:361.
18. National Archives. *Federal Register* 40: Mar 14, 1975, p 11865.
19. 21 CFR 211.72.
20. *Microbiological Evaluation of Filters for Sterilizing Liquids,* vol 4, no 3. Washington, DC: Health Ind Manuf Assoc, 1981.
21. Leahy TJ, et al. *Pharm Technol* 1978; 2:65.
22. Dawson FW, et al. *Nordiska Foreningen for Renlighelsteknik och Rena Rum,* Goteborg, Sweden, 1981, p 5.
23. *Test for Determination of Characteristics of Membrane Filters for Use in Aerospace Liquids (Proposed Tentative Test Method).* Philadelphia: ASTM, June 1965.
24. Reti AR, et al. *Bull Parenteral Drug Assoc* 1977; 31:187.
25. Patel JA, Curtis EG, Phillips GL. *Am J Hosp Pharm* 1972; 29:947.
26. Powell DB. In: Phillips GB, Miller WS, eds. *Industrial Sterilization.* Durham, NC: Duke University Press, 1973, p 79.
27. Runkle RS, Phillips GB, eds. *Microbial Contamination Control Facilities.* New York: Van Nostrand-Reinhold, 1969.
28. *Clean Room and Work Station Requirements: Controlled Environment* (Fed Std No 209B). Washington, DC: USGPO, 24 Apr 1973.

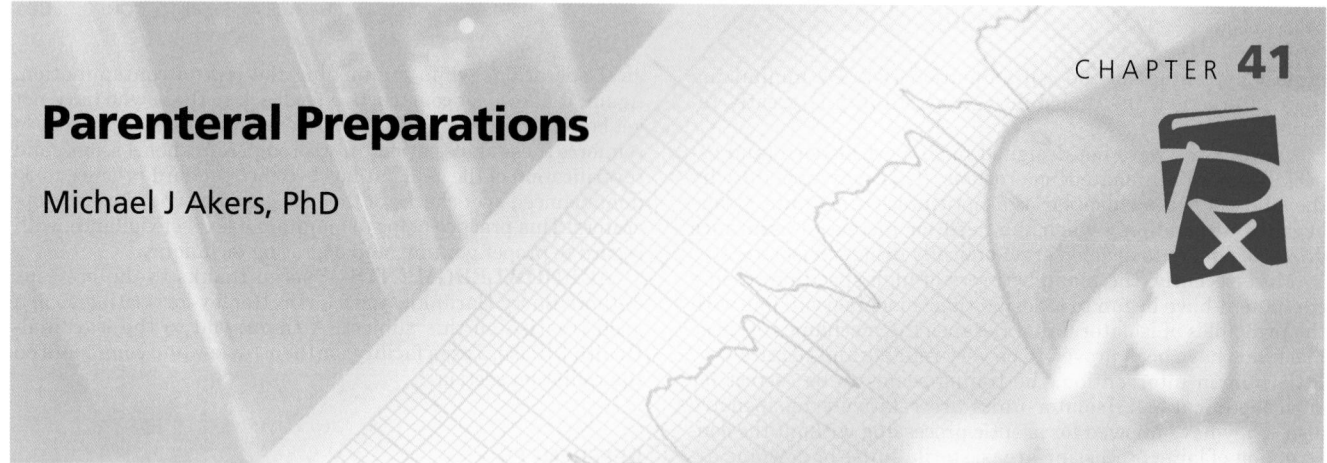

CHAPTER 41

Parenteral Preparations

Michael J Akers, PhD

Parenteral (Gk, *para enteron,* beside the intestine) dosage forms differ from all other drug dosage forms because they are injected directly into body tissue through the primary protective system of the human body, the skin, and mucous membranes. They must be exceptionally pure and free from physical, chemical, and biological contaminants. These requirements place a heavy responsibility on the pharmaceutical industry to practice current good manufacturing practices (cGMPs) in the manufacture of parenteral dosage forms and upon pharmacists and other health care professionals to practice good aseptic practices (GAPs) in dispensing them for administration to patients.

Certain pharmaceutical agents, particularly peptides, proteins, and many chemotherapeutic agents, can only be given parenterally because they are inactivated in the gastrointestinal tract when given by mouth. Parenterally administered drugs are relatively unstable and generally high potent drugs that require strict control of their administration to the patient. Because of the advent of biotechnology, parenteral products have grown in number and usage around the world.

This chapter will focus on the unique characteristics of parenteral dosage forms and the basic principles for formulating, packaging, manufacturing, and controlling the quality of these unique products. The references and bibliography at the end of this chapter contain the most up-to-date texts, book chapters, and review papers on parenteral product formulation, manufacture, and quality control.

OVERVIEW OF UNIQUE CHARACTERISTICS OF PARENTERAL DOSAGE FORMS

Parenteral products are unique from any other type of pharmaceutical dosage form for the following reasons:

- All products must be sterile.
- All products must be free from pyrogenic (endotoxin) contamination.
- Injectable solutions must be free from visible particulate matter. This includes reconstituted sterile powders.
- Products should be isotonic although strictness of isotonicity depends on the route of administration. Products to be administered into the cerebrospinal fluid must be isotonic. Ophthalmic products, while not parenteral, also must be isotonic. Products to be administered by bolus injection by routes other than intravenous (IV) essentially should be isotonic or at least very close to isotonicity. IV infusions must be isotonic.

The author recognizes the long time contributions of Dr. Kenneth Avis. Dr. Avis died in January 1999. Dr. Avis authored this chapter in Remington since 1965. To honor his memory, the author has maintained most of his organization of this chapter with new material and revised information added where appropriate.

- All products must be stable (not only chemically and physically like all other dosage forms, but also "stable" microbiologically, ie, sterility, freedom from pyrogenic and visible particulate contamination must be maintained throughout the shelflife of the product).
- Products must be compatible (if applicable) with IV diluents, delivery systems, and other drug products co-administered.

FORMULATION PRINCIPLES

Parenteral drugs are formulated as solutions, suspensions, emulsions, liposomes, microspheres, nanosystems, and powders to be reconstituted as solutions. This section will describe the components that are commonly used in parenteral formulations focusing on solutions and freeze-dried products. General guidance also will be provided on appropriate selection of the finished sterile dosage form and initial approaches used to develop the optimal parenteral formulation.

VEHICLES

WATER—Since most liquid injections are quite dilute, the component present in the highest proportion is the vehicle. The vehicle of greatest importance for parenteral products is water. Water of suitable quality for compounding and rinsing product contact surfaces may be prepared either by distillation or by reverse osmosis, to meet United States Pharmacopeia (USP) specifications for Water for Injection (WFI). Only by these two methods is it possible to separate adequately various liquid, gas, and solid contaminating substances from water. These two methods for preparation of WFI and specifications for WFI are discussed later in this chapter. With the possible exception of freeze-drying, there is no unit operation more important and none more costly to install and operate than the one for the preparation of WFI.

WATER-MISCIBLE VEHICLES—A number of solvents that are miscible with water have been used as a portion of the vehicle in the formulation of parenterals. These solvents are used primarily to solubilize certain drugs in an aqueous vehicle and to reduce hydrolysis. The most important solvents in this group are ethyl alcohol, liquid polyethylene glycol, and propylene glycol. Ethyl alcohol is used particularly in the preparation of solutions of cardiac glycosides and the glycols in solutions of barbiturates, certain alkaloids, and certain antibiotics. Such preparations usually are given intramuscularly. There are limitations with the amount of these co-solvents that can be administered because of toxicity concerns, greater potential for hemolysis, and potential for drug precipitation at the site of injection.[1] Formulation scientists needing to use one or more of these solvents must consult the literature (eg, reference [2]) and toxicologists to ascertain the maximum amount of co-solvents allowed for their particular product. Several references provide information on concentrations of co-solvents used in approved commercial parenteral products.[3–8]

NON-AQUEOUS VEHICLES—The most important group of non-aqueous vehicles are the fixed oils. The USP provides specifications for such vehicles, indicating that the fixed oils must be of vegetable origin so that they will be metabolized, will be liquid at room temperature, and will not become rancid readily. The USP also specifies limits for the free fatty acid content, iodine value, and saponification value (oil heated with alkali to produce soap, ie, alcohol plus acid salt). The oils most commonly used are corn oil, cottonseed oil, peanut oil, and sesame oil. Fixed oils are used particularly as vehicles for certain hormone (eg, progesterone, testosterone, deoxycorticicosterone) and vitamin (eg, vitamin K, vitamin E) preparations. The label must state the name of the vehicle so that the user may beware in case of known sensitivity or other reactions to it.

SOLUTES

Care must be taken in selecting active pharmaceutical ingredients and excipients to ensure that their quality is suitable for parenteral administration. A low microbial level will enhance the effectiveness of either the aseptic or terminal sterilization process used for the drug product. Likewise, nonpyrogenic ingredients enhance the nonpyrogenicity of the finished injectable product. It is now a common GMP procedure to establish microbial and endotoxin limits on active pharmaceutical ingredients and most excipients. Chemical impurities should be virtually nonexistent in active pharmaceutical ingredients for parenterals, because impurities are not likely to be removed by the processing of the product. Depending on the chemical involved, even trace residues may be harmful to the patient or cause stability problems in the product. Therefore, manufacturers should use the best grade of chemicals obtainable and use its analytical profile to determine that each lot of chemical used in the formulation meets the required specifications.

Reputable chemical manufacturers accept the stringent quality requirements for parenteral products and, accordingly, apply good manufacturing practices to their chemical manufacturing. Examples of critical bulk manufacturing precautions include:

- Using dedicated equipment or properly validated cleaning to prevent cross-contamination and transfer of impurities
- Using WFI for rinsing equipment
- Using closed systems wherever possible for bulk manufacturing steps not followed by further purification
- Adhering to specified endotoxin and bioburden testing limits for the substance.

ADDED SUBSTANCES—The USP includes in this category all substances added to a preparation to improve or safeguard its quality. An added substance may:

- Increase and maintain drug solubility. Examples include complexing agents and surface active agents. The most commonly used complexing agents are the cyclodextrins, including Captisol®. The most commonly used surface active agents are polyoxyethylene sorbitan monolaurate (Tween 20) and polyoxyethylene sorbitans monooleate (Tween 80).
- Provide patient comfort by reducing pain and tissue irritation, as do substances added to make a solution isotonic or near physiological pH. Common tonicity adjusters are sodium chloride, dextrose, and glycerin.
- Enhance the chemical stability of a solution, as do antioxidants, inert gases, chelating agents, and buffers.
- Enhance the chemical and physical stability of a freeze-dried product, as do cryoprotectants and lyoprotectants.
- Enhance the physical stability of proteins by minimizing self aggregation or interfacial induced aggregation. Surface active agents serve nicely in this capacity.
- Minimize protein interaction with inert surfaces such as glass and rubber and plastic. Competitive binders such as albumin and surface active agents are the best examples.
- Protect a preparation against the growth of microorganisms. The

term *preservative* sometimes is applied only to those substances that prevent the growth of microorganisms in a preparation. However, such limited use is inappropriate, being better used for all substances that act to retard or prevent the chemical, physical, or biological degradation of a preparation.

- While not covered in this chapter, other reasons for adding solutes to parenteral formulations include sustaining and/or controlling drug release (polymers), maintaining the drug in a suspension dosage form (suspending agents, usually polymers and surface active agents), establishing emulsified dosage forms (emulsifying agents, usually amphiphilic polymers and surface active agents), and preparation of liposomes (hydrated phospholipids).

Although added substances may prevent a certain reaction from taking place, they may induce others. Not only may visible incompatibilities occur, but hydrolysis, complexation, oxidation, and other invisible reactions may decompose or otherwise inactivate the therapeutic agent or other added substances.[9] Therefore, added substances must be selected with due consideration and investigation of their effect on the total formulation and the container-closure system.

ANTIMICROBIAL AGENTS—The USP states that antimicrobial agents in bacteriostatic or fungistatic concentrations must be added to preparations contained in multiple-dose containers.* They must be present in adequate concentration at the time of use to prevent the multiplication of microorganisms inadvertently introduced into the preparation while withdrawing a portion of the contents with a hypodermic needle and syringe. The USP provides a test for Antimicrobial Preservative Effectiveness to determine that an antimicrobial substance or combination adequately inhibits the growth of microorganisms in a parenteral product.[10] Because antimicrobials may have inherent toxicity for the patient, the USP prescribes maximum volume and concentration limits for those that are used commonly in parenteral products (eg, phenylmercuric nitrate and thimerosal 0.01%, benzethonium chloride and benzalkonium chloride 0.01%, phenol or cresol 0.5%, and chlorobutanol 0.5%).

The above limit rarely is used for phenylmercuric nitrate, most frequently employed in a concentration of 0.002%. Methyl *p*-hydroxybenzoate 0.18% and propyl *p*-hydroxybenzoate 0.02% in combination, and benzyl alcohol 2% also are used frequently. Benzyl alcohol, phenol, and the parabens are the most widely used antimicrobial preservative agents used in injectable products. While the mercurials are still allowed to be used in older products, they are not used for new products because of concerns regarding mercury toxicity. In oleaginous preparations, no antibacterial agent commonly employed appears to be effective. However, it has been reported that hexylresorcinol 0.5% and phenylmercuric benzoate 0.1% are moderately bactericidal. A few therapeutic compounds have been shown to have antibacterial activity, thus obviating the need for added agents.

Antimicrobial agents must be studied with respect to compatibility with all other components of the formula. In addition, their activity must be evaluated in the total formula. It is not uncommon to find that a particular agent will be effective in one formulation but ineffective in another. This may be due to the effect of various components of the formula on the biological activity or availability of the compound; for example, the binding and inactivation of esters of *p*-hydroxybenzoic acid by macromolecules such as polysorbate 80 or the reduction of phenylmercuric nitrate by sulfide residues in rubber closures. A physical reaction encountered is that bacteriostatic agents sometimes are removed from solution by rubber closures.

Protein pharmaceuticals, because of their cost and/or frequency of use, are preferred to be available as multiple dose formulations (eg, human insulin, human growth hormone, interferons, vaccines). However, several proteins are reactive with antimicrobial preservative agents (eg, tissue plasminogen activator, sargramostim, interleukins) and, therefore, are only available as single dosage form units.

---

*The European Pharmacopeia requires multiple-dose products to be bacteriocidal and fungicidal.[10]

Single-dose containers and pharmacy bulk packs that do not contain antimicrobial agents are expected to be used promptly after opening or to be discarded. The ICH/CPMP guidelines† require that products without preservatives must be used immediately (within 3 hours after entering the primary package) or a longer usage period must be justified.

Large-volume, single-dose containers may not contain an added antimicrobial preservative. Therefore, special care must be exercised in storing such products after the containers have been opened to prepare an admixture, particularly those that can support the growth of microorganisms, such as total parenteral nutrition (TPN) solutions and emulsions. It should be noted that while refrigeration slows the growth of most microorganisms, it does not prevent their growth.

BUFFERS are used primarily to stabilize a solution against chemical degradation or, especially for proteins, physical degradation (ie, aggregation and precipitation) that might occur if the pH changes appreciably. Buffer systems employed should normally have as low a buffering capacity as feasible so as not to disturb significantly the body's buffering systems when injected. In addition, the buffer type and concentration on the activity of the active ingredient must be evaluated carefully. Buffer components are known to catalyze degradation of drugs. The acid salts most frequently employed as buffers are citrates, acetates, and phosphates.

ANTIOXIDANTS are required frequently to preserve products because of the ease with which many drugs are oxidized. Sodium bisulfite and other sulfurous acid salts are used most frequently. Ascorbic acid and its salts also are good antioxidants. The sodium salt of ethylenediaminetetraacetic acid (EDTA) has been found to enhance the activity of antioxidants in some cases, apparently by chelating metallic ions that would otherwise catalyze the oxidation reaction.

Displacing the air (oxygen) in and above the solution by purging with an inert gas, such as nitrogen, also can be used as a means to control oxidation of a sensitive drug. Process control is required for assurance that every container is deaerated adequately and uniformly. However, conventional processes for removing oxygen from liquids and containers do not absolutely remove all oxygen. The only approach for completely removing oxygen is to employ isolator technology where the entire atmosphere can be recirculating nitrogen or another non-oxygen gas.

TONICITY AGENTS are used in many parenteral and ophthalmic products to adjust the tonicity of the solution. While it is the goal for every injectable product to be isotonic with physiologic fluids, this is not an essential requirement for small volume injectables that are administered intravenously. However, products administered by all other routes, especially into the eye or spinal fluid, must be isotonic. Injections into the subcutaneous tissue and muscles also should be isotonic to minimize pain and tissue irritation. The agents most commonly used are electrolytes and mono- or disaccharides.

CRYOPROTECTANTS and **LYOPROTECTANTS** are additives that serve to protect biopharmaceuticals from adverse effects due to freezing and/or drying of the product during freeze-dry processing. *Sugars* (non-reducing) such as sucrose or trehalose, *amino acids* such as glycine or lysine, *polymers* such as liquid polyethylene glycol or dextran, and *polyols* such as mannitol or sorbitol all are possible cryo- or lyoprotectants. Several theories exist to explain why these additives work to protect proteins against freezing and/or drying effects.[11,12] Excipients that are preferentially excluded from the surface of the protein are the best cryoprotectants and excipients that remain amorphous during and after freeze-drying serve best as lyoprotectants.

General Guidance for Developing Formulations of Parenteral Drugs

The final formulation of a parenteral drug product depends on understanding the following factors that dictate the choice of

†www.eudra.org/emea/pdfs/CPMP_QWP_159_96.pdf

formulation and dosage form:

1. Route of administration—Injections may be administered by routes such as intravenous, subcutaneous, intradermal, intramuscular, intraarticular, and intrathecal. The type of dosage form (solution, suspension, etc.) will determine the particular route of administration that may be employed. Conversely, the desired route of administration will place requirements on the formulation. For example, suspensions would not be administered directly into the bloodstream because of the danger of insoluble particles blocking capillaries. Solutions to be administered subcutaneously require strict attention to tonicity adjustment, otherwise irritation of the plentiful supply of nerve endings in this anatomical area would give rise to pronounced pain. Injections intended for intraocular, intraspinal, intracisternal, and intrathecal administration require stricter standards of such properties as formulation tonicity, component purity, and limit of endotoxins because of the sensitivity of tissues encountered to irritant and toxic substances.

   If the route of administration must be intravenous, then only solutions or microemulsions can be the dosage form. If the route of administration is to be subcutaneous or intramuscular, then the likely type of dosage form is a suspension or other microparticulate delivery system.

2. Pharmacokinetics of the drug—Rates of absorption (for routes of administration other than intravenous or intra-arterial), distribution, metabolism, and excretion for a drug will have some effect on the selected route of administration and, accordingly, the type of formulation. For example, if the pharmacokinetic profile of a drug is very rapid, modified release dosage formulations may need to be developed. The dose of drug and the dosage regimen are affected by pharmacokinetics so the size (ie, concentration) of dose will also influence the type of formulation and amounts of other ingredients in the formulation. If the dosage regimen requires frequent injections, then a multiple dose formulation must be developed, if feasible. If the drug is distributed quickly from the site injection, complexing agents or viscosity inducing agents may be added to the formulation to retard drug dissolution and transport.

3. Drug solubility—If the drug is insufficiently soluble in water at the required dosage, then the formulation must contain a co-solvent or a solute that sufficiently increases and maintains the drug in solution. If relatively simple formulation additives do not result in a solution, then a dispersed system dosage form must be developed. Solubility also dictates the concentration of drug in the dosage form.

4. Drug stability—If the drug has significant degradation problems in solution, then a freeze-dried or other sterile solid dosage form must be developed. Stability is sometimes affected by drug concentration that, in turn, might affect size and type of packaging system used. For example, if concentration must be low due to stability and/or solubility limitations, then the size of primary container must be larger and this might preclude the use of syringes, cartridges, and/or smaller vial sizes. Obviously, stability dictates the expiration date of the product that, in turn, will determine the storage conditions. Storage conditions might dictate choice of container size, formulation components, and type of container. If a product must be refrigerated, then the container cannot be too large and formulation components must be soluble and stable at colder conditions.

5. Compatibility of drug with potential formulation additives—It is well-known that drug-excipient incompatibilities frequently exist.[9] Initial preformulation screening studies are essential to assure that formulation additives, while possibly solving one problem, will not create another. Stabilizers, such as buffers and antioxidants, while chemically stabilizing the drug in one way, may also catalyze other chemical degradation reactions. Excipients and certain drugs can form insoluble complexes. Impurities in excipients can cause drug degradation reactions. Peroxide impurities in polymers may catalyze oxidative degradation reactions with drugs, including proteins, that are oxygen sensitive.

6. Desired type of packaging—Selection of packaging (type, size, shape, color of rubber closure, label, and aluminum cap) often is based on marketing preferences and competition. Knowing the type of final package early in the development process aids the formulation scientist in being sure that the product formulation will be compatible and elegant in that packaging system.

Table 41-1 provides steps involved in the formulation of a new parenteral drug product. This can also be viewed as a list of questions, the answers of which will facilitate decisions on the final formulation that should be developed.

Table 41-1. Main Steps Involved in the Formulation of a New Parenteral Drug Product

1. <u>Obtain physical properties of active drug substance</u>
   a. Structure, molecular weight
   b. "Practical" solubility in water at room temperature
   c. Effect of pH on solubility
   d. Solubility in certain other solvents
   e. Unusual solubility properties
   f. Isoelectric point for a protein or peptide
   g. Hygroscopicity
   h. Potential for water or other solvent loss
   i. Aggregation potential for protein or peptide

2. <u>Obtain chemical properties of active drug substance</u>
   a. Must have a "validatable" analytical method for potency and purity
   b. Time for 10% degradation at room temperature in aqueous solution in the pH range of anticipated use
   c. Time for 10% degradation at 5°C.
   d. pH stability profile
   e. Sensitivity to oxygen
   f. Sensitivity to light
   g. Major routes of degradation and degradation products

3. <u>Initial formulation approaches</u>
   a. Know timeline(s) for drug product
   b. Know how drug product will be used in the clinic
      i. Single dose vs multiple dose
      ii. If multiple dose, will preservative agent be part of drug solution/powder or part of diluent?
      iii. Shelf life goals
      iv. Combination with other products, diluents
   c. From knowledge of solubility and stability properties, and information from anticipated clinical use formulate drug with components and solution properties that are known to be successful at dealing with these issues. Then perform accelerated stability studies.
      i. High temperature storage
      ii. Temperature cycling
      iii. Light and/or oxygen exposure
      iv. For powders, expose to high humidities
   d. May need to perform several short-term stability studies as excipient types and combinations are eliminated.
   e. Understand need for any special container and closure requirements
   f. Design and implement an initial manufacturing method of the product
   g. Finalize formulation
      i. Need for tonicity adjusting agent
      ii. Need for antimicrobial preservative
   h. Approach to obtain sterile product
      i. Terminal sterilization
      ii. Sterile filtration and aseptic processing

Courtesy of Dr. Eddie Massey and Dr. Alan Fites, Baxter Pharmaceutical Solutions.

ADMINISTRATION

Injections may be classified in six general categories:

1. Solutions ready for injection
2. Dry, soluble products ready to be combined with a solvent just prior to use
3. Suspensions ready for injection
4. Dry, insoluble products ready to be combined with a vehicle just prior to use
5. Emulsions
6. Liquid concentrates ready for dilution prior to administration

When compared with other dosage forms, injections possess select advantages. If immediate physiological action is needed from a drug, it usually can be provided by the intravenous injection of an aqueous solution. Modification of the formulation or another route of injection can be used to slow the onset and prolong the action of the drug. The therapeutic response of a drug is controlled more readily by parenteral administration, since the irregularities of intestinal absorption are circumvented. Also, since the drug normally is administered by a pro-

fessionally trained person, it confidently may be expected that the dose was actually and accurately administered. Drugs can be administered parenterally when they cannot be given orally because of the unconscious or uncooperative state of the patient or because of inactivation or lack of absorption in the intestinal tract. Among the disadvantages of this dosage form are the requirement of asepsis at administration, the risk of tissue toxicity from local irritation, the real or psychological pain factor, and the difficulty in correcting an error, should one be made. In the latter situation, unless a direct pharmacological antagonist is immediately available, correction of an error may be impossible. One other disadvantage is that daily or frequent administration poses difficulties, patients must either visit a professionally trained person or learn to inject themselves. However, the advent of home health care as an alternative to extended institutional care and availability of new medications from biotechnology to treat chronic diseases have mandated the development of programs for training lay persons to administer these dosage forms.

PARENTERAL COMBINATIONS

Most dosage forms, when released to the marketplace by the manufacturer, are consumed by the patient without any significant manipulation of the product. For example, tablets and capsules are ingested in the same form as they were when released by the manufacturer. For many parenteral drug products, this is not the case. For example, products in vials must be withdrawn into a syringe prior to injection and often combined with other products in infusion solutions prior to administration. Freeze-dried products first have to be reconstituted with a specific or nonspecific diluent prior to being withdrawn from the vial. Specifically, it is common practice for a physician to order the addition of a small-volume therapeutic injection (SVI), such as an antibiotic, to large-volume injections (LVIs), such as 1000 mL of 0.9% sodium chloride solution, to avoid the discomfort for the patient of a separate injection. Certain aqueous vehicles are recognized officially because of their valid use in parenterals. Often they are used as isotonic vehicles to which a drug may be added at the time of administration. The additional osmotic effect of the drug may not be enough to produce any discomfort when administered. These vehicles include sodium chloride injection, Ringer's injection, dextrose injection, dextrose and sodium chloride injection, and lactated Ringer's injection.

While the pharmacist is the most qualified health professional to be responsible for preparing such combinations, as is clearly stated in the hospital accreditation manual of the Joint Commission on Accreditation of Healthcare Organizations,[13] interactions among the combined products can be troublesome even for the pharmacist. In fact, incompatibilities can occur and cause inactivation of one or more ingredients or other undesired reactions. Patient deaths have been reported from the precipitate formed by two incompatible ingredients. In some instances incompatibilities are visible as precipitation or color change, but in other instances there may be no visible effect.

The many potential combinations present a complex situation even for the pharmacist. To aid in making decisions concerning potential problems, a valuable compilation of relevant data has been assembled by Trissel[14] and is updated regularly. Further, the advent of computerized data storage and retrieval systems has provided a means to organize and gain rapid access to such information. Further information on this subject may be found in Chapter 42 (*Intravenous Admixtures*).

As studies have been undertaken and more information has been gained, it has been shown that knowledge of variable factors such as pH and the ionic character of the active constituents aids substantially in understanding and predicting potential incompatibilities. Kinetic studies of reaction rates may be used to describe or predict the extent of degradation. Ultimately, a thorough study should be undertaken of each therapeutic agent in combination with other drugs and IV fluids, not only of generic but also of commercial preparations, from the physical, chemical, and therapeutic aspects.

Ideally, no parenteral combination should be administered unless it has been studied thoroughly to determine its effect on the therapeutic value and the safety of the combination. However, such an ideal situation may not exist. Nevertheless, it is the responsibility of the pharmacist to be as familiar as possible with the physical, chemical, and therapeutic aspects of parenteral combinations and to exercise the best possible judgment as to whether or not the specific combination extemporaneously prescribed is suitable for use in a patient.

GENERAL CONSIDERATIONS

An inherent requirement for parenteral preparations is that they be of the very best quality and provide the maximum safety for the patient. Further, the constant adherence to high moral and professional ethics on the part of the responsible persons are the ingredients most vital to achieving the desired quality in the products prepared.

Types of Processes

The preparation of parenteral products may be categorized as small-scale dispensing, usually one unit at a time, or large-scale manufacturing, in which hundreds of thousands of units may constitute one lot of product. The former category illustrates the type of processing that is done in early clinical phase manufacturing or in institutions such as hospital pharmacies. The latter category is typical of the processing done in the later clinical phase and commercial manufacturing in the pharmaceutical industry. Wherever they are made, parenteral products must be subjected to the same basic practices of current Good Manufacturing Practices (cGMPs) and good aseptic processing essential for the preparation of a safe and effective sterile product of highest quality, but the methods used must be modified appropriately for the scale of operation.

The small-scale preparation and dispensing of parenteral products might use sterile components in their preparation. Therefore, the overall process focuses on maintaining rather than achieving sterility in the process steps. In the hospital setting, the final product might have a shelf life measured in hours. However, the extensive movement of patients out of the hospital to home care has modified hospital dispensing of parenteral products, wherein multiple units are made for a given patient, and a shelf life of 30 days or more is required. Such products are sometimes made in hospital pharmacies but increasingly in centers set up to provide this service. A discussion of such processing can be found in the USP general chapter <1206>.

This chapter emphasizes the preparation of parenteral products from nonsterile components in the highly technologically advanced plants of the pharmaceutical industry, using cGMP principles. In the pursuit of cGMP, consideration should be given to:

1. Ensuring that the personnel responsible for assigned duties are capable and qualified to perform them
2. Ensuring that ingredients used in compounding the product have the required identity, quality, and purity
3. Validating critical processes to be sure that the equipment used and the processes followed will ensure that the finished product will have the qualities expected
4. Maintaining a production environment suitable for performing the critical processes required, addressing such matters as orderliness, cleanliness, asepsis, and avoidance of cross contamination
5. Confirming through adequate quality-control procedures that the finished products have the required potency, purity, and quality
6. Establishing through appropriate stability evaluation that the drug products will retain their intended potency, purity, and quality until the established expiration date
7. Ensuring that processes always are carried out in accord with established, written procedures
8. Providing adequate conditions and procedures for the prevention of mix-ups

9. Establishing adequate procedures, with supporting documentation, for investigating and correcting failures or problems in production or quality control
10. Providing adequate separation of quality-control responsibilities from those of production to ensure independent decision-making

The pursuit of cGMP is an ongoing effort that must flex with new technological developments and new understanding of existing principles. Because of the extreme importance of quality in health care of the public, the US Congress has given the responsibility of regulatory scrutiny over the manufacture and distribution of drug products to the FDA (see Chapter 48 for more detail regarding the new drug approval process). Therefore, the operations of the pharmaceutical industry are subject to the oversight of the FDA and, with respect to manufacturing practices, to the application of the cGMPs. These regulations are discussed more fully in Chapter 51 (*Quality Assurance and Control*).

In concert with the pursuit of cGMPs, the pharmaceutical industry has shown initiative and innovation in the extensive technological development and improvement in quality, safety, and effectiveness of parenteral dosage forms in recent years. Examples include developments in:

- Modular facility design and construction
- Container and closure cleaning, siliconization (if applicable), and sterilization
- Sterilization technologies
- Filling technologies
- Aseptic processing technology including barrier isolator technology
- Freeze-drying technologies including automated loading and unloading
- Control of particulate matter
- Automation in weight checking, inspection technologies, and labeling and finishing operations

GENERAL MANUFACTURING PROCESS

The preparation of a parenteral product may be considered to encompass four general areas:

1. Procurement and accumulation of all components in a warehouse area until released to manufacturing
2. Processing the dosage form in appropriately designed and operated facilities
3. Packaging and labeling in a quarantine area to ensure integrity and completion of the product
4. Controlling the quality of the product throughout the process

Procurement encompasses selecting and testing according to specifications of the raw-material ingredients and the containers and closures for the primary and secondary packages. Microbiological purity, in the form of bioburden and endotoxin levels, has become standard requirements for raw materials.

Processing includes cleaning containers and equipment to validated specifications, compounding the solution (or other dosage form), filtering the solution, sanitizing or sterilizing the containers and equipment, filling measured quantities of product into the sterile containers, stoppering (either completely or partially for products to be freeze-dried), freeze-drying, terminal sterilization if possible, and final sealing of the final primary container.

Packaging normally consists of the labeling and cartoning filled and sealed primary containers. The control of quality begins with the incoming supplies, being sure that specifications are met. Careful control of labels is vitally important as errors in labeling can be dangerous for the consumer. Each step of the process involves checks and tests to be sure that the required specifications at the respective step are being met. Labeling and final packaging operations are becoming more automated.

The quality control unit is responsible for reviewing the batch history and performing the release testing required to clear the product for shipment to users. A common FDA citation for potential violation of cGMP is the lack of oversight by the quality control unit in batch testing and review and approval of results.

COMPONENTS

Components of parenteral products include the active ingredient, formulation additives, vehicle(s), and the primary container and closure. Establishing specifications to ensure the quality of each of these components of an injection is essential.

The most stringent chemical-purity requirements normally will be encountered with aqueous solutions, particularly if the product is to be sterilized at an elevated temperature where reaction rates will be accelerated greatly. Dry preparations pose relatively few reaction problems but may require definitive physical specifications for ingredients that must have certain solution or dispersion characteristics when a vehicle is added.

Containers and closures are in prolonged, intimate contact with the product and may release substances into, or remove ingredients from, the product. Rubber closures are especially problematic (sorption, leachables, air and moisture transmission properties) if not properly evaluated for its compatibility with the final product. Assessment and selection of containers and closures are essential for final product formulation, to ensure that the product retains its purity, potency, and quality during the intimate contact with the container throughout its shelf life. Administration devices (syringes, tubing, transfer sets) that come in contact with the product should be assessed and selected with the same care as are containers and closures, even though the contact period is usually brief.

WATER FOR INJECTION (WFI)

Preparation

The source water can be expected to be contaminated with natural suspended mineral and organic substances, dissolved mineral salts, colloidal material, viable bacteria, bacterial endotoxins, industrial or agricultural chemicals, and other particulate matter. The degree of contamination will vary with the source and will be markedly different, whether obtained from a well or from surface sources, such as a stream or lake. Hence, the source water usually must be pretreated by one or a combination of the following treatments: chemical softening, filtration, deionization, carbon adsorption, or reverse osmosis purification. A schematic of a typical process used to convert potable water to Water for Injection is showing in Figure 41-1.

Water for Injection can be prepared by distillation or by membrane technologies (reverse osmosis or ultrafiltration).

The EP (European Pharmacopeia) only permits distillation as the process for producing WFI. The USP and JP (Japanese Pharmacopeia) allow all these technologies to be applied.

Distillation is a process of converting water from a liquid to its gaseous form (steam). Since steam is pure gaseous water, all other contaminants in the feedwater are removed. In general, a conventional still consists of a boiler (evaporator) containing feed water (distilland); a source of heat to vaporize the water in the evaporator; a headspace above the level of distilland, with condensing surfaces for refluxing the vapor, thereby returning nonvolatile impurities to the distilland; a means for eliminating volatile impurities (demister/separation device) before the hot water vapor is condensed; and a condenser for removing the heat of vaporization, thereby converting the water vapor to a liquid distillate.

The specific construction features of a still and the process specifications will have a marked effect on the quality of distillate obtained from a still. Several factors must be considered in selecting a still to produce WFI:

1. The quality of the feed water will affect the quality of the distillate. For example, chlorine in water especially can cause or exacerbate corrosion in distillation units and silica causes scaling within. Controlling the quality of the feed water is essential for meeting the required specifications for the distillate.
2. The size of the evaporator will affect the efficiency. It should be large enough to provide a low vapor velocity, thus reducing the entrainment of the distilland either as a film on vapor bubbles or as separate droplets.
3. The baffles (condensing surfaces) determine the effectiveness of refluxing. They should be designed for efficient removal of the entrainment at optimal vapor velocity, collecting, and returning the heavier droplets contaminated with the distilland.
4. Redissolving volatile impurities in the distillate reduces its purity. Therefore, they should be separated efficiently from the hot water vapor and eliminated by aspirating them to the drain or venting them to the atmosphere.
5. Contamination of the vapor and distillate from the metal parts of the still can occur. Present standards for high-purity stills are that all parts contacted by the vapor or distillate should be constructed of metal coated with pure tin, 304 or 316 stainless-steel, or chemically resistant glass.

The design features of a still also influence its efficiency of operation, relative freedom from maintenance problems, or extent of automatic operation. Stills may be constructed of varying size, rated according to the volume of distillate that can be produced per hour of operation under optimum conditions. Only stills designed to produce high-purity water may be considered for use in the production of WFI. Conventional commercial stills designed for the production of high-purity water are available from several suppliers *(AMSCO, Barnstead, Corning, Kuhlman, Vaponics)*.

There are two basic types of WFI distillation units, the vapor compression still and the multiple effect still.

COMPRESSION DISTILLATION—The vapor-compression still, primarily designed for the production of large volumes of high-purity distillate with low consumption of energy and water, is illustrated diagrammatically in Figure 41-2. To start, the feed water is heated from an external source in the evaporator to boiling. The vapor produced in the tubes is separated from the entrained distilland in the separator and conveyed to a compressor that compresses the vapor and raises its temperature to approximately 107°. It then flows to the steam chest where it condenses on the outer surfaces of the tubes containing the distilland; the vapor is thus condensed and drawn off as a distillate, while giving up its heat to bring the distilland in the tubes to the boiling point. Vapor-compression stills are available in capacities from 50 to 2800 gal/hr *(Aqua-Chem, Barnstead, Meco)*.

MULTIPLE-EFFECT STILLS—The multiple-effect still also is designed to conserve energy and water usage. In prin-

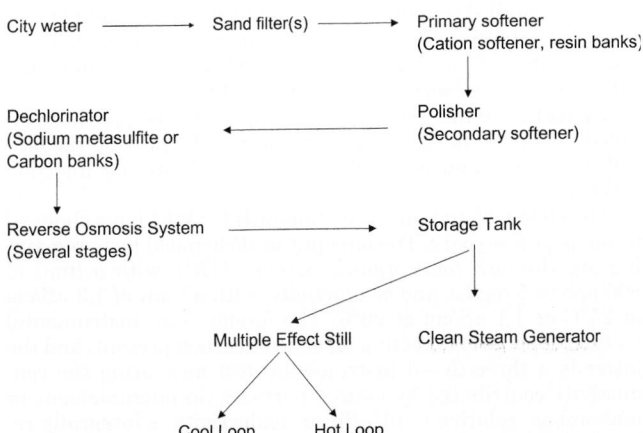

City water   ⟶   Sand filter(s)   ⟶   Primary softener (Cation softener, resin banks)

Dechlorinator (Sodium metasulfite or Carbon banks)

Polisher (Secondary softener)

Reverse Osmosis System (Several stages)   ⟶   Storage Tank

Multiple Effect Still   Clean Steam Generator

Cool Loop   Hot Loop

Figure 41-1. Water for injection system. Example of flow from source to end.

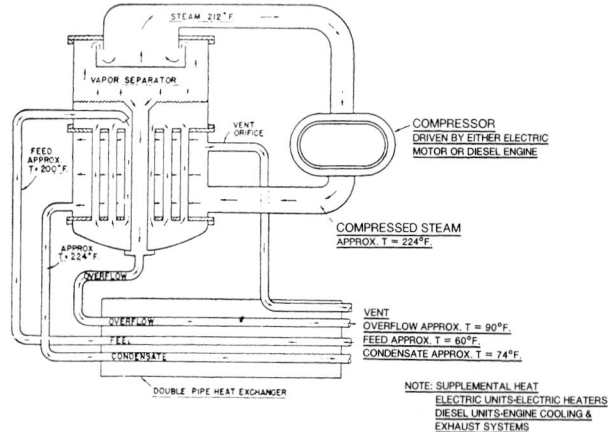

Figure 41-2. Vapor compressor still.

ciple, it is simply a series of single-effect stills or columns running at differing pressures where phase changes of water take place. A series of up to seven effects may be used, with the first effect operated at the highest pressure and the last effect at atmospheric pressure. See a schematic drawing of a multiple-effect still in Figure 41-3. Steam from an external source is used in the first effect to generate steam under pressure from feed water; it is used as the power source to drive the second effect. The steam used to drive the second effect condenses as it gives up its heat of vaporization and forms a distillate. This process continues until the last effect, when the steam is at atmospheric pressure and must be condensed in a heat exchanger.

The capacity of a multiple-effect still can be increased by adding effects. The quantity of the distillate also will be affected by the inlet steam pressure; thus, a 600-gal/hr unit designed to operate at 115 psig steam pressure could be run at approximately 55 psig and would deliver about 400 gal/hr. These stills have no moving parts and operate quietly. They are available in capacities from about 50 to 7000 gal/hr (*AMSCO, Barnstead, Finn-Aqua, Kuhlman, Vaponics*).

REVERSE OSMOSIS (RO)—As the name suggests, the natural process of selective permeation of molecules through a semipermeable membrane separating two aqueous solutions of different concentrations is reversed. Pressure, usually between 200 and 400 psig, is applied to overcome osmotic pressure and force pure water to permeate through the membrane. Membranes, usually composed of cellulose esters or polyamides, are

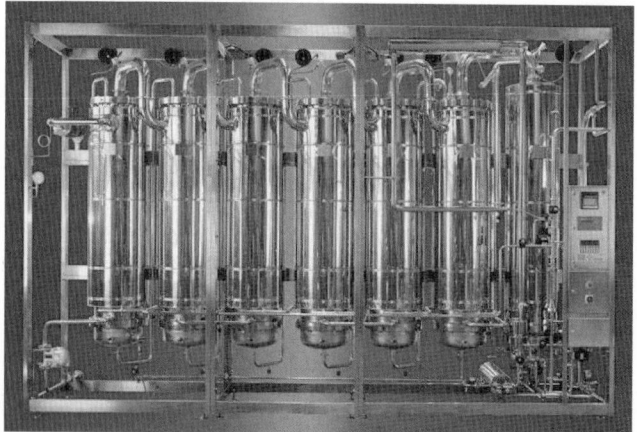

Figure 41-3. Multiple effect still (courtesy, Getinge). See Color Plate 6.

selected to provide an efficient rejection of contaminant molecules in raw water. The molecules most difficult to remove are small inorganic ones such as sodium chloride. Passage through two membranes in series is sometimes used to increase the efficiency of removal of these small molecules and to decrease the risk of structural failure of a membrane to remove other contaminants, such as bacteria and pyrogens.

Several WFI installations utilize both RO and distillation systems for generation of the highest quality water. Since feedwater to distillation units can be heavily contaminated, and, thus, affect the operation of the still, water is first run through RO units to eliminate contaminants. For additional information, see Collentro.[15]

Reverse osmosis systems are available in a range of production sizes (*AMSCO, Aqua-Chem, Finn-Aqua, Meco, Millipore,* etc).

Whichever system is used for the preparation of WFI, validation is required to be sure that the system, consistently and reliably, will produce the chemical, physical, and microbiological quality of water required. Such validation should start with the determined characteristics of the source water and include the pretreatment, production, storage, and distribution systems. All of these systems together, including their proper operation and maintenance, determine the ultimate quality of the WFI.

STORAGE AND DISTRIBUTION—The rate of production of WFI usually is not sufficient to meet processing demands; therefore, it is collected in a holding tank for subsequent use. In large operations, the holding tanks may have a capacity of several thousand gallons and be a part of a continuously operating system. In such instances the USP requires that the WFI be held at a temperature too high for microbial growth. Normally, this temperature is a constant 80°C.

The USP also permits the WFI to be stored at room temperature but for a maximum of 24 hours. Under such conditions, the WFI usually is collected as a batch for a particular use with any unused water being discarded within 24 hours. Such a system requires frequent sanitization to minimize the risk of viable microorganisms being present. The stainless-steel storage tanks in such systems usually are connected to a welded stainless-steel distribution loop supplying the various use sites with a continuously circulating water supply. The tank is provided with a hydrophobic membrane vent filter capable of excluding bacteria and nonviable particulate matter. Such a vent filter is necessary to permit changes in pressure during filling and emptying. The construction material for the tank and connecting lines usually is electropolished 316L stainless steel with welded pipe. The tanks also may be lined with glass or a coating of pure tin. Such systems are very carefully designed and constructed and often constitute the most costly installation within the plant.

When the water cannot be used at 80°C, heat exchangers must be installed to reduce the temperature at the point of use. Bacterial retentive filters should not be installed in such systems because of the risk of bacterial buildup on the filters and the consequent release of pyrogenic substances.

PURITY—While certain purity requirements have been alluded to above, the USP and EP monographs provide the official standards of purity for WFI and Sterile Water for Injection (SWFI).

The chemical and physical standards for WFI have changed in the past few years. The only physical/chemical tests remaining are the new *total organic carbon* (TOC), with a limit of 500 ppb (0.5 mg/L), and *conductivity,* with a limit of 1.3 μS/cm at 25°C or 1.1 μS/cm at 20°C. The former is an instrumental method capable of detecting all organic carbon present, and the latter is a three-tiered instrumental test measuring the conductivity contributed by ionized particles (in microSiemens or micromhos) relative to pH. Since conductivity is integrally related to pH, the pH requirement of 5 to 7 in previous revisions has been eliminated. The TOC and conductivity specifications are now considered to be adequate minimal predictors of the chemical/physical purity of WFI. However, the *wet chemistry* tests still are used when WFI is packaged for commercial distribution and for SWFI.

Biological requirements continue to be, for WFI, not more than 10 colony-forming units (CFUs)/100 mL and 0.25 USP endotoxin units/mL. The SWFI requirements differ in that since it is a final product, it must pass the USP Sterility Test.

WFI and SWFI may not contain added substances. Bacteriostatic Water for Injection (BWFI) may contain one or more

suitable antimicrobial agents in containers of 30 mL or less. This restriction is designed to prevent the administration of a large quantity of a bacteriostatic agent that probably would be toxic in the accumulated amount of a large volume of solution, even though the concentration was low.

The USP also provides monographs giving the specifications for Sterile Water for Inhalation and Sterile Water for Irrigation. The USP should be consulted for the minor differences between these specifications and those for SWFI.

CONTAINERS AND CLOSURES

Injectable formulations are packaged into containers made of glass or plastic. Container systems include ampoules, vials, syringes, cartridges, bottles, and bags (Fig 41-4).

Ampoules are all glass while bags are all plastic. The other containers can be composed of glass or plastic and must include rubber materials such as rubber stoppers for vials and bottles and rubber plungers and rubber seals for syringes and cartridges. Irrigation solutions are packaged in glass bottles with aluminum screw caps.

Table 41-2 provides a generalized comparison of the three compatibility properties—leaching, permeation, and adsorption—of container materials most likely to be involved in the formulation of aqueous parenterals. Further, the integrity of the container/closure system depends upon several characteristics, including container opening finish, closure modulus, durometer and compression set, and aluminum seal application force. Container-closure integrity testing will be discussed in the Quality Assurance and Control section.

CONTAINER TYPES

Glass

Glass is employed as the container material of choice for most SVIs. It is composed principally of silicon dioxide, with varying amounts of other oxides such as sodium, potassium, calcium, magnesium, aluminum, boron, and iron. The basic structural network of glass is formed by the silicon oxide tetrahedron.

Boric oxide will enter into this structure, but most of the other oxides do not. The latter are only loosely bound, are present in the network interstices, and are relatively free to migrate. These migratory oxides may be leached into a solution in contact with the glass, particularly during the increased reactivity of thermal sterilization. The oxides thus dissolved may hydrolyze to raise the pH of the solution and catalyze or enter into reactions. Additionally, some glass compounds will be attacked by solutions and, in time, dislodge glass flakes into the solution. Such occurrences can be minimized by the proper selection of the glass composition.

TYPES—The USP has aided in this selection by providing a classification of glass:

Type I, a borosilicate glass
Type II, a soda-lime treated glass
Type III, a soda-lime glass
NP, a soda-lime glass not suitable for containers for parenterals

Type I glass is composed principally of silicon dioxide (~81%) and boric oxide (~13%), with low levels of the non-network-forming oxides (eg, sodium and aluminum oxides). It is a chemically resistant glass (low leachability) also having a low thermal coefficient of expansion (68×10^{-7} cm/cm-°C).

Types II and III glass compounds are composed of relatively high proportions of sodium oxide (~14%) and calcium oxide (~8%). This makes the glass chemically less resistant. Both types melt at a lower temperature, are easier to mold into various shapes, and have a higher thermal coefficient of expansion than Type I (eg, 90×10^{-7} cm/cm-°C for Type III). While there is no one standard formulation for glass among manufacturers

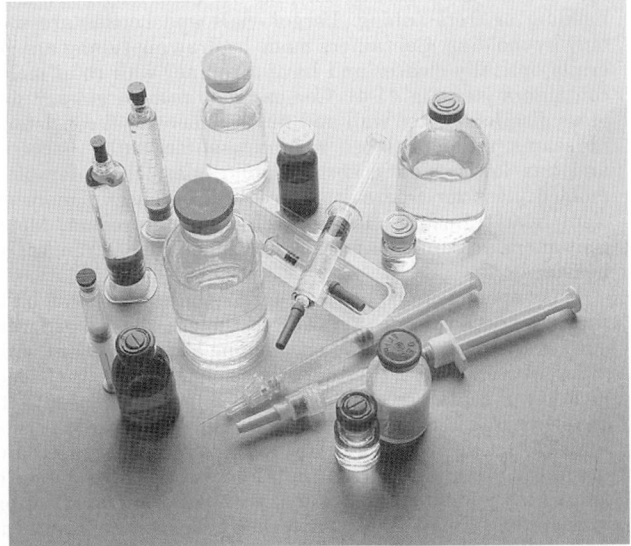
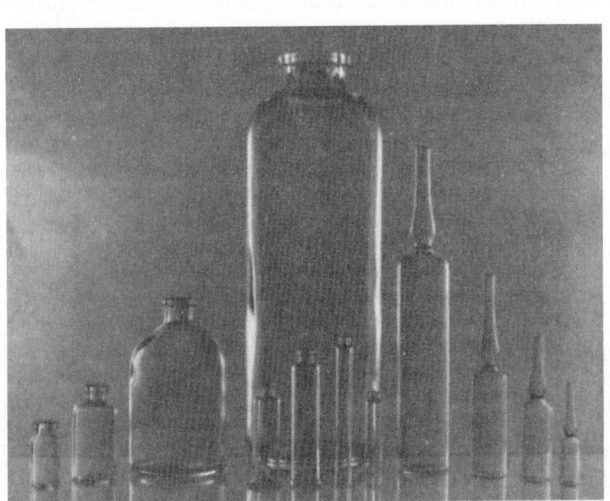

Figure 41-4. Various types of packaging for parenterals (courtesy, Kimble, Baxter).

Table 41-2. Comparative Compatibility Properties of Container Materials

	LEACHING		PERMEATION		ADSORPTION (SELECTIVE) EXTENT[a]
	EXTENT[a]	POTENTIAL LEACHABLES	EXTENT[a]	POTENTIAL AGENTS	
Glass					
Borosilicate	1	Alkaline earth and heavy metal oxides	0	N/A	2
Soda-lime	5	Alkaline earth and heavy metal oxides	0	N/A	2
Plastic polymers					
Polyethylene					
Low density	2	Plasticizers, antioxidants	5	Gases, water vapor, other molecules	2
High density	1	Antioxidants	3	Gases, water vapor, other molecules	2
PVC	4	HCl, especially plasticizers, antioxidants, other stabilizers	5	Gases, especially water vapor and other molecules	2
Polyolefins	2	Antioxidants	2	Gases, water vapor, other molecules	2
Polypropylene	2	Antioxidants, lubricants	4	Gases, water vapor	1
Rubber polymers					
Natural and related synthetic	5	Heavy metal salts, lubricants, reducing agents	3	Gases, water vapor	3
Butyl	3	Heavy metal salts, lubricants, reducing agents	1	Gases, water vapor	2
Silicone	2	Minimal	5	Gases, water vapor	1

[a] Approximate scale of 1 to 5, with 1 as the lowest.

of these USP type categories, Type II glass usually has a lower concentration of the migratory oxides than Type III. In addition, Type II has been treated under controlled temperature and humidity conditions with sulfur dioxide or other dealkalizers to neutralize the interior surface of the container. While it remains intact, this surface will increase substantially the chemical resistance of the glass. However, repeated exposures to sterilization and alkaline detergents will break down this dealkalized surface and expose the underlying soda-lime compound.

The glass types are determined from the results of two USP tests: the Powdered Glass Test and the Water Attack Test. The latter is used only for Type II glass and is performed on the whole container, because of the dealkalized surface; the former is performed on powdered glass, which exposes internal surfaces of the glass compound. The results are based upon the amount of alkali titrated by 0.02 N sulfuric acid after an autoclaving cycle with the glass sample in contact with a high-purity distilled water. Thus, the *Powdered Glass Test* challenges the leaching potential of the interior structure of the glass while the *Water Attack Test* challenges only the intact surface of the container.

Selecting the appropriate glass composition is a critical facet of determining the overall specifications for each parenteral formulation.

In general, the following rules apply with respect to glass leachables:

- Relatively low levels of leachables at pH 4–8
- Relatively high levels of leachables at pH > 9
- Major extractables are silicon and sodium
- Minor extractables include potassium, barium, calcium, and aluminum.
- Trace extractables include iron, magnesium and zinc.
- Treated glass gives less extractables if pH < 8

Type I glass will be suitable for all products, although sulfur dioxide treatment sometimes is used for even greater resistance to glass leachables. Because cost must be considered, one of the other, less-expensive types may be acceptable. Type II glass may be suitable, for example, for a solution that is buffered, has a pH below 7, or is not reactive with the glass. Type III glass usually will be suitable principally for anhydrous liquids or dry substances. However, some manufacturer-to-

manufacturer variation in glass composition should be anticipated within each glass type. Therefore, for highly chemically sensitive parenteral formulations it may be necessary to specify both USP Type and a specific manufacturer.

Schott has developed a technology called Plasma Impulse Chemical Vapor Deposition (PICVD) that coats the inner surface of Type I glass vials with an ultrathin film of silicon dioxide.[16] This film forms a highly efficient diffusion barrier that practically eliminates glass leachables. Such treated glass is especially useful for drug products having high pH values, formulations with complexing agents, or products showing high sensitivity to pH shifts.

PHYSICAL CHARACTERISTICS—Commercially available containers vary in size from 0.5 to 1000 mL. Sizes up to 100 mL may be obtained as ampoules and vials, and larger sizes as bottles. The latter are used mostly for intravenous and irrigating solutions. Smaller sizes also are available as syringes and cartridges. Ampoules, syringes, and cartridges are drawn from glass tubing. The smaller vials may be made by molding or from tubing. Larger vials and bottles are made only by molding. Containers made by drawing tubing are generally optically clearer and have a thinner wall than molded containers (see Fig 41-4). Compared to molded glass, tubing glass also has better wall and finish dimensional consistency, no seams, easier to label, weighs less, facilitates inspection, and has lower tooling costs. Tubing glass is preferable to molded glass for freeze-dried products because of more efficient heat transfer from the shelf into the product. Molded containers are uniform in external dimensions, stronger, and heavier.

Easy-opening ampoules that permit the user to break off the tip at the neck constriction without the use of a file are weakened at the neck by scoring or applying a ceramic paint with a different coefficient of thermal expansion. An example of a modification of container design to meet a particular need is the double-chambered vial (eg, Univial, RediVial, Lyo-ject, InterVialPLUS, Clip'nJect,) designed to contain a freeze-dried product in the lower, and solvent in the upper, chamber. Other examples are wide-mouth ampoules with flat or rounded bottoms to facilitate filling with dry materials or suspensions, and various modifications of the cartridge for use with disposable dosage units.

Glass containers must be strong enough to withstand the physical shocks of handling and shipping and the pressure differentials that develop, particularly during the autoclave sterilization cycle. They must be able to withstand the thermal shock resulting from large temperature changes during processing, for example, when the hot bottle and contents are exposed to room air at the end of the sterilization cycle. Therefore, a glass with a low coefficient of thermal expansion is necessary. The container also must be transparent to permit inspection of the contents.

Preparations that are light-sensitive must be protected by placing them in amber glass containers or by enclosing flint glass containers in opaque cartons labeled to remain on the container during the period of use. It should be noted that the amber color of the glass is imparted by the incorporation of potentially leachable heavy metals, mostly iron and manganese, which may act as catalysts for oxidative degradation reactions. Silicone coatings sometimes are applied to containers to produce a hydrophobic surface, for example, as a means of reducing the friction of a rubber-tip of a syringe plunger.

The size of single-dose containers is limited to 1000 mL by the USP and multiple-dose containers to 30 mL, unless stated otherwise in a particular monograph. Multiple-dose vials are limited in size to reduce the number of punctures for withdrawing doses and the accompanying risk of contamination of the contents. As the name implies, single-dose containers are opened or penetrated with aseptic care, and the contents used at one time. These may range in size from 1000-mL bottles to 1-mL or less ampules, vials, or syringes. The integrity of the container is destroyed when opened, so that the container cannot be closed and reused.

A multiple-dose container is designed so that more than one dose can be withdrawn at different times, the container maintaining a seal between uses. It should be evident that with full aseptic precautions, including sterile syringe and needle for withdrawing the dose and disinfection of the exposed surface of the closure, there is still a substantial risk of introducing contaminating microorganisms and viruses into the contents of the vial. Because of this risk, the USP requires that all multiple-dose vials must contain an antimicrobial agent or be inherently antimicrobial, as determined by the USP *Antimicrobial Preservatives-Effectiveness* tests. There are no comparable antiviral effectiveness tests, nor are antiviral agents available for such use. In spite of the advantageous flexibility of dosage provided by multiple-dose vials, single-dose, disposable container units provide the clear advantage of greater sterility assurance and patient safety.

Because of concerns for user safety and glass particulate matter occurring when glass is broken, glass sealed ampules are no longer glass containers of choice for new SVIs in the United States.

RUBBER CLOSURES

To permit introduction of a needle from a hypodermic syringe into a multiple-dose vial and provide for resealing as soon as the needle is withdrawn, each vial is sealed with a rubber closure held in place by an aluminum cap. Figure 41-5 illustrates how this is done. This principle also is followed for single-dose containers of the cartridge type, except that there is only a single introduction of the needle to make possible the withdrawal or expulsion of the contents.

Rubber closures are composed of multiple ingredients that are plasticized and mixed together at an elevated temperature on milling machines. The elastomer primarily used in rubber closures, plungers, and other rubber items used in parenteral packaging and delivery systems is synthetic butyl or halobutyl rubber. Natural rubber also is used, but if it is natural rubber latex, then the product label must include a warning statement due to the potential for allergic reactions from latex exposure.

The plasticized mixture is placed in molds and vulcanized (cured) under high temperature and pressure. During vulcan-

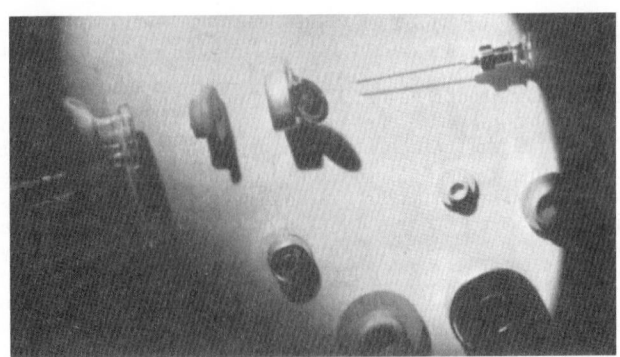

Figure 41-5. Extended view of sealing components for a multiple-dose vial (courtesy, West).

ization the polymer strands are cross-linked by the vulcanizing agent, assisted by the accelerator and activator, so that motion is restricted and the molded closure acquires the elastic, resilient character required for its use. Ingredients not involved in the cross-linking reactions remain dispersed within the compound and, along with the degree of curing, affect the properties of the finished closure. Examples of rubber- closure ingredients are given in Table 41-3.

The physical properties to be considered in the selection of a particular formulation include elasticity, hardness, tendency to fragment, and permeability to vapor transfer. The elasticity is critical in establishing a seal with the lip and neck of a vial or other opening and in resealing after withdrawal of a hypodermic needle from a vial closure. The hardness should provide firmness but not excessive resistance to the insertion of a needle through the closure, while minimal fragmentation of pieces of rubber should occur as the hollow shaft of the needle is pushed through the closure. While vapor transfer occurs to some degree with all rubber formulations, appropriate selection of ingredients makes it possible to control the degree of permeability. Physicochemical and toxicological tests for evaluating rubber closures are described in section <381> in the USP.

The ingredients dispersed throughout the rubber compound may be subject to leaching into the product contacting the closure. These ingredients, examples of which are given in Table 41-2, pose potential compatibility interactions with product ingredients if leached into the product solution, and these effects must be evaluated. Further, some ingredients must be evaluated for potential toxicity. To reduce the problem of leachables, coatings have been applied to the product contact surfaces of

Table 41-3. Examples of Ingredients Found in Rubber Closures

INGREDIENT	EXAMPLES
Elastomer	Natural rubber (latex)
	Butyl rubber
	Neoprene
Vulcanizing (curing) agent	Sulfur
	Peroxides
Accelerator	Zinc dibutyldithiocarbamate
Activator	Zinc oxide
	Stearic acid
Antioxidant	Dilauryl thiodipropionate
Plasticizer/lubricant	Paraffinic oil
	Silicone oil
Fillers	Carbon black
	Clay
	Barium sulfate
Pigments	Inorganic oxides
	Carbon black

closures, with various polymers, the most successful being Teflon. Recently, polymeric coatings have been developed that are claimed to have more integral binding with the rubber matrix, but details of their function are trade secrets.

The physical shape of some typical closures may be seen in Figure 41-5. Most of them have a lip and a protruding flange that extends into the neck of the vial or bottle. Many disk closures are being used now, particularly in the high-speed packaging of antibiotics. Slotted closures are used on freeze-dried products to permit the escape of water vapor, since they are inserted only partway into the neck of the vial until completion of the drying phase of the cycle. Also, the top design of the freeze-dry closure is important to minimize sticking of the closure to the underneath of the dryer shelf after stoppering the vial. Stoppers normally have a small protruding circle at the center of the top of the stopper. Gaps provided within the protruding circle minimize the tendency of the stopper to stick to the freeze-dryer shelf.

The plunger type of rubber is used to seal one end of a syringe or cartridge. At the time of use, the plunger expels the product by a needle inserted through the closure at the distal end of the package. Intravenous solution closures often have permanent holes for adapters of administration sets; irrigating solution closures usually are designed for pouring.

As will be discussed later, rubber closures must be "slippery" in order to move easily through a rubber closure hopper and other stainless steel passages until they are fitted onto the filled vials. Traditionally, rubber materials are "siliconized" (silicone oil or emulsion applied onto the rubber) in order to produce such lubrication. However, advances in rubber closure technologies have introduced closures that do not require siliconization because of a special polymer coating applied to the outer surface of the closure. Examples are the *Daichyo/West* closures (Flurotec) and the *Helvoet* (Omniflex) closures. The *Daichyo* Flurotec coating is a copolymer of tetrafluoroethylene and ethylene.

Plastic

Thermoplastic polymers have been established as packaging materials for sterile preparations such as large-volume parenterals, ophthalmic solutions, and, increasingly, small-volume parenterals. For such use to be acceptable, a thorough understanding of the characteristics, potential problems, and advantages for use must be developed. Three principal problem areas exist in using these materials:

1. Permeation of vapors and other molecules in either direction through the wall of the plastic container
2. Leaching of constituents from the plastic into the product
3. Sorption (absorption and/or adsorption) of drug molecules or ions on the plastic material

Permeation, the most extensive problem, may be troublesome by permitting volatile constituents, water, or specific drug molecules to migrate through the wall of the container to the outside and thereby be lost. This problem has been resolved, for example, by the use of an overwrap in the packaging of IV solutions in PVC bags to prevent the loss of water during storage. Reverse permeation also may occur in which oxygen or other molecules may penetrate to the inside of the container and cause oxidative or other degradation of susceptible constituents. *Leaching* may be a problem when certain constituents in the plastic formulation, such as plasticizers or antioxidants, migrate into the product. Thus, plastic polymer formulations should have as few additives as possible, an objective characteristically achievable for most plastics being used for parenteral packaging. *Sorption* is a problem on a selective basis, that is, sorption of a few drug molecules occurs on specific polymers. For example, sorption of insulin and other proteins, vitamin A acetate, and warfarin sodium has been shown to occur on PVC bags and tubing when these drugs were present as additives in IV admixtures. A brief summary of some of these compatibility relationships is given in Table 41-2.

One of the principle advantages of using plastic packaging materials is that they are not breakable as is glass; also, there is a substantial weight reduction. The flexible bags of polyvinyl chloride or select polyolefins, currently in use for large-volume intravenous fluids, have the added advantage that no air interchange is required; the flexible wall simply collapses as the solution flows out of the bag.

Most plastic materials have the disadvantage that they are not as clear as glass and, therefore, inspection of the contents is impeded. However, recent technologies have overcome this limitation, evidenced by plastic resins such as CZ (polycyclopentane, *Daichyo Seiko*) and Topas COC (cyclic olefin copolymer, *Ticona*). In addition, many of these materials will soften or melt under the conditions of thermal sterilization. However, careful selection of the plastic used and control of the autoclave cycle has made thermal sterilization of some products possible, large-volume parenterals in particular. Ethylene oxide or radiation sterilization may be employed for the empty container with subsequent aseptic filling. However, careful evaluation of the residues from ethylene oxide or its degradation products and their potential toxic effect must be undertaken. Investigation is required concerning potential interactions and other problems that may be encountered when a parenteral product is packaged in plastic. For further details see Chapter 54 (*Plastic Packaging Materials*) and the review article by Jenke.[17]

NEEDLES

Historically, stainless steel needles have been used to penetrate the skin and introduce a parenteral product inside the body. The advent of needleless injection systems (eg, Bioject, AdvantaJet, Medi-ject, Medi-Jector Vision) has obviated the need for the use of needles for some injections (eg, vaccines) and are gaining in popularity over the conventional syringe and needle system. However, needleless injections are generally more expensive, can still produce pain on injection, are potentially a greater source of contamination (and cross-contamination from incessant use), and may not be as efficient in dose delivery.

Needles are hollow devices composed of stainless steel or plastic. Needles are available in a wide variety of lengths, sizes, and shapes. *Needle lengths* range from 1/4 inch to 6 inches. *Needle size* is referred to as its gauge (G), or the outside diameter (OD) of the needle shaft. Gauge ranges are 11 to 32 gauge with the largest gauge for injection usually being no greater than 16 G. 16 G needles have an OD of 0.065 inches (1.65 mm) whereas 32 G have an OD of 0.009 inches (0.20 mm). *Needle shape* includes regular, short bevel, intradermal, and winged. Needle shape typically is defined by one end of a needle enlarged to form a hub with a delivery device such as a syringe or other administration device. The other end of the needle is beveled, meaning that it forms a sharp tip to maximize ease of insertion.

The route of administration, type of therapy, and whether the patient is a child or adult dictate the length and size of needle used.[18] Intravenous injections typically use 1–2 inch 15 to 25 G needles. Intramuscular injections use 1–2 inch 19–22 G needles. Subcutaneous injections use 1/4 to 5/8 inch 24 to 25 G needles. Needle gauge for children rarely is larger than 22 G, usually 25–27 G. Winged needles are used for intermittent heparin therapy. Many different types of therapies, (eg, radiology, anesthesia, biopsy, cardiovascular, ophthalmic, transfusions, tracheotomy) have their own peculiar types of needle preferences.

Needles are purchased either alone (eg, Luer-Lok) to be attached to syringes, cartridge, and other delivery systems, or, for syringes, can be part of the syringe set (stake needle).

PYROGENS (ENDOTOXINS)

Since water and packaging materials are the greatest sources of pyrogenic contamination, this subject will now be covered.

Pyrogens are products of metabolism of microorganisms. The most potent pyrogenic substances (endotoxins) are constituents (lipopolysaccharides, LPS) of the cell wall of gram-negative bacteria (eg, *Pseudomonas* sp, *Salmonella* sp, *Escherichia coli*). Gram-positive bacteria and fungi also produce pyrogens but of lower potency and of different chemical nature. Gram-positive bacteria produce peptidoglycans whereas fungi product β-glucans, both of which can cause non-endotoxin pyrogenic responses. Endotoxins are lipopolysaccharides that typically exist in high molecular weight aggregate forms. However, the monomer unit of LPS is less than 10,000 daltons, enabling endotoxin easily to pass through sterilizing 0.2 micron filters. Studies have shown that the lipid portion of the molecule is responsible for the biological activity. Since endotoxins are the most potent pyrogens and gram-negative bacteria are ubiquitous in the environment, especially water, this discussion focuses on endotoxins and the risk of their presence as contaminants in sterile products.

Pyrogens, when present in parenteral drug products and injected into patients, can cause fever, chills, pain in the back and legs, and malaise. Although pyrogenic reactions are rarely fatal, they can cause serious discomfort and, in the seriously ill patient, shock-like symptoms that can be fatal. The intensity of the pyrogenic response and its degree of hazard will be affected by the medical condition of the patient, the potency of the pyrogen, the amount of the pyrogen, and the route of administration (intrathecal is most hazardous followed by intravenous, intramuscular, and subcutaneous). When bacterial (exogenous) pyrogens are introduced into the body, LPS targets circulating mononuclear cells (monocytes and macrophages) that, in turn, produce pro-inflammatory cytokines such as interleukin-2, interleukin-6, and tissue necrosis factor. Besides LPS, gram-negative bacteria also release many peptides (eg, exotoxin A, peptidoglycan, and muramuyl peptides) that can mimic the activity of LPS and induce cytokine release. The Limulus Amebocyte Lysate (LAL) test, discussed later, can only detect the presence of LPS. It has been suggested that a new test, called Monocyte Activation Test, replace LAL as the official pyrogen test because of its greater sensitivity to all agents that induce the release of cytokines that cause fever and a potential cascade of other adverse physiological effects.[19]

CONTROL OF PYROGENS—In general, it is impractical, if not impossible, to remove pyrogens once present without adversely affecting the drug product. Therefore, the emphasis should be on preventing the introduction or development of pyrogens in all aspects of the compounding and processing of the product.

Pyrogens may enter a preparation through any means that will introduce living or dead microorganisms. However, current technology generally permits the control of such contamination, and the presence of pyrogens in a finished product indicates processing under inadequately controlled conditions. It also should be noted that time for microbial growth to occur increases the risk for elevated levels of pyrogens. Therefore, compounding and manufacturing processes should be carried out as expeditiously as possible, preferably planning completion of the process, including sterilization, within the maximum allowed time according to process validation studies. Aseptic processing guidelines require establishment of time limitations throughout processing for the primary purpose of preventing the increase of endotoxin (and microbial) contamination that subsequently cannot be destroyed or removed.

Pyrogens can be destroyed by heating at high temperatures. A typical procedure for depyrogenation of glassware and equipment is maintaining a dry heat temperature of 250°C for 45 min. Exposure for 650°C for 1 min or 180°C for 4 hr likewise will destroy pyrogens. The usual autoclaving cycle will not do so. Heating with strong alkali or oxidizing solutions will destroy pyrogens. It has been claimed that thorough washing with detergent will render glassware pyrogen-free if subsequently rinsed thoroughly with pyrogen-free water. Rubber stoppers cannot withstand pyrogen-destructive temperatures, so reliance must be placed on an

effective sequence of washing, thorough rinsing with WFI, prompt sterilization, and protective storage to ensure adequate pyrogen control. Similarly, plastic containers and devices must be protected from pyrogenic contamination during manufacture and storage, since known ways of destroying pyrogens affect the plastic adversely. It has been reported that anion-exchange resins and positively charged membrane filters will remove pyrogens from water. Also, although reverse osmosis membranes will eliminate them, the most reliable method for their elimination from water is distillation.

A method that has been used for the removal of pyrogens from solutions is adsorption on adsorptive agents. However, since the adsorption phenomenon also may cause selective removal of chemical substances from the solution, this method has limited application. Other in-process methods for their destruction or elimination include selective extraction procedures and careful heating with dilute alkali, dilute acid, or mild oxidizing agents. In each instance, the method must be studied thoroughly to be sure it will not have an adverse effect on the constituents of the product. Although ultrafiltration now makes possible pyrogen separation on a molecular-weight basis and the process of tangential flow is making large-scale processing more practical, use of this technology is limited, except in biotechnological processing.

SOURCES OF PYROGENS—Through understanding the means by which pyrogens may contaminate parenteral products, their control becomes more achievable. Therefore, it is important to know that water is probably the greatest potential source of pyrogenic contamination, since water is essential for the growth of microorganisms and frequently contaminated with gram-negative organisms. When microorganisms metabolize, pyrogens will be produced. Therefore, raw water can be expected to be pyrogenic and only when it is appropriately treated to render it free from pyrogens, such as WFI, should it be used for compounding the product or rinsing product contact surfaces such as tubing, mixing vessels, and rubber closures. Even when such rinsed equipment and supplies are left wet and improperly exposed to the environment, there is a high risk that they will become pyrogenic. Although proper distillation will provide pyrogen-free water, storage conditions must be such that microorganisms are not introduced and subsequent growth is prevented.

Other potential sources of contamination are containers and equipment. Pyrogenic materials adhere strongly to glass and other surfaces, especially rubber closures. Residues of solutions in used equipment often become bacterial cultures, with subsequent pyrogenic contamination. Since drying does not destroy pyrogens, they may remain in equipment for long periods. Adequate washing will reduce contamination and subsequent dry-heat treatment can render contaminated equipment suitable for use. However, all such processes must be validated to ensure their effectiveness. Aseptic processing guidelines require validation of the depyrogenation process by demonstrating at least 3-log reduction in an applied endotoxin challenge.

Solutes may be a source of pyrogens. For example, the manufacturing of bulk chemicals may involve the use of pyrogenic water for process steps such as crystallization, precipitation, or washing. Bulk drug substances derived from cell culture fermentation will almost certainly be heavily pyrogenic. Therefore, all lots of solutes used to prepare parenteral products should be tested to ensure that they will not contribute unacceptable quantities of endotoxin to the finished product. It is standard practice today to establish valid endotoxin limits on active pharmaceutical ingredients and most solute additives.

The manufacturing process must be carried out with great care and as rapidly as possible, to minimize the risk of microbial contamination. Preferably, no more product should be prepared than can be processed completely within one working day, including sterilization.

The production facility and its associated equipment must be designed, constructed, and operated properly for the manufacture of a sterile product to be achieved at the quality level required for safety and effectiveness. Materials of construction for sterile product production facilities must be "smooth, cleanable, and impervious to moisture and other damage." Further, the processes used must meet cGMP standards. Since the majority of SVIs are aseptically processed (finished product not terminally sterilized), adherence to strict cGMP standards with respect to sterility assurance is essential.

FUNCTIONAL AREAS

To achieve the goal of a manufactured sterile product of exceptionally high quality, many functional production areas are involved: warehousing or procurement, compounding (or formulation), materials (containers, closures, equipment) preparation, filtration and sterile receiving, aseptic filling, stoppering, lyophilization (if warranted) and packaging, labeling, and quarantine. The extra requirements for the aseptic area are designed to provide an environment where a sterile fluid may be exposed to the environment for a brief period during subdivision from a bulk container to individual-dose containers without becoming contaminated. Contaminants such as dust, lint, other particles, and microorganisms normally are found floating in the air, lying on counters and other surfaces, on clothing and body surfaces of personnel, in the exhaled breath of personnel, and deposited on the floor. The design and control of an aseptic area is directed toward reducing the presence of these contaminants so that they are no longer a hazard to aseptic filling.

Although the aseptic area must be adjacent to support areas so that an efficient flow of components may be achieved, barriers must be provided to minimize ingress of contaminants to the critical aseptic area. Such barriers may consist of a variety

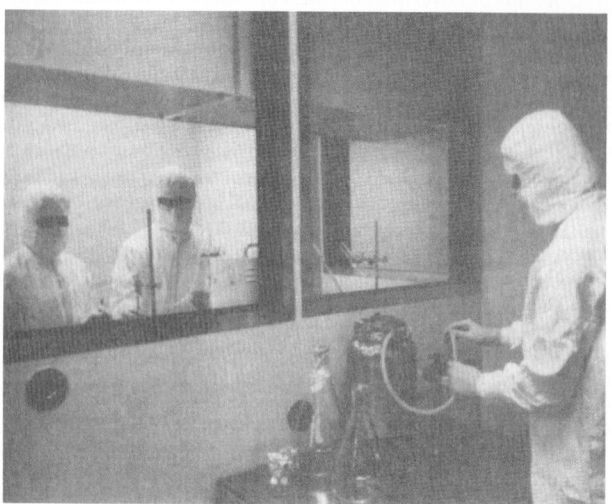

Figure 41-7. Product filtration from the aseptic staging room through a port into the aseptic filling room (courtesy, The University of Tennessee College of Pharmacy).

of forms, including sealed walls, manual or automatic doors, airlock pass-throughs, ports of various types, or plastic curtains. Figure 41-6 shows an example of a floor plan for a clinical supply production facility (selected as an example of a small-scale, noncomplex facility), in which the two fill rooms and the staging area constitute the walled critical aseptic area, access to which is only by means of pass-through airlocks. Adjacent support areas (rooms) consist of glass preparation, equipment wash, capping, manufacturing (compounding), and various storage areas. Figure 41-7 shows an adjacent arrangement with the utilization of a through-the-wall port for passage of a filtrate into the critical aseptic filling room.

FLOW PLAN—In general, the components for a parenteral product flow either from the warehouse, after release, to the compounding area, as for ingredients of the formula, or to the materials support area, as for containers and equipment. After proper processing in these areas, the components flow into the security of the aseptic area for filling of the product in appropriate containers. From there the product passes into the quarantine and packaging area where it is held until all necessary tests have been performed. If the product is to be sterilized in its final container, its passage normally is interrupted after leaving the aseptic area for subjection to the sterilization process. After the results from all tests are known, the batch records have been reviewed, and the product has been found to comply with its release specifications, it passes to the finishing area for final release for shipment. There sometimes are variations from this flow plan to meet the specific needs of an individual product or to conform to existing facilities. Automated operations normally have much larger capacity and convey the components from one area to another with little or no handling by operators.

Clean Room Classified Areas

Because of the extremely high standards of cleanliness and purity that must be met by parenteral products, it has become standard practice to prescribe specifications for the environments in which these products are manufactured (ie, clean rooms). Clean room specifications are summarized in Table 41-4 that compares United States and European classifications

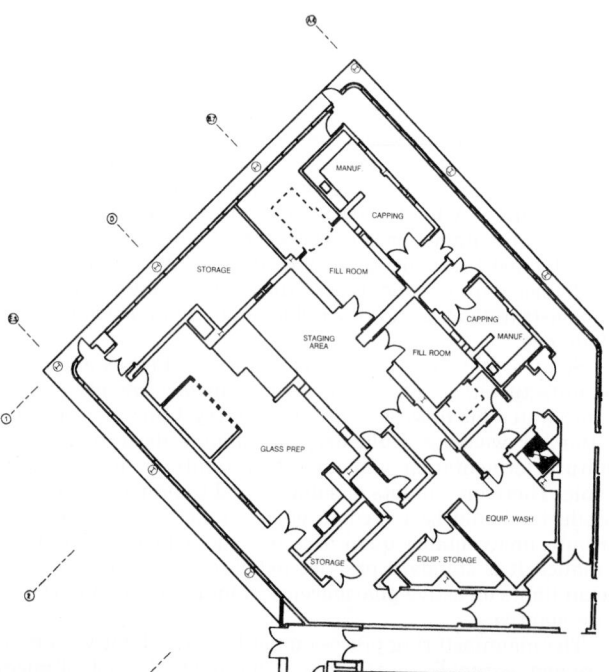

Figure 41-6. Floor plan of aseptic filling rooms and staging room with adjacent support areas (courtesy, Glaxo).

Table 41-4. Clean Room Classifications

EUROPEAN GRADE	UNITED STATES CLASSIFICATION	INTERNATIONAL SOCIETY OF PHARM. ENG. DESCRIPTION	MAX NO. OF PARTICLES per m^3 >/= 0.5 μm	MAX NO. OF PARTICLES per m^3 >/= 5 μm
A	100	Critical	3,500	0
B	100	Clean	3,500	0
C	10,000	Controlled	350,000	2,000
D	100,000	Pharmaceutical	3,500,000	20,000

and clean room designations assigned by the International Society of Pharmaceutical Engineers. The numbers are based on the maximum allowed number of airborne particles/ft^3 or particles/m^3 of 0.5 μm or larger size and, for Europe, 5.0 μm or larger size. The classifications used in pharmaceutical practice normally range from Class 100,000 (Grade D) for materials support areas to Class 100 (Grade A) for aseptic areas. To achieve Class 100 conditions, HEPA filters are required for the incoming air, with the effluent air sweeping the downstream environment at a uniform velocity, normally 90 to 100 ft/min ± 20%, along parallel lines (laminar air flow). HEPA filters are defined as 99.99% or more efficient in removing from the air 0.3 μm particles generated by vaporization of the hydrocarbon Emory 3004.

Because so many parenteral products are manufactured at one site for global distribution, air quality standards in aseptic processing areas must meet both United States and European requirements. European standards differ from United States standards in the following ways:

- Use Grades A, B, C, and D classifications rather than Class X (eg, 100, 1000, etc)
- Use particle and microbial limits per cubic meter rather than per cubic foot
- Require particle measurements at 5 microns in addition to 0.5 microns in Grade A and B areas
- Differentiate area cleanliness dynamically and "at rest"

AIR CLEANING—Since air is one of the greatest potential sources of contaminants in clean rooms, special attention must be given to air being drawn into clean rooms by the heating, ventilating, and air conditioning (HVAC) system. This may be done by a series of treatments that will vary somewhat from one installation to another.

In one such series air from the outside first is passed through a prefilter, usually of glass wool, cloth, or shredded plastic, to remove large particles. Then it may be treated by passage through an electrostatic precipitator (suppliers: *Am*

Air, Electro-Air). Such a unit induces an electrical charge on particles in the air and removes them by attraction to oppositely charged plates. The air then passes through the most efficient cleaning device, a HEPA filter (suppliers: *Am Air, Cambridge, Flanders*).

For personnel comfort, air conditioning and humidity control should be incorporated into the system. The latter is also important for certain products such as those that must be lyophilized and for the processing of plastic medical devices. The clean, aseptic air is introduced into the Class 100 area and maintained under positive pressure, which prevents outside air from rushing into the aseptic area through cracks, temporarily open doors, or other openings.

LAMINAR-FLOW ENCLOSURES—The required environmental control of aseptic areas has been made possible by the use of laminar airflow, originating through a HEPA filter occupying one entire side of the confined space. Therefore, it bathes the total space with very clean air, sweeping away contaminants. The orientation for the direction of airflow can be horizontal (Fig 41-8) or vertical (Fig 41-9), and may involve a limited area such as a workbench or an entire room. Figure 41-9 shows a vial-filling line protected with vertical laminar airflow from ceiling-hung HEPA filters, a Class 100 area. Plastic curtains are installed to maintain the unidirection of airflow to below the filling line and to circumscribe the critical filling portion of the line. The area outside the curtains can be maintained at a slightly lower level of cleanliness than that inside, perhaps Class 1000 or 10,000.

Today, it is accepted that critical areas of processing, wherein the product or product contact surfaces may be exposed to the environment, even for a brief period of time, should meet Class 100 clean room standards.

It must be borne in mind that any contamination introduced upstream by equipment, arms of the operator, or leaks in the filter will be blown downstream. In the instance of horizontal flow this may be to the critical working site, the face of the operator, or across the room. Should the contaminant be, for example, penicillin powder, a biohazard material, or viable microorganisms, the danger to the operator is apparent.

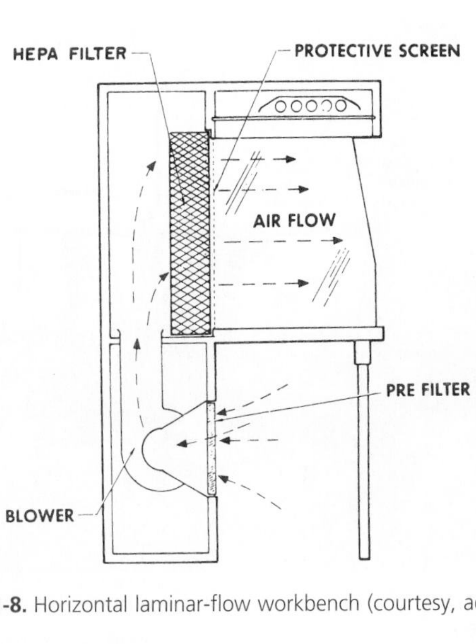

Figure 41-8. Horizontal laminar-flow workbench (courtesy, adaptation, Sandia).

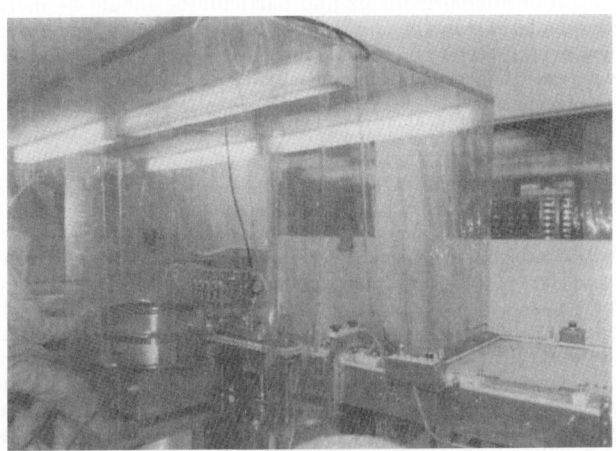

Figure 41-9. Vial filling line under vertical laminar airflow with critical area enclosed within plastic curtains (courtesy, Merck).

Further, great care must be exercised to prevent cross-contamination from one operation to another, especially with horizontal laminar air flow. For most large-scale operations, as shown in Figure 9, a vertical system is much more desirable, with the air flowing through perforations in the countertop or through return louvers at floor level, where it can be directed for decontamination. Laminar-flow environments provide well-controlled work areas only if proper precautions are observed. Any reverse air currents or movements exceeding the velocity of the HEPA-filtered airflow may introduce contamination, as may coughing, reaching, or other manipulations of operators. Therefore, laminar-flow work areas should be protected by being located within controlled environments. Personnel should be attired for aseptic processing, as described below. All movements and processes should be planned carefully to avoid the introduction of contamination upstream of the critical work area. Checks of the air stream should be performed initially and at regular intervals (usually every 6 months) to be sure no leaks have developed through or around the HEPA filters. Workbenches and other types of laminar-flow enclosures are available from several commercial sources (suppliers: *Air Control, Atmos-Tech, Baker, Clean Air, Clestra, Envirco, Flanders, Laminaire, Liberty*).

Clean room design traditionally has Class 100 rooms adjacent to Class 100,000 rooms. Regulatory authorities have raised great concerns about this significant change in air quality from critical to controlled areas. It is now preferable to have an area classified from Class 1000 to Class 10,000 in a buffer area between a Class 100 and Class 100,000 area.

MATERIALS SUPPORT AREA—The area is constructed to withstand moisture, steam, and detergents and is usually a Class 100,000 clean room. The ceiling, walls, and floor should be constructed of impervious materials so that moisture will run off and not be held. One of the finishes with a vinyl or epoxy-sealing coat provides a continuous surface free from all holes or crevices. All such surfaces can be washed at regular intervals to keep them thoroughly clean. These areas should be exhausted adequately so that the heat and humidity will be removed for the comfort of personnel. Precautions must be taken to prevent the accumulation of dirt and the growth of microorganisms because of the high humidity and heat. In this area preparation for the filling operation, such as cleaning and assembling equipment, is undertaken. Adequate sink and counter space must be provided. This area must be cleanable, and the microbial load must be monitored and controlled. Precautions also must be taken to prevent deposition of particles or other contaminants on clean containers and equipment until they have been properly boxed or wrapped preparatory to sterilization and depyrogenation.

COMPOUNDING AREA—In this area the formula is compounded. Although it is not essential that this area be aseptic, control of microorganisms and particulates should be more stringent than in the materials support area. For example, means may need to be provided to control dust generated from weighing and compounding operations. Cabinets and counters should, preferably, be constructed of stainless steel. They should fit snugly to walls and other furniture so that there are no catch areas where dirt can accumulate. The ceiling, walls, and floor should be similar to those for the materials support area.

ASEPTIC AREA—The aseptic area requires construction features designed for maximum microbial and particulate control. The ceiling, walls, and floor must be sealed so that they may be washed and sanitized with a disinfectant, as needed. All counters should be constructed of stainless steel and hung from the wall so that there are no legs to accumulate dirt where they rest on the floor. All light fixtures, utility service lines, and ventilation fixtures should be recessed in the walls or ceiling to eliminate ledges, joints, and other locations for the accumulation of dust and dirt. As much as possible, tanks containing the compounded product should remain outside the aseptic filling area, and the product fed into the area through hose lines. Fig-

ure 41-7 shows such an arrangement. Proper sanitization is required if the tanks must be moved in. Large mechanical equipment that is located in the aseptic area should be housed as completely as possible within a stainless steel cabinet to seal the operating parts and their dirt-producing tendencies from the aseptic environment. Further, all such equipment parts should be located below the filling line. Mechanical parts that will contact the parenteral product should be demountable so that they can be cleaned and sterilized.

Personnel entering the aseptic area should enter only through an airlock. They should be attired in sterile coveralls with sterile hats, masks, goggles, and foot covers. Movement within the room should be minimal and in-and-out movement rigidly be restricted during a filling procedure. The requirements for room preparation and the personnel may be relaxed somewhat if the product is to be sterilized terminally in a sealed container. Some are convinced, however, that it is better to have one standard procedure meeting the most rigid requirements.

ISOLATION (BARRIER) TECHNOLOGY—This technology is designed to isolate aseptic operations from personnel and the surrounding environment. Considerable experience has been gained in its use for sterility testing, with very positive results, including reports of essentially no false-positive test results.[20] In European circles favorable results also have been reported from use in hospital IV admixture programs. Because of such results, experimental efforts in adapting automated, large-scale, aseptic filling operations to isolators has gained momentum.[21,22]

Figure 41-10 illustrates a configuration of an isolator with transparent plastic sides and gloves for operator access to the enclosure. Figure 41-11 illustrates the adaptation of a large-scale filling line to isolator technology. The operations are performed within windowed, sealed walls with operators working through glove ports. The sealed enclosures are presterilized, usually with peracetic acid, hydrogen peroxide vapor, or steam. Sterile supplies are introduced from sterilizable movable modules through uniquely engineered transfer ports or directly from attached sterilizers, including autoclaves and hot-air sterilizing tunnels. Results have been very promising, giving expectation of significantly enhanced control of the aseptic processing environment.[22]

While isolators have been implemented in the industry, progress has been slower than initially anticipated. There are several reasons for this slow growth and acceptance:

- General regulatory and industry caution because of the relative novelty of isolator technology.

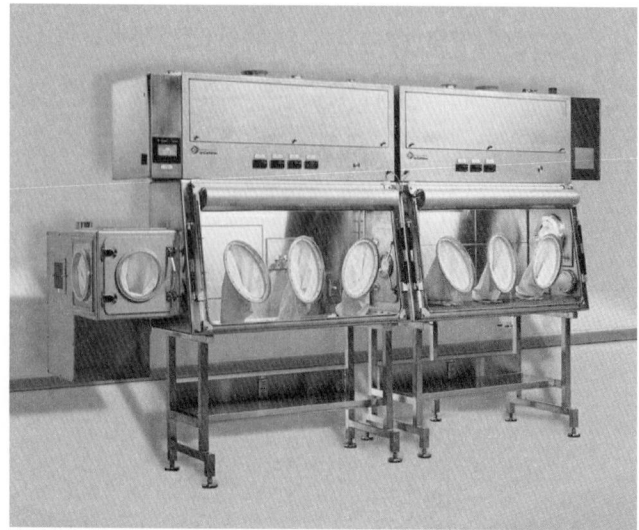

Figure 41-10. Example of an isolator (courtesy, LaCalhene). See Color Plate 7.

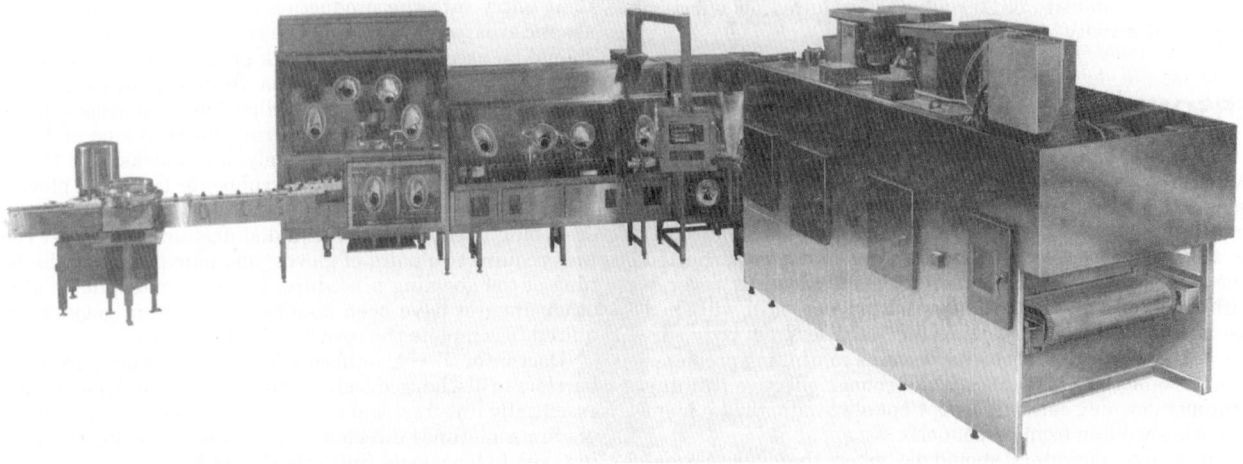

Figure 41-11. Large-scale production line showing, from right to left, container-sterilizing tunnel feeding into isolator enclosing filling and sealing, with access glove ports, and exiting to capper (courtesy, TL Systems).

- Regulatory agencies have insisted so far that isolators be located in classified environments (usually at least Class 100,000). This discouraged investment by some in isolator technology because it was originally thought that classified environments would not be necessary.
- Initial promotion that isolator technology could create a truly sterile environment and, thus, allow a much greater claim for sterility assurance proved not to be true. Isolators tend to have small leaks, particularly at the glove ports and gloves or half suits. The industry has learned the hard way that for aseptic pro-

cessing, sterility assurance levels for isolators are not much greater than conventional Class 100 filling operations.
- Validation of isolators has been more difficult than expected. For example, it is difficult to convince reviewers that contamination will not occur despite constant movement of materials in and out of the isolator, the occasional need to manipulate equipment, and the problem of pinhole leaks. The significantly increased time and resources required to validate and maintain isolators have discouraged many companies from investing in these systems.

MAINTENANCE OF CLEAN ROOMS

Maintaining the clean and sanitized conditions of clean rooms, particularly the aseptic areas, requires diligence and dedication of expertly trained custodians. Assuming the design of the facilities to be cleanable and sanitizable, a carefully planned schedule of cleaning should be developed, ranging from daily to monthly, depending on the location and its relation to the most critical Class 100 areas. Tools used should be non-linting, designed for clean room use, held captive to the area and, preferably, sterilizable.

Liquid disinfectants (sanitizing agents) should be selected carefully because of data showing their reliable activity against inherent environmental microorganisms. They should be recognized as supplements to good housekeeping, never as substitutes. They should be rotated with sufficient frequency to avoid the development of resistant strains of microorganisms. An example of the "three bucket" system used to sanitize facilities is shown in Figure 41-12. One bucket is to remove as much of the remnant of the "dirty" mop or sponge, the second contains a rinse solution to help clean the mop/sponge, while the third bucket contains the sanitizing solution. The sanitizing solution should be rendered sterile prior to use although, of course, once in use, it will no longer be sterile.

It should be noted that ultraviolet (UV) light rays of 237.5 nm wavelength, as radiated by germicidal lamps, are an effective surface disinfectant. But, it must also be noted that they are only effective if they contact the target microorganisms at a sufficient intensity for a sufficient time. The limitations of their use must be recognized, including no effect in shadow areas, reduction of intensity by the square of the distance from the source, reduction by particulates in the ray path, and the toxic effect on epithelium of human eyes. It generally is stated that

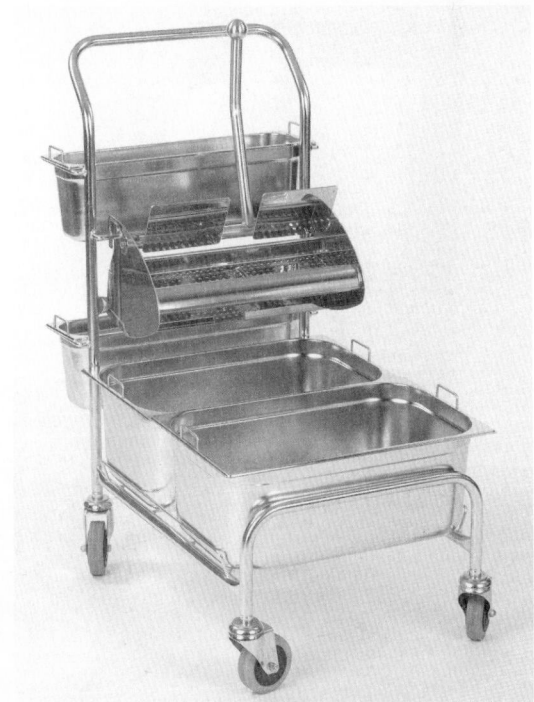

Figure 41-12. Example of a three-bucket assembly used for sanitizing facilities (courtesy, Contec). See Color Plate 8.

an irradiation intensity of 20 μw/cm² is required for effective antibacterial activity.

PERSONNEL

Personnel selected to work on the preparation of a parenteral product must be neat, orderly, and reliable. They should be in good health and free from dermatological conditions that might increase the microbial load. If they show symptoms of a head cold, allergies, or similar illness, they should not be permitted in the aseptic area until their recovery is complete. However, a healthy person with the best personal hygiene still will shed large numbers of viable and nonviable particles from body surfaces.[23] This natural phenomenon creates continuing problems when personnel are present in clean rooms; effective training and proper gowning can reduce, but not eliminate, the problem of particle shedding from personnel.

Aseptic-area operators should be given thorough, formal training in the principles of aseptic processing and the techniques to be employed.[24] Subsequently, the acquired knowledge and skills should be evaluated to assure that training has been effective before they are allowed to participate in the preparation of sterile products. Retraining should be performed on a regular schedule to enhance the maintenance of the required level of expertise. An effort should be made to imbue operators with an awareness of the vital role they play in determining the reliability and safety of the final product. This is especially true of supervisors, since they should be individuals who not only understand the unique requirements of aseptic procedures, but who are able to obtain the full participation of other employees in fulfilling these exacting requirements.

The uniform worn is designed to confine the contaminants discharged from the body of the operator, thereby preventing their entry into the production environment. For use in the aseptic area, uniforms should be sterile. Fresh, sterile uniforms should be used after every break period or whenever the individual returns to the aseptic area. In some plants this is not required if the product is to be sterilized in its final container. The uniform usually consists of coveralls for both men and women, hoods to cover the hair completely, face masks, and Dacron or plastic boots (Fig 41-13). Sterile rubber or latex-free gloves (are also required for aseptic operations, preceded by thorough scrubbing of the hands with a disinfectant soap. Most companies require two pairs of gloves, one pair put on at the beginning of the gowning procedure, the other pair put on after all other apparel have been donned. In addition, goggles are required to complete the coverage of all skin areas.

Dacron or Tyvek uniforms are usually worn, are effective barriers to discharged body particles (viable and nonviable), are essentially lint-free, and are reasonably comfortable. Air showers are sometimes directed on personnel entering the processing area to blow loose lint from the uniforms.

Gowning rooms should be designed to enhance pregowning and gowning procedures by trained operators so that it is possible to ensure the continued sterility of the exterior surfaces of the sterile gowning components. De-gowning should be performed in a separate exit room.

ENVIRONMENTAL CONTROL EVALUATION

As evidenced by the above discussion, manufacturers of sterile products use extensive means to control the environment so that these critical products can be prepared free from contamination. Nevertheless, tests should be performed to determine the level of control actually achieved. Normally, the tests consist of counting viable and nonviable particles suspended in the air or settled on surfaces in the workspace. A baseline count, determined by averaging multiple counts when the facility is operating under controlled conditions, is used to establish the optimal test results expected. During the subsequent monitoring program, the test results are followed carefully for high individual counts, a rising trend, or other abnormalities. If they exceed selected alert or action levels, a plan of action must be put into operation to determine if or what corrective and follow-up measures are required.

The tests used generally measure either the particles in a volume of sampled air or the particles that are settling or are present on surfaces. To measure the total particle content in an air sample, electronic particle counters are available, operating on the principle of the measurement of light scattered from particles as they pass through the cell of the optical system (Suppliers: *Climet, HIAC Royco, Met One, Particle Measuring Systems*). These instruments not only count particles, but also provide a size distribution based on the magnitude of the light scattered from the particle. While a volume of air measured by an electronic particle counter will detect all particles instantly, these instruments cannot differentiate between viable (eg, bacterial and fungal) and nonviable ones. However, because of the need to control the level of microorganisms in the environment in which sterile products are processed, it also is necessary to detect viable particles. These usually are fewer in number than nonviable ones and are only detectable as colony-forming units (CFUs) after a suitable incubation period at, for example, 30° to 35° for up to 48 hours. Thus, test results will not be known for 48 hours after the samples are taken.

Locations for sampling should be planned to reveal potential contamination levels that may be critical in the control of the environment. For example, the most critical process step is usually the filling of dispensing containers, a site obviously requiring monitoring. Other examples include the gowning room, high-traffic sites in and out of the filling area, the penetration

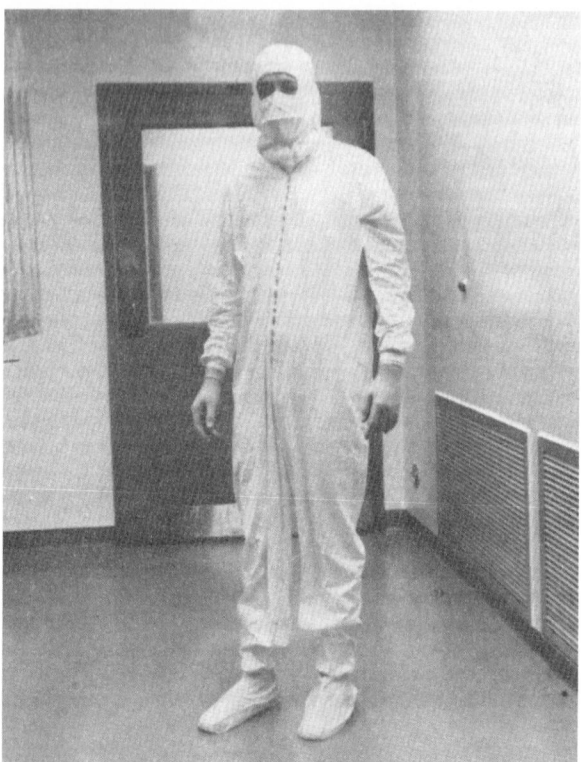

Figure 41-13. Appropriate uniform for operators entering an aseptic filling room (courtesy, Abbott).

of conveyor lines through walls, and sites near the inlet and exit of the air system.

The sample should be large enough to obtain a meaningful particle count. At sites where the count is expected to be low, the size of the sample may need to be increased; for example, in Class 100 areas, Whyte and Niven[25] suggest that the sample should be at least 30 ft³ and, probably, much more. Many firms employ continuous particle monitoring in Class 100 areas to study trends and/or to identify equipment malfunction.

Several air-sampling devices are used to obtain a count of microorganisms in a measured volume of air. A slit-to-agar (STA) sampler (suppliers: *Mattson-Garvin, New Brunswick, Vai*) draws by vacuum a measured volume of air through an engineered slit, causing the air to impact on the surface of a slowly rotating nutrient agar plate (Fig 41-14). Microorganisms adhere to the surface of the agar and grow into visible colonies that are counted as CFUs, since it is not known whether the colonies arise from a single microorganism or a cluster. A centrifugal sampler (supplier: *Biotest*) pulls air into the sampler by means of a rotating propeller and slings the air by centrifugal action against a peripheral nutrient agar strip. The advantages of this unit are that it can be disinfected easily and is portable, so that it can be hand-carried wherever needed. These two methods are used quite widely.

A widely used method for microbiological sampling consists of the exposure of nutrient agar culture plates to the settling of microorganisms from the air. This method is very simple and inexpensive to perform but will detect only those organisms that have settled on the plate; therefore, it does not measure the number of microorganisms in a measured volume of air (a non-quantitative test). Nevertheless, if the conditions of exposure are repeated consistently, a comparison of CFUs at one sampling site from one time to another can be meaningful.[26]

Whyte and Niven suggested that settling plates should be exposed in Class 100 areas for an entire fill (up to 7 to 8 hours) rather than the more common 1 hour. However, excessive dehydration of the medium must be avoided, particularly in the path of laminar-flow air. The European Union GMP guidelines for sterile manufacture of medicinal products suggest an exposure period of not more than 4 hours.

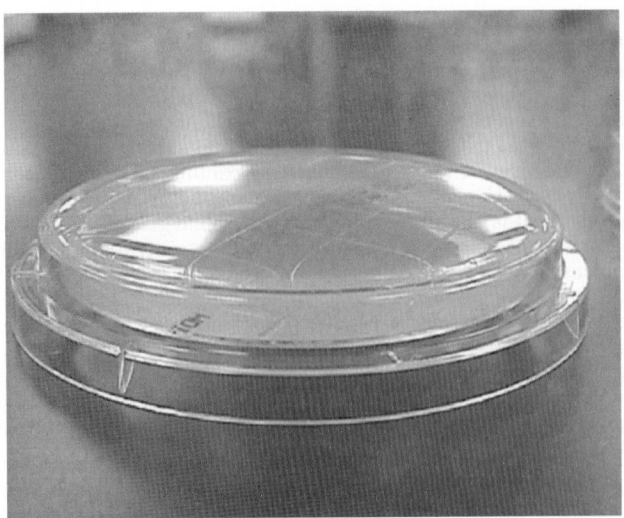

Figure 41-15. Example of a Rodac plate (courtesy, Baxter).

The number of microorganisms on surfaces can be determined with nutrient agar plates having a convex surface (*Rodac Plates*) (Fig 41-15). With these it is possible to roll the raised agar surface over flat or irregular surfaces to be tested. Organisms will be picked up on the agar and will grow during subsequent incubation. This method also can be used to assess the number of microorganisms present on the surface of the uniforms of operators, either as an evaluation of gowning technique immediately after gowning or as a measure of the accumulation of microorganisms during processing. Whenever used, care must be taken to remove any agar residue left on the surface tested.

Further discussion of proposed viable particle test methods and the counts to be accepted will be found in Section <1116> "Microbial Evaluation and Classification of Clean Rooms and Other Controlled Environments" in the USP.

Results from the above tests, although not available until 2 days after sampling, are valuable to keep cleaning, production, and quality-control personnel apprised of the level of contamination in a given area and, by comparison with baseline counts, will indicate when more-extensive cleaning and sanitizing is needed. The results also may serve to detect environmental control defects such as failure in air-cleaning equipment or the presence of personnel who may be disseminating large numbers of bacteria without apparent physical ill effects.

Issues regarding environmental monitoring remain among the most controversial aspects of cGMP regulatory inspections of parenteral manufacturing and testing environments. Regulatory trends include requiring an increase in the number and frequency of locations monitored in the clean room and on clean room personnel, enforcing numerical alert and action limits, and linking environmental monitoring data to the decision to release or reject the batch. It has been pointed out that fully gowned personnel will still release a finite number of microorganisms (typically 10 to 100 CFR per hour) so that it is unreasonable to impose the requirement of zero microbial contamination limits at any location in the clean room.[27]

MEDIA FILL (PROCESS SIMULATION TESTING)— FDA inspections have increasingly focused on media fill studies that truly simulate the production process. The *media fill* or *process simulation test* involves preparation and sterilization (often by filtration) of sterile trypticase soy broth and filling this broth into sterile containers under conditions simulating as closely as possible those characteristics of a filling process for

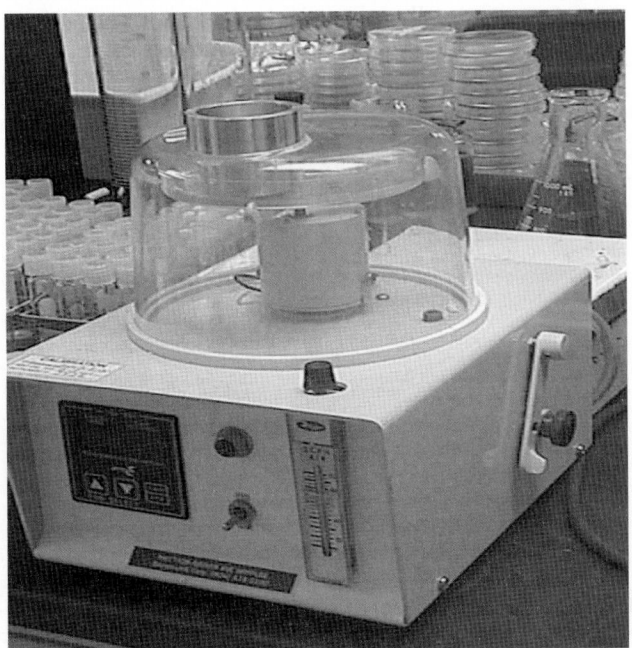

Figure 41-14. Example of slit-to-air sampler (courtesy, Baxter).

a product. The key is designing these studies that simulate all factors that occur during the normal production of a lot. Table 41-5 lists those factors that are given in the FDA Guidelines for Aseptic Processing.[28] The entire lot, normally at least 4750 units, is incubated at temperatures verified to support microbial growth, usually rotating 20° to 25°C storage and 30° to 35°C storage, for at least 14 days and examined for the appearance of growth of microorganisms. The media used must be verified that it is capable of supporting microbial growth. If growth occurs, contamination has entered the container(s) during the processing. To pass the test at 95% confidence, not more than 0.1% of the challenged units may show growth although the current expectation of regulatory agencies is "approaching zero." This evaluation also has been used as a measure of the proficiency of an individual or team of operators. This test is a very stringent evaluation of the efficiency of an aseptic filling process and, by many, is considered to be the most evaluative test available.

Table 41-5. Considerations When Designing Media Fill Studies

- Longest permitted run on processing line
- "Worst case" environmental conditions
- Number and type of normal interventions, atypical interventions, unexpected results, stoppages, equipment adjustments or transfers
- Include lyophilization steps, if applicable
- Aseptic assembly of equipment at start-up and during processing
- Number of personnel involved and their activities
- Number of aseptic additions
- Shift changes, breaks, and gown changes
- Number and type of aseptic equipment disconnections/connections
- Aseptic sample collections
- Line speed and configurations
- Manual weight checks
- Operator fatigue
- Container-closure systems
- Temperature and humidity extremes
- Specific provisions of aseptic processing standard operating procedures (eg, conditions permitted before line clearance is mandated)

PRODUCTION PROCEDURES

The processes required for preparing sterile products constitute a series of events initiated with the procurement of approved raw materials (eg, drugs, excipients, vehicles) and primary packaging components (eg, containers, closures) and ending with the sterile product sealed in its dispensing package. Each step in the process must be controlled very carefully so that the product will have its required quality. To ensure the latter, each process should be validated to be sure that it is accomplishing what it is intended to do. For example, an autoclave sterilization process must be validated by producing data showing that it effectively kills resistant forms of microorganisms; or, a cleaning process for rubber closures should provide evidence that it is cleaning closures to the required level of cleanliness; or a filling process that repeatedly delivers the correct fill volume per container. The validation of processes requires extensive and intensive effort to be successful and is an integral part of cGMP requirements.

CLEANING CONTAINERS AND EQUIPMENT

Containers and equipment coming in contact with parenteral preparations must be cleaned meticulously. It should be obvious that even new, unused containers and equipment will be contaminated with such debris as dust, fibers, chemical films, and other materials arising from such sources as the atmosphere, cartons, the manufacturing process, and human hands. Residues from previous use must be removed from used equipment before it will be suitable for reuse. Equipment should be reserved exclusively for use only with parenteral preparations and, where conditions dictate, only for one product in order to reduce the risk of contamination. For many operations, particularly with biologic and biotechnology products, equipment is dedicated for only one product.

A variety of machines are available for cleaning new containers for parenteral products. These vary in complexity from a small, hand loaded, rotary rinser to large automatic washers capable of processing several thousand containers per hour (Fig 41-16). The selection of the particular type will be determined largely by the physical type of containers, the type of contamination, and the number to be processed in a given period of time.

Validation of cleaning procedures for equipment is another "hot topic" with respect to cGMP regulatory inspections. Inadequate cleaning processes have been a frequent citing by FDA and other regulatory inspectors when inspecting both active ingredient and final product manufacturing facilities. It is incumbent upon parenteral manufacturers to establish scientifically justified acceptance criteria for cleaning validation. If specific analytical limits for target residues are arbitrarily set, this will cause concern for quality auditors. Validation of cleaning procedures can be relatively complicated because of issues with sample methods (eg, swab, final rinse, testing of subsequent batch), sample locations, sensitivity of analytical methods, and calculations used to establish cleaning limits.

CHARACTERISTICS OF MACHINERY—Regardless of the type of cleaning machine selected, certain fundamental characteristics usually are required:

1. The liquid or air treatment must be introduced in such a manner that it will strike the bottom of the inside of the inverted con-

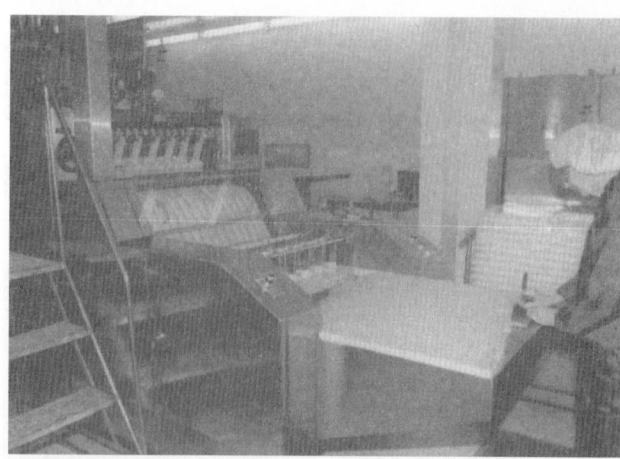

Figure 41-16. Loading end of large conveyor vial washer that subjects inverted vials to a series of cleaning steps before delivery from the far end of the washer. Note the vials in plastic blister packs at right of operator (courtesy, Merck).

tainer, spread in all directions, and smoothly flow down the walls and out the opening with a sweeping action. The pressure of the jet stream should be such that there is minimal splashing and turbulence inside. Splashing may prevent cleaning all areas, and turbulence may redeposit loosened debris. Therefore, direct introduction of the jet stream within the container with control of its flow is required.

2. The container must receive a concurrent outside rinse.
3. The cycle of treatment should provide a planned sequence alternating very hot and cool treatments. The final treatment should be an effective rinse with WFI.
4. All metal parts coming in contact with the containers and with the treatments should be constructed of stainless steel or some other non-corroding and non-contaminating material.

TREATMENT CYCLE—The cycle of treatments to be employed will vary with the condition of the containers to be cleaned. In general, loose debris can be removed by vigorous rinsing with water. Detergents rarely are used for new containers because of the risk of leaving detergent residues. However, a thermal-shock sequence in the cycle usually is employed to aid, by expansion and contraction, loosening of debris that may be adhering to the container wall. Sometimes only an air rinse is used for new containers, if only loose debris is present. In all instances the final rinse, whether air or WFI, must be ultraclean so that no particulate residues are left by the rinsing agent.

Only new containers are used for parenterals. Improvements have been made in maintaining their cleanliness during shipment from the manufacturer through tight, low-shedding packaging, including plastic blister packs, as can be seen stacked on the right of Figure 41-16.

MACHINERY FOR CONTAINERS—The machinery available for cleaning containers embodies the above principles but varies in the mechanics by which it is accomplished. In one manual loading type, the jet tubes are arranged on arms like the spokes of a wheel, which rotate around a center post through which the treatments are introduced. An operator places the unclean containers on the jet tubes as they pass the loading point and removes the clean containers as they complete one rotation. A washer capable of cleaning hundreds of containers an hour, shown in Figure 41-16, uses a row of jet tubes across a conveyor belt. The belt moves the inverted containers past the programmed series of treatments and discharges the clean containers into a sterilizing oven (not shown), which ultimately discharges them through a wall into a clean room for filling.

A continuous automated line operation, capable of cleaning hundreds of containers an hour, is shown in Figure 41-17. The vials are fed into the rotary rinser in the foreground, transferred automatically to the covered sterilizing tunnel in the center, conveyed through the wall in the background, and discharged into the filling clean room.

HANDLING AFTER CLEANING—The wet, clean containers must be handled in such a way that contamination will not be reintroduced. A wet surface will collect contaminants much more readily than will a dry surface. For this reason wet, rinsed containers must be protected, eg, by a laminar flow of clean air until covered, within a stainless steel box, or within a sterilizing tunnel. In addition, microorganisms are more likely to grow in the presence of moisture. Therefore, wet, clean containers should be dry-heat sterilized as soon as possible after washing. Doubling the heating period generally is adequate also to destroy pyrogens; for example, increasing the dwell time at 250° from 1 to 2 hr, but the actual time-temperature conditions required must be validated.

Increases in process rates have necessitated the development of continuous, automated line processing with a minimum of individual handling, still maintaining adequate control of the cleaning and handling of the containers. In Figure 41-17, the clean, wet containers are protected by filtered, laminar-flow air from the rinser through the tunnel and until they are delivered to the filling line.

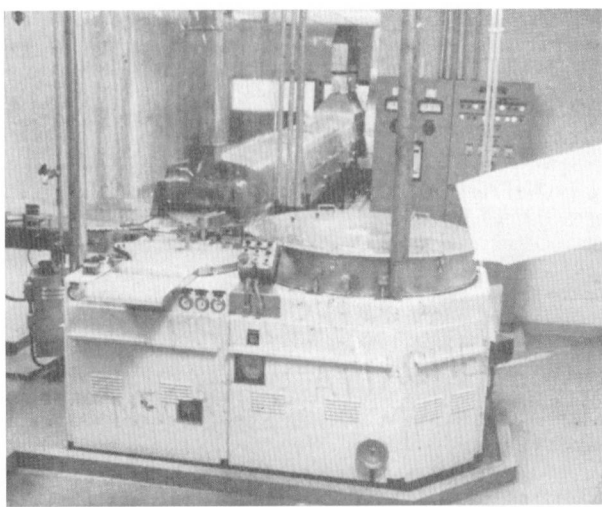

Figure 41-17. Continuous automatic line operation for vials from a rotary rinser through a sterilizing tunnel with vertical laminar-airflow protection of clean vials (courtesy, Abbott).

CLOSURES—The rough, elastic, and convoluted surface of rubber closures renders them difficult to clean. In addition, any residue of lubricant from molding or surface *bloom* of inorganic constituents must be removed. The normal procedure calls for gentle agitation in a hot solution of a mild water softener or detergent. The closures are removed from the solution and rinsed several times, or continuously for a prolonged period, with filtered WFI. The rinsing is to be done in a manner that will flush away loosened debris. The wet closures are carefully protected from environmental contamination, sterilized, usually by steam sterilization (autoclaving), and stored in closed containers until ready for use. This cleaning and sterilizing process also must be validated with respect to rendering the closures free from pyrogens. Actually, it is the cleaning and final, thorough rinsing with WFI that must remove pyrogens, since autoclaving does not destroy pyrogens. If the closures were immersed during autoclaving, the solution is drained off before storage to reduce hydration of the rubber compound. If the closures must be dry for use, they may be subjected to vacuum drying at a temperature in the vicinity of 100°C. Some freeze-dried products require extremely dry closures to avoid desorption of moisture from the closure into the moisture-sensitive powder during storage. This may require drying times of hours following steam sterilization.

The equipment used for washing large numbers of closures is usually an agitator or horizontal basket-type automatic washing machine. Because of the risk of particulate generation from the abrading action of these machines, some procedures simply call for heating the closures in kettles in detergent solution, followed by prolonged flush rinsing. The final rinse always should be with low-particulate WFI. An example of a modern closure processor that washes, siliconizes, sterilizes, and transports closures directly to the filling line is shown in Figure 41-18.

It is also possible to purchase rubber closures already cleaned and lubricated in sterilizable bags supplied by the rubber closure manufacturer.

EQUIPMENT—The details of certain prescribed techniques for cleaning and preparing equipment, as well as of containers and closures, have been presented elsewhere.[29] Here, a few points will be emphasized.

All equipment should be disassembled as much as possible to provide access to internal structures. Surfaces should be scrubbed thoroughly with a stiff brush, using an effective detergent and paying particular attention to joints, crevices, screw threads, and other structures where debris is apt to

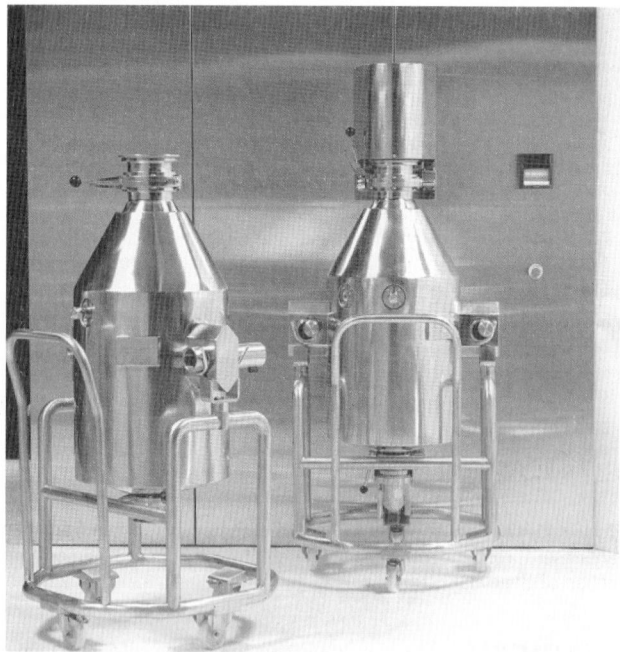

Figure 41-18. Rubber closure processors (courtesy, Getinge USA). See Color Plate 9.

collect. Exposure to a stream of clean steam will aid in dislodging residues from the walls of stationary tanks, spigots, pipes, and similar structures. Thorough rinsing with distilled water should follow the cleaning steps.

Because of the inherent variation in manual cleaning, the difficult accessibility of large stationary tanks and the need to validate the process, computer-controlled systems (usually automated) have been developed and are known as clean-in-place (CIP). Such an approach involves designing the system, normally of stainless steel, with smooth, rounded internal surfaces and without crevices. That is, for example, with welded rather than threaded connections. The cleaning is accomplished with the scrubbing action of high-pressure spray balls or nozzles delivering hot detergent solution from tanks captive to the system, followed by thorough rinsing with WFI. The system often is extended to allow sterilizing-in-place (SIP) to accomplish sanitizing or sterilizing as well.

Rubber tubing, rubber gaskets, and other rubber parts may be washed in a manner such as described for rubber closures. Thorough rinsing of tubing must be done by passing WFI through the tubing lumen. However, because of the relatively porous nature of rubber compounds and the difficulty in removing all traces of chemicals from previous use, it is considered by some inadvisable to reuse rubber or polymeric tubing. Rubber tubing must be left wet when preparing for sterilization by autoclaving.

PRODUCT PREPARATION

The basic principles employed in the compounding of the product are essentially the same as those used historically by pharmacists. However, large-scale production requires appropriate adjustments in the processes and their control.

A master formula would have been developed and be on file. Each batch formula sheet should be prepared from the master and confirmed for accuracy. All measurements of quantities should be made as accurately as possible and checked by a second qualified person. Frequently, formula documents are generated by a computer, and the measurements of quantities of ingredients are computer controlled. Although most liquid preparations are dispensed by volume, they are prepared by

weight, since weighings can be performed more accurately than volume measurements, and no consideration needs to be given to the temperature.

Care must be taken that equipment is not wet enough to dilute the product significantly or, in the case of anhydrous products, to cause a physical incompatibility. The order of mixing of ingredients may affect the product significantly, particularly those of large volume, where attaining homogeneity requires considerable mixing time. For example, the adjustment of pH by the addition of an acid, even though diluted, may cause excessive local reduction in the pH of the product so that adverse effects are produced before the acid can be dispersed throughout the entire volume of product.

Parenteral dispersions, including colloids, emulsions, and suspensions, provide particular problems. In addition to the problems of achieving and maintaining proper reduction in particle size under aseptic conditions, the dispersion must be kept in a uniform state of suspension throughout the preparative, transfer, and subdividing operations.

Proteinaceous solutions are especially "tempermental" when preparing these products. Proteins are usually extremely sensitive to many environmental and processing conditions exposed to during production such as temperature, mixing time and speed, order of addition of formulation components, pH adjustment and control, and contact time with various surfaces such as filters and tubing. Development studies must include evaluation of manufacturing conditions in order to minimize adverse effects of the process on the activity of the protein.

The formulation of a stable product is of paramount importance. Certain aspects of this are mentioned in the discussion of components of the product. Exhaustive coverage of the topic is not possible within the limits of this text, but further coverage is provided in Chapters 39 (*Solutions, Emulsions, Suspensions and Extracts*) and 52 (*Stability of Pharmaceutical Products*). It should be mentioned here, however, that the thermal sterilization of parenteral products increases the possibility of chemical reactions. Such reactions may progress to completion during the period of elevated temperature in the autoclave or be initiated at this time but continue during subsequent storage. The assurance of attaining product stability requires a high order of pharmaceutical knowledge and responsibility.

FILTRATION

After a product has been compounded, it must be filtered if it is a solution. The primary objective of filtration is to clarify a solution. A further step, removing particulate matter down to 0.2 μm in size, would eliminate microorganisms and would accomplish *cold* sterilization. A solution with a high degree of clarity conveys the impression of high quality and purity, desirable characteristics for a parenteral solution.

Filters are thought to function by one or, usually, a combination of the following: (1) sieving or screening, (2) entrapment or impaction, and (3) electrostatic attraction (Fig 41–19). When a filter retains particles by sieving, they are retained on the surface of the filter. Entrapment occurs when a particle smaller than the dimensions of the passageway (pore) becomes lodged in a turn or impacted on the surface of the passageway. Electrostatic attraction causes particles opposite in charge to that of the surface of the filter pore to be held or adsorbed to the surface. It should be noted that increasing, prolonging, or varying the force behind the solution may tend to sweep particles initially held by entrapment or electrostatic charge through the pores and into the filtrate.

Membrane filters are used exclusively for parenteral solutions because of their particle-retention effectiveness, non-shedding property, non-reactivity, and disposable characteristics. However, it should be noted that non-reactivity does not apply in all cases. For example, polypeptide products may show considerable adsorption through some membrane filters, but

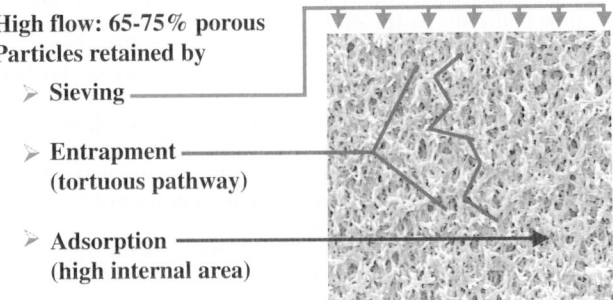

High flow: 65-75% porous
Particles retained by

➢ **Sieving**

➢ **Entrapment**
  (tortuous pathway)

➢ **Adsorption**
  (high internal area)

Figure 41-19. Mechanisms of microbial retention on membrane filters (courtesy, Millipore). See Color Plate 10.

those composed of polysulfone and polyvinylidine difluoride (PVDF) have been developed to be essentially non-adsorptive for these products. The most common membranes are composed of Cellulose esters, Nylon, Polysulfone, Polycarbonate, PVDF, or Polytetrafluoroethylene (Teflon).

Filters are available as flat membranes or pleated into cylinders (Fig 41-20) to increase surface area and, thus, flow rate (suppliers: *Cuno, Gelman, Meissner, Millipore, Pall, Sartorius Schleicher*). Each filter in its holder should be tested for integrity before and after use, particularly if it is being used to eliminate microorganisms. This integrity test usually is performed either as the *bubble-point test* or as the *diffusion or forward flow* test. The bubble point test is commonly used on smaller filters. As the surface area of filters becomes large, diffusion of air through the water-filled pores tends to obscure the bubble point. Therefore, the diffusion test has been developed as an integrity test for filters with large surface areas. A *pressure hold test* also can be applied to large surface area filters. The filter manufacturer will recommend the best integrity test for the filter system in question.

These are tests to detect the largest pore or other opening through the membrane. The basic test is performed by gradually raising air pressure on the upstream side of a water-wet filter. The bubble point test keeps raising pressure until a pressure is obtained where air bubbles first appear downstream is the bubble point. The diffusion or forward flow test raises pressure to some point below the known bubble point pressure, then diffusion flow (usually in mL/min) is measured. These pressures are characteristic for each pore size of a filter and are provided by the filter manufacturer. For example, a 0.2-μm cellulose ester filter will bubble at about 50 psig or a diffusive flow rating of no greater than 13 mL/min at a pressure of 40 psig. If the filter is wetted with other liquids, such as a product, the bubble point will differ and must be determined experimentally. If the bubble point is lower than the rated pressure, the filter is defective, probably because of a puncture or tear, and should not be used.

While membrane filters are disposable and thus discarded after use, the holders must be cleaned thoroughly between uses. Today, clean, sterile, pretested, disposable assemblies for small as well as large volumes of solutions are available commercially.

New evidence is being reported that 0.2 μm filters do not remove all possible microbial contamination,[30] necessitating the need to use certain types of 0.1 μm membrane filters.[31] However, most of the parenteral pharmaceutical industry continues to use 0.2 μm filters although now employing redundant (two 0.2 μm filters side-by-side) filtration systems.

FILLING

During the filling of containers with a product, the most stringent requirements must be exercised to prevent contamination, particularly if the product has been sterilized by filtration and will not be sterilized in the final container. Under the latter conditions the process is called an *aseptic fill* and is validated with media fills. During the filling operation, the product must be transferred from a bulk container or tank and subdivided into dose containers. This operation exposes the sterile product to the environment, equipment, and manipulative technique of the operators until it can be sealed in the dose container. Therefore, this operation is carried out with a minimum exposure time, even though maximum protection is provided by filling under a blanket of HEPA-filtered laminar-flow air within the aseptic area.

Most frequently, the compounded product is in the form of a liquid. However, products are also compounded as suspensions or emulsions and as powders. A liquid is more readily subdivided uniformly and introduced into a container having a narrow mouth than is a solid. Mobile liquids are considerably easier to transfer and subdivide than viscous, sticky liquids, which require heavy-duty machinery for rapid production filling.

Although many devices are available for filling containers with liquids, certain characteristics are fundamental to them all. A means is provided for repetitively forcing a measured volume of the liquid through the orifice of a delivery tube that is introduced into the container. The size of the delivery tube will vary from that of about a 20-gauge hypodermic needle to a tube 1/2 in or more in diameter. The size required is determined by the physical characteristics of the liquid, the desired delivery speed, and the inside diameter of the neck of the container. The tube must enter the neck and deliver the liquid well into the neck to eliminate spillage, allowing sufficient clearance to permit air to leave the container as the liquid enters. The delivery tube should be as large in diameter as possible to reduce the resistance and decrease the velocity of flow of the liquid. For smaller volumes of liquids, the delivery usually is obtained from the stroke of the plunger of a syringe, forcing the liquid through a two-way valve providing for alternate filling of the syringe and delivery of mobile liquids. For heavy, viscous liquids, a sliding piston valve, the turn of an auger in the neck of a funnel, or the oscillation of a rubber diaphragm may be used. For large volumes the quantity delivered usually is measured in the container by the level of fill in the container, the force re-

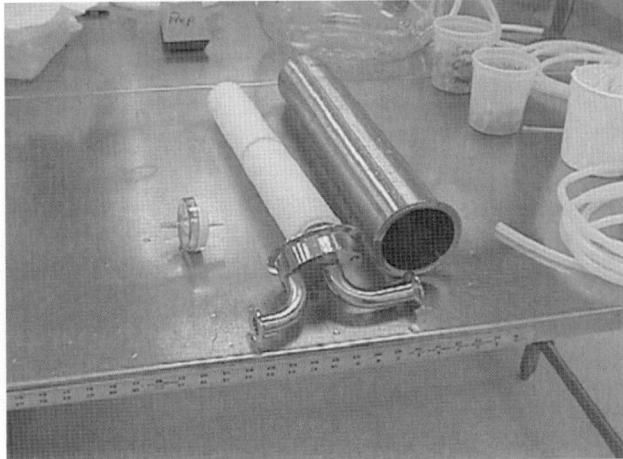

Figure 41-20. Cartridge filter assembly (courtesy, Baxter).

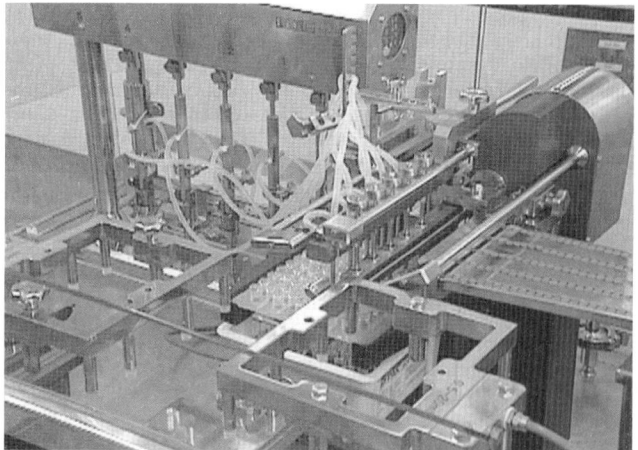

Figure 41-21. Syringe filling machine (courtesy, Baxter). See Color Plate 11.

quired to transfer the liquid being provided by gravity, a pressure pump, or a vacuum pump.

The narrow neck of an ampoule limits the clearance possible between the delivery tube and the inside of the neck. Since a drop of liquid normally hangs at the tip of the delivery tube after a delivery, the neck of an ampoule will be wet as the delivery tube is withdrawn, unless the drop is retracted. Therefore, filling machines should have a mechanism by which this drop can be drawn back into the lumen of the tube. Since the liquid will be in intimate contact with the parts of the machine through which it flows, these must be constructed of non-reactive materials such as borosilicate glass or stainless steel. In addition, they should easily be demountable for cleaning and sterilization.

Because of the concern for particulate matter in injectable preparations, a final filter often is inserted in the system between the filler and the delivery tube. Most frequently this is a membrane filter, having a porosity of approximately 1 μm and treated to have a hydrophobic edge. This is necessary to reduce the risk of rupture of the membrane caused by filling pulsations. It should be noted that the insertion of the filter at this point should collect all particulate matter generated during the process. Only that which may be found in inadequately cleaned containers or picked up from exposure to the environment after passage through the final filter potentially remain as contaminants. However, the filter does cushion liquid flow and reduces the efficiency of drop retraction from the end of the delivery tube, sometimes making it difficult to control delivery volume as precisely as would be possible without the filter.

LIQUIDS—There are three main methods for filling liquids into containers with high accuracy: volumetric filling, time/pressure dosing, and net weight filling. Volumetric filling machines employing pistons or peristaltic pumps are most commonly used.

Stainless steel syringes are required with viscous liquids because glass syringes are not strong enough to withstand the high pressures developed during delivery.

When high-speed filling rates are desired but accuracy and precision must be maintained, multiple filling units often are joined together in an electronically coordinated machine, such as shown in Figures 41-21 and 41-22. When the product is sensitive to metals, a peristaltic-pump filler may be used because the product comes in contact only with silicone rubber tubing. However, there is some sacrifice of filling accuracy.

Time-pressure (or time-gravity) filling machines are gaining in popularity in filling sterile liquids. A product tank is connected to the filling system that is equipped with a pressure sensor. The sensor continuously measures pressure and transmits values to the PLC system that controls the flow of product from tank to filling manifold. Product flow occurs when tubing is mechanically un-pinched and stops when tubing is mechanically pinched. The main advantage of time/pressure filling operations is that these filling apparatuses do not contain mechanical moving parts in the product stream. The product is driven by pressure (usually nitrogen) with no pumping mechanism involved. Thus, especially for proteins that are quite sensitive to shear forces, time/pressure filling is preferable.

Most high-speed fillers for large-volume solutions use the bottle as the measuring device, transferring the liquid either by vacuum or positive pressure from the bulk reservoir to the individual unit containers. Therefore, a high accuracy of fill is not achievable.

The USP requires that each container be filled with a sufficient volume in excess of the labeled volume to ensure withdrawal of the labeled volume and provides a table of suggested fill volumes.

The filling of a small number of containers may be accomplished with a hypodermic syringe and needle, the liquid being drawn into the syringe and forced through the needle into the container. A device for providing greater speed of filling is the Cornwall Pipet *(Becton Dickinson)*. This has a two-way valve

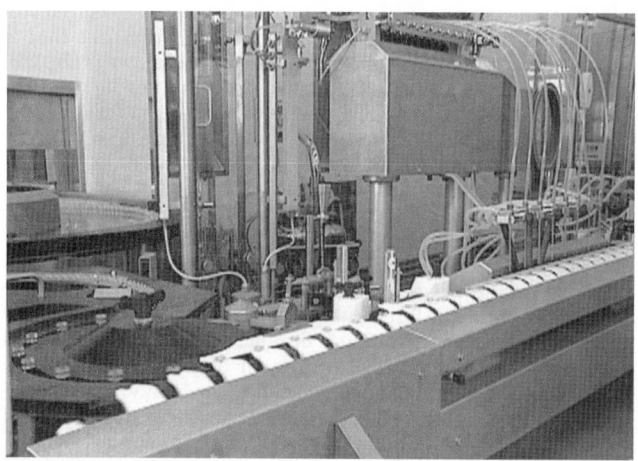

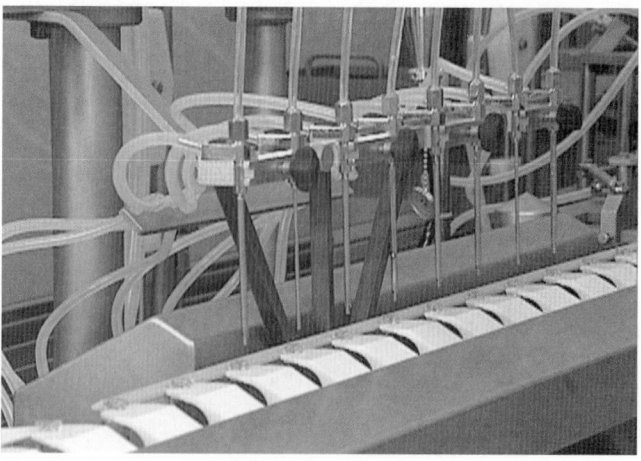

A **B**

Figure 41-22. Vial filling machine, distant and close-up views (courtesy, Baxter). See Color Plate 12.

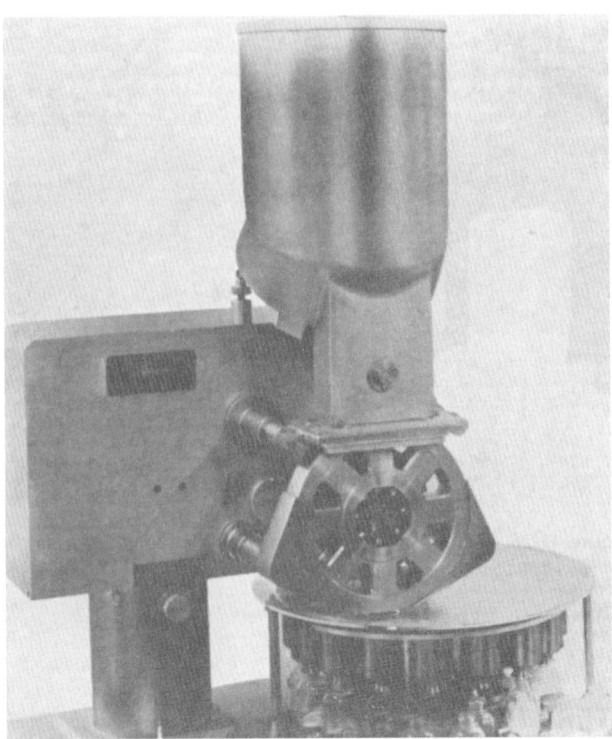

Figure 41-23. Accofil vacuum powder filler (courtesy, Perry).

between the syringe and the needle and a means for setting the stroke of the syringe so that the same volume will be delivered each time. Clean, sterile, disposable assemblies (suppliers: *Burron, Pharmaseal*) operating on the same principle have particular usefulness in hospital pharmacy or experimental operations.

SOLIDS—Sterile solids, such as antibiotics, are more difficult to subdivide evenly into containers than are liquids. The rate of flow of solid material is slow and often irregular. Even though a container with a larger-diameter opening is used to facilitate filling, it is difficult to introduce the solid particles, and the risk of spillage is ever-present. The accuracy of the quantity delivered cannot be controlled as well as with liquids. Because of these factors, the tolerances permitted for the content of such containers must be relatively large.

Some sterile solids are subdivided into containers by individual weighing. A scoop usually is provided to aid in approximating the quantity required, but the quantity filled into the container finally is weighed on a balance. This is a slow process. When the solid is obtainable in a granular form so that it will flow more freely, other methods of filling may be employed. In general, these involve the measurement and delivery of a volume of the granular material that has been calibrated in terms of the weight desired. In the machine shown in Figure 41-23 an adjustable cavity in the rim of a wheel is filled by vacuum and the contents held by vacuum until the cavity is inverted over the container. The solid material then is discharged into the container by a puff of sterile air.

SEALING

AMPOULES—Filled containers should be sealed as soon as possible to prevent the contents from being contaminated by the environment. Ampoules are sealed by melting a portion of the glass neck. Two types of seals are employed normally: tip-seals (bead-seals) or pull-seals.

Tip-seals are made by melting enough glass at the tip of the neck of an ampoule to form a bead and close the opening. These can be made rapidly in a high-temperature gas-oxygen flame. To produce a uniform bead, the ampoule neck must be heated evenly on all sides, such as by burners on opposite sides of stationary ampoules or by rotating the ampoule in a single flame. Care must be taken to adjust the flame temperature and the interval of heating properly to completely close the opening with a bead of glass. Excessive heating will result in the expansion of the gases within the ampoule against the soft bead seal and cause a bubble to form. If it bursts, the ampoule is no longer sealed; if it does not, the wall of the bubble will be thin and fragile. Insufficient heating will leave an open capillary through the center of the bead. An incompletely sealed ampoule is called a *leaker*.

Pull-seals are made by heating the neck of the ampoule below the tip, leaving enough of the tip for grasping with forceps or other mechanical devices. The ampoule is rotated in the flame from a single burner. When the glass has softened, the tip is grasped firmly and pulled quickly away from the body of the ampoule, which continues to rotate. The small capillary tube thus formed is twisted closed. Pull-sealing is slower, but the seals are more sure than tip-sealing. Figure 41-24 shows a machine combining the steps of filling and pull-sealing ampoules.

Powder ampoules or other types having a wide opening must be sealed by pull-sealing. Fracture of the neck of ampoules during sealing may occur if wetting of the necks occurred at the time of filling. Also, wet necks increase the frequency of bubble formation and unsightly carbon deposits if the product is organic.

To prevent decomposition of a product, it is sometimes necessary to displace the air in the space above the product in the ampoule with an inert gas. This is done by introducing a stream of the gas, such as nitrogen or carbon dioxide, during or after filling with the product. Immediately thereafter the ampoule is sealed before the gas can diffuse to the outside. This process should be validated to ensure adequate displacement of air by the gas in each container.

VIALS AND BOTTLES—These are sealed by closing the opening with a rubber closure (stopper). This must be accomplished as rapidly as possible after filling and with reasoned care to prevent contamination of the contents. The large opening makes the introduction of contamination much easier than with ampoules. Therefore, during the critical exposure time the open containers should be protected from the ingress of contamination, preferably with a blanket of HEPA-filtered laminar airflow.

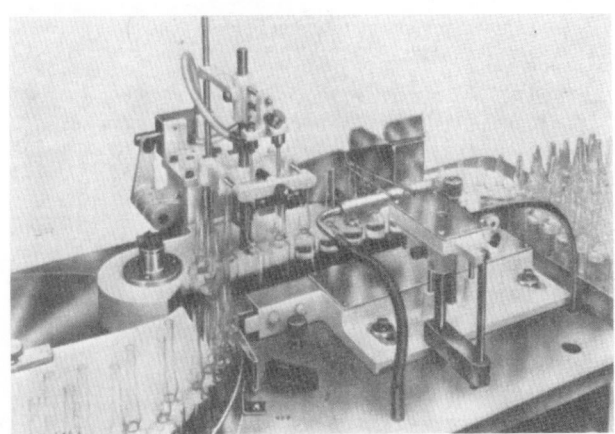

Figure 41-24. Automatic filling and pull-sealing of ampoules (courtesy, Cozzoli).

The closure must fit the mouth of the container snugly enough so that its elasticity will seal rigid to slight irregularities in the lip and neck of the container. However, it must not fit so snugly that it is difficult to introduce into the neck of the container. Closures preferably are inserted mechanically using an automated process, especially with high-speed processing. To reduce friction so that the closure may slide more easily through a chute and into the container opening, the closure surfaces are halogenated or treated with silicone. When the closure is positioned at the insertion site, it is pushed mechanically into the container opening (Fig 41-25). When small lots are encountered, manual stoppering with forceps may be used, but such a process poses greater risk of introducing contamination than automated processes. This is a good test for evaluation aseptic operator aseptic techniques, but not recommended for any product filling and stoppering.

Container-closure integrity testing has become a major focus for the industry because of emphasis by regulatory agencies. Container-closure integrity measures the ability of the seal between the glass or plastic container opening and the rubber closure to remain tight and fit and to resist any ingress of microbial contamination during product shelf life. Container-closure integrity test requirements are covered in USP <1207>, and the various test methods are described by Guazzo.[32]

Rubber closures are held in place by means of aluminum caps. The caps cover the closure and are crimped under the lip of the vial or bottle to hold them in place. The closure cannot be removed without destroying the aluminum cap; it is tamper-proof. Therefore, an intact aluminum cap is proof that the closure has not been removed intentionally or unintentionally. Such confirmation is necessary to ensure the integrity of the contents as to sterility and other aspects of quality.

The aluminum caps are so designed that the outer layer of double-layered caps, or the center of single-layered caps, can be removed to expose the center of the rubber closure without disturbing the band that holds the closure in the container. Rubber closures for use with intravenous administration sets often have a permanent hole through the closure. In such cases, a thin rubber disk overlayed with a solid aluminum disk is placed between an inner and outer aluminum cap, thereby providing a seal of the hole through the closure.

Single-layered aluminum caps may be applied by means of a hand crimper known as the Fermpress (suppliers: *West, Wheaton*). Double- or triple-layered caps require greater force for crimping; therefore, heavy-duty mechanical crimpers (Fig 41-26) are required (suppliers: *Bosch, Cozzoli, Perry, West, Wheaton*).

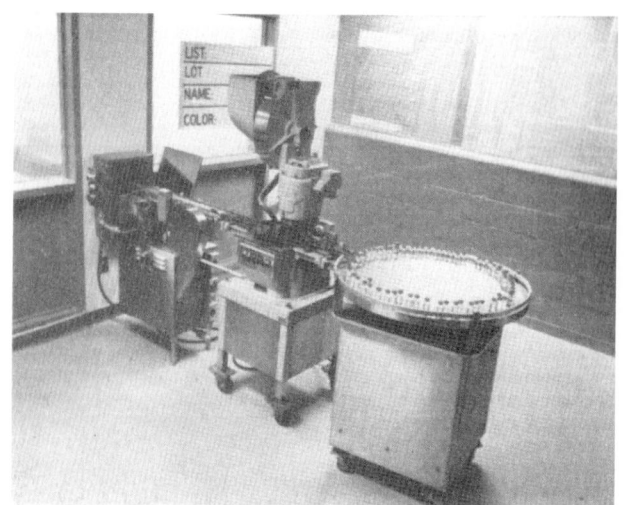

Figure 41-26. Applying aluminum caps to vials at the end of the process line (courtesy, Abbott).

STERILIZATION

Whenever possible, the parenteral product should be sterilized after being sealed in its final container (terminal sterilization) and within as short a time as possible after the filling and sealing have been completed. Since this usually involves a thermal process (although there is a trend in applying radiation sterilization to finished products), due consideration must be given to the effect of the elevated temperature upon the stability of the product. Many products, both pharmaceutical and biological, will be affected adversely by the elevated temperatures required for thermal sterilization. Heat-labile products must, therefore, be sterilized by a non-thermal method, usually by filtration through bacteria-retaining filters. Subsequently, all operations must be carried out in an aseptic manner so that contamination will not be introduced into the filtrate. Colloids, oleaginous solutions, suspensions, and emulsions that are thermolabile may require a process in which each component is sterilized separately and the product is formulated and processed under aseptic conditions.

The performance of an aseptic process is challenging, but technical advances in aseptic processing, including improved automation, use of isolator systems, formulations to include antimicrobial effects, and combinations of limited sterilization with aseptic processing, have decreased the risk of contamination. Therefore, the successes realized should encourage continued efforts to improve the assurance of sterility achievable with aseptic processing. The importance of this is that for many drug solutions and essentially all biopharmaceutical products, aseptic processing is the only method that can be considered for preparing a sterile product.

Interaction among environmental conditions, the constituents in the closure, and the product may result in undesirable closure changes such as increased brittleness or stickiness, which may cause loss of container-closure seal integrity. Thus, shelf life integrity is an important consideration in closure selection and evaluation.

The assessment of aseptic-processing performance is based on the contamination rate resulting from periodic process simulations using media-filling instead of product-filling of containers. A contamination rate no greater than 0.1% at 95% confidence has generally been considered as indicative of satisfactory performance in the industry. However, with current advances in aseptic processing capabilities, lower contamination rates may be achievable.

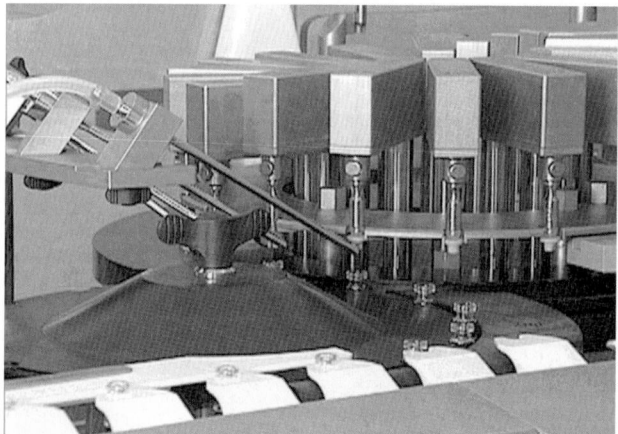

Figure 41-25. Mechanical device for inserting rubber closures in vials (courtesy, Baxter).

Radiation sterilization, as mentioned, is gaining some momentum as an alternative terminal sterilization method. There has been limited understanding of the molecular transformations that may occur in drug molecules and excipients under exposure to the high-energy gamma radiation levels of the process. However, lower energy beta particle (electron beam) radiation has seen some success. There is still significant research that must be accomplished before radiation sterilization is used as a terminal sterilization process. The use of radiation for the sterilization of materials such as plastic medical devices is well established.

Dry-heat sterilization may be employed for a few dry solids that are not affected adversely by the high temperatures and for the relatively long heating period required. This method is applied most effectively to the sterilization of glassware and metalware. After sterilization, the equipment will be sterile, dry, and, if the sterilization period is long enough, pyrogen-free.

Saturated steam under pressure (autoclaving) is the most commonly used and the most effective method for the sterilization of aqueous liquids or substances that can be reached or penetrated by steam. A survival probability of at least 10^{-6} is readily achievable with terminal autoclaving of a thermally stable product. However, it needs to be noted that for terminal sterilization, the assurance of sterility is based upon an evaluation of the lethality of the process, ie, of the probable number of viable microorganisms remaining in product units. However, for aseptic processing, where the components used have been sterilized separately by validated processes and aseptically put together, the level of sterility assurance is based upon an evaluation of the probable number of product units that were contaminated during the process.

Figure 41-27 shows an example of a modern autoclave for sterilization. Since the temperature employed in an autoclave is lower than that for dry-heat sterilization, equipment made of materials such as rubber and polypropylene may be sterilized if the time and temperature are controlled carefully. As mentioned previously, some injections will be affected adversely by the elevated temperature required for autoclaving. For some products, such as dextrose injection, a shortened cycle using an autoclave designed to permit a rapid temperature rise and rapid cooling with water spray or other cooling methods will make it possible to use this method. It is ineffective in anhydrous conditions, such as within a sealed ampoule containing a dry solid or an anhydrous oil. Other products that will not withstand autoclaving temperatures may withstand marginal thermal methods such as tyndallization or pasteurization, eg, 10 to 12 hours at 60°C. These methods may be rendered more effective for some injections by the inclusion of a bacteriostatic agent in the product.

Articles to be sterilized must be properly wrapped or placed in suitable containers to permit penetration of sterilants and provide protection from contamination after sterilization. Sheets or bags made of special steam-penetrating paper or polymeric materials are available for this purpose. Further, containers or bags impervious to steam can be equipped with a microbe-excluding vent filter to permit adequate steam penetration and air exit. Multiple wrapping permits sequential removal of outer layers as articles are transferred from zones of lower to higher environmental quality. The openings of equipment subjected to dry-heat sterilization often are covered with metal or glass covers. Laboratories often used silver-aluminum foil for covering glassware to be used for endotoxin testing. Wrapping materials commonly used for steam sterilization may be combustible or otherwise become degraded under dry-heat sterilization conditions.

The effectiveness of any sterilization technique must be proved (validated) before it is employed in practice. Since the goal of sterilization is to kill microorganisms, the ideal indicator to prove the effectiveness of the process is a resistant form of an appropriate microorganism, normally resistant spores (a biological indicator, or BI). Therefore, during validation of a sterilization process, BIs of known resistance and numbers are used in association with physical-parameter indicators, such as recording thermocouples. Once the lethality of the process is established in association with the physical measurements, the physical measurements can be used for subsequent monitoring of in-use processes without the BIs. Eliminating the use of BIs in direct association with human-use products is appropriate because of the ever-present risk of an undetected, inadvertent contamination of a product or the environment. The number of spores and their resistance in BIs used for validation studies must be accurately known or determined. Additionally, the manner in which BIs are used in validation is critical and must be controlled carefully.

In addition to the data printout from thermocouples, sometimes other physical indicators are used, such as color-change

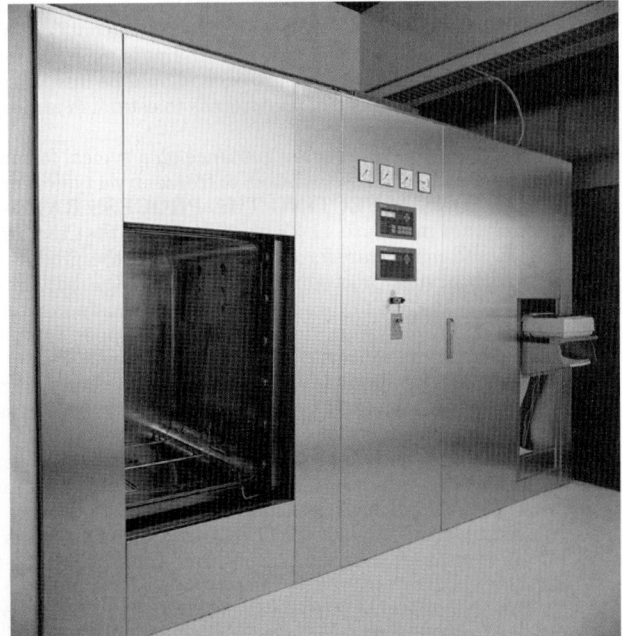
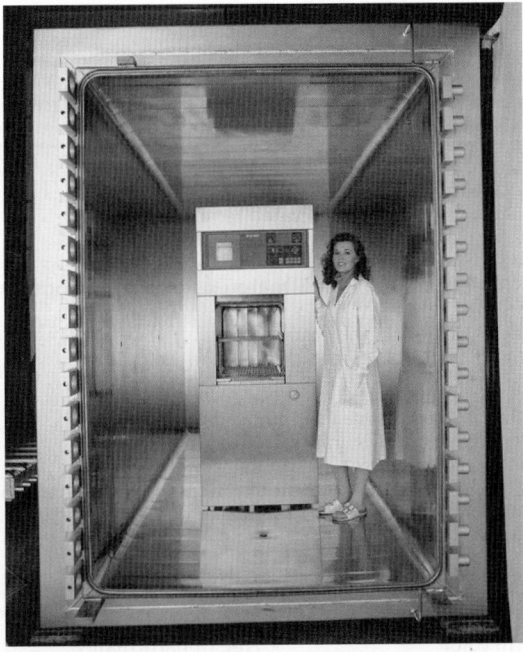

Figure 41-27. Steam sterilizers (small and large) (courtesy, Getinge). See Color Plate 13.

A

B

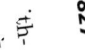
ators, to give visual indication that a package een subjected to a sterilization process. Such ne a part of the batch record to confirm that complished.

concerning methods of sterilization and n be found in Chapter 40 (*Sterilization*). In addition, the USP provides suggestions concerning the sterilization of injections and related materials.

FREEZE-DRYING (LYOPHILIZATION)

Many parenteral drugs, particularly biopharmaceuticals, are too unstable in solution to be available as ready-to-use liquid dosage forms. Such drugs can still be filled as solutions, placed in a chamber where the combined effects of freezing and drying under low pressure will remove the solvent and residual moisture from the solute components, resulting in a dry powder that has sufficient long term stability. The process of freeze-drying has taken on greater prominence in the parenteral industry because of the advent of recombinant DNA technology. Proteins and peptides generally must be freeze-dried for clinical and commercial use. There are other technologies available to produce sterile dry powder drug products besides freeze-drying, such as sterile crystallization or spray-drying and powder filling. However, freeze-drying is by far the most common unit process for manufacturing drug products too unstable to be marketed as solutions.

The term "lyophilization" describes a process to produce a product that "loves the dry state". However, this term does not include the freezing process. Therefore, although lyophilization and freeze-drying are used interchangeably, freeze-drying is a more descriptive term. Equipment used to freeze-dry products are called freeze-dryers or lyophilizers.

Table 41-6 lists the advantages, features, and disadvantages of freeze-drying.

Freeze-drying essentially consists of:

Freezing stage: Freezing the product solution at a temperature below its eutectic (crystalline) or glass transition temperature

Primary drying stage: Removing the solvent (ice) from the product by evacuating the chamber, usually below 0.1torr (100 μm Hg) and subliming the ice onto a cold, condensing surface at a temperature below that of the product, the condensing surface being within the chamber or in a connecting chamber. During primary drying the temperature of the product must remain slightly below its critical temperature, called "collapse temperature." Collapse temperature is

---

Table 41-6. Advantages and Disadvantages of Freeze-Drying and Desirable Characteristics of the Finished Freeze-Dried Dosage Form

Advantages of Freeze-dried Products
1. Product is stored in dry state-few stability problems
2. Product is dried without elevated temperatures
3. Good for oxygen and/or air-sensitive drugs
4. Rapid reconstitution time
5. Constituents of the dried material remain homogenously dispersed
6. Product is process in the liquid form
7. Sterility of product can be achieved and maintained

Disadvantages of Freeze-dried Products
1. Volatile compounds may be removed by high vacuum
2. Single most expensive unit operation
3. Stability problems associated with individual drugs
4. Some issues associated with sterilization and sterility assurance of the dryer chamber and aseptic loading of vials into the chamber

Desired Characteristics of Freeze-Dried Products
- Intact cake
- Sufficient strength
- Uniform color
- Sufficiently dry
- Sufficiently porous
- Sterile
- Free of pyrogens
- Free of particulates
- Chemically stable

---

best measured by visual observation using a freeze-dry microscope that simulates the freeze-drying process. Generally, collapse temperature is similar to the eutectic or glass transition temperature of the product.

Secondary drying stage: Removing bound water from solute(s) to a level that assures long term stability of the product. This is accomplished by introducing heat to the product under controlled conditions, thereby providing additional energy to the product to remove adsorbed water. The temperature for secondary drying should be as high as possible without causing any chemical degradation of the active ingredient. Generally, for small molecules, the highest secondary drying temperature used is 40°C while for proteins it is no more than 30°C.

Figure 41-28 shows a photo and diagram of a small-scale lyophilization system and its functional components. The product may be frozen on the shelf in the chamber by circulating refrigerant (usually silicone) from the compressor through pipes within the shelf. After freezing is complete, which may require several hours, the chamber and condenser are evacuated by the vacuum pump, the condenser surface having been chilled previously by circulating refrigerant from the large compressor.

Heat then is introduced from the shelf to the product under graded control by electric resistance coils or by circulating silicone or glycol. Heat transfer proceeds from the shelf into the product vial and mass transfer (ice) proceeds from the product vial by sublimation through the chamber and onto the condenser. The process continues until the product is dry (usually 1% or less moisture except for some proteins that require a minimum amount of water for conformational stability), leaving a sponge-like matrix of the solids originally present in the product, the input of heat being controlled so as not to degrade the product.

For most pharmaceuticals and biologicals the liquid product is sterilized by filtration before being filled into the dosage container aseptically. The containers must remain open during the drying process to allow water vapor to escape; therefore, they must be protected from contamination during transfer from the filling area to the freeze-drying chamber, while in the freeze-drying chamber, and at the end of the drying process until sealed. Automated loading and unloading of product to and from the freeze-dryer shelves is now state-of-the-art where partially open vials are always under the auspices of Class 100 air and human intervention is eliminated.

Freeze-dryers are equipped with hydraulic or pneumatic internal-stoppering devices designed to push slotted rubber closures into the vials to be sealed while the chamber is still evacuated, the closures having been partially inserted immediately after filling, so that the slots were open to the outside. If internal stoppering is not available or containers such as ampoules are used, filtered dry air or nitrogen should be introduced into the chamber at the end of the process to establish atmospheric pressure.

Table 41-7 provides some guidance on a typical formulation approach and initial cycle chosen to freeze-dry a typical product.

FACTORS AFFECTING THE PROCESS RATE—From the diagram in Figure 41-29, it can be seen that the direction of heat and mass transfer causes the top of the product to dry first with drying proceeding downward to the bottom of the vial. Therefore, as drying proceeds, there exists a three component or layer system in each vial—the upper dry product, the middle sublimation front, and the lower frozen liquid product. As the dried layer increases, it becomes a greater barrier or the source of greatest resistance to the transfer of mass out of the vials. This points out the importance of vial dimensions and volume of product per vial on the efficiency of the freeze-drying process. If large volumes of solution must be processed, the surface area relative to the depth may be increased utilizing larger vials or by using such devices as freezing the container in a slanted position to increase the surface area.

The actual driving force for the process is the vapor pressure differential between the vapor at the surface where drying of the product is occurring (the drying boundary) and that at the surface of the ice on the condenser. The latter is determined by the temperature of the condenser as modified by the insulating

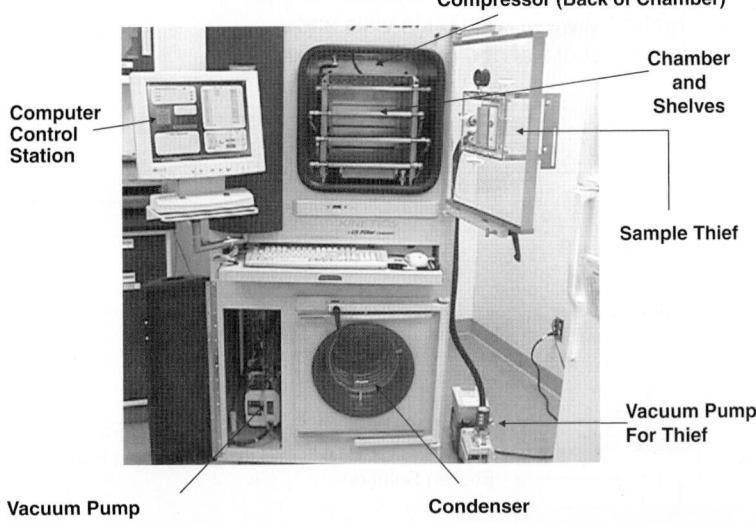

Figure 41-28. Example of a laboratory freeze-dryer (courtesy, Baxter). See Color Plate 14.

effect of the accumulated ice. The former is determined by a number of factors, including:

1. The rate of heat conduction through the container and the frozen material, both usually relatively poor thermal conductors, to the drying boundary while maintaining all of the product below its eutectic temperature
2. The impeding effect of the increasing depth of dried, porous product above the drying boundary
3. The temperature and heat capacity of the shelf itself

The passageways between the product surface and the condenser surface must be wide open and direct for effective oper-ation. The condensing surfaces in large freeze-dryers may be in the same chamber as the product or located in a separate chamber connected by a duct to the drying chamber. Evacuation of the system is necessary to reduce the impeding effect that collisions with air molecules would have on the passage of water molecules. However, the residual pressure in the system must be greater than the vapor pressure of the ice on the condenser or the ice will be vaporized and pulled into the pump, an event detrimental to most pumps.

The amount of solids in the product, the ice crystal size, and their thermal conductance will affect the rate of drying. The

Table 41-7. Practical Aspects of Freeze-Drying

- Have appropriate analytical tools and methods in place for formulation characterization and stability studies
- Depend on literature, previous experience (if none, use consultants), and what is known about the active ingredient, design and develop initial formulations, and conduct preliminary stability and compatibility studies
- Initial formulations should use commonly known excipients used in freeze-drying
  - that produce acceptable cakes with rapid reconstitution times
  - that have known minimal collapse temperatures
  - that provide the desired finished product with respect to nature of the final solid (crystalline or amorphous)
- Solids content should be between 5% and 30% with a target of 10% to 15%
- Should have several initial formulations to evaluate and compare. Usually know the qualitative, but not quantitative composition of additives until after initial comparative stability studies have been conducted
- Determine the maximum allowable temperature permitted during freezing and primary drying
  - Know eutectic, glass transition, and/or collapse temperatures, as appropriate
- Select the appropriate size of vial and product fill volume
- Select the appropriate rubber closure
  - Low water vapor transmission
  - No absorption of oil vapor
  - Top design minimizes sticking to shelf during/after stoppering
- Determine appropriate processing parameters
  - Rate of freezing
  - Set point temperatures during all three phases
  - Need for annealing
  - Pressure during primary drying
  - Pressure during secondary drying
  - Stopper seating conditions (eg, vacuum or gas)

- Optimize formulation and process based on stability information during and after freeze-drying and after storage in dry state
- Use a sample thief attachment for laboratory dryers to remove samples during the freeze-dry cycle in order to measure moisture, potency, or other parameters. Provides information for final selection of type and amount of stabilizer(s), if needed, and the cycle parameters necessary to provide an acceptable final moisture level in product
- Typical freeze-dry formulation components
  - Buffers: Phosphate, citrate, acetate
  - Stabilizers: Sucrose, trehalose, glycine
  - Bulking agents: Mannitol, lactose
  - Collapse temperature modifiers: Polymers, sugars
- Typical freeze-dry cycle (without knowing where to start)
  - Freezing phase
    - After loading, cool to 5°C
    - Decrease shelf temperature to −40°C
    - Hold for 2 hours
  - Primary drying phase
    - Must know collapse temperature(Tc)
    - Set shelf temperature approximately 20°C above Tc but making sure product temperature is 5°C below Tc
    - Maintain chamber pressure at 10% to 30% of vapor pressure of ice at the primary drying temperature (usually 100 to 200 microns)
    - Use temperature probes, pressure rise test, or dewpoint measurement to determine end of primary drying
  - Secondary drying
    - Use moderate to high vacuum (typically 100 microns)
    - Adjust shelf temperature to 25°C to 30°C for proteins; 35°C to 40°C for non proteins and hold for at least 4 hours
    - Adjust shelf temperature to 25°C or 5°C prior to stoppering, neutralizing, and unloading

Temperature difference between chamber and condenser
and pressure differential between solution in vials and
vacuum pump drives ice out of vial and onto the condenser

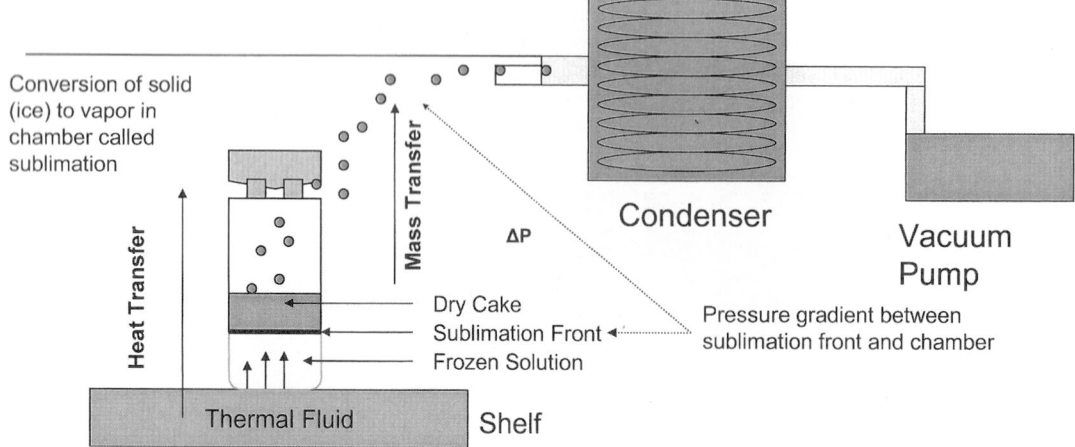

Figure 41-29. Heat and mass transfer in the freeze-dryer. See Color Plate 15.

more solids present, the more impediment will be provided to the escape of the water vapor. The degree of supercooling (how much lower the product temperature goes below its equilibrium freezing point before ice crystals first form) and the rate of ice crystallization define the freezing process and efficiency of primary drying. The larger the size of ice crystals formed, usually as a result of slow freezing, the larger the pore sizes are when the ice sublimes and, consequently, the faster will be the rate of drying. A high degree of supercooling will produce a large number of small ice crystals, a small pore size when the ice sublimes in the dried layer, and a greater resistance to water vapor transport during primary drying. The poorer the thermal conducting properties of the solids in the product, the slower will be the rate of heat transfer through the frozen material to the drying boundary.

The rate of drying is slow, most often requiring 24 hours or longer for completion. The actual time required, the rate of heat input, and the product temperatures that may be used must be determined for each product and then reproduced carefully with successive processes.

FACTORS AFFECTING FORMULATION—The active constituent of many pharmaceutical products is present in such a small quantity that if freeze-dried alone its presence would be hard to detect visually. In fact, the solids content of the original product ideally should be between 5% and 30%. Therefore, excipients often are added to increase the amount of solids. Such excipients are called "bulking agents"; the most commonly used bulking agent in freeze-dried formulations is mannitol. However, most freeze-dried formulations must contain other excipients because of the need to buffer the product and/or to protect the active ingredient from the adverse effects of freezing and/or drying. Thus, buffering agents such as sodium or potassium phosphate, sodium acetate and sodium citrate are commonly used in freeze-dried formulations. Sucrose, trehalose, dextran, and amino acids such as glycine are commonly used lyoprotectants.

Each of these substances contribute to the appearance characteristics of the plug, such as whether dull and spongy or sparkling and crystalline, firm or friable, expanded or shrunken, and uniform or striated. Therefore, the formulation of a product to be freeze-dried must include consideration not only of the nature and stability characteristics required during the liquid state, both freshly prepared and when reconstituted before use, but also the characteristics desired in the dried plug.

MODIFICATIONS IN THE PROCESS AND EQUIPMENT—In some instances a product may be frozen in a bulk container or in trays rather than in the final container and then handled as a bulk solid. Such a state requires a continuation of aseptic processing conditions as long as the product is exposed to the environment.

When large quantities of material are processed it may be desirable to use ejection pumps in the equipment system. These draw the vapor into the pump and eject it to the outside, thereby eliminating the need for a condensing surface. Such pumps are expensive and usually practical only in large installations.

Available freeze-dryers (suppliers: *BOC Edwards, FTS, Hull, Serail, Stokes, Usifroid, Virtis*) range in size from small laboratory units to large industrial models such as the one shown in Figures 41-30 and 41-31. Their selection requires consideration of such factors as

- The tray area required
- The volume of water to be removed
- How the chamber will be sterilized

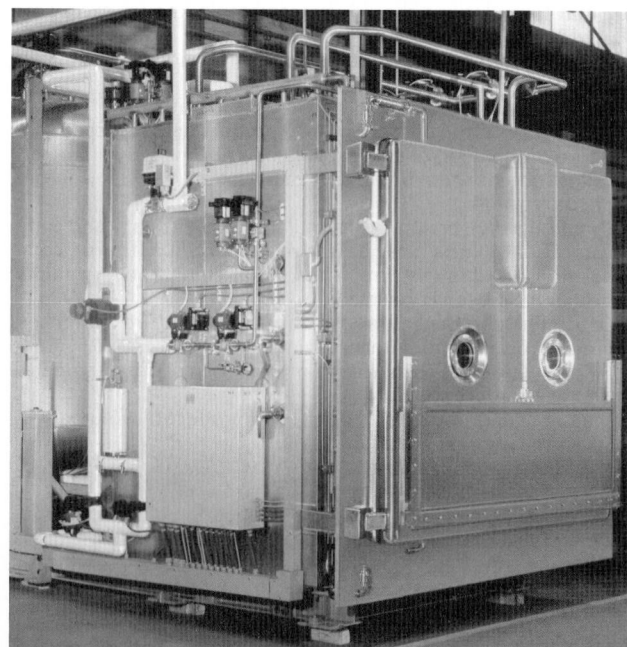

Figure 41-30. Example of a production freeze-dryer (courtesy, Edwards). See Color Plate 16.

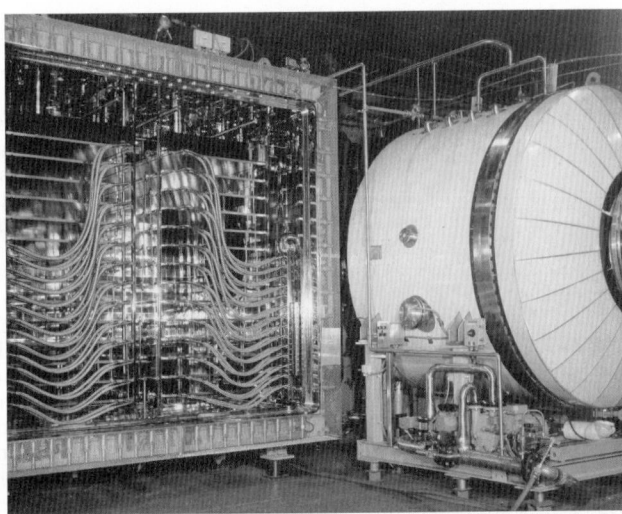

Figure 41-31. Inside view of a production freeze-dryer (courtesy, Edwards). See Color Plate 17.

- Whether internal stoppering is required
- Whether separate freezers will be used for initial freezing and condensation of the product
- The degree of automatic operation desired

Other factors involved in the selection and use of equipment are considered in the literature.[33]

Freeze-drying is being used now for research in the preservation of human tissue and is finding increasing application in the food industry. Most biopharmaceuticals require lyophilization to stabilize their protein content effectively. Therefore, many newer developments in the lyophilization process focus on the requirements of this new class of drug products.

QUALITY ASSURANCE AND CONTROL

The importance of undertaking every possible means to ensure the quality of the finished product cannot be overemphasized. Every component and step of the manufacturing process must be subjected to intense scrutiny to be confident that quality is attained in the finished product. The responsibility for achieving this quality is divided appropriately in concept and practice into Quality Assurance (QA) and Quality Control (QC). QA relates to the studies made and the plans developed for ensuring quality of a product prospectively, with a final confirmation of achievement. QC embodies the carrying out of these plans during production and includes all of the tests and evaluations performed to be sure that quality exists in a specific lot of product.

The principles for achieving quality are basically the same for the manufacture of any pharmaceutical. These are discussed in Chapter 51 (*Quality Assurance and Control*). During the discussion of the preparation of injections in this chapter, mention was made of numerous quality requirements for components and manufacturing processes. Here, only selected tests characteristically required before a finished parenteral product is released are discussed briefly, including sterility, pyrogen, and particulate tests.

STERILITY TEST

All lots of injectables in their final containers must be tested for sterility, except for products that are allowed to apply parametric release.‡ The USP prescribes the requirements for this test for official injections. The FDA uses these requirements as a guide for testing official sterile products. The primary official test is performed by means of filtration, but direct transfer is used if membrane filtration is unsuitable. To give greater as-

surance that viable microorganisms will grow, if present, the USP requires that all lots of culture media be tested for their growth-promotion capabilities. However it must be recognized that the reliability of both test methods has the inherent limitations typical of microbial recovery tests. Therefore, it should be noted that this test is not intended as a thoroughly evaluative test for a product subjected to a sterilization method of unknown effectiveness. It is intended primarily as a check test on the probability that a previously validated sterilization procedure has been repeated or to give assurance of its continued effectiveness. A discussion of sterility testing is given in Chapter 40 (*Sterilization*).

In the event of a sterility-test failure, the immediate issue concerns whether the growth observed came from viable microorganisms in the product (true contamination) or from adventitious contamination during the testing (a false positive). The USP does not permit a retest, unless specific evidence is discovered to suggest contamination occurred during the test. Therefore, a thorough investigation must be launched to support the justification for performing the retest and assessing the validity of the retest results relative to release of the lot of product.

It should be noted that a *lot* with respect to sterility testing is that group of product containers that has been subjected to the same sterilization procedure. For containers of a product that have been sterilized by autoclaving, for example, a lot would constitute those processed in a particular sterilizer cycle. For an aseptic filling operation, a lot would constitute all of those product containers filled during a period when there was no change in the filling assembly or equipment and which is no longer than one working day or shift.

As stated previously, isolator technology has been applied to significantly reduced the incidence of false positives in the conductance of the sterility test. An example of a sterility testing isolator is shown in Figure 41-32. Validation of isolator systems for sterility testing is described in USP <1208>.

---

‡Parametric release means that a lot of product, if terminally sterilized by a well-defined, fully validated sterilization process, has a sterility assurance level sufficient to omit the sterility test for release. [34]

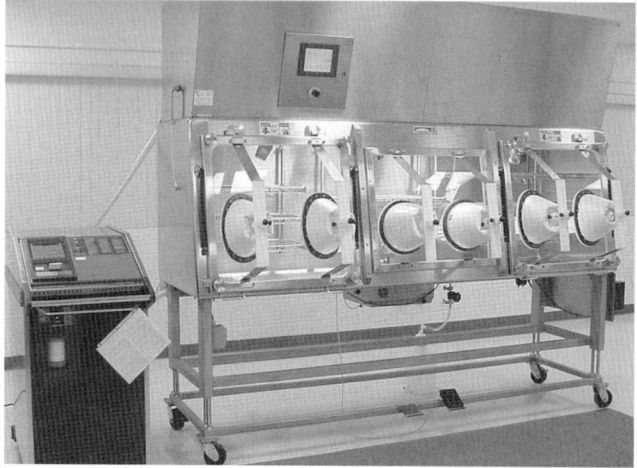

Figure 41-32. Example of an isolator used for sterility testing (courtesy, Baxter). See Color Plate 18.

PYROGEN TEST

The USP evaluates the presence of pyrogens in parenteral preparations by a qualitative fever response test in rabbits, the Pyrogen Test (Section <151>), and by the Bacterial Endotoxins Test (Section <85>). These two USP tests are described in Chapter 40 (*Sterilization*). Rabbits are used as test animals in Section <151> because they show a physiological response to pyrogenic substances similar to that of man. While a minimum pyrogenic dose (MPD), the amount just sufficient to cause a positive USP Pyrogen Test response, sometimes may produce uncertain test results, a content equal to a few times the MPD will leave no uncertainty. Therefore, the test is valid and has continued in use since introduced by Seibert in 1923. It should be understood that not all injections

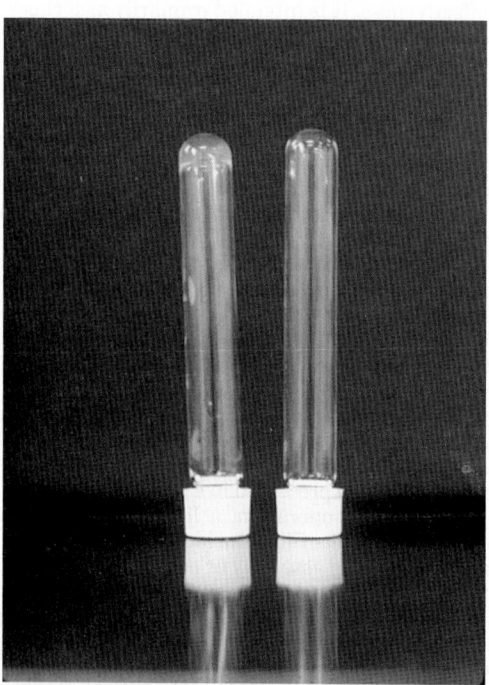

Figure 41-33. Example of positive (left tube) endotoxin test.

may be subjected to the rabbit test, since the medicinal agent may have a physiological effect on the test animal such that any fever response would be masked.

The *Bacterial Endotoxins Test* (BET) is an *in vitro* test based on the formation of a gel or the development of color in the presence of bacterial endotoxins and the lysate of the amebocytes of the horseshoe crab *(Limulus polyphemus)*. The *Limulus Amebocyte Lysate* (LAL) test, as it also is called, is a biochemical test performed in a test tube and is simpler, more rapid, and of greater sensitivity than the rabbit test. An example of a positive endotoxin test result in a test tube is shown in Figure 41-33. Although it detects only the endotoxic pyrogens of gram-negative bacteria, these are the most prominent environmental microbial contaminants likely to invade sterile products. The test has been automated and can determine the quantitative amount of endotoxin in a sample. This test has enabled endotoxin limits to be established on finished products and bulk drug substances and excipients.

To provide standardization for the test, the USP has established a reference standard endotoxin (RSE) against which lots of the lysate are standardized. Thus, the sensitivity of the lysate is given in terms of endotoxin units (EU). Most USP injections now have been given limits in terms of EUs (eg, Bacteriostatic Sodium Chloride Injection, 1.0 EU/mL), thus indicating an increasing priority for the BET in testing for the presence of endotoxin in parenteral products and in medical devices.

PARTICULATE EVALUATION

Particulate matter in parenteral solutions long has been recognized as unacceptable since the user could be expected to conclude that the presence of visible *dirt* would suggest that the product is of inferior quality. Today, it is recognized that the presence of particles in solution, particularly if injected intravenously, can be harmful. While data defining the extent of risk and the effects produced still are limited, it has been shown that particles of lint, rubber, insoluble chemicals, and other foreign matter can produce emboli in the vital organs of animals and man. Further, it has been shown that the development of infusion phlebitis may be related to the presence of particulate matter in intravenous fluids.

The particle size of particular concern has not been clearly delineated, but it has been suggested that since erythrocytes have a diameter of approximately 4.5 μm, particles of more than 5 μm should be the basis for evaluation. This is a considerably smaller particle than can be seen with the unaided eye; approximately 50 μm is the lower limit unless the Tyndall effect is used whereby particles as small as 10 μm can be seen by the light scattered from them.

The USP specifies that good manufacturing practice requires each final container of an injection be subjected individually to a visual inspection and containers in which visible particles can be seen should be discarded. This 100% inspection of a lot of product is designed to prevent the distribution and use of parenterals that contain particulate matter. Therefore, all of the product units from a production line currently are being inspected individually by human inspectors under a good light, baffled against reflection into the eye and against a black-and-white background. This inspection is subject to the limitation of the size of particles that can be seen, the variation of visual acuity from inspector to inspector, their emotional state, eye strain, fatigue, and other personal factors that will affect what is seen. However, it does provide a means for eliminating the few units that normally contain visible particles. Automated inspection machines increasingly are being used today.

The assessment of the level of particulate matter below the visible size of about 50 μm has become an increasingly used QC indicator of process cleanliness in the manufacture of injections. The tests used, however, are destructive of container units. Therefore, they are performed on appropriately selected samples of products. Further, all of these methods require very

Table 41-8. Subvisible Particulate Matter Limits in Injectable Products

COMPENDIA	LVI/SVI	METHOD	$\geq 10 \mu m$	$\geq 25 \mu m$
USP	LVI	Light Blockage	25 part/mL	3 part/mL
		Microscope	12 part/mL	2 part/mL
USP	SVI	Light Blockage	6000 part/contain.	600 part/contain.
		Microscope	3000 part/contain.	300 part/contain.
EP	LVI	Light Blockage	25 part/mL	3 part/mL
	SVI Soln	Light Blockage	6000 part/contain.	600 part/contain.
	SVI Powder	Light Blockage	10000 part/contain.	1000 part/contain.
BP	LVP	Coulter Counter	1000 part/mL $\geq 2 \mu m$	100 part/mL $\geq 5 \mu m$
		Light Blockage	500 part/mL $\geq 2 \mu m$	80 part/mL $\geq 5 \mu m$
JP	LVP	Microscope	20 part/mL	2 part/mL

stringent, ultraclean preparation techniques to ensure accuracy in the counting and sizing of particles only in the product, rather than those that may have been introduced inadvertently during the sample preparation or the testing procedure.

The USP has identified two test methods in <788>, *Particulate Matter in Injections*. All LVIs for single-dose infusion and those SVIs for which the monograph specifies a limit (primarily those commonly added to infusion solutions) are subject to the specified limits given in Table 41–8. The first test to be used is the light obscuration test, which uses an electronic instrument designed to count and measure the size of particles by means of a shadow cast by the particle as it passes through a high-intensity light beam (suppliers: *Climet, HIAC/Royco*). If the injection formulation is not a clear, colorless solution (eg, an emulsion) or it exceeds the limits specified for the light obscuration test, it is to be subjected to the microscopic count test. The latter method consists of filtering a measured sample of solution through a membrane filter under ultraclean conditions and then counting the particles on the surface of the filter, using a microscope and oblique light at 100× magnification. The time requirements for performing the latter test are very long. These standards are being met readily in the US today by the manufacturers of LVIs and the specified SVIs.

Whether or not these standards are realistic toxicologically has not been established; rather, the objective of the compendium is to establish specification limits that would encourage the preparation of clean parenteral solutions, particularly those to be given intravenously.

It also should be realized that administration sets and the techniques used for preparing and administering intravenous infusion fluids may introduce substantial amounts of particulate matter into an otherwise clean solution. Therefore, the pharmaceutical manufacturer, the administration set manufacturer, the pharmacist, the nurse, and the physician must share responsibility for making sure that the patient receives a clean intravenous injection.

CONTAINER/CLOSURE INTEGRITY TEST

Ampoules that have been sealed by fusion must be subjected to a test to determine whether or not a passageway remains to the outside; if so, all or a part of the contents may leak to the outside and spoil the package, or microorganisms or other contaminants may enter. Changes in temperature during storage cause expansion and contraction of the ampoule and contents, and will accentuate interchange if a passageway exists, even if microscopic in size.

This test usually is performed by producing a negative pressure within an incompletely sealed ampoule while the ampoule is submerged entirely in a deeply colored dye solution. Most often, approximately 1% methylene blue solution is employed. After carefully rinsing the dye solution from the outside, color from the dye will be visible within a leaker. Leakers, of course, are discarded.

Vials and bottles are not subjected to such a leaker test because the sealing material (rubber stopper) is not rigid. Therefore, results from such a test would be meaningless. However, assurance of container-closure sealing integrity should be an integral part of product development by developing specifications for the fit of the closure in the neck of the container, the physical characteristics of the closure, the need for lubrication of the closure, and the capping pressure.

Container-closure integrity tests are summarized in Table 41-9.[32]

SAFETY TEST

The National Institutes of Health requires of most biological products routine safety testing in animals. Under the Kefauver-Harris Amendments to the Federal Food, Drug, and Cosmetic Act, most pharmaceutical preparations are now required to be tested for safety. Because it is entirely possible for a parenteral product to pass the routine sterility test, pyrogen test, and chemical analyses, and still cause unfavorable reactions when injected, a safety test in animals is essential, particularly for biological products, to provide additional assurance that the product does not have unexpected toxic properties.

PACKAGING AND LABELING

A full discussion of the packaging of parenteral preparations is beyond the scope of this text. It is essential, of course, that the packaging should provide ample protection for the product against physical damage from shipping, handling, and storage as well as protecting light-sensitive materials from ultraviolet radiation.

PACKAGING—The USP includes certain requirements for the packaging and storage of injections, as follows:

1. The volume of injection in single-dose containers is defined as that which is specified for parenteral administration at one time and is limited to a volume of 1 L.
2. Parenterals intended for intraspinal, intracisternal, or peridural administration are packaged only in single-dose containers.
3. Unless an individual monograph specifies otherwise, no multiple-dose container shall contain a volume of injection more than sufficient to permit the withdrawal and administration of 30 mL.
4. Injections packaged for use as irrigation solutions or for hemofiltration or dialysis or for parenteral nutrition are exempt from the foregoing requirements relating to packaging. Containers for injections packaged for use as hemofiltration or irrigation solutions may be designed to empty rapidly and may contain a volume in excess of 1 L.
5. Injections intended for veterinary use are exempt from the packaging and storage requirements concerning the limitation to single-dose containers and to volume of multiple-dose containers.

LABELING—The labeling of an injection must provide the physician or other user with all of the information needed to ensure the safe and proper use of the product. Since all of this in-

Table 41-9. Container-Closure Integrity Tests

TEST	BASIC PRINCIPLE	ADVANTAGES	DISADVANTAGES
Acoustic Imaging (Sonoscan.com)	Ultrasonic energy focused onto sample submerged in water or other solvent. Echo patterns produce images of package material interior	Visualize delamination, channels Mostly applies to microchip technology	Expensive Sample must be immersed Slow, requires expertise Not for porous materials
Bubble Test	Submerge package in liquid, pressurize and/or temperature cycling to accelerate leakage, improvement sensitivity	Simple Inexpensive Location of leaks can be observed Good troubleshooting technique	Relatively insensitive Operator dependent Wets package seal Qualitative
Gas Tracer Detection (Mocon.com)	Test tracer gas is placed on one side of container seal. Inert carrier gas passed along opposite seal side. Tracer gas is detected either by a coulombic detector (Oxygen) or by photoelectric sensor (Water or Carbon Dioxide). Instruments designed to pierce containers and test package headspace for oxygen or carbon dioxide are another type of gas detection method	Directly relates to package performance Does not pick up false leaks as helium detection can Used on screw-cap bottles, blister packs, polymer and foi pouches	Slow Often fixture dependent
Helium Mass Spectrometry (alcatelvacuum.com) (inficon.com) (varian.com)	Helium is place either inside or outside of the container. Vacuum is applied to seal interface and migrating helium is detected by mass spectrometry	Inert gas Extremely sensitive test Rapid test time Quantitative	May confuse helium diffusion with leakage Expensive and expertise Helium bombing takes time May be destructive
High-Voltage Leak Detection (HVLD) (nikkadensok.com)	High frequency, high voltage is applied to seal container. Increase in conductivity correlated to presence of liquid along the seal	100% automatic inspection Clean, non-destructive Rapid Used for ampoules, vials, syringes, blow/fill/seal containers	Difficult to validate with st'd defects Requires liquid-fill product
Liquid Tracer Tests	Package immersed in solution of tracer chemical or dye. Pressure/vacuum or temperature cycling used to improve sensitivity. Leakage detected visually (dye) or instrumentally (dye or chemical)	Correlates to liquid leakage and microbial ingress Operator independent (instrum method) Inexpensive Simple to perform	Destructive Human variability (dye) Large sample numbers needed Slow
Microbial Challenge	Containers are media filled and the seal is either challenged directly with microorganisms or is allowed to sit in ambient storage environment. Presence of microbial growth is visually confirmed	May provide direct correlation to microbial integrity No special equipment required Airbone challenge best approach for tortuous seal tests Widely used in the industry	Insensitive Expensive in time, storage and resources Slow
Noninvasive Moisture and Oxygen Analysis (foss-nirsystems.com)	Method 1: Moisture by NIR spectroscopy Measures powder moisture inside unopened glass package Method 2: oxygen and moisture Tunable diode laser light passed through package headspace. Frequency of light matched to oxygen or water. Absorbed light proportional to headspace contents	Nondestructive Rapid Sensitive to trace moisure Simple Used for lyophilized and powder filled pdts	Calibration unique for each type of product
Residual Gas Ionization Test (Electro-Technic Pdts)	High voltage, high frequency field is applied to vials sealed under vacuum. The field causes residual gas to glow. Glow intensity is function of vacuum level.	On-line, non-destructive test Rapid Used for lyophilized products	Unknown sensitivity Inconsistencies in results

(continues)

Table 41-9. *Continued*

TEST	BASIC PRINCIPLE	ADVANTAGES	DISADVANTAGES
Residual Seal Force (dynatup.com) (genmap.com)	Vials sealed with closures are compressed at a constant rate of strain. Stress-strain deformation curves generated. Second derivative of the curve = residual seal force	Measures closure forces post compression Non-destructive (plastic cap removed) No human error Qualitative measure; simple	Residual seal force variable Very dependent on rubber material and history
Vacuum/Pressure Decay (packagingtechnologies.com) (wilco.com) (tmelectronics.com)	Change in pressure or vacuum measured inside package (destructive) or outside in a sealed package chamber (nondestructive). Pressure/vacuum change significantly greater than non-leaking package indicative of a reject	Clean Non-destructive (test chamber method) Relevant to shipping/distribution Sensitivity good for leaks >5 microns Rapid test	Difficult to detect leaks <5 mic Some package headspace needed
Visual Inspection (seidenader.de)	Look for leaks	Simple Inexpensive	Insensitive Operator Dependent Qualitative
Weight Change	Container is filled with liquid or dessicant, sealed, stored at various stress conditions, and reweighed over time	Easy Directly relates to closure performance Quantitative Inexpensive	Time consuming Leak location not detected

From Akers MJ, Larrimore DS, Guazzo DM. *Parenteral Quality Control.* New York: Dekker, 2002, pp 310–319.

formation cannot be placed on the immediate container and be legible, it may be provided on accompanying printed matter.

A restatement of the labeling definitions and requirements of the USP for Injections is as follows:

The term *labeling* designates all labels and other written, printed, or graphic matter upon an immediate container or upon, or in, any package or wrapper in which it is enclosed, with the exception of the outer shipping container. The term *label* designates that part of the labeling upon the immediate container.

The label states the name of the preparation, the percentage content of drug of a liquid preparation, the amount of active ingredient of a dry preparation, the volume of liquid to be added to prepare an injection or suspension from a dry preparation, the route of administration, a statement of storage conditions, and an expiration date. The label must state the name of the vehicle and the proportions of each constituent, if it is a mixture; the names and proportions of all substances added to increase stability or usefulness.

Also, the label must indicate the name of the manufacturer or distributor and carry an identifying lot number. The lot number is capable of providing access to the complete manufacturing history of the specific package, including each single manufacturing step. The container label is so arranged that a sufficient area of the container remains uncovered for its full length or circumference to permit inspection of the contents.

Preparations labeled for use as dialysis, hemofiltration, or irrigation solutions must meet the requirements for injections other than those relating to volume and also must bear on the label statements that they are not intended for intravenous injection. Injections intended for veterinary use are so labeled.

REFERENCES

1. Yalkowsky SH, Krzyzaniak JF, Ward GH. *J Pharm Sci* 1998; 87:787.
2. Mottu F, Laurent A, Rufenacht DA, et al: *PDA J Parenteral Sci Tech* 2000; 54:456.
3. Nema S, Washkuhn R, Brendel RJ. *PDA J Parenteral Sci Tech* 1997; 51:166.
4. Powell MF, Nguyen T, Baloian L. *PDA J Parenteral Sci Tech* 1998; 52:238.
5. Strickley RG. *PDA J Parenteral Sci Tech* 1999; 53:324.
6. Strickley RG. *PDA J Parenteral Sci Tech* 2000; 54:69.
7. Strickley RG. *PDA J Parenteral Sci Tech* 2000; 54:152.
8. Kibbe AH, ed. *Pharmaceutical Excipients 2000.* Washington DC: The Pharmaceutical Press, American Pharmaceutical Association, 2000.
9. Akers MJ. *J Pharm Sci* 2002; 91:2283.
10. Sutton SVW, Porter D. *PDA J Parenteral Sci Tech* 2002; 56:300.
11. Carpenter JF, Crowe JH. *Cryobiology* 1988; 25:244.
12. Carpenter JF, Chang BS, Garzon-Rodriquez W, et al. Rational design of stable lyophilized protein formulations: theory and practice. In: Carpenter JF, Manning MC, eds. *Rational Design of Stable Protein Formulations.* New York: Kluwer Academic, 2002, chap 5.
13. Joint Commission on Accreditation of Healthcare Organizations. *The Complete Guide.* Chicago: JCAHO, 1997.
14. Trissel LA. *Handbook on Injectable Drugs,* 12th ed. Bethesda, MD: ASHP, 2003
15. Collentro WV. *Pharmaceutical Water System Design, Operation, and Validation.* Englewood, CO: Interpharm Press (now CRC Press), 1998.
16. Walther M, Rupertus V, Seemann C, et al. *PDA J Pharm Sci Tech* 2002; 56:124.
17. Jenke D. *PDA J Pharm Sci Tech* 2002; 56:332.
18. Turco S, King RE. *Sterile Dosage Forms,* 3rd ed. Philadelphia: Lea & Febiger, 1987.
19. Grandics P. *Pharm Tech* 2000; 25:26.
20. Davenport SM. *J Parenter Sci Technol* 1989; 43:158.
21. Noble N, et al. *Pharm Engr* 1996; 16(4):8.
22. Farquaharson G, Whyte W. *PDA J Pharm Sci Tech* 2000; 54:33.
23. Howorth H. *J Parenteral Sci Tech* 1988; 42:14.
24. Akers MJ. Good aseptic practices: Education and training of personnel involved in aseptic processing. In: Groves MJ, Murty R, eds. *Aseptic Pharmaceutical Manufacturing II.* Englewood, CO: Interpharm Press (now CRC Press), 1995, chap 8.
25. Whyte W, Niven L. *J Parenter Sci Technol* 1986; 40: 182.
26. Whyte W. *PDA J Pharm Sci Technol* 50: 210, 1996.
27. Akers JE. *PDA J Pharm Sci Tech* 2002; 56:283.
28. *Sterile Drug Products Produced by Aseptic Processing—Current Good Manufacturing Practice*—Draft Guidance, August 2003.
29. LeBlanc DA. *Validated Cleaning Technologies for Pharmaceutical Manufacturing,* Boca Raton, FL: CRC Press, 2000.
30. Sundaram S, Eisenhuth J, Howard G Jr, et al. *PDA J Pharm Sci Tech* 2001; 55:65.
31. Sundaram S, Eisenhuth, J, Howard G Jr, et al. *PDA J Pharm Sci Tech* 2002; 55:346.
32. Guazzo D. Container-closure integrity testing. In: Akers MJ, Larrimore D, Guazzo D, eds. *Parenteral Quality Control: Sterility, Pyrogen, Particulate, and Package Integrity Testing.* New York: Marcel Dekker, 2002, chap 4.
33. Nail SL, Jiang S, Chongprasert S, et al: Fundamentals of freeze-drying. In: Nail SL, Akers MJ, eds. *Development and Manufacture of Protein Pharmaceuticals.* New York: Marcel Dekker, 2002, chap 6.
34. PDA Technical Report No. 30. *PDA J Pharm Sci Tech* 53:217.

BIBLIOGRAPHY

Akers MJ, Larrimore D, Guazzo DM. *Parenteral Quality Control*, 3rd ed. New York: Dekker, 2002.

Avis KE. In: *The Theory and Practice of Industrial Pharmacy*, 3rd ed, Lachman L, et al. Philadelphia: Lea & Febiger, 1986, chaps 21 & 22.

Avis KE, Lieberman HA, Lachman L, eds. *Pharmaceutical Dosage Forms: Parenteral Medications,* 2nd ed, vols 1 - 3. New York: Dekker, 1992–1993.

Avis KE, Wagner C, Wu V, eds. *Biotechnology: Quality Assurance and Validation Drug Manufacturing Technology Series,* vol 4. Boca Raton: CRC Press, 1998.

Barber T. *Control of Particulate Matter Contamination in Healthcare Manufacturing.* Englewood, CO: Interpharm Press (now CRC Press), 2000.

Block SS, ed. *Disinfection, Sterilization and Preservation,* 4th ed. Philadelphia: Lea & Febiger, 1991.

Carpenter JF, Manning MC, eds. *Rational Design of Stable Protein Formulations.* New York, Kluwer Academic/Plenum, 2002.

Carleton FJ, Agalloco JP, eds. *Validation of Aseptic Pharmaceutical Processes,* 2nd ed. New York: Dekker, 1998.

Coles T. *Isolation Technology: A Practical Guide.* Englewood, CO: Interpharm Press (now CRC Press), 1999.

Kuhlman H, Coleman D. In: *Sterile Pharmaceutical Products: Process Engineering Applications.* Avis KE, ed. Buffalo Grove, IL: Interpharm Press (now CRC Press), 1995.

Jennings T. *Lyophilization: Introduction and Basic Principles.* Boca Raton: CRC Press, 1999.

Luungqvist B, Reinmuller B. *Clean Room Design: Mimimizing Contamination Through Proper Design.* Boca Raton: CRC Press, 1996.

Meltzer TH. *High Purity Water Preparation for the Semiconductor, Pharmaceutical and Power Industries.* Littleton, CO: Tall Oaks, 1993.

Meltzer TH, Jornitz, MW, eds. *Filtration in the Biopharmaceutical Industry.* New York: Dekker, 1998.

Nail SL, Akers MJ, eds. *Development and Manufacture of Protein Pharmaceuticals.* New York, Kluwers Academic/Plenum, 2002.

Parenteral Drug Association Technical Reports, www.pda.org

Pearson FC III. *Pyrogens.* New York: Dekker, 1985.

Phillips GB, Miller WS, eds. *Industrial Sterilization.* Durham, NC: Duke University Press, 1973.

Swarbrick J, Boylan JC, eds. *Encyclopedia of Pharmaceutical Technology,* 2nd ed. New York: Dekker, 2002.

Turco S, King RE. *Sterile Dosage Forms,* 3rd ed. Philadelphia: Lea & Febiger, 1987.

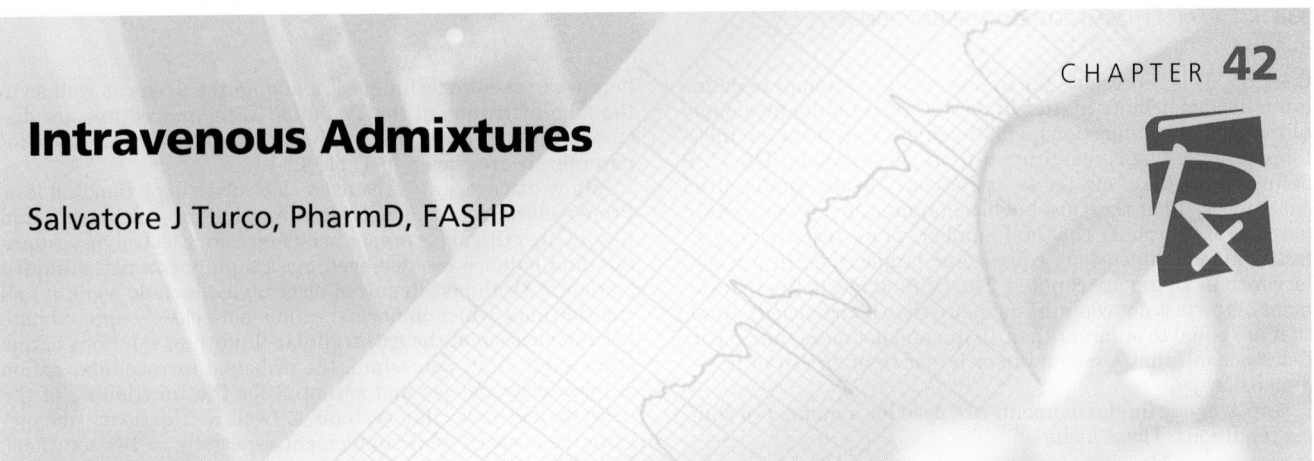

CHAPTER 42

Intravenous Admixtures

Salvatore J Turco, PharmD, FASHP

It has been estimated that 40% of all drugs administered in hospitals are given in the form of injections, and their use is increasing. Part of this increase in parenteral therapy is due to the wider use of intravenous fluids (IV fluids). In the last decade the use of IV fluids has doubled, increasing from 150 million units to 320 million units annually. Not only do IV fluids continue to serve as the means for fluid replacement, electrolyte-balance restoration, and supplementary nutrition, they also are playing major roles as vehicles for administration of other drug substances and in total parenteral nutrition (PN). Intravenous fluids are finding greater use as the means of administering other drugs because of convenience, the means of reducing the irritation potential of the drugs, and the desirability for continuous and intermittent drug therapy.

The techniques for providing PN parenterally have improved steadily in the last decade, and such use is increasing. The use of IV fluids for these purposes requires the compounding of specific intravenous admixtures (parenteral prescriptions) to meet the clinical needs of a given patient. However, the combination of drug substances in an IV fluid can promote parenteral incompatibilities and give rise to conditions not favorable for drug stability. A new area of specialization has been created for hospital pharmacists who can develop the expertise to prepare these solutions—recognizing their compatibility and stability problems and the potential for contamination—and participate in the administration of the solutions. The complex compounding of an order for PN requires knowledgeable personnel capable of making accurate calculations, compounding, and having aseptic technique. The parenteral prescription is becoming increasingly important in hospitals. Centralized admixture programs are now found in 90% of the nation's hospitals with 300 beds or more. Equipment available for administering IV fluids has become more sophisticated and has made possible increased accuracy of dosage and led to the development of new concepts and methods of nutrition and drug therapy.

Electronic mechanical equipment is now commonplace in hospitals. Its use, as well as its sophistication, continues to increase. Newly designed electronic pumps have been developed for hospital ambulatory use. Multichannel pumps have become available for multiple-drug infusion. Over 500,000 implantable infusion ports have been inserted into patients and 100,000 new patients receive these implantable ports each year to accomplish drug therapy. New methods of IV drug delivery systems have been introduced and are constantly evolving. The introduction of patient-controlled analgesia (PCA) is commonplace in hospitals. This technology allows the patient with pain to control the degree of analgesia.

The growth of PN in hospitals has been paralleled by home PN programs. Large numbers of patients conduct parenteral nutrition in the home environment, including those with infectious and neoplastic diseases. More-stringent and more-complete guidelines for the preparation of parenterals in hospitals by pharmacists have been published. These guidelines, promoting sophisticated methods of preparation by the pharmacist, have become recommendations. They are a testament to the importance of parenteral preparation in the institutional setting. Packaging of parenterals in the past 5 years also has undergone dramatic changes. Prefilled, premixed, prefrozen parenterals are now supplied by the manufacturers. Plastic minibags (ADD-Vantage, *Abbott*) have been introduced. Premixed liquids (eg, antibiotics, theophylline, heparin, lidocaine, dopamine) are available from parenteral manufacturers. Multiple-dose containers have been developed to accommodate new methods of preparation of parenterals by the pharmacist. The pharmaceutical industry has responded to the needs of pharmacists by addressing the packaging, labeling, and design requirements necessary to facilitate patient care. The parenteral drug industry continues its efforts to meet higher standards of quality and to ensure the availability of sterile and particulate-free products.

INTRAVENOUS FLUIDS

Large-volume injections intended to be administered by intravenous infusion commonly are called IV fluids and are included in the group of sterile products referred to as large-volume parenterals. These consist of single-dose injections having a volume of 100 mL or more and containing no added substances. Intravenous fluids are packaged in containers having a capacity of 100 to 1000 mL. Minitype infusion containers of 250-mL capacity are available with 50- and 100-mL partial fills for solution of drugs used in the *piggyback* technique (ie, the administration of a second solution through a Y-tube in the administration set of the first intravenous fluid, thus avoiding the need for another injection site). In addition to the IV fluids, this group also includes irrigation solutions and solutions for dialysis.

Intravenous fluids are sterile solutions of simple chemicals such as sugars, amino acids, or electrolytes—materials that easily can be carried by the circulatory system and assimilated. Prepared with Water for Injection USP, the solutions are pyrogen-free. Because of the large volumes administered intravenously, the absence of particulate matter assumes a significant role in view of possible biological hazards resulting from insoluble particles. Absence of particulate matter or clarity of IV fluids is as important at the time of administration following their manipulation in the hospital as it is at the time of manufacture of the injection.

Limits for particulate matter occurring in IV fluids or large-volume injections used for single-dose infusion are defined in the USP. This represents the first regulatory attempt to define limits for particulate matter in parenterals. Limits also apply to multiple-dose injections, small-volume injections, or injections prepared by reconstitution from sterile solids. The USP defines particulate matter as extraneous, mobile, undissolved substances, other than gas bubbles, unintentionally present in parenteral solutions. The total numbers of particles having effective linear dimensions equal to or larger than 10 μm and larger than 25 μm are counted. The IV fluid meets the requirement of the test if it contains not more than 50 particles per mL that are equal to or larger than 10 μm and not more than 5 particles per mL that are equal to or larger than 25 μm in linear dimension.

Intravenous fluids commonly are used for a number of clinical conditions. These include:

Correction of disturbances in electrolyte balance.
Correction of disturbances in body fluids (fluid replacement).
The means of providing basic nutrition.
The basis for the practice of providing PN.
Vehicles for other drug substances.

In both of the latter two cases it has become common practice to add other drugs to certain IV fluids to meet the clinical needs of the patient. Using IV fluids as vehicles offers the advantages of convenience, the means of reducing the irritation potential of the drug, and a method for continuous drug therapy. However, the practice requires that careful consideration be given to the stability and compatibility of additives present in the IV fluids serving as the vehicle. This approach also demands strict ad-

herence to aseptic techniques in adding the drugs as well as in the administration of the IV fluids. These procedures are discussed later in the chapter. The IV fluids commonly used for parenterals are shown in Table 42-1.

Many disease states result in electrolyte depletion and loss. Proper electrolyte concentration and balance in plasma and tissues are critical for proper body function. Electrolyte restoration and balance are achieved most rapidly through administration of IV fluids. Required electrolytes include sodium and chloride ions, which in normal saline more closely approximate the composition of the extracellular fluid than solutions of any other single salt; potassium, the principal intracellular cation of most body tissues and essential for the functioning of the nervous and muscular systems as well as the heart; magnesium, as a nutritional supplement especially in PN solutions; and phosphate ion, important in a variety of biochemical reactions. In addition to the number of standard electrolyte fluids shown in Table 42-1, a large number of combinations of electrolytes in varying concentrations are available commercially. Some of these electrolyte fluids also contain dextrose.

Dextrose Injection 5% (D5/W) is the most frequently used IV fluid, either for nutrition or for fluid replacement. It is slightly hypotonic and administered intravenously into a peripheral vein; 1 g of dextrose provides 3.4 cal, and 1 L of D5/W supplies 170 Kcal. The body uses dextrose at a rate of 0.5 g per kg of body weight per hour. More-rapid administration can result in glycosuria. Therefore, 1 L of D5/W requires 1 1/2 hr for assimilation. The pH range of D5/W can vary from 3.5 to 6.5. The wide range permitted is due to the free sugar acids

Table 42-1. Fluids Used Commonly for IV Use

INJECTION	CONCENTRATION (%)	PH	THERAPEUTIC USE
Alcohol			
with D5/W[a]	5	4.5	Sedative, analgesic, calories
with D5/W in NSS[b]	5		Sedative, analgesic, calories
Amino acid (synthetic)			Fluid and nutrient replenisher
Aminosyn II (Abbott)	3.5, 7, 8.5, 10, 15	5.25	
FreAmine III (B.Braun)	8.5, 10	6.6	
Travasol (Baxter)	3.5, 5.5, 8.5. 10	6.0	
Ammonium chloride	2.14	4.5–6.0	Metabolic alkalosis
Dextran 40			
in NSS	10	5	Priming fluid for plasma volume expander
in D5/W	10	4	Priming fluid for plasma volume expander
Dextran 70			
in NSS	6	5	Plasma volume expander
in D5/W	6	4	Plasma volume expander
Dextrose (glucose, D5/W)	2.5–50	3.5–6.5	Fluid and nutrient replenisher
Dextrose and sodium chloride	Varying concn of dextrose, 5–20, with varying concn of sodium chloride 0.22–0.9	3.5–6.5	Fluid, nutrient, and electrolyte replenisher
Lactated Ringer's (Hartmann's)		6.0–7.5	Systemic alkalizer; fluid and electrolyte replenisher
NaCl	0.6		
KCl	0.03		
CaCl$_2$	0.02		
Lactate	0.3		
Mannitol, also in combination	5	5.0–7.0	Osmotic diuresis
with dextrose or sodium chloride	15		
	20		
Multiple electrolyte solutions, varying combinations of electrolytes, dextrose,		5.5	Fluid and electrolyte replacement
Ringer's		5.0–7.5	Fluid and electrolyte replenisher
NaCl	0.86		
KCl	0.03		
CaCl$_2$	0.033		
Sodium bicarbonate	5	8	Metabolic acidosis
Sodium chloride	0.45, 0.9, 3, 5	4.5–7.0	Fluid and electrolyte replenisher
Sodium lactate	1/6 M	6.3–7.3	Fluid and electrolyte replenisher
Sterile water for injection		5.5	Diluent

[a] 5% Dextrose in water.
[b] Normal saline solution.

Table 42-2. IV Fluid Systems

SOURCE	CONTAINER	CHARACTERISTICS
Baxter	Glass	Vacuum Air tube
Baxter (*Viaflex*)	Plastic	Polyvinyl chloride Flexible Nonvented
B.Braun	Glass	Vacuum Air tube
B.Braun (*Excel*)	Plastic	Flexible
Abbott	Glass	Vacuum Air filter[a]
Abbott (*Lifecare*)	Plastic	Polyvinyl chloride Flexible Nonvented

[a] Part of administration set.

present and formed during the sterilization and storage of the injection. To avoid incompatibilities when other drug substances are added to Dextrose Injection, the possible low pH should be considered in using it as a vehicle. More-concentrated solutions of dextrose are available and provide increased caloric intake with less fluid volume. Being hypertonic, the more concentrated solutions may be irritating to peripheral veins. Highly concentrated solutions are administered in a larger central vein.

Intravenous fluids containing crystalline amino acids can provide biologically usable amino acids for protein synthesis (Chapter 106). Protein contributes to tissue growth, wound repair, and resistance to infection. The protein requirement for the normal adult is 1 g per kg per day; children and patients under stress require greater amounts. Attempts are made to maintain a positive nitrogen balance, indicating that the protein administered is being used properly and not broken down and eliminated through the urine as creatinine and urea, which are normal waste products. In a positive nitrogen balance patients are taking in more nitrogen than they are eliminating. In a negative nitrogen balance there is more nitrogen being eliminated through the urine regularly than is being administered intravenously. This means that tissues are continuing to be torn down, and repair is not necessarily taking place. Amino Acid Injection can afford the total body requirements for proteins by the procedure known as PN (discussed below) or be used for supplemental nutrition by peripheral administration. In addition to the amino acids, these nutritional injections also may contain dextrose, electrolytes, vitamins, and insulin. Fat emulsion (Intralipid, *Baxter*; Liposyn II, *Abbott*) sometimes is used concurrently but usually administered at Y-site. However, new systems such as three-in-one packaging permit mixing of amino acids, carbohydrates, and fat in one container for PN.

Packaging Systems

Containers for intravenous fluids must be designed to maintain solution sterility, clarity (freedom from particulate matter), and nonpyrogenicity from the time of preparation, through storage, and during clinical administration. Container closures must be designed to facilitate insertion of administration sets through which the injections are administered at a regulated flow-rate into suitable veins. IV fluids are available in glass and plastic containers; the latter are made from a flexible plastic material. IV fluids are supplied in 1000-mL, 500-mL and 250-mL sizes in addition to 250-mL capacity containers packaged with 50 or 100 mL of D5/W or sodium chloride injection 0.9% for piggyback use in addition to 0.45% sodium chloride and 2.5% dextrose injections. IV fluids in glass containers are packaged under vacuum, which must be dissipated prior to use. For fluid to leave the IV glass container and flow through the administration set, some mechanism is necessary to permit air to enter the container.

Current flexible plastic systems do not require air introduction to function. Atmospheric pressure pressing on the container forces the fluid to flow.

All glass and plastic containers are single-dose and should be discarded after opening even if not used. Intravenous fluids are packaged with approximately 3% excess fill to allow for removal of air from the administration set and permit the labeled volume to be delivered from the container. The containers are graduated at 20-mL increments on scales that permit the volume in a container to be determined from either an upright or inverted position. Glass containers have aluminum and plastic bands for hanging, while plastic containers have eyelet openings or plastic straps for attachment to IV poles.

Fluids for IV use are available from three sources (*Abbott, Baxter,* and *B.Braun*); all provide both glass and plastic containers. The glass-container systems of *Baxter* and *B.Braun* are similar. The characteristics of current packaging systems are summarized in Table 42-2.

Administration Sets

Administration sets used to deliver fluids intravenously are sterile, pyrogen-free, and disposable. Although these sets are supplied by different manufacturers, each for its own system, they have certain basic components. These usually include a plastic spike to pierce the rubber closure or plastic seal on the IV container, a drip (sight) chamber to trap air and permit adjustment of flow rate, and a length (150 to 450 cm) of polyvinyl chloride (PVC) tubing terminating in a gum-rubber injection port. Non–PVC sets are available for special uses. At the tip of the port is a rigid needle or catheter adapter. An adjustable clamp (screw or roller type) on the tubing pinches the tubing to regulate flow. Since the Y-site port is self-sealing, additional medication can be added to the IV system at these ports of entry. Glass containers that have no air tubes require air-inlet filters designed as part of the administration set (*Abbott*). See Figures 42-1 to 42-6.

Administration Procedures

In the administration of IV fluids, the primary IV container provides for fluid replacement, electrolyte replenishment, drug therapy, or nutrition; the fluid can be infused usually over a 4- to 12-hr period. In some cases an IV fluid is infused slowly for the purpose of keeping the vein open (KVO). This will allow additional drugs to be administered when required. The primary IV fluid also can serve as a vehicle for other drugs to be administered, thus becoming an intravenous admixture (IV drip), and

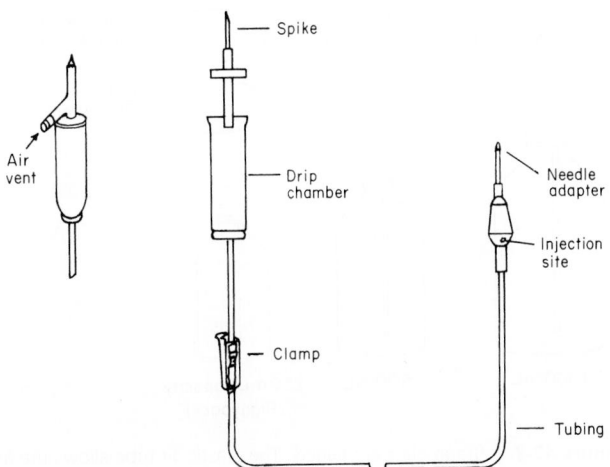

Figure 42-1. Parts of basic administration sets.

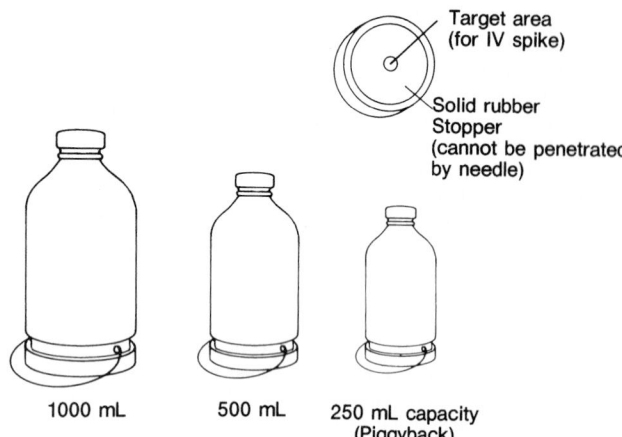

Figure 42-2. Abbott IV glass container. The air venting is provided through the air filter located in the spike of the administration set. See Figure 42-1.

results in continuous blood levels of added drugs once the steady state has been reached.

Incinerated PVC products produce hydrogen chloride gas as a toxic pollutant. Diethylhexylphthalate (DEHP), a component of PVC containers, may leach into the soil in landfills. A number of drugs adsorb on PVC containers, notably nitroglycerin. Some drugs (fat emulsions, blood, Paclitaxel) are known to leach DEHP.

The Excel container is claimed to eliminate or minimize these problems. The plastic film contains no plasticizers and exhibits no leachability. The solution-contact layer of the container is composed of a rubberized copolymer of ethylene and propylene, which is claimed to be clear, nontoxic, and biologically inert. The container is available in 250-mL, 500-mL, and 1-L sizes. Smaller sizes are available in 25, 50, and 100 mL known as PAB containers.

In preparing an IV fluid for administration, the following procedure is used.

The spike adapter of the administration set is inserted into the stopper or seal of the IV container.

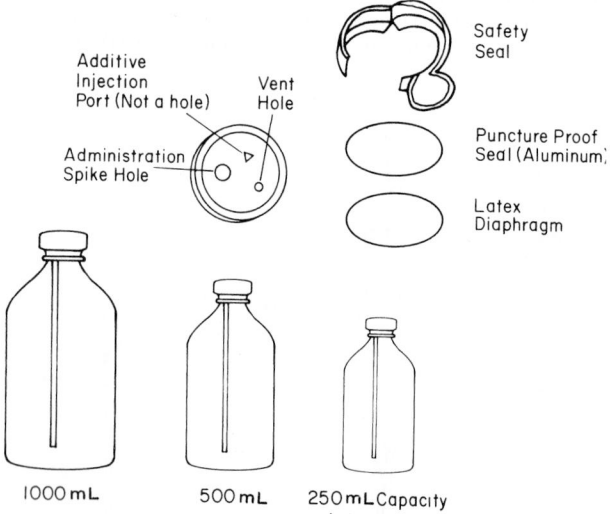

Figure 42-3. B.Braun glass containers. The plastic air tube allows the air to enter the bottle as the fluid is infused into the patient. The spike of the administration set is not vented. See Figure 42-1.

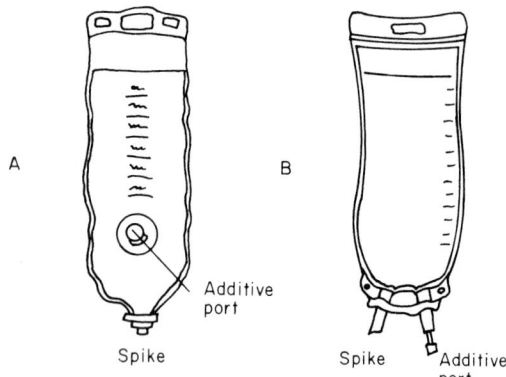

Figure 42-4. *A,* Abbott (Lifecare) polyvinyl chloride flexible container; *B,* Baxter (Viaflex) polyvinyl chloride flexible container. These containers take nonvented administration sets. See Figure 42-1.

The IV fluid is hung on a stand at bedside, and air is purged from the administration set by opening the clamp until fluid comes out of needle. The tubing is then clamped off.

The venipuncture is made by a member of the IV team, floor nurse, or physician.

The infusion rate is adjusted by slowly opening and closing the clamp until the desired drop rate, viewed in the drip chamber, is obtained. The usual running time is 4 to 8 hr (usually 125 mL is delivered in 1 hr). Drugs such as heparin, insulin, lidocaine, or dopamine may be present in the IV drip. When potent drugs are present, the flow rates will vary, depending on the clinical condition of the patient. Sets are calculated to deliver 10, 15, 20, 50, or 60 drops per mL, depending on the manufacturer. Critical drugs are usually administered by electronic pumps.

Intermittent administration of an antibiotic and other drugs can be achieved by any of three methods:

1. Direct IV injection (IV bolus or push)
2. Addition of the drug to a predetermined volume of fluid in a volume-control device
3. Use of a second container (minibottle, minibag) with an already hanging IV fluid (piggybacking)

DIRECT INTRAVENOUS INJECTION—Small volumes (1 to 50 mL) of drugs are injected into the vein over a short period of time (1 to 5 min). The injection also can be made through a resealable Y injection site of an already hanging IV fluid. This method is suitable for a limited number of drugs but too hazardous for most drugs.

VOLUME-CONTROL METHOD—Volume-control sets provide a means for intermittent infusion of drug solutions in precise quantities at controlled rates of flow. These units consist of calibrated, plastic, fluid chambers placed in a direct line under an established primary IV container or more often attached to an independent fluid supply. In either case, the drug to be administered is first reconstituted if it is a sterile solid and injected into the gum-rubber injection port of the volume-control unit. It is then further diluted to 50 to 150 mL with the primary fluid or the separate fluid reservoir. Administration of the total drug-containing solution requires 30 to 60 min and produces a peak concentration in the blood followed by a valley if the dosage is discontinued.

To set up an intermittent IV infusion with a volume-control set, the spike of the volume-control set is inserted into the primary IV fluid or a separate fluid container using aseptic technique. See Figure 42-6.

Air is purged from tubing of the volume-control set by opening the clamps until fluid comes through.

The clamp is opened above the calibrated chamber, and it is filled with 25 to 50 mL fluid from the primary IV container or separate fluid container.

The clamp is closed above the chamber.

The medication is injected through the gum-rubber port of the volume-control unit.

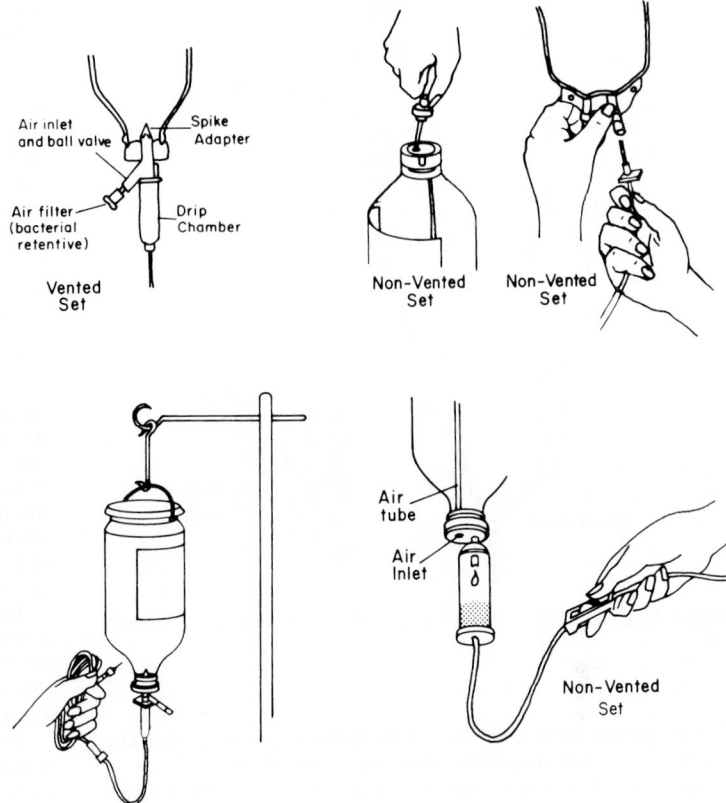

Figure 42-5. Setting up a primary IV fluid for administration.

The clamp above the chamber is opened to complete the dilution to the desired volume (50 to 150 mL), then closed.

Flow commences when the clamp below the volume-control unit is opened.

PIGGYBACK METHOD—The piggyback method (Fig 42-7) refers to the intermittent IV drip of a second admixture drug, through the venipuncture site of an established primary IV system. With this setup the drug can be thought of as entering the vein on *top* of the primary IV fluid, hence the designation *piggyback*. The piggyback technique not only eliminates the need for another venipuncture, but also achieves drug dilution and peak blood levels within a relatively short timespan, usually 30 to 60 min. Drug dilution helps to reduce irritation, and early high serum levels are an important consideration in serious infection requiring aggressive drug therapy. These advantages have popularized the piggyback method of IV therapy, especially for the intermittent administration of antibiotics. In using the piggyback technique, the secondary unit is purged of air, and its needle or blunt cannula inserted into a Y-injection site of the primary set or into the injection site at the end of the primary set.

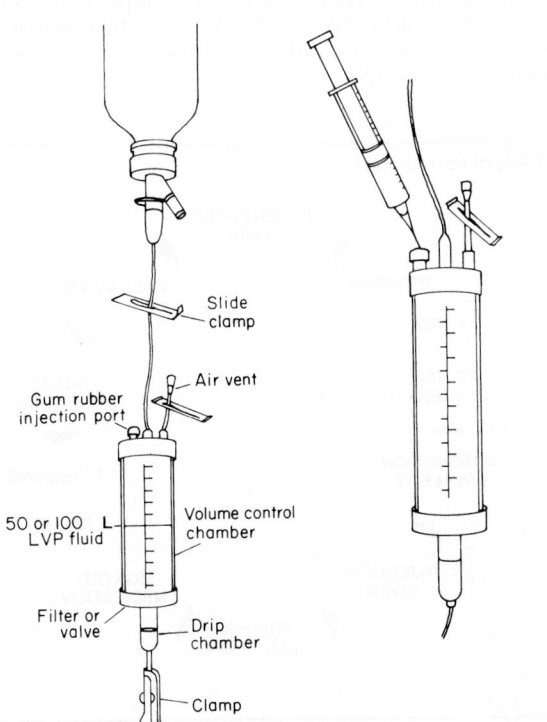

Figure 42-6. Volume control unit for intermittent administration.

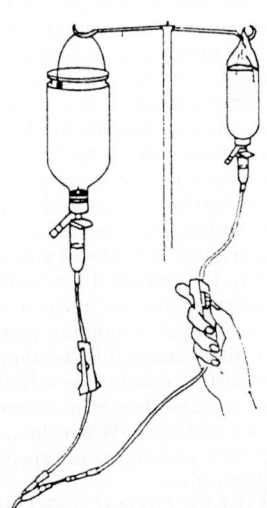

Figure 42-7. Piggyback administration setup.

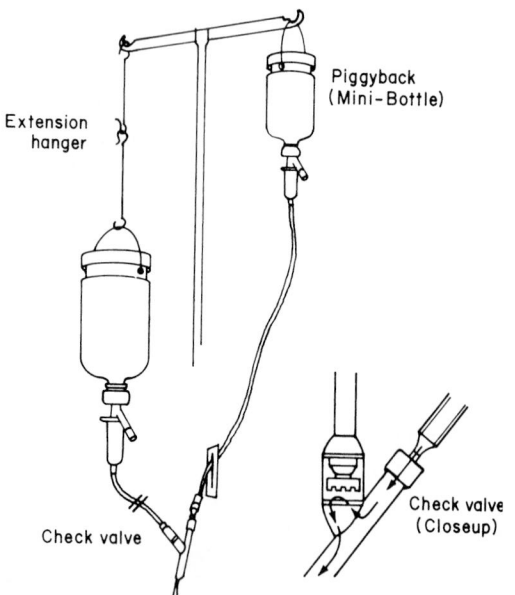

Figure 42-8. Piggyback administration setup with check valve in primary set.

The piggyback infusion is then started. Once it is completed, the primary fluid infusion will be restarted. See Figure 42-7.

Primary IV administration sets are available that have a built-in check valve for use in piggyback administration. When the piggyback is connected to one of these sets and started, the check valve automatically closes off the primary infusion. When the piggyback runs out, the check valve automatically opens, thereby restarting the primary infusion. The check valve works because of pressure differences. To achieve this difference, the primary container is hung lower than the secondary bottle by means of an extension hanger. See Figure 42-8.

Manufacturers have introduced minibottles and minibags prefilled with various antibiotic products; each container is provided with a plastic hanger for direct suspension from an IV pole as the piggyback solution is administered through the resealable gum-rubber injection site or Y-type facility of an existing IV system. Reconstitution of piggyback units requires only the addition of a small volume of compatible diluent. Since reconstitution and administration proceed from the same bottle, no drug transfer is involved, so transfer syringes and additional IV containers are not necessary. Prefilled drug containers offer significant advantages to hospitals. Time-saving, less potential for error and contamination, and convenience are outstanding qualities of this type of packaging. The need exists in hospitals for these types of innovative packaging to help alleviate the critical nursing shortage and reduce the error potential. It is a significant event that drug manufacturers and intravenous fluid manufacturers have combined efforts to achieve optimal packaging for hospital use.

Partial-fill containers available for piggybacking are 250-mL capacity infusion bottles or bags underfilled with 50 or 100 mL D5/W or normal saline. The drug to be administered first is reconstituted in its original parenteral vial and then added by needle and syringe to the partial-fill container. The needle of the piggyback delivery system is inserted into the Y-site or gum-rubber injection port of a hanging primary infusion set. Flow of the primary intravenous fluid is stopped while the drug solution in the partial-fill container is administered (30 to 60 min). After the drug solution has been infused totally, the primary fluid flow is reestablished. When the next dose of drug is required, the piggyback procedure is repeated, replacing the prefilled partial-fill container.

MECHANICAL-ELECTRONIC INFUSION DEVICES— Gravity IV administration systems are affected by many vari-

ables that tend to alter the accuracy of the system. These include variations in the size of the drip-chamber orifice, the viscosity of the solution being administered, plastic cold flow, clamp slippage, final filters, variations in the patient's blood pressure and body movements, clot formation, pressure changes in IV containers' rate of flow, temperature of the IV fluid, changes in the needle, and other factors such as kinked tubing, extravasation, and changes in the height of the IV container. Flow in traditional gravity IV systems is controlled by manual clamps (either screw or roller clamps), which can provide considerable discrepancies in volume delivery. These factors have promoted the development and use of mechanical-electronic infusion devices to control more accurately the administration of IV fluids. This group of devices includes infusion controllers and infusion pumps.

Infusion controllers count drops electronically or extrude volumes of fluid mechanically and electronically. Having no moving components, controllers are less complex than pumps, are usually less expensive, and have fewer maintenance problems. Infusion controllers are gravity-type systems, but the control is regulated automatically rather than manually. In addition to increasing the accuracy of delivery, electronic equipment may be able to detect infiltration of air, empty containers, and excess or deficient flow. Controllers are used less frequently in favor of pumps.

Infusion pumps do not depend on gravity to provide the pressure required to infuse the drug. Pressure is provided by an electric pump that propels a syringe, a peristaltic or roller device, or a cassette. Most pumps are volumetric in that the delivery is measured in milliliters rather than drops.

The quality of patient care has improved with the use of infusion devices. Flow rates can be maintained; therefore parenteral and enteral nutrition can be conducted safely. In addition, accurate drug therapy can be accomplished with adults and children, and *runaways* of IV fluid administration can be eliminated.

PATIENT-CONTROLLED ANALGESIA (PCA)—Usually and traditionally the acute or chronic pain experienced by patients in selected diseases is treated initially by oral narcotics and analgesics. However, many clinical situations preclude oral administration. Typically, the unsatisfied pain from disease has been treated by parenteral analgesics given by the IM or SC route.

This medication cycle from patient complaint to pain relief often can be lengthy. Frequently, the dose administered may be too large or too small, resulting in either sedation or poor pain relief. See Figure 42-9.

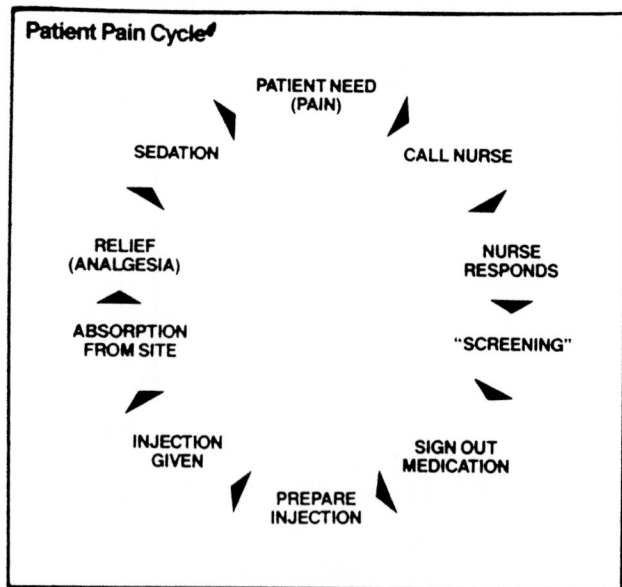

Figure 42-9. Patient pain cycle—sequence of events.[3]

Parenteral drugs given intravenously offer rapid distribution in the body and fast onset of action. The drug undergoes no biotransformation or inactivation and, therefore, allows more precise dose management.

PCA is a system for delivery of IV or SC narcotics by direct patient intervention. This therapy uses a mechanical, electronic, infusion-control device that permits self-administration of analgesics in proportion to the degree of relief desired.

A number of these devices have been developed and are undergoing development at *Bard, Abbott, Deltec, Baxter,* and *Becton Dickinson.* The early devices allowed for patient- triggered IV doses, and later refinement in the microprocessors allowed tailoring of infusions so that additional bolus doses could be given to a baseline infusion. Additional developments have led to ambulatory PCA devices that are small enough to be worn on a belt. An additional design being used is a balloon-powered disposable device (*Baxter*) that operates mechanically from an inflated balloon.

In its simplest terms, PCA allows a patient to initiate an IV infusion of a prescribed narcotic analgesic and maintain a self-regulated small amount of incremental doses needed for controlling a variety of pain-associated medical problems.

The success and popularity of PCA is based upon the inadequacy of conventional IM and IV dosing, such as variables that affect absorption and distribution[1] such as conventional nursing practices, inherent procedural delays in securing medication, and the ultimate administration to the patient.[2] The perception and sensation of pain in any one patient depends upon individual levels of endorphins and other biochemicals in cerebrospinal fluid.[3]

The last several years have seen the increasing use of infusion devices for epidural or intrathecal administration.

PCA eliminates the peak and valley effects of traditional drug therapy (Fig 42-10). Epidural or intrathecal therapy of PCA allows a longer duration of drug action. Kwan[4] reviewed the use of infusion devices for epidural or intrathecal administration.

FINAL-FILTER DEVICES—Particulate matter in IV fluids and IV admixtures can originate from many sources. It can result from the packaging components of the IV fluid, from admixture incompatibilities, from manipulation in preparing the admixture, and even from the administration set itself. Concern about particulate matter led to the design of final-filter devices for attaching to the end of the tubing of the administration set. They afford a final filtration of the IV fluid before it passes through the needle into the vein. The device consists of a plastic chamber containing a membrane or stainless steel filter

with porosities varying from 5 to 0.22 μm. Air lock can be a problem with membrane filters. When wet, membranes with porosities of 0.22 μm and 0.45 μm are impervious to air at normal pressures, and air in the system causes blockage. To prevent this, the filter housing must be purged completely of air prior to use. Newer designs have air eliminators. Using final-filter devices increases medication cost but reduces the biological hazards associated with particulate matter.

Although considerable information is available concerning the clinical use of membrane filters in entrapping particulate matter and microorganisms, little information exists describing drug absorption by the filter. Literature on a limited number of drugs and filter materials indicates that drugs administered in low doses might present a problem with drug bonding to the filter.[5] Solutions containing minute dosages of drugs, 5 mg or less, should not be filtered until sufficient data are available to confirm insignificant absorption. Drugs not recommended to be filtered include all parenteral suspensions, blood and blood products, amphotericin B, digitoxin, insulin, intravenous fat emulsions, mithramycin, nitroglycerin, and vincristine.

Blood is filtered by utilizing blood filters of larger porosity (210 microns).

2 in 1 TPN solutions usually require a 0.22 micron filter.

3 in 1 TPN solutions usually require a 1.2 micron filter.

IV DELIVERY SYSTEMS—*Frozen Premixes*—Baxter provides delivery to hospitals of frozen drug products packaged in PVC containers. These are stored in a freezer in the hospital's pharmacy, thawed, and used when needed. See Figure 42-11A.

Abbott/ADD-Vantage System—Introduced in 1985, the Abbott ADD-Vantage system (Fig 42-11B) has two parts: a plastic IV bag (Abbott) that is filled with solution and a separate glass vial of powder or liquid drug sold by a pharmaceutical manufacturer. The vial is encased in a plastic cover that is removed prior to use. The user locks the vial holding the drug into a chamber at the top of the plastic bag and mixes the drug and solution by externally removing the stopper on the vial which allows drugs to fall into the diluent.

Nutrimix—A dual-compartment container is available from Abbott that allows long-term packaging of amino acids and dextrose mixtures.

Mini-Infuser Pumps for Intermittent IV Drug Delivery—A novel concept in intermittent drug delivery, introduced several years ago, was the Bard-Harvard Mini-Infuser System. This instrument was designed for the administration of antibiotics and other medications delivered intermittently in 40 min or less. This battery-generated, lightweight instrument uses standard disposable syringes and microbore disposable extension sets. Different models are available depending on the volume to be delivered. This instrument provides accuracy, constant flow, convenience, and safety for intermittent drug delivery. See Figure 42-11C.

Introduced and designed for intermittent IV drug delivery, Becton Dickinson's 360 Infusor allows drug delivery intermittently over 60 min or less in a volume dilution of up to 60 mL.

INTERNAL METHODS USED TO ACHIEVE INTRAVASCULAR ACCESS—*Implantable Ports* (Infuse-A-Port, *Infusaid;* Port-A-Cath, *Pharmacia*)—Broviac and Hickman catheters have been used to achieve long-term venous access in a variety of diseases. Although these catheters are widely used, they are associated with some morbidity, which includes fracture of catheters, entrance-site infection, and catheter sepsis. Implantable catheters have been developed to overcome catheter complications and are designed to permit repeated access to the infusion site. The catheters consist of implantable-grade silicone tubing connected to a stainless steel port with a self-sealing septum that allows needle access. The delivery catheter can be placed in a vein, cavity, artery, or the central nervous system (CNS). The system is accessed with a Huber-point needle through the skin into the self-sealing silicone plug positioned in the center of the portal.

The specialized Huber-point needle is designed with an angle bevel that reduces coring and permits easy entry. These

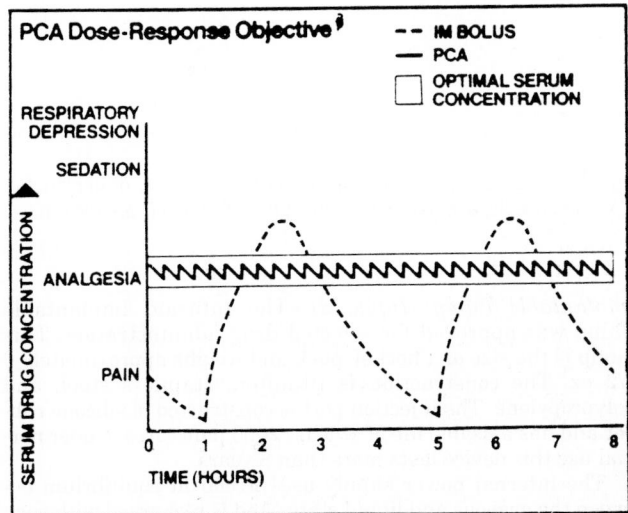

Figure 42-10. Characteristic pattern comparison of IM bolus serum concentration versus PCA.[3]

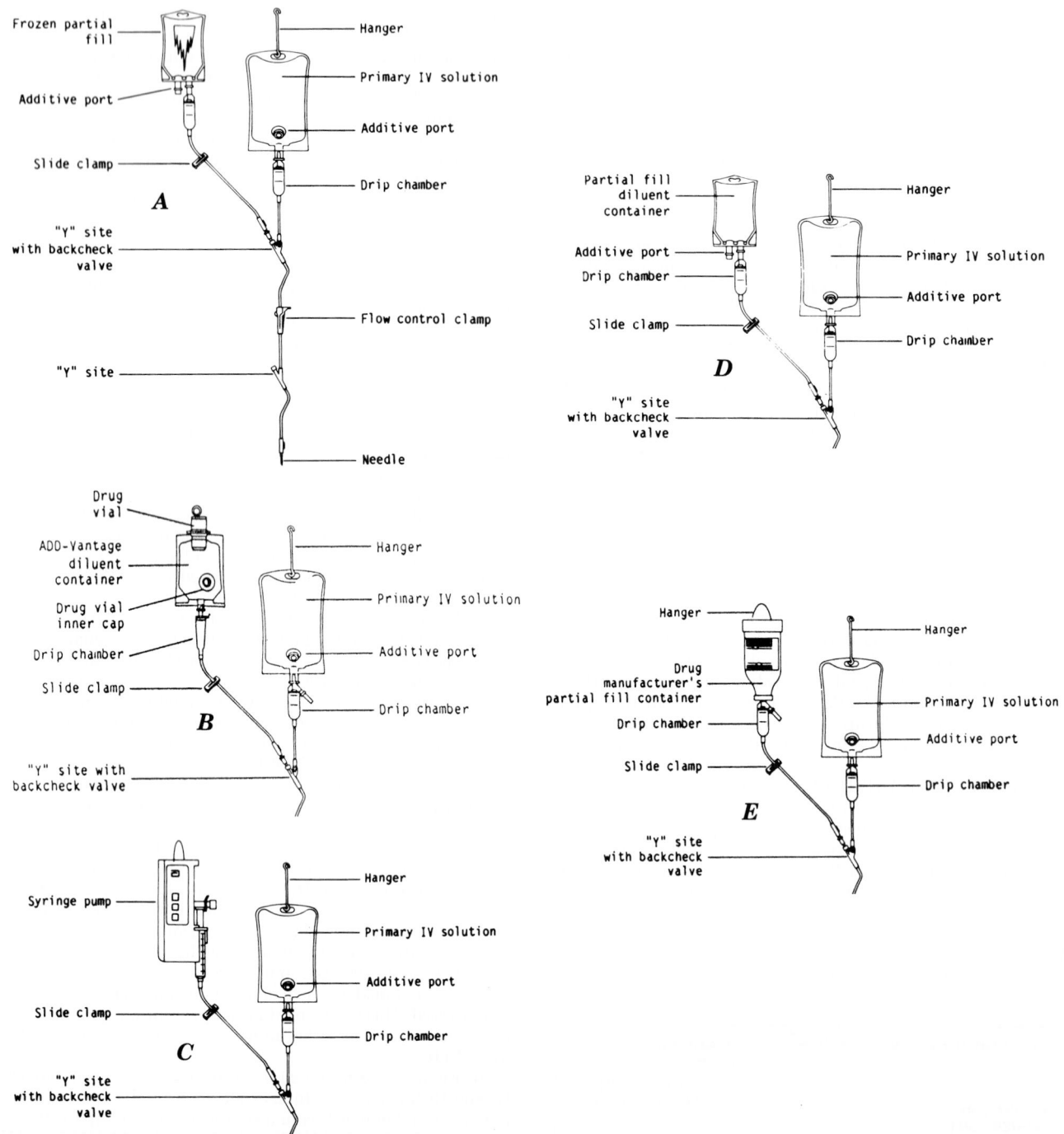

Figure 42-11. Various IV delivery systems. *A,* Frozen partial fill; *B,* ADD-Vantage; *C,* syringe pump; *D,* partial-fill diluent container; *E,* drug manufacturer's partial-fill piggyback (DMP) (courtesy, Abbott). The flow control clamp, "Y" site, needle, and associated tubing for *B* through *E,* are the same as in *A.* (Fig 42-11 is continued on the next page.)

implantable ports can be used for the injection of IV fluids, total parenteral nutrition, chemotherapy, antibiotics, and other drugs.

Some advantages of implantable devices include

The need for a long-term access site to venous, arterial, and spinal systems
An increased dependence on non-hospital treatment of chronic disease states
The direct infusion in a target organ or tumor
A decrease in infection rates that are seen with percutaneous catheters or repeated spinal taps
A greater mobility for the patient (a return to normal function)

Implantable Pump (Infusaid)—The Infusaid Implantable Pump was approved for selected drug administration. This pump is the size of a hockey puck and weighs approximately 6 1/2 oz. The construction is titanium, stainless steel, and polypropylene. The injection port is constructed of silicone rubber and has a usable life of at least 2000 punctures. Under normal use this device lasts more than 8 years.

The internal power supply uses Freon in equilibrium between the gaseous and liquid states and is recharged with each refilling process, thus supplying a power supply for as long as the pump is needed. As the pump is refilled, it compresses the gas back into the liquid state, allowing a fresh supply of energy

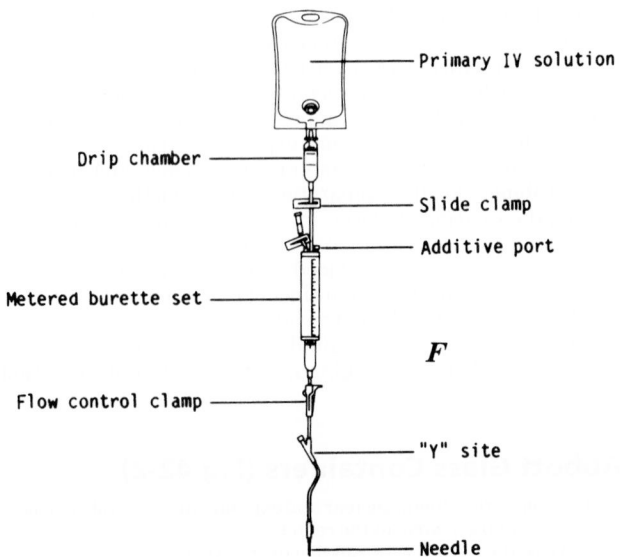

Primary IV solution

Drip chamber

Slide clamp

Additive port

Metered burette set

F

Flow control clamp

"Y" site

Needle

Figure 42-11 (continued). *F*, burette set (courtesy, Abbott).

for the next cycle. The capacity of this pump is 50 mL, which can be administered over a 14-day period. The pump accuracy is stated as over 3%. The cost of one model is approximately $4000.00, not including the surgical implant procedure. The 14-day cycle cannot be altered to any degree.

Model 400 Implantable Drug Delivery System (Infusaid) is designed for long-term therapy in the ambulatory patient. The Model 400 with a 47-mL usable drug volume delivers a precise, continuous flow to a selected organ or site via a soft, nontraumatic, nonthrombogenic, silicone rubber catheter. The Model 400 also features an auxiliary Sideport septum, completely bypassing the pumping mechanism, for delivery of direct bolus injections to the target site. Thus the clinician can easily supplement the continuous infusion with additional drugs, objectively assess the disease state, or monitor catheter location and drug perfusion with the use of radiolabeled microspheres.

INTRAVENOUS ADMIXTURES

When one or more sterile products are added to an IV fluid for administration, the resulting combination is known as an IV admixture. To maintain the characteristics of sterile products, namely, sterility and freedom from particulate matter and pyrogens, it is imperative that they be manipulated in a suitable environment by use of aseptic techniques.

ENVIRONMENT—Proper conditions for aseptic handling can be provided by laminar-flow hoods (see Chapters 40 and 41). Within a laminar-flow hood, air filtered through a HEPA (high-efficiency particulate air) filter moves in a parallel flow configuration at a velocity of 90 fpm. HEPA filters remove 99.97% of all particles larger than 0.3 μm. Since microbial contaminants present in air usually are found on other particulates, removal of the latter results in a flow of air free of both microbial contaminants and particulate matter. The movement of the filtered air in a laminar-flow configuration at a velocity of 90 fpm can maintain the area free of contamination. The flow of air may be in either a horizontal or vertical pattern. In the former case the HEPA filter is located at the back of the hood and the air flows to the front. In vertical flow the air passes through the HEPA filter located in the top of the cabinet and is exhausted through a grated area around the working surface of the hood. Regardless of the type of laminar air flow, the hood must be operated and maintained properly to achieve a satisfactory environment for the preparation of parenteral admixtures.

The hood is situated best in a clean area in which there is little traffic flow past the front of the hood. The inside of the hood is wiped down thoroughly with a suitable disinfectant and allowed to run for at least 30 min before starting manipulations. It is important to remember that the laminar-flow hood is not a means of sterilization. It only maintains an area free of microbial contaminants and particulate matter when it has been prepared, maintained, and used properly by operators with proper aseptic techniques.

Before working in a laminar-flow hood, operators wash their hands thoroughly and scrub them with a suitable disinfectant. Some institutions may require gowning and use of sterile gloves. Sterile gloves can be an asset, but there is always the problem that they can give the operator a false sense of security. Gloved hands can become contaminated as easily as ungloved hands. Additives and IV fluids to be used in the preparation of the admixture, along with suitable syringes, are lined up in the hood in the order they are to be used. The containers must be clean and dust-free. They are inspected for clarity and freedom from cracks. Operators are encouraged to use a lighting device for inspecting IV fluids for particulate matter and cracks. The lighting device should permit the container to be viewed against both a light and a dark background during inspection. If the IV fluid is packaged in plastic containers, pressure is applied to ensure that they are sealed properly and do not leak. Some laboratories disinfect the containers prior to placing them in the hood.

In working within the hood the operators work in the center of the hood, with the space between the point of operation and the filter unobstructed. If the flow of air is blocked, the validity of the laminar flow is destroyed. Articles are arranged within the hood in a manner to prevent clean air from washing over dirty objects and contaminating other objects that must remain sterile. The working area must be at least 6 inches from the front edge of the hood. As the operators stand in front of the hood, their bodies act as a barrier to the laminar air flow causing it to pass around them and create backflow patterns that can carry room air into the front of the hood.

Laminar-flow hoods must be maintained and evaluated periodically to ensure that they are functioning properly. The velocity of air flow can be determined routinely using a velometer. A decrease in the air flow usually indicates a clogged HEPA filter. Some laminar-flow hoods are equipped with pressure gauges indicating pressure in the plenum behind the filter; in these hoods pressure increase also can indicate a clogged filter. Settling plates can be exposed within the hood for given periods of time to determine the presence of microbial contaminants.

The best way to determine the proper functioning of a HEPA filter is to use the dioctylphthalate (DOP) test using the vapor at room temperature. DOP vapor (particles of ;0.3 μm) is allowed to be taken up by the hood through its intake filter. If the HEPA filter is intact and properly installed, no DOP can be detected in the filtered air stream by use of a smoke photometer. Certification services are available through commercial laboratories; the HEPA filters within laminar-flow hoods should be evaluated every 6 months.

ADDITIVES—The additives are injections packaged in ampuls or vials, or sterile solids; the latter are reconstituted with a suitable diluent before addition to the IV fluid. A fresh, sterile, disposable syringe is used for each additive. Before removing a measured volume from an ampul, the container is wiped with a disinfectant solution. If the ampul is scored, the top can be snapped off; if not scored, an ampul file must be used. A sterile syringe is removed from its protective wrapping. The syringe needle with its cover is separated from the syringe aseptically and may be replaced with a sterile aspirating needle. Aspirating needles usually are made from clear plastic and contain a stainless steel or nylon filter with a porosity of 5 μm. The filter will remove glass particles and other particulates from the injection as it is drawn up from the ampul into the syringe. The aspirating needle is replaced with the regular needle. The exact volume is calibrated, and the injection is ready to be added to the IV fluid (see Fig 42-12). In the case of additives packaged in multiple-dose vials, the protective cover is removed and the exposed target area of the rubber closure disinfected. A volume of air, equal to the volume of solution to be removed, is drawn up into the syringe and injected into the air space above the injection within the vial. This facilitates withdrawal of the injection. The solution is drawn into the syringe, the exact dose is measured, and the injection is ready to be added to the IV fluid.

Certain injections are light-sensitive and protected against photolysis by the container packaging. The manufacturer may use amber glass, individual container wrapping, or an amber plastic cover. Many hospital pharmacists use aluminum foil as a protective wrap for light-sensitive drugs during their administration.

In the case of drug substances having poor stability in aqueous solution, the drug is packaged as a sterile solid, either dry-filled or lyophilized. The diluent recommended on the labeling is used to reconstitute the powder; the proper quantity of solution then is removed for addition to the IV fluid. To increase the efficiency of IV admixture programs, a limited number of hospital pharmacists have found it convenient to freeze reconstituted drugs, particularly antibiotics. The stability of reconstituted drugs is somewhat limited. In some cases stability is limited to only a few hours; in many cases, however, reconstituted solutions can be frozen and thawed at the time of use. In the frozen form the stability of the antibiotic solution can be increased. In a number of instances the stability in the frozen form is known and supplied by the manufacturer. Reports have been published on the frozen stability of certain drugs. However, it is unwise to freeze drug solutions without adequate stability studies for guidance. In those cases where published

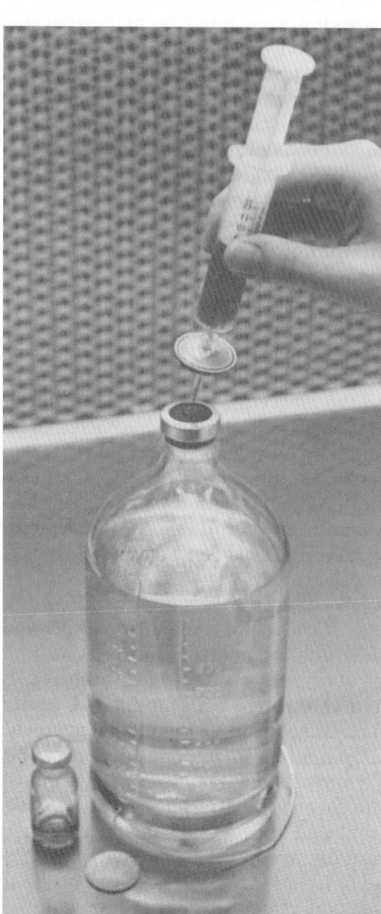

Figure 42-12. Placing an additive into an IV fluid with filtration through a membrane filter (courtesy, Millipore)

information is available, close adherence must be observed as to freezing temperature, storage conditions, and packaging.

There is an increasing awareness of the potential hazard to pharmacists handling antineoplastic drugs.[6] Although the evidence is not conclusive, it appears that measures should be taken to minimize unnecessary exposure.[7,8] These precautions include the use of vertical laminar-flow hoods and biological safety cabinets for the preparation and reconstitution of these agents, the wearing of gloves and masks by the personnel, special labeling of the containers to ensure their proper handling and disposal, and periodic blood studies of personnel involved in preparing admixtures of antineoplastic agents.

The procedure for placing an additive in an IV fluid will vary depending on the type of IV fluid packaging system being used by the hospital. The packaging systems are described in Table 42-2.

Abbott Glass Containers (Fig 42-2)

1. Remove the aluminum tear seal exposing the solid-rubber closure with a target circle in the center.
2. Wipe the closure with suitable disinfectant.
3. Insert the needle of the additive syringe through the target area. The vacuum within the bottle draws in the solution.
4. Gently shake the bottle after each addition, to mix thoroughly.
5. When completed, cover the closure with a plastic protective cap if it is not to be used immediately.

Baxter and McGaw Rigid Glass Containers (Fig 42-3)

1. Remove the aluminum tear seal and the aluminum disk covering the latex diaphragm.
2. Upon exposing the latex diaphragm, note that the latex cover is drawn in over the openings in the rubber closure.
3. The larger of the two holes receives the administration set, the other is the air vent. The triangular indentation can serve as the site for injecting the additives as well as the opening for the administration set.
4. Wipe the diaphragm with a suitable disinfectant and pierce the latex cover to place additive into bottle. The vacuum within the bottle will draw additive from the syringe. Do not remove the diaphragm or the vacuum will dissipate. It will be removed at the time of administration prior to the insertion of the administration set.
5. Gently shake the bottle after each additive.
6. When completed, cover the bottle with a plastic additive cap if the administration set is not to be inserted immediately.

Baxter and Abbott Plastic Container (Fig 42-4)

1. Remove the additive port protective sleeve and swab the injection port plug with a suitable disinfectant.
2. Additives are placed in container by piercing the additive port, mix thoroughly.
3. After each addition, milk the container to ensure adequate mixing.
4. Containers do not contain a vacuum, but vacuum chambers are available for use in conjunction with the flexible plastic container.
5. Protective additive caps are available if the administration set is not inserted immediately.

PHARMACY BULK PACKAGE—The manufactured bulk package is a sterile container for parenteral use that contains many single doses. These containers are intended for use in admixture programs in which large numbers of doses are prepared. It is designed so that the rubber closure is penetrated only once. It is used in laminar-flow hoods. Pharmacy bulk packages are exempt from the USP requirement that multiple-dose containers have a volume not greater than 30 mL. They also have an exemption in that they are not required to have a bacteriostatic agent. Pharmacy bulk packages have special labeling and storage requirements.

PARENTERAL INCOMPATIBILITY—When one or more additives are combined with an IV fluid, their presence together may modify the inherent characteristics of the drug substances present, resulting in a parenteral incompatibility. Parenteral incompatibilities have been divided arbitrarily into three groups: physical, chemical, and therapeutic. The latter is the most difficult to observe because the combination results in undesirable antagonistic or synergistic pharmacological activity. For example, the report that penicillin or cortisone antagonizes the effect of heparin and produces a misleading picture of the anticoagulant effect of heparin represents a therapeutic incompatibility. Physical incompatibilities are observed most easily and can be detected by changes in the appearance of the admixture, such as a change in color, formation of a precipitate, or evolution of a gas.

Physical incompatibilities frequently can be predicted by knowing the chemical characteristics of the drugs involved. For example, the sodium salts of weak acids, such as phenytoin sodium or phenobarbital sodium, precipitate as free acids when added to intravenous fluids with an acidic pH. Calcium salts precipitate when added to an alkaline medium. Injections that require a special diluent for solubilization, such as diazepam, precipitate when added to aqueous solutions because of their low water solubility.

Decomposition of drug substances resulting from combination of parenteral dosage forms is called a chemical incompatibility, an arbitrary classification, since physical incompatibilities also result from chemical changes. Most chemical incompatibilities result from hydrolysis, oxidation, reduction, or complexation and can be detected only with a suitable analytic method.

An important factor in causing a parenteral incompatibility is a change in the acid-base environment.[9] The solubility and stability of a drug may vary as the pH of the solution changes. A change in the pH of the solution may be an indication in predicting an incompatibility, especially one involving drug stability, since this is not necessarily apparent physically. The effect of pH on stability is illustrated in the case of penicillin. The antibiotic remains active for 24 hr at pH 6.5, but at pH 3.5 it is destroyed in a short time. Potassium penicillin G contains a citrate buffer and is buffered at pH 6 to 6.5 when reconstituted with Sterile Water for Injection, Dextrose Injection, or Sodium Chloride Injection. When this reconstituted solution is added to an intravenous fluid such as Dextrose Injection or Sodium Chloride Injection, the normal acid pH of the solution is buffered at pH 6 to 6.5, thus ensuring the activity of the antibiotic.

While it may be impossible to predict and prevent all parenteral incompatibilities, their occurrence can be minimized. The IV admixture pharmacist should be cognizant of the increasing body of literature concerning parenteral incompatibilities. This includes compatibility guides published by large-volume parenteral manufacturers,[10–12] compatibility studies on individual parenteral products by the manufacturer and published with the product as part of the labeling, the study of the National Coordinating Committee on Large-Volume Parenterals,[13] reference books,[14,15] and literature reports of studies with specific parenteral drugs.[16] The pharmacist should encourage the use of as few additives as possible in IV fluids, since the number of potential problems increases as the number of additives increases. Physicians should be made aware of possible incompatibilities, and the pharmacist can suggest alternative approaches to avoid the difficulties. In some instances, incompatibilities can be avoided by selecting another route of administration for one or more of the drugs involved.

QUALITY CONTROL—Each hospital should have written procedures covering the handling and storage, use in preparing admixtures, labeling, and transportation of IV fluids to the floors. In-use clarity and sterility tests should be devised to ensure that IV admixtures retain the characteristics of sterility and freedom from particulate matter. Training and monitoring

personnel involved in preparation of IV admixtures should be done on a regular basis.[17] The efforts of the hospital pharmacy should be no less than those of the industry in following Current Good Manufacturing Practice to ensure the safety and efficacy of these compounded medications.

TOTAL PARENTERAL NUTRITION

Intravenous administration of calories, nitrogen, and other nutrients in sufficient quantities to achieve tissue synthesis and anabolism is called total parenteral nutrition (PN).[18] Originally, the term hyperalimentation was used to describe the procedure, but it is being replaced by PN, the latter being more descriptive for the technique.

The normal caloric requirement for an adult is approximately 2500 per day. If these were to be provided totally by D5/W, approximately 15 L would be required. Each liter contains 50 g dextrose, equivalent to 170 calories. However, it is only possible to administer 3 or 4 L per day without causing fluid overload. To reduce this fluid volume, the concentration of dextrose would have to be increased. By increasing the dextrose to 25%, it is possible to administer five times the calories in one-fifth the volume. D25/W is hypertonic and cannot be administered in large amounts into a peripheral vein without sclerosing the vein.

Dudrick developed the technique for administering fluids for PN by way of the subclavian vein into the superior vena cava where the solution is diluted rapidly by the large volume of blood available, thus minimizing the hypertonicity of the solution. For administration of the PN fluids, a catheter is inserted and retained in place in the subclavian vein. PN is indicated for patients who are unable to ingest food due to carcinoma or extensive burns and patients who refuse to eat, as in the case of depressed geriatrics or young patients suffering from anorexia nervosa and surgical patients who should not be fed orally.

The preferred source for calories in PN fluids is the carbohydrate dextrose. In IV fluid kits commercially available for the preparation of PN solutions, D50/W is provided. On dilution with amino acid injection, the resulting dextrose concentration is approximately 25%. It is this concentration that is administered.

The source of nitrogen in PN fluids is crystalline amino acids (Aminosyn, *Abbott;* FreAmine III, *B.Braun;* Travasol, *Baxter*). The crystalline amino acid injections contain all the essential and nonessential amino acids in the L-form. For optimum use of amino acids and for promoting tissue regeneration, the nitrogen-to-calorie ratio should be 1:150. Calories are needed to provide energy for the metabolism of nitrogen.

Electrolyte requirements vary with the individual patient. The electrolytes present in Amino Acid Injection are given on the label and must be taken into consideration in determining the quantities to be added. Usual electrolyte concentrations are required to fall within the following ranges: sodium, 100 to 120 mEq; potassium, 80 to 120 mEq; magnesium, 8 to 16 mEq; calcium, 5 to 10 mEq; chloride, 100 to 120 mEq; and phosphate, 40 to 60 mEq. It is better to keep a 1:1 ratio between sodium and chloride ions. If the combination of calcium and phosphate ions exceeds 20 mEq, precipitation occurs.

In addition to the electrolytes, the daily requirement for both water-soluble and fat-soluble vitamins may be added, usually in the form of a multivitamin infusion concentrate. Iron should be administered separately from the PN fluids. Trace elements such as zinc, copper, manganese, and chromium are a concern only in long-term cases and can be added when required.

A lack of knowledge concerning preparation of PN admixtures may present a life-threatening hazard to patients. Several deaths have been reported as a result of chemical incompatibility.[19]

Table 42-3. Typical IV Orders (Parenteral Prescriptions)

PRESCRIPTION	COMMENT
1. ℞ NS 1000 mL 125 mL/hr	Sodium Chloride Injection (Normal Saline Solution) 1000 mL, is to be administered at a flow rate of 125 mL per hr. It will require approximately 8 hr.
2. ℞ 1000 D5W + NS + vits 12 hr	Dextrose Injection 5%, 1000 mL, containing 0.9% sodium chloride and container of vitamin B complex with vitamin C is to be administered over a 12-hr period.
3. ℞ 500 D5W + 1/2NS KVO	Dextrose Injection 5%, 500 mL, containing 0.45% sodium chloride is to be administered at a flow rate to keep the vein open (KVO). The flow rate will be approximately 10 mL/hr.
4. ℞ 1000 cc D5W + 1/2NS Add 1 amp vits to each + 100 mg thiamine Each to run 6 hr	Dextrose Injection 5%, 1000 mL, containing 0.45% sodium chloride, the contents of one ampul vitamin B complex with vitamin C and sufficient volume of Thiamine Hydrochloride Injection to give 100 mg thiamine, is to be administered over a 6-hr period (approximately 170 mL/hr). Additional orders of the same can be anticipated.
5. ℞ 1000 cc D5W + 1/2NS + 20 mEq KCl	Dextrose Injection 5%, 1000 mL, is to be provided containing 0.45% sodium chloride and 20 mEq potassium chloride.
6. ℞ 1000 Hyperal + 10 NaCl + 10 KCl + 5 MgSO$_4$ + 10 insulin	1 L of the hospital's basic PN solution is to be provided with the addition of 10 mEq sodium chloride, 10 mEq potassium chloride, 5 mEq magnesium sulfate, and 10 units regular zinc insulin.
7. ℞ 1000 cc PN (FreAmine) + 40 mEq NaHCO$_3$ + 30 mEq KCl + Vits + 5U Reg Insulin to run 80 cc/hr	1 L of the basic PN solution, FreAmine II, is to be provided with the addition of 40 mEq NaHCO$_3$, 30 mEq potassium chloride, the contents of one container vitamin B complex with vitamin C plus 5 units of regular zinc insulin. It is to be administered at the flow rate of 80 mL/hr (approximately 12 hr).
8. ℞ 1000 PN + 40 mEq NaCl + 10 KCl + 10 Insulin + 10 cal gluconate	1 L of the hospital's basic PN solution is to be provided with the addition of 40 mEq sodium chloride, 10 mEq potassium chloride, 10 units regular zinc insulin, and 10 mL Calcium Gluconate Injection.
9. ℞ Cefazolin 500 mg D5W q 6 hr	Cefazolin 500 mg, is reconstituted with Sterile Water for Injection and added to a minibottle containing 100 mL Dextrose Injection 5%. This dose is given every 6 hr using a piggyback technique with a flow rate requiring 30 to 60 min for delivery.
10. ℞ Gentamicin 80 mg IVPB q 8 hr	Gentamicin, 80 mg, is added to a minibag containing 100 mL Dextrose Injection 5%. This dose is given every 8 hr using the piggyback technique (IVPB) with a flow rate requiring at least 80 min (not less than 1 mg/min).

THE PARENTERAL PRESCRIPTION

The physician writes an admixture order or parenteral prescription on a physician's order form located on the patient's chart. A copy of the order is sent to the pharmacy for compounding. It includes the patient's name, room number, the intravenous fluid wanted, additives and their concentrations, rate of flow, starting time, and length of therapy. The order is taken by the technician, nurse, or pharmacist to the pharmacy or sent via pneumatic tube or fax. Orders may be telephoned to the pharmacy; verification with the original order is made on delivery of the admixture. IV orders usually are written for a 24-hr therapy period; the patient's chart is reviewed and new orders are written daily. The order may be for multiple containers, in which case the containers are numbered consecutively. Unlike the extemporaneously compounded prescription, additives are added without regard to final volume of IV fluid. The prescription is checked for proper dose, compatibility, drug

Table 42-4. Product Stability

TRADE NAME	PHYSICAL FORM	SHELF LIFE
Humulin	Liquid solution	2 yr at 2–8°
Protropin	Lyophilized powder	2 yr at 2–8°
Humatrope		
Roferon-A	Lyophilized powder	3 yr at 2–8°
Intron A	Lyophilized powder	2 yr at 2–8°
Activase	Lyophilized powder	2 yr at 2–30°
Recombivax-HB	Liquid solution	
Engerix-B	Liquid solution	
Orthoclone	Liquid solution	1 yr at 2–8°
Epogen	Liquid solution	

Table 42-5. Stability after Reconstitution (Lyophilized Products)

TRADE NAME	SHELF LIFE
Roferon	1 mo at 2–8°
Intron A	1 mo at 2–8°
Humatrope	14 days at 2–8°
Protropin	7 days at 2–8°
Activase	8 hr at 2–30°

Table 42-6. Recombinant Protein Drugs

TRADE NAME	VIAL STRENGTH
Humulin	1000 units
Protropin	5 mg
Humatrope	5 mg
Roferon-A	3 and 18 million units solution
	3 and 18 million units lyo
Intron A	3, 5, 10, 25, and 50 million units
Activase	20, 50 mg
Recombivax HB	5, 10 μg
Engerix-B	20 μg
Orthoclone OKT3	5 μg
Epogen	2, 4, and 10 thousand units

allergies, and stability. Additives usually are given an expiration period of 24 hr from the time of preparation. Drugs such as ampicillin may require shorter expiration periods.

The clerical work for the admixture is prepared. This includes typing the label and preparing the profile worksheet. The profile sheet is filed so that the pharmacist will be alerted when subsequent containers are due for preparation. Charging the patient's account can be done from the profile worksheet or via computer. The label includes the patient's name, room number, bottle number, preparation date, expiration time, and date, intravenous fluid and quantity, additives and quantities, total time for infusion, the milliliters per hour or drops per minute, and space for the name of the nurse who hangs the container. The label will be affixed to the container upside down so that it can be read when hung.

The admixture is prepared by the pharmacist or a supervised technician. In handling sterile products, aseptic techniques as discussed previously must be observed. When completed, a plastic additive cap is affixed before delivery to the floor. The label is applied and checked with the original order. The empty additive containers are checked to confirm the additives present. The admixture is inspected for any color change or particulate matter.

The completed admixture is delivered to the floor. If it is not to be infused immediately (within 1 hr), it is stored under refrigeration; if refrigerated, it must be used within 24 hr. The nurse checks for accuracy of patient's name, drug and concentration, IV fluid, expiration date, time started, and clarity. The infusion of admixtures may run ahead or behind schedule, necessitating that the pharmacist modify the preparation of continued orders. Examples of IV orders are shown in Table 42-3.

PARENTERALS DERIVED BY BIOTECHNOLOGY

In 1993, 14 biotechnology drugs had been approved for clinical use; 21 were in Phase III clinical studies awaiting approval, and over 130 were in various phases of development. The Center for Biologics Evaluation and Review (CBER) had over 3200 Investigational New Drug Applications (INDs) under review. In 1996, 35 biotechnology drugs had been approved for clinical use, with 284 products in testing.

As a result of the stability sensitivities of proteins, the 35 biotechnology pharmaceuticals currently available are all manufactured as parenterals. Many are available as lyophilized parenterals (Table 42-4). Most have limited shelf life after re-

constitution (Table 42-5). All are supplied in low dosage, which attests to their potency (Table 42-6).

For a complete treatment of biotechnology and drugs, see Chapter 49, and for more information on the drug approval process, refer to Chapter 48.

REFERENCES

1. Bennett RL, Griffen WO. *Contemp Surg* 1983; 23:75.
2. Graves DA, et al. *Ann Intern Med* 1983; 99:360.
3. Bivins BA, Baumann TJ. *Patient Controlled Analgesia (PCA): A Clinical Evaluation of Safety and Efficacy in Hospitalized Trauma/Surgery Patients.* Detroit: Depts of Surg and Pharm, Henry Ford Hospital, Dec 1984.
4. Kwan JW. *Am J Hosp Pharm* 1990; 47:18.
5. Turco SJ. *Am J IV Ther Clin Nutr* 1982; 9:6.
6. Zimmerman PF, et al. *Am J Hosp Pharm* 1981; 38:1693.
7. Gallelli JF. *Am J Hosp Pharm* 1982; 39:1877.
8. Valanis BG, et al. *Am J Health-Syst Pharm* 1998; 50:455.
9. Newton DW. *Am J Hosp Pharm* 1978; 35:1213.
10. King JC. *Guide to Parenteral Admixtures.* Berkeley CA: Cutter Laboratories, 1987.
11. Shoup LK, Goodwin NH. *Implementation Guide—Centralized Admixture Program.* Morton Grove, IL: Travenol Laboratories, 1977.
12. Bergman HD. *Drug Intell Clin Pharm* 1977; 11:345.
13. Trissel LA. *Parenteral Drug Information Guide.* Washington, DC: Am Soc Hosp Pharm, 1974.
14. Trissel LA. *Handbook on Injectable Drugs,* 5th ed. Washington, DC: Am Soc Hosp Pharm, 1992.
15. Kobayashi NH, King JC. *Am J Hosp Pharm* 1977; 34:589.
16. Sanders SJ, et al. *Am J Hosp Pharm* 1978; 35:531.
17. Dudrick SJ, Rhoads JE. *Sci Am* 1972; 226:73.
18. *Hazards of Precipitation Associated with Parenteral Nutrition* [Letter]. Rockville, MD: FDA, Apr 18, 1994.

BIBLIOGRAPHY
General

Am J Hosp Pharm 1975; 32:261.
Am J Hosp Pharm 1993; 50:1940.
Am J Health-Syst Pharm. 2000; 57:150.
Avis KE, Akers MJ. *Sterile Preparation for the Hospital Pharmacist.* Ann Arbor, MI: Ann Arbor Sci Publ, 1981.
Flynn EA, Pearson RE, Barker KN. *Am J Health-Syst Pharm* 1997; 54:904.
Int J Pharm Compounding 1997; 1(3):165.
Trissel LA. *Handbook on Injectable Drugs,* 5th ed. Washington, DC: Am Soc Hosp Pharm, 1992.
Turco SJ, King RE. *Sterile Dosage Forms: Their Preparation and Clinical Applications,* 3rd ed. Philadelphia: Lea & Febiger, 1994.

PCA

Buchanan C. *Parenterals* 1986; 4:2.
Graves DA, et al. *Clin Pharm* 1983; 2:49.
White PF. *Semin Anesth* 1985; 4:255.
Williamson J, et al. *Hosp Pharm* 1986; 21:1098.

Implantable Systems

Ecoff E, et al. *NITA* 1983; 4:406.
Fulks KD, Kenady DE. *Hosp Formul* 1987; 22:248.
Gyves J, et al. *Am J Med* 1983; 73:841.
Kwan JW. *Am J Hosp Pharm* 1990; 47:18.
May GS, Davis C. *J Intraven Nurs* 1988; 11:97.
McGovern B, et al. *J Pediatr Surg* 1985; 6:725.
McIntyre KE, et al. *Ariz Med* 1985; 42:308.

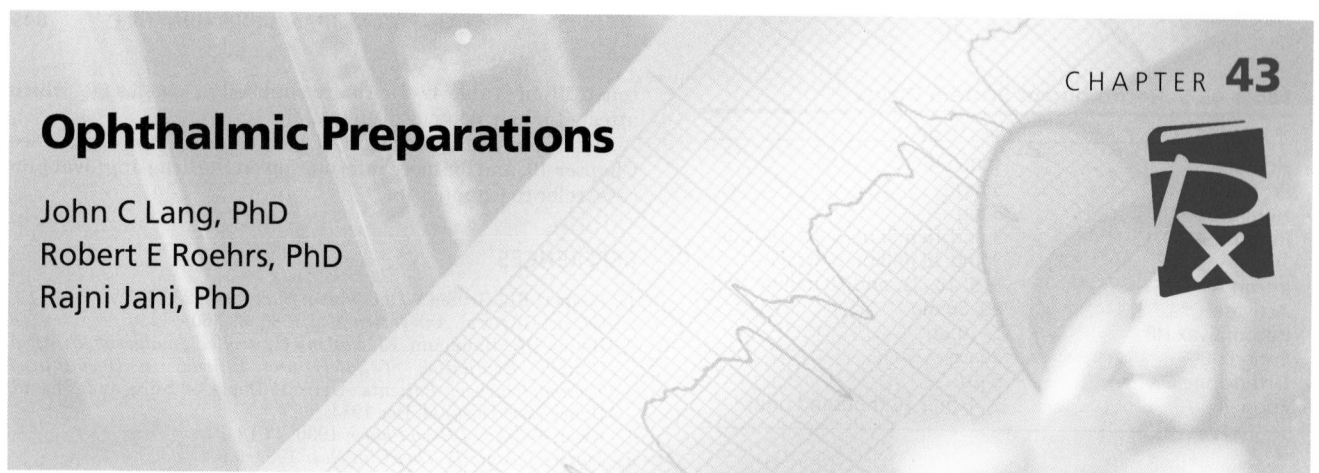

CHAPTER 43

Ophthalmic Preparations

John C Lang, PhD

Robert E Roehrs, PhD

Rajni Jani, PhD

INTRODUCTION[1]

Ophthalmic preparations are specialized dosage forms designed to be instilled onto the external surface of the eye (topical), administered inside (intraocular) or adjacent (periocular such as juxtascleral or subtenon) to the eye, or used in conjunction with an ophthalmic device. The latter include preparations used in conjunction with surgical implantation (such as an intraocular lens), dry eye formulations compatible with a punctal appliance such as a punctal plug, and extends to a variety of solutions utilized in maintenance of contact lenses. The preparations may have any of several purposes, therapeutic, prophylactic or palliative for topically administered agents, but includes mechanical, chemical and biochemical actions of agents used in the care of ocular appliances, and tissue prophylaxis during or following surgery. Because of the dangers associated with their administration, or repetitive administration, intraocular and periocular preparations are restricted to therapeutic applications or surgical adjuncts.

The versatility of dosage forms enables them to be suitable for the function of the preparation. Therapeutically active formulations may be designed to provide extended action for either convenience or reduction in risk of repetitive administration, improved bioavailability of the agent, or improved delivery to a targeted tissue. The residence of an ocular preparation may range from a few seconds needed for tears to clear an irritating substance, to hours for a gel, a gel-forming solution or an ointment, to months or years for an intraocular or periocular dosage form. The preparation may be strictly therapeutic, or may be administered for its prophylaxis. The latter include surgical adjunctives to maintain the health of fragile cells, postsurgical or post-trauma preparations designed to prevent or reduce the likelihood of infection. Another form of prophylaxis, that for a device, is the antisoiling function provided by some contact lens solutions.

Ophthalmic preparations are similar to parenteral dosage forms in their requirement for sterility as well as considerations for osmotic pressure (tonicity), preservation, tissue compatibility, the avoidance of pyrogens in intraocular dosage forms, particulate matter and suitable packaging.

Topical therapeutic dosage forms have customarily been restricted to solutions, suspensions and ointments. But with advances in material science, the range of ophthalmic dosage forms has expanded significantly to include gels, either preformed or spontaneous gels responsive to the ocular environment, and ocular inserts, both forms reducing dosage frequency. These are most often multi-dose products containing suitable preservative(s) to meet compendial preservative effectiveness test (eg, USP,[2] Pharm. Europa,[3] or JP[4]) requirements. Now, however, single-dose units, also referred to as unit-dose products, that are preservative-free preparations generally packaged in form-fill-seal plastic containers with 0.25 mL to up to 0.8 mL, have become available. These unit dose containers are designed to be discarded after a single use or after a single day's use if the container has a reclosable feature and the product is so labeled.

Injections and implants have been developed for intraocular drug delivery. Irrigating solutions and viscoelastic gels are available specifically for adjunctive use in ophthalmic surgery. Specialized formulations are now available for use in the care of contact lenses. The designs of these preparations meeting all of the requirements for safety, efficacy, component compatibility, tissue acceptability, storage, shipping, and shelf life are beyond the scope of this review. Nonetheless, a description of the requirements and the designs for some of these formulations should be illustrative and didactic.

From a historical perspective, preparations intended for treatment of eye disorders can be traced to the writings of the Egyptians, Greeks, and Romans. In the Middle Ages, *collyria* were referred to as materials that were dissolved in water, milk or egg white and used as eyedrops. One such collyrium contained the mydriatic substance belladonna to dilate the pupils of miladys' eyes for cosmetic purpose.

From the time of belladonna collyria, ophthalmic technology progressed at a pharmaceutical snail's pace until after World War II. Prior to WWII and into the 1950s, ophthalmic preparations were mostly compounded by the pharmacist for immediate use. Not until 1953 was there a legal requirement by FDA that all manufactured ophthalmic solutions be sterile. The range of medicinal agents to treat eye disorders was limited as was the state of eye surgery and vision correction, which was limited to eyeglasses. In the past fifty years, a modern pharmaceutical industry specializing in ophthalmic preparations has developed to support the advances in diagnosis and treatment of eye diseases, eye surgery and contact lenses. Because of the variety of ophthalmic products readily available commercially, the pharmacist now is rarely required to compound a patient's ophthalmic prescription. More important, however, is for the pharmacist to appreciate even subtle differences in formulations that may impact efficacy, comfort, compatibility or suitability of a preparation for particular patients.

Currently and in the future, in addition to the advances in dosage-form technology, drug molecules will be designed and optimized specifically for ophthalmic application. New therapies may become available for preventing blindness caused by degenerative disease - including age-related macular degeneration (AMD), macular edema, and diabetic retinopathy. Biotechnological products may also become available to treat causes of multifactorial eye disorders like glaucoma. Such specialized therapeutic agents also will require carefully designed compatible dosage forms.

Because dosage forms are fashioned to complement the requirements of the therapeutic agent, and the latter are selected for their action upon particular tissues in order to modify their function, we will now turn to a description of ocular tissues and their physiology.

ANATOMY AND PHYSIOLOGY OF THE EYE

In many ways the human eye is an ideal organ for studying drug administration and disposition, organ physiology and function. Unlike many bodily organs, most of its structure can be inspected without surgical intervention. Its macroscopic responses can be investigated by direct observation. Its miraculous function so intricate and complex - converting a physical electromagnetic stimulus into a chemical signal that is coupled to distant neurons for signal processing by an electrochemical wave - can be detected by sensitive instruments attached to external tissues. The basis for the function and protection of this important organ that links man to his external environment are the tissues comprising it. The structures to be described are illustrated in Figures 43-1 to 43-3. The first figure[5] provides a horizontal section of the eyeball identifying the major structures and their interrelationships. The second figure[6] shows in greater detail the anterior portion of the eye and eyelids, in vertical section, emphasizing some of the structures associated with tear apparatus. The third figure[6] emphasizes the flow of tears into the nasal structures. This brief introduction will focus on the anatomical structures comprising the eye, and their function.

Eyelids

Eyelids serve two purposes: mechanical protection of the globe and creation of an optimum milieu for the cornea. The inner surfaces of the eyelids and the outermost surfaces of the eye are lubricated by the tears, a composite of secretions from both lacrimal glands and specialized cells residing in both the bulbar (covering the sclera) and palpebral (covering the inner surface of the lids) conjunctiva. The antechamber has the shape of a narrow cleft directly over the front of the eyeball, with pocket-like extensions upward and downward. The pockets are called the superior and inferior fornices (vaults), and the entire space, the cul-de-sac. The elliptical opening between the eyelids is called the palpebral fissure and the corner of the eyes where the eyelids meet are the canthi.

Overview of Structure and Function of the Eyeball

STRUCTURE

The eyeball is housed in the bones of the skull, joined to form an approximately pyramid-shaped housing for the eyeball, called the orbit. The wall of the human eyeball (bulbus, globe) is composed of three concentric layers that envelop the fluid and lenticular core.[7-9]

Outer Fibrous Layer: The outer scleral layer is tough, pliable, but only slightly elastic. The anterior third is covered by the conjunctiva, a clear transparent mucous surface. The most anterior portion of the outer layer forms the cornea, a structure so regular and the water content so carefully adjusted that it acts as a clear, transparent window. It is devoid of blood vessels. Over the remaining two-thirds of the globe the fibrous collagen-rich coat is opaque (the *white* of the eye) and is called the sclera. It contains the microcirculation, which nourishes the tissues of this anterior segment, and is usually white except when irritated vessels become dilated.

The cornea, slightly thicker than the sclera and ranging in thickness from 500 microns to one millimeter, consists of five

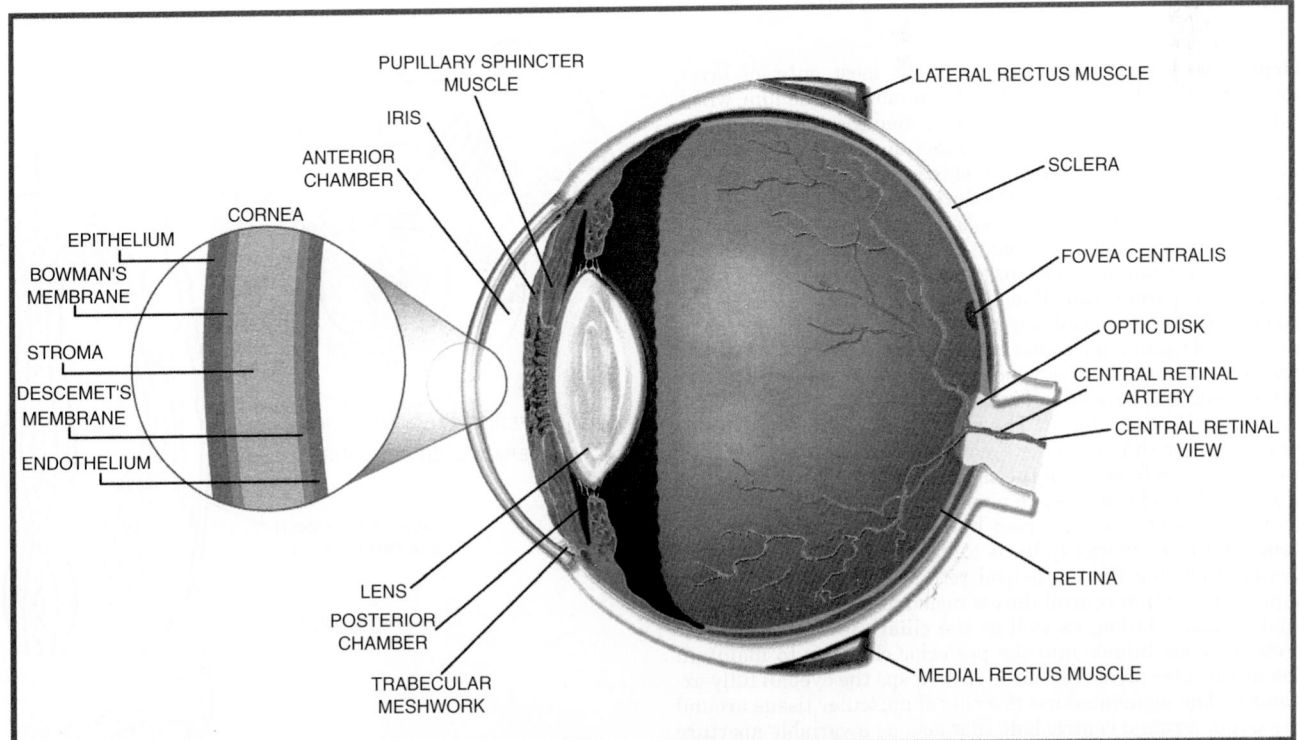

Figure 43-1. A cutaway horizontal section of the eyeball illustrating the important anatomic structures and their interrelationships diagramatically. The different layers of the cornea are illustrated in the magnified view. Relative sizes are suggestive and not proportional. The diameter of a mature eyeball is generally slightly greater than one inch (courtesy, Alcon, Inc., Fort Worth, TX). See Color Plate 19.

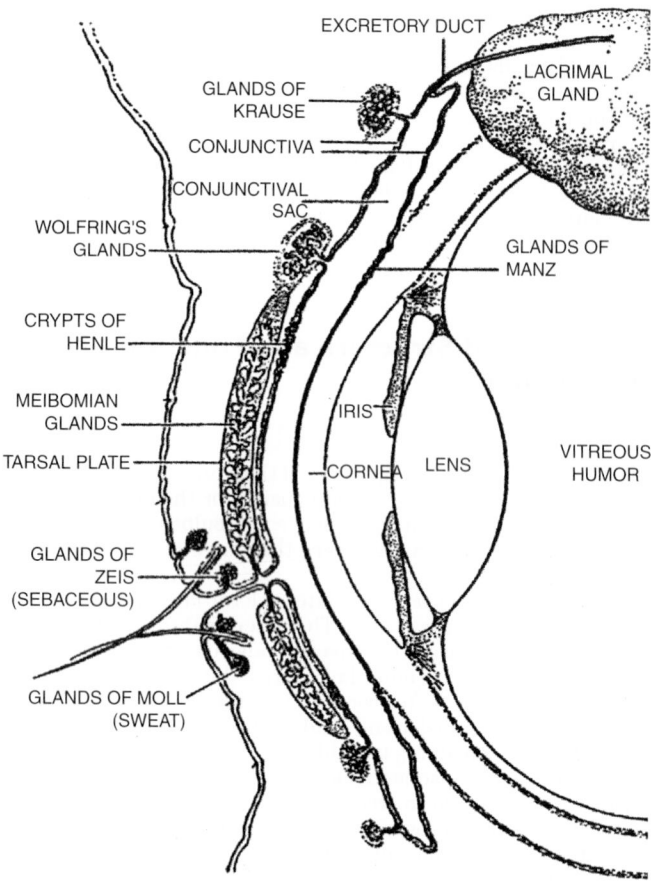

Figure 43-2. The front half of the eye, in vertical section, identifying the important structures associated with cornea and the front of the eye, including the eyelids and the glands associated with tears.

Neural Retina: This innermost layer of the eyeball is a complex tissue that supports the harvesting of light through the action of photoreceptors - nerve cells specialized for distinguishing white from black (rods), or discerning color (cones). In addition, the retina consists of cells that support metabolism (like the heavily pigmented retinal pigmented epithelium, the RPE, which purges photoreceptors of spent molecules and metabolites, and regenerates the *cis*-retinal), provide structure (astrocytes and Mueller cells), or contribute to the primary function of photodetection / signal processing (the ganglion cells that begin to process the electrochemical information transmitted from the photoreceptors).

Ocular Core: Within the globe, the crystalline lens spans the interior fluid-filled center close to the iris and is anchored by zonule fibers to the ciliary body. The lens is composed of a single layer of replicating epithelial cells that with age flatten into layers of long thin crystalline-filled lamellar fibers. The lens is the only tissue in the body that retains all cells ever produced, a fact that contributes to age-related alterations in size, clarity and extensibility. A tough thin transparent membrane called the capsule covers the outermost layer of the lens.

The aqueous and vitreous humors are interposed between the solid structures of the eye. The clear, fluid aqueous humor fills the globe anterior to the lens and is primarily responsible for maintaining correct intraocular pressure. The gel-like vitreous humor accounts for most of the weight of the eye and resides posterior to the lens in direct contact with the retina.

FUNCTION

The eyeball houses the optical apparatus that causes inverted reduced images of the outside world to form on the neural retina.

Dimensional Stability: The optical function of the eye calls for stability of its dimensions, which is provided partly by the fibrous outer coat, but more effectively by the intraocular pressure (IOP), which exceeds the pressure prevailing in the surrounding tissues. This intraocular pressure is the result of a steady production of specific fluid, the aqueous humor, which

identifiable layers. Proceeding from the most anterior layer, these are the hydrophobic stratified squamous epithelium, which is underlaid by Bowman's membrane, then the stroma and Descemet's membrane, and then the innermost layer, the endothelium. The stroma is a hydrophilic elastic network of highly organized connective tissue and is the thickest layer of the cornea. The fibrous collagen-rich Descemet's membrane separates the stroma from the single-squamous-cell layer of endothelium, the location of the pump that keeps the cornea in its relatively dehydrated transparent state. Functionally, the cornea serves as a bi-layer barrier, the hydrophobic epithelium being the primary barrier to hydrophilic molecules, and the hydrophilic stroma, the primary barrier to hydrophobic molecules. A schematic drawing of the cornea is provided in Figure 43-1.

Middle Vascular Layer: The middle vascular layer, or uvea, provides nourishment to the eye and consists, moving from the back of the eye forward, of the choroid, the ciliary body, and the iris. The choroid consists of a pigmented vascular layer, colored by melanocytes and traversed by medium-sized arteries and veins, with the choriocapillaris containing a network of small vessels that nourish the neural retina. The ciliary body contains muscles that control the extension of the lens allowing visual accommodation, as well as the ciliary processes that secrete aqueous humor into the posterior chamber to maintain the intraocular pressure that in turn keeps the eyeball fully expanded. The pigmented iris is a ring of muscular tissue around the pupil, a round centric hole that acts as a variable aperture to control pupil diameter, and thereby the level of light entering the eye. The canal of Schlemm, one of the important paths for outflow of the aqueous humor, resides in the angle of the iris. Bruch's membrane separates the choroid from the retina.

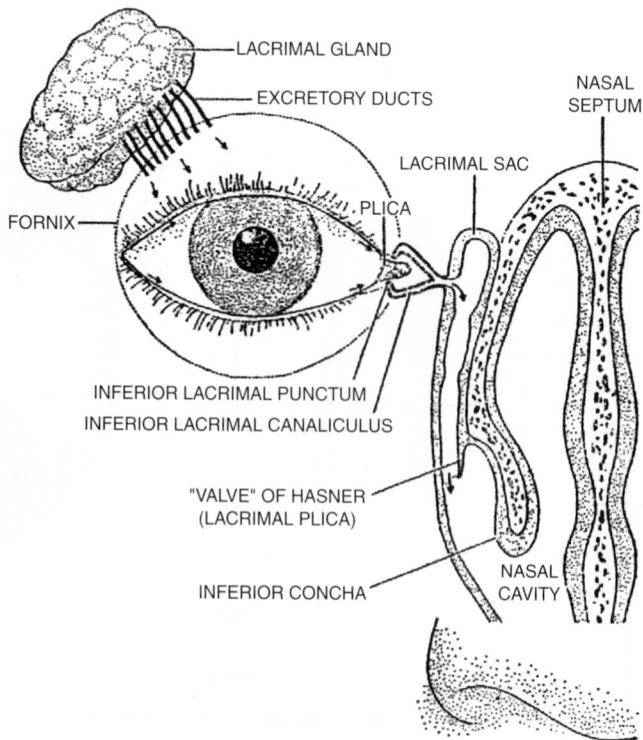

Figure 43-3. The structures associated with the tears and lacrimal flow and access to the nasolacrimal system.

originates from the ciliary processes anterior to the lens and leaves the eye by an intricate system of outflow channels. The resistance encountered during this passage and the rate of aqueous production are the principal factors determining the level of the intraocular pressure. In addition to this hydromechanical function, the aqueous humor acts as a carrier of nutrients, substrates, and metabolites for the avascular tissues of the eye.[10]

Optical Pathway: The optical pathway consists, in sequence, of the precorneal tear film, the cornea, the aqueous humor, the pupil, the crystalline lens, the vitreous humor, and the retina. The chief refraction of light for the eye occurs at the outer surface of the cornea where the index of refraction changes from that of air (1.00) to that of precorneal substance (1.38). After traversing the cornea, light passes through the clear aqueous humor to the pupil, where the amount of light entering the eye is regulated by the pupillary diameter, and to the second refractive element of the eye, the lens, whose variable focal length allows objects both near and far to be brought into focus (accommodation). The shape of the lens, controlled by the muscles of the ciliary body, refracts and focuses the reduced inverted image on the retina. That image is sharp and clear, in part, because of the high transparency of the vitreous humor, which because of its gel-like state keeps debris and cells from entering the pathway for the light. The image formed by the electromagnetic light signal on the neural retina is converted to a chemical signal, changing *cis-* to *trans-* retinal, which in turn is processed by neural cells into an electrochemical signal transported through axons to central nerve bodies. This continuous conversion of the excitation associated with a retinal image to processable information, is integral to the functioning of the retina, and is the reason retinal tissue is amongst the most rapidly metabolizing tissues in the body. The dependence of the neural retina on the metabolic support provided by the underlying cell layer, the RPE, explains why damage to the tissue - such as detachment of the retina or diminished blood supply - can result in nearly immediate and permanent loss of vision.[11]

Tissues Responsible for Refraction: Any alteration in the shape or transparency of the *cornea* interferes with the formation of a clear image; therefore, any pathological process, however slight, may interfere seriously with the resolving power or visual acuity of the eye. Transparency of the cornea is largely attributable to its organized laminar arrangement of cells and fibers and the absence of blood vessels. The normal cornea possesses no blood vessels except at the corneoscleral junction, the limbus. The cornea, therefore, must derive its nutrition by diffusion and must have certain permeability characteristics; it also receives nourishment from the fluid circulating through the chambers of the eye and from the air. The fact that the normal cornea is devoid of blood vessels is an important feature in surgical grafting.

Cloudiness of the cornea may occur as a result of disease (eg, excess pressure in the eyeball, a symptom associated with glaucoma), the presence of scar tissue due to injury, infection, deficiency of oxygen or excess hydration such as may occur during the wearing of improperly fitted contact lenses. A wound of the cornea may heal as an opaque patch that can be a permanent impairment of vision unless it is located in the periphery of the cornea.

The corneal nerves do not supply all forms of sensation to the cornea, but pain and cold are well supplied. The pain fibers have a very low threshold, which makes the cornea one of the most sensitive areas on the surface of the body. It now is agreed that the cornea possesses a true sense of touch; nerve endings supplying the sensation of heat appear to be lacking.

The corneal epithelium provides an efficient barrier against bacterial invasion. Unless its continuity has been broken by an abrasion (a traumatic opening or defect in the epithelium), pathogenic bacteria, as a rule, cannot gain a foothold. Trauma, therefore, plays an important part in most of the infectious diseases of the cornea that occur exogenously. A means of detecting abrasions on the corneal surface is afforded by staining the cornea with sodium fluorescein. Any corneal abrasion is subject to infection.

As with the cornea, any change in the transparency of the *lens* as a result of age or disease can significantly affect visual clarity. Loss of flexibility of the lens can reduce visual accommodation and cause difficulty in focusing on near objects. Also on aging, or as a result of trauma, the lens may generate opacities caused by the oxidation and crosslinking of lens proteins. When cataract surgery is required in order to restore clarity to cloudy vision, the natural lens is removed and replaced by an artificial one. The capsule, though, is preserved so that it may provide scaffolding for the implanted synthetic intraocular lens (IOL).

LACRIMAL SYSTEM—The conjunctival and corneal surfaces are covered and lubricated by a precorneal tear film, a fluid secreted by the conjunctival and lacrimal glands.[11] The clear watery secretion of the lacrimal gland, delivered through a number of fine ducts into the conjunctival fornix, contains numerous salts, glucose, other organic compounds, and approximately 0.7% protein, including the enzyme lysozyme. Small accessory lacrimal glands are situated in the conjunctival fornices. The tear film, compatible with both aqueous and lipid ophthalmic preparations, is composed of a thin outer lipid layer, a thicker middle aqueous layer, and a thin inner mucoid layer. It is renewed during blinking and when blinking is suppressed may dry in patches. It seems to be unaffected by the addition of concentrations of up to 2% sodium chloride to conjunctival fluid. A pH below 4 or above 9 causes derangement of the film. The film affects the movement of contact lenses and forms more easily on hydrophilic than on hydrophobic prostheses.

The innermost mucin-protein layer of the film is especially important in maintaining the stability of the film and is postulated to be held in place by the microvilli of the corneal epithelial cells. Sebaceous Meibomian glands of the eyelids secrete an oily fluid that forms the outer layer of the tears, helps to prevent overflow at the lid margin, and reduces evaporation from the exposed surfaces of the eye.

Spontaneous blinking replenishes the fluid film by pushing a thin layer of fluid ahead of the lid margins as they come together. The excess fluid is directed into the lacrimal lake—a small, triangular area lying in the angle bound by the innermost portions of the lids. The skin of the eyelids is the thinnest in the body and folds easily, thus permitting rapid opening and closing of the palpebral fissures, at velocities of tens of cm /sec. The movement of the eyelids includes a narrowing of the palpebral fissures in a zipper-like action from lateral to medial canthus. This aids transport or movement of fluid toward the lacrimal lake and elimination of unwanted contaminants.

Tears are drained from the lacrimal lake through two small openings, the superior and inferior puncta, which drain into connecting small tubes, the lacrimal canaliculi, which themselves join at the common canaliculus that leads into the upper part of the nasolacrimal duct, the beginning of which is the lacrimal sac, as shown in Figure 43-3 The drainage of tears into the nose does not depend merely on gravity. Fluid enters and passes along the lacrimal canaliculi by capillary action, aided by aspiration resulting from contraction of muscles embedded in the eyelids, and by peristalsis in the muscles near the canaliculi. When the lids close, as in blinking, contraction of the muscle causes dilatation of the upper part of the lacrimal sac and compression of its lower portion. Tears aspirated into the sac are forced down the nasolacrimal duct toward its opening into the nose. As the lids open, the muscle relaxes. The upper part of the sac then collapses and forces fluid into the lower part, which at the same time is released from compression. Thus, the act of blinking exerts a suction force-pump action in removing tears from the lacrimal lake and emptying them into the nasal cavity. Lacrimation is induced reflexively by stimulation of nerve endings of the cornea or conjunctiva. This reflex is abolished by anesthetization of the surface of the eye and by disorders affecting its nerve function.

The normal cul-de-sac is maintained free of pathogenic organisms in part by the chemical action of enzymes, such as lysozyme, which normally destroy saprophytic organisms with limited action against pathogens, and in part by the continuous physical flow of normally sterile secretions, which constantly wash the bacteria, dust, *etc.*, away from the eye down into the nose. In certain diseases or on aging the lacrimal gland, like other glandular structures in the body, may undergo involution, with the result that the lacrimal fluid becomes scanty. Changes in the conjunctival glands may lead to alteration in the character of the secretion so that quality as well as quantity of tears may be abnormal. This can lead to symptoms of dryness, burning, and general discomfort, and ultimately may interfere with visual acuity.

SUMMARY—This brief overview of the structure and function of the eye should provide a basis for understanding the highly integrated tissues comprising this miraculous organ, and suggest the importance of providing medications that in no way impair the balance of functions required for maintaining normal functioning of the eye.

BIOAVAILABILITY

Therapeutic Targets

Bioavailability of pharmacological agents is dictated by ocular structure and physiology just discussed. But bioavailability also is controlled by physical constraints and tissue biochemistry to be discussed in the next subsections, by physical and chemical characteristics of the therapeutic agents and the preparations by which they are presented. The bioavailability and potential efficacy of an agent also is determined by the therapeutic targets, which are governed by disease etiology.

For example, treatment of a superficial infection of the cornea, while possibly requiring sustained delivery in order to provide less frequent administration of antimicrobial therapy, does not involve special considerations of corneal permeation or access to the target tissue. In this circumstance, product design might be directed toward the reduction of any corneal or scleral transport, since these would be regarded as drug lost from the target site. On the other hand a recalcitrant case of uveitis may require both topical and systemic administration of anti-inflammatory agents in order to eliminate the condition. But in this case transport to the uvea, an internal tissue, is desirable.

Chronic diseases associated with aging, like glaucoma, may be amenable to routine administration of a topical medication. The target, however, may be determined by the particular mechanism for treating the disease. For instance, a drug influencing the generation of aqueous humor may target the iris ciliary body, whereas a drug influencing the outflow of aqueous humor might target the trabecular meshwork that opens into the canal of Schlemm. The inherent characteristics of the drug also will determine, in part, any need for sustained delivery. In general, a lipophilic agent will be absorbed readily into the lipophilic corneal epithelium, whereas an ionic or hydrophilic agent will be absorbed more slowly. But corneal permeation may still be a significant barrier to delivery at the target tissue even for a lipophilic drug since transport through the largely aqueous stroma is still required. The capacity of the epithelium for the drug, in part controlled by its partitioning characteristics, may govern any need for sustained administration as well as the dosing regimen. The solubility of the drug, especially for often relatively insoluble hydrophobic lipophilic agents, can limit the size of the reservoir of drug administered, or the exposure to the drug, where the latter is defined as the AUC (the area under the curve in a concentration vs. time plot of drug residence).

Recently treatments for ocular diseases of the deep tissues have invoked techniques more commonly utilized in targeted systemic delivery. For example, the treatment of retinal infection with cytomegalovirus, accompanying end-stage HIV infections, has engendered treatments delivering drug directly to the vitreous humor, either with intracameral injection or an implant. Photodynamic therapy utilizes a radiation—generally light—to activate a drug delivered systemically. Angiostatic agents for the treatment of wet AMD (age-related macular degeneration) are delivered from an implant. As Higuchi years ago and others more recently have described, the rate of delivery from such devices

can be controlled either by the design of the device, drug characteristics (primarily solubility), or a balance of both.[12]

Nonetheless, eye drops remain the most common modality for administration of therapeutic agents, and so considerations of the quantitative relationships governing the balance of effects controlling access of these agents to their target tissues are of significance and will be summarized in the next few sections. The approach will be primarily hydrodynamic,[13,14] though molecular theories are now available to give rationale for the macroscopic transport laws.[15] More intricate transport characteristics, such as those occurring when membranes actively transport the therapeutic agent, are less frequent than simple passive diffusion and for this introduction will be neglected. The approach highlights the interrelationships of phenomena whose subtle control in commercial products improves their efficacy. While transmembrane transport is most relevant to transcorneal delivery, some of the same considerations apply to actives delivered from implants, since these drug reservoirs serve only as a source for the agents that need to traverse tissues or tissue boundaries to reach their target sites.[16]

Corneal Absorption and Drug Access

Physical and Chemical Considerations

Under normal conditions the human tear volume averages about 7 μL.[17] The estimated maximum volume of the cul-de-sac is about 30 μL, with drainage capacity far exceeding lacrimation rate. The outflow capacity accommodates the sudden large volume resulting from the instillation of an eyedrop. Most commercial eyedrops range from 25 to 50 μL in volume.

Within the rabbit cul-de-sac, the drainage rate has been shown to be proportional to the instilled drop volume. Multiple drops administered at intervals produced higher drug concentrations. Ideally, a high concentration of drug in a minimum drop volume is desirable. Patton[18] has shown that approximately equal tear-film concentrations result from the instillation of 5 μL of 1.61×10^{-2} M pilocarpine nitrate or from 25 μL of 1.0×10^{-2} M solution. The 5 μL contains only 38% as much pilocarpine, yet its bioavailability is greater because of decreased drainage loss. Human responses can be expected to be similar, and this is supported by studies of gamma scintigraphy.[19] However, human tear responses are much more significant, and variable, than those in some *in vivo* models. When the therapeutic agents themselves are irritating, excess tearing may occur that may influence bioavailability in affected individuals. There is a practical limit or limits to the concept of minimum dosage volume. There is a difficulty in designing and producing a dropper configuration that will deliver small volumes reproducibly.[20] Also, the patient often cannot detect the administration of such a small volume. This sensation or lack of sensation is particularly apparent at the 5.0 to 7.5-μL dose-volume range.

The concept of dosage-volume drainage and cul-de-sac capacity directly affects the prescribing and administering of separate ophthalmic preparations. The first drug administered may be diluted significantly by the administration of the second. On this basis combination drug products for use in ophthalmology have considerable merit.

While generally not a major concern, an instilled drug can be subject to protein binding in the tear fluid and metabolic degradation by enzymes such as lysozyme. Stability, however, always is a primary consideration, both in the bottle and in the tissues. Rapid conversion of a drug to a metabolite is generally to be avoided unless by design (pro-drugs).

Corneal Absorption

Penetration of drugs administered topically occurs primarily through the cornea. Drugs administered by instillation must penetrate the eye and do so primarily through the cornea. Corneal absorption is generally more effective than scleral or conjunctival absorption, in which drug is removed by circulatory flow into the general circulation. This is also true because most therapeutic agents tend to be reasonably lipophilic. In the case of more hydrophilic materials, which as mentioned earlier are more slowly absorbed into the corneal epithelium, there is evidence to suggest that a scleral route may be more common. A practical example comes from studies of carbonic anhydrase inhibitors,[21] a class of drug used in the treatment of glaucoma.

Many ophthalmic drugs are weak bases and are conveniently applied to the eye as aqueous solutions of their salts. If the molecule is maintained in an ionized state, for example by employing a weakly acidic buffered vehicle, stability of the drug often may be prolonged. If the buffer is weak little discomfort is generally experienced at the time of instillation. Once neutralized by the tears, the fraction of free base may increase and this may be the form of the drug most readily absorbed by the corneal epithelium. Nonetheless, during transport through the hydrophilic stroma, an important fraction of the agent may be ionized. Similarly, the form transported through the endothelium may be the free base and that presented to the ciliary body (one of the sites of pharmacological action) in transport from the aqueous humor may be the ionized salt. This scenario is described simply to suggest the complexity that may be exploited in targeting an ophthalmic drug, as well as complementary considerations involved in providing a preparation capable of the requisite stability for conventional 2-year shelf life.

The cornea can be penetrated by ions to a small, but measurable, degree. Under comparable conditions, the permeabilities are similar for all ions of low molecular weight, which suggests that the passage is through extracellular spaces. The diameter of the largest particles that can pass across the cellular layers seems to be in the range of 10 to 25 Å. Some effort has been directed toward increasing the upper molecular weight limit for water-soluble therapeutic agents by utilizing a class of molecules referred to as penetration, or permeation, enhancers. These molecules are selected for their capacity to increase transiently permeation of larger molecules while producing minimal discomfort or toxicity.

Since highly water-soluble drugs generally penetrate the cornea less readily and since the cornea is known to be a membrane including both hydrophilic and lipophilic barrier layers, most effective penetration is obtained with drugs having both lipophilic and hydrophilic properties. As an example highly water-soluble steroid phosphate esters penetrate the cornea poorly. Better penetration is achieved with the poorly soluble but more lipophilic steroid alcohol; still greater absorption is seen with the steroid acetate form.

Work on transport of drugs through the cornea, dating from the work of Edelhauser,[13] Lee and Robinson in 1976[22] and later in 1990,[23] have indicated the interplay of physical properties that regulate access of drugs to ophthalmic tissues. The hydrodynamic principles are well known and will be outlined here. From the physical chemistry of passive diffusion across a simple membrane capable of sustaining a concentration difference (and discussed in other chapters of this volume), the main mechanism of entry into the eye,

$$J = -D \, dC_m/dx \qquad (1)$$

according to Fick's first law of diffusion, where J is the flux of drug across the membrane (amount per area per time), D is the diffusion coefficient, the derivative of C_m is the spatial concentration gradient in the membrane (at steady-state, constant across the membrane).[24] Even from this simple relationship the consequences of the physical properties of the drug can be inferred. As the solubility of the drug increases the gradient will increase, so the driving force for entry of the agent into the aqueous humor will be increased. Experiment similarly has shown specific characteristics of the diffusion coefficient; namely the diffusion coefficient decreases with increasing molecular size (and hence molecular weight of the compound). So all else being equal, one need balance the increased specificity and targeting of a larger active against the loss in rate of membrane transport. The equation also makes clear that any

means for maintaining the concentration on the donor side of the membrane, thereby sustaining the gradient term for a longer period of time, will increase the mean total flux.

In order to perceive the consequences of partitioning in a more complicated bilayer membrane (a good model for the cornea since the major layers serving as barriers to drug entry are the epithelium and stroma), one need look at the diffusion equation for a bilayer:

$$J \cong \frac{PC_w}{\dfrac{P1_s}{D_s} + \dfrac{1_e}{D_e}} \qquad (2)$$

where P is the distribution coefficient (for example the octanol:water partition coefficient wherein it is a good approximation of the partitioning into the epithelium), the subscripts designate either stroma (s) or epithelium (e), l is the length representing the thickness of the layer, and C_w is the concentration of drug at the donor side of the membrane, *i.e.* in the concentration of drug in the tears.[25] This equation is an approximation to the differential equation. One source of approximation is that it presumes the concentration on the donor side (in the eye, the concentration of active in the tears) is much higher than on the receiver side of the membrane (the concentration in the aqueous humor). From this equation one can observe that as the partitioning increases the effectiveness of the epithelium as a barrier diminishes and is replaced nearly exclusively by the stroma. Similarly, as the partitioning decreases, the epithelium becomes the dominant barrier. Of course, this is just a mathematical representation of an anticipated phenomenon. Clearly there is an advantage to increasing the lipophilicity of the agent in order to improve absorption and transport. A precaution to be kept in mind, however, is that ordinarily when the lipophilicity is increased the aqueous solubility (which C_w may approach) generally decreases. This is an example of the need to balance a number of characteristics, as was mentioned above.

There are circumstances, especially when the drug is sufficiently hydrophilic to limit severely absorption directly into the corneal epithelium, when sustaining the presence and concentration of the drug in the tear volume is important. From the equations for a stirred-tank chemical reactor, which is undergoing a steady-state flow of fluid with a solvent entering and a solution of mixed chemicals flowing from it, one expects

$$C_W(t) = C_I \cdot \exp\left(\frac{-\dot{V}_T \cdot t}{V_T}\right) \qquad (3)$$

where the time dependence of C_w is explicitly indicated, C_I is the initial concentration, V_T is the volume of the reactor (here the tear volume) and its derivative is the rate of flow through the reactor, essentially the rate of tear generation. A number of characteristics of drug delivery are apparent from this equation. One is that if the drug is uncomfortable and increases the rate of tearing, $\dot{V}_T$ in the equation, then the concentration in the tears is depleted more rapidly. Analogously, if the preparation includes a means for retaining a drug carrier in the cul-de-sac, then only a fraction of the drug present is released free into the tears, and $C_w(t)$ no longer changes with time, and until the reservoir is depleted may be approximately constant. Since what is important is the total amount of drug reaching the target tissue over a time period,

$$N_{eff} = A \cdot \int dt \, J(t) \qquad (4)$$

the effect of reducing the loss rate from tear flow may counterbalance the consequence of reducing the total level in the tears. Note, in the circumstance where there is a means for sustaining drug release equations (2) and (3) need to be modified, in any event, since C_I is no longer the total initial concentration but the fraction in the tears that is transportable through the cornea. This introduction should provide some notion of the types of complexity involved in achieving improved delivery of a therapeutic agent! When more is known about the details of ocular function, characteristics of the therapeutic agents and vehicles, it is possible to solve the differential equations numerically in order to improve the design of topically applied medications.[26–28]

This summary would be incomplete if it did not indicate that precisely the approach outlined at the end of the last paragraph is that taken to model and refine the design of preparations used in implants.[29–32] The significance of these activities, ongoing research, is difficult to overstate since the diseases being addressed—AMD, macular edema, diabetic retinopathy - are sight-threatening. The devices used to deliver the drug need to limit invasiveness and restrict frequency of any implanting procedure, providing durations of delivery ranging from months to years. A practical consequence is that the testing period for an implanted device is extended appreciably.

Finally, while the approach described in this section has been primarily macroscopic and phenomenological, microscopic models and calculations of transport based on them have provided additional detail about the molecular features of ocular drug transport. For example, it is generally believed that lipophilic drugs permeate the corneal epithelium by transcellular transport whereas more hydrophilic drugs permeate the corneal epithelium by paracellular transport. A model of these different mechanisms has indicated that the transcellular transport probably is along the lipophilic bilayers of the cell outer membranes, whereas the paracellular transport is probably along the extracellular space, the 'pores' of a macroscopic model.[24] These models provide insight into mechanisms of transport and how these may be manipulated to improve drug delivery while maintaining safety.

TYPES OF OPHTHALMIC DOSAGE FORMS

Ophthalmic products include prescription and OTC drugs, products for the care of contact lenses and products used in conjunction with ocular surgery. This section will focus on the pharmaceutical aspects of the various ophthalmic dosage forms encompassed by these types of products. The therapeutic uses of individual products can be found in several reference books along with the individual products' labeling.[33,34]

Ophthalmic Solutions

These are by far the most common dosage forms for delivering drugs to the eye. By definition, ingredients are completely soluble such that dose uniformity is not an issue and there is little physical interference with vision. The principal disadvantage of solutions is their relatively brief contact time with the drug and the absorbing tissues of the external eye. Contact time may be increased by the inclusion of a viscosity-imparting agent; however, their use is limited to relatively low viscosities so that the eyedrop can be dispensed from the container or eyedropper and to minimize excessive blurring of vision. A viscous solution can produce a residue on the eyelashes and around the eye when any excess spills out of the eye and dries. The residue can usually be easily removed by careful wiping with a moist towel to the closed eye.

Gel-Forming Solutions

Ophthalmic solutions, usually aqueous based, which contain a polymer system that is a low-viscosity liquid in the container and gels on contact with the tear fluid, have increased contact time and can provide increased drug absorption and prolonged duration of therapeutic effect. The liquid to gel phase transition can be triggered by a change in temperature, pH, ionic strength or presence of tear proteins depending on the particular polymer system employed. Timolol maleate gel-forming solutions formulated with specific patented gellan or xanthan gums have clinically demonstrated prolonged duration of IOP-lowering such that their dosing frequency can be reduced from twice to once a day.[35, 36] Review the labeling for commercial gel-forming solutions prior to dispensing for current instructions related to patient administration.

Powders for Solutions

Drugs that have very limited stability in aqueous solution can sometimes be prepared as sterile powders for reconstitution by the pharmacist prior to dispensing to the patient. The sterile powder should be aseptically reconstituted with the accompanying sterile diluent that has been optimized for dissolution, preservation and stability. The pharmacist must convey to the patient any special storage instructions including the expiration dating.

Ophthalmic Suspensions

Suspensions are dispersions of finely divided, relatively insoluble, drug substances in an aqueous vehicle containing suitable suspending and dispersing agents. The vehicle is, among other things, a saturated solution of the drug substance. Because of a tendency of particles to be retained in the cul-de-sac, the contact time and duration of action of a suspension could theoretically exceed that of a solution. The drug is absorbed from solution, and the solution concentration is replenished from retained particles. Each of these actions is a function of particle size, with solubility rate being favored by smaller size and retention favored by a larger size; thus, optimum activity should result from an optimum particle size.

For aqueous suspensions the parameters of intrinsic solubility and dissolution rate must be considered. The intrinsic solubility determines the amount of drug actually in solution and available for immediate absorption upon instillation of the dose. As the intrinsic solubility of the drug increases, the concentration of the drug in the saturated solution surrounding the suspended drug particle also increases. For this reason, any comparison of different drugs in suspension systems should include their relative intrinsic solubilities. The observed differences in their biological activities may be ascribed wholly or in part to the differences in this physical parameter. As the drug penetrates the cornea and the initial saturated solution becomes depleted, the particles must dissolve to provide a further supply of the drug. The requirement here is that the particles must undergo significant dissolution within the residence time of the dose in the eye if any benefit is to be gained from their presence in the dosing system.

For a drug whose dissolution rate is rapid, the dissolution requirement may present few problems, but for a slowly soluble substance the dissolution rate becomes critical. If the dissolution rate is not sufficiently rapid to supply significant additional dissolved drug, there is the possibility that the slowly soluble substance in suspension provides no more drug to the aqueous humor than does a more dilute suspension or a saturated solution of the substance in a similar vehicle. Obviously, the particle size of the suspended drug affects the surface area available for dissolution. Particle size also plays an important part in the irritation potential of the dosing system. This consideration is important, since irritation produces excessive tearing and rapid drainage of the instilled dose, as discussed earlier. It has been recommended that particles be less than 10 μm in size to minimize irritation to the eye. It should be kept in mind, however, that in any suspension system the effects of prolonged storage and changes in storage temperature might cause the smallest particles to dissolve and the largest particles to become larger.

The pharmacist should be aware of two potential difficulties inherent in suspension dosage forms. In the first instance dosage uniformity nearly always requires brisk shaking to distribute the suspended drug. Adequate shaking is a function of the suitability of the suspension formulation but also, and most importantly, patient compliance. Studies have demonstrated that a significant number of patients may not shake the container at all; others may contribute a few trivial shakes. The pharmacist should use a "Shake Well" label and counsel the patient whenever an ophthalmic suspension is dispensed. An improved ophthalmic suspension has been developed for insoluble drugs such as steroids which tend to cake upon settling.[37] The improved suspension controls the flocculation of the drug particles such that they remain substantially resuspended for months and provides for easy resuspension of any settled particles. Nonetheless, the pharmacist also should be aware of the possibility of crystal growth over time. This potential stability problem is especially problematic for drug substances with significant temperature-dependence of their solubility. The majority of suspension products have a "Do Not Freeze" warning on the label because they are likely to agglomerate on freezing and will not be resuspended by simple shaking.

A second and infrequent characteristic of suspensions is the phenomenon of polymorphism or the ability of a substance to exist in several different crystalline forms. A change in crystal structure may occur during storage, resulting in an increase (or decrease) in crystal size and alteration in the suspension characteristics, causing solubility changes reflected in increased or decreased bioavailability. Manufacturers of commercial suspensions take these possibilities into account in the development and testing of the final formulation and the labeled storage conditions.

In some cases a water-soluble drug has been converted to an insoluble form and formulated as a suspension to improve stability or compatibility of the drug or improve its bioavailability or patient tolerance. The insoluble forms of steroids such as prednisolone and dexamethasone have better ocular bioavailability and are considered more potent anti-inflammatories for topical ocular use. A resin-bound form of the beta-blocker betaxolol has been formulated as a suspension and is prepared *in situ* using a carbomer polymer.[38] The novel suspension formulation improves both comfort and ocular bioavailability of betaxolol, the 0.25% suspension therapeutically equivalent to a 0.5% solution.

Ophthalmic Ointments

Ophthalmic ointments are primarily anhydrous and contain mineral oil and white petrolatum as the base ingredients that can be varied in proportions to adjust consistency and the melting temperature. Dosage variability probably is greater than with solutions (although probably not with suspensions). Ointments will interfere with vision and their use is usually limited to bedtime instillation. They remain popular as a pediatric dosage form and for postoperative use. The anhydrous nature of the base enables its use as a carrier for moisture sensitive drugs. The petrolatum base can be made more miscible with aqueous components by the addition of liquid lanolins.

Ointments do offer the advantage of longer contact time and greater total drug bioavailability, albeit with slower onset and time to peak absorption. The relationship describing the availability of finely divided solids dispersed in an ointment base was given by Higuchi,[39] where the amount of solid (drug) released in unit time is a function of concentration, solubility in the ointment base, and diffusivity of the drug in the base.

Ophthalmic Emulsions

An emulsion dosage form offers the advantage of being able to deliver a poorly water-soluble drug in a solubilized form as an eyedrop. The drug is dissolved in a nonaqueous vehicle such as castor oil and emulsified with water using a nonionic surfactant and if needed an emulsion stabilizer. An emulsion with water as the external phase can be less irritating and better tolerated by the patient than use of a purely nonaqueous vehicle. Such an emulsion is used to deliver cyclosporin topically for the treatment of chronic dry eye conditions.[40]

Ophthalmic Gels

Gel-forming polymers such as carbomer have been used to develop aqueous, semi-solid dosage forms which are packaged and administered the same as ointments. The viscous gels have significantly increased topical residence time and can increase drug bioavailability and decrease dosage frequency compared

to solutions. Although they contain a large proportion of water, they can still cause blurring of vision. A carbomer gel of pilocarpine administered at bedtime has been shown to prolong the IOP-lowering effect in patients for up to 24 hours.[41]

Ocular Inserts

Ocular inserts have been developed in which the drug is delivered on the basis of diffusional mechanisms. Such a solid dosage form delivers an ophthalmic drug at a near-constant known rate, minimizing side effects by avoiding excessive absorption peaks. The delivery of pilocarpine by such an insert was commercialized in 1975 (Ocusert Pilo) by *Alza Corporation*. The Ocusert is designed to be placed in the lower cul-de-sac to provide a weekly dose of pilocarpine at which time the system is removed and replaced by a new one. The near zero-order rate delivery is based on the selection of a non-eroding copolymer membrane enclosing the drug reservoir.[42]

Ocular inserts are plagued with some of the same manipulative disadvantages as conventional eyedrops. The insert must be placed in the eye in a manner similar to the insertion of a contact lens. Additionally, the insert, exhausted of its drug content, must be removed from the eye. Such manipulations can be difficult for the elderly patient. Nonetheless, such therapeutic inserts represent a notable commercialized scientific achievement in pharmaceutical sciences. The Ocusert Pilo product is no longer marketed as the drug has largely been replaced in glaucoma therapy by the use of topical beta-blockers.

Ocular inserts that gradually erode in the tear fluid have been studied but not commercially developed as ocular drug delivery systems.[43] In theory, an erodible insert would be advantageous since it would not have to be removed at the end of its therapeutic cycle, would provide precise unit dosing and if anhydrous would not require a preservative. It may also increase ocular bioavailability and reduce the therapeutic dosage and possible systemic effects. The chief disadvantages may be related to patient use issues, control of erosion and drug release rates and sterilization.

An erodible insert is available (Lacrisert) for treatment of dry eye. It is molded in the shape of a rod from a hydroxypropyl cellulose polymer that is the active ingredient. When inserted into the lower cul-de-sac, the polymer imbibes tear fluid and forms a gel-like mass that gradually erodes while thickening the tear film over a period of several hours. The unit dose insert is anhydrous and no preservative is required, beneficial for some sensitive patients.

DRUG ADMINISTRATION

Topical Administration

The instillation of eyedrops remains one of the less precise, yet one of the more accepted means of topical drug delivery. The method of administration is cumbersome at best, particularly for the elderly, patients with poor vision who have difficulty seeing without eyeglasses, and patients with other physical handicaps. Perhaps surprisingly, most patients become quite adept at routine instillation.

The pharmacist should advise each patient to keep the following points in mind to aid in the instillation of eyedrops or ointments:

METHODS OF USE FOR TOPICAL ADMINISTRATION

How to Use Eyedrops

1. Wash hands.
2. With one hand, gently pull lower eyelid down.
3. If dropper is separate, squeeze rubber bulb once while dropper is in bottle to bring liquid into dropper.
4. Holding dropper above eye, drop medicine inside lower lid while looking up; do not touch dropper to eye or fingers.

5. Release lower lid. Try to keep eye open and not blink for at least 30 seconds.
6. If dropper is separate, replace on bottle and tighten cap.

Precautions When Using Eyedrops

- If dropper is separate, always hold it with the tip down.
- Never touch dropper to any surface.
- Never rinse dropper.
- When dropper is at top of bottle, avoid contaminating cap when removed.
- When dropper is a permanent fixture on the bottle, *i.e.*, when supplied by a pharmaceutical manufacturer to the pharmacist, the same rules apply to avoid contamination.
- Never use eye drops that have changed color.
- If you have more than one bottle of the same kind of drops, open only one bottle at a time.
- If you are using more than one kind of drop at the same time, wait several minutes before use of other drops.
- It may be helpful to practice use by positioning yourself in front of a mirror.
- After instillation of drops, do not close eyes tightly and try not to blink more often than usual, as this removes the medicine from the place on the eye where it will be effective.

How to Use Ophthalmic Ointments/Gels

1. Wash hands.
2. Remove cap from tube.
3. With one hand, gently pull lower eyelid down.
4. While looking up, squeeze a small amount of ointment (about 1/4 to 1/2 inch) inside lower lid. Be careful not to touch tip of tube to eye, eyelid, fingers, etc.
5. Close eye gently and roll eyeball in all directions while eye is closed. Temporary blurring may occur.
6. The closed eyelid may be rubbed very gently by a finger to distribute the drug throughout the fornix.
7. Replace cap on tube.

Precautions When Using Ophthalmic Ointments/Gels

- Take care to avoid contaminating cap when removed.
- When opening ointment tube for the first time, squeeze out the first 1/4 inch of ointment and discard, as it may be too dry.
- Never touch tip of tube to any surface.
- If you have more than one tube of the same ointment, open only one at a time.
- If you are using more than one kind of ointment at the same time, wait about 10 minutes before use of another ointment.
- To improve flow of ointment, hold tube in hand several minutes to warm before use.
- It may be helpful in use of the ointment to practice use by positioning yourself in front of a mirror.

Nasalacrimal Occlusion

To limit absorption of topically applied drugs directly into the bloodstream from the highly vascular areas of the nasal cavity, the patient should be instructed to close the eye immediately after eyedrop instillation and place a finger between the eyeball and the nose and apply pressure for several minutes. This will temporarily occlude both superior and inferior canaliculi, preventing nasolacrimal drainage.

Intraocular Preparations

Ophthalmic products introduced into the anterior chamber or vitreous chamber of the internal eye structure are specialized dosage forms requiring additional pharmaceutical considerations in their formulation, packaging and manufacture. They are essentially parenteral-type products requiring both sterility and nonpyrogenicity as well as strict control of particulate matter, being restrictive in formulation to assure they are compatible with sensitive internal tissues critical to visual acuity. In some cases in which the product may be introduced into the ster-

ile field during surgery, sterility of the exterior of the primary package is required. Since preservatives commonly used in topical ophthalmic products can be toxic to sensitive intraocular tissues such as the corneal endothelium, intraocular products are designed and packaged as preservative-free single use products.

Present technologies are summarized in the next subsections, but many novel technologies can be expected in the next several years with the advent of new therapeutics and approaches to delivery for such devastating diseases as AMD, diabetic retinopathy, and cystoid macular edema, diseases of the back of the eye.

IRRIGATING SOLUTIONS

During ocular surgery an irrigating solution is used to maintain hydration and clarity of the cornea providing the surgeon a clear view of the surgical field. The irrigating solution also provides a physiologic medium for removing blood and cellular debris and replacing the natural aqueous intraocular fluid. A balanced salt solution (BSS) is the primary intraocular irrigating solution which includes the key ionic components to maintain corneal endothelial integrity; sodium, potassium, calcium, magnesium and chloride, as well as a neutral to slightly alkaline pH and osmolality of about 305 mOsm.[44] An enriched balanced salt solution (BSS Plus) is also available to provide enhanced physiological compatibility when required in an irrigating solution. The enriched solution contains oxidized glutathione, dextrose and bicarbonate in addition to the critical ionic components.[45] The additional ingredients in the enriched solution require, for maximum shelf-life stability, that the product be packaged in a two-part system to be aseptically reconstituted just prior to its use. Intraocular solutions do not contain a preservative and should be discarded after initial use. These irrigating solutions are also designed to be used without additional additives as there is potential for intraocular toxicity. An acidic epinephrine injection containing sodium bisulfite antioxidant when added to an intraocular irrigating solution and diluted as much as 500-fold has been reported to produce intraocular toxicity.[46]

INTRAOCULAR INJECTIONS

Products approved for direct injection into the eye include miotics and viscoelastics for ocular surgery and two antiviral agents to treat cytomegalovirus retinitis (CMV). The miotics carbachol and acetylcholine are used at the end of cataract surgery to constrict the pupil allowing the iris to cover the implanted intraocular lens. Both products are specially packaged such that the exterior of the primary vial is sterile. This is accomplished by use of a special outer container that is permeable to sterilant gas and prevents contamination of the exterior of the vial.

Solutions with viscoelastic properties are injected into the eye during surgery to provide a mechanical barrier between tissues and allow the eye surgeon more space for manipulation with less potential for trauma to very sensitive intraocular tissues. The primary viscoelastic substance is a highly purified fraction of sodium hyaluronate. Purification is required to remove foreign proteins to be nonantigenic and noninflammatory for intraocular use. The viscoelasticity can be varied by use of different molecular weight fractions and concentrations. Chondroitin sulfate and purified hydroxypropyl methylcellulose are also utilized as viscoelastic and viscoadherent surgical adjuncts. The viscoelastic products are packaged and sterilized such that the primary package can be placed in the sterile surgical field prior to use. Sodium hyaluronate viscoelastic products usually require refrigeration during storage to maintain their integrity.

INTRAVITREAL INJECTIONS/IMPLANTS

Two antivirals have been approved for treatment of the ocular sequelae of AIDS with direct implacement in the vitreous cavity in order to provide high localized ocular therapeutic concentrations. A sterile tablet containing ganciclovir, called a Vitrasert,[47] is implanted by the surgeon in the vitreous cavity where it releases drug over a period of several months and then is removed and replaced with a new tablet. The tablet is formulated with magnesium stearate as the drug carrier and coated with polymers that provide the prolonged drug release. It is important that during handling this polymer coating is not damaged and the special sterile packaging not be compromised. A sterile solution of fomivirsen is also available for intravitreal injection to treat CMV retinitis. It is supplied in single use vials and is injected intravitreally without requiring surgery but must be repeated every 2 to 4 weeks.

JUXTASCLERAL INJECTIONS

Certain disease conditions in the back of the eye are usually untreatable through topical administration to the eye. For example, CME (cystoid macular edema) - associated with trauma, chronic inflammation and diabetes–results in swelling of the macula and, if left untreated, loss of vision. At present there is no effective treatment available for AMD (age-related macular degeneration), whose incidence and severity increases with age resulting in progression from accumulation of proteins and glycosaminoglycans (drusen) to leakage of blood vessels (hemorrhage) and eventual blindness. For such conditions localized intravitreal or juxtascleral injections may be preferable to systemic administration of drugs (either alone or accompanied by laser initiated events such as photodynamic therapy).

Other Modes of Administration

PACKS

These sometimes are used to give prolonged contact of a drug solution with the eye to maximize absorption. Sterile cotton pledgets placed in the lower cul-de-sac have been used in this manner but more recently corneal shields and soft contact lenses developed as bandages have been utilized to protect the cornea during healing.[48] Corneal shields are made of collagen that is cross-linked to control the rate of erosion, usually 12 to 72 hours. Hydrophilic polymers used for soft contact lenses without vision correction have also been utilized as a drug reservoir. The soft lenses remain intact and therefore require removal.

INTRACAMERAL INJECTIONS

Injections may be made directly into the anterior chamber (eg, acetylcholine chloride, alpha-chymotrypsin, carbamylcholine chloride, certain antibiotics, and steroids) or directly into the vitreous chamber (eg, amphotericin B, gentamicin sulfate, and certain steroids).

IONTOPHORESIS

This procedure keeps the solution in contact with the cornea by means of an eyecup bearing an electrode. Diffusion of an ionic drug has imposed on it a driving force generated by a difference in electrical potential, which acts as an electrochemical driving force to transport the drug in the direction of the potential gradient.[49]

SUBCONJUNCTIVAL INJECTIONS

Subconjunctival injections (Fig 43-4)[50] are used frequently to introduce medications that if applied topically either do not penetrate into the anterior segment or penetrate too slowly to attain the concentration required. The drug is injected underneath the conjunctiva and probably passes through the sclera and into the eye by simple diffusion. The most common use of

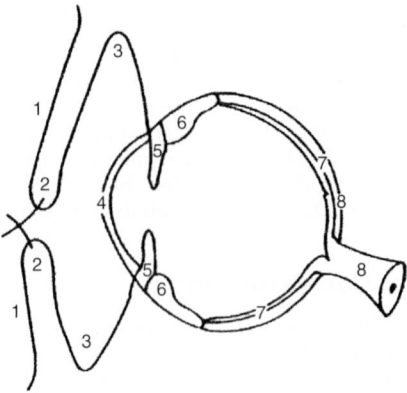

Figure 43-4. The locations for administration and target of therapy. Ointment: regions 1–5. Drops: regions 3–5. Parenteral injections—subconjunctival: regions 4–6, deep subtenons: regions 6–8, retreobulbar: region 8.

subconjunctival injection is for the administration of antibiotics in infections of the anterior segment of the eye. Subconjunctival injections of mydriatics and cycloplegics also are used to achieve maximal pupillary dilation or relaxation of the ciliary muscle. If the drug is injected underneath the conjunctiva and the underlying Tenon's capsule in the more posterior portion of the eye, effects on the ciliary body, choroid, and retina can be obtained.

RETROBULBAR INJECTIONS

Drugs administered by retrobulbar injection (Fig 43-4) may enter the globe in essentially the same manner as the medications given subconjunctivally. The orbit is not well vascularized, and the possibility of significant removal via-bloodstream effects from these injections is remote. In general, such injections are given for the purpose of getting medications (eg, antibiotics, local anesthetics, enzymes with local anesthetics, steroids, vasodilators) into the posterior segment of the globe and to affect the nerves and other structures in that space for a sustained period of time.

PREPARATION

Commerical Manufacture

Pharmaceutical manufacturers provide finished ophthalmic products manufactured and tested for quality according to stringent industrial and governmental standards. The products' sterility and, where required, their nonpyrogenicity as well as other important quality standards are assured by end-product testing of each batch and also the use of validated manufacturing processes developed for each individual product. The products' manufacturing and quality control is governed largely by the Current Good Manufacturing Practice (cGMP) regulations[51] promulgated and enforced by the Food and Drug Administration (FDA). If the product is a new or generic drug or medical device and has received FDA marketing approval, the manufacturer must also meet the requirements specified in the approved application for chemistry, microbiology, manufacturing and quality control. Significant changes to the approved requirements must be submitted and approved by the FDA. For products not requiring prior FDA approval to market such as monographed OTC drug products,[52] the manufacturer must meet the quality standards of applicable USP or NF compendial monographs in addition to the cGMP regulations.

The manufacturer is subject to preapproval inspections and periodic GMP postapproval inspections by FDA. FDA also conducts inspections of the suppliers of active ingredients, both foreign and domestic, and certain inactive ingredients and packaging operations. The manufacture is subject to recalls of batches of product that do not meet quality requirements. In some cases a recall may result not from actual failed test results but from a lack of assurance that the product will continue to meet quality requirements through its shelf life.

Pharmacy Compounding

Compounding of individual patient prescriptions by pharmacists has been and continues in some areas to be an integral part of pharmacy practice. The need to routinely compound sterile ophthalmic products is no longer required with the broad range of commercially manufactured products available today. Most of the new and generic prescription ophthalmic products marketed today have been subjected to FDA's rigorous requirements for proof of safety and efficacy or bioequivalence as well as the above-described manufacturing and quality requirements.

If the pharmacist is requested to compound a prescription for a noncommercial product such as a preservative-free version or pediatric strength, he or she should be well versed in the preparation of sterile products, have the proper equipment and facilities and be knowledgeable about the special requirements for ophthalmic formulations and packaging. Reference information on the standards and technology for pharmacy compounding with special emphasis on preparation of sterile products should be consulted.[53, 54] The pharmacist must also consult the rules and regulations of the applicable state board of pharmacy concerning sterile pharmacy compounding as well as any federal regulatory requirements promulgated by the FDA. Congress included in the 1997 FDA Modernization Act certain legal conditions for which compounding as defined in the Act would be exempt from FDA regulation. The pharmacy compounding section of the Act was subsequently litigated and overturned in its entirety because it contained unconstitutional restrictions on commercial speech. FDA may seek new legislation to address their concerns regarding manufacturing in the guise of compounding. In the meantime, FDA has issued a guidance document on how the Agency intends to regulate pharmacy compounding of human drugs considered to be outside the bounds of traditional pharmacy practice and in violation of the Food, Drug and Cosmetic Act (www.fda.gov/cder/pharmcomp).

STERILIZATION

Common methods of sterilization include moist heat under pressure (autoclave), dry heat, filtration, gas sterilization, and ionizing radiation. Please refer to Chapter 40 where these sterilization procedures are described in detail.

DANGERS OF NONSTERILE MEDICATIONS—The possibility of serious ocular infection resulting from the use of contaminated ophthalmic solutions has been documented amply in the literature. Such solutions have been the cause repeatedly of corneal ulcers and even loss of eyesight. Contaminated solutions have been found in use in physicians' offices, eye clinics, and industrial infirmaries, and dispensed on prescription in community and hospital pharmacies. The microbe most frequently found as a contaminant is the Staphylococcus group. *Pseudomonas aeruginosa* is a less frequent contaminant, and the solution most often found contaminated is sodium fluorescein.

P. aeruginosa (*B. pyocyaneus; Pseudomonas pyocyanea;* blue pus bacillus) is a very dangerous and opportunistic organism that grows well on most culture media and produces both toxins and antibacterial products. The latter tend to kill off other contaminants and allow the *P. aeruginosa* to grow in pure culture. This gram-negative bacillus also grows readily in ophthalmic solutions, which may become the source of extremely serious infections of the cornea. It can cause complete loss of sight in 24 to 48 hr. In concentrations tolerated by tissues of the eye, it seems that all the antimicrobial agents discussed in the following sections may be ineffective against some strains of this organism.

A sterile ophthalmic solution in a multiple-dose container can be contaminated in a number of ways unless precautions are taken. For example, if a dropper bottle is used, the tip of the dropper while out of the bottle can touch the surface of a table or shelf if laid down, or it can touch the eyelid or eyelash of the patient during administration. If the Drop-Tainer (*Alcon*) type of bottle is used, the dropper tip can touch an eyelash or the cap while removed to permit administration, or its edge may touch a table or finger, and that edge can touch the dropper tip as the cap is replaced.

The solution may contain an effective antimicrobial, but the next use of the contaminated solution may occur before enough time has elapsed for all of the organisms to be killed, and living organisms can find their way through an abrasion into the corneal stroma. Once in the corneal stroma, any residual traces of antimicrobial agents are neutralized by tissue components, and the organisms find an excellent culture medium for rapid growth and dissemination through the cornea and the anterior segment of the eye.

OTHER ORGANISMS—*Bacillus subtilis* may produce a serious abscess when it infects the vitreous humor. The pathogenic fungus considered of particular importance in eye solutions is *Aspergillus fumigatus*. Other fungi or molds may be harmful by accelerating deterioration of the active drugs.

With regard to viruses, as many as 42 cases of epidemic keratoconjunctivitis were caused by one bottle of virus-contaminated tetracaine solution. Virus contamination is particularly difficult to control because none of the preservatives now available is virucidal. Moreover, viruses are not removable by filtration. However, they are destroyed by autoclaving. The pharmacist and physician have not been made adequately aware of the dangers of transmitting viral infection via contaminated solutions. This is particularly pertinent to the adenoviruses (Types III and VIII), now believed to be the causative agents of viral conjunctivitis such as epidemic keratoconjunctivitis.

The danger of non-sterile preparations is exponentially increased for products intended to be injected within the eyeball. Endophthalmitis and loss of vision can occur within a short time of onset of a bacterial infection.

Methods

STEAM UNDER PRESSURE—Terminal sterilization by autoclaving is an acceptable, effective method of sterilization; however, the solution or suspension components must be sufficiently heat-resistant to survive the procedure. If sterilization is carried out in the final container, the container also must be able to survive heat and pressure. A recent addition to this technique is the so-called air-over-steam autoclave. This combination allows pressure adjustments to be made during the autoclave cycle. Pressure manipulations permit the autoclave sterilization of materials that while heat-resistant tend to deform (ie, polypropylene containers). The sterilization cycle for a product should be carefully validated and assure that sterilization temperature and time are monitored at the coldest spot of the autoclave load to assure sterility of the product.

FILTRATION—The USP states that sterile membrane filtration under aseptic conditions is the preferred method of sterilization. Membrane filtration offers the substantial advantage of room temperature operation with none of the deleterious effects of exposure to heat or sterilizing gas.

Sterilization by filtration does involve the transfer of the finished sterile product into previously sterilized containers, using aseptic techniques. The membrane filtration equipment itself usually is sterilized as an assembly by autoclaving.

Several types of membrane filtration equipment are available for small-scale processing, as described in Chapter 40.[54] Particular interest has been shown in the Swinney adapter fitted on a syringe and in the *Millipore* Swinnex disposable filter units. Empty sterile plastic *squeeze* containers and sterile plastic filtration units can be purchased directly from the manufacturers, eg, *Wheaton* (polyethylene containers) and *Millipore* (Swinnex filter units). They permit extemporaneous preparation of ophthalmic solutions that have a high probability of being sterile if the work is carried out under aseptic conditions. A supplementary device can permit automatic refilling of the syringe. The filter unit must be replaced after use. To avoid contamination, the pharmacist should fill sterile filtered solutions into pre-sterilized containers closed with appropriate fitments and closure under laminar-flow using aseptic techniques. The Parenteral Drug Association has produced several audio-visual teaching materials for aseptic techniques and processing. The reader should refer to these guidelines for reference.

GAS—Gas sterilization of heat-sensitive materials may be carried out by exposure to ethylene oxide gas in the presence of moisture. Ethylene oxide (EtO) gas for sterilization use is available commercially, diluted with either carbon dioxide or halogenated hydrocarbons. Ethylene oxide sterilization requires careful consideration of conditions required to effect sterility. Temperature and pressure conditions are quite nominal in contrast to wet or dry heat; however, careful control of exposure time, EtO concentration, and moisture is essential.

Gas sterilization requires the use of specialized, but not necessarily elaborate, equipment. Gas autoclaves may range from very large walk-in units to small, laboratory bench–scale units suitable for small hospitals, laboratories, or pharmacies. In using gas sterilization the possibility of human toxicity must be kept in mind. Care should be taken to restrict exposure to ethylene oxide during the loading, venting, and unloading of the sterilizer. Ethylene oxide sterilization produces irritating by-products that remain as residues in or on the articles sterilized. Residues include ethylene glycol and ethylene chlorohydrin (when in contact with chloride ions) in addition to EtO itself. To minimize such residues the sterilized articles should be aerated for at least 72 hr, preferably at 40 to 50°C.

Ambient aeration time for sterilized polyethylene bottles should be about 48 hr. Ethylene oxide is recommended for the sterilization of solid materials that will not withstand heat sterilization. The FDA has recommended maximum residues in the parts per million range for EtO, ethylene glycol, and ethylene chlorohydrin.

Extreme caution should be exercised when using EtO gas sterilization. The previously accepted 12:88 mixture of EtO:Freon has been replaced with 100% EtO for environmental reasons. This gas is explosive and all workers also should be protected from accidental exposure due to concern for carcinogenicity and other toxic reactions to ethylene oxide. This method at present is used as a last resort when no other methods can be used.

RADIATION—Sterilization by exposure to ionizing radiation is an acceptable procedure for components of ophthalmic preparations or indeed for the total product, such as certain ophthalmic ointments. Sources of radiation are twofold and include linear electron accelerators and radioisotopes. The linear accelerators produce high-energy electrons with very little penetrating power. Radioisotopes, particularly ^{60}Co, are employed more widely for sterilization. Sterilization by radiation may produce untoward effects such as chemical changes in product components as well as changes in color or physical characteristics of package components. Gamma sterilization is currently used in place of EtO for sterilizing most of the packaging components. Gamma sterilization of containers may alter the surface characteristics and this can increase degradation of drug molecules and or some of the excipients used in the formulation. Some plastic manufacturers have developed special grades of polypropylene resin that is stabilized to withstand gamma irradiation.

OPHTHALMIC PREPARATION CHARACTERISTICS

CLARITY—Ophthalmic solutions by definition contain no undissolved ingredients and are essentially free from foreign particles. Clarity may be enhanced in some cases by filtration. It is essential that the filtration equipment be clean and well-rinsed so that particulate matter is not contributed to the solution by equipment designed to remove it. Operations performed in clean surroundings, the use of laminar-flow hoods, and proper nonshedding garments will contribute collectively to the preparation of clear solutions essentially free from foreign particles. In many instances clarity and sterility may be achieved in the same filtration step. If viscosity-imparting polymers are used, a polish-filtering step may be required prior to the final filtration.

Both container and closure must be thoroughly clean, sterile, and nonshedding, neither contributing particulate matter to the solution during prolonged contact for the duration of the shelf life. Normally this is established by thorough stability testing, which also will indicate if insoluble particles are generated by drug degradation (by-products with lower solubility). Solution formulations also may contain viscosity imparting polymers that can diminish clarity. In these situations it may be important both to define the visual clarity of the product and monitor its stability. The European Pharmacopoeia describes visual clarity and recommends standards that can be used for clarity specifications.

STABILITY—The stability of a drug in an ophthalmic product depends on a number of factors including the chemical nature of the drug substance, whether it is in solution or suspension, product pH, method of preparation (particularly temperature exposure), solution additives, and type of packaging. A pharmaceutical manufacturer strives for a shelf-life measured in years at controlled room temperature conditions whereas the compounding pharmacist often is not certain about the shelf life of his preparation and thus provides relatively small quantities at one time and assigns a shelf life in terms of days or weeks and may specify refrigerated storage as a further precaution. The attainment of optimum stability often imposes some compromises in the formulation, packaging and preparation of the final product.

The product's pH is often the stability-controlling factor for many drugs. Drugs such as pilocarpine and physostigmine are both active and comfortable in the eye at a pH of 6.8; however, at this pH chemical stability (or instability) can be measured in days or months. With either drug, a substantial loss in chemical stability will occur in less than 1 year. On the other hand, at pH 5 both drugs are stable for a period of several years.

In addition to optimal pH, if oxygen sensitivity is a factor, adequate stability may require inclusion of an antioxidant or special packaging. Plastic packaging, *ie*, the low-density polyethylene containers such as the Drop-Tainer (*Alcon*) that represents a patient convenience, may prove detrimental to stability by permitting oxygen permeation resulting in oxidative decomposition of the drug substance. To develop an epinephrine solution with 2 to 3 years stability in a plastic package requires the use of a pH of about 3 for protection from oxidation whereas an epinephrine borate solution formulated at a pH of about 7, which is more comfortable to the patient, requires an antioxidant system and the use of glass packaging. The prodrug of epinephrine, dipivefrin, significantly increases ocular bioavailability and is effective at one-tenth the concentration of epinephrine. The structure of the chemical derivative protects the active epinephrine portion from oxidation enabling it to be packaged in plastic. However, the prodrug introduces a labile ester linkage and as a result must be formulated at a pH of about 3 to minimize hydrolysis and still can only achieve a room temperature shelf life of less than 18 months.

Pharmaceutical manufacturers conduct comprehensive stability programs to assure the assigned expiration dating for each product. In addition to the standard chemical and physical stability of the pharmaceutical, the stability of the preservative is monitored by chemical means or by actual challenge of the preservative efficacy with appropriate test organisms. Sterility is not a stability parameter per se but each container-closure system can be tested by microbial challenge to assure integrity of the package against environmental contamination prior to opening.

Some of the newer classes of ophthalmic drugs, like prostaglandins, are very hydrophobic and have very low concentrations. For example, in the product Xalatan latanoprost is present at 0.005% and in the product Travatan travoprost is present at 0.004%. Actives at such low concentrations present a challenge for formulators since the loss of even small amounts of drug, eg, from adsorption losses to packaging, may become significant. Pharmacia's Xalatan requires refrigerated storage, and as indicated earlier, temperature cycling also can reduce the concentration of active. It is important for the pharmacist to know the properties of the drug substance so that product quality is maintained throughout the shelf life of the product.

BUFFER AND pH—Ideally, ophthalmic preparations should be formulated at a pH equivalent to the tear fluid value of 7.4. Practically, this seldom is achieved. The large majority of active ingredients used in ophthalmology are salts of weak bases and are most stable at an acid pH. This generally can be extended to suspensions of insoluble corticosteroids. Such suspensions usually are most stable at an acid pH.

Optimum pH adjustment generally requires a compromise on the part of the formulator. The pH selected should be optimized for stability. The buffer system selected should have a capacity adequate to maintain pH within the stability range for the duration of the product shelf life. Buffer capacity is the key in this situation.

It generally is accepted that a low (acid) pH *per se* necessarily will not cause stinging or discomfort on instillation. If the overall pH of the tears, after instillation, reverts rapidly to pH 7.4, discomfort is minimal. On the other hand, if the buffer capacity is sufficient to resist adjustment by tear fluid and the overall eye pH remains acid for an appreciable period of time, then stinging and discomfort may result. Consequently, buffer capacity should be adequate for stability but minimized, so far as possible, to allow the overall pH of the tear fluid to be disrupted only momentarily. Special care in formulating intraocular products is required regarding their pH and buffer capacity. The corneal endothelium can tolerate much less deviation from physiological conditions compared to the external corneal epithelium.[55]

TONICITY—Tonicity refers to the osmotic pressure exerted by salts in aqueous solution. An ophthalmic solution is isotonic with another solution when the magnitudes of the colligative properties of the solutions are equal. An ophthalmic solution is considered isotonic when its tonicity is equal to that of a 0.9% sodium chloride solution (290 mOsm). However, the osmotic pressure of the aqueous intraocular fluid is slightly higher than tears measuring about 305 mOsm.

In actuality the *external* eye is much more tolerant of tonicity variations than was at one time suggested and usually can tolerate solutions equivalent to a range of 0.5 to 1.8% sodium chloride. Given a choice, isotonicity is desirable and particularly is important in intraocular solutions.[56] However, in certain cases a non-isotonic topical product is desirable. Tear fluid in some cases of dry eye (keratoconjunctivitis sicca) is reported to be hypertonic and a hypotonic artificial tear product is used to counteract this condition. Hypertonic ophthalmic products are used to relieve corneal edema and solutions and ointments containing 2% or 5% sodium chloride are available for this use.

The tonicity of ophthalmic (and parenteral) solutions has been investigated intensively over the years. These studies have resulted in the accumulation and publication of a large number of sodium chloride equivalents that are useful in calculating tonicity values. See Chapter 18 for a thorough discussion of the measurement and calculation of tonicity values.

VISCOSITY—Ophthalmic solution and suspension eyedrops may contain viscosity-imparting polymers to thicken the tear film and increase corneal contact time, ie, reduce the rate of tear fluid drainage. For suspensions, the increased viscosity also serves to retard the settling of particles between uses and at the same time maintains their suspension for uniform dosing. However, added viscosity may make initial resuspension more difficult particularly in a suspension that has a tendency to cake during storage. The hydrophilic polymers most often used for these purposes are methylcellulose, hydroxypropyl methylcellulose, hydroxyethyl cellulose and polyvinyl alcohol. They are used at concentrations that produce viscosities in the range of about 5 to 100 cps. These polymers are also used themselves as the active ingredients in artificial tear solutions for their lubrication and moisturizing properties in dry eye therapy. Viscosity agents can have several disadvantages in that they sometimes produce blurring of vision and can leave a residue on the eyelids. These effects are most often seen at the higher end of the viscosity range. The added viscosity can make filtration more difficult particularly for the small pore size filters used to sterilize solutions.

Newer ophthalmic dosage forms such as gel-forming solutions and semi-solid aqueous gels utilize increased viscosity and gel elasticity to improve significantly drug bioavailability and duration of effect. With these advances, the frequency of dosing can be reduced and patient compliance improved. These newer dosage forms utilize novel polymer systems with special rheological properties to enhance their effect. Their complex rheology and intricate dependence on environment, however, increase the complexity of the sterile manufacturing process.

ADDITIVES—Additives or pharmaceutical excipients are used as inactive ingredients in most ophthalmic dosage forms. Because of the need for tissue compatibility, the use of additives is perhaps more limited in ophthalmics, particularly in intraocular products.

The most common inactive ingredient is the product's vehicle. For topical dosage forms, Purified Water USP is used. Because of the requirement for nonpyrogenicity, Water for Injection USP is used for intraocular products. While a mineral oil and petrolatum combination is the vehicle used for ophthalmic ointments, nonaqueous liquids are rarely used in topical eyedrops due to their potential for ocular irritation and poor patient tolerance. Some mineral and vegetable oils have been used for very moisture-sensitive or poorly water-soluble drugs. The purest grade of oil such as those used for parenteral products should be used.

Microbiological preservatives are commonly used in multiple dose topical ophthalmic products and will be discussed in a later section. Other commonly used additives in topical eye products are ingredients to adjust and buffer pH and adjust tonicity in addition to the viscosity agents previously discussed. Ingredients to adjust pH and tonicity and buffer pH are essentially the same as those used in parenteral products. Less commonly used additives are antioxidants such as sodium bisulfite, ascorbic acid and acetylcysteine.

Surfactants are sometimes used in topical eye products for dispersing insoluble ingredients or to aid in solubilization. They are used in the smallest concentration possible to perform the desired function since they can be irritating to sensitive ocular tissues. Nonionic surfactants are used most often since they are generally less irritating than ionic surfactants. Polysorbate 80 is used in the preparation of an ophthalmic emulsion. Polyoxyl 40 stearate and polyethylene glycol have been used to solubilize a drug in an anhydrous ointment so that it can be filter sterilized. Surfactants are often used to stabilize more hydrophobic drugs, for example preventing loss to adsorption on the container walls. For example, a nonionic surfactant like polyoxyl 40 hydrogenated castor oil (HCO-40) has been used to stabilize travoprost, a prostaglandin derivative.[57] Similarly Cremophore EL has been used to stabilize diclofenac in the Voltaren formulation marketed by *Novartis*.

The FDA has published a list of all inactive ingredients used in approved drug products on their Internet website at www.fda.gov/cder. The list includes dosage forms and concentration ranges.

PACKAGING

Currently almost all commercially available ophthalmic products are packaged in plastic containers. Obvious advantages - ease of use, little breakage, less spillage - have led to universal acceptance of these plastic packaging components, consisting of bottle, fitment and closure. Alcon was the first company to introduce these packaging components, identified as a Drop-Tainer for ophthalmic products, in the late 1940s and then saw them adopted by the industry as the standard for packaging topical ophthalmic products. These bottles are generally of low-density polyethylene, either without any colorants or with opacifying agents or other colorants for light protection. Polypropylene or high-density polyethylene resins are also used to meet specific product requirements. The fitments determine drop size of the product and may contain additional features to prevent streaming of product at the time of use. Caps or closures are generally made from polypropylene and basically seal the container to prevent contamination or leakage of the product.

The FDA and other health authorities are also concerned about leachable impurities extracted from either the packaging components themselves or even occasionally from the label adhesives or ink used in printing the labels. Normally as a part of a stability program, actual package-formulation compatibility studies are required, including monitoring any extractables that come out in the product as a function of the duration of storage. Selection of compatible packaging material has become a critical issue for newer drug products, especially those in which the concentration of active is extremely low, like prostaglandins described earlier. The prostaglandin travoprost, the active in Travatan, required re-engineering of the total packaging, starting with the resin (syndiotactic polypropylene) to stabilize the drug, as well as altering size and shape to maintain squeezability of the bottle.[58] Travoprost was found not to be stable when stored in low-density polyethylene containers, the compound being lost to adsorption onto and absorption into surfaces even at room temperature. Consequently, chemical assay of marketed product must be conducted in a manner that does not deplete the concentration.

Specialized containers, like those developed by *Merck* for their Timolol/Pilocarpine combination product, maintain two solutions in different chambers adjusted separately to provide optimal chemical stability. At the time of dispensing the product, fractions of both solutions are combined and reconstituted by the pharmacist. For example, the final Timolol/Pilocarpine product once reconstituted would be at a nearly physiological pH, would provide pilocarpine as stable for one month at room temperature, and will be found comfortable to patients. Alcon also has developed a proprietary package[59] that can keep unstable or reactive components separate during storage, and that permits the pharmacist, at the time of dispensing to the patient, to rupture a diaphragm allowing the disparate fractions to be mixed. After mixing, the product is expected to remain stable for a month at room temperature. This container is designed to handle either liquid/liquid two-part or solid/liquid two-part components.

Pharmacists also should be aware of unit-dose products currently available in form-fill-seal containers that are preservative free. These products are discarded after single use. These products are most suited for patients who are sensitive or allergic to common preservatives and require chronic administration of a product. Specialized manufacturing technology involves melting a plastic resin to form the container walls, filling with the drug solution (usually 0.2 to 0.8 ml), and then sealing to maintain sterility. At the time of use the tip is broken off, the solution is dosed, and then the package is discarded. For technical reasons relating to manufacturing and filling capabilities as well as the need to minimize evaporation rate, these containers contain an excess volume of the product. The disadvantage is that patients may desire to use the entire volume and risk using an accidentally contaminated product. Recently, some unit-dose containers have been modified to allow the product to be recapped after use. These containers are designed and labeled to be discarded after a single day's use (12 hours) in order to reduce the risk of significant contamination yet make them more economical for the patient.

In only a very few instances are glass containers still in use, usually because of stability limitations. Large-volume intraocular solutions of 250 and 500 mL have been packaged in glass, but even these parenteral-type products are beginning to be packaged in specially fabricated polyethylene/polypropylene containers or flexible bags. Type 1 glass vials with appropriate stoppers are used for intraocular ophthalmic products administered by injection. These packaging components should meet the same requirements as parenteral products. Products injected intraocularly also are required to meet endotoxin limits. Readers should refer to the Chapter 41 *Parenteral Preparations* & 42 *Intravenous Preparations* for more details.

Plastic packaging, usually low-density polyethylene, is by no means interchangeable with glass, however. Plastic packaging is permeable to a variety of substances including light and air. The plastic package may contain a variety of extraneous substances such as mold-release agents, antioxidants, reaction quenchers, and the like, which may leach out of the plastic and into the contained solution. Label glues, inks, and dyes also may penetrate polyethylene. Conversely, confined volatile or lipophilic materials may permeate from solution into or through plastic walls. Sterilization, depending on the method, may influence the resin properties; for example gamma irradiation may increase acid extractables or generate sites that may degrade certain drugs. For these products ethylene oxide gas sterilization may be the only remaining option. However, gas sterilization also may degrade active molecules or leave harmful residuals, and certainly requires aeration under forced air to remove the traces of the gas and volatile residues. Whatever process is selected will need to be validated and monitored, assuring the process neither degrades the active nor generates toxic residues.

Patients may be prescribed more than one ophthalmic medication for the same or different conditions and this can lead to confusion as to which medication is for which use. Historically, red caps have been used for mydriatic drops and green caps for miotic drops such as pilocarpine. FDA now requires the use of certain colored caps on several additional types of ophthalmic drugs as a result of a cooperative effort between FDA, the ophthalmic industry and the Academy of Ophthalmology. The intent is to help patients' prevent medication errors and improve patient compliance. The pharmacist should counsel the patient or caregiver about the purpose of the cap color coding and the importance of opening only one container at a time so that the cap is replaced on the correct container. A listing of the current coding is provided in Table 43-1.

Glass containers remain a convenient package material for extemporaneous preparation of ophthalmic solutions. Type 1 glass should be used. The container should be well rinsed with sterile distilled water and may be sterilized by autoclaving. Droppers normally are available presterilized and packaged in a convenient blister pack.

Ophthalmic ointments invariably are packaged in metal tubes with an ophthalmic tip. Such tubes are sterilized conveniently by autoclaving or by ethylene oxide. In rare cases of metal reactivity or incompatibility, tubes lined with epoxy or vinyl plastic may be required.

Table 43-1. Ophthalmic Cap Color Coding

COLOR	PHARMACEUTICAL CLASS
Yellow or Blue	beta-blockers
Grey	non-steroids
Pink	steroids
Brown or Tan	anti-infectives
Orange	carbonic anhydrase inhibitors
Turquoise	prostaglandins
Red	mydriatics
Green	miotics

Regardless of the form of packaging, some type of tamper-evident feature must be used for consumer protection. The common tamper-evident feature used on most ophthalmic preparations is the moisture- or heat-sensitive shrink band. The band should be identified in such a way that its disruption or absence constitute a warning that tampering, either accidental or purposeful, has occurred.

The eyecup, an ancillary packaging device, fortunately seems to have gone the way of the community drinking cup. An eyecup should not be used. Its use inevitably will spread or aggravate eye infections. Pharmacists should not fail to discourage such use just as they should take the time to instruct patients in the proper use and care of eye medications. While ophthalmic administration may seem simple enough, it may be a foreign and difficult task for many people. The suggestions and precautions given elsewhere (under *Types of Dosage Forms*) may be useful in instructing patients.

ANTIMICROBIAL PRESERVATIVES[60]

A preservative is a substance or mixture of substances added to a product formulation to prevent the growth of, or to destroy, microorganisms introduced accidentally once the container is opened for use.[61,62] The preservative is not intended to be a means of preparing a sterile solution. Other appropriate techniques, discussed elsewhere, are to be employed to prepare sterile solutions.

Preservatives are used for topical ophthalmic products packaged in multiple dose containers unless the formulation itself is self-preserving, as is the case with some antimicrobial products like the ophthalmic solution Vigamox (moxifloxacin). FDA regulations (21 CFR 200.50) allow unpreserved ophthalmic liquid products to be packaged in multiple dose containers only if they are packaged and labeled in a manner that affords adequate protection and minimizes the hazards resulting from accidental contamination during patient use. This can be accomplished by using a reclosable container with a minimum number of doses that is to be discarded after 12 hours from initial opening, and so long as the container is labeled appropriately.

Preservatives are not to be used in solutions intended for intraocular use because of the risk of irritation and damage to these delicate tissues, or in chronic topical applications for patients who cannot tolerate preservatives. Unit dose ophthalmic solutions are especially useful for patients sensitive to preservatives yet who require daily medication, such as glaucoma patients or individuals requiring chronic application of palliatives for dry eye. Ophthalmic solutions prepared and packaged for a single application, *i.e.* a unit dose, need not contain a preservative because they are not intended for reuse.

The need for proper control of ophthalmic solutions to prevent serious contamination was recognized in the 1930s. The first preservative recommended for use in ophthalmics was chlorobutanol, as an alternative to daily boiling!

The selection of an ophthalmic preservative can be a rather difficult task, in part because of the relatively small number of suitable candidates. There is, of course, no such thing as an ideal preservative; however, the following criteria may be useful in preservative selection.

1. The agent should have a broad spectrum and be active against gram-positive and gram-negative organisms as well as fungi. The agent should exert a rapid bactericidal activity, particularly against known virulent organisms such as *P. aeruginosa* strains.
2. The agent should be stable over a wide range of conditions including autoclaving temperatures and pH range.
3. Compatibility should be established with other components of the preparation and with package systems.
4. Lack of toxicity and irritation should be established with a reasonable margin of safety.

Preservative substances must be evaluated as a part of the total ophthalmic preparation in the proposed package. Only in this way can the adequacy of the preservative be established.

Criteria for preservative effectiveness in ophthalmic products are official compendial requirements in the USP, Pharm. Europe, and JP. Health authorities expect products will meet these preservative effectiveness criteria throughout their approved shelf lives, in the final packaging, and at the recommended storage conditions.[2-4]

In addition to preservative effectiveness as an immediate measure, its adequacy or stability as a function of time also must be ascertained. This often is done by measuring both chemical stability and preservative effectiveness over a given period of time and under varying conditions.

Many of these test procedures are not completely pertinent to the preparation of an extemporaneous ophthalmic solution. In such a situation the pharmacist must make selections based upon known conditions and physical and chemical characteristics, and should be guided by those used in commercial ophthalmic preparations. In these circumstances it would be prudent to prepare only minimum volumes for short-term patient use.

The choice of preservatives suitable for ophthalmic use is surprisingly narrow. The classes of compounds available for such use are described in Table 43-2.[63] In each case or category there are specific limitations and shortcomings.

QUATERNARY AMMONIUM COMPOUNDS—Benzalkonium chloride (BAC) is a typical quaternary ammonium compound and is, by far, the most common preservative used in ophthalmic preparations. Over 65% of commercial ophthalmic products are preserved with benzalkonium chloride. Despite this broad use the compound has definite limitations. As a cationic surface-active material of high molecular weight it is not compatible with anionic compounds. It is incompatible with salicylates and nitrates and may be inactivated by high-molecular-weight nonionic compounds. Conversely, benzalkonium chloride has excellent chemical stability and very good antimicrobial characteristics. Given the alternative, often it is preferable to modify a formulation to remove the incompatibility, rather than to include a compatible but less effective preservative. The presence of a surfactant, for example, may require higher levels of BAC to achieve an adequate level of preservation.

The literature on benzalkonium chloride is somewhat mixed; however, this is not unexpected given the wide variation in test methods and, indeed, the chemical variability of benzalkonium chloride itself. The official substance is defined as a mixture of alkyl benzyldimethylammonium chlorides including all or some of the group ranging from n-C_8H_{17} through n-$C_{16}H_{33}$. The n-$C_{12}H_{25}$ homolog content is not less than 40% on an anhydrous basis.

Reviews[64] of benzalkonium chloride indicate that it is well suited for use as an ophthalmic preservative. Certain early negative reports have been shown to be quite erroneous; in some cases adverse tissue reactions were attributed to benzalkonium chloride when, in fact, a totally different compound was used as the test material. Although benzalkonium chloride is by far the most common quaternary preservative, others occasionally referred to include benzethonium chloride and cetyl pyridinium chloride. All are official compounds. More recently, quaternary ammonium functionality has been attached to soluble, reasonably high molecular weight polymers. These agents possess good antimicrobial effectiveness with fewer compatibility problems than the official quaternary preservatives.

Search for milder, safer, gentler preservatives for ophthalmic products, specifically artificial tear products and products that are for chronic use, has been a challenge for many companies. Newer preservatives as a result of this research have led to commercial products where these agents are employed as preservatives. Alcon has introduced many lens care and ophthalmic products with Polyquad. Polyquad represents a newer preservative of the same class as, but with less cytotoxicity than BAC. These agents are more effective and are used at a lower concentration than BAC. Their concentration in the product can range from 0.005% to 0.0005% and yet still meet compendial preser-

Table 43-2. Ophthalmic Preservatives[57]

TYPE	TYPICAL STRUCTURE	CONCENTRATION RANGE	INCOMPATIBILTIES
Quaternary ammonium compounds		0.004–0.02%, 0.01% most common	Soaps Anionic materials Salicylates Nitrates
Organic mercurials		0.001–0.01%	Certain halides with phenylmercuric acetate
Parahydroxy benzoates		Maximum 0.1%	Adsorption by macromolecules; marginal activity
Chlorobutanol		0.5%	Stability is pH-dependent; activity concentration is near solubility
Aromatic alcohols		0.5–0.9%	Low solubility in water; marginal activity

vative efficacy requirements. Polyquad has been used widely in many lens care and artificial tear products.

OXIDIZING AGENTS—Systems based on either sodium perborate or a stabilized oxychloro complex (SOC) are being used as preservatives based on their ability to generate a mild oxidative and cytotoxic effect in aqueous media. Sodium perborate produces hydrogen peroxide as the oxidative species and the SOC is a mixture of oxychloro species but primarily made up of chlorite and a trace of chlorine dioxide. Once in the eye the active agents in either system are spontaneously reduced to harmless byproducts and have been marketed as so-called disappearing preservatives in OTC products for dry eye treatment.

ORGANIC MERCURIALS—It generally is stated that phenylmercuric nitrate or phenylmercuric acetate, in 0.002% concentration, should be used instead of benzalkonium chloride as a preservative for salicylates and nitrates and in solutions of salts of physostigmine and epinephrine that contain 0.1% sodium sulfite. The usual range of concentrations employed is 0.002 to 0.004%. Phenylmercuric borate sometimes is used in place of the nitrate or acetate.

Phenylmercuric nitrate has the advantage over some other organic mercurials of not being precipitated at a slightly acid pH. As with other mercurials, it is slow in its bactericidal action, and it also produces sensitization reactions. Phenylmercuric ion is incompatible with halides, as it forms precipitates.

The effectiveness of phenylmercuric nitrate against *P. aeruginosa* is questionable; it has been found that pseudomonads survive after exposure to a concentration of 0.004% for longer than a week.

Development of iatrogenic mercury deposits in the crystalline lens resulting from use of miotic eye drops containing 0.004% phenylmercuric nitrate, 3 times daily, for periods of 3 to 6 years, has been reported. No impairment of vision was found, but the yellowish brown discoloration of the lens capsule is reported to be permanent.

Thimerosal (Merthiolate, *Lilly*) is an organomercurial with bacteriostatic and antifungal activity and is used as an antimicrobial preservative in concentrations of 0.005 to 0.02%. Its action, as with other mercurials, has been reported to be slow.

PARA-HYDROXYBENZOIC ACID ESTERS—Mixtures of methylparaben and propylparaben sometimes are used, mostly in ophthalmic ointments, as antimicrobial preservatives; the concentration of methylparaben is in the range of 0.1 to 0.2%, while that of propylparaben approaches its solubility in water (~0.04%). They are not considered efficient bacteriostatic agents and are slow in their antimicrobial action. Ocular irritation and stinging have been attributed to their use in ophthalmic preparations.

SUBSTITUTED ALCOHOLS AND PHENOLS—Chlorobutanol is stated to be effective against both gram-positive and gram-negative organisms, including *P. aeruginosa* and some fungi. It is broadly compatible with other ingredients and normally is used in a concentration of 0.5%. One of the products of hydrolysis is hydrochloric acid, which causes a decrease in the pH of aqueous solutions. This decomposition occurs rapidly at high temperatures and slowly at room temperature, in un-buffered solutions that were originally neutral or alkaline. Therefore, ophthalmic solutions that contain chlorobutanol should be buffered between pH 5 and 5.5 and generally pack-aged in glass containers. At room temperature it dissolves slowly in water, and although it dissolves more rapidly on heat-ing, loss by vaporization and decomposition is accelerated.

A combination of chlorobutanol and phenylethyl alcohol (0.5% of each) has been reported to be more effective against *P. aeruginosa, Staphylococcus aureus,* and *Proteus vulgaris* than either antimicrobial singly. In addition, dissolving chlorobu-tanol in phenylethyl alcohol before dissolution in water elimi-nated a need for heating the solution.

OVER-THE-COUNTER (OTC) PRODUCTS FOR DRY EYE

Dry eye is a condition that can be an annoying irritation in its mild form, or a painful and destructive pathology in its severe form damaging the corneal surface and interfering with vision. Dry eye can be caused by decreased tear production, increased tear evaporation rate or an abnormality of the tear film that de-creases its natural capacity to protect and lubricate the epithe-lial tissues. It is one of the most common complaints of patients seeking treatment from their eyecare doctor. This condition is somewhat unique in that it is largely treated with OTC mono-graph drug products and the pharmacist is often asked to assist in its selection.[65] These products are variously known as artifi-cial tears, ocular lubricants, demulcents or emollients and are available as solutions, gels or ointments. Also unique is that these dry eye products are often the essential viscous vehicle component of therapeutic ophthalmic products. The composi-tions of the various commercial dry eye products can be found in several reference books.[33, 34]

OTC dry eye products contain water-soluble polymers as ac-tive ingredients that protect and lubricate the mucous mem-brane surfaces of the conjunctiva and cornea providing tempo-rary relief of the symptoms of dryness and irritation. The polymers thicken the tear film and decrease the rate of tear loss in addition to lubricating and protecting the tissues. Mucin is a natural lubricating component of tears and thus dry eye prod-ucts are expected to provide a mucomimetic effect. The active in-gredient demulcent (lubricant) polymers in these products along with their permitted concentrations and labeling are defined in an OTC Monograph issued by FDA.[66] The Monograph does not specify viscosity grades and therefore a wide range of product viscosities are available. The more viscous products can provide longer duration of relief, however, they are also more likely to blur vision and leave a residue of polymer on the eyelids. The OTC products vary in their choice of polymer or combination of polymers, concentrations and viscosity. The majority of OTC dry eye products contain one or more of the following permitted polymers: cellulosics such as hydroxypropyl methylcellulose (hypromellose) or carboxymethylcellulose sodium; polyol liquids such as glycerin, polyethylene glycol, or polysorbate 80; polyvinyl alcohol; or povidone. Dextran 70 can be used only in combination with another permitted demulcent polymer.

The inactive components of OTC dry eye products are simi-lar to those used in therapeutic ophthalmic products and must be selected just as carefully keeping in mind that the Mono-graph products are labeled for use as often as needed and thus must be nonirritating and physiologically compatible. In the moderate to severe forms of dry eye, the product may be dosed as often as every hour and in the especially severe cases as of-ten as every 15 minutes. The preferred vehicle is aqueous for re-plenishing natural tears and dissolving the active and inactive

ingredients. The vehicle is usually adjusted to be isotonic with sodium chloride and in some cases other salts are used as well as nonionic ingredients such as dextrose and mannitiol. Some cases of dry eye have been reported to produce tears that are hypertonic and several products feature a slightly hypotonic formula to restore the natural tear osmotic pressure. The prod-ucts generally are adjusted or buffered to provide a pH of about 7.4 but rarely outside of the range of about 7 to 8.

Some polymers notably polyvinyl alcohol can lead to a more acidic pH upon storage of the solution. The preservative chlorobutanol also produces an acidic pH as it degrades in so-lution. Bicarbonate is included in some products as a more physiological buffer and requires a hermetically-sealed sec-ondary package for stability. Some products include both mono and divalent chloride salts in their vehicles in an attempt to mimic the electrolyte composition of natural tears.

The majority of dry eye products contain a preservative and are packaged in multiple dose plastic ophthalmic containers. As in therapeutic products, benzalkonium chloride is the most widely used preservative. Newer preservatives having im-proved compatibility with ocular tissues such as polyquater-nium-1 (Polyquad) are increasingly being used as well as the so-called "disappearing" preservatives sodium perborate and Purite. Sodium perborate forms hydrogen peroxide which can be irritating in the eye but quickly degrades to oxygen and water. Purite is a stabilized oxychloro complex that degrades to sodium chloride and water when exposed to long wavelength UV light.

Preservative-free products are also available and are gain-ing popularity particularly for patients with chronic dry eye conditions and those that are sensitive to preservatives. These products are packaged in form-fill-seal unit dose containers but due to manufacturing considerations they contain enough prod-uct for several doses but are labeled to be discarded after a sin-gle dose. This has led to the introduction of a modified package that features a reclosable cap and can be used as a small vol-ume multiple dose container for preservative-free products when they are labeled for safety reasons to be discarded no longer than 12 hours after first opening.

The large majority of dry eye products are solution dosage forms administered as eyedrops but there are also available gel-like and ointment dosage forms. Ointments consisting pri-marily of a mixture of petrolatum and mineral oil are used for their emollient properties in dry eye treatment or where there is a defect in lid closing to prevent increased tear evaporation. Lanolin is sometimes added to the base to provide some water miscibility. The ratio of oils can be varied for consistency and melting temperature. The ointments are used primarily as a nighttime medication since they usually cause a blurring of vi-sion. Several products are labeled as gels or liquid gels and are aqueous-based dosage forms containing one or more of the per-mitted lubricant polymers. The gel dosage form identifier is used to designate a more viscous product, however, the dosage directions read the same as for the eyedrop products (instill one or two drops prn) since this dosage statement is the only one permitted for dry eye products marketed using the permitted lubricant polymers under the OTC Monograph.

One disadvantage of most OTC dry eye products is their rel-atively short duration of effect. Several products have become available which incorporate novel delivery system technology into these products to prolong the duration of the lubricant and protectant effects of the Monograph active ingredients. In one product, AquaSite,[67] the polymer polycarbophil is used and in a more recent product, Systane,[68] a modified hydroxypropyl guar polymer is used to form a gel-like matrix when the product com-ponents interact with the tear fluid.

CONTACT LENSES AND THEIR CARE

Historical Background[69–71]

Evidence suggests that the concept of altering corneal power was first envisioned by Leonardo da Vinci early in the sixteen century. In the next century, more than a hundred years later, Rene Descartes described a device, a glass-filled tube in direct contact with the cornea, capable of implementing this concept though it prohibited blinking and so was not a practical solution. In the early nineteenth century the British astronomer Sir John Herschel described the mathematics of these devices and proposed a means of treating very irregular corneas by using a glass capsule filled with a gelatin solution. Not until 1888 was the original concept executed by the artificial eye maker, Albert Muller. He made a glass protective shell for the cornea of a lagophthalmic patient who had carcinoma of the upper lid. The patient wore the device for 20 years, and corneal clarity was maintained.

But, perhaps the first contact lenses, scleral lenses resting on the bulbar conjunctiva beyond the limbal ring, were fabricated and fit by the German ophthalmologist A. E. Fick working in Zurich, Switzerland, late in the nineteenth century. Contact lenses without scleral portions (corneal lenses) were in existence at least as early as 1912, when they were manufactured by Carl Zeiss. Glass prostheses produced by Fick and others, while conceptually a step forward, suffer from reasonably rapid deterioration in the tear fluid. However they had the advantage that the glass was readily wetted by tears.

Experimentation in the twentieth century led J. Dallos, working in Budapest, to perceive the importance of tear flow underneath the contact lens. Dallos also took impressions of human eyes to improve the fidelity of the ground lens to the shape of the cornea. The first contact lenses, scleral lenses, of plastic made in the late 1930s with polymethyl methacrylate (PMMA) from Rohm and Haas are attributed to W. Mullen and T. Obrig. The advantages of durability and weight reduction far outweighed the slight differences in optical properties. And in 1948 K. Tuohy filed a patent for a plastic corneal contact lens. With the advent of PMMA a flush-fitting shell became possible, a concept developed in England in the 1950s by Ridley. The first corneal lenses to have any measure of commercial success were developed in the early '50s by F. Dickinson and W. Sohnges. Its thickness was about 0.2 mm, considered to be a fairly thick lens. Thinner lenses, about 0.1 mm, were introduced in the early '60s.

The first soft contact lenses were made of silicone, an elastomer nearly devoid of water but with good permeability to oxygen and carbon dioxide. However, the first soft contact lenses to be commercialized were of hydroxyethylmethacrylate hydrogels, developed by O. Wichterle and D. Lim in Czechoslovakia in the early '60s. Continuous improvements have progressed to the present day including milestones such as silicone-acrylate rigid gas permeable lenses in the '70s, disposable inexpensive lenses in the 80's, daily disposable and silicone hydrogel lenses in the '90s.

With the advent of commercialized, relatively comfortable and inexpensive corneal contact lenses, the need for lens care products developed beginning in the 1950s, and as summarized below a great variety of functionality has been provided, depending on the requirements of the individual products.

From a regulatory perspective, during the period from approval of the U.S. Food Drug and Cosmetic Act of 1938 (FDCA) until the U.S. Medical Device Amendments to the FDCA of 1976, contact lenses and contact lens care products were regulated as drugs. While during this period a device was defined in the FDCA, many medical devices were thought to be "used for the cure, mitigation, or prevention of disease" leading to their classification as drugs. With increased activity in industry and significance of biomedical devices in maintaining health, Congressional awareness arose of the advantages for greater regulation. The Amendments made provision for three classes of device, with different requirements for each. Those with least risk were assigned to Class I and those associated with increasing risk, to a progressively higher class. If safety and efficacy of a device could be reasonably assured by "general controls" (including restrictions on design, production, storage, maintenance, use, etc.), then the device was assigned to Class I, which may be exempted from the requirement for a 510 (k) but still require company or product registrations. Under the 1976 Amendments, contact lenses and lens care products were reclassified as Class III devices, requiring a premarket approval application (PMA) and approval by the FDA before marketing.

However by 1990, following years of experience with certain devices in the marketplace and recognition that little purpose was being served duplicating regulatory investigation of substantially equivalent safe and effective devices, Congress passed new legislation. The U.S. Safe Medical Devices Act of 1990 authorized reclassification of certain contact lens and lens care products as Class II devices (requiring special controls [a 510 (k) submission and clearance]). The products covered by this reclassification include solutions, dry products, tablets and disinfecting units used in caring for and disinfecting of soft (hydrophilic) and rigid gas permeable contact lenses. In March of 1994, the downclassification of two types of daily-wear contact lenses, from Class III to Class II, was implemented by a rule in the Federal Register. In July of 1997, a similar downclassification of certain contact lens care products, including multi-purpose solutions and in-eye contact lens solutions, was implemented by a rule in the Federal Register. Extended wear contact lenses remain governed by class III regulations.

Contact Lenses, Current Art

As a consequence of these years of development, there is an enormous selection of contact lenses and lens materials currently available to the consumer. There are basically four classes of lenses, and the identification of these classes is both by polymer type and lens characteristics: hard contact lenses, rigid gas permeable contact lenses, soft hydrophilic contact lenses, and silicone-based flexible hydrophobic lenses. These classes are summarized in Table 43-3. Hard contact lenses are generally fabricated from polymethylmethacrylate or polysili-

Table 43-3. Contact Lens Classes, Characteristics, and Support Products

LENS TYPE	CHEMICAL CLASSIFICATION	MAJOR CHARACTERISTICS	TYPICAL SUPPORT PRODUCTS
Hard, rigid, hydrophobic	PMMA (polymethyl methacrylate)	Negligible gas permeability, low water content, medium wettability	Wetting solutions Soaking solutions Cleaning solutions Combination Artificial tears
Soft, flexible, hydrophilic	HEMA (hydroxyethyl methylmethacrylate)	High water content, low gas permeability, good wettability	Cleaning solutions Disinfection solutions
Flexible hydrophobic	Silicone rubber	Good gas permeability; poor wettability	Wetting solutions Cleaning solutions
	Silicone vinylpyrrollidone	Good gas permeability; good wettability	Soaking solutions
Rigid, hydrophilic	CAB (cellulose) acetate butyrate	Good gas permeability; good wettability	Wetting solutions Cleaning solutions Soaking solutions Rewetting solutions

cone acrylate polymers or copolymer blends containing one of these materials. The rigid gas permeable (RGP) contact lenses are generally made from more polarizable and oxygen-permeable materials such as cellulose acetate butyrate, *t*-butyl styrene, or silicone polymers or copolymers. These lenses generally provide superior visual acuity to those of the more flexible soft contact lenses. The U.S. Adopted Names (USAN) designates these hydrophobic lens types with less than 10% water by the suffix *focon*. However, RGPs having low oxygen permeability must be removed after a day's wear, and because of greater lens awareness especially for a new wearer, are recommended to be worn routinely, ie, not intermittently. However, they are durable and the replacement schedule is extended. RGPs with higher oxygen transmissibility tend to be preferred, especially in comparison with hard contact lenses, because the improved exchange of gases assists in maintaining the health of the cornea.

The third class of contact lenses, soft hydrophilic lenses, are fabricated from such a wide variety of materials and their blends and the FDA has grouped them according to two parameters, ionicity and water content (either low or high, less than or greater than 50% water):

- Group I includes the nonionic polymers of low water content such as a Polymacon [a simple poly (hydroxyethylmethacrylate), HEMA],
- Group II includes the nonionic polymers of high water content such as Alphafilcon A (a copolymer of five monomeric units, HEMA, vinyl pyrrolidone, ethylene dimethacrylate, hydroxycyclohexyl methacrylate, and a substituted vinyl carbonate),
- Group III includes ionic polymers of low water content such as Bufilcon (a terpolymer of HEMA, dimethyl oxobutyl acrylamide and the trimethacrylate ester of ethyl t-butane triol with some level of hydrolysis of the esters to the free acid) or Ocufilcon A (a terpolymer with HEMA, methacrylic acid [MA] and ethylene dimethacrylate), and
- Group IV includes ionic polymers of high water content such as a higher water content Ocufilcon B/C or Etafilcon (a terpolymer of HEMA, the salt of MA and the trimethacrylate ester of ethyl *t*-butane triol).

The final class of contact lenses, considered either a group of harder soft lenses or a group of softer RGP lenses with high oxygen solubility and transmission, is the silicone hydrogel lenses. These silicone and fluorosilicone materials are candidates for continuous extended wear applications.

Such diverse functionalities provide distinct properties in addition to water content, ranging from oxygen and metabolite transport, hardness and flexibility, to processability, and to durability and stability. More complete lists of the materials used in contact lens manufacture are available, but in general the USAN designates these hydrophilic lens types with greater than 10% water by the suffix *filcon*.[72–74] While the nomenclature adequately distinguishes monomer components, and the alphabetic trailing designation indicates differences in ratios of monomer units, one must remember that differences in crosslinker (often ethylene glycol dimethacrylate [EGDM]), initiator, catalyst, filler or color additive are not differentiated.

While this is a reasonable overview of the categories of choices for the materials comprising contact lenses, it is still an incomplete list of the properties which otherwise the consumer and his or her practitioner still need to make in selecting a contact lens. In addition to the chemical composition, the following choices need to be made: (1) duration of wear (daily vs. continuous), (2) lens replacement schedule (daily vs. biweekly vs. monthly vs. quarterly), (3) lens design (spherical, toric, bifocal), (4) colored or clear, (5) means of manufacture (lathe-cut or cast-molded), (5) edge design (which can affect lens motion, overall fit, comfort and acuity) and lens thickness, (6) fitting characteristics like the selection available for base curves and lens diameter, and (7) any surface treatment or conditioning. With this multiplicity of choices and the subtlety of competing requirements, the recommendation of the practitioner is vital.

But ultimately, the consumer's metrics—comfort, convenience and cost—also remain significant factors in lens selec-

tion. For some, the soft contact lenses are simply too fragile, and they select an RGP lens. For others, comfort dominates and they choose between the higher-water-content lenses, Groups II and IV. Soft lenses can be worn occasionally, and the blurring associated with the transition to eyeglasses is less troublesome than with hard contact lenses. But comfort and their other advantages have been achieved at a cost, and affects practice. Because Group IV lenses, being anionic, tend to accumulate soil such as protein at a more rapid rate than lenses from other groups, and are more sensitive to ionic strength and may bind absorbable impurities or additives such as preservatives, pollutants, cosmetic ingredients and therapeutic agents, they generally require more care than hard contact lenses or more hydrophobic soft contact lenses.

Replacement frequency also affects the choice of lenses. In America where replacement is biweekly, these disadvantages appear not to be troublesome; however in Europe where replacement schedules run longer, there appears to be a preference for the nonionic lenses with high water content, Group II lenses. However, since most lenses are currently replaced every 14-90 days, the influence of this factor appears to be diminishing. Preference for either of the high-water-content lenses is tempered in those individuals who tend toward dry eyes, since these Group II and IV materials appear to accelerate evaporation rates; and as a consequence patients with drier eyes are more likely to prefer Group I lenses.

In addition to their use in vision correction, soft contact lenses, like collagen shields, are occasionally used for therapeutic purposes, serving as bandages providing protection as in their use in bullous keratopathy (or other forms of corneal edema or other corneal irregularities or sources of cicatrization) or for lid abnormalities, and with ulcers, chemical burns, grafts, or dry eye. They can also be used to sustain the delivery of therapeutic agents, as discussed above. The same preparations used in caring for lenses used for refractive correction will be needed for lenses used for these therapeutic purposes.

In summary, both doctors and consumers have been provided with a broad range of alternatives. Current lens materials and the solutions to maintain them (next section) provide a wide selection of properties suitable for individual ocular health requirements and preferences.

Contact Lenses Care Products

GENERAL CONSIDERATIONS

With the previous two sections for background we are ready to discuss those preparations utilized in the care of these devices. For all of the specialized solutions to be discussed it is generally necessary: (1) to adjust pH, tonicity (osmolality), surface and interfacial tensions, and viscosity, (2) preserve and maintain sterility, (3) assure stability and shelf life, and (4) package and sterilize appropriately. In the US, these solutions are Class II medical devices.[71]

WETTING SOLUTIONS

These are lubricating and cushioning preparations designed to furnish a hydrophilic coating over the characteristically hydrophobic surface of PMMA, silicon, acrylate, and other rigid lens surfaces. Typically, wetting solutions include an acceptable viscosity-imparting agent, a surfactant, and a preservative. The surface-activity and viscosity effects may be obtained from a single compound. Agents commonly used include cellulose derivatives, polyvinyl pyrrolidone, polyvinyl alcohol, and polyethylene glycol derivatives. The need for surface-active agents, which facilitate wetting of lenses and spreading of tears, is greater for hard contact lenses because of their hydrophobic surface characteristics. Preservatives include those acceptable for ophthalmic use, including Polyquad and Dymed.

CLEANING SOLUTIONS

Cleaning solutions commonly are used to remove surface contaminants—lipids, protein, organic salts and the like. Cleaning is accomplished by the use of surfactants that preferably are nonionic or amphoteric. Viscosity-imparting agents generally are not included. Some cleaning agents also include a mild abrasive, silica for RGPs or plastic particles for soft lenses.

Adequate cleaning of hydrophilic lenses is a far more complex and challenging problem than for hard-lens cleaning. Because of their permeability characteristics, contaminants penetrate into the lens structure and may bind chemically or physically to the hydroxyethylmethylmethacrylate (HEMA) or ionic portions of the lens material. Contaminants may be surface films or crystals, amorphous aggregates of protein material, cellular debris, or insoluble inorganic salts.

Cleaning products generally are specific to the lens material and require FDA clearance, with proof of cleaning efficacy and safety. Cleaners are based on surface activity, enzyme action, or even abradant action, in which case the abradant material must be softer than the lens itself. Adequate daily cleaning of hydrophilic lens material can enhance disinfection, but in some cases may not be necessary given the choices of today's powerful disinfecting solutions and enzymatic cleaners, in either a tableted or liquid form. Most recently daily-wear planned replacement lenses have found wide acceptance. Conventionally their successful use is reliant on enzymatic cleaning together with special disinfectants. However, extended wear lenses, soiling at a lower rate, require only rewetting drops.

The significance of adequate cleaning cannot be overstated. Improperly or inadequately cleaned and maintained lenses are perhaps the most important contributors to complications associated with the wear of contact lenses such as discomfort, loss of visual acuity, conjunctivitis and keratitis.

There are two types of cleaning solutions, daily and weekly cleaners. Weekly cleaning solutions may include proteolytic enzymes like *Subtilisin* or a broad-spectrum less-toxic enzyme like pancreatin (which contains protease, lipase and amylase activity), or concentrated surfactants. Daily cleaning solutions achieve cleaning using less aggressive surface active agents and polymers, often nonionic but nonsolubilizing agents that will be less toxic if carried over into the eye. Examples include Tweens and Tyloxapols. A daily cleaning solution containing even a nontoxic enzyme is available (SupraClens).

The goal is to provide thorough cleaning of the lenses, for the benefits described above, without causing any degradation of the lenses.

DISINFECTING SYSTEMS

Disinfection of the first hydrophilic lens approved by the FDA was accomplished using a heating device that generated steam from a saline solution. The latter was either prepared by the user or available from the manufacturer. Subsequent to the so-called thermal systems, requiring heating at 80°C for ten minutes, disinfection solutions were developed that met the requirements for FDA approval while not damaging the more delicate soft lens materials. Because of the sorption characteristics of hydrophilic lens materials, many of the accepted ophthalmic preservatives are unsatisfactory for use in soft-lens disinfecting systems, including the ubiquitous benzalkonium chloride. Once again, however, the use of a quaternary disinfectant covalently bonded to a soluble, relatively high molecular weight polymer has met with some success. These have to a large extent replaced chemical antimicrobial agents like sorbic acid, thimerosal (mercury containing), and hydrogen peroxide amongst many others. Perhaps the most common in current use are a cationic polymer, Polyquad, and a poly biguanide, called PHMB or Dymed.

In addition to possessing satisfactory disinfecting activity, such a preparation must be isotonic, in an acceptable pH range, and nonreactive (nonbinding) with lens materials and, over a normal use period, induce or bring about no physical, chemical, or optical changes in the lens. It is of course sterile and safe for use in the eye, even though direct instillation into the eye is not intended.

SOAKING SOLUTIONS

Soaking or storage solutions, as the name suggests, are used to store and hydrate hard or RGP lenses but, most importantly, to disinfect such lenses. Disinfection should be rapid and as complete as possible making use, once again, of acceptable ophthalmic preservative substances. Soaking solutions typically contain chlorhexidine (gluconate), benzalkonium, or quaternary/polymer compounds enhanced by sodium edetate. Soaking solutions are intended to be rinsed off lenses before insertion.

REWETTING SOLUTIONS

Solutions intended to rewet hard or RGP lenses *in situ* are referred to as rewetting solutions or lubricating drops. Such preparations are intended to reinforce the wetting capacity of the normal tear film. Early products of this type tended to be somewhat viscous wetting solutions acceptable for direct instillation into the eye. More-recent preparations mimic tears more accurately, and their viscosity may be rather low to improve user acceptability, or adjusted to be responsive and to improve retention and duration of the wetting characteristics.

MULTIPURPOSE SOLUTIONS

By combining the actions of two or more of the solutions just described, these products have simplified regimens, improved compliance, generally increased comfort of contact lens products, and greatly increased convenience of using contact lenses. For soft contact lenses multipurpose solutions need combine only the functions of cleaning and disinfection, whereas for a complete multipurpose solution for a hard or RGP lens some level of wetting also need be provided. Suffice it to say that these solutions, which contain an intricate balance of ingredients, have grown in popularity significantly, because of the greatly increased level of convenience they provide. Their efficacy often precludes the need for separate cleaning solutions for many patients.

GUIDELINES FOR SAFETY AND EFFICACY TESTING

The FDA periodically issues or updates guidelines describing recommended test procedures for contact lens–care products. The reader is advised to review the most recent guidelines for appropriate requirements.

Current guidelines cover all lens care products. Applicable guidelines are determined by the type of product (eg, saline solution, cleaning solution, multipurpose solution, rewetting drops) and the claim (eg, disinfection in a regimen vs. a stand-alone process). Safety testing includes determinations of cytotoxicity, oral toxicity, potential for sensitization, and single to multiple exposure in an animal (rabbit) eye. The tests designated depend on the active ingredient (eg, if it is a new entity or has been in previous products) and its concentration (eg, if it is the same or different from that used in a currently approved product). Efficacy of preservation, disinfection and cleaning, compatibility with lens or lens types, and clinical trials are also required with their type and scope dependent on product type, characteristics, ingredients and claims.

SUMMARY

Considerable progress has been made in ophthalmic pharmaceutics and in lens-care products during the last decade. Very substantial advances have been made in designing vehicles and packaging for highly potent actives presented at very low concentrations, in increasing ophthalmic bioavailability and controlling factors influencing ophthalmic drug absorption, in the design of implants and means of delivering them for providing therapeutic agents to the retina and other deep ophthalmic tissues, and in devising robust yet delicately balanced multipurpose solutions for contact lens wearers. Continuing advances in the general field of ophthalmic pharmaceutics and pharmacokinetics can be expected to assist in maintaining and improving ocular health.

ACKNOWLEDGMENTS—The authors gratefully acknowledge insights provided by colleagues, noting especially Masood Chowhan, Michael Christensen, Renee Garofalo, Ralph Larsen, Kiran Randeri, and Denise Rodeheaver.

REFERENCES

1. Hecht G. Ophthalmic preparations. In Gennaro AR, ed. *Remington: The Science and Practice of Pharmacy*, 20th ed. Baltimore: Lippincott Williams & Wilkins, 2000, Chap 43.
2. *Pharmacopeia of the United States,* 26th Revision and the National Formulary 21st Edition, Board of Trustees, 12601 Twinbrook Parkway, Rockville, MD, 2003.
3. *European Pharmacopoeia,* 4th ed. Directorate for the Quality of Medicines of the Council of Europe (EDQM), Council of Europe, 67075 Strasberg Cedex, France, 2001.
4. *Japanese Pharmacopoeia,* 14th ed. Society of Japanese Pharmacopoeia, 2-12-15, Shibuya, Shibuya-Ku, Tokyo, 2001.
5. Alcon, Inc., Fort Worth, TX.
6. Botelho SY. *Sci Am* 1964; 211:80.
7. Slatt BJ, Stein HA. *Ophthalmic Assistant: Fundamentals and Clinical Practice*. St Louis: Mosby, 1983.
8. Vaughan D, Asbury T. *General Ophthalmology*, 11th ed. Los Altos, CA: Lange Medical Publications, 1986.
9. Bron AS, Tripathi RC, Tripathy BJ. *Wolff's Anatomy of the Eye and Orbit*, 8th ed. New York: Chapman and Hall Medical, 1997.
10. Berman ER. *Biochemistry of the Eye*. New York: Plenum Press, 1991.
11. Spaeth GL, ed. *Ophthalmic Surgery Principles and Practice*, 3rd ed. Philadelphia: WB Saunders, 2003.
12. Lee TW-Y, Robinson JR. Controlled-release drug-delivery systems. In Gennaro AR, ed. *Remington: The Science and Practice of Pharmacy*. Baltimore: Lippincott Williams & Wilkins, 2000, Chap 47.
13. Edelhauser HF, Hoffert JR, Fromm PO. *Invest Ophthalmol* 1965; 4:290.
14. Schoenwald RD, Ward RL. *J Pharm Sci* 1983; 72:1266.
15. Edwards A, Prausnitz MR. *Pharm Res* 2001; 18:1497.
16. Lang JC, Roehrs RE, Rodeheaver DP, et al. Design and evaluation of ophthalmic pharmaceutical products. In Banker GS, Rhodes CT, eds. *Modern Pharmaceutics*, 4th ed. New York: Marcel Dekker, 2002.
17. Shell JW. *Surv Ophthalmol* 1982; 26:207.
18. Patton TF. *J Pharm Sci* 1977; 66:1058.
19. Vaidyanathan G, Jay M, Bera RK, et al. *Pharm Res* 1990; 7:1198.
20. Santvliet LV, Ludwig A. *Pharm Ind* 2001; 63:402.
21. Conroy CW, Maren TH. *J Ocul Pharm Ther* 1998; 14:565.
22. Lee VHL, Robinson JR. *J Pharm Sci* 1979; 68:673.
23. Lee VHL. *J Ocul Pharmacol* 1990; 6(2):157.
24. Lang JC, Stiemke MM. Biological barriers to ocular delivery. In Reddy IK, ed. *Ocular Therapeutics and Drug Delivery, A Multidisciplinary Approach*. Technomic Publishing Company, 1996, pp 51–132.
25. Martin AN, Swarbrick J, Cammarata A. *Physical Pharmacy: Physical Chemical Principles in the Pharmaceutical Sciences*. Philadelphia: Lea & Febiger, 1983.
26. United States Patent No. 4,861,760 (Merck Manual).
27. United States Patent No. 5,212,162 (Lang).
28. United States Patent No. 6,174,524 (Bawa).
29. Araie M, Maurice DM. *Exp Eye Res* 1991; 52:27.
30. Missel PJ. *Pharm Res* 2002; 19:1636.
31. United States Patent No. 5,378,475 (Ashton).
32. United States Patent No. 5,416,777 (Yaacobi).
33. Ophthalmic Drug Facts, Facts and Comparisons. St Louis: Mosby, 2003.
34. Physicians Desk Reference for Ophthalmic Medicines, 31st ed, 2003.
35. United States Patent No. 4,861,760 (Manzuel).
36. United States Patent No. 6,174,524 (Bawa).
37. United States Patent No. 5,461,081(Ali).
38. United States Patent No. 4,911,920 (Jani).
39. Higuchi T. *J Pharm Sci* 1961; 50:874.
40. United States Patent No. 5,474,979 (Ding).
41. March WF, Stewart RM, Mandell AI, et al. *Arch Ophthalmol* 1982; 100:1270.
42. Shell JW, Baker RW. *Ann Ophthalmol* 1975; 7:1037.
43. Mitra AK, ed. *Ophthalmic Drug Delivery Systems*. New York: Marcel Dekker, 1993, Chap 17.
44. Edelhauser HF, Van Horn DL, Hyndrink R, et al. *Arch Ophthalmol* 1975; 93:648.
45. Edelhauser HF, Van Horn DL, Gonnering R. *Arch Ophthalmol* 1978; 96:516.
46. Slack JW, Edelhauser HF, Helenek MJ. *Am J Ophthalmol* 1990; 110:77.
47. United States Patent No. 5,378,475 (Smith).
48. Mitra AK, ed. *Ophthalmic Drug Delivery Systems*, 2nd ed. New York: Marcel Dekker, 2003, Chap 10.
49. Mitra AK, ed. *Ophthalmic Drug Delivery Systems*, 2nd ed. New York: Marcel Dekker, 2003, Chap 12.
50. Aronson SD, Elliott JH. *Ocular Inflammation*. St Louis: Mosby, 1972, p 899.
51. Title 21, *Code of Federal Regulations*, Chap 1, Vol 4, Parts 210 & 211.
52. Title 21, *Code of Federal Regulations*, Chap1, Vol 5, Part 330.
53. Allen LV Jr. *The Art, Science and Technology of Pharmaceutical Compounding*, 2nd ed. American Pharmaceutical Association, 2002.
54. *United States Pharmacopeia 26*, Chapter <1206< Sterile Drug Products for Home Use. United States Pharmacopeial Convention, 2003.
55. Gonnering R, Edelhauser HF, Van Horn DL, et al. *Invest Ophthalmol Vis Sci* 1979; 18:373.
56. Edelhauser HF, Hanneken AM, Pederson HJ, et al. *Arch Ophthalmol* 1981; 99:1281.
57. United States Patent Nos. 5,849,792 and 6,011,062 (Schneider).
58. United States Patent No. 6,235,781 (Weiner).
59. United States Patent Nos. 5,474,209 (Valet) and 5,782,345 (Guasch).
60. Block SS. *Disinfection, Sterilization, and Preservation*. Malvern, PA: Lea & Febiger, 1991.
61. Title 21, *Code of Federal Regulations*, Chap 1, Part 200, Subpart C, Section 200.50.
62. *United States Pharmacopeia 26*, Chapter <51> Antimicrobial Effectiveness Testing. United States Pharmacopeial Convention, 2003.
63. Hoover JE. *Dispensing of Medication,* 8th ed. Easton, PA: Mack Publishing Co, 1976, p 237.
64. Mullen W, Shepherd W, Labovitz J. *Surv Ophthalmol* 1973; 17:469.
65. Berardi R, Tietze KJ, Popovich NG, et al: *Handbook of Nonprescription Drugs*, 13th Edition, 546 (2002).
66. Title 21, *Code of Federal Regulations*, Chap 1, Vol 5, Part 349.
67. United States Patent No. 5,188,826 (Chandrasekaran).
68. United States Patent No. 6,403,609 (Asgharian).
69. Mandel RB. *Contact Lens Practice*. Springfield, IL: Charles C Thomas, 1981.
70. Efron N, ed. *Contact Lens Practice*. Boston: Butterworth Heinemann, 2002.
71. Randeri KJ, Quintana RP, Chowhan MA. Lens care products. In Swarbrick J, Boylan JC, eds. *Encyclopedia of Pharmaceutical Technology*, vol 8. New York: Marcel Dekker, 1993, pp 361–402.
72. *Contact Lens Quarterly*. Irvine, CA: Jobson Publishing, Frames Data Inc.
73. *Tyler's Quarterly*, Little Rock, AR: Tyler's Quarterly, Inc.
74. Expert Committee on Nomenclature and Labeling of the USP Council of Experts: *USP and USAN Dictionary*. Rockville, MD: US Adopted Names Council, Rockville, MD.

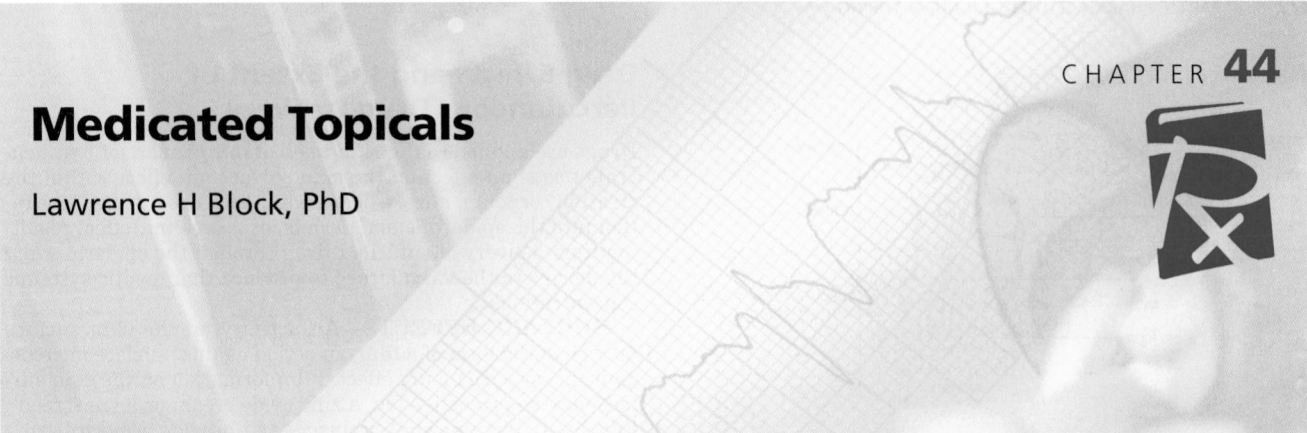

Medicated Topicals

CHAPTER **44**

Lawrence H Block, PhD

The application of medicinal substances to the skin or various body orifices is a concept as old as humanity. The papyrus records of ancient Egypt describe a variety of these medications for external use. Galen described the use in Roman times of a forerunner to today's vanishing creams.

Medications are applied in a variety of forms reflecting the ingenuity and scientific imagination of pharmacists through the centuries. New modes of drug delivery have been developed to remedy the shortcomings of earlier vehicles or, more recently, to optimize drug delivery. Conversely, some external

medications have fallen into disuse because of changes in the practice of medicine.

Medications are applied to the skin or inserted into body orifices in liquid, semisolid, or solid form. Ophthalmics and topical aerosol products will not be discussed in this chapter. Ophthalmic use imposes particle size, viscosity, and sterility specifications that require separate, detailed discussion (see Chapter 43). The complexity of pharmaceutical aerosol systems necessitates their inclusion elsewhere (see Chapter 50).

BIOPHARMACEUTIC ASPECTS OF THE ROUTES OF ADMINISTRATION

EPIDERMAL AND TRANSDERMAL DRUG DELIVERY

The Skin

The skin often has been referred to as the largest of the body organs: an average adult's skin has a surface area of about 2 m². It is probably the heaviest organ of the body. Its accessibility and the opportunity it affords to maintain applied preparations intact for a prolonged time have resulted in its increasing use as a route of drug administration, whether for local, regional, or systemic effects.

Anatomically, human skin may be described as a stratified organ with three distinct tissue layers: the epidermis, the dermis, and the subcutaneous fat layer (Fig 44-1).

Epidermis, the outermost skin layer, comprises stratified squamous epithelial cells. Keratinized, flattened remnants of these actively dividing epidermal cells accumulate at the skin surface as a relatively thin region (about 10 μm thick) termed the *stratum corneum*, or *horny layer*. The horny layer is itself lamellar with the keratinized cells overlapping one another, linked by intercellular bridges and compressed into about 15 layers. The lipid-rich intercellular space in the stratum corneum comprises lamellar matrices with alternating hydrophilic layers and lipophilic bilayers formed during the process of keratinization. The region behaves as a tough but flexible coherent membrane.

The stratum corneum also is markedly hygroscopic—far more so than other keratinous materials such as hair or nails. Immersed in water the isolated stratum corneum swells to about three times its original thickness, absorbing about four to five times its weight in water in the process. The stratum corneum functions as a protective physical and chemical barrier and is only slightly permeable to water. It retards water

loss from underlying tissues, minimizes ultraviolet light penetration, and limits the entrance of microorganisms, medications, and toxic substances from without. The stratum corneum is abraded continuously. Thus, it tends to be thicker in regions more subject to abrasion or the bearing of weight. Its regeneration is provided by rapid cell division in the basal cell layer of the epidermis. Migration or displacement of dividing cells toward the skin surface is accompanied by differentiation of the epidermal cells into layers of flat, laminated plates, as noted above. An acidic film (pH ranging between 4 and 6.5, depending on the area tested) made up of emulsified lipids covers the surface of the stratum corneum.

The dermis apparently is a gel structure involving a fibrous protein matrix embedded in an amorphous, colloidal, ground substance. Protein, including collagen and elastin fibers, is oriented approximately parallel to the epidermis. The dermis supports and interacts with the epidermis, facilitating its conformation to underlying muscles and bones. Blood vessels, lymphatics, and nerves are found within the dermis, though only nerve fibers reach beyond the dermal ridges or papillae into the germinative region of the epidermis. Sweat glands and hair follicles extending from the dermis through the epidermis provide discontinuities in an otherwise uniform integument.

The subcutaneous fat layer serves as a cushion for the dermis and epidermis. Collagenous fibers from the dermis thread between the accumulations of fat cells, providing a connection between the superficial skin layers and the subcutaneous layer.

HAIR FOLLICLES AND SWEAT GLANDS—Human skin is sprinkled liberally with surface openings extending well into the dermis. Hair follicles, together with the sebaceous glands that empty into the follicles, make up the pilosebaceous unit. Apocrine and eccrine sweat glands add to the total.

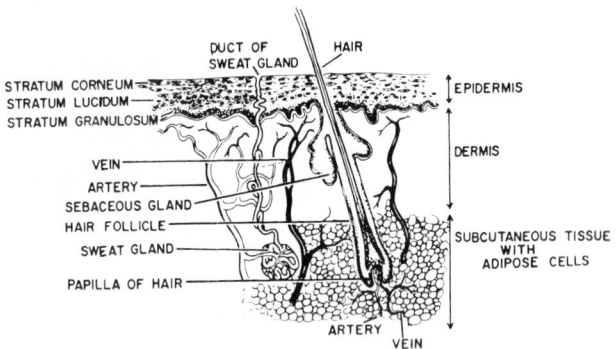

Figure 44-1. Vertical section of human skin.

PILOSEBACEOUS UNITS—Human hair consists of compacted keratinized cells formed by follicles. Sebaceous glands empty into the follicle sites to form the pilosebaceous unit. The hair follicles are surrounded by sensory nerves; thus, an important function of human hair is sensory. Human hair varies enormously within the same individual, even within the same specific body area. Follicular density varies considerably as well, from values of about 250 follicles per cm² for the scalp to 50 per cm², or less, for the thigh and other relatively nonhirsute areas. Follicular density is determined genetically, ie, no new follicles are formed after birth. One characteristic human trait is that although most of the body hairs never develop beyond the rudimentary vellus state, the only hairless areas are confined, primarily, to the palmar and plantar surfaces. Individual hairs can vary in microscopic appearance, diameter, cuticle appearance, and even presence or absence of medulla.

Sebaceous glands are similar anatomically and functionally but vary in size and activity according to location. Population in the scalp, face, and anogenital areas may vary from 400 to 900/cm². Fewer than 100/cm² are found in other areas. Sebaceous glands are richly supplied with blood vessels.

Sebaceous cells synthesize and accumulate lipid droplets. This accumulation results in enlarged cells that fragment to form sebum. Sebum is made up of a mixture of lipids, approximately as shown in Table 44-1.

The sebaceous gland, containing sebum, cell debris, and microorganisms such as *Propionibacterium acnes,* is connected to the pilosebaceous canal by a duct of squamous epithelium. When access to the surface is blocked and bacteria multiply, the result is the comedo of acne.

SWEAT GLANDS—Sweat glands are classified as apocrine and eccrine. Apocrine glands are secretory but are not necessarily responsive to thermal stimulation. Such glands do not produce sweat in the normal sense of the word. Apocrine glands, however, often are associated with eccrine sweat glands, particularly in the axilla.

Eccrine sweat glands are coiled secretory glands, equipped with a blood supply, extending from the dermis to the epidermal surface. Eccrine sweat glands function to regulate heat exchange in man. As such, they are indispensable to survival.

About 3 million eccrine glands are thought to be distributed over the human body. Distribution varies from less than 100 to more than 300/cm². Gland counts after thermal stimulation do not always agree with anatomical counts.

Drug Effects and the Extent of Percutaneous Drug Delivery

Drugs are applied to the skin to elicit one or more of four general effects: an effect on the skin surface, an effect within the stratum corneum, a more deep-seated effect requiring penetration into the epidermis and dermis, or a systemic effect resulting from delivery of sufficient drug through the epidermis and the dermis to the vasculature to produce therapeutic systemic concentrations.

SURFACE EFFECTS—An activity on the skin surface may be in the form of a film, an action against surface microorganisms, or a cleansing effect. Film formation on the skin surface may be protective (eg, a zinc oxide cream or a sunscreen). Films may be somewhat occlusive and provide a moisturizing effect by diminishing loss of moisture from the skin surface. In such instances, the film or film formation *per se* fulfills the objective of product design. The action of antimicrobials against surface flora requires more than simple delivery to the site. The vehicle must facilitate contact between the surface organisms and the active ingredient. Skin cleansers employ soaps or surfactants to facilitate the removal of superficial soil.

STRATUM CORNEUM EFFECTS—Drug effects within the stratum corneum are seen with certain sunscreens; *p*-aminobenzoic acid is an example of a sunscreening agent that both penetrates and is substantive to stratum corneum cells. Skin moisturization takes place within the stratum corneum. Whether it involves the hydration of dry outer cells by surface films or the intercalation of water in the lipid-rich intercellular laminae, the increased moisture results in an apparent softening of the skin. Keratolytic agents, such as salicylic acid, act within the stratum corneum to cause a breakup or sloughing of stratum corneum cell aggregates. This is particularly important in conditions of abnormal stratum corneum such as psoriasis, a disease characterized by thickened scaly plaques.

The stratum corneum also may serve as a *reservoir phase* or depot wherein topically applied drug accumulates due to partitioning into or binding with skin components. This interaction can limit the subsequent migration of the penetrant unless the interaction capacity of the stratum corneum is surpassed by providing excess drug. Examples of drugs that exhibit significant skin interaction include benzocaine, estrogens, scopolamine, and corticosteroids.

EPIDERMAL, DERMAL, LOCAL, AND SYSTEMIC EFFECTS—The penetration of a drug into the viable epidermis and dermis may be difficult to achieve, as noted above. But, once transepidermal permeation has occurred, the continued diffusion of drug into the dermis is likely to result in drug transfer into the microcirculation of the dermis and then into general circulation. Nonetheless, it is possible to formulate drug delivery systems that provide substantial localized delivery without achieving correspondingly high systemic concentrations. Limited studies in man of topical triethanolamine salicylate, minoxidil, and retinoids demonstrate the potential of this approach.

Unwanted systemic effects stemming from the inadvertent transdermal penetration of drugs have been reported for a wide variety of compounds (eg, hexachlorophene, lindane, corticosteroids, or *N,N*-diethyl-*m*-toluamide) over the years. With the commercial introduction of transdermal drug delivery systems for scopolamine, nitroglycerin, clonidine, 17β-estradiol, fentanyl, nicotine, testosterone, lidocaine, and oxybutynin, transdermal penetration is being regarded increasingly as an opportunity rather than a nuisance.

Percutaneous Absorption

Percutaneous absorption involves the transfer of drug from the skin surface into the stratum corneum, under the aegis of a concentration gradient, and its subsequent diffusion through the stratum corneum and underlying epidermis, through the der-

Table 44-1. Composition of Sebum

CONSTITUENTS	% W/W	CONSTITUENTS	% W/W
Triglycerides	57.5	Cholesterol esters	3.0
Wax esters	26.0	Cholesterol	1.5
Squalene	12.0		

mis, and into the microcirculation. The skin behaves as a passive barrier to diffusing molecules. Evidence for this includes the fact that the impermeability of the skin persists long after the skin has been excised. Furthermore, Fick's Law is obeyed in the vast majority of instances.

Molecular penetration through the various regions of the skin is limited by the diffusional resistances encountered. The total diffusional resistance (R_{skin}) to permeation through the skin has been described by Chien as

$$R_{skin} = R_{sc} + R_e + R_{pd}$$

where R is the diffusional resistance, and the subscripts sc, e, and pd refer to the stratum corneum, epidermis, and papillary layer of the dermis, respectively. In addition, resistance to transfer into the microvasculature limits the systemic delivery of drug.

By and large, the greatest resistance to penetration is met in the stratum corneum (ie, diffusion through the stratum corneum tends to be the rate-limiting step in percutaneous absorption).

The role of hair follicles and sweat glands must be considered; however, as a general rule their effect is minimized by the relatively small fractional areas occupied by these appendages. On the other hand, liposomal vehicles and microbead (3 to 10 µm diameter) suspensions appear to accumulate selectively in pilosebaceous and perifollicular areas. In the very early stages of absorption, transit through the appendages may be comparatively large, particularly for lipid-soluble molecules and those whose permeation through the stratum corneum is relatively low. Surfactants and volatile organic solvents such as ethanol have been found to enhance drug uptake via the transfollicular route.

Rather than characterizing drug transfer into and through the skin in terms of the diffusional resistances encountered, one could define permeation in terms of the *pathways* followed by the diffusing species. Drug permeation through the intact skin of humans involves either an intercellular or transcellular path in the stratum corneum, for the most part, rather than the so-called shunt pathways (transglandular or transfollicular routes).

The conventional wisdom is that for the most part, lipophilic compounds transfer preferentially into the lipoidal intercellular phase of the stratum corneum, while relatively more hydrophilic compounds transfer into the intracellular domain of the stratum corneum. One should keep in mind that the often-postulated biphasic character of the horny layer—with hydrophilic cells in a lipophilic matrix—is overly simplistic: the hydrophilic cells themselves are enclosed within lipid bilayer membranes, while the lipophilic matrix comprises intercellular lipids that are, in fact, present in lamellar structures that *sandwich in* hydrophilic layers. As Boddé et al[1] have suggested, the intercellular pathway is *bicontinuous,* consisting of a nonpolar and a polar diffusion pathway between the corneocytes. The implications for dermatopharmacokinetic modeling are clear.

The stratum corneum can be regarded as a passive diffusion membrane but not an inert system; it often has an affinity for the applied substance. The adsorption isotherm is frequently linear in dilute concentration ranges. The correlation between external and surface concentrations is given in terms of the solvent membrane distribution coefficient K_m. The integrated form of Fick's Law is given as

$$J_s = \frac{K_m D C_s}{\delta}$$

and

$$K_p = \frac{K_m D}{\delta}$$

where K_p is the permeability coefficient, J_s is the steady state flux of solute, C_s is the concentration difference of solute across membrane, δ is the membrane thickness,

K_m is the $\dfrac{\text{solute sorbed per cm}^3 \text{ of tissue}}{\text{solute in solution per cm}^3 \text{ of solvent}} = \dfrac{C_m}{C_s}$,

and D is the average membrane diffusion coefficient for solute.

Permeability experiments have shown that the hydrated stratum corneum has an affinity for both lipophilic and hydrophilic compounds. The bifunctional solubility arises from the *hydrophilic* corneocytes and the lipid-rich lamellar structures in the intercellular space. Thus, attempts to predict permeability constants from oil:water or solvent:water partition coefficients have had limited success.

The effect of regional variation on skin permeability can be marked. It has been suggested that one ought to differentiate between two species of horny layer: the palms and soles (up to 600 µm thick), adapted for weight-bearing and friction; and the body horny layer (~10 µm thick), adapted for flexibility, impermeability, and sensory discrimination.

Overall, data suggest the following order for diffusion of simple molecules through the skin: plantar < palmar < arms, legs, trunk, dorsum of hand < scrotal and postauricular < axillary < scalp. Electrolytes in solution penetrate the skin poorly. Ionization of a weak electrolyte substantially reduces its permeability (eg, sodium salicylate permeates poorly compared with salicylic acid). The development of iontophoretic devices in recent years may minimize this problem with ionic penetrants. For any specific molecule, the predictability of regional variations in skin permeability continues to elude investigators. This will continue to be true as long as dermatopharmacokinetic models do not adequately reflect the anisotropicity of the skin's composition and structure, its interactions with the drug and the vehicle, and the physiological parameters that affect transfer.

In Vitro and *In Vivo* Studies

Classically, percutaneous absorption has been studied *in vivo* using radioactively labeled compounds or by *in vitro* techniques using excised human or animal skin. *In vivo* studies in recent years have made use of the skin-stripping method, which permits the estimation of the concentration or amount of the penetrating species as a function of depth of the stratum corneum. Layers of the stratum corneum can be removed or stripped successively away by the repeated application and removal of cellulose adhesive tape strips. Skin penetration of a drug and the effect of additives may be studied and evaluated through analysis of individual skin strips, which provide a profile of skin penetration. Rougier et al[2] have championed the use of the skin-stripping method, in conjunction with short-term exposure to the topically applied penetrant, as a predictor of skin permeation.

Clearly, the evaluation of new chemical entities (NCEs) of indeterminate toxicity mandates *in vitro* testing. A diffusion cell frequently used for *in vitro* experiments is shown in Figure

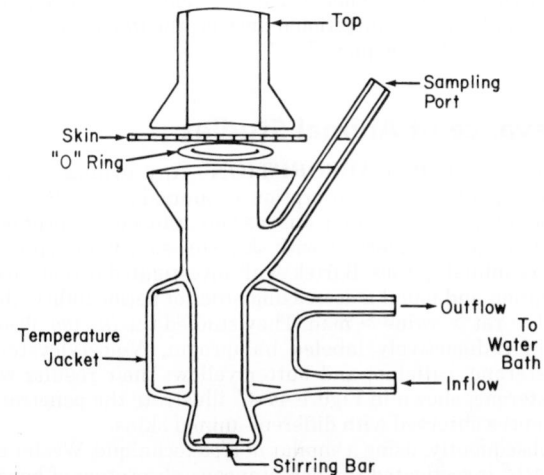

Figure 44-2. Schematic representation of diffusion cell. Top is open to ambient laboratory environment. (From Franz TJ. *J Invest Dermatol* 1975;64:191.)

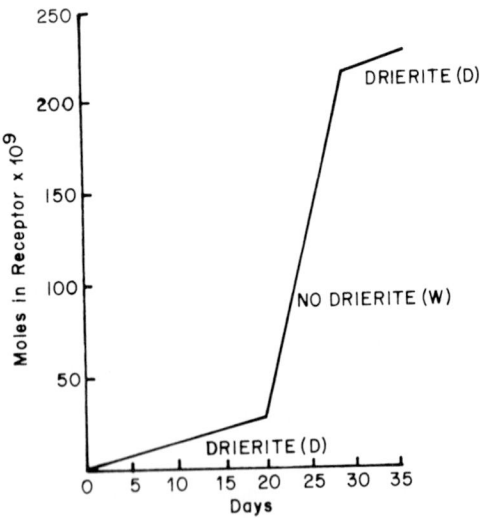

Figure 44-3. Change in cortisone penetration by alternately drying (D) and humidifying (W) the stratum corneum. (From Scheuplein RJ, Ross LW. *J Invest Dermatol* 1974;63:353.)

44-2.[3] In this system, the intact skin or the epidermis is treated as a semipermeable membrane separating two fluid media. The transport rate of a particular drug is evaluated by introducing the drug in solution on the stratum corneum side of the *membrane*, then measuring penetration by periodic sampling and analysis of the fluid across the skin membrane.

Investigators have recognized that transport across an immersed, fully hydrated stratum corneum may not represent the absorption system or rate observed in *in vivo* studies. Percutaneous absorption across a fully hydrated stratum corneum may be an exaggeration. It may be more representative of enhanced absorption that is seen after *in vivo* skin is hydrated by occlusive wrapping.

Using separated epidermal skin mounted in diffusion cells, Scheuplein and Ross[4] varied the atmosphere above the skin strip by use of Drierite to simulate dry conditions and wetted paper strips to simulate the effect of occlusion and observed marked reduction in penetration of cortisone under dry conditions but greatly enhanced penetration on humidifying the stratum corneum (Fig 44-3).[4]

The studies of Scheuplein and Ross,[4] and of Franz,[3] demonstrate that *in vitro* studies of percutaneous absorption under controlled conditions are relevant to *in vivo* drug penetration. As stated by Franz, "whenever a question is asked requiring only a qualitative or directional answer, the *in vitro* technique appears perfectly adequate."

Relevance of Animal Studies

PERCUTANEOUS ABSORPTION—Any evaluation of a study of percutaneous absorption in animals must take cognizance of species variation. Just as percutaneous absorption in man will vary considerably with skin site, so will absorption in various animal species. Bartek et al[5] investigated percutaneous absorption and found a decreasing order of permeability, thus, rabbit > rat > swine > man. They studied the *in vivo* absorption of radioactively labeled haloprogin, *N*-acetylcysteine, testosterone, caffeine, and butter yellow; their results with testosterone, shown in Figure 44-4,[6] illustrate the penetration differences observed with different animal skins.

Subsequently, using a similar *in vivo* technique, Wester and Maibach[7] investigated the percutaneous absorption of benzoic acid, hydrocortisone, and testosterone in the rhesus monkey. Radioactively tagged compounds were applied to the ventral surface of the forearm, and absorption was quantified on the

basis of radioactivity excreted in the urine for 5 days following application. The investigators concluded that the percutaneous penetration of these compounds in the rhesus monkey is similar to that in man and regarded the data as encouraging because of the similarity.

The consensus is that rhesus monkeys and miniature pigs are good *in vivo* models for human percutaneous absorption, while smaller laboratory animals (eg, mouse, rat, rabbit) are not.

It should be stressed again that percutaneous absorption studies in animals, either *in vivo* or *in vitro*, only can be useful approximations of activity in man. The effect of species variation, site variability (about which little is known in animals), skin condition, experimental variables, and, of major importance, the vehicle, must be kept in mind.

As Bronaugh[8] notes, although human skin is preferable for *in vitro* permeation studies, its availability is limited. Additional constraints apply if one is only willing to use freshly obtained viable human skin from surgical specimens or biopsies, as opposed to skin harvested from cadavers.

Concern has been voiced over the notorious variability in barrier properties of excised skin, whether animal or human. Factors responsible for the variability include the source and characteristics of the donor skin (eg, elapsed time from death to harvesting of the skin, age and gender of the donor, health of the skin prior to the donor's death), exposure of the skin to chemicals or mechanical treatment (eg, shaving or clipping prior to harvesting of the skin), etc. The availability of a *living skin equivalent*—comprising a bilayered system of human dermal fibroblasts in a collagenous matrix upon which human corneocytes have formed a stratified epidermis—offers an alternative, less variable, model for evaluating human skin permeation and biotransformation.

Skin-flap methods represent *in vivo* and *in vitro* techniques for evaluating percutaneous absorption in animals or animal models: the general approach entails the surgical isolation of a skin section of an animal such that the blood supply is singular; this ensures that drug can be collected and assayed in the vascular perfusate as it undergoes absorption from the skin surface. The perfused skin flap can be maintained in the intact animal or mounted in an *in vitro* perfusion system, all the while maintaining its viability.

Animals also have been used to detect contact sensitization, measure antimitotic drug activity, measure phototoxicity, and evaluate the comedogenic and comedolytic potential of sub-

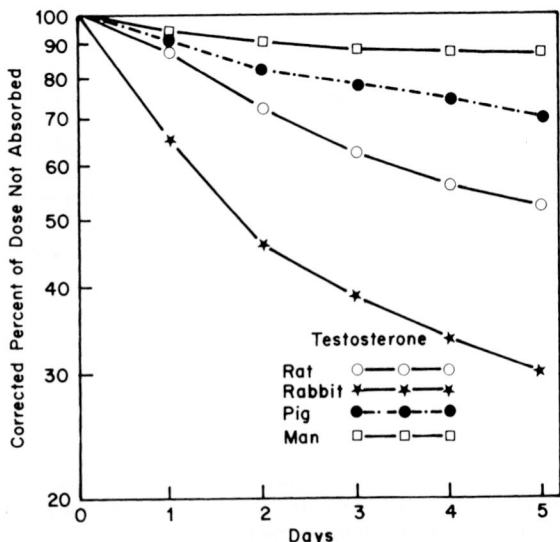

Figure 44-4. Percutaneous absorption of testosterone in rats, rabbits, swine and man for 5 days after application. (From Maibach HI, ed. *Animal Models in Dermatology*. Edinburgh: Churchill Livingstone, 1975.)

stances. In each of these test procedures, be it a safety test or assay model, the animal is considered a substitute for man. It is, therefore, important to realize that the animal is not man, even though man is the ultimate test animal. Animal-testing presents the investigator with unique advantages; lack of appreciation of the variables involved can destroy these advantages.

Mershon and Callahan[9] recorded and illustrated the considerations involved in selecting an animal test model. They interpreted the rabbit irritancy data of several investigators and impressively visualized different possible interpretations of the differing response between rabbit and man.

While the ultimate system for establishing therapeutic efficacy is man, there are specific animal test models that are recognized to be valuable as prehuman-use screens predictive of drug activity in humans. For example, the rat-ear assay and the granuloma-pouch procedure in rats are recognized procedures for the estimation of steroid anti-inflammatory activity.

Lorenzetti[10] tabulated the potency of various topical steroids, comparing the rat-ear-edema assay with potency measured in humans by use of the vasoconstrictor procedure of Stoughton and McKenzie; the results are given in Table 44-2.[11] Animal assay models of this kind, particularly the steroid anti-inflammatory assays, are most useful as preliminary activity screens. The simplicity, safety, and reproducibility of the vasoconstrictor assay in humans recommend it over any corresponding animal procedure. However, a number of concerns have been raised over the years that need to be addressed, particularly if this bioassay is to be used to assess the bioequivalence of topical corticosteroid formulations. These concerns include the linearity of the vasoconstrictor response–drug concentration relationship and the visual assessment of the blanching or vasoconstrictor response.

As the *in vivo* vasoconstrictor response generally approaches a maximum, one must know whether the microcirculation of the skin has exceeded its capacity to respond linearly to the corticosteroid concentration attained in the skin. It may be that only relatively minimal responses will be elicited by relatively high concentrations. At the other end of the response-dose relationship, what is the minimum dose that will produce a reliable, replicable response? Rather than relying on the somewhat subjective visual evaluation of the response, investigators ought to make use of chromometers to provide objective, quantifiable data.

PILOSEBACEOUS UPTAKE—The study of the targeted delivery of drugs to follicles and/or sebaceous glands has become necessary in view of the selective uptake or deposition of antiacne drugs such as tretinoin in pilosebaceous units. Fortunately, the anatomical and physiological correspondence of hamster ear pilosebaceous units to those in humans has facilitated studies of the cutaneous and pilosebaceous disposition of drugs following topical application.[12]

Other Factors Affecting Drug Absorption from the Skin

Percutaneous absorption of a drug can be enhanced by the use of occlusive techniques or by the use of so-called penetration enhancers.

SKIN HYDRATION AND TEMPERATURE—Occluding the skin with wraps of impermeable plastic film such as Saran Wrap prevents the loss of surface water from the skin. Since water is absorbed readily by the protein components of the skin, the occlusive wrap causes greatly increased levels of hydration in the stratum corneum. The concomitant swelling of the horny layer ostensibly decreases protein network density and the diffusional path length. Occlusion of the skin surface also increases skin temperature ($\sim$2 to 3°C), resulting in increased molecular motion and skin permeation.

Hydrocarbon bases that occlude the skin to a degree will bring about an increase in drug penetration. However, this effect is trivial compared with the effects seen with a true occlusive skin wrap. Occlusive techniques are useful in some clinical situations requiring anti-inflammatory activity, and occlusive wrappings are used most commonly with steroids. Since steroid activity can be enhanced so enormously by skin occlusion, it is possible to depress adrenal function unknowingly. Early in the 1960s, McKenzie demonstrated that penetration of steroid could be increased 100-fold by use of occlusion.

Transdermal delivery systems, with their occlusive backing, can effect increased percutaneous absorption as a result of increased skin temperature and hydration.

In experiments with healthy volunteers wearing transdermal nitroglycerin delivery systems, investigators[13] showed that exposure of the surrounding skin area to localized heating or cooling could cause extensive changes in nitroglycerin bioavailability, presumably due to changes in regional cutaneous blood flow and subsequent systemic uptake *(see below)*.

One consequence of occlusion of the skin surface, whether by a transdermal delivery system or a hydrocarbon film, is that an aqueous film may form at the formulation-skin interface. This aqueous film or interphase could result in decreased transfer efficiency, and, in the case of a transdermal delivery system, a loss of adhesion. Accordingly, the suppression of perspiration could enhance vehicle-skin partitioning efficiency and drug permeation.

PENETRATION ENHANCERS—This term has been used to describe substances that facilitate absorption through the skin. While most materials have a direct effect on the permeability of the skin, other so-called enhancers (eg, polyols, such as glycerin and propylene glycol) appear to augment percutaneous absorption by increasing the thermodynamic activity of the penetrant, thereby increasing the effective escaping tendency and concentration gradient of the diffusing species. Penetration enhancers with a direct effect on skin permeability include solvents, surfactants, and miscellaneous chemicals such as urea and *N,N*-diethyl-*m*-toluamide (Table 44-3).[14,15] The mechanism of action of these enhancers is complex since these substances also may increase penetrant solubility. Nonetheless, the predominant effect of these enhancers on the stratum corneum is either to increase its degree of hydration or disrupt its lipoprotein matrix. In either case, the net result is a decrease in resistance to penetrant diffusion. (The formulator should note that the inclusion of a penetration enhancer in a topical formulation mandates additional testing and evaluation to ensure the absence of enhancer-related adverse effects.)

Foremost among the solvents that affect skin permeability is water. As noted above, water is a factor even for *anhydrous* transdermal delivery systems due to their occlusive nature. Due to its safety and efficacy, water has been described as the

Table 44-2. Relative Potency of Anti-Inflammatory Agents

COMPOUND	RAT-EAR EDEMA ASSAY	TOPICAL ANTI-INFLAMMATORY POTENCY HUMAN ASSAY VASOCONSTRICTOR
Dexamethasone	73.2 (49.4–110)	10–20
Dexamethasone 21-acetate	117.3 (85.9–106)	10–20
Prednisolone	2.44 (1.54–7.76)	1–2
Prednisolone 21-acetate	5.43 (4.05–7.70)	3
Betamethasone	97.3 (16.7–141)	3–5
Betamethasone 21-acetate	1072.0 (876–1179)	18–33
Fluorometholone	138.3 (57.9–333)	30–40
Fluorometholone acetate	219.5 (9.15–536)	
Fluprednisolone	31.8 (13.3–76.1)	4–6
Fluprednisolone acetate	61.3 (25.6–147)	
Hydrocortisone	1	1

( ) = 95% confidence limits.
From Maibach HI. In Maibach HI, ed. *Animal Models in Dermatology.*
Edinburgh: Churchill Livingstone, 1975, p 221.

Table 44-3. Penetration Enhancers

Solvents	Dimethyl formamide
Water	Tetrahydrofurfuryl alcohol
Alcohols	*Amphiphiles*
Methanol	L-α -Amino acids
Ethanol	Anionic surfactants
2-Propanol	Cationic surfactants
Alkyl methyl sulfoxides	Amphoteric surfactants
Dimethyl sulfoxide	Nonionic surfactants
Decylmethyl sulfoxide	Fatty acids and alcohols
Tetradecylmethyl sulfoxide	*Miscellaneous*
Pyrrolidones	Clofibric acid amides
2-Pyrrolidone	Hexamethylene lauramide
N-Methyl-2-pyrrolidone	Proteolytic enzymes
N-(2-Hydroxyethyl)	Terpenes and sesquiterpenes
pyrrolidone	α-Bisabolol
Laurocapram	*d*-Limonene
Miscellaneous solvents	Urea
Acetone	*N,N*-Diethyl-*m*-toluamide
Dimethyl acetamide	

Data from Walters KA. In Hadgraft J, Guy RH, eds. *Transdermal Drug Delivery*. New York: Dekker, 1989, p 197; Ghosh TK, Banga AK. *Pharm Technol* 1993; 17(4):62; 1993; 17(5):68.

ultimate penetration enhancer. Other solvents include the classic enhancer, dimethyl sulfoxide (DMSO), which is of limited utility because of its potential ocular and dermal toxicity, its objectionable taste and odor (a consequence of its absorption and subsequent biotransformation), and the need for concentrations in excess of 70% to promote absorption. Analogs of DMSO such as decylmethyl sulfoxide are used currently in some topical formulations. In contrast with other solvents, laurocapram (Azone) has been shown to function effectively at low concentrations (≤5%). Furthermore, laurocapram's effect on skin permeability persists long after a single application, due apparently to its prolonged retention within the stratum corneum.

Surfactants, long recognized for their ability to alter membrane structure and function, can have a substantial effect on skin permeability.[16] However, given the irritation potential of surfactants applied chronically, their utility as penetration enhancers is limited. Their effect on permeability may be complicated further by surfactant/monomer aggregation to form micelles and the concomitant solubilization of the permeant. As the impact of surfactants on skin permeability of a penetrant is problematic, the effect of their inclusion in a formulation should be evaluated using appropriate *in vitro* and *in vivo* studies.

STRATUM CORNEUM BARRIER EFFICACY AND DERMAL CLEARANCE—Even though *in vitro* studies of percutaneous transport may reflect the resistance of the skin to drug diffusion, there is no way such studies can characterize adequately the transfer of diffusing drug into the microvasculature of the dermis and its subsequent transfer into general circulation.

Christophers and Kligman[17] evaluated the dermal *clearance* of ^{22}Na from the midback skin of volunteers following the intradermal injection of ^{22}Na as normal saline solution. The dermal *clearances*, expressed in terms of the half-life for disappearance of radioactivity, are plotted in Figure 44-5.[17] Similar results were obtained with disappearance of skin fluorescence after intradermal injection of sodium fluorescein. The data are indicative of markedly delayed dermal clearance in the aged. This may reflect, in part, a decrease in older subjects in dermal capillary loop density, a decrease in the rate and/or extent of dermal blood perfusion, or an increase in resistance to transfer into the capillaries.

The importance of blood-flow-limited percutaneous absorption was shown by Benowitz et al[18] who documented the effect of the intravenous administration of nicotine, a known cutaneous vasoconstrictor, on the systemic absorption of nicotine administered concurrently in the form of a transdermal delivery

system. Plasma nicotine concentrations rose less rapidly and reached a lower peak at a later time than when nicotine was applied transdermally in the absence of the intravenous nicotine infusion. This raises concerns about the potential cutaneous interactions between vasoconstrictors *or* vasodilators *and* topically applied drugs intended for a systemic effect: bioavailability could be increased or diminished as a result! The assessment of the potency of corticosteroids by corticosteroid-induced skin blanching (ie, vasoconstriction, lends credence to this issue).

On the other hand, Christophers and Kligman[17] demonstrated increased *in vitro* skin permeation by sodium fluorescein in the stratum corneum excised from young and old subjects (Fig 44-6[17]). Thus, the stratum corneum of older subjects may offer less resistance to the penetration of topically applied drugs.

Given the substantial intersubject variations that occur in diffusional resistance and in dermal clearance, it is not surprising that *in vivo* studies of percutaneous absorption often demonstrate marked differences in systemic availability of drugs. Furthermore, the tendency to employ normal, healthy, *young* adults in these studies may not provide data that is indicative of drug permeation through the skin of older subjects or patients.

Roskos, Maibach, and Guy[19] made quantitative measurements of the percutaneous absorption of a number of drugs *in vivo* from the urinary excretion profiles of ^{14}C-radiolabeled drugs in young (18 to 40 years) and old (>65 years) subjects: while permeation of hydrocortisone, benzoic acid, aspirin, and caffeine was significantly lower in older subjects, testosterone and estradiol absorption was comparable in the two groups. Additional comprehensive studies of percutaneous absorption *as a function of age* continue to be warranted.

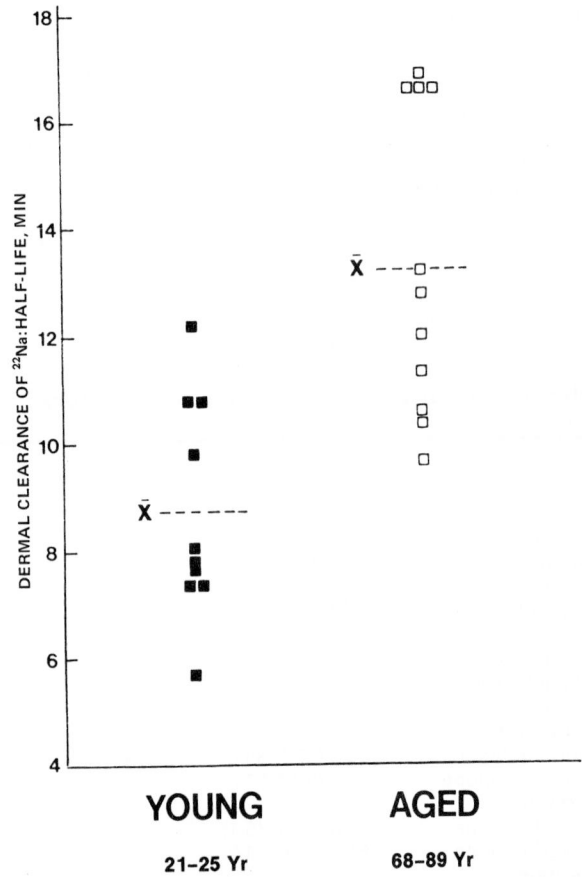

Figure 44-5. Dermal clearance of ^{22}Na in young and aged subjects after intradermal injection. (Data from Christophers E, Kligman AM. In Montagna W, ed. *Advances in the Biology of Skin,* vol 6. Oxford: Pergamon, 1965, p 163.)

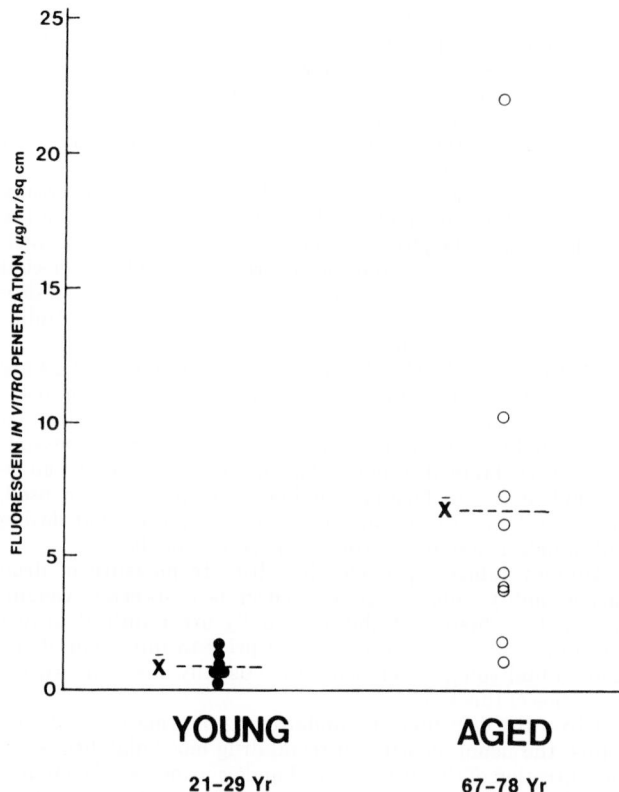

Figure 44-6. Flux of fluorescein through stratum corneum excised from young and aged subjects (Data from Christophers E, Kligman AM. In Montagna W, ed. *Advances in the Biology of Skin*, vol 6. Oxford: Pergamon, 1965, p 163.)

CUTANEOUS BIOTRANSFORMATION—Catabolic enzyme activity in the viable epidermis is substantial. In fact, the viable epidermis is metabolically more active than the dermis. If the topically applied drug is subject to biotransformation during skin permeation, local and systemic bioavailability can be affected markedly. Enzymatic activity in the skin, or for that matter in systemic fluids and tissues, can be taken advantage of to facilitate percutaneous absorption. Sloan and Bodor,[20] for example, synthesized 7-acyloxymethyl derivatives of theophylline that diffuse through the skin far more efficiently than theophylline itself (Fig 44-7[20]) but which are biotransformed rapidly to theophylline. Thus, theophylline delivery to systemic circulation can be enhanced substantially.

Further Considerations for Transdermal Drug Delivery

For a drug to qualify as a candidate for systemic delivery after topical application, it must satisfy requirements in addition to exhibiting good skin permeation. Successful candidates for transdermal drug delivery should be nonirritating and nonsensitizing to the skin. Since relatively little drug may reach systemic circulation over a relatively long time, drug candidates should be relatively potent drugs. In addition, the limitation to relatively potent drugs can ease problems of formulation, since the amount of drug that can be incorporated in the formulation may be limited by physicochemical considerations such as solubility.

In Silico Methods

In recent years, *in silico* or *in numero* modeling or computer simulation of percutaneous absorption has been advocated as a

link between *in vitro* and *in vivo* studies. A number of relatively simplistic dermatopharmacokinetic models have been developed that do provide the formulator with some insight into transdermal drug delivery, in spite of the biological and physicochemical complexity of drug transport into and through the skin. By and large, these models are analogous to the classical pharmacokinetic models that have been employed to assess *in vivo* drug uptake and disposition. Some of the dermatopharmacokinetic models proposed differ from more classically oriented models in that drug transport in the vehicle and in the epidermis, particularly the stratum corneum, is modeled in accordance with Fickian diffusion. Thus, the formulator can anticipate the effect of variables such as the thickness of the applied (vehicle) phase, alterations in drug partitioning between the vehicle and the stratum corneum, and the frequency of reapplication on the overall appearance of drug systemically as a function of time following topical application.

RECTAL ABSORPTION

The bioavailability of rectally administered drugs is a relatively recent concern despite the antiquity of this dosage form; little was known about drug absorption or drug activity via suppository administration until recent years. Rectally instilled preparations, whether suppositories, foams, or solutions (enemas), tend to be confined to the rectum and sigmoid colon if the volume is less than about 50 mL. Foams tend to dissipate or spread to a lesser extent than solutions, particularly large-volume solutions (~100 to 200 mL). Though large-volume fluid formulations—solutions or enemas—may allow drug to reach the ascending colon, substantial intra- and intersubject variation is evident.[21] Literature information indicates that rectal drug absorption from suppositories can be erratic and may be substantially different from absorption following oral administration. With only a few recent exceptions, suppository studies are based on either *in vivo* or *in vitro* data, with few attempts to correlate *in vitro* results with *in vivo* studies.

Major factors affecting the absorption of drugs from suppositories administered rectally are the following: anorectal physiology, suppository vehicle, and the physicochemical properties of the drug.

ANORECTAL PHYSIOLOGY—The rectum is about 150 mm in length, terminating in the anal opening; its surface area is about 200 to 400 cm². In the absence of fecal matter the rec-

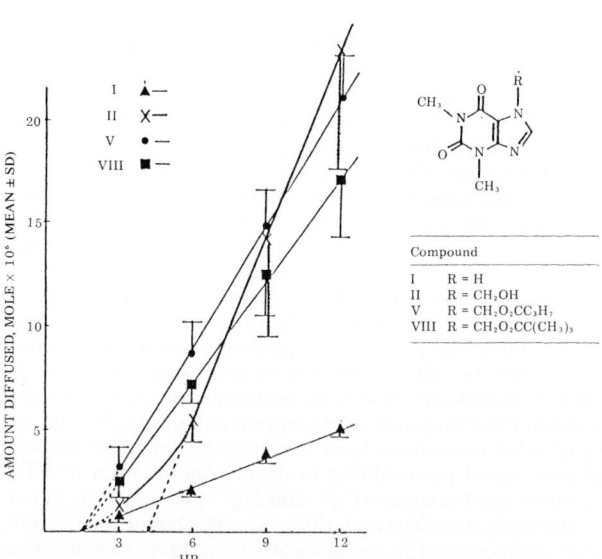

Figure 44-7. Diffusion of theophylline (I) and its derivatives through hairless mouse skin. (From Sloan KB, Bodor N. *Int J Pharm* 1982;12:299.)

tum contains a small amount of fluid (1 to 3 mL) of low buffering capacity. Fluid pH is said to be about 7.2; because of the low buffer capacity pH will vary with the pH of the drug product or drug dissolved in it. Bottger et al [22] studied the influence of pH on the rectal absorption of sodium benzoate in man by the technique of rectal lumen perfusion. This study demonstrates that strong buffers in rectal solutions induce a drastic effect on the pH of the boundary layer, an effect that is not seen if unbuffered solutions are used.

Most rectal suppositories today are torpedo-shaped, with the apex, or pointed end, tapering to the base, or blunt end, following the recommendation of HS Wellcome in 1893 that rectal suppositories should be inserted with the thicker end foremost so that when the anal sphincter contracts, expulsion is prevented. In the intervening 100 years or so, no study has correlated rectal suppository insertion with anorectal physiology until that of Abd-El-Maeboud et al,[23] who found that ease of insertion, retention, and lack of expulsion were enhanced when the suppository was inserted base or blunt end up. This was ascribed to reversed vermicular contractions of the external anal sphincter, which facilitate movement of the suppository upward into the rectum.

The rectal epithelium is lipoidal in character. The lower, middle, and upper hemorrhoidal veins surround the rectum. Only the upper vein conveys blood into the portal system; thus, drugs absorbed into the lower and middle hemorrhoidal veins will bypass the liver. Absorption and distribution of a drug therefore are modified by its position in the rectum, in the sense that at least a portion of the drug absorbed from the rectum may pass directly into the inferior vena cava, bypassing the liver.

Spreading characteristics of rectal formulations may be affected considerably by intraluminal rectal pressure—due, in part, to the weight of abdominal organs and to respiratory activity—and by periodic contractile activity of the rectal wall.[24]

Parrott[25] compared the absorption of salicylates after rectal and oral administration. Using urinary excretion data both aspirin and sodium salicylate were found to be equally bioavailable orally or rectally. Aspirin was released more rapidly from water-miscible suppositories than from the oily type. Conversely, sodium salicylate was released more rapidly from a cocoa butter vehicle.

Based on available data the bioavailability of a drug from a suppository dosage form depends on the physicochemical properties of the drug as well as the composition of the base. The drug-dissolution rate and, where appropriate, the partition coefficient between lipid and aqueous phase should be known.

For suppository formulation, the relative solubility of the drug in the vehicle is a convenient comparison measure. Lipid-soluble drugs present in low concentration in a cocoa butter base will have little tendency to partition and diffuse into rectal fluids. Drugs that are only slightly soluble in the lipid base will partition readily into the rectal fluid. The partition coefficient between suppository base and rectal fluid thus becomes a useful measure. In water-soluble bases, assuming rapid dissolution, the rate-limiting step in absorption would be transport of the drug through the rectal mucosa.

In the absence of evidence of any substantial carrier-mediated uptake mechanisms, the predominant mechanism of colorectal mucosal permeation appears to involve transcellular passage across cell membranes in accordance with the pH-partition hypothesis. Ease of access to the rectal mucosa has encouraged the evaluation of absorption enhancers. A wide variety of substances have been investigated for their ability to enhance rectal permeability to drugs. Agents such as EDTA have been used to chelate Ca^{2+} and Mg^{2+} in the vicinity of paracellular tight junctions and, thus, alter epithelial permeability. Other promoters of rectal absorption (eg, bile salts and nonsteroidal anti-inflammatory agents, including aspirin, salicylic acid and diclofenac) appear to exert their influence by affecting water influx and efflux rates across the rectal mucosa. Surfac-

tants not only may modify membrane permeability but also enhance wetting or spreading of the base and dissolution of the drug. In any event, it should be evident that whatever the mechanism, enhancing the *rectal* absorption of drugs—especially those that undergo presystemic elimination—could result in substantially reduced dosage requirements and decreased risk of adverse reactions.

Clearly, the bioavailability of a drug administered rectally depends on the nature of the drug and the composition of the vehicle or base. The physical properties of the drug can be modified to a degree, as can the characteristics of the base selected as the delivery system. Preformulation evaluations of physicochemical properties then must be confirmed by *in vivo* studies in animals and ultimately in the primary primate, man.

***IN VIVO* RECTAL ABSORPTION STUDIES**—Dogs are probably the animal of choice in evaluating rectal drug availability. (The pig is a closer physiological match, but size and manageability argue in favor of the dog.) Blood and urine samples can be obtained from the dog, and rectal retention can be accomplished with facility. Smaller animals have been used; rabbits, rats, and even mice have been employed, but dosing and sampling become progressively more difficult.

Human subjects provide the ultimate measure of drug bioavailability. Subjects are selected on the basis of age, weight, and medical history. Subjects usually are required to fast overnight and evacuate the bowel prior to initiation of the study. Fluid volume and food intake usually are standardized in studies of this kind.

Given the difficulty of standardizing pharmacological endpoints, the usual measure of rectal drug bioavailability is the concentration of the drug in blood and/or urine as a function of time. A control group using oral drug administration provides a convenient means of comparing oral and rectal drug availability. Such a comparison is meaningful particularly in view of uncertainties and conflicts encountered in the literature. While there is general agreement about drug absorption from the rectum, there is less agreement on dosage adequacy and the relationship between oral and rectal dosage. This state of affairs argues in favor of adequate studies to establish proper dosage and verify bioavailability.

VAGINAL ABSORPTION

Passive drug absorption via the vaginal mucosa, as with other mucosal tissues, is influenced by absorption site physiology, absorption site pH, and the solubility and partitioning characteristics of the drug. The vaginal epithelial surface usually is covered with an aqueous film—emanating from cervical secretions—whose volume, pH, and composition vary with age, stage of the menstrual cycle, and location. Postmenarche, a vaginal pH gradient is evident, with the lowest values (pH ~4) near the anterior fornix and the highest (pH ~5) near the cervix.[26]

Following intravaginal administration, some drug absorption from the intact vaginal mucosa is likely, even when the drug is employed for a local effect. In fact, extensive drug absorption can occur from the vagina. For example, Patel et al[27] reported that plasma propranolol concentrations following vaginal dosing were significantly higher than those after peroral administration of an equivalent dose; a reflection, in part, of decreased first-pass biotransformation following vaginal absorption. Nonetheless, the notion persists that the vaginal epithelium is relatively impermeable to drugs.

The widespread extemporaneous compounding of progesterone vaginal suppositories,[28,29] as well as the marketing of an intrauterine progesterone drug delivery system (Progestasert, *Alza*), has focused interest on systemic drug absorption following intravaginal administration. However, only limited reports of research on *in vitro* and *in vivo* aspects of vaginal absorption have appeared in the literature to date.

DOSAGE FORMS AND DRUG DELIVERY SYSTEMS FOR TOPICAL APPLICATION

The array of formulations and compositions employed for topical application confounds attempts at categorization. Nonetheless, if a distinction is made between drug *dosage forms* and drug *delivery systems*, some clarity emerges. **Dosage forms** contain the active drug ingredient in association with nondrug (usually inert) excipients that comprise the vehicle or formulation matrix. A conventional dosage form tends to be empirical in composition; its formulator's focus tends to emphasize stability and esthetics rather than efficacy. On the other hand, **delivery systems** involve a holistic approach to formulation that is optimized for the drug's relevant biopharmaceutic and pharmacokinetic characteristics in the patient population. Thus, a delivery system is formulated with functionality and efficacy in mind, not just stability and esthetics.

The Skin

In many (if not most) clinical situations, the rate-limiting step is penetration of the drug across the skin barrier (ie, percutaneous penetration through the skin alone). Diffusion of the drug from its vehicle should not be unknowingly the rate-limiting step in percutaneous absorption. Such a rate limitation or control may, of course, be an objective and the endpoint of specific drug optimization, but inappropriate formulation can reduce substantially the effectiveness of a topical drug substance.

In the formulation of a vehicle for topical drug application, many factors must be considered. Drug stability, intended product use, site of application, and product type must be combined in a dosage form or delivery system that will release the drug readily when placed in contact with the skin. Further, the release characteristics of the vehicle depend on the physical-chemical properties of the specific drug substance to be delivered to the skin: drug release from a vehicle is a function of the drug's concentration and solubility in the vehicle, and the drug's partition coefficient between the vehicle and the skin. A vehicle optimized for delivery of hydrocortisone may be quite inappropriate for delivery of a different steroid.

Higuchi (see *Bibliography*) discussed equations describing the rate of release of solid drugs suspended in ointment bases. Ostrenga et al[30] discussed the significance of vehicle composition on the percutaneous absorption of fluocinolone acetonide and fluocinolone acetonide 21-acetate (fluocinonide) (Fig 44-8). These investigators used propylene glycol/isopropyl myristate partition coefficients, *in vitro* (human) skin penetration, and fi-

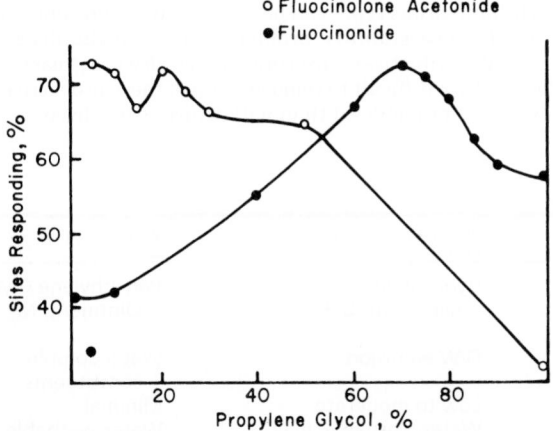

Figure 44-8. *In vivo* response as a function of vehicle composition (24-hour vasoconstriction). (From Ostrenga J, Steinmetz C, Poulsen B. *J Pharm Sci* 1971;60:1175.)

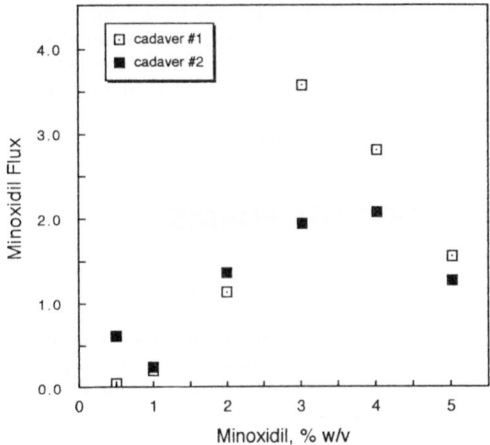

Figure 44-9. Minoxidil flux (x10^4 mg/cm^2/h) through human cadaver skin as a function of minoxidil concentration in the topically applied formulation. (Data from Flynn GL, Weiner ND, et al. *Int J Pharm* 1989;55:229.)

nally *in vivo* vasoconstrictor studies to evaluate formulation variables. They concluded that

"In general, an efficacious topical gel preparation is one in which (a) the concentration of diffusible drug in the vehicle for a given labeled strength is optimized by ensuring that all of the drug is in solution, (b) the minimum amount of solvent is used to dissolve the drug completely and yet maintain a favorable partition coefficient and (c) the vehicle components affect the permeability of the stratum corneum in a favorable manner."

The effect of propylene glycol concentration on *in vivo* vasoconstrictor activity is illustrated strikingly in Figure 44-8, taken from Ostrenga, Steinmetz, and Poulsen.[30]

Experimental work of the kind described by Ostrenga, Steinmetz, and Poulsen provides a means of optimizing drug release from a vehicle and penetration of the drug into the skin. This is a beginning. The formulator must proceed to develop a total composition in which the drug is stable and causes no irritation to sensitive skin areas. Safety, stability, and effective preservative efficacy must be combined with optimum drug delivery in the total formulation.

The work of Flynn, Weiner, and others[31] on the physicochemical stability of topical drug-delivery systems *postapplication* has facilitated the exploration of additional formulation factors that are crucial to the success of topical formulations. Flynn notes that the functionality of topical drug delivery systems stands in stark contrast to those of transdermal drug-delivery systems; while both delivery systems are open systems *kinetically* due to the formulation-skin interface, they differ to a considerable extent *thermodynamically* because most topical formulations are left open to the air postapplication, while transdermal delivery systems are self-contained closed systems.

One study focused on a topical delivery system for minoxidil. The vehicle was 60:20:20 ethanol:propylene glycol:water system, with just enough propylene glycol to maintain 2% minoxidil in solution, following the evaporation of the more volatile ethanol and water. Minoxidil fluxes across human cadaver skin, measured as a function of minoxidil concentration, increased as the initial concentration of drug increased, but only to about 3% (Fig 44-9).[31] At initial minoxidil concentrations greater than 3%, transport was disproportionately low, relative to initial concentration, due to early precipitation of the drug.

Evaporation and loss of volatile formulation components such as water or ethanol postapplication can be expected to affect topical drug-delivery system composition and performance. Flynn et al[31] have shown that so-called nonvolatile excipients (eg, propylene glycol) evaporate after topical application. Skin permeation by excipients also may occur after application leading to further compositional changes in the applied film on the skin surface. The impact of this evaporative and absorptive loss of adjuvants increases as the volume of the applied formulation is reduced. As Flynn et al[31] note, ". . . the momentary compositions, and thus delivery capabilities, of real vehicles are significantly influenced by the amounts applied."

TOPICAL DOSAGE FORMS

OINTMENTS—The USP defines ointments as semisolid preparations intended for external application to the skin or mucous membranes. They usually, but not always, contain medicinal substances. The types of ointment bases used as vehicles for drugs are selected or designed to facilitate drug transfer into the skin. Ointments also contribute emolliency or other quasi-medicinal benefits.

USP Classification and Properties of Ointment Bases

The USP recognizes four general classes of ointment bases: hydrocarbon bases (ie, oleaginous bases), absorption bases, water-removable bases, and water-soluble bases. These various bases are contrasted with one another in Table 44-4. The selection of the optimum vehicle based on the USP classification *per se* may require compromises. For example, stability or drug activity might be superior in a hydrocarbon base; however, patient acceptability is diminished because of the greasy nature of the base. The water solubility of the polyethylene glycol bases may be attractive, but the glycol(s) may be irritating to traumatized tissue. For some drugs, activity and percutaneous absorption may be superior when using a hydrocarbon base; however, it may be prudent to minimize percutaneous absorption by the use of a less occlusive base. In other instances, activity and percutaneous absorption may be enhanced by using a hydrophilic base. These problematic aspects of bioavailability of drugs in topical formulations are discussed above.

HYDROCARBON (OLEAGINOUS) BASES—Hydrocarbon bases are usually petrolatum *per se* or petrolatum modified by waxes or liquid petrolatum to change viscosity characteristics. Liquid petrolatum gelled by the addition of polyethylene also is considered a hydrocarbon ointment base, albeit one with unusual viscosity characteristics.

Hydrocarbon ointment bases are classified as oleaginous bases along with bases prepared from vegetable fixed oils or animal fats. Bases of this type include lard, benzoinated lard, olive oil, cottonseed oil, and other oils. These bases are emollient but generally require addition of antioxidants and other preservatives. They are now largely of historic interest.

Petrolatum USP is a tasteless, odorless, unctuous material with a melting range of 38°C to 60°C; its color ranges from amber to white (when decolorized). Petrolatum often is used externally, without modification or added medication, for its emollient qualities.

Petrolatum used as an ointment base has a high degree of compatibility with a variety of medicaments. Bases of this type are occlusive and nearly anhydrous and thus provide optimum stability for medicaments such as antibiotics. The wide melting range permits some latitude in vehicle selection, and the USP permits addition of waxy materials as an aid in minimizing temperature effects.

Hydrocarbon bases, being occlusive, increase skin hydration by reducing the rate of loss of surface water. Bases of this kind may be used solely for such a skin-moisturizing or emollient effect. Skin hydration on the other hand may increase drug activity as discussed earlier.

A gelled mineral oil vehicle (Plastibase) represents a unique member of this class of bases that comprises refined natural products: When approximately 5% of low-density polyethylene is added to liquid petrolatum and the mixture then heated and subsequently shock-cooled, a soft, unctuous, colorless material resembling white petrolatum is produced. The mass maintains unchanged consistency over a wide temperature range. It neither hardens at low temperatures nor melts at reasonably high temperatures. Its useful working range is between -15° and 60°C. Excessive heat, ie, above 90°C, will destroy the gel structure.

On the basis of *in vitro* studies, drugs may be released faster from a gelled mineral oil vehicle than from conventional petrolatum. This quicker release has been attributed to easier diffusion of drug through a vehicle with lower microscopic viscosity (ie, a vehicle that is essentially a liquid) than through petrolatum.

Despite the advantages hydrocarbon or oleaginous vehicles provide in terms of stability and emolliency, such bases have the considerable disadvantage of greasiness. The greasy or oily material may stain clothing and is difficult to remove. In terms of patient acceptance, hydrocarbon bases (ie, ointments) rank well below emulsion bases such as creams and lotions.

ABSORPTION BASES—Absorption bases are hydrophilic, anhydrous materials or hydrous bases that have the ability to absorb additional water. The former are anhydrous bases, which absorb water to become W/O emulsions; the latter are W/O emulsions, which have the ability to absorb additional water. The word absorption in this context refers only to the ability of the base to absorb water.

Hydrophilic Petrolatum USP is an anhydrous absorption base. Its W/O emulsifying property is conferred by the inclusion of cholesterol. This composition is a modification of the original formulation, which contained anhydrous lanolin. The lanolin was deleted because of reports of allergy; cholesterol was added. Inclusion of stearyl alcohol and wax adds to the physical characteristics, particularly firmness and heat stability.

Absorption bases, particularly the emulsion bases, impart excellent emolliency and a degree of occlusiveness on application. The anhydrous types can be used when the presence of water would cause stability problems with specific drug substances (eg, antibiotics). Absorption bases also are greasy when applied and are difficult to remove. Both of these properties are, however, less pronounced than with hydrocarbon bases.

Table 44-4. Classification and Properties of USP Ointment Bases

	HYDROCARBON BASE	ABSORPTION BASE	WATER-REMOVABLE BASE	WATER-SOLUBLE BASE
Example(s)	White Petrolatum, USP; White Ointment, USP	Hydrophilic Petrolatum, USP; Lanolin, USP	Hydrophilic Ointment, USP	Polyethylene Glycol Ointment, NF
Composition	Hydrocarbons	Anhydrous or W/O emulsion	O/W emulsion	Water-soluble constituents
Occlusiveness	High	Moderate to high	Low to moderate	Minimal
Principal Benefits or Uses	Maintains prolonged contact with application site; emollient effect	Allows incorporation of aqueous solutions; emollient effect	Water-washable; may be diluted with water; allows absorption of serous discharges	Water-washable; no water-insoluble residue

Commercially available absorption bases include Aquaphor (*Beiersdorf*) and Polysorb (*Fougera*). Nivea Cream (*Beiersdorf*) is a hydrated emollient base. Absorption bases, either hydrous or anhydrous, are seldom used as vehicles for commercial drug products. The W/O emulsion system is more difficult to deal with than the more conventional O/W systems, and there is, of course, reduced patient acceptance because of greasiness.

WATER-REMOVABLE (WATER-WASHABLE) BASES— These bases are O/W emulsion bases, commonly referred to as creams, and represent the most commonly used type of ointment base. By far the majority of commercial dermatologic drug products are formulated in an emulsion (or cream) base. Emulsion bases are washable and removed easily from skin or clothing. Emulsion bases can be diluted with water, although such additions are uncommon.

As a result of advances in cosmetic chemistry the formulator of an emulsion base is faced with a bewildering array of potential ingredients. A glance at the cosmetic literature and such volumes as the Cosmetic, Toiletry and Fragrance Association's *International Cosmetic Ingredient Dictionary and Handbook* impresses one with the enormous number and variety of emulsion-base components, particularly surfactants and oil-phase components. Many of these substances impart subtle but distinct characteristics to cosmetic emulsion systems. While desirable, many of these characteristics are not really necessary in drug dosage forms or delivery systems. Furthermore, the likelihood of drug-excipient interactions, either physical or chemical, increases substantially (as does the cost) as the number of formulation components is increased. Thus the formulator of topical products should minimize the number of excipients in the formulation. Nonetheless, emulsion bases typically include antimicrobial preservatives, stabilizers (such as antioxidants, metal chelating agents, or buffers), and humectants (eg glycerin or propylene glycol), in addition to the emulsifiers, in order to ensure stability and efficacy.

Soaps and detergents (ie, emulsifiers) have, overall, a damaging effect on the skin. Both anionic and cationic surfactants can cause damage to the stratum corneum in direct proportion to concentration and duration of contact. Nonionic surfactants appear to have much less effect on the stratum corneum.

WATER-SOLUBLE BASES—Soluble ointment bases, as the name implies, are made up of soluble components or may include gelled aqueous solutions. The latter often are referred to as gels, and in recent years have been formulated specifically to maximize drug availability.

Major components, and in some instances the only components, of water-soluble bases are the polyethylene glycols (PEGs). Patch tests have shown that these compounds are innocuous, and long-term use has confirmed their lack of irritation. PEGs are relatively inert, non-volatile, water-soluble or water-miscible liquids or waxy solids identified by numbers that are an approximate indication of molecular weight. Polyethylene glycol 400 is a liquid superficially similar to propylene glycol, while polyethylene glycol 6000 is a waxy solid.

Polyethylene glycols of interest as vehicles include the 1500, 1600, 4000, and 6000 products, ranging from soft, waxy solids (polyethylene glycol 1500 is similar to petrolatum) to hard waxes. Polyethylene glycols, particularly 1500, can be used as a vehicle *per se;* however, better results often are obtained by using blends of high- and low-molecular-weight glycols, as in Polyethylene Glycol Ointment NF. The water-solubility of polyethylene glycol vehicles does not ensure availability of drugs contained in the vehicle. As hydrated stratum corneum is an important factor in drug penetration, the use of polyethylene glycol vehicles, which are anhydrous and nonocclusive, actually may hinder percutaneous absorption due to dehydration of the stratum corneum.

Aqueous gel vehicles containing water, propylene, and/or polyethylene glycol and gelled with a carbomer or a cellulose derivative also are classed as water-soluble bases. Bases of this kind, sometimes referred to as gels, may be formulated to optimize delivery of a drug, particularly steroids. In such a preparation, propylene glycol is often used for its solvent properties as well as for its antimicrobial or preservative effects.

Gelling agents used in these preparations may be nonionic or anionic. Nonionics include cellulose derivatives, such as methylcellulose or hypromellose (hydroxypropyl methylcellulose). Sodium carboxymethylcellulose is an anionic cellulose derivative.

Carbomers are the USP designation for various polymeric acrylic acids, crosslinked with carbohydrates or polyalcohol derivatives, that are dispersible but insoluble in water. When the acid dispersion is neutralized with a base a clear, stable gel is formed. Carbomers for which monographs appear in the USP include carbomers 910, 934, 934P, 940, 941, and 1342, as well as the more complex carbomer copolymer and carbomer interpolymer.

Other gelling agents employed in topical formulations include sodium alginate and the propylene glycol ester of alginic acid (Kelcoloid). Sodium alginate is a hydrophilic colloid that functions satisfactorily between pH 4.5 and 10; addition of calcium ions will gel fluid solutions of sodium alginate.

Gels can also be formed or stabilized by the incorporation of finely divided solids such as colloidal magnesium aluminum silicate (Veegum) or colloidal (fumed) silicon dioxide (Aerosil, Cab-O-Sil). These inorganic particulates can function as emulsifiers and suspending agents, as well as gellants. Their compatibility with alcohols, acetone, and glycols makes them particularly useful in topical gel formulations.

PREPARATION

Ointment preparation or manufacture depends on the type of vehicle and the quantity to be prepared. The objective is the same (ie, to disperse the drug uniformly throughout the vehicle). Normally, the drug materials are either in finely powdered form or in solution before being dispersed in the vehicle.

Incorporation of Drug by Levigation

The incorporation of a drug powder in small quantities of an ointment (ie, 30-90 g) can be accomplished by using a spatula and an ointment tile (either porcelain or glass). The drug material is levigated thoroughly with a small quantity of the vehicle or a miscible liquid component of the formulation (eg, propylene glycol; light mineral oil) to form a concentrate. The concentrate then is diluted geometrically with the remainder of the base.

If the drug substance is water-soluble it can be dissolved in water and the resulting solution incorporated into the vehicle by use of a small quantity of lanolin if the base is oleaginous. Generally speaking, an amount of anhydrous lanolin equal in volume to the amount of water used will suffice.

On a larger scale, mechanical mixers (eg, Hobart mixers, pony mixers) are used. The drug substance in finely divided form usually is added slowly or sifted into the vehicle contained in the rotating mixer. When the ointment is uniform, the finished product may be processed through a roller mill to ensure complete dispersion and reduce any aggregates.

An alternative procedure involves preparing and milling a concentrate of the drug in a portion of the base. The concentrate then is dispersed in the balance of the vehicle, using a mixer of appropriate size. Occasionally, the base may be melted for easier handling and dispersing. In such cases the drug is dispersed and the base slowly cooled, using continuous agitation to maintain dispersion.

Emulsion Formulations

Emulsions are prepared generally by combining the "oil"-soluble ingredients (eg, petrolatum, waxes, fats) and heating the admixture to about 75°C (ie, a temperature at which the oil-phase ingredients are molten). The "water"-soluble ingredients are combined separately and heated to slightly above 75°C. The aqueous phase then is added to the oil phase, slowly and with constant agitation. When the emulsion is formed, the mixture is allowed to cool, maintaining slow agitation.

At this stage in the process, the medicinal ingredients usually are added as a concentrated slurry, which usually has been milled to reduce any particle aggregates. Volatile or aromatic materials generally are added when the finished emulsion has cooled to about 35°C. At this point, additional water may be added to compensate for any evaporative losses occurring during exposure and transfer at the higher temperatures of emulsion formation.

While the product remains in the tank in bulk, quality-control procedures are performed (ie, for pH, active ingredients, etc). If control results are satisfactory the product is filled into the appropriate containers.

IRRITANCY TESTING OF TOPICAL PRODUCTS

Ointment bases may cause irritant or allergic reactions. Allergic reactions are usually due to a specific base component. Irritant reactions are more frequent and more important, hence a number of test procedures have been devised to test for irritancy levels, both in animals and in man. The consequences of species differences and specificity must be included in the evaluation of animal-test results.

In the past, the most common method for evaluating irritancy was the Draize dermal irritation test in rabbits. In this procedure the test material was applied repeatedly to the clipped skin on the rabbit's back. Endpoints were dermal erythema and/or edema. The assignment of numerical scores for erythema and edema enabled the mathematical and statistical analysis of results.

In the human, a variety of test procedures are used to measure irritancy, sensitization potential, and phototoxicity. Among the most common are the 21-day cumulative irritancy patch test, the Draize-Shelanski repeat-insult patch test, and the Kligman "maximization" test.

21-DAY CUMULATIVE IRRITANCY PATCH TEST—In this test the test compound is applied daily to the same site on the back or volar forearm. Test materials are applied under occlusive tape, and scores are read daily. The test application and scoring are repeated daily for 21 days or until irritation produces a predetermined maximum score. Typical erythema scores range from 0 (no visible reaction) to 4 (intense erythema with edema and vesicular erosion). Usually, 24 subjects are used in this test. Fewer subjects and a shorter application time in days are variants of the test.

DRAIZE-SHELANSKI REPEAT-INSULT PATCH TEST—This test is designed to measure the potential to cause sensitization. The test also provides a measure of irritancy potential. In the usual procedure the test material or a suitable dilution is applied under occlusion to the same site for 10 alternate-day 24-hr periods. Following a 7-day rest period, the test material is applied again to a fresh site for 24 hours. The challenge sites are read on removal of the patch and again 24 hours later. The 0–4 erythema scale is used. A test panel of 100 individuals is common.

KLIGMAN "MAXIMIZATION" TEST—This test is used to detect the contact sensitizing potential of a product or material. The test material is applied under occlusion to the same site for 48-hr periods. Prior to each exposure the site may be pretreated with a solution of sodium lauryl sulfate under occlusion. Following a 10-day interval the test material again is applied to a different site for 48 hours under occlusion. The challenge site may be treated briefly with a sodium lauryl sulfate solution.

The "maximization" test is of shorter duration and makes use of fewer test subjects than the Draize-Shelanski test. The use of sodium lauryl sulfate as a pretreatment increases the ability to detect weaker allergens.

These test methods are adequate to detect even weak irritants and weak contact sensitizers. Positive results, however, do not automatically disqualify the use of a substance as unsafe. The actual risk of use depends on concentration, period of use, and skin condition. Benzoyl peroxide in tests such as the Draize-Shelanski and Kligman "maximization" is a potent sensitizer, yet the incidence of sensitization among acne patients is low.

THE EVOLUTION OF TRANSDERMAL DRUG DELIVERY SYSTEMS

Conventional medicated topicals (eg, creams and ointments) seldom permit substantial systemic uptake of the drug or drugs incorporated therein. This is a consequence, in part, of the limited persistence or residence time of the topical formulation on the skin surface. In effect, a drug does not remain in contact with the absorbing surface long enough for sufficient drug to transfer into the skin and, ultimately, into systemic circulation. Furthermore, there is the concomitant problem of the gradual depletion of drug from the region of the topical formulation immediately adjacent to the skin surface and the corresponding reduction in the concentration gradient for drug transfer from the topical formulation to the skin.

The emergence of adhesive transdermal drug-delivery systems (TDDSs) in the early 1980s permitted skin residence times to increase from hours to days. The novel matrix- or reservoir-formulations employed in these TDDSs also provided for the maintenance of relatively uniform concentrations of diffusible drug in the formulation, thereby preventing the formation of drug-depleted regions within the topical formulation and helping to ensure relatively constant drug-release rates. As noted above, skin occlusion by the water-impermeable backing film of TDDSs further facilitates TDDS systemic efficacy by increasing skin hydration and temperature with a corresponding increase in the rate and extent of skin permeation. The inclusion of skin-penetration enhancers in medicated topicals serves to decrease diffusional resistance and increase transport.

Nonetheless, these—by now—*conventional* TDDSs have their limitations: the increased residence time of occlusive TDDSs on the skin surface leads to an increased incidence of skin maceration and adverse cutaneous reactions. In addition, effective skin permeation is limited to relatively small (<1 kD), lipophilic drug molecules. Thus, increasingly more attention is being placed on alternative TDDSs—eg, electrically modulated systems and mechanical systems—which circumvent the need for partitioning and diffusion of the drug out of the formulation matrix and into and through the skin:

Electrically modulated systems, or *electrotransport* systems, facilitate drug transport by an external electrical field. Electrotransport mechanisms include *iontophoresis, electroosmosis,* or *electroporation.*

Mechanically (physically) *modulated* systems are exemplified by systems employing *phonophoresis* or those using *microneedle arrays* to achieve transdermal drug delivery.

ELECTRICALLY MODULATED DRUG DELIVERY THROUGH THE SKIN[32,33]—For some poorly absorbed (ionic) compounds, parenteral administration appears to be the only viable option for regional or systemic delivery, as chemical penetration enhancers (Table 44-3) often do not function well for these compounds. Given the increased risk of adverse reactions associated with the use of such enhancers, the increased evaluation of iontophoretic devices for the enhancement of topical drug delivery has been of great interest. Iontophoretic drug delivery implies the delivery of ionic drugs into the body by means of an electric current. While the stratum corneum forms the principal barrier to electrical conductivity—due, in part, to its lower water content—the skin also acts as a capacitor. Thus, biological tissues such as the skin provide for a reactive electrical circuit. Ionic transport through the skin in the presence of a uniform electric field can be described, in part, in accordance with the Nernst-Planck equation

$$J_i = -D\frac{dC}{dx} + \frac{DzeEC}{kT}$$

where J_i is the flux of ions across the membrane, C is the concentration of ions with valence z and electron charge e, dC/dx is the concentration gradient, E is the electric field, k is Boltzmann's constant, and T is the absolute temperature. Thus, the ionic flux is the sum of the fluxes that arise from the concentration gradient and the electric field. Given the complexity of the skin's composition, the thickness of the stratum corneum, and the occurrence of electroosmotic effects, the Nernst-Planck equation is only a first approximation of the overall transdermal flux of a solute. Faraday's Law

$$\frac{Q}{t} = \frac{t_j i}{|z|F}$$

further characterizes the iontophoretic flux Q/t in terms of the current i (in amperes) and its duration t (in seconds), the transference number parameter t_j, and the Faraday constant, F. Additional factors that influence the rate and extent of iontophoretic delivery through the skin include pH and ionic strength of the drug solution.

Although iontophoretic techniques have been shown to increase percutaneous absorption of ionizable or ionic drugs (including lidocaine, salicylates, and peptides and proteins such as insulin) markedly, the clinical safety and efficacy of drug-delivery systems employing iontophoretic technology have yet to be evaluated fully.

Problematic aspects of electrotransport include cutaneous irritation or erythema and the effect of the electrical field on the integrity and stability of the formulation. Electrically induced alterations in the formulation generally arise as a result of iontophoresis (due to the increased flux of ions) or electroosmosis (due to the electrically induced convective transport of water molecules and associated electrically neutral solutes).[34,35] The use of pulsed or intermittent current electrotransport systems has been suggested as an alternative to continuous current systems. *Electroporation*—the use of pulsed electrical current to provoke the transient formation of pores in biomembranes—also has been suggested as an alternative, or complement, to iontophoresis. In any event, the potential of electrically modulated drug-delivery systems for the effective transdermal delivery of large, polar or ionic molecules (eg, proteins, peptides, DNA) necessitates continued research in this field. One encouraging advance in this area is the development of flexible wafer-thin arrays of conductive layers or filaments for drug delivery systems that are less bulky and potentially more acceptable to patients.

MECHANICALLY MODULATED DRUG DELIVERY—*Phonophoresis,* or *sonophoresis,* is defined as the movement of drug molecules through the skin under the influence of ultrasound. In general, ultrasound frequencies of 1–3 MHz and intensities of 0.01–2 W/cm^2 have been used with varying degrees of effectiveness,[36] although high-frequency, low-intensity ultrasound has been observed to increase transdermal drug flux and decrease percutaneous diffusional lag times.[37] A more recent analysis of ultrasound-enhanced transdermal transport indicates that low-frequency sonophoresis is much more important than high-frequency sonophoresis in enhancing transport.[38] Various thermal and nonthermal changes have been implicated to explain phonophoretically induced increases in drug transport through the skin. Although the effect of temperature increases on molecular diffusivity and flux is clear, nonthermal effects of ultrasound (eg, cavitation) are less clear. Transient ultrasound-induced cavitation (ie, the generation and oscillation of gas bubbles) in the stratum corneum apparently perturbs barrier permeability and solute transport in the aqueous regions of the stratum corneum. Evidence for this is the lack of correlation between phonophoretic permeability and permeant lipophilicity.

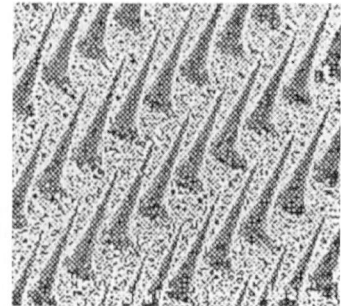

Figure 44-10. Electron micrograph of a microneedle array for transdermal drug delivery (courtesy, Georgia Institute of Technology; ©Georgia Tech Res Corp.).

Silicon microneedle arrays[39] have been proposed recently as painless adjuncts to transdermal delivery systems. The 150-μm long needles (Fig 44-10) can penetrate the stratum corneum, thereby facilitating drug access to the living epidermis and dermis and ultimately to systemic circulation. The needles—prepared by reactive ion etching microfabrication techniques originally developed for integrated circuits—leave holes about 1 μm in diameter when removed from the skin.

SUPPOSITORIES

Suppositories are solid dosage forms of various weights and shapes, usually medicated, for insertion into the rectum, vagina, or urethra. After insertion, suppositories soften, melt, disperse, or dissolve in the cavity fluids.

The use of suppositories dates from the distant past, this dosage form being referred to in writings of the early Egyptians, Greeks, and Romans. Suppositories are suited particularly for administration of drugs to the very young and the very old, a notion first recorded by Hippocrates.

Types

RECTAL SUPPOSITORIES—The USP describes rectal suppositories for adults as tapered at one or both ends and usually weighing about 2 g each. Infant rectal suppositories usually weigh about one-half that of adult suppositories. Drugs having systemic effects, such as sedatives, tranquilizers, and analgesics, are administered by rectal suppository; however, the largest single-use category is probably that of hemorrhoid remedies dispensed over the counter. The 2-g weight for adult rectal suppositories is based on use of cocoa butter as the base; when other bases are used the weights may be greater or less than 2 g.

VAGINAL SUPPOSITORIES—The USP describes vaginal suppositories, or pessaries, as usually globular or oviform and weighing about 5 g each. Vaginal medications are available in a variety of physical forms (eg, creams, gels, or liquids), which depart from the classical concept of suppositories. Vaginal tablets, or inserts prepared by encapsulation in soft gelatin, however, do meet the definition and represent convenience both of administration and manufacture.

URETHRAL SUPPOSITORIES—Urethral suppositories, or bougies, are not described specifically in the USP, either by weight or dimension. Traditional values, based on the use of cocoa butter as a base, are as follows for these cylindrical dosage forms: diameter: 5 mm; length: 50 mm female, 125 mm male; weight: 2 g female, 4 g male. An intraurethral insert containing the prostaglandin alprostadil is available for the treatment of erectile dysfunction. The commercial formulation, described as a sterile micropellet (1.4 mm in diameter and 6 mm long) consisting of the drug and polyethylene glycol 1450 is inserted 3 cm deep into the urethra by use of a hollow applicator.

SUPPOSITORY VEHICLE—The ideal suppository base should meet the following general specifications:

- The base is nontoxic and nonirritating to mucous membranes.
- The base is compatible with a variety of drugs.
- The base melts or dissolves in rectal fluids.
- The base should be stable on storage; it should not bind or otherwise interfere with release or absorption of drug substances.

Rectal suppository bases can be classified broadly into two types: fatty and water-soluble or water-miscible. The traditional cocoa butter vehicle is immiscible with aqueous tissue fluids but melts at body temperature. Water-soluble or water-miscible vehicles also have been used. In general, formulators have been reluctant to use glycerinated gelatin as a rectal suppository base because of its relatively slow dissolution. More typical of this class is the polyethylene glycol vehicle. Drug absorption from such dissimilar bases can differ substantially. Lowenthal and Borzelleca[40] investigated the absorption of salicylic acid and sodium salicylate administered to dogs. The drugs were formulated in a cocoa butter base and in a base composed of polyethylene glycol, synthetic glycerides, and a surfactant. Absorption of salicylic acid and sodium salicylate was about equal from the cocoa butter base; however, salicylic acid gave higher plasma levels than sodium salicylate when the glycol base was used.

SUPPOSITORY BASES

The USP lists the following as usual suppository bases: cocoa butter, cocoa butter substitutes (primarily, vegetable oils modified by esterification, hydrogenation, and/or fractionation), glycerinated gelatin, hydrogenated vegetable oils, mixtures of polyethylene glycols of various molecular weights, and fatty acid esters of polyethylene glycol.

COCOA BUTTER AND OTHER FATTY BASES— Theobroma oil, or cocoa butter, is a naturally occurring triglyceride. About 40% of the fatty acid content is unsaturated. As a natural material there is considerable batch-to-batch variability. A major characteristic of theobroma oil is its polymorphism (ie, its ability to exist in more than one crystal form). While cocoa butter melts quickly at body temperature, it is immiscible with body fluids; this may inhibit the diffusion of fat-soluble drugs to the affected sites. Oleaginous vehicles, such as cocoa butter, seldom are used in vaginal preparations for esthetic reasons: many women consider them messy and prone to leakage.

If, in the preparation of suppositories, the theobroma oil is overheated, ie, heated to about 60°C, molded, and chilled, the suppositories formed will melt below 30°C. The fusion treatment of theobroma oil requires maximum temperatures of 40 to 50°C to avoid a change in crystal form and melting point. Theobroma oil, heated to about 60°C and cooled rapidly, will crystallize in an alpha configuration characterized by a melting point below 30°C. The alpha form is metastable and will slowly revert to the beta form, with the characteristic melting point approaching 35°C. The transition from alpha to beta is slow, taking several days. The use of low heat and slow cooling allows direct crystallization of the more stable beta crystal form.

Certain drugs will depress the melting point of theobroma oil. This involves no polymorphic change, although the net effect is similar. Chloral hydrate is the most important of these substances because its rectal hypnotic dose of 0.5 to 1.0 g will cause a substantial melting-point depression. This effect can be countered by addition of a higher-melting wax, such as white wax or synthetic spermaceti. The amount to be added must be determined by temperature measurements. The effect of such additives on bioavailability also must be considered.

Various cocoa butter substitutes (hard fat, hydrogenated vegetable oil) are available commercially that offer a number of advantages over cocoa butter such as decreased potential for rancidity and phase transition (melting and solidification) behavior tailored to specific formulation, processing, and storage requirements. However, as with cocoa butter, these semisynthetic glyceride mixtures are also subject to polymorphic transformations. Batch-to-batch variations of the physical properties of all of these bases, whether cocoa butter or cocoa butter substitutes, can play havoc with the final products' characteristics. The formulator should ensure that the melting and congealing behavior of these bases and the formulations prepared from them is evaluated thoroughly.

WATER-SOLUBLE OR DISPERSIBLE SUPPOSITORY BASES—Water-miscible suppository bases are of comparatively recent origin. The majority are composed of polyethylene glycols or glycol-surfactant combinations. Water-miscible suppository bases have the substantial advantage of lack of dependence on a melting point approximating body temperature. Problems of handling, storage, and shipping are simplified considerably.

Polymers of ethylene glycol are available as polyethylene glycol polymers (Carbowax, polyglycols) of assorted molecular weights. Suppositories of varying melting points and solubility characteristics can be prepared by blending polyethylene glycols of 1000, 4000, or 6000 molecular weight.

Polyethylene glycol suppositories, while prepared rather easily by molding, cannot be prepared satisfactorily by hand-rolling. The drug-glycol mixture is prepared by melting and then is cooled to just above the melting point before pouring into dry unlubricated molds. Cooling to near the melting point prevents fissuring caused by crystallization and contraction. The USP advises that labels on polyethylene glycol suppositories should instruct patients to moisten the suppository before inserting it.

Water-miscible or water-dispersible suppositories also can be prepared using selected nonionic surfactant materials. Polyoxyl 40 stearate is a white, water-soluble solid melting slightly above body temperature. A polyoxyethylene derivative of sorbitan monostearate is water-insoluble but dispersible. In using surfactant materials, the possibility of drug-base interactions must be borne in mind. Interactions caused by macromolecular adsorption may have a significant effect on bioavailability.

PEG-based water-miscible suppository bases, devised by Collins, Hohmann, and Zopf,[41] are exemplified by a low-melting formulation employing 96% PEG 1000 and 4% PEG 4000 and a more heat-stable formulation with 75% PEG 1000 and 25% PEG 4000. Both may be prepared conveniently by molding techniques.

Water-dispersible bases may include polyoxyethylene sorbitan fatty acid esters. These are either soluble (Tween, Myrj) or water-dispersible (Arlacel), used alone or in combination with other wax or fatty materials. Surfactants in suppositories should be used only with recognition of reports that such materials may either increase or decrease drug absorption.

HYDROGELS—In recent years, hydrogels, defined as macromolecular networks that swell but do not dissolve in water, have been advocated as bases for rectal and vaginal drug delivery. The swelling of hydrogels (ie, the absorption of water) is a consequence of the presence of hydrophilic functional groups attached to the polymeric network. Cross-links between adjacent macromolecules result in the aqueous insolubility of these hydrogels.

The use of a hydrogel matrix for drug delivery involves the dispersal of the drug in the matrix, followed by drying of the system and concomitant immobilization of the drug. When the hydrogel delivery system is placed in an aqueous environment (eg, the rectum or the vagina), the hydrogel swells, enabling the drug to diffuse out of the macromolecular network. The rate and extent of drug release from these hydrogel matrices depend on the rate of water migration *into* the matrix and the rate of drug diffusion *out of* the swollen matrix.

Hydrogels employed for rectal or vaginal drug administration have been prepared from polymers such as polyvinyl alcohol, hydroxyethyl methacrylate, polyacrylic acid, or polyoxyethylene. Although hydrogel-based drug-delivery systems have yet to appear in suppository or insert form commercially, research efforts in this direction are increasing, given their potential for controlled drug delivery, bioadhesion, retention at the site of administration, and biocompatibility.

GLYCERINATED GELATIN—Glycerinated gelatin usually is used as a vehicle for vaginal suppositories. For rectal use a firmer suppository can be obtained by increasing the gelatin content. Glycerinated gelatin suppositories are prepared by dissolving or dispersing the drug substance in enough water to equal 10% of the final suppository weight. Glycerin (70%) then is added and Pharmagel A or B (20%), depending on the drug compatibility requirements. Pharmagel A is acid in reaction, Pharmagel B is alkaline. Glycerinated gelatin suppositories must be formed by molding. The mass cannot be processed by hand-rolling. These suppositories, if not for immediate use, should contain a preservative such as methylparaben and propylparaben.

PREPARATION

Suppositories are prepared by rolling (hand-shaping), molding (fusion), and cold compression.

ROLLED (HAND-SHAPED) SUPPOSITORIES—Hand-shaping suppositories is the oldest and the simplest method of preparing this dosage form. The manipulation requires considerable skill, yet avoids the complications of heat and mold preparation.

The general process can be described as follows:

Take the prescribed quantity of the medicinal substances and a sufficient quantity of grated theobroma oil. In a mortar reduce the medicating ingredients to a fine powder or, if composed of extracts, soften with diluted alcohol and rub until a smooth paste is formed. The correct amount of grated theobroma oil then is added, and a mass resembling a pill mass is made by thoroughly incorporating the ingredients with a pestle, sometimes with the aid of a small amount of wool fat. When the mass has become plastic under the vigorous kneading of the pestle, it quickly is loosened from the mortar with a spatula, pressed into a roughly shaped mass in the center of the mortar, and then transferred with the spatula to a piece of filter paper that is kept between the mass and the hands during the kneading and rolling procedure. By quick, rotary movements of the hands, the mass is rolled to a ball, which immediately is placed on a pill tile. A suppository cylinder is formed by rolling the mass on the tile with a flat board, partially aided by the palm of the other hand, if weather conditions permit. The suppository *pipe* frequently will show a tendency to crack in the center, developing a hollow core. This occurs when the mass has not been kneaded and softened sufficiently, with the result that the pressure of the roller board is not carried uniformly throughout the mass but is exerted primarily on the surface. The length of the cylinder usually corresponds to about four spaces on the pill tile for each suppository, thus making the piece, when cut, practically a finished suppository except for the shaping of the point. When the cylinder has been cut into the proper number of pieces with a spatula, the conical shape is given it by rolling one end on the tile with a spatula, or in some cases even by shaping it with the fingers to produce a rounded point.

COMPRESSION-MOLDED (FUSED) SUPPOSITORIES—This method of suppository preparation also avoids heat. The suppository mass, such as a mixture of grated theobroma oil and drug, is forced into a mold under pressure, using a wheel-operated press. The mass is forced into mold openings, pressure is released, and the mold removed, opened, and replaced. On a large scale, cold-compression machines are hydraulically operated, water-jacketed for cooling, and screw-fed. Pressure is applied via a piston to compress the mass into mold openings.

FUSION OR MELT MOLDING—In this method the drug is dispersed or dissolved in the melted suppository base. The mixture then is poured into a suppository mold, allowed to cool, and the finished suppositories removed by opening the mold. Using this procedure, one to hundreds of suppositories can be made at one time.

Suppository molds are available for the preparation of various types and sizes of suppositories. Molds are made of aluminum alloy, brass, or plastic and are available with from six to several hundred cavities.

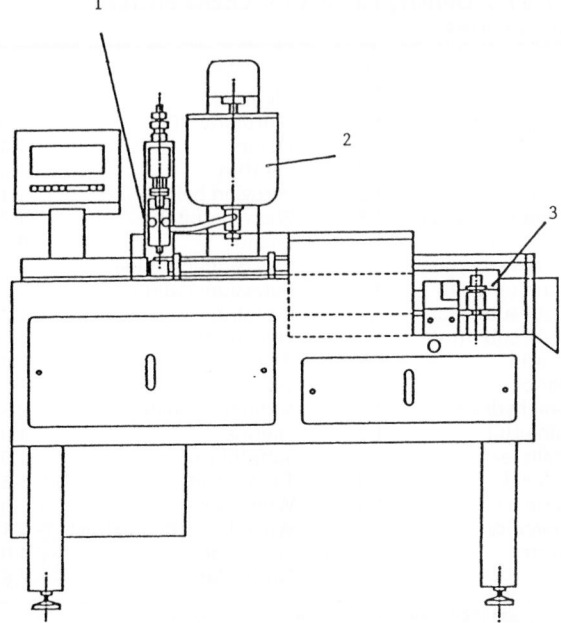

Figure 44-11. A cross-section of the Sarong SpA semiautomatic equipment for the production of suppositories in preformed plastic or foil shells. The fully jacketed piston-type *dosing pump* (1) meters the suppository melt in the jacketed tank (2) into preformed shells that pass directly beneath injection nozzles. The strips of filled preformed shells continue into a cooling chamber (3) prior to sealing and cartoning.

The method of choice for commercial suppository production (Fig 44-11) involves the automated filling of molds or preformed shells by a volumetric dosing pump that meters the melt from a jacketed kettle or mixing tank directly into the molds or shells. Strips of preformed shells pass beneath the dosing pump and are filled successively, passed through cooling chambers (to promote solidification), sealed, and then packaged. Quality control procedures (eg, weight, fill volume, leakage) are conducted readily *online*.

An alternative to the melt-and-pour processes described above is that of injection molding, which has been described by Snipes.[42] This process is distinctive in that it makes use of the injection-molding technique developed for the fabrication of plastics. Polyethylene glycols are the excipients of choice in this process, with polyethylene oxide, povidone, or silicon dioxide added to adjust viscosity or plasticity. Long-chain saturated carboxylic acids also have been added to reduce the hygroscopicity inherent with the use of the polyethylene glycols. Typically, the molten excipient admixture is extruded or injected under pressure into precision-machined multicavity molds, followed by the ejection of the molded units from the mold cavities. Advantages claimed for this method include the wide range of shapes and sizes that can be prepared at very high production rates with great precision.

Suppositories usually are formulated on a weight basis so that the medication replaces a portion of the vehicle as a function of specific gravity. If the medicinal substance has a density approximately the same as theobroma oil, it will replace an equal weight of oil. If the medication is heavier, it will replace a proportionally smaller amount of theobroma oil.

For instance, tannic acid has a density of 1.6 compared with cocoa butter (see Table 44-5).[43,44] If a suppository is to contain 0.1 g tannic acid, then 0.1 g ÷ 1.6, or 0.062 g, cocoa butter should be replaced by 0.1 g of drug. If the blank weight of the suppository is 2.0 g, then 2.0 - 0.062 g, or 1.938 g, cocoa butter is required per suppository. The suppository will actually weigh 1.938 g + 0.1 g, or 2.038 g. Table 44-5 indicates the density fac-

Table 44-5. Density Factors for Cocoa Butter Suppositories

MEDICATION	FACTOR	MEDICATION	FACTOR
Alum	1.7	Menthol	0.7
Aminophylline	1.1	Morphine HCl	1.6
Aminopyrine	1.3	Opium	1.4
Aspirin	1.3	Paraffin	1.0
Barbital	1.2	Peruvian balsam[a]	1.1
Belladonna extract	1.3	Phenobarbital	1.2
Benzoic acid	1.5	Phenol[a]	0.9
Bismuth carbonate	4.5	Potassium bromide	2.2
Bismuth salicylate	4.5	Potassium iodide	4.5
Bismuth subgallate	2.7	Procaine	1.2
Bismuth subnitrate	6.0	Quinine HCl	1.2
Boric acid	1.5	Resorcinol	1.4
Castor oil	1.0	Salicylic acid	1.3
Chloral hydrate	1.3	Sodium bromide	2.3
Cocaine HCl	1.3	Spermaceti	1.0
Digitalis leaf	1.6	Sulfathiazole	1.6
Gallic acid	2.0	Tannic acid	1.6
Glycerin	1.6	White wax	1.0
Ichthammol	1.1	Witch hazel fluidextract	1.1
Iodoform	4.0	Zinc oxide	4.0
		Zinc sulfate	2.8

[a] Density adjusted taking into account white wax in mass.
Data from Davis H. *Bentley's Text-Book of Pharmaceutics,* 7th ed. London: Bailliere, Tindall & Cox, 1961 and Buchi J. *Pharma Acta Helv* 1940;20:403.

tor, or the density compared with cocoa butter, of many substances used in suppositories.

It always is possible to determine the density of a medicinal substance relative to cocoa butter, if the density factor is not available, by mixing the amount of drug for one or more suppositories with a small quantity of cocoa butter, pouring the mixture into a suppository mold and carefully filling the mold with additional melted cocoa butter. The cooled suppositories are weighed, providing data from which a working formula can be calculated as well as the density factor itself.

When using suppository bases other than cocoa butter, such as a polyethylene glycol base, it is necessary to know either the density of the drug relative to the new base or the densities of both the drug and the new base relative to cocoa butter. The density factor for a base other than cocoa butter is simply the ratio of the blank weights of the base and cocoa butter.

For instance, if a suppository is to contain 0.1 g tannic acid in a polyethylene glycol base, then 0.1 g ÷ 1.6 x 1.25, or 0.078 g, polyethylene glycol base should be replaced by 0.1 g drug (the polyethylene glycol base is assumed to have a density factor of 1.25). If the blank weight is 1.75 g for the polyethylene glycol base, then 1.75 g - 0.078 g, or 1.672 g, of base is required per suppository. The final weight will be 1.672 g base + 0.1 g drug, or 1.772 g.

When the dosage and mold calibration are complete the drug-base mass should be prepared using minimum heat. A water bath or water jacket usually is used. The melted mass should be stirred constantly but slowly to avoid air entrapment. The mass should be poured into the mold openings slowly. Prelubrication of the mold will depend on the vehicle. Mineral oil is a good lubricant for cocoa butter suppositories. Molds should be dry for polyethylene glycol suppositories.

After pouring into tightly clamped molds the suppositories and mold are allowed to cool thoroughly using refrigeration on a small scale or refrigerated air on a larger scale. After thorough chilling any excess suppository mass should be removed from the mold by scraping, the mold opened, and the suppositories removed. It is important to allow cooling time adequate for suppository contraction. This aids in removal and minimizes splitting of the finished suppository.

PACKAGING AND STORAGE—Suppositories often are packaged in partitioned boxes that hold the suppositories upright. Glycerin and glycerinated gelatin suppositories often are packaged in tightly closed screwcapped glass containers.

Though many commercial suppositories are wrapped individually in aluminum foil or PVC-polyethylene, strip-packaging is commonplace.

Alternatively, suppositories may be molded directly into their primary packaging. In this operation the form into which the suppository mass flows consists of a series of individual molds formed from plastic or foil. After the suppository is poured and cooled, the excess is trimmed off, and the units are sealed and cut into 3s or 6s as desired. Cooling and final cartoning then can be carried out.

Suppositories with low-melting ingredients are best stored in a cool place. Theobroma oil suppositories, in particular, should be refrigerated.

OTHER MEDICATED APPLICATIONS

Poultices (Cataplasms)

Poultices, or cataplasms, represent one of the most ancient classes of pharmaceutical preparations. A poultice is a soft, moist mass of meal, herbs, seed, etc, usually applied hot in cloth. The consistency is gruel-like, which is probably the origin of the word poultice.

Cataplasms were intended to localize infectious material in the body or to act as counterirritants. The materials tended to be absorptive, which together with heat accounts for their popular use. None is now official in the USP. The last official product was Kaolin Poultice NF IX.

Pastes

The USP defines pastes as semisolid dosage forms that contain one or more drug substances intended for topical application. Pastes are divided into fatty pastes (eg, Zinc Oxide Paste) and those made from a single-phase aqueous gel (eg, Carboxymethylcellulose Sodium Paste). Another official paste is Triamcinolone Acetonide Dental Paste.

The term *paste* is applied to ointments in which large amounts of solids have been incorporated (eg, Zinc Oxide Paste). In the past, pastes have been defined as concentrates of absorptive powders dispersed (usually) in petrolatum or hydrophilic petrolatum. These fatty pastes are stiff to the point of dryness and are reasonably absorptive considering they have a petrolatum base. Pastes often are used in the treatment of oozing lesions, where they act to absorb serous secretions. Pastes also are used to limit the area of treatment by acting both as an absorbent and a physical dam.

Pastes adhere reasonably well to the skin and are poorly occlusive. For this reason, they are suited for application on and around moist lesions. The heavy consistency of pastes imparts a degree of protection and may, in some instances, make the use of bandages unnecessary. Pastes are less macerating than ointments.

Because of their physical properties pastes may be removed from the skin by the use of mineral oil or a vegetable oil. This is particularly necessary when the underlying or surrounding skin is traumatized easily.

Powders

Powders for external use usually are described as dusting powders. Such powders should have a particle size of not more than 150 μm (ie, less than 100-mesh) to avoid any sensation of grittiness, which could irritate traumatized skin. Dusting powders usually contain starch, talc, and zinc stearate. Absorbable Dusting Powder USP is composed of starch treated with epichlorohydrin, with not more than 2.0% magnesium oxide added to maintain the modified starch in impalpable powder form; as it is intended for use as a lubricant for surgical gloves it should be sterilized (by autoclaving) and packaged in sealed paper packets.

The fineness of powders often is expressed in terms of mesh size, with impalpable powders generally in the range of 100- to 200-mesh (149 to 75 μm). Determination of size by mesh analysis becomes increasingly difficult as particle size decreases below 200-mesh.

Dressings

Dressings are external applications resembling ointments, usually used as a covering or protection. Petrolatum Gauze is a sterile dressing prepared by adding sterile, molten, white petrolatum to precut sterile gauze in a ratio of 60 g of petrolatum to 20 g of gauze. Topical antibacterials are available in the form of dressings.

Creams

Creams are viscous liquid or semisolid emulsions of either the O/W or W/O type. Pharmaceutical creams are classified as water-removable bases in the USP and are described under *Ointments*. In addition to ointment bases, creams include a variety of cosmetic-type preparations. Creams of the O/W type include shaving creams, hand creams, and foundation creams; W/O creams include cold creams and emollient creams.

Plasters

Plasters are substances intended for external application, made of such materials and of such consistency as to adhere to the skin and attach to a dressing. Plasters are intended to afford protection and support and/or to furnish an occlusive and macerating action and to bring medication into close contact with the skin. Medicated plasters, long used for local or regional drug delivery, are the prototypical transdermal delivery system.

Plasters usually adhere to the skin by means of an adhesive material. The adhesive must bond to the plastic backing and to the skin (or dressing) with proper balance of cohesive strengths. Such a proper balance provides for removal (ie, adhesive breakage at the surface of application) thus leaving a clean (skin) surface when the plaster is removed.

Contraceptives

In the context of this chapter, contraceptives are considered in the form of creams, jellies, or aerosol foams intended for vaginal use to protect against pregnancy. Contraceptive creams and jellies are designed to melt or spread, following insertion, over the vaginal surfaces. These agents act to immobilize spermatozoa.

Creams and jellies for contraceptive use may contain spermicidal agents such as nonoxynol 9, or they may function by a specific pH effect. A pH of 3.5 or less has an appreciable spermicidal effect. It is important to note that a final *in situ* pH of 3.5 or less is required; thus, the dilution effect and pH change brought about by vaginal fluids must be considered. To achieve the proper pH effect and control, buffer systems composed of acid and acid salts such as lactates, acetates, and citrates are used frequently.

Preservatives in Topical Formulations

Antimicrobial preservative substances are included in ointment formulations to maintain the potency and integrity of product forms and to protect the health and safety of the consumer. The USP addresses this subject in its monograph *Microbiological Attributes of Non-Sterile Pharmaceutical Products*. The significance of microorganisms in nonsterile products should be evaluated in terms of the use of the product, the na-

ture of the product, and the potential hazard to the user. The USP suggests that products applied topically should be tested for the presence of *P aeruginosa* and *S aureus*. In addition, products intended for rectal, urethral, or vaginal administration should be tested for yeasts and molds.

The attributes of an ideal preservative system have been defined by various authors as

- Effective at relatively low concentrations against a broad spectrum or variety of microorganisms that could cause disease or product deterioration
- Soluble in the required concentration
- Nontoxic and nonsensitizing at in-use concentrations
- Compatible with ingredients of the formulation and package components
- Free from objectionable odors and colors
- Stable over a wide range of conditions
- Inexpensive

No preservative or preservative system meets these ideal criteria. In fact, preservative substances once considered most acceptable, if not ideal, now have been questioned. Methylparaben and propylparaben, second and third only to water in frequency of use in cosmetic formulations, have been associated with allergic reactions.

Use of parabens as preservatives in topical products began more than a half-century ago. Animal testing indicated that they virtually are nontoxic and the compounds, usually in combination, became nearly ubiquitous as preservatives in dermatologic and cosmetic products. In spite of concerns about contact sensitization, topical parabens do not appear to constitute a significant hazard to the public based on their low index of sensitization and low overall toxicity.

Alternative preservation substances available for use in topical formulations, together with comments on possible limitations, are given in Table 44-6.[45] It is probably sensible to

Table 44-6. Topical Preservatives: Benefits and Risks

PRESERVATIVES	LIMITATIONS RELATIVE TO USE IN COSMETIC/DERMATOLOGIC FORMULATIONS
Quaternary ammonium compounds	Inactivated by numerous ingredients including anionics, nonionics, and proteins
Organic mercurial compounds	Potentially toxic; many sensitize the skin
	Limited use in formulations used near or in the eye
Formaldehyde	Volatile compound with an objectionable odor
	Irritating to the skin
	High chemical reactivity
Halogenated phenols[a]	Objectionable odor
	Often inactivated by nonionics, anionics or proteins
	Limited gram-negative antibacterial activity
Sorbic acid, potassium sorbate	pH-dependent (can be used only in formulations below the pH of 6.5 to 7.0)
	Higher concentrations are oxidized by sunlight resulting in product discoloration
	Limited antibacterial activity
Benzoic acid, sodium benzoate	pH-dependent (limited to use in formulations with pH of 5.5 or less)
	Replaced by newer antimicrobials because of its limited antimicrobial activity

[a] eg, hexachlorophene, *p*-chloro-*m*-cresol (PCMC), *p*-chloro-*m*-xylenol (PCMX), dichloro-*m*-xylenol (DCMX).

note that with few exceptions, most of these compounds—in contrast to the parabens—do not have a half-century history of use nor have had extensive patch-testing experiments carried out.

Following selection of preservative candidates and preparation of product prototypes, the efficacy of the preservative system must be evaluated. A variety of methods to accomplish this have been proposed. The organism challenge procedure is currently the most acceptable. In this procedure, the test-product formulation is inoculated with specific levels and types of microorganisms. Preservative efficacy is evaluated on the basis of the number of organisms killed or whose growth is inhibited as determined during a specific sampling schedule. Critical to the organism challenge procedure are the selection of challenge microorganisms, the level of organisms in the inoculum, the sampling schedule, and data interpretation.

In addition to efficacy in terms of antimicrobial effects, the preservative system must be assessed in terms of chemical and physical stability as a function of time. This often is done using antimicrobial measurements in addition to chemical analysis.

REFERENCES

1. Boddé HE, van den Brink I, Koerten HK, et al. *J Control Rel* 1991; 15:227.
2. Rougier A, Lotte C. In Shah VP, Maibach HI, eds. *Topical Drug Bioavailability, Bioequivalence, and Penetration.* New York: Plenum Press, 1993, p 163.
3. Franz TJ. *J Invest Dermatol* 1975; 64:191.
4. Scheuplein RJ, Ross LW. *J Invest Dermatol* 1974; 63:353.
5. Bartek MJ, La Bodde JA, Maibach HI. *J Invest Dermatol* 1972; 58:114.
6. Maibach HI, ed. *Animal Models in Dermatology.* Edinburgh: Churchill Livingstone, 1975, p 110.
7. Wester RC, Maibach HI. *J Invest Dermatol* 1976; 67:518.
8. Bronaugh RL. In Kemppainen BW, Reifenrath WG, eds. *Methods for Skin Absorption.* Boca Raton, FL: CRC Press, 1990, p 61.
9. Mershon MM, Callahan JF. In Maibach HI, ed. *Animal Models in Dermatology.* Edinburgh: Churchill Livingstone, 1975, p 36.
10. Lorenzetti OJ. In Maibach HI, ed. *Animal Models in Dermatology.* Edinburgh: Churchill Livingstone, 1975, p 212.
11. Maibach HI. In Maibach HI, ed. *Animal Models in Dermatology.* Edinburgh: Churchill Livingstone, 1975, p 221.
12. Niemiec SM, et al. *Drug Delivery* 1997; 4:33.
13. Flynn GL. In Shah VP, Maibach HI, eds. *Topical Drug Bioavailability, Bioequivalence, and Penetration.* New York: Plenum Press, 1993, p 369.
14. Walters KA. In Hadgraft J, Guy RH, eds. *Transdermal Drug Delivery.* New York: Dekker, 1989, p 197.
15. Ghosh TK, Banga AK. *Pharm Technol* 1993; 17(4):62; 1993; 17(5):68.
16. Scheuplein RJ, Ross LW. *J Soc Cosmet Chem* 1970; 21:853.
17. Christophers E, Kligman AM. In Montagna W, ed. *Advances in the Biology of Skin,* vol 6. Oxford: Pergamon, 1965, p 163.
18. Benowitz NL, et al. *Clin Pharmacol Ther* 1992; 52:223.
19. Roskos KV, Maibach HI, Guy RH. *J Pharmacokin Biopharm* 1989; 17:617.
20. Sloan KB, Bodor N. *Int J Pharm* 1982; 12:299.
21. Wood E, Wilson CG, Hardy JG. *Int J Pharm* 1985; 25:191.
22. Bottger WM, et al. *J Pharmacokinet Biopharm* 1990; 18:1.
23. Abd-El-Maeboud KH, et al. *Lancet* 1991; 338:798.
24. Tukker JJ, de Blaey CJ, Charbon GA. *Pharm Res* 1984; 1:173.
25. Parrott EL. *Pharm Res* 1971; 60:867.
26. Benziger DP, Edelson J. *J. Drug Metab Rev* 1983; 14:137.
27. Patel LG, Warrington SJ, Pearson RM. *Br Med J* 1983; 287:1247.
28. Roffe BD, Zimmer RA, Derewicz HJ. *AJHP* 1977; 34:1344.
29. Allen LV, Stiles ML. *US Pharm* 1988; 13(1):16.
30. Ostrenga J, Steinmetz C, Poulsen B. *J Pharm Sci* 1971; 60:1175.
31. Flynn GL, Weiner ND, et al. *Int J Pharm* 1989; 55:229.
32. Banga AK, Chien YW. *J Control Rel* 1988; 7:1.
33. Burnette RR. In Hadgraft J, Guy RH, eds. *Transdermal Drug Delivery.* New York: Dekker, 1989, p 247.
34. Hsu C-S, Block LH. *Pharm Res* 1996; 13:1865.
35. Ramanathan S, Block LH. *J Contr Rel* 2001; 70:109.
36. Ghosh TK, Banga AK. *Pharm Technol* 1993; 17(3):2.
37. Balsam MS, Sagarin E, eds. *Cosmetics Science and Technology,* 2nd ed, vol. 1. New York: Wiley-Interscience, 1972, p 205.
38. Merino G, Kalia YN, Guy RH. *J Pharm Sci* 2003; 92:1125.
39. Henry S, et al. *J Pharm Sci* 1998; 87:922.
40. Lowenthal W, Borzelleca JF. *J Pharm Sci* 1965; 54:1790.
41. Collins AP, Hohmann JR, Zopf LC. *Am Prof Pharm* 1957; 23:231.
42. Snipes WC. US Pat 5,004,601, Apr 2, 1991.
43. Davis H. *Bentley's Text-Book of Pharmaceutics,* 7th ed. London: Bailliere, Tindall & Cox, 1961, p 569.
44. Buchi J. *Pharm Acta Helv* 1940; 20:403.
45. Lorenzetti OJ, Wernet TC. *Dermatologica* 1977; 154:244.

BIBLIOGRAPHY

Chien YW, ed. *Transdermal Controlled Systemic Medications.* New York: Dekker, 1987.

Chien YW. *Novel Drug Delivery Systems,* 2nd ed. New York: Dekker, 1992.

Flynn GL. In Shah VP, Maibach HI, eds. *Topical Drug Bioavailability, Bioequivalence, and Penetration.* New York: Plenum Press, 1993, p 369.

Frost P, Gomez EC, Zaias N. *Recent Advances in Dermatopharmacology.* New York: Spectrum Publ, 1978.

Glas B, deBlaey CJ, eds. *Rectal Therapy.* Barcelona: JR Prous, 1984.

Guy RH, Hadgraft J. In Maibach H, Lowe R, eds. *Models in Dermatology,* vol 2, 5. Basel: Karger, 1985, p 170.

Higuchi T. *J Soc Cosmet Chem* 1960; 11:85.

Hoover JE, ed. *Dispensing of Medication,* 8th ed. Easton, PA: Mack Publ Co, 1976.

Illel B. *Crit Rev Ther Drug Carrier Systems* 1997; 14:207.

Wenninger JA, ed. *International Cosmetic Ingredient Dictionary and Handbook.* Baltimore: The Cosmetic, Toiletry and Fragrance Assoc, 1998.

Kemppanien BW, Reifenrath WG, eds. *Methods for Skin Absorption.* Boca Raton, FL: CRC Press, 1990.

Maibach HI. *Animal Models in Dermatology.* Edinburgh: Churchill Livingstone, 1975.

Mier PD, Cotton DWK. *The Molecular Biology of Skin.* Oxford: Blackwell, 1976.

Montagna W, Parrakkal PF. *The Structure and Function of the Skin,* 3rd ed. New York: Academic Press, 1974.

Marples MJ. *The Ecology of the Human Skin.* Springfield, IL: Thomas, 1965.

Scranton AB, Peppas NA. *Adv Drug Del Rev* 1993; 11:1.

Walters KA. In Hadgraft J, Guy RH, eds. *Transdermal Drug Delivery.* New York: Dekker, 1989, p 197.

Wester RC, Maibach HI. *Clin Pharmakinet* 1992; 23:253.

CHAPTER 45

Oral Solid Dosage Forms

Edward M Rudnic, PhD

Joseph B Schwartz, PhD

Drug substances most frequently are administered orally by means of solid dosage forms such as tablets and capsules. Large-scale production methods used for their preparation, as described later in the chapter, require the presence of other materials in addition to the active ingredients. Additives also may be included in the formulations to facilitate handling, enhance the physical appearance, improve stability, and aid in the delivery of the drug to the bloodstream after administration. These supposedly inert ingredients, as well as the production methods employed, have been shown in many cases to influence the absorption or bioavailability of the drug substances.[1] Therefore, care must be taken in the selection and evaluation of additives and preparation methods to ensure that the drug-delivery goals and therapeutic efficacy of the active ingredient(s) will not be diminished.

In a number of cases it has been shown that the drug substance's solubility and other physicochemical characteristics have influenced its physiological availability from a solid dosage form. These characteristics include its particle size, whether it is amorphous or crystalline, whether it is solvated or nonsolvated, and its crystalline, or polymorphic form. After clinically effective formulations are obtained, such variations among dosage units of a given batch, as well as batch-to-batch differences, should be reduced to a minimum through proper in-process controls and good manufacturing practices. The recognition of the importance of performance qualification, and validation for both equipment and processes has enhanced assurance in the reproducibility of solid dosage formulations greatly. It is in these areas that significant progress has been made with the realization that large-scale production of a satisfactory tablet or capsule depends not only on the availability of a clinically effective formulation but also on the raw materials, facilities, personnel, documentation, validated processes and equipment, packaging, and the controls used during and after preparation (Fig 45-1).

TABLETS

Tablets may be defined as solid pharmaceutical dosage forms containing drug substances with or without suitable diluents and have been traditionally prepared by either compression, or molding methods. Recently, punching of laminated sheets, electronic deposition methods, and three-dimensional printing methods have been used to make tablets. Tablets have been in widespread use since the latter part of the 19th century, and their popularity continues. The term *compressed tablet* is believed to have been used first by John Wyeth and Brother of Philadelphia. During this same period, molded tablets were introduced to be used as *hypodermic* tablets for the extemporaneous preparation of solutions for injection. Tablets remain popular as a dosage form because of the advantages afforded both to the manufacturer (eg, simplicity and economy of preparation, stability, and convenience in packaging, shipping, and dispensing) and the patient (eg, accuracy of dosage, compactness, portability, blandness of taste, and ease of administration).

Although the basic mechanical approach for most tablet manufacture has remained the same, tablet technology has undergone great improvement and experimentation. Efforts are being made continually to understand more clearly the physical characteristics of powder compaction and the factors affecting the availability of the drug substance from the dosage form after oral administration. Tableting equipment continues to improve in both production speed and the uniformity of tablets compressed. Recent advances in tablet technology have been reviewed.[2–13]

Although tablets frequently are discoid in shape, they also may be round, oval, oblong, cylindrical, or triangular. Other geometric shapes, such as diamonds and pentagons, and hexagons have also been used. They may differ greatly in size and weight depending on the amount of drug substance present and the intended method of administration. Most commercial tablets can be divided into two general classes by whether they are made by compression or molding. Compressed tablets usually are prepared by large-scale production methods, while molded tablets generally involve small-scale operations. The various tablet types and abbreviations used in referring to them are listed below.

COMPRESSED TABLETS (CT)—These tablets are formed by compression and in their simplest form, contain no special coating. They are made from powdered, crystalline, or granular materials, alone or in combination with binders, disintegrants, controlled-release polymers, lubricants, diluents, and in many cases colorants. The vast majority of tablets commercialized today are compressed tablets, either in an uncoated or coated state.

Sugar-Coated Tablets (SCT)—These are compressed tablets surrounded by a sugar coating. Such coatings may be colored and are beneficial in covering up drug substances possessing objectionable tastes or odors and in protecting materials sensitive to oxidation. These coatings were once quite common, and generally lost commercial appeal due to the high cost of process validation. Recently, they have made a comeback due to patient popularity and technical advances.

Film-Coated Tablets (FCT)—These are compressed tablets that are covered with a thin layer or film of a water-soluble material. A number of polymeric substances with film-forming properties may be used. Film coating imparts the same general characteristics as sugar coating,

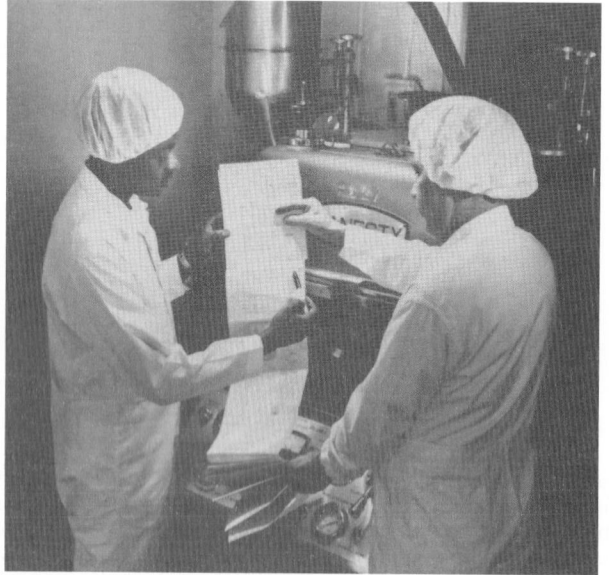

Figure 45-1. Tablet press operators checking batch record in conformance with Current Good Manufacturing Practices (courtesy, Lilly).

with the added advantage of a greatly reduced time period required for the coating operation. Advances in material science and polymer chemistry has made these coatings the first-choice of formulators.

Enteric-Coated Tablets (ECT)—These are compressed tablets coated with substances that resist solution in gastric fluid but disintegrate in the intestine. Enteric coatings can be used for tablets containing drug substances that are inactivated or destroyed in the stomach, for those that irritate the mucosa, or as a means of delayed release of the medication.

Multiple Compressed Tablets (MCT)—These are compressed tablets made by more than one compression cycle. This process is best used when separation of active ingredients is needed for stability purposes, or if the mixing process is inadequate to guarantee uniform distribution of two or more active ingredients.

Layered Tablets—Such tablets are prepared by compressing additional tablet granulation on a previously compressed granulation. The operation may be repeated to produce multilayered tablets of two or three, or more layers. Special tablet presses are required to make layered tablets such as the Versa press *(Stokes/Pennwalt)*.

Press-Coated Tablets—Such tablets, also referred to as dry-coated, are prepared by feeding previously compressed tablets into a special tableting machine and compressing another granulation layer around the preformed tablets. They have all the advantages of compressed tablets (ie, slotting, monogramming, speed of disintegration) while retaining the attributes of sugar-coated tablets in masking the taste of the drug substance in the core tablets. An example of a press-coated tablet press is the *Manesty* Drycota. Press-coated tablets also can be used to separate incompatible drug substances; in addition, they can provide a means of giving an enteric coating to the core tablets. Both types of multiple-compressed tablets have been used widely in the design of prolonged-action dosage forms.

Controlled-Release Tablets (CRT)—Compressed tablets can be formulated to release the drug slowly over a prolonged period of time. Hence, these dosage forms have been referred to as *prolonged-release* or *sustained-release* dosage forms as well. These tablets (as well as capsule versions) can be categorized into three types: (1) those that respond to some physiological condition to release the drug, such as enteric coatings; (2) those that release the drug in a relatively steady, controlled manner; and (3) those that combine combinations of mechanisms to release *pulses* of drug, such as repeat-action tablets. The performance of these systems is described in more detail in Chapter 47. Other names for these types of tablets can be: *Extended Release, Sustained Release, Prolonged Release, Delayed Release*, and in the case of pulsatile tablets, *Repeat Action, Pulsatile Release* or *Pulse Release*.

Tablets for Solution (CTS)—Compressed tablets to be used for preparing solutions or imparting given characteristics to solutions must be labeled to indicate that they are not to be swallowed. Examples of these tablets are Halazone Tablets for Solution and Potassium Permanganate Tablets for Solution.

Effervescent Tablets—In addition to the drug substance, these contain sodium bicarbonate and an organic acid such as tartaric or citric. In the presence of water, these additives react, liberating carbon dioxide that acts as a distintegrator and produces effervescence. Except for small quantities of lubricants present, effervescent tablets are soluble.

Compressed Suppositories or Inserts—Occasionally, vaginal suppositories, such as Metronidazole tablets, are prepared by compression. Tablets for this use usually contain lactose as the diluent. In this case, as well as for any tablet intended for administration other than by swallowing, the label must indicate the manner in which it is to be used.

Buccal and Sublingual Tablets—These are small, flat, oval tablets. Tablets intended for buccal (the space between the lip and gum in the mouth) administration by inserting into the buccal pouch may dissolve or erode slowly; therefore, they are formulated and compressed with sufficient pressure to give a hard tablet. Progesterone tablets may be administered in this way. Some newer approaches have employed materials that act as bioadhesives to increase absorption of the drug.

Some other approaches use tablets that melt at body temperatures. The matrix of the tablet is solidified while the drug is in solution. After melting, the drug is automatically in solution and available for absorption, thus eliminating dissolution as a rate-limiting step in the absorption of poorly soluble compounds. Sublingual tablets, such as those containing nitroglycerin, isoproterenol hydrochloride, or erythrityl tetranitrate, are placed under the tongue. Sublingual tablets dissolve rapidly, and the drug substances are absorbed readily by this form of administration.

MOLDED TABLETS OR TABLET TRITURATES (TT)—Tablet triturates usually are made from moist material, using a triturate mold that gives them the shape of cut sections of a cylinder. Such tablets must be completely and rapidly soluble. The problem arising from compression of these tablets is the failure to find a lubricant that is completely water-soluble.

Dispensing Tablets (DT)—These tablets provide a convenient quantity of potent drug that can be incorporated readily into powders and liquids, thus circumventing the necessity to weigh small quantities. These tablets are supplied primarily as a convenience for extemporaneous compounding and should never be dispensed as a dosage form.

Hypodermic Tablets (HT)—Hypodermic tablets are soft, readily soluble tablets and originally were used for the preparation of solutions to be injected. Since stable parenteral solutions are now available for most drug substances, there is no justification for the use of hypodermic tablets for injection. Their use in this manner should be discouraged, since the resulting solutions are not sterile. Large quantities of these tablets continue to be made, but for oral administration. No hypodermic tablets ever have been recognized by the official compendia.

Compressed Tablets (CT)

For medicinal substances, with or without diluents, to be made into solid dosage forms with pressure, using available equipment, it is necessary that the material, either in crystalline or powdered form, possess a number of physical characteristics. These characteristics include the ability to flow freely, cohesiveness, and lubrication. The ingredients such as disintegrants designed to break the tablet up in gastrointestinal (GI) fluids and controlled-release polymers designed to slow drug release ideally should possess these characteristics or not interfere with the desirable performance traits of the other excipients. Since most materials have none or only some of these properties, methods of tablet formulation and preparation have been developed to impart these desirable characteristics to the material that is to be compressed into tablets.

The basic mechanical unit in all tablet-compression equipment includes a lower punch that fits into a die from the bottom and an upper punch, with a head of the same shape and dimensions, which enters the die cavity from the top after the tableting material fills the die cavity (Fig 45-2). The tablet is formed by pressure applied on the punches and subsequently is ejected from the die. The weight of the tablet is determined by the volume of the material that fills the die cavity. Therefore, the ability of the granulation to flow freely into the die is important in ensuring a uniform fill, as well as the continuous movement of the granulation from the source of supply or feed hopper. If the tablet granulation does not possess cohesive properties, the tablet after compression will crumble and fall apart on handling. As the punches must move freely within the

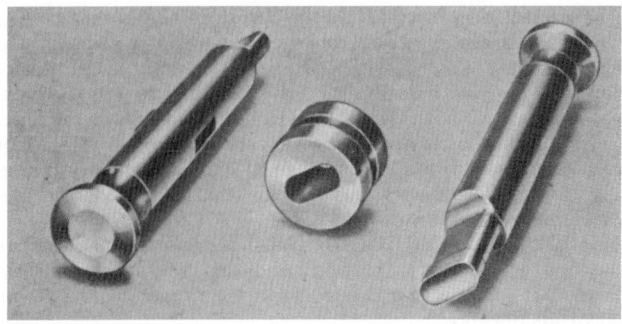

Figure 45-2. Basic mechanical unit for tablet compression: lower punch, die, and upper punch (courtesy, Vector/Colton).

die and the tablet must be ejected readily from the punch faces, the material must have a degree of lubrication to minimize friction and allow the removal of the compressed tablets.

There are three general methods typically used for commercial tablet preparation: the wet-granulation method, the dry-granulation method, and direct compression. The method of preparation and the added ingredients are selected to give the tablet formulation the desirable physical characteristics allowing the rapid compression of tablets. After compression, the tablets must have a number of additional attributes such as appearance, hardness, disintegration ability, appropriate dissolution characteristics, and uniformity, which also are influenced both by the method of preparation and by the added materials present in the formulation. In the preparation of compressed tablets, the formulator also must be cognizant of the effect that the ingredients and methods of preparation may have on the availability of the active ingredients and, hence, the therapeutic efficacy of the dosage form. In response to a request by physicians to change a dicumarol tablet so that it might be broken more easily, a Canadian company reformulated to make a large tablet with a score. Subsequent use of the tablet, containing the same amount of drug substance as the previous tablet, resulted in complaints that larger-than-usual doses were needed to produce the same therapeutic response. On the other hand, literature reports indicate that the reformulation of a commercial digoxin tablet resulted in a tablet that, although containing the same quantity of drug substance, gave the desired clinical response at half its original dose. Methods and principles that can be used to assess the effects of excipients and additives on drug absorption have been reviewed.[2,14,15]

TABLET INGREDIENTS

In addition to the active or therapeutic ingredient, tablets contain a number of inert materials. The latter are known as additives or *excipients*. They may be classified according to the part they play in the finished tablet. The first group contains those that help to impart satisfactory processing and compression characteristics to the formulation. These include diluents, binders, glidants, and lubricants. The second group of added substances helps to give additional desirable physical characteristics to the finished tablet. Included in this group are disintegrants, surfactants, colors, and, in the case of chewable tablets, flavors, and sweetening agents, and in the case of controlled-release tablets, polymers or hydrophobic materials, such as waxes or other solubility-retarding materials. In some cases, anti-oxidants or other materials can be added to improve stability and shelf-life.

Although the term *inert* has been applied to these added materials, it has become apparent that there is an important relationship between the properties of the excipients and the dosage forms containing them. Preformulation studies demonstrate their influence on stability, bioavailability, and the processes by which the dosage forms are prepared. The need for ac-

quiring more information and use standards for excipients has been recognized in a joint venture of the Academy of Pharmaceutical Sciences and the Council of the Pharmaceutical Society of Great Britain. The result is called the *Handbook of Pharmaceutical Excipients*. This reference now is distributed widely throughout the world.[16]

Diluents

Frequently, the single dose of the active ingredient is small, and an inert substance is added to increase the bulk to make the tablet a practical size for compression. Compressed tablets of dexamethasone contain 0.75 mg steroid per tablet; hence, it is obvious that another material must be added to make tableting possible. Diluents used for this purpose include dicalcium phosphate, calcium sulfate, lactose, cellulose, kaolin, mannitol, sodium chloride, dry starch, and powdered sugar. Certain diluents, such as mannitol, lactose, sorbitol, sucrose, and inositol, when present in sufficient quantity, can impart properties to some compressed tablets that permit disintegration in the mouth by chewing. Such tablets commonly are called *chewable tablets*. Upon chewing, properly prepared tablets will disintegrate smoothly at a satisfactory rate, have a pleasant taste and feel, and leave no unpleasant aftertaste in the mouth. Diluents used as excipients for direct compression formulas have been subjected to prior processing to give them flowability and compressibility. These are discussed under *Direct Compression*.

Most formulators of immediate-release tablets tend to use consistently only one or two diluents selected from the above group in their tablet formulations. Usually, these have been selected on the basis of experience and cost factors. However, in the formulation of new therapeutic agents, the compatibility of the diluents with the drug must be considered; eg, calcium salts used as diluents for the broad-spectrum antibiotic tetracycline have been shown to interfere with the drug's absorption from the GI tract. When drug substances have low water solubility, it is recommended that water-soluble diluents be used to avoid possible bioavailability problems. Highly adsorbent substances (eg, bentonite and kaolin) are to be avoided in making tablets of drugs used clinically in small dosage, such as the cardiac glycosides, alkaloids, and the synthetic estrogens. These drug substances may be adsorbed after administration. The combination of amine bases with lactose, or amine salts with lactose in the presence of an alkaline lubricant results in tablets that discolor on aging.

Microcrystalline cellulose (Avicel) usually is used as an excipient in direct-compression formulas. However, its presence in 5–15% concentrations in wet granulations has been shown to be beneficial in the granulation and drying processes in minimizing case-hardening of the tablets and in reducing tablet mottling.

Many ingredients are used for several different purposes, even within the same formulation (eg, cornstarch can be used in paste form as a binder). When added in drug or suspension form, it is a good disintegrant. Even though these two uses are to achieve opposite goals, some tablet formulas use cornstarch in both ways. In some controlled-release formulas, the polymer hydroxypropyl methylcellulose (HPMC) is used both as an aid to prolong the release from the tablet as well as a film-former in the tablet coating. Therefore, most excipients used in formulating tablets and capsules have many uses, and a thorough understanding of their properties and limitations is necessary to use them rationally.

Binders

Agents used to impart cohesive qualities to the powdered material are referred to as binders or granulators. They impart a cohesiveness to the tablet formulation that ensures the tablet remaining intact after compression, as well as improving the free-flowing qualities by the formulation of granules of desired hardness and size. Materials commonly used as binders include starch, gelatin, and sugars such as sucrose, glucose, dextrose, molasses, and lactose. Natural and synthetic gums that have been used include acacia, sodium alginate, extract of Irish moss, panwar gum, ghatti gum, mucilage of isapol husks, carboxymethylcellulose, methylcellulose, polyvinylpyrrolidone, Veegum, and larch arabogalactan. Other agents that may be considered binders under certain circumstances are polyethylene glycol, ethylcellulose, waxes, water, and alcohol.

The quantity of binder used has considerable influence on the characteristics of the compressed tablets. The use of too much binder or too strong a binder will make a hard tablet that will not disintegrate easily and will cause excessive wear of punches and dies. Differences in binders used for CT Tolbutamide resulted in differences in hypoglycemic effects observed clinically. Materials that have no cohesive qualities of their own will require a stronger binder than those with these qualities. Alcohol and water are not binders in the true sense of the word, but because of their solvent action on some ingredients such as lactose, starch, and celluloses, they change the powdered material to granules, and the residual moisture retained enables the materials to adhere together when compressed.

Binders are used both as a solution and in a dry form, depending on the other ingredients in the formulation and the method of preparation. However, several *pregelatinized* starches available are intended to be added in the dry form so that water alone can be used as the granulating solution. The same amount of binder in solution will be more effective than if it were dispersed in a dry form and moistened with the solvent. By the latter procedure, the binding agent is not as effective in reaching and wetting each of the particles within the mass of powders. Each of the particles in a powder blend has a coating of adsorbed air on its surface, and it is this film that must be penetrated before the powders can be wetted by the binder solution. After wetting, a certain period of time is necessary to dissolve the binder completely and make it completely available for use. Since powders differ with respect to the ease with which they can be wetted and their rate of solubilization, it is preferable to incorporate the binding agent in solution. By this technique it often is possible to gain effective binding with a lower concentration of binder.

The direct-compression method for preparing tablets requires a material that is not only free-flowing but also sufficiently cohesive to act as a binder. This use has been described for a number of materials including microcrystalline cellulose, microcrystalline dextrose, amylose, and polyvinylpyrrolidone. It has been postulated that microcrystalline cellulose is a special form of cellulose fibril in which the individual crystallites are held together largely by hydrogen bonding. The disintegration of tablets containing the cellulose occurs by breaking the intercrystallite bonds by the disintegrating medium.

STARCH PASTE—Cornstarch is used widely as a binder. The concentration may vary from 10% to 20%. It usually is prepared as it is to be used, by dispersing cornstarch in sufficient cold purified water to make a 5–10% *w/w* suspension and warming in a water bath with continuous stirring until a translucent paste forms. It has been observed that during paste formation, not all of the starch is hydrolyzed. Starch paste then is not only useful as a binder, but also as a method to incorporate some disintegrant inside the granules.

GELATIN SOLUTION—Gelatin generally is used as a 10–20% solution; gelatin solutions should be prepared freshly as needed and used while warm or they will solidify. The gelatin is added to cold purified water and allowed to stand until it is hydrated. It then is warmed in a water bath to dissolve the gelatin, and the solution is made up to the final volume on a weight basis to give the concentration desired.

CELLULOSIC SOLUTIONS—Various cellulosics have been used as binders in solution form. Hydroxypropyl methylcellulose (HPMC) has been used widely in this regard. Typical of a number of cellulosics, HPMC is more soluble in cold water than hot. It also is more dispersable in hot water than cold. Hence, to obtain a good, smooth gel that is free from lumps or *fisheyes,* it is necessary to add the HPMC in hot, almost boiling water and, under agitation, cool the mixture down as quickly as possible, as low as possible. Other water-soluble cellulosics such as hydroxyethylcellulose (HEC) and hydroxypropylcellulose (HPC) have been used successfully in solution as binders.

Not all cellulosics are soluble in water. Ethylcellulose can be used effectively when dissolved in alcohol or as a dry binder that then is wetted with alcohol. It is used as a binder for materials that are moisture-sensitive.

POLYVINYLPYRROLIDONE—PVP can be used as an aqueous or alcoholic solution, and this versatility has increased its popularity. Concentrations range from 2% and vary considerably.

It will be noted that binder solutions usually are made up to weight rather than volume. This is to enable the formulator to determine the weight of the solids that have been added to the tablet granulation in the binding solution. This becomes part of the total weight of the granulation and must be taken into consideration in determining the weight of the compressed tablet, which will contain the stated amount of the therapeutic agent.

As can be seen by the list of binders in this chapter, most modern binders used in solution are polymeric. Because of this, the flow or spreadability of these solutions becomes important when selecting the appropriate granulating equipment. The rheology of polymeric solutions is a fascinating subject in and of itself and should be considered for these materials.

Lubricants

Lubricants have a number of functions in tablet manufacture. They prevent adhesion of the tablet material to the surface of the dies and punches, reduce interparticle friction, facilitate the ejection of the tablets from the die cavity, and may improve the rate of flow of the tablet granulation. Commonly used lubricants include talc, magnesium stearate, calcium stearate, stearic acid, glyceryl behanate, hydrogenated vegetable oils, and polyethylene glycol (PEG). Most lubricants, with the exception of talc, are used in concentrations below 1%. When used alone, talc may require concentrations as high as 5%. Lubricants are in most cases hydrophobic materials. Poor selection or excessive amounts can result in *waterproofing* the tablets, resulting in poor tablet disintegration and/or delayed dissolution of the drug substance.

The addition of the proper lubricant is highly desirable if the material to be tableted tends to stick to the punches and dies. Immediately after compression, most tablets have the tendency to expand and will bind and stick to the side of the die. The choice of the proper lubricant will overcome this effectively.

The method of adding a lubricant to a granulation is important if the material is to perform its function satisfactorily. The lubricant should be divided finely by passing it through a 60- to 100-mesh nylon cloth onto the granulation. In production this is called *bolting* the lubricant. After adding the lubricant, the granulation is tumbled or mixed gently to distribute the lubricant without coating the particles too well or breaking them down to finer particles. Some research has concluded that the order of mixing of lubricants and other excipients can have a profound effect on the performance of the final dosage form. Thus, attention to the mixing process itself is just as important as the selection of lubricant materials.

These process variables can be seen in the prolonged blending of a lubricant in a granulation. Overblending materially can affect the hardness, disintegration time, and dissolution performance of the resultant tablets.

The quantity of lubricant varies, being as low as 0.1% and, in some cases, as high as 5%. Lubricants have been added to the granulating agents in the form of suspensions or emulsions. This technique serves to reduce the number of operational procedures and thus reduce the processing time.

In selecting a lubricant, proper attention must be given to its compatibility with the drug agent. Perhaps the most widely investigated drug is acetylsalicylic acid. Different talcs varied significantly the stability of aspirin. Talc with a high calcium content and a high loss on ignition was associated with increased aspirin decomposition. From a stability standpoint, the relative acceptability of tablet lubricants for combination with aspirin was found to decrease in the following order: hydrogenated vegetable oil, stearic acid, talc, and aluminum stearate.

The primary problem in the preparation of a water-soluble tablet is the selection of a satisfactory lubricant. Soluble lubricants reported to be effective include sodium benzoate, a mixture of sodium benzoate and sodium acetate, sodium chloride, leucine, and polyethylene glycol/Carbowax 4000. However, it has been suggested that formulations used to prepare water-soluble tablets may represent a number of compromises between compression efficiency and water solubility. While magnesium stearate is one of the most widely used lubricants, its hydrophobic properties can retard disintegration and dissolution. To overcome these waterproofing characteristics, sodium lauryl sulfate sometimes is included. One compound found to have the lubricating properties of magnesium stearate without its disadvantages is magnesium lauryl sulfate. Its safety for use in pharmaceuticals has not been established.

Glidants

A glidant is a substance that improves the flow characteristics of a powder mixture. These materials always are added in the dry state just prior to compression (ie, during the lubrication step). Colloidal silicon dioxide Cab-o-sil *(Cabot)* is the most commonly used glidant and generally is used in low concentrations of 1% or less. Talc (asbestos-free) also is used and may serve the dual purpose of lubricant/glidant.

It is especially important to optimize the order of addition and the mixing process for these materials, to maximize their effect and to make sure that their influence on the lubricant(s) is minimized.

Disintegrants

A disintegrant is a substance or a mixture of substances added to a tablet to facilitate its breakup or disintegration after administration. The active ingredient must be released from the tablet matrix as efficiently as possible to allow rapid dissolution. Materials serving as disintegrants have been classified chemically as starches, clays, celluloses, algins, gums, and cross-linked polymers.

The oldest and still the most popular disintegrants are corn and potato starch that have been well dried and powdered. Starch has a great affinity for water and swells when moistened, thus facilitating the rupture of the tablet matrix. However, others have suggested that its disintegrating action in tablets is due to capillary action rather than swelling; the spherical shape of the starch grains increases the porosity of the tablet, thus promoting capillary action. Starch, 5%, is suggested, but if more rapid disintegration is desired, this amount may be increased to 10% or 15%. Although it might be expected that disintegration time would decrease as the percentage of starch in the tablet increased, this does not appear to be the case for tolbutamide tablets. In this instance, there appears to be a critical starch concentration for different granulations of the chemical. When their disintegration effect is desired, starches are added to the powder blends in the dry state.

A group of materials known as *super disintegrants* have gained in popularity as disintegrating agents. The name comes from the low levels (2–4%) at which they are completely effective. Croscarmellose, crospovidone, and sodium starch glycolate represent examples of a cross-linked cellulose, a cross-linked polymer, and a cross-linked starch, respectively.

The development of these disintegrants fostered new theories about the various mechanisms by which disintegrants

work. Sodium starch glycolate swells 7- to 12-fold in less than 30 sec. Croscarmellose swells 4- to 8-fold in less than 10 sec. The starch swells equally in all three dimensions, while the cellulose swells only in two dimensions, leaving fiber length essentially the same. Since croscarmellose is the more efficient disintegrating agent, it is postulated that the rate, force, and extent of swelling play an important role in those disintegrants that work by swelling. Cross-linked PVP swells little but returns to its original boundaries quickly after compression. Wicking, or capillary action, also is postulated to be a major factor in the ability of cross-linked PVP to function.[17–19]

In addition to the starches, a large variety of materials have been used and are reported to be effective as disintegrants. This group includes Veegum HV, methylcellulose, agar, bentonite, cellulose and wood products, natural sponge, cation-exchange resins, alginic acid, guar gum, citrus pulp, and carboxymethylcellulose.[20] Sodium lauryl sulfate in combination with starch also has been demonstrated to be an effective disintegrant. In some cases the apparent effectiveness of surfactants in improving tablet disintegration is postulated as due to an increase in the rate of wetting.

The disintegrating agent usually is mixed with the active ingredients and diluents prior to granulation. In some cases it may be advantageous to divide the starch into two portions: one part is added to the powdered formula prior to granulation, and the remainder is mixed with the lubricant and added prior to compression. Incorporated in this manner, the starch serves a double purpose; the portion added to the lubricant rapidly breaks down the tablet to granules, and the starch mixed with the active ingredients disintegrates the granules into smaller particles. Veegum has been shown to be more effective as a disintegrator in sulfathiazole tablets when most of the quantity is added after granulation and only a small amount before granulation. Likewise, the montmorillonite clays were found to be good tablet disintegrants when added to prepared granulations as powder. They are much less effective as disintegrants when incorporated within the granules.

Factors other than the presence of disintegrants can affect the disintegration time of compressed tablets significantly. The binder, tablet hardness, and the lubricant have been shown to influence the disintegration time. Thus, when the formulator is faced with a problem concerning the disintegration of a compressed tablet, the answer may not lie in the selection and quantity of the disintegrating agent alone.

The evolution of carbon dioxide is also an effective way to cause the disintegration of compressed tablets. Tablets containing a mixture of sodium bicarbonate and an acidulant such as tartaric or citric acid will effervesce when added to water. Sufficient acid is added to produce a neutral or slightly acidic reaction when disintegration in water is rapid and complete. One drawback to the use of the effervescent type of disintegrator is that such tablets must be kept in a dry atmosphere at all times during manufacture, storage, and packaging. Soluble, effervescent tablets provide a popular form for dispensing aspirin and noncaloric sweetening agents.

Coloring Agents

Colors in compressed tablets serve functions other than making the dosage form more esthetic in appearance. Color helps the manufacturer to control the product during its preparation, as well as serving as a means of identification to the user. The wide diversity in the use of colors in solid dosage forms makes it possible to use color as an important category in the identification code developed by the AMA to establish the identity of an unknown compressed tablet in situations arising from poisoning.

All colorants used in pharmaceuticals must be approved and certified by the FDA. For several decades colorants have been subjected to rigid toxicity standards, and as a result, a number of colorants have been removed from an approved list of Food, Drug and Cosmetic Act (FD&C) colors, or *delisted*. Several have

Table 45-1. Colors Approved for Use in the US in Oral Dosage Forms[a,b]

COLOR	OTHER NAMES	COLOR INDEX (CI 1971)	USE RESTRICTION (US)
FD&C Red 40	Allura red	16035	FDA certification on each lot of dye
D&C Red 33	Acid fuchsin D Naphtalone red B	17200	ADI 0–0.76 mg
D&C Red 36			ADI 0–1.0 mg
Canthaxanthinin	Food orange 8	40850	None
D&C Red 22	Eosin Y	45380	FDA certification on each lot of dye
D&C Red 28	Phloxine B	45410	FDA certification on each lot of dye
D&C Red 3	Erythrosine	45430	FDA certification on each lot of dye
Cochineal extract	Natural red 4 Carmine	75470	None
Iron oxide—red	—	77491	ADI 0–5 mg elemental iron
FD&C Yellow 6	Sunset yellow FCF Yellow orange 5	15985	None
FD&C Yellow 5	Tartrazine	19140	Label declaration and FDA certification on each lot of dye
D&C Yellow 10	Quinoline yellow WS	47005	FDA certification on each lot of dye
Beta-carotene	—	40800	
Iron oxide—yellow	—	77492	ADI 0–5 mg elemental iron
FD&C BLue 1	Brilliant blue FCF	42090	FDA certification on each lot of dye
FD&C Blue 2	Indigotine Indigo carmine	73015	None
FD&C Green 3	Fast green FCF	42035	FDA certification on each lot of dye
Iron oxide—black	—	77499	ADI 0–5 mg elemental iron
Caramel	Burnt sugar	—	None
Titanium dioxide	—	77891	None

[a] Abbreviations: ADI, acceptable daily intake (per kg body weight); CI, color index numbers of 1971 (US); D&C, Drug and Cosmetic Dyes (US); FD&C, Food, Drug and Cosmetic Dyes (US); FDA, Food and Drug Administration (US).
[b] As of February, 1988 and subject to revision.

been listed as well. The colorants currently approved in the US are listed in Table 45-1. Each country has its own list of approved colorants, and formulators must consider this in designing products for the international market.[21]

Any of the approved, certified, water-soluble FD&C dyes, mixtures of the same, or their corresponding lakes may be used to color tablets. A color lake is the combination by adsorption of a water-soluble dye to a hydrous oxide of a heavy metal resulting in an insoluble form of the dye. In some instances multiple dyes are used to give a purposefully heterogeneous coloring in the form of speckling to compressed tablets. The dyes available do not meet all the criteria required for the ideal pharmaceutical colorants. The photosensitivity of several of the commonly used colorants and their lakes has been investigated, as well as the protection afforded by a number of glasses used in packaging tablets.

Another approach for improving the photostability of dyes has been in the use of ultraviolet-absorbing chemicals in the tablet formulations with the dyes. The Di-Pac line *(Amstar)* is a series of commercially available colored, direct-compression sugars.

The most common method of adding color to a tablet formulation is to dissolve the dye in the binding solution prior to the granulating process. Another approach is to adsorb the dye on starch or calcium sulfate from its aqueous solution; the resultant powder is dried and blended with the other ingredients. If the insoluble lakes are used, they may be blended with the other dry ingredients. Frequently during drying, colors in wet granulations migrate, resulting in an uneven distribution of the color in the granulation. After compression, the tablets will have a mottled appearance due to the uneven distribution of the color. Migration of colors may be reduced by drying the granulation slowly at low temperatures and stirring the granulation while it is drying. The affinity of several water-soluble, anionic, certified dyes for natural starches has been demonstrated; in these cases this affinity should aid in preventing color migration.

Other additives have been shown to act as dye-migration inhibitors. Tragacanth (1%), acacia (3%), attapulgite (5%), and talc (7%) were effective in inhibiting the migration of FD&C Blue No 1 in lactose. In using dye lakes, the problem of color migration is avoided since the lakes are insoluble. Prevention of mottling can be helped also by the use of lubricants and other additives that have been colored similarly to the granulation prior to their use. The problem of mottling becomes more pronounced as the concentration of colorants increases. Color mottling is an undesirable characteristic common to many commercial tablets.

Flavoring Agents

In addition to the sweetness that may be afforded by the diluent of the chewable tablet, eg, mannitol or lactose, artificial sweetening agents may be included. Formerly, the cyclamates, either alone or in combination with saccharin, were used widely. With the banning of the cyclamates and the indefinite status of saccharin, new natural sweeteners are being sought. Aspartame *(Pfizer),* has found applications in pharmaceutical formulations. Sweeteners other than the sugars have the advantage of reducing the bulk volume, considering the quantity of sucrose required to produce the same degree of sweetness. Being present in small quantities, they do not affect markedly the physical characteristics of the tablet granulation.

POWDER COMPACTION

Compressed tablets became a commercially viable and efficient dosage form with the invention of tablet machines. In 1843 William Brockendon, a British inventor, author, artist, and watchmaker, received British Patent #9977 for *Shaping Pills, Lozenges, and Black Lead by Pressure in Dies.*[22] In over 150 years of tablet manufacture, the basic process has not changed. Surprisingly, improvements have been made only with regards to speed of manufacture and quality control.

The process of compaction has several identifiable phases. As can be seen in Figure 45-3, when powders undergo compression (a reduction in volume), the first process to occur is a consolidation of the powders. During this consolidation phase, the powder particles adopt a more efficient packing order. The second phase of the compaction process is elastic, or reversible de-

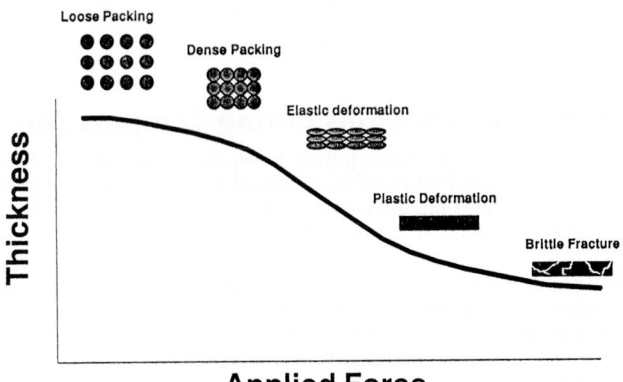

Figure 45-3. The stages of powder compaction.

formation. If the force were to be removed during this phase, the powder would recover completely to the efficiently packed state. For most pharmaceutical powders, this phase is very short in duration and very difficult to identify on most instrumented tablet presses. The third phase of compaction is plastic, or irreversible, deformation of the powder bed. It is this phase of the compaction process that is the most critical in tablet formation. If too much force is applied to the powder, brittle fracture occurs. If the force was applied too quickly, fracture and de-bonding during stress relaxation can occur.

In 1950, Stewart reported on the importance of plastic flow and suggested that if a material has significant plastic flow under compression, it will be more likely to form a compact.[23] David and Augsburger evaluated stress-relaxation data, using the Maxwell model of viscoelastic behavior in an attempt to quantify the rate of plastic deformation of some direct compression excipients.[24] Jones has used the term *contact time* to describe the total time for which a moving punch applies a detectable force to the die contents during the compression and decompression event, excluding ejection.[25]

Rees and Rue evaluated three parameters: stress relation during compaction, effect of contact time on tablet density, and rate of application of diametrical compression on tablet deformation.[26]

Jones[25] outlined numerous techniques to evaluate the compactability of powders. Because of the completeness of his review, these parameters are discussed below.

Tablet Strength—Compression Pressure Profile

Most formulators use tablet *hardness,* or tensile strength, as a measure of the cohesiveness of a tablet. With even the simplest of instrumented tablet presses, it is possible to plot tensile strength versus the force applied to the tablet. Figure 45-4 illustrates such a plot. These plots can be useful in identifying forces that can cause fracture and can lead to a quick, tangible assessment of the compatibility of the formulation. However, there are many limitations to this method, as these plots cannot predict *lamination* or *capping*. In addition, the cohesiveness of a tablet can change upon storage, in either a positive or negative direction.

Tablet Friability

This test is discussed later in the chapter, and there have been many suggestions about how they should be performed. Many formulators believe this is an important indicator of cohesiveness but is of limited value in predicting failure in the field.

Changes in Bed Density during Compression

As applied stress (force) increases, elastic and plastic deformation of the particles occurs, which results in plastic flow and a reduction in inter- and intraparticulate void spaces. This lowers the overall compact density.

For highly cohesive systems, the reduction in void space may yield a compact of sufficient strength for insertion into a capsules shell. However, the inherent cohesiveness for most drugs and excipients is not suitable alone for tablet manufacture.

The Heckel equation is given below; K can be considered equal to the reciprocal of the mean yield pressure, and A is a function of the original compact volume and is related to the densification and particle rearrangement prior to bonding.

$$\text{Log } [1/(1 - D)] = KP + A$$

where D is the relative density at pressure P, and K and A are constants.

Hersey and Rees[28] have classified Heckel plots into two categories. Figure 45-5 shows both types of Heckel plots. Type 2 differs from Type 1 in that above a certain pressure a single linear relationship occurs irrespective of the initial bed density.

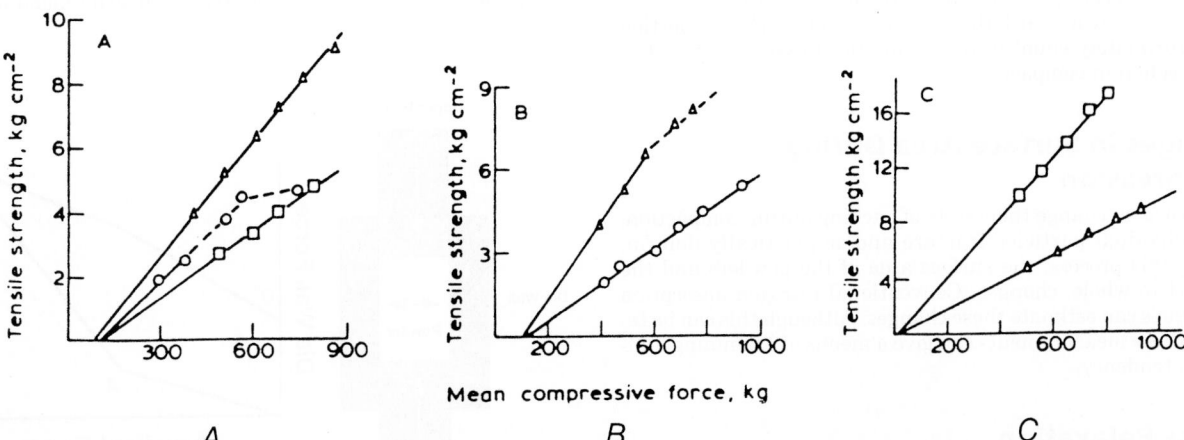

Figure 45-4. Tensile strength of compacts prepared from different crystal forms. *A:* Barbitone (104–152 μm)—○, Form I; □, Form II; △, Form III. *B:* Sulfathiazole (104–152 μm)—○, Form I; △, Form II. *C:* Aspirin (250–353 μm)—△, Form I; □, Form IV. (From Summers MP, Enever RP, Carless JE. *J Pharm Sci* 1977; 66:1172.)

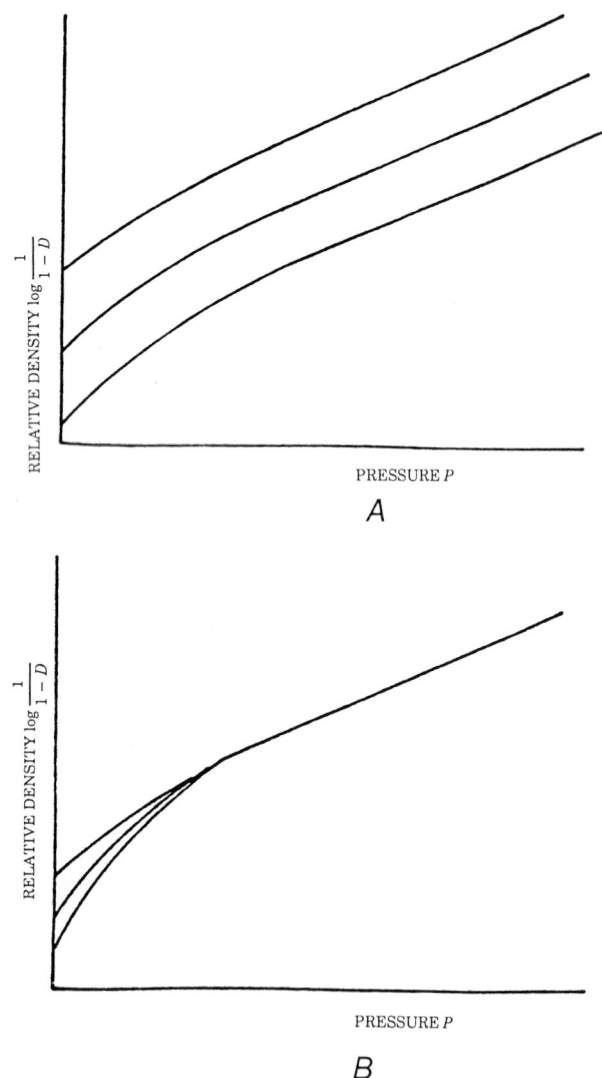

Figure 45-5. Heckel plots. *A:* Type I. *B:* Type II. (From Jones TM. *Acta Pharm Tech* 1978.)

This is independent of particle size and is probable due to fragmentation of particles and their subsequent compaction by plastic deformation. For Type 1 materials, no such fracture occurs, but adjacent particles simply deform plastically.

The pressure at which the plots transition to a linear portion is approximately equal to the minimum pressure required to form a coherent compact.

Changes in Surface Area During Compression

Bulk powders change their state of packing during compaction, and individual particles fracture and/or plastically deform. During this process, the surface area of the powders and the compact in whole, changes. Conventional nitrogen absorption techniques can estimate these changes. Although this can be tedious, these measurements can give a means of examining lamination tendency.

Stress Relaxation

The experimental technique consists of holding the compression process at a point of maximum compression and observing the compression force over various periods of time. By increas-

ing the duration of this period (dwell time), plastic flow is maximized, and tablet strength increases.

Stress Transmissions during Compression

If the stresses in the upper punch, lower punch, and die wall are monitored, as in Figure 45-6, a general plot can be constructed showing the relationship between these forces. The elastic limit is reached at point *A*. At point *B,* the applied force is released, and the transmitted force on the wall of the die falls rapidly. The upper punch ceases to contact the powder/compact at point *C,* where the transmitted force falls rapidly to a residual force, point *D*. The force needed to eject the tablet from the die must be greater than the residual force holding it to the sides of the die. Therefore, residual forces tend to be proportional to ejection forces. In addition, these plots can give a good assessment of the elastic component of the compaction process of a powder.

Work and Compaction

Force-displacement (*F-D*) curves are useful in determining the *work* involved in forming a compact. Curves, such as shown in Figure 45-7,[29] represent the work of the compression process, but all compacts expand somewhat during decompression, and this force is transferred back to the punch. Therefore, by performing a second compression of the compact, the second result can be subtracted from the first for a *corrected F-D curve*. The corrected curve represents the work associated with plastic deformation during powder compaction, as well as a determination of the work of friction of the die wall and the work of elastic deformation.

GRANULATION METHODS

Wet Granulation

The most widely used and most general method of tablet preparation is the wet-granulation method. Its popularity is due to the greater probability that the granulation will meet all the physical requirements for the compression of good tablets. Its chief disadvantages are the number of separate steps involved, as well as the time and labor necessary to carry out the procedure, especially on a large scale. The steps in the wet method are weighing, mixing, granulation, screening the damp mass, drying, dry screening, lubrication, and compression. The equipment involved depends on the quantity or size of the batch. The active ingredient, diluent, and disintegrant are mixed or blended well. For small batches the ingredients may be mixed in stainless steel bowls or mortars. Small-scale blending also

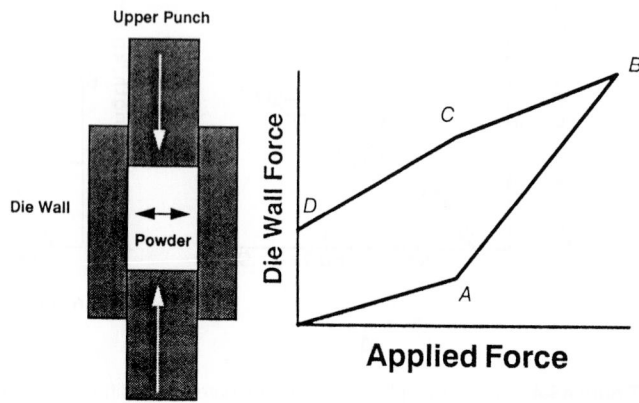

Figure 45-6. Transmitted stresses during tablet compaction.

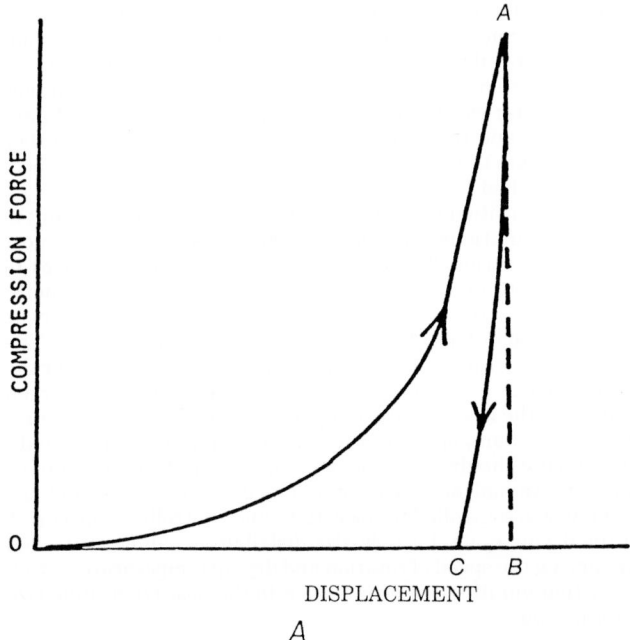

A

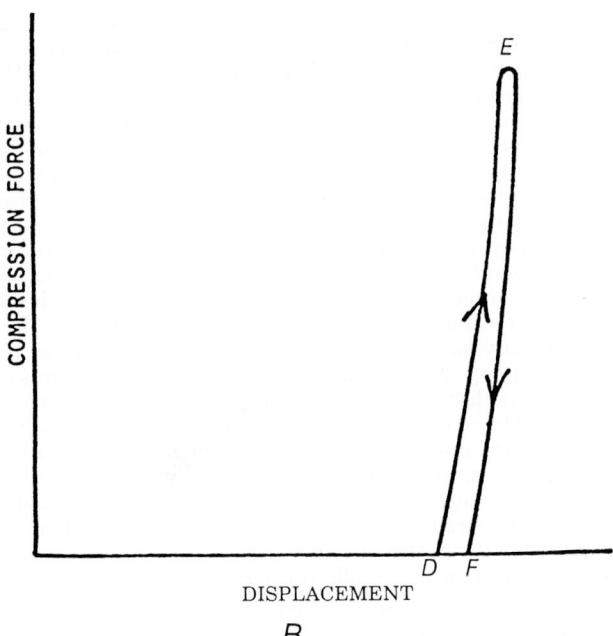

B

Figure 45-7. Typical forces. *A:* Displacement (F–D) curve; *B:* displacement (F–D), second compression. (From Jones TM. *Acta Pharm Tech* 1978.)

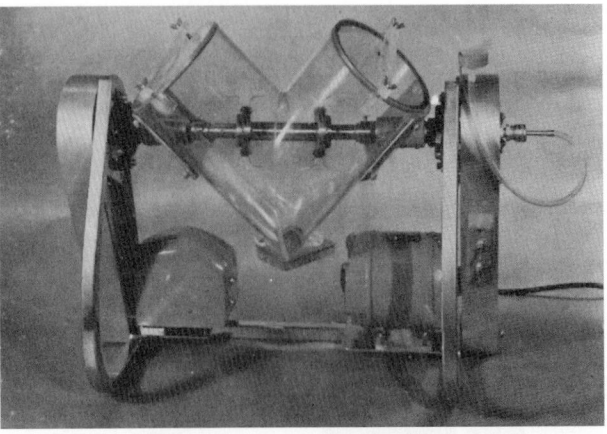

Figure 45-8. Twin-shell blender for solids or liquid-solids blending (courtesy, Patterson-Kelley).

the Glen mixer and the Hobart mixer) have served this function in the pharmaceutical industry for many years (Fig 45-9). On a large scale, ribbon blenders also are employed frequently and may be adapted for continuous-production procedures. Mass mixers of the sigma-blade type have been used widely in the pharmaceutical industry.

Highly popular are the high-speed, high-shear mixers such as the Diosna, Fielder, Lodige/Littleford, and Baker-Perkins. For these mixers a full range of sizes are available. The processing of granulations in these machines is generally faster than in conventional granulators. However, control over the process is critical, and scale-up issues may become extremely important.[30] Fluid-bed granulation (discussed below) also is gaining wide acceptance in the industry. For both of these types of processing, slight modifications to the following procedures are required.

can be carried out on a large piece of paper by holding the opposite edges and tumbling the material back and forth. The powder blend may be sifted through a screen of suitable fineness to remove or break up lumps. This screening also affords additional mixing. The screen selected always should be of the same type of wire or cloth that will not affect the potency of the ingredients through interaction. For example, the stability of ascorbic acid is affected deleteriously by even small amounts of copper, thus care must be taken to avoid contact with copper or copper-containing alloys.

For larger quantities of powder, the Patterson-Kelley twin-shell blender and the double-cone blender offer a means of precision blending and mixing in short periods of time (Fig 45-8). Twin-shell blenders are available in many sizes from laboratory models to large production models. Planetary mixers (eg,

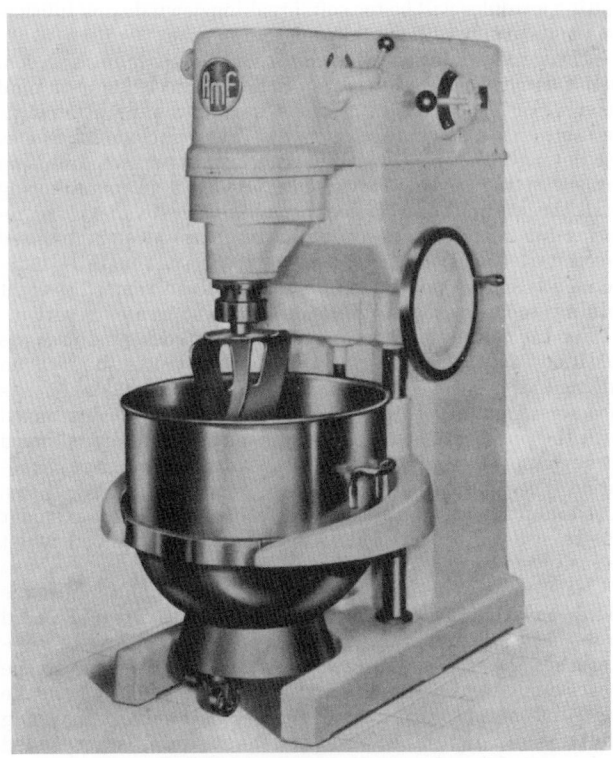

Figure 45-9. The Glen powder mixer (courtesy, Am Machine).

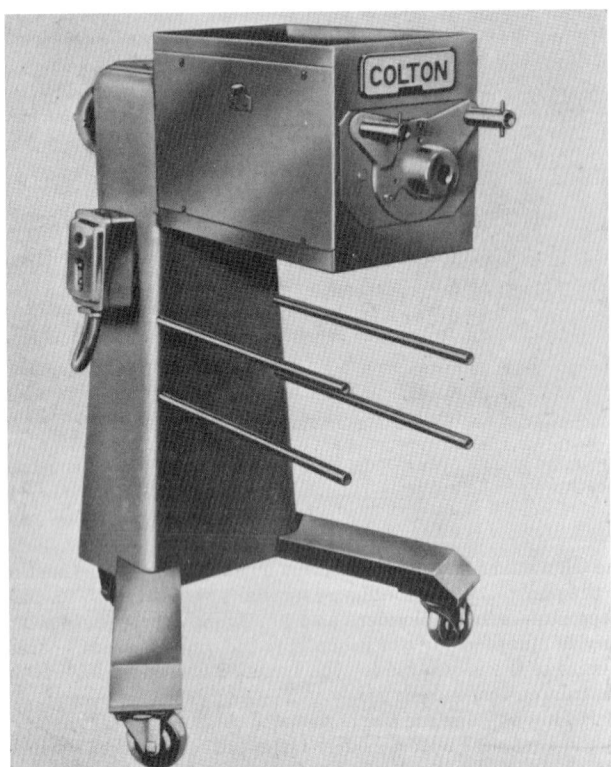

Figure 45-10. Rotary granulator and sifter (courtesy, Vector/Colton).

Solutions of the binding agent are added to the mixed powders with stirring. The powder mass is wetted with the binding solution until the mass has the consistency of damp snow or brown sugar. If the granulation is over-wetted, the granules will be hard, requiring considerable pressure to form the tablets, and the resultant tablets may have a mottled appearance. If the powder mixture is not wetted sufficiently, the resulting granules will be too soft, breaking down during lubrication and causing difficulty during compression.

The wet granulation is forced through a 6- or 8-mesh screen. Small batches can be forced through by hand using a manual screen. For larger quantities, one of several comminuting mills suitable for wet screening can be used. These include the Stokes oscillator, Colton rotary granulator, Fitzpatrick comminuting mill, or Stokes tornado mill. See Figure 45-10. In comminuting mills the granulation is forced through the sieving device by rotating hammers, knives, or oscillating bars. Most high-speed mixers are equipped with a chopper blade that operates independently of the main mixing blades and can replace the wet milling step, ie, can obviate the need for a separate operation.

For tablet formulations in which continuous production is justified, extruders such as the Reitz extruder have been adapted for the wet-granulation process. The extruder consists of a screw mixer with a chamber where the powder is mixed with the binding agent, and the wet mass gradually is forced through a perforated screen, forming threads of the wet granulation. The granulation then is dried by conventional methods. A semiautomatic, continuous process using the Reitz extruder has been described for the preparation of the antacid tablet Gelusil *(Warner-Lambert/Pfizer)*.

Moist material from the wet milling step traditionally was placed on large sheets of paper on shallow wire trays and placed in drying cabinets with a circulating air current and thermostatic heat control. See Figure 45-11. While tray drying was the most widely used method of drying tablet granulations in the past, fluid-bed drying is now considered the standard. In drying tablet granulation by fluidization, the material is suspended and agitated in a warm air stream while the granulation is maintained in motion. Drying tests comparing the fluidized bed

and a tray dryer for a number of tablet granulations indicated that the former was 15 times faster than the conventional method of tray drying. In addition to the decreased drying time, the fluidization method is claimed to have other advantages such as better control of drying temperatures, decreased handling costs, and the opportunity to blend lubricants and other materials into the dry granulation directly in the fluidized bed. See Figure 45-12.[31]

The application of microwave drying and infrared drying to tablet granulations has been reported as successful for most granulations tried. These methods readily lend themselves to continuous granulation operations. The study of drying methods for tablet granulations led to the development of the Rovac dryer system by Ciba/Novartis pharmacists and engineers. The dryer is similar in appearance to the cone blender except for the heating jacket and vacuum connections. By excluding oxygen and using the lower drying temperatures made possible by drying in a vacuum, opportunities for degradation of the ingredients during the drying cycle are minimized. A greater uniformity of residual moisture content is achieved because of the moving bed, controlled temperature, and controlled time period of the drying cycle. Particle-size distribution can be controlled by varying the speed of rotation and drying temperature as well as by comminuting the granulation to the desired granule size after drying.

In drying granulations it is desirable to maintain a residual amount of moisture in the granulation. This is necessary to maintain the various granulation ingredients, such as gums, in a hydrated state. Also, the residual moisture contributes to the reduction of the static electric charges on the particles. In the selection of any drying process, an effort is made to obtain a uniform moisture content. In addition to the importance of moisture content of the granulation in its handling during the manufacturing steps, the stability of the products containing moisture-sensitive active ingredients may be related to the moisture content of the products.

Previously it was indicated that water-soluble colorants can migrate toward the surface of the granulation during the drying process, resulting in mottled tablets after compression. This is also true for water-soluble drug substances, resulting in tablets unsatisfactory as to content uniformity. Migration can be reduced by drying the granulation slowly at low temperatures or using a granulation in which the major diluent is present as granules of large particle size. The presence of microcrystalline cellulose in wet granulations also reduces migration tendencies.

After drying, the granulation is reduced in particle size by passing it through a smaller-mesh screen. Following dry screening, the granule size tends to be more uniform. For dry granulations the screen size to be selected depends on the diameter of the punch. The following sizes are suggested:

Tablets up to ³⁄₁₆ inch diameter, use 20-mesh
Tablets ⁷⁄₃₂ to ⁵⁄₁₆ inch, use 16-mesh
Tablets ¹¹⁄₃₂ to ¹³⁄₃₂ inch, use 14-mesh
Tablets ⁷⁄₁₆ inch and larger, use 12-mesh

For small amounts of granulation, hand screens may be used and the material passed through with the aid of a stainless steel spatula. With larger quantities, any of the comminuting mills

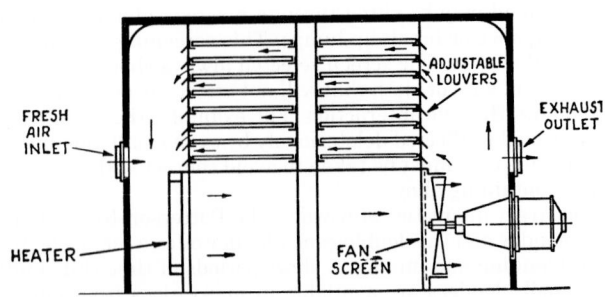

Figure 45-11. Cross-section of tray dryer.

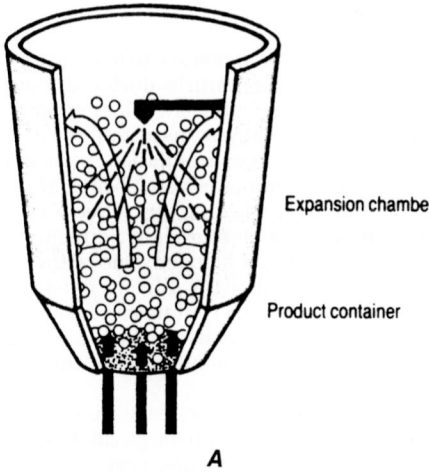

Expansion chamber

Product container

A

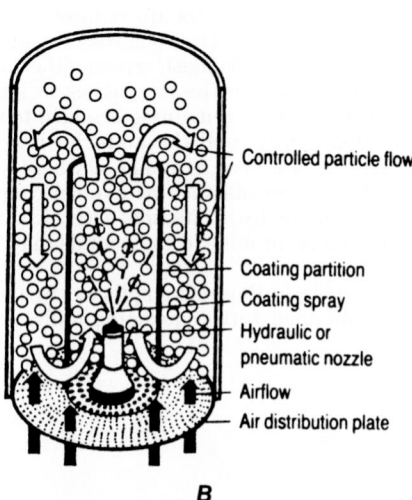

Controlled particle flow

Coating partition

Coating spray

Hydraulic or
pneumatic nozzle

Airflow

Air distribution plate

B

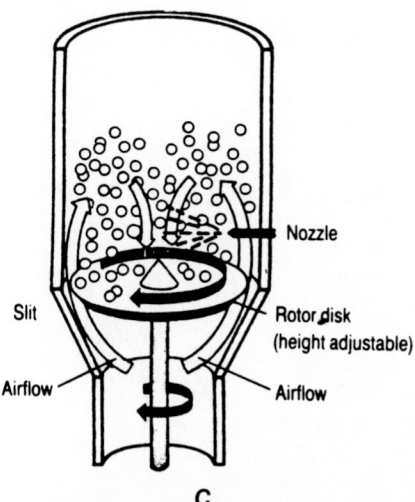

Nozzle

Slit

Rotor disk
(height adjustable)

Airflow

Airflow

C

Figure 45-12. Three versions of fluidized-bed granulation and drying. *A:*
Top-spray method used in conventional fluid-bed granulation coaters; *B:*
bottom-spray method used in Wurster air-suspension columns; *C:* tangential-spray method used in rotary fluid-bed coaters/granulators. (Courtesy, Aster Publ, adapted from Mehta AM. *Pharm Technol* 1988; 12:46.)

with screens corresponding to those just mentioned may be
used. Note that the smaller the tablet, the finer the dry granulation to enable more uniform filling of the die cavity; large granules give an irregular fill to a comparatively small die cavity.
With compressed tablets of sodium bicarbonate, lactose, and
magnesium trisilicate, a relationship has been demonstrated
between the particle size of the granulated material and the disintegration time and capping of the resultant tablets. For a sulfathiazole granulation, however, the particle-size distribution
did not appear to influence hardness or disintegration.

After dry granulation, the lubricant is added as a fine powder. It usually is screened onto the granulation through 60- or
100-mesh nylon cloth to eliminate small lumps as well as to increase the covering power of the lubricant. As it is desirable for
each granule to be covered with the lubricant, the lubricant is
blended with the granulation very gently, preferably in a
blender using a tumbling action. Gentle action is desired to
maintain the uniform granule size resulting from the granulation step. It has been claimed that too much fine powder is not
desirable because fine powder may not feed into the die evenly;
consequently, variations in weight and density result. Fine
powders, commonly designated as *fines,* also blow out around
the upper punch and down past the lower punch, making it necessary to clean the machine frequently. Fines, however, at a
level of 10–20%, traditionally are sought by the tablet formulator. The presence of some fines is necessary for the proper filling of the die cavity. Now, even higher concentrations of fines
are used successfully in tablet manufacture. Most investigators
agree that no general limits exist for the amount of fines that
can be present in a granulation; it must be determined for each
specific formula.

Many formulators once believed (and some still believe) that
overblending resulted in an increased amount of fines and,
hence, caused air entrapment in the formula. The capping and
laminating of tablets associated with overblending lubricants
was thought to be caused by these air pockets. Most scientists
now recognize that a more plausible explanation has to do with
the function of the lubricants themselves. Since the very nature
of a lubricant tends to make surfaces less susceptible to adhesion, overblending prevents the intergranular bonding that
takes place during compaction.

Fluid-Bed Granulation

A new method for granulating evolved from the fluid-bed drying technology described earlier. The concept was to spray a
granulating solution onto the suspended particles, which then
would be dried rapidly in the suspending air. The main benefit
from this system is the rapid granulation and drying of a batch.
The two main firms that developed this technology are *Glatt*
and *Aeromatic (now NIRO).* The design of these systems is basically the same with both companies (see Fig 45-12). In this
method, particles of an inert material or the active drug are
suspended in a vertical column with a rising air stream; while
the particles are suspended, the common granulating materials
in solution are sprayed into the column. There is a gradual particle buildup under a controlled set of conditions resulting in a
tablet granulation that is ready for compression after the addition of the lubricant. An obvious advantage exists, since granulating and drying can take place in a single piece of equipment.
It should be noted, however, that many of the mixers discussed
previously can be supplied with a steam jacket and vacuum and
can provide the same advantage.

In these systems a granulating solution or solvent is sprayed
into or onto the bed of suspended particles. The rate of addition
of the binder, temperature in the bed of particles, temperature
of the air, volume, and moisture of the air all play an important
role in the quality and performance of the final product. Many
scientists feel that this method is an extension of the wet-granulation method, as it incorporates many of its concepts. However anyone who has developed a formulation in a fluid-bed

system knows that the many operating parameters involved make it somewhat more complex.[31] In addition to its use for the preparation of tablet granulations, this technique also has been proposed for the coating of solid particles as a means of improving the flow properties of small particles. Researchers have observed that, in general, fluid-bed granulation yields a less dense particle than conventional methods, and this can affect subsequent compression behavior. A large-scale fluid-bed granulation process has been described for Tylenol *(McNeil)*. Methods for the preparation of compressed tablets have been reviewed in the literature.[32]

The *Merck* facility at Elkton, VA was the first completely automated tablet production facility in the world. The entire tablet-manufacturing process based on a wet-granulation method was computer-controlled. By means of a computer, the system weighed the ingredients, blended, granulated, dried, and lubricated to prepare a uniform granulation of specified particle size and particle-size distribution. The computer directed the compression of the material into tablets with exacting specifications for thickness, weight, and hardness. After compression, the tablets were coated with a water-based film coating. The computer controlled and monitored all flow of material. The plant represented the first totally automated pharmaceutical manufacturing facility. However, due to shifting market trends and the burdens of process validation and changes to processes, totally automated processes are generally not used today. Instead, many production operations focus on computer-controlled and monitored unit operations, such as seen in various tableting machines and granulators today. See Figure 45-13.

Equipment suppliers work closely with individual pharmaceutical companies in designing specialized and unique systems.

Dry Granulation

When tablet ingredients are sensitive to moisture or are unable to withstand elevated temperatures during drying, and when the tablet ingredients have sufficient inherent binding or cohesive properties, slugging may be used to form granules. This method is referred to as dry granulation, precompression, or double-compression. It eliminates a number of steps but still includes weighing, mixing, slugging, dry screening, lubrication, and compression. The active ingredient, diluent (if required), and part of the lubricant are blended. One of the constituents, either the active ingredient or the diluent, must have cohesive properties. Powdered material contains a considerable amount of air; under pressure this air is expelled, and a fairly dense piece is formed. The more time allowed for this air to escape, the better the tablet or slug.

When slugging is used, large tablets are made as slugs because fine powders flow better into large cavities. Also, producing large slugs decreases production time; 7/8 to 1 in are the most practical sizes for slugs. Sometimes, to obtain the pressure that is desired the slug sizes are reduced to 3/4 in. The punches should be flat-faced. The compressed slugs are comminuted through the desirable mesh screen either by hand or, for larger quantities, through the Fitzpatrick or similar comminuting mill. The lubricant remaining is added to the granulation and blended gently, and the material is compressed into tablets. Aspirin is a good example of where slugging is satisfactory. Other materials such as aspirin combinations, acetaminophen, thiamine hydrochloride, ascorbic acid, magnesium hydroxide, and other antacid compounds may be treated similarly.

Results comparable to those accomplished by the slugging process also are obtained with compacting mills. In the com-

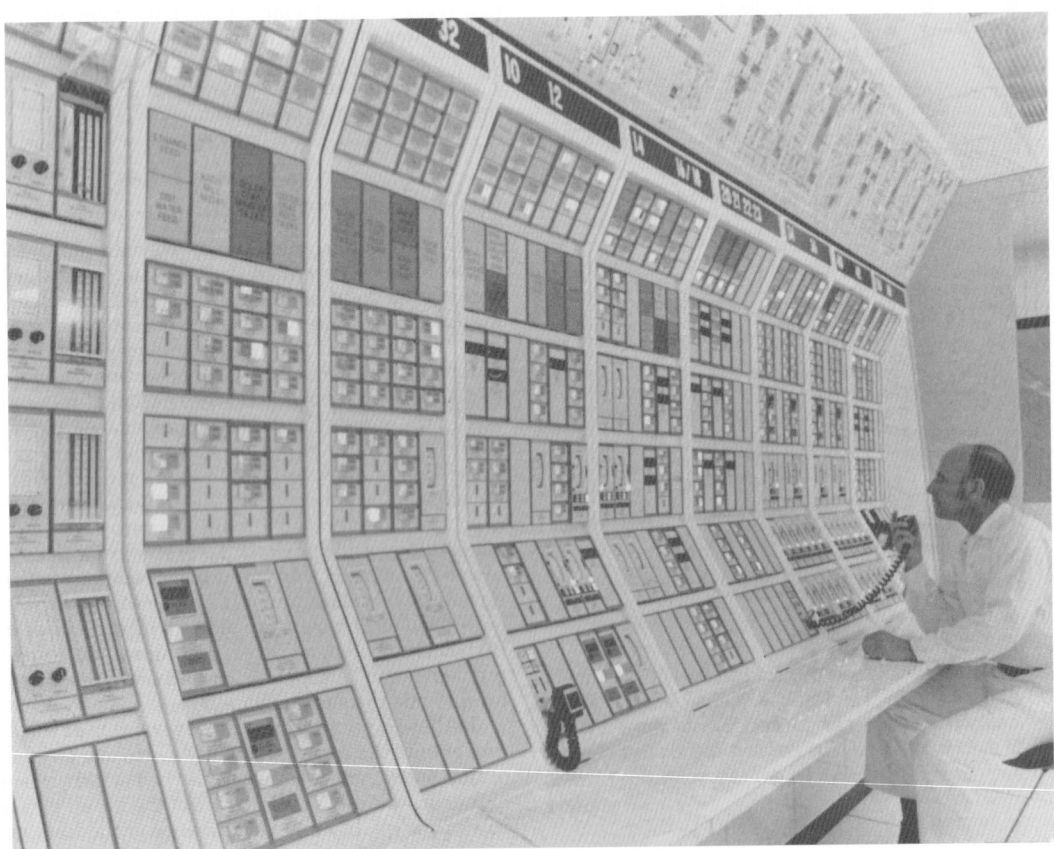

A

Figure 45-13. Fixed automated processes in the 1980s have given way to flexible micro-processor controlled unit operations. **a.** Computer control room for the first large-scale computer-controlled tablet manufacturing facility (courtesy, Merck).

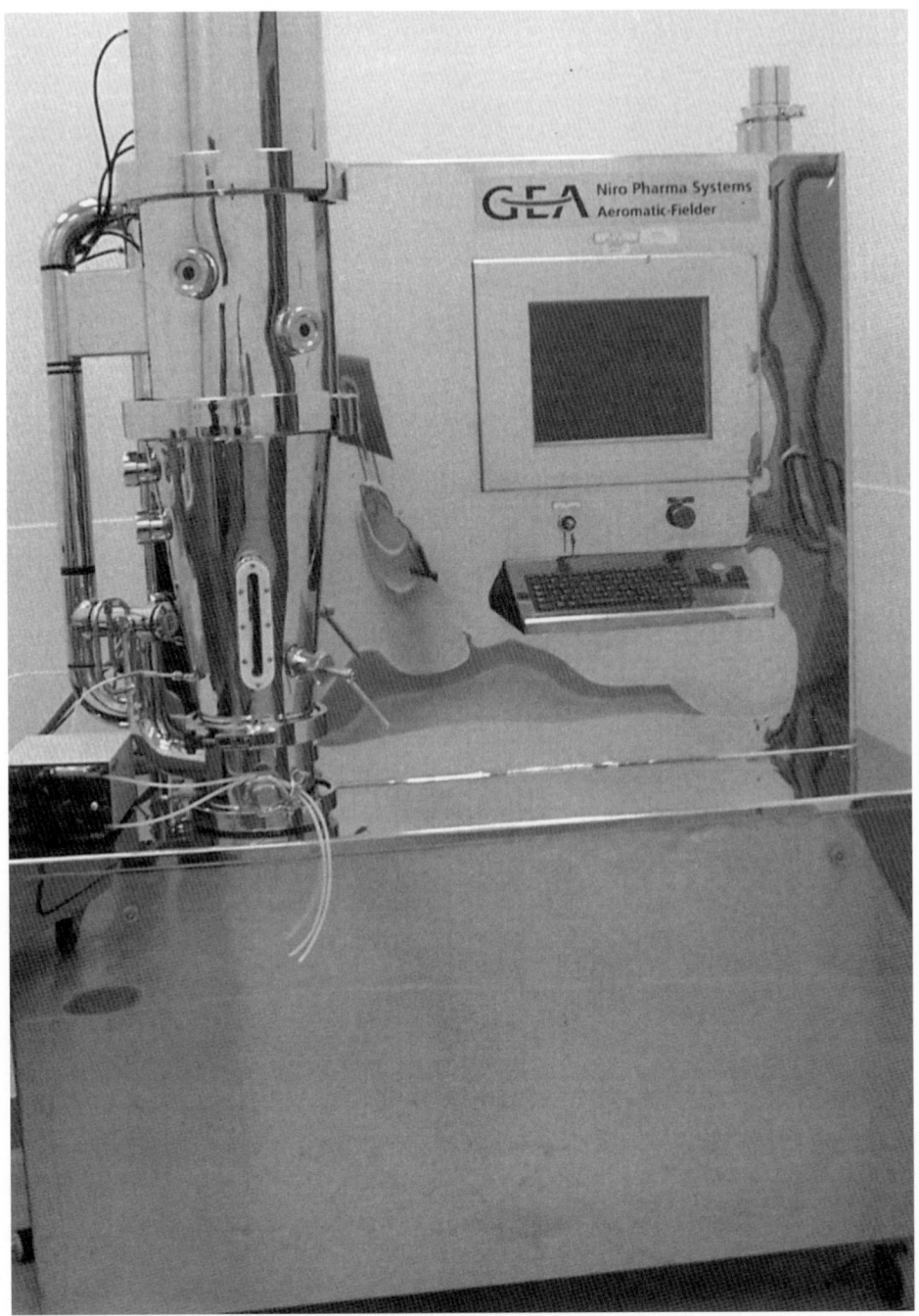

Figure 45-13. *(continued)* **b.** Computer-controlled/monitored coating.

paction method the powder to be densified passes between high-pressure rollers that compress the powder and remove the air. The densified material is reduced to a uniform granule size and compressed into tablets after the addition of a lubricant. Excessive pressures that may be required to obtain cohesion of certain materials may result in a prolonged dissolution rate. Compaction mills available include the Chilsonator *(Fitzpatrick),* Roller Compactor *(Vector),* and the Compactor Mill *(Allis-Chalmers).*

Direct Compression

As its name implies, direct compression consists of compressing tablets directly from powdered material without modifying the physical nature of the material itself. Formerly, direct compression as a method of tablet manufacture was reserved for a small group of crystalline chemicals having all the physical characteristics required for the formation of a good tablet. This group includes chemicals such as potassium salts (chlorate, chloride, bromide, iodide, nitrate, permanganate), ammonium chloride, and methenamine. These materials possess cohesive and flow properties that make direct compression possible.

Since the pharmaceutical industry constantly is making efforts to increase the efficiency of tableting operations and reduce costs by using the smallest amount of floor space and labor as possible for a given operation, increasing attention is being given to this method of tablet preparation. Approaches being used to make this method more universally applicable include the introduction of formulation additives capable of im-

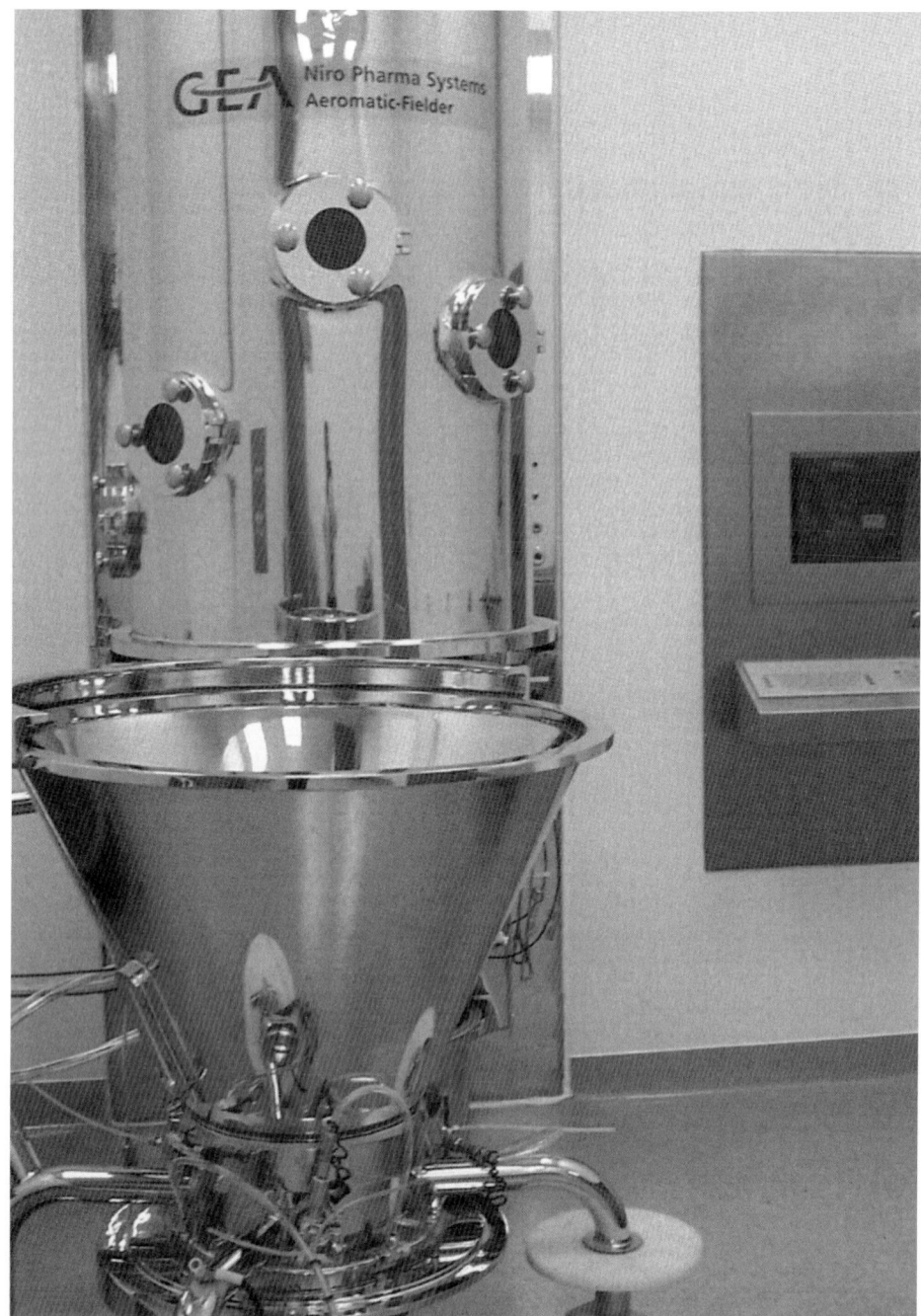

Figure 45-13. *(continued)* **c.** Computer-controlled/monitored granulation.

parting the characteristics required for compression and the use of force-feeding devices to improve the flow of powder blends.

For tablets in which the drug itself constitutes a major portion of the total tablet weight, it is necessary that the drug possess those physical characteristics required for the formulation to be compressed directly. Direct compression for tablets containing 25% or less of drug substances frequently can be used by formulating with a suitable diluent that acts as a carrier or vehicle for the drug.[32–34]

Direct-compression vehicles or carriers must have good flow and compressible characteristics. These properties are imparted to them by a preprocessing step such as wet granulation, slugging, spray drying, spheronization, or crystallization. These vehicles include processed forms of most of the common diluents including dicalcium phosphate dihydrate, tricalcium

phosphate, calcium sulfate, anhydrous lactose, spray-dried lactose, pregelatinized starch, compressible sugar, mannitol, and microcrystalline cellulose. These commercially available direct-compression vehicles may contain small quantities of other ingredients (eg, starch) as processing aids. Dicalcium phosphate dihydrate (Di-Tab, *Stauffer*) in its unmilled form has good flow properties and compressibility. It is a white, crystalline agglomerate insoluble in water and alcohol. The chemical is odorless, tasteless, and nonhygroscopic. Since it has no inherent lubricating or disintegrating properties, other additives must be present to prepare a satisfactory formulation.

Compressible sugar consists mainly of sucrose that is processed to have properties suitable for direct compression. It also may contain small quantities of dextrin, starch, or invert sugar. It is a white crystalline powder with a sweet taste and complete water solubility. It requires the incorporation of a suitable lu-

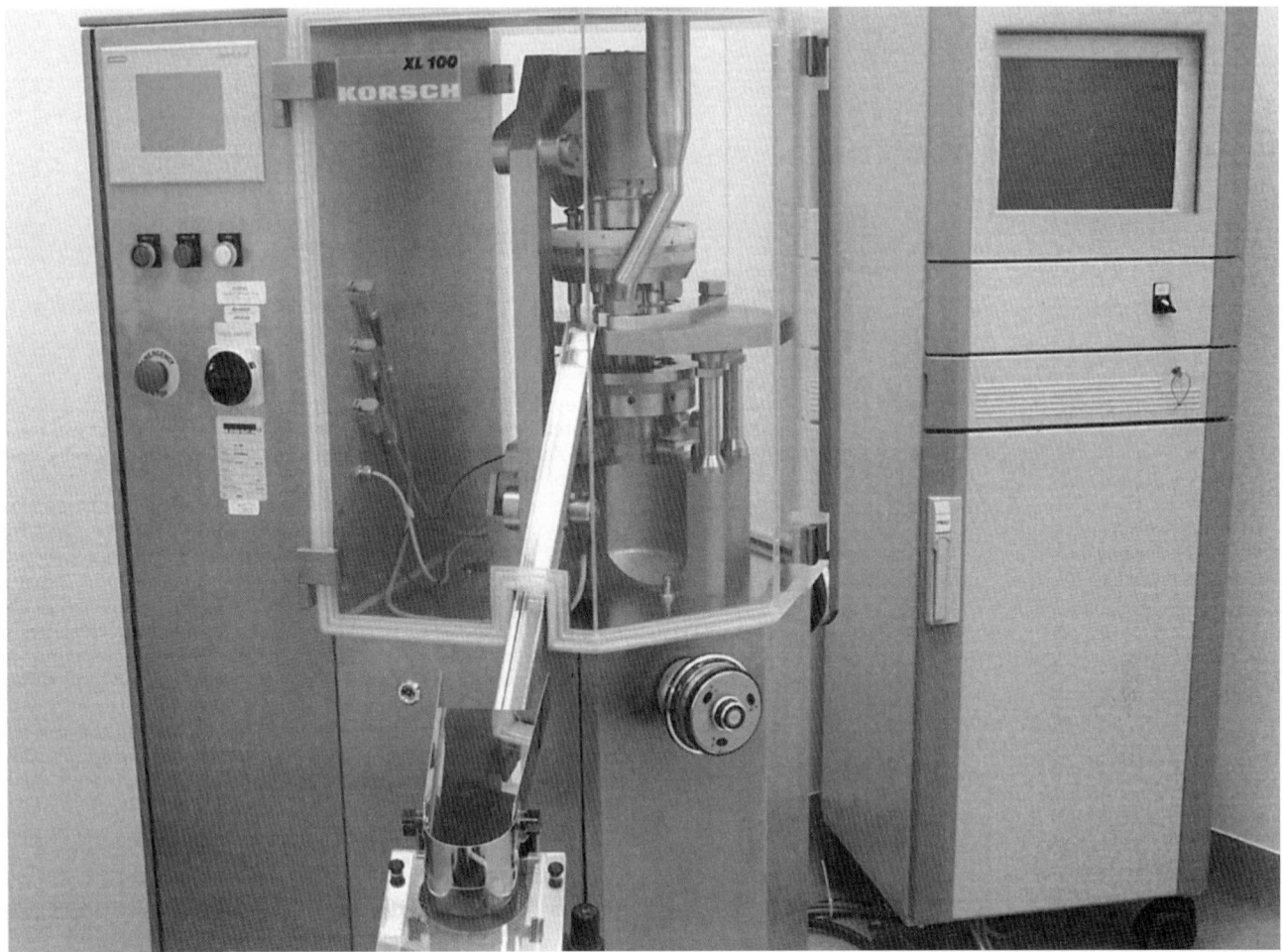

Figure 45-13. *(continued)* **d.** Computer-controlled/monitored tableting.

bricant at normal levels for lubricity. The sugar is used widely for chewable vitamin tablets because of its natural sweetness. One commercial source is Di-Pac *(Amstar)* prepared by the cocrystallization of 97% sucrose and 3% dextrins. Some forms of lactose meet the requirements for a direct-compression vehicle. Hydrous lactose does not flow, and its use is limited to tablet formulations prepared by the wet-granulation method. Both anhydrous lactose and spray-dried lactose have good flowability and compressibility and can be used in direct compression provided a suitable disintegrant and lubricant are present. Mannitol is a popular diluent for chewable tablets because of its pleasant taste and mouth feel resulting from its negative heat of solution. In its granular form *(ICI Americas)* it has good flow and compressible qualities. It has a low moisture content and is not hygroscopic.

The excipient that has been studied extensively as a direct compression vehicle is microcrystalline cellulose (Avicel, *FMC*). This nonfibrous form of cellulose is obtained by spray-drying washed, acid-treated cellulose and is available in several grades that range in average particle size from 20 to 100 μm. It is water-insoluble, but the material has the ability to draw fluid into a tablet by capillary action; it swells on contact and thus acts as a disintegrating agent. The material flows well and has a degree of self-lubricating qualities, thus requiring a lower level of lubricant than other excipients.

Forced-flow feeders are mechanical devices, available from pharmaceutical equipment manufacturers, designed to deaerate light and bulky material. Mechanically, they maintain a steady flow of powder moving into the die cavities under moderate pressure. By increasing the density of the powder,

higher uniformity in tablet weights is obtained. See Figure 45-14.

Recently, many companies have reversed their optimism for some direct-compression systems. Some formulations made by direct compression were not as *forgiving* as the older wet-granulated products were. As raw material variations occurred, especially with the drug, many companies found themselves with poorly compactable formulations. Interest in direct compression also is stimulating basic research on the flowability of powders with and without additives.

Related Granulation Processes

SPHERONIZATION—Spheronization, a form of pelletization, refers to the formation of spherical particles from wet granulations. Since the particles are round, they have good flow properties when dried. They can be formulated to contain sufficient binder to impart cohesiveness for tableting. Spheronization equipment such as the Marumerizer *(Luwa)* and the CF-Granulator *(Vector)* are commercially available for small-scale manufacture, on up to commercial sized equipment. A wet granulation containing the drug substance, diluent (if required), and binder, is passed first through an extruding machine to form rod-shaped cylindrical segments ranging in diameter from 0.5 to 12 mm. The segment diameter and the size of the final spherical particle depend on the extruder screen size. After extrusion the segments are placed into the Marumerizer where they are shaped into spheres by centrifugal and frictional forces on a rotating plate (see Fig 45-15). The

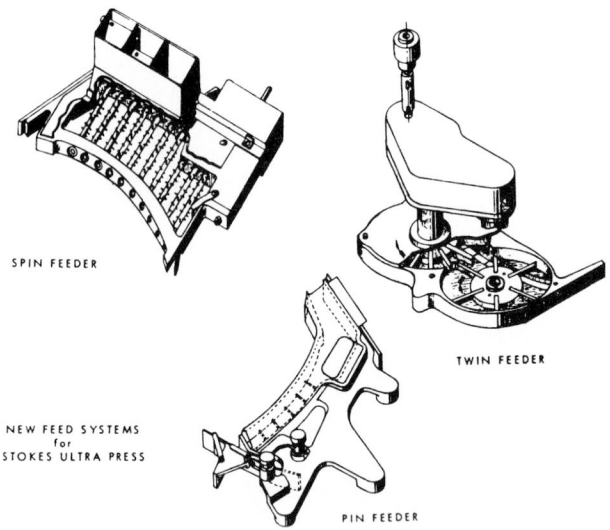

Figure 45-14. Feeding devices designed to promote flow of granulations for high-speed machines (courtesy, Stokes/Pennwalt).

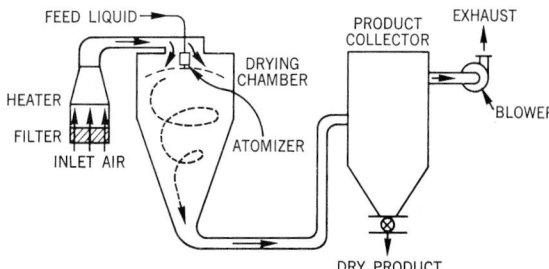

Figure 45-16. Typical spray-drying system (courtesy, Bowen Eng).

pellets then are dried by conventional methods, mixed with suitable lubricants, and compressed into tablets or used as capsule-fill material. Microcrystalline cellulose has been shown to be an effective diluent and binder in granulations to be spheronized.[35–38] The advantages of the process include the production of granules, regular in shape, size, and surface characteristics; low friability resulting in fewer fines and less dust; and the ability to regulate the size of the spheres within a narrow particle-size distribution.

Spheres also can be produced by fluid-bed granulation techniques and by other specialized equipment such as the CF-Granulator *(Vector)*. These processes, however, must begin with crystals or nonpareil seeds followed by buildup. Exact results, such as sphere density, are different for the various methods and could be important in product performance. These processes can be run as batches or continuously.

SPRAY-DRYING—A number of tableting additives suitable for direct compression have been prepared by the drying process known as spray-drying. The method consists of bringing together a highly dispersed liquid and a sufficient volume of hot air to produce evaporation and drying of the liquid droplets. The feed liquid may be a solution, slurry, emulsion, gel, or paste, provided it is pumpable and capable of being atomized. As shown in Figure 45-16, the feed is sprayed into a current of warm filtered air. The air supplies the heat for evaporation and

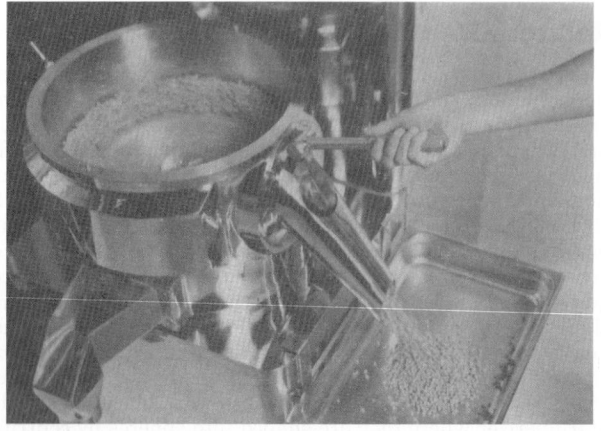

Figure 45-15. The inside of a QJ-400 Marumerizer (courtesy, Luwa).

conveys the dried product to the collector; the air is then exhausted with the moisture. As the liquid droplets present a large surface area to the warm air, local heat and transfer coefficients are high.

The spray-dried powder particles are homogeneous, approximately spherical in shape, nearly uniform in size, and frequently hollow. The latter characteristic results in low bulk density with a rapid rate of solution. Being uniform in size and spherical, the particles possess good flowability. The design and operation of the spray-dryer can vary many characteristics of the final product, such as particle size and size distribution, bulk and particle densities, porosity, moisture content, flowability, and friability. Among the spray-dried materials available for direct compression formulas are lactose, mannitol, and flour. Another application of the process in tableting is spray-drying the combination of tablet additives as the diluent, disintegrant, and binder. The spray-dried material then is blended with the active ingredient or drug, lubricated, and compressed directly into tablets.

Since atomization of the feed results in a high surface area, the moisture evaporates rapidly. The evaporation keeps the product cool and as a result the method is applicable for drying heat-sensitive materials. Among heat-sensitive pharmaceuticals successfully spray-dried are the amino acids; antibiotics as aureomycin, bacitracin, penicillin, and streptomycin; ascorbic acid; cascara extracts; liver extracts; pepsin and similar enzymes; protein hydrolysates; and thiamine.[39]

Frequently, spray-drying is more economical than other processes, since it produces a dry powder directly from a liquid and eliminates other processing steps as crystallization, precipitation, filtering or drying, particle-size reduction, and particle classifying. By the elimination of these steps, labor, equipment costs, space requirements and possible contamination of the product are reduced. Intrinsic factor concentrate obtained from hog mucosa previously was prepared by *Lederle/American Home Products*, using a salt-precipitation process followed by a freeze-drying. By using spray-drying it was possible to manufacture a high-grade material by a continuous process. The spherical particles of the product facilitated its subsequent blending with vitamin B_{12}. Similar efficiencies have been found in processes producing magnesium trisilicate and dihydroxyaluminum sodium carbonate; both chemicals are used widely in antacid preparations.

Encapsulation of chemicals also can be achieved using spray-drying equipment. The process is useful in coating one material on another to protect the interior substance or to control the rate of its release. The substance to be coated can be either liquid or solid but must be insoluble in a solution of the coating material. The oil-soluble vitamins, A and D, can be coated with a variety of materials such as acacia gum to prevent their deterioration. Flavoring oils and synthetic flavors are coated to give the so-called dry flavors.

SPRAY-CONGEALING—Also called spray-chilling, spray-congealing is a technique similar to spray-drying. It consists of melting solids and reducing them to beads or powder by spraying the molten feed into a stream of air or other gas. The same basic equipment is used as with spray-drying, although

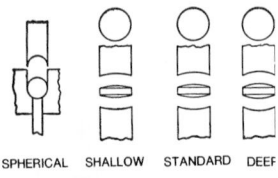

Figure 45-17. Concave punches.

no source of heat is required. Either ambient or cooled air is used, depending on the freezing point of the product. For example, monoglycerides and similar materials are spray-congealed with air at 50°F. A closed-loop system with refrigeration cools and recycles the air. Using this process, drugs can be dissolved or suspended in a molten wax and spray-congealed; the resultant material then can be adapted for a prolonged-release form of the drug.

Among the carbohydrates used in compressed tablets, mannitol is the only one that possesses high heat stability. Mannitol melts at 167° and, either alone or in combination with other carbohydrates, can be fused and spray-congealed. Selected drugs have been shown to be soluble in these fused mixtures, and the resultant spray-congealed material possesses excellent flow and compression characteristics.

TABLET MACHINES

As mentioned previously, the basic mechanical unit in tablet compression involves the operation of two steel punches within a steel die cavity. The tablet is formed by the pressure exerted on the granulation by the punches within the die cavity, or cell. The tablet assumes the size and shape of the punches and die used. See Figures 45-17 and 45-18. While round tablets are used more generally, oval, capsule-form, square, triangular, or other irregular shapes may be used. Likewise, the curvature of the faces of the punches determines the curvature of the tablets. The diameters generally found to be satisfactory and frequently referred to as standard are as follows: ³⁄₁₆, ⁷⁄₃₂, ¼, ⁹⁄₃₂, ⁵⁄₁₆, ¹¹⁄₃₂, ⁷⁄₁₆, ½, ⁹⁄₁₆, ⅝, ¹¹⁄₁₆, and ¾ in. Punch faces with ridges are used for compressed tablets scored for breaking into halves or fourths, although it has been indicated that variation among tablet halves is significantly greater than among intact tablets. However, a patented formulation[40] for a tablet scored to form a groove that is one-third to two-thirds the depth of the total tablet thickness is claimed to give equal parts containing substantially equal amounts of the drug substance. Tablets, engraved or embossed with symbols or initials, require punches with faces embossed or engraved with the corresponding designs. See Figures 45-19 and 45-20. The use of the tablet sometimes determines its shape; effervescent tablets are usually large, round, and flat, while vitamin tablets frequently are prepared in capsule-shaped forms. Tablets prepared using deep-cup punches appear to be round and when coated take on the appearance of pills. Veterinary tablets often have a bolus shape and are much larger than those used in medical practice.

The quality-control program for punches and dies, frequently referred to as tooling, instituted by large pharmaceutical companies, emphasizes the importance of their care in modern pharmaceutical production. To produce physically perfect compressed tablets, an efficient punch-and-die program must be set up. Provisions for inspection of tooling, parameters for cost-per-product determination, product identification, and tooling specifications must all be considered. A committee of the Industrial and Pharmaceutical Technology Section of the APhA Academy of Pharmaceutical Sciences established a set of dimensional specifications and tolerances for standard punches and dies.[41]

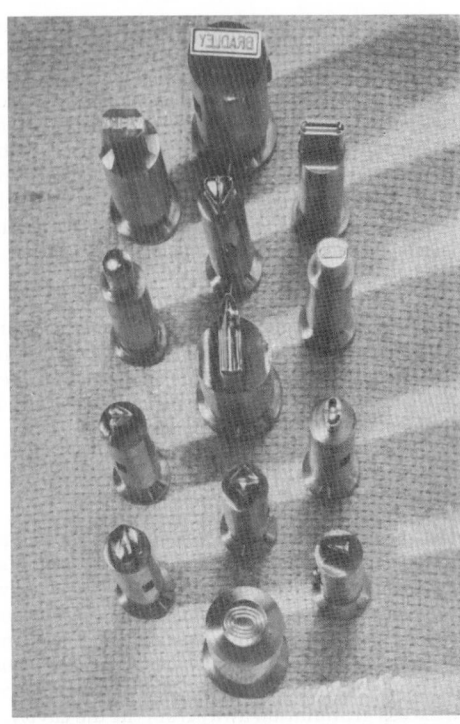

Figure 45-19. Collection of punches (courtesy, Stokes/Pennwalt).

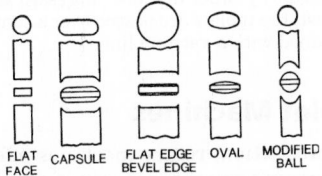

Figure 45-18. Specially shaped punches.

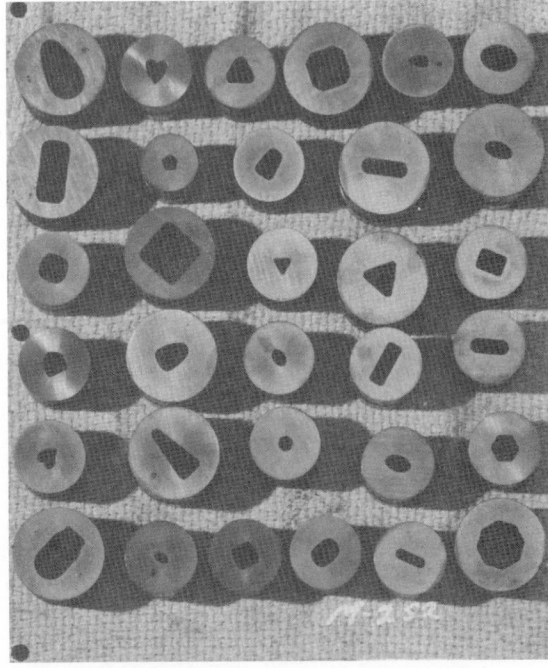

Figure 45-20. Collection of dies (courtesy, Stokes/Pennwalt).

Regardless of the size of the tableting operation, the attention that must be given to the proper care of punches and dies should be noted. They must be highly polished and kept free from rust and imperfections. In cases in which the material pits or abrades the dies, chromium-plated dies have been used. Dropping the punches on hard surfaces will chip their fine edges. When the punches are in the machine, the upper and lower punches should not be allowed to contact each other; otherwise, a curling or flattening of the edges will result that is one of the causes of capping. This is especially necessary to observe in the case of deep-cup punches.

When the punches are removed from the machine, they should be washed thoroughly in warm soapy water and dried well with a clean cloth. A coating of grease or oil should be rubbed over all parts of the dies and punches to protect them from the atmosphere. They should be stored carefully in boxes or paper tubes.

Single-Punch Machines

The simplest tableting machines available are those having the single-punch design. A number of models are available as outlined in Table 45-2. While most of these are power-driven, several hand-operated models are available. Compression is accomplished on a single-punch machine as shown in Figure 45-21. The feed shoe filled with the granulation is positioned over the die cavity, which then fills. The feed shoe retracts and scrapes all excess granulation away from the die cavity. The upper punch lowers to compress the granulation within the die cavity. The upper punch retracts, and the lower punch rises to eject the tablet. As the feed shoe returns to fill the die cavity, it pushes the compressed tablet from the die platform. The weight of the tablet is determined by the volume of the die cavity; the lower punch is adjustable to increase or decrease the volume of granulation, thus increasing or decreasing the weight of the tablet.

For tablets having diameters larger than 1/2 inch, sturdier models are required. This is also true for tablets requiring a high degree of hardness, as in the case of compressed lozenges. The heavier models are capable of much higher pressures and are suitable for slugging.

OPERATION OF SINGLE-PUNCH MACHINES—In installing punches and dies in a single-punch machine, insert the lower punch first by lining up the notched groove on the punch with the lower punch setscrew and slipping it into the smaller bore in the die table; the setscrew is not tightened yet. The lower punch is differentiated from the upper punch in that it has a collar around the punch head. Slip the die over the punch head so that the notched groove (with the widest area at the top) lines up with the die setscrew. Tighten the lower punch setscrew after seating the lower punch by pressing on the punch with the thumb. Tighten the die setscrew, making certain that the surface of the die is flush with the die table. Insert the upper punch, again lining up the grooved notch with the upper punch setscrew. To be certain that the upper punch is seated securely, turn the machine over by hand with a block of soft wood or wad of cloth between the upper and lower punches. When the punch is seated, tighten the upper punch setscrew. Adjust the pressure so that the upper and lower punches will not come

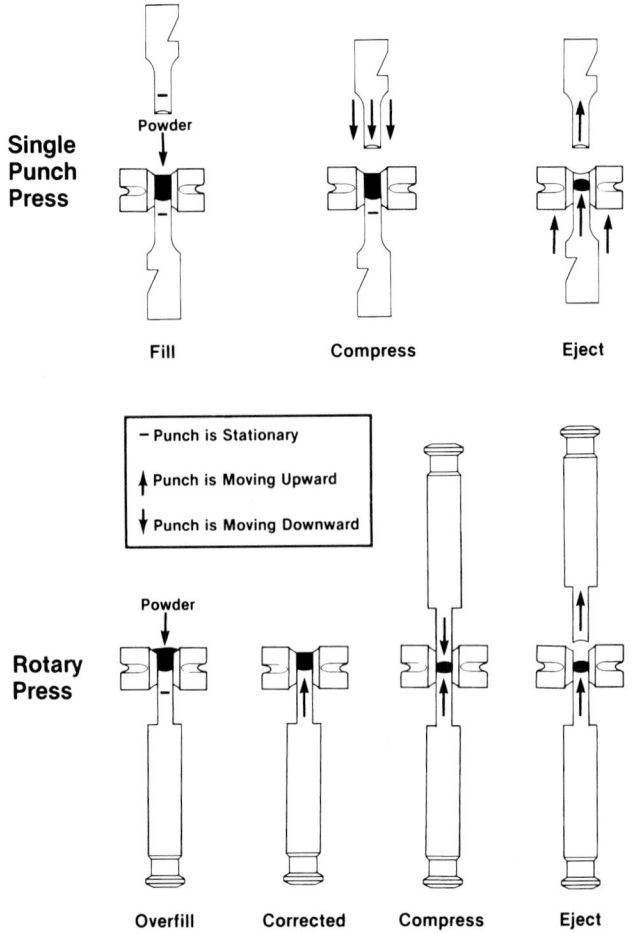

Figure 45-21. The steps associated with single-punch and rotary tablet machines.

in contact with each other when the machine is turned over. Adjust the lower punch so that it is flush with the die table at the ejection point. Install the feed shoe and hopper.

After adding a small amount of granulation to the hopper, turn the machine over by hand and adjust the pressure until a tablet is formed. Adjust the tablet weight until the desired weight is obtained. The pressure will have to be altered concurrently with the weight adjustments. It should be remembered that as the fill is increased the lower punch moves farther away from the upper punch, and more pressure will have to be applied to obtain comparable hardness. Conversely, when the fill is decreased, the pressure will have to be decreased. When all the adjustments have been made, fill the hopper with granulation and turn on the motor. Hardness and weight should be checked immediately, and suitable adjustments made if necessary. Periodic checks should be made on the tablet hardness and weight during the running of the batch, at 15- to 30-min intervals.

When the batch has been run off, turn off the power and remove loose dust and granulation with the vacuum cleaner. Release the pressure from the punches. Remove the feed hopper and the feed shoe. Remove the upper punch, the lower punch, and the die. Clean all surfaces of the tablet machine, and dry well with clean cloth. Cover surfaces with thin coating of grease or oil prior to storage.

As tablets are ejected from the machine after compression, they usually are accompanied by powder and uncompressed granulation. To remove this loose dust, the tablets are passed over a screen, which may be vibrating, and cleaned with a vacuum line.

Rotary Tablet Machines

For increased production, rotary machines offer great advantages. A head carrying a number of sets of punches and dies revolves continuously while the tablet granulation runs from the

Table 45-2. Single-Punch Tablet Machines

MACHINE MODEL	MAXIMUM TABLET DIAMETER (INCHES)	PRESS SPEED (TABLETS/MIN)	DEPTH OF FILL (INCHES)
Stokes-Pennwalt equipment[a]			
511-5	½	40–75	⁷⁄₁₆
206-4	1¾	10–40	1¹⁄₁₆
530-1	2	12–48	1⅝
525-2	3	16–48	2
Manesty equipment (Thomas Eng)			
Hand machine	½	100	⁷⁄₁₆
Model F3	⅞	85	1¹¹⁄₁₆
Model 35T[a]	3	36	2¼

[a] Widely used for veterinary boluses.

hopper, through a feed frame and into the dies placed in a large, steel plate revolving under it. This method promotes a uniform fill of the die and therefore an accurate weight for the tablet. Compression takes place as the upper and lower punches pass between a pair of rollers, as can be seen in Figure 45-21. This action produces a slow squeezing effect on the material in the die cavity from the top and bottom and so gives a chance for the entrapped air to escape. The lower punch lifts up and ejects the tablet. Adjustments for tablet weight and hardness can be made without the use of tools while the machine is in operation. Figure 45-22 shows a high speed press. Figure 45-23 shows the tooling in a 16-station rotary press in the positions of a complete cycle to produce 1 tablet per set of tooling. One of the factors that contributes to the variation in tablet weight and hardness during compression is the internal flow of the granulation within the feed hopper.

On most rotary machine models there is an excess pressure release that cushions each compression and relieves the machine of all shocks and undue strain. The punches and dies can be removed readily for inspection, cleaning, and inserting different sets to produce a great variety of sizes and shapes. Many older presses have been modernized with protective shields to prevent physical injury and to comply with OSHA standards (Fig 45-24). It is possible to equip the machine with as few punches and dies as the job requires and thus economize on installation costs. For types of rotary machines available, see Table 45-3.

OPERATION OF ROTARY MACHINES—Before inserting punches and dies, make certain that the pressure has been released from the pressure wheel. The die holes should be cleaned thoroughly, making certain that the die seat is completely free of any foreign materials. Back off all die locks, and loosely insert dies into the die holes, then tap each die securely into place with a fiber of soft metal rod through the upper punch holes. After all the dies have been tapped into place, tighten each die lockscrew progressively and securely. As each screw is tightened the die is checked to see that it does not project above the die table. Insert the lower punches through the hole made available by removing the punch head. Turn the machine by hand until the punch bore coincides with the plug hole. Insert each lower punch in its place progressively. Insert the upper punches by

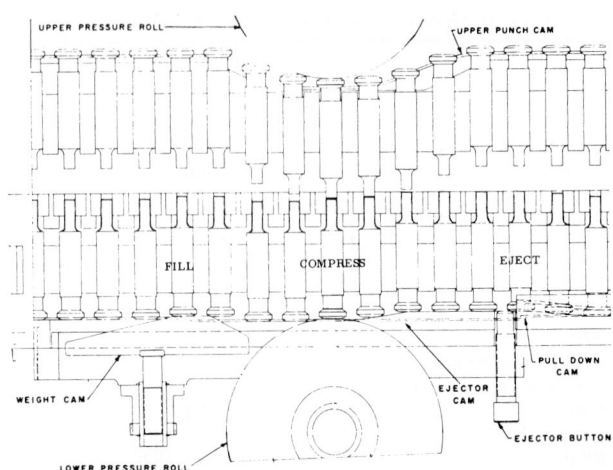

Figure 45-23. Tooling for a 16-station rotary press showing positions of the cycle required to produce one tablet per set of tooling (courtesy, Vector/Colton).

dropping them into place in the head. Each punch (upper and lower) should be coated with a thin film of mineral oil before insertion into the machine. Adjust the ejection cam so that the lower punch is flush with the die table at the ejection point.

After insertion of the punches and dies, adjust the machine for the tablet weight and hardness. The feed frame should be attached to the machine along with the feed hopper. Add a small amount of the granulation through the hopper and turn over the machine by hand. Increase the pressure by rotating the pressure wheel until a tablet is formed. Check the weight of the tablet and adjust the fill to provide the desired tablet weight. Most likely more than one adjustment of the fill will be necessary before obtaining the acceptable weight. When the fill is decreased, the pressure must be decreased to provide the same hardness in the tablet. Conversely, when the fill is increased, the pressure must be increased to obtain comparable hardness.

Fill the hopper with the granulation and turn on the power. Check tablet weight and hardness immediately after the mechanical operation begins, and make suitable adjustments, if necessary. Check these properties routinely and regularly at 15- to 30-min intervals while the machine is in operation. When the batch has been run, turn off the power. Remove the hopper and feed frame from the machine. Remove loose granulation and dust with a vacuum line. Remove all pressure from the wheel. Remove the punches and dies in the reverse order of that used in setting up the machine. First, remove the upper punches individually,

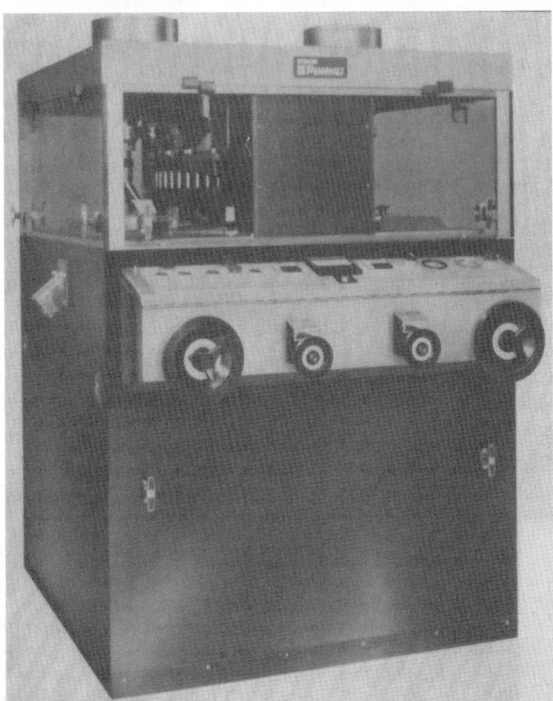

Figure 45-22. Model 747 High Speed Press, double-sided rotary compacting press designed to produce at speeds over 10,000/min (courtesy, Stokes/Pennwalt).

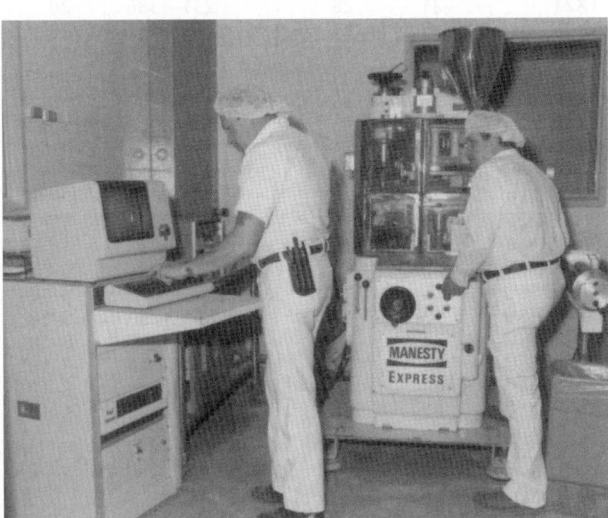

Figure 45-24. Research technicians use an instrumented tablet press to develop processes at Schering-Plough.

Table 45-3. High-Speed Rotary Tablet Machines

MACHINE MODEL	TOOL SETS	MAXIMUM TABLET DIAMETER (INCHES)	PRESS SPEED (TABLETS/MIN)	DEPTH OF FILL (INCHES)
Vector-Colton equipment				
2216	16	5/8	1180	3/4
240	16	7/8	640	13/16
250	12	1 1/4	480	1 1/8
260	25	1 3/16	1450	1 3/8
	31	1	1800	1 3/8
	33	15/16	1910	1 3/8
	43	5/8	2500	1 3/8
270	25	1 3/8	450	2 3/4
Stokes/Pennwalt equipment				
Manesty equipment (Thomas Eng)				
B3B	16	5/8	350–700	11/16
	23	7/16	500–1000	11/16
BB3B	27	5/8	760–1520	11/16
	33	7/16	924–1848	11/16
	35	5/8	1490–2980	11/16
	45	7/16	1913–3826	11/16
D3B	16	1	260–520	13/16
Key equipment				
DC-16	16	15/16	210–510	13/16
BBC	27	5/8	1025–2100	11/16
	35	5/8	1325–2725	11/16
	45	7/16	1700–3500	11/16
Cadpress	37	15/16	850–3500	13/16
	45	5/8	2000–6000	11/16
	55	7/16	2500–7500	11/16
Fette equipment (Raymond Auto)		(mm)		(mm)
Perfecta 1000	28	16	2100	18
	33	13	2475	18
Perfecta 2000	29	25	2175	22
	36	16	3600	18
	43	13	4300	18
Courtoy equipment (AC Compact)				
R-100	24	25	285–2260	20
	30	19	356–2850	20
	36	13	550–440	16
Kikusui equipment				
Hercules	18	37	180–540	16
	21	26	210–630	16
	29	25	290–870	16
Virgo	19	16	418–1330	16
	24	11	528–1680	16
Killian equipment				
TX21	21	28	231–1386	20
TX25	25	22	275–2166	20
TX30	30	16	330–3150	20
TX21D	21	25	231–1826	20
TX30A	30	16	330–3150	16
TX40A	40	13	440–4200	16
Korsch equipment				
PH 250/20	20	25	240–1640	22
PH 250/25	25	16	270–2700	18
PH 250/30	30	13	315–3233	18
Elizabeth-Hata equipment				
AP-15-SSU	15	17	300–1050	8–18
AP-18-SSU	18	13	360–1260	8–18
AP-22-SSU	22	11	440–1540	8–18
AP-32-SSU	32	17	640–2240	8–18
AP-38-MSU	38	13	760–2660	8–18
AP-45-MSU	32	11	900–3150	8–18
Vector-Colton equipment				
2247	33	5/8	3480	3/4
	41	7/16	4300	3/4
	49	7/16	5150	3/4
Magna	66	22/32	10,560	3/4
	74	1/2	11,840	3/4
	90	7/16	14,400	3/4

MACHINE MODEL	TOOL SETS	MAXIMUM TABLET DIAMETER (INCHES)	PRESS SPEED (TABLETS/MIN)	DEPTH OF FILL (INCHES)
Stokes/Pennwalt equation				
552-2	35	5/8	800–3200	1 1/16
328-4	45	3/4	1600–4500	1 3/8
610	65	7/16	3500–10,000	1 1/16
747	65	7/16	3000–10,000	1 1/16
	53	5/8	2900–8100	1 1/16
	41	15/16	2150–6150	1 1/16
Direct Triple Compression Type				
580-1	45	7/16	525–2100	1 1/16
580-2	35	5/8	400–1600	1 1/16
610	65	7/16	3500–10,000	1 1/16
	53	5/8	2900–8100	1 1/16
Manesty equipment (Thomas Eng)				
Betapress	16	5/8	600–1500	1 1/16
	23	7/16	860–2160	1 1/16
Express	20	1	800–2000	13/16
	25	5/8	1000–2500	1 1/16
	30	7/16	1200–3000	1 1/16
Unipress	20	1	970–2420	13/16
	27	5/8	1300–3270	1 1/16
	34	7/16	1640–4120	1 1/16
Novapress	37	1	760–3700	13/16
	45	5/8	900–4500	1 1/16
	61	7/16	1220–6100	1 1/16
BB3B	35	5/8	1490–2980	1 1/16
BB4	27	5/8	900–2700	1 1/16
	35	5/8	1167–3500	1 1/16
	45	7/16	1500–4500	1 1/16
Rotapress				
Mark IIA	37	1	710–3550	13/16
	45	5/8	1640–8200	1 1/16
	61	7/16	2200–11,100	1 1/16
Mark IV	45	1	2090–6000	13/16
	55	5/8	2550–7330	1 1/16
	75	7/16	3500–10,000	1 1/16
Fette tool systems		(mm)		(mm)
PT 2080	29	25	435–2900	18
	36	16	540–4100	18
	43	16	645–4900	18
PT 2090IC	22	34	1760	18
	29	25	2900	18
	36	16	4140	18
	43	13	5160	18
	47	11	6110	18
PT 3090IC	37	34	5920	18
	49	25	7840	18
	61	16	9760	18
P 3100	37	25	5618	22
	45	16	8100	18
	55	13	9900	18
Courtoy equipment (AC Compact)				
R-200	43	25	750–5833	20
	55	19	916–8500	20
	65	13	1083–10,000	16
Kikusui equipment				
Libra	36	16	900–2520	16
	45	11	1125–3150	16
	49	8	1225–3430	16
Gemini	55	16	2200–7700	16
	67	11	2680–9380	16
	73	8	2920–10,200	16
Elizabeth-Hata equipment				
AP-45-LDU	45	17	1800–6300	8–18
AP-55-LDU	55	13	2200–7700	8–18
AP-65-LDU	65	11	2600–9100	8–18
AP-71-LDU	71	11	2840–9940	8–18
51-XLDU	51	17	2040–7140	8–18
65-XLDU	61	13	2440–8540	8–18

then the lower punches, and finally the dies. Wash each punch and die in alcohol and brush with a soft brush to remove adhering material. Dry them with a clean cloth, and cover them with a thin coating of grease or oil before storing.

High-Speed Rotary Tablet Machines

The rotary tablet machine has evolved gradually into models capable of compressing tablets at high production rates. See Figures 45-22, 45-25, and 45-26. This has been accomplished by increasing the number of stations, ie, sets of punches and dies, in each revolution of the machine head, improving feeding devices, and on some models installing dual compression points. In Figure 45-26, the drawing shows a rotary machine with dual compression points. Rotary machines with dual compression points are referred to as double rotary machines, and those with one compression point, single rotary. In the diagram, half of the tablets are produced 180° from the tablet chute. They travel outside the perimeter and discharge with the second tablet production. While these models are mechanically capable of operating at the production rates shown in Table 45-3, the actual speed still depends on the physical characteristics of the tablet granulation and the rate that is consistent with compressed tablets having satisfactory physical characteristics. The main difficulty in rapid machine operation is ensuring adequate filling of the dies. With rapid filling, dwell time of the die cavity beneath the feed frame is insufficient to ensure the requirements of uniform flow and packing of the dies. Various methods of force-feeding the granulation into the dies have been devised to refill the dies in the very short dwell time permitted on the high-speed machine. These devices are illustrated in Figure 45-14. Presses with triple compression points (see Table 45-3) permit the partial

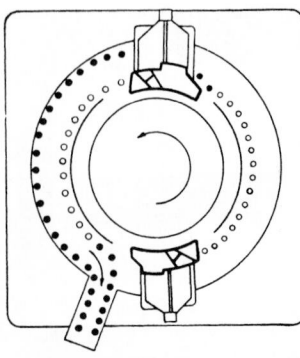

Figure 45-26. The movement of tablets on die table of a double rotary press (courtesy, Vector/Colton).

compaction of material before final compaction. This provides for partial deaeration and particle orientation of material before final compression. This helps in the direct compacting of materials and reduces laminating and capping due to entrapped air.

Multilayer Rotary Tablet Machines

The rotary tablet machines also have been developed into models capable of producing multiple-layer tablets; the machines are able to make 1-, 2-, or 3-layer tablets (Versa Press, *Stokes/Pennwalt*). Stratified tablets offer a number of advantages. Incompatible drugs can be formed into a single tablet by separating the layers containing them with a layer of inert material. It has permitted the formulation of time-delay medication and offers a wide variety of possibilities in developing color combinations that give the products identity.

Originally, the tablets were prepared by a single-compression method. The dies were filled with the different granulations in successive layers, and the tablet was formed by a single compression stroke. The separation lines of the tablets prepared by this method tended to be irregular. In the machines now available for multilayer production the granulation receives a precompression stroke after the first and second fill, which lightly compacts the granulation and maintains a well-defined surface of separation between each layer. The operator is able to eject either precompressed layer with the machine running at any desired speed for periodic weight and analysis checks.

Other multiple-compression presses can receive previously compressed tablets and compress another granulation around the preformed tablet. An example of a press with this capability is the Manesty Drycota *(Thomas/Manesty)*. Pressure-coated tablets can be used to separate incompatible drug substances and also to give an enteric coating to the core tablets.

Capping and Splitting of Tablets

The splitting or capping of tablets is one of great concern and annoyance in tablet making. It is quite difficult to detect while the tablets are being processed but can be detected easily by vigorously shaking a few in the cupped hands. A slightly chipped tablet does not necessarily mean that the tablet will cap or split.

There are many factors that may cause a tablet to cap or split:

Excess *fines* or powder, which traps air in the tablet mixture.
Deep markings on tablet punches. Many designs or *scores* on punches are too broad and deep. Hairline markings are just as appropriate as deep, heavy markings.

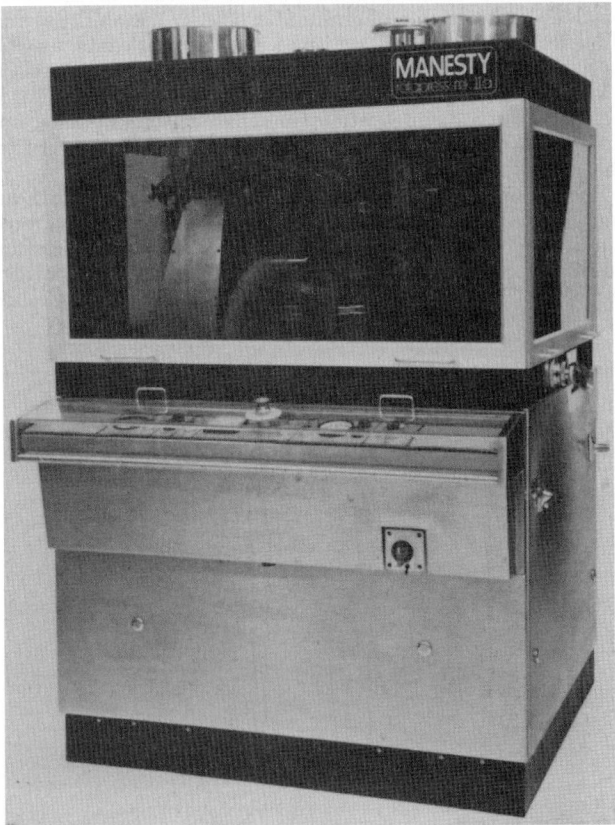

Figure 45-25. Rotapress Mark IIA. Designed for improvements in sound reduction, operator safety, cleanliness, and operational convenience; note the control panel on front of machine (courtesy, Thomas/Manesty).

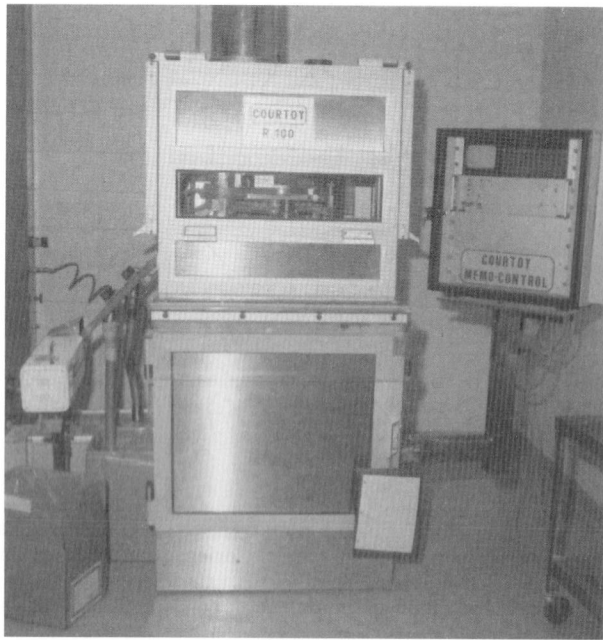

Figure 45-27. Courtoy R-100 with computer-controlled operation.

Worn and imperfect punches. Punches should be smooth and buffed. Nicked punches often cause capping. The development of fine feather edges on tablets indicates wear on punches.

Worn dies. Dies should be replaced or reversed. Dies that are chrome-plated or have tungsten carbide inserts wear longer and give better results than ordinary steel dies.

Too much pressure. By reducing the pressure on the machines the condition may be corrected.

Unsuitable formula. It may be necessary to change the formula.

Moist and soft granulation. This type of granulation will not flow freely into the dies, thus giving uneven weights and soft or capped tablets.

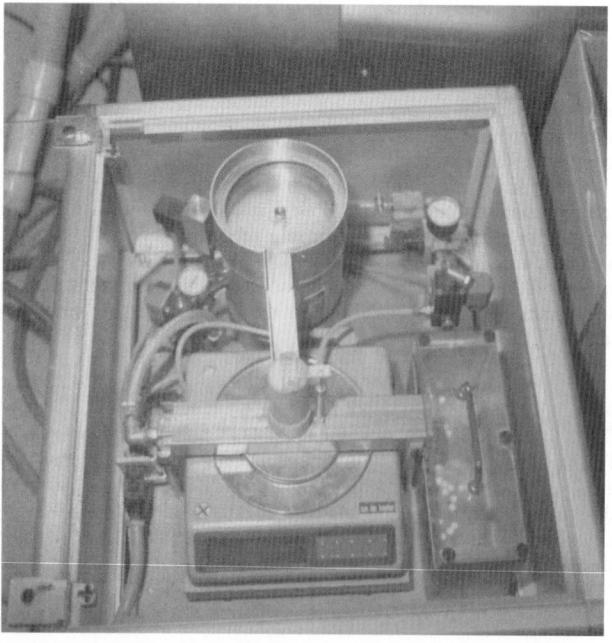

Figure 45-28. Direct weighing of tablets produced gives actual weight feedback for the controller of the Courtoy R-100 (seen in the bottom left of Fig 45-27).

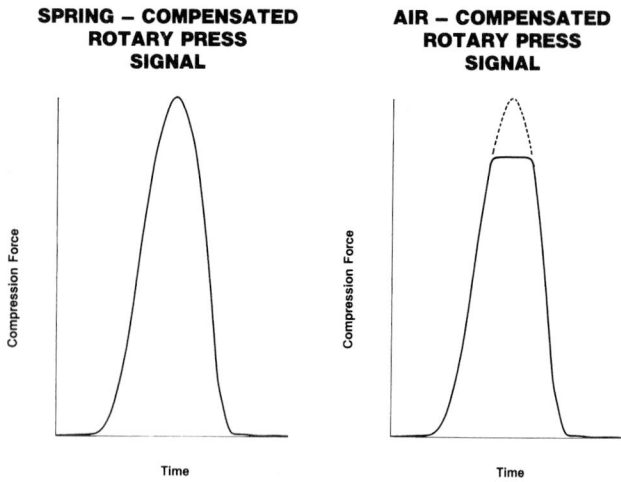

Figure 45-29. Force-time curves for two types of tablet press.

Poorly machined punches. Uneven punches are detrimental to the tablet machine itself and will not produce tablets of accurate weight. One punch out of alignment may cause one tablet to split or cap on every revolution.

Instrumented Tablet Presses

Compressional and ejectional forces involved in tablet compression can be studied by attaching strain gauges to the punches and other press components involved in compression. The electrical output of the gauges has been monitored by telemetry or use of a dual-beam oscilloscope equipped with camera.[42,43] Instrumentation permits a study of the compaction characteristics of granulations, their flowabilities, and the effect of formulation additives, such as lubricants, as well as differences in tablet press design, as shown in Figures 45-27 to 45-30. Physical characteristics of tablets, such as hardness, friability, disintegration time, and dissolution rate, are influenced not only by the nature of the formulation but by the compressional force as well.

As can be seen in Figures 45-29 and 45-30, the rate and duration of compaction forces can be quantified. The rate of force application has a profound effect on powder consolidation within the die and, hence, efficiency of packing and powder compaction. The rate of release of force, or *decompression* has

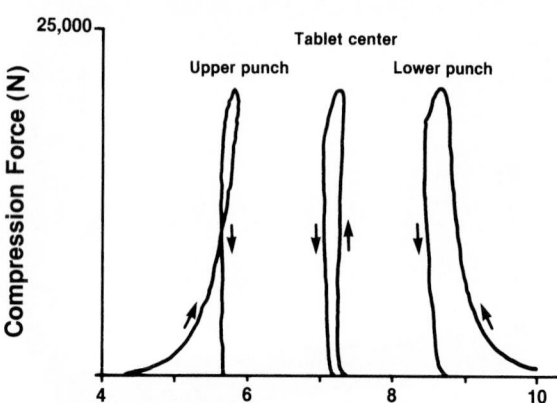

Figure 45-30. Plot showing the upper and lower punch forces as functions of the position of the punch face within the die. A biaxial force/displacement curve also shown is a plot of the position of the tablet center as a function of the compression force.

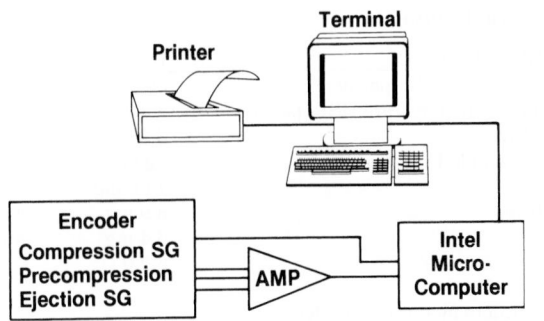

Figure 45-31. Schematic of an instrumentation system using a microcomputer as developed by Schering-Plough.

a direct effect on the ability of the tablet to withstand relaxation. A prominent hypothesis, fostered by Hiestand[44,45] and later Luenberger[46], suggested that capping and laminating of tablets is caused by too-rapid stress relaxation or decompression. This explains why slowing a tablet press and using tapered dies is useful in such situations. Most prominent pharmaceutical scientists have embraced this theory and largely have discounted air entrapment as a cause of capping and laminating.

Figure 45-30 presents an interesting set of plots. Walter and Augsburger reported that as compaction force rises, the steel tooling actually compresses in accommodation to the forces applied. The forces used to produce a tablet are considerable and should be monitored and understood.[47] Therefore, definition of the compressional force and duration of force (dwell time) giving a satisfactory tablet for a formulation provides an in-process control for obtaining both tablet-to-tablet and lot-to-lot uniformity (see Figs 45-24 and 45-31).

Instrumentation has led to the development of on-line, automatic, electromechanical tablet weight-control systems capable of continuously monitoring the weights of tablets as they are produced. Units are available commercially (Thomas Tablet Sentinel *(Thomas Eng);* Fette Compression Force Monitor *(Raymond Auto);* Vali-Tab *(Stokes / Pennwalt))* and are applicable to single or rotary tablet machines. Most commercial presses today can be delivered with some sort of instrumentation attached. When tablet weights vary from preset limits, the monitor automatically will adjust the weight control mechanism to reestablish weights within acceptable limits. If the difficulty continues, the unit will activate an audible warning signal or an optional shut-down relay on the press (see Figs 45-27 and 45-28). Most production-model tablet presses come equipped with complete instrumentation (optional) and with options for statistical analysis and print out of compression/ejection signals. The techniques and applications of press instrumentation have been reviewed.[48,49]

Contamination Control

While good manufacturing practices used by the pharmaceutical industry for many years have stressed the importance of cleanliness of equipment and facilities for the manufacture of drug products, the penicillin contamination problem resulted in renewed emphasis on this aspect of manufacturing. Penicillin, as either an airborne dust or residual quantities remaining in equipment, is believed to have contaminated unrelated products in sufficient concentrations to cause allergic reactions in individuals hypersensitive to penicillin who received these products. This resulted in the industry spending millions of dollars to change or modify buildings, manufacturing processes, equipment, and standard operating procedures to eliminate penicillin contamination.

With this problem has come renewed emphasis on the dust problem, material handling, and equipment cleaning in dealing with drugs, especially potent chemicals. Any process using chemicals in powder form can be a dusty operation; the preparation of compressed tablets and encapsulation fall in this category. In the design of tablet presses attention is being given to the control and elimination of dust generated in the tableting process. In the Perfecta press shown in Figure 45-32, the pressing compartment is completely sealed off from the outside environment, making cross-contamination nearly impossible. The pressing compartment can be kept dust-free by the air supply and vacuum equipment developed for the machine. It removes airborne dust and granular particles that have not been compressed, thus keeping the circular pressing compartment and the upper and lower punch guides free of dust.

Drug manufacturers have the responsibility to make certain that microorganisms present in finished products are unlikely to cause harm to the patient and will not be deleterious to the product. An outbreak of *Salmonella* infections in Scandinavian countries was traced to thyroid tablets that had been prepared from contaminated thyroid powder. This concern eventually led to the establishment of microbial limits for raw materials of animal or botanical origin, especially those that readily support microbial growth and are not rendered sterile during subsequent processing. Harmful microorganisms when present in oral products include *Salmonella* spp, *Escherichia coli*, certain *Pseudomonas* spp such as *P aeruginosa,* and *Staphylococcus aureus.* The compendia have microbial limits on raw materials such as aluminum hydroxide gel, cornstarch, thyroid, acacia, and gelatin.

These represent examples of the industry's efforts to conform with the intent of current good manufacturing practice as defined by the FDA.

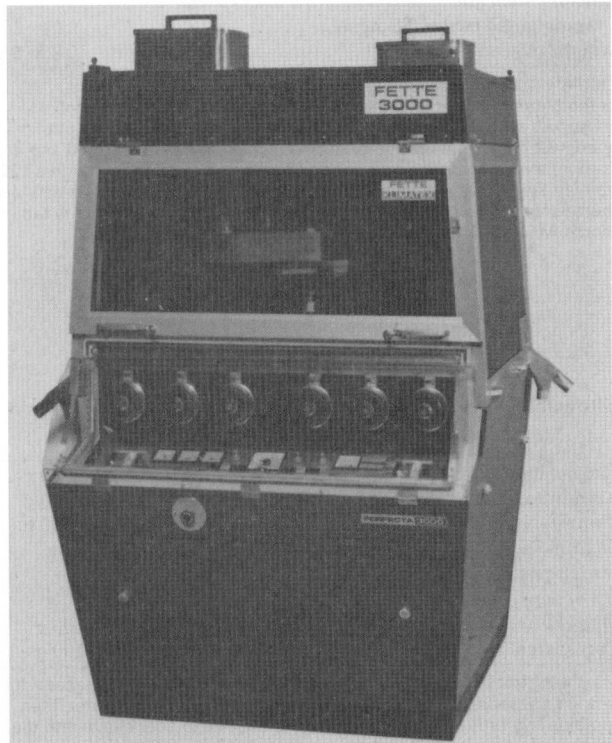

Figure 45-32. Fette Perfecta 3000 high-speed tablet press with pressing compartment completely sealed off from outside environment, making cross-contamination impossible (courtesy, Raymond Auto).

Tablet Formulations

WET GRANULATION

CT Acetaminophen, 300 mg

INGREDIENTS	IN EACH	IN 10,000
Acetaminophen	300 mg	3000 g
Polyvinylpyrrolidone	22.5 mg	225 g
Lactose 61.75 mg 617.5 g		
Alcohol SD3A—200 proof	4.5 mL	45 L
Stearic acid	9 mg	90 g
Talc	13.5 mg	135 g
Cornstarch	43.25 mg	432.5 g

Blend acetaminophen, polyvinylpyrrolidone, and lactose together; pass through a 40-mesh screen. Add the alcohol slowly, and knead well. Screen the wet mass through a 4-mesh screen. Dry the granulation at 50° overnight. Screen the dried granulation through a 20-mesh screen. Bolt the stearic acid, talc, and cornstarch through a 60-mesh screen prior to mixing by tumbling with the granulation. Compress, using 7/16-inch standard concave punch. Ten tablets should weigh 4.5 g (courtesy, *Abbott*).

CT Ascorbic Acid USP, 50 mg

INGREDIENTS	IN EACH	IN 7000
Ascorbic acid USP (powder No. 80)[a]	55 mg	385 g
Lactose	21 mg	147 g
Starch (potato)	13 mg	91 g
Ethylcellulose N 100 (80–105 cps)	16 mg	112 g
Starch (potato)	7 mg	49 g
Talc	6.5 mg	45.5 g
Calcium stearate (impalpable powder)1 mg		7 g
Weight of granulation		836.5 g

[a] Includes 10% in excess of label claim.

Granulate the first three ingredients with ethylcellulose (5%) dissolved in anhydrous ethyl alcohol, adding additional anhydrous alcohol to obtain good, wet granules. Wet-screen through a #8 stainless steel screen and dry at room temperature in an air-conditioned area. Dry-screen through a #20 stainless steel screen and incorporate the remaining three ingredients. Mix thoroughly and compress. Use a flat, beveled, ¼-inch punch. Twenty tablets should weigh 2.39 g.

Chewable Antacid Tablets

INGREDIENTS	IN EACH	IN 10,000
Magnesium trisilicate	500 mg	5000 g
Aluminum hydroxide, dried gel	250 mg	2500 g
Mannitol	300 mg	3000 g
Sodium saccharin	2 mg	20 g
Starch paste, 5%	qs	qs
Oil of peppermint	1 mg	10 g
Magnesium stearate	10 mg	100 g
Cornstarch	10 mg	100 g

Mix the magnesium trisilicate and aluminum hydroxide with the mannitol. Dissolve the sodium saccharin in a small quantity of purified water, then combine this with the starch paste. Granulate the powder blend with the starch paste. Dry at 140°F and screen through 16-mesh screen. Add the flavoring oil, magnesium stearate, and corn starch; mix well. Age the granulation for at least 24 hr and compress, using a ⅝-inch, flat-face, bevel-edge punch (courtesy, *Atlas*).

CT Hexavitamin

INGREDIENTS	IN EACH	IN 7000
Ascorbic acid USP (powder)[a]	82.5 mg	577.5 g
Thiamine mononitrate USP (powder)[a]	2.4 mg	16.8 g
Riboflavin[a]	3.3 mg	23.1 g
Nicotinamide USP (powder)[a]	22 mg	154 g
Starch	13.9 mg	97.4 g
Lactose	5.9 mg	41.2 g
Zein	6.4 mg	45 g
Vitamin A acetate	6250 U	
Vitamin D_2[a] (use Pfizer crystalets medium granules containing 500,000 U vitamin A acetate and 50,000 U vitamin D_2/g)	625 U	87.5 g
Magnesium stearate		7.5 g
Weight of granulation		1050 g

[a] Includes the following in excess of label claim: ascorbic acid 10%, thiamine mononitrate 20%, riboflavin 10%, nicotinamide 10%, and vitamin A acetate–vitamin D_2 crystalets 25%.

Thoroughly mix the first six ingredients and granulate with zein (10% in ethyl alcohol, adding additional alcohol if necessary to obtain good, wet granules). Wet-screen through a #8 stainless steel screen and dry at 110 to 120°F. Dry-screen through a #20 stainless steel screen and add the vitamin crystalets. Mix thoroughly, lubricate, and compress. Ten tablets should weigh 1.50 g. Coat with syrup.

CT Theobromine-Phenobarbital

INGREDIENTS	IN EACH	IN 7000
Theobromine	325 mg	2275 g
Phenobarbital	33 mg	231 g
Starch	39 mg	273 g
Talc	8 mg	56 g
Acacia (powder)	8 mg	56 g
Stearic acid	0.7 mg	4.9 g
Weight of granulation		2895.9 g

Prepare a paste with the acacia and an equal weight of starch. Use this paste for granulating the theobromine and phenobarbital. Dry and put through a 12-mesh screen, add the remainder of the material, mix thoroughly, and compress into tablets, using a 13/32-inch concave punch. Ten tablets should weigh 4.13 g.

FLUID-BED GRANULATION

CT Ascorbic Acid USP, 50 mg

INGREDIENTS	IN EACH	IN 10,000
Ascorbic acid USP (powder no 80)[a]	55 mg	550 g
Lactose	21 mg	210 g
Starch (potato)	13 mg	130 g
Ethylcellulose N100 (80–105 cps)	16 mg	160 g
Starch (potato)	7 mg	70 g
Talc	6.5 mg	65 g
Calcium stearate	1 mg	10 g
Weight of granulation		1195.0 g

[a] Includes 10% in excess of claim.

Add the first three ingredients to the granulator. Mix for 5 to 15 min or until well mixed. Dissolve the ethylcellulose in anhydrous ethanol and spray this solution and any additional ethanol into the fluidized mixture. Cease spraying when good granules are produced. Dry to approximately 3% moisture. Remove the granules and place them in a suitable blender. Sequentially add the remaining three ingredients with mixing steps in between each addition. Compress, using a flat, beveled, 1/4-inch punch. Twenty tablets should weigh 2.39 g.

Sustained-Release (SR) Procainamide Tablets

INGREDIENTS	IN EACH	IN 10,000
Procainamide	500 mg	5000 g
HPMC 2208, USP	300 mg	3000 g
Carnauba wax	60 mg	600 g
HPMC 2910, USP	30 mg	300 g
Magnesium stearate	4 mg	40 g
Stearic acid	11 mg	110 g
Talc	5 mg	50 g
Weight of granulation		9100 g

Place the first three ingredients in the granulator and mix for 5 to 15 min. Dissolve the HPMC in water (mix in hot water, then cool down) and spray into the fluidized mixture. Dry to approximately 5% moisture. Sequentially add the last three ingredients, with mixing steps in between each addition. Compress, using capsule-shaped tooling. Ten tablets should weigh 9.1 g.

DRY GRANULATION

CT Acetylsalicylic Acid

INGREDIENTS	IN EACH	IN 7000
Acetylsalicylic Acid (crystals 20-mesh)	0.325 g	2275 g
Starch		226.8 g
Weight of granulation		2501.8 g

Dry the starch to a moisture content of 10%. Thoroughly mix this with the acetylsalicylic acid. Compress into slugs. Grind the slugs to 14- to 16-mesh size. Recompress into tablets, using a $^{13}/_{32}$-inch punch. Ten tablets should weigh 3.575 g.

CT Sodium Phenobarbital

INGREDIENTS	IN EACH	IN 7000
Phenobarbital sodium	65 mg	455 g
Lactose (granular, 12-mesh)	26 mg	182 g
Starch	20 mg	140 g
Talc	20 mg	140 g
Magnesium stearate	0.3 mg	2.1 g
Weight of granulation		919.1 g

Mix all the ingredients thoroughly. Compress into slugs. Grind and screen to 14- to 16-mesh granules. Recompress into tablets, using a $^{9}/_{32}$-inch concave punch. Ten tablets should weigh 1.3 g.

CT Vitamin B Complex

INGREDIENTS	IN EACH	IN 10,000
Thiamine mononitrate[a]	0.733 mg	7.33 g
Riboflavin[a]	0.733 mg	7.33 g
Pyridoxine hydrochloride	0.333 mg	3.33 g
Calcium pantothenate[a]	0.4 mg	4 g
Nicotinamide	5 mg	50 g
Lactose (powder)	75.2 mg	752 g
Starch	21.9 mg	219 g
Talc	20 mg	200 g
Stearic acid (powder)	0.701 mg	7.01 g
Weight of granulation		1250 g

[a] Includes 10% in excess of label claim.

Mix all the ingredients thoroughly. Compress into slugs. Grind and screen to 14- to 16-mesh granules. Recompress into tablets, using a ¼-inch concave punch. Ten tablets should weigh 1.25 g.

Sufficient tartaric acid should be used in these tablets to adjust the pH to 4.5.

DIRECT COMPRESSION

APC Tablets

INGREDIENTS	IN EACH	IN 10,000
Aspirin (40-mesh crystal)	224 mg	2240 g
Phenacetin	160 mg	1600 g
Caffeine (anhyd USP gran)	32 mg	320 g
Compressible sugar (Di-Pac[a])	93.4 mg	934 g
Sterotex	7.8 mg	78 g
Silica gel (Syloid 244[b])	2.8 mg	28 g

[a] Amstar.
[b] Davison Chem.

Blend ingredients in a twin-shell blender for 15 min and compress on a $^{13}/_{32}$-inch standard concave punch (courtesy, Amstar).

CT Ascorbic Acid USP, 250 mg

INGREDIENTS	IN EACH	IN 10,000
Ascorbic Acid USP (Merck, fine crystals)	255 mg	2550 g
Microcrystalline cellulose[a]	159 mg	1590 g
Stearic acid	9 mg	90 g
Colloidal silica[b]	2 mg	20 g
Weight of granulation		4250 g

[a] Avicel-PH-101.
[b] Cab-O-Sil.

Blend all ingredients in a suitable blender. Compress, using $^{7}/_{16}$-inch standard concave punch. Ten tablets should weigh 4.25 g (courtesy, FMC).

Breath Freshener Tablets

INGREDIENTS	IN EACH	IN 10,000
Wintergreen oil	0.6 mg	6 g
Menthol	0.85 mg	8.5 g
Peppermint oil	0.3 mg	3 g
Silica gel (Syloid 244[a])	1 mg	10 g
Sodium saccharin	0.3 mg	3 g
Sodium bicarbonate	14 mg	140 g
Mannitol USP (granular)	180.95 mg	1809.5 g
Calcium stearate	2 mg	20 g

[a] Davison Chem.

Mix the flavor oils and menthol until liquid. Adsorb onto the silica gel. Add the remaining ingredients. Blend and compress on $^{5}/_{16}$-inch, flat-face bevel-edge punch to a thickness of 3.1 mm (courtesy, Atlas).

Chewable Antacid Tablets

INGREDIENTS	IN EACH	IN 10,000
Aluminum hydroxide and magnesium carbonate, codried gel[a]	325 mg	3250 g
Mannitol USP (granular)	675 mg	6750 g
Microcrystalline cellulose[b]	75 mg	750 g
Corn starch	30 mg	300 g
Calcium stearate	22 mg	220 g
Flavor	qs	qs

[a] Reheis F-MA-11.
[b] Avicel

Blend all ingredients in a suitable blender. Compress, using a 5/8-inch, flat-face, bevel-edge punch (courtesy, Atlas).

Chewable Multivitamin Tablets

INGREDIENTS	IN EACH	IN 10,000
Vitamin A USP (dry, stabilized form)	5000 USP units	50 million units
Vitamin D dry, stabilized form)	400 USP units	4 million units
Ascorbic Acid USP	60.0 mg	600 g
Thiamine Hydrochloride USP	1 mg	10 g
Riboflavin USP	1.5 mg	15 g
Pyridoxine Hydrochloride USP	1 mg	10 g
Cyanocobalamin USP	2 μg	20 mg
Calcium Pantothenate USP	3 mg	30 g
Niacinamide USP	10 mg	100 g
Mannitol USP (granular)	236.2 mg	2362 g
Cornstarch	16.6 mg	166 g
Sodium saccharin	1.1 mg	11 g
Magnesium stearate	6.6 mg	66 g
Talc USP	10 mg	100 g
Flavor	qs	qs

Blend all ingredients in a suitable blender. Compress, using a ⅜-inch, flat-face, bevel-edge punch (courtesy, *Atlas*).

CT Ferrous Sulfate

INGREDIENTS	IN EACH	IN 7000
Ferrous Sulfate USP (crystalline)	0.325 g	2275 g
Talc		0.975 g
Sterotex		1.95 g
Weight of granulation		2277.93 g

Grind to 12- to 14-mesh, lubricate, and compress. Coat immediately to avoid oxidation to the ferric state with 0.410 gr of tolu balsam (dissolved in alcohol) and 0.060 gr of salol and chalk. Use a deep, concave, ¹¹⁄₃₂-inch punch. Ten tablets should weigh 3.25 g.

CT Methenamine

INGREDIENTS	IN EACH	IN 7000
Methenamine (12- to 14-mesh crystals)	0.325 g	2275 g
Weight of granulation		2275 g

Compress directly, using a ⁷⁄₁₆-inch punch. Ten tablets should weigh 3.25 g.

CT Phenobarbital USP, 30 mg

INGREDIENTS	IN EACH	IN 10,000
Phenobarbital	30.59 mg	305.9 g
Microcrystalline cellulose[a]	30.59 mg	305.9 g
Spray-dried lactose	69.16 mg	691.6 g
Colloidal silica[b]	1.33 mg	13.3 g
Stearic acid	1.33 mg	13.3 g
Weight of granulation		1330 g

[a] Avicel-PH-101.
[b] QUSO F-22.
Screen the phenobarbital to break up lumps and blend with the microcrystalline cellulose. Add spray-dried lactose and blend. Finally, add the stearic acid and colloidal silica; blend to obtain a homogeneous mixture. Compress, using a ⁹⁄₃₂-inch, shallow, concave punch. Ten tablets should weigh 1.33 g (courtesy, *FMC*).

Molded Tablets or Tablet Triturates (TT)

Tablet triturates are small, discoid masses of molded powders weighing 30 to 250 mg each. The base consists of lactose, β-lactose, mannitol, dextrose, or other rapidly soluble materials. It is desirable in making tablet triturates to prepare a solid dosage form that is rapidly soluble; as a result they are generally softer than compressed tablets.

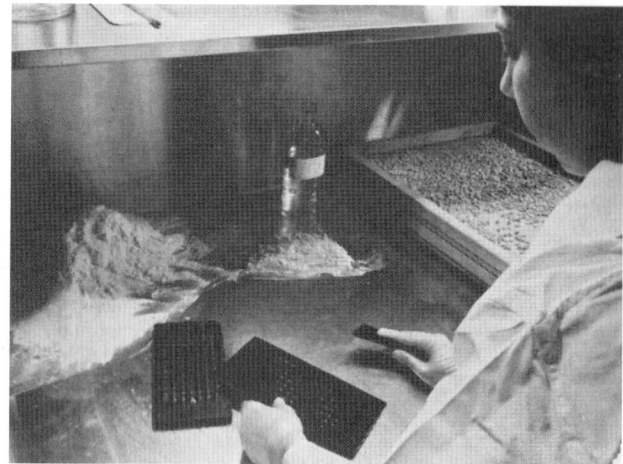

Figure 45-33. Hand-molding tablet triturates (courtesy, Merck).

This type of dosage form is selected for a number of drugs because of its rapidly dissolving characteristic. Nitroglycerin in many concentrations is prepared in tablet triturate form since the molded tablet rapidly dissolves when administered by placing under the tongue. Potent alkaloids and highly toxic drugs used in small doses are prepared as tablet triturates that can serve as dispensing tablets to be used as the source of the drug in compounding other formulations or solutions. Narcotics in the form of hypodermic tablets originally were made as tablet triturates because they rapidly dissolve in sterile water for injection prior to administration. Today with stable injections of narcotics available, there is no longer any justification for their use in this manner. Although many hypodermic tablets currently are made, they are used primarily for oral administration.

Tablet triturates are made by forcing a moistened blend of the drug and diluent into a mold, extruding the formed mass, which is allowed to dry. This method is essentially the same as it was when introduced by Fuller in 1878. Hand molds may vary in size, but the method of operation is essentially the same. Molds consist of two plates made from polystyrene plastic, hard rubber, nickel-plated brass, or stainless steel. The mold plate contains 50 to 500 carefully polished perforations. The other plate is fitted with a corresponding number of projecting pegs or punches that fit the perforations in the mold plate. The mold plate is placed on a flat surface, the moistened mass is forced into the perforations, and the excess is scraped from the top surface. The mold plate is placed over the plate with the corresponding pegs and lowered. As the plates come together, the pegs force the tablet triturates from the molds. They remain on the tops of the pegs until dry, and they can be handled (see Fig 45-33). In some hand molds, as shown in Figure 45-34, the pegs are forced down onto the plate holding the moist trituration.

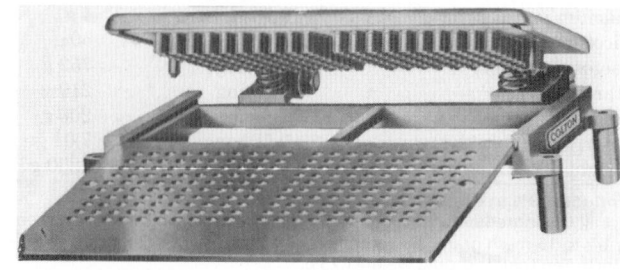

Figure 45-34. Tablet triturate mold (courtesy, Vector/Colton).

FORMULATION

In developing a formula it is essential to know the blank weight of the mold that is to be used. To determine this, the weight of the diluent that exactly fills all the openings in the mold is determined by experiment. This amount of diluent is weighed and placed aside. The total amount of the drug required is determined by multiplying the number of perforations in the plate used in the previous experiment by the amount of drug desired in each tablet. The comparative bulk of this medication is compared with that of an equal volume of diluent and that quantity of diluent is removed and weighed. The drug and the remaining diluent are mixed by trituration, and the resulting triturate is moistened and forced into the openings of the mold. If the perforations are not filled completely, more diluent is added, its weight noted, and the formula written from the results of the experiments.

It is also permissible in the development of the formula to weigh the quantity of medication needed for the number of tablets represented by the number of perforations in the mold, triturate with a weighed portion (more than 1/2) of the diluent, moisten the mixture, and press it into the perforations of the mold. An additional quantity of the diluent is moistened immediately and also forced into the perforations in the plate until they are filled completely. All excess diluent is removed, the trial tablets are forced from the mold, then triturated until uniform, moistened again, if necessary, and remolded. When these tablets are dried thoroughly and weighed, the difference between their total weight and the weight of medication taken will indicate the amount of diluent required and accordingly supply the formula for future use for that particular tablet triturate.

PREPARATION

The mixed powders are moistened with a proper mixture of alcohol and water, although other solvents or moistening agents such as acetone, petroleum benzin, and various combinations of these may be used in specific cases; the agent of choice depends on the solvent action that it will exert on the powder mixture. Often the moistening agent is 50% alcohol, but this concentration may be increased or decreased depending on the constituents of the formula. Care must be used in adding the solvent mixture to the powder. If too much is used, the mass will be soggy and will require a long time to dry, and the finished tablet will be hard and slowly soluble; if the mass is too wet, shrinkage will occur in the molded tablets; finally, a condition known as creeping will be noticed. Creeping is the concentration of the medication on the surface of the tablet caused by capillarity and rapid evaporation of the solvent from the surface. Because molded tablets by their very nature are quite friable, an inaccurate strength in each tablet may result from creeping if powder is lost from the tablet's surface. On the other hand, if an insufficient amount of moistening agent is used, the mass will not have the proper cohesion to make a firm tablet. The correct amount of moistening agent can be determined initially only by experiment.

HAND-MOLDING TABLET TRITURATES

In preparing hand-molded tablets place the mold plate on a glass plate. The properly moistened material is pressed into the perforations of the mold with a broad spatula, exerting uniform pressure over each opening. The excess material is removed by passing the spatula at an oblique angle, with strong hand pressure, over the mold to give a clean, flat surface. The material thus removed should be placed with the remainder of the unmolded material.

The mold with the filled perforations should be reversed and moved to another clean part of the plate where the pressing operation with the spatula is repeated. It may be necessary to add more material to fill the perforations completely and uniformly. The mold should be allowed to stand in a position so that part of the moistening agent will evaporate equally from both faces. While the first plate is drying, another mold can be prepared. As soon as the second mold has been completed, the first mold should be sufficiently surface-dried so that the pegs will press the tablets from the mold with a minimum of sticking.

To remove the tablets from the mold, place the mold over the peg plate so that the pegs and the perforations are in juxtaposition. The tablets are released from the mold by hand pressure, which forces the pegs through the perforations. The ejected tablets are spread evenly in single layers on silk trays and dried in a clean, dust-free chamber with warm, circulating air. If only a small quantity of tablet triturates is made and no warm-air oven is available, the tablet triturates may be dried to constant weight at room temperature.

MACHINE-MOLDING TABLET TRITURATES

Tablet triturates also can be made using mechanical equipment. The automatic tablet triturate machine illustrated in Figure 45-35 makes tablet triturates at a rate of 2500/min. For machine-molding, the powder mass need not be as moist as for plate-molding, since the time interval between forming the tablets and pressing them is considerably shorter. The moistened mass passes through the funnel of the hopper to the feed plates below. In this feed plate are four holes having the same diameter as the mouth of the funnel. The material fills one hole at a time and, when filled, revolves to a position just over the mold plate. When in position the weighted pressure foot lowers and imprisons the powder. At the same time a spreader in the sole of the pressure foot rubs it into the mold cavities and evens it off so that the triturates are smooth on the surface and are of uniform density. When this operation is completed, the mold passes to the next position, where it registers with a nest of punches or pegs that eject the tablets from the mold plate onto a conveyor belt. The conveyor belt sometimes is extended to a length of 8 or 10 ft. under a battery of infrared drying lamps to hasten the setting of the tablets for more rapid handling. This method of drying can be used only if the drug is chemically stable to these drying conditions.

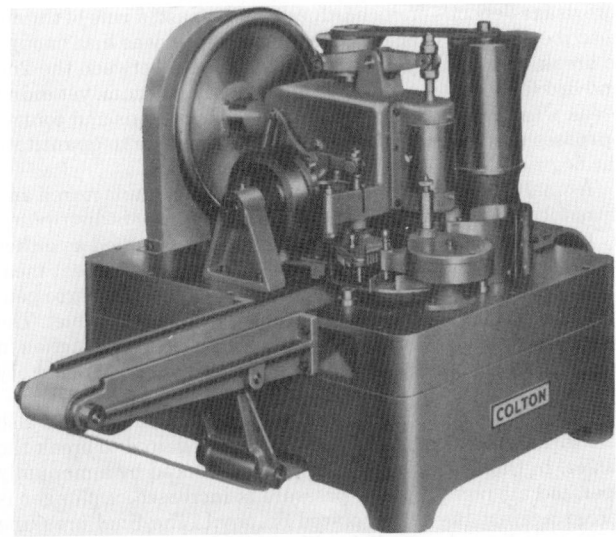

Figure 45-35. Automatic tablet triturate machine (courtesy, Vector-Colton).

COMPRESSED TABLET TRITURATES

Frequently, tablet triturates are prepared on compression tablet machines using flat-face punches. When solubility and a clear solution are required, water-soluble lubricants must be used to prevent sticking to the punches. The granulations are prepared as directed for ordinary compressed tablets; lactose generally is used as the diluent. Generally, tablet triturates prepared by this method are not as satisfactory as the molded type regarding their solubility and solution characteristics.

TABLET CHARACTERISTICS

Compressed tablets may be characterized or described by a number of specifications. These include the diameter size, shape, thickness, weight, hardness, disintegration time, and dissolution characteristics. The diameter and shape depend on the die and the punches selected for the compression of the tablet. Generally, tablets are discoid in shape, although they may be oval, oblong, round, cylindrical, or triangular. Their upper and lower surfaces may be flat, round, concave, or convex to various degrees. The concave punches (used to prepare convex tablets) are referred to as shallow, standard, and deep cup, depending on the degree of concavity (see Figs 45-17 to 45-20). The tablets may be scored in halves or quadrants to facilitate breaking if a smaller dose is desired. The top or lower surface may be embossed or engraved with a symbol or letters that serve as an additional means of identifying the source of the tablets. These characteristics along with the color of the tablets tend to make them distinctive and identifiable with the active ingredient that they contain.

The remaining specifications assure the manufacturer that the tablets do not vary from one production lot to another. In the case of new tablet formulations their therapeutic efficacy is demonstrated through clinical trials, and it is the manufacturer's aim to reproduce the same tablet with the exact characteristics of the tablets that were used in the clinical evaluation of the dosage form. Therefore, from the control viewpoint these specifications are important for reasons other than physical appearance.

Tablet Hardness

The resistance of the tablet to chipping, abrasion, or breakage under conditions of storage, transportation, and handling before usage depends on its hardness. In the past, a rule of thumb described a tablet to be of proper hardness if it was firm enough to break with a sharp snap when it was held between the 2nd and 3rd fingers and using the thumb as the fulcrum, yet didn't break when it fell on the floor. For obvious reasons and control purposes a number of attempts have been made to quantitate the degree of hardness.

A small and portable hardness tester was manufactured and introduced in the mid-1930s by *Monsanto*. It now is distributed by the Stokes Div *(Pennwalt)* and may be designated as either the Monsanto or Stokes hardness tester. The instrument measures the force required to break the tablet when the force generated by a coil spring is applied diametrically to the tablet. The force is measured in kilograms and when used in production, a hardness of 4 kg is considered to be minimum for a satisfactory tablet.

The Strong-Cobb hardness tester introduced in 1950 also measures the diametrically applied force required to break the tablet. In this instrument the force is produced by a manually operated air pump. As the pressure is increased, a plunger is forced against the tablet placed on anvil. The final breaking point is indicated on a dial calibrated into 30 arbitrary units. The hardness values of the Stokes and Strong-Cobb instruments are not equivalent. Values obtained with the Strong-Cobb tester have been found to be 1.6 times those of the Stokes tester.

Another instrument is the Pfizer hardness tester, which operates on the same mechanical principle as ordinary pliers. The force required to break the tablet is recorded on a dial and may be expressed in either kilograms or pounds of force. In an experimental comparison of testers the Pfizer and the Stokes testers were found to check each other fairly well. Again the Strong-Cobb tester was found to give values 1.4 to 1.7 times the absolute values on the other instruments.

The most widely used apparatus to measure tablet hardness or crushing strength is the Schleuniger apparatus, also known as the Heberlein, distributed by *Vector*. This and other, newer, electrically operated test equipment eliminate the operator variability inherent in the measurements described above. Newer equipment is also available with printers to provide a record of test results. See Figure 45-36.

Manufacturers, such as *Key, Van Kel, Erweka,* and others, make similar hardness testers.

Hardness (or more appropriately, crushing strength) determinations are made throughout the tablet runs to determine the need for pressure adjustments on the tableting machine. If the tablet is too hard, it may not disintegrate in the required period of time or meet the dissolution specification; if it is too soft, it will not withstand the handling during subsequent processing such as coating or packaging and shipping operations.

A tablet property related to hardness is *friability,* and the measurement is made by use of the Roche friabilator. Rather than a measure of the force required to crush a tablet, the instrument is designed to evaluate the ability of the tablet to withstand abrasion in packaging, handling, and shipping. A number of tablets are weighed and placed in the tumbling apparatus where they are exposed to rolling and repeated shocks resulting from freefalls within the apparatus. After a given number of rotations the tablets are weighed, and the loss in weight indicates the ability of the tablets to withstand this type of wear (Fig 45-37).

Recent research has proposed that there are at least three measurable hardness parameters that can give a clue to the compatibility and intrinsic strength of powdered materials. These include bonding strength, internal strain, and brittleness. Hiestand proposed indices to quantify these parameters, and they are listed in Table 45-4 for a number of materials.

The higher the bonding index, the stronger a tablet is likely to be. The higher the strain index, the weaker the tablet. Since the two parameters are opposite in their effect on the tablet, it is possible for a material (such as Avicel) to have a relatively high strain index, but yet have superior compaction properties because of an extraordinary bonding potential. The higher the brittleness index, the more friable the tablet is likely to be. For

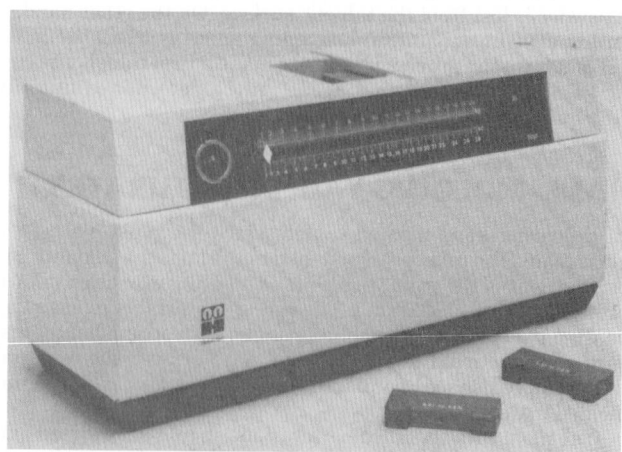

Figure 45-36. The Schleuniger or Heberlein tablet hardness tester shown with calibration blocks (courtesy, Vector).

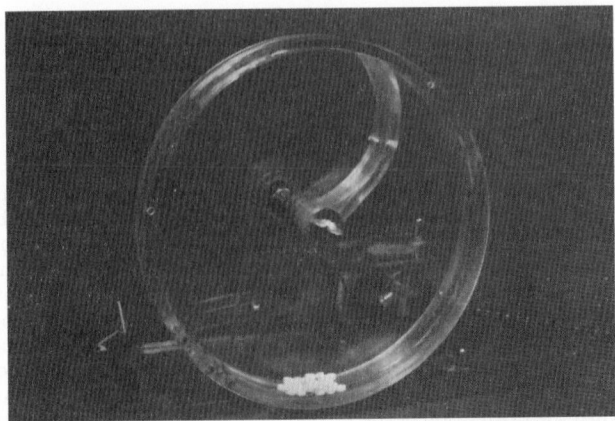

Figure 45-37. The Roche friabilator (courtesy, Hoffmann-LaRoche).

a more detailed discussion of this subject, the reader is directed to References 22, 37, 38.

A similar approach is taken by many manufacturers when they evaluate a new product in the new market package by sending the package to distant points and back using various methods of transportation. This is called a *shipping test*. The condition of the product on its return indicates its ability to withstand transportation handling.

Tablet Thickness

The thickness of the tablet from production-run to production-run is controlled carefully. Thickness can vary with no change in weight because of difference in the density of the granulation and the pressure applied to the tablets, as well as the speed of tablet compression. Not only is the tablet thickness important in reproducing tablets identical in appearance but also to ensure that every production lot will be usable with selected packaging components. If the tablets are thicker than specified, a given number no longer may be contained in the volume of a given size bottle. Tablet thickness also becomes an important characteristic in counting tablets using filling equipment. Some filling equipment uses the uniform thickness of the tablets as a counting mechanism. A column containing a known number of tablets is measured for height; filling is accomplished by continually dropping columns of tablets of the same height into bottles. If thickness varies throughout the lot, the result will be variation in count. Other pieces of filling equipment can malfunction because of variation in tablet thickness, since tablets above specified thickness may cause wedging of tablets in previously adjusted depths of the counting slots. Tablet thickness is determined with a caliper or thickness gauge that measures the thickness in millimeters. Plus or minus 5% may be allowed, depending on the size of the tablet.

Table 45-4. Hiestand Compaction Indices for a Number of Materials

MATERIAL	BONDING INDEX	STRAIN INDEX	BRITTLENESS INDEX
Aspirin	1.5	1.11	0.16
Dicalcium phosphate	1.3	1.13	0.15
Lactose anhydrous	0.8	1.40	0.27
Avicel pH 102	4.3	2.20	0.04
Corn starch	0.4	2.48	0.26
Sucrose NF	1.0	1.45	0.35
Erythromycin dihydrate	1.9	2.13	0.98

Uniformity of Dosage Forms

TABLET WEIGHT—The volumetric fill of the die cavity determines the weight of the compressed tablet. In setting up the tablet machine the fill is adjusted to give the desired tablet weight. The weight of the tablet is the quantity of the granulation that contains the labeled amount of the therapeutic ingredient. After the tablet machine is in operation the weights of the tablets are checked routinely, either manually or electronically, to ensure that proper-weight tablets are being made. This has become rather routine in most manufacturing operations with newer, electronically controlled tablet presses. The USP has provided tolerances for the average weight of uncoated compressed tablets. These are applicable when the tablet contains 50 mg or more of the drug substance or when the latter comprises 50% or more, by weight, of the dosage form. Twenty tablets are weighed individually, and the average weight is calculated. The variation from the average weight in the weights of not more than two of the tablets must not differ by more than the percentage listed below; no tablet differs by more than double that percentage. Tablets that are coated are exempt from these requirements but must conform to the test for content uniformity if it is applicable.

AVERAGE WEIGHT	PERCENT DIFFERENCE
130 mg or less	10
More than 130 mg through 324 mg	7.5
More than 324 mg	5

CONTENT UNIFORMITY—To ensure that every tablet contains the amount of drug substance intended, with little variation among tablets within a batch, the USP includes the content uniformity test for certain tablets. Due to the increased awareness of physiological availability, the content uniformity test has been extended to monographs on all coated and uncoated tablets and all capsules intended for oral administration where the range of sizes of the dosage form available includes a 50 mg or smaller size, in which case the test is applicable to all sizes (50 mg and larger and smaller) of that tablet or capsule. The official compendia can be consulted for the details of the test. Tablet monographs with a content uniformity requirement do not have a weight variation requirement.

Tablet Disintegration

It is recognized generally that the *in vitro* tablet disintegration test does not necessarily bear a relationship to the *in vivo* action of a solid dosage form. To be absorbed, a drug substance must be in solution, and the disintegration test is a measure only of the time required under a given set of conditions for a group of tablets to disintegrate into particles. Generally, this test is useful as a quality-assurance tool for conventional (non-sustained-release) dosage forms. In the present disintegration test the particles are those that will pass through a 10-mesh screen. In a comparison of disintegration times and dissolution rates or initial absorption rates of several brands of aspirin tablets, it was found that the faster-absorbed tablets had the longer disintegration time. Regardless of the lack of significance as to *in vivo* action of the tablets, the test provides a means of control in ensuring that a given tablet formula is the same as regards disintegration from one production batch to another. The disintegration test is used as a control for tablets intended to be administered by mouth, except for tablets intended to be chewed before being swallowed or tablets designed to release the drug substance over a period of time.

Exact specifications are given for the test apparatus, inasmuch as a change in the apparatus can cause a change in the results of the test. The apparatus consists of a basket rack holding six plastic tubes, open at the top and bottom; the bottom of the tubes is covered with 10-mesh screen. See Figure 45-38. The basket rack is immersed in a bath of suitable liquid, held at 37°C,

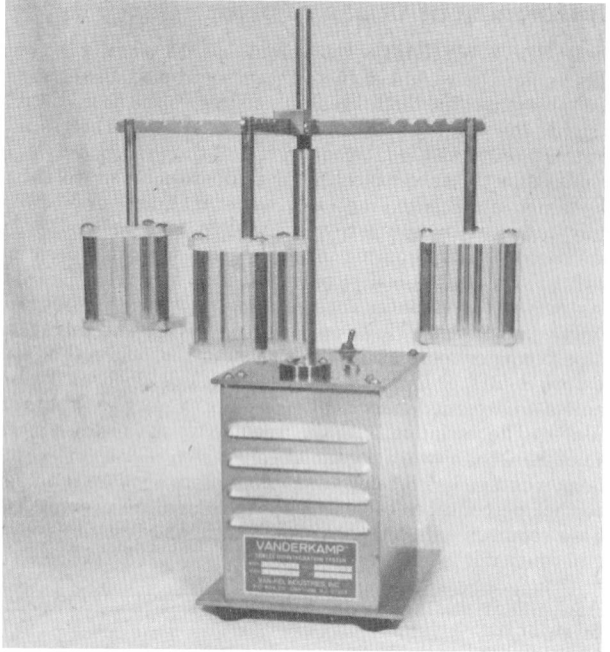

Figure 45-38. Vanderkamp tablet disintegration tester (courtesy, VanKel).

sublingual tablets, such as CT Isoproterenol Hydrochloride, the disintegration time is 3 min. For the exact conditions of the test, consult the USP.

Dissolution Test

For certain tablets the monographs direct compliance with limits on dissolution rather than disintegration. Since drug absorption and physiological availability depend on having the drug substance in the dissolved state, suitable dissolution characteristics are an important property of a satisfactory tablet. Like the disintegration test, the dissolution test for measuring the amount of time required for a given percentage of the drug substance in a tablet to go into solution under a specified set of conditions is an *in vitro* test. It is intended to provide a step toward the evaluation of the physiological availability of the drug substance, but as described currently, it is not designed to measure the safety or efficacy of the tablet being tested. Both the safety and effectiveness of a specific dosage form must be demonstrated initially by means of appropriate *in vivo* studies and clinical evaluation. Like the disintegration test, the dissolution test does provide a means of control in ensuring that a given tablet formulation is the same as regards dissolution as the batch of tablets shown initially to be clinically effective. It also provides an *in vitro* control procedure to eliminate variations among production batches. Refer to Chapter 35 for a complete discussion of dissolution testing.

Validation

In this era of increasing regulatory control of the pharmaceutical industry, manufacturing procedures cannot be discussed without the mention of some process-validation activity. By way of documentation, product testing, and perhaps in-process testing as well, manufacturers can demonstrate that their formulas and processes perform in the manner expected and that they do so reproducibly.

Although the justification for requiring validation is found in the regulations relating to *Current Good Manufacturing Practices for Finished Pharmaceuticals* as well as other sources, there is still much room for interpretation, and the process varies from one company to another. General areas of agreement appear to be that

The validation activity must begin in R&D and continue through product introduction.
Documentation is the key.
In general, three batches represent an adequate sample for validation.

The FDA has rejected historical data or *retrospective validation.* They require that new products be validated from beginning to end, a process called *prospective validation.*

preferably in a 1-L beaker. The rack moves up and down in the fluid at a specified rate. The volume of the fluid is such that on the upward stroke the wire mesh remains at least 2.5 cm below the surface of the fluid and descends to not less than 2.5 cm from the bottom on the downward stroke. Tablets are placed in each of the six cylinders along with a plastic disc over the tablet unless otherwise directed in the monograph. The endpoint of the test is indicated when any residue remaining is a soft mass with no palpably soft core. The plastic discs help to force any soft mass that forms through the screen.

For compressed, uncoated tablets the testing fluid is usually water at 37°, but in some cases the monographs direct that Simulated Gastric Fluid TS be used. If one or two tablets fail to disintegrate, the test is to be repeated using 12 tablets. Of the 18 tablets then tested, 16 must have disintegrated within the given period of time. The conditions of the test are varied somewhat for coated tablets, buccal tablets, and sublingual tablets. Disintegration times are included in the individual tablet monograph. For most uncoated tablets the period is 30 min, although the time for some uncoated tablets varies greatly from this. For coated tablets up to 2 hr may be required, while for

---

CAPSULES

Capsules are solid dosage forms in which the drug substance is enclosed in either a hard or soft, soluble container or shell of a suitable form of gelatin. The soft gelatin capsule was invented by Mothes, a French pharmacist, in 1833. During the following year DuBlanc obtained a patent for his soft gelatin capsules. In 1848 Murdock patented the two-piece hard gelatin capsule. Although development work has been done on the preparation of capsules from methylcellulose, starch and calcium alginate, gelatin, because of its unique properties, remains the primary composition material for the manufacture of capsules. The gelatin used in the manufacture of capsules is obtained from collagenous material by hydrolysis. There are two types of gelatin, Type A, derived mainly from pork skins by acid processing, and Type B, obtained from bones and animal skins by

alkaline processing. Blends are used to obtain gelatin solutions with the viscosity and bloom strength characteristics desirable for capsule manufacture.[50]

The encapsulation of medicinal agents remains a popular method for administering drugs. Capsules are tasteless, easily administered, and easily filled either extemporaneously or in large quantities commercially. In prescription practice the use of hard gelatin capsules permits a choice in prescribing a single drug or a combination of drugs at the exact dosage level considered best for the individual patient. This flexibility is an advantage over tablets. Some patients find it easier to swallow capsules than tablets, therefore preferring to take this form when possible. This preference has prompted pharmaceutical manufacturers to market the product in capsule form, even though the product already has been produced in tablet form. While the industry prepares approximately 75% of its solid dosage forms as compressed tablets, 23% as hard gelatin capsules, and 2% as soft elastic capsules, market surveys have indicated a consumer preference of 44.2% for soft elastic capsules, 39.6% for tablets, and 19.4% for hard gelatin capsules.[51]

HARD GELATIN CAPSULES

The hard gelatin capsule, also referred to as the dry-filled capsule (DFC), consists of two sections, one slipping over the other, thus completely surrounding the drug formulation. The classic capsule shape is illustrated in Figure 45-39. These capsules are filled by introducing the powdered material into the longer end or body of the capsule and then slipping on the cap. Hard gelatin capsules are made largely from gelatin, FD&C colorants, and sometimes an opacifying agent such as titanium dioxide; the USP permits the gelatin for this purpose to contain 0.15% sulfur dioxide to prevent decomposition during manufacture. Hard gelatin capsules contain 12–16% water, but the water content can vary depending on the storage conditions. When the humidity is low, the capsules become brittle; if stored at high humidities, the capsules become flaccid and lose their shape. Storage in high-temperature areas also can affect the quality of hard gelatin capsules. Gelatin capsules do not protect hygroscopic materials from atmospheric water vapor, as moisture can diffuse through the gelatin wall.

Companies having equipment for preparing empty hard gelatin capsules include *Lilly, Parke-Davis, Scherer,* and *SmithKline.* The latter's production is mainly for its own use; the others are suppliers to the industry. With this equipment, stainless steel pins, set in plates, are dipped into the gelatin solution, which must be maintained at a uniform temperature and an exact degree of fluidity. If the gelatin solution varies in viscosity, it correspondingly will decrease or increase the thickness of the capsule wall. This is important since a slight variation is sufficient to make either a loose or a tight joint. When the pins have been withdrawn from the gelatin solution, they are rotated while being dried in kilns through which a strong blast of filtered air with controlled humidity is forced. Each capsule is stripped, trimmed to uniform length and joined, the entire process being mechanical. Capsule-making equipment is illustrated in Figures 45-40 and 45-41. These show the stainless steel pins being dipped into the gelatin solutions and then being rotated through the drying kiln.

Capsules are supplied in a variety of sizes. The hard, empty capsules (Fig 45-39) are numbered from 000, the largest size that can be swallowed, to 5, which is the smallest. Larger sizes are available for use in veterinary medicine. The approximate capacity for capsules from 000 to 5 ranges from 600 to 30 mg, although this will vary because of the different densities of powdered drug materials.

Commercially filled capsules have the conventional oblong shape illustrated, with the exception of capsule products by *Lilly* and *SmithKline,* which are of distinctive shape. For Lilly

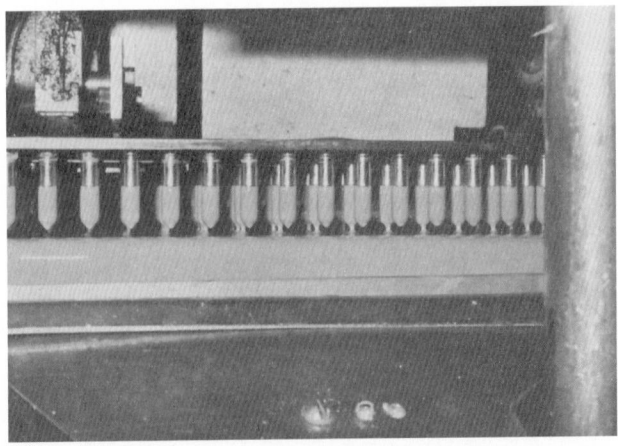

Figure 45-40. Manufacture of hard gelatin capsules by dipping stainless steel pins into gelatin solutions (courtesy, Lilly).

products, capsules are used in which the end of the base is tapered to give the capsule a bullet-like shape; products encapsulated in this form are called *Pulvules.* The *SmithKline* capsules differ in that both ends of the cap and body are angular, rather than round.

After hard gelatin capsules are filled and the cap applied, there are a number of methods used to ensure that the capsules will not come apart if subjected to vibration or rough handling, as in high-speed counting and packaging equipment. The capsules can be spot-welded by means of a heated metal pin pressed against the cap, fusing it to the body, or they may be banded with molten gelatin laid around the joint in a strip and dried. Colored gelatin bands around capsules have been used for many years as a trademark by *Parke-Davis* for their line of capsule products, *Kapseals.* Another approach was used in the *Snap-Fit* and *Coni-Snap* capsules. A pair of matched locking rings are formed into the cap and body portions of the capsule. Prior to filling, these capsules are slightly longer than regular capsules of the same size. When the locking rings are engaged after filling, their length is equivalent to that of the conventional capsule.

Following several tampering incidents, many pharmaceutical companies now use any number of locking and sealing technologies to manufacture and distribute these very useful dosage forms safely. Unfortunately, tamper-resistant packaging has become standard for capsule products.

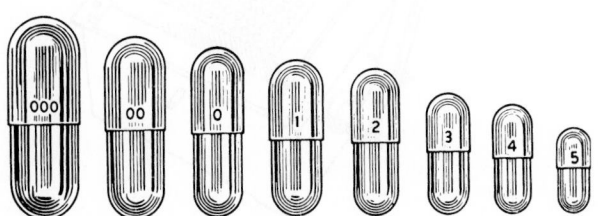

Figure 45-39. Hard gelatin capsules showing relative sizes (courtesy, Parke-Davis).

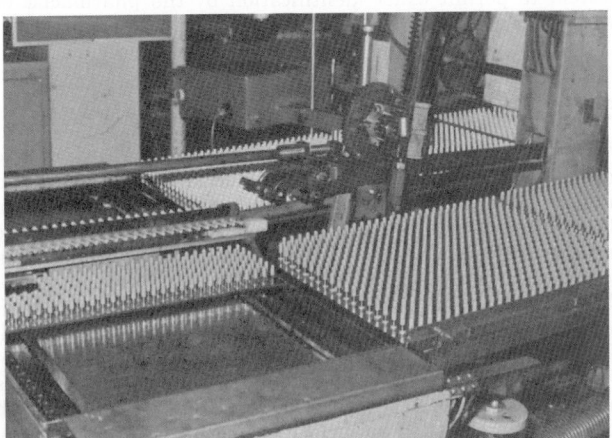

Figure 45-41. Formed capsules being dried by rotating through a drying kiln (courtesy, Lilly).

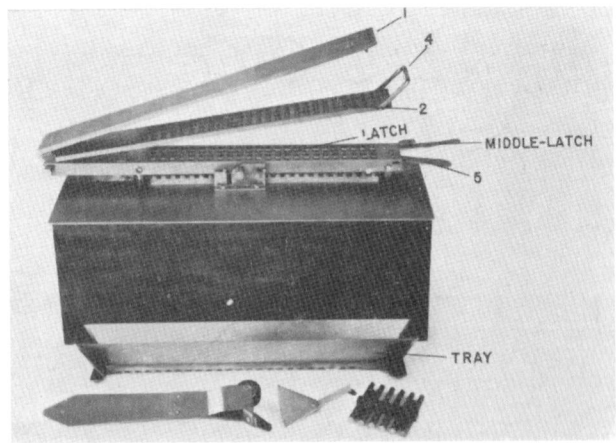

Figure 45-42. Hand-operated capsule machine (courtesy, Chemi-Pharm).

It is usually necessary for the pharmacist to determine the size of the capsule needed for a given prescription through experimentation. The experienced pharmacist, having calculated the weight of material to be held by a single capsule, often will select the correct size immediately. If the material is powdered, the base of the capsule is filled and the top is replaced. If the material in the capsule proves to be too heavy after weighing, a smaller size must be taken and the test repeated. If the filled capsule is light, it is possible that more can be forced into it by increasing the pressure or, if necessary, some of the material may be placed in the cap. This is not desirable as it tends to decrease the accuracy of subdivision and it is much better to select another size, whose base will hold exactly the correct quantity. In prescription filling it is wise to check the weight of each filled capsule.

In addition to the transparent, colorless, hard gelatin capsule, capsules are also available in various transparent colors such as pink, green, reddish brown, blue, yellow, and black. If they are used, it is important to note the color as well as the capsule size on the prescription so that in the case of renewal the refilled prescription will duplicate the original. Colored capsules have been used chiefly by manufacturers to give a specialty product a distinctive appearance. Titanium dioxide is added to the gelatin to form white capsules or to make an opaque, colored capsule. In addition to color contrasts, many commercial products in capsules are given further identification by markings, which may be the company's name, a symbol on the outer shell of the capsule, or banding. Some manufacturers mark capsules with special numbers based on a coded system to permit exact identification by the pharmacist or physician.

Extemporaneous Filling Methods

When filling capsules on prescription, the usual procedure is to mix the ingredients by trituration, reducing them to a fine and uniform powder. The principles and methods for the uniform distribution of an active medicinal agent in a powder mixture are discussed in Chapter 37. Granular powders do not pack readily in capsules, and crystalline materials, especially those that consist of a mass of filament-like crystals such as the quinine salts, are not fitted easily into capsules unless powdered. Eutectic mixtures that tend to liquefy may be dispensed in capsules if a suitable absorbent such as magnesium carbonate is used. Potent drugs given in small doses usually are mixed with an inert diluent such as lactose before filling into capsules. When incompatible materials are prescribed together, it is sometimes possible to place one in a smaller capsule and then enclose it with the second drug in a larger capsule.

Usually, the powder is placed on paper and flattened with a spatula so that the layer of powder is not greater than about ⅓ the length of the capsule that is being filled. This helps to keep both the hands and capsules clean. The cap is removed from the selected capsule and held in the left hand; the body is pressed repeatedly into the powder until it is filled. The cap is replaced and the capsule is weighed. In filling the capsule the spatula is helpful in pushing the last quantity of the material into the capsule. If each capsule has not been weighed, there is likely to be an excess or a shortage of material when the specified number of capsules have been packed. This condition is adjusted before dispensing the prescription.

A number of manual filling machines and automatic capsule machines are available for increasing the speed of the capsule-filling operation. Figure 45-42 illustrates a capsule-filling machine that was known formerly as the Sharp & Dohme machine. This equipment is now available through *ChemiPharm*. Many community pharmacists find this a useful piece of apparatus, and some pharmaceutical manufacturers use it for small-scale production of specialty items. The machine fills 24 capsules at a time with the possible production of 2000 per day. Entire capsules are placed in the machine by hand; the lower plate carries a clamp that holds the capsule bases and makes it possible to remove and replace the caps mechanically. The plate holding the capsule bases is perforated for three sizes of capsules. The powder is packed in the bases; the degree of accuracy depends on the selection of capsule size and the amount of pressure applied in packing. The hand-operated machine (Model 300, *ChemiPharm*) illustrated in Figure 45-43 has a production capacity of 2000 capsules per hour. The machine is made for a single capsule size and cannot be changed over for other sizes. A different machine is required for any additional capsule size. Its principle of operation is similar to that of the Sharp & Dohme machine.

Machine Filling Methods

Large-scale filling equipment for capsules operates on the same principle as the manual machines described above, namely the filling of the base of the capsule. Compared with tablets,

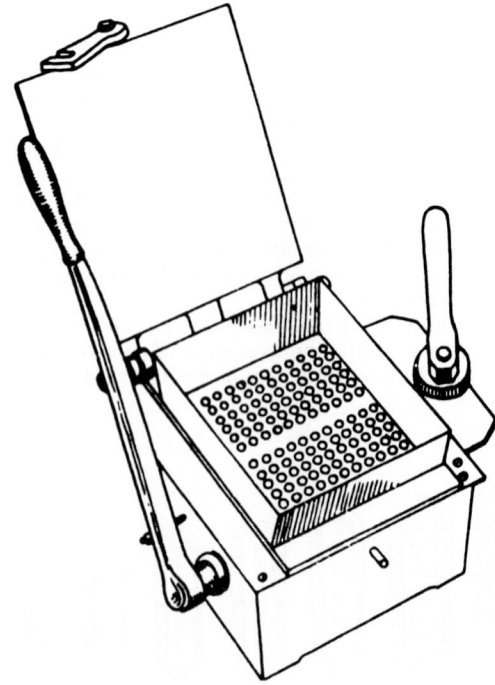

Figure 45-43. Hand-operated capsule machine, Model 300 (courtesy, ChemiPharm).

Table 45-5. Capsule Fill Chart
CAPSULE FILL WEIGHTS (MG) BASED ON SIZE AND DENSITY

POWDER DENSITY (g/ml)	CAPSULE VOLUME (mL)									
	0.95	0.78	0.68	0.54	0.5	0.37	0.3	0.25	0.21	0.13
	CAPSULE SIZE									
	00	0el	0	1el	1	2	3	4el	4	5
0.3	285	234	204	162	150	111	90	75	63	39
0.4	380	312	272	216	200	148	120	100	84	52
0.5	475	390	340	270	250	185	150	125	105	65
0.6	570	468	408	324	300	222	180	150	126	78
0.7	665	546	476	378	350	259	210	175	147	91
0.8	760	624	544	432	400	296	240	200	168	104
0.9	855	702	612	486	450	333	270	225	189	117
1.0	950	780	680	540	500	370	300	250	210	130
1.1	1045	858	748	594	550	407	330	275	231	143
1.2	1140	936	816	648	600	444	360	300	252	156
1.3	1235	1014	884	702	650	481	390	325	273	169
1.4	1330	1092	952	756	700	518	420	350	294	182
1.5	1425	1170	1020	810	750	555	450	375	315	195

powders for filling into hard gelatin capsules require a minimum of formulation efforts. The powders usually contain diluents such as lactose, mannitol, calcium carbonate, or magnesium carbonate. Since the flow of material is of great importance in the rapid and accurate filling of the capsule bodies, lubricants such as the stearates also are used frequently.

Because of the absence of numerous additives and manufacturing processing, the capsule form is used frequently to administer new drug substances for evaluation in initial clinical trials. However, it is now realized that the additives present in the capsule formulation, like the compressed tablet, can influence the release of the drug substance from the capsule. Tablets and capsules of a combination product containing triamterene and hydrochlorothiazide in a 2:1 ratio were compared clinically. The tablet caused approximately twice as much excretion of hydrochlorothiazide and three times as much triamterene as the capsule.[52]

Most equipment operates on the principle by which the base of the capsule is filled and the excess is scraped off. Therefore, the active ingredient is mixed with sufficient volume of a diluent, usually lactose or mannitol, to give the desired amount of the drug in the capsule when the base is filled with the powder mixture. The manner of operation of the machine can influence the volume of powder that will be filled into the base of the capsule; therefore, the weights of the capsules must be checked routinely as they are filled. See Table 45-5.

Semiautomatic capsule-filling machines manufactured by *Parke-Davis* and *Lilly* are illustrated in Figures 45-44 and 45-45. The Type 8 capsule-filling machine performs mechanically under the same principle as the hand filling of capsules. This includes separation of the cap from the body, filling the body half, and rejoining the cap and body halves.

Empty capsules are taken from the bottom of the capsule hopper into the magazine. The magazine gauge releases one

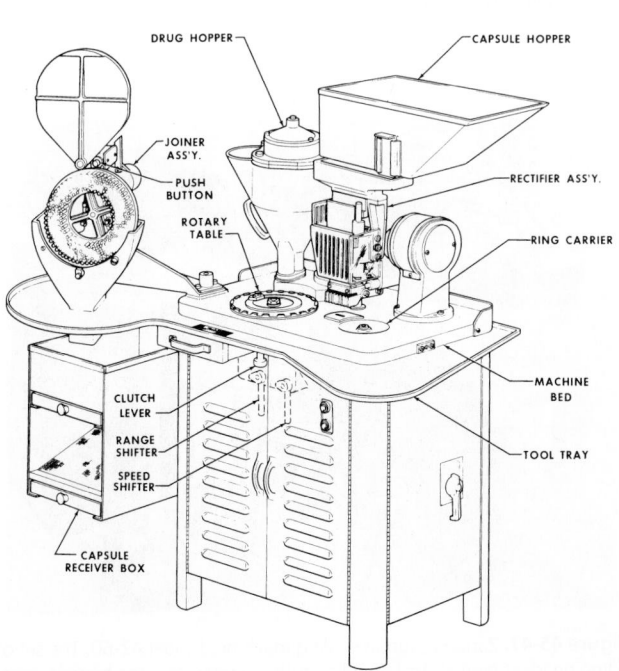

Figure 45-44. Schematic of Type 8 capsule-filling machine (courtesy, Parke-Davis).

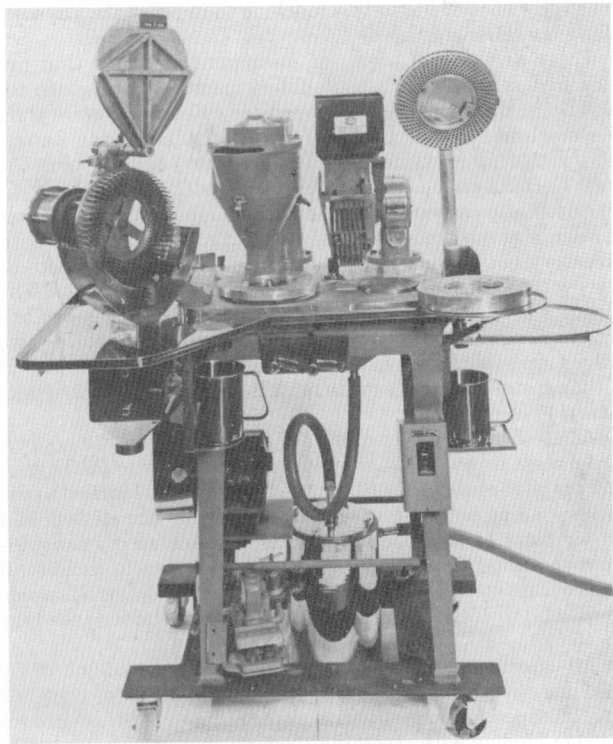

Figure 45-45. Type 8 capsule-filling machine (courtesy, Lilly).

capsule from each tube at the bottom of each stroke of the machine. Leaving the magazine, the capsules drop onto the tracks of the raceway and are pushed forward to the rectifying area with a push blade. The rectifier block descends, turning the capsules in each track, cap up, and drops them into each row of holes in the capsule-holding ring assembly.

As the capsules fall into the holding ring, the cap half has a seat on the counter bore in each hole for the top ring. The body half is pulled by vacuum down into the bottom ring. When all rows in the ring assembly are full, the top ring, filled with caps only, is removed and set aside for later assembly. The body halves now are located in the bottom ring, ready for filling.

The ring holding the body halves is rotated at one of eight speeds on the rotary table. The drug hopper is swung over the rotating ring, and the auger forces drug powder into the open body cavities. When the ring has made a complete revolution and the body halves have been filled, the hopper is swung aside. The cap-holding ring is placed over the body-holding ring and the assembly is ready for joining. The capsule-holding ring assembly is placed on the joiner and the joiner plate is swung down into position to hold the capsules in the ring. The peg ring pins are entered in the holes of the body holding ring and tapped in place by the air cylinder pushing the body halves back into the cap halves.

The holding-ring assembly is now pushed by hand back onto the peg ring away from the joiner plate, thus pushing the capsules out of the holding-ring assembly. The joined capsules then fall through the joiner chute into the capsule receiver box. The capsule receiver box screens the excess powder from the capsules and delivers them to any convenient container.

Many companies use the Type 8 capsule-filling equipment for small-scale manufacture and clinical supplies for investigational use because of its ease of operation, low cost, and extreme flexibility. A Type 8 capsule filling machine will produce approximately 200,000 capsules per day. This, of course, depends upon the operator and the type of material being filled. For this machine, a mathematical model has been developed that describes the effect of selected physical powder properties as well as mechanical operating conditions on the capsule-filling operation. While the Type 8 capsule-filling machine has been in existence for many years, recent modifications have been made to this machine to improve the capsule-filling operations.

There are several pieces of equipment available that are classified as automatic capsule-filling machines. These are automatic in the sense that one operator can handle more than one machine. In this category are the Italian-made Zanasi (*United Machinery*) and MG-2 (*Supermatic*) models, plus the West German–made Hoefliger & Karg models (*Bosch*).

Automatic capsule machines are capable of filling either powder or granulated products into hard gelatin capsules. With accessory equipment these machines also can fill pellets or place a tablet into the capsule with the powder or pellets. The capsules are fed at random into a large hopper. They are oriented as required and transferred into holders where the two halves are separated by suction. The top-half and bottom-half of the capsules are in separate holders, which at this stage take diverting directions.

A set of filling heads collects the product from the hopper, compresses it into a soft slug, and inserts this into the bottom half of the capsule. After filling, each top-half is returned to the corresponding bottom-half. The filled capsules are ejected, and an air blast at this point separates possible empty capsules from the filled. The machines can be equipped to handle all sizes of capsules. Depending upon the make and model, speeds from 9000 to 150,000 units per hour can be obtained (see Figs 45-46 to 45-48).

All capsules, whether they have been filled by hand or by machine, will require cleaning. Small quantities of capsules may be wiped individually with cloth. Larger quantities are rotated or shaken with crystalline sodium chloride. The capsules then are rolled on a cloth-covered surface.

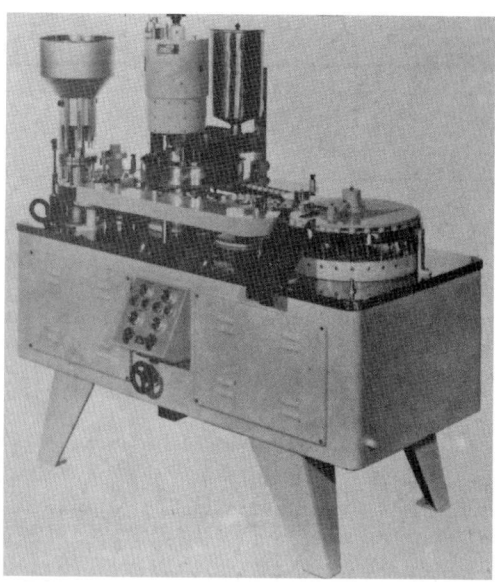

Figure 45-46. MG-2, automatic capsule-filling machine (courtesy, Supermatic).

Uniformity of Dosage Units

The uniformity of dosage forms can be demonstrated by either of two methods, weight variation or content uniformity. Weight variation may be applied when the product is a liquid-filled, soft, elastic capsule or when the hard gelatin capsule contains 50 mg or more of a single active ingredient comprising 50% or more, by weight, of the dosage form. See the official compendia for details.

Disintegration tests usually are not required for capsules unless they have been treated to resist solution in gastric fluid (enteric-coated). In this case they must meet the requirements for disintegration of enteric-coated tablets. For certain capsule dosage forms a dissolution requirement is part of the monograph. Procedures used are similar to those employed in the case of compressed tablets.

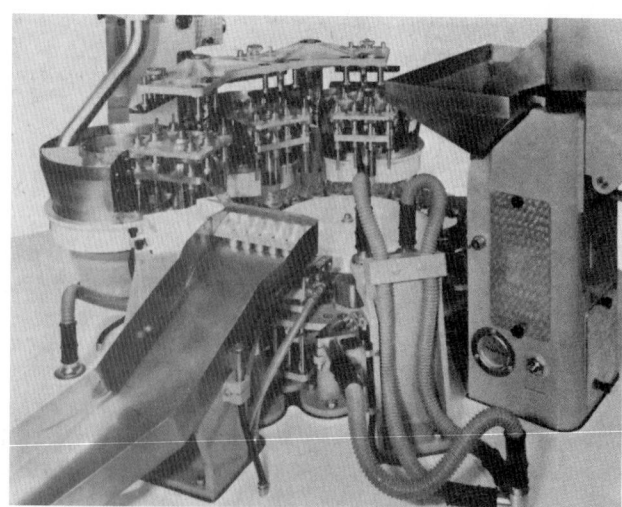

Figure 45-47. Zanasi automatic filling machine, Model AZ-60. The set of filling heads shown at the left collects the powder from the hopper, compresses it into a soft slug, and inserts it into the bottom half of the capsule (courtesy, United Machinery).

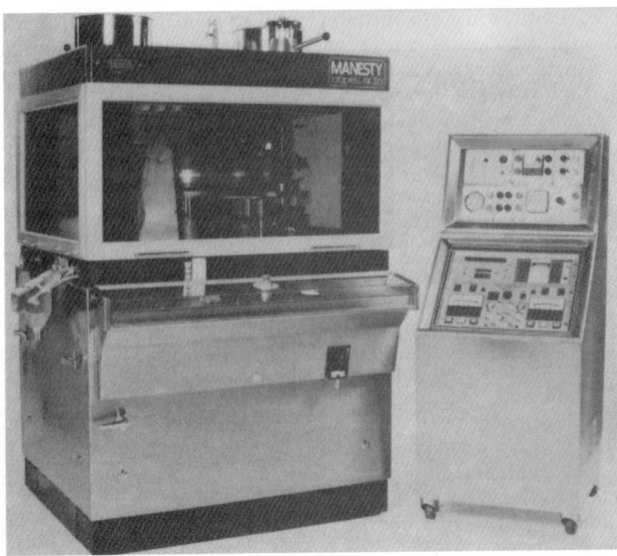

Figure 45-48. Hoefliger & Karg automatic capsule-filling machine, Model GFK 1200 (courtesy, Amaco).

SOFT ELASTIC CAPSULES

The soft elastic capsule (SEC) is a soft, globular, gelatin shell somewhat thicker than that of hard gelatin capsules. The gelatin is plasticized by the addition of glycerin, sorbitol, or a similar polyol. The soft gelatin shells may contain a preservative to prevent the growth of fungi. Commonly used preservatives are methyl- and propylparabens and sorbic acid. When the suspending vehicle or solvent can be an oil, soft gelatin capsules provide a convenient and highly acceptable dosage form. Large-scale production methods generally are required for the preparation and filling of soft gelatin capsules.

Formerly, empty soft gelatin capsules were available to the pharmacist for the extemporaneous compounding of solutions or suspensions in oils. Commercially filled soft gelatin capsules come in a wide choice of sizes and shapes; they may be round, oval, oblong, tubular, or suppository-shaped. Some sugar-coated tablets are quite similar in appearance to soft gelatin capsules. The essential differences are that the soft gelatin capsule has a seam at the point of closure of the two halves, and the contents can be liquid, paste, or powder. The sugar-coated tablet will not have a seam but will have a compressed core.

Oral SEC dosage forms generally are made so that the heat seam of the gelatin shell opens to release its liquid medication into the stomach less than 5 min after ingestion. Its use is being studied for those drugs poorly soluble in water having bioavailability problems. When used as suppositories, it is the moisture present in the body cavity that causes the capsule to come apart at its heat-sealed seam and to release its contents.

Plate Process

In this method a set of molds is used. A warm sheet of prepared gelatin is laid over the lower plate, and the liquid is poured on it. A second sheet of gelatin is carefully put in place, and this is followed by the top plate of the mold. The set is placed under the press where pressure is applied to form the capsules, which are washed off with a volatile solvent to remove any traces of oil from the exterior. This process has been adapted and is used for encapsulation by *Upjohn*. The sheets of gelatin may have the same color or different colors.

Rotary-Die Process

In 1933 the rotary-die process for elastic capsules was perfected by Robert P Scherer.[53] This process made it possible to improve the standards of accuracy and uniformity of elastic gelatin capsules and globules.

The rotary-die machine is a self-contained unit capable of continuously and automatically producing finished capsules from a supply of gelatin mass and filling material, which may be any liquid, semiliquid, or paste that will not dissolve gelatin. Two continuous gelatin ribbons, which the machine forms, are brought into convergence between a pair of revolving dies and an injection wedge. Accurate filling under pressure and sealing of the capsule wall occur as dual and coincident operations; each is delicately timed against the other. Sealing also severs the completed capsule from the net. The principle of operation is shown in Figure 45-49. See also Figure 45-50.

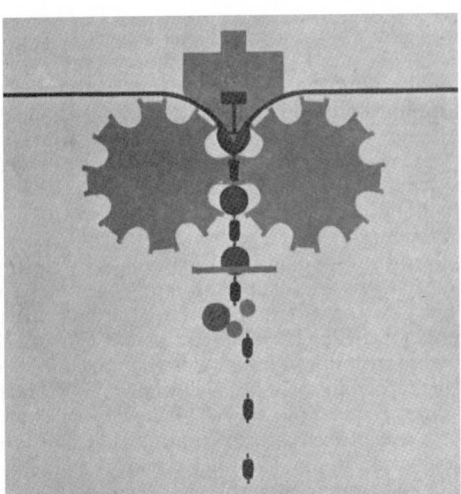

Figure 45-49. Rotary-die elastic capsule filler.

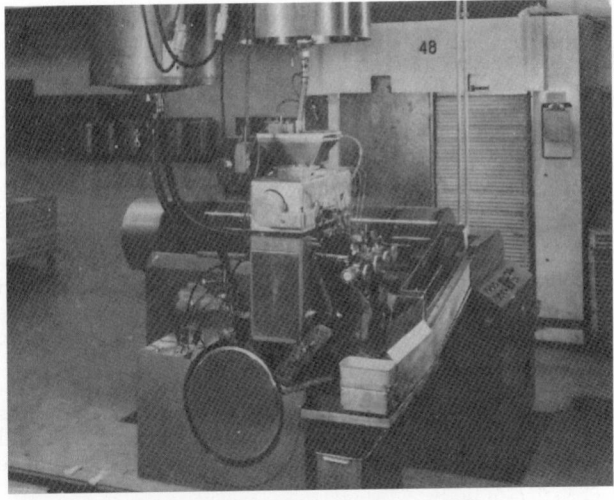

Figure 45-50. Scherer soft elastic capsule machine (courtesy, Scherer).

By this process the content of each capsule is measured individually by a single stroke of a pump so accurately constructed that plunger travel of 0.025 inch will deliver 1 <minim> (apoth). The Scherer machine contains banks of pumps so arranged that many capsules may be formed and filled simultaneously. All pumps are engineered to extremely small mechanical tolerances and to an extremely high degree of precision and similarity. All operations are controlled on a weight basis by actual periodic checks with a group of analytical balances. Individual net-fill weights of capsules resulting from large-scale production vary no more than ±1 to 3% from theory, depending upon the materials used.

The rotary-die process makes it possible to encapsulate heavy materials such as ointments and pastes. In this manner solids can be milled with a vehicle and filled into capsules. When it is desirable to have a high degree of accuracy and a hermetically sealed product, this form of enclosure is suited ideally.

The modern and well-equipped capsule plant is completely air conditioned, a practical necessity for fine capsule production. Its facilities and operations include the availability of carbon dioxide at every exposed point of operation for the protection of oxidizable substances before encapsulation. Special ingredients also have been used in the capsule shell to exclude light wavelengths that are destructive to certain drugs.

Norton Capsule Machine

This machine produces capsules completely automatically by leading two films of gelatin between a set of vertical dies. These dies as they close, open, and close are in effect a continual vertical plate forming row after row of pockets across the gelatin film. These are filled with medicament and, as they progress through the dies, are sealed, shaped, and cut out of the film as capsules, which drop into a cooled solvent bath.

Accogel Capsule Machine

Another means of soft gelatin encapsulation uses the Accogel machine and process which were developed at *Lederle*. The Accogel, or Stern machine, uses a system of rotary dies but is unique in that it is the only machine that successfully can fill dry powder into a soft gelatin capsule. The machine is available to the entire pharmaceutical industry by a lease arrangement and is used in many countries of the world. It is extremely versatile, not only producing capsules with dry powder but also encapsulating liquids and combinations of liquids and powders. By means of an attachment, slugs or compressed tablets may be enclosed in a gelatin film. The capsules can be made in a variety of colors, shapes, and sizes.

Microencapsulation

As a technology, microencapsulation is placed in the section on capsules only because of the relationship in terminology to mechanical encapsulation described above. The topic is also discussed in Chapter 47 (Extended-release and Targeted Drug Delivery Systems) of this text. Essentially, microencapsulation is a process or technique by which thin coatings can be applied reproducibly to small particles of solids, droplets of liquids, or dispersions, thus forming microcapsules. It can be differentiated readily from other coating methods in the size of the particles involved; these range from several tenths of a micrometer to 5000 μm in size.

A number of microencapsulation processes have been disclosed in the literature.[54] Some are based on chemical processes and involve a chemical or phase change; others are mechanical and require special equipment to produce the physical change in the systems required.

A number of coating materials have been used successfully; examples of these include gelatin, polyvinyl alcohol, ethylcellu-

lose, cellulose acetate phthalate, and styrene maleic anhydride. The film thickness can be varied considerably, depending on the surface area of the material to be coated and other physical characteristics of the system. The microcapsules may consist of a single particle or clusters of particles. After isolation from the liquid manufacturing vehicle and drying, the material appears as a free-flowing powder. The powder is suitable for formulation as compressed tablets, hard gelatin capsules, suspensions, and other dosage forms.

The process provides answers for problems such as masking the taste of bitter drugs, a means of formulating prolonged-action dosage forms, a means of separating incompatible materials, a method of protecting chemicals against moisture or oxidation, and a means of modifying a material's physical characteristics for ease of handling in formulation and manufacture.

Among the processes applied to pharmaceutical problems is that developed by the National Cash Register Co (NCR). The NCR process is a chemical operation based on phase separation or coacervation techniques. In colloidal chemistry, coacervation refers to the separation of a liquid precipitate, or phase, when solutions of two hydrophilic colloids are mixed under suitable conditions.

The NCR process, using phase separation or coacervation techniques, consists of three steps:

1. Formation of three immiscible phases: a liquid manufacturing phase, a core material phase, and a coating material phase.
2. Deposition of the liquid polymer coating on the core material.
3. Rigidizing the coating, usually by thermal, cross-linking, or desolvation techniques, to form a microcapsule.

In Step 2, the deposition of the liquid polymer around the core material occurs only if the polymer is absorbed at the interface formed between the core material and the liquid vehicle phase. In many cases physical or chemical changes in the coating polymer solution can be induced so that phase separation (coacervation) of the polymer will occur. Droplets of concentrated polymer solution will form and coalesce to yield a two-phase, liquid-liquid system. In cases in which the coating material is an immiscible polymer or insoluble liquid polymer, it may be added directly. Also monomers can be dissolved in the liquid vehicle phase and, subsequently, polymerized at the interface.

Equipment required for microencapsulation by this method is relatively simple; it consists mainly of jacketed tanks with variable-speed agitators. Figure 45-51 shows a typical flow diagram of a production installation.

Other Oral Solid Dosage Forms

PILLS

Pills are small, round, solid, dosage forms containing a medicinal agent and are intended for oral administration. Pills were formerly the most extensively used oral dosage form, but they have been replaced largely by compressed tablets and capsules. Substances that are bitter or unpleasant to the taste, if not corrosive or deliquescent, can be administered in this form if the dose is not too large.

Formerly, pills were made extemporaneously by the community pharmacist whose skill at pill-making became an art. However, the few pills that are now used in pharmacy are prepared on a large scale with mechanical equipment. The pill formulas of the NF were introduced largely for the purpose of establishing standards of strength for the well-known and currently used pills. Hexylresorcinol Pills consist of hexylresorcinol crystals covered with a rupture-resistant coating that is dispersible in the digestive tract. It should be noted that the official hexylresorcinol pills are prepared not by traditional methods but by a patented process, the gelatin coating being sufficiently tough that it cannot be broken readily, even when chewed. Therefore,

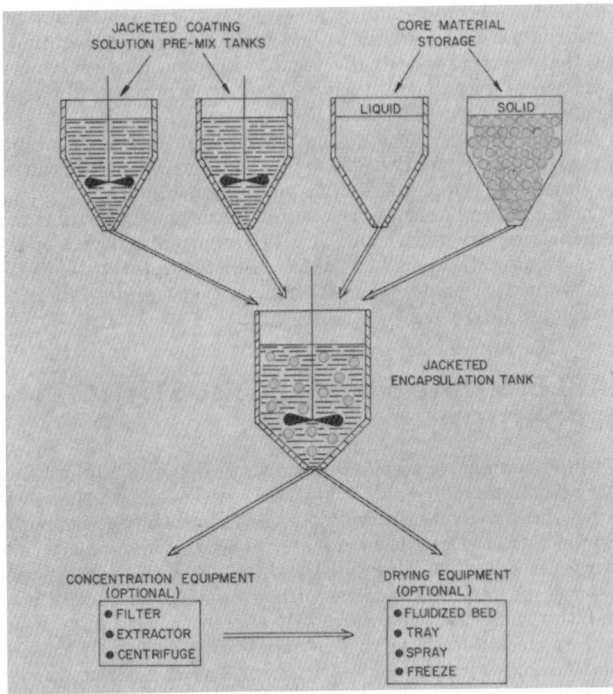

Figure 45-51. Production installation for the microencapsulation process (courtesy, NCR).

the general method for the preparation of pills does not apply to hexylresorcinol pills.

Previous editions of this text should be consulted for methods of pill preparation.

TROCHES

These forms of oral medication, also known as *lozenges* or *pastilles,* are discoid-shaped solids containing the medicinal agent in a suitably flavored base. The base may be a hard sugar candy, glycerinated gelatin, or the combination of sugar with sufficient mucilage to give it form. Troches are placed in the mouth, where they slowly dissolve, liberating the active ingredient. The drug involved can be an antiseptic, local anesthetic, antibiotic, antihistaminic, antitussive, analgesic, or a decongestant.

Formerly, troches were prepared extemporaneously by the pharmacist. The mass is formed by adding water slowly to a mixture of the powdered drug, powdered sugar, and a gum until a pliable mass is formed. Powdered acacia in 7% concentration gives sufficient adhesiveness to the mass. The mass is rolled out and the troche pieces cut out using a cutter, or else the mass is rolled into a cylinder and divided. Each piece is shaped and allowed to dry before dispensing.

If the active ingredient is heat-stable, it may be prepared in a hard candy base. Syrup is concentrated to the point at which it becomes a pliable mass, the active ingredient is added, and the mixture is kneaded while warm to form a homogeneous mass. The mass is worked gradually into a pipe form having the diameter desired for the candy piece, and the lozenges are cut from the pipe and allowed to cool. This is an entirely mechanical operation with equipment designed for this purpose.

If the active ingredient is heat-labile, it may be made into a lozenge preparation by compression. The granulation is prepared in a manner similar to that used for any compressed tablet. The lozenge is made using heavy compression equipment to give a tablet that is harder than usual, as it is desirable for the troche to dissolve or disintegrate slowly in the mouth. In the formulation of the lozenge the ingredients are chosen that will promote its slow-dissolving characteristics. Compression is

gaining in popularity as a means of making troches and candy pieces because of the increased speeds of compression equipment. In cases in which holes are to be placed in troches or candy pieces, core-rod tooling is used (Fig 45-52). Core-rod tooling includes a rod centered on the lower punch around which the troche is compressed in the die cavity. The upper punch has an opening in its center for the core rod to enter during compression. It is evident that maximum accuracy is needed to provide alignment as the narrow punches are inserted into the die.

CACHETS

Related to capsules, inasmuch as they provide an edible container for the oral administration of solid drugs, cachets formerly were used in pharmacy. They varied in size from ¾ to ⅛ inch in diameter and consisted of two concave pieces of wafer made of flour and water. After one section was filled with the prescribed quantity of the medicinal agent, they were sealed tightly by moistening the margins and pressing them firmly together. When moistened with water, their character was changed entirely; they became soft, elastic, and slippery. Hence, they could be swallowed easily by floating them on water.

PELLETS

The term pellet is sometimes applied to small, sterile cylinders about 3.2 mm in diameter by 8 mm in length, which are formed by compression from medicated masses.[55] Whenever prolonged and continuous absorption of testosterone, estradiol, or desoxycorticosterone is desired, pellets of these potent hormones may be used by implantation.

MEDICATED CHEWING GUM

Chewing gum has been a widely popular form of confection that has its roots in ancient times. Only recently has its use as a drug delivery system become mainstream. Worldwide, there are commercially available chewing gums for use in smoking cessation, pain relief, and motion sickness. Chewing gum can also offer an advantage for localized delivery of drugs in the mouth, and is now being evaluated for these uses.[56–60]

Gums can be manufactured by a variety of mixing processes that incorporate several components into a sheet of product,

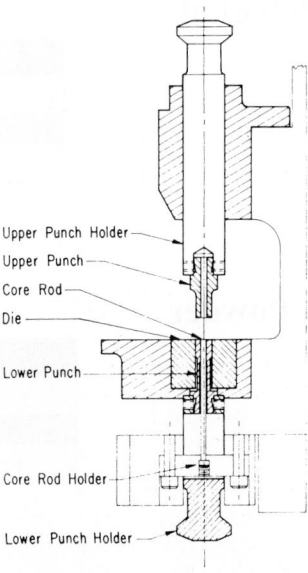

Figure 45-52. Core-rod tooling for compressing troches or candy pieces with hole in center (courtesy, Vector/Colton).

Table 45-6. Formula of a Medicated Chewing Gum

COMPONENT	CONENTRATION (%W/W)
Drug	0–40
Gum Base	20–45
Sweeteners	30–60
Softeners	0–10
Flavor(s)	1–5
Color(s)	0–1

whereby the units are stamped or cut from the rolled out sheet. A typical formulation for a chewing gum might be considered in Table 45-6.

Chewing gums can be made by compression and other processes, but the predominant method in use today is mixing, rolling and stamping of the finished units. After the finished units are completed, they can be film or sugar coated for better mouth feel or taste improvement.

RAPIDLY DISSOLVING TABLETS

Recently, a number of fast-dissolving tablets have been produced to rapidly deliver drugs for a variety of applications. One of the first solid dosage forms, Zydis (RP Scherer) used lyophilized technology to prepare the powder to dissolve quickly on the tongue. Since then, numerous technologies have been developed to give quick dissolution of the active in the mouth. Other technologies such as Lyoc (Farmalyoc), WOW-Tab (Yamanouchi), Flash-Dose (Biovail), Orasolv (CIMA) and DuraSolv

(CIMA) have been used in commercialized products. There are some comparable benefits to one technology over the others, but the objective is still the same. These products have had some acceptance, and will have a place in formularies for years to come.

The challenges these dosage forms have had is durability during shipping, and changes to the drug substance that can occur during the lyophilization or manufacturing process. In addition, these products are best suited for drugs where there is a demonstrable benefit from very fast onset of activity of the drug. To date, there have been few clinical studies to show the significance of benefit of these products over standard immediate-release products.

TABLETS MADE BY ELECTROSTATIC DEPOSITION

The most common example of electrostatic deposition takes place every day in the office photocopy machine. The basic principle of electrostatic deposition is well-founded in basic physics: opposite charges attract. Deposition of material occurs when a pattern of charges is established on the substrate where the deposition is desired, and very fine particles with an opposite charge is placed near the substrate. The Sarnoff Research Laboratories developed an electro-static method of depositing and thereby coating solid surfaces with powder in a dry form. This technology was initially developed for phosphorus coating for cathode ray tubes, and was first applied to the manufacture of tablets by Delsys Corporation, now merged with Elan Corporation.[61–65]

Figure 45-53 illustrates this process. A substrate is chosen as the base for the deposit of particles. The charging is done us-

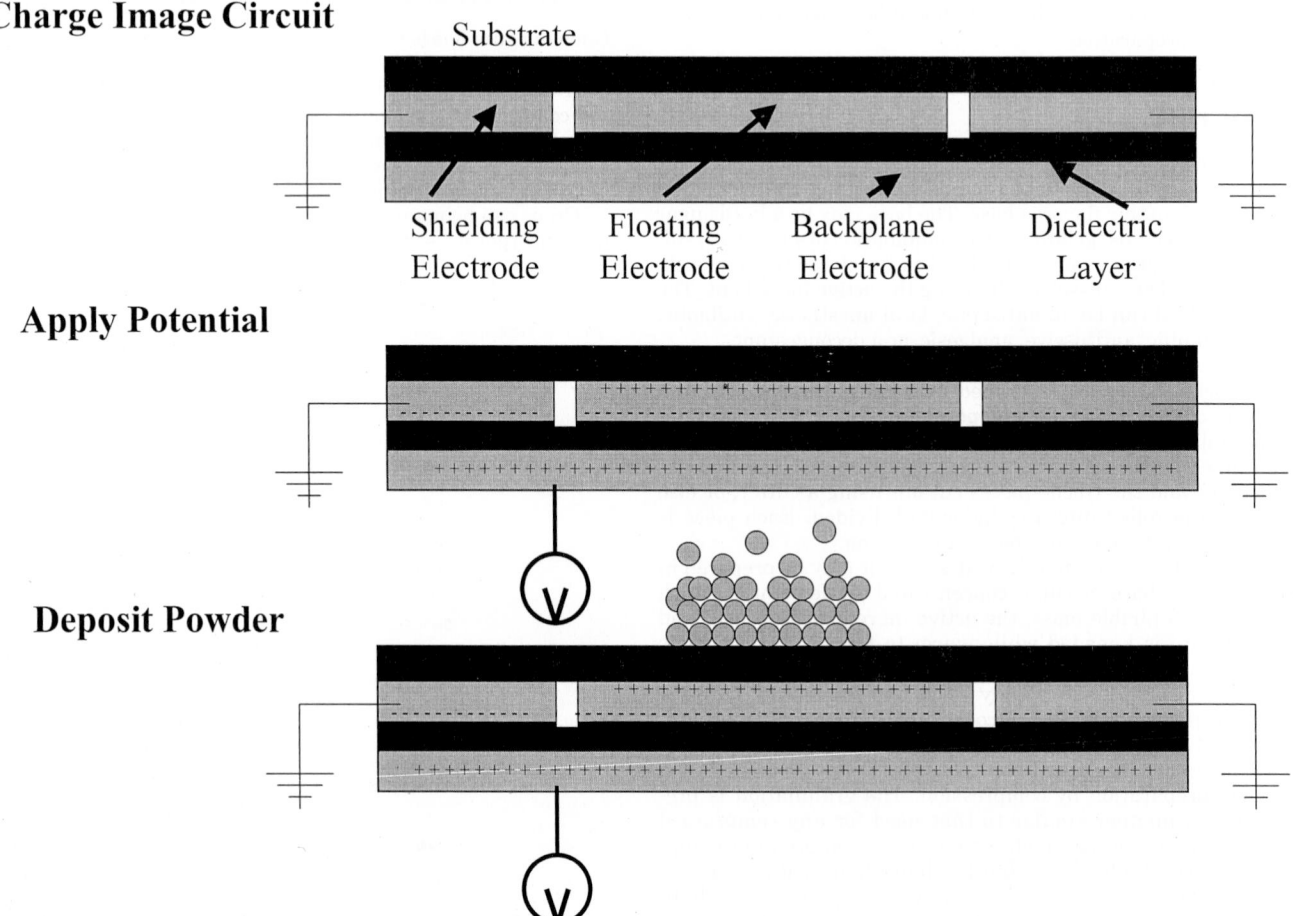

Figure 45-53. Electrostatic powder deposition process.

ing a three-layer structure that has a conducting backplane electrode, an insulating layer and a patterned conducting top electrode. Application of a positive voltage to the backplane electrode establishes a positive surface charge in the electrode. Charges that mirror the backplane charges are induced in the conductive top electrodes. In the floating electrodes, negative mirror charges induced by the backplane electrode leave uncompensated positive charges in the top surface of the floating electrode. By controlling the amount and strength of these positive charges, the rate of deposition and porosity of the resulting solid can be controlled.

The electrostatic process has several potential applications. First, the uniformity of ultra low dose drugs could be precisely achieved. Drugs with significant stability or incompatibility problems could be easily addressed without separate operations. Because little or no excipients are used in this process, the cost, storage and movement of materials in the modern manufacturing facility may be reduced significantly. In addition, it may be possible to have a final formulation designed and finalized much earlier in the development process. Currently, there are no commercial tablets using this technology, but one can imagine the considerable issues associated with the scale-up, validation and implementation of this technology.

THREE-DIMENSIONAL PRINTING OF TABLETS

Another technology that has been adapted for the manufacture of tablets is three-dimensional printing, called 3DP by Therics Corporation, the company to first apply this technology to pharmaceuticals. The technology is quite similar to ink-jet printer technology. It was improved by engineers at the Massachusetts Institute of Technology, and later at Therics.

Figures 45-54 and 45-55 illustrate three-dimensional printing.[66] In Figure 45-54, the basic system is shown. Powder is spread into a tray and binder droplets are precisely sprayed onto a substrate to form virtually any shape or design. A piston holding the unit changes position for each pass of the dispensing module, allowing for a build-up of the tablet. The process is repeated over and over until the desired shape is obtained. Using a tray that can accommodate many hundreds of powder wells, and hundreds of dispensing modules would be required to make this unit suitable for commercial manufacture. To this date, there are no commercial tablets made from this technology. However, it's versatility and complete freedom for design of novel solid dosage forms make this technology fascinating. Figure 45-55 illustrates this point showing a design on the computer screen, with a tablet completed next to it. In the cutaway section can be seen many programmed

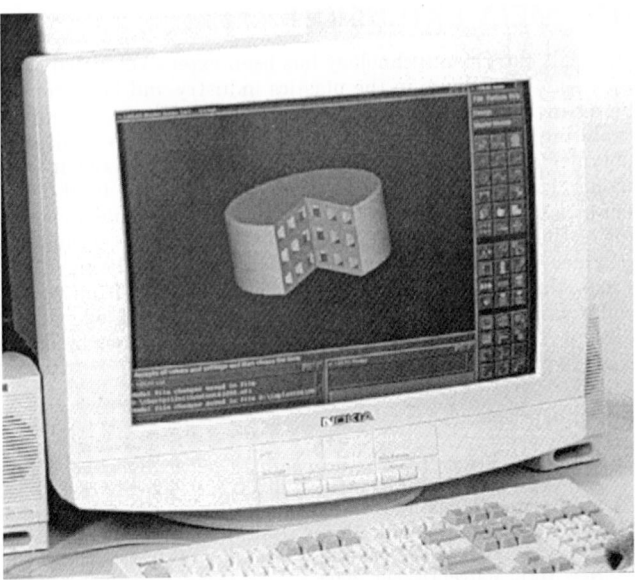

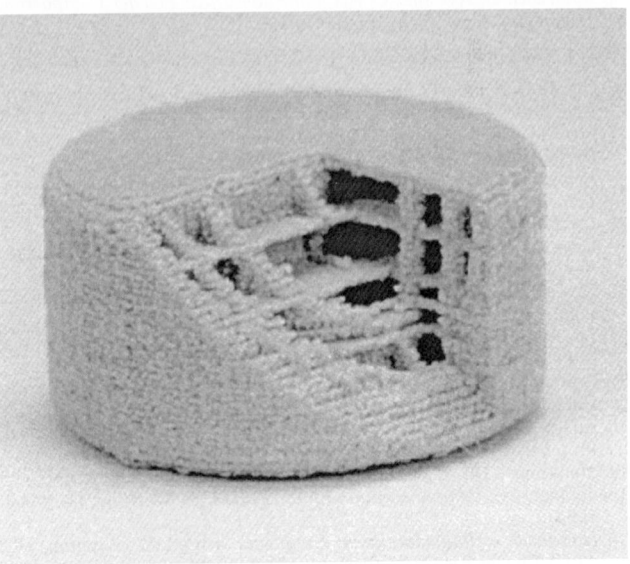

Figure 45-55. Design versatility of three-dimensional printing.

walls and empty compartments "constructed" within the confines of the tablet.

Three-dimensional printing technology has all of the advantages of electrostatic powder deposition, but has many more practical applications.

WEB-COATED SYSTEMS

In the early 1980s, Roche laboratories developed a system whereby sheets of a substrate were coated with drug and binder solution.[62] A number of sheets were then laminated, or glued together to form a complex, multi-layered sheet containing drug and various binder/excipient systems. The final laminate sheet was then punched to produce many dosage forms. This system was quite flexible, and was capable of producing various types of controlled-release, and combination products. However, due to it's impracticality, it was abandoned by Roche in the mid-1980s. It remains an important development, and is instructive from a historical perspective.

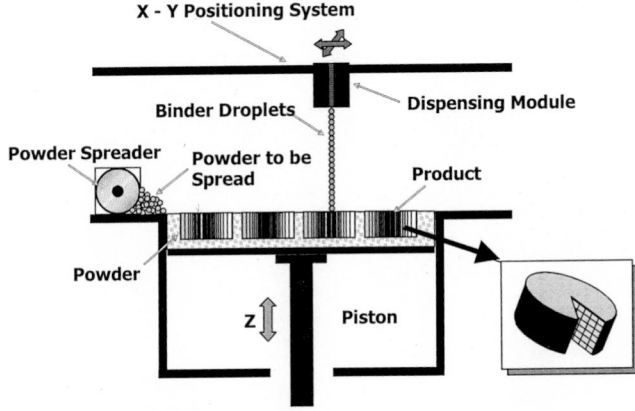

Figure 45-54. Three-dimensional printing process.

HOT-MELT EXTRUSION

Hot-melt extrusion technology has been extensively used as a processing technique in the plastics industry and is currently being investigated in the pharmaceutical arena as a novel tableting method. The process involves the active, suitable polymeric carrier, and other excipients being mixed in the molten state and then extruded through a die. The final product may take the form of a film, pipe, tube, or granule, depending on the shape of the die. A matrix is formed due to the melted polymer acting as a thermal binder. In addition to being anhydrous, this technology offers the advantage of tableting poorly compressible materials and manufacturing sustained-release tablets. The thermal stability of each material must be sufficient to withstand the production process.

REFERENCES

1. Rowland M, Tozer TN. *Clinical Pharmacokinetics: Concepts & Applications.* Baltimore: Lippincott Williams & Wilkins, 1995.
2. Kottke MK, Rudnic EM. In BankerGS, Rhodes CT, eds. *Modern Pharmaceutics.* New York: Marcel Dekker, 2002.
3. Rathbone MJ, et al, eds. *Modified Release Drug Delivery Technology.* New York: Marcel Dekker, 2003.
4. Alderborn G, Nystrom C, eds. *Pharmaceutical Powder Compaction Technology.* New York: Marcel Dekker, 1996.
5. Parikh DM, ed. *Pharmaceutical Granulation Technology.* New York: Marcel Dekker, 1997.
6. Carstensen JT. *Pharmaceutical Principles of Solid Dosage Forms.* Lancaster: Technomic Publishers, 1993.
7. McGinity JW. *Aqueous Polymeric Coatings for Pharmaceutical Dosage Forms.* New York: Dekker, 1989.
8. Lieberman HA, Lachman L, eds. *Pharmaceutical Dosage Forms: Tablets,* vols I, II, and III. New York: Dekker, 1980, 1981, 1982, 2nd rev 1989.
9. Evans AJ, Train D. *A Bibliography of the Tableting of Medicinal Substances.* London: Pharmaceutical Press, 1963.
10. Evans AJ. *A Bibliography of the Tableting of Medicinal Substances.* London: Pharmaceutical Press, 1964.
11. Lachman L, et al. *The Theory and Practice of Industrial Pharmacy,* 3rd ed. Philadelphia: Lea & Febiger, 1988.
12. Banker G, Rhodes CT. *Modern Pharmaceutics,* 4th ed. New York: Dekker, 2002.
13. Ansel HC. *Introduction to Pharmaceutical Dosage Forms,* 3rd ed. Philadelphia: Lea & Febiger, 1981.
14. Monkhouse DC, Lach JL. *Can J Pharm Sci* 1972; 7:29.
15. de Boer, AG. *Drug Absorption Enhancement,* Switzerland: Harwood, 1994.
16. *Handbook of Pharmaceutical Excipients,* 4th ed. Washington, DC: APhA/Pharm Soc Great Brittain, APhA, 2003.
17. Rudnic EM, Kanig JL, Rhodes CT. *J Pharm Sci* 1985; 74:647.
18. Rudnic EM, et al. *Drug Dev Ind Pharm* 1982; 8:87.
19. Kanig JL, Rudnic EM. *Pharm Technol* 1984; 8:50.
20. Rudnic EM, et al. *Drug Dev Ind Pharm* 1981; 7:347.
21. *Capsugel List of Colorants for Oral Drugs.* Basel: Capsugel AG, 1988.
22. Foley VL, Belcastro PF. *Pharm Technol* 1987; 9:110.
23. Stewart A. *Engineering* 1950; 169:203.
24. David ST, Augsburger LL. *J Pharm Sci* 1977; 66:155.
25. Jones TM. In Poldermand J, ed. *Formulation and Preparation of Dosage Forms.* North Holland: Elsevier, 1977, p 29.
26. Rees JE, Rue PJ. *J Pharm Pharmacol* 1987; 30:601.
27. Summers MP, Enever RP, Carless JE. *J Pharm Sci* 1977; 66:1172.
28. Hersey JA, Rees JE. In *Particle Size Analysis.* Groves MJ, Wyatt-Sargent JL, eds. London: Soc Anal Chem, 1970.
29. Jones TM. *Acta Pharm Tech* 1978.
30. Chowhan ZT. *Pharm Technol* 1988; 12:46.
31. Mehta AM. *Pharm Technol* 1988; 12:46.
32. Mendes RW, Roy SB. *Pharm Technol* 1978; 2:35.
33. Wurster DE. *J APhA Sci Ed* 1960; 49:82.
34. Mendes RW, Roy SB. *Pharm Technol* 1978; 2(9):61.
35. Malinowski HJ, Smith WE. *J Pharm Sci* 1974; 63:285.
36. Woodruff CW, Nuessle NO. *J Pharm Sci* 1972; 61:787.
37. O'Connor RE, Holinej J, Schwartz JB. *Am J Pharm* 1984; 156:80.
38. O'Connor RE, Schwartz JB. *Drug Dev Ind Pharm* 1985; II:1837.
39. Newton JM. *Mfg Chem Aerosol News* 1966; 37(Apr):33.
40. U.S. Pat 3,883647, May 13, 1975.
41. *Tableting Specification Manual.* Washington DC: APhA, 1981.
42. Knoechel EL et al. *J Pharm Sci* 1967; 56:116.
43. Wray PE. *Drug Cosmet Ind* 1969; 105(3):53.
44. Hiestand EN, Smith DP. *Powder Tech* 1984; 38:145.
45. Hiestand EN, *et al. J Pharm Sci* 1977; 66:510.
46. Luenberger H. *Int J Pharm* 1982; 12:41.
47. Walter JT, Augsburger LL. *Pharm Technol* 1986; 10:26.
48. Schwartz JB. *Pharm Technol* 1981; 5(9):102.
49. Marshall K. *Pharm Technol* 1983; 7(3):68.
50. Jones BE. *Mfg Chem Aerosol News* 1969; 40(Feb):25.
51. Delaney R. *Pharm Exec* 1982; 2(3):34.
52. Tannenbaum PJ et al. *Clin Pharmacol Ther* 1968; 9:598.
53. Ebert WR. *Pharm Technol* 1977; 1(10):44.
54. Madan PL. *Pharm Technol* 1978; 2(9):68.
55. Cox PH, Spanjers F. *Pharm Weekbl* 1970; 105:681.
56. Rassing MR, Jacobsen J. In Rathbone MJ, et al, eds. *Modified Release Drug Delivery Technology.* New York: Marcel Dekker, 2003, p 419.
57. U.S. Patent 5,338,809, 1993.
58. Christrup LL. *Arch Pharm Chem* 1986; 14:30.
59. U.S. Patent 4,740,376, 1987.
60. European Patent 486,563, 1990.
61. Chrai SS et al. *Pharm Technol* 1998; 12(4).
62. U.S. Patent 5,714,007, 1998.
63. U.S. Patent 5,753,302, 1998.
64. U.S. Patent 5,788,814, 1998.
65. U.S. Patent 5,642,727, 1998.
66. U.S. Patent 4,197,289, 1980.

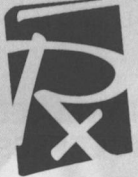

CHAPTER 46

Coating of Pharmaceutical Dosage Forms

Stuart C Porter, PhD

Any introduction to tablet coating must be prefaced by an important question—*Why coat tablets?*—since in many instances, the coating is applied to a dosage form that already is functionally complete. In attempting to answer this question, if one examines the market, it will become apparent that a significant proportion of pharmaceutical solid dosage forms are coated. The reasons for this range from the esthetic to a desire to control the bioavailability of the drug, and include:

1. Protecting the drug from its surrounding environment (particularly air, moisture, and light) in order to improve stability
2. Masking unpleasant taste and odor
3. Making it easier for the patient to swallow the product
4. Improving product identity, from the manufacturing plant, through intermediaries, and to the patient
5. Facilitating handling, particularly in high-speed packaging/filling lines, and automated counters in pharmacies, where the coating minimizes cross-contamination due to dust elimination
6. Improving product appearance, particularly where there are noticeable visible differences in tablet core ingredients from batch to batch
7. Reducing the risk of interaction between incompatible components. This would be achieved by using coated forms of one or more of the offending ingredients (particularly active compounds)
8. Improving product robustness, since coated products generally are more resistant to mishandling (eg, abrasion, attrition)
9. Modifying drug release, as in enteric-coated, repeat-action and sustained-release products.

EVOLUTION OF THE COATING PROCESS—Tablet coating is perhaps one of the oldest pharmaceutical processes still in existence. Historically, the literature cites Rhazes (850–932 AD) as being one of the earliest *tablet coaters,* having used the mucilage of psyllium seeds to coat pills that had an offending taste. Subsequently, Avicenna[1] was reported to have used gold and silver for pill coating. Since then, there have been many references to the different materials used in *tablet coating.* White[2] mentioned the use of finely divided talc in what was at one time popularly known as *pearl coating,* while Kremers and Urdang[3] described the introduction of the gelatin coating of pills by Garot in 1838.

An interesting reference[4] reports the use of waxes to coat poison tablets. These waxes, being insoluble in all parts of the gastrointestinal tract, were intended to prevent accidental poisoning (the contents could be utilized by breaking the tablet prior to use).

While earlier coated products were produced by individuals working in pharmacies, particularly when extemporaneous compounding was the order of the day, that responsibility now has been assumed by the pharmaceutical industry. The earliest attempts to apply coatings to pills yielded variable results and usually required the handling of single pills. Such pills would have been mounted on a needle or held with a pair of forceps and literally dipped into the coating fluid, a procedure that

would have to be repeated more than once to ensure that the pill was coated completely. Subsequently, the pills were held at the end of a suction tube, dipped, and then the process repeated for the other side of the pill. Not surprisingly, these techniques often failed to produce a uniformly coated product.[5]

Initially, the first sugar-coated pills seen in the US were imported from France about 1842[5]; while Warner, a Philadelphia pharmacist, became among the first indigenous manufacturers in 1856.[6]

Pharmaceutical pan-coating processes are based on those used in the candy industry, where techniques were highly evolved, even in the Middle Ages. Today most coating pans are fabricated from stainless steel, while early pans were made from copper, because drying was effected by means of an externally applied heat source. Current thinking, even with conventional pans, is to dry the coated tablets with a supply of heated air and remove the moisture and dust-laden air from the vicinity of the pan by means of an air-extraction system.

Pan-coating processes underwent little further change until the late 1940s and early 1950s, with conventional pans being the mainstay of all coating operations up to that time. However, in the last 50 years there have been some significant advances made in coating-process technology, mainly as a result of a steady evolution in pan design and associated ancillary equipment.

Interestingly, in the early years of this development, an entirely new form of technology evolved, namely that of film coating. Recognizing the deficiencies of the sugar-coating process, advocates of film coating were achieving success by using polymer based coatings dissolved in highly volatile organic solvents.

These solvents circumvented the problems often associated with the poor drying capabilities of conventional equipment and enabled production quotas to be met with significant reductions in processing times and materials used. The disadvantage of this approach, however, always has been associated with the fact that the solvents used were often flammable and toxic.

Advances that occurred with equipment design, begun with the development of the Wurster[7] process and continued by the evolution of side-vented pans, have resulted in the gradual emergence of coating processes in which drying efficiency can be maximized. Thus, while film coating began as a process using inefficient drying equipment, relying on highly volatile coating formulations for success, it has evolved into one in which the processing equipment is a major factor in ensuring that rapid drying occurs. Improved drying capabilities have permitted common use of aqueous film-coating formulations.

Advances in equipment design also have benefited the sugar-coating process, where, because of current Good Manufacturing Practices (cGMP) and to maintain product uniformity and performance, the trend has been toward using fully automated processes. Nonetheless, film coating tends to dominate as the process of choice for tablet coating.

PHARMACEUTICAL COATING PROCESSES

Basically, there are four major techniques for applying coatings to pharmaceutical solid dosage forms: (1) sugar coating, (2) film coating, (3) microencapsulation, and (4) compression coating.

Although it could be argued that the use of mucilage of psylium seed, gelatin, etc, as already discussed, was an early form of film coating, *sugar coating* is regarded as the oldest method for tablet coating and involves the deposition from aqueous solution of coatings based predominantly on sucrose as a raw material. The large quantities of coating material that are applied and the inherent skill often required of the operators combine to result in a long and tedious process. The introduction of improved formulations and processing techniques has resulted, however, in a significant reduction in processing times (from several days to less than 1 day).

Film coating, the deposition of a thin polymeric film onto the dosage form from solutions that were originally organic-solvent-based, but which now rely much more on water as the prime solvent, has proven to be a popular alternative to sugar coating, to the extent that this latter process has all but been superceded.

Microencapsulation is a modified form of film coating, differing only in the size of the particles to be coated and the methods by which this is accomplished. This process is based on either mechanical methods such as pan coating, air-suspension techniques, multiorifice centrifugal techniques, and modified spray-drying techniques, or physicochemical ones involving coacervation-phase separation, in which the material to be coated is suspended in a solution of the polymer. Phase separation is facilitated by the addition of a nonsolvent, incompatible polymer or inorganic salts or by altering the temperature of the system.

Compression coating involves the use of modified tabletting machines that allow the compaction of a dry coating around a tablet core produced on the same machine. The main advantage of this type of coating process is that it eliminates the use of any solvent, whether aqueous or organic in nature. However, this process is mechanically complex and has not proven popular as a method for coating tablets. Compression technology has, in recent times, been readopted as a means of applying special coatings for novel drug-delivery applications.

Sugar Coating of Compressed Tablets

While the term *sugar* is somewhat generic and lends itself to describing a range of carbohydrate materials, sugar coating relies primarily on the use of sucrose. The main reason is that sucrose is one of the few materials that produces smooth, high-quality coatings that are essentially dry and tack-free at the end of the process. While the popularity of sugar coating has certainly declined, this process is still used by many companies that have invested in the complete modernization of the process. In spite of certain inherent difficulties associated with the sugar-coating process, products that have been expertly sugar coated still remain among the most elegant available.

Since sugar coating is a multistep process, where esthetics of the final coated product is an important goal, it has been, and still is in many companies, highly dependent on the use of skilled manpower. For these reasons, the sugar-coating process is often protracted and tedious. However, processing times have been reduced gradually in the last few decades through process modification, typically involving thin sugar-coating procedures, and by means of automation.

The sugar-coating process can be subdivided into six main steps: (1) sealing, (2) subcoating, (3) smoothing, (4) color coating, (5) polishing, and (6) printing.

SEALING—The sealing coat is applied directly to the tablet core for the purpose of separating tablet ingredients (primarily the drug) from water (which is a major constituent of the coating formulation) in order to achieve good product stability. A secondary function is to strengthen the tablet core. Sealing coats usually consist of alcoholic solutions (approximately 10–30% solids) of resins such as shellac, zein, cellulose acetate phthalate, or polyvinyl acetate phthalate.

Historically, shellac has proven to be the most popular material, although it can cause impaired bioavailability due to a change in resin properties on storage. A solution to this problem has been to use a shellac-based formulation containing a measured quantity of polyvinylpyrrolidone (PVP).[8]

The quantities of material required to be applied as a sealing coat will depend primarily on tablet and batch size. However, another important factor is tablet porosity, since highly porous tablets will tend to soak up the first application of solution, thus preventing it from spreading uniformly across the surface of every tablet in the batch. Thus, one or more further applications of resin solution may be necessary to ensure that the tablet cores are sealed effectively.

Since most sealing coats develop a degree of tack (stickiness) at some time during the drying process, it is usual to apply a dusting powder to prevent tablets from sticking together or to the pan. A common dusting powder is asbestos-free talc. Overzealous use of talc may cause problems, firstly, by imparting a high degree of slip to the tablets, thus preventing them from rolling properly in the pan, and secondly by creating a surface that, at the beginning of the subsequent subcoating stage, is very difficult to wet. Such poor wetting often results in uneven subcoat buildup, particularly on the tablet edges. If there is a tendency for either of these problems to occur, one solution is to replace part or all of the talc with some other material such as terra alba, which will form a slightly rougher surface. Use of talc now is being frowned upon because of its potential carcinogenicity.

If it is necessary to prepare a delayed-release (enteric-coated) product, this can be achieved by making additional applications of the seal-coat solution. Under these circumstances, however, it is more preferable to use sealcoating formulations based on synthetic polymers such as polyvinyl acetate phthalate or cellulose acetate phthalate, rather than shellac.

SUBCOATING—Subcoating is a critical operation in the sugar-coating process that can have a marked effect on ultimate tablet quality. Sugar coating is a process that often leads to a 50 to 100% weight increase, and it is at the subcoating stage that most of the buildup occurs.

Historically, subcoating has been achieved by the application of a gum-based solution to the sealed tablet cores, and once this solution has been distributed uniformly throughout the tablet mass, it is followed by a liberal dusting of powder, which serves to reduce tack and facilitate tablet buildup. This procedure of application of gum solution, spreading, dusting, and drying is continued until the requisite buildup has been achieved. Thus, the subcoating is a sandwich of alternate layers of gum and powder. Some examples of binder solutions are shown in Table 46-1 and those of dusting powder formulations in Table 46-2.

Table 46-1. Binder Solution Formulations for Subcoating

	A, % W/W	B, % W/W
Gelatin	3.3	6.0
Gum acacia (powdered)	8.7	8.0
Sucrose	55.3	45.0
Water	to 100.0	to 100.0

Table 46-2. Dusting Powder Formulations for Subcoating

	A, % W/W	B, % W/W
Calcium carbonate	40.0	—
Titanium dioxide	5.0	1.0
Talc (asbestos-free)	25.0	61.0
Sucrose (powdered)	28.0	38.0
Gum acacia (powdered)	2.0	—

While this approach has proved to be very effective, particularly where there is difficulty in covering edges, if care is not taken, a *lumpy* subcoat will be the result. Also, if the amount of dusting powder applied is not matched to the binding capacity of the gum solution, not only will the ultimate coating be brittle, but also dust will collect in the back of the pan, a factor that may contribute to excessive roughness. An alternative approach, particularly when using an automated dosing system, involves the application of a suspension subcoat formulation. With this type of formulation, the powdered materials responsible for coating buildup are dispersed in the gum-based solution. A typical formulation is shown in Table 46-3. This approach allows the solids loading to be matched more closely to the binding capacity of the base solution and often permits the less-experienced coater to achieve satisfactory results.

SMOOTHING—Depending on how successfully the subcoat was applied, it may be necessary to smooth out the tablet surface further prior to application of the color coating. Smoothing usually can be accomplished by the application of a simple syrup solution (approximately 60–70% sugar solids).

Often, the smoothing syrups contain a low percentage of titanium dioxide (1–5%) as an opacifier. This can be particularly useful when the subsequent color-coating formulation uses water-soluble dyes as colorants, since it makes the surface under the color coating more reflective, resulting in a brighter, cleaner final color.

COLOR COATING—This stage is often the most critical to the successful production of a sugar-coating product and involves the multiple application of syrup solutions (60–70% sugar solids) containing appropriate coloring materials. The types of coloring materials used can be divided into two categories: dyes or pigments. The distinction between the two simply is one of solubility in the coating fluid. Since water-soluble dyes behave entirely differently from water-insoluble pigments, the application procedure used in the color coating of tablets will depend on the type of colorant chosen.

When used by a skilled artisan, water-soluble dyes produce the most elegant sugar-coated tablets, since it is possible to obtain a cleaner, brighter final color. However, since water-soluble dyes are migratory colorants (that is to say, moisture that is removed from the coating on drying will cause migration of the colorant, resulting in a nonuniform appearance), great care must be exercised in their use, particularly when dark color shades are required. Such care can be achieved by applying small quantities of colored syrup that are just sufficient to wet the surface of every tablet in the batch, and then allowing the tablets to dry slowly. It is essential that each application be allowed to dry thoroughly before subsequent applications are made, otherwise moisture may become trapped in the coating and may cause the tablets to *sweat* on standing.

The final color obtained may be the result of up to 60 individual applications of colored syrup. This factor, combined with the need to dry each application slowly and thoroughly, results in very long processing times (eg, assuming 50 applications are made, which can take between 15 and 30 min each, the coloring process can take up to 25 hours to complete). The more recent introduction of preformulated dye-based coloring systems has obviated many of these problems.

Tablet color coating with pigments, as advocated by Tucker et al,[9] offers some significant advantages. First of all, since pigment colors are water-insoluble, they present no problems of migration since the colorant remains where it is deposited. In addition, if the pigment is opaque or is combined with an opacifier such as titanium dioxide, the desired color can be developed much more rapidly, thus resulting in a thinner color coat. Since each color-syrup application now can be dried more rapidly, fewer applications are required, and significant reductions can be made in both processing times and costs.

Although pigment-based color coatings are by no means foolproof, they will permit more abuse than a dye color-coating process and are easier to use by less-skilled coating operators. Pharmaceutically acceptable pigments can be classified either as inorganic pigments (eg, titanium dioxide, iron oxides) or certified lakes. Certified lakes are produced from water-soluble dyes using a process known as *laking,* whereby each dye molecule is bonded to the surface of a suitable insoluble substrate (such as alumina hydrate, a material chemically very similar to the aluminum hydroxide used in many antacid formulations).

Certified lakes, particularly when used in conjunction with an opacifier such as titanium dioxide, provide an excellent means of coloring sugar coatings and permit a wide range of shades to be achieved. However, the incorporation of pigments into the syrup solution is not as easy as with water-soluble dyes, since it is necessary to ensure that the pigment is wetted completely and dispersed uniformly. Thus, the use of pigment color concentrates, which are commercially available, is usually beneficial.

POLISHING—Sugar-coated tablets are, by nature, very dull in appearance, and thus need to be polished to achieve a final elegance. Polishing is achieved by applying mixtures of waxes (beeswax, carnauba wax, candelila wax, or hard paraffin wax) to the tablets in a polishing pan. Such wax mixtures may be applied as powders or as dispersions in various organic solvents.

PRINTING—To identify sugar-coated tablets (in addition to shape, size, and color) often it is necessary to print them, either before or after polishing, using pharmaceutical branding inks, by means of the process of *offset rotogravure.*

SUGAR-COATING PROBLEMS—Various problems may be encountered during the sugar coating of tablets. It must be remembered that any process in which tablets are kept tumbling constantly can cause problems if the tablets are not strong enough to withstand the applied stress. Tablets that are too soft or have a tendency to laminate may break up and the fragments adhere to the surface of otherwise good tablets.

Sugar-coating pans exhibit inherently poor mixing characteristics. If care is not exercised during the application of the various coating fluids, non-uniform distribution of coating material can occur, resulting in an unacceptable range of sizes of finished tablets within the batch.

Overzealous use of dusting powders, particularly during the subcoating stage, may result in a coating being formed in which the quantity of fillers exceeds the binding capacity of the polymer used in the formulation, creating soft coatings or those with increased tendency to crack.

Irregularities in appearance are not uncommon and occur either as the result of color migration during drying when water-soluble dyes are used or of *washing back* when overdosing

Table 46-3. Typical Suspension Subcoating Formulation

	% W/W
Distilled water	25.0
Sucrose	40.0
Calcium carbonate	20.0
Talc (asbestos-free)	12.0
Gum acacia (powdered)	2.0
Titanium dioxide	1.0

of colored syrups causes the previously dried coating layers to be redissolved. Rough tablet surfaces will produce a *marbled* appearance during polishing, since wax buildup occurs in the small depressions in the tablet surface.

Film Coating of Solid Dosage Forms

Film coating is a process that involves the deposition of a thin, but uniform, film onto the surface of the substrate. Unlike sugar coating, film coating is a very flexible process that allows a broad range of products (eg, tablets, powders, granules, non-pareils, capsules) to be coated. Film coatings essentially are typically applied continuously to a moving mass of product, usually by means of a spray technique, although manual application procedures have been used.

Historically, film coating was introduced in the early 1950s to combat the shortcomings of the then predominant sugar-coating process. Film coating has proved successful as a result of the many advantages offered, including

1. Minimal weight increase (typically 2–3% of tablet core weight)
2. Significant reduction in processing times
3. Increased process efficiency and output
4. Increased flexibility in formulations
5. Improved resistance to chipping of the coating

In the early years of film coating, the major process advantages resulted from the greater volatility of the organic solvents used; however, the use of such organic solvents has created many potential problems, including

1. Flammability hazards
2. Toxicity hazards
3. Concerns over environmental pollution
4. Cost (relating either to minimizing items 1 to 3 or to the cost of the solvents themselves)

However, since the initial introduction of film coating, significant advances have been made in process technology and equipment design. The emphasis has changed from a process needing highly volatile organic solvents (in order to facilitate rapid drying) to one where even a relatively slow drying solvent such as water can be accommodated through significant improvements in the drying capabilities of the processing equipment used.

Thus, there has been a transition from conventional pans to side-vented pans and fluid-bed equipment, and consequently from the problematic organic solvent-based process to an aqueous one.

FILM COATING RAW MATERIALS—The major components in any film-coating formulation consist primarily of a polymer, plasticizer, colorant, and solvent (or vehicle).

Ideal properties for the polymer include solubility in a wide range of solvent systems to promote flexibility in formulation, an ability to produce coatings that have suitable mechanical properties, and appropriate solubility in gastrointestinal fluids such that drug bioavailability is not compromised.

Cellulose ethers are often the preferred polymers in film coating, particularly hydroxypropyl methylcellulose. Suitable substitutes are hydroxypropyl cellulose, which may produce slightly tackier coatings, and methylcellulose, although this polymer has been reported to retard drug dissolution.[10] Alternatives to the cellulose ethers are acrylic copolymers (eg, methacrylate and methyl methacrylate copolymers) and vinyl polymers (eg, polyvinyl alcohol).

For most film-coating applications, where there is no intent to modify drug-release characteristics, polymers are typically used as solutions in either water (preferred) or organic solvents.

Many of the commonly used polymers are available in a range of molecular-weight grades, a factor that also must be considered in the selection process. Molecular weight may have an important influence on various properties of the coating system, such as solution viscosity and mechanical strength and flexibility of the resultant film.

The incorporation of a plasticizer into the formulation improves the flexibility of the coating, reduces the risk of the film cracking, and potentially improves adhesion of the film to the substrate. To ensure that these benefits are achieved, the plasticizer must show a high degree of compatibility with the polymer and be retained permanently in the film, if the properties of the coating are to remain consistent on storage. Examples of typical plasticizers include glycerin, propylene glycol, polyethylene glycols, triacetin, acetylated monoglyceride, citrate esters (eg, triethyl citrate), or phthalate esters (eg, diethyl phthalate).

Colorants usually are used to improve the appearance of the product as well as to facilitate product identification. Additionally, certain physical properties of the coating (eg, its performance as a moisture barrier) may be improved. As in the case of sugar coating, colorants can be classified as either water-soluble dyes or insoluble pigments.

The use of water-soluble dyes is precluded with organic solvent-based film coating because of the lack of solubility in the solvent system. Thus, the use of pigments, particularly aluminum lakes, provides the most useful means of coloring film-coating systems. Although it may seem obvious to use water-soluble dyes in aqueous formulations, the use of pigments is preferred, since:

1. They are unlikely to interfere with bioavailability[11] as do some water-soluble dyes.
2. They help to reduce the permeability of the coating to moisture.[12]
3. They serve as bulking agents to increase the overall solids content in the coating dispersion without dramatically increasing viscosity.
4. They tend to be more light stable.

The major solvents used in film coating typically belong to one of these classes: alcohols, ketones, esters, chlorinated hydrocarbons, and water. Solvents perform an important function in the film-coating process, since they aid in the application of the coating to the surface of the substrate. Good interaction between solvent and polymer is necessary to ensure that optimal film properties are obtained when the coating dries. This initial interaction between solvent and polymer will yield maximum polymer chain extension, producing films having the greatest cohesive strength and, thus, the best mechanical properties. An important function of the solvent systems also is to ensure a controlled deposition of the polymer onto the surface of the substrate so that a coherent and adherent film coat is obtained.

Although it is very difficult to give typical examples of film-coating formulations, since these will depend on the properties of the materials used, such formulations usually are based on 5–20% (w/w) coating solids in the requisite vehicle (with the higher concentration range preferred for aqueous formulations), of which 60–70% is polymer, 6–7% is plasticizer, and 20–30% is pigment.

Modified-Release Film Coatings

Film coatings can be applied to pharmaceutical products to modify drug release. The USP describes two types of modified-release dosage forms, namely those that are *delayed release* and those that are *extended release*. Delayed-release products often are designed to prevent drug release in the upper part of the gastrointestinal (GI) tract. Film coatings used to prepare this type of dosage form are commonly called *enteric coatings*. Extended-release products are designed to extend drug release over a period of time, a result that can be achieved by the application of a *sustained-* or *controlled-release* film coating.

ENTERIC COATINGS—Enteric coatings generally remain intact in the stomach but will dissolve and release the contents of the dosage form once it reaches the small intestine. The purpose of an enteric coating is to delay the release of drugs that are inactivated by the stomach contents, (eg, pancreatin, erythromycin, and substituted benzimidazole compounds that are proton pump inhibitors) or may cause nausea or bleeding by irritating the gastric mucosa (eg, aspirin, steroids). In addition, such coatings can be used to give a simple repeat-action effect in which additional drug that has been applied over the enteric coat is released in the stomach, while the remainder, being protected by the coating, is released further down the gastrointestinal tract.

The action of enteric coatings results from a difference in composition of the respective gastric and intestinal environments in regard to pH and enzymatic properties. Although there have been repeated attempts to produce coatings that are subject to intestinal enzyme breakdown, this approach is not popular, since enzymatic decomposition of the film is rather slow. Thus, most currently used enteric coatings are weak acids that remain undissociated in the low pH environment of the stomach but readily ionize when the pH rises to about 5. The most effective enteric polymers are polyacids having a pK_a of 3 to 5. Coatings that respond to enzymatic breakdown are now being considered as protective coatings suitable for the colonic delivery of polypeptide drugs.

Historically, the earliest enteric coatings used formalin-treated gelatin, but this approach was unreliable, since the polymerization of gelatin could not be controlled accurately and often resulted in failure to release the drug, even in the lower intestinal tract. Another early candidate was shellac, but again the main disadvantage resulted from further polymerization that occurred on storage, often resulting in failure to release the active contents. Pharmaceutical formulators now prefer to use synthetic polymers to prepare more effective enteric coatings.

One of the oldest synthetic polymers used for enteric coating is cellulose acetate phthalate (CAP). However, a pH greater than 6 usually is required to allow the coating to dissolve, and thus a significant delay in drug release may ensue. It also is relatively permeable to moisture and gastric fluid compared with most enteric polymers. Additionally, this polymer is very susceptible to hydrolytic decomposition in which phthalic and acetic acids are split off, resulting in a change in polymer properties, and thus enteric coating performance.

Other useful polymers include polyvinyl acetate phthalate (PVAP, which is less permeable to moisture and gastric fluid, more stable to hydrolysis, and able to ionize at a lower pH); hydroxypropyl methylcellulose phthalate (HPMCP, which has properties similar to PVAP); acrylic copolymers, such as methacrylic acid–methacrylic acid ester copolymers (some of which have a high dissociation constant[13]); cellulose acetate trimellitate (CAT, which has properties similar to CAP); carboxymethyl ethylcellulose (CMEC); and hydroxypropyl methylcellulose acetate succinate (HPMCAS).

In recent years, acrylic copolymers have evolved as the most preferred (in terms of performance and global acceptability) materials for designing enteric coating formulations.

Since enteric coating polymers are, by nature, insoluble in water (except at high pH), their use in aqueous coating systems has required the adaptation of so-called latex technology that has resulted in the creation of either liquid polymer dispersions or dry powder coating systems that can readily be dispersed in water prior to use.

SUSTAINED-RELEASE COATINGS—The concept of sustained release formulations was developed to eliminate the need for multiple dosage regimens, particularly for those drugs requiring reasonably constant blood levels over a long period of time. In addition, it also has been adopted for those drugs that need to be administered in high doses, but where too rapid a release is likely to cause undesirable side effects (eg, the ulceration that occurs when potassium chloride is released rapidly in the gastrointestinal tract).

Formulation methods used to obtain the desired drug release rate from sustained-action dosage forms include

1. Increasing the particle size of the drug
2. Embedding the drug in a matrix
3. Coating the drug or dosage form containing the drug
4. Forming complexes of the drug with materials such as ion-exchange resins

Only those methods that involve some form of coating fall within the scope of this chapter. A discussion of other controlled release drug delivery systems can be found in Chapter 47

(Extended-Release and Targeted Drug Delivery Systems). The mechanisms of drug release from film-coated products are also provided.

Materials that have been found suitable for producing sustained-release coatings include

1. Mixtures of waxes (eg, beeswax, carnauba wax) with glyceryl monostearate, stearic acid, palmitic acid, glyceryl monopalmitate, and cetyl alcohol. These provide coatings that are dissolved slowly or broken down in the GI tract.
2. Shellac and zein. These polymers remain intact until the pH of gastrointestinal contents becomes less acidic.
3. Ethylcellulose, which provides a membrane around the dosage form and remains intact throughout the gastrointestinal tract. However, it does permit water to permeate the film, dissolve the drug, and diffuse out again.
4. Acrylic resins, which behave similarly to ethylcellulose as a diffusion-controlled drug-release coating material
5. Cellulose acetate (diacetate and triacetate)
6. Silicone elastomers

As with enteric coatings, many of the synthetic polymers suitable for sustained-release film-coating applications are available as aqueous polymer dispersions (often called latexes or pseudolatexes) that can be used in aqueous coating processes.[14]

Various methods have been used to prepare sustained-release products using film-coating techniques. Examples include the application of suitable film coatings to:

1. Dried granules (either irregular or spheronized)
2. Drug-loaded beads (or nonpareils)
3. Drug crystals
4. Drug/ion-exchange-resin complexes
5. Tablets (including mini tablets[15])

In the first four examples, the final coated particles can be either filled into two-piece hard-gelatin capsules or compacted into tablets. Additionally, coated drug/ion-exchange-resin complexes may be dispersed in viscous liquids to create liquid suspensions. A comprehensive overview of the coating of multiparticulate dosage forms has been given by Ghebre-Sellassie.[16]

An interesting application of the film-coated, sustained-release tablet is the elementary osmotic pump. In this device, a tablet core (formulated to contain osmotically active ingredients) is film coated with a semi-permeable membrane. This membrane is subsequently *pierced* with a laser to create a delivery orifice. Once such a device is ingested, the infusion of water generates an osmotic pressure within the coated tablet that *pumps* the drug out through the orifice.

With sustained-release products, one must remain aware constantly of the fact that the final dosage forms typically contain drug loadings that are sufficiently high to cause problems if the entire dose is released quickly. This phenomenon, commonly called *dose-dumping,* can be avoided only if:

1. The film coating is mechanically sound and will resist rupture on ingestion of the dosage form.
2. Sufficient coating is applied uniformly across the surface of the material that is to be coated.
3. The dosage form is not chewed or crushed prior to ingestion.

FILM-COATING PROBLEMS

As with sugar coating, problems may occur during, or subsequent to, the film-coating process. The tablets being coated may not be sufficiently robust or may have a tendency to *laminate* while being coated. Since film coats are relatively thin, their ability to hide defects is significantly less than that of sugar coating. Hence, tablets that have poor resistance to abrasion (ie, they exhibit high friability characteristics) can be problematic, since imperfections may readily be apparent after coating. It is very important to identify tablets with suspect properties, whether mechanical or performance related (eg, poor dissolution), prior to a coating process, since subsequent recovery or reworking of tablets may be extremely difficult after a coating has been applied.

Various process-related problems can occur during the application of a film coating. One example is *picking,* which is a consequence of the fluid delivery rate exceeding the drying capacity of the process, causing tablets to stick together and subsequently break apart. Another example, *orange peel* or *roughness,* is usually the result of premature drying of atomized droplets of solution, or it may be a consequence of spraying too viscous a coating solution such that effective atomization is difficult.

Mottling, or lack of color uniformity, can result from uneven distribution of color in the coating, a problem often related to the use of soluble dyes in aqueous film coating, when color migration can occur, either by evolution of residual solvent in the film or by migration of plasticizer in which the colorant may be soluble. The use of pigments in the film-coating process minimizes the incidence of this latter objection considerably. However, uneven color also can result from inadequate dispersion of the pigments in the coating solution.

Finally, some major problems occur as the result of internal stresses that develop within the film as it dries. One example is *cracking,* which occurs when these stresses exceed the tensile strength of the film. This problem may be compounded by the existence of post compaction strain relaxation (a phenomenon that can occur with certain types of tablet formulations, such as those containing ibuprofen, after ejection from the die during the tabletting process), which causes tablets to expand. Another example is *logo-bridging* (ie, bridging of monograms present in the surface of the tablet core), which occurs when the internal stresses are able to overcome the adhesive bonds formed between the coating and the tablet surface, causing the film to pull away so that legibility of the monogram is lost. An understanding of the properties of the various ingredients used in the film-coating formulation and how these ingredients interact with one another can allow the formulator to avoid many of these internal-stress-related problems.[17]

COATING PROCEDURES AND EQUIPMENT

COATING PANS—Sugar coating historically has involved the ladling of the various coating fluids onto a cascading bed of tablets in a conventional coating pan (Fig 46-1) fitted with a means of supplying drying air to the tablets and an exhaust to remove moisture and dust-laden air from the pan.

Typically, after the requisite volume of liquid has been applied, some time is allowed for the tablets to mix and the liquid to be dispersed fully throughout the batch. To facilitate the uniform transfer of liquid, the tablets often are *stirred* by hand, or in larger pans, by means of a rake, to overcome mixing problems often associated with *dead spots,* an inherent problem seen with conventional pans. Finally, tablets are dried by blowing air onto the surface of the tablet bed. Thus, sugar coating is a sequential process consisting of consecutive cycles of liquid application, mixing, and drying.

During the early history of film coating, the equipment used was adapted essentially from that already employed for sugar coating. Although ladling of coating liquids during the film-coating process has been practiced, usually the liquid is applied using a spray technique. Spray equipment used is essentially of two types:

1. Airless (or hydraulic) spray, where the coating liquid is pumped under pressure to a spray nozzle with a small orifice and atomization of the liquid occurs as it expands rapidly on emerging from the nozzle. This is analogous to the effect achieved when one places one's finger over the end of a garden hose.
2. Air spray, where liquid is pumped, under little or no pressure, to the nozzle and is subsequently atomized by means of a blast of compressed air that makes contact with the stream of liquid as it passes through the nozzle aperture.

Airless-spray techniques typically are used in large-scale film-coating operations employing organic solvents, while air-spray techniques are more effective in either a small-scale laboratory set-up or aqueous film-coating operations.

Spray application enables finely atomized droplets of the coating solution to be delivered across the surface of the moving tablet mass in a manner that achieves uniform coverage while preventing adjacent tablets from sticking together as the coating solution is rapidly dried. While all the events that take place during the spray application process occur continuously and concurrently, the overall picture can be more simply represented as shown in Figure 46-2.

The spray process can be operated either intermittently or continuously. In the early years of film coating, the lack of adequate drying conditions inside the coating apparatus, together with the preference for using airless coating techniques (with their inherently higher delivery rates) with organic solvent-based formulations typically required the use of intermittent spray procedures. This technique allowed excess solvent to be removed during the nonspray part of the cycle and thus reduced the risk of *picking* and the tendency for tablets to stick together. However, in later years, improvements in drying capabilities have resulted in the preferred use of continuous spray procedures, as this permits uniform coatings to be applied in a shorter process.

As indicated previously, pan equipment initially was completely conventional in design and, with the exception of the addition of spray-application equipment, was similar to that used in sugar coating. Fortunately, film-coating formulations were based on relatively volatile organic solvents, which enabled acceptable processing times to be achieved in spite of the relative deficiencies of the air-handling systems. However, such equipment did not produce a completely enclosed system, a fact that

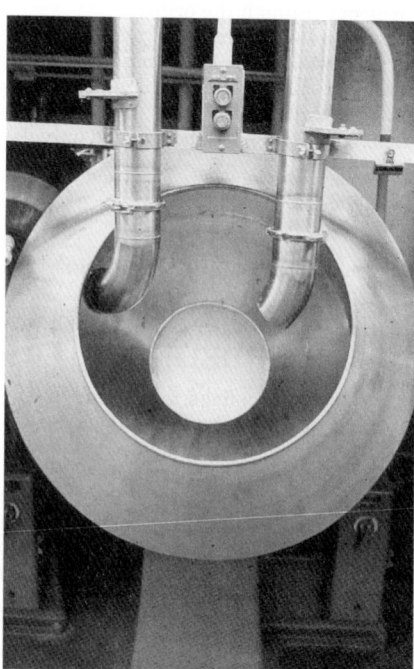

Figure 46-1. Typical equipment set-up for conventional sugar coating.

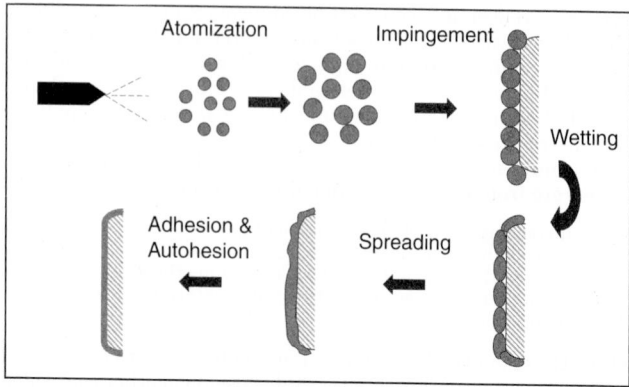

Figure 46-2. The film-coating process.

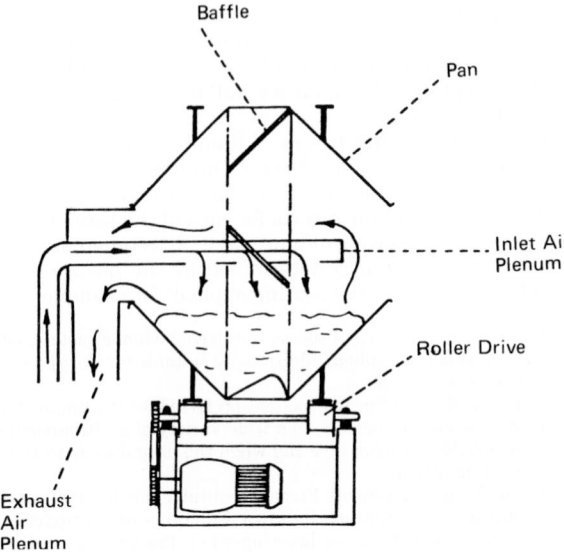

Figure 46-3. A Pellegrini coating pan.

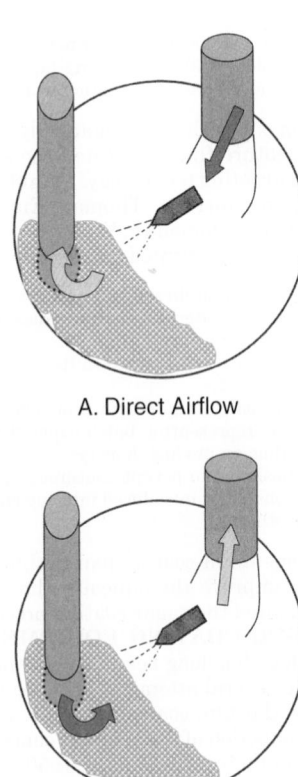

Figure 46-4. Upgraded conventional coating pans. **A.** Direct airflow. **B.** Reverse airflow.

made effective solvent containment extremely difficult to achieve. Although conventional pans possessed acceptable properties with regard to mixing of the tablet mass in the sugar-coating process (particularly as this could be augmented by manual stirring of the tablets during processing), they were less suited to meet the more rigorous demands of the film-coating process, even when some simple baffle system was installed.

The introduction of aqueous film coating in the latter part of the twentieth century presented a more serious challenge to the continued use of conventional processing equipment. Limitations in both drying and mixing capabilities potentially signified a dramatic increase in processing times while substantially compromising product quality and long-term stability. Fortunately, these problems have been eliminated as coating-pan design has evolved and improved.

Although considerable experimentation has taken place with the geometric design of conventional equipment, a substantial change came with the introduction of the Pellegrini coating pan (Fig 46-3), a somewhat angular pan that rotates on a horizontal axis. Pan design, and installation of an integral baffle system, ensures that more uniform mixing is achieved. Additionally, since the services are introduced through the rear opening, the front can potentially be closed off to produce an enclosed coating system. Although drying air is still applied only to the surface of the tablet bed, the other advantages derived from the basic overall design ensure that the Pellegrini pan is more suitable for film coating than the conventional equipment previously discussed. Pellegrini pans are available with capacities ranging from the 10-kg laboratory scale-up to 1000 kg for high-output production.

Considering the drying inefficiencies in pan where most of the drying takes place only on the surface of the tablet bed, several attempts have been made to improve air exchange, particularly within the tablet bed. The schematic shown in Figure 46-4 conceptually describes the basis for equipment designed to improve the drying capabilities exhibited by more conventional coating equipment.

Two such types of equipment, both based on the Pellegrini style of coating pan, are supplied by GS and Nicomac. In both cases, an air plenum fitted with a perforated *boot* is immersed into the cascading bed of product being coated. A second air plenum is also led inside the coating pan. With this type of design, either a *direct* or a *reverse airflow* plan can be used.

A major advance in pan coating technology was the introduction of the side-vented pan concept, an innovation developed by Eli Lilly. This concept, formally designated as the Accela-cota, has formed the basis for a wide range of *side-vented*

coating pan designs, a schematic of which is shown in Figure 46-5. The salient features of side-vented coating pans are:

1. An angular pan (fitted with an integral baffle system) that rotates on a horizontal axis.
2. A coating system that is completely enclosed.

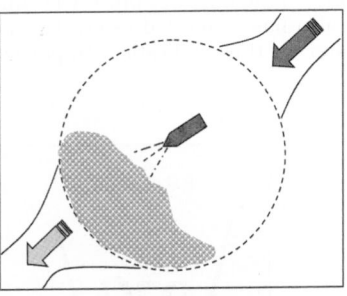

A. Direct Airflow

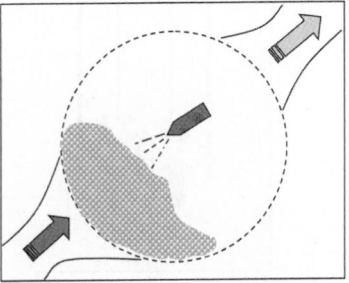

B. Reverse Airflow

Figure 46-5. Side-vented coating pans. **A.** Direct airflow. **B.** Reverse airflow.

3. A perforated pan that allows drying air to be pulled through a cascading bed of tablets while the coating liquid is applied to the tablet surface using a spray-atomization technique.

Side-vented coating pans exhibit dramatically improved drying characteristics, a feature that facilitated the successful adoption of aqueous film-coating technology. Manufacturers of sidevented coating pans include Thomas Engineering, BWI Manesty, O'Hara, Glatt, Dumoulin, Vector Freund, and Driam.

Ongoing trends with side-vented coating pans have produced:

1. Designs that permit multidirectional air flow.
2. Fully automated, computerized coating processes (especially for production-scale coating purposes).
3. Effective clean-in-place (CIP) systems that facilitate compliance with GMPs.
4. Laboratory-scale coating equipment provided with interchangeable coating pans representing batch capacities in the range of 3–40 kg (depending on product density).
5. Coating pans designed to permit continuous processing (where the product is constantly introduced into one end and flows, fully coated, out the other).

Although improvements in coating-pan design have predominately occurred to improve the aqueous film-coating process, they have also benefited the sugar-coating process.

FLUIDIZED-BED COATING EQUIPMENT—Fluid-bed processing technology has long been used in the pharmaceutical industry. While several attempts have been made to apply this technology to the film-coating process, a major success came with the introduction of the Wurster concept (a schematic of which is shown in Figure 46-6) in the 1950s.

At a time when organic-solvent-based coating formulations were still primarily used, the Wurster process was extremely popular for coating a variety of pharmaceutical dosage forms, especially tablets. Although fluid-bed processing inarguably exhibits the most effective drying characteristics of any film-coating process, the introduction of aqueous coating formulations initially created waning interest in using the Wurster process for coating tablets. A major factor in this trend undoubtedly was related to the increased potential (compared with use of coating pans) for tablet breakage in the fluid-bed process. During the last 30 years, however, resurgent interest in the Wurster process has occurred as a result of the growing demand for applying film coatings to pellets, granules, and powders (so-called *multiparticulates*) when producing modified-release dosage forms.

The suitability of the fluid-bed process for film coating multiparticulates also has generated interest in processes other than the Wurster for this application. In particular, modifica-

tions of the spray granulation process (often termed the *topspray coating process*) and a rotary process (often called the *tangential spray process*) have both been used for the film coating of multiparticulates. Schematics for all these processes also are shown in Figure 46-6.

Three major manufacturers of fluid-bed processing equipment (Glatt Air Techniques, Vector Corporation, and GEA) all have adopted a principle in which a basic processing unit is designed to accept modular inserts for each of the three fluid-bed coating processes shown in Figure 46-6. Selection of a particular type of insert often is determined by the nature and intended functionality of the coating applied; for example

1. Granulator Top-Spray Process—preferred when a taste-masking coating is being applied; additionally suitable for the application of hot-melt coatings.
2. Wurster, Bottom-Spray Process—preferred for the application of modified-release coatings to a wide variety of multiparticulates; also suitable for drug layering when the drug dose is in the low-to-medium range.
3. Rotor, Tangential-Spray Process—suitable for the application of modified-release film coatings to a wide range of multiparticulate products; ideal for drug layering when the dose is medium to high; also useful as a spheronizing process for producing spheres from powders.

While the general trend has been to use equipment employing this modular concept, an innovative approach to fluid-bed film coating was introduced by Hüttlin, who created a design known as the Kugel coater.[18]

POTENTIAL FOR TOTALLY AUTOMATED COATING SYSTEMS—Over the course of time, the pharmaceutical industry has witnessed a general transition away from manually operated sugar-coating processes, requiring total operator involvement, to film-coating ones where operator intervention is infrequent. Increasing familiarity with, and understanding of, tablet coating as a unit process, and a desire to ensure compliance with GMPs, ultimately have increased the desire to achieve reproducible and consistent conformity to design specifications for every batch of product made. Achievement of such an objective is clearly compromised if the idiosyncrasies of individual operators are allowed to have a major impact on final product quality (in its broadest sense).

Total automation of a well designed and validated process can provide a solution to these problems. Automation involves the development of a process in which all the important variables (and requisite constraints) are predetermined. These variables, once adequately defined, can then be used as the ba-

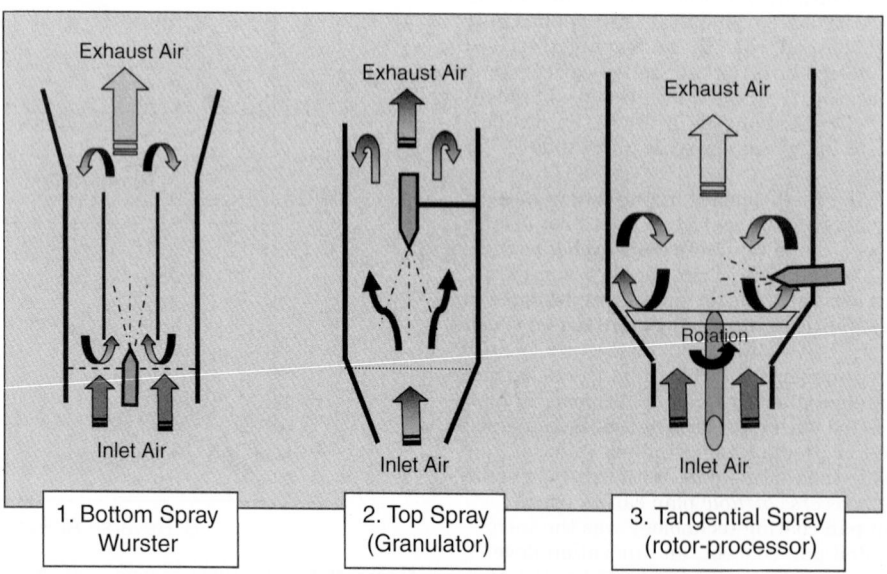

Figure 46-6. Three basic processes used for fluid-bed film coating.

sis for creating a process where ultimate control and monitoring of each critical process parameter can be accomplished through use of either a microprocessor or a central computer system. However, such a system will only be as good as those peripheral devices used to detect critical process conditions (eg, such as air flow, temperature, humidity, application volumes, or delivery rates), and the rate at which the control systems can respond to changes so that the process can be maintained within defined process limits.

Since a sugar-coating process always has been highly operator dependent, removal of much of the operator intervention could be achieved by automation. Automation has, however, been complex because of the various sequences that occur and the variety of coating fluids used in a single sugar-coating process. That it has been accomplished is evidenced by the number of commercially available systems that have been introduced.[19] The technology for automated control of both sugar- and film-coating processes has become very refined, and most major equipment suppliers are able to offer a coating process that is automated to various degrees (depending on end-user preferences).

QUALITY CONTROL OF COATED TABLETS

The most important aspects of coated tablets that must be assessed from a quality-control standpoint are appearance characteristics and drug availability. From the appearance standpoint, coated tablets must be shown to conform, where applicable, to some color standard, otherwise the dispenser and the consumer may assume that differences have occurred from previous lots, signifying a changed or substandard product. In addition, because of the physical abuse that tablets, both in their uncoated and coated forms, receive during the coating process, it is essential to check for defects such as chipped edges, picking, etc, and ensure that they do not exceed predetermined limits.

Often, to identify the products, coated tablets may be imprinted (particularly with sugar-coated tablets) or bear a monogram (commonly seen with tablets that are film-coated). The clarity and quality of such identifying features must be assessed. The failure of a batch of coated tablets to comply with such preset standards may result in 100% inspection being required or the need for the batch to be reworked.

Batch-to-batch reproducibility for drug availability is of paramount importance; consequently each batch of product should be submitted to some meaningful test such as a dissolution test. Depending on the characteristics of the tablet core to be coated, tablet coatings can modify the drug release profile, even when not intended (unlike the case of enteric- or controlled-release products). Since this behavior may vary with each batch coated (being dependent, for example, on differences in processing conditions or variability in raw materials used), it is essential that this parameter be assessed, particularly in products that are typically borderline (refer to Chapter 45 *Oral Solid Dosage Forms*).

STABILITY TESTING OF COATED PRODUCTS

The stability-testing program for coated products will vary depending on the dosage form and its composition. Many stability-testing programs are based on studies that have disclosed the conditions a product may encounter prior to end use. Such conditions usually are referred to as normal and include ranges in temperature, humidity, light, and handling conditions. The conditions to be employed in modern stability-testing programs often conform to the guidelines established by the International Committee on Harmonization (ICH). A more detailed discussion on the stability of pharmaceutical products may be found in Chapter 52.

Limits of acceptability are established for each product for qualities such as color, appearance, availability of drug for absorption, and drug content. The time over which the product retains specified properties, when tested at normal conditions, may be defined as the *shelf life*. The container for the product may be designed to improve the shelf life. For example, if the color in the coating is light-sensitive, the product may be packaged in an amber bottle and/or protected from light by using a paper carton. When the coating is friable, resilient material such as cotton may be incorporated in both the top and bottom of the container, and if the product is affected adversely by moisture, a moisture-resistant closure may be used and/or a desiccant may be placed in the package. The shelf life of the product is determined in the commercial package tested under normal conditions.

The stability of the product also may be tested under exaggerated conditions. This usually is done for the purpose of accelerating changes so that an extrapolation can be made early, concerning the shelf life of the product. Although useful, highly exaggerated conditions of storage can supply misleading data for coated dosage forms. Any change in drug release from the dosage form is measured *in vitro,* but an *in vivo* measurement should be used to confirm that drug availability remains within specified limits over its stated shelf life. This confirmation can be obtained by testing the product initially for *in vivo* availability and then repeating at intervals during storage at normal conditions for its estimated shelf life (or longer).

Interpretation of stability data for coated, modified-release products should be undertaken with extreme care, since the diffusion characteristics of polymeric films can change significantly under exaggerated temperature conditions. This change may be confounding when trying to predict their diffusion characteristics under more moderate conditions and thus can prove misleading when predicting shelf life.

When elevated-temperature stability studies are conducted on products coated with aqueous polymeric dispersions (latexes or pseudolatexes), the data obtained might be more indicative of morphological changes that have occurred in the film. Such changes may result from partial destruction of the film when coated material adheres together in the container and subsequently is broken apart; additionally, these changes might result from further coalescence of the coating (which can occur when the coating is not coalesced completely during the coating process).

Stability tests usually are conducted on a product at the time of development, during the pilot phase and on representative lots of the commercial product. Stability testing must continue for the commercial product as long as it remains on the market because subtle changes in a manufacturing process and/or a raw material can have an impact on the shelf life of a product.

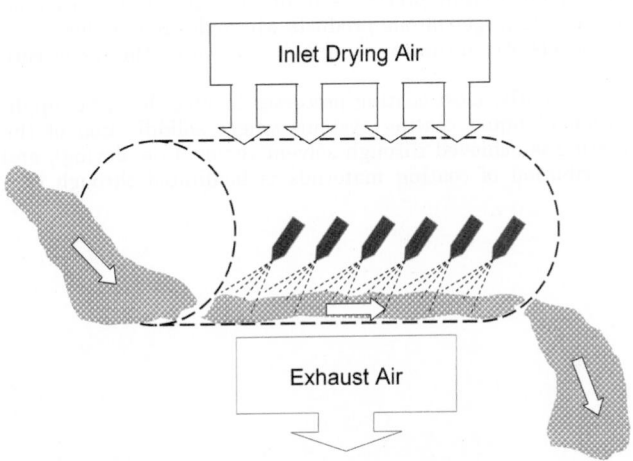

Figure 46-7. Continuous film-coating process.

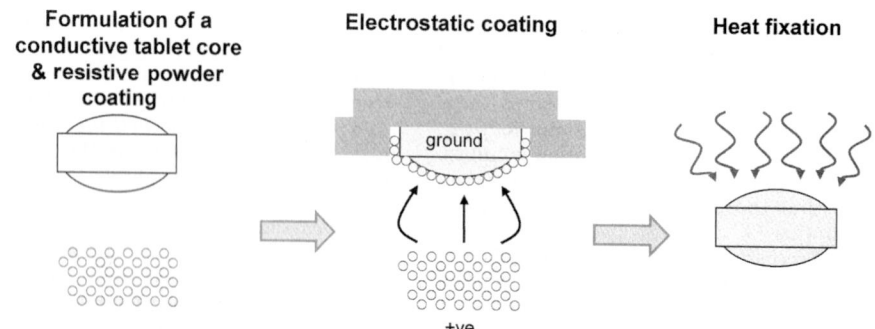

Figure 46-8. Electrostatic powder coating process.

RECENT TRENDS IN PHARMACEUTICAL COATING TECHNOLOGY

There is an inherent conservatism expressed by pharmaceutical manufacturers towards accepting major changes in raw materials (ie, non-active ingredients) and processing technologies. Thus, change tends to be evolutionary rather than revolutionary. Still, some interesting events have occurred over the last decade.

Of particular note is the growing interest in *Process Analytical Technology*. This has resulted in bringing many analytical procedures out of the laboratory and closer to the manufacturing process with which they may be associated. The desire here is to introduce, ideally as an on-line control function, specific analytical techniques that can be used to enhance the quality of the final coated products. One example is the use of near infrared techniques that can be used to analyze coated product in such a way that, for example, product moisture contents, drug contents, amount of coating applied, and even, to some extent, drug release rates can be predicted before that product is discharged from the coating process.

Another advance involves the increasing acceptance of continuous film coating processes, as described by Mancoff[20] and Pentecost.[21] Current continuous processes are based on the concept of a stretched side-vented coating pan, where uncoated product is introduced at one end, passes by a whole bank of spray guns, and emerges from the other end fully coated (Fig 46-7). The advantages of this type of process include:

1. Increasing output (typical outputs are in the range of 500 to 1000 kg h^{-1}), compared to common batch processes which might coat a 250 kg batch in one to two hours, while a 500kg batch might be coated in three to four hours.
2. Reducing residence time in a process where product is typically exposed to stressful conditions (attrition, high humidities and temperatures) from several hours to about 15 minutes.
3. Improving uniformity of distribution of coating materials.

Continuous coating processes of this type are usually reserved for coating large-volume products where desired applied coating levels are in the range of 3–4% (based on the tablet core weight).

Currently, most coating processes involve the spray application of liquid coating systems where solidification of the coating is achieved through solvent removal (ie, drying), and distribution of coating materials is facilitated through con-

stant motion of the material being coated. A more revolutionary approach to film coating, also based on a continuous process, involves the electrostatic deposition of powder coating systems to the surface of tablets (and fusing the coating through application of heat) using principles that are based on electrophotography (photocopying). In this process, described by Staniforth et al[22] and illustrated in Figure 46-8, tablets are coated individually one side at a time. The advantages of this type of process are:

1. No solvents (aqueous or organic) are used.
2. The coating is deposited onto tablets in a much more precise manner than can be achieved with any other existing pharmaceutical coating process.
3. Novel imaging can be achieved.
4. Tablet surfaces can be only partially coated, thus facilitating applications involving novel drug delivery.

REFERENCES

1. Urdang G. *What's New,* 1943, pp 5–14; through *JAPhA* 1945; 34:135
2. White RC. *JAPhA* 1922; 11: 345.
3. Kremers E, Urdang G. *History of Pharmacy.* Philadelphia: Lippincott, 1940, p 20, 319.
4. Anon. *JAMA* 1920; 84: 829.
5. Wiegand TS. *Am J Pharm* 1902; 74: 33.
6. Warner WR Jr. *Ibid* 1902; 74: 32.
7. Wurster DE. (Wisconsin Alumni Research Foundations) US Pat 2,648,609 (1953).
8. Signorino CA. US Pat 3,738,952 and 3,741,795 (June, 1973).
9. Tucker SJ, et al. *JAPhA* 1958; 47: 849.
10. Schwartz JB, Alvino TP. *J Pharm Sci* 1976; 65: 572.
11. Prillig EB. *Ibid* 1969; 50: 1245.
12. Porter SC. *Pharm Tech* 1980; 4: 67.
13. Delporte JP, Jaminet F. *J Pharm Belg* 1976; 31: 38.
14. Chang RK, Hsiao CH, Robinson JR. *Pharm Tech* 1987; 11: 56.
15. Butler J, et al. *Pharm Tech* 1998; 22(3): 122.
16. Ghebre-Sellassie I, ed. *Multiparticulate Oral Drug Delivery.* New York: Dekker, 1994.
17. Rowe RC. *J Pharm Pharmacol* 1981; 33: 423.
18. Huklin H. *Drugs Made in Germany* 1985; 28: 147
19. Praade DJ, ed. *Automation of Pharmaceutical Operations.* Springfield, OR: Pharm Tech Publ, 1983.
20. Mancoff WO. *Pharm Tech Yearbook* 1998; 12
21. Pentecost B. *Proceedings of TechSource® Coating Technology 99* 1999, Atlantic City.
22. Staniforth JN, Reeves LA, and Page T. *Proceedings of the 13th Annual Meeting & Exposition of AAPS* 1998, San Francisco.

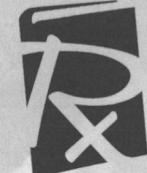

Extended-Release and Targeted Drug Delivery Systems

Xuan Ding, B Med

Adam WG Alani, M Sc

Joseph R Robinson, PhD

The goal of any drug delivery system is to provide a therapeutic amount of drug to a proper site in the body so that the desired drug concentration can be achieved promptly and then maintained. That is, the drug-delivery system should deliver drug at a rate dictated by the needs of the body over a specified period of time. This idealized objective points to the two aspects most important to drug delivery, namely, *spatial placement* and *temporal delivery*. Spatial placement relates to targeting drugs to specific organs, tissues, cells, or even subcellular compartments; whereas temporal delivery refers to controlling the rate of drug delivery to the target site. An appropriately designed controlled drug delivery system can be a major advance toward solving these two problems. It is for this reason that the science and technology responsible for development of controlled drug delivery has been, and continues to be, the focus of a great deal of attention in both industrial and academic laboratories. The history of controlled delivery technology can be divided roughly into three time periods. From 1950 to 1970 is the period of extended drug release. A number of systems containing hydrophobic polymers and waxes were fabricated with drugs into dosage forms with the aim of maintaining drug levels and, hence, drug action for an extended period of time. However, a lack of understanding of anatomic and physiologic barriers impeded the development of efficient delivery systems. From 1970 to 1990, research mainly focused on determining the needs in controlled drug delivery and on understanding the barriers for various routes of administration. Zero-order release was emphasized in controlled drug delivery. Interest in drug targeting accelerated during this period as well. The rapid progress in biotechnology and molecular biology promoted drug delivery research in the 1980s and early 1990s. Post 1990, the modern era of controlled drug delivery technology, represents the period in which an attempt at drug optimization was emphasized. In the past two decades, considerable effort has been expended on developing novel polymeric carriers, biomacromolecule delivery systems, etc.[1] Currently, numerous products formulated for various routes of administration and claiming sustained or controlled drug delivery, exist on the market. The bulk of research has been directed toward oral dosage forms that satisfy the temporal aspect of drug delivery. In addition, some of the newer approaches under investigation may allow for spatial placement as well.

CONVENTIONAL DRUG THERAPY

To gain an appreciation for the value of controlled drug therapy, it is useful to review some fundamental aspects of conventional drug delivery. Consider single dosing of a hypothetical drug that follows a simple one-compartment pharmacokinetic model for disposition. Depending on the route of administration, a conventional dosage form of the drug can produce a drug blood level versus time profile similar to that shown in Figure 47-1. The term *drug blood level* refers to the concentration of drug in blood or plasma, but the concentration in any tissue could be plotted on the ordinate. It can be seen from this figure that administration of a drug by either intravenous injection or an extravascular route (eg, orally, intramuscularly, or rectally) does not maintain drug blood levels within the therapeutic range for an extended period of time. The short duration of action is due to the inability of conventional dosage forms to control temporal delivery. If an attempt is made to maintain drug blood levels in the therapeutic range for longer periods by, for example, increasing the initial dose of an intravenous injection, as shown by the dotted line in Figure 47-1, toxic levels may be produced at early time points. Obviously, this approach is undesirable and unsuitable. An alternative approach is to administer the drug repetitively using a constant dosing interval, as in a multiple-dose therapy. This is shown in Figure 47-2 for the oral route. In this case the therapeutic drug blood level reached and the time required to reach that level depend on the dose and the dosing interval.

There are several potential problems inherent in multiple-dose therapy:

1. If the dosing interval is not appropriate for the biological half-life of the drug, large peaks and valleys in the drug blood level may result. For example, drugs with short half-lives require frequent dosing to maintain constant therapeutic levels.
2. The drug blood level may not be within the therapeutic range at sufficiently early time points, an important consideration for certain disease states.
3. Patient noncompliance with the multiple-dosing regimen can result in failure of this approach.

In many instances, potential problems associated with conventional drug therapy can be overcome. When this is the case, drugs given in conventional dosage forms by multiple dosing can produce the desired drug blood level for extended periods of time. Frequently, however, these problems are significant enough to make drug therapy with conventional dosage forms less desirable than modified-release drug therapy. This fact, coupled with the intrinsic inability of conventional dosage forms to achieve spatial placement, is a compelling stimulus for development of controlled drug delivery systems.

MODIFIED-RELEASE DRUG THERAPY

Terminology

Currently, most modified-release delivery systems fall into the following four categories:

1. Delayed-release
2. Extended-release

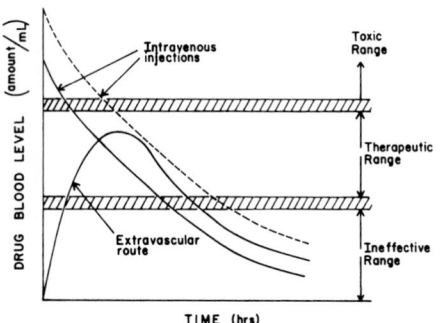

Figure 47-1. Typical drug blood level versus time profiles for intravenous injection or an extravascular route of administration.

3. Site-specific targeting
4. Receptor targeting

Delayed-release systems are either those that use repetitive, intermittent dosing of a drug from one or more immediate-release units incorporated into a single dosage form, or an enteric delayed release system. Examples of delayed-release systems include repeat-action tablets and capsules, and enteric-coated tablets where timed release is achieved by a barrier coating.

Extended-release systems include any dosage form that maintains therapeutic blood or tissue levels of the drug for a prolonged period. If the system can provide some actual therapeutic control, whether this is temporal or spatial or both, of drug release in the body, it is considered a controlled delivery system. This explains why extended-release is not equivalent to controlled-release.

Site-specific and *receptor targeting* refer to targeting a drug directly to a certain biological location. In the case of site-specific release, the target is adjacent to or in the diseased organ or tissue; for receptor release, the target is the particular drug receptor within an organ or tissue. Both of these systems satisfy the spatial aspect of drug delivery requirement and are also considered controlled drug delivery systems.

Controlled drug delivery can be defined as delivery of the drug at a predetermined rate and/or to a location according to the needs of the body and disease states for a definite time period. A controlled delivery system must fulfill one or several of the following requirements[2]:

1. *Extend drug action at a predetermined rate* by maintaining a relatively constant, effective drug level in the body with concomitant minimization of undesirable side effects that may be associated with a sawtooth kinetic pattern of conventional release.
2. *Localize drug action* by placing a controlled delivery system (usually rate-controlled) adjacent to or in a diseased tissue or organ.
3. *Target drug action* by using carriers or chemical derivatives to deliver a drug to a particular target cell type.
4. *Provide a physiologically/therapeutically based drug release system.* In other words, the amount and the rate of drug release are determined by the physiological/therapeutic needs of the body.

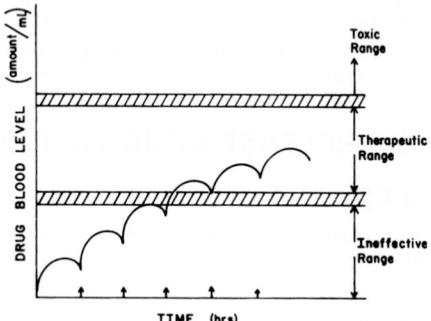

Figure 47-2. Typical drug blood level versus time profile following oral multiple-dose therapy.

Recently, a novel modification of drug delivery systems has emerged from the pharmaceutical industry. A *fast-dissolve drug delivery system* consists of a solid dosage form that dissolves or disintegrates in the oral cavity without the need of water or chewing. Among commercial products, fast dissolution or disintegration is achieved by forming an open matrix network containing the active ingredient (Zydis, *Eli Lilly*), by incorporating saliva-activated effervescent agents (OraSolv, *Cima*), or by using a mixture of a disintegrating agent and a swelling agent (Flashtab, *Prographarm*).[3]

Potential Advantages

All modified-release products share the common goal of improving drug therapy over that achieved with their conventional counterparts. There are several potential advantages of modified-release systems over conventional dosage forms, as shown in Table 47-1.

Patient compliance has been recognized as a necessary and important component in the success of all self-administered drug therapies. Minimizing or eliminating patient compliance is an obvious advantage of extended-release therapy. Because of the nature of its release kinetics, an extended-release system should be able to use less total drug over the time course of therapy than a conventional preparation. The advantages of this are a decrease or elimination of both local and systemic side effects, less potentiation or reduction in drug activity with chronic use, and minimization of drug accumulation in body tissues with chronic dosing.

The most important reason for modified-release drug therapy is improved efficiency in treatment (ie, optimized therapy). By obtaining constant or some other pattern of drug blood levels from an extended-release system, the desired therapeutic effect can be obtained promptly and maintained for a prolonged period of time. Reducing or eliminating fluctuations in the drug blood level allows better disease state management. In addition, the method by which extended release is achieved can improve the bioavailability of some drugs. For example, drugs susceptible to enzymatic inactivation or bacterial decomposition can be protected by encapsulation in polymeric systems suitable for extended release. For drugs that have a specific window for absorption, increased bioavailability can be achieved by localizing the extended-release delivery system in certain regions of the gastrointestinal tract. Improved efficiency in treatment also can take the form of a special therapeutic effect not possible with a conventional dosage form.

The last potential advantage listed in Table 47-1 (ie, economic savings) can be examined from two points of view. Although the initial unit cost of most extended-release delivery systems usually is greater than that of conventional dosage forms because of the special nature of these products, the average cost of treatment over an extended time period may be

Table 47-1. Potential Advantages of Modified-Release Drug Therapy

1. Avoid patient compliance problems
2. Employ less total drug
   a. Minimize or eliminate local side effects
   b. Minimize or eliminate systemic side effects
   c. Obtain less potentiation or reduction in drug activity with chronic use
   d. Minimize drug accumulation with chronic dosing
3. Improve efficiency in treatment
   a. Cure or control condition more promptly
   b. Improve control of condition (ie, reduce fluctuation in drug level)
   c. Improve bioavailability of some drugs
   d. Make use of special effects (eg, sustained-release aspirin for morning relief of arthritis by dosing before bedtime)
4. Economic savings

lower. Economic savings also may result from a decrease in nursing time/hospitalization, less lost work time, etc.

DRUG PROPERTIES RELEVANT TO EXTENDED-RELEASE FORMULATION

The design of extended-release delivery systems is subject to several variables of considerable importance. Among these are the route of drug administration, the type of delivery system, the disease being treated, the patient, the length of therapy, and the properties of the drug. Each of these variables is inter-related, which imposes additional constraints upon the design of the delivery system. Of particular interest to the scientist designing the system are the constraints imposed by the properties of the drug. It is these properties that have the greatest effect on the behavior of the drug in the delivery system and in the body. The properties of a drug are conveniently described as being either physicochemical or biological. Obviously, there is no clear-cut distinction between these two categories, since the biological properties of a drug are a function of its physicochemical properties. For this discussion, however, those attributes that can be determined from *in vitro* experiments will be considered physicochemical properties. Biological properties resulting from typical pharmacokinetic studies on the absorption, distribution, metabolism, and elimination (ADME) characteristics of a drug and from pharmacodynamic studies will be covered in the next section.

Among all the physicochemical properties, solubility and membrane permeability are recognized as fundamental parameters controlling the rate and extent of drug absorption. A *Biopharmaceutic Drug Classification,* proposed by Amidon et al,[4] defines four cases of oral therapeutic products based on these two attributes:

1. High solubility-high permeability drugs.
2. Low solubility-high permeability drugs.
3. High solubility-low permeability drugs.
4. Low solubility-low permeability drugs.

Solubility and permeability play an influential role in the performance of conventional products; their role is even greater in extended-release systems.

Aqueous Solubility and pKa

It is well known that for a drug to be absorbed, it must dissolve in the aqueous phase surrounding the site of administration and then partition into the absorbing membrane. The aqueous solubility of a drug influences its dissolution rate, which in turn establishes its concentration in solution and, hence, the driving force for diffusion across membranes. Dissolution rate is related to aqueous solubility, as shown by the *Noyes-Whitney equation* that, under sink conditions, is

$$dC/dt = k_D A C_s \qquad (1)$$

where dC/dt is the dissolution rate, k_D is the dissolution rate constant, A is the total surface area of the drug particles, and C_s is the aqueous saturation solubility of the drug. The dissolution rate is constant only if A remains constant, but the important point to note is that the initial rate is directly proportional to C_s. Therefore, the aqueous solubility of a drug can be used as a first approximation of its dissolution rate. Drugs with low aqueous solubility have low dissolution rates and usually suffer oral bioavailability problems.

The aqueous solubility of weak acids or bases is governed by the pKa of the compound and the pH of the medium. For a weak acid

$$S_t = S_0 (1 + Ka/[H^+]) = S_0 (1 + 10^{\,pH-pKa}) \qquad (2)$$

where S_t is the total solubility (both the ionized and unionized forms) of the weak acid, S_0 is the solubility of the unionized form,

Ka is the acid dissociation constant, and $[H^+]$ is the hydrogen ion concentration in the medium. Similarly, for a weak base

$$S_t = S_0 (1 + [H^+]/Ka) = S_0 (1 + 10^{\,pKa-pH}) \qquad (3)$$

where S_t is the total solubility (both the conjugate acid and free-base forms) of the weak base, S_0 is the solubility of the free-base form, and Ka is the acid dissociation constant of the conjugate acid. Equations 2 and 3 predict that the total solubility of a weak acid or base with a given pK$_a$ can be affected by the pH of the medium.

Considering the pH-partition hypothesis, the importance of Equations 2 and 3 relative to drug absorption is evident. The pH-partition hypothesis simply states that the unionized form of a drug will be absorbed preferentially, in a passive manner, through membranes. Since weakly acidic drugs exist primarily in the unionized form in the stomach (pH = 1 to 2), their absorption will be excellent in such an acidic environment. On the other hand, weakly basic drugs exist primarily in the ionized form (conjugate acid) at the same site, and their absorption will be poor. In the upper portion of the small intestine, the pH is more basic (pH = 5 to 7), and the reverse will be expected for weak acids and bases. The ratio of Equation 2 or 3 written for either the pH of the gastric or intestinal fluid and the pH of blood is indicative of the driving force for absorption based on pH gradient. For example, consider the ratio of the total solubility of aspirin in the blood and gastric fluid

$$R = (1 + 10^{\,pHb-pKa})/(1 + 10^{\,pHg-pKa}) \qquad (4)$$

where pH$_b$ is the pH of blood (pH 7.4), pH$_g$ is the pH of the gastric fluid (pH 2), and the pKa of aspirin is about 3.4. Substituting these values into Equation 4 gives a value for R of $10^{3.8}$, indicating that aspirin is readily absorbed within the stomach. The same calculation for intestinal pH (about 7) yields a ratio close to 1, indicating less driving force for aspirin absorption within the small intestine. Ideally, the release of an ionizable drug from an extended-release system should be programmed in accordance with the variation in pH of the different segments of the gastrointestinal tract so that the amount of preferentially absorbed forms, and thus the plasma level of the drug, will be approximately constant throughout the time course of drug action.

In general, extremes in aqueous solubility of a drug are undesirable for formulation into an extended-release product. A drug with very low solubility and a slow dissolution rate will exhibit dissolution-limited absorption and yield an inherently sustained blood level. In most instances, formulation of such a drug into an extended-release system may not provide considerable benefits over conventional dosage forms. Even if a poorly soluble drug were considered a candidate for formulation into an extended-release system, a constraint would be placed on the type of delivery system that could be used. For example, any system relying on diffusion of the drug through a polymer as the rate-limiting step in release would be unsuitable for a poorly soluble drug, since the driving force for diffusion is drug concentration in the polymer or solution, and this concentration would be low. For a drug with very high solubility and a rapid dissolution rate, it is often quite difficult to decrease its dissolution rate and slow its absorption. Preparing a slightly soluble form of a drug with normally high solubility is one possible method for producing extended-release dosage forms.

Partition Coefficient

Between the time when a drug is administered and when it is eliminated from the body, it must diffuse through a variety of biological membranes that act primarily as lipid-like barriers. A major criterion in evaluation of the ability of a drug to penetrate these lipid membranes (ie, its membrane permeability) is its apparent oil/water partition coefficient, defined as

$$K = C_O/C_W \qquad (5)$$

where C_O is the equilibrium concentration of all forms of the drug in an organic phase at equilibrium, and C_W is the equilibrium concentration of all forms in an aqueous phase. A frequently used solvent for the organic phase is 1-octanol. In general, drugs with extremely large values of K are very oil-soluble and will partition into membranes quite readily. The relationship between tissue permeation and partition coefficient for the drug generally is defined by the *Hansch correlation*, which describes a parabolic relationship between the logarithm of the activity of a drug or its ability to be absorbed and the logarithm of its partition coefficient, as shown in Figure 47-3. The explanation for this relationship is that the activity of a drug is a function of its ability to cross membranes and interact with the receptor. As a first approximation, the more effectively a drug crosses membranes, the greater its activity. There is also an optimum partition coefficient for a drug in which it most effectively permeates membranes and thus shows greatest activity. Values of the partition coefficient below this optimum result in decreased lipid solubility, and the drug will remain localized in the first aqueous phase it contacts. Values larger than the optimum result in poorer aqueous solubility but enhanced lipid solubility, and the drug will not partition out of the lipid membrane once it gets in. The value of K at which optimum activity is observed is approximately 1000/1 in n-octanol/water. Drugs with a partition coefficient that is higher or lower than the optimum are, in general, poorer candidates for formulation into extended-release dosage forms.

Drug Stability

Of importance for oral dosage forms is the loss of drug through acid hydrolysis and/or metabolism in the gastrointestinal tract. Since a drug in the solid state undergoes degradation at a much slower rate than a drug in suspension or solution form, it would seem possible to improve significantly the relative bioavailability of a drug that is unstable in the gastrointestinal tract by placing it in a slowly available extended-release form. For those drugs that are unstable in the stomach, the most appropriate controlling unit would be one that releases its contents only in the intestine. The reverse is the case for those drugs that are unstable in the environment of the intestine; the most appropriate controlling unit in such a case would be one that releases its contents only in the stomach. However, it is very difficult for a delivery system to release its contents in a specific region of the gastrointestinal tract. Thus, drugs with significant stability problems in any particular area of the gastrointestinal tract are less suitable for formulation into extended-release systems that deliver their contents uniformly over the length of the gastrointestinal tract. Delivery systems that remain localized in a certain area of the gastrointestinal tract (eg, a bioadhesive drug-delivery system) and act as reservoirs for drug release are preferred for drugs that not only suffer from stability problems but have other bioavailability problems. Under some circumstances, extended-release drug delivery systems may provide benefits for highly unstable drugs. As mentioned earlier, the drug may be protected from enzymatic degradation by incorporation into an enteric-coated dosage form.

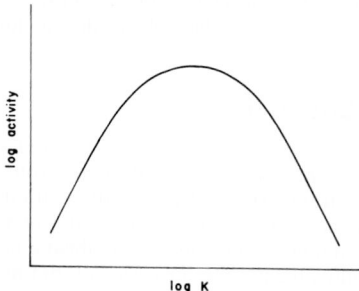

Figure 47-3. Typical relationship between drug activity and partition coefficient, K, generally known as the Hansch correlationship.

The presence of metabolizing enzymes at the site of absorption is not necessarily a negative factor in extended-release formulation. Indeed, the prodrug approach to drug delivery takes advantage of the presence of these enzymes to regenerate the parent molecule of an inactive drug derivative.

Molecular Size and Diffusivity

As previously discussed, a drug must diffuse through a variety of biological membranes during its time course in the body. In addition to diffusion through these biological membranes, drugs in many extended-release systems must diffuse through a rate-controlling polymeric membrane or matrix. The ability of a drug to diffuse in polymers, its so-called diffusivity (diffusion coefficient D), is a function of its molecular size (or molecular weight). For most polymers, it is possible to relate $\log D$ empirically to some function of molecular size as

$$\log D = -s_v \log v + k_v = -s_M \log M + k_m \quad (6)$$

where v is molecular volume, M is molecular weight, s_v, s_M, k_v, and k_m are constants. The value of D thus is related to the size and shape of the cavities as well as size and shape of drugs. Generally, values of the diffusion coefficient for intermediate-molecular-weight drugs (ie, 150 to 400 Da) through flexible polymers range from 10^{-6} to 10^{-9} cm²/sec, with values on the order of 10^{-8} being most common.[5] A value of approximately 10^{-6} is typical for these drugs through water as the medium. For drugs with a molecular weight greater than 500 Da, their diffusion coefficients in many polymers frequently are so small that they are difficult to quantify (ie, less than 10^{-12} cm²/sec). Thus, high-molecular-weight drugs should be expected to display very slow release kinetics in extended-release devices using diffusion through polymeric membranes or matrices as the releasing mechanism.

Protein Binding

Distribution of the drug into the extravascular space is governed by the equilibrium process of dissociation of the drug from the bound plasma proteins (eg, albumin). The drug-protein complex can serve as a reservoir in the vascular space for extended drug release to extravascular tissues, but only for those drugs that exhibit a high degree of binding. Thus, the protein-binding characteristics of a drug can play a significant role in its therapeutic effect, regardless of the type of dosage form. Extensive binding to plasma proteins may result in a long half-life of elimination for the drug; such drugs generally do not require an extended-release dosage form. On the other hand, drugs that exhibit a high degree of binding to plasma proteins also might bind to biopolymers in the gastrointestinal tract, which could have an influence on drug delivery.

The main attractive forces responsible for binding are van der Waals forces, hydrogen bonding, and electrostatic forces. In general, charged compounds have a greater tendency to bind a protein than uncharged compounds because of electrostatic effects. The presence of a hydrophobic moiety on the drug molecule also increases its binding potential. Some drugs that exhibit greater than 95% protein binding at therapeutic levels are amitriptyline, bishydroxycoumarin, diazepam, diazoxide, dicumarol, and novobiocin.

PHARMACOKINETIC AND PHARMACODYNAMIC CONSIDERATIONS

Release Rate and Dose[6]

Conventional dosage forms include solutions, suspensions, capsules, tablets, emulsions, aerosols, foams, ointments, and suppositories. For purposes of this discussion, these dosage forms can be considered to release their active ingredients into an absorption pool immediately. This is illustrated by the following simple kinetic scheme:

$$\text{Dosage Form} \xrightarrow[\substack{\text{drug release}}]{k_r} \text{Absorption Pool} \xrightarrow[\substack{\text{absorption}}]{k_a} \text{Target Area} \xrightarrow[\substack{\text{elimination}}]{k_e}$$

The absorption pool represents a solution of the drug at the site of absorption, and the terms k_r, k_a, and k_e are first-order rate constants for drug release, absorption, and overall elimination, respectively. Immediate release from a conventional dosage form implies that $k_r >>> k_a$ or, alternatively, that absorption of drug across a biological membrane, such as the intestinal epithelium, is the rate-limiting step in delivery of the drug to its target area. For nonimmediate-release dosage forms, $k_r <<< k_a$, that is, release of drug from the dosage form is the rate-limiting step. This causes the above kinetic scheme to reduce to

$$\text{Dosage Form} \xrightarrow[\substack{\text{drug release}}]{k_r} \text{Target Area} \xrightarrow[\substack{\text{elimination}}]{k_e}$$

Essentially, the absorptive phase of the kinetic scheme becomes insignificant compared with the drug release phase. Thus, the effort to develop a nonimmediate-release delivery system must be directed primarily to altering the release rate by affecting the value of k_r. This has been attempted in many ways, as discussed later in this chapter.

Although it is not necessary or desirable to maintain a constant level of drug in the blood or target tissue for all therapeutic cases, this is the ideal starting goal of an extended-release delivery system. In fact, in some cases optimum therapy is achieved by providing oscillating, rather than constant, drug levels. An example of this is antibiotic therapy, where the activity of the drug is required only during the growth phase of the microorganism.

The ideal goal in designing an extended-release system is to deliver drug to the desired site at a rate according to the needs of the body (ie, a self-regulated system based on feedback control). However, this is a difficult assignment. Although some attempts have been made to achieve this goal, such as with the self-regulating insulin pump, there is no commercial product representing this type of system as yet. In the absence of feedback control, we are left with a simple extending effect. The pivotal question is at what rate a drug should be delivered to maintain a constant blood drug level. This constant rate should be the same as that achieved by continuous intravenous infusion where a drug is provided to the patient at a constant rate just equal to its rate of elimination. This implies that the rate of delivery must be independent of the amount of drug remaining in the dosage form and constant over time. That is, release from the dosage form should follow zero-order kinetics, as shown by

$$k_r^0 = \text{Rate In} = \text{Rate Out} = k_e \cdot C_d \cdot V_d \qquad (7)$$

where k_r^0 is the zero-order rate constant for drug release (amount/time), k_e is the first-order rate constant for overall drug elimination (time^{-1}), C_d is the desired drug level in the body (amount/volume), and V_d is the volume of the space in which the drug is distributed. The values of k_e, C_d, and V_d needed to calculate k_r^0 are obtained from appropriately designed single-dose pharmacokinetic studies. Equation 7 provides the method to calculate the zero-order release rate constant necessary to maintain a constant drug blood or tissue level for the simplest case, where drug is eliminated by first-order kinetics. For many drugs, however, more complex elimination kinetics and other factors affecting their disposition are involved. This in turn affects the nature of the release kinetics necessary to maintain a constant drug blood level. It is important to recognize that while zero-order release may be desirable theoretically, non-zero-order release may be equivalent clinically to constant release in many cases. Aside from the extent of intra- and intersubject variation is the observation that for many drugs, modest changes in drug tissue levels do not result

in an improvement in clinical performance. Thus, a nonconstant drug level may be indistinguishable clinically from a constant drug level.

To achieve a therapeutic level promptly and sustain the level for a given period of time, the dosage form generally consists of two parts: an initial priming dose, D_i, that releases drug immediately, and a maintenance or sustaining dose, D_m. The total dose, W, thus required for the system is

$$W = D_i + D_m \qquad (8)$$

For a system in which the maintenance dose releases drug by a zero-order process for a specified period of time, the total dose is

$$W = D_i + k_r^0 T_d \qquad (9)$$

where T_d is the total time required for extended release from one dose. If the maintenance dose begins release of drug at the time of dosing ($t = 0$), it will add to that which is provided by the initial dose, thus increasing the initial drug level. In this case a correction factor is needed to account for the added drug from the maintenance dose

$$W = D_i + k_r^0 T_d - k_r^0 T_p \qquad (10)$$

The correction factor $k_r^0 T_p$ is the amount of drug provided during the period from $t = 0$ to the time of the peak drug level, T_p. No correction factor is needed if the dosage form is constructed in such a fashion that the maintenance dose does not begin to release drug until time T_p.

It already has been mentioned that a perfectly invariant drug blood or tissue level versus time profile is the ideal starting goal of an extended-release system. The way to achieve this, in the simplest case, is use of a maintenance dose that releases its drug by zero-order kinetics. However, satisfactory approximations of a constant drug level can be obtained by suitable combinations of the initial dose and a maintenance dose that releases its drug by a first-order process. The total dose for such a system is

$$W = D_i + (k_e C_d / k_r) V_d \qquad (11)$$

where k_r is the first-order rate constant for drug release (time^{-1}), and k_e, C_d, and V_d are as defined previously. If the maintenance dose begins releasing drug at $t = 0$, a correction factor is required just as in the zero-order case. The correct expression in this case is

$$W = D_i + (k_e C_d / k_r) V_d - D_m k_e T_p \qquad (12)$$

To maintain drug blood levels within the therapeutic range over the entire time course of therapy, most extended-release drug delivery systems are, like conventional dosage forms, administered as multiple rather than single doses. For an ideal extended-release system that releases drug by zero-order kinetics, the multiple dosing regimen is analogous to that used for a constant intravenous infusion. For those extended-release systems having release kinetics other than zero-order, the multiple dosing regimen is more complex, and its analysis is beyond the scope of this chapter; Welling and Dobrinska[7] provide a more detailed discussion about this subject.

Since an extended-release system is designed to alleviate repetitive dosing, it naturally will contain a greater amount of drug than a corresponding conventional form. The typical administered dose of a drug in a conventional dosage form will give some indication of the total amount of drug needed in an extended-release preparation. For those drugs requiring large conventional doses, the volume of the sustained dose may be too large to be practical or acceptable, depending on the route of administration. The same may be true of drugs that require a large release rate from the extended-release system (eg, drugs with short half-lives). For the oral route, the volume of the product is limited by patient acceptance. For the intramuscular, intravenous, or subcutaneous routes, the limitation is tolerance of the drug at the injection site. For very potent drugs, incorporation of large amounts of drug is potentially dangerous if the system fails to control drug release.

Absorption

The rate, extent, and uniformity of absorption of a drug are important factors when considering its formulation into an extended-release system. Since the rate-limiting step in drug delivery from an extended-release system is its release from a dosage form, rather than absorption, a rapid rate of drug absorption relative to its release is essential if the system is to be successful. As stated previously, $k_r <<< k_a$. This becomes most critical in the case of oral administration. Assuming that the transit time of a drug through the absorptive area of the gastrointestinal tract is between 9 and 12 hr, the maximum absorption half-life should be 3 to 4 hr.[8] This corresponds to a minimum absorption rate constant k_a value of 0.17 to 0.23 hr^{-1} necessary for about 80–95% absorption over a 9- to 12-hr transit time. For a drug with a very slow rate of absorption (ie, $k_a << 0.17$ hr^{-1}), the above discussion implies that a first-order release rate constant k_r less than 0.17 hr^{-1} is likely to result in unacceptably poor bioavailability in many patients. Therefore, slowly absorbed drugs will be difficult to be formulated into extended-release systems where the criterion $k_r <<< k_a$ must be met.

The extent and uniformity of the absorption of a drug, as reflected by its bioavailability and the fraction of the total dose absorbed, may be quite low for a variety of reasons. This is usually not a prohibitive factor in its formulation into an extended-release system. Some possible reasons for a low extent of absorption are poor water solubility, low partition coefficient, acid hydrolysis and metabolism, or site-specific absorption. The last reason is also responsible for nonuniformity of absorption. Many of these problems can be overcome by an appropriately designed extended-release system, as exemplified by the discussion under *Potential Advantages of Modified-Release Drug Therapy*.

Distribution

When designing extended-release systems, it is desirable to have as much information as possible regarding drug disposition. In actual practice, decisions usually are based on only a few pharmacokinetic parameters, one of which is the volume of distribution (V_d) as given in Equation 7. The distribution of a drug into vascular and extravascular spaces in the body is an important factor in its overall elimination kinetics. This, in turn, influences the formulation of that drug into an extended-release system, primarily by restricting the magnitude of the release rate and the dose size that can be employed.[6] At present, calculation of these quantities is based primarily on one-compartment pharmacokinetic models. A description of estimation of these quantities based on multicompartment models is beyond the scope of this chapter. However, the main considerations that need to be dealt with will be presented if a two-compartment model is operative.

Two parameters that are used to describe the distribution characteristics of a drug are its apparent volume of distribution and the ratio of drug concentration in tissue to that in plasma at steady state, the so-called T/P ratio. The apparent volume of distribution is merely a proportionality constant that relates drug concentration in the blood or plasma to the total amount of drug in the body. The magnitude of the apparent volume of distribution can be used as a guide for additional studies and as a predictor for a drug-dosing regimen and hence the need to employ an extended-release system. For drugs that obey a one-compartment model, the apparent volume of distribution is

$$V = dose/C_0 \quad (13)$$

where C_0 is the initial drug concentration immediately after an intravenous bolus injection, but before any drug has been eliminated. The application of this equation is based on the assumption that the distribution of a drug between plasma and tissues takes place instantaneously. This is rarely a good assumption, and it is usually necessary to invoke multi-compartment models to account for the finite time required for the drug

to distribute fully throughout the available body space. In the case of a two-compartment model, it has been shown that the best estimate of total volume of drug distribution is given by the apparent volume of distribution at steady state[9]:

$$V_{ss} = (1 + k_{12}/k_{21})V_1 \quad (14)$$

where V_1 is the volume of the central compartment, k_{12} is the rate constant for distribution of drug from the central to the peripheral compartment, and k_{21} is that from the peripheral to the central compartment. As its name implies, V_{ss} relates drug concentration in the blood or plasma at steady state to the total amount of drug in the body during repetitive dosing or constant-rate infusion. The use of Equation 14 is limited to those instances where a steady-state drug concentration in both compartments has been reached; at any other time, it tends to overestimate or underestimate the total amount of drug in the body.

To avoid the ambiguity inherent in the apparent volume of distribution as an estimator of the amount of drug in the body, the T/P ratio also can be used. If the amount of drug in the central compartment, P, is known, the amount of drug in the peripheral compartment, T, and hence the total amount of drug in the body can be calculated by

$$T/P = k_{12}(k_{21} - \beta) \quad (15)$$

Here, β is the slow disposition rate constant. The important point to note is that the T/P ratio estimates the relative distribution of drug between compartments, whereas V_{ss} estimates the extent of distribution in the body. Both parameters contribute to an estimation of the distribution characteristics of a drug, but their relative importance in this respect is open to debate.

Metabolism

The metabolic conversion of a drug to another chemical form usually can be considered in the design of an extended-release system for that drug. As long as the location, rate, and extent of metabolism are known and the rate constant(s) for the process(es) are not too large, successful extended-release products can be developed.

There are two factors associated with the metabolism of some drugs, however, which present problems for their use in extended-release systems. One is the ability of the drug to induce or inhibit enzyme synthesis, which may result in a fluctuating drug blood level with chronic dosing. The other is a fluctuating drug blood level due to intestinal (or other tissue) metabolism or through hepatic first-pass effect. Examples of drugs that are subject to intestinal metabolism upon oral dosing are hydralazine, salicylamide, nitroglycerin, isoproterenol, chlorpromazine, and levodopa. Examples of drugs that undergo extensive first-pass hepatic metabolism are propoxyphene, nortriptyline, phenacetin, propranolol, and lidocaine.

Elimination and Biological Half-Life

The rate of elimination of a drug is described quantitatively by its biological half-life, $t_{1/2}$, which is related to its apparent volume of distribution (V) and its systemic clearance (Cl):

$$t_{1/2} = 0.693V/Cl = 0.693V \cdot AUC/dose \quad (16)$$

Cl is equal to the ratio of an intravenously administered dose to the total area under the drug blood level versus time curve (AUC).

To achieve extended-release drug delivery, it is desirable to have zero-order drug input. Under steady state, rate in = rate out, then

$$R_0 = C_{ss}Cl \quad (17)$$

This equation shows that the input rate of an extended-release system is determined solely by steady-state concentration C_{ss} and systemic clearance. Half-life, a common pharmacokinetic parameter, is not directly needed to determine the input rate.

Similarly, volume of distribution is also not a major consideration in designing extended-release delivery systems, although a larger volume of distribution often requires a higher drug load to achieve a therapeutic blood level. However, half-life does play a role in determining the benefits of formulating a drug into an extended-release dosage form. A drug with a short half-life requires frequent dosing, and this makes it a desirable candidate for an extended-release formulation. On the other hand, a drug with a long half-life is dosed at greater time intervals, and thus there is less need for an extended-release system. Practically, it is difficult to define precise upper and lower limits for the value of half-life of a drug that best suits extended-release formulation. In general, a drug with a half-life of less than 2 hr probably should not be used, since such systems will require unacceptably large release rates and large doses. At the other extreme, drugs with half-lives longer than 8 hours are usually not suitable candidates for extended-release dosage forms because they do not provide benefits over conventional dosage forms. In addition, half-life may be useful in determining the dosing interval of an extended-release dosage form. Some examples of drugs with half-lives less than 2 hr are ampicillin, cephalexin, cloxacillin, furosemide, levodopa, penicillin G, and propylthiouracil. Examples of those with half-lives greater than 8 hr are dicumarol, diazepam, digitoxin, digoxin, guanethidine, phenytoin, and warfarin.

Efficacy and Safety

There may not exist a direct correlation between the pharmacokinetics (PK) and pharmacodynamics (PD) of a drug. In other words, it may be difficult to predict the effect of a drug based only on pharmacokinetic data. As a result, a PK/PD model may be required to obtain a rational design of an extended-release dosage form. Typically, a graded response can be represented by

$$E = PC + E_0 \qquad (18)$$

where P is a proportionality constant, C is the plasma concentration, and E_0 is the baseline effect. In some cases, a more satisfactory relationship is obtained by using

$$E = P \log C + E_0 \qquad (19)$$

In fact, in most cases, the relationship is much more complex than a simple linear one, and sometimes it can be represented only by an expression closely related to enzyme kinetics.

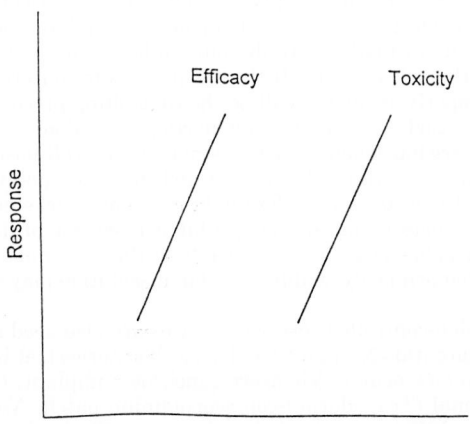

Figure 47-4. Relationship between pharmacological and toxicological responses and concentration. The relative distance between efficacy and toxicity is the therapeutic index of the drug substance. (From Park K, ed. *Controlled Drug Delivery: Challenges and Strategies.* Washington DC: American Chemical Society, 1997, p 589.)

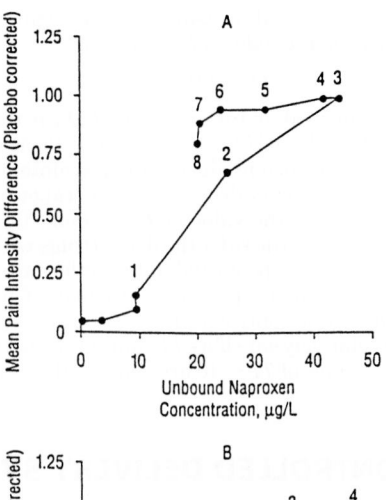

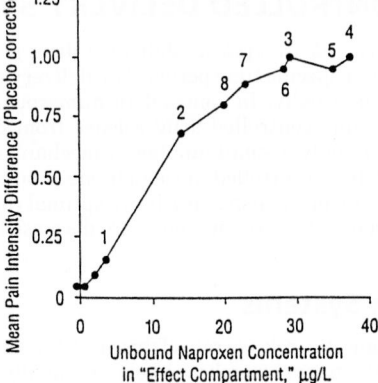

Figure 47-5. Relationship between the mean pain index and concentration of the analgesic index. Obviously, there is a hysteresis in A. However, this clockwise hysteresis is removed when an effect compartment is introduced. (From Rowland M, Tozer TN. *Clinical Pharmacokinetics: Concepts and Applications,* 3rd ed. Baltimore: Lippincott Williams & Wilkins, 1995, p 360.)

$$E = E_0 + (E_{max} C^n)/(E_{50}{}^n + C^n) \qquad (20)$$

where E_{max} is the maximal effect, E_{50} is the drug concentration to produce 50% of a maximal effect, and n is a constant. This equation is sometimes subject to variability. Patients differ widely in their values of E_{50} and n for a given drug. Figure 47-4[10] shows a typical response-concentration relationship. Hysteresis may often be found in response-concentration relationships when there is a delayed response due to a slow distribution phase. In this case, an effect compartment model may be useful to correlate the response and concentration (Fig 47-5A and B[11]). A constant blood level by zero-order release does not necessarily produce a constant pharmacological effect. Nitroglycerin is a good example for illustrative purposes. A constant level of nitroglycerin can lead to tolerance and result in a decreased pharmacological response. Hence, an "off" period is required for adequate nitroglycerin therapy. To conclude, it is necessary to have a thorough knowledge of the relationship between concentration and effect and its dependence on disease and time profile of drug input to have a more rational design of extended-release delivery systems.

There are very few drugs whose specific therapeutic concentrations are known. Instead, a therapeutic concentration range is listed, with increasing toxic effects expected above this range and a falloff in desired therapeutic response observed below the range. For some drugs, the incidence of side effects, in addition to toxicity, is believed to be a function of plasma concentration.[12] An extended-release system can, at times, minimize side effects for a particular drug by controlling its plasma concentration and using less total drug over the time course of therapy.

The most widely used measure of the margin of safety of a drug is its therapeutic index, TI, defined as

$$TI = TD_{50}/ED_{50} \qquad (21)$$

where TD_{50} is the median toxic dose and ED_{50} is the median effective dose. The value of TI varies from as little as unity, where the effective dose is also producing toxic symptoms, to several thousand. For very potent drugs, whose therapeutic concentration range is narrow, the value of TI is small. In general, the larger the value of TI, the safer the drug. Drugs with very small values of TI usually are poor candidates for formulation into extended-release products, primarily because of technological limitations of precise control over release rates. A drug is considered to be relatively safe if its TI value exceeds 10. Examples of drugs with values of $TI < 10$ are some barbiturates and cardiac glycosides.

RATE-CONTROLLED DELIVERY SYSTEMS

Rate-controlled release systems deliver a drug at a predetermined rate for a specific time period. The delivery can be either systemically or locally. In contrast to numerous commercial products claiming controlled drug release from delivery systems, there are only a small number of mechanisms by which the release rate is controlled, although one product may combine two or more mechanisms to achieve optimal control. In this section, the commonly used methods are discussed.

Diffusion Systems

In these systems, the release rate of drug is determined by its diffusion through an inert membrane barrier, usually an insoluble polymer. There are basically two types of diffusion devices: *reservoir devices*, in which a core of drug is surrounded by a polymeric membrane, and *matrix devices*, in which dissolved or dispersed drug is distributed uniformly in an inert polymeric matrix.

RESERVOIR DEVICES—The release of drug from a reservoir device is governed by *Fick's first law of diffusion*

$$J = -DdC_m/dx \qquad (22)$$

where J is the flux of drug across a membrane in the direction of decreasing concentration (amount/area-time), D is the diffusion coefficient of the drug in the membrane (area/time), and dC_m/dx is the change in concentration of drug in the membrane over a distance x. If it is assumed that the drug on either side of the membrane is in equilibrium with the respective surface layer of the membrane, as shown in Figure 47-6[13], then the concentration just inside the membrane surface can be related to the concentration in the adjacent region by the expressions:

$$K = C_{m(0)}/C_{(0)} \text{ at } x = 0 \qquad (23)$$

$$K = C_{m(l)}/C_{(l)} \text{ at } x = l \qquad (24)$$

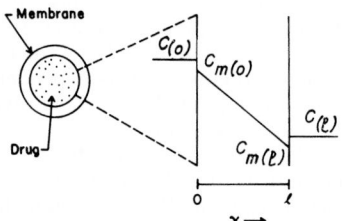

Figure 47-6. Reservoir diffusion device. $C_{m(0)}$ and $C_{m(l)}$ represent concentrations of drug at the inside surfaces of the membrane and $C_{(0)}$ and $C_{(l)}$ represent concentrations in the adjacent regions. (From Langer R, Wise D, eds. *Medical Applications of Controlled Release Technology.* Boca Raton, FL: CRC Press, 1985, p 171.)

Table 47-2. Reservoir Diffusion Products

PRODUCTS	ACTIVE INGREDIENT(S)	MANUFACTURER
Nico-400	Nicotinic acid	Jones
Nitro-Bid	Nitroglycerin	Hoechst Marion Roussel
Cerespan capsules	Papaverine HCl	Rorer
Nitrospan capsules	Nitroglycerin	Rorer
Measurin tablets	Acetylsalicylic acid	Sanofi-Winthrop
Bronkodyl S-R capsules	Theophylline	Sanofi-Winthrop

where K is the partition coefficient. Assuming that D and K are constant, Equation 22 can be integrated to give

$$J = DK\Delta C/l \qquad (25)$$

where ΔC is the concentration difference across the membrane.

If the activity of the drug inside the reservoir is maintained constant and the value of K is less than unity, zero-order release can be achieved. This is the case when the drug is present as a solid (ie, its activity is unity). Depending on the shape of the device, the equation describing drug release will vary. Only the simplest geometry, that of a rectangular slab or sandwich, is presented here. For the slab geometry, the equation describing release is

$$dM_t/dt = ADK\Delta C/l \qquad (26)$$

where M_t is the mass of drug released at time t, dM_t/dt is the steady-state release rate at time t, A is the surface area of the device. Similar equations can be written for cylindrical or spherical geometric devices. To obtain a constant drug-release rate, it is necessary to maintain constant area, diffusion path length, concentration, and diffusion coefficient. In other words, all the terms on the right hand side of Equation 26 are held constant. This is often not the case in actual practice because one or more of the above terms will change in the product. Swelling or contraction of the polymer membrane causes a change in the diffusion length and diffusion coefficient of the drug through the membrane.

Diffusion reservoir devices have been some of the widely used and most successful oral systems. Common methods used to develop reservoir-type devices include microencapsulation of drug particles and film coating of tablets (see Chapter 46, *Coating of Pharmaceutical Dosage Forms*). In most cases, particles coated by microencapsulation form a system in which the drug is contained in the coating film as well as in the core of the microcapsule. Drug release usually involves a combination of dissolution and diffusion, with dissolution being the process that controls the release rate. If the encapsulating material is selected properly, diffusion will be the controlling process. Some materials used as the membrane barrier coat, alone or in combination, are hardened gelatin, methyl- or ethylcelluloses, polyhydroxymethacrylate, hydroxypropylcellulose, polyvinylacetate, and various waxes. Examples of some marketed orally dosed products using an encapsulated reservoir of drug are shown in Table 47-2. Drug release from these products probably is based primarily on diffusion, but dissolution may occur as well.

Diffusion-controlled reservoir devices are also used in other routes: parental (Norplant subdermal levonorgestrel implant, *Wyeth-Ayerst*), ocular (Vitrasert ganciclovir implant, *Chiron*), transdermal (Transderm-Scop scopolamine patch, *Novartis*), and vaginal (Estring estradiol vaginal ring, *Pharmacia*).

MATRIX DEVICES—The rate of release of a drug dispersed as a solid in an inert matrix has been described by Higuchi.[14,15] Figure 47-7 depicts the physical model for a planar slab. In this model, it is assumed that the solid drug dissolves from the surface layer of the device first; when this layer becomes exhausted of drug, the next layer begins to be depleted by dissolution and diffusion through the matrix to the external

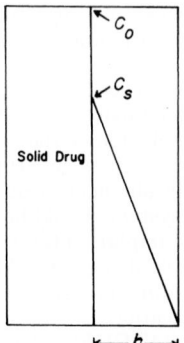

Figure 47-7. Physical model used for a planar-slab matrix-diffusion device.

solution. In this fashion, the interface between the region containing dissolved drug and that containing dispersed drug moves into the interior as a front. The assumptions made in deriving the mathematical model are

1. A pseudo-steady state is maintained during release.
2. The total amount of drug present per unit volume in the matrix, C_0, is substantially greater than the saturation solubility of the drug per unit volume in the matrix, C_s (ie, excess solute is present).
3. The release medium is a perfect sink at all times.
4. Drug particles are much smaller in diameter than the average distance of diffusion.
5. The diffusion coefficient remains constant.
6. No interaction occurs between the drug and the matrix.

Based on Figure 47-7, the change in the amount of drug released per unit area, dM, with a change in the depleted zone thickness, dh, is

$$dM = C_0\,dh - (C_s/2)dh \qquad (27)$$

However, based on Fick's first law

$$dM = (D_mC_s/h)dt \qquad (28)$$

where D_m is the diffusion coefficient in the matrix. If Equations 27 and 28 are equated, solved for h, and that value of h substituted back into the integrated form of Equation 28, an equation for M is obtained

$$M = [C_s D_m (2C_0 - C_s)t]^{1/2} \qquad (29)$$

Similarly, a drug released from a porous or granular matrix is described by

$$M = [C_a D_s (\varepsilon/T)(2C_0 - \varepsilon C_a)t]^{1/2} \qquad (30)$$

where ε is porosity of the matrix, T is tortuosity, C_a is the solubility of the drug in the release medium, and D_s is the diffusion coefficient of drug in the release medium. In this system, drug is leached from the matrix through channels or pores.

For purposes of data treatment, Equations 29 and 30 are conveniently reduced to

$$M = kt^{1/2} \qquad (31)$$

where k is a constant, so that a plot of the amount of drug released versus the square root of time should be linear if release of the drug from the matrix is diffusion-controlled. The release rate of drug from such a device is not zero-order, since it decreases with time, but as previously mentioned, this may be clinically equivalent to constant release for many drugs.

The three major types of materials used in the preparation of matrix devices are insoluble plastics, hydrophilic polymers, and fatty compounds. Plastic matrices that have been investigated include methyl acrylate–methyl methacrylate, polyvinyl chloride, and polyethylene. The Gradumet tablet *(Abbott)* was an example of a dosage form using a plastic matrix. Hydrophilic

polymers include methylcellulose, hydroxypropylmethylcellulose, sodium carboxymethylcellulose, and carbopol 934. Fatty compounds include various waxes such as carnauba wax and glyceryl tristearate.

The most common method of preparation is to mix the drug with the matrix material and then compress the mixture into tablets. In the case of wax matrices, the drug generally is dispersed in molten wax, which is then congealed, granulated, and compressed into cores. In any extended-release system, it is necessary for a portion of the drug to be available immediately as a priming dose and the remainder to be released in a sustained fashion. This is accomplished in a matrix tablet by placing the priming dose in a coat of the tablet. The coat can be applied by press coating or by conventional pan or air suspension coating. Some marketed matrix diffusion products for oral dosing are listed in Table 47-3. Similar to reservoir devices, matrix devices are also used to deliver drugs in other routes: parental (Compudose subdermal estradiol implant, *Elanco*) and transdermal (Deponit nitroglycerin patch, *Schwarz Pharma*).

DIFFUSION-CONTROLLED IMPLANTS—Implants are most commonly used for parental administration over a significantly prolonged period of time (days to years). Norplant *(Wyeth-Ayerst)* is a commercially available levonorgestrel implant system, indicated for the prevention of pregnancy for as long as 5 yr. Although implants possess such evident advantages as convenience and compliance, concerns over body responses to a foreign material often raise biocompatibility and safety issues. Application of biocompatible polymers to the construction of implants for achieving better control over the duration of drug activity and precision of dosing actually started with the discovery of the silicone elastomer. The rate of drug release was found to be controlled by the thickness and surface area of the membrane as well as polarity of the penetrant. Toward the end of the 1960s, a concentrated effort was made to expand the silicone elastomer-based implantable therapeutic system technology to other biocompatible polymers, in an attempt to control the release of water-soluble molecules. Some of these systems include a microporous membrane made from an ethylene/vinyl acetate copolymer for the ocular delivery of pilocarpine, a biodegradable (lactic/glycolic acid) copolymer for subcutaneous and intramuscular controlled administration of narcotic antagonists, a bioerodible polysaccharide polymer for delivery of anti-inflammatory steroids, hydrogel for subcutaneous controlled administration of estrus-synchronizing agents, or implantable therapeutic systems activated by osmotic pressure, vapor pressure, magnetism, etc.

In both types of implants made of nondegradable polymer (ie, reservoir devices and matrix devices), drug release is governed by diffusion.

In reservoir devices, the drug is encapsulated within a compartment that is enclosed by a rate-limiting polymeric membrane. The drug reservoir may contain either solid drug particles or a dispersion of solid drug in a liquid- or solid-type dispersing medium. The polymeric membrane may be fabricated from a homogeneous or a heterogeneous nonporous polymeric material or a microporous or semipermeable membrane.

Table 47-3. Matrix Diffusion Products

PRODUCTS	ACTIVE INGREDIENT(S)	MANUFACTURER
Gradumet tablets		Abbott
Desoxyn	Methamphetamine	
Ferro-Gradumet	Ferrous sulfate	
Tral	Hexocyclium methylsulfate, Phenobarbital	
Lontab tablets		
PBZ-SR	Tripelennamide HCl	Novartis
Procan SR	Procainamide HCl	Pfizer
Choledyl SA	Oxtriphylline	Pfizer

Drug encapsulation may be accomplished by molding, encapsulation, microencapsulation, or other techniques.

The drug release (dQ/dt) from this type of implantable therapeutic systems is defined by

$$dQ/dt = C_R\,(^1\!/P_m + {}^1\!/P_d) \tag{32}$$

where C_R is the drug concentration in the reservoir compartment; P_m and P_d are the permeability coefficients of the rate-controlling membrane and of the hydrodynamic diffusion layer existing on the surface of the membrane, respectively. P_m and P_d are defined as

$$P_m = (K_{m/r}\,D_m)/\delta_m \tag{33}$$

$$P_d = (K_{a/m}\,D_a)/\delta_d \tag{34}$$

where $K_{m/r}$ and $K_{a/m}$ are the partition coefficients for the interfacial partitioning of drug molecules from the reservoir to the membrane and from the membrane to the aqueous diffusion layer, respectively; D_m and D_a are the diffusion coefficients in the membrane and in the aqueous diffusion layer, respectively; and δ_m and δ_d are the thickness of the membrane and of the aqueous diffusion layer, respectively.

Substituting Equation 33 and Equation 34 for P_m and P_d in Equation 32 and then integrating gives

$$Q/t = [(K_{m/r}\,K_{a/m}\,D_a\,D_m)C_R\,]/\ [(K_{m/r}\,D_m\,\delta_d) + (K_{a/m}\,D_a\,\delta_m)] \tag{35}$$

that defines the rate of drug release at steady state from a membrane permeation-type extended-release drug delivery device. Since the drug reservoir consists of solid drug particles or a solid drug suspension, C_R in the system remains constant. Hence, the release rate from reservoir-type diffusion-controlled implant does not vary with time (zero-order release kinetics). Examples of this type of implantable therapeutic systems are Alza's Progestasert IUD and Ocusert.[16]

In matrix diffusion-type extended-release drug delivery, drug particles are homogeneously dispersed throughout a lipophilic or hydrophilic polymer matrix. The dispersion may be accomplished by blending the drug with a viscous liquid polymer or a semisolid polymer at room temperature, followed by cross-linking of the polymer or by mixing drug particles with a melted polymer at an elevated temperature. Dispersion also can be achieved by dissolving the drug particles and/or the polymer in an organic solvent followed by mixing and evaporation of the solvent in a mold at an elevated temperature or under vacuum.

The rate of drug release from this type of delivery device is not constant and is defined by

$$dQ/dt = [(AC_p\,D_p)/2t]^{1/2} \tag{36}$$

where A is the initial drug loading dose dispersed in the polymer matrix; C_p and D_p are the solubility and diffusivity of the drug molecules in the polymer, respectively. Integration of Equation 36 gives

$$Q/t^{1/2} = (2AC_p\,D_p)^{1/2} \tag{37}$$

that defines the flux of drug release at steady state from a matrix diffusion-type drug-delivery device. Thus a matrix system provides decreasing release with time (square root of time-release kinetics). Examples of this type of implantable therapeutic system are the contraceptive vaginal ring[17] and Compudose implant (*Elanco*).[18]

Drug release kinetic of a matrix system can be improved by using reservoir/matrix hybrid-type polymeric implants so that release approximates the constant release from a reservoir system. Examples of this hybrid system are Syncro-Mate-C implant (*Sanofi-CEVA*) and Implanon (*Organon*).[19] In the former, an estradiol valerate suspension is dispersed in millions of individually sealed microreservoirs; then the mixture of microreservoirs is placed in a silicone polymer tube for *in situ* polymerization and molding. Drug molecules initially diffuse through the microreservoir membrane and then through the silicone polymer coating membrane. In the latter, 3-ketodesogestrel is dispersed in a polymer matrix; this polymer matrix is then coated with another rate-limiting polymeric membrane.

Implants typically are placed subcutaneously to control drug release via various mechanisms. Both nonbiodegradable polymers, such as silicone elastomer (polydimethylsiloxane), and biodegradable polymers, such as poly(caprolactone), poly(lactic acid) (PLA), or poly(glycolic acid), can be used. An ideal implantable therapeutic system should be biostable, biocompatible with minimal tissue-implant interactions, nontoxic, noncarcinogenic, and removable if required. Also, the system should release drug at a constant, programmed rate for a predetermined duration of medication.

TRANSDERMAL PATCHES—The transdermal route offers several advantages over other methods of delivery. Although the skin, particularly the stratum corneum, presents a barrier to most drug absorption, it provides a large (1–2 m^2) and accessible surface area for drug diffusion. Additionally, transdermal administration, as compared to other routes, is fairly noninvasive. Patients are quite willing to accept the use of a simple-looking "patch" as it can be conveniently applied and removed. Over the past two decades, the challenge of transdermal drug delivery has been acknowledged by pharmaceutical scientists. The intensity of interest in the potential biomedical applications of transdermal controlled drug administration is demonstrated by increasing research activity in the development of various types of transdermal therapeutic systems for long-term continuous infusion of therapeutic agents, including antihypertensive, antianginal, analgesic, steroidal, and contraceptive drugs. Although transdermal delivery is currently limited to relatively few drugs, it has achieved considerable commercial success. Success in developing these drugs (ie, nitroglycerin, scopolamine, estradiol, testosterone, nicotine, clonidine, fentanyl, and the estrogen-progestin combination) into transdermal products lies in the fact that all these drugs are very potent and require no more than 20mg/day for effective therapy. A discussion of the fundamental aspects of transdermal drug absorption can be found in Chapter 44, *Medicated Topicals*.

Current transdermal patches can be classified into four types:

1. Membrane-modulated system represented by Transderm-Scop (Scopolamine, *Novartis*).
2. Adhesive dispersion-type system represented by Deponit (nitroglycerin, *Schwarz Pharma*).
3. Matrix dispersion-type system represented by Nitrodur (nitroglycerin, *Schering*).
4. Microreservoir system represented by Nitrodisc (nitroglycerin, *Roberts*).

In a *membrane-modulated system*, the drug reservoir is totally encapsulated in a shallow compartment molded from a drug-impermeable backing and a rate-controlling polymeric membrane. The drug molecules are released only through the rate-controlling polymeric membrane. The rate-limiting membrane can be microporous or nonporous. On the external surface of the membrane, a thin layer of drug-compatible, hypoallergenic, adhesive polymer (eg, silicone or polyacrylate adhesive) may be applied to achieve intimate contact of the transdermal system with the skin. The rate of drug release from this type of drug-delivery system can be tailored by varying the polymer composition, permeability coefficient, or thickness of the rate-limiting membrane and adhesive. A representation of these systems is shown in Figure 47-8.

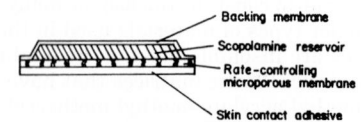

Figure 47-8. Transdermal device for delivery of scopolamine.

An *adhesive dispersion-type system* lacks the permeation-controlling membrane. In this system the drug reservoir is formulated by directly dispersing the drug in an adhesive polymer and then spreading the medicated adhesive, by solvent casting, onto a flat sheet of drug-impermeable backing membrane to form a thin drug-reservoir layer. On top of the drug-reservoir layer, layers of nonmedicated, rate-controlling adhesive polymer of constant thickness are applied to produce an adhesive diffusion-controlled drug delivery system.

In a *matrix dispersion-type system*, the drug reservoir is formed by homogeneously dispersing the drug in a hydrophilic or lipophilic polymer matrix, and then the medicated polymer is molded into a medicated disc with a defined surface area and controlled thickness. The disc is then glued onto an occlusive baseplate in a compartment fabricated from a drug-impermeable backing. The adhesive polymer is spread along the circumference to form a strip of adhesive rim around the medicated disc. Release rate is controlled by diffusion from the matrix.

In a *microreservoir system*, the drug reservoir is formed by first suspending the drug particles in an aqueous solution of water-soluble polymer and then dispersing it homogeneously in a lipophilic polymer by high-shear mechanical force to form a large number of unleachable, microscopic spheres of drug reservoirs. This thermodynamically unstable dispersion is stabilized quickly by immediately cross-linking the polymer *in situ,* which produces a medicated polymer disc with a constant surface area and a fixed thickness. This medicated disc is positioned at the center and surrounded by an adhesive rim. Release of the drug from this type of drug-delivery device follows either an interfacial partition or a matrix diffusion-controlled process.

Dissolution Systems

As mentioned earlier in this chapter, a drug with a slow dissolution rate will yield an inherently sustained blood level. In principle, then, it would seem possible to prepare extended-release products by controlling the dissolution rate of drugs that are highly water-soluble. This can be done by preparing an appropriate salt or derivative, by coating the drug with a slowly soluble material, or by incorporating it into a tablet with a slowly soluble carrier. Ideally, the surface area available for dissolution must remain constant to achieve a constant release rate. This is, however, difficult in practice.

The dissolution process can be considered diffusion-layer-controlled, where the rate of diffusion from the solid surface to the bulk solution through an unstirred liquid film is the rate-determining step. In this case the dissolution process at steady state is described by the Noyes-Whitney equation

$$dC/dt = k_D A(C_s - C) = (D/h)A(C_s - C) \qquad (38)$$

where dC/dt is the dissolution rate, k_D is the dissolution rate constant, A is the total surface area, C_s is the saturation solubility of the solid, and C is the concentration of solute in the bulk solution. The dissolution-rate constant, k_D, is equal to the diffusion coefficient, $D,$ divided by the thickness of the diffusion layer, h. The above equation predicts a constant dissolution rate if the surface area, diffusion coefficient, diffusion layer thickness, and concentration difference are kept constant. However, as dissolution proceeds, all of these parameters may change, especially surface area. For spherical particles, the change in area can be related to the weight of the particle; under the assumption of sink conditions, Equation 38 becomes the cube-root dissolution equation

$$w_0^{1/3} - w^{1/3} = k_D't \qquad (39)$$

where k_D' is the cube-root dissolution-rate constant, and w_0 and w are initial weight and weight of the amount remaining at time t, respectively.

Two common formulations relying on dissolution to determine release rate of drug are shown in Figure 47-9. Most products fall into two categories: *encapsulated/reservoir dissolution systems* and *matrix dissolution systems.*

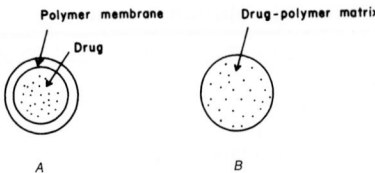

Figure 47-9. Systems using dissolution. **A.** Encapsulated formulation in which drug release is determined by thickness and dissolution rate of the polymer membrane. **B.** Matrix formulation in which drug release is determined by dissolution rate of the polymer.

Encapsulated dissolution systems can be prepared either by coating particles or granules of drug with slowly soluble polymers whose thicknesses vary or by microencapsulation. Microencapsulation can be accomplished by using phase separation, interfacial polymerization, heat-fusion, or solvent-evaporation. The coating materials may be selected from a wide variety of natural and synthetic polymers, depending on the drug to be coated and the release characteristics desired. The most commonly used coating materials include gelatin, carnauba wax, shellac, cellulose acetate phthalate, and cellulose acetate butyrate. Drug release from microcapsules is a mass-transport phenomenon and can be controlled by adjusting the size of microcapsules, thickness of coating materials, and the diffusivity of core materials. The thickness can be varied from less than 1 μm to 200 μm by changing the amount of coating material from 3% to 30% of the total weight. If only a few different thicknesses are used, usually three or four, drugs will be released at different, predetermined times to give a delayed-release effect (ie, repeat-action). If a spectrum of different thicknesses is employed, a zero-order release of the drug can be obtained from the dosage form as a whole. Microcapsules commonly are filled into capsules and rarely tableted as their coatings tend to disrupt during compression. A partial list of some marketed products relying primarily on encapsulated dissolution is shown in Table 47-4.

A matrix dissolution device is prepared by compressing the drug with a slowly soluble polymer carrier into a tablet form. There are two general methods of preparing drug-wax particles: congealing and aqueous dispersion. In the congealing method, drug is mixed with a wax material and either spray-congealed or congealed and screened. In the aqueous dispersion method, the drug-wax mixture is simply sprayed or placed in water, and the resulting particles are collected. Matrix tablets are also made by direct compression of a mixture of drug, polymer, and excipients. Examples of marketed orally administered products relying primarily on matrix dissolution are listed in Table 47-5. In a matrix dissolution device, the decrease in drug release due to decreased size of the matrix can be partially offset by constructing a nonlinear concentration profile in the polymer matrix (eg, the core of the dissolution matrix contains more drug than the outer layer [Adalat nifedipine tablet, *Bayer*]).[20] Matrix dissolution devices are also widely used in parenteral therapy (eg, Zoladex subcutaneous implant for delivery of goserelin [*AstraZeneca*]).

Table 47-4. Encapsulated Dissolution Products

PRODUCTS	ACTIVE INGREDIENT(S)	MANUFACTURER
Spansule capsules		GlaxoSmithKline
Dexedrine	Dextroamphetamine sulfate	
Hispril	Diphenylpyraline HCl	
Thorazine	Chlorpromazine HCl	
Sequel capsules		
Artane	Trihexyphenidyl	Lederle
Diamox	Acetazolamide	Wyeth-Ayerst
Ferro-sequels	Ferrous fumarate, Docusate sodium	Lederle

Table 47-5. Matrix Dissolution Products

PRODUCTS	ACTIVE INGREDIENT(S)	MANUFACTURER
Extentab tablets		Whitehall-Robins
Dimetane	Brompheniramine maleate	
Quinidex	Quinidine sulfate	
Timespan tablets		
Mestinon	Pyridostigmine bromide	ICN
Repetab tablets		Schering-Plough
Chlor-Trimeton	Chlorpheniramine maleate	
Demazin	Dexchlorpheniramine maleate, Pseudoephedrine HCl	
Trilafon	Perphenazine	

Osmotic Systems

Osmotic pressure can be employed as the driving force to generate a constant release of drug, provided a constant osmotic pressure is maintained and a few other features of the physical system are constrained. A tablet consists of a core of an osmotically active drug, or a core of an osmotically inactive drug, in combination with an osmotically active salt surrounded by a semipermeable membrane containing a small orifice, as shown in Figure 47-10A.[21] The membrane allows free diffusion of water but not drug. When the tablet is exposed to water or any fluid in the body, water will flow into the tablet because of the osmotic pressure difference, and the volume flow rate, dV/dt, of water into the tablet is

$$dV/dt = (kA/h)(\Delta\pi - \Delta P) \qquad (40)$$

where k, A, and h are the membrane permeability, area, and thickness, respectively, $\Delta\pi$ is the osmotic pressure difference, and ΔP is the hydrostatic pressure difference. If the orifice is sufficiently large, the hydrostatic pressure difference is small compared with the osmotic pressure difference, and Equation 40 becomes

$$dV/dt = (kA/h)\Delta\pi \qquad (41)$$

Thus, the volume flow rate of water into the tablet is determined by permeability, area, and thickness of the membrane. The drug will be pumped out of the tablet through the orifice at a controlled rate, dM/dt, equal to the volume flow rate of water into the tablet multiplied by the drug concentration, C_s:

$$dM/dt = (dV/dt)C_s \qquad (42)$$

The release rate will be constant until the concentration of drug inside the tablet falls below saturation.

Several modifications of the osmotic pressure-controlled drug delivery system have been developed. A layer of bioerodible polymer can be applied to the external surface of the semipermeable membrane. As a result, the system consists of two compartments separated by a movable piston, as shown in Figure 47-10B.[22] For a system that does not have an orifice, hydraulic pressure is built up inside as the gastrointestinal fluid is imbibed, until the wall ruptures and the contents are released to the environment.

The advantage of the osmotic system is that it only requires osmotic pressure to be effective and is essentially independent of the environment. The drug release rate can be predetermined precisely regardless of pH changes through the gastrointestinal tract. Some materials used as the semipermeable membrane include polyvinyl alcohol, polyurethane, cellulose acetate, ethylcellulose, and polyvinyl chloride. Drugs that have demonstrated successful release from an osmotic system *in vivo* after oral dosing are potassium chloride and acetazolamide. Osmosis is also successfully used to consistently release drug from an implant, such as *Alza*'s Alzet miniosmotic pump and Duros pump.

Mechanical Systems[19]

Mechanically driven pumps are commonly used to precisely control the infusion rate of a drug in the clinics. Externally programmable pumps can facilitate zero-order and intermittent drug release. Pumps made of biocompatible and long-lasting titanium also can be implanted intraperitoneally, even intraarterially or intrathecally with proper surgical procedures.

The Infusaid pump is a fixed-rate (nonprogrammable) implantable infusion pump using vapor pressure activation theory, in which the vapor chamber contains a fluid that vaporizes at body temperature and creates a vapor pressure. Under the vapor pressure, a bellows moves upward and forces release of the drug.

The SynchroMed implantable pump allows the infusion rate of drug solution to be programmed by a portable computer with special software that transmits instructions to the pump. The pump is driven by a step motor, controlled by signals from the microprocessor, and is capable of delivering infusate at varying rates. The programmer even provides delivery patterns that are characteristic of various doses at different times. The SynchroMed pump is approved for a variety of uses including chemotherapy, management of cancer pain, osteomyelitis and spasticity. The MiniMed pump delivers insulin intraperitoneally. Insulin infused into the peritoneum is absorbed faster and more completely than by subcutaneous injection. In this pump, a solenoid-motor controlled piston drives insulin through a delivery catheter. The pumping rate can be programmed to deliver the desired insulin dose.

Swelling Systems

In these systems, drug is dispersed throughout the polymer and has difficulty in diffusing out of the polymer matrix. *In vivo*, biological fluid diffuses into the matrix and causes its outer polymer region to swell, allowing release of the drug entrapped inside the polymer at a predictable rate. This release mechanism and osmosis-induced drug release are summarized as solvent activation by Langer.[23]

Hydrogel-constructed swelling systems are attractive because they can achieve spatial placement of a dosage form in the gastrointestinal tract as well as extended release. Gastric emptying is a size-dependent process. Particles greater than 10

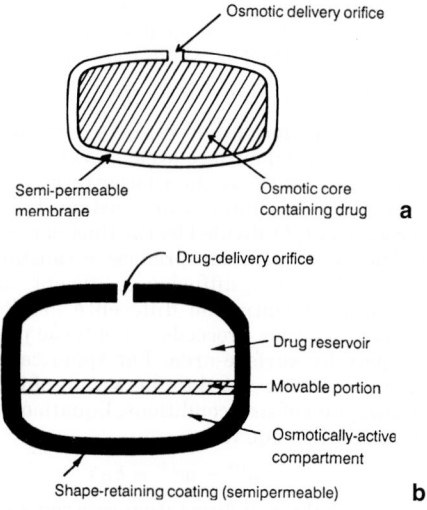

Figure 47-10. Osmotic pressure-controlled drug-delivery systems **A.** An osmotic tablet. (From Robinson JR, ed. *Sustained and Controlled Release Drug Delivery Systems.* New York: Dekker, 1978, p 557.) **B.** A system with two compartments separated by movable partition. (From Robinson JR, Lee VHL, eds. *Controlled Drug Delivery,* 2nd ed. New York: Dekker, 1987, p 373.)

mm are unable to be released into the duodenum and thus retained in the stomach. Hence, a dosage form with a larger size may be beneficial in prolonging retention time in the stomach. However, a dosage form with too big a size is difficult for patients to swallow and, more importantly, the dosage form must dissolve/degrade to be discharged. Hydrogel can absorb up to 100 times its dry weight of water. Thus it is retained because of its large size caused by swelling and expanding. In addition, the adhesive property of swollen hydrogel can further increase residence time of the dosage form.

Erosion-Controlled Systems

In these systems, drug is dispersed throughout the polymer, and the rate of drug release depends on the erosion rate of the polymer. However, some diffusion of the drug from the polymer may also occur. Degradation of the polymer *in vivo* makes long-term accumulation impossible. Therefore an implant made of degradable polymers does not require surgical removal. However, the surface area over which drug release occurs changes as a function of time, which makes zero-order release unlikely.

To maximize control over release, it is often desirable for a system to degrade only from its surface. Poly(lactic-co-glycolic acid) (PLGA), the most commonly used degradable polymer, however, displays bulk erosion with significant degradation in the matrix interior. In a surface-eroding system, the drug release rate is proportional to the polymer erosion rate and can be controlled by changing system thickness and total drug content. Surface erosion eliminates the possibility of dose dumping, thus improving device safety. Surface erosion can be achieved when the degradation rate of the polymer matrix surface is much faster than the rate of water penetration into the matrix bulk. Theoretically, the polymer should be hydrophobic with water-labile linkages connecting monomers. One example is the safe and successful local delivery of nitrosoureas by intracerebrally implanting polyanhydride disks containing the drug.[23]

Controlled Release by Stimulation

MAGNETISM-ACTIVATED IMPLANTS—In this system, drug and small magnetic beads are dispersed throughout a polymer matrix. Upon exposure to biological fluid, drug is released slowly by diffusion. When the system is under the influence of an external magnetic field, drug is released at a much higher rate. This is probably due to movement of the dispersed magnetic beads that squeeze out the drug through pores on the polymer surface. Rate of drug release from these systems can be changed by manipulating the orientation and the strength of the magnetic field or by modifying the mechanical properties of the polymer matrix. Kost and Langer[24] showed that insulin release from poly(ethylene-co-vinyl acetate) matrix bearing magnetic beads could be triggered by using an oscillating magnetic field. This device demonstrated a significant reduction in glucose level when implanted in diabetic rats.

ELECTRICITY-MODULATED SYSTEMS—*Iontophoresis*, primarily used in transdermal delivery, is the facilitated movement of ions across a membrane under the influence of an externally applied electric field. The mechanism of iontophoresis is based on the physical phenomenon "like charges repel and opposite charges attract." Figure 47-11[25] gives a schematic description of an iontophoretic system. Positively charged drugs are placed at the positive pole, while negatively charged peptides are placed at the negative pole. Repulsion of "like charges" and attraction of opposite charges push the drug across the membrane. Iontophoretic delivery of ionic species can be described by the following equation[26]:

$$J^{isp} = J^p + J^e + J^c \qquad (43)$$

where J^p, J^e, J^c represent the passive skin permeation flux, the electrically driven skin permeation flux, and the convective

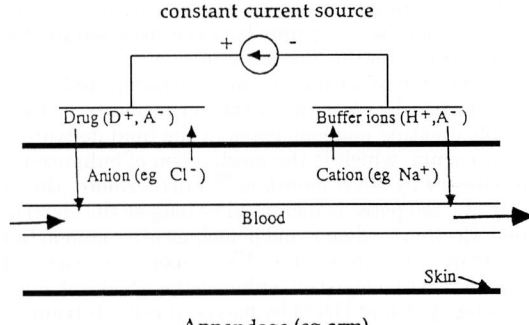

Figure 47-11. An iontophoretic system. (From Singh P, Maibach HI. *Crit Rev Ther Drug Carrier Sys* 1994; 11:161.)

flow-driven skin permeation flux, respectively. Because of the presence of J_p and J_c, facilitation of delivery of neutral molecules is also possible using iontophoresis.

Figure 47-12[27] gives a schematic representation of an iontophoretic transdermal patch. Generally speaking, an iontophoretic patch consists of three components:

1. An aqueous *drug reservoir* that is usually a biocompatible gel or adsorbent-pad material.
2. A *return reservoir* that completes the circuit. Typically, this circuit is a saline formulation.
3. An *electronic controller* that is programmable to give a complicated dosing pattern.

There are two profiles of applying electric current: continuous and pulsatile. Pulsatile application is more efficient in facilitating peptide delivery.[28] An electric field with direct current applied continuously to the stratum corneum causes electrochemical polarization, which operates against the applied field and results in a decrease in the magnitude of the effective current across the skin. This greatly decreases the efficiency of iontophoretic drug delivery. When the current is applied periodically (on and off), it presents an opportunity for the skin to depolarize during the "off" state. Each cycle starts in a state with no residual polarization. Pulsatile profile also enables the skin to tolerate much higher voltage and stronger current.

Iontophoresis carries a number of advantages. It is simple and noninvasive so that patients are willing to accept it. Moreover, electronically controlled patches allow complex dosing regimens according to the individual need of the patients. While most delivery systems are limited to small, nonpolar, lipophilic molecules, iontophoresis can facilitate transport of charged and high-molecular-weight drugs (eg, protein and peptide drugs). As a versatile technique, iontophoresis may be useful for local drug delivery in several areas of medicine other than dermatology, such as dentistry, ophthalmology, and otolaryngology. Local irritation and erythema are two common adverse effects of iontophoresis. Generally, the side effects are

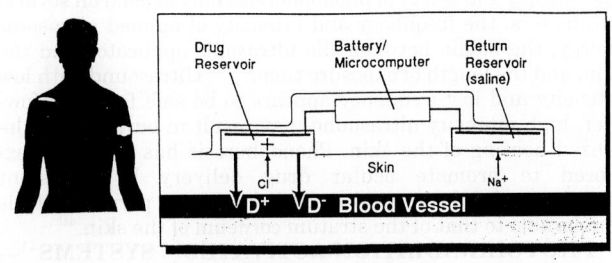

- Drug ions are repelled from the reservoir of similar polarity
- Drug ions compete for current with extraneous ions
- Drug flux is proportional to applied current

Figure 47-12. The components of an iontophoretic patch. (From Green PG. *J Controlled Release* 1996; 41:33.)

mild; however, iontophoresis may not be useful in emergency situations as there is a lag time between drug administration and its appearance in the bloodstream.

Short-term (micro- or milliseconds) exposure to brief, high-intensity electrical pulses increases permeability of the skin, presumably creating aqueous pores in the lipid network of the stratum corneum, which is the mechanism of enhanced transdermal delivery by *electroporation*.[29] Furthermore, the size of the newly created pores is increased as long as the electric field is applied. Erythma, edema, and petechiae are common but presumably transient side effects. Electroporation was initially used by molecular biologists to enhance the uptake of biomacromolecules (eg, plasmid DNA) by bacterial cells. Intramuscular electroporation gene delivery has found potential in treating various diseases including tumors, renal diseases and anemia.[30]

Electricity also can be used to modulate drug release from polymeric delivery systems by mechanisms such as solubilization of a polymer complex and modification of polymer swelling/deswelling. The small solute release can be enhanced during deswelling by a squeezing mechanism, whereas large molecule release can be increased during the swelling process. Kwon et al[31] reported a novel polymeric system. Reacting to a small electric current, the system changed from a solid state to solution by distintegrating the insoluble polymer complex into the two water-soluble composite polymers: polyethyloxazoline and poly(methacrylic acid) (PMAA). The insoluble polymer complex formed by intermolecular hydrogen bonding between carboxyl and oxazoline groups below pH 5, but dissociated above pH 5.4. The disintegration of the polymer complex was attributed to unionization and ionization of the carboxyl group of PMAA at different pHs. A pulsatile pH change induced by a step function of electric current could facilitate the disintegration, resulting in modulated release of such drugs as insulin.

ULTRASOUND-MODULATED SYSTEMS—In general, ultrasound-controlled polymeric delivery systems are simple devices designed for subcutaneous implantation. Miyazaki et al[32] studied the releases of bovine insulin from ethylenevinyl alcohol copolymer matrices and reservoir-type drug delivery systems. When the devices implanted in diabetic rats were exposed to ultrasound (1W/cm^2 for 30 min), a sharp drop in blood glucose levels was observed, indicating a rapid release of insulin from the implants. Drug carrier matrices can be made of either erodible or nonerodible polymers. Kost et al[33] observed that both polymer erosion and drug release were increased when the systems were exposed to ultrasound. Ultrasound can enhance permeation of water into the degradable polymer matrix, leading to exposure of labile linkage for hydrolysis and mechanical shear stress caused by the micro liquid jet produced by cavitation phenomenon.[34] Drug release was also enhanced in nonerodible systems where the release was diffusion dependent. However, the mechanism is not fully understood yet.

Phonophoresis is ultrasound-activated migration of drug molecules through the skin. Its enhancement mechanism is not clear; however, a combination of thermal, mechanical, or cavitational effects are thought to be involved in this process.[35,36] The efficacy and safety of phonophoresis may depend on several parameters: the frequency and intensity of applied ultrasonic energy, the media between the ultrasonic applicator and the skin, and the length of exposure time.[37–39] Ultrasound with low intensity and low frequency appears to be safe for use. However, high-intensity ultrasound may result in burns due to localized heating of the skin. Phonophoresis has also been explored to promote ocular drug delivery by transient modification of the corneal epithelium, whose permeability is comparable to that of the stratum corneum of the skin.[40]

PHOTOIRRADIATION-ACTIVATED SYSTEMS[41]— Photoresponsive polymers can be prepared by incorporation of photosensitive compounds such as azobenzene, stilbene, spiropyren, and rhodopsin into a polymeric backbone. These polymers are used for photochemical control of permeation of various solutes, such as metal salts, proteins, amino acids, etc.

Modulation of protein permeation was achieved by UV irradiation.[42] Cross-linked random copolymers of hydroxyethyl methacrylate with a monomer containing azobenzene groups in the side chain slightly changed swelling levels by cis-trans isomerization of the azobenzene group to effectively control permeation of large molecules.

THERMORESPONSIVE DELIVERY SYSTEMS—These systems are constructed from thermosensitive hydrogels that exhibit phase transition when temperature is raised to a critical value called the *lower critical solution temperature (LCST)*. The phase transition is characterized by a dramatic change in polymer volume accompanied by a significant change in the release rate of the drug formulated into the polymeric system. Thermosensitivity of hydrogels originates from polymer-water interactions, especially hydrophobic-hydrophilic balancing effects and the configuration of side groups; and/or polymer-polymer interaction. Poly[N-isopropylacrylamide (NIPAAm)] hydrates below its LCST (32°C) and dehydrates above the LCST. Thermosensitive polymers composed of NIPAAm and various comonomers with different hydrophilicity have been synthesized. A study on the effect of comonomers on the LCST of the polymers revealed that the anionic acrylic acid caused the highest LCST elevation, followed by the cationic N,N-dimethylaminoethyl methacrylate, and nonionic acrylamide comonomers; while the hydrophobic butylmethacrylate (BMA) led to decreased LCST.[43] When such a swollen hydrogel loaded with drug is transferred to a medium kept at T > LCST, it delivers the drug because the gel collapses on warming through its LCST. Initially, the temperature gradient across the gel causes a burst of surface drug, with formation of a skin and buildup of hydrostatic pressure inside the gel. This pressure will squeeze the fluid containing the drug since a collapsing or desorbing polymer gel matrix/swollen gel front moves rapidly into the interior of the gel. There are two different consequences associated with thermosensitive hydrogels when temperature is raised to the LCST. In the case of the copolymers of NIPPAm with more hydrophobic comonomers, such as BMA, increased temperature over the LCST hinders delivery of the drug due to formation of a dense skin layer.[44,45] This may be advantageous in sustaining drug action, since the hydrogel has adhesive properties and can be retained at the absorption site for an extended period of time. Moreover, slowing of drug release, because of the dense skin layer, provides an extended-release property. On the contrary, an increase in temperature over the LCST can lead to increased delivery. In this case, the drug is squeezed out of the gel with shrinking and the release rate is accelerated. This system has potential application in the control of inflammatory or hyperpyretic reactions. These situations are usually associated with an increase in body temperature. When the temperature is over the LCST, the increased delivery of the anti-inflammatory drug from the gel can alleviate the symptoms promptly.

Recently, Kim's research group[46] synthesized a series of thermosensitive, biodegradable hydrogels composed of poly(ethyleneoxide) and poly(L-lactic acid) block copolymer. An aqueous solution of these copolymers exhibits temperature-dependent reversible gel-sol transitions. The hydrogel can be loaded with bioactive molecules in the aqueous phase at an elevated temperature (around 45°C), where they form a solution. In this form, the polymer is injectable. On subcutaneous injection and subsequent rapid cooling to body temperature, the loaded copolymer forms a gel that can act as an extended-release matrix for the drug.

pH-SENSITIVE DELIVERY SYSTEMS—pH sensitive polymers have either weakly acidic or basic groups covalently attached to a polymer backbone; therefore the charge density of the polymer depends on pH and ionic composition of the environment. Changing the pH of the environment will cause swelling or deswelling of the polymer, which affects the drug release rate from devices or matrices made of these polymers. pH-sensitive polymers containing free carboxyl groups, eg, hydroxypropylmethyl cellulose phthalate and poly(methyl methacrylate), have been employed in developing enteric coating in conventional oral dosage forms. They are impermeable at low pH, but disintegrate at neutral pH. Polymers composed of hydroxyethyl methacrylate and dimethylaminoethyl methacrylate are involved in controlled delivery of insulin from a reservoir containing a saturated solution of insulin.[47] The membrane consists of a hydrogel polymer with a pendant amine group entrapped with glucose oxidase. In the presence of glucose, the following reaction can take place:

$$\text{Glucose} + H_2O + O_2 \rightarrow \text{Gluconate} + H_2O + H^+$$

The hydrogen ions decrease the pH and lead to protonation of the amine groups. The charged amine groups repel each other, which results in increased swelling and subsequently release of insulin. Permeability of the membrane to insulin is controlled by the insulin level. A pH-sensitive bioerodible polymer such as poly(orthoester) is based on the same principle.[48] Insulin is trapped in the polymer matrix rather than surrounded by a membrane. Protonation of the amine group, triggered by the glucose/glucose oxidase reaction, results in an increase in erosion, with concomitant release of insulin.

SELF-REGULATED DELIVERY SYSTEMS[49]—Self-regulated or feedback-controlled systems should be capable of adjusting drug release according to physiological needs or feedback information (eg, insulin delivery in response to blood glucose level of the patient). Self-regulated delivery systems can be divided into two types: *modulated devices* and *triggered devices*. A modulated device releases a drug continuously at a rate controlled by the concentration of a specific external chemical (eg, hydrogen ion, glucose). A triggered device does not have basal drug release. The drug is only released at a preprogrammed rate when the system is activated by a specific external moiety (eg, metal ion, antibody).

One example of modulated devices for insulin delivery is the pH-sensitive polymeric system utilizing glucose oxidase reaction, which has been described earlier. The solubility of trilysyl insulin is a function of pH.[50] There is a large change in its solubility between pH 5 and 7. The glucose oxidase reaction can alter the pH of the local environment, which leads to increased solubility and dissolution rate. This forms the basis for *solubility-controlled delivery of insulin*.

Lectin-Glycosylated Insulin-Controlled Device is based on competitive binding between glycosylated insulin and glucose to a saccharide-binding substrate, concanavalin A (Con-A). The glycosylated insulin complexed with Con-A can be displaced from the complex in direct proportion to glucose levels. This forms a controlled delivery system for insulin. Due to immunogenicity, Con-A can be cross-linked to minimize its leakage from the device into the plasma. Because the delayed "off" response could lead to hypoglycemia, microspheres were prepared to accelerate the response process since their large surface areas allow rapid diffusion of insulin and glucose.[51]

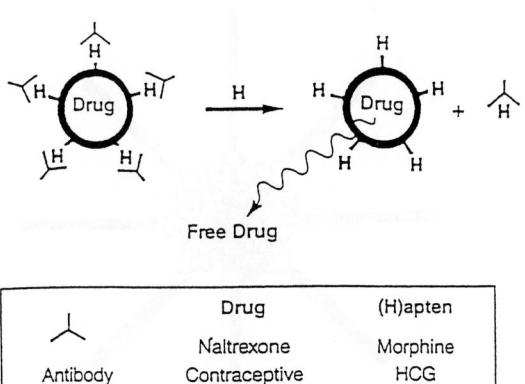

Figure 47-13. Hapten-antibody device. (From Pitt CG, et al. *J Controlled Release* 1985; 2:363.)

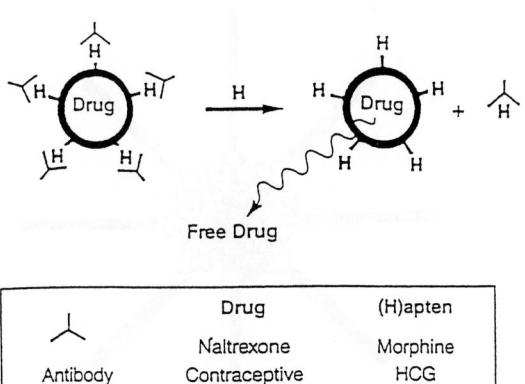

Figure 47-14. Chelation-enhanced hydrolysis device. (From Pitt CG, et al. *J Controlled Release* 1984; 1:3.)

Some hydrogels such as copolymers of acrylamide and allyl glucose can undergo a phase transition in response to glucose concentration.[52] At physiological pH, Con-A exists as a tetramer with four binding sites for glucose. The glucose-containing polymer chains are physically cross-linked by Con-A to form a gel. Free glucose can compete against polymer-bound glucose for the binding sites on Con-A. This competitive binding may result in loosening the network structure and transformation from a gel to a solution. This transition can control the release rate of insulin.

Triggered devices were developed based on hapten-antibody interactions and chelation-enhanced hydrolysis. In the system involving the former mechanism, the drug was enclosed in a membrane that bore haptens conjugated with antibodies (Fig 47-13[53]). The antibodies blocked access of esterase to the polymer, preventing enzyme-induced polymer erosion and concomitant release of the drug. Drug release, accompanying polymer erosion, was triggered by displacement of antibodies from the membrane in the presence of free haptens. Systems using the latter mechanism may be useful in delivery of chelating agents. Metal ions can accelerate hydrolysis of carboxylic esters, phosphate esters, and amides. This enhancement results from complexation of the metal to the ester carbonyl group as shown in Figure 47-14[54]. Release rate of the chelating agent is influenced by the concentration of target metal.

TARGETED DELIVERY SYSTEMS

Targeted drug delivery implies selective and effective localization of drug into the target(s) at therapeutic concentrations with limited access to nontarget sites. A targeted drug delivery system is preferred in the following situations[55]:

1. Pharmaceutical: drug instability, low solubility.
2. Pharmacokinetic: short half-life, large volume of distribution, poor absorption.
3. Pharmacodynamic: low specificity, low therapeutic index.

Targeted drug delivery may provide maximum therapeutic activity by preventing drug degradation or inactivation during transit to the target sites. Meanwhile, it can protect the body from adverse effects because of inappropriate disposition, and minimize toxicity of potent drugs by reducing dose. An ideal targeted delivery system should be nontoxic, biocompatible, biodegradable, and physicochemically stable *in vivo* and *in vitro*. The preparation of the delivery system must be reasonably simple, reproducible, and cost-effective.[56]

Colloidal Drug Carriers

Colloidal drug-delivery systems include micro- and nanoparticles, macromolecular complexes (eg, lipoproteins), liposomes, and niosomes. In many cases, colloidal carriers are used to improve stability of the drug either in biological fluids or in the formulation, to develop extended-release systems with targeting features, and/or to enhance the therapeutic efficacy and reduce drug toxicity by modifying the distribution and controlling the disposition of the drug. Colloidal particles larger than 1 μm are microparticles. Although they are considered as carriers of an earlier generation that can deliver the active agent to the target, because of their size and thus tendency to occlude needles and capillaries, microparticles are not suitable for administration by general routes, such as intravenous injection. Lipoproteins have been suggested as potential drug carriers for several reasons [56]: (a) they are natural and thus nonimmunogenic; (b) they are not rapidly cleared by the reticuloendothelial system (RES), but endocytosed by a variety of cells expressing lipoprotein receptors on the surface; (c) they are capable of solubilizing lipophilic drugs in their apolar inner core, and carrying amphilic drugs in the outer phospholipid coat; and (d) drugs in the core appear not to affect the binding of surface ligands to various cells. However, the involvement of lipoproteins, especially low-density lipoprotein (LDL), in the pathogenesis of certain cardiovascular disorders makes them less desirable drug carriers. Niosomes are vesicles made of nonionic surfactants (eg, polyglycerol alkylethers, glucosyl dialkylthers, and polyoxyethylene alkylethers). Niosomes can be prepared by similar techniques as those used for liposomes. Their *in vivo* behavior is also similar to that of liposomes: prolonging the circulation of entrapped drug and increasing local concentration at the target site. Niosomes have demonstrated their potential as carriers of the cytotoxic agent doxorubicin.[57]

NANOPARTICLES—A nanoparticle is a submicroscopic solid particle with a size ranging from 10 nm to 1 μm. The size of a nanoparticle allows it to be administered intravenously with little risk of embolism. Materials used in the preparation of nanoparticles are sterilizable, nontoxic, and biodegradable; examples are albumin, ethylcellulose, casein, gelatin, polyesters, polyanhydrides, and polyalkyl cyanoacrylates. They can be prepared from emulsion, micelles, interfacial polymerization, preformed polymers, and coacervation.

Nanoparticles have been successfully applied to medical diagnostics by taking advantage of their rapid uptake by the RES and sequestration by liver Kupffer's cells. For example, nanoparticles loaded with radioisotopic technetium-99m can be used to image hepatic pathologies.[58] The RES consists of phagocytic cells designed to cleanse the bloodstream of bacteria, viruses, cell debris, and other unwanted foreign particles. Such specific cellular processing of nanoparticles points to the possibility of using nanoparticles to target drugs to the liver and phagocytic cells. "Macrophage-evading" or long-circulating nanoparticles may find more applications in experimental and clinical medicine. One expectation is to provide a long-circulating drug reservoir where controlled release of the drug into the vascular compartment can be achieved. To prolong the circulation, nanoparticles should be small enough (≤200 nm) or deformable to escape the simple filtration in the spleen; whereas long-circulating rigid large particles can find the application as splenotropic agents.[59] Besides size, the surface of nanoparticles can be modified to avoid opsonization. Opsonization is the adsorption of protein capable of interacting with specific surface receptors on phagocytic cells. *PEGylation* (ie, attaching polyethylene glycol [PEG] to the particles) is perhaps the most explored approach to avoiding protein adsorption. PEG can be adsorbed or covalently linked to the surface of particles. The PEG chains exposed on the particle surfaces confer hydrophilicity to the particles and thus effectively suppress the binding of opsonins through hydrophobic interaction. PEG is also believed to sterically hinder opsonins from interaction. However, the current technology is not yet sophisticated enough to effectively circumvent rapid clearance of nanoparticles by the RES. The complex processes of gradual nanoparticle degradation within the vasculature and drug release into the circulation have not been well understood. At present, few nanoparticles exist as extended-release systems for delivery of the entrapped drug over a period of days. Much more research focuses on long-circulating nanoparticles as targeted drug delivery systems. Capillary permeability of nanoparticles is found to increase when the endothelial integrity is perturbed during inflammation and in certain cancers. The permeable vascular endothelia in lymph nodes and bone marrow are also capable of removing small-sized particles from the circulation.[60,61] Hence, nanoparticles can promise targeted delivery to inflammation

sites such as arthritic joints, to solid tumors, and to hematological malignancies simply because of size exclusion/permeation effect. Attachment of specific ligands that are recognized by nonphagocytic cells through ligand-receptor interaction onto the surface of macrophage-evading particle, expands the targeting spectrum of nanoparticles within the vasculature. Ligand-mediated drug targeting is discussed later in this section.

Block copolymer micelles are among the newest nanoparticles currently under investigation. Copolymers are polymers composed of several different monomeric units. Block copolymers are defined as polymers composed of terminally connected structures. Unlike random polymers, functions can be distinctly designed for each monomeric segment that forms a domain in block copolymer micelles. The features of each monomeric segment can be modified without affecting the others because of separation from other monomeric units. Block copolymers are subdivided into three types, AB-type, ABA type, and $(AB)_n$ multisegments. AB-type copolymers are the most appropriate candidates for the formation of polymeric micelle drug carriers in terms of size, aggregation number, and micelle stability. Usually, the AB-type block copolymers are composed of both hydrophilic poly(ethylene oxide) (PEO) and hydrophobic blocks such as poly(propylene oxide) (PPO), which allows the polymers to self-assemble as micelles in an aqueous media with hydrophobic cores and highly hydrated outer shells. Therefore, a key function of copolymer micelles is to solubilize hydrophobic drugs, such as taxol.[62] Hydrophobic drugs can be incorporated into the hydrophobic core by covalent or noncovalent interaction. The structure of drug-loaded polymeric micelles is shown in Figure 47-15.[63] The polymeric micelle has a diameter of about 20 to 40 nm based on atomic force microscopy, dynamic light scattering measurement, and transmission electron microscopy.[64–66] This

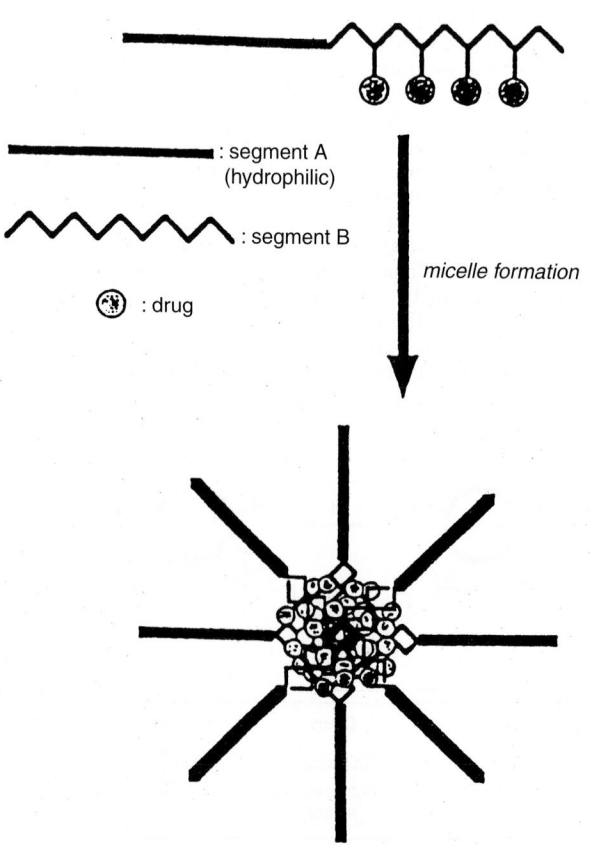

Figure 47-15. Design of micelle-forming polymeric drug. (From Yokoyama M. *Crit Rev Ther Drug Carrier Sys* 1992; 9:213.)

size is very important for the micelle to escape clearance because it is believed that the RES recognition and elimination is lower for particles under 100 nm. Hence, polymeric micelles could be long-circulating in the blood because of their small size as well as hydrophilic shell. Prolonged circulation allows polymeric micelles to accumulate at solid tumors as a result of the so-called enhanced permeability and retention (EPR) effect.[67] Micelles based on PEO-block-PLA or PEO-block-PLGA can gradually release drugs.[68–70] Release of the drug from PEO-block-PLA micelles may be controlled by degradation of PLA.[69] The stability of micelle, micelle core hydrophobicity, and the spacer groups used in binding the drugs to polymer backbones all can play roles in controlling drug release. In other words, a drug-independent delivery system can be designed with its release rate or pattern dictated by the carrier. Other promising biological properties have been discovered with block copolymer micelles, including inhibition of P-glycoprotein responsible for multidrug resistance in cancer cells by PEO-block-PPO-block-PEO micelles,[71] enhancement of drug transport across the blood-brain barrier by the same block micelles,[72] and reduction of self-aggregation and toxicity of amphotericin B by PEO-block-poly(beta-benzyl-l-aspartate) micelles.[73]

LIPOSOMES—When phospholipids are dispersed gently in an aqueous medium, they swell, hydrate, and spontaneously form multilamellar, concentric, bilayer vesicles with layers of aqueous media separating the lipid bilayers. These systems commonly are referred to as multilamellar liposomes, or multilamellar vesicles (MLVs), and can have diameters as large as 4 μm. Sonication or solvent dilution of MLVs results in the formation of small unilamellar vesicles (SUVs) with diameters below 80-100 nm, containing an aqueous solution in the core. Liposomes bear many resemblances to cellular membranes and have been widely used to study membrane behavior and membrane-mediated processes. It probably remains the most extensively studied class of carrier systems as well because of the advantages listed in Table 47-6.[56]

The drug-loading capacity varies among different types of liposomes. For example, MLVs are moderately efficient at trapping solutes, but SUVs are extremely inefficient. However, SUVs offer the advantage of homogeneity and reproducibility in size distribution. A compromise between size and trapping efficiency is offered by large unilamellar vesicles (LUVs). In addition to liposome characteristics, drug entrapment is also dependent on the physicochemical properties of the drug itself, the phospholipids, and other additives used. Polar drugs are trapped in the aqueous space, and nonpolar drugs bind to the lipid bilayer of the vesicle. Polar drugs are released when the bilayer is broken or by permeation, but nonpolar drugs remain affiliated with the bilayer unless it is disrupted by temperature or exposure to lipoproteins. Loading of cationic (or anionic) drugs can be significantly improved by using liposomes containing anionic (or cationic) lipids. Macromolecules such as proteins, polysaccharides, and nucleic acids also can be incorporated into liposomes. More recent studies of liposomal drug delivery have focused on their potential for cellular delivery of biomacromolecules.

Liposomes can interact with cells by four different mechanisms[74]:

1. Endocytosis by phagocytic cells of the RES.
2. Adsorption to the cell surface either by nonspecific hydrophobic or electrostatic forces or by specific interactions with cell-surface components.
3. Fusion with the plasma cell membrane by insertion of the lipid bilayer of the liposome into the plasma membrane, with simultaneous release of liposomal content into the cytoplasm.
4. Transfer of liposomal lipids to cellular or subcellular membranes, or vice versa, without any association of the liposome contents.

Often it is difficult to determine what mechanism is operative, and more than one may operate at the same time.

The fate and disposition of intravenously injected liposomes depend on their physical properties, such as size, fluidity, and surface charges. They may persist in tissues for hours or days, depending on their composition, and their half-lives in the blood range from minutes to several hours. Because of their size, liposomes can exit only in places where large openings or pores exist in the capillary endothelia, such as the sinusoids of the liver or the spleen. Thus, these organs are the predominate sites of uptake. In general, this *in vivo* behavior limits the potential targeting of liposomes to only those organs and tissues accessible to their large size. These include the blood, liver, spleen, bone marrow, and lymphoid organs. Liposomes also can accumulate within leaky vasculature of solid tumors, which encourages many researchers to explore liposomal delivery of chemotherapeutics to tumors. Similar to polymeric nanoparticles, long-circulating PEGylated liposomes that can evade the rapid uptake by the RES are usually more successful than unprotected liposomes in this task.[75–77] Active targeting with drug-entrapped liposomes can be achieved by appending ligands to the carrier systems. For example, immunoliposomes are constructed by attaching antibodies to the drug-loaded liposome surface. Such delivery systems can be directed to groups of cells that express specific antigenic receptors. LDL, folate, and carbohydrate determinants, whose receptors are often overexpressed on the surface of certain malignant cells, also appear on the lists for construction of ligand-conjugated liposomes.

Numerous books, book chapters, and review articles have been dedicated to liposomal drug delivery. The interested reader can go to *Liposome Technology*, edited by Gregoriadis,[78] for preparation, analysis, drug loading, and biological properties of liposomes. *Medical Applications of Liposomes*, edited by Lasic and Papahadjopoulos,[79] summarizes the most important and promising usages of liposomes in medicine.

Ligand-Mediated Targeting

Ligand-mediated targeting has emerged as a novel approach to targeting vascular compartment (first-order), cellular (second-order), or intracellular (third-order) levels.

The ligands explored so far to selectively deliver carrier systems or drugs to cells include antibodies, complements, interleukins, lectins, lipoproteins, polypeptides (eg, insulin, growth factors), transferrin, folate, CAM (cell adhesion molecules), viral proteins, etc. These molecules specifically bind to antigens, carrier molecules, or receptors on the cell surfaces. Appropriate targets expressing these surface recognition molecules for ligand-mediated interactions are immune cells (lymphocytes, leukocytes, macrophages and other phagocytic cells including Kupffer's cells of liver, microglia of brain, Langerhans' cells of skin), endothelial cells, epithelia of the gastrointestinal tract, hepatocytes, certain malignant cells, etc. Thus, ligand-conjugated delivery systems can macroscopically target a variety of organs and specific compartments: vasculature, lymphatics, liver, gastrointestinal tract, brain, and solid tumors.

Ligands are often covalently or noncovalently associated with the drug or the surface of the carrier. Labeling macromolecules with gold particles could stimulate nonspecific interactions involved in the noncovalent association of ligand to

Table 47-6. Advantages of Liposomes as Drug Carriers

1. Biologically inert and completely biodegradable
2. Nontoxic, nonantigenic, and nonpyrogenic
3. Producible with various sizes, compositions, and surface properties
4. Entrap a wide variety of hydrophilic and lipophilic drugs
5. Protect entrapped drugs from enzymatic degradation or deactivation from the external media
6. Offer new possibilities of drug targeting by releasing drugs at the site of liposome destruction

macromolecular drugs or carrier systems.[80] One of the most popular methods of noncovalent conjugation is utilizing natural strong binding of avidin or streptividin to biotin (association constant 10^{15} M^{-1}). Biotinylated ligands can be associated with avidin- or streptividin-attached carrier systems to construct a targeted delivery system. Most studies of ligand-drug/carrier conjugates have employed covalent conjugation. Chemical cross-linking agents are used commonly to attach a drug/carrier to a ligand by reacting with appropriate groups (eg, amine, carbonyl, or sulfhydryl) available on both species. Among the cross-linking agents used are carbodiimide, glutaraldehyde, bisazobenzidine, cyanuric chloride, diethylmalonimidate, and various mixed anhydrides.

Cellular uptake of drugs bound to ligands mostly relies on receptor-mediated endocytosis. Binding of ligand to receptor on the cell surface leads to subsequent internalization of receptor-ligand complex. Upon arrival into the endosome, a specific intracellular compartment to store and process ligand-receptor complex, ligand-drug conjugates may dissociate from the receptors and are directed to the lysosome for degradation. In some cases, ligand-drug conjugates are transported through the cell with the receptors, and the conjugates are released by exocytosis at a different surface locus of the cell from where they originate (transcytosis). A successful ligand-mediated targeted delivery system would be efficiently transported to the target cells, rapidly internalized, processed in the acidic endosomes and lysosomes, and eventually diffuse into the cytosol or specific action sites, such as the nucleus, with functional integrity. The lysosomal membrane is a natural barrier to macromolecular ligands and sizable ligand-drug conjugates, and only low-molecular-weight degradation products are liberated to the cytosol. To avoid the degradation from lysosomes, endosomolytic agents (eg, chloroquine) can be used to break the endosomes containing the conjugates and liberating their contents directly into the cytosol. Or the conjugate could be engineered to become an "artificial virus" whose coat proteins undergo a conformational change at low pH and expose their fusogenic components to fuse with the wall of the endosomes, releasing their contents into the cytosol. Lysosomal degradation may be reduced by neutralizing the acidic pH necessary for hydrolase activity (eg, ammonium chloride, monensin), or directly inhibiting hydrolases with leupeptin. However, all these approaches are usually inappropriate for *in vivo* applications.

Although targeted delivery, with probably the highest specificity at cellular and subcellular levels, can be achieved through ligand-receptor interaction, receptor targeting does have several limitations as suggested by Feener and King.[81] First, the competition of endogenous ligands against exogenously delivered ligands for the same receptor binding sites may substantially reduce the availability of cell-surface receptors to the delivered conjugates. Drug targeting via an antireceptor antibody may eliminate the competition as the antibody may occupy a different site. Second, exogenous ligands, typically a hormone, a growth factor or a transporter protein, may interfere with normal physiological processes and/or elicit undesirable biological and immunological responses. This problem can be encountered when delivering drugs across the blood brain barrier with insulin or transferrin as a ligand. Systemic delivery of insulin puts nondiabetic patients at risk of hypoglycemia. This potential can be overcome by using a proteolytic fragment of insulin maintaining high affinity for receptor binding yet possessing minimal effect on glucose homeostasis.[82] Exogenous supply of transferrin may disturb transport of ferrous ions into the central nervous system. Transferrin receptor antibody could be a solution to this problem. Third, certain natural ligands may exhibit relatively low specificity by binding multiple receptor types that are differentially expressed in various cells. Antireceptor antibodies provide a means to specifically target certain types of receptors.

Among all the ligands discussed above, antibodies are probably the most outstanding candidates due to their excellent binding affinity and specificity. Antibodies have been exten-sively explored as carriers in cancer diagnosis and therapy when certain specificities expressed on tumor cells, referred to as membrane-bound tumor-associated antigens (TAAs), are discovered and characterized. Currently, monoclonal antibodies of defined class and antigenic specificity can be obtained in a highly purified form from hybridoma cells, which renders construction of antibody-chemotherapeutic conjugates and immunotoxins accomplishable. To improve specificity of action and to aid cellular penetration, antibody fragments rather than the whole antibody molecule are used for drug targeting. Consequently, the molecular size decreases from 150 kD for an entire IgG molecule, to 50 kD for a Fab' fragment, or to 27 kD for a single-chain Fv protein.[83] Fragments of small size, such as Fv protein, can be readily fused with therapeutic entities to construct recombinant proteins with inherent targeting functionality.

A novel strategy to deliver cytotoxic drugs to tumor cells is known as ADEPT (antibody directed enzyme prodrug therapy). In such a system, the enzyme β-glucuronidase is covalently immobilized or coupled to the surface of antibody-attached liposomes; then, when the nontoxic and pharmacologically inactive prodrug epirubicin glucuronide is administered simultaneously, it is converted by the enzyme to the potent antitumor reagent epirubicinin at the vicinity of tumor cells.[84] GDEPT (Gene-directed EPT) differs from ADEPT in that the gene encoding the prodrug-activating enzyme rather than the enzyme itself is delivered into the target cells, which actually makes the tumor or virus-infected cells themselves manufacture the enzyme *in situ*. One apparent advantage of this approach over conventional antibody-drug conjugation is that the formation of active derivatives in close proximity of the target cells could result in higher cellular but lower systemic level of active drugs and thus further reduce systemic toxicity.

As another novel approach, bispecific antibodies have been proposed for cancer or HIV immunotherapy. A bispecific protein, made of a chimeric combination of an antitumor or an anti-gp120 (a glycoprotein expressed on the surface of HIV-infected cells) antibody with an anti-lymphocyte antibody, could redirect T-lymphocytes to lyse tumor cells or HIV-infected cells.[85] One drawback of antibody (and possibly its fragment) targeting is immunogenicity.

Folate, in principle, offers several advantages over antibodies as a targeting ligand. As a vitamin necessary to cell growth and metabolism, folate is presumably nonimmunogenic. It has good stability as well. Furthermore, it is highly specific for tumors as the elevated expression of folate receptor has frequently been identified in various types of human cancers.[86] The interested reader is directed to the exhaustive review by Reddy and Low[87] about folate-mediated tumor targeting.

Another group of macromolecules that can serve in tumor targeting is carbohydrate determinants. Carbohydrate determinants are glycoprotein or glycolipid cell-surface components that are critical in cell-cell recognition, interaction, and adhesion. These markers are often upregulated on the surface of tumor-associated endothelial cells and play an important role in angiogenesis and metastasis of cancers.

Resealed Erythrocytes

The mature erythrocytes serve only as hemoglobin carriers in the blood circulation. It was thought that if therapeutic agents could be entrapped and replace hemoglobin in the viable erythrocytes, the cells may turn into efficient drug delivery systems. Several methods have been employed to incorporate drugs into erythrocytes, including hypoosmotic lysis, electrical breakdown, endocytosis, membrane perturbation with amphotericin B, and lipid fusion.[88] Hypoosmotic lysis is the most commonly used. In this process, erythrocytes first swell to about one and a half times their normal size in a hypotonic medium and the membrane ruptures, resulting in the formation of pores with diameters of 20 to 50 nm. The pores allow equilibration of the intracellular and extracellular solutions. If the ionic strength of the medium then is adjusted to isotonicity and the cells are incubated at 37°C, the pores will close and cause the erythrocyte to "reseal." Using this technique with a drug present in the extracellular solution, it is possible to entrap up to 40% of the drug inside the resealed erythrocyte and to use this system for targeted delivery via intravenous injection. A variety of biomacromolecules ranging in size from 5000 to 600,000 Da, such as I-asparaginase, insulin, heparin, can be entrapped in erythrocytes.[56] Drug may release from erythrocyte carriers by phagocytosis, diffusion through the cell membrane, or by a specific transport system.[89] Considerable control of drug release can be achieved by modifying polar or charged substituents of the entrapped molecules. The rate of diffusion decreases with increased polarity of entrapped molecules. Prolonged release is possible by entrapment of potent transporter protein inhibitor with the drug.[90] The advantages of using resealed erythrocytes as drug carriers are that they are biodegradable, fully biocompatible, and nonimmunogenic; they exhibit flexibility in circulation time depending on their physicochemical properties; the entrapped drug is shielded from immunological detection; and chemical modification of drug is not required.

The assessment of resealed erythrocytes for use in targeted delivery has been facilitated by studies on the behavior of normal and modified reinfused erythrocytes. They are removed from the circulation by the RES, especially by cells in the spleen and the liver. In general, normal aging erythrocytes, slightly damaged erythrocytes (eg, treated with low concentrations of gluteraldehyde), and those coated lightly with antibodies are recognized by the spleen after intravenous reinfusion, but heavily damaged or modified erythrocytes are removed from the circulation by the liver. This suggests that resealed erythrocytes can be targeted selectively to either the liver or the spleen, depending on their membrane characteristics. In addition to coating with antibodies, removal of portions of cell-surface carbohydrates reduces the circulating half-life. The ability of resealed erythrocytes to deliver drug to the liver or the spleen can be viewed as a disadvantage in that other organs and tissues are inaccessible. Thus the application of this system to targeted delivery may be limited mainly to diseases of these organs and hematological disorders, including tumors, Leishmaniasis, leukemia, thromboembolism, etc. Resealed erythrocytes are also suitable for carrying drugs whose action sites are on these organs; insulin is one example of this case.

Bioadhesives

The success of drug delivery to various mucosal tissues of the body, for either local action or systemic absorption, largely depends on the degree of contact between the drug delivery system and the tissue surface and residence time. Residence time for most musosal routes is less than an hour and typically of the order of minutes, unless some form of adhesive is incorporated in the delivery system.

A bioadhesive can be defined as a substance that can adhere to a biological substrate and remain there for an extended period of time. If the biological substrate is mucus, then the bioadhesive is referred to as a mucoadhesive. Basically, a bioadhesive is used to localize a delivery system to a specific area for local action or to increase contact time at the absorption site so that bioavailability can be improved. Typical increases in residence time by using bioadhesives are given in Table 47-7[91].

Bioadhesion can be regarded as a two-step process.[92] The first step involves establishment of intimate contact that is governed by surface characteristics, composition of the mucoadhesive, mucin, and the applied force or pressure. The second step involves formation of secondary bonds between the adhesive and the mucin-epithelial surfaces. Secondary bonding includes hydrogen bonding as well as electrostatic and hydrophobic interactions. Mucin consists of a protein backbone with pendant sugar groups at appropriate locations. Many of these sugar

Table 47-7. Approximate Clearance Time of Applied Suspensions for Selected Areas of the Body

ROUTE	RESIDENCE TIME WITHOUT BIOADHESIVE	RESIDENCE TIME WITH BIOADHESIVE
Ocular (human)	1–2 min	12–15 hr
Nasal (human)	2–60 min	6–12 hr
Buccal (human)	2–30 min	6–10 hr
Intestine (dog)	1–3 hr	6–10 hr
Vaginal (human)	30–90 min	3–4 days

groups terminate in a sialic or sulfonic acid residue. They carry anionic charges as a result. Mucin can be regarded as a polyelectrolyte with a high charge density holding a large amount of water. The expanded nature of mucin and polymer allows interpenetration that results in an increase in contact area and establishment of physical entanglement between mucin and the mucoadhesive polymer. Physical entanglement can strengthen the network and increase contact area that in turn increases the formation of secondary bonds. Usually, bioadhesive polymers contain a number of hydrophilic groups such as carboxyl, hydroxyl, amide, and sulfate. These groups interact with mucin or epithelial tissues primarily through hydrogen bonding and to a lesser extent through hydrophobic and electrostatic interactions. These groups also allow the polymers to swell after absorbing water and thus maximize the number of adhesion sites. Polycarbophil with thiol groups is able to form disulfide bonds with mucin and thus exhibits significantly stronger adhesive property. When a delivery system containing such modified polycarbophil and carboxymethyl cellulose was used to administer insulin orally to mice, the hypoglycemic effect lasted up to 80 hours.[93] Typically, bonding between the polymer and mucin is strong enough to prevent detachment, so removal is mainly through mucin turnover. It is believed that water-insoluble polymers with light cross-linking are preferred because they are not removed from the site of application by dissolution.

There are a number of limitations associated with bioadhesive polymers: fouling of the bioadhesive sites of the polymer before reaching the desired target and rapid mucus turnover making long-term secure adhesion impossible. Eichman and Robinson[94] showed that effervescence possessing mucus-stripping effect may potentially improve the performance of bioadhesives.

Bioadhesive delivery systems have been tried in various routes of administration. Some measure of success has been achieved in vaginal delivery. *Columbia Laboratories* introduced Crinone and Advantage-S to the market using a gel containing the bioadhesive polycabophil developed by Robinson et al.[95] The gel adheres to the vaginal tissue for 3 to 4 days and hence serves as a platform for delivery of progesterone or spermicide nonoxynol-9. The major obstacle for ocular drug delivery is the rapid loss of drug because of tear turnover, making the eye a target for bioadhesive systems in order to prolong the residence time. One drawback of these systems, especially gel-like formulations, is that they spread on the cornea surface, causing blurred vision. Bioadhesive microparticles may be attractive for intranasal delivery of peptides and vaccines, especially when combined with penetration enhancers.[96] However, for the buccal route, because of low mucosal permeability, coadministration of bioadhesives and penetration enhancers is recommended for protein and peptide delivery.

The bioadhesive properties of a broad spectrum of polymers in rat and human gastrointestinal tracts have been studied.[97,98] These polymers showed good bioadhesion *in vivo* and *in vitro* in rats, but unfortunately the results in human were disappointing and there is no clear explanation at this time. Second-generation bioadhesives take advantage of specific receptor-mediated interaction between various lectins, bacterial fimbriae and the sugar groups in the mucus or on the epithelial surface. Lectins or fimbriae can be attached to the surfaces of drug-loaded micro- or nanoparticles to provide a bioadhesive system. One concern with these exogenous biological macro-molecules is immunogenicity and toxicity. Safe adhesive delivery systems may be developed using nontoxic tomato lectin.

Prodrugs

A prodrug is a compound formed by chemical modification of a biologically active compound that will liberate the active compound *in vivo* by enzymatic or chemical processes. The primary purposes for designing prodrugs are improving physicochemical properties of drugs to overcome formulation problems, and altering biological properties to enhance their efficacy and to reduce their toxicity. To be useful in targeted delivery, a prodrug must be activated by enzyme or chemical agents near the target site to provide a sufficient supply of parent drug *in situ*. Furthermore, the active parent drug must remain at the target site and not sneak into the systemic circulation, which could cause adverse effects. However, chemically activated prodrugs frequently experience conversion before reaching the target site, which makes them unsuitable for targeted delivery.

Brain targeting remains one of the greatest challenges because the blood-brain barrier is highly impermeable to numerous polar drugs. The most famous prodrug for targeted delivery to the brain is L-3,4-dihydroxyphenylalanine (L-dopa) for Parkinson's disease, a degenerative brain disorder. In this case, L-dopa is transported into the brain, where it is converted to the active drug dopamine by aromatic amino acid decarboxylase. With more and more potent therapeutics identified to treat various brain disorders, effective delivery systems that can accommodate many drugs are desperately needed. A prodrug carrier system developed by Bodor and Simpkins[99] is based on the observation that certain dihydropyridines can easily enter the brain, where they are oxidized to the pyridinium ion whose permeation through the blood-brain barrier is very low. The ionic species formed in the peripheral tissues are rapidly cleared by kidney or biliary secretion. Chemical or enzymatic cleavage of the ester bond on the pyridinium ion slowly releases the conjugated drug in the brain. More lipophilic prodrugs also can be developed to conquer the comparably impermeable stratum corneum of the skin and corneal epithelia of the eye.[100,101]

Prodrugs for oral administration are designed primarily to increase intestinal absorption or to reduce such local side effects as gastric irritation by aspirin. Azo-prodrugs, such as sulphasalazine, olsalazine and balsalazide, have long been used in managing inflammatory disorders of the colon. After entry into the large intestine, the active species, 5-ASA, is released from the prodrug after the cleavage of the azo-linkage. More recently, a number of prodrugs have been developed to target steroid anti-inflammatory agents to the colon. The colonic activation of these prodrugs is based on the colonic microflora producing a wide array of glycosidases.[102] These glycosidases are capable of hydrolyzing glycosides and polysaccharides. The glucoside prodrug of dexamethasone has demonstrated comparable efficacy and reduced side effects with lower doses in experimental animals.[103,104]

In most cases, the prodrug approach is attempted for site-specific drug delivery. However, prodrugs can be used to control the drug release in a limited sense. Consider a water-soluble drug that is modified to a water-insoluble prodrug. The prodrug will have a slower dissolution rate in an aqueous medium than the parent drug, and thus the appearance of the parent drug in plasma will be delayed. This is observed with theophylline prodrug, 7,7'-succinyldytheophylline.

DELIVERY OF BIOTECHNOLOGY PRODUCTS

Being charged macromolecules, proteins and nucleic acids exhibit similar biological properties: limited diffusion from the site of administration, rapid clearance from the circulation by enzymatic degradation, inability to penetrate biological membranes, etc. An extensive search for efficient delivery of these two major biotechnology products is encouraged for several reasons. Proteins and peptides continue to be the most potent therapeutics with high specificity. Their sophisticated functions are derived from their complex structures, thus satisfactory "mimicry" with small molecules is no easy to achieve if possible at all. Unlike conventional treatments, most of which provide symptomatic alleviation, gene therapy eliminates genetic defects that cause a variety of diseases including genetic disorders, cancers and cardiovascular diseases, that is, gene therapy promises "cure" in a sense.

Protein and Peptide Drug Delivery

Despite the enormous success of synthetic peptides and biotechnology products to date, much effort continues to be exerted on controlled delivery of peptide drugs via convenient and noninvasive routes of administration.

Basically, low bioavailability of protein and peptide drugs can be attributed to:

1. *Low permeability of absorbing tissue to the drug.* There are two transport pathways for protein and peptide absorption across the mucosal membrane: transcellular (across cells) and paracellular (between cells). Proteins and peptides are charged molecules that cannot penetrate the lipophilic plasma membrane easily (transcellular transport). Meanwhile, paracellular transport through the tight junctions is also fairly limited because of their large molecular sizes (> 500 Da).

2. *Physicochemical instability caused by enzymatic degradation, molecular interaction.* Enzymatic degradation not only affects the fraction absorbed but also half-lives of peptides in the body. The exopeptidases (ie, aminopeptidase and carboxypeptidase) cleave the peptide bond either at the amino or carboxyl terminus of a peptide chain. The endopeptidases (eg, trypsin, chymotrypsin) function within the peptide chains and maintain certain substrate selectivity. Proteins tend to aggregate themselves or interact with various components in the biological milieu, which dramatically affect their biological activity, absorption and biodistribution.

3. *Short residence time of the dosage form at the absorption site.* In most cases, contact time of the delivery system with the absorbing surface is too short to allow therapeutic levels to be maintained over an extended period of time. Short residence time leads to incomplete absorption and failure to maintain sustained drug action.

Table 47-8[105] gives some general methods for enhancing protein delivery. All these methods are essentially based on conquest of the enzymatic and permeation barrier to peptide absorption.

Table 47-8. General Methods for Enhancing Protein Delivery

Increasing absorption
1. Use of prodrugs
2. Chemical modification of the primary structure
3. Incorporation into liposomes or other encapsulation material
4. Coadministration with chemical enhancers
5. Use of physical methods such as iontophoresis and phonophoresis
6. Targeting to specific tissues

Minimizing metabolism
1. Chemical modification of the primary structure
2. Covalent attachment to a polymer
3. Incorporation into liposomes of other encapsulation material
4. Coadministration with an enzyme inhibitor
5. Targeting to specific tissues

Prolonging half-life
1. Protection with polymers, liposomes
2. Use of bioadhesives
3. Targeting to specific tissues

From Wearley LL. *Crit Rev Ther Drug Carrier Sys* 1991; 8:331.

PENETRATION ENHANCEMENT—Penetration of peptides into biological membranes can be enhanced by physical methods or with the assistance of penetration enhancers. The physical approaches proposed for peptide drug delivery (ie, ionophoresis and phonophoresis) are used mainly in transdermal delivery and have been discussed in a previous section. Penetration enhancers are chemical entities that facilitate transport of coadministered substances across biological membranes. The classification of penetration enhancers is shown in Table 47-9.[106] Basically, penetration enhancers adopt one or more of the following mechanisms to improve membrane permeability to peptides:

1. Enhancing transcellular transport by extracting membrane components or increasing its fluidity.
2. Enhancing paracellular transport.
   a. Chelating calcium ions to open tight junctions.
   b. Inducing high osmotic pressure that transiently opens tight junctions.
   c. Introducing agents to disrupt the biochemical structure of tight junctions.
3. Altering mucus structure and rheology to facilitate drug diffusion.
4. Modifying the physical properties of the drug-enhancer entity, eg, forming ion pairs with charged molecules, reducing aggregation of peptides.

The major concern with penetration enhancers to facilitate transport of peptides is their toxicity because most of them act by nonspecific membrane-disrupting mechanisms. For example, some surfactants and bile salts, such as sodium dodecyl sulfate and deoxycholate, can alter brush border membrane and change intestinal permeability and intestinal secretion.[107] In fact, few penetration enhancers have been approved by the FDA because of the safety issue. A good penetration enhancer should only inflict minimal, localized, transient, and rapidly reversible damage to the absorbing tissue. A series of amino acid

Table 47-9. Classification of Penetration Enhancers

1. *Surfactants*	Acylcholines
Ionic	Caprylic acids
Sodium lauryl sulfate	Acylcarnitines
Sodium laurate	Sodium caprate
Polyoxyethylene-20-cetylether	4. *Chelating agents*
Laureth-9	EDTA
Sodium dodecylsulfate (SDS)	Citric acid
Dioctyl sodium sulfosuccinate	Salicylates
Nonionic	5. *Sulfoxides*
Polyoxyethylene-9-lauryl ether (PLE)	Dimethyl sulfoxide (DMSO)
Tween 80	Decylmethyl sulfoxide
Nonylphenoxypoly-oxyethylene(NP-POE)	6. *Polyols*
Polysorbates	Propylene glycol
2. *Bile salts and derivatives*	Polyethylene glycol
Sodium glycocholate	Glycerol
Sodium deoxycholate	Propanediol
Sodium taurocholate	7. *Monohydric alcohols*
Sodium taurodihydro-fusidate (STDHF)	Ethanol
Sodium glycodihydro-fusidate	2-Propanol (isopropyl alcohol)
3. *Fatty acids and derivatives*	8. *Others (Nonsurfactants)*
Oleic acid	Urea and its derivatives
Caprylic acid	Unsaturated cyclic ureas
Mono(di)glycerides	Azone (1-dodecylazacycloheptan-2-one) (laurocapram)
Lauric acids	Cyclodextrin
	Enamine derivatives
	Terpenes
	Liposomes
	Acyl carnitines and cholines

From Swarbrick J, Boylan JC, eds. *Encyclopedia of Pharmaceutical Technology*, New York, Dekker, 1999, p 1.

Table 47-10. Peptidase Inhibitors

INHIBITOR	PEPTIDASE(S) INHIBITED
Antipain	Cathepsin A, B, papain, trypsin
Leupeptin	Cathepsin B, papain, serine proteinases
Chymostatin	Chymotrypsin (and cysteine proteinases)
Pepstatin	Carboxypeptidases, pepsin, renin, cathepsin B
Bestatin	Leucine aminopeptidase, aminopeptidase B
Amastatin	Aminopeptidase A
PHPFHLFVF	Renin
Alpha-1-antitrypsin	Neutrophil elastase

derivatives with low molecular weight, developed by *Emisphere Technologies*, exhibited their ability to dramatically enhance oral absorption of various peptide drugs, including human growth hormone and insulin, without obvious toxicity.[108,109] The exact mechanism adopted by these compounds has not yet been elucidated. It is speculated that they may modify the conformation of these peptides and thus make the peptides more lipophilic and absorbable.[108] A common complaint associated with penetration enhancers is irritation, especially for transdermal and nasal routes.[110,111] However, irritation is a very complicated phenomenon that may result from the interaction among vehicle, penetration enhancers, buffers, etc. Also, this response is very subjective and varies among individuals.

PROTEASE INHIBITORS—Protease inhibitors are employed, hopefully, to overcome the enzymatic degradation. Some of the proteases and their inhibitors are shown in Table 47-10.[112,113] However, proteins and peptides are subject to multiple routes of degradation. Coadministration of a single enzyme inhibitor does not necessarily result in improved bioavailability. It is necessary to have a thorough understanding of the enzymatic degradation pathway and distribution of the responsible enzymes before this approach can be used successfully in designing a delivery system for proteins and peptides. In addition, the extent of improvement of delivery with this approach largely depends on the relative contribution of enzymatic degradation to the overall barriers. If mucosal permeability and/or short residence time are the major limitations, enzyme inhibitors alone may not necessarily improve the delivery. Rather, a combination of protease inhibitors and penetration enhancers or a protease inhibitor possessing penetration enhancement function (eg, bestatin) may be more useful.

CHEMICAL MODIFICATION— Chemical modification of the primary structure of a peptide could lead to improvement on enzymatic stability and/or mucosal penetration. One example is desmopressin (DDAVP tablets, *Aventis*) for neural diabetes insipidus. It differs structurally from the natural vasopressin in two positions: β-mercaptopropionic acid instead of hemicystine in position 1 and D-arginine in place of L-arginine in position 8. It was found that the cyclic structure accounted for metabolic stability and high membrane permeability of cyclosporin. Cyclization using "chemical linkers" was proposed to stabilize oligopeptides and improve their lipophilicity by reducing their charges and hydrogen bonding potential.[114,115] The linkers were designed to be susceptible to esterase metabolism, leading to release of the peptides. The apparent drawback of this approach is requiring the synthesis of a new chemical entity, which may lead to altered efficacy and/or toxicity. Additionally, modification becomes much more difficult with large peptides. The cyclic prodrug was predicted to be possible for peptides with up to 8 or 9 amino acids.

Chemical modification of peptide drugs is also explored for the purpose of improving their pharmacokinetic profiles and/or reducing their immunogenicity. PEG modification seemingly is able to increase the plasma half-life of protein and reduce the immunogenicity dramatically.[116] A possible mechanism is that the PEGylated protein is too large for glomerular filtration.

PEG may also sterically hinder the protein's interaction with cellular receptors required for metabolism and elimination. PE-Gylated adenosine deaminase (PEG-ADA) was the first such product approved for use in ADA-deficiency.

BIOADHESIVES—Bioadhesives allow close contact of peptides to the mucous lining, while at the same time minimizing transit so that a high concentration gradient across the membrane can be maintained for an extended period of time. Moreover, localizing the delivery system to a small area permits penetration enhancers and enzyme inhibitors to be used at lower concentrations. This may lessen toxicity and irritation. Harris and Robinson[98] demonstrated that bioadhesives could enhance peptide delivery in ocular and nasal routes because their major barrier was short residence time. When mucosal permeability and/or enzymatic degradation are major limitations, such as the gastrointestinal route, bioadhesives possessing inherent penetration-enhancing effects and/or protease inhibition may be beneficial. Polycarbophil and other polyacrylic acid-based polymers are able to chelate calcium ions in physiological buffers.[117] This may lead to opening of tight junctions that are calcium dependent, with an associated increase in paracellular transport. Moreover, polyacrylate is proposed to chelate bivalent cations that are essential to normal enzyme activity. Nevertheless, this inhibitory effect may be still too weak to protect peptides from enzymatic degradation. Recently, multifunctional matrices have been proposed as a promising strategy for oral peptide delivery.[118] These matrices are based on polymers that possess bioadhesive properties, penetration-enhancing effect, enzyme-inhibiting ability, and/or high buffer capacity. Polyacrylates, cellulose derivatives, and chitosans can be chemically modified to improve certain properties and subsequently serve as the construct materials of the matrices. For example, bioadhesive and penetration-enhancing properties can be improved by the covalent attachment of thiol moieties to these polymers. Conjugation of protease inhibitors enables the matrices to protect peptide drugs against enzymatic degradation. Consequently, multifunctional matrices are capable of overcoming almost all the barriers to the peptide drug absorption simultaneously, leading to substantial improvement of bioavailability.

NANO(MICRO)PARTICLES—Encapsulation can protect a peptide against enzymatic degradation and achieve controlled release as well. There are two subtypes of nano(micro)particles. Nano(Micro)capsules are vesicular systems in which drug molecules are surrounded by a membrane. Nano(Micro)spheres are matrix systems in which drug molecules are dispersed throughout the particle. There are a number of methods for preparing nano(micro)particles such as solvent evaporation, organic phase separation, interfacial polymerization, emulsion polymerization, and spray drying. The choice of methods depends on the physicochemical characteristics and stability of the proteins and peptides.

Among numerous biodegradable or bioerodible polymers used for nano(micro)particles, PLGA-based microspheres have proved useful for controlled delivery of several peptides and proteins. The injectable PLGA microsphere of leuprolide acetate, used for prostate cancer, provides controlled release of the peptide over 30 days.[23] Since diffusivity of a protein or peptide is commonly very low, biodegradation of the polymer allows release of peptides from the nano(micro)particles. The possible mechanisms for release of proteins and peptides are[119]:

1. Polymer erosion or degradation
2. Self-diffusion through pores
3. Release from the polymer surface
4. Pulsed delivery initiated by stimulation, such as application of an oscillating magnetic or sonic field

Mechanism 2 is not as important as 1 because usually the drug-loading efficiency is low, which means the concentration gradient is not high enough for the peptide to be released by passive diffusion. Mechanisms 1 and 3 are the most important processes. An initial burst is frequently observed because of solubilization of free drug near the surface that is followed by dis-

integration of the matrix. In other words, the release pattern is biphasic, with an initial high release rate followed by a quiescent period and then a period of significant release due to degradation of the polymer. Mechanism 4 has been applied to control the release rate of insulin. The release pattern is controlled by a magnetic field that alters the structure of polymer chains, resulting in increased drug release.[120] Release rates are subject to protein particle size and loading, protein solubility and molecular weight, polymer composition and molecular weight, and dimensions and shape of the matrix.[121–124] One persistent problem of this approach is that, when encapsulated proteins remain in the body for a long time, they tend to denature or aggregate as a result of exposure to moisture at 37°C. This can cause a loss of biological activity and/or changes in immunogenicity.

GENE DELIVERY

It suffices to say that the success of gene therapy largely relies on an efficient and safe delivery system. Currently, gene delivery can be divided into two categories: viral and nonviral. Viral infection involves highly specific processes for targeting the virus to cells in the body and trafficking viral DNA into the nucleus. In a viral delivery system, the gene encoding viral functions are replaced by that encoding therapeutic function within infectious viral particles. The ability of the virus to infect the target cell and direct gene expression is kept intact. The major concern with viral gene delivery is immunogenicity. The residual viral elements can be immunogenic, cytopathic, and/or recombinogenic.

In the nonviral approach, the genetic materials are considered as chemical entities or pharmaceutical products and particulate carriers are used in their delivery. In general, a nonviral gene delivery system comprises plasmid DNA complexed and condensed by a polycationic agent. The polycation can be a cationic lipid, a liposome composed of cationic lipids, a cationic polymer (eg, polylysine, polyethyleneimine), or a positively charged protein (eg, histones). Viral vectors are superior to nonviral systems in terms of transfection efficiency. Although nonviral systems can protect DNA from nuclease degradation, the lesser ability to overcome various systemic barriers listed in Table 47-11[125] presents substantial challenges to their use in gene delivery. Additionally, the ionic interaction of positively surface-charged plasmid/polycation complex with plasma proteins can result in particle destabilization, characterized by aggregation of particles and/or premature release of DNA.

CATIONIC LIPIDS—Liposomes are the most classic and traditional nonviral carriers in gene delivery because they are biodegradable, and ligands can be incorporated for cell-specific targeting. Cationic liposomes are typically composed of charged and neutral lipids. DOPE and cholesterol are the most frequently used neutral lipids. Nucleic acids can be complexed with cationic liposomes by charge interaction. Freeze fracture[126] and cryoelectron microscopy[127] studies established that complexes resemble aggregated spherical particles surrounded by interwound DNA. Complexes with optimal activity usually contain a slight excess of net positive charge that is capable of

Table 47-11. Biological Barriers to Plasmid/Polycation Particles

1. Particle instability in the blood circulation
2. Particle opsonization and rapid clearance by the RES
3. Extravasation, particularly in organs with continuous endothelia
4. Poor cellular internalization
5. Endosomal entrapment and subsequent delivery to lysosomes for degradation
6. Poor uncoupling of DNA and carrier in the cytoplasm
7. Inefficient uptake into the nucleus

efficient binding with the negatively charged cell surface. The complexes are then internalized by endocytosis, and induce a "flip-flop" of anionic lipids normally present on the cytoplasmic face of the membrane bilayer. The oligonucleotides are displaced from the cationic lipid by the anionic lipid that diffuses into the monolayer and subsequently released into the cytoplasm.[128] However, electron microscope studies[129] showed that plasmids complexed with DMRIE liposomes were endocytosed and remained in vesicles or endosomes. No plasmids were found free in the cytosol. Furthermore, the perinuclear endosomes or vesicles fused to generate large aggregates without releasing their contents. pH-sensitive liposomes have been shown to enhance gene delivery efficiency because they are able to fuse with lipid membranes in the acidic environment of the endosomes, thus facilitating the endosomal release of encapsulated gene-expression systems into the cytoplasm of transfected cells.[130] Proteoliposomes, also known as virosomes or chimerasomes, contain reconstituted viral envelope protein that can facilitate the cellular entry and fusion with the endosomal membranes.[131]

Cationic lipids are capable of interacting electrostatically with the negatively charged phosphate backbone of DNA, neutralizing the charge, and promoting condensation of DNA into a compact structure. The complexes usually are formed in combination of DOPE or cholesterol. This complex is not a liposome, but rather a condensed nanoparticle formed by ionic interaction between the negatively charged DNA and cationic lipids and subsequent hydrophobic interactions between the lipids. The mechanism of gene transfer is hypothesized as fusion of the complex with the plasma membrane followed by entry into the cell. It is not clear whether endocytosis is involved in the process. The complex is then fused with an endosome. Endosomal disruption induced by neutral lipids results in release of DNA into the cytoplasm followed by transport of DNA into the nucleus.[132,133]

POLYMERS—Formulations of plasmid DNA with polymers such as polyvinylpyrrolidone (PVP) and polyvinyl alcohol show enhanced stability, retention, and dispersion of DNA. It has been shown that PVP derivatives facilitate dispersion of DNA in muscles.[134] They also protect DNA against degradation by forming hydrogen bonds followed by creating a hydrophobic coating of DNA that improves stability. Moreover, the enhanced cellular uptake of DNA, probably through hydrophobic interaction with the cell membrane, is also evident.

Although DNA can be condensed by neutral polymers, cationic polymers usually provide more efficient gene delivery. Starburst polyamidoamine dentrimer is a highly branched spherical polymer whose surface has a uniform positive charge. Dendrimers can condense plasmids through electrostatic interactions of their terminal primary amines with the DNA phosphate groups. It can allow very efficient gene delivery with a reduced cytotoxicity (compared to polylysine) to a variety of cell types in vitro.[135] Polethylenimine (PEI) can also give very high transfection efficiency in vitro. PEI may enhance the intracellular trafficking of plasmids by buffering the endosomal compartments, thus preventing degradation of DNA and facilitating release of plasmids via osmotic swelling and rupture. Chitosan is a biodegradable polysaccharide and able to interact with the phosphate groups of DNA. In general, the cationic polymers are capable of forming more homogeneously small and stable complexes, but these complexes show lower levels of transgene expression than lipid-DNA complexes.

Recently, a number of targeted gene delivery systems have been developed by conjugating various ligands to cationic polymers or lipids. The targeting ligands include antibodies, asialoglycoprotein, transferrin, insulin, growth factors, folate, and integrin peptides containing RGD (arginine-glycine-aspartate) motif.[136]

PEPTIDE-BASED GENE DELIVERY[137]—Positively charged synthetic peptides such as poly-L-lysine (PLL) can form small stable complexes with plasmids; however, a PLL/plasmid complex exhibits low transfection efficiency. Peptide-based delivery systems are designed to improve the bioavailability of the therapeutic gene to the target cells. Their major components are:

1. A condensing function mediated by a cationic peptide, such as PLL, histones, protamine, or poly-L-ornithine
2. A receptor-binding function mediated by a peptide or polysaccharide, glycolipid ligand
3. An endosomolytic peptide (eg, synthetic analog of influenza hemaglutinin protein active moiety[138]) or an amphiphilic membrane associating peptide JTS-1[139]
4. A nuclear localization signal peptide to enhance nuclear entry of the plasmid

All these features could make such a peptide-based delivery construct as efficient as viruses but without their limitations.

NOVEL DELIVERY SYSTEMS

Tissue Engineered Delivery Systems[140,141]

Extended-release implants have direct applications to tissue engineering. For instance, a biocompatible polymer matrix or microsphere loaded with growth factors can be implanted at a desired tissue site, where it releases the soluble factors directly into the interstitial space of the tissue. The diffusible agent can affect the survival or function of damaged cells within the local tissue, or provide a signal that elicits cell proliferation or migration within the tissue. Controlled growth factor delivery systems also can be conjugated with biocompatible matrices or porous scaffolds that provide morphological guides for the assembly of regeneration tissue. These matrices are typically implanted at a specific anatomic location where they serve multiple roles. The matrix functions to create and maintain a space in vivo. It also serves as a scaffold to support migration, proliferation, and differentiation of healthy cells from the surrounding tissues. As cells invade the matrix, they encounter the growth factor that is either released from or entrapped within the matrix. Saltzman et al[142] have developed a similar system that uses nerve growth factor-loaded PLGA microparticles to prevent the degradation of cholinergic neurons in the brain.

By physically entrapping a plasmid carrying the gene for an active fragment of human parathyroid hormone within a bovine collagen matrix, Bonadio et al[143] created a moldable three-dimensional porous sponge called a gene activated matrix (GAM) to enhance regeneration of bone tissue in dogs after defect injuries. Here, the collagen carrier serves as a scaffold that holds the plasmid in situ. After the endogenous fibroblasts arrive at the scaffold, the cells start the process of tissue repair and regeneration. Therefore, by taking advantage of the natural tendency of fibroblasts to grow into the wound, GAM allows for physical targeting of these cells for direct in vivo plasmid gene transfer.

Stent implantation has emerged as a new standard angioplasty procedure. The major limitation of coronary stenting is in-stent restenosis. Optimization of stent characteristics could provide improvement to a very limited extent. Preventive or therapeutic agents given systemically may not reach sufficient levels in injured arteries to impact significantly on the restenosis process. Local delivery of drugs from drug-eluting stents allows for drug application at the precise site in a timely manner. Restenosis therapeutics are usually incorporated into eluting polymeric matrices that are subsequently used to coat the stents. Polymers used for such drug delivery vehicles include PVP/cellulose esters, PVP/polyurethane, polymethylidenemaloleate, PLA-co-PLGA, PEG, polyethylenevinyl alcohol, polydimethylsiloxane, etc. Rapamycin-coated Bx Velocity stent (Cordis), coated with a 50:50 mixture of polyethylenevinyl acetate and polybutylmethacrylate containing 30% rapamycin by weight, have appeared to be very effective in preventing restenosis. A stent also can be used as a platform for cell-based gene transfer, which would provide a significant advantage in terms of site-specific gene expression in the vasculature.

Panetta et al[144] presented a stable *in vivo* transgene expression in the vasculature for over 4 weeks, using a mesh-stent coated with fibronectin as an excellent platform for adherent porcine smooth muscle cells.

ENCAPSULATED CELLS

The principle of cell encapsulation is to develop a capsule with sufficient permeability to nutrient and oxygen for the transplanted cells as well as proteins, polypeptides, hormones, or neurotransmitters secreted by the entrapped cells (insulin in the case of islet cells); at the same time, the capsule shall effectively restrict the entry of immune cells and antibodies that would cause rejection. Various polymers have been used for such a semipermeable capsule. These include polyelectrolyte complexes of cellulose sulphate, photo-crosslinked PEG hydrogels, agarose, copolymers and terpolymers of 2-hydroxyethyl methacrylate, methyl methacrylate and dimethylaminoethyl methacrylate, alginate-poly(L-lysine)-alginate complex, and N-isopropylacrylamide (NIPAAm)-based copolymers. As diabetes continues to be a worldwide medical concern, encapsulated islet cells are regarded as the most promising treatment of the disease. Different immunoisolated cell capsules can be classified as vascular and extravascular. In a vascular device, a tubular membrane enveloping islet cells is grafted directly to the vasculature, mimicking the natural islet environment. Its disadvantages include thrombosis at anastomosis sites and the surgical risk associated with device implantation and retrieval. Extravascular devices can be further classified as microcapsule and macrocapsule. The former involves the envelopment of a single or a small number of islets into a microsphere. The latter is often referred to as an *artificial pancreas*. Compared to microencapsulation, macroencapsulation may better simulate the natural environment of the cells as well as more efficiently protect them from rejection. The macrocapsule is also easier to reseed or remove, and more stable. However, larger transplant volume, longer diffusion distances, limited specific surface area, and the aggregation of the entrapped islet cells may impede diffusion of nutrients and oxygen to the central portion of the islets, thus causing necrosis and malfunction of implanted islets.

The refillable biohybrid artificial pancreas, being developed by Bae's group,[145] has several unique features: a thermally reversible extracellular matrix made of NIPAAm hydrogel copolymers; a long-term biocompatible immunoprotective membrane with improved chemical, mechanical and transport stability; and oxygen carriers and biospecific stimulant polymers added to the extracellular matrix. The extracellular matrix primarily serves to immobilize the cells to prevent their aggregation and necrosis and to provide an acceptable physicochemical environment for cell adherence and growth. To replace and refill the device, the polymer matrix can be cooled and redissolved below its gelation temperature. The used solution is withdrawn and a fresh islet/polymer suspension is injected into the device. At body temperature, the polymer forms a gel to immobilize the cells. Oxygen carriers are added to improve the function and viability of immunoisolated islets. Sulfonylurea grafted polymers can stimulate insulin secretion through interaction with its receptors on the islet cell membrane, so the number of islets can be reduced, resulting in reduced volume of the artificial pancreas.

Based on the same principle, cellular implants have attracted interest in extended-release drug delivery to the central nervous system. Examples are encapsulated dopamine-producing cells and glial cell line-derived neurotrophic factor (GDNF)-producing cells implanted in the striatum and the nigra substantia, respectively for Parkinson's disease, encapsulated trophic factor-producing cells for Alzheimer's disease, Huntington's disease, and amylotropic lateral sclerosis.[146]

MICROCHIP DELIVERY SYSTEMS[147]

Microchips can provide controlled release of single or multiple chemical substances on demand. A representation of microchip

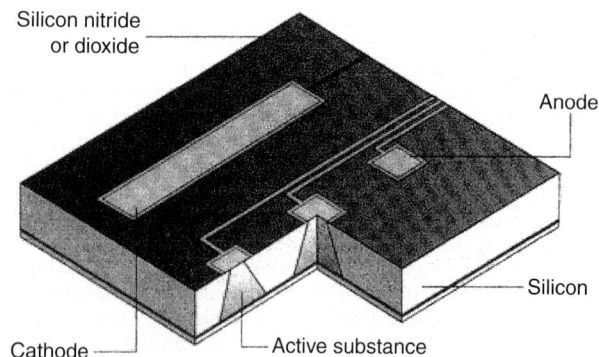

Figure 47-16. Multi-reservoir drug-delivery microchip. (From La Van DA, et al. *Nature Rev Drug Discovery* 2002; 1:77.)

delivery systems is shown Figure 47-16.[148] The system consists of a substrate containing multiple reservoirs capable of holding chemicals in a solid, liquid, or gel form. Each reservoir is capped with a conductive membrane (eg, gold) and wired with the final circuitry controlled by a microprocessor. The central processor controls the exact time and amount of the drug release by controlling the dissolution of the gold membrane. A microchip as small as 2 mm by 2 mm could accommodate over 1000 reservoirs.

Microchip delivery systems have a number of advantages: simplicity of release mechanism, accuracy, complex release patterns, potential for local delivery, stability enhancement, storage and release of multiple chemicals. Microchips are biocompatible and small enough for implantation. The release time could be extended for years depending on the number of reservoirs in the microchip.

The silicone chip is made of non-degradable materials; therefore the chip has to be retrieved at the end of the treatment. The chip is brittle and unfixable, which could cause injuries and aggravation. For some reason the device may fail to operate, requiring surgical intervention to correct. The usage of the chip as a self-regulating release device is limited by biosensors because a specific biosensor is required for an individual disease.

MICROFABRICATED MICRONEEDLES

As mentioned earlier, transdermal administration is fairly restrictive to a majority of therapeutic agents due to extreme impermeability of the stratum corneum. Microfabricated microneedles have the potential to significantly promote transdermal delivery of a large variety of drugs. A microneedle array patch (Fig 47-17[148]) consists of hollow microneedles, which are long and strong enough to penetrate the stratum corneum, but short enough not to stimulate nerves in deeper tissues. Once a drug molecule crosses the stratum corneum, it can rapidly diffuse through the deeper tissue and be taken up by the underlying blood capillaries. Such a patch can dramatically enhance the transdermal delivery without causing pain.[149]

POWDERED DRUG DELIVERY[150]

Dermal and oral powdered drug delivery systems (*PowderJect Technologies*) use the energy from a transient helium gas jet to accelerate and deliver particulate ("powdered") drugs into the skin and mucosal sites, respectively. In the dermal PowderJect, drug particles entrained within a supersonic flow of gas reach velocities sufficient for penetrating the stratum corneum. High-velocity powder injection provides needle- and pain-free delivery of small and large molecules. This technology delivers limited dose (approximately 6 mg), although usually it is adequate

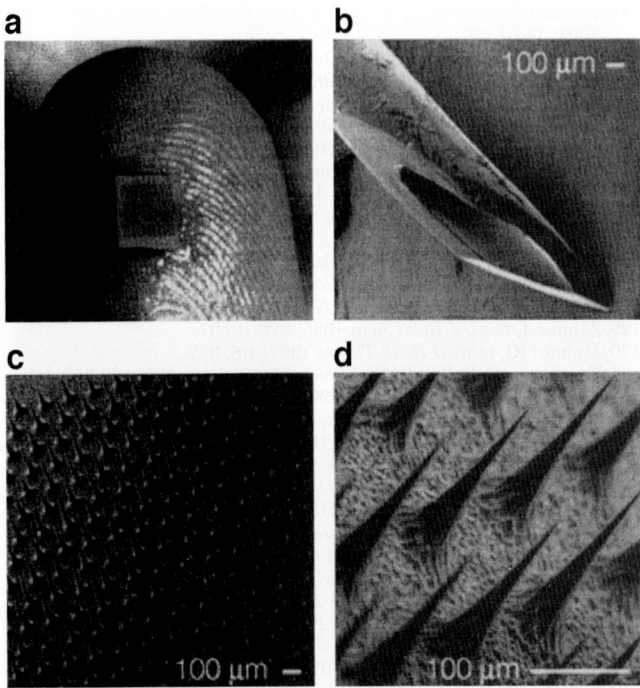

Figure 47-17. Micromachined needles and needle arrays. These images show the design of a needle array for painless transdermal drug delivery. For scale, a conventional hypodermic needle (panel B) is also shown. (From La Van DA, et al. *Nature Rev Drug Discovery* 2002; 1:77.)

to potent drugs. The physical requirements of powders for injection are unique, including particle size range, maximum density and inherent particle strength. Therefore, formulation and methods of characterization and processing are different from those for conventional products.

REFERENCES

1. Robinson JR. In: Park K, ed. *Controlled Drug Delivery: Challenges and Strategies.* Washington DC, American Chemical Society, 1997, p 1.
2. Li VHK, et al. In: Robinson JR, Lee VHL, eds. *Controlled Drug Delivery,* 2nd ed. New York, Dekker, 1987, p 3.
3. Habib W, et al. *Crit Rev Ther Drug Carrier Sys* 2000; 17(1):61.
4. Amidon GL, et al. *Pharm Res* 1995; 12(3):413.
5. Burnette RR. In: Robinson JR, Lee VHL, eds. *Controlled Drug Delivery,* 2nd ed. New York: Dekker, 1987, p 95.
6. Robinson JR, Eriksen SP. *J Pharm Sci* 1966; 55:1254.
7. Welling PG, Dobrinska MR. In: Robinson JR, Lee VHL, eds. *Controlled Drug Delivery,* 2nd ed. New York, Dekker, 1987, p 253.
8. Gibaldi M, Perrier D. *Pharmacokinetics,* 2nd ed. New York: Dekker, 1982, p 189.
9. Riegelman S, et al. *J Pharm Sci* 1968; 57:128.
10. Mayer PR. In: Park K, ed. *Controlled Drug Delivery: Challenges and Strategies.* Washington, DC: American Chemical Society, 1997, p 589.
11. Rowland M, Tozer TN. *Clinical Pharmacokinetics: Concepts and Applications,* 3rd ed. Baltimore: Lippincott Williams & Wilkins, 1995, p 360.
12. Wagner JG. *Am J Pharm* 1969; 141:5.
13. Park K, et al. In: Langer R, Wise D, eds. *Medical Applications of Controlled Release Technology.* Boca Raton, FL: CRC Press, 1985, p 171.
14. Higuchi T. *J Pharm Sci* 1961; 50:874.
15. Higuchi T. *J Pharm Sci* 1963; 52:1145.
16. Chien YW. *Novel Drug Delivery Systems,* 2nd ed. New York: Dekker, 1992, p 1.
17. Chien YW. *Novel Drug Delivery Systems.* 2nd ed. New York: Dekker, 1992, p 43.
18. Hsieh DST, Smith N, Chien YW. In: Meyers WE, Dunn RL, eds. *Proceedings 11th International Symposium on Controlled Release of Bioactive Materials.* Chicago: Controlled Release Society, 1984, p 134.
19. Sah H, Chien YW. In: Hillery AM, Lloyd AW, Swarbrick J, eds. *Drug Delivery and Targeting for Pharmacists and Pharmaceutical Scientists.* London: Taylor & Francis, 2001, p 83.
20. Hillery AM. In: Hillery AM, Lloyd AW, Swarbrick J, eds. *Drug Delivery and Targeting for Pharmacists and Pharmaceutical Scientists.* London: Taylor & Francis, 2001, p 63.
21. Chandrasekaran SK, et al. In: Robinson JR, ed. *Sustained and Controlled Release Drug Delivery Systems.* New York: Dekker, 1978, p 557.
22. Hui HW, et al. In: Robinson JR, Lee VHL, eds. *Controlled Drug Delivery,* 2nd ed. New York: Dekker, 1987, p 373.
23. Langer R. *Science* 1990; 249(4976):1527.
24. Kost J, Langer R. *J Biomed Mater Res* 1987; 21:1367.
25. Singh P, Maibach HI. *Crit Rev Ther Drug Carrier Sys* 1994; 11:161.
26. Chien YW, et al. *J Controlled Release* 1990; 13:263.
27. Green PG. *J Controlled Release* 1996; 41:33.
28. Chien YW, et al. *Ann NY Acad Sci* 1987; 507:32.
29. Asbill CS, et al. *Crit Rev Ther Drug Carrier Sys* 2000; 17(6):621.
30. Li S, Benninger M. *Curr Gene Ther* 2002; 2(1):101.
31. Kwon IC, et al. *Nature* 1991; 354:291.
32. Miyazaki S, et al. *J Pharm Pharmcol* 1988; 40:716.
33. Kost J, et al. *Markromol Chem Makrom Symp* 1988; 19:275.
34. Liu LS, et al. *Macromolecules* 1992; 25:511.
35. Mitragotri S, et al. *Science* 1995; 269:850.
36. Mitragotri S, et al. *J Pharm Sci* 1995; 84:697.
37. Hippius M, et al. *Exp Toxicol Pathol* 1998; 50:450.
38. Hippius M, et al. *Int J Clin Pharmacol Ther* 1998; 36:107.
39. Asano J, et al. *Biol Pharm Bull* 1997; 20:288.
40. Sasaki H, et al. *Crit Rev Ther Drug Carrier Sys* 1999; 16(1):85.
41. Bae YH. In: Park K, ed. *Controlled Drug Delivery: Challenges and Strategies.* Washington, DC: America Chemical Society, 1997, p 147.
42. Ishihara K, Shinohara I. *J Polym Sci Polym Lett Ed* 1984; 22:515.
43. Feil H, et al. *Macromolecules* 1992; 25:5528.
44. Hoffman AS, et al. *J Controlled Release* 1986; 4:213.
45. Dong LC, Hoffman AS. *J Controlled Release* 1986; 4:223.
46. Jeong B, et al. *Nature* 1997; 388:860
47. Albib G, et al. *J Controlled Release* 1984; 2:153.
48. Heller J, et al. *J Controlled Release* 1990; 13:295.
49. Heller J. In: Park K, ed. *Controlled Drug Delivery: Challenges and Strategies.* Washington, DC: American Chemical Society, 1997, p 127.
50. Fishel-Ghodsian F, et al. *Proc Natl Acad Sci USA* 1988; 85:2403.
51. Kim SW, Jacobs HA. *Drug Dev Ind Pharm* 1994; 20:575
52. Obaidat AA, Park K. *Pharm Res* 1996; 13:989.
53. Pitt CG, et al. *J Controlled Release* 1985; 2:363.
54. Pitt CG, et al. *J Controlled Release* 1984; 1:3.
55. Tomlinson E. *J Pharm Technol Prod Manuf* 1983; 4:49.
56. Kumar V, Banker GS. In: Banker GS, Rhodes CT, eds. *Modern Pharmaceutics,* 4th ed. New York: Dekker, 2002, p 529.
57. Rogerson A, et al. *J Pharm Pharmacol* 1988; 40(5):337.
58. Oppenheim RC. *J Steroid Biochem* 1975; 6:182.
59. Moghimi SM, et al. *Biochem Biophys Res Commun* 1991; 177(2):861.
60. Moghimi SM. *Adv Drug Delivery Rev* 1995; 17(1):61.
61. Moghimi SM, Bonnemain B. *Adv Drug Delivery Rev* 1999; 37(1–3):295.
62. Zhang X, et al. *Int J Pharm* 1996; 132:195.
63. Yokoyama M. *Crit Rev Ther Drug Carrier Sys* 1992; 9:213.
64. Cammas S, et al. *J Controlled Release* 1997; 48:157.
65. Xu R, et al. *Macromolecules* 1991; 24:87.
66. Khan TN, et al. *Eur Polym J* 1987; 23:191.
67. Maeda H, et al. *Bioconj Chem* 1992; 3:351.
68. Kwon G, et al. *Langmuir* 1993; 9:945.
69. Piskin E, et al. *J Biomater Sci Polym Ed* 1995; 7:359.
70. Peracchia MT, et al. *J Controlled Release* 1997; 46:223.
71. Alakhov VY, et al. *Bioconj Chem* 1996; 7:209.
72. Miller DW, et al. *Bioconj Chem* 1997; 8:649.
73. Yu BG, et al. *J Controlled Release* 1998; 56(1–3):285.
74. Margolis LB. In: Gregoriadis G, ed. *Liposomes as Drug Carriers: Recent Trends and Progress,* New York: Wiley, 1988, p 75.
75. Gill PS, et al. *J Clin Oncol* 1995; 13(4):996.
76. Harrison M, et al. *J Clin Oncol* 1995; 13(4):914.
77. Drummond DC, et al. *Pharmacol Rev* 1999; 51(4):691.
78. Gregoriadis G, ed. *Liposome Technology,* 2nd ed. Boca Raton, FL: CRC Press, 1993.
79. Lasic DD, Papahadjopoulos D, eds. *Medical Applications of Liposomes.* Amsterdam: Elsevier, 1998.
80. Gee B, et al. *J Histochem Cytochem* 1991; 39(6):863.
81. Feener EP, King GL. *Adv Drug Delivery Rev* 1998; 29:197.
82. Fukuta M, et al. *Pharmacol Res* 1994; 11:1681.
83. Cho BK, et al. *Bioconjug Chem* 1997; 8:338.

84. Vingerhoeds MH, et al. *FEBS Lett* 1993; 336:485.
85. Fanger MW, et al. *Crit Rev Immunol* 1992; 12:101.
86. Sudimack J, Lee FJ. *Adv Drug Delivery Rev* 2000; 41:147.
87. Reddy JA, Low PS. *Crit Rev Ther Drug Carrier Sys* 1998; 15:587.
88. Jain S, Jain NK. *Pharmazie* 1998; 1:5.
89. Eichler HC, et al. *Adv Biosci* 1987; 67:11.
90. Jarvis SM, et al. *Biochem J* 1980; 190:373.
91. Yang X, Robinson JR. In: Okano T, ed. *Biorelated Functional Polymers and Gels: Controlled Release and Applications in Biomedical Engineering*, San Diego: Academic Press, 1998, p 135.
92. Gu J M, et al. *Crit Rev Ther Drug Carrier Sys* 1988; 5:21.
93. Marschutz MK, et al. In: *Proceedings International Symposium on Controlled Release of Bioactive Materials*. Paris: Controlled Release Society, 2000, p 27.
94. Eichman JM, Robinson JR. *Pharm Res* 1998; 15:761.
95. Robinson JR, Bolonga WJ. *J Controlled Release* 1994; 28:87.
96. Dondeeti P, et al. *Int J Pharm* 1995; 122:91.
97. Park K, Robinson JR. *Int J Pharm* 1984; 19:107.
98. Harries D, Robinson JR. *Biomaterials* 1990; 11:652.
99. Bodor N, Simpkins JW. *Science* 1983; 221:65.
100. Lipp R, et al. *Pharm Res* 1998; 15(9):1419.
101. Kawakami S, et al. *J Pharm Sci* 2001; 90(12):2113.
102. Friend DR, Tozer TN. *J Controlled Release* 1992; 19:109.
103. Tozer TN, et al. *Pharm Res* 1991; 8:445.
104. Haeberlin B, et al. *Pharm Res* 1993; 10:1553.
105. Wearley LL. *Crit Rev Ther Drug Carrier Sys* 1991; 8:331.
106. Yang X, Robinson JR. In: Swarbrick J, Boylan JC, eds. *Encyclopedia of Pharmaceutical Technology*. New York: Dekker, 1999, p 1.
107. Gullikson GW, et al. *Gastroenterology* 1977; 73:501.
108. Milstein SJ, et al. *J Controlled Release* 1998; 53:259.
109. Wu SJ, Robinson JR. *Pharm Res* 1999; 16(8):1266.
110. Aungst BJ. *Pharm Res* 1989; 6:244.
111. Geppeti P, et al. *Br J Pharmacol* 1988; 93:509.
112. Lee VHL, Traver RD, Taub ME. In: Lee VHL, ed. *Peptide and Protein Drug Delivery*. New York: Dekker, 1991, p 303.
113. Junginger HE. *Acta Pharm Technol* 1990; 36:110.
114. Gangwar S, et al. *Drug Discovery Today* 1997; 2:148.
115. Shan D, et al. *J Pharm Sci* 1997; 86:765.
116. Katre N. *Adv Drug Delivery Rev* 1993; 10:91.
117. Kriwet B, Kissel T. *Int J Pharm* 1996; 127:135.
118. Bernkop-Schnurch A, Walker G. *Crit Rev Ther Drug Carrier Sys* 2001; 18(5):459.
119. Couvreur P, Puisieux F. *Adv Drug Delivery Rev* 1993; 10:141.
120. Saslawski O, et al. *Life Sci* 1988; 42:1521.
121. Bawa R, et al. *J Controlled Release* 1985; 1:259.
122. Hsu T, Langer R. *J Biomed Mater Res* 1985; 19:445.
123. Ogawa Y, et al. *Chem Pharm Bull* 1988; 36:1502.
124. Saltzman WM, Langer R. *Biophys J* 1989; 55:163.
125. Pouton CW. In: Rolland A, ed. *Advanced Gene Delivery: From Concepts to Pharmaceutical Products*. Amsterdam: Harwood Academic Publishers, 1999, p 65.
126. Sternberg B, et al. *FEBS Lett* 1994; 356:361.
127. Gustaffson J, et al. *Biochem Biophys Acta* 1995; 1235:305.
128. Zelphati O, Szoka FC Jr. *Proc Natl Acad Sci USA* 1996; 93:11493.
129. Zabner J, et al. *J Biol Chem* 1995; 270:18997.
130. Mahato RI, et al. *J Drug Target* 1997; 4:6, 337.
131. Tomlinson E, Rolland AP. *J Controlled Release* 1996; 39:357.
132. Mahato RI, et al. *Pharm Res* 1997; 14:853.
133. Zabner J. *Adv Drug Delivery Rev* 1997; 27:17.
134. Mumper RJ, et al. *Pharm Res* 1996; 13:701.
135. Hill IR, et al. *Biochem Biophys Acta* 1999; 1427:161.
136. Anwer K, et al. *Crit Rev Ther Drug Carrier Sys* 2000; 17(4):377.
137. Mahato RI, Tomlinson E. In: Hillery AM, Lloyd AW, Swarbrick J, eds. *Drug Delivery and Targeting for Pharmacists and Pharmaceutical Scientists*. London: Taylor & Francis, 2001, p 371.
138. Wagner E, et al. *Proc Natl Acad Sci USA* 1992; 89:6099.
139. Fominaya J, et al. *J Gene Med* 2000; 2(6):455.
140. Saltzman WM, Olbricht WL. *Nature Rev Drug Discovery* 2002; 1:177.
141. Regar E, et al. *Br Med Bull* 2001; 59:227.
142. Mahoney MJ, Saltzman WM. *Nature Biotech* 2001; 19:934.
143. Bonadio J, et al. *Nature Med* 1999; 5:753.
144. Panetta CJ, et al. *Hum Gene Ther* 2002; 13(3):433.
145. Hou QP, Bae YH. *Adv Drug Delivery Rev* 1999; 35:271.
146. Emerich DF, Winn SR. *Crit Rev Ther Drug Carrier Sys* 2001; 18(3):265.
147. Santini JT, et al. *Nature* 1999; 397:335.
148. La Van DA, et al. *Nature Rev Drug Discovery* 2002; 1:77.
149. Kaushik S, et al. *Anesth Analg* 2001; 92:502.
150. Burkoth TL, et al. *Crit Rev Ther Drug Carrier Sys* 1999; 16(4):331.

CHAPTER 48

The New Drug Approval Process and Clinical Trial Design

Dennis W Raisch, RPh, PhD

Linda A Felton, PhD

The research and development efforts needed to ensure the safety and efficacy of new drugs are complex, time consuming, and financially risky. Thousands of compounds undergo extensive testing for every one new chemical that receives marketing approval.[1] Research and development costs for each new drug product are estimated to be over $800 million.[2] It has been reported that only 30% of drugs that reach the marketplace generate sufficient revenue to recover the average cost of its development.[3] This chapter discusses the various stages of new drug development and approval in the United States with a focus on clinical trial design and methodology. Readers are encouraged to refer to specific FDA guidance documents for more detailed information (www.fda.gov/cder/guidance/index.htm).

FOOD AND DRUG ADMINISTRATION

The Food and Drug Administration (FDA) oversees the new drug approval process in the United States. Other countries have similar regulatory bodies. The FDA was created as the result of multiple deaths associated with a diethylene glycol-based sulfanilamide product. This solvent was used to enhance the aqueous solubility of the antibiotic. Diethylene glycol, however, is a highly toxic agent used in antifreeze solutions, and numerous deaths resulted from the ingestion of the product. Based on these tragic events, Congress passed the Food, Drug, and Cosmetic Act of 1938, which established FDA as the regulatory authority overseeing the development of new drug products.[4] The Act required disclosure of the ingredients and formulation, assay methods, manufacturing processes, and all animal and human testing to the FDA prior to distribution of the product.

While the Act of 1938 required new drug products to be safe, efficacy standards were not established until another tragedy in the early 1960s. Thalidomide, a synthetic sedative/tranquilizer, had been sold in Europe at that time without a prescription and was viewed as a possible alternative to the more toxic barbiturates.[5] Prior to approval of thalidomide by the FDA, several incidences of toxicity in Europe were reported. Severe birth defects were noted when the drug was administered to pregnant women, the most common being phocomelia or arrested limb development. These events brought about the Kefauver-Harris Amendments of 1962, which strengthened existing laws and emphasized the need for the safety of approved drugs.[6] These Amendments required manufacturers to establish both safety and efficacy of new drug products prior to approval and required investiga-

tors to file Investigational New Drug Applications (INDs) prior to testing all drugs in humans. As a side note, thalidomide is currently approved in the United States for the treatment and prevention of painful skin lesions associated with erythema nodosum leprosum. Other potential uses of this drug under investigation include several types of cancer, Crohn's disease, and autoimmune deficiency-associated diseases.[5,7]

The role of the FDA is to promote and protect the health of Americans. A multidisciplinary staff consisting of pharmacists, physicians, pharmacologists, chemists, statisticians, attorneys, and other scientists as well as administrative personnel is employed at the FDA to achieve this goal. The FDA consists of several Centers, each designated with specific responsibilities. The Center for Food Safety and Applied Nutrition oversees food and cosmetic products. The Center for Veterinary Medicine is responsible for animal feed and drugs. The safety and efficacy of medical devices are covered under the Center for Devices and Radiological Health. This Center also oversees radiation-emitting devices such as cellular telephones. The Center for Biologics Evaluation and Research (CBER) supervises biologics. Finally, the Center for Drug Evaluation and Research (CDER) is responsible for drugs and drug products. In addition to reviewing the safety and efficacy of all prescription and over-the-counter drug products prior to marketing, CDER is responsible for monitoring drug safety after initial market approval and has the authority to withdraw from the market drugs posing significant health risks. CDER provides health care professionals and consumers with drug-related information and screens television, radio, and print ads for truthfulness and balance.

OVERVIEW OF THE DRUG APPROVAL PROCESS

As mentioned previously, drug discovery and development is a complex and expensive endeavor. The next several sections of this chapter discuss the various phases of the new drug development and approval process in the United States. While focused specifically on CDER and new drugs/drug products, similar requirements exist for biologics and medical devices. The development process is divided into two sections: (1) preclinical testing (lead compound selection and animal testing of new chemicals) and (2) clinical testing (administration of new chemicals to humans). A schematic of these steps is shown in Figure 48-1.

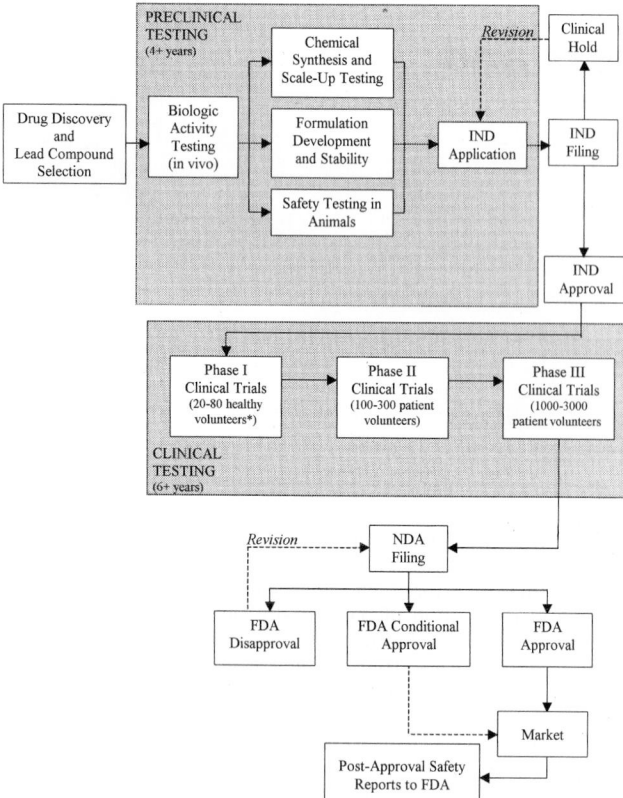

Figure 48-1. The new drug approval process in the United States. *For life-threatening illnesses such as cancer, patients enrolled in Phase I studies may suffer from the disease.

Drug Discovery and Lead Compound Selection

Pharmaceutical companies generally begin the discovery process by targeting a broad disease category (ie, cancer or cardiovascular disease) or a specific disease state (breast cancer or hypertension). A chemical with potential therapeutic benefit(s), known as a lead compound, must first be identified and researchers use various high-throughput assay techniques to rapidly screen large numbers of chemicals for biological activity.

Random screening, as the name implies, requires biological testing of a large variety of diverse compounds from existing chemical libraries. While less up-front financial investment is needed, thousands of compounds may be screened and tested before one agent with significant biochemical activity is identified. A more mechanism-based drug design is targeted synthesis, where researchers focus on one step in a disease process as the target for drug intervention. While an extensive knowledge of the disease state is required, this more directed approach increases the likelihood of successfully identifying a lead compound. In combinatorial chemistry, one compound is used as a base chemical and various functional groups are randomly added to enhance biological activity. This technique is a more expensive, more complex method of identifying potential lead agents. Another method to enhance biological activity is drug modeling, where computers are used to manipulate virtual structures and calculate protein binding capabilities. Although initial costs are significant, drug modeling techniques show a great deal of promise for future drug discovery as more research is conducted to identify biochemical pathways. Generally, combinations of these discovery techniques are used to identify lead compounds. Future discovery techniques will likely rely on the field of functional proteomics and identification of the biological roles of proteins coded by various genes.[8]

Preclinical Testing

A multidisciplinary team of researchers works to determine many of the lead compound's critical properties. This team may continue to work with the compound throughout the entire development process or the development responsibilities may be transferred to another group of scientists during the clinical testing phase. Preclinical testing includes:

- Discovery testing to ensure biological activity in vivo
- Chemical synthesis and scale-up to ensure adequate quantities of high purity can be made
- Formulation development and stability testing to characterize various chemical properties, develop the initial drug delivery system, and determine the stability of the compound (see Chapter 38, *Property-based Design and Preformulation*)
- Animal safety testing to ensure limited toxicities of the lead agent

At this stage of the development process, good laboratory practices (GLPs) are followed. These regulations, set forth in Title 21 of the Code of Federal Regulations (CFR) Section 58, provide standards for the design and conduct of preclinical studies. Qualifications of personnel are specified and requirements for standard operating procedures are established.

During discovery testing, the specifics of the compound's properties, such as the mechanism of action in animal models, compound specificity, duration of action, and structure-activity relationships, are determined. Adequate quantities of the new chemical compound must be produced at a high level of purity. Impurities present at concentrations greater than 0.1% must be characterized and tested for toxicity. The physicochemical properties of the active compound are determined, and the drug delivery system to be used in human testing begins to be developed during this preclinical testing phase. Animal testing provides initial data regarding the absorption, distribution, metabolism, and excretion (ADME) in a living system. Possible side effects and toxicities are noted. Toxicity studies of at least the same duration as the proposed human testing and a minimum of 2 weeks must be completed. Active and inactive metabolites must be characterized. Often times the most appropriate animal model to predict human response is not known, thus toxicity studies are conducted in at least two animal species, one rodent and one nonrodent, to obtain a comprehensive view of the potential toxicity. Early ADME or toxicity problems may be corrected by slight modifications in the new chemical entity.

Animals should be given the new drug product by the same route as intended for humans. Certain dosage forms, such as aerosol, nasal, or buccal delivery systems, may be difficult to administer to animals. In these circumstances, alternative drug delivery routes may be used, and the selected route of administration should ensure sufficient exposure to the new chemical entity. During animal safety testing, dosing studies are conducted, and the highest no-effect dose is determined. In addition to dose, plasma concentrations of the drug are followed, and noted toxicities are correlated to dose and/or blood concentration.

Generally, once discovery testing shows therapeutic promise, the chemical synthesis, formulation development, and animal safety testing occur concurrently (see Fig 48-1). While resources may be wasted on earlier failures, successful candidates will be ready for human testing earlier. The administration of drugs in humans at the earliest time possible ultimately saves valuable resources, as highly toxic compounds can be eliminated while lead agents and alternative compounds are developed.

Additional preclinical studies are conducted during clinical testing to support larger trials and eventually the marketing of the drug product. Formulation development continues throughout the development process and the data gained from both animal and human testing allow for optimization of the drug delivery system. It is imperative to identify and resolve formulation problems early in the development process, as unresolved problems will surely re-emerge later, costing the company both time and money as clinical testing is delayed. More chronic animal exposure experiments are generally conducted to support further clinical testing.

PRE-IND MEETINGS

Pre-IND meetings may be held prior to submission of an Investigational New Drug application (IND) and at the request of the sponsor during these early stages of product development to discuss testing plans and data requirements. These meetings are generally useful when a drug has been developed overseas, and a great deal of preclinical and clinical data is readily available. During pre-IND meetings, the sponsor and FDA should agree on the acceptable phase of the initial clinical investigation. Clinical data from other countries may eliminate the need for Phase I human safety testing. FDA guidance documents provide an overview of procedures for requesting formal meetings. These meetings are not intended to replace informal discussions with the FDA.

Investigational New Drug Application (IND)

An Investigational New Drug application (IND) must be filed with the FDA and approved prior to administering new drug products to humans. In 21 CFR Section 312, the guidelines for preapproval of all clinical testing are specified. The name and chemical description of the active, a list of active and inactive components, and the manufacturers of these components must be provided. The method of preparation and the dosage form to be administered must be specified. The IND includes all preclinical animal data and the names and locations of the investigators who will be performing the planned clinical trials. Data from clinical trials conducted in other countries should also be included if available. The FDA has 30 days from receipt of the IND to decide if the proposed clinical trial should proceed. The protocol(s) conducted under the IND must be approved by each facility's Institutional Review Board (IRB, described more fully in a subsequent section of this chapter).

Upon receipt, the IND is assigned to one of the various divisions of CDER and the application thoroughly reviewed. If the investigator is not contacted within 30 days, the trial may proceed. Reviewers at FDA may place a clinical hold on the clinical trials at any time. A clinical hold effectively prevents human testing under the IND, until FDA concerns have been adequately addressed. Reasons for placing an IND under a clinical hold include unreasonable or significant risk of illness or injury to trial subjects, insufficient information to assess patient risks, inadequate qualifications of the clinical investigators, or a misleading, erroneous, or incomplete Investigator's Brochure (a document that contains all relevant information about the drug). Revisions to clinical protocols, as well as new protocols or substudies are submitted to the FDA as amendments to the IND. In addition, progress reports regarding the trial must also be provided annually.

It should be noted that not all clinical trials require an IND. A sponsor proposing a trial with a commercially available, FDA-approved drug product is exempt from these IND requirements if the trial (1) is not intended to be submitted to the FDA to support labeling changes or a new indication; (2) is not intended to support a major change in advertising; and (3) does not involve a route of administration, dose, or patient population that significantly increases the risk of the drug. An IND is not required if the trial is exempt according to the above criteria regardless of whether a placebo (inert or inactive treatment) is employed as a control group. Independent investigators rather than pharmaceutical companies often conduct these types of clinical trials.

Clinical Investigations

Clinical investigations involve the administration of a drug to humans. This segment of the drug development process requires substantial financial and time commitments.[9] Figure 48-2 shows the considerable increase in development costs associated with the initiation of clinical trials. Human testing is divided into four phases, each phase having specific objectives. The following sections discuss the various phases of clinical testing.

PHASE I CLINICAL TRIALS

The first series of experiments performed in humans occurs during Phase I clinical testing. A small number of generally healthy volunteers (approximately 20-80 people) are exposed to the new drug product in closely monitored trials, primarily to assess the compound's safety. For the investigation of drugs to treat life-threatening diseases, such as cancer or Acquired Immune Deficiency Syndrome (AIDS), patients afflicted with the disease may be enrolled.[10] In Phase I trials, the starting dose is generally low, often 1/10 of the highest no-effect dose in the animal models. After the initial treatment is completed, additional subjects may be recruited and administered higher doses to determine the maximum dose tolerated without significant side effects. During this phase of testing, preliminary ADME data of the parent drug and all metabolites should be evaluated. Sufficient data regarding pharmacokinetic and pharmacological effects are also obtained to be used in designing future Phase II trials.

PHASE II CLINICAL TRIALS

Phase II clinical testing shifts the focus of the trials from safety to efficacy. In comparison to Phase I trials, a larger number of people (100-300 patients) are enrolled in the trial and the majority of these participants suffer from the target illness. Side effects from the new drug product are also investigated. These clinical trials are closely monitored and well-controlled (see Clinical Trial Planning and Design section). Failure during Phase II testing is common, as the human body is more complex than the test tube. Clinical protocols for Phase II trials must be sent to the FDA as amendments to the IND prior to beginning the trials.

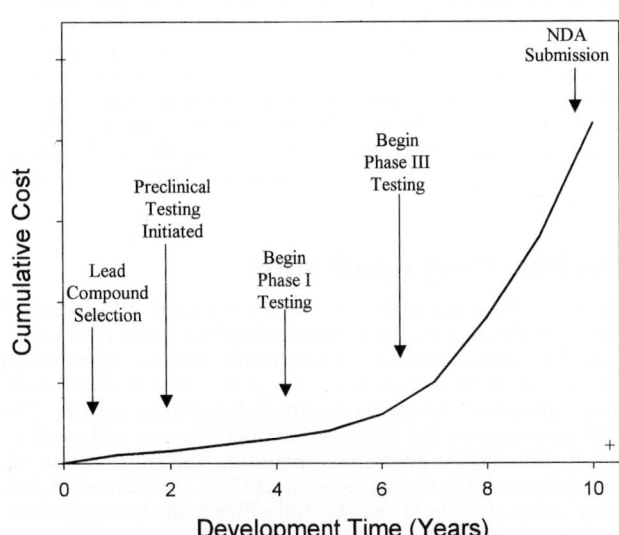

Figure 48-2. Relationship between the time devoted to new drug development and dollars invested. Adapted from Lakings DB. Nonclinical drug development: Pharmacology, drug metabolism, and toxicology. In: Guarino RA, ed. *New Drug Approval Process*. 2000, New York: Marcel Dekker, 2002; pp 17–54.

PHASE III CLINICAL TRIALS

At the end of Phase II testing, sponsors are encouraged to meet with the FDA. These meetings generally involve review of the acceptability of past trials, the design of future trials, and the general drug development plan. Scientists at the FDA carefully review preclinical and clinical data in evaluating proposed Phase III protocols. Specific areas of the proposed Phase III trials that are scrutinized include the inclusion/exclusion criteria, dosing regimens, methods and timing of data collection, duration of treatment and follow-up assessment, blinding of the drug products and plans for maintaining the blind, plans to assess compliance with protocol, identification of primary outcome variables, and methods to account for dropouts. Addressing these key areas of proposed Phase III protocols is expected to limit the bias of trial results. The overall goal of the meeting is a good-faith agreement between the sponsor and FDA regarding data required for submission of a New Drug Application (NDA).

Phase III clinical trials are the longest, most comprehensive trials regarding efficacy and safety of new compounds. Significantly larger numbers (1000-3000) of patients who are afflicted with the target illness are tested. Patients are often recruited, tested, and monitored by several major hospitals and clinics throughout the country. Phase III trials may also be conducted internationally. In addition to determining efficacy, these trials monitor adverse reactions. The new drug may be compared to existing therapeutic regimens (ie, comparator products) or to placebo. The final market formulation for the drug product should be optimized prior to the start of these Phase III trials. Compounds that successfully complete Phase III testing have a 95% chance of being approved by the FDA.[10]

Prior to the completion of Phase III testing and NDA submission, sponsors are encouraged to meet again with the appropriate review division of the FDA. These meetings help establish the appropriate format of the submission so that the review proceeds smoothly and determine if additional animal or human trials are necessary. The meeting should be held sufficiently in advance of the tentative NDA filing date to allow ample time to incorporate recommended changes or perform additional trials.

PHASE IV CLINICAL TESTING

Phase IV trials are post-approval clinical trials designed for one of several reasons. The FDA may mandate Phase IV testing in a specific patient population to further assess efficacy and side effects. Companies may also choose to conduct additional clinical tests to more fully understand how their product compares to other commercially available therapeutic regimens. Since duration of exposure is often limited during Phase III testing, Phase IV trials may be required to assess long-term safety of the drug.

The New Drug Application

Once the Phase III trials have been completed, all preclinical and clinical data are compiled and submitted to the FDA for review. The NDA process is the last hurdle prior to approval and marketing. A NDA document is typically hundreds of thousands of pages containing highly detailed information. The FDA also reviews the proposed product labeling and package insert. Regulation guidelines including the information required for an NDA are provided in 21 CFR 314 Subpart B. Primary items include (1) safety and efficacy of the drug treatment(s); (2) components of drug product(s); (3) description of methods and controls used in manufacturing the active ingredient and the drug delivery system and its packaging; and (4) proposed labeling. According to CDER, the time for a NDA review has been reduced from a median of 22 months in 1992 to approximately 15 months in 2000 (www.fda.gov/cder/reports/reviewtimes/default.htm). The faster review times have been attributed to the Prescription Drug User Fee Act (PDUFA) of 1992 (www.fda.gov/cder/pdufa/default.htm). In 2002, 78 NDAs were approved by the FDA, including 17 new chemical entities.[11]

When a NDA is submitted, relevant sections of the document are distributed to the appropriate reviewers and evaluated first for completeness. If the document is sufficiently complete, the NDA is accepted for review and assigned a priority status. NDAs for new chemical entities are classified as either 'P' for priority review or 'S' for standard review. A 'P' rating is given to new drug products with improved therapeutic effects, safety, and/or side effects in comparison to currently marketed drugs. NDAs assigned a 'P' rating are expected to be reviewed in a more timely manner than those assigned an 'S' rating. If the NDA is deemed too incomplete to review, it is not filed. The decision to accept the NDA is made within 60 days of the date of submission.

Once the NDA is accepted, detailed evaluation continues and the FDA has 180 days from submission to complete the review. Each reviewer submits written comments of his assigned section and makes a recommendation. The NDA may also be presented to an Advisory Committee for comment. All documents are then compiled and ultimately submitted to the Director of the Office of Drug Evaluation. The FDA may approve the product for market, approve with specific conditions attached (Conditional Approval), or disapprove the drug product. Primary reasons for disapproval include lack of demonstrated safety and efficacy, issues with the manufacturing/processing procedures, or false/misleading labeling. If not approved, a letter is sent to the sponsor detailing deficiencies in the application. If the NDA is approved, an approval letter along with a draft of the product labeling is sent to the sponsor. The label is generally a combination of the draft submitted by the sponsor and revisions provided by the reviewing section of the FDA. Standardized labeling requirements are provided in 21 CFR Section 201.57.

Prior to NDA approval, the FDA conducts an inspection of the sponsor's facilities to ensure compliance with current Good Manufacturing Practices (cGMPs) as set forth in 21 CRF Parts 210 and 211. These cGMPs are minimal industry standards and procedures established to ensure consistent quality of manufactured drug products. Pre-approval inspections are conducted within 45 days of the NDA acceptance. If deficiencies are noted during an inspection, a letter (FDA Form 483) is sent to the sponsor delineating the problems. Once the deficiencies are resolved, the company must provide written certification and the FDA will clear the application within 45 days if the corrections are adequate. As this step is often critical in the approval process, companies often hold mock pre-approval audits.

Abbreviated New Drug Application (ANDA)

In addition to approving new drug products for the United States, the FDA is charged with the approval of generic drug products (21 CFR Part 314). This work is accomplished through CDER's Office of Generic Drugs. A generic drug product must be bioequivalent in comparison to an approved proprietary drug product. The review process for generic drugs is specifically focused on bioequivalence testing rather than safety and efficacy. Thus, conventional clinical testing is not required. To be considered bioequivalent, both the rate and extent of drug absorption must be within established parameters in comparison to the reference drug. In vivo (within a biological system) bioequivalence testing is required for most tablet and capsule dosage forms. Applicants may request a waiver from performing in vivo bioequivalence studies for certain drug products where bioavailability may be established by submitting (1) a formulation comparison for products whose bioavailability is evident (eg, oral solutions, injectables) or (2) comparative dissolution. The FDA provides guidance on establishing bioequivalency and Chapter 53 (*Bioavailability and Bioequivalency Testing*) discusses bioequivalency in greater detail. If any portion of the application is not acceptable, a letter of deficiency is issued which details the insufficiencies and requests additional information and data to resolve these concerns. A tentative approval letter delaying the marketing of the generic product may be issued if approval of the generic occurs prior to the expiration date of patents or exclusivities of the reference drug product.

Rapid Access to New Drug Products

As a result of the demand for more rapid access to new drug products, the FDA has written several regulations and policies specifically designed for drugs intended to treat severely debilitating or life-threatening illnesses. Subpart E (21 CFR 312.80-.88) regulations expedite the development and approval process. Subpart H (21 CFR 314.500-.550) allows the FDA to approve a new drug based on a surrogate endpoint (laboratory finding or physical sign that may not be a direct measure of patient response, yet is considered likely to predict therapeutic benefit). Treatment INDs (21 CFR 312.34) are intended to make drugs that are relatively far along in the development process available to seriously ill patients and are typically made available during Phase III clinical trials. The parallel track is an FDA policy focused on patients with clinically significant illnesses related to human immunodeficiency virus (HIV) diseases who cannot be enrolled in ongoing treatments trials (ie, do not meet inclusion criteria, are too severely ill, enrollment is completed, etc). These patients may receive treatment in an open-label design before safety and efficacy have been established.

ORPHAN DRUG APPROVAL

Orphan drugs are defined as drugs used to treat rare diseases or conditions that affect less than 200,000 people in the United States. Orphan drugs go through the same FDA review process previously described. However, the review is generally expedited through FD&C Act Subpart E, as the majority of orphan drugs are used in the treatment of serious or life-threatening disease. The process by which a company can file an application for orphan drug designation is described in 21 CFR Section 316.20. Due to the substantial drug development costs, this class of drugs provides limited opportunities for companies to recoup their investments. The United States federal government through the Orphan Drug Act of 1983 established tax incentives, reduced user fees, and exclusivity agreements to encourage research in the orphan diseases.[12] Grants are also available through the FDA to support clinical research and annual requests for applications may be found in the Federal Register. From 1983 to 1995, 121 drugs have been brought to market in the US under the Act.[12]

Over-The-Counter Drug Approval

The approval process for over-the-counter (OTC) drugs is considerably different from prescription medications and the review is not held to the same standards as a NDA. The first phase of the approval process involves an advisory panel consisting of a multidisciplinary group of scientists that review data provided by manufacturers and other previously published research. The findings are submitted to the FDA and these reports are subsequently summarized in the Federal Register. Interested parties are given an opportunity to comment. Next, the FDA reviews all statements and publishes a tentative final monograph. The FDA also publishes the nature of comments received and provides further opportunity for feedback. Then, the final monograph is published in the Federal Register and goes into effect one year after publication. The monographs

establish conditions under which OTC drugs are generally recognized as safe and effective and are not misbranded. By following a monograph, a company can then market an OTC drug without additional FDA approval. For any unsubstantiated claims that a company wishes to make (ie, claims not approved in the monograph), data must be presented to the FDA to justify revision of the monograph or the sponsor may submit a NDA.

POST-APPROVAL ACTIVITIES

Safety Monitoring

After a NDA has been granted and marketing of the drug product is initiated, drug safety is still monitored. Sponsors of the NDA must submit reports of adverse events periodically. For newly approved drugs, these reports are filed quarterly for the first three years then annually. For adverse events that are considered serious and unexpected (ie, fatal or life-threatening, permanently disabling, or requiring or prolonging hospitalization), the sponsor must provide a written report to the FDA within 15 days of receipt of the information. The FDA's MedWatch program encourages health-care providers to directly report serious adverse reactions to drugs to the FDA (www.fda.gov/medwatch). The program also provides alerts to practitioners regarding actions and recommendations by the FDA. Serious adverse events may require minor labeling changes or the addition of warning or precaution statements. If serious safety concerns arise, FDA may withdraw approval of the NDA. Often times an FDA Advisory Committee reviews the NDA in light of the new data prior to an official NDA withdrawal. In some instances, manufacturers have withdrawn drug products prior to FDA action.[13] Periodic, random inspections of drug production facilities are conducted by FDA to ensure conformance with regulations and current Good Manufacturing Practices (see 21 CFR Sections 210 and 211).

Changes to an Approved Product

Any change made to an FDA-approved drug product, including component or composition, chemical synthesis, analytical methods, manufacturing site, manufacturing process, batch size, or labeling, must be submitted to the FDA. Some of the so-called scale-up and post approval changes (SUPAC) require FDA approval prior to the implementation of the change. Depending on the type of change made and the impact the change may have on the quality of the drug product, notification to the FDA may be done through annual reports or supplemental new drug applications (SNDA).

CLINICAL TRIAL PLANNING AND DESIGN

Once pre-clinical testing has been completed, the company will determine whether to pursue further development of the drug, often based on the attractiveness and competitiveness of the pharmaceutical.[14] First, the pharmacological profile must be such that the product will be equal to or better than existing competitors in regards to therapeutic effect. Second, the drug should address an unmet medical need or improve therapy in a population of individuals. The incidence of morbidity and mortality associated with the illness impacts medical need. Third, the market potential must be sufficient to sustain profitability. The number of patients who might change from other therapies to the new therapy is considered. Fourth, risk factors for drug development are assessed. Potential risk is impacted by the pharmacological profile, specifically the efficacy and toxicity of the drug. Fifth, the potential expenses associated with activities required to continue development of the drug are considered. Sixth, the success in the marketplace is estimated. Success is determined by the number of competitors, whether the drug is the first in its class, and the potential for patients to change from other competing products. Once the pharmaceutical company determines that the product has good potential for success, clinical trials are planned and conducted to move the product forward. The remaining sections of this chapter discuss the clinical trial process for pharmaceutical development and subsequent therapeutic research of marketed products.

Selecting Trial Objectives

The trial objectives vary depending upon the phase of the trial. Objectives for Phase I trials are limited to determining toxicity at a range of dosages. Phase I trials of treatments for terminal illnesses such as cancer chemotherapy or human immunosuppressive virus may also involve efficacy assessment. Objectives of Phase II and III trials are usually based upon clinical efficacy of the product in an increasingly large sample of patients, respectively. Phase IV trials generally assess efficacy and side effects in specific patient populations.

A statement of trial objectives should include, at minimum, the approach of the trial (eg, to compare, assess, evaluate), the specific disease, the types of patients, drug therapy(ies) and dosages being studied, the purpose (eg, safety, efficacy, pharmacokinetic properties) and the clinical endpoints to be measured (eg, biologic measure, rate of cure, cost effectiveness).[15] Clinical trial objectives drive the entire project, from determination of sample size, to recruitment, to measurement of effects of the drug. They also determine feasibility of the trial, because trial duration and costs are directly impacted by the objective under consideration. Objectives involving ultimate outcomes such as mortality or hospitalizations can require durations of several years as well as large sample sizes and multiple trial sites. Trial objectives limited to pharmacokinetic or clinical measurements may be conducted over a shorter time period, at a single site, and with a small number of patients. Generally, broader objectives have more generalizability and, thus, greater clinical implications.

Often several trial objectives are of interest. When this is the case, the clinical question that is most crucial becomes the primary objective and the others become secondary objectives. Selecting the primary objective is important because determination of sample size and data analyses techniques is based upon it. Although secondary objectives should be assessed in regards to sample size, it is understood that sample size may be inadequate to address all of them. Data collection procedures and statistical analyses are established from the trial objectives during planning.

Occasionally results indicate no significant difference in the primary objective, yet the secondary objectives are significant. An example is the DIG trial, where no significant differences in the primary objective of all-cause mortality were found between the digoxin versus placebo treatments, but there were significant differences in rates of and days of hospitalization, and quality of life.[16] Thus, secondary objectives can be very important and should be well-described prior to the conduct of the trial.

Trial Designs

Various designs are used in clinical trials, and the most suitable may be related to the testing phase of the research trial. During Phase I trials, all patients receive the drug, thus an unblinded, open label trial is suitable. In Phase II through III trials, clinical efficacy trial objectives usually dictate that the drug is compared to placebo (inactive treatment) or an alternative therapy. Usually patients receive one of the treatments during the entire course of the trial. This is referred to as a parallel design. Depending upon the objectives of the trial, the treatments may vary by drug, combinations of drug therapy, or dosage levels. In some parallel trials the same patients may receive various dosages of a drug therapy over time. A factorial design is a type of parallel design used to compare different types and combinations of drug therapy. It allows comparisons between single drug therapies and the combination of the two drugs combined. Factorial designs answer several clinical questions with one trial but are complex and must include sufficient sample sizes to detect differences between all treatment options. An example is the Veterans Affairs Cooperative Studies Program trial of terazosin, an alpha blocker, and finasteride, an anti-androgen, for benign prostatic hypertrophy.[17] The research question included comparisons between each drug and each drug versus placebo plus the combination of both drugs versus the other three therapies.

Another type of trial is the crossover design. Crossover designs allow for patients to receive more than one drug treatment or dosage level during the course of the trial. The assumption with a crossover design is that the drug therapy does not have a carry-over effect between the different treatment periods. Usually there is a "washout" period between drug treatment periods, where patients receive a placebo or no medication. The length of time for the "washout" period is dependent upon the duration of action or rate of elimination of the trial drug(s). A key issue to be addressed in crossover designs is whether the washout period is sufficient to eliminate potential carryover effects of the drug(s). If a drug may have long-term effects after it is discontinued, the crossover design is inappropriate. In crossover designs, the type or dosage of therapy may be randomly assigned to allow for detection of crossover effects (Table 48-1). During the washout period, trial data and clinical measures are collected to assess impact of the previous treatments. These measures are considered baseline data for subsequent treatments. Crossover designs are efficient in regards to numbers of patients required to collect a great deal of scientific data. Repeated measures statistical analyses are used to account for the potential impact of collecting data in the same patients over time and different treatments.

In postmarketing surveillance (Phase IV) trials, nonexperimental (observational) designs are used. These include epidemiologic designs such as case-control or cohort studies in which drug therapy is not assigned by the researcher.[18]

Controlling for Bias

A critical component of a clinical trial is control of the intervention being studied. Control occurs primarily at three levels: assignment of patients to the interventions, application of the intervention, and measurement of the trial outcomes.

Table 48-1. Patient Treatment Regimens in a Crossover Design with Three Treatments and Washout Periods

PATIENT	FIRST TREATMENT	WASHOUT PERIOD	SECOND TREATMENT	WASHOUT PERIOD	THIRD TREATMENT
1	A	Placebo or no treatment	B	Placebo or no treatment	C
2	A		C		B
3	B		C		A
4	B		A		C
5	C		B		A
6	C		A		B

ASSIGNMENT OF INTERVENTION

Ability to control assignment is important because cause and effect relationships between drug therapy and clinical outcomes can then be established. Unless the assignment is controlled, confounding variables may affect the outcomes measured in the trial. Control of assignment of interventions is usually accomplished through randomization, whereby patients are assigned to treatment groups by chance. A randomization scheme generated by a computer program or from random numbers lists is often used to assure that assignment to treatment intervention is unbiased.

In most trials, patients have an equal chance of receiving each treatment. However, some trials are designed to have imbalance in treatment assignment. For example, if previous clinical research indicates one treatment is likely to be superior, more patients may be randomly assigned to that treatment (for example 2:1 or 3:1). Specific statistical analysis techniques are used to adjust for the differences in sample size.

Stratified randomization is used to adjust for potential differences in response between specific patient groups or trial sites. The characteristic of concern (eg, type or severity of disease, gender, age, race, or study site) is determined, and then patients are randomized within their stratification group. This assures that equal numbers of patients with these characteristics are assigned to each trial treatment. For example, after stratified randomization, equal proportions of patients in each treatment group would be male or over age 65, etc.

Block randomization is also used in clinical trials. The sample size for a specific number of patients is established so that, as randomization occurs, at regular intervals equal numbers of patients are assigned to each treatment group. This procedure avoids an imbalance in enrollment between the treatment groups as the trial progresses. Often, the sizes of the blocks of trial patients are randomly varied (eg, 8, 4, 16, 12), to help prevent site personnel from guessing patient treatment assignment.

APPLICATION OF INTERVENTIONS

The protocol is used to control the application of the intervention during a clinical trial. Unless the interventions are provided similarly to all patients between and within each treatment group, variations in outcomes may be due to differences in how the intervention was administered. Protocols are designed to address most potential contingencies that occur during the trial, including requirements for dosage adjustments associated with varying patient conditions. Protocol adherence is monitored throughout the trial. Deviations from the protocol are documented and discussed by individuals administering the trial. Clinical site personnel may need to be retrained regarding the protocol or, if deviations are common, the protocol may need revision. In multi-center trials, repeated deviations by a particular site may result in disciplinary action such as removal from participation in the trial.

MEASUREMENT OF TRIAL OUTCOMES

Control of the measurement of trial outcomes is also critical to decrease bias. This is accomplished in several manners. If a special type of measurement tool or instrument is used to measure outcomes, training of all trial personnel regarding use of the instrument is performed prior to trial start-up. Training usually includes an assessment tool to determine whether personnel are using the instrument(s) uniformly. To eliminate the impact of different laboratory procedures, a centralized laboratory for analysis of specimens is often used. Another method is to have a centralized group review and analyze assessments conducted at the trial site(s). When the determination of a trial outcome (endpoint) involves medical judgment, a centralized endpoints committee is used. The endpoints committee reviews the data and determines whether the outcome assessment has

been correctly identified and attributed to treatment. The endpoints committee is composed of specialists in the medical subject of the research.

Selecting the Trial Population

Patients are selected for clinical trials using inclusion and exclusion criteria. For Phase I trials, healthy volunteers are generally enrolled (with the exception of drug trials for the treatment of life-threatening diseases). In contrast, patients with the disease are enrolled in Phase II and III trials, and the goal is to select patients to participate in the trial who will likely benefit from the treatment. Inclusion criteria are also used to identify patient groups specified by the trial objectives. Exclusion criteria are used to eliminate patients who might be harmed by treatment, who are unlikely to survive the entire trial period due to nonrelated health problems, or those who should not receive the drug treatment due to allergy, concomitant illness, or a contraindication.

Sample Size

Determination of sample size is a critical aspect of clinical trial design. Sample size is based upon four factors: the expected difference in clinical outcomes between the treatments, the level of error in measurement of clinical outcomes, the alpha level, and the power desired for the trial. Table 48-2 depicts the interrelationships between these four concepts and sample size in clinical trials.

The size of the difference between treatments is predicted based upon the difference that is considered "clinically important" and results of previous research. The question to consider is: How great a difference in the outcome is needed for a clinician to consider changing from standard (or placebo) therapy to the new treatment? Medical specialists are consulted to answer this question. If the intervention is unlikely to achieve this difference in outcomes, then the trial is infeasible. If the difference selected is so small that it is unlikely to change clinical practice, the trial will be inefficient or superfluous.

The "clinically important" difference is adjusted by the level of inherent error in measurement of the outcome. For clinical outcomes that are parametric measures, which have a definite 0 and are mathematically uniform across the scale of measurements, this is expressed as standard deviation, or the inter-related terms, variance or standard error. The "clinically important" difference in outcomes is divided by the amount of inherent error in measurement of outcomes to determine effect size of the treatment expected.

The statistical alpha level is also incorporated into sample size analysis. Alpha is equivalent to Type I error which is defined as the chance of accepting the conclusion that treatments are different when the two treatments are equal. Generally, an alpha level of 0.05 is accepted for medical research. This is equivalent to 5 chances in 100 of making the wrong conclusion that there is a difference between the treatments.

Table 48-2. Interrelationships Between Factors Used to Determine Sample Size in Clinical Trials

	IMPACT ON SAMPLE SIZE	
FACTOR IN CALCULATING SAMPLE SIZE	INCREASE IN FACTOR	DECREASE IN FACTOR
Clinically-important difference between treatments	↓	↑
Inherent error in measurement of outcome	↑	↓
Statistical alpha level	↓	↑
Desired power level	↑	↓

Beta level is known as the chance of a Type II error. Type II error is the chance of concluding that no difference exists between the treatments, when one truly exists. In medical research, beta levels of 0.1 or 0.2 are generally acceptable. This can be interpreted as 10 to 20 chances in 100 that no difference is found by the trial when one truly exists. Power of the trial is 1.00 − beta. The concept of power can be interpreted as: the likelihood of finding a difference when one truly exists. Thus, power levels between 80% and 90% are usually considered sufficient in medical research.

Sample size estimation requires consideration of several scientific aspects of the trial. Since all four factors must be balanced in this calculation, there are usually several potential alternative sample size scenarios developed before a decision regarding sample size is reached. Planning the appropriate sample size is critical to the success of the trial. An inadequate sample size may cause the trial to have insufficient power to detect a significant difference. An excessive sample size results in unnecessary costs and additional risks for patients exposed to ineffective treatment.

Feasibility of Conducting the Trial

Feasibility is dependent upon the trial purpose, the intended application of trial results, and access to trial sites and patients. Generally, the question of feasibility comes down to overall trial cost and timeline, which are intertwined with the primary objective and the sample size required to complete the trial. If the trial purpose is extensive and the results are intended to be generalizable across a broad population, the sample size will be large. Prevention of disease events may require long observation periods, significantly lengthening trial duration and, thus, costs. If the trial population is transient, it may be difficult to perform sufficient patient follow-up over long time periods.

Another aspect of trial purpose that impacts feasibility is the type of outcome. Outcomes of mortality often require lengthy observation periods, depending upon the baseline mortality rate of the trial population. Furthermore, outcomes that are intended to be generalizable across a wide range of patients need to have broad inclusion criteria and few exclusion criteria, to assure that all relevant types of patients are represented in the trial. Lastly, the trial outcome measurements directly affect the type and quantity of data required, as well as additional testing requirements specific for the trial.

Access to trial patients impacts feasibility of conducting the clinical trial. Prior to trial initiation, the number of available patients in a health system is estimated, along with the percentage likely to meet inclusion criteria and enroll. These values are used to determine the number of patients required for recruitment. The rate of estimated enrollment is frequently much greater that actual enrollment.[19] Increasing the number of trial sites can enhance access, but with substantial cost. Many pharmaceutical companies outsource this portion of the drug development process to contract research organizations (CROs). CROs can help identify and provide access to patients. Proper management of outsourcing projects can provide a cost-efficient method for new drug development, saving a pharmaceutical company time, space, and manpower.

Drug Product Design and Blinding

Blinding involves the disguising of drug therapy to the patient and health professionals to minimize the introduction of bias into the trial. It is often an essential characteristic of a controlled trial. Blinding is categorized as single, double, or triple. Single blinding indicates that only the patient is unaware of which treatment group they are assigned. Double blinding indicates that both the patient and the health professional evaluating the effect and collecting data are unaware of trial drug assignment. Triple blinding indicates additional blinding of the

biostatistician and Data Safety and Monitoring Board, who assess the comparative safety and efficacy of the treatments during the trial.

Blinding is achieved by developing dosage forms of active and placebo (inert ingredients only) that are indistinguishable in regards to size, shape, color, odor, weight, and other characteristics. Blinding generally requires some type of manipulation of the dosage form, and common techniques and considerations for blinding drug products are displayed in Table 48-3.[20] Ideally, the manufacturer produces a matching placebo (or active comparator) for each drug using a similar formulation, but without the active ingredient. However, it may not be economical or timely for the pharmaceutical company to do so. In these cases the researcher may need to develop matching drug products. Irrespective of the technique used, blinding must not significantly alter the drug release characteristics, the physical stability of the dosage form, or the chemical stability of the active component.[21] In vitro tests for dissolution and potency may be needed to ensure the blinding technique does not affect the performance of the dosage form. In addition, labeling is used to assure that different drugs or dosages used in the trial are indistinguishable.

When factorial designs are used, blinding of each drug product is required. Although it is sometimes possible to make matching dosage forms with each study drug, it is more common to use a "double dummy" approach. This method involves the preparation of a separate matching placebo for each drug product used in the trial. For example, a patient may take two placebo products, an active and placebo combination, or two active drug products. A disadvantage of the double dummy method is that, for drugs used in multiple daily doses, patients must take a large number of dosage forms each day, which can affect patient adherence with the therapeutic regimen.

Trial Drug Packaging

Packaging trial drugs involves creativity as well as consideration of the scientific aspects of the trial. Drugs are packaged to (1) meet trial design requirements, (2) maintain the blinding, (3) minimize the chances for dosing errors, (4) enhance patient adherence to the therapeutic regimen, and (5) maintain drug potency/stability. Package sizes (eg, count per bottle and number of bottles per kit) are designed to meet trial requirements of dosage adjustments, clinical visit periods, visit windows, and dosing frequency. For example, in the DIG trial[16] patients were dosed from 0.125 mg to 0.5 mg (1 to 4 tablets) per day, depending upon clinical response. Patient clinic visits were scheduled for every 4 months ± 14 days. Patients taking 1 or 2 tablets daily were dispensed 1 bottle of 270 dosage units (0.125 mg digoxin or matching placebo tablets) whereas 2 bottles were dispensed to patients taking 3 or 4 tablets per day. Therefore, the package size of 270 tablets was sufficient to meet the requirements of all dosage levels used in the trial for the maximum 134-day visit window.

Clinical trial drug packaging helps to maintain the blinding of the drug through assuring that package style and labeling are exactly equivalent between the different drugs and their matching placebos. Each package is labeled with unique bottle numbers or patient therapy numbers to assure that the therapy matches the treatment assignment. A database is maintained which provides the correspondence between the bottle or therapy number and treatment assignment. Bottle or therapy number assignments can be provided to clinical trial personnel through pre-determined lists or through real-time methods such as telephone assignment systems or web-based programs.

Complicated dosage regimens must occasionally be accommodated in trial drug packaging designs. For example, a patient may receive induction (ramp-up) dosing, taper dosing, or individualized dosing with multiple dosage adjustments during a trial. For oral dosage forms, blister cards can accommodate

Table 48-3. Techniques and Considerations for Blinding of Drug Products

TYPE OF ORIGINAL DOSAGE FORM	TECHNIQUE	CONSIDERATIONS
Tablet	Removal of markings	• Time consuming and manually intensive • Still must match size/shape/color of tablet • Process may alter release properties of a film coating
	Over-encapsulation	• Time consuming and manually intensive • Patients may open capsule and discover original dosage form
	Grinding and re-tableting	• Properties of new dosage form may be different from original form, affecting patient response • Complexity in developing new formulation
	Grinding and encapsulating	• Properties of new dosage form may be different from original, potentially affecting patient response. • Assuring blend uniformity of grinded dosage form while encapsulating • Manually intensive, unless automated encapsulating equipment is available
	Tablet overcoating	• Tablets are developed to match original dosage form • Preserves original dosage form • Pharmaceutical testing (ie,. dissolution) can help verify similarity to original dosage • Cannot be used for embossed tablets
Capsules	Removal of markings	• Time consuming and manually intensive • Still must match size/shape/color of capsule
	Over-encapsulating Grinding and re-encapsulating	• Same as above tablets • Capsule shells from original dosage form may be visible in manufactured product
	Removing ingredients from capsule shells and encapsulating	• Manually intensive • Time consuming • Most capsules are difficult to open
Oral solutions	Matching solution without active ingredient	• Taste and odor may be unique to active ingredient • Discoloration of active ingredient over time may occur and cause unblinding
Injectables	Matching solution without active ingredient Blinding just prior to administration	• May be difficult to obtain in same packaging and labeling • Differences in odor or color • Unblinded pharmacy personnel prepare injectable dosage form • Additional opportunity for communication of actual treatment to trial personnel
Topical, including skin patches	Matching product without active ingredient	• Difficult to match packaging, unless prepared by manufacturer • Odor, texture, or color may differ between products

Adapted from Carney CF, Killeen MJ, Galloway-Ludwig S. *Pharm Eng* 1995; 15(3):42.

these alternatives, while helping to minimize dosing errors. For example in a trial comparing clozapine versus haloperidol, blister card dosing allowed for combinations of active and placebo capsules to be included in each daily dosing regimen.[16,23] Since patients received dosages based upon symptoms of schizophrenia, dosages could range from 100 to 1200 mg per day for clozapine or from 5 to 30 mg for haloperidol. Patients received from 4 to 9 matching capsules daily with combinations of active and placebo capsules of 3 strengths of clozapine (12.5 mg, 25 mg, or 100 mg) and one strength of haloperidol (5 mg) or placebo. Patients randomized to clozapine or haloperidol received matching placebo capsules of the other drug. The use of combinations of active and placebo capsules allowed for blinded dosing adjustments to be made as well as induction and taper dosing. Through a computerized assignment system, specific cards were assigned according to the clinical criteria established in the protocol. Once the card was assigned, dosage errors were minimized because all patients took the same number of capsules daily regardless of drug treatment.

Blister card dosage packages can also help improve adherence with orally administered drug, because dosage times can be specified on the cards. In addition, the cards provide direct and timely feedback to patients and clinical trial personnel regarding adherence. Pharmaceutical potency and stability are further considerations for clinical trial drug packaging. Any drug product not stored in the original manufacturers' packages should be subjected to periodic, scheduled testing (potency, dissolution) to verify stability during the clinical trial.

Regulations Governing the Conduct of Clinical Trials

Prior to initiation of any trial among human subjects, approval must be obtained from the investigator's local institutional review board (IRB). Composed of experts and laymen with varying backgrounds, IRB committees critically review clinical protocols to ensure patient safety and institutional, regulatory, and professional acceptability. IRBs also assess the trial protocol regarding scientific validity and whether the study involves unwarranted risks to the patients. The IRB also will determine if the protocol includes appropriate patient populations and whether inducements to participate in the trial are reasonable and non-coercive. Approval signals that the IRB has determined that the trial is appropriate and does not involve undue risks to the participant. IRB approval must be renewed annually for the trial to continue.

A critical aspect of clinical trial conduct is informed consent from participants. Participants must be informed of all aspects of the trial including the rationale and previous research, potential risks and benefits, treatment alternatives, the likelihood of being randomized to a particular treatment, discomforts associated with the trial, that they may voluntarily dis-enroll at any time, and their rights for future treatment should they be affected adversely by the trial. Informed consent documents must be at a reading level understandable by patients. IRB committees review and approve these documents. In addition to written informed consent, the trial must be discussed verbally with the patient. Each page must be initialed and dated by the patient and clinical personnel, as well as signatures on the final page of the document. A copy of this legal document is given to the patient as well maintained in patient records throughout the trial.

In April 2003, the Health Insurance Portability and Accountability Act of 1996 (HIPAA) was implemented. This act provides that patients be informed of their rights to maintain the privacy of their health information. Data collection for clinical trials is impacted by HIPAA in that patients must be informed of their rights and provided written consent to researchers to access their medical records. Researchers must verify that they will not allow data collected during the trial to be distributed with patient-identifiable information. HIPPA requirements can be addressed within the informed consent process. More information is available at www.cms.hhs.gov/hipaa.

GOOD CLINICAL PRACTICE MONITORING

FDA regulations governing the conduct of clinical trials, referred to as Good Clinical Practices (GCP), are specified in 21 CFR Sections 50, 56, 312, and 314. In addition, the International Conference on Harmonization has established guidelines to assure patient safety during clinical trials at an international level (www.ich.org). GCP training is necessary for all personnel who are involved in the conduct of a clinical trial.

In addition to addressing patient safety, GCP regulations also help protect against fraud and falsification of trial data. There are significant incentives to health care professionals to assure that patients are enrolled and complete all follow-up visits and that positive trial results are achieved. These incentives include direct financial gain because some trial sponsors reimburse based upon per capita enrollment and/or per follow-up visit. In addition, future funding may be discontinued if results are negative. Sometimes clinical researchers may have financial investments in the company sponsoring the trial. There are also academic pressures to achieve positive results, as trials with positive results tend to more likely be published in prestigious journals. Failure to attempt to publish negative results has been considered a form of scientific misconduct.[24] Fraud and falsification of data have been identified in published literature.[25,26]

The GCP monitoring of clinical trials involves outside reviewers who monitor trial conduct and data collection. Reviewers are specially trained to match trial data with source documentation (data that is not collected as part of the trial) to identify fraud and falsification of data. GCP monitoring is required for any trial that will be used commercially to gain FDA approval or change the labeling or advertising of a drug product. FDA inspections of study sites are also conducted after completion of the trial to verify the appropriate conduct of the trial and the veracity of its results. The FDA requires that all trial records be maintained and accessible at the trial sites for a minimum of 2 years after marketing or change in labeling of a drug product. If marketing or change in labeling is not pursued, records must be maintained for 2 years after completion of the study and FDA notification.

Monitoring and Reporting Adverse Events during Clinical Trials

Safety data are important outcomes of clinical trials. Due to randomization, blinding, and placebo control, trials can provide unbiased reports of prevalence and incidence rates of adverse events. FDA regulations specify how adverse events should be reported. Serious adverse events (SAEs) are defined as those that result in death, are life threatening, cause hospitalization or prolong hospitalization, cause cancer or congenital abnormalities, or require extensive treatment to prevent hospitalization. Unexpected adverse events are defined as events that are

not previously identified as associated with the drug by nature of the event, its severity, or its frequency. Unexpected SAEs must be reported to the FDA within 7 calendar days of disclosure to the trial sponsor. They also must be reported to site investigators who are required to report them to their local IRB. SAEs are summarized in the IND annual report that is submitted to the FDA. Furthermore, SAEs resulting in patient's termination from the trial are summarized in the IND annual report. All clinical and subjective information relevant to the event are reported in the SAE reports. For ongoing SAEs, follow-up reports are completed.

Other adverse events (AEs) are also collected regularly during clinical trials. Although these are less severe, they provide important information regarding the impact of drug therapy. AEs are usually coded to a common glossary, so that, although clinicians may use different descriptors for similar events, the events can be consolidated. The FDA has adopted the Medical Dictionary for Drug Regulatory Affairs (MedDRA) as the standard coding system for AE reports. AEs can be categorized by type of event, severity, relatedness to study treatment, intervention used to treat the event, and outcome. Comparisons of incidence rates (number of events per person-years) between drug treatment groups are specified in clinical trial publications. AE data from a minimal number of patients are required for NDAs. However, the limited number of patients exposed at the approval stage, usually about 3000 to 5000, is insufficient for determination of rare adverse events.[27] Thus, postmarketing studies of adverse events are used to identify rare events. The reporting of unusual AEs to the FDA during clinical trials help provide additional data on rare events.

For trials over 1 year in duration, monitoring of the results of the trial is conducted periodically. An impartial group, such as a Data Safety and Monitoring Board (DSMB), provides this oversight. Monitoring usually includes both clinical efficacy and adverse events. Interim reports are usually provided to the DSMB group in a blinded format so that although the treatment groups are compared, the DSMB cannot determine which group is better or worse in terms of efficacy or adverse events. The DSMB has the power to recommend discontinuance of the trial and will do so if there is clear evidence that it may be detrimental to patients assigned to one of the treatment groups if the trial is continued. This may be due to strong evidence of efficacy or safety differences between the groups. Interim statistical analyses that are provided in DSMB reports are preplanned and included in the overall plan for statistical testing.[28]

Overview of Statistical Analysis of Clinical Trial Data

It is not possible to provide comprehensive descriptions of statistical methodologies in this chapter; the reader is referred to statistical textbooks for further information.[29,30] However, certain general statistical issues will be discussed in brief.

Good clinical research will always be conducted using an intention to treat analysis (ITA).[31] This means that even if the patient has stopped taking the medication, did not complete the assigned treatment, or has been switched to an active alternative therapy, the data from the patient is included in the original treatment group to which the patient was randomized. The impact of ITA is to lessen the likelihood of finding a difference between the treatments. However, the ITA is more analogous to what happens outside of the clinical trial situation. Patients typically do not fully comply with therapy or may change therapies. Thus ITA is a key statistical feature of clinical trials.

Adjustment for multiple comparisons is another statistical consideration of clinical trials. The adjustment involves lowering the statistical boundary at which the researcher will consider the results significantly different. When the same data are used for multiple statistical tests, such as in provision of multiple reports to the DSMB, there is an increased likelihood that a significant difference will be found by chance. If one considers alpha = 0.05 to be acceptable, this means the researcher is willing to accept a 1 in 20 chance that a significant finding will be in error. By doing multiple tests, for example four tests on the same data, the alpha level changes to 4/20 or 1 in 5. A conservative adjustment of alpha for multiple tests is Bonferroni correction, which involves dividing the alpha level by the number of tests. For example, performing four tests at an overall alpha = 0.05 would change to alpha = 0.0125, thus the researcher would not consider the result significant unless the statistical finding was $p \le 0.0125$.

Another statistical consideration in clinical trials is subgroup analysis. Once the data are obtained, researchers sometimes re-analyze data from many different perspectives, for example, dividing the data into several different patient groups. Pre-planned comparisons, such as those in secondary objectives, are acceptable. However, results of comparisons conducted post-hoc should be interpreted cautiously, especially if based upon trends in the data, as the findings may be misleading. Some potential causes of the deceptive findings are: (1) the trial was not designed to assure there was adequate sample size for the subgroup analysis, (2) potentially confounding variables were not measured or controlled, and (3) insufficient theoretical underpinnings for the test. The number of subgroup analyses should be minimized, and if results of subgroup analyses are published, these limitations should be clearly stated as speculative.

SUMMARY

In the United States, new drug products must be shown to be safe and effective before they are approved by the FDA for marketing. This chapter outlined the various stages involved in new drug development, including the milestones of IND and NDA submission. The costs associated with the development of new drug products are substantial and the most significant expenditures occur during clinical testing. Thus, the design and conduct of clinical trials are critical to successful drug product development. Several considerations in clinical trial design have been highlighted. The reader is encouraged to refer to specific FDA guidance documents and other referenced materials for further information.

REFERENCES

1. Cato A, Sutton L, Cato AE. *Current challenges and future directions of drug development.* In: Cato AE, ed. *Clinical Drug Trials and Tribulations.* New York: Marcel Dekker, 2002; pp 1-19.
2. DiMasi JA, Hansen RW, Grabowski HG. *J Health Econ* 2003; 22:151.
3. Grabowski HG, Vernon J, DiMasi J. *Pharmacoeconomics* 2002; 20(suppl 3):11.
4. Wax PM. *Ann Intern Med* 1995; 122(6):456.
5. Matthews SJ, McCoy C. *Clin Ther* 2003; 25(2):342.
6. Goyan JE. *Drug Intell Clin Pharm* 1983; 17(7–8):566.
7. Calabrese L, Fleischer AB. *Am J Med* 2000; 108(6):487.
8. Roepstorff P. *Curr Opin Biotech* 1997; 8:6.
9. Lakings DB. Nonclinical drug development: Pharmacology, drug metabolism, and toxicology. In: Guarino RA, ed. *New Drug Approval Process.* 2000, New York: Marcel Dekker, 2002; pp 17–54.
10. Lu C, et al. *Clin Cancer Res* 2003; 9(6):2085.
11. Boothby LA, Doering PL. *Drug Topics* 2003; 147:80.
12. Shulman SR, Manocchia M. *Pharmacoeconomics* 1997; 12(3):312.
13. Chaudhry MU, Simmons DL. *J Ark Med Soc* 2001; 98(1):16.
14. Sedkacek HH, Sapienza AM, Eid V. *Ways to Successful Strategies in Drug Research and Development.* New York: VCH Publishers, 1996; pp 49–90.
15. Spilker B. Establishing clinical trial objectives. In: *Guide to Clinical Trials.* New York: Raven Press, 1991 pp 10–14.
16. Digitalis Investigation Group. *N Engl J Med* 1997; 336(8):525.
17. Lepor H, et al. *N Engl J Med* 1996; 335(8):533.
18. Elwood M. *Critical Appraisal of Epidemilogical Studies and Clinical Trials.* 2nd ed. New York: Oxford University Press, 2000.
19. DeSantis P, Gross LS, DeLuca S. *Prog Cardiovasc Nurs* 1997; 12(3):24.
20. Carney CF, Killeen MJ, Schulteis WM. *Pharm Eng* 1997; 17(2):48.
21. Felton LA, Wiley CJ. *Drug Dev Ind Pharm* 2003; 29(1):9.
22. Carney CF, Killeen MJ, Galloway-Ludwig S. *Pharm Eng* 1995; 15(3):42.
23. Rosenheck R, et al. *N Engl J Med* 1997; 337(12):809.
24. Chalmers I. JAMA 1990; 263(10):1405.
25. Bivens LW, Macfarlane DK. *N Engl J Med* 1994; 330(20):1461.
26. Buyse M, et al. *Stat Med* 1999; 18(24):3435.
27. Ahmad SR. *J Gen Intern Med* 2003; 18(1):57.
28. Rademaker AW. *Contemp Urol* 1994; 6(2):43.
29. Norleans MX. *Statistical Methods for Clinical Trials.* New York: Marcel Dekker, 2001; p 257.
30. Cleophas TJ, Zwinderman AH, Cleophas TF. *Statistics Applied to Clinical Trials,* 2nd ed. Boston: Kluwer Academic, 2002; p 210.
31. Sabin CA, Lepri AC, Phillips AN. *HIV Clin Trials* 2000; 1(2):31.

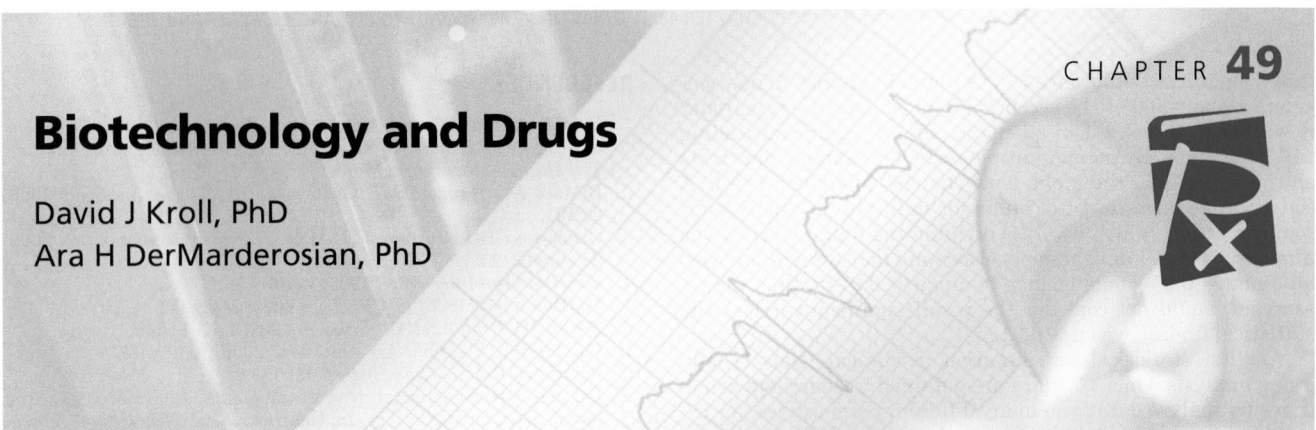

CHAPTER 49

Biotechnology and Drugs

David J Kroll, PhD

Ara H DerMarderosian, PhD

In medical and pharmaceutical history, the last 30 years ultimately will be regarded as the dawn of the age of biotechnology. Previously rare or even unattainable pharmaceuticals can now be produced in useful quantities by harnessing the power of molecular biology. Interestingly, the term *biotechnology* was first coined in 1919 by the Hungarian engineer, Károly (Karl) Ereky, to describe how products could be produced from raw materials with the aid of living organisms as agriculture began to join forces with industry following World War I.[1] Hence, biotechnology is not a new concept. Humans have been manipulating living organisms over the millennia to solve problems and improve the quality of life. But today, especially in the context of science and health, the term biotechnology is used interchangeably with "genetic engineering." The concept of DNA manipulation is central to most modern references to biotechnology.

The practical realization of this technology has followed from our ability to now detect, isolate, produce, and characterize the various proteins that coordinate the numerous functions essential to human life and health. Processes that precede or are causative in pathophysiology cannot only be identified, but also now manipulated in an attempt to restore normal function. This relatively new methodology involves the synergism of discoveries in recombinant DNA methodology, DNA alteration, gene-splicing, genetic engineering, immunology, and immunopharmacology, with advances in automation and data analysis to create a cogent, high-technology industry. Overall, biotechnology has led to the creation of new products for home and industry, improvement of agricultural yields, diagnosis of genetic disorders, and the enhancement of our medical arsenal against disease. The publications in February 2001, of the virtually complete sequence of the human genome[2,3] will certainly accelerate the application of these technologies. While the close of the last millennium has clearly witnessed the benefits resulting from the proliferation of biotechnology-derived products, new questions have arisen regarding issues of ethics and pharmacoeconomics. Nonetheless, it is clear that the benefits of biotechnology already have far outweighed the drawbacks.

BACKGROUND

As biotechnology-derived pharmaceuticals have become commonplace in healthcare, pharmacy practitioners should have a detailed knowledge of the manufacture and use of these newer agents.[4,5] As a backdrop to understanding modern biotechnology, it will be instructive to review some of the basic biological milestones that precede it. Table 49-1 provides a compilation of milestones in biotechnology, both in general and as they relate specifically to the pharmaceutical sciences. It is clear that technology is proceeding at a rate that is already threatening to bypass our ability to manage the ethical dilemmas presented by

these advances. Fortunately, visionaries such as Nobel laureate James Watson have used their positions to encourage the proper and ethical use of genetic information and technology. As the initial director of the publically funded Human Genome Project, Watson announced 15 years ago a plan to set aside 3% of the project budget (now 5%) devoted to ethical, legal, and social implications (ELSI) research, a decision he recently deemed, "probably the smartest thing I did."[6]

Nature has for some 3.5 billion years been conducting what we may call natural genetic experiments. These include mutation (random heredity alteration), crossing-over (breakage and exchange of corresponding segments of homologous chromosomes), and recombination at meiosis (fertilization). These processes all have contributed to the current diversity of life on this planet. In addition, it is well known that humans have been manipulating genetic characteristics of different species for over 10,000 years through inbreeding and cross-breeding experiments. To cite a few examples, one can point to the modern robust strains of wheat or corn, which are a far cry from their puny ancestors. Similarly, the varied breeds of dogs, cats, poultry, and cattle may be mentioned. These manipulative efforts continue, and in less than a lifetime, the development of larger and sweeter oranges, seedless watermelons, and flamboyant ornamental plants has occurred. Also familiar are such hybridizations as the tangelo (crossing the tangerine and the grapefruit) and the mule (crossing a donkey and a horse).

All cell structures and functions begin with proteins, and the code for building the proteins is found in deoxyribonucleic acid (DNA). This is why the discovery of the double-helix structure of DNA by Watson and Crick, in 1953, fundamentally began the unraveling of the mystery of cell processes. (The 50th anniversary of publication of their model was celebrated in 2003, with some exceptional retrospective documentation published in print and on the Internet by Cold Spring Harbor Laboratory and the journals, *Science* and *Nature*). DNA, the genetic blueprint of an organism, is made up of building blocks known as nucleotides (molecules containing a sugar, nitrogen-containing purine or pyrimidine bases, and a phosphate group) that are connected in a very long ladder-like structure. When this rubber-like twisted-ladder structure is coiled tightly, it is referred to as a two-stranded, or double, helix.

There are four different nucleotides (containing the bases adenine, cytosine, guanine, and thymidine) with a total of about 3 billion nucleotide units in the human genome, tightly packed into chromosomes. These include the genetic code for a large number of genes, originally estimated at 100,000 in the human but downgraded to roughly 30,000 as a result of the Human Genome Project. Each of these genes controls the synthesis of a protein made up of a long strand of 50 to 3000 amino acids. Nirenberg and Matthei, in 1961, and others later, elucidated how the nucleotide sequence of a gene regulates the particular

Table 49-1. Milestones in Biotechnology

The recent explosion of growth in the development and application of biotechnology may be traced to a number of successive, discrete, milestone discoveries and events.

1. X-ray diffraction data and proposed double-helix model for the 3-dimensional structure of DNA (RE Franklin and MH Wilkins; JD Watson and FH Crick, 1952–1953).
2. Site-specific recognition and cleavage of DNA by restriction endonucleases (W Arber, 1962; M Meselson and R Yuan, 1968; HO Smith, 1970; D Nathans, 1971).
3. Determination of the genetic code (M Nirenberg, S Ochoa, and P Leder, 1966; HG Khorana, 1966).
4. Identification of DNA ligase (M Gellert, 1967).
5. Identification of RNA-directed DNA polymerase (reverse transcriptase) (HM Temin and S Mizutani, 1970; D Baltimore, 1970).
6. DNA cloning techniques (HW Boyer, S Cohen, and P Berg, 1971–1972).
7. Formal discussions on emerging rDNA technologies (Gordon Conference on Nucleic Acids, June 1973).
8. Asilomar Conference and self-imposed standards for rDNA research (Feb 1975).
9. Hybridoma created (C Milstein and G Kohler, 1975).
10. Recombinant Advisory Committee (RAC) issues guidelines (1976).
11. DNA sequence technologies (F Sanger, 1977; W Gilbert, 1977).
12. US Supreme Court rules that microorganisms are patentable (General Electric *superbug*, 1980).
13. US approval of first diagnostic kit using MAb technology (anti-C3d BioClone: Ortho Diagnostics, 1981).
14. US approval of first ethical pharmaceutical produced by using rDNA technologies (Humulin (human insulin): Genentech and Eli Lilly & Co, 1982).
15. Expression of a foreign gene in plants (bacterial antibiotic resistance gene expressed in tobacco plants: Monsanto Co. Washington University and Max Planck Institute, 1982).
16. The polymerase chain reaction (PCR) methodology enables targeted amplification of DNA sequences (KB Mullis; Cetus Corp., 1983, use of thermostable DNA polymerase, 1988).
17. FDA approval of first recombinant vaccine (for hepatitis B virus; Chiron Corp., 1986).
18. US Patent and Trademarks Office issues first patent for genetically engineered mammal (transgenic mouse: P Leder and Harvard University, 1988).
19. Formal launch of Human Genome Project, 1990
20. First human gene therapy patient (for adenosine deaminase deficiency, WF Anderson, 1990)
21. Dolly the sheep becomes the first cloned mammal (I Wilmut, 1997)
22. Simultaneous publication of human genome sequence by Human Genome Project and Celera Genomics, 2001

---

sequence in which the 20 different amino acids will be united to produce a particular protein. A single codon is made up of units of three adjacent nucleotides; each codon specifies one amino acid. The arrangement of codons in the DNA, following transcription into messenger RNA (mRNA), determines the sequence of amino acids that will form a particular protein. The detailed understanding of how these genes and their proteins govern basic cellular processes is the underpinning of molecular biology and biotechnology.

Because each of the major organs of the body (brain, liver, blood, tissue, etc) has a specified set of tasks to perform, certain specific sets of genes in each organ (collection of specialized cells) must be activated and deactivated, that is, turned *on* and *off* as needed. Following the directions laid down by the genetic code of DNA and mediated by mRNA, each cell type continuously produces a unique and characteristic array of proteins. Each cell type maintains a complement of transcriptional activating and repressing proteins whose actions balance to create the specific gene expression profile of a particular tissue. Moreover, epigenetic processes such as gene methylation and histone acetylation status also contribute to tissue-specific gene expression. Expressed proteins are then secreted into the extracellular milieu, while many are used within the cell itself. The number of possible biosynthetic permutations is very high if one considers that a typical protein can be made up of some 500 amino acids and, further, that every one of these sites may be occupied by any one of 20 different amino acids. It is likely that over the long periods of evolution of each organism, given the vast array of possible combinations of these amino acids, a multitude of unique proteins with all sorts of optimized functions have developed.

The concept that genetic information flows from DNA to RNA to proteins has become a fundamental milestone of modern biology. Thus, with the discovery of reverse transcriptase (from an RNA virus) by Temin and Baltimore, in 1970, which could convert its own genomic RNA into double-stranded RNA, a second milestone was reached. Modern biotechnology relies heavily on this enzyme. Examples of cellular catalysts,

or enzymes, include those that are involved in the digestion of food, and others that produce the chemical building blocks of cell life such as sugars and lipids, hormones for organism regulation, fuel for energy production, and important molecules such as DNA.

Proteins also make up the cell cytoskeleton providing an organized three-dimensional structure. They permit directed transport and movement of molecules throughout the cell. They are embedded in the outer cell membrane and pump nutrients and ions across the membranes. They serve as receptor sites for hormones that finitely adjust the functions of the cell according to changing bodily needs. Another group of proteins regulates gene activities by binding to DNA and activating or repressing gene transcription. Still other proteins, and their smaller fragments (peptides), are secreted by cells as neurotransmitters or hormones like insulin. Some serve as carrier molecules like hemoglobin, the body's oxygen carrier.

As is well recognized, these hormones and various related peptide molecules hold enormous power, and because they can act on numerous specific cell surface receptors, they can influence virtually all bodily functions from the nervous system to the immune system. It is obvious that their selectivity, potency, and often-desired evanescent effects on selective target cells make them enormously attractive candidates as a new generation of drugs in the *magic bullet* concept of Paul Ehrlich. Further, when administered parenterally, hormones have the potential to reach target receptors on the surface of cells, without the need to penetrate membranes. Not unlike the normal bodily processes, they can bind to cell surface receptors and activate the cell's particular function. An example of one such approach is seen with the anticancer drug interleukin-2, which can stimulate some immune cells to attempt to overcome cancerous cell growth.

The body's specific defense response to invading organisms is due to the immune system. Normally, phagocytes called to a site of inflammation induced by pathogens mount a generalized attack response. Indiscriminately, they engulf cellular debris as well as anything recognized as foreign. Occasionally, however, this is not enough, and illness ensues. At this point, several more focused counterattacks proceed by the three types of white blood cells known as macrophages, T lymphocytes, and B lymphocytes. The key features of the immune system are specificity (the ability to focus on specific pathogens) and memory (the ability to recognize and respond rapidly to previously encountered infections). About 1% of the blood cells are white blood cells. The ones that are central to the immune responses are

B Cells—Lymphocytes that produce antibodies (antibody-mediated immune response).

Macrophages—Phagocytic cells that alert helper T cells of the presence of pathogens.

Helper T Cells—*Master switches* of the immune system that stimulate the rapid division of both killer T cells and B cells.

Suppressor T Cells—Lymphocytes with regulatory functions; ie, they slow down or prevent immune responses.

Killer T Cells and Natural Killer (NK) Cells—Lymphocytes that directly destroy body cells that already have been infected by pathogens (or cancer cells).

Memory Cells—A group of the T cell and B cell population that was produced during the primary encounter with a pathogen but was not used in the battle. These circulate through the body ready to respond rapidly to later attacks by the same organisms.

As a further refinement in the understanding of the immune system, several key weapons are involved in the process. These include the antibodies, which are circulating freely or membrane-bound receptor molecules that bind specific foreign invaders and thereby tag them for destruction by the complement system or phagocytes. There are the perforin proteins, which are secreted by certain T cells and kill their cellular targets by punching holes in them. Finally, there are the lymphokines and interleukins that are secretions by which white blood cells communicate with each other. Thus, the immune system has two fighting branches with specificity, and often both are employed against infections and antigens in general. The T cells dominate one part of the system, and when they are activated it is referred to as a *cell-mediated* response. The B cells dominate the other branch, and events associated with their activation are referred to as *antibody-mediated* response.

An edition of *Science*[4] was devoted to the frontiers in biotechnology for the 1990s. It provided articles on new shortcuts of immediate practicality and great interest in understanding the human genome via expressed sequence tags (ESTs) of complementary DNA that has uncovered a large number of new genes (mainly in the brain). Similarly, *lighthouses* have been developed along the chromosomes to guide the way for sequencing dim restriction maps. DNA research using the polymerase chain reaction (PCR) has become a powerful tool in forensic and research applications.

New publications described how modern metabolic engineering has brought intermediary metabolism back to life through techniques involving enhancing copies of a gene at a rate-controlling point, adding a gene to remove a poisonous product, or adding several genes to introduce a new pathway into an organism that stops short of the desired product. This metabolic engineering has had numerous practical results in addition to helping develop new theories. DNA technology has been applied to metabolic pathways so that branch point control problems can be solved. Even the insertion of similar enzymes from different species into the studied organism has introduced new flexibility and better metabolic characteristics into the older organism.

This issue also covered the recent developments of the vaccinia virus, so that it now can serve as a molecular vehicle for carrying foreign genes into other organisms. As a means for research, this recombinant vaccinia vector has served as a vehicle for producing live vaccines that would otherwise be difficult to produce. Also discussed is the use of monoclonal antibodies in diagnosis and therapy. The monoclonal antibody OKT3 has been approved by the FDA for treatment of acute renal allograph rejection. Antibody power has been enhanced by attachment of a biological poison such as ricin, a cytotoxin such as calicheamicin, or a physical agent such as an alpha emitter. The latter can be used to damage tissue adjacent to that with which the antibody interacts. These are all good examples of combined basic research followed by rapid practical application.

BIOTECHNOLOGY DRUGS

In terms of drug therapy, the body's ability to remember and identify previous infections already has been exploited through the vaccination technique. This relatively simple procedure involves injecting the person with a weakened or killed pathogen that induces an effective immune response without causing the disease. The procedure gives a lasting immunity through the formation of the memory cells mentioned above. Continued advantage of these natural phenomena (normal immunization through infection) is being taken through the application of molecular biology and biotechnology. Among the recent and significant developments are the novel vaccines (eg, Recombivax HB *(Merck)*, a hepatitis B vaccine), which are highly specific antibodies that are intended to act like *magic bullets*, and protein drugs that are duplicates of the chemical messages or secreted factors (interleukin-2) through which immune cells communicate with each other. Figure 49-1 shows the production of a genetically engineered vaccine.

As of 2003 it can be said that more biotechnology medicines are in development than ever before. Holmer[7] reported in the 2002 survey of the Pharmaceutical Research and Manufacturers of America (PhRMA) that over the next decade or so, we will see the results of this biotechnology research infrastructure in the forms of cures and treatments for many age-old diseases. These advances will serve to complement the 95 biotechnology products already FDA-approved for therapeutic indications.

This 2002 survey of the PhRMA showed that 371 biotechnology medicines and vaccines are in human clinical trials or are at the FDA awaiting final approval; in 1988 (the first year of the survey) there were 81 biotechnology products, in 1991 there were 132, in 1993 there were 143, and in 1996 there were 284. Even more striking, biotechnology medicines comprise onethird of *all* drugs currently in clinical trials. The growth rate of the industry has increased dramatically, to 77% between the last two surveys and by 100% between 1993 and 1996. This rate of growth has not escaped Wall Street, but investors are now somewhat cautious because of some failures and corporate scandals that have terminated the programs of some companies. The 10–40% annual returns on biotechnology stocks seen in the late 90s had all but evaporated by 2000. However, long-awaited successes in some key therapeutic areas (ie, anti-angiogenic therapies for cancer) has rekindled investor enthusiasm for pharmaceutical biotechnology as the sector is on target to post a nearly 60% return in 2003.

Further study of the 371 biotechnology products now in development showed 144 companies now engaged in treatments for nearly 200 diseases. Fully 48% of the products were in development for cancer treatment, and another 13% are for treating or preventing infectious diseases excluding AIDS/HIV, 7% for autoimmune disorders, and 6% for AIDS/HIV and related disorders. In the mid-1990s, the fastest growing category of biotechnology products had been gene therapy; however, the death of an 18-year-old Phase I gene therapy trial participant, Jesse Gelsinger in 1998 led to a sober reassessment of strategies, precautions, and controls in such trials.[8] The currently fastest growing segments are monoclonal antibodies and vaccines. Vaccine targets are cancer, AIDS, rheumatoid arthritis, and multiple sclerosis. Monoclonal antibodies have also been instrumental in treating various forms of cancer and autoimmune disorders. Product candidates that are nearly approved also are increasing. The number of products in Phase III clinical studies has nearly tripled since 1993 (from 33 to 87). A total of 95 products have been approved by the FDA as of 2002.

Interestingly, several products are being tested for the first time against certain diseases: the common cold due to rhinovirus, Huntington's disease, Parkinson's disease, sickle cell anemia, lupus nephritis, and osteoporosis. In addition, all of

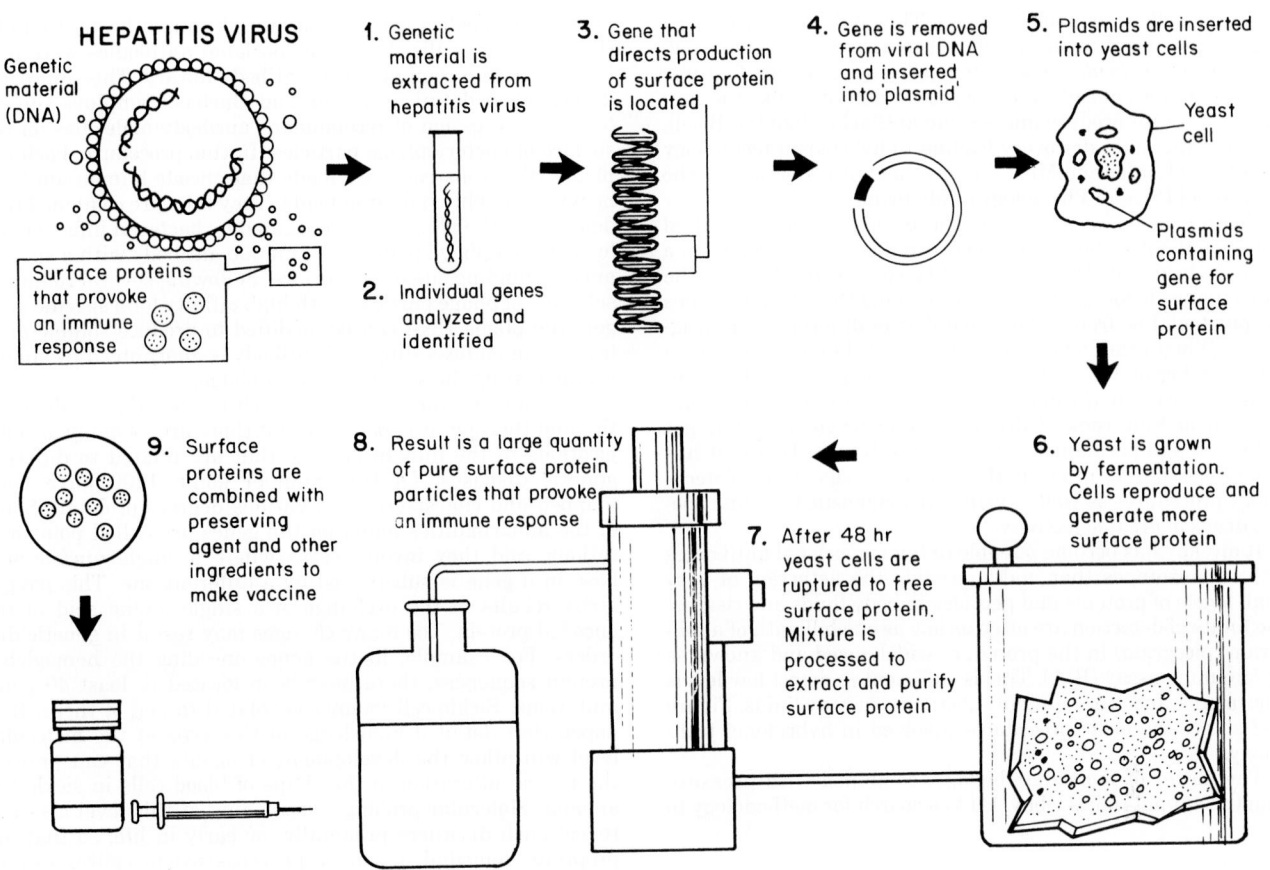

Figure 49-1. Making a genetically engineered vaccine.

these data show that the US pharmaceutical industry continues to hold a worldwide lead in biotechnology research, drugs, and patents. The 1999 figures of the US Office of Patents and Trademarks reveal that the US was the country of origin for 63% of the biotechnology patents issued that year. Japan followed with 13%, the United Kingdom with 10%, and Germany with 7%. With the explosive growth of products in development, space limitations allow us to display only already approved biotechnology products in Appendix A. A glossary of terms also is provided.

All of these agents have been made possible through the biotechnology techniques that allow the isolation, identification, and production of normally minute amounts of proteinaceous *signal agents* found in the extracellular fluids of the body. Once the composition and sequence of amino acids is determined for a protein, that protein can be reproduced in the laboratory. Even better, the protein precursor, DNA, now can be analyzed readily and sequenced, allowing another organism to use that part of the code that determines the protein. This has been made possible through the discovery and use of restriction enzymes by HO Smith, which make specific reproducible cuts along DNA strands. Frederick Sanger et al devised procedures for quickly determining the nucleotide sequence of DNA fragments. This allowed the identification of the DNA sequence of complete genes. Also, the discovery of reverse transcriptase by Temin et al became important in biotechnology because it allowed the mass production of genes from mRNA, which led to increased production of a desired protein. Through these procedures it became possible to determine the amino acid sequence of entire proteins via inference of the genetic code.

The 1972–1973 landmark experiments of Stanley Cohen, Herbert Boyer, and Paul Berg applied this technology to produce recombinant plasmid DNA molecules for propagation in *E*

coli and are recognized as the first creation of a genetically engineered organism capable of producing proteins from another species. This hybrid plasmid now could be grown in the common and rapidly producing bacterium, *E coli*. A plasmid is a circular DNA molecule that carries a few genes that the bacterium perpetuates and is replicated in addition to its own normal chromosomes. More than any other technique, this really heralded the birth of recombinant DNA (hybrid DNA is produced by joining pieces of DNA from different sources; also designated rDNA) technology. This permitted, for the first time, rapid isolation of unique proteins and their mass production by rapidly growing microorganisms. In addition, new organisms having specifically inserted and desired characteristics could be engineered for medical, agricultural, and ecological uses.

Another important aspect of recombinant DNA technology is the use of antibodies in biotechnology, therapy, and diagnosis. Antibodies are produced by plasma cells (B cells) and are made up of four protein chains interconnected by disulfide bonds. The surface of the antibody possesses a highly specific indentation, or *lock* that can recognize the specific foreign particle (key) with which it complexes or binds. It long has been known that different antibodies are produced in each individual for their particular immunological experience with antigens. Hence, perhaps millions of different antibodies may be found in any given individual. For a long time it was not known how the B cells were capable of producing this diversity of antibodies that possessed the ability to recognize almost every possible foreign invader. It also was not known whether each B cell secreted a single or many different antibodies.

Fortunately, through the early *clone selection* theory of Mac-Farlane Burnet in 1957 came the idea that one cell produces only one type of antibody. And, in 1975, Kohler and Milstein devised a method of growing very large numbers of antibody-producing cells from a single B cell. They did this by the ingenious technique of fusing the B cell to a myeloma cancer cell. The resulting *hybridoma* (Fig 49-2) retained two main features from its two parent cells. It could grow indefinitely like the cancer cell, yet also produce and secrete antibodies like the B cell. This was the main discovery leading to hybridoma technology and earned Kohler and Milstein (together with Niels Jerne) the 1984 Nobel Prize in Physiology or Medicine.

The antibodies produced by these hybridomas are called monoclonal antibodies (MAbs) because they are derived from a single hybrid cell. Using the ability to identify directly the genes that code for antibodies, it was found that the antibodies are put together from a large number of different gene fragments. When combined in different ways they can produce a large number of different antibodies. Those portions of the antibody that contain the antigen-binding site are coded by a combination of hundreds of different gene fragments that get reshuffled and permanently fixed in the B cells. Hence, it has become possible to produce MAbs as key reagents in biotechnology procedures as well as exquisite diagnostic tools and specific drugs of great selectivity.

It already has become possible to tag monoclonal antibodies with radioisotopes that make possible the detection of very small levels of proteins and peptides in body fluids and tissues. The limits of detection are often as low as one billionth of a milligram (picogram) in the procedure widely used and known as radioimmunoassay (RIA). This is sufficient to detect low levels of hormones and other protein substances in body fluids. Figure 49-2 shows the basic procedures involved in hybridoma technology.

The power of molecular biology, combined with pressure from the animal rights lobby, led to a search for methodology to produce antibodies without the use of animal hosts. In 1989, this goal was realized when monoclonal antibodies were first isolated from a combinatorial antibody library. This approach, described in detail by Rader and Barbas,[9] employs the selectable expression of recombinant antibody molecules on the surface of bacteriophage particles. In this procedure, bacteriophage DNA constructs are made that encode human antibody heavy- and light-chain fragments. They then are combined randomly, and the phage are propagated by bacterial infection, allowing each phage to display a unique antibody with a specific antigen-binding site on its surface. Following several rounds of selection of phage particles with high affinity for a specific antigen, the phage DNA can be modified to produce soluble antibodies. An endless supply of antibody is guaranteed by simply repropagating the selected bacteriophage.

Another exciting area of research is that of gene diagnostics and therapy. It is believed that there are as many as 4000 locations in the human genome that are related to different genetic diseases. Of this number some 1200 have been mapped and characterized to various degrees of detail. Some of the abnormalities found on the genes are called point mutations, and they involve cases where a single nucleic acid base in a gene is substituted by a different one. This irregularity results in the exchange of a single amino acid in the encoded protein. Too many changes may result in genetic disorders. For example, in the genes encoding the hemoglobin protein sequences, there have been located at least 40 point mutations. Sickle-cell anemia is related to one of these. It is hoped that detailed knowledge of this type at the molecular level will allow the development of agents that can prevent the typical alteration in the shape of blood cells in sickle-cell anemia. Molecular probing or screening at this level also will reveal such disorders prenatally, or early in life, so that appropriate remedial action or preventative measures can be instituted (*viz,* gene therapy). Figure 49-3 shows how genetic defects may be detected.

Pharmacogenomics, or pharmacogenetics, is another research area that has sprung from the observation of mutations in key genes among a subset of the population that confer relative resistance or hypersensitivity to certain drugs. In the pharmacogenomic context, these mutations are more commonly referred to as polymorphisms and are often observed in genes encoding drug metabolizing enzymes, transporters, receptors, or other drug targets. These variations in DNA sequence are often single-nucleotide polymorphisms (SNPs) and can occur in either the coding region of a gene causing an amino acid change, or in the regulatory region of a gene thereby causing an alteration in the absolute amount of protein produced. For example, a patient with a polymorphism in one or both copies of a gene encoding a drug-inactivating enzyme would be at risk for exaggerated pharmacological action and potential toxicity for that drug. These pharmacogenetic differences are likely at the heart of most of the heterogeneity of drug responses observed among large populations and have significant impact on the ordinary practice of medicine and in clinical trials. Specific examples of known polymorphisms and the altered effects they confer are delineated in an excellent review article[10] from a premier PharmD pharmacogenomics expert and a table is available online at http://www.sciencemag.org/feature/data/1044449.shl.

Advances in DNA technology also have made this procedure more rapid, particularly when looking for any one of many individual mutations within a single gene that can give rise to disease. This technology, called high-density DNA affinity arrays,[11] or microarrays, is becoming more widespread and financially accessible to even small research institutions. Individual DNA targets that each contain one of these mutations are adsorbed onto a glass substrate in an array pattern and then hybridized with a fluorescently labeled probe generated from the gene expressed in the individual being tested. Another adaptation of this technology is to investigate the relative expression level of genes implicated in various disease processes. Some diseases are not due to gene mutations, but rather to

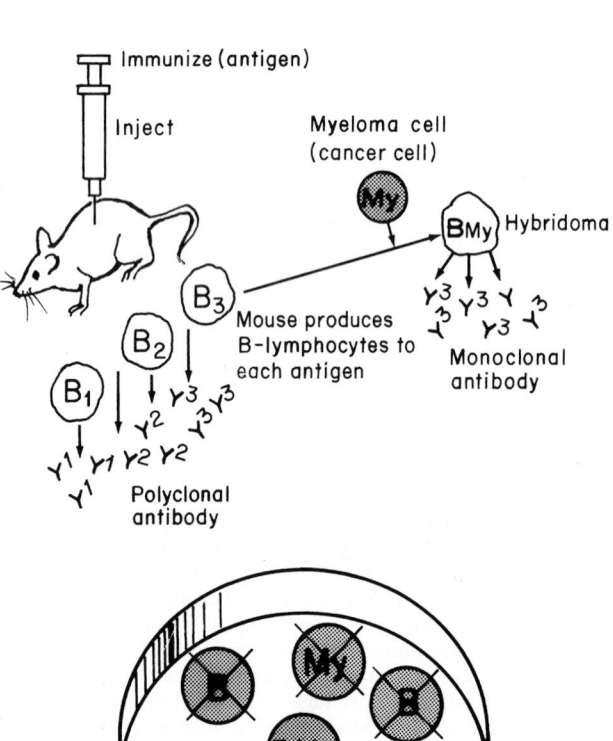

Figure 49-2. Hybridoma manufacture (courtesy, Armour Pharm).

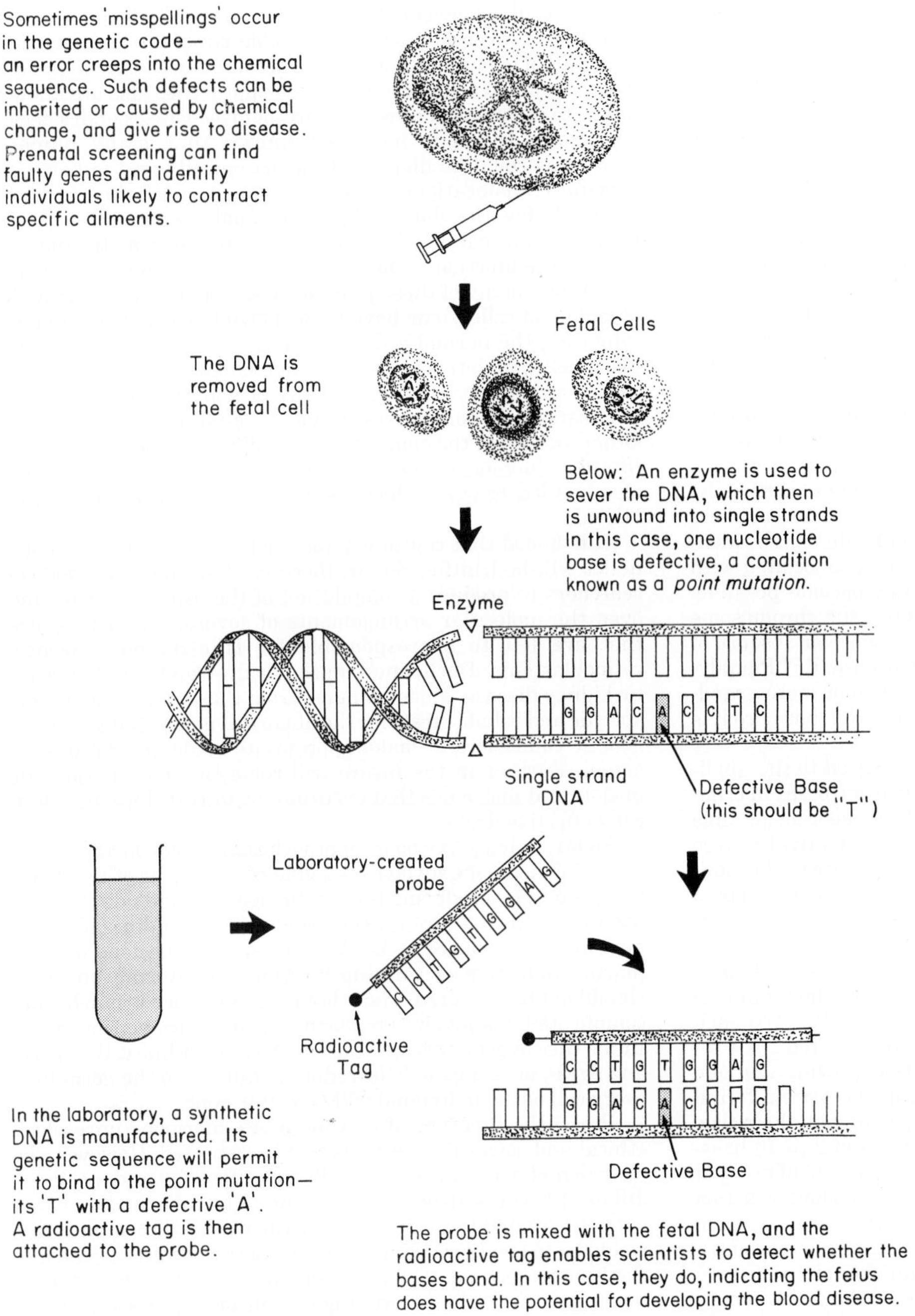

Sometimes 'misspellings' occur in the genetic code— an error creeps into the chemical sequence. Such defects can be inherited or caused by chemical change, and give rise to disease. Prenatal screening can find faulty genes and identify individuals likely to contract specific ailments.

Fetal Cells

The DNA is removed from the fetal cell

Below: An enzyme is used to sever the DNA, which then is unwound into single strands In this case, one nucleotide base is defective, a condition known as a *point mutation*.

Enzyme

G G A C A C C T C

Single strand DNA

Defective Base (this should be "T")

Laboratory-created probe

Radioactive Tag

In the laboratory, a synthetic DNA is manufactured. Its genetic sequence will permit it to bind to the point mutation— its 'T' with a defective 'A'. A radioactive tag is then attached to the probe.

C C T G T G G A G
G G A C A C C T C

Defective Base

The probe is mixed with the fetal DNA, and the radioactive tag enables scientists to detect whether the bases bond. In this case, they do, indicating the fetus does have the potential for developing the blood disease.

Figure 49-3. Searching for genetic defects.

abnormal over- or underproduction of certain regulatory proteins. DNA arrays permit the screening of literally thousands of genes in a single experiment by comparing genes expressed in normal versus diseased individuals. In fact, the expressed mRNAs from the entire human genome can now be screened on two commercially available "chips" and the race is on for the first manufacturer to put the entire expressed human genome on a single chip. Availability of such technology is expected to allow early diagnosis of many diseases that are due to multiple genetic abnormalities, such as cancer. In one specific case of diffuse B-cell lymphoma patients, microarrays have been used to subclassify the disease to understand which patients will respond best to chemotherapy.[12] In this manner, patients at greatest risk can be given the most aggressive therapy, while those at lower risk can be spared unnecessary toxicity. Microarrays of gene expression can also be applied in drug discovery; a recent application of this technology has been used to

predict the general therapeutic classes into which psychotropic medications fall.[13]

One drawback to microarrays in diagnosis and drug treatment is that gene expression is not always predictive of the amount of protein produced. Moreover, it completely ignores post-translational modification of proteins that can vastly influence biological responses. With advances in mass spectrometry instrumentation, the field of proteomics has emerged as the next means to secure a snapshot of cellular activities and correlate the pattern with specific drug responses or disease processes. Researchers at the US Food and Drug Administration and the National Institutes of Health have recently shown the power of proteomics in early detection of ovarian cancer using simple blood samples.[14] It was demonstrated that cancerous alterations in organ function causes an altered profile of proteins in serum, allowing this disease to be caught long before patients are symptomatic and with a high degree of accuracy, thereby minimizing the false-positive rate associated with many clinical diagnostic tests. The pharmacy practitioner is wisely advised to keep abreast of developments in proteomic technologies as these advances are quite likely to influence other therapeutic areas with equal magnitude.

As the ability to determine genetic defects that cause a variety of disorders emerges, health care will improve. However, society must develop policies governing the use and misuse of this information. Baum has reviewed this problem and provides information on some of genetic screening's serious implications. For instance, the use of DNA fingerprinting bothers some observers who question the reliability of such an analysis carried out on a large scale. Results may affect civil liberties, insurability, guilt or innocence, etc. The 1996 Health Insurance Portability and Accountability Act (HIPAA) prohibits group health insurance providers from using genetic information for determining eligibility or setting premiums, but provides no protection for the millions of Americans with individual insurance policies.[15]

As the technique known as restriction fragment length polymorphism (RFLP) analysis develops,[2] it provides markers throughout the genome that vary among individuals. The identification of particular RFLPs that are tightly associated with genes responsible for certain diseases has become possible. Thus, RFLPs provide markers that identify the chromosome that carries the defective gene. But the presence or absence of the marker does not necessarily indicate disease. RFLP analysis must be performed on both parents or two or more grandparents to determine the status of a disorder. Furthermore it is an expensive and complex analysis.

In the mid-1990s, public attention was raised to the applications of genetic polymorphisms for forensic purposes in criminal investigations. However, RFLP analysis has considerable drawbacks for this purpose. The need for relatively large amounts of nondegraded DNA and the time necessary for multiple allelic comparisons led to a search for other methods of individual genotyping. The most popular recent technology[9] analyzes interindividual differences in the variable number of tandem repeats (VTNRs), or *DNA fingerprinting,* as it is known to the lay public. A similar name for the same method is amplified fragment length polymorphisms (AMP-FLPs). We each possess in our genome a variable number of repeated DNA sequences that, when measured in combination, provide a unique *fingerprint* of our DNA. These repeated sequences are referred to as minisatellites or microsatellites, depending on their size, and are often made up of repeated sequences of 2 to 70 base-pair-length monomeric sequences. Since the location of many of these polymorphisms is known, the polymerase chain reaction (PCR) can be used to amplify these repeated sequences from even the extremely small amounts of blood, tissue, or semen found at crime scenes. Depending on the number of satellite sequences analyzed, the individual source of the DNA can be identified with near absolute certainty. So useful is this technique that it was employed in 1994 to positively identify the remains of the Romanovs, using mitochondrial DNA isolated from the bones of the Russian royal family who were murdered by the Bolsheviks in 1918.[16]

So, while many tests will be devised to predict genetic risk factors for complex diseases, what one does with the knowledge remains to be worked out, and undoubtedly society will grapple with this issue for many years to come. Even the magazine *Consumer Reports* provides the lay person with a guide to genetic screening and discusses who's testing what, the possible problem of genetic discrimination, genetic screening's limited powers of prediction, the role of genetic tests in preemployment screening, the presence of few legal safeguards, how some inherited adult-onset disorders may be preempted, remembering that genetic testing is a tool, knowing that the demand for genetic services likely will increase, the role of individual decisions, the pace of change, how to prepare for genetic testing, etc.

The major diseases of mankind owe much of their origin to heredity, so that it will be exciting in the decades to come to see how molecular biotechnological techniques will allow for early detection, prevention, or even possible cures for many of the maladies of old age such as cardiovascular disease, Alzheimer's disease, diabetes, and cancer. These approaches also are allowing us to understand previous unrecognized causes of diseases. For many years, it has been known that many human leukemias could be diagnosed microscopically on the basis of specific translocations, or rearrangements, of the chromosomes. Today, the abnormal proteins made as a result of these translocations can be identified. Look[17] provides a striking review on the function of these aberrant proteins in leukemogenesis. While many of these proteins lead to uncontrolled growth of leukemia cells, some have been shown to cause leukemia by inhibiting the normal cell death that usually occurs in white blood cell populations. This had led to our reclassification of cancer as a disease not necessarily of abnormal cell division, but instead, in some cases, of loss of appropriate cell death. Other articles in the same 1997 issue of *Science* deal with more frontiers in cancer research, showing that molecular biology also has led to our understanding of how cancer can be prevented.

It is hoped that continued approaches based on reverse genetics will be fruitful. So far, these methods have allowed researchers to produce a compilation of the exact locations and even the molecular arrangements of several defective genes that are felt to be responsible for Huntington's disease, retinoblastoma, Duchenne's muscular dystrophy, and polycystic kidney disease, among others. From these studies will come specific and reliable tests for the abnormal genes that will allow genetic counselors to make appropriate recommendations for action. Further in the future will come the new therapeutic models and molecules that eventually will translate into clinically effective drugs.

So far, at least two basic approaches in *genetic medicine* can be envisioned. One involves possible replacement of the defective protein by producing it biotechnologically outside the body (eg, insulin, as has already been done with Humulin *(Lilly),* human insulin produced by DNA). The same can be done with replacing defective or missing enzymes or altering one that should not be produced. The other basic approach is much more complicated and involves replacing the defective gene entirely. In the case of gene therapy that involves germ-line cells (sperm and eggs), once a gene is introduced stably into the germ line, every cell of the individual will bear this gene.

Presently, this type of therapy poses enormous unresolved ethical and scientific questions and is restricted. However, the inclusion of genes in somatic cells (specific body organ cells) is different because these genomes cannot be inherited and stay with the treated individual. One of the ways to accomplish this would be to use *harmless* viruses to insert a corrected gene into the human genome. Unfortunately, in most cases, it is not yet understood how the inserted gene will be expressed in these tissues, only where and when they are needed. Some ways to circumvent these difficulties have been found, but they are limited. For example, one way to produce tissue specificity is to take out the tissues to be altered, insert the corrected gene, and place the corrected cells back into the body. Alternatively, tissue-specific genetic control elements have been identified and can be used to restrict expression of the recombinant gene.

So far, bone marrow cells can be handled in this manner, and they have been the first somatic cell type submitted to clinical testing of this gene-transfer technique. In one example, the goal is the treatment of an inborn disease affecting bone marrow function and involving an enzyme (adenosine deaminase) deficiency that produces severe weakening of the immune system.

One of the goals in biochemistry and pharmacology is to understand the molecular features of cell receptors. These are the *locks* into which the *keys* (drugs) fit that alter or control the function of the cell. While now there exists the capability to determine the basic genetic code and thus learn the sequence of the amino acids that make up the protein, its spatial configuration still is not known. This is called the tertiary structure of the protein, the functional form of the protein after the proper folding of a simple straight-chain of amino acids.

The novel combination of x-ray crystallography, molecular mechanics, calculations, and supercomputers are brought to bear to reveal the folded or three-dimensional arrangement. From this 3-D picture of the *lock*, researchers can design specifically shaped drugs that fit the active sites of the folded protein. This computational chemistry methodology is a leap forward and truly a rational approach in drug design. In like manner, the possibility of cloning *receptor sites* of specific design and function provides the pharmacologist with excellent *in vitro* test systems for pharmacological screening and understanding of the mechanisms of actions of drugs. For example, the solution of the x-ray crystal structure of the HIV protease has led to the rapid development of four FDA-approved drugs that have revolutionized our treatment of AIDS. A similar approach with thymidylate synthase was used to produce a unique inhibitor of this enzyme for cancer chemotherapy.[18]

In the past few years, several publications have dealt specifically with the pharmacist's role in implementing pharmaceutical care with regard to biotechnology agents. Tami and Evens[19] recently presented an overview on the evaluation of biotechnology products. The authors first discuss the manufacturing, pharmacokinetics, and stability issues that we present in greater detail forthcoming. They specifically made the point that biotechnology product costs often can account for 10% of a pharmacy's total budget. In addition, they discuss pharmacoeconomic studies, availability of alternative agents, concomitant drug costs, special pharmacy procedures, reimbursement, and manufacturer's support. Pharmacists are a particularly important link in assisting patients with reimbursement issues for these expensive drugs.

UNIQUE PHARMACEUTICAL CHALLENGES OF BIOTECHNOLOGY-DERIVED THERAPEUTICS

The transition of biotechnology from theory to pharmaceutical practicality has posed a whole new series of challenges to those involved in drug development. With classical small molecules possessing formula weights less than 1000, a series of chemical compounds normally are screened for a particular pharmacological activity and assessed for specificity. The results of these findings then guide fine-tuning of the chemical entity. As advances in combinatorial chemistry are now generating thousands of compounds in a given class, the rate-limiting step in drug development has shifted to high-throughput screening technologies. Natural products are also regaining prominence in drug discovery because they often possess greater molecular diversity than can be obtained with combinatorial compound libraries. It is now rare that pharmaceutical formulation and drug-delivery problems limit the success of small molecules.

In contrast, macromolecular agents (eg, recombinant proteins and vaccines, antisense DNA, gene therapy constructs) already have the advantage, in theory, of possessing inherent selectivity for a particular biological process. By and large, the limitation to the utility of these agents rests with problems related to drug delivery and stability. In fact, it is no surprise that most biotechnology drugs currently approved in the US act at extracellular sites and/or in compartments that are easily accessible, such as the blood-forming elements. In addition, each type of biotechnology agent also is subjected to unique considerations based on our emerging biological understanding of each system. The discussion that follows attempts to address the obstacles to successful therapeutic use of biotechnology products.

Recombinant proteins almost exclusively constitute the currently approved list of biotechnology-derived agents in the US.[7] These proteins usually have resulted from a search for endogenous agents acting by a newly identified physiological mecha-

nism (such as the stimulation of red blood cell production by erythropoietin manufactured in the kidney). Since the therapeutic administration of a recombinant molecule that mimics an endogenous protein carries with it a naturally inherent specificity, it is no surprise that development times for these agents has been considerably shorter than for most conventional small molecules. The probability of regulatory success with recombinant proteins also has been more favorable.[20] While a new, small, organic molecule may have a 10% chance of achieving NDA status, this percentage is near 40% for recombinant proteins. When compared with conventional small molecules, recombinant products reaching the clinical trials in Phase I (25% versus 71%) or Phase III (66% versus 93%) are much more likely to become successful therapeutic agents. Nonetheless, Cho and Juliano[21] state,

"The main challenge encountered in development is not so much identifying a bioactive molecule but, rather, how to maintain a therapeutically meaningful concentration of the macromolecule in the vicinity of its target for the desired period of time."

Recombinant protein drugs are produced in various host cells from carefully designed expression systems. For monoclonal antibodies, production is enabled by the highly specialized hybridoma systems described earlier. But for the bulk of the other recombinant protein drugs, the exploitation of any one of these protein *factories* begins in a similar fashion. As addressed earlier in the section on gene splicing, the complementary DNA encoding a particular protein product is spliced (or subcloned) into a circular DNA vector. This recombinant vector contains gene regulatory sequences that enable highly efficient transcription and translation of the recombinant gene once the construct is introduced into the appropriate host.

The choice of host system (bacteria, yeast, or mammalian cells) depends highly on the biological requirements of the protein. One major consideration is whether the protein product requires glycosylation, the specific addition of certain sugars, for biological activity.[20] Bacteria like *E coli* are unable to conjugate such carbohydrates onto recombinant proteins, but yeast possesses a limited ability for glycosylation. However, mammalian cell systems such as Chinese hamster ovary cells have the full complement of glycosyltransferase enzymes. For molecules such as the interferons and filgrastim (G-CSF), glycosylation is not necessary for biological activity; therefore these proteins can be produced in less expensive *E coli* systems. However, erythropoietin requires mammalian glycosylation and must be produced in the more costly Chinese hamster ovary cell system. Hamilton and colleagues[22] have recently reported the heroic engineering of the yeast *Pichia pastoris* to encode the entire complement of human N-glycosylation enzymes while deleting the yeast's own glycosylation pathways. Such an organism might represent a more cost-effective host for future manufacture of human therapeutic proteins requiring glycosylation.

These modern protein expression systems have several advantages over trying to isolate the corresponding protein from the organs or tissues of other mammals. First, immune reactivity to a nonhuman protein (human insulin versus porcine insulin) is largely obviated (with exceptions described later). Also, protein drugs can be produced that could never be made by conventional methods (interferons, G-CSF) or in quantities previously only available in limited amounts (insulin, growth hormone). Finally, the protein is inherently free of potentially pathogenic human viruses (factor VIII or hepatitis vaccines), although treatments to destroy any zoonotic pathogens are often employed in subsequent processing.

As the biotechnology drug sector has matured, manufacturers have begun to follow conventional, small-molecule pharmaceuticals in the production of second-generation agents with improved bioavailability and/or safety. While the cynic might argue that these innovations are merely spurred by pending patent expiration of first-in-class agents, it seems that most second-generation biotech drugs represent true advances. For example, the treatment of anemia due to kidney disease or cancer chemotherapy has been improved by increasing the bioavailability of erythropoietin in the second-generation drug, darbepoietin. Recognizing that N-linked oligosaccharides are essential to the activity of erythropoietin, scientists altered two amino acid residues to accept two additional sialic acid chains. The resulting darbopoietin molecule possesses a 3-fold improvement in serum half-life (26.3 hr relative to 8.5 hr for erythropoietin). This alteration reduces the number of injections necessary for patients to maintain therapeutic hemoglobin levels. While regimens vary by patient and indication, the general rule has been that if a patient had been stabilized previous with three erythropoietin injections per week, only one weekly injection of darbopoietin is now required. From the standpoint of patient quality of life and burden on pharmacy and nursing staff, less frequent dosing has a number of significant advantages.

While scale-up of recombinant protein expression and purification is becoming more routine, these drugs present other challenges not seen with small molecule agents. Issues of proper protein folding, formulation, and stability are proving as labor-intensive as the initial cloning of the gene itself. Betaseron (human recombinant interferon β) required modification of one amino acid to enhance the yield of properly disulfide-linked protein after renaturation processing.[20] This processing modification reflects another advantage of recombinant protein expression that can be employed quite easily, so long as the pharmacological activity of the protein is not compromised. In fact, optimizing the cDNA sequence (and the resulting encoded amino acids) of a recombinant product has resulted recently in the approval of consensus interferon, a single molecule that incorporates the combined activities of multiple interferons.

Manipulation of the expressed gene also can involve the deletion of regions dispensable for biological activity, to optimize therapeutic utility. Human tissue plasminogen activator (tPA) has been used since 1987 for thrombolytic therapy following myocardial infarction. However, tPA is poorly soluble and must be administered in relatively high concentrations, since it is cleared rather rapidly from plasma. Structure-function analysis of individual tPA protein domains allowed the construction of a smaller molecule (reteplase or recombinant plasminogen activator; rPA) that possesses superior solubility and also can be manufactured in *E coli*.

The effects of changes in protein formulation or amino acid substitutions can now be assessed rapidly as a result of advances in protein analytical methodology. Protein secondary structure can be monitored quickly and accurately by such techniques as circular dichroism (CD) spectroscopy and Fourier-transformed infrared spectroscopy (FTIR). This technology has been quite useful in that the structural fidelity of the protein drug can be ensured prior to the initiation of more costly pharmacological evaluation. FTIR also has the advantage of being able to detect protein structure in the lyophilized state, greatly facilitating the optimization of formulations capable of maximal stability.

Pharmacokinetic evaluation of recombinant proteins is also an emerging field of significant relevance to pharmacy.[23] Since most protein drugs cannot be given orally, the impact of other routes of administration must be assessed. It also must be appreciated that for most biotechnologically derived agents, there is a preexisting and nonconstant concentration of the corresponding endogenous molecule present in plasma. Bioanalytical techniques for monitoring concentrations of the agent require optimization for specificity. Unfortunately the specificity of any one method often depends on the particular matrix in which analysis is performed (blood, urine, or the initial formulation).

In addition, the prediction that recombinant human molecules would not be immunogenic has not proven to be the case.[23] Antibodies to several recombinant drugs now are known, but not all neutralize the pharmacological activity of the agent and, in some cases, they can decrease clearance of the agent. These factors obviously complicate the interpretation of pharmacokinetic data. The immunogenicity of a particular protein also may depend on the route of administration. Protein aggregation, known to occur after subcutaneous or intramuscular injection, leads to a greater antigenic response than soluble

protein. Finally, the influence of the lymphatic system on protein pharmacokinetics should not be underestimated. After subcutaneous administration, absorption via the lymphatics becomes quantitatively more important than that of blood capillaries as the molecular weight of the drug increases. Since several recombinant protein drugs act primarily through the lymphatics (interferons and interleukins), blood concentrations may be irrelevant to pharmacological activity.

Obviously, there remain immunologic concerns in any instance when a recombinant analog of an endogenous protein is fashioned into a drug product. Known as neoantigenicity, altered protein structure due to amino acid changes, chimeric products (ie, humanized mouse monoclonal antibodies), or fusion with other constituents could trigger antibody-mediated inactivation of the therapeutic molecule as well as its endogenous counterpart. In some instances, the very same modification in one context can result in the opposite effect in another. For example, *E coli* asparaginase had been used to treat certain leukemias based on the observation of their need for the amino acid asparagine. However, some patients experienced immunological reactions to the bacterial protein, and a new product was produced, pegaspargase, where the enzyme was modified by covalent attachment of polyethylene glycol (PEG) molecules. This approach, now known as PEGylation, is also known to improve the bioavailability of a number of proteins by reducing their renal clearance.[24] However, this same strategy used to reduce antigenicity in one context recently caused an immunogenic response with another product, megakaryocyte derived growth factor or thrombopoietin. This product had been in development to treat bleeding disorders due to platelet loss in some disease and with chemotherapy and a PEGylated form being tested in normal volunteers caused inactivating antibodies to be made to their own endogenous thrombopoietin.[24] This example should serve as a reminder that protein modifications do not always have the intended consequences.

The future of recombinant biological agents continues to evolve. To date, most approved agents have been recombinantly expressed, naturally occurring proteins. To a limited extent, some approved agents represent our venture into *protein engineering,* in which chimeric or fusion proteins (immunotoxin conjugates) or mutated or deleted proteins (consensus interferon and rPA) have been developed as a result of our experiences with first-generation agents. A number of other biotechnology approaches are currently under investigation, often in human clinical trials, and their success remains to be fully realized. These agents include antisense RNA and DNA, small interfering RNA (siRNA), ribozymes, aptamers, and gene therapy.

In 1978, the first *in vitro* experiments in which *antisense DNA* was used for specific repression of gene expression opened the door to the opportunity to block disease-causing genes selectively. The antisense nucleotide approach is based on the use of short oligonucleotides (10–20 base pairs) complementary to a specific mRNA whose protein product is implicated in a disease such as cancer or viral infection.[25] Binding of the antisense molecule to its target mRNA is then believed to inhibit protein translation by interfering with ribosomal function. In addition, the resulting DNA-RNA duplex recruits the activity of RNase H, a ubiquitous enzyme that degrades the RNA itself. This approach meets the two crucial criteria in the design of any successful therapeutic agent: the identification of a target implicated in disease etiology and the ability to find a molecule capable of high affinity and selectivity for the target. Although problems of stability, delivery, and specificity have somewhat dulled the initial promise of these agents, several second-generation antisense molecules are in late clinical trials, and the first antisense drug (to prevent blindness due to cytomegalovirus infections in HIV-positive patients) was approved in 1997.

All antisense DNA molecules in these trials possess a modified phosphodiester backbone in which one of the nonbridging oxygens on the phosphate has been replaced with sulfur. The resulting phosphorothioate molecules possess enhanced stability to DNA-degrading nucleases, enabling *in vivo* administration, and effectively penetrate cells and bind target mRNAs.

However, there are numerous reports of antisense efficacy, particularly in inhibiting cancer and other abnormal cell growth, that are due to nonantisense mechanisms.[26] These nonantisense actions may be due to the fact that phosphorothioates have enhanced affinity for polyanions including heparin, growth factors (bFGF, PDGF, EGF, and VEGF), and enzymes required for cell growth (PKC and phospholipase A_2). Other non-sequence-specific actions of phosphorothioates *in vivo* may be due to their enhancement of immune system function by increasing production of immunoglobulins and interferons and by activation of natural killer cell activity. It should be noted that these nonspecific actions may not necessarily be deleterious, especially when the target mRNA is viral or involved in cancer. Nonetheless, antisense molecules with other backbones or backbone combinations currently are being evaluated for greater specificity for their target mRNAs.

Another encouraging adaptation of antisense therapies is an approach that takes advantage of the Nobel prize–winning discovery of Thomas Cech and Sidney Altman, who demonstrated that certain RNA molecules possess an enzymatic RNA-degrading activity. The RNAs, called *ribozymes,* are directed toward a specific disease-causing RNA by the sequence homology used by antisense molecules. However, the promise of ribozymes relates to their catalytic nature; one ribozyme molecule can lead to the destruction of thousands of target RNA molecules. In addition, ribozyme technology appears to possess greater specificity over some antisense nucleotides. Nonetheless, the instability of RNAs as therapeutic agents is one hurdle that must be overcome before the promise of ribozymes can be fully realized.

Other RNA technologies also being investigated take advantage of the three-dimensional nature of RNA molecules. Aptamers are RNA molecules specifically selected for high affinity to certain molecular targets. *In vitro* selectivity of these molecules is quite impressive; affinity-selected RNAs can distinguish between theophylline and caffeine, hypoxanthine molecules that differ by only one methyl group.[27] The hope is that such selectivity can be applied to closely related enzymes (ie, COX-1 and COX-2) or receptor family subtypes.

The most recent, highly-hyped technology to emerge in the late 1990s is the use of small, double-stranded RNA molecules to specifically turn off expression of genes involved in pathogenesis (reviewed in [28]). In 1998, this pathway was first shown to exist in an invertebrate model dear to geneticists, the worm *C elegans.* Shortly thereafter, it was recognized that mammalian cells possess a similar regulatory mechanism for silencing endogenous genes called RNA interference (RNAi). But most commonly, the pathway seems to exist to fight retroviral infections whereby a type III RNase enzyme (appropriately called "Dicer") is activated to cleave viral RNA genomes into 21–28 basepair fragments which then hybridize to other copies of viral RNA to catalyze their degradation. Based on these observations, small, interfering RNA molecules (siRNA) could be synthesized and have now been shown in a number of systems to selectively "knockdown" gene expression. A number of companies have sprung up hoping to exploit this technology in treating viral diseases, especially HIV/AIDS, and other disorders caused by overactivity of an enzyme or protein. The challenges facing siRNA technology are not dissimilar from those of antisense oligonucleotides, focusing primarily on efficient delivery of the molecules or expression vectors capable of producing the siRNA molecules intracellularly. Another problem is specificity and the potential for "off-target" gene silencing. Researchers using microarray technology have recently published conflicting reports on this issue with one showing alterations in dozens of genes using a single targeted siRNA while another group observes no off-target silencing across 20,000 human genes studied.[29,30] As with other revolutionary technologies that propose to realize Ehrlich's dream of the magic bullet, only time and experience will determine the true clinical utility of these agents.

Until the unexpected death of Jesse Gelsinger in a Phase I recombinant adenovirus trial in 1998, the next wave of products seemed destined to be directed toward *gene therapy.*[31] Many different approaches constitute gene therapy, but the most common is to attempt to replace a nonfunctioning or mutated gene product by the directed expression of a new, nonmutated copy of that gene. In other cases, genes are being introduced to make drug therapy more effective (eg, HSV thymidine kinase, p53) or gene therapy is combined with other aforementioned approaches (eg, intracellular expression of antisense RNA to the K-*ras* oncogene). In general, the DNA encoding these new genes is encoded on a plasmid molecule or is part of a retroviral vector that can infect cells with the appropriate desirable gene without causing viral disease. (The Gelsinger case points out that the recombinant virus might still be lethal via other mechanisms.) Delivery methods for these gene sources usually either exploit the DNA delivery tactic of the virus itself or employ cationic liposomal complexes with the DNA to mask the plasmid's negative charge. Obviously, there is substantial concern over the use of modified retroviruses or adeno-associated viruses as gene delivery systems for fear that important host cell genes might be disrupted if the viral DNA is integrated into the host genome. Cationic liposomal strategies have made substantial leaps in the last several years, but their efficiency of gene delivery pales in comparison with viral delivery. Nonetheless, liposome/DNA complexes are amenable to lyophilization and reconstitution, and advances are being made in maximizing the efficiency of these stabilized preparations.[32]

Finally, a new area has emerged for the potential application of biotechnology products against bioterrorism. Following the September 11, 2001 terrorist attacks in New York, Washington, DC, and Pennsylvania and the subsequent anthrax scare, Congress earmarked $37 billion toward homeland defense of which $6 billion is targeted to developing biodefense strategies. A little-known provision of new FDA guidelines are that counter-terrorism agents are eligible for expedited review, as seen now for drugs to treat AIDS or cancer. Biotechnological approaches have already been proposed for both the detection and treatment for biological agents most likely to be used in terrorist attacks.

PHARMACOGNOSTICAL APPLICATIONS

In regard to the applications of biotechnology in pharmacognosy (drugs from natural sources) Cordell[33] reports that major efforts in this field are under way in Germany, Japan, and the People's Republic of China. These countries are attempting to use manipulated plant-cell cultures to produce otherwise difficult to extract natural products. In Germany, which has a substantial number of efficacious prescription natural products not available in the US, the pharmaceutical industry and government have joined together to form an institute designed specifically to produce natural products commercially through cell-free systems and gene technology of medicinal plants. One company in Japan reported that it can produce ginseng extract, identical in chemical composition with that from mature 6-year-old root, in 20,000-gal fermenters.

Davies summarized the application of genetic engineering to the production of pharmaceuticals. He pointed out that new drugs traditionally have come from natural product sources, usually followed by improved growing techniques or chemical synthesis. However, while the plant or microorganism strain-improvement procedures have resulted in up to 1000-fold increases in yield, the techniques largely have been empirical. Furthermore, these methods have virtually no genetic or biochemical pedigree for successive improvements.

The organisms currently used to produce antibiotics (eg, penicillin and tetracycline) on a commercial scale are the same species as those originally collected from the natural state and really have been modified only through forced genetic manipulations (by virtue of the media, etc), based on strain improvement. Of paramount importance is the fact that while gene cloning and recombinant DNA techniques have been successful for proteins and peptides, the higher plants and microbes producing antibiotics have not been manipulated similarly. This is because an entirely different situation exists when more complex genetic and biochemical processes need to be manipulated. As discussed later, there are also some regulatory assurances that remain to be met, particularly in using transgenic plants as a source of pharmaceuticals.

Antibiotics and alkaloids usually are biosynthesized through multistep pathways possessing complex biogenesis and regulatory circuits. The numerous genes involved in the synthesis of a simple antibiotic are not necessarily present as a single genetic linkage group. Thus, cloning the genes needed would require numerous operations, often without the advantage of selective procedures to detect the presence of the cloned genes. Similarly, the same technical problems associated with multiple components of antibiotic synthesis apply to the genetic engineering of improved yields of many secondary metabolites like alkaloids from plants. Further complicating the issue is that suitable host-vector systems need to be developed fully for the application of recombinant DNA techniques to plants. However, if there is a single rate-limiting step in the pathway of antibiotic biosynthesis, it might be possible to clone the gene for this step by selecting for increased antibiotic production by *shotgun* cloning back into the producing organism.

An alternative way to achieve increased levels of antibiotic production might be to clone appropriate genes on multicopy or high-expression vectors. Another idea would be to engineer antibiotic-producing organisms to produce hybrid or specifically modified antibiotics. This would result in several model compounds that might have more desirable or better properties than the parent antibiotic. For example, Hailes[34] outlined the directed biotransformation of opiate analogs including morphine and hydromorphone using genetically engineered bacteria and discussed the application of this method toward biosynthesis of novel alkaloids. Marsden[35] reported the engineering of broader substrate specificity into a macrolide antibiotic-producing polyketide synthase from the erythromycin producer, *Saccharopolyspora erythraea*. These investigators modified the carboxylic acid acceptor unit of this multicomponent enzyme complex to utilize over 40 alternative branched-chain starter carboxylic acids (as opposed to the two straight chain acids uti-

lized normally). In doing so, a vast number of novel, macrolide antibiotics can now be synthesized.

In the case of plant tissue culture, many compounds such as secondary metabolites have been produced with yields that are equal to or greater than that of parent plants. Staba[36] reports on at least 30 natural products that have been generated through plant-cell culture. Among these are included several well-known, but still difficult to obtain, drugs such as diosgenin-derived steroid hormone precursors, the opium alkaloids, digitalis glycosides, several different essential oils, and the *Catharanthus* alkaloids, vincristine, and vinblastine. However, it has been pointed out that these methods still are not economical when compared with the traditional methods used currently, *viz,* direct extraction from whole plant materials.

Thus far, only one Asiatic drug, known as shikonin (from *Lithospermasm erythrorhizon*), has been produced through plant-cell culture methodology in greater quantities and with substantially lower costs than usual extraction procedures.[37] Certainly, continued efforts expended in the biotechnological manipulation of plant genes will prove more successful as research continues in this area. Table 49-2[38] shows established hairy root cultures (the result of genetic transformation of the plant by *Agrobacterium rhizogenes*) and examples of secondary product formation.

Finally, even though many efforts are oriented toward the cheap, controlled, pharmaceutical production of secondary plant products, it should be remembered that this new approach can offer a valuable system for basic plant biosynthesis. These techniques offer a means quite suitable for physiological studies as well as for genetic manipulation. For once, it will be possible to have a powerful tool for the study of the control of gene expression at both the cellular and whole plant or organ levels. Beyond this, the increased efficiency with which biosynthetic pathways for desired compounds may be expressed makes plant DNA promising material as a source of mRNA for cloning operations directed at the transfer of specific plant enzymes into microorganisms.[38]

Awad[39] has provided an overview on plant biotechnology that he feels is a field fertile for pharmaceutical research. In addition to providing two tables listing both microorganisms and plants that have been used in agricultural, horticultural, and

Table 49-2. Established Hairy Root Cultures with Examples of Secondary Product Formation

FAMILY	SPECIES	MAJOR SECONDARY PRODUCTS
Solanaceae	*Atropa belladonna*	Atropine
	Datura stramonium	Hyoscyamine
	Hyoscymus muticus	Hyoscyamine
	Nicotiana rustica	Nicotine, anatabine
	N tabacum	Nicotine, anatabine
	N hesperis	Nicotine, anabasine
	N cavicola	Nicotine, nornicotine
	Scopolia japonica	Hyoscyamine
	Solanum laciniatum	Steroidal alkaloids
Apocynaceae	*Catharanthus roseus*	Ajmalicine, serpentine, vindolinine, catharanthine
Chenopodiaceae	*Beta vulgaris*	Betacyanin, betaxanthin
Polygonaceae	*Polygonum hydropiper*	
Boraginaceae	*Lithospermum erythrorhizon*	Shikonin
Compositae	*Tagetes patula*	Thiophenes
Rubiaceae	*Cinchona ledgeriana*	Quinoline alkaloids

From Hamill J, Parr A, Robins R, et al. *Bio/Technology* 1987; 5:800.

pharmaceutical research in biotechnology, he shows the major groups of compounds of commercial importance that are derived from plants. These include pharmaceuticals (alkaloids, steroids, anthraquinones), enzymes (papain), latex (rubber), waxes (jojoba, carnuba), pigments (food dyes), oils (olive oil, corn oil, etc), agrochemicals (pyrethrins), cosmetic substances (essential oils and perfumes), food additives (flavor compounds, nonnutritive sweeteners), and gums (gum acacia and tragacanth). He perceives the major trends in plant biotechnology to include plant-microbe interactions, gene delivery and manipulation, diversity of gene engineering, and microbial and plant secondary metabolites.

Constabel [40] reviewed medicinal plant biotechnology as a revolutionary methodology useful in enhancing the formation and accumulation of desirable natural products and a possible product-modification method. He describes advances in micropropagation that involve plant regeneration from *in vitro* cultured cells. Here the multiplication factor can be high and of great advantage to speed up slow-growing important medicinal plants. Recent studies with ipecac (*Cephaelis ipecacuanha*) yielded 100 plantlets per shoot-tip explant per year or 600 plantlets per axenic shoot. Similarly, *Digitalis lanata* cultivars with high cardenolide content were obtained by inbreeding and subsequent crossing of selected genotypes. The isolation and *in vitro* culture of shoot tips led to the formation of adventitious shoots. Following short- and long-term culture, rooting of these shoots on solid medium established plantlets that were transferred to soil. The cardenolide yields equaled those of the parent plants.

Similar studies showed that axenic shoot-tip cultures also can be stored for long periods of time and even be cryopreserved for gene banks. Some studies also are focusing on overcoming somaclonal variation, so that stable, high-yield chemovariants can be developed. In terms of enhancement of productivity, gene technology has allowed true transgenic plants. Their uniqueness is shown as a change, ie, enhancement, in plant performance (insect resistance, herbicide) and productivity (storage proteins, pigmentation). Transgenic cell cultures of drug plants with modified or increased productivity and microorganisms producing phytochemicals are conceivable and may further increase the feasibility of phytochemical production by *in vitro* methods. Already key enzymes for biosynthetic pathways in plants have been identified and related to isolated DNA clones and genes. Schell described plant biotechnology as a powerful tool to use plant resources and to improve the environmental impact of agriculture. He described how transgenic plants can be developed to promote insect tolerance, virus resistance, and tolerance to fungal diseases in crop plants. Critics of plant biotechnology raise legitimate concerns over the potential immunogenicity of foreign proteins expressed in foodstuffs. The European Union nations have been particularly opposed to the marketing of these so-called "Frankenfoods" but these genetically engineered food crops have now grown to represent more than 40% of the corn and soybeans harvested annually. Similarly reviewed are the enhancement of stress tolerance, development of hybrid seeds, and improvement of nutritional-quality plants. For example, Miller and Ackerman[41] also provided new perspectives on food biotechnology, describing tomatoes that are rot resistant and animal foods being modified by genetic means.

Plant biotechnology has also been used to omit products that are undesirable in a particular crop. Of greatest pharmaceutical relevance is the presence of caffeine in the coffee plant.[42] Those who wish to avoid the hypertensive and CNS-stimulating effects of this methylxanthine must resort to coffee products that have been decaffeinated by chemical processes that either employ organic solvents which also remove some components of flavor and aroma. However, Japanese researchers[43] have now succeeded in using RNA interference technology to downregulate one of the three N-methyltransferase enzymes required for caffeine biosynthesis in the non-commercial plant, *Coffea cenephora*. The resulting transgenic plants exhibited a 50–70% decrease in caffeine content. The remaining challenge is to cross these plants with the more economically important *Coffea arabica* and achieve a 97% reduction in caffeine content as required in the US for "decaffeinated" labeling.

The use of transgenic plants or animals in producing recombinant proteins for pharmaceutical use is called "pharming," a term accepted in the 2001 release of the *The Columbia Encyclopedia*. A 2003 survey by the Pew Initiative on Food and Biotechnology revealed that while 81% of Americans favored tinkering with plant genes to produces medicines, only half felt comfortable making transgenic animals for the same purpose. Proponents of transgenic plants as pharmaceutical sources point out that production of recombinant proteins requires a specialized facility costing $300–$500 million and roughly 5 years of set-up. In contrast, transgenic plant or animal scale-up can be done on the scale of tens of millions of dollars and in half the time. However, no recombinant product produced in plants or animals has yet made it to market, and only three plant-produced products are currently in clinical trials. The industry has suffered numerous setbacks,[44] not the least of which relate to concerns on the contamination of food crops with plant-made pharmaceuticals, particularly since some companies are using plants to produce orally-active vaccines. In late 2002, a Texas plant biotechnology company was cited for twice contaminating soybean crops in Nebraska and Iowa with transgenic corn harboring either a pig vaccine or a human protease inhibitor. Plants clearly hold great promise for producing biotechnology drugs, but several hurdles must be overcome before this idea is practically implemented.

PHARMACOLOGICAL APPLICATIONS

Pharmacologically directed biotechnological methodology also holds much promise for the medical field. Even before completion of the Human Genome Project, genes had been isolated for literally dozens of neurochemical receptor drug targets, ion channels, and transporters. With these sequences in hand, target proteins could be produced in vitro or in cellular systems for high-throughput drug screening. Not only do these expressed proteins provide tools for identifying drug molecules active against a certain system, but the availability of other similar gene sequences enable determination of molecular specificity (eg, dopamine D2 antagonism vs dopamine D1 antagonism). Moreover, these potent drug discovery technologies are no longer exclusive to pharmaceutical companies. Academic researchers in the neuropharmacology area now have access to recombinant protein screening services of the National Institute for Mental Health (NIMH) for novel CNS-active agents. Through an NIMH contract, Drs. Linda Brady and Bryan Roth at Case Western Reserve University maintain cellular systems for assaying drug activity against over 70 neurochemical receptors and transporters. In fact, this system has recently been used in an attempt to resolve the controversy over the active antidepressant component(s) of extracts from the herbal remedy, St. John's wort.[45]

It should be mentioned that long before their testing as therapeutic agents, antisense oligonucleotides were used experimentally to advance our understanding of physiology and pharmacology. As an example, Pasternak and Standifer[46] have outlined their exploitation of antisense molecules in elucidating the functional biology of opioid receptor subtypes. Using antisense molecules to down-regulate certain opioid receptor subtypes (or mRNA-splicing variants of the same receptors), these investigators have been able to differentiate between receptors responsible for morphine-induced spinal analgesia, morphine-induced supraspinal analgesia, and the supraspinal analgesia induced by the active glucuronide conjugate of morphine. A similar approach has been used to investigate dopamine, muscarinic acetylcholine, and NMDA receptors.

Huber[47] provides an excellent review on the therapeutic opportunities involving cellular oncogenes because of the novel approaches fostered by biotechnology. Oncogenes can serve as novel therapeutic targets for cancer diagnosis, prognosis, and treatment. Marx[48] provides another perspective on oncogenes by detailing advancements made in our understanding of tumor suppressor genes whose function is inactivated in carcinogenic progression. Tumor suppressor genes are obviously excellent candidates for reintroduction strategies in treating cancer.

PHARMACEUTICAL MANUFACTURING APPLICATIONS

The use of genetically modified bacteria also has played a part in increasing the efficiency of producing certain pharmaceutically important synthetic organic compounds. For example, researchers have isolated a gene from a species of *Corynebacterium* that codes for 2,5-diketo-D-glucose reductase. This particular enzyme catalyzes the conversion of 2,5-diketo-D-glucose to 2-keto-L-gulose, which is an intermediate in ascorbic acid (vitamin C) production. The scientists successfully have inserted the gene into *Erwinia herbicola* bacteria, via a plasmid. Unchanged *E herbicola* has the ability to ferment D-glucose into 2,5-diketo-D-glucose. Inserting the new gene provides the changed bacterium with the ability to ferment D-glucose to 2-keto-L-gulose in one step. The second step involved in the production of vitamin C is base- or acid-catalyzed cyclization of 2-keto-L-gulose to the acid. Thus, the genetic engineering process saves at least four steps, compared with the previous procedure. The older Keichstein-Grussner process involves six steps in the synthesis of ascorbic acid.[49]

ORGANIC SYNTHESIS APPLICATIONS

In an interesting synthesis application, Iverson and Lerner[50] report on sequence-specific peptide cleavage catalyzed by an antibody. The monoclonal antibodies necessary for this procedure were produced by immunizing with a Co(III) triethylenetetramine (trien)-peptide hapten capable of catalyzing specific hydrolysis of the Gly-Phe bond of peptide substrates at a neutral pH with a metal complex cofactor. As a group, these antibodies are able to bind trien complexes of not only Co(III), but also numerous other metals. At least six peptides were studied as possible substrates with these antibodies as well as various metal complexes. The results of these studies demonstrate the feasibility of using cofactor-assisted catalysis in an antibody-binding site to achieve successful results in difficult chemical transformations.

MORAL AND ETHICAL QUESTIONS

On the matter of moral and ethical questions of biotechnology applications in medicine, numerous articles appear periodically[8,15,51] to debate the issue. Francis Collins, Director of the National Human Genome Research Institute (NHGRI) has written,

"It is estimated that all of us carry dozens of glitches in our DNA–so establishing principles of fair use of this information is important for all of us."

There are many questions such as

Does genetic testing constitute invasion of privacy?
Will there be an increase in abortions that discriminate against the *genetically unfit*?
Should those destined to be stricken with a fatal genetic disease be informed of their fate, especially if there is no remedy available?
Will these decisions become mandated legally and ultimately demean humans or create a new underclass of the genetically less-fortunate?
Should gene therapy be used only for treating disease or also for *improving* an individual's genetic legacy?

Currently, most protections on the use of genetic information are regulated at the state level, resulting in uneven application across the population. Senators Jeffords and Daschle recently outlined their respective views on the passage of federal laws that protect the collection and use of genetic information, particularly relating to employment and health insurance.[15] The Human Genome Project's ELSI program (Ethical, Legal, and Social Implications of Human Genetics Research) is now charged with addressing issues that appear as daunting as the sequencing of the genome itself. The benefits of biotechnology in disease prevention and treatment are numerous and the decoding of the human genome will continue to produce new opportunities to improve our quality of life. But as with all technological advances, safeguards are required to prevent discriminatory and unethical use of this new information.

REFERENCES

1. Bud R. *Nature* 1989; 337:10.
2. Lander ES, Linton LM, Birren B, et al. *Nature* 2001; 409:860.
3. Venter JC, Adams MD, Myers EW, et al. *Science* 2001; 291:1304.
4. Broder S, Caplan A, Evans WE. *J Am Pharm Assoc (Wash)* 2003; 42:S22.
5. Roth RI, Fleischer NM. *J Am Pharm Assoc (Wash)* 2002; 42:692.
6. Maher B. *The Scientist 2003.*
7. Holmer A. Pharmaceutical Research and Manufacturers of America (PhRMA). Washington, DC, 2002:1 - 48.
8. Somia N, Verma IM. *Nat Rev Genet* 2000; 1:91.
9. Rader C, Barbas CF, 3rd. *Curr Opin Biotechnol* 1997; 8:503.
10. Evans WE, Relling MV. *Science* 1999; 286:487.
11. Chee M, Yang R, Hubbell E, et al. *Science* 1996; 274:610.
12. Rosenwald A, Wright G, Chan WC et al. *N Engl J Med* 2002; 346:1937.
13. Gunther EC, Stone DJ, Gerwien RW et al. *Proc Natl Acad Sci U S A* 2003; 100:9608.
14. Petricoin EF, Ardekani AM, Hitt BA, et al. *Lancet* 2002; 359:572.
15. Jeffords JM, Daschle T. *Science* 2001; 291:1249.
16. Gill P, Ivanov PL, Kimpton C, et al. *Nat Genet* 1994; 6:130.
17. Look AT. *Science* 1997; 278:1059.
18. Jackson RC. *Semin Oncol* 1997; 24:164.
19. Tami J, Evens RP. *Pharmacotherapy* 1996; 16:527.
20. Buckel P. *Trends Pharmacol Sci* 1996; 17:450.
21. Cho MJ, Juliano R. *Trends Biotechnol* 1996; 14:153.
22. Hamilton SR, Bobrowicz P, Bobrowicz B, et al. *Science* 2003; 301:1244.
23. Toon S. *Eur J Drug Metab Pharmacokinet* 1996; 21:93.
24. Sheffield WP. *Curr Drug Targets Cardiovasc Haematol Disord* 2001; 1:1.
25. Agrawal S. *Trends Biotechnol* 1996; 14:376.
26. Stein CA. *Trends Biotechnol* 1996; 14:147.
27. Gold L, Polisky B, Uhlenbeck O, et al. *Annu Rev Biochem* 1995; 64:763.
28. McManus MT, Sharp PA. *Nat Rev Genet* 2002; 3:737.
29. Jackson AL, Bartz SR, Schelter J, et al. *Nat Biotechnol* 2003; 21:635.
30. Chi JT, Chang HY, Wang NN, et al. *Proc Natl Acad Sci U S A* 2003; 100:6343.
31. Blau HM, Springer ML. *N Engl J Med* 1995; 333:1204.
32. Anchordoquy TJ, Carpenter JF, Kroll DJ. *Arch Biochem Biophys* 1997; 348:199.
33. Cordell G. *American Druggist* 1987; 96:96.
34. Hailes AM, French CE, Rathbone DA, et al. *Ann N Y Acad Sci* 1996; 799:391.
35. Marsden AF, Caffrey P, Aparicio JF, et al. *Science* 1994; 263:378.
36. Staba J. *Journal of Natural Products* 1995; 48:203.
37. Fujita Y, Hara Y, Suga C, et al. *Plant Cell Reports* 1981; 1:61.
38. Hamill J, Parr A, Robins R, et al. *Bio/Technology* 1987; 5:800.
39. Awad A. Ohio Northern University, Ada, OH, 1987.
40. Constabel F. *Planta Med* 1990; 56:421.
41. Miller H, Ackerman S. *FDA Consum* 1990:8.
42. Ashihara H, Crozier A. *Trends Plant Sci* 2001; 6:407.
43. Ogita S, Uefuji H, Yamaguchi Y, et al. *Nature* 2003; 423:823.
44. Whitehouse D. *BBC Science and Technology News,* 2002.
45. Butterweck V, Nahrstedt A, Evans J, et al. *Psychopharmacology (Berl)* 2002; 162:193.
46. Pasternak GW, Standifer KM. *Trends Pharmacol Sci* 1995; 16:344.
47. Huber BE. *Faseb J* 1989; 3:5.
48. Marx J. *Science* 1994; 266:1942.
49. Anonymous. *Chemical and Engineering News* 1985; 6:6.
50. Iverson BL, Lerner RA. *Science* 1989; 243:1184.
51. Roberts L. *Science* 1989; 243:1134.

BIBLIOGRAPHY
General

Antebi E, Fishlock D. *Biotechnology, Strategies for Life.* Cambridge MA: MIT Press, 1986: 239.

Collins FS, Green ED, Guttamacher AE, et al. *Nature* 2003; 422:835.

Drews J. *Arzneimittelforsch* 1995; 45(8):934.

Schlumberger HD, Stadler P. *Arzneimittelforsch* 1997; 47(1):106.

Schonfeld E. *Fortune* 1997; (Nov 10):293.

Starr C, Taggart R. *Biology, the Unity and Diversity of Life*, 5th ed. Belmont, CA: Wadsworth Publ, 1989.

Wiseman A, ed. *Principles of Biotechnology*, 2nd ed. New York: Surrey University Press (Chapman & Hall), 1988.

Drugs, Medicine and Pharmacy

Anon. *Am J Pharm Educ* 1991;55.

Brenner MK. *N Engl J Med* 1996; 335:337.

Davies JE. In Krongsgaard P, Brøgger Christensen S, Kofod H, eds. *Natural Products and Drug Development* (Alfred Benzon Symp 20). Copenhagen: 1984, p 65.

Fix JA. *Pharm Res* 1996; 13(12):1760.

Galbraith WM. *Prog Clin Biol Res* 1987; 235:3.

Illum L, Davis SS. *Curr Opin Biotechnol* 1991; 2:254,

Hollingshead A. *Springer Semin Immunopathol* 1989; 9:856.

Szkrybalo W. *Pharm Res* 1987; 4:361.

Vermeij P, Blok D. *Pharma World Sci* 1996; 18(3):87.

Plants

Anon. *Chem Eng News* 1984; 16(Oct):29.

Baum R. *Chem Eng News* 1987; (Aug 10).

Pareilliux A. *Ann Pharm Fr* 1987; 45:155.

Powell K. *Nat Biotechnol* 2003; 21:965.

Schell J. In Baba S, et al, eds. *National Resources and Human Health—Plants of Medicinal and Nutritional Value* (Proc 1st WHO Symp on Plants and Health for All: Sci Advance, Kobe, Japan, 26–28 Aug 1991). New York: Elsevier, 1992:49.

Yoxen E. *The Gene Business. Who Should Control Biotechnology.* New York: Oxford University Press, 1983, p 230. [*Note:* This reference provides a detailed analytical study of the corporate agenda for biotechnology. It is a readable account of how genetic engineering evolved from a pure science into a profitable business. The structure and function of the multinational gene business, the effects to date, and the economic, scientific, social, and political implications are examined in detail.)

Biotechnology Medicines Approved and in Development

The content of this chart has been obtained through government and industry sources, based on the latest information. Chart is current as of September 27, 2002. The information may not be comprehensive. For more specific information about a particular product, contact the individual company directly. This table on the entire series of "New Medicines in Development" is available on PhRMA's web site at http://www.phrma.org. Provided as a Public Service by PhRMA. Founded in 1958 as the Pharmaceutical Manufacturers Association.

Copyright © 2002 by the Pharmaceutical Manufacturers Association, with permission.

PRODUCT NAME	COMPANY	INDICATION (DATE OF US APPROVAL)
Actimmune interferon gamma-1b	Genentech, San Francisco, CA	Management of chronic granulomatous disease (12/90) Osteopetrosis (2/00)
Activase alteplase (recombinant)	Genentech, South San Francisco, CA	Acute myocardial infarction (11/87) acute massive pulmonary embolism (6/90) acute myocardial infarction, accelerated infusion (4/95) ischemic stroke within 3 to 5 hours of symptom onset (6/96)
AcuTect Tc-99m apticide	Berlex Laboratories, Montville, NJ	Scintigraphic imaging of acute venous thrombosis in the lower extremities of patients who have signs and symptoms of acute venous thrombosis (9/98)
Adagen injection pegademase bovine	Enzon, Bridgewater, NJ	Treatment of severe combined immunodeficiency disease (SCID) (9/90)
Alferon N interferon alfa-n3 (injection)	Interferon Sciences, New Brunswick, NJ	Genital warts (10/89)
Apligraf graftskin	Novartis Pharmaceuticals, East Hanover, NJ	Treatment of venous leg ulcers (5/98)
Aranesp darbopoietin alfa	Amgen, Thousand Oaks, CA	Treatment of anemia in chronic renal failure (9/01) Treatment of chemotherapy-induced anemia (7/02)
Argatroban	GlaxoSmithKline, Philadelphia, PA/Res. Triangle Park, NC Texas Biotechnology, Houston, TX	Heparin-induced thrombocytopenia (HIT) syndrome (6/00)
Avonex beta interferon 1a (recombinant)	Biogen, Cambridge, MA	Relapsing multiple sclerosis (5/96)
BeneFIX recombinant human factor IX	Wyeth Pharmaceuticals, Philadelphia, PA	Treatment of hemophilia B (2/97)
Betaseron recombinant interferon beta-1b	Berlex Laboratories, Wayne, NJ Chiron, Emeryville, CA	Relapsing, remitting multiple sclerosis (8/93)
BioTropin human growth hormone	Bio-technology General, Iselin, NJ	Growth deficiency in children (5/95)
Campath alemtuzumab	Berlex Laboratories, Montville, NJ ILEX Oncology, San Antonio, TX	treatment of B-cell chronic lymphocytic leukemia (B-CLL) in patients who have been treated with alkylating agents and who have failed fludarabine therapy (5/01)
Carticel autologous cultured chondrocytes	Genzyme Tissue Repair, Cambridge, MA	Repair of clinically significant, symptomatic cartilaginous defects of the femoral condyle (medial, lateral, or trochlear) caused by acute or repetitive trauma (8/97)
CEA-Scan technetium-99m-arcitumomab	Immunomedics, Morris Plains, NJ	presence, location and detection of recurrent and metastatic colorectal cancer (6/96)
Cerezyme imiglucerase (recombinant)	Genzyme, Cambridge, MA	Gaucher's disease (5/94)
Comvax haemophilus b conjugate (meningococcal protein conjugate) and hepatitis b recombinant vaccine	Merck, Whitehouse Station, NJ	vaccination of infants beginning at two months of age against both invasive *Haemophilus influenzae* type b diseases (Hib) and hepatitis B (10/96)
DACS SC stem cell enrichment device	Dendreon, Seattle, WA	Rescue therapy following high-dose chemotherapy (8/99)
Eliteck rasburicase	Sanofi-Synthelabo, New York, NY	Prophylaxis for chemotherapy-induced hyperuricemia, treatment of cancer-related hyperuricemia (7/02)

continued

PRODUCT NAME	COMPANY	INDICATION (DATE OF US APPROVAL)
Enbrel etanercept	Amgen, Thousand Oaks, CA Wyeth Pharmaceuticals, Philadelphia, PA	Moderate to severe rheumatoid arthritis (11/98) Moderate to severe active juvenile rheumatoid arthritis (5/99) Disease modification of active rheumatoid arthritis and psoriatic arthritis (1/02)
Engerix-B hepatitis B vaccine (recombinant)	GlaxoSmithKline, Philadelphia, PA/Res. Triangle Park, NC	Hepatitis B (9/89)
EPOGEN epoetin alfa (rEPO)	Amgen, Thousand Oaks, CA	Treatment of anemia associated with chronic renal failure, including patients on dialysis and not on dialysis, and anemia in Retrovir-treated HIV-infected patients (6/89) treatment of anemia caused by chemotherapy in patients with non-myeloid malignancies (4/93) prevention of anemia associated with surgical blood loss, autologous blood donation adjuvant (12/96) anemia in children with chronic renal failure who are currently undergoing dialysis (11/99)
PROCRIT epoetin alfa (rEPO)	Ortho Biotech, Raritan, NJ	Treatment of anemia associated with chronic renal failure, including patients on dialysis and not on dialysis, and anemia in Retrovir-treated HIV-infected patients (6/90) treatment of anemia caused by chemotherapy in patients with non-myeloid malignancies (4/93) prevention of anemia associated with surgical blood loss, autologous blood donation adjuvant (12/96) anemia in children with chronic renal failure who are currently undergoing dialysis (11/99) [PROCRIT was approved for marketing under Amgen's epoetin alfa PLA. Amgen manufactures the product for Ortho Biotech.] Under an agreement between the two companies, Amgen licensed to Ortho Pharmaceutical the U.S. rights to epoetin alfa for indications for human use excluding dialysis and diagnostics.
Follistim recombinant follicle-stimulating hormone	Organon, West Orange, NJ	infertility (10/97)
GenoTropin somatotropin (rDNA origin) for injection	Pharmacia, Peapack, NJ	Short stature in children due to growth hormone deficiency (8/95) Growth failure due to Prader-Willi syndrome (6/00) Long-term treatment of growth failure in children born small for gestational age (7/01)
Geref human growth hormone-releasing factor	Serono, Rockland, MA	Evaluation of the ability of the somatotroph of the pituitary gland to secrete growth hormone (12/90) Pediatric growth hormone deficiency (10/97)
GlucaGen glucagon (rRNA origin) for injection	Novo Nordisk Pharmaceuticals, Princeton, NJ	Treatment of hypoglycemia and for use as a diagnostic aid (6/98)
Gonal-F recombinant follicle-stimulating hormone (r-FSH)	Serono, Rockland, MA	Female infertility (9/97)
Helixate FS antihemophilic factor (recombinant)	Aventis Behring, King of Prussia, PA	Treatment of hemophilia A (6/00)
Hepsera adefovir dipivoxil	Gilead Sciences, Foster City, CA	Treatment of chronic hepatitis B (9/02)
Herceptin trastuzumab	Genentech, South San Francisco, CA	Treatment of HER2 overexpressing metastatic breast cancer (9/98)
Humalog insulin lispro	Eli Lilly, Indianapolis, IN	Diabetes (10/82)
Humatrope somatotropin (rDNA origin) for injection	Eli Lilly, Indianapolis, IN	Human growth hormone deficiency in children (3/87)

continued

PRODUCT NAME	COMPANY	INDICATION (DATE OF US APPROVAL)
Humulin human insulin (recombinant DNA origin)	Eli Lilly, Indianapolis, IN	Diabetes (10/82)
Infergen interferon alfacon-1	Amgen, Thousand Oaks, CA	Treatment of chronic hepatitis C viral infection (10/97)
Intron A interferon alfa-2b (recombinant)	Schering-Plough, Kenilworth, NJ	Hairy cell leukemia (6/86), genital warts (6/88), Kaposi's sarcoma (11/88), hepatitis C (2/91), hepatitis B (7/92), malignant melanoma (12/95), follicular lymphoma in conjunction with chemotherapy (11/97)
Kineret anakinra	Amgen, Thousand Oaks, CA	Signs and symptoms of rheumatoid arthritis (11/01)
KoGENate antihemophiliac factor (recombinant)	Bayer, West Haven, CT	Treatment of hemophilia A (2/93)
KoGENate-FS rFVIII	Bayer, West Haven, CT	Hemophilia A (6/00)
Leukine sargramostim (GM-CSF)	Berlex Laboratories, Montville, NJ	Autologous bone marrow transplantation (3/91), neutropenia resulting from chemotherapy in acute myelogenous leukemia (9/95), allogenic bone marrow transplantation (11/95), peripheral blood progenitor cell mobilization and transplantation (12/95)
LYMErix Lyme disease vaccine (recombinant OspA)	GlaxoSmithKline, Philadelphia, PA/Rsch. Triangle Park, NC	Prevention of Lyme disease (12/98)
Mylotarg gemtuzumab ozogamicin for injection	Wyeth Pharmaceuticals, Philadelphia, PA	Treatment of patients 60 years and older in first relapse with CD33-positive acute myeloid leukemia (AML) who are not considered candidates for cytotoxic chemotherapy (5/00)
Natrecor nesiritide	Scios, Sunnyvale, CA	Acute decompensated congestive heart failure (8/01)
Neulasta pegfilgrastim	Amgen, Thousand Oaks, CA	Chemotherapy-induced neutropenia (1/02)
Neumega oprelvekin	Wyeth Pharmaceuticals, Philadelphia, PA	Prevention of severe chemotherapy-induced thrombocytopenia (11/97)
NEUPOGEN filgrastim (rG-CSF)	Amgen, Thousand Oaks, CA	Chemotherapy-induced neutropenia (2/91), autologous or allogenic bone marrow transplantation (6/94), chronic severe neutropenia (12/94), support peripheral blood progenitor cell transplantation (12/95), acute myelogenous leukemia (4/98)
Norditropin somatropin (rDNA origin) for injection	Novo Nordisk Pharmaceuticals, Princeton, NJ	Treatment of growth failure in children due to inadequate growth hormone secretion (5/95)
Novolin 70/30 70% NPH human insulin isophane suspension & 30% regular human insulin (rDNA origin)	Novo Nordisk Pharmaceuticals, Princeton, NJ	Insulin-dependent diabetes mellitus (6/91)
Novolin L Lente human insulin zinc suspension (rDNA origin)	Novo Nordisk Pharmaceuticals, Princeton, NJ	Insulin-dependent diabetes mellitus (6/91)
Novolin N NPH human insulin isophane suspension (rDNA origin)	Novo Nordisk Pharmaceuticals, Princeton, NJ	Insulin-dependent diabetes mellitus (7/91)
Novolin R regular human insulin (rDNA origin)	Novo Nordisk Pharmaceuticals, Princeton, NJ	Insulin-dependent diabetes mellitus (6/91)
NovoLog insulin aspart (rDNA origin) injection	Novo Nordisk Pharmaceuticals, Princeton, NJ	Treatment of adult diabetes mellitus (6/00)
NovoLog Mix 70/30 70% insulin aspart (rDNA origin) protamine suspension and 30% insulin aspart (rDNA origin) injection	Novo Nordisk Pharmaceuticals, Princeton, NJ	Treatment of adult diabetes mellitus (11/01)
NovoSeven coagulation factor VIIa (recombinant)	Novo Nordisk Pharmaceuticals, Princeton, NJ	Treatment of bleeding episodes in hemophilia A or B patients with inhibitors to factor VIII or factor IX (3/99)
Nutropin somatropin (rDNA origin) for injection	Genentech, South San Francisco, CA	Growth failure in children due to chronic renal insufficiency, growth hormone inadequacy in children (3/94), Turner's syndrome (12/96), growth hormone inadequacy in adults (12/97)
Nutropin AQ somatropin (injection/liquid)	Genentech, San Francisco, CA	Growth failure in children caused by chronic renal insufficiency

continued

PRODUCT NAME	COMPANY	INDICATION (DATE OF US APPROVAL)
		Growth hormone inadequacy in children (12/95), Turner's syndrome (12/96), growth hormone inadequacy in adults (12/97)
Nutropin Depot somatropin (rDNA origin) for injection (suspension)	Alkermes, Cambridge, MA Genentech, South San Francisco, CA	Growth failure in children due to chronic renal insufficiency, growth hormone inadequacy in children (3/94), Turner's syndrome (12/96), growth hormone inadequacy in adults (12/97)
OncoScint CR/OV satumomab pendetide	CYTOGEN, Princeton, NJ	Detection, staging, and follow-up of colorectal and ovarian cancers (12/92)
Oncospar PEG-L-asparaginase	Enzon, Bridgewater, NJ	First-line treatment of acute lymphoblastic leukemia (2/94)
Ontak denileukin diftitox	Ligand Pharmaceuticals, San Diego, CA Seragen, Hopkinton, MA	Persistent or recurrent cutaneous T-cell lymphoma (2/99)
ORTHOCLONE OKT 3 muromonab-CD3	Ortho Biotech, Raritan, NJ	Reversal of kidney transplant rejection (6/86), reversal of liver and heart transplant rejection (6/93)
PEG-Intron A interferon alfa-2b	Enzon, Bridgewater, NJ Schering-Plough, Kenilworth, NJ	Hepatitis C (8/01)
Proleukin aldesleukin (interleukin 2)	Chiron, Emeryville, CA	Renal cell carcinoma (5/92)
ProstaScint capromab pentetate	CYTOGEN, Princeton, NJ	Detection, staging and follow-up of prostate adenocarcinoma (10/96)
Protropin somatrem for injection	Genentech, San Francisco, CA	Human growth hormone deficiency in children (10/85)
Pulmozyme DNase dornase alpha	Genentech, San Francisco, CA	Cystic fibrosis (12/93), management of advanced cystic fibrosis (12/96)
Rebetron ribavirin/interferon alfa-2b, recombinant combination	Schering-Plough, Kenilworth, NJ	Treatment of chronic hepatitis C in patients who have relapsed following alpha interferon therapy (6/98), treatment of chronic hepatitis C in patients with compensated liver disease previously untreated with alpha interferon therapy (12/99)
Rebif interferon beta-1a	Serono, Rockland, MA	Relapsing forms of multiple sclerosis (3/02)
Recombinate antihemophiliac factor rAHF (recombinant)	Baxter Healthcare, Deerfield, IL Wyeth Pharmaceuticals, Philadelphia, PA	Prevention and control of bleeding episodes in patients with hemophilia A (12/92)
RECOMBIVAX HB hepatitis B vaccine (recombinant), MSD	Merck, Whitehouse Station, NJ	Hepatitis B prevention (7/86)
ReFacto antihemophilic factor VIII (recombinant)	Wyeth Pharmaceuticals, Philadelphia, PA	Hemophilia A (3/00)
Refludan lepirudin (rDNA) for injection	Berlex Laboratories, Montville, NJ	Heparin-induced thrombocytopenia type II (3/98)
Regranex becaplermin	Ortho-McNeil Pharmaceuticals, Raritan, NJ	Chronic diabetic ulcers (12/97)
Remicade infliximab	Centocor, Malvern, PA	Short-term use in Crohn's disease (8/98), reduction in signs and symptoms in rheumatoid arthritis (11/99), inhibit the progression of structural damage in patients with rheumatoid arthritis (1/01), improve physical function in rheumatoid arthritis (2/02), long-term remission-level control of Crohn's disease (7/02)
ReoPro abciximab	Centocor, Malvern, PA Eli Lilly, Indianapolis, IN	Antiplatelet prevention of blood clots in the setting of high risk percutaneous transluminal coronary angioplasty (12/94), refractory unstable angina when percutaneous coronary intervention is planned (11/97)
Retavase reteplase	Centocor, Malvern, PA	Treatment of acute myocardial infarction (10/96)
Rituxan ritixmab	Genentech, South San Francisco, CA IDEC Pharmaceuticals, San Diego, CA	Treatment of relapsed or refractory low-grade or follicular CD20-positive B-cell non-Hodgkin's lymphoma (11/97)
Roferon-A interferon alfa-2a (recombinant)	Roche, Nutley, NJ	Hairy cell leukemia (6/86), AIDS-related Kaposi's sarcoma (11/88), chronic myelogenous leukemia (11/95), hepatitis C (11/96)

continued

PRODUCT NAME	COMPANY	INDICATION (DATE OF US APPROVAL)
Saizen somatropin (rDNA origin) for injection	Serono, Rockland, MA	Pediatric growth hormone deficiency (11/96)
Serostim somatropin (rDNA origin) for injection	Serono, Rockland, MA	Treatment of AIDS-associated catabolism/wasting (8/96), pediatric HIV failure to thrive (2/98)
Simulect basiliximab	Novartis Pharmaceuticals, East Hanover, NJ	Prevention of renal transplant rejection (5/98)
Synagis palivizumab	MedImmune, Gaithersburg, MD	Respiratory syncytial virus (6/98)
Thymoglobulin thymocyte globulin (rabbit)	SangStat, Menlo Park, CA	Prevention of kidney transplant rejection (12/98)
Thyrogen thyrotropin alfa for injection	Genzyme, Cambridge, MA	Detection and treatment of thyroid cancer (11/98)
TNKase tenecteplase	Genentech, South San Francisco, CA	Acute myocardial infarction (6/00)
Velosulin BR buffered regular human insulin injection (rDNA origin)	Novo Nordisk Pharmaceuticals, Princeton, NJ	Treatment of diabetes mellitus (7/99)
Verluma nofetumomab	DuPont Merck Pharmaceutical, Billerica, MA	Detection of small-cell lung cancer (8/96)
Viread tenofovir disoproxil	Gilead Sciences, Foster City, CA	HIV infection (10/01)
Vistide cidofovir injection	Gilead Sciences, Foster City, CA	Cytomegalovirus retinitis in AIDS patients (6/96)
Visudine verteporfin	QLT, Vancouver, British Columbia	Minimally classic age-related macular degeneration (4/00)
Vitravene fomviren sodium injectable	Ciba Vision, Duluth, GA Isis Pharmaceuticals, Carlsbad, CA	Treatment of cytomegalovirus retinitis in patients with AIDS (8/98)
Xigris drotrecogin alfa	Eli Lilly, Indianapolis, IN	Severe sepsis (11/01)
Zenapax daclizumab	Roche, Nutley, NJ Protein Design Labs, Fremont, CA	Prevention of acute kidney transplant rejection (12/97)
Zevalin ibritumomab	IDEC Pharmaceuticals, San Diego, CA	Treatment of relapsed or refractory low grade, follicular, or transformed B-cell non-Hodgkin's lymphoma (2/02)

A Guide to Understanding the New Biotechnology[a]

Appendix A lists a large number of major types of therapeutic products produced using genetic engineering. Many of these terms are new or unfamiliar to all but specialists. To help understand them, the following is an explanation of these new classes of products and the therapeutic benefits they may provide:

ANTICOAGULANTS/THROMBOLYTIC AGENTS—Inappropriate or unnecessary clotting of the blood is responsible for more deaths than cancer. The body's own clot-dissolving process begins with formation of the enzyme plasmin. Substances that activate plasmin are found in the body only in minute amounts. As a result of biotechnology, sufficient quantities of these substances are available and are being developed.

COLONY-STIMULATING FACTORS—The production of white blood cells is controlled by proteins called colony-stimulating factors (CSFs). Cancer chemotherapy and inherited disorders are among the causes of low white blood counts, which lower resistance to infection. CSFs are being investigated not only as a way to counteract low white blood cell counts generally but also as a way to produce specific types of white blood cells. In addition, there is hope that CSFs can stimulate the body to produce additional bone marrow as well as cause some cancer cells to stop dividing.

DISMUTASES—Dismutase, an enzyme, is important in organ transplantation and in treating heart attack when tissues have been deprived of blood for a short time. When the blood flow is restored to the transplanted organ or to the heart muscle after a clot is dissolved, the cells in the organ can be damaged by the excessively oxygen-rich blood. Dismutases prevent this *reperfusion injury* by allowing the oxygen-deprived tissues to recover their normal state in a more orderly manner.

ERYTHROPOIETIN (EPO)—Kidney disease often impairs the body's ability to produce this hormone, causing anemia, a deficiency in red blood cell production. Frequent blood transfusions or restoration of the missing hormone, EPO, can add more red blood cells to correct chronic anemia. Since transfusions may expose those who receive them to infectious agents, such as hepatitis and AIDS, EPO may provide major gains in safety and efficiency. Through genetic engineering, it is now possible to obtain EPO in large amounts, a development of great importance to the 225,000 Americans who rely on kidney dialysis machines. Researchers also are looking into ways to use EPO to treat other types of anemia, including those resulting from arthritis and the side effects of the AIDS drug Retrovir (AZT). Further, since EPO can cause a tenfold increase in red cell production, it is possible that blood banks may be turned into blood farms.

HUMAN GROWTH HORMONE—Our growth is regulated by human growth hormone (hGH) secreted by the pituitary gland. A child whose body produces insufficient hGH will be limited to an adult height of about 4 feet. It is estimated that as many as 15,000 American children suffer from hGH deficiency. Beginning in the late 1950s, such children were treated with hGH extracted from cadaver pituitaries. This not only was extraordinarily expensive but also exposed the children to the risk of infection from viral contamination of the hormone. Now, genetic engineering technology makes available pure supplies of hGH. Research is continuing to find other beneficial applications of this new product.

INTERFERONS—In 1957 it was discovered that a glycoprotein naturally produced by the cells apparently could interfere with the ability of a virus to reproduce after it invaded the body. By the mid-1970s it appeared that this protein, interferon, might also curtail the spread of certain types of cancer. The application of recombinant DNA techniques provided sufficient interferon for useful research. While much more needs to be learned about the interferons, they hold great promise. The alpha group has proved effective against hairy cell leukemia, once a lethal disease. It normalizes blood counts and controls tumor growth in 90% of patients. Alpha interferon is being investigated and has approval applications at FDA for other cancers.

INTERLEUKINS—In the 1960s it was discovered that interleukin, a natural substance occurring in the body, transmits signals between types of white blood cells, or leukocytes. While the full therapeutic potential of the interleukins is only beginning to be explored, interleukin-2 has been used to fight cancer. A patient's T cells, specialized white blood cells involved in ridding the body of diseased cells, are exposed to interleukin outside the patient's body, to activate them against the cancer. The activated T-cells are then given back to the patient, where they are much more effective in finding and destroying the cancer cells.

MONOCLONAL ANTIBODIES—Antibodies, often referred to as the body's missile defense system, are large protein molecules produced by white blood cells. They seek out and destroy harmful foreign substances. Such foreign cells are recognized by telltale surface proteins, called antigens. After the invader has been destroyed, the antibodies remain in the blood, on instant alert should a similar antigen arrive. Antibodies also are useful in matching donors and recipients in organ transplantation, in blood typing, and in measuring and identifying hormones, toxins, and various antigens in blood and fluids. In addition to their extraordinary diagnostic capability, monoclonals can be used alone for a pinpoint attack on a cancerous cell or to mop up cancerous cells remaining after conventional chemotherapy. They also can be enlisted as porters (adjuvants or adjuncts) to transport drugs, toxins, or radioactive particles to such cells.

PEPTIDES—Proteins are made of simple organic molecules called amino acids. When the amino acids are *knitted* together, they form peptide links. As more amino acids are combined, the chain of the peptide becomes longer. At a certain point, when about 40 or 50 amino acids are joined together, the peptide becomes a protein. Thus, peptides and proteins only differ by the length of their amino acid chain. The body often uses peptides as special messenger substances for specific purposes such as increasing heart beat or body temperature and turning on or off a cell that secretes an important substance. Because peptides are smaller, they travel around the body more efficiently than larger proteins. Once the peptide reaches its target and does its job, it is broken down easily by the body to stop the process. Scientists also have learned that only portions of a protein are involved in biological activity. By making the peptide portion of the protein that shows biological activity, a number of peptide drugs have been discovered.

TUMOR NECROSIS FACTOR—As far back as the 1700s, a few physicians noted that cancer regression sometimes ac-

[a] Courtesy, PhRMA, 1996.

companied an infection. In 1975 it was learned that in response to some bacterial infections, the body produces peptides that permit cells to transmit signals to one another. One such intercellular messenger, tumor necrosis factor (TNF), triggers the deployment of immune defenses that can destroy tumors. By damaging the blood vessels that nourish the tumor, it is, in effect, starved to death. Research continues on how it works and how best to control it.

VACCINES—When a virus or other germ invades the body, its immune system produces antigens to protect it by attaching to the protein coat on the surface of the virus. Genetic engineering allows large-scale production of the protein components of a virus. A vaccine using only the protein coat of the virus will still activate antigen production to neutralize the real, full virus. The *protein coat* vaccine is incapable of reproducing like the virus and therefore cannot cause the disease.

Glossary[a]

ACTINIC KERATOSES–Roughness and thickening of the skin caused by overexposure to the sun's ultraviolet rays. It can degenerate into a skin cancer called squamous cell carcinoma.

ADENOCARCINOMA—Technical name for a malignant tumor derived from a gland or glandular tissue, or a tumor of which the gland-derived cells form gland-like structures. Examples include most cancers of the colon, breast, pancreas, and kidney and many of the other organs.

ADJUNCT—An auxiliary treatment that is secondary to the main treatment.

ADJUVANT—Substance or drug that aids another substance in its action.

AIDS—Acquired immune deficiency syndrome.

ALLOGENEIC (transplantation)–Refers to having cell types that are distinct and cause reactions in the immune system.

AMYLOIDOSIS–A disease in which amyloid, an unusual protein that normally isn't present in the body, accumulates in various tissues. There are many forms of the disease. In primary amyloidosis, the cause isn't known, but it is associated with abnormalities of plasma cells. In secondary amyloidosis, the disease is secondary to another disease, such as tuberculosis. A third form is hereditary and affects nerves and certain organs.

AMYOTROPHIC LATERAL SCLEROSIS (ALS)—Also known as Lou Gehrig's disease, the most common of the motor neuron diseases, a group of rare disorders in which the nerves that control muscular activity degenerate within the brain and spinal cord, causing weakness and wasting of the muscles.

ANAPLASTIC ASTROCYTOMAS—Fast-growing primary brain tumors that originate in nerve tissue. They can produce signs of abnormal brain function, such as weakness, loss of sensation and an unsteady gait.

ANGIOPLASTY—A technique to open up blocked coronary arteries with a catheter tube.

ANKYLOSING SPONDYLITIS–An inflammatory disorder of unknown cause that primarily affects the spine. The vertebrae may fuse together and form a rigid back that is impossible to bend. The arthritis may involve large joints, such as the hip.

ANTISENSE—An antisense drug is the mirror, or complementary image, of a small segment of messenger RNA (mRNA), the substance that carries instructions *(sense)* from the genes to the cell's protein-making machinery. The antisense drug readily binds to the mRNA strand, keeping it from transmitting its instructions to the cell and thus inhibiting the production of an unwanted protein.

ATOPIC DERMATITIS—A chronic form of eczema characterized by an intensely itchy skin rash occurring in people who have an inherited tendency toward allergies, such as asthma or allergic rhinitis. It is common in babies, often appearing between the ages of 2 and 18 months.

AUTOLOGOUS (TRANSFUSION; TRANSPLANTATION)—An autologous blood transfusion uses the patient's own blood. An autologous transplantation refers to a graft in which the donor and recipient areas are in the same individual.

B- AND T-CELL LYMPHOMAS—Cancers caused by proliferation of the two principal types of white blood cells, B and T lymphocytes.

BIOTECHNOLOGY—The collection of industrial processes that involve the use of biological systems. For some of the industries, these processes involve the use of genetically engineered organisms. For the purpose of this chart, only those products that involve recombinant DNA, monoclonal antibody/hybridoma, continuous cell lines, cellular therapy, and gene therapy technology are included.

CLOTTING FACTORS—Proteins involved in the normal clotting of blood.

CLONE—A group of genetically identical cells or organisms asexually descended from a common ancestor. All cells in the clone have the same genetic material and are exact copies of the original. An additional molecular biological use of the word is to refer to a DNA plasmid construct used as the source for generation of protein/peptide pharmaceuticals.

CMV (CYTOMEGALOVIRUS)—A DNA virus related to the herpes virus, affecting mostly neonatal infants and immunocompromised individuals. CMV is sexually transmitted and can occur without symptoms or result in mild flu-like symptoms. As an opportunistic infection in AIDS patients, it can cause *CMV retinitis,* an inflammation of the retina that can lead to blindness if left untreated.

COLITIS—Inflammation of the colon or large intestine.

COLONY STIMULATING FACTOR (CSF)–Protein responsible for the production of white blood cells.

CONGESTIVE HEART FAILURE—The end result of many different types of heart disease. The heart cannot pump blood out normally. This results in congestion (water and salt retention) in the lungs, swelling in the extremities, and reduced blood flow to body tissues.

CROHN'S DISEASE–A subacute chronic gastrointestinal disorder, involving the small intestine, characterized by deep patchy ulcers that may cause fistulas and a narrowing and thickening of the bowel.

CYSTIC FIBROSIS—A genetic disorder of the exocrine glands that causes abnormal mucous secretions that obstruct glands and ducts in various organs, particularly the lungs. It is the most common fatal hereditary disorder of US Caucasians and the most common cause of chronic lung disease in children and young adults.

CYTOKINES—Substances secreted usually by cells of the immune system that can produce an effect on other cells. Chemically consist of protein hormones. Are normally involved in common and pathological functions of the immune system.

DYSPLASIA—Any abnormality of growth, such as abnormal cell features including the size, shape, and rate of multiplication of cells.

ENDOGENOUS—Arising from within the body.

ENZYME REPLACEMENT THERAPY—A therapeutic procedure in which an isolatable or genetically engineered protein is used to replace a defective or missing human enzyme.

EX VIVO—Occurring outside the body.

FUSION GENE—Made up of two or more gene-coding DNA molecules commonly fused together via DNA ligase enzyme or by a modification of the polymerase chain reaction. This results in a union of individual genetic elements that can be used in genetic engineering of a recombinant molecule designed to produce a polypeptide coded by the combined gene units.

---

[a] Compiled from past and current PMA/PhRMA surveys.

GENOME—The entire DNA capable of expressing all the genetic information in the cell.

GAUCHER'S DISEASE—A group of inherited diseases caused by a lack of, or deficient amount of, an enzyme *(gluco-cerebrosidase)* that causes an accumulation of effects throughout the body that usually results in death.

GENE THERAPY—Therapy at the intracellular level to replace or inactivate the effects of disease-causing genes or to augment normal gene functions to overcome disease.

GRAFT VS HOST DISEASE (GVHD)—A complication in bone marrow transplants in which immune system cells attack the transplant recipient's tissue.

GROWTH FACTORS—Factors responsible for regulating cell proliferation (rapid and repeated reproduction), function, and differentiation.

HEMOPHILIA A AND B—Hemophilia A, the *classic* hemophilia, is a genetic bleeding disorder caused by deficiency of the coagulation factor VIII. Hemophilia B, or *Christmas* disease, is caused by deficiency of coagulation factor IX.

HEMATOLOGICAL NEOPLASMS—Tumors of the blood-forming organs.

HEPATITIS–Inflammation of the liver with accompanying liver cell damage or death, caused most often by viral infection, eg, hepatitis A, B, and C.

HERPES SIMPLEX 2—A strain of herpes virus that may lie dormant in nerve tissue and can be reactivated to produce painful sores of the anus or genitals.

HIV—Human immunodeficiency virus (the virus that causes AIDS).

HUMAN PAPILLOMAVIRUS (HPV)—Viral agent of warts, believed to be contagious, affecting only the skin's topmost layer. Associated with human cervical cancer, since the cervix contains keratin-expressing cells.

HUNTINGTON'S DISEASE—Huntington's chorea is an uncommon, inherited disease in which degeneration of the basal ganglia results in rapid, jerky, involuntary movements and dementia (progressive mental impairment). Symptoms do not usually appear until age 35 to 50.

HYBRIDOMA—A cell culture consisting of a clone of fused cells of different kinds, eg, mouse myeloma cells and lymphocytes. A cell that produces antibody can be rendered *immortal* by fusing it with a tumor cell (see *Monoclonal*).

INFLAMMATORY BOWEL DISEASE—Term for inflammatory disorders affecting the small and/or large intestine.

INTERFERON—A glycoprotein naturally produced by cells that interferes with the ability of a virus to reproduce after it invades the body. Interferon potentially might also curtail the spread of certain types of cancer.

IN VIVO—Within the body.

ISCHEMIA—Insufficient supply of blood to an organ or tissue, which can cause damage such as an *ischemic stroke.*

IV—Intravenous.

KAPOSI'S SARCOMA—A rare, malignant skin tumor, which occurs in some AIDS patients. It can be accompanied by fever, enlarged lymph nodes, and gastrointestinal problems.

LEUKEMIA—Form of cancer in which the white blood cells are dedifferentiated and grow abnormally.

LUPUS NEPHRITIS—Inflammation of the kidney(s) caused by systemic lupus erythematosus.

LYMPHOKINE—Cytokine derived from a lymphocyte.

LYMPHOMA—Cancer in which the cells of lymphoid tissue, found mainly in the lymph nodes and spleen, multiply unchecked. Lymphomas fall into two categories: One is called *Hodgkin's disease,* characterized by a particular kind of abnormal cell. All others are called *non-Hodgkin's lymphomas,* which vary in their malignancy according to the nature and activity of the abnormal cells.

MONOKINE—Cytokine derived from a monocyte, usually a macrophage.

MALARIA VIVAX—Vivax is one of the four species of the genus *Plasmodium* responsible for human malaria, which is transmitted from human to human by the bite of infected female *Anopheles* mosquitoes.

MALIGNANT MELANOMA—A cancer made up of pigmented (usually brown-colored) skin cells anywhere in the body.

METASTASES—Secondary cancers that have spread from the primary or original cancer site.

MONOCLONAL—Derived from a single cell; pertaining to a single clone. *Monoclonal antibodies* are produced from hybrid cells by use of hybridoma technology; these antibodies can be traced back to production by a single cell.

MULTIPLE MYELOMA—A malignant condition characterized by uncontrolled proliferation of plasma cells (a class of white blood cells) in bone marrow. Symptoms include pain and destruction of bone tissue, numbness and paralysis, kidney damage, anemia, and frequent infections. The condition is rare and affects those of middle to older age groups.

MULTIPLE SCLEROSIS (MS)—Progressive disease of the central nervous system in which scattered patches of the covering of nerve fibers (myelin) in the brain and spinal cord are destroyed. Symptoms range from numbness and tingling to incontinence and paralysis.

MYELODYSPLASTIC SYNDROMES—A group of acquired blood disorders, often referred to as *preleukemia,* which ultimately are fatal, as patients usually succumb to infections or bleeding.

MYELOGENOUS LEUKEMIA—One of the many forms of cancer of the blood-forming organs in the bone marrow. The blood cells are not complete and do not function properly.

MYOCARDIAL INFARCTION—Damage to the heart muscle caused by stoppage or impairment of blood flow to the heart, also known as a heart attack.

NECROTIZING FASCIITIS–An extremely severe form of cellulites (bacterial skin infection) that destroys infected tissue under the skin. Some refer to it as the "flesh-eating disease."

NEUROBLASTOMA—A tumor of the adrenal glands or sympathetic nervous system. Neuroblastomas are the most common extracranial (outside the skull) solid tumor of childhood.

NEUTROPENIA—Caused by an abnormally low neutrophil count (certain white blood cells), leaving a patient vulnerable to bacterial infections.

ONCOLYTIC VIRUSES–The use of viruses to preferettially infect and kill cancer cells while not harming healthy cells. Oncolytic refers to lysis or breakdown of cancer cells through the process of apoptosis. There are many methods of oncolytic virus therapy, all of which involve the virus becoming active in cancer cells that have specific genetic and metabolic transformations.

OSTEOMYELITIS—Infection of bone and bone marrow, usually caused by bacteria.

OXYGEN TOXICITY IN PREMATURE NEONATES—Incomplete development of the lungs in premature babies causes damage from high oxygen levels.

PARKINSON'S DISEASE—Chronic neurological disease of unknown cause, characterized by tremors, rigidity, and an abnormal gait. There is an imbalance of dopamine and acetylcholine, brain neurotransmitters. Some patients with advanced disease develop dementia. It is a common chronic disease of later life.

PERIPHERAL NEUROPATHY—Disease, inflammation, or damage to the peripheral nerves, which connect the central nervous system to the sense organs, muscles, glands, and internal organs.

PERTUSSIS—Also called *whooping cough,* which mainly affects infants and young children.

PHASE I—Safety testing and pharmacological profiling in humans.

PHASE II—Effectiveness testing in humans.

PHASE III—Extensive clinical trials in humans.

PRADER-WILLI SYNDROME–A genetic disorder characterized by short stature, mental retardation, abnormally small hands and feet, hypogonadism, and uncontrolled appetite leading to extreme obesity.

PROPHYLAXIS—Preventive treatment; intended to preserve health and prevent the spread of disease.

PSEUDOMONAS INFECTIONS—Refers to infections caused by a genus of bacteria called *Pseudomonas.*

PULMONARY EMBOLISM—A blood clot that obstructs the pulmonary artery, which transports blood from the heart to the lungs. More than 90% of pulmonary emboli originate as clots in the deep veins of the lower extremities (deep vein thromboses). They can result in sudden death.

RECOMBINANT DNA—The hybrid DNA produced by joining pieces of DNA from different sources. Usually designated as rDNA.

RECOMBINANT SOLUBLE RECEPTORS—Synthetic version of cellular receptors manufactured with recombinant DNA technology, used as decoys to attract pathogens that otherwise would bind to cellular receptors and cause disease. They are *soluble* because they are freestanding and not attached to cells.

RESPIRATORY SYNCYTIAL VIRUS DISEASE (RSV)—One of the most important causes of lower respiratory tract disease in children, accounting for more than 90% of cases of bronchiolitis.

RENAL ALLOGRAFT REJECTION—Rejection of a transplanted kidney.

RENAL FAILURE—Kidney failure.

RHINITIS—Inflammation of the membranes of the nose.

SEPSIS—A condition associated with the presence of bacteria in the blood. *Gram-negative sepsis* is caused by a particular kind of bacteria.

SEPTIC SHOCK—Blood poisoning due to reaction to toxins made by bacteria. The effects of shock include a sudden drop in blood pressure and changes in heart rate and temperature.

SCLERODERMA—Shrinkage and hardening of the skin anywhere in the body.

STROKE (CEREBRAL THROMBOSIS)—Usually caused by atherosclerosis, a blood clot obstructs a major blood vessel of the brain, resulting in death or serious brain damage.

THALASSEMIA—An inherited blood disorder in which the abnormal production of hemoglobin causes fragile and broken blood cells leading to anemia.

THROMBOCYTOPENIA—A reduction in the number of platelet cells in the blood, which causes a tendency to bleed, especially from the smaller blood vessels.

TISSUE PLASMINOGEN ACTIVATOR (TPA)—tPA is a substance produced in small amounts by the inner lining of blood vessels that prevents abnormal blood clotting by converting plasminogen (an inactive protein in the blood) to the active enzyme plasmin.

TURNER'S SYNDROME—Females born with a missing X chromosome are characterized by shortness of stature, webbed neck, absence or very retarded development of secondary sexual characteristics, absence of menstruation, narrowing of the aorta, eye and bone abnormalities, some mental retardation, and infertility.

UNSTABLE ANGINA—An accelerating pattern of chest pain in cases of previously stable angina, which is caused by insufficient oxygen in the heart muscle.

VENOUS STASIS—Diminished or complete stoppage of blood flow through one or more veins.

WASTING SYNDROMES—Any number of conditions, such as anorexia and cachexia, resulting in a loss of body mass, notably protein.

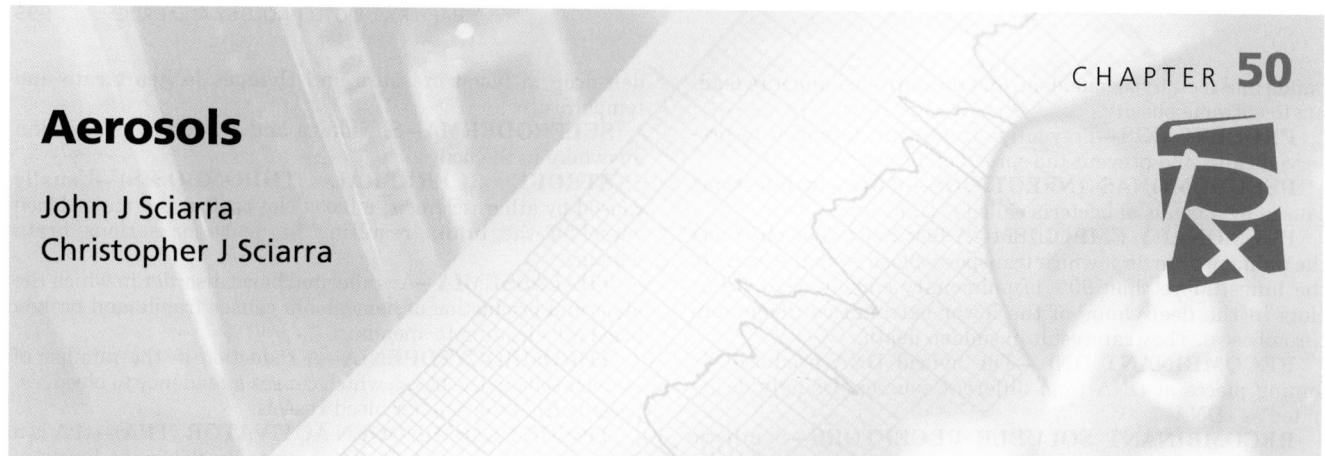

CHAPTER 50

Aerosols

John J Sciarra
Christopher J Sciarra

Inhalation therapy has been used for many years, and there has been a resurgence of interest in delivery of drugs by this route of administration. The number of new drug entities delivered by the inhalation route has increased over the past 5 to 10 years. This type of therapy also has been applied to delivery of drugs through the nasal mucosa, as well as through the oral cavity for buccal absorption. Originally, this type of therapy was used primarily to administer drugs directly to the respiratory system (treatment of asthma); inhalation therapy is now being used for drugs to be delivered to the bloodstream and finally to the desired site of action. Proteins (insulins), steroids, cardiac agents, immunizing agents, etc, are being developed for delivery in this manner.

Drugs administered via the respiratory system (inhalation therapy) can be delivered either orally or nasally. Further, these products can be developed as a:

nebulizer/atomizer
dry powder inhaler
nasal inhaler
metered dose aerosol inhaler

Drugs delivered via a nebulizer/atomizer are generally formulated as aqueous solutions (or suspensions) and are inhaled by the patient through an atomizer, nebulizer, or other similar devices. These products are not included in this chapter.

Dry powders have been used for inhalation therapy for over 75 years. The active ingredients were packaged in capsules, representing a single dose of drug. The capsule was punctured and a small amount of powder fell into a chamber while the patient inhaled. The procedure was repeated until all of the powder was inhaled. While these dry powders were somewhat popular during the early 1940s–1950s, they fell into disuse with the introduction of the aerosol metered dose inhaler, which became available around 1955. This first generation MDI was formulated with chlorofluorocarbons (CFC), was compact, and contained epinephrine hydrochloride or albuterol as the active ingredient. These MDIs quickly became the dosage form of choice for inhalation therapy, especially for the treatment of asthmatics. With the phase out of CFC's starting in 1996, dry powders containing about 25–30 to 60 doses of active ingredient were developed and became commercially available from 2000 to 2003. Several dry powder inhalers currently available include salmeterol, fluticasone, and budesonide. Mometasone dry powder inhaler is available in Europe while insulin dry powder inhaler is presently in the final stages of development and submitted to the Food and Drug Administration for review. These dry powder inhalers do not contain a propellant. These consist of active, very potent drugs that are dispensed from a specially designed package. An accurate amount of drug as a dry powder is released while the patient inhales deeply. The dry powder

will then travel to the lungs along with the inspired air. The technology of dry powders is not a part of this chapter.

The nasal metering drug delivery system produces an aqueous spray consisting of active ingredient and excipients. The drugs used can act locally within the nasal mucosa or systemically by passing the nasal mucosa and enter the general circulation system. This occurs via numerous capillary vessels present in the mucosa. These nasal sprays can also be formulated similar to MDIs using propellants and a nasal adapter. The latter type of nasal inhaler is included in this chapter.

The development of the metered-dose inhaler (MDI) in the mid 1950s made possible a convenient dosage form for the delivery of medication to the respiratory system. Atomizers and nebulizers were cumbersome to use and in many instances did not offer convenience of use, so that administration of drugs by atomizers/nebulizers was generally left to hospital or at-home use. While many improvements were made to these nebulizers and atomizers, they lacked the convenience of use especially as to their portability and use outside of a hospital and/or home setting.

Metered Dose Inhalers consists of a pressurized container filled with active ingredient, excipients and propellant, and a metered-dose valve. The pressurized container is placed within an oral adapter (mouthpiece), and when the unit is dispensed, an exact amount of drug is expelled in the proper particle size distribution to achieve maximum deposition of drug into the lungs. The aerosol dosage form (MDI) has become the dosage form of choice for delivery of drugs to the lungs. Metered dose inhalers are formulated as solutions or suspensions of active drug in a mixture of solvents, dispersing agents, and liquefied gas propellants.

Topical pharmaceutical aerosols can be formulated as a spray, foam, and semisolid and can be used to deliver therapeutic agents topically to the skin surface, rectally, and vaginally. They consist of a liquid, emulsion, or semisolid concentrate and liquefied gas or compressed gas propellant. Each of these systems is discussed in later parts of this chapter.

Many therapeutically active ingredients have been administered or applied to the body by means of the aerosol dosage form. This dosage form has been used orally to dispense a variety of agents such as budesonide, salmeterol xinafoate, fluticasone propionate, fenoterol, epinephrine hydrochloride, albuterol, albuterol sulfate, metaproterenol sulfate, cromolyn sodium, flunisolide hemihydrate, ipratropium bromide, beclomethasone dipropionate, and triamcinolone acetonide. These MDIs were formulated using a CFC propellant and are currently in widespread use in the United States even though the use of CFCs has been phased out throughout the world. Some exemptions have been granted to Third World Countries and "essential use" exemption has been granted to MDIs, which were commercially available prior to the year 2000.

Oral aerosols have been used mainly for the symptomatic treatment of asthma as well as for the treatment of several other ailments. These aerosols have been readily accepted by both physician and patient.

ADVANTAGES—One of the main reasons for the rapid and widespread acceptance of the MDI dosage form for the administration of therapeutically active agents is that it affords many distinct advantages to the user. These advantages have been described by various investigators and, for MDIs, include:

Rapid onset of action

Circumvention of the first-pass effect and avoidance of degradation in the GI tract

Lower dosage that will minimize adverse reactions, especially in the case of steroid therapy where most of the steroid reaches the respiratory tract and less is swallowed

Dose titration to individual needs and ideal for prn medication

Alternate route when therapeutic agent may interact chemically or physically with other medicinals needed concurrently

Viable alternative when the drug entity exhibits erratic pharmacokinetics upon oral or parenteral administration

Container and valve closure are tamperproof

The pressure package is convenient and easy to use. Medication is dispensed in a ready-to-use form at the push of a button. There is generally no need for further handling of the medication. Since the medication is sealed in a tamperproof pressure container, there is no danger of contamination of the product with foreign materials, and at the same time, the contents can be protected from the deleterious effects of both air and moisture. Easily decomposed drugs, such as epinephrine, lend themselves to this type of package as oxygen is excluded from the headspace.

Sterility is always an important consideration with certain pharmaceutical and medicinal preparations. While initial sterility is generally no problem to the manufacturer, there is concern for the maintenance of the sterility of the package during use as, for example, with ophthalmic preparations. When necessary, the aerosol package can be prepared under aseptic conditions, and sterility be maintained throughout the life of the product. For those products requiring regulation of dosage, a metering valve can be used. An accurately measured dose of therapeutically active drug can be administered quickly and, in the case of drugs for inhalation, buccal or nasal application, in the proper particle-size range.

There are many advantages to the administration of medicinal agents by inhalation, buccally and nasally. Response to drugs administered by inhalation, buccally and nasally, is prompt, often very specific and with minimal side effects, faster in onset of activity than drugs given orally and, with most drugs, approaches intravenous therapy in rapidity of action. Drugs that normally are decomposed in the GI tract can be administered safely by inhalation, buccally and nasally. The use of the self-pressurized aerosol package makes this type of therapy simple, convenient, and acceptable, compared with the use of atomizers and nebulizers, which are bulky and require cleaning.

DEFINITIONS—The term *aerosol* is used to denote various systems ranging from those of a colloidal nature to systems consisting of *pressurized packages*. Aerosols have been defined as colloidal systems consisting of very finely subdivided liquid or solid particles dispersed in and surrounded by a gas. Originally, the term *aerosol* referred to liquid or solid particles having a specific size range, but this concept has fallen into disuse.

The present-day definition refers to those products that depend upon the power of a liquefied or compressed gas to dispense the active ingredient(s) in a finely dispersed spray, foam, or semisolid. Pump systems that also dispense the active ingredient(s) in the form of a finely dispersed mist (although of greater particle size) often are classified as aerosols. These pump systems generally are used to dispense medication intranasally.

In 1978, the use of certain chlorofluorocarbons (CFCs) was curtailed by the FDA, EPA, and CPSC. These restrictions applied to the use of Propellants 11, 12, and 114 (CFCs) for use in all aerosol products. Exemptions were granted to MDIs and a few other essential uses. Because of these restrictions, new valve systems and dispensing systems, which allowed greater use of liquefied hydrocarbons and compressed gases, were developed for non-MDIs. While newer HFA propellants were developed for use with MDIs, CFC propellants still can be used to produce medicinal aerosols that are currently commercially available in the US. These regulatory requirements are discussed in greater detail in the *Propellant* section of this chapter.

MODE OF OPERATION

Liquefied-Gas Systems

Liquefied gases have been used widely as propellants for most aerosol products. These compounds are useful for this purpose, since they are gases at room temperature and atmospheric pressure. However, they can be liquefied easily by lowering the temperature (below the boiling point) or by increasing the pressure. The compounds chosen generally have boiling points below 70°F (21°) and vapor pressures between 14 and 85 psia at 70°F (21°). When a liquefied-gas propellant is placed into a sealed container, it immediately separates into a liquid and a vapor phase.

Since these materials are liquefied gases, some of the molecules will leave the liquid state and enter the vapor state. As molecules enter the vapor state, a pressure gradually develops. As the number of molecules in the vapor state increases, the pressure also will increase. An equilibrium soon is attained between the number of molecules changing from a liquid to a vapor and from a vapor to a liquid. The pressure at this point is referred to as the vapor pressure (expressed as psia) and is characteristic for each propellant at any given temperature. The term psig (pounds/square inch gauge) represents the uncorrected gauge pressure and is to be distinguished from psia (pounds per square inch absolute), which is corrected to include atmospheric pressure (0 psig, which equals 14.7 psia). This vapor pressure is exerted equally in all directions and is independent of the quantity of liquefied gas present.

The pressure exerted against the liquid phase is sufficient to push the latter up a dip tube and against the valve. In cases when there is no dip tube (MDIs) the container is used in the inverted position so that the liquid phase is in direct contact with the valve. When the valve is opened, the liquid phase is emitted and comes into contact with the warm air at atmospheric pressure. The liquid propellant immediately reverts to the vapor state, since its boiling point is substantially below room temperature. As the contents of the container are expelled, the volume within the container occupied by the vaporized propellant increases, causing a temporary fall in pressure. However, as soon as the pressure decreases, a sufficient number of molecules change from the liquid state to the vapor state and restore the original pressure. When a compressed gas is used as the propellant, the relationship is quite different, and there is a drop in pressure as the contents are used.

TWO-PHASE SYSTEM—This is the simplest of all aerosol systems. It consists of a solution or a suspension of active ingredients in liquid propellant or a mixture of liquid propellant and solvent. Both a liquid and a vapor phase are present, and when the valve is depressed, liquid propellant containing dissolved active ingredients and other solvents are released. Depending on the nature of the propellants used, the quantity of propellant present, and the valve mechanism, a fine mist or wet spray is produced because of the large expansion of the propellant at room temperature and atmospheric pressure. This system is used to formulate aerosols for inhalation or nasal application.

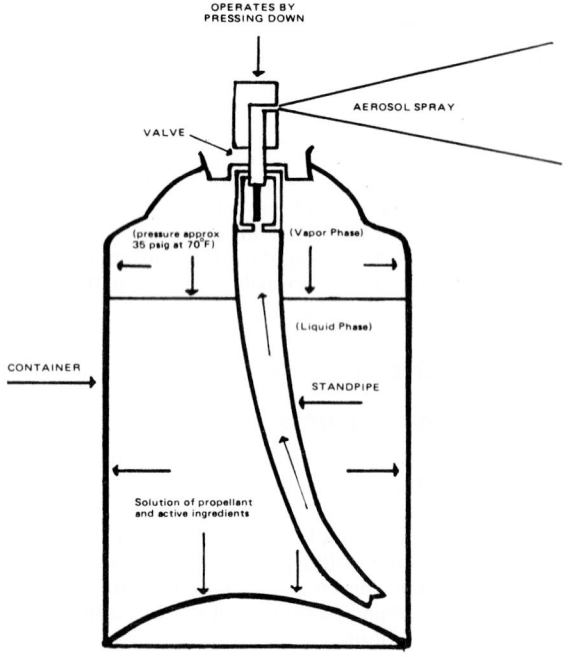

Figure 50-1. Cross-section of a typical space or surface-coating aerosol spray.

Fluorocarbon propellants, primarily trichloromonofluoromethane (P-11), dichlorodifluoromethane (P-12), and dichlorotetrafluoroethane (P-114), are used for MDIs provided that they currently have been approved under an NDA or ANDA. All new products must use other fluorocarbon propellants that are environmentally acceptable, a hydrocarbon propellant, or a compressed gas. The section dealing with propellants indicates those that are useful for this purpose.

A *space spray* generally contains from 2 to 20% active ingredients and from 80 to 98% propellant. While the pressure of space sprays is in the range of 30 to 40 psig, the particles that are produced range from less than 1 to 50 μm. These particles remain suspended in air for relatively long periods of time. Space insecticides, room deodorants, and vaporizer sprays are examples of this type of system. MDIs formulated with a non-CFC propellant will generally have a internal pressure of about 50 to 70 psig.

A *surface-coating spray* (a relatively wet or coarse spray) can be achieved by decreasing the amount of low-boiling propellants and increasing the ratio of active ingredients and solvents. The product concentrate can vary from 20 to 75%, and the propellant from 25 to 80%. Particles are produced ranging in size from 50 to 200 μm. Products such as hair sprays, residual insecticides, perfumes, colognes, paints, protective coatings, and topical

sprays are formulated in this manner. The pressure of this system is generally lower than that in the space spray.

Figure 50-1 shows a cross-section of a typical space or surface-coating aerosol spray.

The liquefied gas propellants widely used for MDIs include those shown in Table 50-1. Combinations of these propellants are used to achieve the desired spray characteristics. In certain instances the nature of the product will determine the propellant combination. Dispersion or suspension sprays used for MDIs are similar to space sprays in that they are two-phase systems, in which the active ingredients are either dissolved or suspended, in the liquid propellant phase. At the present time Propellants 12, 12/11, or 12/114, are used for these inhalation aerosols that are exempted from the CFC ban. Propellant 134a is used to formulate the only non-CFC MDIs approved by the FDA for use in the U.S. Propellant 227 also can be used to formulate aerosols with a non-CFC propellant. Their properties are shown in Table 50-2. Propellant 152a can be used in topical aerosols along with hydrocarbons, dimethyl ether (DME), and compressed gases. The properties of these propellants are included in Tables 50-3 to 50-5.

THREE-PHASE SYSTEM—This system is useful for topical pharmaceutical aerosols in that it allows a greater use of liquid components not miscible with the propellants. Water is not miscible with liquefied-gas propellants and, in many instances, presents a problem, since active ingredients are soluble in water. With the increased emphasis upon the decrease of volatile organic compounds (VOCs) in all products, these systems are finding increased use. These problems have been overcome to a large extent by use of the three-phase system. Depending on the nature of the formulation, one of the following two systems may be employed. Dimethyl ether is most useful for products containing large amounts of water.

Two-Layer System—In this system the liquid propellant, the vaporized propellant, and the aqueous solution of active ingredients make up the three phases. Since the liquid propellant and water are not miscible, the liquid propellant will separate as an immiscible layer. When a hydro alcohol mixture is used, the propellant and hydro alcohol solution will mix and form a single layer. When this propellant is of the fluorocarbon type, being denser than water, it will fall to the bottom of the container. Hydrocarbons, on the other hand, are lighter than water and, when used in this manner, will float on top of the aqueous layer. A spray is produced by the mechanical action of an exceedingly small valve orifice through which the liquid and some vaporized propellant are forced by the vapor pressure of the propellant. The vapor layer is replaced continuously by vaporization of the liquid layer of propellant. This action results in the maintenance of a constant vapor pressure in the headspace.

An important characteristic of this system is that the propellant layer can be adjusted by varying the components so its specific gravity is almost equal to, but does not exceed, that of the hydroalcoholic phase. The propellant floats on top of the hydro alcoholic phase and, when shaken, is dispersed easily. When the valve is depressed, sprays are produced of varying

Table 50-1. Properties of Fluorocarbons (CFCs)

PROPERTY		TRICHLOROMONOFLUOROMETHANE	DICHLORODIFLUOROMETHANE	DICHLOROTETRAFLUOROETHANE
Molecular formula		CCl_3F	CCl_2F_2	$CClF_2CClF_2$
Numerical designation		11	12	114
Molecular weight		137.28	120.93	170.93
Boiling point (1 atm)	°F	74.7	−21.6	38.39
	°C	23.7	−29.8	3.55
Vapor pressure (psia)	70°F	13.4	84.9	27.6
	130°F	39.0	196.0	73.5
Liquid density (g/mL)	70°F	1.485	1.325	1.468
	130°F	1.403	1.191	1.360
Solubility in water (weight %)	77°F	0.11	0.028	0.013

Table 50-2. Properties of Hydrofluorocarbons (HFCs)

PROPERTY		TETRAFLUOROETHANE	HEPTAFLUOROPROPANE
Molecular formula		CF_3CH_2F	CF_3CHFCF_3
Numerical designation		134a	227
Molecular weight		102	170
Boiling point (1 atm)	°F	−15.0	−3.2
	°C	−26.2	−16.5
Vapor pressure (psig)	70°F	71.1	43 at (20°)
	130°F	198.7	—
Liquid density (g/mL)	21.1°	1.22	1.41
Flammability		Nonflammable	Nonflammable
Solubility in water	% w/w	0.150	0.058

Table 50-3. Properties of Hydrochlorofluorocarbons (HCFCs)

PROPERTY		DIFLUOROETHANE
Molecular formula		CH_3CHF_2
Numerical designation		152a
Molecular weight		66.1
Boiling point (1 atm)	°F	−12.0
	°C	−11.0
Vapor pressure (psia)	70°F	63.0
	130°F	176.3
Liquid density (g/mL)	70°F	0.91
	130°F	—
Solubility in water (weight %)	77°F	<1.0

Table 50-4. Properties of Hydrocarbons and Ethers

PROPERTY	PROPANE	ISOBUTANE	N-BUTANE	DIMETHYL ETHER
Molecular formula	C_3H_8	C_4H_{10}	C_4H_{10}	CH_3OCH_3
Molecular weight	44.1	58.1	58.1	46.1
Boiling point (°F)	−43.7	10.9	31.1	−13
Vapor pressure (psig at 70°F)	110.0	30.4	16.5	63.0
Liquid density (g/mL at 70°F)	0.50	0.56	0.58	0.66
Flash point (°F)	−156	−117	−101	—

Table 50-5. Properties of Compressed Gases

PROPERTY	CARBON DIOXIDE	NITROUS OXIDE	NITROGEN
Molecular formula	CO_2	N_2O	N_2
Molecular weight	44	44	28
Boiling point °F	−109[a]	−127	−320
Vapor pressure, psia, 70°F	852	735	492[b]
Solubility in water,[c] 77°F	0.7	0.5	0.014
Density (gas) g/mL	1.53	1.53	0.96699

[a] Sublimes
[b] At the critical point (−233°F)
[c] Volume of gas at atmospheric pressure soluble in one volume of water.

characteristics depending on the nature of the formulation. This system is designed to dispense pressurized products efficiently and economically using relatively small amounts of hydrocarbon, HFA, or HCFC propellants.

The vapor phase of the propellant and the product concentrate enter the mixing chamber in the actuator through separate ducts or channels. The vaporized propellant enters, moving at tremendous velocity, while the product is forced into the actuator by the pressure of the propellant. It is at this point that product and vapor are mixed with violent force, resulting in a uniform, finely dispersed spray. Depending on the configuration of the valve and actuator, either a dry or a wet spray can be obtained.

Water-based aerosols developed for use in this system have the advantage that the chilling effect associated with liquefied-gas systems is eliminated. Since only vaporized propellant is dispensed, less propellant is required in the container. With greater use of water as a solvent for active ingredients a greater range of products can be developed. Because the use of volatile organic compounds (VOCs) is now being curtailed, water is being used, when possible, as an alternative to some solvents such as alcohol. The use of P-152a and/or DME as a propellant also helps to reduce the VOC content of some aerosols such as hairsprays. Table 50-3 and Table 50-4 illustrates the properties of these propellants.

Foam System—Foam aerosols, which often are classified separately, consist of three-phase systems in which the liquid propellant, which normally does not exceed 10 to 15% by weight, is emulsified with the propellant. When the valve is depressed, the emulsion is forced through the nozzle, and in the presence of warm air and at atmospheric pressure; the entrapped propellant reverts to a vapor and whips the emulsion into a foam. The use of a dip tube is optional with this type of system, and when present, the container is designed for upright use. For those containers where the dip tube is omitted, the container must be inverted prior to use.

Foam valves have been developed that are applicable to both types of packages. Foam products operate at a pressure of about 30 to 45 psig at 70°F (21°) and generally contain about 4% to 7% propellant, depending upon the nature of the propellant. Hydrocarbon propellants are used at the lower percentage, since their density is much lower than that of their fluorocarbon counterparts. A typical foam-type aerosol can be seen in Figure 50-2. Shave creams, suntan foams, as well as several topical dermatological aerosols have been formulated as foam aerosols. Generally, a blend of propane/isobutane or propane/isobutane/butane or isobutane alone is used for foam aerosols.

Some foams use P-152a as the propellant, since this propellant will produce a somewhat more stable foam and is less flammable than hydrocarbons. It is also possible to use the non-CFC propellants for foams. Depending on the formulation, some aerosols use nitrous oxide, carbon dioxide, or a mixture of both as the propellant. Contraceptive foam aerosols are formulated with a hydrocarbon, generally A-31, as the propellant.

Compressed-Gas Aerosols

Aerosols using compressed gases as the propellant are finding increased use. These propellants, especially nitrogen, carbon dioxide, and nitrous oxide, are acceptable for use with pharmaceuticals. Compressed gases are used to dispense the product as a solid stream, wet spray, or foam. These aerosol products use an inert gas such as nitrogen, carbon dioxide, or nitrous oxide as the propellant. The gas is compressed in the container, and it is the expansion of the compressed gas that provides the push or the force necessary to expel the contents from the container. As the contents of the container are expelled, the volume of the gas will increase, causing a drop in pressure according to Boyle's law. This enables one to calculate the drop in pressure as the contents of a compressed-gas aerosol are used. Table 50-5 indicates some of the more important properties of these compressed gases. Depending upon the nature of the formulation and the type of compressed gas used, the product may be dispensed as a semisolid, foam, or spray.

Semisolid Dispensing—The concentrate generally is semisolid in nature, and since the gas is insoluble and immiscible with the concentrate, the product is dispensed in its original form. This system is applicable to the dispensing of dental creams, hairdressings, ointments, creams, cosmetic creams, foods, and other products. Compressed-gas aerosols operate at a substantially higher initial pressure of 90 to 100 psig at 70°F (21°). This pressure is necessary to ensure adequate pressure for the dispensing of most of the contents from the container. The amount of product retained in the unit after exhaustion of the pressure varies with the viscosity of the product and loss of pressure due to seepage of gas during storage. Since the concentrate generally is semisolid in nature and the dispensing characteristics depend largely on the viscosity of the product and the pressure within the container, the viscosity of the product concentrate must be adjusted accordingly.

Foam Dispensing—Soluble compressed gases such as nitrous oxide and carbon dioxide can be used to produce a foam when used with emulsion products. This system is typical for whipped creams and toppings and several pharmaceutical and veterinary products. When this system is used, the gas dissolved in the concentrate will be evolved and cause a whipping of the emulsion into a foam. To facilitate the formation of a foam this system is shaken prior to use, to disperse some of the gas throughout the product concentrate.

Spray Dispensing—This system is similar to a space or surface spray except that a compressed gas is used as the propellant. Since these gases do not possess the dispersing power of the liquefied gases, a mechanical breakup actuator is used. The product is dispensed as a wet spray and is applicable to solutions of medicinal agents in aqueous solvents.

Another application for this type of system is found in the contact lens saline solutions. These consist of a normal saline solution packaged in an aluminum aerosol container and pressurized with nitrogen. Since these solutions may come in contact with the eye, they are sterilized using cobalt-60 gamma irradiation.

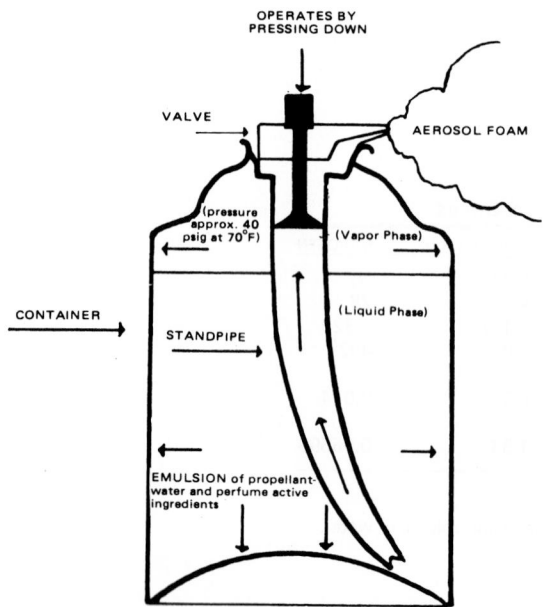

OPERATES BY
PRESSING DOWN

VALVE

AEROSOL FOAM

CONTAINER

(pressure approx. 40 psig at 70°F)

(Vapor Phase)

(Liquid Phase)

STANDPIPE

EMULSION of propellant-water and perfume active ingredients

Figure 50-2. Foam-type aerosol.

Barrier-Type Systems

These systems separate the propellant from the product itself. The pressure on the outside of the barrier serves to push the contents from the container. The following types are available.

PISTON TYPE—Since it is difficult to empty the contents of a semisolid from an aerosol container completely, a piston-type aerosol system has been developed. This uses a polyethylene piston fitted into an aluminum container. The product is placed into the upper portion of the container. The pressure from nitrogen (about 90 to 100 psig) or a liquefied gas pushes against the other side of the piston, and when the valve is opened, the product is dispensed. The piston scrapes against the sides of the container and dispenses most of the product concentrate. The piston-type aerosol system is shown in Figure 50-3. This system has been used successfully to package cheese spreads, cake decorating icings, and some ointments and creams. Since the products that use this system are semisolid and viscous, they are dispensed as a lazy stream rather than as a foam or spray. This system is limited to viscous materials, since limpid liquids, such as water or alcohol, will pass between the wall of the container and the piston. The piston type system has also been used to formulate post-foaming type gels.

PLASTIC-BAG AND BAG-IN-BAG TYPE—This system consists of a collapsible plastic bag fitted into a standard, three-piece, tinplate or aluminum container as shown in Figure 50-4. The product is placed within the bag, and the propellant is added through the bottom of the container. Since the product is placed into a plastic bag, there is no contact between the product and the container wall except for any product that may escape by permeation through the plastic bag. A variation of this system is shown in Figure 50-5. The valve and a collapsed inner bag is inserted into a container. A compressed or liquefied gas is added at the same time as the valve/bag is inserted and then the valve is crimped. The product is forced through the valve and into the bag. The bag expands and will compress the propellant resulting in an increase in pressure. As the valve is opened, the product will be dispensed. Ointments, creams, and gels can be packaged in this system.

Limpid liquids, such as water, can be dispensed as either a stream or a fine mist, depending on the type of valve used, while semisolid substances are dispensed as a stream. To prevent the gas from pinching the bag and preventing the dispensing of product, the inner plastic bag is accordion-pleated.

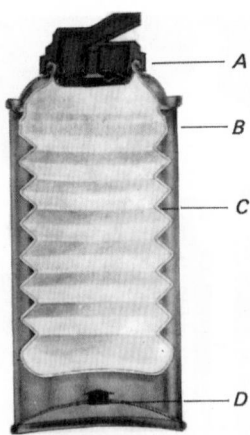

Figure 50-4. Plastic Bag Aerosol System.

This system can be used for a variety of different pharmaceutical and nonpharmaceutical systems, including topical pharmaceutical products as a cream, ointment, or gel.

A modification of the barrier system dispenses the product as a gel that will then foam. By dissolving a low-boiling liquid such as isopentane or pentane in the product, a foam will result when the product is placed on the hands and the warmth of the hands will cause vaporization of the solvent. This system, as well as the piston system, is used in post foaming shave gels.

CAN-IN-CAN SYSTEMS—Figure 50-6 illustrates a system consisting of an aluminum can into which an aluminum thin-walled can has been inserted. This inner can is glued to the outer can at the neck and forms a gas-tight seal. Then, the neck of the can is fabricated. The propellant (liquid or compressed) is added through a small opening in the bottom of the can that is sealed with a rubber plug. A recent addition to this system includes replacement of the inner aluminum pouch with an inner plastic bag made of organic polymers. Sufficient space remains between this bag and the walls and the bottom of the outer container to accommodate sufficient propellant to evacuate the product completely. Systems illustrated by Figure 50-6 can be used with a continuous or metered dose valve to dispense medicated solutions, gels, creams, and lotions.

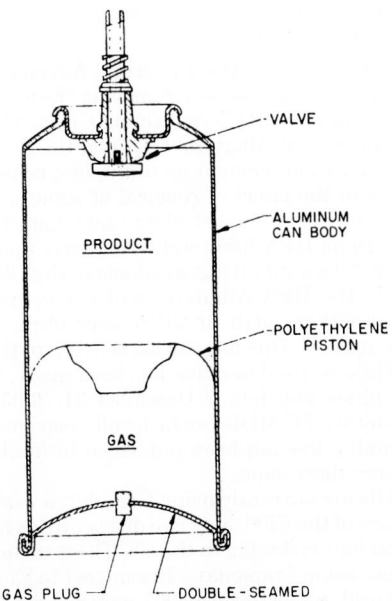

Figure 50-3. Free-piston aerosol system.

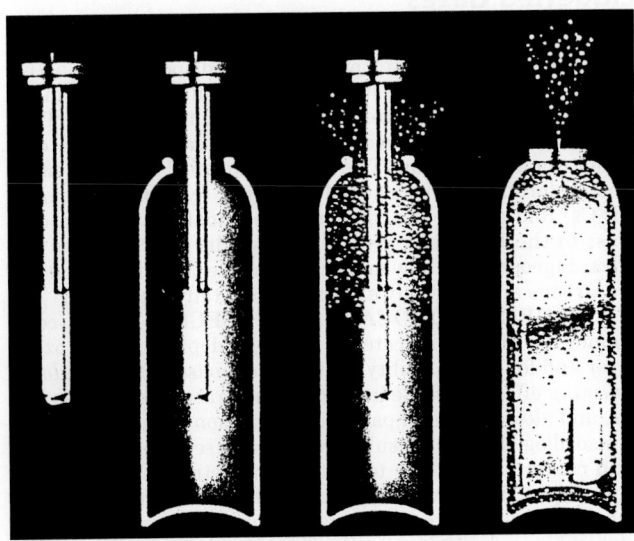

Figure 50-5. Bag-in Can System–ABS (courtesy, CCL Container, Aerosol Division).

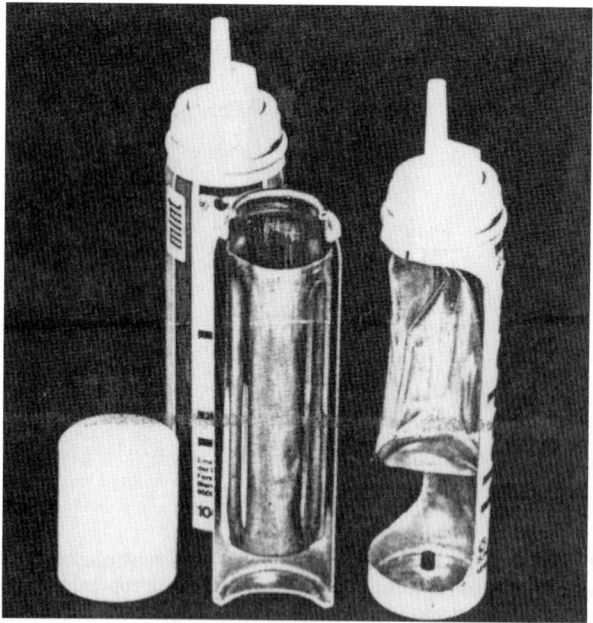

Figure 50-6. Cross-section of the Lechner barrier pack. It consists of a rigid or flexible inner bag that can be evacuated more than 95%, depending upon the viscosity of the product (courtesy, Lechner GMBH).

PROPELLANTS

The propellant generally is regarded as the *heart* of the aerosol package. In addition to supplying the necessary force to expel the product, the propellant must also act as a solvent and diluent and has much to do with determining the characteristics of the product as it leaves the container. Various chemical compounds have been used as aerosol propellants.

Compounds useful as propellants can be classified as:

Liquefied gases
Chlorofluorocarbons (CFC)
Hydrochlorofluorocarbons (HCFC)
Hydrofluorocarbons (HFC)
Hydrocarbons (HC)
Hydrocarbon ethers
Compressed gases

Liquefied Gases

The liquefied-gas compounds have widespread use as propellants, since they are extremely effective in dispersing the active ingredients into a fine mist or foam, depending on the form desired. In addition, they are relatively inert and nontoxic. They have the added advantage that the pressure within the container remains constant. Two types of liquefied gases are used. The chlorofluorocarbons (CFCs) and hydrofluorocarbons (HFCs) find greater use since they are nonflammable in contrast to the flammable hydrocarbons. The hydrocarbons are advantageous since they are less expensive than any of the fluorocarbons and generally are environmentally acceptable.

CHLOROFLUOROCARBONS (CFCS)—These compounds have been implicated in causing a depletion of the ozone layer and for responsibility for the *greenhouse* or for the *global warming* effect (increase in earth's temperature, rising sea levels, and altered rainfall patterns). Depletion of the ozone layer is also alleged to have resulted in an increase in the incidence of skin cancer. This is due to a greater penetration of the ozone layer by the skin-cancer-causing UV radiation from the sun (the ozone layer will prevent these rays from penetrating the earth's atmosphere). In 1974, the Environmental Protection Agency (EPA), Consumer Product Safety Commission (CPSC), and the FDA promulgated a *ban* on the use of chlorofluorocarbons,

namely Propellants 11, 12, and 114, in most aerosol products. Certain pharmaceutical aerosols for inhalation use (MDIs) were exempted from this ban. According to the Montreal Agreement reached in 1988, beginning in 1989, the production of these propellants was restricted worldwide. Starting January 1, 1996, worldwide production of CFCs was reduced to only the amount needed for certain exempted uses that included MDIs for the treatment of asthma and chronic obstructive pulmonary disease (COPD). CFC propellants are used in all of the metered dose inhalers in the US. MDIs have been classified by the Environmental Protection Agency and Food and Drug Administration as "essential use" and as such are exempted from the ban on the use of CFCs. The EPA granted allocation of CFC 11, 12, and 114 to those manufacturers of MDI inhalers currently being sold so that these products can continue to be manufactured and available in the US marketplace. At the present time, no firm date has been issued by the EPA as to when CFCs will no longer be available; however, EPA regulations prohibit the granting of a CFC allocation for any MDI classified as essential use and not approved by the FDA prior to December 31, 2000. Essentially this ruling prevents the development and sale of a generic version of these CFC containing MDIs. MDIs containing Albuterol are the only MDI products available in generic form. All other CFC propelled MDIs can continue to be sold in the marketplace free from generic product competition.

Generic MDI products containing Albuterol and those containing Epinephrine have been developed since the late 1990s and are currently marketed by generic pharmaceutical companies. No other generic version of an MDI product is available in the US.

In the latter part of the 1990s, FDA issued a ruling to encourage the development of ozone-friendly propellants (HFAs) so that essential use designation could be removed. This ruling allowed for the removal of essential use designation from existing MDIs containing CFCs if the following conditions are met:

- At least one non-CFC product with the same active drug is marked with the same route of administration, for the same indication, and with approximately the same level of convenience of use as the CFC product containing that active moiety (while these alternatives are not required to be MDIs, the presumption is that HFA-MDIs would most easily fit criteria compared to, for example, dry powder inhalers);
- Supplies and production capacity for the non-CFC products(s) exist or will exist at levels sufficient to meet patient need;
- Adequate US postmarketing use data are available for the non-CFC product(s); and
- Patients who medically required the CFC product are adequately served by the non-ODS product(s) containing that active moiety and other available products.

The FDA Pulmonary-Allergy Drugs Advisory Committee met on June 10, 2004 to consider removing "Essential Use" designation for Albuterol MDI's containing CFCs. The committee was in agreement that Albuterol MDI met the first three criteria but were not in agreement as to the last criteria. Concern was raised as to the effect of removal of Albuterol MDIs containing CFCs from the market place and what effect their replacement with an HFA Albuterol would have upon the cost to the consumer. Albuterol MDI is available in the US as a generic product while the HFA Albuterol will not be available as a generic until either 2010 or 2015 depending upon which patent(s) are upheld. This has caused concern to the committee members. While no final decision has been made, the FDA has suggested a phase out date of December 31, 2005 after which date no Albuterol CFC MDIs can be legally marketed in the US. This rule making has not been published in final form and is currently under discussion.

While MDIs are currently being formulated with a HFC propellant in place of the CFC, only two drug entities have received FDA approval for marketing in the US. These include Albuterol and Beclomethosone Propionate. In contrast to Europe and the rest of the world, almost every CFC metered dose inhaler has been replaced with a HFC propellant. These replacements will be discussed in greater detail in another section of this chapter.

Since the early 1990s topical aerosol products have been reformulated using a hydrocarbon or a compressed gas propellant in place of the CFC. Compressed gasses, hydrocarbon, and HFC propellants are the suggested alternative propellant.

Since CFC propellants are in widespread use for most of the MDIs currently in use, the properties of the CFCs remain important and are covered in the next section of this chapter. Other than some of the specific properties of the CFCs and the HFCs, the principles of use in dosage form development remain essentially the same.

Liquefied gases provide a nearly constant pressure during packaging operations and have a large expansion ratio. Several of the fluorinated hydrocarbons have an expansion ratio of about 240, that is, 1 mL of liquefied gas will occupy a volume of approximately 240 mL if allowed to vaporize. Dimethyl ether has a value over 350. On the other hand, compressed gases expand only to the extent of 3 to 10 times the original volume.

The physicochemical properties of these compounds are of prime importance in the formulation and manufacture of aerosol products. The solvent power, stability, and lack of reactivity of the propellants have made them extremely useful for this purpose.

Nomenclature—To refer easily to the fluorinated hydrocarbons a relatively simple system of nomenclature was developed some time ago by the refrigeration industry. A numerical designation is used to identify each propellant.

All propellants are designated by three digits (000). When the first digit is zero, the propellant is designated by the last two digits and zero is assumed to be the first digit (ex: Propellant 011 is Propellant 11).

The first digit is one less than the number of carbon atoms in the compound. When there are only two digits, (0) is understood to be the first digit and indicates a methane derivative. When this first digit is (1), the propellant is an ethane derivative, when (2) it is propane, and when (3) it is a butane derivative.

The second digit is one more than the number of hydrogen atoms in the compound.

The last digit represents the number of fluorine atoms.

The number of chlorine atoms (for CFCs) in the compound is found by subtracting the sum of the fluorine and the hydrogen atoms from the total number of atoms that can be added to saturate the carbon chain.

In the case of isomers, each has the same number, and the most symmetrical one is indicated by the number alone. As the isomers become more and more asymmetrical, the letter a, b, c, etc, follows the number.

For cyclic compounds, a C is used before the number.

The use of this system can be exemplified as follows:

For CFC 114–Dichlorotetrafluoroethane

Propellant 114 is an ethane derivative, has no hydrogens, and contains 4 fluorine atoms.

Since 6 atoms are required to saturate the carbon chain, of necessity there must be 2 chlorine atoms. These can be arranged in two different ways; however, since there is no letter following the numerical designation, the symmetrical structure refers to Propellant 114.

Propellant 114   Propellant 114a

For CFC 11–Trichloromonofluoromethane

The designation is 0 for methane (first digit)
1 for number of fluorine atoms (third digit)
1 for one more than number of hydrogen atoms (second digit)
3 chlorine atoms required to saturate molecule.

Propellant 11

For HFC-227–Heptafluoropropane

The designation is 2 for propane (first digit)
7 for number of fluorine atoms (third digit)
2 for one more than number of hydrogen atoms (second digit)

Since there is no letter following the third digit, the one H atom must be on the #2 carbon as this is the most symmetrical configuration.

Propellant 227

For HFC-134a–Tetrafluoroethane

The designation is 1 for ethane (first digit)
4 for number of fluorine atoms (third digit)
3 for one more than number of hydrogen atoms (second digit)

There are two possibilities for the 2 hydrogen atoms (one on each carbon or two on one carbon). Since this designation has an "a" following the last digit, it is the unsymmetrical compound.

Propellant 134a

Physical Properties—Table 50-1 shows some of the more useful physicochemical properties of CFC propellants. Propellants 11, 12, and 114 are included in the latest issue of the USP/NF and the British Pharmacopoeia. Specifications for these propellants, hydrocarbons, as well as the HFCs, HCFCs and compressed gases can be found in the *Handbook of Pharmaceutical Excipients*, Fourth Edition.

From a solubility standpoint, the CFC, HFC, and HCFC propellants, which are nonpolar, are miscible with most nonpolar solvents over a wide range of temperature. They also are capable of dissolving many substances. For the most part the propellants are not miscible with water, although the degree of miscibility depends on the individual propellants. A cosolvent such as ethanol, 2-propanol, or DME, must be used when water is present, to produce a clear solution. However, when one considers that these propellants are used for metered-dose aerosols, the choice of cosolvent is extremely limited and, in many cases, to the use of ethyl alcohol. The alternative is to form an emulsion for topical aerosol pharmaceuticals.

One of the most important physicochemical properties of a propellant is its vapor pressure, which may be defined as the pressure exerted by a liquid in equilibrium with its vapor. When the vapor pressure exceeds atmospheric pressure, boiling and vaporization take place. However, if the vaporized molecules are prevented from leaving the container (by placing the propellant into a sealed container), they will fill the head space and eventually cause an increase in pressure. The pressure developed at equilibrium is the vapor pressure. The vapor pressure of a liquefied gas is independent of the quantity used but is influenced by temperature changes. Assuming ideal behavior for the liquefied gas, the effect of temperature on the vapor pressure can be calculated from

$$\log P = -\frac{\Delta H_{vap}}{2.303\,RT}$$

where P is the vapor pressure, H is the heat of vaporization, R is the gas constant (generally 1.987 cal deg^{-1} mole^{-1}), and T is the absolute temperature.

Since

$$\ln P = -\frac{\Delta H_{vap}}{RT} + C$$

a plot of $\log P$ versus $1/T$ should yield a straight line, and from this the heat of vaporization may be calculated.

$$\Delta H_{vap}\ (cal\ mole^{-1}) = -(slope)(2.303R)$$

These equations can be used to predict the behavior of pure propellants at elevated temperatures. When one considers that an aerosol preparation consists of a propellant and solvents or mixtures of these, the vapor pressure considerations are somewhat different. By mixing various propellants such as Propellants 11 and 12 or Propellants 12 and 114, a range of vapor pressures is obtained. This is not possible when the HFCs are used, since the range in pressure between P-134a and P-227 is relatively small (about 26 psig compared with about 70 psig between P-11 and P-12). The vapor pressure of a mixture of propellants may be calculated from Raoult's law, which states that the *vapor pressure of a solution is dependent upon the vapor pressure of the individual components. For ideal solutions, the vapor pressure is equal to the sum of the mole fractions of each component present times the vapor pressure of the pure compound at the desired temperature.*

Mathematically, this law may be expressed as

$$p_A = \frac{n_A}{n_A + n_B} p_A{}^\circ = N_A p_A{}^\circ$$

where p_A = partial vapor pressure of Component A, $p_A{}^\circ$ = vapor pressure of pure Component A, n_A = mols of Component A, n_B = moles of Component B, and N_A = mol fraction of Component A.

$$p_B = \frac{n_B}{n_B + n_A} p_B{}^\circ = N_B p_B{}^\circ$$

The total vapor pressure of the system is obtained by

$$P_{total} = p_A + p_B$$

When the mole fraction of one component is large, the other component has a small mol fraction, and as such, it does not appreciably affect the vapor pressure. This system approaches ideal behavior.

When the components are of similar physical and chemical nature, the experimentally determined values and the calculated values are approximately the same. In the case of the fluorinated hydrocarbons, the deviation from ideal behavior is not great, and the results are approximately equal or within 5%. When other solvents are present, such as alcohols, the vapor pressures can be calculated in a similar manner.

Chemical Properties—The fluorinated hydrocarbons have been widely used as aerosol propellants because they generally are considered to be chemically inert. From the standpoint of formulation, the only chemical property that need be considered is hydrolysis in regard to Propellant 11. While addition of fluorine to a carbon atom generally increases stability, a propellant such as trichloromonofluoromethane may undergo hydrolysis with the formation of hydrochloric acid. Propellant 11 is not used with aqueous products, as hydrolysis will occur; Propellant 114 generally is used instead. For topical and cosmetic aerosols, hydrocarbons, or hydrochlorofluorocarbons are used (Propellants 152b, or DME). Propellants 134a and 227 have properties similar to those of P-12 except for their solubility characteristics.

HYDROCARBONS—Hydrocarbon propellants have replaced CFCs for topical pharmaceutical aerosols. Their low-order toxicity makes them suitable, while their flammability tends to limit their use. With the development of newer types of dispensing valves, the flammability hazard has been reduced considerably. The advantage of hydrocarbons is their greater range of solubility and a lower cost than CFCs. To date they represent a readily available replacement for CFCs as propellants, provided that the flammability hazard can be reduced.

The HFC propellant used for MDIs are also applicable to topical aerosol pharmaceuticals with the added advantage of nonflammability.

In addition to having the proper vapor pressure, hydrocarbons have other properties that make them useful as propellants. Their density of less than 1 and their immiscibility with water make them useful in the formulation of three-phase (two-layer) aerosols. Being lighter than water, the hydrocarbon remains on top of the aqueous layer and serves to push the contents out of the container. Not being halogenated, hydrocarbons generally possess better solubility characteristics than the fluorinated hydrocarbons.

As with CFCs, a range of pressures can be obtained by mixing various hydrocarbons in varying proportions. As the composition of the hydrocarbons is likely to vary somewhat, depending on their source, blending of hydrocarbons must be based on the final pressure desired and not on the basis of a stated proportion of each component, whose pressure will depend on its purity. Table 50-6 lists some commonly used blends that are commercially available.

Finally, it should be indicated that the hydrocarbons are characterized further by their extreme chemical stability. They are not subject to hydrolysis, making them useful with water-based aerosols. They will react with the halogens but only under severe conditions.

Alternative Propellants (HCFCs and HFCs)

Many pharmaceutical aerosols were developed originally using chlorofluorocarbons (CFCs) 11, 12, and 114. These propellants have found widespread use because of their inertness, nonflammability, and nontoxicity. Unfortunately, the CFCs have been implicated in depleting the ozone layer, and their use as aerosol propellants has practically been eliminated, except for exempted medical uses which included MDIs.

Topical pharmaceutical aerosols have been successfully reformulated with Propellants 152a, DME, hydrocarbons, and compressed gases. Suitable valves are available that, together with modifications in formulation and propellant blends, produce topical aerosol pharmaceuticals that are satisfactory and acceptable.

Several new liquefied-gas materials have been developed to replace the CFCs as refrigerants and foaming agents and in other nonpharmaceutical uses. Propellant 134a and Propellant 227 have been developed as substitutes for Propellant 12 in MDIs and have survived many of the short- and long-term toxicity studies. To date, no suitable replacement has been found for Propellants 11 and 114. Propellant 114 is not essential for use with MDIs, but most of the present suspension formulations require a minimum amount of Propellant 11. Propellant 11 is used to form a slurry with the active ingredient and dispensing agent. This is impossible to accomplish with Propellants 134a and P-227 (unless these propellants are chilled well below their boiling point and handled as a cold fill). Propellant 11 also has been used to dissolve the surfactants that have been used with CFC MDIs. The HFCs are extremely poor solvents and will not dissolve a sufficient amount of the currently used

Table 50-6. Commonly Used Hydrocarbon Blends

DESIGNATION[a]	PRESSURE (psig AT 70°F)	COMPOSITION (mol %)		
		n-BUTANE	PROPANE	ISOBUTANE
A-108	108 ± 4	Traces	99	1
A-31	31 ± 2	3	1	96
A-17	17 ± 2	98	Traces	2
A-24	24 ± 2	49.2	0.6	50
A-40	40 ± 2	2	12	86
A-46	46 ± 2	2	20	78
A-52	52 ± 2	2	28	70
A-70	70 ± 2	1	51	48

[a] Designations used by Phillips Chemical Co, Bartlesville, OK.
Other designations include: Aeron—Diversified CPC International, Inc., Channahon, IL

FDA-approved surfactants (oleic acid, sorbitan trioleate, and soya lecithin).

It also has been noted that some of the currently used valves are not compatible with these newer HFC propellants. The gaskets and sealing compounds used in metered-dose valves may present compatibility problems to the formulator; however, other gasket materials (EPDM) have been developed and found to be satisfactory. Several of the critical properties of these newer propellants are shown in Table 50-2. Additional details about their use in formulation of MDIs is included in a later part of this chapter.

Compressed Gases

The compressed gases such as nitrogen, nitrous oxide, and carbon dioxide have been used as aerosol propellants. Depending on the nature of the formulation and the valve design, the product can be dispensed as a fine mist, foam, or semisolid. However, unlike the liquefied gases, the compressed gases possess little, if any, expansion power and will produce a fairly wet spray and foams that are not as stable as liquefied-gas foams. This system has been used for the most part to dispense food products and for nonfoods, to dispense the product in its original form as a semisolid. Compressed gases have been used in products such as dental creams, hair preparations, ointments, and aqueous antiseptic and germicidal aerosols and are extremely useful in contact lens cleaner saline solution and barrier systems.

CONTAINERS
Metal

TIN-PLATED STEEL—To produce an aerosol container that was light and relatively inexpensive, tin-plated steel was used for aerosol containers. This resulted in the large-scale production of aerosol containers. For certain products the tin affords sufficient protection, so that no further treatment is necessary. For additional protection to either the drug product or container, a coating, usually organic in nature, may consist of an oleoresin, phenolic, vinyl, or epoxy coating. The liner (single or double coat) is added to the container prior to fabrication; that is, it is applied to the flat sheets of tin plate.

ALUMINUM—Many MDIs and pharmaceutical aerosols use an aluminum container. Aluminum containers (sometimes referred to as canisters) are produced by an impact extrusion process so that the container is seamless. These containers are extremely strong and will withstand relatively high pressures. A variety of different aluminum aerosol containers ranging in size from 10 mL to 45 fl oz is available. While aluminum is less reactive than other metals used in can manufacture, added resistance can be obtained by coating the inside of the container with organic materials such as epoxy, vinyl, phenolic, or polyamide resins. Many of the MDIs will use an anodized or nonanodized internal surface, with or without an organic inner coating. Most of the aluminum containers for MDIs formulated with an HFC propellant are coated with an organic inner coating.

GLASS—For pharmaceuticals and medicinals, glass is preferred because of the absence of incompatibilities, as well as for its esthetic value. The use of glass containers is limited to those products having a lower pressure and lower percentage of propellant. While glass is basically stronger than most metallic containers, a potential hazard is present if, and when, the container is dropped with subsequent breakage. Two types of glass aerosol containers are available. The uncoated glass container has the advantage of decreased cost and high clarity. The contents can be viewed at all times. The plastic-coated glass containers are protected by a plastic coating that prevents the glass from shattering in the event of breakage. The plastic coated glass container is used for some topical and MDI aerosols.

VALVES

Probably the most basic part of any aerosol or pressurized package is the valve mechanism through which the contents of the package are emitted. Together with the formulation, the valve determines the performance of a pressurized package. The interaction of these two components is such that one cannot readily be discussed without reference to the other.

The primary purpose of the valve is to regulate the flow of product from the container. It provides a means of discharging the desired amount when needed and prevents loss at other times. The valve also exerts a major effect on the character of the dispensed product. For example, a product formulated to produce a foam can be dispensed as a spray or as a wet stream by the use of different actuators or push buttons on the valve. The selection of proper propellants also governs whether a foam, spray, or wet stream will be produced.

Continuous-Spray Valves

Figure 50-7 illustrates the basic subcomponents used in aerosol valves. A fully assembled valve is shown in Figure 50-8.

A small hole about 0.013 to 0.020″ in diameter sometimes is placed in the valve body as seen in Figure 50-7. This allows the escape of a small quantity of vaporized propellant along with the product. This gives a greater degree of dispersion to the emitted spray as well as cleaning the valve orifices following discharge. However, since a greater amount of propellant is used than with nonvapor-tap systems, care must be exercised during formulation of the product to take this into account. One may also note a change in spray pattern from start to finish because of the change in propellant composition that takes place as the contents are used. Vapor-tap valves are used with powder aerosols, water-based aerosols, aerosols containing suspended materials, and other agents that would tend to clog the valve. They currently are used with hydrocarbon aerosols since

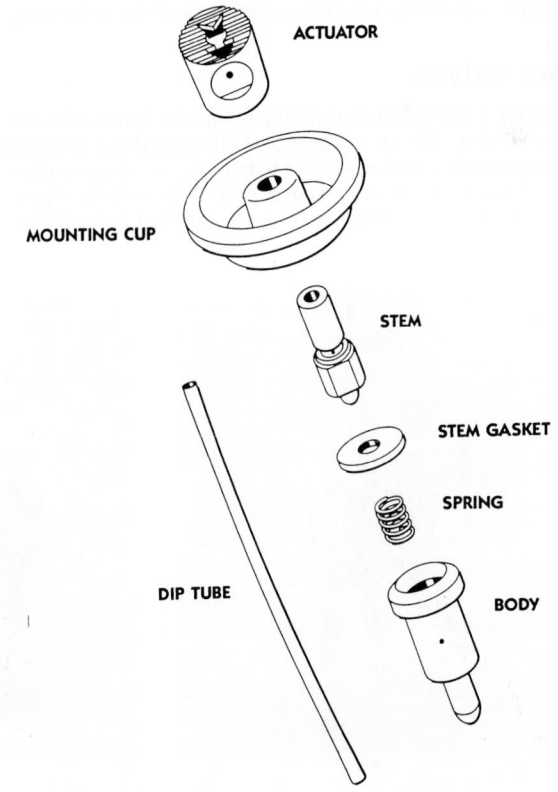

Figure 50-7. Continuous-spray aerosol valve, showing subcomponents used for sprays, foams, and semisolids (courtesy, Precision Valve).

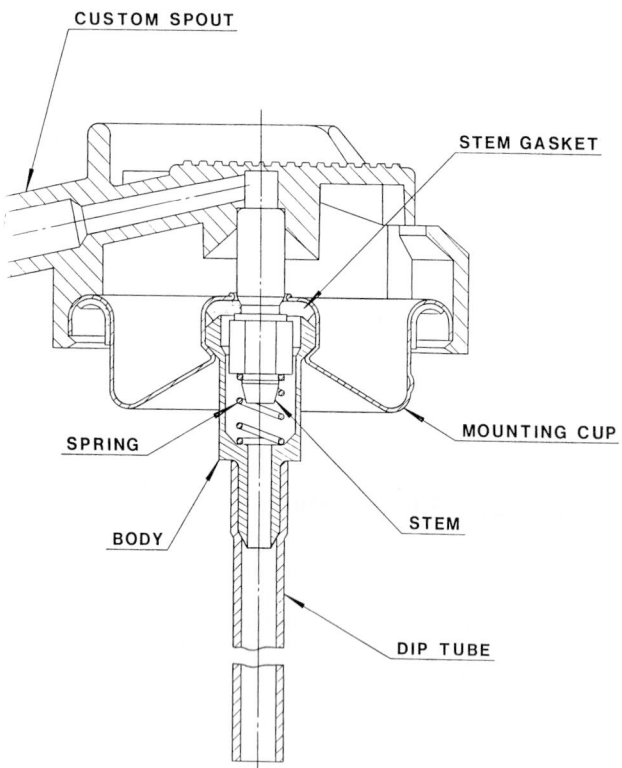

Figure 50-8. Assembled continuous-spray valve (courtesy, Precision Valve).

the flame extension of the spray can be reduced substantially through use of a vapor-tap valve. This is accomplished by balancing the size of the vapor-tap opening and the valve orifice.

Foam Valves

Valves for foam or aerated products usually have only one expansion orifice, the one at the seat. Following this is a single expansion chamber that serves as a delivery nozzle or applicator. It is sufficiently large in volume to permit immediate expansion of the pressurized product to form the familiar ball of foam. As demonstrated earlier, the same formulation will be discharged as a solid stream when dispensed with a valve and actuator having small orifices and expansion chambers. Under these latter conditions, the ball of foam will begin to develop where the stream impinges on a surface. This rather interesting performance is used in some pressurized surgical soaps on the market. These products are preferred for use by surgeons and other operating room personnel since when applied; the foam breaks down easily and is rubbed into large areas of the hands and arms. Another similar product contains ethyl alcohol made into a similar foam and is used as a skin disinfectant or sprayed onto instruments, etc.

Because of their large openings, foam valves may lend themselves to use with viscous materials such as syrups, creams, and ointments. Foam valves also have been used to dispense rectal and vaginal foams. Metered valves are discussed later in this chapter.

ACTUATORS

The actuator provides a rapid and convenient means for releasing the contents from a pressurized container. It provides the additional functional use in allowing the product to be dispensed in the desired form, that is, a fine mist, wet spray, foam, or solid stream. Mechanical breakup actuators are used for three-phase or compressed-gas aerosols. In addition, special actuators are available for use with pharmaceutical and medicinal aerosols that allow dispensing of products into the mouth, nose, throat, vagina, or eye.

PACKAGING

Two methods have been used to package aerosol products. Unlike nonaerosol products, part of the manufacturing of necessity takes place during the filling operation. The propellant and product concentrate must be brought together in a way, which ensures uniformity of product.

Depending on the nature of the product concentrate, the aerosol can be filled by a cold-filling or a pressure-filling process. There are advantages and disadvantages to both methods, and there are many factors that must be considered before deciding which process to use. Since aerosol packaging is a very specialized procedure; many of the pharmaceutical aerosols are manufactured and packaged at commercial contract filling facilities. A typical unit used to fill MDIs in the laboratory is shown in Figure 50-9, while Figure 50-10 and 50-10a illustrates

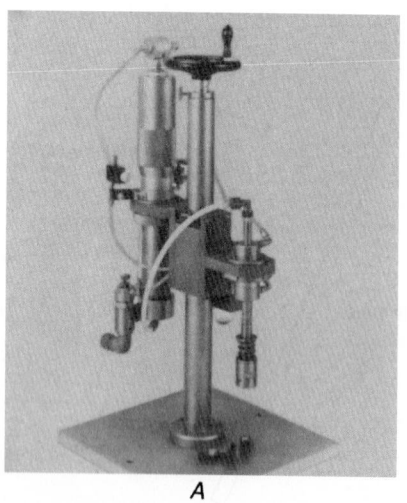

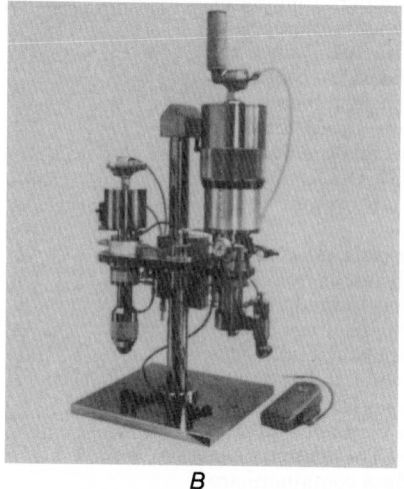

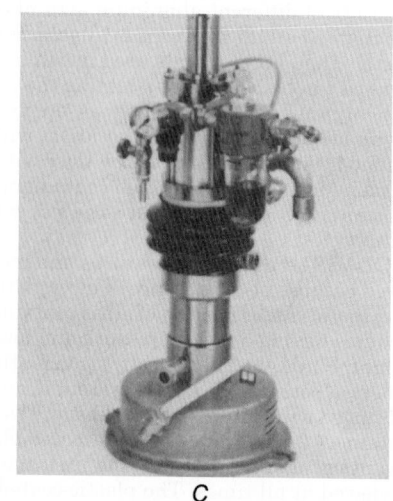

Figure 50-9. Aerosol laboratory and pilot-sized filling equipment. *A*, Product filler. *B*, Crimper and pressure filler for propellant. *C*, Propellant pump (courtesy, Pamasol Willi Mader AG).

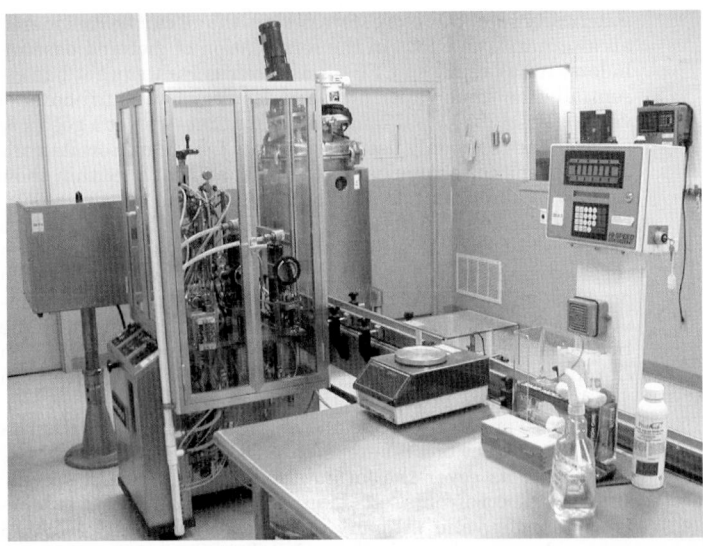
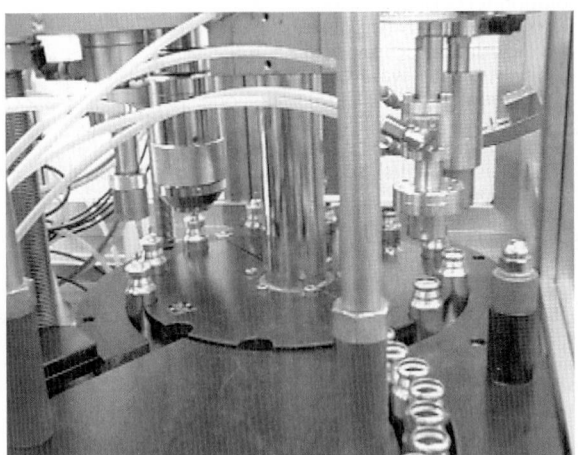

A   B

Figure 50-10. (A) Commercial Aerosol filling and packaging Pamasol line for MDIs (courtesy, Sciarra Laboratories, Inc.) (B) Detail of crimping and pressure filling head.

a typical Pamasol aerosol packaging line for MDIs. Figure 50-11 shows a Terco filling and packaging line for topical pharmaceutical aerosols.

APPLICATIONS

Aerosol technology has been applied to the formulation of products containing therapeutically active ingredients. A pharmaceutical aerosol may be defined as an aerosol product containing therapeutically active ingredients dissolved, suspended, or emulsified in a propellant or a mixture of solvent and propellant and intended for oral or topical administration or for administration into the nose, eye, ear, rectum, or vagina.

MDIs are intended for administration as fine, solid particles or as liquid mists via the respiratory system or nasal passages. They are used for their local action in the nasal areas, throat, and lungs, as well as for prompt systemic effect when absorbed from the lungs into the bloodstream (inhalation therapy). The particle size must be considerably below 10 μm and, in most instances, should be between 3 and 6 μm for maximum therapeutic response.

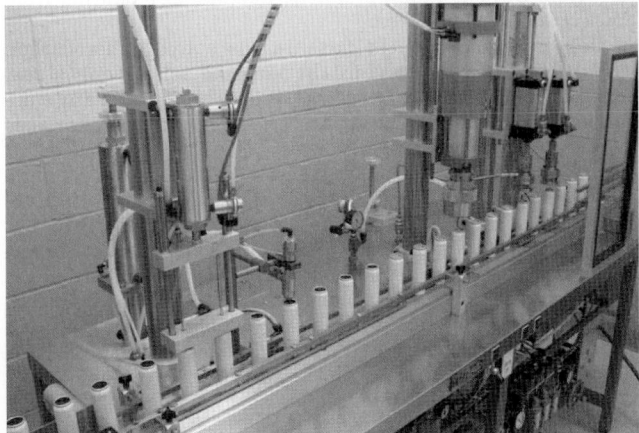

Figure 50-11. Aerosol filling and packaging Terco line for Topical Aerosols (courtesy, Sciarra Laboratories, Inc.)

An alternative definition of this dosage form includes: *Pharmaceutical aerosols are products that are packaged under pressure and contain therapeutically active ingredients that are released upon actuation of an appropriate valve system. They are intended for topical application to the skin as well as local application into the nose (nasal aerosols), mouth (lingual aerosols) or lungs (inhalation aerosols).*

Aerosol Formulation

Topical pharmaceuticals may be formulated as aerosols using solutions, suspensions, emulsions, powders, and semisolid preparations while MDIs are formulated as solutions or suspensions. Table 50-7 illustrates the basic formulation of aerosol products for use as metered-dose inhalants.

SOLUTION AEROSOLS—Topical aerosols consist of a solution of active ingredients in pure propellant or a mixture of propellant and solvents. The solvent is used to dissolve the active ingredients and/or retard the evaporation of the propellant. Solution aerosols are relatively easy to formulate, provided the ingredients are soluble in the propellant. However, the propellants are nonpolar in nature and in most cases are poor solvents for some of the commonly used medicinal ingredients. Through use of a solvent that is miscible with the propellant, one can achieve varying degrees of solubility of the active ingredient. For topicals, (isopropyl alcohol, isopropyl myristate, polyethylene glycols, etc.) ethyl alcohol has found the greatest use, although some other solvents may be of limited value. For those substances that are insoluble in the propellant or propellant/solvent system, a dispersion or suspension can be produced. In this case the drug must be micronized so that the particles are less than 10 μm in average diameter.

The usual fluorocarbon propellants used in currently available MDIs are blended as indicated in Table 50-7 or used alone when appropriate. Propellant 11 is used often when solubility of the drug and solvents presents a problem, as it is a better solvent than either Propellant 12, 114, 134a, or 227. Additionally, Propellant 11 may be required to prepare a suitable slurry when preparing a dispersion aerosol. Generally the propellant represents upward of 60 weight-percent of the final formulation and, in most cases, may be as high as 99.9%. Propellant 12 may be used alone or in combination as indicated. The proportion of each propellant is varied to obtain the desired pressure within the container and the proper particle-size distribution.

Table 50-7. Metered-Dose Inhalants (Solution and Suspensions): Prototype Formulation

Solution (CFC, HFC)[a]
  Active ingredient(s): solubilized
  Antioxidants: ascorbic acid
  Solvent blends: water, ethanol, glycols
  Propellants: 12/11, 12/114 or 12 alone; 134a, 227, 134a/227
Suspensions (CFC)
  Active ingredient(s): micronized and suspended
  Dispersing agent(s): sorbitan trioleate, oleyl alcohol, oleic acid, lecithin, etc.
  Propellants: 12/11, 12/114, 12 or 12/114/11
Suspensions (HFC)[a]
  Active ingredient(s): micronized and suspended
  Solvent: ethanol
  Dispersing agent(s): sorbitan trioleate, oleyl alcohol, oleic acid, lecithin, etc.
  Propellants: 134a, 227, 134a/227
or
  Active ingredient(s): micronized and suspended
  Propellants: 134a, 227, 134a/227

---

[a] The reader is directed to the patent literature to ensure that the formulations are not covered by a patent.

Topical pharmaceutical solutions are formulated using the hydrocarbon propellants, butane, isobutene, and propane. Although butane and isobutene can be used individually, the hydrocarbons are generally used as a blend as shown in Table 50-6. Other non-MDIs are formulated as aqueous solutions (eye care, etc.) and utilize nitrogen as the propellant. These are packaged as a conventional aerosol or utilize a barrier system.

DISPERSIONS OR SUSPENSIONS (POWDER AEROSOLS)—These aerosols are similar to solution aerosols except that the active ingredients are suspended or dispersed throughout the propellant or propellant and solvent phase. This system is useful with antibiotics, steroids, and other poorly soluble compounds. Problems associated with the formulation of this system include agglomeration, caking, particle-size growth, and valve clogging. Some of these problems have been overcome through use of lubricants such as isopropyl myristate, sorbitan trioleate, oleic acid, or other substances that provide slippage between particles of the compound as well as lubricating component parts of the valve. Surfactants also have been used to disperse the particles. The use of dispersing agents such as sorbitan trioleate, oleic acid, or lecithin is useful in keeping the suspended particles from agglomerating. Thought also should be given to both the particle size and the moisture content of the powder. The moisture content should be kept between 100 and 300 ppm or less, depending upon the type of product, and the propellants and solvents must be dried by passing them through a drying agent. The particle size for metered-dose inhalants should remain in the micrometer range and should be between 2 and 8 μm or less, with a mass median diameter of between 3 and 6 μm.

FORMULATION OF MDIS USING HFCS AS THE PROPELLANT:

Several new environmentally acceptable propellants are available worldwide as replacements for CFCs in MDI inhalers. Among the alternatives is Tetrafluoroethane (HFC 134a), which is available as Dymel 134a/P from *DuPont Fluoroproducts;* Solkane 134a pharma from *Solvay;* and Zephex 134a from *Ineos Fluor.*

Tetrafluoroethane (P-134a) is a hydrofluorocarbon (HFC) or hydrofluoroalkane (HFA) aerosol propellant (contains hydrogen, fluorine, and carbon) as contrasted to a CFC (chlorine, fluorine, and carbon). The lack of chlorine in the molecule and the presence of hydrogen reduce the ozone depletion activity to practically zero, therefore, tetrafluoroethane can be considered an alternative to CFCs in the formulation of metered dose inhalers. It has replaced CFC-12 as a refrigerant since it has essentially the same vapor pressure. Its very low Kauri-butanol value and solubility parameter indicate that it is not a good solvent for the commonly used surfactants for MDIs. Sorbitan trioleate, sorbitan sesquioleate, oleic acid, and soya lecithin show limited solubility in tetrafluoroethane and the amount of surfactant that actually dissolves may not be sufficient to keep a drug readily dispersed. Tetrafluoroethane has been used as a replacement for CFCs in MDIs containing Albuterol. Two such products containing Albuterol Sulfate and one product containing Beclomethasone Dipropionate are currently available in the US. Outside the US, this propellant has found greater use in Europe and the rest of the world, where many MDIs have been developed using Tetrafluoroethane.

The use of tetrafluoroethane as a propellant for MDIs has been the subject of numerous patents throughout the world. These patents cover the formulation of MDIs, use of specific surfactants, cosolvents, etc. Many of these formulation patents are no longer valid in many countries of the world. The US patents have not been challenged to date.

US Patent No. 5,605,674 claims *a self-propelling aerosol formulation which may be free from CFCs which comprises a medicament, 1,1,1,2-tetrafluoroethane, a surface active agent, and at least one compound having a higher polarity than 1,1,1,2-tetrafluoroethane.*

The formulator is referred to the patent literature prior to formulating an MDI with tetrafluoroethane and/or heptafluoropropane (P-227) as the propellant. The use of an HFC as the propellant may also requires a change in manufacturing procedure that necessitates a redesign of the filling and packaging machinery for an MDI.

One commercially available MDI is Proventil HFA *(Schering),* which contains albuterol sulfate suspended in ethanol, oleic acid, and tetrafluoroethane (P-134a). Each actuation delivers 108 μg of albuterol sulfate equivalent to 90 μg of albuterol from the mouthpiece. To date this MDI and one containing beclomethasone propionate are the only non-CFC MDI available in the United States. Similar versions of this product are available in the United Kingdom and the rest of the world. In 1998, 3M released Qvar for sale in the United Kingdom. This MDI contains beclomethasone in solution form. Since the respiratory fraction of the product is substantially higher than the current CFC product, according to the literature, a 200-μg dose of Qvar achieved a total beclomethasone level comparable to a 400-μg dose of the CFC-containing beclomethasone formulation. An NDA for Qvar has since been approved by the FDA and Qvar MDI is now available commercially in the US.

Another replacement for CFCs in metered dose inhalers is Heptafluoropropane (P-227), which is available as Dymel 227 ea/P from *DuPont Fluoroproducts;* Solkane 227 pharma from *Solvay;* and Zephex 227ea.

Heptafluoropropane is classified as a hydrofluorocarbon (HFC) aerosol propellant since the molecule consists only of carbon, fluorine, and hydrogen atoms. It does not contain any chlorine and consequently does not affect the ozone layer, nor does it have an effect upon global warming. It is therefore considered as an alternative propellant to CFCs for metered dose inhalers. The vapor pressure is somewhat lower than that of tetrafluoroethane and dichlorodifluoromethane, but considerably higher than the vapor pressure used to formulate most MDIs. Similar to tetrafluoroethane, heptafluoropropane is not a good solvent or medicinal agents used in the formulation of MDIs. Its use as a propellant is included in US Patent 5,605,674.

Although there are no MDIs formulated with this propellant currently available in the US, the rest of the world–including Europe and Asia–have many MDIs that contain P-227. There are several MDIs formulated with P-227 currently under review by the FDA.

EMULSIONS—An emulsion system is useful for a great variety of topical pharmaceutical products. Since these systems contain a relatively small amount of propellant (4 to 10%), there is little if any chilling effect. Active ingredients that may be irritating if inhaled can be used as a foam. Depending on the nature of the formulation and the manner in which the product is to be used, the foam is aqueous or nonaqueous and can be stable or quick-breaking.

Emulsions can be dispensed from an aerosol container as a spray, stable foam, or quick-breaking foam, depending on the type of valve used and the formulation. Two types of emulsions can be formulated for use in an aerosol. A W/O emulsion is one in which the water phase is dispersed throughout the oil phase; an O/W emulsion is one in which the water is the continuous phase.

If the product concentrate is dispersed throughout a propellant, the system behaves similarly to a W/O emulsion. However, since the propellant is in the external phase, the product is dispersed as a wet stream rather than as a foam. When the propellant is in the internal phase (O/W), a foam will be produced. The consistency and stability of the foam can be modified by choice of surfactants and solvents used.

Many water-based aerosols are of the W/O type, in which the propellant is in the external phase. Stable shave-cream foams, on the other hand, are produced by keeping the propellant in the internal phase.

The stable foam is similar to a shaving-cream formulation into which therapeutically active ingredients are incorporated. The foam is dispensed and rubbed into the skin or affected area. By substituting glycols and glycol derivatives for the water in an emulsion, a nonaqueous foam is obtained. The foam stability can be varied by the choice of surfactant, solvent, and propellant. It has been suggested that these foams are applicable to ointment bases, rectal and vaginal medication, and burn preparations.

A quick-breaking foam allows convenient and efficient application of medication. In certain instances the product was dispensed as a foam that quickly collapsed. This was useful in covering large areas with no rubbing necessary to disperse the medication. These quick-breaking foams consist of alcohol, surfactant, water, and propellant.

Container and Valve Components

PHARMACEUTICAL CONTAINERS—Aluminum is used as the material of construction for most metered-dose aerosols. While aluminum can be used without an internal organic coating for certain aerosol formulations, many containers are available that have been anodized or may have an internal coating made from an epoxy, epoxy phenolic, or polyamide resin.

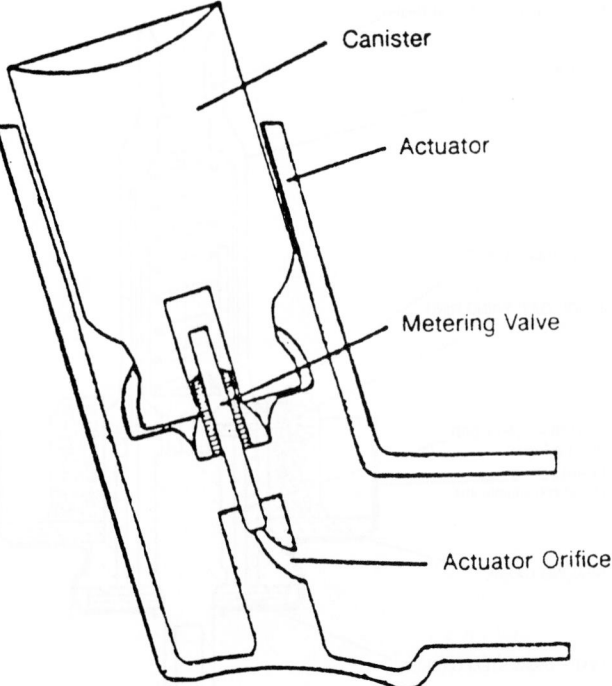

Figure 50-13. Typical metered-dose aerosol delivery system.

Aluminum containers are produced with a 20-mm opening so as to receive the standard metered 20mm and non-metered valves. These canisters are used for MDIs and are fitted with a 20mm metered dose valve. Albuterol made with a CFC will utilize a non-anodized aluminum canister while other MDIs use an anodized canister or one, which has been coated internally with an organic liner. A variety of openings ranging from 13 to 20 mm are available for special and customized applications. Aluminum containers are manufactured from a *slug* of aluminum and are seamless; therefore, there is virtually no danger of leakage. Figure 50-12 shows a typical aluminum container used for MDIs.

PHARMACEUTICAL VALVES—A typical metered-dose aerosol delivery system is illustrated in Figure 50-13. Metering valves fitted with a 20-mm ferrule are used with the above containers for all metered-dose inhalation, nasal aerosols, and oral products.

The metering valve delivers a measured amount of product and the amount delivered is reproducible not only for each dose delivered from the same package but from package to package. Two basic types of metering valves are available, one for inverted use and the other for upright use. Generally, valves for upright use contain a thin capillary dip tube and are used with solution-type aerosols. On the other hand, suspension or dispersion aerosols use a valve for inverted use that does not contain a dip tube. Figures 50-14 and 50-15 illustrate both types of valves and are typical of those commercially available.

An integral part of these valves is the metering chamber that directly is responsible for the delivery of the desired amount of therapeutic agent. The size of the chamber can be varied, so that from about 25 to 150 μL of product can be delivered per actuation. Most of the products commercially available use dosages in the range of 25 to 75 μL. The chamber is sealed via the metering and stem gasket. In the actuated position, the stem gasket will allow the contents of the metering chamber to be dispensed while the metering gasket will seal off any additional product from entering the chamber. In this manner the chamber always is filled and ready to deliver the desired amount of therapeutic agent.

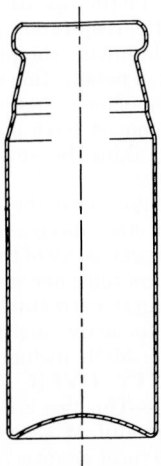

Figure 50-12. Typical aluminum aerosol container, cut-edge type used with an O ring (courtesy, Presspart).

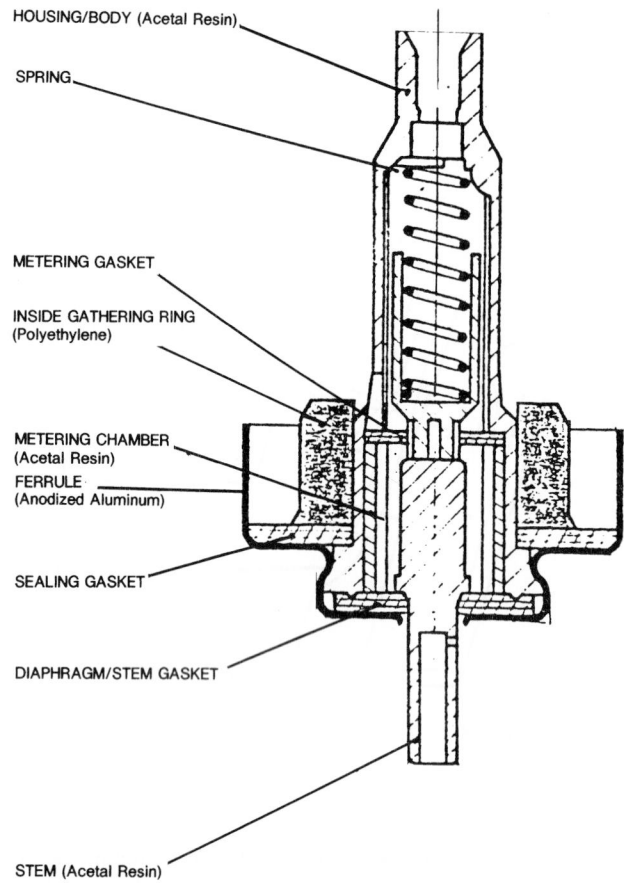

Figure 50-14. Metering valve—inverted (courtesy, Valois).

These valves should retain their prime over fairly long periods of time. However, it is possible for the material in the chamber to return slowly to the main body of product in the event the container is stored upright (for those used in the inverted position). The degree to which this can occur varies with the construction of the valve and the length of time between actuations.

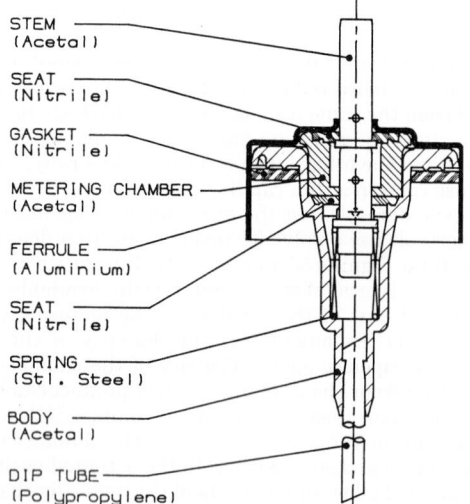

Figure 50-15. 20-mm metered-dose valve showing the subcomponent parts and metering chamber. It is used in the upright position (courtesy, Bespak).

Both types of valves currently are used on commercially available oral inhalation aerosols. During the development stage, the compatibility of the valves should be determined with the exact formulation to be used, to determine the accuracy of the metered dose in regard to doses delivered from the same container of product and from different containers. Additionally, one should ensure that there is no interaction between the various valve subcomponents and the formulation. If distortion or elongation of some of the plastic subcomponents occurs, this may result in leakage, inaccurate dosage, and/or decomposition of the active ingredients.

There also have been instances in which the therapeutic agent was adsorbed or absorbed onto the various plastic components, and a lower than normal dose of the active ingredient was dispensed. For these reasons, one must not only determine the total weight of product dispensed per dose but also the actual amount of active ingredient in each dose. Some test procedures use the results obtained by taking 10 doses of material and determining the average amount present in one dose. When possible and when the analytical procedure permits detection of fairly small amounts of active ingredients present per dose, multiple single-dose assays should be performed. Using the average of 10 doses may fail to reveal problems of variations in each of the individual doses dispensed.

Evaluation of MDIs and Topical Pharmaceuticals

Various tests have been devised to ensure the integrity of the aerosol package. These aerosol products are said to be tamperproof, since they cannot be opened and closed in the usual manner. Because these products are all under pressure, it is very difficult to add any foreign material to the product once the entire package is assembled. This also makes it rather difficult to obtain suitable samples for an analysis. Special sampling procedures and test methods have been developed and are used to determine the suitability of the product.

Topical pharmaceutical aerosols do not present any special problems other than the sampling procedure. The USP includes several tests under the specific monographs for the topical aerosols. These include delivery rate, leak testing, microbial limit test, and assay. While several of these products are dispensed as sprays, no special emphasis or consideration is given to the particle size of the droplets or particles emitted. The spray may be defined as a fine, dry, or wet spray. Of special interest for topical spray products is the concern that some of the smaller particles may be inhaled by the user.

MDIs require a greater amount of testing since the metered valve, oral adapter, and the formulation are collectively responsible for delivering the therapeutically active ingredient to the appropriate site in the respiratory passages. This assumes that the patient will administer the product properly, so that both the dose and depth of penetration of the medication can be ensured. Unfortunately, this is not always done. Both the physician and the pharmacist have provided a most valuable service to the patient by taking the time to demonstrate the correct use of these inhalers.

Many of the tests required for the evaluation of MDIs are similar to those used for other dosage forms. These include description, identification, and assay of the active ingredient; microbial limits; moisture content; net weight, degradation products and impurities (if any); extractables; and any other tests deemed appropriate for the active ingredient.

Other tests specific for MDIs include:

DOSE UNIFORMITY OVER THE ENTIRE CONTENTS–(MDIS ONLY)—This test is described in the USP/NF and determines the amount of active ingredient delivered through the mouthpiece (oral adapter) per a specified number of actuations (dose taken by patient).

LEAKAGE RATE—This test is also available in the USP/NF and is used to estimate the weight loss over a 1-yr period. Since

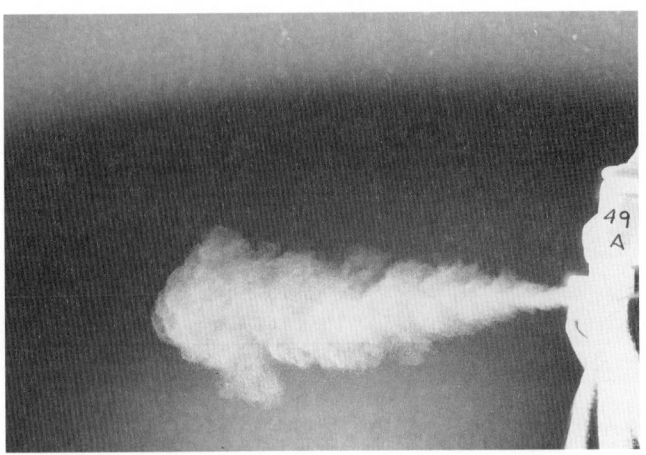

Figure 50-16. Plume emitted from a solution type MDI.

there are several sealing gaskets present in a metered-dose valve, this test determines the integrity of the gaskets as well as the proper crimping of the valve onto the container.

TOTAL NUMBER OF DISCHARGES PER CONTAINER—This is defined as the number of actuations per container and is not less than the label claim.

SPRAY PATTERN AND/OR PLUME GEOMETRY— This test evaluates the type of spray pattern emitted for the MDI and relates to the characteristics of the metering valve and oral adapter as well as to the formulation. Figure 50-16 illustrates a typical cloud or plume emitted from a solution type MDI.

It is beyond the scope of this chapter to discuss these tests in greater detail. The reader is referred to the USP/NF for specifics on each test. However, particle-size distribution is covered in greater detail because of its relationship to deposition of particles of drug in the respiratory system.

Particle-Size Distribution

Particle-size distribution is probably one of the most important characteristics of an MDI. To be effective, the particles emitted from the spray must be below 10 μm and in most cases between 2 and 8 μm in diameter. Several methods are available for the determination of the particle-size distribution for MDIs. A common method includes a cascade impactor that depends upon the principle of carrying particles in a stream of air through a series of consecutively smaller jet openings. The heavier and larger-diameter particles are impacted on a slide under the larger opening, and as the openings get smaller, the velocity of the stream increases and the next larger particles are deposited on the next slides. Figure 50-15 illustrates a cascade impactor that can be used to indicate the particle-size distribution of MDIs.

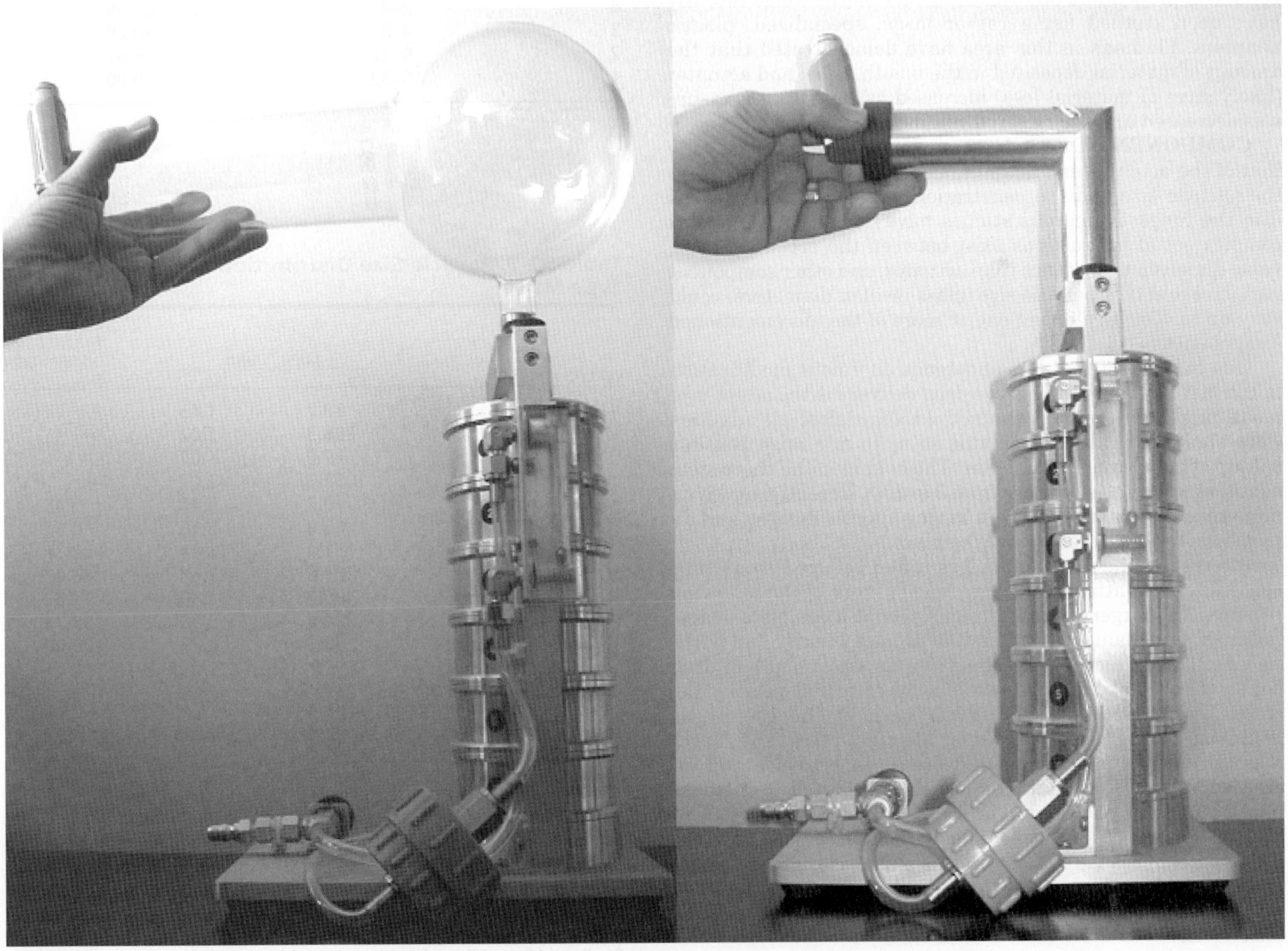

Figure 50-17. Cascade impactor (Impaq AS-6) used for particle-size distribution of MDIs (left-fitted with a 1000ml sampling throat; right-fitted with USP throat).

Figure 50-18 and Table 50-8 give a typical analysis of a suspension MDI. Table 50-9 gives a full analysis of the particle size for a solution MDI. Other methods include the use of a microscope or instrumentation based on the use of laser technology. The reader is referred to the USP/NF for a more comprehensive review of this subject.

FORMULATION FACTORS—Included among formulation factors are the physicochemical characteristics of the active ingredients, the particle size and shape of the drug, the type and concentration of surface-active agent used, and, to some extent, the vapor pressure and the metered volume of propellants. In terms of physicochemical properties, the lipoidal solubility and pulmonary absorption rates of the active ingredient are of utmost importance. Another physicochemical factor governing the biopharmaceutics of a drug is its dissolution characteristics in pulmonary fluids. Drugs having a rapid dissolution rate in pulmonary fluids predictably produce much more intense and rapid onset of action, having a shorter duration than their less soluble derivatives. Therapeutic agents that exhibit very poor solubility in pulmonary fluids are to be avoided, since they are likely to serve as irritants and precipitate bronchial spasms.

The selection of the appropriate surface-active agent (required in most pressurized inhalation suspension aerosols) is another important consideration, since the surfactant will influence droplet evaporation, particle size, and overall hydrophobicity of the particles reaching the respiratory passageways and pulmonary fluids. Solubility of these dispersing agents or surfactants is limited when formulating with an HFC propellant. Ethyl alcohol has been added to increase their solubility.

The effects of propellant vapor pressure and the metered volume of propellants on drug deposition in the lungs recently have been studied using rather large, specialized, plastic adapters. Findings in this area have demonstrated that the amount of material deposited in the mouth, tube, and actuator (likely sites of material loss) increased as the vapor pressure was decreased and the metered volume increased.

COMPONENT DESIGN—Component design, specifically that of the actuator and adapter, also has been shown to alter the particle size and the penetration and deposition of drugs into the lungs. Numerous studies have demonstrated that a complex set of interactions exist between the actuation type, valve dimensions, distance from actuator, and other component variables and that particle size (mass median diameters) could vary up to 40% by altering one or more of the aforementioned components.

One component that has undergone enormous modification in the last few years to improve drug delivery is the adapter or mouthpiece. Up to about the mid 1970s, almost all adapters were short and rather simplistic so as to minimize possible holdup of material in the adapter. The holdup in the short-stem adapters averages anywhere from 5 to 20%. Recently, however, numerous customized adapters having specific designs and dimensions have entered the marketplace.

Interest in the larger adapters (often referred to as tube spacers) can be attributed to any one or more of the following reasons. The larger adapter designs permit a complete evaporation of propellant, reducing initial droplet velocity and particle size. This reduction of particle size improves depth of drug penetration into the lungs, while a lower initial velocity decreases product impaction to the back of the esophagus (whiplash effect), common to short-stem adapters. The larger adapter designs also permit a decrease in pressure and increased volume flow that also has been reported to increase penetration of particles into the lungs. It should be pointed out that the larger tube spacers are not without problems. They are inconvenient because of their size, are expensive, and are somewhat difficult to clean. They also present the manufacturer with the problem of assessing product holdup in a rather complex device.

ADMINISTRATION TECHNIQUES—The metered-inhalation aerosol dosage form, although popular, generally is

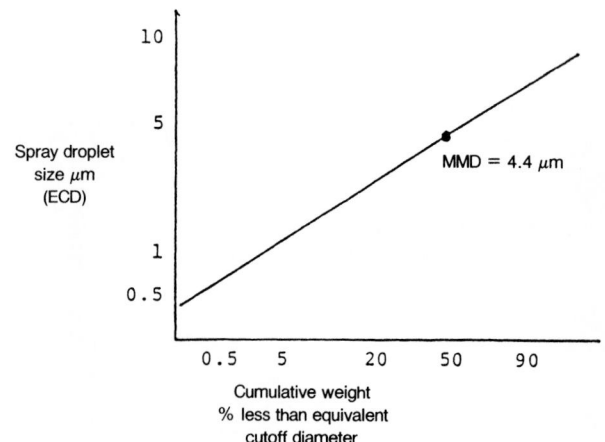

Figure 50-18. Log probability plot of data from the cascade impactor (MMD, mass median diameter).

Table 50-8. Cumulative Particle-Size Distribution

SLIDE NO.	PARTICLE SIZE (μM)	CUMULATIVE PARTICLE SIZE DISTRIBUTION (%)
Filter	Less than 0.5	0.55
6	0.5–1	5.35
5	1–2	18.98
4	2–4	61.59
3	4–8	90.20
2	8–16	96.67
1	16–32	100.00

Table 50–9. Particle Size Distribution of Solution Type MDI

COLLECTION UNIT	MASS FOUND		CUMULATIVE PARTICLE SIZE DISTRIBUTION %
	μg	%	
Valve stem	38.7	1.43	—
Mouthpiece	298.3	11.02	—
Collar	27.6	1.02	—
Induction Port	1057.8	39.07	—
Filder—(0.3 μm)	70.2	5.46	5.46
Stage 6—(0.5 μm)	66.3	5.16	10.61
Stage 5—(1.0 μm)	151.4	11.77	22.39
Stage 4—(2.0 μm)	303.8	23.64	46.02
Stage 3—(4.0 μm)	408.8	31.80	77.83
Stage 2—(8.0 μm)	204.4	15.90	93.73
Stage 1—(16.0 μm)	80.6	6.27	100.00
Total A	2300.7		
Total B	1285.4		
Total C	2707.8		
Total R	1204.7		

Respirable Dose (μg) = 120.47
Respirable Fraction = 52.36%
Mass Median Aerodynamic Diameter (MMAD) (μm) = 1.95
Geometric Standard Deviation (GSD) = 2.81
Mass Balance = 99.73%

A = Total Mass of Drug found on the collar, induction port, filter, and stages 1–6.
B = Total Mass of Drug found on the filter and stages 1–6.
C = Total Mass of Drug found on the valve stem, mouthpiece, collar induction port, filter and stage 1–6.
R = Total Mass of Drug found on stages 2–6 and filter.

considered one of the most complicated to use drug-delivery systems currently marketed by the pharmaceutical industry. It is viewed by many as being only slightly simpler to use than an injectable, since inhalation products often require up to 10 to 15 maneuvers by the patient during use. Failure of the patient to perform any one of these maneuvers correctly may alter significantly the deposition of the drug into the appropriate portion of the lungs.

Differences in the directions for use of each inhalation product are a result of the product formulation and actuator design that the manufacturer deemed most appropriate for the particular product. In light of this, it is not surprising to find patients who require two or more aerosol inhalation products or who are constantly changing their medication (such as the asthmatic patient) occasionally experiencing difficulties in complying with the suggested method of application.

These problems present a unique opportunity for the pharmacist to counsel the patient on the correct use of these inhalers. Several manufacturers will provide placebo inhalers for this purpose. Others will provide videotapes that can be used by the pharmacist and other health professionals to teach the correct use of these inhalers. Brown bag and senior citizen programs, health seminars, and other similar programs can provide a suitable audience for group presentations. However, the most successful programs are conducted on a one-to-one basis in the privacy of the pharmacy.

Many attempts have been made to overcome these problems and increase the efficacy of this dosage form. A breath- activated inhaler has been developed by 3M Pharmaceuticals and is used as an integral part of their pirbuterol acetate inhalation aerosol. They found that in a study of 70 patients, the use of the breath-activated inhaler increased the efficient use of these inhalers from 50 to 91%. These patients were given both written and verbal instructions. Reading instructions alone increased the efficiency from 39 to 63%. Many other devices, including tube spacers, breath activated, and electronic devices have been under study for numerous years. To date none of these units have become commercially available other than one breath activated (Maxair Autohaler–3M) and one spacer (Azmacort Inhalation Aerosol–*Aventis Pharmaceuticals*).

Tube spacers also increase the efficiency of drug delivery via MDIs. These spacers permit atomization of the delivered dose in a confined chamber or bag and eliminate the need for the precise synchronization of actuations and deep breathing with inspiration. Triamcinolone acetonide MDI is available as an MDI and is fitted with a tube spacer instead of the conventional short-stem actuators. Figure 50-19 illustrates several metered-dose aerosols with short-stem actuators. Patients must check with their physician before using these spacers, since the particle- size distribution of the drug being dispersed through one of these spacers may be substantially

different from those emitted from a short-stem actuator. Certainly, the deposition pattern will change, and the efficiency of the delivered dose reaching the proper pulmonary airways will be increased.

NEWER DEVELOPMENTS

At present, there is much interest in developing MDIs for a variety of conditions including asthma, emphysema, diabetes, aids, cancer, heart disease, and cystic fibrosis. Many of these compounds have been developed using biotechnology processes, and their delivery to the respiratory system via an MDI is an extremely challenging undertaking. With the introduction of newer, alternative propellants, the challenge becomes even greater and presents a unique opportunity for the delivery of these compounds. There is very little interest by manufacturers of currently available MDIs formulated with a CFC to convert the existing therapeutic agents to a HFC product. As indicated previously, Albuterol and Beclomethasone Propionate are the only two drug entities available in the US with a HFC propellant. It is doubtful if any others will ever be converted to a HFC. Manufacturers are currently discovering newer therapeutic agents for development as an MDI using the environmental acceptable HFA propellant. Several "second generation steroids" are currently under development and are formulated with a HFA propellant.

The valve and container suppliers are cooperating with the industry to develop much-needed hardware to accommodate this change. At present, there is no specific scheduled date when manufacturers can no longer use CFCs for their metered dose inhalers. As long as CFCs remain available, the changeover will continue at the current slow pace.

BIBLIOGRAPHY

Burke GP, Poochikian G, Botstein P. *J Aerosol Med* 1991; 4:265.
Dalziel SM, Creazzo JA. *Spray Technology and Marketing* 2003; 13(6):20.
Hickey AJ. *Pharmaceutical Inhalation Aerosol Technology.* New York: Dekker, 1992.
Johnsen M. *The Aerosol Handbook,* 2nd ed. Caldwell, NJ: Wayne E Dorland Co, 1982.
Johnsen MA. *Spray Marketing and Technology* 2001; 11(5):42.
Johnsen MA. *Spray Marketing and Technology* 2001; 11(10):22.
Johnsen MA. *Spray Marketing and Technology* 2001; 11(11):36.
Johnsen MA. *Spray Marketing and Technology* 2002; 12(2):41.
Leskovsek N. *Drug Delivery Technology* 2003; 3(7):30.
Purewal TS, Greenleaf DJ. *Medicinal Aerosol Formulations,* US Pat 5,605,674, Feb 25, 1997.
Robinson G. *Spray Technology and Marketing* 2003; 13(6):16.
Sanders P. *Handbook of Aerosol Technology,* 2nd ed. Malabar, FL: Robert E Krieger Publ, 1987.
Sciarra CJ, Sciarra JJ. Monographs on aerosol propellants. In *Handbook of Pharmaceutical Excipients,* 4th ed. Rowe RC, Sheskey PJ, Weller PJ, ed. London, UK: AphA and the Pharmaceutical Press, 2003, p 93, 147, 149, 211, 215, 274, 278, 408, 410, 646.
Sciarra JJ, Sciarra CJ. Aerosols. In Gennaro AR, ed. *Remington: The Science and Practice of Pharmacy,* 20th ed. Philadelphia, PA: Lippincott Williams and Wilkins, 2000, p 963.
Sciarra JJ. Aerosol suspensions and emulsions. In Liebermann H, Rieger M, Banker G, eds. *Pharmaceutical Dosage Forms: Disperse Systems,* vol 2, 2nd ed. New York: Marcel Dekker Inc, 1996, p 319.
Sciarra JJ. Pharmaceutical aerosols. In Banker GS, Rhodes CT, eds. *Modern Pharmaceutics,* 3rd ed, New York: Marcel Dekker Inc, 1996, p 547.
Sciarra JJ, Sciarra CJ. "Aerosols". In Kirk-Othmer Encyclopedia of Chemical Technology, 2001. <http://jws-edck,interscience,wiley, com:8095/articles/aeroscia.a01/abstract.html>.
Sciarra JJ. The next generation of metered dose inhalers. *US Pharm* 1997; 22(7):37.
Sciarra CJ, Sciarra JJ. Validation of Inhalation Aerosols. In Nash RA, Wachter, AH. ed. *Pharmaceutical Process Validation,* 3rd ed. New York: Marcel Dekker Inc, 2003, p 329.
Sciarra CJ, Sciarra JJ. *Spray Technology and Marketing* 2003; 13(6):25.
Strobach DR. *Aerosol Age* 1988; 33(7):32.
USP 26/NF21. *Physical Tests and Determination: <601> Aerosols, Metered Dose Inhalers, and Dry Powder Inhalers.* 2002, p 2105.

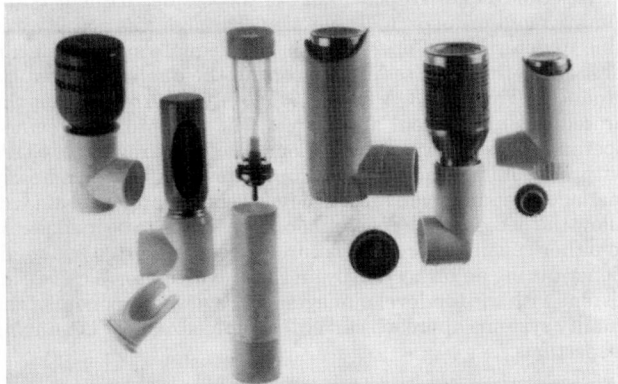

Figure 50-19. Medicinal aerosols with short oral applicators.

CHAPTER 51

Quality Assurance and Control

John H Parker, PhD

John E Enders, PhD, MBA

The pharmaceutical industry, as a vital segment of the healthcare system, conducts research and manufactures and markets pharmaceutical and biological products and medical devices used for the acute/chronic treatment and diagnosis of disease. Recent advances in drug discovery, primarily in the field of biotechnology and in the required controls over manufacturing processes, are presenting new challenges to the control of quality and to the systems that operate internally in the industry. The external regulations established by the federal Food and Drug Administration (FDA) and other regulatory bodies also add to these challenges. The evolving role of the industrial quality professional requires more extensive education including food and drug law, business, as well as the traditional science/technology coursework.

The pursuit of quality is being approached through the application of quality systems such as Total Quality Management (TQM) and continuous improvement, whereby management and labor join forces to build quality into products while helping to ensure the company's financial success. This changed emphasis is directed toward defect prevention (proactive) rather than defect detection (after the fact).

Quality assurance (QA) and quality control (QC) groups develop and follow standard internal operating procedures directed toward assuring the quality, safety, purity, and effectiveness of drug products. The FDA has issued a primary regulation to the industry entitled *Current Good Manufacturing Practice for Finished Pharmaceuticals* (commonly referred to as the cGMPs or GMPs). Numerous guidelines have been issued relative to specific dosage forms and operations such as aseptic manufacturing, validation and stability testing, etc., which impose significant compliance requirements. These guidelines also serve as the basis for compliance investigations conducted by the FDA and are used in regulatory agency inspections of facilities and operations. Recently, emphasis is being placed on the inspection of quality systems as part of the regulatory pre-approval program when reviewing submissions relative to New Drug Applications (NDAs) and Biological License Applications (BLAs).

QA AND QC: ORGANIZATION/ RESPONSIBILITIES

Industry, to ensure compliance with these government regulations and with their own internal policies and procedures, has developed very sophisticated quality organizations with well-defined responsibilities. It has been accepted that QA and QC have different functions within an organization; although both are considered part of the Quality Unit as identified in 21CFR. QC most commonly functions to test and measure material and product. QA establishes systems for ensuring the quality of the product. Firms must decide upon the exact roles they wish QC and QA to perform in operations and put these definitions in writing.

QA Functions and Responsibilities

The QA department within any organization, because of its responsibilities, normally will report to a relatively high-level administrator within a company, depending on its size. In smaller companies they may report to the chief executive officer or the president. In larger corporations they will sometimes report to the president or executive vice-president or chief of operations. In any case, however, responsibility for quality, as currently dictated by FDA, ultimately resides with top management.

In all cases QA will be independent of the economic issues associated with manufacturing and distribution of the product. The QA department is responsible for ensuring that the quality policies adopted by a company are followed. In some organizations, QA serves as the primary contact with regulatory agencies and is the final authority for product acceptance (release) or rejection. It is customary for QA to play a major role in the identification and preparation of the necessary policies and standard operating procedures (SOPs) relative to the control of quality. Where it has responsibility for final product release, it must determine that the product meets all the applicable specifications and that it was manufactured according to internal standards and cGMPs. QA departments now tend to work as a team member with the other functional groups within the firm rather than simply to serve a police function, a largely outdated role of QA.

A second major responsibility of the QA department is the quality monitoring or audit function. Through this activity it is able to determine if operations have adequate systems, facilities, and written procedures to control the quality of products produced. Thus, the QA function not only determines that the procedures are current and correct, but that properly trained operators are following them. Combining this review of SOPs with an audit of facilities and operations will give company management an inside report on its level of compliance and will allow the necessary changes and/or corrections to be made prior to either causing a product failure or being reported as a deficiency during an inspection by an FDA investigator. This is consistent with the top-level management review component of the quality systems approach currently emphasized by FDA during inspections.

Senior management of a company looks to the QA function to assess operations continually and to advise and guide them toward full compliance with all applicable internal and external regulations. Organizationally, the Quality Department(s) should report, as directed by the GMPs, to someone other than the person responsible for production.

QC Functions and Responsibilities

Quality Control is responsible for the day-to-day control of quality within a company. This department is staffed with scientists and technicians responsible for the sampling and analytical testing of incoming raw materials and inspection of packaging components, including labeling. They conduct in-process testing when required, perform environmental monitoring, and inspect operations for compliance. Finally, they conduct the required tests on finished dosage form. QC is also responsible for monitoring product quality through distribution, including testing of product complaint samples, evaluating product stability, etc.

Many companies have the heads of QC and production report to a common higher level of management, but with QC being independent of production. This higher-level management may be the same or different individuals, but it allows independent operation of both functions without direct conflict arising when reaching a final decision on the acceptability of final products.

The analytical control laboratory must be staffed with persons who are trained academically and are, through experience, capable of performing the often complex analyses used to evaluate the acceptability of the materials tested. The equipment and instrumentation in the laboratory must be suitable for performing the testing in an accurate and efficient manner. Detailed specifications must be available, as well as validated test methods against which products and raw materials will be evaluated. The specifications detail the limits for acceptance of the article, based on identified critical parameters.

The testing and acceptance of only high-quality raw materials is essential for the production of uniformly acceptable products. Quality Control plays a major role in the selection and qualification of vendors from whom these materials are purchased. Testing of representative samples is required, and in many cases, an audit of the vendor's operation is necessary to determine their suitability and degree of compliance with GMPs and other relevant standards prior to their being approved. The vendor audit frequently is organized by QA, with technical support from research, QC, and manufacturing.

At various critical in-process steps in production, it may be necessary to sample and test product against criteria previously established. Often, in-process alert or action levels will be identified for the critical in-process parameters as a means of process control. These alert or action levels are normally set such that they are more restrictive than the final acceptance limits, but serve as an in-process control by providing early warnings of conditions that could lead to an out-of-control situation and thus will allow timely corrective action before such conditions occur. Trending of analytical data is also useful in providing early warning signals that the process is moving out of control. It should be noted, however, that materials, which have reached the alert or action level criteria, are still acceptable for use in manufacturing, since they have not exceeded an out-of-limit rejection level.

Quality Control is responsible, as part of its testing and inspection functions, for monitoring the environmental conditions under which products are manufactured and/or held. Different levels of control are established depending on the intended use of the dosage form. Parenteral and ophthalmic products must be produced in a controlled environment that is designed to ensure their sterility. Monitoring of air and water systems is critical in confirming that they are being controlled and that the levels of particulates, microbial matter, and other contaminants are within pre-established limits. The USP contains monographs and specifications on Water Used for Pharmaceutical Purposes. Formerly, the Federal Government Standard 209E, *Airborne Particulate Cleanliness Classes in Cleanrooms and Clean Zones,* established acceptable limits for particulates in a controlled environment, but is no longer considered applicable to the pharmaceutical industry. Federal standards are currently not enforced for environmental quality, but guidance is available in the FDA Concept Paper, Sterile Drug Products Produced by Aseptic Processing–Draft, published on September 27, 2002. In addition, reference is made to the Baseline Pharmaceutical Engineering Guide, Vol. 3, Sterile Manufacturing Facilities, published by the International Society of Pharmaceutical Engineering (ISPE) in partnership with the FDA, in June 2000. Generally, conditions listed as Class 100 (or equivalent) are maintained in areas where parenteral products are filled into clean, sterile containers. Class 100 is defined as an area that can be controlled to contain fewer than 100 particles, 0.5 μm and larger, per cubic foot of air. In addition, manufacturers must establish limits for the presence of viable microorganisms in the environment and appropriately monitor the air quality in the filling area.

Another major element of control is the environmental monitoring of the areas in which nonsterile products are manufactured, such as liquids, tablets, and capsules. The objective here is first to determine an acceptable level of particulates and microbial contaminates and then to control them to this level. If particulate levels are found to be excessive, steps must be taken to bring them within acceptable limits so as not to compromise the quality of the product. This monitoring and control of the environment will further ensure the quality and stability of the product by preventing the products from being exposed to a hostile environment.

Control of packaging components, especially those that come into direct contact with a product, is required. These materials must be inspected and tested against rigid specifications to ensure that they meet predetermined functional standards. This includes evaluation of compatibility of the product with the packaging materials. Labeling is understandably a critical component, not just in its original design and acceptance, but also with regard to secure storage and issuance to ensure accountability. Furthermore, final product labeling must be 100% inspected to ensure that it is correct.

TOTAL QUALITY MANAGEMENT/TOTAL PRODUCT QUALITY

The production of quality pharmaceutical products requires embracing the principles of Total Quality Management (TQM). Although the term TQM has fallen out of favor in recent years and has been replaced by other, though similar designations, such as Total Product Quality (TPQ), the principles of TQM will serve to improve productivity and customer satisfaction. The quality function is part of a team composed of research, production, marketing/sales, and customer service. In the competitive markets of today, it is critical to improve quality and service continually while minimizing costs and maximizing resource utilization to help contain overall health care costs. The concept of TQM requires the total commitment of senior-level management and supervision of all departments, operators, suppliers, and customers. Its basic principle is one of continually striving for process improvement that begins with product development and only concludes when feedback and follow-up have been completed on customer complaints and suggestions. In many firms the QA Department has the responsibility to organize and implement programs with these objectives in mind.

Quality must be designed into products, beginning with research and development phases. Product quality criteria are established, and detailed specifications are written. Meticulous, written procedures must be prepared for production and control, and processes must be rigorously validated. Raw materials must be characterized and then purchased from reputable, approved suppliers to ensure that, when the materials are incorporated into the finished dosage form, they will provide products of uniformly high quality. Facilities must be designed, constructed, and controlled to provide the proper stable environment for protecting the integrity of products. Equipment must be selected that is efficient and can be cleaned readily and sanitized, to aid in preventing cross- contamination of one product with another. Personnel must be trained properly so that their personal habits, clothing, and job performance do not compromise product quality. The directions that they use must be in writing, approved by responsible individuals, and strictly followed. Training programs must be thoroughly documented and include an evaluation of mastery of the procedures employed.

Distribution departments are responsible for controlling the shipping and handling of products, using inventory-control systems based on the *first in–first out* principle. They select modes of distribution that will protect products from adverse handling or environmental conditions while in transit to distribution points and to customers. Furthermore, they must maintain accurate records of distribution to ensure that any product recall, if required, will be effectively and thoroughly conducted.

The marketing department must be sensitive to the customer's needs and be responsive to complaints. The quality department should be kept informed of real or potential problems as reported from the marketplace so that they may conduct investigations of product complaints, as appropriate, to determine the cause of the condition described in the complaint.

Involved with each of the operations described above, QA is ever present and gives approval only after assessing and being assured that the entire production process has been completed satisfactorily and that all the aspects of the GMPs have been satisfied.

In the pharmaceutical industry, TQM or the equivalent system, therefore, can be looked upon as a combined team effort to develop, produce, market, distribute, and control products that are safe and will be effective for the time they remain in the marketplace. Such a program ultimately will assure the professional dispenser and the final consumer that each lot of every product conforms to certain specifications and that each unit has met all the requirements, both internal and external, of the industry and will fulfill the declarations made in its labeling.

DOCUMENTATION

The saying, "If it wasn't documented, it wasn't done," describes the linkage between written records of action taken and the quality operation. These written documents include those found in the product-development phase as well as those associated with the actual manufacture and testing of individual batches. The former will consist of research and development reports, technology transfer reports, and the validation records required when the FDA conducts its pre-approval investigations. Elements of these documents will include raw material and final product specifications along with appropriate validated test methods, technology-transfer documents, and production scale-up support data. Specific critical pieces of equipment must be identified along with the process and product qualification/validation records. The *Master Production Batch Record* (MPBR) is often the document that facilitates the orderly transition from product and process development to commercial-scale production, since it is the document that captures the process as described by the product development documentation.

The *Production Batch Record* (PBR), an exact copy of the approved MPBR, is used along with written SOPs to produce individual batches of product that are assigned specific code or lot numbers. The PBR provides a historical record of every step,

beginning with the receipt of raw materials and package components and continuing through each phase of production. Recording charts or computer printouts of significant operations such as autoclaving, drying, air-particulate monitoring, lyophilizing, etc, become part of the batch history. After a batch has been completed, including final analytical and physical testing, there is one final additional step that must be completed prior to approving the batch for distribution. All documentation relating to the production of the specific batch is given a final review. This is often a two-step process in which each of the required documents is checked for accuracy and completeness by manufacturing. Any discrepancy must then be investigated and a written explanation made. This is followed by a final review by QA to ensure that all documents are complete and that all issues have been appropriately resolved. Only after this final review by QA has been completed satisfactorily may the batch be approved for release. Once the batch has been approved, accurate distribution records are required, to trace the batch in the marketplace, which would facilitate, if the need arose, recalling the batch.

QUALITY IN PHARMACEUTICAL BIOTECHNOLOGY

Because of the physical/chemical nature of the proteinaceous products derived from pharmaceutical biotechnology, unique quality considerations prevail that are associated with early research and development synthesis, clinical product scale-up, and commercial manufacture. The reason that this is particularly challenging becomes more evident when some gross differences between biological therapeutic agents and chemical drug products are examined. In contrast to small-molecule pharmaceuticals, biotechnology-derived drugs are obtained from living organisms and often consist of complex mixtures of protein and other substances, often heat labile, and, finally, highly susceptible to microbiological contamination. In the context of this discussion, pharmaceutical biotechnology products are defined to include proteins and peptides produced by recombinant DNA (rDNA) techniques and monoclonal antibody/hybridoma (Mab) technology. The former refers to the fact that these products are often produced by microorganisms or mammalian cells containing hybrid DNA, most often produced by joining pieces of DNA from different sources to gain the appropriate expressed product; the latter involves production of a single clone from hybrid cells, using hybridoma technology that fuses different cells to make the desired antibody. See also Chapter 49, *Biotechnology and Drugs*. In general, the object of the pharmaceutical biotechnology manufacturing process is to produce a product essentially free of contamination. The attributes that the product should possess are sterility and the absence of pyrogens, unwanted organisms, by-products of the manufacturing process, and degradation by-products. The same requirements for adherence to cGMPs exist throughout the production process for recombinant proteins and monoclonal antibodies as apply to other pharmaceutical products.

Consideration must also be given to the design of the delivery system for the biotechnology-derived drug, especially because of the lability of many of these products. In accomplishing this task, often the more conventional manufacturing processes may be employed such as sterile filtration, aseptic handling, and, in some instances, lyophilization. However, for many of these products, new delivery systems are being evaluated as described below.

Characterization of the products produced by pharmaceutical biotechnology is a rapidly changing technical challenge, but tremendous advances have been made in the past few years. The FDA considers many of these products to be well characterized and has changed the approach to license approval with this improved understanding of product specifications in mind. Bogdansky[1] outlines QC or testing considerations that address the structure, potency, and purity of proteins and the analysis of contaminants resulting from the manufacturing process or degradation. Full characterization includes physical and chemical stability. Satisfactory stability of the product is a requirement for controlled manufacture and an acceptable shelf life following distribution.

CONTEMPORARY ISSUES

As a demonstration of the pace of change in the pharmaceutical industry, technologies that were on the cutting edge as recently as 5 years ago have become rather commonplace, as organizations routinely employ them to increase productivity and reduce costs while maintaining product quality.

Statistical process control permits improved real-time control, thereby reducing end-product failures. Qualification and potential certification of suppliers of goods and services adds to the thrust of building in quality and allows the reduction in inventory costs by following just-in-time purchasing and receipt principles. Finally, in practically all facets of research, development, and operations, automation and computerization, including robotics, are work methods that have an impact on our daily lives by increasing productivity and raising the standards of quality by enhancing reproducibility. This application of computerized manufacturing and control has led to increasingly rigorous requirements for the appropriate design and validation of computer-controlled processes. This is evident in the publishing of 21CFR part 11 and GAMP4, which describe the requirements for electronic records and signatures and validation respectively. It should be noted, however, that in January 2003, draft guidance from FDA on these matters was withdrawn, accompanied by a statement from FDA that the approach to these issues is changing. New FDA guidance is expected to be forthcoming in the not-too-distant future.

Today, the pace of change in the pharmaceutical industry continues unabated. There is increased emphasis on analytical chemistry as it relates to the entire drug discovery, development, and manufacturing sequence. This, coupled with new clues as to potential drug targets uncovered through the Human Genome Project and new approaches to computer modeling of potential drug compounds, has led to many new candidates for development. This is evident in the new drug submissions made by industry to the FDA and in the depth and complexity of the review process associated with these new compounds. More technically sophisticated instrumental methods of analysis, assisted by computer interfacing, provide greater sensitivity along with the ability to analyze the results more efficiently and effectively. From these advances flows the requirement for more stability-indicating assay methods as well as increased emphasis on the impurities in drug substances and products, such as organic volatile impurities and even ordinary impurities. Taken as a whole, accurate mass balance of the parent compound, degradents, and impurities is an expectation. Compendia such as the USP are including these concepts in general chapters and individual drug monographs. The evolution of high-pressure liquid chromatography (HPLC) methods, and other even more sensitive technologies, and the wide acceptance of these techniques has increased the trend toward painstakingly thorough characterization of products, so that it is becoming the exception rather than the rule. Additionally, HPLC facilitates the recent focus on optical purity through chiral separation to support improvements in asymmetric synthesis, with the intent of producing the single, therapeutically active compound.

The move toward the elimination of tests that require animals is exemplified by the replacement of the rabbit pyrogen test with the bacterial endotoxin (LAL) method. It may be expected that similar chemical and biochemical approaches will be developed to eliminate the use of animal testing in pre-clinical drug evaluation and toxicological testing as well.

The concept of parametric release of end-product is being applied on the basis of complete knowledge and control of all phases of the process including such things as information on suppliers, process and product validation, operator training, and thorough process knowledge coupled with statistical process controls. The sum of these prospectively managed and controlled quality activities results in greater real-time control and, hence, a diminished need for end-product confirmatory testing.

In the operations area, newer types of dosage forms, such as liposomes and transdermal devices, are demanding innovative manufacturing and control procedures and practices. Novel routes of administration such as pulmonary inhalation for the administration of insulin are also being explored. Automation and computerization continue to increase manufacturing yields and concomitant tighter tolerances. As a result, there is a renewed interest in functional testing of raw materials, to keep up with these manufacturing advances.

All of these advances will, no doubt, be refined with the passage of time and continuing diligent efforts on the part of industrial professionals and regulators. This will lead to ever-new issues affecting the industrial quality professional and, hence, the challenge and reward of such an exciting endeavor.

FDA MODERNIZATION

The FDA Modernization Act (FDAMA) of 1997 was introduced with the intent of improving the review process and thereby making new drug products available to the public faster than in the past. This effort continues both in form and detail and, in general, has shortened the review and approval timeline. A recent decision by FDA to merge many of the product categories regulated by the Center for Biologics (CBER) into the Center for Drugs (CDER) is intended to further expedite the review process. See Chapter 48 for more information on the new drug approval process.

GMP REGULATIONS

In March 1979, the FDA issued revised GMP regulations. These regulations, still in effect today, present the minimum requirements to be met by industry when manufacturing, packaging, and holding human and veterinary drugs.

The FD&C Act states that a drug is deemed to be adulterated unless the methods used in its manufacture, processing, packing, and holding, as well as the facilities in which it was produced and the controls used during its production, conform to the GMPs so that the drug will meet the safety requirements of the Act and that it has the correct identity and strength to meet the quality and purity characteristics that it is represented to possess. Through the intervening years additional regulations and guidelines have been issued to supplement the original drug GMPs such as those for the *Good Manufacturing Practice for the Manufacture, Packing, Storage and Installation of Medical Devices* and *Good Laboratory Practice (GLPs) for Controlling and Conducting Human Clinical Studies.* Additionally, guidelines have been issued relating to the *Manufacture and Control of Large Volume Parenteral Solutions, Control of Sterile Products Produced by Aseptic Processing, Inspections of Bulk Pharmaceutical Chemicals,* and an *Inspection Guide for Quality Control Laboratories,* as well as on many other topics. A number of other guidelines or concept papers have been prepared by various organizations within the industry itself, such as the Pharmaceutical Manufacturers Association (PhRMA), the Parenteral Drug Association (PDA), the International Society of Pharmaceutical Engineering (ISPE), and others. A partial listing is provided in the *Bibliography.*

The current GMP regulations and these additional guides and guidelines should be read and understood thoroughly by those involved in or interested in pursuing QC and QA responsibilities. The scope of the present regulation is given in the following outline, along with a brief interpretation of each subpart.

REFERENCES

1. Bogdansky FM. *Pharm Technol* 1987; (Sep): 72.

BIBLIOGRAPHY

Human and Veterinary Drugs—Current Good Manufacturing Practice for Finished Pharmaceuticals. 21 CFR 211: 2002.

Airborne Particulate Cleanliness Classes in Cleanrooms and Clean Zones (Fed Std 209E). Washington, DC: GSA, 1992.

Quality System Regulation in the Manufacturing of Medical Devices. 21 CFR 820: 2002.

Good Laboratory Practice for Non-clinical Laboratory Studies. 21 CFR 58: 2002. Rockville, MD: USP/NF, USPC.

Validation of Steam Sterilization Cycles (Tech Monogr #1). Philadelphia: PDA, 1978.

Validation of Dry Heat Processes Used for Sterilization and Depyrogenation (Tech Monogr #3). Philadelphia: PDA, 1981.

Sterile Pharmaceutical Packaging: Compatibility and Stability (Tech Rep #5). Philadelphia: PDA, 1984.

Fundamentals of a Microbiological Environment Monitoring Program (Tech Rep #13). Philadelphia: PDA, 1990.

Current Practices in the Validation of Aseptic Processing—1992 (Tech Rep #17). Philadelphia: PDA, 1993.

Process Simulation Testing for Aseptically Filled Products-1996 (Tech Rep # 22). Philadelphia: PDA, 1996.

Technical Report: Process Simulation Testing for Aseptically Filled Products (Tech Rep #22). Philadelphia: PDA, 1996.

Points to Consider for Aseptic Processing–2003 (Supplement Volume 57, #2). Philadelphia: PDA, 2003

Guideline on Sterile Products Produced by Aseptic Processing. Rockville, MD: FDA, Jun 1987.

Sterile Drug Products Produced by Aseptic Processing–Draft. Rockville, MD: FDA, Sep 2002.

Concepts and Principles for the Validation of Computer Systems Used in the Manufacture and Control of Drug Products. *Proc PMA Sem* Apr 1986.

Risk-Based Approach to 21 CFR Part 11–ISPE White Paper. Tampa, FL: ISPE, 2003.

Points to Consider in the Manufacture and Testing of Monoclonal Antibody Products for Human Use. Rockville, MD: FDA, Feb 1997.

Points to Consider on Plasmid DNA Vaccines for Preventive Infectious Disease Indications. Rockville, MD: FDA, Dec 1996.

Huxsoll JF. *Quality Assurance for Biopharmaceuticals*. New York: Wiley, 1994.

Guide to Inspection of Bulk Pharmaceutical Chemicals. Rockville, MD: FDA, Sep 1992.

FDA Website [http://www.fda.gov] has many current guidance documents available for review and/or downloading.

GMP Training Organizations Website [http://gmptraining.com/news.html] has links to several organizations including DIA, ISPE, and PDA for current information on quality issues.

Other Websites providing useful references: [http://www.ispe.org/; http://www.diahome.org; http://www.raps.org/; http://www.pda. org/;]

Current Good Manufacturing Practices

CFR Title 21 Food and Drugs

PART 211 CURRENT GOOD MANUFACTURING
PRACTICE FOR FINISHED PHARMACEUTICALS

SUBPART A GENERAL PROVISIONS

211.3 (Definitions) The scope of the regulations are explained for human prescription and OTC drug products including drugs used to produce medicated animal feed. Reference is made to Part 210.3 of the chapter that gives definitions for all significant terms used in the regulations.

SUBPART B ORGANIZATION AND PERSONNEL

211.22 (Responsibilities of QC unit) Highlighted here is the assignment to the QC unit of total responsibility for ensuring that adequate systems and procedures exist and are followed to ensure product quality.

211.25 (Personnel qualifications) Personnel, either supervisory or operational, must be qualified by training and experience to perform their assigned tasks.

211.28 (Personnel responsibilities) The obligations of personnel engaged in the manufacture of drug products concerning their personal hygiene, clothing, and medical status are defined.

211.34 (Consultants) The qualifications of consultants must be sufficient for the project to which they are assigned.

SUBPART C BUILDINGS AND FACILITIES

Buildings and facilities can be considered acceptable only if they are suitable for their intended purpose and can be maintained. Construction concepts, such as air handling systems, lighting, eating facilities, and plumbing systems including water, sewage and toilet facilities, are outlined.

211.42 (Design and construction features)

211.44 (Lighting)

211.46 (Ventilation, air filtration, air heating and cooling)

211.48 (Plumbing)

211.50 (Sewage and refuse)

211.52 (Washing and toilet facilities)

211.56 (Sanitation)

211.58 (Maintenance)

SUBPART D EQUIPMENT

Equipment must be designed, constructed, of adequate size, suitably located, and able to be maintained and cleaned to be considered suitable for its intended use. Reference is made to the use of automatic equipment, data processors, and computers, highlighting the need for input/output verification and for proper calibration of recorders, counters, and other electrical or mechanical devices.

211.63 (Equipment design, size, and location)

211.65 (Equipment construction)

211.67 (Equipment cleaning and maintenance)

211.68 (Automatic, mechanical, and electronic equipment)

211.72 (Filters) Special note is made that the only filters to be used are those that do not release fibers into products.

SUBPART E CONTROL OF COMPONENTS AND DRUG PRODUCT CONTAINERS AND CLOSURES

211.80 (General requirements) Written procedures must be available that describe the receipt, identification, storage, handling, sampling, testing, and approval or rejection of components (raw materials) and drug products.

211.82 (Receipt and storage of untested components, drug product containers, and closures)

211.84 (Testing and approval or rejection of components, drug product containers, and closures)

211.86 (Use of approved components, drug product containers, and closures) These shall be rotated so that the oldest approved stock is used first.

211.87 (Retesting of approved components, drug product containers, and closures) Materials that are subject to deterioration during storage should be retested at an appropriate time based on stability profiles.

211.89 (Rejected components, drug product containers, and closures) These shall be identified and controlled to prevent their use in manufacturing.

211.94 (Drug product containers and closures) Containers and closures (product contact materials) must protect the product and must be nonreactive with or additive to the product, suitable for their intended use, and controlled using written procedures.

SUBPART F PRODUCTION AND PROCESS CONTROLS

211.100 (Written procedures; deviations) Written standard operating procedures (SOPs) for each production process and control procedure are necessary. Any deviation from an SOP must be investigated, recorded, and approved prior to final product acceptance.

211.101 (Charge-in of components) The procedures used to formulate a batch shall be written and followed.

211.103 (Calculation of yield) Actual yields and theoretical yields shall be determined. All products are to be formulated to provide not less than 100% of the required amount of active ingredient. Records are to be maintained of each component and the quantity, which is incorporated into a batch.

211.105 (Equipment identification) Equipment shall be properly identified.

211.110 (Sampling and testing of in-process materials and drug products) Significant in-process steps are to be identified and appropriate sampling, testing, and approvals obtained before proceeding further in the production cycle. Rejected material must be controlled.

211.111 (Time limitations on production) If required, time limitations will be placed on in-process steps.

211.113 (Control of microbiological contamination) Appropriate procedures are to be prepared for the control and prevention of microbiological contamination. The sterilization process must be validated.

211.115 (Reprocessing) Reprocessing of product is allowed providing there are written procedures covering the methods and QC unit review to be used.

SUBPART G PACKAGING AND LABELING CONTROL

211.122 (Materials examination and usage criteria) Labeling and packaging materials are to be received, identified, stored, sampled, and tested following detailed written procedures.

211.125 (Labeling issuance) Strict control shall be exercised over labeling for use in drug product labeling operations

211.130 (Packaging and labeling operations) There shall be written procedures designed to ensure that correct labels, labeling, and packaging materials are used for drug products. Special controls must be exercised over labeling to ensure that only the correct labels are issued to packaging for a specific product and that the quantities used are reconciled with the quantity issued.

211.132 (Tamper-resistant packaging requirements for over-the-counter (OTC) human drug products) Provides details of tamper-resistant packaging.

211.134 (Drug product inspection) Packaged and labeled products shall be inspected for correct labels.

211.137 (Expiration dating) Following appropriate stability studies at prescribed temperature conditions, products on the market shall bear an expiration date to ensure that they are used within their expected shelf life.

SUBPART H HOLDING AND DISTRIBUTION

211.142 (Warehousing procedures) Describes the requirements for warehousing holding product under appropriate conditions of light, temperature, and humidity.

211.150 (Distribution procedures) Written procedures describing product distribution shall be prepared

SUBPART I LABORATORY CONTROLS

211.160 (General requirements) Describes the general requirements for laboratory control mechanisms.

211.165 (Testing and release for distribution) Concerns written procedures in the form of specifications, standards, sampling plans, and test procedures that are used in a laboratory for controlling components and finished drug products. Acceptance criteria for sampling and approval shall be adequate to support release of product for distribution.

211.166 (Stability testing) There shall be a written testing program designed to assess the stability characteristics of drug products. The results of this testing shall be used in assigning appropriate storage conditions and expiration dates.

211.167 (Special testing requirements) Special testing requirements are given for sterile and/or pyrogen-free ophthalmic ointment and controlled-release dosage form products.

211.170 (Reserve samples) Reserve sample quantity and retention times are described.

211.173 (Laboratory animals) Animals used in any testing shall be maintained and controlled in a manner suitable for use.

211.176 (Penicillin contamination) Drug products cannot be marketed if, when tested by a prescribed procedure, found to contain any detectable levels of penicillin.

SUBPART J RECORDS AND REPORTS

211.180 (General requirements) Describes record retention time and availability for inspection.

211.182 (Equipment cleaning and use log) A written record of major equipment cleaning, maintenance, and use shall be included in major equipment logs.

211.184 (Component, drug product container, closure, and labeling records) Deals with the issues of the receipt, testing, and storage of components, drug product containers, and closures. Details the various records and documents that should be generated during the manufacture of drug products and that are to be available for review.

211.186 (Master production and control records) A master production record must be prepared for each drug product, describing all aspects of its manufacture, packaging, and control. Individual batch records are derived from this approved master.

211.188 (Batch production and control records) Calls for batch production and control records with information about the production and control of each batch

211.192 (Production record review) All drug product batch records shall be reviewed and approved by the QC unit (QA/QC) before the batch is released.

211.194 (Laboratory records) Complete records of any laboratory testing shall be maintained to include raw data, test procedures and results, equipment calibration, and stability testing.

211.196 (Distribution records) Distribution records include warehouse shipping logs, invoices, bills of lading, and all documents associated with distribution. These records should provide all the information necessary to trace lot distribution to facilitate product retrieval if necessary.

211.198 (Complaint files) Records of complaints received from consumers and professionals are to be maintained along with the report of their investigation and response.

SUBPART K RETURNED AND SALVAGED DRUG PRODUCTS

211.204 (Returned drug products) Records are to be maintained of drug products returned from distribution channels and the reason for their return. These data can be used as part of the total lot accountability, should the need arise, to trace its distribution and/or for its recall.

211.208 (Drug product salvaging) Drug products that have been stored improperly are not to be salvaged.

CHAPTER 52

Stability of Pharmaceutical Products

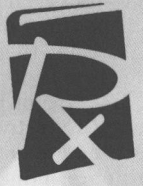

Patrick B O'Donnell, PhD

Allan D Bokser, PhD

Stability of a pharmaceutical product may be defined as the capability of a particular formulation, in a specific container/closure system, to remain within its physical, chemical, microbiological, therapeutic, and toxicological specifications. Assurances that the packaged product will be stable for its anticipated shelf life must come from an accumulation of valid data on the drug in its commercial package. These stability data involve selected parameters that, taken together, form the stability profile. Pharmaceutical products are expected to meet their specifications for identity, purity, quality, and strength throughout their defined storage period at specific storage conditions.

The stability of a pharmaceutical product is investigated throughout the various stages of the development process. The stability of a drug substance is first assessed in the preformulation stage. At this stage, pharmaceutical scientists determine the drug substance and its related salts stability/compatibility with various solvents, buffered solutions, and excipients considered for formulation development. Optimization of a stable formulation of a pharmaceutical product is built upon the information obtained from the preformulation stage and continues during the formulation development stages.

Typically, the first formulation development stage is the preparation of a "first in human" formulation which is often a non-elegant formulation optimized for short-term dose-ranging clinical studies. The second major formulation development stage occurs to support Phase II and early Phase III clinical studies. The pharmaceutical product developed at this stage is usually the prototype for the commercial product. Therefore, the pharmaceutical product will be formulated based in part on the stability information obtain from the previous formulations and must meet stability requirements for longer-term clinical studies. The final formulation development stage is for the commercial pharmaceutical product. In addition to building on the clinical requirements of the drug, the commercial pharmaceutical product must also incorporate the commercial or the final market image of the product, which includes the container closure system. The stability of this product must be demonstrated to the appropriate regulatory agencies in order to assign an expiration date for the product.

Once a pharmaceutical product has gained regulatory approval and is marketed, the pharmacist must understand the proper storage and handling of the drug. In some cases, a pharmacist may need to prepare stable compounded preparations from this product. It is the responsibility of the pharmacist, via the information of the manufacturer, to instruct the patient in the proper storage and handling of the drug product. The impact of a drug product with a poor stability profile could delay approval, affect the safety and efficacy of the drug, and/or cause product recall.

Much has been written about the development of a stable pharmaceutical product. Comprehensive treatments of all aspects of pharmaceutical product stability has been published by Lintner,[1] Connors et al,[2] and more recently Carstensen[3]. This chapter will outline the appropriate steps from preformulation to drug approval to assure that the pharmaceutical product developed is stable. Requirements for compounded products will also be discussed.

The USP defines the stability of a pharmaceutical product as "extent to which a product retains, within specified limits, and throughout its period of storage and use (ie, its shelf-life), the same properties and characteristics that it possessed at the time of its manufacture." There are five types of stability that must be considered for each drug.

Type of Stability	Conditions Maintained Throughout the Shelf-Life of the Drug Product
Chemical	Each active ingredient retains its chemical integrity and labeled potency, within the specified limits.
Physical	The original physical properties, including appearance, palatability, uniformity, dissolution, and suspendability are retained.
Microbiological	Sterility or resistance to microbial growth is retained according to the specified requirements. Antimicrobial agents that are present retain effectiveness within the specified limits.
Therapeutic	The therapeutic effect remains unchanged.
Toxicological	No significant increase in toxicity occurs.

Stability of a drug also can be defined as the time from the date of manufacture and packaging of the formulation until its chemical or biological activity is not less than a predetermined level of labeled potency and its physical characteristics have not changed appreciably or deleteriously. Although there are exceptions, 90% of labeled potency generally is recognized as the minimum acceptable potency level. Expiration dating is defined, therefore, as the time in which a drug product in a specific packaging configuration will remain stable when stored under recommended conditions.

An expiration date, which is expressed traditionally in terms of month and year, denotes the last day of the month. The expiration date should appear on the immediate container and the outer retail package. However, when single-dose containers are packaged in individual cartons, the expiration date may be placed on the individual carton instead of the immediate product container. If a dry product is to be reconstituted at the time of dispensing, expiration dates are assigned to both the dry mixture and the reconstituted product. Tamper-resistant packaging is to be used where applicable.

One type of time-related stability failure is a decrease in therapeutic activity of the preparation to below labeled content. A second type of stability failure is the appearance of a toxic substance, formed as a degradation product upon storage of the formulation. The numbers of published cases reflecting this second type are few. However, it is possible, though remote, for both types of stability failures to occur simultaneously within the same pharmaceutical product. Thus, the use of stability studies with the resulting application of expiration dating to pharmaceuticals is an attempt to predict the approximate time at which the probability of occurrence of a stability failure may reach an intolerable level. This estimate is subject to the usual Type 1 or alpha error (setting the expiration too early so that the product will be destroyed or recalled from the market appreciably earlier than actually is necessary) and the Type 2 or beta error (setting the date too late so that the failure occurs in an unacceptably large proportion of cases). Thus, it is obligatory that the manufacturer clearly and succinctly define the method for determining the degree of change in a formulation and the statistical approach to be used in making the shelf-life prediction. An intrinsic part of the statistical methodology must be the statements of value for the two types of error. For the safety of the patient a Type 1 error can be accepted, but not a Type 2 error.

REGULATORY REQUIREMENTS

Stability study requirements and expiration dating are covered in the Current Good Manufacturing Practices (cGMPs),[4] the USP,[5] and the FDA guidelines.[6]

GOOD MANUFACTURING PRACTICES—The GMPs[4] state that there shall be a written testing program designed to assess the stability characteristics of drug products. The results of such stability testing shall be used to determine appropriate storage conditions and expiration dating. The latter is to ensure that the pharmaceutical product meets applicable standards of identity, strength, quality, and purity at time of use. These regulations, which apply to both human and veterinary drugs, are updated periodically in light of current knowledge and technology.

COMPENDIA—The compendia also contain extensive stability and expiration dating information. Included are a discussion of stability considerations in dispensing practices and the responsibilities of both the pharmaceutical manufacturer and the dispensing pharmacist. It now is required that product labeling of official articles provide recommended storage conditions and an expiration date assigned to the specific formulation and package. Official storage conditions as defined by the USP 26[5] are as follows: *Cold* is any temperature not exceeding 8°C, and *refrigerator* is a cold place where the temperature is maintained thermostatically between 2 and 8°C. A *freezer* is a cold place maintained between −25 and −10°C. *Cool* is defined as any temperature between 8 and 15°C, and *room temperature* is that temperature prevailing in a working area. *Controlled room temperature* is that temperature maintained thermostatically between 20 and 25°C. *Warm* is any temperature between 30 and 40°C, while *excessive heat* is any heat above 40°C. Should freezing subject a product to a loss of potency or to destructive alteration of the dosage form, the container label should bear appropriate instructions to protect the product from freezing. When no specific storage instructions are given in a USP monograph, it is understood that the product's storage conditions shall include protection from moisture, freezing, and excessive heat.

As is noted above in USP 26, the definition of controlled room temperature was a "temperature maintained thermostatically between 20 and 25°C (68 and 77°F)." This definition was

established to harmonize with international drug standards efforts. The usual or customary temperature range is identified as 20 to 25°C, with the possibility of encountering excursions in the 15 to 30°C range and with the introduction the mean kinetic temperature (MKT).

The mean kinetic temperature is calculated using the following equation:

$$T_k = \left[\frac{\Delta H/R}{-In\left(\dfrac{e^{-\Delta H/RT_1} + e^{-\Delta H/RT_2} + \ldots + e^{-\Delta H/RT_{n-1}} + e^{-\Delta H/RT_n}}{n} \right)} \right]$$

in which T_k is the mean kinetic temperature; ΔH is the heat of activation, 83.144 kJ·mole^{-1}; R is the universal gas constant, 8.3144×10^{-3} kJ·mole^{-1}·degree^{-1}; T_1 is the value for the temperature (in degrees Kelvin [°K]) recorded during the first time period, T_2 is the value for the temperature recorded during the second time period, eg, second week; T_{n-1} is the value of the second to last time period, and T_n is the value for the temperature recorded during the nth time period. Typically, the time period is in days or weeks. The mean kinetic temperature determines the thermal exposure of a material. This allows an acceptable estimation to assess if a temperature excursion (or series of excursions) adversely affected a material.

FDA Guidelines provide recommendations for:

1. The design of stability studies to establish appropriate expiration dating periods and product storage requirements
2. The submission of stability information for investigational new drugs, biologicals, new drug applications, and biological product license applications

Thus, the guidelines represent a framework for the experimental design and data analysis as well as the type of documentation needed to meet regulatory requirements in the drug-development process.

Table 52-1. Stability Protocols

CONDITIONS	MINIMUM TIME PERIOD AT SUBMISSION
Long-term testing 25°C ± 2°C/60% ± 5% RH	12 mo
Accelerated testing 40°C ± 2°C/75% ± 5% RH	6 mo
Alternate testing[a] 30°C ± 2°C/65% ± 5% RH	12 mo

[a]Required if *significant change* occurs during 6-mo storage under conditions of accelerated testing.

Example Stability Pull Schedule for a Solid Oral Dose for Zone I and II

STORAGE CONDITIONS	DURATIONS (MONTHS)								
	0	1	3	6	9	12	18	24	36
25°C/60% RH	R*		X	X	X	X, Y	X	X	X
30°C/65% RH			O	O	O	O			
40°C/75% RH		X	X	X, Y					

*From Release testing if testing is within 30 days of stability set down.

R = Release Tests
    Appearance (visual)
    Identity
    Assay (HPLC)
    Impurities (HPLC)
    Dissolution (USP <711>)
    Moisture Content (Karl
      Fischer)
Uniformity of Dosage Unit
O = Pull and test only after
    40°C/75% is out of
    specification
    Appearance (visual)
    Assay (HPLC)
    Impurities (HPLC)
    Dissolution (USP <711>)

X = Tests at Every Stability Pull
    Appearance (visual)
    Assay (HPLC)
    Impurities (HPLC)
    Dissolution (USP <711>)

Y = Additional tests periodically
    performed
    Moisture Content (Karl
      Fischer)

FDA Guidelines, however, has been reevaluated and revised significantly in the last few years, with the aim of harmonizing the technical requirements for the registration of pharmaceuticals worldwide. The International Conference on Harmonization of Technical Requirements for Registration of Pharmaceuticals for Human Use (ICH) is a unique project that brought together regulatory authorities and experts from the pharmaceutical industry from three regions of the world; Europe, Japan, and the US. The first conference (ICH1) took place in November 1991 in Brussels, and the second conference (ICH2) in Orlando, FL, in October 1993. These conferences provided an open forum for discussion and resulted in the creation of an extensive set of guidelines dealing with the many aspects of safety, quality, and efficacy of medicinal products. The ICH Harmonized Tripartite Guideline provides a general indication on the requirements for *Stability Testing of New Drug Substances and Products.* The main thrust of the stability guideline centers around criteria for setting up stability protocols, shown in Table 52-1 and the example Stability Pull Schedule.

The guidelines were published in a draft form in the *Federal Register,* April 16, 1993. The final guidelines were published in 1994, with implementation of the guidelines occurring with Registration Applications after January 1, 1998. Revision 1 of the guidance was published in August 2001. Online computer can now access a complete listing of FDA publications and guidances. To view the publications, go to http://www.fda.gov/cder/guidance/index.htm.

PRODUCT STABILITY

Many factors affect the stability of a pharmaceutical product and include the stability of the active ingredient(s), the potential interaction between active and inactive ingredients, the manufacturing process, the dosage form, the container-liner-closure system, and the environmental conditions encountered during shipment, storage and handling, and length of time between manufacture and usage.

Classically, pharmaceutical product stability evaluations have been separated into studies of chemical (including biochemical) and physical stability of formulations. Realistically, there is no absolute division between these two arbitrary divisions. Physical factors, such as heat, light, and moisture, may initiate or accelerate chemical reactions, while every time a measurement is made on a chemical compound. Physical dimensions are included in the study.

In this treatment, physical and chemical stability are discussed along with those dosage form properties that can be measured and are useful in predicting shelf life. The effect of various physical and chemical phenomena of pharmaceuticals also is treated.

Knowledge of the physical stability of a formulation is very important for three primary reasons. First, a pharmaceutical product must appear fresh, elegant, and professional, for as long as it remains on the shelf. Any changes in physical appearance such as color fading or haziness can cause the patient or consumer to lose confidence in the product. Second, since some products are dispensed in multiple-dose containers, uniformity of dose content of the active ingredient over time must be ensured. A cloudy solution or a broken emulsion can lead to a non-uniform dosage pattern. Third, the active ingredient must be available to the patient throughout the expected shelf life of the preparation. A breakdown in the physical system can lead to non-availability or "dose dumping" of the medication to the patient. In the case of metered-dose inhaler pulmonary aerosols, particle aggregation may result in inadequate lung deposition of the medication.

The chemical causes of drug deterioration have been classified as incompatibility, oxidation, reduction, hydrolysis, racemization, and other mechanisms. In the latter category, decarboxylation, deterioration of hydrogen peroxide and hypochlorites, and the formation of precipitates have been included.

PHARMACEUTICAL DOSAGE FORMS

As the various pharmaceutical dosage forms present unique stability problems, they are discussed separately in the following section.

TABLETS—Stable tablets retain their original size, shape, weight, and color under normal handling and storage conditions throughout their shelf life. In addition, the *in vitro* availability of the active ingredients should not change appreciably with time.

Excessive powder or solid particles at the bottom of the container, cracks or chips on the face of a tablet, or appearance of crystals on the surface of tablets or on container walls are indications of physical instability of uncoated tablets. Hence, the effect of mild, uniform, and reproducible shaking and tumbling of tablets should be studied. The recommended test for such studies is the determination of tablet friability as described in the USP. Tablet Friability <1216> describes the recommended apparatus and the test procedure. After visual observation of the tablets for chips, cracks, and splits, the intact tablets are sorted and weighed to determine the amount of material worn away by abrasion. In general a maximum weight loss of not more than 1% of the weight of the tablets being tested is considered acceptable for most products. The results of these tests are comparative rather than absolute and should be correlated with actual stress experience. Packaged tablets also should be subjected to cross-country shipping tests as well as to various *drop tests.*

Tablet hardness (or resistance to crushing or fracturing) can be assessed by commercially available hardness testers. As results will vary with the specific make of the test apparatus used, direct comparison of results obtained on different instruments may not necessarily be made. Thus, the same instrument should be used consistently throughout a particular study.

Color stability of tablets can be followed by an appropriate colorimeter or reflectometer with heat, sunlight, and intense artificial light employed to accelerate the color deterioration. Caution must be used in interpreting the elevated temperature data, as the mechanism for degradation at that temperature may differ from that at a lower temperature. It is not always proper to assume that the same changes will occur at elevated temperatures as will be evidenced later at room temperature. Cracks, mottling, or tackiness of the coating indicates evidence of instability of coated tablets.

For tablets containing the more insoluble active ingredients, the results of dissolution tests are more meaningful than disintegration results for making bioavailability predictions. Dissolution-rate tests should be run in an appropriate medium such as artificial gastric and/or intestinal fluid at 37°. When no significant change (such as a change in the polymorphic form of the crystal) has occurred, an unaltered dissolution-rate profile of a tablet formulation usually indicates constant *in vivo* availability.

Uniformity of weight, odor, texture, drug and moisture contents, and humidity effect also are studied during a tablet stability test.

GELATIN CAPSULES—Hard gelatin capsules are the type used by pharmaceutical manufacturers in the production of the majority of their capsule products. The pharmacist in the extemporaneous compounding of prescriptions may also use hard gelatin capsules. Soft gelatin capsules are prepared from shells of gelatin to which glycerin or a polyhydric alcohol such as sorbitol has been added to render the gelatin elastic or plastic-like. Gelatin is stable in air when dry but is subject to microbial decomposition when it becomes moist or when it is maintained in aqueous solution. Normally hard gelatin capsules contain between 13% and 16% moisture. If stored in a high humidity environment capsule shells may soften, stick together, or become distorted and lose their shape. On the other hand, in an environment of extreme dryness gelatin capsules may harden and crack under slight pressure. Gelatin capsules should be protected from sources of microbial contamination.

Encapsulated products, like all other dosage forms, must be packaged properly.

Because moisture may be absorbed or released by gelatin capsules depending on the environmental conditions, capsules offer little physical protection to hygroscopic or deliquescent materials enclosed within a capsule when stored in an area of high humidity. It is not uncommon to find capsules packaged in containers along with a packet of desiccant material as a precautionary measure.

Both hard and soft gelatin capsules exposed to excessive heat and moisture may exhibit delayed or incomplete dissolution due to cross-linking of the gelatin in the capsule shell. The cross-linking of gelatin capsules is an irreversible chemical reaction. Cross-linking may also occur in capsules that are exposed to aldehydes and peroxides. Although cross-linked capsules may fail dissolution due to pellicle formation, digestive enzymes will dissolve the capsules. For hard or soft gelatin capsules that do not conform to the dissolution specification, the dissolution test may be repeated with the addition of enzymes. Where water or a medium with a pH less than 6.8 is specified as the medium in the individual monograph, the same medium specified may be used with the addition of purified pepsin that results in an activity of 750,000 units or less per 1000 mL. For media with a pH of 6.8 or greater, pancreatin can be added to produce not more than 1750 USP units of protease activity per 1000 mL.

SUSPENSIONS—A stable suspension can be redispersed homogeneously with moderate shaking and can be poured easily throughout its shelf life, with neither the particle-size distribution, the crystal form, nor the physiological availability of the suspended active ingredient changing appreciably with time.

Most stable pharmaceutical suspensions are flocculated; that is, the suspended particles are bonded together physically to form a loose, semi rigid structure. The particles are said to uphold each other while exerting no significant force on the liquid. Sedimented particles of a flocculated suspension can be redispersed easily at any time with only moderate shaking.

In nonflocculated suspensions, the particles remain as individuals unaffected by neighboring particles and are affected only by the suspension vehicle. These particles, which are smaller and lighter, settle slowly, but once they have settled, often form a hard, difficult-to-disperse sediment. Nonflocculated suspensions can be made acceptable by decreasing the particle size of the suspended material or by increasing the density and viscosity of the vehicle, thus reducing the possibility of settling.

When studying the stability of a suspension, first determine with a differential manometer if the suspension is flocculated. If the suspension is flocculated, the liquid will travel the same distance in the two side arms. With nonflocculated suspensions, the hydrostatic pressures in the two arms are unequal; hence, the liquids will be at different levels.

The history of settling of the particles of a suspension may be followed by a Brookfield viscometer fitted with a Helipath attachment. This instrument consists of a rotating T-bar spindle that descends slowly into the suspension as it rotates. The dial reading on the viscometer is a measure of the resistance that the spindle encounters at various levels of the sedimented suspension. This test must be run only on fresh, undisturbed samples.

An electronic particle counter and sizer, such as a Coulter counter, or a microscope may be used to determine changes in particle-size distribution. Crystal form alterations may be detected by microscopic, near-IR or Raman examination and, when suspected, must be confirmed by x-ray powder diffraction.

All suspensions should be subjected to cycling temperature conditions to determine the tendency for crystal growth to occur within the suspension. Shipping tests, ie, transporting bottles across the country by rail or truck are also used to study the stability of suspensions.

SOLUTIONS—A stable solution retains its original clarity, color, and odor throughout its shelf life. Retention of clarity of a solution is a main concern of a physical stability program. As visual observation alone under ordinary light is a poor test of clarity, a microscope light should be projected through a diaphragm into the solution. Undissolved particles will scatter the light, and the solution will appear hazy. While the Coulter counter also can be used, light-scattering instruments are the most sensitive means of following solution clarity.

Solutions should remain clear over a relatively wide temperature range such as 4 to 47°C. At the lower range an ingredient may precipitate due to its lower solubility at that temperature, while at the higher temperature the flaking of particles from the glass containers or rubber closures may destroy homogeneity. Thus, solutions should be subjected to cycling temperature conditions.

The stability program for solutions also should include a study of pH changes, especially when the active ingredients are soluble salts of insoluble acids or bases. Among other tests are observations for changes in odor, appearance, color, taste, light-stability, redispersibility, suspendibility, pourability, viscosity, isotonicity, gas evolution, microbial stability, specific gravity, surface tension, and pyrogen content, in the case of parenteral products.

When solutions are filtered, the filter medium may absorb some of the ingredients from the solution. Thus, the same type of filter should be used for preparing the stability samples as will be used to prepare the production-size batches.

For dry-packaged formulations reconstituted prior to use, the visual appearance should be observed on both the original dry material and on the reconstituted preparation. The color and odor of the cake, the color and odor of the solution, the moisture content of the cake, and the rate of reconstitution should be followed as a part of its stability profile.

EMULSIONS—A stable emulsion can be redispersed homogeneously to its original state with moderate shaking and can be poured at any stage of its shelf life. Although most of the important pharmaceutical emulsions are of the oil in water (O/W) type, many stability test methods can be applied to either an O/W or water in oil (W/O) emulsion.

Two simple tests are used to screen emulsion formulations. First, heating to 50 to 70°C and observing its gross physical stability either visually or by turbidimetric measurements can determine the stability of an emulsion. Usually the emulsion that is the most stable to heat is the one most stable at room temperature. However, this may not be true always, because an emulsion at 60°C may not be the same as it is at room temperature. Second, the stability of the emulsion can be estimated by the *coalescence time* test. Although this is only a rough quantitative test, it is useful for detecting gross differences in emulsion stability at room temperature.

Emulsions also should be subjected to refrigeration temperatures. An emulsion stable at room temperature has been found to be unstable at 4°C. It was reasoned that an oil-soluble emulsifier precipitated at the lower temperature and disrupted the system. An emulsion chilled to the extent that the aqueous base crystallizes is damaged irreversibly.

The ultracentrifuge also is used to determine emulsion stability. When the amount of separated oil is plotted against the time of centrifugation, a plateau curve is obtained. A linear graph results when the oil flotation (creaming) rate is plotted versus the square of the number of centrifuge revolutions per minute. The flotation rate is represented by the slope of the line resulting when the log distance of emulsion-water boundary from the rotor center is plotted against time for each revolution per minute.

For stability studies, two batches of an emulsion should be made at one time on two different sizes of equipment. One should be a bench-size lot and the other a larger, preferably production-size, batch. Different types of homogenizers produce different results, and different sizes of the same kind of homogenizer can yield emulsions with different characteristics.

OINTMENTS—Ointments have been defined as high-viscosity suspensions of active ingredients in a non-reacting vehicle. A stable ointment is one that retains its homogeneity throughout its shelf-life period. The main stability problems observed in ointments are *bleeding* and changes in consistency due to aging or changes in temperature. When fluid components such as mineral oil separate at the top of an ointment, the phenomenon is known as *bleeding* and can be observed visually. Unfortunately, as there is no known way to accelerate this event, the tendency to *bleed* cannot be predicted.

An ointment that is too soft is messy to use, while one that is very stiff is difficult to extrude and apply. Hence, it is important to be able to define quantitatively the consistency of an ointment. This may be done with a penetrometer, an apparatus that allows a pointed weight to penetrate into the sample under a measurable force. The depth of the penetration is a measure of the consistency of an ointment. Consistency also can be measured by the Helipath attachment to a high-viscosity viscometer or by a Burrell Severs rheometer. In the latter instrument, the ointment is loaded into a cylinder and extruded with a measured force. The amount extruded is a measure of the consistency of the ointment.

Ointments have a considerable degree of structure that requires a minimum of 48 hours to develop after preparation. As rheological data on a freshly made ointment may be erroneous, such tests should be performed only after the ointment has achieved equilibrium. Slight changes in temperature (1 or 2°C) can affect the consistency of an ointment greatly; hence, rheological studies on ointments must be performed only at constant and controlled temperatures.

Among the other tests performed during the stability study of an ointment are a check of visual appearance, color, odor, viscosity, softening range, consistency, homogeneity, particle-size distribution, and sterility. Undissolved components of an ointment may change in crystal form or in size with time. Microscopic examination or an x-ray diffraction measurement may be used to monitor these parameters.

In some instances it is necessary to use an ointment base that is less than ideal, to achieve the required stability. For example, drugs that hydrolyze rapidly are more stable in a hydrocarbon base than in a base containing water, even though they may be more effective in the latter.

TRANSDERMAL PATCHES—A typical transdermal patch consists of a protective backing, a matrix containing active drug, an adhesive that allows the patch to adhere to the skin, and a release liner to protect the skin adhering adhesive. Therefore, the transdermal patch must deliver drug as labeled, adhere properly to both the backing and to the patient's skin. In addition, the transdermal patch must be pharmaceutically elegant through the shelf life of the product. For a transdermal patch, this means that the release line peels easily with minimal transfer of adhesive onto the release liner and that the adhesive does not ooze from the sides of the patch. Therefore, the typical stability related tests for transdermal patches are, appearance, assay, impurities, drug release USP<724> and, backing peel force.

METERED-DOSE AEROSOLS DRUG PRODUCTS—A metered dose inhalation product consists of an aerosol can containing a propellant, a drug and a mouthpiece used to present an aerosolized drug to the patient. There are many drug contact components in a metered-dose inhalation product. Therefore, the drug may be in contact with materials that could allow plasticizer leach into the drug. The typical stability related tests for metered-dose aerosols include appearance, assay, impurities, plume geometry, emitted dose, particle size distribution of the emitted dose, and number of doses per unit. In addition, stability studies on leachables may be required. Shelf life of metered-dose aerosols drug products may also be dependent on the orientation that the drug product is stored. Typically most canisters type product are tested at least in the upright orientation.

DRY-POWDERED INHALATION PRODUCTS—A dry-powdered inhalation product consists of drug with excipients delivered in a dry powdered form. The delivery system for a dry-powdered inhalation product may be a separate device or integrated with the active. A dry-powdered dosage must reproducibly deliver a specific amount of drug at a particle size that can be deposited into the lungs. Particles too large will get trapped in the throats and particles too small will just be carried out of the lungs on the next expiration. The typical stability related tests for dry powder inhalation products include appearance, assay, impurities, emitted dose, particle size distribution of the emitted dose, and water content.

NASAL INHALATION PRODUCTS—A nasal inhalation product consists of drug with excipients delivered from a delivery system. The delivery system for a nasal inhalation product may be a separate device or integrated with the active. A nasal inhalation product must reproducibly deliver a specific amount of drug at a particle size and plume that can be deposited into the nasal membrane. Particles too large will not be absorbed into nasal membrane or run out of the nose; and poor spray pattern will deposit the drug ineffective in the nasal cavity. The typical stability related tests for nasal inhalation products include appearance, assay, impurities, spray content uniformity, particle (droplet) size distribution of the emitted dose, spray pattern or /and plume geometry, leachables, weight loss and preservative content. Sterility and microbial testing may be required periodically for stability testing.

INCOMPATIBILITY

Typically, physicochemical stability is assessed at the preformulation stage of development. A drug substance candidate is treated with acid, base, heat, light, and oxidative conditions to assess its inherit chemical stability. Binary mixtures of the drug substance with individual excipients are also investigated at the preformulation stage. These tests are performed to determine the drug substance sensitivity to degrade or react with common pharmaceutical excipients. The most common reactions observed for drug substances from these tests include: hydrolysis, epimerization (racemization), decarboxylation, dehydration, oxidation, polymerization, photochemical decomposition, and addition. All drug substances have the potential to degrade by at least one of the reactions mentioned above. With an understanding of the stability/reactivity of a drug substance in the preformulation stage, it is possible to formulate the drug product to minimize drug decomposition. Numerous examples are described in other sections of this book, and the literature is replete with illustrations.

While undesirable reactions between two or more drugs are said to result in a *physical, chemical,* or *therapeutic* incompatibility, physical incompatibility is somewhat of a misnomer. It has been defined as a physical or chemical interaction between two or more ingredients that leads to a visibly recognizable change. The latter may be in the form of a gross precipitate, haze, or color change.

On the other hand, a chemical incompatibility is classified as a reaction in which a visible change is not necessarily observed. Since there is no visible evidence of deterioration, this type of incompatibility requires trained, knowledgeable personnel to recognize it.

A therapeutic incompatibility has been defined as an undesirable pharmacological interaction between two or more ingredients that leads to

1. Potentiation of the therapeutic effects of the ingredients
2. Destruction of the effectiveness of one or more of the ingredients
3. Occurrence of a toxic manifestation within the patient.

REACTION KINETICS

An understanding of reaction kinetics is important in determining the shelf life of a product.

CHEMICAL REACTIONS

The most frequently encountered chemical reactions, which may occur within a pharmaceutical product, are described below.

OXIDATION-REDUCTION—Oxidation is a prime cause of product instability, and often, but not always, the addition of oxygen or the removal of hydrogen is involved. When molecular oxygen is involved, the reaction is known as auto-oxidation because it occurs spontaneously, though slowly, at room temperature.

Oxidation, or the loss of electrons from an atom, frequently involves free radicals and subsequent chain reactions. Only a very small amount of oxygen is required to initiate a chain reaction. In practice, it is easy to remove most of the oxygen from a container, but very difficult to remove it all. Hence, nitrogen and carbon dioxide frequently are used to displace the headspace air in pharmaceutical containers to help minimize deterioration by oxidation.

As an oxidation reaction is complicated, it is difficult to perform a kinetic study on oxidative processes within a general stability program. The redox potential, which is constant and relatively easy to determine, can, however, provide valuable predictive information. In many oxidative reactions, the rate is proportional to the concentration of the oxidizing species but may be independent of the concentration of the oxygen present. The rate is influenced by temperature, radiation, and the presence of a catalyst. An increase in temperature leads to an acceleration in the rate of oxidation. If the storage temperature of a preparation can be reduced to 0 to 5°C, usually it can be assumed that the rate of oxidation will be at least halved.

The molecular structures most likely to oxidize are those with a hydroxyl group directly bonded to an aromatic ring (eg, phenol derivatives such as catecholamines and morphine), conjugated dienes (eg, vitamin A and unsaturated free fatty acids), heterocyclic aromatic rings, nitroso and nitrite derivatives, and aldehydes (eg, flavorings). Products of oxidation usually lack therapeutic activity. Visual identification of oxidation, for example, the change from colorless epinephrine to its amber colored products, may not be visible in some dilutions or to some eyes.

Oxidation is catalyzed by pH values that are higher than optimum, polyvalent heavy metal ions (eg, copper and iron), and exposure to oxygen and UV illumination. The latter two causes of oxidation justify the use of antioxidant chemicals, nitrogen atmospheres during ampul and vial filling, opaque external packaging, and transparent amber glass or plastic containers.

Trace amounts of heavy metals such as cupric, chromic, ferrous, or ferric ions may catalyze oxidation reactions. As little as 0.2 mg of copper ion per liter considerably reduces the stability of penicillin. Similar examples include the deterioration of epinephrine, phenylephrine, lincomycin, isoprenaline, and procaine hydrochloride. Adding chelating agents to water to sequester heavy metals and working in special manufacturing equipment (eg, glass) are some means used to reduce the influence of heavy metals on a formulation. Parenteral formulations should not come in contact with heavy metal ions during their manufacture, packaging, or storage.

Hydronium and hydroxyl ions catalyze oxidative reactions. The rate of decomposition for epinephrine, for example, is more rapid in a neutral or alkaline solution with maximum stability (minimum oxidative decomposition) at pH 3.4. There is a pH range for maximum stability for any antibiotic and vitamin preparation, which usually can be achieved by adding an acid, alkali, or buffer.

Oxidation may be inhibited by the use of antioxidants, called negative catalysts. They are very effective in stabilizing pharmaceutical products undergoing a free-radical-mediated chain reaction. These substances, which are easily oxidizable, act by possessing lower oxidation potentials than the active ingredient. Thus, they undergo preferential degradation or act as chain inhibitors of free radicals by providing an electron and receiving the excess energy possessed by the activated molecule.

The ideal antioxidant should be stable and effective over a wide pH range, soluble in its oxidized form, colorless, nontoxic, nonvolatile, nonirritating, effective in low concentrations, thermostable, and compatible with the container-closure system and formulation ingredients.

The commonly used antioxidants for aqueous systems include sodium sulfite, sodium metabisulfite, sodium bisulfite, sodium thiosulfate, and ascorbic acid. For oil systems, ascorbyl palmitate, hydroquinone, propyl gallate, nordihydroguaiaretic acid, butylated hydroxytoluene, butylated hydroxyanisole, and alpha-tocopherol are employed.

Synergists, which increase the activity of antioxidants, are generally organic compounds that complex small amounts of heavy metal ions. These include the ethylenediamine tetraacetic acid (EDTA) derivatives, dihydroethylglycine, and citric, tartaric, gluconic, and saccharic acids. EDTA has been used to stabilize ascorbic acid, oxytetracycline, penicillin, epinephrine, and prednisolone.

Reduction reactions are much less common than oxidative processes in pharmaceutical practice. Examples include the reduction of gold, silver, or mercury salts by light to form the corresponding free metal.

HYDROLYSIS—Drugs containing esters (eg, cocaine, physostigmine, aspirin, tetracaine, procaine and methyldopa), amides (eg, dibucaine), imides (eg, amobarbital), imines (eg, diazepam) and lactam (eg, penicillins, cephalosporins) functional groups are among those prone to hydrolysis.

Hydrolysis reactions are often pH dependent and are catalyzed by either hydronium ion or hydroxide ions (specific-acid or specific-base catalysis, respectively). Hydrolysis reactions can also be catalyzed by either a Brønsted acid or a Brønsted base (general-acid or general-base catalysis, respectively). Sources of Brønsted acid or base include buffers and some excipients. Sometimes, it is necessary to compromise between the optimum pH for stability and that for pharmacological activity. For example, several local anesthetics are most stable at a distinctly acid pH, whereas for maximum activity they should be neutral or slightly alkaline. Small amounts of acids, alkalines, or buffers are used to adjust the pH of a formulation. Buffers are used when small changes in pH are likely to cause major degradation of the active ingredient.

Obviously, the amount of water present can have a profound effect on the rate of a hydrolysis reaction. When the reaction takes place fairly rapidly in water, other solvents sometimes can be substituted. For example, barbiturates are much more stable at room temperature in propylene glycol–water than in water alone.

Modification of chemical structure may be used to retard hydrolysis. In general, as it is only the fraction of the drug in solution that hydrolyzes, a compound may be stabilized by reducing its solubility. This can be done by adding various substituents to the alkyl or acyl chain of aliphatic or aromatic esters or to the ring of an aromatic ester. In some cases less-soluble salts or esters of the parent compound have been found to aid product stability. Steric and polar complexation have also been employed to alter the rate of hydrolysis. Caffeine reduces the rate of hydrolysis and thus promotes stability by complexation with local anesthetics such as benzocaine, procaine, or tetracaine.

Esters and β-lactams are the chemical bonds that are most likely to hydrolyze in the presence of water. For example, the acetyl ester in aspirin is hydrolyzed to acetic acid and salicylic acid in the presence of moisture, but in a dry environment the hydrolysis of aspirin is negligible. The aspirin hydrolysis rate increases in direct proportion to the water vapor pressure in an environment.

The amide bond also hydrolyzes, though generally at a slower rate than comparable esters. For example, procaine (an ester) will hydrolyze upon autoclaving, but procainamide will not. The amide or peptide bond in peptides and proteins varies in the labiality to hydrolysis. The lactam and azomethine (or imine) bonds in benzodiazepines are also labile to hydrolysis. The major chemical accelerators or catalysts of hydrolysis are adverse pH and specific chemicals (eg, dextrose and copper in the case of ampicillin hydrolysis).

The rate of hydrolysis depends on the temperature and the pH of the solution. A much-quoted estimation is that for each 10°C rise in storage temperature, the rate of reaction doubles or triples. As this is an empiricism, it is not always applicable.

When hydrolysis occurs, the concentration of the active ingredient decreases while the concentration of the decomposition products increases. The effect of this change on the rate of the reaction depends on the order of the reaction. With zero-order reactions the rate of decomposition is independent of concentration of the ingredient. Although dilute solutions decompose at the same absolute rate as more concentrated solutions, the more dilute the solution, the greater the proportion of active ingredient destroyed in a given time; ie, the percentage of decomposition is greater in more dilute solutions. Increasing the concentration of an active ingredient that is hydrolyzing by zero-order kinetics will slow the percentage decomposition.

With first-order reactions, which occur frequently in the hydrolysis of drugs, the rate of change is directly proportional to the concentration of the reactive substance. Thus, changes in the concentration of the active ingredient have no influence on the percentage decomposition.

The degradation of many drugs in solution accelerates or decelerates exponentially as the pH is decreased or increased over a specific range of pH values. Improper pH ranks with exposure to elevated temperature as a factor most likely to cause a clinically significant loss of drug, resulting from hydrolysis and oxidation reactions. A drug solution or suspension, for example, may be stable for days, weeks, or even years in its original formulation, but when mixed with another liquid that changes the pH, it degrades in minutes or days. It is possible that a pH change of only one unit (eg, from 4 to 3 or 8 to 9) could decrease drug stability by a factor of ten or greater.

A pH-buffer system, which is usually a weak acid or base and its salt, is a common excipient used in liquid preparations to maintain the pH in a range that minimizes the drug degradation rate. The pH of drug solutions may also be either buffered or adjusted to achieve drug solubility. For example, pH in relation to pKa controls the fractions of the usually more soluble ionized and less soluble nonionized species of weak organic electrolytes.

INTERIONIC (ION N+ −ION N−) COMPATIBILITY— The compatibility or solubility of oppositely charged ions depends mainly on the number of charges per ion and the molecular size of the ions. In general, polyvalent ions of opposite charge are more likely to be incompatible. Thus, an incompatibility is likely to occur upon the addition of a large ion with a charge opposite to that of the drug.

As many hydrolytic reactions are catalyzed by both hydronium and hydroxyl ions, pH is an important factor in determining the rate of a reaction. The pH range of minimum decomposition (or maximum stability) depends on the ion having the greatest effect on the reaction. If the minimum occurs at about pH 7, the two ions are of equal effect. A shift of the minimum toward the acid side indicates that the hydroxyl ion has the stronger catalytic effect and *vice versa* in the case of a shift toward the alkaline side. In general, hydroxyl ions have the stronger effect. Thus, the minimum is often found between pH 3 and 4. The influence of pH on the physical stability of two-phase systems, especially emulsions, is also important. For example, intravenous fat emulsion is destabilized by acidic pH.

DECARBOXYLATION—Pyrolytic solid-state degradation through decarboxylation usually is not encountered in pharmacy, as relatively high heats of activation (25 to 30 kcal) are required for the reaction. However, solid p-aminosalicylic acid undergoes pyrolytic degradation to m-aminophenol and carbon dioxide. The reaction, which follows first-order kinetics, is highly pH-dependent and is catalyzed by hydronium ions. The decarboxylation of p-aminobenzoic acid occurs only at extremely low pH values and at high temperatures.

Some dissolved carboxylic acids, such as p-aminosalicylic acid, lose carbon dioxide from the carboxyl group when heated. The resulting product has reduced pharmacological potency. β-Keto decarboxylation can occur in some solid antibiotics that have a carbonyl group on the β-carbon of a carboxylic acid or a carboxylate anion. Such decarboxylations will occur in the following antibiotics: carbenicillin sodium, carbenicillin free acid, ticarcillin sodium, and ticarcillin free acid.

RACEMIZATION—Racemization, or the action or process of changing from an optically active compound into a racemic compound or an optically inactive mixture of corresponding R (*rectus*) and S (*sinister*) forms, is a major consideration in pharmaceutical stability. Optical activity of a compound may be monitored by polarimetry and reported in terms of specific rotation. Chiral HPLC has been used in addition to polarimetry to confirm the enantiomeric purity of a sample.

In general, racemization follows first-order kinetics and depends on temperature, solvent, catalyst, and the presence or absence of light. Racemization appears to depend on the functional group bound to the asymmetric carbon atom, with aromatic groups tending to accelerate the process.

EPIMERIZATION—Members of the tetracycline family are most likely to incur epimerization. This reaction occurs rapidly when the dissolved drug is exposed to a pH of an intermediate range (higher than 3), and it results in the steric rearrangement of the dimethylamino group. The epimer of tetracycline, epitetracycline, has little or no antibacterial activity.

PHOTOCHEMICAL REACTIONS

Photolytic degradation can be an important limiting factor in the stability of pharmaceuticals. A drug can be affected chemically by radiation of a particular wavelength only if it absorbs radiation at that wavelength and the energy exceeds a threshold. Ultraviolet radiation, which has a high energy level, is the cause of many degradation reactions. Exposure to, primarily, UV illumination may cause oxidation (photo-oxidation) and scission (photolysis) of covalent bonds. Nifedipine, nitroprusside, riboflavin, and phenothiazines are very labile to photo-oxidation. In susceptible compounds, photochemical energy creates free radical intermediates, which can perpetuate chain reactions.

If the absorbing molecule reacts, the reaction is said to be photochemical in nature. When the absorbing molecules do not participate directly in the reaction, but pass their energy to other reacting molecules, the absorbing substance is said to be a photosensitizer.

As many variables may be involved in a photochemical reaction, the kinetics can be quite complex. The intensity and wavelength of the light and the size, shape, composition, and color of the container may affect the velocity of the reaction.

The photodegradation of chlorpromazine through a semiquinone free-radical intermediate follows zero-order kinetics. On the other hand, alcoholic solutions of hydrocortisone, prednisolone, and methylprednisolone degrade by reactions following first-order kinetics.

Colored-glass containers most commonly are used to protect light-sensitive formulations. Yellow-green glass gives the best protection in the ultraviolet region, while amber confers considerable protection from ultraviolet radiation but little from infrared. Riboflavin is best protected by a stabilizer that has a hydroxyl group attached to or near the aromatic ring. The photodegradation of sulfacetamide solutions may be inhibited by an antioxidant such as sodium thiosulfate or metabisulfite.

A systematic approach to photostability testing is recommended covering, as appropriate, studies such as tests on the drug substance, tests on the exposed drug product outside of the immediate pack; and if necessary, tests on the drug product in the immediate pack. ICH Q1B discusses the minimum requirements for assessing photostability. Drug substance is first assessed by exposing sample powder having a depth of not more than 3 mm to an overall illumination of not less than 1.2 million lux hours and an integrated near ultraviolet energy of not less than 200 watt hours/square meter. If the drug substance shows sensitivity to photodegrations, then the drug product will need to be tested as well. The testing of drug product uses the same light exposure that was used to test drug substance. The drug product should be tested directly exposed to light and in its container closure system.

ULTRASONIC ENERGY

Ultrasonic energy, which consists of vibrations and waves with frequencies greater than 20,000 Hz, promotes the formation of free radicals and alters drug molecules. Changes in prednisolone, prednisone acetate, or deoxycorticosterone acetate suspensions in an ultrasonic field have been observed spectrometrically in the side chain at C-17 and in the oxo group of the A ring. With sodium alginate, in an ultrasonic field, it has been reported that above a minimum power output, degradation increased linearly with increased power.

IONIZING RADIATION

Ionizing radiation, particularly gamma rays, has been used for the sterilization of certain pharmaceutical products. At the usual sterilizing dose, 2.5 mRad, it seldom causes appreciable chemical degradation. In general, formulations that are in the solid or frozen state are more resistant to degradation from ionizing radiation than those in liquid form. For example, many of the vitamins are little affected by irradiation in the solid state but are decomposed appreciably in solution. On the other hand, both the liquid- and solid-state forms of atropine sulfate are affected seriously by radiation.

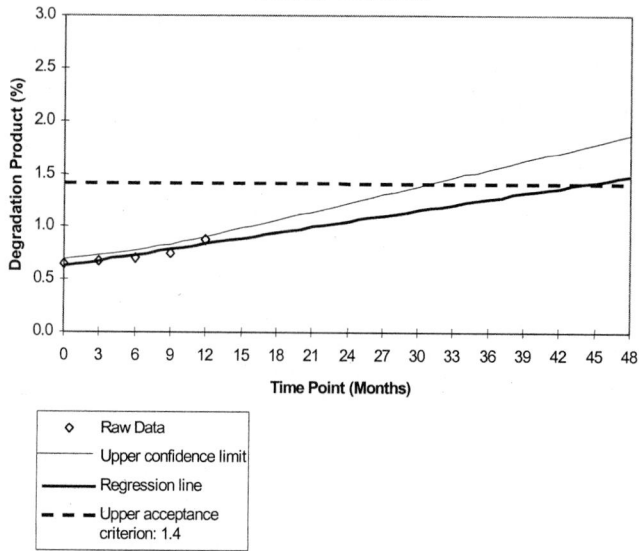

Shelf Life Estimation with Upper Acceptance Criterion Based on a Degradation Product at 25C/60%RH

Figure 52-2. Typical one-sided shelf-life estimation plot.

PREDICTING SHELF LIFE

ICH Recommended Evaluation

The shelf life of a commercial drug product must be determined in the commercial container closure at the defined storage conditions. ICH requires at least 12 months stability data at the time of NDA submission. Most products require at least 24 months to be commercially viable. The ICH Q1E recommends how the 12 months data may be used to predict long-term stability. Figures 52-1 and 52-2 show trending graphs with double-sided and single-sided 95% confidence limits plots, respectively.

Figure 52-1 shows a plot of 12 months of assay (potency) results versus time. The acceptance criteria for this test have a lower and an upper limit of 95% and 105%, respectively. The extrapolated line from this data set intersects the lower acceptance limit at about 35 months. However, there is always statistical uncertainty when extrapolating a data set. The 95% confidence limit is used to take this uncertainty into account. The lower 95% confidence intersects the lower acceptance limit at about 29 months. Therefore, this product would be assessed an expiration date of 29 months.

Figure 52-2 shows a plot of 12 months of degradation product results. In this case, the acceptance criterion is an upper limit of not more than 1.4%. The extrapolated line from this data set intersects the acceptance limit at about 44 months. The upper 95% confidence limit curve intersects the acceptance limit at about 30 months. Therefore, this product would be assessed an expiration date of 30 months. The expiration of a product is the time where the confidence line intersects with the acceptance limit. Trend analysis of data need only be performed on test data that shows a change related to time.

Approximations in Assessing Product Stability—Estimation of Temperature Effect

In early development, a shelf life prediction of a clinical material, especially a Phase I material, may be based on a very limited amount of sample and limited amount of time to make the evaluation. One way to estimate long-term storage for a material is by extrapolating data from studies performed at elevated conditions. An understanding of potential activation energy is needed to estimate long-term stability. Many may have heard

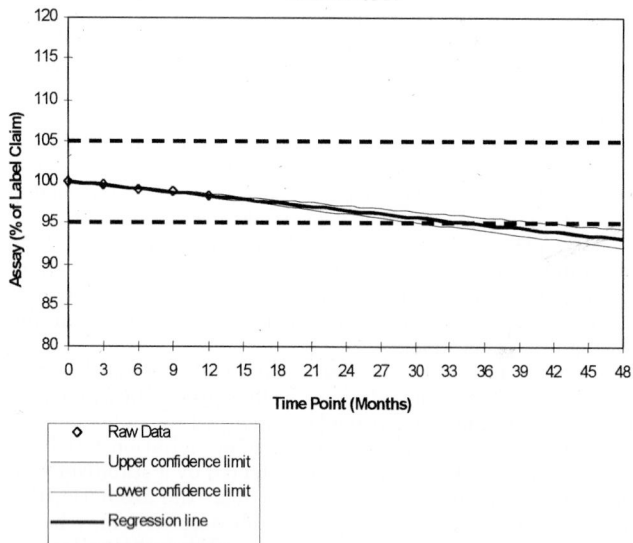

Shelf Life Estimation with Upper and Lower Acceptance Criteria Based on Assay at 25C/60%RH

Figure 52-1. Typical two-sided shelf-life estimation plot.

of the estimate that for every 10°C decrease in storage temperature the shelf-life doubles. This is only true, however, if the activation energy of the reaction(s) that causes degradation is 15 kcal/moles. The activation energy, E_a, for many chemical processes related to the degradation of a drug substance/product is typically within the range of 10 to 25 kcal/moles.

The equation below shows a way of calculating the $Q_{\Delta T}$ value that may be used to estimate the affect of temperature on shelf life.

$$Q_{\Delta T} = \exp\left[\frac{E_a}{R}\left(\frac{\Delta T}{T + \Delta T(T)}\right)\right] \quad (1)$$

where, $Q_{\Delta T}$ is a factor (multiplier/divisor) used to estimate the change in the reaction rate constant with change in temperature, ΔT. E_a is the activation energy established for a reaction

An approximation for the change in reaction rate constants due to the temperature effects are shown in the table below.

Ea (kcal/mole)	Q_5 (25 to 30°C)	Q_{10} (25 to 35°C)	Q_{15} (25 to 40°C)
10	1.32	1.73	2.24
15	1.52	2.27	3.36
20	1.75	2.99	5.04
25	2.01	3.93	7.55

Therefore, the old rule of thumb that a reaction rate doubles with every 10°C is only true if the reaction has an activation energy between 10 to 15 kcal/mole (Q_{10} = 1.73 and 2.27, respectively). Q_{15} is useful for understanding the relationship of ICH accelerated temperature of 40°C has with controlled room temperature at 25°C. Materials made and packaged for clinical studies are usually tested at an accelerated condition in order to predict that the packaged material will be stable for the duration of the clinical study. A material stable for one month at accelerated temperature (40°C) supports that the material stored at room temperature should be stable for at least 3 months. This true only when the activation energy of the degradation process is about 15 kcal/mole (Q_{15} factor = 3.36) [In other words, a reaction at 40°C should be 3.36 times faster than the same reaction at 25°C; or the reaction will take 3.36 times longer at 25°C than at 40°C)].

The technique of estimating the shelf life of a formulation from its accumulated stability data has evolved from examining the data and making an educated guess through plotting the time-temperature points on appropriate graph paper and crudely extrapolating a regression line to the application of rigorous physical-chemical laws, statistical concepts, and computers to obtain meaningful, reliable estimates.

A simple means of estimating shelf life from a set of computer-prepared tables has been described by Lintner et al.[6] This system was developed to select the best prototype formulation on the basis of short-term stability data and predict both estimated and minimum shelf-life values for the formulation. It is a middle-ground approach between the empirical methods and the modern, rigorous statistical concepts. All calculations can be made readily by hand, and the estimated values can be obtained easily from appropriate tables. The system assumes that

1. Shelf-life predictions can be made satisfactorily for lower temperatures using the classical Arrhenius model from data obtained at higher temperatures.
2. The energy of activation of the degradation reaction is between 10 and 20 kcal/mol (this is a safe assumption, as Kennon[8] has noted that rarely are drugs with energies of activation below 10 kcal/mol used in pharmacy, and for values as high as 20 kcal/mol, the error in the shelf-life prediction will be on the conservative side).
3. The rate of decomposition will not increase beyond that already observed.
4. The standard deviation of the replicated assays is known or can be estimated from the analytical data.

This concept further assumes that the degradation reaction follows zero- or pseudo-zero-order kinetics. For data corresponding to a zero-, first-, or second-order degradation pattern, it is impossible to distinguish one order from another with usual analytical procedures, when the total degraded material is not large. In addition, shelf-life calculations assuming zero-order kinetics are more conservative than those for higher orders.

This middle-ground system is useful in creating the experimental design for the stability study. The formulator has the opportunity to study various combinations of parameters to try to optimize the physical-statistical model. One can check the effect of improving the assay standard deviation, running additional replicates, using different time points, and assuming various degradation rates and energies of activation on the stability of the test formulation.

McMinn and Lintner later developed and reported on an information-processing system for handling product stability data.[9] This system saves the time of formulators in analyzing and interpreting their product stability data, in addition to minimizing the amount of clerical help needed to handle an ever-increasing assay load. For products such as those of vitamins, for example, where large overages are required, the statistical portions of this advanced technique aid the manufacturer to tailor the formula composition to obtain the desired and most economical expiration dating.

This system stores both physical and chemical data and retrieves the information in three different formats (one of which was designed specifically for submitting to regulatory agencies). It analyzes single-temperature data statistically by analysis of covariance and regression or multiple-temperature data by weighted or unweighted analysis using the Arrhenius relationship; provides estimates of the shelf life of the preparation with the appropriate confidence intervals; preprints the assay request cards that are used to record the results of the respective assay procedures and to enter the data into the system; and produces a 5-yr master-stability schedule as well as periodic 14-day schedules of upcoming assays.

As mentioned above, a portion of the advanced system analyzes the stability data obtained at a single temperature by analysis of covariance and regression. This analysis is based on the linear (zero-order) model

$$Y_{ij} = \beta_i X_{ij} + \alpha_i + \varepsilon_{ij} \quad (2)$$

where Y_{ij} is the percentage of label of the jth stability assay of the ith lot, X_{ij} is the time in months at which Y_{ij} was observed, β_i and α_i are the slope and intercept, respectively, of the regression line of the ith lot, and ε_{ij} is a random error associated with Y_{ij}. The random errors are assumed to be identically and independently distributed normal variables with a zero mean and a common variance, σ^2.

A summary of the regression analysis for each individual lot and for the combination of these lots, plus a summary of the analyses of covariance and deviation from regression is prepared by the computer.

Because the computer combines, or pools, the stability data from the individual lots, irrespective of the statistical integrity of this step, the pooled data are examined for validity by the F test. The mean square of the regression coefficient (slope) is divided by the mean square of the deviation within lots, and similarly, the adjusted mean (y intercept) is divided by the common mean square to give the respective F ratios. The latter values then are compared with the critical 5% F values. When the calculated F values are smaller than the critical F values, the data may be combined, and the pooled data analyzed.

A printout for the combined lots as well as for each individual lot provides the estimated rate of degradation and its standard error in percentage per month for each ingredient. The *Student t* value is calculated from these estimates and tested for significance from zero. When the t value is significant, the printout contains an estimate of the shelf life with the appropriate confidence interval. When the t value is not significantly different from zero, estimates of the minimum and projected shelf-life values are made. In addition, coordinates of the calculated least-squares regression line with appropriate confidence limits for the mean and individual predicted assays are printed.

Plots of the resulting least-squares line containing the individual data points also are printed by the computer. For the calculation of X_0, $\hat{Y}$ equals $\bar{Y} + \hat{\beta}(X_0 - \bar{X}..)$, where $\hat{\beta}$ is the least-squares estimate of the slope, and $\bar{X}..$ is the mean time of assay. The sample variance for this estimate, $S^2(\hat{Y})$ is equal to

$$S_{y \cdot x}^2 \left[\frac{1}{N} + \left[\frac{(X_0 - \bar{X}..)^2}{\sum(X_{ij} - \bar{X}..)^2} \right] \right] \quad (3)$$

where N is the number of assays. The 95% confidence interval is equal to $Y \pm t_{0.05S}(\hat{Y})$.

For cases in which the slope of the best fitting line is positive and significantly different from zero (resulting, eg, from solvent evaporation), the statement "no degradation has been detected and hence no shelf-life estimate is made" is printed. When the computed line has a positive slope but not significantly different from zero, only the minimum shelf-life value is calculated.

Traditionally, extensive stability data are collected at the recommended storage temperatures (usually refrigerator and/or room temperature) to be placed on the label of the package. However, elevated-temperature data are very valuable in determining the shelf life of a product. In practice, multiple levels of thermal stress are applied to the formulation so that appropriate shelf-life estimates can be made for normally expected marketing conditions. In cases in which data from accelerated studies are used to project a tentative expiration date that is beyond the date supported by actual shelf-life studies, testing must continue until the tentative expiration date is verified.

The effect of temperature variation on the rate of a reaction can be expressed by an integrated form of the Arrhenius equation

$$k = s e - E_A / RT \quad (4)$$

where, k is the rate constant, E_A is the energy of activation in kcal/mole, R is the universal gas constant of 1.987 cal/deg mole, T is the temperature in degrees in Kelvin, and S is a constant that is related to the specific reaction.

$$\log \frac{k_2}{k_1} = \frac{E_a}{2.303R} \left(\frac{T_2 - T_1}{T_2 * T_1} \right) \quad (5)$$

where, k_1 is the rate constant at temperature T_1 and k_2 is the rate constant at temperature T_2.

A weighted modification of this model has been incorporated into the previously described computerized system. Each printout contains a statement concerning the acceptability of the Arrhenius assumption with its appropriate probability level, the slope and intercept for the Arrhenius line, the estimated apparent energy of activation with its 95% confidence limits, plus the estimated shelf-life values at selected temperatures.

The analysis of first-order stability data is based on the linear model

$$Y_{ij} = \alpha_i + \beta_i X_{ij} + \varepsilon_{ij} \quad (6)$$

where Y_{ij} is the natural logarithm of the assay value for the jth observation of the ith temperature, X_{ij} is the elapsed time in months for the assay sample for the ith temperature, β_i and α_i are the slope and intercept, respectively, and ε_{ij} is a random error associated with Y_{ij}. The errors are assumed to be distributed identically and independently, normally with a zero mean and variance σ^2.

For orders other than first, Y_{ij} represents the concentration raised to the power of 1 minus the order.

The estimated rate constant (ie, the negative slope) is

$$-b_i = -\sum_j (Y_{ij} - Y_i)(X_{ij} - X_i)/\sum_j(X_{ij} - X_i)^2 \quad (7)$$

The standard error of the estimated rate constant is

$$S_{-b_i} = \frac{S(X/Y)}{\left[\sum(X_{ij} - X_i)^2 \right]^{1/2}} \quad (8)$$

where $S(Y/X)$, the residual standard error, is equal to

$$S(X/Y) =$$

$$\left\{ \frac{1}{N-2} \left[\sum_{j=1}^{12} (Y_{ij} - Y_i)^2 - \frac{[\sum(X_{ij} - X_i)(Y_{ij} - Yi)^2]}{\sum(X_{ij} - X_i)^2} \right] \right\}^{\frac{1}{2}} \quad (9)$$

According to the Arrhenius relationship, faster degradation occurs at the higher temperatures; hence, assays for the high-temperature data usually are run more often but for a shorter period of time. The effect of simple least-squares analysis of this type of data is to force the Arrhenius equation through the low temperature data and essentially ignore the high-temperature information. Thus, much more credence is placed in the point estimates of the low temperature than is warranted. In addition, the usual confidence limits on extrapolated degradation rates at refrigerator or room temperature cannot be made validly. For these reasons, Bentley[10] presented a method based on a weighted least-squares analysis to replace the unweighted approximation. He also developed a statistical test for the validity of the Arrhenius assumption, which is computed easily from the results of the unweighted method.

To make shelf-life estimates from elevated temperature data, two storage temperatures are obviously the minimum. As the accuracy of the extrapolation is enhanced by using additional temperatures, a minimum of four different temperatures is recommended for most product stability studies. With the current use of computers to do the bulk of stability calculations, including weighted least-squares analysis, the temperatures and storage conditions need not be selected for arithmetic convenience.

It is not necessary to determine the mechanism of the degradation reaction. In most cases, it is necessary only to follow some property of degradation and to linearize this function. Either the amount of intact drug or the amount of a formed degradation product may be followed. It usually is impractical to determine the exact order of the reaction. With assay errors in the range of 2 to 5%, at least 50% decomposition must occur before the reaction order can be determined. As the loss with pharmaceuticals generally is less, zero-order kinetics should be assumed, unless the reaction order is known from previous work. In any case, replication of stability assays is advisable.

The batches of drugs used for a stability study should be representative of production run material or at least material of a known degree of purity. The quality of the excipients also should be known, as their impurities or even their moisture content can affect product stability deleteriously. Likewise, the samples of the formulation taken for the stability study must be representative of the lot.

Specific, stability-indicating assay methods must be used, to make meaningful shelf-life estimates. The reliability and specificity of the test method on the intact molecule and on the degradation products must be demonstrated.

ADDITION OF OVERAGE

The problem of declining potency in an unstable preparation can be ameliorated by the addition of an excess or overage of the active ingredient. Overages, then, are added to pharmaceutical formulations to keep the content of the active ingredient within the limits compatible with therapeutic requirements, for a predetermined period of time.

The amount of the overage depends upon the specific ingredient and the galenical dosage form. The International Pharmaceutical Federation has recommended that overages be limited to a maximum of 30% over the labeled potency of an ingredient.

PHARMACEUTICAL CONTAINERS

The official standards for containers apply to articles packaged by either the pharmaceutical manufacturer or the dispensing pharmacist unless otherwise indicated in a compendial monograph. In general, repackaging of pharmaceuticals is inadvisable. However, if repackaging is necessary, the manufacturer of the product should be consulted for potential stability problems.

A pharmaceutical container has been defined as a device that holds the drug and is, or may be, in direct contact with the preparation. The immediate container is described as that which is in direct contact with the drug at all times. The liner and closure traditionally have been considered to be part of the container system. The container should not interact physically or chemically with the formulation so as to alter the strength, quality, or purity of its contents beyond permissible limits.

The choice of containers and closures can have a profound effect on the stability of many pharmaceuticals. Now that a large variety of glass, plastics, rubber closures, tubes, tube liners, etc are available, the possibilities for interaction between the packaging components and the formulation ingredients are immense. Some of the packaging elements themselves are subject to physical and chemical changes that may be time-temperature dependent.

Frequently, it is necessary to use a well-closed or a tight container to protect a pharmaceutical product. A *well-closed container* is used to protect the contents from extraneous solids or a loss in potency of the active ingredient under normal commercial conditions. A *tight container* protects the contents from contamination by extraneous materials, loss of contents, efflorescence, deliquescence, or evaporation and is capable of tight re-closure. When the packaging and storage of an official article in a well-closed or tight container is specified, water-permeation tests should be performed on the selected container.

In a stability program, the appearance of the container, with special emphasis on the inner walls, the migration of ingredients onto/into the plastic or into the rubber closure, the migration of plasticizer or components from the rubber closure into the formulation, the possibility of two-way moisture penetration through the container walls, the integrity of the tac-seal, and the back-off torque of the cap, must be studied.

GLASS—Traditionally, glass has been the most widely used container for pharmaceutical products to ensure inertness, visibility, strength, rigidity, moisture protection, ease of re-closure, and economy of packaging. While glass has some disadvantages, such as the leaching of alkali and insoluble flakes into the formulation, these can be offset by the choice of an appropriate glass. As the composition of glass may be varied by the amounts and types of sand and silica added and the heat treatment conditions used, the proper container for any formulation can be selected.

According to USP 26, glass containers suitable for packaging pharmacopeial preparations may be classified as either Type I, Type II, Type III, or type NP. Containers of Type I borosilicate glass are generally used for preparations that are intended for parenteral administration, although Type II treated soda-lime glass may be used where stability data demonstrates its suitability. Containers of Type III and Type NP are intended for packaging articles intended for oral or topical use.

New, unused glass containers are tested for resistance to attack by high-purity water by use of a sulfuric acid titration to determine the amount of released alkali. Both glass and plastic containers are used to protect light-sensitive formulations from degradation. The amount of transmitted light is measured using a spectrometer of suitable sensitivity and accuracy.

Glass is generally available in flint, amber, blue, emerald green, and certain light-resistant green and opal colors. The blue-, green-, and flint-colored glasses, which transmit ultraviolet and violet light rays, do not meet the official specifications for light-resistant containers.

Colored glass usually is not used for injectable preparations, since it is difficult to detect the presence of discoloration and particulate matter in the formulations. Light-sensitive drugs for parenteral use usually are sealed in flint ampuls and placed in a box. Multiple-dose vials should be stored in a dark place.

Manufacturers of prescription drug products should include sufficient information on their product labels to inform the pharmacist of the type of dispensing container needed to maintain the identity, strength, quality, and purity of the product. This brief description of the proper container, e.g., light- resistant, well-closed, or tight, may be omitted for those products dispensed in the manufacturer's original container.

PLASTICS—Plastic containers have become very popular for storing pharmaceutical products. Polyethylene, polystyrene, polyvinyl chloride, and polypropylene are used to prepare plastic containers of various densities to fit specific formulation needs.

Factors such as plastic composition, processing and cleaning procedures, contacting media, inks, adhesives, absorption, adsorption, and permeability of preservatives also affect the suitability of a plastic for pharmaceutical use. Hence, biological test procedures are used to determine the suitability of a plastic for packaging products intended for parenteral use and for polymers intended for use in implants and medical devices. Systemic injection and intracutaneous and implantation tests are employed. In addition, tests for nonvolatile residue, residue on ignition, heavy metals, and buffering capacity were designed to determine the physical and chemical properties of plastics and their extracts.

The high-density polyethylene (HDPE) containers, which are used for packaging capsules and tablets, possess characteristic thermal properties, a distinctive infrared absorption spectrum, and a density between 0.941 and 0.965 g/cm^3. In addition, these containers are tested for light transmission, water-vapor permeation, extractable substances, nonvolatile residue, and heavy metals. When a stability study has been performed to establish the expiration date for a dosage form in an acceptable high-density polyethylene container, any other high-density polyethylene container may be substituted provided that it, too, meets compendial standards and that the stability program is expanded to include the alternative container.

Materials from the plastic itself can leach into the formulation, and materials from the latter can be absorbed onto, into, or through the container wall. The barrels of some plastic syringes bind various pharmaceutical preservatives. However, changing the composition of the syringe barrel from nylon to polyethylene or polystyrene has eliminated the binding in some cases.

A major disadvantage of plastic containers is the two-way permeation or *breathing* through the container walls. Volatile oils and flavoring and perfume agents are permeable through plastics to varying degrees. Components of emulsions and creams have been reported to migrate through the walls of some plastics, causing either a deleterious change in the formulation or collapse of the container. Loss of moisture from a formulation is common. Gases, such as oxygen or carbon dioxide in the air, have been known to migrate through container walls and affect a preparation.

Solid dosage forms, such as penicillin tablets, when stored in some plastics, are affected deleteriously by moisture penetration from the atmosphere into the container.

Single unit does packaging in the form of blister packages are often used to package capsule and tablet dosage forms. A typical blister package is comprised of a polymeric film that is molded to have a cavity into which the dosage form is placed. The polymer film is then heat bonded to a paper backed foil liner.

As with plastic bottles, the blister package will allow a certain amount of moisture vapor permeation to occur, and this must be a consideration when selecting the type of film used for the package. The choice of packaging materials used depends on the degree to which the product needs to be protected from light, heat and moisture. Each material has different resistance to each of these elements and will affect the shelf life and storage conditions of the packaged pharmaceutical.

Polyvinylchloride (PVC) offers the least resistance to moisture vapor permeation. Polyvinylidenechloride (PVdC) has characteristics similar to PVC but offers superior resistance to moisture vapor permeation. Aclar, which is a polychlorotrifluoroethylene (PVC-CTFE) film has the lowest water vapor permeability and thus offers the best protection from moisture.

METALS—The pharmaceutical industry was, and to a degree still is, a tin stronghold. However, as the price of tin constantly varies, more-collapsible aluminum tubes are being used. Lead tubes tend to have pinholes and are little used in the industry.

A variety of internal linings and closure fold seals are available for both tin and aluminum tubes. Tin tubes can be coated with wax or with vinyl linings. Aluminum tubes are available with epoxy or phenolic resin, wax, vinyl, or a combination of epoxy or phenolic resin with wax. As aluminum is able to withstand the high temperatures required to cure epoxy and phenolic resins adequately, tubes made from this metal presently offer the widest range of lining possibilities.

Closure fold seals may consist of unmodified vinyl resin or plasticized cellulose and resin, with or without added color.

Collapsible tubes are available in many combinations of diameters, lengths, openings, and caps. Custom-use tips for ophthalmic, nasal, mastitis, and rectal applications also are available. Only a limited number of internal liners and closure seals are available for tubes fitted with these special-use tips.

Lined tubes from different manufacturers are not necessarily interchangeable. While some converted resin liners may be composed of the same base resin, the actual liner may have been modified to achieve better adhesion, flow properties, drying qualities, or flexibility. These modifications may have been necessitated by the method of applying the liner, the curing procedure, or, finally, the nature of the liner itself.

CLOSURES

The closures for the formulations also must be studied as a portion of the overall stability program. While the closure must form an effective seal for the container, the closure must not react chemically or physically with the product. It must not absorb materials from the formulation or leach its ingredients into the contents.

The integrity of the seal between the closure and container depends on the geometry of the two, the materials used in their construction, the composition of the cap liner, and the tightness with which the cap has been applied. Torque is a measure of the circular force, measured in inch-pounds, which must be applied to open or close a container. When pharmaceutical products are set up on a stability study, the formulation must be in the proposed market package. Thus, they should be capped with essentially the same torque to be used in the manufacturing step.

Rubber is a common component of stoppers, cap liners, and parts of dropper assemblies. Sorption of the active ingredient, preservative, or other formulation ingredients into the rubber and the extraction of one or more components of the rubber into the formulation are common problems.

The application of an epoxy lining to the rubber closure reduces the amount of leached extractives but essentially has no effect on the sorption of the preservative from the solution.

Teflon-coated rubber stoppers may prevent most of the sorption and leaching.

REFERENCES

1. Lintner CJ. *Quality Control in the Pharmaceutical Industry,* vol 2. New York: Academic, 1973, p 141.
2. Connors KA, Amidon GL, Stella JV. *Chemical Stability of Pharmaceuticals,* 2nd ed. New York: Wiley, 1986.
3. Carstensen, JT. *Drug Stability Principles and Practices.* New York: Marcel Dekker, 1990
4. *Current Good Manufacturing Practice, 21 CFR 211.*
5. USP 26, 2003
6. *Guideline for Submitting Documentation for the Stability of Human Drugs and Biologics.* FDA, Center for Drugs and Biologics. Office of Drug Research Review, Feb 1987.
7. Lintner CJ, et al. *Am Perfum Cosmet* 1970; 85(12):31.
8. Kennon L. *J Pharm Sci* 1964; 53:815.
9. McMinn CS, Lintner CJ. (Oral presentation), APhA Acad Pharm Sci Mtg Ind Pharm Tech Sec. Chicago, May 1973.
10. Bentley DL. *J Pharm Sci* 1970; 59:464.

BIBLIOGRAPHY

Analysis. San Diego, Academic Press, 2001, Chap 13.
Carstensen, JT. *Drug Stability: Principles and Practices,* 2nd ed. New York: Marcel Dekker, 1995.
Cha J, Ranweiler JS, Lane PA. Stability studies. In Ahuja S, Scypinski S, eds. *Handbook of Modern Pharmaceutical Analysis.* San Diego: Academic Press, 2001.
Connors KA, Amidon GL, Stella VJ. *Chemical Stability of Pharmaceuticals.* New York: Wiley, 1986.
Documentation Practices: A Complete Guide to Document Development and Management for GMP and ISO9000 Compliant Industries. C DeSain, Advanstar Comm Inc, 1998.
Florence AT, Attwood D. *Physicochemical Principles of Pharmacy,* 2nd ed. New York: Chapman and Hall, 1988, Chap 4.
Florey K. *STP Pharma* 1986; 2:236.
Grimm W, Krummen K. *Stability Testing in the EC, Japan and the USA.* Stuttgart: Wiss. Verl.-Ges, 1993.
ICH Q1A (R): Stability Testing of New Drug Substances and Products. Step 4 Draft, 2003.
ICH Q1B: Photostability Testing of New Drug Substances and Products, 1996.
ICH Q1C: Stability Testing of New Dosage Forms, 1996.
ICH Q1D: Bracketing and Matrixing Designs for Stability Testing of New Drug Substances and Products. Step 4, 2003.
ICH Q1E: Evaluation OF Stability Data. Step 4, Draft, 2003.
ICH Q1F: Stability Data Package for Registration Applications in Climatic Zones III and IV, 2003.
Irwin WJ. *Kinetics of Drug Decomposition: Basic Computer Solutions.* Amsterdam: Elsevier, 1990.
Lachman L, et al. *The Theory and Practice of Industrial Pharmacy,* 3rd ed. Philadelphia: Lea & Febiger, 1986.
USP 24, Section <1077>, 1999.
Wagner JG, ed. *Biopharmaceutics and Relevant Pharmacokinetics.* Hamilton, IL: Hamilton Press, 1971.
Wells, JI. *Pharmaceutical Preformulation: The Physicochemical Properties of Drug Substances.* Chinchester: Ellis Horwood, 1988, Chap 5.
Windheuser JJ, ed. *The Dating of Pharmaceuticals.* Madison, WI: University Extension, University of Wisconsin, 1970.

CHAPTER 53

Bioavailability and Bioequivalency Testing

Henry J Malinowski, PhD

Steven B Johnson, PharmD

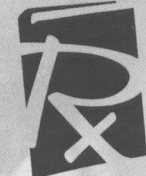

Oral solid dosage forms, tablets and capsules, are prescribed widely and are a very effective means of providing drugs to patients. A basic assumption is that when an oral solid dosage form is used by a patient, the drug from the dosage form is released, dissolves, and is absorbed promptly and consistently. Drug product quality is needed for this to be a valid assumption. In addition, many drugs are incompletely absorbed, due to factors relating to the drug, dosage form, and human physiology in the gastrointestinal tract. Optimal and consistent absorption of such drugs needs to be assured. Bioavailability and bioequivalence become important considerations in assuring optimal drug absorption. Major aspects of these areas are the topics covered in this chapter.

The bioavailability of a drug in an oral solid dosage form can be affected by numerous factors including food, changes in the metabolism of the drug due to drug interactions, gastrointestinal transit time, and changes in release characteristics of the drug from the dosage form (especially for modified release products). Changes in bioavailability can be thought of in terms of changes in exposure to the drug, which, if substantial, can relate to safety and efficacy concerns.

Bioequivalence is an important consideration in several key situations involving lot to lot consistency, innovator to generic product therapeutic equivalence, and situations where a marketed product undergoes changes in certain aspects including formulation, manufacturing process, and dosage strength.

In this chapter, bioavailability and bioequivalence topics are emphasized. Chemical equivalence, lot-to-lot uniformity of physicochemical characteristics, and stability equivalence are other factors that are important, as they too can affect product quality.

GENERAL CONCEPTS

Regarding bioavailability and bioequivalence, it is best to start with the basic concepts and factors that can affect the bioavailability of a drug and consider how these can influence bioequivalence and the clinical outcome of drug treatment. At the outset, the terms used in this chapter require careful definition, since, as in any area, some terms have been used in many different contexts by different authors.

Bioavailability is a term that indicates measurement of both the rate of drug absorption and total amount (extent) of drug that reaches the general circulation from an administered dosage form. It is specific to the active drug substance as contrasted to metabolites.

Equivalence is more a general, relative term that indicates a comparison of one drug product with another or with a set of established standards. Equivalence may be defined in several ways:

Chemical equivalence indicates that two or more dosage forms contain the same labeled quantities (plus or minus specified range limits) of the drug.

Clinical equivalence occurs when the same drug from two or more dosage forms gives identical *in vivo* effects as measured by a pharmacological response or by control of a symptom or disease.

Therapeutic equivalence implies that two brands of a drug product are expected to yield the same clinical result. The FDA specifically uses the term therapeutic equivalence in the evaluation of multisource prescription drug products.

Bioequivalence indicates that a drug in two or more similar dosage forms reaches the general circulation at the same relative rate and the same relative extent (ie, that the plasma level profiles of the drug obtained using the two dosage forms are the same).

Pharmaceutical equivalence refers to two drug products with the same dosage form and same strength.

THERAPEUTIC EQUIVALENCE EVALUATIONS

The FDA publication *Approved Drug Products with Therapeutic Equivalence Evaluations* identifies drug products approved on the basis of safety and effectiveness. In addition, this list contains therapeutic equivalence evaluations for approved multisource prescription drug products. These evaluations have been prepared to serve as public information and advice to state health agencies, physicians, and pharmacists to promote public education in the area of drug product selection and to foster containment of health-care costs.

To help contain drug costs, virtually every state has adopted laws and/or regulations that encourage the substitution of drug products. These state laws generally require either that substitution be limited to drugs on a specific list (the positive formulary approach) or that substitution be permitted for all drugs except those prohibited by a particular list (the negative formulary approach). Because of the number of requests for FDA assistance in preparing both positive and negative formularies, it became apparent that the FDA could not serve the needs of each state on an individual basis. The agency also recognized that providing a single list based on common criteria would be preferable to evaluating drug products on the basis of differing definitions and criteria in various state laws. The therapeutic equivalence evaluations in this publication reflect FDA's application of specific criteria to the approved multisource prescription drug products.

FDA classifies as therapeutically equivalent those products that meet the following general criteria:

1. They are approved as safe and effective.
2. They are pharmaceutical equivalents in that they (1) contain identical amounts of the same active drug ingredient in the same dosage form and route of administration and (2) meet compendial

or other applicable standards of strength, quality, purity, and identity.
3. They are bioequivalent in that (1) they do not present a known or potential bioequivalence problem, and they meet an acceptable *in vitro* standard, or (2) if they do present such a known or potential problem, they are shown to meet an appropriate bioequivalence standard.
4. They are adequately labeled.
5. They are manufactured in compliance with Current Good Manufacturing Practice regulations.

This concept of therapeutic equivalency applies only to drug products containing the same active ingredient(s) and does not encompass a comparison of different therapeutic agents used for the same condition. The FDA considers drug products to be therapeutically equivalent if they meet the criteria outlined above, even though they may differ in certain other characteristics such as shape, scoring configuration, release mechanisms, packaging, excipients, expiration date/time, and minor aspects of labeling (eg, the presence of specific pharmacokinetic information). The FDA believes that products classified as therapeutically equivalent can be substituted with the full expectation that the substituted product will produce the same clinical effect and safety profile as the prescribed product.

Methods for Determining Bioequivalence

Bioequivalence usually involves human testing but sometimes may be demonstrated using an *in vitro* bioequivalence standard, especially when such an *in vitro* test has been correlated with human *in vivo* bioavailability data. In other situations, bioequivalence may sometimes be demonstrated through comparative clinical trials or pharmacodynamic studies.

The FDA has categorized (21CFR320.24) various *in vivo* and *in vitro* approaches that may be utilized to establish bioequivalence. In descending order of accuracy, sensitivity and reproducibility these are:

1. An *in vivo* test in humans in which the active drug substance, as well as active metabolites when appropriate, is measured in plasma.
2. An *in vitro* test that has been correlated with human *in vivo* bioavailability data. This approach is most likely for oral extended release products and is described in detail in an FDA Guidance.
3. An *in vivo* test in animals that has been correlated with human bioavailability data.
4. An *in vivo* test in humans, where urinary excretion of the active drug substance, as well as active metabolites when appropriate, is measured.
5. An *in vivo* test in humans in which an appropriate acute pharmacological effect is measured.
6. Well-controlled clinical trials in humans that establish the safety and efficacy of the drug product, for establishing bioavailability. For bioequivalence, comparative clinical trials may be considered. This approach is the least accurate, sensitive, and reproducible approach and should be considered only if other approaches are not feasible.
7. A currently available *in vitro* test, acceptable to FDA, that ensures bioavailability. This approach is intended only when *in vitro* testing is deemed adequate, but no *in vitro in vivo* correlation has been established. It also can relate to considerations involving the Biopharmaceutics Classification System (BCS).

Most bioequivalence studies involve the direct measurement of the parent drug, as described in (1) above. Bioequivalence testing in animals is not a recommended approach due to possible differences in metabolism, gastrointestinal physiology, weight, and diet.

Minimizing the Need for Bioequivalence Studies

To minimize the need for human testing for bioequivalence, various approaches have been suggested:

1. *Situation where no changes are made for an approved, marketed product*–If a drug product has been adequately tested and ap-

proved for marketing, and if no changes in the manufacturing of the product are made, it is reasonable to assume that all subsequent batches of the product would be expected to be bioequivalent to the original product. If subsequently manufactured batches meet all tests of quality, including the dissolution test, no further human bioequivalence testing is needed.

2. *Situation where changes are made for an approved, marketed drug product*–Depending on the degree of change, bioequivalence may sometimes need to be reconfirmed. Although it is somewhat difficult to categorize such major changes, this issue has been addressed in a series of FDA Guidances Related to Scale-Up and Post-Approval Changes (SUPAC).

3. *Situation where human bioequivalence testing may not be needed for initial approval or for major post-approval changes*–Drug characteristics related to solubility and permeability may allow a reasonable expectation that the drug is unlikely to be subject to significant bioavailability problems. For such drugs, *in vitro* dissolution testing may be adequate, in lieu of *in vivo* testing. These concepts are described in the Biopharmaceutics Classification System (BCS). This classification system provides a scientific framework for classifying drugs based on aqueous solubility and intestinal permeability. In addition, criteria for rapid dissolution are described (not less than 85% dissolved in 30 minutes, using mild agitation and physiological media). The BCS permits waivers of in vivo bioequivalence testing for high solubility, high permeability drugs (Class I), which are formulated into immediate release dosage forms having rapid dissolution. A basic concept behind the BCS is that solutions of drugs are thought to have few bioavailability or bioequivalence issues. Dosage forms that contain high solubility drugs that exhibit rapid dissolution behave similar to solutions when either a solution or the highly soluble drug is in the stomach. Particularly for such drugs that are, in addition, highly permeable (well absorbed), the likelihood of bioavailability issues is quite small and, consequently, in vivo bioequivalence testing for such drugs is thought to be unnecessary. Similarly for oral solutions, in vivo bioequivalence testing is not necessary.

Additional Information

A significant factor related to drug bioavailability is the fact that many times drug is administered not as a solution but as a solid dosage form. Optimal bioavailability might be expected from a solution, since drug must first dissolve to be absorbed, but considerations such as drug stability, unpalatable taste, and desired duration of action (for controlled-release drug products) may prevent the use of a solution dosage form.

DOSAGE FORMS—In the dose titration of any patient the objective is, in conceptual terms, to attain and maintain a blood level that exceeds the minimum effective level required for response but does not exceed the minimum toxic (side-effect) level. This is shown graphically in Figure 53-1. There are several major absorption factors that can affect the general shape of this blood-level curve and thus drug response.

The Dose of the Drug Administered—The blood levels will rise and fall in proportion to the dose administered.

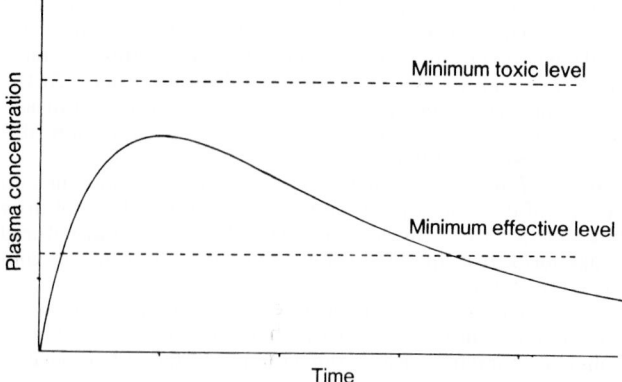

Figure 53-1. Typical plasma-level curve of a drug with effective and toxic (side-effect) profile levels defined.

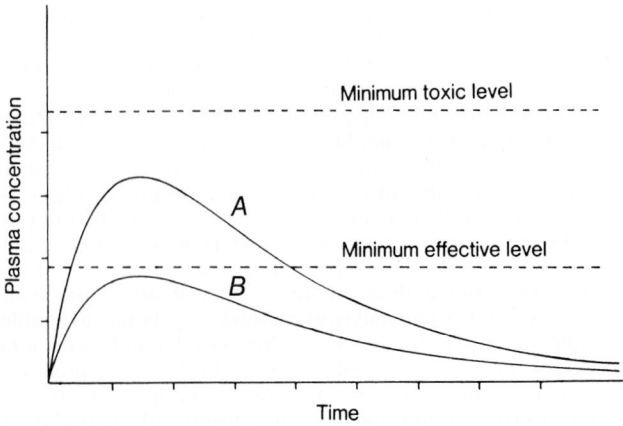

Figure 53-2. Effect of the extent of drug absorption from a dosage form on drug-plasma levels and efficacy. The extent of absorption from dosage form *B* is 50% of that from dosage form *A*.

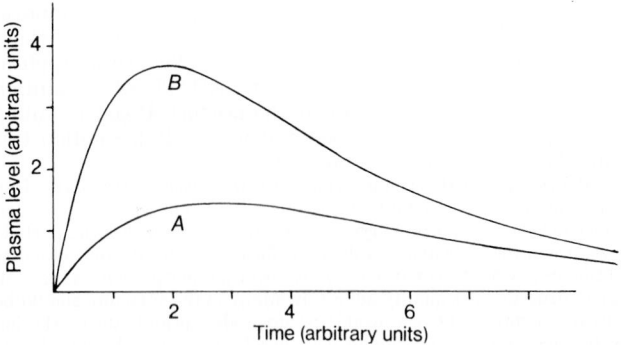

Figure 53-4. Computer simulation of the plasma-level curves for two dosage forms of the same drug assuming that the rate and extent of drug absorption for dosage form *A* were 50% and 50%, respectively, of those for dosage form *B*.

The Amount of Drug Absorbed from a Given Dosage Form—This involves the same principle as the first factor but is brought about by a different process. The effect of having only one half of the drug absorbed from a dosage form is equivalent to lowering the dose (Fig 53-2).

The Rate of Absorption of the Drug—If absorption from the dosage form is more rapid than the rate of absorption that gave the profile in Figure 53-1, minimum toxic (side-effect) levels may be exceeded. If absorption from the dosage form is sufficiently slow, minimum effective levels may never be attained (Fig 53-3).

A Combination of These Last Two Factors—This is also possible (Fig 53-4) and is probably the most likely situation in real life.

In any of these instances, the time course and extent of clinical response to the drug may be altered because of changes in dose or rate and extent of absorption.

Both factors, rate and extent of drug absorption, can be affected by the dosage form in which the drug is contained. The effect of rate of absorption may be intentional, as in controlled-release products, or unintentional, as brought about by, for example, a change in the composition and/or method of manufacture of the dosage form.

The choice of the inactive ingredients (excipients) used to prepare a dosage form is up to the individual manufacturer. It is through these changes, in composition and manufacturing technique, that unintended changes in bioavailability and bioequivalence may occur. Revalidation of bioequivalence may be needed for major changes in the manufacturing process, whereas small changes may not raise significant bioavailability concerns. In situations involving minor changes in the manufacturing process, comparative dissolution testing of the original and reformulated product provides adequate documentation of continued product quality, if the resulting dissolution profiles are similar. These considerations apply to all drug manufacturers, both innovator and generic companies. A description of the formulation of dosage forms and the factors that must be considered is given in Chapter 38.

DISSOLUTION—For a drug to be absorbed, it must first go into solution. In Figure 53-5, the steps in the dissolution and absorption of a tablet or capsule dosage form are outlined. Similar profiles could be obtained for any solid or semisolid dosage form, including oral suspensions, parenteral suspensions, and suppositories. The theory and mechanics of drug dissolution rate are described in detail in Chapter 35. The physical characteristics of the drug and the composition of the tablet (dosage form) can have an effect on the rates of disintegration, deaggregation, and dissolution of the drug. As such, these can affect the rate of absorption and resultant blood levels of the drug.

An important aspect of product quality for marketed oral solid dosage forms relates to dissolution testing. Nearly all of the dosage forms actually used by patients will be from lots that have not directly undergone human bioavailability testing. It is previous batches of these products that would have been tested in humans. Once adequate product quality has been established by bioavailability testing, subsequent batches manufactured using the same formulation, equipment, and process are likely to be bioequivalent to the original batch tested in humans. This is an important concept in the regulatory control of product quality and is where *in vitro* testing such as assay, content uniformity, tablet hardness, and dissolution are involved. Among these several *in vitro* tests, dissolution testing is probably the most important, related to bioavailability. As part of the drug approval process, a dissolution test procedure is established for all oral solid dosage forms. These dissolution tests are incorporated in the

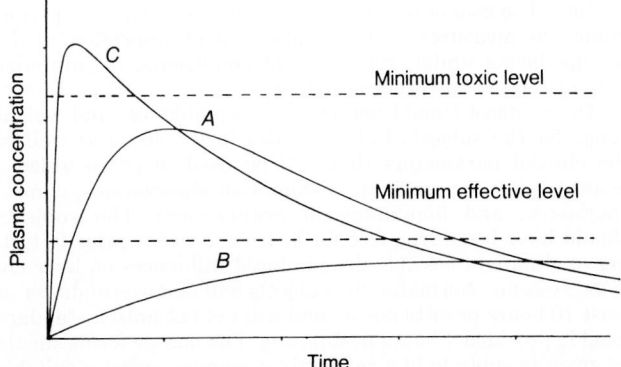

Figure 53-3. Effect of the rate of drug absorption from a dosage form on the plasma-level profile and efficacy. The rates of absorption from dosage forms *B* and *C* and 1/10 and 10 times those from dosage form *A*.

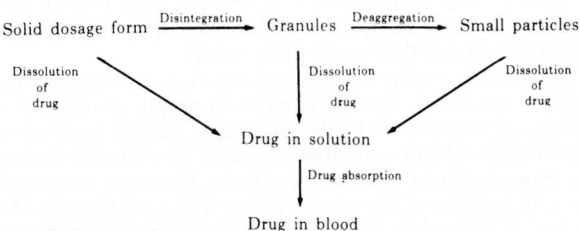

Figure 53-5. Sequence of events involved in the dissolution and absorption of a drug from a solid oral dosage form.

United States Pharmacopeia (USP) and apply both to innovator and generic drug products. All marketed batches of these drug products must meet the Abbreviated New Drug Application (ANDA)/New Drug Application (NDA)/USP dissolution tests throughout the shelf life of the product. Products failing their approved dissolution test and/or a USP dissolution test must be removed from the market.

Properties of the Drug—The physical characteristics of the drug that can alter bioavailability are discussed in Chapters 38 and 57 and consist of the polymorphic crystal form, choice of the salt form, particle size, use of the hydrated or anhydrous form, wettability, and solubility of the drug. Chapter 38 also discusses several other properties that can affect drug product quality adversely. Many of these factors should be discovered during the testing of the drug product prior to the marketing of the dosage form and should not, therefore, affect unknowingly the bioavailability of the drug product.

Properties of the Dosage Form—The various components of the solid or semisolid dosage form, other than the active ingredient, are discussed in Chapter 45. Only an overview, for tablet dosage forms, is given here. In addition to the active ingredient, a tablet product usually will contain the following types of inactive ingredients.

Glidants are used to provide a free-flowing powder from the mix of tablet ingredients, so that the material will flow when used on a tablet machine.

Binders provide a cohesiveness to the tablet. Too little binder will produce tablets that do not maintain their integrity; too much may affect adversely the release (dissolution rate) of the drug from the tablet.

Fillers are used to give the powder bulk so that an acceptably sized tablet is produced. Most commercial tablets weigh from 100 to 500 mg, so it is obvious that for many potent drugs the filler constitutes a large portion of the tablet. Binding of drug to the fillers may occur and affect bioavailability.

Disintegrants are used to cause the tablets to disintegrate when exposed to an aqueous environment. Too much will produce tablets that may disintegrate in the bottle because of atmospheric moisture; too little may be insufficient for disintegration to occur and may thus alter the rate and extent of release of the drug from the dosage form.

Lubricants are used to enhance the flow of the powder through the tablet machine and to prevent sticking of the tablet in the die of the tablet machine after the tablet is compressed. Lubricants are usually hydrophobic materials such as stearic acid, magnesium, or calcium stearate. Too little lubricant will not permit satisfactory tablets to be made; too much may produce a tablet with a water-impervious hydrophobic coat, which can inhibit the disintegration of the tablet and dissolution of the drug.

BIOEQUIVALENCE TESTING

The awareness of the potential for clinical differences between otherwise chemically equivalent drug products has been brought about by a multiplicity of factors that include, among others, better methods for clinical efficacy evaluation, development of techniques to measure microgram or nanogram quantities of drugs in biological fluids, improvements in the technology of dosage form formulation and physical testing, awareness of reported clinical inequivalencies in the literature, increased costs of classical clinical evaluation, the objective and quantitative nature of bioavailability tests, and the increase in the number of chemically equivalent products on the market because of patent expirations on the wonder drugs of the 1950s and 1960s as well as the Drug Price Competition and Patent Term Restoration Act of 1984, which established the generic drug approval procedures that are in place today.

The increase in the number of drugs that are available from multiple sources frequently has placed people involved in the delivery of health care in the position of having to select one from among several marketed products. As with any decision, the more pertinent the data available, the more comfortable one is in arriving at the final decision. The need to make these choices, in light of the potential for *in vivo* inequivalency among products or different batches of a given product, has increased the demand for quantitative data on the therapeutic equivalence of similar drug products. Bioequivalence testing represents one alternative solution to clinical testing for efficacy and

is the means by which generic drugs are approved for marketing as well as the means by which the product quality of all drug products is maintained in situations involving major changes in formulation or manufacturing process.

Requirements for bioequivalence data on drug products should be applied reasonably. For example, with single-supplier drugs, bioequivalence testing is not an issue as far as brand-switching but can be a means of assessing changes between clinical and to-be-marketed formulations. In this context, the reason for bioequivalence testing should not be forgotten (ie, it is used as a surrogate, in certain situations, for the clinical evaluation of drug products). Bioequivalence data cannot be required if bioanalytical methodology is not available. However, in a number of cases, pharmacodynamic data may provide a more sensitive, objective evaluation of a product's therapeutic equivalence than clinical testing, and this can be an alternative approach in the absence of bioanalytical methodology.

Basic pharmacokinetic evaluation of bioavailability data is not necessary to show bioequivalence of two drug products. Pharmacokinetics has its major utility in the prediction or projection of dosage regimens and/or in providing a better understanding of observed drug reactions or interactions that result from the accumulation of drug in some specific site, tissue, or compartment of the body. The basis of the conclusion that two drug products are bioequivalent must be that the responses observed (blood, serum or plasma level, urinary excretion, or pharmacological response) for one drug product are essentially the same as the responses observed for the second drug product. The easy, but relatively rare, decisions in the evaluation of the bioequivalence of two drug products are those in which the two products are exactly superimposable (definitely bioequivalent) and those in which the two products differ in their bioequivalence parameters by a large amount, such as 50% or more (definitely not bioequivalent). Statistical evaluation of the data is necessary for all situations, particularly for data between these two extremes.

Evaluation of Bioequivalence Data

The following sections highlight some of the tests that should be considered when evaluating data from bioequivalence studies. The topics discussed are directed specifically toward plasma level evaluations. With minor modifications, the approaches outlined can be used for urinary excretion measurements or for suitable, quantitative, pharmacological response measurements.

Bioequivalence studies are usually conducted in healthy adults under standardized conditions. Most often, single doses of the test and reference product will be evaluated. However, in selected cases, multiple-dose regimens may be used (eg, when patients are used and they cannot be discontinued from a medication). The goal of the study is to evaluate the *in vivo* performance, as measured by rate and extent of absorption, of the dosage forms under standardized conditions, to minimize patient-related and other variability.

The protocol should define the acceptable age and weight range for the subjects to be included in the study as well as the clinical parameters that will be used to characterize a healthy adult (eg, physical examination observations, clinical chemistry, and hematological evaluations). The subjects should have been drug-free for at least 2 weeks prior to testing to eliminate possible drug-induced influences on liver enzyme systems. Normally, the subjects will fast overnight for at least 10 hours prior to dosing and will not eat until a standard meal is provided 4 hours post-dosing. The dosage forms should be given to subjects in a randomized manner, using a suitable crossover design, so that possible daily variations are distributed equally between the dosage forms tested. The protocol should define sample collection times and techniques to collect the biological fluid. The method of sample storage should also be defined.

Bioequivalence Assessment and Data Evaluation

Several parameters are used to provide a general evaluation of the overall rate and extent of absorption of a drug. An analysis of all characteristics is required before one can implicate any one factor or parameter as indicating bioequivalence or lack of bioequivalence. It is implicit that the analytical methodology used for analysis of drug in the samples is specific, sensitive, and precise.

The plasma concentration-time curve is the focal point of bioequivalence assessment and is obtained when serial blood samples, taken after drug administration, are analyzed for drug concentration. The concentrations are plotted on the ordinate (y-axis) and the times after drug administration that the samples were obtained, on the abscissa (x-axis).

A drug product is administered orally at time zero, and the plasma drug concentration at this time clearly should be zero. As the product passes through the gastrointestinal (GI) system (stomach, intestine), it must go through the sequence of events depicted in Figure 53-5. As the drug is absorbed, increasing concentrations of the drug are observed in successive samples until the maximum concentration is achieved. This point of maximum concentration (C_{max}) is called the peak of the concentration-time curve. If a simple model describes the pharmacokinetics of the drug tested, the peak concentration represents approximately the point in time when absorption and elimination of the drug have equalized.

The section of the curve to the left of the peak represents the absorption phase (or absorption and distribution), during which absorption predominates over elimination. The section of the curve to the right of the peak is called the elimination phase, during which elimination predominates over absorption. It should be understood that elimination begins as soon as the drug appears in the bloodstream and continues until all of the drug has been eliminated. Elimination is classically the log-linear portion of the curve. Absorption continues for some period of time into the elimination phase, for as long as there is drug (in gradually decreasing amounts) available for absorption in the GI tract.

One must recognize that elimination of the drug includes all processes of elimination of the drug, involving urinary excretion as well as metabolism by various tissues and organs. The *efficiency* of metabolism and urinary excretion will determine the shape of the elimination phase of the curve.

Bioequivalence studies normally are performed in healthy, adult volunteers under rigid conditions of fasting and activity because the objective is to obtain quantitative information on the influence of pharmaceutical formulation variables on the drug product's absorption. Drug blood-level profiles, therefore, allow quantification of the rate and extent of drug absorption and are critical in establishing the comparative efficiency of two drug products in delivering the drug to the systemic circulation.

Suggestions that bioequivalence studies should be performed in a disease-state population are not tenable if the object of the study is to assess drug formulations, unless safety considerations prohibit administration of the drug to healthy volunteers. If, on the other hand, the purpose is to determine the effect of disease on the efficiency of absorption of the drug product, then one must use the disease-state population. The reasoning is obvious. To ensure that any differences observed in the drug blood-level profiles are attributable to formulation factors, as much as possible, one must hold all other variables constant (ie, food, activity, and state of disease).

One need not be limited to drug blood-level profiles, but in a similar manner, may obtain cumulative urinary drug amount–time profiles. Drug concentration is determined in the urine at specified time intervals, and the amount excreted per interval is determined by multiplying the concentration by the volume of urine obtained in that interval. The amounts per interval then are combined, and ultimately the total amount excreted in the urine is obtained. This value is analogous to the area under the blood concentration-time curve. However, one limitation to this method is that rate cannot be readily determined. A typical cumulative urinary drug amount–time profile for several nitrofurantoin products is presented in Figure 53-6.

In assessing the bioequivalence of drug products, one must quantitate the rate and extent of absorption, which can be determined by evaluating parameters, derived from the blood-level concentration-time profile. Three parameters describing a blood level curve are considered important in evaluating the bioequivalence of two or more formulations of the same drug. These are the peak-height concentration, the time of the peak concentration, and the area under the blood (serum or plasma) concentration-time curve.

PEAK-HEIGHT CONCENTRATION—The peak of the blood level-time curve represents the highest drug concentration achieved after oral administration. It is reported as an amount per volume measurement (eg, micrograms/milliliter, units/milliliter, or grams/100 mL). The importance of this parameter is illustrated in Figure 53-7, where the blood concentration-time curves of two different formulations of a drug are represented. A line has been drawn across the curve at 4 µg/mL. Suppose that the drug is an analgesic and 4 µg/mL is the minimum effective concentration (MEC) of the drug in blood. If the blood concentration curves in Figure 53-7 represent the blood levels obtained after administration of equal doses of two formulations of the drug and it is known that analgesia would not be produced unless the MEC was achieved or exceeded, it becomes clear that formulation A would be expected to provide pain relief, while formulation B, even though it is well absorbed regarding extent of absorption, might be ineffective in producing analgesia.

On the other hand, if the two curves represent blood concentrations following equal doses of two different formulations of the same cardiac glycoside, and 4 µg/mL now represents the

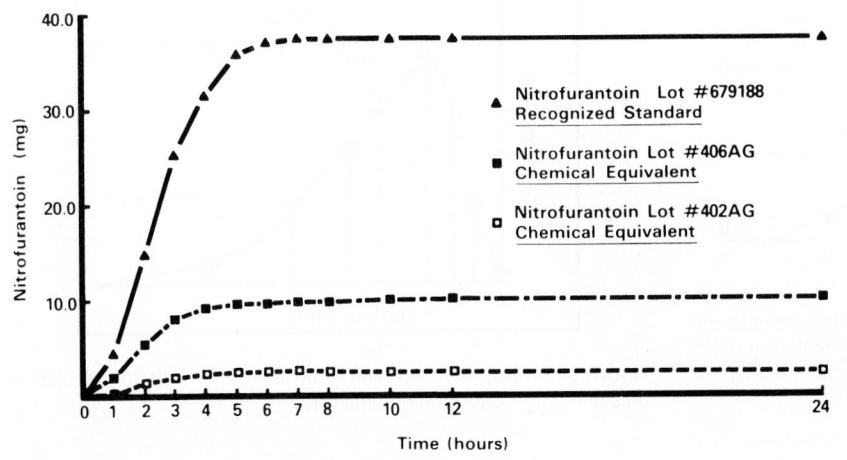

Figure 53-6. Average cumulative amounts of nitrofurantoin excreted form three lots of two commercially available products after a single oral dose of 100 mg of nitrofurantoin.

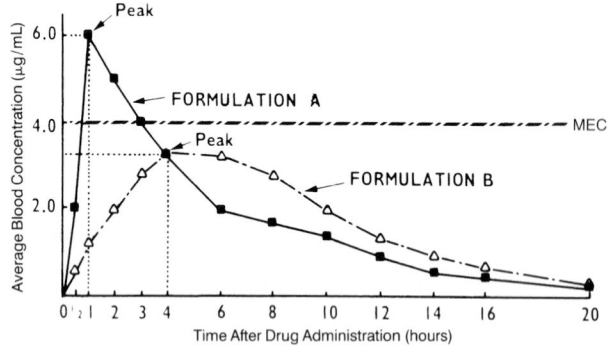

Figure 53-7. Blood concentration-time curves obtained for two different formulations of the same drug, demonstrating relationship of the profiles to the minimum effective concentration (MEC).

Table 53-1. Using the trapezoidal rule to calculate area under the concentration time curve. $AUC_{(0-\infty)}$ is used for bioequivalence analyses when the $AUC_{(0-t)}$ makes up $\geq 80\%$ of the $AUC_{(0-\infty)}$. $AUC_{(0-t)}$ is used when the $AUC_{(0-t)}$ makes up $< 80\%$ of the $AUC_{(0-\infty)}$. When drugs with long half-lives, such as levothyroxine, are evaluated, $AUC_{(0-t)}$ is used and is truncated at 48 or 72 hours.

Area under the concentration-time curve from time zero to time t (AUC_{0-t})

1. Plot the concentration-time data for each subject;
2. Divide the curve into trapezoids by drawing vertical lines from each data point to the x-axis;
3. Calculate the area of the trapezoids using the following formula:
   - $AUC_{(t2-t1)} = [(C_2 + C_1)(t_2 - t_1)] / 2$
4. $AUC_{(0-t)}$ is then calculated by summing the individual areas to the time of the last concentration:
   - $AUC_{(0-t)} = AUC_{(t2-t1)} + AUC_{(t3-t2)} + ... + AUC_{(tn-(tn-1))}$

Area under the concentration-time curve from time zero to infinity ($AUC_{0-\infty}$)

5. To calculate $AUC_{(0-\infty)}$, the tail region of the curve must be added to the $AUC_{(0-t)}$:
   - $AUC_{(0-\infty)} = AUC_{(0-t)} + AUC$ "tail"
6. AUC "tail" $= C_t / \lambda_z$, where:
   - C_t is the last detectable concentration, and
   - λ_z is the terminal elimination rate constant (see Figure 58-9)

---

minimum toxic concentration (MTC) and 2 µg/mL represents the MEC (Fig 53-8), formulation A, although effective, may also present safety concerns, while formulation B produces concentrations well above the MEC but never reaches toxic levels.

TIME OF PEAK CONCENTRATION—The second parameter of importance is the measurement of the length of time necessary to achieve the maximum concentration after drug administration. This parameter is called the time of peak blood concentration (T_{max}). In Figure 53-7, for formulation A, the time necessary to achieve peak blood concentration is 1 hour. For formulation B, T_{max} is 4 hours. This parameter is related closely to the rate of absorption of the drug from a formulation and may be used as a simple measure of rate of absorption but is normally not evaluated statistically.

To illustrate the importance of T_{max}, suppose that the two curves in Figure 53-8 now represent two formulations of an analgesic and that in this case the minimum effective concentration is 2 µg/mL. Formulation A will achieve the MEC in 30 minutes; formulation B does not achieve that concentration until 2 hours. Formulation A would produce analgesia much more rapidly than formulation B and would probably be preferable as an analgesic agent. On the other hand, if one were more interested in the duration of the analgesic effect than on the time of onset, formulation B would present more prolonged activity, maintaining serum concentrations above the MEC for a longer time (8 hours) than formulation A (5.5 hours).

AREA UNDER THE CONCENTRATION-TIME CURVE—The third, and sometimes the most important, parameter for evaluation, is the area under the serum, blood, or plasma concentration-time curve (AUC). This area is reported in amount/volume times time (eg, µg/mL × hr or g/100 mL × hr) and can be considered representative of the amount of drug absorbed following administration of a single dose of the drug.

Although several methods exist for calculating area under the concentration time curve (AUC), the trapezoidal rule method is most often used. This method assumes a linear function, $y = bt + a$, and its accuracy increases as the number of appropriate sampling intervals are increased. Table 53-1 and Figure 53-9 describes the process for calculating the AUC using the trapezoidal rule.

Returning to Figure 53-8, the curves, although much different in shape, have approximately the same areas (A = 34.4 µg/mL × hr; B = 34.2 µg/mL × hr), and both formulations can be considered to deliver the same amount of drug to the systemic circulation. Thus, one can see that AUC should not represent the only criterion on which bioequivalence is judged. All the results, as a composite, must be considered in reaching a decision about bioequivalence; no single parameter serves this purpose.

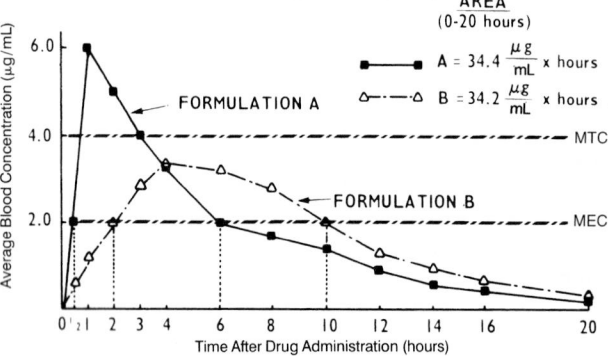

Figure 53-8. Blood concentration-time curves obtained for two different formulations of the same drug, demonstrating relationship of the profiles to the minimum toxic concentration (MTC) and the minimum effective concentration (MEC).

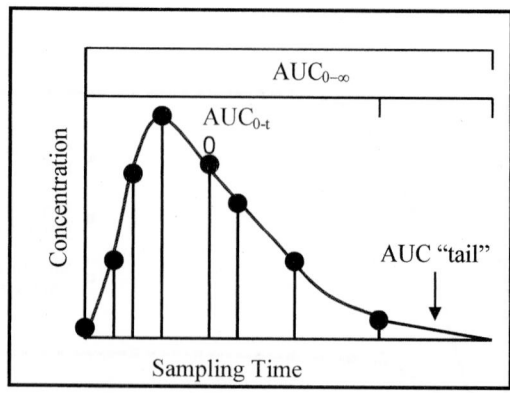

Figure 53-9. Graphical depiction using trapezoidal rule for calculating area under the concentration-time curve.

Criteria for Bioequivalence

Under the *Drug Price Competition and Patent Term Restoration Act of 1984,* manufacturers seeking approval to market a generic drug must submit data demonstrating that the drug product is bioequivalent to the pioneer (innovator) drug product. A major premise underlying the 1984 law is that bioequivalent drug products are therapeutically equivalent and, therefore, interchangeable.

The standard bioequivalence study is conducted in a crossover fashion in a small number of volunteers, usually with 24 to 36 healthy adults. The number of subjects appropriate for a bioequivalence study can be determined on the basis of previous knowledge of the drug's variability. In general, the number of subjects should be sufficient to detect 20% differences in the measured parameters, with 80% certainty. Single doses of the test and reference drugs are administered, and blood or plasma levels of the drug are measured over time. Characteristics of these concentration-time curves, such as the area under the curve (AUC) and the peak blood or plasma concentration (C_{max}) are examined by statistical procedures.

Bioequivalence of different formulations of the same drug substance involves equivalence with respect to the rate and extent of drug absorption. Two formulations whose rate and extent of absorption differ by $\pm 20\%$ or less are generally considered bioequivalent. The use of the $\pm 20\%$ criteria is based on a medical decision that for most drugs, a $\pm 20\%$ difference in the concentration of the active ingredient in blood will not be clinically significant.

To verify, for a particular pharmacokinetic parameter, that the $\pm 20\%$ criteria are satisfied, two one-sided statistical tests are carried out using the log-transformed data from the bioequivalence study. In order to interpret the statistical results, the log-transformed data must first be back-transformed. When the log-transformed data are back-transformed, the $\pm 20\%$ now becomes $-20\%/+25\%$. One test is used to verify that the lower bound of the 90% confidence interval of the average response for the generic product is no more than 20% below that of the innovator product; the other test is used to verify that the upper bound of the 90% confidence interval of the average response for the generic product is no more than 25% above that for the innovator product. The current practice is to carry out each of the two one-sided tests at the 0.05 level of significance.

Computationally, the two one-sided tests are carried out by computing a 90% confidence interval. For approval of ANDAs, in most cases, the generic manufacturer must show that a 90% confidence interval for the ratio of the mean response (usually AUC and C_{max}) of its product to that of the innovator is within the limits of 0.8 and 1.25, after the log-transformed data has been back-transformed. If the true average response of the generic product in the population is near 20% below, or 25% above, the innovator average, one or both of the confidence limits is likely to fall outside the acceptable range, and the product will fail the bioequivalence test. Thus, an approved product is likely to differ from the innovator by far less than this quantity. These same criteria are applied to other bioequivalence situations such as post-approval changes in innovator or generic products.

The current practice of carrying out two one-sided tests at the 0.05 level of significance ensures that if the two products truly differ by as much as or more than is allowed by the equivalence criteria, there is no more than a 5% chance that they will be approved as equivalent. This reflects the fact that the primary concern from the regulatory point of view is the protection of the patient against a conclusion of bioequivalence if this does not hold true. The results of a bioequivalence study usually must be acceptable for more than one pharmacokinetic parameter. As such, a generic product that truly differs by $\pm 20\%$ or more from the innovator product with respect to one or more pharmacokinetic parameters would have less than a 5% chance of being approved. Different statistical criteria may be used when bioequivalence is demonstrated through comparative

clinical trials, pharmacodynamic studies, or comparative *in vitro* methodology.

Using the two one-sided test procedures, when two drug products differ by more than 12–13% in means, they are unlikely to pass the bioequivalence confidence interval criteria of 80–125%. A study of more than 200 approved generic drugs indicated a mean bioavailability difference of only 3.5% existed. Although somewhat larger differences might meet the bioequivalence criteria, the reality is that, for generic drug products approved by FDA, observed differences have been quite small.

Fed Bioequivalence Studies

Food has been shown to alter the bioavailability of some drugs, and this alteration can have a negative impact on the interpretation of bioequivalence results between test and reference products. As a result, bioequivalence studies are usually conducted under fasting conditions. However, in some instances a fasting study may not be reasonable for a particular drug because of safety considerations or perhaps because of the drug's intended clinical indication. In these situations, a fed bioequivalence study is sometimes acceptable. A fed bioequivalence study is similar to the standard bioequivalence study except that following an overnight fast, the test and reference products are administered 30 minutes after the start of a standardized meal. The FDA currently recommends a high-fat, high-calorie meal as described in an FDA Guidance. The composition of this meal is described in Table 53-2. The same statistical criteria, as used for the standard bioequivalence study, are observed for the resultant fed bioequivalence study data.

Average Bioequivalence

The standard *in vivo* bioequivalence study design is based on administration of the test and reference products on separate occasions to healthy subjects, either in single or multiple doses, with random assignment to the two possible sequences of drug product administration. Samples of plasma or blood are analyzed for drug and/or metabolite(s) concentrations, and pharmacokinetic parameters are obtained from the resulting concentration-time curves. Parameters are analyzed statistically to determine if the test and reference products yield comparable values. Statistical analysis for pharmacokinetic parameters, such as area under the curve (AUC) and peak concentration (C_{max}), is based on the two one-sided tests procedure, which determines whether the average values for pharmacokinetic parameters measured after administration

Table 53-2. The FDA Standardized High-Fat Test Meal Composition

The example test meal would be two eggs fried in butter, two strips of bacon, two slices of toast with butter, four ounces of hash brown potatoes, and eight ounces of whole milk. Substitutions in this test meal can be made as long as the meal provides a similar amount of calories from protein, carbohydrate, and fat and has a comparable meal volume and viscosity.

MEAL COMPOSITION	ENERGY (kcal)
Protein	150
Carbohydrate	250
Fat	500–600

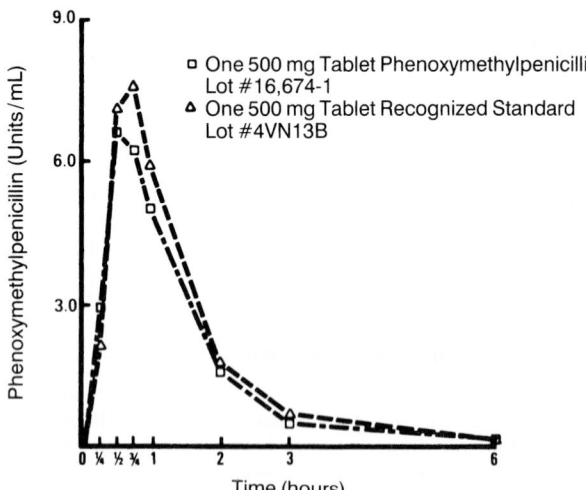

Figure 53-10. Average serum concentration of phenoxymethyl penicillin following oral administration of 500 mg given as one tablet of recognized standard (Δ) or of test product, research lot (□).

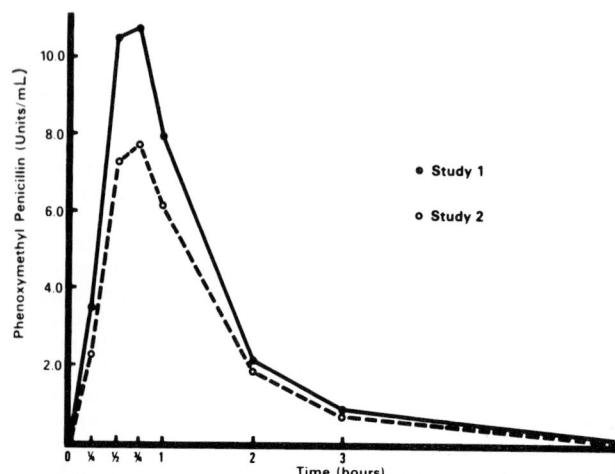

Figure 53-12. Average serum concentration of phenoxymethyl-pencillin following a single oral 500-mg dose of recognized standard, in two different subject populations.

of the test and reference products are comparable (ie, average bioequivalence). This procedure involves the calculation of a 90% confidence interval for the ratio of the averages of the test and reference product. To establish bioequivalence, the calculated confidence interval must fall within a bioequivalence limit, usually 80–125% for the ratio of the product averages. In addition to this general approach for determining bioequivalence, a 2001 FDA Guidance provides specific recommendations for (1) logarithmic transformation of pharmacokinetic data, (2) methods to evaluate sequence effects, and (3) methods to evaluate outlier data.

Population and Individual Bioequivalence

Statistically, the average bioequivalence approach focuses on the comparison of population averages of a bioavailability metric of interest and not on the variability of the metric for the test and reference products. In addition, average bioequivalence cannot describe a subject-by-formulation interaction, that is, the variation that may be present among individuals in the average test and reference difference. In contrast, population and

individual bioequivalence approaches include comparisons of both averages and variability of the study metric. The population bioequivalence approach assesses the total variability of the metric in the population. The individual bioequivalence approach assesses the within-subject variability as well as the subject-by-formulation interaction. However, due to statistical and study design issues with population and individual bioequivalence, respectively, the FDA has deferred recommending these analyses methods.

Study Design

AVERAGE OR POPULATION BIOEQUIVALENCE—A conventional, nonreplicated crossover design, such as the standard two-formulation, two-period, two-sequence crossover design, may be used to generate data for assessment of population bioequivalence. Replicated-crossover designs or parallel designs also may be used.

INDIVIDUAL BIOEQUIVALENCE—Three important parameters, the within-subject variability for the test and reference metric and subject-by-formulation interaction variability components, are integral components of the individual bioequivalence criterion. A replicated-crossover design of the bioequivalence study should be used to estimate these parameters.

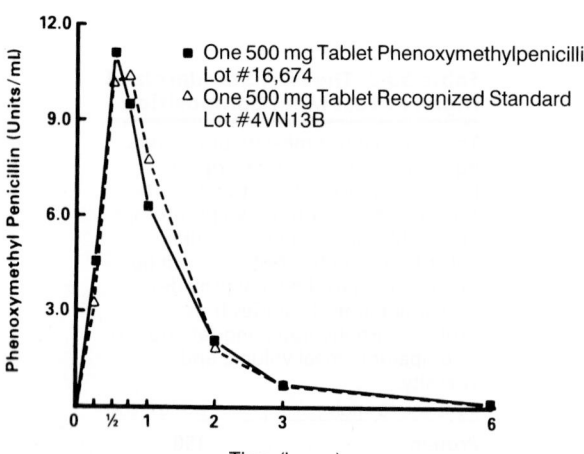

Figure 53-11. Average serum concentration of phenoxymethyl-pencillin following oral administration of 500 mg given as one tablet of recognized standard (Δ) or of test product full mfg lot (■).

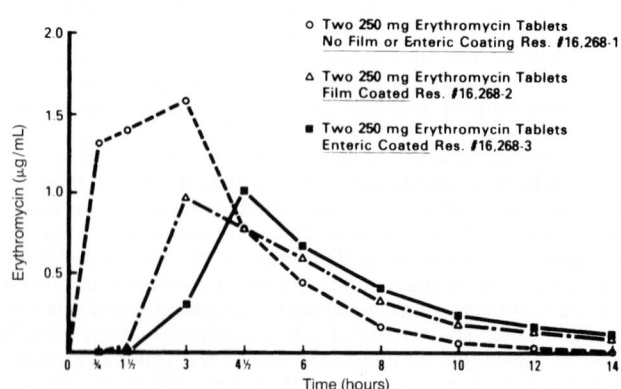

Figure 53-13. Average serum erythromycin concentration administered in 500-mg doses as three different tablet dosage forms. The results were obtained from 21 healthy adult subjects following an overnight fast of 12 hr before, and 2 hr after, drug administration.

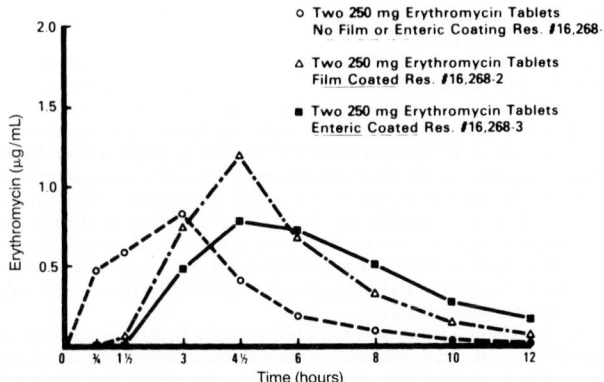

Figure 53-14. Average serum erythromycin concentration administered in 500-mg doses as three different tablet dosage forms. The results were obtained from 12 healthy adult subjects with only a 2-hr fast before drug administration.

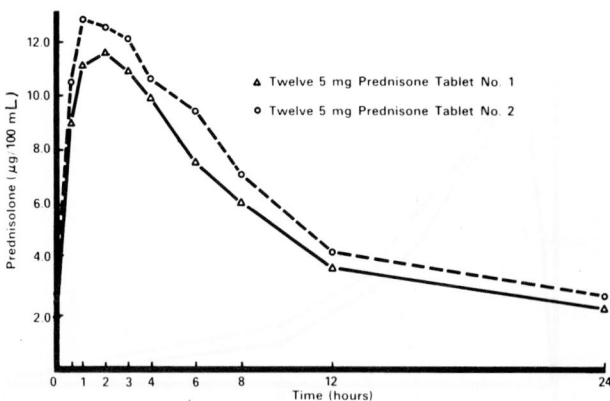

Figure 53-16. Average plasma prednisolone levels following 60 mg of prednisone administered to 24 normal adults as a single oral dose of 125-mg prednisone tablets from two different manufacturers. Plasma levels were determined by a competitive protein-binding assay.

Further information related to current FDA recommendations regarding the design and analysis of bioequivalence studies is available on the internet at http://www.fda.gov/cder/, under *Regulatory Guidance Documents*.

PITFALLS ASSOCIATED WITH CROSS-STUDY COMPARISONS—This is a situation in which the blood concentration-time curve of a drug product in one study is compared with the blood concentration-time curve of that drug product in another study. There are several reasons why such cross-study comparisons are not recommended and may lead to false conclusions. However, if no other data are available, and if important comparisons must be made, cross study comparison may be informative, keeping in mind the possible limitations. The following examples, used to illustrate these three points, are taken from actual bioavailability data.

Different Subject Population—In Figure 53-10, a research lot of potassium phenoxymethyl penicillin was compared with the appropriate reference standard for that product. The research lot drug was found to be bioequivalent, with average peak-serum concentrations differing by 8% and the area differing by only 9%. In another study conducted with a full-manufacture lot of the test product, the same lot of the reference standard potassium phenoxymethyl penicillin was used.

The results of this study are shown in Figure 53-11. Again, the two products were found to be bioequivalent, as the peak and area parameters differed by less than 5%. In these two studies, identical test conditions were used, and the same analytical procedure and laboratory was employed. However, if one compares the plasma levels for the reference standard lot found in Figure 53-10 with the levels for the same lot of tablets in the study in Figure 53-11, sizable differences in blood levels are found, as shown in Figure 53-12.

The average peak serum levels for this lot of tablets were found to be 8.5 and 12.5 units/mL in the two respective studies, a difference of approximately 31%. Likewise, the average AUC was found to differ by approximately 21%. Such apparent differences are solely the result of cross-study comparisons and are not due to differences in actual bioavailability.

The same lot of reference standard tablets was used in both studies. Hence, the difference must be due to the experimental variables that occur normally from study to study. The major difference between the two studies was the subject population involved. In the first study, healthy adult male prison volunteers were used, whereas in the second study, there were 17 females and 7 males in a hospital clinic, also described as normal, healthy volunteers. An appreciable difference in sex distribution was obvious when comparing these studies. Adjustments for body weight and surface area alone did not correct for the apparent discrepancies in peak concentration or blood level AUC. It is difficult to deter-

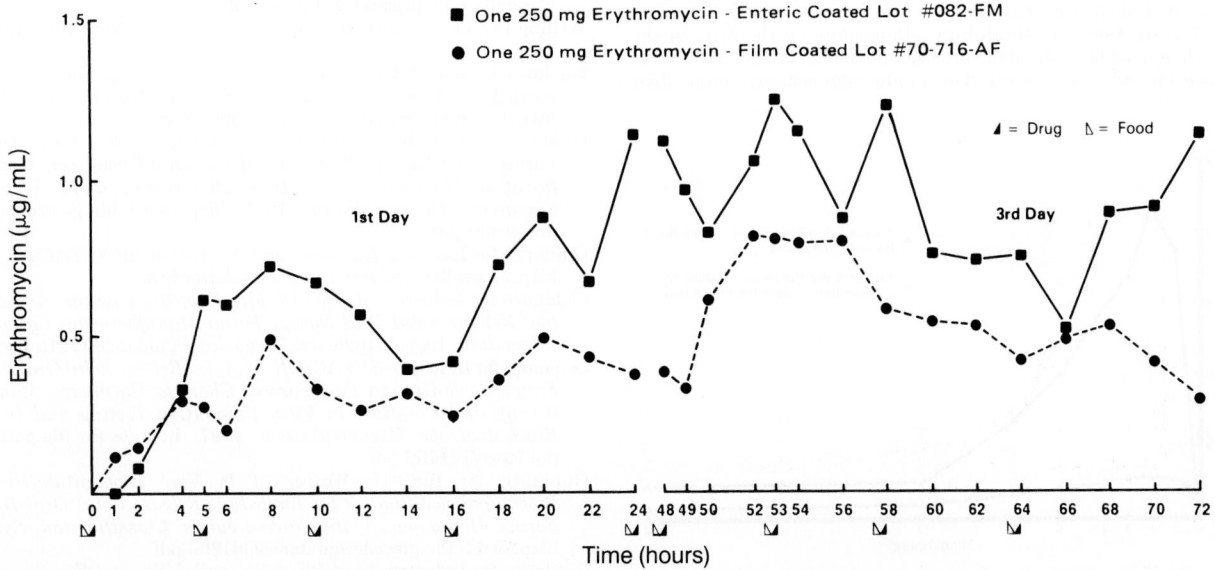

Figure 53-15. Average serum erythromycin concentration-time profiles from drug administered in two different tablet dosage forms. The results were obtained from 24 healthy adult subjects, following administration of 250 mg, four times a day, with meals and at bedtime.

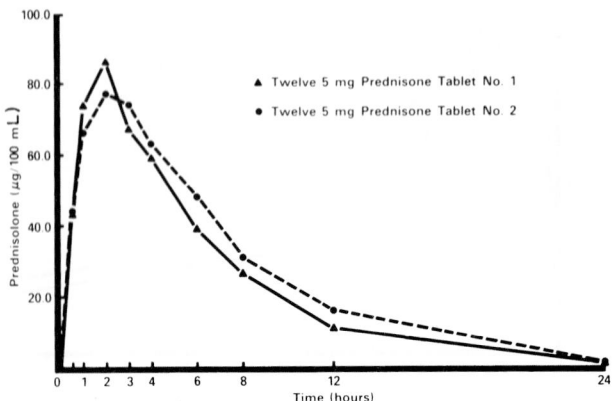

Figure 53-17. Average plasma prednisolone levels following 60 mg of prednisone administered to 24 normal adults as a single oral dose of 125-mg prednisone tablets from two different manufacturers. Plasma levels were determined by a radioimmunoassay procedure.

mine the exact factors that caused the observed differences. This example should serve as a note of caution in comparing bioavailability values of peak concentration and area under the curve from different studies.

Different Study Conditions—Parameters such as the food or fluid intake of the subject before, during, and after drug administration can have dramatic effects on the absorption of certain drugs. Figure 53-13 shows the results of a three-way crossover test in which the subjects were fasted 12 hours overnight and 2 hours after drug administration of an uncoated tablet, a film-coated tablet, or an enteric-coated tablet of erythromycin.

The results of this study suggest that the uncoated tablet is superior to both the film-coated and enteric-coated tablets in terms of blood level performance. These results also suggest that neither film coating nor enteric coating is necessary for optimal blood-level performance. Figure 53-14 shows results with the same tablets when the study conditions were changed to only a 2-hr preadministration fast with a 2-hr postadministration fast. In this case, the blood levels of the uncoated tablet were depressed markedly, while the film-coated and enteric-coated tablets showed relatively little difference in blood levels.

From this second study, it might be concluded that film coating appears to impart the same degree of acid stability as an enteric coating. This might be acceptable if only one dose of the antibiotics was required. However, Figure 53-15 shows the results of a multiple-dose study in which the enteric-coated tablet and the film-coated tablet were administered four times a day, immediately after meals. The results show that the film coating does not impart the degree of acid stability that the enteric coating does when the tablets are administered immediately after food in a typical clinical situation.

Different Assay Methodology—Depending on the drug under study, there may be more than one assay method available. For example, some steroids can be assayed by a radioimmunoassay, competitive

protein-binding, gas-liquid chromatography, or indirectly by a 17-hydroxycorticosteroid assay.

Figures 53-16 and 53-17 show the results of a comparison of prednisone tablets using a competitive protein-binding method and a radioimmunoassay, respectively. The serum concentration-time curves resulting from each method lead to the same conclusion, that the products are bioequivalent. However, Figure 53-18 shows a comparison of the absolute values obtained by the two assay methods with the same product.

Obviously, the wrong conclusion would have been reached if one product had been assayed by one method and the other product by the other method and the results had been compared. Even in cases in which only one assay method is employed, there are numerous modifications with respect to technique among laboratories that could make direct comparisons difficult.

The backbone of any bioavailability study involving plasma (or urine) levels of drug, in addition to good study design and subject controls, is the analytical methodology used to determine the levels of a drug. In most cases, one probably can assume that the precision and reliability of the method employed in a given study have been established to a sufficient degree to make the results of the study internally consistent. As demonstrated, major problems arise when, without careful evaluation of the analytical methodology employed, one attempts to compare the data of studies from different laboratories. Even with similar analytical methodology performed by the same laboratory, it would be unreasonable to expect agreement, using the same dosage form, closer than 20% to 25% for plasma levels from one study to the next.

Under the best conditions, cross-study comparisons are relatively insensitive, and at worst they can be misleading. Cross-study comparisons certainly cannot be used to make decisions or estimate differences in drug products with the generally acceptable sensitivity of difference detection of 20% or less.

BIBLIOGRAPHY

Abdou HM. *Dissolution, Bioavailability and Bioequivalence*. Easton, PA: Mack Publishing Co, 1989.

Amidon GL, Robinson JR, Williams RL. *Scientific Foundations for Regulating Drug Product Quality*. Alexandria, VA: AAPS Press, 1997.

Chow S-C. *Design and Analysis of Bioavailability and Bioequivalence Studies*. New York: Dekker, 1992.

Marston SA, et al. Evaluation of direct curve comparison metrics applied to pharmacokinetic profiles and relative bioavailability and bioequivalence. *Pharm Res* 14:1363, 1997.

Schuirmann DJ. A comparison of the two one-sided tests procedure and the power approach for assessing the bioequivalence of average bioavailability. *J Pharmacokinet Biopharm* 1987; 15:657.

Shah VP, Maibach HI. *Topical Drug Bioavailability, Bioequivalence and Penetration*. New York: Plenum, 1993.

Shargel L, Yu AB. *Applied Biopharmaceutics and Pharmacokinetics*. Norwalk, CT: Appleton & Lange, 1993.

Welling PG, et al. *Pharmaceutical Bioequivalence*. New York: Dekker, 1991.

Guidance for Industry - Extended Release Oral Dosage Forms: *Development, Evaluation, and Application of In Vitro / In Vivo Correlations*. http://www.fda.gov/cder/guidance/1306fnl.pdf

Guidance for Industry–Immediate Release Solid Oral Dosage Forms–*Scale-Up and Postapproval Changes: Chemistry, Manufacturing, and Controls, In Vitro Dissolution Testing, and In Vivo Bioequivalence Documentation*. 1995. http://www.fda.gov/cder/guidance/cmc5.pdf

Guidance for Industry–*Questions and Answers about SUPAC-IR*. 1997. http://www.fda.gov/cder/guidance/qaletter.htm

Guidance for Industry–*SUPAC-IR/MR: Immediate Release and Modified Release Solid Oral Dosage Forms Manufacturing Equipment Addendum*. 1999. http://www.fda.gov/cder/guidance/1721fnl.pdf

Guidance for Industry–*SUPAC-MR: Modified Release Solid Oral Dosage Forms Scale-Up and Postapproval Changes: Chemistry, Manufacturing, and Controls; In Vitro Dissolution Testing and In Vivo Bioequivalence Documentation*. 1997. http://www.fda.gov/cder/guidance/1214fnl.pdf

Guidance for Industry–*Waiver of In Vivo Bioavailability and Bioequivalence Studies for Immediate-Release Solid Oral Dosage Forms Based on a Biopharmaceutics Classification System*. http://www.fda.gov/cder/guidance/3618fnl.pdf

Guidance for Industry–*Food-Effect Bioavailability and Fed Bioequivalence Studies*. 2002. http://www.fda.gov/cder/guidance/5194fnl.doc

NTI Letter. *Therapeutic Equivalence of Generic Drugs Response to National Association of Boards of Pharmacy*. 1997. http://www.fda.gov/cder/news/ntiletter.htm

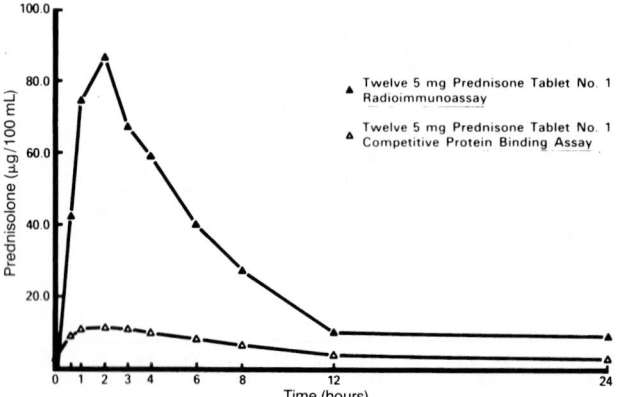

Figure 53-18. Average plasma prednisolone profiles from drug administered as a single 60-mg dose to 24 normal adults. Plasma levels were determined by both a competitive protein-binding assay and a radioimmunoassay.

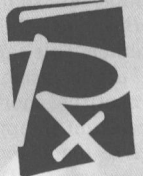

CHAPTER 54

Plastic Packaging Materials

Barrett E Rabinow, PhD

Theodore J Roseman, PhD

As defined by the American Society for Testing and Materials (ASTM), a plastic is a material that contains as an essential ingredient one or more polymeric organic substances of large molecular weight, is solid in its finished state and at some stage in its manufacture or processing into finished articles can be shaped by flow. The large-molecular-weight organic substance is called a polymer.

The use of plastics in the health care industry has grown at a very rapid rate since the 1960s. This phenomenal growth is due primarily to the wide flexibility in choice of properties offered by plastics. However, because of the wide range of properties of plastics, judicious selection must be made for the intended application.

Prior to the recognition of the potential use of plastics in health care practice, glass was the predominate material used in the primary packaging of pharmaceutical products. Glass has a definite advantage in being a relatively unreactive and an inert substance (although leachable aluminum and glass particles or delamination have occasionally posed problems). As such, it can be used in contact with many critical products, either dry or liquid. It provides excellent protection against water vapor and gas permeation, and it can withstand steam sterilization (autoclaving) without incurring physical distortion. Two definite disadvantages of glass in the field of packaging, however, are its fragility and weight. Because of these negative aspects, coupled with the many positive attributes of plastics, significant inroads for the use of plastic in pharmaceutical packaging have been made. Today, for example, plastics are being used in the following primary packaging areas, where in the 1960s only glass could be considered: syringes, bottles, vials, and ampules.

There are many other significant medical uses that, without the use of plastics, would never have been technically feasible. A few examples include indwelling catheters, prosthetic devices, tracheotomy tubes, unit dose packaging, and flexible containers for intravenous, irrigation, and inhalation solutions, as well as for the collection of blood. An additional use for plastics is in secondary container packaging (ie, packaging that is not in direct contact with the product itself). This particular use normally involves plastic films of various types and thicknesses used for tamper-proof overwrapping, whereas the previously mentioned devices normally are fabricated by molding or extrusion of the finished part.

Selection of the appropriate materials for a packaging application should be performed with an understanding of the intended overall design of the package. The requirements should be specified with regard to customer usage, regulatory approval, marketing presentation, toxicological considerations, manufacturability, sterility, and, very importantly, protection of the pharmaceutical product or device during transportation, storage, and use. These functional requirements then must be analyzed in terms of the stress requirements they impose on the material, permitting translation of those requirements into material properties. A target material profile is developed by assigning required values of design and performance properties that predict or correlate with the container functions. Likely candidate materials are determined by comparing their properties with the property profile derived from the functional requirements. A prototype is built and tested via functionally oriented tests such as maintenance of product stability, simulated usage and storage tests, and customer focus groups. These concepts are embodied in ISO 11607.[1] Material properties affecting functional performance are described below.

MATERIAL PROPERTIES

Mechanical Properties

Important mechanical properties in plastic packaging materials are:

Tensile strength—the maximum force needed to pull apart a specimen of material, divided by its cross-sectional area. Elongation is the percentage change over original length at breaking point and measures a film's ability to stretch.

Impact strength—a measure of the ability to withstand shock-loading, in which a specimen receives a blow from a swinging pendulum, for example. Fracture will occur if the impact force exceeds the limit of elasticity of the material. Glass, for example, has a much lower impact strength than many plastics, although it has appreciable tensile strength.

Tear strength—measured both as the force necessary to initiate a tear and force to propagate a tear. Propagation of tear is undesirable in shipping sacks but desirable in tear tapes. Orientation of the material can affect results, because the polymer chains can be aligned along a particular direction during manufacturing, thus conferring greater strength in that direction.

Stiffness—the resistance of bending where deflection against a load can be measured.

Flex resistance to the development of pinholing and fracture, when subjected to repeated flexing or creasing, is important in shipping applications. Unsupported aluminum foil, unless it is heavy gauge, is prone to this failure mode.

Coefficient of friction or *slip*—relates to the ease with which one material will slide over another. Passage of films through packaging machinery requires high slip to prevent binding and is important in form–fill-seal operations.

Blocking—the tendency of two adjacent layers of film to stick together. This can create difficulties during manufacturing.

Fatigue resistance, or the ability to withstand the imposition of repetitive short-time stress or deformation without cracking, is relevant in applications involving continual cyclical loading, such as toggle mechanisms, gear teeth of a pump, or peristaltic compression of IV tubing.

Creep failure occurs when a plastic is subjected to a constant static load; it deforms quickly and elastically (reversibly) to a predicted strain value and then continues to deform at a slower rate indefinitely. Rupture may eventually occur. Creep is both temperature and time dependent. The design life of the package thus plays a role, because both strength and stiffness may be time related. The loss of torque of a static bottle-closure system over time or deformation of plastic IV tubing under constant compression are examples.

Other properties of plastics may affect their usage in a particular application. For example, low-temperature mechanical behavior is important if a plastic is exposed to freezing temperatures during its use, since the impact strength of certain plastics decreases in the frozen state. The density of plastics, which varies between 0.8 and 1.8 g/cm^3, is an important property, since lower-density materials will produce more items per unit weight. Additionally, the melting point, which may extend over a range of temperatures, is important for determining processing temperatures, heat sterilizability, ability to hot-fire a product, and heat-sealing characteristics.

Additional mechanical properties are characteristic of component subsystems or of the entire package:

Hot tack—the ability of a heat seal to remain intact as it cools down from its sealing temperature, thus preserving package integrity.

Abrasion and shock test measures the interactive effects of abrasion and shock on a form-fill-seal package.

Optical Properties

Important optical properties in plastic packaging materials are:

Light transmission—the ratio of the intensity of a light source measured with the film interposed to the intensity without the film. It gives no indication of image distortion or blurring.

Clarity—the degree of distortion of an object seen through the film.

Haze—a measure of milkiness caused by light scattering by surface imperfections or film inhomogeneities such as crystallites, voids, cross-linked materials, and undissolved additives. Haze obscures visibility for product inspection.

Gloss—measures specular reflection, or the reflectance of light as a mirror reflects. This parameter indicates the ability to produce a sharp image of any light source, giving rise to a pleasing sparkle of the film.

Electrical Properties

Electrical properties can be important, as for the dissipation of static charge in the operating room. This was previously of greater concern when ether was used more widely as an anesthetic and poured from a bottle, resulting in a potential fire hazard. More importantly, static electricity is a hazard to electronic equipment and devices. In addition, dirt and dust are attracted by static to the surface and increase the chance of contamination.

PHYSICOCHEMICAL PROPERTIES

Mass Transfer

Many pharmaceutical preparations must be protected adequately from oxygen, water vapor, carbon dioxide, and other permeants. An effervescent tablet requires a barrier to moisture, for example, whereas an oil-based product must be protected from oxygen-induced oxidation. Unlike glass, plastics are permeable. Barrier properties indicate permeability to water vapor, oxygen, carbon dioxide, etc. In addition, components of the product can permeate through the package. Examples include stabilizing agents such as parabens or antibacterials, flavorants, water vapor, and oils.

Permeation through a plastic barrier depends on the composition of the plastic, permeation area, thickness of the barrier, partial pressure differential of the permeant across the barrier, and time. Fick's law of diffusion describes these phenomena mathematically. Permeation through a plastic also can be affected greatly by additives and the crystalline structure of the plastic. Specific additives, primarily plasticizers, can increase the permeation rate greatly. Highly crystalline plastics such as polypropylene generally exhibit low water-permeation rates. An increase in the size (eg, diameter, molar volume) of a penetrant in a series of chemically similar penetrants generally leads to an increase in solubility and a decrease in diffusion coefficient. Since the permeability coefficient is related to the product of these, its variation with penetrant size is often much less.[2]

As a guide, the approximate relative permeation rates for water vapor, oxygen, and carbon dioxide through the more commonly used plastics in packaging are given in Table 54-1.[3] More extensive compilations of permeation rates for a variety of migrating molecules can be found in the *Polymer Handbook.*[4] The total ingress of gas into a package can be divided into contributions from the separate components, for example, permeation through the lid, bottle, and outer protective overpouch and gross leakage through microscopic cracks and pinholes. This analysis can be performed kinetically to verify container integrity or to resolve manufacturing problems.[5]

Chemical Attack

Resistance to acids, alkalies, fats, solvents, water, and light are important if compatibility with these materials is required. Some plastics are incompatible with plasticizers used with PVC polymers, lipid emulsions, detergents, or antiseptic solutions. Iodine-containing liquids permanently stain many polyolefin compounds after a brief exposure. Absorption of the migrating

Table 54-1. Permeability Rates of Selective Plastic Packaging Materials

PLASTIC	G/100 IN^2/ 24 HR/MIL @ 37.8°C WATER VAPOR	CC/100 IN^2/MIL/24 HR/ ATM @ 25°C OXYGEN	CARBON DIOXIDE
Nylon			
Type 6	16–22	2.6	10–12
Type 12	4	34–92	153–336
Polyethylene terephthalate	1.0–1.3	3.0–6.0	15–25
Polyethylene			
Low density	1.0–1.5	500	2700
Medium density	0.7	250–535	1000–2500
High density	0.3	185	580
Polypropylene	0.7	150–240	500–800
Polystyrene	7–10	250–350	900
Vinyl			
Nonplasticized	2–5	4–30	4–30
Plasticized	15–40	600	20–500
Vinyl chloride-acetate copolymer			
Nonplasticized	4	15–20	40–70
Plasticized	5–8	20–150	70–800
Polyvinylidene chloride	0.2–0.6	0.8–6.9	3.8–44
Polycarbonate	11	300	1075

From *Modern Plastics Encyclopedia,* vol 64. New York: McGraw-Hill, 1987, p. 554.

chemical forces the polymer chains apart, swells the plastic, and causes stress cracking. This can occur, as well, from solvents used to solvent-bond plastic components.

Rubber exposed to ozone, as from electrostatic dust precipitators, will lose elasticity and become brittle. In this case, chemical reaction of the ozone with the polymer backbone is responsible. Another failure mode involves simply the leaching of components, such as silicone lubricant from rubber syringe plungers, into the contained solution. This increases the particulate burden and can form a visual haze. In some instances pigmentation used in the plastic is attacked chemically and leached by the product.

In the case of plastics used in direct contact with a product— in either dry or liquid form—the length of time that the medication and the container are in contact may determine if problems such as discoloration, leaching, and absorption or adsorption of a constituent of the product may arise. It is possible that both the product and the package containing it could change significantly from the time of manufacture. Lack of visual indication of a reaction at the onset of a stability study does not imply that the reaction(s) was not occurring during the early stages of storage.

In certain instances, a specific set of storage parameters must exist before a reaction is initiated. For many drugs, generally the higher the temperature and humidity in the storage area, the more rapid the chemical attack. For many IV solutions in flexible plastic containers, however, shelf life is limited by water-vapor loss, which is diminished in the presence of high humidity. Other factors that may affect the plastic packaging and product are pH, surface treatment of the plastic, container configuration, type of polymer used, method of package preparation, light transmission, and means of assembly or sterilization.[6]

Theory and experiment have been developed sufficiently to permit prediction of the maximal accumulation of leachables in solution without waiting for the results of shelf-life stability studies. This expedites product development and addresses material/solution compatibility concerns. Accumulation of a leachable material from a container into solution can be limited by any of four physical factors[7]:

1. The initial amount of leachable material present in the container material (total available pool, TAP)
2. The solubility limit of the leachable material in the solution phase
3. The equilibrium partitioning of the leachable component between the container and the solution
4. The rate of migration of the leachable component from the container into solution

The TAP, solubility limit, and equilibrium partitioning can be evaluated for each identified leachable substance. These characteristics then can be used to identify the process that would limit the accumulation of leachable chemicals. The lowest value found determines the limiting accumulation and identifies the limiting mechanism. The solubility limit, equilibrium partitioning, and rate of migration may restrict actual solution accumulation below the total available pool estimate. Kinetic control produces the minimum accumulation estimate, since no matter how fast the rate of migration, a leachable component cannot accumulate in excess of what is thermodynamically available. As an example, the equilibrium solution accumulation of a leachable material, C_e, is given by

$$C_e = (TAP \times W_c)/[(W_c \times E_b) + V_s]$$

where TAP is the µg leachable/g of film, W_c is the weight of the container (in grams), V_s is the solution volume (in liters), and E_b is the equilibrium partitioning constant, the ratio of the concentration of solute in the film to that in water at equilibrium. This can be calculated from the more familiar, and referenced, solvent-solvent partition coefficients. This methodology also can be used to predict the extent of the reverse process, that of adsorption of solution components (drugs or antimicrobial agents) into the plastic.[8]

The concept of solid/liquid partition coefficients is discussed in Chapter 33, *Chromatography*. Similarly, liquid/liquid partition coefficients are discussed in Chapter 36, *Separation*. Additional consideration of failure modes for pharmaceutical applications may be found in Chapter 52, *Stability of Pharmaceutical Products*.

Safety Testing

Numerous testing procedures must be followed to ensure the safety of use of any plastic. Among these are biological, chemical, physical, and pharmacological assessments. A greater degree of safety testing is warranted as the extent of contact of the material with the body increases. Thus, an IV solution container is studied in greater depth than is secondary packaging. Medical devices that are left intact in the human body for prolonged periods of time (vascular grafts, cartilage replacements, pacemakers, or prosthetics) are studied most extensively. Their reactivity and degree of safety and toxicity must be determined. In all cases, it is imperative that the plastic and its processing procedure provide a nonreactive and nontoxic end product.

The official compendia provide procedures for performing certain biological and physicochemical tests on plastic containers; for details, see the United States Pharmacopeia (USP). The principles of these tests are described in the following sections.

BIOLOGIC TESTING PROCEDURES—USP General Chapter <87> and <88> Biological Reactivity determine the suitability of plastic materials intended for use in fabricating containers or accessories for both parenteral and ophthalmic preparations. The procedures for the former determine the reaction of living animal tissues and normal animals to implanted portions of the plastic or injected extracts prepared from it. Depending on the use of the plastic, other biological tests may be performed, such as pyrogenicity, blood compatibility, antigenicity, suitability for use in cardiovascular devices, gene-toxicity reaction, and tissue-toxicity testing.

PHYSIOCHEMICAL TESTING PROCEDURES— Many chemical and physical tests are applied to plastics, the particular ones used depending on the intended applications of the substances. USP General Chapter <661> Physicochemical Testing specifies the physical and chemical properties of plastics used as containers, based on tests with extracts prepared by heating samples with Water for Injection at 70° for 24 hr. Portions of the extract are used to determine Nonvolatile Residue, Residue on Ignition, Heavy Metals, and Buffering Capacity or Reaction, official limits for each of which are specified. Also described is a procedure for determining the light transmission of plastics, with limits for maximum transmission. USP General Chapter <381> Elastomeric Closures and <661> and <671> Moisture Permeation are relevant for the final container/closure system fabricated from the materials. Drug contacting materials must also meet the chemical standards embodied in 21 CFR Part 175 and Part 177 Indirect Food Additives Section. Additionally, the Food and Drug Administration (FDA) has published a guidance document, "Container Closure Systems for Packaging Human Drugs and Biologics," dated May 1999.

The actual product/package should be evaluated under simulated use conditions, including shipping and storage, to ensure product integrity throughout its shelf life. Potential incompatibilities between the primary plastic container and secondary packaging should be addressed to anticipate adulteration of the product. Prolonged exposure to ultraviolet light has been shown to enhance the migration of certain additives that in turn can accelerate the aging characteristics of the plastic and decrease the shelf life of the product. In some instances, incompatibilities that might occur readily can be detected visually; in others, sophisticated extraction techniques must be followed to ascertain the effects storage conditions may have had. For this reason, well-planned stability studies need to be established.

Desirable features used for health care packaging are transparency, thermal stability, physical strength, formability, sealability, biological barrier, radiation resistance, and disposability. Usually one cannot find all the desired properties in a single material, but two or more plastics can be combined into a composite packaging material.

Failure Mode Analysis

After development and subsequent distribution of plastic-packaged items, functional problems may occur occasionally. Resolution of these problems requires analysis of the causative-failure mode. This involves problem isolation, segregating the problem material to a particular batch, for example, to identify potential causative factors. The failed parts are subjected to mechanical, microscopic, and chemical analysis for further determination of how they differ from acceptable parts. The analytical techniques chosen are dictated by the observed mode of failure.

Physical tests, such as mechanical, electrical, and optical determinations, can be performed quickly, and control values exist in the form of manufacturers' specifications, which are readily available. As the problem becomes more precisely focused, more specific and often elaborate testing is performed to isolate the cause further. For example, reduced stiffness of a part may be attributable to lowered molecular weight of the plastic. Microscopic analysis is rapid, and a skilled analyst often can identify the problem as a pinhole, improper seal, delamination of a composite material, or foreign material acting as a stress fracture initiator.

Chemical analysis of impurities that may cause bloom or prevent seal formation is often time consuming because of the tiny amounts present, the large variety of potential compounds, and a lack of control information from the supplier. The expense and variety of chemical instrumentation available requires judicious selection of the approach to be used.

CLASSIFICATION

There are over 100 different polymer types available for use that can be classified further into two subcategories. These are identified as thermoplastics and thermosets (thermosetting plastics). Thermoplastics consist of those plastics that normally are rigid at operating temperatures but can be remelted and reprocessed. Thermosets consist of those plastics that, when subjected to heat, normally will become infusible or insoluble, and as such cannot be remelted.

ADDITIVES AND MODIFIERS

Thermoplastics can be modified greatly and have their properties enhanced by the addition of specific additives. As chemicals may act synergistically, any two safe additives may have the potential to produce undesirable effects when combined. For these reasons, the FDA requires that these blends or combinations be evaluated totally, prior to marketing in product form. Chemical, pharmacological, and biological tests should be conducted to establish safety. Problems involving additives include migration to the surface of molded parts and leaching into aqueous solutions. Additives used routinely in thermoplastic formulations are discussed below.

Lubricants are used to assist processing of the plastic during the molding or extrusion operation, facilitating flow in contact with metal surfaces. A commonly used lubricant in the case of polyethylene is zinc stearate. The quantities employed vary from formulation to formulation.

Stabilizers are used to retard or prevent degradation of the polymer by heat and light during manufacturing as well as to improve its aging characteristics. Common stabilizer families include organometallic compounds, fatty acid salts, and inorganic oxides.

Antioxidants are a special type of stabilizer used to retard oxidation, by inhibiting formation of free radicals. Examples are aromatic amines, hindered phenolics, thioesters, and phosphites. Combinations of antioxidants with other additives may result in undesirable chemical reactions. Recent technology permits introduction of a desiccant directly into plastic packaging for protection of moisture-sensitive products. The process involves entraining a desiccant in the polymer stream for molding into a container wall. It is intended for medical diagnostic and test-strip kits, effervescent drugs, and nutritional products.[9] Some work also has been done with adding the antioxidant vitamin E to plastic packaging,[10] permitting food to taste fresh for longer times. Oxygen scavengers can be incorporated directly into films, closure liners, and container walls and customized to the required oxygen-absorbing capacity.[11]

Plasticizers are used to achieve softness, flexibility, and melt flow during processing. They are used commonly in plastic materials such as vinyls, cellulosics, and propionates. The most common are high boiling liquids, usually phthalates, of which dioctyl phthalate is the most popular.

Antistatic agents are used to prevent the buildup of static charges on the plastic surface.

Slip agents are added primarily to polyolefins (polyethylene and polypropylene) to reduce the coefficient of friction of the material. These particular chemicals result in antitack and antiblock characteristics in the end product.

Dyes and pigments are added to impart color.

Surface treatments of film, by corona discharge or deposition of thin layers of other plastics, improve such properties as ink adherence, adherence to other films, heal sealability, or gas barrier.

PROCESSING

Besides the addition of additives, the manner in which a plastic is formed into the desired configuration can affect the end properties. It is important that process parameters, such as temperature, pressure, and time, be controlled rigidly to ensure batch-to-batch uniformity for plastic objects. If process parameters are not controlled adequately, such deleterious effects on plastic properties as thermal degradation, piece-part stresses, and incorrect physical dimensions may result. Process thermal degradation of a plastic can affect the leaching characteristics of the plastic object, its permeation characteristics, and its long-term stability during the shelf life of the pharmaceutical product. Piece-part stresses may be relieved when the pharmaceutical package is subjected to certain environmental conditions, resulting in package failure during the shelf life of the product. Small stress fractures in the flange of thermoformed trays, introduced during the thermoforming process, for example, may compromise sterility.

The more common plastic-processing methods employed for pharmaceutical packaging components follow.

Injection Molding

Injection molding is an intermittent process, the plastic being heated to a melted or viscous state and then forced into a cavity (mold) at high pressure. The melted material cools in the cavity and solidifies. The mold is then opened and the part removed. A wide range of thermoplastic and several thermosetting materials can be injection molded. Besides threads on bottle caps, very intricate configurations can be obtained by injection molding of plastics.

Extrusion

Extrusion is a continuous process, the plastic being heated to a melted or viscous state and forced under pressure through a die, resulting in a configuration of desired shape. A slit-shaped die will result in a plastic sheet, and a circular die will yield a tube of plastic. The extruded profile is cooled to a solid state, generally by spraying with or immersion in water, or by using chilled rolls for film material. A wide range of thermoplastic materials can be extruded. Typical extruded profiles used by the pharmaceutical industry are packaging films and medical tubing. Plastic packaging film also is formed by blow extrusion, an extruded tube being blown into a large cylinder and then slit after cooling.

Besides simply imparting a new shape to the molten plastic, the manufacturing process can preferentially orient the molecular chains in a given direction, by stretching the plastic. This in turn affects physical properties such as clarity and impact strength, as the chains are oriented along the load-bearing direction. Crystallites can be formed and oriented to yield increases in strength, albeit at reduction in elongation at break. Barrier properties are improved for polypropylene. Biaxially oriented film has balanced properties if the same extent of stretching is used in each direction. In cast film, orientation in the machine direction is achieved by feeding the film through a series of rolls running at gradually increasing speeds. Rolls are heated sufficiently to bring the film to suitable temperature below the melting point. Transverse orientation is obtained by use of a tenter frame, which has two divergent endless belts fitted with clips. These grip the film, so that as it travels forward, it is drawn transversely at the required draw ratio. Uniaxial orientation is used for high-performance tape.

Composite Film Manufacture

Multilayer plastic structures permit incorporation of disparate properties not otherwise obtainable from one material. These include tailoring of gas barrier, heat sealability, strength, and adhesion to other materials such as paper. They are made by the basic methods of coating, lamination, and coextrusion. Coatings are applied to films as dispersions, as solutions in organic solvents, or as molten material. In metallization, coatings of aluminum are applied by vaporization of the molten metal under vacuum and condense on moving film. Lamination is the most versatile process, permitting joining together of paper and foil, in addition to thermoplastics. Preformed dissimilar films are joined together with heat and adhesives, such as vinyl acetate or polyurethanes. Coextrusion is less expensive than lamination, where applicable, forming the composite structure without separately creating the component webs. From multiple extruders, separate streams of different molten polymers are simultaneously fed to a die that joins them while preventing their intermixing.

Blow Molding

The plastic is heated to a melted or viscous state and formed into a hollow cylinder (parison) either by extrusion or injection molding. If extruded, the parison is cut to the required length and transferred to the blowing cavity (mold). The bottom of the parison is pinched off by the mold, and air is blown into the parison, expanding the viscous plastic to the walls of the cavity, thus forming the desired container shape. The melted material cools in the cavity and solidifies. The mold is opened, and the container removed. Pharmaceutical bottles are blow molded from a wide range of thermoplastic materials, among which polyethylene and polypropylene predominate.

Solvent Casting

A liquid suspension of rubber is deposited on an endless belt, and the solvent is vaporized. The belt carries the rubber material through a heat cabinet to cure it, whereupon the film is stripped off the belt, cooled, and wound onto reels.

Compression Molding

Compression molding is used for thermosetting materials and is an intermittent process. The thermosetting material (powder or a tablet preform) is placed into a heated cavity (mold). The material melts and flows to fill the cavity. The mold is held under pressure until the thermosetting material cures, after which the mold is opened and the part removed. As with injection molding, very intricate configurations can be obtained by compression molding of thermosetting materials.

TYPES AND USES

The following types of plastics are used commonly in healthcare practice; several of their properties and end uses are indicated.

Thermoplastics

The following are used commonly in injection molding, blow molding, extrusion, and fabricated sheeting.

POLYETHYLENE—This polymer, PE, has the molecular structure $(CH_2)_n$ and is the most pervasively used because it affords essential properties for the least cost. The properties of polyethylene vary according to molecular weight and type: low-density (LDPE) or branched, and high-density (HDPE) or linear. The length and number of side-chain branches determine the degree of crystallinity and density. The linear type has a more regular molecular structure, hence is more crystalline, and therefore is stronger, stiffer, more heat resistant, less permeable to gases, and more resistant to oils than LDPE. Additionally, as crystallinity and density increase, opacity, tensile strength, surface hardness, and chemical resistance increase. Silicone oil and surfactants, however, can act as stress-crack agents, leading to crack formation in stressed areas, as the permeants spread apart the polymeric chains.

Both LDPE and HDPE have relatively low water absorption, excellent electrical resistance, and high resistance to most solvents and chemicals and are tasteless and odorless. PE is thus well suited to many applications in which only moderate-to-low heat exposure will be encountered. Its use ranges from containers for liquid or dry products to both laminated and unsupported films for sterile-device packaging and to molded parts for a variety of devices and equipment. Unsupported polyethylene is used for shrink wrapping, stretch wrapping, skin packaging, and bags.

With more tightly packed molecules HDPE has better moisture-barrier properties with less elongation (better tensile strength) than LDPE. It is used widely, when rigidity and barrier properties are preferred, for bottles of solid dosage form products. However, LDPE is used when flexibility is required, for squeeze bottles of sprays and drops, as well as drum liners for bulk solid drugs. Blown films of LDPE have very low haze and high gloss, whereas HDPE films have higher haze, because of crystal-induced light scattering, and are semiglossy. The less crystalline LDPE has a lower melting point with broader melting range than does HDPE and, therefore, is easier to heat seal. The low melting point, however, negates steam sterilization for LDPE, unlike HDPE.

Polyethylene is used as a primary packing film, but its use as a sealant, through the application of heat and pressure, is more important. This application requires strong seals to be made at low temperature that have good hot tack (ie, to maintain seal integrity as the temperature cools). For this purpose, linear low density polyethylene (LLDPE)is used. This resin has reduced side chain branching and combines the clarity and density of LDPE with the toughness of HDPE. These characteristics arise from the molecular structure, resulting from the reaction of HDPE with unsaturated comonomers such as butene, hexene, or octene. The incompatibility of these two types of polymers inhibits the sealant layer from forming a complete bond, by reducing the number of available bonding sites and thereby reducing the interfacial adhesion. On the other hand, by narrowing the molecular weight range of LLDPE, one can produce film with the same strength at a lower gauge, thus saving cost.[12]

ETHYLENE-VINYL ACETATE (EVA)—Addition of vinyl acetate comonomer to ethylene reduces polymer crystallinity, improving clarity, low-temperature flexibility and toughness, impact strength, and stress-crack and flex-crack resistance and reducing hardness. Melting and heat-seal temperatures are lowered, as are the barrier properties. Increased vinyl acetate concentration also increases polarity, resulting in increased tackiness and adhesion to a variety of substrates. The copolymer also can be cross-linked (chemical bonds form between the polymer chains) by either radiation or addition of organic peroxides. This increases the melting temperature, permitting autoclaving as a sterilization option. Adding vinyl acetate softens the material, resulting in a smoother surface. The copolymer EVA is used in tip protectors, where flex resistance is required, and for low-temperature IV bags.

The two main characteristics controlled in the copolymerization of vinyl acetate and ethylene are crystallinity and molecular weight. Molecular weight is controlled by the addition of radical chain-transfer agents. As the molecular weight of EVA increases, so does the melt viscosity, heat-seal strength, toughness, flexibility, stress-crack resistance, and hot-tack strength. One of the leachables is acetic acid, resulting from the hydrolysis of the acetate esters.

POLYPROPYLENE—Propylene (PP) is clearer than HDPE, and it is stronger, stiffer, and more heat resistant than LDPE. This material is available as the highly crystalline, isotactic polypropylene and the higher-impact grades of atactic and syndiotactic types. *Isotactic* refers to a plastic with the organic groups (R) on the same side of the polymer chain. *Syndiotactic* refers to the alternation of organic groups above and below the polymer chain, and *atactic* signifies no regular sequences of the groups.

Polypropylene is used widely for packaging of solid dosage products. Injection-molded bottles, for example, can be made either with separate lids or with integrally molded lids, which exhibit high flexural strength. Compared to PE, PP offers better resistance to oils, odors, and less tendency to absorb antimicrobial agents agents from bactericidal solutions.

Polypropylenes can be modified with polyethylene or rubber to improve their impact resistance. Higher levels of ethylene lower stiffness and improve clarity. Biaxial orientation also will improve its clarity and mechanical properties, but is difficult to heat seal. It is, however, the nonoriented cast copolymer that is most used for health care packaging. Devices made of this material can be sterilized with steam and ethylene oxide but not radiation, unless modified polypropylenes are used.

The low density polypropylene offers an economic advantage, as more molds can be made from a given weight of the material. Nucleating agents may be added to speed the rate of crystallization, thus shortening the molding cycle, resulting in more economical manufacturing processes and cheaper products.

Because polypropylene is largely chemically resistant, it cannot be solvent bonded. It can, nevertheless, be heat bonded. Bonding by use of adhesives requires surface pretreatment using corona, plasma or flame, or chemical etching. It can be made heat sealable by applying a coating of polyvinylidene chloride or ethylene-polypropylene copolymer.

CYCLIC OLEFIN COPOLYMERS—Cyclic Olefin Copolymers (COCs) represent a new resin family. The resulting films for blister packs combine a high moisture barrier with the easy forming and sealing properties of polyolefins such as PE. A co-extruded PP/COC structure offers a gas and water vapor transmission rate equivalent to polyvinylidene dichloride without the halogens.[13]

POLYVINYL CHLORIDE—Polyvinyl chloride (PVC) commonly called vinyl, is next to HDPE the most widely used plastic for drug packaging, largely because of clarity, low cost, and great fabrication flexibility. The term vinyl comes from the monomer structural group (CH_2=CH—), which has many derivatives, such as vinyl chloride (CH_2=$CHCl$), vinyl acetate (CH_2=$COCOCH_3$), and vinylidene chloride (CH_2=CCl_2, Saran). With this group of vinyl compounds, many polymers are made either as homopolymers of themselves or as copolymers with other vinyl derivatives or other monomeric materials. For example, polyvinylidene chloride (PVDC) resins are, for the most part, copolymers of vinylidene chloride with vinyl chloride, acrylonitrile, and acrylate esters. These are used primarily where high barrier properties to moisture, oxygen, and other chemicals are required.

The versatile vinyl plastics are used to prepare materials ranging from soft, flexible sheeting to rigid, hard tubing. The great variety of PVC resins, with their wide range of physical properties, led to the development of many applications of this material in the fields of pharmacy and medicine. It is used in the manufacture of blood bags, examination gloves, IV solution containers, and pump tubing. An unplasticized form is used in the fabrication of rigid parts for devices. Because unplasticized PVC has glass-like clarity, is inexpensive, and has excellent thermoformability, it makes an appealing blister pack, where it has a dominant market position for the plastic component. It finds limited use in packaging devices because it turns brown when exposed to radiation sterilization and is too heat sensitive for steam sterilization, and degassing ethylene oxide is too lengthy. However, more than 25% of all plastic-based medical devices used in hospitals are made of PVC, because of its weldability, cost, response to heat and pressure, and versatility.[14]

PVC is used in clear bottles rather than HDPE for reasons of better clarity, gloss, better odor barrier, or absorption of fewer flavor components. HDPE, however, can be autoclaved and does not require the extensive additive package of PVC, involving antioxidants, etc.[15]

Flexible PVC has excellent impact and flex-crack resistance at room temperature. As the temperature is lowered, the material becomes stiffer, resulting in decreased flex-crack resistance and impact strength. The type and amount of plasticizer determines the temperature at which the failure mode changes from ductile to a brittle failure. For flexible medical applications such as IV bags and tubing, the plasticizer DEHP (di(2-ethylhexyl)phthalate) is used most often. Because it can leach into solution, the safety of DEHP has been studied extensively throughout the years. No long-term exposure problems have been identified.[16]

Cyclohexanone can be used to bond PVC to most materials. When bonded to DEHP-noncompatible materials, such as polycarbonate and impact-grade polystyrene, a barrier adhesive must be used.

POLYSTYRENE (PS)—This polymer is one of the oldest and most widely used plastics. Its clarity, stiffness, thermoformability and cheap cost are responsible for its use in manufacture of pharmaceutical bottles and tubes, which do not require a gas barrier.

PS has relatively low heat resistance and is attacked by a number of chemical agents, such as phthalate plasticizers in vinyl polymers, resulting in crazing (microcracks). It is available in a clear crystal grade and an increasingly popular rubber-modified impact-resistant grade, in which polystyrene is copolymerized with acrylonitrile and butadiene. The crystal versions craze during most ethylene oxide cycles, but impact grades withstand both gas and radiation sterilization. Polystyrene cannot, however, be autoclaved. While this polymer is inexpensive, the lack of impact strength in the conventional grade and poor optical properties in impact-modified grades limit its use in more demanding applications. Use in drug packaging is also declining because of its poor gas barrier and solvent resistance.

TYVEK (*DUPONT*)—This is a nonwoven, spun-bonded polyethylene that appears white, smooth, and water repellent and offers high tear strength as well as good porosity for sterilization. It is the preferred material for lidding of trays. However, it is expensive and has poor print quality, and its web varies in thickness and density. It can be used for autoclaving up to 137°. Prior to thermal disintegration, it will become translucent, indicating that its properties have been compromised. A new, nonwoven polypropylene, Securon, withstands steam sterilization over 153°.[17]

IONOMER—Ionomer is used as an inner ply in laminates, offering good heat sealing (even when the seal area is contaminated by liquid or powder) over a wide temperature range for LDPE and oriented PP. Heat sealing usually can proceed faster than by using alternate materials. Ionomers are clear, semiflexible, tough materials with good abrasion resistance, all of which are features valued in sachet and pouch packs. Their expense limits application to those areas such as seal integrity or enhanced puncture resistance where the additional cost can be justified.

Chemically, ionomers are the sodium or zinc salts of ethylene/methacrylic acid polymers. The ionic cross-links occur randomly along the long-chain polymer molecules to produce solid-state properties usually associated with polymers of high molecular weight. Heating ionomers to normal thermoplastic-processing temperatures, however, diminishes these ionic forces, allowing the material to be melt processed in conventional molding and extrusion equipment. The long-chain, semicrystalline hydrocarbon polymer imparts polyolefinic character, chemical inertness, thermal stability, and low water-vapor transmission.

FLUORINE-CONTAINING POLYMERS—Fluoropolymer-Aclar Film (polymonochlorotrifluoroethylene, PCTFE) has extremely low transmission of moisture, is transparent, and can be heat sealed, laminated, printed, thermoformed, metallized, and sterilized. Because it is the most expensive plastic used in the pharmaceutical industry, it is employed only where the most demanding barrier properties are required. Laminated Aclar/PVC sheet is used widely in thermoformed blister packs for moisture-sensitive solid dosage forms.

POLYTETRAFLUOROETHYLENE—Polytetrafluoroethylene (PTFE) or Teflon offers exceptional chemical resistance, compelling its use as a liner for rubber stoppers to protect the package contents from adulteration by stopper components.

POLYURETHANE FOAMS—Polyurethane foams are formed by polymerization in the presence of a foaming agent, which evolves carbon dioxide, and have been used as a replacement for cotton wool in tablet containers. The polyurethane is however light sensitive, thus limiting application to opaque containers or tinted to hide light-catalyzed discoloration.

NYLONS—Nylon is the generic designation for a class of polyamides containing repeating amide groups (—CONH—) connected to methylene units (—CH$_2$—) in the structure of the polymer. They are characterized by good chemical resistance to most solvents and chemicals, with the exception of strong solutions of certain mineral acids, phenolic compounds, and strong oxidizers. Nylons can be used in the fabrication of precision parts and adapters for devices and equipment. Aerosol valves, for example, have a low wear requirement that is satisfied by nylon's low friction-bearing surfaces. Nylon also is used in the manufacture of certain high end packaging films and laminates, providing clarity and imparting excellent resistance to puncture and abrasion. Because of high cost, poor moisture barrier properties, and poor sterilization survival (it wrinkles during autoclaving and degrades upon irradiation) its success in form/fill/seal food-packaging applications has not made an impact on health-care packaging.

POLYETHYLENE TEREPHTHALATE (PET)—PET is prepared from ethylene glycol and either terephthalic acid or the dimethyl ester of terephthalic acid. Its chemical structure is p-HO(COC$_6$H$_4$COOCH$_2$CH$_2$O)$_n$H. PET exists in an amorphous state, an oriented and partially crystalline state, and a highly crystalline state. Most applications require orientation and/or crystallization to take advantage of the dramatically increased strength and improved serviceability at high temperatures that

result. PET polymers offer many advantages to the container and packaging field. Among those are its high strength, excellent clarity, low transmission rate to gas and water vapor, and sterilizability by all major modes. PET bottles are used for a wide variety of foods and beverages, as well as pharmaceutical containers. Use of PET and glycol modified PET (PETG) for liquid oral dosage form containers is described in detail in the USP.[18] Heavier gauge, semirigid, unoriented polyester is used in the manufacture of blister packs.

POLYCARBONATES—These are formed by condensation of polyphenols such as bisphenol-A with phosgene. The polymers are transparent thermoplastics (although opacifiers are added for some applications), with high strength and high temperature resistance. Because they are expensive, their use is limited to specialty applications where dimensional stability or high-impact resistance are valued, such as in rigid, transparent, blood oxygenator housings. The polycarbonates have hardness properties similar to those of metals and are being used to replace metals in numerous industrial applications. Their use is increasing, partly because of their ability to withstand radiation sterilization.

Creep-resistance is good over a broad range of temperatures, and parts can be molded consistently to tolerances of 0.002 inch/inch. They can be heat or solvent sealed, facilitating fabrication procedures, but this advantage also renders them susceptible to phthalate crazing, when placed in contact with plasticized vinyls.

ACRYLICS—This class includes the polymethacrylates, polyacrylates, and copolymers of acrylonitrile. There are many variations in this class, mainly concerned with the combinations of methacrylate and acrylate esters, as well as acrylonitrile. These plastics are characterized by clarity and unusual optical properties, low water absorption, good electrical resistivity, excellent weatherability, and fair tensile strength. Their heat resistance is low, and care should be taken to keep them below temperatures of 200°F, at which they tend to soften. Acrylics find considerable use in a multiplicity of devices employed in today's hospitals and clinics. A specific application is in the adapters used in solution-administration sets and blood-collection sets.

CELLULOSICS—To be used as a thermoplastic without charring, cellulose must be modified. The range of modification available permits a wide variety of physical characteristics, including toughness, surface gloss, good clarity, good scuff resistance, and high gas permeability. To achieve these properties, the cellulosic alcohol groups are esterified with acetate, butyrate, and/or propionate. Butyrate and propionate are chosen over acetate for applications requiring low-temperature impact strength and dimensional stability. Extruded butyrate and propionate sheeting have good gage uniformity, surface quality, brilliance, and visual effects. Propionate is selected over butyrate and acetate when increases in hardness, tensile strength, and stiffness are important. Increased plasticizer level lowers hardness, stiffness, and tensile strength but increases impact strength. Combined esters such as cellulose acetate propionate and cellulose acetate butyrate are especially popular for medical applications. This family of cellulosics is used in articles such as tubing and special trays for urological or spinal procedures, membranes in dialyzers and some filters, and IV buret housings.

Thermosets

The following are some of the commonly used compression-molded, thermosetting compounds. These plastics are used when good dimensional and temperature stability are required. Parts are fabricated by means of compression-molding techniques. The formaldehyde plastics are obtained by condensation reactions between formaldehyde and substances such as melamine, phenol, and urea.

As a family, the formaldehydes have been found to be of most use in the pharmaceutical industry as closures for glass and/or plastic containers. By virtue of high resistance to heat, they are used in specific applications where the molded part requires sterilization by steam.

Elastomeric polymers are characterized by high stretchability. This characteristic arises from an extensive, highly crosslinked, thee dimensional structure of the polymer. The more cross links, the stronger and stiffer the product. A greater frequency of unsaturated bonds in the polymer affords greater elasticity, but also poorer resistance to water and oil. The resulting mechanical properties of compressibility and resealability are desirable for parenteral container closures. Compressibility permits sealing of small irregularities in mating surfaces and reclosability affords improved sterility control following puncture after a hypodermic needle has been withdrawn. Butyl and chlorobutyl rubber are used primarily for these applications because of their additional feature of resistance to permeation by oxygen and water vapor. The addition of natural rubber is added to the formulation when better coring resistance to multiple needle penetration is desired.

Following their molding, the stoppers may be glazed by chorination or siliconized to reduce their coefficient of friction. To minimize chemical interaction with container contents, a teflon coating may also be applied.

MELAMINE FORMALDEHYDE—This family of plastics exhibits good-to-excellent dimensional stability. When used in the manufacture of closures, high torque strength and good impact strength are obtained. These plastics also exhibit good resistance to oils, grease, and many organic solvents.

PHENOL FORMALDEHYDE—This type of plastic provides good scratch-resistant parts. It exhibits very low shrinkage and low water-absorption properties. It is, however, a relatively brittle plastic.

UREA FORMALDEHYDE—This plastic exhibits good dimensional stability as well as good strength properties. Articles produced from this material are highly rigid and provide good resistance to alcohols, oils, grease, and some of the weaker acids. These properties permit use for injection-molded heads for collapsible tubes used to contain liquid-based topical products.

APPLICATIONS

Composite materials, incorporating several components or plies, are used often to obtain the numerous advantages of multiple materials, all of which are unavailable from just one component. A stable material forming the bulk of the film is selected, such as PET, which is very popular for flexible packaging, providing dimensional and thermal stability. To this can be added protective coatings, such as barrier materials affording protection from oxygen, water vapor, and gasses. Also available are sealant layers permitting the package to be heat sealed and bonding layers to accommodate printing inks and to bond the various layers together in multiple-ply extrusions or laminations.

HEALTH CARE DEVICE PACKAGING—This is designed to protect medical devices during sterilization and shipping. The material porosity required for steam or ethylene oxide gas sterilization must be considered in conjunction with the need for maintaining a bacterial barrier following sterilization. Some candidate materials must be rejected because they cannot survive the sterilization mode. For example, PVC, unless specially stabilized, turns brown when subjected to radiation sterilization. Polypropylene becomes brittle only months following radiation exposure.

A satisfactory vent bag consists of a porous Tyvek pouch incorporated into a 3-mil or thicker LDPE bag. This permits rapid in- and out-gassing of ethylene oxide, minimizing expensive sterilization and hold-storage times. The thickness represents a compromise between cost and performance, because thinner bags tend to tear, thus occasioning repacking and resterilizing.

For products requiring better protection than that afforded by a flexible pouch, tray packages can be used. Thermoformed trays

are the dominant form of sterile packaging, popular because of strict infection-control standards. These may be either preformed or formed on-line. The latter uses thermoform/fill/seal machinery that first unwinds a web of flexible material from a reel, and then heats a section of it, forming it into a container. This is then filled with product and sealed on-line in one continuous operation. Inexpensive PVC or the higher-barrier PETG copolyester often is considered for the blister tray, because of thermoforming capability, appearance, toughness, and dimensional stability. Denesting agents as additives are critical for thermoformed trays, which require materials characterized by high gloss and a high coefficient of friction.[19]

The blister tray subsequently is sealed to a Tyvek or paper lid. Either lidding material is a sterile barrier and permits steam to penetrate the package. Paper may yellow and embrittle, however, during autoclaving. Furthermore, paper is hygroscopic and changes dimension in response to changes in humidity. This can lead to seal failure, as the lidding can pull away from the tray.

Clamshell packaging also affords stronger, infection-resistant containers. Transparency of both blister and clamshell packages allows the user to inspect the contents visually prior to breaking the seal, thus eliminating waste created from opening the wrong package.[20]

Heat-seal coating technology is important to ensure a reliably sterile product. Modified PE often is used for the heat-seal coating. Sealant properties of PE can be modified, depending upon the product requirements, by branching the polymer chain, which decreases its crystallinity and hence density. By decreasing density, the sealing range, elongation, stress-flex resistance, elasticity, and impact strength increase. As density increases, the following properties increase: sealing temperature, tensile strength, stiffness, hardness, barrier properties, and chemical resistance.

The seal occurs as the melt zones of the plastic are forged together to allow the polymer chains to cross the interface and form a bond. Package leaks can arise form poor uniformity of the heat-source application, and bubble and pore formation from foaming of moisture due to improperly dried plastics. Additionally, poor control of mechanical pressure applied during the melting process can result in squeezing the molten plastic out of the melt zone. Hermeticity is measured by dye-penetrant, bubble-emission, pressure decay, microbial-ingress, radioactive, and mass spectrometer systems.[21]

For packaging products high in alcohol content, EMA (ethylene methacrylic acid) copolymers may be used because of their ability to seal despite contact with organic contaminants in the seal area. For bonding to metal foils, PE must be made more hydrophilic. This is accomplished by copolymerizing hydrophobic ethylene with the more hydrophilic EAA (ethylene acrylic acid), EMA, or ionomer. Polypropylene also can be modified by the incorporation of random ethylene monomers in the polymer chain. This confers rubbery character to the sealant, increasing impact strength and flexibility.

Reduction of costs and increased requirements for validation drive technology trends in the packaging area. The future will see reduced material being used or a shift to less expensive materials where possible. The following are examples of these trends: shift from semi-rigid to flexible packaging for IV catheters; thick flexible to thin flexible packaging for syringes; nylon to polyolefin for dressings; coated products to uncoated products; and clean peel to fiber tear for syringes and needles.[22]

BLISTER PACKAGING—This type, for solid dosage forms, uses tray technology similar to that described above, except that the compartments are smaller. It involves forming a heat-softened plastic film into or around a deep-drawn, pocketed mold to make a plastic tray (thermoforming), filling with a solid dosage-form product and sealing with push-through or peelable covering. The forming film, covering, and product must flow at the right rates without sticking. Appropriate heat and pressure must be applied to ensure that permanent sealing will be formed that will protect the product throughout its shelf life. A critical property of the seal is hot tack, resistance of creep while warm, because as the package is ejected from the heat-seal jig, the still-warm bond line must support its entire weight.[23] It comprises two components: the melt strength of the seal layer at the temperature of the seal and the interfacial adhesion of the sealant layer to the opposite web.

Choice of film thickness affects both material costs and barrier properties. Other considerations are machineability, production rates, depth of the blister, wall thickness and uniformity of the blister, and sealing properties. Unplasticized, or rigid, PVC is the most common material for forming film because it is thermoformed easily, has glass-like clarity, is inexpensive, has high flexural strength, good chemical resistance, low permeability to fats, oils, easy tintability, and has barrier properties that are adequate for many drugs. The typical film thickness of 250 μm (10 mil) can be increased by applying a 25 to 50 μm coating of PVDC (polyvinylidene chloride) that increases the water vapor barrier properties 5- to 10-fold.

For better protection, films are made from PVC and CTFE (chlorotrifluoroethylene, Aclar). Such films are 15-fold less permeable to moisture than is PVC of comparable thickness. Maximal protection from water vapor is provided by biaxially oriented polyamide/aluminum/PVC (nylon-Al-PVC) that gives barrier properties that are immeasurably low. Aluminum makes the material more recyclable. The cost is comparable to that of PVDC-coated PVC. Other materials such as PP, PS, or PET have been tried for blister packs but have not achieved commercial success because of technical difficulties, poor barrier properties, or economic issues. The highest degree of protection is afforded by an all-foil package, which is cold-formable. The aluminum layer consists of several very thin layers rather than a single thick one to ensure that pinholes do not go all the way through the foil.[24] Nondestructive blister inspection devices are used to check for leaks in a 30 s vacuum test cycle.

For blister lidding, the selection of material structures depends on product fragility and whether the blister must be child resistant (CR). Polyester/foil is selected for CR applications. For non-CR applications, lidding material is usually aluminum/paper for fragile products or preprinted aluminum for sturdy products.[25] A standard 25-μm thickness of aluminum is considered to be pinhole free and represents an optimum combination of cost and product protection. The hardness of the aluminum can be optimized either for facilitating a push-through opening or hindering it, if a child-proof feature is desired. Lidding material also is perforated along the sealed seams to prevent it from being peeled from the formed film in one piece. The lidding material has a printing primer on one side and a heat-sealing lacquer on the other, which faces the product and forming film. A value-added feature is a peel-off-push-through foil, offered by a paper-polyester-aluminum laminate. The paper/PET laminate first is peeled from the aluminum, and then the tablet is pushed through the aluminum.[26]

Strip and sachet packaging are other unit-type packs used for tablets, capsules, powders, etc. Multidose packs for solid dosage forms can be made from PS, PVC, polyester, PP, or HDPE. The latter two are preferred for their better barrier properties toward moisture. All can be made child resistant and tamper evident/resistant using innovative closure systems reflecting the versatility of plastic materials. To discourage children from biting a package, a non-toxic bittering agent can be added to the paper side of the blister. To combat counterfeiting, 2D and 3D holographic security paper can be incorporated into blister laminate structures.[27] A paperboard-based sleeve-blister card combines compliance assistance with child resistance, tamper evidence, and elder friendliness. A die-cut hinge in the outer sleeve releases a folded paperboard encased film/foil blister slide card, which can be printed with dosage instructions to aid compliance.[28]

COLLAPSIBLE TUBES AND FLEXIBLE POUCHES— These are used to contain viscous and liquid-based topical products. They usually are constructed of metal or metal-lined, low-

density polyethylene, or a laminated material. Tubes are fabricated by rolling and heat-sealing flat stock into a continuous tube, then trimming to length and attaching the head by injection molding. Metal tubes are airtight, light-proof, and impermeable and offer superior protection. Plastic tubes are lightweight, leakproof, and relatively nonbreakable. In contrast to collapsible metal tubes that flatten as the product is removed, plastic tubes have memory that permits them to retain their original shape after squeezing. Laminate squeeze tubes offer the advantages of plastic with barrier properties close to those of metal. For some applications, an internal liner is used, shielding the product from the seam of the tube, which can cause crystallization.[29]

INTRAVENOUS (IV) SOLUTIONS—Compared with glass bottles, plastic packaging offers nonbreakability and light weight, affording easier transport and handling. Additionally, flexible packaging permits collapsibility, which provides greater protection from aerial contamination. Also, squeezing the bag with a pressure cuff enables rapid administration of large fluid quantities in emergency situations. This puts a burst-strength requirement on both the material and the quality of the seals. A container designed to keep products separated before mixing features a frangible seal between two or more pouch compartments that keeps multiple injectable solutions apart until just before use. [30]

Because of its transparency, durability, autoclavability, and manufacturability at an economical cost, PVC has been a material of choice. The realities of shipping require pinhole resistance. This is offered by flexible, high-yield strength materials like plasticized vinyl, rather than stiffer, more brittle materials like unmodified polyolefins. The polar nature of PVC permits rapid radiofrequency sealing of the bag, incorporating the port tubes for an IV administration set and medication sites. A polyolefin overwrap is used as a water-vapor barrier to prevent excessive moisture loss through the plasticized PVC.

Automatic packaging of IV solutions can be accomplished with an aseptic form (blow molding)-fill-seal system for rigid containers or a seal-fill-seal system for flexible containers. The latter requires preformed plastic film, which is reel-fed onto a forming manifold and side-sealed to form a tube, which is then filled. After incorporating fitments and closures, the final seal is made, and the completed container is cut from the web of material. The materials used are primarily polyethylene, polypropylene, and polyolefin, modified with rubber to increase yield strength for flexible containers. Composite materials may be used, incorporating a heat-seal layer facing the solution, an economical bulk layer for strength, and a polyester outside layer for scuff resistance and glossy appearance.[31] Additional considerations for IV container materials may be found in the chapters on parenteral preparations and intravenous admixtures.

PHARMACEUTICAL COIL—Coil material is placed into bottles of solid oral dosage forms to prevent damage during shipping and handling. These materials include cotton, rayon, polyester, or an HDPE plastic spring. Purified rayon filler is a fibrous form of bleached, regenerated cellulose. Purified polyester filler contains a number of additives (eg, antistatic, antiabrasives, lubricants) and therefore could leach residues. But it has the advantage that it does not contain water, as do the other hydrophilic polymeric materials.[32]

COATING MEDICAL DEVICES—Medical devices that are exposed to body fluids are often coated for protection against corrosion or for lubricity to surfaces. In one process, Parylene C, the low molecular weight dimer of para-chloro-xylylene is vapor deposited under vacuum on the device part, where it immediately polymerizes by a free radical process. Typical anticorrosion applications include blood pressure sensors, cardiac-assist devices, prosthetic components, bone pins, electronic circuits, ultrasonic transducers, bone-growth stimulators, and brain probes. Applications to promote lubricity include mandrels, injections needles, cannulae, and catheters.[33]

STERILIZATION

For plastic medical devices and packaging materials, a number of sterilizing agents have been used, including (1) steam, (2) gas, and (3) irradiation (cobalt and electron discharge). Of these agents, steam can be used on only a few polymers because of their inability to withstand heat without distortion. The following commonly used plastic types generally can withstand steam sterilization at temperatures of 121° C: polypropylene, high-density polyethylene, polycarbonate, PVC for certain applications, and all thermosets.

The most commonly used procedure for sterilizing plastic devices is gas sterilization. Some of the gases available are (1) 100% ethylene oxide, (2) 88%/12% mixtures of Freon and ethylene oxide, and (3) 80%/20% or 90%/10% mixtures of carbon dioxide and ethylene oxide.

Gas sterilization cannot be used for containers of aqueous products because side-reaction products such as ethylene glycol and 2-chloroethanol are formed. Ethylene oxide itself is carcinogenic. It also can react with body proteins and certain material leachables to form immunogenic compounds that can elicit hypersensitivity reactions. For this reason, regulatory permissible limits have been established for residual levels of ethylene oxide. To meet these limits, packaged products are degassed prior to shipping or use. Degassing properties depend upon geometry, heat history, storage conditions, contact with other plastics, and type of secondary packages used. Because of this complexity, degassing hold times must be determined for each product.

Newer gas sterilization technologies also have been developed. These include vaporized hydrogen peroxide, plasma processes such as Plazlyte and Sterrad, and chloride dioxide as well as PureBright, an intense, pulsed-light process. These modalities may afford a wider availability of materials compatible with these processes.[34]

Irradiation can cause degradation or cross-linking of certain polymers. This is particularly serious for polypropylene. Although a radiation-stable form of PP has been developed, it may not be suitable for multiple sterilizations.[35] PVC loses hydrochloric acid upon irradiation, decomposing into unstable fragments, which may then cross-link. This dehydrochlorination leads to the formation of conjugated double bonds, which impart yellow discoloration to the plastic. As part of the additive package to make PVC more radiation resistant, blue dyes are added to mask the yellow coloration. Radical-chain terminators also are added to minimize chain scission. Plastic packaging films, based on the total amount of radiolysis products, may be ranked in order of decreasing stability as polystyrene, polyester, PTFE, nylon, PVDC, PC, PP, HDPE, and LDPE.[36] As cobalt 60 becomes depleted, it may require increased exposure times to produce the same dose level. These longer exposure times can increase oxidative degradation on the packaging.[37] Certain polymers like polyethylene acquire improved tensile and impact strength because of the cross-linking attendant with radiation. The effect upon composite materials may not necessarily correlate with the properties of the individual components. Thus, the loss of strength of a cellulosic film may not be noticed if the film is supported by polyethylene or foil. The suitability of packaging materials subjected to various sterilization methods is discussed further in the chapter on sterilization.

QUALITY-CONTROL CONSIDERATIONS

The selection and approval of a polymer type (and a specific compound within that type) is as important as the need to check it routinely against the criteria used in its selection. The following basic areas of control and/or procedures are recommended regarding an ongoing quality-control program.

Tissue-cell toxicity testing (or a similar toxicity test) should be conducted to provide assurance that the material being used is nontoxic or falls within the toxicity range originally specified.

Characterization analysis should be conducted to provide assurances that the proper polymer type is used and that the physical parameters have not been altered, which in turn could affect the function of the product/package. Such techniques as infrared spectrometric analysis, density, melt-flow, and thermal and rheological tests can assist in providing the necessary assurances.

Any plastic part or package should be inspected routinely on an incoming basis for dimensional and attribute variables against statistically accepted sampling plans such as MIL-STD-105D.

ENVIRONMENTAL CONSIDERATIONS

Disposal is a critical issue, as the volume of solid waste continues to increase and the capacity of landfill sites dwindles. Hospitals are coming under increasing pressure as communities frown upon incineration and disposal costs escalate. Of the total municipal waste generated, plastic packaging accounts for only 4% by weight. While paper accounts for 50% and glass about 25%, plastics draw much of the concern of environmentalists, because of their persistence (nondegradability) in landfill sites. Additionally, plastics are increasingly displacing conventional packaging materials, and on a volume basis, bulky and resilient plastic bottles constitute more of a problem than their weight percentage would imply. The problem is being addressed from a number of standpoints.

Disposal is a complex issue, involving both economics and regulatory requirements. Often the plastic selection alternatives depend upon many factors, such as the mode of disposal or incineration versus landfill. For example, PVC has come under attack because it forms hydrochloric acid when incinerated, necessitating expensive scrubbing systems to neutralize the acid. Dioxins also may be formed if the incineration system is not optimized. If incineration will not be used to dispose of the medical waste for a given location, however, these objections become irrelevant for the particular case.

A global trend to eliminate solvents and volatile organic compounds (VOCs) is leading to interest in packaging with UV-curable inks. The faster drying times associated with this technology helps increase throughput.[38]

In response to their customers, hospital supply manufacturers are reducing the amount of packaging material accompanying their products. Some are working with hospitals to establish successful recycling efforts. This requires convenience of collection, viable reprocessing technology, markets for waste-derived products, and good economics. The individual plastic resins must be sorted prior to being reprocessed for relatively undemanding, nonpackaging applications such as fiberfill. Under some circumstances, homogeneous resins, such as the PET in beverage bottles, can be recycled more easily than composite materials, because of this sorting issue. Plastics manufacturers can, however, incorporate scrap into one of the component layers of some composite materials, making such items potentially recyclable. Recycling of PVC infusion containers is hampered by the difficulties involved in separating metal and rubber components, disinfecting, and drying the products to render them suitable for processing.[14] Nevertheless, the industry is investing in sorting technology and reclamation capacity to create commercially viable recycling programs.[39]

There is a trend toward elimination of folding carton dispensers. These are being replaced with polyethylene bagged shipments, used in conjunction with reusable bins in the hospital central supply rooms and pharmacies, to reduce both cost and waste. In the mail service prescription industry, air bubble mailers are preferred to corrugated ones because of the savings in postage, labor, and incorporation of interior cushioning.

SUMMARY

Before the selection of a plastic for a packaging application is made, all the functional and safety requirements must be specified. These requirements are restated in terms of engineering and scientific material-testing parameters. Candidate materials are reviewed and selected on the basis of the most economical solution that addresses the critical needs. Within each polymer class, properties may be altered to an extent by modifying molecular weight, copolymerizing with other polymers, or blending in particular additives. Often, composite materials are used to combine the advantages of the individual components. Proper sterilization procedures, including adequate degassing, must be identified to obtain a sterile product that is nontoxic. Once designed, the product/package must demonstrate physical and chemical stability in formal stability studies over the shelf life of the product. An ongoing quality assurance program should be designed to ensure that packaging- product requirements are maintained. After use, disposal of the packaging is becoming more of an issue from economic and environmental standpoints. For more specific and in-depth information, consult the *Bibliography*.

REFERENCES

1. ISO 11607. *Packaging for Terminally Sterilized Medical Devices.*
2. Comyn J, ed. *Polymer Permeability.* New York: Elsevier, 1985.
3. *Modern Plastics Encyclopedia,* vol 64. New York: McGraw-Hill, 1987, p 554.
4. Yasuda H, Stannett V. In: Brandrup J, Immergut EH, eds. *Polymer Handbook,* 2nd ed. New York: Wiley, 1975.
5. Rabinow B, Payton R, Raghavan N. *J Pharm Sci* 1986; 75: 808.
6. Wang YJ, Chien YW. *Sterile Pharmaceutical Packaging: Compatibility and Stability* (Tech Rpt #5). Philadelphia: PDA, 1984.
7. Sanchez IC, Chang SS, Smith LE. *Polymer News* 1980; 6:249.
8. Jenke DR, et al. *Int J Pharm* 1992; 78:115.
9. *Mod Plastics* 1997; (May).
10. *Business Wire* 1996; (Jul 9).
11. Forcinio H. *Pharm Technol* 1999; (Nov):30.
12. *Med Device & Diag Ind* 1998; (Aug).
13. Forcinio H. *Pharm Technol* 2000; (May):26
14. *Med Device Technol* 1991; (Jun).
15. Jenkins WA, Osborn, KR. *Packaging Drugs and Pharmaceuticals.* Lancaster, PA: Technomic Publishing, 1993, p 113.
16. Van Dooren AA. *Pharm Weekbl [Sci]* 1991; 13(3):109.
17. *Pharm Med Pkg News* 1995; (Mar).
18. USP/NF. Rockville, MD: USPC, 661.
19. *Pkg Week* 1997; (Apr 24).
20. Smith RC Jr, ed. *Medical & Healthcare Marketplace Guide,* 12th ed. IDD Enterprises, 1996.
21. *Med Device & Diag Ind* 2000; (Jan):186.
22. *Med Device Technol* 1999; (April):26.
23. Pilchuk R. *Pharm Technol* 2000; (Nov):68.
24. Pilchuk R. *Pharm Technol* 2000; (Nov):68.
25. Forcinio H. *Pharm Technol* 2000; (Jun):24.
26. Reiterer F. *Pharm Technol* 1991; (Mar):74.
27. Forcinio H. *Pharm Technol* 1999; (Nov):30.
28. Forcinio H, *Pharm Technol* 2000; (Jun):24
29. *Pharm Med Pkg News* 1996; (Feb).
30. Forcinio H. *Pharm Technol* 1999; (Jan):28.
31. Lambert P. *Pharm Technol* 1991; (Apr): 48.
32. Taborsky CJ, Mehta U, Kusz M, et al. *Pack Technol* 2000; (Mar):44.
33. *Med Plast and Biomat* 1996; (Mar).
34. *Pkg Week* 1997; n41(Apr 24):17.
35. *Pharm Med Pkg News* 1996; (Sep).
36. *Pkg Technol Eng* 1996; (Jun).
37. Dyke D. *Med Device & Diag Ind* 1996; (Jan).
38. *Pkg Week* 1997; n41(Apr 24):17.
39. *J Vinyl Technol* 1991; 13(2).

BIBLIOGRAPHY

Briston JH. *Plastic Films,* 3rd ed. New York: Wiley, 1988.
Brostow W, Corneliussen RD. *Failure of Plastics.* New York: Macmillan, 1986.
Comyn J, ed. *Polymer Permeability.* New York: Elsevier, 1985.
Crank J, Park GS, eds. *Diffusion in Polymers.* New York: Academic, 1968.
Dean DA. *The Packaging of Pharmaceuticals* (Int Pkg Conf, CONEX 85 (Oct 22–25, 1985), vol 1. Beijing: China Pkg Technol Assoc, 1985, p 287.
Dean DA. *Plastics in Pharmaceutical Packaging.* England: Antony Rowe Ltd, 1990.
Dean DA , Evans ER, Hall IH. *Pharmaceutical Packaging Technology.* New York: Taylor and Francis, 2000.
Finlayson KM. *Plastic Film Technology, High Barrier Plastic Films for Packaging,* vol 1. Lancaster, PA: Technomic Publ Co, 1989.
Jenkins WA, Osborn KR,.*Packaging Drugs and Pharmaceuticals.* Lancaster, PA: Technomic Publishing, 1993.
Modern Plastics Encyclopedia, vol 68. New York: McGraw-Hill, 1992.
Osborn KR, Jenkins WA, *Plastic Films.* Lancaster, PA: Technomic Publishing, 1992.
Yasuda H, Stannett V. Permeability coefficients. In *Polymer Handbook,* 2nd ed, Brandrup J, Immergut EH, eds. New York: Wiley, 1975.
Rodriguez F. *Principles of Polymer Systems,* 2nd ed. New York: Hemisphere, 1982.
Wiley Encyclopedia of Packaging Technology. New York: Wiley, 1986.

CHAPTER 55

Pharmaceutical Necessities

William J Reilly, Jr, RPh, MBA

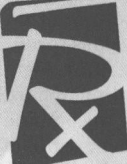

The practice of pharmacy is an ever-evolving profession that has changes occurring regularly. The costs associated with discovering new compounds are increasing at such a rapid rate that many in healthcare and government don't think is capable of being maintained. The Food and Drug Administration has levied the largest fines in its history over the last couple of years on manufacturers who have failed to comply with what is known as current Good Manufacturing Procedures. The government's approval of new products is in a downward trend, this being a result of companies wanting to provide more information in the filings and the FDA frequently issuing 'not approvable' letters, requiring the sponsor company to conduct additional studies. At the community level, more independent pharmacies are closing their doors or selling their patient lists to national or regional chains. Hospital settings are seeing a greater degree of mergers so that economics are more favorable.

In addition to the profession, pharmacy education has undergone dramatic changes in the United States since the last edition of the *Remington* was published. Now the PharmD degree is the entry-level degree for everyone wanting to practice pharmacy. With this degree, the focus on the clinical aspects of pharmacy has an even greater emphasis on the educational process. Much of this is at the expense of basic pharmaceutics and in some instances, because of course loads, electives such as industrial pharmacy courses are not conveniently taken by students. The pharmaceutical industry used to be able to hire graduates with pharmacy degrees for positions in production, quality control, and dosage-form development because of the breadth of understanding the graduate had of pharmaceutical processes. Unfortunately, gaining this understanding is becoming increasingly difficult unless a student pursues an advanced degree in industrial pharmacy or pharmaceutics.

Regardless of what is happening within the profession, the educational system or the industry, it is imperative that pharmacists in all practice settings know it is their obligation to understand what is used to prepare a medication, whether by commercial means or by extemporaneously compounding it in a practice setting. This chapter does not address the legal aspects of community compounding by a pharmacist, nor does it explain all the specifics of formulating a product for commercial manufacturing. The intent of this information is to inform the practicing pharmacist and other interested individuals in understanding commercial formulations which ingredients are necessary for creating a drug product. These substances, known as excipients, are useful in both the community and commercial settings, although they might be used differently. The excipients described include antioxidants and preservatives, emulsifying and suspending agents, ointment bases, solvents, and miscellaneous ingredients. A more detailed review of these excipients and their commercial applicability to dosage-form development can be found in the *Handbook of Pharmaceutical Excipients* (Rowe, Sheskey, and Weller, eds.) as well as other chapters in this edition of *Remington*.

ANTIOXIDANTS AND PRESERVATIVES

An antioxidant is a substance capable of inhibiting oxidation, which may be added for this purpose to pharmaceutical products subject to deterioration by oxidative processes, as for example the development of rancidity in oils and fats or the inactivation of some medicinals in the environment of their dosage forms. A preservative is, in the common pharmaceutical sense, a substance that prevents or inhibits microbial growth, which may be added to pharmaceutical preparations for this purpose to avoid consequent spoilage of the preparations by microorganisms. Both antioxidants and preservatives have many applications in making medicinal products.

ALCOHOL—page 1080.
BENZALKONIUM CHLORIDE—page 1626.
BENZETHONIUM CHLORIDE—page 1627.
BENZYL ALCOHOL—page 1627.

BUTYLATED HYDROXYANISOLE

Phenol, (1,1-dimethylethyl)-4-methoxy-, Tenox BHA

$$\text{OH} \quad \text{C(CH}_3)_3 \quad \text{OCH}_3$$

tert-Butyl-4-methoxyphenol [25013-16-5] $C_{11}H_{16}O_2$ (180.25).

Preparation—By an addition interaction of *p*-methoxyphenol and 2-methylpropene. US Pat 2,428,745.

Description—White or slightly yellow, waxy solid having a faint, characteristic odor.

Solubility—Insoluble in water; 1 g in 4 mL alcohol, 2 mL chloroform or 1.2 mL ether.

Uses—An antioxidant in cosmetics and pharmaceuticals containing fats and oils.

BUTYLATED HYDROXYTOLUENE

Phenol, 2,6-bis(1,1-dimethylethyl)-4-methyl-, Butylated Hydroxytoluene Crystalline; Tenox BHT

2,6-Di-*tert*-butyl-*p*-cresol [128-37-0] $C_{15}H_{24}O$ (220.35).

Preparation—By an addition interaction of *p*-cresol and 2- methylpropene. US Pat 2,428,745.

Description—White, tasteless crystals with a mild odor; stable in light or air; melts at 70°C.

Solubility—Insoluble in water; 1 g in 4 mL alcohol, 1.1 mL chloroform, or 1.1 mL ether.

Uses—An antioxidant employed to retard oxidative degradation of oils and fats in various cosmetics and pharmaceuticals.

CHLOROBUTANOL

2-Propanol, 1,1,1-trichloro-2-methyl-, Chlorbutol; Chlorbutanol; Acetone Chloroform; Chloretone

$(CCl_3)C(CH_3)_2OH$

1,1,1-Trichloro-2-methyl-2-propanol [57-15-8] $C_4H_7Cl_3O$ (177.46); *hemihydrate* [6001-64-5] (186.46).

Preparation—Chloroform undergoes chemical addition to acetone under the catalytic influence of powdered potassium hydroxide.

Description—Colorless to white crystals of a characteristic, somewhat camphoraceous odor and taste; anhydrous melts about 95°C; hydrous melts about 76°C; boils with some decomposition between 165° and 168°C.

Solubility—1 g in 125 mL water, 1 mL alcohol or about 10 mL glycerin; freely soluble in chloroform, ether, or volatile oils.

Incompatibilities—The anhydrous form must be used to prepare a clear solution in liquid petrolatum. It is decomposed by alkali; ephedrine is sufficiently alkaline to cause its breakdown with the formation of ephedrine hydrochloride, which will separate from a liquid petrolatum solution. It is only slightly soluble in water, hence alcohol must be used to dissolve the required amount in certain vehicles. Trituration with antipyrine, menthol, phenol, and other substances produce a soft mass.

Uses—Topically, as a solution in clove oil as a dental analgesic. It has local anesthetic potency to a mild degree and has been employed as an anesthetic dusting powder (1 to 5%) or ointment (10%). It has antibacterial and germicidal properties. When administered orally, it has much the same therapeutic use as chloral hydrate. Hence, it has been employed as a sedative and hypnotic. It has been taken orally to allay vomiting due to gastritis.

DEHYDROACETIC ACID

Keto form: 2H-Pyran-2,4(3H)-dione, 3-acetyl-6-methyl-,

(keto form)　　　　(enol form)

Enol form: 3-acetyl-4-hydroxy-6-methyl-2*H*-pyran-2-one [520-45-6] (keto), [771-03-9] (enol) $C_8H_8O_4$ (168.15).

Preparation—By fractional distillation of a mixture of ethyl acetoacetate and sodium bicarbonate, maintaining almost total reflux conditions, allowing only ethanol to be removed. The residue is distilled under vacuum. *Org Syn Coll III:* 231, 1955.

Description—White to creamy-white crystalline powder melting about 110°C with sublimation.

Solubility—1 g dissolves in 25 g acetone, 18 g benzene, 5 g methanol, or 3 g alcohol.

Uses—Preservative.

ETHYLENEDIAMINE

1,2-Ethanediamine

$H_2NCH_2CH_2NH_2$

Ethylenediamine [107-15-3] $C_2H_8N_2$ (60.10).

Caution—Use care in handling because of its caustic nature and the irritating properties of its vapor.

Note—It is strongly alkaline and may readily absorb carbon dioxide from the air to form a nonvolatile carbonate. Protect it against undue exposure to the atmosphere.

Preparation—By reacting ethylene dichloride with ammonia, then adding NaOH and distilling.

Description—Clear, colorless, or only slightly yellow liquid, with an ammonia-like odor and strong alkaline reaction; miscible with water and alcohol; anhydrous boils 116 to 117°C and solidifies at about 8°C; volatile with steam; a strong base and readily combines with acids to form salts with the evolution of substantial heat.

Uses—A pharmaceutical necessity for Aminophylline Injection. It is irritating to skin and mucous membranes. It also may cause sensitization characterized by asthma and allergic dermatitis.

ETHYL VANILLIN—page 1064.
GLYCERIN—pages 1081 and 1423.
HYPOPHOSPHOROUS ACID—page 1086.
PHENOL—page 1087.
PHENYLETHYL ALCOHOL page 1066.
PHENYLMERCURIC NITRATE—see RPS-19, page 1270.

POTASSIUM BENZOATE

Benzoic Acid, Potassium Salt

[582-25-2] $C_7H_5KO_2$ (160.21) (anhydrous).

Description—Crystalline powder.

Solubility—Soluble in water or alcohol.

Uses—Preservative.

POTASSIUM METABISULFITE

Dipotassium Pyrosulfite

[16731-55-8] $K_2S_2O_5$ (222.31).

Description—White crystals or crystalline powder with an odor of SO_2. Oxidizes in air to the sulfate. May ignite on powdering in a mortar if too much heat develops.

Solubility—Freely soluble in water; insoluble in alcohol.

Uses—Antioxidant.

POTASSIUM SORBATE

2,4-Hexadienoic Acid, *(E,E)-*, Potassium Salt; 2,4-Hexadienoic Acid, Potassium Salt; Potassium 2,4-Hexadienoate

Potassium *(E,E)*-sorbate; potassium sorbate [590-00-1] [24634-61-5] $C_6H_7KO_2$ (150.22).

Preparation—Sorbic acid is reacted with an equimolar portion of KOH. The resulting potassium sorbate may be crystallized from aqueous ethanol. US Pat 3,173,948.

Description—White crystals or powder with a characteristic odor; melts about 270°C with decomposition.

Solubility—1 g in 4.5 mL water, 35 mL alcohol, >1000 mL chloroform, or >1000 mL ether.

Uses—A water-soluble salt of sorbic acid used in pharmaceuticals to inhibit the growth of molds and yeast. Its toxicity is low, but it may irritate the skin.

SASSAFRAS OIL—page 1069.
SODIUM BENZOATE—see RPS-19, page 1271.

SODIUM BISULFITE

Sulfurous acid, monosodium salt; Sodium Hydrogen Sulfite; Sodium Acid Sulfite; Leucogen

Monosodium sulfite [7631-90-5] $NaHSO_3$ and sodium metabisulfite ($Na_2S_2O_5$) in varying proportions; yields 58.5 to 67.4% of SO_2.

Description—White or yellowish white crystals or granular powder with the odor of sulfur dioxide; unstable in air.

Solubility—1 g in 4 mL water; slightly soluble in alcohol.

Uses—An antioxidant and stabilizing agent. Epinephrine hydrochloride solutions may be stabilized by the addition of small quantities of the salt. It also is used to help solubilize kidney stones. It is useful for removing permanganate stains and for solubilizing certain dyes and other chemicals.

SODIUM METABISULFITE

Disulfurous acid, disodium salt

Disodium pyrosulfite [7681-57-4] $Na_2S_2O_5$ (190.10).

Preparation—Formed when sodium bisulfite undergoes thermal dehydration. It also may be prepared by passing sulfur dioxide over sodium carbonate.

Description—White crystals or white to yellowish crystalline powder with an odor of sulfur dioxide; on exposure to air and moisture, it is slowly oxidized to sulfate.

Solubility—1 g in 2 mL water; slightly soluble in alcohol; freely soluble in glycerin.

Uses—A reducing agent. It is used in easily oxidized pharmaceuticals, such as epinephrine hydrochloride and phenylephrine hydrochloride injections, to retard oxidation.

SORBIC ACID

2,4-Hexadienoic acid, *(E,E)-, 2,4-Hexadienoic acid*

$$\text{H}_3\text{C}-\text{CH}=\text{CH}-\text{CH}=\text{CH}-\text{COOH} \qquad (6)$$

(E,E)-Sorbic acid; Sorbic acid [22500-92-1] [110-44-1] $C_6H_8O_2$ (112.13).

Preparation—By various processes. Refer to US Pat 2,921,090.

Description—Free-flowing, white, crystalline powder, with a characteristic odor; melts about 133°C.

Solubility—1 g in 1000 mL water, 10 mL alcohol, 15 mL chloroform, 30 mL ether, or 19 mL propylene glycol.

Uses—A mold and yeast inhibitor. It also is used as a fungistatic agent for foods, especially cheeses.

THIMEROSAL—see RPS-19, page 1271.

COLORING, FLAVORING, AND DILUTING AGENTS

The use of properly colored and flavored medicinal substances, although offering no particular therapeutic advantage, is of considerable importance psychologically. A water-clear medicine is not particularly acceptable to most patients and, in general, is thought to be inert. Many very active medicinal substances are quite unpalatable, and the patient may fail to take the medicine simply because the taste or appearance is objectionable. Disagreeable medication can be made both pleasing to the taste and attractive by careful selection of the appropriate coloring, flavoring, and diluting agents. Therefore, judicious use of these substances is important in securing patient cooperation in taking or using the prescribed medication and continued compliance with the prescriber's intent.

Coloring Agents or Colorants

Coloring agents may be defined as compounds employed in pharmacy solely for the purpose of imparting color. They may be classified in various ways (eg, inorganic or organic). For the purpose of this discussion two subdivisions are used: *Natural Coloring Principles* and *Synthetic Coloring Principles*. The members of these groups are used as colors for pharmaceutical preparations, cosmetics, and foods and as bacteriological stains and diagnostic agents.

NATURAL COLORING PRINCIPLES

Natural coloring principles are obtained from mineral, plant, and animal sources. They are used primarily for artistic purposes; as symbolic adornments of natives; as colors for foods, drugs, and cosmetics; and for other psychological effects.

Mineral colors frequently are termed pigments and are used to color lotions, cosmetics, and other preparations, usually for external application. Examples are Red Ferric Oxide and Yellow Ferric Oxide, titanium dioxide, and carbon black.

The term pigment also is applied generically to plant colors by phytochemists. Many plants contain coloring principles that may be extracted and used as colorants (eg, chlorophyll). Anattenes are obtained from annatto seeds and give yellow-to-orange water-soluble dyes. Natural beta-carotene is a yellow color extracted from carrots and used to color margarine. Alizarin is a reddish yellow dye obtained from the madder plant. The indigo plant is the source of a blue pigment called indigo. Flavones, such as riboflavin, rutin, hesperidin, and quercetin, are yellow pigments. Saffron is a glycoside that gives a yellow color to drugs and foods. Cudbear and red saunders are two other dyes obtained from plants. Most plant colors now have been characterized and synthesized, however,

and those with the desirable qualities of stability, fastness, and pleasing hue are available commercially as synthetic products.

Animals have been a source of coloring principles from the earliest periods of recorded history. For example, Tyrian purple, once a sign of royalty, was prepared by air oxidation of a colorless secretion obtained from the glands of a snail *(Murex brandaris)*. This dye now is known to be 6,6'-dibromoindigo, and has been synthesized, but cheaper dyes of the same color are available. Cochineal from the insect *Coccus cacti* contains the bright-red coloring principle carminic acid, a derivative of anthraquinone. This dye is no longer used in foods and pharmaceuticals because of *Salmonella* contamination.

SYNTHETIC COLORING PRINCIPLES

Synthetic coloring principles date from 1856 when WH Perkin accidentally discovered mauveine, also known as a Perkin's purple, while engaged in unsuccessful attempts to synthesize quinine. He obtained the dye by oxidizing aniline containing *o*- and *p*-toluidines as impurities. Other discoveries of this kind followed soon after, and a major industry grew up in the field of coal-tar chemistry.

The earliest colors were prepared from aniline, and for many years all coal-tar dyes were called aniline colors, irrespective of their origin. The coal-tar dyes include more than a dozen well-defined groups among which are nitroso-dyes, nitro-dyes, azo-dyes, oxazines, thiazines, pyrazolones, xanthenes, indigoids, anthraquinones, acridines, rosanilines, phthaleins, quinolines, and others. These in turn are classified, according to their method of use, as acid dyes and basic dyes, or direct dyes and mordant dyes.

Certain structural elements in organic molecules, called chromophore groups, give color to the molecules, eg, azo (—N═Noj), nitroso (—N═O), nitro (—NO₂), azoxy (—N═N(O)—), carbonyl (>C═O), and ethylene (>C═C<). Other such combinations augment the chromophore groups, eg, methoxy, hydroxy, and amino groups and are known as auxochromes.

STABILITY—Most dyes are relatively unstable chemicals because of their unsaturated structures. They are subject to fading because of light, metals, heat, microorganisms, oxidizing and reducing agents, plus strong acids and bases. In tablets, fading may appear as spotting and specking.

USES—Most synthetic coloring principles are used in coloring fabrics and for various artistic purposes. They also find application as indicators, bacteriological stains, diagnostic aids, reagents in microscopy, etc.

Many coal-tar dyes originally were used in foodstuffs and beverages without careful selection or discrimination between those that were harmless and those that were toxic and without any supervision as to purity or freedom from poisonous constituents derived from their manufacture.

After the passage of the Food and Drugs Act in 1906, the US Department of Agriculture established regulations by which a few colors came to be known as permitted colors. Certain of these colors may be used in foods, drugs, and cosmetics, but only after certification by the Food and Drug Administration (FDA) that they meet certain specifications. From this list of permitted colors may be produced, by skillful blending and mixing, other colors that may be used in foods, beverages, and pharmaceutical preparations. Blends of certified dyes must be recertified.

The word permitted is used in a restricted sense. It does not carry with it the right to use colors for purposes of deception, even though they are permitted colors, for all food laws have clauses prohibiting the coloring of foods and beverages in a manner so as to conceal inferiority or to give a false appearance of value.

The certified colors are classified into three groups: FD&C dyes, which legally may be used in foods, drugs, and cosmetics; D&C dyes, which legally may be used in drugs and cosmetics; and external D&C dyes, which legally may be used only in externally applied drugs and cosmetics. There are specific limits for the pure dye, sulfated ash, ether extractives, soluble and insoluble matter, uncombined intermediates, oxides, chlorides, and sulfates. As the use status of these colors is subject to change, the latest regulations of the FDA should be consulted to determine how they may be used—especially since several FD&C dyes formerly widely used have been found to be carcinogenic even when pure and, therefore, have been banned from use.

The Coal-Tar Color Regulations specify that the term externally applied drugs and cosmetics means drugs and cosmetics that are applied only to external parts of the body and not to the lips or any body surface covered by mucous membrane. No certified dye, regardless of its category, legally may be used in any article that is to be applied to the area of the eye.

Lakes are calcium or aluminum salts of certified dyes extended on a substrate of alumina. They are insoluble in water and organic solvents and hence are used to color powders, pharmaceuticals, foods, hard candies, and food packaging.

The application of dyes to pharmaceutical preparations is an art that can be acquired only after an understanding of the characteristics of dyes and knowledge of the composition of the products to be colored has been obtained. Specific rules for the choice or application of dyes to pharmaceutical preparations are difficult to formulate. Each preparation may present unique problems.

Preparations that may be colored include most liquid pharmaceuticals, powders, ointments, and emulsions. Some general hints may be offered in connection with solutions and powders, but desired results usually can be obtained only by a series of trials. In general, an inexperienced operator tends to use a much higher concentration of the dye than is necessary, resulting in a dull color. The amount of dye present in any pharmaceutical preparation should be of a concentration high enough to give the desired color and low enough to prevent toxic reactions and permanent staining of fabrics and tissues.

Liquids (Solutions)—The dye concentration in liquid preparations and solutions usually should come within a range of 0.0005% (1 in 200,000) and 0.001% (1 in 100,000), depending upon the depth of color wanted and the thickness of column to be viewed in the container. With some dyes, concentrations as low as 0.0001% (1 in 1,000,000) may have a distinct tinting effect. Dyes are used most conveniently in the form of stock solutions.

Powders—White powders usually require the incorporation of 0.1% (1 in 1000) of a dye to impart a pastel color. The dyes may be incorporated into the powder by dry-blending in a ball mill or, on a small scale, with a mortar and pestle. The dye is incorporated by trituration and geometric dilution. Powders also may be colored evenly by adding a solution of the dye in alcohol or some other volatile solvent having only a slight solvent action on the powder being colored. When this procedure is employed, the solution is added in portions, with thorough mixing after each addition, after which the solvent is allowed to evaporate from the mixture.

Many of the syrups and elixirs used as flavoring and diluting agents are colored. When such agents are used, no further coloring matter is necessary. The use of colored flavoring agents is discussed in a subsequent section. However, when it is desired to add color to an otherwise colorless mixture, one of the agents described in the first section may be used.

INCOMPATIBILITIES—FD&C dyes are mainly anionic (sodium salts) and hence are incompatible with cationic substances. Since the concentrations of these substances are generally very low, no precipitate is evident. Polyvalent ions such as calcium, magnesium, and aluminum also may form insoluble compounds with dyes. A pH change may cause the color to change. Acids may release the insoluble acid form of the dye.

Flavoring Agents

FLAVOR

The word flavor refers to a mixed sensation of taste, touch, smell, sight, and sound, all of which combine to produce an infinite number of gradations in the perception of a substance. The four primary tastes—sweet, bitter, sour, and saline—appear to result partly from physicochemical and partly from psychological action. Taste buds (Fig 55-1), located mainly on the tongue, contain very sensitive nerve endings that react, in the presence of moisture, with the flavors in the mouth, and as a result of physicochemical activity, electrical impulses are produced and transmitted via the seventh, ninth, and tenth cranial nerves to the areas of the brain that are devoted to the perception of taste. Some of the taste buds are specialized in their function, giving rise to areas on the tongue that are sensitive to only one type of taste. The brain, however, usually perceives taste as a composite sensation, and accordingly, the components of any flavor are not readily discernible. Children have more taste buds than adults and hence are more sensitive to tastes.

Taste partly depends on the ions that are produced in the mouth, but psychologists have demonstrated that sight (color) and sound also play a definite role when certain reflexes become conditioned through custom and association of sense perceptions. Thus, in the classic experiments of Pavlov demonstrating conditioned reflexes, the ringing of a bell or the showing of a circle of light caused the gastric juices of a dog to flow, although no food was placed before it, and much of the enjoyment derived from eating celery is due to its crunchy crispness as the fibrovascular bundles are crushed. The effect of color is just as pronounced; oleomargarine is unpalatable to most people when it is uncolored, but once the dye has been incorporated, gourmets frequently cannot distinguish it from butter. Color and taste must coincide (eg, cherry flavor is associated with a red color).

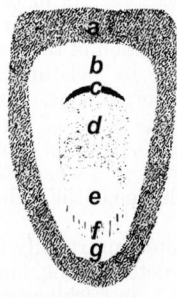

Figure 55-1. Upper surface of the tongue. *a,* Taste receptors for all tastes; *b,* sweet, salty, and sour; *c,* salty and sour; *d,* sour only; *e,* no taste sensation; *f,* sweet and sour; *g,* bitter, sweet, and sour. (Adapted from Crocker EC. *Flavor.* New York: McGraw-Hill, 1945, p 22.)

Persons suffering from a head cold find their food much less palatable than usual because their sense of smell is impaired, and if the nostrils are held closed, raw onions taste sweet, and it is much easier to ingest castor oil and other nauseating medicines. The volatility of a substance is an important factor that is influenced by the warmth and moisture of the mouth, since the more volatile a compound, the more pronounced its odor. The sense of smell detects very minute amounts of material and is usually much more sensitive in detecting the presence of volatile chemicals, but the tongue is able to detect infinitesimal amounts of some vapors if it is protruded from the mouth so that solution of the gases in the saliva may take place. In this manner traces of sulfur dioxide can be detected in the air, since it dissolves in the saliva and creates a sour taste.

Flavors described as hot are those that exert a mild counterirritant effect on the mucosa of the mouth; those that are astringent and pucker the mouth contain tannins and acids that produce this effect by reacting with the lining of the mouth, and wines possess a bouquet because of the odor of the volatile constituents. Indian turnip (Jack-in-the-pulpit) owes its flavor largely to the stinging sensation caused by the minute acicular crystals of calcium oxalate that penetrate the mucous membrane.

Other physiological and physical factors that also may affect taste are coarseness or grittiness due to small particles (eg, ion-exchange resins). Antidiarrheal preparations have a chalky taste. Menthol imparts a cool taste because it affects the coldness receptors. Mannitol gives a cool sensation when it dissolves because its negative heat of solution will cause the temperature to drop. For this reason, mannitol often is used as the base for chewable tablets.

There is a definite threshold of taste for every substance, which varies somewhat with the individual and with the environment. Experienced chefs taste their delicacies at the temperature at which they will be served, since heat and cold alter the flavor of many preparations. Thus, lemon loses its sour taste entirely at an elevated temperature, and other flavors become almost nonvolatile, tasteless, and odorless when cooled sufficiently. In addition to the influence of temperature, the sensitivity of each individual must be considered. For example, it has been determined by experiment that the amount of sugar that can just be detected by the average individual is about 7 mg. However, this amount cannot be tasted by some, and it is definitely sweet to others.

People are more sensitive to odor than to taste. There are about 10,000 to 30,000 identifiable scents, of which the average person can identify about 4000. Women are more sensitive to odors than men. Additional insights can be obtained by reading Beauchamp GK, et al: *Tasting and Smelling*, (New York: Academic, 1997) and Cagan RH, et al: *Neural Mechanisms in Taste* (Boca Raton, FL: CRC Press, 1989).

PRESERVATION OF FLAVORS—Most monographs of official products contain specific directions for storage. Proper methods of storage are essential to prevent deterioration, which in many instances results in destruction of odor and taste. Under adverse conditions undesirable changes occur because of one or a combination of the following: enzymatic activity, oxidation, change in moisture content, absorption of odors, activity of microorganisms, and effects of heat and light. In certain products some of the changes wrought by these factors are desirable, as when esters are formed because of the activity of enzymes and when blending and mellowing results from the interchange of the radicals of esters (transesterification).

One method for protecting readily oxidizable substances, such as lemon oil, from deteriorating, and thus preserving their original delicate flavor, is to microencapsulate them by spray-drying. The capsules containing the flavors then are enclosed in various packaged products (eg, powdered gelatins) or tablets, which are flavored deliciously when the capsule is disintegrated by mixing and warming with water or saliva.

CORRELATION OF CHEMICAL STRUCTURE WITH FLAVOR AND ODOR—The compounds employed as flavors in vehicles vary considerably in their chemical structure, ranging from simple esters (methyl salicylate), alcohols (glycerin), and aldehydes (vanillin) to carbohydrates (honey) and the complex volatile oils (anise oil). Synthetic flavors of almost any desired type are now available. These frequently possess the delicate flavor and aroma of the natural products and also the desirable characteristics of stability, reproducibility, and comparatively low cost. Synthetic products such as cinnamaldehyde and benzaldehyde, first officially recognized when several of the essential oils became scarce during World War II, have been used widely.

There is a close relationship between chemical structure and taste. Solubility, the degree of ionization, and the type of ions produced in the saliva definitely influence the sensation interpreted by the brain.

Sour taste is caused by hydrogen ions, and it is proportional to the hydrogen ion concentration and the lipid solubility of the compound. It is characteristic of acids, tannins, alum, phenols, and lactones. Saltiness is due to simultaneous presence of anions and cations (eg, KBr, NH_4Cl, and sodium salicylate). High-molecular-weight salts may have a bitter taste. Sweet taste is due to polyhydroxy compounds, polyhalogenated aliphatic compounds, and α-amino acids. Amino and amide groups, especially if the positive effect is balanced by the proximity of a negative group, may produce a sweet taste. Sweetness increases with the number of hydroxy groups, possibly because of increased solubility. Imides such as saccharin and sulfamates such as cyclamates are intensely sweet. Cyclamates have been removed from the market because they reportedly cause bladder tumors in rats. Free bases such as alkaloids and amides such as amphetamines give bitter tastes. Polyhydroxy compounds with a molecular weight greater than 300, halogenated substances, and aliphatic thio compounds also may have bitter tastes. Unsaturation frequently bestows a sharp, biting odor and taste on compounds.

No precise relationship between chemical structure and odor has been found. There are no primary odors, and odors blend into each other. Polymerization reduces or destroys odor, high valency gives odor, and unsaturation enhances odor. A tertiary carbon atom often will give a camphoraceous odor, esters and lactones have a fruity odor, and ketones have a pleasant odor. Strong odors often are accompanied by volatility and chemical reactivity.

SELECTION OF FLAVORS

The proper selection of flavors for disguising nauseating medicines aids in their ingestion. Occasionally, sensitive patients have become nauseated sufficiently to vomit at the thought of having to take disagreeable medication, and it is particularly difficult to persuade children to continue to use and retain distasteful preparations. There is a need to know the allergies and idiosyncrasies of the patient; thus, it is foolish to use a chocolate-flavored vehicle for the patient who dislikes the flavor or who is allergic to it, notwithstanding the fact that this flavor is generally acceptable.

FLAVORING METHODOLOGY

Each flavoring problem is unique and requires an individual solution. The problem of flavoring is further complicated because flavor and taste depend on individual preferences. In solving flavoring problems the following techniques have been used:

Blending—Fruit flavors blend with sour taste; bitter tastes can be blended with salty, sweet, and sour tastes; salt reduces sourness and increases sweetness; chemicals such as vanillin, monosodium glutamate, and benzaldehyde are used for blending.

Overshadow—Addition of a flavor whose intensity is longer and stronger than the obvious taste (eg, methyl salicylate, glycyrrhiza, and oleoresins).

Physical—Formation of insoluble compounds of the offending drug (eg, sulfonamides); emulsification of oils; effervescence (eg, magnesium citrate solution); high viscosity of fluids to limit contact of drug with the tongue; and mechanical procedures such as coating tablets are physical methods to reduce flavoring problems.

Chemical—Absorption of the drug on a substrate or formation of a complex of the drug with ion-exchange resins or complexing agents.

Physiological—The taste buds may be anesthetized by menthol or mint flavors.

Flavors, as used by the pharmacist in compounding prescriptions, may be divided into four main categories according to the type of taste that is to be masked, as follows:

Salty Taste—Cinnamon syrup has been found to be the best vehicle for ammonium chloride and other salty drugs such as sodium salicylate and ferric ammonium citrate. In a study of the comparative efficiency of flavoring agents for disguising salty taste, the following additional vehicles were arranged in descending order of usefulness: orange syrup, citric acid syrup, cherry syrup, cocoa syrup, wild cherry syrup, raspberry syrup, glycyrrhiza elixir, aromatic elixir, and glycyrrhiza syrup. The last-named is particularly useful as a vehicle for the salines by virtue of its colloidal properties and the sweetness of both glycyrrhizin and sucrose.

Bitter Taste—Cocoa syrup was found to be the best vehicle for disguising the bitter taste of quinine bisulfate, followed, in descending order of usefulness, by raspberry syrup, cocoa syrup, cherry syrup, cinnamon syrup, compound sarsaparilla syrup, citric acid syrup, licorice syrup, aromatic elixir, orange syrup, and wild cherry syrup.

Acrid or Sour Taste—Raspberry syrup and other fruit syrups are especially efficient in masking the taste of sour substances such as hydrochloric acid. Acacia syrup and other mucilaginous vehicles are best for disguising the acrid taste of substances such as capsicum, since they tend to form a colloidal protective coating over the taste buds of the tongue. Tragacanth, unlike acacia, may be used in an alcoholic vehicle.

Oily Taste—Castor oil may be made palatable by emulsifying with an equal volume of aromatic rhubarb syrup or with compound sarsaparilla syrup. Cod liver oil is disguised effectively by adding wintergreen oil or peppermint oil. Lemon, orange, and anise or combinations of these are also useful. It is better to mix most of the flavor with the oil before emulsifying it, and then the small remaining quantity can be added after the primary emulsion is formed.

Those flavors that are most pleasing to the majority of people are associated with some stimulant of a physical or physiological nature. This may be a CNS stimulant such as caffeine, which is the reason so many enjoy tea and coffee as a beverage, or it may be a counterirritant such as one of the spices that produce a *biting* sensation or an agent that *tickles* the throat such as soda water. Sherry owes its sharp flavor to its acetaldehyde content, and some of the volatile oils contain terpenes that are stimulating to the mucous surfaces.

SELECTION OF VEHICLES

Too few pharmacists realize the unique opportunity they have in acquainting physicians with a knowledge of how to increase both the palatability and efficacy of their prescribed medicines through the judicious selection of vehicles. Because of the training pharmacists receive, their knowledge of the characteristics of various pharmaceuticals and therapeutic agents and their technique and skill in preparing elegant preparations are well developed, so that they are qualified admirably to advise concerning the proper use of vehicles.

A large selection of flavors is available as well as a choice of colors, so that one may prescribe a basic drug for a prolonged period but by changing the vehicle from time to time, the taste and appearance are so altered that the patient does not tire of the prescription or show other psychological reactions to it.

The statement of the late Dr Bernard Fantus that "the best solvent is the best vehicle" helps to explain the proper use of a flavoring vehicle. For example, a substance that is soluble in alcohol (eg, phenobarbital) will not leave an alcoholic vehicle readily to dissolve in the aqueous saliva.

WATERS—These are the simplest of the vehicles and are available with several flavors. They contain no sucrose, a fact to be considered at times, since sucrose under certain circumstances may be undesirable. They are likewise nonalcoholic, another fact that frequently influences vehicle selection.

ELIXIRS—These have added sweetness that waters lack, and they usually contain alcohol, which imparts an added sharpness to the flavor of certain preparations, making the latter more pleasing to the taste. Elixirs are suitable for alcohol-soluble drugs.

SYRUPS—These vehicles, like elixirs, offer a wide selection of flavors and colors from which to choose. Their specific value, however, lies particularly in the fact that they are intensely sweet and contain little or no alcohol, a combination that makes them of singular value as masking agents for water-soluble drugs.

Vehicles consisting of a solution of pleasantly flavored volatile oils in syrup or glycerin (1:500) have been employed successfully in producing uniform and stable preparations. These vehicles are prepared by adding 2 mL of the volatile oil, diluted with 6 mL of alcohol, to 500 mL of glycerin or syrup, which has been warmed gently. The solution is added a little at a time with continuous shaking; then sufficient glycerin or syrup is added to make 1000 mL and mixed well.

Alcohol solutions of volatile oils are sometimes used as stock solutions for flavoring pharmaceuticals.

A listing of substances, most of them official, used as flavors, flavored vehicles, or sweeteners, is given in Table 55-1. Additional information on flavoring ingredients may be obtained in

Table 55-1. Flavoring Agents

Acacia syrup	Lavender oil
Anethole	Lemon oil
Anise oil	Lemon tincture
Aromatic elixir	Mannitol
Benzaldehyde	Methyl salicylate
Benzaldehyde elixir, compound	Nutmeg oil
Caraway	Orange, bitter, elixir
Caraway oil	Orange, bitter, oil
Cardamom oil	Orange flower oil
Cardamom seed	Orange flower water
Cardamom spirit, compound	Orange oil
Cardamom tincture, compound	Orange peel, bitter
Cherry juice	Orange peel, sweet, tincture
Cherry syrup	Orange spirit, compound
Cinnamon	Orange syrup
Cinnamon oil	Peppermint
Cinnamon water	Peppermint oil
Citric acid	Peppermint spirit
Citric acid syrup	Peppermint water
Clove oil	Phenylethyl alcohol
Cocoa	Raspberry juice
Cocoa syrup	Raspberry syrup
Coriander oil	Rosemary oil
Dextrose	Rose oil
Eriodictyon	Rose water
Eriodictyon fluidextract	Rose water, stronger
Eriodictyon syrup, aromatic	Saccharin
Ethyl acetate	Saccharin calcium
Ethyl vanillin	Saccharin sodium
Fennel oil	Sarsaparilla syrup, compound
Ginger	Sorbitol solution
Ginger fluidextract	Spearmint
Ginger oleoresin	Spearmint oil
Glucose	Sucrose
Glycerin	Syrup
Glycyrrhiza	Thyme oil
Glycyrrhiza elixir	Tolu balsam
Glycyrrhiza extract	Tolu balsam syrup
Glycyrrhiza extract, pure	Vanilla
Glycyrrhiza fluidextract	Vanilla tincture
Glycyrrhiza syrup	Vanillin
Honey	Wild cherry syrup
Iso-Alcoholic elixir	

Burdock GA, *Fenaroli's Handbook of Flavor Ingredients,* Cleveland: CRC, 1994.

ACACIA SYRUP—page 1070.

ANISE OIL

Aniseed Oil; Star Anise Oil

The volatile oil distilled with steam from the dried, ripe fruit of *Pimpinella anisum* Linné (Fam *Umbelliferae*) or from the dried, ripe fruit of *Illicium verum* Hooker filius (Fam *Magnoliaceae*).

Note—If solid material has separated, carefully warm the oil until it is completely liquefied, and mix it before using.

Constituents—The official oil varies somewhat in composition, depending upon whether it was obtained from *Pimpinella anisum* or the star anise, *Illicium verum.* Anethole is the chief constituent of both oils, occurring to the extent of 80 to 90%. Methyl chavicol, an isomer of anethole, and anisic ketone [$C_{10}H_{12}O_2$] also are found in both oils, as are small amounts of many other constituents.

Description—Colorless or pale yellow, strongly refractive liquid, having the characteristic odor and taste of anise; specific gravity 0.978 to 0.988; congeals not below 15.

Solubility—Soluble in 3 volumes of 90% alcohol.

Uses—Extensively as a flavoring agent, particularly for licorice candies. It has been given as a carminative in a dose of about 0.1 mL.

AROMATIC ELIXIR—page 1071.

BENZALDEHYDE

Artificial Essential Almond Oil

Benzaldehyde [100-52-7] C_7H_6O (106.12).

Preparation—By the interaction of benzal chloride with lime in the presence of water. Benzal chloride is obtained by treating boiling toluene with chlorine.

Description—Colorless, strongly refractive liquid, with an odor resembling that of bitter almond oil and a burning aromatic taste; affected by light; specific gravity 1.041 to 1.046; boils about 180°C, solidifies about -56.5°C, and on exposure to air it gradually oxidizes to benzoic acid.

Solubility—Dissolves in about 350 volumes of water; miscible with alcohol, ether, chloroform, or fixed and volatile oils.

Uses In place of bitter almond oil for flavoring purposes; it is much safer than the latter because it contains no hydrocyanic acid. It also is used extensively in perfumery and in the manufacture of dyestuffs and many other organic compounds, such as aniline, acetanilid, or mandelic acid.

Compound Benzaldehyde Elixir—Preparation: Dissolve benzaldehyde (0.5 mL) and vanillin (1 g) in alcohol (50 mL); add syrup (400 mL), orange flower water (150 mL), and sufficient purified water, in several portions, shaking the mixture thoroughly after each addition, to make the product measure 1000 mL; then filter, if necessary, until the product is clear. Alcohol Content: 3 to 5%.

Uses—A useful vehicle for administering bromides and other salts, especially when a low alcoholic content is desired.

CARDAMOM SEED

Cardamom Fruit; Cardamom; Ceylon or Malabar Cardamom

The dried ripe seed of *Elettaria cardamomum* (Linné) Maton (Fam. *Zingiberaceae*). It should be removed recently from the capsule.

Constituents—A volatile oil, the yield of which is 1.3% from Malabar Ceylon Seeds and 2.6% from Mysore-Ceylon Seeds. Fixed oil is present to the extent of 10%, also starch, mucilage, etc.

Uses—A flavor. For many years it was employed empirically as a carminative.

Cardamom Oil—The volatile oil distilled from the seed of *Elettaria cardamomum* (Linné) Maton (Fam *Zingiberaceae*). Varieties of the oil contain d-α-terpineol $C_{10}H_{17}OH$, both free and as the acetate; 5 to 10% cineol $C_{10}H_{18}O$; and limonene $C_{10}H_{16}$. The Ceylon Oil, however, contains the alcohol 4-terpineol (4-carbomenthenol) $C_{10}H_{17}OH$, the terpenes, terpinene and sabinene, and acetic and formic acids, probably combined as esters. Description and solubility: Colorless or very pale yellow liquid possessing the aromatic, penetrating, and somewhat camphoraceous odor of cardamom and a persistently pungent, strongly aromatic taste; affected by light; specific gravity 0.917 to 0.947. Miscible with alcohol; dissolves in 5 volumes of 70% alcohol. Uses: A flavor.

CHERRY SYRUP—page 1070.

CINNAMON

Saigon Cinnamon; True Cinnamon; Saigon Cassia

The dried bark of *Cinnamomum loureirii* Nees (Fam. *Lauraceae*). It contains, in each 100 g, not less than 2.5 mL of volatile oil.

Uses—A flavoring used as a carminative. Formerly, it was used as a carminative.

Cinnamon Oil (Cassia Oil; Oil of Chinese Cinnamon)—The volatile oil distilled with steam from the leaves and twigs of *Cinnamomum cassia* (Nees) Nees ex Blume (Fam *Lauraceae*), rectified by distillation; contains not less than 80%, by volume, of the total aldehydes of cinnamon oil. Cinnamaldehyde is the chief constituent. Description and solubility: Yellowish or brownish liquid, becoming darker and thicker on aging or exposure to the air, with the characteristic odor and taste of cassia cinnamon; specific gravity 1.045 to 1.063. Soluble in an equal volume of alcohol, 2 volumes of 70% alcohol, or an equal volume of glacial acetic acid. Uses: A flavor. It formerly was used in a dose of 0.1 mL for flatulent colic.

COCOA SYRUP—page 1070.
CORIANDER—page 1069.
DENATONIUM BENZOATE—page 1085.

ETHYL VANILLIN

Benzaldehyde, 3-ethoxy-4-hydroxy-, Bourbanal; Ethovan; Vanillal; Vanirome

3-Ethoxy-4-hydroxybenzaldehyde [121-32-4] $C_9H_{10}O_3$ (166.18).

Preparation—By reacting *o*-ethoxyphenol with formaldehyde and *p*-nitrosodimethylaniline in the presence of aluminum and water.

Description—Fine, white or slightly yellowish crystals; odor and taste similar to those of vanillin; affected by light; solutions are acid to litmus; melts about 77°C.

Solubility—1 g in about 100 mL water at 50°C; freely soluble in alcohol, chloroform, ether, or solutions of fixed alkali hydroxides.

Uses—A flavor, like vanillin, but stronger.

EUCALYPTUS OIL

The volatile oil distilled with steam from the fresh leaf of *Eucalyptus globulus* Labillardiére or of some other species of *Eucalyptus* (Fam *Myrtaceae*). It contains not less than 70% of $C_{10}H_{18}O$ (*eucalyptol*).

Constituents—The most important constituent is eucalyptol (cineol). Other compounds include d-α-pinene, globulol, pinocarveol, pinocarvone, and several aldehydes.

Description—Colorless or pale yellow liquid, with a characteristic, aromatic, somewhat camphoraceous odor, and a pungent, spicy, cooling taste; specific gravity 0.905 to 0.925 at 25°C.

Solubility—Soluble in 5 volumes of 70% alcohol.

Uses—A flavoring agent and an expectorant in chronic bronchitis. It also has bacteriostatic properties. This oil may be toxic.

FENNEL OIL

The volatile oil distilled with steam from the dried ripe fruit of *Foeniculum vulgare* Miller (Fam *Umbelliferae*).

Note—If solid material has separated, carefully warm the oil until it is completely liquefied, and mix it before using.

Constituents—Anethole $C_{10}H_{12}O$ is the chief constituent, occurring to the extent of 50 to 60%. Some of the other constituents are d-pinene, phellandrene, dipentene, fenchone, methylchavicol, anisaldehyde and anisic acid.

Description—Colorless or pale yellow liquid, with the characteristic odor and taste of fennel; specific gravity 0.953 to 0.973; congealing temperature is not below 3°C.

Solubility—Soluble in 8 volumes of 80% alcohol or in 1 volume of 90% alcohol.

Uses—A flavoring agent. It formerly was employed in a dose of 0.1 mL as a carminative.

GLYCYRRHIZA

Licorice Root; Liquorice Root; Sweetwood; Italian Juice Root; Spanish Juice Root

The dried rhizome and roots of *Glycyrrhiza glabra* Linné, known in commerce as Spanish Licorice, or of *Glycyrrhiza glabra* Linné var *glandulifera* Waldstein et Kitaibel, known in commerce as Russian Licorice, or of other varieties of *Glycyrrhiza glabra* Linné, yielding a yellow and sweet wood (Fam. *Leguminosae*).

Constituents—This well-known root contains 5 to 7% of the sweet principle glycyrrhizin, or glycyrrhizic acid, which is 50 times as sweet as cane sugar. There also is present an oleoresinous substance to which it's slight acidity is due. If alcohol or an alkali is used as a menstruum for the root and the preparation is not treated to deprive it of acridity, it will have a disagreeable aftertaste. For this reason boiling water is used for its extraction in both the extract and the fluid-extract.

Description—The USP/NF provides descriptions of Unground Spanish and Russian Glycyrrhizas, Histology, and Powdered Glycyrrhiza.

Uses—Valuable in pharmacy chiefly for its sweet flavor, it is one of the most efficient substances known for masking the taste of bitter substances, like quinine. Acids precipitate the glycyrrhizin and should not be added to mixtures in which glycyrrhiza is intended to mask disagreeable taste. Most of the imported licorice is used by tobacco manufacturers to flavor tobacco. It also is used in making candy.

Pure Glycyrrhiza Extract (Pure Licorice Root Extract)—Preparation: Moisten 1000 g of glycyrrhiza, in granular powder, with boiling water, transfer it to a percolator, and percolate with boiling water until the glycyrrhiza is exhausted. Add enough diluted ammonia solution to the percolate to impart a distinctly ammoniacal odor, then boil the liquid under normal atmospheric pressure until it is reduced to a volume of about 1500 mL. Filter the liquid, and immediately evaporate the filtrate until the residue has a pilular consistency. Pure extract of glycyrrhiza differs from the commercial extract in that it is almost completely soluble in aqueous mixtures. The large amount of filler used in the commercial extract to give it firmness renders it unfit to use as a substitute for the pure extract. Description: Black, pilular mass having a characteristic, sweet taste. Uses: A flavoring agent. One of the ingredients in Aromatic Cascara Sagrada Fluidextract.

Glycyrrhiza Fluidextract (Licorice Root Fluidextract); Liquid Extract of Liquorice—Preparation: To 1000 g of coarsely ground glycyrrhiza add about 3000 mL of boiling water, mix and allow to macerate in a suitable, covered percolator for 2 hr. Then allow the percolation to proceed at a rate of 1 to 3 mL/min, gradually adding boiling water until the glycyrrhiza is exhausted. Add enough diluted ammonia solution to the percolate to impart a distinctly ammoniacal odor, then boil the liquid actively under normal atmospheric pressure until it is reduced to a volume of about 1500 mL. Filter the liquid, evaporate the filtrate on a steam bath until the residue measures 750 mL, cool, gradually add 250 mL of alcohol and enough water to make the product measure 1000 mL, and mix. Alcohol Content: 20 to 24%, by volume. Uses: A pleasant flavor for use in syrups and elixirs to be employed as vehicles and correctives.

GLYCYRRHIZA ELIXIR—page 1071.
GLYCYRRHIZA SYRUP—page 1071.
HONEY—page 1092.
HYDRIODIC ACID SYRUP—page 1071.
ISO-ALCOHOLIC ELIXIR—page 1091.

LAVENDER OIL

Lavender Flowers Oil

The volatile oil distilled with steam from the fresh flowering tops of *Lavandula officinalis* Chaix ex Villars (*Lavandula vera* DeCandolle) (Fam *Labiatae*) or produced synthetically. It contains not less than 35% of esters calculated as $C_{12}H_{20}O_2$ (linalyl acetate).

Constituents—It is a product of considerable importance in perfumery. Linalyl acetate is the chief constituent. Cineol appears to be a normal constituent of English oils. Other constituents include amyl alcohol, d-borneol (small amount); geraniol, lavandulol ($C_{10}H_{18}O$); linalool; nerol; acetic, butyric, valeric, and caproic acids (as esters); traces of d-pinene, limonene (in English oils only), and the sesquiterpene caryophyllene; ethyl n-amyl ketone; an aldehyde (probably valeric aldehyde), and coumarin.

Description—Colorless or yellow liquid, with the characteristic odor and taste of lavender flowers; specific gravity 0.875 to 0.888.

Solubility—1 volume in 4 volumes of 70% alcohol.

Uses—Primarily as a perfume. It formerly was used in doses of 0.1 mL as a carminative.

LEMON OIL

The volatile oil obtained by expression, without the aid of heat, from the fresh peel of the fruit of *Citrus limon* (Linné) Burmann filius (Fam *Rutaceae*), with or without the previous separation of the pulp and the peel. The total aldehyde content, calculated as citral ($C_{10}H_{16}O$), is 2.2 to 3.8% for California-type oil, and 3.0 to 5.5% for Italian-type oil.

Note—Do not use oil that has a terebinthine odor.

Constituents—From the standpoint of odor and flavor, the most noteworthy constituent is the aldehyde citral, which is present to the extent of about 4%. About 90% of d-limonene is present; small amounts of l-α-pinene, β-pinene, camphene, β-phellandrene, and γ-terpinene also occur. About 2% of a solid, nonvolatile substance called citroptene, limettin, or lemon-camphor, which is dissolved out of the peel, also is present. In addition, there are traces of several other compounds: α-terpineol; the acetates of linalool and geraniol; citronellal, octyl, and nonyl aldehydes; the sesquiterpenes bisabolene and cadinene, and the ketone methylheptenone.

When fresh, the oil has the fragrant odor of lemons. Because of the instability of the terpenes present, the oil readily undergoes deterioration by oxidation, acquiring a terebinthinate odor.

Description—Pale yellow to deep yellow or greenish yellow liquid, with the characteristic odor and taste of the outer part of fresh lemon peel; specific gravity 0.849 to 0.855.

Solubility—In 3 volumes of alcohol; miscible in all proportions with dehydrated alcohol, carbon disulfide, or glacial acetic acid.

Uses—A flavor in pharmaceutical preparations and in certain candies and foods.

METHYL SALICYLATE

Benzoic acid, 2-hydroxy-, methyl ester; Gaultheria Oil; Wintergreen Oil; Betula Oil; Sweet Birch Oil; Teaberry Oil; Artificial Wintergreen Oil; Synthetic Wintergreen Oil

Methyl salicylate [119-36-8] $C_6H_4(OH)COOCH_3$ (152.15); produced synthetically or obtained by maceration and subsequent distillation with steam from the leaves of *Gaultheria procumbens* Linné (Fam *Ericaceae*) or from the bark of *Betula lenta* Linné (Fam *Betulaceae*).

Note—It must be labeled to indicate whether it was made synthetically or distilled from either of the plants mentioned above.

Preparation—Found naturally in gaultheria and betula oils and in many other plants, but the commercial product is usually synthetic, made by esterifying salicylic acid with methyl alcohol in the presence of sulfuric acid, and distilling.

Description—Colorless, yellowish, or reddish liquid, with the characteristic odor and taste of wintergreen; specific gravity (synthetic), 1.180 to 1.185, (from gaultheria or betula), 1.176 to 1.182; boils between 219 and 224°C with some decomposition.

Solubility—Slightly soluble in water; soluble in alcohol or glacial acetic acid.

Uses—A pharmaceutical necessity and counterirritant (local analgesic). As a pharmaceutical necessity, it is used to flavor the official Aromatic Cascara Sagrada Fluidextract and it is equal in every respect to wintergreen oil or sweet birch oil. As a counterirritant, it is applied to the skin in the form of a liniment, ointment, or cream; care should be exercised since salicylate is absorbed through the skin.

Caution—Because it smells like wintergreen candy, it is ingested frequently by children and has caused many fatalities. Keep out of the reach of children.

MONOSODIUM GLUTAMATE

Glutamic acid, monosodium salt, monohydrate

[142-47-2] $C_5H_8NNaO_4H_2O$ (187.13)

Preparation—From the fermentation of beet sugar or molasses or by hydrolysis of vegetable proteins.

Description—White, crystalline powder. The pentahydrate effloresces in air to form the monohydrate.

Solubility—Very soluble in water; sparingly soluble in alcohol.

Uses—Flavoring agent and perfume.

NUTMEG OIL

Myristica Oil NF; East Indian Nutmeg Oil; West Indian Nutmeg Oil

The volatile oil distilled with steam from the dried kernels of the ripe seeds of *Myristica fragrans* Houttuyn (Fam Myristicaceae).

Constituents—It contains about 80% of d-pinene and d-camphene; 8% of dipentene; about 6% of the alcohols d-borneol, geraniol, d-linalool, and terpineol; 4% of myristicin; 0.6% of safrol; 0.3% of myristic acid free and as esters; 0.2% of eugenol and isoeugenol; and traces of the alcohol terpineol-4, a citral-like aldehyde, and several acids, all present as esters.

Description—Colorless or pale yellow liquid with the characteristic odor and taste of nutmeg; specific gravity (East Indian Oil) 0.880 to 0.910, (West Indian Oil) 0.854 to 0.880.

Solubility—In an equal amount of alcohol; 1 volume of East Indian Oil in 3 volumes of 90% alcohol; 1 volume of West Indian Oil in 4 volumes of 90% alcohol.

Uses—Primarily as a flavoring agent. It is used for this purpose in Aromatic Ammonia Spirit. The oil also is employed as a flavor in foods, certain alcoholic beverages, dentifrices, and tobacco; to some extent, it also is used in perfumery. It formerly was used as a carminative and local stimulant to the GI tract in a dose of 0.03 mL. In overdoses, it acts as a narcotic poison. This oil is very difficult to keep and if even slightly terebinthinate is unfit for flavoring purposes.

ORANGE OIL

Sweet Orange Oil

The volatile oil obtained by expression from the fresh peel of the ripe fruit of *Citrus sinensis* (Linné) Osbeck (Fam *Rutaceae*). The total aldehyde content, calculated as decanal ($C_{10}H_{20}O$), is 1.2 to 2.5%.

Note—Do not use oil that has a terebinthine odor.

Constituents—Consists of d-limonene to the extent of at least 90%; in the remaining 5 to 10% are the odorous constituents, among which, in samples of American origin, are n-decylic aldehyde, citral, d-linalool, n-nonyl alcohol, and traces of esters of formic, acetic, caprylic and capric acids.

In addition to most of these compounds, Italian-produced oil contains d-terpineol, terpinolene, α-terpinene, and methyl anthranilate.

Kept under the usual conditions it is very prone to decompose and rapidly acquires a terebinthine odor.

Description—Intensely yellow-orange or deep orange liquid, which possesses the characteristic odor and taste of the outer part of fresh sweet orange peel; specific gravity 0.842 to 0.846.

Solubility—Miscible with dehydrated alcohol or carbon disulfide; dissolves in an equal volume of glacial acetic acid.

Uses—A flavoring agent in elixirs and other preparations.

ORANGE FLOWER WATER—page 1070.

SWEET ORANGE PEEL TINCTURE

Preparation—From sweet orange peel, which is the outer rind of the naturally colored, fresh, ripe fruit of *Citrus sinensis* (Linné) Osbeck (Fam *Rutaceae*), by Process M. Macerate 500 g of the sweet orange peel (exclude the inner, white portion of the rind) in 900 mL of alcohol, and complete the preparation with alcohol to make the product measure 1000 mL. Use talc as the filtering medium.

The white portion of the rind must not be used, as the proportion of oil, which is only in the yellow rind, is reduced, and the bitter principle hesperidin is introduced.

Alcohol Content—62 to 72%.

Uses—A flavor, used in syrups, elixirs, and emulsions. This tincture was introduced to provide a delicate orange flavor direct from the fruit instead of depending upon orange oil, which so frequently is terebinthinate and unfit for use. The tincture keeps well.

COMPOUND ORANGE SPIRIT

Contains, in each 100 mL, 25 to 30 mL of the mixed oils.

Orange Oil	200 mL
Lemon Oil	50 mL
Coriander Oil	20 mL
Anise Oil	5 mL
Alcohol, a sufficient quantity, to make 1000 mL	

Mix the oils with sufficient alcohol to make the product measure 1000 mL.

Alcohol Content—65 to 75%.

Uses—A flavor for elixirs. An alcoholic solution of this kind permits the uniform introduction of small proportions of oils and also preserves orange and lemon oils from rapid oxidation. The pharmacist should buy these two oils in small quantities, since the spirit is made most satisfactorily from oils taken from bottles not previously opened. This will ensure that delicacy of flavor that should always be characteristic of elixirs.

ORANGE SYRUP

Syrup of Orange Peel

Contains, in each 100 mL, 450 to 550 mg of citric acid ($C_6H_8O_7$).

Sweet Orange Peel Tincture	50 mL
Citric Acid (anhydrous)	5 g
Talc	15 g
Sucrose	820 g
Purified Water, a sufficient quantity, to make 1000 mL	

Triturate the talc with the tincture and citric acid, and gradually add 400 mL of purified water. Then filter, returning the first portions of the filtrate until it becomes clear, and wash the mortar and filter with enough purified water to make the filtrate measure 450 mL. Dissolve the sucrose in this filtrate by agitation, without heating, and add enough purified water to make the product measure 1000 mL. Mix and strain.

Note—Do not use syrup that has a terebinthine odor or taste or shows other indications of deterioration.

Alcohol Content—2 to 5%.

Uses—A pleasant, acidic vehicle.

PEPPERMINT

American Mint; Lamb Mint; Brandy Mint

Consists of the dried leaf and flowering top of *Mentha piperita* Linné (Fam *Labiatae*).

Uses—The source of green color for Peppermint Spirit (see RPS-19 page 902). The odor of fresh peppermint is due to the presence of about 2% of a volatile oil, much of which is lost on drying the leaves in air. It is cultivated widely both in the US and France. It formerly was used as a carminative.

Peppermint Oil—The volatile oil distilled with steam from the fresh overground parts of the flowering plant *Mentha piperita* Linné (Fam *Labiatae*), rectified by distillation and neither partially nor wholly dementholized. It yields not less than 5% of esters, calculated as menthyl acetate $C_{12}H_{22}O_2$, and not less than 50% of total menthol $C_{10}H_{20}O$, free and as esters. Constituents: This is one of the most important of the group of volatile oils. The chief constituent is Menthol (page 1285), which occurs in the levorotatory form; its ester, menthyl acetate, is present in a much smaller amount. Other compounds that are present include the ketone menthone, piperitone, α-pinene, l-limonene, phellandrene, cadinene, menthyl isovalerate, isovaleric aldehyde, acetaldehyde, menthofuran, cineol, an unidentified lactone $C_{10}H_{16}O_2$, and probably amyl acetate.

Description and Solubility—Colorless or pale yellow liquid, with a strong, penetrating odor of peppermint and a pungent taste, followed by a sensation of cold when air is drawn into the mouth; specific gravity 0.896 to 0.908; 1 volume dissolves in 3 volumes of 70% alcohol. Uses: A flavoring agent, carminative, antiseptic, and local anesthetic. It also is used extensively as a flavor in candy, chewing gum, etc.

PEPPERMINT SPIRIT—see RPS-19, page 902.
PEPPERMINT WATER—page 1070.

PHENYLETHYL ALCOHOL

Benzeneethanol; 2-Phenylethanol

Phenethyl alcohol [60-12-8] $C_8H_{10}O$ (122.17); occurs in a number of essential oils such as those of rose, neroli, hyacinth, carnation, and others.

Description—Colorless liquid with a rose-like odor and a sharp, burning taste; solidifies at −27°C; specific gravity 1.017 to 1.020.

Solubility—1 g in 60 mL water or <1 mL alcohol, chloroform, or ether; very soluble in fixed oils, glycerin, or propylene glycol; slightly soluble in mineral oil.

Uses—Introduced for use as an antibacterial agent in ophthalmic solutions, but it is of limited effectiveness.

It is used in flavors, as a soap perfume, and in the preparation of synthetic oils of rose and similar flower oils. It is also a valuable perfume fixative.

ROSE OIL

Otto of Rose; Attar of Rose

The volatile oil distilled with steam from the fresh flowers of *Rosa gallica* Linné, *Rosa damascena* Miller, *Rosa alba* Linné, *Rosa centifolia* Linné, and varieties of these species (Fam *Rosaceae*).

Constituents—From the quantitative standpoint the chief components are the alcohols geraniol ($C_{10}H_{18}O$) and l-citronellol ($C_{10}H_{20}O$). The sesquiterpene alcohols farnesol and nerol occur to the extent of 1% and 5 to 10%, respectively. Together, the four alcohols constitute 70 to 75% of the oil. Phenylethyl alcohol, which constitutes 1% of the oil, is an important odoriferous constituent. Other compounds present are linalool, eugenol, nonyl aldehyde, traces of citral, and two solid hydrocarbons of the paraffin series.

Description and Solubility—A colorless or yellow liquid, which has the characteristic odor and taste of rose; at 25°C, a viscous liquid;

on gradual cooling it changes to a translucent, crystalline mass, which may be liquefied easily by warming; specific gravity 0.848 to 0.863 at 30°C, compared with water at 15°C; 1 mL mixes with 1 mL of chloroform without turbidity; on the addition of 20 mL of 90% alcohol to this solution, the resulting liquid is neutral or acid to moistened litmus paper and deposits a crystalline residue within 5 min on standing at 20°C.

Uses—Principally as a perfume. It is recognized officially for its use as an ingredient in Rose Water Ointment and cosmetics.

STRONGER ROSE WATER

Triple Rose Water

A saturated solution of the odoriferous principles of the flowers of *Rosa centifolia* Linné (Fam *Rosaceae*), prepared by distilling the fresh flowers with water and separating the excess volatile oil from the clear, water portion of the distillate.

Note—When diluted with an equal volume of purified water, it may be supplied when Rose Water is required.

Description—Nearly colorless and clear liquid that possesses the pleasant odor and taste of fresh rose blossoms; must be free from empyreuma, mustiness, and fungal growths.

Uses—An ingredient in Rose Water Ointment. It sometimes is prepared extemporaneously from concentrates or from rose oil, but such water is not official and rarely compares favorably with the fresh distillate from rose petals.

SACCHARIN

1,2-Benzisothiazol-3(2H)-one, 1,1-dioxide; Gluside; *o*-Benzosulfimide

1,2-Benzisothiazolin-3-one 1,1-dioxide [81-07-2] $C_7H_5NO_3S$ (183.18).

Preparation—Toluene is reacted with chlorosulfonic acid to form *o*-toluenesulfonyl chloride, which is converted to the sulfonamide with ammonia. The methyl group then is oxidized with dichromate, yielding *o*-sulfamoylbenzoic acid, which, when heated, forms the cyclic imide.

Description—White crystals or a white crystalline powder; odorless or with a faint aromatic odor; in dilute solution it is intensely sweet; solutions are acid to litmus; melts between 226 and 230°C.

Solubility—1 g in 290 mL water, 31 mL alcohol, or 25 mL boiling water; slightly soluble in chloroform or ether; readily dissolved by dilute solution of ammonia, solutions of alkali hydroxides, or solutions of alkali carbonates, with the evolution of CO_2.

Uses—A sweetening agent in Aromatic Cascara Sagrada Fluidextract and highly alcoholic preparations. It is an intensely sweet substance. A 60-mg portion is equivalent in sweetening power to approximately 30 g of sucrose. It is used as a sweetening agent in vehicles, canned foods, and beverages and in diets for diabetics to replace the sucrose. The relative sweetening power of saccharin is increased by dilution.

SACCHARIN CALCIUM

1,2-Benzisothiazol-3(2H)-one, 1,1-dioxide, calcium salt, hydrate (2:7) Calcium *o*-Benzosulfimide

1,2-Benzisothiazolin-3-one 1,1-dioxide calcium salt hydrate (2:7) [6381-91-5] $C_{14}H_8CaN_2O_6S_2$ • 31/2 H_2O (467.48); anhydrous [6485-34-3] (404.43).

Preparation—Saccharin is reacted with a semimolar quantity of calcium hydroxide in aqueous medium, and the resulting solution is concentrated to crystallization.

Description—White crystals or a white, crystalline powder; odorless or with a faint aromatic odor; and an intensely sweet taste even in dilute solutions; in dilute solution it is about 300 times as sweet as sucrose.

Solubility—1 g in 2.6 mL water or 4.7 mL alcohol.

Uses See Saccharin.

SACCHARIN SODIUM

1,2-Benzisothiazol-3(2H)-one, 1,1-dioxide, sodium salt, dihydrate; Soluble Saccharin; Soluble Gluside; Sodium *o*-Benzosulfimide

1,2-Benzisothiazolin-3-one 1,1-dioxide sodium salt dihydrate [6155-57-3] $C_7H_4NNaO_3S$ • 2 H_2O (241.19); *anhydrous* [128-44-9] (205.16).

Preparation—Saccharin is dissolved in an equimolar quantity of aqueous sodium hydroxide, and the solution is concentrated to crystallization.

Description—White crystals or a white crystalline powder; odorless or with a faint aromatic odor, and an intensely sweet taste even in dilute solutions; in dilute solution it is about 300 times as sweet as sucrose; in powdered form it usually contains about 1/3 the theoretical amount of water of hydration because of efflorescence.

Solubility—1 g in 1.5 mL water or 50 mL alcohol.

Uses—Same as Saccharin but has the advantage of being more soluble in neutral aqueous solutions.

SORBITOL

Sionin; Sorbit; D-Sorbitol; D-Glucitol; Sorbo

D-Glucitol [50-70-4] $C_6H_{14}O_6$ (182.17); it may contain small amounts of other polyhydric alcohols.

Preparation—Commercially by reduction (hydrogenation) of certain sugars, such as glucose.

Description—White, hygroscopic powder, granules, or flakes, with a sweet taste; the usual form melts about 96°C.

Solubility—1 g in about 0.45 mL of water; slightly soluble in alcohol, methanol, or acetic acid.

Uses—An osmotic diuretic given intravenously in 50% (w/v) solution to diminish edema, lower cerebrospinal pressure, or reduce intraocular pressure in glaucoma; used as a laxative, sweetener, humectant, plasticizer and, in 70% (w/w) solution, as a vehicle.

Sorbitol Solution—a water solution containing, in each 100 g, 69 to 71 g of total solids consisting essentially of D-sorbitol and a small amount of mannitol and other isomeric polyhydric alcohols. The content of D-sorbitol $C_6H_8(OH)_6$ in each 100 g is not less than 64 g. Description: Clear, colorless, syrupy liquid, with a sweet taste and no characteristic odor; neutral to litmus; specific gravity not less than 1.285; refractive index at 20 1.455 to 1.465. Uses: It is not to be injected. It has been used as a replacement for propylene glycol and glycerin.

SPEARMINT

Spearmint Leaves; Spearmint Herb; Mint

The dried leaf and flowering top of *Mentha spicata* Linné (*Mentha viridis* Linné) (Common Spearmint) or of *Mentha cardiaca* Gerard ex Baker (Scotch Spearmint) (Fam *Labiatae*).

Fresh spearmint is used in preparing mint sauce and also the well-known mint julep. The volatile oil is the only constituent of importance in this plant; the yield is from 1/2 to 1%.

Uses A flavoring agent.

Spearmint Oil—the volatile oil distilled with steam from the fresh overground parts of the flowering plant *Mentha spicata* or *Mentha cardiaca;* contains not less than 55%, by volume, of $C_{10}H_{14}O$ (carvone, 150.22). The chief odoriferous constituent is the ketone l-carvone. American oil also contains dihydrocarveol acetate [$CH_3COOC_{10}H_{17}$], l-limonene [$C_{10}H_{16}$], a small amount of phellandrene [$C_{10}H_{16}$], and traces of esters of valeric and caproic acids.

Description and Solubility—Colorless, yellow, or greenish yellow liquid, with the characteristic odor and taste of spearmint; specific gravity 0.917 to 0.934. Soluble in 1 volume of 80% alcohol, but upon further dilution may become turbid. Uses: Primarily as a flavoring agent. It also has been used as a carminative in doses of 0.1 mL.

SUCROSE

α-D-Glucopyranoside, β-D-fructofuranosyl-, Sugar; Cane Sugar; Beet Sugar

Sucrose [57-50-1] $C_{12}H_{22}O_{11}$ (342.30); a sugar obtained from *Saccharum officinarum* Linné (Fam *Gramineae*), *Beta vulgaris* Linné (Fam *Chenopodiaceae*), and other sources. It contains no added substances.

Preparation—Commercially from sugar cane, beat root, and sorghum. Originally, sugar cane was the only source, but at present the root of *Beta vulgaris* is used largely in Europe, and to an increasing degree in this country, for making sucrose.

The sugar cane is crushed, and the juice amounting to about 80% is expressed with roller mills. The juice, after defecation with lime and removal of excess of lime by carbonic acid gas, is run into vacuum pans for concentration, and the saccharine juice is evaporated in this until it begins to crystallize. After the crystallization is complete, the warm mixture of crystals and syrup is run into centrifuges, in which the crystals of raw sugar are drained and dried. The syrup resulting as a by-product from raw sugar is known as molasses. Raw beet sugar is made by a similar process but is more troublesome to purify than that made from sugar cane.

The refined sugar from either raw cane or beet sugar is prepared by dissolving the raw sugar in water, clarifying, filtering, and finally decolorizing the solution by passing it through bone-black filters. The water-white solution finally is evaporated under reduced pressure to the crystallizing point and then forced to crystallize in small granules that are collected and drained in a centrifuge.

Description—Colorless or white crystals, crystalline masses or blocks, or a white, crystalline powder; odorless; sweet taste; stable in air; solutions neutral to litmus; melts with decomposition from 160 to 185°C; specific gravity of about 1.57; specific rotation at 20°C not less than +65.9; unlike the other official sugars (dextrose, fructose, and lactose), it does not reduce Fehling's solution even in hot solutions; also differs from these sugars in that it is darkened and charred by sulfuric acid in the cold, is fermentable, and in dilute aqueous solutions, it ferments into alcohol and eventually acetic acid.

Sucrose is hydrolyzed by dilute mineral acids, slowly in the cold and rapidly on heating, into one molecule each of dextrose or levulose. This process is known technically as inversion and the product is referred to as invert sugar the term inversion being derived from the change, through the hydrolysis, in the optical rotation from dextro of sucrose to levo of the hydrolyzed product. The enzyme invertase also hydrolyzes sucrose.

Solubility—1 g in 0.5 mL water, 170 mL alcohol, or slightly more than 0.2 mL boiling water; insoluble in chloroform or ether.

Uses—Principally as a pharmaceutical necessity for making syrups and lozenges. It gives viscosity and consistency to fluids.

Intravenous administration of hypertonic solutions has been employed chiefly to initiate osmotic diuresis. Such a procedure is not completely safe, and renal tubular damage may result, particularly in patients with existing renal pathology. Safer and more effective diuretics are available.

CONFECTIONER'S SUGAR

Sucrose ground together with corn starch to a fine powder; contains 95.0 to 97.0% sucrose.

Description—Fine, white, odorless powder; sweet taste; stable in air; specific rotation not less than +62.6.

Solubility—The sucrose portion is soluble in cold water; this is entirely soluble in boiling water.

Uses—A pharmaceutical aid as a tableting excipient and sweetening agent. See also Sucrose.

SYRUP—page 1071.

TOLU BALSAM

Tolu

A balsam obtained from *Myroxylon balsamum* (Linné) Harms (Fam *Leguminosae*).

Constituents—Up to 80% resin, about 7% volatile oil, 12 to 15% free cinnamic acid, 2 to 8% benzoic acid, and 0.05% vanillin. The volatile oil is composed chiefly of benzyl benzoate, and benzyl cinnamate, ethyl benzoate, ethyl cinnamate, a terpene called tolene (possibly identical with phellandrene), and the sesquiterpene alcohol farnesol also have been reported to be present.

Description—Brown or yellowish brown, plastic solid; transparent in thin layers and brittle when old, dried, or exposed to cold temperatures; pleasant, aromatic odor resembling that of vanilla and a mild, aromatic taste.

Solubility—Nearly insoluble in water or solvent hexane; soluble in alcohol, chloroform, or ether, sometimes with slight residue or turbidity.

Uses—A vehicle, flavoring agent, and stimulating expectorant as a syrup. It is also an ingredient of Compound Benzoin Tincture (page 1280).

Tolu Balsam Syrup [Syrup of Tolu; Tolu Syrup]—Preparation: Add tolu balsam tincture (50 mL, all at once) to magnesium carbonate (10 g) and sucrose (60 g) in a mortar, and mix intimately. Gradually add purified water (430 mL) with trituration, and filter. Dissolve the remainder of the sucrose (760 g) in the clear filtrate with gentle heating, strain the syrup while warm, and add purified water (qs) through the strainer to make the product measure 1000 mL. Mix thoroughly. Note: May be made also in the following manner: Place the remaining sucrose (760 g) in a

suitable percolator, the neck of which nearly is filled with loosely packed cotton, moistened after packing with a few drops of water. Pour the filtrate, obtained as directed in the formula above, upon the sucrose, and regulate the outflow to a steady drip of percolate. When all of the liquid has run through, return portions of the percolate, if necessary, to dissolve all of the sucrose. Then pass enough purified water through the cotton to make the product measure 1000 mL. Mix thoroughly. Alcohol Content: 3 to 5%. Uses: Chiefly for its agreeable flavor in cough syrups. Dose: 10 mL.

Tolu Balsam Tincture [Tolu Tincture]—Preparation: With tolu balsam (200 g), prepare a tincture by Process M using alcohol as the menstruum. Alcohol Content: 77 to 83%. Uses: A balsamic preparation employed as an addition to expectorant mixtures; also used in the preparation of Tolu Balsam Syrup.

VANILLA

Vanilla Bean

The cured, full-grown, unripe fruit of *Vanilla planifolia* Andrews, often known in commerce as Mexican or Bourbon Vanilla, or of *Vanilla tahitensis* JW Moore, known in commerce as Tahiti Vanilla (Fam *Orchidaceae*); yields not less than 12% of anhydrous extractive soluble in diluted alcohol.

Constituents—Contains a trace of a volatile oil, fixed oil, 4% resin, sugar, vanillic acid, and about 2.5% vanillin (see below). This highest grade of vanilla comes from Madagascar; considerable quantities of the drug also are produced in Mexico.

Uses—A flavor.

Note—Do not use if it has become brittle.

Vanilla Tincture [Extract of Vanilla]—Preparation: Add water (200 mL) to comminuted vanilla (cut into small pieces, 100 g) in a suitable covered container, and macerate during 12 hr, preferably in a warm place. Add alcohol (200 mL) to the mixture of vanilla and water, mix well, and macerate about 3 days. Transfer the mixture to a percolator containing sucrose (in coarse granules, 200 g), and drain; then pack the drug firmly, and percolate slowly, using diluted alcohol (qs) as the solvent. If the percolator is packed with an evenly distributed mixture of the comminuted vanilla, sucrose, and clean, dry sand, the increased surface area permits more efficient percolation. This tincture is unusual in that it is the only official one in which sucrose is specified as an ingredient. Alcohol Content: 38 to 42%. Uses: A flavoring agent. See Flavors, page 1061.

VANILLIN

Benzaldehyde, 4-hydroxy-3-methoxy-,

4-Hydroxy-3-methoxybenzaldehyde [121-33-5] $C_8H_8O_3$ (152.15).

Preparation—From vanilla, which contains 2 to 3%. It also is found in many other substances, including tissues of certain plants, crude beet sugar, asparagus, and even asafetida. Commercially, it is made synthetically. While chemically identical with the product obtained from the vanilla bean, flavoring preparations made from it never equal in flavor the preparation in which vanilla alone is used, because vanilla contains other odorous products. It is synthesized by oxidation processes from either coniferin or eugenol, by treating guaiacol with chloroform in the presence of an alkali, and by other methods.

Description—Fine, white to slightly yellow crystals, usually needle-like, with an odor and taste suggestive of vanilla; affected by light; solutions are acid to litmus; melts 81 to 83°C.

Solubility—1 g in about 100 mL water, about 20 mL glycerin, or 20 mL water at 80°C; freely soluble in alcohol, chloroform, ether, or solutions of the fixed alkali hydroxides.

Incompatibilities—Combines with glycerin, forming a compound that is almost insoluble in alcohol. It is decomposed by alkali and is oxidized slowly by the air.

Uses—Only as a flavor. Solutions of it sometimes are sold as a synthetic substitute for vanilla for flavoring foods, but it is inferior in flavor to the real vanilla extract.

WATER—page 1070.
WATER PURIFIED—page 1070.
WILD CHERRY SYRUP—page 1069.

OTHER FLAVORING AGENTS

Anise NF [Anise Seed; European Aniseed; Sweet Cumin]—The dried ripe fruit of *Pimpinella anisum* Linné. It contains about 1.75% of volatile oil. Uses: A flavor and carminative.

Ceylon Cinnamon—The dried inner bark of the shoots of coppiced trees of *Cinnamomum zeylanicum* Nees (Fam *Lauraceae*); contains, in each 100 g, not less than 0.5 mL volatile oil. Uses: A carminative and flavor.

Clove—The dried flower-bud of *Eugenia caryophyllus* (Sprengel) Bullock et Harrison (Fam *Myrtaceae*). It contains, in each 100 g, not less than 16 mL of clove oil. Uses: An aromatic in doses of 0.25 g and as a condiment in foods.

Coriander—The dried ripe fruit of *Coriandrum sativum* Linné (Fam *Umbelliferae*); yields not less than 0.25 mL volatile coriander oil/100 g. Uses: Seldom used alone, but sometimes is combined with other agents, chiefly as a flavor. It also is used as a condiment and flavor in cooking.

Eucalyptol [Cineol; Cajeputol] C10H18O (154.25)—Obtained from eucalyptus oil and from other sources. Colorless liquid, with a characteristic aromatic, distinctly camphoraceous odor and a pungent, cooling, spicy taste; 1 volume is soluble in 5 volumes of 60% alcohol; miscible with alcohol, chloroform, ether, glacial acetic acid, or fixed or volatile oils; insoluble in water. Uses: Primarily as a flavoring agent. Locally it is employed for its antiseptic effect in inflammations of the nose and throat and in certain skin diseases. It sometimes is used by inhalation in bronchitis.

Fennel [Fennel Seed]—The dried ripe fruit of cultivated varieties of *Foeniculum vulgare* Miller (Fam *Umbelliferae*); contains 4 to 6% of an oxygenated volatile oil and 10% of a fixed oil. Uses: A flavor and carminative.

Ginger NF [Zingiber]—The dried rhizome of *Zingiber officinale* Roscoe (Fam *Zingiberaceae*), known in commerce as Jamaica Ginger, African Ginger and Cochin Ginger. The outer cortical layers often are removed either partially or completely. Constituents: A pungent substance, gingerol; volatile oil (Jamaica Ginger, about 1%; African Ginger, 2 to 3%), containing the terpenes d-camphene and β-phellandrene and the sesquiterpene zingiberene; citral cineol and borneol. Uses: A flavoring agent. It formerly was employed in a dose of 600 mg as an intestinal stimulant and carminative in colic and in diarrhea.

Ginger Oleoresin—Yields 18 to 35 mL of volatile ginger oil/100 g of oleoresin. Preparation: Extract the oleoresin from ginger, in moderately coarse powder, by percolation, using either acetone, alcohol, or ether as the menstruum.

Glycyrrhiza Extract [Licorice Root Extract; Licorice]—An extract prepared from the rhizome and roots of species of *Glycyrrhiza* Tournefort ex Linné (Fam *Leguminosae*). Description: Brown powder or in flattened, cylindrical rolls, or in masses; the rolls or masses have a glossy black color externally and a brittle, sharp, smooth, conchoidal fracture; the extract has a characteristic sweet taste that is not more than very slightly acrid. Uses: A flavoring agent.

Lavender [Lavendula]—The flowers of *Lavandula spica* (*Lavandula officinalis* or *Lavandula vera*); contains a volatile oil with the principal constituent l-linalyl acetate. Uses: A perfume.

Lemon Peel USP, BP [Fresh Lemon Peel]—The outer yellow rind of the fresh ripe fruit of *Citrus limon* (Linné) Burmann filius (Fam *Rutaceae*); contains a volatile oil and hesperidin. Uses: A flavor.

Lemon Tincture USP [Lemon Peel Tincture]—Preparation: From lemon peel, which is the outer yellow rind of the fresh, ripe fruit of *Citrus limon* (Linné) Burmann filius (Fam Rutaceae), by Process M, 500 g of the peel being macerated in 900 mL alcohol, and the preparation being completed with alcohol to make the product measure 1000 mL. Use talc as the filtering medium. The white portion of the rind must not be used, as the proportion of oil, which is found only in the yellow rind, is reduced, and the bitter principle, hesperidin, introduced. Alcohol Content: 62 to 72%. Uses: A flavor, its fineness of flavor being ensured as it comes from the fresh fruit, and being an alcoholic solution it is more stable than the oil.

Myrcia Oil [Bay Oil; Oil of Bay]—The volatile oil distilled from leaves of *Pimenta racemosa* (Miller) JW Moore (Fam *Myrtaceae*); contains the phenolic compounds eugenol and chavicol. Uses: In the preparation of bay rum as a perfume.

Orange Oil, Bitter—The volatile oil obtained by expression from the fresh peel of the fruit of *Citrus aurantium* Linné (Fam *Rutaceae*); contains primarily *d*-limonene. Pale yellow liquid with a characteristic aromatic odor of the Seville orange; if it has a terebinthinate odor, it should not be dispensed; refractive index 1.4725 to 1.4755 at 20°C. It differs little from Orange Oil except for the botanical source. Miscible with anhydrous alcohol and with about 4 volumes alcohol. Uses: A flavor.

Orange Peel, Bitter [Bitter Orange; Curacao Orange Peel; Bigarade Orange]. The dried rind of the unripe but fully grown fruit of *Citrus aurantium* Linné (Fam *Rutaceae*). Constituents: The inner part of the peel from the bitter orange contains a volatile oil and the glycoside hesperidin ($C_{28}H_{34}O_{15}$). This, upon hydrolysis in the presence of H_2SO_4, yields hesperetin ($C_{16}H_{14}O_6$), rhamnose ($C_6H_{12}O_5$), and D-glucose ($C_6H_{12}O_6$). Uses: A flavoring agent. It has been used as a bitter.

Orange Peel, Sweet USP—The fresh outer rind of the non-artificially-colored, ripe fruit of *Citrus sinensis* (Linné) Osbeck (Fam *Ru-*

taceae); the white inner portion of the rind is to be excluded. Contains a volatile oil but no hesperidin, since the glycoside occurs in the white portion of the rind. Uses: A flavor.

Orris [Orris Root; Iris; Florentine Orris]—The peeled and dried rhizome of *Iris germanica* Linné, including its variety *florentina* Dykes (*Iris florentina* Linné), or of *Iris pallida* Lamarck (Fam *Iridaceae*); contains about 0.1 to 0.2% of a volatile oil (orris butter), myristic acid and the ketone irone; irone provides the fragrant odor of orris. Uses: A perfume.

Pimenta Oil [Pimento Oil; Allspice Oil]—The volatile oil distilled from the fruit of *Pimenta officinalis* Lindley (Fam *Myrtaceae*). Uses: A carminative and stimulant and also as a condiment in foods.

Rosemary Oil—The volatile oil distilled with steam from the fresh flowering tops of *Rosmarinus officinalis* Linné (Fam *Labiatae*); yields not less than 1.5% of esters calculated as bornyl acetate ($C_{12}H_{20}O_2$) and not less than 8% of total borneol ($C_{10}H_{18}O$), free and as esters. Constituents: The amount of esters, calculated as bornyl acetate, and of total borneol, respectively, varies somewhat with its geographical source. Cineol is present to the extent of about 19 to 25%, depending on the source. The terpenes d- and l-α-pinene, dipentene, and camphene, and the ketone camphor also occur in this oil. Description and Solubility: Colorless or pale yellow liquid, with the characteristic odor of rosemary and a warm, camphoraceous taste; specific gravity 0.894 to 0.912. Soluble in 1 volume of 90% alcohol, by volume, but upon further dilution may become turbid. Uses: A flavor and perfume, chiefly, in rubefacient liniments such as Camphor and Soap Liniment.

Sassafras—The dried bark of the root of *Sassafras albidum* (Nuttall) Nees (Fam *Lauraceae*). Uses: Principally because of its high content of volatile oil that serves to disguise the taste of disagreeable substances. An infusion (sassafras tea) formerly was used extensively as a home remedy, particularly in the southern states.

Sassafras Oil—The volatile oil distilled with steam from Sassafras. Uses: A flavor by confectioners, particularly in hard candies. Either the oil or safrol is used as a preservative in mucilage and library paste, being far superior to methyl salicylate for this purpose. Since the oil is antiseptic, it sometimes is employed in conjunction with other agents for local application in diseases of the nose and throat; safrol also is used in this way.

Wild Cherry [Wild Black Cherry Bark]—The carefully dried stem bark of *Prunus serotina* Ehrhart (Fam *Rosaceae*), free of borke and preferably having been collected in autumn. Constituents: A glucoside of d-mandelonitrile (C_6H_5 • CHOH • CN) known as prunasin, the enzyme emulsin, tannin, a bitter principle, starch, resin, etc. In the BP and the English literature this drug has been termed Virginian Prune—a literal but incorrect translation of the older botanical name, *Prunus virginiana*. Uses: A flavoring agent, especially in cough preparations. It is an ingredient in Wild Cherry Syrup. As with bitter almond, contact with water, in the presence of emulsin, results in the production of benzaldehyde and HCN. All preparations of wild cherry should be made without heat, to avoid destruction of the enzyme that is responsible for the production of the free active principles.

Diluting Agents

Diluting agents (vehicles or carriers) are indifferent substances that are used as solvents for active medicinals. They are of primary importance for diluting and flavoring drugs that are intended for oral administration, but a few such agents are designed specifically for diluting parenteral injections. The latter group is considered separately.

The expert selection of diluting agents has been an important factor in popularizing the specialties of compounding pharmacists. Since a large selection of diluting agents is available in a choice of colors and flavors, prescribers have the opportunity to make their own prescriptions more acceptable to the patient. The best diluting agent is usually the best solvent for the drug. Water-soluble substances, for example, should be flavored and diluted with an aqueous agent, and alcohol-soluble drugs with an alcoholic vehicle. Thus, the diluting agents presented herein are divided into three groups on the basis of their physical properties: aqueous, hydroalcoholic, and alcoholic.

AQUEOUS DILUTING AGENTS

Aqueous diluting agents include aromatic waters, syrups, and mucilages. Aromatic waters are used as diluting agents for water-soluble substances and salts but cannot mask the taste of very disagreeable drugs. Some of the more common flavored aqueous agents and the official forms of water are listed below.

ORANGE FLOWER WATER

Stronger Orange Flower Water; Triple Orange Flower Water

A saturated solution of the odoriferous principles of the flowers of *Citrus aurantium* Linné (Fam *Rutaceae*), prepared by distilling the fresh flowers with water and separating the excess volatile oil from the clear, water portion of the distillate.

Description—Should be nearly colorless, clear, or only faintly opalescent; the odor should be that of the orange blossoms; it must be free from empyreuma, mustiness, and fungoid growths.

Uses—A vehicle flavor and perfume in syrups, elixirs, and solutions.

PEPPERMINT WATER

A clear, saturated solution of peppermint oil in purified water, prepared by one of the processes described under Aromatic Waters (page 749).

Uses—A carminative and flavored vehicle.

TOLU BALSAM SYRUP—page 1068.

WATER

Water [7732-18-5] H_2O (18.02).

Drinking water, which is subject to EPA regulations with respect to drinking water and which is delivered by the municipal or other local public system or drawn from a private well or reservoir, is the starting material for all forms of water covered by Pharmacopeial monographs.

Drinking water may be used in the preparation of USP drug substances (eg, in the extraction of certain vegetable drugs and in the manufacture of a few preparations used externally) but not in the preparation of dosage forms or in the preparation of reagents or test solutions. It is no longer the subject of a separate monograph (in the USP), inasmuch as the cited standards vary from one community to another and generally are beyond the control of private parties or corporations.

PURIFIED WATER

Water obtained by distillation, ion-exchange treatment, reverse osmosis, or any other suitable process; contains no added substance.

Caution—Do not use this in preparations intended for parenteral administration. For such purposes, use Water for Injection, Bacteriostatic Water for Injection, or Sterile Water for Injection, page 1070.

Preparation—From water complying with EPA regulations with respect to drinking water. A former official process for water, when prepared by distillation, is given below. The pharmacist who is preparing sterile solutions and must have freshly distilled water of exceptionally high grade, not only free from all bacterial or other microscopic growths but also free from the products of metabolic processes resulting from the growth of such organisms in the water, advantageously may follow this plan. The metabolic products commonly are spoken of as pyrogens and usually consist of complex organic compounds that cause febrile reactions if present in the solvent for parenteral medicinal substances.

DISTILLATION PROCESS

Water   1000 vol.
To make   750 vol.

Distill the water from a suitable apparatus provided with a block-tin or glass condenser. Collect the first 100 volumes and reject this portion. Then collect 750 volumes and keep the distilled water in glass-stoppered bottles that have been rinsed with steam or very hot distilled water immediately before being filled. The first 100 volumes are discarded to eliminate foreign volatile substances found in ordinary water, and only 750 volumes are collected, since the residue in the still contains concentrated dissolved solids.

Description—Colorless, clear liquid, without odor or taste.

Uses—A pharmaceutical aid (vehicle and solvent). It must be used in compounding dosage forms for internal (oral) administration as well as sterile pharmaceuticals applied externally, such as collyria and dermatological preparations, but these must be sterilized before use.

Whenever water is called for in official tests and assays, this must be used.

WATER FOR INJECTION

Water purified by distillation or by reverse osmosis. It contains no added substance.

Caution—It is intended for use as a solvent for the preparation of parenteral solutions. For parenteral solutions that are prepared under aseptic conditions and are not sterilized by appropriate filtration or in the final container, first render it sterile and thereafter protect it from microbial contamination.

Description—Clear, colorless, odorless liquid.

Uses—Vehicle and solvent

BACTERIOSTATIC WATER FOR INJECTION

Sterile water for injection containing one or more suitable antimicrobial agents

Note—Use it with due regard for the compatibility of the antimicrobial agent or agents it contains with the particular medicinal substance that is to be dissolved or diluted.

Uses—Sterile vehicle for parenteral preparations.

STERILE WATER FOR INJECTION

WATER FOR PARENTERALS

Water for injection sterilized and suitably packaged. It contains no antimicrobial agent or other added substance.

Description—Clear, colorless, odorless liquid.

Uses—For the preparation of all aqueous parenteral solutions including those used in animal assays.

STERILE WATER FOR IRRIGATION

Water for injection that has been sterilized and suitably packaged. It contains no antimicrobial agent or other added substance.

Description—Clear, colorless, odorless liquid.

Uses—An irrigating solution.

SYRUPS USED AS DILUTING AGENTS

Syrups are useful as diluting agents for water-soluble drugs and act both as solvents and flavoring agents. The flavored syrups usually consist of simple syrup (85% sucrose in water) containing appropriate flavoring substances. Glycyrrhiza Syrup is an excellent vehicle for saline substances because of its colloidal properties, sweet flavor, and lingering taste of licorice. Acacia Syrup is valuable in disguising the taste of urea. Fruit syrups are especially effective for masking sour tastes. Aromatic Eriodictyon Syrup is the diluting agent of choice for masking the bitter taste of alkaloids. Cocoa Syrup and Cherry Syrup are good general flavoring agents.

ACACIA SYRUP

Acacia, granular or powdered	100 g
Sodium Benzoate	1 g
Vanilla Tincture	5 mL
Sucrose	800 g
Purified Water, a sufficient quantity to make	1000 mL

Mix the acacia, sodium benzoate, and sucrose; then add 425 mL of purified water and mix well. Heat the mixture on a steam bath until solution is completed. When cool, remove the scum, and add the vanilla tincture and sufficient purified water to make the product measure 1000 mL and strain, if necessary.

Uses—A flavored vehicle and demulcent.

CHERRY SYRUP

Syrupus Cerasi

Cherry Juice	475 mL
Sucrose	800 g
Alcohol	20 mL
Purified Water, a sufficient quantity to make	1000 mL

Dissolve the sucrose in cherry juice by heating on a steam bath, cool, and remove the foam and floating solids. Add the alcohol and sufficient purified water to make 1000 mL and mix.

Alcohol Content—1 to 2%.

Uses—A pleasantly flavored vehicle that is particularly useful in masking the taste of saline and sour drugs.

COCOA SYRUP

Cacao Syrup; Chocolate-flavored Syrup; Chocolate Syrup

Cocoa	180 g
Sucrose	600 g
Liquid Glucose	180 g
Glycerin	50 mL
Sodium Chloride	2 g
Vanillin	0.2 g
Sodium Benzoate	1 g
Purified Water, a sufficient quantity to make	1000 mL

Mix the sucrose and the cocoa, and to this mixture gradually add a solution of the liquid glucose, glycerin, sodium chloride, vanillin, and sodium benzoate in 325 mL of hot purified water. Bring the entire mixture to a boil, and maintain at boiling temperature for 3 min. Allow to cool to room temperature, and add sufficient purified water to make the product measure 1000 mL.

Note—Cocoa containing not more than 12% nonvolatile, ether- soluble, extractive (fat) yields a syrup having a minimum tendency to separate. Breakfast cocoa contains over 22% fat.

Uses—A pleasantly flavored vehicle.

SYRUP

Simple Syrup

Sucrose	850 g
Purified Water, a sufficient quantity, to make	1000 mL

May be prepared by using boiling water or, preferably, without heat, by the following process:

Place the sucrose in a suitable percolator the neck of which is nearly filled with loosely packed cotton, moistened, after packing, with a few drops of water. Pour carefully about 450 mL of purified water upon the sucrose, and regulate the outflow to a steady drip of percolate. Return the percolate, if necessary, until all of the sucrose has dissolved. Then wash the inside of the percolator and the cotton with sufficient purified water to bring the volume of the percolate to 1000 mL, and mix.

Specific Gravity—Not less than 1.30.

Uses—A sweet vehicle, sweetening agent, and as the basis for many flavored and medicated syrups.

OTHER SYRUPS USED AS DILUTING AGENTS

Glycyrrhiza Syrup USP [Licorice Syrup]—Preparation: Add fennel oil (0.05 mL) and anise oil (0.5 mL) to glycyrrhiza fluidextract (250 mL) and agitate until mixed. Then add syrup (qs) to make the product measure 1000 mL, and mix. Alcohol Content: 5 to 6%. Incompatibilities: The characteristic flavor is destroyed by acids because of precipitation of the glycyrrhizin. Uses: A flavored vehicle, especially adapted to the administration of bitter or nauseous substances.

Hydriodic Acid Syrup—Contains, in each 100 mL, 1.3 to 1.5 g HI (127.91). Preparation: Mix diluted hydriodic acid (140 mL) with purified water (550 mL), and dissolve dextrose (450 g) in this mixture by agitation. Add purified water (qs) to make the product measure 1000 mL, and filter. Caution: It must not be dispensed if it contains free iodine, as evidenced by a red coloration. Description: Transparent, colorless, or not more than pale straw-colored, syrupy liquid; odorless, with a sweet, acidulous taste; specific gravity about 1.18; hydriodic acid is decomposed easily in simple aqueous solution (unless protected by hypophosphorous acid), free iodine being liberated, and if taken internally, when in this condition, it is irritating to the alimentary tract. The dextrose used in this syrup should be of the highest grade obtainable.

Incompatibilities—The reactions of the acids as well as those of the water-soluble iodide salts. Oxidizing agents liberate iodine; alkaloids may be precipitated. Uses: Traditionally as a vehicle for expectorant drugs. Its therapeutic properties are those of the iodides. Dose: Usual, 5 mL.

Wild Cherry Syrup USP—Preparation: Pack wild cherry (in coarse powder, 150 g), previously moistened with water (100 mL), in a cylindrical percolator, and add water (qs) to leave a layer of it above the powder. Macerate for 1 hr, then proceed with rapid percolation, using added water, until 400 mL of percolate is collected. Filter the percolate, if necessary, add sucrose (675 g) and dissolve it by agitation, then add glycerin (150 mL), alcohol (20 mL), and water (qs) to make the product measure 1000 mL. Strain if necessary. It may be made also in the following manner: The sucrose may be dissolved by placing it in a second percolator as directed for preparing Syrup, and allowing the percolate from the wild cherry to flow through it and into a graduated vessel containing the glycerin and alcohol, until the total volume measures 1000 mL. Note: Heat is avoided, lest the enzyme emulsin be inactivated. If this should happen, the preparation would contain no free HCN, upon which its action as a sedative for coughs mainly depends. For a discussion of the chemistry involved, see Wild Cherry. Alcohol Content: 1 to 2%. Uses: Chiefly as a flavored vehicle for cough syrups.

MUCILAGES USED AS DILUTING AGENTS

Mucilages are also suitable as diluting agents for water-soluble substances, and are especially useful in stabilizing suspensions and emulsions.

The following mucilage used for this purpose is described under Emulsifying and Suspending Agents.

ACACIA MUCILAGE—page 1072.

HYDROALCOHOLIC DILUTING AGENTS

Hydroalcoholic diluting agents are suitable for drugs soluble in either water or diluted alcohol. The most important agents in this group are the elixirs. These solutions contain approximately 25% alcohol. Medicated elixirs that have therapeutic activity in their own right are not included in this section. Listed below are the common, non-medicated elixirs that are used purely as diluting agents or solvents for drugs.

AROMATIC ELIXIR

Simple Elixir

Orange Oil	2.4 mL
Lemon Oil	0.6 mL
Coriander Oil	0.24 mL
Anise Oil	0.06 mL
Syrup	375 mL
Talc	30 g

Alcohol, Purified Water, each, a sufficient quantity, to make 1000 mL

Dissolve the oils in alcohol to make 250 mL. To this solution add the syrup in several portions, agitating vigorously after each addition, and afterward add, in the same manner, the required quantity of purified water. Mix the talc with the liquid, and filter through a filter wetted with diluted alcohol, returning the filtrate until a clear liquid is obtained.

Alcohol Content—21 to 23%.

Uses—A pleasantly flavored vehicle, employed in the preparation of many other elixirs. The chief objection to its extensive use is the high alcohol content (about 22%), which at times may counteract the effect of other medicines.

OTHER HYDROALCOHOLIC DILUTING AGENTS

Glycyrrhiza Elixir [Elixir Adjuvants; Licorice Elixir]—Preparation: Mix glycyrrhiza fluidextract (125 mL) and aromatic elixir (875 mL) and filter. Alcohol Content: 21 to 23%. Uses: A flavored vehicle.

FLAVORED ALCOHOLIC SOLUTIONS

Flavored alcoholic solutions of high alcoholic concentration are useful as flavors to be added in small quantities to syrups or elixirs. The alcohol content of these solutions is approximately 50%. There are two types of flavored alcoholic solutions: tinctures and spirits. Only non-medicated tinctures and spirits are used as flavoring agents.

LEMON TINCTURE—page 1069.
ORANGE SPIRIT, COMPOUND—page 1066.
ORANGE PEEL, SWEET, TINCTURE—page 1066.

DILUTING AGENTS FOR INJECTIONS

Injections are liquid preparations, usually solutions or suspensions of drugs, intended to be injected through the skin into the body. Diluting agents used for these preparations may be aqueous or non-aqueous and must meet the requirements for sterility and also of the pyrogen test. Aqueous diluting agents include such preparations as Sterile Water for Injection and various sterile, aqueous solutions of electrolytes and/or dextrose. Non-aqueous diluting agents are generally fatty oils of vegetable origin, fatty esters, and polyols such as propylene glycol and polyethylene glycol. These agents are used to dissolve or dilute oil-soluble substances and to suspend water-soluble substances when it is desired to decrease the rate of absorption and, hence, prolong the duration of action of the drug substances. Preparations of this type are given intramuscularly. See *Parenteral Preparations*, page 802.

CORN OIL

Maize Oil

The refined fixed oil obtained from the embryo of *Zea mays* Linné (Fam *Gramineae*).

Preparation—Expressed from the Indian corn embryos or germs separated from the grain in starch manufacture.

Description—Clear, light yellow, oily liquid with a faint characteristic odor and taste; specific gravity 0.914 to 0.921.

Solubility—Slightly soluble in alcohol; miscible with ether, chloroform, benzene, or solvent hexane.

Uses—Main official use is as a solvent and vehicle for injections. It is used as an edible oil substitute for solid fats in the management of hypercholesterolemia. Other uses include making soaps and for burning.

It is a semidrying oil and therefore unsuitable for lubricating or mixing paint.

COTTONSEED OIL

Cotton Seed Oil; Cotton Oil

The refined fixed oil obtained from the seed of cultivated plants of various varieties of *Gossypium hirsutum* Linné or of other species of *Gossypium* (Fam *Malvaceae*).

Preparation—Cotton seeds contain about 15% oil. The testae of the seeds are first separated, and the kernels are subjected to high pressure in hydraulic presses. The crude oil thus has a bright red to blackish red color. It requires purification before it is suitable for medicinal or food purposes.

Description—Pale yellow, oily liquid with a bland taste; odorless or nearly so; particles of solid fat may separate below 10°C; solidifies at about 0 to −5°C; specific gravity 0.915 to 0.921.

Solubility—Slightly soluble in alcohol; miscible with ether, chloroform, solvent hexane, or carbon disulfide.

Uses—Officially as a solvent and vehicle for injections. It is sometimes taken orally as a mild cathartic in a dose of 30 mL or more. Taken internally, digestible oils retard gastric secretion and motility and increase the caloric intake. It also is used in the manufacture of soaps, oleomargarine, lard substitutes, glycerin, lubricants, and cosmetics.

ETHYL OLEATE

(Z)−9−Octadecenoic acid, ethyl ester

$$HC—CH_2(CH_2)_6COOC_2H_5$$
$$\|$$
$$HC—CH_2(CH_2)_6CH_3$$

Ethyl oleate [111−62−6] $C_{20}H_{38}O_2$ (310.52).

Preparation—Among other ways, by reacting ethanol with oleoyl chloride in the presence of a suitable dehydrochlorinating agent.

Description—Mobile, practically colorless liquid, with an agreeable taste; specific gravity 0.866 to 0.874; acid value not greater than 0.5; iodine value 75 to 85; sterilized by heating at 150°C for 1 hr; properties similar to those of almond and arachis oils, but is less viscous and more rapidly absorbed by the tissues; boils about 207°C.

Solubility—Does not dissolve in water; miscible with vegetable oils, mineral oil, alcohol, or most organic solvents.

Uses—A vehicle for certain intramuscular injectable preparations.

PEANUT OIL

Arachis Oil; Groundnut Oil; Nut Oil; Earth−Nut Oil

The refined fixed oil obtained from the seed kernels of one or more of the cultivated varieties of *Arachis hypogaea* Linné (Fam *Leguminosae*).

Description—Colorless or pale yellow, oily liquid, with a characteristic nutty odor and a bland taste; specific gravity 0.912 to 0.920.

Solubility—Very slightly soluble in alcohol; miscible with ether, chloroform, or carbon disulfide.

Uses—A solvent in preparing oil solutions for injection. It also is used for making liniments, ointments, plasters, and soaps, as a substitute for olive oil.

SESAME OIL

Teel Oil; Benne Oil; Gingili Oil

The refined fixed oil obtained from the seed of one or more cultivated varieties of *Sesamum indicum* Linné (Fam *Pedaliaceae*).

Description—Pale yellow, almost odorless, oily liquid with a bland taste; specific gravity 0.916 to 0.921.

Solubility—Slightly soluble in alcohol; miscible with ether, chloroform, solvent hexane, or carbon disulfide.

Uses—A solvent and vehicle in official injections. It is used much like olive oil both medicinally and for food. It does not readily turn rancid. It also is used in the manufacture of cosmetics, iodized oil, liniments, ointments, and oleomargarine.

EMULSIFYING AND SUSPENDING AGENTS

An emulsion is a two−phase system in which one liquid is dispersed in the form of small globules throughout another liquid that is immiscible with the first liquid. Emulsions are formed and stabilized with the help of emulsifying agents, which are surfactants and/or viscosity−producing agents. A suspension is defined as a preparation containing finely divided insoluble material suspended in a liquid medium. The presence of a suspending agent is required to overcome agglomeration of the dispersed particles and to increase the viscosity of the medium so that the particles settle more slowly. Emulsifying and suspending agents are used extensively in the formulation of elegant pharmaceutical preparations for oral, parenteral, and external use. For the theoretical and practical aspects of emulsions the interested reader is referred to Chapter 39 *(Solutions, Emulsions, Suspensions, and Extracts)*.

ACACIA

Gum Arabic

The dried gummy exudate from the stems and branches of *Acacia senegal* (Linné) Willdenow or of other related African species of *Acacia* (Fam *Leguminosae*).

Constituents—Principally calcium, magnesium, and potassium salts of the polysaccharide *arabic acid,* which on acid hydrolysis yields L-arabinose, L-rhamnose, D-galactose, and an aldobionic acid containing D-glucuronic acid and D-galactose.

Description—Acacia: Spheroidal tears up to 32 mm in diameter or angular fragments of white to yellowish white color; translucent or somewhat opaque; very brittle; almost odorless; produces a mucilaginous sensation on the tongue. Flake Acacia: White to yellowish white, thin flakes. Powdered Acacia: White to yellowish white, angular microscopic fragments. Granular Acacia: White to pale yellowish white, fine granules. Spray-dried Acacia: White to off-white compacted microscopic fragments or whole spheres.

Solubility—Insoluble in alcohol, but almost completely soluble in twice its weight of water at room temperature; the resulting solution flows readily and is acid to litmus.

Incompatibilities—Alcohol or alcoholic solutions precipitate acacia as a stringy mass when the alcohol amounts to more than about 35% of the total volume. Solution is effected by dilution with water. The mucilage is destroyed through precipitation of the acacia by heavy metals. Borax also causes a precipitation that is prevented by glycerin. It contains calcium and, therefore, possesses the incompatibilities of this ion.

It contains a peroxidase that acts as an oxidizing agent and produces colored derivatives of aminopyrine, antipyrine, cresol, guaiacol, phenol, tannin, thymol, vanillin, and other substances. Among the alkaloids affected are atropine, apomorphine, cocaine, homatropine, hyoscyamine, morphine, physostigmine, and scopolamine. A partial destruction of the alkaloid occurs in the reaction. Heating the solution of acacia for a few minutes at 100°C destroys the peroxidase and the color reactions are avoided.

Uses—Extensively as a suspending agent for insoluble substances in water, in the preparation of emulsions and for making pills and troches.

It is used for its demulcent action in inflammations of the throat or stomach.

Its solutions should not be used as a substitute for serum protein in the treatment of shock and as a diuretic in hypoproteinemic edema, since it produces serious syndromes that may result in death.

Acacia Mucilage [Mucilage of Gum Arabic]—Preparation: Place acacia (in small fragments, 350 g) in a graduated bottle having a wide mouth and a capacity not greatly exceeding 1000 mL, wash the drug with cold purified water, allow it to drain, and add enough warm purified water in which benzoic acid (2 g) has been dissolved, to make the product measure 1000 mL. After stoppering, lay the bottle on its side, rotate it occasionally, and when the acacia has dissolved, strain the mucilage. It also may be prepared as follows: dissolve benzoic acid (2 g) in purified water (400 mL) with the aid of heat, and add the solution to powdered or granular acacia (350 g), in a mortar, triturating until the acacia is dissolved. Then add sufficient purified water to make the product measure 1000 mL, and strain if necessary. This second method is primarily for extemporaneous preparation. Uses: A demulcent and a suspending agent. It also has been employed as an excipient in making pills and troches and as an emulsifying agent for cod liver oil and other substances. Caution—It must be free from mold or any other indication of decomposition.

AGAR

Agar-Agar; Vegetable Gelatin; Gelosa; Chinese or Japanese Gelatin

The dried, hydrophilic, colloidal substance extracted from *Gelidium cartilagineum* (Linné) Gaillon (Fam *Gelidiaceae*), *Gracilaria confervoides* (Linné) Greville (Fam *Sphaerococcaceae*) and related red algae (Class *Rhodophyceae*).

Constituents—Chiefly of the calcium salt of a galactan mono-(acid sulfate).

Description—Usually in bundles of thin, membranous, agglutinated strips or in cut, flaked, or granulated forms; may be weak yellowish orange, yellowish gray to pale yellow or colorless; tough when damp, brittle when dry; odorless or with a slight odor; produces a mucilaginous sensation on the tongue. Also supplied as a white to yellowish white or pale-yellow powder.

Solubility—Insoluble in cold water; soluble in boiling water.

Incompatibilities—Like other gums, it is dehydrated and precipitated from solution by alcohol. Tannic acid causes precipitation; electrolytes cause partial dehydration and decrease in viscosity of sols.

Uses—A relatively ineffective bulk-producing laxative used in a variety of proprietary cathartics. In mineral oil emulsions it acts as a stabilizer. It also is used in culture media for bacteriological work and in the manufacture of ice cream, confectioneries, etc.

ALGINIC ACID

Alginic acid [9005-32-7] (average equivalent weight 200); a hydrophilic colloidal carbohydrate extracted with dilute alkali from various species of brown seaweeds *(Phaeophyceae)*.

Preparation—Precipitates when an aqueous solution of *Sodium Alginate* is treated with mineral acid.

Description—White to yellowish white, fibrous powder; odorless or practically odorless, and tasteless; pH (3 in 100 dispersion in water) 1.5 to 3.5; pK_a (0.1 N NaCl, 20°C) 3.42.

Solubility—Insoluble in water or organic solvents; soluble in alkaline solutions.

Uses—A tablet binder and emulsifying agent. It is used as a sizing agent in the paper and textile industries.

SODIUM ALGINATE

Alginic acid, sodium salt; Algin; Kelgin; Manucol; Norgine

Sodium alginate [9005-38-3] (average equivalent weight 220); the purified carbohydrate product extracted from brown seaweeds by the use of dilute alkali. It consists chiefly of the sodium salt of alginic acid, a polyuronic acid composed of beta-D-mannuronic acid residues linked so that the carboxyl group of each unit is free while a glycosidic linkage shields the aldehyde group.

Description—Nearly odorless and tasteless, coarse or fine powder, yellowish white in color.

Solubility—Dissolves in water, forming a viscous, colloidal solution; insoluble in alcohol or in hydroalcoholic solutions in which the alcohol content is greater than about 30% by weight; insoluble in chloroform, ether, or acids, when the pH of the solution becomes lower than about 3.

Uses—A thickening and emulsifying agent. This property makes it useful in a variety of areas. For example, it is used to impart smoothness and body to ice cream and to prevent formation of ice particles.

BENTONITE

Wilhinite; Soap Clay; Mineral Soap

Bentonite [1302-78-9]; a native, colloidal, hydrated aluminum silicate.

Occurrence—Bentonite is found in midwestern United States and Canada. Originally called Taylorite after its discoverer in Wyoming, its name was changed to bentonite after its discovery in the Fort Benton formation of the Upper Cretaceous of Wyoming.

Description—Very fine, odorless powder with a slightly earthy taste, free from grit; the powder is nearly white, but may be pale buff or cream colored.

The US Geological Survey has defined bentonite as transported stratified clay formed by the alteration of volcanic ash shortly after deposition. Chemically, it is $Al_2O_3 \cdot 4SiO_2 \cdot H_2O$ plus other minerals as impurities. It consists of colloidal crystalline plates, of less than microscopic dimensions in thickness, and of colloidal dimensions in breadth. This fact accounts for the extreme swelling that occurs when it is placed in water, since the water penetrates between an infinite number of plates. A good specimen swells 12 to 14 times its volume.

Solubility—Insoluble in water or acids, but it has the property of adsorbing large quantities of water, swelling to approximately 12 times its original volume, and forming highly viscous thixotropic suspensions or gels. This property makes it highly useful in pharmacy. Its gel-forming property is augmented by the addition of small amounts of alkaline substances, such as magnesium oxide. It does not swell in organic solvents.

Incompatibilities—Acids and acid salts decrease its water- absorbing power and thus cause a breakdown of the magma. Suspensions are most stable at a pH above 7.

Uses—A protective colloid for the stabilization of suspensions. It also has been used as an emulsifier for oil and as a base for plasters, ointments, and similar preparations.

Bentonite Magma—Preparation: Sprinkle bentonite (50 g), in portions, on hot purified water (800 g), allowing each portion to become thoroughly wetted without stirring. Allow it to stand with occasional stirring for 24 hr. Stir until a uniform magma is obtained, add purified water to make 1000 g, and mix. The magma may be prepared also by mechanical means such as by use of a blender, as follows: Place purified water (about 500 g) in the blender, and while the machine is running, add bentonite (50 g). Add purified water to make up to about 1000 g or up to the operating capacity of the blender. Blend the mixture for 5 to 10 min, add purified water to make 1000 g, and mix. Uses: A suspending agent for insoluble medicaments.

CARBOMER

Carboxy polymethylene; polyacrylic acid; acrylic acid polymer; carboxyvinyl polymer

A synthetic high-molecular-weight cross-linked polymer of acrylic acid; contains 56% to 68% of carboxylic acid (-COOH) groups. The viscosity of a neutralized preparation (2.5 g/500 mL water) is 30,000 to 40,000 centipoise.

Description—White, fluffy powder with a slight, characteristic odor; hygroscopic; pH (1 in 100 dispersion) about 3; specific gravity about 1.41.

Solubility—neutralized with alkali hydroxides or amines); dissolves in water, alcohol, or glycerin.

Uses—A thickening, suspending, dispersing and emulsifying agent for pharmaceuticals, cosmetics, waxes, paints, and other industrial products.

CARRAGEENAN

Carrageenan [9000-07-1]; Chondrus; Irish Moss

Preparation—The hydrocolloid extracted with water or aqueous alkali from certain red seaweeds of the class *Rhodophyceae,* and separated from the solution by precipitation with alcohol (methanol, ethanol, or isopropanol) or by drum-roll drying or freezing.

Constituents—It is a variable mixture of potassium, sodium, calcium, magnesium, and ammonium sulfate esters of galactose and 3,6-anhydrogalactose copolymers, the hexoses being alternately linked α-1,3 and β-1,4 in the polymer. The three main types of copolymers present are *kappa*-carrageenan, *iota*-carrageenan, and *lambda*-carrageenan, which differ in the composition and manner of linkage of monomeric units and the degree of sulfation (the ester sulfate content for carrageenans varies from 18% to 40%). *Kappa*-carrageenan and *iota*-carrageenan are the gelling fractions; *lambda*-carrageenan is the nongelling fraction. The gelling fractions may be separated from the nongelling fraction by addition of potassium chloride to an aqueous solution of carrageenan. Carrageenan separated by drum-roll drying may contain mono- and di-glycerides or up to 5% of polysorbate 80, used as roll-stripping agents.

Description—Yellow-brown to white, coarse to fine powder; odorless; tasteless, producing a mucilaginous sensation on the tongue.

Solubility—All carrageenans hydrate rapidly in cold water, but only *lambda*-carrageenan and sodium carrageenans dissolve completely. Gelling carrageenans require heating to about 80°C for complete solution when potassium and calcium ions are present.

Uses—In the pharmaceutical and food industries as an emulsifying, suspending, and gelling agent.

CARBOXYMETHYLCELLULOSE SODIUM

Carbose D; Carboxymethocel S; CMC; Cellulose Gum

Cellulose, carboxymethyl ether, sodium salt [9004-32-4]; contains 6.5 to 9.5% of sodium (Na), calculated on the dried basis. It is available in several viscosity types: low, medium, high, and extra high.

Description—White to cream-colored powder or granules; the powder is hygroscopic; pH (1 in 100 aqueous solution) about 7.5.

Solubility—Easily dispersed in water to form colloidal solutions; insoluble in alcohol, ether, or most other organic solvents.

Uses—Suspending agent, tablet excipient, or viscosity-increasing agent. In tablet

POWDERED CELLULOSE

Cellulose [9004-34-6] $(C_6H_{10}O_5)_n$; purified, mechanically disintegrated cellulose prepared by processing alpha cellulose obtained as a pulp from fibrous plant materials.

Description—White, odorless substance, consisting of fibrous particles, which may be compressed into self-binding tablets that disintegrate rapidly in water; exists in various grades, exhibiting degrees of fineness ranging from a free-flowing dense powder to a coarse, fluffy, non-flowing material; pH (supernatant liquid of a 10 g/90 mL aqueous suspension after 1 hr) 5 to 7.5.

Solubility—Insoluble in water, dilute acids, or nearly all organic solvents; slightly soluble in NaOH solution (1 in 20).

Uses—Tablet diluent, adsorbent, or suspending agent.

CETYL ALCOHOL—page 1078.

CHOLESTEROL

Cholest-5-en-3-ol, (3β)-, Cholesterin

Cholest-5-en-3β-ol [57-88-5] $C_{27}H_{46}O$ (386.66).

A steroid alcohol widely distributed in the animal organism. In addition to cholesterol and its esters, several closely related steroid alcohols occur in the yolk of eggs, the brain, milk, fish oils, wool fat (10 to 20%), etc. These closely resemble it in properties. One of the methods of commercial production involves extraction of it from the unsaponifiable matter in the spinal cord of cattle, using petroleum benzin. Wool fat also is used as a source.

Description—White or faintly yellow, almost odorless pearly leaflets or granules; usually acquires a yellow to pale tan color on prolonged exposure to light or to elevated temperatures; melts 147 to 150°C.

Solubility—Insoluble in water; 1 g slowly dissolves in 100 mL alcohol or about 50 mL dehydrated alcohol; soluble in acetone, hot alcohol, chloroform, dioxane, ether, ethyl acetate, solvent hexane, or vegetable oils.

Uses—To enhance incorporation and emulsification of medicinal products in oils or fats. It is a pharmaceutical necessity for Hydrophilic Petrolatum in which it enhances water-absorbing capacity. See Chapter 21.

DOCUSATE SODIUM—page 1308.

GELATIN

White Gelatin

A product obtained by the partial hydrolysis of collagen derived from the skin, white connective tissues, and bones of animals. Gelatin derived from an acid-treated precursor is known as Type A and exhibits an isoelectric point between pH 7 and 9, while gelatin derived from an alkali-treated precursor is known as Type B and exhibits an isoelectric point between pH 4.7 and 5.2.

Gelatin for use in the manufacture of capsules in which to dispense medicines or for the coating of tablets may be colored with a certified color, may contain not more than 0.15% of sulfur dioxide, may contain a suitable concentration of sodium lauryl sulfate and suitable antimicrobial agents, and may have any suitable gel strength that is designated by Bloom Gelometer number.

Regarding the special gelatin for use in the preparation of emulsions, see Emulsions.

Description—Sheets, flakes, shreds, or a coarse-to-fine powder; faintly yellow or amber in color, the color varying in depth according to the particle size; slight, characteristic bouillon-like odor; stable in air when dry, but is subject to microbial decomposition when moist or in solution.

Solubility—Insoluble in cold water, but swells and softens when immersed in it, gradually absorbing from 5 to 10 times its own weight of water; soluble in hot water, acetic acid, or hot mixtures of glycerin or water; insoluble in alcohol, chloroform, ether, or fixed and volatile oils.

Uses—In pharmacy, to coat tablets and form capsules, and as a vehicle for suppositories. It also is recommended as an emulsifying agent. See under Emulsions in Chapters 20 and 39, also Suppositories; and Absorbable Gelatin Sponge. It also has been used as an adjuvant protein food in malnutrition.

GLYCERYL MONOSTEARATE—page 1078.

HYDROXYETHYL CELLULOSE

Cellulose, 2-hydroxyethyl ether; Cellosize; Natrosol

Cellulose hydroxyethyl ether 9004-62-0.

Preparation—Cellulose is treated with NaOH and then reacted with ethylene oxide.

Description—White, odorless, tasteless, free-flowing powder; softens at about 137°C; refractive index (2% solution) about 1.336; pH about 7; solutions are nonionic.

Solubility—Dissolves readily in cold or hot water to give clear, smooth, viscous solutions; partially soluble in acetic acid; insoluble in most organic solvents.

Uses—Resembles carboxymethylcellulose sodium in that it is a cellulose ether, but differs in being nonionic, and hence, its solutions are unaffected by cations. It is used pharmaceutically as a thickener, protective colloid, binder, stabilizer, and suspending agent in emulsions, jellies and ointments, lotions, ophthalmic solutions, suppositories, and tablets.

HYDROXYPROPYL CELLULOSE

Cellulose, 2-hydroxypropyl ether; Klucel

Cellulose hydroxypropyl ether [9004-64-2].

Preparation. elevated temperature and pressure.

Description—Off-white, odorless, tasteless powder; softens at 130°C; burns out.\ completely about 475°C in N_2 or O_2; refractive index (2% solution) about 1.337; pH (aqueous solution) 5 to 8.5; solutions are nonionic.

Solubility—Soluble in water below 40°C (insoluble above 45°C); soluble in many polar organic solvents.

Uses—A broad combination of properties useful in a variety of industries. It is used pharmaceutically as a binder, granulation agent, and film-coating in the manufacture of tablets; an alcohol-soluble thickener and suspending agent for elixirs and lotions; and a stabilizer for emulsions.

HYDROXYPROPYL METHYLCELLULOSE

Cellulose, 2-hydroxypropyl methyl ether

Cellulose hydroxypropyl methyl ether [9004-65-3], available in grades containing 16.5 to 30.0% of methoxy and 4.0 to 32.0% of hydroxypropoxy groups, and thus in viscosity and thermal gelation temperatures of solutions of specified concentration.

Preparation—The appropriate grade of methylcellulose (see below) is treated with NaOH and reacted with propylene oxide at elevated temperature and pressure for a reaction time sufficient to produce the desired degree of attachment of methyl and hydroxypropyl groups by ether linkages to the anhydroglucose rings of cellulose.

Description—White to slightly off-white, fibrous or granular, free-flowing powder.

Solubility—Swells in water and produces a clear to opalescent, viscous, colloidal mixture; undergoes reversible transformation from sol to gel on heating and cooling, respectively. Insoluble in anhydrous alcohol, ether, or chloroform.

Uses—A protective colloid that is useful as a dispersing and thickening agent, and in ophthalmic solutions to provide the demulcent action and viscous properties essential for contact-lens use and in artificial-tear formulations. Also used in the preparation of sustained release matrix tablets and as a film coating material.

LANOLIN, ANHYDROUS—page 1077.

METHYLCELLULOSE

Cellulose, methyl ether; Methocel

Cellulose methyl ether [9004-67-5]; a methyl ether of cellulose containing 27.5 to 31.5% of methoxy groups.

Preparation—By the reaction of methyl chloride or of dimethyl sulfate on cellulose dissolved in sodium hydroxide. The cellulose methyl ether so formed is coagulated by adding methanol or other suitable agent and centrifuged. Since cellulose has 3 hydroxyl groups/glucose residue, several methylcelluloses can be made that vary in, among other properties, solubility and viscosity. Types useful for pharmaceutical application contain from 1 to 2 methoxy radicals/glucose residue.

Description—White, fibrous powder or granules; aqueous suspensions neutral to litmus; stable to alkali and dilute acids.

Solubility—Insoluble in ether, alcohol, or chloroform; soluble in glacial acetic acid or in a mixture of equal parts of alcohol and chloroform; swells in water, producing a clear to opalescent, viscous colloidal solution; insoluble in hot water and saturated salt solutions; salts of minerals, acids, and particularly polybasic acids, phenols, and tannins coagulate its solutions, but this can be prevented by the addition of alcohol or of glycol diacetate.

Uses—A synthetic substitute for natural gums that has both pharmaceutical and therapeutic applications. Pharmaceutically, it is used as a dispersing, thickening, emulsifying, sizing, and coating agent. It is an ingredient of many nose drops, eye preparations, burn medications, cosmetics, tooth pastes, liquid dentifrices, hair fixatives, creams, and lotions. It functions as a protective colloid for many types of dispersed substances and is an effective stabilizer for oil-in-water emulsions.

Therapeutically, it is used as a bulk laxative in the treatment of chronic constipation. Taken with 1 or 2 glassfuls of water, it forms a colloidal solution in the upper alimentary tract; this solution loses water in the colon, forming a gel that increases the bulk and softness of the stool. The gel is bland, demulcent, and nonirritating to the GI tract. Once a normal stool develops, the dose should be reduced to a level adequate for maintenance of good function. Although it takes up water from the GI tract quite readily, methylcellulose tablets have caused fecal impaction and intestinal obstruction when taken with a limited amount of water. It also is used as a topical ophthalmic protectant, in the form of 0.5 to 1% solution serving as artificial tears or a contact-lens solution applied to the conjunctiva, 0.05 to 0.1 mL at a time, 3 or 4 times a day as needed.

OLEYL ALCOHOL

9-Octadecen-1-ol, *(Z)-*, Aldol 85

$$HC-CH_2(CH_2)_7OH$$
$$HC-CH_2(CH_2)_6CH_3$$

(Z)-9-Octadecen-1-ol [143-28-2] $C_{18}H_{36}O$ (268.48); a mixture of unsaturated and saturated high-molecular-weight fatty alcohols consisting chiefly of oleyl alcohol.

Preparation—One method reacts ethyl oleate with absolute ethanol and metallic sodium (*Org Syn Coll III*: 673, 1955).

Description—Clear, colorless to light yellow, oily liquid; faint characteristic odor and bland taste; iodine value between 85 and 90; hydroxyl value between 205 and 215.

Solubility—Soluble in alcohol, ether, isopropyl alcohol, or light mineral oil; insoluble in water.

Uses—A *pharmaceutical aid* (emulsifying agent or emollient).

POLYVINYL ALCOHOL

Ethenol, homopolymer

$$\left[CH_2-\underset{OH}{CH} \right]_n$$

Vinyl alcohol polymer [9002-89-5] $(C_2H_4O)_n$.

Preparation—Polyvinyl acetate is approximately 88% hydrolyzed in a methanol-methyl acetate solution using either mineral acid or alkali as a catalyst.

Description—White to cream-colored powder or granules; odorless.

Solubility—Freely soluble in water; solution effected more rapidly at somewhat elevated temperatures.

Uses—A suspending agent and emulsifier, either with or without the aid of a surfactant. It commonly is employed as a lubricant and protectant in various ophthalmic preparations, such as decongestants, artificial tears, and contact-lens products.

POVIDONE

2-Pyrrolidinone, 1-ethenyl-, homopolymer; Polyvinylpyrrolidone; PVP

$$\left[CHCH_2 \right]_n$$

1-Vinyl-2-pyrrolidinone polymer [9003-39-8] $(C_6H_9NO)_n$; a synthetic polymer consisting of linear 1-vinyl-2-pyrrolidinone groups, the degree of polymerization of which results in polymers of various molecular weights. It is produced commercially as a series of products having mean molecular weights ranging from about 10,000 to about 700,000. The viscosity of solutions containing 10% or less is essentially the same as that of water; solutions more concentrated than 10% become more viscous, depending upon the concentration and the molecular weight of the polymer used. It contains between 12 to 13% nitrogen.

Preparation—1,4-Butanediol is dehydrogenated thermally with the aid of copper to γ-butyrolactone, which then is reacted with ammonia to form 2-pyrrolidinone. Addition of the latter to acetylene yields vinylpyrrolidinone (monomer), which is polymerized thermally in the presence of hydrogen peroxide and ammonia.

Description—White to creamy white, odorless powder, hygroscopic; pH (1 in 20 solution) 3 to 7.

Solubility—Soluble in water, alcohol, or chloroform; insoluble in ether.

Uses—A dispersing and suspending agent in pharmaceutical preparations. Also used as a binder in wet granulation processes.

PROPYLENE GLYCOL MONOSTEARATE

Octadecanoic acid, monoester with 1,2-propanediol

1,2-Propanediol monostearate [1323-39-3]; a mixture of the propylene glycol mono- and diesters of stearic and palmitic acids. It contains not less than 90% monoesters of saturated fatty acids, chiefly propylene glycol monostearate ($C_{21}H_{42}O_3$) and propylene glycol monopalmitate ($C_{19}H_{38}O_3$).

Preparation—By reacting propylene glycol with stearoyl chloride in a suitable dehydrochlorinating environment.

Description—White, wax-like solid or white, wax-like beads or flakes; slight, agreeable, fatty odor and taste; congeals not lower than 45°C; acid value not more than 2; saponification value 155 to 165; hydroxyl value 150 to 170; iodine value not more than 3.

Solubility—Dissolves in organic solvents such as alcohol, mineral or fixed oils, benzene, ether, or acetone; insoluble in water but may be dispersed in hot water with the aid of a small amount of soap or other suitable surface-active agent.

Uses—A surfactant. It is particularly useful as a dispersing agent for perfume oils or oil-soluble vitamins in water, and in cosmetic preparations.

SILICON DIOXIDE, COLLOIDAL—page 1089.

SODIUM LAURYL SULFATE

Sulfuric acid monododecyl ester sodium salt; Irium; Duponol C; Gardinol WA

Sodium monododecyl sulfate [151-21-3]; a mixture of sodium alkyl sulfates consisting chiefly of sodium lauryl sulfate. The combined content of sodium chloride and sodium sulfate is not more than 8%.

Preparation—The fatty acids of coconut oil, consisting chiefly of lauric acid, are catalytically hydrogenated to form the corresponding alcohols. The latter are then esterified with sulfuric acid (sulfated) and the resulting mixture of alkyl bisulfates (alkylsulfuric acids) is converted into a mixture of sodium salts by reacting with alkali under controlled conditions of pH.

Description—Small, white or light yellow crystals having a slight, characteristic odor.

Solubility—1 g in 10 mL water, forming an opalescent solution.

Incompatibilities—Reacts with cationic surface-active agents with loss of activity, even in concentrations too low to cause precipitation. Unlike soaps, it is compatible with dilute acids and calcium and magnesium ions.

Uses—An emulsifying, detergent, and wetting agent in ointments, tooth powders, and other pharmaceutical preparations, and in the metal, paper, and pigment industries.

SORBITAN ESTERS

Spans

Sorbitan esters (monolaurate [1338-39-2]; monooleate [1338-43-8]; monopalmitate [26266-57-9]; monostearate [1338-41-6]; trioleate [26266-58-0]; tristearate [26658-19-5]).

Preparation—Sorbitol is dehydrated to form a hexitan that is then esterified with the desired fatty acid which are polyethylene glycol ethers of sorbitan fatty acid esters.

Description—Monolaurate: Amber, oily liquid; may become hazy or form a precipitate; viscosity about 4250 cps; HLB number 8.6; acid number 7.0 max; saponification number 158 to 170; hydroxyl number 330 to 358. Monooleate: Amber liquid; viscosity about 1000 cps; HLB number 4.3; acid number 8.0 max; saponification number 145 to 160; hydroxyl number 193 to 210. Monopalmitate: Tan, granular waxy solid; HLB number 6.7; acid number 4 to 7.5; saponification number 140 to 150; hydroxyl number 275 to 305. Monostearate: Cream to tan beads; HLB number 4.7; acid number 5 to 10; saponification number 147 to 157; hydroxyl number 235 to 260. Trioleate: Amber, oily liquid; viscosity about 200 cps; HLB number 1.8; acid number 15 max; saponification number 170 to 190; hydroxyl number 55 to 70. Tristearate: Tan, waxy beads; HLB number 2.1; acid number 12 to 15; saponification number 176 to 188; hydroxyl number 66 to 80.

Solubility—Monolaurate: Soluble in methanol or alcohol; dispersible in distilled water and hard water (200 ppm); insoluble in hard water (20,000 ppm). Monooleate: Soluble in most mineral or vegetable oils; slightly soluble in ether; dispersible in water; insoluble in acetone. Monopalmitate: Dispersible in distilled water or hard water (200 ppm); soluble in ethyl acetate; insoluble in cold distilled water or hard water (20,000 ppm). Monostearate: Soluble (above melting point) in vegetable oils or mineral oil; insoluble in water, alcohol, or propylene glycol. Trioleate: Soluble in mineral oil, vegetable oils, alcohol, or methanol; insoluble in water. Tristearate: Soluble in isopropyl alcohol; insoluble in water.

Uses—Nonionic surfactants used as emulsifying agents in the preparation of water-in-oil emulsions.

STEARIC ACID—page 1079.

STEARYL ALCOHOL

1-Octadecanol [112-92-5] $C_{18}H_{38}O$ (270.50); contains not less than 90% of stearyl alcohol, the remainder consisting chiefly of cetyl alcohol [$C_{16}H_{34}O = 242.44$].

Preparation—Through the reducing action of lithium aluminum hydride on ethyl stearate.

Description—White, unctuous flakes or granules having a faint, characteristic odor and a bland taste; melts 55 to 60°C.

Solubility—Insoluble in water; soluble in alcohol, chloroform, ether, or vegetable oils.

Uses—A surface-active agent used to stabilize emulsions and increase their ability to retain large quantities of water. See Hydrophilic Ointment (page 1078); Hydrophilic Petrolatum (page 1078).

TRAGACANTH

Gum Tragacanth; Hog Gum; Goat's Thorn

The dried gummy exudation from *Astragalus gummifer* Labillardiére or other Asiatic species of *Astragalus* (Fam *Leguminosae*).

Constituents—60 to 70% bassorin and 30 to 40% soluble gum *(tragacanthin)*. The bassorin swells in the presence of water to form a gel, and tragacanthin forms a colloidal solution. Bassorin, consisting of complex methoxylated acids, resembles pectin. Tragacanthin yields glucuronic acid and arabinose when hydrolyzed.

Description—Flattened, lamellated, frequently curved fragments or straight or spirally twisted linear pieces 0.5 to 2.5 mm in thickness; white to weak-yellow in color; translucent; horny in texture; odorless; insipid, mucilaginous taste. When powdered, it is white to yellowish white.

Introduced into water, tragacanth absorbs a certain proportion of that liquid, swells very much, forms a soft adhesive paste, but does not dissolve. If agitated with an excess of water, this paste forms a uniform mixture; but in the course of 1 or 2 days the greater part separates and is deposited, leaving a portion dissolved in the supernatant fluid. The finest mucilage is obtained from the whole gum or flake form. Several days should be allowed for obtaining a uniform mucilage of the maximum gel strength. A common adulterant is Karaya Gum, and the USP has introduced tests to detect its presence.

Solubility—Insoluble in alcohol.

Uses—A suspending agent in lotions, mixtures, and extemporaneous preparations and prescriptions. It is used with emulsifying agents largely to increase consistency and retard creaming. It is sometimes used as a demulcent in sore throat, and the jelly-like product formed when the gum is allowed to swell in water serves as a basis for pharmaceutical jellies, eg, Ephedrine Sulfate Jelly. It also is used in various confectionery products. In the form of a glycerite, it has been used as a pill excipient.

Tragacanth Mucilage—Preparation: Mix glycerin (18 g) with purified water (75 mL) in a tared vessel, heat the mixture to boiling, discontinue the application of heat, add tragacanth (6 g) and benzoic acid (0.2 g), and macerate the mixture during 24 hr, stirring occasionally. Then add enough purified water to make the mixture weigh 100 g, stir actively until of uniform consistency, and strain forcibly through muslin. Uses: A suspending agent for insoluble substances in internal mixtures. It is also a protective agent.

XANTHAN GUM

Keltrol

A high-molecular-weight polysaccharide gum produced by a pure-culture fermentation of a carbohydrate with *Xanthomonas campestris*, then purified by recovery with isopropyl alcohol, dried and milled; contains D-glucose and D-mannose as the dominant hexose units, along with D-glucuronic acid and is prepared as a sodium, potassium, or calcium salt; yields 4.2 to 5% carbon dioxide.

Preparation—See above and US Patents 3,433,708 and 3,557,016.

Description—White or cream-colored, tasteless powder with a slight organic odor; powder and solutions stable at 25°C or less; does not exhibit polymorphism; aqueous solutions are neutral to litmus.

Solubility—1 g in about 3 mL alcohol; soluble in hot or cold water.

Uses—A hydrophilic colloid to thicken, suspend, emulsify, and stabilize water-based systems.

OTHER EMULSIFYING AND SUSPENDING AGENTS

Malt—The partially germinated grain of one or more varieties of *Hordeum vulgare* Linné (Fam *Gramineae*) and contains amylolytic enzymes. Yellowish or amber-colored grains, with a characteristic odor and a sweet taste. The evaporated aqueous extract constitutes malt extract.

Malt Extract—The product obtained by extracting malt, the partially and artificially germinated grain of one or more varieties of *Hordeum vulgare* Linné (Fam *Gramineae*). Uses: An infrequently used emulsifying agent.

OINTMENT BASES

Ointments are semisolid preparations for external application to the body. They should be of such composition that they soften, but not necessarily melt, when applied to the skin. Therapeutically, ointments function as protectives and emollients for the skin, but are used primarily as vehicles or bases for the topical application of medicinal substances. Ointments also may be applied to the eye or eyelids.

Ideally, an ointment base should be compatible with the skin, stable, permanent, smooth and pliable, nonirritating, nonsensitizing, inert, and readily able to release its incorporated medication. Since there is no single ointment base that possesses all these characteristics, continued research in this field has resulted in the development of numerous new bases. Indeed, ointment bases have become so numerous as to require classification. Although ointment bases may be grouped in several ways, it is generally agreed that they can be classified best according to composition. Hence, the following four classes are recognized here: oleaginous, emulsifiable, emulsion bases, and water-soluble.

For completeness, substances are included that, although not used alone as ointment bases, contribute some pharmaceutical property to one or more of the various bases.

Oleaginous Ointment Base and Components

The oleaginous ointment bases include fixed oils of vegetable origin, fats obtained from animals, and semisolid hydrocarbons obtained from petroleum. The vegetable oils are used chiefly in ointments to lower the melting point or to soften bases. These oils can be used as a base in themselves when a high percentage of powder is incorporated.

The vegetable oils and the animal fats have two marked disadvantages as ointment bases: their water-absorbing capacity is low and they have a tendency to become rancid. Insofar as vegetable oils are concerned, the second disadvantage can be overcome by hydrogenation, a process that converts many fixed oils into white, semisolid fats or hard, almost brittle, waxes.

The hydrocarbon bases comprise a group of substances with a wide range of melting points so that any desired consistency and melting point may be prepared with representatives of this group. They are stable, bland, and chemically inert and will mix with virtually any chemical substance. Oleaginous bases are excellent emollients.

WHITE OINTMENT

Ointment USP; Simple Ointment

White Wax	50 g
White Petrolatum	950 g
To make	1000 g

Melt the white wax in a suitable dish on a water bath, add the white petrolatum, warm until liquefied, then discontinue the heating and stir the mixture until it begins to congeal. It is permissible to vary the proportion of wax to obtain a suitable consistency of the ointment under different climatic conditions.

Uses—An emollient and vehicle for other ointments.

YELLOW OINTMENT

Yellow Wax	50 g
Petrolatum	950 g
To make	1000 g

Melt the yellow wax in a suitable dish on a steam bath, add the petrolatum, warm until liquefied, then discontinue the heating and stir the mixture until it begins to congeal. It is permissible to vary the proportion of wax to obtain a suitable consistency of the ointment under different climatic conditions.

Uses—An emollient and vehicle for other ointments. Both white and yellow ointments are known as simple ointment. White ointment should be used to prepare white ointments and yellow ointments should be used to prepare colored ointments when simple ointment is prescribed.

CETYL ESTERS WAX

Synthetic Spermaceti

A mixture consisting primarily of esters of saturated fatty alcohols (C_{14} to C_{18}) and saturated fatty acids (C_{14} to C_{18}). It has a saponification value of 109 to 120 and an acid value of not more than 5.

Description—White to off-white, somewhat translucent flakes; crystalline structure and pearly luster when caked; faint odor and a bland, mild taste; free from rancidity; specific gravity 0.820 to 0.840 at 50°C; iodine value not more than 1; melts 43 to 47°C.

Solubility—Insoluble in water; practically insoluble in cold alcohol; soluble in boiling alcohol, ether, chloroform, or fixed and volatile oils; slightly soluble in cold solvent hexane.

Uses—A replacement for spermaceti used to give consistency and texture to ointments, eg, Cold Cream and Rose Water Ointment.

OLEIC ACID

(Z)-9-Octadecenoic acid; Oleinic Acid; Elaic Acid

$$HC-CH_2(CH_2)_6COOH$$
$$\parallel$$
$$HC-CH_2(CH_2)_6CH_3$$

Oleic acid [112-80-1] obtained from tallow and other fats and consists chiefly of (Z)-9-octadecenoic acid (282.47). Oleic acid used in preparations for internal administration is derived from edible sources.

It usually contains variable amounts of the other fatty acids present in tallow, such as linolenic and stearic acids.

Preparation—Obtained as a by-product in the manufacture of the solid stearic and palmitic acids used in the manufacture of candles, stearates, and other products. The crude oleic acid is known as red oil, the stearic and palmitic acids being separated by cooling.

Description—Colorless to pale yellow, oily liquid; lard-like odor and taste; specific gravity 0.889 to 0.895; congeals at a temperature not above 10°C; pure acid solidifies at 4°C; at atmospheric pressure it decomposes when heated at 80 to 100°C; on exposure to air it gradually absorbs oxygen, darkens, and develops a rancid odor.

Solubility—Practically insoluble in water; miscible with alcohol, chloroform, ether, benzene, or fixed and volatile oils.

Incompatibilities—Reacts with alkali to form soaps. Heavy metals and calcium salts form insoluble oleates. Iodine solutions are decolorized by formation of the iodine addition compound of the acid. It is oxidized to various derivatives by nitric acid, potassium permanganate, and other agents.

Uses—Classified as an emulsion adjunct, which reacts with alkalis to form soaps that function as emulsifying agents; it is used for this purpose in such preparations as Benzyl Benzoate Lotion and Green Soap. It also is used to prepare oleate salts of bases.

PARAFFIN

Paraffin Wax; Hard Paraffin

A purified mixture of solid hydrocarbons obtained from petroleum.

Description—Colorless or white, more or less translucent mass with a crystalline structure; slightly greasy to the touch; odorless and tasteless; congeals 47 to 65°C.

Solubility—Freely soluble in chloroform, ether, volatile oils, or most warm fixed oils; slightly soluble in dehydrated alcohol; insoluble in water or alcohol.

Uses—Mainly, to increase the consistency of some ointments.

PETROLATUM

Yellow Soft Paraffin; Amber Petrolatum; Yellow Petrolatum; Petroleum Jelly; Paraffin Jelly

A purified mixture of semisolid hydrocarbons obtained from petroleum. It may contain a suitable stabilizer.

Preparation—The residuums as they are termed technically, which are obtained by the distillation of petroleum, are purified by melting, usually treating with sulfuric acid and then percolating through recently burned bone black or adsorptive clays; this removes the odor and modifies the color. Selective solvents are also sometimes employed to extract impurities.

It has been found that the extent of purification required to produce Petrolatum and Light Mineral Oil of official quality removes antioxidants that are naturally present, and the purified product subsequently has a tendency to oxidize and develop an offensive odor. This is prevented by the addition of a minute quantity of α-tocopherol or other suitable antioxidant, as is now permissible.

Description—Unctuous mass of yellowish to light amber color; not more than a slight fluorescence after being melted; transparent in thin layers; free or nearly free from odor and taste; specific gravity 0.815 to 0.880 at 60°C; melts between 38 and 60°C.

Solubility—Insoluble in water; almost insoluble in cold or hot alcohol or in cold dehydrated alcohol; freely soluble in benzene, carbon disulfide, chloroform, or turpentine oil; soluble in ether, solvent hexane, or in most fixed and volatile oils, the degree of solubility in these solvents varying with the composition of the petrolatum.

Uses—A base for ointments. It is highly occlusive and therefore a good emollient, but it may not release some drugs readily.

WHITE PETROLATUM

White Petroleum Jelly; White Soft Paraffin

A purified mixture of semisolid hydrocarbons obtained from petroleum, and wholly or nearly decolorized. It may contain a suitable stabilizer.

Preparation—In the same manner as petrolatum, the purification treatment being continued until the product is practically free from yellow color.

Description—White or faintly yellowish, unctuous mass; transparent in thin layers, even after cooling to 0°C; specific gravity 0.815 to 0.880 at 60°C; melts 38 to 60°C.

Solubility—Similar to that described under Petrolatum.

Uses—Similar to yellow petrolatum but often is preferred because of its freedom from color. It is employed as a protective, as a base for ointments and cerates, and to form the basis for burn dressings. See Petrolatum Gauze (page 1278).

Absorbent Ointment Bases

The term absorbent is used here to denote the water-absorbing or emulsifying properties of these bases and not to describe their action on the skin. These bases, sometimes called emulsifiable ointment bases, are generally anhydrous substances that have the property of absorbing (emulsifying) considerable quantities of water and still retaining their ointment-like consistency. Preparations of this type do not contain water as a component of their basic formula, but if water is incorporated, when and as desired, a W/O emulsion results. The following official products fall into this category.

LANOLIN ANHYDROUS

Anhydrous Lanolin; Wool Fat USP; Refined Wool Fat

Lanolin that contains not more than 0.25% of water.

Constituents—Contains the sterols cholesterol [$C_{27}H_{45}OH$] and oxycholesterol, as well as triterpene and aliphatic alcohols. About 7% of the alcohols are found in the free state, the remainder occurring as esters of the following fatty acids: carnaubic, cerotic, lanoceric, lanopalmitic, myristic, and palmitic. Some of these are found free. The emulsifying and emollient actions of lanolin are due to the alcohols that are found in the unsaponifiable fraction when lanolin is treated with alkali. Constituting approximately one-half of this fraction and known as lanolin alcohols, the latter is composed of cholesterol (30%), lanosterol (25%), cholestanol (dihydrocholesterol) (3%), agnosterol (2%), and various other alcohols (40%).

Preparation—By purifying the fatty matter (suint) obtained from the wool of the sheep. This natural wool fat contains about 30% of free fatty acids and fatty acid esters of cholesterol and other higher alcohols. The cholesterol compounds are the important constituents, and to secure these in a purified form, many processes have been devised. In one of these the crude wool fat is treated with weak alkali and the saponified fats and emulsions are centrifuged to secure the aqueous soap solution, from which, on standing, a layer of partially purified wool fat separates. This product is further purified by treating it with calcium chloride and then dehydrated by fusion with unslaked lime. It is finally extracted with acetone, and the solvent subsequently separated by distillation. This differs from lanolin in that the former contains practically no water.

Description—Yellow, tenacious, unctuous mass; slight, characteristic odor; melts between 36 and 42°C.

Solubility—Insoluble in water but mixes without separation with about twice its weight of water; sparingly soluble in cold alcohol; more soluble in hot alcohol; freely soluble in ether or chloroform.

Uses—An ingredient of ointments, especially when an aqueous liquid is to be incorporated. It gives a distinctive quality to the ointment, increasing absorption of active ingredients and maintaining a uniform consistency for the ointment under most climatic conditions. However, it has been omitted from many ointments on the recommendation of dermatologists who have found that many patients are allergic to this animal wax.

HYDROPHILIC PETROLATUM

Cholesterol	30 g
Stearyl Alcohol	30 g
White Wax	80 g
White Petrolatum	860 g
To make	1000 g

Melt the stearyl alcohol, white wax, and white petrolatum together on a steam bath, then add the cholesterol and stir until it completely dissolves. Remove from the bath, and stir until the mixture congeals.

Uses—A protective and water-absorbable ointment base. It will absorb a large amount of water from aqueous solutions of medicating substances, forming a W/O type of emulsion. See Chapter 44 *(Medicated Topicals)*.

Emulsion Ointment Bases and Components

Emulsion ointment bases are actually semisolid emulsions. These preparations can be divided into two groups on the basis of emulsion type: emulsion ointment base water-in-oil (W/O) type and emulsion ointment base oil-in-water (O/W) type. Bases of both types will permit the incorporation of some additional amounts of water without reducing the consistency of the base below that of a soft cream. However, only O/W emulsion ointment bases can be removed readily from the skin and clothing with water. W/O emulsions are better emollients and protectants than are O/W emulsions. W/O emulsions can be diluted with oils.

CETYL ALCOHOL

Cetostearyl Alcohol; Palmityl Alcohol; Aldol 52

CH$_3$(CH$_2$)$_{14}$CH$_2$OH

1-Hexadecanol [124-29-8] C$_{16}$H$_{34}$O (242.44); a mixture of not less than 90% of cetyl alcohol, the remainder chiefly stearyl alcohol.

Preparation—By catalytic hydrogenation of palmitic acid or saponification of spermaceti, which contains cetyl palmitate.

Description—Unctuous, white flakes, granules, cubes, or castings; faint characteristic odor and a bland, mild taste; melts 45 to 50°C; not less than 90% distills between 316 and 336°C.

Solubility—Insoluble in water; soluble in alcohol, chloroform, ether, or vegetable oils.

Uses—Similar to Stearyl Alcohol (page 1076). It also imparts a smooth texture to the skin and is used widely in cosmetic creams and lotions.

COLD CREAM

Petrolatum Rose Water Ointment USP

Cetyl Esters Wax	125 g
White Wax	120 g
Mineral Oil	560 g
Sodium Borate	5 g
Purified Water	190 mL
To make about	1000 g

Reduce the cetyl esters wax and the white wax to small pieces, melt them on a steam bath with the mineral oil, and continue heating until the temperature of the mixture reaches 70°C. Dissolve the sodium borate in the purified water, warmed to 70°C, and gradually add the warm solution to the melted mixture, stirring rapidly and continuously until it has congealed.

If the ointment has been chilled, warm it slightly before attempting to incorporate other ingredients (see USP for allowable variations).

Uses—Useful as an emollient, cleansing cream, and ointment base. It resembles *Rose Water Ointment,* differing only in that mineral oil is used in place of almond oil and omitting the fragrance. This change produces an ointment base that is not subject to rancidity as is one containing a vegetable oil. This is a W/O emulsion.

GLYCERYL MONOSTEARATE

Octadecanoic acid, monoester with 1,2,3-propanetriol

Monostearin [31566-31-1]; a mixture chiefly of variable proportions of glyceryl monostearate [C$_3$H$_5$(OH)$_2$C$_{18}$H$_{35}$O$_2$ = 358.56] and glyceryl monopalmitate [C$_3$H$_5$(OH)$_2$C$_{16}$H$_{31}$O$_2$ = 330.51].

Preparation—Among other ways, by reacting glycerin with commercial stearoyl chloride.

Description—White, wax-like solid or occurs in the form of white, wax-like beads, or flakes; slight, agreeable, fatty odor and taste; does not melt below 55°C; affected by light.

Solubility—Insoluble in water, but may be dispersed in hot water with the aid of a small amount of soap or other suitable surface-active agent; dissolves in hot organic solvents such as alcohol, mineral or fixed oils, benzene, ether, or acetone.

Uses—A thickening and emulsifying agent for ointments. See *Ointments* (page 1076).

HYDROPHILIC OINTMENT

Methylparaben	0.25 g
Propylparaben	0.15 g
Sodium Lauryl Sulfate	10 g
Propylene Glycol	120 g
Stearyl Alcohol	250 g
White Petrolatum	250 g
Purified Water (qs)	1000 g

Melt the stearyl alcohol and the white petrolatum on a steam bath, and warm to about 75°C. Add the other ingredients, previously dissolved in the water and warmed to 75°C, and stir the mixture until it congeals.

Uses A water-removable ointment base for the so-called washable ointments. This is an O/W emulsion.

LANOLIN

Hydrous Wool Fat

The purified, fat-like substance from the wool of sheep, *Ovis aries* Linné (Fam *Bovidae*); contains 25% to 30% water.

Description—Yellowish white, ointment-like mass, with a slight, characteristic odor; when heated on a steam bath it separates into an upper oily and a lower water layer; when the water is evaporated a residue of *Lanolin* remains that is transparent when melted.

Solubility—Insoluble in water; soluble in chloroform or ether with separation of its water of hydration.

Uses—Largely as a vehicle for ointments, for which it is admirably adapted on account of its compatibility with skin lipids. It emulsifies aqueous liquids. Lanolin is a W/O emulsion.

ROSE WATER OINTMENT

Cold Cream; Galen's Cerate

Cetyl Esters Wax	125 g
White Wax	120 g
Almond Oil	560 g
Sodium Borate	5 g
Stronger Rose Water	25 mL
Rose Oil	0.2 mL
Purified Water (qs)	1000 g

Reduce the cetyl esters wax and the white wax to small pieces, melt them on a steam bath, add the almond oil, and continue heating until the temperature of the mixture reaches 70°C. Dissolve the sodium borate in the purified water and stronger rose water, warmed to 70°C, and gradually add the warm solution to the melted mixture, stirring rapidly and continuously until it has cooled to about 45°C. Incorporate the rose oil.

It must be free from rancidity. If the ointment has been chilled, warm it slightly before attempting to incorporate other ingredients (see USP for allowable variations).

History—Originated by Galen, the famous Roman physician-pharmacist of the 1st Century AD; was known for many centuries by the name of *Unguentum* or *Ceratum Refrigerans*. It has changed but little in proportions or method of preparation throughout many centuries.

Uses—An emollient and ointment base. It is a W/O emulsion.

STEARIC ACID

Octadecanoic acid; Cetylacetic Acid; Stearophanic Acid

Stearic acid [57-11-4]; a mixture of stearic acid [$C_{18}H_{36}O_2 = 284.48$] and palmitic acid [$C_{16}H_{32}O_2 = 256.43$], which together constitute not less than 90.0% of the total content. The content of each is not less than 40.0% of the total.

Purified Stearic Acid USP is a mixture of the same acids that together constitute not less than 96.0% of the total content, and the content of $C_{18}H_{36}O_2$ is not less than 90.0% of the total.

Preparation—From edible fats and oils (see exception below) by boiling them with soda lye, separating the glycerin, and decomposing the resulting soap with sulfuric or hydrochloric acid. The stearic acid subsequently is separated from any oleic acid by cold expression. It also is prepared by the hydrogenation and subsequent saponification of olein. It may be purified by recrystallization from alcohol.

Description—Hard, white or faintly yellowish, somewhat glossy and crystalline solid, or a white or yellowish white powder; an odor and taste suggestive of tallow; melts about 55.5°C and should not congeal at a temperature below 54°C; the purified acid melts at 69 to 70°C and congeals between 66 and 69°C; slowly volatilizes between 90 and 100°C.

Solubility—Practically insoluble in water; 1 g in about 20 mL alcohol, 2 mL chloroform, 3 mL ether, 25 mL acetone, or 6 mL carbon tetrachloride; freely soluble in carbon disulfide; also soluble in amyl acetate, benzene, or toluene.

Incompatibilities—Insoluble stearates are formed with many *metals*. Ointment bases made with stearic acid may show evidence of drying out or lumpiness due to such a reaction when zinc or calcium salts are compounded therein.

Uses—In the preparation of sodium stearate, which is the solidifying agent for the official glycerin suppositories; in enteric tablet coating; ointments; and for many commercial products, such as toilet creams, vanishing creams, solidified alcohol, etc. (when labeled solely for external use, it is exempt from the requirement that it be prepared from edible fats and oils).

Water-Soluble Ointment Bases and Components

Included in this section are bases prepared from the higher ethylene glycol polymers (PEGs). These polymers are marketed under the trademark of Carbowax. The polymers have a wide range in molecular weight. Those with molecular weights ranging from 200 to 700 are liquids; those above 1000 are wax-like solids. The polymers are water-soluble, nonvolatile, and unctuous agents. They do not hydrolyze or deteriorate and will not support mold growth. These properties account for their wide use in washable ointments. Mixtures of PEGs are used to give bases of various consistency, such as very soft to hard bases for suppositories.

GLYCOL ETHERS AND DERIVATIVES

This special class of ethers is of considerable importance in pharmaceutical technology. Both mono- and polyfunctional compounds are represented in the group. The simplest member is ethylene oxide, [$-CH_2CH_2-O$], the internal or cyclic ether of the simplest glycol, ethylene glycol [$HOCH_2CH_2OH$]. External

mono- and diethers of ethylene glycol $ROCH_2CH_2OH$ and $ROCH_2CH_2OR$ are well known largely because of research done by Union Carbide.

PREPARATION—In the presence of NaOH at temperatures of the order of 120 to 135°C and under a total pressure of about 4 atmospheres, ethylene oxide reacts with ethylene glycol to form compounds having the general formula $HOCH_2(CH_2OCH_2)_nCH_2OH$, commonly referred to as condensation polymers and termed polyethylene (or polyoxyethylene) glycols. Other glycols besides ethylene glycol function in a similar capacity, and the commercial generic term adopted for the entire group is polyalkylene (or polyoxyalkylene) glycols.

NOMENCLATURE—It is to be noted that these condensation polymers are bifunctional; ie, they contain both ether and alcohol linkages. The compound in which $n = 1$ is the commercially important diethylene glycol [$HOCH_2CH_2OCH_2CH_2OH$], and its internal ether is the familiar dioxane [$-CH_2CH_2OCH_2CH_2-O$]. The mono- and diethers derived from diethylene glycol have the formulas $ROCH_2CH_2OCH_2CH_2OH$ and $ROCH_2CH_2OCH_2CH_2OR$. The former is commonly termed Carbitols and the latter Cellosolves.

Polyethylene glycols are differentiated in commercial nomenclature by adding a number to the name, which represents the average molecular weight. Thus, polyethylene glycol 400 has an average molecular weight of about 400 (measured values for commercial samples range between 380 and 420), corresponding to a value of n for this particular polymer of approximately 8. Polymers have been produced in which the value of n runs into the hundreds. Up to n = approximately 15, the compounds are liquids at room temperature, and viscosity and boiling point increase with increasing molecular weight. Higher polymers are waxy solids and are termed commercially Carbowaxes.

It should be observed that the presence of the two terminal hydroxyl groups in the polyalkylene glycols makes possible the formation of both ether and ester derivatives, several of which are marketed products.

USES—Because of their vapor pressure, solubility, solvent power, hygroscopicity, viscosity, and lubricating characteristics, the polyalkylene glycols or their derivatives function in many applications as effective replacements for glycerin and water-insoluble oils. They find considerable use as plasticizers, lubricants, conditioners, and finishing agents for processing textiles and rubber. They also are important as emulsifying agents and as dispersants for such diverse substances as dyes, oils, resins, insecticides, and various types of pharmaceuticals. In addition, they are employed frequently as ingredients in ointment bases and in a variety of cosmetic preparations.

POLYETHYLENE GLYCOLS

Poly(oxy-1,2-ethanediyl), α-hydro-φ-hydroxy-, Carbowaxes; Atpeg

$$H-[OCH_2CH_2-]_nOH$$

Polyethylene glycols [25322-68-3].

Preparation—Ethylene glycol is reacted with ethylene oxide in the presence of NaOH at temperatures in the range of 120 to 135°C under pressure of about 4 atm.

Description—Polyethylene glycols 200, 300, 400, and 600 are clear, viscous liquids at room temperature. Polyethylene glycols 900, 1000, 1450, 3350, 4500, and 8000 are white, waxy solids. The glycols do not hydrolyze or deteriorate under typical conditions. As their molecular weight increases, their water solubility, vapor pressure, hygroscopicity, and solubility in organic solvents decrease; at the same time, freezing or melting range, specific gravity, flash point, and viscosity increase. If these compounds ignite, small fires should be extinguished with carbon dioxide or dry-chemical extinguishers and large fires with alcohol-type foam extinguishers.

Solubility—All members of this class dissolve in water to form clear solutions and are soluble in many organic solvents.

Uses—These possess a wide range of solubilities and compatibilities, which make them useful in pharmaceutical and cosmetic preparations. Their blandness renders them highly acceptable for hair dressings, hand lotions, sun-tan creams, leg lotions, shaving creams, and skin creams (eg, a peroxide ointment that is stable may be prepared using these compounds, while oil-type bases inactivate the peroxide). Their use in washable ointments is discussed under Ointments (page 1076). They also are used in making suppositories, hormone creams, etc. See Polyethylene Glycol Ointment (below) and Glycol Ethers (above). The liquid polyethylene glycol 400 and the solid polyethylene glycol 3350, used in the proportion specified (or a permissible variation thereof) in the official Polyethylene Glycol Ointment, provide a water-soluble ointment base used in the formulation of many dermatological preparations. The solid, waxy, water-soluble glycols often are used to increase the viscosity of liquid polyethylene glycols and to stiffen ointment and suppository bases. In addition, they are used to compensate for the melting point-lowering effect of other agents, ie, chloral hydrate, etc, on such bases.

Polyethylene Glycol Ointment USP—Preparation: Heat polyethylene glycol 3350 (400 g) and polyethylene glycol 400 (600 g) on a water bath to 65°C. Allow to cool, and stir until congealed. If a firmer preparation is desired, replace up to 100 g of polyethylene glycol 400 with an equal amount of polyethylene glycol 3350. If 6 to 25% of an aqueous solution is to be incorporated in this ointment, replace 50 g of polyethylene glycol 3350 by 50 g of stearyl alcohol. Uses: A water-soluble ointment base.

POLYOXYL 40 STEARATE

Poly(oxy-1,2-ethanediyl), α-hydro-φ-hydroxy-, octadecanoate; Myrj

$RCOO(C_2H_4O)_nH$ ($RCOO$ is the stearate moiety; n is approximately 40).

Polyethylene glycol monostearate [9004-99-3]; a mixture of monostearate and distearate esters of mixed polyoxyethylene diols and corresponding free glycols, the average polymer length being equivalent to about 40 oxyethylene units. Polyoxyethylene 50 Stearate is a similar mixture in which the average polymer length is equivalent to about 50 oxyethylene units.

Preparation—One method consists of heating the corresponding polyethylene glycol with an equimolar portion of stearic acid.

Description—White to light-tan waxy solid; odorless or has a faint fat-like odor; congeals between 37 and 47°C.

Solubility—Soluble in water, alcohol, ether, or acetone; insoluble in mineral or vegetable oils.

Uses—Contains ester and alcohol functions that impart both lyophilic and hydrophilic characteristics to make it useful as a surfactant and emulsifier. It is an ingredient of some water-soluble ointment and cream bases.

POLYSORBATES

Sorbitan esters, poly(oxy-1,2-ethanediyl) derivs; Tweens

[Sum of w, x,y, and z is 20; R is (C₁₁H₂₃)COO]

Sorbitan esters, polyoxyethylene derivatives; fatty acid esters of sorbitol and its anhydrides copolymerized with a varying number of moles of ethylene oxide. The NF recognizes Polysorbate 20 (structure given above), a laurate ester; Polysorbate 40, a palmitate ester; Polysorbate 60, a mixture of stearate and palmitate esters; and Polysorbate 80, an oleate ester.

Preparation—These important nonionic surfactants are prepared starting with sorbitol by (1) elimination of water-forming sorbitan (a cyclic sorbitol anhydride); (2) partial esterification of the sorbitan with a fatty acid such as oleic or stearic acid, yielding a hexitan ester known commercially as a Span; and (3) chemical addition of ethylene oxide, yielding a Tween (the polyoxyethylene derivative).

Description—Polysorbate 80: Lemon- to amber-colored, oily liquid; faint, characteristic odor; warm, somewhat bitter taste; specific gravity 1.07 to 1.09; pH (1:20 aqueous solution) 6 to 8.

Solubility—Polysorbate 80: Very soluble in water, producing an odorless and nearly colorless solution; soluble in alcohol, cottonseed oil, corn oil, ethyl acetate, methanol, or toluene; insoluble in mineral oil.

Uses—Because of their hydrophilic and lyophilic characteristics, these nonionic surfactants are very useful as emulsifying agents, forming O/W emulsions in pharmaceuticals, cosmetics, and other types of products. Polysorbate 80 is an ingredient in Coal Tar Ointment and Solution. See Glycol Ethers (page 1079).

PHARMACEUTICAL SOLVENTS

The remarkable growth of the solvent industry is attested by the more than 300 solvents now being produced on an industrial scale. Chemically, these include a great variety of organic compounds, ranging from hydrocarbons through alcohols, esters, ethers, and acids to nitroparaffins. Their main applications are in industry and the synthesis of organic chemicals. Comparatively few, however, are used as solvents in pharmacy, because of their toxicity, volatility, instability, and/or flammability. Those commonly used as pharmaceutical solvents are described in this section.

ACETONE

2-Propanone; Dimethyl Ketone

CH_3COCH_3

Acetone [67-64-1] C_3H_6O (58.08).

Caution—It is very flammable. Do not use where it may be ignited.

Preparation—Formerly obtained exclusively from the destructive distillation of wood. The distillate, consisting principally of methanol, acetic acid, and acetone was neutralized with lime, and the acetone was separated from the methyl alcohol by fractional distillation. Additional quantities were obtained by pyrolysis of the calcium acetate formed in the neutralization of the distillate.

It now is obtained largely as a by-product of the butyl alcohol industry. This alcohol is formed in the fermentation of carbohydrates such as corn starch, molasses, etc, by the action of the bacterium Clostridium acetobutylicum (Weizmann fermentation), and it is always one of the products formed in the process. It also is obtained by the catalytic oxidation of isopropyl alcohol, which is prepared from propylene resulting from the cracking of crude petroleum.

Description—Transparent, colorless, mobile, volatile, flammable liquid with a characteristic odor; specific gravity not more than 0.789;

distills between 55.5 and 57°C; congeals about -95°C; aqueous solution neutral to litmus.

Solubility—Miscible with water, alcohol, ether, chloroform, or most volatile oils.

Uses—An antiseptic in concentrations above 80%. In combination with alcohol it is used as an antiseptic cleansing solution. It is employed as a menstruum in the preparation of oleoresins in place of ether. It is used as a solvent for dissolving fatty bodies, resins, pyroxylin, mercurials, etc, and also in the manufacture of many organic compounds such as chloroform, chlorobutanol, and ascorbic acid.

ALCOHOL

Ethanol; Spiritus Vini Rectificatus; S. V. R.; Spirit of Wine; Methylcarbinol

Ethyl alcohol [64-17-5]; contains 92.3 to 93.8%, by weight (94.9 to 96.0%, by volume), at 15.56°C (60°F) of C_2H_5OH (46.07).

Preparation—Has been made for centuries by fermentation of certain carbohydrates in the presence of zymase, an enzyme present in yeast cells. Usable carbohydrate-containing materials include molasses, sugar cane, fruit juices, corn, barley, wheat, potato, wood, and waste sulfite liquors. As yeast is capable of fermenting only D-glucose, D-fructose, D-mannose, and D-galactose, it is essential that more complex carbohydrates, such as starch, be converted to one or more of these simple sugars before they can be fermented. This is accomplished variously, commonly by enzyme- or acid-catalyzed hydrolysis.

The net reaction that occurs when a hexose, glucose for example, is fermented to alcohol may be represented as

$$C_6H_{12}O_6 \equiv 2\,C_2H_5OH + 2\,CO_2$$

but the mechanism of the process is very complex. The fermented liquid, containing about 15% alcohol, is distilled to obtain a distillate containing 94.9% C_2H_5OH, by volume. To produce absolute alcohol, various processes dehydrate the 95% product.

Hydration of ethylene, abundant supplies of which are available from natural and coke oven gases, from waste gases of the petroleum industry, and other sources may produce it also. In another synthesis acetylene is hydrated catalytically to acetaldehyde, which then is hydrogenated catalytically to ethyl alcohol.

Description—Transparent, colorless, mobile, volatile liquid; slight but characteristic odor; burning taste; boils at 78°C but volatilizes even at a low temperature, and is flammable; when pure, it is neutral toward all indicators; specific gravity at 15.56 (the US Government standard temperature for Alcohol) not above 0.816, indicating not less than 92.3% of C_2H_5OH by weight, or 94.9% by volume.

Solubility—Miscible with water, acetone, chloroform, ether, or many other organic solvents.

Incompatibilities—This and preparations containing a high percentage of alcohol will precipitate many inorganic salts from an aqueous solution. Acacia generally is recipitated from a hydroalcoholic medium when the alcohol content is greater than about 35%.

Strong oxidizing agents such as chlorine, nitric acid, permanganate, or chromate in acid solution react, in some cases violently, with it to produce oxidation products.

Alkali cause a darkening in color because of the small amount of aldehyde usually present in it.

Uses—In pharmacy principally for its solvent powers. It also is used as the starting point in the manufacture of many important compounds, like ether, chloroform, etc. It also is used as a fuel, chiefly in the denatured form.

It is a CNS depressant. Consequently, it occasionally has been administered intravenously for preoperative and postoperative sedation for patients in whom other measures are ineffective or contraindicated. The dose employed is 1 to 1.5 mL/kg. Its intravenous use is a specialized procedure and should be employed only by one experienced in the technique of such use.

It is used widely and abused by lay persons as a sedative. It has, however, no medically approved use for this purpose. Moreover, alcohol potentiates the CNS effects of numerous sedative and depressant drugs. Hence, patients taking certain prescription drugs or OTC medications should not use it.

Externally, it has a number of medical uses. It is a solvent for the toxicodendrol causing ivy poisoning and should be used to wash the skin thoroughly soon after contact. In a concentration of 25% it is employed for bathing the skin for the purpose of cooling and reducing fevers. In high concentrations it is a rubefacient and an ingredient of many liniments. In a concentration of 50% it is used to prevent sweating in astringent and anhidrotic lotions. It also is employed to cleanse and harden the skin and is helpful in preventing bedsores in bedridden patients. In a concentration of 60 to 90% it is germicidal. At optimum concentration (70% by weight) it is a good antiseptic for the skin (local anti-infective) and also for instruments. It also is used as a solvent to cleanse the skin splashed with phenol. High concentrations of it often are injected into nerves and ganglia for the relief of pain, accomplishing this by causing nerve degeneration.

DENATURED ALCOHOL

An act of Congress, June 7, 1906, authorizes the withdrawal of alcohol from bond without the payment of internal revenue tax, for the purpose of denaturation and use in the arts and industries. This is ethyl alcohol to which has been added such denaturing materials as to render the alcohol unfit for use as an intoxicating beverage. It is divided into two classes, namely, completely denatured alcohol and specially denatured alcohol, prepared in accordance with approved formulas prescribed in Federal Industrial Alcohol Regulations 3.

Completely Denatured Alcohol—This term applies to ethyl alcohol to which has been added materials (methyl isobutyl ketone, pyronate, gasoline, acetaldol, kerosene, etc) of such nature that the products may be sold and used within certain limitations without permit and bond.

Specially Denatured Alcohol—This alcohol is intended for use in a greater number of specified arts and industries than completely denatured alcohol, and the character of the denaturant or denaturants used is such that specially denatured alcohol may be sold, possessed, and used only by those persons or firms that hold basic permits and are covered by bond.

Uses—Approximately 50 specially denatured alcohol formulas containing combinations of more than 90 different denaturants are available to fill the needs of qualified users. Large amounts of specially denatured alcohols are used as raw materials in the production of acetaldehyde, synthetic rubber, vinegar, and ethyl chloride as well as in the manufacture of proprietary solvents and cleaning solutions. Ether and chloroform can be made from suitably denatured alcohols, and formulas for the manufacture of Iodine Tincture, Green Soap Tincture, and Rubbing Alcohol are set forth in the regulations.

Specially denatured alcohols also are used as solvents for surface coatings, plastics, inks, toilet preparations, and external pharmaceuticals. Large quantities are used in the processing of such food and drug products as pectin, vitamins, hormones, antibiotics, alkaloids, and blood products. Other uses include supplemental motor fuel, rocket and jet fuel, antifreeze solutions, refrigerants, and cutting oils. Few products are manufactured today that do not require the use of alcohol at some stage of production. Specially denatured alcohol may not be used in the manufacture of foods or internal medicines when any of the alcohol remains in the finished product.

DILUTED ALCOHOL

Diluted Ethanol

A mixture of alcohol and water containing 41.0 to 42.0%, by weight (48.4 to 49.5%, by volume), at 15.56°C, of C_2H_5OH (46.07).

Preparation

Alcohol	500 mL
Purified Water	500 mL

Measure the alcohol and the purified water separately at the same temperature, and mix. If the water and the alcohol and the resulting mixture are measured at 25°C, the volume of the mixture will be about 970 mL.

When equal volumes of alcohol and water are mixed together, a rise in temperature and a contraction of about 3% in volume take place. In small operations the contraction generally is disregarded; in larger operations it is very important. If 50 gal of official alcohol are mixed with 50 gal of water, the product will not be 100 gal of diluted alcohol, but only 96 1/4 gal, a contraction of 3 3/4 gal. US *Proof Spirit* differs from this and is stronger; it contains 50%, by volume, of absolute alcohol at 15.56°C (60°F). This corresponds to 42.5% by weight and has a specific gravity of 0.9341 at the same temperature. If spirits have a specific gravity lower than that of proof spirit (0.9341), they are said to be above proof; if greater, below proof.

It also may be prepared from the following:

Alcohol	408 g
Purified Water	500 g

Rules for Dilution—The following rules are applied when making an alcohol of any required lower percentage from an alcohol of any given higher percentage:

I. By Volume—Designate the volume percentage of the stronger alcohol by V and that of the weaker alcohol by v.

Rule—Mix v volumes of the stronger alcohol with purified water to make V volumes of product. Allow the mixture to stand until full contraction has taken place and until it has cooled, then make up the deficiency in the V volumes by adding more purified water.

Example—An alcohol of 30% by volume is to be made from an alcohol of 94.9% by volume.—Take 30 volumes of the 94.9% alcohol, and add enough purified water to produce 94.9 volumes at room temperature.

II. By Weight—Designate the weight-percentage of the stronger alcohol by W and that of the weaker alcohol by w.

Rule—Mix w parts by weight of the stronger alcohol with purified water to make W parts by weight of product.

Example—An alcohol of 50% by weight is to be made from an alcohol of 92.3% by weight.—Take 50 parts by weight of the 92.3% alcohol, and add enough purified water to produce 92.3 parts by weight.

Description—As for Alcohol except its specific gravity is 0.935 to 0.937 at 15.56°C, indicating that the strength of C_2H_5OH corresponds to that given in the official definition.

Uses—A solvent in making tinctures, fluid-extracts, extracts, etc. Its properties already have been described fully in connection with the various preparations. Its value consists not only in its antiseptic properties, but also in its possessing the solvent powers of both water and alcohol. See Alcohol.

CHLOROFORM—page 1085.

GLYCERIN

1,2,3-Propanetriol; Glycerol

$$\text{HOCH}_2\text{CHCH}_2\text{OH} \quad \overset{\text{OH}}{\underset{|}{}}$$

Glycerol [56-81-5] $C_3H_8O_3$ (92.09).

Chemically, it is the simplest trihydric alcohol. It is worthy of special note because the two terminal alcohol groups are primary, whereas the middle one is secondary. Thus this becomes the first polyhydric alcohol that can yield both an aldose (glyceraldehyde) and a ketose (dihydroxyacetone).

Preparation

1. By saponification of fats and oils in the manufacture of soap.
2. By hydrolysis of fats and oils through pressure and superheated steam.
3. By fermentation of beet sugar molasses in the presence of large amounts of sodium sulfite. Under these conditions a reaction takes place expressed as

$$C_6H_{12}O_6 \rightarrow C_3H_5(OH)_3 + CH_3CHO + CO_2$$
$$\text{Glucose} \qquad \text{Glycerin} \qquad \text{Acetaldehyde}$$

4. Glycerin is now prepared in large quantities from propylene, a petroleum product. This hydrocarbon is chlorinated at about 400°C to form allyl chloride, which is converted to allyl alcohol. Treatment of the unsaturated alcohol with hypochlorous acid (HOCl) yields the chlorohydrin derivative. Extraction of HCl with soda lime yields 2,3-epoxypropanol, which undergoes hydration to glycerin.

Description—Clear, colorless, syrupy liquid with a sweet taste and not more than a slight, characteristic odor, which is neither harsh nor disagreeable; when exposed to moist air it absorbs water and also such gases as H_2S and SO_2; solutions are neutral; specific gravity not below 1.249 (not less than 95% $C_3H_5(OH)_3$); boils at about 290°C under 1 atm, with decomposition, but can be distilled intact in a vacuum.

Solubility—Miscible with water, alcohol, or methanol; 1g in about 12 mL ethyl acetate or about 15 mL acetone; insoluble in chloroform, ether, or fixed and volatile oils.

Incompatibilities—An explosion may occur if it is triturated with strong oxidizing agents such as chromium trioxide, potassium chlorate, or potassium permanganate. In dilute solutions the reactions proceed at a slower rate, forming several oxidation products. Iron is an occasional contaminant of it and may be the cause of a darkening in color in mixtures containing phenols, salicylates, tannin, etc.

With boric acid or sodium borate, it forms a complex, generally spoken of as glyceroboric acid, which is a much stronger acid than boric acid.

Uses—One of the most valuable products known to pharmacy by virtue of its solvent property. It is useful as a humectant in keeping substances moist, owing to its hygroscopicity. Its agreeable taste and high viscosity adapt it for many purposes. Some modern ice collars and ice bags contain it and water hermetically sealed within vulcanized rubber bags. The latter are sterilized by dipping in a germicidal solution and are stored in the refrigerator until needed. It also has some therapeutic uses. In pure anhydrous form, it is used in the eye to reduce corneal edema and to facilitate ophthalmoscopic examination. It is used orally as an evacuant and, in 50 to 75% solution, as a systemic osmotic agent.

ISOPROPYL ALCOHOL—pages 221 and 1629.

METHYL ALCOHOL

Methanol; Wood Alcohol

CH_3OH

Methanol [67-56-1] CH_4O (32.04).

Caution—It is poisonous.

Preparation—By the catalytic reduction of carbon monoxide or carbon dioxide with hydrogen. A zinc oxide–chromium oxide catalyst is used commonly.

Description—Clear, colorless liquid; characteristic odor; flammable; specific gravity not more than 0.790; distills within a range of 63.5 and 65.7°C.

Solubility—Miscible with water, alcohol, ether, benzene, or most other organic solvents.

Uses—A solvent for non-ingested preparations. It is toxic. Ingestion may result in blindness; vapors also may cause toxic reactions.

METHYL ISOBUTYL KETONE

2-Pentanone, 4-methyl-, $(CH_3)_2CHCH_2COCH_3$ [108-10-1]; contains not

less than 99% of $C_6H_{12}O$ (100.16).

Description—Transparent, colorless, mobile, volatile liquid; faint, ketonic and camphoraceous odor, distills between 114 and 117°C.

Solubility—Slightly soluble in water; miscible with alcohol, ether, or benzene.

Uses—A denaturant for rubbing alcohol and also a *solvent* for gums, resins, nitrocellulose, etc. It may be irritating to the eyes and mucous membranes, and, in high concentrations, narcotic.

MONOETHANOLAMINE

Ethanol, 2-amino-, Ethanolamine; Ethylolamine

$HOCH_2CH_2NH_2$ [141-43-5] C_2H_7NO (61.08).

Preparation—This alkanolamine is prepared conveniently by treating ethylene oxide with ammonia.

Description—Clear, colorless, moderately viscous liquid; distinctly ammoniacal odor; affected by light; specific gravity 1.013 to 1.016; distills between 167 and 173°C.

Solubility—Miscible in all proportions with water, acetone, alcohol, glycerin, or chloroform; immiscible with ether, solvent hexane, or fixed oils; dissolves many essential oils.

Uses—A *solvent* for fats, oils, and many other substances, it is a pharmaceutical necessity for Thimerosal Solution (see RPS-17 page 1173). It combines with fatty acids to form soaps that find application in various types of emulsions such as lotions, creams, etc.

PROPYLENE GLYCOL

$CH_3CH(OH)CH_2OH$

1,2-Propanediol [57-55-6 $C_3H_8O_2$] (76.10).

Preparation—Propylene is converted successively to its chlorohydrin (with HOCl), epoxide (with Na_2CO_3), and glycol (with water in presence of protons).

Description—Clear, colorless, viscous, and practically odorless liquid; slightly acrid taste; specific gravity 1.035 to 1.037; completely distills between 184 and 189°C; absorbs moisture from moist air.

Solubility—Miscible with water, alcohol, acetone, or chloroform; soluble in ether; dissolves many volatile oils; immiscible with fixed oils.

Uses—A solvent, preservative, and humectant. See Hydrophilic Ointment (page 1078).

TROLAMINE

Ethanol, 2,2′,2″-nitrilotris-, Triethanolamine

2,2′,2″-Nitrilotriethanol [102-71-6] $N(C_2H_4OH)_3$ (149.19); a mixture of alkanolamines consisting largely of triethanolamine, containing some diethanolamine [$NH(C_2H_4OH)_2$ = 105.14] and monoethanolamine [$NH_2C_2H_4OH$ = 61.08].

Preparation—Along with some mono- and diethanolamine, by the action of ammonia on ethylene oxide.

Description—Colorless to pale yellow, viscous, hygroscopic liquid; slight odor of ammonia; aqueous solution is very alkaline; melts about 21°C; specific gravity 1.120 to 1.128; a strong base and readily combines even with weak acids to form salts.

Solubility—Miscible with water or alcohol; soluble in chloroform; slightly soluble in ether or benzene.

Uses—In combination with a fatty acid, eg, oleic acid (see Benzyl Benzoate Lotion, 748), as an emulsifier. See Monoethanolamine.

WATER—page 1070.

OTHER PHARMACEUTICAL SOLVENTS

Alcohol, Dehydrated, BP, PhI [Dehydrated Ethanol; Absolute Alcohol]—Transparent, colorless, mobile, volatile liquid; characteristic odor; burning taste; specific gravity not more than 0.798 at 15.56°C; hygroscopic, flammable and boils about 78°C. Miscible with water, ether, or chloroform. *Uses:* A pharmaceutical solvent, antimicrobial preservative and penetration enhancer for topical preparations.

MISCELLANEOUS PHARMACEUTICAL NECESSITIES

The agents listed in this section comprise a heterogeneous group of substances with both pharmaceutical and industrial applications. Pharmaceutically, some of these agents are used as diluents, enteric coatings, excipients, and filtering agents and as ingredients in products considered in other chapters. Industrially, some of these agents are used in various chemical processes, in the synthesis of other chemicals, and in the manufacture of fertilizers, explosives, etc.

ACETIC ACID

Acetic acid; a solution containing 36 to 37%, by weight, of $C_2H_4O_2$ (60.05).

Preparation—By diluting with distilled water an acid of higher concentration, such as the 80% product, or more commonly glacial acetic acid, using 350 mL of the latter for the preparation of each 1000 mL of acetic acid.

Description—Clear, colorless liquid, having a strong characteristic odor and a sharply acid taste; specific gravity about 1.045; congeals about -14°C; acid to litmus.

Solubility—Miscible with water, alcohol, or glycerin.

Uses—In pharmacy as a solvent for making diluted acetic acid. It also is used as a starting point in the manufacture of many other organic compounds, eg, acetates, acetanilid, sulfonamides, etc. It is official primarily as a pharmaceutical necessity for the preparation of Aluminum Subacetate Solution.

DILUTED ACETIC ACID

Dilute Acetic Acid

A solution containing, in each 100 mL, 5.7 to 6.3 g of $C_2H_4O_2$.

Preparation

Acetic Acid	158 mL
Purified Water, a sufficient quantity to make	1000 mL

Mix the ingredients.

Note—This acid also may be prepared by diluting 58 mL of glacial acetic acid with sufficient purified water to make 1000 mL.

Description—Essentially the same properties, solubility, purity, and identification reactions as Acetic Acid, but its specific gravity is about 1.008, and it congeals about -2°C.

Uses—Bactericidal to many types of microorganisms and occasionally is used in 1% solution for surgical dressings of the skin. A 1% solution is spermicidal. It also is used in vaginal douches for the management of Trichomonas, Candida, and Haemophilus infections.

GLACIAL ACETIC ACID

Concentrated Acetic Acid; Crystallizable Acetic Acid; Ethanolic Acid; Vinegar Acid

CH_3COOH

Glacial acetic acid [64-19-7] $C_2H_4O_2$ (60.05).

Preparation—This acid is termed glacial because of its solid, glassy appearance when congealed. In one process it is produced by distillation of weaker acids to which has been added a water-entraining substance such as ethylene dichloride. In this method, referred to as azeotropic distillation, the ethylene dichloride distills out with the water before the acid distills over, thereby effecting concentration of the latter.

In another process the aqueous acid is mixed with triethanolamine and heated. The acid combines with the triethanolamine to form a triethanolamine acetate. The water is driven off first; then, at a higher temperature, the triethanolamine compound decomposes to yield this acid.

A greater part of the acid now available is made synthetically from acetylene. When acetylene is passed into this acid containing a metallic catalyst such as mercuric oxide, ethylidene diacetate is produced, which yields, upon heating, acetic anhydride and acetaldehyde. Hydration of the former and air oxidation of the latter yields this acid.

Description—Clear, colorless liquid; pungent, characteristic odor; when well diluted with water, it has an acid taste; boils about 118°C; congeals at a temperature not lower than 15.6°C, corresponding to a minimum of 99.4% of CH_3COOH; specific gravity about 1.05.

Solubility—Miscible with water, alcohol, acetone, ether, or glycerin; insoluble in carbon tetrachloride or chloroform.

Uses—A caustic and vesicant when applied externally and is often sold under various disguises as a corn solvent. It is an excellent solvent for fixed and volatile oils and many other organic compounds. It is used primarily as an acidifying agent.

ALUMINUM

Aluminum Al (26.98); the free metal in the form of finely divided powder. It may contain oleic acid or stearic acid as a lubricant. It contains not less than 95% Al and not more than 5% Acid-insoluble substances, including any added fatty acid.

Description—Very fine, free-flowing, silvery powder free from gritty or discolored particles.

Solubility—Insoluble in water or alcohol; soluble in hydrochloric and sulfuric acids or in solutions of fixed alkali hydroxides.

Uses—A protective. An ingredient in Aluminum Paste.

ALUMINUM MONOSTEARATE

Aluminum, dihydroxy (octadecanoato-*O*-)-,

Dihydroxy (stearato) aluminum [7047-84-9]; a compound of aluminum with a mixture of solid organic acids obtained from fats, and consists chiefly of variable proportions of aluminum monostearate and aluminum monopalmitate. It contains the equivalent of 14.5 to 16.5% of Al_2O_3 (101.96).

Preparation—By interaction of a hydroalcoholic solution of potassium stearate with an aqueous solution of potassium alum, the precipitate being purified to remove free stearic acid and some aluminum distearate simultaneously produced.

Description—Fine, white to yellowish white, bulky powder; faint, characteristic odor.

Solubility—Insoluble in water, alcohol, or ether.

Uses—A pharmaceutical necessity used in the preparation of Sterile Procaine Penicillin G with Aluminum Stearate Suspension.

STRONG AMMONIA SOLUTION

Stronger Ammonia Water; Stronger Ammonium Hydroxide Solution; Spirit of Hartshorn

Ammonia [1336-21-6]; a solution of NH_3 (17.03), containing 27.0 to 31.0% (w/w) of NH_3. Upon exposure to air it loses ammonia rapidly.

Caution—Use care in handling it because of the caustic nature of the Solution and the irritating properties of its vapor. Cool the container well before opening, and cover the closure with a cloth or similar material while opening. Do not taste it, and avoid inhalation of its vapor.

Preparation—Ammonia is obtained commercially chiefly by synthesis from its constituent elements, nitrogen and hydrogen, combined under high pressure and at high temperature in the presence of a catalyst.

Description—Colorless, transparent liquid; exceedingly pungent, characteristic odor; even when well diluted it is strongly alkaline to litmus; specific gravity about 0.90.

Solubility—Miscible with alcohol.

Uses—Only for chemical and pharmaceutical purposes. It is used primarily in making ammonia water by dilution and as a chemical reagent. It is too strong for internal administration. It is an ingredient in Aromatic Ammonia Spirit.

BISMUTH SUBNITRATE

Basic Bismuth Nitrate; Bismuth Oxynitrate; Spanish White; Bismuth Paint; Bismuthyl Nitrate

Bismuth hydroxide nitrate oxide [1304-85-4] $Bi_5O(OH)_9(NO_3)_4$ (1461.99); a basic salt that, dried at 105°C for 2 hr, yields upon ignition not less than 79% of Bi_2O_3 (465.96).

Preparation—A solution of bismuth nitrate is added to boiling water to produce the subnitrate by hydrolysis.

Description—White, slightly hygroscopic powder; suspension in distilled water is faintly acid to litmus (pH about 5).

Solubility—Practically insoluble in water or organic solvents; dissolves readily in an excess of hydrochloric or nitric acid.

Incompatibilities—Slowly hydrolyzed in *water* with liberation of nitric acid; thus, it possesses the incompatibilities of the acid. Reducing agents darken it with the production of metallic bismuth.

Uses—A pharmaceutical necessity in the preparation of milk of bismuth. It also is used as an astringent, adsorbent, and protective; however, its value as a protective is questionable. This agent, like other insoluble bismuth salts, is used topically in lotions and ointments.

BORIC ACID

Boric Acid (H_3BO_3); Boracic Acid; Orthoboric Acid

Boric acid [10043-35-3] H_3BO_3 (61.83).

Preparation—Lagoons of the volcanic districts of Tuscany formerly furnished the greater part of this acid and borax of commerce. Borax is now found native in California and some of the other western states; calcium and magnesium borates are found there also. It is produced from native borax or from the other borates by reacting with hydrochloric or sulfuric acid.

Description—Colorless scales of a somewhat pearly luster, or crystals, but more commonly a white powder slightly unctuous to the touch; odorless and stable in the air; volatilizes with steam.

Solubility—1 g in 18 mL water, 18 mL alcohol, 4 mL glycerin, 4 mL boiling water, or 6 mL boiling alcohol.

Uses—A buffer, and it is this use that is recognized officially. It is a very weak germicide (local anti-infective). Its nonirritating properties make its solutions suitable for application to such delicate structures as the cornea of the eye. Aqueous solutions are employed as an eyewash, mouth wash, and for irrigation of the bladder. A 2.2% solution is isotonic with lacrimal fluid. Solutions, even if they are made isotonic, will hemolyze red blood cells. It also is employed as a dusting powder, when diluted with some inert material. It can be absorbed through irritated skin, eg, infants with diaper rash.

Although it is not absorbed significantly from intact skin, it is absorbed from damaged skin and fatal poisoning, particularly in infants, has occurred with topical application to burns, denuded areas, granulation tissue, and serous cavities. Serious poisoning can result from oral ingestion of as little as 5 g. Symptoms of poisoning are nausea, vomiting, abdominal pain, diarrhea, headache, and visual disturbance. Toxic alopecia has been reported from the chronic ingestion of a mouth wash containing it. The kidney may be injured, and death may result. Its use as a preservative in beverages and foods is prohibited by national and state legislation. There is always present the danger of confusing it with dextrose when compounding milk formulas for infants. Fatal accidents have occurred. For this reason boric acid in bulk is colored, so that it cannot be confused with dextrose.

It is used to prevent discoloration of physostigmine solutions.

CALCIUM HYDROXIDE

Slaked Lime; Calcium Hydrate

Calcium hydroxide [1305-62-0] $Ca(OH)_2$ (74.09).

Preparation—By reacting freshly prepared calcium oxide with water.

Description—White powder; alkaline, slightly bitter taste; absorbs carbon dioxide from the air, forming calcium carbonate; solutions exhibit a strong alkaline reaction.

Solubility—1 g in 630 mL water or 1300 mL boiling water; soluble in glycerin or syrup; insoluble in alcohol; the solubility in water is decreased by the presence of fixed alkali hydroxides.

Uses—In the preparation of Calcium Hydroxide Solution.

CALCIUM HYDROXIDE TOPICAL SOLUTION

Calcium Hydroxide Solution; Lime Water

A solution containing, in each 100 mL, not less than 140 mg of $Ca(OH)_2$ (74.09).

Note—The solubility of calcium hydroxide varies with the temperature at which the solution is stored, being about 170 mg/100 mL at 15°C and less at a higher temperature. The official concentration is based upon a temperature of 25°C.

Preparation

Calcium Hydroxide	3 g
Purified Water	1000 mL

Add the calcium hydroxide to 1000 mL of cool, purified water, and agitate the mixture vigorously and repeatedly during 1 hr. Allow the excess calcium hydroxide to settle. Dispense only the clear, supernatant liquid.

The undissolved portion of the mixture is not suitable for preparing additional quantities of the solution.

The object of keeping limewater over undissolved calcium hydroxide is to ensure a saturated solution.

Description—Clear, colorless liquid; alkaline taste; strong alkaline reaction; absorbs carbon dioxide from the air, a film of calcium carbonate forming on the surface of the liquid; when heated, it becomes turbid, owing to the separation of calcium hydroxide, which is less soluble in hot than in cold water.

Uses—It is too dilute to be effective as a gastric antacid. It is employed topically as a protective in various types of lotions. In some lotion formulations it is used with olive oil or oleic acid to form calcium oleate, which functions as an emulsifying agent. The USP classes it as an astringent.

CALCIUM STEARATE

Octadecanoic acid, calcium salt

Calcium stearate [1592-23-0]; a compound of calcium with a mixture of solid organic acids obtained from fats, and consists chiefly of variable proportions of stearic and palmitic acids [calcium stearate, $C_{36}H_{70}CaO_4$ = 607.03; calcium palmitate, $C_{32}H_{62}CaO_4$ = 550.92]; contains the equivalent of 9 to 10.5% of CaO (calcium oxide).

Preparation—By precipitation from interaction of solutions of calcium chloride and the sodium salts of the mixed fatty acids (stearic and palmitic).

Description—Fine, white to yellowish white, bulky powder; slight, characteristic odor; unctuous and free from grittiness.

Solubility—Insoluble in water, alcohol, or ether.

Uses—A lubricant in the manufacture of compressed tablets. It also is used as a conditioning agent in food and pharmaceutical products. Its virtually nontoxic nature and unctuous properties makes it ideal for these purposes.

CALCIUM SULFATE

Sulfuric acid, calcium salt (1:1); Gypsum; Terra Alba

Calcium sulfate (1:1) [7778-18-9] $CaSO_4$ (136.14); dihydrate [10101-41-4] (172.17).

Preparation—From natural sources or by precipitation from interaction of solutions of calcium chloride and a soluble sulfate.

Description—Fine, white to slightly yellow-white, odorless powder.

Solubility—Dissolves in diluted HCl; slightly soluble in water.

Uses—A diluent in the manufacture of compressed tablets. It is sufficiently inert that few undesirable reactions occur in tablets made with this substance. It also is used for making plaster casts and supports.

CARBON TETRACHLORIDE

Methane, tetrachloro-, Tetrachloromethane

Carbon tetrachloride [56-23-5] CCl_4 (153.82).

Preparation—One method consists of catalytic chlorination of carbon disulfide.

Description—Clear, colorless liquid; characteristic odor resembling that of chloroform; specific gravity 1.588 to 1.590; boils about 77°C.

Solubility—Soluble in about 2000 volumes water; miscible with alcohol, acetone, ether, chloroform, or benzene.

Uses—Officially recognized as a solvent. Formerly it was used as a cheap anthelmintic for the treatment of hookworm infections, but it causes severe injury to the liver if absorbed.

CARNAUBA WAX

Obtained from the leaves of *Copernicia cerifera* Mart (Fam *Palmae*).

Preparation—Consists chiefly of myricyl cerotate with smaller quantities of myricyl alcohol, ceryl alcohol, and cerotic acid. It is obtained by treating the leaf buds and leaves of *Copernicia cerifera,* the so-called Brazilian Wax Palm, with hot water.

Description—Light-brown to pale-yellow, moderately coarse powder; characteristic bland odor; free from rancidity; specific gravity about 0.99; melts about 84°C.

Solubility—Insoluble in water; freely soluble in warm benzene; soluble in warm chloroform or toluene; slightly soluble in boiling alcohol.

Uses—A pharmaceutical aid used as a polishing agent in the manufacture of coated tablets.

CELLULOSE ACETATE PHTHALATE

Cellulose, acetate, 1,2-benzenedicarboxylate

Cellulose acetate phthalate [9004-38-0]; a reaction product of the phthalic anhydride and a partial acetate ester of cellulose. When dried at 105°C for 2 hr, it contains 19 to 23.5% of acetyl (C_2H_3O) groups and 30 to 36.0% of phthalyl (o-carboxybenzoyl, $C_8H_5O_3$) groups.

Preparation—Cellulose is esterified by treatment with acetic and phthalic acid anhydrides.

Description—Free-flowing, white powder; may have a slight odor of acetic acid.

Solubility—Insoluble in water or alcohol; soluble in acetone or dioxane.

Uses—An enteric tablet-coating material. Coatings of this substance disintegrate because of the hydrolytic effect of the intestinal esterases, even when the intestinal contents are acid. *In vitro* studies indicate that cellulose acetate phthalate will withstand the action of artificial gastric juices for long periods of time but will disintegrate readily in artificial intestinal juices.

MICROCRYSTALLINE CELLULOSE

Cellulose [9004-34-6]; purified, partially depolymerized cellulose prepared by treating alpha cellulose, obtained as a pulp from fibrous plant material, with mineral acids.

Preparation—Cellulose is subjected to the hydrolytic action of 2.5 N HCl at the boiling temperature of about 105°C for 15 min, whereby amorphous cellulosic material is removed and aggregates of crystalline cellulose are formed. These are collected by filtration, washed with water and aqueous ammonia, and disintegrated into small fragments, often termed cellulose crystallites, by vigorous mechanical means such as a blender. US Pat 3,141,875.

Description—Fine, white, odorless, crystalline powder; consists of free-flowing, non-fibrous particles.

Solubility—Insoluble in water, dilute acids, or most organic solvents; slightly soluble in NaOH solution (1 in 20).

Uses A tablet diluent and disintegrant and dry binder. It can be compressed into self-binding tablets that disintegrate rapidly when placed in water.

Microcrystalline Cellulose and Sodium Carboxymethylcellulose, co-processed—A colloid-forming, attrited mixture of sub-micron microcrystalline cellulose and sodium carboxymethylcellulose. Description and Solubility: Tasteless, odorless, white to off-white, coarse to fine powder; pH (dispersion) 6 to 8; swells in water, producing, when dispersed, a white, opaque dispersion or gel. Insoluble in organic solvents or dilute acids. Uses: Pharmaceutical aid (suspending agent). Resultant viscosities vary depending upon the grade used and the type of CMC present.

POWDERED CELLULOSE—pages 1074 and 1278.

CHLOROFORM

Methane, trichloro-,

Trichloromethane [67-66-3] $CHCl_3$ (119.38); contains 99 to 99.5% $CHCl_3$, the remainder consisting of alcohol.

Caution—Care should be taken not to vaporize it in the presence of a flame, because of the production of harmful gases (hydrogen chloride and phosgene).

Preparation—Made by the reduction of carbon tetrachloride with water and iron and by the controlled chlorination of methane.

The pure compound readily decomposes on keeping, particularly if exposed to moisture and sunlight, resulting in formation of phosgene (carbonyl chloride $COCl_2$) and other products. The presence of a small amount of alcohol greatly retards or prevents this decomposition; hence, the requirement that it contain 0.5 to 1% of alcohol. The alcohol combines with any phosgene, forming ethyl carbonate, which is non-toxic.

Description—Clear, colorless, mobile liquid; characteristic, ethereal odor; burning, sweet taste; not flammable, but its heated vapors burn with a green flame; affected by light and moisture; specific gravity 1.474 to 1.478, indicating 99 to 99.5% of $CHCl_3$; boils about 61°C; not affected by acids but is decomposed by alkali hydroxide into alkali chloride and sodium formate.

Solubility—Soluble in 210 volumes of water; miscible with alcohol, ether, benzene, solvent hexane, acetone, or fixed and volatile oils.

Uses—An obsolete inhalation anesthetic. Although it possesses advantages of non-flammability and great potency, it rarely is used because of the serious toxic effects it produces on the heart and liver. Internally, it has been used, in small doses, as a carminative. Externally, it is an *irritant* and when used in liniments it may produce blisters.

It is categorized as a pharmaceutical aid. It is used as a preservative during the aqueous percolation of vegetable drugs to prevent bacterial decomposition in the process of manufacture. In most instances it is evaporated before the product is finished. It is an excellent solvent for alkaloids and many other organic chemicals and is used in the manufacture of these products and in chemical analyses.

CITRIC ACID

1,2,3-Propanetricarboxylic acid, 2-hydroxy-,

$$
\begin{array}{c}
CH_2COOH \\
| \\
HOCCOOH \\
| \\
CH_2COOH
\end{array}
$$

Citric acid [77-92-9] $C_6H_8O_7$ (192.12); *monohydrate* [5949-29-1] (210.14).

Preparation—Found in many plants. It formerly was obtained solely from the juice of limes and lemons and from pineapple wastes. Since about 1925 the acid has been produced largely by fermentation of sucrose solution, including molasses, by fungi belonging to the *Aspergillus niger* group, theoretically according to the following reaction

$$
\underset{\text{Sucrose}}{C_{12}H_{22}O_{11}} + \underset{\text{Oxygen}}{3O_2} \rightarrow \underset{\text{Citric Acid}}{2H_3C_6H_5O_7} + \underset{\text{Water}}{3H_2O}
$$

but in practice there are deviations from this stoichiometric relationship.

Description—Colorless, translucent crystals, or a white, granular to fine crystalline powder; odorless; strongly acid taste; the hydrous form effloresces in moderately dry air but is slightly deliquescent in moist air; loses its water of crystallization at about 50°C; dilute aqueous solutions are subject to molding (fermentation), oxalic acid being one of the fermentation products.

Solubility—1 g in 0.5 mL water, 2 mL alcohol, or about 30 mL ether; freely soluble in methanol.

Uses—In the preparation of Anticoagulant Citrate Dextrose Solution, Anticoagulant Citrate Phosphate Dextrose Solution, Citric Acid Syrup, and effervescent salts. It also has been used to dissolve urinary bladder calculi and as a mild astringent.

COCOA BUTTER

Cacao Butter; Theobroma Oil; Oil of Theobroma

The fat obtained from the roasted seed of *Theobroma cacao* Linné (Fam *Sterculiaceae*).

Preparation—By grinding the kernels of the *chocolate bean* and expressing the oil in powerful, horizontal hydraulic presses. The yield is about 40%. It also has been prepared by dissolving the oil from the unroasted beans by the use of a volatile solvent.

Constituents—Chemically, it is a mixture of stearin, palmitin, olein, laurin, linolein, and traces of other glycerides.

Description—Yellowish, white solid; faint, agreeable odor; bland (if obtained by extraction) or chocolate-like (if obtained by pressing) taste; usually brittle below 25°C; specific gravity 0.858 to 0.864 at 100°C/25°C; refractive index 1.454 to 1.458 at 40°C.

Solubility—Slightly soluble in alcohol; soluble in boiling dehydrated alcohol; freely soluble in ether or chloroform.

Uses—Valuable in pharmacy for making suppositories by virtue of its low fusing point and its property of becoming solid at a temperature just below the melting point. See Suppositories (page 883). In addition to this use, it is an excellent emollient application to the skin when inflamed; it also is used in various skin creams, especially the so-called skin foods. It also is used in massage.

DENATONIUM BENZOATE

Benzenemethanaminium N-2-(2,6-dimethylphenyl)amino-2-oxoethyl-N,N-diethyl-, benzoate;

Benzyldiethyl (2,6-xylylcarbamoyl)methylammonium benzoate [3734-33-6] $C_{28}H_{34}N_2O_3$ (446.59).

Preparation—2-(Diethylamino)-2',6'-xylidide is quaternized by reaction with benzyl chloride. The quaternary chloride then is treated with methanolic potassium hydroxide to form the quaternary base that, after filtering off the KCl, is reacted with benzoic acid. The starting xylidide may be prepared by condensing 2,6-xylidine with chloroacetyl chloride and condensing the resulting chloroacetoxylidide with diethylamine. US Pat. 3,080,327.

Description—White, odorless, crystalline powder; an intensely bitter taste; melts about 168°C.

Solubility—1 g in 20 mL water, 2.4 mL alcohol, 2.9 mL chloroform, or 5000 mL ether.

Uses—A denaturant for ethyl alcohol.

DEXTRIN

British Gum; Starch Gum; Leiocom

Dextrin [9004-53-9] $(C_6H_{10}O_5)_n$.

Preparation—By the incomplete hydrolysis of starch with dilute acid or by heating dry starch.

Description—White or yellow, amorphous powder (white: practically odorless; yellow: characteristic odor); dextrorotatory; $[\alpha]_D^{20}$ generally above 200°C; does not reduce Fehling's solution; gives a reddish color with iodine.

Solubility—Soluble in 3 parts of boiling water, forming a gummy solution; less soluble in cold water.

Uses—As a tablet diluent and an emulsifier in semi-solids.

DEXTROSE

Anhydrous Dextrose; Dextrose Monohydrate; Glucose; D(+)-Glucose; α-D(+)-Glucopyranose; Medicinal Glucose; Purified Glucose; Grape Sugar; Bread Sugar; Cerelose; Starch Sugar; Corn Sugar

D-Glucose monohydrate [5996-10-1] $C_6H_{12}O_6 \cdot H_2O$ (198.17); anhydrous [50-99-7] (180.16). A sugar usually obtained by the hydrolysis of starch.

Preparation—See Liquid Glucose (page 1086).

Description—Colorless crystals or a white, crystalline or granular powder; odorless; sweet taste; specific rotation (anhydrous) +52.5 to +53; anhydrous dextrose melts at 146°C; dextrose slowly reduces alkaline cupric tartrate TS in the cold and rapidly on heating, producing a red precipitate of cuprous oxide (difference from *sucrose*).

Solubility—1 g in 1 mL of water or 100 mL of alcohol; more soluble in boiling water or boiling alcohol.

Uses—See Dextrose Injection (page 1323). It also is used, instead of lactose as a supplement to milk for infant feeding.

DICHLORODIFLUOROMETHANE

Methane, dichlorodifluoro-, CCl_2F_2

Dichlorodifluoromethane [75-71-8] CCl_2F_2 (120.91).

Preparation—Carbon tetrachloride is reacted with antimony trifluoride in the presence of antimony pentafluoride.

Description—Clear, colorless gas; faint, ethereal odor; vapor pressure at 25°C about 4883 torr.

Uses—A propellant (No 12).

DICHLOROTETRAFLUOROETHANE

Ethane, 1,2-dichloro-1,1,2,2-tetrafluoro-, $CClF_2CClF_2$

1,2-Dichlorotetrafluoroethane [76-14-2] $C_2Cl_2F_4$ (170.92).

Preparation—By reacting 1,1,2-trichloro-1,2,2-trifluoroethane with antimony trifluorodichloride [SbF_3Cl_2], whereupon one of the 1-chlorine atoms is replaced by fluorine. The starting trichlorofluoroethane may be prepared from hexachloroethane by treatment with SbF_3Cl_2 (Henne AL: *Org Reactions II:* 65, 1944).

Description—Clear, colorless gas; faint, ethereal odor; vapor pressure at 25°C about 1620 torr; usually contains 6 to 10% of its isomer, $CFCl_2$-CF_3.

Uses—A propellant (No 114 and 114a).

EDETIC ACID

Glycine, N,N'-1,2-ethanediylbis[N-(carboxymethyl)], $(HOOCCH_2)_2NCH_2CH_2N(CH_2COOH)_2$

(Ethylenedinitrilo)tetraacetic acid [60-00-4] $C_{10}H_{16}N_2O_8$ (292.24).

Preparation—Ethylenediamine is condensed with sodium monochloroacetate with the aid of sodium carbonate. An aqueous solution of the reactants is heated to about 90°C for 10 hr, then cooled and acidified with HCl whereupon the acid precipitates. US Pat. 2,130,505.

Description—White, crystalline powder; melts with decomposition above 220°C.

Solubility—Very slightly soluble in water; soluble in solutions of alkali hydroxides.

Uses—A metal complexing agent. The acid, rather than any salt, is the form most potent in removing calcium from solution. It may be added to shed blood to prevent clotting. It also is used in pharmaceutical analysis and the removal or inactivation of unwanted ions in solution. Salts of the acid are known as edetates. See Edetate Calcium Disodium (page 1343) and Edetate Disodium (page 1343).

ETHYLCELLULOSE

Cellulose ethyl ether [9004-57-3]; an ethyl ether of cellulose containing 44 to 51% of ethoxy groups. The medium-type viscosity grade contains less than 46.5% ethoxy groups; the standard-type viscosity grade contains 46.5% or more ethoxy groups.

Preparation—By the same general procedure described on page ____ for Methylcellulose except that ethyl chloride or ethyl sulfate is employed as the alkylating agent. The 45 to 50% of ethoxy groups in the official ethylcellulose corresponds to from 2.25 to 2.61 ethoxy groups/$C_6H_{10}O_5$ unit, thus representing from 75 to 87% of the maximum theoretical ethoxylation, which is 3 ethoxy groups/$C_6H_{10}O_5$ unit.

Description—Free-flowing, white to light tan powder; forms films that have a refractive index of about 1.47; aqueous suspensions are neutral to litmus.

Solubility—The medium type is freely soluble in tetrahydrofuran, methyl acetate, chloroform, or mixtures of aromatic hydrocarbons with alcohol; the standard type is freely soluble in alcohol, methanol, toluene, chloroform, or ethyl acetate; both types are insoluble in water, glycerin, or propylene glycol.

Uses—A tablet binder and for film-coating tablets and drug particles.

GELATIN—page 1074.

LIQUID GLUCOSE

Glucose; Starch Syrup; Corn Syrup

A product obtained by the incomplete hydrolysis of starch. It consists chiefly of dextrose [D-(+)-glucose, $C_6H_{12}O_6$ = 180.16] dextrins, maltose, and water.

Preparation—Commercially by the action of very weak H_2SO_4 or HCl on starch.

One of the processes for its manufacture is as follows: The starch, usually from corn, is mixed with 5 times its weight of water containing less than 1% of HCl, the mixture is heated to about 45°C and then transferred to a suitable reaction vessel, into which steam is passed under pressure until the temperature reaches 120°C. The temperature is maintained at this point for about 1 hr or until tests show complete disappearance of starch. The mass is then heated to volatilize most of the hydrochloric acid, sodium carbonate or calcium carbonate is added to neutralize the remaining traces of acid, the liquid is filtered, then de-

colorized in charcoal or bone-black filters, as is done in sugar refining, and finally concentrated in vacuum to the desired consistency.

When made by the above process, it contains about 30 to 40% of dextrose mixed with about an equal proportion of dextrin, together with small amounts of other carbohydrates, notably maltose. By varying the conditions of hydrolysis, the relative proportions of the sugars also vary.

If the crystallizable dextrose is desired, the conversion temperature is higher, and the time of conversion longer. The term glucose, as customarily used in the chemical or pharmaceutical literature, usually refers to dextrose, the crystallizable product.

The name grape sugar sometimes is applied to the solid commercial form of dextrose because the principal sugar of the grape is dextrose, although the fruit has never been used as a source of the commercial supply.

Description—Colorless or yellowish, thick, syrupy liquid; odorless, or nearly so; sweet taste; differs from sucrose in that it readily reduces hot alkaline cupric tartrate TS, producing a red precipitate of cuprous oxide.

Solubility—Miscible with water; sparingly soluble in alcohol.

Uses—As an ingredient of Cocoa Syrup (page 1070), as a tablet binder and coating agent, and as a diluent in pilular extracts; it has replaced glycerin in many pharmaceutical preparations. It is sometimes given per rectum as a food in cases when feeding by stomach is impossible. It should not be used in the place of dextrose for intravenous injection.

HYDROCHLORIC ACID

Chlorhydric Acid; Muriatic Acid; Spirit of Salt

Hydrochloric acid [7647-01-0] HCl (36.46); contains 36.5 to 38.0%, by weight, of HCl.

Preparation—By the interaction of NaCl and H_2SO_4 or by combining chlorine with hydrogen. It is obtained as a by-product in the manufacture of sodium carbonate from NaCl by the Leblanc process in which common salt is decomposed with H_2SO_4. HCl is also a by-product in the electrolytic production of NaOH from NaCl.

Description—Colorless, fuming liquid; pungent odor; fumes and odor disappear when it is diluted with 2 volumes of water; strongly acid to litmus even when highly diluted; specific gravity about 1.18.

Solubility—Miscible with water or alcohol.

Uses—Officially classified as a pharmaceutical aid that is used as an acidifying agent. It is used in preparing Diluted Hydrochloric Acid.

HYPOPHOSPHOROUS ACID

Phosphoric acid

Hypophosphorous acid [6303-21-5] HPH_2O_2 (66.00); contains 30 to 32% by weight, of H_3PO_2.

Preparation—By reacting barium or calcium hypophosphite with sulfuric acid or by treating sodium hypophosphite with an ion-exchange resin.

Description—Colorless or slightly yellow, odorless liquid; solution is acid to litmus even when highly diluted; specific gravity about 1.13.

Solubility—Miscible with water or alcohol.

Incompatibilities—Oxidized on exposure to air and by nearly all oxidizing agents. Mercury, silver, and bismuth salts are reduced partially to the metallic state as evidenced by a darkening in color. Ferric compounds are changed to ferrous.

Uses—An antioxidant in pharmaceutical preparations.

ISOPROPYL MYRISTATE

Tetradecanoic acid, 1-methylethyl ester

$CH_3(CH_2)_{12}COOCH(CH_3)_2$

Isopropyl myristate [110-27-0] $C_{17}H_{34}O_2$ (270.45).

Preparation—By reacting myristoyl chloride with 2-propanol with the aid of a suitable dehydrochlorinating agent.

Description—Liquid of low viscosity; practically colorless and odorless; congeals about 5°C and decomposes at 208°C; withstands oxidation and does not become rancid readily.

Solubility—Soluble in alcohol, acetone, chloroform, ethyl acetate, toluene, mineral oil, castor oil, or cottonseed oil; practically insoluble in water, glycerin, or propylene glycol; dissolves many waxes, cholesterol, or lanolin.

Uses—Pharmaceutical aid used in cosmetics and topical medicinal preparations as an emollient, as a lubricant, and to enhance absorption through the skin.

KAOLIN—page 1313.

LACTIC ACID

Propanoic acid, 2-hydroxy-, 2-Hydroxypropionic Acid; Propanoloic Acid; Milk Acid

$CH_3CH(OH)COOH$

Lactic acid [50-21-5] $C_3H_6O_3$ (90.08); a mixture of lactic acid and lactic acid lactate ($C_6H_{10}O_5$) equivalent to a total of 85 to 90%, by weight, of $C_3H_6O_3$.

Discovered by Scheele in 1780, it is the acid formed in the souring of milk, hence the name *lactic*, from the Latin name for milk. It results from the decomposition of the lactose (milk sugar) in milk.

Preparation—A solution of glucose or of starch previously hydrolyzed with diluted sulfuric acid is inoculated, after the addition of suitable nitrogen compounds and mineral salts, with *Bacillus lactis*. Calcium carbonate is added to neutralize the lactic acid as soon as it is formed, otherwise the fermentation stops when the amount of acid exceeds 0.5%. When fermentation is complete, as indicated by failure of the liquid to give a test for glucose, the solution is filtered, concentrated, and allowed to stand. The calcium lactate that crystallizes is decomposed with dilute sulfuric acid and filtered with charcoal. The lactic acid in the filtrate is extracted with ethyl or isopropyl ether, the ether is distilled off, and the aqueous solution of the acid is concentrated under reduced pressure.

Description—Colorless or yellowish, nearly odorless, syrupy liquid; acid to litmus; absorbs water on exposure to moist air; when a dilute solution is concentrated to above 50%, lactic acid lactate begins to form; in the official acid the latter amounts to about 12 to 15%; specific gravity about 1.20; decomposes when distilled under normal pressure but may be distilled without decomposition under reduced pressure.

Solubility—Miscible with water, alcohol, or ether; insoluble in chloroform.

Uses—In the preparation of Sodium Lactate Injection (page 1341). It also is used in babies' milk formulas, as an acidulant in food preparations, and in 1 to 2% concentrations in some spermatocidal jellies. A 10% solution is used as a bactericidal agent on the skin of neonates. It is corrosive to tissues on prolonged contact. A 16.7% solution in flexible collodion is used to remove warts and small cutaneous tumors.

LACTOSE

D-Glucose, 4-*O*-β-D-galactopyranosyl-, Milk Sugar

Lactose [63-42-3] $C_{12}H_{22}O_{11}$ (342.30); monohydrate [10039-26-6] (360.31); a sugar obtained from milk.

Preparation—From skim milk, to which is added diluted HCl to precipitate the casein. After removal of the casein by filtration, the reaction of the whey is adjusted to a pH of about 6.2 by addition of lime, and heating coagulates the remaining albuminous matter; this is filtered out and the liquid set aside to crystallize. Animal charcoal is used to decolorize the solution in a manner similar to that used in purifying sucrose.

Another form of lactose, known as β-lactose, also is available on the market. It differs in that the D-glucose moiety is β instead of α. It is reported that this variety is sweeter and more soluble than ordinary lactose and for that reason is preferable in pharmaceutical manufacturing where lactose is used. Chemically, β-lactose does not appear to differ from ordinary α-lactose. It is manufactured in the same way as α-lactose up to the point of crystallization, then the solution is heated to a temperature above 93.5°C, the temperature at which the α form is converted to the β variety. The β form occurs only as an anhydrous sugar, whereas the α variety may be obtained either in the anhydrous form or as a monohydrate.

Description—White or creamy white, hard, crystalline masses or powder; odorless; faintly sweet taste; stable in air, but readily absorbs odors; pH (1 in 10 solution) 4 to 6.5; specific rotation +54.8 to +55.5.

Solubility—1 g in 5 mL water or 2.6 mL boiling water; very slightly soluble in alcohol; insoluble in chloroform or ether.

Uses—A diluent in tablet formulation. The amorphous and monohydrate forms are used in wet granulation processing of materials, whereas the spray-dried anhydrous type is usually used in direct compression formulations. It is generally an ingredient of the medium used in penicillin production. It is used extensively as an addition to milk for infant feeding.

MAGNESIUM CHLORIDE

Magnesium chloride hexahydrate [7791-18-6] $MgCl_2 \cdot 6H_2O$ (203.30); anhydrous [7786-30-3] (95.21).

Preparation—By treating magnesite or other suitable magnesium minerals with HCl.

Description—Colorless, odorless, deliquescent flakes or crystals, which lose water when heated to 100°C and lose HCl when heated to 110°C; pH (1 in 20 solution in carbon dioxide-free water) 4.5 to 7.

Solubility—Very soluble in water; freely soluble in alcohol.

Uses—Electrolyte replenisher; pharmaceutical necessity for hemodialysis and peritoneal dialysis fluids.

MAGNESIUM STEARATE

Octadecanoic acid, magnesium salt

Magnesium stearate [557-04-0]. A compound of magnesium with a mixture of solid organic acids obtained from fats, which consists chiefly of variable proportions of magnesium stearate and magnesium palmitate. It contains the equivalent of 6.8 to 8.0% MgO (40.30).

Description—Fine, white, bulky powder; faint, characteristic odor; unctuous, adheres readily to the skin and free from grittiness.

Solubility—Insoluble in water, alcohol, or ether.

Uses—A lubricant in the manufacture of compressed tablets.

MEGLUMINE

D-Glucitol, 1-deoxy-1-(methylamino)-,

$$HOCH_2-\underset{\underset{OH}{|}}{\overset{\overset{H}{|}}{C}}-\underset{\underset{OH}{|}}{\overset{\overset{H}{|}}{C}}-\underset{\underset{H}{|}}{\overset{\overset{OH}{|}}{C}}-\underset{\underset{OH}{|}}{\overset{\overset{H}{|}}{C}}-CH_2NHCH_3$$

1-Deoxy-1-(methylamino)-D-glucitol [6284-40-8] $C_7H_{17}NO_5$ (195.21).

Preparation—By treating glucose with hydrogen and methylamine under pressure and in the presence of Raney nickel.

Description—White to faintly yellowish white, odorless crystals or powder; melts about 130°C.

Solubility—Freely soluble in water; sparingly soluble in alcohol.

Uses—In forming salts of certain pharmaceuticals, surface-active agents and dyes. See Diatrizoate Meglumine Injections (page 1263), Iodipamide Meglumine Injection (page 1264) and Iothalamate Meglumine Injection (page 1266).

LIGHT MINERAL OIL

Light Liquid Petrolatum NF XII; Light Liquid Paraffin; Light White Mineral Oil

A mixture of liquid hydrocarbons obtained from petroleum. It may contain a suitable stabilizer.

Description—Colorless, transparent, oily liquid, free, or nearly free, from fluorescence; odorless and tasteless when cold, and develops not more than a faint odor of petroleum when heated; specific gravity 0.818 to 0.880; kinematic viscosity not more than 33.5 centistokes at 40°C.

Solubility—Insoluble in water or alcohol; miscible with most fixed oils, but not with castor oil; soluble in volatile oils.

Uses—Officially recognized as a vehicle. Once it was used widely as a vehicle for nose and throat medications; such uses are now considered dangerous because of the possibility of lipoid pneumonia. It sometimes is used to cleanse dry and inflamed skin areas and to facilitate removal of dermatological preparations from the skin. It should never be used for internal administration because of leakage. See Mineral Oil (page 1308).

NITRIC ACID

Nitric acid [7697-37-2] HNO_3 (63.01); contains about 70%, by weight, of HNO_3.

Preparation—May be prepared by treatment of sodium nitrate (Chile saltpeter) with sulfuric acid, but usually produced by catalytic oxidation of ammonia.

Description—Highly corrosive fuming liquid; characteristic, highly irritating odor; stains animal tissues yellow; boils about 120°C; specific gravity about 1.41.

Solubility—Miscible with water.

Uses—Acidifying agent

NITROGEN

Nitrogen [7727-37-9] N_2 (28.01); contains not less than 99%, by volume, of N_2.

Preparation—By the fractional distillation of liquefied air.

Uses—A diluent for medicinal gases. Pharmaceutically, is employed to replace air in the containers of substances that would be affected adversely by air oxidation. Examples include its use with fixed oils, certain vitamin preparations, and a variety of injectable products. It also is used as a propellant.

PHENOL

Carbolic Acid

C_6H_5OH

Phenol [108-95-2] C_6H_6O (94.11).

Preparation—For many years made only by distilling crude carbolic acid from coal tar and separating and purifying the distillate by repeated crystallizations; it now is prepared synthetically.

One process uses chlorobenzene as the starting point in the manufacture. The chlorobenzene is produced in a vapor phase reaction, with benzene, HCl, and oxygen over a copper catalyst, followed by hydrolysis with steam to yield HCl and phenol (which is recovered).

Description—Colorless to light pink, interlaced, or separate, needle-shaped crystals, or a white or light pink, crystalline mass; characteristic odor; when undiluted, it whitens and cauterizes the skin and mucous membranes; when gently heated, phenol melts, forming a highly refractive liquid; liquefied by the addition of 10% of water; vapor is flammable; gradually darkens on exposure to light and air; specific gravity 1.07; boils at 182°C; congeals not lower than 39°C.

Solubility—1 g in 15 mL water; very soluble in alcohol, glycerin, chloroform, ether, or fixed and volatile oils; sparingly soluble in mineral oil.

Incompatibilities—Produces a liquid or soft mass when triturated with camphor, menthol, acetanilid, acetophenetidin, aminopyrine, antipyrine, ethyl aminobenzoate, methenamine, phenyl salicylate, resorcinol, terpin hydrate, thymol, and several other substances including some alkaloids. It also softens cocoa butter in suppository mixtures.

It is soluble in about 15 parts of water; stronger solutions may be obtained by using as much glycerin as phenol. Only the crystallized form is soluble in fixed oils and liquid petroleum, the liquefied form is not all soluble because of its content of water. Albumin and gelatin are precipitated by it. Collodion is coagulated by the precipitation of pyroxylin. Traces of iron in various chemicals such as alum, borax, etc, may produce a green color.

Uses—A caustic, disinfectant, topical anesthetic, and pharmaceutical necessity as a preservative for injections, etc. At one time widely used as a germicide and still the standard against which other antiseptics are compared, it has few legitimate uses in modern medicine. Nevertheless, it is still used in several proprietary antiseptic mouthwashes, hemorrhoidal preparations, and burn remedies. In full strength, a few drops of the liquefied form may be used to cauterize small wounds, dog bites, snake bites, etc. It commonly is employed as an antipruritic, in the form of phenolated calamine lotion (1%), phenol ointment (2%), or a simple aqueous solution (0.5 to 1%). It has been used for sclerosing hemorrhoids, but more effective and safer drugs are available. A 5% solution in glycerin is used in simple earache. Crude carbolic acid is an effective, economical agent for disinfecting excrement. It is of some therapeutic value as a fungicide, but more effective and less toxic agents are available. If accidentally spilled, it should be removed promptly from the skin by swabbing with alcohol.

Liquefied Phenol [Liquefied Carbolic Acid]—Phenol maintained in a liquid condition by the presence of 10.0% of water. It contains not less than 89.0%, by weight, of C_6H_6O. Note—When it is to be mixed with a fixed oil, mineral oil, or white petrolatum, use the crystalline Phenol, not Liquefied Phenol. Preparation: Melt phenol (a convenient quantity) by placing the unstoppered container in a steam bath and applying heat gradually. Transfer the liquid to a tared vessel, weigh, add 1 g of purified water for each 9 g of phenol, and mix thoroughly. Description: Colorless liquid, which may develop a red tint upon exposure to air and light; characteristic, somewhat aromatic odor; when undiluted it cauterizes and whitens the skin and mucous membranes; specific gravity about 1.065; when it is subjected to distillation, the boiling temperature does not rise above 182°C, which is the boiling temperature of phenol; partially solidifies at about 15°C. Solubility: Miscible with alcohol, ether, or glycerin; a mixture of liquefied phenol and an equal volume of glycerin is miscible with water. Uses: Its therapeutic uses are described above under Phenol. It is a pharmaceutical necessity for Phenolated Calamine Lotion (see RPS-18 page 762).

PHOSPHORIC ACID

Orthophosphoric Acid; Syrupy Phosphoric Acid; Concentrated Phosphoric Acid

Phosphoric acid [7664-38-2] H_3PO_4 (98.00); contains 85 to 88%, by weight, of H_3PO_4.

Preparation—Phosphorus is converted to phosphorus pentoxide P_2O_5 by exposing it to a current of warm air, then the P_2O_5 is treated with water to form phosphoric acid. The conversion of the phosphorus to the pentoxide takes place while the phosphorus, distilling from the phosphorus manufacturing operation, is in the vapor state.

Description—Colorless, odorless liquid of a syrupy consistency; specific gravity about 1.71.

Solubility—Miscible with water or alcohol, with the evolution of heat.

Uses—To make the diluted acid and as a weak acid in various pharmaceutical preparations. Industrially, it is used in dental cements and in beverages as an acidulant.

Diluted Phosphoric Acid [Dilute Phosphoric Acid]—Contains, in each 100 mL, 9.5 to 10.5 g of H_3PO_4 (98.00). Preparation: Mix phosphoric acid (69 mL) and purified water (qs) to make 1000 mL. Description and Solubility: Clear, colorless, odorless liquid; specific

gravity about 1.057. Miscible with water or alcohol. Uses: A pharmaceutical necessity. It also has been employed in lead poisoning and in other conditions in which it is desired to administer large amounts of phosphate and at the same time produce a mild acidosis. It has been given in the dosage of 60 mL a day (5 mL/hr) under carefully controlled conditions.

POTASSIUM METAPHOSPHATE

Metaphosphoric acid (HPO₃), potassium salt

Potassium metaphosphate [7790-53-6] KPO_3 (118.07); a straight-chain polyphosphate, having a high degree of polymerization; contains the equivalent of 59 to 61% P_2O_5.

Preparation—By thermal dehydration of monopotassium phosphate (KH_2PO_4).

Description—White, odorless powder.

Solubility—Insoluble in water; soluble in dilute solutions of sodium salts.

Uses—Buffering agent

MONOBASIC POTASSIUM PHOSPHATE

For the full monograph, see page 1340.

Comments—A component of various buffer solutions. Medicinally, it has been used as a urinary acidifier.

PUMICE

Pumex

A substance of volcanic origin, consisting chiefly of complex silicates of aluminum, potassium, and sodium.

Description—Very light, hard, rough, porous, grayish masses or a gritty, grayish powder of several grades of fineness; odorless, tasteless, and stable in the air.

Three powders are available:

Pumice Flour or Superfine Pumice—Not less than 97% passes through a No 200 standard mesh sieve.

Fine Pumice—Not less than 95% passes through a Number 150 standard mesh sieve, and not more than 75% passes through a Number 200 standard mesh sieve.

Coarse Pumice—Not less than 95% passes through a No 60 standard mesh sieve, and not more than 5% passes through a No 200 standard mesh sieve.

Solubility—Insoluble in water and is not attacked by acids or alkali hydroxide solutions.

Uses—A filtering and distributing medium for pharmaceutical preparations. Because of its grittiness the powdered form is used in certain types of soaps and cleaning powders and also as a dental abrasive.

PYROXYLIN

Cellulose, nitrate; Soluble Guncotton

Pyroxylin [9004-70-0]; a product obtained by the action of a mixture of nitric and sulfuric acids on cotton, which consists chiefly of cellulose tetranitrate ($C_{12}H_{16}N_4O_{18}$)ₙ.

Note—The commercially available form is moistened with about 30% of alcohol or other suitable solvent. The alcohol or solvent must be allowed to evaporate to yield the dried substance described in the *USP*.

Preparation—Shönbein, in 1846, found that nitric acid acts on cotton and produces a soluble compound. It subsequently was proved that this substance belongs to a series of closely related nitrates in which the nitric acid radical replaces the hydroxyl of the cellulose formula. Taking the double empirical formula for cellulose C12H20O10 and indicating replacement of four of the OH groups thus usually indicates this

$$C_{12}H_{20}O_{10} + 4HNO_3 \rightarrow C_{12}H_{16}O_6(NO_3)_4 + 4H_2O$$
Cellulose   **Cellulose**
                           Tetranitrate

The compound used in preparing collodion is a varying mixture of the di-, tri-, tetra-, and pentanitrates, but is mainly tetranitrate. The hexanitrate is the true explosive guncotton and is insoluble in ether, alcohol, acetone, or water.

Description—Light yellow, matted mass of filaments, resembling raw cotton in appearance but harsh to the touch; exceedingly flammable, burning, when unconfined, very rapidly and with a luminous flame; when kept in well-closed bottles and exposed to light, it is decomposed with the evolution of nitrous vapors, leaving a carbonaceous residue.

Solubility—Insoluble in water; dissolves slowly but completely in 25 parts of a mixture of 3 volumes of ether and 1 volume of alcohol; soluble in acetone or glacial acetic acid and precipitated from these solutions by water.

Uses—A pharmaceutical necessity for collodion.

ROSIN

Resina; Colophony; Georgia Pine Rosin; Yellow Pine Rosin

A solid resin obtained from *Pinus palustris* Miller and from other species of *Pinus* Linné (Fam *Pinaceae*).

Constituents—American rosin contains sylvic acid $[C_{20}H_{30}O_2]$, α-, β-, and γ-abietic acids $[C_{20}H_{30}O_2]$, γ-pinic acid (from which α- and β-pinic acids are gradually formed), and resene. Some authorities also include pimaric acid $[C_{30}H_{20}O_2]$ as a constituent. French rosin is called galipot.

Description—Sharply angular, translucent, amber-colored fragments, frequently covered with yellow dust; fracture brittle at ordinary temperatures, shiny and shallow conchoidal; odor and taste are slightly terebinthinate; easily fusible and burns with a dense, yellowish smoke, specific gravity 1.07 to 1.09

Solubility—Insoluble in water; soluble in alcohol, ether, benzene, glacial acetic acid, chloroform, carbon disulfide, dilute solutions of sodium hydroxide and potassium hydroxide, or some volatile and fixed oils.

Uses—A pharmaceutical necessity for Zinc-Eugenol Cement. Formerly, and to some extent still, used as a component of plasters, cerates, and ointments, to which it adds adhesive qualities.

PURIFIED SILICEOUS EARTH

Purified Kieselguhr; Purified Infusorial Earth; Diatomaceous Earth; Diatomite

A form of silica $[SiO_2]$ [7631-86-9] consisting of the frustules and fragments of diatoms, purified by boiling with acid, washing, and calcining.

Occurrence and Preparation—Large deposits of this substance are found in Virginia, Maryland, Nevada, Oregon, and California, usually in the form of masses of rocks, hundreds of feet in thickness. Under the microscope it is seen to consist largely of the minute siliceous frustules of diatoms. It must be purified carefully in a manner similar to that directed for Talc (page 1091) and thoroughly calcined. The latter treatment destroys the bacteria that are present in large quantities in the native earth.

Description—Very fine, white, light-gray or pale-buff mixture of amorphous powder and lesser amounts of crystalline polymorphs, including quartz and cristobalite; gritty, readily absorbs moisture and retains about four times its weight of water without becoming fluid.

Solubility—Insoluble in water, acids, or dilute solutions of alkali hydroxides.

Uses—Introduced into the USP as a distributing and filtering medium for aromatic waters; also suitable for filtration of elixirs. Like talc, it does not absorb active constituents.

COLLOIDAL SILICON DIOXIDE

Silica [7631-86-9] SiO_2 (60.08); a submicroscopic fumed silica prepared by the vapor-phase hydrolysis of a silicon compound.

Description—Light, white, non-gritty powder of extremely fine particle size (about 15 nm).

Solubility—Insoluble in water or acids (except hydrofluoric); dissolved by hot solutions of alkali hydroxides.

Uses—A tablet moisture scavenger or glidant and as a suspending and thickening agent in non-solid preparations (coatings, semi-solids, liquids).

SODA LIME

A mixture of calcium hydroxide and sodium or potassium hydroxide or both.

It may contain an indicator that is inert toward anesthetic gases such as ether, cyclopropane, and nitrous oxide and that changes color when the soda lime no longer can absorb carbon dioxide.

Description—White or grayish white granules; if an indicator is added, it may have a color; absorbs carbon dioxide and water on exposure to air.

Uses—Neither a therapeutic nor a pharmaceutical agent. It is a reagent for the absorption of carbon dioxide in anesthesia machines, oxygen therapy, and metabolic tests. Because of the importance of the proper quality for these purposes it has been made official and standardized.

SODIUM BORATE

Sodium Tetraborate; Sodium Pyroborate; Sodium Biborate

Borax [1303-96-4] $Na_2B_4O_7 \cdot 10H_2O$ (381.37); anhydrous [1330-43-4] $Na_2B_4O_7$ (201.22).

Preparation—Found in immense quantities in California as a crystalline deposit. The earth, which is strongly impregnated with borax, is lixiviated (leached); the solution is evaporated and crystallized.

Calcium borate, or "cotton balls" also occurs in the borax deposits of California, and sodium borate is obtained from it by double decomposition with sodium carbonate.

Description—Colorless, transparent crystals, or a white, crystalline powder; odorless; the crystals often are coated with white powder because of efflorescence; solution alkaline to litmus and phenolphthalein; pH about 9.5.

Solubility—1 g in 16 mL water, 1 mL glycerin, or 1 mL boiling water; insoluble in alcohol.

Incompatibilities—Precipitates many metals as insoluble borates. In aqueous solution it is alkaline and precipitates aluminum salts as aluminum hydroxide, iron salts as a basic borate, and ferric hydroxide and zinc sulfate as zinc borate and a basic salt. Alkaloids are precipitated from solutions of their salts. Approximately equal weights of glycerin and boric acid react to produce a decidedly acid derivative generally called glyceroboric acid. Thus, the addition of glycerin to a mixture containing it overcomes incompatibilities arising from an alkaline reaction.

Uses—As a pharmaceutical necessity, it is used as an alkalizing agent and as a buffer for alkaline solutions. Its alkalizing properties provide the basis for its use in denture adhesives and its buffering action for its use in eyewash formulations.

SODIUM CARBONATE

Carbonic acid, disodium salt, monohydrate; Monohydrated Sodium Carbonate USP

Disodium carbonate monohydrate [5968-11-6] $Na_2CO_3 \cdot H_2O$ (124.00); anhydrous [497-19-8] (105.99).

Preparation—The initial process for its manufacture was devised by Leblanc, a French apothecary, in 1784, and consists of two steps: first, the conversion of common salt [NaCl] into sodium sulfate by heating it with sulfuric acid and, second, the decomposition of the sulfate by calcium carbonate (limestone) and charcoal (coal) at a high temperature to yield this salt and calcium sulfide. The carbonate then is leached out with water.

It currently is prepared by the electrolysis of sodium chloride, whereby sodium and chlorine are produced, the former reacting with water to produce sodium hydroxide and this solution treated with carbon dioxide to produce the salt. The process is used most extensively in localities where electric power is very cheap.

The monohydrated form is made by crystallizing a concentrated solution of this salt at a temperature above 35°C (95°F) and stirring the liquid so as to produce small crystals. It contains about 15% water of crystallization.

Soda ash is a term designating a commercial quality of the anhydrous salt. Its annual production is very large, and it has a wide variety of applications, among which are the manufacture of glass, soap, and sodium salts; it also is used for washing fabrics.

Description—Colorless crystals or a white, crystalline powder; stable in air under ordinary conditions; when exposed to dry air above 50°C it effloresces, and at 100°C it becomes anhydrous; decomposed by weak acids, forming the salt of the acid and liberating carbon dioxide; aqueous solution alkaline to indicators (pH about 11.5).

Solubility—1 g in 3 mL water or 1.8 mL boiling water; insoluble in alcohol.

Incompatibilities—Acids, acid salts, and acidic preparations cause its decomposition. Most metals are precipitated as carbonates, hydroxides, or basic salts. Alkaloids are precipitated from solutions of their salts.

Uses—Occasionally, for dermatitides topically as a lotion; it has been used as a mouthwash and a vaginal douche. It is used in the preparation of the sodium salts of many acids. The *USP* recognizes it as a pharmaceutical aid used as an alkalizing agent.

SODIUM HYDROXIDE

Caustic Soda; Soda Lye

Sodium hydroxide [1310-73-2] NaOH (40.00); includes not more than 3% Na_2CO_3 (105.99).

Caution—Exercise great care in handling it, as it rapidly destroys tissues—

Preparation—By treating sodium carbonate with milk of lime or by the electrolysis of a solution of sodium chloride as explained under Potassium Hydroxide (page 1287). It now is produced largely by the latter process. See also Sodium Carbonate, above.

Description—White, or nearly white, fused masses, small pellets, flakes, sticks, and other forms; hard and brittle and shows a crystalline fracture; exposed to the air, it rapidly absorbs carbon dioxide and moisture; melts at about 318°C; specific gravity 2.13; when dissolved in water or alcohol or when its solution is treated with an acid, much heat is generated; aqueous solutions, even when highly diluted, are strongly alkaline.

Solubility—1 g in 1 mL water; freely soluble in alcohol or glycerin.

Incompatibilities—Exposed to air, it absorbs carbon dioxide and is converted to sodium carbonate. With fats and fatty acids it forms soluble soaps; with resins it forms insoluble soaps. See Potassium Hydroxide (page 1287).

Uses—Too alkaline to be of medicinal value but occasionally used in veterinary practice as a caustic. It is used extensively in pharmaceutical processes as an alkalizing agent and is generally preferred to potassium hydroxide because it is less deliquescent and less expensive; in addition, less of it is required, since 40 parts of it are equivalent to 56 parts of KOH. It is a pharmaceutical necessity in the preparation of Glycerin Suppositories.

SODIUM STEARATE

Octadecanoic acid, sodium salt

Sodium stearate [822-16-2] $C_{18}H_{35}NaO_2$ (306.47) consists chiefly of sodium stearate and sodium palmitate $C_{16}H_{31}NaO_2 = 278.41$).

Preparation—Stearic acid is reacted with an equimolar portion of NaOH.

Description—Fine, white powder, soapy to the touch; usually has a slight, tallow-like odor; affected by light; solutions are alkaline to phenolphthalein TS.

Solubility—Slowly soluble in cold water or cold alcohol; readily soluble in hot water or hot alcohol.

Uses—Officially, a pharmaceutical aid used as an emulsifying and stiffening agent. It is an ingredient of glycerin suppositories. In dermatological practice it has been used topically in sycosis and other skin diseases.

STARCH

Corn Starch; Wheat Starch; Potato Starch

Starch [9005-25-8] consists of the granules separated from the mature grain of corn *Zea mays* Linné (Fam *Gramineae*) or of wheat *Triticum aestivum* Linné (Fam *Gramineae*) or from tubers of the potato *Solanum tuberosum* Linné (Fam *Solanaceae*).

Preparation—In making starch from corn, the germ is separated mechanically, and the cells softened to permit escape of the starch granules. Permitting it to become sour and decomposed generally does this, stopping the fermentation before the starch is affected. On the small scale, making a stiff ball of dough and kneading it while a small stream of water trickles upon it may make it from wheat flour. It is carried off with the water, while the gluten remains as a soft, elastic mass; the latter may be purified and used for various purposes to which gluten is applicable. Commercially, its quality largely depends on the purity of the water used in its manufacture. It may be made from potatoes by first grating them, and then washing the soft mass upon a sieve, which separates the cellular substances and permits the starch granules to be carried through. It then must be washed thoroughly by decantation, and the quality of this starch also depends largely on the purity of the water that is used in washing it.

Description—Irregular, angular, white masses or fine powder; odorless; slight, characteristic taste. Corn starch: Polygonal, rounded, or spheroidal granules up to about 35 μm in diameter, which usually have a circular or several-rayed central cleft. Wheat starch: Simple lenticular granules 20 to 50 μm in diameter and spherical granules 5 to 10 μm in diameter, striations faintly marked and concentric. Potato starch: Simple granules, irregularly ovoid or spherical, 30 to 100 μm in diameter, and small spherical granules 10 to 35 μm in diameter; striations well marked and concentric.

Solubility—Insoluble in cold water or alcohol; when it is boiled with about 20 times its weight of hot water for a few minutes and then cooled, a translucent, whitish jelly results; aqueous suspension neutral to litmus.

Uses—Has absorbent and demulcent properties. It is used as a dusting powder and in various dermatological preparations; also as a pharmaceutical aid (filler, binder, and disintegrant). Note—Starches obtained from different botanical sources may not have identical properties with respect to their use for specific pharmaceutical purposes, eg, as a tablet-disintegrating agent. Therefore, types should not be interchanged unless performance equivalency has been ascertained.

Under the title Pregelatinized Starch, the NF recognizes starch that has been processed chemically or mechanically to rupture all or part of the granules in the presence of water and subsequently dried. Some types may be modified to render them compressible and flowable.

STORAX

Liquid Storax; Styrax; Sweet Gum; Prepared Storax

A balsam obtained from the trunk of *Liquidambar orientalis* Miller, known in commerce as Levant Storax, or of *Liquidambar styraciflua* Linné, known in commerce as American Storax (Fam *Hamamelidaceae*).

Constituents—The following occur in both varieties: styracin (cinnamyl cinnamate), styrol (phenylethylene, C_8H_8), α- and β-storesin (the cinnamic acid ester of an alcohol called storesinol), phenylpropyl cinnamate, free cinnamic acid, and vanillin. In addition to these, Levant storax contains ethyl cinnamate, benzyl cinnamate, free storesinol, isocinnamic acid, ethylvanillin, styrogenin, and styrocamphene. This variety yields from 0.5 to 1% of volatile oil; from this have been isolated styrocamphene, vanillin, the cinnamic acid esters of ethyl, phenylpropyl, benzyl, and cinnamyl alcohols, naphthalene, and styrol.

The American variety contains, in addition to the aforementioned substances common to both varieties, styaresin (the cinnamic acid ester of the alcohol styresinol, an isomer of storesinol) and styresinolic acid. It yields up to 7% of a dextrorotatory volatile oil, the composition of which has not been investigated completely; styrol and traces of vanillin have been isolated from it.

Description—Semi-liquid, grayish to grayish brown, sticky, opaque mass, depositing on standing a heavy dark brown layer (Levant storax); or a semisolid, sometimes a solid mass, softened by gently warming (American storax); transparent in thin layers; characteristic odor and taste; more dense than water.

Solubility—Insoluble in water, but soluble, usually incompletely, in an equal weight of warm alcohol; soluble in acetone, carbon disulfide, or ether, some insoluble residue usually remaining.

Uses—An expectorant but is used chiefly as a local remedy, especially in combination with benzoin; eg, it is an ingredient of Compound Benzoin Tincture. It may be used, like benzoin, to protect fatty substances from rancidity.

SUCROSE OCTAACETATE

α-D-Glucopyranoside, 1,3,4,6-tetra-O-acetyl-β-D-fructofuranosyl-, tetraacetate

Sucrose octaacetate [126-14-7] $C_{28}H_{38}O_{19}$ (678.60).

Preparation—Sucrose is subjected to exhaustive acetylation by reaction with acetic anhydride in the presence of a suitable condensing agent such as pyridine.

Description—White, practically odorless powder; intensely bitter taste; hygroscopic; melts not lower than 78°C.

Solubility—1 g in 1100 mL water, 11 mL alcohol, 0.3 mL acetone, or 0.6 mL benzene; very soluble in methanol or chloroform; soluble in ether.

Uses—A denaturant for alcohol.

SULFURATED POTASH

Thiosulfuric acid, dipotassium salt, mixed with potassium sulfide ($K_2(S_x)$); Liver of Sulfur

Dipotassium thiosulfate mixture with potassium sulfide (K_2S_x) [39365-88-3]; a mixture composed chiefly of potassium polysulfides and potassium thiosulfate. It contains not less than 12.8% S (sulfur) in combination as sulfide.

Preparation—By thoroughly mixing 1 part of sublimed sulfur with 2 parts of potassium carbonate and gradually heating the mixture in a covered iron crucible until the mass ceases to swell and is melted completely. It then is poured on a stone or glass slab and, when cold, is broken into pieces and preserved in tightly closed bottles. When the heat is regulated properly during its production, the reaction is represented approximately by

$$3K_2CO_3 + 8S = 2K_2S_3 + K_2S_2O_3 + 3CO_2$$

As this product rapidly deteriorates on exposure to moisture, oxygen, and carbon dioxide, it is important that it be prepared recently to produce satisfactory preparations.

Description—Irregular pieces, liver-brown when freshly prepared, changing to a greenish yellow; decomposes upon exposure to air; an odor of hydrogen sulfide and a bitter, acrid, alkaline taste; even weak acids cause the liberation of H_2S from sulfurated potash; 1 in 10 solution light brown in color and alkaline to litmus.

Solubility—1 g in about 2 mL water, usually leaving a slight residue; alcohol dissolves only the sulfides.

Uses—Extensively in dermatological practice, especially in the official White Lotion or *Lotio Alba* (page 1283). It is used as an opacifier.

The equation for the reaction of the potassium trisulfide in preparing the lotion is

$$ZnSO_4 + K_2S_3 \equiv ZnS + 2S + K_2SO_4$$

TALC

Talcum; Purified Talc; French Chalk; Soapstone; Steatite

A native, hydrous magnesium silicate, sometimes containing a small proportion of aluminum silicate.

Occurrence and Preparation—The native form, called soapstone or French chalk, is found in various parts of the world. An excellent quality is obtained from deposits in North Carolina. Deposits of a high grade, conforming to the USP requirements, also are found in Manchuria. The native form usually is accompanied by variable amounts of mineral substances. These are separated from it by mechanical means, such as flotation or elutriation. It then is powdered finely, treated with boiling dilute HCl, washed well, and dried.

Description—Very fine, white, or grayish white crystalline powder, unctuous to the touch, adhering readily to the skin, and free from grittiness.

Uses—Officially, as a dusting powder and pharmaceutical aid; in both categories it has many specific uses. Its medicinal use as a dusting powder depends on its desiccant and lubricant effects. When perfumed, and sometimes medicated, it is used extensively for toilet purposes under the name talcum powder; for such use it should be in the form of an impalpable powder. When used as a filtration medium for clarifying liquids, a coarser powder is preferred to minimize passage through the pores of the filter paper; for this purpose it may be used for all classes of preparations with no danger of adsorption or retention of active principles. It is used as a lubricant in the manufacture of tablets and as a dusting powder when making handmade suppositories. Although it is used as a lubricant for putting on and removing rubber gloves, it should not be used on surgical gloves because even small amounts deposited in organs or healing wounds may cause granuloma formation.

TARTARIC ACID

Butanedioic acid, R-(R*,R*) 2,3-dihydroxy-,

```
        COOH
         |
   H —— C —— OH
         |
  HO —— C —— H
         |
        COOH
```

L-(+)-Tartaric acid [87-69-4] $C_4H_6O_6$ (150.09).

Preparation—From argol, the crude cream of tartar (potassium bitartrate) deposited on the sides of wine casks during the fermentation of grapes, by conversion to calcium tartrate, which is hydrolyzed to tartaric acid and calcium sulfate.

Description—Large, colorless or translucent crystals, or a white granular to fine crystalline powder; odorless; acid taste; stable in the air; solutions acid to litmus; dextrorotatory.

Solubility—1 g in 0.8 mL water, 0.5 mL boiling water, 3 mL alcohol, or 250 mL ether; freely soluble in methanol.

Uses—Chiefly, as the acid ingredient of preparations in which it is neutralized by bicarbonate, as in effervescent salts and the free acid is completely absent or present only in small amounts in the finished product. It also is used as a buffering agent.

TITANIUM DIOXIDE—page 1293.

TRICHLOROMONOFLUOROMETHANE

Methane, trichlorofluoro-, CFCl₃

Trichlorofluoromethane [75-69-4] CCl_3F (137.37).

Preparation—Carbon tetrachloride is reacted with antimony trifluoride in the presence of a small quantity of antimony pentachloride. The reaction produces a mixture of CCl_3F and CCl_2F_2, which readily is separable by fractional distillation.

Description—Clear, colorless gas; faint, ethereal odor; vapor pressure at 25°C is about 796 torr; boils about 24°C.

Solubility—Practically insoluble in water; soluble in alcohol, ether, or other organic solvents.

Uses—A propellant.

TYLOXAPOL

Phenol, 4-(1,1,3,3-tetramethylbutyl)-, polymer with formaldehyde and oxirane

[R is $CH_2CH_2O(CH_2CH_2O)_mCH_2CH_2OH$; m is 6 to 8; n is not more than 5]

p-(1,1,3,3-Tetramethylbutyl)phenol polymer with ethylene oxide and formaldehyde [25301-02-4].

Preparation—p-(1,1,3,3-Tetramethylbutyl)phenol and formaldehyde are condensed by heating in the presence of an acidic catalyst, and the polymeric phenol thus obtained is reacted with ethylene oxide at elevated temperature under pressure in the presence of NaOH. US Pat. 2,454,541.

Description—Amber, viscous liquid; may show a slight turbidity; slight aromatic odor; specific gravity about 1.072; stable at sterilization temperature and in the presence of acids, bases, and salts; oxidized by metals; pH (5% aqueous solution) 4 to 7.

Solubility—Slowly but freely soluble in water; soluble in many organic solvents, including acetic acid, benzene, carbon tetrachloride, carbon disulfide, chloroform, or toluene.

Uses—A nonionic detergent that depresses both surface tension and interfacial tension. It also is used in contact-lens-cleaner formulations.

ISO-ALCOHOLIC ELIXIR

Iso-Elixir

Low-Alcoholic Elixir
High-Alcoholic Elixir of each a calculated volume
Mix the ingredients.

LOW-ALCOHOLIC ELIXIR

Compound Orange Spirit	10 mL
Alcohol	100 mL
Glycerin	200 mL
Sucrose	320 g
Purified Water qs	1000 mL
Alcohol Content—8 to 10%.	

HIGH-ALCOHOLIC ELIXIR

Compound Orange Spirit	4 mL
Saccharin	3 g
Glycerin	200 mL
Alcohol, a sufficient quantity, to make	1000 mL
Alcohol Content—73 to 78%.	

Uses Intended as a general vehicle for various medicaments that require solvents of different alcoholic strengths. When it is specified in a prescription, the proportion of its two ingredients to be used is that which will produce a solution of the required alcohol strength.

The alcoholic strength of the elixir to be used with a single liquid galenical in a prescription is approximately the same as that of the galenical. When galenicals of different alcoholic strengths are used in the same prescription, the elixir to be used is to be of such alcoholic strength as to secure the best solution possible. This generally will be found to be the average of the alcoholic strengths of the several ingredients.

For non-extractive substances, the lowest alcoholic strength of the elixir that will yield a perfect solution should be chosen.

UREA

For the full monograph, see page 1424.

Comments—A protein denaturant that promotes hydration of keratin and mild keratolysis in dry and hyperkeratotic skin. It is used in 2 to 20% concentrations in various dry-skin creams.

OTHER MISCELLANEOUS PHARMACEUTICAL NECESSITIES

Bucrylate [Propenoic acid, 2-cyano-, 2-methylpropyl ester; Isobutyl 2-cyanoacrylate [1069-55-2] $C_{80}H_{11}NO_2$ (153.18)]—Preparation: One method reacts isobutyl 2-chloroacrylate with sodium cyanide. Uses: Surgical aid (tissue adhesive).

Ceresin [Ozokerite; Earth Wax; Cerosin; Mineral Wax; Fossil Wax] A hard, white odorless solid resembling spermaceti when purified, occurring naturally in deposits in the Carpathian Mountains, especially in Galicia. It is a mixture of natural complex paraffin hydrocarbons. Melts between 61 and 78°C; specific gravity 0.91 to 0.92; stable toward oxidizing agents. Soluble in 30% alcohol, benzene, chloroform, petroleum, benzin, or hot oils. Uses: Substitute for beeswax; in dentistry, for impression waxes.

Ethylenediamine Hydrate BP, PhI [$H_2NCH_2CH_2NH_2 \cdot H_2O$]—Clear, colorless or slightly yellow liquid with an ammoniacal odor and characteristic alkaline taste; solidifies on cooling to a crystalline mass (mp 10°C); boils 118 to 119°C; specific gravity about 0.96; hygroscopic and absorbs CO_2 from the air; aqueous solutions alkaline to litmus. Miscible with water or alcohol; soluble in 130 parts of chloroform; slightly soluble in benzene or ether. Uses: In the manufacture of aminophylline and in the preparation of aminophylline injections. See Ethylenediamine (page 1059).

Ferric Oxide, Red—Contains not less than 90% Fe_2O_3. Heating native ferric oxide or hydroxide at a temperature that will yield a product of the desired color makes it. The temperature and time of heating, the presence and kind of other metals, and the particle size of the oxide govern the color. A dark-colored oxide is favored by prolonged heating at high temperature and the presence of manganese. A light-colored oxide is favored by the presence of aluminum and by finer particle size. Uses: Imparting color.

Ferric Oxide, Yellow—Contains not less than 97.5% Fe_2O_3. It is prepared by heating ferrous hydroxide or ferrous carbonate in air at a low temperature. Uses: Imparting color.

Honey NF [Mel; Clarified Honey; Strained Honey]—The saccharine secretion deposited in the honeycomb by the bee, *Apis mellifera* Linné (Fam *Apidae*). It must be free from foreign substances such as parts of insects, leaves, etc, but may contain pollen grains. Honey is one of the oldest of food and medicinal products. During the 16th and 17th Centuries it was recommended as a cure for almost everything. Constituents: invert sugar (62–83%), sucrose (0–8%), and dextrin (0.26–7%). Description: thick, syrupy liquid of a light yellowish to reddish brown color; translucent when fresh but frequently becomes opaque and granular through crystallization of dextrose; characteristic odor and a sweet, faintly acrid taste. Uses: A sweetening agent.

Polacrilin Potassium—Methacrylic acid polymer with divinylbenzene, potassium salt [39394-76-5]; Amberlite IRP-88. Prepared by polymerizing methacrylic acid with divinylbenzene, and the resulting resin is neutralized with KOH. Dry, buff-colored, odorless, tasteless, free-flowing powder; stable in light, air, and heat; insoluble in water. Uses: Pharmaceutical aid (tablet disintegrant ion exchange resin for controlled release liquids).

Poloxalene—Glycols, polymers, polyethylene-polypropylene [9003-11-6]. Polypropylene glycol is reacted with ethylene oxide. Uses: Pharmaceutical aid (surfactant).

Sodium Thioglycollate [Sodium Mercaptoacetate; $HSCH_2COONa$]—Hygroscopic crystals that discolor on exposure to air or iron. Freely soluble in water; slightly soluble in alcohol. *Uses:* Reducing agent in Fluid Thioglycollate Medium for sterility testing.

PART 6

Pharmacokinetics and Pharmacodynamics

Paul Beringer, PharmD, BCPS
Associate Professor, Department of Pharmacy
USC School of Pharmacy
Los Angeles, CA

CHAPTER 56

Diseases: Manifestations and Pathophysiology

Martin C Gregory, BM, BCh, DPhil

Michael B Strong, MD

This chapter provides a brief overview of certain basic information about some major diseases, the objective being to prepare students and practitioners of pharmacy for more effective service as drug information specialists and consultants on drug therapy.

We include symptoms and signs, pathophysiology, etiology and epidemiology of the diseases. Some discussion of relevant physiology, biochemistry, anatomy, and pathology serves to provide a better understanding of the diseases. Clinical features and means of diagnosis are discussed. Some conditions are discussed more extensively than others; many are not discussed at all. This uneven treatment is the result of variables such as state of knowledge, frequency of disease, applicability of drug therapy and space constraints. For additional information the reader should refer to textbooks of medicine or to textbooks of basic science disciplines for amplification of the introductory material provided here.

HEART DISEASE

Atherosclerosis

This is the single most important cause of mortality in the US because it is involved in the development of ischemic heart disease and cerebrovascular disease.

Normal Anatomy and Physiology—Arterial walls have three layers: the intima, media, and adventitia. The intima is composed of endothelial cells; the media of smooth muscle cells, and the adventitia of collagen, elastic fibers, fibroblasts, and some smooth muscle cells.

Arteries are not inert conduits, but metabolically complex structures that regulate their own caliber and perform many endothelial cell functions, including local inhibition of blood clotting and maintenance of cellular integrity. Throughout life, arteries withstand tremendous physical forces. Areas of particular stress, friction, and turbulence include bifurcations and openings of branch arteries.

Epidemiology—In all populations studied, early changes of atherosclerosis have been seen in young individuals who died of unrelated causes. Mortality and morbidity is more common in men than premenopausal women. After menopause, the differences decrease. The incidence of atherosclerotic disease also is different in various nationalities. The mortality from atherosclerotic disease in North Americans and Scots is twice that of Swedes. The incidence is low in Japanese and in native Africans. The incidence of atherosclerotic disease in immigrants to the US is similar to that of native Americans rather than to that of age-matched individuals who did not migrate. Primary relatives of individuals who become symptomatic from atherosclerotic disease before 50 years are likely to develop symptomatic atherosclerotic disease at an earlier age.

Etiology—Although the etiology is not known, clinical and epidemiological studies suggest that many factors contribute to the disease process. The two most important risk factors are advancing age and male sex. Other significant factors include diabetes mellitus, plasma cholesterol level, arterial blood pressure, cigarette smoking, and plasma homocysteine.

Other risk factors associated with a high incidence of atherosclerotic disease include diet, lack of physical activity, obesity, and heredity. The role of a competitive aggressive personality (Type A) is debated. These factors may not be independent of the others already listed.

Pathology—Atherosclerosis is a patchy thickening and hardening of arterial walls that is characterized in the early stages by streaks of cholesterol and other lipids ("fatty streaks") and later by atheromas. Atheromas consist of a fibrous cap that covers proliferating smooth muscle cells. When advanced they contain a necrotic core of lipids and proteins, the lesions initially involve the intima and progress to involve the media. Rupture of the fibrous cap precipitates thrombosis of the vessel.

Pathophysiology—The mechanism for the development is poorly understood, but increased stress associated with increased blood pressure and turbulent flow may foster development of lesions. The actual initiating event in the intima is unknown, but minute tears in this layer occur and may be important. Platelet aggregation and changes in endothelial permeability and fibrin deposition are important in the development of the atheroma.

These changes may induce smooth muscle proliferation in the intima with subsequent lipid accumulation. Another hypothesis advocates lipid deposition as the inciting and most important event. Later, fibrosis, calcification, hemorrhage, ulceration, and thrombosis develop causing eventual rupture or further lumen narrowing causing tissue blood flow to be critically reduced.

Blood lipids (cholesterol and triglycerides) are carried in combination with phospholipids and proteins, as lipoproteins. Acceleration of atherosclerosis correlates best with elevations of the LDL fraction (low-density lipoprotein), which is rich in cholesterol and poor in triglycerides. Elevation of the HDL fraction (high-density lipoprotein) protects against atherosclerosis.

Symptoms and Signs—Manifestations of atherosclerotic disease depend on the location and degree of impairment of blood flow to an organ. Atherosclerotic disease presents as sudden death (probably due to a ventricular arrhythmia), angina pectoris, myocardial infarction, cerebrovascular accident, dissecting aneurysm, thrombosis of a major vessel, ischemic renal disease, or peripheral vascular disease. Only those that are not discussed elsewhere will be discussed here. Peripheral vascular disease may cause intermittent claudication (pain in the legs precipitated by exercise and relieved by rest), leg pain at night, atrophy, and weakness of leg muscles, loss of pulses in the feet, neuropathy, extreme sensitivity to cold and eventually, dry gangrene. Atherosclerosis of the mesenteric vessels may cause abdominal pain that is precipitated by eating (abdominal angina), weight loss, diarrhea, and steatorrhea. Thrombosis of these vessels will cause bowel infarction. The diagnosis of atherosclerotic disease usually is based on symptoms and signs of reduced organ perfusion. Noninvasive studies and angiography are often helpful in defining the sites of vessel narrowing.

Coronary Artery Disease

This disease (CAD) also is referred to as ischemic heart disease (IHD). Inadequate oxygen supply for myocardial demand is caused most commonly by coronary artery atherosclerotic disease. Other causes of decreased oxygen delivery to the myocardium include coronary embolism, coronary ostial stenosis in tertiary syphilis, and coronary artery spasm. Anemia, carboxyhemoglobinemia, and hypoxemia from lung disease can also reduce the oxygen-carrying capacity of the blood. Perfusion and O_2 delivery of the myocardium is decreased in hypotension. Myocardial oxygen demand is increased with exertion, myocardial hypertrophy, thyrotoxicosis, and beriberi. In the majority of cases of CAD, atherosclerosis is the underlying disorder.

Normal Anatomy—Arteries from the aorta nourish the myocardium. The right coronary artery supplies the right atrium, right ventricle, left atrium, posterior septum, AV node and, in over 50% of individuals, the SA node. The left coronary artery branches into two arteries. The circumflex supplies the anterolateral, lateral, posterolateral, inferior lateral, and inferior wall of the left ventricle, left atrium and, in about 45% of individuals, the SA node. The left anterior descending supplies the anterior, anterolateral, and apical left ventricular wall, the septum, and the right ventricle adjacent to the septum.

Normal Physiology—Under normal resting conditions, the myocardium extracts about 70% of the available oxygen from the coronary blood flow. This is in contrast to resting skeletal muscle, which extracts only 25% of available oxygen. Unlike skeletal muscle, the myocardium is capable of anaerobic metabolism for only a short time and cannot incur an oxygen debt. Increased myocardial oxygen demand must be met by increased coronary blood flow. The myocardium normally receives 5% of cardiac output. The normal heart can increase coronary blood flow by fivefold by a combination of coronary vasodilatation due to an autoregulatory process and increasing cardiac output. Blood flow to the myocardium occurs almost exclusively during diastole. Local tissue hypoxia results in potent vasodilatation and may increase coronary blood flow. Local tissue factors are more important than neuronal factors in regulating vasodilatation.

Systolic and diastolic wall tension, fraction of the cardiac cycle time spent in systole, and myocardial contractility determine myocardial oxygen consumption. The systolic wall tension (T) is determined by the systolic ventricular pressure (P), the radius (r) of the ventricular cavity and wall thickness (h) (T = P r/2h). The greater the cavity size and pressure, the greater the tension. Aortic diastolic pressure (afterload) partly determines the ventricular systolic pressure. The fraction of time spent in systole is determined by heart rate and ejection time. Oxygen demand of the myocardium depends on the amount of work the muscle must perform.

Pathology—Most atherosclerotic lesions occur in the proximal portion of the coronary arteries, because this is not a small vessel disease. Lesions in the left anterior descending artery are usually within 3 cm of the bifurcation of the left main coronary artery. Lesions in the right coronary artery usually occur within 6 to 8 cm of the ostium. A lesion that occludes less than 50% of the lumen of the vessel usually does not produce symptoms.

Pathophysiology—As the lumen of the vessels begins to narrow, blood flow decreases. Vessels distal to the obstruction dilate to maintain flow, presumably in response to hypoxia. When the obstruction reaches a critical size, the distal vessels become dilated permanently.

Ischemia causes changes in the biochemical, electrical, and mechanical properties of the heart. Myocardium normally oxidizes glucose and free fatty acids completely to carbon dioxide and water. In ischemia, lactate, pyruvate and other metabolic products accumulate in the myocardium. Ischemia also alters the electrical properties of the heart and decreases the membrane potential. Decreased conduction velocity and altered action potential duration result; thus arrhythmias may occur. Ischemia causes decreased contractility transiently, and necrosis causes irreversible loss of contractility. Ischemia may cause asymmetry and asynchrony of ventricular contraction.

The location of the lesion is important because this determines the size and location of the ischemia. The presence of collateral vessels may prevent the development of permanent injury. Unfortunately, the only known stimulus for collateral vessel formation is ischemia. A sudden decrease in lumen size, as with thrombosis or hemorrhage, is a catastrophic event as collateral vessels have not yet formed and therefore cannot provide an alternative source of oxygen. There is a group of people in whom coronary artery spasm plays a role in ischemic heart disease with or without fixed atherosclerotic lesions. How ischemia produces pain is unknown.

Angina pectoris is classified according to its frequency, severity, and precipitating event. Unstable angina describes a syndrome of attacks of recent onset or of increasing frequency, severity, or duration, or occurring with less exercise or at rest. Myocardial infarction and arrhythmias are more likely to develop during periods of unstable angina. Stable angina describes a clinical picture of little-varying attacks. Nocturnal angina occurs during sleep and may be associated with either dreams and rapid eye movement (REM) sleep or increased venous return in a patient with congestive failure. Prinzmetal angina is atypical angina. It occurs at rest, is associated with ventricular arrhythmias, and is thought to be due to coronary artery spasm.

Symptoms and Signs—CAD may present as ventricular arrhythmias or myocardial infarction, which will be discussed below. The other manifestation of CAD is angina pectoris, which is a clinical syndrome that results from transient myocardial ischemia but with no evidence of permanent damage.

The patient with angina pectoris usually describes the chest discomfort as heaviness, pressure, tightness, or squeezing. The patient often will not use the word "pain" or may ascribe his symptoms to indigestion. The substernal discomfort may radiate to the left arm, throat, jaw, shoulder, back, or abdomen. The discomfort typically is precipitated by exercise and also, but less often, by eating, emotional upset, exposure to cold, or cigarette smoking. Rest relieves it. The episodes usually last longer than 1 minute and not longer than 30 minutes.

Diagnosis—The diagnosis of angina is made from the history. The physical examination of these patients may be normal between attacks. Evidence of ischemia on EKG stress testing is inversion of T waves and depression of the S-T segment. Angiography and a therapeutic response to nitroglycerin may be helpful in establishing the diagnosis. Other causes of chest pain such as other forms of heart disease, gastrointestinal, and musculoskeletal disease must be considered in the differential diagnosis.

Ischemic heart disease is the leading cause of death among males over 35 years of age in the US and accounts for one-third of male deaths before age 65. The chief prognostic factors are the state of left ventricular function and the extent of the atherosclerotic disease.

Myocardial Infarction

Acute myocardial infarction (AMI) may be totally asymptomatic, can be fatal, or cause a variety of complications.

Pathology—The coronary arteries show thrombosis in approximately 90% of cases; thrombosis is central to the pathogenesis of AMI. Infarction is death of myocardial tissue. Most infarctions involve the endocardial layer. If the area of necrosis exceeds 3 cm in diameter, the infarct is likely to be transmural. Twenty-four hours after the infarction occurs, myocardial fibers show clumping, coagulation, and interstitial edema. By the 4th day the area is necrotic and shows fatty change and phagocytosis of fibers by neutrophils. Between the 4th and 10th days the area shows distinct fatty change, may contain hemorrhage, and is maximally soft. By the 10th day vascularized scar tissue begins to replace the infarct. The infarction heals completely by the 6th to 8th week.

Symptoms and Signs—Chest pain is usually the presenting complaint. It is described as severe, excruciating, deep, heavy, squeezing or crushing. No precipitating cause for the pain may be identified. The pain is similar to the pain of angina pectoris but is more severe, lasts longer, and is not relieved by rest or sublingual nitroglycerin. The pain may wax and wane. In 25% of patients, the substernal pain radiates to the arms; the pain also may radiate to the jaw, neck, abdomen, and back. Weakness, diaphoresis, nausea, vomiting, light-headedness, marked anxiety, and a sense of doom accompany the pain. The patient attempts in vain to find a comfortable position. In 15–20% of patients, AMI may be asymptomatic, particularly in diabetics. Elderly persons may complain of dyspnea rather than pain. Other presentations of MI include syncope, confusion, arrhythmias, and hypotension. Greater than 50% of the deaths following MI occur within the first 24 hours and are due to arrhythmias.

Physical examination typically discloses an anxious patient who is sweating and has cool extremities. Auscultation of the heart may reveal decreased heart sounds, S3, S4, or the murmur of mitral regurgitation. Temperature may be elevated to 38°.

Laboratory examination may reveal an increased white blood count to 15,000/mm^3. Enzymes released from damaged myocardial cells are used to diagnose AMI. The serum concentrations of these enzymes follow a characteristic pattern, with creatine (CK) and aspartate aminotransferase (AST) rising and falling quickly while lactic acid dehydrogenase (LDH) rises later and remains elevated longer. Measurement of serum troponin I has largely supplanted these enzyme measurements because of its greater sensitivity, specificity, and more rapid appearance after the infarction.

The EKG initially shows T-wave inversion and S-T segment elevation. When the infarct is transmural, Q-waves appear. Infarction also may cause decreased voltage in the precordial leads.

Complications—Arrhythmias are the most common cause of deaths in the early stages of AMI. Ventricular arrhythmias are the most ominous, and ventricular fibrillation is the most common fatal arrhythmia. Coronary care units that prevent or aggressively treat arrhythmias have decreased mortality from this complication.

Cardiac failure is now the primary cause of death in hospitalized patients with AMI. If greater than 40% of the myocardium is destroyed, the prognosis is poor.

Mitral regurgitation may occur as a result of rupture or dysfunction of the papillary muscles. This may decrease cardiac output and contribute to cardiac failure.

Thromboembolism contributes to the cause of death in some cases. Mural thrombosis may develop on the endocardium of the left ventricle. Emboli from this thrombus may cause strokes or a new AMI. Deep venous thrombosis may develop in the legs and embolize to the lungs (pulmonary embolism).

Rupture of the infarct may occur during the first week when the infarcted area is weakest. The blood pressure falls rapidly and the patient loses consciousness. The EKG may not change immediately. Cardiac tamponade occurs as the pericardium fills with blood. This complication is almost always fatal. The septum may rupture leading to left-to-right shunting. A pansystolic murmur is heard, and cardiac output decreases.

A weakening of the ventricular wall is called a ventricular aneurysm. When the remaining myocardium contracts, the aneurysm bulges. Because this portion of the wall has lost contractility, cardiac output decreases and congestive heart failure may develop. Systemic embolism may arise from a mural thrombus in the aneurysm. Arrhythmias are common with ventricular aneurysm and portend a poor prognosis.

Pericarditis may develop 2 to 3 days after the infarction. Pericardial pain is usually sharp, knife-like, and substernal. It may radiate to the neck and shoulders, is relieved by leaning forward, and is worsened by deep breathing. A pericardial friction rub may be heard. The pericarditis usually resolves with the healing of the infarct.

Heart Failure

This is defined as an inability of the heart, under normal filling conditions, to pump blood at a rate sufficient to meet the metabolic demands of the tissues. The inability to pump blood can be due to various abnormalities in the myocardium, coronary circulation, or heart valves. When the heart pumps blood at an insufficient rate, the kidneys retain salt and water and fluid accumulates in interstitial spaces. Thus, the term congestive heart failure usually is used. However, not all types of fluid overload or congestion are due to heart failure. Other causes of fluid overload include nephrotic syndrome, renal failure, liver disease, and starvation. Heart failure may develop acutely or chronically and may be mild to severe. Severe heart failure is synonymous with cardiogenic shock.

Normal Physiology—Function of the heart as a pump depends upon the number of functioning muscle fibers and their length at the onset of contraction. The end diastolic volume (EDV), which is referred to as preload, the cardiac impedance or afterload against which the blood is ejected, and the intrinsic myocardial activity or the contractile state determine fiber length. Heart rate and the stroke volume determine cardiac output (CO). The normal stroke volume (SV) is 70 ml, and the normal end systolic volume is 5 to 60 ml. SV is described by the equation: end diastolic volume minus end systolic volume.

The heart contracts in two phases. In the isovolumic phase, the length of the fiber remains constant while the pressure increases. When the left ventricular pressure reaches aortic diastolic pressure, the ejection phase occurs, during which contraction occurs as the fibers shorten. Heart rate determines filling time for the ventricles. With a normal heart, cardiac output remains stable between 50 to 180 beats/min. The afterload or the resistance against which the heart works influences cardiac output—the higher the resistance, the lower the CO.

Normally, the heart will pump out the blood that flows into it so that cardiac output is equal to venous return. Cardiac output can be increased within certain limits by autonomic stimulation, hypertrophy of the heart muscle, and an increase in blood volume. The heart has tremendous reserve capacity and can increase CO by increasing both heart rate and stroke volume.

The Frank-Starling relation describes the relationship between the stroke volume, diastolic volume or filling pressure and the length of the fibers at the end of diastole. The Frank-Starling relation also describes the ability of the heart to adapt to changing amounts of inflowing blood.

Within physiological limits, the more the chamber is filled, the greater the quantity of blood that will be pumped. If the muscle fibers are stretched by volume, the muscle contracts with greater force, thereby increasing CO. Increased contractility results from sympathetic stimulation, and decreased contractility indicates a failing heart. This relationship shows that for a given end diastolic volume, the ventricles receive and eject a higher stroke volume when contractility is increased and a lower stroke volume when contractility is decreased.

Etiology—Processes that cause the heart to fail are those that increase the work of the heart, usually over many years, or that damage the myocardial fibers. As a result, cardiac output decreases. The most common cause of left ventricular failure is systemic hypertension. Stenotic (narrow) valves lead to heart failure sooner than incompetent (leaky) ones. Congenital defects may result in increased cardiac work. Cardiomyopathies, atherosclerotic coronary disease, and myocardial infarction damage muscle fibers and impair contractility. Tachyarrhythmias and atrial-ventricular dissociation reduce ventricular filling and ventricular arrhythmias decrease contractility. Pericarditis may impair ventricular filling. The most-common cause of right heart failure is left heart failure. Pulmonary embolism may precipitate acute right ventricular failure. Cor pulmonale is right heart failure due to pulmonary hypertension, which can occur as a complication of hypoxemia from lung disease.

Increased metabolic demands or decreased oxygen-carrying capacity of the blood may exceed cardiac reserve. Causes of high-output heart failure (see below) include hyperthyroidism, anemia, A-V fistulas, pregnancy, infections (particularly pulmonary infection), and beriberi.

Pathophysiology—The majority of cases of congestive heart failure (CHF) are due to low-output failure as occurs in hypertension, atherosclerotic heart disease, or valvular disease. Less commonly, the cardiac output is greater than normal, high-output heart failure. This is due to the metabolic demands of the tissue being increased greatly or the oxygen-carrying capacity of the blood being decreased greatly. Hyperthyroidism and pregnancy are causes of increased metabolic demands of the tissues. Anemia, arteriovenous fistulas, and hypoxemia are examples of decreased oxygen delivery.

Compensatory Mechanisms of Low Cardiac Output—When cardiac output falls, reflexes occur immediately. The baroreceptors sense the decreased arterial pressure and increase sympathetic tone while decreasing parasympathetic tone. This increases the force of contraction of the heart, increases heart rate, raises mean systemic arterial pressure, and increases venous return. These reflexes are maximal at 30 sec after a drop in arterial pressure.

Redistribution of blood flow occurs resulting in maintenance of blood flow to the myocardium and brain. Blood flows to the skin and skeletal muscle are decreased greatly by norepinephrine-induced vasoconstriction. Blood flow also is decreased to the kidneys in CHF.

Decreased cardiac output reduces the glomerular filtration rate because of both decreased renal blood flow and sympathetic vasoconstriction of afferent renal arterioles. Blood flow within the kidneys is redistributed by the vasoconstriction to the medulla at the expense of the cortex. Renin production by the juxtaglomerular apparatus is increased in response to decreased blood flow. Renin cleaves angiotensinogen to angiotensin I which is converted by angiotensin converting enzyme (ACE) to angiotensin II. Angiotensin II is a potent peripheral vessel constrictor and stimulator of aldosterone secretion by the adrenal cortex. Aldosterone promotes the retention of sodium and water by the distal convoluted renal tubule, causes expansion of the blood volume and accumulation of fluid in interstitial spaces. Aldosterone may have other harmful effects because blockade of its effects prolongs survival in heart failure. Serum sodium remains normal or is decreased, although total body sodium is increased.

Increased blood volume and increased systemic blood pressure increase venous return to the heart. Eventually, the heart can no longer keep pace with the increased venous return. In mild heart failure, the increased fluid volume helps to increase cardiac output by applying some stretch to the myocardial fibers. In severe heart failure, the amount of fluid overload becomes so great that the fibers are stretched beyond the limits of efficient contraction and the fibers descend to a lower Frank-Starling curve. A greater end-diastolic pressure is necessary to maintain CO on this lower curve. The increase in left ventricular end diastolic pressure (LVEDP) is transmitted as increased hydrostatic pressure to the pulmonary veins, capillaries, and arteries. Eventually, the increased pressure in the pulmonary arteries causes the right ventricle to fail. Increased right ventricular end diastolic pressure translates into increased hydrostatic pressure in the systemic veins and capillaries.

Edema Formation—Most of the fluid accumulation in interstitial spaces results from increases in capillary hydrostatic pressures. The colloidal osmotic (oncotic) pressure of the blood that holds fluid in the vascular compartment is about 25 to 30 mmHg. When the hydrostatic pressure in the capillaries exceeds 25 mmHg, fluid is pushed into the interstitial spaces. CHF involves fluid retention in both the intra- and extravascular space. Fluid retention also results in distention of the venous reservoirs in the liver and spleen. When LVEDP exceeds 25 mmHg, the pressure transmitted to the pulmonary capillaries causes pulmonary edema. Oxygen does not diffuse efficiently in alveoli filled with edema fluid so hypoxemia results.

Symptoms and Signs—Patients with left ventricular failure most commonly complain of a sensation of shortness of breath (dyspnea). Initially, the dyspnea is present only on exertion (DOE), but the amount of activity necessary to precipitate dyspnea progressively lessens until the patient is dyspneic at rest. Orthopnea is the sensation of breathlessness that occurs in the recumbent position and may be relieved by elevating the head on several pillows or by sitting. Paroxysmal nocturnal dyspnea (PND) is severe dyspnea occurring at night that awakens the patient with a sensation of smothering. PND usually is accompanied by coughing and/or wheezing. The patient may produce frothy pink sputum.

Patients with left ventricular failure also may experience fatigue, weakness, and alterations in mental status such as confusion, difficulty in concentrating, impaired memory, headache, insomnia, and anxiety.

Physical examination of the patient with left heart failure reveals a person who may have lost considerable body mass. The patient may be unable to lie flat during the examination. The pulse may be weak, although the blood pressure remains normal until very late in the course. The extremities will be pale and cool. Cyanosis of the lips and nailbeds may be present. Examination of the heart reveals tachycardia and S3 gallop. Moist crepitant inspiratory crackles over the lung bases in moderately severe CHF and over the entire lung fields in pulmonary edema are heard. Chest radiograph shows the enlarged heart and signs of pulmonary venous congestion.

Patients with right ventricular failure complain of weight gain and the accumulation of fluid. A 10% gain in body weight may occur before pitting edema occurs. In ambulatory patients the edema is symmetrical in the ankles and legs. Since gravity influences the distribution of the edema, the buttocks and sacrum may be edematous in bedfast patients. Anasarca is massive body fluid overload including generalized edema, ascites, and pleural effusions. As fluids accumulate in the pleural cavity, the patient may develop dyspnea. Patients experience an increased girth as fluid accumulates in the peritoneal cavity. The liver may become enlarged and tender, and there may be right upper quadrant pain. Anorexia, nausea, and abdominal fullness occur. The patient becomes jaundiced as impairment of liver function becomes severe.

Physical examination of the patient with severe right-sided heart failure will reveal pleural effusions, ascites, jugular venous distension, hepatomegaly, splenomegaly, and pitting edema. Urine volume will be decreased, and prerenal azotemia may be present.

Valvular Heart Disease

This disease occurs when the heart valves become damaged and no longer will open or close properly. If fibrous scar tissue forms or calcium deposits on the valve, the valve becomes stenotic and no longer opens easily. If the valve leaflets shrink or do not oppose each other properly when closing, due to scarring or are destroyed by infection, the valve no longer is competent and blood flows in a retrograde fashion. A single valve may be both stenotic and incompetent. More than one valve may be involved. The consequences of valvular disease include congestive heart failure, arrhythmias, and systemic emboli. The hallmark of valvular disease is a murmur—a noise representing turbulence of blood flow across the valve.

Normal Anatomy and Physiology—The valves between the atria and the ventricles, tricuspid on the right side and mitral on the left side, are large and normally offer little resistance to flow. The semilunar valves, the aortic and pulmonic, are smaller. The atrioventricular valves are supported by chordae tendineae, but the semilunar valves are not. All valves open and close passively in response to pressure gradients.

The opening and closing of the valves cause the heart sounds. The first sound ("lub") occurs at the beginning of systole and represents the closure of the mitral and tricuspid valves. The second sound ("dup") is heard at the beginning of diastole and signals closure of the aortic and pulmonic valves. In normal individuals, the second sound may be split because the aortic and pulmonic valves do not close simultaneously. The first sound is loud when the mitral valve leaflets are far apart at the onset of ventricular systole. This occurs in mitral stenosis and tachycardia of any cause. A loud second sound indicates an increased pressure, as in systemic and pulmonary hypertension. A third heart sound (S3) is caused by blood flowing into the ventricles early in diastole, particularly into the dilated ventricles of CHF. A fourth heart sound (S4) also emanates from the ventricles late in diastole, but is caused by forceful atrial contraction thrusting blood into ventricles whose compliance is decreased, as in hypertensive heart disease.

Etiology—Formerly most valvular lesions followed rheumatic fever. Now the causes are more varied and include congenital lesions such as a bicuspid aortic valve, which may become significantly stenotic only in adult life as it calcifies. Another congenital condition is mitral valve prolapse, in which the mitral valve is redundant and billows into the left atrium during systole.

A number of systemic diseases are associated with valvular lesions: seronegative spondylitides, polycystic kidney disease, and Marfan's syndrome are examples. Acute bacterial endocarditis can attack previously normal valves and destroy them rapidly. The aortic and tricuspid valves are particularly vulnerable, especially in intravenous drug users. Subacute bacterial endocarditis also damages valves, but it usually alights on previously abnormal valves.

An increasingly common cause of mitral and tricuspid insufficiency is dilatation of the valve ring from chronic fluid overload as in CHF and end-stage renal disease.

Pathology—In acute rheumatic fever, the valve leaflets become swollen and thickened and small bead-like nodules develop along the valve closure lines and on the chordae. These nodules are composed of fibrin, platelets, and white blood cells. The inflammation may subside with the acute attack or develop into a subacute or chronic process. The inflammation leads to erosion of the endothelial surface and deposition of collagen by fibroblasts. The fibrous scarring during organization leaves a permanently thickened, distorted, rigid valve. Contraction of the scar results in shortening of the leaflets and distortion of the architecture of the valve. The edges of the deformed valve fail to fit together during closure causing valvular incompetence. The chordae also may be involved in scarring and shortening. Fibrous adhesions may occur across the cusp edges. Irregular fibrous thickening and scarring also are associated with calcification. Adhesions and calcification increase the rigidity of the valve and cause stenosis. Stenosis and the uneven surface are associated with increased turbulence of flow across the valve.

MITRAL STENOSIS (MS)

Pathophysiology—The normal area of the mitral valve is 4 to 6 cm^2 in adults. Symptoms of MS occur when the area is reduced to 1.5 cm^2. If the valve is stenotic, greater pressures are required to pump the blood from the left atrium to the left ventricle. Normally mean pressure in the left atrium is 12 mmHg. A valve orifice less than 1 cm^2 requires a pressure of 25 mmHg in the left atrium to pump the blood into the left ventricle. The elevated atrial pressure is transmitted back into the pulmonary veins, capillaries, and arteries. Pulmonary arteries develop medial hypertrophy and intimal thickening, which leads to high resistance and pulmonary hypertension. Alveolar fibrosis may occur also. When the pressure in the pulmonary capillaries exceeds the osmotic pressure of blood, pulmonary edema develops although the patient does not have left ventricular failure and left ventricular end diastolic pressure is normal. Eventually, the right heart fails.

Left ventricular output may be normal or decreased. The flow across the valve depends on heart rate as well as size of the opening. Increasing heart rate decreases the time available for flow across the mitral valve.

Symptoms and Signs—Two decades usually elapse between the initial attack of rheumatic fever and the development of the symptoms and signs of MS. Most patients become symptomatic during the fourth decade of life. Once the symptoms occur, the prognosis is poor with death occurring in 2 to 5 years unless the valve is replaced. Symptoms begin with dyspnea and cough during extreme exertion, but over the years the amount of exercise necessary to produce symptoms decreases until dyspnea occurs at rest. Orthopnea and paroxysmal nocturnal dyspnea may occur. With longstanding MS, atrial arrhythmias are common.

Extensive fibrosis of the alveolar walls and pulmonary capillary thickening lead to decreased vital capacity, total lung capacity, maximum breathing capacity and oxygen uptake. V/Q mismatching occurs. Decreased compliance of the lung increases the work of breathing and increases the sensation of breathlessness. Hemoptysis results from rupture of small vessels in the bronchioles.

Patients with MS, particularly those with atrial fibrillation, are likely to embolize thrombi from the left atrium to the brain, kidneys, spleen, or extremities.

The physical examination of patients with MS often discloses cyanosis of the lips and nails, and signs of right heart failure. The first heart sound is accentuated. The opening snap of the mitral valve may be heard. A low-pitched rumbling diastolic murmur is characteristic of mitral stenosis. Chest radiograph shows an enlarged left atrium, pulmonary arteries, and right ventricle, as well as markings of increased pulmonary venous pressure. EKG shows signs of left atrial enlargement and may disclose an atrial arrhythmia. Echocardiogram, the most useful noninvasive test shows inadequate valve separation, thickened leaflets, and left atrial enlargement.

MITRAL INSUFFICIENCY (MR)

Pathophysiology—When the mitral valve leaks, blood flows from the left ventricle in two directions: into the aorta and back into the left atrium. Left ventricular end diastolic volume increases. As left ventricular function deteriorates, left ventricular end diastolic pressure increases and cardiac output eventually falls.

Symptoms and Signs—Patients present with symptoms of decreased cardiac output such as fatigue, dyspnea, weakness, and, perhaps, cachexia. Palpitations due to atrial arrhythmias may be felt. If pulmonary vascular resistance is increased, right heart failure results. If pulmonary pressures are high the patient may complain of orthopnea, DOE, and PND. The symptoms of MR are less episodic than those of MS.

Physical examination discloses a loud murmur that may radiate to the axilla. The murmur is usually pansystolic in MR caused by rheumatic heart disease, but it may be shorter if the MR is caused by mitral valve prolapse or ischemia. The EKG reveals evidence of left ventricular and/or right ventricular hypertrophy, left atrial enlargement and, in chronic cases, atrial fibrillation. Chest x-ray may show extreme left atrial enlargement and left ventricular enlargement. Echocardiogram shows left atrial enlargement, a hyperdynamic left ventricle, failure of coaption of the mitral valve leaflets, and a regurgitant jet on color Doppler examination. Calcifications of the mitral valve may be seen on chest radiograph.

AORTIC STENOSIS

Pathophysiology—Aortic stenosis causes obstruction to the flow of blood from the left ventricle. Cardiac output is maintained by the generation of increased pressures by the left ventricle. The left ventricle responds to this situation by developing concentric hypertrophy without dilatation if the obstruction develops gradually. The diameter of the normal aortic orifice is 3 to 3.5 cm^2, and a reduction to 0.5 to 1.0 cm^2 is critical.

The patient initially develops symptoms during exercise because cardiac output cannot be increased to meet the oxygen demands of exercise. Later, as the left ventricle begins to fail, cardiac output cannot be maintained at rest.

Symptoms and Signs—Aortic stenosis may exist for years before symptoms develop. The onset of symptoms for rheumatic aortic stenosis is usually in the 4th or 5th decade. The characteristic symptoms are fatigue, exertional dyspnea, angina, and syncope. The syncope is usually exertional and occurs when cardiac output cannot be increased. Reduced cerebral blood flow may cause syncope. An arrhythmia also may result in decreased cardiac output and syncope. Very late in the course of the disease, the patient has the symptoms and signs of left ventricular failure and, finally, in the preterminal phase, symptoms and signs of right heart failure.

When aortic stenosis occurs with mitral stenosis, less blood fills the left ventricle so less of a pressure gradient develops across the aortic valve. The left ventricle does not hypertrophy as much, and less angina occurs. When aortic stenosis occurs with mitral stenosis, the patient has more of the symptoms and signs of mitral stenosis.

On physical examination of the patient with aortic stenosis, an ejection click may be heard as well as closure of the aortic valve if the valve is not calcified The pulmonary valve may close before the aortic valve resulting in paradoxical splitting of the second heart sound. A systolic ejection murmur, which begins after the first heart sound, increases in intensity reaching a peak in the middle of the ejection period and decreases in intensity until closure of the aortic valve is heard. The ejection murmur thus is referred to as crescendo decrescendo.

Once the patient has become symptomatic, the prognosis is poor with 80% mortality at 4 years. Congestive heart failure accounts for mortality in up to two-thirds of the patients, and its onset suggests an average prognosis of 1 1/2 years. Ten to 20% of the patients die from an arrhythmia.

AORTIC INSUFFICIENCY (AI)

Pathophysiology—In AI a fraction of the stroke volume flows retrograde into the left ventricle so that cardiac output decreases. To compensate for the decrease in cardiac output, left ventricular end diastolic volume increases to allow for greater stroke volume. The left ventricle dilates to accommodate the increased end diastolic volume. Eventually, left ventricular function fails, and cardiac output decreases.

Symptoms and Signs—A patient who develops AI is usually asymptomatic for 10 to 20 years. The first symptom is an uncomfortable awareness of the heart beat particularly in the supine position or during exertion or emotional upset. Next, exertional dyspnea develops as a sign of decreased cardiac reserve. Later, signs of left ventricular failure appear. The patient may complain of chest pain due to pounding of the chest wall. Typical or atypical angina may develop, may be prolonged, and will not respond to nitroglycerin. Finally, symptoms and signs of systemic fluid overload and right heart failure appear. The cause of death may be pulmonary edema. Syncope is rare.

Physical examination of patients with AI reveals an increased systolic pressure and decreased diastolic pressure with a wide pulse pressure. A diastolic high-pitched blowing decrescendo murmur is heard. The murmur becomes louder and longer as the AI worsens. EKG shows left ventricular enlargement. Chest radiograph shows left ventricular enlargement and dilatation of the ascending aorta. Echocardiography shows left atrial and left ventricular enlargement and high frequency fluttering of the mitral valve.

The prognosis in decompensated AI is poor. Surgical correction is necessary before left ventricular deterioration occurs.

TRICUSPID STENOSIS

Pathophysiology—Tricuspid stenosis presents an obstruction to outflow from the right atrium and results in an increased end-diastolic pressure in the right atrium. The increased right atrial pressure causes backup of blood and congestion in the systemic circulation. Cardiac output decreases because of decreased return to the left atrium.

Symptoms and Signs—The patient presents with the symptoms and signs of right heart failure. A diastolic murmur is characteristic of tricuspid stenosis.

TRICUSPID INSUFFICIENCY

Pathophysiology—Some blood from the right ventricle flows back into the right atrium leading to enlargement of the right atrium and increased right atrial pressure. The increased right atrial pressure leads to systemic venous congestion.

Symptoms and Signs—The patient with advanced tricuspid insufficiency exhibits the signs of right heart failure and decreased cardiac output. A blowing systolic murmur is heard in tricuspid insufficiency. Atrial fibrillation may be present.

Disorders of Cardiac Rhythm (Electrophysiology)

Dysrhythmias ("arrhythmias") are irregularities in the heart rhythm that result from disturbances in the generation or conduction of the impulse. Certain dysrhythmias occur in the absence of any detectable disease of the heart. Other dysrhythmias occur characteristically in certain diseases of the heart or with toxic amounts of drugs. Predisposing factors for the development of a dysrhythmia include ischemic heart disease, congestive heart failure, hypoxemia, electrolyte imbalance, acidosis, and treatment with certain drugs such as sympathomimetics or antiarrhythmic drugs. The treatment of a dysrhythmia may be difficult unless all predisposing factors are corrected.

Normal Physiology—The conduction of an impulse through the myocardium proceeds in an orderly fashion so that both atria contract together shortly before both ventricles. The heart rate normally is controlled by the SA node, which fires at 60 to 100 beats/min. The electrophysiology of the pacemaker dictates that the faster pacemaker controls the heart rate: SA node 60 to 100/minute; AV node 40 to 60/minute; ventricular pacemaker 20 to 40/minute.

An impulse is conducted from the SA node through the atria to the AV node. Atrial depolarization causes the P wave of the EKG. The AV node slows the impulse so that the atria may contract to fill the ventricles. The impulse then proceeds down the common bundle of His, the bundle branches and into the Purkinje fibers. The QRS complex of the EKG is caused by ventricular depolarization and the T wave is caused by ventricular repolarization.

Pathophysiology—Many dysrhythmias result from a decrease or increase in automaticity of myocardial tissue. Increased automaticity may result from a more-rapid rate of depolarization, more-negative threshold potential, less-negative resting potential, or a combination of these alterations. A decreased automaticity results from the opposite situations. Conduction disturbances, particularly slowing or failure of propagation, also may cause dysrhythmias. Conduction disturbances are caused electrophysiologically by low resting potential, a slowly rising action potential and delayed recovery from depolarization.

Many paroxysmal tachycardias are due to reentrant phenomena (ie, a circus movement) in which an impulse is propagated continually in a circuit of excitable tissue. Such circuits may exist because of structural abnormalities, such as a bypass tract, or because of functional abnormalities of diseased heart tissue. When a critically timed impulse comes to two potential pathways with different refractory periods, it may be blocked down one pathway but conducted down the second. The impulse can then be conducted up the initially refractory pathway in a retrograde direction and back down the second pathway, thus setting up the circus movement.

Dysrhythmias may have various or no effects on the individual. Significant changes in the heart rate may impair cardiac output. In pathologic bradycardia, cardiac output fails to increase during conditions of increased demand such as exercise, infection, or stress. In tachycardia the synchrony of atrial-ventricular contraction may be lost or the time for ventricular filling may be decreased so that cardiac output is decreased.

Heart rate is a determinant of myocardial oxygen consumption. Coronary artery blood flow to the ventricles occurs only in diastole. Tachycardia increases cardiac oxygen demand while decreasing supply.

Pathophysiology and Symptoms and Signs of Common Arrhythmias—Sinus bradycardia is a heart rate of less than 60 beats/minute with the impulse originating in the sinus node. Sinus bradycardia occurs in individuals who are in excellent physical condition, have increased parasympathetic tone, intracerebral pressure or hypothyroidism, or in patients with SA node dysfunction due to degenerative or ischemic heart disease.

Sinus arrest refers to total cessation of sinus node activity. This may occur because of complete sinoatrial block (interference of conduction between sinus node and atrium) or loss of automaticity. There is a pause of at least 3 seconds between two P waves on the EKG. Causes of sinus arrest include excessive vagal stimulation, ischemic heart disease, and digitalis toxicity.

Sinus arrhythmia usually is not a dysrhythmia but a normal change in heart rate (less than 10% variation in length of adjacent sinus cycles) that occurs with respiration. Heart rate increases during inspiration and decreases during expiration.

Sinus tachycardia is a heart rate of greater than 100 beats/minute with the impulse originating in the sinus node. Usually sinus tachycardia is less than 140 beats/minute. The etiologies of sinus tachycardia include anxiety, fever, anemia, blood loss, thyrotoxicosis, pregnancy, pheochromocytoma, hypoxemia, various drugs, and electrolyte disturbances.

Premature atrial depolarizations (PADs) are ectopic atrial beats. Usually PADs are of little significance, although they may precede a more serious atrial arrhythmia. The rhythm with PADs is usually irregular. The P wave is abnormal in PADs or may be hidden in the T wave. A PAD may be confused with a premature ventricular contraction. The etiology of PADs is related to stimulation by nicotine, caffeine, or sympathomimetics or the deranged electrophysiology of failing atria.

Paroxysmal supraventricular tachycardia (PSVT) is a sudden attack of atrial tachycardia that is sustained by reentry. The heartbeat is regular and 140 to 250 beats/minute. This is a benign arrhythmia unless the rate is very rapid. PSVT occurs in young people with no obvious cardiac disease, and the precipitating event is usually emotional upset, trauma, fatigue, indigestion, stimulant drugs, or alcohol ingestion. The patient may become very anxious because of prominent palpitations. PSVT may end abruptly, spontaneously, or be terminated by carotid massage or medications. The prognosis for PSVT is excellent unless the rapid rate results in CHF, angina, or myocardial infarction.

Atrial flutter is a regular rhythm with an atrial rate of 250 to 350, usually 300 beats/min. The ventricular rate is 75 to 150 beats/minute reflecting AV block. The rhythm is sustained by reentry. The EKG shows sawtooth flutter waves instead of P waves. Atrial flutter occurs in patients with ischemic heart disease, mitral stenosis, thyrotoxicosis, hypertension, atrial septal defect, and hypoxemia due to chronic lung disease.

Atrial fibrillation is an arrhythmia in which the atria do not contract. The atrial rate is 400 to 600, and the ventricular rate is 80 to 180. The ventricular rate, which is slower than the atrial rate because of AV block, is usually rapid and irregularly irregular. The EKG shows fibrillating undulations instead of P waves. Because the atria do not contract, cardiac output is decreased, and the symptoms and signs of congestive heart failure may be seen. Blood stagnates in the fibrillating atria, and thrombi may form and embolize to either the lungs or the systemic cir-

culation. The patient also may complain of palpitations due to the irregular rhythm. Paroxysmal atrial fibrillation may precede the onset of permanent atrial fibrillation in patients with mitral stenosis, constrictive pericarditis, ischemic heart disease, CHF, and thyrotoxicosis.

Premature ventricular depolarizations (PVDs) are beats that originate in an ectopic ventricular pacemaker. No P waves precede the QRS complex, which appears widened and bizarre. PVDs are a benign arrhythmia when they occur in young people without underlying heart disease. The precipitating factors in these individuals include the consumption of caffeine, nicotine or alcohol, emotional stress, and reflexes from the GI tract. PVDs may be a more serious arrhythmia when their frequency increases, they occur in pairs or runs, occur on the T wave, or originate from multiple foci. In these cases, the arrhythmia may precede ventricular tachycardia or ventricular fibrillation. PVDs are associated with ischemic heart disease, myocardial infarction, and digitalis intoxication.

Ventricular tachycardia is an arrhythmia with a rate of 150 to 250 and a regular rhythm. The rhythm originates from an ectopic focus or occurs by a reentrant mechanism. The P wave is often independent of the QRS complex (A-V dissociation). Cardiac output is decreased markedly, and the patient is usually unconscious if the arrhythmia is sustained. Ventricular fibrillation may originate from ventricular tachycardia. Common causes of ventricular tachycardia are an acute myocardial infarction, chronic ischemic heart disease, digitalis, and Type 1 antiarrhythmic drug toxicity. Ventricular tachycardia rarely occurs in a healthy individual.

Ventricular fibrillation is an irregular chaotic rhythm that is associated with no cardiac output and death if the arrhythmia is prolonged. The EKG reveals disorganized waveforms.

Abnormalities of Conduction

Normally the AV node delays the impulse from the atria. In pathologic conditions, the impulse may be delayed abnormally or blocked completely.

First-degree (1°) heart block is a dysrhythmia that usually requires no treatment. In 1° heart block, the delay of atrial impulses by the AV node is prolonged (PR interval is greater than 0.20 sec). Each atrial impulse is conducted through the AV node and results in a ventricular impulse. First-degree heart block can result from any inflammatory or degenerative disease of the heart, ischemic heart disease, and multiple medications. In healthy persons, an increase in vagal tone may result in 1° heart block.

Second-degree (2°) heart block is a dysrhythmia in which the atrial rate is greater than the ventricular rate. Mobitz Type 1 (Wenckebach) is progressive lengthening of the PR interval until an atrial impulse is not conducted to the ventricle and the corresponding QRS does not occur. The dropped ventricular beat may occur after every 2nd beat, 2:1 block or less frequently. The block may disappear during exercise or with a decrease in vagal stimulation. The atrial rate is regular while the ventricular rate is irregular. Mobitz Type 1 block is caused by ischemic heart disease, disease that involves the AV node, and by increases in vagal tone. The dysrhythmia requires no treatment unless cardiac output is impaired.

Mobitz Type 2 is a more serious block of the lower His bundle complex that may progress to complete heart block. The EKG shows a normal or increased PR interval that remains constant. QRS complexes may be dropped after the P wave on a 2:1, 3:1, 4:1, or irregular basis. Mobitz Type 2 block occurs in myocardial infarction, chronic ischemic heart disease, myocarditis, and in sclerosing diseases of the myocardium.

Complete or third degree (3°) heart block involves a normal P wave that is unrelated to QRS complexes. The atrial impulse is blocked completely from conducting into the ventricles, and the CO is maintained by the ventricles' own pacemakers. Digitalis toxicity, myocardial infarction, and degeneration of the conduction tissue cause third degree heart block. The prognosis for 3° heart block depends on whether the patient is symptomatic and the exact site of the block. Treatment is by pacemaker insertion.

Syncopal episodes due to bradydysrhythmias with resultant decreased CO are known as the Stokes-Adams-Morgagni syndrome.

Hypertension

This means abnormally elevated blood pressure. It may refer to increased pressure in any blood vessel, such as pulmonary or portal hypertension. However, it usually refers to an elevated systemic arterial blood pressure. Hypertension is not a disease but is a physical finding. Hypertension is defined as a systolic blood pressure (SBP) of greater than 140 or a diastolic blood pressure (DBP) of greater than 90 mmHg: an elevation of either SBP or DBP defines the presence of hypertension. Prehypertension, SBP 120-139 or DBP 80-89, may also merit treatment, because above 120/80 the frequency of complications due to hypertension rises significantly. Isolated systolic hypertension (SBP > 140 with DBP < 90) also may occur, particularly in the elderly. Above the age of 50, increased cardiovascular complications are more strongly associated with elevations of SBP than of DBP.

Normal Physiology—Blood pressure is determined by cardiac output and peripheral resistance (BP = CO × PR). Cardiac output is determined by stroke volume and heart rate (CO = SV × HR). Vascular resistance is inversely proportional to the 4th power of the internal radius of the blood vessels, according to the law of Poiseuille ($R \propto \dfrac{length}{r4}$). Therefore, variations in the internal lumen of blood vessels profoundly affect the blood pressure. Blood pressure varies throughout the day in any individual and is affected by physical activity, emotional upset, and other factors.

Epidemiology—Approximately 20% of the population in the US has hypertension. The incidence depends on age, race, and gender. For example, Blacks at any age have twice the incidence of hypertension as Caucasians. Hypertension is slightly more common in males than in females.

Etiology—Between 5 and 10% of the cases have an identifiable cause, and these are called secondary hypertension. Causes include renal disease, renovascular disease, endocrine disorders, and coarctation of the aorta, which will be discussed below. The remaining 90 to 95% of the cases have no known cause and are called idiopathic, primary, or essential. The etiology of essential hypertension is probably multifactorial and may involve a number of abnormalities in physiological regulatory systems. The pressure receptors in the cardiovascular system, ie, baroreceptors, may become reset at a higher pressure in response to chronic stress, overactivity of the sympathetic nervous system, or heredity. The kidneys may retain too much salt and water in response to alter reflexes that tend to maintain abnormal intravascular fluid volumes. Statistical evidence correlates the incidence of hypertension with the quantity of dietary sodium chloride. Approximately 30% of patients with hypertension are salt-sensitive; their blood pressure falls significantly with salt restriction.

Systolic hypertension most commonly occurs in elderly individuals and diabetics with stiff, noncompliant blood vessels, ie, atherosclerosis. Systolic hypertension also occurs in situations of increased cardiac output such as anemia, fever, beriberi, aortic valve insufficiency, arteriovenous fistulas, and thyrotoxicosis.

Pathophysiology—Hypertension is a major risk factor for atherosclerosis and cardiovascular complications such as CHF, AMI, and angina pectoris (see previous discussions). Sustained hypertension results in damage to the target organs: the eyes, brain, heart, and kidneys.

Damage to the eyes has been classified by Keith, Wagener, and Barker. Grades I and II retinopathy correlate well with duration of hypertension, while Grades III and IV correspond to severity. Grade I: Arteriolar narrowing with mild depression of the venule by the crossing arteriole. Grade II: Greater arteriolar narrowing and compression of the venule by the crossing arteriole (AV nicking). Grade III: Arteriolar spasm, hemorrhages, and exudates. Grade IV: all other findings, plus papilledema. Hypertensive retinopathy leads to visual disturbances.

Damage to the brain results from cerebral edema, thrombosis, and hemorrhage (see discussion of strokes). Strokes are 12 times more common in hypertensive patients. The stroke may be small and result in focal signs or a large, fatal, cerebral hemorrhage.

The heart compensates for the increased work imposed by the increased afterload with left ventricular hypertrophy. Eventually, left ventricular function deteriorates; the chamber dilates and left ventricular failure occurs (see previous discussion of heart failure). Mortality from hypertensive congestive heart failure is 50% in 5 years. Hypertension accelerates coronary atherosclerotic heart disease and increases myocardial oxygen consumption. Angina pectoris and myocardial infarction are more common in hypertensive patients (see previous discussion of CAD).

Hypertension causes intimal and muscular hypertrophy of afferent arterioles. Malignant hypertension causes fibrinoid necrosis in the afferent arterioles and rapid deterioration if renal function. Eventually renal failure occurs (see the discussion of chronic failure below).

Symptoms and Signs—Hypertension per se causes no symptoms or signs unless the BP is very high. The symptoms and signs of essential hypertension are secondary to target organ damage. For example, retinopathy causes scotomas, blurred vision, and finally, blindness. In severe accelerated hypertension, CNS symptoms may include lethargy, confusion, increased neuromuscular irritability, convulsions, and coma. Damage to the heart results in angina pectoris or the symptoms and signs of CHF or AMI. The symptoms and signs of chronic renal failure are described later.

Elevated blood pressure may be an incidental finding during routine physical examination. The diagnosis of hypertension is based on documentation of increased blood pressure on several independent readings unless target-organ damage is already present. Adequate treatment of hypertension reduces its mortality and morbidity.

SECONDARY HYPERTENSION—This presently accounts for only 5–10% of the cases. It may be cured or ameliorated if the underlying disorder is treated successfully.

Renal vascular hypertension is mediated by the renin-angiotensin system. Renal blood flow is decreased by renal artery stenosis secondary to fibromuscular dysplasia or atherosclerosis. The renal artery lesion may be either unilateral or bilateral. The decreased renal blood flow is sensed by the juxtaglomerular apparatus, which secretes renin. Renin cleaves angiotensinogen to angiotensin I (a decapeptide). Converting enzyme in the pulmonary circulation converts angiotensin I to angiotensin II. Angiotensin II (an octapeptide) constricts blood vessels and stimulates aldosterone production. Aldosterone stimulates the retention of sodium and water and the excretion of potassium by the distal convoluted tubule. Renal parenchymal disease also is associated with hypertension; the mechanism is not understood well. The decreased excretion of sodium and water that occurs in renal failure results in volume expansion that contributes to hypertension.

Endocrine disorders cause hypertension by the production of hormone by tumors or hyperplasia of endocrine glands. Hypertension is seen in Cushing's syndrome, primary hyperaldosteronism, and hyperparathyroidism (see later discussion of these disorders). A very rare cause of hypertension is a tumor of the adrenal gland known as pheochromocytoma, which secretes excessive quantities of norepinephrine and epinephrine. Elevations of blood pressure are often episodic. Accompanying symptoms of excessive catecholamines include acute pounding headache, tachycardia, and sweating. Administration of oral contraceptives can rarely cause hypertension. Estrogens increase hepatic synthesis of renin substrate and angiotensin-I. The hypertension reverts to normal when the oral contraceptives are discontinued.

Coarctation of the aorta is a congenital malformation of the aorta exulting in a narrow area in the aorta, usually in the arch, Alterations in hemodynamics lead to a decreased renal blood flow, which activates the renin-angiotensin system.

PULMONARY DISEASES

Normal Physiology

Respiration involves all the processes in the transfer of oxygen from the air to the mitochondria of cells and of carbon dioxide from the cells back to the air. Four major steps are involved in respiration: ventilation, alveolar diffusion, transport, and tissue diffusion.

Ventilation is the functioning of the lungs to move air in and out to maintain the appropriate concentrations of oxygen and carbon dioxide in the alveoli. The process of ventilation requires proper functioning of the respiratory center in the brainstem, the peripheral nerves to the muscles, the muscles such as the diaphragm, the intercostals, the abdominals and others, and the lungs themselves. Spirometry is a technique that is used to measure the ventilatory functioning of the lungs.

For purposes of measuring lung function, the lung is divided arbitrarily into various volumes and capacities. Tidal Volume (TV) is the amount of air moved in and out of the lungs during a normal breath. The amount of air remaining in the lungs after a maximal exhalation is called the Residual Volume (RV). The level to which the lung volumes return after a normal breath is called the Functional Residual Capacity (FRC). If one takes a maximal inspiration, filling the lungs with as much air (or gases) as possible, one then reaches the Total Lung Capacity (TLC). The Vital Capacity (VC) is the maximum amount of air that can be exhaled following a maximal inspiration. The VC represents the ability of the subject to change the size of the thoracic cavity; ie, the bellows function of the lung. Age, sex, size, and disease may affect the vital capacity. When the vital capacity is forcibly exhaled, the measurement is called the Forced Vital Capacity (FVC). The rate of exhaling the FVC is measured at time intervals, ie, Forced Expiratory Volume in one second (FEV_1), FEV_2, etc. The volume exhaled during the timed interval may be expressed as percentage of the vital capacity (FEV_1/FVC). This value is useful in assessing the severity of obstructive airway disease. The measurement of the airflow during the middle 50% of the VC is relatively independent of patient effort and is useful in determining the mechanical properties of the lung. This is called the Forced Expiratory Flow (FEF) from 25% to 75% of the VC, (FEV25–75%). This measurement is a sensitive spirometric measurement for the detection of early obstructive lung disease.

Each breath contains a portion of air that does not come in contact with a gas-exchanging membrane, such as the air in the large conducting airways. This is called dead space. The larger the dead space, the smaller the proportion of each breath which reaches a gas exchanging membrane and this affects the alveolar and arterial content of oxygen (O_2) and carbon dioxide (CO_2). In a steady state, the amount of CO_2 eliminated from the lung per minute is equal to the amount of CO_2 produced by the body. Since the partial pressure of CO_2 in the artery ($PaCO_2$) is almost equal to the partial pressure of CO_2 in the alveoli ($PACO_2$), the measurement of $PaCO_2$ assesses the adequacy of alveolar ventilation. An elevated $PaCO_2$ (>42 mmHg) means alveolar hypoventilation and a decreased $PaCO_2$ means alveolar hyperventilation.

Alveolar Diffusion—Gases are exchanged across the alveolar-pulmonary capillary membranes. The ability for this diffusion to occur depends on (1) the surface area of the alveoli, (2) the gradient between the partial pressures of gases in the alveoli and those in the blood, (3) the condition of the membranes, and (4) the amount of hemoglobin in the red blood cells. When a person breathes 100% oxygen, the gradient between the partial pressure of O_2 in the alveoli and that in the blood is so great the oxygen reaches the blood very rapidly regardless of reduction in surface area, changes in diffusion, or decreases in hemoglobin concentration. Under normal circumstances, the partial pressure of oxygen in the arteries (PaO_2) approximates the partial pressure of oxygen in the alveolus (PAO_2). The difference in these measurements, the alveolar-arterial oxygen gradient ($P(A-a)O_2$) is a measurement of the efficiency of the lungs in transferring oxygen into the blood. A normal $P(A-a)O_2$ is 10 to 15 mmHg in young people. This value increases with age.

Transport in the Blood—The maximum amount of oxygen that the blood can carry is called oxygen capacity and is determined by the amount of hemoglobin in the blood. One gram of hemoglobin can carry 1.39 ml of oxygen. The presence of hemoglobin increases the oxygen-carrying capacity of the blood by 30- to 100-fold. Normally 97% of the oxygen is carried bound to hemoglobin. The actual amount of oxygen carried, which is usually less than the oxygen capacity, is the oxygen content. The oxyhemoglobin saturation (SaO_2) is the O_2 content divided into O_2-carrying capacity × 100 and is expressed as a percentage. The oxygen content can be calculated from the oxygen saturation and the hemoglobin content. The best measurement of tissue oxygenation is O_2 delivery, which is the product of cardiac output and O_2 content. A patient with normal lungs but with extremely low hemoglobin would have a normal PaO_2 because the amount of O_2 dissolved in the plasma would be normal but the blood actually would be carrying little O_2 to the tissues because of the decreased carrying capacity. Also, the oxygen-carrying capacity of hemoglobin may be affected by physiological conditions that change the pH or temperature of the blood.

Hypoxemia

This refers to decreased amounts of oxygen in the arterial blood. There are five general mechanisms for its development.

Low Inspired-Oxygen Tension—This is not a disease but the result of the person breathing air that has less than the normal amount of oxygen. Such conditions exist at high altitudes and in some deep mines where methane may replace oxygen. As long as the lungs are normal, the $P(A-a)O_2$ will be normal. Ventilation remains normal or may be increased so the elimination of CO_2 is normal or increased.

Primary Hypoventilation—This condition occurs when the lungs no longer move air in and out to maintain appropriate concentrations of gases. The lungs themselves may or may not be normal. Primary hypoventilation may be caused by abnormalities in the respiratory centers, the peripheral nerves to the muscles, the muscles of respiration, or the chest wall. If the lungs are normal, the PaO_2 will be essentially normal but the $PaCO_2$ will be increased indicating inadequate alveolar ventilation. Drugs suppressing the ventilation centers are probably the most-common cause of primary hypoventilation.

Mismatching of Ventilation to Perfusion (V/Q Abnormalities)—If each alveolus were perfused with the appropriate amount of blood for maximum gas exchange, the ventilation-to-perfusion ratio would equal one. Normally, in the erect position, there is excess ventilation to perfusion in the apices of the lung and excess perfusion to ventilation at the lung bases. At the apex V/Q = 3 and at the bases V/Q = 0.6. In normal individuals the overall V/Q = 0.8. Airflow obstruction decreases ventilation while perfusion remains unchanged. In this situation the V/Q ratio is less than normal. If blood flow to an area is restricted while ventilation remains normal, the V/Q ratio is very high. When no ventilation is present but perfusion is normal, V/Q = 0; this is defined as a true shunt. When there is no perfusion but ventilation is normal, V/Q = ∞ _, this is defined as dead space. High V/Q ratios do not decrease the PaO_2 as ventilation is more than adequate to supply O_2 to the capillaries, which have decreased blood flow. However, low V/Q ratios do characterize hypoxemia, as ventilation is inadequate to oxygenate the relatively increased blood flow to that area. V/Q mismatching, which is the most common cause of hypoxemia, may be corrected by allowing the patient to breathe 100% oxygen for 10 to 15 minutes. This is because replacing nitrogen (which is normally 79% of the gas in the alveolus) with oxygen raises alveolar PO_2. Also V/Q mismatching results in an increased $P(A-a)O_2$. Low V/Q ratios, which occur normally at the lung bases, probably account for much of the normal $P(A-a)O_2$. Chronic bronchitis, emphysema, asthma, and many other lung diseases cause hypoxemia by affecting ventilation and lowering the V/Q ratios in many areas of the lung.

True Right-to-Left Shunting—This occurs when venous blood goes from the right heart through the pulmonary circulation without contacting a gas-exchanging surface (ventilated alveolus). Such a situation exists in pulmonary arteriovenous malformations where the pulmonary capillaries are bypassed, in the adult respiratory distress syndrome, in atelectasis where alveoli are airless, and in pneumonia and pulmonary edema where the air in the alveoli is replaced by fluid. Since the blood is not in contact with an alveolar membrane that can exchange oxygen, breathing 100% oxygen will not correct hypoxemia that results from right-to-left shunting.

Diffusion Defects—Diffusion defects are caused by thickened alveolar membranes. This is not a cause of significant hypoxemia in a resting patient but probably does play a role during exercise. Breathing 100% oxygen may increase the gradient across the alveolar membrane sufficiently to overcome a diffusion defect.

Airflow Obstructive Disease

Obstructive disorders, the most common diseases of the lungs, are characterized by an increase in airway resistance. Alterations in resistance may be acute or chronic, reversible or irreversible.

CHRONIC BRONCHITIS—Chronic bronchitis is a disease associated with excessive tracheobronchial mucus production sufficient to cause daily cough with expectoration of sputum for at least 3 months/year for 2 consecutive years. Chronic bronchitis is a clinical diagnosis that is made after other pulmonary diseases are excluded. Emphysema is defined as distention of the airspaces distal to the terminal bronchioles with destruction of the alveolar septa. The diagnosis of emphysema is based on anatomical alterations and frequently is made at autopsy. However, the entity can be considered to be present on the basis of certain physiological studies. These two diseases, although distinct processes, are often present simultaneously.

Etiology—The etiologies of these diseases have not been delineated clearly, although a variety of host and environmental factors have been implicated. Respiratory infections with viruses, *Mycoplasma*, and bacteria may play a role in the development of chronic bronchitis. Cigarette smoking correlates with the prevalence and severity of chronic bronchitis and emphysema and is by far the most common cause. Currently, these diseases occur more commonly in males over 35 years, although the incidence in females is increasing, paralleling the increase in cigarette smoking by women. Air pollution has been incriminated in the etiology of both chronic bronchitis and emphysema. Also, people who work in occupations associated with dusts and noxious gases have a higher incidence of chronic bronchitis. The hereditary deficiency of the enzyme alpha-1-antitrypsin is associated with the development of severe emphysema relatively early in life in both men and women.

Pathology—Chronic bronchitis is associated with hyperplasia and hypertrophy of the mucus-producing glands in the large airways. In the small airways, there is goblet-cell hyperplasia, mucosal and submucosal inflammation and edema, peribronchial fibrosis, and intraluminal mucus plugs. Ciliated cells are lost. Emphysema is classified according to the pattern of involvement distal to the terminal bronchioles. Centrilobular or centroacinar emphysema involves the respiratory bronchioles. Panacinar emphysema involves the respiratory bronchioles, the alveolar ducts, the alveoli, and their blood supply. Both forms of emphysema often occur in a single patient, although one form may predominate.

Pathophysiology—Both chronic bronchitis and emphysema can exist without clinically significant airflow obstruction. However, using sophisticated pulmonary function testing, early disease can be detected in young smokers. Both diseases result in narrowing of the airways with increased airway resistance and decreased FEF rates. Due to the altered pressure-airflow relationships, the work of breathing is increased in chronic bronchitis and emphysema. In both diseases, the TLC and RV are increased. The hypoxemia results from ventilation to perfusion mismatching. The $PaCO_2$ may be normal, be decreased because of hyperventilation, or be elevated in severe disease or during an acute exacerbation. The chronic hypoxia leads to pulmonary vascular constriction and pulmonary artery hypertension. The chronic increased afterload on the right heart ultimately leads to right heart failure (cor pulmonale). Other sequelae of severe hypoxemia include polycythemia and alteration of the patient's mental status

Symptoms and Signs—Dyspnea on exertion and functional disability result from severe airway obstruction with its increased work of breathing.

PREDOMINANT EMPHYSEMA—These patients have a long history of exertional dyspnea with little cough or sputum production. The typical patient is thin, uses accessory muscles to breathe, is tachypneic, with prolonged expiration through pursed lips, frequently leans forward when sitting, has a hyperresonant percussion note, and has diminished breath sounds by auscultation. The chest radiograph reveals low and flattened diaphragms and signs of hyperinflation. The clinical course is progressive, severe dyspnea for which little can be done. Resting blood gases become abnormal late in the course of the disease.

PREDOMINANT BRONCHITIS ALONG WITH EMPHYSEMA—The typical patient has an impressive history of cough and sputum production for many years. Acute exacerbations increase in frequency, duration, and severity over the years. After each episode, the patient's baseline status may have deteriorated slightly. The presenting complaints may include cough, sputum production, exertional dyspnea, or peripheral edema secondary to right heart failure. This patient is usually overweight, cyanotic, and only slightly tachypneic. On auscultation coarse rhonchi and wheezes may be heard throughout the lung fields. Arterial blood gas analysis reveals hypoxia and hypercapnia. The VC is normal or only slightly decreased while the FEF rates are low. Some of these patients develop emphysema with the resultant symptoms. A patient with chronic bronchitis may experience many episodes of acute respiratory failure usually precipitated by a respiratory tract infection.

Reversible Airway Obstruction

BRONCHIAL ASTHMA OR REACTIVE AIRWAYS DISEASE—This is defined as a disease characterized by increased responsiveness of the trachea, bronchi, and bronchioles to various stimuli and is manifested by widespread narrowing of the airways that changes in severity either spontaneously or as a result of therapy.

Etiology and Epidemiology—Asthma affects at least 2% of the population. About one-half of the cases develop before age 10 and another third develop before age 40. Childhood asthma occurs in males predominantly (2:1), but after age 30 there is no sex difference.

Because of the diversity of the disease, the classification of asthma is difficult. Allergic or extrinsic asthma usually is found in individuals with a history or a family history of atopy or allergic diseases such as rhinitis, urticaria, and eczema. Allergic asthma, which accounts for 25% of the cases, tends to be seasonal and occurs more commonly in children and young adults. Nonseasonal allergic asthma may be due to antigens such as animal dander, molds, and dust. In another group of patients, ingestion of aspirin or nonsteroidal anti-inflammatory agents may aggravate the asthma. Asthma also may occur during times of heavy industrial air pollution, physical exercise, or emotional upset. Pulmonary infections, congestive heart failure, pulmonary embolism, and treatment with cholinergic agents or beta-adrenergic blockers may also provoke asthma. Asthma that occurs without an identifiable cause is labeled intrinsic or idiosyncratic.

Pathology—The hallmarks of acute asthma are over distention of the lungs, gelatinous plugs in the bronchioles, hypertrophy of the bronchial smooth muscle, mucosal edema, denudation of the surface epithelium, pronounced thickening of the basement membranes, and infiltration of the bronchial wall with inflammatory cells, particularly eosinophils and mast cells. Emphysematous changes are usually absent.

Pathophysiology—In those with allergic asthma, bronchoconstriction and alterations in bronchial secretions are the result of an immediate hypersensitivity reaction. In this response the interaction of antigen and antibody, particularly IgE, causes the release of chemical mediators from sensitized mast cells in the lungs. The mediators include histamine, leukotrienes, platelet-activating factor, eosinophil chemotactic factor of anaphylaxis (ECF-A), and neutrophil chemotactic factor of anaphylaxis (NCF-A). Secondary mediators include prostaglandins and bradykinin. These mediators constrict bronchial smooth muscle and increase vascular permeability.

Adenylate cyclase catalyzes the formation of the cyclic nucleotide, cyclic 3′,5′-adenosine monophosphate (cyclic AMP; cAMP), from adenosine triphosphate (ATP). cAMP is an intracellular mediator that inhibits the release of the chemical mediators. An increase in the concentration of cAMP causes relaxation of bronchial smooth muscle. It is thought that bronchoconstriction in asthmatics might result from a defect in cAMP as a result of nonresponsiveness to endogenous catecholamines due to downregulation of receptors. Catecholamines stimulate adenyl cyclase to increase the intracellular concentration of cAMP.

A second cyclic nucleotide, cyclic 3′,5′-guanosine monophosphate (cyclic GMP; cGMP), opposes the action of cAMP. Actions that are facilitated by cAMP are suppressed by cGMP and vice versa. cGMP promotes the release of bronchoconstrictor substances from mast cells. Guanylate cyclase catalyzes the synthesis of cGMP in response to stimulation by acetylcholine.

Symptoms and Signs—Symptoms include dyspnea, chest tightness, cough, and wheezing. Some patients with asthma do not wheeze and may have only dyspnea and/or cough. The symptoms are episodic and frequently occur at night. In asthma, the contraction of bronchial smooth muscle and the presence of mucosal edema and thick, tenacious mucus result in airflow obstruction. Hypoxemia is present during an acute severe attack. Blood-gas analysis usually shows decreased $PaCO_2$ and respiratory alkalosis. Normal or elevated levels of carbon dioxide during an acute episode should be viewed as impending respiratory failure. Clinical symptoms and signs are unreliable for judging tissue oxygenation. When severe symptoms persist for days or weeks, or fail to respond to basic therapy, the condition is known as status asthmaticus. Eosinophilia in sputum and blood suggests but is not specific for asthma. The chest radiograph shows hyperinflation and is not diagnostic.

Restrictive Lung Disease

This is a general term applied to a wide spectrum of diseases with a decrease in total lung capacity. In advanced cases, other lung volume components also are reduced. Most patients with restrictive lung diseases have intrinsic structural and functional abnormalities of the lung, which cause a stiff lung. Stiffness of the lungs is defined by a decrease in lung compliance or change in lung volume per unit change in pressure. A few of patients have normal lungs but have reduced lung volumes because of abnormalities of the chest wall, pleura, or abdomen.

Pathology—Although some restrictive lung diseases have unique pathology, many have similar nonspecific end-stage changes. Such changes may include pulmonary fibrosis of the alveolar septa, peribronchiolar fibrosis, mononuclear inflammatory cell infiltrate, smooth muscle proliferation within the interstitium, metaplasia of the alveolar lining cells, and vascular obliteration with pulmonary hypertension.

Etiology—Restrictive lung disease may be acute or chronic. An example of an acute, reversible restrictive lung disease is pulmonary edema. Chronic restrictive lung diseases are diverse. In asbestosis, hypersensitivity pneumonitis, drug- or toxin-induced lung injury, the etiology is known, as it is for lung disease associated with sarcoid, collagen vascular disease, or other well-defined systemic illnesses. In pulmonary alveolar proteinosis, desquamative interstitial pneumonitis (DIP), and idiopathic pulmonary fibrosis, the cause is not known.

Symptoms and Signs—The hallmark of all restrictive lung diseases is dyspnea, a sensation of shortness of breath. This results from the increased work of breathing caused by stiff lungs. In addition, airflow resistance is increased because patients breathe at low lung volumes, which allows small airways to close. Tachypnea and a nonproductive cough are common findings. Although fine crackles may be heard, auscultatory findings are usually minimal compared to the degree of pathological changes. Patients with extensive fibrosis may experience recurrent pneumothorax. Pulmonary hypertension advancing to cor pulmonale may be seen as a late sequel. This complication is caused either by obliteration of the pulmonary vascular bed or by increased pulmonary resistance due to hypoxemia.

The chest x-ray in restrictive lung diseases may show decreased lung volumes and increased interstitial markings. Arterial blood gases often reveal hypoxemia and hypocapnia.

Abnormalities on physiological testing include an increased alveolar-arterial oxygen gradient and a decreased diffusion capacity.

Adult Respiratory Distress Syndrome

This syndrome (ARDS) is a common cause of acute respiratory failure in a hospitalized patient. Its hallmark is damage to the pulmonary capillaries and alveolar epithelium leading to increased permeability and acute pulmonary edema. The etiology of this syndrome is multiple and includes shock, infection, near drowning, drug and toxin exposure, acute pancreatitis, and aspiration pneumonia. Despite the wide spectrum of diseases that may lead to ARDS, there is a similar clinical picture in all cases. Acute respiratory failure is accompanied by a diffuse infiltrate on chest x-ray and physiological disturbances of restrictive lung disease. On pathology there is edema, hemorrhage, hyaline membranes, inflammatory cells, and fibrosis.

Deep Venous Thrombosis and Pulmonary Embolism

Both deep venous thrombosis (DVT) and pulmonary embolism (PE) are significant causes of mortality and morbidity. Together they form a spectrum referred to as venous thromboembolism (VTE). The most important factor for decreasing morbidity and mortality is the prevention of DVT.

Normal Anatomy and Physiology—Veins are thin-walled vessels composed mainly of collagen with some smooth muscle and little elastic tissue. They normally contain a large proportion of the circulating blood but at significantly lower pressures than arteries. The venous system of the lower extremities is composed of the deep, superficial and communicating veins.

Blood return from lower extremities depends on the contraction of skeletal muscles, especially in the calves. Valves prevent retrograde flow of blood in the veins. These valves are present even in very small and their number decreases in the proximal veins. Valves are composed of elastic and collagen tissue and operate passively in response to pressure changes.

The lung has two arterial blood supplies. The pulmonary artery exits from the right ventricle, immediately divides into the right and left branches, and carries deoxygenated blood from the systemic venous system to the lungs for gas exchange. The bronchial arteries branch off the aorta and carry oxygenated blood to the supporting tissue of the lung.

Normally, clots do not form within the vascular system. The smooth endothelial surface of the blood vessels and a negatively charged protein layer on the endothelial surface that repels platelets are probably the most important factors in preventing clot formation. Two factors prevent excessive clotting. Approximately 85% of the thrombin formed is adsorbed to the fibrin threads, which prevents the spread of the thrombin. The remaining thrombin is inactivated in 20 min by combining with antithrombin III.

Plasma normally contains a protein called plasminogen which, when activated, forms plasmin. Plasmin is a proteolytic enzyme that digests fibrin, fibrinogen, prothrombin, and Factors V, VIII, and XII. The process that activates plasminogen is understood poorly. Plasminogen is incorporated in all blood clots and is involved in dissolution of intravascular clots.

Epidemiology—It is difficult to estimate the incidence of DVT. The incidence of PE has been estimated as high as 500,000 cases/year and is the cause of at least 50,000 deaths/year in the US. On autopsy, PE is found in 20 to 25% of deaths in general hospitals, 25% of deaths in nursing homes and as many as 50% of deaths due to congestive heart failure. The risk of VTE is increased markedly in individuals over 40 years. It is postulated that the diagnosis of PE is missed frequently in elderly chronically ill patients.

Etiology—A number of conditions and situations have been associated with increased risk of VTE. These include prolonged bed rest, immobilization, cancers (particularly adenocarcinomas of the pancreas, lungs, or prostate), polycythemia vera, congestive heart failure, administration of estrogens, the postpartum state, orthopedic injuries, major surgery, trauma, chemical irritations, and infections. Approximately 85% of pulmonary embolic episodes are caused by DVT.

Pathophysiology—Over 100 years ago, Virchow described three factors that promote venous thrombosis: stasis, hypercoagulability, and vessel wall factors. Increased platelet adhesiveness and aggregation also may be involved.

Stasis occurs at various sites in veins. The edges of the valves cause turbulent blood flow with eddy formation and stasis. Areas adjacent to the valves and the junctions of tributaries also are areas of stasis. Dilated veins (varicose veins) or previously damaged veins may have sluggish flow and incompetent valves. Lack of pumping of the blood in the veins by skeletal muscle contraction or compression of the veins by the muscle mass may explain the increased risk of DVT during bed rest or immobilization, and part of the increased risk during surgery. In polycythemia vera the blood is viscous and prone to stasis. Congestive heart failure also may increase the stasis of blood in the lower limbs. The stasis may allow the activation of factors as well as inhibit the dilution or removal of activated factors.

Various risk factors for VTE are associated with hypercoagulable states. Cancers are thought to increase production of Factors V, VIII, IX, and XI, release tissue thromboplastin from necrotic tumor, and decrease the efficiency of the fibrinolytic system. Trauma and surgery may increase plasma concentration of fibrinogen and procoagulants, increase platelet adhesiveness, and decrease fibrinolysis. Estrogens increase the production of Factors I, II, VIII, IX, and X, increase platelet adhesiveness, and decrease the activity of antithrombin III. Estrogens also dilate veins and promote stasis. Congenital abnormalities of the coagulation cascade predispose strongly to VTE, often recurrent. These include the Factor V Leiden mutation, the prothrombin 20201A mutation, and congenital deficiencies of protein C and protein S.

Increasing age predisposes individuals to thrombosis because of increased stasis caused by venous dilatation, malfunction of venous valves, decreased skeletal muscle mass, decreased physical activity, and decreased cardiac output. Increased Factor VIII and decreased antithrombin III activity enhance coagulation.

If the vessel wall is disrupted, collagen is exposed and/or tissue thromboplastin is released. Exposed collagen and the extrinsic system activate the intrinsic coagulation system via tissue thromboplastin. Platelets adhere to the exposed collagen, aggregate to form a platelet plug and release platelet Factor III. Platelet Factor III is similar to tissue thromboplastin in that it initiates the extrinsic coagulation system. Platelet Factor III also can activate Factors VIII, IX, XI, and XII. The end product of coagulation is the thrombus, which is composed of fibrin, trapped serum, and blood cells. The clot itself initiates a vicious cycle that promotes more clotting. The clot extends until it reaches an area of faster-flowing blood.

The most-feared form of DVT involves the iliofemoral veins, since thrombi here are most likely to result in large emboli to the lungs.

When an embolus lodges in a pulmonary artery, the area being ventilated but not perfused. The area is now dead space. The alveoli transiently constrict due to hypocapnia. Surfactant is lost and atelectasis develops in 24 to 48 hours. Hypoxemia usually develops. In massive PE, pulmonary hypertension may result and lead to acute right heart failure. Whether lung infarction occurs depends on the size of the embolus and the dual pulmonary blood flow. Many emboli are dissolved quickly by the fibrinolytic system. Recanalization may occur in 1 week. Some vessels, however, remain totally occluded with resultant loss of lung function.

Symptoms and Signs—DVT may present as swelling of the calf or thigh with edema of the lower extremity. The area over the thrombosis may be tender, warm, and erythematous. The thrombosed vein may be felt as a hard cord. Physical maneuvers of the limb or walking may worsen the pain. However, in many cases of DVT no symptoms or signs are present. More than 50% of patients with symptoms and signs normally attributed to DVT do not have VTE. The diagnosis of DVT is made conclusively by phlebography, but this invasive test is difficult to obtain quickly, is painful, and may cause phlebitis. Noninvasive evaluation is most practically carried out with Doppler flow studies. Elevated plasma levels of D-dimer are suggestive of VTE, and this test is becoming increasingly used. DVT can lead to PE, the postphlebitic syndrome (edema, pain, increased pigmentation, eczema, induration, and ulceration) or recurrence of DVT.

The symptoms and signs of PE depend on the size of the embolus and the presence of infarction. The classic presentation of PE is the sudden onset of dyspnea. If infarction occurs, pleuritic chest pain and hemoptysis also may be present. Hypoxemia and an increased alveolar-arterial oxygen gradient may be seen. Physical examination may or may not demonstrate the signs of DVT. Crackles, local wheezes, and a pleural friction rub may be heard on auscultation. Tachycardia and tachypnea are seen. Signs of acute right heart failure can be seen in massive PE. However, the physical examination may be completely normal. Laboratory examination is not diagnostic. The chest radiograph is often normal but may show a pleural effusion and/or infiltrate and/or changes in size or disappearance of blood vessels. A ventilation perfusion scan may give presumptive evidence for the diagnosis of PE. The test is associated with false negatives if the area involved is small or false positives if other lung diseases are present. Pulmonary arteriography is the most accurate method used to diagnose PE. CT angiography is somewhat more specific than ventilation-perfusion scanning and may even replace pulmonary angiography when the findings are definite.

Cystic Fibrosis

This is a disease with diverse clinical manifestations characterized by abnormal exocrine gland secretions. It presents in childhood; with improved methods of detection in mild cases and better treatment, more adults are followed now for this disease.

Etiology and Epidemiology—Cystic fibrosis is an autosomal recessive disease carried by a gene on the long arm of chromosome 7 that codes for cystic fibrosis transmembrane regulatory protein (CFTR), a protein with a predicted molecular weight of 170 kD. There is one common mutation, the Δ508 mutation, accounting for 70% of mutations, and over 1000 less common ones. Cystic fibrosis affects both sexes equally and occurs predominantly in Caucasians. In the past, cystic fibrosis was considered a fatal disease of childhood. With better techniques for earlier detection and improved methods of treatment, the median life expectancy has risen to 32 years.

Pathophysiology—Defects in CFTR protein, the chloride channel in the membrane of epithelial cells, impair cAMP-dependent chloride secretion by respiratory epithelium. Epithelial secretions become thick and difficult to clear. The high chloride concentration in secretions impairs bactericidal activity and predisposes to infection, particularly with Pseudomonas.

Symptoms and Signs—The initial manifestation may be intestinal obstruction in the newborn secondary to abnormally thick meconium. Early in life pulmonary complications develop. Thick, tenacious mucus results in bronchial obstruction with subsequent atelectasis and infection. The initial bacterial pathogens, including *S. aureus*, are replaced later by *P. aeruginosa* and other gram-negative organisms. Death in cystic fibrosis is usually due to overwhelming pulmonary infection and respiratory failure. With longer survivals, cor pulmonale and recurrent hemoptysis are seen more frequently.

Pancreatic insufficiency develops in approximately 80% of patients and causes malabsorption characterized by steatorrhea and deficiencies of vitamin B12, and the fat-soluble vitamins. Some patients experience recurrent bouts of pancreatitis. Biliary cirrhosis develops in approximately 10% of patients. The incidence of gallstones is increased. Most male patients are sterile because of a malformation or blockage of the vasa deferentia. Secondary sex characteristics are normal. The fertility rate among females is approximately one-fifth that of a control population. The reason for this is probably the increased viscosity of the cervical mucus.

The best initial diagnostic test is the sweat test. There is usually a 3- to 5-fold increase in the concentration of chloride in the sweat of patients with cystic fibrosis. The level of sweat electrolytes does not correlate with severity of disease. The sweat test is a difficult test to perform correctly and must be obtained in a reliable, experienced laboratory.

GASTROENTEROLOGY

Esophagus

The esophagus is a muscular, hollow tube, which extends from the pharynx to the stomach. Its major function is to transport food from the oropharynx to the stomach. It has a sphincter at both the top and the bottom end. The upper esophageal sphincter maintains a zone of high pressure between the oropharynx and the body of the esophagus. The sphincter pressure increases with respiration and prevents inspired air from entering the gastrointestinal tract. It also acts as a barrier against the regurgitation of esophageal contents into the pharynx. The lower esophageal sphincter (LES) consists of highly specialized muscles, which is tonic in the resting state. It thus maintains a zone of high pressure between the esophagus and stomach. Its major function is to prevent reflux of gastric contents into the esophagus.

The two most specific symptoms of esophageal disease are dysphagia and heartburn. Dysphagia is the sensation of food sticking in the esophagus. It always indicates esophageal disease. Dysphagia may be of two types—to solids only, indicating a mechanical disorder such as stricture or tumor, or to both solids and liquids, indicating a motility such as diffuse spasm of achalasia. Heartburn refers to a burning discomfort that typically migrates from the abdomen up the retrosternal area of the chest. Less common symptoms are chest pain and odynophagia (painful swallowing and regurgitation).

Normal Physiology—The esophagus is a muscular organ that actively transports food by means of peristaltic waves. Swallowing involves the propulsion of a bolus of food from the oropharynx through the relaxed upper esophageal sphincter. Primary peristaltic waves then transport the bolus through the esophagus and past the LES, which relaxes in response to peristalsis. Secondary peristalsis is the same as primary peristalsis, but is initiated by a bolus of material in the body of the esophagus, such as occurs with the reflux of gastric contents. Tertiary contractions are nonpropulsive, nonperistaltic waves that, for the most part, are pathologic and interfere with normal transport of food through the esophagus. Tertiary contractions are associated with dysphagia to solids and liquids and, in some patients, pain.

The regulation of esophageal function is complex and modulated by the swallowing center in the brain. Afferent impulses from the pharynx and the esophagus are mediated by the vagus nerve. The efferent impulses also are mediated vagally through cholinergic fibers splayed around the esophagus in a myenteric network known as the plexus of Auerbach. The resting tone of the esophageal body is maintained largely by cholinergic stimulation, although sympathetic innervation probably plays some regulatory role. The resting pressure of the LES is maintained by specialized circular, smooth muscle. Relaxation of the LES is mediated by a balanced cholinergic-adrenergic stimulated release of noncholinergic, nonadrenergic neurotransmitters. The resting pressure of the LES is modified by a number of factors. Factors known to increase the LES pressure are certain G-I hormones such as gastrin; foods such as a protein meal; drugs such as bethanechol, metoclopramide, erythromycin, cisapride, and domperidone; and increased gastric pH that occurs with eating. Factors known to decrease LES pressure are the GI hormones secretin and cholecystokinin; foods such as fat; certain drugs such as caffeine, alcohol, anticholinergics, calcium channel blockers, and theophylline; and a decreased gastric pH that occurs with fasting.

DISEASES OF THE ESOPHAGUS

GASTROESOPHAGEAL REFLUX DISEASE—

Pathophysiology—This is the most common disorder of the esophagus and refers to the reflux of gastric content into the esophagus with subsequent injury to the esophageal mucosa. Gastroesophageal reflux disease (GERD) is caused, in most people, by an incompetent LES such that either the resting pressure (normally 12 to 20 mmHg) is decreased or, more commonly, the LES relaxes inappropriately allowing gastric contents to reflux into the esophagus. The gastric contents (primarily acid and to some extent bile) then damage the squamous epithelium of the esophagus. In some patients, a defect in secondary peristalsis caused by smoking, or a defect in gastric emptying caused by diabetes or a gastric stapling operation, may contribute. Inflammation of the mucosa and thickening of the basal layer of epithelial cells characterize esophagitis. In some patients, erosions and ulcerations may occur. In most patients, a hiatus hernia, a bulging of the stomach into the chest cavity, occurs, but its role in the pathophysiology of GERD is thought to be relatively minor. Nevertheless, it is unusual to see severe GERD in the absence of a hiatus hernia.

Symptoms and Signs—The major symptom of GERD is heartburn, a retrosternal burning pain that migrates up the chest from the epigastrium. It is accompanied sometimes by an acid or bile taste in the back of the throat or a profusion of watery saliva (water brash). Typically' the heartburn is aggravated by overeating, bending, straining, or lying down after eating. Dysphagia may occur with GERD, either secondary to esophageal spasm (causing liquid and solid dysphagia) or due to stricture (causing dysphagia to solids only).

Diagnosis—The diagnosis of GERD depends on the demonstration of esophagitis by endoscopy with biopsy and the demonstration of reflux of acid into the esophagus by direct measurement of pH in the distal esophagus with an esophageal pH probe. The treatment of GERD has two phases: (1) healing the esophageal mucosa, and (2) preventing recurrence. Since the injury is mediated by acid, the hallmark of therapy is acid reduction. This can be achieved with H2 receptor antagonists (cimetidine, famotidine, nizatidine, ranitidine) or proton pump inhibitors (lansoprazole and omeprazole). In general, the proton pump inhibitors (PPIs) are approximately 50% more effective for treating all grades of esophagitis to healing and are thus the treatment of choice. After 8 weeks of therapy, PPIs will heal 90–95% of patients with mild disease and 80–90% of patients with severe disease, while H2RAs heal 50% of patients with mild disease and 20% of patients with severe disease. The prokinetic drugs, metoclopramide and cisapride, despite addressing the underlying problem of lower esophageal sphincter dysfunction, do not have sufficient healing rates, have a narrow therapeutic index and are not FDA approved as primary therapy for GERD.

For most patients (ie, 90%), GERD is a lifetime disease requiring a lifetime of therapy. This can only be achieved with the proton pump inhibitors. Prokinetic drugs, because of their narrow therapeutic index and propensity for tachyphylaxis, have not been shown to maintain healing adequately. The H2RAs, because of tachyphylaxis, also do not maintain healing. To date, the only drugs shown to maintain healing above 80% are full dose proton pump inhibitors—either lansoprazole or omeprazole.

ESOPHAGEAL STRICTURE—Strictures of the esophagus may be benign or malignant. Chronic GERD or the ingestion of toxic materials such as lye usually causes benign strictures. They are manifested anatomically by a symmetric narrowing of the esophagus that can be seen either by barium swallow or esophagoscopy. They are manifested clinically by dysphagia to solids only. Malignant strictures are caused either by esophageal squamous cell carcinoma or adenocarcinoma arising from the stomach or metaplastic columnar epithelium in the esophagus (so-called Barrett's esophagus). Malignant strictures are usually irregular and asymmetric on barium swallow or endoscopy and can be diagnosed by esophageal biopsy. They usually are associated with rapidly worsening dysphagia to solids along with weight loss.

DIFFUSE ESOPHAGEAL SPASM—This is a motility disorder of the esophagus characterized by frequent and severe tertiary contractions. It occurs predominantly in elderly patients, but may be seen secondary to other disorders of the esophagus such as GERD. It is manifested clinically by intermittent dysphagia to solids and liquids and/or chest pain. Swallowing hot or cold drinks frequently precipitates the symptoms. Barium swallow or manometry makes the diagnosis.

ACHALASIA—This is a motility disorder of the esophagus characterized by an increase in lower esophageal sphincter pressure and an absence of primary peristalsis. Pathophysiologically, achalasia is caused by a loss of the myenteric plexus. This may occur as a primary defect of unknown etiology or as a secondary defect due to invasive carcinoma of the lower esophagus or infestation from Trypanosoma cruzi, the cause of Chaga's disease. The diagnosis is made by manometry, which demonstrates an increase in the LES pressure, incomplete relaxation of the LES, and a total absence of primary and secondary peristaltic waves. Tertiary contractions may be seen. There is also a characteristic x-ray appearance with the body of the esophagus dilated and tapering down to a closed esophageal sphincter (so-called "bird beak" appearance). The disorder is seen more commonly in young people in their teens and twenties, but may be seen at any age. The patients typically are afflicted with intermittent dysphagia to solids and liquids. They may have regurgitation in the supine position with choking and coughing from aspiration. Weight loss occurs as the symptoms become more severe and more continuous.

Stomach and Duodenum

The main function of the stomach is to receive ingested food and then present it to the small bowel in tiny particles suitable for digestion and subsequent absorption. The first step in this process is expansion of the stomach (so-called receptive relaxation) to accommodate the ingested liquid and solid food (chyme) without an increase in gastric pressure. The stomach then mixes, emulsifies, acidifies, and meters the chyme into the small bowel. This is achieved through gastric motility. The proximal and distal portions of the stomach have separate and distinct roles in motility. The proximal stomach receives and stores solids and is primarily responsible for the transfer of emulsified foodstuffs from the body of the stomach to the duodenum. The properties that allow this to occur are receptive relaxation (the ability to relax and receive food stuffs without increasing intragastric pressure), accommodation (the ability to distend to a large size without an increase in intragastric pressure), and contraction. The contraction waves of the proximal stomach are slow and sustained. They act to force solid meal components from the proximal to the distal portion of the stomach.

The main function of the distal stomach is to retain and grind foodstuffs and to prevent reflux of duodenal content back into the stomach. The motor activity of the distal stomach is characterized by peristaltic waves sweeping downward toward the pylorus. These contractions are lumen-obliterating such that solid particles are retropelled for further emulsification. Only when the particles are smaller than 1 mm in diameter will they pass into the duodenum. The motor function of the stomach is regulated largely by the vagus nerve.

The stomach also has a major secretory function. It secretes acid, pepsin, and intrinsic factor. The function of gastric acid is not entirely clear, but it does not play a particularly important role in digestion; rather, it seems to function more as a barrier to toxins and bacteria in the environment. It also plays a minor role in pH homeostasis. There are two types of acid secretion-basal and stimulated. Basal acid secretion occurs continuously and independently of external stimuli. It is characterized by a circadian rhythm in which acid secretion is highest from about 10 pm until midnight and lowest from about 4 am until 8 am. This pattern of acid secretion is responsible for one of the characteristic features of peptic ulcer disease, which is nighttime waking with pain when acid secretion is high and unneutralized by food.

Stimulated acid secretion, on the other hand, occurs in response to the sight, smell, and ingestion of food. This acid secretion is stimulated by acetylcholine, the neurotransmitter of the vagus nerve; the hormone gastrin, secreted by G cells in the gastric antrum and histamine, secreted by enterochromafin cells in the wall of the stomach. Acid secretion is turned off by prostaglandin E, somatostatin, and some yet to be identified enterokinase. During most of the day, the food that stimulates acid secretion also neutralizes it, keeping the pH between 4 and 5. However, when the stomach is empty, approximately 2 to 3 hours after eating, the pH again drops and ulcer patients tend to get pain that is relieved by eating or antacids.

The epithelium of the stomach, duodenum, and esophagus is protected from autodigestion by hydrochloric acid by means of a mucosal defense system. The most characteristic feature of this system is the secretion of mucous and bicarbonate. Bicarbonate is secreted by epithelial cells in the stomach and duodenum and is separated from luminal acid by a layer of mucous, which also is secreted by epithelial cells. These cells are largely under the influence of prostaglandin E_1. Thus, the net effect of prostaglandin E_1 is to decrease acid secretion and increase mucosal defense. This is another example of the adaptive or protective effects of prostaglandins in the body.

The function of the duodenum is to receive gastric contents and to mix them with secretions from the pancreas and gallbladder, which serve to digest (pancreatic enzymes) and solubilize (bile) the nutrients received from the stomach.

DISEASES OF THE STOMACH AND DUODENUM—

The major diseases of the stomach and duodenum are gastritis, gastric ulcer, duodenitis, and duodenal ulcer, all of which are in some way related to gastric acid.

PEPTIC ULCER DISEASE—Peptic ulcer disease is a spectrum of diseases consisting of gastritis, gastric ulcer, and duodenal ulcer. They are among the most frequently encountered disorders of the gastrointestinal tract. Common to these disorders as well as gastric cancer is gastritis, an inflammation of the epithelial surface and gastric glands of the stomach. The most common cause of gastritis and thus of ulcer disease and gastric cancer, is *Helicobacter pylori* infection.

Epidemiology—Peptic ulcer disease is on the decline in the developed world, having peaked early in the century, and probably reflecting the improved sanitary conditions that reduce the spread of enteric infections such as H pylori. Nevertheless, the point prevalence is still 1%, and the lifetime incidence 10%.

Symptoms and Signs—The clinical presentation of ulcer disease is characteristic and is a reflection of the pH in the stomach. Thus, the typical burning epigastric pain occurs on an empty stomach, ie, 2–3 hours after eating and is relieved by eating. It also occurs in the late evening and early morning hours when acid secretion is high and the acid is unneutralized by eating. Ulcer disease may also present with its complications of bleeding (manifested by hematemesis, melena, or anemia), obstruction (manifested by early satiety and weight loss), and penetration/perforation (manifested by persistent epigastric pain, back pain, and fever). These are the so-called alarm manifestations of ulcer disease and should always preclude empiric treatment and dictate further work-up.

Pathophysiology—Ulcer disease occurs whenever there is an increase in acid secretion (eg, Zollinger-Ellison syndrome) or a decrease in mucosal defense (eg, non-steroidal anti-inflammatory therapy) or a combination of both (eg, *H pylori* infection). *H pylori* causes approximately 70% of ulcer disease in the developed world and more than 90% of ulcer disease in the undeveloped world. NSAIDs cause 5–10% of duodenal ulcers and 20–25% of gastric ulcers. Twenty to 30% of ulcer disease is idiopathic.

H pylori is a unique organism that is exquisitely well adapted to the gastric environment and, in fact, cannot exist outside an acidified environment. It is a gram-negative, flagellated spirochete. The flagella allow it to burrow through the mucous layer of the stomach and attach to the epithelial surface. It is a facilitative acidophile, meaning it can adjust its cytoplasmic pH to its surrounding environment. It is also microaerophilic making it highly adaptive to the interface of the oxygen-reduced environment of the gastric lumen and the oxygen-enriched environment of the gastric mucosa. Finally, it has the unique enzyme, urease, which splits urea into bicarbonate and ammonia, thus creating an alkalinized ammonia shell to interface with the acidified gastric lumen.

The pathogenesis of *H pylori* ulcer disease is only partially understood. It appears that 70–80% of ulcers are associated with *H pylori*, but that only 10% of *H pylori* infected individuals develop ulcers. Thus, host factors and co-factors are important in the pathogenesis. In general, there appear to be two patterns of infection. The first is characterized by diffuse antral gastritis that leads to increased acid secretion, secondary gastric metaplasia of the duodenum, duodenal ulcer in the gastric metaplasia, and in some patients, formation of lymphomas in the antrum. The second type of infection is a patchy atrophic gastritis involving the antrum and fundus of the stomach. It leads to gastric atrophy, decreased acid secretion, intestinal metaplasia of the stomach followed by gastric ulcer, and in some patients, gastric adenocarcinoma.

In summary, *H pylori* accounts for 70–80% of ulcers, almost 100% of gastric mucosal lymphomas and 90% of gastric cancer. The World Health Organization has classified *H pylori* as a class I (ie, definite) carcinogen and estimates that eradication of *H pylori* would lead to a 90% reduction in gastric cancer worldwide.

Diagnosis—The diagnosis of peptic ulcer disease is best made by endoscopy. Helicobacter infection can be diagnosed by gastric biopsy, a pH color indicator test based on the production of ammonium by urease in Helicobacter-infected patients or by a serum antibody test. A radioisotope test based on the urease reaction has recently been developed. In this test, the patient ingests 14C urea. If urease (ie, H pylori) is present, the urea is converted to ammonium and carbon dioxide with the 14CO2 blown off in the breath. The specificity and sensitivity of this test are both greater than 95%.

The treatment of acid peptic disease is (1) acid reduction to heal the ulcer and relieve symptoms and (2) prevention of recurrence by treating the underlying cause, either NSAIDs or *H pylori*.

Acid reduction may be achieved with H2 receptor antagonists (cimetidine, famotidine, nizatidine, or ranitidine) or proton pump inhibitors (lansoprazole, omeprazole). The proton pump inhibitors are far superior and in the case of *H pylori* disease raise the pH to sufficient levels to improve antibiotic efficacy. Either discontinuing the NSAID or increasing mucosal resistance with the prostaglandin E1 analog, misoprostil can prevent NSAID-induced ulcers. *H pylori* ulcers can be prevented by antibiotic therapy. It should be noted that *H pylori* is an organism of great genetic diversity with a high mutation rate. It is therefore important to use multiple antibiotics. It is also important to keep the gastric pH above 5 in order to create an optimum environmental pH for the antibiotics. This can only be achieved with proton pump inhibitors given twice daily. The most widely used antibiotics are metronidazole, amoxicillin,

and clarithromycin. It should be noted, however, that metronidazole has a 40% drug resistance rate. The best eradication rates at the time of publication have been achieved with lansoprazole (30 mg bid) or omeprazole (40 mg bid) and amoxicillin (1 g bid) and clarithromycin (500 mg bid). This will change as the organism evolves. Development of a prophylactic/therapeutic vaccine is underway.

GASTRIC CANCER—The two major types of gastric cancer are adenocarcinoma and lymphoma, both of which are seen most commonly with *H pylori* infections.

Adenocarcinoma occurs almost exclusively in the presence of gastric atrophy caused by either environmental gastritis (mostly *H pylori*) or autoimmune gastritis (pernicious anemia). It is usually, clinically silent until well advanced at which time patients present with weight loss (96%), pain (70%), vomiting (50%), anorexia (25%), early satiety (10%), hematemesis (10%), or dysphagia. Diagnosis is made by endoscopy with biopsy. The treatment is surgical with a 5-year survival rate of only 5–10%.

Lymphoma is the second most common malignancy in the stomach. The stomach is ordinarily devoid of lymphatic tissue, thus, lymphomas comprise less than 5% of all gastric malignancies. Most lymphomas are derived from mucosa-associated lymphoid tissue (MALT) and are B cell tumors. More than 90% are associated with *H pylori*. They may be associated with abdominal discomfort, nausea, vomiting, weight loss, or hemorrhage. Low-grade tumors regress after *H pylori* eradication. More advanced tumors require surgical resection followed by combined radiation therapy and chemotherapy.

Pancreas

The pancreas is located in the retroperitoneal space at approximately the level of the 2nd and 3rd lumbar vertebrae. The head of the pancreas fits into the C-loop, ie, the second portion of the duodenum. The body extends across the spine behind the stomach, and the tail lies in the hilus of the spleen. The pancreas has both exocrine and endocrine function.

Normal Physiology—The endocrine functions of the pancreas are mediated by hormones secreted by the islets of Langerhans. These cells account for less than 1% of the total mass of the pancreas and are scattered erratically throughout the gland. Within the islets are four distinct types of cells. The beta cells comprise 80% of the islet cell mass and secrete insulin. Alpha cells are found in the periphery of the islets and make up 16% of its mass. They secrete glucagon. Delta cells secrete somatostatin and the newly recognized polypeptide cells secrete yet to be identified products.

Pancreatic exocrine function is mediated by bicarbonate and digestive enzymes secreted into the intestine. Bicarbonate is secreted by the intralobular ductal cells. It provides an appropriate pH environment for pancreatic enzymes and protects the duodenal mucosa from acid from the stomach. There are more than 15 digestive enzymes that have been identified to date. These are produced in the pancreatic acinar cells. The most important are lipase, which cleaves triglycerides to form fatty acids and monoglycerides; amylase, which is responsible for the digestion of complex carbohydrates; and trypsinogen, which activates various protease enzymes that break down complex proteins.

Water and bicarbonate secretion are mediated by secretin, a 27 amino acid peptide secreted by S cells in the upper small intestine. Secretin release is induced by acidification of the duodenum. Pancreatic enzyme release is mediated by cholecystokinin, a 33 amino acid polypeptide release from mucosal cells in the upper small intestine in response to amino acids and triglycerides. Other hormones also are thought to play a role in pancreatic secretion although their precise function is not understood.

DISEASES OF THE PANCREAS

ACUTE PANCREATITIS—Acute pancreatitis is an acute inflammation of the pancreas. Gallstones and alcohol are the most common causes. Hyperlipidemia is an important and increasingly recognized cause of acute pancreatitis. It usually is associated with lipoprotein lipase deficiency and causes the most severe form of acute pancreatitis. Triglyceride levels are generally over 1000 mg/L in these patients. Other causes include trauma, vasculitis, infections (mumps and Coxsackie virus are the most common), spider bites and drugs (azathioprine, steroids, and thiazides are the most common).

The most common symptoms of pancreatitis are pain, nausea, and vomiting. The pain is usually mid-epigastric and bores through to the back. Fever may be present.

The diagnosis of acute pancreatitis is based on the clinical presentation and supported by a marked elevation of serum amylase or lipase. The white count usually is elevated, and mild jaundice may be present. X-rays of the abdomen usually show a dilated loop of bowel (so-called sentinel loop) near the pancreas. CT scan shows swelling of the pancreas.

Treatment of acute pancreatitis is supportive. Intravenous fluids are required. Nasogastric suction may be necessary to decrease nausea and vomiting. Pain is alleviated with narcotics. When patients are infected, antibiotics are given.

CHRONIC PANCREATITIS—Chronic pancreatitis is a chronic, relapsing inflammation of the pancreas that is manifested by recurrent episodes of abdominal pain, steatorrhea, and diabetes. The most important cause is alcoholism. The disease may be insidious in onset and present only with its end-stage manifestations of steatorrhea and diabetes. Bulky, foul-smelling, light-colored stools characterize steatorrhea. Malnutrition ensues from fat malabsorption, negative nitrogen balance, and diabetes. Malnutrition may be associated with weakness, anorexia, and signs of specific nutritional deficiencies. These include pathological bone fractures from vitamin D deficiency, bruising, and bleeding from vitamin K deficiency, night blindness from vitamin A deficiency, and muscle wasting and edema from protein deficiency. Pain may be a prominent feature of the disease. The treatment of chronic pancreatitis is directed toward the prevention of malnutrition and, if present, the relief of pain. Nutrition is restored with the use of good diet and pancreatic replacement enzymes. Pain management is very difficult in these patients because many are addicted. Narcotics should be avoided. There is evidence that pancreatic enzyme replacement relieves pain in some patients.

PANCREATIC TUMORS—There are two major types of pancreatic tumors: adenocarcinomas arising from ductular epithelium and islet cell tumors arising from cells in the islets of Langerhans. Adenocarcinoma of the pancreas is usually insidious in onset with nonspecific symptoms such as weight loss, mild abdominal pain, and back pain. Jaundice due to obstruction of the common bile duct ultimately ensues. Occasionally, systemic manifestations such as migratory thrombophlebitis, erythema multiforme, thrombocytosis, and fever of unknown origin occur. Pancreatic adenocarcinoma is almost invariably incurable at the time of diagnosis.

Patients with islet cell tumors frequently exhibit symptoms and signs related to the tumor secretory products. For example, hyperinsulinemia may produce hyperphagia, weight gain, and mental changes. Hypergastrinemia may be associated with aggressive ulcer disease. These tumors are frequently difficult to locate, often eluding CT scan and angiography. They are diagnosed most commonly based on the clinical history and measurement of their secretory products.

CYSTIC FIBROSIS—Cystic fibrosis is an inherited, autosomal recessive disease seen in about 1 in 1500 to 2000 live births. Severe pulmonary disease predominates, but there are also gastrointestinal manifestations, particularly steatorrhea with malnutrition. (See Respiratory section.)

Colon

The colon, or large bowel, is a 3- to 4-foot long tubular organ. It extends around the periphery of the abdominal cavity. Its primary functions are the reabsorption of water and electrolytes and the storage of feces for evacuation at a convenient time.

Normal Physiology—Approximately 1500 to 2000 ml of liquid chyme reaches the ileocecal valve each day. This is the net volume following ingestion, absorption, and secretion from the upper GI tract. The intestinal bolus empties slowly through the ileocecal valve into the cecum. In the ascending and transverse colon, the ring-like contractions further delay the movement of chyme. Sodium, followed by water, is absorbed actively in this part of the bowel, transforming the chyme into a soft, fecal mass. In the transverse and descending colon, tonic contractions carry the globular mass downstream, often propelling it distances that reach 1/3 the length of the colon. These mass movements frequently occur as part of the gastrocolic reflex after eating. Defecation is initiated by distention of the rectum by the fecal mass. If the urge to

defecate is resisted, the stimulus gradually diminishes, and sometimes constipation ensues. The colon's contribution to water balance in the intestine is relatively minor. Approximately 10 L of fluid enters the gut daily. This consists of oral intake of 2 L, saliva of 1 L, gastric juice of 2 L, bile of 1 L, pancreatic juice of 2 L, and jejunal secretions of 2 L. Of this amount, 8 to 9 L are reabsorbed in the small intestine. Another 1 to 2 L is reabsorbed in the colon, leaving 100 to 160 ml to be excreted daily as stool. It follows that the volume of the stool aids in defining the site of bowel dysfunction, which results in diarrhea.

Large-volume diarrhea, ie, greater than 1 L per day, is usually due to a disorder of the small intestine, whereas small-volume diarrhea, consisting of less than 1 L per day, is usually of colonic origin. Diarrhea and constipation are difficult to define because the frequency and volume of defecation varies greatly among individuals and in varying parts of the world depending on the diet. In general, normal bowel activity is defined as between three bowel movements per day and three bowel movements per week.

SYMPTOMS OF DYSFUNCTION

CONSTIPATION—Constipation generally denotes the infrequent or difficult evacuation of feces. It is a symptom of a problem rather than a medical disorder itself. By far the most common cause is irritable bowel syndrome, but it also occurs in association with hypothyroidism, hyperparathyroidism, hypercalcemic states, neurological disorders, and psychiatric disorders and in association with many drugs. Minor episodes of constipation may occur with changes in diet, particularly a decrease in fiber intake, and with alterations in daily routines such as travel and decreased physical activity. It also may occur in disorders of anal function that accompany neuromuscular disorders of the anal area. The law of Laplace ($t = P.r$) describes the important relationship between the tension in the muscle wall (t), the radius of the bowel lumen (r), and the pressure in the lumen (P). It forms the rationale for treatment of constipation with increased fiber. The important point is that increased muscle contraction, particularly in the colon, increases intraluminal pressure and retards the forward movement of feces, thus increasing the contact time for the reabsorption of water and the hardening of the stool. An increased fiber diet increases luminal diameter, thus decreasing intraluminal pressure and allowing more forward flow of the feces. Thus, fiber-containing laxatives form the most physiological basis for relieving constipation.

DIARRHEA—Diarrhea is defined as increased frequency or decreased consistency of bowel movements. It usually is classified as either of small bowel or large bowel origin. Small bowel diarrhea is usually large volume, consisting of large rushes and is associated with periumbilical cramping. Colonic diarrhea is small volume consisting of small spurts and associated with hypogastric cramping. Diarrhea is classified further as osmotic or secretory. Osmotic diarrhea is typically smaller volume, aggravated by eating and partially relieved by fasting. Secretory diarrhea is usually large volume and persists with fasting. It is possible to distinguish osmotic and secretory diarrhea by measuring stool osmolality. However, the logistics of such an examination make it difficult at best and almost routinely inaccurate in most clinical settings.

The major causes of osmotic diarrhea are inflammatory bowel disease, intestinal lactase deficiency, and various infections. The major causes of secretory diarrhea, which is uncommon, are villous adenoma and the various hormonal syndromes from non-GI tumors that secrete peptides that stimulate intestinal water secretion.

DISEASES OF THE COLON

IRRITABLE BOWEL SYNDROME—Irritable bowel syndrome is the most common chronic G-l disorder in the western world affecting close to 20% of those living in the US. It is characterized by intermittent abdominal pain, bloating, complaints of excess gas, food intolerance, and disordered bowel function consisting of either diarrhea or constipation or, most typically, both. The symptoms are thought to be the consequence of altered bowel motility, although specific disorders of motility have not been identified. The pain typically occurs in the lower abdomen or the left- or right-upper quadrant. It is intermittent and often relieved by bowel movement or passage of flatus. It does not awaken the patient at night. When the pain occurs under the left coastal margin, it is known as splenic flexure syndrome, and when it occurs under the right costar mar gin, it is known as hepatic flexure syndrome. The diagnosis is made primarily on the basis of symptoms. It frequently occurs during stressful periods in people s lives or with changes in lifestyle with subsequent alterations in diet, particularly a change to diets that are low in fiber. It also is seen frequently with pharmacologic therapy, especially drugs with anticholinergic activity such as tricyclic antidepressants or major tranquilizers. Patients less than 30 years of age can be treated without diagnostic *workup*, but for those over 30, sigmoidoscopy and microscopic stool exam should be included. It is also important in these patients to rule out intestinal lactase deficiency.

The treatment of irritable bowel syndrome is reassurance, dietary modification to a regular high-fiber diet and fiber supplementation with bulk laxatives. Occasionally, antidepressants are needed for patients who are depressed. It is desirable to avoid antidepressants with anticholinergic activity in such patients.

DIVERTICULOSIS AND DIVERTICULITIS—Diverticula are acquired herniations of the mucosa through the muscular layers of the bowel. Diverticulitis is inflammation in a diverticulum resulting from microperforation. Diverticula may be the ultimate expression of irritable bowel syndrome and are rare before age 35 but present in 40–50% of people over 70. They are most common in the sigmoid colon, which has the highest intraluminal pressure. Diverticula are usually asymptomatic although they occasionally bleed. The treatment of diverticulosis consists of a high-fiber diet as used in the management of irritable bowel syndrome.

Diverticulitis, resulting from a perforation of a diverticulum, occurs in only 10–20% of people with diverticula. It manifests with acute, left lower-quadrant abdominal pain, fever, and constipation. Barium enema or colonoscopy usually makes diagnosis. The treatment of diverticulitis consists of the administration of antibiotics and, initially, a low residue diet consisting of enteral formulas. Once recovery occurs, the treatment is the same as that for diverticulosis.

ULCERATIVE COLITIS—Ulcerative colitis is a chronic disease of unknown etiology. It is an immune-mediated disease, but it is not known what triggers the immune response. The disease occurs predominantly in adults, 20 to 50 years of age, but may be seen at any age. It is more common in women, Caucasians, and Jews and in those who reside in urban settings. It is rare among Africans, Asians, and North American Indians

The pathology of the disease is very characteristic. The mucosa of the rectum and bowel is edematous with a bloody purulent exudate. The rectum is virtually always involved with the disease, having a tendency to spread from the rectum to more proximal areas in a continuous pattern.

Bloody diarrhea is the most characteristic presentation of ulcerative colitis. The stool also may be purulent. Diarrhea with as many as 20 to 30 bowel movements per day is common. Lower abdominal pain, hematochezia, and fever also occur. Laboratory data usually show leukocytosis and anemia. Diagnosis is made by sigmoidoscopy with mucosal biopsy.

The clinical course of ulcerative colitis is variable but intractable. Spontaneous remission does occur but, in general, the course of the disease is one of exacerbations and remissions. It is a lifetime disease. Because of the risk of colon cancer and the superimposition of complications, most patients have a total colectomy within the first 10 years of the onset of disease.

Complications include perforation with peritonitis, toxic megacolon resulting from a dilated functionless bowel, and adenocarcinoma of the colon. The risk of adenocarcinoma increases with age. It is about 2–3% at 10 years and 20–25% after 20 years of disease. The diagnosis of carcinoma in the presence of ulcerative colitis is difficult because the symptoms of ulcerative colitis mask the symptoms of carcinoma. Because of the difficulty in diagnosing colon cancer in patients with ulcerative col-

itis, the diagnosis often is delayed, and the mortality rate is greater than 50%.

Extracolonic manifestations also occur and include erythema nodosum, pyoderma gangrenosum, uveitis, iritis, and a variety of liver diseases including chronic hepatitis and primary sclerosing cholangitis, which, ultimately, usually requires liver transplant.

The treatment of ulcerative colitis consists of drugs that reduce the inflammation. These include corticosteroids, azathioprine, and methotrexate. In addition, intestinally acting preparations of salicylate such as azulfidine, olsalazine, and mesalamine are used. The latter drugs are particularly useful in reducing the frequency of flare-ups of disease. The ultimate treatment, however, is total colectomy with ileo-anal pull through.

CROHN'S DISEASE (GRANULOMATOUS COLITIS)—Crohn's disease is a granulomatous inflammation that affects both the colon and small bowel. When it involves only the colon, it is frequently indistinguishable from ulcerative colitis. Like ulcerative colitis, the etiology is unknown, but immune mechanisms appear to be important. The clinical and laboratory features of Crohn's colitis are indistinguishable from ulcerative colitis. Distinction is made by bowel biopsy, which may show the characteristic granulomatous inflammation. When that inflammation is not present, Crohn's may be indistinguishable from ulcerative colitis for several years. The complications of Crohn's colitis are the same as those for ulcerative colitis.

The medical treatment of Crohn's colitis is the same as that for ulcerative colitis. However, in Crohn's colitis, every effort is made to preserve the colon, since surgery has a tendency to chase the disease up the bowel. Surgery in Crohn's disease is indicated only for complications such as perforation and stricture.

POLYPOID LESIONS OF THE COLON—Colonic polyps are very common. The adenomatous polyp is the most important polyp, affecting more than 20% of the population. Because of the frequency with which it occurs and because it is the precursor of colon cancer, adenomatous polyps are the targets of colon cancer screening.

Colonic adenomatous polyps are seen in 5–15% of the general population over 45 years of age, and prevalence increases with age. Adenomas usually are found during screening examinations for colon cancer, but may also present with symptoms of rectal bleeding, abdominal pain or diarrhea. Most patients with polyps will have 1 to 3, but as many as 50 may be seen. Most are pedunculated and can be removed through the colonoscope by snare electrocautery. Following removal, they tend to recur and thus, follow-up examinations are important.

COLON CANCER—Malignant lesions of the colon include adenocarcinoma, lymphoma, sarcoma, carcinoid tumors, and, rarely, metastatic tumors. However, 95% of colon malignancies are adenocarcinomas. There are approximately 150,000 new cases with 60,000 deaths per year in the US. It is the second most common cause of cancer death in men (following lung) and women (following breast). One in 20 Americans will develop this malignancy. The incidence of colon cancer increases with age and is most common in the seventh decade.

Both environmental and genetic factors have been implicated in the cause of colon cancer. A high incidence has been linked to low dietary fiber intake and high animal fat consumption. An increased prevalence of colon cancer in relatives of colon cancer patients indicates that genetic factors are also important.

Colon cancer may cause blood in the stools, a change in bowel habits, abdominal pain, and/or weight loss. In most patients, however, the symptoms are late. Thus, most cancers are not resectable for cure by the time they become symptomatic. Because of the frequency of colon cancer and its curability when detected early, routine screening is indicated. The current recommendations for screening include yearly rectal exam after age 40, stool Hemoccult testing yearly after age 50, and proctoscopic exam at age 50 and every 3 to 5 years thereafter. Widespread screening has been shown to reduce the death rate from colon cancer.

Liver

The liver is responsible for the synthesis of cholesterol, bile salts, phospholipids and various proteins. It also stores and transforms carbohydrates. A major function of the liver is the detoxification and excretion of exogenous substances.

Amino acids are synthesized by the liver to tissue and plasma proteins, especially albumin. It also synthesizes nonessential amino acids as well as all of the coagulation factors except Factor 8. Glucose is stored in the liver as glycogen. A visible function of the liver is its conjugation of bilirubin, a product of hemoglobin degradation. The liver converts bilirubin to a polar form that can be excreted in bile and to some extent in the urine. Failure to metabolize bilirubin results in jaundice, a yellow discoloration of the skin and sclera that is a common symptom of liver disease.

Virtually all lipid-soluble exogenous substances are metabolized in the liver. This function is carried out largely by hydroxylation by the mixed-function oxidases, followed by conjugation. This process is responsible for most drug metabolism and is at the heart of many drug interactions.

The liver is unique in having two blood supplies. The veins from the GI tract and spleen form the portal vein, which perfuses the liver and normally accounts for about 70% of its blood supply. The liver also receives arterial blood from the hepatic artery. Approximately one-fifth of cardiac output normally flows through the liver.

The liver has a limited number of ways of responding to injury. These include acute hepatitis, chronic hepatitis, and fibrosis and tumor formation. In addition, there are a number of storage diseases of the liver. The remarkable ability of the liver to regenerate spares it from end-organ failure in most of these diseases.

DISEASES OF THE LIVER

ACUTE HEPATITIS—Acute hepatitis is caused by either viruses or toxins. The most important causes of acute hepatitis in the US are hepatitis A, B, and C viruses. The important drugs causing hepatitis are halothane, isoniazid and acetaminophen. The various types of viral hepatitis are compared in Table 56-1.

HEPATITIS A—Hepatitis A virus was first identified in 1973. Type A hepatitis occurs in epidemics, particularly in younger people. There is, however, a disturbing trend toward an increased age of acquisition. This is particularly problematic because hepatitis A virus, while causing a mild, flu-like illness in children, causes a very serious illness in middle-aged and older adults.

In the typical clinical course, a prodrome of malaise, anorexia, headache, mild fever, and alteration of taste occurs 6 to 8 weeks after exposure. Soon after, the patient notices dark urine, light stool, and some right-upper quadrant discomfort. Jaundice may follow after a few days. It is noteworthy that only a small percentage of patients actually become jaundiced; thus, the illness tends to be missed and attributed to flu. While hepatitis A occasionally becomes fulminant and causes death, the overwhelming majority of patients, (ie, greater than 99%) recover without sequelae.

HEPATITIS B—The hepatitis B virus was discovered in the mid 1970s. Hepatitis B virus is a DNA virus that has a tendency to cause chronic disease. The acute illness is indistinguishable from other types of viral hepatitis, but about 10% of patients develop a chronic hepatitis with some of these going on to ultimately develop cirrhosis or hepatocellular carcinoma. The primary mode of transmission throughout the world is vertical (ie, from infected mother to newborn infant), but in the US, the primary modes of transmission are sexual and IV drug abuse.

There is now an effective vaccine for hepatitis B. At present, only people at high risk of acquiring the disease are being vaccinated, but it is hoped that universal vaccination will be underway soon.

HEPATITIS C—Hepatitis C virus is the major cause of transfusion-associated hepatitis, although transfusion is not the major mode of spread. Over 50% of cases are acquired by an unknown mode of transmission. The clinical course of hepatitis C virus is indistinguishable from other forms of viral hepatitis, although it tends to be milder. The most characteristic feature of this illness is its propensity to become chronic. At least 70% of patients who are infected, ultimately developing chronic disease, and about 20% of these ultimately going on to develop liver failure or liver cancer.

There is no vaccine to prevent hepatitis C. There is some evidence, however, that treating the acute illness with alpha-interferon reduces the incidence of chronic disease.

PREVENTION OF VIRAL HEPATITIS

Hepatitis A—Optimum control lies in good general hygiene, safe disposal of feces, and identification of epidemics. Immune serum globulin is effective in preventing or modifying type A hepatitis in over 50% of those exposed. A worrisome feature, however, is that with the declining incidence of hepatitis A in the young population, less and less of the pooled immune specific globulin is effective in preventing hepatitis A. A hepatitis A vaccine has been developed and should be available commercially in the near future.

Table 56-1. Comparison of Types of Hepatitis

FEATURE	A	B	C	D	E
Virus	RNA	DNA	RNA	RNA	RNA
Incubation					
Range (days)	15–50	30–150	15–160	30–150	20–40
Mean (days)	30	75	50		27
Transmission					
Fecal-oral	Yes	No	Min[a]	?	Yes
Household	Yes	Min[a]	Min[a]	?	Yes
Vertical	No	Yes	? Min[a]	?	?
Blood	Rare	Yes	Yes	Yes	No
Sexual	No	Yes	Min[a]	?	?
Carrier state	No	Yes	Yes	Yes	No
Risk of chronic hepatitis	No	10%	70%–90%	Yes	No
Risk of liver cancer	No	Yes	Yes	?	No
Prevention					
Vaccine	Yes	Yes	No	No	No
Immunoglobulin	Yes	Yes	No	No	?
Mortality rate	≈0.15%	≈1%	≈0.5%	High	0.5%–1.5%

[a] Min = minimal.

Hepatitis B—Avoidance of multiple sexual partners and IV drug use is the most useful way of preventing hepatitis B. Hepatitis B immune specific globulin (HBIG) appears to be effective in preventing hepatitis B in about 75% of cases. There is also an effective vaccine for preventing hepatitis B (Energix B or Recombivax BB).

Hepatitis C—There is no known mechanism for preventing hepatitis C. Pooled immune globulin is not effective. There is as yet no vaccine.

Chronic Hepatitis—Chronic hepatitis is the pathological and clinical manifestation of a heterogeneous group of disorders, both genetic and acquired. What they have in common is a chronic inflammatory reaction directed against the hepatocyte. By far the most common causes are hepatitis B and C viruses, which account for 70–80% of cases in most series. Autoimmune chronic hepatitis, Wilson's disease, and drugs account for the remainder. The disorders can be distinguished on the basis of several serological tests. Our understanding of these diseases has evolved largely over the past 20 years and was propelled by the discovery of the hepatitis viruses.

Chronic infection with hepatitis B is the most important worldwide cause of chronic hepatitis. The liver injury results from an inflammatory immune attack against hepatocytes. In most patients, the hepatitis B virus itself is not cytopathic. The infected cells are not eliminated, allowing the attack to continue. In the usual circumstance, the hepatocyte expresses cell surface markers (in this case HBcAg and HLA Class I antigen). Primed lymphocytes then attack the infected hepatocytes. The expression of the HLA markers is stimulated by interferon. There is now considerable evidence that patients with chronic hepatitis B are deficient in interferon and, by inference, unable to express HLA markers that would attract an appropriate lymphocyte response. This deficiency is probably genetic in some populations and acquired in others. The acquired deficiency occurs as a consequence of transfection of chromosome 9 at the site that codes for interferon.

The discovery of interferon deficiency in chronic hepatitis B has led to the successful use of interferon as therapy in some of these patients. Approximately half of the patients respond with a loss of viral replication, a reduction in inflammation and, in some cases, a loss of the markers of hepatitis B infection including HBsAg. In general, patients with aminotransferase enzyme (ALT or AST) levels of 100 to 200, DNA levels of less than 100 and positive HBeAg respond best. The treatment is 5 million units subcutaneously daily for 6 months. At about the 12th or 14th week, one can expect to see a flare-up of the hepatitis. This is a good sign and usually associated with conversion of HBeAg to anti-HBe and loss of viral replication. The response, when obtained, usually is prolonged with a relapse rate of only 2–3% per year.

WILSON'S DISEASE—Wilson's disease is an autosomal recessive disorder of copper metabolism that manifests primarily as either neuropsychiatric disease or liver disease. It has a gene frequency of 1/200 and a disease frequency of 1/30,000. More than 30 different mutations on chromosome 13 have been found. Wilson's disease usually presents prior to age 30, although several patients in their 50s and 60s have been reported. For reasons that are unknown, children tend to have predominantly hepatic involvement while adolescents and adults have the neuropsychiatric manifestations. The hepatic manifestations include fulminant hepatitis, chronic hepatitis, and cirrhosis. Hepatocellular carcinoma is virtually unknown in Wilson's patients. Approximately 25% of patients have evidence of involvement of more than one organ system at the time of diagnosis. The characteristic laboratory features include moderately elevated aminotransferase enzymes (2–5 fold), normal or near normal alkaline phosphatase and absence or near absence of the copper carrier protein, ceruloplasmin. The role of ceruloplasmin in the pathogenesis of Wilson's disease is unknown. The ceruloplasmin gene, however, is on chromosome 3, rather than 13, and thus the deficiency of ceruloplasmin is probably a secondary feature. The underlying pathophysiology, whatever the mechanism, is an inability to excrete biliary copper that accumulates in various tissues leading to the characteristic clinical features consisting of neuropsychiatric changes including behavioral change, psychosis, extrapyramidal signs, and cerebellar or pseudobulbar signs. Corneal rings known as Kayser-Fleischer rings are virtually pathognomonic. However, they are frequently not present in younger patients with liver disease. Other manifestations of Wilson's disease include proximal renal tubular dysfunction, osteopenia, osteoarthropathy, and hemolysis.

The diagnosis is based on finding disturbances in copper metabolism including decreased or absent serum ceruloplasmin, urinary copper excretion of greater than 100 mg per day

and hepatic copper concentration of greater than 250 μg/g of liver tissue.

Untreated Wilson's disease is fatal. The treatment consists of chelation therapy with D-penicillamine and is lifelong. Patients who develop fulminant hepatitis die unless they receive a liver transplant. Patients with chronic hepatitis eventually progress to cirrhosis despite treatment and eventually require liver transplantation.

AUTOIMMUNE CHRONIC HEPATITIS—This is also a heterogeneous group of disorders that can be distinguished on the basis of serological tests. It is not yet known, however, whether the different types of autoimmune hepatitis have different courses or response to treatment. It is less common than chronic hepatitis B or C. The typical clinical features are female predominance, young age, association with autoantibodies and other autoimmune disorders, presence of hyperglobulinemia, and virtually universal response to corticosteroids. It is associated with HLA phenotypes B8 and DR3. Interestingly, patients with either autoimmune or viral chronic hepatitis that is associated with other autoimmune disorders are more likely to be DR4 phenotype. The disease usually is progressive with development of cirrhosis and liver failure within a few years. Corticosteroids greatly improve the prognosis of autoimmune chronic hepatitis. The initial steroid therapy is titered to the serum aminotransferase enzyme levels. Patients should be maintained on low-dose steroids indefinitely after the initial response. Azathioprine may be used for a steroid-sparing effect.

Wilson's disease is a rare cause of chronic hepatitis. It usually occurs before age 30, but several patients in their 50s and 60s have been reported. For reasons that are not known, patients have predominantly either the liver or the neuropsychiatric form of the disease. In children, hepatic involvement tends to dominate, while in adolescents and adults the neuropsychiatric disease tends to dominate. Approximately 25% of patients have evidence of involvement of more than one organ system at the time of diagnosis. The consequence of missing the diagnosis is disastrous with virtually all patients subsequently developing acute liver failure. Patients with Wilson's disease tend to have normal or near-normal serum alkaline phosphatase and alanine (ALA) levels. They also tend to have periportal Mallory's hyaline on liver biopsy, unlike other forms of chronic active hepatitis (CAI1). Early intervention with chelation therapy (D-penicillamine) leads to stabilization and improvement in the liver disease. Development of fulminant hepatic failure is always fatal and an indication for emergency liver transplantation.

The final cause of chronic hepatitis among the major categories is drug-induced. A number of drugs have been reported including methyldopa, nitrofurantoin, isoniazid, ketoconazole, and acetaminophen Women appear to be more susceptible, and there is frequently a background of autoimmune disease. The clinical presentation mimics autoimmune chronic hepatitis. The treatment is drug withdrawal.

CIRRHOSIS—Cirrhosis (Gk, kirrhos = yellow) is defined as a diffuse increase in fibrous tissue within the liver plus the presence of regenerative nodules. The fibrosis is the result of active fibrogenesis. The fibrogenesis generally is thought to be stimulated by cytokines released during inflammation and necrosis. Virtually all chronic liver diseases ultimately can end with cirrhosis. The fibrous tissue leads to a distortion of the architecture of the liver with loss of normal function. Even though regeneration of hepatocytes occurs, the distorted architecture compromises their overall function.

By far the most common cause of cirrhosis in this country is alcohol consumption. Other causes include chronic active hepatitis of all types, primary biliary cirrhosis, hemochromatosis, Wilson's disease, and alpha-1 antitrypsin deficiency. The typical patient with alcoholic cirrhosis has consumed approximately a pint of whiskey per day for 15 years. However, the majority of patients who drink this much alcohol never develop cirrhosis. It probably is determined genetically whether or not cirrhosis occurs. In the case of alcoholic cirrhosis, only about 20% of patients who are alcoholic develop cirrhosis.

The clinical presentation of cirrhosis is related primarily to the development of portal hypertension and the loss of hepatocellular function.

Portal hypertension results from the resistance of flow through the liver. The increased pressure in the portal system is transmitted within that system, especially the coronary vein leading to esophageal varices, the gastric veins leading to gastric varices, and the inferior mesenteric vein leading to hemorrhoids. When the pressure reaches a certain level, these veins tend to burst, causing gastrointestinal hemorrhage. This is particularly true for the esophageal varices.

Another manifestation of cirrhosis is ascites, the accumulation of fluid in the abdominal cavity. The pathophysiology of ascites formation is complex, but the two most important features appear to be an increase in hydrostatic pressure in the portal circulation as the consequence of portal hypertension and decreased oncotic pressure due to the development of hypoalbuminemia. The hypoalbuminemia is caused by decreased synthesis of albumin by hepatocytes and the loss of albumin from the surface of the liver. This results in decreased oncotic pressure in the circulation (from decreased albumin synthesis) and increased oncotic pressure in the free peritoneal space (from albumin in the perinatal space). These factors in combination favor fluid accumulation in the abdominal space. The loss of fluid from the intravascular space causes secondary hyperaldosteronism, which activates the renin angiotensin system causing the kidneys to retain sodium and water. Thus, a vicious cycle is formed, all directed toward fluid retention.

Porto-systemic encephalopathy (PSE) is another manifestation of cirrhosis and is characterized by a spectrum of decreased mental and neurologic function. PSE is thought to occur because of the failure of the liver to remove noxious products of protein metabolism, particularly ammonia. Typical symptoms include sleep reversal, hypersomnia, apathy, personality changes, and intellectual deterioration. There may be neurological abnormalities such as slurred speech, asterixis, and exaggerated deep-tendon reflexes. The diagnosis is made on the basis of the clinical presentation and a characteristic delta wave pattern on electroencephalogram.

Other clinical features include the manifestations of excess feminization due to the toxic effect of alcohol on testicular function and the failure of the liver to metabolize estrogen. The net effect of excess feminization is spider angioma, palmar erythema, Dupuytren's contracture, parotid enlargement, gynecomastia, and testicular atrophy.

Symptoms and Signs—The most characteristic manifestations of cirrhosis are jaundice and ascites. However, an insidious onset characterized by weakness, fatigue, anorexia, and ultimately the signs of PSE, including sleep reversal, apathy, forgetfulness, confusion, euphoria, and personality changes, may occur. Social graces are often lost. Stupor and coma eventually ensue. Neurological findings, at this time, might include asterixis, slurred speech, muscle rigidity, hyperreflexia, and occasionally, localizing neurological signs. Primary biliary cirrhosis may have some unique features such as pruritus, dark urine, pale stools, steatorrhea, and xanthelasma.

Laboratory abnormalities include hyperbilirubinemia, hypoalbuminemia, prolonged prothrombin time, hyponatremia, and mildly elevated AST and ALA levels. Pancytopenia may be present. In primary biliary cirrhosis, the serum alkaline phosphatase is elevated markedly as is the serum cholesterol. Antimitochondrial antibodies are present in the serum.

The clinical course of cirrhosis is usually relentlessly downward. In alcoholic patients, this downward course may continue despite abstinence. The fatal event is usually bleeding from esophageal varices or an infection.

There is no specific curative treatment for any form of cirrhosis. However, the prognosis in alcoholic cirrhosis is improved by abstinence. The prognosis in autoimmune chronic active hepatitis is improved by continuous low-dose corticosteroid therapy. A preliminary study has shown methotrexate to be partially effective in the treatment of primary biliary cirrhosis. The cirrhosis of hemochromatosis is treated by iron removal by phlebotomy, but there is little evidence that once the patient has become cirrhotic that the prognosis is improved. The prognosis of Wilson's disease is improved with copper chelation therapy with D-peni-

cillamine. Preliminary studies have shown that the course of chronic hepatitis B may be improved with alpha-interferon therapy. Nevertheless, liver transplantation remains the treatment of choice for patients with end-stage liver disease.

Gallbladder and Gallstones

The gallbladder stores and concentrates bile. It is the usual site of gallstone formation.

Normal Physiology—The gallbladder fills passively with bile secreted by the liver. The filling process is facilitated by the secretion of bile and the closing of the sphincter of Oddi between meals, which enables the gallbladder to fill with bile, concentrate the bile, and then contract after meals to empty into the intestine where the bile solubilizes lipids for ultimate digestion and absorption. The gallbladder contracts and empties its concentrated bile in response to cholecystokinin released from the duodenal mucosa during a meal.

Bile is the major secretory product of the liver. It is composed of water in which small amounts of cholesterol, phospholipids, and bile salts are solubilized. It also contains bilirubin, which gives bile its characteristic yellow color. Bile is increasingly concentrated as it proceeds through the biliary tree and is concentrated 10- to 20-fold in the gallbladder, which absorbs water. Cholesterol is insoluble in water but is dissolved in bile by incorporation into mixed micelles and small vesicles. Mixed micelles are composed of bile acids, which are detergents, and lecithin, which together solubilize cholesterol. There is a limit to the quantity of cholesterol that can be dissolved in micelles. If this quantity is exceeded, cholesterol precipitates, which predisposes to gallstone formation.

Bile acids are synthesized from cholesterol in liver cells. The primary bile acids, cholic acid and chenodeoxycholic acid, are conjugated in the liver, excreted into the bile, and eventually reach the small intestine, where they participate in the solubilization of lipids. About one-third of the primary bile acids secreted into bile are converted by intestinal bacteria to the secondary bile acids, lithocholic acid and deoxycholic acid, which are lost in the stool. The remaining primary bile acids are reabsorbed in the terminal ileum and returned to the liver to be recycled—the enterohepatic circulation. This mass of recirculating bile acids, called the bile acid pool, recirculates approximately twice with each meal. Most of the reabsorption takes place in the last 100 cm of the terminal ileum, leaving a high concentration of bile acids to participate in digestion in the jejunum and proximal ileum. Loss of the last 100 cm of the terminal ileum, as occurs with surgery or regional enteritis (Crohn's disease), leads to malabsorption of fats, decreased fat absorption, and diarrhea (induced by bile acids in the colon).

CHOLELITHIASIS (GALLSTONES)—Gallstones are classified according to their composition: cholesterol, pigment, and mixed. Mixed stones are by far the most common. They are predominantly cholesterol but also contain bile pigments, calcium salts, and protein. They probably have a pathogenesis similar to that of pure cholesterol stones. They are often multiple, with a brown center, hard shell, and faceted surface. Pigment stones contain bile pigment such as bilirubinate. They are black, round to amorphous, and hard. Two-thirds of gallstones in the US are predominantly cholesterol.

Epidemiology—An estimated 24 million Americans have gallstones. In those over age 65, the incidence approaches 30%. Cholesterol and mixed stones are three times more common in women of child-bearing age than in men. The incidence is increased in individuals who are obese, elderly, multiparous, or cirrhotic. The incidence exceeds 70% in women of some Native American tribes.

Pathophysiology—The pathogenesis of cholesterol gallstone formation has been clarified. Failure of cholesterol-volatilization leads to precipitation and potentially to a gallstone. Normal people may secrete iatrogenic bile (supersaturated with cholesterol) during fasting when bile acid secretion is minimal but not all people develop gallstones. Nevertheless, certain defects have been identified in patients with cholesterol gallstones. Lean people with gallstones tend to have reduced biliary secretion of bile acids and phospholipids. Obese people secrete excessive quantities of cholesterol into bile. Some individuals have a contracted bile acid pool because their bile acid loss exceeds the maximum rate of liver synthesis of bile acids. For example resection or chronic inflammatory disease of the ileum may cause the net loss of bile acids as may the chronic ingestion of the binding resin, cholestyramine.

Once a crystal is formed as a result of cholesterol precipitation from bile, the crystal may grow or several crystals may aggregate. This phase of gallstone formation is poorly understood. Nucleating factors exist in bile and appear to foster precipitation of cholesterol crystals. The process of gallstone growth appears to involve the entrapment of crystals by gallbladder mucus, and the process may be fostered by impaired gallbladder emptying.

Information regarding pigment stone formation is scarce. Many patients have increased bilirubin production as a result of chronic hemolysis. Thus, the liver conjugates and excretes increased quantities of bilirubin. Beta-glucuronidase in bile may deconjugate bilirubin, making it less soluble in bile and possibly fostering precipitation.

Gallstones cause morbidity by irritating the gallbladder mucosa directly (cholecystitis) or by impacting in the cystic duct. They also may pass into and obstruct the common duct.

Symptoms and Signs—Most patients with gallstones are asymptomatic. The characteristic symptom is epigastric pain that may lateralize to the right side and radiate to the tip of the right scapula. The pain is a severe, aching sensation that is not influenced by body position. The pain begins rapidly, grows in intensity, and disappears rather abruptly. The duration of pain is variable but usually is about 2 to 6 hours. Nausea and vomiting may accompany the pain. Jaundice may appear in several days if the stones remain in the common bile duct. Fever and chills often occur with acute cholelithiasis because of infection in the biliary tree. Sepsis may occur. The symptoms of flatulence, bloating, and fatty food intolerance, frequently attributed to gallbladder disease, are not characteristic of gallbladder disease and are more likely due to irritable bowel syndrome.

Physical examination in the acute case reveals tenderness, muscle guarding, and rigidity over the area of the gallbladder. A mass is rarely palpable. Serum levels of alkaline phosphatase and bilirubin may be increased; WBC count is elevated in infection. Ultrasound discloses gallstones in most cases.

RENAL DISEASE

Normal Physiology—The kidneys receive about 20% of the resting cardiac output. From this torrential blood flow, the one million glomeruli in each kidney create an ultrafiltrate (glomerular filtrate) at a rate of 120 ml/minute. The glomerular filtrate contains all small molecules in the same concentration as they are dissolved in the plasma but does not allow the escape of large molecules (protein). Each glomerulus is connected to a renal tubule. The tubule reabsorbs about 99% of the glomerular filtrate and most of the dissolved solutes, returning to the bloodstream what is required for maintenance of the internal environment and allowing any excess to escape into the urine. Waste products such as urea and creatinine are reabsorbed to a much lesser extent or not at all and are thus preferentially eliminated. Relevant details of physiology are included in the appropriate sections below.

Glomerular Disease

As might be expected from the physiology above, disease of the glomeruli tends to reduce glomerular filtration rate and to allow leakage of protein into the urine. Common features of glomerular disease thus include fluid overload, hypertension, proteinuria, and renal failure. Diabetes is the most common cause of glomerular disease in western countries. Most other forms of glomerulonephritis (GN) involve immunologically mediated inflammation of the glomeruli in both kidneys symmetrically. GN must be differentiated from interstitial nephritis, which is inflammation of the connective tissue surrounding the glomeruli and tubules.

DIABETIC NEPHROPATHY

Definition/Overview—Diabetic nephropathy is characterized clinically by a stereotyped march from normality to subtle increase in glomerular filtration rate (hyperfiltration) to excretion of albumin in minimally increased quantities (microalbuminuria) to heavy urinary protein loss, and eventually decline of renal function to uremia.

Epidemiology—In the absence of effective treatment, 25–45% of patients with type 1 or type 2 diabetes will develop nephropathy during their lifetime. Certain groups (Native Americans) not only have a higher prevalence of diabetes than average, but also a greater likelihood of developing nephropathy

Pathology and Pathogenesis—Glycosylation of tissue proteins appears to lie at the root of the microvascular damage in diabetic nephropathy. High blood pressure and activation of cytokines including TGF-β magnifies the damage. By electron microscopy, uniform thickening of the glomerular basement membrane, diffuse expansion of the mesangium, and later the appearance of glomerular nodules (Kimmelstiel-Wilson lesion) characterize diabetic nephropathy.

Symptoms and Signs—Typically symptoms and signs develop late in the evolution of the renal disease. Hypertension, proteinuria, nephrotic syndrome, and chronic renal failure (see descriptions below).

GLOMERULONEPHRITIS

Etiology—Glomerulonephritis has diverse causes. Several potential immunological mechanisms can give rise to glomerulonephritis. For example, in Goodpasture syndrome or antiglomerular basement membrane nephritis, an endogenous antigen attaches to the basement membrane of glomerular capillaries and incites a destructive inflammatory nephritis. In lupus nephritis and postinfectious glomerulonephritis, antigen-antibody complexes deposit and initiate inflammation. In lupus nephritis, the antigen is DNA; in postinfectious glomerulonephritis, the antigen is a protein associated with the organism infecting some other part of the body; streptococcal antigen is a well-researched example. In IgA nephropathy, the immune mechanism is not clear. Broadly similar glomerular damage can also occur from non-immunological mechanisms, for example in vasculitis and hereditary nephritis (Alport syndrome).

Epidemiology—Glomerulonephritis is the leading cause of chronic renal failure after diabetes. IgA nephropathy is the most common cause of glomerulonephritis worldwide and is particularly common in Asians. Glomerulonephritis occurs in two-thirds of patients with lupus.

Pathology—Diverse types of histological damage reflect the diverse etiologies. In acute GN, such as poststreptococcal, the glomeruli are swollen, infiltrated with PMNs, and there is proliferation of endothelial and epithelial glomerular cells. In severe cases, epithelial crescents form in Bowman's capsule. In immune complex GN granular, nodular, or "lumpy bumpy" deposits of immunoglobulin are found in the glomeruli. In antiglomerular basement membrane nephritis, immunofluorescence microscopy shows antibodies in a linear pattern along the capillary walls of the glomeruli.

The pathological classification of chronic GN includes IgA nephropathy, membranoproliferative, membranous, focal or diffuse proliferative and rapidly progressive GN. A description of the histopathological features of these forms of GN is beyond the scope of this chapter.

Pathophysiology—All cases of GN are the result of immune reactions. Many cases involve formation of antibodies against circulating extrarenal antigens. These antibodies are usually IgG and also circulate in the blood. Antigen-antibody complexes are formed when a critical ratio of antibody to antigen is reached in the blood. The complexes become trapped in the glomeruli during filtration, hence the name immune complex glomerulonephritis. The process actually is more complex than simple trapping and involves dysfunction of the mesangial cells, the reticuloendothelial cells in the glomeruli that normally remove foreign materials. The antigen-antibody complexes in the glomeruli activate the complement cascade via the classic or alternate pathways. Activation of complement also activates Factor XII and the clotting system, which leads to the deposition of fibrin. Factor XII also activates the kinin system, which causes release of chemotactic factors, and substances that increase permeability of blood vessels. The inflammatory reaction with the release of lysosomal enzymes damages the glomeruli. Fibrosis ensues.

The remaining 5% of cases of GN are due to the development of antibodies against glomerular basement membrane. These antibodies also are active against alveolar basement membrane. The inflammatory reaction is responsible for the damage to the glomeruli and alveoli.

Symptoms and Signs—The hallmarks of GN are gross or microscopic hematuria (RBCs in the urine), hypertension, proteinuria, and facial, periorbital, and pedal edema. Edema is also part of the nephrotic syndrome and will be discussed below. Glomerulonephritis also may be associated with hypertension, fatigue, anorexia, and congestive symptoms such as orthopnea and dyspnea on exertion. The urine also may contain RBC casts, WBCs, granular or hyaline casts, and epithelial debris. Chronic GN eventually leads to the symptoms and signs of chronic renal failure.

Oliguria, "coke-colored" or "smoky" urine, bilateral steady flank pain, and malaise typically herald the onset of acute poststreptococcal glomerulonephritis. Edema develops in a few days unless salt and fluid are restricted.

The prognosis of acute poststreptococcal GN is excellent in children: 90% recover completely, although the urinary signs may persist for 1 year. The prognosis for chronic GN is variable. Some forms progress slowly while others deteriorate rapidly to chronic renal failure.

Nephrotic Syndrome

This is not a single disease but a constellation of abnormalities that occur when the glomerular capillary wall becomes permeable to protein.

Normal Physiology—Only small quantities of protein are filtered by normal glomeruli, a situation largely explained by the barriers to protein filtration and the nature of plasma proteins. The normal glomerular capillary wall is almost impermeable to protein. The endothelium is not a barrier, but the glomerular basement membrane prevents filtration of large proteins and blood cells. The negative charge on the glomerular basement membranes repels protein molecules. Thus, only proteins with a molecular weight of less than 40,000 may be filtered normally by the glomeruli, and the tubules reabsorb these proteins so that insignificant quantities of protein appear in the urine.

Etiology—Any glomerular disease that damages the basement membrane and allows leakage of protein may cause the syndrome. The most common cause of nephrotic syndrome in children is minimal change disease. In adults diabetes mellitus is far and away the most common cause; other causes include glomerulonephritis, amyloidosis, collagen vascular diseases, and nephrotoxins such as mercury, gold, anticonvulsant drugs, and penicillamine. Tubular disorders may cause mild to moderate proteinuria but do not cause nephrotic syndrome.

Pathophysiology—Large quantities of protein, mainly albumin, are lost in the urine in nephrotic syndrome. In adults the proteinuria is at least 3 to 4 g/day but may be as high as 30 to 40 g/day. Some filtered protein is degraded by tubules. Thus, measured proteinuria underestimates the total protein loss. Albumin synthesis by the liver can contend with a 15 g/day loss if dietary protein intake is adequate. When the loss exceeds the synthetic capacity of the liver, hypoalbuminemia occurs. Hypoalbuminemia results in a decreased oncotic pressure within blood vessels. Decreased oncotic pressure causes a decrease in fluid reabsorption in the venous capillaries resulting in edema. Loss of vascular fluid volume causes hypotension. The kidneys respond to the fall in blood pressure and volume by retaining sodium and water via the renin-angiotensin system. Up to 20 L of water may be retained in a futile attempt to restore blood volume, as the retained water simply becomes more edema fluid. Proteinuria leads to cast formation in the tubules. These may be hyaline, granular or waxy.

Hypercholesterolemia and hypercoagulability arise from overproduction of apolipoproteins and coagulation factors respectively Lipiduria also occurs, but not as a consequence of hyperlipidemia.

Symptoms and Signs—The classical symptoms and signs are proteinuria (greater than 3.5 g/m^2/day), hypoalbuminemia, and edema. The edema may be dependent and occur in the feet and ankles, or accumulate in compliant periorbital and facial tissue. The edema occasionally involves the entire body, a condition known as anasarca. Hyperlipidemia and lipiduria may or may not be present and are not essential for the diagnosis. Complications of nephrotic syndrome include hypotension and possibly shock, intravascular fluid overload or depletion, protein malnutrition, and a predisposition to thrombosis.

The prognosis is related to the prognosis of the underlying cause. However, the syndrome due to any cause may be fatal if fluid overload is not corrected.

Renal Failure

Renal failure is the inability of the kidney to perform its usual physiological functions and maintain homeostasis.

Renal failure may be classified as acute, subacute or chronic, depending on the time course.

Normal Physiology—The kidneys perform many functions. The fluid volume and serum osmolality are maintained by regulation of both sodium and water excretion. The pH of body fluids is maintained within narrow limits, normally 7.40 ± 0.04. The kidneys excrete many waste products.

The normal glomerular filtration rate (GFR) is 125 ml/minute and decreases with increasing age. The kidneys have a remarkable ability to adjust their excretion of water and solutes. They can excrete 20% of the glomerular filtrate if blood volume is expanded, which means that water intake could be as high as 35 L/day. The daily osmolar load obligates a urine output of 400 to 500 ml. The kidneys can excrete as much as 500 mEq of sodium/day or maintain sodium balance if intake of sodium is limited to 5 mEq/day. The kidneys normally excrete 50 to 80 mEq of potassium/day. The kidneys cannot produce urine virtually free of potassium, as they can in the case of sodium. This usually poses no problem as any mixed diet contains potassium, but it may prevent the kid-

neys from correcting hypokalemia if there are ongoing losses from the GI tract.

A person ingesting 70 g of protein forms 40 to 60 mEq of acid/day. The range of blood pH compatible with life is 6.9 to 7.6 but the normal range is much narrower. One half of the acid is excreted as titratable acid: $HPO_4^{2-} + H^+ \rightarrow H_2PO_4^-$. The other half is excreted by ammonia formation: $H^+ + NH_3 \rightarrow NH_4^+$. Filtered bicarbonate is reabsorbed completely unless the patient is alkalemic. The kidneys are responsible for excreting other waste products. Approximately 20% of filtered phosphate is excreted in the urine. A diet of 80 g of protein/day results in the formation of 20 grams of urea, which is excreted. The blood level of urea (blood urea nitrogen, BUN) is normally maintained below 20 mg/dl. The kidneys also excrete uric acid, magnesium, calcium, and other substances to maintain homeostasis.

The kidneys have several endocrine or metabolic functions. They produce erythropoietin, which regulates the red-blood-cell mass and renin, which regulates blood pressure and sodium and water balance. The kidneys degrade insulin and gastrin. The kidneys also participate in vitamin D metabolism and thus calcium homeostasis by converting a derivative of vitamin D, 25-hydroxycholecalciferol, to the biologically active form, I,25-dihydroxycholecalciferol.

ACUTE RENAL FAILURE—This is most commonly due to acute tubular necrosis (ATN) but also may be due to hypovolemia (prerenal azotemia) or to obstruction of the ureters, bladder or urethra. All excretory renal function can be lost within a few days.

Etiology—ATN is due most commonly to ischemia or toxins. Any event that leads to shock and intense vasoconstriction within the renal vascular bed may lead to it. Hemorrhage, hypotension during anesthesia, burns, sepsis, crush injuries, massive intravascular hemolysis, heart surgery requiring extracorporeal oxygenation, and childbirth may cause it. Toxins that may cause ATN include aminoglycoside antibiotics, radiographic contrast media, bichloride of mercury, carbon tetrachloride, ethylene glycol, methanol, myoglobin from crush injuries, and hemoglobin from intravascular hemolysis. Some cases have no identifiable cause.

Pathology—Ischemia causes patchy necrosis of the tubular epithelial cells and basement membrane. Other areas of the tubule may appear normal. Toxins cause diffuse necrosis of the tubular endothelial cells but do not injure the basement membrane. The glomeruli are spared in ATN unless the injury is severe and prolonged. The lesions are reversible if the patient survives.

Pathophysiology—Immediately after the injury renal blood flow may be reduced by as much as 50% by arteriolar constriction. Fluid filtered by the glomeruli leaks back into the interstitium through damaged tubules. The subsequent edema of the interstitium increases interstitial hydrostatic pressure, which further decreases renal blood flow and causes the tubules to collapse. Casts of degenerating epithelial cells block urine flow in the lumens and cause further increases in interstitial fluid. The kidneys can no longer maintain homeostasis by the excretion of sodium, water, and waste products.

Symptoms and Signs—Oliguria (urine volume of less than 400 to 500 ml/day) usually is the first sign of ATN but may not appear until several days after the injury. The composition of the urine formed is little changed from glomerular filtrate, but also contains protein and RBCs. The sodium concentration of the urine is fixed at about 50 mEq/L. BUN begins to rise and acidemia and hyperkalemia develop. If fluid therapy is not managed appropriately, hyponatremia and edema develop. The patient complains of nausea and lethargy. Death may occur within a few days because of acidosis and/or hyperkalemia.

During the second week, nausea, somnolence, weakness and thirst ensue. The BUN continues to rise and acidosis, edema, hyponatremia, and hyperkalemia worsen. Complications are common during this phase. Pulmonary edema, congestive heart failure, and hypertension may develop because of fluid overload. Hyperkalemia may cause cardiac arrhythmias. Metabolic encephalopathy, possibly due to urea, hyponatremia, and hypocalcemia results in neurological deterioration, convulsions, and coma. Anemia due to decreased RBC production, increased RBC destruction and dilution appears in the second week. Nosocomial infection is the most common cause of death in this phase.

During the recovery phase, urine volume increases daily. The BUN may continue to rise until urine volume has exceeded 1000 ml/day for several days. Polyuria (urine volume of greater than 3000 ml/day) may develop. Weight loss is rapid as the edema resolves. Since the tubules may not yet be able to conserve water, sodium or potassium, dehydration, hyponatremia and hypokalemia may develop. The diuresis may continue for 1 to 3 weeks. The GFR may never return to normal, but the symptoms and signs of renal failure resolve.

CHRONIC RENAL FAILURE—CRF is a loss of kidney function that occurs over a number of years. Azotemia is the accumulation of nitrogenous waste products in the blood caused by renal failure. Uremia refers to the symptoms and signs caused by CRF when renal function is less than about 10% of normal.

Etiology—Many diseases can destroy renal parenchymal tissue and result in CRF. These include chronic glomerulonephritis, hypertension, diabetes mellitus, polycystic kidney disease, analgesic nephropathy, nephrocalcinosis, reflex nephropathy, chronic pyelonephritis, obstructive uropathy, and interstitial nephritis. In certain patients, more than one disease may have caused the CRF. In some cases it is not possible to establish the cause.

Pathophysiology—CRF develops because the number of functioning nephrons decreases below that necessary to maintain homeostasis. Uremia and end stage renal disease (ESRD) occur when 90–95% of the nephrons are destroyed. As renal function deteriorates, hypertrophy occurs in the remaining nephrons and the amount of solute and water excreted per nephron may increase. Compensatory mechanisms eventually are overwhelmed by even the normal daily intake of water, sodium, potassium, acid, and nitrogen. Uremia, electrolyte disturbances, and fluid overload ensue.

The earliest renal impairment is the loss of ability to concentrate urine. This is due partially to the increased solute load per nephron. The patient then must increase water intake to prevent dehydration. The diurnal pattern of water excretion is reversed.

Most patients develop a tendency to retain salt and water early in the course of CRF. In a few forms of renal failure, salt wasting occurs because the kidneys are unable to conserve sodium even when sodium intake is restricted. The osmotic diuresis of the solute load causes an obligatory sodium loss. Hyponatremia and hypovolemia may occur and worsen renal failure by reducing the GFR. Salt-wasting eventually ceases and the kidneys are then unable to excrete dietary sodium. Sodium and water retention then results in edema and hypertension.

Serum potassium is normal during the early stages of renal failure. Renin-angiotensin-induced production of aldosterone stimulates potassium excretion and the osmotic diuresis further enhances potassium excretion. Eventually, the urine volume may fall below 500 ml/day, and serum potassium will begin to rise. Acidosis worsens hyperkalemia by causing the movement of potassium out of cells.

As renal function deteriorates, ability to form ammonia and therefore to excrete hydrogen is impaired. Ability to reabsorb filtered bicarbonate is also impaired. Acidosis ensues.

The percentage of phosphate excreted decreases as the GFR declines. The increased serum phosphate level and other factors described below cause a drop in the serum calcium level. Hypocalcemia stimulates the production of parathyroid hormone, which increases renal excretion of phosphate and resorption of calcium from bones. When the GFR reaches less than 20 ml/minute, the increased serum PTH level is no longer effective in increasing phosphate excretion.

Hypocalcemia is due to other factors besides the increased serum phosphate. Hypoalbuminemia reduces the quantity of carrier proteins for calcium. Absorption of calcium from the GI tract is impaired because of lack of 1,25-dihydroxyvitamin D, the active metabolite of vitamin D. The ionized fraction of serum calcium is decreased because ions such as sulfate, phosphate, and citrate bind the calcium.

Magnesium levels usually do not rise until the GFR is below 30 ml/minute. Uric acid levels rise, but not usually above 10 mg/dl, and gouty arthritis is uncommon.

Urea is poorly excreted in CRF, and the BUN rises. The magnitude of the rise correlates poorly with the symptoms of uremia except for the gastrointestinal symptoms. Increased quantities of urea are excreted into the intestinal lumen, presumably contributing to irritation and ulceration.

Other presumably toxic substances accumulate in uremia. These include indoles, phenols, amino acids, organic acids, and derivatives of guanidine. The accumulation of carotene-like pigments results in sallow skin color.

A normochromic normocytic anemia parallels the severity of the azotemia. Decreased RBC production occurs because erythropoietin deficiency and iron deficiency due to chronic GI blood loss. The anemia of chronic disease also is found in these patients. (See Hematology section.)

Several complications may occur. A bleeding tendency is caused by platelet dysfunction. The accumulation of guanidinosuccinic acid may be responsible for loss of platelet adhesiveness and aggregation. Osteomalacia occurs in part because vitamin D is not converted to the active metabolite, 1,25-dihydroxyvitamin D. Hypertension is exacerbated by fluid retention. A peripheral demyelinating neuropathy, mostly in the legs, results in decreased nerve conduction and impairment of motor and sensory function. Pericarditis may or may not cause chest pain and occasionally causes pericardial tamponade or constriction.

Renal-failure patients are predisposed to infections because of poor nutrition, pulmonary edema, lack of physical activity, vascular insuffi-

ciency, and indwelling tubes and catheters. Repeated transfusions increase the risk of viral hepatitis.

Symptoms and Signs—The onset of renal failure is insidious. The first symptoms may be polyuria or nocturia or both. Hypertension and anemia are common early signs, but lack specificity. As renal function deteriorates, the symptoms and signs relate to the organ systems -involved.

Fluid accumulation produces the symptoms and signs of edema, congestive heart failure, and hypertension. Hyponatremia causes inability to concentrate, drowsiness, lethargy, psychotic disturbances, stupor, and coma. Hyperkalemia may cause cardiac arrhythmias. Acidosis contributes to nausea, fatigue, malaise, and dyspnea, and causes Kussmaul respiration. Hypocalcemia may result in tremor, muscle twitching, muscle cramps and convulsions. The increased PTH level leads to the erosive and cystic changes and bone pain of osteitis fibrosa cystica. Phosphate deposition in the skin contributes to severe itching; in the eyes, to conjunctivitis; in the blood vessels, to gangrene; and around the joints, to pain. Hypermagnesemia results in drowsiness, muscle weakness, and coma.

Ammonia formation from urea in the GI tract contributes to the unpleasant taste, anorexia, nausea, vomiting, and hiccups. Pericarditis may cause pain and be detected by hearing a friction rub. Pulmonary congestion from hypervolemia may cause dyspnea and hypoxemia. Urea in sweat precipitates on the skin and is known as "uremic frost."

The symptoms and signs of anemia are seen when the hematocrit falls below 15–20%. Patients with renal failure experience ecchymoses, epistaxis, and oozing of blood from mucous membranes due to coagulation abnormalities.

Neuropathy causes numbness, tingling, muscular weakness and, on occasion, paralysis.

The symptoms and signs of uremia progressively worsen. Renal failure is fatal unless the patient is treated by hemo- or peritoneal dialysis or receives a renal transplant.

Acid-Base and Fluid and Electrolyte Disturbances

Acid-base and fluid and electrolyte disturbances can be caused by a wide variety of diseases, including the kidney disorders previously discussed in this section. They also may be caused by gastrointestinal (eg, severe diarrhea), pulmonary (eg, chronic obstructive lung disease), or metabolic (eg, diabetes) disorders. The defects observed with these diseases have been described in earlier sections of this chapter.

Normal Physiology—A number of mechanisms act to maintain normal plasma pH (7.35 to 7.45), one of which is the chemical buffering by extra and intracellular buffer systems. These include hemoglobin, plasma proteins, and the carbonic acid-bicarbonate buffer system. Hydrogen ions ($H+$) migrate into or out of cells in exchange for potassium ($K+$) to maintain electrical neutrality. The respiratory system contributes through the exchange of carbon dioxide (an acid-former). Lastly, the kidneys help to maintain normal pH through the elimination or retention of $H+$ and bicarbonate (HCO_3^-). Each of these mechanisms acts to maintain a constant HCO_3^-:CO_2 ratio of approximately 20:1. As long as this ratio is maintained, the pH will be 7.4 (see Chapter 17).

The human body is composed largely of water. Fifty to 60% of total body weight is water. Body water is distributed between the intracellular space (intracellular fluid or ICF) and the extracellular space (extracellular fluid or ECF). Two-thirds of all body water is contained in the ICF and the remaining one-third in the ECF. The ECF is further divided into intravascular fluid (IVF) and interstitial fluid, which contain one-fourth and three-fourths of the ECF, respectively. Electrolytes are unequally divided between ICF and ECF. Potassium is the major ICF cation, and phosphate and organic ions are the ICF anions. Sodium is the major ECF cation, and chloride and bicarbonate are the ECF anions. Although water moves readily in and out of cells, electrolytes do not, often requiring active transport. Although electrolyte composition differs between the ICF and ECF, osmolality is equal.

Water homeostasis is regulated by the interrelationships between water intake, kidney function, and water loss through the lungs, skin, and GI tract. A decrease in ECF volume or an increase in osmotic pressure of plasma both stimulate water intake. The kidneys act to preserve water homeostasis through their relationship to antidiuretic hormone (ADH), which was discussed under **Endocrinology**. ADH release is under the control of both osmotic and volume factors. Increased osmotic pressure or decreased ECF volume stimulates increased ADH production and secretion. The glomerular filtration rate (GFR) is normally 125 ml/minute. The GFR is affected by renal blood flow, hydrostatic pressure in Bowman's space, and plasma protein concentration. Essentially everything in the plasma, except protein, is filtered. The kidney tubules both reabsorb and secrete solutes via active transport and passive diffusion. Almost all water (90%) and electrolytes initially filtered are reabsorbed by active transport in the tubules and Henle's loop. Ammonia and urea are secreted into the filtrate.

Pathophysiology—Acid-base disorders may be divided into respiratory acidosis and alkalosis and metabolic acidosis and alkalosis. *Respiratory acidosis* is associated with disorders that cause an impairment of gas exchange and thus CO_2 retention. Arterial blood gases (ABGs) show a decreased pH, elevated pCO_2 (dissolved CO_2 gas) and elevated bicarbonate. *Respiratory alkalosis* is caused by conditions that result in hyperventilation with an abnormally large loss of CO_2. ABGs reflect an increased pH and decreased PCO_2 and HCO_3-. *Metabolic acidosis* occurs as a result of either the addition of acid or a loss of bicarbonate. Acids may be endogenous, as in the case of diabetic ketoacidosis, or exogenous, as in the case of methanol ingestion. Bicarbonate may be lost through diarrhea or through the kidneys as in renal tubular acidosis. ABGs show low pH, HCO_3-, and PCO_2. Calculation of the anion gap ($Na+ - Cl^- + HCO_3$-) is helpful in determining whether metabolic acidosis is due to addition of acid or loss of $HCO3$-. The normal anion gap is 10 to 12 mEq/L and is elevated when acidosis is due to addition of organic acid. *Metabolic alkalosis* usually is due to the loss of acid ($H+$) but may occur occasionally with excessive HCO_3- ingestion. Elevated pH and HCO_3- characterize it.

Once one of the above conditions occurs, the body compensates. For example, in cases of metabolic acidosis, the body compensates with increased respiratory activity, thus removing CO_2 and thereby blunting the fall in pH.

The causes of fluid and electrolyte imbalances are many. Such derangements may be interrelated, occurring together, or may occur independently. Fluid losses occur with gastrointestinal disorders such as vomiting and diarrhea. In such cases, electrolytes are lost with the water. In others, the losses of electrolytes and water are not proportional resulting in hypo- or hyperosmolality. In the various renal disorders, a number of fluid and electrolyte shifts are common. In the diuretic phase of acute tubular necrosis, large volumes of fluid are lost due to lack of reabsorption. In nephrotic syndrome, large shifts of water are often involved. This water is not lost necessarily from the body but may be lost from the vascular compartment, frequently in the form of edema. In addition to the fluid shifts, electrolyte disturbances ensue. Secondary to decreased renal blood flow and thus, decreased glomerular filtration rate, the renin-angiotensin system is activated causing further fluid retention. The specific renal diseases associated with fluid and electrolyte disturbances have been described in greater detail earlier in this section.

Symptoms and Signs—Signs of volume depletion include postural hypotension and tachycardia and decreased jugular venous pressure. Less reliable signs include decreased skin turgor, dry mucous membranes, and cloudy sensorium. Severe hypovolemia can result in shock. Fluid excess may be manifested by hypertension or peripheral or pulmonary edema. Of all electrolyte disturbances, only two of the more serious, those involving $K+$, will be discussed here. Others have been discussed in previous sections. Signs of hyperkalemia include muscle weakness and cardiac dysrhythmias. Severe hyperkalemia results in cardiac standstill. Hypokalemia also may be reflected as muscle weakness. Abdominal distress may occur from impaired intestinal smooth muscle mobility. Abdominal distention and depressed deep tendon reflexes may be evident. Cardiac rhythm disturbances also occur with hypokalemia.

The measurement of ABGs, plasma electrolytes, urine volume, and electrolytes are all helpful in assessing a patient with acid-base or fluid and electrolyte disorders, but the most helpful information frequently comes from careful physical examination (blood pressure, pulse rate, and jugular venous pressure).

NEUROLOGY

Epilepsy and Convulsive Disorders

Epilepsy is a chronic disorder of cerebral function. It may be defined as a paroxysmal disturbance of CNS function that is recurrent, stereotyped in character, and associated with excessive neuronal discharge that is synchronous and self-limited. The episodic manifestations of epilepsy are dependent on the portion(s) of the CNS involved.

Epidemiology—A total of 0.5–1% of the population suffers from epilepsy.

Epilepsy can begin at almost any age. However, the age of onset often is related to the etiology of the seizure disorder. One example is that of generalized absence seizures or petit mal, which typically present in early childhood.

Etiology—Epilepsy is a symptom complex that has many causes. In many cases, the precipitating factor(s) or cause of the seizure disorder is not apparent, and the condition is referred to as idiopathic. Severe hypoxia, genetic metabolic defects, developmental brain defects, and perinatal injuries can lead to seizures in newborns and infants. Certain metabolic disorders such as hypoglycemia, hypocalcemia, and vitamin B6 deficiency also can lead to seizures during infancy. Brain infections such as meningitis and encephalitis can trigger seizures during childhood. Seizures during childhood are less often caused by tumors, toxins, vascular disease, degenerative disease, or trauma.

In young adults, head trauma is a major cause of seizures. Likewise, ruling out the presence of a brain tumor is important for anyone over the age of 20. In patients over the age of 50, cerebrovascular disease is the most identified cause of seizures. In certain forms of epilepsy, genetic predisposition plays a role. Individuals with a first-degree relative with epilepsy are at a somewhat greater risk than the normal population of developing a seizure disorder. Despite our growing understanding of the disorder itself, an etiological diagnosis cannot be made with certainty in about two-thirds of epileptic patients.

In all age groups, a wide variety of drugs can provoke seizures.

Pathology—Various lesions in the brain, such as congenital lesions, gliotic scars, abnormal vascularization, and degenerative brain disease in the elderly have been associated with epilepsy in some patients and not in others. Even when the clinical information suggests that a seizure is of focal origin, it is not always possible to identify the epileptogenic lesion.

Pathophysiology—The convulsion results from sudden hypersynchronization of electrical discharge in neuronal networks in an apparently normal or a diseased cerebral cortex. The mechanisms and reasons for the discharge are not well understood. One hypothesis is that a group of diencephalic neurons normally exerts a constant inhibitory influence on cortical neurons, thereby preventing excessive activation. In epilepsy, the neurons are deafferented, supersensitive, and susceptible to activation or depolarization by a variety of stimuli. Seizures may result from a reduction of inhibitory neurotransmission mediated by the neurotransmitter gamma-aminobutyric acid (GABA) or by enhancement of the excitatory neurotransmitter system mediated by glutamate and aspartate.

During a seizure, consciousness may be unaffected, lost completely, or altered but not completely lost. Patients may experience only minor interruptions in their motor activity or they may experience intense muscular activation that leads to motor behavior characteristic of generalized tonic-clonic seizures.

Symptoms and Signs—The frequency of seizures within individual patients can vary from as few as one per year to dozens per day depending on the particular seizure type. Thus, the need for accurate diagnosis of the seizure type is of more than just theoretical interest. Since there are so many different seizure types, each of which may require a different therapeutic approach, an accurate diagnosis permits the clinician to select the most appropriate anticonvulsant drug while avoiding the use of contraindicated drugs. The International Classification of Epileptic Seizures classifies seizure types as either partial or generalized.

Partial seizures generally are categorized as simple, complex, or secondarily generalized and would include those traditionally called focal motor and temporal lobe seizures. Partial seizures all begin from a discrete brain region and may or may not be preceded by an aura. An aura consists of sensations or experiences often recognized by the patient as a warning of an impending seizure. Partial seizures may or may not involve loss of consciousness.

The symptoms of simple partial seizures result from abnormal discharges originating in specific areas of the cortex, and often remain unilateral regardless of whether the seizure is motor, somatosensory, psychic, autonomic, or a combination. The aura of a simple partial seizure may include somatosensory symptoms or hallucinations (eg, tingling, light flashes, or buzzing); autonomic symptoms including epigastric sensation, pallor, sweating, flushing, piloerection, and pupillary dilation; or psychic symptoms.

One form of a simple partial seizure is that traditionally known as *Jacksonian*. It usually begins with twitching of the fingers of one hand, the face, or one foot. The movement then spreads (marches) to other muscles along the same side of the body. If the movements generalize to include both sides of the body and the patient loses consciousness, the seizure is said to have become secondarily generalized. One type of a partial seizure with complex symptomatology is traditionally known as a psychomotor seizure.

In a complex partial seizure, consciousness is lost. Complex partial seizures are associated often with a lesion in the temporal lobe. The patient acts as though he/she were conscious, although he/she is amnesic. The patient may continue an activity or perform tasks but may not be able to respond to questions or commands. The seizure often is preceded by an aura. Motor activity due to the seizure may include chewing, lip-smacking, and tonic spasms of the extremities.

Generalized seizures, on the other hand, involve both hemispheres from the beginning. Consciousness is lost at the outset, and patients experiencing generalized seizures usually do not experience aura or display focal motor manifestations. The two most widely recognized generalized seizure disorders include generalized tonic-clonic (formerly grand mal) and generalized absence (formerly petit mal). Generalized tonic-clonic seizures are characterized by a sudden loss of consciousness, a cry, falling, tonic then clonic movements of the muscles, and incontinence of sphincters. After the motor seizure has ceased, the patient may be unconscious for many minutes. On awakening, the patient may complain of a headache. Generalized absence seizures almost always begin between 4 and 12 years of age. They are characterized by a brief loss of consciousness lasting for a few seconds. The child typically displays a blank facial expression and may or may not display a characteristic blinking of the eyelids. Absence seizures are almost always associated with a typical EEG abnormality of spike and slow wave discharges of approximately 3 Hz. Other generalized seizures include myoclonic seizures, clonic seizures, tonic seizures, and atonic seizures.

The International Classification of Epilepsies and Epileptic Syndromes takes into consideration the fact that some patients with epilepsy display more than one seizure type. After all, seizures are only a symptom of the underlying disorder. The prognosis is often a product of the epileptic syndrome whose diagnosis depends on numerous factors including family history, age of onset, rate of progression, presence or absence of neurological impairment and interictal EEG abnormalities, and a patient's response to pharmacological treatment. In this respect, the epileptic syndrome generally is classified according to whether an individual patient's seizures are localization-related (focal, local, partial) or generalized and whether they are idiopathic or symptomatic. They may be classified further as to anatomical localization (eg, frontal lobe, Rolandic, occipital, or temporal epilepsy). To date, more than 50 epileptic syndromes have been proposed.

The diagnosis of epilepsy is based on the clinical history and the EEG. The first steps to an accurate diagnosis usually involve obtaining an accurate and complete history from the patient as well as from a witness. A detailed physical exam is followed by an even more in-depth neurological exam. The EEG can provide precise information that may be useful for classifying the seizure type. It is characteristically abnormal during a seizure but may be normal between seizures. Specialized diagnostic procedures may include computerized tomography and magnetic resonance imaging. These two noninvasive techniques can be useful in identifying a particular brain lesion that may have led to the development of a patient's seizure disorder. Intensive monitoring employing closed circuit television and EEG recording is an expensive procedure that should be considered when a patient's seizures are not responsive to drug therapy. This latter procedure also can be helpful in determining whether difficult-to-diagnose seizures are nonepileptic in nature.

Parkinsonism

This disease, also called paralysis agitans, is a disorder of the extrapyramidal system that originally was described in 1817. James Parkinson described a syndrome that consisted of a resting tremor, rigidity, postural abnormalities, and bradykinesia, but spared the senses and intellect.

Normal Physiology—The basal ganglia normally control postural tone and provide the background adjustments for intentional movements. The dopaminergic pathway from the caudate nucleus to the thalamus inhibits the inhibition of voluntary movement. The cholinergic pathway opposes this pathway, which is excitatory for the inhibition of voluntary movement. A dopaminergic pathway inhibits the cholinergic pathway in the caudate nucleus from the substantia nigra.

Epidemiology—Parkinsonism usually occurs in middle or late life, though it rarely is seen in young people. The prevalence of this disease is estimated to be between 59 and 353 cases per 100,000 in various populations worldwide, resulting in 300,000 to 400,000 cases in this country.

Etiology—Although the actual cause of Parkinson's disease remains undetermined, there is accumulating evidence that multiple genetic and environmental factors interact to cause damage to extrapyramidal dopamine neurons. It is believed that 70–80% of these neurons must be lost before symptoms of Parkinson's disease become evident. Many of the persons who survived the pandemic of von Economo encephalitis in 1918 and 1922 developed Parkinsonism 20 to 30 years later. Psychoactive drugs such as the phenothiazines and butyrophenones can cause a syndrome similar to Parkinsonism. Infections, tumors, and certain chemicals and drugs may cause an identical but reversible disorder. The term Parkinson's disease is reserved for paralysis agitans of unknown cause.

Autosomal recessive and sporadic juvenile cases are often caused by mutations in the parkin gene located at 6q25.2–27.

Pathology—Melanin is lost from nerve cells in the brainstem, particularly in the substantia nigra, and accompanied by extensive loss of dopaminergic nerve cells and reactive gliosis. Intracytoplasmic inclusion bodies, Lewy bodies, also can be found in surviving neurons in the affected areas.

Pathophysiology—Loss of inhibition and the unbalance of opposing pathways in the thalamus and caudate nucleus result in the movement difficulties of Parkinsonism. The origin of the tremor is less clear. Decreased dopamine is found in the substantia nigra, caudate nucleus, and putamen.

Symptoms and Signs—The clinical features are characteristic. There is often a prodromal phase consisting of nonspecific symptoms, such as fatigue, musculoskeletal pain, declining performance, and depression. Within 1 to 2 years, more definitive symptoms appear. The typical tremor occurs at rest and lessens with voluntary movement. The tremor may involve the hands, legs, lips, tongue, and eyelids when the eyes are closed. In the early stages of the disease, the tremor is unilateral but becomes bilateral later in the course. The tremor occurs at a frequency of 4 to 8 cycles/second. The hand tremor is described as "pill rolling."

In the early stage of the disease, there is bradykinesia as all movement is slowed. Later, the patient has particular difficulty initiating movement. Finally, there is absence of movement or akinesia. The spontaneous movements of posture change, such as arm swinging while walking, disappear. The face becomes expressionless and is known as mask-like facies. The voice becomes monotonous. The posture is stooped. Because the patient cannot make reflex adjustments to the posture changes of walking, "he walks with quick shuffling steps at an accelerating pace, as if attempting to catch up with his center of gravity." Passive movement of the extremities elicits "lead pipe rigidity" because both flexors and extensors are contracted or "cog wheel" motion from the superimposition of tremor on rigidity.

Anxiety and tension aggravate the symptoms. The patient also may have seborrhea, excessive sweating, and salivation.

Eventually the patient is incapacitated by the rigidity, and the tremor disappears. The clinical course is one of gradual deterioration.

Stroke Syndromes

A stroke is a process involving one or more blood vessels in the brain, which results in the sudden and dramatic development of a focal neurological deficit. The deficit reflects the location and size of brain injury. Three separate entities are recognized: transient ischemic attack (TIA), stroke in evolution, and completed stroke. While TIAs are transient, evolving and completed strokes are not.

Etiology—The vast majority of strokes are caused by atherosclerotic thrombosis of the cerebral arteries. Embolism from the heart or ulcerated atherosclerotic plaques in the carotid arteries also causes them. Cerebral hemorrhages are due most often to hypertension but also may be due to the rupture of an aneurysm. Less frequent causes include trauma, excessive anticoagulation, hypercoagulable disorders, and inflammatory diseases of cerebral blood vessels.

Normal Physiology—The effects of the blood vessel occlusion relate to the location and availability of collateral or anastomotic blood flow. The circle of Willis provides collateral circulation and protects the brain from ischemia that would otherwise result from occlusion of a carotid or vertebral artery. Retrograde flow from the external carotid may prevent damage when the internal carotid is occluded. Collaterals for the vertebral artery exist. Other anastomoses may prevent or lessen damage if the lesion is distal to the circle of Willis.

Pathophysiology—Infarction results from occlusion of arteries of the brain as elsewhere in the body (see the discussion of atherosclerosis). Thrombotic stroke results when a thrombus develops on an atherosclerotic plaque: the lumen of the vessel is narrowed or may be occluded completely, and collaterals are insufficient to preserve function. Extension of the thrombus may block collateral blood flow. Dural sinus (venous) thrombosis may cause hemorrhagic infarction.

Cerebral embolism most commonly originates from a thrombus in the heart, particularly during atrial fibrillation. Other sources of embolic strokes are mural thrombi that occur after myocardial infarction and pieces of intra-arterial thrombi. The emboli usually lodge at bifurcations.

Intracranial hemorrhage is the third most frequent cause of stroke. Intracranial hemorrhage is due most commonly to hypertension, rupture of saccular aneurysm, and bleeding disorders. Cerebral hemorrhages due to hypertension involve a penetrating artery and occur within the brain tissue. Adjacent tissue is compressed and displaced by the mass of blood. Saccular aneurysms or berry aneurysms are thin-walled blisters protruding from the arteries of the circle of Willis or major branches of the circle at bifurcations. Developmental defects in the media of the arteries cause the aneurysms, which are composed of intima and adventitia. The defect in the wall structure is congenital, but enlargement and eventual rupture occur during later life, reaching a peak at 35 to 65 years. Rupture of the aneurysm results in bleeding into the subarachnoid space and occasionally into the brain as well.

Symptoms and Signs—The location of the lesion determines the nature of the deficit. Lesions in the carotid system result in unilateral signs of hemiplegia, hemihypoesthesia, hemianopia, aphasia, and agnosia. Lesions in the basilar system result in bilateral signs, motor and sensory deficit, brainstem deficit, and variable cranial nerve abnormalities. Cerebellar infarction results in severe dizziness, nausea, vomiting, ataxia, and nystagmus.

In most cases of thrombotic stroke, a TIA has occurred previously. A TIA due to temporary or partial occlusion of all or part of the carotid or middle cerebral artery system may consist of hemiplegia, hemiparesthesia, monocular blindness, or other focal signs, depending on the area of brain affected. A TIA due to temporary or partial occlusion of the vertebral-basilar system consists of dizziness, diplopia, numbness, impaired vision, and dysarthria. A TIA usually lasts for about 10 minutes but may last from a few seconds up to 24 hours. Between the TIAs, the patient may have no neurological deficit. A bruit may be heard over the carotid arteries if they are severely atherosclerotic.

A thrombotic stroke begins suddenly but may progress over several days. Parts of the body may become involved in a stepwise fashion. A completed stroke is defined as 18 to 24 hours without progression for the carotid system and 72 hours without progression for the vertebral-basilar system.

Prognosis in a thrombotic stroke is difficult to predict. Comatose patients have a poor prognosis. Improvement generally occurs as functions are taken over by other parts of the brain or when edema surrounding an infarct subsides. If improvement has not begun by the second week, prognosis is poor. Any deficit that remains at the end of 6 months is likely to be permanent.

Embolic strokes develop the most rapidly and are fully developed within minutes. No warning symptoms precede an embolic stroke. Focal deficits such as motor aphasia, receptive aphasia, or a sensorimotor paralysis may occur. The ultimate prognosis depends upon the correction of the underlying disease.

Cerebral hemorrhage due to hypertension occurs without warning and evolves over hours. It occurs more commonly and at a younger age in blacks. The symptoms and signs depend on the site and size of the hemorrhage. Hemorrhage is most common in the putamen, where it causes hemiplegia, hemisensory loss, homonymous visual loss, and aphasia when the lesion is on the dominant side. Severe headache and vomiting occur at the onset. A total of 85% of patients with cerebral hemorrhages due to hypertension do not survive the first 8 hours. A CT scan reliably detects intracerebral and intracerebellar hemorrhages of 1 cm or more if the study is performed within 2 weeks of the hemorrhage.

Rupture of a saccular aneurysm may present with sudden unconsciousness with or without preceding excruciating headache. There are no lateralizing neurological signs when the blood is confined to the subarachnoid space. The hemorrhage tends to recur if surgical correction is not carried out or is unsuccessful. Prognosis is poor if the patient is comatose; however, if the patient awakes, recovery is likely.

Headache

The three major types of primary headaches are migraine, cluster, and tension-type headaches. Migraine is divided into migraine with and without aura, (formerly called classic and common migraine respectively).

Epidemiology—Migraine affects about 12% of the population. It is four times as common in women, and frequently runs on families. Tension-type headache is several times more common than migraine.

Pathogenesis and Pathophysiology—The pathogenesis of migraine has been exhaustively investigated, but remains incompletely understood. An abnormality of the trigeminal nerve vasculature provoked by release of nitric oxide appears central, but other mediators, such as serotonin likely also play a role.

Tension-type headaches are not a result of scalp or neck muscle contraction. Their pathogenesis is debated but shares some features with migraine.

Symptoms and Signs—Migraine with aura occurs in three stages, prodrome, aura, and headache. The first stage or prodrome lasts from hours to days and may involve changes in mood or appetite and fluid retention. The prodrome may be unapparent or not recognized. The aura is most commonly visual (blurred or cloudy vision, scotomas, and/or flashes of light), but vertigo, chills, tremors, unilateral numbness, aphasia, photophobia, or pallor also may occur. As the aura subsides, the patient experiences a severe, throbbing headache, which initially is unilateral in most cases. Nausea, vomiting, diarrhea, chills, tremors, and perspiration also may occur at this time. During recovery the pain decreases markedly, but the head is tender and exhaustion is present. The migraine without aura lacks the aura phase, but the actual headache may last longer (more than 2 hours) than in migraine with aura.

Cluster headaches are usually unilateral, nonthrobbing, and are more common in males. The patient experiences excruciating pain lasting 20 to 90 minutes. Autonomic features such as nasal stuffiness, rhinorrhea, tearing, and pupillary changes frequently accompany the pain. Bouts may follow one another several times a day for 4 to 8 weeks, not to recur again for 6 to 12 months,

Tension-type headaches may cause intermittent, recurrent, or constant pain. Patients may describe scalp soreness with pain on combing their hair, band-like pain or tightness, and pressure.

Neuromuscular Disease

GUILLAIN-BARRE SYNDROME

This acute inflammatory demyelinating polyneuropathy results in flaccid paralysis with spontaneous recovery.

Epidemiology—Annual incidence is 0.6 to 2.4 cases/100,000/year. It is now the most common cause of flaccid paralysis.

Etiology—The cause of most cases of Guillain-Barre syndrome is unknown. Most cases follow within 3 months of an acute respiratory or gastrointestinal illness, most commonly campylobacter. Cases have been associated with many other infections or medical illnesses.

Pathophysiology—Pathological changes observed in patients who die of Guillain-Barre syndrome include perivascular lymphocytic infiltrates usually associated with demyelination of the affected nerves. Infiltrates also may occur in the liver, spleen, lymph nodes, and heart. Although the pathogenesis is unclear, the syndrome may involve a cell-mediated immunological reaction directed at peripheral nerves.

Symptoms and Signs—The principal symptom is muscle weakness of both proximal and distal limbs. The weakness may advance to muscles of the trunk. While loss of sensation is unusual, paresthesias often occur. Affected patients are afebrile. In severe cases, the respiratory system may be affected, requiring ventilator support. Death is rare, and complete recovery occurs in the majority of cases. Examination of the cerebrospinal fluid shows few cells but a distinct elevation in CSF protein. Nerve conduction studies show slowed motor nerve conduction with temporal dispersion and prolonged distal latencies.

MYASTHENIA GRAVIS

This is a disease characterized by muscle fatigability and weakness most prominently affecting the muscles of the eye and cranium.

Incidence and Epidemiology—The incidence is 1 in 20,000 in the general population. All age groups are affected with females in the 20- to 40-year age group predominating.

Etiology and Pathophysiology—While the underlying cause remains a mystery, the physiological defect has been clarified. The disease is due to a reduction in number and effectiveness of acetylcholine receptors at the motor and plate. This reduction is secondary to an autoimmune mechanism that destroys the receptors. In experimental models, massive phagocytic infiltration of motor end plates with large areas of postsynaptic membrane destruction and associated decrease in acetylcholine receptors is observed. This process results in the denervation of muscle fibers. There are other forms of myasthenia that are not associated with disturbed immunity, including inherited deficiencies in biosynthesis of acetylcholine or its receptors.

Symptoms and Signs—The typical clinical presentation includes drooping eyelids, aphasia, and the inability to perform usually simple muscular functions. Early in the disease, only a few muscles are affected. Neuromuscular fatigue is a cardinal sign: patients are unable to sustain or repeat muscular movements.

Electromyography is a useful diagnostic technique and shows a rapid decline in the amplitude of muscle action potentials with repetitive muscle contraction. Other tests used in diagnosis include the use of anticholinesterase agents and the detection of antibodies to acetylcholine receptors, which can be demonstrated in 90% of patients with myasthenia gravis.

MULTIPLE SCLEROSIS

A number of neurological disorders are characterized by the degeneration of the myelin sheath of nerve fibers. Of these, only multiple sclerosis (MS) will be discussed. Other dieases falling into this classification include acute disseminated encephalomyelitis (postvaccinial and postinfectious encephalomyelitis) and acute hemorrhagic leukoencephalitis.

Normal Physiology—Many of the nerve fibers of the body are covered with a layer of lipid material called myelin. This myelin sheath is interrupted at intervals by spaces termed nodes of Ranvier. Myelinated nerves are found in great number in cranial and spinal processes and in the white matter of the brain and spinal cord. The myelin sheath facilitates rapid nerve impulse conduction.

Etiology and Epidemiology—The etiology is unclear although several epidemiological factors may offer some clues. This disease is rare between the equator and latitudes 30° to 35° north and south. It occurs more frequently with increasing latitude. MS is more common in some families, suggesting simultaneous exposure to some etiological agent or perhaps a hereditary factor. These factors suggest, to some, an infectious etiology with a resultant autoimmune response.

Pathophysiology—The pathologic lesions vary in size and appearance but always include or reflect demyelination. The lesions ("plaques") occur throughout the white matter of the CNS. They are located most commonly in subpial and periventricular white matter of the cerebrum, optic nerves, cerebellum, brainstem, and spinal cord. The associated pathophysiological change is a decrease in speed of nerve impulse conduction. Symptoms worsen with age, reflecting the ongoing nature of the disease.

Symptoms and Signs—While most patients present with evidence of spinal cord or brainstem involvement, about 40% present with only optic neuritis. The former presentation may include paresthesias, numbness, or weakness in an asymmetrical distribution. Diplopia, nystagmus, and cerebellar ataxia also may occur. The latter presentation may include partial or complete blindness in one or both eyes, scotomas, or pain with eye movement. This disease progresses with time with interspersed exacerbations and eventually may result in quadraplegia and coma. The usual patient survives 20 years or more from the time of the initial diagnosis. Magnetic resonance imaging (MRI) scans are the most sensitive means of detecting lesions. Cerebral spinal fluid may contain oligoclonal bands, myelin basic protein, or elevated IgG. Visual, somatosensory, or brainstem auditory evoked potentials may be abnormal and assist in the diagnosis.

Dementia

This is a generic term referring to a syndrome of declining cognitive function. The clinical course of the disorder is extremely variable, and the causes are probably multiple. About 70% of progressive dementias are believed to be due to Alzheimer's disease (AD).

Pathophysiology—Many types of dementia involve structural disease of the cerebrum and diencephalon. Degeneration and loss of nerve cells with secondary changes in the cerebral white matter often are observed. These changes may occur in one or many parts of the brain. AD is characterized by neurofibrillary tangles and senile plaques, found prominently in the hippocampus and association cortex. While the underlying etiology is often undetectable, dementia with its various lesions may be due to identifiable disorders such as chronic hydrocephalus, syphilis, and certain virus infections.

Symptoms and Signs—The initial presentation is quite variable. Symptoms include irritability, lack of interest, distractibility, unclear thinking, loss of memory, and wide mood swings. As the disorder progresses, incontinence, aphasia, and speech disorders often develop. Eventually, the patient becomes unable to care for himself and apparently has no interest in doing so. The course is variable with progression occurring over months or years. It should be stressed that the disease may be due to a wide variety of disorders, many of which are treatable. Therefore, a detailed diagnostic effort is warranted.

RHEUMATOLOGY

Normal Physiology—Joints allow movement of one bone upon another. The ends of the bones are covered with hyaline cartilage, and diarthrodial joints are covered by collagenous tissue called the joint capsule. The synovial membrane lines the joint space side of the joint capsule. The synovial membrane is a relatively acellular, highly vascular, delicate membrane that secretes the synovial fluid. Cartilage, which is avascular, derives its nutrition from the synovial fluid. Various inflammatory diseases, trauma, and degeneration may involve the joint.

Rheumatoid Arthritis

Rheumatoid arthritis (RA) is a systemic autoimmune disorder of unknown etiology. It is characterized by chronic, symmetric, and erosive destruction of the peripheral joints. The severity of the joint disease may fluctuate over time, but generally, joint destruction and deformity are the end results of this disease. There are also common manifestations of this disease affecting other body systems. For instance, subcutaneous nodules, pulmonary nodules and fibrosis, vasculitis, pericarditis, and episcleritis of the eye, are just some of the examples of extra-articular involvement.

Epidemiology—Approximately 3 million people in the US have RA. The onset is most common in the 3rd and 4th decades but may affect all age groups, including children. Women develop the disease more commonly than men do by a ratio of 2.5:1. The prevalence of disease increases with age for both males and females.

Etiology—The etiology is unknown. Histocompatibility typing has proven that a predisposition for the disease is inherited. Unknown environmental factors may play a role in the development of RA. Viruses and bacteria are suspected as possible causes, although to date there is no convincing evidence to support their etiologic role.

Pathophysiology—The disease is characterized by inflammation of the synovium. Infiltration by mononuclear leukocytes occurs along with edema, vascular congestion, and fibrin deposition. As a result of chronic inflammation, the synovium thickens, and forms large villi, which protrude into the joint space. This is referred to as a pannus. The pannus erodes the underlying cartilage and bone. The inflammatory process and destruction of normal joint anatomy results in weakening of tendons, ligaments, and other supporting structures. This leads to instability and partial dislocation (subluxation) of the joint.

Rheumatoid nodules, characteristic of RA, are found most commonly in subcutaneous tissue over pressure points such as the extensor surface of the forearms. However, they also may be found in the lung, heart, or vocal cords. Microscopically, the nodules contain a central area of necrosis surrounded by palisading epitheloid cells and chronic inflammatory cells. Severe RA also may be complicated by vasculitis involving multiple organs.

Antibodies against immunoglobulin G (IgG) are found in the serum and synovial fluid of most patients with RA. The antibodies are of the IgM, IgG, and IgA classes of immunoglobulins and are called rheumatoid factors. Chronic antigenic stimulation is thought to induce production of these antibodies. The exact role of rheumatoid factor in the development of RA has not been demonstrated. However, immunologic mechanisms do appear to play a role in the pathogenesis of RA. Immune complexes of immunoglobulins, rheumatoid factor, and complement generate vasoactive and chemotactic substances in the joint. Lysosomal enzymes, which cause tissue injury, are released after phagocytic cells ingest the immune complexes. It is the release of these vasoactive substances and enzymes that are primarily responsible for the joint erosion and destruction that characterizes this disease.

Symptoms and Signs—The onset is usually insidious. Fatigue, weakness, joint stiffness, arthralgias, and myalgias may precede signs of joint inflammation. The joints gradually become tender, swollen, hot, and painful. Joint stiffness, particularly after a prolonged period of rest ("gelling"), is a major complaint of patients with RA. Morning stiffness is a particular and almost universal complaint of patients with RA. In contrast to the rather brief (5–10 minutes) of gelling seen in patients with osteoarthritis, the morning stiffness of RA is prolonged, sometimes lasting in excess of 1 hour.

Nearly all patients with RA will have synovitis of the wrist, metacarpophalangeal joints (MCP), and proximal interphalangeal joints (PIP) of the hands. Typically the distal interphalangeal joints (DIP) are spared. The cervical spine is frequently involved but interestingly, disease of the thoracic and lumbar spine is exceptionally rare. Other commonly affected joints are the shoulders, elbows, hips, knees, ankles, and metatarsophalangeal joints (MTP) of the feet.

The hypertrophied synovium of involved joints may be palpated. Muscle weakness and atrophy often parallel the severity of the joint disease. Range of motion, especially extension, becomes limited and can lead to flexion contractures. Swan-neck, boutonniere, and cock-up toes are terms used to describe the deformities of the hands and feet. Ulnar deviation of the fingers can occur.

Duration of morning stiffness, which usually is measured in hours, may be used to monitor disease activity. Other indicators include grip strength, time required to walk a certain distance, number and clinical assessment of joints involved, and radiographs demonstrating erosion of bone, loss of joint space, and soft-tissue swelling.

RA is a systemic disease involving multiple organ systems besides the joints. Rheumatoid nodules are found in 20% of RA patients. Less than 5% of the patients have vasculitis. However, the vasculitis may be severe and can result in peripheral neuropathy, nail-fold thrombi, digital gangrene, and leg ulcers. The most common ocular manifestation is keratoconjunctivitis sicca (Sjögren's syndrome); episcleritis also may occur. In the lungs, interstitial fibrosis, rheumatoid nodules, and pleural effusions are seen. Inflammation of the pericardium may cause pericarditis. Rarely this may result in cardiac tamponade. Rheumatoid nodules on the heart valves may lead to murmurs and nodules in the heart muscle that can cause electrical conduction disturbances.

Patients with severe arthritis may develop Felty's syndrome. Felty's syndrome was originally described as RA, splenomegaly, leukopenia, and leg ulcers. However, subsequent observations have shown that there is an additional association with lymphadenopathy and thrombocytopenia.

Mild to moderate anemia that is normochromic or hypochromic is found in patients with RA. The severity of the anemia parallels the activity of the disease. The defect is thought to be in iron utilization in hemoglobin synthesis (see anemia of chronic disease).

Other abnormal laboratory tests include a high erythrocyte sedimentation rate, which may be used to monitor disease activity. The latex aggregation test for IgM rheumatoid factor is positive in 70–80% of patients. Unfortunately, other diseases of chronic inflammation also are associated with a positive rheumatoid factor test, therefore, it is not specific to RA despite its name. Analysis of the synovial fluid, while not diagnostic, typically shows neutrophils (10,000–50,000/mm³) and elevated protein levels.

Diagnosis—The highly variable clinical course of RA makes prognosis difficult in individual patients. Spontaneous remissions and exacerbations are characteristic. Remissions occur most frequently in the early stages of the disease. Some patients may experience a complete remission with little or no joint deformity. Others have a chronically progressive course over many years with development of varying degrees of joint damage. A smaller group, 10–15%, has a relentless destructive course that results in severe deformities and crippling. The unpredictable course of RA also makes evaluation of therapy particularly difficult and contributes to the quackery seen in this field.

The diagnosis of RA is based on the clinical picture of symmetrical inflammatory arthritis usually involving small joints, characteristic radiograph changes, and a positive rheumatoid factor test. Other causes of inflammatory arthritis are Reiter's syndrome, psoriatic arthritis, and systemic lupus erythematosus. Arthritis associated with inflammatory bowel disease must be excluded. The arthritis associated with Lyme disease or hepatitis B may mimic RA. Degenerative joint disease may occur simultaneously.

Degenerative Joint Disease

Loss of joint cartilage and hypertrophy of bone characterize degenerative joint disease (DJD), also known as osteoarthritis (OA).

Epidemiology—Approximately 40 million Americans have radiographic evidence of DJD, but many have no symptoms attributable to the disease. The prevalence of DJD increases with age, 85% of people 75 years or older have characteristic radiographic changes. DJD is a major cause of disability. Severe osteoarthritis of the knee is more likely to result in disability than significant involvement of any other joint.

There are racial and gender differences in both the prevalence and pattern of joint involvement for DJD. For example, Caucasians have a higher rate of hip osteoarthritis than do Blacks, Native Americans, or Asian races. Women are twice as likely as men to have OA of the knees, and Black women twice as likely as Caucasian women.

Etiology—Evidence indicates that heavy use of a joint, so-called "wear and tear" may play a role in initiating the degeneration of cartilage. In other patients, degenerative changes occur when infection, acute trauma, excessive use, or congenital deformities have damaged the car-

tilage. The precise mechanisms of cartilage loss in DJD are unknown. Obesity has also been linked to increased prevalence of OA, especially of the knee. Likewise, genetic factors seem to have additional roles in the development of DJD. For instance, in a woman with DJD of her distal interphalangeal joints (Heberden's nodes), her mother is twice as likely and her sister three times as likely to have the same findings than the mother or sister of an unaffected woman. The mechanism of transmission appears to be autosomal dominant in women and recessive in men.

Pathophysiology—Degenerative joint disease essentially develops in two settings: when there is normal cartilage and bone but abnormal stress or excessive loads placed on the joint which cause the tissues to fail; and when there is a normal applied stress but the underlying joint tissues are defective. DJD may be classified as either primary or secondary. No predisposing cause can be identified in primary DJD. Causes of secondary DJD include infection, trauma, fractures, unusual use, and damage by inflammation as in RA, and congenital abnormalities. In addition, acromegaly, alkaptonuria, hemochromatosis, and chrondrocalcinosis are predisposing factors for secondary DJD.

In either case, histologically degenerative changes are seen in cartilage as progressive loss of metachromasia, which is evidence of proteoglycan loss. Chondrocytes increase in number and form clusters. The surface of the cartilage loosens, flakes off, and fissures form as deeper layers become involved. The cartilage may be lost completely. The bone at joint margins responds by osteophyte formation and hypertrophy. The subchondral bone, which has lost the covering cartilage, becomes dense, smooth, and glistening (eburnation). Cystic areas may develop below the joint surface. Inflammation of the synovium and joint capsule is usually mild.

Collagen fibers and proteoglycans give normal cartilage the properties of compressibility and elasticity. The proteoglycan molecules bind large numbers of water molecules that are released when the cartilage is compressed and are regained when the force is removed. The proteoglycan content of DJD cartilage is diminished and the molecular species is altered.

In contrast to normal adult cartilage, the chrondrocytes proliferate. The chrondrocytes are continuously rebuilding the cartilage matrix in DJD. The amount of hydrolases is increased. As the disease progresses, the destruction exceeds the rate of repair, resulting in a net loss of cartilage. Cartilage laid down during the rebuilding process is of the type normally found in tendons and skin but not in bone. Simultaneously, the subchondral bone sclerosis and marginal bone overgrowths (spurs) develop.

Symptoms and Signs—Pain in the joints particularly with motion or weight bearing is characteristic of DJD. Joint stiffness occurs after rest and quickly subsides after resuming movement. The duration of morning stiffness is measured in minutes rather than hours as in RA.

Examination of the joints reveals decreased range of motion, local tenderness, bony enlargement, but usually no heat or erythema. DJD commonly involves the distal interphalangeal (DIP) joints, in contrast to RA. Bony enlargement of the DIP joints is called Heberden's nodes. Enlargement of the proximal interphalangeal (PIP) joints is known as Bouchard's nodes. DJD involvement of the spine may cause compression of spinal nerve roots by the bony spurs, which can lead to a variety of complaints. DJD of the hips and knees may be the most disabling form of the disease.

Diagnosis—There is no laboratory abnormality characteristic of DJD. The diagnosis is based on symptoms and signs and the radiographic changes of joint space narrowing and bony spur formation.

Crystal-Induced Arthritis: Gout and Pseudogout

Several distinct diseases are characterized by crystal deposition in and about joint spaces. This deposition can lead to acute inflammation of the joint. Gout is a disorder of sodium urate deposition whereas pseudogout is characterized by deposition of calcium pyrophosphate dihydrate crystals. Recently, a form of arthritis has been attributed to hydroxyapatite deposition.

Epidemiology—Contrary to folklore, gout is not related to socioeconomic class. Few individuals with gout consume excessive quantities of purine-containing foods. Primary gout is a disease primarily of the adult male with a peak incidence in the 5th decade. Only 10–15% of cases occur in females, and these are usually in the postmenopausal group. Hyperuricemia is found in 5% of all asymptomatic persons at least one time during adulthood. However, fewer than one in five will develop clinically evident crystal deposition.

Diabetes mellitus, obesity, hypertension, coronary and cerebral atherosclerosis, and hypertriglyceridemia all occur more frequently among gouty patients for unknown reasons.

Etiology—The etiology of gout is either the overproduction or the underexcretion of uric acid. Overproduction may be primary and due to enzyme deficiencies in the metabolic pathway for purines; or may be secondary due to increased purine turnover as in hemolytic or myeloproliferative diseases. Occasionally, increased dietary consumption may cause increased levels as can ethanol abuse. Uric acid underexcretion may be caused by diminished renal function, interaction with various medications, or may be idiopathic.

Calcium pyrophosphate dihydrate crystal deposition disease (CPPD) is due to hereditary causes, trauma, or may be associated with certain metabolic diseases such as hemochromatosis, hypothyroidism, hyperparathyroidism, and amyloidosis,

Pathophysiology—The rates of production and elimination of uric acid determine the amount of uric acid in the body. Exogenous (dietary) and endogenous purines are oxidized to uric acid and eliminated. Of the uric acid eliminated, the kidney excretes two-thirds and the gastrointestinal tract excretes the remainder. The two most important processes in the development of hyperuricemia are abnormalities of endogenous purine production and of uric acid excretion by the kidneys. The majority of patients with gout have a defect of uric acid clearance through the kidneys. Specific enzyme abnormalities that have been identified include decreased hypoxanthine-guanine phosphoribosyltransferase and increased PP-ribose-P synthetase, which result in the overproduction of uric acid.

Uric acid is filtered by glomeruli, but 98% of the filtered amount is reabsorbed by the tubules. The majority of the uric acid excreted (80–85%) is secreted actively into the urine by the renal tubules. The exact reason for undersecretion of uric acid by the tubules is unknown. Metabolic acidosis or increased acid load as occurs in chronic renal failure after a prolonged fast or with ethanol ingestion, inhibits the secretion of uric acid.

Hyperuricemia is defined statistically as a serum uric acid level of above 7.5 mg per 100 ml for males and above 6.6 mg per 100 ml for females using the automated colorimetric method of determination. The risk of developing gout correlates with the serum uric acid level. Gout is rare in patients with uric acid levels of less than 7 mg per 100 ml, whereas 83% of patients with a uric acid level greater than 9 mg per 100 ml develop gout. Although the exact reason for the sudden attack of gout in a hyperuricemic patient is unknown, acute attacks may be precipitated by acute fluctuations in serum uric acid level and trauma to the joint. The likelihood of developing gout increases with age.

When urate crystal precipitate in the joint fluid, they are able to stimulate an intense inflammatory reaction. Neutrophils infiltrate the joint space attempting to remove the foreign crystals. During this process, they release bradykinin, proteases, interleukins, and other inflammatory mediators. The clinical result is a swollen, painful, red joint.

The pathognomonic lesion of gout is the tophus, which is sodium urate deposit surrounded by a foreign-body reaction. The water-soluble crystals are anisotropic (negatively birefringent) when viewed under a polarized light microscope. Sodium urate is deposited in cartilage, epiphyseal bone, periarticular structures, and kidneys. Common sites for tophi include the earlobe, the olecranon, and patellar bursas and tendons. Urate deposits in the joints result in cartilage degeneration synovial proliferation and pannus formation, destruction of subchondral bone, proliferation of marginal bone, and fibrous or bony ankylosis.

Sodium urate crystals are found in the medulla of the kidneys with interstitial inflammatory or vascular reaction. The interstitial inflammation, which may be acute or chronic, results in tubular damage.

Acquired hyperuricemia occurs in patients with polycythemia vera, secondary polycythemia, leukemia, lymphoma, multiple myeloma, chronic hemolytic anemia, and after radiation or chemotherapy for a variety of cancers. Both overproduction and undersecretion of uric acid play roles in the development of secondary gout. Serum and urinary levels of uric acid tend to be higher than in primary gout. Drugs that interfere with secretion of uric acid, such as the thiazide diuretics, also may cause secondary gout. Chronic renal disease may cause hyperuricemia, but gouty arthritis usually is not seen. Patients who have had lead intoxication may develop gout due to damage to the kidneys.

The pathophysiology of CPPD is similar to that described for gout excepting that the inflammatory response is not generally as intense.

Symptoms and Signs—Primary gout has three manifestations: asymptomatic hyperuricemia, acute gouty arthritis (which recurs after asymptomatic intervals), and chronic gouty arthritis. For unknown reasons many patients with hyperuricemia never develop gouty arthritis, urolithiasis, or renal damage.

Acute Gouty Arthritis—The onset of the attack is abrupt and typically involves the great toe, although the instep, ankle, or knee may be involved. The pain is intense or excruciating. Fever may be present. The initial attack usually subsides in a few days to a few weeks, and recovery is complete.

The interval following the initial attack may be from a few weeks to many years. Later, the attacks become more frequent, may involve more joints, and are often more severe.

Chronic Gouty Arthritis—Without treatment and after many years, visible tophi develop, permanent joint destruction occurs, and symptoms become chronic. The tophi are relatively painless. However, there is progressive stiffness and persistent aching of affected joints. Destruction of joints and large tophi may lead to grotesque deformities and crippling. The tophi may ulcerate and extrude the chalky sodium urate.

Urolithiasis—Uric acid stones occur in approximately 20% of patients with gout. The development of urolithiasis may precede the acute attack of gout. A predisposing factor to urate renal stone formation is the excretion of acidic urine throughout the day.

Calcium Pyrophosphate Dihydrate Deposition Disease—CPPD is characterized by chondrocalcinosis and acute attacks of pseudogout. The prevalence increases with age. Associations with other diseases such as hemochromatosis, hyperparathyroidism, ochronosis, Wilson's disease, and hypothyroidism have been demonstrated. Pseudogout describes acute inflammatory arthritis in which positively birefringent rhomboid crystals of CPPD are identified on synovial fluid analysis. By far the most commonly involved joint is the knee. Between attacks the joint may be entirely asymptomatic or show changes of osteoarthritis. Radiographic evidence of calcinosis in cartilage and other joint-related structures usually is found.

Hydroxyapatite crystals have been described recently in the synovial fluid of acutely inflamed joints. They are not resolvable by light microscopy and require electron microscopic or microanalytic techniques for identification. The knee and shoulder are most commonly involved.

Diagnosis—The diagnosis of gout requires the examination of affected joint fluid or tophus material under a polarizing microscope, which will reveal the presence of negatively birefringent, yellow, needle-shaped crystals. In CPPD, the crystals are rod-shaped and show a weakly positive or no birefringence by polarizing, compensated microscopy. Patients with CPPD will also commonly have linear densities noted in the articular cartilage of affected joints on x-ray.

Systemic Lupus Erythematosus

This condition is a multisystem disease of unknown etiology that predominately affects young women but can affect men and women of all ages. It often is viewed as the prototypic autoimmune disease in which antibodies are formed against one's own tissues.

Epidemiology—Systemic lupus erythematosus (SLE) is most commonly seen in women between ages 15 and 40, although all ages may be affected. Females predominate over males 5:1. In the United States, Blacks and Hispanics have a higher incidence of disease compared with Caucasians. There is also a strong familial pattern with first-degree relatives of patients having a higher likelihood of disease.

Etiology—Although many potential etiologies, (eg, viral infections) have been proposed, none have been clearly substantiated. A small percentage of patients given procainamide or hydralazine develop a syndrome, which mimics SLE.

Pathophysiology—Antibodies are formed against one's own DNA. These autoantibodies bind the antigen (DNA) and complement, forming immune complexes which, when deposited in various organs, cause injury. The cause for the formation of these antibodies remains unknown.

Symptoms and Signs—The manifestations of SLE are multiple and involve several body systems. The most frequently involved areas are: skin, musculoskeletal, renal, neurological, and hematological.

Skin Manifestations—The most recognized manifestation of SLE is the malar or "butterfly rash" of the face. This is an erythematous elevated rash across the nose and cheeks. SLE may also cause a discoid rash. Discoid lesions begin as erythematous papules or plaques that may scale and become hypopigmented in the center. They may eventually produce scarring. Patients with SLE are frequently photosensitive to sun exposure. Ulcers of the mucous membranes including the mouth and vagina are often seen as well.

Musculoskeletal Manifestations—Arthritis and arthralgias are the most common presenting symptoms and signs of SLE. The arthritis may involve any joint but most often involves the small joints of the hands, wrists, and knees. Generally involvement of the joints is symmetrical. The arthritis is not destructive or erosive, in contrast to rheumatoid arthritis.

Renal Manifestations—Nephritis is suspected by the finding of proteinuria, hematuria, casts, or elevated serum creatinine. The glomerulonephritis may be of several different types. Renal destruction can be rapid and severe in some cases.

Neurological Manifestations—Neuropsychiatric signs and symptoms include seizures, strokes, peripheral neuropathies, cranial neuropathies, intractable headaches, organic brain syndrome, and psychosis.

Hematological Manifestations—Anemia, leukopenia, lymphopenia, and thrombocytopenia are common findings in patients with SLE. The anemia may be due to chronic inflammation, renal disease, or drugs. However, the most significant is a hemolytic anemia due to antibodies directed against red cell antigens. A variety of clotting abnormalities have been described in patients with SLE. The most common of these is lupus anticoagulant. The name is paradoxical as these patients do have a prolonged PTT and yet generally form both venous and arterial clots causing DVT, PE, and arterial thrombosis. Recurrent fetal loss is associated with the presence of lupus anticoagulant.

Other common manifestations found in patients with SLE include serositis meaning inflammation of the serosa of various internal organs. Most often this involves pericarditis, pleurisy, or peritonitis. Splenomegaly and non-specific lymphadenopathy are also frequent findings.

Laboratory abnormalities may include leukopenia, anemia, thrombocytopenia, false-positive serological test for syphilis, abnormal urinary sediment, and proteinuria, antinuclear antibodies (ANA), antibodies against double-stranded DNA, and hypocomplementemia.

Diagnosis—No single test establishes the diagnosis of SLE. Rather, the diagnosis is classically made by the finding of four of eleven possible criteria as established by the American Rheumatologic Association though finding two or three criteria may be sufficient in some cases. The criteria are a combination of many of the above noted physical manifestations and laboratory findings. Most patients with SLE with have a positive ANA.

Scleroderma

Scleroderma is a disease of unknown etiology characterized by fibrosis of the skin and internal organs.

Epidemiology—Scleroderma is a rare disease estimated to have a prevalence of between 19 and 75/100,000. The peak incidence is in the 5th decade of life. Females are affected more commonly than males, and Black females more commonly than Caucasian.

Etiology—The etiology of scleroderma is unknown.

Pathophysiology—This disease is characterized by increased fibrous tissue disposition and obliteration of small vessels in many organs. Lymphocytic and monocytic cell infiltration is frequently seen in the skin early in the disease. Later, the skin is relatively acellular. The vascular lesions are characterized by widespread endothelial abnormalities and an exuberant proliferation of the vascular intima.

Symptoms and Signs—The first symptoms for most patients are Raynaud's phenomenon, swelling or puffiness of the fingers or hands. The skin of hands typically becomes swollen and then firm, thickened, and leathery in appearance. Gradually, this sclerosis of the skin progresses to involve the face and trunk. Fibrosis of the lungs, GI tract, heart, and kidneys is a later finding. Patients also may manifest one or more of a collection of findings referred to as "CREST" (calcinosis, Raynaud's phenomenon, esophageal involvement, sclerodactyly, and telangiectasis). The most-feared complication of scleroderma is malignant hypertension with rapid onset of renal failure.

Diagnosis—The diagnosis of scleroderma is made clinically. There is no laboratory test available to secure the diagnosis.

Polymyositis and Dermatomyositis

Polymyositis (PM) and dermatomyositis (DM) are idiopathic inflammatory diseases of the skeletal muscle. Dermatomyositis also has skin involvement and is often associated with underlying malignancy.

Epidemiology—Both polymyositis and dermatomyositis are rare conditions with an estimated prevalence of 1/100,000 in the general population. Female outnumber males 2:1. The peak incidence is in the 5th decade of life.

Etiology—The etiology of both PM and DM is unknown. However, there is an association with both conditions and malignancy. Patients with PM and DM have been shown to have an underlying malignant tumor 9% and 15% of the time, respectively. Nearly all tumor types can be associated with PM and DM, although there may be a higher incidence of ovarian, lung, pancreatic, gastric, cervical, bladder, and non-Hodgkin lymphoma.

Pathophysiology—The myositis is characterized by both degenerating and regenerating muscle fibers with a mononuclear cell infiltrate. Several antibodies directed at cytoplasmic RNA synthetases, ribonucleoproteins, and other cytoplasmic proteins have been identified. Unfortunately, these can also be found in other autoimmune disorders and none is specific for either PM or DM.

Symptoms and Signs—Muscle weakness is generally the presenting symptom. It is usually slow in onset and gradually progressive. Often patients will have some symptoms for several months before seeking medical attention. The weakness is most often in the proximal muscle groups and symmetrical. Myalgias and muscle tenderness occur in about half of patients. Muscle atrophy is not usually present until late in the disease even when there is severe weakness.

PM and DM may overlap with features of other connective tissue diseases, particularly scleroderma and systemic lupus erythematosus. Raynaud's phenomena, inflammatory arthritis, fever, and weight loss may also be evident.

In DM, there are several characteristic rashes that distinguish it from PM, although the rash may be transient and may have resolved by the time the patient presents with weakness. The most common rash seen is Gottron's sign. This is a violaceous, erythematous, symmetrical rash that occurs on the extensor surfaces of the metacarpophalangeal and interphalangeal joints of the hands. Similar lesions can occur over the elbows and knees.

The heliotrope rash is a reddish-purple rash that occurs on the eyelids and often has associated swelling of the eyelid. Periungual erythema, abnormal nail-bed capillary loops, and cracking of the skin of the tips of the fingers may also be seen.

Diagnosis—The diagnosis is suspected in patients with proximal muscle weakness, elevated muscle enzymes, and abnormal electromyogram. Confirmation is by muscle biopsy showing inflammation and necrosis. The presence of the skin rash distinguishes DM from PM.

Vasculitis

This is a term used to describe inflammatory changes in blood vessels that can lead to necrosis, thrombosis, and obliteration of the involved vessels. Vasculitis can be a manifestation of an underlying systemic disease or constitute the primary process. Understanding of the vasculitides has been hampered by the lack of a universally accepted and clear classification system. Classifications have been based on clinical, histopathological, and etiological considerations. A major obstacle to classification is the fact that vasculitis is a manifestation of several diseases, and most individual cases do not fit precisely into a well-defined category.

Since vasculitis can involve all organs, a multitude of clinical expressions is seen. Many patients have constitutional complaints such as fever, malaise, anorexia, weight loss, myalgias, and arthralgias. Other features include glomerulonephritis, ischemic heart disease, peripheral neuropathy (mononeuritis multiplex) or CNS involvement, pulmonary infiltrates or effusions, ischemic bowel disease, and rash. Laboratory tests usually suggest a nonspecific inflammatory reaction (eg, elevated erythrocyte sedimentation rate). Diagnosis is based on the clinical presentation in conjunction with biopsy and angiographic results.

POLYARTERITIS NODOSA primarily involves medium-sized vessels and is characterized by infiltration of the vessels with polymorphonuclear leukocytes. In a majority of cases, the etiology is unknown but a few patients have hepatitis B antigenemia. The vessel injury may be mediated through deposition of immune complexes of hepatitis B antigen, antibody, and complement, with resultant damage by neutrophils drawn to the lesions by chemotaxis.

HYPERSENSITIVITY ANGIITIS is a small-vessel vasculitis predominantly involving the skin. It appears to be a manifestation of an allergic reaction to an exogenous (drug, infection) or endogeneous (tumor) antigen. The histopathology is described as "leukocytoclastic angiitis," which is vasculitis with neutrophils and their nuclear dust, extravasated red blood cells, and fibrinoid necrosis of the vessel wall.

WEGENER'S GRANULOMATOSIS is characterized by granulomatous vasculitis of the upper respiratory tract (sinusitis, nasal ulcerations, otitis media), lower respiratory tract (cavitary and nodular infiltrates), and glomerulonephritis. There may also be a variable degree of small vessel involvement.

GIANT-CELL ARTERITIS (also called temporal arteritis) is characterized by segmental involvement of large vessels (primarily branches of the carotid artery) with a mononuclear infiltrate including giant cells and destruction of the internal elastic lamina. The most dreaded complication of giant-cell arteritis is sudden blindness due to ischemic optic neuritis.

ENDOCRINOLOGY

Endocrine glands are organs that secrete hormones directly into the blood. The major endocrine glands are the anterior pituitary, posterior pituitary, thyroid, adrenals, parathyroids, pancreas, and ovaries or testes. The anterior pituitary gland controls the function of the other glands with the exception of the parathyroids, pancreas, and posterior pituitary. The hypothalamus and the central nervous system control the pituitary. Hormones regulate metabolism. Endocrine disorders arise when there is excess or a deficiency of a hormone. Most patients with endocrine dysfunction can be treated successfully.

The Hypothalamus

This organ is responsible for the integration of the central nervous system and endocrine system and is particularly related to the physiological response to stress.

Normal Physiology—See Chapter 64.

Anterior Pituitary Disorders

The pituitary gland is located at the base of the brain in the sella turcica. The cells of the anterior lobe secrete the hormones described below.

Normal Physiology—See Chapter 64.

Epidemiology—Tumors of the anterior pituitary account for 6–18% of all brain tumors. The peak incidence is age 40 to 50 years. There is a similar incidence in men and women with the exception of prolactin secreting tumors, which are more common in women.

Etiology—Pituitary adenomas originate from one of the adenohypophyseal cell types of the pituitary gland. Some forms are associated with certain inherited disorders though the majority arise spontaneously.

Pathophysiology—Tumors that cause increased production of TSH, ACTH, GH, and prolactin develop in the anterior pituitary. Only a few tumors that produce increased amounts of gonadotropins have been identified. A tumor that secretes excess TSH is a rare cause of hyperthyroidism. A tumor may secrete excess ACTH and result in Cushing's disease.

Growth hormone-secreting tumors cause gigantism or acromegaly. If the tumor occurs before puberty and closure of the epiphyseal plate, gigantism with generalized overgrowth of the skeleton and soft tissue occurs. After puberty, a GH-secreting tumor causes acromegaly, which is characterized by overgrowth of bone and cartilage in the distal parts of the body such as the face, head, hands, and feet. Acromegaly also is associated with early osteoarthritis, psychological disturbances, glucose intolerance, and hypertension.

Prolactin-secreting tumors, the most common of the functioning pituitary tumors, cause galactorrhea and amenorrhea.

Sheehan's syndrome is destruction of the pituitary due to hypotension during delivery. The clinical manifestations of panhypopituitarism depend on whether the destruction occurs pre- or post puberty. Prepubertal destruction results in stunted growth and lack of sexual development, and may result in thyroid and adrenal insufficiency. Postpubertal destruction results in gonadal, thyroid, and adrenal insufficiency. Large tumors of the pituitary may also lead to generalized destruction and panhypopituitarism.

Symptoms and Signs—Pituitary tumors may cause headaches, loss of temporal visual fields, bilateral hemianopia, loss of visual acuity, and blindness. The other symptoms and signs relate to the excess or lack of hormone(s).

Diagnosis—The diagnosis of these pituitary disorders is made by the determination of serum levels of the respective hormones combined with imaging (usually MRI) of the pituitary gland.

Posterior Pituitary Disorders

The posterior pituitary secretes ADH and oxytocin.

Normal Physiology—See Chapter 64.

DIABETES INSIPIDUS (DI)—Central diabetes insipidus is a disorder due to decreased production of anti-diuretic hormone (ADH) also known as vasopressin. A decrease in the responsiveness of the kidneys to ADH is called nephrogenic diabetes insipidus.

Epidemiology—No specific epidemiological pattern is described.

Etiology—The most common causes of central DI are neurosurgery or trauma, primary tumors (craniopharyngioma, meningioma, lymphoma), metastatic tumor (breast, lung), infiltrative diseases (sarcoid, histiocytosis X), and idiopathic DI. Rarely, central DI is transmitted as an inherited disorder in an autosomal dominant pattern.

Pathophysiology—Without ADH, the kidney is not able to adequately concentrate the urine. This results in increased urine flow and may lead to dehydration. Typically, the thirst mechanism is stimulated and polydipsia ensues. Hypernatremia occurs if the increase in fluid intake is not sufficient to compensate for the loss of free water.

Diagnosis—Central DI must be distinguished from other causes of polyuria and polydipsia. This can be done by using the water restriction test and serially monitoring urine osmolality, volume, and serum sodium concentration.

Symptoms and Signs—The hallmark of diabetes insipidus is polyuria with excessive thirst and polydipsia. In severe forms, the urine volume is 16 to 24 L/day. Micturition may be required every half-hour, day or night. Urine osmolality is low and urine specific gravity is less than 1.005. If intake does not equal output, the patient may become dehydrated severely.

SYNDROME OF INAPPROPRIATE ADH SECRETION (SIADH)—This is caused by continual release of ADH regardless of plasma osmolality.

Epidemiology—SIADH is typically a disease of adults.

Etiology—Increased and unregulated ADH secretion may be caused by CNS disorders such as stroke, hemorrhage, infection, trauma, or psychosis. Several drugs are known to enhance the secretion of ADH or its effect. Drugs commonly associated with SIADH are chlorpropamide, carbamazepine, cyclophosphamide, SSRIs, anti-psychotics, and some chemotheraputic agents. Pain especially following surgery can lead to increased ADH secretion. Lung diseases (pneumonia, Tb, asthma) and HIV also cause SIADH.

Pathophysiology—Increased levels of ADH acts to interfere with the excretion of free water by the kidneys. This leads to progressive dilution of the serum. Hyponatremia is the result of this dilution and can lead to mental status changes, especially in the elderly.

Symptoms and Signs—Ingested fluids are retained, so that volume expansion and dilutional hyponatremia occur. The patient complains of weight gain, weakness, lethargy, and mental confusion. The serum sodium is low, as is plasma osmolality, and the urine is concentrated.

Diagnosis—The combination of hyponatremia, hypo-osmolality, and urine osmolality above 100 mOsmol/kg establishes the diagnosis of SIADH. Generally the urine sodium will be above 40meq/L.

Thyroid Disorders

The thyroid gland, which is located in the anterior neck, secretes thyroid hormones that control a number of metabolic processes.

Normal Physiology—For the biosynthesis and actions of the thyroid hormones, see Chapter 64.

Disorders that affect serum proteins can affect the amount of bound T3 or T4 but not the metabolic status of the patient. Actions of thyroid hormone include maintenance of body temperature and weight, control of skin texture, stimulation of protein catabolism, stimulation of heart rate and myocardial contractility, increased metabolism of cholesterol, and proper functioning of the CNS. At the tissue level the actions of thyroid hormone are synergistic with those of epinephrine.

HYPOTHYROIDISM—This is a state of deficient thyroid hormone production. Cretinism is hypothyroidism that begins at birth and results in developmental abnormalities and severe mental retardation. Myxedema is severe hypothyroidism with the accumulation of hydrophilic mucopolysaccharides in the dermis.

Epidemiology—The prevalence of hypothyroidism is estimated at 0.1–2% of the population. Women are affected 5 to 8 times more often then men.

Etiology—Various mechanisms may cause hypothyroidism. The most common etiology is autoimmune destruction of the thyroid gland (Hashimoto's thyroiditis). Other causes are inherited defects in thyroid hormone synthesis, dietary deficiency of iodine, and disruption of TSH production by the pituitary. The treatment of hyperthyroidism by either surgery or radioactive iodide usually results in hypothyroidism.

Pathophysiology—The lack of thyroid hormone leads to decrease in overall metabolic rate, changes in skin and hair, and affects on some neurological function. The replacement of thyroid hormone generally restores all of these functions.

Symptoms and Signs—The cretin is constipated and somnolent and has a hoarse cry and feeding problems. Physical abnormalities include short stature, coarse features, protruding tongue, broad flat nose, widely set eyes, a protuberant abdomen, and an umbilical hernia. The child is mentally retarded.

Hypothyroidism in adults is insidious in onset. Complaints include cold intolerance, lethargy, constipation, menorrhagia, slowing of intellectual and motor activity, a modest weight gain, dry hair that falls out, dry skin, stiff aching muscles and a deep-hoarse voice. Patients with myxedema have a dull expressionless face, sparse hair, periorbital puffiness, a large tongue, and pale, cool, rough, doughy skin. Coma is a poor prognostic sign.

Physical examination of patients with hypothyroidism is remarkable for the skin changes, bradycardia, and prolonged relaxation phase of deep tendon reflexes. Goiter is caused by hyperplasia of the thyroid gland because of excessive stimulation by TSH in conditions where there is a defect in thyroid hormone synthesis.

Diagnosis—The most sensitive indicator of thyroid function is the TSH level. As thyroid hormone levels fall, the pituitary responds by increasing the production of TSH. Elevated TSH levels are the hallmark of primary hypothyroidism. In some cases, direct measurement of the thyroid hormone level is required.

HYPERTHYROIDISM—This is a state of excess thyroid hormone production and may arise from several different etiologies.

Epidemiology—Graves' disease is the most common form of hyperthyroidism. It is the most common autoimmune disorder with a prevalence of 0.5/1000. Females are 5 to 10 times more likely to have Graves' disease than males. The peak incidence is 40 to 60 years. There is a similar occurrence in Caucasians and Asians, but it is less common in Blacks.

Etiology—There are several causes of hyperthyroidism. The most common, Graves' disease, is caused by autoantibodies to the thyrotropin (TSH) receptor (TSHR-Ab) that activate the receptor, thereby stimulating thyroid hormone synthesis and secretion and thyroid growth (causing a diffuse goiter). Graves' disease is also associated with ophthalmopathy.

Toxic adenoma and toxic multinodular goiter are conditions in which there is focal or diffuse hyperplasia of the thyroid follicular cells, which leads to overproduction of thyroid hormone. Increased iodine load (such as with IV contrast) can lead to hyperthyroidism. Rarely, hyperthyroidism results from a TSH secreting tumor.

Pathophysiology—The excess thyroid hormone leads to increased metabolism, tremor, weight loss, tachycardia, etc. that are characteristic of the disease. In Graves' disease, there is also an increase in the retro-orbital fat that leads to the exophthalmos that is seen.

Symptoms and Signs—Patients with hyperthyroidism may complain of a goiter, a fine tremor particularly when the fingers are spread, increased nervousness, emotional instability, increased sweating, heat intolerance, weight loss, palpitations, weakness, increased appetite, diarrhea, nausea, vomiting, dyspnea, and amenorrhea. Physical examination reveals wasting of muscles, sinus tachycardia, atrial arrhythmias, and perhaps congestive heart failure. The skin is warm, moist, and velvety and the hair, fine and silky. The goiter is usually diffuse, and a bruit may be heard over the gland.

In Graves' disease, the patient also may complain of decreased lacrimation, eye redness, and a sensation of sand in the eyes. The ocular signs include the characteristic stare and frightened facies, infrequent blinking, lid lag, failure of convergence, and failure to wrinkle the brow on upward gaze. Varying degrees of ophthalmoplegia and proptosis occur. Corneal ulceration may occur as a complication. The exophthalmos is usually bilateral.

Diagnosis—The diagnosis of hyperthyroidism is made by detecting depressed levels of TSH and an elevated level of thyroid hormone (except in rare cases of a TSH producing tumor). Radioactive thyroid scans are useful for differentiating hyperthyroidism caused by autoimmune stimulation from autonomously functioning adenoma or goiter. Antibodies to the TSH receptor can also be detected in the serum of affected individuals.

Adrenal Disorders

The adrenal glands produce three principal hormones. Disorders may involve excess or a deficiency of any one or a combination of the hormones. The disorders may be primary, in the adrenal gland, or secondary, due to a problem outside the adrenal gland.

Normal Physiology—See Chapter 64.

CUSHING'S SYNDROME—Cushing's syndrome refers to the presence of excess glucocorticoids.

Epidemiology—ACTH producing adenoma (Cushing's disease) is the most common cause of Cushing's syndrome (other than iatrogenic administration of corticosteroids). There is a female predominance with a female to male ratio of 8:1. The age range is most frequently 20 to 40 years. Ectopic ACTH producing tumors (oat cell carcinoma of the lung) occur 3 times more commonly in males. Cortisol-producing tumors of the adrenal gland occur equally in males and females but are rare with a prevalence of only 2/million in the general population.

Etiology—Cushing's disease is the result of increased cortisol production due to bilateral adrenal hyperplasia caused by an ACTH-producing tumor of the pituitary gland, which acts independently of feedback mechanisms. This accounts for 68% of cases. Nonendocrine tumors, such as bronchogenic carcinoma, bronchial adenoma and pancreatic carcinoma secrete an ACTH-like peptide that causes the syndrome in 15% of cases. Adrenal adenomas or carcinomas are the cause 9% and 8% of the time.

Pathophysiology—Increased levels of glucocorticoids lead to the symptoms and signs that are seen in Cushing's disease and are similar regardless of the underlying mechanism.

Symptoms and Signs—The syndrome is characterized by truncal obesity, hypertension, weakness and fatigability, hirsutism, amenorrhea, purple abdominal striae, edema, and osteoporosis. Approximately 80% of patients have the first four symptoms and signs.

The symptoms and signs of the syndrome are secondary to the excess cortisol. Increased cortisol levels promote the deposition of adipose tissue in the face (the moon facies), in the interscapular area (the buffalo hump), and in the mesenteric bed (the truncal obesity). The obesity is modest, not extreme. Mobilization of protein from peripheral supporting tissue results in muscle weakness, fatigability, osteoporosis, striae, ecchymoses, and easy bruising. Because of increased hepatic gluconeogenesis and insulin resistance, glucose intolerance or diabetes mellitus occurs. Hypertension is almost always present. Marked emotional changes from irritability, emotional instability, and euphoria to severe depression and psychosis occur. Amenorrhea, acne, and hirsutism are seen in females. Acne is seen in both sexes.

Laboratory tests reveal a mild neutrophilic leukocytosis, normal serum sodium, hypokalemia, metabolic alkalosis, and increased serum glucose with intermittent glycosuria. Radiographs show generalized osteoporosis, particularly of the spine and pelvis, and perhaps compression fractures of the vertebrae.

Diagnosis—The diagnosis of the syndrome is based on elevated serum levels of cortisol. Dexamethasone in sufficient doses can suppress ACTH release and subsequently cortisol production in the syndrome due to a pituitary tumor, but will not affect cortisol secretion in the syndrome due to other causes. Patients with an adrenal tumor have increased serum cortisol but decreased serum ACTH.

PRIMARY HYPERALDOSTERONISM—This is due to excessive production of aldosterone independent of angiotensin II.

Epidemiology—The prevalence is estimated to be 0.5% of all hypertensive patients. It occurs in all age groups but most commonly in the 3rd or 4th decades. Conn's syndrome (adrenal adenoma producing aldosterone) occurs twice as often in females than males.

Etiology—Conn's syndrome is primary hyperaldosteronism due to an adrenal adenoma. Approximately 60% of primary aldosteronism is due to an adrenal adenoma, 30% due to bilateral adrenal hyperplasia and the remainder to carcinoma, nodular hyperplasia, or undetermined causes. Secondary hyperaldosteronism occurs in states of overstimulation of the renin-angiotensin system such as in renal vascular hypertension or in hepatic cirrhosis, nephrotic syndrome, or congestive heart failure in which there is a decrease in the intravascular volume.

Pathophysiology—Excess production of mineralocorticoids, primarily aldosterone, leads to sodium retention and hypokalemia due to the effects of these hormones on the kidneys. This results in volume overload and hypertension most commonly.

Symptoms and Signs—The hallmarks of the disease are hypokalemia, hypertension, and volume expansion. The hypokalemia leads to muscle weakness and fatigue, particularly in the legs, and EKG changes. Hypokalemia may predispose to the development of pyelonephritis. The patients complain of polyuria and polydipsia.

Diagnosis—The diagnosis is based on a normal renin levels and elevated urine aldosterone level from a 24-hour collection.

PRIMARY ADRENAL INSUFFICIENCY (ADDISON'S DISEASE)—This is a disease originally described by Addison, which refers to the autoimmune destruction of the adrenal gland with the resultant loss of sufficient cortisol production.

Epidemiology—The prevalence of Addison's disease has been reported to be 39 to 60/million of the general population. The mean age is 40 years.

Etiology—The adrenal glands are destroyed. Approximately 90% of the glands must be destroyed before clinical manifestations occur. Chronic granulomatous infections such as tuberculosis or fungal infection or acute infections such as meningococcemia can cause the destruction. Most cases are due to atrophy of the adrenal glands, which is immunologically mediated and may have a genetic predisposition.

Pathophysiology—Destruction of the adrenal gland is mediated by autoantibodies. Cortisol, which is vitally important for the metabolism of carbohydrates and protein, control of the immune system, and control of vasopressin, is not produced in adequate amounts. Often there is accompanying autoimmune disease of the thyroid or other endocrine glands. In autoimmune adrenalitis, the adrenal medulla,which is the portion of the gland responsible for the production of epinephrine, is usually spared. However, the synthesis of epinephrine depends on high local cortisol concentration. This may lead to inadequate production of epinephrine under physiological stress conditions.

Symptoms and Signs—This disease presents as progressive fatigability, weakness, anorexia, nausea, vomiting, weight loss, increased skin and mucosal pigmentation, and hypotension. Other symptoms include those due to hypoglycemia and abdominal pain, diarrhea, constipation, salt craving, and syncope. Hyperkalemia and hyponatremia due to lack of aldosterone are typically present. The most prominent symptom is fatigue. The hyperpigmentation is brown, tan, or bronze in both exposed and nonexposed areas and particularly over pressure points or in skin creases. The hyperpigmentation results from the over production of ACTH by the pituitary in an effort to stimulate cortisol release from the adrenal gland. ACTH binds to melanocortin-1 receptors in addition to its effects on the adrenal gland and this leads to the hyperpigmentation that is seen clinically.

Diagnosis—A serum cortisol level obtained between 8 am and 9 am is useful to rule out the presence of adrenal insufficiency if the level is >19 μg/dl. Levels <3μg/dl are indicative of the disease. All other patients need dynamic testing. This consists of corticotropin stimulation testing and measurement of serum ACTH levels.

SECONDARY ADRENAL INSUFFICIENCY—This is an ACTH deficiency caused by pituitary destruction or pituitary atrophy secondary to prolonged administration of exogenous corticosteroids. The patient has the same symptoms and signs as the patient with primary adrenal insufficiency (above) but not the hyperpigmentation. ACTH deficiency due to pituitary destruction usually occurs along with other hormone deficiencies. Generally, hypotension is not as problematic because the release of aldosterone is more dependent on Angiotensin II than on ACTH. For this same reason, hyperkalemia is not seen in secondary adrenal insufficiency.

The diagnosis of secondary adrenal insufficiency is made by the finding of low morning cortisol levels and is confirmed by using the insulin-induced hypoglycemia test and following the rise of cortisol in response to hypoglycemia. With secondary adrenal insufficiency, this response will me minimal or absent. A second test known as the short metyrapone test is also available.

ADRENAL CRISIS—This is a state of acute adrenal insufficiency and is life-threatening. Adrenal crisis should be suspected in any patient with unexplained catecholamine-resistant hypotension, especially if they have hyperpigmentation, vitiligo, scanty axillary and pubic hair, hyponatremia, or hyperkalemia.

Etiology—Stress, surgery, trauma, or infection may precipitate acute adrenal insufficiency in a patient who has been chronically adrenally insufficient. Adrenal hemorrhage due to septicemia or anticoagulants or rapid withdrawal of exogenous steroids may precipitate an acute adrenal crisis in a patient with previously normal adrenal function.

Pathophysiology—The symptoms and signs are due to the relative lack of cortisol and catecholamines under conditions of physiological stress.

Symptoms and Signs—The symptoms and signs of chronic adrenal insufficiency become severe and intractable. The nausea, vomiting and abdominal pain are difficult to control and contribute to the dehydration. Somnolence is profound. The blood pressure is low, and the patient may die of hypovolemic shock.

Diagnosis—Finding low serum cortisol levels in a patient with physiological stress makes the diagnosis. A cortisol level of >25 μg/dl in a patient requiring intensive care probably rules out adrenal insufficiency however, a safe cutoff is unknown. A "normal" cortisol level in an acutely ill patient does not exclude this diagnosis, as the level may be normal but insufficient for the physiological state of the patient.

Diabetes Mellitus

This is a disorder of glucose metabolism that results from an absolute or relative lack of insulin and of complications that include accelerated atherosclerosis, retinopathy, nephropathy, and neuropathy. The interrelationship between the glucose intolerance and the vascular disease has not been defined clearly. Type 1 diabetes (insulin-dependent diabetes, formerly called "juvenile onset diabetes") is believed to be an autoimmune disorder. It is characterized by marked insulin deficiency and rapid onset. Late onset and a diminished insulin response characterize type 2 diabetes (also called noninsulin-dependent diabetes, formerly adult onset diabetes).

Epidemiology—This is a disease that occurs worldwide with about 4.2 million diabetics in the US. The incidence is higher in relatives of diabetics, people older than 45 years, and those who are currently or were obese.

Etiology—Both types have a genetic predisposition, which is more obvious in the case of Type 2 diabetes. Destruction of the pancreas by chronic pancreatitis, hemochromatosis, or carcinoma results in diabetes. Other endocrine disorders, such as Cushing's syndrome, hyperpituitarism, and hyperthyroidism, are associated with the disease. Glucose intolerance may occur during pregnancy or times of excessive stress, and at times with the administration of glucocorticosteroids, thiazides, and oral contraceptives.

Pathophysiology—The beta cells of the pancreas are decreased in number or are degranulated in diabetes. The reduction in number of beta cells corresponds to the lack of insulin. In Type 1 diabetes, there are no beta cells. In Type 2 diabetes, only about one-half of them are present. In some cases, these cells are infiltrated with lymphocytes, suggesting an autoimmune mechanism for Type 1 diabetes. The presence of anti-islet antibodies also supports an autoimmune hypothesis in Type 1 diabetes.

The atherosclerosis that occurs in diabetes is the same as the atherosclerosis previously discussed, but it occurs as frequently in females as males and at an earlier age. In the kidneys, nodular glomerulosclerosis (Kimmelstiel-Wilson's) is seen, which is the deposition of glycoprotein in ball-like masses in the mesangial regions of the capillary tufts. Diffuse glomerulosclerosis, which is the deposition of glycoprotein in the mesangium, also is seen, as well as tubular basement membrane thickening. The earliest finding of diabetic retinopathy is microaneurysms. Proliferative retinopathy (the formation of new blood vessels around the optic disk) occurs with long-standing diabetes. Repeated hemorrhages cause scar formation that may lead to retinal detachment. The changes of hypertensive retinopathy also are seen in diabetics with hypertension.

The lack of insulin results in a peripheral underutilization and a hepatic overproduction of glucose, which leads to hyperglycemia. Insulin facilitates the entry of glucose into cells of adipose tissue and muscle, stimulates fat synthesis in cells, and induces protein synthesis. See Chapter 50. The lack of glucose in muscle cells leads to glycogenolysis and the release of amino acids for gluconeogenesis. Lack of insulin and glucose in adipose tissue impairs triglyceride synthesis and promote the release of free fatty acids. The liver metabolizes free fatty acids to ketones, which are used by muscles for energy, to a limited extent. Lack of insulin also results in hepatic overproduction of glucose from glycogenolysis and gluconeogenesis. Another hormone, glucagon, is increased in diabetes. Glucagon effects oppose insulin physiologically.

Hyperglycemia results in glycosuria when the serum level of glucose exceeds the renal threshold for reabsorption of glucose. The osmotic diuresis results in polyuria and polydipsia and may result in dehydration. Excess ketones also are excreted in the urine, as strong acids. This results in urinary loss of bicarbonate and potassium and dehydration.

Normally insulin is released only in response to a glucose load such as a carbohydrate-containing meal. Serum insulin levels rise within 15 to 20 minutes after eating. Patients with Type 1 diabetes do not produce insulin. Those with Type 2 diabetes produce too little insulin and produce it too late to prevent hyperglycemia. Obese people have hypertrophied adipose cells, which, because of their size, are less sensitive to the action of insulin.

The vascular complications of diabetes mellitus have been related to the hyperglycemia. It is postulated that glycoprotein is deposited in the capillaries when glucose levels are elevated. Formation of cataracts and neuropathy are thought to occur because glucose is metabolized to sorbitol by aldose reductase in hyperglycemia. The sorbitol causes osmotic swelling and damage.

Symptoms and Signs—The onset of Type 1 diabetes is sudden and characterized by polyuria, polydipsia, polyphagia, weight loss, decreased muscle strength, irritability, and perhaps a return of bed-wetting. Often the initial presentation may be ketoacidosis. About one-third of these patients have a remission shortly after the onset of the diabetes.

The remission may last for weeks to 1 year, and the patient does not require insulin during this time. After the remission, Type 1 diabetics require insulin for the remainder of their lifetime. They are very sensitive to the effects of insulin and physical activity. Both hypoglycemia and ketoacidosis punctuate their course.

The clinical presentation of Type 2 diabetes may be the insidious onset of weight loss, nocturia, vascular complications, decreased or blurred vision, fatigue, anemia, or symptoms and signs of neuropathy. The disease may be diagnosed from an elevated glucose level without any symptoms. Type 2 diabetics usually are not prone to ketoacidosis. The majority of Type 2 diabetics respond to weight loss.

Diagnosis—The diagnosis of diabetes mellitus is based on the documentation of elevated fasting blood sugar, elevated blood glucose 2 hours after a meal, or an abnormal glucose tolerance test. Diet, physical activity, age, underlying diseases, and drugs influence the accuracy of a glucose tolerance test.

Complications of Diabetes—*Ketoacidosis* occurs in diabetic patients who develop high levels of glucose and ketones plus metabolic acidosis. The usual cause is lack of compliance with insulin therapy but ketoacidosis may be the first episode for an undiagnosed diabetic or a manifestation of an infection. The symptoms and signs of ketoacidosis include nausea, vomiting, abdominal pain, and air hunger (Kussmaul breathing - heavy labored breathing as a compensatory mechanism to the decreased pH). The dehydration may be severe. Oliguria and hypotension may be present. Hyperglycemia, decreased bicarbonate, hypokalemia, azotemia, and acidosis may be seen on laboratory evaluation.

Hyperglycemic hyperosmolar nonketotic coma occurs in Type 2 diabetics. The patients are usually elderly and have some renal impairment. Polyuria and polydipsia precede neurological manifestations. The patient presents with hyperpyrexia, hypotension, tachycardia, hyperventilation, and the signs of dehydration. Hyperreflexia, mild disorientation, confusion, seizures, or coma reflect the intracellular dehydration of the CNS. Laboratory examination is remarkable for increased serum osmolality and hyperglycemia without ketosis or hypernatremia.

Retinopathy occurs in the majority of diabetics after many years of the disease. Venous dilatation, the formation of microaneurysms and small hemorrhages into the retina occur but do not interfere with vision. Hemorrhages into the vitreous cause temporary blindness. Retinal detachment occurs due to repeated hemorrhages and scar formation. Secondary hemorrhagic glaucoma occurs in proliferative retinopathy. Diabetes is the second leading cause of blindness. Cataracts also are associated with the disease.

Neuropathy may result from the sorbitol pathway or from ischemia resulting from the vascular disease. Diabetic neuropathy most frequently involves the peripheral nerves but can involve any nerve. Manifestations of diabetic neuropathy include sexual dysfunction in the male, gastric atony, nocturnal diarrhea, fecal incontinence, orthostatic hypotension, neurogenic bladder, paresthesias, and loss of sensation.

Diabetic ulcers and gangrene result from the neuropathy, the vascular disease, or both. The painless foot is more prone to injury. The ischemic foot is less likely to heal. The patient usually has a history of intermittent claudication, nocturnal leg pain and cramps, loss of hair, and muscle atrophy. Both feet and legs usually become involved.

Nephropathy typically occurs with diabetes of 15 years or more duration and usually occurs along with the other complications. The first sign of diabetic nephropathy is mild proteinuria. Later, the nephrotic syndrome may appear, and renal function deteriorates or progressive renal failure occurs without the nephrotic syndrome. Diabetic nephropathy may cause hypertension. Urinary tract infections and pyelonephritis are more common in the diabetic and may contribute to the renal failure.

Disorders of Calcium Metabolism

These disorders may relate to dysfunction of the parathyroid glands or to vitamin D deficiency.

Normal Physiology—Calcium and phosphate homeostasis is maintained by parathyroid hormone (PTH), vitamin D, and calcitonin. The normal serum calcium varies only slightly for an individual. Dietary vitamin D or that produced in the skin by sunlight is inactive. Vitamin D must be hydroxylated at the 25-position by the liver and at the 1-position by the kidneys to form the active 1,25-dihydroxycholecalciferol. Parathyroid hormone is necessary for the hydroxylation in the kidneys. Parathyroid hormone and vitamin D work together to stimulate gastrointestinal absorption of calcium, bone resorption, and renal reabsorption of calcium. The actions of vitamin D and parathyroid hormone are opposed by calcitonin. Parathyroid hormone promotes the excretion of phosphate by the kidneys. Vitamin D promotes phosphate absorption from the gastrointestinal tract. See also Chapters 64 and 65.

PRIMARY HYPERPARATHYROIDISM—This is an overproduction of PTH with increased serum calcium and decreased serum phosphate.

Epidemiology—Primary hyperparathyroidism is the most common cause of hypercalcemia. It occurs in 0.2% of women over age 65 years and 0.1% of men in that same age group. The majority of cases are sporadic, although there are some with a hereditary cause.

Etiology—Most cases are caused by benign adenomas of one parathyroid gland (80% of cases). Other cases are caused by chief cell hyperplasia in all four parathyroid glands, and a few are caused by carcinoma of the parathyroids. Nonendocrine neoplasms without metastases to the bone that secrete PTH-related peptide cause pseudohyperparathyroidism.

Pathophysiology—The increased level of PTH leads to increased bone resorption, calcium absorption by the gut, and reabsorption in the kidneys resulting in hypercalcemia.

Symptoms and Signs—The majority of patients with primary hyperparathyroidism are asymptomatic, and the diagnosis is discovered after routine screening demonstrates elevated serum calcium.

Some patients present with recurrent nephrolithiasis that leads to urinary tract obstruction, recurrent urinary-tract infections, a predisposition to pyelonephritis, and chronic renal failure. The stones are usually either calcium oxalate or calcium phosphate. Nephrocalcinosis or deposition of calcium in the renal parenchyma also can occur as a result of hyperparathyroidism. Nephrocalcinosis may lead to chronic renal failure. The effect of increased levels of PTH on the bone results in decreased number of trabeculae, increased osteoclasts, and replacement of normal bone by fibrous tissue, which is known as osteitis fibrosa cystica. The hands and skull are affected most commonly. Radiographs show phalangeal resorption.

Increased serum calcium can result in mental status changes from mild personality disturbances to severe psychotic disorders, obtundation, and coma. Proximal muscle weakness, easy fatigability, and muscle atrophy are caused by increased serum calcium. Patients with hyperparathyroidism have a high incidence of duodenal ulcers that may be related to the increased serum calcium.

Other causes of hypercalcemia, such as osteolytic metastases from various malignancies, prostaglandins from various cancers without metastases to the bone, vitamin D intoxication, milk-alkali syndrome, and prolonged immobilization must be excluded. The serum level of PTH is not elevated in these situations.

Diagnosis—Finding an elevated level of PTH in the presence of hypercalcemia makes the diagnosis.

SECONDARY HYPERPARATHYROIDISM—This occurs in situations in which serum calcium levels fall and the parathyroids are intact. Chronic renal failure causes secondary hyperparathyroidism. The failing kidney is not able to hydroxylate vitamin D to the active form resulting in low serum calcium levels. The parathyroid glands secrete more PTH in an effort to stimulate more vitamin D hydroxylation and more bone resorption. Thus, osteitis fibrosa cystica is a part of the bone disease of chronic renal failure. The serum calcium level is normal, although the serum phosphate and PTH levels are high.

HYPOPARATHYROIDISM—The production of PTH is decreased. Pseudohypoparathyroidism is a resistance of the renal tubules to the action of PTH. Serum calcium is low, and serum phosphate and PTH are high.

Etiology—Hypoparathyroidism is caused most commonly by surgical removal or damage to the glands. A congenital absence of PTH occurs rarely. Pseudohypoparathyroidism is an X-linked inherited disorder.

Symptoms and Signs—Hypocalcemia causes neuromuscular irritability, which is manifested by tingling and numbness around the lips, and of the hands and feet. Tetany and convulsions are the most serious manifestations of hypocalcemia.

The patient with pseudohypoparathyroidism is of short stature and has short metacarpals and metatarsals. The serum PTH level is high. In addition to the symptoms and signs of hypocalcemia, these patients may have resorption of bone and soft tissue calcifications as in primary hyperparathyroidism.

OSTEOMALACIA AND RICKETS—This is due to defective mineralization of the normal bone matrix. Osteomalacia refers to the disorder that occurs after the bones have ceased growing; rickets refers to the disorder in growing bones.

Etiology—The defect is a deficiency of vitamin D. Vitamin D deficiency may result from consumption of a deficient diet, inadequate exposure to the sun, intestinal malabsorption of vitamin D (a fat-soluble vitamin), chronic acidosis, renal tubular defects, and therapy with anti-convulsants.

Pathophysiology—A precise concentration of calcium and phosphate is required for mineralization of bone matrix. A deficiency of vitamin D results in decreased absorption of calcium and phosphate from the gastrointestinal tract. Hypocalcemia stimulates the production of PTH, which increases calcium resorption from the bone and phosphate excretion by the kidneys. Mineralization cannot occur because of the decreased calcium and decreased phosphate.

Symptoms and Signs—A child with rickets has skeletal deformities, an increased susceptibility to bone fractures, muscular weakness, hypotonia, delayed dental eruption, defects in the enamel of the teeth, and in severe cases, tetany. Adults with osteomalacia have skeletal pain, bone tenderness, muscular weakness, and fractures of the bones with minimal trauma.

Diagnosis—X-rays of the bones show typical findings. In children, there will be widening of the epiphyseal growth plates, a frayed appearance of the metaphysis, and cupping and widening of the metaphyses. In adults, the radiographic findings are similar to those found in patients with osteoporosis—a generalized loss of bone density with thinning of the cortex.

Serum levels of vitamin D and vitamin D metabolites can assist in the diagnosis.

OSTEOPOROSIS—This is not a disorder of calcium metabolism. The amount of calcium per unit mass of bone is normal in osteoporosis, but the amount of bone is decreased. The condition occurs with aging as bone resorption exceeds bone formation. It occurs in the spine leading to back pain, collapse of vertebrae, and deformity of the spine. Long bones and hips are also susceptible to the disease with subsequent ease of fracture.

The Hyperlipoproteinemias

These result from disturbances in the synthesis or degradation of lipoproteins. The morbidity and mortality associated with this family of disease result from the ability of abnormally high lipoprotein levels to cause atherosclerosis and pancreatitis. Primary lipoproteinemias are due to disorders in lipoprotein metabolism and have a genetic basis, while secondary hyperlipoproteinemias occur because of a concurrent disease such as diabetes mellitus or hypothyroidism. As a complete discussion of all hyperlipoproteinemias is not possible here, only two of the more common primary types, familial hypercholesterolemia and familial hypertriglyceridemia, will be presented.

Normal Physiology—The physiological role of the lipoproteins is to transport lipids (ie, triglycerides, and cholesterol esters) through plasma. Lipoproteins are comprised of triglycerides, cholesterol, phospholipids, and protein (apoprotein). Various lipoproteins differ in the quantity of these components and thus density and size. Lipids are transported in the body by lipoproteins through exogenous and endogenous pathways.

In the exogenous pathway, dietary lipids are incorporated into chylomicrons that are transported to adipose and muscle tissue where the triglycerides are removed. The remainder of the chylomicron, or remnant particle, is transported to the liver for further metabolism.

The endogenous pathway has its base primarily in the liver, where carbohydrates and other substrates are converted to triglycerides. The liver secretes these triglycerides into the blood as very low-density lipoproteins (VLDL). These particles are handled in much the same way as chylomicrons except that after removal of the triglycerides by adipose tissue, a further transformation occurs. Most of the protein is removed, yielding low-density lipoprotein (LDL), which is composed chiefly of cholesterol. These LDL particles supply cholesterol for various uses, including cell-membrane composition and glucocorticoid synthesis. In addition, some LDL particles are degraded by the reticuloendothelial system. As the cells of this system turn over, cholesterol is released and incorporated into the high-density lipoprotein (HDL). Certain components of the HDL apoprotein are transferred to VLDL, and cholesterol is transported back to the liver, a major site of cholesterol synthesis.

FAMILIAL HYPERCHOLESTEROLEMIA—

Epidemiology—This common type affects approximately 1 in 500 individuals in the general population.

Etiology—Familial Hypercholesterolemia (FH) is caused by an autosomal defect in the gene that codes for the LDL receptor. A rare autosomal recessive form is caused by a defect in an adaptor protein for the LDL receptor or for a ligand on the LDL receptor.

Pathophysiology—The defects occurring with this disorder are an inability to bind and/or transport LDL into cells for subsequent catabolism and regulation of cholesterol-synthesizing mechanisms. Thus plasma LDL is elevated. More is taken up by the reticuloendothelial system resulting in accumulations in various locations in the body. These accumulations are called xanthomas. LDL also infiltrates the walls of blood vessels, ultimately resulting in atherosclerosis.

Symptoms and Signs—Patients have high LDL blood levels from birth and throughout life. The chief manifestation is myocardial infarction, which results from coronary atherosclerosis. Myocardial infarctions may occur as early as the 1st decade in homozygotes and generally by the 3rd or 4th decade in heterozygotes. Xanthomas, a common sign of this disorder, increase in frequency with age. They tend to occur in tendons and the eyelids. With the homozygous form of this disease, xanthomas also may form in the skin over the knees, elbows, and buttocks as well as between fingers. High plasma cholesterol (or LDL) yet normal triglyceride levels suggest the diagnosis.

Diagnosis—The diagnosis of FH requires elevated cholesterol levels with usually normal triglycerides and genetic or cellular confirmation of a defect in the LDL receptor. Supportive evidence is the presence of premature coronary artery disease in a first-degree relative or two or more second-degree relatives.

FAMILIAL HYPERTRIGLYCERIDEMIA—This disease involves elevated blood levels of VLDL with resultant hypertriglyceridemia.

Epidemiology—Familial hypertriglyceridemia occurs in approximately 1 in 500 persons.

Etiology—This is caused by an autosomal dominant disorder. It is often associated with obesity, insulin resistance, hyperglycemia, hypertension, and hyperuricemia. The underlying disorder is a mutation in the lipoprotein lipase gene (LPL).

Pathophysiology—The underlying defect is one of several inactivating mutations in the gene for LPL. The incidence of diabetes mellitus and obesity is higher in this patient population and both contribute to the hypertriglyceridemia.

Symptoms and Signs—These patients usually exhibit hyperglycemia, hyperinsulinism, and obesity in addition to hypertriglyceridemia. Such findings usually are not manifested until after puberty. As with familial hypercholesterolemia, atherosclerosis is frequent and may lead to myocardial infarction. Unlike in hypercholesterolemia, xanthomas are not common. In addition to the inherent complications of diabetes and obesity, both contribute to this condition and thus to the atherosclerosis. The diagnosis is suggested by the finding of elevated plasma triglycerides with normal cholesterol levels. Some patients have elevated chylomicron levels in addition to the increased VLDL.

HEMATOLOGY

Normal Physiology-Hematopoiesis—Blood is an organ that performs many functions. It is the transport system for the body. Oxygen, glucose, amino acids, and fats are transported to cells for metabolism. Waste products of metabolism are transported to organs for excretion. Hormones transported by blood regulate the functions of organs and tissues. Blood cells and proteins are responsible for host defenses against infection and cancer. Blood also has the self-preserving function of hemostasis or clot formation. Blood is composed of red blood cells (RBCs), white blood cells (WBCs), platelets, and plasma.

In the embryo, the yolk sac is the blood-forming organ until about 3 months of gestation. The liver and spleen then become the blood-forming organs. These organs do not normally continue to form blood cells after birth. The bone marrow becomes a hematopoietic organ at 6 months of gestation and continues so after birth. An adult has active bone marrow in the axial skeleton whereas hematopoiesis during childhood also occurs in the long bones. With age the bone marrow in the long bones becomes progressively replaced by fat. In disease states where the need for red blood cells (RBCs) is increased greatly, bone marrow may revert to the infant pattern, increasing RBC production 5- to 8-fold. When this compensatory mechanism is exceeded, the spleen and liver may assume some hematopoietic functions. The fetus makes hemoglobin F, which carries oxygen more efficiently at low oxygen tensions. At birth hemoglobin F is replaced largely by hemoglobin A, although production of hemoglobin F continues throughout life, especially in certain diseases. The fetus has a high RBC count, which falls at birth since the increased number of RBCs is no longer needed.

Blood cells follow certain principles of maturation. Bone-marrow stem cells are pluripotent and can become a RBC, WBC, or platelet. During maturation, the size of a blood cell decreases. Young cells are capable of protein synthesis while mature cells, except lymphocytes and macrophages, are not. The nucleus in a young cell is large and contains loose fine chromatin. A mature cell has a small nucleus without nucleoli and with dense chromatin.

The reticulocyte is the next-to-last step of maturation of the red blood cell. The nucleus is absent in the reticulocyte, but some RNA and ribosomes are still present. These are absent in mature RBCs. Reticulocytes are seen in the peripheral circulation and normally compose 1% of the RBCs. A normal RBC has a life span of 120 days. The production of red blood cells is stimulated by erythropoietin, which is synthesized, in part, in the kidneys in response to hypoxia. Androgens also increase RBC production probably through their effect on erythropoietin.

White blood cells (WBC) are the second component of blood and are primarily responsible for immune functions. The earliest white blood cells evolve along a differentiation line to become several different cell types, each with a distinct function. These include: polymorphonuclear cells (PMNs), lymphocytes, eosinophils, monocytes, and basophiles.

Platelets are small cellular entities that are involved in hemostasis. They are responsible for initiating blood clotting and help form a physical plug at a bleeding site. The precursor cell in the bone marrow is a megakaryocyte.

Plasma contains various proteins. The most abundant of these is albumin. The various coagulation proteins are also found in plasma.

Hematological disorders can affect any or several of these components of blood.

Anemia

Anemia is defined as a decrease in the number of red blood cells. This may occur as a result of RBC loss (bleeding), RBC destruction, or decreased RBC production.

PERNICIOUS ANEMIA—This is a defect in RBC production caused by lack of vitamin B12.

Epidemiology—Pernicious anemia is most commonly seen in people of Northern European decent and African-Americans. It is uncommon in Asian people. The average age of onset is 60 years and is rare under age 30 years. The incidence is substantially increased in patients with autoimmune diseases such as Graves', thyroiditis, vitiligo, adrenal insufficiency, and hypoparathyroidism.

Etiology—Most cases are caused by autoimmune destruction of the parietal cells of the stomach that make a protein known as intrinsic factor which is responsible for permitting absorption of vitamin B12 by the ileum. A total of 90% will have anti-parietal cell antibodies, and 60% have antibodies directed at intrinsic factor as well.

Other causes of vitamin B12 deficiency include total gastrectomy, stomach damage due to corrosives, intestinal malabsorption due to inflammatory disease, resection of the ileum, and competition for vitamin B12 by bacterial overgrowth or the fish tapeworm.

Pathophysiology—It is characterized by lack of intrinsic factor secretion, and consequent atrophy of the gastric mucosa. As a result, vitamin B12, which is needed for proper RBC production, is not absorbed by the ileum of the small intestine. This leads to the decreased production of RBCs by the bone marrow. Those that are produced are characteristically larger than normal RBCs (macrocytic).

Vitamin B12 is also important for normal neurological function. Lack of vitamin B12 leads to demyelination of nerves followed by axonal degeneration.

Symptoms and Signs—The nonspecific symptoms and signs of anemia occur and because of defects in epithelial cells a red, sore, glazed tongue is seen. The neurological abnormalities consist of numbness, tingling, and loss of vibratory sense in the extremities, loss of position sense, loss of fine coordination, spasticity, irritability, memory loss, and mild depression. The GI complaints include anorexia and significant weight loss. Examination of the blood shows oval macrocytes. The red blood cells may be shaped bizarrely (poikilocytosis) and of different sizes (anisocytosis). The reticulocyte count is decreased. The nuclei of the neutrophils may have five or more lobes (hypersegmentation), and there may be mild to moderate neutropenia and thrombocytopenia, with the platelets also bizarre in appearance. The bone marrow shows the megaloblasts, erythroid hyperplasia, abnormal mitoses in the red cell series, large leukocytes with bizarrely shaped nuclei, and decreased numbers of megakaryocytes.

Diagnosis—Macrocytic anemia with low vitamin B12 levels makes the diagnosis.

FOLIC-ACID DEFICIENCY ANEMIA—This is a megaloblastic anemia due to folic-acid deficiency that may be confused with vitamin B12 deficiency anemia.

Etiology—Most cases are due to an inadequate diet. Folic-acid deficiency is seen frequently in alcoholics. A dietary deficiency also may be combined with increased demand, as in pregnancy, hemolytic anemia,

hemoglobinopathies, or myelofibrosis. Malabsorption of folic acid occurs in inflammatory small bowel diseases. Certain drugs such as methotrexate, pyrimethamine, triamterene, pentamidine, trimethoprim, and nitrous oxide inhibit conversion of folic acid to its biologically active form. Oral contraceptives, barbiturates, phenytoin, and ethanol have been associated with megaloblastic anemia that responds to treatment with folic acid.

Symptoms and Signs—In addition to the other symptoms and signs of anemia, the patient with folic-acid deficiency may appear wasted. Diarrhea is a prominent complaint. No neurological deficits are attributed to folic-acid deficiency.

ANEMIA OF CHRONIC DISEASE—This is seen in association with a number of chronic inflammatory or infectious diseases.

Pathophysiology—The problem involves a defect that prevents transport of iron from storage depots. The impaired RBC production along with a mildly reduced RBC survival leads to the development of anemia.

Symptoms and Signs—The anemia is usually normocytic normochromic but may be microcytic normochromic or even hypochromic. The serum iron is low, and the total iron binding capacity (TIBC) is normal or low. The saturation index is greater than 10%. The serum ferritin level is normal to high. Increased amounts of iron are stored in the bone-marrow reticuloendothelial system.

Diagnosis—The combination of low serum iron, normal or low TIBC, and an underlying inflammatory or infectious process is adequate for the diagnosis.

ANEMIA OF RENAL FAILURE—This anemia is usually severe and multifactorial in origin.

Pathophysiology—The kidneys are the source of erythropoietin, and production of erythropoietin is decreased in chronic renal failure. The anemia also may be due to iron deficiency because blood is lost from the gastrointestinal and genitourinary tracts in uremia. A hemolytic anemia occurs possibly because of toxins in the blood. Bone marrow is suppressed by the accumulation of toxins.

Symptoms and Signs—Anemia is usually severe, with hematocrit values of 15–30%. However, patients are not as symptomatic as the severity of the anemia would suggest. The anemia is normochromic normocytic unless iron deficiency is also present.

Diagnosis—Typically a low serum erythropoietin level is detected in the presence of renal failure.

HEMOLYTIC ANEMIAS—These involve the destruction of RBCs in the blood stream or by macrophages in the liver and spleen.

Etiology—Hemolysis may be caused by a variety of factors. Antibodies may develop toward RBCs as a result of sensitization, exposure to drugs, infections, or spontaneously. Excessive external trauma, such as marching or jogging, or excessive internal trauma such as occurs with a prosthetic cardiac valve may cause hemolysis. Toxins from the venom of a cobra, the brown recluse spider, and *Clostridium welchii* cause hemolysis. Infections of the RBCs with malaria and bacteremia due to pneumococcus, *Staphylococcus*, and *E coli* cause hemolysis. The RBCs may be made defectively because of an inherited error or have hereditary errors in metabolic enzyme systems.

AUTOIMMUNE HEMOLYTIC ANEMIA—This is characterized by development of IgG or IgM antibodies against the patient's own RBCs.

Etiology and Epidemiology—The disease can occur at any age and may be idiopathic or occur in association with another immune disorder such as lymphoma, chronic lymphocytic leukemia, or systemic lupus erythematosus.

Pathophysiology—The RBCs are coated with an antibody that is directed at one of the many RBC surface antigens. The RBCs are then destroyed in the spleen.

Symptoms and Signs—The anemia ranges from mild to severe. The reticulocyte count is increased. Spherocytes are seen on the peripheral blood smear. Bilirubin is increased. The course is variable but may end in fatal massive hemolysis. The direct Coombs' test is positive. This test uses specific antisera to detect IgG, IgM, or C3 coating the circulating RBCs.

Diagnosis—The diagnosis is based on the evidence of hemolysis (anemia, elevated bilirubin, low haptoglobin) and a positive direct Coombs' test.

DRUG-INDUCED IMMUNE HEMOLYTIC ANEMIA—Three types may occur. Methyldopa induces an autoimmune hemolytic anemia identical to the idiopathic form. The antibody is an IgG against components of the Rh antigen. The direct Coombs' test is positive in about 15% of patients who take methyldopa. There is extravascular hemolysis.

Penicillin and cephalosporins produce a hemolytic anemia by serving as a hapten. The hapten forms a complex with the RBC and antibodies are produced against the drug-red blood cell complex. The hemolysis is extravascular. The direct Coombs' test is positive.

Quinine and quinidine cause hemolysis by the "innocent bystander" mechanism. The drug forms a complex with plasma proteins and IgG and IgM antibodies form against the drug-protein complex. The antibody-drug-plasma protein complex settles on the RBC and fixes complement. C3 remains attached to the RBC. The direct Coombs' test is positive. Intravascular hemolysis occurs. Hemoglobin appears in the urine and acute tubular necrosis may result. See also Chapter 45.

HEMOLYTIC ANEMIA DUE TO HEXOSE MONO-PHOSPHATE SHUNT DEFECTS—Glucose metabolism via the hexose monophosphate shunt increases several times when the RBC is exposed to oxidants. The shunt generates glutathione to protect the sulfhydryl group of the hemoglobin from oxidation. Oxidized hemoglobin precipitates in RBCs, forming Heinz bodies. The spleen removes RBCs with Heinz bodies from the circulation. The most common defect in the hexose monophosphate shunt is a hypofunction of glucose 6-phosphodehydrogenase (G6PD) of which there are more than 100 variants. The G6PD gene is located on the X chromosome (sex-linked trait).

Epidemiology—The two most clinically significant forms of G6PD deficiency occur in blacks who originated in Central Africa, and in Eastern Mediterraneans, particularly Sephardic Jews.

Pathophysiology—Some patients with G6PD deficiency are only symptomatic when the RBCs are subject to the stress of infections or oxidants including drugs such as sulfonamides, antimalarials, or nitrofurantoin Heterozygous women have two populations of cells, one with normal enzyme concentration and one deficient.

Symptoms and Signs—Within a few hours of infection or exposure to a drug, the patient has acute hemolysis. Generally, the older RBCs are deficient in G6PD and are destroyed. Therefore, the hemolysis is self-limited even if the exposure to the oxidant continues. The Mediterranean form is characterized by more severe hemolysis. The patient has a decreased hematocrit, increased level of unconjugated bilirubin and hemoglobinuria. A test for G6PD will be falsely negative if done shortly after a hemolytic crisis.

Diagnosis—Deficiency of G6PD can be determined directly by analyzing RBCs in suspected individuals.

SICKLE-CELL ANEMIA—This is the most common conjoint hemolytic anemia. It is due to the substitution of valine for glutamic acid on the β-chain of hemoglobin, which results in hemoglobin S (HbS).

Epidemiology—Approximately 8% of Black Americans are heterozygous or carry the sickle-cell trait. The disease or homozygous form is seen in 0.15% of Black American children.

Etiology—The disorder is inherited according to Mendelian genetics, so that one-fourth of the offspring from heterozygous parents are homozygous, one-fourth are normal and one-half are heterozygous.

Pathophysiology—RBCs must be able to withstand distortion of shape in order to traverse the capillary circulation. RBCs that contain HbS change from biconcave discs to elongated crescent shaped (sickle) cells on deoxygenation. The sickled cells obstruct capillary blood flow, resulting in tissue hypoxia, further deoxygenation of RBCs, and further sickle formation. A small area of ischemia may become a large area of infarction as the process continues. Formation of sickle cells is initially a reversible process, but with time RBC-membrane damage occurs and the sickle formation becomes irreversible. Patients who are homozygous also have 2–20% hemoglobin F, which prevents polymerization of hemoglobin S. RBCs with a high concentration of hemoglobin F do not irreversibly sickle. Any condition that causes hypoxia or dehydration of RBCs increases sickle-cell formation. HbS has decreased affinity for oxygen so the oxygen content of the blood is decreased. Sickled cells are removed from the circulation by the spleen and have an average life span of 15 days.

Symptoms and Signs—Individuals with the sickle-cell trait, but not the disease, usually do not have significant clinical problems. Severe hypoxia is necessary to cause a sickle-cell crisis in these individuals. A person who is homozygous for sickle-cell anemia develops symptoms at about 6 months when much of the hemoglobin F has been replaced. Initial symptoms may be impairment of growth and development. Later, a severe hemolytic anemia develops.

The mortality and morbidity of sickle-cell anemia is related to recurrent episodes of vascular occlusion. A crisis is an episode of sickle-cell formation resulting in severe pain in the chest, abdomen, joints, or other sites. An infection or exposure to cold resulting in vasospasm or conditions that lead to dehydration may precipitate a crisis. The crisis may be mistaken for an "acute abdomen." Chronic organ damage results from recurrent crises. Lung function is decreased because of recurrent pulmonary infarcts. CHF results from the chronic severe anemia, hypoxemia, and pulmonary hypertension. Gallstones develop because of increased bilirubin turnover. Hepatic infarcts may become hepatic abscesses. The hypertonic, hypoxic, acidosis renal medulla is most susceptible to infarction. After repeated infarctions, the ability to concentrate urine is lost. Papillary necrosis also occurs. Prolonged hematuria may result in iron-deficiency anemia. Osteomyelitis may develop in bony infarcts. Aseptic necrosis of the femur occurs. Retinal infarcts, vitreous hemorrhage, and retinal detachment occur. Chronic skin ulcers are seen on lower extremities. Cerebral vascular occlusion can result in stroke, seizures, or coma. With repeated splenic infarcts, splenic function becomes impaired so susceptibility to infection, particularly pneumococcal, increases.

Diagnosis—The diagnosis is made by finding HbS on hemoglobin electrophoresis.

BLOOD DYSCRASIAS

Blood dyscrasia is a term used to indicate a general disorder of the blood. The most common blood dyscrasias include aplastic anemia, agranulocytosis, and thrombocytopenia. Many drugs and chemicals have been cited as the causative agents in blood dyscrasias.

APLASTIC ANEMIA—This term is actually a misnomer. A more accurate description is pancytopenia resulting from damaged pluripotent stem cells. All three cell types—RBCs, WBCs, and platelets—are affected. It is characterized by an acellular or hypocellular bone marrow.

Epidemiology—The overall incidence of aplastic anemia is estimated at 5 to 10 cases per million persons. There are approximately 1000 new cases annually in the United States. Young adults (15–30 years) and the elderly (>60 years) are the most commonly affected.

Etiology—A number of drugs and chemicals have been associated with its production including benzene, chloramphenicol, phenylbutazone, gold, and cancer chemotherapeutic agents. Radiation, infectious hepatitis, and other diseases may also be associated with the condition. Approximately one-half of the cases have no identifiable cause, but recent evidence suggests that many may be due to increased activity of suppressor lymphocytes.

Pathophysiology—The pathogenesis of aplastic anemia is only partially understood. In general, there is one of two pathologic processes that lead to the pancytopenia seen: (1) an acquired intrinsic stem cell defect or (2) an immune-mediated suppression of the bone marrow stem cells.

Symptoms and Signs—The patient complains of progressive weakness and fatigue, mild bleeding from mucous membranes, ecchymoses, and petechiae. The usual signs of infection are not present even though an infection may exist. Symptoms and signs of anemia are present.

Examination of the blood reveals a severe normochromic, normocytic anemia with no reticulocytes. The WBC count is low and is comprised mostly of lymphocytes. There is no increase in bilirubin unless liver disease also is present.

Diagnosis—Bone marrow biopsy is required to make the diagnosis of aplastic anemia.

AGRANULOCYTOSIS—This is characterized by a marked reduction or disappearance of neutrophilic granulocytes in the peripheral blood. Severe neutropenia is defined as less than 500 polymorphonuclear leukocytes (PMNs)/mm^3. The incidence of infection directly correlates with the number of PMNs.

Etiology—Various drugs may cause agranulocytosis, including cancer chemotherapeutic agents, thiouracils, phenothiazines, sulfonamides, or thiazide diuretics.

Pathophysiology—Several mechanisms convey a decreased number of circulating PMNs. Drugs used in cancer chemotherapy as well as radiation will decrease predictably the production of PMNs. This interference with production is usually reversible when the agent is discontinued, unless precursor cells in the bone marrow have been destroyed. Other drugs decrease production of PMNs in an unpredictable fashion and by an unknown mechanism. These drugs include the phenothiazines, sulfonamides, and thiouracils. The decrease in PMNs occurs about 10 days after initiation of therapy with the drug. When the drug is withdrawn the WBC count returns to normal. In some cases the drug may be readministered without problems.

Neutropenia may also result from increased destruction of PMNs. In severe infections the rate of PMN use may exceed the rate of production. Aminopyrine is the prototype for drug-induced granulocytopenia via the "innocent bystander" mechanism. The drug serves as a hapten with plasma proteins, and antibodies are formed against the drug protein complex. The antibody-drug-protein complex settles on the granulocyte and fixes complement. The WBC is removed from the circulation by the spleen. Initially, with increased destruction, production increases but eventually the bone marrow is not able to keep pace.

Symptoms and Signs—The patient may have fever, chills, severe prostration, severe sore throat, and oral ulcers. There is no accumulation of pus at the sites of infection.

Diagnosis—The diagnosis is made by finding an absolute neutrophil count of <500/mm^3 on a CBC with differential.

THROMBOCYTOPENIA—A blood dyscrasia characterized by a platelet count of less than 100,000/mm^3. Spontaneous bleeding may occur when the count is less than 20,000/mm^3.

Etiology—Thrombocytopenia is caused by one of three mechanisms—decreased production in the bone marrow, increased splenic sequestration, or increased destruction of platelets in the blood stream. There are several causes in each of these categories.

Pathophysiology—*Decreased marrow production.* The most common causes of decreased platelet production are processes that result in infiltration of the marrow. Lymphoma, leukemia, and other tumors can invade the marrow and crowd and reduce the number of megakaryocytes. A number of drugs, such as cancer chemotherapeutic agents, gold, ethanol, thiazides, and sulfonamides, can decrease production of platelets through direct toxic effects on the megakaryocytes.

Splenic sequestration. One third of the platelet mass is normally sequestered in the spleen. Disease states causing splenomegaly such as portal hypertension, splenic infiltration with tumor, or storage diseases such as Gaucher's, cause this percentage of sequestered platelets to increase resulting in lower numbers of circulating platelets.

Accelerated destruction. Destruction of platelets may be immunologic or non-immunologic. The most common immune-mediated causes are viral or bacterial infections, drugs, and idiopathic thrombocytopenic purpura (ITP). Drugs may act as haptens and induce formation of antibodies against the drug-platelet complex. These include quinidine, quinine, analgesics, antibiotics, sedatives, and sulfonamides. Heparin causes thrombocytopenia in approximately 10–15% of patients treated with this agent. The mechanism is generally the formation of a drug-antibody complex binding to the platelet.

Non-immunological mechanisms for platelet destruction may be due to abnormal vessels, fibrin thrombi, and intravascular prostheses. Patients with vasculitis have abnormal vessels that cause platelet destruction. Disseminated intravascular coagulation (DIC), hemolytic-uremic syndrome (HUS), and thrombotic thrombocytopenic purpura (TTP) are all examples of diseases that cause intravascular fibrin thrombi that destroy platelets. Patients with prosthetic heart valves may have low platelet counts from mechanical sheering of the platelets.

Symptoms and Signs—The patient complains of petechiae, purpura, and ecchymoses over the back, upper chest, and limbs and of mucosal bleeding. Blood-filled bullae are found in the mouth. Bleeding may occur from any mucosal surface. Spontaneous bleeding may occur, which may last for several days. The most serious site of bleeding is into the brain. Bleeding time is prolonged.

Diagnosis—Simply finding a low platelet count makes the diagnosis of thrombocytopenia. The underlying cause may require a bone marrow biopsy or antibody titers. Splenomegaly found on physical exam my also provide a clue to the underlying process.

DISORDERS OF HEMOSTASIS

Blood-clotting disorders may result from a defect in any of the steps of coagulation. They may be mild or severe. The coagulation defect may be inherited or acquired.

Normal Physiology—When a blood vessel is cut, two events occur to prevent blood loss—platelet plug formation and blood coagulation. Platelets adhere to the injured vessel surfaces and also aggregate to each other. During adherence and aggregation, platelets assume bizarre shapes with many protruding processes or pseudopodia that overlap.

The next step in hemostasis is blood coagulation. Either the intrinsic or extrinsic coagulation pathway is activated by the surfaces of the injured vessel or by substances liberated by the traumatized tissue or platelets. This process is complete within less than 10 minutes. The clot is composed of a fibrin meshwork with entrapped red blood cells, platelets, and serum. The final step in hemostasis is clot retraction, which expresses the serum from the clot and physically draws the torn edges of the blood vessels together. Clot retraction occurs within 1 hour. Clots that form in repairing an injured blood vessel are replaced later by scar tissue. Other clots dissolve.

IDIOPATHIC THROMBOCYTOPENIC PURPURA (ITP)—This usually occurs in young women. An acute idiopathic thrombocytopenic purpura may occur in children following a URI.

Epidemiology—Acute ITP following a viral illness accounts for 90% of cases of thrombocytopenia in children. Most adults with ITP have a more indolent disease that affects women more commonly than men (3:1). Typically it is seen in patients age 20 to 40 years.

Etiology—Acute ITP in children is caused by antibodies directed against viral antigens that cross react with platelet antigens. Adult ITP is an idiopathic autoimmune disorder.

Pathophysiology—IgG, which sensitizes platelets for sequestration by the spleen or liver, develops so that platelet life span is shortened.

Symptoms and Signs—Consists of purpura over the limbs, upper chest and back, and mucosal bleeding. The onset is sudden. No adenopathy, fever, or malaise is associated with the bleeding. The bone marrow shows a normal or increased number of megakaryocytes. The platelet count is low. The bleeding time is prolonged.

Diagnosis—ITP is primarily a diagnosis of exclusion.

HEMOPHILIA A—This is due to an inherited deficiency of Factor VIII activity.

Epidemiology and Etiology—This is a sex-linked recessive trait that occurs in one in 10,000 people. Males and, rarely, homozygous females have the disease.

Pathophysiology—Factor VIII is a large glycoprotein found in trace amounts in normal plasma. It has three components: clot-promoting or antihemophiliac factor activity, antigen, and the von Willebrand factor (VWF). The defect is a deficiency of clot-promoting activity. It may be a defect in the activity of Factor VIII rather then the amount.

Symptoms and Signs—In severe hemophilia, bleeding is often spontaneous, whereas in milder cases excessive bleeding may occur only after injury or surgery. The severity of the bleeding depends on the degree of Factor VIII deficiency. Spontaneous bleeding occurs into joints and muscles. Recurrent hemarthroses are characteristic of the disease and result in permanent joint damage and deformity. Bleeding into the urogenital or gastrointestinal tracts also occurs. Hemorrhage may occur into any organ and may be fatal. Patients with severe hemophilia do not have a normal life span.

Tests of platelet function, bleeding time, and platelet count are normal. The prothrombin time is normal, but the partial thromboplastin time is prolonged.

Diagnosis—An assay finding a low Factor VIII level makes the diagnosis.

HEMOPHILIA B—This is due to an inherited deficiency of Factor IX activity.

Epidemiology—This is a rare sex-linked form of hemophilia.

Pathophysiology and Symptoms and Signs—These are similar to those of hemophilia A.

VON WILLEBRAND'S DISEASE—This is due to an inherited deficiency in von Willebrand Factor (VWF) activity.

Epidemiology—This autosomal dominant condition may be the most common inherited bleeding disorder.

Pathophysiology—VWF is the high molecular-weight component of the Factor VIII complex. VWF supports platelet interaction with the subendothelium. It also carries Factor VIII coagulation activity and prevents its elimination. Defective VWF causes unpaired platelet adhesion and decreased Factor VIII levels.

Symptoms and Signs—Bleeding usually is in mucocutaneous sites. Homozygotes may have symptoms and signs as severe as those in hemophilia. Heterozygotes are often asymptomatic. The bleeding time is prolonged.

Diagnosis—Patients with von Willebrand's disease will have a low Factor VIII level along with an abnormal VWF antigen and ristocetin cofactor assay

VITAMIN K DEFICIENCY—This results in deficiencies of Factors II, VII, IX, and X. Vitamin K is a fat-soluble vitamin found in leafy green vegetables. Stores of vitamin K are limited and deficiency develops in 1 to 3 weeks if intake is stopped.

Etiology and Pathophysiology—Vitamin K deficiency is multifactorial in etiology and involves decreased absorption due to decreased bile acids, impaired intestinal absorption due to inflammatory bowel disease, and changes or decreases in the gut flora, which synthesize vitamin K.

Symptoms and Signs—They are those of bleeding seen in other coagulopathies. The prothrombin time and partial thromboplastin time are prolonged.

Liver disease results in coagulopathy due to decreased synthesis of all factors except Factor VIII. Also, removal by the liver of proteases or enzymes that inactivate the clotting factors is decreased, causing a consumption coagulopathy. The symptoms and signs of the coagulopathy due to liver disease are similar to those of other coagulopathies. The prothrombin time and partial thromboplastin time are prolonged. In addition, hemostasis is further impaired by thrombocytopenia and platelet dysfunction.

Diagnosis—Patients with vitamin K deficiency will have a prolonged prothrombin time (PT), a normal or prolonged activated partial thromboplastin time (PTT), normal bleeding time, and normal platelet count. Confirmation is made by normalization of the PT and PTT following administration of Vitamin K.

DERMATOLOGY

Normal Anatomy and Physiology—The skin is the largest organ in the body. The functions of the skin include sensation, temperature control, prevention of water loss or penetration, synthesis of vitamin D, and protection from organisms and irritants. The skin is composed of three layers: the epidermis, the dermis, and the hypodermic or subcutaneous tissue. The outer layer of the epidermis is the stratum corneum or horny layer. The cells of the stratum corneum are keratinized fully and are without nuclei or granules. In the process of keratinization, the cells from the basal layer migrate upward, flatten, lose water, and fill with keratin. This process normally requires 28 days from formation of a daughter cell (through mitotic division of a cell in the basal layer of the epidermis) until that cell is shed at the surface of the stratum corneum. The cells of the stratum corneum normally are shed invisibly as scales.

The dermis is composed of connective tissue in which are found blood vessels, lymphatics, nerves, arrectores pilorum muscles, fibroblasts, mast cells, and dermal appendages—hair follicles, sebaceous glands, and sweat glands. Elastin and collagen embedded in mucopolysaccharide give the skin its elasticity. Blood vessels in the papillae of the dermis bring nutrients to the avascular epidermis. Sebaceous glands are attached to hair follicles and produce sebum that lubricates the skin and may help prevent water loss. Sebum also has some antiseptic and antifungal properties. Hairs and nails are specialized structures composed of modified types of keratin. The subcutaneous tissues are composed of connective tissue and fat.

Certain microorganisms may be found on the skin as normal flora. Other microorganisms transiently may colonize the skin.

Acne Vulgaris

This is a common disease, which affects teenagers primarily and has, as the characteristic lesions, the open comedo (blackhead) and closed comedo. Most patients have only mild acne and never consult a physician, although they may spend large sums of money on OTC acne aids. In severe forms, acne may lead to extensive scarring. Even the milder forms may cause considerable psychological distress for the patients.

Epidemiology—Acne vulgaris is the most common disorder of the skin in the US. It affects over 17 million patients annually and accounts for 10% of all patient visits to a primary care physician. Almost everyone has some acne during the adolescent years. It may continue in some people until 30 to 40 years of age or appear postmenopausally in women. Administration of certain drugs, such as corticosteroids, halogens, androgens, lithium, and anticonvulsants may result in acne. Acne also may be associated with certain occupations in which tars, oil, and chlorinated hydrocarbons come in contact with the skin. The application of certain cosmetics, including moisturizers, has been associated with acne.

Etiology—The etiology is multifactorial. Heredity plays a role. Androgenic simulation of sebum production by the sebaceous glands at puberty is important, but the main factor in precipitating acne appears to be occlusion of the ducts draining sebaceous glands. There is no scientific evidence that diet commonly plays a role in the development of acne. Anxiety, fatigue, heat, and humidity probably do aggravate acne.

Pathophysiology—The characteristic lesions are the open comedo (blackheads) and closed comedo (whiteheads), which are sebaceous glands that have become plugged with sebum and keratin debris. The black color is he result of oxidation of pigment granules in shed cells forming the plug. When the epidermis covers the opening of the sebaceous gland so that oxidation cannot occur, the lesion is known as a whitehead. Comedones are not inflamed. When they become inflamed, other lesions are formed: papules, pustules, and nodular-cystic lesions.

Acne most commonly occurs on the oily areas of the skin, primarily the face, ears, neck, and upper trunk. Healed acne may result in atrophic, pitted, or hypertrophic scars.

Androgens cause sebaceous glands to mature and to produce large quantities of sebum. Both males and females produce androgens. The sebaceous glands respond to very low levels of androgens. Obstruction of flow of sebum from the sebaceous gland to the surface of the skin results in a comedo. Increased amounts of sebum, as well as increased viscosity of sebum and keratin debris, contribute to the obstruction. Chronic obstruction of the sebaceous gland leads to follicular dilatation (enlarged pores). Sebum is composed of triglycerides, waxes, cholesterol, squalene, and minute amounts of free fatty acids. Normally, sebum is not inflammatory. However, bacterial flora in the follicle hydrolyze the triglycerides to free fatty acids, which are extremely irritating and initiate the inflammatory process. In addition, propionibacterium acnes, an anaerobic bacterium that is a normal component of skin flora, thrives on the increased production of sebum. *P acnes* then release chemotactic factors, which enhance the inflammatory process. The inflamed follicle may rupture and spread the process to the adjacent dermis causing increased inflammation via a foreign-body reaction.

Symptoms and Signs—The comedones and other lesions, including scars, are the physical abnormalities of acne. The course is usually chronic throughout adolescence until hormonal balance is achieved, usually in the early 20s. Occasional flares are common during the course. The objective of treatment is to clear the lesions, prevent scarring, and minimize psychological distress.

Diagnosis—Diagnosis is by clinical exam and identification of the classical lesions.

Psoriasis

This is a chronic disease characterized by epidermal hyperplasia and a greatly accelerated rate of epidermal turnover. The lesions are characteristically red, slightly raised, and scaly. Though psoriasis is usually a minor disorder, generalized forms and systemic manifestations also occur.

Epidemiology—Approximately 1–3% of individuals in the US have some form of psoriasis. A higher incidence occurs in Northern European countries, while the disease is rare or absent among Native Americans, Western Africans, Japanese, and Eskimos. Males and females are affected equally. Peak incidence occurs in early and middle adulthood but psoriasis may occur at any time during life.

Etiology—The etiology is unknown. Heredity is thought to play a role, transmission being autosomal dominant with incomplete penetrance or multifactorial. Frequently, the first lesions are associated with previous injury to the site, which is known as the Koebner phenomenon.

Environmental factors such as decreased humidity may aggravate psoriasis.

Pathophysiology—The histopathological changes include parakeratosis (retention of nuclei in cells in the keratin layer), hyperkeratosis (increased thickness of the keratin layer), hypogranulosis (loss of the granular layer), elongation of the epidermal rete ridges, pustules with surrounding intercellular edema (spongiform pustules), and papillomatosis (increased height of the dermal papillary pegs) with thinning of the suprapapillary epidermis. There is an inflammatory infiltrate in the upper dermis and proliferation of small blood vessels in the papillae (vascular ectasia). Mitotic figures are seen in the bottom three cell layers of the epidermis rather than just in the basal layer.

The characteristic change is the markedly shortened rate of turnover and accelerated production of the epidermal cells. Instead of the normal 28 days from cell division in the basal layers until the cell is shed from the stratum corneum, in psoriasis it takes only 3 to 4 days for this to occur. The mechanism for this and the other symptoms and signs of psoriasis is not understood at this time.

Symptoms and Signs—The lesions of psoriasis are discrete or confluent erythematous plaques and papules covered with white or silvery scales. The lesions are characteristically found on the extensor surfaces such as the elbows and knees and also on the back and scalp. However, any area of skin can be involved. Nails commonly are involved with pitting and ridging, while mucous membranes rarely are involved. The lesions may be localized or generalized and are usually asymptomatic but may cause discomfort from burning and itching. Auspitz sign is characteristic (punctate bleeding that occurs when psoriatic scales are removed). The onset of psoriasis is usually insidious, although it may be explosive. The clinical course is chronic and recurring with periods of remission. Spontaneous cures rarely occur. Most cases are only cosmetically disfiguring. Some forms such as psoriatic erythroderma and pustular psoriasis may be life threatening. Although pustular psoriasis looks like an infection, the lesions are sterile. A form of arthritis that resembles rheumatoid arthritis, but affects the distal joints is associated with psoriasis in some cases. There are no characteristic laboratory abnormalities of psoriasis.

Diagnosis—Diagnosis is by clinical exam and identification of the classical lesions.

Allergic Skin Diseases

URTICARIA (HIVES)—Urticaria is a skin reaction composed of transient wheals (edematous papules and plaques, usually pruritic). Urticaria may be acute or chronic. Immediate reactions occur within 1 to 60 minutes of exposure to the antigen and are manifested by generalized pruritus and urticaria. IgE is the mediator of immediate reactions. These reactions are the most dangerous, since they may be associated with laryngeal edema and/or anaphylaxis. Accelerated reactions occur within 1 to 72 hours of contact with the antigen and also are manifested by generalized urticaria and pruritus. An exanthem is seen rarely with this type of reaction. A late reaction may occur from 3 to 21 days after exposure to the antigen. The urticaria in this case may subside even though the exposure to the antigen is not terminated because of the development of IgG and IgA blocking antibodies. Chronic urticaria lasts longer than 30 days and is rarely IgE mediated. The etiology is unknown in 80–90% of the cases. Emotional stress often exacerbates this condition.

Epidemiology—Approximately 15–23% of the population will experience at least one episode of urticaria. Young adults are afflicted most frequently by the acute form. The chronic form, lasting longer than 4 weeks, usually is seen in patients over 35 years. Individuals with urticaria, or their family members, are likely to be allergic to a number of antigens and also suffer from seasonal rhinitis, asthma, and atopic dermatitis.

Etiology—Urticaria can be caused by IgE or complement mediated reactions usually in response to an antigen. Common antigens are food (milk, eggs, shellfish, nuts, wheat), drugs (penicillin), and parasites.

Urticaria is also caused in some individuals by physical stimuli. Cold urticaria occurs most often in children or young adults. These individuals develop urticarial lesions when the skin contacts extremely cold stimuli such as ice. Similarly, exposure to sunlight may cause urticaria in others. Urticaria may also result from exercise to the point of sweating, prolonged pressure on the skin, or vibration.

Hereditary angioedema is a severe form of recurrent, episodic urticaria that is inherited in an autosomal dominant pattern. This form is characterized by low levels of C1 esterase inhibitor.

Urticaria has also been associated with some connective tissue disorders such as SLE or Sjögren's syndrome. Often this is a sign of underlying urticarial vasculitis. Some bacterial infections, and underlying occult malignancy may also cause urticaria.

Pathophysiology—Urticaria may develop as a result of several different processes, although all involve liberation of histamine from mast cells in the dermis. Systemic exposure to an antigen may result in formation of IgE antibodies toward that antigen. The antibodies are fixed to mast cells in the dermis and lungs and to circulating basophiles. The interaction of antigen and antibody results in liberation of histamine and other mediators (prostaglandin E and kinins). These substances cause arteriolar dilatation and increased capillary permeability in the skin. Histamine is degraded quickly in tissues so urticaria seldom lasts for more than 48 hours. A degranulated mast cell is refractory to further stimulation until histamine granules reform.

Other antibodies may be involved in the liberation of histamine and mediator substances from mast cells. IgG and IgM may be formed against antigens. These antibodies, when they interact with antigens, may activate the complement cascade, which results in histamine release. Cold and solar urticaria are mediated by antibodies (IgE) that are only active at decreased temperature or upon exposure to light.

Histamine may be released from mast cells by nonimmunological mechanisms. Certain chemicals stimulate mast cells directly to liberate histamine. These chemicals include drugs such as morphine, codeine, dextrans, and crayfish toxin or snake venom. Direct physical pressure may also cause release of histamine from mast cells.

Symptoms and Signs—Urticarial lesions are well-circumscribed discrete wheals with erythematous raised serpiginous borders and blanched centers. The lesions, which involve only the superficial layer of the skin may be scattered, localized, or may coalesce. The patient will complain of intense pruritus or burning. Urticaria alone is seldom life threatening, but it may indicate a future anaphylactic reaction. Skin testing is usually of little value in these individuals in that they are allergic to numerous antigens. The acute form usually lasts less than 6 weeks. The chronic form may last for years but usually does not last for life.

Diagnosis—Diagnosis is by clinical exam and identification of the classical lesions.

ATOPIC DERMATITIS (ECZEMA)—Eczema is chronic pruritic inflammatory skin disease of the epidermis and dermis. It is usually associated with a personal or family history of hayfever, asthma, allergic rhinitis, or atopic dermatitis. Atopic dermatitis is characterized by itching. The appearance and distribution of the lesions depends on the age of onset.

Epidemiology—The onset is typically early in life, often in the first 2 months and by 1 year of age in 60% of cases. There is a slight male predominance. Over two thirds of patients have a personal or family history of allergic rhinitis, hay fever, or asthma.

Etiology—The etiology is unknown. Those with onset in early childhood tend to improve after a period of time. Irritants, excessive bathing, wide temperature variation, low humidity, and nervous tension may aggravate the condition.

Pathophysiology—Pathological changes are those of nonspecific dermatitis. Epidermal vesicles due to intercellular edema, parakeratosis, acanthosis, and an inflammatory infiltrate of the epidermis and dermis are seen in acute atopic dermatitis. In the chronic form, hyperkeratosis, parakeratosis, acanthosis, and a lymphocytic infiltrate of the thickened upper dermis are seen.

The mechanisms for the development are not understood. Various immunological hypotheses have been put forth to explain the development of atopic dermatitis, but none of these explains all cases. Some patients with the disease have elevated levels of IgE and perhaps elevated levels of IgG and IgM. It also occurs commonly in immune-deficient individuals and may be due to an impairment of delayed hypersensitivity or impaired phagocytosis. Depressed IgA also has been reported in atopic patients.

Symptoms and Signs—Infant-type atopic dermatitis (infantile eczema) begins during the first few months of life, perhaps as a reaction to food, although this is controversial. The eruption may be local or generalized, acutely inflamed, vesicular or popular, and spreads rapidly. The scalp, face, trunk, extremities, and diaper area are frequently involved. There is considerable oozing and crusting associated with the lesions along with intense pruritus. The skin may become infected secondarily. The child usually outgrows the disease spontaneously at 2 to 3 years.

Childhood-type atopic dermatitis may be a recurrence of infant type or may be the first appearance of the disease. In contrast to the vesicles and oozing of the infant type, these lesions are dried, lichenified plaques and patches. The lesions also are more localized in the childhood type and are found on the flexor surfaces and the face, neck, feet, genitalia, and scalp. Again, there is intense pruritus. The disease may clear or persist into adulthood.

In adult type atopic dermatitis, the lesions consist of chronic lichenified patches, which are intensely pruritic and may be hyperpigmented. Commonly flexures and the creases of the neck and eyelids are involved as well as the same areas as in the childhood type. The clinical course is chronic and characterized by spontaneous exacerbations and remissions. Eventually, the disease fades.

ALLERGIC CONTACT DERMATITIS—This is an extremely common skin disease caused by direct contact with the substance and the development of delayed hypersensitivity. Primary irritant contact dermatitis is caused by contact with noxious agents such as acids or corrosives or excessive contact with soap and water. The inflammatory skin reaction that results from such a contact occur in all individuals exposed to these agents and does not involve the development of hypersensitivity.

Epidemiology—Many patients have this disease, which affects any age group and is equally common in both sexes.

Etiology—Substances capable of forming a stable bond with cutaneous proteins and being transported to a lymph node are allergens for contact dermatitis. These include Rhus (poison ivy and poison oak), ragweed preservatives, solvents, rubber, low-molecular-weight polymers, metals, particularly nickel, and medications.

Pathophysiology—The chemical group binds to skin protein and is transported to the lymph nodes. Cellular proliferation occurs in the paracortical area of the lymph nodes. Small lymphocytes become sensitized to the antigen within 7 to 10 days of the first exposure. The sensitized lymphocytes react with the antigen and release soluble chemotactic factors, which attract other lymphocytes and macrophages into the area. Also, the sensitized lymphocytes release migratory inhibitory factors that inhibit the movement of macrophages and other cells away from the area lysosomal enzymes released from the macrophages result in skin destruction. On subsequent exposures, reaction will occur within 24 to 48 hours.

Symptoms and Signs—The distribution of the lesions is characteristic the rash occurs where the allergen comes in contact with the skin. The scalp is rarely involved. The lesions begin as intense, relatively limited areas of erythema that are soon associated with edema. Papules and vesicles form, with subsequent oozing and weeping. Sometimes the lesions are bullous. The erythema lessens and is replaced with crusting and scaling. Pruritus in varying degrees of severity is always present. If contact with the allergen is eliminated, healing occurs in 1 to 3 weeks. With chronic exposure, a chronic contact dermatitis may develop with thickening, fissuring, scaling, and hyperpigmentation of the area. Vesiculation is minimal in the chronic form. Intense itching and burning may result in excoriation and secondary infection. The disease will recur if there is another contact with the allergen

Diagnosis—Diagnosis may be made via patch testing, although the patient may react to a variety of allergens including some, which he/she is not allergic to.

PHOTOALLERGIC REACTION—Uncommon delayed hypersensitivity reactions that require three factors: light, skin, and an allergen. Distribution is limited to the areas exposed to light. Photoallergic reactions must be distinguished from the more common phototoxic reaction, which occurs when a photosensitizing substance ingested or applied externally, plus minimal exposure to sunlight or artificial lighting, results in an exaggerated sunburn in 6 to 18 hours. No immunologic mechanisms are involved in phototoxic reactions, which can occur with the first exposure to the substance. Pigment is protective in the phototoxic reaction and tanning results as the reaction subsides.

Epidemiology—These reactions are rare but occur predominantly in males (7:1) and in the age group of 40 to 60 years. Pigment and dark skin are not protective for this reaction.

Etiology—Numerous drugs, chemicals, and cosmetics can cause both phototoxic and photoallergic reactions.

Pathophysiology—The energy of light depends on the wavelength in the electromagnetic spectrum. A molecule, when exposed to light, may dissipate the absorbed energy as heat or may undergo one of numerous photochemical reactions including chemical-bond formation. The chemical and the cutaneous protein are the antigen for the development of delayed hypersensitivity.

Symptoms and Signs—A photoallergic reaction occurs as an urticarial or eczematous eruption in the areas of sun exposure. The initial eruption will not be seen until 7 to 10 days after the first exposure but occurs within 24 to 48 hours on subsequent exposures. No tanning occurs as the reaction subsides. The reaction may recur with each re-exposure. Photopatch testing may make the diagnosis.

Adverse Reactions to Drugs as Manifested by the Skin

Cutaneous reactions are among the most common adverse reactions to drugs. The significance of these reactions varies from minor to life threatening. Nonallergic drug reactions of the skin include alopecia, purpura, secondary infections, and phototoxic reactions. Allergic reactions include urticaria, the rash seen with serum sickness, allergic contact dermatitis, and photoallergic reactions as already discussed. In addition, several less-common but potentially more serious reactions may occur.

EXFOLIATIVE ERYTHRODERMA SYNDROME—Exfoliative erythroderma syndrome (EES) is a serious, and at times life-threatening reaction of the skin characterized by generalized erythema and scaling associated with fever and generalized lymphadenopathy. It may be a reaction to a drug or may be an extension of a preexisting skin disorder.

Epidemiology—Exfoliative erythroderma syndrome is almost always seen in patients over age 50 years and is more common in males.

Etiology—EES is seen as a generalized spreading of a drug reaction, psoriasis, contact dermatitis, seborrheic dermatitis, atopic der-

matitis, or in association with leukemia or lymphoma. In 10–20% of patients no underlying cause can be identified.

Pathophysiology—The pathophysiology is entirely unknown.

Symptoms and Signs—There is a generalized erythematous eruption with scaling involving the entire skin surface. In extensive exfoliative erythroderma syndrome, the metabolic demand is such that the patient develops negative nitrogen balance, edema, hypoalbuminemia, and loses muscle mass. Serious water and electrolyte imbalance can result from the greatly increased loss of water through the skin. The cause and complications determine the course. The erythroderma syndrome persists in patients with malignancy. If psoriasis, atopic dermatitis, or other skin diseases cause EES, improvement occurs over 8 to 10 months. Prognosis is better if the etiological factor can be removed. Approximately 30% of patients with EES die.

Diagnosis—The finding of generalized skin erythema and scaling make the diagnosis.

ERYTHEMA MULTIFORME—This is a characteristic skin disorder that occurs as a result of a systemic allergic reaction to various agents. The syndrome may include only a few typical skin lesions or become a more severe illness known as Stevens-Johnson syndrome.

Epidemiology—Erythema multiforme most often affects patients age 20 to 30 years, although 50% of cases are in patients under age 20 years.

Etiology—Infectious agents including herpes virus and *Mycoplasma* pneumoniae, drugs (especially penicillin, aspirin, phenytoin, allopurinol, and sulfonamides), and malignancy may cause this condition. More than 50% of cases are idiopathic.

Pathophysiology—Histopathologically, the changes seen are those of spongiotic dermatitis with epidermal necrosis, ballooning, and vacuolar alteration. An associated superficial perivasculitis and interface lymphohistiocytic infiltrate is present. This disease is probably antigen-antibody-mediated.

Symptoms and Signs—The lesions may be papules, macules, urticaria, vesicles, or bullae. The type of lesion may change as the disease progresses. The lesions are symmetrical in distribution and are found most commonly on extensor surfaces, the backs and palms of hands, and the tops and soles of feet. Both mucous membranes and skin are involved in the severe form. The lesions begin as a bright redness that extends peripherally as the center pales, becomes firm, and may contain bullae. These classical lesions are called target lesions because of their appearance, but do not always occur in the disease. In Stevens-Johnson syndrome, the skin, conjunctiva, and mucous membranes are involved. This reaction includes toxemia, prostration, high fever, cough, and inflammation of the lungs. The disease usually resolves within a few weeks after the inciting agent is removed although the severe form may be fatal.

Diagnosis—The diagnosis is made by the finding of the typical skin lesions on physical exam and supported by skin biopsy.

Skin Infections

IMPETIGO—This is a common superficial bacterial infection of the skin that may arise in normal skin or as a secondary infection of dermatitis, intertrigo, infestations, other infections, or trauma.

Epidemiology—Impetigo occurs primarily in children and young adults.

Etiology—The causative organisms are beta hemolytic streptococci and coagulase-positive staphylococci. In secondary forms, gram-negative organisms also may be found. The lesions may be autoinoculable and are somewhat contagious.

Pathophysiology—Impetigo is caused by the invasion of the superficial layers of the skin by the offending organism.

Symptoms and Signs—The disease begins as a macule that progresses to a vesicle covering about 2 to 3 cm^2 in area. The vesicle, which is located just below the stratum corneum, becomes a pustule filled with polymorphonuclear leukocytes. The pustule ruptures and may spread the bacteria to the adjacent skin. The lesion then becomes denuded and seeps. The seropurulent fluid quickly dries, forming the characteristic friable honey-colored crust of the disease.

Diagnosis—The diagnosis is made by the identification on physical exam of the typical lesions and may be confirmed by Gram's stain and culture.

Mycotic Infections

Dermatophytoses are mycotic infections of the skin that involve the epidermis, nails, and hair. The diseases differ as to causative organism, area affected, mode of transmission, and response to therapy. These infections may occur in any age group.

Tinea capitis usually occurs in prepubertal children and may occur in epidemics in schools or institutions. The lesions are found on the scalp and appear as scaly, crusted patches with the hair broken off close to the scalp. Inflammation and deeper lesions may occur and may result in scarring alopecia. The fungus is of the Microsporum genus.

Tinea corporis is classic ringworm. The lesions occur anywhere on the glabrous skin of the body. A papule begins and spreads centrifugally as a scaly red rim with central clearing. The border of the lesions may contain vesicles. The causative organisms are of the *Microsporum* and *Trichophyton genera*.

Tinea cruris is known more commonly as "jock itch." The lesions begin as a symmetrical scaly red eruption of the groin and inner thighs. Chronic lesions are browner in color. The lesions have specific margins and the margins are more inflamed than the center. Severe pruritus accompanies the eruption. The fungus belongs to either *Epidermophyton* or *Trichophyton* genus. Heat and humidity are aggravating factors for the development of Tinea cruris. This condition must be distinguished from a similar eruption that is caused by another fungus, *Candida albicans*.

Tinea pedis (athlete's foot) is perhaps the most common of the dermatophytoses. Darkness, heat, and humidity predispose an individual to the development of this infection. *Trichophyton mentagrophytes* causes an inflammatory eruption with vesicles and weeping. *Trichophyton rubrum* causes a dry, scaly eruption.

Tinea unguum is a fungal infection of the nails; most commonly the toe nails. The nails become yellow in color, brittle, thickened and raised by the underlying debris. Infections of the nails are difficult to eradicate.

Diagnosis—The diagnosis of any of the mycotic skin infections depends on the physical findings during examination. It is confirmed by skin scrapings and microscopic examination revealing the invading fungus.

INFECTIOUS DISEASES

Urinary Tract Infections

Urinary tract infection (UTI) refers to bacteria multiplying in the urinary tract. It is the most common bacterial infection seen in the US. UTIs are broadly divided into complicated and uncomplicated UTIs.

An uncomplicated UTI, exemplified by cystitis, is a UTI in an anatomically normal urinary tract. Complicated UTIs are those infections of the urinary tract that are associated with a condition that increases the risk of treatment failure. These conditions may include anatomical abnormalities of the urinary tract or the presence of a catheter.

Acute pyelonephritis is a bacterial infection of the kidney. It primarily arises under one of two circumstances. First, if there is vesicoureteral reflux of infected urine. This is a potential long-term problem that can result in recurrent episodes of infection and is due to an anatomical abnormality. Second, a normal urinary tract may become infected with an uropathogenic strain of *E coli* whose *P fimbriae* permit ascent of the urethra without being washed out. This demands adequate immediate treatment but is not a long-term hazard.

Prostatitis and urethritis are infections of the prostate gland and urethra, respectively. Prostatitis often requires a longer course of therapy for complete eradication of the infection.

Each of these infections may be asymptomatic but each has characteristic symptoms and signs.

All urinary tract infections may be either acute or chronic.

Normal Anatomy and Physiology—The urinary tract is a closed system for drainage of urine from kidneys to bladder and eventually to the outside via the urethra. Under normal circumstances the entire urinary tract except for the anterior urethra is sterile. Various defense mechanisms prevent infection in the urinary tract.

The outward flow of urine serves to wash out organisms. This is probably the most important defensive mechanism and can clear 99% of organisms experimentally inoculated into the bladder. Urinary tract anatomy prevents retrograde flow of urine. Valves at the ureterovesical junction prevent reflux of urine from bladder into the ureters and thence the kidneys. Females have a shorter urethra than males (4 cm versus 12 cm), which contributes to the much higher incidence of urinary tract infections in women. Also organisms from the adjacent vagina or rectum colonize the urethra in women easily.

The urine itself has certain characteristics that discourage bacterial growth. These include an acidic pH (5.5), as bacteria prefer a more alkaline medium (pH = 6 to 8); low osmolality, usually below that required for optimal bacterial growth; and the presence of urea and weak organic acids. Prostatic secretions also are probably antibacterial.

The kidney is particularly susceptible to infection because of the hypertonic state of the papillae and medulla. This leads to impairment of leukocyte migration, complement activity, and phagocytosis, as well as development of spheroplasts or protoplasts by bacteria, which make them less susceptible to antibiotics.

Epidemiology—The incidence of urinary tract infections depends on the age, sex, sexual activity, and underlying diseases in the population. Women have a 10–20% lifetime risk of a UTI. The annual incidence is around 1% until adolescence and rises to 10% by age 50. Incidence is much lower in celibate women and higher during pregnancy. A total of 20% of pregnant women with bacteriuria develop acute pyelonephritis. In infancy, the rate of UTIs in males, usually associated with a structural anomaly, exceeds that of females. Urinary obstruction from an enlarged prostate accounts for the rate in elderly men being even higher than that in women. Men under 50 years rarely have UTI unless they are uncircumcised, have an anatomic abnormality of the urinary tract, engage in unprotected insertive anal intercourse, or have AIDS with a CD4 T cell count under 200/µl. Long-term indwelling catheters facilitate entry of uropathogens and hinder their clearance.

Etiology—Most UTIs are caused by gram-negative organisms that normally inhabit the large intestine. *Escherichia coli* accounts for 85% of first urinary tract infections. Other organisms, including *Klebsiella*, *Enterobacter*, *Proteus*, and *Pseudomonas*, are seen less commonly. Instrumentation of the urinary tract is a predisposing factor for development of an infection, particularly with *Proteus* or *Pseudomonas*. *Neisseria gonorrhoeae*, *Chlamydia*, and vaginal organisms may cause urethritis.

Pathophysiology—Bacteria that ascend the urinary tract through the urethra cause most urinary tract infections. This ascent is easier in the shorter urethra of females. The anterior urethra is normally colonized by bacteria from the large intestine in females. The trauma to the female urethra that occurs during sexual intercourse can result in the entrance of bacteria in to the bladder. Instrumentation of the lower urinary frequently results in infection. Bacteriuria commonly occurs within 24 to 48 hours after the placement of an indwelling urinary catheter. The rate of acquisition of catheter-associated bacteriuria is 2–6% per day for each day of catheterization.

Normally, flow of urine washes out any bacteria that enter the bladder. However, certain conditions interfere with this flow and therefore predispose the individual to the development of UTIs. Tumors, stones, strictures, bladder diverticulum, anatomical abnormalities, and prostatic hypertrophy may impede flow of urine. Structural abnormalities, as well as a neurogenic bladder, may prevent complete emptying of the bladder and allow bacteria to remain and multiply in the residual urine.

Conditions that allow retrograde flow of urine increase the incidence of infection. In vesicoureteral reflux, urine from the bladder is forced up the ureters and perhaps into the renal parenchyma by increased pressure in the bladder during voiding. Urethrovesical reflux may draw contaminated urine back into the bladder from the urethra during coughing, sneezing, or laughing. In pregnancy the urine flow is obstructed partially by the enlarged uterus. This results in dilation of the ureters and decreased peristaltic activity of the bladder, allowing for reflux.

Certain uropathogenic strains of *E coli* possess adhesins that bind to receptors on the surface of urinary epithelium. These adhesins allow *E coli* to resist being "washed out" from the urinary tract. The best known form of adhesion is by *P fimbriae* on the bacterial cell wall. *P fimbriae* attach to the carbohydrate moiety of a glycolipid in the epithelial cell. It is adhesion to this receptor that is apparently interrupted by substances in cranberry juice.

Rarely, UTIs may be caused by the hematogenous spread of bacteria from other sites. This usually involves seeding of the kidney by staphylococci.

Symptoms and Signs—Urethritis is accompanied by symptoms related to micturition, including urgency and dysuria. Cystitis is characterized by symptoms of frequency, urgency, dysuria, and perhaps pain or pressure in the lower abdomen. Systemic symptoms or signs are uncommon with cystitis. Acute pyelonephritis is manifested by symptoms that develop over a few hours to 2 days, including aching pain in the lumbar region (flank pain), fever to 39°, shaking chills, nausea, vomiting, and local symptoms of urgency and dysuria. On physical examination, there may be tenderness over the kidney in the area of the costovertebral angle.

The urinalysis in a UTI may show bacteria, leukocytes, red blood cells, and epithelial debris. White blood cell casts indicate pyelonephritis.

In patients with acute urinary tract infections, the symptoms may resolve with or without therapy. Acute pyelonephritis may resolve spontaneously or recur over many years. Patients without underlying disease usually do not have continuing asymptomatic bacteriuria. However, for patients with stones, obstruction, reflux, or other anatomical abnormalities, eradication of the organism is difficult. These patients are at risk of septicemia or recurrent urinary tract infections that are often caused by persistence of the same organisms.

Diagnosis—Microscopy of the urine for leukocytes suffices to diagnose a UTI in most circumstances. Ten or more leukocytes/high-powered field is considered abnormal. If complicated UTI is suspected or if infections have been resistant to therapy, culture and sensitivity of the urine are indicated. The culture is taken from a midstream, clean-voided, urine specimen. The adequacy of the collection can be judged by the absence of squamous epithelial cells or multiple organisms on culture. Squamous epithelial cells and multiple organisms indicate contamination. If fewer than 1000 bacterial colonies/ml of urine are cultured, significant infection is present as the bacteria are probably contaminants from the urethra or perineal areas. If between 10^3 and 10^4 organisms/ml of urine is cultured, interpretation depends on the apparent degree of contamination of the specimen and the plausibility of the organism cultured: often the culture should be repeated. If there are more than 10^5 organisms/ml of urine, the diagnosis of a UTI will be correct in 80% of the cases. When urine is obtained from the bladder, ureters, or renal pelvis by sterile technique, the presence of any number of bacteria indicates a UTI.

The extent of the diagnostic workup of a patient with a UTI depends on whether it is the first infection, the age and sex of the patient and the presence of underlying disease. Male children and adult men presenting with a second UTI should receive a complete evaluation to rule out anatomical abnormalities. A female in the childbearing years may be diagnosed on the basis of urinalysis and gram stain of bacteria in the urine if this is the first infection. Cultures are obtained in other situations. Recurrent UTIs require a complete diagnostic workup in certain circumstances.

Sexually Transmitted Disease

Sexually transmitted disease (STD) refers to a disease acquired through sexual activity. There are many diseases in this category, and STD refers to no specific one; therefore, the term is confusing.

GONORRHEA (GC)—This is an extremely common disease that is transmitted by genital, anal-genital, or oral-genital contact.

Epidemiology—Gonorrhea is pandemic in the US, particularly in poor urban settings. The highest incidence is in persons aged 15 to 24 years, minorities, and persons living in the Southeastern United States. Historically, gonorrhea has been reported more commonly in men. This difference has been ascribed to the higher prevalence of asymptomatic disease in women. However, since 1980 there has been a decreased incidence in homosexual men coupled with better case finding in women that has resulted in a near equal rate of disease for both men and women in the US currently.

Etiology—Gonorrhea is caused by the fastidious, nonspore-forming gram-negative diplococcus, *Neisseria gonorrhoeae*. This organism requires precise conditions for growth. It dies quickly on a dry swab, survives only briefly on a moist towel, and does not grow at room temperature. Certain strains of *N gonorrhoeae* are resistant to penicillin and tetracycline. There are no nonhuman reservoirs of gonorrhea.

Pathophysiology—After an infected person inoculates gonococci onto a mucous membrane, local invasion occurs. The hallmark of GC is copious, yellow pus. Common sites of inoculation are the pharynx, urethra, cervix, and anus. The incubation period for gonorrhea is 3 to 5 days. Once inoculated in the genital tract, the infection may ascend, particularly in the female. However, in men, epididymitis and prostatitis are rare. In the female, the gonococcus does not survive well in the uterus but does infect the fallopian tubes in about 15% of cases. This may cause scarring and later sterility. About 1–3% of affected adults develop gonococcemia; two-thirds of these are females. Distant sites of infection include joints, meninges, and heart valves.

Symptoms and Signs—Clinical manifestations of gonorrhea depend on the site and duration of infection and whether there has been local or systemic spread.

A profuse, purulent, yellow urethral discharge associated with dysuria and frequency develops in 90–95% of infected males. If untreated, the urethritis will resolve in 8 weeks. Anorectal infections are usually asymptomatic but may produce anorectal burning or itching, tenesmus, and a bloody, mucopurulent, rectal discharge. These symptoms may subside without treatment. Pharyngeal infections may produce an exudative tonsillitis but are most commonly asymptomatic.

Only 5–10% of infected females develop symptoms, which include dysuria, frequency, increased vaginal discharge, abnormal menstrual bleeding, and anorectal discomfort. The symptoms of urethritis may be confused with a urinary tract infection, and the increased vaginal discharge may be attributed to vaginitis. Vaginitis and UTI may occur concomitantly with GC. Lower abdominal tenderness and pain suggest pelvic inflammatory disease. Fever chills, nausea, vomiting, and leukocytosis may also occur. Physical examination reveals signs of pelvic peritonitis.

Gonococcemia may be the first sign of disseminated infection and includes fever, polyarthralgias and skin lesions that usually are located on the distal extremities. The skin lesions may be papular, petechial, pustular, hemorrhagic, or necrotic. Tenosynovitis or a septic arthritis of a single, large joint or of several joints usually follows but may precede symptoms and signs of gonococcemia. The synovial fluid is purulent, and joint destruction occurs very rapidly without proper treatment.

Diagnosis—Diagnosis of gonorrhea in a male is made on a gram stain of the urethral discharge by the presence of gram-negative diplococci within leukocytes. If gram-negative diplococci are seen but are extracellular, a culture is required for diagnosis. The diagnosis of gonorrhea in females is made by culture of the cervix. The anal canal and pharynx should also be cultured in women and homosexual men. Blood cultures are unlikely to be positive for gonococcus 48 hours after the onset of gonococcemia.

SYPHILIS—Syphilis is a chronic systemic infection that is seen in three stages: primary, secondary, and tertiary, that progress over many years. In untreated syphilis, degeneration eventually occurs in the central nervous and cardiovascular systems.

Epidemiology—The incidence of syphilis has increased over the past decade. The incidences of tertiary and congenital syphilis had been declining since 1943 but rose in epidemics in 1982 and 1990. As with other sexually transmitted diseases, syphilis is more common among indigent nonwhites living in urban areas, illicit drug users, homosexuals, and patients infected with HIV.

Etiology—Syphilis is caused by the spirochete *Treponema pallidum*, a spiral-shaped organism that is not seen under an ordinary light microscope but that can be visualized using the dark-field technique. The organisms have not been cultured because their growth requirements are so precise. The only naturally occurring host for *T pallidum* is man.

Pathophysiology—Nearly all cases of syphilis are acquired by sexual contact with infectious lesions. Syphilis may be acquired rarely by nonsexual personal contact, contact with contaminated fomites, blood transfusions, and in utero. The spirochete penetrates intact mucous membranes or abraded skin and enters the lymphatics and blood within a few hours. The average incubation time for syphilis is 21 days; however, it ranges from 10 to 90 days depending on the size of the inoculum.

The immune response to infection with *T pallidum* begins with the migration to the site of infection by polymorphonuclear cells that coincide with the formation and eventual resolution of the primary chancre. Antibodies also form that can be detected relatively early in most infected patients. Despite this immune response, without treatment widespread dissemination of organisms occurs which leads to the secondary and tertiary stages of the disease.

Symptoms and Signs—The hallmark of *primary syphilis* is the chancre. The chancre begins as a papule, which rapidly becomes eroded and forms an ulcer that is generally painless. The chancre is most commonly found on the external genitalia or the anal canal but can be located anywhere. This primary chancre heals spontaneously in 2 to 6 weeks. The chancre is highly infectious. Approximately 25% of patients with untreated disease will progress to secondary syphilis.

Secondary syphilis appears approximately 6 weeks after the chancre has healed and is characterized by appearance of nonpruritic red or pink macules on the trunk and proximal extremities. In about 1 to 2 months, red papular lesions also appear that may progress to pustular or necrotic lesions. The lesions are widespread and may involve the palms, soles, face, and scalp. The papules may scale, but vesicles are not seen. Lymphadenopathy and headache are common. Just as in primary syphilis, the manifestations of secondary syphilis typically resolve spontaneously even in the absence of therapy. Occasionally, patients may experience relapsing secondary syphilis for up to five years after the initial episode.

Tertiary syphilis may occur 1 to 30 years after the primary infection. It is not necessary for individuals to have experience clinically symptomatic primary syphilis prior to the development of tertiary symptoms. The most common manifestations of tertiary syphilis are central nervous system involvement, cardiovascular disease, and gummatous syphilis.

Central nervous system involvement is manifested primarily in one of three ways and is seen in 5% of patients. First, meningovascular syphilis may erupt 5 to 10 years after the primary infection and involves inflammation of the pia and the arachnoid. There may be either focal or widespread symptoms. Second, general paresis reflects widespread parenchymal damage to the brain. It causes changes in personality, affect, intellect, judgment, orientation, calculating ability, and insight. There will likely be hyperactive reflexes, difficulty with speech, and small irregular pupils that react to near, but not to light. General paresis is seen about 20 years after infection. Third, tabes dorsalis is due to demyelination of the posterior columns, dorsal roots, and dorsal-root ganglia of the spinal cord. Symptoms and signs include ataxia, wide-based gait, foot-slap, paresthesias, and bladder disturbances. There may be impotence and loss of position, deep pain, and temperature sensations. Trophic degeneration of joints and ulcers of the feet may develop as a result of loss of pain sensation. Tabes dorsalis occurs 25 to 30 years after infection.

Cardiovascular syphilis generally begins 15 to 30 years after the initial infection. Classically the aorta is involved with resulting dilation of the aorta (aneurysm). The aortic valve may also become incompetent with regurgitation of blood through the weakened valve. The onset is generally insidious, and most patients present with an asymptomatic murmur or sometimes with congestive heart failure. The coronary arteries may also be compromised and coronary thrombosis may occur.

Gummas are granulomatous, nodular lesions that may occur anywhere but are most common on the skin or in the bones. Gummas involving the internal organs may appear as mass lesions. Gummas are rare but are being seen more frequently in HIV-infected individuals.

In HIV-coinfected people, persistent chancres, secondary infection, and early neurosyphilis may be more common.

GENITAL HERPES—Genital Herpes or herpes genitalis is a common sexually transmitted disease in the US. It occurs in acute (primary) and recurrent forms.

Epidemiology—Genital herpes has reached epidemic proportions in this country, and the rate of occurrence seems to be increasing. The peak incidence is during the sexually active years, although all age groups are affected. Herpes infections occur in all socioeconomic groups. Recurrent episodes may be more frequent than primary ones. Genital herpes is the most common ulcerative sexually transmitted disease.

Pathophysiology—Genital herpes is contracted primarily through sexual contact with an individual who has an active infection. The primary infection consists of grouped vesicles on an inflamed base. It is spread by lymphatics, blood, and ascending sensory nerves. The virus resides in dorsal root ganglia and periodically descends to the skin to cause lesions. Causes of reactivation from the latent stage are not clear. It is often difficult to identify primary cases of herpes genitalia, since many cases are asymptomatic. Recurrent episodes generally are shorter in duration, less severe, and less likely to be associated with systemic involvement than are primary cases.

Symptoms and Signs—A prodromal stage usually precedes the appearance of skin lesions. Symptoms during this phase may include pain, tingling sensations, or itching. Usually, within 24 hours, lesions appear that initially are papular and rapidly progress through vesicular, ulcer, and crusting stages in an otherwise asymptomatic patient. Systemic involvement may occur in neonates and immunocompromised patients.

A typical primary episode lasts 2 to 3 weeks, whereas recurrent cases are much shorter (5–10 days). Recurrent disease is more likely to occur in patients with a more severe initial episode, a prior recurrence, a history of sexually transmitted disease, younger age, and immunosuppression. While lesions often are limited to the genitals and perineal area, they also may occur on the thighs and buttocks.

Etiology—Herpes Simplex Virus Type 2 (HSV-2) causes the vast majority of cases of genital herpes. A very small number may be caused by Herpes Simplex Virus Type 1 (HSV-1) or a concurrent infection with both types. HSV is a DNA virus and is identified through cultures and serological testing for antibodies to the virus.

Diagnosis—The diagnosis of herpes genitalis is made through history, physical exam, and culture of scrapings or biopsies. Serological

techniques can help in the diagnosis of a primary infection though these generally take 4 to 6 weeks to become positive.

Respiratory Tract Infections

These infections are the most common of acute illnesses. Etiologic agents include viruses, bacteria, *Mycoplasma*, and rarely other organisms. Lower respiratory tract infections usually indicate an impairment of host defenses.

Normal Anatomy and Physiology—A number of organisms normally colonize the nasopharynx (normal flora). Most of these organisms are not pathogenic and return after antibiotic therapy. Normal flora may inhibit growth of pathogenic organisms. Potential pathogens often colonize the upper respiratory tract; although they will not often result in infection to the individual, they may transmit disease to others (eg, meningococcus). Transient colonizers may become infectious in some individuals. Anaerobic organisms constitute 90% of the normal flora of the upper respiratory tract. Also, normal flora does not usually extend below the larynx. The lower respiratory tract is sterile in healthy people.

The lungs are protected from infection by several defense mechanisms. The lining of the respiratory tract is composed of sticky surfaces on which particles adhere. Particles larger than 5 μm are usually filtered efficiently and do not reach the alveoli. The lungs also have mechanisms to remove particles that reach the bronchi or alveoli. Coughing and sneezing are natural defenses for removing particles. Ciliated epithelial cells line the lower respiratory tract. Mucus secretion by goblet cells to trap particles and suspend them for transport by the cilia. This mucociliary transport system is the most important means for clearing particles. Macrophages located in alveoli can engulf particles. Specific antibodies and other soluble factors, such as lactoferrin and lysozyme, also contribute to clearance. If a particle cannot be removed or destroyed within the lung, a granuloma forms around it to wall it off.

Environmental factors such as air pollution, cigarette smoking, drugs such as alcohol and anesthetics, and various disease states such as congestive heart failure and leukemia can suppress the normal defensive mechanisms of the lung.

UPPER RESPIRATORY TRACT INFECTIONS—

Epidemiology—URIs follow seasonal variation, with the incidence being highest in winter and lowest in summer. This type of virus infection is transmitted mainly through the coughing and sneezing of infectious aerosolized droplets, but transmission occurs principally through contamination of hands and objects by nasal secretions and saliva. Infection depends on the size of the inoculum and the response of the host.

Etiology—Approximately 95% of upper respiratory tract infections are due to viruses. More than 150 serotypes, representing 12 groups of viruses, have been associated with URIs. Rhinoviruses cause 40% of respiratory illness; adenoviruses cause 2 to 10%, with the remainder being caused by respiratory syncytial virus (RSV), coronavirus, or influenza viruses. *Mycoplasma*, *Chlamydia*, and at times bacteria primarily cause the remaining 5% of URIs with Streptococci being the most common of these.

Pathophysiology—Respiratory viruses cause mucosal sloughing and consequently decreased lung defense mechanisms. This predisposes to serious bacterial infections, although this suprainfection occurs in only a minority of patients.

Symptoms and Signs—The symptoms and signs of a viral URI are familiar and are known as the "common cold." These include a coryzal syndrome characterized by nasal stuffiness and discharge, sneezing, moderate sore throat, and mild constitutional symptoms. Fever may or may not be present. Children with rhinoviruses may develop bronchitis, bronchiolitis, and pneumonia. Both children and adults with adenovirus, respiratory syncytial virus, or influenza viruses may develop lower respiratory infection.

Diagnosis—The diagnosis of URI is made on clinical grounds. Rarely is any additional testing required as these are primarily self-limiting viral infections for which there is no specific therapy. Occasionally, such as in cases of suspected influenza or RSV, nasal/throat washings for viral culture might be considered to confirm the diagnosis when antiviral therapy has been initiated.

STREPTOCOCCAL INFECTIONS—Streptococcal infections are important because of the seriousness of the acute illness as well as the late complications that are not infective but are mediated immunologically. Acute respiratory tract infections with streptococci may manifest as streptococcal pharyngitis, scarlet fever, or pneumonia. The late complications include acute rheumatic fever, rheumatic heart disease, and acute glomerulonephritis.

Epidemiology—Streptococcal infections occur throughout the population. Respiratory streptococcal infections are more common during the colder months. Scarlet fever is usually a disease of children between 6 months and 10 years. Infants less than 3 months rarely have streptococcal infections. Streptococcal pharyngitis occurs commonly among children and young adults. As many as 20% of the population are asymptomatic carriers of Group A streptococcus. A streptococcal URI may be spread by inhalation of respiratory secretions. Epidemics of streptococcal URIs occur.

Etiology—Streptococci are gram-positive cocci that tend to form chains. Three groups have been identified by their ability to hemolyze red cells in culture media by the enzymes streptolysin O and S. Alpha streptococci (or viridans streptococci), beta hemolytic streptococci, and gamma-nonhemolytic streptococci are the three groups. There are 13 serologic types of streptococci designated by the letters A to O. Most bacterial URIs are caused by Group A streptococci. The late complications of rheumatic fever and glomerulonephritis have been attributed only to Group A streptococci.

Pathophysiology—Streptococci are inhaled into the nasopharynx and normally are cleared by defense mechanisms or become transient colonizers. The size of the inoculum, the virulence of the organism, the presence of type-specific immunity, and the defense mechanisms of the host determine if an infection is to occur. Type-specific immunity lasts for years.

Symptoms and Signs—Streptococcal infections present a variable clinical syndrome, and as many as 40% of individuals may be asymptomatic. The incubation period usually lasts 3 to 5 days. The onset is acute, and the illness includes fever, chills, headache, sore throat, anorexia, malaise and, in children, nausea and vomiting. Symptoms reach a maximum in 1 to 2 days. Swallowing worsens the sore throat, hoarseness is present, and nasal stuffiness, nasal discharge, and a nonproductive cough may occur. Earache is common. Scarlet fever is streptococcal pharyngitis followed by a rash with circumoral pallor.

Patients with streptococcal pharyngitis may be mildly to moderately ill, with fever to 40°. Tachycardia and a diffusely red posterior pharynx and soft palate are common. The uvula is edematous. Characteristically, there is an exudate on the tonsils, which may be scraped off without bleeding. The nasal discharge is thick, mucopurulent, and may contain blood.

The clinical course of a streptococcal URI is short with the fever resolving in 3 to 4 days or 5 to 9 days in adults and children, respectively. If scarlet fever develops, exfoliation of the epithelium begins as the rash fades.

Diagnosis—A positive rapid optical immunoassay or throat culture for Group A beta-hemolytic streptococci in the setting of the characteristic history, symptoms and signs makes the diagnosis of streptococcal pharyngitis.

PNEUMONIA—Pneumonia is an infection in the alveoli that only occurs when impairment of host defenses allows the organism access to alveoli and the infectious process cannot be contained. Pneumonia occurs more frequently in individuals with underlying chronic cardiopulmonary disease, immunologic compromise, habitual cigarette smoking, or alcoholism, although it is not uncommon is otherwise healthy individuals. It is also more likely in individuals who recently had a viral pneumonia or general anesthesia.

Epidemiology—Community-acquired pneumonia is the 6th most common cause of death in the US and the most common infectious cause with approximately 6 million cases annually. Approximately 5–60% of the population are asymptomatic carriers of the pneumococcus, depending on the season. The infection is more prevalent in winter and spring. Nearly 500,000 patients with pneumonia are admitted to hospital each year with more than half of these being patients over the age of 65 years. However, the incidence of pneumonia is actually highest among persons younger than age 65 years. The incidence of pneumococcal pneumonia has changed little, although the mortality has decreased greatly with the advent of antibiotics except in the elderly where the mortality rate continues to rise. *Pneumococcus* accounts for 30–60% of community-acquired for which a cause is found. Atypical organisms are felt to be present in up to 25% of cases and may be found as single causative organisms but not infrequently can also be found as mixed infections with other bacteria. *Staphylococcus* is uncommon as a cause of pneumonia except in patients who are hospitalized or those who have had influenza recently. Anaerobic bacteria are often the causes of pneumonia in patients with impairment of swallowing who aspirate oral contents into the lung.

All causes of pneumonia are more frequent in patients with underlying lung disease such as chronic bronchitis or emphysema.

Etiology—Pneumonia may be caused by bacteria, atypical organisms (*Mycoplasma*, *Chlamydia*), or viruses. Rarely fungi are causes of pneumonia. Bacterial causes of pneumonia are the most common. *Pneumococcus (Streptococcus pneumoniae)*, the most frequent bacterial cause of pneumonia, is a gram-positive encapsulated coccus that usually grows in pairs, hence the name diplococcus. Other common bacterial causes are *Haemophilus influenzae*, *Moraxella catarrhalis*, enteric gram-negative organisms, *Staphylococcus aureus*, *Legionella pneumoniae*, and anaerobic bacteria. However, a specific etiology can be identified in approximately 50–60% of cases.

Pneumonia is broadly divided into community-acquired pneumonia and hospital-acquired pneumonia. This division allows for differentiation in terms of expected pathogens, diagnostic approach, expected mortality, and treatment.

Community-acquired pneumonia has traditionally been divided into broad categories of "typical" verses "atypical" pneumonia. This classification was based on clinical presentation, patient demographics, and chest x-ray findings and was felt to provided clues to likely underlying pathogens. However, recent data has shown that this classification is inaccurate and not useful.

Pathophysiology—Bacterial pneumonia occurs when pathogens are aspirated or inhaled into the lungs and the normal defense mechanisms fail in their ability to promptly remove the offending organisms. Bacteria that are aspirated into the lung and usually lodge in the right-lower, right-middle, or left-lower lobe, where they multiply rapidly. The response to the multiplying organisms involves transudation of fluid into the alveoli, which becomes a growth medium for the organism and a mode for local spread to other alveoli, segments, lobules, lobes, and pleura. Polymorphonuclear leukocytes migrate to the site of infection to phagocytose the bacteria. Macrophages appear later to clean up the fibrin and debris. Antibodies against the *Pneumococcus* or other bacteria enhance phagocytosis and cause organisms to agglutinate and adhere to the alveolar wall, thus slowing spread of the infection. Bacteremia is usually transient. The most common complication is the migration of infection to the pleural space causing the formation of an empyema. Lung abscess formation and spread of infection to distant sites such as meninges, pericardium, or joints are other complications but are less common.

Symptoms and Signs—The clinical course of pneumococcal pneumonia is classic. A URI syndrome may precede the pneumonia by a few days. The onset is abrupt, and patients often can state the hour of onset. In 80% of patients, there is a sudden shaking chill and a rapid rise in temperature with tachycardia and tachypnea. In 75% of patients, pleuritic chest pain and a productive cough develop. The sputum is mucoid and pink or rusty in color. Dyspnea is a common complaint. The patient will appear acutely ill but will not complain of nausea, headache, or malaise. If untreated, the symptoms and signs last for 7 to 10 days. Then there is diaphoresis, a sudden drop in temperature, and dramatic improvement. Circulatory collapse and heart failure are common in fatal cases. With other bacterial causes of pneumonia, the onset of symptoms may be more insidious, but fever, productive cough, and dyspnea are still typically present regardless of the underlying pathogen.

On physical examination, breath sounds are decreased, and crackles and rhonchi are present. The chest radiograph shows a homogeneous density in the affected areas. There is a leukocytosis with 70–90% of the WBC being mature or immature polymorphonuclear leukocytes, the "shift to the left." Blood culture is positive in only 10–20% of cases. Gram stain of the sputum shows many PMNs and gram-positive cocci usually in pairs in cases of pneumococcal pneumonia. The Gram stain is less sensitive and specific for other bacterial etiologies.

Poor prognostic signs include leukopenia, bacteremia, multilobar involvement, extrapulmonary infection, underlying systemic disease, and circulatory collapse. The fatality rate in pneumococcal pneumonia is about 5% despite appropriate treatment.

Diagnosis—The diagnosis of pneumonia is suspected by the clinical findings of cough, fever, and dyspnea. A chest x-ray confirms the clinical suspicion. No other specific tests are available for diagnosis. However, an elevated WBC, sputum Gram stain, blood culture, serological tests, and low oxygen saturation can assist in determining prognosis and/or etiology.

MYCOPLASMA—Mycoplasma pneumoniae, (previously called pleuropneumonia-like organisms (PPLO) or Eaton's agent), causes asymptomatic infections, upper respiratory infections, and pneumonia. Mycoplasma pneumonia has been called atypical pneumonia or walking pneumonia, to distinguish it from pneumococcal pneumonia, but the clinical distinction is not crisp.

Epidemiology—The infection is spread by inhalation of respiratory secretions and is characterized by occurrence among many family members or in large numbers of people living in crowded environments such as military bases and college dormitories. *Mycoplasma* infections are common among children and young adults. Traditionally *Mycoplasma* has been felt to be rare in older adults. However, recent data shows that the incidence rises consistently with age. *Mycoplasma* pneumoniae accounts for 15–20% of all pneumonias. *Mycoplasma* infections are more common in the winter.

Etiology—*Mycoplasma* is a unique organism of extremely small size. Instead of a cell wall, a unit membrane surrounds each *Mycoplasma*. Lacking cell walls, *Mycoplasma* resistant to β-lactam antibiotics. *Mycoplasma* frequently may be found as normal flora in the upper respiratory tract.

Symptoms and Signs—The incubation period for *Mycoplasma* varies from 9 to 12 days. The disease begins as a URI that progresses to bronchitis and subsequently to pneumonia in 3–10% of cases. A nonproductive cough is the most characteristic symptom. In cases of pneumonia, the cough may become productive of blood-tinged sputum later in the course. Headache, general malaise, muscle aches, nasal congestion, and sore throat are common.

The clinical course of the disease is variable. Fever may persist for 2 weeks in untreated cases. The pneumonia is usually multilobar and may be bilateral. Lower lobes are involved more commonly than upper lobes. The infiltrate is less dense than in bacterial pneumonia and often is of an interstitial pattern. The physical findings on chest examination usually are much less striking than the severity of disease noted on the chest radiograph.

Complications are rare even without treatment.

Diagnosis—The diagnosis, as with other forms of pneumonia, is based on the history and clinical picture and the chest radiograph. There is a minimal increase in WBC count without a "shift to the left." Lymphocytosis with atypical forms may be present. Cold agglutinins are positive in 50% of the cases after the second week of the illness. A rise in specific antibodies to *Mycoplasma* is a more sensitive and specific test. It takes 2 to 4 weeks to culture *Mycoplasma*.

SEVERE ACUTE RESPIRATORY SYNDROME (SARS)—

Epidemiology—In early 2003, a new, virulent, and apparently highly contagious URI appeared in Guangdong Province of China and has spread to other countries in South East Asia and to Toronto, Canada.

Etiology—The causative agent appears to be a coronavirus.

Pathology—Diffuse alveolar damage and consolidation.

Symptoms and Signs—Patients present with high fever, dry cough, rigor, dyspnea, malaise, and headache. Examination of the chest shows crackles and dullness to percussion. Lymphopenia is common. The chest x-ray shows progressive consolidation.

Diagnosis—Diagnosis is based on the clinical picture in a patient who has been in an endemic area or who has had contact with known cases. Serological tests and culture methods are being developed.

Tuberculosis

Tuberculosis (TB) is a bacterial infection that has greatly decreased in prevalence in the US but remains a threat. Although TB can involve many organs, pulmonary TB is the most common.

Epidemiology—Since the beginning of the 20th century the incidence of TB has been declining in the US, but this decline was punctuated by an increase around 1980 when there was an influx of refugees from Indochina. A second rise of about 20% followed in 1985–92, largely in HIV-infected people. In 1997, under 20,000 cases were reported, an all-time low. Microepidemics often occur in nursing homes and families.

Tubercle bacilli are aerosolized as droplets during coughing by a person with cavitary disease. After evaporation, droplet nuclei, which are 1 to 5 μm in diameter, can reach the alveoli and establish an infection in a susceptible host. The infectivity of a patient is related to the severity of the disease, the number of bacilli in the lesion, and the closeness and length of the contact. An infected person is considered no longer contagious after about 2 weeks of appropriate chemotherapy.

Etiology—*Mycobacterium tuberculosis* is a rod-shaped organism that requires high oxygen tension for optimum growth and produces no toxins or enzymes. The organism has unique staining properties due to the lipid composition of the cell wall. Carbol-fuchsin stain does not wash off with acid, hence the name "acid fast." The bacilli can be cultured.

Pathophysiology—Tubercle bacilli are inhaled and deposited in peripheral alveoli throughout the lung. Before the infection can be contained by a local cellular response, the bacilli are drained to lymph nodes in the hilum and then disseminated throughout the body by the bloodstream.

Sites that are seeded by bacilli include the apices of the lungs, the kidneys, the growing ends of bones, and other areas of high oxygen tension. Cellular immunity involving lymphocyte, macrophages, and giant cells develops in several weeks. Once cellular immunity develops, the reaction forms granulomas at the sites of infection, and in time caseous necrosis may develop in these granulomas. During caseation, cytotoxic material released from T lymphocytes destroys the bacilli as well as the surrounding tissue. The sites then heal by resolution, fibrosis, and calcification. In some cases the immunity is inadequate, and overwhelming infection develops. Healed lesions still contain viable tubercle bacilli. These may remain dormant for the life of the individual. In 10% of cases, these lesions develop into clinical disease sometime after the initial infection.

Symptoms and Signs—The initial infection of primary TB usually produces few symptoms or signs. The incubation period is 4 to 8 weeks. Mild fever and malaise may occur as tuberculin hypersensitivity develops. In some cases, especially in a child less than 3 years, an overwhelming infection may result from the primary infection.

Pulmonary tuberculosis usually occurs after a period of dormancy in a previously infected individual. The onset is insidious. The patient may be asymptomatic with a routine chest radiograph leading to the diagnosis. Fever to 40° may occur in the late afternoon or evening. Night sweats are common. General malaise, fatigue, irritability, and weight loss may occur. A cough, productive of green or yellow sputum that may be blood-streaked is common. When cavitation occurs, highly infectious material spills into the bronchi and is coughed up.

Spread of pulmonary tuberculosis to the pleura results in pleuritic chest pain and the formation of a pleural effusion as part of the inflammatory reaction. The presence of a large effusion may compromise lung function and result in the complaint of dyspnea. Tuberculosis also can spread from the lung or the lymph nodes into the pericardium where the same inflammatory process occurs. A friction rub may be heard. Later, the inflamed pericardium may scar down, calcify, restrict cardiac motion, and present as congestive heart failure.

During the dissemination phase, bacilli are seeded in the kidneys, bone, adrenals, and meninges. At each site the same inflammatory process occurs with caseation and liquefaction. If the infection cannot be contained, local spread may occur. Tuberculosis in the kidneys may result in infection of the rest of the genitourinary tract and present as cystitis, epididymitis, or prostatitis. In females, tuberculosis of the fallopian tubes and uterus may result in abdominal pain, vaginal discharge, sterility, or ectopic pregnancy. Spondylitis may result in localized back pain or compression of the spinal cord. Tuberculosis of the adrenal glands may cause total destruction of the glands and result in Addison's disease. Tuberculous meningitis also is seen. Symptoms and signs include headache, restlessness, irritability, nausea, vomiting, and stiffness of the neck. A change in mentation may be the only sign of the disease.

Miliary tuberculosis is a massive dissemination of tubercle bacilli throughout the body. Lesions are found in the liver, spleen, bone marrow, and other organs (which do not have a high oxygen tension) in addition to the previously mentioned sites of typical spread. The symptoms and signs are nonspecific and include dyspnea, weight loss, weakness, fever, night sweats, and gastrointestinal disturbances. Death is certain unless appropriate treatment is instituted promptly.

Diagnosis—The diagnosis of tuberculosis rests on the use of a skin test with tuberculin, which is the protein fraction of the tubercle bacilli. However, this test cannot discriminate between dormant and active disease. Sensitized lymphocytes accumulate at the site of intradermal injection of tuberculin. Five tuberculin units are injected and the skin test is read in 48 to 72 hours. The criterion for a positive test depends on the age of the patient, degree of exposure, and HIV status. False negative tests occur in 15–20% of patients with clinical tuberculosis. The skin test does not become positive until the development of cellular immunity. In patients with a decreased number of lymphocytes, an overwhelming infection, a pleural effusion, or a fever, the skin test may be falsely negative. The chest radiograph also is essential to the diagnosis of pulmonary tuberculosis. It shows multinodular infiltrates, with or without cavitation, in one or both upper lobes. The Ziehl-Neelsen stain for acid-fast bacilli has been largely supplanted by fluorescent staining methods and nucleic acid amplification techniques: the latter require less than 6 hours, but are expensive. Sputum also may be cultured for the organisms. With modern BACTEC radiometric culture systems, growth can often be detected within 10 days.

Nontuberculous Mycobacterial Disease

Many mycobacteria live freely in our environment and are not generally pathogenic unless host defenses are impaired. They have become important causes of disease in patients with AIDS.

Epidemiology—*M avium* is ubiquitous and is particularly found in water sources and wet environments. *M kansasii* is concentrated in the urban midwest of the US. Person-to-person transmission has never been shown, but infection is extremely common. Skin testing indicates that at least 40 million Americans have been infected, but few of these became ill.

Etiology—*Mycobacterium avium* differs from *M tuberculosis* in growth rate, colony morphology and pigment formation, DNA composition, and pathogenicity. It is readily seen with conventional acid-fast staining.

Pathophysiology—Pulmonary infection is the most common site. Infection is presumably by inhalation. Generally the disease progresses slowly, but occasionally it advances rapidly. In patients with AIDS dissemination is common.

Symptoms and Signs—Patients with AIDS usually present with fever. The liver and spleen may be enlarged. The organism can be readily grown from many sites including blood. Organisms grow within 5 days in appropriate liquid media, and DNA probes permit rapid species identification.

Infections Of the GI Tract

VIRAL HEPATITIS—See Gastroenterology section.

INFECTIOUS DIARRHEA—

Normal Anatomy and Physiology—The gastrointestinal tract has several defenses against infection. Gastric acid keeps the stomach sterile. If intragastric pH increases, fewer pathogens are needed to establish an infection. The remainder of the gastrointestinal tract has a normal bacterial flora that inhibits the growth of other organisms. The flora of the large intestine is composed predominantly of anaerobes. Some species of the normal flora produce short-chain fatty acids or antibiotics such as clostin that prevent the growth of pathogens. Other members of the normal flora compete with pathogens for nutrients. Antibiotics that suppress normal flora predispose to bacterial infection. Cells that produce mucus line the gastrointestinal tract. This mucus forms a barrier to bacterial invasion of the gut wall. Locally produced IgA antibodies and antibodies produced elsewhere, such as IgG, enhance phagocytosis of bacteria within the GI tract. Motility of the gastrointestinal tract moves organisms out and thus prevents infections. Diarrhea increases transit and rids the body of organisms. Antimotility agents interfere with this defense.

Diarrhea is defined as an increase in numbers of stools per day and/or an increase in stool volume. Acute diarrhea is sudden in onset, lasts for less than 2 weeks, and usually is caused by an infectious agent. Chronic diarrhea is of longer duration and usually is due to noninfectious gastrointestinal disease.

Epidemiology—The transmission of the causative agent is by the fecal-oral route in most cases. Contaminated objects, hands, food, and water may transmit the agent. The incidence of infectious diarrhea in the general population has been estimated to be approximately 20 to 40 cases per 100 person years. Foodborne diseases account for roughly 76 million cases, 325,000 hospitalizations, and 5000 deaths in the US annually. These rates are most likely underestimates, as many patients do not seek medical attention.

Etiology—Bacterial toxins, bacterial organisms, viruses, or parasites may cause diarrhea. Diarrhea need not be caused by a pathogen but may be due to changes in normal flora or by normal colonic flora reaching the small intestine. Bacteria that commonly cause diarrhea by the production of toxins include enterotoxigenic *Escherichia coli*, *Staphylococcus*, *Clostridium perfringens*, and *Clostridium difficile*. Bacterial diarrhea is caused by *Shigella*, *Salmonella*, *Campylobacter jejuni*, and *Yersinia enterocolitica* in the US and *Vibrio cholerae* in other countries. Reovirus-like agent (Norwalk agent), echo, and coxsackie viruses commonly cause diarrhea, whereas influenza viruses do not. Parasites include *Entamoeba histolytica* and *Giardia lamblia* as common causes of diarrhea. The frequency of identifying an organism is 2–40%.

Pathophysiology—Viral diarrhea may cause villous shortening in the small intestine, an increase in the number of crypt cells, and widening of the lamina propria. Diarrhea caused by bacterial invasion results in hyperemia, leukocyte infiltration, and frank ulceration of the bowel wall. *Entamoeba histolytica* produces an inflammatory colitis similar to ulcerative colitis except for the presence of the parasite and larger, flask-shaped ulcers of the colonic mucosa. Bacteria may cause diarrhea via enterotoxin-induced hypersecretion or invasion of the gut wall by the bacteria. Enterotoxins stimulate adenyl cyclase in the mucosal cells of the intestine that results in massive secretion of fluid and electrolytes into the bowel lumen. Mucosal integrity is preserved and absorption is normal. In bacterial invasion, the damage to the mucosa results in defective absorption. Giardia probably produces diarrhea by the same

mechanism since invasion of the small bowel occurs. *C difficile* causes pseudomembranous colitis (antibiotic-associated colitis).

Symptoms and Signs—Systemic symptoms including fever, headache, anorexia, vomiting, malaise, and myalgias may accompany diarrhea regardless of the etiology except when toxins are ingested.

Twelve to 24 hours after eating food contaminated by *Clostridium perfringens* or *Staphylococcus*, diarrhea with abdominal pain, cramps and nausea, but no vomiting or systemic symptoms occurs. The diarrhea contains no pus or blood. Recovery occurs in 12 to 24 hours.

In diarrhea in which the mucosa is invaded by organisms, such as Shigella or Salmonella, systemic symptoms occur along with lower abdominal cramps, tenesmus, and rectal urgency. Pus and erythrocytes or gross blood are found in the stool. Shigella causes explosive diarrhea and fever. The disease is usually self-limited with the fever subsiding in 4 days and the diarrhea subsiding in 1 wk. Shigella also produces a neurotoxin that may cause seizures in children. Salmonella produces a less acute clinical picture.

Enterotoxigenic *E coli*, frequently the causative agent in "turista" or "traveler's diarrhea," may produce mild or severe symptoms. The incubation period is 24 to 48 hours, and the diarrhea lasts for 2 to 7 days. The stools contain no blood and few white blood cells.

Nausea and vomiting and other systemic symptoms usually accompany viral diarrhea. The diarrhea is usually mild, recovery occurs in 48 hours, but malabsorption due to lactase deficiency may persist for several weeks. No red blood cells or white blood cells are seen in examination of the stool.

The prognosis of acute infectious diarrhea is usually excellent when treated with adequate fluid replacement. Complications are rare except in infants or extremely debilitated patients who are unable to tolerate the dehydration. Pseudomembranous colitis usually responds promptly to discontinuation of the causative antibiotic, although some cases require treatment with an antibiotic directed at *C difficile*.

Diagnosis—Diagnosis of the specific cause of infectious diarrhea is frequently made on clinical grounds alone as the majority of cases are self-limited. In cases where there is persistent fever, bloody diarrhea, or symptoms lasting for more than 4 days, a stool culture can be useful. Stool examination for the presence of WBCs is also beneficial to exclude non-infectious or non-inflammatory causes. With the proper history, stool analysis for *C difficile* toxin is beneficial as there is specific therapy for this condition. Likewise, when suspected by history, a stool examination for ova and parasites may yield a specific diagnosis.

Central Nervous System Infection

Meningitis and encephalitis are medical emergencies requiring rapid diagnosis and specific therapy. While meningitis involves only the leptomeninges, encephalitis involves the brain tissue itself and also may involve the meninges.

Normal Anatomy and Physiology—The central nervous system is composed of the brain and spinal cord. These structures are enveloped by the meninges, a three-layered fibrous structure within which flows the cerebral spinal fluid. This is a closed structure and is normally sterile.

Epidemiology—There are between 30,000 and 40,000 cases of meningitis annually in the US. People of any age may become infected; however, the frequency of infection and the type of organism varies with age. The highest incidence is found in neonates who are primarily infected with Group B streptococcus during the birth process. Gram-negative bacteria, enterococci, and *Listeria monocytogenes* are also seen. From age 1 month to 23 months *Streptococcus pneumoniae* and *Neisseria meningitidis* are the most common organisms. From age 2 to 8, *N meningitidis* accounts for more than half of all cases with *S pneumoniae* being second in frequency. *Haemophilus influenzae* type b used to have a high rate of infection in this age group but vaccination has dramatically curtailed this organism. In adults up to age 60, *S pneumoniae* and *N meningitidis* are most common. Over age 60, *S pneumoniae* still accounts for most cases but *Listeria monocytogenes* is also common.

Meningitis is most common in the winter and spring. The lowest incidence is noted in the summer months. Epidemics are uncommon in the US but are still seen in developing countries worldwide.

Etiology—Bacteria often cause meningitis with the most common pathogens in most age groups being *Streptococcus pneumoniae*, *Haemophilus influenzae*, and *Neisseria meningitidis*. In neonates, *Escherichia coli* and Group B streptococci are common. Viruses such as enteroviruses and mumps virus also cause meningitis. Fungal meningitis occurs predominantly in immunocompromised patients. Viruses such as mumps and herpes viruses are the usual cause of concomitant encephalitis.

Pathophysiology—Meningitis most commonly results from the colonization of the nasopharynx with potential pathogens, which gain access to the CNS by mucosal invasion. Other causes are direct extension of bacteria through skull fractures caused by trauma. Also, hematological spread of bacteria associated with cases of endocarditis or UTI for example is known to occur. Immunocompromise from HIV, asplenia, corticosteroid use, etc. predisposes to meningitis.

Bacteria that cause meningitis have the ability to invade the mucosa of the nasopharynx as opposed to other normal flora. This leads to transient bacteremia. Generally, the immune system is able to clear these bacteremic episodes before infection begins. However, circumstances that allow for large numbers of bacteria to invade and escape rapid clearance can lead to infection of the CSF. When infection of the CSF occurs, the organisms multiply rapidly. This initiates an intense inflammatory host response. It is the inflammatory response that is responsible for most of the symptoms and signs of meningitis that are seen clinically.

Symptoms and Signs—Systemic manifestations of CNS infection include fever, irritability, and somnolence. A single seizure prior to diagnosis is not uncommon. Nuchal rigidity and headache are often present. The headache is usually described as severe and generalized. Frequently there is hypersensitivity to light and/or sounds. Nuchal rigidity may not be a specific complaint but usually can be found on physical exam. It is manifested by inability of the patient to touch their chin to their chest with either passive or active flexion of the neck. Changes in mental status, seizures, and other focal neurological signs can be seen but usually are later findings.

Diagnosis—The definitive diagnosis of meningitis usually depends on analysis of CSF obtained through lumbar puncture. Every patient should have a lumbar puncture unless contraindicated. Of note however, antibiotic therapy should be given promptly in suspected cases even if the lumbar puncture has not been obtained. In classical bacterial meningitis, CSF glucose is decreased, protein is increased, and white blood cells (predominantly polymorphonuclear cells) and bacteria are present. These findings are quite variable in viral and fungal meningitis, however. Blood cultures are positive in at least half of the cases of bacterial meningitis and can be useful diagnostically especially when CSF cannot be obtained prior to the administration of antibiotics. Similar CSF findings also may be present with encephalitis. These patients often have more severe CNS dysfunction with symptoms such as coma and paresis. A culture of brain material obtained through biopsy is often necessary to identify clearly the etiologic agent in encephalitis.

Infective Endocarditis

This is an infection of the heart valves or the endocardial lining of the heart wall. The etiologic agent is most commonly bacterial but may be fungal. Based on the clinical course the endocarditis is said to be either acute or subacute (duration greater than 6 weeks).

Normal Anatomy and Physiology—The heart valves are fibrous tissue structures that have no intrinsic blood supply. As a result, infection of these valves does not generate a host immune response to the infection (ie, migration of PMNs to the site of infection). As a result, antibiotics are essentially the only treatment for endocarditis. Bacterial or fungal infection of the valves form clusters of organisms known as vegetations that can often be seen by echocardiography.

Epidemiology—A total of 10,000 to 15,000 new cases of infective endocarditis occur annually in the US. There is a male predominance for endocarditis. More than half of patients are in over the age of 60. Endocarditis is uncommon in children. Risk factors for the development of endocarditis are IV drug use, prosthetic heart valves, and structural heart disease (especially rheumatic heart disease).

Etiology—Endocarditis can be classified in three categories: native valve endocarditis, endocarditis in IV drug abusers, and prosthetic valve endocarditis. These categories are associated with different infecting organisms. Endocarditis can also be classified as acute or subacute. Acute disease is caused by *Staphylococcus aureus* infecting native, normal heart valves. It is aggressive and rapidly destructive. It is fatal within 6 weeks if not treated. Subacute endocarditis is usually caused by viridans streptococci on damaged heart valves and is much more indolent in its course.

Native valve endocarditis may be caused by any organism but most commonly is due to viridans streptococci (55%), enterococci, and *S aureus*. Most patients will have some prior damage to the heart valves (eg, rheumatic, age-related degeneration); however, *S aureus* can attack normal valves.

Endocarditis in IV drug users is due to *S aureus* in more than 50% of the cases. Streptococci, enterococci, gram-negative organisms, and fungi also are seen. Polymicrobial infections can also be seen in this population. Unlike native valve endocarditis, IV drug users have infection of the tricuspid valve 50% of the time.

Prosthetic valve endocarditis is divided into early-onset (<60 days from placement of the prosthetic valve) and late-onset (>60 days). *S epidermidis* and *S aureus* constitute more than 50% of the cases of early-onset disease with gram negatives and fungi also being common. Late-onset disease is most frequently caused by streptococci or other organisms that are indigenous flora.

A group of gram-negative fastidious organisms known as the HACEK group (Haemophilus, Actinobacillus, Cardiobacterium, Eikenella, Kingella) are responsible for "culture negative" endocarditis. Although it is possible to grow these organisms in culture, special growth conditions are generally required making the diagnosis more difficult.

Pathophysiology—In subacute endocarditis, the congenital or acquired abnormal valve causes flow disturbances that injure the endocardial lining of the heart valves or wall. This area of injury becomes a focus of thrombus formation, which is seeded with bacteria during transient periods of bacteremia. Dental work or manipulation of either the gastrointestinal or genitourinary tracts with endoscopes, catheters, and surgical instruments can cause bacteremia with indigenous flora. The mass of adherent thrombus and organisms is known as a vegetation. Vegetations grow, erode the valve, and may create myocardial abscesses. Fragments can break off as emboli. Acute endocarditis results from direct attack of normal valves by aggressive organisms that can destroy valves rapidly. Abscess formation and disruption of cardiac conducting tissue is more common in acute endocarditis. Emboli are also more common in acute endocarditis especially with *S aureus*.

Endocarditis is associated with injury to many organs. The pathophysiology involves emboli (both septic and sterile) from the heart focus and immune complexes. In the setting of chronic infection with continued stimulation of the immune system, immune complexes of antibody and antigen form and deposit in various organs, thereby initiating a potentially harmful inflammatory response. Some manifestations of emboli and immune complex deposition are described in the following section.

Symptoms and Signs—Subacute endocarditis often begins with non-specific constitutional complaints. Fever, sweats, anorexia, malaise, myalgias, and arthralgias are prominent. These symptoms often persist and the patient may receive several courses of antibiotics, a practice that interferes with correct diagnosis.

A previous heart murmur may change or a new murmur may occur. Petechiae may appear in the optic fundi, conjunctiva, mucosal surfaces, or skin. Subungual splinter hemorrhages are a feature of this disease as are peculiar lesions on the hands and fingertips (Janeway lesions and Osler's nodes). In acute endocarditis, skin pustules occur. Arthritis and osteomyelitis, splenomegaly, and retinal lesions may develop. Renal manifestations (flank pain, hematuria) may be secondary to renal infarction by emboli or immune complex-mediated glomerulonephritis. Pulmonary infiltrates caused by septic emboli may occur with right-sided endocarditis. Cardiac conduction defects or congestive heart failure may develop as the infection erodes into the conduction system or chordae tendineae, respectively. Stroke, seizures, or meningitis resulting from emboli are seen more commonly in patients with acute bacterial endocarditis.

Diagnosis—No single test makes the diagnosis of endocarditis. Rather, a constellation of findings from history, physical exam, blood cultures, and echocardiogram are required. Of these however, positive blood cultures are of paramount importance. Culture negative endocarditis is possible but is rare.

Because of the difficulty in making an accurate diagnosis, criteria have been established to assist clinicians with suspected cases. These criteria are divided into major and minor criteria. The presence of two major or one major and three minor or five minor criteria is highly associated with endocarditis. The major criteria focus on the presence of multiple positive blood cultures and echocardiogram evidence of valvular vegetations or paravalvular abscess.

Acquired Immunodeficiency Syndrome

This syndrome (AIDS) is a condition characterized by the development of life-threatening opportunistic infection or malignancies in a patient with severe depression of the T-cell-mediated immune system caused by infection with human immunodeficiency virus (HIV). AIDS was first described as a specific entity in the US in 1981, and its frequency and mortality since have increased geometrically. As of December 2000, a total of 58 million individuals have become infected with HIV, and 21.8 million have died since the beginning of the epidemic. A total of 36.1 million are now living with HIV/AIDS, and 90% of these persons are living in developing countries with over 25 million in sub-Saharan Africa alone. Half of those infected are women and less than 25 years of age. In the year 2000, 5.3 million people became newly infected (2.2 million women and 600,000 children). It is estimated that worldwide there are 15,000 people who become infected daily.

Epidemiology—In the US, AIDS was first described in 1981 in previously healthy homosexual men with *Pneumocystis carinii* pneumonia and Kaposi's sarcoma. In the US, the number of cases of AIDS has risen steadily over the past 20 years to over 750,000 total cases and 430,000 deaths. While the incidence of new cases peaked in the late 1980s, there are still approximately 45,000 new cases annually. The number of persons currently living with HIV infection or AIDS in the US is estimated to be approximately 920,000 and 320,000, respectively. Historically most cases have been in homosexual men and intravenous drug users, with different proportions in different areas. Currently, the proportion of cases is still most common in homosexual men. However, the number of new cases infected heterosexually has now surpassed the number infected by injection drug use.

Advances in the treatment of HIV have caused a marked reduction in the number of deaths in the US and Western Europe. From 1996 to 1999 the number of deaths due to AIDS decreased by 50%. However, this trend slowed from the latter part of 1998 through 2000.

Etiology—AIDS is a syndrome that results from infection with either the HIV-1 or HIV-2 virus. HIV-1 was discovered to be the causative agent for AIDS in 1984, 3 years after the first reports of the disease. In 1986, a second type of HIV called HIV-2 was isolated from AIDS patients in West Africa. Both HIV-1 and HIV-2 have the same mode of transmission and cause the same immunodeficient syndrome. However, persons infected with HIV-2 seem to develop immunodeficiency more slowly and have a milder clinical syndrome. There are only a few reported cases of HIV-2 in the US at this time.

The human retroviruses all share certain important functional features. Like all retroviruses, they produce reverse transcriptase that produces a DNA copy of the RNA material of the virus. They also are unusually trophic for T4 lymphocytes. All retroviruses that cause human disease tend to live silently within their target cells until they are activated to replicate. The HIV viruses, but not the other human retroviruses, attach to the CD4 receptor of their target cells, which are principally T4 lymphocytes and monocytes/macrophages.

Pathophysiology—HIV has been isolated from the blood, semen, vaginal fluid, urine, and tears of AIDS patients. Blood, semen, and vaginal fluid are believed to contain sufficient viruses for transmission. Thus, sexual contact, injection of blood or blood products, and birth to an infected mother are well-established modes of transmission. Casual contact with infected individuals has not been found to transmit HIV.

Sexual transmission presently is the predominant mode of transmission. Receptive anal intercourse is more effective than other forms of sexual activity in transmitting HIV in homosexual men. Vaginal intercourse is largely responsible for transmission from men to women and from women to men. Intravenous inoculation of infected blood accounts for transmission of the virus among intravenous drug abusers who share needles. Inoculation of blood or blood products such as Factor VIII or XI concentrates has transmission infection in patients who have received such products and have not engaged in other risky activities. With current blood screening methods, the risk of transmitting HIV by a blood transfusion is estimated at between 1:40,000 and 1:225,000. Approximately 50% of babies born to infected mothers appear to develop HIV infections. Perinatal transmission occurs in utero or during delivery. Breast-feeding possibly transmits the virus as well.

Pathogenesis AIDS results from the infection and subsequent destruction of T4-lymphocytes by HIV. T4 lymphocytes play a key role in maintaining cellular immunity; their depletion leads to a multitude of abnormalities, which collectively undermine the immune response to infections. The infections often are lethal. The virus also infects other cells and promotes the development of certain tumors.

The activities and features of the viruses and T4 lymphocytes are central to understanding the pathogenesis of AIDS. HIV penetrates cells that contain CD4 receptors. Within the cytoplasm of the cell, the reverse transcriptase of the virus produces a DNA copy of its RNA genetic information. The DNA copy then is integrated into the genome of

the host cell. A latency period ensues, after which immune activation results in viral replication and release from the cell, a process that destroys it.

T4 lymphocytes are the main target of HIV. T4 lymphocytes are responsible for inducing nearly every aspect of the immune response, including cytotoxic cells, suppressor cells, macrophages, B cells, natural killer cells, and even bone-marrow progenitor cells. Thus, replication of the virus leads in turn to depletion of the T4 lymphocytes and impairment of a multitude of immune responses.

Other cells with CD4 receptors also may be infected, including monocytes and macrophages. The monocytes are important in the pathogenesis of AIDS. Unlike T4 lymphocytes, the virus does not kill them rapidly. The monocytes thus harbor HIV and disseminate it to brain, bone marrow, and other organs.

Most of the clinical manifestations of AIDS result from opportunistic infections such as *Pneumocystis carinii* pneumonia, toxoplasmosis, cryptococcal meningitis, disseminated mycobacterium avium intracellulare cytomegalovirus, candida esophagitis, and several others. Other clinical manifestations result from the release of cytotoxins and growth factors from infected cells. Dementia in AIDS patients is fostered or caused by cytokines released from HIV-infected macrophages or monocytes rather than by HIV infection of neurons. Similarly, Kaposi's sarcoma appears to be due to the release of tumor-promoting factors from infected cells.

Symptoms and Signs—Infection by HIV usually is followed in a few days by an illness lasting 2 to 3 weeks. Symptoms include malaise, fever, weakness, rash, myalgia, and headache. The patient is then asymptomatic for several months or even several years. During this period antibodies to HIV can be detected in nearly all patients, but the virus and the clinical picture are in a period of latency. When HIV is activated and replicates, the number of T4 lymphocytes declines, and symptoms and signs begin to appear. Over 5 to 10 years after infection, 25–50% of persons will progress to overt AIDS without treatment. Most patients first experience fatigue, anorexia, weight loss, and unexplained fever. Chronic lymph node enlargement, particularly in the neck, is common. Diarrhea often ensues. Nonproductive cough and dyspnea often herald the presence of opportunistic pneumonia. A host of neuropsychiatric symptoms may occur, including confusion, headache, seizures, focal weakness, personality changes, and impaired memory. This is an abbreviated list since every organ may be involved. The possible clinical expressions are vast.

Diagnosis—The diagnosis of HIV infection is made by the detection of the HIV virus using any of the following methods: detecting antibodies to the virus, detecting the viral p24 antigen, detecting viral nucleic acid, or culturing the virus from tissue or blood. The most widely used of these methods is the serology test for antibodies. Antibodies to HIV are first detectable 6 to 12 weeks after infection though may be delayed as much as 6 months.

AIDS is a clinical definition. In 1993 the criteria for AIDS was re-defined. Patients are now classified as having AIDS if they have any of several clinical diseases known as "AIDS indicator conditions" and/or a CD4 count of less than 200/mm^3. AIDS indicator conditions are mostly opportunistic or recurrent infections that have become associated with advanced HIV disease.

BIBLIOGRAPHY

Mandell GL, Douglas RG, Bennett JE, eds. Mandell, Douglas, and Bennett's Principles and Practices of Infectious Diseases, 5th ed. Philadelphia: Churchill Livingstone, 2000.

Callen JP et al, eds. Dermatological Signs of Internal Disease, 3rd ed. Philadelphia: WB Saunders, 2002.

Kelley WN, et al, eds. Textbook of Internal Medicine, 3rd ed. Philadelphia: Lippincott-Raven, 1997.

Felig P, Frohman LA, eds. Endocrinology and Metabolism, 4th ed. New York: McGraw-Hill, 2001.

Klippel JH, Weyand CM, Crofford LJ, et al, eds. Primer on the Rheumatic Diseases, 12th ed. Atlanta: Arthritis Foundation, 2001.

Kjeldsberg CR, ed. Practical Diagnosis of Hematologic Disorders, 3rd ed. Chicago: ASCP Press, 2000.

George RB, et al, eds. Chest Medicine: Essentials of Pulmonary and Critical Care medicine, 4th ed. Philadelphia: Lippincott Williams and Wilkins, 2000.

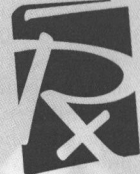

CHAPTER 57

Drug Absorption, Action, and Disposition

Michael R Franklin, PhD

Donald N Franz, PhD

Although drugs differ widely in their pharmacodynamic effects and clinical applications; in penetration, absorption, and usual route of administration; in distribution among the body tissues; and in disposition and mode of termination of action, there are certain general principles that help explain these differences. These principles have both pharmaceutic and therapeutic implications. They facilitate an understanding of both the features that are common to a class of drugs and the differences among the members of that class.

For a drug to act it must be absorbed, transported to the appropriate tissue or organ, penetrate to the responding cell surface or subcellular structure, and elicit a response or alter ongoing processes. The drug may be distributed simultaneously or sequentially to a number of tissues, bound or stored, metabolized to inactive or active products, or excreted. The history of a drug in the body is summarized in Figure 57-1. Each of the processes or events depicted relates importantly to therapeutic and toxic effects of a drug and to the mode of administration, and drug design must take each into account. Since the effect elicited by a drug is its *raison d'être, drug action,* and *effect* are discussed first in the text that follows, even though they are preceded by other events.

DRUG ACTION AND EFFECT

The word *drug* imposes an action-effect context within which the properties of a substance are described. The description of necessity must include the pertinent properties of the recipient of the drug. Thus, when a drug is defined as an analgesic, it is implied that the recipient reacts to a noxious stimulus in a certain way, called pain. (Studies indicate that pain is not simply the *perception* of a certain kind of stimulus but rather, a *reaction* to the perception of a variety of kinds of stimuli or stimulus patterns.) Both because the pertinent properties are locked into the complex and somewhat imprecise biological context and because the types of possible response are many, descriptions of the properties of drugs tend to emphasize the qualitative features of the effects they elicit. Thus, a drug may be described as having analgesic, vasodepressor, convulsant, antibacterial, etc, properties. The specific effect (or use) categories into which the many drugs may be placed are the subject of Chapters 64 through 89 and are not elaborated upon in this chapter. However, the description of a drug does not end with the enumeration of the responses it may elicit. There are certain intrinsic properties of the drug-recipient system that can be described in quantitative terms and that are essential to the full description of the drug and to the validation of the drug for specific uses. Under *Definitions and Concepts* below, certain general terms are defined in qualitative language; under *Dose-Effect Relationships,* the foundation is laid for an appreciation of some of the quantitative aspects of pharmacodynamics.

DEFINITIONS AND CONCEPTS

In the field of pharmacology, the vocabulary that is unique to the discipline is relatively small, and the general vocabulary is that of the biological sciences and chemistry. Nevertheless, there are a few definitions that are important to the proper understanding of pharmacology. It is necessary to differentiate among action, effect, selectivity, dose, potency, and efficacy.

ACTION VS EFFECT—The *effect* of a drug is an *alteration of function* of the structure or process upon which the drug acts. It is common to use the term *action* as a synonym for effect. However, action precedes effect. *Action* is the *alteration of condition* that brings about the effect.

The final effect of a drug may be far removed from its site of action. For example, the diuresis subsequent to the ingestion of ethanol does not result from an action on the kidney but instead from a depression of activity in the region of the hypothalamus, which regulates the release of antidiuretic hormone from the posterior pituitary gland. The alteration of hypothalamic function is, of course, also an effect of the drug, as is each subsequent change in the chain of events leading to diuresis. The action of ethanol was exerted only at the initial step, each subsequent effect being then the action to a following step.

MULTIPLE EFFECTS—No known drug is capable of exerting a single effect, although a number are known that appear to have a single mechanism of action. Multiple effects may derive from a single mechanism of action. For example, the inhibition of acetylcholinesterase by physostigmine will elicit an effect at every site where acetylcholine is produced, is potentially active, and is hydrolyzed by cholinesterase. Thus, physostigmine elicits a constellation of effects.

A drug also can cause multiple effects at several different sites by a single action at only one site, providing that the function initially altered at the site of action ramifies to control other functions at distant sites. Thus, a drug that suppresses steroid synthesis in the liver may not only lower serum cholesterol, impair nerve myelination and function, and alter the condition of the skin (as a consequence of cholesterol deficiency) but also may affect digestive functions (because of a deficiency in bile acids) and alter adrenocortical and sexual hormonal balance.

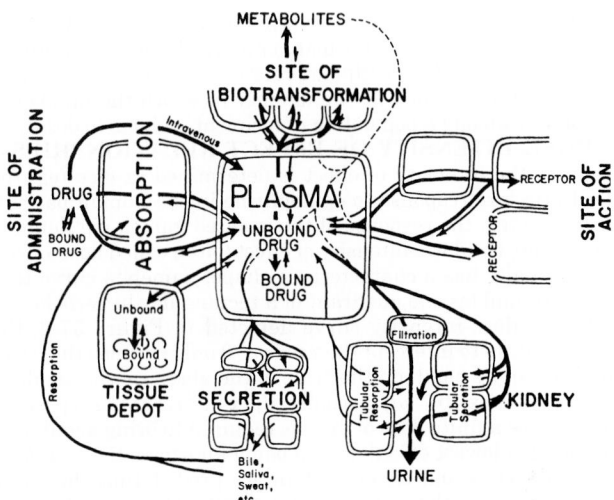

Figure 57-1. The absorption, distribution, action, and elimination of a drug (arrows represent drug movement). Intravenous administration is the only process by which a drug may enter a compartment without passing through a biological membrane. Note that drugs excreted in bile and saliva may be resorbed.

Although a single action can give rise to multiple effects, most drugs exert multiple actions. The various actions may be related, as for example, the sympathomimetic effects of phenylephrine that accrue to its structural similarity to norepinephrine and its ability to exert sympathetic responses, or the actions may be unrelated, as with the actions of morphine to interfere with the release of acetylcholine from certain autonomic nerves, block some actions of 5-hydroxytryptamine (serotonin), and release histamine. Many drugs bring about immunological (allergic or hypersensitivity) responses that bear no relation to the other pharmacodynamic actions of the drug.

SELECTIVITY—Despite the potential most drugs have for eliciting multiple effects, one effect is generally more readily elicitable than another. This differential responsiveness is called *selectivity*. It usually is considered to be a property of the drug, but it is also a property of the constitution and biodynamics of the recipient subject or patient.

Selectivity may come about in several ways. The subcellular structure (receptor) with which a drug combines to initiate one response may have a higher affinity for the drug than that for some other action. Atropine, for example, has a much higher affinity for muscarinic receptors that subserve the function of sweating than it does for the nicotinic receptors that subserve voluntary neuromuscular transmission, so that suppression of sweating can be achieved with only a tiny fraction of the dose necessary to cause paralysis of the skeletal muscles. A drug may be distributed unevenly, so that it reaches a higher concentration at one site than throughout the tissues generally; chloroquine is much more effective against hepatic than intestinal (colonic) amebiasis because it reaches a much higher concentration in the liver than in the wall of the colon. An affected function may be much more critical to, or have less reserve in, one organ than in another, so that a drug will be predisposed to elicit an effect at the more critical site. Some inhibitors of dopa decarboxylase (which is also 5-hydroxytryptophan decarboxylase) depress the synthesis of histamine more than that of either norepinephrine or 5- hydroxytryptamine (serotonin), even though histidine decarboxylase is less sensitive to the drug, simply because histidine decarboxylase is the only step and, hence, is rate-limiting in the biosynthesis of histamine. Dopa decarboxylase is not rate limiting in the synthesis of either norepinephrine or 5-hydroxytryptamine until the enzyme is nearly completely inhibited. Another example of the determination of selectivity by the

critical balance of the affected function is that of the mercurial diuretic drugs. An inhibition of only 1% in the tubular resorption of glomerular filtrate usually will double urine flow, since 99% of the glomerular filtrate is normally resorbed. Aside from the question of the possible concentration of diuretics in the urine, a drug-induced reduction of 1% in sulfhydryl enzyme activity in tissues other than the kidney usually is not accompanied by an observable change in function. Selectivity also can be determined by the pattern of distribution of inactivating or activating enzymes among the tissues and by other factors.

DOSE—Even the uninitiated person knows that the dose of a drug is the amount administered. However, the appropriate dose of a drug is not some unvarying quantity, a fact sometimes overlooked by pharmacists, official committees, and physicians. The practice of pharmacy is entrapped in a system of fixed-dose formulations, so that fine adjustments in dosage are often difficult to achieve. Fortunately, there is usually a rather wide latitude allowable in dosages. It is obvious that the size of the recipient individual should have a bearing upon the dose, and the physician may elect to administer the drug on a body-weight or surface-area basis rather than as a fixed dose. Usually, however, a fixed dose is given to all adults, unless the adult is exceptionally large or small. The dose for infants and children often is determined by one of several formulas that take into account age or weight, depending on the age group of the child and the type of action exerted by the drug. Infants, relatively, are more sensitive to many drugs, often because systems involved in the inactivation and elimination of the drugs may not be developed fully in the infant.

The nutritional condition of the patient, the mental outlook, the presence of pain or discomfort, the severity of the condition being treated, the presence of secondary disease or pathology, and genetic and many other factors affect the dose of a drug necessary to achieve a given therapeutic response or to cause an untoward effect (Chapter 61). Even two apparently well-matched normal persons may require widely different doses for the same intensity of effect. Furthermore, a drug is not always employed for the same effect and, hence, not in the same dose. For example, the dose of a progestin necessary for an oral contraceptive effect is considerably different from that necessary to prevent spontaneous abortion, and a dose of an estrogen for the treatment of the menopause is much too small for the treatment of prostatic carcinoma.

From the above, it is evident that the wise physician knows that *the dose of a drug* is not a rigid quantity but rather that which is necessary and can be tolerated and individualizes the regimen accordingly. The wise pharmacist also recognizes that official or manufacturer's recommended doses are sometimes quite narrowly defined and should serve only as a useful guide rather than as an imperative.

POTENCY AND EFFICACY—The *potency* of a drug is the reciprocal of dose. Thus, it will have the units of persons/unit weight of drug or body weight/unit weight of drug, etc. Potency generally has little utility other than to provide a means of comparing the relative activities of drugs in a series, in which case *relative potency,* relative to some prototypic member of the series, is a parameter commonly used among pharmacologists and in the pharmaceutical industry.

Whether a given drug is more potent than another has little bearing on its clinical usefulness, provided that the potency is not so low that the size of the dose is physically unmanageable or the cost of treatment is higher than with an equivalent drug. If a drug is less potent but more selective, it is the one to be preferred. Promotional arguments in favor of a more potent drug thus are irrelevant to the important considerations that should govern the choice of a drug. However, it sometimes occurs that drugs of the same class differ in the maximum intensity of effect; that is, some drugs of the class may be less efficacious than others, irrespective of how large a dose is used.

Efficacy connotes the property of a drug to achieve the desired response, and *maximum efficacy* denotes the maximum achievable effect. Even huge doses of codeine often cannot achieve the relief from severe pain that relatively small doses

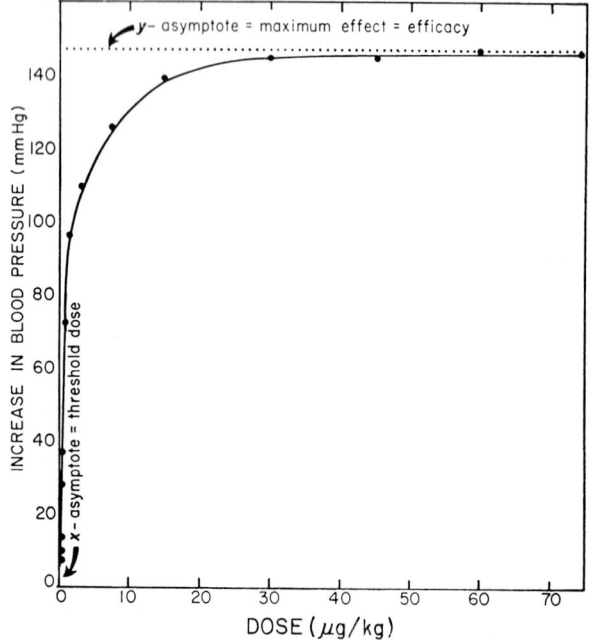

Figure 57-2. The relationship of the intensity of the blood-pressure response of the cat to the intravenous dose of norepinephrine.

of morphine can; thus, codeine is said to have a lower maximum efficacy than morphine. Efficacy is one of the primary determinants of the choice of a drug.

DOSE-EFFECT RELATIONSHIPS

The importance of knowing how changes in the intensity of response to a drug vary with the dose is virtually self-evident. Both the physician, who prescribes or administers a drug, and the manufacturer, who must package the drug in appropriate dose sizes, must translate such knowledge into everyday practice. Theoretical or molecular pharmacologists also study such relationships in inquiries into mechanism of action and receptor the-

ory It is necessary to define two types of relationships: (1) dose-intensity relationship, ie, the manner in which the intensity of effect in the individual recipient relates to dose, and (2) dose-frequency relationship, ie, the manner in which the number of responders among a population of recipients relates to dose.

DOSE–INTENSITY OF EFFECT RELATIONSHIPS— Whether the intensity of effect is determined *in vivo* (eg, the blood-pressure response to epinephrine in the human patient) or *in vitro* (eg, the response of the isolated guinea pig ileum to histamine), the dose–intensity of effect (often called dose-effect) curve usually has a characteristic shape, namely a curve that closely resembles one quadrant of a rectangular hyperbola.

In the dose-intensity curve depicted in Figure 57-2, the curve appears to intercept the x axis at 0 only because the lower doses are quite small on the scale of the abscissa, the smallest dose being 1.5×10^{-3} μg. Actually, the x intercept has a positive value, since a finite dose of drug is required to bring about a response, this lowest effective dose being known as the *threshold dose*. Statistics and chemical kinetics predict that the curve should approach the y axis asymptotically. However, if the intensity of the measured variable does not start from zero, the curve possibly may have a positive y intercept (or negative x intercept), especially if the ongoing basal activity before the drug is given is closely related to that induced by the drug.

In practice, instead of an asymptote to the y axis, dose-intensity curves nearly always show an upward concave foot at the origin of the curve, so that the curve has a lopsided sigmoid shape. At high doses, the curve approaches an asymptote that is parallel to the x axis, and the value of the asymptote establishes the maximum possible response to the drug, or *maximum efficacy*. However, experimental data in the regions of the asymptotes generally are too erratic to permit an exact definition of the curve at very low and very high doses. The example shown represents an unusually good set of data.

Because the dose range may be 100- or 1000-fold from the lowest to the highest dose, it has become the practice to plot dose-intensity curves on a logarithmic scale of abscissa (ie, to plot the log of dose versus the intensity of effect). Figure 57-3 is such a semilogarithmic plot of the same data used in Figure 57-2. In the figure the intensity of effect is plotted both in absolute units (at the left) or in relative units, as percentages (at the right).

Although no new information is created by a semilogarithmic representation, the curve is stretched in such a way as to facilitate the inspection of the data; the comparison of results

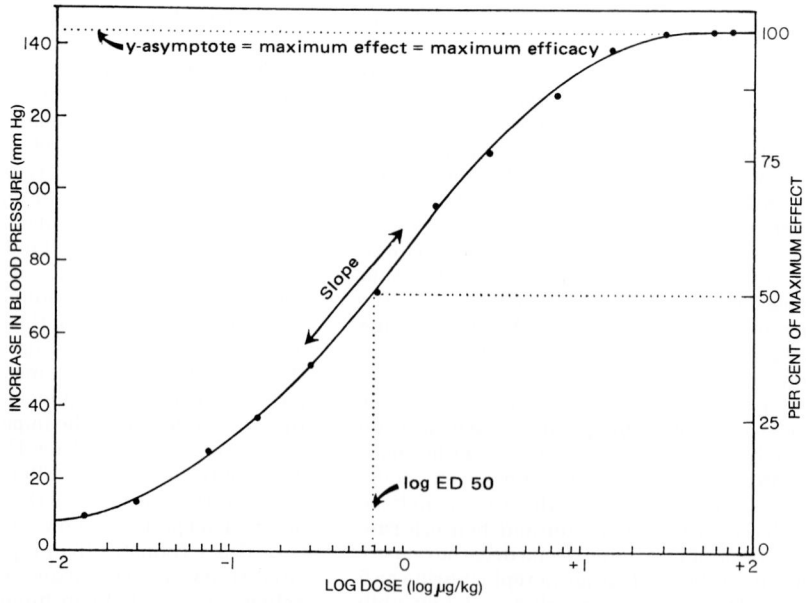

Figure 57-3. The relationship of the intensity of the blood-pressure response of the cat to the log of the intravenous dose of norepinephrine.

from multiple observations and the testing of different drugs also is rendered easier. In the example shown, the curve is essentially what is called a *sigmoid curve* and is nearly symmetrical about the point that represents an intensity equal to 50% of the maximal effect (ie, about the midpoint). The symmetry follows from the rectangular hyperbolic character of the previous Cartesian plot (see Fig 57-2). The semilogarithmic plot reveals better the dose-effect relationships in the low-dose range, which are lost in the steep slope of the Cartesian plot. Furthermore, the data about the midpoint are almost a straight line; the nearly linear portion covers approximately 50% of the curve. The slope of the linear portion of the curve or, more correctly, the slope at the point of inflection, has theoretical significance (see *Drug Receptors and Receptor Theory*).

The upper portion of the curve approaches an asymptote, which is the same as that in the Cartesian plot. If the response system is completely at rest before the drug is administered, the lower portion of the curve should be asymptotic to the *x* axis. Both asymptotes and the symmetry derive from the law of mass action.

Dose-intensity curves often deviate from the ideal configuration illustrated and discussed above. Usually, the deviate curve remains sigmoid but not extended symmetrically about the midpoint of the *linear* segment. Occasionally, other shapes occur. Deviations may derive from multiple actions that converge upon the same final effector system, from varying degrees of metabolic alteration of the drug at different doses, from modulation of the response by feedback systems, from nonlinearity in the relationship between action and effect, or from other causes.

It is frequently necessary to identify the dose that elicits a given intensity of effect. The intensity of effect that is generally designated is 50% of maximum intensity. The corresponding dose is called the *50% effective dose,* or *individual ED50* (see Fig 57-3). The use of the adjective *individual* distinguishes the ED50 based upon the intensity of effect from the median effective dose, also abbreviated ED50, determined from frequency of response data in a population (see *Dose-Frequency Relationships,* this chapter).

Drugs that elicit the same quality of effect may be compared graphically. In Figure 57-4, five hypothetical drugs are compared. Drugs *A, B, C,* and *E* all can achieve the same maximum effect, which suggests that the same effector system may be common to all. *D* possibly may be working through the same effector system, but there are no *a priori* reasons to think this is so. Only *A* and *B* have parallel curves and common slopes. Common slopes are consistent with, but in no way prove, the idea that *A* and *B* not only act through the same effector system but also by the same mechanism. Although drug-receptor theory (see *Drug Receptors and Receptor Theory*) requires that the curves of identical mechanism have equal slopes, examples of exceptions are known. Furthermore, mass-law statistics require that all simple drug-receptor interactions generate the same slope; only when slopes depart from this universal slope in accordance with distinctive characteristics of the response system do they provide evidence of specific mechanisms.

The relative potency of any drug may be obtained by dividing the ED50 of the standard, or prototypic, drug by that of the drug

in question. Any level of effect other than 50% may be used, but it should be recognized that when the slopes are not parallel, the relative potency depends upon the intensity of effect chosen. Thus, the potency of *A* relative to *C* (see Fig 57-4) calculated from the ED50 will be smaller than that calculated from the ED25.

The low maximum intensity inducible by *D* poses even more complications in the determination of relative potency than do the unequal slopes of the other drugs. If its dose-intensity curve is plotted in terms of percentage of its own maximum effect, its relative inefficacy is obscured, and the limitations of relative potency at the ED50 level will not be evident. This dilemma underscores the fact that drugs can be compared better from their entire dose-intensity curves than from a single derived number like ED50 or relative potency.

Drugs that elicit multiple effects will generate a dose-intensity curve for each effect. Even though the various effects may be qualitatively different, the several curves may be plotted together on a common scale of abscissa, and the intensity may be expressed in terms of percentage of maximum effect; thus, all curves can share a common scale of ordinates in addition to a common abscissa. Separate scales of ordinates could be employed, but this would make it harder to compare data.

The selectivity of a drug can be determined by noting what percentage of maximum of one effect can be achieved before a second effect occurs. As with relative potency, selectivity may be expressed in terms of the ratio between the ED50 for one effect and that for another effect, or a ratio at some other intensity of effect. As with relative potency, difficulties follow from nonparallelism. In such instances, selectivity expressed in dose ratios varies from one intensity level to another.

When the dose-intensity curves for a number of subjects are compared, it is found that they vary considerably from individual to individual in many respects; eg, threshold dose, midpoint, maximum intensity, and sometimes even slope. By averaging the intensities of the effect at each dose, an average dose-intensity curve can be constructed.

Average dose-intensity curves enjoy a limited application in comparing drugs. A single line expressing an average response has little value in predicting individual responses unless it is accompanied by some expression of the range of the effect at the various doses. This may be done by indicating the standard error of the response at each dose. Occasionally, a simple scatter diagram is plotted in lieu of an average curve and statistical parameters. An average dose-intensity curve also may be constructed from a population in which different individuals receive different doses; if sufficiently large populations are employed, the average curves determined by the two methods will approximate each other.

It is obvious that the determination of such average curves from a population large enough to be statistically meaningful requires a great deal of work. Retrospective clinical data occasionally are treated in this way, but prospective studies infrequently are designed in advance to yield average curves. The usual practice in comparing drugs is to employ a quantal (all-or-none) endpoint and plot the frequency or cumulative frequency of response over the dose range, as discussed below.

DOSE–FREQUENCY OF RESPONSE RELATIONSHIPS—When an endpoint is truly all-or-none, such as death, it is an easy matter to plot the number of responding individuals (eg, dead subjects) at each dose of drug or intoxicant. Many other responses that vary in intensity can be treated as all-or-none if simply the presence or absence of a response (eg, cough or no cough, convulsion or no convulsion) is recorded, without regard to the intensity of the response when it occurs. When the response changes from the basal or control state in a less abrupt manner (eg, tachycardia, miosis, rate of gastric secretion), it may be necessary to designate arbitrarily some particular intensity of effect as the endpoint. If the endpoint is taken as an increase in heart rate of 20 beats/min, all individuals whose tachycardia is less than 20 beats/min would be recorded as nonresponders, while all those with 20 or above would be recorded as responders. When the percentage of responders in the population is plotted against the dose, a characteristic dose-response curve, more

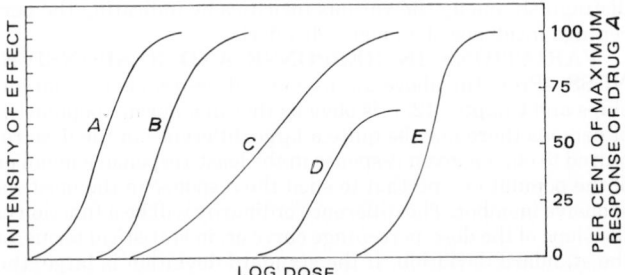

Figure 57-4. Log dose–intensity of effect curves of five different hypothetical drugs (see text for explanation).

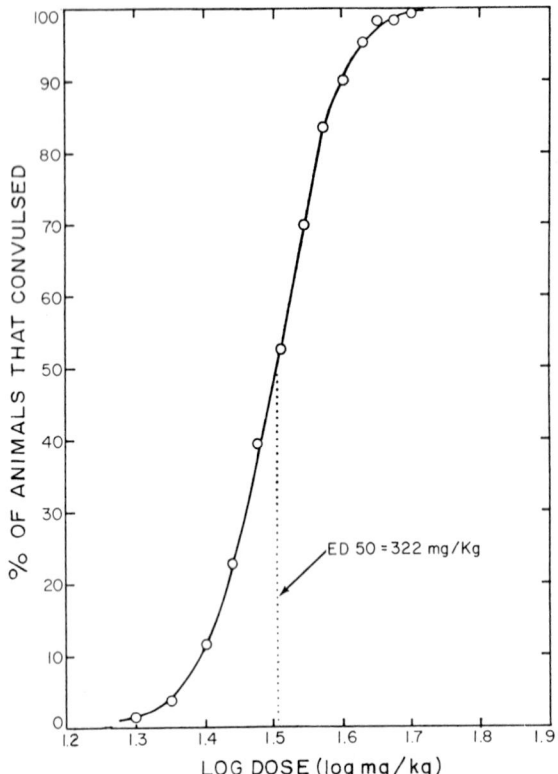

Figure 57-5. The relationship of the number of responders in a population of mice to the dose of pentylenetetrazole.

properly called a *dose–cumulative frequency* or *dose-percentage* curve, is generated. Such a curve is, in fact, a cumulative frequency-distribution curve, the percentage of responders at a given dose being the frequency of response.

Dose–cumulative frequency curves are generally of the same geometric shape as dose-intensity curves (namely, sigmoid) when frequency is plotted against log dose (Fig 57-5). The tendency of the cumulated frequency of response (ie, percentage) to be linearly proportional to the log of the dose in the middle of the dose range is called the *Weber-Fechner law,* although it is not invariable, as a true natural law should be. In many instances, the cumulative frequency is simply proportional to dose rather than log dose. The Weber-Fechner law applies to either dose-intensity or dose–cumulative frequency data. The similarity between dose-frequency and dose-intensity curves may be more than fortuitous, since the intensity of response will usually have an approximately linear relationship to the percentage of responding *units* (smooth muscle cells, nerve fibers, etc) and, hence, is also a type of cumulative frequency of response. These are the same kind of statistics that govern the law of mass action.

If only the increase in the number of responders with each new dose is plotted, instead of the cumulative percentage of responders, a bell-shaped curve is obtained. This curve is the first derivative of the dose–cumulative frequency curve and is a *frequency-distribution* curve. The distribution will be symmetrical—ie, *normal* or Gaussian (see Chapter 12)—only if the dose–cumulative frequency curve is symmetrically hyperbolic. Because most dose–cumulative frequency curves are more nearly symmetrical when plotted semilogarithmically (ie, as log dose), dose–cumulative frequency curves are usually *log-normal.*

Since the dose-intensity and dose–cumulative frequency curves are basically similar in shape, it follows that the curves have similar defining characteristics, such as ED50, maximum effect (maximum efficacy), and slope. In dose–cumulative frequency data, the ED50 *(median effective dose)* is the dose to which 50% of the population responds (see Fig 57-5). If the fre-

quency distribution is normal, the ED50 is both the arithmetic mean and the median dose and is represented by the midpoint on the curve; if the distribution is log-normal, the ED50 is the median dose but not the arithmetic mean dose. The efficacy is the cumulative frequency summed over all doses; it is usually, but not always, 100%. The slope is characteristic of both the drug and the test population. Even two drugs of identical mechanism may give rise to different slopes in dose-percentage curves, whereas in dose-intensity curves the slopes are the same.

Statistical parameters (such as standard deviation), in addition to ED50, maximum cumulative frequency (efficacy) and slope, characterize dose–cumulative frequency relationships (see Chapter 12).

There are several formulations for dose–cumulative frequency curves, some of which are employed only to define the linear segment of a curve and to determine the statistical parameters of this segment. For the statistical treatment of dose-frequency data, see Chapter 12. One simple mathematical expression of the entire log-symmetrical sigmoid curve is

$$\log \text{dose} = K + f \log \left(\frac{\% \text{ response}}{100\% - \text{response}} \right) \quad (1)$$

where percentage response may be either the percentage of maximum intensity or the percentage of a population responding. The equation is thus basically the same for both log normal dose-intensity and log normal dose-percentage relationships. *K* is a constant that is characteristic of the midpoint of the curve, or ED50, and $1/f$ is characteristically related to the slope of the linear segment, which, in turn is closely related to the standard deviation of the derivative log-normal frequency-distribution curve.

The comparison of dose-percentage relationships among drugs is subject to the pitfalls indicated for dose-intensity comparisons, namely, that when the slopes of the curves are not the same (ie, the dose-percentage curves are not parallel), it is necessary to state at which level of response a potency ratio is calculated. As with dose-intensity data, potencies generally are calculated from the ED50, but potency ratios may be calculated for any arbitrary percentage response. The expression of selectivity is, likewise, subject to similar qualifications, inasmuch as the dose-percentage curves for the several effects are usually nonparallel.

The term *therapeutic index* is used to designate a quantitative statement of the selectivity of a drug when a therapeutic and an untoward effect are being compared. If the untoward effect is designated *T* (for toxic) and the therapeutic effect, *E,* the therapeutic index may be defined as TD50/ED50 or a similar ratio at some other arbitrary levels of response. The TD and the ED are not required to express the same percentage of response; some clinicians use the ratio TD1/ED99 or TD5/ED95, based on the rationale that if the untoward effect is serious, it is important to use a most-severe therapeutic index in passing judgment upon the drug. Unfortunately, therapeutic indices are known in man for only a few drugs.

There will be a different therapeutic index for each untoward effect that a drug may elicit and, if there is more than one therapeutic effect, a family of therapeutic indices for each therapeutic effect. However, in clinical practice, it is customary to distinguish among the various toxicities by indicating the percentage incidence of a given side effect.

VARIATIONS IN RESPONSE AND RESPONSIVENESS—From the above discussion of dose-frequency relationships and Chapter 12, it is obvious that in a normal population of persons there may be quite a large difference in the dose required to elicit a given response in the least-responsive member of the population and that to elicit the response in the most-responsive member. The difference ordinarily will be a function of the slope of the dose-percentage curve or, in statistical terms, of the standard deviation. If the standard deviation is large, the extremes of responsiveness of responders are likewise large.

In a normal population, 95.46% of the population responds to doses within two standard deviations from the ED50 and

99.73% within three standard deviations. In log-normal populations, the same distribution applies when standard deviation is expressed as log dose.

In the population represented in Figure 57-5, 2.25% of the population (two standard deviations from the median) would require a dose more than 1.4 times the ED50; an equally small percentage would respond to 0.7 of the ED50. The physician who is unfamiliar with statistics is apt to consider the 2.25% at either extreme to be abnormal reactors. The statistician will argue that these 4.5% are within the normal population and that only those who respond well outside the normal population, at least three standard deviations from the median, deserve to be called abnormal.

Irrespective of whether the criteria of abnormality that the physician or the statistician obtain, the term *hyporeactive* applies to those individuals who require abnormally high doses and *hyperreactive* to those who require abnormally low doses. The terms *hyporesponsive* and *hyperresponsive* also may be used. It is incorrect to use the terms hyposensitive and hypersensitive in this context; *hypersensitivity* denotes an allergic response to a drug and should not be used to refer to hyperreactivity. The term *supersensitivity* correctly applies to hyperreactivity that results from denervation of the effector organ; it is often more definitively called denervation supersensitivity. Sometimes hyporeactivity is the result of an immunochemical deactivation of the drug, or *immunity*. Hyporeactivity should be distinguished from an increased dose requirement that results from a severe pathological condition. Severe pain requires large doses of analgesics, but the patient is not a hyporeactor; what has changed is the baseline from which the endpoint quantum is measured. The responsiveness of a patient to certain drugs sometimes may be determined by the history of previous exposure to appropriate drugs.

Tolerance is a diminution in responsiveness as use of the drug continues. The consequence of tolerance is an increase in the dose requirement. It may be due to an increase in the rate of elimination of drug (as discussed elsewhere in this chapter), to reflex or other compensatory homeostatic adjustments, to a decrease in the number of receptors or in the number of enzyme molecules or other coupling proteins in the effector sequence, to exhaustion of the effector system or depletion of mediators, to the development of immunity, or to other mechanisms. Tolerance may be gradual, requiring many doses and days to months to develop, or acute, requiring only the first or a few doses and only minutes to hours to develop. Acute tolerance is called *tachyphylaxis*.

Drug resistance is the decrease in responsiveness of microorganisms, neoplasms, or pests to chemotherapeutic agents, antineoplastics, or pesticides, respectively. It is not tolerance in the sense that the sensitivity of the individual microorganism or cancer cell decreases; rather, it is the survival of normally unresponsive cells, which then pass the genetic factors of resistance on to their progeny.

Patients who fail to respond to a drug are called *refractory*. Refractoriness may result from tolerance or resistance, but it also may result from the progression of pathological states that negate the response or render the response incapable of surmounting an overwhelming pathology. Rarely, it may result from a poorly developed receptor or response system.

Sometimes a drug evokes an unusual response that is *qualitatively* different from the expected response. Such an unexpected response is called a *meta-reaction*. A not uncommon *meta*-reaction is a central nervous system (CNS) stimulant rather than depressant effect of phenobarbital, especially in women. Pain and certain pathological states sometimes favor *meta*-reactivity. Responses that are different in infants or the aged from those in young and middle-aged people are not *meta*-reactions if the response is usual in the age group. The term *idiosyncrasy* also denotes *meta*-reactivity, but the word has been so abused that it is recommended that it be dropped. Although hypersensitivity may cause unusual effects, it is not included in *meta*-reactivity.

DRUG RECEPTORS AND RECEPTOR THEORY

Most drugs act by combining with some key substance in the biological milieu that has an important regulatory function in the target organ or tissue. This biological partner of the drug goes by the name *receptive substance* or *drug receptor*. The receptive substance is considered mostly to be a cellular constituent, although in a few instances it may be extracellular, as the cholinesterases are, in part. The receptive substance is thought of as having a special chemical affinity and structural requirements for the drug. Drugs such as emollients, which have a physical rather than chemical basis for their action, obviously do not act upon receptors. Drugs such as demulcents and astringents, which act in a nonselective or nonspecific chemical way, also are not considered to act upon receptors, since the candidate receptors have neither sharp chemical nor biological definition. Even antacids, which react with the extremely well defined hydronium ion, cannot be said to have a receptor, since the reactive proton has no permanent biological residence.

Because of early preoccupation with physical theories of action and the classical and illogical dichotomy of chemical and physical molecular interaction, there is a reluctance to admit receptors for drugs such as general anesthetics, certain electrolytes, etc, which generally are not accepted to combine selectively with distinct cellular or organelle membrane constituents. The word receptor often is used inconsistently and intuitively. However, the term is a legitimate symbol for that biological structure with which a drug interacts to initiate a response. Ignorance of the identities of many receptors does not detract from, but rather increases, the importance of the term and general concept.

Once a receptor is identified, it frequently is no longer thought of as a receptor, although such identification may afford the basis of profound advances in receptor theory. Since the effects of anticholinesterases are derived only indirectly from inhibition of cholinesterase and no drugs are known that stimulate the enzyme, it may be argued that it is not a receptor. Nevertheless, a number of drugs ultimately act indirectly through the inhibition of such modulator enzymes, and it is important for the theoretician to develop models based upon such indirect interrelations.

Enzymes, of course, readily suggest themselves as candidates for receptors. However, there is more to cellular function than enzymes. Receptors may be membrane or intracellular constituents that govern the spatial orientation of enzymes, gene expression, compartmentalization of the cytoplasm, contractile or compliant properties of subcellular structures, or permeability and electrical properties of membranes. For nearly every cellular constituent there can be imagined a possible way for a drug to affect its function; therefore, few cellular constituents can be dismissed *a priori* as possible receptors. All the receptors for neurotransmitters and autonomic agonists are membrane proteins with agonist-binding groups projecting into the extracellular space. The transducing apparatus, whereby an occupied receptor elicits a response, is called a *coupling system*. Excitatory neurotransmitters in the CNS, and ACh receptors elsewhere, are coupled to ion channels that, when opened, permit the rapid ingress, especially of sodium ions. Each ion channel is composed of five subunits, and each subunit has four transmembrane, spanning regions. GABA (γ-aminobutyric acid) and glycine are coupled to inhibitory chloride channels. Each of these receptors is composed of pentameric proteins, each of which has two to four different types of subunits. Benzodiazepine receptors are coupled to the GABA-receptor. Beta-adrenergic receptors, histamine (H2) receptors, and a number of receptors for polypeptide hormones interact with a stimulatory GDP/GTP-binding protein (G-protein) that can activate the enzyme adenylate cyclase. The cyclase then produces 3′,5′-cyclic AMP (cAMP), which, in turn, activates protein kinases. Other receptors interact with inhibitory G-proteins. Some receptors couple to guanylate cyclase.

Alpha-adrenergic α_1, some muscarinic (M_1 and M_3), and various other receptors couple to the membrane enzyme, phospholipase-C, which cleaves inositol phosphates from phosphoinositides. The cleavage product, 1,4,5-inositol triphosphate (IP_3), then causes an increase in intracellular calcium, whereas the product, diacylglycerol (DAG), activates kinase-C. There are a number of other less ubiquitous coupling systems. Substances such as cAMP, cGMP, IP_3, and DAG are called *second messengers*.

It has been found that there may be several different receptors for a given agonist. Differences may be shown not only in the types of coupling systems and effects but also by differential binding of agonists and antagonists, desensitization kinetics, physical and chemical properties, genes and amino acid sequences. The differentiation among receptor subtypes is called *receptor classification*. Receptor subtypes are designated by Greek or Arabic alphabetical prefixes and/or numerical subscripts. There are at least two each of beta-adrenergic, histaminergic, serotoninergic, GABAergic, and benzodiazepine receptors; three each of muscarinic and alpha-adrenergic; and five of opioid receptor subtypes.

OCCUPATION AND OTHER THEORIES

Drug-receptor interactions are governed by the law of mass action. However, most chemical applications of mass law are concerned with the rate at which reagents disappear or products are formed, whereas receptor theory usually concerns itself with the fraction of the receptors combined with a drug. The usual concept is that only when the receptor actually is occupied by the drug is its function transformed in such a way as to elicit a response. This concept has become known as the *occupation theory*. The earliest clear statement of its assumptions and formulations is often credited to Clark in 1926, but both Langley and Hill made important contributions to the theory in the first two decades of the 20th century.

In all receptor theories, the terms agonist, partial agonist, and antagonist are employed. An *agonist* is a drug that combines with a receptor to initiate a response.

In the classical occupation theory, two attributes of the drug are required: (1) *affinity*, a measure of the equilibrium constant of the drug-receptor interaction, and (2) *intrinsic activity*, or *intrinsic efficacy* (not to be confused with efficacy as intensity of effect), a measure of the ability of the drug to induce a positive change in the function of the receptor.

A *partial agonist* is a drug that can elicit some but not a maximal effect and that antagonizes an agonist. In the occupation theory it would be a drug with a favorable affinity but a low intrinsic activity.

A *competitive antagonist* is a drug that occupies a significant proportion of the receptors and thereby preempts them from reacting maximally with an agonist. In the occupation theory the prerequisite property is affinity without intrinsic activity.

A *noncompetitive antagonist* may react with the receptor in such a way as not to prevent agonist-receptor combination but to prevent the combination from initiating a response, or it may act to inhibit some subsequent event in the chain of action-effect-action-effect that leads to the final overt response.

The mathematical formulation of the receptor theories derives directly from the law of mass action and chemical kinetics. Certain assumptions are required to simplify calculations. The key assumption is that the intensity of effect is a direct linear function of the proportion of receptors occupied. The correctness of this assumption is most improbable on the basis of theoretical considerations, but empirically it appears to be a close enough approximation to be useful. A second assumption

upon which formulations are based is that the drug-receptor interaction is at equilibrium. Another common assumption is that the number of molecules of receptor is negligibly small compared with that of the drug. This assumption is undoubtedly true in most instances, and departures from this situation greatly complicate the mathematical expression of drug-receptor interactions.

The first clearly stated mathematical formulation of drug-receptor kinetics was that of Clark.[1] In his equation

$$Kx^n = \frac{y}{100 - y} \qquad (2)$$

where K is the affinity constant, x is the concentration of drug, n is the molecularity of the reaction, and y is the percentage of maximum response. Clark assumed that y was a linear function of the percentage of receptors occupied by the drug, so that y could also symbolize the percentage of receptors occupied. When the equation is rearranged to solve for y

$$y = \frac{100Kx^n}{1 + Kx^n} \qquad (3)$$

A Cartesian plot of this equation is identical in form to that shown in Figure 57-2. When y is plotted against $\log x$ instead of x, the usual sigmoid curve is obtained. Thus, it may be seen that the dose-intensity curve derives from mass action equilibrium kinetics, which in turn derive from the statistical nature of molecular interaction. The fact that dose-intensity and dose-percentage curves have the same shape shows that they involve similar statistics.

If Equation 2 is put into log form

$$\log K + n \log x = \log \frac{y}{100 - y} \qquad (4)$$

a plot of $\log y/100 - y$ against $\log x$ then will yield a straight line with a slope of n; n is theoretically the number of molecules of drug that react with each molecule of receptor. At present, there are no known examples in which more than one molecule of agonist combines with a single receptor, hence, n should equal 1, universally. Nevertheless, n often deviates from 1. Deviations occur because of cooperative interactions among receptors *(cooperativity), spare receptors* (see below), amplifications in the response system *(cascades),* receptor coupling to more than one sequence (eg, to both adenylate cyclase and calcium channels), and other reasons. In these departures from $n = 1$, the slope becomes a characteristic of the mechanism of action and response system.

The probability that a molecule of drug will react with a receptor is a function of the concentration of both drug and receptor. The concentration of receptor molecules cannot be manipulated as the concentration of a drug can. But, as each molecule of drug combines with a receptor, the population of free receptors is diminished accordingly. If the drug is a competitive antagonist, it will diminish the probability of an agonist-receptor combination in direct proportion to the percentage of receptor molecules preempted by the antagonist. Consequently, the intensity of effect will be diminished. However, the probability of agonist-receptor interaction can be increased by increasing the concentration of agonist, and the intensity of effect can be restored by appropriately larger doses of agonist. Addition of more antagonist will again diminish the response, which can, again, be overcome or *surmounted* by more agonist.

Clark showed empirically and by theory that as long as the ratio of antagonist to agonist was constant, the concentration of the competitive drugs could be varied over an enormous range without changing the magnitude of the response (Fig 57-6). Since the presence of competitive antagonist only diminishes the probability of agonist-receptor combination at a given concentration of agonist and does not alter the molecularity of the reaction, it also follows that the effect of the competitive antagonist is to shift the dose-intensity curve to the right in proportion to the amount of antagonist present; neither shape nor slope of the curve is changed (Fig 57-7).

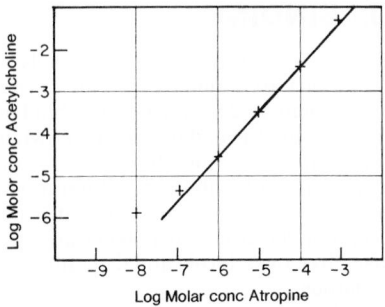

Figure 57-6. Direct proportionality of the dose of agonist (acetylcholine) to the dose of antagonist (atropine) necessary to cause a constant degree of inhibition (50%) of the response of the frog heart. (Adapted from Clark AJ. *J Physiol (London)* 1926; 61:547.)

Many refinements of the Clark formula have been made, but they will not be treated here; details and citations of relevant literature can be found in various works on receptors cited in the *Bibliography*. Several refinements are introduced to facilitate studies of competitive inhibition. The introduction of the concepts of intrinsic activity[2] and efficacy[3] required appropriate changes in mathematical treatment.

Another important concept has been added to the occupation theory, namely the concept of *spare receptors*. Clark assumed that the maximal response occurred only when the receptors were completely occupied, which does not account for the possibility that the maximum response might be limited by some step in the action-effect sequence subsequent to receptor occupation. Work with isotopically labeled agonists and antagonists and with dose-effect kinetics has shown that the maximal effect sometimes is achieved when only a small fraction of the receptors are occupied. The mathematical treatment of this phenomenon has enabled theorists to explain several puzzling observations that previously appeared to contradict occupation theory.

The classical occupation theory fails to explain several phenomena satisfactorily, and it is unable to generate a realistic model of intrinsic activity and partial agonism. A rate theory, in which the intensity of response is proportional to the rate of drug-receptor interaction instead of occupation, was proposed to explain some of the phenomena that occupation theory could not, but the rate theory was unable to provide a realistic mechanistic model of response generation, and it had other serious limitations as well.

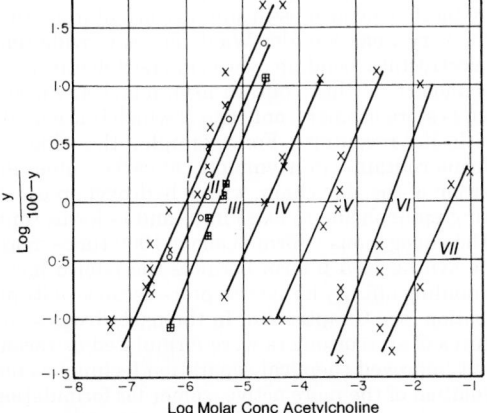

Figure 57-7. Effect of an antagonist to shift the log dose-intensity curve to the right without altering the slope. The effector is the isolated heart. *I:* no atropine; *II:* atropine, 10^{-8} M; *III:* 10^{-7} M; *IV:* 10^{-6} M; *V:* 10^{-5} M; *VI:* 10^{-4} M; *VII:* 10^{-3} M; *Y:* % of maximum intensity of response. The function log $y/(100 - y)$ converts the log dose-intensity relationship to a straight line. (Adapted from Clark AJ. *J Physiol (London)* 1926; 61:547.)

The phenomena that neither the classical occupation nor the rate theory could explain can be explained by various theories in which the receptor can exist in at least two conformational states, one of which is the active one; the drug can react with one or more conformers. In a *two-state model*[4]

$$R \rightleftharpoons R^*$$

where R is the inactive and R* is the active conformer. The agonist combines mainly with R*, the partial agonist can combine with both R and R*, and the antagonist can combine with R, the equilibrium being shifted according to the extent of occupation of R and R*. Other variations of occupation theory treat the receptor as an aggregate of subunits that interact cooperatively.[5]

MECHANISMS OF DRUG ACTION

Drugs are distributed to many or all parts of the body by the circulation. However, they do not act everywhere; they would have extremely limited usefulness if they did. Clinically useful drugs act only on certain existing biological systems. Although drugs cannot create new systems, some drugs can temporarily or permanently damage existing functional systems that are susceptible to them, thereby producing toxic effects. Almost all drugs act more or less *selectively* on large specific proteins, glycoproteins, or lipoproteins located on the cell membrane or in the cell cytoplasm, nuclei, or other intracellular organelles. These specific proteins are referred to as *receptors*. Although they often are regarded as drug receptors, they are in reality receptors for *endogenous* substances that mediate normal biological and physiological regulatory processes.

Virtually all cells of the body have multiple receptors, since they are regulated by a variety of endogenous substances that act continuously, intermittently, or only occasionally. Similarly, cells theoretically can be influenced by a variety of drugs that act on the different receptors that the cells contain. The chemical nature of many of the endogenous substances that activate receptors is known, but new ones continue to be identified and sought. For example, the former mystery of why animals have receptors for morphine, which is produced by some species of poppy plants, was solved when endogenous opioid peptides were identified in the brain and some peripheral tissues in the mid-1970s.

Drugs that selectively activate receptors and produce the same *effects* normally produced by a respective endogenous substance are called *agonists*. Drugs that selectively block receptors are called *antagonists* because they antagonize, or block, the normal effects of the respective endogenous substance. Pure antagonists do not activate their receptors. Some experimental drugs stimulate or activate certain enzymes, but none are useful therapeutic agents because their effects are too widespread. Forskolin is one such example; it directly stimulates the enzyme adenylyl cyclase to synthesize cyclic AMP, which is a second messenger in many cellular systems throughout the body.

On the other hand, many very useful therapeutic drugs are *enzyme inhibitors*, which selectively inhibit the normal activity of only one type of enzyme, thereby reducing the ability of the enzyme to act on its normal biochemical substrate. In this context, the enzymes are the drug receptors. Although the chemical nature of receptors and enzymes and their interactions with drugs was often vague in the past, the application of new techniques in molecular biology, biochemistry, and pharmacology since the mid-1980s has made unprecedented progress in defining the structures of receptors and enzymes and the consequences of drug-receptor interactions.

TYPES OF TARGETS FOR DRUG ACTION

Drug *effects* are the result of drug *actions*. Drug action may be defined as the drug-receptor interaction, whereas drug effects are the consequences of that action. For example, the interaction of epinephrine with β-receptors in the heart sets into motion a cascade of intracellular events (actions) that lead to increases in heart rate and strength of contraction (effects). The interaction of epinephrine with α-receptors in the vasculature sets into motion a cascade of intracellular events (actions) that lead to vasoconstriction and increased blood pressure (effects).

Typical responses that involve drug-receptor interactions are those that involve agonist or antagonist interactions at a receptor. Agonists also can act through various transduction mechanisms to produce a variety of intracellular changes that alter cellular activity. Transduction mechanisms are considered in more detail near the end of this section. Agonist actions may be direct, as with acetylcholine acting on the nicotinic receptors at the neuromuscular junction to briefly open sodium channels. This produces rapid depolarization of skeletal muscle, leading to muscle contraction. Drugs also can act directly on ion channels to block their activity. For example, lidocaine *(Xylocaine)* and other local anesthetics block sodium channels in nerve fibers (axons) so that the conduction of action potentials is blocked, and the area served by those nerve fibers is anesthetized. Drugs also can act directly on ion channels to modulate their activity. The benzodiazepines, characterized by diazepam *(Valium)*, produces multiple effects (sedation, hypnosis, anticonvulsant and antianxiety activity, and muscle relaxation) by *modifying* the actions of GABA on its receptors in the CNS. GABA is the predominant inhibitory neurotransmitter in the CNS, and it acts on GABA$_A$-receptor complexes by opening chloride channels on neurons to hyperpolarize them and render them less excitable. The benzodiazepines act on a different receptor on the GABA$_A$-receptor complex to enhance the actions of GABA on its receptors, thereby rendering target neurons even less excitable.

Many drugs act by inhibiting enzymes so that they cannot perform their normal functions as efficiently. One such drug, omeprazole *(Prilosec)*, reduces the ability of parietal cells in the stomach to produce hydrochloric acid by inhibiting the enzyme, or proton pump, H^+, K^+-ATPase, which is found only in these parietal cells. It is used to facilitate healing of peptic ulcers and control esophageal reflux (heartburn). The body's normal enzymes also can convert false substrates into active drugs. For example, α-methyldopa *(Aldomet)* is converted into α-methylnorepinephrine by the enzymes that normally synthesize dopamine and norepinephrine from dopa. α-Methylnorepinephrine acts on brain receptors to reduce sympathetic activity to blood vessels, thereby reducing blood pressure in hypertensive patients. Antimetabolites used to treat cancer are also false substrates, which are similar in structure to endogenous metabolites involved in cell-cycle reactions but function abnormally to interfere with synthesis of essential metabolites. Some drugs are, or have been, designed to be inactive until they are converted, usually by liver drug-metabolizing enzymes such as cytochrome P450, to active drug; the inactive drug is called a *prodrug.*

Various *carriers* are used by cells to take up neurotransmitters that have been released. The actions of dopamine released from dopamine nerve terminals in the brain are terminated by reuptake into the nerve terminals by a dopamine carrier. The dopamine then is reused for neurotransmission. If the carrier is blocked by a reuptake blocker such as cocaine, dopamine concentrations between the nerve terminals and the dopamine receptors build up for a time and produce greater effects.

Finally, antibiotics and antiviral, antifungal, and antiparasitic drugs owe their selectivities to selective actions on certain biochemical processes that are essential to the offending organism but are not shared by the mammalian host. The penicillins and related antibiotics interfere with the synthesis of rigid cell walls by growing bacteria, but mammalian cells are contained only by plasma membranes and, therefore, are not affected by penicillins. Antiparasitic drugs target enzymes found only in parasites, enzymes that are indispensable only in parasites, or biochemical functions with different pharmacological properties in the parasite and the host.

RECEPTOR BINDING

Drugs that bind to certain receptors selectively at pharmacological concentrations are known as *receptor ligands;* they can be agonists or antagonists. Many drugs also bind nonselectively to nonreceptor proteins throughout the body where they exert no pharmacological actions or effects. Many drugs bind to plasma proteins, especially albumin. Albumin-bound drug can act as a reservoir for free drug, with which it is in equilibrium, and competition among drugs for plasma protein binding can lead to increased free drug levels and drug interactions as they displace one another.

Drugs and endogenous ligands or substrates bind selectively to certain receptors because of both a chemical attraction and a proper *fit* to the protein. The lock-and-key analogy provides a useful concept of proper fit. Carried a step further, an agonist fits the lock and turns it, but an antagonist only fits the lock but cannot turn it; yet, it does block entry of the agonist key. Generally, a number of drugs with both characteristics can combine with the same receptor. The study of structure-activity relationships among similar drugs and their receptors always has been an important and fruitful approach of both pharmacology and medicinal chemistry. Highly selective drugs tend to bind to only one or several closely related receptors. However, some drugs can combine with and activate or inactivate a number of different receptors that have similar structures, thereby diminishing selectivity and magnifying side effects.

The types of chemical bonds by which drugs bind to their receptors are, in decreasing order of bond strength: covalent, ionic, hydrogen, hydrophobic, and van der Waals bonds. Relatively few drugs form covalent bonds with their receptors. Covalent bonds are *irreversible* and very long-lasting; new receptors or enzymes must be synthesized to restore function, and this process takes a week or two. Most drugs rely on combinations of the other weaker bonds to bind tightly but *reversibly* to receptors. For example, the binding of acetylcholine, a relatively simple molecule, to nicotinic receptors at the neuromuscular junction, involves ionic, hydrogen, and van der Waals bonds, with ionic and hydrogen bonds being the most important. It is no accident that receptor-binding drugs are partially ionized at body pH, because receptor proteins also are partially ionized. Drugs and proteins contain positively charged nitrogen groups and negatively charged carboxyl groups that strongly attract one another and usually provide the initial drug-receptor bonds. Hydrogen bonds, formed between bound hydrogen atoms and oxygen, nitrogen, fluoride, or sulfur atoms, further orient the drug molecule to its receptor to enhance the proper fit. One or several hydrogen bonds can be involved. Hydrophobic bonds form among nonpolar ring structures (eg, benzene) or chains of methylene groups to stabilize orientation further. Finally, the very weak van der Waals forces provide some additional, electrostatic bonding over very short distances.

Drug molecules that contain asymmetrical carbon atoms can exist as stereoisomers, only one of which is oriented to bond well with its receptors. For example, the side chain of epinephrine contains an asymmetrical carbon atom in the alpha position of the side chain, with a hydroxyl group attached, permitting epinephrine to exist in D- and L- forms (mirror images). The endogenous L-form is about 1000 times more potent than the synthesized D-form because the L-form has a much greater binding affinity for its receptors because of its preferred configuration (see Chapter 28). In the past, drugs synthesized as mixtures of stereoisomers were formulated as racemic mixtures, but improved chemical separation techniques now often allow isolation of the more active isomer for formulation.

RECEPTOR STRUCTURE AND FUNCTION

The number of receptors and their subtypes continues to grow at a rapid pace as a result of identifying new endogenous ligands and applying advancing techniques to study them. Despite this large number, most receptors can be classified structurally and functionally into only a few basic types that are described below. No attempt is made to provide detailed descriptions of individual receptors within each category. Rather, one or two examples will suffice for each, with brief reference to some prominent types that are therapeutically relevant.

VOLTAGE-SENSITIVE CHANNELS—While not generally classified as receptors, voltage-sensitive channels contain receptors that are acted upon by drugs or toxins to block or modify their normal function. The voltage-sensitive sodium channels in axons allow initiation and conduction of action potentials in response to a voltage change in the plasma membrane. When sodium channels open, sodium ions rush into the cytoplasm, thereby causing depolarization and propagation of the action potential. The crucial component of the sodium channel is a single protein composed of a chain of about 2000 amino acids and called the α subunit. Several β subunits with minor roles are also associated with the α subunit. The α subunit has four repeating domains composed of about 250 amino acids each, and each domain contains six, α-helical, 22–to 25–amino acid, transmembrane, spanning segments. Each domain forms one of four clusters of the six membrane-spanning regions to encircle the sodium channel so formed. On end, the channel resembles 24 cylinders neatly arranged around the sodium channel that, at rest, is charged positively due to positive charges on the four transmembrane helices that surround the channel. Upon activation, these particular helices are thought to rotate upward, thereby moving the positive charges away from the channel and allowing the positive sodium ions to rush through. The channel remains open for only about 1 msec because the voltage changes attract a protein loop of the channel in the cytoplasm to shut the channel like a tether ball. Local anesthetics block the sodium channel from the cytoplasmic side by binding to receptors inside the channel. Several neurotoxins block from the outside.

Axons are repolarized by brief (~1 msec) opening of voltage-activated potassium channels that are constructed similarly to sodium channels but are composed of four identical subunits of peptide that associate in the membrane to form the potassium channel. Each subunit spans the membrane six times. It probably functions much like the sodium channel, including inactivation by a tether-ball segment of cytoplasmic peptide. Quinidine, an antiarrhythmic drug, will block this potassium channel in the heart.

Voltage-activated calcium channels of the L-type are composed of five similar protein subunits that assemble across heart muscle and vascular smooth muscle membranes to form the calcium channel. Its arrangement in the membrane is similar to that of the sodium and potassium channels. Calcium channel blockers such as verapamil *(Calan)* and nifedipine *(Procardia)* are used to treat several cardiovascular conditions by virtue of their ability to block calcium channels in the heart and blood vessels.

LIGAND-ACTIVATED ION CHANNELS—The best-characterized ligand-activated ion channel is the nicotinic receptor complex at the neuromuscular junction. As the name implies, these channels are activated by receptor ligands, in this case acetylcholine. The nicotinic receptor complex is composed of five subunit proteins with similar structures that associate across the plasma membrane to form a sodium channel. The receptor complex is formed from two α and one each of β, γ, and δ subunits (Fig 57-8). In contrast to the voltage-activated ion channels, each of the five proteins crosses the membrane only four times. The two α subunits contain the nicotinic receptors, which acetylcholine activates, and both must be activated to open the sodium channel to 6.5 Å for about 4 msec. The receptors can be blocked by neuromuscular blocking agents such as curare. The nicotinic receptors on autonomic ganglia are similar in structure but are composed of a different set of subunits, which accounts for the long-known differences in selective antagonists at the two sites.

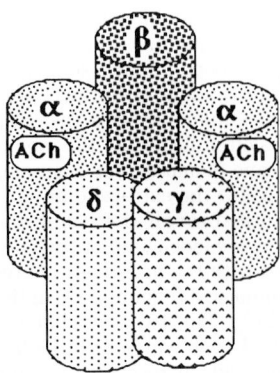

Figure 57-8. Nicotinic receptor complex.

Other ligand-activated ion channels, GABA$_A$, glycine, and glutamate, have structures that are similar to that of the nicotinic receptor complex. GABA and glycine channels are chloride channels, which permit chloride influx into neurons to produce hyperpolarization and decreased neuronal excitability. Glutamate channels are primarily sodium channels, and they also contain modifying receptors for glycine and polyamines. The GABA$_A$-receptor complex contains receptors not only for GABA but also separate receptors for benzodiazepines (eg, *Valium*), barbiturates, and steroids, which modify the actions of GABA on the chloride channel. The convulsant activity of strychnine is due solely to its ability to block glycine receptors, primarily in the brainstem and spinal cord.

G PROTEIN–COUPLED RECEPTORS—These receptors comprise a very large family of receptors that are activated by monoamines (epinephrine, norepinephrine, dopamine, and serotonin), acetylcholine (muscarinic receptors), opioids, and a host of active peptides including a number of hormones. Structurally, these receptors are single proteins, most of which are composed of chains of 350 to 550 amino acids and cross the plasma membrane seven times in a *serpentine* arrangement (Fig 57-9). Each

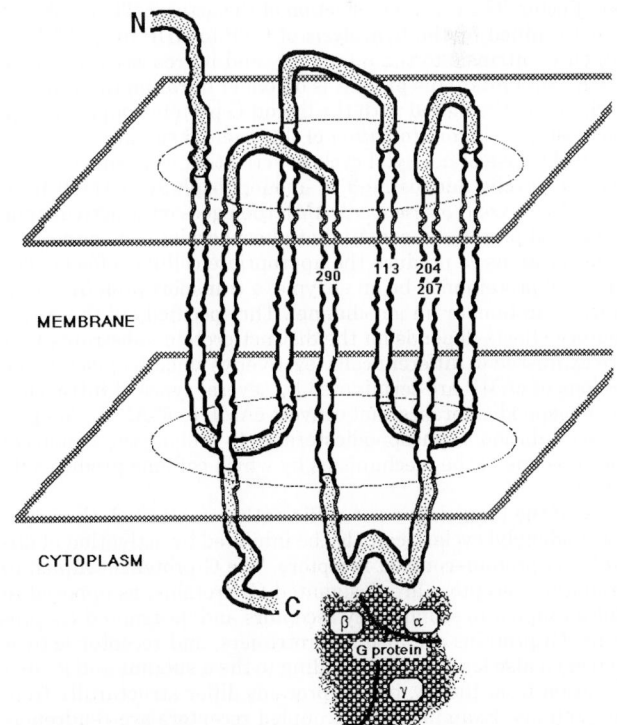

Figure 57-9. G-Protein coupled receptor complex.

of the seven transmembrane domains is composed of 22 to 30 amino acids configured into an α-helix. The third of three intracellular (cytoplasmic) loops is much longer than the other two and is responsible for coupling with the G proteins. Rather than residing at the extracellular surface of the receptor, the actual receptor-binding sites often lie *within* the membrane between the seven transmembrane domains. For example, the β-adrenergic receptor lies 11 Å below the extracellular surface, or about one-third of the distance through the membrane. The positively charged nitrogen on the side chain of the epinephrine molecule forms an ionic bond with the negatively charged carboxyl group on an aspartate amino acid (residue 113) in the third transmembrane domain (TM3). The two catechol hydroxyl groups of epinephrine form hydrogen bonds with the free hydroxyl groups of two serine amino acids at residues 204 and 207 in TM5, and the aromatic ring of epinephrine forms a hydrophobic bond with that of a phenylalanine at residue 290 in TM6. The location of G protein-coupled receptors within the membrane underscores the importance of *size and configuration* in the molecular structure of both agonists and antagonists for these receptors. Some negatively charged and peptide ligands do bind to an extracellular domain, however.

Among some families of G protein-coupled receptors there is considerable structural homology; ie, the same amino acids and the same sequences make up large portions of a number of different receptors. Consequently, a number of antagonist receptor ligands bind to these similar arrangements of amino acids in the transmembrane domains. For example, many of the antipsychotic drugs (neuroleptics) are antagonists not only at dopamine receptors, where they are thought to exert their therapeutic effects, but also at α₁-adrenergic, serotonin, histamine, and muscarinic receptors, thereby producing hypotension, sedation, blurred vision, dry mouth, and constipation as side effects.

The G proteins closely associated with the third cytoplasmic loop of the receptors are heterotrimers composed of three different subunits, α, β, and γ. Upon receptor activation, the α subunit exchanges a bound GDP for a GTP and dissociates from the βγ subunits to activate a membrane enzyme such as adenylyl cyclase or to influence an ion channel. In some cases, the βγ subunits may interact with the same or a different intracellular effector. The duration of action of the active GTP–α subunit is determined by the hydrolysis of GTP to GDP by a GTPase, which is intrinsic to the α subunit, and its reassociation with the βγ subunits. This process is of longer duration than the association of the ligand with the ligand-G protein-coupled receptor, resulting in *amplification* of the original signal.

In the case of adenylyl cyclase activation, this enzyme synthesizes cyclic adenosine-3′,5′-monophosphate (cAMP) from ATP. As a *second messenger,* cAMP then goes on to activate one or several protein kinase As that phosphorylate one or several other proteins to produce the appropriate cellular effects. The targeted protein may be an enzyme, a transport protein, a contractile protein, or an ion channel. The specificity of these regulatory effects depends on the distinct protein substrates that are expressed in different cells (eg, liver vs smooth muscle). The actions of cAMP are terminated by several types of intracellular phosphodiesterases that convert cAMP to 5'-AMP. Competitive inhibition of phosphodiesterases to prolong the actions of cAMP is one of the mechanisms by which caffeine produces its effects.

As if the foregoing is not sufficiently complicated, the activity of adenylyl cyclase can also be inhibited by activation of different G protein–coupled receptors. The G proteins coupled to inhibitory receptors are designated Gi proteins, as opposed to those coupled to stimulatory receptors and designated Gs proteins. Gi proteins are also heterotrimers, and receptor activation of Gi also leads to GTP binding to the α subunit and its dissociation from the βγ, but Gi proteins differ structurally from Gs proteins. Examples of Gs-coupled receptors are β-adrenergic, dopamine-1, histamine-2, glucagon, and ACTH. Examples of Gi-coupled receptors are α₂-adrenergic, dopamine-2, mus-

carinic, and opioid. A number of different Gs and Gi protein-coupled receptors can exist on the same cell, so that the activity of adenylyl cyclase can be fine-tuned between zero and maximum.

Another important group of G protein–coupled receptors activate the enzyme phospholipase C (PLC) to hydrolyze a minor component of the plasma membrane, phosphatidylinositol-4,5-biphosphate, into two second messengers, diacylglycerol (DAG) and inositol-1,4,5-triphosphate (IP3). In contrast to the cAMP systems, receptors coupled to PLC are only excitatory. Examples are α₁-adrenergic, muscarinic, Substance P, and thyrotropin-releasing hormone receptors. The second messenger DAG is confined to the membrane, where it activates a protein kinase C, of which nine distinct types have been identified. The other second messenger, IP3, diffuses through the cytosol to release calcium from intracellular stores. Calcium is involved in many cellular regulatory activities including activation of calcium-calmodulin, which regulates the activities of other enzymes including other kinases. The kinases in turn phosphorylate enzymes, ion channels, or other proteins to produce cellular effects. When the phosphoinositide and cAMP signaling systems coexist, they can oppose or complement one another in complex ways.

A third second-messenger system uses cyclic guanosine-3′,5′-monophosphate (cGMP) in intestinal mucosa and vascular smooth muscle. It is synthesized from GTP by activation of guanylyl cyclase and activates protein kinase G, which then dephosphorylates myosin light chains in vascular smooth muscle, thereby producing muscle relaxation. Agonists, eg, acetylcholine and histamine, cause the release of nitric oxide from vascular endothelial cells, which then diffuses into the smooth muscle cells to activate guanylyl cyclase. A direct receptor-mediated activation is produced by atrial natriuretic factor (ANF), a blood-borne peptide hormone. In this case, the receptor domain is outside the membrane and is connected through a single transmembrane domain to the intracellular guanylyl cyclase enzyme, which is activated by receptor binding.

TYROSINE KINASE–LINKED RECEPTORS—These receptors are composed of an extracellular receptor domain, a *single* transmembrane domain, and an intracellular catalytic domain that catalyzes phosphorylation of tyrosine residues on target proteins. Some receptors are composed of single proteins, whereas others are assembled from two subunits (eg, insulin receptors). Activation of insulin receptors triggers increased uptake of glucose and amino acids and regulates metabolism of glycogen and lipids in the cell. The catalytic actions persist for a number of minutes after insulin leaves the binding site. Several growth factors also exert their complex cellular effects by activating tyrosine kinase or similar receptors. Growth factors trigger changes in membrane transport and other metabolic events including regulation of DNA synthesis.

INTRACELLULAR RECEPTORS THAT CONTROL DNA TRANSCRIPTION—Activation of intracellular receptors for steroids (glucocorticoids, mineralocorticoids, sex steroids, vitamin D) and thyroid hormones stimulates the transcription of certain genes by binding to specific DNA sequences in the nucleus. The receptors generally are composed of a single protein with a ligand-binding domain, a DNA-binding domain, and a transcription-activating domain. In the inactivated state, the receptor protein is bound to another protein, a heat shock protein (hsp 90), which dissociates upon activation by a hormone, permitting DNA binding and transcription of mRNA, which then is translated into new protein. This process typically takes several hours, and the effects can last for days or weeks if there is a slow turnover of the newly synthesized proteins. A similar process accounts for the induction of drug-metabolizing enzymes in the liver by certain drugs and other chemicals. In this process, formation of a heterodimeric complex between a second protein and the ligand-bound receptor is required for DNA binding.

ENZYME INHIBITION—Enzymes are very large, complex proteins or associated proteins that evolved to catalyze specific biochemical reactions that are essential to normal cellular function. A number of very selective drugs exert their effects by inhibiting particular enzymes, so that their abilities to process their normal substrates are blocked or impaired. Enzyme inhibitors can produce competitive blockade at a substrate or cofactor binding site on the enzyme. For example, the stimulant effect of digitalis glycosides on cardiac muscle contraction is mediated by competitive inhibition of a sodium pump, Na^+,K^+-ATPase, which leads indirectly to an increase in intracellular calcium to interact with contractile proteins. Other enzyme inhibitors act noncompetitively at allosteric sites (sites remote from the substrate binding site), which prevent the enzyme from performing its catalytic function. For example, aspirin binds irreversibly to a site on cyclooxygenase that is remote from the binding site for arachidonic acid, which is normally converted to prostaglandins by the enzyme. The binding of related drugs such as ibuprofen (*Advil*) is reversible. Irreversible inhibition by the formation of covalent bonds between a drug and an enzyme is typically long lasting because new enzyme must be synthesized to restore function.

RECEPTOR REGULATION—The regulation of receptor numbers or density is normally constant, as synthesis keeps pace with degradation of the proteins. However, continuous stimulation of receptors with agonists can lead to desensitization or *down-regulation* of receptor sensitivity or number. Desensitization can occur rapidly without a change in receptor number, whereas down-regulation usually implies a decline in receptor number. For example, excess use of β-adrenergic agonists for treating bronchial asthma can lead to loss of receptor sensitivity to the agonist, caused by changes in coupling mechanisms to the G proteins. Chronic blockade of receptors can lead to *up-regulation,* which, in some cases, is due to synthesis of new receptors. An example is chronic blockade of β-adrenergic receptors in the heart, in which new β-receptors are synthesized, leading to supersensitivity upon abrupt withdrawal of the blocker. Another form of supersensitivity is demonstrated by denervation of skeletal muscle, which is followed by a proliferation of nicotinic receptors within and adjacent to the neuromuscular junction.

ABSORPTION, DISTRIBUTION, AND EXCRETION

No matter by which route a drug is administered it must pass through several to many biological membranes during the processes of absorption, distribution, biotransformation, and elimination. Since membranes are traversed in all of these events, this section begins with a brief description of biological membranes and membrane processes and the relationship of the physicochemical properties of a drug molecule to penetration and transport.

STRUCTURE AND PROPERTIES OF MEMBRANES

The concept that a membrane surrounds each cell arose shortly after the cellular nature of tissue was discovered. The biological and physicochemical properties of cells seemed in accord with this view. Microchemical, x-ray diffraction, electron microscopic, nuclear magnetic resonance, electron spin resonance, and other investigations have established the nature of the plasma, mitochondrial, nuclear, and other cell membranes. The description of the plasma membrane that follows is much oversimplified, but it will suffice to provide a background for an understanding of drug penetration into and through membranes.

STRUCTURE AND COMPOSITION—The cell membrane has been described as a bimolecular layer of lipid material entrained between two parallel monomolecular layers of protein. However, the protein does not make continuous layers, but rather is sporadically scattered over the surfaces, like icebergs; ie, much of the protein is below the surface. In Figure 57-10 the lipid layers are represented as a somewhat orderly, closely packed, lamellar array of phospholipid molecules associated tail-to-tail, each *tail* being an alkyl chain or steroid group, and the *heads* being polar groups, including the glycerate moieties, with their polar ether and carbonyl oxygens and phosphate with attached polar groups. In reality, the lamellar portion is probably not so orderly, since its composition is quite complex. Chains of fatty acids of different degrees of saturation and cholesterol cannot array themselves in simple parallel arrangements. Furthermore, the polar heads will assume a number of orientations depending upon the substances and groups involved. Moreover, the lamellar portion is penetrated by large globular proteins, the interior of which, like the lipid layers, has a high hydrophobicity, and some fibrous proteins.

The plasma membrane appears to be asymmetrical. The lipid composition varies from cell type to cell type and perhaps from site to site on the same membrane. There are, for example, differences between the membrane of the endoplasmic reticulum and the plasma membrane, even though the membranes are co-

extensive. Where membranes are double, the inner and outer layers may differ considerably; the inner and outer membranes of mitochondria have been shown to have strikingly different compositions and properties. Some authorities have expressed doubt as to the existence of the protein layers in biological membranes, although the evidence is preponderantly in favor of at least an outer glycoprotein coat. Sugar moieties also are attached to the outer proteins, most often to the asparagine residue. These sugar moieties are important to cellular and immunological recognition and adhesion and have other functions as well.

The cell membrane appears to be perforated by water-filled pores of various sizes, varying from about 4 to 10 Å, most of which are about 7 Å. Probably all major ion channels are through the large globular proteins that traverse the membrane. Through these pores pass inorganic ions and small organic molecules. Since sodium ions are more hydrated than potassium and chloride ions, they are larger and do not pass as freely through the pores as potassium and chloride. The vascular endothelium appears to have pores at least as large as 40 Å, but these seem to be interstitial passages rather than transmembrane pores. Lipid molecules small enough to pass through the pores may do so, but

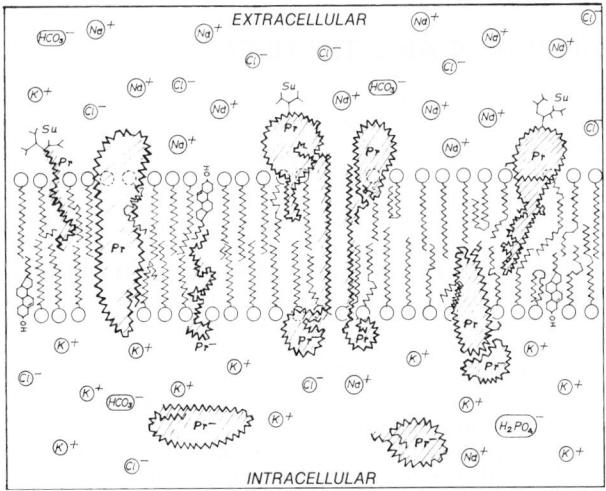

Figure 57-10. Simplified cross section of a cell membrane (components are not to scale). The lipid interior of the lamellar portion of the membrane consists of various phospholipids, fatty acids, cholesterol, and other steroids. Ions are indicated to illustrate differences in size relative to the channel. *Pr*, protein; *Su*, sugar.

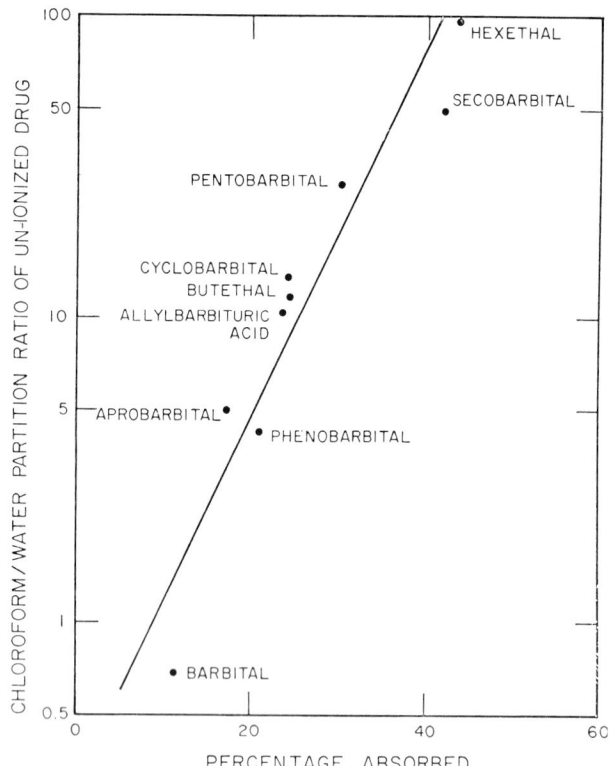

Figure 57-11. The relationship of absorption of the un-ionized forms of drugs from the colon of the rat to the chloroform:water partition coefficient. (From Schanker LS. *Adv Drug Res* 1964; 1:71.)

the pH of gastric fluid. Nevertheless, when a drug is a weak acid or base, the un-ionized form, with a favorable partition coefficient, passes through a biological membrane so much more readily than the ionized form that for all practical purposes, only the un-ionized form is said to pass through the membrane. This has become known as the *principle of nonionic diffusion.*

This principle is the reason that only the concentrations of the un-ionized form of the barbiturates are plotted in Figure 57-11.

For the purpose of further illustrating the principle, Table 57-1 is provided.[7] In the table, the permeability constants for penetration into the cerebral spinal fluid of rats are higher for un-ionized drugs than for ionized ones. The apparent excep-

tions—barbital, sulfaguanidine, and acetylaminoantipyrine—may be explained by the dipolarity of the un-ionized molecules. With barbital, the two lipophilic ethyl groups are too small to compensate for the considerable dipolarity of the un-ionized barbituric acid ring; also it may be seen that barbital is appreciably ionized, which contributes to the relatively small permeability constant. Sulfaguanidine and acetylaminoantipyrine are both very polar molecules. Mecamylamine also might be considered an exception, since it shows a modest permeability even though strongly ionized; there is no dipolarity in mecamylamine except in the amino group.

Absorption of Drugs

Absorption is the process of movement of a drug from the site of application into the extracellular compartment of the body. Inasmuch as there is a great similarity among the various membranes that a drug may pass through to gain access to the extracellular fluid, it might be expected that the particular site of application (or *route*) would make little difference to the successful absorption of the drug. In actual fact, it makes a great deal of difference; many factors, other than the structure and composition of the membrane, determine the ease with which a drug is absorbed. These factors are discussed in the following sections, along with an account of the ways that drug formulations may be manipulated to alter the ability of a drug to be absorbed readily.

ROUTES OF ADMINISTRATION

Drugs may be administered by many different routes. The various routes include oral, rectal, sublingual or buccal, parenteral, inhalation, and topical. The choice of a route depends upon both convenience and necessity.

ORAL ROUTE—This is obviously the most convenient route for access to the systemic circulation, providing that various factors do not militate against this route. Oral administration does not always give rise to sufficiently high plasma concentrations to be effective; some drugs are absorbed unpredictably or erratically; patients occasionally have an absorption malfunction. Drugs may not be given by mouth to patients with GI intolerance or who are in preparation for anesthesia or who have had GI surgery. Oral administration also is precluded in coma.

RECTAL ROUTE—Drugs that ordinarily are administered by the oral route usually can be administered by injection

Table 57-1. Rates of Entry of Drugs in CSF and the Degrees of Ionization of Drugs at pH 7.4[7]

DRUG/CHEMICAL	% BINDING TO PLASMA PROTEIN	PK$_a$[a]	% UN-IONIZED AT pH 7.4	PERMEABILITY CONSTANT (P min^{-1}) ± S.E.
Drugs mainly ionized at pH 7.4				
5-Sulfosalicylic acid	22	(strong)	0	<0.0001
N-Methylnicotinamide	<10	(strong)	0	0.0005 ± 0.00006
5-Nitrosalicylic acid	42	2.3	0.001	0.001 ± 0.0001
Salicylic acid	40	3.0	0.004	0.006 ± 0.0004
Mecamylamine	20	11.2	0.016	0.021 ± 0.0016
Quinine	76	8.4	9.09	0.078 ± 0.0061
Drugs mainly un-ionized at pH 7.4				
Barbital	<2	7.5	55.7	0.026 ± 0.0022
Thiopental	75	7.6	61.3	0.50 ± 0.051
Pentobarbital	40	8.1	83.4	0.17 ± 0.014
Aminopyrine	20	5.0	99.6	0.25 ± 0.020
Aniline	15	4.6	99.8	0.40 ± 0.042
Sulfaguanidine	6	>10.0[b]	>99.8	0.003 ± 0.0002
Antipyrine	8	1.4	>99.9	0.12 ± 0.013
N-Acetyl-4-aminoantipyrine	<3	0.5	>99.9	0.012 ± 0.0010

[a] The dissociation constant of both acids and bases is expressed as the pK$_a$, the negative logarithm of the acidic dissociation constant.
[b] Sulfaguanidine has a very weakly acidic group (pK$_a$ > 10) and two very weakly basic groups (pK$_a$ 2.75 and 0.5). Consequently, the compound is almost completely undissociated at pH 7.4.

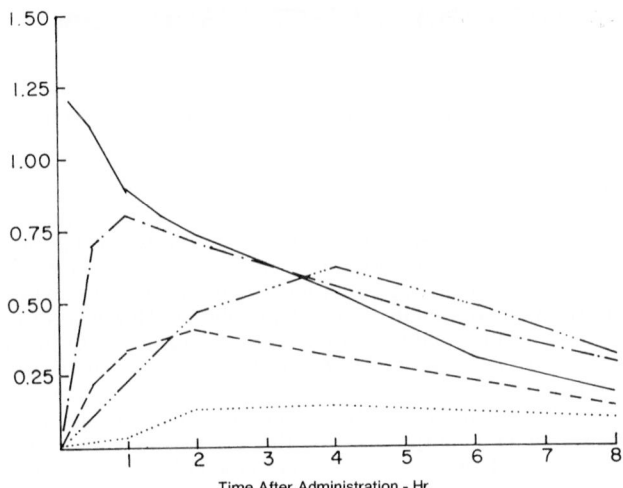

Figure 57-12. Blood concentration in mg/100 mL of theophylline (ordinate) following administration to humans of aminophylline in the amounts and by the routes indicated. Doses: per 70 kg. Theophylline-ethylenediamine by various routes:———intravenous, 0.5 g;—·—·—retention enema, 0.5 g;—•••—•••—oral tablets-Pl, 0.5 g; - - - oral tablets-Pl, 0.3 g; •••• rectal suppository, 0.5 g. (Adapted Truitt EB, et al. *J Pharmacol Exp Ther* 1950; 100:309.)

or by the alternative *lower enteral* route, through the anal portal into the rectum or lower intestine. With regard to the latter, *rectal suppositories* or *retention enemas* formerly were used quite frequently, but their popularity has abated somewhat, owing to improvements in parenteral preparations. Nevertheless, they continue to be valid and, sometimes, very important ways of administering a drug, especially in pediatrics and geriatrics. In Figure 57-12[8] the availability of a drug by retention enema may be compared with that by the intravenous and oral routes and rectal suppository administration. It is apparent that the retention enema may be a very satisfactory means of administration but that rectal suppositories may be inadequate when rapid absorption and high plasma levels are required. The illustration is not intended to lead the reader to the conclusion that a retention enema always will give more prompt and higher blood levels than the oral route, for converse findings for the same drug have been reported,[9] but rather to show that the retention enema may offer a useful substitute for the oral route.

SUBLINGUAL OR BUCCAL ROUTE—Even though an adequate plasma concentration eventually may be achievable by the oral route, it may rise much too slowly for use in some situations when a rapid response is desired. In such situations parenteral therapy usually is indicated. However, the patients with angina pectoris may get quite prompt relief from an acute attack by the *sublingual* or *buccal* administration of nitroglycerin, so that parenteral administration may be avoided. When only small amounts of drugs are required to gain access to the blood, the buccal route may be very satisfactory, providing the physicochemical prerequisites for absorption by this route are present in the drug and dosage form. Only a few drugs may be given successfully by this route.

PARENTERAL ROUTES—These routes, by definition, include any route other than the oral-GI (enteral) tract, but in common medical usage the term excludes topical administration and includes only various hypodermic routes. Parenteral administration includes the intravenous, intramuscular, and subcutaneous routes. Parenteral routes may be employed whenever enteral routes are contraindicated (see above) or inadequate.

The *intravenous* route may be preferred on occasion, even when a drug may be well absorbed by the oral route. There is no delay imposed by absorption before the administered drug reaches the circulation, and blood levels rise virtually as rapidly as the time necessary to empty the syringe or infusion bottle. Consequently, the intravenous route is the preferred route when an emergency calls for an immediate response.

In addition to the rapid rise in plasma concentration of drug, another advantage of intravenous administration is the greater predictability of the peak plasma concentration, which, with some drugs, can be calculated with a fair degree of precision. Smaller doses generally are required by the intravenous than by other routes, but this usually affords no advantage, inasmuch as the sterile injectable dosage form costs more than enteric preparations, and the requirements for medical or paramedical supervision of administration also may add to the cost and inconvenience.

Because of the rapidity with which drug enters the circulation, dangerous side effects to the drug may occur, which are often not extant by other routes. The principal untoward effect is a depression of cardiovascular function, which is often called *drug shock.* Consequently, some drugs must be given quite slowly to avoid vasculotoxic concentrations of drug in the plasma. Acute, serious, allergic responses also are more likely to occur by the intravenous route than by other routes.

Many drugs are too irritant to be given by the oral, intramuscular, or subcutaneous route and must, of necessity, be given intravenously. However, such drugs also may cause damage to the veins (phlebitis) or, if extravasated, cause necrosis (slough) around the injection site. Consequently, such irritant drugs may be diluted in isotonic solutions of saline, dextrose, or other media and given by slow infusion, providing that the slower rate of delivery does not negate the purpose of the administration in emergency situations.

Absorption by the *intramuscular route* is relatively fast, and this parenteral route may be used when an immediate effect is not required but a prompt effect is desirable. Intramuscular deposition also may be made of certain repository preparations, rapid absorption not being desired. Absorption from an intramuscular depot is more predictable and uniform than from a subcutaneous site.

Irritation around the injection site is a frequent accompaniment of intramuscular injection, depending upon the drug and other ingredients. Because of the dangers of accidental intravenous injection, medical supervision generally is required. Sterilization is necessary.

In *subcutaneous* administration the drug is injected into the connective tissue just below the skin. Absorption is slower than by the intramuscular route but, nevertheless, may be prompt with many drugs. Often, however, absorption by this route may be no faster than by the oral route. Therefore, when a fairly prompt response is desired with some drugs, the subcutaneous route may not offer much advantage over the oral route, unless for some reason the drug cannot be given orally.

The slower rate of absorption by the subcutaneous route is usually the reason why the route is chosen, and the drugs given by this route are usually those in which it is desired to spread the action out over a number of hours, to avoid either too intense a response, too short a response, or frequent injections. Examples of drugs given by this route are insulin and sodium heparin, neither of which is absorbed orally, and both of which should be absorbed slowly over many hours. In the treatment of asthma, epinephrine usually is given subcutaneously to avoid the dangers of rapid absorption and consequent dangerous cardiovascular effects. Many repository preparations, including tablets or pellets, are given subcutaneously. As with other parenteral routes, irritation may occur. Sterile preparations also are required. However, medical supervision is not required always and self-administration by this route is customary with certain drugs, such as insulin.

Intradermal injection, in which the drug is injected into, rather than below, the dermis, is rarely employed, except in certain diagnostic and test procedures, such as screening for allergic or local irritant responses.

Occasionally, even by the intravenous route, it is not possible, practical, or safe to achieve plasma concentrations high enough so that an adequate amount of drug penetrates into special compartments, such as the cerebrospinal fluid, or various cavities, such as the pleural cavity. The brain is especially difficult to penetrate with water-soluble drugs. The name *blood-brain barrier* is applied to the impediment to penetration. When drugs do penetrate, the choroid plexus often secretes them back into the blood very rapidly, so that adequate levels of drugs in the cerebrospinal fluid may be difficult to achieve. Consequently, *intrathecal* or *intraventricular* administration may be indicated.

Body cavities such as the pleural cavity normally are wetted by a small amount of effusate that is in diffusion equilibrium with the blood and, hence, is accessible to drugs. However, infections and inflammations may cause the cavity to fill with serofibrinous exudate that is too large to be in rapid diffusion equilibrium with the blood. *Intracavitary* administration, thus, may be required. It is extremely important that sterile, nonirritating preparations be used for intrathecal or intracavitary administration.

INHALATION ROUTE—Inhalation may be employed for delivering gaseous or volatile substances into the systemic circulation, as with most general anesthetics. Absorption is virtually as rapid as the drug can be delivered into the alveoli of the lungs, since the alveolar and vascular epithelial membranes are quite permeable, blood flow is abundant, and there is a very large surface for absorption.

Aerosols of nonvolatile substances also may be administered by inhalation, but the route is used infrequently for delivery into the systemic circulation because of various factors that contribute to erratic or difficult-to-achieve blood levels. Whether or not an aerosol reaches and is retained in pulmonary alveoli depends critically upon particle size. Particles larger than 1 μm in diameter tend to settle in the bronchioles and bronchi, whereas particles smaller than 0.5 μm fail to settle and mainly are exhaled. Aerosols are employed mostly when the purpose of administration is an action of the drug upon the respiratory tract itself. An example of a drug commonly given as an aerosol is isoproterenol, which is employed to relax the bronchioles during an asthma attack.

TOPICAL ROUTE—Topical administration is employed to deliver a drug at, or immediately beneath, the point of application. Although occasionally enough drug is absorbed into the systemic circulation to cause systemic effects, absorption is too erratic for the topical route to be used routinely for systemic therapy. However, various transdermal preparations of nitroglycerin and clonidine are employed quite successfully for systemic use. Some investigations with aprotic solvent vehicles such as dimethyl sulfoxide (DMSO) also have generated interest in topical administration for systemic effects. A large number of topical medicaments are applied to the skin, although topical drugs are also applied to the eye, nose, throat, ear, vagina, etc.

In man, percutaneous absorption probably occurs mainly from the surface. Absorption through the hair follicles occurs, but the follicles in man occupy too small a portion of the total integument to be of primary importance. Absorption through sweat and sebaceous glands generally appears to be minor. When the medicament is rubbed on vigorously, the amount of the preparation that is forced into the hair follicles and glands is increased. Rubbing also forces some material through the stratum corneum without molecular dispersion and diffusion through the barrier. Rather large particles of substances such as sulfur have been demonstrated to pass intact through the stratum corneum. When the skin is diseased or abraded, the cutaneous barrier may be disrupted or defective, so that percutaneous absorption may be increased. Since much of a drug that is absorbed through the epidermis diffuses into the circulation without reaching a high concentration in some portions of the dermis, systemic administration may be preferred in lieu of, or in addition to, topical administration.

FACTORS THAT AFFECT ABSORPTION

In addition to the physicochemical properties of drug molecules and biological membranes, various factors affect the rate of absorption and determine, in part, the choice of route of administration.

CONCENTRATION—It is self-evident that the concentration, or, more exactly, the thermodynamic activity, of a drug in a drug preparation will have an important bearing upon the rate of absorption, since the rate of diffusion of a drug away from the site of administration is directly proportional to the concentration. Thus, a 2% solution of lidocaine will induce local anesthesia more rapidly than a 0.2% solution. However, drugs administered in solid form are not absorbed necessarily at the maximal rate (see *Physical State of Formulation and Dissolution Rate,* below).

After oral administration the concentration of drugs in the gut is a function of the dose, but the relationship is not necessarily linear. Drugs with a low aqueous solubility (eg, digitoxin) quickly saturate the GI fluids, so that the rate of absorption tends to reach a limit as the dose is increased. The peptizing and solubilizing effects of bile and other constituents of the GI contents assist in increasing the rate of absorption but are in themselves somewhat erratic. Furthermore, many drugs affect the rates of gastric, biliary, and small intestinal secretion, which causes further deviations from a linear relationship between concentration and dose.

Drugs that are administered subcutaneously or intramuscularly also may not always show a direct linear relationship between the rate of absorption and the concentration of drug in the applied solution, because osmotic effects may cause dilution or concentration of the drug, if the movement of water or electrolytes is different from that of the drug. Whenever possible, drugs for hypodermic injection are prepared as isotonic solutions. Some drugs affect the local blood flow and capillary permeability, so that at the site of injection there may be a complex relationship of concentration achieved to the concentration administered.

PHYSICAL STATE OF FORMULATION AND DISSOLUTION RATE—The rate of absorption of a drug may be affected greatly by the rate at which the drug is made available to the biological fluid at the site of administration. The intrinsic physicochemical properties, such as solubility and the thermodynamics of dissolution, are only some of the factors that affect the rate of dissolution of a drug from a solid form. Other factors include not only the unavoidable interactions among the various ingredients in a given formulation but also deliberate interventions to facilitate dispersion (eg, comminution, Chapter 38 and dissolution, Chapter 35) or retard it (eg, coatings, Chapter 46 and slow-release formulations, Chapter 47). There also are factors that affect the rate of delivery from liquid forms. For example, a drug in a highly viscous vehicle is absorbed more slowly from the vehicle than a drug in a vehicle of low viscosity; in oil-in-water emulsions the rate depends upon the partition coefficient. These manipulations are the subject of biopharmaceutics (see Chapter 47).

AREA OF ABSORBING SURFACE—The area of absorbing surface is an important determinant of the rate of absorption. To the extent that the therapist must work with the absorbing surfaces available in the body, the absorbing surface is not subject to manipulation. However, the extent to which the existing surfaces may be used is subject to variation. In those rare instances in which percutaneous absorption is intended for systemic administration, the entire skin surface is available.

Subsequent to subcutaneous or intramuscular injections, the site of application may be massaged to spread the injected fluid from a compact mass to a well-dispersed deposit. Alternatively, the dose may be divided into multiple small injections, although this recourse is generally undesirable.

The different areas for absorption afforded by the various routes account, in part, for differences in the rates of absorption by those routes. The large alveolar surface of the lungs allows extremely rapid absorption of gases, vapors, and properly aerosolized solutions; with some drugs the rate of absorption may be nearly as fast as with intravenous injection. In the gut the small intestine is the site of the fastest, and hence most, absorption because of the small lumen and highly developed villi and microvilli; the stomach has a relatively small surface area, so that even most weak acids are absorbed predominately in the small intestine despite a pH partition factor that should favor absorption from the stomach (see *The pH Partition Principle*).

VASCULARITY AND BLOOD FLOW—Although the thermal velocity of a freely diffusible, average drug molecule is on the order of meters per second, in solution the rate at which it will diffuse away from a reference point will be much slower. Collisions with water and/or other molecules that cause a random motion, and the forces of attraction between the drug and water or other molecules, slow the net mean velocity.

The time taken to traverse a given distance is a function of the square of the distance; on average it would take about 0.01 sec for a net outward movement of 1 μm, 1 sec for 10 μm, 100 sec for 100 μm, etc. In a highly vascular tissue, such as skeletal muscle, in which there may be more than 1000 capillaries/mm^2 of cross-section, a drug molecule would not have to travel more than a few microns, hence less than a second on average, to reach a capillary from a point of extravascular injection.

Once the drug reaches the blood, diffusion is not important to transport and the rate of blood flow determines the movement. The velocity of blood flow in a capillary is about 1 mm/sec, which is 100 times faster than the mean net velocity of drug molecules 1 mm away from their injection site. The velocity of blood flow is even faster in the larger vessels. Overall, less than a minute is required to distribute drug molecules from the capillaries at the injection site to the rest of the body.

From the above discussion it follows that absorption is most rapid in the vascular tissues. Drugs are absorbed more rapidly from intramuscular sites than from less vascular subcutaneous sites, etc. Despite the small absorbing surface for buccal or sublingual absorption, the high vascularity of the buccal, gingival, and sublingual surfaces favors an unexpectedly high rate of absorption. Because of hyperemia, absorption will be faster from inflamed than from normal areas, unless the presence of edema lengthens the mean distance between capillaries and, thus, negates the effects of hyperemia on absorption.

Vasoconstriction may have a profound effect upon the rate of absorption. When a local effect of a drug is desired, as in local anesthesia, absorption away from the infiltered site may be impeded greatly by vasoconstrictors included in the preparation. Unwanted vasoconstriction sometimes may cause serious problems. For example, on World War II battlegrounds many wounded soldiers were given subcutaneous morphine without evident effect. As a result, injections were sometimes repeated more than once. When the patient was removed to the field hospital, toxic effects would occur suddenly. The explanation is that cold-induced vasoconstriction occurred in the field; when the patient was warmed in the hospital, vasodilation would result and the victim would be flooded with drug. Shock also contributes to the effect, since during shock the blood flow is diminished, and there also may be a superimposed vasoconstriction; repair of the shock condition then facilitates absorption.

Extravascularly injected molecules too large to pass through the capillary endothelium will, of necessity, enter the systemic circulation through the lymph. Thus, the lymph flow may be important to the absorption of a few drugs.

MOVEMENT—A number of factors combine so that movement at the site of injection increases the rate of absorption. In the intestine, segmental movements and peristalsis aid in dividing and dispersing the drug mass. The continual mixing of the chyme helps keep the concentration maximal at the mucosal surface. The pressures developed during segmentation and peristalsis also may favor a small amount of filtration. Movement at the site of hypodermic injection also favors absorption, since it tends to force the injected material through the tissue, increasing the surface area of drug mass and decreasing the mean distance to the capillaries. Movement also increases the flow of blood and lymph. The selection of a site for intramuscular injection may be determined by the amount of expected movement, according to whether the preparation is intended as a fast-acting or a repository preparation.

GASTRIC MOTILITY AND EMPTYING—The motility of the stomach is more important to the rate at which an orally administered drug is passed on to the small intestine than it is to the rate of absorption from the stomach itself, since for various reasons noted above, absorption from the stomach is usually of minor importance.

The average emptying time of the unloaded stomach is about 40 min, and the half-time is about 10 min, though it varies according to its contents, reflex, and psychological factors, and the action of certain autonomic drugs or disease. The effect of food to delay absorption is due, in part, to its action to prolong emptying time. The emptying time causes a delay in the absorption of drug, which may be unfavorable or favorable according to what is desired. In the case of therapy with antacids, gastric emptying is a nuisance, since it removes the antacid from the stomach where it is needed.

SOLUBILITY AND BINDING—The dissolution of drugs of low solubility is generally a slow process. Indeed, low solubility is the result of a low rate of departure of drug molecules from the undispersed phase. Furthermore, since the concentration around the drug mass is low, the concentration gradient from the site of deposition to the plasma is small, and the rate of diffusion is low, accordingly.

When it is desired that a drug have a prolonged action but not a high plasma concentration, a derivative of low solubility is often sought. The *insoluble* estolates and other esters of several steroids have durations of action of weeks because of the slow rates of absorption from the sites of injection. Insoluble salts or complexes of acidic or basic drugs also are employed as repository preparations; for example, the procaine salt of penicillin G has a low solubility and is used in a slow-release form of the antibiotic.

The solubility of certain macromolecules depends critically on the ionization of substituent groups. When they are amphiprotic, they are least soluble at their isoelectric pH. Insulin is normally soluble at the pH of the extracellular fluid, but by combining insulin with the right proportion of a basic protein, such as protamine, the isoelectric pH can be made to be approximately 7.4 from 5.1, and the complex can be used as a low-solubility, prolonged-action drug. For more details, see Chapter 77.

Some drugs may bind with natural substances at or near the site of application. The strongly ionized mucopolysaccharides in connective tissue, ground substance, and mucous secretions of the gut retard the absorption of a number of drugs, especially large cationic or polycationic molecules. In the gut, the binding is the least at low pH, which should favor absorption of large cations from the stomach; however, absorption from the stomach is slow (see above), so that the absorption of large cations occurs mainly in the upper duodenum where the pH is still relatively low. Pharmacologically inactive quaternary ammonium compounds sometimes are included in an oral preparation of a quaternary ammonium drug for the purpose of saturating the binding sites of mucin and other mucopolysaccharides and, thereby, enhancing the absorption of drug.

In addition to mucopolysaccharides in mucous secretions, food in the GI tract binds many drugs and slows absorption. Antacids, especially aluminum hydroxide plus other basic aluminum compounds and magnesium trisilicate, bind amine and ammonium drugs and interfere with absorption.

DONNAN EFFECT—The presence of a charged macromolecule on one side of a semipermeable membrane (impermeable to the macromolecule) will alter the concentration of permeant ionized particles according to the Donnan equilibrium. Accordingly, drug molecules of the same charge as the macromolecule will be constrained to the opposite side of the membrane. The presence of appropriately charged macromolecules not only will influence the distribution of drug ions in accordance with the Donnan equation but also increase the rate of transfer of the drug across the membrane, because of mutual ionic repulsion. This effect is sometimes used to facilitate the absorption of ionizable drugs from the GI tract. The Donnan effect also operates to retard the absorption of drug ions of opposite charge; however, the mutual electrostatic attraction of a macromolecule and drug ion generally results in actual binding, which is more important than the Donnan effect.

VEHICLES AND ABSORPTION ADJUVANTS—Drugs that are to be applied topically to the skin and mucous membranes often are dissolved in vehicles that are thought to enhance penetration. For a long time it was thought that oleaginous vehicles promoted the absorption of lipid-soluble drugs. However, the role and effect of the vehicle has proven to be quite complex. In the skin at least five factors are involved:

1. The effect of the vehicle to alter the hydration of the keratin in the barrier layer.
2. The effect of the vehicle to promote or prevent the collection of sweat at the surface of the skin.
3. The partition coefficient of the drug in a vehicle-water system.
4. The permeability of the skin to the undissolved drug.
5. The permeability of the skin to the vehicle.

The effect of the vehicle to aid in the access of the drug to the hair follicles and sebaceous glands also may be involved, although in man the follicles and glands are probably ordinarily of minor importance to absorption.

A layer of oleaginous material over the skin prevents the evaporation of water, so that the stratum corneum may become macerated and more permeable to drugs. In dermatology it is sometimes the practice to wrap the site of application with plastic wrap or some other waterproof material for the purpose of increasing the maceration of the stratum corneum. However, the layer of perspiration that forms under an occlusive vehicle may become a barrier to the movement of lipid-soluble drugs from the vehicle to the skin, but it may facilitate the movement of water-soluble drugs. Conversely, polyethylene glycol vehicles remove the perspiration and dehydrate the barrier, which decreases the permeability to drugs; such vehicles remove the aqueous medium through which water-soluble drugs may pass down into the stratum corneum but at the same time facilitate the transfer of lipid-soluble drugs from the vehicle to the skin.

Even in the absence of a vehicle, it is not clear what physicochemical properties of a drug favor cutaneous penetration, high lipid-solubility being a prerequisite, according to some authorities, and an ether-water partition coefficient of approximately one, according to others. Yet, the penetration of ethanol and dibromomethane are nearly equal, and other such enigmas exist. It is not surprising, then, that the effects of vehicles are not altogether predictable.

A general statement might be made that if a drug is quite soluble in a poorly absorbed vehicle, the vehicle will retard the movement of the drug into the skin. For example, salicylic acid is 100 times as permeant when absorbed from water than from polyethylene glycol, and pentanol is five times as permeant from water as from olive oil. Yet, ethanol penetrates five times faster from olive oil than from either water or ethanol, all of which denies the trustworthiness of generalizations about vehicles.

For several decades there has been much interest in certain highly dielectric, aprotic solvents, especially dimethyl sulfoxide (DMSO). Such substances generally prove to be excellent solvents for both water- and lipid-soluble compounds and for some compounds not soluble in either water or lipid solvents. The extraordinary solvent properties probably are due to a high polarizability and van der Waals bonding capacity, a high degree of polarization (dipole moment), and a lack of association through hydrogen bonding. As a vehicle, DMSO greatly facilitates the permeation of the skin and other biological membranes by numerous drugs, including such large molecules as insulin. The mechanism is understood poorly. Such vehicles have a potential for many important uses, but they are at present only experimental, pending continuing investigations on toxicity.

From time to time, a claim is made that a new ingredient of a tablet or elixir enhances the absorption of a drug, and a comparison of plasma levels of the old and new preparations seems to support the claim. Upon further investigation, however, it may be revealed that the new so-called absorption adjuvant is replacing an ingredient that previously bound the drug or delayed its absorption; thus, the new *adjuvant* is not an adjuvant but rather it is only a nondeterrent.

OTHER FACTORS—A number of other, less well-defined factors affect the absorption of drugs, some of which may operate, in part, through factors already cited above. Disease or injury has a considerable effect upon absorption. For example, debridement of the stratum corneum increases the permeability to topical agents, meningitis increases the permeability of the blood-brain barrier, biliary insufficiency decreases the absorption of lipid-soluble substances from the intestine, and acid-base disturbances can affect the absorption of weak acids or bases. Certain drugs, such as ouabain, that affect active transport processes may interfere with the absorption of certain other drugs. The condition of the *ground substance,* or *intracellular cement,* probably bears on the absorption of certain types of molecules. Hyaluronidase, which depolymerizes the mucopolysaccharide ground substance, can be demonstrated to facilitate the absorption of some, but not all, drugs from subcutaneous sites.

Drug Disposition

The term *drug disposition* is used here to include all processes that tend to lower the plasma concentration of drug, as opposed to drug absorption, which elevates the plasma level. Consequently, the distribution of drugs to the various tissues is considered under *Disposition*. Some authors use the term disposition synonymously with elimination, that is, to include only those processes that decrease the amount of drug in the body. In the present context, disposition comprises three categories of processes: distribution, biotransformation, and excretion.

DISTRIBUTION, BIOTRANSFORMATION, AND EXCRETION

The term *distribution* denotes the partitioning of a drug among the numerous locations where a drug may be contained within the body. *Biotransformations* are the alterations in the chemical structure of a drug that are imposed upon it by the life processes. *Excretion* is, in a sense, the converse of absorption, namely, the transportation of the drug or its products out of the body. The term applies whether or not special organs of excretion are involved.

Distribution

The body may be considered to comprise a number of *compartments:* enteric (GI), plasma, interstitial, cerebrospinal fluid, bile, glandular secretions, urine, storage vesicles, cytoplasm or intracellular space, etc. Some of these *compartments,* such as urine and secretions, are open-ended, but since their contents relate to those in the closed compartments, they also must be included.

At first thought, it may seem that if a drug was distributed passively (ie, by simple diffusion) and the plasma concentration could be maintained at a steady level, the concentration of a drug in the water in all compartments ought to become equal. It is true that some substances, such as ethanol and antipyrine, are distributed nearly equally throughout the body water, but they are more the exception than the rule. Such substances are mainly small, uncharged, nondissociable, highly water-soluble molecules.

The condition of small size and high water solubility allows passage through the pores without the necessity of carrier or active transport. Small size also places a limit on van der Waals binding energy and configurational complementariness, so that binding to proteins in plasma, or cells, is slight. The presence of a charge on a drug molecule makes for unequal distribution across charged membranes, in accordance with the Donnan distribution (see below). Dissociability causes unequal distribution when there is a pH differential between compartments, as discussed under *The pH Partition Principle* (see below). Thus, even if a drug is distributed passively, its distribution may be uneven throughout the body. When active transport into, or rapid biotransformation occurs within, some compartments, uneven distribution also is inevitable.

THE pH PARTITION PRINCIPLE—An important consequence of nonionic diffusion is that a difference in pH between two compartments will have an important influence upon the partitioning of a weakly acidic or basic drug between those compartments. The partition is such that the un-ionized form of the drug has the same concentration in both compartments, since it is the form that is freely diffusible; the ionized form in each compartment will have the concentration that is determined by the pH in that compartment, the pK and the concentration of the un-ionized form. The governing effect of pH and pK on the partition is known as the *pH partition principle*.

To illustrate the principle, consider the partition of salicylic acid between the gastric juice and the interior of a gastric mucosal cell. Assume the pH of the gastric juice to be 1, which it occasionally becomes. The pK_a of salicylic acid is 3 (Martin[10] provides one source of pK values of drugs). With the Henderson-Hasselbalch equation (see Chapter 17) it may be calculated that the drug is only 1% ionized at pH 1. (The relationship of ionization and partition to pH and pK has been formulated in several different ways, but the student may calculate the concentrations from simple mass law equations. More sophisticated calculations and reviews of this subject are available.[6,11–16]) The intracellular pH of most cells is about 7. Assuming the pH of the mucosal cell to be the same, it may be calculated that salicylic acid will be 99.99% ionized within the cells. Since the concentration of the un-ionized form is theoretically the same in both gastric juice and mucosal cells, it follows that the total concentration of the drug (ionized + un-ionized) within the mucosal cell will be 10,000 times greater than that in gastric juice. This is illustrated in Figure 57-13. Such a relatively high intracellular concentration can have important osmotic and toxicological consequences.

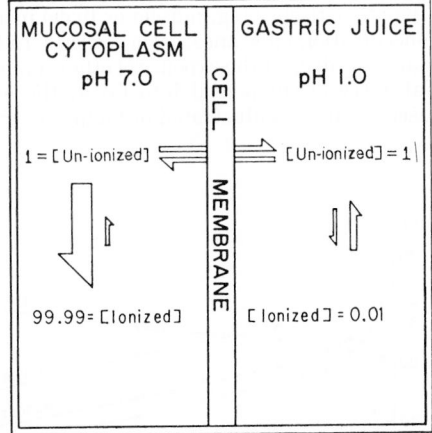

Figure 57-13. Hypothetical partition of salicylic acid between gastric juice and the cytoplasm of a gastric mucosal cell. It is assumed that the ionized form cannot pass through the cell membrane. The intragastric concentration of salicylic acid is arranged arbitrarily to provide unit concentration of the un-ionized form. *Bracketed values,* concentration; *arrows,* relative size depicts the direction in which dissociation-association is favored at equilibrium.

Had the drug been a weak base instead of an acid, the high concentration would have been in the gastric juice. In the small intestine, where the pH may range from 7.5 to 8.1, the partition of a weak acid or base will be the reverse of that in the stomach, but the concentration differential will be lower, because the pH differential from lumen to mucosal cells, etc, will be lower. The reversal of partition as the drug moves from the stomach to the small intestine accounts for the phenomenon that some drugs may be absorbed from one GI segment and returned to another. The weak base atropine is absorbed from the small intestine, but because of pH partition, it is *secreted* into the gastric juice.

The pH partition of drugs has never been demonstrated to be as marked as that illustrated in Figure 57-13 and in the text. Not only do many drug ions probably pass through the pores of the membrane to a significant extent, but also some may pass through the lipid phase, as explained above for the morphinans and mecamylamine. Furthermore, ion-pair formation in carrier transport also bypasses nonionic diffusion. All processes that tend toward an equal distribution of drugs across membranes and among compartments will cause further deviations from theoretical predictions of pH partition.

ELECTROCHEMICAL AND DONNAN DISTRIBUTION—A drug ion may be distributed passively across a membrane in accordance with the membrane potential, the charge on the drug ion, and the Donnan effect. The relationship of the membrane potential to the passive distribution of ions is expressed quantitatively by the Nernst equation (Eq 7) and already has been discussed. Barring active transport, pH partition, and binding, the drug will be said to be distributed according to the electrical gradient or to its *equilibrium* potential. If the membrane potential is 90 mV, the concentration of a univalent cation will be 30 times as high within the cell as without; if the drug cation is divalent, the ratio will be 890. The distribution of anions would be just the reverse. If the membrane potential is but 9 mV, the ratio for a univalent cation will be only 1.4 and for a divalent cation only 2.0. It thus can be seen how important membrane potential may be to the distribution of ionized drugs.

It was pointed out under *Membrane Potentials,* that large potentials derive from active transport of ions but that small potentials may result from Donnan distribution. Donnan membrane theory is discussed in Chapter 20. According to the theory, the ratio of intracellular/extracellular concentration of a permeant univalent anion is equal to the ratio of extracellular/intracellular concentration of a permeant univalent cation. A more general mathematical expression that includes ions of any valence is

$$\left(\frac{A_i}{A_e}\right)^{1/Z_a} = \left(\frac{C_e}{C_i}\right)^{1/Z_c} = r \tag{8}$$

where A_i is the intracellular and A_e the extracellular concentration of anion, Z_c is the valence of cation, Z_a is the valence of anion, C_i is the intracellular and C_e the extracellular concentration of cation, and r is the Donnan factor. The value of r depends upon the average molecular weight and valence of the macromolecules (mostly protein) within the cell and the intracellular and extracellular volumes. Since the macromolecules within the cell are charged negatively, the cation concentration will be higher within the cell; that is, $C_i > C_e$. Since a Donnan distribution results in a membrane potential, the distribution of drug ion also will be in keeping with the membrane potential.

The Donnan distribution also applies to the distribution of a charged drug between the plasma and interstitial compartment, because of the presence of anionic proteins in the plasma. Equation 8 applies by changing the subscript i to p, for plasma, and e to i, for interstitial. The Donnan factor, r, for plasma–interstitial space partition is about 1.05:1.

BINDING AND STORAGE—Drugs frequently are bound to plasma proteins (especially albumin), interstitial substances, intracellular constituents, and bone and cartilage. If binding is

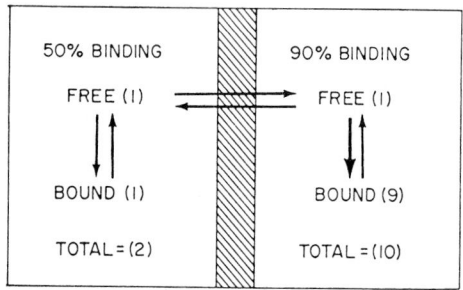

Figure 57-14. Distribution of a drug between two compartments in which the degrees of binding to protein differ. The percentage of binding is indicated. Only the unbound drug can pass through the membrane. *Bracketed values:* concentration. (From Schanker LS. *Pharmacol Rev* 1961; 14:501.)

extensive and firm, it will have a considerable impact upon the distribution, excretion, and sojourn of the drug in the body. Obviously, a drug that is bound to a protein or any other macromolecule will not pass through the membrane in the bound form; only the unbound form can negotiate among the various compartments.

The partition among compartments is determined by the binding capacity and binding constant in each compartment. As long as the binding capacity exceeds the quantity of drug in the compartment, the following equation generally applies:

$$\log D_b = \log K + a \log D_f$$

where D_b is the concentration of bound drug, D_f is the concentration of free drug, and a and K are constants characteristic of the drug and binding macromolecule. The equation is that of a Freundlich isotherm. As the binding capacity is approached, the relationship no longer holds. For a nondissociable drug at equilibrium, D_f will be the same in all communicating compartments, so that it would be possible to calculate the partition if K and a are known for each compartment. Except for plasma, the values of K and a are generally unknown, but the percentage bound is often known.

From the percentage bound, the partition also can be calculated, as in Figure 57-14.[12] However, the logarithmic relationships shown in Equation 9 serve as a reminder that the percentage bound changes with the concentration, so that the partition will vary with the dose. If the drug is a weak acid or base, the un-ionized free form negotiates among the compartments, but the ionized form is often the more firmly bound, and calculations must take into account the dissociation constant and the different Ks and as of the ionized and un-ionized forms.

It is misbelieved commonly that binding in the plasma interferes with the activity of a drug and the intracellular binding in a responsive cell increases activity or toxicity. Both binding in plasma and in the tissues decreases the concentration of free drug, but this is easily remedied by adjusting the dose to give a sufficient concentration for pharmacological activity. The distribution and activity of the free form are not affected by binding. The principal effect of binding is to increase the initial dose requirement for the drug and create a reservoir of drug from which the drug may be withdrawn as the free form is excreted or metabolized. However, if the binding is extremely firm and release is slow, the rate of release may not be enough to sustain the free form at a level sufficient for pharmacological activity; in such instances the bound drug cannot be considered a reserve.

The effect of binding upon the sojourn of a drug may be considerable. For example, quinacrine, which may be concentrated in the liver to as much as several thousand times the concentration in plasma, may remain in the body for months. Some iodine-containing, radiopaque, diagnostic agents are bound strongly to plasma protein and may remain in the plasma for as long as 2 yr. In pathological conditions, such as nephrosis, diabetes, or cirrhosis, in which plasma protein levels may be

decreased, the plasma protein binding, loading dose, and duration of action all may be decreased.

If a drug is bound to a functional macromolecule, binding may relate to pharmacological activity and toxicity, providing that the binding is at a critical center of the macromolecule. The binding by nucleic acids of certain antimalarials, such as quinacrine, undoubtedly contributes to the parasiticidal actions as well as to toxicity.

Most drugs are bound to proteins by relatively weak forces, such as van der Waals (London, Keesom, or Debye) forces, or hydrogen or ionic bonds. Consequently, binding constants generally are small, and binding is usually readily reversible. The larger the molecule, the greater the van der Waals bonding, so that large drug molecules are more likely to be bound strongly than are small ones.

Just as shape and the nature of functional groups are important to drug-receptor combination, so they also are to binding. Drugs of similar shape and/or chemical affinities may bind at the same sites on a binding protein and hence compete with one another. For example, phenylbutazone displaces warfarin from human plasma albumin, which may cause an increase in the anticoagulant effect of warfarin. Some drugs also may displace protein-bound endogenous constituents. For example, sulfisoxazole displaces bilirubin from plasma proteins; in infants with kernicterus the freed bilirubin floods the CNS and causes sometimes fatal toxicity.

Depending on the lipid-water partition coefficient, a drug may be taken up into fatty tissue. The ratio of concentration in fat to that in the plasma, will not be the same as dictated by the partition coefficient, because of the content of water and nonlipids in adipose tissue, and because electrolytes and other solutes alter the dielectric constant and hence solubilities from those of pure water. Lipoproteins and even nonpolar substituents on plasma proteins also take up lipid-soluble molecules, so that solubility in plasma can be considerably higher than that in water. The relatively high solubility of ether in plasma makes plasma a pool for ether, the filling of which delays the onset of anesthesia. However, ether and other volatile anesthetics are taken up gradually into the adipose tissue, which acts as a store of the anesthetic. The longer the anesthetic is administered, the greater the store, and the longer it takes for anesthesia to terminate when inhalation has been discontinued.

Another notable substance that is taken up readily into fat is thiopental. Even though there is a high solubility of this barbiturate in fat, the low rate of blood flow in fat limits the rate of uptake. Because the blood flow in the brain is very high, thiopental rapidly enters brain tissue. However, it soon equilibrates with the other tissues, and the brain concentration falls as that in the other tissues (eg, muscle or liver) increases. As the brain concentration falls, anesthesia ceases. Gradually, the fat accumulates the drug at the expense of other compartments. The gradual entry of thiopental into fat at the expense of plasma, muscle, or liver is illustrated in Figure 57-15.

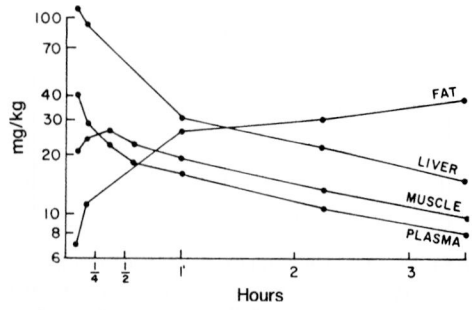

Figure 57-15. Predisposition of thiopental for fat; 25 mg/kg was given to a dog. After a brief sojourn in the more vascular tissues, thiopental gradually transfers to fat, where the lipid-soluble drug dissolves in fat droplets. (From Brodie BB, Hogben CA. *J Pharm Pharmacol* 1957; 9:345.)

NONEQUILIBRIUM AND REDISTRIBUTION—Thus far, the distribution of drugs has been discussed mainly as though equilibrium or steady-state conditions exist after a drug is absorbed and distributed. However, since most drugs are administered at intervals and the body content of drug rises and falls with absorption and biotransformation-excretion, neither a true equilibrium among the body compartments nor a steady state exist.

The term equilibrium is used misleadingly to describe the conditions that exist when the plasma concentration and the concentration in a tissue are equal, as exemplified at the point of intersection of the curves for plasma and muscle or plasma and fat in Figure 57-15. But such *equilibrium* with fat occurs much later than *equilibrium* with muscle, so that no true equilibrium really exists among all the compartments. Furthermore, the crossover point for plasma and any one tissue is not necessarily an equilibrium point, because the rates of ingress and egress from the tissue are not necessarily equal when the internal and external concentrations are equal, since there are numerous factors that make for unequal distribution (pH partition, Donnan effect, electrochemical distribution, active transport, binding, etc).

A study of Figure 57-15 shows that the distribution of thiopental continually changed during the 3.5 hr of observation. At the end of the period, the content in fat was still increasing, while that in each of the other compartments was decreasing. This time-dependent shift in partition is called *redistribution*. Eventually, the content in fat would have reached a peak, which would represent as nearly a true equilibrium point as could be achieved in the dynamic situation where biotransformation and a slight amount of excretion of the drug was taking place. Once the concentration in the fat had reached its peak, its content would have declined in parallel with that in the other tissues, and the partition among the compartments would have remained essentially constant. Redistribution, then, takes place only until the concentration in the slowest-filling compartment reaches its peak, so long as the kinetics of elimination are constant.

An index of distribution known as the *volume of distribution* (amount of drug in the body divided by plasma concentration) is of considerable usefulness in pharmacokinetics but is of limited value in defining the way in which a drug is partitioned in the body.

The word *space* often is used synonymously with volume of distribution. It is employed especially when the distributed substance has a volume of distribution that is essentially identical to a physical real space or body compartment. *N*-acetyl-4-aminoantipyrine is distributed evenly throughout the total body water and is not bound to proteins or other tissue constituents. Thus, the acetylaminoantipyrine space, or volume of distribution, coincides with that of total body water. Inulin, sucrose, sulfate, and a number of other substances essentially are confined to extracellular water, so that an inulin space, for example, measures the extracellular fluid volume. Evans blue is confined to the plasma, so that the Evans blue space is the plasma volume. Such space measurements with standard space indicators are a necessary part of studies on the distribution of drugs, since it is desirable to compare the volume of distribution of a drug with the physiological spaces.

Biotransformations

Most drugs are acted upon by enzymes in the body and converted to metabolic derivatives called metabolites. The process of conversion is called *biotransformation*. Metabolites are usually more polar and less lipid-soluble than the parent drug because of the introduction of oxygen into the molecule, hydrolysis to yield more highly polar groups, or conjugation with a highly polar substance. As a consequence, metabolites often show less penetration into tissues and less renal tubular resorption than the parent drug, in accordance with the principle of the low penetration of polar and high penetration of lipid-soluble substances. For similar reasons, metabolites, particularly conjugates, are usually less active than the parent drug and often inactive. Even if they are appreciably active, they generally are excreted more rapidly. Therefore, the usual net effect of biotransformation may be said to be one of *inactivation* or *detoxication*.

There are, however, numerous examples in which biotransformation does not result in inactivation.

There are also examples in which the parent drug has little or no activity of its own but is converted to an active metabolite: parathion, malathion, and certain other anticholinesterases require metabolic activation; inactive chloroguanide is converted to an active triazine derivative; phenylbutazone is hydroxylated to the antirheumatic hydroxyphenylbutazone; inactive pentavalent arsenicals are reduced to their active trivalent metabolites, and there are other examples of an activating biotransformation.

When a delayed or prolonged response to a drug is desired or an unpleasant taste or local reaction is to be avoided, it is a common pharmaceutical practice to prepare an inactive or nonoffending precursor, such that the active form may be generated in the body. This practice has been termed *drug latentiation*. Chloramphenicol palmitate, dichloralphenazone, and the estolates of various steroid hormones are examples of deliberately latentiated drugs. Because inactive metabolites do not always result from biotransformation, the term detoxication should not be used as a synonym for biotransformation.

Biotransformations take place principally in the liver, although the kidney, skeletal muscle, intestine, or even plasma may be important sites of the enzymatic attack of some drugs. Biotransformations in plasma are mostly hydrolytic.

ENDOPLASMIC RETICULUM AND MICROSOMAL SYSTEM—Many biotransformations in the liver occur in the *endoplasmic reticulum*. The endoplasmic reticulum is a tubular system that courses through the interior of the cell but also appears to communicate with the interstitial space, and its membrane is continuous with the cell membrane. Some of the reticulum is lined with ribonucleoprotein particles, called ribosomes, which are engaged in protein synthesis; this is the *rough* endoplasmic reticulum. The smooth endoplasmic reticulum lacks such a granular appearance. The endoplasmic reticulum is invested heavily with numerous enzymes, which biotransform many drugs and some endogenous substances.

When a broken-cell homogenate of the liver is prepared, the reticulum becomes fragmented, and the fragments form vesicular structures called *microsomes*. Although the microsomes are artifacts, it is often the practice to refer to drug metabolism as occurring in microsomes rather than in the endoplasmic reticulum.

The microsomal system is peculiar in that both oxidations and reductions usually require the reducing cofactor, reduced nicotinamide adenine dinucleotide phosphate (NADPH). This is because microsomal oxidations proceed by way of the introduction of oxygen rather than by dehydrogenation, and NADPH is essential to reduce one of the atoms of oxygen. The drug first binds to an oxidized cytochrome P450. The drug-cytochrome complex then is reduced by NADPH–cytochrome P450 reductase; the reduced complex then combines with oxygen, after which the metabolite is released and oxidized cytochrome P450 is regenerated. Cytochrome P450 is a generic term for a superfamily of enzymes.[17]

The general designation of the cytochromes P450 is *CYP* followed by number (the family) and letter (the subfamily) subdivisions. The classification is based on amino acid sequence homology. To belong to the same family, the homology must be greater than 40% and to the same subfamily greater than 59%. The form is indicated by a number that is based upon the chronological discovery order. The major human forms involved in drug metabolism are CYP1A1 and CYP1A2, CYP2A6, CYP2B6, CYP2C8, CYP2C9/10, CYP2C18/19, CYP2D6, CYP2E1, CYP3A4, CYP3A5, and CYP3A7. In concentration, CYP3As comprise 40% of the liver P450, CYP2Cs comprise 25%, and CYP1A2 about 15%. Despite its limited concentration (2%), CYP2D6 metabolizes about one-fourth of currently used drugs and is widely tested for because of a genetic polymorphism in which 5 to 10% of the population are poor metabolizers. The different isozymes present in humans, together with which drugs they metabolize, are of increasing importance in understanding drug interactions and toxicities and individual responses to standardized doses.

In addition to cytochrome P450, the endoplasmic reticulum contains flavoprotein monooxygenases, which are also responsible for the oxidative metabolism of drugs. The mechanism of oxidation differs from that of cytochrome P450, and their substrate (any drug containing a nucleophilic heteroatom) selectivity is much less. *FMO3* is the major human liver form.

Some of the enzymes of the microsomal system are quite easily *induced;* that is, a drug may increase considerably the activity of the enzyme by increasing the biosynthesis of the enzyme. An increase in the amount of endoplasmic reticulum sometimes occurs concomitantly with enzyme induction.

The mechanism of induction is best documented for polycyclic aromatic hydrocarbon (Ah)-type inducers but is thought to be similar for all agents; however, it involves different receptors, which interact with different regulatory elements on the DNA (Fig 57-16). The cytosol contains proteins that have a high affinity for the inducing agents. In normal drug therapy, the drug (D) enters the liver cell and, if adequately metabolized, is discharged as metabolites. Inefficient clearance from the cell, possibly due to high dosage, results in accumulation (ie, excess), and some is able to bind to the protein, which has a high affinity for the accumulating drug. When the inducing agent binds to its receptor, there is a conformational change (for an Ah receptor, chaperone proteins are displaced) allowing the receptor-inducer complex to translocate into the nucleus, link with additional nuclear factors, and initiate the transcription of mRNA to a limited number of proteins, by binding to DNA regions termed a drug-response element (DRE) (xenobiotic response element for the Ah receptor complex) that activate gene transcription. (For polycyclic aromatic hydrocarbons, the activated genes including specific isozymes of cytochrome P450, glutathione S-transferase, and UDP-glucuronosyltransferase.) These mRNA molecules move out of the nucleus and are translated into new proteins on the ribosomes attached to the endoplasmic reticulum.

The drug-metabolizing enzymes differ in their ability to be induced. For cytochrome P450s, CYP1A2 is induced preferentially by polycyclic aromatic hydrocarbons and other chemicals contained in cigarette smoke and charcoal-broiled meats, as well as by components in cruciferous vegetables. CYP2A6 is induced by barbiturates as are CYP2C9 and CYP3A4. CYP2C9, CYP2C19, and CYP3A4 are all induced by rifampicin, but CYP3A4 is additionally induced by many drugs including carbamazepine, phenytoin, glucocorticoids (dexamethasone), clotrimazole, sulfinpyrazone, and macrolide antibiotics such as troleandomycin. CYP2E1 can be induced by ethanol and isoniazid. There are no known inducers of CYP2D6.

Treatment of an experimental subject with phenobarbital will increase the rate of metabolism of phenobarbital, which necessitates larger and more frequent doses of the drug to maintain a constant sedative effect. Moreover, phenobarbital may induce an increased metabolism of some other, but not all, barbiturates as well as some unrelated drugs, such as strychnine and warfarin. Oddly, warfarin does not induce its own biotransformation readily.

Induction may create therapeutic problems. For example, the use of phenobarbital during treatment with warfarin increases the dose requirement for warfarin. If the physician is unaware of this interaction and fails to increase the dose, the patient may suffer a thrombotic episode. If the dose of warfarin has been increased and the phenobarbital is then discontinued, the rate of metabolism of warfarin may drop to its previous level, so that the patient is overdosed, with hemorrhagic consequences. Some drugs inhibit rather than induce the microsomal enzymes, which reduces the dose requirement and may lead to toxicity. Cimetidine is an example of a drug that inhibits the hepatic metabolism of a number of other drugs.

The activity of the microsomal biotransformation enzymes is affected by many factors other than the presence of drugs. Age, sex, nutritional states, pathological conditions, and genetic factors are among the influences that have been identified. Age, particularly, has received considerable attention. Infants have a poorly developed microsomal biotransformation system, which accounts for the low dose requirement for morphine and also explains the high toxicity of chloramphenicol in infants.

The activity and selectivity of the microsomal biotransformation system varies greatly from species to species, so that care must be exercised in extrapolating experimental findings in laboratory animals to man.

TYPES OF BIOTRANSFORMATIONS—Biotransformations may be *degradative,* wherein the drug molecule is diminished to a smaller structure, or *synthetic,* wherein one or more atoms or groups may be added to the molecule. Very few drugs are degraded completely. However, it is more useful to categorize biotransformations with respect to *metabolic* (nonconjugative) biotransformations and conjugative biotransformations. The former is called Phase I and the latter, Phase II. In Phase I, pharmacodynamic activity may be lost; however, active and chemically reactive intermediates also may be generated. The polarity of the molecule may or may not be increased sufficiently to increase excretion markedly. In Phase II, metabolites from Phase I may be conjugated, and sometimes the original drug may be conjugated, thus bypassing Phase I. Phase II generates metabolites of high polarity, which are excreted readily.

Biotransformations may be placed into four main categories: (1) oxidation, (2) reduction, (3) hydrolysis, and (4) conjugation. Oxidation, reduction, and hydrolysis comprise Phase I. Conjugation comprises Phase II.

Oxidation—Oxidation is more common than any other type of biotransformation. Oxidations that occur primarily in the liver microsomal system include side-chain hydroxylation; aromatic hydroxylation; deamination (which is oxidative and results in the intermediate formation of RCHO); N-, O-, and S-dealkylation (which probably involves hydroxylation of the alkyl group followed by oxidation to the aldehyde); and sulfoxide formation.

Oxidations that occur elsewhere, other than the microsomes, are generally dehydrogenations followed by the addition of oxygen or water. Examples are the oxidation of alcohols by alcohol dehydrogenase, the oxidation of aldehyde by aldehyde dehydrogenase, and the deamination of monoamines by monoamine oxidase and diamines by diamine oxidase.

Reduction—Reductions are relatively uncommon. They mainly occur in liver microsomes, but they occasionally take place in other tissues. Examples are the reduction of nitro and nitroso groups (as in chloramphenicol, nitroglycerin, and organic nitrites), of the azo group (as in prontosil), and of certain aldehydes to the corresponding alcohols.

Hydrolysis—Hydrolysis is a common biotransformation among esters and amides. Esterases are located in many structures besides the microsomes. For example, cholinesterases are found in plasma, erythrocytes, liver, nerve terminals, junctional interstices, and postjunctional structures, and procaine esterases are found in plasma. Various phosphatases and sulfatases also are distributed widely in tissues and plasma, although few drugs are appropriate substrates. The hydrolytic deamidation of meperidine occurs primarily in the hepatic microsomes.

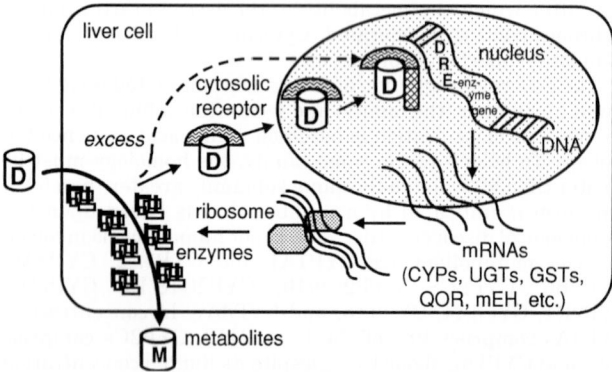

Figure 57-16.

The hydrolysis of epoxides, often generated by cytochrome P450 oxidations, to form dihydrodiols is an important detoxification reaction.

Desulfuration, in which oxygen may replace sulfur, takes place in the liver. Thiopental is converted in part to pentobarbital by desulfuration, and parathion is transformed to paraoxon.

Dehalogenation of certain insecticides and various halogenated hydrocarbons may take place, principally in the liver but not in the microsomes.

Conjugation—A large number of drugs, or their metabolites, are conjugated. Conjugation is the biosynthetic process of combining a chemical compound with a highly polar and water-soluble natural substance to yield a water-soluble, usually inactive, product. Conjugations generally involve either esterification, amidation, mixed anhydride formation, hemiacetal formation, or etherization.

Glucuronic acid is the most frequent partner to the drug in conjugation. Actually, the drug reacts with uridine diphosphoglucuronic acid rather than with simple glucuronic acid. The drug or drug metabolite combines at the number 1 carbon (aldehyde end) and not at the carboxyl end of glucuronic acid. The hydroxyl group of an alcohol or a phenol attacks the number 1 carbon of the pyran ring to replace uridine diphosphate. The product is a hemiacetal-like derivative. Since the product is not an ester, the term *glucuronide* is appropriate. Rarely, thiols and amines may form analogous glucuronides.

Carboxyl compounds form esters, appropriately called glucuronates, in replacing the uridine diphosphate. *Sulfuric acid* is also a frequent conjugant, especially with phenols and to a lesser extent with simple alcohols. The sulfurated product is called an *ethereal sulfate.*

Occasionally sulfuric acid conjugates with aromatic amines to form *sulfamates. Phosphoric acid* also conjugates with phenols and aromatic amines. The conjugation of benzoic acid with glycine to yield hippuric acid is a classical example of an *amidation* conjugative process.

Many electrophilic compounds conjugate with the nucleophilic tripeptide, glutathione. Through a series of enzymatic reactions, the γ-glutamyl and glycyl residues are removed, the remaining cysteine conjugate is *N*-acetylated, and the product spontaneously dehydrates to form a mercapturic acid.

Amidations with amino acids are less frequent than *acetylation,* partly because few drugs are carboxylic compounds. Aromatic amines and occasionally aliphatic amines or heterocyclic nitrogen frequently are acetylated. Acetyl-CoA is the biological reagent rather than acetic acid itself. Unlike most other conjugates, the acetylate (amide) is usually less water-soluble than the parent compound. The acetylation of the para-amino group of the sulfonamides is a prime example of this type of conjugation.

Although most conjugations occur in the liver, some occur in the kidney or in other tissues.

Many amines, especially derivatives of β-phenylethylamine and heterocyclic compounds, are methylated in the body. The products are usually biologically active, sometimes more so than the parent compound. *N-Methylation* may occur in the cytoplasm of the liver and elsewhere, especially in chromaffin tissue in the case of phenylethylamines.

Phenolic compounds may be *O*-methylated. *O-Methylation* is the principal route of biotransformation of catecholamines such as epinephrine and norepinephrine, the methyl group being introduced on the *meta*-hydroxy substituent. Both *N*- and *O*-methylation require *S*-adenosylmethionine.

All the drug conjugation reactions are catalyzed by specialized enzymes present in multiple forms. Glucuronidation is catalyzed by UDP-glucuronosyltransferases, *UGTs,* located in the endoplasmic reticulum. UGTs are classified in two major classes, UGT1As and UGT2Bs, based on amino acid homology, but the two classes also differ in substrate selectivity, with UGT1As preferring planar drugs and UGT2Bs preferring bulkier molecules. As with cytochrome P450s, these enzymes are inducible, and the two classes differ in their response to various drugs and other chemicals.

Sulfation is catalyzed by sulfotransferases, *SULTs,* located in the cytoplasm. The many isozymes exhibit substrate selectivity, and some differ in thermal stability. Unlike most major drug-metabolizing enzymes, SULTs are refractory to induction by drugs.

Glutathione conjugations are catalyzed by glutathione-*S*-transferases, *GSTs,* also located in the cytoplasm. The multiple isozymes are designated into four major classes: alpha, mu, pi and theta. The isozymes have relatively low substrate (electrophile) selectivity. Methylation reactions are catalyzed by cytoplasmic *O*-, *N*-, and *S*-methyltransferases, and each exists in multiple forms.

Acetylation is catalyzed by cytoplasmic *N*-acetyltransferases, *NAT*1, and in the liver, *NAT*2. NAT2 exhibits a genetic polymorphism, giving *fast and slow* acetylator phenotypes with differing incidences in various populations (slow is high in Middle Eastern, low in Asian).

Excretion

Some drugs are not biotransformed in the body. Others may be biotransformed, but their products still remain to be eliminated. It follows that excretion is involved in the elimination of all drugs and/or their metabolites. Although the kidney is the most important organ of excretion, some substances are excreted in bile, sweat, saliva, or gastric juice or from the lungs.

RENAL EXCRETION—The excretory unit of the kidney is called the *nephron* (Fig 57-17). There are several million nephrons in the human kidney. The nephron is essentially a filter funnel, called *Bowman's capsule,* with a long stem, called a *renal tubule.* It also is recognized now that the collecting duct is functionally a part of the nephron. The *blood vessels* that invest the capsule and the tubule are also an essential part of the nephron.

Bowman's capsule is packed with a tuft of branching interconnected capillaries *(glomerular tuft),* which provide a large surface area of capillary endothelium *(filter paper)* through which fluid and small molecules may filter into the capsule and begin passage down the tubule. The glomerular tuft, together with Bowman's capsule, constitute the *glomerulus.* The glomerular capillary endothelium and the supporting layer of Bowman's capsule have channels ranging upward to 40 Å. Consequently, all unbound crystalloid solutes in plasma, and even a little albumin, pass or are forced by pressure into the glomerular filtrate.

The postglomerular vessels, which lie close to the tubules, are critically important to renal function in that substances resorbed from the filtrate by the tubule are returned to the blood along these vessels. The tubule is not straight but rather first

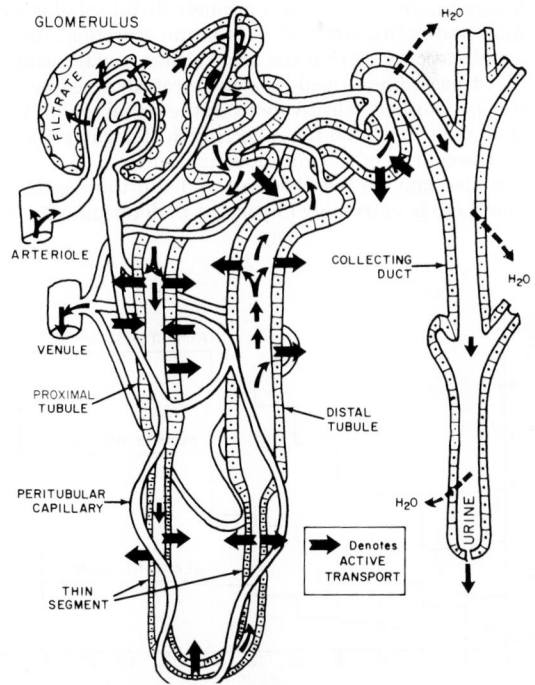

Figure 57-17. Diagram of a mammalian nephron. Note how the lower loops of the postglomerular capillaries course downward and double back along with the tubule. This allows countercurrent distribution to maintain hyperosmolar urine within the thin segment.

makes a number of convolutions (called a *proximal convoluted tubule*), then courses down and back up a long loop (called the *loop of Henle*), makes more convolutions (the *distal convoluted tubule*) and finally joins the collecting duct. The loop of Henle is divided into a *proximal (descending) tubule*, a thin segment and a *distal (ascending) tubule*.

As the glomerular filtrate passes through the proximal tubule, some solute may be resorbed *(tubular resorption)* through the tubular epithelium and returned to the blood. Resorption occurs in part by passive diffusion and in part by active transport, especially with sodium and glucose. Chloride follows sodium obligatorily.

In the proximal region, the tubule is quite permeable to water, so that resorbed solutes are accompanied by enough water to keep the resorbate isotonic. Consequently, although the filtrate becomes diminished in volume by approximately 80% in the proximal tubule, it is not concentrated.

Some *acidification* occurs in the proximal tubule as the result of carbonic anhydrase activity in the tubule cells and the diffusion of hydronium ions into the lumen. In the lumen the hydronium ion reacts with bicarbonate ion, which is converted to resorbable nonionic CO_2.

There is also active transport of organic cations and anions into the lumen *(tubular secretion)*, each by a separate system. These active transport systems are extremely important in the excretion of a number of drugs; for example, penicillin G is secreted rapidly by the anion transport system, and tetraethyl-lammonium ion by the cation transport system. Probenecid is an inhibitor of anion secretion and, hence, decreases the rate of loss of penicillin from the body.

As the filtrate travels through the thin segment it becomes concentrated, especially at the bottom, as a result of active resorption and a countercurrent-distribution effect enabled by the recurrent and parallel arrangement of the ascending segment, the parallel orientation of the collecting duct, and the similar recurrent geometry of the associated capillaries.

In the thick segment of the ascending loop of Henle, both sodium and chloride are transported actively.

In the distal tubule, sodium resorption occurs partly in *exchange* for potassium *(potassium secretion)* and for hydronium ions. Adrenal mineralocorticoids promote distal tubular sodium resorption and potassium and hydronium secretion. *Ammonia secretion* also occurs, so that the urine either may be acidified or alkalinized, according to acid-base and electrolyte requirements.

Water is resorbed selectively from the distal end of the distal convoluted tubule and the collecting ducts; water resorption is under the control of the antidiuretic hormone.

Drugs also may be resorbed in the distal tubule; the pH of the urine there is extremely important in determining the rate

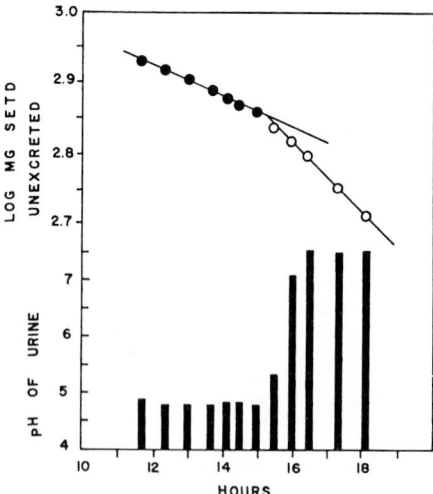

Figure 57-19. The effect of urinary pH on the excretion of sulfaethidole in a human subject after oral administration of 2 g. *Bars* (lower half): urinary pH; *circles* (open and closed, top): log of the amount of drug remaining in the body; *negative slopes* (of lines defined by the circles): a function of the rate constant of excretion. Note the abrupt increase in rate when the urinary pH is changed from acidic to neutral or slightly alkaline. (From Kostenbauder HB, et al. *J Pharm Sci* 1962; 51:1084.)

of resorption, in accordance with the principle of non-ionic diffusion and pH partition. The pH of the tubular fluid also affects the tubular secretion of drugs.

As an example of the importance of urinary pH, in humans the secondary amine mecamylamine is excreted more than four times faster when the urinary pH is below 5.5 than when it is above 7.5; Figure 57-18 illustrates the effect of urinary pH on the excretion of this amine. The effect of urinary pH on the excretion of a weak acid, sulfaethidole, is shown in Figure 57-19.

The urinary pH and, hence, drug excretion may fluctuate widely according to the diet, exercise, drugs, time of day, and other factors. Obviously, the excretion of weak acids and bases can be controlled partly with acidifying or alkalinizing salts, such as ammonium chloride or sodium bicarbonate, respectively. Comparative studies on potency and efficacy in man have demonstrated the importance of controlling urinary pH. Urinary pH is important only when the drug in question is a weak acid or base of which a significant fraction is excreted. The plasma levels will change inversely to the excretory rate. For example, it has been shown clinically with quinidine that alkalinization of the urine not only decreases the urine concentration but also increases the plasma concentration and toxicity.

The collecting duct also resorbs sodium and water, secretes potassium, and acidifies and concentrates the urine. Antidiuretic hormone (ADH) controls the permeability to water of both the collecting duct and the distal tubule.

Renal clearance and the kinetics of renal elimination are discussed in Chapter 58.

BILIARY EXCRETION AND FECAL ELIMINATION— Many drugs are secreted into the bile and then pass into the intestine. A drug that is passed into the intestine via the bile may be reabsorbed and not lost from the body. A drug conjugate entering the intestine may be deconjugated by enzymes and the parent drug reabsorbed. This cycle of biliary secretion and intestinal resorption is called *enterohepatic circulation*. Examples of drugs enterohepatically circulated are morphine, and the penicillins. The biliary secretory systems greatly resemble those of the kidney tubules. The enterohepatic system may provide a considerable reservoir for a drug.

If a drug is not absorbed completely from the intestine, the unabsorbed fraction will be eliminated in the feces. An unabsorbable drug that is secreted into the bile will likewise be eliminated in the feces. Such fecal elimination is called *fecal*

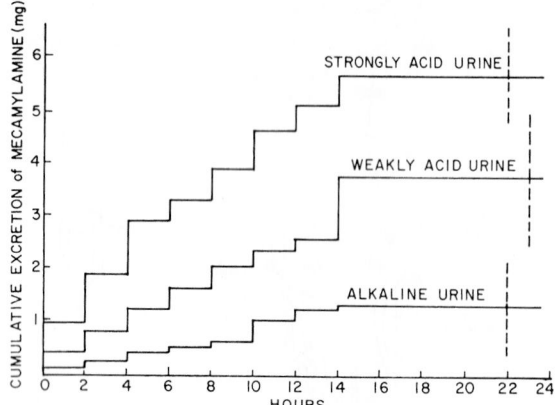

Figure 57-18. The effect of urinary pH on the mean cumulative excretion in man of mecamylamine during the first day after oral administration of 10 mg. *Vertical broken lines:* standard deviation. (From Milne MD, et al. *Clin Sci* 1957; 16:599.)

excretion. Only rarely are drugs secreted into the intestine through the succus entericus (intestinal secretions), although a number of amines are secreted into gastric juice.

ALVEOLAR EXCRETION—The large alveolar area and high blood flow make the lungs ideal for the excretion of appropriate substances. Only volatile liquids or gases are eliminated from the lungs. Gaseous and volatile anesthetics essentially are eliminated completely by this route. Only a small amount of ethanol is eliminated by the lungs, but the concentration in the alveolar air is related so constantly to the blood alcohol concentration that the analysis of expired air is acceptable for legal purposes. The high aqueous solubility and relatively low vapor pressure of ethanol at body temperature account for the reten-

tion of most of the substance in the blood. Carbon dioxide from those drugs that are partly degraded also is excreted in the lungs.

PHARMACOKINETICS

Pharmacokinetics is the science that treats the rate of absorption, extent of absorption, rates of distribution among body compartments, rate of elimination, and related phenomena. Because of its importance, Chapters 58 and 59, *Basic Pharmacokinetics* and *Clinical Pharmacokinetics,* have been devoted to the subject.

DRUG INTERACTION AND COMBINATION

Frequently a patient may receive more than one drug concurrently. Case records show that surgical patients commonly receive more than 10 drugs, and the patient is often under the influence of several drugs at once. Multiple-drug administration also is common for patients hospitalized for infections and other disorders. Furthermore, a patient may be suffering from more than one unrelated disorder that demands simultaneous treatment with two or more drugs. In such instances, interactions are unsolicited and often unexpected.

In addition to the administration of drugs concurrently for their independent and unrelated effects, drugs are sometimes administered concurrently deliberately to make use of expected interactions.

TYPES OF INTERACTION AND REASONS FOR COMBINATION THERAPY

A drug may affect the response to another drug in a quantitative way. On one hand, the intensity of either the therapeutic effect, or side effect, may be augmented or suppressed. On the other hand, a qualitatively different effect may be elicited. The mechanisms of such interactions are many and are not always well understood. A drug may not necessarily affect either the quality or initial intensity or effect of another drug, but may cause significant to profound changes in the duration of action. The nature of this type of interaction generally is understood fairly well, although it may not yet have been ascertained for any particular drug combination. The deliberate use of combined interacting drugs is most valid when the mechanism of the interaction is understood and the combined effects are both quantifiable and predictable. The rationales of drug combination and the principles involved are discussed below.

COMBINATIONS TO INCREASE INTENSITY OF RESPONSE OR EFFICACY—Sometimes the basis for the action of one drug to increase the intensity of response to another is well understood, but often the reason for a positive interaction is obscure. A terminology has arisen that frequently is not only enlightening as to mechanisms and principles but which also is somewhat confusing.

Drugs that elicit the same quality of effect and are mutually interactive are called *homergic,* regardless of whether there is anything in common between the separate response systems. Thus, the looseness of the term admits a pressor response consequent to an increase in cardiac output to be homergic with one resulting from arteriolar constriction, even though there is not one common responsive element, the blood pressure itself being but a passive indicator. However, homergic drugs usually have in common at least part of a response system. Thus, both norepinephrine and vasopressin stimulate some of the same vascular smooth muscle, even though they do not excite the same receptors.

Two homergic drugs can be agonists of the same receptor, so that the entire response system is common to both. Such drugs are called *homodynamic.* As discussed under *Drug Receptors*

and Receptor Theory, homodynamic drugs will generate dose–intensity of effect curves with parallel slopes but not necessarily with identical maxima or efficacies, if one of the drugs is a partial agonist.

From mass-law kinetics and dose-effect data of the separate drugs, it is possible to predict the combined effects of two agonists to the same receptor. If both drugs are full agonists, theory predicts that an EDx of Drug A added to an EDy of Drug B should elicit the same effect as an EDy of Drug A added to an EDx of Drug B. An example is shown in Figure 57-20. Dose-percentage data with homodynamic drugs can be treated in the same way.[21]

Drugs whose combined effects fit the above conditions are called *additive*. If the response to the combination exceeds the expected value for additivity, the drugs are considered to be *supra-additive*. Purely homodynamic drugs do not show supra-additivity; however, if one drug in the pair has an additional action to affect the concentration or penetration of the other or to prime the response system in some way, two agonists to the same receptor may exhibit supra-additivity. Two homergic drugs are *infra-additive* if their combined effect is less than expected from additivity. As with supra-additivity, infra-additivity must involve an action elsewhere than on a common receptor.

Two drugs are said to be *summative* if a dose of drug that elicits response x added to a dose of another drug that elicits response y gives the combined response $x + y$. Very little significance usually can be attached to summation. Unless the dose-intensity curve of each drug is linear, rather than log-linear,

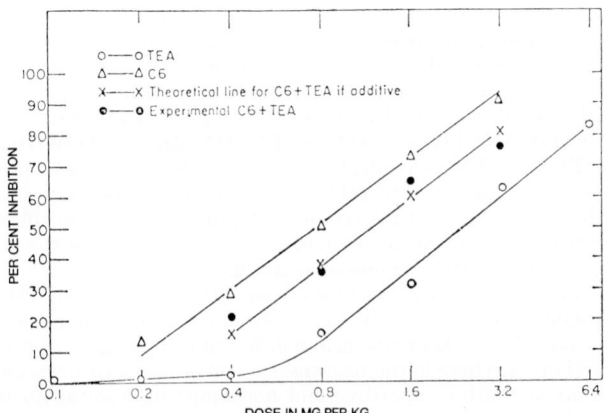

Figure 57-20. Additive inhibitory effects of tetraethylammonium (TEA) and hexamethonium (C6) on the superior cervical ganglion of the cat. The theoretical line for additivity was calculated on the basis that an increment of TEA added to an *EDx* of C6 should have the same effect as if it were added to an *EDx* of TEA. When TEA and C6 were administered together, an equal amount of each was given. The dose is the sum of the doses of the two components. (From Harvey SC. *Arch Intern Pharmacodyn* 1958; 114:232.)

summation cannot be predicted from the two curves. When summation does occur with the usual clinical doses of two drugs, it almost never occurs over the entire dose range; indeed, if the dose of each of the two drugs is greater than an ED50, summation is theoretically impossible unless it is possible to increase the maximal response. At best, summation is an infrequent clinical finding, limited to one or two doses.

Two drugs are said to be *heterergic* if the drugs do not cause responses of the same quality. When heterergy is positive, ie, the response to one drug is enhanced by the other, *synergism* is said to occur. The word often has been used to describe any positive interaction, but it should be used only to describe a positive interaction between heterergic drugs. The term *potentiation* has been used synonymously with synergism, but misuse of the term has led to the recommendation that the term be dropped. Synergism is often the result of an effect to interfere with the elimination of a drug and, thus, to increase the concentration; synergism also may result from an effect on penetration or on the responsivity of the effector system. Examples of a synergistic effect, in which responsivity is enhanced, are the action of adrenalcorticoids to enhance the vasoconstrictor response to epinephrine and the increase of epinephrine- induced hyperglycemia consequent to impairment by theophylline of the enzymatic destruction of the cAMP that mediates the response.

In clinical practice two homodynamic drugs rarely are coadministered for the purpose of increasing the response, since a sufficient dose of either drug should be able to achieve the same effect as a combination of the two. Most clinical combinations with positively interacting drugs involve heterergic drugs.

COMBINATIONS TO DECREASE INDIVIDUAL DOSES AND TOXICITY—When homodynamic drugs are coadministered, it is usually for the purpose of decreasing toxicity. If the toxicities of two homodynamic drugs are infra-additive, the toxicity of combined partial doses of the two drugs often will be less than with full doses of either drug. This principle is valid for trisulfapyrimidines mixture (see RPS-18, page 1181).

COMBINATIONS TO ATTACK A DISEASE COMPLEX AT DIFFERENT POINTS—With many diseases, more than one organ or tissue may be affected or events at more than one locus may bear upon the ultimate perturbation. For example, in duodenal ulcer, psychic factors appear to increase activity in the vagus nerve, which modulates gastric secretion, so that it is rational to explore the effects of sedatives, ganglionic blocking drugs, antimuscarinic drugs, and antacids, singly and in combination. In heart failure the decrement in renal plasma flow and changes in aldosterone levels promote the retention of salt and water, so that diuretics and digitalis usually are employed concomitantly. Pain, anxiety, and agitation or depression are frequent accompaniments of various pathological processes, so that it is to be expected that analgesics, tranquilizers, sedatives, or antidepressives frequently will be given at the same time, along with other drugs intended to correct the specific pathology.

COMBINATIONS TO ANTAGONIZE UNTOWARD ACTIONS—The side effects of a number of drugs can be prevented or suppressed by other drugs. An antagonist may compete with the drug at the receptor that initiates the side effect, depress the side-effector system at a point other than the receptor, or stimulate an opposing system.

Antagonism at the receptor is *competitive antagonism* if the antagonist attaches at the same receptor group as the agonist (see page 1104). Antagonism at a different receptor group or inhibition elsewhere in the response system is *noncompetitive antagonism*. Both competitive and noncompetitive antagonism are classified as *pharmacological antagonism*. The stimulation of an opposing system is *physiological antagonism*.

Examples of pharmacological antagonism are the use of atropine to suppress the muscarinic effects of excess acetylcholine consequent to the use of neostigmine and the use of antihistaminics to prevent the effects of histamine liberated by tubocurarine. Examples of physiological antagonism are the use of amphetamine to correct partially the sedation caused by anticonvulsant doses of phenobarbital and the ad-

ministration of ephedrine to correct hypotension resulting from spinal anesthesia.

COMBINATIONS THAT AFFECT ELIMINATION—Only a few drugs presently are used purposefully to elevate or prolong plasma levels by interfering with elimination, although continued interest in such drugs probably will increase the number.

Probenecid, which already has been mentioned to antagonize the renal secretion of penicillin, was introduced originally for this purpose. However, because penicillin G is inexpensive and available in repository forms as well as oral forms (obviating the need for injection), it is less imperative to retard the excretion of penicillin. The low, nonallergenic toxicity of penicillin permits very large doses to be given without concern for the high plasma concentrations that result, which also means that there is little necessity for increasing the biological half-life of the drug. Consequently, probenecid is not used routinely today in combination with penicillin.

The use of vasoconstrictors to increase the sojourn of local anesthetics at the site of infiltration continues, but few other clinical examples of the deliberate use of one drug to interfere with either the distribution or elimination of another can be cited. Nevertheless, the subject of the effect of one drug on the elimination of another has become immensely active. Innumerable drugs affect the fate of others, and the therapist must be aware of such interactions.

Drugs that induce cytochrome P450s and other drug- metabolizing enzymes enhance the elimination of drugs that are metabolized by the liver. There would be very little point ordinarily in soliciting combinations that would shorten the duration of action or lower plasma levels, unless it were to reduce an overdosage. However, since such combinations are used unwittingly or unavoidably, this type of interaction is of great clinical importance.

Drugs that inhibit cytochrome P450 will, of course, reduce the metabolism of a wide range of additional drugs and serve to prolong or elevate plasma concentration.

COMBINATIONS TO ALTER ABSORPTION—In the section *Vehicles and Absorption Adjuvants*, it was mentioned that certain substances facilitate the absorption of others. The use of such absorption adjuvants generally is included under the subject of formulation rather than under drug combination. Although drugs that increase blood flow, motility, etc, have an effect to increase the rate of absorption, the use of such drugs so far has not proved to be very practical. When it is desired to slow the absorption of drugs, various physical or physicochemical means prove to be more effective and less troublesome than drug combinations.

Fixed Combinations of Drugs

Concomitant treatment with two or more drugs frequently is unnecessary, and generally, it immeasurably complicates therapy and the evaluation of response and toxicity. Nevertheless, it is often warranted, even essential, and cannot be condemned categorically. However, with fixed-dose or fixed-ratio combinations, in which the drugs are together in the same preparation, there are certain disadvantages, except for a few rare instances such as trisulfapyrimidines.

The disadvantages are as follows: patients differ in their responsivity or sensitivity to drugs, and adjustments in dosage or dose-interval may be necessary. If adjustment of only one component of the mixture is required, it is undesirable that the schedule of the second component be adjusted obligatorily, as it is in a fixed combination. According to which way the dose is adjusted, either toxicity or loss of the therapeutic effect may result. Furthermore, when adverse effects to either component occur, both drugs must be discontinued. The fixed combination denies the physician flexible control of therapy. Especially when one component in a mixture is superfluous yet potentially toxic, as is often the case, the promotion of fixed combinations is reprehensible. However, the separate administration of drugs used in combination often complicates treatment for patients, who, in an outpatient situation and sometimes in the hospital, may not take all of their medication or may take it at inappropriate intervals. The resulting consequences may be worse than those of fixed combinations in certain instances. Consequently, a summary dismissal of fixed combinations is unwarranted. Rather, the fundamentals of pharmacokinetics and clinical experience must be brought together with biopharmaceutics to analyze present combinations and to predict possible new allowable combinations.

DANGERS IN MULTIPLE-DRUG THERAPY

Some objections to fixed-dose combinations were stated above. Also the unanticipated effects of drug combinations have been touched upon, particularly with respect to effects upon elimination. But it should be made clear that more is at stake than simply the biological half-life of a drug. An example is given of the grave clinical consequences of the effect of phenobarbital enhancing the biotransformation of warfarin. Other examples of dangerous interactions, such as the effect of several antidepressants in greatly synergizing catecholamines, may be cited. Even some antibiotics antagonize each other and increase mortality.

In addition to the obvious pitfalls posed by the interactions themselves, the use of multiple-drug therapy fosters careless diagnosis and a false sense of security in the number of drugs employed. Multiple-drug therapy should never be employed without a convincing indication that each drug is beneficial beyond the possible detriments or without proof that a therapeutically equivocal combination is definitely harmless. Finally, the expense to the patient warrants consideration.

REFERENCES

1. Clark AJ. *J Physiol (London)* 1926; 61:547.
2. Ariens EJ, ed. *Molecular Pharmacology,* vol 1. New York: Academic, 1964, p 176.
3. Stephenson RP. *Br J Pharmacol* 1956; 11:379.
4. Rang HP. *Br J Pharmacol* 1973; 48:475.
5. Colquhoun D. In: Rang HP, ed. *Drug Receptors.* Baltimore: University Park, 1973.
6. Schanker LS. *Adv Drug Res* 1964; 1:71.
7. Brodie BB, et al. *J Pharmacol Exp Ther* 1960; 130:20.
8. Truitt EB, et al. *J Pharmacol Exp Ther* 1950; 100:309.
9. Lillehei JP. *JAMA* 1968; 205:531.
10. Martin AN, et al. *Physical Pharmacy,* 2nd ed. Philadelphia: Lea & Febiger, 1969, pp 247, 253.
11. Jacobs MH. *Cold Spring Harbor Symp Quant Biol* 1940; 8:30.
12. Schanker LS. *Pharmacol Rev* 1961; 14:501.
13. Brodie BB, Hogben CA. *J Pharm Pharmacol* 1957; 9:345.
14. Hogben CA. *Fed Proc* 1960; 19:864.
15. Albert A. *Pharmacol Rev* 1952; 4:136.
16. Ariens EJ, et al. In: *Molecular Pharmacology,* vol 1. Ariens EJ, ed. New York: Academic, 1964, p 7.
17. Nelson DR, et al. *DNA Cell Biol* 1993; 12:1.
18. Milne MD, et al. *Clin Sci* 1957; 16:599.
19. Kostenbauder HB, et al. *J Pharm Sci* 1962; 51:1084.
20. Harvey SC. *Arch Intern Pharmacodyn* 1958; 114:232.
21. Weaver LC, et al. *J Pharmacol Exp Ther* 1955; 113:359.

BIBLIOGRAPHY

Anders MW. *Bioactivation of Foreign Compounds.* New York: Academic, 1985.
Bend JR, Serabjit-Singh CJ, Philpot RM. The pulmonary uptake accumulation and metabolism of xenobiotics. *Annu Rev Pharmacol Toxicol* 1985; 25:97.
Benford D, et al. *Drug Metabolism: From Molecules to Man.* New York: Taylor & Francis, 1987.
Bertolino M, Llinas R. The central role of voltage activated and receptor operated calcium channels in neuronal cells. *Annu Rev Pharmacol Toxicol* 1992; 32:399.
Black JW, et al, eds. *Perspectives on Receptor Classification.* New York: Liss, 1987.
Boelsterli U. *Mechanistic Toxicology: The Molecular Basis of How Chemicals Disrupt Biological Targets.* New York: Taylor and Francis, 2003
Caldwell J, Jakoby WB. *Biological Basis of Detoxification.* New York: Academic, 1983.
Coulson CJ. *Mechanisms of Drug Action.* New York: Taylor & Francis, 1987.
Dean PM. *Molecular Foundations of Drug-Receptor Interaction.* Cambridge: Cambridge University Press, 1987.
Denison MS, Nagy SR. Activation of the aryl hydrocarbon receptor by structurally diverse exogenous and endogenous chemicals *Annu Rev Pharmacol Toxicol* 2003; 43:309.
Ding X, Kaminsky LS. Human extrahepatic cytochromes P450: function in xenobiotic metabolism and tissue selective chemical toxicity in the respiratory and gastrointestinal tract. *Annu Rev Pharmacol Toxicol* 2003; 43:149.
Finean JB, Michell RH, eds. *Membrane Structure.* Amsterdam: Elsevier/North Holland, 1981.
Gibson GG, Skett PL. *Introduction to Drug Metabolism,* 2nd ed. London: Chapman & Hall, 1994.
Gilman AG. G proteins: transducers of receptor generated signals. *Annu Rev Biochem* 1987; 56:615.
Lewis DFV. *Guides to Cytochromes P450.* New York: Taylor & Francis, 2002.
Gregoriadis G, Senior J. *Targeting of Drugs with Synthetic Systems.* New York: Plenum, 1986.
Hulme EC, Birdsall NJM, Buckley NJ. Muscarinic receptor subtypes. *Annu Rev Pharmacol Toxicol* 1990; 30:633.
Ioannides C, ed. *Cytochromes P450, Metabolic and Toxicological Aspects.* Boca Raton, FL: CRC Press, 1996.
Jakoby WB, et al, eds. *Metabolic Basis of Detoxification.* New York: Academic, 1982.
Kalow W. Pharmacogenetics in biological perspective. *Pharmacol Rev* 1997; 49:369
Karlin A. Anatomy of a receptor. *Neurosci Comment* 1983; 1:111.
Kenakin TP. The classification of drugs and drug receptors in isolated tissues. *Pharmacol Rev* 1984; 36:165.
Kenakin TP. *Pharmacological Analysis of Drug Receptor Interaction.* New York: Raven Press, 1987.
La Du B, et al. *Fundamentals of Drug Metabolism and Drug Disposition.* Baltimore: Williams & Wilkins, 1971.
Lamble JW, Abbott AC, eds. *Receptors Again!* Amsterdam: Elsevier, 1984.
Lefkowitz RJ, ed. *Receptor Regulation.* London: Chapman & Hall, 1981.
Levine RR. *Pharmacology: Drug Actions and Reactions,* 4th ed. Boston: Little, Brown, 1990.
Limbird LE. *Cell Surface Receptors: A Short Course on Theory and Methods.* Boston: Nijhoff, 1986.
Loh HH, Smith AP, Birnbammer L. Molecular characterization of opioid receptors G proteins in signal transduction. *Annu Rev Pharmacol Toxicol* 1990; 30:123.
Martonosi AN. *Membranes and Transport.* New York: Plenum, 1982.
Meyer UA. Drugs in special patient groups: clinical importance of genetics in drug effects. In: Melman KL, et al, eds. *Clinical Pharmacology,* 3rd ed. New York: McGraw-Hill, 1992.
Mulder GJ, ed. *Conjugation Reactions in Drug Metabolism.* New York: Taylor & Francis, 1990.
Mulder GJ: Glucuronidation and its role in regulation of biological activity of drugs. *Annu Rev Pharmacol Toxicol* 1992; 32:25.
Nguyen T, Sherratt PJ, Pickett CB. Regulatory mechanisms controlling gene expression mediated by the antioxidant response element *Annu Rev Pharmacol Toxicol* 2003; 43:233.
O'Dowd BF, et al. Structure of the adrenergic and related receptors. *Annu Rev Neurosci* 1989; 12:67.
Olson RW, Venter JC, eds. *Benzodiazepine/GABA Receptors and Chloride Channels.* New York: Liss, 1986.
Ortiz de Montellano PR, ed. *Cytochrome P450. Structure, Mechanism, and Biochemistry,* 3rd ed. New York: Kluwer Academic Plenum, 2003.
Parkinson A. Biotransformation of xenobiotics. In: *Casarett and Doull's Toxicology: The Basic Science of Poisons,* 6th ed. New York: McGraw Hill, 2001.
Post G, Crooke ST, eds. *Mechanisms of Receptor Regulation.* New York: Plenum, 1986.
Pratt WB, Taylor P. *Principles of Drug Action.* New York: Churchill Livingstone, 1986.
Putney JW Jr, ed. *Phosphoinositides and Receptor Mechanisms.* New York: Liss, 1986.
Roche EB, ed. *Bioreversible Carriers in Drug Design.* New York: Pergamon, 1987.
Roth SH, Miller KW, eds. *Molecular and Cellular Mechanisms of Anesthetics.* New York: Plenum, 1986.

Sandler M, ed. *Enzyme Inhibitors As Drugs.* Baltimore: University Park, 1980.

Schmucker DL. Aging and drug disposition. *Pharmacol Rev* 1985; 37:133.

Schou JS, et al, eds. *Drug Receptors and Dynamic Processes in Cells.* New York: Raven, 1986.

Stein WD. *Transport and Diffusion Across Cell Membranes.* Orlando: Academic, 1986.

Stoughton RB. Percutaneous absorption of drugs. *Annu Rev Pharmacol Toxicol* 1989; 29:55.

Stroud RM. Acetylcholine receptor structure. *Neurosci Comment* 1983; 1:124.

Sueyoshi T, Negishi M. Phenobarbital response elements of cytochrome P450 genes and nuclear receptors. *Annu Rev Pharmacol Toxicol* 2001; 41:123.

Testa, B, ed. *Advances in Drug Research,* vols 14, 15. London: Academic, 1985, 1986.

Thummel KE, Wilkinson GR. In vitro and in vivo drug interactions involving human CYP3A. *Annu Rev Pharmacol Toxicol* 1998; 38:389.

Triggle DJ, Janis RA. Calcium channel ligands. *Annu Rev Pharmacol Toxicol* 1987; 27:347.

Tukey RH, Strassburg CP. Human UDP-glucuronosyltransferases: metabolism, expression and disease. *Annu Rev Pharmacol Toxicol* 2000; 40:581.

Venter JC, Harrison LC, eds. *Molecular and Chemical Characterization of Membrane Receptors.* New York: Liss, 1984.

Wardle EN. *Cell Surface Science in Medicine and Pathology.* New York: Elsevier, 1985.

Yamazaki M, Suzuki H, Sugiyama Y. Recent advances in carrier mediated hepatic uptake and biliary excretion of xenobiotics. *Pharmacut Res* 1996; 13:497.

Zaki Y, et al. Opioid receptor types and subtypes: the δ receptor as a model. *Annu Rev Pharmacol Toxicol* 1996; 36:379.

CHAPTER 58

Basic Pharmacokinetics and Pharmacodynamics

Raymond E Galinsky, PharmD

Craig K Svensson, PharmD, PhD

The goal of pharmacotherapy is to provide optimal drug therapy in the treatment or prevention of disease. A major barrier to the achievement of this goal is the large variability in pharmacological effect that is observed following drug administration (Fig 58-1).[1] The ability to implement drug therapy in a safe and rational manner necessitates an understanding of the factors that cause this variability. One of the most important factors is the concentration of drug that is achieved at the site of action.

THE CRITICAL NATURE OF THE CONCENTRATION VERSUS EFFECT RELATIONSHIP

The quantitative response to a drug depends highly on the concentration of drug at the site of action. In most situations, one cannot quantify drug concentration at the actual site of action. Rather, drug concentrations are measured in an easily accessible site that is believed to be in equilibrium with the site of action (eg, blood or one of its components). Figure 58-2[2] provides a good illustration of a drug whose pharmacological effect is particularly sensitive to changes in blood concentration. Numerous studies have been published that substantiate the critical nature of the concentration-effect relationship for a wide variety of drugs.

It is recognized now that drug therapy may be optimized by designing regimens that account for the concentration of a drug necessary to achieve a desired pharmacological response. However, there is often significant difficulty in achieving such target concentrations. In particular, it often is observed that if a fixed dose of a drug is administered to a group of individuals, the drug concentration measured in plasma can vary widely. For example, the peak concentration of 6-mercaptopurine achieved in a group of 20 patients who received a standard 1 mg/m² dose is shown in Figure 58-3.[3] The concentrations ranged from 0 to 660 ng/mL. Taken together, this suggests that variability in drug concentration is a major source of variability in drug effect, and there may be a significant degree of variability among individuals in the drug concentrations produced by a given dose of drug.

A basic understanding of the factors that control drug concentration at the site of action is important for the optimal use of drugs. This is the area of study referred to as *pharmacokinetics,* which is the study of the time course of drug absorption, distribution, metabolism, and elimination.

DRUG CONCENTRATION VERSUS TIME PROFILE

Blood (or its components, plasma or serum) represents the most frequently sampled fluid used to characterize the pharmacokinetics of drugs. Drug concentration in the blood is the sum of several processes (Fig 58-4).[4] Initially, visual characterization of the processes controlling the concentration of drug in the blood can be made by constructing a drug concentration versus time profile (ie, a plot of drug concentration in the blood versus time). As can be seen from Figure 58-5, several useful pieces of information can be derived from such a profile. For example, the time at which the peak concentration occurs can be approximated and the peak concentration quantified. If the minimum concentration needed to maintain a desired effect is known, the onset and duration of effect also can be approximated. While useful information can be drawn casually from a simple graph as depicted in Figure 58-5, a more rigorous description of the pharmacokinetics of a drug is necessary to achieve the accuracy in dosage regimen design required for the safe and effective use of drugs. This higher degree of accuracy necessitates the development of mathematical models for describing the time course of absorption, distribution, metabolism, and elimination.

PHARMACOKINETIC MODELS

One of the primary objectives of pharmacokinetic models is to develop a quantitative method to describe the relationship of drug concentration or amount in the body as a function of time. The complexity of the pharmacokinetic model will vary with the route of administration, the extent and duration of distribution into various body fluids and tissues, the processes of elimination, and the intended application of the pharmacokinetic model. Often, numerous potential mathematical models exist for a particular drug. In such cases, the simplest model that will adequately and accurately describe the pharmacokinetics of the drug is the model that should be chosen.

There are a wide variety of potential uses for pharmacokinetic models, which include

1. Prediction of drug concentration in blood/plasma or tissue.
2. Calculation of a dosage regimen.
3. Quantitative assessment of the effect of disease on drug disposition.
4. Elucidation of the mechanism of disease-induced alterations in drug disposition.
5. Determination of the mechanism for drug-drug interactions.
6. Prediction of drug concentration versus effect relationships.

There are three primary types of pharmacokinetic models: compartmental, noncompartmental, and physiological.

Compartmental models describe the pharmacokinetics of drug disposition by grouping body tissues that are kinetically indistinguishable and describe the transfer of drug between body tissues in terms of rate constants.

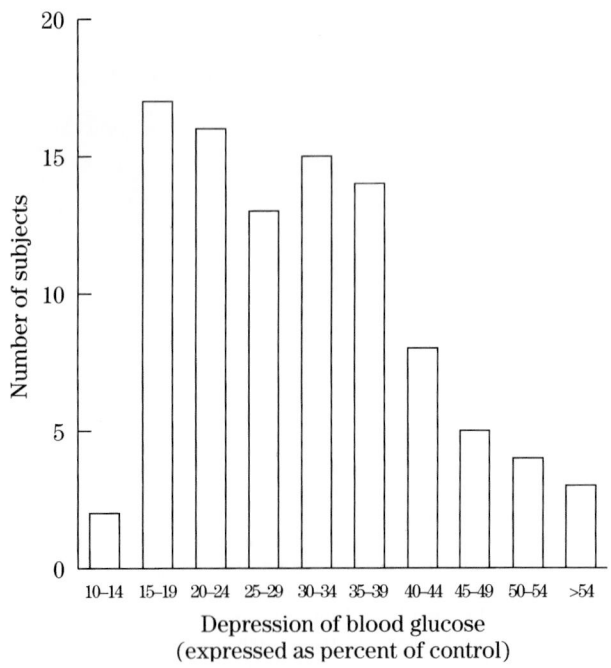

Figure 58-1. Decrease in blood glucose in 97 subjects 30 min after an intravenous dose of 1 g of tolbutamide. Note the large variability observed after the equivalent dose was administered in this group. (Data from Swerdloff RS, et al. *Diabetes* 1967; 16:161.)

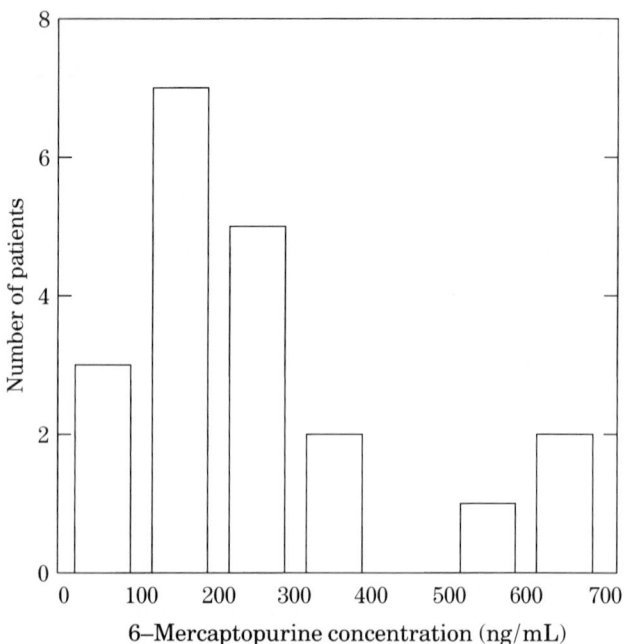

Figure 58-3. Distribution of peak 6-mercaptopurine concentrations achieved in a group of 20 patients receiving an oral dose of 1 mg/m². (Data from Sulh H, et al. *Clin Pharmacol Ther* 1986; 40:604.)

Noncompartmental models describe the pharmacokinetics of drug disposition using time- and concentration-averaged parameters.

Physiological models attempt to describe drug disposition in terms of realistic physiological parameters, such as blood flow and tissue-partition coefficients.

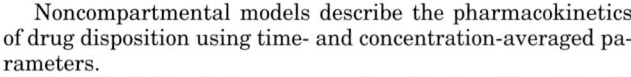

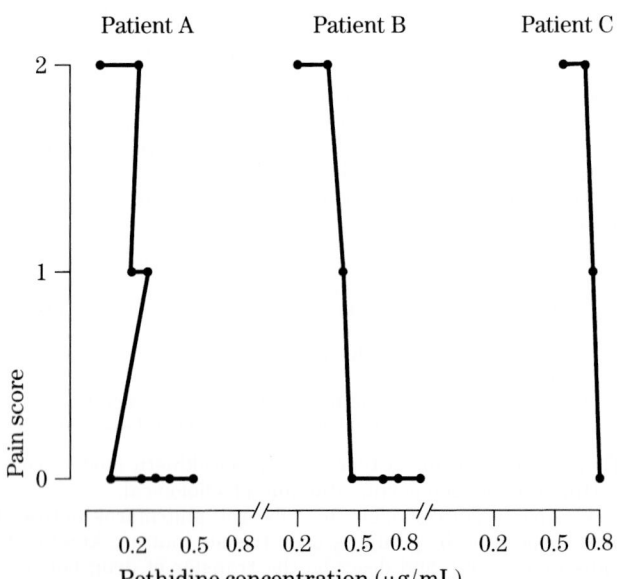

Figure 58-2. Blood-pethidine concentration-response curves for three individual patients, illustrating a typical range in interpatient responses. (From Edwards DJ, et al. *Clin Pharmacokinet* 1982; 7:421.)

RATES AND ORDERS OF REACTIONS

Many pharmacokinetic models use parameters that are analogous to rate constants in chemical kinetics. For example, consider the case of a drug (D) that is metabolized to a metabolite (M).

$$D \rightarrow M$$

This reaction may be described as a function of either the disappearance of the drug or as a function of the appearance of the metabolite. If the *amount* of the drug that is converted to a metabolite is a constant with respect to time, the reaction is said to be *zero-order* and is expressed as

$$\frac{-dD}{dt} = k_0 \tag{1}$$

where K_0 is the zero-order rate constant with units of mass per time (eg, mg/min). A plot of the time-course of the amount of the drug in the body that is converted to a metabolite by zero-order kinetics is shown in Figure 58-6. Integration of Equation 1 yields an equation for a straight line, which describes the amount of the drug in the body at any time (t):

$$\text{Amount}_t = -k_0 t + \text{Amount}_{t=0} = -k_0 t + \text{Dose} \tag{2}$$

Zero-order rate processes typically are found when an enzyme or transport system becomes saturated and the rate process becomes constant and cannot be increased by increases in the concentration of substrate. Zero-order rate processes are typical of constant-rate intravenous infusions and prolonged-release dosage forms.

If the amount of the drug in the body is converted to a metabolite at a rate that is a constant *fraction* of the amount of the drug in the body, the conversion of D to M is said to be a first-order reaction described by

$$\frac{dD}{dt} = -kD \tag{3}$$

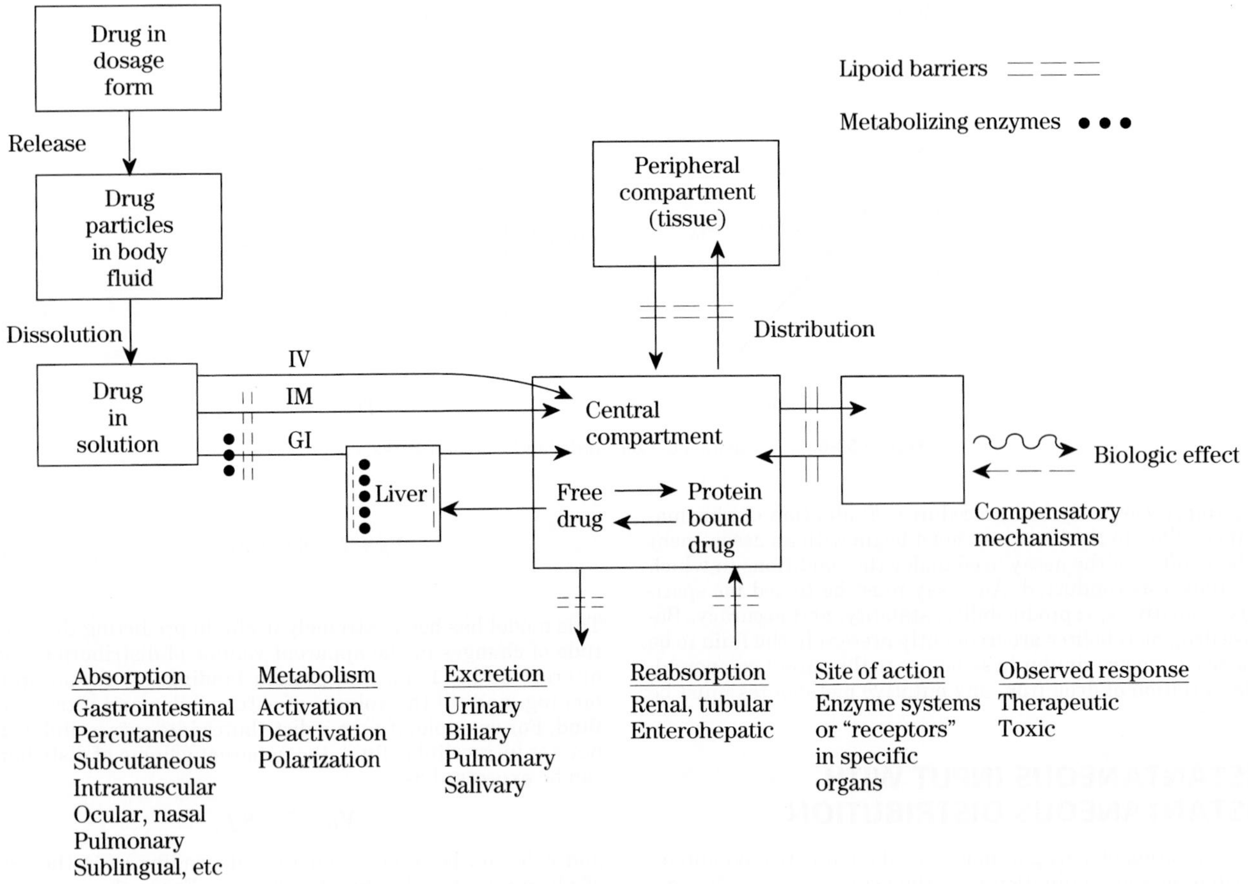

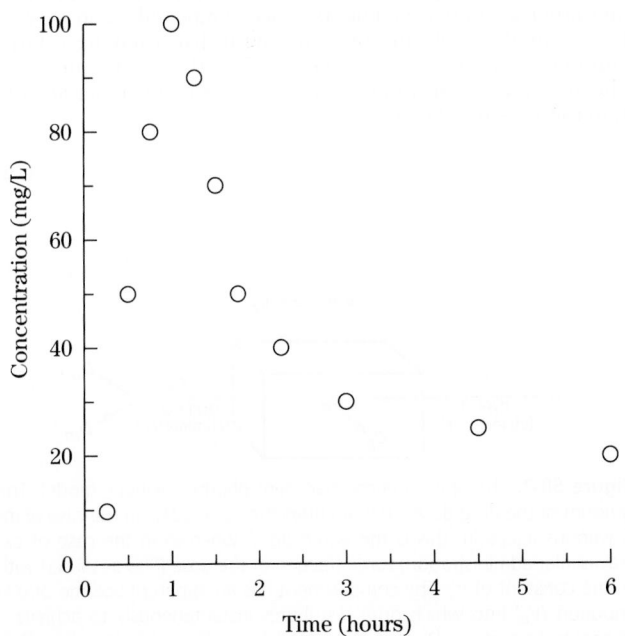

Figure 58-4. Diagram illustrating the factors that influence onset, duration, and intensity of drug effects. Note that the drug must dissolve before being absorbed and that it passes across many lipoid barriers and some metabolizing systems before reaching the site of action. (From Barr WH. *Am J Pharm Educ* 1968; 52:958.)

Figure 58-5. Hypothetical plot of drug-concentration data after oral administration of a drug.

where k is the first-order rate constant expressed in units of reciprocal time (eg, min^{-1}). Rearrangement of Equation 3 leads to

$$\frac{dD}{D} = -k dt \tag{4}$$

and integration of this expression yields

$$\int_0^t \frac{dD}{D} \Rightarrow \ln D = -kt + \ln D_0 \tag{5}$$

where ln is the natural logarithm. This equation also can be expressed in the exponential form

$$D_t = D_0 e^{-kt} \tag{6}$$

Graphically, the integrated form usually is expressed in terms of $\log_{10}$ rather than in natural logarithms (see Fig 58-6):

$$\log D = \frac{-kt}{2.303} + \log D_0 \tag{7}$$

ANALYTICAL CONSIDERATIONS

Any discussion of pharmacokinetics presumes that the drug concentrations can be determined with a high degree of accuracy and precision. One of the most frequent causes of high variability in pharmacokinetic parameters is poor data resulting

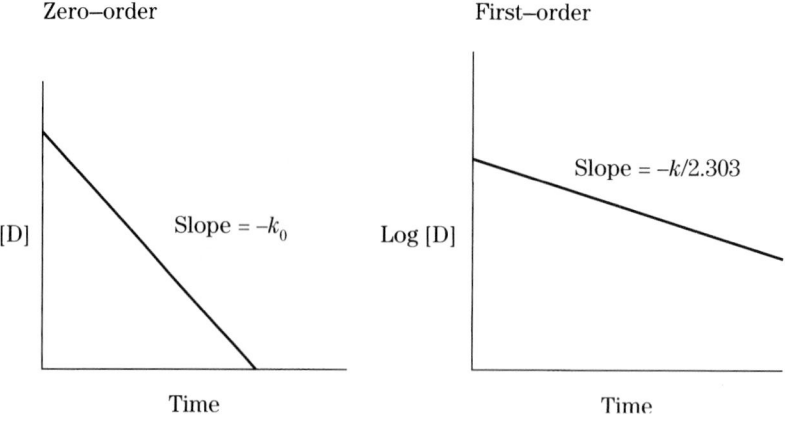

Figure 58-6. Plots illustrating a zero-order and a first-order reaction.

from imprecise analytical procedures. Evaluation of pharmacokinetic data in the literature must begin with an assessment of the validity of the assay used under the conditions in which the study was conducted. An assay must be tested for specificity, sensitivity, reproducibility, stability, and accuracy. Because drug metabolites are frequently present in the fluid to be measured and are similar in structure to the parent compound, differentiation of drug from any putative metabolites must be ensured.

INSTANTANEOUS INPUT WITH INSTANTANEOUS DISTRIBUTION

The disposition of a drug from its site of administration and its distribution and elimination from the body occurs via the vascular system. Most drugs are low-molecular-weight compounds of sufficient lipophilicity that they are able to distribute readily into the intra- and extracellular fluid compartments in the body. The transfer of drug from the circulation to these fluid compartments and then into tissues is called distribution. The pharmacokinetic parameter *volume of distribution* is a proportionality constant that relates drug concentration in a reference fluid, typically plasma, to the amount of drug distributed throughout the body.

$$\text{Volume of distribution } (V_D)$$
$$= \frac{\text{Amount of drug in body } (D_B)}{\text{Drug concentration } (Cp)} \quad (8)$$

Drugs that distribute widely to tissues will have large volumes of distribution and low plasma concentrations relative to the dose administered, whereas drugs that are highly bound to plasma proteins (eg, warfarin, phenylbutazone) or do not readily enter cells (eg, amikacin) will have low volumes of distribution and high plasma concentrations relative to the administered dose.

Øie and Tozer[5] have developed a physiological model for expression of the apparent volume of distribution, which takes into account the extracellular water, including plasma- and protein-binding of the drug in both plasma and tissue. For an average 70-kg male, total body water is about 42 L, of which 3 L is plasma and 12 L is extracellular fluid space. Moreover, 55–60% of the albumin in the extracellular space is found outside of plasma. Thus, for drugs that are largely bound to albumin, the apparent volume of distribution can be expressed as

$$V_D = 7 + 8f_u + V_T \left[\frac{f_u}{f_{u_T}} \right] \quad (9)$$

where f_u is the fraction of the drug in plasma that is unbound (often referred to as the *free fraction*), f_{uT} is the free fraction of drug in tissue, and V_T is the volume of intracellular tissue water. Equation 9 can be simplified further to

$$V_D = 7 + 8f_u + 27 \left[\frac{f_u}{f_{u_T}} \right] \quad (10)$$

This model has been extremely useful in predicting the magnitude of changes in the apparent volume of distribution due to alterations in (1) plasma protein binding, (2) tissue protein binding, and (3) the volume of extracellular and intracellular fluid. For example, if a drug distributes into extracellular fluid but not intracellular fluid, the apparent volume of distribution can be expressed as

$$V_D = 7 + 8f_u \quad (11)$$

and will vary between 7 and 15 L, depending upon the extent of plasma protein binding to albumin. For such a compound, with a relatively small volume of distribution, alterations in the plasma protein binding will not produce proportional changes in the apparent volume of distribution. Indeed, as reported by Williams et al,[6] the free fraction of tolbutamide in plasma increases in patients with cirrhosis by 28%, from 0.068 to 0.087, yet the apparent volume of distribution increases less than 10%, from 0.15 to 0.164 L/kg. Conversely, drugs with a volume of distribution greater than total body water indicate drug distribution and binding to tissue proteins and other cellular components. Such compounds also may be bound highly to plasma proteins. With drugs having a large volume of distribution (>50–100 L), the contribution of plasma and extracellular water space can be ignored, and Equation 3 simplifies to

$$V_D = 27 \left[\frac{f_u}{f_{u_T}} \right] \quad (12)$$

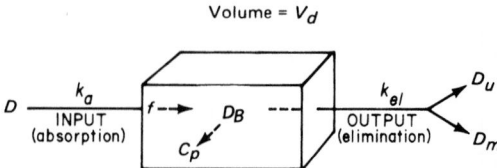

Figure 58-7. The open one-compartment pharmacokinetic model. The amount of the drug dose (D) that enters the body is D_B; in the case of intravenous injection, this is the entire dose, whereas in the case of extravascular administration, some fraction of the dose (F) is absorbed with a rate constant of k_a. The compartment has an apparent volume of distribution (V_d) into which drug distributes instantaneously to achieve a concentration of C_p. Drug is eliminated from the compartment with a rate constant k_{el}. D_u is the amount excreted into urine, feces, bile, expired air, sweat, milk, etc; D_m is the amount of drug metabolized.

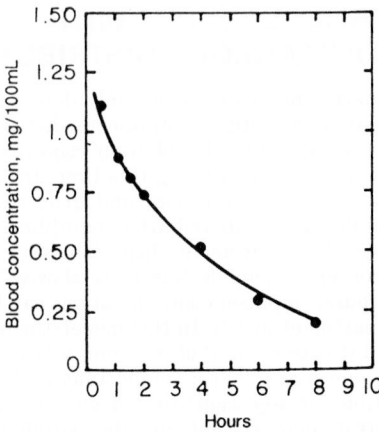

Figure 58-8. Elimination curve of average blood levels of theophylline in 11 human subjects after intravenous administration of 0.5 g aminophylline per 70 kg to each. (Data from Truitt EB Jr, et al. *J Pharmacol Exp Ther* 1950; 100:309.)

Changes in the plasma or plasma-free fraction will produce proportional changes in the apparent volume of distribution. For example, a twofold increase in the free fraction of drug in tissue, f_{uT}, will decrease the apparent volume of distribution by twofold. Less drug will be distributed to tissue, reflected by an increase in plasma concentrations. The volume necessary to account for the total amount of drug in the body will appear to have been decreased.

Once a drug is in the vascular system, it is transported by the blood to tissues where it can be eliminated from the circulation by distribution into tissue, metabolism by the tissue, or excretion from the tissue (see Fig 58-4). All of these processes lower the plasma concentration of drug. Each separate process may be described by a first-order rate constant, and the overall change in the plasma concentration is the net effect of all of these parallel, competing, first-order processes.

Intravenous injection of a drug that has nearly instantaneous distribution and first-order elimination can be described by an open one-compartment model (Fig 58-7). The body behaves as if it were a homogeneous compartment. In the one-compartment model, distribution is very rapid and can be considered instantaneous and is, therefore, ignored. After intravenous administration the plasma concentration declines exponentially according to

$$C = C_0 e^{-\lambda t} \qquad (13)$$

where C_0 is the initial concentration and λ is the overall elimination rate constant. Such an exponential elimination of theophylline given intravenously, is shown in Figure 58-8.[7] According to Equation 13, if the data of Figure 58-8 are plotted on semilog paper, a straight line should result, and such a plot is shown in Figure 58-9. Several derived data can be obtained from a plot of log concentration versus time. Extrapolation to zero time (ie, the y-intercept) gives an estimated theoretical concentration in plasma at time zero, from which the apparent volume of distribution (V_D) can be estimated by simply dividing the dose by C_0. It is a theoretical concentration because neither the injection nor distribution are actually instantaneous.

The *half-life* of a drug is the time required to reduce the amount of drug in the body or the plasma concentration by 50%. For a first-order process, the half-life is constant and is independent of the starting value of the amount of drug in the body (or plasma concentration). The plasma half-life, $t_{1/2}$, can be determined directly from the graph or from the elimination rate constant, λ or k_{el}, by means of the relationship

$$t_{1/2} = \frac{0.693}{\lambda} = \frac{0.693}{k_{el}} \qquad (14)$$

As shown, the half-life is related inversely to the elimination rate constant. When the elimination rate constant, k_{el}, is determined from the slope of the concentration versus time plot, one must keep in mind that the data need to be plotted on a semilog scale. From Figure 58-9, the k_{el} is determined to be 0.22 hr^{-1}. This is the instantaneous rate constant and indicates that 22% of the theophylline in the body is lost per hour. The rate constant for elimination (see Fig 58-7) is shown without reference to the route of elimination. It must be recognized that k_{el} represents the overall elimination by all competing, parallel pathways and is equal to the sum of the rate constants that define the various simultaneous (ie, parallel) contributory processes (eg, metabolism, renal excretion, or biliary secretion). Thus, the overall rate constant, $k_{el} = k_1 + k_2 + k_3 + \dots k_N$, where $k_1 + k_2 + k_3 + \dots k_N$ are the rate constants of the separate contributory processes.

Half-life is a clinically useful pharmacokinetic parameter in that it indicates when the next dose of a drug needs to be administered and is therefore helpful in designing an optimal dosing regimen. The half-life also is useful in determining

1. The fluctuation of plasma concentrations between doses;
2. The time required to reach steady-state equilibrium after beginning continuous drug administration; and
3. The persistence of drug in the system once drug administration has ceased.

Under some conditions, it is not possible to obtain plasma concentration data over sufficient time to obtain accurate estimates of the half-life for designing dosage regimens. The elimination rate constant, and hence the half-life, may be estimated from the excretion rate of unchanged drug. Because the first-order elimination rate constant is independent of the amount of drug in the body, the instantaneous excretion rate, dD_u/dt is directly proportional to the total amount of drug in the body.

$$\frac{dD_u}{dt} = k_e D_B \qquad (15)$$

where D_B and D_u are the amount of drug in the body at time zero and the amount of drug excreted in the urine, respectively, and k_e is the urinary excretion rate constant. A plot of log dD_u/dt versus time yields a straight line with slope of $-k_e/2.3$. One also may estimate the half-life from urinary excretion data using the cumulative amount of drug excreted (sigma-minus) method. Using this approach

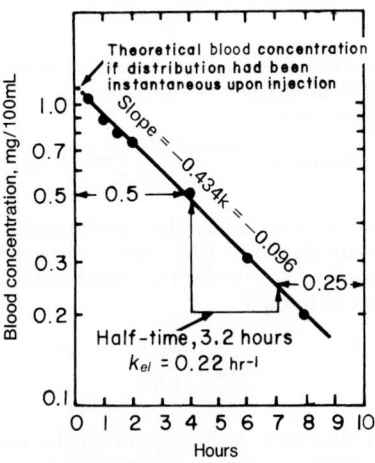

Figure 58-9. Semilog plot of the elimination curve in Figure 58-8. Note the log scale of the ordinate.

$$D_u = D_B \frac{k_u}{k_{el}} (1 - e^{-k_{el}t}) \qquad (16)$$

k_u/k_{el} represents the fraction of the drug in the body that eventually is excreted in urine as unchanged drug and D_u^∞ represents the total amount of unchanged drug excreted in urine. A plot of the log of the amount of drug remaining to be excreted $(D_u^\infty - D_u)$ versus time yields a slope equal to $-k_e /2.303$. This method requires collecting urine for at least 6 to 8 half-lives to achieve an accurate measure of D_u^∞.

For a drug eliminated by first-order kinetics, the elimination rate constant, k_{el}, can be expressed as the fraction of the volume of distribution that is presented to an eliminating organ and cleared of drug per unit time *(clearance)* relative to the total volume of distribution, V_D. Thus, k_{el} represents the fractional removal rate of drug from the system, and the elimination rate constant can be expressed in terms of clearance and volume of distribution:

$$\frac{\text{Clearance}}{V_D} = \text{Elimination-rate constant } (k_{el}) \qquad (17)$$

As written in Equation 17, the elimination rate constant (and hence, plasma half-life) is a dependent parameter that, by itself, is not always the most reliable indicator of drug removal from the body. Disease or altered physiology (eg, aging, pregnancy) can alter protein binding, thereby affecting the apparent volume of distribution, or alter organ function, thereby affecting clearance, but these changes may not be reflected by changes in the half-life. For example, the volume of distribution may be altered due to changes in tissue or plasma protein binding, independent of specific organ function (clearance). In this instance, the half-life of a drug may be changed, but clearance could remain constant. Although a useful parameter, one must always bear in mind that half-life is a dependent or derived parameter that does not reliably reflect irreversible removal of drug from the body. A more accurate way to express half-life (Equation 14) therefore is

$$t_{1/2} = 0.693 \frac{V_D}{CL} \qquad (18)$$

Clearance is the most useful pharmacokinetic indicator of irreversible loss of drug from the body and refers to a volume of fluid from which drug appears to be removed in a given amount of time. Clearance also can be expressed as the quotient of overall rate of elimination of a drug relative to the drug concentration at a particular organ of elimination,

$$\text{Clearance} = \frac{\text{Rate of elimination}}{\text{Concentration}} \qquad (19)$$

and, if time-averaged over the time course of plasma concentrations, drug clearance can be expressed as

$$\text{Clearance} = \frac{\text{Amount of drug removed}}{AUC} \qquad (20)$$

where AUC is the area under the concentration-versus-time curve. Total body clearance, CL_T, also can be estimated as the quotient of dose and area under the concentration-versus-time curve from zero to infinity.

$$CL_T = \frac{\text{Dose}_{IV}}{AUC_0^\infty} \qquad (21)$$

Total body clearance is the sum of all the separate clearances that contribute to drug elimination

$$CL_T = CL_{RENAL} + CL_{HEPATIC} + CL_{OTHER} \qquad (22)$$

INSTANTANEOUS INPUT WITH NONINSTANTANEOUS DISTRIBUTION

The one-compartment model adequately describes the pharmacokinetics of drugs with instantaneous distribution. However, for some compounds, distribution requires some finite time to reach equilibrium. During this time, the drug undergoes distribution and elimination, and drug concentrations decrease rapidly. When distribution equilibrium is established, the loss of drug from the body is due to elimination, and plasma concentrations decline more slowly. This biexponential time-course of plasma concentrations can be described by a two-compartment model. In this model, the body appears to behave as if it is comprised of two compartments, a central compartment and a peripheral compartment. By convention, drug absorption (or injection) and drug elimination occur from the central compartment and the peripheral compartment is closed and communicates with the environment only through the central compartment (Fig 58-10). The movement of drug between compartments following rapid intravenous injection with elimination from the central compartment can be described by

$$\frac{dD_1}{dt} = k_{21}D_2 - k_{12}D_1 - k_{10}D_1$$

and

$$\frac{dD_2}{dt} = k_{12}D_1 - k_{21}D_2 \qquad (23)$$

where D_2 is the amount of drug in the peripheral or tissue compartment, D_1 is the amount of drug in the central compartment, k_{21} and k_{12} are the apparent first-order intercompartmental distribution rate constants, and k_{10} or k_{el} is the apparent first-order elimination rate constant from Compartment 1.

After intravenous injection of a drug that obeys two-compartment pharmacokinetics, the plasma concentration de-

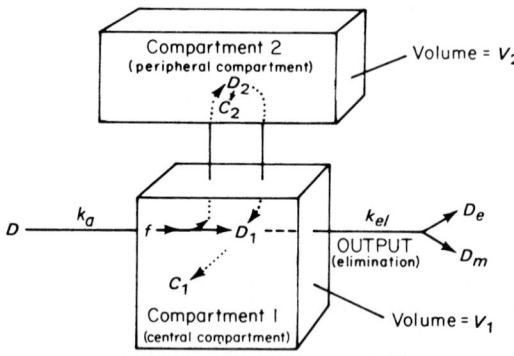

Figure 58-10. Diagram of open two-compartment pharmacokinetic model. The amount of dose that enters the body for an intravenous injection is the entire dose, and administration is instantaneous. The amount of dose absorbed from an extravascular dose is $F D$, where F is the fraction of dose absorbed with a rate constant, k_a. Some of the absorbed drug enters Compartment 2 with a first-order rate constant of k_{12} and is returned to Compartment 1 with a first-order rate constant of k_{21}. D_1 is the amount of drug in Compartment 1, and D_2 in Compartment 2; C_1 and C_2 are the respective concentrations in Compartments 1 and 2 $(C_1 = C_p)$. Drug is eliminated from Compartment 1 with a first-order rate constant, k_{el}, which, however, is obscured by the lag in transfer of drug from Compartment 2 to Compartment 1. D_u is the amount excreted into urine, feces, expired air, sweat, milk, etc; D_m is the amount of drug metabolized. The relative volumes V_1 and V_2 may vary greatly, V_1 sometimes being the larger and other times the smaller.

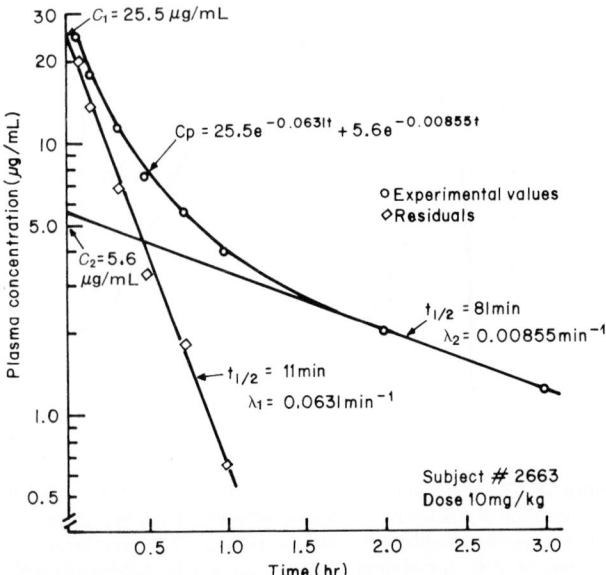

Figure 58-11. Resolution of the plasma concentration curve for pralidoxime into its distribution and elimination components after intravenous administration. Note that plasma concentration is plotted on a logarithmic scale. The time constant for the elimination phase is determined from the slope, $-0.434 \lambda_2$; it is a hybrid constant and λ_2 is not the same as k_{el} (see text). Likewise, the time constant for distribution, λ_1, is obtained from the slope, $-0.434\lambda_1$, of the distribution line; λ_1 is also a hybrid constant. (From Gibaldi M, Perrier D. *Pharmacokinetics,* 2nd ed. New York: Dekker, 1982.)

clines in a complex biexponential fashion. When plotted on semilog graph paper, the separate processes of distribution and elimination can be identified by the method of residuals (Fig 58-11).[8] Figure 58-11 shows such a resolution of the biexponential decay into the two components of distribution and elimination. From the slopes and intercepts of the residuals, the plasma concentration, C, at any time, t, can be described as the sum of two exponentials, namely

$$C = C_1 e^{-\lambda_1 t} + C_2 e^{-\lambda_2 t} \qquad (24)$$

where

$$C_1 = \frac{Dose(\lambda_1 - k_{21})}{V_1(\lambda_1 - \lambda_2)} \qquad (25)$$

and

$$C_2 = \frac{Dose(k_{21} - \lambda_2)}{V_1(\lambda_1 - \lambda_2)} \qquad (26)$$

Distribution is more rapid than elimination, such that at some point, the first term in Equation 24, $C_1 e^{\lambda_1}{}_1 t$ approaches zero and the biological half-life can be determined from the slope of the terminal phase

$$t_{1/2} = \frac{0.693}{\lambda_2} \qquad (27)$$

$C1$, $C2$, λ_1, and λ_2 are hybrid constants, representing the intercepts, $C1$, $C2$, and slopes, λ_1, λ_2, of the two exponential phases, which can be obtained by computer-fitting the biexponential data. The zero-time intercept of the central compartment, V_1, and the actual pharmacokinetic parameters k_{12}, k_{21}, and k_{el} can be derived from the hybrid rate constants using the following relationships. At time $t = 0$

$$C_0 = C_1 + C_2; V_1 = \frac{Dose}{C_1 + C_2} \qquad (28)$$

The hybrid rate constants, λ_1 and λ_2, can be defined using the following two equations:

$$\lambda_1 \lambda_1 = k_{21} k_{el} \qquad (29)$$

$$\lambda_1 + \lambda_1 = k_{12} + k_{21} + k_{el} \qquad (30)$$

Thus

$$k_{el} = \frac{\lambda_1 \lambda_2}{k_{21}} \qquad (31)$$

$$k_{21} = \frac{C_1 \lambda_2 + C_2 \lambda_1}{\lambda_1 - \lambda_2} \qquad (32)$$

$$k_{12} = \lambda_1 + \lambda_2 - k_{21} - k_{el} \qquad (33)$$

The reader is referred to Gibaldi and Perrier (see *Bibliography*) for a more in-depth derivation of these expressions. The slope of the final phase of biexponential disposition, λ_2, can be related to the elimination-rate constant, k_{el}, by

$$\lambda_2 = f_C k_{el} \qquad (34)$$

where f_C is the fraction of the drug that is in the central compartment after distribution equilibrium has been achieved. After distribution, the fraction of the drug in the central compartment is a constant.

$$f_C = \frac{k_{21} - \lambda_2}{k_{21} + k_{12} - \lambda_2} \qquad (35)$$

The terminal disposition constant, λ_2, reflects disposition from the entire body and is a function of distribution and elimination. The rate constant, k_{el}, represents only elimination from the theoretical central compartment.

The volume of distribution, V_D, can be determined in a two-compartment system; however, the estimation is complicated by the noninstantaneous nature of the distribution phase between the two compartments and results in the apparent volume of distribution being time-dependent. From Equation 18, it can be seen that the volume of distribution of the central compartment, V_1, can be obtained following administration of an intravenous dose, D_{IV}, of drug from

$$V_1 = \frac{D_{IV}}{C_1 + C_2} \qquad (36)$$

Clearance can be calculated from the product of k_{el} and V_1, and the volume of the central compartment can be expressed as

$$V_1 = \frac{D_{IV}}{k_{10}[AUC]_{0 \to \infty}} \qquad (37)$$

The most accurate method of estimating the volume of distribution is to estimate the steady-state volume of distribution. The volume of distribution at the steady state, V_{SS}, represents the steady state with respect to distribution of the drug from the central compartment to the tissue compartments and is not altered by changes in drug elimination or clearance. The total amount of the drug in the body at the steady state is the sum of the amounts in all compartments, thus

$$V_{SS} = V_1 + \frac{k_{12}}{k_{21}} V_1 \qquad (38)$$

Notice that V_{SS} is independent of the elimination rate constant, k_{el}, and λ_2.

The volume of distribution by area, V_β, is an alternate method of estimating the apparent volume of distribution and relies on the assumption that the plasma and the amount of drug in the body decline in parallel during the postdistributive phase.

$$V_\beta = \frac{V_1 k_{ei}}{\lambda_2} \qquad (39)$$

The least accurate method of estimating the volume of distribution for a drug that follows biexponential elimination kinetics is by extrapolation, V_{EXTRAP}, because changes in distribution can alter the estimation of the hybrid intercept, C_2.

$$V_{EXTRAP} = \frac{D_{IV}}{C_2} \qquad (40)$$

Distribution to various tissues depends upon both blood flow to that tissue and the rate of uptake (effective partition coefficient) into a particular tissue and its cells. The overall pattern of drug distribution is governed by both tissue perfusion and diffusion of drug within tissues. Tissues with the highest blood flow, such as liver, kidney, and brain, equilibrate more rapidly than tissues that are perfused less well, such as skin and fat. Once in the tissue vasculature, drug distribution into tissue is controlled largely by diffusional barriers of cell membranes. Rowland and Tozer (see *Bibliography*) present a useful expression for the first-order rate constant for distribution of drug into tissue.

$$k_{TISSUE} = \frac{(Q/V_{TISSUE})}{k_{PARTITION}} \qquad (41)$$

where $k_{PARTITION}$ is the equilibrium distribution ratio of tissue and venous drug concentration, Q is tissue blood flow, V_{TISSUE} is the tissue volume, and the quotient of Q and V_{TISSUE} is the tissue perfusion rate. The time to reach tissue equilibrium is the reciprocal of Equation 41. For a poorly perfused tissue such as fat, the $k_{PARTITION}$ may be quite high and the Q/V_{TISSUE} low, resulting in a long time to reach tissue equilibrium. Even for highly perfused tissues, such as the brain, the distribution of some drugs may be quite variable and will depend upon diffusion across cell membranes. In this case, distribution is said to be diffusion-rate-limited and will depend upon both the oil-to-water partition coefficient and the degree of ionization at physiological pH.

For most drugs, distribution usually occurs more rapidly than elimination, resulting in complete distribution before most of the drug has been eliminated. For some drugs, once injected, distribution is so rapid that the overall plasma-concentration time-course represents elimination (see Fig 58-7). Thus, both administration and distribution appear to be instantaneous, and the pharmacokinetics can be modeled by the simplest one-compartment model (see Fig 58-7). For such a drug, the volume of distribution can be calculated as the quotient of the intravenous dose and the extrapolated plasma concentration at time zero, C_0.

CONTINUOUS INPUT

It is sometimes desirable to administer a drug continuously to maintain constant plasma concentration. This is often the case for drugs with very rapid elimination or for those that have a low therapeutic index. Continuous input commonly is thought of in terms of intravenous infusion; however, sustained-release oral dosage forms and delivery of drugs through the skin from patches also are examples of continuous input, and the pharmacokinetics of drug administration is similar for all systems with continuous input.

With constant intravenous infusion, the plasma concentration rises in a logarithmic fashion and eventually reaches a plateau (Fig 58-12).[8] The time to reach the plateau or steady-state concentration is determined by the elimination rate constant. The rate of change of drug in the body (D_B) during a constant rate infusion (R_0) is the difference between the zero-order infusion rate and the first-order elimination rate.

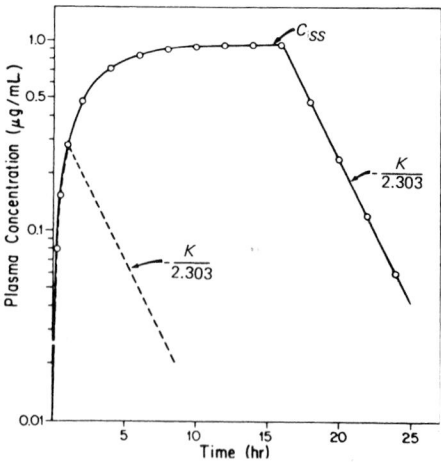

Figure 58-12. Semilogarithmic plot of plasma concentration during and after cessation of a constant intravenous infusion of a drug in a one-compartment system. Whether infusion is stopped prior to the attainment of a plateau or after, the plasma concentration will fall log-linearly with a slope of $-0.434k_{el}$. In the figure, K is k_{el} and $1/2.303 = 0.434$. C_{ss} is the steady-state concentration, C_p^{ss}. (From Gibaldi M, Perrier D. *Pharmacokinetics*, 2nd ed. New York: Dekker, 1982.)

$$\frac{dD_B}{dt} = R_0 - (k_{el} \cdot D_B) \qquad (42)$$

The plasma concentration (C) at any time during the constant infusion is

$$C = \frac{R_0}{CL_T}(1 - e^{-k_{el}t_{inf}}) \qquad (43)$$

where t_{inf} equals the time of the infusion. As the time of the infusion increases, the exponential expression approaches zero, and the concentration approaches steady state. At steady state, the rate of infusion is equal to the rate of elimination, and the simplified expression can be expressed as

$$C_{SS} = \frac{R_0}{CL_T} \qquad (44)$$

The fraction of the steady state that is achieved in some time, t_{inf}, after the start of the infusion can be calculated as

$$\frac{C}{C_{SS}} = (1 - e^{-k_{el}t_{inf}}) \qquad (45)$$

and can be expressed in terms of half-lives as

$$\frac{C}{C_{SS}} = (1 - 2^{-n}) \qquad (46)$$

where n is the ratio of infusion time and half-life. For example, when the infusion time equals three half-lives ($n = 3$), the concentration is at 87.5% of the steady state, and when the infusion has lasted for four half-lives ($n = 4$), the concentration has achieved 93.75% of the steady state. Theoretically, one never reaches steady-state conditions because this is an exponential process; however, for clinical purposes one can assume, with little error, that steady-state concentrations are achieved within four to five half-lives.

If a drug has a relatively long half-life and the therapeutic situation demands rapid attainment of therapeutic plasma concentrations, it is sometimes desirable to give a loading dose at the beginning of the constant-rate infusion. The loading dose should approximate the amount of drug in the body at steady state. If the apparent volume of distribution and target concentration is known, the loading dose can be calculated simply as

$$Dose_{LOADING} = (\text{Target concentration})(V_D) \qquad (47)$$

The plasma concentration is the sum of the contributions from the loading dose and the infusion and can be estimated at any time after the loading dose has been given and infusion started from

$$C = \frac{Dose_{LOADING}}{V_D}(e^{-k_{el}t}) + \frac{R_0}{CL_T}(1 - e^{-k_{el}t_{inf}}) \tag{48}$$

and if the half-life of the drug is known, the loading dose can be estimated from the quotient of infusion rate, R_0, and elimination rate constant, k_{el}. For some drugs, such as lidocaine, the entire loading dose cannot be given in a single bolus injection because there is a significant distribution phase. In such a case, fractional loading-dose schemes can be used in which the loading dose is divided into several smaller bolus doses and given during the beginning of the infusion.

Finally, it should be noted that whether or not a loading dose is given, the attainment of steady state is determined by the elimination half-life and not by the rate of the infusion or the use of bolus loading doses to achieve concentrations rapidly.

MULTIPLE-DOSE ADMINISTRATION

Continuous administration of a drug is often impractical, and multiple-dose regimens are used to maintain the concentration of a drug within an acceptable range that mimimizes the development of toxicity and avoids loss of efficacy. Usually, the dose of a drug is administered with a constant dose interval, referred to as τ. Some features of a multiple dosage scheme are shown in Figure 58-13. The drug is administered at a fixed dose and a fixed interval. Each successive dose is administered before the previous dose has been eliminated entirely, and thus drug accumulation occurs. As with the constant intravenous infusion, the time to reach a steady-state fluctuation depends upon the elimination half-life and not on the size of the dose or the dosing interval. In Figure 58-13, the dose, D, is administered at a dosing interval equal to the half-life. After the first dose is given, the amount of drug in the body is equal to that dose. When the next dose is given, the amount of drug in the body is

equal to $D + 0.5D$. At the end of each dose interval, the total amount of drug in the body is half of the postinjection peak and is the sum of the amount remaining from all of the previous doses. The maximum, $C_{MAX,SS}$, and minimum, $C_{MIN,SS}$, concentrations at steady state are described by

$$C_{MAX,SS} = \frac{Dose/V_D}{(1 - e^{-k_{el}\tau})} \tag{49}$$

and

$$C_{MIN,SS} = C_{MAX,SS}e^{-k_{el}\tau} \tag{50}$$

The concentration at the midpoint of a dosing interval at the steady state is a time-averaged concentration, C_{AV}, over the entire dosing interval and is described by

$$C_{AV} = \frac{D_{IV}}{V_D k_{el}\tau} = \frac{1.44t_{1/2}D_{IV}}{\tau} \tag{51}$$

NONCOMPARTMENTAL ANALYSIS FOLLOWING INSTANTANEOUS INPUT

There are numerous disadvantages associated with viewing drug disposition from a compartmental perspective, not the least of which is the lack of physiological relevance of such models. Noncompartmental models have been developed and are generally the *preferred* method for assessing overall drug disposition, in part because parameters such as volume of distribution and clearance can be calculated directly from the data, without computer fitting. Moreover, parameters estimated by these methods generally are less sensitive to variability in the data. Noncompartmental methods characterize drug disposition using time- and concentration-averaged parameters and have been described by Jusko.[9] This analysis also is known as nonparametric analysis and assumes that all processes are first-order and that the parameters of the model reflect steady-state behavior. A primary tool used in this methodology is that of statistical moments.[10]

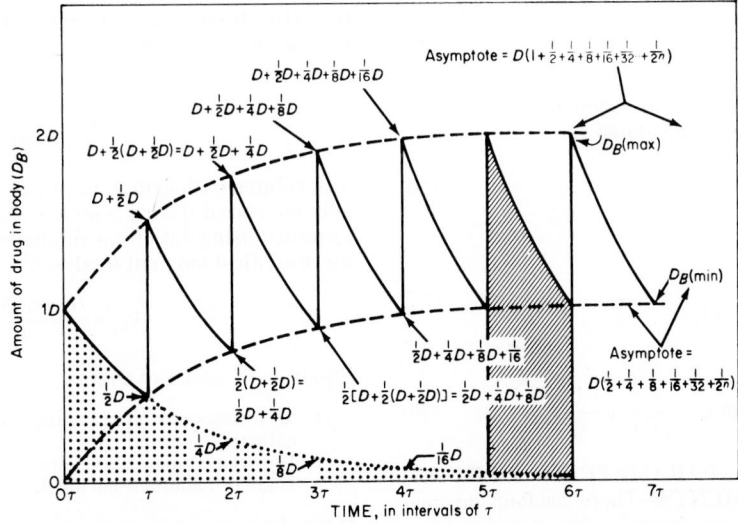

Figure 58-13. The accumulation of drug in the body during a regimen of multiple dosing. Dose, *D,* is administered intravenously at intervals, τ, equal to the half-life, $t_{1/2}$. Thus, after each dose, the amount in the body, D_B, has decreased to half the previous peak amount at the time each dose is administered. When the cumulated amount in the body after injection reaches 2*D,* the body content will fluctuate from 2*D* to 1*D* during each dose interval thereafter. Approximately five half-lives are required before this leveling off (plateau) of the body content occurs. The stippled area is the area under the elimination curve of a single injection, if no second dose had been given. The cross-hatched area is the area under the curve during a single-dose interval at steady state. The two areas are equal.

STATISTICAL MOMENTS—The use of statistical moments in the analysis of the time-course of drug concentrations is especially useful because it frees the investigator from the use of such models as the compartmental, which often are derived empirically and do not represent physiological events.

The time-course of drug concentration in blood generally can be viewed as a statistical distribution curve and described in a similar manner as any other array of data. A moment is simply a mathematical description of a discrete distribution of data. In the field of statistics, for example, the sample size (n), mean, and variance are the zero (M_0), first (M_1) and second (M_2) moments, respectively, for an array of data. In physics, for example, weight, center of mass, and moment of inertia represent (M_0), (M_1), and (M_2), respectively.

In statistics, the mean of a population is estimated by the sample mean. Similarly, in pharmacokinetics one may calculate estimates of the true function that describes the drug concentration versus time using statistical moments. Assume the existence of a theoretical relationship for $C(t)$ as a function of time. The nonnormalized moments, S_r, where $r = 0, 1, 2, \ldots,$ m^{th} moment, about the origin are calculated as

$$S_r = \int_0^\infty t^r C(t)\, dt \quad (r = 0, 1, 2, \ldots m) \tag{52}$$

Hence

$$S_0 = \int_0^\infty C(t)\, dt = AUC \tag{53}$$

$$S_1 = \int_0^\infty t C(t)\, dt = AUMC \tag{54}$$

where $AUMC$ is the area under the $C \cdot t$ versus time curve, whereas S_0 and S_1 are the zero and first nonnormalized moments, respectively. These two parameters, AUC and $AUMC$, are derived from the drug concentration versus time data and are used to calculate the pharmacokinetic parameters of interest.

The use of noncompartmental methods requires a means of determining the AUC. While several methods are available for such determinations, the simplest is the use of the trapezoidal rule.[11] This permits calculation of the AUC or the $AUMC$ from zero to the time of the last sample (t^n). However, it generally is necessary to determine the area from zero to infinity. If one assumes that there is log-linear decline from t^n to infinity, then

$$AUC_{t^n}^\infty = \int_{t^n}^\infty C\, dt = \frac{C^n}{\lambda_Z} \tag{55}$$

where λ_Z is the slope of the terminal exponential. Thus, the AUC from zero to infinity can be calculated as

$$AUC_0^\infty = AUC_0^{t^n} + \frac{C^n}{\lambda_Z} \tag{56}$$

for the $AUMC$

$$AUMC_{t^n}^\infty = \frac{C^n}{(\lambda_Z)^2} + \frac{t^n C^n}{\lambda_Z} \tag{57}$$

and

$$AUMC_0^\infty = AUMC_\infty^{t^n} + \frac{C^n}{(\lambda_Z)^2} + \frac{t^n C^n}{\lambda_Z} \tag{58}$$

PHARMACOKINETIC PARAMETERS DERIVED FROM STATISTICAL MOMENTS—There are four parameters of primary interest that are derived using statistical moments, the most important of which is clearance. A conceptual consideration of clearance is provided by considering an organ through which blood containing a drug flows.

where Q_{IN}, Q_{OUT}, C_A, and C_V are the blood flow in and out and the concentration of the drug in arterial and venous blood, respectively. If $C_V < C_A$, the organ is capable of elimination and is referred to as a clearing organ, or an organ of elimination. The elimination of a drug can be described using mass balance considerations:

$$\text{Rate of the drug entering the organ} = QC_A \tag{59}$$

$$\text{Rate of the drug leaving the organ} = QC_V \tag{60}$$

Rate of elimination of the drug

$$= QC_A - QC_V = Q(C_A - C_V) \tag{61}$$

The ratio of the rate of drug elimination and the rate at which the drug enters the organ is defined as the *extraction ratio, E*.

$$E = \frac{\text{Rate of elimination}}{\text{Rate of entry}} = \frac{Q(C_A - C_V)}{QC_A} = \frac{(C_A - C_V)}{C_A} \tag{62}$$

The extraction ratio is a measure of the efficiency with which an organ eliminates a drug. From this parameter, the organ clearance of a drug can be described as

$$CL_T = QE = \frac{Q(C_A - C_V)}{C_A} \tag{63}$$

Recall that clearance is defined as the volume of blood from which all of the drug would appear to be removed per unit time. By analogy to the definition of organ clearance, one can define the total or systemic clearance as the ratio of overall elimination rate, dX/dt, to drug concentration in blood, C:

$$CL_T = \frac{dX/dt}{C} \tag{64}$$

Integrating from zero to infinity yields

$$CL_T = \frac{\int_0^\infty \frac{dX}{dt}\, dt}{\int_0^\infty C\, dt} \tag{65}$$

where the numerator is the total amount of the drug ultimately eliminated (the IV dose) and the denominator is the AUC from zero to infinity. Thus, the total clearance is the quotient of intravenous dose and the AUC from zero to infinity.

$$CL_T = \frac{Dose_{IV}}{AUC_0^\infty} \tag{66}$$

The volume of distribution at the steady-state, V_{SS}, most reliably measured during a steady-state infusion, now can be determined using data from single-dose experiments and employing statistical moment analysis.[12]

$$V_{SS} = \frac{(Dose_{IV})(AUMC)}{(AUC)^2} \tag{67}$$

Equation 67 assumes that

1. All processes involved in drug disposition (eg, distribution, elimination) are linear.
2. The drug is administered to and eliminated via the sampling site.
3. There is instantaneous input.

If the drug is administered via a short infusion, the volume of distribution at the steady state can be estimated from

$$V_{SS} = \frac{(R_0 T)(AUMC)}{(AUC)^2} - \frac{R_0 T^2}{2(AUC)} \tag{68}$$

where R_0 is the rate of infusion and T is the duration of the infusion.

Another important pharmacokinetic parameter that can be determined using statistical moment analysis is the *systemic availability, F,* which is a measure of the fraction of the administered dose that reaches the systemic circulation following oral administration. This parameter can be calculated as

$$F = \frac{AUC_{PO}Dose_{IV}}{AUC_{IV}Dose_{PO}} \quad (69)$$

where AUC_{PO} and $Dose_{PO}$ are the oral area under the concentration-versus-time curve and oral dose, respectively.

When administering a drug, the amount administered in terms of gross weight (eg, mg, g, or μ g) often is considered. It is, however, probably more appropriate to focus on *molecules* when considering pharmacokinetic and pharmacodynamic events. Even the administration of a relatively small dose of drug may represent a large number of molecules. Consider the administration of 1 mg of a drug with a molecular weight of 300 daltons. The number of molecules in this dose is approximately 2×10^{18}. Instantaneous administration of the entire dose will result in drug molecules spending various amounts of time in the body. After the intravenous injection of a drug, one can imagine that some of the drug molecules are eliminated immediately, whereas some of the molecules require a longer time to be eliminated, and some molecules even require a very long time to be eliminated. The time spent in the body, for a given molecule, is its residence time. The *mean residence time, MRT,* is the sum of all the residence times divided by the number of molecules. A conceptual understanding of this can be gained from the following example.

Assume a child receives 20 dimes for his birthday and immediately places them in his piggy bank. Over the next month, he periodically removes one or more dimes from the piggy bank to purchase candy. Specifically, 3 days after placing the coins in his bank, he removes 5 dimes, on day 10 he removes 4 dimes, on day 21 he removes 6 dimes, and on day 30 he removes 5 dimes. At the 30th day after placing the coins in his bank, all of the coins have been removed. Hence, the *elimination* of dimes from the bank is complete. The *MRT* of dimes in the piggy bank is simply the sum of the times that coins spend in the bank divided by the number of dimes placed in the bank:

$$MRT =$$
$$\frac{\begin{matrix} 3+3+3+3+3+10+10+10+10+21+21 \\ +21+21+21+21+30+30+30+30+30 \end{matrix}}{20}$$

$$MRT = \frac{3*5 + 10*4 + 21*6 + 30*5}{20}$$

$$MRT = 16.55 \text{ days}$$

This provides a relationship with which one can determine the *MRT* for any given number of drug molecules, A_i, which spend a given amount of time in the body of, t_i, thus

$$MRT = \frac{\sum_{i=1}^{n} A_i t_i}{A_{TOTAL}} \quad (70)$$

where *n* equals the total number of residence times. The mean rate of drug leaving the body relative to the total amount eliminated also can be expressed in terms of concentration.

$$MRT = \frac{\int_0^\infty tC(t)\,dt}{\int_0^\infty C(t)\,dt} = \frac{AUMC}{AUC} \quad (71)$$

Equation 71 is not a definition of *MRT*, rather it is the derived expression from which one can calculate *MRT* when clearance is constant. The mean residence time assumes instantaneous administration, and therefore, it is technically incorrect to calculate the mean residence time following an oral dose using the

quotient of $AUMC_{PO}$ and AUC_{PO}. When calculated in this manner, it often is stated that the *MRT* is a function of the route of administration. Actually, *MRT* is *independent* of the route of administration because the mean time that molecules reside in the body is not influenced by the route of administration.[13] However, the interpretation of the ratio of *AUMC* and *AUC* does change as a function of administration because this ratio only yields the *MRT* when the input is instantaneous.

A better way to express the route dependence of the *AUMC/AUC* is to refer to this ratio as the *mean transit time, MTT*. The *MTT* is the average time required for drug molecules to leave a kinetic system after administration. Thus, because an IV bolus assumes instant input,

$$AUMC_{IV}/AUC_{IV} = MRT = MTT_{IV} \quad (72)$$

whereas

$$AUMC_{PO}/AUC_{PO} = MTT_{PO} = MTT_{IV} + MAT$$
$$= MRT + MAT \quad (73)$$

where *MAT* is the mean absorption time. Thus, for oral absorption, the *AUMC/AUC* provides an *MTT* in the kinetic system that is composed of the gastrointestinal (GI) tract and the body. The *MRT* also can be calculated as the quotient of the V_{SS} and clearance. Finally, one can relate the *MRT* to the elimination half-life by considering the situation in which a drug displays monoexponential decline. The *MRT* can be written as

$$MRT = \frac{AUMC}{AUC} = \frac{C_0/\lambda^2}{C_0/\lambda} = \frac{1}{\lambda} \quad (74)$$

and represents the time required for 63.2% of an intravenous dose to be eliminated from the body.

ABSORPTION

If a drug is administered intravenously in a single, rapid injection, the process of absorption is bypassed. The time for this injection is typically so short compared with other pharmacokinetic processes that it is ignored. As previously described for a one-compartment model, peak plasma concentration and distribution equilibrium are achieved instantaneously. This is depicted in Figure 58-14A.[14] In the model for the figure, there is no elimination, and the concentration remains constant following administration. With a constant intravenous infusion (B), the concentration rises rectilinearly so long as the infusion is maintained at a constant, zero-order rate. With other routes of administration, there are delays in the appearance of drug in the vascular system because the drug must be absorbed from the site of administration (oral, intramuscular, subcutaneous, rectal). Drug absorption depends upon both the physicochemical properties of the drug (pK$_a$, dosage form, partition coeffi-

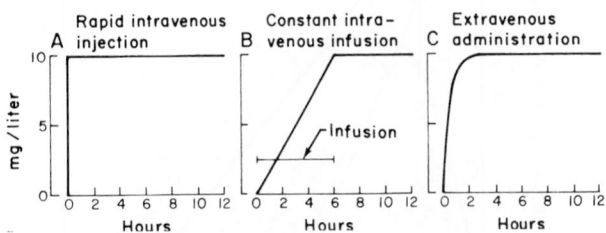

Figure 58-14. Time-concentration curves for injection *(A)*, infusion *(B)*, and extravenous *(C)* administration of drug in the one- compartment model. The volume of the compartment is 100 L (V_d = 100 L); the amount of drug administered in each instance is 1000 mg. Drug elimination has been set to zero, so that the time- concentration curve for each model of administration can be examined without the complication of simultaneous elimination. (Adapted from Bigger JT. *Am J Med* 1975; 58:479.)

cient) and the physiology of the site of absorption (surface area, blood flow). Most drugs are absorbed by simple diffusion, and the kinetics are first-order. Zero-order absorption occurs for some processes that are saturable and for sustained-release dosage forms. Absorption and elimination of a drug are a sequential process, and the rate of change of drug in the body is the difference between the rate of uptake (absorption) and rate of efflux (elimination). For a drug that is absorbed by a first-order process and eliminated by a first-order process, with instantaneous distribution, the rate of change of the amount of drug in the body can be expressed as

$$\frac{dD_B}{dt} = RATE_{IN} - RATE_{OUT} \tag{75}$$

For a drug that is absorbed from the GI tract, the rate of change of the amount of drug in the body is

$$\frac{dD_B}{dt} = Fk_aD_{GI} - kD_{BODY} \tag{76}$$

The time-course of absorption and elimination is shown in Figure 58-15.[7] The plasma concentration at any time t is equal to

$$C = \frac{k_aD_0F}{V_D(k_a - k_{el})}\left(e^{-k_{el}t} - e^{-k_at}\right) \tag{77}$$

where F is the fraction of the dose, D_0, that is absorbed from the GI tract and k_{el} and k_a are the first-order rate constants for elimination and absorption, respectively. The time to reach the maximum concentration, t_{MAX}, can be determined from

$$t_{MAX} = \frac{2.3\log(k_a/k)}{k_a - k} \tag{78}$$

and this time substituted into Equation 77 will determine the maximum concentration, C_{MAX}. The rising phase of the plot (see Fig 58-15) is not log-linear because absorption and elimination are occurring simultaneously. At C_{MAX}, the absorption rate is equal to the elimination rate, and after absorption is complete, the plot declines in a log-linear manner. This log-linear line described by the elimination phase, when extrapolated to zero time, yields a theoretical zero-time concentration. The absorption rate constant, k_a, can be obtained from the difference between the empirical curve and the extrapolated line using the

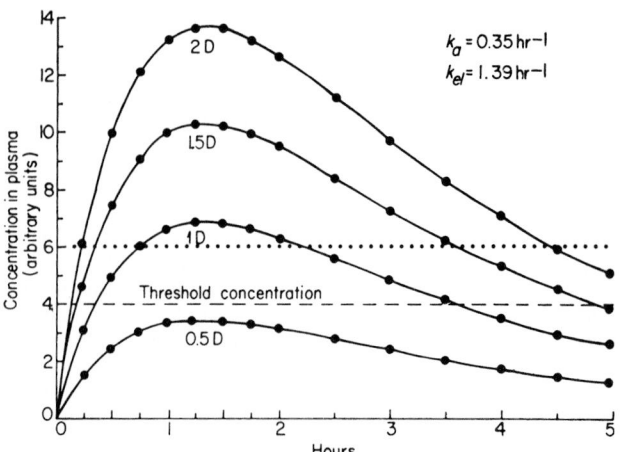

Figure 58-16. The effect of the size of the dose of a drug on the peak concentration, time of peak concentration, and duration of action. The data were calculated from a one-compartment model.

method of residuals. This is a commonly used technique in pharmacokinetics to separate a curve into its component parts and is often referred to as *feathering, stripping,* or *peeling* the curve. The reader is referred to Gibaldi and Perrier (see *Bibliography*) for a more comprehensive discussion with examples of the application of this technique.

That the peak concentration should vary with the dose is self-evident from Equations 77 and 78 and from Figure 58-16. The time of the peak concentration is the same for all doses. The time to peak concentration can be affected by both the absorption rate and the elimination rate. In Figure 58-17, the effect of altering the absorption rate on the time to peak concentration is shown. With faster absorption, the time to peak concentration occurs earlier and is higher than with slower absorption. Figure 58-18 shows the effect of altering the elimination rate constant on the t_{MAX}. With a rapid elimination rate (shorter half-life), the peak concentration occurs sooner and is lower than with slower elimination (longer half-life).

The maximum concentration at the steady state for an oral regimen is given by

$$C_{MAX,SS} = \frac{FDose}{V_D}\left(\frac{1}{1 - e^{-k\tau}}\right)e^{-kt_{PEAK}} \tag{79}$$

The minimum concentration at the steady state is

$$C_{MIN,SS} = \frac{k_aFD}{V(k_a - k)}\left(\frac{1}{1 - e^{-k\tau}}\right)e^{-k\tau} \tag{80}$$

To design multiple oral dosing regimens, the equations that describe the maximum and minimum concentrations at the steady state are somewhat unwieldy. In clinical practice, values for k_a are not always readily available, and in such instances the equations for the maximum and minimum concentrations at the steady state following intravenous administration will generally suffice as long as one recalls that because absorption is not instantaneous, the peak concentration and time to peak concentration will not occur immediately.

ORGAN-SPECIFIC CLEARANCE

The total clearance of a drug from the body almost always involves more than one organ of elimination. The anatomy of the human body is such that the clearance from the composite clearing organs occurs in parallel and is, therefore, additive. For example, if a drug is eliminated solely by hepatic and renal elimination, the total clearance, CL_T, of the drug is given as

$$CL_T = CL_H + CL_R \tag{81}$$

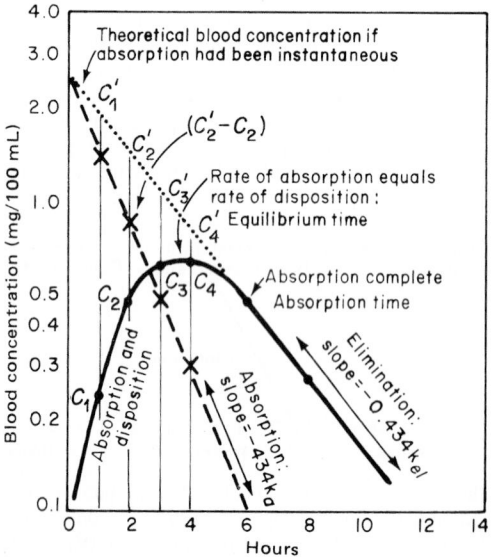

Figure 58-15. Kinetics of absorption and disposition of theophylline in a human subject after oral administration of 0.5 g of aminophylline per 70 kg. Blood concentration is plotted on a log scale. (Data from Truitt EB Jr, et al. *J Pharmacol Exp Ther* 1950; 100:309.)

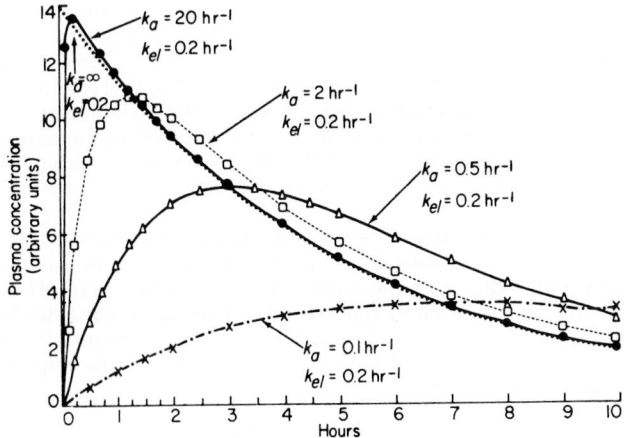

Figure 58-17. The effect of differences in the rate of absorption of drugs on the peak concentration, time of peak concentration, and sojourn in the body. The rate of elimination is the same for all curves. The dotted line ($k_a = \infty$) is approximately what the concentration curve would be, had the drug been given intravenously. The data were calculated from a one-compartment model.

where CL_H and CL_R are the hepatic and renal clearance, respectively. Measurement of the total amount of drug excreted unchanged in urine, D_U, after an intravenous dose, D_{IV}, allows the calculation of the fraction of the drug eliminated renally, F_r, where

$$F_r = \frac{D_U}{D_{IV}} \qquad (82)$$

The renal clearance, CL_R, may be determined as the product of total clearance and the fraction of the drug eliminated by the kidney. If the liver is the only other eliminating organ, the hepatic clearance is given by

$$CL_H = CL_T - CL_R \rightarrow (1 - F_r)CL_T \qquad (83)$$

One exception to the principle of the additivity of organ clearances is pulmonary drug elimination. This exception is because the lung is in circulatory series with the rest of the body organs such that 100% of cardiac output passes through the lungs. Few drugs exhibit significant elimination by the lungs so that this exception is rarely of concern in the overall assessment of drug elimination.

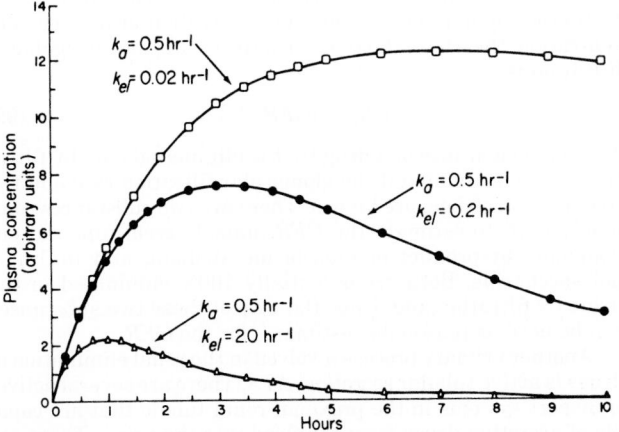

Figure 58-18. The effect of differences in the rate of elimination of drugs on the peak concentration, time of peak concentration, and sojourn in the body. The rate of absorption is the same for all curves. The data were calculated from a one-compartment model.

HEPATIC CLEARANCE—It was shown previously that the ratio of the rate of drug elimination and the rate at which drug enters the organ of elimination is defined as the extraction ratio, E, and is a measure of the efficiency with which an organ eliminates a given drug. One can define the organ clearance of a drug as the product of blood flow to the organ, Q, and the extraction ratio, and for hepatic clearance the equation becomes

$$CL_H = Q_H E \qquad (84)$$

where Q_H is the hepatic blood flow. While an initial examination of this simplistic model for hepatic clearance would suggest that CL_H is directly proportional to Q_H, this conclusion is not correct because E varies inversely with Q_H. Specifically, as Q_H increases, E decreases. This observation indicates that a more complex model of hepatic clearance is necessary if quantitative and qualitative predictions of hepatic drug clearance are to be made. In particular, this parameter must be described in terms that are physiologically independent.

Numerous models have been proposed and tested to describe the hepatic clearance of drugs. While a discussion of the advantages and disadvantages of the various models proposed is beyond the scope of this chapter, the *venous equilibrium* model of hepatic clearance has shown substantial utility in the prediction of both pathophysiological and drug-induced changes in hepatic clearance. For a good discussion of the various models of hepatic clearance, see the review by Morgan and Smallwood.[15] In the venous equilibrium model, the hepatic extraction is described by

$$E = \frac{f_{ub}CL_{u,int}}{Q_H + f_{ub}CL_{u,int}} \qquad (85)$$

where f_{ub} and $CL_{u,int}$ are the unbound fraction in blood and the unbound intrinsic hepatic clearance, respectively. The unbound intrinsic clearance reflects the ability of the liver to remove drug from blood in the absence of other confounding factors, such as Q_H and f_{ub}. Since it has already been shown that hepatic clearance is the product of Q_H and E

$$CL_H = \frac{(Q_H)(f_{ub}CL_{u,int})}{Q_H + f_{ub}CL_{u,int}} \qquad (86)$$

This model for hepatic clearance provides a powerful tool for predicting changes in drug clearance and, subsequently, steady-state drug concentrations, when certain limiting conditions are met. In particular

When $Q_H >> f_{ub}\,CL_{u,int}$, CL_H

can be approximated by $f_{ub}\,CL_{u,int}$ $\qquad (87)$

When $Q_H << f_{ub}\,CL_{u,int}$, CL_H can be approximated by Q_H $\quad (88)$

Compounds with a high $f_{ub}CL_{u,int}$ are said to exhibit perfusion rate–limited elimination; that is, their elimination rate will be rate-limited by hepatic blood flow. Compounds with a low $f_{ub}CL_{u,int}$ are said to be perfusion rate-independent. These limiting conditions allow us to place many drugs into classifications that exhibit similar pharmacokinetics. For example, agents with an $f_{ub}CL_{u,int} < 0.2$ L/min can be classified as low intrinsic clearance drugs, whereas those with an $f_{ub}CL_{u,int} > 5$ L/min are defined as exhibiting a high intrinsic clearance (Table 58-1).

The venous equilibrium model also serves as a useful tool in the assessment of the impact of changes in protein binding on hepatic clearance. Recall in Equation 87 that for a drug exhibiting a low intrinsic clearance, changes in protein binding will result in proportional changes in hepatic clearance. This type of drug is said to exhibit *restrictive clearance;* that is, only the free (or unbound) drug is available for clearance by the liver. High intrinsic clearance drugs, on the other hand, are said to exhibit *nonrestrictive clearance.*

These relationships provide important insight into the effect of changes in protein-binding on the steady-state concentration

Table 58-1. Examples of Drugs with Low and high Intrinsic Clearances That Are Eliminated Largely by Hepatic Metabolism

LOW $f_{ub}CL_{u,int}$ (<0.2 L/min)	HIGH $f_{ub}CL_{u,int}$ (>5.0 L/min)
Antipyrine	Chlorpromazine
Barbiturates	Encainide
Diazepam	Meperidine
Digitoxin	Metoprolol
Isoniazid	Organonitrates
Phenytoin	Propafenone
Theophylline	Propranolol
Tolbutamide	Tricyclic antidepressants
Warfarin	Verapamil

of drugs. Consider the case of a drug being administered as a constant-rate intravenous infusion. As described previously

$$C_{ss} = R_0/CL_T \rightarrow R_0/CL_H \qquad (89)$$

for a drug solely eliminated by the liver. In the case of a drug with a low intrinsic clearance, Equation 89 can be simplified to

$$C_{ss} = R_0/(f_{ub}CL_{u,int}) \qquad (90)$$

If f_{ub} were to be increased, for example, by displacement from protein-binding sites, the steady-state concentration would decrease. This may lead one to the conclusion that the infusion rate needs to be increased to maintain the original steady-state concentration. However, one needs to examine the effects of altered physiology on the free or unbound drug concentration, $C_{u,ss}$

$$C_{u,ss} = f_{ub}C_{ss} \rightarrow C_{ss} = C_{u,ss}/f_{ub} \qquad (91)$$

substituting for C_{ss} in Equation 90 and solving for $C_{u,ss}$ yields

$$C_{u,ss} = R_0/CL_{u,int} \qquad (92)$$

It can be seen that the steady-state concentration of unbound (active) drug is independent of changes in the free fraction, and no dosage adjustment would be necessary. This conclusion also is valid following the oral administration of a drug with a low intrinsic clearance.

In contrast, for a drug with a high intrinsic clearance, a change in f_{ub} will result in a proportional change in the steady-state unbound drug concentration during a constant-rate infusion.

An additional consideration, which must be accounted for with high intrinsic clearance drugs, is the impact of the first-pass effect. When a drug is absorbed from the stomach and small intestine, the venous blood from the sites of absorption enters into the portal venous flow. This results in all of the absorbed drug passing through the liver prior to entry into the systemic circulation. For drugs that exhibit a high intrinsic clearance, the consequence of presystemic hepatic metabolism is a substantial reduction in the systemic availability of the drug when administered orally. This phenomenon explains the marked discrepancy between an oral and an intravenous dose of a given drug required to achieve identical plasma concentrations. For example, the therapeutic dose of propranolol ranges between 1 and 6 mg intravenously, whereas the oral doses necessary to achieve therapeutic effect range from 40 to 200 mg.

The systemic availability, F, of a drug that is absorbed completely from the GI tract after oral administration is the fraction of the absorbed dose that escapes extraction and is given as

$$F = 1 - E \qquad (93)$$

Rearranging Equation 85 and substituting for E in Equation 93 yields

$$F = \frac{Q_H}{Q_H + f_{ub}CL_{u,int}} \qquad (94)$$

Similar to the limiting conditions described for CL_H, one can define two limiting conditions for systemic availability, F. Specifically, when $Q_H << f_{ub}CL_{u,int}$, F approaches 1.0, whereas when $Q_H << f_{ub}CL_{u,int}$, F approaches zero. These limiting conditions indicate that a drug with a high $f_{ub}CL_{u,int}$ will exhibit low systemic availability after oral administration, because of extensive first-pass metabolism. On the other hand, drugs with a low $f_{ub}CL_{u,int}$ will not be subject to significant first-pass metabolism.

Generally, the parameter most commonly determined to assess overall drug availability after oral administration is the area under the drug concentration-versus-time curve, AUC. Recall from Equation 67 that the total clearance is equal to the quotient of intravenous dose and AUC from zero to infinity. If the drug is eliminated entirely by metabolism, the hepatic clearance is defined as

$$CL_H = \frac{Dose_{IV}}{AUC_{IV}} = \frac{FDose_{PO}}{AUC_{PO}} \qquad (95)$$

Substituting Equation 86 for CL_H and Equation 94 for F yields

$$\frac{(Q_H)(f_{ub}CL_{u,int})}{Q_H + f_{ub}CL_{u,int}} = \left(\frac{Dose_{PO}}{AUC_{PO}}\right)\left(\frac{Q_H}{Q_H + f_{ub}CL_{u,int}}\right) \qquad (96)$$

Simplifying,

$$f_{ub}CL_{u,int} = Dose_{PO}/AUC_{PO} \qquad (97)$$

Thus, for a high intrinsic hepatic clearance drug, the AUC_{PO} is independent of Q_H. Additionally, the steady-state AUC for unbound drug is independent of the free fraction. For a more in-depth discussion of these concepts on hepatic clearance, see the paper by Wilkinson and Shand.[16]

RENAL CLEARANCE—Physiologists studied the renal clearance of endogenous and exogenous substances long before the use of clearance concepts became *popular* in pharmacokinetics. Indeed, the basis for the understanding of drug clearance in pharmacokinetics has its roots in the decades of work by renal physiologists. Moreover, there are significant differences in the complexity of processes involved in hepatic and renal handling of drugs. In the kidney, there are three primary processes (and one minor process) responsible for the renal elimination of drugs, namely filtration, secretion, and reabsorption (and metabolism), respectively. Each of the major processes are affected by common, yet unique, determinants.

The rate of filtration in the kidney for a drug is given as

$$\text{Rate of filtration} = (GFR)(C_u) \qquad (98)$$

where GFR is the glomerular filtration rate and C_u is the previously defined free-drug concentration. The clearance by filtration is the quotient of the rate of filtration at a given concentration; therefore, the renal clearance, CL_R, of a drug due to filtration is

$$CL_R = (GFR)(f_u) \qquad (99)$$

The renal clearance of a drug that is eliminated only by filtration can be estimated if the glomerular filtration rate and the free fraction of drug are known. There are two substances commonly used to estimate the GFR, namely creatinine, an endogenous by-product of muscle metabolism, and inulin, a polysaccharide. Both are essentially 100% eliminated in the urine by filtration and, thus, the CL_T of these two substances can be used as reasonable estimates for the GFR.

Another primary process involved in the renal elimination of drugs is active tubular secretion, ATS. There are several active-transport systems in the proximal renal tubule that are capable of excreting drugs from the flood into the urine. There appears to be a multiplicity of systems for the ATS of cations and anions. Whenever the renal clearance is greater than the product of the GFR and the free fraction, there must be net tubular secretion in addition to clearance by filtration. The renal clearance due to ATS, which is CL_{ATS}, is given as

$$CL_{ATS} = \frac{(Q_{RP})(f_u CL_{u,s,int})}{Q_{RP} + f_u CL_{u,s,int}} \tag{100}$$

where QRP and $CL_{us,int}$ represent effective renal plasma flow and unbound intrinsic secretory clearance, respectively. Similar to the situation described for hepatic clearance, drugs may exhibit a high or low intrinsic secretory clearance. The impact of changes in plasma protein–binding on renal clearance would substantially differ between these two situations.

For drugs that undergo both filtration and ATS, the renal clearance is simply the sum of the clearance due to filtration and the clearance due to secretion

$$CL_R = (f_u)(GFR) + CL_{ATS} \tag{101}$$

In addition to these two processes, some drugs undergo tubular reabsorption, whereby some fraction of the drug excreted into the urine by filtration and secretion is reabsorbed into the body. Therefore, the full expression for renal clearance, taking into account all three processes, is given by

$$CL_R = (f_u)(GFR) + CL_{ATS} - F_{TR}((f_u)(GFR) + CL_{ATS})$$
$$\text{or } CL_R = (1 - F_{TR})((f_u)(GFR) + CL_{ATS}) \tag{102}$$

where F_{TR} is the fraction undergoing tubular reabsorption.

These relationships provide the basis for determining the primary mechanisms involved in the renal handling of a given drug. Specifically, determination of the ratio of renal clearance and that of inulin provides a clinically useful means to determine the processes that are primarily responsible for renal excretion. If the ratio is equal to 1, the drug would appear to be filtered exclusively by the kidney. Both ATS and TR also could be occurring, but at equal rates (an unlikely occurrence). If the ratio of renal clearance to inulin clearance is greater than 1, it is clear that the drug is undergoing net tubular secretion as well as filtration. Similarly, if the ratio is less than 1, the drug must be undergoing net tubular reabsorption.

Assessment of the mechanisms for the renal excretion of specific drugs is important because different factors will alter CL_R. For example, if a drug undergoes net tubular secretion, other drugs secreted by the same transport processes may compete for secretory sites, resulting in an overall decrease in the renal excretion of the drug. Alternatively, if a drug undergoes tubular reabsorption and is a weak acid (eg, salicylate) or a weak base (eg, amphetamine), the renal clearance may be altered by manipulation of the urine pH or urine flow. See the review by Tucker[17] for a description of the methods for calculation of CL_R.

PROTEIN-BINDING—Drugs circulating in the blood may bind reversibly to a number of components including plasma proteins. This reversible binding may be described by simple mass-law relationships.

$$[D_{unbound}] + [P] \leftrightarrow [D - P] \tag{103}$$

where $[D_{unbound}]$, $[P]$, and $[D - P]$ are the molar concentrations of the free drug, the protein to which the drug binds, and the drug-protein complex, respectively. It is obvious from this relationship that the amount of drug-protein complex formed is a function both of the concentration of the drug and protein and the affinity between the protein and the drug. Thus, changes in the protein concentration may alter binding, as may changes in the total drug concentration. For most drugs and their respective binding proteins, the concentration of protein far exceeds the concentration of drug, such that the fraction of drug that is bound to protein is independent of drug concentration in plasma or blood.

Because plasma proteins often have a molecular size that restricts their passage across cell membranes and capillary walls, drugs that are bound to plasma proteins are restricted similarly. Thus, plasma protein-binding can have a marked effect on the distribution and elimination of drugs. It is a basic tenet of pharmacology that only the unbound (free) drug is pharmacologically active, because it is assumed that the unbound drug is able to traverse biological membranes and reach the site of drug action. While there have been few direct tests of this hypothesis, those investigations that have been conducted support the assumption that the free drug is the principal pharmacologically active species.

There are several methods by which drug protein-binding may be described quantitatively, though the most frequent and useful is the free fraction, f_u. The f_u can be determined as

$$fu = \frac{C_u}{C_u + C_B} = \frac{C_u}{C_t} \tag{104}$$

where C_u is the concentration of unbound or free drug, C_B is the concentration of drug bound to protein, and C_T is the concentration of total drug (bound plus free). Obviously, f_u can range from 0 to 1. This relationship provides a means by which free drug *in vivo* can be calculated if the total concentration and the free fraction are known.

$$C_u = (C_T)(f_u) \tag{105}$$

Recognizing changes in protein-binding is important because it may substantially alter the pharmacokinetics of a drug. The previous section described the impact of protein-binding on clearance, referenced to total drug concentration. Protein-binding changes also may result in alterations in other pharmacokinetic parameters. The volume of distribution at the steady state can be expressed as

$$V_{ss} = V_{blood} + V_{TW}\frac{f_u}{f_{u_T}} \tag{106}$$

where V_{TW} is the volume of tissue water and f_{uT} is the free fraction of drug in tissue. From the relationship in Equation 106 (which is analogous to Equation 12, for drugs with a volume of distribution >50 L), it is clear that a decrease in protein-binding (ie, an increase in f_u) will result in an increase in the V_{SS}. The impact of changes in f_u on the half-life of a drug with a large volume of distribution can be assessed from Equation 18 and either Equations 87 or 88. The impact resulting from a change in protein-binding of a drug depends upon the magnitude of such binding alterations on both V_{SS} and CL_T.

The two major drug-binding proteins in plasma are albumin and α^1-acid glycoprotein (AAG). Albumin is the major protein both in plasma and in the extracellular space outside of plasma and is present in concentrations ranging from 3.5 to 5.5 g/dL in normal, healthy individuals. Albumin is the primary binding protein for acidic drugs, such as salicylate, tolbutamide, or warfarin. Numerous diseases can result in marked reductions in the concentration of albumin, including nephrotic syndrome, severe burns, liver disease, malnutrition, and some chronic inflammatory conditions.[18] Thus, disease is most likely to produce an increase in f_u for those drugs highly bound to albumin.

The substance AAG belongs to the family of *acute-phase reactants*, endogenous substances that are markedly increased in concentration secondary to some type of stress. While normal AAG concentrations range from 80 to 120 mg/dL, concentrations may increase above 300 mg/dL in patients experiencing major stress, such as surgery, trauma, or burns. More-moderate elevations of AAG have been observed in patients following a myocardial infarction or in inflammatory diseases such as Crohn's disease. The increase in AAG concentration results in a decrease in f_u, and AAG is the major binding protein for many basic, lipophilic drugs.

A major source of drug interactions is competition for protein-binding sites. Each albumin molecule contains at least four different drug-binding sites, two of which are the sites where most drugs that bind to albumin interact with the other molecule. If two drugs bind to the same site on a protein, they may compete with each other for binding. Thus, the addition of a drug to the existing therapeutic regimen of a patient may result in displacement of existing bound drug molecules from their protein-binding sites. However, as described in the *Hepatic Clearance* section of this chapter, these types of interactions rarely are clinically significant (ie, these interactions do not significantly alter the free-drug concentration). Hence, while protein-binding interactions are probably the most widely reported drug interaction, they rarely necessitate alterations in drug therapy (citation Benet and Hoerner, CPT.

DOSE- AND TIME-DEPENDENT PHARMACOKINETICS

Up to this point, the processes for drug absorption, distribution, metabolism, and elimination have been assumed to be characterized by first-order rate constants, and the general concepts and equations presented are applicable to a wide variety of drugs, with modification. Moreover, with any of the pharmacokinetic models (compartmental, noncompartmental, or physiological), a number of basic assumptions apply, in particular, the principle of superposition holds. In other words, measurements of the concentration of drug plasma, urinary excretion of unchanged drug, or amount of metabolite recovered in bile increase proportionally with increases in dose. When these measurements or other observations are corrected for dose, the values are identical or superimposable. Thus, the pharmacokinetic parameters V_D, CL_T, and F remain constant with respect to time and with dose or concentration.

But the processes controlling the disposition of drugs are biological and therefore involve processes that are mediated by specialized carriers or enzymes. Under some conditions, these processes can become saturated, and changes in dose may produce nonproportional changes (eg, in concentration, amount of metabolite(s) produced, etc.) Table 58-2 delineates some of the various causes of nonlinear pharmacokinetic behavior.

Nonlinearity is a term applied to all situations in which a semilogarithmic plot of plasma concentration versus time data cannot be resolved completely into log-linear components (ie, first-order processes). There are a wide variety of causes for nonlinearity, such as capacity-limited metabolism, capacity-limited absorption, saturable first-pass metabolism, changes in blood supply to the site of absorption and/or the organ of elimination, low or erratic dissolution or release rates from dosage forms, low solubility of the drug, or drug-induced changes in organ function or body temperature. Nonlinear drug disposition primarily has been determined by measuring the pharmacokinetics at several dosage levels. When a capacity-limited enzyme metabolism is the source of the nonlinearity, the Henri-Michaelis-Menten equation

$$Velocity = \frac{V_{MAX}C_{ss}}{K_M + C_{ss}} \qquad (107)$$

can be applied to assess the velocity versus substrate (drug) concentration relationship. There are several techniques for the determination of the direct cause of nonlinearity in drug kinetics, including direct calculation of CL_T, CL_{ORAL}, F, V_{SS}, and V_1. Most commonly, lack of superposition (disproportionate increase in AUC with increasing dose) is an indication of nonlinearity in the system.

PROTEIN-BINDING—When the amount of drug bound to plasma proteins approaches saturation, the percentage of the drug that is unbound may vary considerably with increasing dose. Under the conditions of saturation, for example, after a salicylate overdose, the f_u may vary considerably with the total amount of drug in the body and hence, certain pharmacokinetic parameters, such as apparent volume of distribution, will be influenced.

TIME-DEPENDENT KINETICS—Carbamazepine is a drug with low-to-intermediate intrinsic clearance, which also induces an increase in the activity of the biotransforming enzyme system by which it is metabolized. This increase will increase total clearance and decrease half-life. Because such autoinduction of metabolism does not occur until several dose-intervals of repetitive dosing, the pharmacokinetics vary with time and are called time-dependent. *Allosteric* (feedback)

Table 58-2. Examples of Mechanisms for Dose- and Time-Dependent Pharmacokinetics (Nonlinear Drug Disposition)

KINETIC PROCESS AND MECHANISM	EXAMPLES
Gastrointestinal absorption	
Saturable transport	Riboflavin, penicillins
Intestinal metabolism	Salicylamide
Biotransformation	
Saturable metabolism	Phenytoin, salicylate
Product inhibition	Phenytoin (rat)
Cosubstrate depletion	Acetaminophen
Plasma protein-binding	Prednisolone, disopyramide
Renal excretion	
Glomerular filtration/ protein-binding	Naproxen
Tubular secretion	p-Aminohippuric acid, mezlocillin
Tubular reabsorption	Riboflavin, cephapirin
Biliary excretion	
Biliary secretion	Iodipamide, BSP
Enterohepatic cycling	Cimetidine, isotretinoin
Tissue distribution	
Plasma protein-binding	Prednisolone, ceftriaxone
Hepatic uptake	Indocyanine green, warfarin (rat)
CSF transport	Benzylpenicillins
Cellular uptake	Methicillin (rabbit)
Tissue-binding	Cyclosporine, dideoxyinosine (rat)

inhibition by accumulated metabolites of a drug, or an effect of a drug to impair its route of elimination, also will cause dose- and time-dependent changes in pharmacokinetics. Drugs that cause the depletion of some slowly replaceable intermediary factor, such as the depletion of norepinephrine by reserpine or the depletion of inorganic sulfate by acetaminophen, will manifest time-dependent effects.

DOSE-DEPENDENT KINETICS—When the elimination route is saturated by either capacity-limited metabolism or capacity-limited renal excretion, it is evident that the total clearance of a drug will decrease and the half-life will increase with increases in doses. Examples of important drugs that demonstrate dose-dependent kinetics are salicylic acid, phenylbutazone, probenecid, levodopa, phenytoin, heparin, and dicumarol. Ethanol obeys essentially zero-order elimination kinetics at blood concentrations above 0.02 to 0.04%, which is a fact of considerable social and legal importance.

Salicylic acid is one of the most interesting examples of dose-dependent kinetics from multiple sources. Salicylic acid is eliminated from the body by at least five, parallel, competing processes.[19] Two of these are saturable processes for the formation of salicyluric acid (the glycine conjugate of salicylic acid) and salicylphenol glucuronide. The other three processes of elimination, excretion of unchanged salicylic acid in urine and formation of gentisic acid and salicyl glucuronide are first-order processes. The half-life of salicylic acid increases from about 3 hr to over 20 hr as the dose is increased upward from 300 mg to 10 g. At low doses, the half-life is about 3 hr, the apparent volume of distribution is approximately 9L, and a total clearance can be estimated to be 2 L/hr. The binding of salicylic acid to albumin also is capacity-limited (saturable), and saturation occurs even at therapeutic (low) doses of the drug. Therefore, as the amount of salicylic acid in the body increases, the $CL_{u,int}$ decreases, whereas the f_u increases. These two effects tend to oppose each other, such that the total clearance of salicylic acid remains relatively unchanged within the anti-inflammatory range of unbound concentrations (between 10 and 60 mg/L; Fig 58-19).[20] Finally, the renal excretion of salicylic acid ($pK_a = 3.5$) can be increased by increasing urinary pH, resulting in a decrease in renal tubular reabsorption (data not shown). The toxicological consequences of a salicylic acid overdose are well known, but it is not always appreciated that as the concentration of salicylic acid increases, the total amount of drug in the body increases out of proportion to the total plasma concentration.

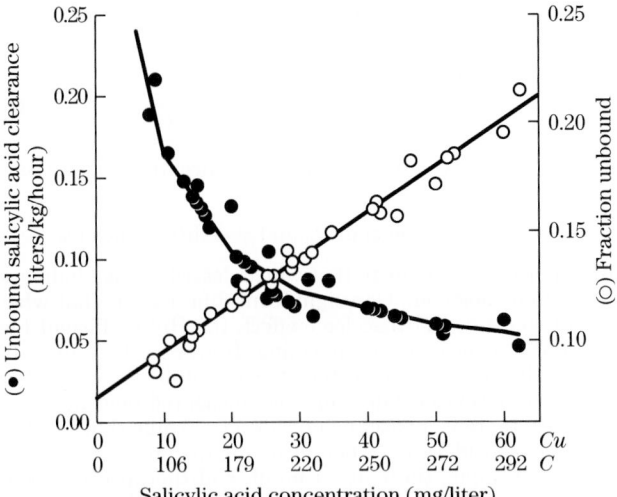

Figure 58-19. The clearance of unbound drug (●), determined under steady-state conditions, and the fraction unbound in plasma (○) vary inversely with each other as the salicylic acid concentration is increased. The corresponding total plasma salicylic acid concentrations are superimposed on the linear scale of the concentration of unbound drug; 1 mg/L = 7.2 micromolar. (Redrawn from Furst DE, Tozer TN, Melmon KL. *Clin Pharmacol Ther* 1979; 26:380.)

STEREOCHEMICAL CONSIDERATIONS

Chiral drugs constitute approximately 60% of the drugs that are currently commercially available. Most of these are marketed as racemic mixtures. These facts obviously indicate the importance of understanding the impact of stereochemistry on both pharmacokinetics and pharmacodynamics. While it has long been appreciated that optical isomers often differ in the potency of pharmacological or toxic effect, it is only recently that significant attention has been paid to the influence of chirality on pharmacokinetic processes involved in absorption, distribution, and elimination. This is primarily due to the previous lack of analytical methodology required to separate drug enantiomers. The recent development of reasonably inexpensive methods for the separation of stereoisomers has led to a more comprehensive assessment of the pharmacokinetics of drugs that are administered as racemic mixtures.

Enantiomers possess identical physical and chemical properties, despite significant differences in spatial configuration. Thus, biological processes that are passive in nature (and thereby depend only upon physical and chemical characteristics of the molecule) do not display selectivity for one isomer over another. In contrast, biological processes that require the interaction of a drug molecule with a macromolecule (such as protein-binding or metabolism) may exhibit stereoselectivity. This knowledge permits some generalizations about when pharmacokinetic processes may differ between enantiomers.

ABSORPTION—Since most drugs are absorbed by passive diffusion, most will not exhibit stereoselective alterations in absorption. Drugs that are absorbed by a carrier-mediated or active process may display such stereoselectivity. Indeed, demonstration of stereoselective absorption would be strong evidence that a drug is absorbed via a carrier-mediated process.

PROTEIN-BINDING—Drug association with plasma proteins requires interaction of a small molecule with a macromolecule, which depends upon the spatial configuration of both components. It should not be surprising, therefore, that plasma protein-binding has been found to exhibit stereoselectivity for some drugs, including disopyramide, ibuprofen, mexilitene, propranolol, and verapamil.

METABOLISM—Biotransformation requires the interaction of a drug with an enzyme, an interaction in which spatial arrangement is critical. Many drugs that undergo metabolism

exhibit stereoselective hepatic clearance. For example, the oral clearance of verapamil (a high intrinsic clearance drug) displays profound stereoselectively such that the oral clearance ratio of the R to S isomers is approximately 4.

RENAL EXCRETION—Filtration in the kidney is a passive process; however, if a drug exhibits stereoselective protein-binding, one might anticipate that the drug enantiomers would exhibit differential filtration rates. Active tubular secretion, being an active process, also may demonstrate stereoselectively for some drugs. Indeed, numerous drugs, including chloroquine, disopyramide, and terbutaline, have been found to be secreted stereoselectively by the kidney. While passive tubular reabsorption would not be expected to show stereoselective effects, active reabsorption may demonstrate these effects as has been shown for certain endogenous substances such as glucose and amino acids.

KINETICS OF PHARMACOLOGIC EFFECT

In addition to considering the relationship between drug concentration and time, proper design of therapeutic regimens often necessitates an understanding of the relationship between concentration and response. These two relationships can be combined to produce a time course of pharmacologic response, and this is referred to as pharmacodynamics. This area of investigation provides important quantitative information regarding the onset, duration, and intensity of pharmacologic effect often in relation to drug concentration. Full characterization of these elements can involve the development of pharmacokinetic-pharmacodynamic models. Modeling the kinetics of effect requires an understanding of the mechanism of pharmacologic action, of which there are many. These include receptor stimulation (eg, β_2-adrenoceptor agonists), receptor antagonism (eg, H_1-histamine receptor antagonists), transporter inhibition (probenecid, diuretics), enzyme inhibitors (eg, angiotensin converting enzyme), substrate replacement (eg, thyroxine, testosterone), non-receptor-mediated drug action (eg, chelation) and chemotherapy (eg, antibiotics).

Clinically useful information can often be derived from relatively simplistic models. The relationship between drug response and concentration is usually graded, that is, the rise in concentration results in a progressively increasing magnitude of effect (Fig 58-20). There is essentially always a ceiling, or maximum, to the intensity of effect, such that further increases in drug concentration will not result in additional increases in the intensity of pharmacologic response. In practice, plasma concentrations rarely, if ever, reach the maximum effect because toxicities often develop. Thus, only the linear portion of the concentration-effect curve may be observed. The placement of the curve along the *x*-axis may vary among compounds, resulting in differences in the potency the drugs. Moreover, the steepness of the curve (the rate at which the intensity of the effect changes as a function of concentration) will vary among drug responses. For some drugs, such as narcotic agonists, a small change in the drug concentration can result in marked changes in drug effect (see Fig 58-20).

There are certain agents that appear to exhibit an all-or-none response. Rather than the typical graded increase in effect as concentration increases, these compounds exhibit a threshold of response that once reached result in the detection in the response. While a given individual's response to the drug is identified by the presence or absence of the effect, the fraction of subjects in a sample population responding will increase as the concentration of drug is increased. A good example of this is seen in the conversion to normal sinus rhythm in patients with atrial fibrillation treated with an antiarrhythmic agent (Fig 58-21). In this instance, there is variation within the patient population in the concentration that must be achieved to convert a specific patient from atrial fibrillation to normal sinus rhythm. Thus, the higher the concentration achieved in a patient, the more likely they are to exhibit the pharmacologic effect.

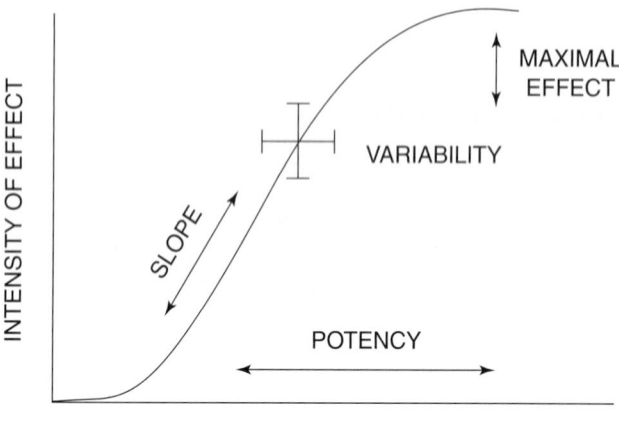

Figure 58-20. A graded pharmacologic response to a drug, showing a progressive increase in the intensity of effect as concentration increases, until the maximal effect is achieved when effect is plotted as a function of the log concentration. (Redrawn from Nies AS, Spielberg SP, Principles of Therapeutics, In: *Goodman and Gilman's The Pharmacologic Basis of Therapeutics*, 9th edition, Hardman JG, Limbird LE, Molinoff PB, Ruddon RW (eds). McGraw Hill, San Francisco, 1996.)

Although visual inspection of concentration-response graphs can yield much useful information, rigorous comparisons between agents requires a more quantitative analysis of concentration response data. The models that are used for such analyses are highly dependent upon the mechanism of action of the drug. In general, the mechanisms of pharmacologic agents can be divided into three categories: direct acting reversible agents, indirect acting reversible agents, and irreversibly acting agents.

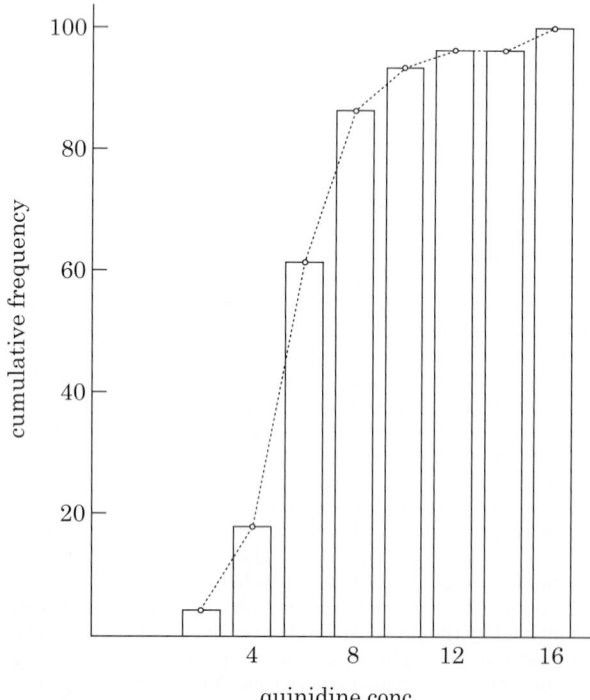

Figure 58-21. Cumulative frequency of conversion to normal sinus rhythm (expressed as percent of patients) as a function of quinidine concentration in a group of subjects with atrial fibrillation treated with the antiarrhythmic quinidine. (Redrawn from Gibaldi M, *Biopharmaceutics and Clinical Pharmacokinetics*, 4th edition, Lea & Febiger, 1991.)

INTENSITY OF EFFECT—The intensity (or magnitude) of pharmacologic effect is given as

$$Intensity\ of\ Effect = \frac{E_{max} \times C^{\gamma}}{EC_{50}{}^{\gamma} + C^{\gamma}} \quad (108)$$

where E_{max} = maximum effect, EC_{50} = concentration necessary to achieve 50% E_{max},

C = concentration of drug, and γ = Hill coefficient.$_x$

This equation is similar to that which describes the binding of oxygen to hemoglobin. One significant difference is that when used to quantify pharmacologic effect, the Hill coefficient has no physical or mechanistic meaning. However, the larger the value of the Hill coefficient, the steeper will be the concentration-response relationship. For some measured pharmacologic responses, there is a baseline physiological value that must be taken into consideration when modeling the pharmacologic effect. For example, there are a number of therapeutic agents that induce methemoglobinemia after ingestion. There is, however, a low level of methemoglobin (1-2%) in drug-naïve subjects that needs to be accounted for in modeling the intensity of effect of agents that induce methemoglobinemia. Equation 108 can be adjusted to account for baseline effect:

$$Intensity\ of\ Effect = \frac{E_0 + E_{max} \times C^{\gamma}}{EC_{50}{}^{\gamma} + C^{\gamma}} \quad (109)$$

where E_0 = baseline effect.

Such a quantitative approach permits comparison of the intensity of drug effect between various agents. For example, while the antimicrobial agent dapsone is widely reported to cause methemoglobinemia in patients treated with the drug, the antimicrobial agent sulfamethoxazole is rarely associated with methemoglobinemia; despite the fact that both form a reactive hydroxylamine metabolite and that sulfamethoxazole is administered at much higher doses than dapsone. It was unclear whether this difference was due to differences in the potency of their respective hydroxylamine metabolite or due differences in the pharmacokinetics of the drugs and/or metabolites. This question was addressed by comparing the ability of the two hydroxylamine metabolites for forming methemogobin when incubated with human erythrocytes *in vitro* and modeling the effects using Equation 109.[21] As shown in Table 58-3, the maximal effect of the two metabolites studied were similar, but the potency (EC_{50}) of dapsone hydroxylamine was 20-fold greater than that of sulfamethoxazole hydroxylamine.

DURATION OF EFFECT—A measurable pharmacologic effect will be observable as soon as drug concentration reaches the minimal effect concentration (MEC). The duration of effect is determined by how long the concentration remains above the MEC, which is influenced by the dose administered and the rate of elimination of the drug. Consider the linear range of the log concentration-effect curve, such that $0.2E_{max} < E < 0.8E_{max}$. The effect within this boundary may be expressed as

$$E = m\log C + r \quad (110)$$

Table 58-3. Pharmacodynamics of Dapsone Hydroxylamine (DNOH) and Sulfamethoxazole Hydroxylamine (SNOH) Induced Methemoglobin Formation in Human Erythrocytes

	DNOH	SNOH
E_{max} (%)	26 (5)	463 (105)
EC_{50} (μM)	89 (4)	84 (5)

Data from Reilly TP, et al. *J Pharmacol Exp Ther* 199; 288:951.

where m = slope of E versus log C plot and r = constant. This equation can be rearranged, such that

$$\log C = \frac{E - r}{m} \quad (111)$$

Recall that for a drug exhibiting instantaneous distribution, following instantaneous administration

$$\log C = \log C_0 - \frac{\lambda}{2.303} t \quad (112)$$

The maximal effect elicited by this dose, E_m, will occur when $C = C_0$. Thus,

$$\log C_0 = \frac{E_m - r}{m} \quad (113)$$

Substituting the equivalents in Eq. 111 and 113 into Eq. 112 yields

$$E = E_m = \frac{m\lambda}{2.303} t \quad (114)$$

Thus, the intensity of effect should decline at a constant rate that is a function of the elimination rate constant and the slope of the response versus log concentration curve. It should be noted that though the decrease in concentration is first-order, the decrease in effect is zero-order. But how can we quantify the actual duration of action following a given dose of a drug? Recall from Equation 13 that

$$C = C_0 e^{-\lambda t}$$

Expressed in terms of dose

$$C = \frac{D_{iv}}{V_d} e^{-\lambda t} \quad (115)$$

The duration time (t_d) is that time at which the plasma concentration drops just below the MEC, such that

$$MEC = \frac{D_{iv}}{V_d} e^{-\lambda t} \quad (116)$$

Solving to duration time

$$t_d = \frac{1}{\lambda} [\log D_{iv} - \log (MEC)V_d] \quad (117)$$

DIRECT ACTING, REVERSIBLE AGENTS—It could be argued that few, if any, drugs are truly 'direct acting.' Most drugs interact with a receptor that produces the effect. Sometimes this interaction results in a cascade of events that ultimately produce the measured pharmacologic response. Thus, it might be appropriate to designate a category of drugs as *rapid acting, reversible agents*. The drug-receptor interaction is easily reversible, the pharmacological effect is easily reversible, and the time course of the effect is not delayed with respect to the time course of the drug-receptor interaction. For example, the β_1-adrenoceptor antagonists (metoprolol) and the suppression of exercise-induced heart rate. There is a reversible (ie, non-covalent) interaction with a cellular macromolecule, which, as a consequence of the binding of the drug, stimulates a cellular response. This can expressed as

$$C \leftrightarrow C_R + R \leftrightarrow C_R - R \Rightarrow RESPONSE$$

where C = concentration in plasma, C_R = concentration at receptor site, R = receptor, $C_R - R$ = drug receptor complex.

The intensity and duration of response can be readily quantified by measuring the 'response' at several different concentrations.

INDIRECT ACTING, REVERSIBLE AGENTS—For many drugs, the response measured clinically is several steps removed from the initial biochemical effect of the drug. The time course of the effect therefore lags behind the time course of concentrations. In these circumstances, there may appear to be no direct association or relationship between the concentration of the drug in blood or plasma and the pharmacologic response.

$$C \leftrightarrow C_R + R \leftrightarrow C_R - R \Rightarrow (\Rightarrow \Rightarrow \Rightarrow) RESPONSE$$

and "$\Rightarrow$" represents a 'transduction' of the response that may depend on several factors including the rate of turnover and trafficking of endogenous substrates or other mediators of drug effect. In this instance, the drug-receptor interaction may not easily be reversible and the pharmacologic effect is prolonged, such as the acetylation by aspirin of the serine moiety at the active site of cyclooxygenase. For some drugs with an indirect pharmacologic response, the drug-receptor interaction is easily reversible but the pharmacologic effect is prolonged. An example might be corticosteroids which bind with nuclear receptor proteins resulting in RNA transcription and protein synthesis.

A classic example of an indirect pharmacologic response is the oral anticoagulant warfarin (Fig. 58-22). In this instance, the dissociation between the pharmacologic effect and the concentration is readily understood by a consideration of the mechanism action. Warfarin inhibits the synthesis of the vitamin K-dependent factors that determine the prothrombin time. However, there is a time lag for this effect to be observed since circulating clotting factors must be degrading by the normal metabolic processes before an anticoagulant effect is observed. Thus, the turnover rate of the clotting factors and not the time course of warfarin concentrations, becomes key determinant for the onset, duration and offset of effect. This was accounted for by models that incorporated the endogenous degradation and synthesis rates of the clotting factors, thereby providing a good relationship between the concentration and 'true' pharmacologic effect.[22]

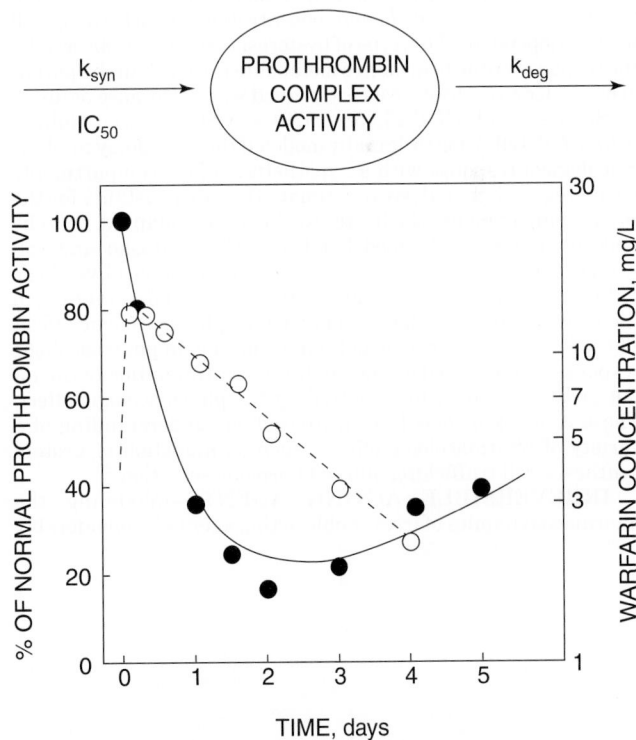

Figure 58-22. Time course of plasma warfarin concentration (top panel) and pharmacologic response, measured as % decrease in normal prothrombin activity (bottom panel). Note that the pharmacologic effect does not become evident until the concentration has reduced substantially from its maximal value. (Redrawn from Nagashima R, et al. *Clin Pharmacol Ther* 1969; 10:22.)

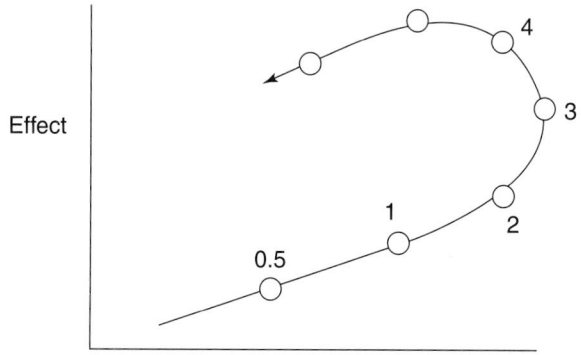

Figure 58-23. A counterclockwise hysteresis is observed following administration of a drug that exhibits non-instantaneous distribution and for which the site of action is in the slowly equilibrating tissues. Open circles represent a single effect measurement at a given concentration, and numbers indicate time (in hours) that measurements were made.

If distribution of a drug to its site of action is delayed, a counterclockwise hysteresis curve can be observed when plotting the effect versus plasma concentration after a dose of the drug, particularly when administered via a slow infusion (Fig 58-23). Thus, the intensity of effect observed for a given concentration shortly after administration (while concentrations are rising) is less than the intensity observed at that same concentration during the decline in concentration. This is due to the fact that during the distribution phase most of the drug is in the rapidly equilibrating tissues (ie, the central compartment), while in the latter time periods the larger fraction of the drug is in the slowly equilibrating tissues (ie, the peripheral compartment). Hence, the relationship between effect and *plasma* concentration for such a drug will be time dependent. This type of hysteresis can also be observed if the response is due to an active metabolite rather than the parent drug. A clockwise hysteresis is observed when tolerance occurs.

Sheiner et al (*CPT* 25:358, 1979) and Sheiner and Holford (*Clin PK* 6:429, 1982) originally modeled the time delay in pharmacological response with a hypothetical 'effect compartment.' Using regression analysis to estimate the rate constants for the 'effect compartment,' the hysteresis loop was collapsed, thereby making it possible to model indirect effects. Jusko and colleagues[24] have developed a series of comprehensive physiologic indirect response models that incorporate an understanding of the mechanism(s) producing a particular pharmacologic effect. These indirect response models envision a given pharmacologic response that is based on the inhibition or stimulation of the input or the output factors controlling the pharmacologic effect. These complex models have increased our understanding of a variety of pharmacologic effects, such as induction of protein synthesis, cell trafficking, altered hormone secretion.[23]

IRREVERSIBLE ACTING AGENTS—Modeling the pharmacodynamics of irreversible acting agents is considerably more complex, but has been successfully accomplished. The most intensely studied agents are those used in the treatment of cancer or infections. Modeling the ability of such agents to kill tumor or bacterial cells necessitates incorporation of cell-cycle kinetics. Such models have been useful in determining whether agents are best administered infrequently at high doses or in continuous exposure regimens.

REFERENCES

1. Swerdloff RS, et al. *Diabetes* 1967; 16:161.
2. Edwards DJ, et al. *Clin Pharmacokinet* 1982; 7:421.
3. Sulh H, et al. *Clin Pharmacol Ther* 1986; 40:604.
4. Barr WH. *Am J Pharm Educ* 1968; 52:958.
5. Øie S, Tozer TN. *J Pharm Sci* 1979; 68:1203.
6. Williams RL, et al. *Clin Pharmacol Ther* 1977; 21:301.
7. Truitt EB Jr, et al. *J Pharmacol Exp Ther* 1950; 100:309.
8. Gibaldi M, Perrier D. *Pharmacokinetics,* 2nd ed. New York: Dekker, 1982, pp 30, 276, 441.
9. Jusko WJ. In *Applied Pharmacokinetics:. Principles of Therapeutic Drug Monitoring,* 3rd ed. Evans WE, Schentag JJ, Jusko WJ, eds. Spokane, WA: Applied Therapeutics, 1992, 2-1.
10. Nuesch EA. *Drug Metab Rev* 1984; 15:103.
11. Yeh KC, Kwan KC. *J Pharmacokinet Biopharm* 1978; 6:79.
12. Benet LZ, Galeazzi RL. *J Pharm Sci* 1979; 68:1071.
13. Karol MD. *Biopharm Drug Dispos* 1990; 11:179.
14. Bigger JT. *Am J Med* 1975; 58:479.
15. Morgan DJ, Smallwood RA. *Clin Pharmacokinet* 1990; 18:61.
16. Wilkinson GR, Shand DG. *Clin Pharmacol Ther* 1975; 18:377.
17. Tucker GT. *Br J Clin Pharmacol* 1981; 12:761.
18. Svensson CK, et al. *Clin Pharmacokinet* 1986; 11:450.
19. Levy G, Tsuchuya T. *N Engl J Med* 1972; 287:430.
20. Furst DE, Tozer TN, Melmon KL. *Clin Pharmacol Ther* 1979; 26:380.
21. Reilly TP, et al. *J Pharmacol Exp Ther* 1999; 288:951.
22. Nagashima R, et al. *Clin Pharmacol Ther* 1969; 10:22.
23. Sharma A, Jusko WJ. *Br J Clin Pharmacol* 1998; 45:229.
24. Jusko WJ, Ko HC. *Clin Pharmacol Ther* 1994; 56:406.

BIBLIOGRAPHY

Evans WE, Schentag JJ, Jusko WJ. *Applied Pharmacokinetics. Principles of Therapeutic Drug Monitoring,* 3rd ed. Spokane, WA: Applied Therapeutics, 1992.
Gibaldi M. *Biopharmaceutics and Clinical Pharmacokinetics,* 4th ed. Philadelphia: Lea & Febiger, 1991.
Gibaldi M, Perrier D. *Pharmacokinetics,* 2nd ed. New York: Dekker, 1982.
Pecile A, Rescigno A. *Pharmacokinetics. Mathematical and Statistical Approaches to Metabolism and Distribution of Chemicals and Drugs.* New York: Plenum Press, 1988.
Pratt WB, Taylor P. *Principles of Drug Action. The Basis of Pharmacology,* 3rd ed. New York: Churchill Livingstone, 1990.
Reidenberg MM, Erill S, eds. *Drug-Protein Binding,* Esteve Found Symp I. New York: Praeger, 1986.
Rowland M, Tozer TN: *Clinical Pharmacokinetics. Concepts and Applications,* 3rd ed. Philadelphia: Lea & Febiger, 1995.
Shargel L, Yu ABC. *Applied Biopharmaceutics and Pharmacokinetics,* 4th ed. Norwalk, CT: Appleton & Lange, 1999.
Winter ME. *Basic Clinical Pharmacokinetics,* 3rd ed. Spokane, WA: Applied Therapeutics, 1994.

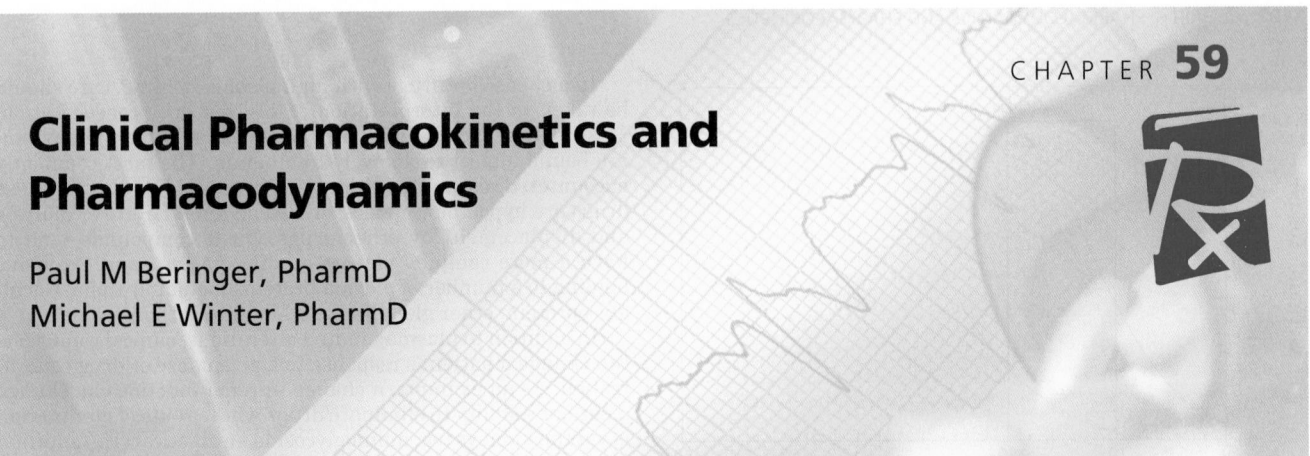

CHAPTER 59

Clinical Pharmacokinetics and Pharmacodynamics

Paul M Beringer, PharmD

Michael E Winter, PharmD

In Chapter 58, the basic principles of pharmacokinetics were presented. Clinical pharmacokinetics is the discipline in which basic pharmacokinetic principles are applied to the development of rational dosage regimens. In this chapter, the concepts of pharmacokinetics are placed into perspective with the development of individualized drug dosage regimens. The clinical significance of drug absorption, distribution, and elimination and influence of disease states on these processes are emphasized. Examples are given of the ways pharmacokinetic principles can be applied in the calculation and adjustment of dosage regimens designed to fit the pharmacokinetic and pharmacodynamic properties of drugs and specific disease states that alter drug disposition. The principles of therapeutic drug monitoring and the rational use of this clinical science in the management of patients also are discussed.

Overview of Clinical Pharmacokinetics

The application of pharmacokinetic principles to patient care can aid the clinician in making rational drug use decisions. However, knowing the relationship between the time course of drug concentration and the pharmacologic effect is critical to the application of pharmacokinetic principles and the interpretation of plasma drug concentrations in the patient care setting.

As a general rule traditional pharmacokinetic research is an intensive study of a limited number of subjects resulting in very precise pharmacokinetic and pharmacodynamic parameter estimates. Clinical pharmacokinetics, on the other hand, is usually limited to very few and sometimes no plasma drug concentrations, requiring the clinician to make an educated guess about key elements of drug disposition and the drug use process. In the research setting, it is common to obtain 10 or more samples for drug concentration measurements within a single dosing interval. In the clinical setting, it is uncommon to obtain more than two or three samples for a patient during a hospitalization or within a year for ambulatory care patients.

Therefore, understanding the usual manner in which drugs are absorbed, distributed, and eliminated as well as the known factors that alter drug disposition and which of these elements is most likely to be altered in the individual patient is key to the clinician's ability to effectively use pharmacokinetics. A basic knowledge of pharmacokinetics provides guidance to the clinician when selecting a drug product, dosing regimen, the anticipated onset of drug effect, and determining an appropriate sampling strategy if drug concentrations are to be obtained.

Drugs with Narrow Versus Wide Therapeutic Range

The therapeutic range is a concentration range that is likely to result in the desired clinical or therapeutic response with an acceptable risk or likelihood of developing a toxic response. For every drug, there is a therapeutic range, but it is those drugs in which the minimum concentration that is likely to result in the desired drug effect is relatively close to the higher drug concentration that is likely to result in a toxic response. The therapeutic index is the ratio of the maximum desired concentration relative to the minimum desired concentration. The application of pharmacokinetic principles may be limited in the use of some drugs. Drugs that have a wide therapeutic index may not require precise dose adjustments when drug disposition is altered and a simple approximation may be satisfactory to limit the probability of toxicity and assure efficacy. Other drugs may have a complex series of biological events that result in an obscure relationship between the pharmacologic effects and the drug dose or drug concentration making it difficult to apply the usual pharmacokinetic principles to the daily care of a patient.

Drugs with a narrow therapeutic range, however, tend to lend themselves to careful dose adjustments and plasma drug concentration monitoring to help ensure optimal patient outcomes. For those drugs that are monitored with plasma drug concentrations, there is usually a *Normal Therapeutic Range* that attempts to define the drug concentrations where the benefit to risk ratio is optimal (Fig 59-1). While the Normal Therapeutic Range is important, it is only a guide, and it is the patient and not the drug concentration that is therapeutic or toxic. There are patients with an optimal clinical outcome whose plasma drug concentrations fall outside the usual range and others who develop unacceptable side effects or toxicities when drug concentrations are within or even below the usual Therapeutic Range.

Plasma Protein Binding and the Therapeutic Range

One potential factor that can change the Normal Therapeutic Range is alterations in plasma protein binding. In most cases, clinical laboratories use assay procedures that measure and report the total plasma drug concentration, ie, the drug concentration that is bound to plasma protein and the unbound plasma drug concentration. It is only the unbound drug in plasma that can cross into the tissue where the receptors are located.

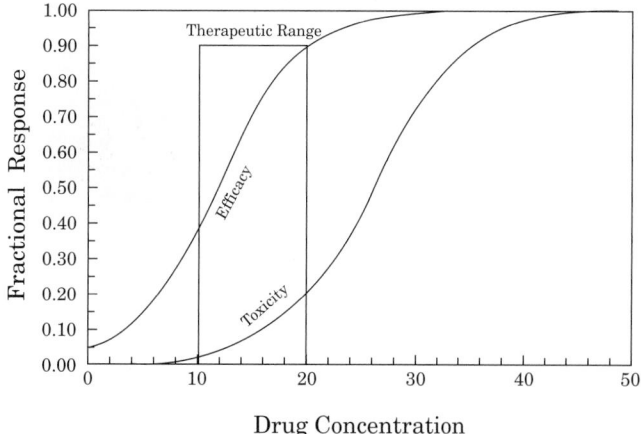

Figure 59-1. "Normal therapeutic range." The "normal therapeutic range" defines the region of drug concentrations where the probability of a positive therapeutic response is good and the risk for development of a significant dose-related adverse effect is acceptable. For most agents the normal therapeutic range is quite wide; however, for certain agents there is a relatively narrow therapeutic range and monitoring of drug concentrations may be necessary to maximize the potential for efficacy and minimize the risk of toxicity.

Therefore, it is the unbound drug concentration that is proportional to the tissue and receptor drug concentration and the pharmacodynamic response (Fig 59-2). Any change in plasma protein binding would be expected to alter the potential for any plasma drug concentration, reported as both bound and unbound drug, to result in a toxic or therapeutic response. Many drugs have significant binding to plasma proteins and the relationship between the unbound drug concentration and the total drug concentration is referred to as the free fraction or fu.

$$\text{fu} = \frac{\text{Unbound Drug Concentration}}{\text{Total Drug Concentration}} \quad (1)$$

or

Unbound Drug Concentration =
$$\text{(fu)(Total Drug Concentration)} \quad (2)$$

Any factor that alters plasma protein binding will result in an altered free fraction (fu'). Therefore, when interpreting assayed drug concentrations with altered plasma binding, the clinician should make some type of adjustment when using the assayed drug concentration.

One approach is to calculate a normal plasma binding drug concentration:

Normal Plasma Binding
Drug Concentration

$$\left(\frac{\text{fu}'}{\text{fu}}\right)\left(\begin{array}{c}\text{Assayed Drug Concentration}\\ \text{with}\\ \text{Altered Plasma Binding}\end{array}\right) = \quad (3)$$

and then compare the normal plasma binding drug concentration to the normal therapeutic range to evaluate the drug's potential for either efficacy or toxicity

An alternative approach is to calculate an adjusted therapeutic range:

$$\begin{array}{c}\text{Adjusted}\\ \text{Therapeutic Range}\end{array} = \left(\frac{\text{fu}}{\text{fu}'}\right)\text{(Normal Therapeutic Range)} \quad (4)$$

and compare this adjusted therapeutic range to the assayed drug concentration with altered plasma binding to evaluate the drug's potential for either efficacy or toxicity.

In any case for drugs with high plasma binding, care should be taken in the interpretation of assayed drug concentration. Most weak acid drugs with high plasma binding (eg, phenytoin) are bound almost exclusively to albumin. The most commonly encountered reasons for alterations in plasma binding for these drugs are hypoalbuminemia, end stage renal failure or dialysis and displacement by other drugs. Basic compounds tend to have a more complex plasma-binding pattern and extensive binding to a number of plasma proteins including alpha-1-acid-glycoprotein, other globulins and albumin is common.

In addition to plasma binding alterations, clinical conditions can change a patient's response to a given dose or drug concentration. As an example, a change in renal function can change a patient's ability to eliminate drugs whose route of elimination is via the kidneys (eg, aminoglycoside antibiotics). The addition of a new drug that either inhibits the elimination or metabolism (eg, amiodarone when added to a patient receiving digoxin) or induces metabolism (eg, carbamazepine inducing the metabolism of warfarin) can alter the relationship between the drug dosing regimen and the resultant drug concentrations and drug effect. In addition, alterations in electrolyte or acid base balance might alter the potential of a drug to produce toxicity (eg, hypokalemia in a patient receiving digoxin). While the normal therapeutic range is usually thought of as fixed upper and lower boundaries, there are many situations that require the clinician to make adjustments in dosing regimens and target drug concentrations. Knowing both the drug's pharmacokinetic and pharmacodynamic characteristics allow the clinician to design drug regimens that have an optimal chance of producing a beneficial outcome for the patient.

Absorption, Distribution, and Elimination

In the application of pharmacokinetics to the clinical practice setting, the ability to estimate a patient's absorption, distribution, and elimination characteristics is an important step in initiating drug therapy. For many drugs, clinicians simply learn the "usual" dose and use that dose for all patients. In a number of situations, knowing the principles behind the usual dose allows the clinician to make adjustments in drug therapy for those patients where therapeutic problems, toxicity or lack of efficacy, are likely to occur.

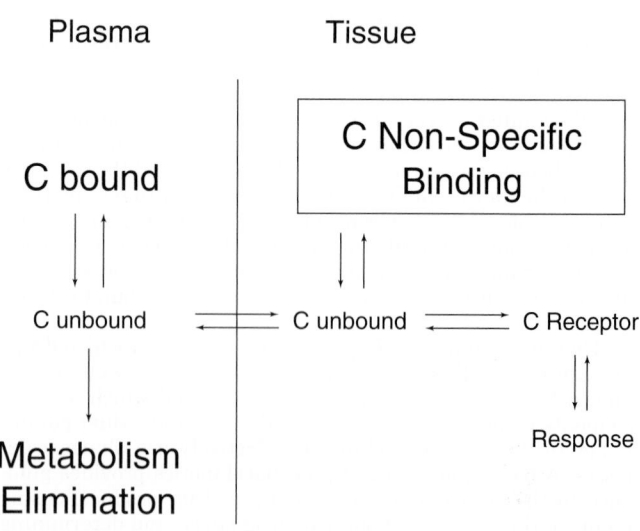

Figure 59-2. Note that it is the unbound drug concentration (C unbound) that is able to cross into the tissue and equilibrate with the tissue binding sites and the drug receptor. While C bound may be a significant percentage of the plasma drug pool, in most cases very little drug is in plasma and therefore C bound represents relatively little of the total drug in the body.

Absorption/Bioavailability

The absorption of a drug is a key element in determining a drug-dosing regimen. The extent of absorption is referred to as bioavailability and is usually expressed as either a fraction (F) or percent of an administered drug that is available to produce a pharmacologic effect. An F value of 1 represent 100% of an administered dose is bioavailable. Most drugs when given by the intravenous route are assumed to be 100% bioavailable (F of 1.0). Absorption by other routes of administration (oral, rectal, etc) may or may not be complete. A number of factors influence the bioavailability of a drug.

To be orally absorbed, drugs must have a reasonable degree of water solubility so that they can dissolve in the gastrointestinal (GI) fluids. In addition, they must also have some lipid solubility characteristics so that the drug can cross the lipid membranes of the cell wall in the GI tract and enter the general circulation and eventually cross the cell walls of other tissues in the body. Aminoglycoside antibiotics are an example of a drug class whose water solubility is so high (lipid solubility very low) that they are not absorbed to any significant extent when administered by the oral route and must be given parenterally to achieve systemic effects.

Drugs that are unstable in the GI tract may have low bioavailability because they are broken down or decompose before they can be absorbed. The proton pump inhibitors (eg, omeprazole) are an example of a drug class that is unstable in the gastric acid and are administered orally as an enteric-coated tablet. In addition, although some drugs are absorbed, they are metabolized by the enzymes in the gut wall or the liver prior to reaching the systemic circulation. Lidocaine is an example of a drug that is metabolized so extensively as it passes through the liver following oral absorption that effective systemic effects require parenteral administration. Extensive hepatic metabolism following oral absorption is referred to as a *First Pass Effect* (see Chapter 58 *Hepatic Clearance*). Recently a greater appreciation for the impact of drug transporters on oral bioavailability of a number of compounds has been realized. In particular, the xenobiotic transporter P-glycoprotein has been shown to significantly affect the oral bioavailability of cyclosporine and other large hydrophobic compounds. Similar to the knowledge gained by studying the CYP450 enzymes responsible for metabolism of commonly prescribed drugs, knowledge of the substrate specificity of P-glycoprotein is integral to predicting the bioavailability of drugs that are substrates for this transporter.

Bioavailability or F, refers only to the extent of absorption. The rate of drug absorption can also be in important factor in drug administration. Extended release tablets and capsules are often designed for the drug to be slowly released from the dosage form so that drug absorption is relatively constant over the entire dosing interval. As a result these types of oral dosage forms tend to produce relatively little fluctuation in the plasma drug concentrations within a dosing interval. While this may be ideal for a drug with a narrow therapeutic index, these drug products may not be useful when relatively rapid drug onset is desired. In addition the drug release characteristics are usually designed to be consistent with a specific dosing interval. If a drug product is designed to be absorbed over 12 hours, extending the doing interval to 24 hours may result in unacceptable swings in plasma concentrations.

Patients with certain gastrointestinal diseases may have a very short gastrointestinal transit time and thereby limiting the use of some extended release drug products. One example of a slowly absorbed drug with a limited bioavailability is phenytoin in the newborn. While not designed as an extended release product, phenytoin is so limited in its water solubility that several hours are required for complete absorption following oral administration. The newborn child has such a short GI transit time that when infants are changed from parenteral to equal oral doses of phenytoin, the plasma concentrations almost always decline dramatically because of a limited oral bioavailability.

Volume of Distribution (V)

Following absorption, drugs distribute throughout the body. Each drug has its own characteristics that result in an apparent volume of distribution (V) and can be expressed mathematically as:

$$\text{Volume of Distribution} = \frac{\text{Amount of Drug in the Body}}{\text{Plasma Concentration}}$$

or

$$V = \frac{\text{Amount of Drug in the Body}}{C} \tag{5}$$

where V is the volume of distribution and C is the plasma drug concentration. As can be seen from the equation above, volume of distribution is the volume required to account for the drug assuming the tissues have the same concentration as plasma. Volume of distribution is an important pharmacokinetic parameter when calculating the loading dose required to rapidly increase the plasma drug concentration to some desired concentration:

$$\text{Loading Dose} = \frac{(C)(V)}{F}$$

where C is the desired plasma concentration and F the bioavailability. In some cases, there may be drug already present and only a partial or incremental loading dose is needed to achieve the desired C_{Target}.

$$\frac{\text{Incremental}}{\text{Loading Dose}} = \frac{(C_{\text{Target}} - C_{\text{Initial}})(V)}{F} \tag{6}$$

In the above equation C_{Target} is the desired concentration following and C_{Initial} is the drug concentration just prior to the incremental loading dose.

Body Composition and Volume of Distribution

Volume of distribution is most often reported as L/kg. The applicability of this L/kg value assumes that the physical characteristics of the patient are similar to the study population. Patients who are obese, emaciated, or have extensive third spacing of fluid (ascites or edema) may have an altered volume of distribution based on total body weight. Therefore some assessment of body composition is important when making initial estimates of V.

OBESE VERSUS IDEAL BODY WEIGHT—When patients are obese the most common approach is to calculate the patient's Ideal Body Weight (IBW):

$$\text{IBW}_{\text{males}} = 50\text{ kg} + 2.3(\text{Height in inches} > 60) \tag{7}$$

$$\text{IBW}_{\text{Females}} = 45\text{ kg} + 2.3(\text{Height in inches} > 60) \tag{8}$$

IBW in the above equations is in kg, and it is this weight that is generally assumed to represent a "non-obese" weight. When the volume of distribution is known to correspond best to ideal or non-obese weight, it is the IBW that should be used for obese patients. As a practical approach, if a patient who weighs more than their IBW, most clinicians consider the patient to be clinically obese only if the patient is greater than 120% of their IBW:

$$\text{Clinically Obese} = \left(\frac{\text{Patient's Weight}}{\text{IBW}}\right)100 > 120 \tag{9}$$

There are a few drugs that either part or all of the excess adipose weight in the clinically obese patient is used in calculating the apparent volume of distribution. Care should be taken to carefully evaluate the patient's weight as well as the characteristics of the specific drug in question.

EXCESS THIRD SPACE FLUID (EDEMA AND ASCITES)—Some patients have extensive edema or ascites. This fluid accumulates in the interstitial space between the vasculature and the intracellular compartment or the peritoneal cavity. The degree to which a patient's vascular volume and/or intracellular volume can change is limited. Therefore, in most cases, significant changes in body water occur in the intraperitoneal and interstitial or third space. Depending on the drug's distribution characteristics the presence of third space fluid may alter how the apparent volume of distribution is calculated. In most cases, the presence of third space fluid is evaluated by changes in weight, with 1 kg of weight gain representing 1 liter of third space fluid. Alternatively, an experienced clinician can often approximate in patients with ascites or edema the number of excess third space liters present.

One method that can be used to account for any third space fluid is to calculate the contribution that one would expect for each liter (kg) of excess edema or ascites. The apparent V for each liter can be calculated by multiplying the fraction of unbound drug in plasma (fu) times the number of liters of excess third space fluid.

$$V_{\text{Excess 3rd space fluid}} = (fu)(\text{Liters of Excess 3}^{\text{rd}}\text{ Space Fluid})\quad(10)$$

The units of V are liters. The liters of excessive third space fluid gain are usually estimated by subtracting the patient's current weight from their usual weight in kilograms. Care should be taken to evaluate whether or not the weight gain is in fact *excess* third space fluid. Usually this is accomplished by determining the time course of the weight gain. Muscle mass and adipose weight gain generally takes many months, but third space weight gain can occur over weeks, days, or even a few hours. The presence of or change in the patient's edema or ascites is also a factor that should be considered when estimating excess third space fluid gain. As an example, a patient who gains 10 kg of weight in 2 days may have been initially dehydrated and simply replaced a fluid deficit rather than have gained 10 L of *excess* third space fluid. On the other hand if the patient has extensive edema before gaining the 10 kg, the amount of excess third space fluid may be much more than the most recent 10 kg weight gain would suggest.

In most cases the amount of excess fluid gained is in the range of 5 to 10 L and is seldom more than 20 L. Because the contribution of 5 to 20 L is not significant for most drugs, the weight used in calculating the volume of distribution need only consider the patient's usual weight. However, if the volume of distribution is small and plasma protein binding is low (fu approaches 1), then excess third spacing of fluid should be considered in the calculation. This would be accomplished by first calculating the patient's weight without the excess third space weight and using the *non-excess third space weight* to calculate the patient's V in the usual way. In addition, Equation 10 above can be used to determine the additional contribution of $V_{\text{Excess 3rd space fluid}}$. The sum of these two values would be the most reasonable value to use for the patient's volume of distribution.

Digoxin and aminoglycoside antibiotics are two drugs that represent the extremes. Digoxin has a fu of approximately 0.9 and a V of approximately 500 L (7 L/Kg). If a patient accumulated 10 liters of excessive third space fluid, the increase in V would only be 9 L [ie, (0.9) (Liters of Excess 3rd Space Fluid)]. This increase in V is less than 2% of the total volume of distribution and therefore not clinically significant. It is important to note that the patient's weight without the excess third space fluid should be used to calculate the volume of distribution for digoxin and most other drugs with a large volume of distribution. Aminoglycoside antibiotics also have a fu of approximately 0.9 but the usual V is approximately 15 to 20 liters. Therefore, the increase in V of 9 L associated with 10 liters of excess third space fluid would be significant and would be incorporated in the calculation of V.

Two Compartment Volume Of Distribution

While it is often useful to think of the body as a single compartment, in reality we are made of hundreds if not thousands of individual spaces into which a drug distributes. However, for most drugs the volume of distribution can be conceptualized into two individual compartments. An initial first volume (V_1) consisting of plasma and other rapidly equilibrating tissues and a second more slowly equilibrating volume (V_2) (Fig 59-3).

LOCATION OF TARGET ORGAN—The two-compartment model has two important clinical implications. First is related to the location of the target organ for clinical response (therapeutic or toxic). Some drugs have an end organ for clinical response (efficacy or toxicity) that equilibrates very rapidly with plasma. Therefore, large doses administered rapidly into the smaller first compartment will result in elevated drug concentrations and have the potential for causing drug toxicity. It is also possible to give a smaller first dose that achieves an initial therapeutic concentration and response that is quickly lost as the drug concentration declines during distribution into the larger volume. Drugs whose target organ respond as though it were located in the initial volume of distribution must be administered in such a way as to avoid the transiently elevated drug concentrations during the administration process. This is most common when drugs are administered by the intravenous route. Most drugs have a maximum recommended rate of infusion. Usually this rate is designed to allow drug distribution to take place as the drug is being infused. Occasionally it is recommended to divide a dose into portions that are administered at set intervals, again allowing for distribution to be completed before the next part of the dose is administered. For some drugs, the intravenous administration rate has to be controlled because of an agent in the injectable dosage form that has the potential for toxicity. As an example, penicillin is most commonly available as the potassium salt. While rapid injection of penicillin itself can be potentially harmful, it is the potassium that is probably the most dangerous and the reason for controlling the infusion rate of IV potassium penicillin. When drugs

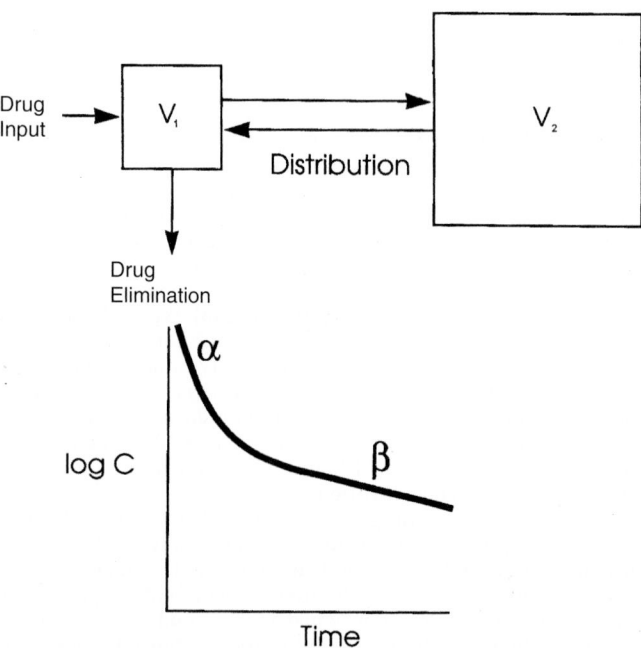

Figure 59-3. Drug first enters the body into V_1. The initial rapid decrease in drug concentration (α phase) is primarily due to drug moving into the larger more slowly equilibrating V_2. the more slowly declining drug concentrations (β phase) are primarily due to drug being eliminated from the body.

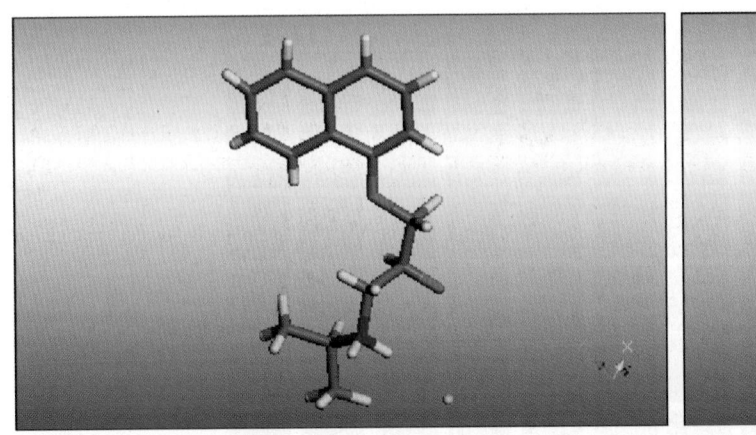

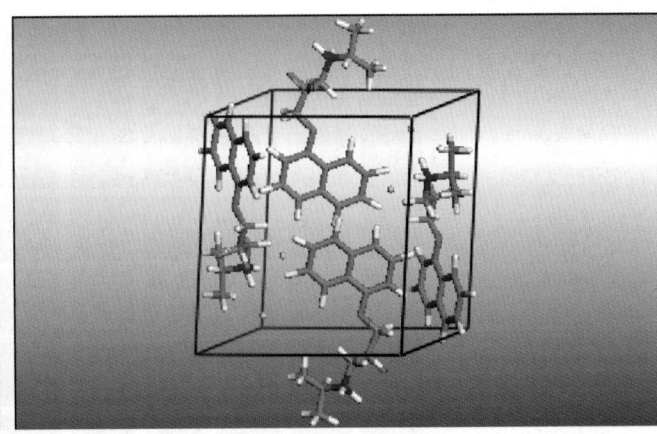

Color Plate 1. Figure 34-32. The 3-dimensional molecular structure of d,l-propranolol hydrochloride provides information about the molecular conformation and bonding whereas the its packing arrangement within the crystallographic unit cell is useful in understanding the physical properties of the crystalline form.

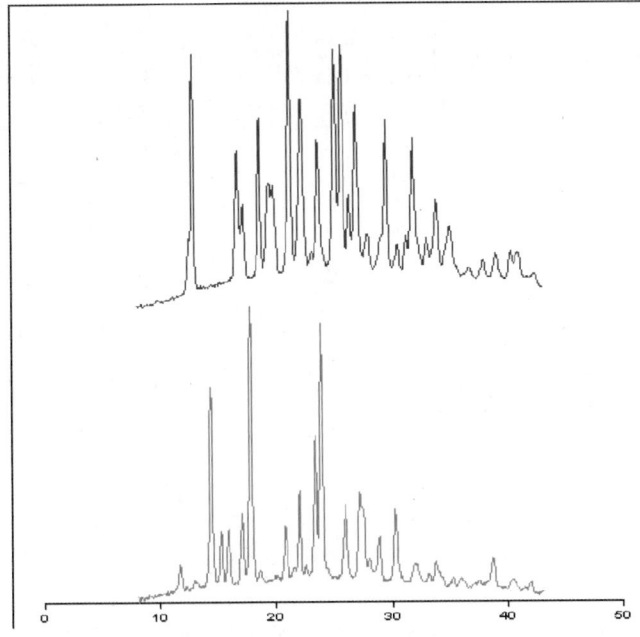

Color Plate 2. Fre 34-35. The x-ray powder diffraction patterns of two polymorphic forms of d,l-propranolol hydrochloride indicate differences in molecular arrangements within their different crystal lattices.

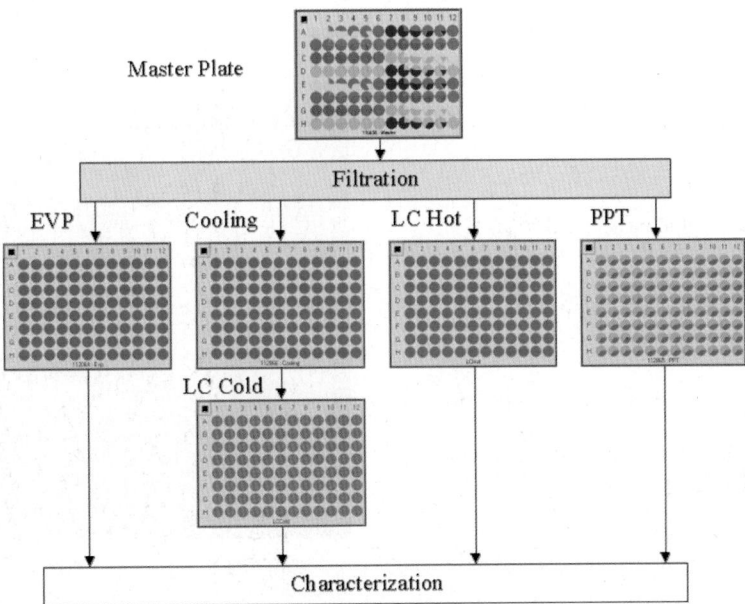

Color Plate 3. Figure 34-44. Design for the crystallization process for polymorphic form screening demonstrates hot filtration of the crystallization solution and its transfer to three crystallization plates and two plates for solubility determination.

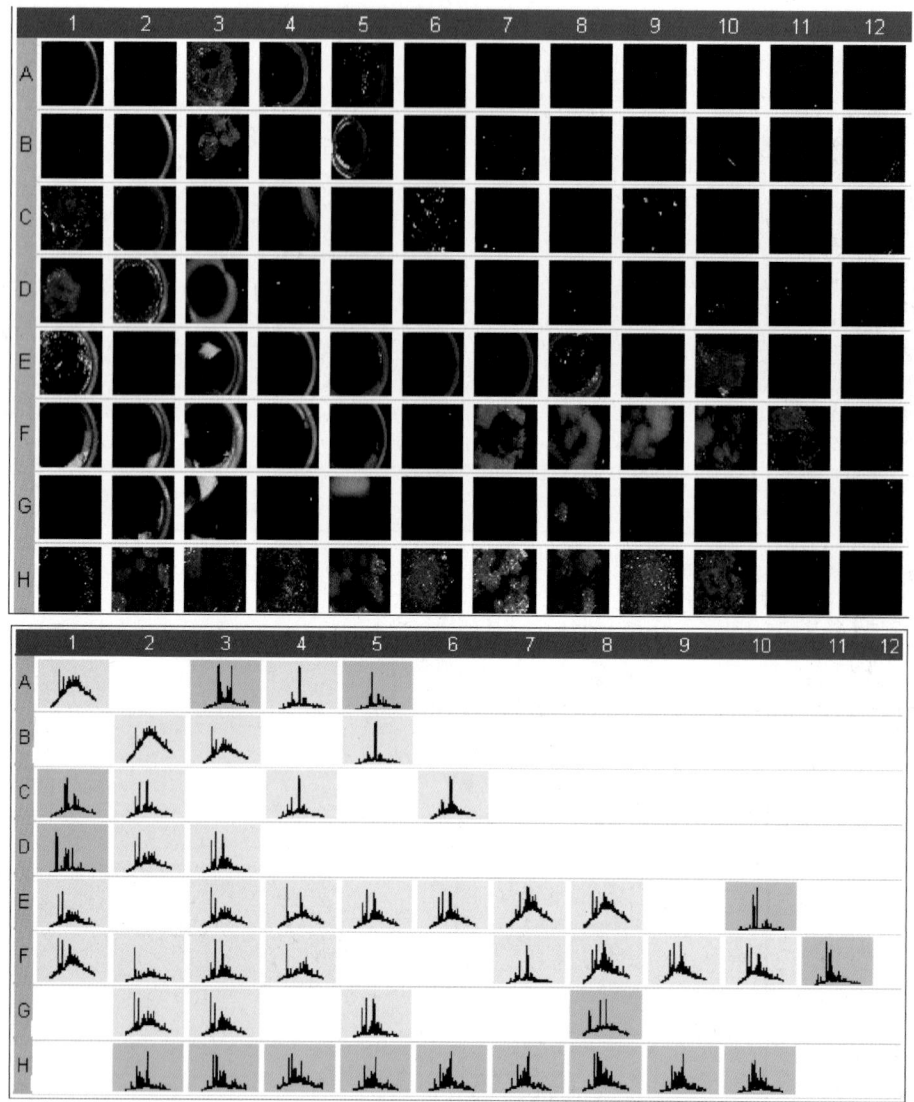

Color Plate 4. Figure 34-45. Birefringence images and powder diffraction patterns collected from the evaporative crystallization plate in the HTS of d,l-propranolol hydrochloride indicates two polymorphic crystal forms and their location within the 96-well plate, thus enabling correlation of crystallization chemistry with the crystal form obtained.

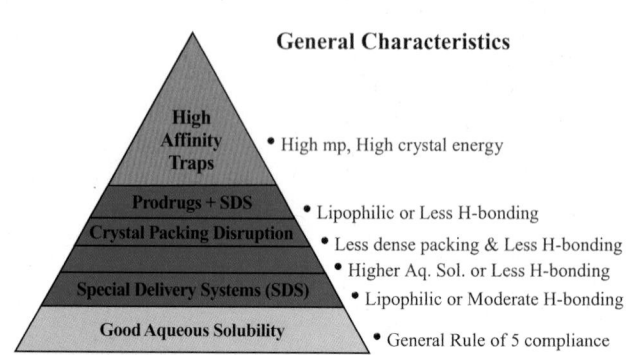

Color Plate 5. Figure 38-7. Possible and physiological-negative drug spaces.

General Characteristics

- High mp, High crystal energy
- Lipophilic or Less H-bonding
- Less dense packing & Less H-bonding
- Higher Aq. Sol. or Less H-bonding
- Lipophilic or Moderate H-bonding
- General Rule of 5 compliance

High Affinity Traps

Prodrugs + SDS
Crystal Packing Disruption

Special Delivery Systems (SDS)

Good Aqueous Solubility

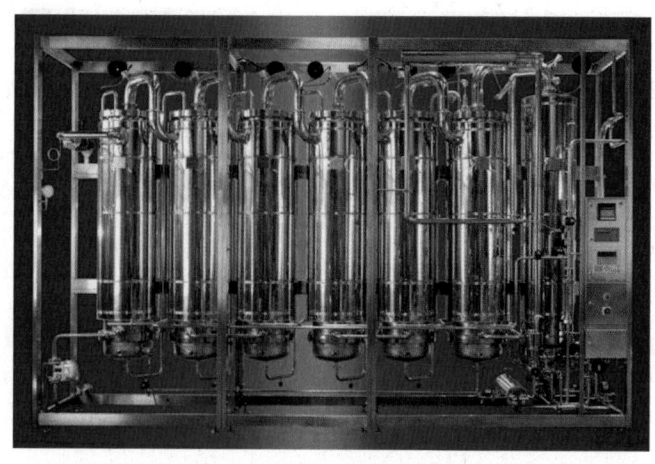

Color Plate 6. Figure 41-3. Multiple effect still (courtesy, Getinge).

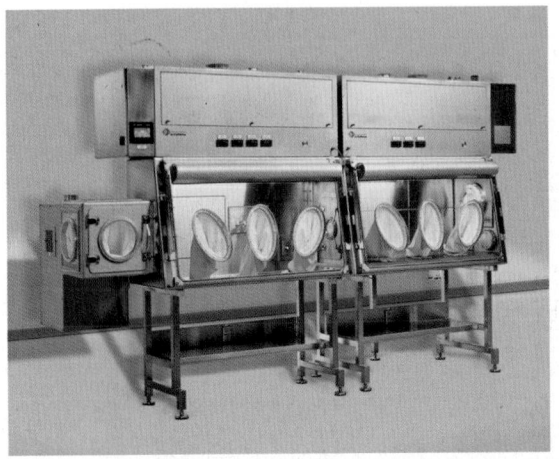

Color Plate 7. Figure 41-10. Example of an isolator (courtesy, LaCalhene).

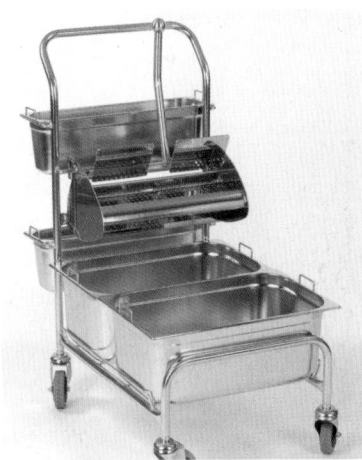

Color Plate 8. Figure 41-12. Example of a three-bucket assembly used for sanitizing facilities (courtesy, Contec).

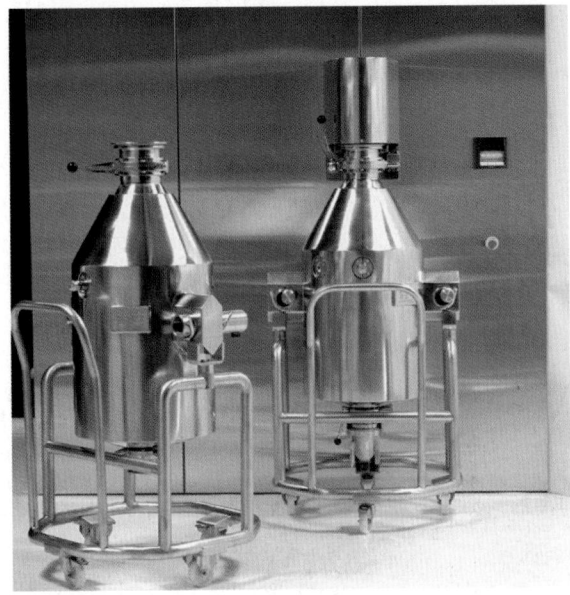

Color Plate 9. Figure 41-18. Rubber closure processors (courtesy, Getinge USA).

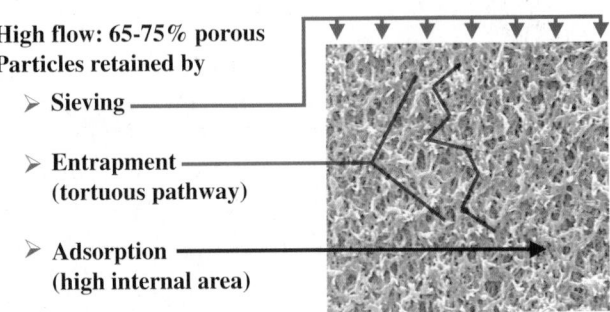

High flow: 65-75% porous
Particles retained by

➢ **Sieving**

➢ **Entrapment**
 (tortuous pathway)

➢ **Adsorption**
 (high internal area)

Color Plate 10. Figure 41-19. Mechanisms of microbial retention on membrane filters (courtesy, Millipore).

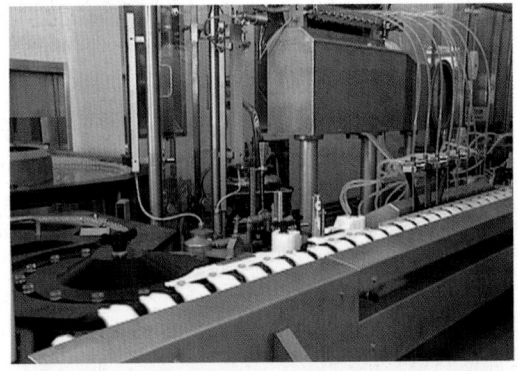

A

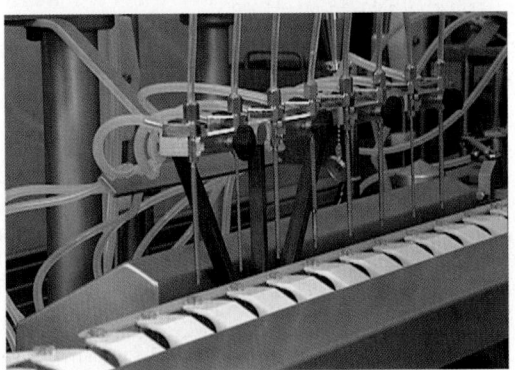

B

Color Plate 12. Figure 41-22. Vial filling machine, distant and close-up views (courtesy, Baxter).

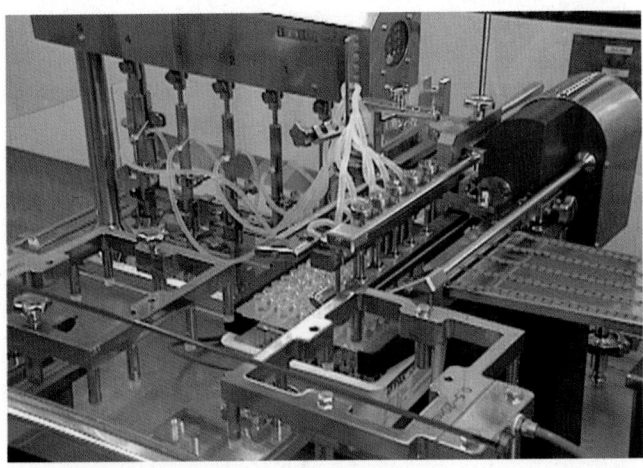

Color Plate 11. Figure 41-21. Syringe filling machine (courtesy, Baxter).

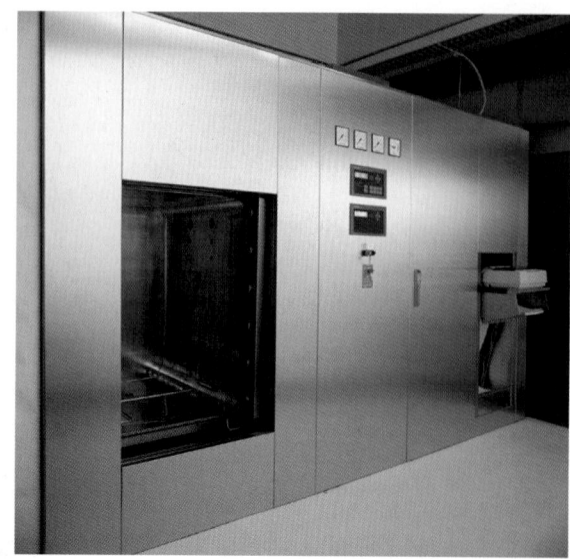
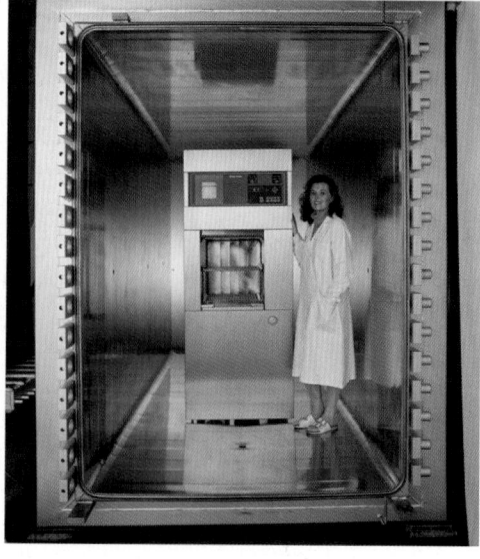

A

B

Color Plate 13. Figure 41-27. Steam sterilizers (small and large) (courtesy, Getinge).

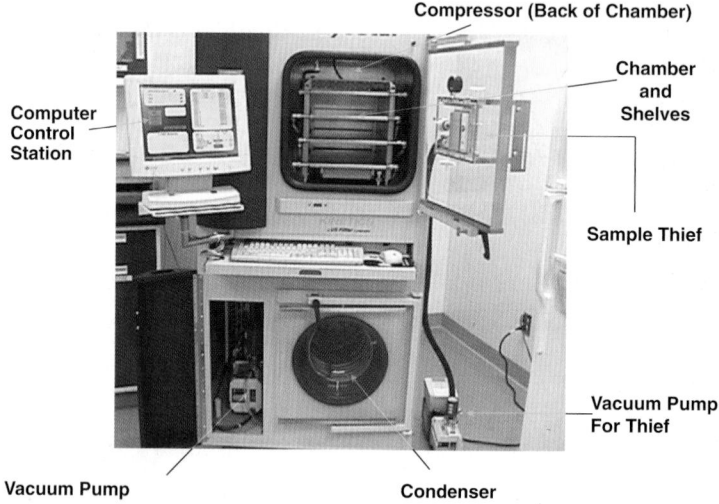

Compressor (Back of Chamber)

Chamber
and
Shelves

Computer
Control
Station

Sample Thief

Vacuum Pump
For Thief

Vacuum Pump

Condenser

Color Plate 14. Figure 41-28. Example of a laboratory freeze-dryer (courtesy, Baxter).

Temperature difference between chamber and condenser
and pressure differential between solution in vials and
vacuum pump drives ice out of vial and onto the condenser

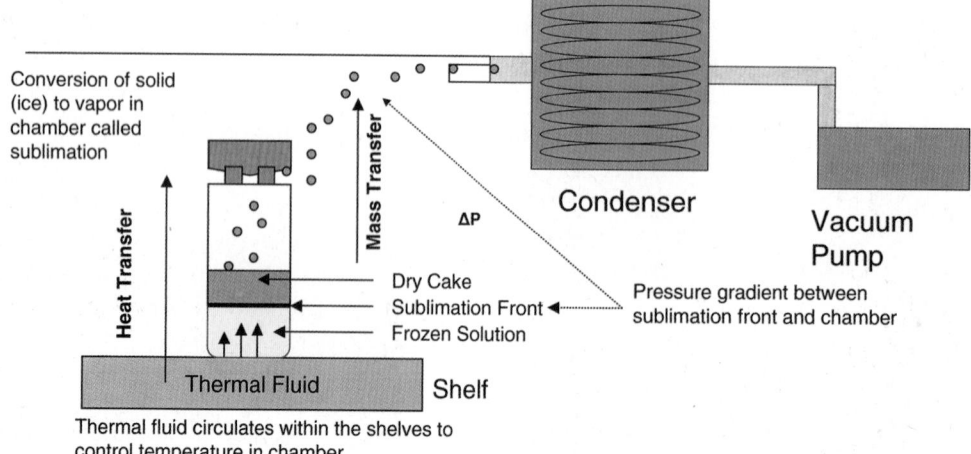

Conversion of solid
(ice) to vapor in
chamber called
sublimation

Heat Transfer

Mass Transfer

ΔP

Condenser

Vacuum
Pump

Dry Cake
Sublimation Front
Frozen Solution

Pressure gradient between
sublimation front and chamber

Thermal Fluid   Shelf

Thermal fluid circulates within the shelves to
control temperature in chamber

Color Plate 15. Figure 41-29. Heat and mass transfer in the freeze-dryer.

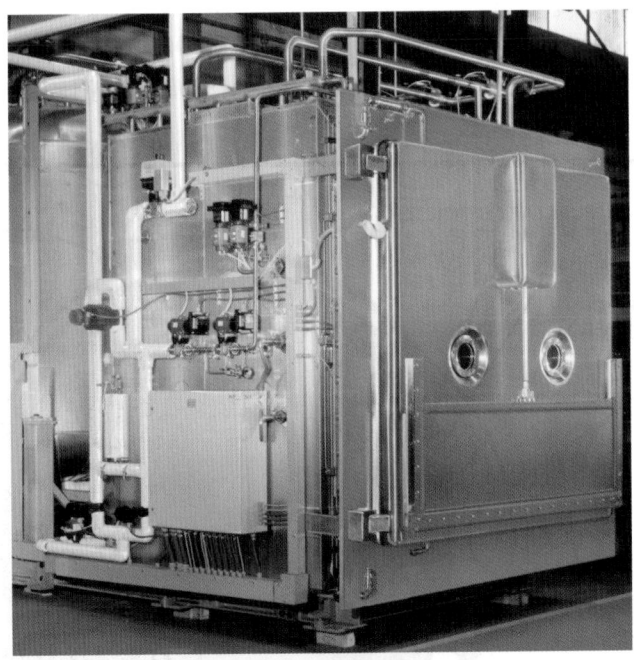

Color Plate 16. Figure 41-30. Example of a production freeze-dryer (courtesy, Edwards).

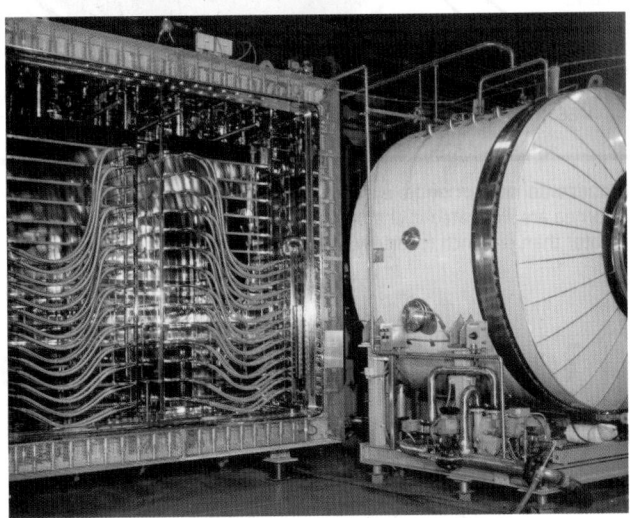

Color Plate 17. Figure 41-31. Inside view of a production freeze-dryer (courtesy, Edwards).

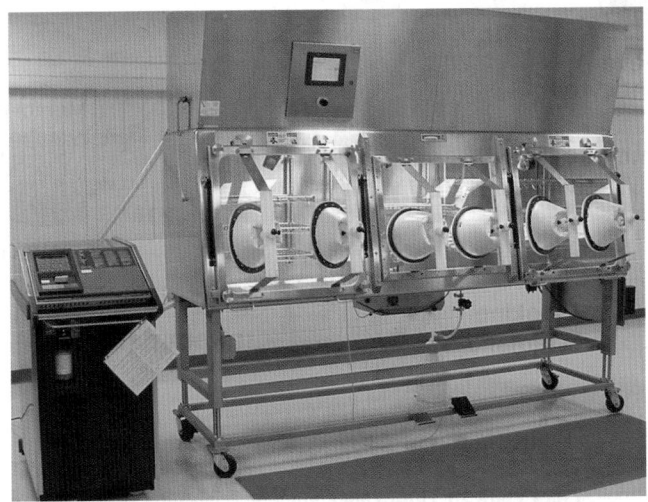

Color Plate 18. Figure 41-32. Example of an isolator used for sterility testing (courtesy, Baxter).

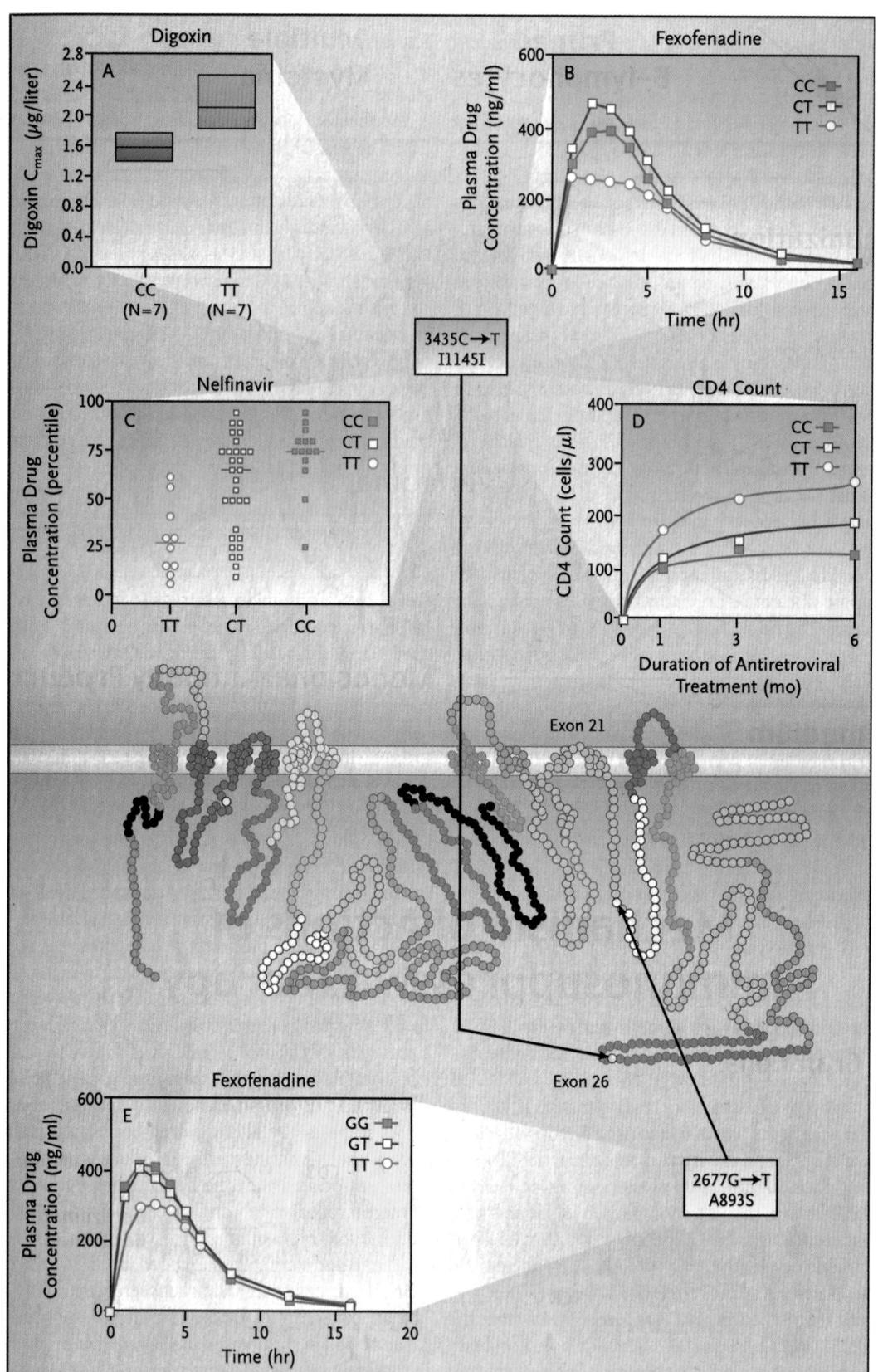

Color Plate 23. Figure 62-3. Functional consequences of genetic polymorphisms in the human p-glycoprotein transporter gene (*MDR1* or *ABCB1*). The schematic of the human P-glycoprotein was adapted from Kim RB, Leake BF, Choo EF, et al. *Clin Pharmacol Ther* 2001; 70:189, with each circle representing an amino acid and each color a different exon encoding the corresponding amino acids. Two SNPs in the human *ABCB1* gene have been associated with altered drug disposition (Panels A,B,C,E) or altered drug effects (Panel D) in humans. The synonymous SNP in exon 26 (nucleotide 3435 C>T SNP), has been associated with higher digoxin oral bioavailability in patients homozygous for the T nucleotide[167] (Panel A), but lower plasma concentrations after oral does of fexofenadine[170] (Panel B) and nelfinavir[171] (Panel C). This SNP has also been linked to better CD4 cell recovery in HIV infected patients treated with nelfinavir and other antiretroviral agents (Panel D).[171] The SNP at nucleotide 2766 (G>T) has been associated with lower fexofenadine plasma concentrations in patients homozygous for the T nucleotide at position 2766(Panel E).[170] Panels A-E have been adapted from the original reports of Kim RB, Leake BF, Choo EF, et al. *Clin Pharmacol Ther* 2001; 70: 189; Hoffmeyer S, Burk O, von Richter O, et al. *Proc Natl Acad Sci U S A* 2000; 97: 3473. and Fellay J, Marzolini C, Meaden ER, et al. *Lancet* 2002; 359: 30. (From Evans WE, McLeod HL. *N Engl J Med* 2003; 348:538.)

are administered orally, the absorption process is usually sufficiently slow so that elevated concentrations in the initial volume of distribution are limited. Digoxin and lithium are two exceptions, but fortunately both drugs have the end organ or response located in the tissue compartment and the transiently elevated concentrations in the initial volume of distribution do not result in an augmented clinical response.

For drugs that have the end organ for response in the deeper more slowly equilibrating volume, administration rate is not usually very critical. Digoxin is an example of a drug where the end organ for response, in this case the myocardium, is in the deep compartment. However, it is still a common clinical practice to divide large loading doses because digoxin has a significant potential for toxicity. The loading doses are divided so that the patient can be evaluated and the remaining part of the loading dose withheld if adverse events are observed.

Clearance

Clearance (CL) is a measure of the body's potential to eliminate drug. Clearance is expressed as volume/time and can be thought of as the proportionality constant between the average steady-state drug concentration (Css ave) and the rate of drug administration. At steady state the rate of drug administration must equal the rate of drug elimination.

$$\text{Rate of Administration} = \text{Rate of Elimination}$$

$$\text{Rate of Administration} = (CL)(\text{Css ave})$$

If the Rate of Administration is expressed as F Dose/τ, where F is the bioavailability, Dose is the amount of drug administered, and τ is the interval between doses we have the following:

$$\text{F Dose}/\tau = (CL)(\text{Css ave}) \tag{11}$$

This equation can be rearranged to calculate the desired dose necessary to achieve a desired Css ave if CL and F are known and a dosing interval τ is selected.

$$\text{Dose} = \frac{(CL)(\text{Css ave})(\tau)}{F} \tag{12}$$

Alternatively, if a dose has been prescribed, the anticipated Css ave can be calculated.

$$\text{Css ave} = \frac{\text{F Dose}/\tau}{CL} \tag{13}$$

Clearance is often expressed as L/day, L/hr, or mL/min. To allow adjustment for size, clearance values are usually expressed as L/hr per kg or L/hr per m^2. There is some evidence that clearance values are best adjusted using surface area of m^2, but in clinical practice this is usually limited to patients who are substantially different from the usual 70 kg or 1.73 m^2 adult, and there is no representative patient population for a more direct comparison.

The two primary elimination pathways are elimination of unchanged drug by the renal route and hepatic metabolism.

CREATININE CLEARANCE (CLCR) AND RENAL CLEARANCE (CL$_{Renal}$)—Renal elimination parallels renal function, and the most common measure of renal function is creatinine clearance (CLcr). The equation by Cockcroft and Gault is the most common method of estimating CLcr or renal function:

$$\text{CLcr for males (ml/min)} = \frac{(140 - \text{Age})(\text{Weight})}{(72)(\text{SCrss})} \tag{14}$$

$$\text{CLcr for females (ml/min)} = (0.85)\frac{(140 - \text{Age})(\text{Weight})}{(72)(\text{SCrss})} \tag{15}$$

where age is in years, weight in kg, and SCrss is the steady-state plasma creatinine in mg/dL. There are a number of assumptions inherent in the above equations. First is that the plasma creatinine is stable and not rising or falling (ie, at steady state and the patient not receiving dialysis), and the second is that the patient's muscle mass is average for his/her age, weight, and sex. In obese patients, IBW should be used in the equation to calculate CLcr. Also if a patient has extensive third spacing of fluid, that weight should not be included in the patient's weight, and for those patients who weigh less than their IBW, their actual and not IBW should be used.

Once a patient's CLcr is known or estimated, then maintenance dose adjustments can be made based on the degree of renal impairment and the fraction of the total clearance that is renal. In addition, the impact of adding to a patient's regimen a drug that can inhibit the secretion or reabsorption of a renally eliminated drug should be considered.

In some instances, it is appropriate to collect urine to directly measure creatinine clearance. The urine is collected usually over a 24-hour period, the creatinine concentration in plasma is measured, and the patient's creatinine clearance calculated by the following equation:

$$\text{CLcr (mL/min)} = \frac{(U)(V)}{(P)} \tag{16}$$

where U is the urine concentration of creatinine in mg/dL, V is the urine volume in mL divided by the collection time in minutes. In the above equation, P is in units of mg/dL and is analogous to the value of SCrss in Equation 14 or 15 above. The value of (U)(V) is the production rate of creatinine and analogous to the 140 - Age, Weight and 72 in Equations 14 and 15. The advantage of obtaining a urine collection to measure creatinine clearance is that it is a direct measurement and does not make an assumption about creatinine production as do the methods that do not utilize a urine collection (eg, Equations 14 and 15).

There are two major disadvantages of 24-hour urine collections for creatinine clearance. The first and most obvious is that the information required to make clinical decisions may be unacceptably delayed because of the time required to collect the patient's urine. The second is that urine collections are often inaccurate. It is common for patients and even health care professionals to inadvertently discard a portion of the urine during the collection process or on occasion to collect for longer than the time listed on the collection document.

Whenever a creatinine collection is obtained, it is important to evaluate whether or not the collection appears to be adequate or complete. Although there are a number of methods that could be used, the most straightforward is to compare the CLcr from the 24-hour urine collection to the CLcr calculated from Equation 14 or 15 above. If the two values are in close agreement, it is usually a good indication that the patient is average in terms of their muscle mass, creatinine production, and the collection was properly obtained. However, if the two values are substantially different, one of the values is more likely to be the better estimate of the patient's renal function. Because both the urine collection and Equations 14 and 15 use the same value for the plasma creatinine, the difference has to be in either the accuracy of the 24-hour urine collection or the inherent assumptions in Equations 14 or 15 about the patient's muscle mass and creatinine production.

In most cases where there are significant differences, the 24-hour collection CLcr is lower than the value calculated by Equation 14 or 15. This is because the most common error is either not collecting all of the urine in the 24-hour collection period or that Equations 14 or 15 over-predicts the patient's muscle mass and creatine production. Therefore if the patient has a reasonably normal body stature and muscle mass, it is likely that Equation 14 or 15 would be the better estimate of the patient's renal function. On the other hand, if a patient is very thin and emaciated with a lower than average muscle mass, it is likely that the 24-hour collection is the better estimate of the patient's renal function. There are other possibilities, but the examples above are the most common scenarios.

Once creatinine clearance is known, CL_{Renal} can be calculated by multiplying the patient's creatinine clearance by a "factor" or ratio of the usual drug clearance to CLcr. As an example, procainamide CL_{Renal} is about 3 times CLcr and so a patient's creatinine clearance would be multiplied by 3 to obtain an estimate of renal clearance for procainamide. Aminoglycosides have a CL_{Renal} that is approximately equal to CLcr while the factor for phenobarbital is so small that CLcr is not considered in calculating the clearance of phenobarbital.

HEPATIC CLEARANCE ($CL_{Hepatic}$)—Hepatic metabolism or $CL_{Hepatic}$ usually represents the conversion of active drug into a more polar and inactive compound by changing one or more of the functional groups on the compound. Hepatic clearance is a function of both the number and the quality of the hepatic enzymes. Clearly there are a number of factors that influence the liver's ability to metabolize drugs. Genetic composition as well as environmental factors and disease play a role in a patient's hepatic metabolic capabilities. Currently genetic profiles are not commonly available, but there are a number of drugs that are known to either inhibit or induce hepatic metabolism and we are learning more about which enzymes are responsible.

Accurate assessment of hepatic function and a patient's ability to metabolize drugs is difficult. Elevated plasma enzymes such as alanine aminotransferase (ALT), aspartate aminotransferase (AST), and alkaline phosphatase (Alk Phos) represent ongoing liver damage but are a poor reflection of function. More direct but still relatively unreliable predictors of hepatic dysfunction and decreased drug metabolism are an increased plasma bilirubin (Bili), decreased plasma albumin (Alb), and an increased prothrombin time (PT). These three biological indicators are useful in that they each represent a metabolic function of the liver. However, there are a number of factors that influence each of these laboratory tests. As an example, a patient with a low plasma albumin may have a gastroenteropathy or nephritis and have a low albumin because of a protein wasting problem and not because of decreased hepatic synthesis. Similarly, a high PT may be due to warfarin and not a reflection of a patient's hepatic metabolic capacity for drugs. Patients with severe liver failure and cirrhosis would be expected to have an elevated bilirubin and prothrombin time as well as a decreased plasma albumin. However, the presence of these abnormal laboratory test, even in the face of obvious liver disease, are not always good predictors of the extent to which a patient's ability to metabolize drugs will be decreased. Similarly congestive heart failure is known to be associated with decreased metabolism of a number of drugs. The exact mechanism of this disease-drug interaction is not known but is assumed to be secondary to either decreased hepatic blood flow or an increase in portal pressure and thereby a decrease in the ability of the hepatic enzymes to function properly.

In most clinical settings, when there is evidence of significant hepatic dysfunction the tendency is to assume that the patient's hepatic capacity is approximately half normal. Clearly this "yes" or "no" approach to estimating the presence and the extent of hepatic disease on drug metabolism leaves much to be desired. Unfortunately, with few exceptions, this is the state of the art in clinical pharmacokinetics with regard to hepatic metabolism.

OTHER CLEARANCE MECHANISMS—Renal elimination of unchanged drug and hepatic metabolism are the most common routes of elimination. However, on occasion other elimination pathways play an important role. As an example, succinylcholine is hydrolyzed and inactivated (cleared from the body in a pharmacokinetic sense) by butyrylcholinesterase enzymes located in the liver and to a significant extent in the circulating in plasma. There are other examples of in-vivo and in-vitro drug interactions that essentially act as a clearance mechanism. Aminoglycoside antibiotics with a primary amine group (eg, gentamicin) can form a covalent bond with beta-lactam antibiotics (eg, penicillin) and as a result the aminoglycoside is inactivated. This interaction is not very rapid, and significant inactivation of an aminoglycoside antibiotic only occurs when the aminoglycoside and beta-lactam antibiotic are mixed in the same IV bag or in-vivo when the two drugs are administered to a patient with end-stage renal failure. In these types of patients, the additional "clearance" can be equivalent to as much as 5 mL/min. Other potential routes of elimination are via dialysis, either hemo- or peritoneal. Some drugs are significantly removed by dialysis and care should be taken to adjust the initial dosing regimen for patients with very poor renal function and to determine if any supplemental doses would be required because of the dialysis process.

The overall approach to using pharmacokinetics and assessment of a patient's renal and hepatic function needs to be combined with the urgency of the clinical situation, the available options, and the consequences of either drug toxicity or a therapeutic failure.

Drug-Drug Interactions

With today's trend towards polypharmacy, drug-drug interactions are common and can result in therapeutic misadventures. Care should be taken to evaluate how adding or removing a drug from a patient's regimen will affect the absorption, distribution, and elimination of the other drugs the patient may be taking. Knowing the direction of the interaction (ie, increase or decrease), the time course of the onset, and the magnitude of the interaction are all important considerations when evaluating drug-drug interaction. Understanding the specifics of a drug-drug interaction helps the clinician know how and when to monitor the patient and the probable adjustments in the dosing regimen that will be necessary. As an example, both quinidine and amiodarone will approximately double a patient's steady state digoxin concentration. The doubling in the steady state digoxin concentration is due to the fact that quinidine and amiodarone both reduce by half the total clearance of digoxin; however, quinidine has a half-life of about 6 hours and accumulates to steady state within 1 day. In addition, quinidine reduces the volume of distribution digoxin, and as a result digoxin concentrations will increase rapidly within 24 hours following the initiation of quinidine therapy. Amiodarone, on the other hand, has a very long half-life and appears to have little influence on the volume of distribution for digoxin. Therefore, the increase in digoxin concentrations following the addition of amiodarone occurs over 1 to 2 weeks. Understanding these differences in how quinidine and amiodarone affect digoxin's volume of distribution vs. clearance helps to explain the difference in clinical management when either quinidine or amiodarone are added to a patient's therapy. When quinidine is initiated, a daily dose of digoxin is usually withheld to blunt the rapid rise in digoxin due to the decrease in volume of distribution, and the maintenance dose is halved to compensate for the reduction in clearance in an attempt to maintain the same digoxin concentration at steady state. In contrast, when amiodarone is added to a patient's regimen, the usual practice is to simply reduce the digoxin maintenance dose in half to compensate for the reduction in clearance.

Again knowing which parameter is affected, in which direction the parameter will be altered, and the time course as well as the expected magnitude of the change will provide the clinician with a logical approach to dealing with the drug-drug interaction.

Elimination Rate Constant (K) and Half-Life (t 1/2)

In physical chemistry, the K or rate constant is the independent parameter that controls the rate of change in a reaction. In the physiologic model used in clinical pharmacokinetics, CL and V are the independent parameters and the relationship of CL to V that controls the rate of change of drug in the body. The fractional rate of change or K constant has the units of inverse time, usually hours^{-1} or days^{-1}) and its relationship to CL and V is represented in the following equation.

$$K = \frac{CL}{V} \qquad (17)$$

or

$$CL = (K)(V) \qquad (18)$$

Note that although Equation 18 appears to represent CL as a function of K and V, it is Equation 17 that represents the true dependence of K on CL and V.

Half-life is a common clinical tool and is related to K or CL and V in the following way:

$$t\,1/2 = \frac{0.693}{K} \qquad (19)$$

and

$$t\,1/2 = \frac{0.693\,V}{CL} \qquad (20)$$

The half-life of a drug is the time required for half of the drug to be eliminated from the body or the time required for a drug concentration to decline by half (Fig 59-4). This definition assumes a single compartment volume of distribution and that CL and V are constant values, independent of dose or concentration. The utility of half-life is in estimating the rate of change of drug within the body. When a drug is administered at a consistent dosing rate, the drug will accumulate to 50% of steady state after one t 1/2, 75% after 2 t 1/2 and after 3.3 t 1/2's will be at 90% of the final steady-state or plateau value. Similarly during decline, after one t 1/2 50% will be eliminated (50% remaining), after two t 1/2's 75% will be eliminated (25% remaining) and after 3.3 t 1/2's 90% will be eliminated (10% remaining). The equation that predicts drug accumulation towards steady-state assuming continuous input (see PK models section) is as follows:

$$C_t = \frac{(F)(Dose/\tau)}{CL}(1 - e^{-Kt}) \qquad (21)$$

where $\dfrac{(F)(Dose/\tau)}{CL}$ represents the eventual Css ave, and (1-e^{-Kt}) represents the fraction of steady-state achieved after t hours of

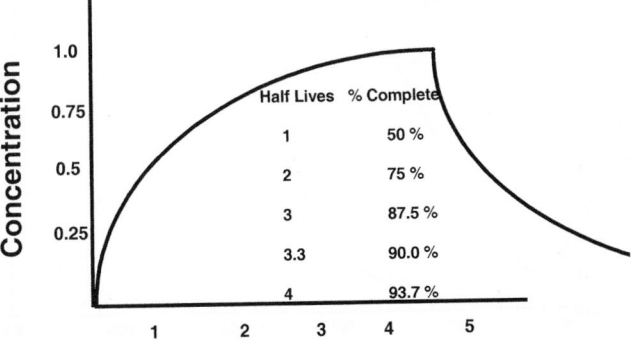

Time: Number of Half Lives

Figure 59-4. Drug Accumulation and Decline. The ascending curve represents drug concentration accumulating towards steady-state and the descending curve represents drug concentration declining after the drug is discontinued. After one t 1/2 the drug is at 50% of steady-state, two t 1/2's 75% and 3.3 t 1/2's 90-% of steady-state. In the declining phase the drug concentration declines to half of the previous concentration in each t 1/2 after 3.3 t 1/2's 90% of the drug will have been eliminated.

input at a rate of (F)(Dose/τ). Alternatively the concentration of drug remaining some time t later can be expressed by the following:

$$C_2 = (C_1)(e^{-Kt}) \qquad (22)$$

where C_1 is the initial concentration, e^{-Kt} is the fraction remaining at t hours later, and C_2 is the remaining concentration. Equation 22 assumes that CL and V are constant, that the V behaves as a one-compartment model and that there is no additional drug input between C_1 and C_2. Clearly an equation can become complex when it is composed of a series of equations representing the concentration at C_1. Take for example a drug that is infused for 10 hours and then the infusion is discontinued and 5 hours later a drug concentration is to be calculated. This could be accomplished by using Equation 21 to calculate the concentration (C_t) at the end of the 10-hour infusion and then substituting that value for C_1 in Equation 22 and calculating the value of C_2 5 hours later. Alternatively Equations 21 and 22 could be combined as follows:

$$C_2 = \frac{(F)(Dose/\tau)}{CL}(1 - e^{-K\,10\,hours})(e^{-K\,5\,hours}) \qquad (23)$$

Either approach is reasonable, but equations can become somewhat complex depending on the number of dose manipulations that are made and the time when the drug concentration is to be calculated.

INDIVIDUALIZED DRUG DOSING REGIMENS

The goal of clinical PK/PD is to develop individualized drug therapy regimens to maximize the likelihood of therapeutic success. The doses utilized in clinical practice typically are derived from phase II/III clinical trials in which the safety and efficacy of an agent are evaluated. The information from clinical trials as well as preclinical work from animal and in-vitro studies provides data on the doses necessary to obtain concentrations in the "usual therapeutic range." As discussed previously, the therapeutic range defines the range of concentrations in which most patients have a therapeutic effect and a low incidence of toxicity; however, for drugs exhibiting a narrow therapeutic index, it may be necessary to more precisely define the dosage regimen for an individual based on (1) patient factors (severity of disease), (2) concentrations achievable at site of drug action (distribution, elimination), and (3) the level of sensitivity to the drug (pharmacodynamics). For example, it is widely recognized that higher doses of the aminoglycoside antibiotics are necessary in the treatment of sepsis versus a urinary tract infection. The high mortality rate from sepsis requires early aggressive therapy in order to control the infection before serious end organ damage occurs. Higher doses are also necessary where penetration into the site of the infection is reduced (ie, pneumonia or meningitis), whereas lower doses would be appropriate when renal function is compromised. These differences can be characterized and are based on knowledge of the pharmacokinetics of the drug being administered. Over the past decade, our understanding of the pharmacodynamics of drugs has improved significantly. This recognition stemmed from the observation that despite achievement of concentrations in the desired range, not all patients exhibit the same clinical response. Subsequently, a number of studies have evaluated the relationship between measures of drug exposure (Cmax, AUC), measures of disease sensitivity (eg, minimum inhibitory concentration for bacteria), and clinical outcomes (efficacy and toxicity). For the aminoglycoside antibiotics, it has been shown that the bactericidal activity and clinical improvement is correlated with the peak to MIC ratio (Fig 59-5). According to this analysis, the probability of normalizing the temperature and leukocyte count is maximized when the peak/MIC ratio exceeds 10. Therefore, higher doses would be necessary for

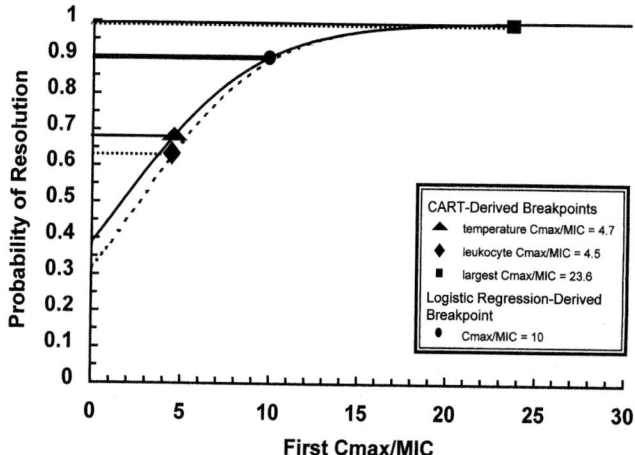

Figure 59-5. Probability of clinical improvement with aminoglycoside therapy based on the pharmacodynamic endpoint of Cmax:MIC. Resolution of temperature and leukocyte count is optimal in patients in whom the Cmax:MIC exceeds 10. (From Kashuba et al. *Antimicrob Agents Chemother* 1999; 43:623.)

treating infections involving less susceptible organisms (ie, *P. aeruginosa* vs. *E. coli*). Similarly, the probability of experiencing an adverse reaction has been linked to measures of drug exposure. The probability of a nephrotoxic event is associated with the daily AUC (>100 mg x h/L for gentamicin and tobramycin) and concomitant use of other nephrotoxic agents. In particular, in the presence of vancomycin, the amount of aminoglycoside exposure as measured by 24-hr AUC to maintain a similar risk for nephrotoxicity as aminoglycoside monotherapy is significantly reduced (Fig 59-6). Therefore, lower doses may be required when the aminoglycosides are prescribed in combination with other potentially nephrotoxic agents (ie, vancomycin). The importance of these observations is that truly individualized drug therapy cannot be established without consideration of patient factors, pharmacokinetics and pharmacodynamics, and weighing their relative importance.

Methods for Dosage Individualization

Numerous methods for dosage individualization have been described in the literature and can be grouped based on their level of precision in achieving specific concentration goals. Dosage individualization for drugs that have a relatively wide therapeutic range is typically performed using nomograms incorporating an assessment of patient demographics (ie, weight) and clinical characteristics (ie, renal function). Since renal function and weight are the principal covariates affecting the pharmacokinetics of drugs that are predominately renally cleared (ie, vancomycin), they are frequently incorporated into nomograms to reduce the variability in drug exposure between individuals within the population when compared with fixed dosing regimens (ie, vancomycin 1 gm q12h). The use of dosing nomograms such as these are most applicable for the "average" patient whose pharmacokinetics can be easily predicted based on estimates of variables such as weight and renal function. In contrast, in clinical situations where the pharmacokinetics of the drug is likely to differ significantly from the "average" patient or if the risk of therapeutic failure or toxicity is great, then a more precise measure of dosing is necessary. The aminoglycoside antibiotics are an example of a class of drugs that often meet this latter category. For many years, it has been recognized that there is a relatively narrow range of concentrations that result in efficacy and avoidance of toxicity. As a result, it is vital to determine the dose that will maximize the probability

of efficacy while minimizing the risk of serious toxicity. Similar to vancomycin, weight and renal function are important variables in describing the pharmacokinetics within an individual. Therefore nomograms incorporating these factors are widely used in clinical practice to individualize the dose. However, in addition, factors such as third space fluid (edema, ascites), obesity, certain clinical conditions (ie, cystic fibrosis, burns, spinal cord injury) can alter the pharmacokinetics of the aminoglycosides. It is under these circumstances that more sophisticated PK/PD methods may be required to individualize the dosing regimen.

The use of models to determine the optimal dose using patient demographics and clinical characteristics are often referred to as *a-priori* dosing since the dosage prediction is done before direct measures of drug disposition are available (ie, measured drug concentrations). Most clinical laboratories are capable of quantifying the amount of certain drugs (drugs exhibiting a narrow therapeutic range) in biological fluids (ie, plasma), which enables a more direct assessment of the appropriateness of a dosing regimen. *A-posteriori* dosing refers to development of a revised dosing regimen based on feedback from measured drug concentrations. The drug concentration data along with the dosing history is incorporated into the PK model to determine the revised PK parameters and then are utilized to calculate a revised dosing regimen to achieve the desired concentrations.

PHARMACOKINETIC MODELS

Compartmental pharmacokinetic models, in particular the linear one-compartment open model (see *Basic PK/PD* chapter), have been extensively studied and applied to the individualization of a number of drugs used in clinical practice (aminoglycosides, procainamide, theophylline, valproic acid, vancomycin etc.). The advantage of this model is its simplicity enabling determination of dosage regimens using a handheld calculator. The disadvantage of this model is that many drugs do not exhibit instantaneous distribution. If drug levels are drawn to check the accuracy of the predictions the levels need to be appropriately timed to avoid the distribution phase. Alternatively, multicompartmental models have been employed to more accurately describe the disposition of drugs such as digoxin that exhibit a significant distribution phase. The availability of computers facilitates the relatively complex calcula-

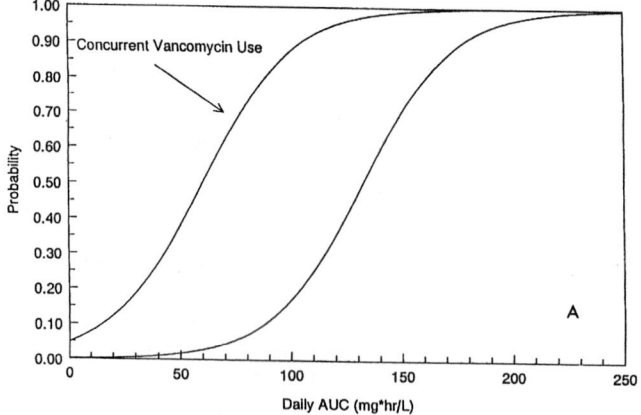

Figure 59-6. Probability of experiencing a nephrotoxic event while receiving gentamicin or tobramycin according to Daily AUC (mg x hr/L). The probability of a nephrotoxic event increases significantly when the daily AUC exceeds 100 mg x h/L. The risk is compounded by the concomitant administration of vancomycin as evidenced by a left shift in the probability curve. (From Rybak et al. *Antimicrob Agents Chemother* 1999; 43:1549.)

tions necessary to determine the revised pharmacokinetic parameters necessary to individualize the dose. The disadvantage of the multicompartment models is that typically more assay measurements are needed in order to provide good estimates of the additional PK parameters needed to describe these models. While multiple plasma concentration measurements are commonly obtained in the drug development process, typically in the clinical setting we are limited to fewer samples (eg, peak and trough). As a result, the linear one-compartment model is the most commonly employed model for predicting and revising drug dosage regimens in the clinical setting.

Steady State

In the clinical setting typically multiple doses of a medication are given to the patient, which necessitates the use of models taking into consideration potential drug accumulation. The dose and dosing interval determine the rate of drug administration $[(F)(Dose/\tau)]$ and help to establish the type of drug input process that would be most appropriate. Drugs that are administered with a dosing interval that is much shorter than the drug t 1/2 (eg, $\tau \leq$ 1/3 t 1/2) can usually be modeled as a continuous infusion as represented by Equation 13 described previously.

Continuous input

$$Css\ ave = \frac{F\ Dose/\tau}{CL} \qquad (13)$$

As can be seen in Figure 59-7, when the τ is very short compared to the drug t 1/2, the difference between the peak and trough concentration is very small (<20%), and all concentrations within the dosing interval are a good representation of the Css ave. This assumption that all drug concentrations are an approximation of Css ave when $\tau \leq$ 1/3 t 1/2 is based on a one compartment model and is not valid when drug concentrations are obtained during the distribution phase.

The dosage form is also important in terms of evaluating the drug input process. For many orally administered drugs, absorption is relatively rapid, and peak concentrations will occur within 1 to 2 hours. As an example, if a drug is administered every 12 hours as a non-sustained-release product, it might be thought of as an intermittent dose and modeled with Equation

24, which is the one-compartment intermittent bolus equation that assumes instantaneous absorption and distribution. The input may be considered instantaneous even if administered orally or as a short infusion as long as the absorption/input is short relative to the elimination half-life (ie,<1/6 t1/2 ~ 10% drug loss during absorption/input). In the example, figure the drug was absorbed or infused over 1 hour and had an elimination half-life of 6 hours.

Intermittent Bolus (t_{in} <1/6 t1/2)

$$C_{ss_t} = \frac{\dfrac{(F)Dose}{V_D}}{(1 - e^{-k_{el}\tau})}\ e^{-k_{el}t} \qquad (24)$$

where Css_t is the steady-state drug concentration at any time t after the Dose or Css max concentration.

However, if absorption is slow or a sustained-release dosage form is used, the drug input process may be more appropriately thought of as a continuous process. As an example, if a drug product is administered every 12 hours as a sustained-release dosage form with an absorption time of approximately 12 hours (time of absorption equal to τ), there would be very little change in the drug concentration within the dosing interval. The drug concentrations could therefore be modeled as a continuous infusion using Equation 13.

In contrast, the input may not be considered instantaneous when administered as a short infusion or orally if the input is considered long relative to the elimination half-life (ie, $\geq$1/6 t1/2). For example, if the same drug product with a 12-hour absorption time were administered with a dosing interval of 24 hours, the drug concentration time curve would be most appropriately modeled by Equation 25 as follows:

Intermittent Infusion ($t_{in} \geq$ 1/6 t1/2)

$$C_{ss_t} = \frac{\dfrac{(F)(Dose/t_{in})}{CL_T}(1 - e^{k_{el}t_{in}})}{(1 - e^{-k_{el}\tau})}\ e^{-kt} \qquad (25)$$

where $Dose/t_{in}$ is the rate of infusion, t_{in} is the duration of the infusion, and t is the time from the end of the infusion to when the drug concentration at steady state (Css_t) is obtained.

Loading Dose

As can be seen readily from the figures (Figs 59-8 and 59-9), it may take only a few doses if $\tau \gg$ t1/2 or many doses if $\tau \ll$ t1/2 for concentrations to reach steady. Under these circumstances, it may be clinically beneficial to administer a loading dose to rapidly achieve therapeutic concentrations. As discussed previously, the incorporation of the initial concentration into the loading dose equation (Equation 6) to account for any existing drug in the body that may be present prior to administration of the loading dose should be considered.

PK/PD DOSAGE ADJUSTMENT

Drug Dosing in Renal Disease

Dosage adjustment of drugs in patients with renal impairment should be based on a knowledge of the pharmacokinetic parameters of the drug and, when indicated, on monitoring of plasma drug concentration. The aim of individualizing dosing regimens for patients with impaired elimination is to maintain plasma concentrations similar to that of patients with normal elimination and, thus, to avoid unnecessary toxicity or loss of efficacy.

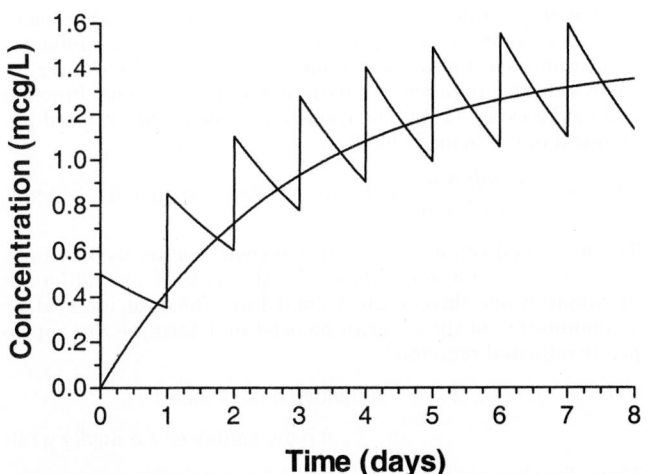

Figure 59-7. Serum concentration time profile for a drug administered as a continuous infusion. Continuous input model can also be assumed if the input time is less than one-third of a half-life.

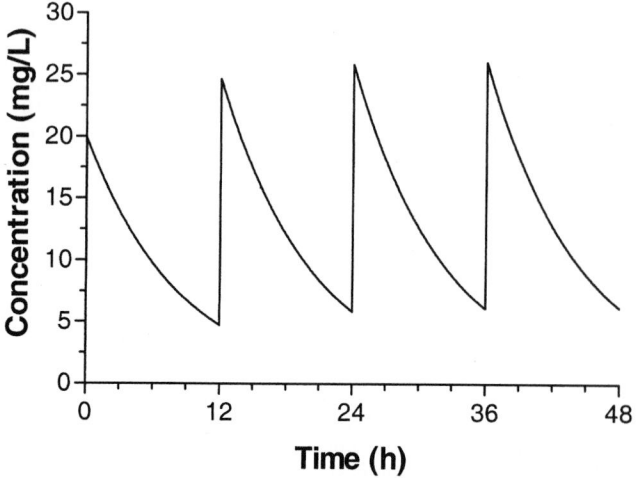

Figure 59-8. Serum concentration time profile for a drug administered as an intermittent bolus dose. Bolus input can also be assumed if the input time is less than one-sixth of a half-life.

In Chapter 58 it can be seen that $C_{ss(ave)}$ is a direct function of dose (D) and bioavailability (F) and an inverse function of the dosing interval (τ) and clearance. In the patient with impaired elimination or decreased clearance, $C_{ss(ave)}$ will increase until a new steady state is achieved. If clearance is impaired markedly or if the therapeutic index of the drug is small, toxicity may occur.

It is apparent from the same equation that either an appropriate decrease in dose or increase in the dosing interval will offset a decrease in elimination, and a $C_{ss(ave)}$ can be attained that is similar to that in a nonimpaired patient.

In the patient with renal impairment, individualization of drug therapy requires knowledge of the degree of impairment and its effect on drug elimination, to choose a proper dose or dosing interval to achieve a desired $C_{ss(ave)}$. As discussed above, the endogenous creatinine clearance is usually the most practical index of GFR, and it is used widely (with the limitations indicated) to determine the degree of renal impairment in a patient with renal disease.

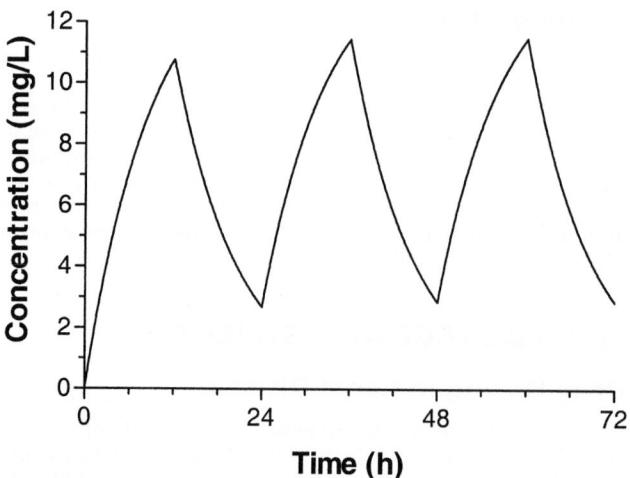

Figure 59-9. Serum concentration time profile for a drug administered as an intermittent infusion dose. The intermittent infusion model (zero order input) can also be assumed for most oral dosage forms where the input time exceeds one-sixth of a half-life.

In the literature, there are a variety of nomograms and equations available to aid in calculating dosage regimens for patients with renal impairment as discussed previously. Each is based on a set of assumptions that provide limitations to its use. Therefore, a nomogram or an equation used to determine a dose of a drug to be given to a patient with renal impairment must be used only as a guideline and, when possible, should be used along with monitoring of plasma drug concentration, when indicated, and careful clinical observation to ensure optimal therapy.

The fractional drug clearance in patients with renal insufficiency (F_{CL}) can be estimated from the relationship of the creatinine clearance in the renally impaired patient, the creatinine clearance of normal persons, and the fractional renal and nonrenal clearance of drug in patients with normal renal function according to the equation:

$$F_{CL} = \left[\frac{(CL_{cr})_I}{(CL_{cr})_N} (fe) \right] + (1 - fe) \qquad (26)$$

$$F_{CL} = (Fractional\ renal\ clearance) + (Fractional\ extrarenal\ clearance)$$

where F_{CL} is the fractional drug clearance in a patient with renal insufficiency, $(Cl_{cr})_N$ is the normal creatinine clearance, $(Cl_{cr})_I$ is the creatinine clearance in the patient, and fe (is the fraction of drug excreted unchanged in the urine in patients with normal renal function. The creatinine clearance in normal 70 kg individuals is typically in the range of 100–120 ml/min. If the patient's body size differs significantly from 70 kg then the creatinine clearance estimate should be normalized to 70 kg. Values for fe are readily available in the product information for most currently marketed drugs.

An example of how this PK dosage adjustment method can be applied is as follows. Insofar as the maintenance dose is concerned, the dosage regimen for the patient in renal failure can be modified by adjusting the dose, the dosage interval, or a combination of both according to the calculated dose fraction.

$$(D/\tau_{ri}) = (D/\tau)_n (F_{CL}) \qquad (27)$$

$$\begin{bmatrix} \text{Adjusted} \\ \text{regimen in} \\ \text{renal disease} \end{bmatrix} = \begin{bmatrix} \text{Regimen} \\ \text{in normal} \\ \text{renal function} \end{bmatrix} \times \begin{bmatrix} \text{fractional} \\ \text{drug} \\ \text{clearance} \end{bmatrix}$$

where (D/τ_{ri}) is the dose and dosing interval in renal insufficiency, $(D/\tau)_n$ is the usual dose and interval for normal persons, and the fractional drug clearance is the value determined from the equation as described above. An example of an adjustment in a ganciclovir dosage regimen for a patient with an impaired creatinine clearance of 35 mL/min is as follows: the usual ganciclovir dosage regimen in a patient with normal renal function is 5 mg/kg every 12 hr. The fraction of ganciclovir excreted unchanged in the urine is 0.90.

$$F_{CL} = \left[\frac{(35\ ml/\text{min})}{(120\ ml/\text{min})} (0.9) \right] + (1 - 0.9) = 0.26 + 0.1 = 0.36$$

The fractional renal and extrarenal clearance totals 0.36 indicating that the dosage regimen for this patient should be approximately one-third of the normal dose. The dose, interval, or a combination of the two can be used to determine the appropriate adjusted regimen.

$$(D/\tau_{ri}) = (D/\tau)_n (F_{CL}) = 5\text{mg/kg}/0.5\ \text{days}\ (0.36) =$$

$$3.6\ \text{mg/kg/day or } 1.8\ \text{mg/kg q12h}$$

Thus, for this patient with impaired renal function, a once-a-day dose of 3.6 mg/kg or 1.8 mg/kg q12h is likely to maintain therapeutic plasma concentrations. The decision to adjust the dose or the dosage interval also should be individualized. Fluctuations in plasma concentrations of ganciclovir will be lower if the dosage interval remains 12 rather than 24 hours. However, for some drugs there may be a therapeutic reason to achieve a higher peak plasma concentration by administering a higher dose less frequently (eg, once-daily aminoglycosides). As mentioned above, this or any other nomogram or calculation for dosage adjustment is only an approximation. Once the dosage adjustment has been made, careful clinical observation and, when indicated, monitoring of plasma concentrations is warranted. Since the loading dose depends primarily on the V, a change only in clearance does not typically necessitate a change in the loading dose.

Adjustments Based on Targeted Concentration and/or Pharmacodynamic Response/Surrogates

OBTAINING CLINICAL DATA—Adjustment in a patient's drug regimen requires a careful assessment of the relationship between the drug dosing regimen, laboratory data and the patient's clinical response.

DOSING REGIMEN—Knowing the dose, dosage form, frequency of administration, and duration of a drug regimen is an important piece of information. Clearly an accurate history of the patient's drug intake is one of the key elements required for pharmacokinetic interpretation. The dose of each drug administered as well as the dosage form is important. The route of administration can alter the bioavailability (F) for a number of drugs. Some drugs have a low oral bioavailability that must be considered when the route of drug administration is changed from the intravenous to the oral route.

Linking the drug input characteristics and the pharmacokinetic properties of the drug to the appropriate equation is an important step in the data gathering process.

The duration of drug therapy for a specific regimen is important in determining whether or not steady state has been obtained. As previously indicated, when a patient is receiving a dose at a constant interval, 90% of steady state will be achieved after 3.3 half-lives. While 90% of steady state is probably a reasonable approximation, many clinicians use 4 to 5 half-lives as the time required for steady state to be achieved. This is because in clinical practice the drug's t 1/2 in an individual patient may be shorter or longer than the usual value. Using 4 to 5 t 1/2 as the time required to achieve steady state helps to ensure that steady state has been achieved and decreases the chances that a false assumption about steady state will be made. (See revision of parameters.)

MONITORING EFFICACY AND TOXICITY—In the clinical setting, there are a number of factors that should be considered when evaluating a patient's response to drug therapy. Efficacy of the drug is usually focused on the disease or symptom being treated. As an example in the treatment of an infection, a reduction in a patient's fever, and a decrease in the inflammatory process would be signs of efficacy. Depending on the site of the infection, the inflammatory symptoms could range from swelling and erythema for soft tissue infections to pain or burning on urination for cystitis to mental acuity or headache for central nervous system infections. In addition, laboratory data such as a reduction in white blood cell count could also be used to monitor efficacy. For patients who are being treated for arrhythmias, suppression of the arrhythmia is often the goal and can be monitored by something as simple as taking a patient's pulse and noting that the rhythm is regular (eg, even beats with no intermittent pauses) and the rate is not excessively slow (bradycardia) or rapid (tachycardia). In other arrhythmias, electrocardiograms are used to evaluate a patient's response to therapy. Efficacy in the case of seizures is often the frequency and character of the patient's seizures. Approximately half of the patients with epilepsy are seizure-free, but the other half are only partially controlled with drug therapy.

Monitoring toxicity is equally important. Most of the drug for which pharmacokinetic calculations and plasma drug concentrations are used as an aid to determining dosing regimens have a narrow therapeutic index and or have significant toxicities. For many drugs, the order of drug toxicity is not progressive from what a clinician might consider to be "mild" to "serious." As an example, while gastrointestinal symptoms (anorexia, nausea, or vomiting) are perhaps the most commonly reported digoxin toxicities, some patients may initially present with a life-threatening ventricular arrhythmia.

The aminoglycoside antibiotics are an example of a drug that requires dose adjustment in patients with altered renal function, and plasma drug concentrations can be used to help assure that the patient is not put at additional risk for further nephrotoxicity.

Optimal Sampling Times

DRUG INPUT AND DISTRIBUTION PHASE—In almost all cases, obtaining plasma samples for drug concentrations during or shortly after the administration of a drug is not advisable. When drugs are administered by the intravenous route, there is a distribution phase that is transient and will result in either invalid or at best more complicated pharmacokinetic and clinical interpretations when employing a one-compartment model. For most drugs, the distribution phase is relatively short, and distribution is complete within 1 hour after the end of the drug infusion. Digoxin is an exception and following IV administration at least 4 hours is required for equilibrium to be attained between the plasma and more slowly equilibrating deeper compartment. Some drugs may equilibrate more rapidly and aminoglycoside antibiotics following a 30-minute infusion will distribute within 30 minutes. Clearly, sampling during the IV administration of a drug is not advisable and results in drug concentrations that are, in the clinical setting, useless.

Most drugs following oral administration are absorbed at a rate that is sufficiently slow so that the two-compartment distribution phase is not observed. Two exceptions to the limited distribution phase following oral administration are digoxin and lithium. Following oral administration, digoxin requires at least 6 hours for absorption and distribution to be complete, and lithium takes even longer. In addition, following oral administration, the onset of absorption is often delayed and/or the rate of absorption is sufficiently altered so that drug samples obtained shortly after the administration of an oral dose are difficult to interpret. For this reason, for most orally administered drugs, the preferred time to sample is at the trough. On occasion sampling at the middle of the interval is acceptable and is most common when sustained-release products are used or the trough occurs at a time that would be very inconvenient to obtain a sample.

NON-STEADY STATE—In most clinical settings, routine samples for therapeutic drug monitoring are obtained at steady state or more than 3 to 5 half-lives after starting or changing the maintenance regimen. In some cases, however, it may be advisable to obtain drug samples prior to steady state. Early sampling may allow the clinician to detect the unusual patient who is accumulating the drug rapidly and will, at steady state, have very high and potentially dangerous drug concentrations or the patient who can clear the drug unusually well and would have an unnecessarily prolonged time with low and non-therapeutic concentrations.

As a general rule drug samples obtained within 2 half-lives of starting therapy are useful only for assessing the patient at that time. If the drug concentration is unacceptably high, it might indicate that drug administration should be stopped to allow the drug concentration to decline. If the drug concentration is unacceptably low, it might indicate that an incremental loading dose should be administered to rapidly move the drug concentration into the desired concentration range. If the drug concentration is within a reasonable range, however, it does not mean that the maintenance regimen is appropriate because drug samples obtained within the first 2 half-lives of starting or changing therapy are not useful for revising clearance and predicting steady-state concentrations.

Drug concentrations obtained after 2 half-lives but before 3.3 to 5 half-lives do contain some information about clearance and steady state but generally require more complex, non-steady state pharmacokinetic calculations and are most easily done using a computer program.

STEADY STATE—At steady state, most plasma samples for routine monitoring are obtained at specific times that allow pharmacokinetic interpretation. As previously discussed, no sample should be obtained during the drug administration/-absorption or distribution time. In addition, comparing the expected or usual drug t 1/2 and the dosing interval as well as the dosage form type (rapid vs. sustained) helps to determine the optimal time for obtaining samples.

For drugs that are administered with a dosing interval that is less than 1/3 of the drug's t 1/2 or if the dosage form is designed to release the drug over the entire dosing interval (Fig 59-7), then a single sample obtained at almost any time is acceptable so long as the absorption and distribution phase is avoided. However, for simplicity these drugs are usually recommended to be sampled at the trough or just before a dose. In some cases, sampling at the trough is not convenient, and midpoint sampling may be acceptable. Under these conditions, all of the drug concentrations within the dosing interval are assumed to be a close approximation of the Css ave concentration, making clearance the pharmacokinetic parameter of interest.

For drugs that are administered with a dosing interval that is more than 1/3 of a t 1/2 but less than one t 1/2 (Fig 59-8), it is usually recommended that a single trough concentration be obtained. Additional samples only increase the cost and do not usually increase substantially the amount of pharmacokinetic information that can be determined. Pharmacokinetic manipulations to calculate clearance require a literature estimate of volume of distribution. While the peak and trough concentrations are not a good direct approximation of Css ave, it is still clearance that is the pharmacokinetic parameter most responsible for determining both the steady state peak and trough drug concentrations when the dosing interval is less than t 1/2.

When the dosing interval exceeds t 1/2 and especially when the dosing interval is several t 1/2's (Fig 59-9), both volume of distribution and clearance play an important role in determining the steady-state peak and trough concentrations. Therefore, if both peak and trough concentrations are of clinical interest, two samples are required. In the clinical setting, the most common drugs following this type of dosing and plasma monitoring routine are the aminoglycoside antibiotics. In most cases, it is recommended to obtain a "peak sample" sometime after the distribution phase is complete, usually 30 minutes to 1 hour after the end of the infusion and trough concentrations within 30 minutes of the next dose. For convenience, it is common for the trough concentration to be obtained before a dose and then the peak after the dose. Although an accurate time of sampling is always appropriate, the short t 1/2 of the aminoglycoside antibiotics makes recording the time of sampling especially important.

DETERMINATION OF REVISED (A POSTERIORI) PK PARAMETERS—Once drug concentrations are obtained they need to be analyzed to determine the appropriateness of the current dosage regimen in achieving the desired goals (ie, peak, AUC). Several different methods have been described for analyzing such data and include log-linear regression, non-linear regression, and maximum *a posteriori* Bayesian analysis.

Log-Linear Regression—Log-linear regression analysis is used most widely in the clinical setting due to its simplicity requiring only a handheld calculator to determine the revised parameters. This method of analysis was first proposed for dosage individualization of aminoglycosides by Sawchuk and Zaske for use in the clinical setting. This method is based on the observation that for drugs for which the disposition can be adequately described using a one-compartment model, the concentrations decline in a log-linear relationship. As illustrated in the figure below (Fig 59-10), the concentrations decline in a nonlinear fashion when plotted on a linear scale; however, if plotted on a natural logarithm scale, the concentrations decline in a linear fashion. The importance of this observation is that the elimination rate constant can be readily determined from slope = K.

In the clinical setting typically we are able to obtain a peak and trough concentration to assess the adequacy of the dosing regimen. These concentrations can then be utilized to revise our estimates for the elimination rate constant using the aforementioned log-linear model as demonstrated below. The half-life can then be calculated from the revised K *using equation 19 as described earlier.*

Revise K and $T\ 1/2$:

$$K = \frac{\ln \dfrac{C_1}{C_2}}{\Delta t} \qquad (28)$$

$$t\ 1/2 = \frac{0.693}{K} \qquad (19)$$

The estimated volume of distribution can then be revised using the one compartment model substituting values for the dose, measured drug concentration, revised elimination rate constant, and time within the dosing interval that the drug concentration was obtained relative to the start of the dose. The revised clearance estimate can then be calculated from the revised K and V.

Revise V and CL:

$$V_d = \frac{\dfrac{(F)\text{Dose}}{C_1}}{1 - e^{-K\tau}}\, e^{-Kt} \qquad (29)$$

$$CL = (K)\,(V) \qquad (18)$$

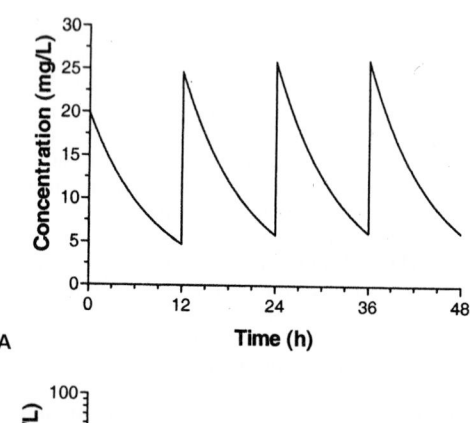

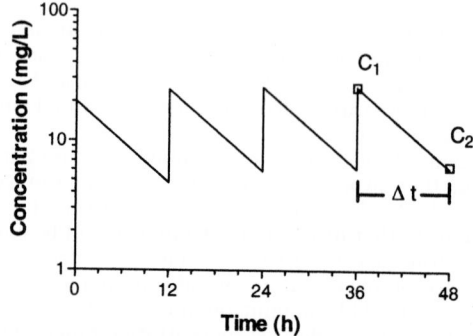

Figure 59-10. Nonlinear (a) and log-linear (b) decline in concentrations.

As stated earlier, the simplicity of this model accounts for its widespread use in clinical practice. One significant limitation of this model is that it requires that the levels to be analyzed are all within the same dosing interval or are obtained at steady state with the same dosing regimen. Therefore, this method cannot be used in situations where multiple sets of drugs levels are available or when the levels are from different dosing intervals under non steady state conditions.

Nonlinear Regression—Nonlinear regression analysis is a tool available in many statistical and commercially available pharmacokinetic software programs. This method employs regression analysis on the unaltered drug concentration data (ie, no log transformation). The parameter values that are identified using this method are those that result in the minimum error between the fitted and measure concentration data. The advantage of this type of analysis is that multi-compartmental models can be utilized to fit the data if necessary. In addition, data from multiple dosing intervals obtained under steady state or non-steady state conditions can be analyzed. One limitation to this method is that the revised parameters are determined based on the best fit to the measured drug concentration data without regard to the expected or a priori estimates of the parameters. Since many different combinations of the parameters might equally well explain the data it is possible to identify parameter values which are well described by the model but may not correlate well with values from the population particularly if the data is sparse (ie, single peak and trough concentrations).

Maximum A Posteriori Bayesian—MAP Bayesian analysis is a data analysis tool which seeks to identify the parameter values that best fit the measured data (similar to nonlinear regression) and which are most likely given the prior expectations for the values within the population. The initial parameter values utilized in the data fitting are those obtained from prior pharmacokinetic studies performed in similar types of patients. Additional iterations are performed to identify the parameter values that minimize the residual error between the fitted and measured drug concentrations as well as the difference between the revised and expected parameter values. Therefore, MAP Bayesian analysis is thought to provide the most likely estimates of the parameters. Similar to nonlinear regression, multicompartmental models can be utilized to fit the data if necessary, and data from multiple dosing intervals obtained under steady state or nonsteady state conditions can be analyzed.

CASE STUDIES

Digoxin Case History

TY is a 70-year-old, 5 foot 7 inch, 77 kg man who was admitted to the Coronary Care Unit for CHF and atrial fibrillation. He is in stable condition, but because of his rapid ventricular response it is decided that he should receive an IV loading dose of digoxin followed by an oral maintenance dose with the target digoxin concentration of 1.5 mcg / mL.

TY has lower extremity edema, and review of his previous records indicates that one month ago his weight was 69 kg.

Laboratory:

Na^+	134 mEq/L	HCT	36 %	AST	28 IU/L
Cl^-	101 mEq/L	Hgb	12.2 gm/dL	ALT	55 IU/L
K^+	4.4 mEq/L	WBC	5.4 K/mcL	TSH	3 mIU/mL
HCO_3	23 mEq/L	Plts	170 /mm^3	T. Bili	0.6 mg/dL
BUN	41 mg/dL	Albumin	3.9 gm/dL	Gluc	119 mg/dL
SCr	3.2 mg/dL				

In order to calculate the expected pharmacokinetic parameters, clearance (CL), volume of distribution (V), half-life (t 1/2), and the elimination rate constant (K) we first need to evaluate the patient's weight. At 5 feet 7 inches and 77 kg TY would not be considered to be obese. However TY's current weight of 77 kg when compared to his weight 1 month ago of 69 kg suggests that he has approximately 8 liters of third space fluid (77 − 69 = 8). The assumption that the weight gain is all excess third space fluid is based on the presence of lower extremity edema and that an 8-kg increase in either muscle mass or adipose tissue in one month is unlikely.

When calculating creatinine clearance and digoxin's CL and V, it is the non-obese, non-excess third space fluid weight that should be used. Therefore for TY, we will use his weight of 69 kg.

In order to calculate the CL and V for digoxin, we will first calculate TY's creatinine clearance using Equation 14:

$$\text{Clcr for males (ml/min)} = \frac{(140 - \text{Age})(\text{Weight})}{(72)(\text{SCrss})}$$

$$= \frac{(140 - 70 \ years)(69 \ kg)}{(72)(3.2 \ mg/dL)}$$

$$= 21 \ ml/min$$

or

$$= \frac{21 \ ml/min}{69 \ kg}$$

$$= 0.30 \ mL/min/kg$$

Using this estimate of Clcr of 0.3 mL/min/kg for T.Y. and the following equation for $V_{Digoxin}$:

$$V_{Digoxin} = [(3.12)(CL_{cr}) + 3.84](weight)$$

where $V_{Digoxin}$ is liters, CL_{cr} is mL/min/kg, weight is kg of non-obese, non-excess third space fluid weight. Substituting the appropriate values for TY, we calculate a $V_{Digoxin}$ of 330 L.

$$V_{Digoxin} = [(3.12)(0.3) + 3.84](69)$$

$$= [0.94 + 3.84](69)$$

$$= [4.78](69)$$

$$= 330 \ L$$

Note that this value of 330 L for $V_{Digoxin}$ is smaller than the commonly quoted value of approximately 500 L. The lower estimate is because of TY's decreased renal function. The reason for the smaller $V_{Digoxin}$ in patients with decreased renal function is not known but is assumed to be the result of decreased tissue binding of digoxin.

We can estimate TY's $CL_{Digoxin}$ using the equation below.

$$CL_{Digoxin} = [(0.88)(CL_{cr}) + 0.33](weight)$$

$CL_{Digoxin}$ is mL/min, Cl_{cr} is in mL/min/kg and weight is the non-obese, non- excess third space fluid weight. This equation is indicated for patients with congestive heart failure. Substituting the appropriate values for TY, we calculate a $CL_{Digoxin}$ of 41 mL/min.

$$CL_{Digoxin} = [(0.88)(0.3) + 0.33](69)$$

$$= [0.264 + 0.33](69)$$

$$= [0.594](69)$$

$$= 41 \ mL/min$$

While the $CL_{digoxin}$ of 41 mL/min could be used to calculate a digoxin maintenance dose, units of L/day would be more convenient, given that the dosing interval of digoxin is usually one day. The conversion to L/day is as follows:

$$CL \ in \ L/day = CL \ in \ mL/min \left(\frac{1440 \ min/day}{1000 \ mL/L} \right)$$

$$= 41 \ mL/min \left(\frac{1440 \ min/day}{1000 \ mL/L} \right)$$

$$= 59 \ L/day$$

Using the values for $V_{Digoxin}$ and $CL_{digoxin}$ we can now calculate the t 1/2 and K for digoxin in TY.

$$t \ 1/2 = \frac{0.693 \ V}{CL}$$

$$= \frac{0.693(330 \ L)}{59 \ L/day}$$

$$= 3.9 \ days$$

and

$$K = \frac{CL}{V}$$

$$K = \frac{59 \ L/day}{330 \ L}$$

$$= 0.179 \ day^{-1}$$

Now that we have the expected pharmacokinetic parameters for digoxin in TY, we can calculate a loading dose and maintenance dose to achieve and maintain a steady-state digoxin concentration of 1.5 mcg/L.

To calculate the loading dose we would use Equation 6.

$$\text{Loading Dose} = \frac{(C)(V)}{F}$$

By substituting 330 L for V, 1.5 mcg/L for C, and 1 for F, assuming the loading dose is to be administered by the intravenous route, we calculate a loading dose of approximately 500 mcg.

$$\text{Loading Dose} = \frac{(C)(V)}{F}$$

$$= \frac{(1.5 \ \text{mcg/L})(330 \ \text{L})}{1}$$

$$= 495 \ mcg \ \text{or} \approx 500 \ mcg$$

Digoxin is one of the drugs whose end organ for response, in this case the myocardium, responds as though it were located in the deeper more slowly equilibrating tissue compartment. The loading dose is usually divided so that one-half of the total loading dose is administered followed by one fourth and then the final one-fourth. The interval between the loading dose increments is usually from 1 to 6 hours, depending on the clinical urgency. Dividing the loading dose and waiting for it to distribute into the tissue allows the clinician to evaluate the patient's clinical response (toxicity or efficacy) before subsequent portions of the loading dose are administered. If the patient developed toxicity or achieved the desired therapeutic goal before the entire loading dose had been administered the remaining part of the loading dose would be withheld.

To estimate the daily dose necessary to maintain TY's digoxin steady-state concentration at 1.5 mcg/L we would use Equation 12 below.

$$\text{Dose} = \frac{(CL)(Css \ ave)(\tau)}{F}$$

Using the equation above to calculate the maintenance dose required is appropriate based on the t 1/2 of almost 4 days and the dosing interval of 1 day. Under these conditions, there should be relatively little fluctuation in the digoxin concentrations within the 1 day dosing interval. Substituting 59 L/day for CL, 1.5 mcg/L for Css ave, 1 day for τ, and 0.7 for F, assuming that the daily digoxin dose will be administered orally as tablets, we calculate a maintenance dose of 126.4 mcg/day.

$$\text{Dose} = \frac{(CL)(Css \ ave)(\tau)}{F}$$

$$= \frac{(59 \ \text{L/day})(1.5 \ \text{mcg/L})(1 \ day)}{0.7}$$

$$= 126.4 \ mcg/day$$

Given that a daily dose of 126.4 mcg would be difficult to administer, the patient would be given 125 mcg (0.125 mg) of digoxin daily.

To monitor for efficacy the patient's heart rate and symptoms of congestive heart failure would be closely followed. In addition the patient would also be monitored for symptoms of toxicity (eg, nausea or vomiting, anorexia, visual changes, or a new cardiac arrhythmia). If digoxin concentrations are to be obtained, care should be taken to avoid the distribution phase (no sampling for digoxin levels within 4 hours of an intravenous dose or 6 hours of an oral dose). In addition because of the expected t 1/2 of approximately 4 days any sample obtained before 12 to 20 days (3 to 5 t 1/2's) should be viewed with caution as steady state may not yet have been achieved.

Aminoglycoside Case History

DS, a 65-year-old, 5 foot 5 inch, 62 kg woman, is hospitalized and recovering from total hip replacement surgery. On postoperative day 5, she develops shortness of breath and becomes febrile. A chest x-ray is performed, and she is diagnosed with a nosocomial-acquired pneumonia. She is initiated empirically on cefepime 2 gm intravenously q12h and tobramycin 440 mg intravenously over 1 hour q24h.

Pertinent Laboratory values:

BUN	14 mg/dL	SCr	1.0 mg/dL	WBC	16.2 K/mcL

Is the current tobramycin regimen appropriate? In order to assess the current dosing regimen it is necessary to calculate the predicted (a priori) pharmacokinetic parameters. As discussed previously, the aminoglycosides can be adequately described using a one-compartment linear model. Since aminoglycosides are almost exclusively excreted unchanged in the urine the clearance is typically approximated by creatinine clearance.

DS's ideal body weight can be estimated using equation 8:

$$\text{IBW} = 45 + 2.3 \ [\text{Ht (in)} - 60]$$

$$= 45 + 2.3 \ (65 - 60)$$

$$= 56.5$$

Since DS's actual weight is only 110% of her ideal body weight, it would be reasonable to assume she is not obese, and therefore we can utilize her actual body weight in estimating the clearance and volume of distribution of tobramycin.

Therefore, the tobramycin clearance can be estimated using equation 15:

$$\text{Clcr for females (ml/min)} = (0.85) \frac{(140 - Age)(Weight)}{(72)(SCrss)}$$

$$= (0.85) \frac{(140 - 65 \ \text{years})(62 \ \text{kg})}{(72)(1.0 \ \text{mg/dL})}$$

$$= 55 \ \text{ml/min}$$

This estimated creatinine clearance indicates that DS has mild renal insufficiency (normal creatinine clearance ~ 100–120 ml/min/70kg), which is most likely due to an age related decline in renal function. This estimate of renal function can be used then to estimate tobramycin clearance. The clearance is then converted from ml/min to L/hr for convenience since the dosing interval is usually 8, 12, or 24 hours.

$$\text{CL}_{\text{Tobramycin}} \text{ (L/hr)} = \text{CLcr (ml/min)} \left(\frac{60 \ \text{min/hr}}{1000 \ \text{ml/L}} \right)$$

$$= 55 \ \text{ml/min} \ (0.06)$$

$$= 3.3 \ \text{L/hr}$$

The volume of distribution of tobramycin approximates extracellular fluid volume and therefore can be estimated based on 25% of a patient's normal weight. If the patient is significantly obese (ie, >120% of ideal body weight) or exhibits significant third spaced fluid (edema or ascites), then these need to be taken into consideration in estimating the volume of distribution as follows:

$$\text{Vd}_{\text{Tobramycin}} = 0.25 \ \text{L/kg (IBW)} + 0.1 \ (\text{TBW} - \text{IBW}) + 1 \ (\text{kg of fluid excess})$$

where IBW is the ideal body weight (equation 8), TBW is the total non-fluid weight, and the kg of fluid excess is typically estimated from the difference between the patients current weight and admission weight.

Since DS is not obese and does not exhibit significant third space fluid, her volume of distribution can be estimated as follows:

$$\text{V}_{\text{Tobramycin}} = 0.25 \ \text{L/kg [Wt (kg)]}$$

$$= 0.25 \ \text{L/kg (62 kg)}$$

$$= 15.5 \ \text{L}$$

The elimination rate constant and half-life can then be calculated using the following equations:

$$K(h^{-1}) = \frac{CL}{V} = \frac{3.3 \text{ L/hr}}{15.5 \text{ L}} = 0.21 \text{ h}^{-1}$$

$$T1/2(\text{h}) = \frac{0.693}{K} = \frac{0.693}{0.21 \text{ h}^{-1}} = 3.3 \text{ h}$$

The predicted steady state peak and trough tobramycin concentrations can be predicted using the intermittent bolus equation 24.

$$C_{SS_1} = \frac{\dfrac{(F)(Dose)}{V}}{(1 - e^{-K\tau})} e^{-Kt_1}$$

where C_{SS_1} is the steady state plasma concentration at time (t_1) from the end of infusion, to the time of sampling, and τ is the dosing interval.

$$Peak = \frac{\dfrac{(1)(440 mg)}{15.5 L}}{(1 - e^{-(0.21 \text{h}^{-1})(24\text{h})})} e^{-(0.21 \text{h}^{-1})(1\text{h})} = 23.1 \text{ mg/L}$$

This peak concentration is therapeutic based on the target of > 10 times breakpoint for susceptibility; MIC = 2mcg/mL. The trough concentration can be calculated using the same equation or by decaying the peak concentration to the time of the trough assuming monoexponential decay.

$$\text{Trough} = \text{Peak } e^{-Kt}$$

$$\text{Trough} = 23.1 mg/L(e^{-(0.21 \text{h}-1)(23\text{h})}$$

$$\text{Trough} = 0.17 \text{ mg/L}$$

Trough concentrations <0.5 mcg/mL are typically below the limit of assay detection and are therefore not useful for assessing the degree of drug exposure. Therefore, midpoint or concentrations obtained greater then 2 to 3 half-lives from the peak concentration may be more useful is determining the level of drug exposure (ie, AUC_{24}).

$$AUC_{24} = \frac{Dose_{24}}{CL}$$

$$AUC_{24} = \frac{440 mg}{3.3 L/hr} = 133 \text{ mg} \times \text{h/L}$$

This measure of drug exposure exceeds the target of 70–100 mg x h/L and may place the patient at increased risk for toxicity. Exposure for elderly with seemingly normal renal function (normal SCr) is much greater than for younger patients given the equivalent doses due to age-related decline in renal function. While extended interval dosing may still be appropriate, the actual dose administered may need reduction to achieve similar levels of drug exposure. Since the dose and concentrations are linearly related, a revised dose and peak estimate can be determined using a proportional adjustment.

To achieve a target AUC_{24} of ~100 the dose should be:

$$C_{New} = C_{Observed}\left(\frac{Target\ AUC}{Observed\ AUC}\right)$$

or

$$Dose_{New} = Dose_{Old}\left(\frac{Target\ AUC}{Observed\ AUC}\right)$$

$$Dose_{New} = 440 mg\left(\frac{100 mgxh/L}{133 mgxh/L}\right)$$

$$= 330 \text{ mg given intravenously q24h}$$

$$C_{New} = 23.1 mg/L\left(\frac{100 mgxh/L}{133 mgxh/L}\right) = 17.3 \text{ mg/L}$$

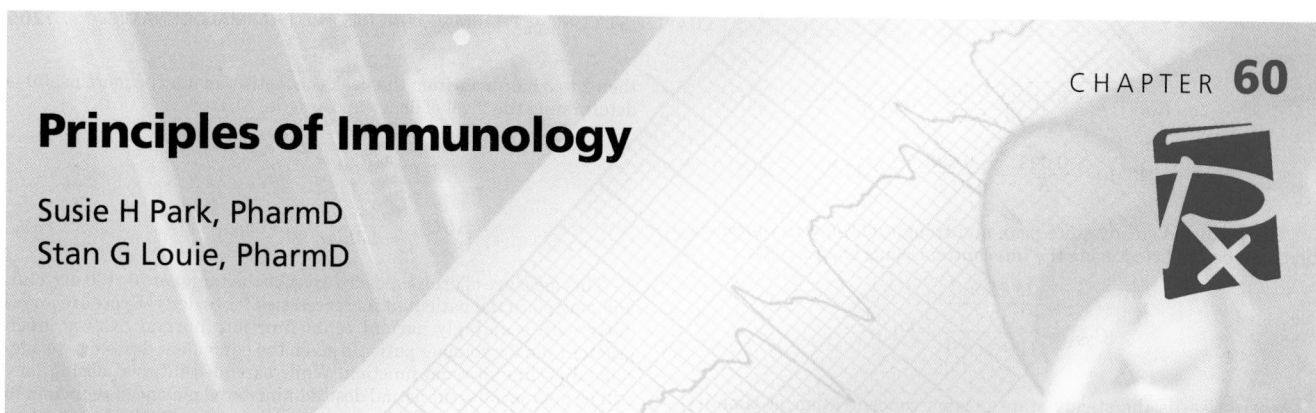

CHAPTER **60**

Principles of Immunology

Susie H Park, PharmD
Stan G Louie, PharmD

Our lives are filled with stresses and problems, and yet the effort to perform the cellular and biochemical processes required for survival are closely regulated. The regulation of normal physiological activity is called homeostasis, which is activated or "inducible" in times of stress and down regulated to basal levels when the stress is eliminated. One component of this complex system is a defense mechanism more commonly known as the "immune system."

The immune system is a network of defense mechanisms classified as the humoral and cellular compartment. The humoral and cellular compartment can be further subdivided into three distinctive classes know as antibodies, complement factors, and cytokines. However the humoral compartment cannot function alone, rather, it must coordinate its activities with the cellular compartment. The combination of the two compartments will orchestrate an effective defense against any foreign intrusion. The cellular compartment is often divided into regulatory and effector components. The regulatory role is primarily carried out by T-lymphocytes bearing the cell differentiating cluster-4 (CD4+), which elaborates cytokines that in turn can regulate immune function. The effector component of the immune system is made up of cytotoxic T-lymphocytes (CTLs) and natural killer cells (NKCs) where they have the capacity to kill foreign organisms (Table 60-1).

Cellular immunity is not restricted to lymphocytes. Close coordination with myeloid cells such as macrophages, neutrophils, basophils, and eosinophils is necessary in response to specific antigenic challenges. Macrophages function primarily as scavengers, seeking out antigens that have traversed the barrier defenses such as the skin and mucosal membranes. Macrophages are important in the eradication of fungal and bacterial infections, and control of tumor proliferation. Neutrophils, basophils, and eosinophils all have granules in the cytoplasm and are grouped as granulocytes. Neutrophils are important in suppressing bacterial and fungal infections, where a reduction in the number of neutrophils will predispose the individual to life-threatening infections. Eosinophils are important components in response to allergens; however, they are also important in immune response against parasitic infections. This chapter will highlight the various functions of the immune system and how the various components work together to orchestrate a defense. An overview will also be presented on the biological consequence(s) that may occur when one of the compartment(s) is not functioning sufficiently.

LYMPHOID ORGANS

The various organs that make up the immune system include the bone marrow, thymus gland, spleen, and lymph nodes.

These organs are connected by a network of lymphatic vessels, filled with lymphatic fluid and cellular elements that allow immune elements to circulate from one organ to another. The lymphatic system is similar to the circulatory system; however, the lymphatic fluid is devoid of erythrocytes. The lymphatic fluid contains high levels of leukocytes, important in response to local infections and antigenic intrusion.

Circulating cells found in the blood and lymphatic fluid are all derived from a common parental source, the pluripotent stem cells (PSCs), which reside in the marrow of long bone and the pelvis. It is estimated that PSCs make up only 0.1% of all the cells found in the marrow, yet they provide a continuous supply of cells found in the circulatory system. The ability to produce seemingly unlimited number of cells is achieved through a unique capacity called *self-renewal*. In this process, the stem cell is able to divide into two daughter cells, where one cell will further undergo the maturation and differentiation process to form circulating cells. In contrast, the second daughter cell will maintain quiescent and rejoin the pool of stem cells. Self-renewal will maintain the number of parental cells and allow the stem cells to constantly replenish the various cells found in the circulation.

A more intriguing question is what regulates the type of cells being produced. It appears that the maturation and differentiation processes are under strict control of hematopoietic cytokines or growth factors. Cytokines can influence the formation and function of either myeloid or lymphoid progenitor cells, where the binding of one cytokine can down regulate other cytokine receptors, thus preferentially regulating the maturation process. The maturation of lymphoid progenitor is influenced by the presence of lymphokines and interferons, whereas the formation of myeloid progenitor cells are influenced by programmed myeloid growth factors or colony stimulating factors (CSFs) such as erythropoietin (EPO), thrombopoietin (TPO), granulocyte-macrophage CSF (GM-CSF), granulocyte-CSF (G-CSF), and macrophage-CSF (M-CSF) (Table 60-2).

The thymus is the primary lymphoid tissue that regulates differentiation and maturation of lymphocytes. In this role, immature lymphocytes (CD3+) that enter into the circulation migrate into the thymus. In the thymic environment, a number of cytokines, growth factors, and interactions with the basement membrane will initiate cellular maturation and differentiation.

In organ ablation studies, the specific role of the thymus has been delineated. In mature mice whose thymus was removed, profound cellular immunodeficiency developed. Significantly lowered number of circulating lymphocytes was a hallmark of these mice when compared to mice with intact thymus. In genetically engineered-athymic mice that were transplanted with thymus, functional T-lymphocytes were identified in the blood.

1206

Table 60-1. Types of Lymphocytes

TYPES OF LYMPHOCYTES	SURFACE MARKER	FUNCTIONS
T-lymphocytes		
Helper T-lymphocytes	CD4	Regulate the activation of the immune cascade
• TH₁	CD4	Regulate cellular immunity
• TH₂	CD4	Regulate humoral immunity
Suppressor T-lymphocytes	CD8	Down-regulate the immune cascade
Cytotoxic T-lymphocytes	CD8	Cellular cytotoxic activity
Natural killer Cells	NK 1.1	Antibody dependent cellular cytotoxic
B-lymphocytes	CD19	Antibody production
	CD24	

However, mice that received shammed transplants developed viral infections and malignancies.

The spleen is the largest lymphatic organ in the body and is located just below the diaphragm stretching from the middle to the left side of the abdomen. It serves as a filter, where reticular and macrophage-like cells line the vascular sinusoids. The spleen plays an important role in host defense against microorganisms that have penetrated barrier defense. Antigens that are found in the circulation will be filtered within the confines of the spleen. While in the spleen, the antigen will encounter a rapid and intense immune response. In addition to its ability to remove antigens, the spleen is important in eliminating old circulating cells. The numbers of B-lymphocytes, the cells that produce antibodies, found in the spleen explain why it is an important antibody-producing organ.

Lymphatic fluid circulates through the lymphatic vessels and a series of bean-shaped lymphatic tissue called lymph nodes. Lymph nodes are comprised of lymphatic vessels that lead into a connective tissue network that is filled with lymphocytes and macrophages. These connective tissue complexes are produced by reticular cells, which are specialized fibroblasts. Similar to other lymphatic tissues, lymph nodes function as a biological filter, where lymphatic fluids flow through them. Antigens and microorganisms found in the lymphatic fluid will be trapped within the connective tissue lattice. The presence of foreign intrusion will activate lymphocytes and macrophages residing within the confines of the lymph nodes and will induce proliferation of the cells and activate the inflammatory process. In the event of intense immune response, there can be noticeable enlargement of the lymph node and is referred to as lymphadenopathy.

HUMORAL IMMUNITY

Antibodies

The presence of antibodies in all fluids and secretion demonstrate its role in preventing antigenic intrusion. Antibodies are glycoproteins that can neutralize any foreign antigen. Immunoglobulins or antibodies exist in two forms, cellular and soluble forms. The cell-associated antibodies are expressed on the surfaces of resting B-lymphocytes and serve as antigen receptors. In contrast, the soluble form neutralizes foreign agents and activates the immune cascade.

CLASSES OF ANTIBODIES—Antibodies can be divided into five categories that are designated as immunoglobulin A (IgA), immunoglobulin D (IgD), immunoglobulin E (IgE), immunoglobulin G (IgG), and immunoglobulin M (IgM). The difference among the various immunoglobulins is in the nature of polypeptides that makes the entire complex. Immunoglobulin typically has identical heavy chains but different light chains. This difference in immunoglobulin structure is called isotypic variation. However, immunoglobulins from different individuals may be different due to genetic variations. These changes are referred to as allotypic variation and are usually minor and involve only one or two amino acids along the constant region (Fc) along the immunoglobulin complex. Although not important in terms of immune response, they are important as markers for the study of immunogenetics and for the detection of genetic diseases.

IgA is the major secretory antibody and is found in all physiological fluids such as tears, saliva, gastrointestinal fluids, milk, and mucous. IgA neutralizes microorganisms and toxins before such pathogens can cross epithelia. IgD exists predominantly on the surface of B-lymphocytes, and is present in very low concentration (<0.1 mg/mL) in the serum. The half-life of IgD is less than 3 days. The physiological role of IgD is not well delineated, but these antibodies act like antigenic receptors able to stimulate B-lymphocyte after antigen binding. In contrast, IgE is found almost exclusively on the surface of mast cells. Upon binding to an antigen molecule, IgE can cross-link to each other on the surface of the mast cell and stimulate the release of many allergic mediators. In addition, IgE is elevated when the host encounters a parasitic infection.

IgG is the most abundant immunoglobulin found in the serum, where normal serum concentration is 15 mg/mL, accounting for 75% of total serum immunoglobulin. The half-life of IgG is approximately 3 weeks and is dependent on the presence of antigens. IgG is capable of crossing the placenta and the immature intestinal epithelium to provide immunity to the fetus and the newborn infant.

IgG is the most important antibody in the serosal immunity. IgG has a high affinity to antigen and IgG-antigen complexes can be recognized by complement factors and by Fc (fragment constant)-receptors on the surface of phagocytes. In both cases, IgG binding leads to the elimination of antigen-bearing cells. More importantly, IgG binding facilitates natural killer cell (NKC) activity that is more commonly called antibody-dependent cell mediated cytotoxicity (ADCC). In this process, NKCs with receptors for the Fc region of IgG will attach onto the antibody and elicit its biological activity by secreting cytotoxins.

The polymeric IgM is found in the pentameric and hexameric form in the blood, where the structure is formed through disulfide linkages between the immunoglobulin moieties and a polypeptide J chain. Although IgM can exist in the monomeric form, this form is found only on the surfaces of B cells. IgM is

Table 60-2. Myeloid Cytokines

FACTOR	CLASS	NO. AMINO ACID	MW (KDA)	BIOLOGICAL ACTIVITY
IL-3 Multi-CSF	I	133	14–28	Influence differentiation of immature progenitors of RBC, monocytes, granulocytes, and platelets
GM-CSF	I	127	14–35	Influence differentiation of mature progenitors of RBC, monocytes, granulocytes, and platelets
G-CSF	II	174	18.8	Terminal differentiation of neutrophils
M-CSF	II	256, 554, 438		Terminal differentiation of monocytes
EPO	II	165	30	Terminal differentiation of RBC
TPO or MDGF	II	332		Terminal differentiation of platelets

lymphocytes derived from the bursa of Fabricius, thus giving rise to the name B-lymphocytes. In humans, the ontogeny of B-lymphocytes starts in bone marrow, where stem cells form lymphocyte progenitors. These progenitor cells will differentiate and mature into plasma cells. Following antigenic challenge, circulating B-lymphocytes serve as the progenitor to plasma cells and will produce immunoglobulin type M or IgM. Subsequent antigenic exposure to the same antigen can induce the expression of immunoglobulin type G (IgG), A (IgA), or E (IgE).

Other immune cells include those that are classified as myeloid cells, which include granulocytes, monocytes, erythrocytes, and platelets. These cells have a wider variety of biological activities as compared to lymphocytes. A subpopulation of myeloid cells called granulocytes and monocytes are important in host defense. Morphologically, granulocytes have pigmented granules in the cytoplasm. Other distinctive morphologies include multi-lobed nuclei. In contrast, macrophages have an unsegmented nuclei and lack granules in the cytoplasm. Biologically, granulocytes and monocytes work in concert to eliminate foreign intrusion, particularly bacteria, parasites, and fungi.

Granulocytes are subdivided into eosinophils, neutrophils, and basophils. Eosinophils have granules filled with histamine that are released during allergic reactions. The release of histamine results in vasodilatation and pulmonary constriction that prevent more antigens from entering the body. Although eosinophils play an important role in allergic reactions, they are also important in resisting parasitic infections. Similar to eosinophils, basophils provide an inflammatory response to allergic reactions, however, the exact role of these cells is still unclear.

The most prominent granulocyte is the neutrophil, which plays a crucial role in the defense against bacterial and fungal infections. When the absolute neutrophil counts (ANC) drops below 500 cells/mm^3, an individual may become more susceptible to life-threatening infections. Most notable of these infections is gram-negative bacteremia, which is responsible for the majority of deaths associated with severe neutropenia. In the presence of foreign organisms, neutrophils will produce and secrete hydrogen peroxide (H_2O_2), which has anti-infective properties. The presence of H_2O_2 will also serve as an intracellular signal and increase transcription of stimulating cytokine production, which will initiate the immune cascade. The immune system can also be activated through the presence of nitric oxide, which has vascular dilation activity. Similar to neutrophils, macrophages are essential in the eradication of bacterial and fungal pathogens. Macrophages are antigen-presenting cells (APCs), which ingest or phagocytose and break down the antigen into recognizable fragments for immune recognition. This serves as one type of activating signal to stimulate naïve T-lymphocytes.

IMMUNE ACTIVATION

Once an antigen has penetrated the barrier defense, the immune response usually results in non-specific antibodies and complement factors binding. This coating process is also known as *opsonization*, which serves two purposes: (1) neutralize the antigen and (2) recruit cells to the affected site. After the antibody has attached onto the antigen, a conformation change within the structure of the antibody will allow cells with antibody receptors to attach onto it.

Once the antigen is recognized by antigen-presenting cells (APC), primed B-lymphocytes or mature monocytes/macrophages and then internalized via phagocytosis or endocytosis, it is degraded into smaller fragments inside an intracellular compartment, an endosome. The degradation of the antigen will make it recognizable to lymphocytes when the antigen is presented along with class II major histocompatibility complex (MHC) (Fig 60-1). Antigen fragment-MHC class II

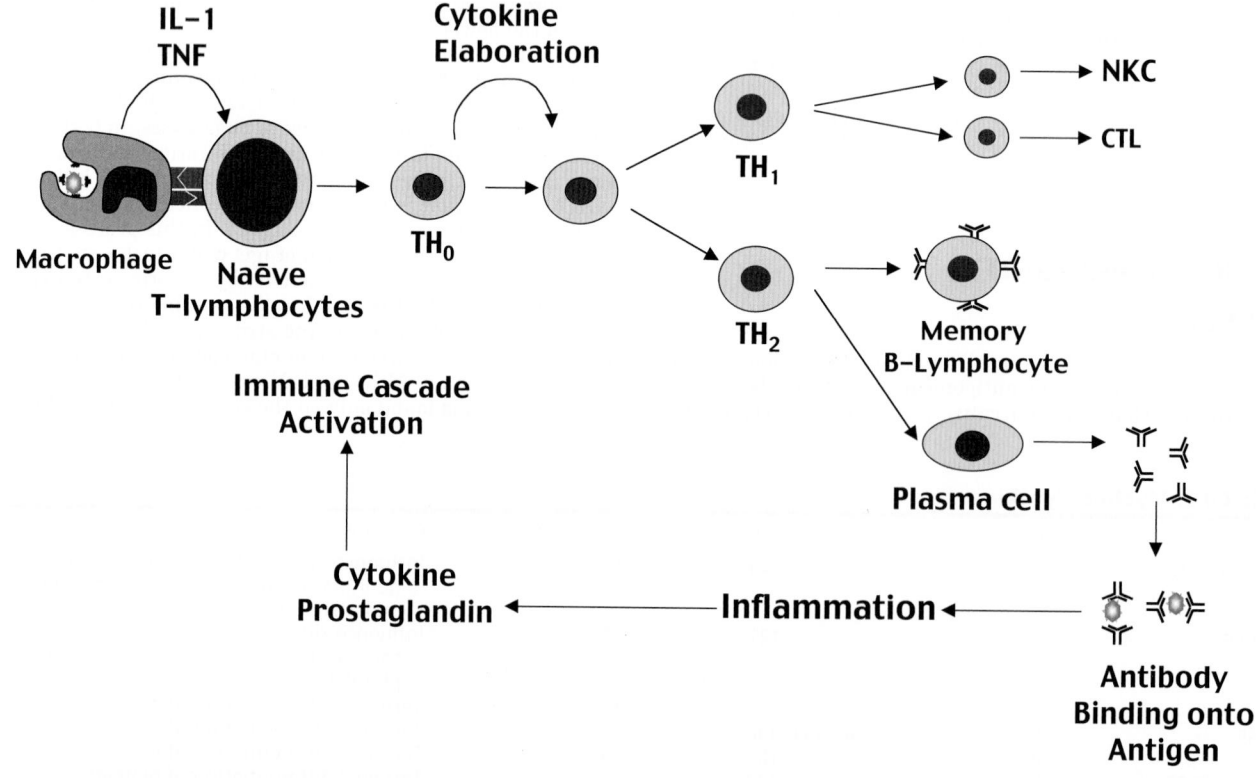

Figure 60-1. Immune activation cascade. See Color Plate 20.

the first antibody produced by the fetus and is also the first antibody to respond when presented with a new antigen challenge. In the primary response against a new antigen, the appearance of IgM in the blood precedes that of IgG. The production of IgM decreases when the production of IgG increases. Therefore, IgM in the serum amounts only about 1.5 mg/mL with a half-life in the blood of less than a week. Usually, the affinity of each antigen-binding site in IgM is lower than that in IgG because specificity has not been defined. However, the multivalent attachment of pentameric IgM provides it with very high affinity toward the surface of antigen-bearing microbials. The antigen-IgM complex can activate the complement system, but unlike IgG complexes, it cannot activate macrophage-mediated cytotoxicity.

Complement Factors

Serum has been shown to have some bacteriolytic properties; however, it was found that this antibacterial activity was lost following heat inactivation. This heat-labile activity was later called alexin. The biological activity of alexin could be restored by the addition of a second component that Paul Ehrlich called *non-immune serum*. Since alexin worked in complement with antibodies, he reasoned that alexin should be renamed as *complement factor*.

What is now known is that antibodies can recognize pathogens through antibody-antigen interaction. Antibody binding cannot only neutralize the antigen, but it can also activate the immune cascade. However, antibody binding rarely results in cytotoxic effects where the organism is killed by the addition of antibodies alone. At first, this appears incongruous with the above observation, where humoral-mediated immunity can induce cytotoxicity. It has been shown that antibodies must work in conjunction with complement factors to initiate cellular lysis of the targeted cell.

Complement factors are a group of serum glycoproteins, designated as C1 to C9. Unlike antibodies, complement factors require some assembly before it is able to carry out its functions. Complement factors will form a pore-like complex that allows intracellular contents to leak into extracellular space. The complement cascade is activated in response to ADCC. Although the complement-mediated immunity usually works in conjunction with antibodies, it can act independently of antibodies.

The complement cascade can be initiated by two distinct pathways, which are classified as the classical and alternative cascade pathways. The classical pathway is initiated when antibody binding onto the antigen causes a structural change in the Fc region of the antibody. This structural change in the Fc will activate C1. The activation of one factor will activate subsequent factors, finally forming the pore-like complex that will allow intracellular leakage to occur.

C1 consists of six C1q subunits with six binding sites at one end and is held together by the six long fibrous peptides at the other end, an arrangement that resembles six tulips held together by tightening their six stems. In addition, there are two C1r and two C1s molecules associated with the "stem" structure. The six C1q binding sites can interact with the Fc domains of antibody-antigen complexes. The six binding units in C1q can form a cross linkage between two IgG molecules. IgM molecules are the only isotype of immunoglobulins other than IgGs that are also recognized by C1q. Since IgM molecules consist of five immunoglobulin units, C1q can bind more than one Fc domain in each IgM molecule.

Upon C1q binding onto the Fc portion of IgG or IgM molecule, the C1r proenzyme is activated. Activated C1r can in turn convert C1s to an active enzymatic form, which can initiate the classic complement pathway. C4 is the first complement component that is activated by C1s. Activation of C4 will cause the glycoprotein to split and form two polypeptides, where the shorter component is referred to as C4a and the larger component is designated as C4b.

C4b is an activated enzyme capable of converting C2 to the active form, C2b. This polypeptide has enzymatic activity. When C2b is combined with C1s, C2a, and C4b, they form a complex known as C3 convertase, which converts C3 into C3a and C3b. The formation of C3b is an important step for both the alternative and the classic complement pathways. C3b is able to bind onto target cell membrane that has antibody-antigen complex together with C2a and C4b. The binding of C3b can enhance the phagocytosis of the target cell by phagocytes with C3b receptors present on the surface. The membrane bound complex of C4b, C2b, and C3b is called the C5 convertase, which produces a membrane-bound C5b fragment by cleaving off a small C5a fragment from C5 component.

During the activation process from C1 to C5, three small polypeptide fragments are generated: C3a, C4a, and C5a. While these three peptides are not directly involved in complement complex formation, they are important in the induction of inflammatory responses. C3a, C4a, and C5a are called anaphylatoxins because they are able to bind onto mast cells and basophils, thus stimulating degranulation. Mediators released by the granules can activate anaphylactic responses such as smooth muscle contraction. The anaphylactic response is inactivated by carboxypeptidase B, which removes the carboxyl terminal arginine residue of anaphylatoxins. In addition to anaphylaxis, C5a also acts as a factor of chemotaxis and an activator of neutrophils. However, the chemotactic activity of C5a is not reduced by the action of carboxypeptidase B.

Unlike factors C1 to C5, complement components following C5b in either the classical or the alternative pathway do not require modification or activation. Thus, intact C6, C7, and C8 molecules aggregate sequentially around C5b to form a membrane-associated complex, which, in turn, polymerizes C9 molecules to form a transmembrane channel. This transmembranous channel, known as the membrane attack complex (MAC), consists of an average of 15 molecules of C9 and acts as a pore to cause the leakage of electrolytes and other cytoplasmic components from the antigen-bearing cells. Eventually, the target cells are killed by this cytolytic action.

CELLS OF THE IMMUNE SYSTEM

Each cell plays an important role in maintaining homeostasis of the body. As stated above, there are various types of lymphocytes, which are divided as either B or T lymphocytes. B-lymphocytes will mature to form plasma cells that have the capacity to produce and secrete antibodies. The activity of T-lymphocytes include both regulatory and effector type activity. In contrast, myeloid cells are important in maintaining homeostasis and cell defenses.

In the early 1960s, lymphocytes isolated from lymph nodes were found to attack and destroy target cells from other animals. When these lymphocytes were introduced into tumor-bearing mice, the size of the neoplasm was reduced. In addition, these cells were able to eradicate virally infected cells, whereby giving rise to the name cytoxic T-lymphocytes (CTLs). CTLs are one of two types of effector cells that are found in humans. The second effector cell is named natural killer cells (NKCs). Unlike CTLs, this subpopulation of lymphocytes are able to attack and destroy tumor cells without prior sensitization, thus giving rise to the name *natural killer* cells. The cellular origin of NKCs has not been clearly defined. Despite this, there is little controversy regarding the role of NKC in the immune system, where the primary role of NKCs is to eliminate antibody-coated pathogen by ADCC. On the surface of NKC are receptors for the constant region of antibodies or Fcγ receptors, which allow these cells to attach onto antibody-coated or opsonized pathogenic organisms. NKCs carry out their cytotoxic function through the release of cytotoxins.

Chick embryos whose lymphoid tissue was ablated developed into chickens that were unable to produce adequate concentrations of immunoglobulins. This was attributed to a reduction of

complexes expressed on the surface of APC are easily recognized by both B- and T-lymphocytes with surface-binding antigen recognizing moieties and T-cell receptors, respectively. B- and T-lymphocytes may bind to an identical portion of the antigen fragment, but at different distinct sites. Thus, it is not unusual for most antigen molecules possessing multiple antigenic recognition sites.

Helper T lymphocytes (CD4+ cells), the cornerstone of immune activation, will only recognize antigens when they are presented on the membrane of the APC. This is to prevent producing an immune response against its own antigen. In order for the T-lymphocytes to recognize the antigen, MHC class II protein must also accompany the processed antigen. Processed antigen presentation to T-lymphocytes must also be accompanied by a co-stimulus, which includes B7 binding onto CD28. B7 is present on APC, whereas CD28 is found on the surface of CD4 cells. In the absence of this costimulation with B7/CD28, T-lymphocytes are anergic and will enter a state where it is unresponsive to antigen stimulation. In the anergic state where B7/CD28 interaction is absent, T-lymphocyte activation can utilize a secondary pathway where cytokine activation will serve as the co-stimulus.

Cytokine expression occurs as the antigen is being processed. Activation of the immune system occur when there is increased expression of interleukin-2 (IL-2) and the number of IL-2 receptors found on the surfaces of T-lymphocytes. Thus the production of IL-2 not only increases the activity of CTLs and NKC, but also of itself (autocrinic activation). This will enable autocrinic expansion, where ligand produced by the induced cells can also utilize cytokines they produce themselves. The activation of T-lymphocytes will not only increase expression of IL-2, but there is also a substantial increase in the primary inflammatory cytokines IL-1 and TNF. Similar to IL-1, IL-2 is both a paracrinic and autocrinic factor. Paracrinic factors are stimulatory cytokines that are stimulating neighboring cells. Whereas autocrinic factors are factors that are produced by the cell, which can also be utilized by the cell itself to further enhance its proliferation and/or stimulation.

There are various monocyte-derived cytokines, most notable are the primary inflammatory mediators like IL-1 and tumor necrosis factor-alpha (TNF-α). CD4+ cell activation will in turn initiate immune activation resulting in synthesis of IL-1, this will expand the number of committed progenitor stem cells. Additionally, activated CD4+ cells also produce IL-2, which will expand the population of helper-T-lymphocytes and cytotoxic T-lymphocytes, and suppress T-lymphocytes, natural killer cells, and B-lymphocytes.

There are two major types of T Helper (TH) cells that are designated as TH_1 and TH_2. TH_1 regulates cellular immunity, whereas TH_2 regulates humoral immunity. The regulation of cellular immunity is controlled by TH_1 through expression of IL-2, IL-12, and IFN-γ. These cytokines will modulate CTLs and NKCs, where IL-2 and IL-12 will increase their cytotoxic effects, respectively. IFN-γ is a cytokine synergistic with both IL-2 and IL-12, and is able to increase expression of MHC I on target cells.

In contrast, TH_2 regulate humoral immunity through expression of IL-4, IL-5, IL-6, and IL-10. IL-4 is able to induce the production of TH_2 cells, eosinophils, and mast cells. An increase in IgE expression is seen after IL-4 administration. In the process of activating both eosinophils and humoral immunity, IL-4 and IL-10 are also able to suppress the induction and function of TH_1 cells.

IL-1 can also stimulate the recruitment of cells to the affected site. There are two ways this can be accomplished: (1) demargination of cell immune cells adhering onto the vascular walls, and (2) stimulation of the maturation and differentiation of stem cells to increase production of circulating cells. In addition, IL-1 is also able to induce expression of CSFs and lymphokines, which regulate the differentiation, proliferation, and maturation of myeloid cells.

T-lymphocyte activation will also enhance the expression of IL-2, which was originally named T-cell growth factor (TCGF).

IL-2 is a pleiotropic factor that can activate CTLs, TH lymphocytes, B-lymphocytes, and NK cells. The expression of IL-2 receptor, or IL-2R, is one indicator that the cells are activated. In order for IL-2 to exert its activity, it must first bind onto a receptor and thus activate a series of intracellular signals resulting in cellular activation.

IMMUNE DISORDERS

Inability to respond adequately to an antigen intrusion is usually considered an immunodeficiency, whereby the immune system is unable to neutralize or eliminate the pathogen. However, immune dysfunction is often the term that is used when immunodeficiency is partially impaired. Immunodeficiency occurs when one or more immune compartments are significantly affected. Immunodeficiency disorders are characterized by partial (specifically humoral or cellular) or complete impairment of immune response to an antigenic challenge. These disorders can be classified as humoral (B-cell mediated), cellular (T-cell mediated), combined immunodeficiency, phagocytic dysfunction disorders, and complement deficiencies.

The emergence of acquired immunodeficiency syndrome (AIDS) has highlighted the importance of an intact immune system. Various causes of immunodeficiency include chemical-, autoimmune-, malignancy-, and viral-induced syndromes. These disparate causes accentuate the paradigm that the various components of the immune system must work in concert to orchestrate a defense against foreign invasion.

Immunodeficiencies occur in either the humoral or cellular compartment of the immune system. Humoral immunodeficiency includes individuals who produce either inadequate quantity of antibodies or non-functional antibodies. Pre-term infants and patients with chronic lymphoblastic leukemia (CLL) are examples of individuals who may have low concentrations of antibodies or hypogammaglobulinemia. These individuals are susceptible to pyrogenic bacterial infections. Alternatively, patients with cellular immunodeficiency such as patients with cyclic neutropenia, severe combined immunodeficiency (SCID), and HIV are susceptible to non-bacterial forms of opportunistic infections. Advances in our understanding of the immune system have led to the emergence of therapies that increase patient survival.

Humoral Immune Dysfunction

Individuals who have depressed levels of either antibodies or complements are associated with increased risk of bacterial infections. The reduction of these humoral factors will impair the ability to opsonize pathogens such as *Streptococcus pneumoniae* or *Haemophilus influenzae*. Reduced levels of immunoglobulin may account for the inability to neutralize antigens and recruit cellular response. However, patients with multiple myeloma have high levels of antibodies, yet these patients are susceptible to recurrent pneumococcal infections. In this situation, the issue of antigen specific antibodies is illustrated where both antibody concentration and specificity are crucial to eliminate infections.

X-LINKED AGAMMAGLOBULINEMIA—The importance of B-lymphocytes in the immune system is highlighted in B-cell dysfunction disorders. One disorder is X-linked agammaglobulinemia (X-LA), which is an autosomal recessive genetic disorder found primarily in males. The hallmark manifestation of X-LA is low levels of IgG. This is attributed to a defect in normal lymphopoiesis. Pre-B-lymphocytes isolated from X-LA patients are unable to form mature plasma cells, thus they are unable to produce antibodies. Two possible causes of this disorder are the inability to form lymphoid progenitor cells and/or to produce inadequate cytokine signals that are required for differentiation.

Patients with X-LA are usually diagnosed relatively young, usually between 5 and 36 months of age. Clinically, these patients develop recurrent bacterial sinusitis or pulmonary infections caused by *Streptococcus* sp., *Staphylococcus* sp., *Escherichia coli*, and *Haemophilus influenzae*. Although these infections are common in this age range, X-LA patients are also susceptible to viral and protozoal infections despite having an adequate number of circulating T-cells with normal function. The inability to produce specific antibodies against a foreign organism will reduce immune response. The loss of antibody production will also reduce the cellular response and more specifically, ADCC.

SELECTIVE IGA DEFICIENCY—IgA deficiency (IgA-D) is the most common primary immunodeficiency where patients with IgA-D may not have any clinical manifestation, due to the capacity to yet compensate for IgA deficiency. Patients with primary IgA-D normally have low IgA concentration (<5 mg/dL). Inadequate IgG and IgM compensation may manifest as recurrent infections, gastrointestinal disorders, autoimmune syndromes, allergic diseases, and malignancies.

The actual pathogenesis of IgA-D is not well delineated, however, there is evidence suggesting that patients with this disorder also have a defect in HLA-A1, HLA-B8, and HLA-D expression. There is also a decrease in the number of circulating B-lymphocytes in these patients. These B-cells are able to synthesize IgA but are unable to secrete the immunoglobulins across the epithelium into extracellular space. This would suggest that IgA-D is a disorder caused by the inability to secrete the immunoglobulin.

COMMON VARIABLE IMMUNODEFICIENCY—Common variable immunodeficiency (CVID) is a primary B-lymphocyte deficiency syndrome that is characterized by low levels of serum IgG <250 mg/dL. Unlike IgA-D, low antibody levels may be seen in one or more classes. Paradoxically, low levels of IgG are not accompanied by a reduction of B-cell levels. In this disorder, circulating B-cells can be low, normal, or above normal, suggesting the cause of this disorder may be due to inadequate immunoglobulin synthesis or secretion. Other causes of CVID have been attributed to increased numbers of suppressor T-lymphocytes. This could be a consequence of the failure to adequately stimulate B-lymphocyte maturation. These findings led to the thought that CVID may be caused by viruses, such as Epstein-Barr virus (EBV). Clinical presentation of these patients support the viral-mediated etiology because these patients may develop an autoimmune defect, increases in autoantibodies, and viral-associated hypogammaglobulinemia.

CELLULAR IMMUNODEFICIENCY SYNDROMES—In contrast to humoral immunodeficiency, patients with T-cell immunodeficiencies are susceptible to viral and fungal infections. They are at risk for severe reactions to childhood disease such as varicella zoster (Chicken pox) and measles. These individuals are also at risk of developing acute infections following vaccination with live attenuated vaccines because of inadequate immune capacity to prevent subacute infection from increasing its virulence. In addition, they are more likely to develop graft versus host disease (GvHD) after transfusion contaminated with lymphocytes or allogeneic bone marrow transplantation.

DiGeorge syndrome is a T-lymphocyte immunodeficiency caused by abnormal pharyngeal pouch developmental. This normally occurs between the 6th to 10th weeks of gestation that may affect thymus, parathyroid, thyroid, heart, and certain facial features. Absence or partial absence of thymus in the newborn can inhibit T-lymphocyte development. The thymus is vital in T-lymphocyte maturation. Immature T-cells migrate from the bone marrow to the thymus. In the thymic environment, various signals and cytokines will regulate T-lymphocyte maturation and differentiation. Thus patients with DiGeorge syndrome are unable to produce mature and functional T-lymphocytes. This is evident by the lack of T-cell receptor (TCR) found in the peripheral blood lymphocytes (PBL) from patients with DiGeorge syndrome, suggesting even the most primitive

T-cells are not developed due to the loss of thymic functions. Although antibody levels are oftentimes normal in these patients, they may have difficulties in producing T-cell dependent antibodies, such as specific IgG.

In contrast, Wiskott-Aldrich syndrome (WAS) is a chromosomal autosomal recessive immunodeficiency found primarily in males. WAS is caused by the inability to produce antibodies directed against polysaccharide antigens. As a consequence, abnormal granules are found in the macrophages and platelets in WAS patients. The macrophages are unable to process antigen for presentation to naive T-cells, thus leading to immunodeficiency in both B- and T-lymphocytic lineages.

At birth, WAS patients have normal lymphocyte counts but develop a decline in circulating lymphocytes with aging. More specifically, lymphocyte decline is accompanied by a drop in the number of helper T-cells along with an abnormal CD4/CD8 ratio. Furthermore, these lymphocytes do not respond to antigenic stimuli. In later stages, WAS patients can clinically present with markedly reduced T- and B-cells, low serum immunoglobulin, anergic response to exposed antigens, and recurrent infections.

Severe combined immunodeficiency disease (SCID) is another autosomal recessive disorder. Patients with SCID have profound immunodeficiency in both T- and B-cell lineages, thus have frank lymphopenia, where lymphocytes bearing CD3, CD4, and CD8 are significantly diminished or even absent. As the name describes, lymphopenia is not restricted to T-lymphocytes; circulating B-cell may also be absent. This condition will render afflicted individuals susceptible to opportunistic infections such as *Pneumocystis carinii* pneumonia (PCP). The only treatment for SCID is allogeneic transplantation for reconstituting the immune system using donor bone marrow. The identification of the specific genetic defect that causes this disorder has enabled researchers to develop methods to deliver the gene into stem cells, where the introduction of the wild type gene may ameliorate the effect of this deadly disorder.

Similar to SCID, patients with adenosine deaminase (ADA) deficiency have severe immunodeficiency. ADA is an enzyme that catalyzes the conversion of adenosine and 2'-deoxyadenosine (dAdo) to inosine and 2'-deoxyinosine, resulting in the accumulation of dAdo in body fluids and tissue. dAdo is phosphorylated to deoxy-ATP which can act as an inhibitor of DNA synthesis, resulting in cellular death. The principle site where ADA deficiency causes damage is in T-lymphocytes; however, B-cells are also affected. The molecular mechanism of ADA deficiency has been tracked to either a point mutation or deletion of the ADA gene.

The identification of a genetic mutation in patients with ADA deficiency has provided important insights into the strategies to treat this disorder. One such therapy includes bone marrow transplantation where the allogeneic stem cells have functional ADA gene. Unfortunately, allogeneic BMT has significant morbidity associated with it. Thus, other therapeutic modalities must be developed. Irradiated red blood cells (RBCs) transfusions, a rich supply of ADA, have been used to treat patients with the deficiency. Other alternatives have included bovine ADA conjugated with polyethylene glycol (PEG-ADA), which has proven to be effective in reducing levels of dAdo. PEG-ADA provides several advantages over irradiated RBCs because it eliminates the transfusion related adverse effects. In addition, PEG conjugation prolongs ADA elimination thus decreasing the frequency of administration.

CHRONIC GRANULOMATOUS DISEASE—One genetic disorder that reduces phagocytic activity is chronic granulomatous disease (CGD) syndrome, where macrophages accumulate particles in large granules in their cytoplasms. These granules are fused to each other but are unable to digest the ingested material. CGD is a rare X-linked or autosomal genetic disorder that affects phagocytic activity in the host defense. More specifically, these individuals with CGD have a defect in the NADPH oxidase system that is important in host defense against various microorganisms. The resultant effect is decreased production of superoxide radicals, which is an important component of microbicidal mechanism. A reduction of superoxide formation can lead to recurrent serious life-threatening infections and granuloma formation. The most commonly encountered recurrent infections are catalase positive microorganisms such as *Staphylococcus aureus* and *Aspergillus* sp. Other organisms that are frequently encountered in CGD patients include *Serratia marcescens*, *Pseudomonas cepacia*, *Klebsiella* sp., *Escherichia coli* and *Nocardia* sp.

CGD is a heterogeneous disorder that is characterized by a disorder of phagocytic oxidative metabolism. CGD can occur as a result of defects in either the cytosolic or membrane component of the NADPH oxidase system. Estimates suggest that 60% of patients have a defect in the membrane oxidase system. Patients with cytosolic defects are linked to patients with autosomal recessive traits. The majority of these patients have a defect in 47 kDa cytosolic protein of the cytochrome b-558.

AUTOIMMUNE DISORDERS

The immune system normally responds specifically against foreign antigen while sparing host tissue, thus able to discriminate between self and foreign antigens. In autoimmune disorders, there are aberrations altering the ability to distinguish between foreign and self-antigens, thus permitting the immune system to attack host tissues. Occasionally, these aberrations may be initiated by infection, while at other times antigens from the infectious organisms may have structural similarities to host cellular surface markers. This can lead to immune cross reactivity, also known as immune mimicry.

There are various autoimmune disorders that are defined by the affected tissue or organ. Regardless of tissue or organ, autoimmunity is a condition where the immune system recognizes these tissues as foreign. Inflammatory bowel syndrome, systemic lupus erythematosus, diabetes mellitus, and rheumatoid arthritis are all diverse examples of autoimmune disorders (Table 60-3).

TYPE I DIABETES—Type I diabetes, or insulin-dependent diabetes mellitus, is a disease in which the selective destruction of insulin-producing β cells of the pancreatic islets of Langerhans by specific T cells results in insulin deficiency. This disease is seen almost entirely in people under the age of 30 years and peaks at age of onset between 10 and 14 years. Unlike most of the autoimmune disorders, type I diabetes occurs mostly in males.

RHEUMATOID ARTHRITIS—Rheumatoid arthritis is a complex, pathological inflammatory condition whereby autoantibodies, called rheumatoid factors such as anti-IgM, are formed against IgG. The resultant IgG:IgM immune complexes cause inflammation of the small joints of the hands and feet. This will lead to immune activation causing an increase in inflammatory cytokines such as TNF and IL-1. Individuals may experience stiffness and joint pain, accompanied by signs of articular inflammation, including swelling, warmth, erythema, as well as tenderness on palpation.

HASHIMOTO'S THYROIDITIS—Hashimoto's thyroiditis, also known as chronic thyroiditis, is an inflammatory disorder that leads to progressive destruction of the thyroid gland and symptoms of altered thyroid function. Autoantibodies to tissue-specific antigens such as thyroid peroxidase and thyroglobulin are found in very high levels in the thyroid gland for a chronic period of time. This leads to an inflammatory process that leads to fibrosis of the gland and the development of a goiter.

SYSTEMIC LUPUS ERYTHEMATOSUS—Systemic Lupus Erythematosus (SLE) is a chronic inflammatory disease that involves multiple organ systems and follows a course of alternating episodes of exacerbations and remissions. The hallmark of SLE is autoantibody production directed against double-stranded DNA. These autoantibodies are also directed against other components of the cell nucleus such as histones and ribonuclear proteins. It is the complexes of these autoantibodies and their antigen that damage tissues by activating complement. Some of the clinical features associated with SLE include the classic "butterfly" rash on the cheeks, polyarthralgia, avascular bone necrosis, myalgias, pleuritic chest pain, dyspnea, glomerulonephritis, anemia, leukopenia, and thrombocytopenia.

HYPERSENSITIVITY AND ALLERGIC REACTIONS

Hypersensitivity reactions are immune responses to environmental antigens resulting in symptomatic reactions upon secondary exposure to the same antigen, more commonly referred to as "allergen." Hypersensitivity reactions are classified as type I to IV. Types I, II, and III are antibody-mediated reactions, whereas Type IV reaction is cell-mediated. Each type of hypersensitivity reaction, however, is unique and is summarized in Table 60-4.

Hypersensitivity Types

Type I hypersensitivity reaction is the most common category of allergic reaction and is commonly referred to as immediate or anaphylactic immune response. As the name describes, this hypersensitivity occurs after antigen (eg, pollen) binds onto IgE found on the surfaces of mast cells. Re-exposure to the same allergen will result in a cross-linking of the cell-bound IgE leading to degranulation, thus releasing its contents that include histamines and prostaglandins. Rapid release of these mediators causes profound vasodilation, increased capillary permeability, and contraction of smooth muscle. Other clinical manifestations include the development of urticaria, allergic rhinitis, angioedema, and even anaphylaxis. Systemic anaphylaxis, or anaphylactic shock, represents an extreme example of type I hypersensitivity and is considered an acute, life-threatening immunologic reaction manifesting as diffuse erythema, bronchospasm, laryngeal edema, circulatory collapse, suffocation due to tracheal swelling, hyperperistalsis, hypotension, or cardiac arrhythmias. Symptoms of anaphylaxis can develop rapidly, often reaching peak severity within 5 to 30 minutes of following allergen exposure. These clinical manifestations are primarily mediated by rapid release of eosinophil mediators such as histamine, chemotactic factor of anaphylaxis (ECF-A), and prostaglandins. Other factors include the production of slow-reacting substance of anaphylaxis (SRS-A), a group of leukotrienes produced during the anaphylactic reaction.

Type II hypersensitivity reaction is classified as cytotoxic reactions that is initiated by antibody directed against antigens found on the cell membrane of a given target cell (eg, erythrocytes, leukocytes). Antibody binding activates the complement cascade, whereby the antibody (ie, IgG or IgM) attaches to the antigen at the Fab region whereby acting as a bridge in order to complement through the Fc region. This composes a membrane attack complex which subsequently damages the cell membrane.

Table 60-3. Examples of Autoimmune Disorders

AFFECTED TISSUE OR ORGAN	AUTOIMMUNE DISORDER
Thyroid	Grave's disease or thyroiditis
Vasculature	Goodpasture's disease
Islet of Langerhans	Diabetes mellitus
Myocardial cells	Myocarditis
Platelets	Idiopathic thrombocytopenia purpura
Red blood cells	Systemic lupus erythematosus
Joints and synovium	Rheumatoid arthritis
Intestinal cells	Crohn's disease or ulcerative colitis
Skin	Dermatitis and psoriasis

Table 60-4. Four Different Types of Hypersensitivity Reactions

TYPE	I	II	III	IV
Name	Immediate; Anaphylactic	Cytotoxic	Immune Complex	Delayed
Mediator	Antibody: IgE	Antibodies: IgG, IgM	Antibody: IgG	Cellular
Antigen	Atopic	Cell membrane-associated	Soluble	Tissue-associated
Target tissues	Smooth muscle	Blood	Kidneys	Varies
Target cell	Mast cells	Erythrocytes	Endothelium	Macrophages
Mediators	Histamines, leukotrienes	Complements	Complements, vasodilators	Interleukins
Mechanism	IgE antibody is induced by an allergen and binds to mast cells and basophils. When exposed to the allergen again, the allergen cross-links the bound IgE, leading to an induction of degranulation and the release of mediators (eg, histamine).	Antigens on a cell surface combine with antibody. Complement-mediated lysis then occurs.	Antigen-antibody immune complexes are deposited into tissue leading to complement is activation. Polymorphonuclear cells are attracted to the site. This causes release of lysosomal enzymes, resulting in tissue damage.	Helper T lymphocytes sensitized by an antigen release lymphokines after subsequent contact with the same antigen. Lymphokines induce inflammation and activate macrophages, which lead to the release of mediators.
Examples	Hay fever Anaphylaxis	Blood transfusion reactions	Serum sickness	Contact dermatitis
Other Characteristics	The most common form of allergic reaction			

Immune complex hypersensitivity, or Type III hypersensitivity reaction, is caused by the formation of soluble antibody-antigen complexes that aggregate in blood or tissue. These complexes adhere to various sites such as the endothelium of blood vessels subsequently leading to tissue damage. Conditions associated with immune complex include serum sickness and the Arthus reaction. Serum sickness occurs when foreign serum or serum proteins like antilymphocyte immunoglobulin derived from animals such as rabbit, goat, and horse enters the host. The recipient may then develop chills, fever, arthralgias, and nephritis. These symptoms subside as the immune system removes these agents which it recognizes as antigens. Arthus reaction is a cutaneous reaction following subcutaneously or intradermally administration leading to immune response with IgG disposition to the affected site. This leads to complement activation and phagocytic cells producing a local inflammatory response. Deposits of antigen, antibody and complement form on vessel walls, leading to polymorphonuclear cell infiltration and aggregation of platelets. Ultimately, this can lead to vessel occlusion and tissue necrosis.

Unlike the other reactions previously described, Type IV hypersensitivity reaction is a cell-mediated reaction, in particular by T-lymphocytes. Type IV hypersensitivity reaction is commonly referred to as delayed-type hypersensitivity since an immune response may not occur until hours or even days after initial contact with the triggering agent. The reaction commonly lasts several days. A classic example of this particular type of hypersensitivity reaction is allergic contact dermatitis. Antigen is processed by antigen-presenting cells and presented on MHC class II molecules, which interacts with antigen-specific T helper cells which recognized it, thus stimulates the production of IL-1 and up-regulates T lymphocyte synthesis of IL-2 and IFN-γ. These induced cytokines act on vascular endothelium and recruit the infiltration of inflammatory cells, particularly macrophages. This causes fluid and protein accumulation and consequently, local tissue destruction and lesions ensue. Acute lesions are characterized by erythema, pruritus, and vesicle formation.

Allergic Drug Reactions

Drugs are commonly implicated in causing hypersensitivity reactions (Table 60-5). Antibody-mediated hypersensitivity reactions (ie, anaphylactic, cytotoxic, serum sickness) are involved in drug allergy. Either the drug molecule itself, or its metabolite, can elicit the allergic response upon re-exposure to the identical drug. Some medications (eg, aspirin) directly stimulate mast cells. Low-molecular-weight molecules (eg, penicillin, phenytoin) become antigenic via haptenation, a chemical process by which the drug molecule reacts with host proteins in order to become immunogenic and stimulate an antibody response.

Prevention of anaphylactic reactions due to drug hypersensitivity is vital. It is important to take a complete history of a patient's past medication use and note any reactions to medications that may have induced an allergic response. Prudent clinical knowledge, and its application to medications that commonly cause allergic reactions and those agents that cross-react with them, is essential. Diagnosis of drug hypersensitivity can be accomplished via three main methods (Table 60-6): (1) in vivo skin testing for immediate reaction to a suspected agent, (2) in vitro analysis of drug-specific IgE from a person's affected blood, (3) oral challenge testing. Treatment of anaphylaxis consists of maintaining airway, breathing, and circulation control by using agents such as epinephrine and implementing supportive care.

Table 60-5. Agents Associated with Causing Allergic Reactions

AGENT/DRUG CLASS	EXAMPLES
Antibiotics	Penicillin
	Sulfonamides
	Isoniazid
Anesthetics	Propofol
Antiarrhythmics	Quinidine
	Procainamide
Antihypertensives	Hydralazine
	Methyldopa
Antipsychotics	Phenothiazine
Anti-Inflammatory Agents	Acetyl-salicylic acid
	Indomethacin
	Ibuprofen
	Naproxen
	Celecoxib
Proteins/Peptides	Insulin
Antibodies	Antisera
	Monoclonal
	Immunoglobulins
Muscle relaxants	Chlorzoxazone
	Metaxalone
Other	Monosodium glutamate

Table 60-6. Methods for Testing Drug Allergy

IMMUNOLOGIC REACTION TYPE	IN VIVO	IN VITRO
I	Immediate skin prick; intradermal	RAST ELISA
II	(none)	Coombs
III	Intradermal Arthus test	RAST ELISA
IV	Patch test	Lymphocyte proliferation

RAST = radioallergosorbent assay.
ELISA = enzyme-immunosorbent assay.

NEUROIMMUNOLOGY

The field of psychoneuroimmunology (PNI) explores the complex relationship between the nervous and immune systems. Neurology and immunology are converging as the role of neuroimmune interactions between neurotransmitters and cytokines has intertwined in health and diseases. Examples include depression, schizophrenia, anxiety, Alzheimer's disease, autoimmune disorders, chronic fatigue syndrome, stress, and sickness behavior. This section will address some of these disorders in the context of neuroimmunological dysregulation in relation to changes in behavior.

The common factors that link the two areas of study in explaining the pathophysiology of these disorders are cytokines. These pleiotropic proteins are the chemical messengers between cells that can function as both immunomodulators as well as neuromodulators. They mediate brain function as well as regulate the immune system. In addition, specific cytokines can induce the expression of neurochemical, neuroimmune, and neuroendocrine elements. Neurotropic cytokines can be secreted by cells found in the brain; these include astrocytes and microglia (immunocompetent cells within the brain). Along with secreting these cytokines, neuronal cells are also found to express receptors for the cytokines, suggesting that they are responsive to them. It was originally thought that large molecules such as cytokines could not cross the blood–brain barrier (BBB), an anatomical and functional separation between brain parenchyma and peripheral tissues that consists of vascular endothelium, basement membrane, neuroglial membrane, and glial perivascular feet. Elaborated cytokines, regardless of the source, can exert their effects on the brain via indirect and direct routes. Peripheral tissues are innervated by the peripheral and autonomic nervous systems and can send direct signals to the brain via peripheral nerves. Brain vasculature can send signals through secondary messengers such as nitric oxide (NO) or prostanoids (any group of complex fatty acids derived from arachidonic acid, including prostaglandins and the thromboxanes). These types of secondary signals are elaborated in response to cytokine activation. These secondary messengers mediate the effects of the immune molecules on brain function. Finally, cytokines can directly act on the brain by crossing the BBB or after entering an area of the brain that lacks a BBB. Cytokines released by activated immune cells influence activation of the hypothalamic-pituitary-adrenal (HPA) axis and are, in turn, influenced by glucocorticoid secretion (Table 60-7). More-

Table 60-7. Biological, Behavioral, and Psychiatric Effects of Cytokines

CYTOKINE	BIOLOGICAL ACTIVITY	PHYSIOLOGICAL EFFECTS	PSYCHIATRIC EFFECT	NEURO-TRANSMITTER EFFECTS	SECRETION SUPPRESSED BY
Proinflammatory					
TNF-α	Cytotoxic Activates T cells Pyrogenic Antitumor Septic Shock	Stimulates activity of the HPA axis	Somnolence Anorexia Cognition	Increases catecholamines	Glucocorticoids
IL-1	Activates T, B, and endothelial cells Induces acute phase proteins Pyrogenic Hematopoiesis	Stimulates activity of the HPA axis Modulates many central monoamine activity	Somnolence Confusion Delusions Sickness behavior Stress	Serotonin Dopamine Norepinephrine	
IL-6	Activates T cells Produces Immuno-globulin-G Induces acute phase proteins Pyrogenic Hematopoiesis	Stimulates activity of the HPA axis Differentiates and promotes growth of neuronal cells Increases serotonin and mesocortical dopamine activity in the hippocampus and prefrontal cortex	Somnolence Depression Psychosis Stress	Serotonin Dopamine Norepinephrine	Glucocorticoids
Inflammatory					
IL-2 (T cell growth factor)	Activates T, B, and natural killer cells Antitumor	Increases hypothalamic and hippocampal norepinephrine utilization Increases dopamine turnover in the prefrontal cortex	Depression Psychosis Confusion Delirium Memory Cognition	Dopamine Norepinephrine Acetylcholine	
IFN-γ	Activates macrophages Enhances expression of MHC Induces acute phase proteins Pyrogenic Antitumor	Neuromodulation	Fatigue Depression Suicidal ideation Psychosis Cognitive impairment	Serotonin	

over, central nervous system functioning during an immune response is modulated not only by cytokines from the periphery, but also by cytokines that are synthesized in the brain. Genes that encode for many of the cytokines and cytokine receptors are often constitutively expressed in the brain in response to immune system molecules or the cytokine itself. Within the central nervous system, cytokines can then induce changes in brain monoaminergic and cholinergic neural pathways. Cytokines modulate centrally mediated responses such as neurologic and neuroendocrine changes including the activation of the HPA axis. Cytokine receptors are localized with high densities in the hippocampus and hypothalamus of the brain.

Psychiatric Disturbances

Exogenous cytokines can influence certain behaviors such as sleep and eating, as well as modify mood states. Cytokines used therapeutically are associated with a number of adverse drug reactions including depression, mania, anxiety, irritability, decreased concentration, confusion, psychosis, and suicidal ideation. Interferons, in particular, have been implicated in causing many of these psychiatric disturbances in a dose-dependent fashion. In addition, interleukins and tumor necrosis factor-α have also been associated with causing psychological adverse effects. Since the severity of these effects appears to be dose-dependent and are reversible when the cytokine is discontinued, this would represent a causal relationship. The mechanism by which cytokines produce neuropsychiatric effects, in part, is caused by their ability to alter levels of neurotransmitters in certain areas of the brain. It is the relationship between cytokines and neurotransmitters that may explain certain behavioral disturbances.

Alzheimer's Disease

Inflammatory processes have been implicated in Alzheimer's dementia (AD) since epidemiology studies have demonstrated a lower incidence of AD in those patients using anti-inflammatory agents. Other correlative evidence includes elevated levels of inflammatory mediators in the brains of AD patients. Data suggests that inflammatory processes may initiate or enhance the pathological process that leads to the development of cerebral amyloid that may eventually lead to neuronal death. Acute phase proteins, such as α-1-antichymotrypsin, are elevated in the cerebrospinal fluid (CSF) of AD patients and appear to become integrated into the amyloid deposits that are characteristic of the pathophysiology of AD. Moreover, there are elevated levels of IL-1 and IL-6 in the serum of AD patients and IL-6 has been observed in plaques. Moreover, both of these cytokines induce the synthesis of β-amyloid precursor protein by human astrocytoma cells.

Schizophrenia

Immune abnormalities, found in some forms of schizophrenia, may reflect immunoregulation dysfunction in either the etiology or pathogenesis of this psychiatric disorder. The idea that the immune process is involved in a psychotic disorder such as schizophrenia correlates with the fact that psychosis is associated with the autoimmune disease, systemic lupus erythematosus. Schizophrenia has a chronic but episodic course similar to that seen in many autoimmune disorders. Earlier investigations have reported an elevation of serum immunoglobulin levels, abnormally large lymphocytes, and antibody to the brain in schizophrenic patients. More current research has focused on investigating specific cytokine abnormalities. Findings of altered interleukin regulation have been regarded as confirmation that schizophrenia has an autoimmune etiology, at least in part. Conclusive findings illustrate a decrease in IL-2 production in untreated schizophrenics as well as a decreased production of

IL-2 correlating with clinical variables such as more negative symptoms of schizophrenia (eg, flat and inappropriate affect, cognitive deficit, alogia) and a younger age of onset of the illness. Notably, this decrease in IL-2 production is found especially in paranoid schizophrenics. This suggests that low IL-2 production occurs at an early stage in the course of schizophrenia and that IL-2 production may serve as a marker for a subtype of illness of severity of schizophrenia. Low IL-2 production may be the result of the inability of T lymphocytes to produce more IL-2 or the decreased number of T-cells that secret IL-2, as well as to the intrinsic disorder of T-cells. However, there have also been investigations that suggest an increase in IL-2 production. Furthermore, there are high concentrations of IL-2 receptors in the hippocampus and striatum; therefore it is proposed that IL-2 serves as a neuromodulator possibly by increasing dopaminergic neurotransmission. The actual effects of this postulate are unknown at this time.

In addition to changes in IL-2 production, the observation has been made that there are elevated serum levels of IL-6 in schizophrenia. There is also an association with serum IL-6 and the state of schizophrenia in which acutely ill patients appear to have higher levels than patients in remission. In order to explain decreases in IL-2 with concomitant increases in IL-6 in schizophrenic patients, it is thought that there is an imbalance with the $TH_1:TH_2$ with a shift to the TH_2 system. These findings that represent evidence of an autoimmune pathogenesis are gaining more acceptance. More investigations, however, are needed to ascertain the correlation between IL-2 and IL-6 changes and the severity of the symptoms of schizophrenia.

Major Depression

Evidence that immunological disturbance of acute phase proteins (ie, significantly increased haptoglobulin) and cellular immune response in patients with depression comes from the observation that there is a significant decrease in lymphocyte proliferation in response to a mitogen, in severely and moderately depressed patients. Acute phase proteins are mediated by the pro-inflammatory cytokines, mainly IL-1, IL-6, and TNF. It has been reported that serum and plasma concentrations of immunoglobulins (IgA, IgM) and C3 and C4 complement are also changed in depressed patients. Furthermore, there is much clinical and experimental data to support the relationship between cytokines and depressive symptoms, such as depressed mood, decreased appetite, anhedonia, psychomotor retardation, changes in sleep patterns, fatigue, and cognitive deficits. Depression increases the production of proinflammatory cytokines from activated macrophages in the periphery and brain, including IL-1, TNF and IL-6. The consequence of the hypersecretion of these cytokines results in the malfunctioning of noradrenergic and serotonergic neurotransmission in the brain. There is evidence that IL-1 can activate the serotonin transporter, whereby increasing reuptake of serotonin into the presynaptic neuron and decreasing the amount of serotonin in the synaptic cleft. Likewise, IL-2 alters the functional activity of the central noradrenergic system. Serotonin and norepinephrine are two of the primary neurotransmitter deficits found in depressed patients. Other findings include high CSF concentrations of IL-Iβ and lower IL-6 in depressed patients. With respect to the effects that antidepressant medications have on cytokines, selective serotonin reuptake inhibitor (SSRI) administration has been associated with an increase in IL-10, a decrease in the synthesis of IFN-γ, and a decrease in the release of IL-6. Moreover, the tricyclic antidepressant (TCA), desipramine, impairs the secretion of both IL-1 and TNF; paroxetine, an SSRI, and venlafaxine, a serotonin and norepinephrine reuptake inhibitor, do not. Whatever the alteration in cytokine production and levels, HPA axis changes induced by these cytokines are found in depressed patients. Research on cytokine regulation in depression is rather controversial. Despite the amount of research currently done in an attempt to describe the relationship between the immune-endocrine-neurotransmitter systems, further investigation is required to measure these changes (in serum, plasma, CSF) and to correlate them to the severity of depressive illness and treatment response.

Effects and Responses to Stress

Stress in humans influences cytokine production and function by activating the HPA axis and increasing circulating glucocorticoids. It is generally stated that stress is "immunosuppressive." Specifically, induced stress and emotional distress leads to decreased IFN-γ and IL-6 and increased IL-2, as well as other effects on additional cytokines. Studies have concluded that the explanation for the changes in cytokine secretion is that stress induces an increase in the ratio TH_1/TH_2. An excessive HPA response to inflammation can mimic a condition of stress or hypercortisolemia, whereby increasing susceptibility to viral and bacterial infections

IMMUNOTHERAPEUTICS

Cancer

Immunotherapy is now an established modality in the treatment of several types of cancers, including malignant melanoma, renal cell carcinoma, multiple myeloma, and carcinoid tumor. Immunologically based anticancer therapy is based on two different types of strategies: (1) immune activation leading to specific tumor cytotoxicity, and (2) antibody therapy on tumor specific antigens.

Immunostimulants to enhance immune response against tumors have used cytokines that regulate immune response. Cytokines such as interferons (IFNs) and interleukins (ILs) are commonly used in this scenario. Although myeloid cytokines such as colony-stimulating factors (CSFs) have been investigated, their antitumor activity appears to be limited. The rationale to this disparity in biological activity is due in part to the role of cytotoxic lymphocytes (CTLs) and natural killer cells in tumor clearance. These effector cells play a major role in tumor suppression.

IFN is a family of cytokines that can induce cellular production of antiviral agents and thus block viral replication. Since a close relationship with viral infections and oncogenesis exists, it stands to reason that IFN, which can inhibit viral replication, may be able to inhibit cancer proliferation. Alpha IFN, or IFN-α, is the most frequently used biological agent used in cancer. It is approved for a broad range of cancers such as hairy cell leukemia, chronic myeloid leukemia, and AIDS-related Kaposi's sarcoma. The mechanism by which IFN-α exerts antitumor activity have included suppression of oncogenic viruses, inhibition of oncogenes, and stimulation of cytotoxic T-lymphocytes. In addition, IFN-α appears to have anti-neovascularization activity, thus it can reduce the formation of new blood vessels critical in tumor progression.

IFN-α is a key component of chronic myeloid leukemia (CML), a slowly progressing blood disorder with a number of clinical phases. Patients typically present in the chronic phase and later they develop transformation into the accelerated and blastic phase of the disease where the disease becomes resistant to conventional chemotherapy. As the disease progresses, production and function of white blood cells and platelets diminish, thus infections and spontaneous bleeding and bruising may ensue. Approximately 10% to 20% of patients who use IFN-α, alone or in combination, have complete cytogenetic response with no evidence of bcr-abl translocation (the etiological event in CML), suggesting response to therapy. These patients often times are disease-free beyond 10 years, however, maintenance of therapy with interferon is required to maintain this clinical status.

IFN-α is also used frequently in AIDS-related Kaposi's sarcoma (KS). This is the most prevalent form of KS with increasing incidence as patients become immunodeficient. KS usually presents with cutaneous lesion(s) but may present as lesions lining the mucocutaneous tracts such as the oropharynx, lungs and gastrointestinal system. Cytotoxic treatment is often given concomitantly with IFN in order to stimulate the immune system and make treatment more effective.

Recombinant human IL-2 (rhIL-2) is another lymphokine with potent antitumor activity. IL-2 is a potent stimulator of CTLs and NKCs, both responsible for immune response to the presence of cancers. Although it is approved for renal cell carcinoma and malignant melanoma, IL-2 has been used to augment a number of standard cytotoxic chemotherapy regimens.

Renal cell carcinoma (RCC) is diagnosed in approximately 30,000 individuals annually in the US, where more than 40% have metastases at the time of detection. rhIL-2 is able to activate CTLs which are able to suppress progression of the disease. When rhIL-2 is combined with IFN-α, there appears to be no additional benefit as compared to high-dose rhIL-2 alone.

Another role of rhIL-2 includes the development of therapeutic cancer vaccines directed against melanoma, breast and prostate cancers. This strategy stimulates the immune system to direct its attack against cells overexpressing a specific antigen found in cancer cells. This has taken the form of priming the patient's own immune system to directly attack their own tumors, or more commonly referred to as *therapeutic vaccines*. The use of therapeutic vaccines may be used alone or in combination with interleukins or interferons which can act as immune stimulators or adjuvants.

Currently there are a number of monoclonal antibodies used in the cancer arena. The production of monoclonal antibodies is summarized in Figure 60-2. Monoclonal antibodies that are used as therapeutic agents include Herceptin and Rituxan which are mainstays for breast cancer and non-Hodgkin's lymphoma. Other monoclonal antibodies have recently received FDA approval suggesting that this therapeutic platform will be an avenue by which new drugs will be developed.

Organ Transplantation

Allograft transplantation is now more commonly employed as a modality in patients with end stage organ failure. Visceral organs such as heart, liver, lung, and kidney are commonly harvested from donors and subsequently transplanted into recipients. The surgical transplantation of organs procured from donors with different types of antigens present an immunological obstacle. The immune system of the recipient will recognize the newly transplanted organ as a foreign antigen and thus will mount an immunological response. Crucial to the survival of the transplanted organ is immunosuppression allowing the transplanted organ to thrive in such a new and hostile environment. Immunosuppression must be balanced to preserve immune function in order to prevent intrusion of unwanted foreign antigens.

Initiation of immune response against allograft can be from one of many types of circulating cells including neutrophils, lymphocytes, and macrophages. These cells can infiltrate into grafted tissues and stimulate cytokine release and promote vascular endothelial injury. The resultant immune activation will lead to more tissue destruction, hemorrhage and ultimately organ failure.

Although allograft rejections are often categorized as an immunological response against the graft, there are various types of rejections which vary significantly. In clinical transplantation, three main types of rejection may occur: hyperacute, acute, and chronic. Regardless of the type of rejection, warning signs include fever, flu-like symptoms, hypertension, edema or sudden weight gain, changes in heart rate, and shortness of breath.

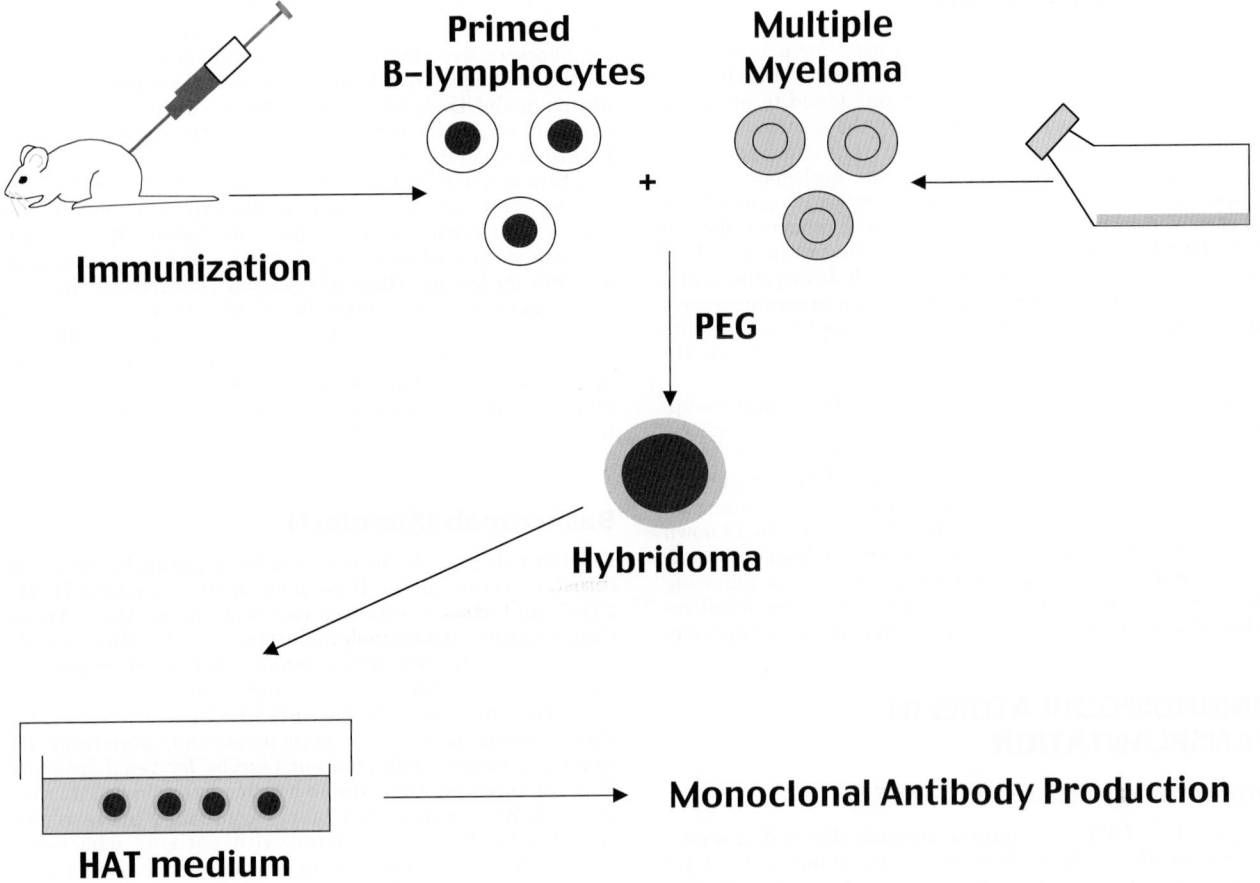

Figure 60-2. Production of monoclonal antibodies. See Color Plate 21.

TYPES OF GRAFT REJECTION

Hyperacute Rejection

Hyperacute rejection can occur within minutes to days of following surgical organ transplantation. One factor that may predispose an individual to hyperacute rejection is the presence of preformed IgG antibodies directed against class I HLA of the allograft. Organ vitality and function is lost as a result of antibody deposition and complement activation, which will ultimately result in vascular destruction and organ failure. Transplanted kidneys are most susceptible to hyperacute rejection, since patients with end stage renal dysfunction often present with chronic anemia requiring multiple red blood cell transfusion. Blood transfusions have been correlated with enhanced production of IgG. However, hyperacute rejection can be prevented by detecting the antibody with simple crossmatching prior to transplantation, and it is now rare. In addition, chronic anemia can be managed with the administration of erythropoietin which is a myeloid growth factor that enhances the production of erythrocytes.

Acute Rejection

Acute graft rejection is the most common form which is most frequently encountered within the first 6 months after transplantation. This type of allograft rejection is mediated by T-lymphocyte infiltration into allograft tissue that leads to in situ clonal expansion. Tissue destruction will then ensue, and thus cause organ failure. Of all of the mechanisms of rejection, acute graft rejection is most responsive to immunosuppressive drugs

Chronic Rejection

Chronic rejection is the term used when allograft function slowly deteriorates. Histological evidence of chronic rejection include intimal hypertrophy and fibrosis. Chronic rejection has been well characterized in heart transplants, where it presents similar to progressive coronary artery disease. In lung transplants, chronic graft rejection can present as bronchiolitis obliterans. In kidney transplantation, the onset of chronic rejection manifests similar to progressive interstitial fibrosis, tubular atrophy, and glomerular ischemia. The liver appears to be less affected by chronic rejection, but when it does occur, biliary epithelium is lost, eventually leading to hyperbilirubinemia and graft failure. The etiology of chronic rejection is unclear, however, there is evidence suggesting that chronic rejection may represent a low-grade acute rejection. This type of rejection may be a consequence of organ injury during the organ procurement and preservation process. This process appears to be independent of the type of organ that is transplanted and present. Progressive intimal hypertrophy of the small to medium-sized arteries occurs, that in turn leads to interstitial fibrosis, atrophy, and eventual failure of the organ transplant. Although chronic rejection is most likely to occur later in the post-transplantation course, it may develop as early as 6 to 12 months after transplantation. Unfortunately, there is no standard treatment for chronic rejection.

ANTIREJECTION AGENTS

Immunosuppressive agents have been used for a number of years in organ transplantation with little success. This changed with the advent of cyclosporine which was found to preferentially suppress lymphocytes by inhibiting the synthesis of IL-2 (Fig 60-3). Since then, a number of immunosuppressive regimens have been developed around cyclosporine and cyclosporine-like compounds. Other cyclosporine agents have been classified as calcineurin, which exert its pharmacological activity by inhibiting intracellular signals that ultimately lead to IL-2 synthesis. Other immunophilins include tacrolimus and sacrolimus, which are both macrolides with immunosuppressive activity. Similar to cyclosporine, these immunophilins bind onto intracellular enzymes and terminate the signals to activate IL-2 transcription.

Immunophilins are often coupled with other immunosuppressants such as corticosteroid and antimetabolites. Corticosteroids such as prednisone induce apoptosis of activated T-lymphocytes. In addition, corticosteroids can block lymphocyte activation through increased expression of an intracellular inhibitor, more commonly known as Ikb. Ikb binds onto a known nuclear factor, NFkb, which in turn activates T-lymphocytes to replicate and stimulate cytokine activation. In the following section, immunomodulators are discussed in more detail regarding their biological activity to prevent acute graft rejection.

IMMUNOMODULATORS IN TRANSPLANTATION

Muromonab(Orthoclone OKT3)

Muromonab, or OKT3, is a murine antibody directed against a glycoprotein (the 20-kilodalton side chain) found on the CD3 complex which is present in all active circulating T-cells. The binding of muromonab onto CD3 interaction initially results in a transient activation of T-cells with release of cytokines, but ultimately block T-cell proliferation and differentiation. As a consequence, nearly all functional T-cells are eliminated transiently from the peripheral circulation. Muromonab bound T-lymphocytes are cleared from circulation through monocyte mediated phagocytosis found in the reticuloendothelial system. Muromonab-CD3 is 68% to 95% effective in reversing rejection, which is especially beneficial for patients experiencing renal failure induced by cyclosporine.

Muromonab-CD3 has also been shown to be effective in reversing acute cardiac and hepatic allograft rejection in patients who are unresponsive to high doses of steroids. Reversal rates in acute cardiac allograft rejection have been reported at 83% and 90% for hepatic allograft rejection. Additionally, investigational trials have shown it to be effective in pancreas and lung transplant rejection resistant to steroid or other therapy. However, when used for prophylaxis, it does not reduce the incidence of rejection or prolong graft survival. OKT3 has also been investigated for use in multiple sclerosis and psoriasis vulgaris, but is not FDA-approved for these indications.

Basiliximab (Simulect)

Basiliximab is a chimeric monoclonal antibody (IgG$_{1\kappa}$) produced by recombinant DNA technology, targeting IL-2R or CD25 and thus inhibiting the binding of IL-2. Through chimerization, basiliximab maintains a high affinity for the α subunit of the IL-2R complex, which is selectively expressed on the surface of activated T-lymphocytes, only.

A study involving 348 patients who were also receiving cyclosporine microemulsion and corticosteroids were randomized to receive either basiliximab or placebo for renal transplant. Patients receiving basiliximab had reduction in the number of patients who experienced biopsy-confirmed acute rejection episodes by 28% as compared with patients who received placebo. Serious adverse events associated with basiliximab occurred in 54% of patients as compared to 61% of patients receiving placebo. There was no difference in the incidence of infection between basiliximab and placebo where incidences were 75% and 73%, respectively.

Mechanism of Actions of Immunosuppressive Therapy

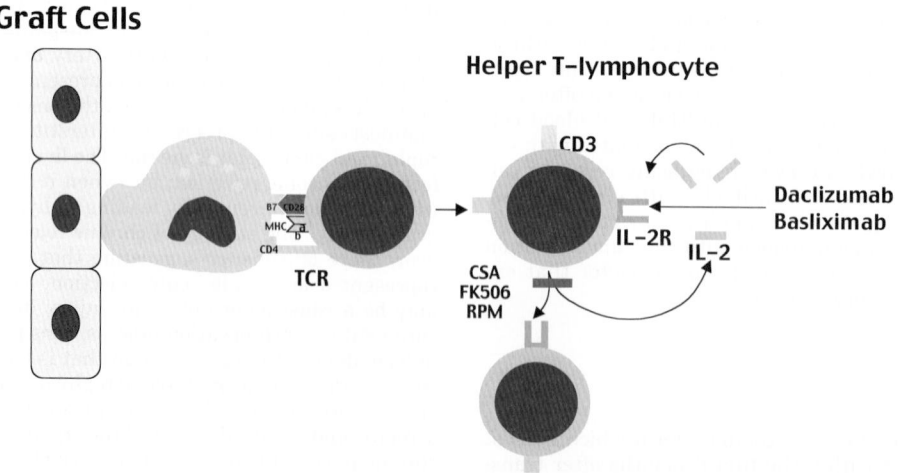

Figure 60-3. Immunosuppressants' mechanism of actions. See Color Plate 22.

Daclizumab (Zenapax)

Daclizumab is another chimeric IgG$_1$ monoclonal antibody directed against the α subunit of the IL-2R. Daclizumab binds to lymphocytes expressing CD25 but does not activate them. Two phase III international, multicenter, double blinded, placebo-controlled studies involving 535 patients receiving their first cadaveric renal transplant were performed to evaluate efficacy and safety. Daclizumab was administered every 14 days for a total of five doses and was given with either double (cyclosporine and prednisone) or triple (cyclosporine, prednisone, and azathioprine) therapy. Two hundred and seventy-five patients were enrolled in the double therapy and 260 patients were enrolled in the triple therapy. Daclizumab resulted in a significant reduction in the incidence of biopsy-proven acute rejection during the 6 months and the year after transplantation (p > 0.001) and a significantly lower dose of steroids were required as compared with placebo. Daclizumab was not associated with any immediate side effects.

HUMAN IMMUNODEFICIENCY VIRUS

Human immunodeficiency virus (HIV) infection is an infectious disorder in which the progression of disease will ultimately lead to lysis of infected cells, such as lymphocytes and monocytic cells. Progressive lysis of these cells without adequate compensation will lead to a clinical state more commonly known as acquired immunodeficiency syndrome (AIDS). In this clinical state, there is reduced immune capacity as evident by low levels of regulatory Helper T-lymphocytes or CD4+ cells. Clinically, these patients will be unable to immunologically respond to normally non-pathogenic organisms, where the development of disease is more commonly referred to as *opportunistic infections*.

Efforts to enhance the immune system have been previously explored in concert with the development of recombinant hemopoietic growth factors. A number of these factors can modulate immune activities and have been tested in patients infected with HIV. In the following sections, the use of interleukins, interferons and myeloid growth factors (aka colony stimulating factors or CSFs) in HIV infected patients will be reviewed.

Immunomodulators in HIV

INTERLEUKIN-2—Interleukin-2 (IL-2) is a T-lymphocyte growth factor that enhances immune response against viral infection such as Epstein Barr virus (EBV) and cytomegalovirus (CMV). Clinically, T-lymphocytes isolated from HIV-infected patients were found to have lower levels of IL-2 expression when compared to non-infected individuals. It was thought that the reduction of IL-2 expression may lower the capacity to expand T-cells, thus accounting for reduced antigenic response. Clinical trials to test the effectiveness of recombinant IL-2 (rIL-2) to enhance immune capacity in HIV were initiated. Despite more than ten years of experience, there is still no conclusive evidence regarding its benefit in HIV infected patients.

Initial data with regard to rIL-2 in HIV was encouraging, where this lymphokine was able to enhance expansion of CD4+ cells. This enthusiasm was hampered when IL-2 was found to stimulate HIV replication, which was attributed to its ability to stimulate the HIV transactivatory (*tat*) gene, leading to increased viral proliferation. Moreover, IL-2 can induce expression of other inflammatory factors such as interleukin-1 (IL-1) and tumor necrosis factor (TNF), which can in turn activate *tat* expression.

High doses of rhIL-2 administered as an intermittent continuous infusion with antiretroviral agents, T-lymphocytes isolated from these patients had an increased expression of IL-2 receptor (IL-2R). As expected, HIV patients treated with rIL-2 had increased CD4+ levels that were 50% above their baseline levels. However, elevation of CD4 counts appeared to be based on baseline CD4 counts. Clinical response was seen only in patients with an intact immune system, defined as baseline CD4 levels above 200 cells/mm^3. CD4 elevation was blunted in patients whose CD4 counts were below 200 cells/mm^3, where CD4 elevation was seen in only 20% in patients. Analysis of patients whose baseline CD4 was below 100 cells/mm^3 further supported the hypothesis that initial immune capacity is crucial in response to rhIL-2 therapy. Patients with baseline CD4 below 200 cells/mm^3 did not benefit from rhIL-2 administration where CD4 elevation was in this category.

GRANULOCYTE-MACROPHAGE COLONY STIMULATING FACTOR—The myeloid factors have also been investigated in humans for their abilities to enhance immune response. Initially, recombinant granulocyte-macrophage colony stimulating factor (rhGM-CSF) was given to AIDS patients with leukopenia. The administration of rhGM-CSF resulted in a dose-dependent increase in circulating white blood cell count, in particular neutrophils, eosinophils, and monocytes. rhGM-CSF administration reversed neutrophil dysfunction, where neutrophils isolated from rhGM-CSF patients were compared to neutrophils prior to drug administration demonstrated enhance neutrophil activities. This includes increased neutrophil chemotaxis toward f-Met-Leu-Phe, a chemoattractant, and superoxide production (an indicator of cytotoxic activity). Although a transient lymphocyte elevation was seen in a few patients, rhGM-CSF did not alter the CD4/CD8 ratio. Similar to rhIL-2, rhGM-CSF also activated replication of HIV, thus limiting it use in this scenario.

There were studies suggesting that GM-CSF can activate HIV replication, thus serum p24 levels were measured. In patients receiving rhGM-CSF, a notable increase of HIV p24 (HIV protein with molecular weight of 24 kilodalton) was observed suggesting that GM-CSF can enhance HIV replication. The p24 levels returned to baseline after cessation of rhGM-CSF. Despite an increase in p24, no clinical signs of HIV progression were noted. Therefore, the co-administration of antiviral agents should be encouraged in HIV patients who are receiving rhGM-CSF support.

Recently, rhGM-CSF was used in HIV patients in combination with antiretroviral therapy. In a phase II trial, rhGM-CSF was able to down-regulate HIV chemokine receptor expression in monocyte/macrophage, which is critical for HIV infection of CD4+ cells. The thought is that a down regulation of chemokine receptors will reduce the HIV infection leading to enhancement of the immune system. In a follow-up phase III trial, the presence of rhGM-CSF along with highly active antiretroviral therapy (HAART) led to a substantial increase CD4+ cells after 6 months of therapy. More importantly, rhGM-CSF prevented the need to change antiretroviral regimens due to viral failures as defined by detectable levels of HIV. This study suggests that the concomitant administration of rhGM-CSF at 250 μg three times a week may make antiretroviral therapy more effective. This antiviral activity is based on the theory that low levels of sargramostim inhibit the expression of chemokine receptor vital for viral entry into CD4 cells.

INTERFERONS—The first interferon (IFN) was first isolated back in 1957, when lymphocytes that were exposed to inactivated viruses produced a soluble factor capable of inhibiting viral replication. This ability to "interfere" with viral or "virion" replication gave rise to its name, interferon. IFNs released from virus-infected cells are able to bind onto receptors found on neighboring cells, and activated defenses against potential viral intrusion. Intracellularly, IFN induces the expression 2'-5' oligo adenylate synthetase, which in turn can activate ribonucleases and protein kinase. These enzymes are capable of inhibiting viral protein synthesis, and thus preventing viral proliferation and integration into potential target cells. IFN treated cells are able to prevent HIV infection, which suggests that IFN can activate the immune system to prevent serious infections such as HIV and hepatitis C virus as well. Unfortunately, resistance against viral infection is short lived, which was found to be correlated with the levels of IFN found in the blood. Since these types of cytokines have low circulating levels, the protection against new viral infection is limited.

Abbreviations:

CSA=Cyclosporine

FK506=Tacrolimus

RPM=Rapamycin=Sirolimus

BIBLIOGRAPHY

Davies D, Halablab M, Clarke J, et al. *Infection and Immunity.* Philadelphia: Taylor & Francis, 1999.

Janeway C, Travers P. *Immunobiology,* 3rd ed. New York: Current Biology/Garland, 1997.

Kuby J. *Immunology.* New York: Freeman, 1997.

Roitt I, Brostoff J, Male D. *Immunology,* 5th ed. St. Louis: Mosby, 1998.

Stites D, Terr A, Parslow T. *Medical Immunology,* 9th ed. Norwalk, CT: Appleton & Lange, 1997.

Shen WC, Louie SG. *Immunology for Pharmacy Students.* Philadelphia: Gordon & Breach: 1998.

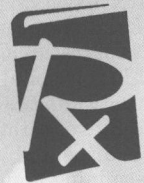

CHAPTER 61

Adverse Drug Reactions and Clinical Toxicology

Robert Middleton, PharmD

Drug availability and use have risen steadily for the last several decades. In 1961, only 656 drugs were marketed in the United States. By 1989, this number had increased to 8,000, and by 2003 more than 11,700 drugs are marketed in the United States.[1, 2] A total of 60% of the world's drugs are first introduced in the US,[3] and an average of 30 new molecular entities (ie, a new chemical entity marketed for the first time in the US) have been approved each year from 1993 to 2002,[4] a 42% increase over the period from 1975 to 1985.[1] Two thirds of patient visits to a physician result in a prescription,[3] resulting in 3.3 billion outpatient prescriptions filled in 2001.[5] In that same year, prescription pharmaceutical sales totaled $208 billion.[5] Prescription drug spending is projected to approach $4 billion by 2011.[6] Additionally, consumers are using an increasing number of over-the-counter medicines, dietary supplements, and "natural" or alternative products.

Medications unquestionably have provided tremendous benefits to society. Whether preventing childhood illness through vaccination, treating or preventing infections with antimicrobials, or forcing cancer into remission with antineoplastic agents, the benefits of modern drug therapy are immense. However, such therapy is not without risk. Encephalitis has been associated with vaccines; allergic reactions to antimicrobials are well documented; and antineoplastic agents can severely impair a patient's immune system, exposing them to life-threatening infections. The negative and undesirable effects of drug therapy are adverse drug reactions or ADRs.

All medical products, whether drugs, biologicals, diagnostic agents (eg, radiocontrast dye), natural products, or nutritional agents can cause adverse reactions. These reactions may be caused by the drug itself or one of its metabolites; from an interaction between two or more drugs or between a drug and food; or may be caused by an excipient in the product, such as a dye or preservative. Some reactions occur with most or all drugs in the class, so called "class effects," for example cough from angiotensin converting enzyme inhibitors. Other reactions are unique to the drug. Among antibiotics, chloramphenicol causes aplastic anemia, a reaction rarely seen with other antimicrobials. Some drugs can affect multiple organ systems; for example, amiodarone may cause pulmonary fibrosis, dermatological reactions, hyper- or hypothyroidism, ophthalmologic changes, and arrhythmias. Adverse effects from other drugs can be highly specific, for example, toxicity from aminoglycoside antibiotics is limited primarily to the kidney and vestibular/cochlear systems. And while drugs and biologicals marketed in the US are required to be proven safe and effective, safe does not mean risk-free. Thus, the decision to use any medicinal product is always the result of examining its risk to benefit ratio.

What is an ADR?

Although there are many definitions of an adverse drug reaction,[7,8,9] an internationally accepted description is that of the World Health Organization (WHO):

"A response to a drug that is noxious and unintended, and that occurs at doses normally used in humans for the prophylaxis, diagnosis, or therapy of disease or for the modification of physiological function."[10]

Notably, this definition tacitly excludes the failure of a drug to have its intended effect (ie, a therapeutic failure), and situations of drug abuse, drug overdose, or poisonings.

It is important to distinguish an *adverse drug reaction* from an *adverse drug event (ADE)*. While the two terms have been used interchangeably, the differences are important. An adverse drug reaction is the result of the intrinsic properties of the drug and cannot be prevented. An adverse drug event is an injury resulting from medical intervention related to a drug[11] and includes ADRs, but also includes preventable reactions, including those caused by human error. The WHO definition of an ADR does not necessarily include drugs administered or taken in error or given by an erroneous method.

Tremendous attention has been paid to adverse medical events and medical errors, which includes adverse drug events, largely as a result of the Institute of Medicine publication *To Err is Human: Building a Safer Health System.*[12] This report reviewed and summarized the literature on medical errors in the US health care system and concluded that between 44,000 and 98,000 deaths occur annually as a result of preventable medical mistakes. Drug-related errors account for an estimated 7,000 of these deaths.

As progress is made toward better assessment and management of drug risk, the line between adverse drug reactions and adverse drug events blurs. While much of the research in recent years has been on identifying risk factors for adverse drug events and ADE prevention, much of what is learned can apply to ADRs as well. Indeed, comprehensive management of drug risk requires that adverse drug reactions and adverse drug events be considered equally. To this end, FDA has identified four sources of risk from medical products: known side effects (both avoidable and unavoidable), medication errors, product defects, and "remaining uncertainties," which include side effects not yet known or reported, long-term effects, and unstudied uses and unstudied populations.[13] *All* sources of risk must be considered and evaluated to truly improve drug safety. While the focus of this chapter will be on adverse drug reactions, references to adverse drug events are made throughout.

How Common Are ADRs?

An exact incidence rate for adverse drug reactions is difficult to determine for several reasons. Different trials and national reporting programs have used differing definitions of an ADR, resulting in varying reporting rates. Differing means of gathering ADR data (eg, computerized vs manual surveillance), differing areas of research (eg, all hospitalized patients vs a specific unit within a hospital vs an ambulatory setting), differences in reporting statistics (eg, adverse reactions may be reported as a percentage, a rate per unit of time, or a rate per number of doses dispensed), underreporting of reactions, and difficulty in determining numerators and denominators for drug exposure and drug use, all lead to heterogeneous results and difficulty in defining a precise figure or comparing figures.

To address some of these issues, a meta-analysis of published studies of adverse drug reactions in hospitalized patients was conducted.[14] Thirty-nine studies meeting predetermined criteria were reviewed, and an overall incidence of serious and fatal ADRs was determined. The authors included only prospective trials and excluded "possible" ADRs in an effort to improve the quality of the data (ie, only definite ADRs were studied). Notably, only trials that used the WHO definition of an ADR were included and trials that reported adverse events from medication errors were excluded. The overall incidence of serious ADRs (defined as an ADR that required hospitalization, prolonged hospitalization, was permanently disabling, or resulted in death) was found to be 6.7%. The incidence of fatal ADRs was 0.32%. Based upon 1994 hospitalization figures, the authors estimated that over 2 million hospitalized patients experienced a serious ADR during that year; in over 1.5 million of these cases the ADR was the cause of hospitalization. Additionally 76,000–106,000 deaths due to ADRs were projected, making ADRs between the 4th and 6th leading cause of death in the US for that time period. The range of ADRs occurring during hospitalization reported from other trials varies tremendously between 1.5 and 43.5%,[1] as does the number of deaths from ADRs (200–200,000 annually[15]). Interestingly, the aforementioned Institute of Medicine report[12] estimated between 44,000 and 98,000 deaths annually from *all* medical errors, making fatality from adverse drug reactions possibly more common than fatality from all medical errors combined.

The frequency of ADRs in non-hospital settings is less well reported but is becoming increasingly available, often as part of medical error research. For example, a study of nursing home residents examined the incidence and preventability of adverse drug events.[16] Of the adverse drug events documented, 50% were considered nonpreventable and therefore adverse drug reactions resulting in an ADR rate of 0.94 per 100 resident months. Based upon these figures, 175,000 ADRs may occur in US nursing homes annually. A review of drug misadventuring[1] noted between 2% and 50% of ambulatory patients experienced an ADR; a more recent trial reported a much lower rate, 0.19%, of all hospital outpatient visits were due to an adverse drug reaction.[17]

The occurrence of ADRs in the non-adult population is also less well studied than in the adult age group. However, studies in vulnerable populations such as pediatrics and the elderly are increasing. One trial of adverse drug events in hospitalized pediatric patients found 5.3 nonpreventable adverse drug reactions per 1000 patient-days,[18] while 15.1 ADRs per 1000 children was reported through a network of pediatricians seeing patients in an ambulatory setting.[19] A trial in ambulatory Medicare enrollees found the overall adverse drug event rate to be 50.1 per 1000 person-years; of these events, 72% were nonpreventable ADRs (36.3 ADRs per 1000 patient-days).[20]

A largely unexplored and poorly quantified area is adverse reactions to alternative or "natural" products, the use of which may rival that of traditional medicines. Numerous reports document the toxicities of such products. For example, several deaths and complications have been reported with ephedra,[21] and hepatotoxicity has been described with chaparral.[22] Because herbal products are considered dietary supplements and not drugs, manufacturers are not required to seek premarket approval from the Food and Drug Administration (FDA), perform a risk-benefit analysis, or perform safety surveillance af-

ter the product is launched. In fact, it is FDA and not the product sponsor that is tasked with proving the safety, or lack thereof, of alternative products, which is the reverse of the requirements for drugs and biologicals. To assist with this assessment, the Institute of Medicine has proposed a framework for FDA to evaluate the safety of dietary supplements.[23]

How Costly Are ADRs?

The cost associated with ADRs is considerable and takes many forms. Studies have consistently shown that patients experiencing an ADR have longer hospitalizations, sometimes doubling the length of stay, relative to the non-affected population.[24–28] Not surprisingly, the cost of hospitalization for such patients is greater as more resources are used to manage and treat drug-induced illnesses.[27,28] One matched case-control study at a tertiary care hospital found the cost of hospitalization for patients experiencing an adverse drug reaction to be $2200 greater relative to control patents who did not experience an ADR.[28] Similar results have been found in other trials.[29] FDA has estimated that if the incidence of hospitalizations related to adverse drug reactions can be reduced by just 2%, the annual cost savings to the nation would be $368 million.[30] In addition to the direct increase in the cost of hospitalization, there is the cost to patients themselves in terms of lost time at work, decreased productivity, and possibly permanent disability. Patients or their families may utilize legal means to seek financial remuneration if a serious ADR is experienced. Litigation costs can be significant and place a burden on the court system, individual practitioners, and health care institutions. For example, there were greater than 4,200 lawsuits filed against the maker of troglitazone (Rezulin), after it was linked to hepatotoxicity and several deaths.[31] Although uncommon, some manufacturers have filed for bankruptcy as a result of ADR-related litigation.[32] Additionally, litigation influences liability and malpractice insurance costs for health care providers and institutions, contributing to the malpractice insurance crisis experienced in several states.[33] A final consideration is the cost of lost confidence and distrust of health care providers and the health care system. A patient's fear of drug-related harm may cause delays in seeking medical assistance at some future point when it is truly needed, possibly causing prolonged illness and severe outcome. The total annual cost to the nation of ADRs is difficult, if not impossible, to quantify but is certainly quite large and is likely in the billions of dollars.[28,34,35]

Classification of Adverse Drug Reactions

Adverse drug reactions have historically been placed into two broad classes: A and B.[8,36] Type A reactions are common and predictable with most identified prior to marketing. Type A reactions are dose related and result directly from the pharmacological action of the drug, but can be due to drug-drug interactions, drug-food interactions, or concomitant illness as well. About 80% of all ADRs fall into this category. Although type A reactions are common and have high morbidity, they usually have low mortality. Examples of type A reactions include hypoglycemia from oral sulfonylureas, tachycardia from albuterol, or diarrhea from an antibiotic. By contrast, type B reactions are uncommon, cannot be predicted, are not dose-related, and have no relation to the pharmacological action of the drug. In most cases, the mechanisms involved in type B reactions are unknown. Although rare in occurrence, mortality from type B reactions can be high. These reactions predominantly affect the liver, skin, and hematopoietic systems. Type B reactions include hypersensitivity reactions such as anaphylaxis from penicillin, idiosyncratic reactions such as malignant hyperthermia from an antipsychotic, and pseudoallergic reactions such as flushing and hypotension from vancomycin. Type B reactions may be influenced by genetic and environmental factors and are frequently not discovered until after a drug is marketed.

Additional classifications, types C, D, E, and F have been suggested.[8,36] Type C reactions are uncommon, dose- and time-related, and associated with the cumulative dose of the drug. Prolonged corticosteroid administration causing adrenal suppression and benzodiazepine dependence are examples of type C reactions. Type D reactions are rare, delayed in onset and are usually dose-related. Examples include carcinogenesis, teratogenesis, and tardive dyskinesia from antipyschotic agents. Type E reactions are withdrawal symptoms. These generally occur shortly after stopping the drug and are uncommon; opiate withdrawal is an example of this reaction type. Last, a type F reaction is an unexpected failure of therapy. These reactions are common, dose-related, and may result from drug-drug interactions. Note that type F reactions may not be considered an ADR under the WHO definition.

ADRs can also be classified according to their onset or severity. The timing of the reaction can be acute (occurring within 1 hour of exposure), subacute (occurring within 24 hours of exposure), or latent (appearing 2 or more days after drug exposure). Reaction severity may be mild (bothersome but not requiring treatment or a change in therapy), moderate (requiring a change in therapy, treatment, or continued hospitalization), or severe or significant. FDA defines significant reactions as those that are fatal, life-threatening, permanently or significantly disabling, require or substantially prolong hospitalization, results in a congenital abnormality, or require an intervention to prevent permanent impairment or damage.

Risk Factors for ADRs

Many factors appear to increase the likelihood of an adverse drug reaction, including age, multiple medications, duration of drug exposure, gender, concurrent illness, narrow therapeutic index drugs, and genetics. Recognition of these risk factors is important in ultimately leading to their prevention.

AGE—The very young and the very old are particularly vulnerable to ADRs. Young children, especially neonates, lack fully developed organs for drug metabolism and elimination. As children grow, drug dosing can be affected by changes in body weight, drug distribution, and drug elimination. Many reports have shown the incidence of ADRs increases with increasing age, being the highest in the very elderly.[37,38] Age-related changes in body composition and organ function, such as decreased liver and kidney function, and increased sensitivity to medications predispose the elderly patient to drug toxicity. Additionally, this population tends to use more drugs and have more illnesses than younger age groups.[39] Last, neither pediatrics nor geriatrics is generally included in the clinical trials conducted to gain drug approval. Thus, experience is limited in these populations.

CONCURRENT MEDICINES—Taking multiple prescription medicines, over-the-counter drugs, and/or alternative or natural products increases the risk of experiencing an adverse drug reaction. The number and severity of adverse reactions increase disproportionately with the number of drugs taken, and some trials have found that the best predictor of ADRs is the number of concurrent medicines. One study over an 18-month period found that patients who experienced an ADR had almost three times the drug exposures as those who did not.[40] Clearly the potential for drug-drug interactions increases as the number of medical products used rises.

DURATION OF THERAPY—The greater the degree of drug exposure, the greater the likelihood an ADR will occur. This is particularly true for already predisposed persons (the very young and very old), and or those with existing organ dysfunction such as renal or hepatic failure.

GENDER—Females have a 1.5- to 1.7-fold greater risk of developing an ADR compared to males.[41] A review of drug safety over a 10-year period found that almost three-quarters of the reactions reported were in women.[42] Numerous explanations for these disparities have been suggested, including over-dosing, gender-based differences in pharmacokinetics and pharmacodynamics, differences in immunological and hormonal makeup, women are more likely to report adverse events than men, or women take more medications than men.[41] Women are another group that as historically been poorly represented in clinical trials.

COMORBID CONDITIONS—Patients with concurrent medical problems are more likely to experience an adverse drug reaction than comparatively healthy persons. Illnesses such as congestive heart failure, malnutrition, obesity, hepatitis, cirrhosis, or diabetes can alter the pharmacokinetics and pharmacodynamics of drugs, leading to drug accumulation and toxicity. Additionally, such patients are typically using multiple medicines, further increasing their risk.

NARROW THERAPEUTIC INDEX DRUGS—Again noting that the majority of ADRs are dose-related, those drugs with little separation between therapeutic and toxic concentrations are highly associated with adverse reactions. Examples include aminoglycosides, anticonvulsants, digoxin, heparin, theophylline, and warfarin.

ETHNICITY AND GENETICS—It is well known that there are inherited or genetic differences to drug response. Responses may vary from minimal effect to the desired therapeutic response to an untoward result, manifested as an ADR. Some, but not all, of this variability can be attributed to differences in the genes encoding for drug-metabolizing enzymes, drug transporters, or drug targets. In fact, adverse drug reactions are often the clinical events that ultimately lead to discovery of such genetic variations. The study of these differences is called pharmacogenetics.[43] Pharmacogenetics can influence drug therapy in one of three ways.[43] First are genetic polymorphisms that are associated with altered drug metabolism. Increased or decreased drug metabolism can alter the concentration of a drug and/or its metabolites, whether active, inactive, or toxic. For example, 5–10% of the population carries two decreased activity alleles for the drug-metabolizing enzyme CYP2D6. These "poor metabolizers" can have a higher frequency of toxicity from antidepressants metabolized via this enzyme because of decreased elimination and drug accumulation. A recent study found that 59% of the drugs cited in ADR studies are metabolized by at least one enzyme with a variation known to cause poor drug metabolism.[44] Second, genetic variations can produce unexpected or idiosyncratic reactions, such as hemolytic anemia in persons with a deficiency in glucose-6-phosphate dehydrogenase. Last, genetic variation in a drug target or transporter can alter the clinical response and frequency of toxicity. For example, 1–2% of the population may have mutations in the genes encoding for cardiac ion channels, predisposing them to sudden cardiac death due to long-QT syndrome after exposure to antiarrhythmics or certain drugs such as terfenadine.

Reporting Requirements and Hospital-Based Adverse Drug Reaction Monitoring

Institutional settings play an important role in monitoring and reporting adverse drug reactions and having a program for this function is a requirement for gaining accreditation by the Joint Committee on Accreditation of Healthcare organizations (JCAHO). Development and coordination of the program commonly falls to the pharmacy department, although the most effective programs involve all disciplines.[45] An ADR program must have the following basic components: (a) a definition of an ADR that clearly describes what is a reportable adverse drug reaction; (b) a method of monitoring and reporting adverse drug reactions; (c) a system for evaluating reactions for severity, causality, and preventability; and (d) a system for using the results of the ADR program. The guidelines published by the American Society of Health-System Pharmacists (ASHP) provide a detailed explanation of each of these components.[9]

Hospital-based programs use several methods for detecting adverse reactions, including retrospective chart review, concurrent surveillance, and prospective monitoring. JCAHO requires hospitals to have a concurrent monitoring system in place, while ASHP recommends both concurrent and prospective monitoring programs. In particular, prospectively identifying high-risk drugs and high-risk patients and utilizing knowledge of the risk factors for ADRs can help with the monitoring and ultimately the prevention of adverse reactions. Concurrent monitoring, particularly when coupled with ongoing advances in information technology, is clearly superior to retrospective monitoring of adverse drug reactions.[28]

Once reported, an adverse reaction is evaluated for its severity, causality, and preventability. Determining the causality of a drug reaction (ie, the likelihood that the drug in question is the reason for the reaction) is somewhat arbitrary but usually assigns the probability to one of a few categories such as definite, likely, possible, and unlikely. Several algorithms are available, some complex, to assist with this assessment, but often clinicians must rely upon clinical judgment, literature review, and communication with the manufacturer or other health professionals to make a determination. Regardless of the method used, assessing the causal relationship involves several elements: the timing between drug administration and the appearance of the reaction (also called the temporal or chronological relationship); (b) whether the drug was withdrawn or a specific antidote administered with improvement in the symptoms (positive dechallenge); (c) whether the drug was reintroduced or the dose increased with recurrence or worsening of the symptoms (positive rechallenge); (d) whether the reaction has been previously described or reported; (e) whether objective data (eg, drug levels, other laboratory findings) support that the reaction is an ADR; and (f) whether the reaction has an alternative etiology, ie, can it be explained by an existing condition or another agent? Many algorithms use a weighted scoring system, allocating points for responses to questions about each of these areas.[46] Perhaps the most widely used algorithm is that by Naranjo et al.[47] The reaction must also be categorized by its severity as previously described.

It is becoming increasingly important to also assess the *preventability* of an ADR and criteria for making such a determination have been published.[48] As noted, drug errors resulting in adverse reactions account for significant morbidity and mortality. Determining which ADRs are preventable and at what point in the medication process an error occurred will help to identify ways to improve the medication system.

Information gained from ADR programs should be shared with all health care providers and should be integrated into hospital quality assurance and performance improvement programs. In some institutions a dedicated Drug Safety Committee or Medication Safety Committee may oversee this function, in others it falls to the Pharmacy and Therapeutics Committee.

Drug Development and Its Relation to Adverse Drug Reactions

As noted above, all drugs and biologicals marketed in the US must be shown to be safe and effective. FDA, based upon information submitted by the pharmaceutical sponsor or developer, evaluates the data supporting these outcomes. The drug is approved if its benefits, as it's intended to be used in the proposed population, outweigh its foreseeable risks. The tolerance for toxicity is higher for drugs that treat serious or life-threatening illnesses, such as antineoplastic drugs.

Safety and efficacy data are generated in the preclinical animal and toxicology studies and the premarketing human testing that all drugs and biologicals are required to undergo, known as phase I, II, and III testing.[49] Phase I trials are generally focused on drug safety. Studies are usually conducted in healthy volunteers and assess the most common acute side effects and evaluate the size of doses subjects can safely take

without a high frequency of adverse reactions. Phase II trials involve small numbers of patients with the disease to be treated. Although the primary focus of these trials is efficacy, safety data on short-term use are also gathered. Phase III trials involve several hundred to several thousand patients with the primary goals of confirming drug efficacy and safety at the doses to be used once the drug is marketed.

It's important to note that the overall safety goal of prelicensure research is not to identify every ADR that may occur, but instead to establish the common dose-related effects that might be expected from its approved use, whether predictable or not. Most drugs approved by FDA are done so with a few thousand patient exposures, which may be sufficient to detect a reaction occurring in 1 of every 500–1000 patients.[50] However, for idiosyncratic reactions, rare side-effects (for example occurring in 1 in 10,000 patients), or reactions that may require a long induction period, premarketing clinical trials generally do not enroll enough subjects to detect such reactions and are too short in duration. But there are other limitations that prevent establishing a drug's entire toxicity profile before it's approved for use.[51,52] Since the aim of premarketing trials is to show drug efficacy, such trials frequently exclude patients with complicated medical histories, significant comorbid conditions, or those who are receiving other drugs, since this may hinder establishing the drug's effectiveness. Therefore, the type and frequency of ADRs that will occur once the drug is used in a broader population using differing medications is unknown. Drug companies also generally seek drug approval for a single indication. Once marketed, the drug may be used to treat entirely different illnesses or diseases from what was studied. Premarketing trials have also historically excluded pediatric patients, pregnant or breast-feeding women, and elderly patients; how these populations will react to new drugs is frequently unknown. Significant headway has been made in addressing this last shortcoming, however, with rules adopted in 1997 and 1998 requiring pediatric safety data on new drugs, a specific "Geriatric use" section in the labeling of all drugs and biologicals, and the requirement that guidance documents be developed on the inclusion of women and minorities in clinical trials.[53,54]

Recognizing the limitations of prelicensure studies, the FDA frequently requires that a drug manufacturer conduct one or more *postmarketing* phase IV trials as a condition of drug approval. Such trials are designed to further evaluate drug safety and efficacy, often in specific populations (eg, children), confirm safety in the target population and look for chronic effects from prolonged use.[52] However, one report suggests that phase IV trials are rarely completed as required, calling into question the ability of the FDA to monitor and enforce compliance with this requirement.[55]

Drug-Development: Toxicokinetics and Toxicodynamics

Early in drug development, the toxicity of a candidate compound must be assessed to determine if further development and progression to human trials is warranted. This typically involves administration of doses that are several-fold higher than the human pharmacological dose eventually used. Such research obviously cannot be performed in humans, so *preclinical* (sometimes called *nonclinical*) toxicity studies in animals are undertaken. However, the majority of animal toxicity data generated during preclinical studies cannot be extrapolated to humans without an understanding of the pharmacokinetics and pharmacodynamics involved. The kinetics of a compound when given at toxic doses is termed *toxicokinetics*. More specifically, toxicokinetics is the study of the absorption, distribution, metabolism, and excretion (ADME) of a xenobiotic (a foreign, natural, or synthetic chemical) at higher than therapeutic doses resulting in toxicity or excessive exposure.[56] The study of the relationship between the toxic levels of xenobiotics and the ultimately observed clinical illness is *toxicodynamics*.[56,57] Toxicokinetics and toxicodynamics are areas of increasing importance in drug development and risk assessment that are relevant to the prediction of ADRs and their management. Although the WHO definition of an ADR excludes drug overdose and poisoning (ie, situations typically resulting in toxic drug exposure), toxicokinetic data gained during preclinical and toxicology testing in animals is relevant to treatment in humans. Furthermore, toxicokinetic and toxicodynamic studies are a prerequisite for all drugs submitted to FDA for approval, a requirement that extends globally as well as a result of the International Conference on Harmonization (see International Drug Monitoring).[58]

Although toxicokinetics follows many of the same principles and mathematical models as pharmacokinetics,[56] it is important to note the differences between these two disciplines. The essential difference is that the kinetics of a compound is frequently altered when that compound is administered at toxic doses compared to pharmacological doses. For example, high doses can alter drug solubility in the intestinal tract, leading to precipitation and differing patterns of absorption. High drug doses can overwhelm or saturate many processes, eg, enzymatic metabolism, protein binding, and active tubular secretion, leading to non-linear kinetics. The altered kinetics of a drug taken or administered at toxic levels may ultimately lead to cellular toxicity, manifested as the clinical symptoms of poisoning or overdose.[59]

The ultimate goal of toxicokinetic (TK) and toxicodynamic (TD) studies is to relate the adverse reactions from drug toxicity observed in animals (both short term and long term) to safety and toxicity in humans, as well as to formulate strategies to manage human toxicity.[60,61] TK/TD data are used in a variety of ways to meet this goal.[62] For example, researchers may use initial TK/TD data to validate the choice of animal species and to provide information that will help in the design of subsequent experiments to provide animal safety data. Selecting the animal species that most closely models human toxicokinetics and pharmacokinetics is key to determining the safe starting dose of a candidate drug for human trials. TK data may be used to modify dose administration (ie, the dose administered, the route of administration, the time of administration, frequency of administration, dosage form, etc.). Clinicians use TK/TD data to assist in establishing the margin of safety between preclinical safety trials and human trials and to determine the mechanism of toxicity. Pharmacokineticists use TK/TD data to help design pharmacokinetic studies to validate human safety and efficacy. Pathologists may use TK data to relate the pathology found on necropsy (eg, lesions) to drug exposure and to determine the target organs for toxicity that will eventually be part of the adverse drug reaction monitoring in future trials. Reproduction and developmental toxicologists use TK data to aid in dose selection for reproduction and teratology studies, which will assist in monitoring for Type D (long-term) reactions in humans. Although much of the TK/TD data are discovered in preclinical animal trials, such data are in fact generated and refined throughout the entire drug development process, including postmarketing drug safety surveillance, which will be discussed later. Interested readers are referred to more in-depth discussions on the increasing role of toxicokinetics and toxicodynamics in drug development[63,64] and to references that describe fundamental toxicokinetic and toxicodynamic principles and models.[56,61,65]

Drug Development: Pharmacogenomics

As noted earlier, genetics plays an important role in drug response. Pharmacogenomics harnesses the information gained from genome-wide research, notably the Human Genome Project, to understand the inherited differences in drug response between individuals as well as to optimize drug therapy based upon a person's specific genetic information.[43,66] Applying advances in pharmacogenomics to drug development means there is the potential to stop many adverse reactions that are currently considered nonpreventable. The implication is that determining *a priori* an individual's genetic makeup, coupled with the knowledge of a drug's pharmacology may allow drug selection that optimizes the desired clinical response while reducing the risk of an adverse drug reaction. Additionally, coupling genetic advances with toxicokinetics is leading to the emerging field of *toxicogenomics*,[67] providing a genetic understanding for the response to toxic drug exposure. Undoubtedly as information on pharmacogenomics, pharmacogenetics, and toxicogenomics grows, drug developers will conduct trials in populations with specific genotypes and phenotypes to develop a clearer understanding of the ADRs that may be anticipated and how best to avoid them. Readers are referred to Chapter 62 for a more in depth discussion of pharmacogenetics and pharmacogenomics.

POSTMARKETING SAFETY SURVEILLANCE— The previously mentioned problems in detecting ADRs during premarket drug testing are well recognized by FDA. Additionally, drug approval times have become increasingly shorter[50] and critically important drugs can reach the market quickly by shortening the length of time required for premarket testing or eliminating some phases of testing altogether.[68] Thus, drugs can be marketed with less and less knowledge of their full toxicity profile. Accordingly, significant effort has been made to observe drugs after their approval to monitor their continued safety. This effort, termed *postmarketing safety surveillance*, also falls under the authority of FDA. The goals of the postmarketing surveillance system are to detect potential adverse drug reactions that were not seen in prelicensure trials as well as problems that may arise when a drug is used in ways or in populations that were not studied or anticipated. Postmarketing surveillance also provides an opportunity to ascertain toxicokinetic and toxicodynamic parameters in situations of human poisoning and drug overdose that were not possible during drug development. Such data assist clinical toxicologists in developing treatment strategies and can lead to revised drug labeling, requests by FDA for further safety assessment, or to phase IV postmarketing trials. Readers are referred to Chapter 103 on poison control and to detailed toxicokinetic references for more information.[56,57,65]

FDA utilizes a passive system for postmarketing safety surveillance that relies upon voluntary reporting of ADRs from health professionals and consumers, mandatory reporting by drug manufacturers, and reports from ongoing clinical trials. Manufacturers must file within 15 days of their detection or notification reports of any serious reaction not listed in the current product labeling, and any reports of drug overdose, cancer, or congenital defects. In addition to these "15-day" reports, manufacturers must submit periodic reports at least annually and as often as quarterly that describe serious labeled reactions and all nonserious reactions, as well as any reports of an increased frequency of serious, labeled reactions and deaths, beyond what might be anticipated from increased drug use alone.[69]

Supplementing the manufacturer reports are voluntary reports from health professionals and consumers via the MedWatch program, which was started in 1993 under the Centers for Drug Evaluation and Research (CDER) at FDA. Although postmarketing surveillance by health professionals was established prior to this, MedWatch was designed to emphasize the responsibility of health care providers to identify and report adverse reactions related to the use of not only drugs and biologics, but to medical devices and certain nutritional products as well. Importantly, causality is not a prerequisite for MedWatch reporting; *suspicion* that a medical product may be related to a serious event is sufficient reason to submit a MedWatch report.

While health professionals are encouraged to report any ADR considered significant, not every ADR need be reported. To do so would overwhelm FDA resources and reduce its ability to identify significant reactions. FDA is most interested in reports of serious reactions, defined as any event that is fatal, life-threatening, is permanently or significantly disabling, requires or prolongs hospitalization, results in a congenital abnormality, or requires an intervention to prevent permanent impairment

In the first quarter of 2003, FDA proposed many additional far-reaching changes to drug safety, safety monitoring, and safety reporting.[94,97,98] Among these were:

- Mandating bar code labeling on all prescription and OTC drugs, biologicals, and vaccines.
- Adopting a new internationally accepted definition for *suspected* adverse drug reaction (SADR). Adoption of this definition will require reporting of a reaction unless the drug company is *certain* that the product is not the cause, thus increasing the number of reports made to FDA and improving safety signal generation.
- Requiring that greater emphasis be devoted to serious SADRs that have the potential for significant impact on the public health, with less importance and resources placed on non-serious SADRs. Additionally, more detailed information will be required for reports of serious SADRs increasing the value of such reports.
- Requiring reports of all unexpected reactions for which a determination of serious or nonserious cannot be made.
- Mandating reporting of medically significant reactions, whether expected or unexpected, and whether or not considered serious such as those that may jeopardize the patient and/or require medical or surgical intervention to treat the patient.
- Mandating reporting of safety findings from animal or human studies, or other information, that is sufficient to consider changes in product administration.
- Establishing postmarketing periodic safety update reports that conform to international standards and use internationally accepted terminology to describe and classify SADRs.
- Requiring submission from industry of spontaneously reported individual cases of serious, expected SADRs that occur *outside* the US (current rules only require reporting of such cases if they occur domestically).
- Requiring that a health care professional at the company speak *directly* to the initial reporter of an SADR when additional information is needed.
- Requiring that a licensed physician at the pharmaceutical company be responsible for the content and medical interpretation of postmarketing safety reports submitted to FDA.
- Requiring companies to submit to FDA, within 15 calendar days, all reports they receive of actual or potential *medication errors* occurring in the US whether they resulted in a serious SADR, nonserious SADR, or no SADR at all. This also includes potential medication errors that do not involve a patient but instead describe information or a complaint about packaging, labeling, or similar product names.

These changes will be adopted internationally. Once implemented, the net effect will be to improve the prevention of medication errors and enable FDA to more quickly identify adverse reactions associated with the use of drugs and biologicals and to take more timely action to reduce patient harm.

International ADR Monitoring

FDA is a member of the World Health Organization (WHO) Programme for International Drug Monitoring. The program houses the Global Database on Adverse Drug Reactions and, similar to FDA's AERS, the data collected are used to generate early warning signals of potential adverse reactions. Currently over 70 countries participate in the program that was established in 1968 with the goal of increasing early recognition of new and unexpected adverse reactions. Additionally, the program offers guidance and training courses on pharmacovigilance and establishes internationally accepted definitions for terms used in ADR reporting.[99] FDA and the US pharmaceutical industry also have had substantial input into the development of the standards proposed by the International Conference on Harmonisation of Technical Requirements for Registration of Pharmaceuticals for Human Use (ICH) and in the World Health Organization's Council for International Organization of Medical Sciences (CIOMS) drug safety working groups. In addition to efforts to harmonize the drug and biological product application process worldwide, these proposals establish international standards for safety reporting (including terminology used in reports, format of reports, and timing of reports) developed jointly by the US, the European Union, Canada, Switzerland, and Japan to improve the quality, consistency, and usefulness of these reports. Many of the proposed enhancements to the US pre- and postmarketing safety programs noted above are a direct result of participation in ICH. As the pharmaceutical industry becomes an increasingly global enterprise, participation in international drug safety endeavors will become increasingly important.

Summary

Drug use continues to increase in the US and will likely do so for many years to come. While drug therapy offers tremendous benefits, it does so with the potential for patient harm. Adverse drug reactions are a significant cause of morbidity and mortality and have a significant financial, emotional, and societal impact. ADRs are part of a spectrum of drug safety that includes adverse drug events that may be due to medical error. There are numerous risk factors for developing ADRs; the role genetics plays in drug response is being increasingly recognized and will likely have an impact on future drug development and testing. Progress is being made toward comprehensive risk management that addresses both ADRs and ADEs. Postmarketing safety monitoring of drugs is essential, as not all reactions a drug may cause are known at the time of its approval. Institutional settings can play a significant role in monitoring for ADRs. Although postmarketing surveillance has functioned as intended, significant improvements are needed to make drug therapy safer. Several initiatives are underway that will meet this goal.

REFERENCES

1. Manasse HR Jr. *Am J Hosp Pharm* 1989; 46:929.
2. Remarks by Mark B. McClellan, MD, PhD, Commissioner of Food and Drugs, U.S. Food and Drug Administration, to the Generic Pharmaceutical Association, January 29, 2003. Available at http://www.fda.gov/oc/speeches/2002/gpha.html. Accessed February 15, 2003.
3. Keynote address by Mark B. McClellan, MD, PhD, Commissioner of Food and Drugs, U.S. Food and Drug Administration, for Health Services and Outcomes Research Conference, Houston, Texas, November 25, 2002. Available at http://www.fda.gov/oc/speeches/2002/healthservice.html. Accessed February 15, 2003.
4. US Food and Drug Administration. Approval times for priority and standard NMEs calendar years 1993–2002. Available at http://www.fda.gov/cder/rdmt/NMEapps93-02.htm. Accessed February 15, 2003.
5. Pharmaceutical sales continue upward momentum in 2001. *Drug Topics* 2002; (April 1):62.
6. Drug and formulary trends. *Formulary* 2003; 38:28.
7. Karch FE, Lasagna L. *JAMA* 1975; 234:1236.
8. Edwards IR, Aronson JK. *Lancet* 2000; 356:1255.
9. American Society of Health-Systems Pharmacists. *Am J Health-Syst Pharm* 1995; 52:417.
10. World Health Organization. International Drug Monitoring: The Role of National Centres. Geneva, Switzerland: World Health Organization 1972. Technical Report Series No. 498.
11. Bates DW, Cullen DJ, Laird N, et al. *JAMA* 1995; 274:29.
12. Kohn LT, Corrigan JM, Donaldson MS, eds. *To Err is Human: Building a Safer Health System.* Washington, D.C.: National Academy Press, Institute of Medicine Committee on Quality of Health Care in America; 1999.
13. Task Force on Risk Management. U.S. Department of Health and Human Services, Food and Drug Administration. Managing the risks from medical product use. Creating a risk management framework. May 1999. Available at http://www.fda.gov/oc/tfrm/Tableofcontents.htm. Accessed November 12, 2002.
14. Lazarou J, Pomeranz BH, Corey PN. *JAMA* 1998; 279:1200.
15. Chyka PA. *Am J Med* 2000; 109:122.
16. Gurwitz JH, Field TS, Avorn J, et al. *Am J Med* 2000; 109:87.
17. Aparasu RR, Helgeland DL. *Manag Care Interface* 2000; 13:70.
18. Kaushal R, Bates DW, Landrigan C, et al. *JAMA* 2001; 285:2114.
19. Menniti-Ippolito F, Raschetti R, Da Cas R, et al. *Lancet* 2000; 355:1613.
20. Gurwitz JH, Field TS, Harrold LR, et al. *JAMA* 2003; 289:1107.
21. Haller CA, Benowitz NL. *N Engl J Med* 2000; 343:1833.
22. Sheikh NM, Philen RM, Love LA. *Arch Intern Med* 1997;157:913.

23. Committee on the Framework for Evaluating the Safety of Dietary Supplements. Proposed Framework for Evaluating the Safety of Dietary Supplements—For Comment (2002). Available at http://books.nap.edu/books/NI000760/html/index.html. Accessed January 23, 2003.
24. Melmon KL. *N Engl J Med* 1974; 284:1361.
25. Miller RR. *Am J Hosp Pharm* 1973; 30:584.
26. Gardner P, Watson LJ. *Clin Pharmacol Ther* 1970; 11:802.
27. Wu WK, Pantaleo N. *Am J Health-Syst Pharm* 2003; 60:253.
28. Classen DC, Pestotnik SL, Evans RS, et al. *JAMA* 1997; 277:301.
29. Suh DC, Woodall BS, Shin SK, et al. *Ann Pharmacother* 2000; 34:1373.
30. Department of Health and Human Services. FDA announces proposed rule to improve safety reporting for human drugs and biological products. Available at http://www.fda.gov/oc/initiatives/barcode-sadr/fs-sadr.html. Accessed March 25, 2003.
31. Ly P. Diabetes drug suit could set tone nationwide. MD drug suit could set tone for 4,200 in U.S. The Washington Post, December 31, 2001. Available at http://www.washingtonpost.com/ac2/wp-dyn?pagename=article&node=&contentId=A42754-2001Dec30&notFound=true. Accessed January 25, 2003.
32. Willig SH. A view from the US courtroom. In Strom BL, ed. *Pharmacoepidemiology*. New York: Churchill Livingstone, 1989, pp 85–103.
33. Associated Press. States consider solutions to malpractice insurance crisis. The Kansas City Star, February 3, 2003. Available at http://www.kansascity.com/mld/kansascity/business/5068585.htm. Accessed February 15, 2003.
34. Manasse HR Jr. *Am J Hosp Pharm* 1989; 46;1141.
35. Johnson JA, Bootman JL. *Arch Intern Med* 1995; 155:1949.
36. Gruchalla RS. *Lancet* 2000; 356:1505.
37. Faich GA, Knapp D, Dreis M, et al. *JAMA* 1987; 257:2068.
38. Faich GA, Dreis M, Tomita D. *Arch Intern Med* 1988; 148:785.
39. Williams B. Geriatric therapy. In Koda-Kimble MA, Young LY, eds. *Applied Therapeutics. The Clinical Use of Drugs*, 7th ed. Philadelphia: Lippincott Williams & Wilkins, 2001, pp 97-1–97-20.
40. Classen DC, Pestotnik SL, Evans RS, et al. *JAMA* 1991; 266:2847.
41. Rademaker M. *Am J Clin Dermatol* 2001; 2:349.
42. Tran C, Knowles SR, Liu BA, et al. *J Clin Pharmacol* 1998; 38:1003.
43. Meyer UA. *Lancet* 2000; 356:1667.
44. Phillips KA, Veenstra DL, Oren E, et al. *JAMA* 2001; 286:2270.
45. Prosser TR, Kamysz PL. *Am J Hosp Pharm* 1990; 47:1334.
46. Blanc S, Leuenberger P, Berger JP, et al. *Clin Pharmacol Ther* 1979; 25:493.
47. Naranjo CA, Busto U, Sellers EM, et al. *Clin Pharmacol Ther* 1981; 30:239.
48. Hartwig SC, Siegel J, Schneider PJ. *Am J Hosp Pharm* 1992; 49:2229.
49. Trenter ML, ed. *From Test Tube to Patient: Improving Health Through Human Drugs*. US Food and Drug Administration, Center for Drug Evaluation and Research, September, 1999. Available at http://www.fda.gov/cder/audiences/default.htm. Accessed February 5, 2003.
50. Friedman MA, Woodcock J, Lumpkin MM, et al. *JAMA* 1999; 281:1728.
51. Porta MS, Hartzema AG. *Drug Intell Clin Pharm* 1987; 21:741.
52. Smith Rogers A. *Drug Intell Clin Pharm* 1987; 21:915.
53. Nordenberg T. Pediatric drug studies: protecting pint-sized patients. *FDA Consumer Magazine* May-June 1999. Available at http://www.fda.gov/fdac/features/1999/399_kids.html. Accessed January 15, 2003.
54. Remarks by Jane E. Henney, MD, Commissioner of Food and Drugs, U.S. Food and Drug Administration, to Howard University. Health issues and concerns of women of color: a call to action "marching to a different drummer: health policy looking to the new millennium." April 29, 1999. Available at http://www.fda.gov/oc/speeches/Henney499.html. Accessed December 3, 2002.
55. Sasich LD, Lurie P, Wolfe SM. The drug industry's performance in finishing postmarketing research (phase IV) studies. Available at http://www.citizen.org/publications/release.cfm?ID=6721. Accessed February 27, 2003.
56. Howland MA. In Goldfrank LR, Flomenbaum NE, Lewin NA, et al, eds. *Goldfrank's Toxicologic Emergencies*, 7th ed. New York: McGraw-Hill, 2002, pp166–185.
57. Baud FJ, Borron SW, Bismuth C. *Toxicol Lett* 1995; 82–83;785.
58. Cayen MN. *Toxicol Pathol* 1995; 23:148.
59. Welling PG. *Toxicol Pathol* 1995; 23:143.
60. Noda K. *J Toxicol Sci* 1998; 23 (suppl 2): 214.
61. Dixit R, Riviere J, Krishnan K, et al. *J Toxicol Environ Health B Crit Rev* 2003; 6:1.
62. Dahlem AM, Allerheiligen SR, Vodicnik MJ. *Toxicol Pathol* 1995; 23:170.
63. Zhong WZ, Williams MG, Branstetter DG. *Curr Drug Metab* 2000; 1:243.
64. Baldrick P. *Drug Discov Today* 2003; 8:127.
65. Medinsky MA, Valentine JL. Toxicokinetics. In Klaassen CD, ed. *Casarett and Doull's Toxicology. The Basic Science of Poisons*, 6th ed. New York: McGraw-Hill, 2001, pp 225–237.
66. Evans WE, McLeod HL. *N Engl J Med* 2003; 348:538.
67. Boorman GA, Anderson SP, Casey WM, et al. *Toxicol Pathol* 2002; 30:15.
68. Nightingale SL. *JAMA* 1988; 260:2980.
69. Baum C, Anello C. The spontaneous reporting system in the United States. In Strom BL, ed. *Pharmacoepidemiology*. New York: Churchill Livingstone, 1989, pp 107–118.
70. Brewer T, Colditz GA. *JAMA* 1999; 281:824.
71. Vaccine Adverse Event Reporting System, US Food and Drug Administration, Centers for Biologics Evaluation and Research. Available at http://www.fda.gov/cber/vaers/vaers.htm. Accessed December 20, 2002.
72. Levy S. *Drug Topics*. September 16, 2002:20.
73. Strom BL (ed). *Pharmacoepidemiology*, 3rd ed. Sussex: John Wiley, 2000.
74. Pharmacovigilance Working Group, Centers for Drug Evaluation and Research and Centers for Biologicals Evaluation and Research, U.S. Food and Drug Administration. Concept Paper: Risk assessment of observational data: good pharmacovigilance practices and pharmacoepidemiologic assessment. March 3, 2002. Available at http://www.fda.gov/cber/meetings/rmcncpt3.htm. Accessed March 31, 2003.
75. Kaufman DW, Shapiro S. *Lancet* 2000; 356;1339.
76. Meadows M. *FDA Consumer Magazine* (online edition). January-February 2002; 36(1). Available at http://www.fda.gov/fdac/features/2002/102_drug.html. Accessed December 1, 2002.
77. Bupropion for depression. *Med Lett Drugs Ther* 1989; 31:97.
78. Piazza-Hepp TD, Kennedy DL. *Am J Health-Syst Pharm* 1995; 52:1436.
79. Office of Drug Safety, Center for Drug Evaluation and Research, Food and Drug Administration. Annual Report FY 2001. Available at http://www.fda.gov/cder/Offices/ODS/AnnRep2001/annual-report2001.htm. Accessed November 5 2002.
80. Is the FDA approving drugs too fast? *BMJ* 1998; 317:899.
81. Lasser KE, Allen PD, Woolhandler SJ, et al. *JAMA* 2002; 287:2215.
82. Postmarketing drug dosage changes of NMEs approved between 1980–1999. *Formulary* 2002; 37:513.
83. CDER/CBER Risk Assessment Working Group. Concept Paper: Premarketing risk assessment. March 3, 2003. Available at http://www.fda.gov/cder/meeting/riskmanagement.htm. Accessed March 31, 2003.
84. Wood AJJ. *N Engl J Med* 2000; 342:1824.
85. Martin RM, Kapoor KV, Wilton LV, et al. *BMJ* 1998; 317:119.
86. Bates DW. *JAMA* 1998; 279:1216.
87. Rogers AS, Israel E, Smith CR, et al. *Arch Intern Med* 1988; 148:1596.
88. Chyka PA, McCommon SW. *Drug Saf* 2000; 23:87.
89. Uhl K, Honig P. *Pharmacoepidemiol Drug Saf* 2001; 10:205.
90. Weatherby LB, Walker AM, Fife D, et al. *Pharmacoepidemiol Drug Saf* 2001; 10:209.
91. Weatherby LB, Nordstrom BL, Fife D, et al. *Clin Pharmacol Ther* 2002; 72:735.
92. CDER/CBER Risk Assessment Working Group. Concept Paper: Risk management programs. March 3, 2003. Available at http://www.fda.gov/cder/meeting/riskmanagement.htm. Accessed March 31, 2003.
93. Chen RT. *Lancet* 1995; 345:1369.
94. Department of Health and Human Services. FDA announces new framework for 21st century patient safety programs. Available at http://www.fda.gov/oc/initiatives/barcode-sadr/fs-future.html. Accessed March 27, 2003.
95. Berlin JA, Colditz GA. *JAMA* 1999; 281:830.
96. Wood AJ, Stein CM, Woosley R. *N Engl J Med* 1998; 339:1851.
97. Department of Health and Human Services. FDA announces proposed rule to improve safety reporting for human drugs and biological products. March 13, 2003. Available at http://www.fda.gov/oc/initiatives/barcode-sadr/fs-sadr.html. Accessed March 27, 2003.
98. Department of Health and Human Services. Secretary Thompson announces steps to reduce medication errors. FDA proposals for medication bar coding and safety reporting will improve patient safety. March 13, 2003. Available at http://www.hhs.gov/news/press/2003pres/20030313.html. Accessed March 27, 2003.
99. WHO Collaborating Centre for International Drug Monitoring, the Uppsala Monitoring Centre. Available at http://www.who-umc.org/. Accessed January 20, 2003.

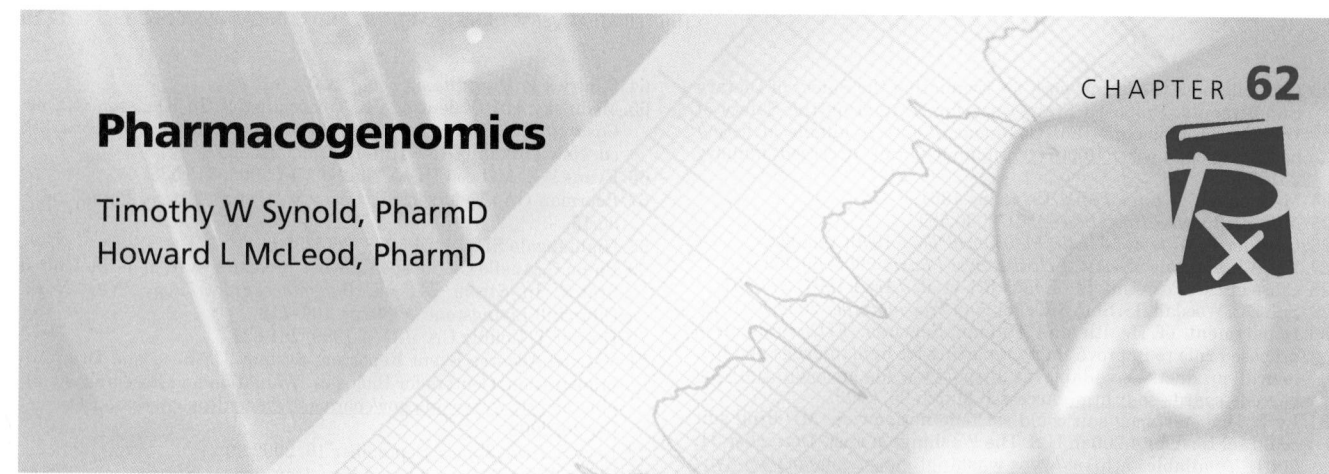

CHAPTER 62

Pharmacogenomics

Timothy W Synold, PharmD

Howard L McLeod, PharmD

Administering an identical dose of the same medication to apparently similar patients can often lead to quite different clinical responses. While variable response to drugs will be influenced by many environmental and demographic factors such as age, concomitant medications, kidney or liver function, and diet, there remains a significant degree of variation that cannot be explained by external causes. This suggests that a major component of inter-individual differences in drug response is inheritable. In fact, it has been proposed that genetics may account for 20–95% of variability in drug disposition and effects.[1] There are now several examples where inter-individual differences in drug response have been traced to heritable genetic variations (genetic polymorphisms) in genes encoding drug metabolizing enzymes, drug transporters, or drug targets.[2–4] While it is clearly important to identify environmental factors that influence the effect of medications, inherited determinants of drug response remain stable for an individual's lifetime, can effect agents across number of different drug classes, and the effects can be profound.

Clinical observations of inherited differences in the effects of drugs were first documented in the 1950s,[5–7] and led to the early development of the field of *pharmacogenetics*. More recently, as a result of the successful sequencing of the entire human genome and the development of genome wide analysis techniques, pharmacogenetics has been redefined by a broad spectrum of academia and industry, giving rise to *pharmacogenomics*. The goal of pharmacogenomics is to elucidate the inherited basis for inter-individual differences in drug response, using genome-wide approaches to identify the genetic polymorphisms that determine an individual's response to specific medications. In addition to conventional targeted genetic studies to identify functional variants, the field includes such diverse areas as RNA-based microarray analysis and genome-wide DNA analysis to identify the major genetic sites (loci) associated with altered drug effects.

Because a key principle in the practice of pharmacotherapy is the optimization of drug treatment through the identification of those patient-specific variables that affect the likelihood of a clinical response or toxicity, this chapter will focus on the examination of the genetic basis of differences in drug response. The discussion will center on well-described examples of variations in specific human genes that are involved in drug disposition and effect. However, in order to provide an adequate context for the specific examples, one must start with a brief background on the history and principles of modern genomics. Finally, technological considerations, along with current and future applications of pharmacogenomics will be examined.

THE HUMAN GENOME

The Human Genome Project

In 1990, the Human Genome Project was officially initiated in the United States under the direction of the National Institutes of Health and the U.S. Department of Energy with a 15-year, $3 billion plan for completing the genome sequence of humans. This enormous multi-national effort was undertaken by a number of public and private laboratories, known collectively as the International Human Genome Sequencing Consortium (IHGSC). The IHGSC first announced a draft sequence of the human genome in 2000, and by April of 2003, the entire 3.1 gigabases that makes up the human genome was essentially complete.[8,9] In other words, greater than 99% of what can be done with current technology was done, and virtually all of the bases were identified in their proper order. Political leaders from the United States, Britain, China, France, Germany, and Japan issued a joint proclamation honoring their scientists who worked on the project, hailing their work as one of the most significant scientific breakthroughs of modern times.

While much is now known about the structure the human genome, many mysteries remain. It is known, for instance, that less than 2% of the human genome are sequences that actually code for proteins, while over 50% represents repetitive sequences of several types, whose function is less well understood.[8] Moreover, it is still not known precisely how many genes the human genome contains. Current data indicate that the human genome includes approximately 30,000 to 35,000 genes—a number that is substantially smaller than was previously thought.[8] Only about half these genes have recognizable DNA-sequence patterns, or motifs, that suggest their possible function. Furthermore, while it was once dogma that one gene encodes one protein, it now appears that, through the mechanism of alternative splicing, more than 100,000 different proteins can be derived from these 30,000 to 35,000 genes.[9] In addition to alternative splicing, a number of "epigenetic" phenomena, such as methylation, phosphorylation, and histone modification, can alter the effect of a gene.[10–12] Furthermore, a complex array of molecular signals allows specific genes to be "turned on" (expressed) or "turned off" in specific tissues and at specific times. It is widely accepted that every human gene contains inherited genetic variants or mutations.[13] Mutations known to cause disease have been identified in approximately 1000 genes. However, it is likely that nearly all human genes are capable of causing disease or altering response to drug treatment if their function is altered significantly.

Variation in the Human Genome

One characteristic of the human genome with medical and social relevance is that, on average, two unrelated persons share over 99.9% of their DNA sequences.[13] However, given that more than 3 billion base pairs constitute the human genome, this means that the DNA sequences of two unrelated individuals differ at millions of bases. Since a person's genotype represents the blending of parental genotypes, we are each thus heterozygous at about 3 million genetic loci. Many efforts are currently under way, in both the academic and commercial sectors, to catalogue these variants, commonly referred to as "single-nucleotide polymorphisms" (SNPs), and to correlate these specific genotypic variations with specific phenotypic variations relevant to health.

The Single Nucleotide Polymorphism (SNP) Consortium was established in 1999 as a collaboration of several companies and institutions within the larger IHGSC to produce a public resource of genetic variation in the human genome. SNPs, as the name implies, are single nucleotide changes in the DNA sequence that are present in the genome, and therefore, represent inheritable genetic variations. More than 1.4 million SNPs were identified in the initial sequencing of the human genome,[13] with over 60,000 of these in the regions encoding for the proteins, and it is anticipated that >10 million common SNPs will ultimately be identified. Some of these SNPs have already been associated with significant changes in the metabolism or effects of medications and are beginning to make their way into clinical medicine as important molecular diagnostic tools.[2–4] Because most drug effects are determined by the complex interplay of gene products that influence both the pharmacokinetics and pharmacodynamics of medications, pharmacogenomics is increasingly focused on polygenic determinants of drug effects, including inherited difference in drug targets (eg, receptors) and drug disposition (eg, metabolizing enzymes, transporters). The human genes involved in many pharmacogenetic traits have now been identified, their molecular mechanisms detailed and their clinical importance more clearly defined. In some cases, SNP–phenotype correlations occur as a direct result of the influence of the SNP on health. However, more commonly, the SNP is merely a marker of biologic diversity that happens to correlate with health because of its proximity to the genetic factor that is the actual cause of the clinical phenotype.[14] In this sense, the term "proximity" is only a rough measure of physical closeness. More specifically, proximity means that, as genetic material has passed through 5000 generations from our common ancestral pool, recombination between the SNP and the actual genetic factor has occurred only rarely. In genetic terminology, the SNP and the actual genetic factor are said to be in linkage disequilibrium.[15,16]

As an extension of the current efforts to catalogue individual SNPs and correlate them to phenotype, efforts are being made to map and use haplotypes.[14–16] Whereas a SNP represents a single-base variant, a haplotype represents a considerably longer sequence of nucleotides (averaging about 25,000 bases), that tend to be inherited together.[15,17] SNPs and haplotypes will be the key to the association studies (ie, studies of affected persons and control subjects) necessary to identify the genetic factors in complex, common diseases, just as family studies have been important to the identification of the genes involved in monogenic conditions. Also, until whole-genome sequencing of individual patients becomes feasible clinically, the identification of SNPs and haplotypes will prove instrumental in efforts to use genomic medicine to individualize health care.

Types of Genetic Variations

There are a number of ways to categorize genetic changes or mutations. One is according to the causative mechanism, whereas another is according to their functional effect. When classified according to the mechanism, point mutations—that is, a change in a single DNA base in the sequence—are the most common. There are many types of point mutations. One type is a missense mutation, or a substitution that encodes for an alternative amino acid, because of the way in which it changes the three-base sequence, or codon, for the amino acid. Nonsense mutations are typically a more dramatic type of point mutation that changes the codon to a "stop" codon, a codon that causes the termination of the protein instead of producing an amino acid. Another type of genetic change is the frame-shift mutation, which changes the way the cell's transcription machinery reads the sequence of the gene downstream from the site of the mutation, often leading to a premature stop codon.

In terms of functional effect, rather than mechanism, most variants in the human-genome sequence have no apparent phenotypic effect. Among these are silent mutations, which replace one base with another, so that the resultant codon still encodes for the same amino acid. Also, mutations may not change the behavior of the resulting protein if the altered codon substitutes one amino acid for another that produces very little change in the function of the protein. These are referred to as "conservative mutations." In contrast, nonconservative mutations replace an amino acid with a very different one and are more likely to affect the phenotype.

Although genetic mutations can result in altered protein function by a variety of means, the most common is loss of function. Loss-of-function mutations alter the phenotype of the affected individual by decreasing the quantity or the functional activity of a protein. Typically, loss of function mutations are the most easily identified due to their "all-or-none" phenotypic outcome. Therefore, examples of heritable genetic changes involving loss of function are plentiful. For instance, mutations in the glucose-6-phosphate dehydrogenase (G6PD) gene on the X chromosome decreases the functional activity of the enzyme, leading to acute hemolytic anemia if a male (who would have only one copy of the X chromosome) with the mutation is exposed to certain drugs, including sulfonamides, primaquine, and nitrofurantoins.[18] Furthermore, since genes involved in metabolism do not exist merely to handle pharmacologic agents, variants that cause severe G6PD deficiency also lead to hemolytic anemia when affected males ingest fava beans (favism), since the enzyme is also important in the degradation of a toxic component of the beans.[19,20] Additional well described examples of loss of function mutations in drug metabolizing enzymes include cytochrome P450 2D6 (CYP2D6),[21,22] thiopurine methyltransferase (TPMT),[23,24] and dihydropyrimidine dehydrogenase (DPD).[25,26] Alternatively, some mutations can result in a gain of function, whereby the protein can take on some new function or is simply more highly expressed. While fewer gain of function mutations have been identified, likely due to the subtlety of their phenotypic effects, some examples include mutations in the genes that cause such neurologic disorders as Huntington's disease and spinocerebellar ataxia which appear to lead to neuropathologic abnormalities by producing proteins with abnormally improved function.[27,28] Gain-of-function mutations are often dominantly inherited, since a single copy of the mutant gene is sufficient to alter function.

Although it was previously assumed that mutations in the approximately 98.5% of the genome that does not code for proteins do not affect the phenotype, several recent examples of non-coding mutations with important phenotypic implications have changed this perception. Indeed, while the vast majority of these "non-coding" mutations do not affect protein function, other so called "regulatory mutations" may ultimately prove as important in the variability of drug metabolism and etiology of common diseases as the coding region variants. Such regulatory mutations act by altering the expression of a gene, and therefore, the level of its protein product. For instance, a regulatory mutation could lead to the loss of expression of a gene, to unexpected expression in a tissue in which it is usually silent, or to a change in the time at which it is expressed. Examples of regulatory mutations associated with disease include those in the flanking region of the *FMR1* gene (causing fragile X syndrome),[29] a regulatory site of the type I collagen gene (increasing the risk of osteoporosis),[30] and an intronic regulatory site of the calpain-10 gene (increasing the risk of type 2 diabetes mellitus).[31] More recently, a regulatory mutation with important implications for drug metabolism has been identified in the gene that encodes cytochrome P450 3A5 (Schuetz Nat. Med. 2001).[32]

GENETIC POLYMORPHISMS INFLUENCING DRUG DISPOSITION

Metabolism typically converts a drug to metabolites that are more water soluble and thus more easily excreted.[33] Metabolism can also convert prodrugs into therapeutically active compounds, and it may even result in the formation of toxic metabolites. Pathways of drug metabolism are classified as either phase I reactions (ie, oxidation, reduction, and hydrolysis) or phase II conjugation reactions (eg, acetylation, glucuronidation, sulfation, and methylation).[33] The names used to refer to these pathways for drug metabolism are purely historical, so phase II reactions can precede phase I reactions. However, both types of reactions typically convert relatively lipid-soluble drugs into relatively inactive and more water-soluble metabolites, allowing for more efficient systemic elimination.

Approximately 40 years ago, the finding that impairment in the hydrolysis of the muscle relaxant succinylcholine by butyrylcholinesterase was an inherited trait served as a seminal event in the development of the field of pharmacogenetics. Approximately 1 in 3500 white subjects is homozygous for the gene encoding an atypical form of the enzyme butyrylcholinesterase.[5] Individuals who have this inherited trait are relatively unable to hydrolyze succinylcholine, thus prolonging the drug-induced muscle paralysis and resulting apnea. At almost the same time as the discovery of inherited variability in butyrylcholinesterase activity, it was determined that genetic variability in the phase II metabolic inactivation by N-acetylation could result in striking differences in half-life and plasma concentrations of drugs metabolized by *N*-acetyltransferase. Such drugs include the antituberculosis agent isoniazid,[34] the antihypertensive agent hydralazine,[35,36] and the antiarrhythmic drug procainamide,[37] and this genetic variation had clinical consequences in each of these cases.[38] These early examples of the influence of inheritance on the clinical effects of a drug set the stage for subsequent studies of genetic variation in other pathways of drug biotransformation.

The subsequent elucidation of functional polymorphisms in *CYP2D6* represents an excellent example of both the potential clinical implications of pharmacogenetics and the process by which pharmacogenetic research led from the phenotype to an understanding of molecular mechanisms at the level of the genotype. Similar approaches were subsequently applied to other phase I drug metabolizing enzymes, including CYP2C19, CYP2C9, DPD, and CYP3A5. While it is now known that polymorphisms exist in every human gene involved in drug metabolism, the functional and clinical implications of most of these genetic variants are still under investigation. Table 62-1 lists selected examples of clinically relevant genetic variations involving drug-metabolizing enzymes and transporters. While for most of the genes listed in this table, the molecular basis of inherited variation in the drug-metabolizing enzymes has been determined, in some cases, the polymorphism has been found to be associated with a clinically important phenotype without an understanding of the underlying molecular mechanism. There are more than 30 families of drug metabolizing enzymes in humans,[2,39] and essentially all have genetic variants, many of which translate into changes in the proteins they encode. In the discussion that followings, several of the most well described phenotype/genotype associations within the area of drug metabolism and transport are presented, along with some examples of how the ever increasing knowledge of the pharmacogenomics of drug disposition might be applied in the future.

Pharmacogenetics of Phase I Drug Metabolism

CYTOCHROME P4502D6—The cytochrome P450 enzyme CYP2D6 is probably the most extensively studied polymorphic drug metabolizing enzyme in humans and was the first to be characterized at the molecular level.[40] As was common in the pre-genomics era, the discovery of inherited differences in CYP2D6 activity was in part serendipitous, initially stemming from an investigator's own personal experience with marked hypotension following a dose of the antihypertensive agent debrisoquine. Subsequent studies determined that a significant proportion of the general population had an impaired ability to hydroxylate, and therefore, inactivate debrisoquin. Approximately 5–10% of white subjects were found to have a relative deficiency in their ability to oxidize debrisoquin.[41] These individuals also had an impaired ability to metabolize the antiarrhythmic and oxytocic drug sparteine.[42] Subjects who were considered "poor metabolizers" of these two drugs had lower urinary concentrations of metabolites and higher plasma concentrations of the parent drug than did subjects who were "extensive metabolizers." Furthermore, the drugs had exaggerated effects in the poor metabolizers, and family studies demonstrated that poor oxidation of debrisoquin and sparteine was inherited as an autosomal recessive trait.[41,42] In other words, subjects with poor debrisoquin metabolism had inherited two copies of a gene or genes that encoded an enzyme with either decreased CYP2D6 activity or one with no activity at all. Over 30 medications have now been identified as substrates for CYP2D6, and it has been shown that this genetic polymorphism translates into either exaggerated or diminished drug effects, depending on whether the enzyme inactivates (eg, nortriptyline, fluoxetine) or activates (eg, codeine) the medication.[43-45]

A plot of the ratio of urinary debrisoquin to 4-hydroxydebrisoquin—a so-called metabolic ratio—is shown in Figure 62-1. The higher the metabolic ratio, the less the metabolite is excreted. Therefore, subjects with poor metabolism are shown at the far right of the graph, with a few subjects at the far left of the frequency distribution who are now classified as having ultrarapid metabolism.[46,47] Therefore, individuals with genetic variants of *CYP2D6* can have either a slow or rapid acetylator phenotype. Debrisoquin and sparteine represent "probe drugs"—compounds that could be used to classify subjects as having either poor metabolism or extensive metabolism. That strategy, the administration of a probe compound metabolized by a genetically polymorphic enzyme, has become a standard technique used in many pharmacogenetic studies. Unfortunately, even though it is useful for research purposes, the approach is not easily adapted for the routine clinical laboratory. Furthermore, phenotypic studies involving probe drugs are often unreliable due to the many sources of error that accompany pharmacokinetic research, as well as the concern over a lack of substrate specificity. Therefore, the application of molecular genetic techniques to pharmacogenetics not only has made it possible to determine underlying molecular mechanisms responsible for genetic polymorphisms, but also has created the possibility of high-throughput clinical tests that can be performed with DNA isolated from a single blood sample. This approach can then easily be adapted for routine diagnostic use in clinical laboratories.

The application of molecular genetic techniques resulted in the cloning of a complementary DNA (cDNA) and the gene encoding CYP2D6.[48,49] Those advances, in turn, made it possible to characterize a series of genetic variants that led to either low levels of CYP2D6 activity or no activity. The genetic changes ranged from single-nucleotide polymorphisms that altered the

Table 62-1. Genetic Polymorphisms in Genes that Can Influence Drug Metabolism and Transport

ENZYME	SUBSTRATE	CLINICAL CONSEQUENCE OF POLYMORPHISM
Phase I enzymes		
CYP1A1	Benzo(a)pyrene, phenacetin	Possible increased or decreased cancer risk
CYP1A2	Acetaminophen, amonafide, caffeine, paraxanthine, ethoxyresorufin, propanalol, fluvoxamine	Decreased theophylline metabolism
CYP1B1	Estrogen metabolites	Possible increased cancer risk
CYP2A6	Coumarin, nicotine, halothane	Decreased nicotine metabolism and cigarette addiction
CYP2B6	Cyclophosphamide, aflatoxin, mephenytoin	Significance unknown
CYP2C8	Retinoic acid, paclitaxel	Significance unknown
CYP2C9	Tolbutamide, warfarin, phenytoin, NSAIDS	Anitcoagulant effect of warfarin
CYP2C19	Mephenytoin, omeprazole, hexobarbital, mephobarbital, propranolol, proquanil, phenytoin	Peptic ulcer response to omeprazole
CYP2D6	Beta blockers, antidepressants, antipsychotics, codeine, debrisoquin, dextromethorphan, encainide, flecainide, fluoxetine, guanoxan, methoxy-amphetamine, phenacetin, propafenone, sparteine	Tardive dyskinesia from antipsychotics; narcotic side effects, efficacy and dependence; imipramine dose requirement; beta blocker effects
CYP2E1	Acetaminophen, ethanol	Possible effect on alcohol consumption; possible increased cancer risk
CYP3A4/3A5/3A7	Macrolides, cyclosporine, tacrolimus, calcium channel blockers, midazolam, terfenadine, lidocaine, dapsone, quinidine, triazolam, etoposide, teniposide, lovastatin, alfentanil, tamoxifen, steroids, benzo(a)pyrene	Tacrolimus dose requirement in pediatric cardiac transplant patients
Aldehyde dehydrogenase	Cyclophosphamide, vinyl chloride	SCE frequency in lymphocytes
Alcohol dehydrogenase	Ethanol	Increased alcohol consumption and dependence
Dihydropyrimidine dehydrogenase (DPD)	5-fluorouracil	Increased 5-fluorouracil toxicity
NQO1 (DT-diaphorase)	Ubiquinones, menadione, mitomycin C	Menadione-associated urolithiasis; decreased tumor sensitivity to mitomycin C; possible increased cancer risk
Phase II Enzymes		
N-acetyltransferase (NAT1)	Aminosalicylic acid, aminobenzoic acid, sulfamethoxazole	Possible increased cancer risk
N-acetyltransferase (NAT2)	Isoniazid, hydralazine, sulfonamides, amonifide, procainamide, dapsone, caffeine	Hypersensitivity to sulfonamides; amonafide toxicity; hydralazine-induced lupus; isoniazid neurotoxicity and hepatitis
Glutathione transferase (GSTM1, M3, T1)	Busulfan, aminochrome, dopachrome, adrenochrome, noradrenochrome	Possible increased cancer risk; cisplatin induced ototoxicity
Glutathione transferase (GSTP1)	13-cis retinoic acid, busulfan, ethacrynic acid, epirubicin	Possible increased cancer risk
Sulfotransferases	Steroids, acetaminophen, tamoxifen estrogens, dopamine	Possible increased or decreased cancer risk; clinical outcome in women receiving tamoxifen for breast cancer
Catechol-O-methyltransferase	Estrogens, levodopa, ascorbic acid	Decreased response to amphetamine; substance abuse; levodopa response
Thiopurine methyltransferase	Mercaptopurine, thioguanine, azathioprine	Thiopurine toxicity and efficacy; risk of second cancers
UDP-glucuronosyl-transferase (UGT1A1)	Irinotecan, troglitazone, bilirubin	Irinotecan glucuronidation and toxicity
UDP-glucuronosyl-transferase (UGT2B)	Opiods, morphine, naproxen, ibuprofen, epirubicin	Significance unknown
Transport Proteins		
Bile salt export pump (BSEP)	Bile acid conjugates	Increased risk of intrahepatic cholestasis of pregnancy
Multidrug resistance gene 1 (MDR1)	Several anticancer agents, most CYP3A4 substrates, digoxin	Decreased p-glycoprotein expression and increased digoxin bioavailability
Organic anion transporter (OATP)	Pravastatin, benzylpenicillin	Decreased total and renal clearance of pravastatin
Organic cation transporter 1 (OCT1)	Serotonin, dopamine, creatinine, procainamide, desipramine, amantidine	Significance unknown
MDR-related proteins (MRP's)	Glutathione, glucuronide and sulfate conjugates, nucleoside antiviral agents	Significance unknown

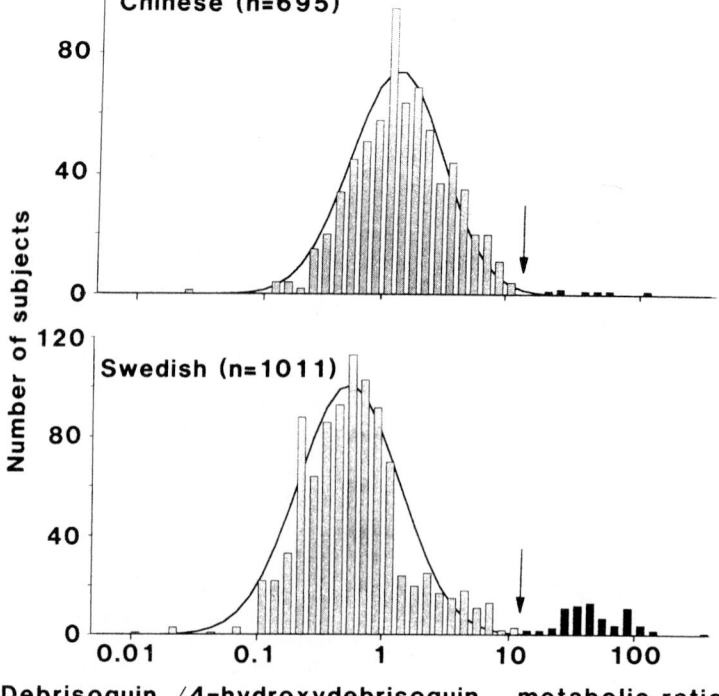

Figure 62-1. Frequency distribution of debrisoquin urinary metabolic ratios. Urinary metabolic ratios of debrisoquin to its metabolite, 4-hydroxydebrisoquin, are shown for 695 Chinese subjects and 1011 Swedish subjects. The arrows indicate the cutoff point between subjects with poor metabolism as a result of decreased or absent CYP2D6 activity and subjects with extensive metabolism. (From Bertilsson L, Lou YQ, Du YL, et al. *Clin Pharmacol Ther* 1992; 51:388.)

amino acid sequence of the encoded protein to single-nucleotide polymorphisms that altered RNA splicing or even deletions of the *CYP2D6* gene.[50] In addition, some subjects with very rapid CYP2D6-mediated metabolism have been shown to have multiple copies of the *CYP2D6* gene.[46] Such subjects may theoretically have an inadequate therapeutic response to standard doses of the drugs metabolized by CYP2D6. Although the occurrence of multiple copies of the *CYP2D6* gene is relatively infrequent among northern Europeans, in East African populations, the frequency can be as high as 29 percent.[51] In total, more than 75 *CYP2D6* alleles have now been described.

CYTOCHROME P4502C SUBFAMILY—In humans, the CYP2C subfamily of cytochrome P450's account for approximately 18% of the CYP content in the liver and catalyzes roughly 20% of the CYP-mediated metabolism of drugs.[52] Historically, the first polymorphism discovered in the CYP2C subfamily was a well-described deficiency in the ability to metabolize the anticonvulsant drug mephenytoin.[53] As in the case of CYP2D6, the inherited nature of the variability in metabolism was first identified phenotypically using a model substrate. Population studies performed in the 1980s using mephenytoin as the probe drug determined that individuals could be segregated into two phenotypic groups, extensive metabolizers (EMs) or poor metabolizers (PMs).[54] The PM trait is autosomal recessive, and is present in 3–5% of Caucasians and 12–23% of Asian populations.[55] Subsequent investigations determined that the inherited variability in the metabolism of mephenytoin was due to genetic variations in the gene coding for CYP2C19. In addition to mephenytoin, CYP2C19 catalyzes the metabolism of several proton pump inhibitors such as omeprazole,[56,57] diazepam,[58] thalidomide,[59] and some barbiturates.[60,61] Furthermore, CYP2C19 is partially responsible for the inactivation of propranolol,[62] as well as the metabolic activation of the antimalarial drug proquanil.[63] At least seven different inactivating mutations in *CYP2C19* have been described, including null mutations that prevent the expression of the protein, as well as single amino acid changes that effect the catalytic activity of the protein.[55]

CYP2C19 catalyzes the 5-hydroxylation of omeprazole, and the metabolism of omeprazole has been found to correlate closely with the metabolism of mephenytoin.[56] Following a single dose of omeprazole, the plasma area under the concentration time curve (AUC) is significantly higher in *CYP2C19* PMs than EMs. The significant increase AUC is because PM individuals have a 10-fold lower oral clearance of omeprazole. Furthermore, it has also been shown that *CYP2C19* genotype predicts the likelihood of cure of *H pylori* infection in peptic ulcer patients receiving omeprazole and amoxicillin. In one study, the cure rate was 100% in patients homozygous for the PM genotype, 60% in heterozygous PM/EM patients, and 29% in homozygous EM patients.[64] Patients with the homozygous PM genotype had markedly highly plasma omeprazole concentrations and higher gastric pH, leading to higher antibacterial activity of amoxicillin. Several other proton pump inhibitors are also metabolized by CYP2C19, and therefore, their activity may also be dependent on *CYP2C19* genotype.[65–67]

The anti-anxiolytic agent diazepam is demethylated by CYP2C19. Plasma diazepam half-lives are dramatically longer in individuals who are homozygous for the defective *CYP2C19*2* allele compared to those who are homozygous for the wildtype allele. Furthermore, the half-life of the desmethyldiazepam metabolite is also longer in the *CYP2C19* PMs.[68] Asian populations have been reported to have slower diazepam metabolism than Caucasians, which has been attributed to the high frequency of the *CYP2C19*2* allele in Asians.[58] As a result, diazepam induced toxicity may occur as a result of slower metabolism, and it has, therefore, been recommended that care be used when dosing diazepam in Asian individuals.

CYP2C9 is the major CYP2C subfamily member in the liver and is primarily responsible for the oxidative metabolism of many clinically important compounds, including warfarin,[69] phenytoin,[70] tolbutamide,[71] glipizide,[72] and losartan.[73] As with CYP2C19, multiple genetic variants of *CYP2C9* have been described. Six distinct polymorphisms, designated *CYP2C9*1, *2, *3, *4, *5,* and *6,* have been identified in the sequence for the CYP2C9 protein, with *CYP2C9*1* considered the wild type allele and the others as variants.[74] Because they were identified first, the *CYP2C9*2* and *3* alleles have undergone the most thorough *in vitro* and *in vivo* investigation of the known variants. In contrast, considerably less is known about the more recently identified *4, *5 and *6 alleles. The variant *2 and *3 alleles are found quite commonly in Caucasians (roughly 35%), however, they are significantly less prevalent in African-American and Asian populations.[74] In vitro data have consistently demonstrated that the CYP2C9*2 and *3 alleles are associated with reduced enzymatic oxidation of a variety of 2C9 substrates compared with CYP2C9*1.[75,76,77,78] In addition, multiple in vivo investigations and clinical case reports have associated genotypes expressing the CYP2C9*2 and *3 alleles with significant reductions in the metabolism and clearance of selected CYP2C9 substrates.[55]

Genetic polymorphisms in CYP2C9 have been linked to both toxicity and dosage requirements for optimal anticoagulation with warfarin.[79] Patients with CYP2C9 genetic variants *2 and *3 have a higher risk of acute bleeding complications than patients with a wild-type genotype,[80] and require 15–30% lower maintenance doses of warfarin to achieve the target INR.[79–81] Because warfarin dosing can be titrated to a clear effect endpoint (ie, INR), genotyping CYP2C9 is not widely used in clinical practice. However, the recent demonstration that patients with a variant CYP2C9 genotype take a median of 95 days longer to achieve stable dosing compared with the wild-type group, providing an important example of how genotype studies can reduce the time a patient is receiving inadequate warfarin therapy.[79] In addition, the inclusion of these CYP2C9 SNPs among a panel of several thousand genotypes determined in a single genetic test, as discussed below, may allow the utilization of CYP2C9 genotype to select the optimal starting dose of warfarin.

DIHYDROPYRIMIDINE DEHYDROGENASE—Another important example of the pharmacogenetics of phase I drug metabolism involves metabolism of the antineoplastic agent fluorouracil. In the mid-1980s, fatal central nervous system toxicity developed in several patients after treatment with standard doses of fluorouracil.[82,83] The patients were shown to have an inherited deficiency of dihydropyrimidine dehydrogenase (DPD), an enzyme that metabolizes fluorouracil and endogenous pyrimidines. While the exact frequency of DPD deficient patients is unknown, severe fluorouracil toxicity occurs in individuals with reduced DPD activity (below 100 pmol/min/mg protein). Several variant alleles for the gene encoding DPD have now been described that place patients at risk for toxic effects when they are exposed to standard doses of fluorouracil.[84] Approximately 3% of the general population are thought to carry heterozygous mutations that inactivate DPD, and 0.1% are homozygous for the inactivating mutations. Total DPD deficiency (ie, homozygous mutants) is associated with severe neurological disorders due to impaired endogenous pyrimidine metabolism.[85] However, individuals who are heterozygous for the inactivating mutation exhibit no phenotype until challenged with fluorouracil. Therefore, pharmacogenetics of DPD and its effect on the metabolism of fluorouracil serve as an excellent illustration of the importance of genetic variation in the context of drug therapy. Indeed, inherited variability in the response to drugs is most critical in the case of an agent with a narrow therapeutic index. Fluoruracil-induced toxicity can be life threatening in patients with severe DPD deficiency, and prospective determination of DPD genotype may be useful for identifying those individuals at high risk for unacceptable toxicity.

CYTOCHROME P4503A SUBFAMILY—The human CYP3A subfamily plays a critical role in the metabolism of more drugs than any other phase I enzyme.[86] CYP3A enzymes are expressed in the liver and small intestine and thus contributes to oral absorption, first-pass, and systemic metabolism.[87] Although CYP3A expression has been shown to vary by as much as 40-fold in the liver and small intestine,[88] CYP3A-dependent in vivo drug clearance appears to be normally distributed, suggesting that the wide inter-individual variability is the result of complex interaction between genes and environment. The expression of the CYP3A enzymes are highly inducible,[89] and therefore, the wide range in enzyme activity levels may be due to factors such as variable homeostatic

control mechanisms, up- or down-regulation by environmental factors (eg, alcohol, concomitant drugs, or diet), and genetic polymorphisms.

Unlike other human P450s (eg, CYP2D6) there is no evidence of a deleted or 'null' allele for CYP3A4. However, more than 30 SNPs have been identified in the CYP3A4 gene.[88] Generally, variants in the coding regions of CYP3A4 occur at allele frequencies of <5% and appear as heterozygous with the wild-type allele. These coding variants may contribute to, but are not likely to be the major cause, of inter-individual differences in CYP3A-dependent clearance. The most common variant in CYP3A4, CYP3A4*1B, is an A392G transition in the promoter region referred to as the nifedipine response element.[90] Although the results of one clinical study indicated that the CYP3A4*1B polymorphism may be associated with a slower oral clearance of cyclosporine,[91] the functional impact of the CYP3A4*1 polymorphism on CYP3A4-mediated drug metabolism remains controversial.[92] In contrast, there are several reports about its association with various disease states including prostate cancer,[93] secondary leukemias,[94] and early puberty.[95] Linkage disequilibrium between CYP3A4*1B and another CYP3A allele (CYP3A5*1) may be the true cause of the clinical phenotype.[96]

In contrast to CYP3A4, clinically relevant genetic variation in CYP3A5 has been demonstrated. CYP3A5 is polymorphically expressed in adults with detectable expression in about 10–20% in Caucasians, 33% in Japanese, and 55% in African Americans.[32] The primary cause for its variable expression is a mutation (CYP3A5*3) that confers low CYP3A5 expression as a result of improper mRNA splicing and reduced translation of a functional protein.[32] The CYP3A5*3 allele frequency varies from approximately 50% in African Americans to 90% in Caucasians. Functionally, microsomes from a homozygous CYP3A5*3/*3 liver contains very low CYP3A5 protein and displays reduced catalytic activity towards the model substrate midazolam.[97] Additional intronic or exonic mutations (CYP3A5*5, *6, and *7) also alter splicing and result in premature stop codons or exon deletions.[88] While several CYP3A5 coding variants have been described, they occur at relatively low allelic frequencies and their functional significance has not yet been established. Because CYP3A5 is the primary extrahepatic CYP3A isoform, its polymorphic expression has be implicated in disease risk and the metabolism of endogenous steroids or drug in tissues other than liver (eg, lung, kidney, prostate, breast, leukocytes). Furthermore, the presence of CYP3A5 genotype has been linked to tacrolimus dose requirements to maintain adequate immunosuppression in solid organ transplant patients.[98,99]

CYP3A7 is the form of CYP3A enzyme expressed in fetal liver during development. Although hepatic expression appears to be significantly down-regulated after birth, CYP3A7 protein and mRNA have been detected in some adults.[100] Recently, increased CYP3A7 mRNA expression has been associated with the replacement of a 60 nucleotide fragment of the CYP3A7 promoter with the corresponding region from the CYP3A4 promoter (CYP3A7*1C allele).[101] This promoter "swap" results in increased gene expression due to enhanced transcriptional activation through the transfer of the pregnane X receptor (PXR) response element. PXR signaling serves as a central regulator of inducible CYP3A expression, as well as several other genes involved in drug detoxification.[89] Polymorphisms have recently been identified in PXR,[102,103] suggesting that the observed variability in CYP3A enzymatic activity may, in part, be due to inherited differences in the upstream signaling proteins that control induction of gene expression.

The genetic basis for polymorphic expression of CYP3A5 and CYP3A7 has now been established. Substrate specificity and tissue distribution of these enzymes can differ from that of CYP3A4, such that the impact of variability in CYP3A5 and CYP3A7 expression on drug disposition will be both drug and tissue dependent. In addition to genetic variation, other factors that may affect CYP3A expression include tissue-specific splicing, variable control of gene transcription by endogenous molecules (circulating hormones) and exogenous molecules (diet or environment), and genetic variations in proteins that may regulate constitutive and inducible CYP3A expression (nuclear receptors). Thus, the complex regulatory pathways may confound evaluation of the effect of individual CYP3A genetic variations on drug disposition, efficacy and safety. However, because of the major contribution of the CYP3A subfamily to the metabolism of drugs, it is critically important that the genetic and epigenetic factors involved in the variability in this pathway be better understood.

Pharmacogenetics of Phase II Drug Metabolism

N-ACETYLTRANSFERASE—The *N*-acetylation of isoniazid represents one of the earliest examples of inherited variation in phase II drug metabolism. Wide inter-individual variability exists in the rates at which isoniazid acetylated.[34] The original population studies demonstrated that the rate of isoniazid acetylation is an inherited trait, with individuals being classified as either slow or rapid acetylators (Fig 62-2). The distribution of the acetylator phenotype shows a striking ethnic variation.[104] For example, the proportion of slow acetylators in the Japanese population is about 10%, in the Chinese population about 20%, and among Caucasians about 60%. Molecular cloning studies demonstrated that there are two N-acetyltransferase (*NAT*) genes in humans, *NAT1* and *NAT2*.[105] The NAT2 protein is the specific protein isoform that acetylates isoniazid. Seven missense (G191A, T341C, A434C, G590A, A803G, A845C, and G857A) and four silent (T111C, C282T, C481T, and C759T) substitutions have been identified thus far in the *NAT2* coding sequence.[106] To date, 27 unique *NAT2* alleles have been identified in humans, with *NAT2*4* considered the wildtype allele since it does not contain any of the known substitutions. However, *NAT2*4* is not the most common allele in many ethnic groups, including Caucasians and Africans. *NAT2* alleles containing the G191A, T341C, A434C, G590A, and/or G857A missense substitutions are associated with slow acetylator phenotype, while the other known nucleotide changes do not appear to affect enzyme activity.[107] Laboratory investigations

on the recombinant proteins demonstrate that multiple mechanisms exist for the reduction in enzyme activity, including altered catalytic activity, decreased protein expression, and protein instability.[108,109] Striking ethnic differences exist in the frequencies of these missense substitutions in various ethnic populations, and these differences correspond to ethnic differences in frequency of the slow acetylator phenotype.

Isoniazid is metabolized to acetylisoniazid via NAT2.[107] Acetylisoniazid undergoes further chemical hydrolysis to acetylhydrazine, which is then metabolized by CYP2E1 to a hepatotoxic intermediate. Importantly, the hydrolysis product acetylhydrazine is also acetylated by NAT2 to form a non-toxic metabolite. Acute or chronic hepatitis is a commonly encountered toxicity in patients receiving isoniazid-containing regimens for tuberculosis, with a reported incidence as high as 36%.[38] Several studies have investigated the relationship between acetylator status and the risk of hepatitis.[110–112] While the earliest of these studies suggested that rapid acetylators might have an increased risk of drug-induced hepatitis, several more recent studies concluded that slow acetylators have a greater susceptibility to developing hepatotoxicity. Most of the studies conducted to date have used phenotyping to determine acetylator status, however, at least one recent study using genotyping confirmed the association between slow acetylator status and increased risk of hepatitis.[113] Because of this important genotype/phenotype relationship, it has been recommended that patients determined to be slow acetylators be monitored more regularly during therapy for signs of overt hepatotoxicity.

The anticancer agent amonafide represents an example of how one might use pharmacogenetic information to guide the drug development process.[114] Amonafide is a DNA intercalating agent and topoisomerase II inhibitor that is extensively metabolized to active and inactive metabolites. Acetylation of amonafide by NAT2 results in a metabolite of similar potency compared to the parent drug.[115] During the initial clinical trials, it was determined that the pharmacokinetics of amonafide was highly variable. Because of the importance of NAT2 to the disposition of amonafide, these early investigations also included phenotyping for acetylator status. It was demonstrated that the production of the acetylated metabolite was a major determinant of myelosuppression, since fast acetylators had significantly greater toxicity than slow acetylators.[116] Interestingly, the area under the plasma concentration-time curve of amonafide was significantly greater in the fast acetylators, who would have been expected to have a higher clearance and a lower area under the plasma concentration-time curve. This appeared to be an unusual finding compared with other drugs metabolized by *N*-acetylation. For most drugs, slow acetylators are at greater risk of adverse reactions. This unexpected finding was shown to be due to inhibition of parent amonafide oxidation by *N*-acetylamonafide.[116] Once the relationship between acetylator status and myelosuppression was identified, subsequent studies prospectively dosed amonafide based on each individual's acetylator status.[117] Although the clinical development of amonafide was later abandoned due to a lack of anti-tumor activity and unacceptable toxicity, it still serves as an example of how clinical decisions regarding drug therapy may ultimately be guided by genetic considerations.

In addition to their role in the metabolism of clinically administered drugs, phase I and II metabolizing enzymes are thought to play an important role in host defense against environmental toxins. Several well known environmental carcinogens, such as aromatic amines and heterocyclic amines, are present in cigarette smoke and cooked meats.[118] Aromatic and heterocyclic amines have been shown to induce tumors in multiple experimental models. Following *N*-oxidation, *N*-hydroxy-aromatic and *N*-hydroxy-heterocyclic amines are further activated by the *N*-acetyltransferases to unstable acetoxy intermediates, which react spontaneously with DNA to form carcinogenic DNA adducts.[119] Thus, it has been hypothesized that *NAT1* and *NAT2* genotype may be related to an individual's

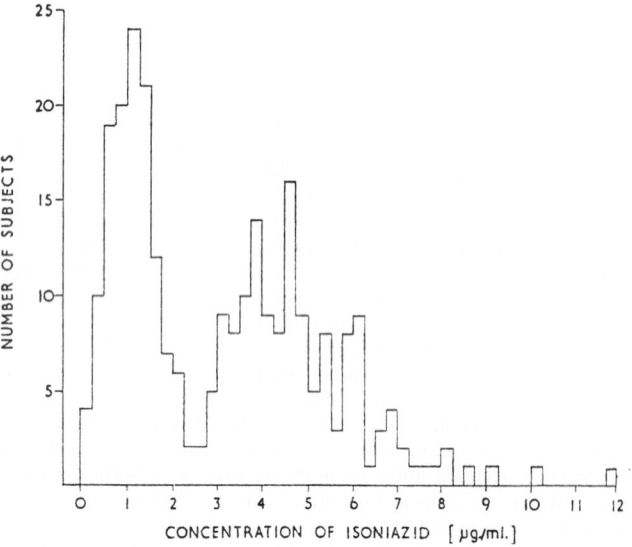

Figure 62-2. Frequency distribution of isoniazid acetylation. Plasma isoniazid concentrations were measured in 267 subjects 6 hours after an oral dose. The bimodal distribution in the rate of acetylation is due to genetic polymorphism within the *N*-acetyltransferase 2 gene. (From Price Evans DA, Manley KA, McKusick VA *BMJ* 1960; 2:485.)

risk of environmentally induced cancers. While several epidemiological studies suggest that *NAT1* and *NAT2* genotype may contribute to ones predisposition to cancers,[120–123] there is a great deal of inconsistency in the published results. These inconsistencies are likely due to the difficulty one has in controlling for all of the possible contributory aspects of an epidemiologic study. Factors such as population differences in carcinogen exposures, genotyping and/or phenotyping methods, insufficient sample sizes, and the confounding effects of other susceptibility genes and factors all lead to noise in the final conclusions. Associations between slow *NAT2* acetylator genotypes and bladder cancer and between rapid *NAT2* acetylator genotypes and colorectal cancer are the most consistently reported associations.[119] Although individual risks associated with *NAT1* and/or *NAT2* genotypes are generally small, they increase when combined with measures of aromatic and heterocyclic amine carcinogen exposures. Ethnic differences in *NAT1* and *NAT2* genotype frequencies may be a factor in observed differences in cancer incidence. Large-scale molecular epidemiological studies that investigate the role of *NAT1* and *NAT2* genotypes together with other genetic susceptibility gene polymorphisms and biomarkers of carcinogen exposure are critical to improve our understanding of the role of the *NAT1* and *NAT2* acetylation polymorphisms in cancer risk.

THIOPURINE METHYLTRANSFERASE—One of the most mature examples of applied clinical pharmacogenomics involves the genetic polymorphism of thiopurine methyltransferase (TPMT). TPMT catalyzes the S-methylation of the thiopurine agents azathioprine, mercaptopurine, and thioguanine.[124] These agents are used for a wide range of indications, including childhood leukemia, rheumatoid arthritis, inflammatory bowel disease, dermatologic disorders, and solid organ transplantation. The cytotoxic mechanism of these agents is mediated via the incorporation of thioguanine nucleotides (TGN) into DNA. Thiopurines are themselves inactive prodrugs that require activation to TGN to exert cytotoxicity.[125] Metabolic activation is a complex process catalyzed by multiple enzymes, the first of which is hypoxanthine phosphoribosyl transferase. Alternatively, these agents can be inactivated via oxidation by xanthine oxidase or methylation by TPMT. In bone marrow, TPMT is the only inactivation pathway for the thiopurines. Furthermore, TPMT activity is highly variable and polymorphic, such that approximately 90% of individuals have high enzyme activity, 10% have intermediate activity, and 0.3% have low or no detectable activity.[126,127] Family studies have shown that TPMT activity is inherited as an autosomal codominant trait. As a result, patients who inherit TPMT deficiency accumulate excessive cellular concentrations of TGN, predisposing them to potentially fatal hematological toxicity.[128]

The molecular basis for polymorphic TPMT activity has been determined for the majority of individuals with this observed deficiency.[129] At least 8 TPMT variant alleles have been identified, with 3 of the alleles (*TPMT*2, *TPMT*3A, *TPMT*3C) accounting for about 95% of patients with intermediate or low enzyme activity. The mutant allele *TPMT*2 is defined by a single nucleotide transversion (G238C) in the coding sequence, leading to an amino acid substitution at codon 18 (Ala>Pro).[130] *TPMT*3A contains two nucleotide transition mutations (G460A and A719G), leading to amino acid substitutions at codon 154 (Ala>Thr) and codon 240 (Tyr>Cys),[131] whereas *TPMT*3C contains only the A719G transition mutation.[131,132] All three alleles are associated with lower enzyme activity, owing to decreased protein stability and enhanced rates of protein degradation.[23]

Phenotypic deficiency in TPMT activity is a fairly rare event. Furthermore, studies in Caucasian, African, and Asian populations have revealed that the frequency of these mutant *TPMT* alleles differs among various ethnic populations. In Caucasians, *TPMT*3A is the most common mutant *TPMT* allele (3.2–5.7% of *TPMT* alleles), whereas *TPMT*3C has an allele frequency of 0.2–0.8% and *TPMT*2 represents 0.2–0.5% of *TPMT* alleles.[24,125] East and West African populations have a frequency of mutant alleles similar to that of Caucasians, but all mutant alleles in the African populations are *TPMT*3C.[133] Among African Americans, *TPMT*3C is the most prevalent allele, but *TPMT*2 and *TPMT*3A are also found, reflecting the integration of Caucasian and African-American genes in the US population.[134] In Asian populations, *TPMT*3C is the predominant mutant allele.

The presence of *TPMT*2, *TPMT*3A, or *TPMT*3C is predictive of phenotype. In other words, patients who are heterozygous for these alleles have intermediate activity, and subjects homozygous for these alleles are TPMT deficient.[24,134] In addition, compound heterozygotes (*TPMT*2/3A, *TPMT*3A/3C) are also TPMT deficient, as would be expected.[24] Whereas most studies have used erythrocytes as a surrogate tissue for measuring TPMT activity, studies have also shown that TPMT genotype determines TPMT activity in leukemia cells,[127,135] as would be expected for germline mutations. Therefore, the enthusiasm for TPMT pharmacogenetics has been stimulated by the finding that TPMT genotype identifies patients who are at risk of toxicity from mercaptopurine or azathioprine. Numerous studies have shown that TPMT-deficient patients are at very high risk of developing severe hematopoietic toxicity when treated with conventional doses of thiopurines,[136,137] while others have shown that patients who are heterozygous at the TPMT gene locus are at intermediate risk of dose-limiting toxicity.[138–140] In a study of 67 patients treated with azathioprine for rheumatic disease, six patients (9%) were heterozygous for mutant TPMT alleles,[138] and therapy was discontinued in five of the six patients because of low white blood cell counts within one month of starting treatment. In contrast, patients with wild-type TPMT received therapy for a median of 39 weeks without complications compared with a median of 2 weeks in patients heterozygous for mutant TPMT alleles.[138] A second study in Japanese patients with rheumatic disease receiving azathioprine recently confirmed the importance of a heterozygous TPMT genotype for predicting toxicity.[140] Furthermore, TPMT-deficient patients with acute lymphoblastic leukemia were able to tolerate full doses of mercaptopurine for only 7% of scheduled weeks of therapy, whereas heterozygous and homozygous wild-type leukemia patients tolerated full doses for 65% and 84% of scheduled weeks of therapy, respectively.[139] Collectively, these studies demonstrate that the influence of TPMT genotype on hematopoietic toxicity is most dramatic for homozygous mutant patients, but is also of clinical relevance for heterozygous individuals, who represent about 10% of patients treated with these medications. TPMT deficiency has also been linked to a higher risk of second malignancies among patients with acute lymphoblastic leukemia, including topoisomerase-inhibitor-induced acute myeloid leukemia[141,142] and radiation-induced brain tumors.[143] Therefore, knowledge of a patient's genotypic TPMT status permits patient-specific dosages that reduce the risk of acute toxicity from thiopurine medications and may identify those at higher risk of second malignancies.

URIDINE DIPHOSPHATE-GLUCURONOSYLTRANSFERASES—Uridine diphosphate-glucuronosyltransferases (UGTs) are microsomal phase II enzymes that catalyze the glucuronidation of numerous endogenous and exogenous substrates.[144] Human UGTs are further classified into UGT1 and UGT2 families.[145] The UGT1 gene consists of at least 13 unique forms with a variable exon 1 and common exons 2 to 5. As a result, the UGT1 subfamily is further classified into multiple isoforms, ie, UGT1A1, UGT1A3, UGT1A4, up to UGT1A12. The UGT1A1 isoform is responsible for the conjugation of bilirubin,[146] along with the glucuronidation of irinotecan and troglitazone.[147] Clinically relevant polymorphisms in UGT1A1 are associated with familial hyperbilirubinemic syndromes such as Crigler-Najjar syndromes type I (CN-I) and type II (CN-II), and Gilbert's syndrome. CN-I syndrome is a rare disorder associated with severe unconjugated hyperbilirubinemia.[148] Patients with CN-I syndrome have absent or reduced UGT1A1 activity with correspondingly high serum levels of unconjugated bilirubin.[149,150] Gilbert's syndrome is a more mild form of chronic unconjugated hyperbilirubinemia, with serum bilirubin levels usually <3 mg/dl, although higher levels are sometimes seen.[150] A wide ethnic variation in the incidence of Gilbert's syndrome has been reported, ranging from 0.5 to 19% in various groups.[151,152,153] Gilbert's syndrome is typically associated with a polymorphism in the regulatory region of the UGT1A1 promoter. A variant (TA)$_7$TAA sequence in the UGT1A1 promoter, instead of wildtype (TA)$_6$TAA, results in reduced UGT1A1 expression levels and lower enzymatic activity.[154,152] In addition the (TA)$_7$ alleles, three other alleles with five, six, or eight TA repeats [(TA)$_5$, (TA)$_6$, and (TA)$_8$] have been identified.[155] The (TA)$_5$ and (TA)$_8$ alleles are primarily present in African populations, and occur at much lower frequencies than the (TA)$_6$ and (TA)$_7$ alleles.

UGT1A1 plays several roles in the metabolic inactivation of the anticancer drug irinotecan. Irinotecan (CPT-11) is a camptothecin derivative used in the treatment of metastatic colorectal cancer. Irinotecan is a prodrug, since it requires activation by carboxylesterases to SN-38 (7-ethyl-10-hydroxycamptothecin) in order to exert its antitumor activity mediated by the inhibition of topoisomerase I. SN-38 is in turn glucuronidated to form the inactive SN-38 glucuronide (SN-38G).[156] SN-38 is associated with severe episodes of diarrhea occurring shortly after irinotecan therapy.[157] Because of its extensive biliary excretion,[158] SN-38 is secreted directly into the lumen of gastrointestinal tract, resulting in high local tissue exposures to this very toxic compound. Glucuronidation of SN-38 to the inactive SN-38G via UGT1A1 protects against irinotecan-induced intestinal toxicities due to increased conversion to the inactive SN-38G and increased renal elimination of the more polar conjugated form.[159] Patients with the (TA)$_7$ polymorphism have significantly lower rates of SN-38 glucuronidation rates than those with the wildtype allele. In addition, more severe diarrhea is seen in patients who are either heterozygous or homozygous for the (TA)$_7$ sequence.[160] The association between UGT1A1 genotype and risk of irinotecan-induced diarrhea might be exploited in the future in order to prospectively identify those individuals with a greater susceptibility to chemotherapy induced gastrointestinal toxicity.

Pharmacogenetics of Drug Transporters

Although passive diffusion accounts for some drug and metabolite distribution, increased emphasis is being placed on understanding the role of membrane transporters in absorption of oral medications across the gastrointestinal tract, excretion into the bile and urine, distribution of drug into "therapeutic sanctuaries," such as the brain and testes, and transport into sites of action, such as cardiovascular tissue, tumor cells, and infectious microorganisms. The most widely studied class of membrane transporters belong to the adenosine triphosphate (ATP)-binding-cassette (ABC) family of membrane transporters, which share many physicochemical characteristics. ABC family members include P-glycoprotein, MRP1-6 (multidrug resistance proteins), OCT (organic cation transporter), OAT (organic anion transporter), and SPGP (sister of Pgp). While it has been established that Pgp is not an essential protein for life, since genetically engineered mice lacking the protein appear normal until they are challenged with toxic compound, Pgp function is critical to the cellular and systemic clearance of many commonly used pharmacologic agents. Moreover, other members of the ABC family play critical physiologic roles in transport of endogenous substances, such as bilirubin and glutathione conjugates, as well as some medications. Although polymorphisms in ABC family members have been have been reported,[161] and such genetic variation may have functional significance for drug absorption and elimination, the full clinical relevance of polymorphisms in drug transporters has yet to be fully elucidated.

ABCB1 (MDR1)—Transport proteins play an important role in regulating the absorption, distribution and excretion of many medications. The many members of the ABC family of transporters are among the most extensively studied proteins involved in drug disposition and effect.[162] Among these, Pgp is the 170 kd transmembrane protein encoded by the human *ABCB1* gene (also named *MDR1*). The principal function of Pgp is the energy-dependent cellular efflux of a wide variety of substrates, including bilirubin, several anti-cancer drugs, cardiac glycosides, immunosuppressive agents, glucocorticoids, HIV-1 protease inhibitors, and many other medications.[161–163] As a result of the striking overlap in substrate specificity between Pgp and CYP3A4, it is believed that this transporter plays a role in the bioavailability and/or biliary excretion of more drugs than any other. The relatively high expression of Pgp in normal tissues involved in drug uptake and elimination suggests that it plays a vital role in excreting xenobiotics and metabolites into urine, bile, and the intestinal lumen.[164] Furthermore, Pgp in the blood-brain barrier has been shown to limit CNS accumulation of many drugs, including digoxin, ivermectin, vinblastine, dexamethasone, cyclosporine A, domperidone, and loperamide.[165,166]

Pgp expression is highly variable among individuals, the molecular basis of which is still being explored. Among the many possible explanations for this observed variability in Pgp expression and function may be inherited differences in the *ABCB1* gene. Figure 62-3 graphically depicts the functional consequences of polymorphisms in *ABCB1*. A synonymous SNP (ie, a SNP that does not change the amino acid encoded) in exon 26 (3435C>T) has been identified, and despite the fact that the 3435C>T polymorphism does not result in an amino acid substitution, the variant has been associated with decreased duodenal Pgp expression. Patients who are homozygous for the variant allele had more than two-fold lower duodenal Pgp levels compared to patients with the homozygous wildtype genotype.[167] Furthermore, laboratory studies have demonstrated that the rate of in vitro efflux of the Pgp substrate rhodamine in CD56+ natural killer cells is significantly higher in subjects homozygous for wildtype 3435C compared to those homozygous for the 3435T variant.[168] A clinical pharmacokinetic study of digoxin, a known Pgp substrate, also demonstrated significantly higher oral bioavailability in subjects with the 3435TT genotype (Fig 62-3A), consistent with the hypothesis that lower duodenal Pgp expression results in increased oral drug absorption.[169] However, results of other pharmacokinetic studies have shown that the 3435TT genotype is associated with lower plasma concentrations of fexofenadine[170] (Fig 62-3B) and nelfinavir[171] (Fig 62-3C), contradicting the hypothesis that this polymorphism results in increased oral bioavailability.

To further confuse the issue of the functional importance of the 3435C>T polymorphism, it has also been shown that the recovery of CD4 count in HIV infected patients receiving protease inhibitors was significantly greater and more rapid in patients with the wildtype TT genotype than in patients with either CT or CC genotypes[171] (Fig 62-3D), despite lower plasma levels of the protease inhibitors. It is not mechanistically clear how greater efficacy (CD4 recovery) could be linked to a polymorphism associated with lower plasma drug concentrations.

Recently, a second, non-synonymous polymorphism (ie, a SNP causing an amino acid change) was identified in exon 21 (2677G>T) of ABCB1. The 2677T variant allele, resulting in a alanine to serine amino acid substitution, has been associated with increased Pgp function *in vitro* and lower plasma fexofenadine plasma concentrations[170] (Fig 62-3E). Interestingly, the 3435T allele has been shown to be in incomplete linkage disequilibrium with the 2677T allele. In other words, individual who inherit the 3435T allele have a reasonable probability of also inheriting the 2677T allele, with their potentially opposite effects on drug transport. Recently, results from renal transplant patients receiving the immunosuppressive agent tacrolimus, demonstrated that the dose required to achieve

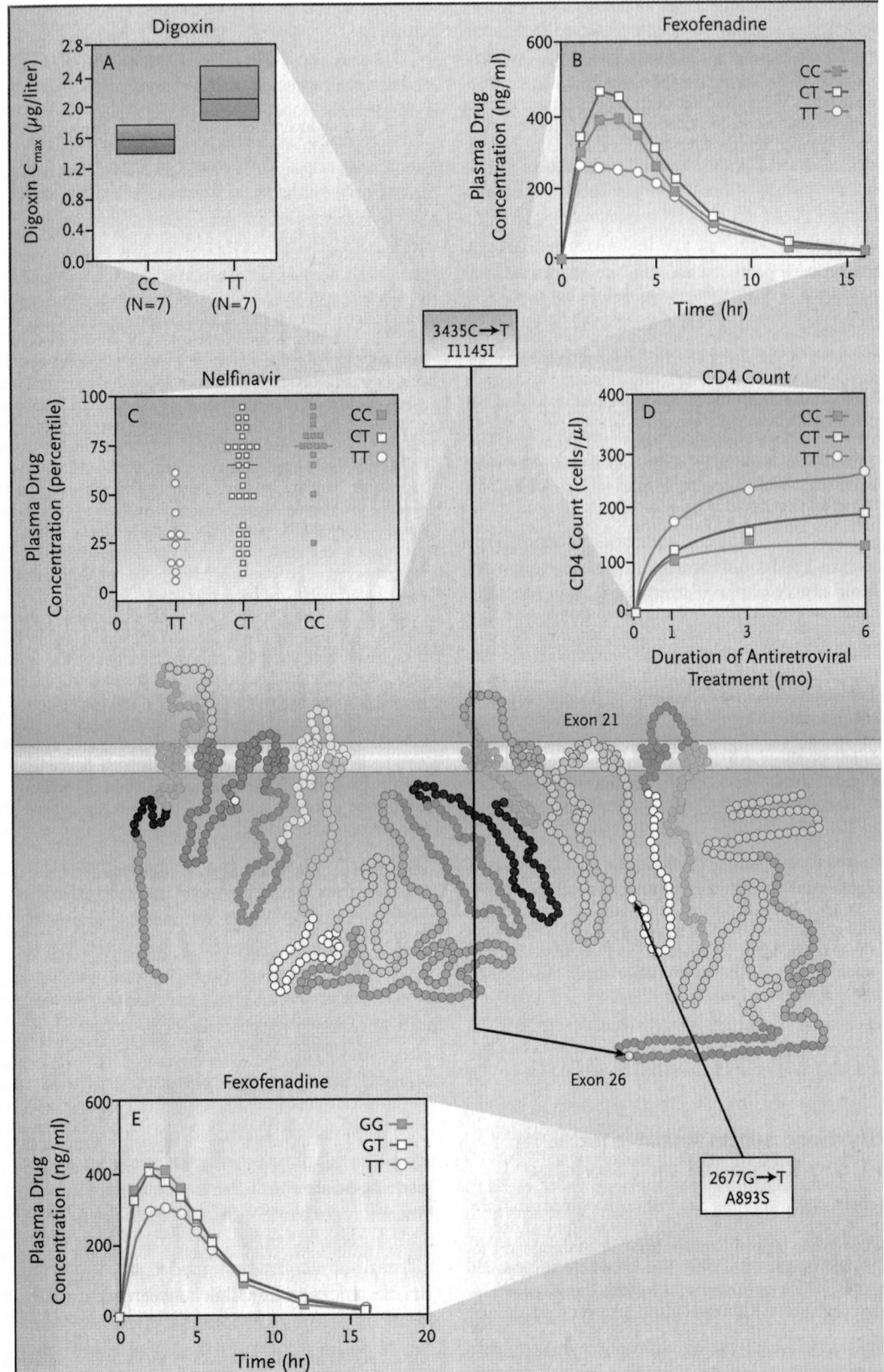

Figure 62-3. Functional consequences of genetic polymorphisms in the human p-glycoprotein transporter gene (*MDR1* or *ABCB1*). The schematic of the human P-glycoprotein was adapted from Kim RB, Leake BF, Choo EF, et al. *Clin Pharmacol Ther* 2001; 70:189, with each circle representing an amino acid and each color a different exon encoding the corresponding amino acids. Two SNPs in the human *ABCB1* gene have been associated with altered drug disposition (Panels A,B,C,E) or altered drug effects (Panel D) in humans. The synonymous SNP in exon 26 (nucleotide 3435 C>T SNP), has been associated with higher digoxin oral bioavailability in patients homozygous for the T nucleotide[167] (Panel A), but lower plasma concentrations after oral does of fexofenadine[170] (Panel B) and nelfinavir[171] (Panel C). This SNP has also been linked to better CD4 cell recovery in HIV infected patients treated with nelfinavir and other antiretroviral agents (Panel D).[171] The SNP at nucleotide 2766 (G>T) has been associated with lower fexofenadine plasma concentrations in patients homozygous for the T nucleotide at position 2766(Panel E).[170] Panels A-E have been adapted from the original reports of Kim RB, Leake BF, Choo EF, et al. *Clin Pharmacol Ther* 2001; 70: 189; Hoffmeyer S, Burk O, von Richter O, et al. *Proc Natl Acad Sci U S A* 2000; 97: 3473. and Fellay J, Marzolini C, Meaden ER, et al. *Lancet* 2002; 359: 30. (From Evans WE, McLeod HL. *N Engl J Med* 2003; 348:538.) See Color Plate 23.

optimal immunosuppression was correlated with *ABCB1* genotype.[99] In patients one month after tacrolimus introduction, dose requirements were 40% higher in 2677T homozygotes than wild-type patients, consistent with the finding that the 2677T variant results in increased Pgp activity. Similar results have been seen in pediatric cardiac transplant patients.[98] The results of haplotype analyses suggest that both the 2677T and 3435T polymorphisms might be associated with tacrolimus dose requirements. The potential co-segregation of polymorphisms with opposite effects on protein function may explain the conflicting results reported when the investigators look only at the contribution of one genetic variant and not both. The pharmacogenomics of *ABCB1*, therefore, serves a good example of the importance of considering multiple polymorphisms within the same gene (or haplotype) when evaluating the relationship between genotype and phenotype.

ORGANIC ION TRANSPORTERS—Organic anion transporter polypeptides (OATPs) and organic cation transporters (OCTs) are two major classes of secretory transporters expressed differentially in the kidney, liver, blood-brain barrier, lung, heart, intestine, placenta, and testis.[172] OATPs are mainly important for the hepatic uptake of large organic anions, organic cations and uncharged substrates,[173] whereas OCTs mediate uptake of predominantly small organic cations and anions in liver and kidney.[174] The many different members of the OATP family have partially overlapping and partially distinct substrate preferences for organic solutes such as bile salts, steroid conjugates, thyroid hormones, anionic oligopeptides, drugs, and toxins.[172] Although significant progress has been made in the characterization of these important classes of transporters at the molecular level, there is still much to learn about the functional and clinical importance of genetic variations in these secretory pathways. However, several non-synonymous variants in the OATP-C gene have recently been identified, and individuals with certain commonly occurring polymorphisms have a reduced clearance of the cholesterol-lowering agent pravastatin.[175–177] While the example of pravastatin represents the first report of a genotype/phenotype association within the organic anion transporter family, this highlights the potential for other important associations between genetic variants of transporters and clinical outcome. In addition, the paucity of published data regarding the pharmacogenomics of drug transporters underscores how little is currently known about many of the most important pathways of drug elimination and distribution.

GENETIC POLYMORPHISMS IN DRUG TARGETS

Genetic Polymorphisms Associated with Effects on Drug Response and Toxicity

There has recently been growing interest in determining genetic variations in drug targets, with the overall goal of defining their impact on drug efficacy and/or toxicity. A drug target, in this context, is defined as either the direct protein target of a drug (eg, a receptor or enzyme), proteins involved in a pharmacologic response (eg, signal transduction proteins or downstream proteins), or proteins associated with disease risk or pathogenesis that is somehow altered by the drug. The major objective of drug target pharmacogenomics research is to identify the inherited basis for interindividual variability in drug response and toxicity, particularly when the variability is not explained by differences in pharmacokinetics. Although studies of the pharmacogenetics of drug metabolism date back to the 1950s, the literature on drug target pharmacogenetics essentially began in the mid to late 1990s. In addition, the field of pharmacogenetics is moving from a monogenic (single gene or pharmacogenetic) to a polygenic (multiple genes or pharmacogenomic) approach, largely because of the acknowledgement that most drug effects are due to the complex interaction be-

tween several genes involved in both pharmacokinetics and cellular drug response. Furthermore, this shift towards a polygenic focus has been greatly facilitated by the recent development of new molecular tools for high throughput genotyping.

Most of the early pharmacogenetic studies of therapeutic drug targets focused on a single polymorphism within a single gene, with the gene of interest being the direct target of the drug. Although single polymorphism drug target studies have identified numerous associations between polymorphisms and the anticipated alteration in drug response, such studies have also been somewhat disappointing with respect to the lack of consistency of the findings. For example, the insertion/deletion polymorphism of the angiotensin converting enzyme (ACE) gene is one of the most extensively studied of all the drug target polymorphisms.[3] The homozygous deletion (DD) genotype has been associated with increased ACE activity and heterozygous ACE genotypes have been associated with various clinical effects of ACE inhibitors, including renoprotective effects,[178] blood pressure reduction,[179] left ventricular hypertrophy reduction,[180,181] and improvements in endothelial function.[182] However, the results of studies are not always in agreement since some investigators have found no association between response and ACE genotype,[180] some have shown that the homozygous insertion (II) genotype is associated with better drug response,[183,184] and others have shown that the DD genotype is associated with the best response.[181–185]

Drug target genes for which clinically relevant polymorphisms have been identified are listed in Table 62-2. The table includes examples of polymorphisms that have associated with both altered therapeutic drug response and risk of drug-induced toxicity. In addition to examples of polymorphisms in genes that encode for proteins that are direct targets of a drug (eg, β_2-adrenergic receptor), there are several examples where the genetic variant has an indirect effect on drug response (eg, apolipoprotein E). In other words, the polymorphism occurs in a gene that encodes a protein that is not a direct drug target for the therapeutic response nor involved in drug clearance or disposition. However, the genetic variation still results in altered response to drug treatment. Unlike many of the gene-therapeutic drug response associations, gene-drug toxicity relationships tend to be more robust across studies. In this case, when a drug known to cause a certain adverse event is given to an individual with a particular genetic polymorphism that has been associated with the adverse event, the result is a marked increase in the degree or risk of toxicity. For example, the use of oral contraceptive in patients with Factor V or prothrombin mutations leads to a significantly higher risk of a thrombotic event than in patients with the mutation alone or with oral contraceptive use alone.[186] Similarly, gene mutations in cardiac potassium and sodium channels that are associated with long QT syndrome are also associated with increased risk of clarithromycin-induced Torsade de Pointes.[187] The relative predictability of the relationship between a given polymorphism and drug-induced toxicity represents a useful therapeutic paradigm. Indeed, the clinical utility of pharmacogenomics of drug targets may emerge most rapidly as a valuable molecular diagnostic tool to identify those individuals who are most at risk for an adverse drug effect. The potential importance of direct target polymorphisms is illustrated below by the β_2-adrenergic receptor, while the apolipoprotein E gene represents an example of how polymorphisms can result in indirect effects on drug response. Finally, the relatively recent discovery of a genetic variation in thymidylate synthase is discussed as an example of how pharmacogenomics may ultimately be used to optimize drug therapy.

β_2-ADRENERGIC RECEPTOR—The β_2-adrenergic receptor is a G protein–coupled receptor that interacts with endogenous catecholamines and various medications. These receptors are widely distributed and play an important role in regulating cardiac, vascular, pulmonary, and metabolic functions.[188] Studies of the many physiologic functions of the β_2-adrenergic receptor in humans have revealed substantial interpatient variation in receptor function and responsiveness to stimulation. In the heart, activation of β_2-adrenergic receptor

Table 62-2. Genetic Polymorphisms in Genes that Can Influence Drug Response and Toxicity

GENE/PROTEIN	DRUG	CONSEQUENCE OF POLYMORPHISM
ACE	ACE inhibitors (eg, enalapril)	Renoprotective effects; blood pressure reduction; left ventricular mass reduction; endothelial function improvement; ACE inhibitor induced cough
Bradykinin B2 receptor	ACE inhibitors	ACE inhibitor induced cough
β₂-adrenergic receptor	β₂-agonists (eg, albuterol)	Bronchodilation; susceptibility to agonist-induced desensitization; cardiovascular effects (eg, increased heart rate, peripheral vasodilation)
Gs protein α	β-blockers (eg, propranolol)	Antihypertensive effect
ACE	Fluvastatin	Lipid changes (decreased LDL and apoliprotein B); progression/regression of atherosclerotic lesions
Platelet FC receptor (FCRII)	Heparin	Heparin induced thrombocytopenia
Glycoprotein IIIa subunit of glycoprotein IIb/IIIa receptor	Aspirin/glycoprotein IIb/IIIa inhibitors (eg, abciximab)	Antiplatelet effect
ALOX5	Leukotriene biosynthesis inhibitors (eg, ABT-761- zileuton-derivative)	Improvement in FEV₁
Estrogen receptor	Conjugated estrogens	Bone mineral density increases
Sufonylurea receptor	Sulfonylureas (eg, tolbutamide)	Sulfonylurea-induced insulin release
Inositol-p1p	Lithium	Response of manic depression
Dopamine receptors (D2, D3, D4)	Antipsychotics (eg, haloperidol, clozapine, thioridazine)	Antipsychotic response (D2, D3, D4); antipsychotic-induced tardive dyskinesia and acute akathisia (D3); (D3); hyperprolactinemia (D2)
Dopamine receptor	Levodopa and dopamine	Drug induced hallucinations
5HT2A, 5HT6	Antipsychotics (eg, clozapine)	Clozapine response; typical antipsychotic response and long term outcomes
G protein β3	Antidepressants (various)	Response to antidepressant therapy
Seratonin transporter (5-HTT)	Antidepressants (eg, clomipramine, fluoxetine, paroxetine, fluvoxamine)	5-HT neurotransmission antidepressant response
Ryanodine receptor	Anesthetics (eg, halothane)	Malignant hyperthermia
Thymidylate synthase	5-fluorouracil	Response to 5-fluorouracil based therapy
Ion channels (HERG, KvLQT1, Mink, MiRP1)	Erythromycin, terfenadine, cisapride, clarithromycin, quinidine	Increased risk of drug-induced Torsade de pointes
Methylguanine methyltransferase	Carmustine	Response of glioma to carmustine methyltransferase
Cholesterol ester transfer protein (CETP)	Statins	Slowing of progression of atherosclerosis by pravastatin
HLA-B*5701	Abacavir	Hypersensitivity reaction

results in an increased rate and force of cardiac muscle, whereas β₂-adrenergic receptor stimulation in the lungs acts to relax airway smooth muscle. Influences on lipolysis in subcutaneous fat have also been described, possibly through regulation of lipid mobilization, energy expenditure, and glycogen breakdown. Several polymorphisms in the β₂-adrenergic receptor have been identified, and their effects on β₂-agonist mediated response have been the focus of multiple investigations.

Understanding the molecular basis for variability in the β₂-adrenergic receptor has been facilitated by the identification of five distinct single nucleotide polymorphisms, each associated with either altered expression, down regulation, or coupling of the receptor.[188] Alteration at amino acid 16 (Arg>Gly) appears to have relevance in pulmonary disease, with patients homozygous for Arg exhibiting a greater response to β₂-agonist medications.[189,190] For example, the FEV₁ response to oral albuterol is 6.5-fold higher in patients with an Arg/Arg genotype at amino acid 16 compared with Gly/Gly patients, even though similar plasma drug concentrations are achieved.[189] In contrast, the alteration at codon 27 (Gln>Glu) does not appear to influence lung function, but there is an association between the Gln/Gln genotype and an increased incidence of obesity.[191,192] This relationship appears to be more prominent in men and can be overcome with exercise.[191]

While the β₂-adrenergic receptor alleles for amino acid 16 (frequency 0.61) and 27 (frequency 0.43) are relatively common and have been investigated thoroughly for their clinical relevance, a third much less common allele has been studied for in vivo function. A variation at amino acid 164 (Thr>Ile) with an allele frequency of 0.05 has been associated with probability of survival in patients with congestive heart failure.[193] Patients with congestive heart failure and the Thr/Ile genotype have a

significantly poorer one-year survival rate compared to those with Thr/Thr (42 vs. 76%). Moreover, patients with the Thr/Ile genotype show blunted cardiac beta(2)-AR responsiveness, which may help explain the decreased survival of patients with this genotype in the setting of congestive heart failure.[194] The potential clinical importance of the Thr>Ile variant has led to the suggestion that patients with the Ile164 polymorphism and heart failure should be considered as candidates for early aggressive intervention or cardiac transplantation.

Although the three genetic variants discussed represent the most widely studied β₂-adrenergic receptor polymorphisms, at least 13 distinct variant alleles have been identified.[195] As a result of the many possible receptor genotypes, the importance of haplotype structure versus individual SNPs in determining receptor function and pharmacological response has been investigated. Interestingly, out of a possible 8,192 unique β₂-adrenergic receptor haplotypes, only 12 distinct haplotypes have been observed among subjects from several different ethnic groups.[195] Subsequent assessment of the relationship between response to β-agonist therapy in asthma patients and genetic variation revealed a better association of haplotype and bronchodilator response, than could be found with any single polymorphism.[195] This is not surprising, as haplotype structure in the case of a gene with many polymorphisms in varying degrees of linkage disequilibrium should be a better predictor of phenotypic consequences than any ony variant. Examples such as the β₂-adrenergic receptor has provided the impetus to develop simple but robust molecular methods to determine haplotype structure for many important genes in patients.[196]

APOLIPOPROTEIN E—Human apolipoprotein E (apoE) plays an important role in lipid metabolism and neurobiology through its interactions with the low density lipoprotein (LDL) receptor and cell surface heparin sulfate proteoglycans.[197–200] ApoE exists as three major genetic variants, apoE2, apoE3, and apoE4, each differing by a cysteine or arginine at amino acids 112 and 158. ApoE3, the most common variant, contains cysteine at 112 and arginine at 158, whereas apoE2 contains two cysteines and apoE4 contains two arginines.[201] These differences have profound effects on both the physical stability and biological function of apoE.[202] For example, while both apoE3 and apoE4 bind to the LDL receptor with high affinity, apoE2 exhibits defective LDL receptor binding.[6] In addition, the presence of the apoE4 allele is associated with elevated plasma cholesterol levels and an increased risk for both coronary artery and Alzheimer's disease.[203–205]

In addition to the increased risk of disease, genetic variability in apoE also appears to have a predictive role in the response to drug treatment in patients with Alzheimer's disease and those receiving lipid lowering therapy.[206–209] In a study of the acetylcholinesterase inhibitor tacrine for patients with Alzheimer's disease, 83% of individuals without the apoE4 genotype showed improvement in total response and cognitive response after 30 weeks of drug treatment compared to only 40% of patients with the apoE4 genotype.[210] However, the greatest individual improvement in this particular study was seen in a patient with the unfavorable apoE4 genotype, underscoring that a single gene will not always be predictive of response to a given treatment.[210] Indeed, additional studies have indicated that the interaction between tacrine therapy and apoE genotype was strongest for women, suggesting that the complexity of efficacy prediction goes beyond analysis of one gene.[211] Although the molecular basis for an association between apolipoprotein genotype and tacrine efficacy has not been elucidated, it has been postulated that apoE4 plays a role in cholinergic dysfunction in Alzheimer's disease in a way that cannot be consistently overcome by therapy with acetylcholinesterase inhibitors such as tacrine. A randomized, placebo controlled study of the noradrenergic/vasopressinergic agonist S12024 in patients with Alzheimer's disease found the greatest protection of cognition in patients with the apoE4 genotype.[212] Should these results be confirmed, it may offer a rational approach for prospective selection of initial therapy for Alzheimer's disease, with S12024 or similar medications being recommended for patients with the apoE4 genotype.

In addition to the association between apoE genotype and response drug therapy for Alzheimer's disease, phenotypic and genotypic analyses have shown an association between apoE status and response to lipid lowering medications.[209,213,214] Most studies have demonstrated that patients with the apoE2 genotype have the greatest decrease of LDL cholesterol after drug therapy (E2 > E3 > E4). The association has been observed after treatment with a wide range of lipid lowering agents, including probocol, gemfibrozil, and many different HMG CoA-reductase inhibitors (ie, "statins").[209] However, a significant influence of apoE genotype on response to lipid lowering agents has not been observed in all studies.[209] In addition, although apoE4 genotype was associated with less reduction in total cholesterol and LDL and a smaller increase in HDL after fluvastatin therapy, there was no apparent influence of genotype on coronary artery disease progression or clinical events.[215] Thus, prospective clinical evaluations with robust clinical endpoints and sufficient sample size are needed to better quantitate the benefit of apoE genotype in the treatment of hyperlipidemia. The potential utility of apoE genotype must be balanced by concerns that it could be used by insurance companies, health systems, and federal programs to identify those at 'high risk' for development of Alzheimer's disease, coronary artery disease, and possibly other illnesses.[208]

THYMIDYLATE SYNTHASE—Thymidylate synthase (TS) is a key enzyme in the synthesis of pyrimidine nucleotides, by catalyzing the methylation dUMP to dTMP. The TS reaction is the sole source of *de novo* thymidylate in the cell and is essential for DNA replication.[216] The critical role of TS in nucleotide metabolism has made it an important target for a variety of anticancer drugs including 5-fluorouracil and the 5-fluorouracil <prodrug>, capecitabine, and to a lesser extent methotrexate.[216,217] Inhibition of TS by these agents causes tumor cell death depleting the intracellular pool of dTTP. Despite their clinical utility, resistance to TS inhibitors is an all too common problem. Fluoropyrimidine resistance arises through a variety of mechanisms, including elevated TS protein expression resulting from increases in *TS* transcription and translation.[218–221] A polymorphism within the 5'-untranslated region of the *TS* gene, consisting of tandem repeats of a 28 base pair fragment, has been implicated in modulating TS mRNA expression and TS mRNA translational efficiency.[222] Although there have been reports of four, five, and nine repeats within certain African and Asian populations, the vast majority of individual human *TS* alleles harbor either a double repeat (*2R*) or a triple repeat (*3R*) for this polymorphism, creating genotypes of *2R/2R*, *2R/3R*, and *3R/3R*.[223,224] Individuals that are homozygous for the *3R* have been shown to have elevated levels of TS mRNA and protein in their tumors compared with *2R* homozygotes.[225]

In recent pharmacogenomic studies evaluating the impact of TS polymorphisms on the clinical outcome in patients with locally-advanced or metastatic colorectal cancer treated with 5-fluorouracil based chemotherapy regimens, patients with the 3R/3R polymorphism showed no significant response or survival benefit from chemotherapy, whereas those with the 2R/2R or 2R/3R genotype showed significant better responses and gains in survival time from treatment.[226,227] In addition, it has been shown that patients with metastatic colon cancer treated with the 5-fluorouracil prodrug capecitabine who are homozygous for the 3R allele have a dramatically poorer probability of a response to treatment.[228] Additional data in children with acute lymphoblastic leukemia (ALL) indicates that TS polymorphisms are associated with response to treatment, as well as risk of disease, for other cancers.[229,230] Children with the 3R/3R genotype have been shown to have a poorer clinical outcome following treatment for ALL. Methotrexate, one of the key drugs in treatment regimens for ALL, is metabolized intracellularly to long-chain methotrexate polyglutamates, which then act as inhibitors of TS. Therefore, association between *TS* genotype and outcome in ALL makes sense mechanistically. The growing number of independent clinical investigations that point to a strong relationship between *TS* polymorphisms and outcome in patients with cancer has led some clinicians to recommend routine screening of *TS* genotypes to help guide therapeutic decisions. In the case of colon cancer, where there are now several active drugs to choose from when designing a treatment regimen, the ability to use genetic information to help decide which drug therapy might be best for each individual represents a clinically useful application of pharmacogenomics.

APPLIED PHARMACOGENOMICS

Technological Considerations

Although the examples provided in this chapter serve to illustrate the clinical importance of single nucleotide polymorphisms, for many of the genes that play a role in the regulation of drug activity, the true functional impact of genetic variations is not known. Furthermore, even for genes for which the genetic variants have been fully characterized with respect to function, results of genotype-phenotype investigations can be contradictory. For example, in the case of the drug transport gene MDR1, the 3435C>T has been associated with lower duodenal expression of the transport protein and either higher (eg, digoxin)[167] or lower (eg, fexofenadine)[170] drug concentrations in patients following oral dosing. Such contradictory results may be due to the presence complex multi-gene interactions so that the analysis of a single gene locus is not sufficient to explain the clinical outcome. Indeed, it is clear that in most cases, drug disposition and effect are complex processes involving multiple genetic pathways. Therefore, considerable time and effort has now been invested in the production of large libraries of single nucleotide polymorphisms[231] that can be investigated for a possible association with drug response. These efforts include nonprofit ventures (eg, The SNP Consortium) that release all information to the public free of charge, as well as private SNP libraries from a number of biotech companies (eg, Genset, Celera Genomics, Incyte). SNPs may serve as both physical landmarks and as genetic markers whose transmission can be followed from generation to generation. According to theoretical models, if the genotype of a group of individuals with a certain phenotype (eg, poor drug clearance) and a group with a different phenotype (eg, rapid drug clearance) are studied, certain genotypes may be consistently associated with those individuals who have the disease. Owing to linkage disequilibrium, alleles of genetic markers in close proximity to the actual phenotype modifying mutation are often found to be associated with the phenotype in question, even though they themselves are not involved in the phenotype itself. This molecular/population genetic approach also provides a strategy to identify genes associated with other phenotypes, such as drug toxicity or therapeutic benefit. This approach can be used for genome-wide mapping in which no genes or genomic regions are assumed to be associated with the drug effect under investigation.

The number of subjects and the numbers of markers needed for such a study depend on the level of contribution of the specific locus to the complex trait. In other words, a single causative mutation is easier to find than an alteration that is one of several contributors to the phenotype. It has been estimated that 60,000 markers, at 50-kb spacing, are needed to cover the genome in an association study of 1,000 individuals (eg, 500 patients with toxicity and 500 patients tolerating therapy).[129] If 1,000 individuals were to be genotyped for 60,000 markers, 60,000,000 genotyping assays would have to be completed. This approach would require a dramatic advance in high throughput genotyping techniques in order to be used in a timely and cost-efficient manner. An alternative, more practical approach uses an educated guess as to which of the genes in the human genome are likely to be important contributors to a given clinical phenotype.[232] This "candidate gene approach" narrows the search to the most likely informative polymorphisms in these genes. Such an approach is especially useful for classes of agents with clearly defined biochemistry, allowing for rational candidate gene selection. The candidate gene approach substantially reduces the number of loci under evaluation, but may miss important genes with no anticipated role in the particular phenotype in question. It is through efforts such as these that the next wave of pharmacogenetic predictive tools will emerge, requiring extensive in vitro and in vivo functional analyses to determine the role of each specific SNP in selecting optimal drug therapy.

Although the principles of pharmacogenomics have been around for decades, the more recent rapid development of the field has been the direct result of new technological advances in high throughput DNA and mRNA analysis and in the processing of these large data sets in an efficient manner. The most dramatic change has been the introduction of gene arrays for the simultaneous assessment of multiple genes. Initial studies used robotics-based systems to "imprint" a series of genes onto a silicone-coated glass slide. By labeling the mRNA of interest with a fluorescent probe, a correlation could be found between the fluorescence intensity emitted by each gene and the level of gene expression. The gene array approach has been modified to use large gene clones from the Human Genome Project, smaller fragments for specific genes, and cDNA derived from differential expression projects. The arrays are currently constructed on nylon filters or glass slides, with slides allowing greater density of genes per experiment and nylon generally being more reproducible. Improvements in robotics and fluid physics has allowed for the ability to evaluate up to 64,000 genes on a single 1-inch by 1 inch slide. The gene expression arrays have enabled a degree of genomic analysis not feasible in the recent past. It is estimated that the quantity of data available from a single array containing 64,000 genes (generated in approximately 48 hours) would have taken a researcher over 20 years to complete by Northern blot analysis.

As in the case of gene expression analysis, the ability to obtain information on patient genotype in a rapid manner has also greatly improved in the past few years. Strategies such as fluorescence energy transfer detection, fluorescence polarization, real-time PCR, time-of-flight mass spectrometry, oligonucleotide ligation/flow cytometry, HPLC fragment analysis, and mini-sequencing have all been used to increase the throughput of genotype information from genomic DNA. Currently, analysis of 1,000 to 5,000 genotypes per day is routine in many pharmacogenomics laboratories, with automated multiplex assays extending this to 100,000 genotypes per day. While the ideal approach for rapid genotyping is not yet clear, a large amount of effort is currently being expended to test various approaches in the clinical setting. However, as the speed and efficiency with which genotyping can be performed increases, the need for improved methods of data analysis becomes critical.

Computational biology, or bioinformatics, has been instrumental in the development of pharmacogenomics. The gene expression arrays and high throughput genotyping techniques generate a large amount of data in a single experiment, much more than can be evaluated using commonly available spreadsheets or manual approaches. Therefore, software has been developed that not only captures the experimental data, but includes the comparison of results with existing genome databases, generation of dendrograms for sequence homology, and pattern recognition to pull together genotypes with similar patterns of expression, as part of the initial algorithm. This provides the investigator with a powerful and comprehensive output on which rapid interpretation and implementation of data can be made.

The development of glass and nylon membrane microarrays has revolutionized the way gene expression is evaluated in all areas of medicine, including pharmacology. Initial studies focused on gene expression along biologic pathways and provided an increased understanding of the regulation of cellular proliferation and the cell's response to nutrient stimulation.[233] Gene expression arrays have also been used in the molecular classification of disease and have highlighted the great genetic heterogeneity among cells with histologically similar appearance.[234,235] For example, gene expression profiling has been used to identify subclasses of patients with diffuse large B-cell lymphoma (DLBCL). The clinical heterogeneity of DLBCL is such that 40% of patients respond well to current therapy, whereas the remainder eventually die of their disease. By using a "lymphochip" containing 17,856 genes that are preferentially expressed in lymphoid cells, investigators have demonstrated the presence of two molecularly distinct forms of the disease: germinal center B-like DLBCL and activated B-like DLBCL. More importantly, patients with germinal center B-like DLBCL have a superior overall survival following chemotherapy than those with activated B-like DLBCL.[234] Based on each individual's gene expression profile, a patient with activated B-like DLBCL will not benefit from standard therapy, and experimental treatment approaches should be considered. Alternatively, a patient with germinal center B-like DLBCL may be currently "over treated" because of their "good risk" status, and treatment strategies with more manageable side-effect profiles may need to be considered. As the basic understanding of the underlying molecular biology of diseases such as DLBCL increases, gene profiling will become more sophisticated, allowing for the discrimination of many more subclasses with associated differences in outcome and best clinical management.

Molecular Diagnostics for Optimizing Drug Therapy

Just as gene expression array analysis may someday allow investigators to define a genetic "therapeutic signature" for specific agents and diseases, "SNP" arrays have been developed to facilitate the rapid and efficient genotyping of individuals across a wide range of genetic pathways. While both *de novo* (static) and post-treatment (dynamic) analysis of gene expression in normal and disease tissues are used for gene expression analysis, array-based genotyping is required only once, since a persons genotype is stable throughout their lifetime. In this regard, automated systems are currently being developed to allow the rapid determination of an individual's genotype for genes that are known to be involved in the pathogenesis of their disease, in the metabolism and disposition of medications, and in the critical targets of drug therapy. This strategy is illustrated by Fig 62-4, which depicts various genes that one might choose to include on a SNP assay to help guide drug selection and drug dosing for patients with acute lymphoblastic leukemia (ALL).[236] It has previously been shown that polymorphisms in drug-metabolizing enzymes can have a significant effect on toxicity and efficacy of medications used to treat patients with ALL,[237] and that individualization of drug dosages can improve clinical outcome. Moreover, it has been established that the genotype of leukemic blasts is an important prognostic variable that can be used to guide the intensity of treatment.[238] Furthermore, genetic polymorphisms are known to exist for various cytokines and other determinants of host susceptibility to infection, as well as polymorphisms in cardiovascular, endocrine, and other receptors that may be important determinants of an individual's susceptibility to drug toxicity. Therefore, by putting all of these polymorphic genes on a single ALL "SNP chip," one would potentially have a valuable molecular diagnostic tool that would allow the rapidly and objective selection of optimal drug therapy for each individual.

The potential is enormous for pharmacogenomics to yield a powerful set of molecular diagnostics that will become routine tools by which clinicians select medications and drug doses for individual patients. Furthermore, unlike essentially all biochemical tests (serum creatinine, bilirubin, etc), a patient's genotype would only need to be determined once for a given gene, because it will not change. Using the amount of DNA that can be isolated from a few milliliters of blood, it is possible to determine thousands of genotypes. Currently available techniques such as primer extension followed by minisequencing (eg, Pyrosequencing), allele-specific signal (eg, Taqman, fluorescence polarization, molecular beacons) or mass spectrometry (eg, Sequenome) have brought high throughput genotyping within the reach of most clinical scientists. Ultimately, the process will be to collect a single blood sample from each patient (DNA can be stored for decades), submit a small aliquot for analysis of a panel of genotypes (eg, 20,000 SNPs in 5,000 genes), and test for those that are important determinants of drug disposition and effects. Patient-specific genotyping results will need to be stored in a secure electronic repository that can be queried as new treatment decisions are made. These genotyping results will not be easily interpreted if reported as a list of SNPs, rather will need to be formatted and interpreted according to the patient's diagnosis and treatment options. These new tools will not replace the more conventional biochemical tests that are now routinely used to assess organ function and disease progression, rather they will complement these tests, and provide additional tools for selecting medications that are optimal for each patient. It is likely that clinical pharmacists will have an increasingly important role in the safeguarding and interpretation of pharmacogenetic data.

The translation of pharmacogenetics into clinical practice is already underway, but will continue to evolve for decades to come. There are currently several examples where genotypes are already being used prospectively for the selection of medications and drug doses.[2,239,240] At present, these clinical applications are limited to medications with narrow therapeutic indices, such as anticancer agents, and for genes with discrete, well described functional polymorphisms (eg, TPMT, DPD, and UGT1A1), but as additional pharmacogenomic relationships are identified, the use of genetically-targeted therapy will expand to include a broad range of medications. The field of

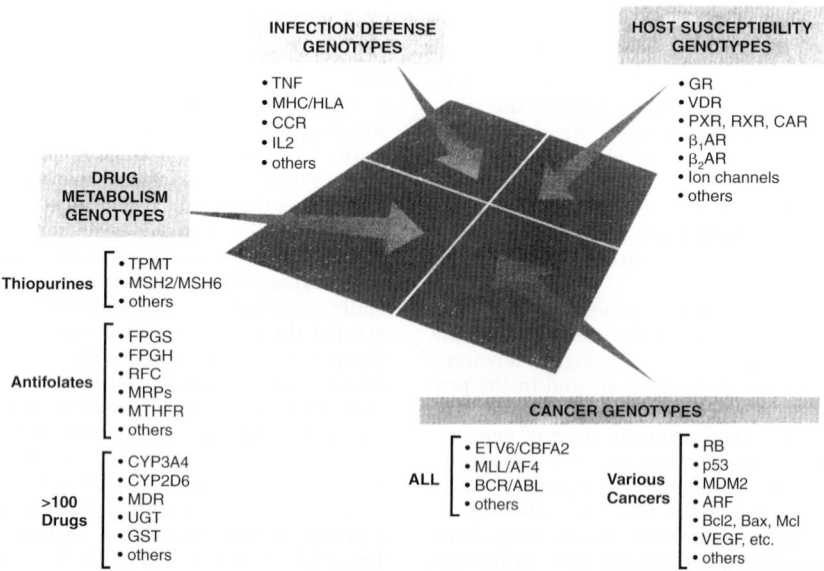

Figure 62-4. Molecular diagnostics of pharmacogenomic traits. DNA arrays are being made for automated, high-throughput detection of functionally important mutations in genes that are important determinants of drug effects, such as drug-metabolizing enzymes, drug targets (receptors), disease pathogenesis, and other polymorphic genes that influence an individual's susceptibility to drug toxicities or environmental exposures (such as pathogens, carcinogens, and others). This figure exemplifies components of a potential diagnostic DNA array for genes that could influence a patient's response to chemotherapy for acute lymphoblastic leukemia, including genes that determine drug metabolism, disease sensitivity, and the risk of adverse effects of treatment (cardiovascular or endocrine toxicities, infections, and so forth). (Reprinted with permission from Evans WE, Relling MV. *Science* 1999; 286:487. Copyright 1999 AAAS.)

pharmacogenomics is growing rapidly, fueled by dozens of genomic companies, academic centers and large pharmaceutical companies that are incorporating pharmacogenomic studies into clinical trials during the earliest stages of drug development.[241,242] Furthermore, several biotechnology companies are working to develop more efficient and less expensive high throughput methods for determining genotypes and haplotypes. In the future, the greatest challenge will not be the ability to determine an individual's genotype (or haplotype), rather it will be the strategy for precisely determining the associations between the genetic determinants and drug response.

Pharmacogenomics and Drug Development

The rapid acceleration of growth in the field of pharmacogenomics has been heavily influenced by the pharmaceutical industry and its desire for a more rational drug development process.[242] Potential industrial applications of pharmacogenomics extend from identification of novel targets against which new therapies can be designed to speeding up the clinical development and approval process. As a result, many companies have invested enormous human and financial resources in the area of pharmacogenomics with the goal determining the role genetic variability in human disease. The pharmaceutical industry is currently utilizing both human and mouse SNP arrays in an attempt to find specific genes or genomic loci that are associated with disease. Once identified, the genetic determinant of a particular disease becomes the target for new drug development. Similar approaches are also being conducted using gene expression arrays, where disease tissue is used to produce mRNA for comparison with normal reference tissue. The goal of these approaches is sometimes referred to as "gene hunting," and arrays covering the broadest range of known and unknown genes are the most useful. Important genetic variants may either be putative modulators of the disease phenotype or represent novel mechanisms of disease pathogenesis. Furthermore, pharmacogenomics has the potential to streamline the drug development process, by decreasing the number of patients required to show efficacy in early clinical trials.[243] If, for example, a certain genotype is shown to be associated with a higher probability of response to a given investigational drug, one would require fewer subjects with that particular genotype to show a benefit compared to a trial that included individuals with all the possible genotypes.

Gene expression arrays are also being applied to define the mechanism of action for new compounds or to screen for direct influence of an agent on a specific pathway. Targeted agents developed in the most mechanistically guided program can often lead to surprises during *in vivo* evaluation. For example, inhibitors of HMG-CoA reductase, initially developed as cholesterol lowering agents, were subsequently found to inhibit farnesyl transferase activity in the cell-signaling pathway of the ras oncogene.[244] Using gene expression arrays, one can generate a profile of the changes in gene expression in response to a drug, thereby yielding a greater understanding of mechanisms of action. Gene expression arrays can also be used during screening of candidate compounds. By constructing arrays for genes involved in a pathway of interest, *in vivo* gene expression dynamics can be used as a quantifiable measure of drug activity. This results a more rational approach to optimization of drug therapy and design of new agents based on actual *in vivo* observations in patients, rather than by animal models or theory alone.

Pharmacogenomics as a Public Health Tool

Although the promise of pharmacogenomics is enormous, it is likely to have the greatest initial benefit for patients in developed countries, owing to expense, availability of technology and the focus of initial research. However, pharmacogenomics will ultimately be a useful tool throughout the world. It has long been appreciated that there are ethnic variations in disease risk, disease incidence, and response to treatment.[245] In addition, as discussed in this chapter, the frequency distribution of polymorphisms in most of the human genes studied differ among various racial groups. Therefore, one approach to applying pharmacogenomics to public health is through SNP allele frequency analysis in defined populations. For example, analysis of TPMT genotype in world populations suggests that TPMT-mediated toxicity from azathioprine or mercaptopurine would likely be lower in Japanese or Chinese populations than Caucasians.[125] In contrast, a higher frequency of the TPMT mutant allele is found in the Ghanaian and Kenyan populations,[125] suggesting that these racial groups would be at a greater risk for thiopurine-induced toxicity. Moreover, even greater ethnic diversity has been demonstrated for other polymorphic drug-metabolizing enzymes (eg, NAT2, CYP2D6, CYP2C19), and such will likely be the case for other traits like direct or indirect drug targets. Therefore, by combining the understanding of associations between genetic variability and drug response or toxicity with the knowledge about the ethnic distribution of various polymorphisms, public health officials will be able to make broad recommendations about the safe and appropriate use of medications in each of the world's populations. This general approach will have broad applications to the development of clinical practice guidelines and national formularies in developing countries.

While in theory using the knowledge of ethnic differences will be important to most of the world's populations, such an approach is significantly limited in geographic regions with extensive genetic mixing. For example, it is known that the African American population has a great degree of geographic and social mixing that provide a basis for wide genetic heterogeneity. This is illustrated in by a comparison of TPMT mutations between African American and West African populations. Although the *TPMT *3C* allele is the most frequently observed variant in both populations, it represents 100% of the mutant alleles in West Africans and 52% in African Americans.[133,134] Interestingly, the remaining African American mutant alleles are the *TPMT*2* and *TPMT*3A*[134] alleles that are common in Caucasians. Therefore, great care must be taken when applying pharmacogenomics to public health issues, and testing at the genetic level in each patient will remain the most definitive approach.

A number of issues influencing the development of pharmacogenomics include several that are of a practical or nonscientific nature. One important limitation to the broad application of pharmacogenomics is the availability of inexpensive gene expression arrays, cost-effective high throughput genotyping, and disseminated bioinformatics resources. Currently, there is considerable growth in the number of companies offering both genomics analysis on a fee-for-service basis and the equipment for user-maintained instruments. As technology and competition bring down the high initial capital costs of array and genotype systems, the potential for general application of these approaches will be further enhanced. Currently, the technology for gene expression and genotype assessment is only affordable in the pharmaceutical research and development setting or in the context of funded academic research. A thorough pharmacoeconomic analysis will ultimately be required to justify and direct the future scope of pharmacogenomics for clinical medical practice. However, once an individual's genotype has been correctly determined, it does not need to be repeated and can be stored for a multitude of potential applications. One can certainly envision a time in the future when each individual will have their genetic information recorded in a secure database, accessible only to authorized health care providers, to be used for disease risk assessment or as a guide in therapeutic decision-making. For example, this potentially web-based compilation of an individuals' genotype could be used by the clinical pharmacist when making recommendations regarding the choice of medications, appropriate dosing, or risk of potential side effects.

Absolutely critical to the future application of pharmacogenomics to clinical medicine, is the protection of the patients' right to privacy. While patient confidentiality is at the very heart of good medical care, genetic information adds a new layer of ethical complexity. In addition to pharmacogenomic data, an individuals' genotype contains features that will ultimately be associated with many other measures of outcome such as the risk of some future illness. While this information may be useful with respect to screening or chemopreventative strategies, a patient may want to keep such genetic data confidential. As a result, the ethics of genetic testing is currently an active area for discussion and debate. A system of trust and internal control has historically been utilized to prevent the inappropriate use of genetic information. Although this approach has been generally successful, with breach of trust being a rare event, the field of bioethics is now focused on prevention of potential or theoretical abuses of genetic information against individuals. Most of the discussion and debate centers around what information is needed, who should have access, and how should the information be used. Ethical issues such as these are obviously challenging, since the insurance carrier paying for the genetic testing will be the same entity that could potentially use the information to identify disease or therapy risks that could in turn be used to restrict or deny future coverage. However, while such patient confidentiality issues represent a significant challenge to the ultimate application of genetic testing, it is generally acknowledged that the potential gains from pharmacogenomics, in terms of patient well-being and cost of healthcare, heavily outweigh the risks. Indeed, the promise of pharmacogenomics is such that society must eventually find a way to ensure that the risk of exploitation does not overshadow the public good that will come from putting such powerful information in the hands of knowledgeable health care providers and those involved in the discovery of new approaches to disease treatment and prevention.

REFERENCES

1. Kalow W, Tang BK, Endrenyi L. *Pharmacogenetics* 1998; 8:283.
2. Evans WE, Relling MV. *Science* 1999; 286:487.
3. Evans WE, Johnson JA. *Annu Rev Genomics Hum Genet* 2001; 2:9–39.
4. Evans WE, McLeod HL. *N Engl J Med* 2003; 348:538.
5. Kalow W. *Lancet* 1956; 221:576.
6. Hughes HB, Biehl JP, Jones AP, et al. *Am Rev Tuberc* 1954; 70:266.
7. Carson PE, Flanagan CL, Ickles CE, et al. *Science* 1956; 124:484.
8. Venter JC. *Science* 2003; 299:1183.
9. Lander ES, Linton LM, Birren B, et al. *Nature* 2001; 409:860.
10. Issa JP, Baylin SB. *Nat Med* 1996; 2:281.
11. Lewin B. *Cell* 1998; 93:301.
12. Wolffe AP, Matzke MA. *Science* 1999; 286:481.
13. Sachidanandam R, Weissman D, Schmidt SC, et al. *Nature* 2001; 409:928.
14. Hoehe MR. *Pharmacogenomics* 2003; 4:547.
15. Wall JD, Pritchard JK. *Nat Rev Genet* 2003; 4:587.
16. Stephens JC, Schneider JA, Tanguay DA, et al. *Science* 2001; 293:489.
17. Salisbury BA, Pungliya M, Choi JY, et al. *Mutat Res* 2003; 526:53.
18. Eichelbaum M, Evert B. *Clin Exp Pharmacol Physiol* 1996; 23:983.
19. Mareni C, Repetto L, Forteleoni G, et al. *J Med Genet* 1984; 21:278.
20. Vives Corrons JL, Pujades A. *Hum Genet* 1982; 60:216.
21. Evans WE, Relling MV, Rahman A, et al. *J Clin Invest* 1993; 91:2150.
22. Saxena R, Shaw GL, Relling MV, et al. *Hum Mol Genet* 1994; 3:923.
23. Tai HL, Krynetski EY, Schuetz EG, et al. *Proc Natl Acad Sci U S A* 1997; 94:6444.
24. Yates CR, Krynetski EY, Loennechen T, et al. *Ann Intern Med* 1997; 126:608.
25. Meinsma R, Fernandez-Salguero P, van Kuilenburg AB, et al. *DNA Cell Biol* 1995; 14:1.
26. Wei X, McLeod HL, McMurrough J, et al. *J Clin Invest* 1996; 98:610.
27. Coles R, Caswell R, Rubinsztein DC. *Hum Mol Genet* 1998; 7:791.
28. Tachikawa M, Nagai Y, Nakamura K, et al. *J Hum Genet* 2002; 47:275.
29. Bontekoe CJ, Bakker CE, Nieuwenhuizen IM, et al. *Hum Mol Genet* 2001; 10:1693.
30. Bernad M, Martinez ME, Escalona M, et al. *Bone* 2002; 30:223.
31. Horikawa Y, Oda N, Cox NJ, et al. *Nat Genet* 2000; 26:163.
32. Kuehl P, Zhang J, Lin Y, et al. *Nat Genet* 2001; 27:383.
33. Wilkinson GR. 2001; 10th edition: 3.
34. Price Evans DA, Manley KA, McKusick VA. *BMJ* 1960; 2:485.
35. Timbrell JA, Harland SJ, Facchini V. *Clin Pharmacol Ther* 1980; 28:350.
36. Timbrell JA, Harland SJ, Facchini V. *Clin Pharmacol Ther* 1981; 29:337.
37. Reidenberg MM, Drayer DE, Levy M, et al. *Clin Pharmacol Ther* 1975; 17:722.
38. Drayer DE, Reidenberg MM. *Clin Pharmacol Ther* 1977; 22:251.
39. Ingelman-Sundberg M, Oscarson M, McLellan RA. *Trends Pharmacol Sci* 1999; 20:342.
40. Gonzalez FJ, Skoda RC, Kimura S, et al. *Nature* 1988; 331:442.
41. Mahgoub A, Idle JR, Dring LG, et al. *Lancet* 1977; 2:584.
42. Eichelbaum M, Spannbrucker N, Steincke B, et al. *Eur J Clin Pharmacol* 1979; 16:183.
43. Dalen P, Dahl ML, Ruiz ML, et al. *Clin Pharmacol Ther* 1998; 63:444.
44. Fjordside L, Jeppesen U, Eap CB, et al. *Pharmacogenetics* 1999; 9:55.
45. Poulsen L, Brosen K, Arendt-Nielsen L, et al. *Eur J Clin Pharmacol* 1996; 51:289.
46. Johansson I, Lundqvist E, Bertilsson L, et al. *Proc Natl Acad Sci U S A* 1993; 90:11825.
47. Lovlie R, Daly AK, Molven A, et al. *FEBS Lett* 1996; 392:30.
48. Gonzalez FJ, Vilbois F, Hardwick JP, et al. *Genomics* 1988; 2:174.
49. Kimura S, Umeno M, Skoda RC, et al. *Am J Hum Genet* 1989; 45:889.
50. Ingelman-Sundberg M, Evans WE. *Pharmacogenetics* 2001; 11:553.
51. Aklillu E, Persson I, Bertilsson L, et al. *J Pharmacol Exp Ther* 1996; 278:441.
52. Rendic S, Di Carlo FJ. *Drug Metab Rev* 1997; 29:413.
53. Kupfer A, Branch RA. *Clin Pharmacol Ther* 1985; 38:414.
54. Wilkinson GR, Guengerich FP, Branch RA. *Pharmacol Ther* 1989; 43:53.
55. Goldstein JA. *Br J Clin Pharmacol* 2001; 52:349.
56. Balian JD, Sukhova N, Harris JW, et al. *Clin Pharmacol Ther* 1995; 57:662.
57. Andersson T, Miners JO, Veronese ME, et al. *Br J Clin Pharmacol* 1993; 36:521.
58. Wan J, Xia H, He N, et al. *Br J Clin Pharmacol* 1996; 42:471.
59. Ando Y, Fuse E, Figg WD. *Clin Cancer Res* 2002; 8:1964.
60. Hadama A, Ieiri I, Morita T, et al. *Ther Drug Monit* 2001; 23:115.
61. Kobayashi K, Kogo M, Tani M, et al. *Drug Metab Dispos* 2001; 29:36.
62. Ward SA, Walle T, Walle UK, et al. *Clin Pharmacol Ther* 1989; 45:72.
63. Ward SA, Helsby NA, Skjelbo E, et al. *Br J Clin Pharmacol* 1991; 31:689.
64. Furuta T, Ohashi K, Kamata T, et al. *Ann Intern Med* 1998; 129:1027.
65. Sohn DR, Kwon JT, Kim HK, et al. *Clin Pharmacol Ther* 1997; 61:574.
66. Tanaka M, Ohkubo T, Otani K, et al. *Clin Pharmacol Ther* 2001; 69:108.
67. Ishizaki T, Chiba K, Manabe K, et al. *Clin Pharmacol Ther* 1995; 58:155.
68. Bertilsson L. *Clin Pharmacokinet* 1995; 29:192.
69. Rettie AE, Korzekwa KR, Kunze KL, et al. *Chem Res Toxicol* 1992; 5:54.
70. Bajpai M, Roskos LK, Shen DD, et al. *Drug Metab Dispos* 1996; 24:1401.
71. Miners JO, Birkett DJ. *Methods Enzymol* 1996; 272:139.
72. Kidd RS, Straughn AB, Meyer MC, et al. *Pharmacogenetics* 1999; 9:71.
73. Stearns RA, Chakravarty PK, Chen R, et al. *Drug Metab Dispos* 1995; 23:207.
74. Lee CR, Goldstein JA, Pieper JA. *Pharmacogenetics* 2002; 12:251.
75. Dickmann LJ, Rettie AE, Kneller MB, et al. *Mol Pharmacol* 2001; 60:382.
76. Tracy TS, Hutzler JM, Haining RL, et al. *Drug Metab Dispos* 2002; 30:385.
77. Rettie AE, Haining RL, Bajpai M, et al. *Epilepsy Res* 1999; 35:253.
78. Gill HJ, Tjia JF, Kitteringham NR, et al. *Pharmacogenetics* 1999; 9:43.
79. Higashi MK, Veenstra DL, Kondo LM, et al. *JAMA* 2002; 287:1690.
80. Aithal GP, Day CP, Kesteven PJ, et al. *Lancet* 1999; 353:717.
81. Taube J, Halsall D, Baglin T. *Blood* 2000; 96:1816.
82. Tuchman M, Stoeckeler JS, Kiang DT, et al. *N Engl J Med* 1985; 313:245.

83. Diasio RB, Beavers TL, Carpenter JT. *J Clin Invest* 1988; 81:47.
84. Gonzalez FJ, Fernandez-Salguero P. *Trends Pharmacol Sci* 1995; 16:325.
85. Berger R, Stoker-de Vries SA, Wadman SK, et al. *Clin Chim Acta* 1984; 141:227.
86. Hustert E, Haberl M, Burk O, et al. *Pharmacogenetics* 2001; 11:773.
87. Cholerton S, Daly AK, Idle JR. *Trends Pharmacol Sci* 1992; 13:434.
88. Lamba JK, Lin YS, Schuetz EG, et al. *Adv Drug Deliv Rev* 2002; 54:1271.
89. Lehmann JM, McKee DD, Watson MA, et al. *J Clin Invest* 1998; 102:1016.
90. Sata F, Sapone A, Elizondo G, et al. *Clin Pharmacol Ther* 2000; 67:48.
91. Min DI, Ellingrod VL. *Ther Drug Monit* 2003; 25:305.
92. Spurdle AB, Goodwin B, Hodgson E, et al. *Pharmacogenetics* 2002; 12:355.
93. Paris PL, Kupelian PA, Hall JM, et al. *Cancer Epidemiol Biomarkers Prev* 1999; 8:901.
94. Felix CA, Walker AH, Lange BJ, et al. *Proc Natl Acad Sci U S A* 1998; 95:13176.
95. Kadlubar FF, Berkowitz GS, Delongchamp RR, et al. *Cancer Epidemiol Biomarkers Prev* 2003; 12:327.
96. Floyd MD, Gervasini G, Masica AL, et al. *Pharmacogenetics* 2003; 13:595.
97. Paulussen A, Lavrijsen K, Bohets H, et al. *Pharmacogenetics* 2000; 10:415.
98. Zheng H, Webber S, Zeevi A, et al. *Am J Transplant* 2003; 3:477.
99. Macphee IA, Fredericks S, Tai T, et al. *Transplantation* 2002; 74:1486.
100. Lacroix D, Sonnier M, Moncion A, et al. *Eur J Biochem* 1997; 247:625.
101. Burk O, Tegude H, Koch I, et al. *J Biol Chem* 2002; 277:24280.
102. Hustert E, Zibat A, Presecan-Siedel E, et al. *Drug Metab Dispos* 2001; 29:1454.
103. Zhang J, Kuehl P, Green ED, et al. *Pharmacogenetics* 2001; 11:555.
104. Lin HJ, Han CY, Lin BK, et al. *Am J Hum Genet* 1993; 52:827.
105. Blum M, Grant DM, McBride W, et al. *DNA Cell Biol* 1990; 9:193.
106. Grant DM, Hughes NC, Janezic SA, et al. *Mutat Res* 1997; 376:61.
107. Grant DM, Blum M, Meyer UA. *Xenobiotica* 1992; 22:1073.
108. Blum M, Demierre A, Grant DM, et al. *Proc Natl Acad Sci U S A* 1991; 88:5237.
109. Deguchi T, Mashimo M, Suzuki T. *J Biol Chem* 1990; 265:12757.
110. Dickinson DS, Bailey WC, Hirschowitz BI, et al. *J Clin Gastroenterol* 1981; 3:271.
111. Gent WL, Seifart HI, Parkin DP, et al. *Eur J Clin Pharmacol* 1992; 43:131.
112. Singh J, Arora A, Garg PK, et al. *Postgrad Med J* 1995; 71:359.
113. Huang YS, Chern HD, Su WJ, et al. *Hepatology* 2002; 35:883.
114. Innocenti F, Iyer L, Ratain MJ. *Drug Metab Dispos* 2001; 29:596.
115. Felder TB, McLean MA, Vestal ML, et al. *Drug Metab Dispos* 1987; 15:773.
116. Ratain MJ, Mick R, Berezin F, et al. *Clin Pharmacol Ther* 1991; 50:573.
117. Ratain MJ, Mick R, Berezin F, et al. *Cancer Res* 1993; 53:2304.
118. Cascorbi I, Brockmoller J, Roots I. *Int J Clin Pharmacol Ther* 2002; 40:562.
119. Hein DW. *Mutat Res* 2002; 506–507:65.
120. Costa S, Medeiros R, Vasconcelos A, et al. *J Cancer Res Clin Oncol* 2002; 128:678.
121. Fretland AJ, Doll MA, Zhu Y, et al. *Cancer Detect Prev* 2002; 26:10.
122. Firozi PF, Bondy ML, Sahin AA, et al. *Carcinogenesis* 2002; 23:301.
123. Wikman H, Thiel S, Jager B, et al. *Pharmacogenetics* 2001; 11:157.
124. Krynetski EY, Tai HL, Yates CR, et al. *Pharmacogenetics* 1996; 6:279.
125. McLeod HL, Krynetski EY, Relling MV, et al. *Leukemia* 2000; 14:567.
126. Weinshilboum RM, Sladek SL. *Am J Hum Genet* 1980; 32:651.
127. McLeod HL, Relling MV, Liu Q, et al. *Blood* 1995; 85:1897.
128. Schutz E, Gummert J, Mohr F, et al. *Lancet* 1993; 341:436.
129. McLeod HL, Evans WE. *Annu Rev Pharmacol Toxicol* 2001; 41:101.
130. Krynetski EY, Schuetz JD, Galpin AJ, et al. *Proc Natl Acad Sci U S A* 1995; 92:949.
131. Tai HL, Krynetski EY, Yates CR, et al. *Am J Hum Genet* 1996; 58:694.
132. Loennechen T, Yates CR, Fessing MY, et al. *Clin Pharmacol Ther* 1998; 64:46.
133. Ameyaw MM, Collie-Duguid ES, Powrie RH, et al. *Hum Mol Genet* 1999; 8:367.
134. Hon YY, Fessing MY, Pui CH, et al. *Hum Mol Genet* 1999; 8:371.
135. Coulthard SA, Howell C, Robson J, et al. *Blood* 1998; 92:2856.
136. Lennard L, Van Loon JA, Weinshilboum RM. *Clin Pharmacol Ther* 1989; 46:149.
137. Evans WE, Horner M, Chu YQ, et al. *J Pediatr* 1991; 119:985.
138. Black AJ, McLeod HL, Capell HA, et al. *Ann Intern Med* 1998; 129:716.
139. Relling MV, Hancock ML, Rivera GK, et al. *J Natl Cancer Inst* 1999; 91:2001.
140. Ishioka S, Hiyama K, Sato H, et al. *Intern Med* 1999; 38:944.
141. Relling MV, Yanishevski Y, Nemec J, et al. *Leukemia* 1998; 12:346.
142. Bo J, Schroder H, Kristinsson J, et al. *Cancer* 1999; 86:1080.
143. Relling MV, Rubnitz JE, Rivera GK, et al. *Lancet* 1999; 354:34.
144. Burchell B. *Am J Pharmacogenomics* 2003; 3:37.
145. Mackenzie PI, Owens IS, Burchell B, et al. *Pharmacogenetics* 1997; 7:255.
146. Owens IS, Ritter JK, Yeatman MT, et al. *J Pharmacokinet Biopharm* 1996; 24:491.
147. Ando Y, Saka H, Asai G, et al. *Ann Oncol* 1998; 9:845.
148. Jansen PL, Bosma PJ, Chowdhury JR. *Prog Liver Dis* 1995; 13:125.
149. Seppen J, Bosma PJ, Goldhoorn BG, et al. *J Clin Invest* 1994; 94:2385.
150. Sampietro M, Iolascon A. *Haematologica* 1999; 84:150.
151. Owens D, Evans J. *J Med Genet* 1975; 12:152.
152. Monaghan G, Ryan M, Seddon R, et al. *Lancet* 1996; 347:578.
153. Monaghan G, Foster B, Jurima-Romet M, et al. *Pharmacogenetics* 1997; 7:153.
154. Bosma PJ, Chowdhury JR, Bakker C, et al. *N Engl J Med* 1995; 333:1171.
155. Beutler E, Gelbart T, Demina A. *Proc Natl Acad Sci U S A* 1998; 95:8170.
156. Jinno H, Tanaka-Kagawa T, Hanioka N, et al. *Drug Metab Dispos* 2003; 31:108.
157. Araki E, Ishikawa M, Iigo M, et al. *Jpn J Cancer Res* 1993; 84:697.
158. Atsumi R, Suzuki W, Hakusui H. *Xenobiotica* 1991; 21:1159.
159. Gupta E, Lestingi TM, Mick R, et al. *Cancer Res* 1994; 54:3723.
160. Ando Y, Saka H, Ando M, et al. *Cancer Res* 2000; 60:6921.
161. Brinkmann U, Roots I, Eichelbaum M. *Drug Discov Today* 2001; 6:835.
162. Borst P, Evers R, Kool M, et al. *J Natl Cancer Inst* 2000; 92:1295.
163. Choo EF, Leake B, Wandel C, et al. *Drug Metab Dispos* 2000; 28:655.
164. Thiebaut F, Tsuruo T, Hamada H, et al. *Proc Natl Acad Sci U S A* 1987; 84:7735.
165. Rao VV, Dahlheimer JL, Bardgett ME, et al. *Proc Natl Acad Sci U S A* 1999; 96:3900.
166. Schinkel AH, Wagenaar E, Mol CA, et al. *J Clin Invest* 1996; 97:2517.
167. Hoffmeyer S, Burk O, von Richter O, et al. *Proc Natl Acad Sci U S A* 2000; 97:3473.
168. Hitzl M, Drescher S, van der KH, et al. *Pharmacogenetics* 2001; 11:293.
169. Sakaeda T, Nakamura T, Horinouchi M, et al. *Pharm Res* 2001; 18:1400.
170. Kim RB, Leake BF, Choo EF, et al. *Clin Pharmacol Ther* 2001; 70:189.
171. Fellay J, Marzolini C, Meaden ER, et al. *Lancet* 2002; 359:30.
172. van Montfoort JE, Hagenbuch B, Groothuis GM, et al. *Curr Drug Metab* 2003; 4:185.
173. Hagenbuch B, Meier PJ. *Biochim Biophys Acta* 2003; 1609:1.
174. Koepsell H. *Annu Rev Physiol* 1998; 60:243.
175. Tirona RG, Leake BF, Merino G, et al. *J Biol Chem* 2001; 276:356.
176. Nozawa T, Nakajima M, Tamai I, et al. *J Pharmacol Exp Ther* 2002; 302:804.
177. Nishizato Y, Ieiri I, Suzuki H, et al. *Clin Pharmacol Ther* 2003; 73:554.
178. van Essen GG, Rensma PL, de Zeeuw D, et al. *Lancet* 1996; 347:94.
179. Nakano Y, Oshima T, Watanabe M, et al. *Am J Hypertens* 1997; 10:1064.
180. Cannella G, Paoletti E, Barocci S, et al. *Kidney Int* 1998; 54:618.
181. Sasaki M, Oki T, Iuchi A, et al. *J Hypertens* 1996; 14:1403.
182. Prasad A, Narayanan S, Husain S, et al. *Circulation* 2000; 102:35.
183. Jacobsen P, Rossing K, Rossing P, et al. *Kidney Int* 1998; 53:1002.
184. Kohno M, Yokokawa K, Minami M, et al. *Am J Med* 1998; 106:544.
185. Perna A, Ruggenenti P, Testa A, et al. *Kidney Int* 2000; 57:274.
186. Martinelli I, Sacchi E, Landi G, et al. *N Engl J Med* 1998; 338:1793.
187. Napolitano C, Schwartz PJ, Brown AM, et al. *J Cardiovasc Electrophysiol* 2000; 11:691.
188. Liggett SB. *J Allergy Clin Immunol* 2000; 105:S487.
189. Lima JJ, Thomason DB, Mohamed MH, et al. *Clin Pharmacol Ther* 1999; 65:519.

190. Tan S, Hall IP, Dewar J, et al. *Lancet* 1997; 350:995.
191. Large V, Hellstrom L, Reynisdottir S, et al. *J Clin Invest* 1997; 100:3005.
192. Meirhaeghe A, Helbecque N, Cottel D, et al. *Lancet* 1999; 353:896.
193. Liggett SB. *Pharmacology* 2000; 61:167.
194. Brodde OE, Buscher R, Tellkamp R, et al. *Circulation* 2001; 103:1048.
195. Drysdale CM, McGraw DW, Stack CB, et al. *Proc Natl Acad Sci U S A* 2000; 97:10483.
196. McDonald OG, Krynetski EY, Evans WE. *Pharmacogenetics* 2002; 12:93.
197. Mahley RW. *Science* 1988; 240:622.
198. Weisgraber KH. *Adv Protein Chem* 1994; 45:249.
199. Al Haideri M, Goldberg IJ, Galeano NF, et al. *Biochemistry* 1997; 36:12766.
200. de Knijff P, Havekes LM. *Curr Opin Lipidol* 1996; 7:59.
201. Weisgraber KH, Rall SC, Jr., Mahley RW. *J Biol Chem* 1981; 256:9077.
202. Morrow JA, Segall ML, Lund-Katz S, et al. *Biochemistry* 2000; 39:11657.
203. Davignon J, Gregg RE, Sing CF. *Arteriosclerosis* 1988; 8:1.
204. Strittmatter WJ, Roses AD. *Annu Rev Neurosci* 1996; 19:53.
205. Weisgraber KH, Mahley RW. *FASEB J* 1996; 10:1485.
206. Gerdes LU, Gerdes C, Kervinen K, et al. *Circulation* 2000; 101:1366.
207. Ordovas JM, Lopez-Miranda J, Perez-Jimenez F, et al. *Atherosclerosis* 1995; 113:157.
208. Issa AM, Keyserlingk EW. *Can J Psychiatry* 2000; 45:917.
209. Siest G, Bertrand P, Herbeth B, et al. *Clin Chem Lab Med* 2000; 38:841.
210. Poirier J, Delisle MC, Quirion R, et al. *Proc Natl Acad Sci U S A* 1995; 92:12260.
211. Farlow MR, Lahiri DK, Poirier J, et al. *Neurology* 1998; 50:669.
212. Richard F, Helbecque N, Neuman E, et al. *Lancet* 1997; 349:539.
213. Nestruck AC, Bouthillier D, Sing CF, et al. *Metabolism* 1987; 36:743.
214. Ballantyne CM, Herd JA, Stein EA, et al. *J Am Coll Cardiol* 2000; 36:1572.
215. Watanabe J, Kobayashi K, Umeda F, et al. *Diabetes Res Clin Pract* 1993; 20:21.
216. Rustum YM, Harstrick A, Cao S, et al. *J Clin Oncol* 1997; 15:389.
217. Pinedo HM, Peters GF. *J Clin Oncol* 1988; 6:1653.
218. Johnston PG, Lenz HJ, Leichman CG, et al. *Cancer Res* 1995; 55:1407.
219. Lenz HJ, Leichman CG, Danenberg KD, et al. *J Clin Oncol* 1996; 14:176.
220. Rooney PH, Stevenson DA, Marsh S, et al. *Cancer Res* 1998; 58:5042.
221. Leichman CG. *Oncology (Huntingt)* 1998; 12:43.
222. Horie N, Aiba H, Oguro K, et al. *Cell Struct Funct* 1995; 20:191.
223. Marsh S, McKay JA, Cassidy J, et al. *Int J Oncol* 2001; 19:383.
224. Marsh S, Collie-Duguid ES, Li T, et al. *Genomics* 1999; 58:310.
225. Kawakami K, Omura K, Kanehira E, et al. *Anticancer Res* 1999; 19:3249.
226. Iacopetta B, Grieu F, Joseph D, et al. *Br J Cancer* 2001; 85:827.
227. Pullarkat ST, Stoehlmacher J, Ghaderi V, et al. *Pharmacogenomics J* 2001; 1:65.
228. Park DJ, Stoehlmacher J, Zhang W, et al. *Int J Colorectal Dis* 2002; 17:46.
229. Lauten M, Asgedom G, Welte K, et al. *Haematologica* 2003; 88:353.
230. Krajinovic M, Costea I, Chiasson S. *Lancet* 2002; 359:1033.
231. Kwok PY, Gu Z. *Mol Med Today* 1999; 5:538.
232. Emahazion T, Jobs M, Howell WM, et al. *Gene* 1999; 238:315.
233. Ross DT, Scherf U, Eisen MB, et al. *Nat Genet* 2000; 24:227.
234. Alizadeh AA, Eisen MB, Davis RE, et al. *Nature* 2000; 403:503.
235. Golub TR, Slonim DK, Tamayo P, et al. *Science* 1999; 286:531.
236. Evans WE, Relling MV. *Science* 1999; 286:487.
237. Krynetski EY, Evans WE. *Am J Hum Genet* 1998; 63:11.
238. Evans WE, Relling MV, Rodman JH, et al. *N Engl J Med* 1998; 338:499.
239. Evans WE, Johnson JA. *Annu Rev Genomics Hum Genet* 2001; 2:9.
240. McLeod HL, Evans WE. *Annu Rev Pharmacol Toxicol* 2001; 41:101.
241. Lindpaintner K. *Clin Chem Lab Med* 2003; 41:398.
242. Lesko LJ, Salerno RA, Spear BB, et al. *J Clin Pharmacol* 2003; 43:342.
243. Fijal BA, Hall JM, Witte JS. *Control Clin Trials* 2000; 21:7.
244. Rowinsky EK, Windle JJ, Von Hoff DD. *Clin Oncol* 1999; 17:3631.
245. Wood AJ. *Ther Drug Monit* 1998; 20:525.
246. Bertilsson L, Lou YQ, Du YL, et al. *Clin Pharmacol Ther* 1992; 51:388.

CHAPTER 63

Pharmacokinetics/Pharmacodynamics in Drug Development

G L Drusano, MD

Developing drugs requires a long, expensive process of discovery and preclinical development followed by clinical trials resulting in the submission of a package of data to a regulatory agency that will ultimately lead to licensure of that product for sale.

The goal of drug development is to find a dose of a drug for a specific indication that attains the desired therapeutic outcome while engendering a low probability of the patient experiencing a toxic event. Pharmacokinetics and pharmacodynamics can straightforwardly lead to attaining this goal. Indeed, in the last one to two decades there has been a marked increase in our understanding of the relationship between drug exposure and response. This is related to wider availability of the appropriate mathematical modeling methodologies. The application of these techniques in the time-line of drug development is presented in Figure 63-1.

The clearest example of employing a pharmacokinetic/pharmacodynamic approach to drug development can be seen in the area of anti-infective agents. Part of the reason for this is that these drugs are unique in that we are not attempting to dock a molecule into a receptor in the human body. Rather, the target of drug action and the site to which we are attempting to bind the drug is a receptor in the pathogen of interest. This has several important consequences.

The first is toxicity. Anti-infective targets are chosen specifically so that they have little sequence homology to similar mammalian targets. A straightforward example is the topoisomerase enzymes seen in bacteria but also in man. The fluoroquinolone antimicrobials have a 100- to 1000-fold difference in the concentrations necessary for microbiological effect relative to activity for topoisomerase targets in man.[1] In contrast, there is often a narrow therapeutic index, for example, between normal human cells and cancerous cells, meaning that oncologic chemotherapy is often (but not always) saddled with considerable toxicity.

The other important consequence is the ease with which pharmacodynamic relationships can be developed both preclinically as well as in clinical trials. The reason is that almost always (Hepatitis C is currently an exception to the rule) one can straightforwardly grow the pathogen of interest *in vitro* and determine a measure of drug exposure that will affect the growth of the pathogen in some standardized way. For example, for viruses, we can measure an EC_{50}, a drug concentration that will cause a 50% downturn in the number of rounds of replication per unit time. For bacteria, we can measure indices such as MICs or MBCs, that are defined as drug concentrations that will keep the bacteria from growing enough over an 18- to 24-hour period to cause turbidity in the growth medium (MIC) or to cause the number of bacteria to be reduced by 1000 fold over the 18–24 hour time frame (MBC). This ability to measure the difficulty a drug will encounter inhibiting or killing different pathogens allows the drug exposure necessary to achieve different endpoints to be normalized across pathogens. In contrast, if one were to try

to develop an anti-hypertensive agent, the true between-patient variability in the affinity with which a drug will bind to the receptor cannot currently be measured. Certainly, in the near future, the widespread use of phamacogenomic profiling, looking, for example, for specific single nucleotide polymorphisms (SNPs) or deletions will allow identification of patients likely to respond less well to therapy. Currently, however, this true between-patient variance in receptor affinity is completely unobserved variability.

Creating a Pharmacodynamic Relationship

MEASURE OF DRUG EXPOSURE—The process of creating a pharmacodynamic relationship starts with the idea of linking some measure of drug exposure to the outcome of interest. There are a number of measures of drug exposure that can be employed. Some of the most common are Peak concentration, Area Under the concentration-time Curve (AUC) and Time > Threshold. Many other measures of drug exposure are possible (eg, trough concentrations), but are usually related in some way to those mentioned above.

The critical idea behind which of these metrics is most closely linked to a specific measure of outcome is that the shape of the concentration-time curve may have an impact on the outcome measure. For example, for agents where the range of concentration that mediates minimal effect to that which mediates maximal effect is small, Time > Threshold will be the most useful metric for exposure. That is because higher concentrations will not produce significantly more effect than moderate concentrations. The overall effect will then be maximized by maintaining the drug concentration above the level that produces the degree of effect that is required. In contrast, many drugs are quite concentration-dependent in the effect that they produce. Here, much more effect will be produced at higher concentrations with much less being produced as concentrations decline. This will produce a situation where the total drug exposure will be linked to effect and AUC will be the most useful measure of drug exposure. Peak concentrations may be seen as linked to effect when an irreversible event occurs, such as covalent binding to a receptor that only occurs above a specific concentration. Here, only peak concentrations will produce enough exposure to have the binding occur in the appropriate time frame. This is the rarest situation seen in the development of pharmacodynamic relationships. Peak concentrations can also appear to be linked to outcome when there is a mixture of populations of sensitive and less sensitive targets present. This will be discussed in greater detail below under the topic of suppression of emergence of resistance.

For the development of such relationships for anti-infective agents, the exposure measures are normalized to the measure

Drug Discovery and Preclinical Development

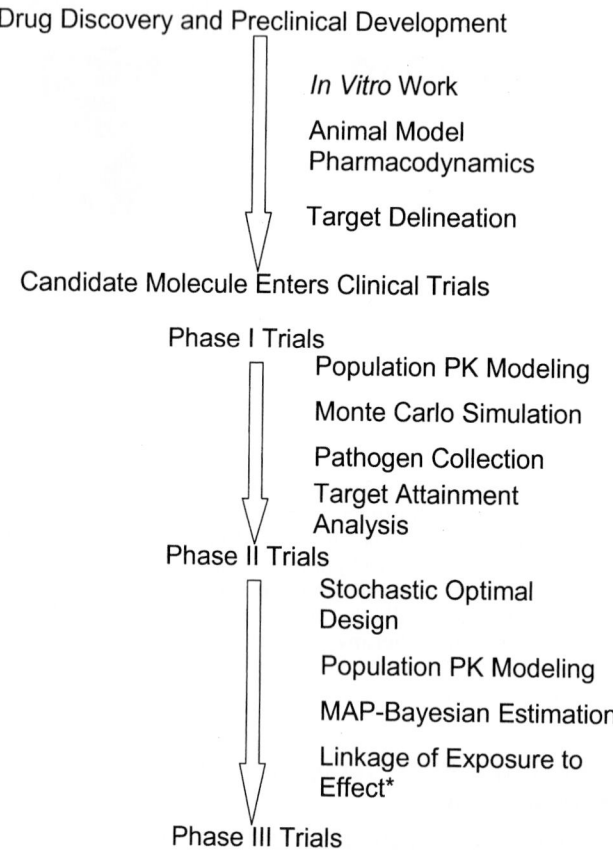

Figure 63-1. Use of pharmacodynamics in the drug development process.

of susceptibility of the pathogen to the drug being studied (eg, MIC, EC_{50}). This produces a hybrid measure that explicitly depends on the drug exposure, but also on the pathogen being studied. So we can now measure Time > MIC, AUC/MIC ratio, or Peak Concentration/MIC ratio.

As an example of the shape of the curve having an impact on the effect developed by drug exposure, the β-lactam antibiotic imipenem/cilastatin was studied in a neutropenic mouse thigh infection model by Fluckiger, Segessenmann, and Gerber.[2] The actual idea that the shape of the curve can affect the endpoint measured was popularized by the laboratory of Craig,[3–5] but arguably the clearest demonstration was by Fluckiger.[2] In this study, the effect of a dose of drug was determined on the number of organisms present at the primary infection site. In parallel, a second cohort of animals received the same drug dose, but on a highly fractionated basis, so that the resultant concentration-time curve had a much lower peak concentration, but remained above the MIC for a much longer time interval. The AUC/MIC ratios developed in the two cohorts were nearly identical. The results are shown in Figure 63-2. The number of organisms killed was much greater when the Time > MIC was longer. This indicates that there was no benefit derived from the high peak concentrations developed in the first group and that keeping the drug concentrations in excess of the MIC was the effect driver in this circumstance.

An example of exactly the opposite linkage can be seen with fluoroquinolone antimicrobials, as well as other agents like aminoglycosides, or the new anti-MRSA agent, daptomycin. For these drugs, there is a clear relationship between drug concentration and the rate of organism kill that is engendered. In

this circumstance, AUC/MIC ratio is the exposure variable most closely linked to outcome.

In a study by Louie et al,[6] a mouse thigh infection model study was performed using methodology similar to that described above, but without the massive dose fractionation. An exposure-response curve was described (Fig 63-3). On the steep part of the curve Q 24 hour, Q 12 hour, and Q 6 hour administration schedules were studied, so that the 24-hour AUC was the same for each group (same AUC/MIC ratio), but that the once daily dosing group had the highest Peak concentrations (and hence Peak concentration/MIC ratio) while the Q 6 hour dosing group attained the longest Time > M IC. When the results for these groups were tested for differences by analysis of variance, no differences could be discerned (Table 63-1). This indicates that for daptomycin, AUC/MIC ratio is the exposure variable most closely linked to outcome.

CHOOSING THE TARGET—In the examples given above, a microbiological endpoint was chosen. This is because we were dealing with animal model systems. It is important to recognize that in the drug development process, there will be a progression from a preclinical stage to the performance of clinical trials to document safety and efficacy.

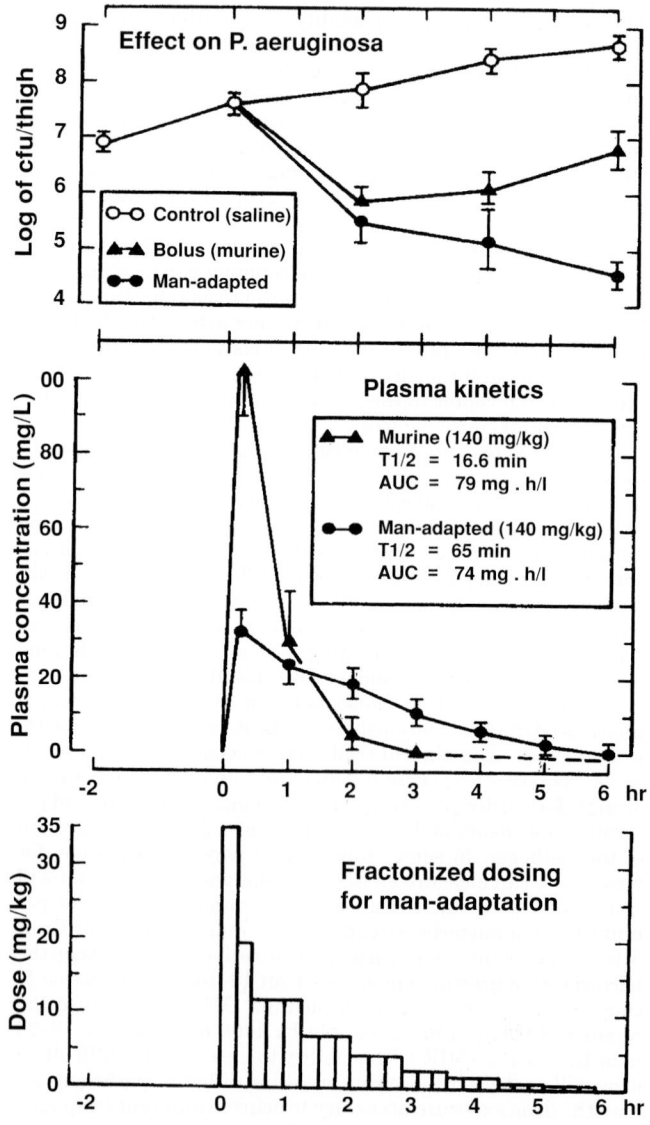

Figure 63-2. Effect of the shape of the concentration-time curve on the ability of imipenem-cilastatin to kill *P aeruginosa* in a mouse thigh infection model. (From Fluckiger U, Segessenmann C, Gerber AU. *Antimicrob Agents Chemother* 1991; 35:1905.)

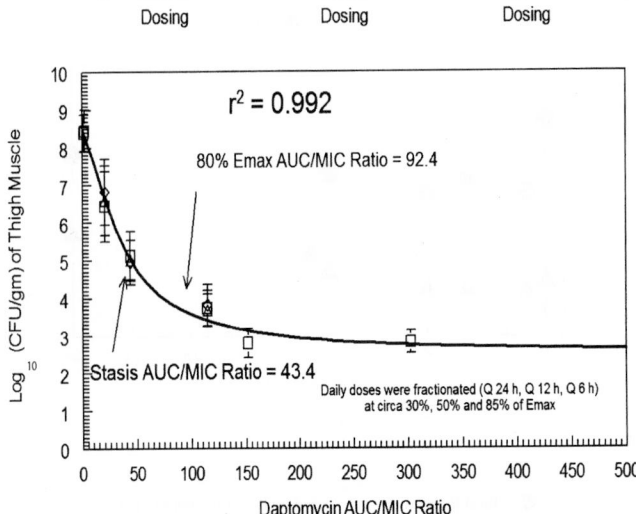

Figure 63-3. Relationship between the 24-h AUC/MIC ratio of dapto-mycin and log10 CFU of *S. aureus* per gram of thigh muscle (mean ± 1 SD) when the total daily dose of daptomycin is given as one dose in 24 h, two equally divided doses every 12 h, or four equally divided doses every 6 h. The total daily doses of 2.5, 5.6, and 15.0 mg of daptomycin/kg resulted in AUC/MIC ratios of approximately 21, 44, and 115, respectively. The AUC/MIC ratio for a given total daily dose was similar regardless of whether a total daily dose was administered as one, two, or four equally divided doses over 24 h. (From Louie A, Kaw P, Liu W, et al. *Antimicrob Agents Chemother* 2001; 45:845.)

Prior to the inception of clinical trials, animal model and *in vitro* systems are required for the determination of the true pharmacodynamically linked effect variable (eg, AUC/MIC ratio, Time > MIC). After the start of clinical trials, we can examine either clinical or microbiological endpoints. These endpoints can be dichotomous in nature (succeed/fail, eradication/persistence) or can be continuous (microbiological quantitative repetitive sampling from an infection site). The target that is chosen in either of these circumstances will determine, to a great degree, the dose that is required to attain the target.

In the preclinical circumstance, one can examine the ability of a regimen (dose and schedule) to kill organisms at a primary infection site (as above, Figs 63-2 and 63-3). Alternatively, one could examine a mortality endpoint. In either circumstance, the model system could be developed so that the animal was either normal or rendered immunocompromised. In each instance, this will change the interpretation of the endpoint chosen and, in the case of an immunocompromised animal system, will require a larger drug exposure to achieve whatever endpoint is desired. The reason to perform these studies in immunocompromised animals is twofold. First, it is a conservative measure of the drug exposure required to achieve whatever target is desired. It is a more direct measure of "bug versus drug." Second, and perhaps as important, it is much easier to find strains of pathogens that will grow in whatever model is being used. In the presence of the full immune system of the animal, many pathogens will self-clear over the period of observation in the no-treatment control group. This renders the interpretation of the experiment much more difficult.

It is also important to recognize that the animal system being employed should accurately reflect the local pharmacokinetics of the drug for the indication being sought. While a mouse thigh infection model may accurately represent the ability of the drug to kill organisms in a skin/skin structure infection, the lessons learned and exposure targets derived would not be helpful if the drug were going to be studied for a meningitis indication in clinical trials.

This also raises the issue of what endpoint will be chosen. Do we wish merely to shut off organism growth or to kill the organism at the primary infection site to a specific degree (eg, 1 $\log_{10}$ (CFU/g) kill, 2 $\log_{10}$ (CFU/g) kill, 80% of maximal kill). Figure 63-3 demonstrates that an AUC/MIC ratio of 43.4 is required to shut off growth of the organism, whereas attaining 80% of the maximal bacterial kill for this strain of *Staphylococcus aureus* requires a larger exposure, with an AUC/MIC ratio of 92.4. For a relatively uncomplicated skin and skin structure infection, attaining an exposure target that will result in organism stasis is likely all that is required. However, for a complicated skin and skin structure infection, particularly if bacteremia would be likely, an exposure target that would drive some high percentage of the maximal bacterial kill (80–90% of maximal kill) would be more appropriate. This choice of target is crucial to the successful choice of an appropriate drug dose for clinical trial.

SUPPRESSION OF EMERGENCE OF RESISTANCE AS AN ENDPOINT—Until recently, little has been done with suppression of emergence of resistance as an endpoint for the choice of drug dose. The key idea underlying the problem of emergence of resistance is the population burden of bacterial cells at an infection site relative to the inverse of the mutational frequency to resistance. If the population burden exceeds the inverse of the mutation frequency, there will be a high probability (but not a certainty) that organisms bearing a resistance mechanism will already be present. The larger the burden relative to the frequency, the higher will be the probability. This means there will be multiple populations of organisms present at the time that drug therapy is initiated. It is not surprising that the population bearing a resistance mechanism will respond quite differently to the pressure of drug therapy than will the population without this mechanism. Again, as above, the example used will be from the anti-infective literature, but the lessons are clearly applicable in the realm of oncolytic chemotherapy.

In Figure 63-4 Panels A-D, the effect of different doses (including a no-treatment control) of the fluoroquinolone levofloxacin on the total and resistant populations of *Pseudomonas aeruginosa* is displayed.[7] As the effect was determined at multiple time points, it allowed the effect of the drug concentrations on the two populations to be modeled simultaneously for all regimens.[7] This allowed a calculation of dose to maximally amplify the resistant population as well as a dose to hold the number of clones in the resistant population steady. These doses were then studied prospectively over a longer time frame (24 versus 48 hours) as a validation of the modeling result. This is displayed in Figure 63-5.

This is the first prospective validation that a target drug exposure can be derived to suppress the amplification of mutant subpopulations. This makes the point that the choice of the exposure target is flexible and is a choice that should be made with great care if the drug is to achieve the hoped-for results when it enters clinical trials. If the toxicity profile of the drug allows it, a suppression of resistance endpoint may be wise, as it will extend the lifetime of the drug.

CHOOSING A DRUG DOSE FROM PRECLINICAL PLUS PHASE I DATA—Once the appropriate animal or *in*

Table 63-1. *Staphylococcus aureus* **Densities in Thigh Muscles of Mice That Were Treated With Various Doses of Daptomycin, Administered in One, Two, or Four Divided Doses**

Staphylococcus aureus Densities
($\log_{10}$ (CFU/g) + 1 Standard Deviation) with:

TOTAL DOSAGE (MG/KG)	1 DOSE	2 DIVIDED DOSES[b]	4 DIVIDED DOSES[c]	P VALUE[a]
2.5	6.54 ± 0.98	6.83 ± 0.88	6.61 ± 0.93	0.64
5.6	5.12 ± 0.66	4.96 ± 0.59	5.02 ± 0.52	0.73
15.0	3.73 ± 0.48	3.82 ± 0.55	3.68 ± 0.43	0.59

[a]Statistical testing was performed by analysis of variance. A P value of <0.05 was considered statistically significant.
[b]One-half of the single dose was administered at 0 hour and then 12 hours later.
[c]One-quarter the single dose was administered at 0 hour and then 6, 12 and 18 hours later.

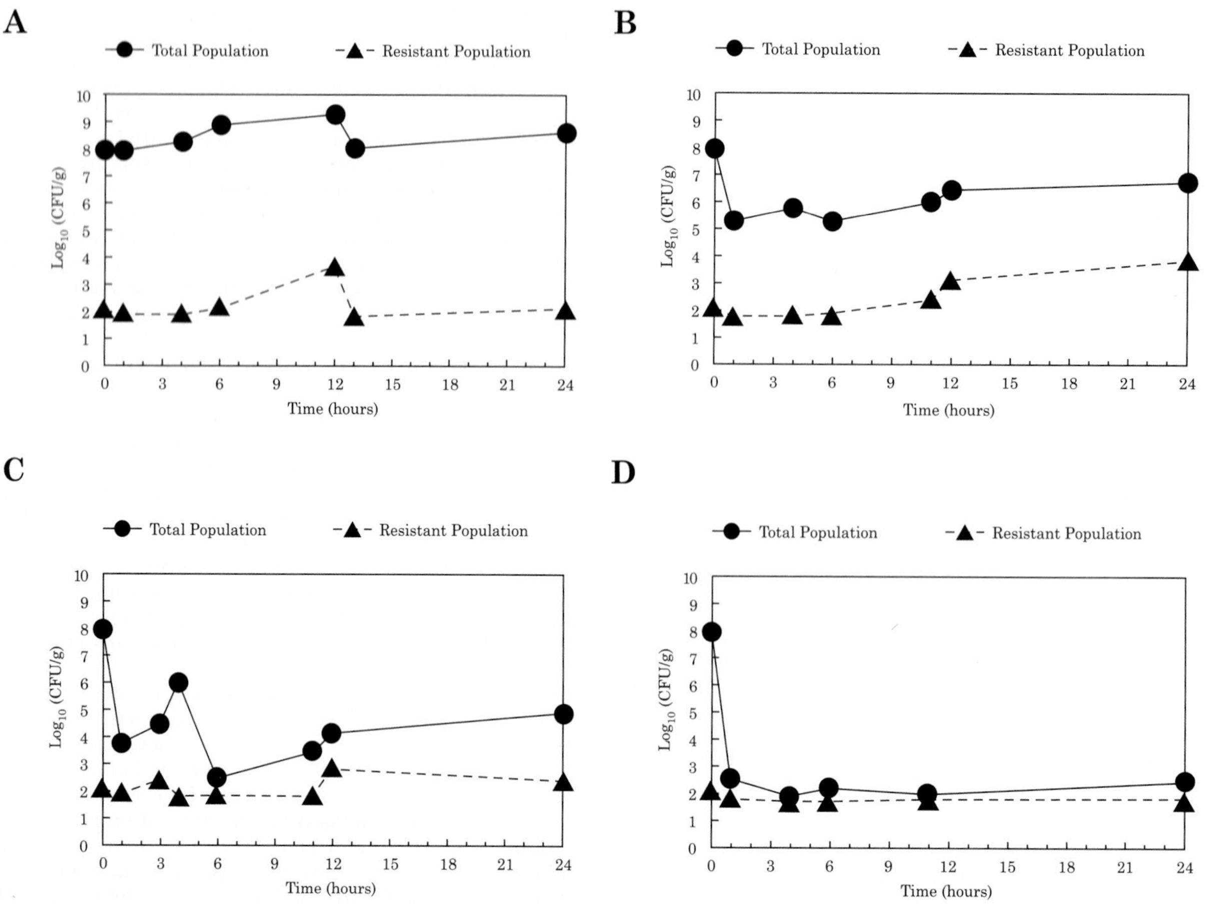

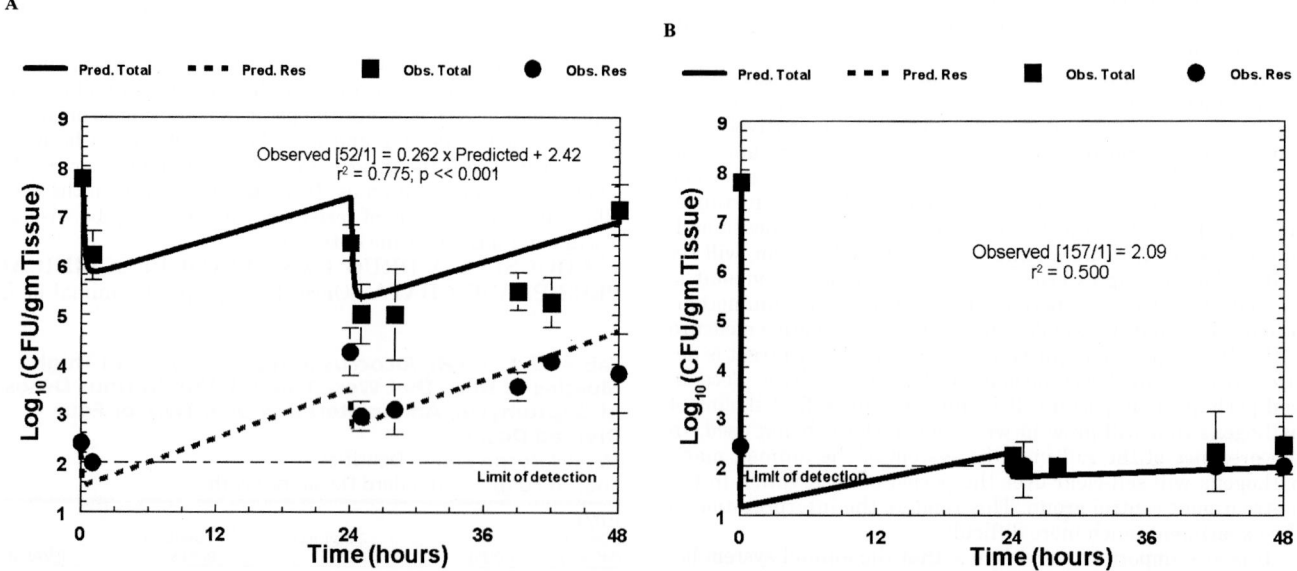

Figure 63-4. Effect of 4 drug doses of levofloxacin on the total and resistant bacterial populations of Pseudomonas aeruginosa over 24 hours. Drug doses were 0, 90, 215, and 600 mg/kg (Figure 63-3, panels A-D, respectively). The 90 mg/kg dose allowed amplification of the resistant population by almost 2 $\log_{10}$ (CFU/g). The 215 mg/kg dose allowed only minimal resistant mutant amplification. (From Jumbe N, Louie A, Leary R, et al. *The Journal of Clinical Investigation* 2003; 112(2):275. Reproduced with permission from the American Society for Clinical Investigation.).

Figure 63-5. Model validation. The emergence of resistance model developed in this study was prospectively evaluated and validated by generating response predictions for doses not previously studied that would (A) encourage selection of resistance or (B) suppress emergence of resistance. An exposure of an AUC/MIC ratio of 157/1 was calculated to prevent emergence of resistance. Experiments were performed to 48, not 24 hours as in the studies performed to generate parameter estimates, using model predicted conditions. Levofloxacin dosing occurred at time 0 and at 24 hours. The lines are model predictions (not best-fit curves). (■) represents experimental measurements of the total population. (•) represents experimental measurements of the resistant subpopulation. The model predicted changes in the resistant mutant population well at both exposures. (From Jumbe N, Louie A, Leary R, et al. *The Journal of Clinical Investigation* 2003; 112(2):275. Reproduced with permission from the American Society for Clinical Investigation.).

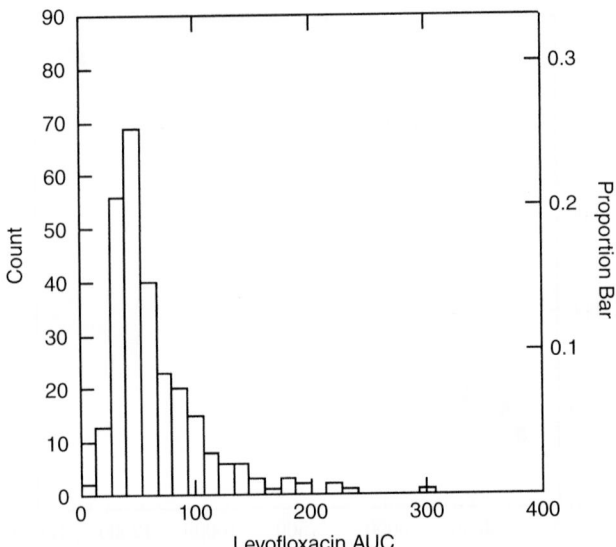

Figure 63-6. The distribution of Area Under the concentration-time Curve (AUC) values for 272 patients receiving 500 mg of levofloxacin for the therapy of community-acquired infections.

vitro models have been chosen and the drug studied in these systems, the linked pharmacodynamic variable will have been elucidated and the exposure target(s) identified for the indications that are to be sought for the drug. A critical issue is how to employ the pharmacodynamic information to allow the "correct" dose of drug to be chosen for clinical trial(s).

The ability of a specific dose of drug to attain the desired exposure target is influenced by a small number of factors. These are (*i*) The true between-patient variability in drug pharmacokinetics; (*ii*) The variability in the MIC of the drug for the pathogens of interest (ie, those pathogens that are likely causes of the diseases for which indications are being sought); (*iii*) The protein binding of the agent being studied. Each of these factors will be examined in turn.

PHARMACOKINETIC VARIABILITY—True between-patient variability in pharmacokinetics clearly exists. The same dose of drug will produce very different drug concentration profiles if given to a large number of patients. We can account for some portion of this variance by measuring covariates such as age, sex, weight, height, creatinine clearance, etc. However, even after examining these and other covariates, there will still be true, residual between-patient variance. Accounting for this variability plays an important role in determining the correct dose for clinical trials. The basic idea is that whatever dose is chosen, it should be adequate to attain the desired exposure target in a very high proportion of the population of interest.

It is important to obtain an idea of the degree of variability of the drug exposure achieved when a fixed dose of drug is administered. Preston et al[8] studied 272 patients with community-acquired infections who received the fluoroquinolone antibiotic levofloxacin. In this study, all patients had a serum creatinine that was <2.0 mg/dl. Figure 63-6 shows the variability in AUC achieved in these patients with a fixed dose of drug. In this relatively normal community-based population there was a >10-fold range of AUCs observed.

It is unusual to have such a rich data set early on in drug development. The usual reality is to have anywhere between 12 and 60 volunteers who have had the drug's pharmacokinetics studied. These study subjects represent a very biased estimator of how the drug will be handled in the population of interest, most of whom will be older and, by definition, sicker than the normal volunteer population. Nevertheless, if these data can be employed to choose a drug dose, it will almost certainly be a conservative choice.

Monte Carlo simulation is a mathematical technique that allows prior knowledge of the central tendency of a parameter

and its distribution to be employed to set up a sampling distribution. That is, we can take a large number of samples (eg, 1,000, 10,000, 30,000) from the "known" prior distribution of parameter values. These can be used to calculate Peak concentrations, AUC values, or Time > Threshold. It provides the opportunity to perform large clinical trials "*in silico.*" These measures of drug exposure then can be employed to determine how often a specific drug dose will produce an exposure that will attain the exposure target value for a specific MIC.

MICROBIOLOGICAL VARIABILITY—Usually the pathogen(s) of interest for a specific indication have a broad range of values. It is obvious that for whatever range of drug exposures are achieved by a specific dose, it will be more difficult to achieve the exposure target for an organism with a higher MIC value.

Luckily, the determination of the range of MIC values for organisms that are causative pathogens for the indications being studied is relatively straightforward to obtain.

PROTEIN BINDING—As a rule, only non-protein bound drug is active. This has been most clearly seen in two studies, one of bacteria[9] and one of HIV.[10]

Merriken, Briant, and Rolinson[9] examined a group of isoxazolyl penicillins for their activity against *Staphylococcus aureus*. There were 7 molecules studied. Each was chosen because it had the same MIC for the challenge strain of Staphylococcus and had very similar pharmacokinetics, but had very different protein binding that ranged from 30% bound to >97% bound. When examined in a mouse model, the effect of the drug was related to the free fraction of the drug concentration (Fig 63-7).

For HIV, Bilello et al[10] examined a highly bound (ca 90%) HIV-1 protease inhibitor and examined the impact of protein binding *in vitro*. In a transitive logic set of experiments, the impact in free fraction of the major drug binding protein for this agent (α-1 acid glycoprotein) was determined. In Figure 63-8A, it is demonstrated that increasing the amount of binding protein over the physiologic range of 0.5–1.5 mg/ml decreases the free fraction in a quantitative manner. In was also demonstrated (Fig 63-8B) that lower free amounts of drug were associated with less cell-associated drug. Finally, the lower cell-associated

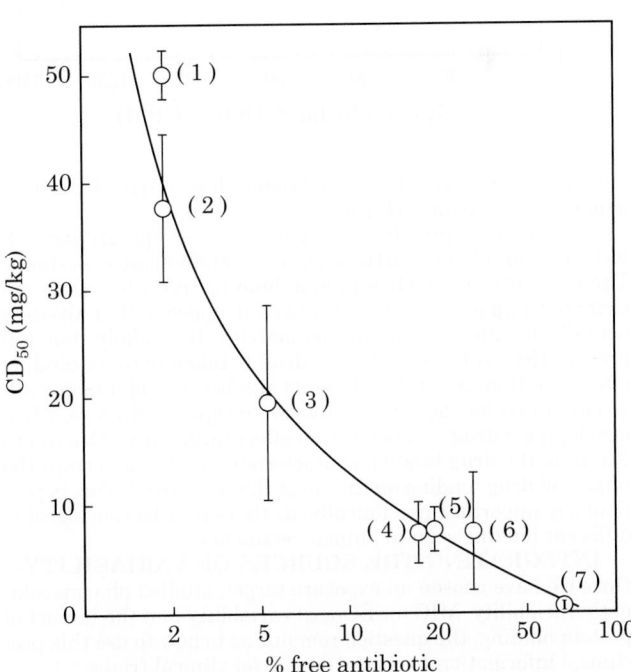

Figure 63-7. The effect of protein binding on the microbiological activity of 7 isoxazolyl penicillins as determined in a mouse model of Staphylococcal intraperitoneal infection. (From Merriken DJ, Briant J, Rolinson GN. *J Antimicrob Chemother* 1983; 11:233.)

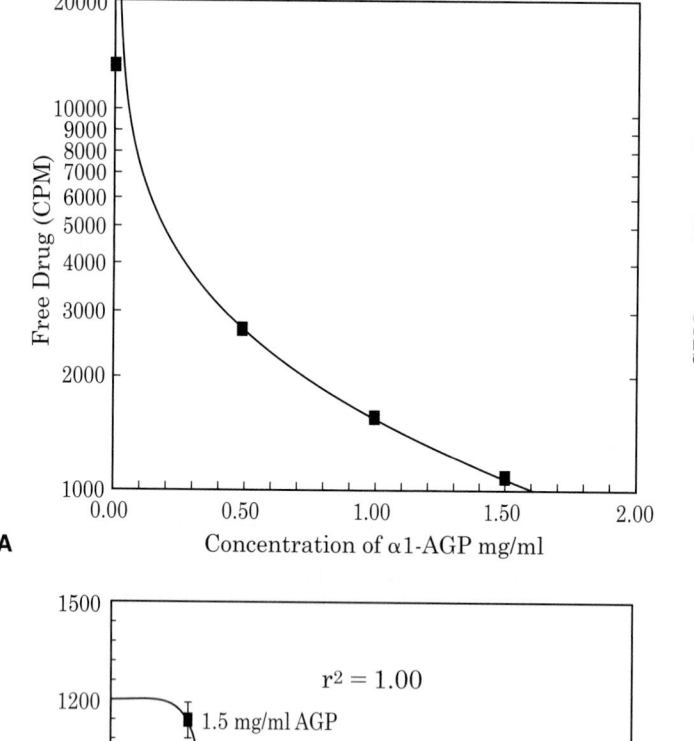

A

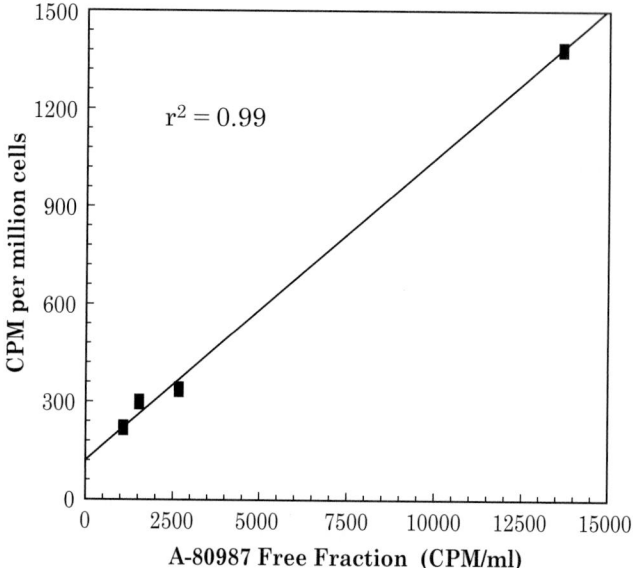

B

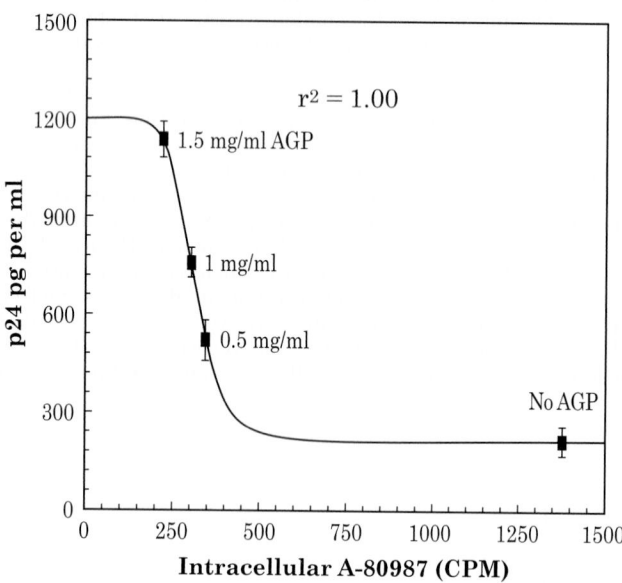

C

Figure 63-8. Effect of protein binding on the antiviral activity of a HIV-1 protease inhibitor. In (A), increasing amounts of the major binding protein (α-1 acid glycoprotein) results in a deceasing amount of unbound drug. In (B), the decrease in unbound drug is shown to be associated with decreased cellular penetration. In (C), it is shown that decreased amounts of intracellular drug is associated with decreased antiviral effect. Together, these experiments demonstrate that protein binding has a major impact on virological activity.

amounts of drug were shown to produce less antiviral effect, in a quantitative fashion (Fig 63-8C).

Clearly, then, protein binding has a major, quantitative effect on drug effect, particularly in microbiological systems. There are instances when protein binding has a less than anticipated impact on effect or where it appears that there is actually no effect of binding on activity. It is likely (but unproven) that in these instances drug is taken onto its binding effect site from its protein-binding site because of a major difference in K_d for the drug for the two receptors. Even so, when developing a drug and picking an effect target, it is wise to understand the drug binding characteristics and to ascertain the impact of drug binding on the effect that is desired. This is particularly important preclinically, as there may be considerably different binding seen in animal versus man.

INTEGRATING THE SOURCES OF VARIABILITY—

Once we have chosen an exposure target, studied pharmacokinetic variability, MIC (or $EC_{50/95}$) variability and the impact of protein binding, the question remains as to how to use this preclinical information to choose dose(s) for clinical trials.

Our group (11–14) developed the use of Monte Carlo simulation to integrate these disparate sources of variability. In the paradigm developed, a population pharmacokinetic study is performed. The measure of central tendency (usually, but not necessarily the mean parameter values) and dispersion (full or

major diagonal covariance matrix) are employed to generate a Monte Carlo simulation for specific drug doses. These generated values are then corrected for protein binding, as a function of the measured impact of binding on effect. Then the fraction of the simulated population that attains the desired exposure target is determined for different values of MIC (or $EC_{50/95}$). In so doing, clear breakpoint values for pathogen drug susceptibility can be determined for a specific dose of drug. Because we have information regarding the distribution of MIC (or $EC_{50/95}$) values, the overall response of the population can be determined by taking a weighted average over the product of the range of target attainment rates and MIC (or $EC_{50/95}$) values.

An example of this technique validated with a prospective study was performed with an HIV-1 non-nucleoside reverse transcriptase inhibitor [NNRTI].[14] The target agreed upon was keeping trough free drug concentrations above the EC_{90} of HIV. Preclinical study demonstrated that addition of purified binding proteins to the medium increased the EC_{50} value by 7.6-fold. In addition, other preclinical studies demonstrated that there was approximately a 10-fold change in drug concentration between the EC_{50} and the EC_{90}. Therefore, a 76-fold adjustment was made to the simulated trough concentrations of the drug for doses of 50 mg, 100 mg, and 200 mg. Finally, preliminary preclinical data indicated that different wild-type HIV isolates all had EC_{50} values less than 10 nM. In Figure 63-9A, the target

A

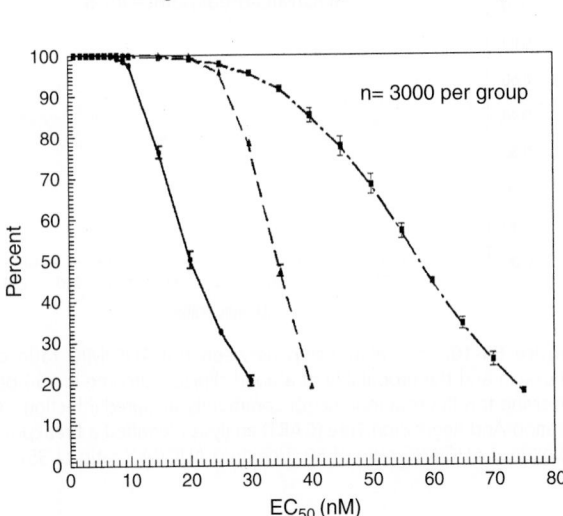

Percentage of Simulated Subjects with Trough
Free Drug of GW420867X > 10XEC$_{50}$ of HIV
50 mg
100 mg
200 mg
n= 3000 per group
Percent
EC$_{50}$ (nM)

Figure 63-9. In (A), three different doses of an experimental non-nucleoside reverse transcriptase inhibitor keep free drug in excess of the EC$_{90}$ of HIV for the whole dosing interval to the same extent, as long as the EC$_{50}$ is less than 10 nM. As is demonstrated in (B), this leads to equipotent antiretroviral activity in a Phase I/II randomized, double-blind clinical trial.

Log$_{10}$ Plasma HIV-1 RNA from Baseline, copies/mL
GW420867X Alone
GW420867X+ZDV+3TC
Placebo
GW420867X 50mg
GW420867X 100mg
GW420867X 200mg
Days

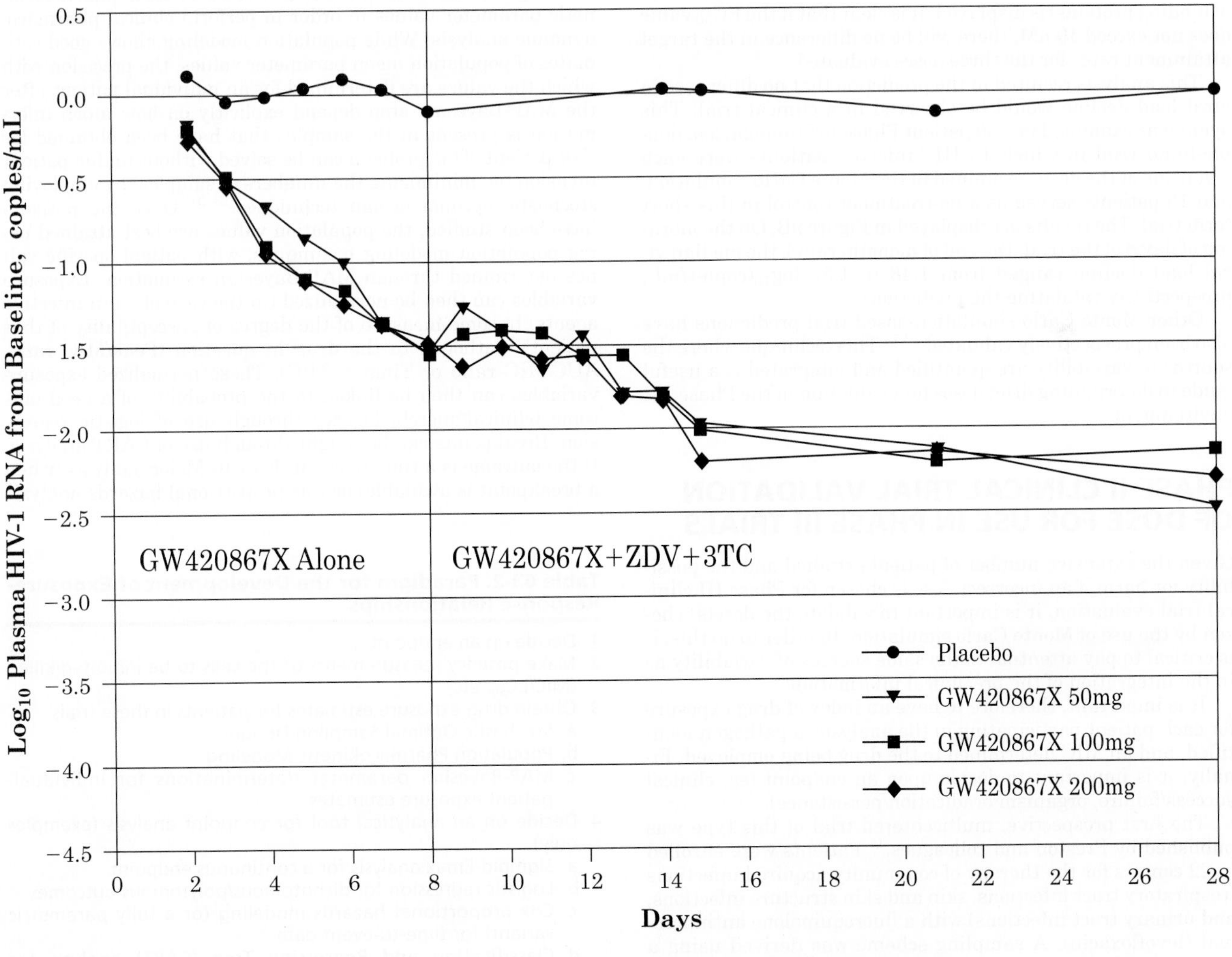

B

Levofloxacin Clinical Outcome
Probability of Clinical Success

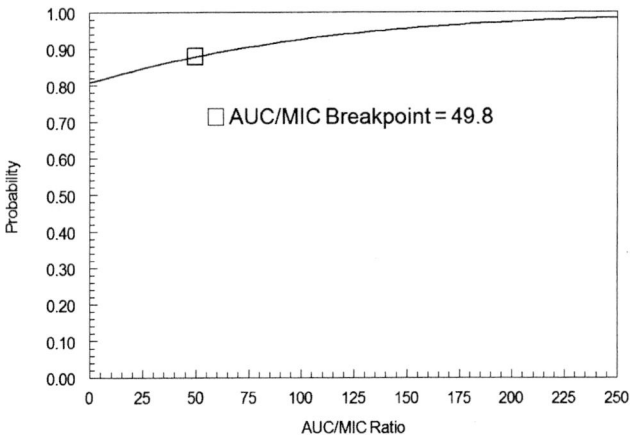

Figure 63-10. The relationship between the AUC/MIC ratio of levofloxacin and the probability of a good clinical outcome in 134 patients receiving this fluoroquinolone for community-acquired infections. Classification And Regression Tree (CART) analysis identified a breakpoint of a total drug AUC/MIC ratio of 50 (free drug AUC/MIC ratio of 35).

attainment rate by EC_{50} values (not determined in the presence of binding proteins) is displayed. It is clear that if the EC_{50} value does not exceed 10 nM, there will be no difference in the target attainment rates for the three doses evaluated.

This analysis resulted in the prediction that no difference in viral load decline would be observed in a clinical trial. This agent was examined in a 60 patient Phase I/II randomized, double-blind trial in which 15 HIV-infected patients were each given one of the doses examined in the Monte Carlo simulation, and 15 patients served as a no-treatment control in this short term trial. The results are displayed in Figure 9B. On the morning of day 8 of the trial (the end of monotherapy), the median viral load decline ranged from 1.48 to 1.52 $\log_{10}$(copies/ml), prospectively validating the predictions.

Other Monte Carlo simulation-based trial predictions have also been prospectively validated.[12,13] This technique where the sources of variability are quantified and integrated is a useful guide to determining drug doses for evaluation in the Phase I/II environment.

PHASE II CLINICAL TRIAL VALIDATION OF DOSE FOR USE IN PHASE III TRIALS

Given the extensive number of patients studied and the possibility for harm if an incorrect dose is chosen for Phase III clinical trial evaluation, it is important to validate the dose(s) chosen by the use of Monte Carlo simulation. In order to do this, it is critical to pay attention to the same sources of variability as in the integration of the preclinical information.

It is important, therefore to have an index of drug exposure for each patient participating in the analysis, a pathogen identified, and an MIC determined to the drug being employed. Finally, it is important to decide upon an endpoint (eg, clinical success/failure, organism eradication/persistence).

The first prospective, multicentered trial of this type was published by Preston and colleagues.[15] Patients were enrolled in 22 centers for the therapy of community-acquired infections (respiratory tract infections, skin and skin structure infections, and urinary tract infections) with a fluoroquinolone antimicrobial (levofloxacin). A sampling scheme was derived using a stochastic D-optimal sampling technique. There were 272 patients who had pharmacokinetic data collected. These data

were analyzed employing a non-parametric population modeling technique (NPEM II program of Schumitzky and Jelliffe). Individual estimates of exposure were calculated for each patient by obtaining patient-specific pharmacokinetic parameter values employing Maximum A-posteriori Probability (MAP) Bayesian parameter estimation. Of these patients, there were 134 patients with a documented outcome and identified pathogen that had a levofloxacin MIC. For clinical outcome, both Peak/MIC ratio as well as AUC/MIC ratio could be linked to outcome. As there has been considerable preclinical data linking AUC/MIC ratio to fluoroquinolone effect, this relationship will be presented in Figure 63-10. The breakpoint AUC/MIC value, determined by Classification and Regression Tree (CART) analysis, was 49.8. This was for total drug. The free drug value would be 34.9. A mouse thigh infection model developed in our laboratory examined levofloxacin for the therapy of *Streptococcus pneumoniae*.[16] The value for an organism kill of 1 log10(cfu/g) was 29.4 for a free drug AUC/MIC ratio. The free drug AUC/MIC value associated with a good outcome determined in a separate clinical study by Ambrose only for *Streptococcus pneumoniae* for two fluoroquinolones (levofloxacin and gatifloxacin) was 27.2–33.7.[17] All these determinations are in excellent concordance.

What is clear is that it is possible to identify targets for desired drug action preclinically and to bridge between animal and man employing Monte Carlo simulation techniques. Further, it is also clear that these findings are robust. They have been validated in clinical trials. The paradigm for clinical validation is simple. It is set forth in Table 63-2. It is important to obtain good individual-patient estimates of their pharmacokinetic parameter values in order to perform clinical pharmacodynamic analysis. While population modeling allows good estimates of population mean parameter values, the precision with which the values are determined for an individual patient after the MAP-Bayesian step depend explicitly on how much information is present in the samples that have been obtained for *that* patient. This problem can be solved without undue patient invasion (ie, minimizing the numbers of samples) by employing stochastic optimal design techniques.[18–21] Once the patients have been studied, the population values are best attained using population modeling techniques, with patient-specific values determined through MAP-Bayesian estimation. Exposure variables can then be normalized (in the case of anti-infective agents) to some measure of the degree of susceptibility of that patient's pathogen to the drug in question (Peak/MIC ratio, AUC/MIC ratio or Time > MIC). These normalized exposure variables can then be linked to the probability of a good outcome (clinical/microbiological) through use of logistic regression. Breakpoints can be sought through use of CART analysis. If the outcome is a time-to-event, Kaplan-Meier analysis (when a breakpoint is available) or Cox proportional hazards analysis

---

Table 63-2. Paradigm for the Development of Exposure-Response Relationships

1. Decide on an endpoint
2. Make potency measurements of the cells to be inhibited/killed (MIC/EC$_{50}$, etc)
3. Obtain drug exposure estimates for patients in these trials
   a. Stochastic Optimal Sampling Design
   b. Population Pharmacokinetic Modeling
   c. MAP-Bayesian parameter determinations for individual-patient exposure estimates
4. Decide on an analytical tool for endpoint analysis (examples only)
   a. Sigmoid-Emax analysis for a continuous endpoint
   b. Logistic regression for dichotomous/polytomous outcomes
   c. Cox proportional hazards modeling (or a fully parametric variant) for time-to-event data
   d. Classification and Regression Tree (CART) analysis for breakpoint determination

(for a continuous variable) can be employed. If the outcome is a continuous variable (eg, viral load determination), some variant of a sigmoid-Emax effect model can be employed to link exposure to effect.

Determination of a pharmacodynamically linked variable pre-clinically with an exposure target combined with a target attainment analysis from Phase I/II data will allow identification of a dose for Phase III trials. Validation of this outcome in a (relatively) small Phase II trial will provide confidence that the dose chosen for large, Phase III clinical trial investigation is optimal for the effect target desired. This will maximize the speed of drug development and minimize drug failure.

REFERENCES

1. Albertini S, Chetalat AA, Miller B, et al. *Mutagenesis* 1995; 10:343.
2. Fluckiger U, Segessenmann C, Gerber AU. *Antimicrob Agents Chemother* 1991; 35:1905.
3. Gerber AU, Craig WA, Brugger HP, et al. *J Infect Dis* 1982; 146:691.
4. Vogelman B, Gudmundsson S, Leggett J, et al. *J Infect Dis* 1988; 158:831.
5. Leggett JE, Fantin B, Ebert S, et al. *J Infect Dis* 1989; 159:281.
6. Louie A, Kaw P, Liu W, et al. *Antimicrob Agents Chemother* 2001; 45:845.
7. Jumbe N, Louie A, Leary R, et al. *J Clin Invest* 2003; 112:275–285.
8. Preston SL, Drusano GL, Berman AL, et al. *Antimicrob Agents Chemother* 1998; 42:1098.
9. Merriken DJ, Briant J, Rolinson GN. *J Antimicrob Chemother* 1983; 11:233.
10. Bilello JA, Bilello PA, Stellrecht K, et al. *Antimicrob Agents Chemother* 1996; 40:1491.
11. FDA Anti-Infective Drug Products Advisory Committee. October 15, 1998.
12. Drusano GL, Preston SL, Hardalo C, et al. *Antimicrob Agents Chemother* 2001; 45:13.
13. Drusano GL, Bilello JA, Preston SL, et al. *J Infect Dis* 2001; 183:1126.
14. Drusano GL, Moore KHP, Kleim JP, et al. *Antimicrob Agents Chemother* 2002; 46:913.
15. Preston SL, Drusano GL, Berman AL, et al. *J Am Med Assoc* 1998; 279:125.
16. Tumbe NL, Louie A, Liu W, Miller MA, Drusano GL. 40th Interscience Conference on Antimicrobial Agents and Chemotherapy, Abstract 291, 2000.
17. Ambrose PG, Grasela DM, Grasela TH, et al. *Antimicrob Agents Chemother* 2001; 45:2793.
18. Drusano GL, Forrest A, Snyder MJ, et al. *Clin Pharmacol Therapeut* 1988; 44:232.
19. Drusano GL, Forrest A, Plaisance KI, et al. *Clin Pharmacol Therapeut* 1989; 45:635.
20. Drusano GL, Forrest A, Yuen JA, et al. *J Clin Pharmacol* 1994; 34:967.
21. Tam VH, Preston SL, Drusano GL. *Antimicrob Agents Chemother* 2003; 47:2888–2891.

PART 7

Pharmaceutical and Medicinal Agents

Steven Gelone, PharmD
Consultant
AGE Consultants
Wyndmoor, PA

Alfonso R Gennaro, PhD
Professor Emeritus of Chemistry
University of the Sciences in Philadelphia
Philadelphia, PA

Diagnostic Drugs and Reagents

Elaine D Mackowiak, PhD, RPh

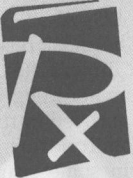

Optimum treatment of a patient begins after a physician makes a diagnosis. This process usually begins with a discussion between patient and physician regarding symptoms the patient is experiencing. The physician performs a physical examination of the patient and then decides if further tests are required for diagnosis.

Biological samples such as blood, urine, or tissue biopsy may be required for in vitro analysis that may use chemical reagents and scientific instruments. However, accurate analysis depends on the purity of reagents and proper functioning and calibration of any instrumentation. The United States Pharmacopeia/National Formulary publishes standards for reagents used in testing.

Certain diagnostic procedures require the administration of drugs to the patient for determining the functional status of organs and tissues within the body, in vivo tests. Some diagnostic drugs are not metabolized as they pass through the body; inulin is a classic example of this type of diagnostic drug. Inulin is administered intravenously and filtered by the glomeruli. It is not reabsorbed or secreted by the renal tubules and is excreted unchanged. Measurement of inulin in the urine provides information about the glomerular filtration rate of the kidney, thereby providing information about the status of kidney function. The incidence of adverse drug effects to inulin is very low.

Other drugs must undergo rather extensive processes in the body before they provide the information needed for diagnosis. For example, iopanoic acid is administered orally after consumption of a fat-free meal the evening before the scheduled examination of gallbladder function. Iopanoic acid is absorbed from the gastrointestinal tract, concentrating in the gallbladder. The next morning the patient has an x-ray study of the gallbladder, cholecystography. Iopanic acid is eventually excreted in the feces and urine. Adverse effects from ingestion of iopanoic acid are mild, usually nausea and diarrhea, but allergic reactions may occur.

Cholecystography requires that the drug possesses radiopaque properties. A radiopaque drug absorbs x-rays so that the organ, in this case the gallbladder, can be visualized and distinguished from other structures in the abdomen. Body structures can be examined using radioactive drugs, which provide their own source of ionizing radiation to produce images. Newer techniques using magnetic resonance and ultrasound have been developed that produce images. Some studies may require the administration of drugs, but each imaging modality requires drugs with different physical properties.

The physician's order for any diagnostic test must balance the benefit of the procedure with the risk to the patient. Factors the physician considers before ordering any diagnostic test are: (1) the type of information needed, (2) the sensitivity and specificity of the procedure, (3) potential adverse effects associated with the procedure, (4) concomitant diseases of the patient, (5) current drug therapy of the patient, and (6) cost of the procedure. MF Roizen expressed these concerns by writing, "In this era of cost efficiency, the best method for both patient and practice survival is to perform the tests and assessments that provide more benefit for the patient than risk."[1]

The inter-relationship of these factors may be understood more clearly by examining some specific examples. Generally, in vitro tests may be perceived to be safer than in vivo tests. Obtaining a urine sample for analysis is a simple procedure without adverse effects. However, obtaining a biopsy sample of kidney for examination, an in vivo test, has a greater risk of adverse effects because of the invasive nature of obtaining the sample.

Any in vivo test requiring the administration of a drug possesses several factors that could cause adverse effects. The most serious adverse effect is, of course, an anaphylactic allergic reaction to the drug. Diagnostic drugs that are most likely to cause allergic reactions are those containing protein or iodine. All parenteral drugs used as contrast media for studies utilizing x-rays contain iodine. These drugs are also called contrast agents, radiopaques, or roentgenographic drugs.

Other adverse effects from drugs administered parenterally, chemotoxic effects, are related to factors such as osmolality, viscosity, hypertonicity, inherent toxicity of the drug, route of administration, rate of administration, total dose, concentration of drug, and formulation of the drug. Osmolality of drugs used as contrast media is of particular concern for the radiopaque drugs. High osmolality drugs have a greater risk of producing adverse drug reactions (ADRs) than low osmolality drugs.

Osmolality depends on the number of particles of drug in solution and its molecular size. The first iodinated contrast drugs developed were all ionic monomers, having high osmolality when compared to plasma, about 1500 to 1800 milliosmols (mOsm) per kilogram. They are either sodium or meglumine salts with the anionic portion of the molecule containing a tri-iodinated aromatic ring. These high osmolality contrast agents (HOCA), sodium or meglumine diatriazoate, meglumine iodipamide, and meglumine iothalamate, are also known as ratio 1.5 drugs. This ratio is determined by dividing the number of iodine atoms in the molecule by the number of particles in solution. The chemical structure of sodium diatriazoate contains 3 atoms of iodine and consists of 2 particles in solution, producing a ratio of 1.5. Iothalamate is a representative of 1.5 ratio drugs.

Because of the high incidence of ADRs associated with the HOCAs, lower osmolality contrast agents (LOCA) were developed. These drugs include iohexol, iopamidol, iopromide, and ioversol, which are all nonionic monomeric drugs. In solution these drugs have one particle containing 3 atoms of iodine in the molecule. These LOCAs are known as ratio 3.0 drugs and have an osmolality of 600 to 850 mOsm per kilogram. However, not all ratio 3.0 drugs are nonionic monomers. Ioxaglate sodium or meglumine is an ionic dimer molecule, also having a ratio of 3.0 (6 iodine atoms divided by 2 particles; and is considered to be a LOCA.

The most recently developed drugs in this group are non-ionic dimers that are nearly iso-osmolar with plasma, about 290 mOsm per kilogram. Iodixanol was the first drug of this type to be approved in the United States. Although dimers have lower osmolality, they have greater viscosity, which may limit their use in some situations, for example, greater difficulty in administration through small arterial catheters.

ADRs associated with contrast media may be described as mild, moderate, or severe. Mild reactions include flushing or feeling of warmth after injection, itchy skin, mild rash, or diaphoresis. Moderate ADRs include extensive rash or hives, nausea, bronchoconstriction, dyspnea, and edema of the larynx. Severe ADRs include hypotension, shock, pulmonary edema, cardiac arrhythmias, nephrotoxicity, respiratory depression and deaths.[2]

Mild to moderate ADRs may be greatly reduced or prevented by pretreating patients sensitive to radiopaque drugs with antihistamines or corticosteroids. The risk of severe ADRs from HOCAs in the normal population is rather low, ranging from 0.025% to 0.1%, and the risk of fatalities is about 10 times lower.[2] The risk of nephrotoxicity, a very serious ADR is much higher in patients with diabetes and pre-existing renal disease. It is estimated that the use of contrast media causes about 10% of the cases of hospital-acquired acute renal failure, which occurs in about 5% to 7% of all hospitalized patients.[3,4] Risk of ADRs associated with contrast media is greatly reduced for all patients by adequately hydrating them using either 0.45% or 0.9% normal saline administered intravenously prior to performing contrast studies.

Risks of all ADRs can be reduced by using low osmolality or iso-osmolar contrast media. However, these agents currently cost about 10 times more than HOCAs and are used for patients categorized as high risk. A randomized, double-blind, prospective study by Aspelin et al reported that use of iodixanol, an iso-osmolar drug, had an incidence of 3% for nephrotoxocity in sample of high-risk patients undergoing coronary angiography compared with 26% in patients who received iohexol, a LOCA.[5]

Diseases associated with increased risk of adverse effects in patients receiving intravascular iodine contrast agents are severe cardiovascular disease, multiple myeloma, diabetes mellitus, homozygous sickle-cell disease, and pheochromocytoma. There are reports of thyroid storm following the use of these drugs in patients with hyperthyroidism. Thyroid testing of patients receiving iodinated contrast media should be delayed for a week or more because levels of iodine may be detected for days or even weeks in some patients after imaging procedures.

Storage conditions may affect solutions containing high concentrations of drug, causing precipitation of the drug in the vial or ampoule. Gentle agitation or mild heating should result in re-solution of the drug. If any particulate remains or if there is a color change in the solution, the drug should be discarded.

Drugs used for magnetic resonance imaging (MRI) also present a risk for chemotoxic ADRs. Many MRI drugs are hyperosmolar and hypertonic compared to plasma, but the volume of drug administered is less than that needed in radiopaque studies. Thus, the osmotic load is much less than the iodine contrast media, producing fewer ADRs. Risk of allergic reactions or sensitivity to MR drugs is low, but remains a concern.

MR images are created when protons present in tissues align themselves in a magnetic field depending on the nuclear magnetic moment to produce a nuclear spin energy state. A second magnetic field is produced by pulsed radiofrequency to induce nuclear resonance. The time it takes for the protons to return to the lower energy state is the relaxation time. The relaxation time varies from tissue to tissue, creating signals that are detected by a receiver coil and analyzed by a computer to produce an image. MR-enhancing drugs must contain one or more unpaired electrons. Currently approved MR drugs (also known as paramagnetic or supramagnetic agents) contain one of the following atoms in their structure: manganese (Mn^{2+}), iron (Fe^{3+}), or gadolinium (Gd^{3+}).

Additional precautions must be followed in patients with deoxygenated sickle erythrocytes, hemolytic anemias, cardiovascular disease, and renal or hepatic impairment.

Ultrasound diagnostic drugs are relatively new agents in diagnostic imaging. The FDA approved the first ultrasound drug, 5% human albumin microspheres, for cardiac imaging in 1995. Ultrasound studies use non-ionizing electromagnetic waves in the low megahertz range. Ultrasound waves produced in a transducer head are projected into a patient and reflected from tissue surfaces back to the transducer, much like radar waves. The transducer receives the ultrasound waves, converts them into signals, which are interpreted by a computer, producing an image.

Ultrasound contrast studies require very small particles, microspheres. Drugs used currently for cardiac studies consist of human albumin or lipid coated microspheres containing perflutren gas. ADRs include headache, dizziness, palpitations, and potential serious cardiopulmonary effects. Protein containing drugs have a higher risk of producing allergic reactions.

Technical advances made in the various modalities used for imaging the human body have been accompanied by the introduction of new drugs to enhance image formation to improving diagnostic information available to physicians. This chapter reviews the radiopaque, magnetic resonance, and ultrasound drugs.

This chapter also includes drugs used frequently to evaluate other physiological states or diagnose diseases by either in vivo *or* in vitro methods, including many self-care diagnostic aids. However, tests for identifying organisms for infectious diseases are not included in this chapter. Readers desiring the most complete information for identification of micro-organisms should refer to *The Manual of Clinical Microbiology*,[6] or *Manual of Commercial Methods in Clinical Microbiology*.[7] This chapter also does not include the many tests that are performed in clinical laboratories or doctors' offices.

Advances in the application computer technology and biotechnology methods have added a great number of diagnostic tests or devices available for patients to use at home. Patients who desire to be more pro-active about their health care have created a growing market for these devices. For example, at one time patients with diabetes mellitus could only monitor blood glucose and urinary ketones, but now they can measure blood glucose, blood ketones, and hemoglobin A1c. Other OTC devices are available to monitor blood cholesterol, predict ovulation, determine pregnancy, detect occult blood in the urine and feces, detect protein and leuckocytes in the urine, and detect the use of illicit drugs. This chapter includes a discussion of selected devices that are used frequently as self-care in vitro diagnostic aids.

DIAGNOSTIC IMAGING DRUGS

ROENTGENOGRAPHIC DRUGS (X-RAY CONTRAST AGENTS)

The discovery of x-rays by Wilhem Conrad Roentgen in 1895 gave physicians a tool that allowed them to view the inside of the body, thus improving their ability to make a more accurate diagnosis of a patient's illness. Physicians were using x-rays and urethral catheters with metal inside them for examining the urinary tract by 1905.[8]

Oral administration of bismuth and barium salts were used to produce images of the gastrointestinal tract, and by 1906, the technique of retrograde pyelography using bismuth subnitrate or colloidal silver was developed. Toxicities associated with these drugs led to the use of thorium salts (a radioactive element) as imaging agents in 1915. The use of sodium or potassium iodide as a contrast agent was proposed in 1918, but the concentrations needed for good images produced numerous toxicities.[8]

The mid-1920s saw the introduction of compounds composed of pyridine with iodine or arsenic substituents as therapy for infectious diseases, especially syphilis. One of these iodinated pyridine compounds was selectively concentrated and excreted by the kidneys, and it was eventually developed as an imaging agent for the urinary tract. Intravenous examination of the urinary tract using substituted pyridines became an integral part of medical practice by the end of the decade.[8]

Adverse reactions to contrast agents were a significant problem. The search for safer drugs resulted in the development of tri-iodinated benzoic acid compounds that produced better quality images with fewer adverse effects. Development continued to improve the safety profile of these drugs throughout the decade of the 1950s. The first drugs developed were ionic, monomeric salts that had either sodium or meglumine (N-methylglucamine) as the cation. Meglumine salts produce less pain at the site of injection and less vasodilation during arteriography, both advantages; however, they increase urine output, a disadvantage during venography. Sodium salts are less viscous, an advantage in reducing administration problems, but they are more toxic to the blood brain barrier and heart. Efforts to improve benefit to risk profiles for imaging agents led to the use of mixtures of the two salts in varying ratios, depending on the organ system to be visualized.[8]

Although much safer than earlier drugs, the high osmolality of the ionic monomeric contrast agents (HOCA) compared to plasma and their hypertonicity contribute significantly to their adverse effects. Lower osmolality contrast agents (LOCA) were developed in the 1960s and 1970s by creating dimers of ionic monomeric agents or by synthesizing nonionic contrast agents. The newest compounds, which have almost the same osmolality as plasma, are nonionic dimer compounds. The LOCA and iso-osmolality drugs are considerably more expensive than the older agents and are used in patients who are at a greater risk of adverse effects, particularly for patients with renal impairment, diabetes mellitus, and those undergoing *coronary angiography* studies. Patients with multiple myeloma, homozygous sickle-cell disease, and pheochromocytoma are also at higher risk for adverse effects. Iodinated drugs must be used with caution in patients allergic or sensitive to iodine or any other components of the drug.

The drugs in this section are listed in alphabetical order by their generic name because some drugs are used to visualize several organ systems depending on their concentrations. Each drug's description includes the concentration used for each organ system. Only barium sulfate and organic iodine compounds are used as radiopaque drugs.

BARIUM SULFATE

Sulfuric acid, barium salt (1:1); Synthetic or Artificial Barytes

Barium sulfate (1:1)
[7727-43-7] $BaSO_4$ (233.39).

Caution—When Barium Sulfate is prescribed, the title always should be written out in full to avoid confusion with the poisonous barium sulfide or barium sulfite.

Preparation—Barium sulfate precipitates when an aqueous solution containing barium ion is mixed with a solution containing sulfate ion. It also can be obtained by suitable purification of native barium sulfate.

Description—Fine, white, bulky powder, free from grittiness; odorless; tasteless; its suspension in water is neutral to litmus paper.

Solubility—Practically insoluble in water; solutions of acids or alkalies, or organic solvents.

Comments—Primary contrast agent for visualizing the esophagus, stomach, small and large intestines. Barium sulfate is available as either a powder for suspension or suspensions with different concentrations. The particle size in the suspension and the concentration of the final preparation are important determinants in the ability of barium sulfate to adhere to the mucosal wall of the digestive system. High-density

preparations (>200% w/v) are preferred for the stomach, medium density (100–200% w/v) for the esophagus, and low density (<100% w/v) for the small intestine. Barium sulfate of medium density is administered as an enema for visualization of the large intestine (colon).[9]

If barium sulfate is used alone, the study is referred to as a single contrast study. Studies using air or carbon dioxide force the particles in the suspension against the mucosal wall for optimum visualization and are referred to as double-contrast studies. Sodium bicarbonate and tartaric acid may be administered with barium sulfate when carbon dioxide serves as the second contrast medium. Barium sulfate is usually used for *fluoroscopy*, but it is also used for *computed tomography* (CT) of the gastrointestinal tract.

Preparations intended for oral use are available in several flavors to improve palatability of barium suspensions. Stabilizers are added to prevent flocculation of the particles, such as gelatin; and, simethicone is added to prevent bubbles from forming during the procedure.[9]

Severe adverse effects are rare. Common adverse effects include bowel disturbances, either constipation or diarrhea. Known contraindications for the use of barium sulfate are intestinal obstruction, perforation of the gastrointestinal tract, tracheoesophageal fistula, and sensitivity to barium sulfate formulations.

DIATRIZOATE MEGLUMINE

Benzoic acid, 3,5-bis(acetylamino)-2,4,6-triiodo-, compound with 1-deoxy-1-(methylamino)-D-glucitol (1:1); Cystografin, Cystografin Dilute, Hypaque Meglumine (30 and 60%), Reno-30, Reno-60, Reno-DIP

1-Deoxy-1-(methylamino)-L-glucitol 3,5-diacetamido-2,4,6-triiodobenzoate (salt)
[131-49-7] $C_7H_{17}NO_5.C_{11}H_9I_3N_2O_4$ (809.13).

Preparation—Diatrizoic acid is reacted with an equimolar quantity of methylglucamine (meglumine), usually in water for injection, to produce a solution of the required concentration.

Description—A clear, colorless solution.

Comments—Different concentrations are used for visualizing several organs. A 60% solution is used for *excretory urography, cerebral angiography, peripheral arteriography, venography operative and postoperative cholangiography, percutaneous transhepatic cholangiography, splenoportography, arthrography, discography, urography,* and enhancement of *computed tomography* of the brain and body. *Retrograde pyelography* is performed using a 30% solution whereas *retrograde cystourethrography* may be performed with either a 30% or 18% solution. Cystografin and Cystografin Dilute are only used for retrograde studies and are not to be injected intravascularly. Reno-DIP, a 30% solution of diatrizoate, may be used for drip infusion *pyelography*, lower extremity *venography*, and *computed tomography* of the brain and body.

Diatrizoate meglumine is contraindicated for use in intrathecal procedures, and must be used with great caution in patients who are allergic or sensitive to diarizoate salts. Severe adverse effects to ionic iodinated contrast agents include inhibition of blood coagulation, acute renal failure, myocardial infarction, and stroke. Patients who have multiple myeloma, pheochromocytoma, or are homozygous for sickle-cell disease are at greater risk for adverse effects. Extreme caution should be used in patients with renal or hepatic impairment or disease. Safety for use in pregnancy has not been established.

DIATRIZOATE MEGLUMINE AND DIATRIZOATE SODIUM

Hypaque-76, Gastrografin, MD-Gastroview, MD-76R, RenoCal-76, Renografin-60

A sterile solution of diatrizoate meglumine and diatrizoate sodium in water for injection, or a sterile solution of diatrizoic acid in water for injection prepared with the aid of NaOH and meglumine. It may contain small amounts of suitable buffers and of edetate calcium disodium or edetate disodium as a stabilizer. When intended for intravascular use, it contains no antimicrobial agents.

Description—Clear, colorless to pale yellow, slightly viscous liquid; may crystallize at room temperature or below.

Comments—Designed to combine the lower toxicity of the meglumine salt with the lower viscosity and higher iodine content of the sodium salt. Two concentrations are in current use. Intravenous products with 76 in the trade name contain 66% of the meglumine salt and 10% of the sodium salt. They are used as contrast agents for *angiocardiography, aortography, angiography, excretion urography, peripheral* *arteriography, nephrotomography* (RenoCal-76 only), *venography* (Hypaque-76 only*), ventriculography,* and *computed tomography.*

Renografin-60 contains 52% of the meglumine salt and 8% of the sodium salt of diatrizoate. It is indicated for use in *urography, angiography, arteriography, venography, cholangiography, splenoportography, arthrography, discography,* and *computed tomography.*

A solution containing 66% of diatrizoate meglumine and 10% of diatrizoate sodium (Gastrografin, *Bracco*) is used as a contrast medium for radiographic examination of the GI tract following oral or rectal administration. This preparation is used when the use of barium is not feasible or is potentially dangerous. It may also be used for *computed tomography* studies.

These diatrizoate salt combinations have the same contraindications and warnings as diatrizoate meglumine and daitrizoate sodium. The safety of the oral solution in pregnancy has not been established. It is usually tolerated well; occasionally, diarrhea occurs.

DIATRIZOATE MEGLUMINE AND IODIPAMIDE MEGLUMINE

Sinografin

A sterile, aqueous, clear to pale yellow solution of diatrizoate meglumine equivalent to 40% diatrizoic acid and iodipamide meglumine equivalent to 20% iodipamide, containing approximately 38% bound iodine.

Comments—A radiopaque medium indicated for *hysterosalpingography.* Intrauterine administration provides immediate visualization of the uterus and uterine tubes. Any contrast agent spilled into the peritoneal cavity is absorbed within 20 to 60 minutes. Use of this drug is contraindicated during pregnancy, within 6 months of a terminated pregnancy, and within 30 days following curettage or conization. The procedure should not be performed during the menstrual period or if the patient has a genital tract infection. Precautions, adverse effects, and contraindications are similar to those for other iodinated diagnostic agents.

DIATRIZOATE SODIUM

Benzoic acid, 3,5-bis(acetylamino)-2,4,6-triiodo-, monosodium salt; Hypaque Sodium 50% Injection, Hypaque Sodium (powder)

[737-31-5] $C_{11}H_8I_3N_2NaO_4$ (635.90).

Preparation—Diatrizoic acid is reacted with an equimolar quantity of NaOH, usually in water for injection, to produce a solution of the required concentration.

Comments—A radiopaque agent with uses, profile of toxicity, and precautions similar to those for *Diatrizoate Meglumine.* It contains somewhat more iodine (59.87%) than the meglumine salt (47.01%). Solutions are considerably less viscous than those prepared from diatrizoate meglumine. Diatrizoate sodium if used in *coronary angiography* is more likely to cause serious cardiac arrhythmias than is the meglumine salt.

Indications for the use of diatrizaote sodium include *excretory urography, angioangiography, aortography, cholangiography, hysterosalpingography, splenoportography,* and *computed tomography.*

DIATRIZOIC ACID

Benzoic acid, 3,5-bis (acetylamino)-2,4,6-triiodo-

anhydrous [117-96-4] $C_{11}H_9I_3N_2O_4$ (613.92); *dihydrate* [50978-11-5] (649.95).

Preparation—Derived from benzoic acid by (1) nitration to the 3,5-dinito acid, (2) reduction by means of stannous chloride or other reducing agent to the corresponding diamino acid, (3) iodination with iodine monochloride in acetic acid to the 2,4,6-triiodo derivative, or (4) acetylation of the amino groups by use of acetic anhydride.

Description—White powder; odorless.

Solubility—Very slightly soluble in water or alcohol; soluble in dimethylformamide or alkali hydroxide solutions.

Comments—Radiopaque component of *Diatrizoate Meglumine Injection, Diatrizoate Meglumine and Diatrizoate Sodium Injection, Diatrizoate Sodium Injection,* and *Diatrizoate Sodium Oral Solution.*

ETHIODIZED OIL

Ethiodol

A sterile iodine addition product of the ethyl ester of the fatty acids of poppy seed oil, containing 35.2% to 38.9% organically combined iodine. [8008-53-5] (no molecular weight given).

Preparation—By saponifying poppy seed oil and subjecting the resulting fatty acids to iodination and subsequent esterification with ethanol.

Description—Straw-colored to amber-colored, oily liquid; may have an alliaceous odor.

Solubility—Insoluble in water; soluble in acetone, chloroform, or ether.

Comments—A contrast agent used in *hysterosalpingography* and *lymphography.* Contraindications for *hysterosalpingography* are the same as for other iodine contrast agents as well as the following: pregnancy, presence of intrauterine bleeding, pelvic inflammatory disease, cervical erosion, and 30 days after conization.

Contradications for *lymphography* include right-to-left cardiac shunt, advanced pulmonary disease, and patients who have had radiation therapy to the lungs. Subclinical pulmonary embolism may occur that is usually transient in nature. Pregnancy category is C, and it is unknown if ethiodized oil appears in breast milk.

IODIPAMIDE

Benzoic acid, 3,3'-[(1,6-dioxo-1,6-hexanediyl)diimino]bis[2,4,6-triiodo; Cholografin

3,3–(Adipoyldiimino)bis[2,4,6-triiodobenzoic acid] [606-17-7] $C_{20}H_{14}I_6N_2O_6$ (1139.76).

Preparation—From benzoic acid by (1) nitration to 3-nitrobenzoic acid, (2) reduction by means of stannous chloride or other reducing agent to 3-aminobenzoic acid, (3) iodination with iodine monochloride in acetic acid to the 2,4,6-triiodo derivative, or (4) acylation of the amino group with adipoyl chloride [ClCO(CH₂)₄COCl].

Description—White, crystalline powder; nearly odorless.

Solubility—Very slightly soluble in water, chloroform, or ether; slightly soluble in alcohol.

Comments—Radiopaque component of *Iodipamide Meglumine Injection.*

IODIPAMIDE MEGLUMINE

Benzoic acid, 3,3'-[(1,6-dioxo-1,6-hexanediyl)diimino]bis2,4,6-triiodo-, compound with 1-deoxy-1-(methylamino)-D-glucitol (1:2); Cholografin Meglumine

1-Deoxy-1-(methylamino)-D-glucitol3,3'-(adipoyldiimino)bis[2,4,6-triiodobenzoate] (2:1) (salt) [3521-84-4] $C_{20}H_{14}I_6N_2O_6.2C_7H_{17}NO_5$ (1530.19).

Preparation—Iodipamide is reacted with a double equimolar quantity of methylglucamine (meglumine), using sufficient water for injection to produce a solution of the required concentration.

Description—Clear, colorless to pale yellow, slightly viscous liquid.

Comments—For *intravenous cholangiography* and *cholecystography* as follows: visualization of the gallbladder and biliary ducts in the differential diagnosis of acute abdominal conditions; visualization of the biliary ducts especially in patients with symptoms after cholecystectomy; and visualization of the gallbladder in patients unable to take oral contrast media or to absorb media from the gastrointestinal tract. The contrast agent appears in the bile within 10 to 15 minutes after injection, and the biliary ducts are visualized within 25 minutes; the gallbladder begins to fill within 1 hour, maximum filling occurs within 2 to 2.5 hours.

Adverse reactions and contraindications are similar to those common to iodine containing compounds.

IODIXANOL

1,3-Benzenedicarboxamide, 5,5'-[(2-hydroxy-1,3-propane diyl)bis(acetylimino)]bis[N,N'-bis(2,3-dihydroxypropyl)-2,4,6-triiodo-; Visipaque

[92339-11-2] $C_{35}H_{44}I_6N_6O_{15}$ (1550.18).

Preparation—Eur Pat Appl EP 108,538 (1984) See *CA* 1984; 101:151,599g,

Description—Melts about 250°–250°; I_2 content 49.1%; a 50% aqueous solution (w/v) d 1.26; viscosity 8.7 cP @ 37°. Osmolality 290 mOsm/kg water, pH 7.2-7.6.

Solubility—Soluble in water.

Comments—A dimeric, isomolar, nonionic, iodine contrast agent used for both intra-arterial and intravenous administration. Intra-arterial Visipaque 320 is used for *angiocardiography (left ventriculography* and *selective coronary arteriography), peripherial arteriography, visceral artiography,* and *cerebral arteriography.* Visipaque 270 is only approved for *intra-arterial digital subtraction angiography.* Both concentrations are used intravenously for *computer tomography* of the head, and body, and *excretory urography;* Visipaque 270 is also approved for *peripheral venography.*

Iodixanol is isosmolar with plasma and is preferred to the hyperosmolar contrast agents in patients at increased risk for adverse effects, such as acute renal failure. The same warnings and precautions must be taken with iodixanol as with other iodinated contrast agents. Iodixanol is pregnancy category B, and it is not known if is excreted in human milk.

IOHEXOL

1,3-Benzenedicarboxamide, 5-[acetyl(2,3-dihydroxypropyl)amino]-N,N-bis(2,3-dihydroxypropyl)-2,4,6-triiodo-, Omnipaque 140, 180, 240, 300, and 350 (Note: The numerical values indicate the concentration of organically bound iodine in mg/mL, not the concentration of drug/mL.)

[66108-95-0] $C_{19}H_{26}I_3N_3O_9$ (821.14).

Preparation—US Pat 4,250,113.

Description—White crystals; melts at about 176°.

Solubility—Soluble in water to form stable solutions.

Comments—A nonionic, water-soluble, radiographic contrast medium used in different concentrations. The lowest concentration, Omnipaque 140, has 140 mg of iodine per mL, and is 1.1 times the osmolality of plasma. Omnipaque 350 has an osmolality that is 3 times higher than plasma. Omnipaque 180, 240, and 300 are indicated for intrathecal use for *myelography* (lumbar, thoracic, cervical, total columnar) and for contrast enhancement in *computed tomography* (CT) for *myelography, cisternography,* and *ventriculography.*

Contraindications for intrathecal use include known hypersensitivity to iohexol. Patients with infections that could cause bacteremia should not undergo *myelography* with iohexol. Intrathecal administration of corticosteroids is contraindicated with iohexol use. In addition to the usual warnings and precautions for use of iodinated contrast agent, the package insert warns about possible idiosyncratic reactions in patients who may have a history of sensitivity to iodine, other contrast agents, bronchial asthma, hay fever, and food allergies.[10] Iohexol is pregnancy category B, and it is not known if is secreted in breast milk.

Caution is advised in patients with a history of epilepsy, severe cardiovascular disease, chronic alcoholism, or multiple sclerosis. Drugs that lower seizure threshold, especially phenothiazine derivatives, including those used for their antihistaminic or anti-nauseant properties, are not recommended for use with iohexol. Others drugs to be avoided include monoamine oxidase (MAO) inhibitors, tricyclic antidepressants, CNS stimulants, psychoactive drugs described as analeptics, major

tranquilizers, or antipsychotic drugs. Such medications should be discontinued at least 48 hours prior to *myelography,* should not be used for the control of nausea or vomiting during or after *myelography,* and should not be resumed for at least 24 hours after procedure.

Iohexol also may be administered intravascularly and is distributed in the extracellular fluid and excreted unchanged by glomerular filtration. Intravascular administration is used in *computed tomography* imaging of the head and total body as well as for *angiocardiography, arteriography, digital subtraction, peripheral angiography,* and *excretory urography.*

Iohexol may be injected directly into body cavities for a variety of procedures including *arthrography, hysterosalpingography, herniography, voiding cystourethrography, endoscopic retrograde pancreatography,* and *cholangiopancreatography.*

IOMEPROL

1,3-Benzendicarboxamide, N,N'- bis (2,3-dihydroxypropyl)-5-[(hydroxyacetyl)methylamino]-2,4,6-triiodo-, Iomeron

[78649-41-9] $C_{17}H_{22}I_3N_3O_8$ (777.09).

Preparation—US Pat 4,352,788.

Description—Crystalline powder; melts about 290°.

Solubility—Very soluble in water or methanol; poorly soluble in ethanol; insoluble in chloroform.

Solution Properties

mg I_2/mL	Conc drug mg/mL	$d^{20}/_4$	$\eta^{20}/_D$	Osmolality 37° (mOsmol/Kg water)
150	303.6	1.166	1.3828	0.27
300	607.3	1.329	1.4327	0.52
400	809.7	1.446	1.4660	0.72

Comments—This drug is available in over 40 countries, but has not been approved for use in the United States by the FDA. It is a tri-iodinated, nonionic contrast agent intended for examination of the brain and liver by *computed tomography.*

IOPAMIDOL

(S)- N,N'-bis[2-Hydroxy-1-(hydroxymethyl)ethyl]-2,4,6-triiodo-5-lact-amidoisophtpalamide. Isovue 128, 200, 250, 300, and 370; Isovue-M 200, Isovue-M 300 (Note: The numerical values indicate the concentration of organically bound iodine in mg/mL, not the concentration of drug/mL.)

1,3-Benzenedicarboxamide,(S)-N,N'-bis[2-hydroxy-1-(hydroxymethyl) ethyl]-5-[(2-hydroxy-1-oxopropyl)amino]-2,4,6-triiodo-,
[60166-93-0] $C_{17}H_{22}I_3N_3O_8$ (777.09).

Preparation—See US Pat 4,001,323.

Description—White, odorless crystals; decomposes at about 300° without melting.

Solubility—Very soluble in water or methanol; soluble in boiling ethanol; practically insoluble in chloroform.

Comments—Only Isovue-M 200 and Isovue-M 300 are used administered by intrathecal injection for *myelography, (lumbar, thoracic, cervical, total columnar,* and *contrast enhancement of CT cisternography* and *ventriculography.* They are nonionic contrast agent that have osmolalities greater than plasma and cerebrospinal fluid and are more hypertonic than plasma and cerebrospinal fluid.

Iopamidol is absorbed rapidly into the blood from the cerebrospinal fluid, following intrathecal administration. It appears in plasma within 1 hour but does not bind to plasma protein. It is excreted by the kidneys and eliminated within 48 hours.

Iopamidol should not be administered with any other drugs, and contraindications and precautions are the same as for other iodine contrast agents. It should be administered with caution in patients with increased intracranial pressure, a history of convulsive disorders, severe cardiovascular disease, chronic alcoholism, or multiple sclerosis and in elderly patients. Other adverse reactions include headache, nausea, and back and leg pain. It is pregnancy category B and not known if it appears in breast milk.

The lowest concentration, iopamidol 128 mg I/mL, has the same osmolality as plasma and is approved for use during *intra-arterial digital subtraction angiography*. Selective *visceral arteriography* and *aortography, pediatric angiocardiography*, and *coronary arteriography* and *ventriculography* are performed using the highest concentration, iopamidol 370 mg I/mL. Iopamidol 250, 300, and 370 mg I/mL are indicated during *excretory urography*, while iopamidol 250 and 300 mg I/mL are used for *computed tomography* of the head and body. *Cerebral arteriography* is performed using Iopamidol 300 mg I/mL, and *peripheral venography* is performed using Iopamidol 200 mg I/mL.

IOPANOIC ACID

Benzenepropanoic acid, 3-amino-α-ethyl-2,4,6-triiodo-, Telepaque

3-Amino-α-ethyl-2,4,6-triiodohydrocinnamic acid.
[96-83-3] $C_{11}H_{12}I_3NO_2$ (570.93).

Preparation—A mixture of *m*-nitrobenzaldehyde, butyric anhydride, and sodium butyrate is heated in xylene to effect a Perkin condensation yielding *m*-nitro-α-ethylcinnamic acid. The acid is reduced with hydrogen in the presence of Raney nickel. The resulting *m*-amino-α-ethylhydrocinnamic acid is iodinated with iodine monochloride in acetic acid solution.

Description—Cream-colored powder; tasteless or nearly so; faint characteristic odor; affected by light; melts with decomposition between 152° and 158°.

Solubility—Insoluble in water; soluble in alcohol, chloroform, or ether; soluble in solutions of alkali hydroxides or carbonates.

Comments—Administered as oral tablets for *cholecystography* and *cholangiography*. It is absorbed rapidly from the GI tract, concentrated in the gallbladder, and subsequently excreted, approximately two-thirds through the GI tract and one-third through the kidneys. About 50% of an administered dose is excreted within 24 hours and the remainder in about 5 days.

Iopanoic acid has low toxicity, causing nausea, diarrhea, and rarely, dysuria. Hypersensitivity reactions involving the skin and mucous membranes and a systemic serum sickness-type reaction have been reported. It is contraindicated in patients with acute nephritis and uremia, since it is eliminated by the kidneys. It should not be administered when disorders of the GI tract exist that prevent absorption of the drug. Its safety in pregnant women has not been evaluated.

The patient has a fat-free evening meal followed by administration of the drug approximately 14 hours before the time scheduled for *roentgenography*. Immediately after the roentgen examination, the patient is given a high-fat meal, causing the gallbladder to contract via stimulation of the hormone, cholecystokinin from the intestinal mucosa. This permits visualization of the patency of the extrahepatic ducts.

IOPHENDYLATE

Benzenedecanoic acid, iodo-x-methyl-, ethyl ester

[1320-11-2] $C_{19}H_{29}IO_2$ (416.34).

Comments—*NOTE: This drug appears in USP 26 and NF 21 but the manufacturer has discontinued the product. It has been replaced by the low-osmolality nonionic contrast media.*

IOPROMIDE

1,3-Benzenedicarboxamide, *N, N*′-bis(2,3-dihydroxypropyl)-2,4,6-triiodo-5-[(methoxyacetyl)amino]-*N*-methyl-, Ultravist 150, 240, 300, and 370

[73334-07-3] $C_{18}H_{24}I_3N_3O_8$ (791.11).

Preparation—US Pat 4,364,921 (1982).

Description—Colorless solid; non-ionic and stable in aqueous solution. Iodine content 48.1%.

Solubility—Very soluble in water.

Comments—A nonionic, sterile, clear, colorless solution used by intravascular injection. Iopromide 150 mg I/mL is used *for intra-arterial digital subtraction angiography*; the 240I/mL for *peripheral venography*; the 300 mg I/mL for *cerebral arteriography, peripheral arteriography*, and *computed tomography of the head and body*, and *excretory urography*; and the 370 mgI/mL for *coronary arteriography, left ventriculography, visceral angiography*, and *aortography*.

Adverse effects include pain at injection site and back, nausea, vomiting, chest pain, headache, dizziness, drowsiness, confusion, dyspnea, and altered vision and taste perception in addition to allergic and sensitivity warnings. It is pregnancy category B, and it is not known if it appears in breast milk.

IOTHALAMATE MEGLUMINE

Benzoic acid, 3-(acetylamino)-2,4,6-triiodo-5-[(methylamino)carbonyl]-, compound with 1-deoxy-1-(methylamino)-D-glucitol (1:1); Conray (60%), Conray 30, Conray 43, Cysto-Conray II (17.2%)

[13087-53-1] $C_{11}H_9I_3N_2O_4 \cdot C_7H_{17}NO_5$ (809.13).

Preparation—Iothalamic acid is reacted with an equimolar quantity of methylglucamine (meglumine), using sufficient water for injection to produce a solution of the required concentration.

Comments—A radiopaque medium used *parenterally* as a 30%, 43%, or 60% solution for *urography*; as a 30% or 60% solution for *angiography* and *computed tomography*; as a 43% or 60% solution for *venography*; as a 43% solution for *pyelography* and *cystourethrography*; and, as a 60% solution for *cholangiography, arteriography, ventriculography*, and *arthrography*. Cysto-Conray II, a 17.2% solution, is indicated for *cystography* and *cystourethrography*.

Iothalamate Meglumine is contraindicated in patients with a known allergy or sensitivity to salts of iothalamic acid and should not be used for urography in patients with anuria. Intravenous urography is hazardous to patients with multiple myeloma, anuria, progressive uremia, renal failure, and deaths have occurred. It is pregnancy category B, and it is excreted unchanged in breast milk. Bottle feedings should be used for 24 hours after the drug is administered.

IOTHALAMATE MEGLUMINE AND IOTHALAMATE SODIUM

Comments—*NOTE: Still listed in the USP 26 and NF 21, but the manufacturer discontinued the product.*

IOTHALAMATE SODIUM

Benzoic acid, 3-(acetylamino)-2,4,6-triiodo-5-[(methylamino)carbonyl]-, monosodium salt; Conray 400

[1225-20-3] $C_{11}H_8I_3N_2NaO_4$ (635.90).

Preparation—Iothalamic acid is reacted with an equimolar quantity of NaOH, using sufficient water for injection to produce a solution of the required concentration.

Comments—For *intravascular angiocardiography, aortography, excretory urography*, and enhancement of *computerized tomography*. It is contraindicated in cerebral angiography, and in patients with sensitivity to iothalamic acid. Its adverse effects and precautions are similar to those for other iodinated diagnostic agents.

IOTHALAMIC ACID

Benzoic acid, 3-(acetylamino)-2,4,6-triiodo-5-[(methylamino)carbonyl]-

[2276-90-6] $C_{11}H_9I_3N_2O_4$ (613.92).

Preparation—By oxidizing *m*-xylene with potassium permanganate, condensing the resulting isophthalic acid with an equimolar quantity of methylamine, and iodinating with iodine monochloride in acetic acid.

Description—White powder; odorless.

Solubility—Slightly soluble in water or alcohol; soluble in solutions of alkali hydroxides.

Comments—Radiopaque component for *Iothalamate Meglumine Injection, Iothalamate Meglumine and Iothalamate Sodium Injection,* and *Iothalamate Sodium Injection.*

IOVERSOL

1,3-Benzenedicarboxamide, *N,N'*-bis(2,3-dihydroxypropyl)-5-[(hydroxyacetyl)-(2-hydroxyethyl)amino]-2,4,6-triiodo-,Optiray 160, 240, 300, 320, and 350. (Note: The numerical values indicate the concentration of organically bound iodine in mg/mL, not the concentration of drug/mL.)

[87771-40-2] $C_{18}H_{24}I_3N_3O_9$ (807.12).

Preparation—See US Pat 4,396,598.

Solubility—Soluble in water.

Description—A nonionic, water-soluble, radiographic contrast medium used in different concentrations having osmolalities that range from 1.2 (Optiray 160) to 2.8 (Optiray 350) times that of plasma and are hypertonic under conditions of use.

The lowest concentration of ioversol, 160mg I/mL, is only indicated for *intra-arterial digital subtraction angiography* (IA-DSA). Only the highest concentration of ioversol, 350 mg I/mL, is indicated for *intravenous digital subtraction angiography*. Ioversol 350, 320, 300, and 240 mg I/mL are indicated for *venography, computed tomography of the head and body, and intravenous urography*. Ioversol 350, 320 and 240 mg I/mL are indicated for *peripheral arteriography*; the 320, 300 and 240 mg I/mL for *cerebral arteriography*; the 350 and 320 mg I/mL for *coronary arteriography and left ventriculography*; and the 320 mg I/mL for *visceral and renal arteriography and aortography*.

Caution must be exercised in patients with severely impaired renal function, combined renal and hepatic disease, severe thyrotoxicosis, myelomatosis, or anuria, particularly when large doses are administered. Intravenously administered iodine-containing radiopaque media are potentially hazardous in patients with multiple myeloma or other paraproteinemia, particularly in those with therapeutically resistant anuria. Arterial injection should never be made following the administration of vasopressors, since they strongly potentiate neurological effects. Extreme caution must be used if patient is known or suspected to have pheochromocytoma because a hypertensive crisis could occur. It is pregnancy category B and it is not known if it appears in breast milk.

IOXAGLATE MEGLUMINE AND IOXAGLATE SODIUM
Hexabrix

A mixture of ioxaglate meglumine 39.3% [59018-13-2] $C_{24}H_{21}N_5O_9 \cdot C_7H_{17}O_5$ (1464.10) and ioxaglate sodium 19.6% ([67992-58-9]

$C_{24}H_{20}I_6N_5NaO_8$ (1290.87)). The structure for the meglumine adduct is depicted above. The other component of Hexabrix is the sodium salt of the benzoic acid moiety of ioxaglate.

Comments—A radiopaque medium containing 32% iodine for *urography, arthrography, angiography, angiocardiography, arteriography, aortography, venography, hysterosalpingography,* and *computerized tomography*. Its precautions, drug interactions, adverse reactions, and clinical procedures are similar to those for other iodine-containing radiopaque agents. It is pregnancy category B and is excreted unchanged in breast milk. Bottle feeding is advised for 24 hours after the administration of the drug.

MAGNETIC RESONANCE CONTRAST AGENTS

The majority of MR contrast agents are gadolinium chelates. These compounds don't cross the intact blood-brain barrier, making them important drugs for evaluating the brain. They are eliminated by passive glomerular filtration through the kidney. Gadolinium, a lanthanide metal, is relatively inert and produces few adverse effects.

Although most MR contrast agents are hypertonic and of higher osmolality than plasma, they have a lower risk of adverse effects, especially renal toxicity, than radiopaque contrast agents. The magnetic field can alter the alignment of the iron in hemoglobin in patients with sickle-cell disease and hemolytic anemias, possibly causing vaso-occlusive effects.

FERUMOXIDES

Ferumoxides; Feridex, Endodorm (as IV injection)

[119683-68-0]

Preparation—See US Pat 4,770,183 (1988).

Description—A colloidal suspension of super paramagnetic cores of non-stoichiometric magnetite coated with dextran. The injection is black to red-brown.

Osmolality – 340 mOsm/Kg, d. = 1.04. *Mag Res Imaging* 1995; 13:661.

Comments—A colloid that is taken up by reticuloendothial cells and used primarily for *visualization of the liver*. It is contraindicated in patients with known allergic or hypersensitivity reactions to parenteral iron, parenteral dextran, parenteral iron-dextran, or parenteral iron-polysaccharide preparations.

Adverse effects include anaphylactic-like reactions, hypotension, acute severe back, leg or groin pain or generalized body pain, dyspnea and other respiratory symptoms, angioedema, and urticaria. It is pregnancy category C, and it is not known if it appears in breast milk.

FERUMOXIL

Ferumoxsil; GastroMARK

Preparation—US Pat 4,554,088 (1985).

Description—Colloidal particles of supermagnetic, non-stoichiometric magnetite coated (bonded to) with siloxane. The injection is a dark brown slightly viscous suspension. Osmolality; 250 mOsm/kg of water.

Comments—A dark brown to orange-brown oral suspension, consisting of silicone-coated particles of supramagnetic iron oxide approximately 0.4 microns that is used to enhance visualization of the bowel.

The usual dose of 600 mL, containing 105 mg of iron, is administered orally after a patient has fasted for at least 4 hours. Refrigeration of the drug before use may improve its taste; it should be shaken for at least 1 minute before administration. Absorption of iron from the gastrointestinal tract depends on existing iron stores in each patient and unabsorbed drug is excreted in the feces. Absorbed iron is metabolized by the hematopoietic system, becoming incorporated into hemoglobin in erythrocytes or stored as ferritin. The amount of silicone absorbed or metabolized in humans is unknown.[11]

Ferumoxsil is contraindicated for patients with known or suspected bowel obstruction or perforation and with a known allergy to the drug or any of its components.

Adverse drug reactions include nausea, vomiting, abdominal pain, and diarrhea. Patients who have a history of hiatal hernia, esophageal reflux, nausea, vomiting, abdominal pain and inflammatory bowel disease may not be able to tolerate administration of ferumoxsil. Less frequently seen adverse effects include fever, chills, postoperative ileus, itching, rash, stomatitis, paresthesia of the oral cavity, taste alteration, and edema of the hands and feet. It is pregnancy category B. Iron is known to appear in breast milk, but it is not know if ferumoxsil is excreted in human milk.

GADODIAMIDE

Gadolinium, [5,8-bis(carboxymethyl)-11-[2-(methylamino)-2-oxo-ethyl]-3-oxo-2,5,8,11-tetraazatridecane-13-oato(3-)-, Omniscan, Gd-DTPA-NMA

[131319-48-5] (anhydrous); [122795-43-1] (with water of hydration and coordination).

Preparation—US Pat 4,687,659 (1987).

Description—A non-ionic, low osmolar, paramagnetic chelate.

Injection; (37°, 0.5 M) 789 mOsm/Kg water; d = 1.13. Partition coefficient (butanol/water) -2.1.

Solubility—Water soluble.

Comments—Gadodiamide injection is a sterile, colorless to slightly yellow, clear, nonionic extracellular enhancing agent for magnetic resonance imaging. It is used to visualize lesions with abnormal vascularity in the brain, spine, and associated tissues. It also is used to detect lesions with abnormal vascularity within the thoracic, abdominal, pelvic cavities, and the retroperitoneal space, but it is not used for cardiac studies.

It should be used with caution in patients with sickle cell anemia because deoxygenated sickle erythrocytes line up perpendicular to the magnetic field in in vitro studies. This phenomenon could cause vaso-occlusive complications. Gadodiamide has not been properly evaluated in other types of hemolytic anemias. It is pregnancy category C, and it is not known if it is excreted in human breast milk.

Gadodiamide should be used with caution in patients who are hypersensitive or allergic to it. Its osmolality is 2.8 times greater than plasma, and it is hypertonic. Adverse reactions most commonly include nausea, headache, dizziness, vasodilation, worsening of migraine headaches, ataxia, and seizures.

GADOPENTETATE DIMEGLUMINE

Gadolinate (2-), [N,N-bis[2-[bis(carboxymethyl)amino]-ethyl]glycinato(5-)-, dihydrogen, compound with 1-deoxy-1-(methylamino)-D-glucitol (1:2); Magnevist, Gd-DTPA

[86050-77-3] $C_{14}H_{20}GdN_3O_{10} \cdot 2C_7H_{17}NO_5$ (938.00).

Preparation—See US Pat 4,687,659.

Solubility—Very soluble in water.

Comments—An ionic contrast drug for magnetic resonance imaging (MRI) that detects abnormal vascularity in the brain, head, and neck regions, and in the body, excluding the heart. Adverse reactions most frequently include headache, nausea, coldness at site of injection, and hypotension. Patients with a history of allergy or hypersensitivity-like problems should be monitored closely during the procedure and for several hours after the drug is administered. The drug may cause anaphylaxis, seizures, paresthesias, dizziness, weakness, vomiting, stomach pain, rashes, and urticaria. The drug has an osmolality that is 6.9 greater than plasma and is hypertonic.

Gadopentetate dimeglumine should be used with caution in patients at risk for developing thrombotic syndromes and hemolytic anemias. In vitro studies showed that deoxygenated sickle erythrocytes become aligned perpendicular to the magnetic field that may cause vaso-occlusive complications. It is pregnancy category C, and it is not known if it appears in human breast milk but it is excreted in lactating rats.

GADOTERIDOL

Gadolinium, [10-(2-hydroxypropyl)-1,4,7,10- tetraazacyclodecane-1,4,7-triacetato(3-)-N^1,N^4,N^7,N^{10},O^1,O^4,O^7,O^{10}]-, ProHance

[120066-54-8] $C_{17}H_{29}GdN_4O_7$ (558.68).

Preparation—US Pat 4,885,363 (1989).

Description—Non-ionic, low osmolality, paramagnetic chelate. Microcrystalline needles (clumped) from acetone:methanol; melting about 225°. Inorg Chem 1991: 30; 1265. **Injection**: Osmolality at 37°, 630 mOsm/Kg water; d^{25} 1.137.

Solubility—(mg/mL) Water 737; methanol 119; 2-propanol 41; DMF 10.1; acetonitrile 6.1; methylene chloride 5.2; ethyl acetate 0.5; acetone 0.4, hexane 0.2; toluene 0.3. At pH 7, log P = −3.68 (octanol/water); −1.98 (butanol/water).

Comments—The injection is a nonionic, clear, colorless to slightly yellow paramagnetic drug used to visualize lesions in the head and neck. It should not be used if discolored, and must be used immediately after being withdrawn into a syringe. Gadoteridol does not cross the intact blood-brain barrier but will appear in lesions with abnormal vascularity, or in areas where the blood-brain barrier is disrupted. It is excreted via glomerular filtration but dosing adjustments haven't been evaluated in patients with renal or hepatic impairment.

Gadoteridol has an osmolality 2.2 times greater than plasma. Its predominate adverse effects are nausea and taste perversion. More severe adverse effects that occur less frequently include facial edema, pain at the injection site, neck rigidity, and vasovagal reactions. It is pregnancy category C, and it is not known if it is excreted in human milk.

GADOVERSETAMIDE

Gadolinium, [8,11-bis(carboxymethyl-14-[2-[(2-methoxy-ethyl)amino]-2-oxoethyl]-6-oxo-2-oxa-5,8,11,14-tetraazahexa-decan-16-oato(3-)]-, OptiMARK

[131069-91-5] $C_{20}H_{34}GdN_5O_{10}$ (661.76).

Preparation—US Pats 5,130,120; 5,137,711; 5,508,388.

Description—Non-ionic, paramagnetic chelate; contains labile water. Log P (butanol/water) −1.93. **Injection**: Osmolality (37°) 1110 mOsmol/Kg water; d^{25} 1.160

Comments—A nonionic gadolinium chelate of diethyelentriamine pentaacetic acid bismethoxyethylamide used to enhance visualization of abnormal vascularity in the brain, spine and associated tissues, and liver. It is a clear, colorless to slightly yellow solution with an osmolality that is 3.9 times that of plasma.

Gadoversetamide is administered intravenously and is contraindicated in patients known to be allergic to gadolinium or versatamide. It should be used cautiously if patients have sickle cell anemia because deoxygenated erythrocytes align in a perpendicular manner in the magnetic field, which could cause vaso-occlusive complications. It should be used with caution in patients with renal impairment because it is excreted primarily in the urine.

Adverse effects include headache, vasodilation, abnormal taste, dizziness, nausea, parathesia, body pain, and flu-like symptoms. It is pregnancy category C, and nursing women are advised to use bottle feedings for 72 hours after the drug is administered.

MANGAFODIPIR TRISODIUM

Trisodium trihydrogen (OC-6-13)-[[N, N′-1,2-ethane-diylbis[N-[[3-hydroxy-2-methyl-5-[(phosphonooxy)methyl]-4-pyridinyl]methyl]glycinato]](8-)manganate(6-), Teslascan

[140678-14-4] $C_{22}H_{27}MnN_4O_{14}P_2$ (757.32).

Preparation—US Pat 4,933,456 and Inorg Chem 1989; 28:447.

Description—Pale yellow, hygroscopic crystals, d 1.537. A 0.01 mmol/mL aqueous infusion is a clear, bright yellow solution, pH 7.5.

Solubility—(g/mL) water (0.46), methanol (0.23); practically insoluble in ethanol, acetone or chloroform.

Comments—A sterile, clear, yellow solution of a complex of param-agnetic manganese and fodipir, a chelating agent that is nearly iso-os-molar with plasma. It is injected intravenously to detect, localize, char-acterize, and evaluate lesions of the liver.

Mangafodipir trisodium is contraindicated in patients allergic or hy-persensitive to manganese, fodipir, or any of the inert ingredients in the drug. Mangafodipir trisodium should be used with caution in patients who cannot tolerate nausea and vomiting and in patients with renal or hepatic impairment because the drug is eliminated via urine and bile.[12]

Common adverse effects include pain at the site of injection, headache, nausea, vomiting, abdominal pain, and generalized body dis-comfort described as warmth, flushing, pressure, pain, and/or cold. It is pregnancy category C, and the extent of its secretion in milk varies. Nursing women are advised to bottle-feed, but the package insert has no specific time recommendation.

ULTRASOUND CONTRAST AGENTS

Ultrasound agents that are administered intravenously in-crease the reflectivity of blood and act as echo-enhancing agents because they increase the radiofrequency signal received by the transducers in the ultrasound unit. These drugs must be smaller than the diameter of capillaries, less than 8 μm. The micro-bubbles of gases used for ultrasound studies must be coated to stabilize them or they will collapse and dissolve in blood in less than a second, too short a time for their detection.

Contraindications for intravenous use of ultrasound agents include right-to-left cardiac shunts that could lead to pul-monary emboli formation, and allergic or sensitivity reactions to the drug or its coating.

PERFLUTREN LIPID MICROSPHERES

Propane, octafluoro-, Gaseous component of Definity, Optison

Perfluoropropane, [76-19-7] C_3F_8 (188.02).

Description—The dosage form consists of a sterile suspension of perfluoropropane encapsulated in lipid or protein microspheres.

Comments—A sterile, clear, colorless, non-pyrogenic liquid that af-ter activation in a specialized vial results in an opaque, milky white sus-pension of perflutren lipid microspheres. It is used in echocardiography to enhance imaging of the left ventricular endocardial borders.

The drug is stored at 2° to 8° C and warmed to room temperature be-fore it is activated in its special mixing vial. The activation reaction re-quires 45 seconds and must be continuously shaken. The drug should be

administered within 5 minutes of activation or the suspension must be re-suspended by hand agitation. The drug is stable for 12 hours after ac-tivation and is maintained at room temperature.[13]

The microspheres ranges in size from 1.1 to 43.3 μm. Perflutren gas diffuses out of the microspheres after it is injected and is not metabo-lized in the body. It could not be detected in the blood or expired air 10 minutes after injection. The lipid microspheres are metabolized to free fatty acid.

Perflutren lipid microspheres are contraindicated in patients aller-gic or sensitive to perflutren or in patients who have right-to-left cardiac shunts, bi-directional shunts, or transient right-to-left shunts because microspheres could enter the arterial circulation, bypassing filtration and trapping in the capillaries of the lungs.

Common adverse effects include headache, back and renal pain, flushing and feeling of warmth, and nausea. It is pregnancy category B, and studies have not been done to determine if it is excreted in human breast milk.

PERFLUTREN [PROTEIN-TYPE A MICROSPHERES]

Human serum albumin with perflutren, a stable gas, which is chemically Propane, octafluoro-, Optison

Comments—A sterile, nonpyrogenic suspension of human serum albumin microspheres with perflutren that is used in echocardiography to enhance imaging of the left ventricular endocardial borders. The drug is in two distinct layers in a vial, an upper white layer and a lower clear layer, and is stored at temperatures between 2° to 8° C but must not be frozen.

Gentle mixing produces a milky, white, homogeneous, opaque sus-pension that is injected intravenously. If any clear liquid remains after mixing, the drug should not be used. The drug must be injected within 1 minute after formation of the white, opaque suspension.[14]

The microspheres ranges in size from 3.0 to 4.5 μm. Perflutren gas diffuses out of the microspheres after it is injected, producing an acous-tic impedance lower than blood. Perflutren is not metabolized in the body, and about 96% is exhaled unchanged from the lungs within 10 minutes of its injection. The human serum microspheres are eliminated after metabolism by the same biological pathways as normal albumin.[14]

Perflutren protein-type A microspheres should not be administered to patients who are allergic or sensitive to blood, blood products, or al-bumin. This drug must be used with caution in patients who have right-to-left cardiac shunts, bi-directional shunts, or transient right-to-left shunts because microspheres could enter the arterial circulation, by-passing filtration and trapping in the capillaries of the lungs.

Caution must also be used if the drug is to be administered to pa-tients with severe emphysema, pulmonary vasculitis, previous pul-monary emboli, respiratory distress syndrome, or severe liver disease. It is pregnancy category C, and no studies have been done to determine its excretion in human breast milk.

Common adverse effects include headache, nausea, vomiting, flush-ing and feeling of warmth, pain at the site of injection, dizziness, and al-tered taste.

NON-IMAGING IN VIVO DIAGNOSTIC DRUGS

Drugs in this category are listed based on the physiological sys-tem to be evaluated.

CARDIOVASCULAR SYSTEM

ADENOSINE
See page 1362 for full monograph.

Comments—An endogenous nucleoside that is in all cells of the body. It is a potent peripheral vasodilator used during *myocardial per-fusion stress scintigraphy* studies in patients who are unable to exercise. It produces a more reliable and more potent vasodilation than dipyra-midole.

Contraindications include allergy or sensitivity to adenosine, second or third degree AV block, sinus node disease, asthma, and other bron-choconstrictive diseases.

Adverse reactions include flushing, chest discomfort, dyspnea, headache, throat, neck or jaw discomfort, gastrointestinal discomfort, dizziness, ST segment depression, first- and second-degree heart block, and hypotension. It is pregnancy category C.

Adenosine has a half-life of less than 10 seconds. Methylxanthines, like theophylline and caffeine, are competitive antagonists that can be used to reverse severe adverse effects when they are administered in-travenously.

DOBUTAMINE
See Chapter 70, *Sympathomimetic Drugs* for full monograph.

Comments—Dobutamine is a sympathomimetic amine that pro-duced inotropic and chronotropic effects in the heart. It is used during *myocardial perfusion stress scintigraphy* in patients who can't exercise. It is only used when adenosine or dipyridamole cannot be used as phar-macological stress agents because of dobutamine's severe adverse ef-fects. These effects include chest pain, ST-T segment ECG changes, ven-tricular ectopy, headache, flushing, dyspnea, and parathesis.

DIPYRIDAMOLE

Persantine

Comments—A vasodilator used during *myocardial perfusion stress scintigraphy* as an alternative to exercise in patients who cannot exer-cise adequately when it is administered intravenously. Dipyridamole indirectly increases of endogenous adenosine by blocking uptake and/or by inhibiting the enzymes adenosine deaminase and phosphodiesterase.

INDOCYANINE GREEN

1*H*-Benz[*e*]indolium, 2-[7-[1,3-dihydro-1,1-dimethyl-3-(4-sulfobutyl)-2*H*-benz[*e*]indol-2-ylidene]-1,3,5-heptatrienyl]-1,1-dimethyl-3-(4-sulfobutyl)-, hydroxide, inner salt, sodium salt; Cardio-Green

[3599-32-4] $C_{43}H_{47}N_2NaO_6S_2$ (774.98).

Preparation—By reacting 1,1,2-trimethyl-3-(4-sulfobutyl)-1*H*-benz[*e*]indolium hydroxide inner salt (I) with a bis(Schiff base) derived from glutaconic aldehyde. The starting indolium compound (I) is prepared by heating 1,1,2-trimethyl-1*H*-benz[*e*]indole with 4-hydroxy-1-butanesulfonic acid δ-sulfone. Details for preparing these tricarbocyanine dyes are provided in US Pats 2,251,286 and 2,895,955.

Description—Dark green, blue-green, olive brown, dark blue, or black powder; odorless or with a slight odor; solutions are deep emerald-green; pH (1 in 200 solution) about 6; unstable in solution. When reconstituted with its diluent, indocyanine remains stable for 8 to 10 hours.

Solubility—Soluble in water or methanol; practically insoluble in most other organic solvents.

Comments—To determine *cardiac output, hepatic function,* and *liver blood flow.* It also has been used to measure *plasma volume* and *regional blood flow* in various organs including the kidneys, eyes, and lungs. Following intravenous injection, the distribution volume is relatively constant among individuals and approximates the plasma volume, because tissue binding is negligible and the fraction of unbound drug in blood is very small. It is so highly bound to plasma proteins, particularly alpha lipoproteins, that it does not distribute extravascularly, and its clearance is not limited by binding.

Indocyanine green should be used with caution in patients allergic or sensitive to it or to iodine because the product contains a small quantity of sodium iodide. Radioactive iodine uptake studies should be delayed for at least 1 week following its use. Its safety in pregnancy has not been established.

ENDOCRINE SYSTEM

Adrenal Gland Function

Both corticotropin (ACTH) and cosyntropin are used to diagnose adrenocortical insufficiency. Cosyntropin may be preferred and/or used as a screening test because it has a lower incidence of allergic or sensitivity reactions and can provide a result within 30 minutes. For a definitive diagnosis, the 24-hour infusion test using corticotropin test is required.

CORTICOTROPIN—page 1439.

Pheochromocytoma Diagnosis

The *overproduction and secretion of catecholamines* from tumors found most often in the adrenal medulla are diagnosed by collecting a 24-hour urine sample and measurement of free or metabolized catecholamines. When the results of this test are equivocal, either clonidine or glucagon may act as aids in the diagnosis.

Clonidine—Clonidine normally suppresses catecholamine level in the plasma, but has little effect in patients with pheochromocytoma.

Glucagon—Glucagon increases circulating catecolamines; phentolamine has also been used in the manner.

Pancreatic Gland Function

The pancreas has both an endocrine and exocrine function. Pancreatic exocrine function tests are described in the gastrointestinal section. An oral glucose tolerance test is used to *diagnose diabetes mellitus.* Devices for measuring blood glucose levels appear in the section on in vitro self-care devices.

TOLBUTAMIDE SODIUM

Orinase Diagnostic

Comments—A single intravenous dose of tolbutamide sodium is useful in the diagnosis of functioning *insulinomas.* Patients consume a diet of 150 to 300 g of carbohydrates for 3 days before the test. A fasting blood glucose levels is obtained before the injection of tolbutamide sodium. Several blood samples are withdrawn over a period of 180 minutes after the injection.

Adverse effects include venospasm, thrombophlebitis, and hypoglycemia, especially in nondiabetic patients. Tolbutamide is contraindicated in patients allergic or sensitive to it, other sulfonylurea drugs, or sulfonamides.

Salicylates and other drugs that produce hypoglycemia should not be administered in the 3 days before the test. It is not recommended for use in pregnant women, and it has a pregnancy category of C. It appears in breast milk, and infants should be temporarily bottle-fed.

Parathyroid Function

TERIPARATIDE ACETATE

L-Phenylalanine, L-valyl-L-seryl-L-α-glutamyl-L-isoleucyl-L-glutaminyl-L-leucyl-L-methionyl-L-histidyl-L-asparaginyl-L-leucylglycyl-L-lysyl-L-histidyl-L-leucyl-L-asparaginyl-L-seryl-L-methionyl-L-α-glutamyl-L-arginyl-L-valyl-L-α-glutamyl-L-tryptophyl-L-leucyl-L-arginyl-L-lysyl-L-leucyl-L-glutaminyl-L-α-aspartyl-L-valyl-L-histidyl-L-asparaginyl-, acetate (salt) hydrate

[99294-94-7] $C_{181}H_{291}N_{55}O_{51}S_2.xH_2O.yC_2H_4O_2$.

Description—A synthetic polypeptide composed of 34 amino acids of the terminal fragment of human parathyroid hormone.

Comments—It is used to distinguish between *hypocalcemia* due to *hypoparathyroidism* and *pseudohypoparathyroidism* but not between these conditions and normal. Adverse effects include headache, nausea, dizziness, leg cramps, and diarrhea. Hypertensive crisis, hypocalcemia convulsions, and tingling of the extremities also have been reported. It is pregnancy category C, and no clinical studies have been done to determine if it is secreted in breast milk.

Pituitary Function

ARGININE HYDROCHLORIDE

See RPS-20, page 1818 for full monograph.

Comments—Intravenous infusion of arginine HCl stimulates the release of growth hormone in patients with competent *pituitary function.*

CORTICORELIN OVINE TRIFLUATE

Acthrel

Corticotropin-releasing factor (sheep), trifluoroacetate salt; CRF, CRH. [121249-14-7] $C_{205}H_{339}N_{59}O_{63}S$ (4670.36).

Preparation—See *Science* 1981; 213:1394.

Comments—Approved as an orphan drug for differentiating between the *pituitary gland and ectopic sources of production of ACTH* in patients who have ACTH-dependent Cushing's syndrome. Patients who have primary Cushing's syndrome experience a rise in plasma ACTH and cortisol, whereas patient who have ectopic sources of ACTH do not.

Adverse reactions include flushing of the head and neck, dyspnea, tachycardia, tightness in the chest, hypotension, and decreased blood pressure. It is pregnancy category C and not known if it appears in breast milk.

GONADORELIN HYDROCHLORIDE

Factrel

$$5-oxoPro-His-Trp-Ser-Tyr-Gly-Leu-Arg-Pro-Gly-NH_2 \quad \cdot \quad xHCl$$
$$1 \quad\;\; 2 \quad\; 3 \quad\; 4 \quad 5 \quad\; 6 \quad\; 7 \quad\; 8 \quad 9 \quad 10$$

Luteinizing hormone–releasing factor hydrochloride (LH-RH); [51952-41-1] $C_{55}H_{75}N_{17}O.xHCl$ (1182.33 for the free base—the *hydrochloride* may be either the mono- or dihydrochloride or a mixture of the two.)

Preparation—Isolated from the hypothalamus of pigs or sheep. The industrial preparation is described in German Pat 2,213,737. Now available as synthetic luteinizing hormone-releasing factor that is identical to the natural compound.

Description—The base is a white to very pale yellowish powder containing not less than 85% active peptide and not more than 6% acetic acid.

Comments—A diagnostic agent used for evaluating *hypothalamic-pituitary gonadotropic* function. The test should be conducted in the absence of other drugs that directly affect pituitary secretion of the gonadotropins, including preparations that contain androgens, estrogens, progestins, or glucocorticoids.

Adverse reactions include headache, nausea, lightheadedness, and abdominal discomfort. Localized swelling and pruritus may occur at the site of injection. Safety for use during pregnancy has not been established.

METYRAPONE

2-methyl-1,2-di-3-pyridinyl-1-propanone; Metopirone

[54-36-4] $C_{14}H_{14}N_2O$ (226.28).

Preparation—Methyl 3-pyridyl ketone is reduced electrolytically to the corresponding pinacol, 2,3-bis(3-pyridyl)-2,3-butanediol; heating with a strong inorganic acid results in dehydration of the pinacol with subsequent rearrangement to form metyrapone. US Pat 2,966,493.

Description—White to light-amber, fine, crystalline powder; characteristic odor; darkens on exposure to light.

Solubility—Sparingly soluble in water; soluble in methanol or chloroform; forms water-soluble salts with acids.

Comments—A synthetic compound that inhibits 11-β -hydroxylation in the biosynthesis of cortisol, corticosterone, and aldosterone. It is used to test for *hypothalamic- pituitary* function in patients suspected of hypopituitarism and Cushing's syndrome. Primary adrenal insufficiency must be excluded before the test is performed. Metyrapone blocks the enzymatic step that leads to cortisol and corticosterone synthesis in normal individuals, and produces an intense stimulation of ACTH secretion, followed by a marked increase in urinary excretion of 17-hydroxycorticosteroids. In patients with abnormal pituitary function, the ability to increase ACTH production is lacking, and no significant increase in 17-hydroxy-corticosteroids is seen.

There are two methods for performing the test. A single dose of metyrapone may be administered at midnight, and a blood sample is taken at 8 o'clock the next morning. A multi-dose test is performed over a 6-day period.

Adverse effects include anorexia, nausea, abdominal discomfort, diarrhea, dizziness, vertigo, headache, sedation, and allergic rash. The drug is contraindicated in patients with adrenal cortical insufficiency. Both hypo- and hyperthyroidism may interfere with the test, causing reduced response to metyrapone. Corticosteroids, estrogen, acetaminophen, and phenytoin alter the results obtained in the test and should not be used during the testing period.

SERMORELIN ACETATE

Somatoliberin (human pancreatic islet), acetate (salt), hydrate; Geref

$$H-Tyr-Ala-Asp-Ala-Ile-Phe-Thr-Asn-Ser-Tyr-Arg-Lys-Val-$$
$$1 \quad 2 \quad\; 3 \quad\; 4 \quad 5 \quad\; 6 \quad\; 7 \quad\; 8 \quad 9 \quad 10 \quad 11 \quad 12 \quad 13$$

$$Leu-Gly-Gln-Leu-Ser-Ala-Arg-Lys-Leu-Leu-Gln-Asp-Ile-$$
$$14 \quad 15 \quad 16 \quad 17 \quad 18 \quad 19 \quad 20 \quad 21 \quad 22 \quad 23 \quad 24 \quad 25 \quad 26$$

$$Met-Ser-Arg-NH_2 \quad \cdot \quad xC_2H_4O_2 \cdot yH_2O$$
$$27 \quad 28 \quad 29$$

[114466-38-5] $C_{149}H_{246}N_{44}O_{42}S.xC_2H_4O_2.yH_2O$.

Preparation—See US Pat 4,703,035.

Comments—A diagnostic agent that directly *stimulates the pituitary gland to secrete growth hormone*. It is used in the differential diagnosis of growth hormone deficiency. It may also be used in treatment of *growth hormone deficiency*.

Adverse reactions include irritation at site of injection, warmth, flushing, nausea, vomiting, taste alterations, and chest tightness. No studies are available that evaluate its safety in pregnancy.

Thyroid Function

PROTIRELIN

L-prolinamide, 5-oxo-L-propyl-L-histidyl-;

Thyrotropin-releasing factor [24305-27-9] $C_{16}H_{22}N_6O_4$ (362.39).

Preparation—Protirelin obtained from most mammals appears to be identical and is apparently not species specific. A review of synthetic methods is found in *Methods Enzymol* 1975; 37: 408.

Solubility—Highly purified material is partially soluble in chloroform and very soluble in methanol.

Comments—An adjunct in the diagnostic assessment of *thyroid function* and *pituitary or hypothalamic dysfunction*. It is a synthetic tripeptide believed to be structurally identical to the naturally occurring thyrotropin-releasing hormone produced by the hypothalamus. Following intravenous administration, the $T_{1/2}$ is approximately 5 minutes; TSH levels reach a peak in 20 to 30 minutes and decline slowly over a period of 3 hours to baseline levels.

Adverse effects occur in about 50% of patients and include hypertension or hypotension with or without syncope and breast enlargement. Other reactions include nausea, urge to urinate, flushing, lightheadedness, bad taste, abdominal discomfort, headache, and dry mouth. Safety has not been determined during pregnancy.

THYROTROPIN ALFA

Thyrogen

Comments—An adjunct used in determining serum thyroglobulin in patients with well-differentiated thyroid cancer.

GASTROINTESTINAL TRACT

Gallbladder

SINCALIDE

Caerulein, 1-de(5-oxo-L-proline)-2-de-L-glutamide-5-L-methionine; Kinevac

$$SO_3H$$
$$|$$
$$Asp-Tyr-Met-Gly-Trp-Met-Asp-Phe-NH_2$$
$$1 \quad\; 2 \quad\; 3 \quad\; 4 \quad 5 \quad\; 6 \quad\; 7 \quad\; 8$$

[25126-32-3] $C_{49}H_{62}N_{10}O_{16}S_3$ (1143.27).

Sincalide is the synthetic C-terminal octapeptide of cholecystokinin.

Description—White, lyophilized powder.

Solubility—Very slightly soluble in water; practically insoluble in alcohol.

Comments—A synthetic fragment of cholecystokinin that stimulates contraction of the gallbladder and increases intestinal motility. It is most frequently used during imaging studies such as *cholecystography or ultrasonography* to stimulate the gallbladder to contract and release bile instead of a fatty meals because of its fast action, usually 5 to 15 minutes. It may be used to obtain a *specimen of gallbladder bile for analysis* in conjunction with secretin to *stimulate pancreatic secretion* for analysis. It may also be used to increase movement of barium sulfate through the intestine during *roentgenograpghy or fluoroscopy*.

Adverse reactions include mild, transient, abdominal discomfort and an urge to defecate, and occasional dizziness, flushing, and nausea. It is pregnancy category B and not known if it appears in breast milk.

Liver Function

INDOCYANINE GREEN

Most evaluations of liver function tests utilize liver enzyme activity. However, liver function and blood flow can be evaluated by the intravenous injection of indocyanine green, an agent *not* taken up by any organ other than the liver. The intrinsic clearance of bound and unbound drug is high, hepatic extraction ratios in man vary from 50% to 80%. It is not metabolized but is eliminated entirely by active uptake into hepatic parenchymal cells. It is transported to bile, excreted in the small intestine, and not reabsorbed; consequently, it imparts a green color to the stool.

Indocyanine green has very low toxicity, is easily analyzed in low concentrations, is not metabolized, and has a plasma-disappearance rate-curve that is nearly exponential. It is injected intravenously in one arm, and 20 minutes later, 6 mL of venous blood is withdrawn from the opposite arm. A sample of serum is read in a photometer at 800 to 810 nm. Retention of 4% of the dye indicates normal liver function, while retention of greater quantities indicates hepatic dysfunction.

Intestinal Absorption

XYLOSE

D-**Xylose; Wood Sugar**

β-D-Xylopyranose [2460-44-8] $C_5H_{10}O_5$ (150.13).

Preparation—Prepared from corn cobs by distilling with 8% sulfuric acid; *J Am Chem Soc* 1919; 41: 1002.

Description—White, monoclinic prisms or needles melting at about 144°; very sweet taste; pK_a 12.14.

Solubility—1 g in 0.8 mL water; soluble in hot alcohol or pyridine.

Comments—The dextrorotatory form of this 5-carbon monosaccharide (Wood Sugar) is used for evaluating *intestinal absorption* in both adults and children. Malabsorption may occur in any disease that affects the small bowel directly or indirectly, including conditions such as celiac sprue, tropical sprue, lymphoma, small bowel ischemia, blind loop syndrome, short bowel syndrome, Whipple's gastroenteritis, amyloid disease of the gut, Crohn's disease, radiation enteritis, cow's milk protein intolerance (postchallenge), and certain parasitic diseases such as giardiasis, coccidiosis, and ascariasis.

The xylose test indicates the degree impairment in patients with signs and symptoms of malabsorption, and can also be used to monitor or evaluate therapy. Blood and urine samples may be collected, and analyses of these samples provide a better indication of any abnormalities. There are no known contraindications to the use of xylose for the evaluation of intestinal absorption.

Stomach

GASTRIC ACID TEST

Normal functioning of the gastrointestinal tract depends, in part, on the *ability of the stomach to secrete gastric acid*. The absence of hydrochloric acid in the stomach is essential in diagnosing of pernicious anemia and is frequently associated with gastric cancer. The presence of hydrochloric acid is useful in the diagnosis of certain peptic ulcer conditions. The absence of gastric acid excludes peptic esophagitis as a possible diagnosis in many cases.

The volume of acid secreted by the stomach varies greatly in normal individuals as well as in individuals with pathological states. It is usually important only to establish the presence or absence of free hydrochloric acid in the stomach. The gastric stimulants used for this purpose follow.

HISTAMINE PHOSPHATE—page 1543.

PENTAGASTRIN

L-**Phenylalaninamide**, *N*-**[(1,1-dimethylethoxy)carbonyl]-β-alanyl-**
L-**tryptophyl-**L-**methionyl-**L-**α-aspartyl-; Peptavlon**

N-Carboxy-β-alanyl-L-tryptophyl-L-methionyl-L-aspartylphenyl-L-alaninamide, *N-tert*-butyl ester [5534-95-2] $C_{37}H_{49}N_7O_9S$ (767.90).

Description—Fine colorless needles; melts at about 230° with decomposition.

Solubility—Soluble in dimethylsulfoxide or dimethylformamide; slightly soluble in alcohol or dilute solutions of ammonia; practically insoluble in water, ether, or benzene.

Comments—A diagnostic agent used to evaluate *gastric acid secretory function*. It is useful in testing for *anacidity* in patients with suspected pernicious anemia, atrophic gastritis, or gastric carcinoma; for *hypersecretion* in patients with possible duodenal ulcer or postoperative stomach ulcer; for the diagnosis of Zollinger-Ellison tumor; and for determining the adequacy of acid-reducing operations for peptic ulcer. Acid secretion is increased within 10 minutes after intradermal injection and reaches a peak in most patients within 20 to 30 minutes, persisting for 60 to 80 minutes. Plasma half-life is reported to be less than 1 minute. Excessive doses may inhibit gastric acid secretion.

It is contraindicated in patients hypersensitive to the drug and should be used with caution in patients with pancreatic, hepatic, or biliary disease. Adverse reactions include abdominal pain, nausea, vomiting, flushing, tachycardia, dizziness, faintness, lightheadedness, drowsiness, blurred vision, and headache. Its use in pregnant women and children has not been studied.

GASTRIC UREASE TEST (*HELIOBACTER PYLORI TEST*)

Pytest

Comment—Patients infected with *H pylori* produce gastric urease, an enzyme that releases carbon dioxide from urea. Patients ingest urea that is labeled with radioactive carbon-14 orally. The patient breathes into a device that collects the expired breath and the [14]carbon dioxide present in the sample is measured in a liquid scintillation counter.

Pancreas (Exocrine Function)

BENTIROMIDE

Benzoic acid, (*S*)4-[[2-(benzoylamino)-3-(4-hydroxyphenyl)-1-oxopropyl]- amino]-; Chymex

[37106-97-1] $C_{23}H_{20}N_2O_5$ (404.42).

Preparation—See *J Med Chem* 1972; 15: 1098.

Description—White crystals; melts at about 240°.

Comments—Used to diagnose exocrine pancreatic insufficiency and to monitor the adequacy of enzyme replacement therapy in patients with exocrine pancreatic insufficiency. Pancreatic chymotrypsin selectively cleaves para-aminobenzoic acid (ABA) from bentiromide following oral administration. ABA is absorbed rapidly under normal GI function, conjugated by the liver, and excreted in the urine in about 6 hours. If approximately 50% of the ABA content of bentiromide (170 mg in 500 mg) is collected in the 6-hour urine sample, it indicates normal exocrine pancreatic function, gastric emptying, and intestinal and kidney function. This test is a simple, noninvasive test shown to produce reliable, reproducible results in the diagnosis of pancreatic insufficiency.

Adverse effects are transient and relatively infrequent; diarrhea, headache, flatulence, nausea, vomiting, and weakness are the most frequent. Safety and efficacy in children over 6 years have not been established. The drug should not be used during pregnancy or in nursing mothers unless clearly needed. Drugs and foods that are metabolized to primary arylamines, and multiple vitamins should be discontinued at least 3 days prior to the drug's administration.

SECRETIN

SecreFlo

[1393-25-5] $C_{130}H_{220}N_{44}O_{41}$ (no molecular weight was given).

Description—A polypeptide hormone, secreted by the duodenal mucosa and to a lesser extent by the upper jejunal mucosa, which stimulates secretion of water and bicarbonate from the pancreas. As isolated from porcine mucosa and purified, it consists of 27 amino acid units from 12 different amino acids. It has been synthesized (Bodanszky et al, *J Am Chem Soc* 1967; 89:685, 6753). It is the synthetic, C-terminal, octapeptide fragment of cholecystokinin. The hormone supplied for diagnostic use is of porcine origin as a sterile, refined, freeze-dried powder, stable for 2 years when stored in its original, unopened vial at 2° to 7° C; it is unstable in solution.

Comments—Used *to diagnosis pancreatic exocrine disease and gastrinoma (Zollinger-Ellison syndrome)*. It may be combined with sincalide as a diagnostic aid for chronic pancreatic function or carcinoma. Intravenous injection of the hormone in persons with normal pancreatic secretion increases the bicarbonate content and volume of secretion from the pancreas. Reduced secretory volume and diminished bicarbonate concentration are signs of pancreatic insufficiency. Reduction is volume only indicates pancreatic duct obstruction while bicarbonate only reductions indicate pancreatic inflammatory disease.

A double-lumen tube is passed through the mouth after a 12- to 15-hour fast, under fluoroscopic guidance so that a proper placement of the proximal tube in the gastric antrum and of the distal tube beyond the papilla of Vater is accomplished. Constant suction is applied to both outlets of the tube throughout the test. After a control period of collection of fluid for 10 to 20 minutes, 0.2 μg of drug is injected intravenously over a period of 1 minute to test for allergic reactions. If none occurs, the full dose of drug is injected. Secretions from the duodenum are collected every 15 minutes for 1 hour and analyzed for volume variations and bicarbonate concentrations.

Secretin is contraindicated in patients with an allergic or sensitivity to the drug and is administered with caution in patients with a history of atopic asthma. It should not be used in patients with acute pancreatitis until the episode has resolved itself.

LYMPHATIC SYSTEM

ISOSULFAN BLUE

Ethanaminium, *N*-[4-[[4-(diethylamino)-phenyl(2,5-disulfophenyl)methylene]-2,5-cyclohexadien-1-ylidene]-*N*-ethyl-, hydroxide, inner salt, sodium salt; Lymphazurin

Colour Index: Sulphan Blue; CI no 42045 (often confused with Patent Blue V, CI no 42051) [68238-36-8] $C_{27}H_{31}N_2NaO_6S_2$ (566.68).

Preparation—By condensation of 4-formylbenzene-1,3-disulfonic acid and *N,N*-diethylaniline. See *Colour Index v4, 1971*.

Description—Violet powder; aqueous solutions are blue, and the color is stable over a wide range of pH if protected from light.

Solubility—Soluble in water (1 in 20); partially soluble in alcohol.

Comments—An adjunct to *lymphography* for visualization of the lymphatic system draining the area in which it is injected. It has no known pharmacological action. Allergic-type adverse effects occur in about 1.5% of patients and include localized swelling and pruritus of the hands, abdomen, and neck. Edema of the face and glottis, respiratory distress, and shock have been reported. These reactions are more likely to occur in patients with a history of hypersensitivity. Its safe use during pregnancy and lactation, as well as in children, has not been established.

NEUROMUSCULAR SYSTEM

The following drugs are used in the *diagnosis of myasthenia gravis*.

EDROPHONIUM CHLORIDE— page 1395.
NEOSTIGMINE METHYLSULFATE—page 1395.

PULMONARY SYSTEM

Bronchial Airway Hyperactivity

METHACHOLINE CHLORIDE— page 1391.

Comments—A parasympathomimetic (cholinergic) agent that is only administered by inhalation for the *diagnosis of bronchial airway hyperactivity* in subjects who do not display symptoms of asthma. Asthmatics are significantly more sensitive to inhaled methacholine chloride than are healthy subjects. The difference in response provides the pharmacological basis for this diagnostic test. It should not be used in patients with epilepsy or cardiovascular, peptic ulcer, or thyroid disease; likewise, it is contraindicated in patients with urinary tract obstruction.

Adverse effects after *inhalation* include headache, throat irritation, lightheadedness, and itching. The safety of the test during pregnancy and lactation and in children under 5 years has not been established.

REPRODUCTIVE SYSTEM

UTERINE CAVITY (SEE DEXTRAN MONOGRAPH page 1322.)

Dextran 70 (32% *W/V*) in Dextrose (10% *W/V*), Hyskon

Comments—intended for use as an aid with the hysteroscope in the distension of the *uterine cavity* and in irrigating and visualizing its surfaces.

SPECIAL SENSES

Ophthalmic Diagnostic Aids

FLUORESCEIN SODIUM

Spiro[isobenzofuran-1(3*H*),9'-[9*H*]xanthene]-3-one, 3',6'-dihydroxy-, disodium salt; Resorcinolphthalein Sodium, Soluble Fluorescein, Uranin, Uranine Yellow

Colour Index: Acid Yellow 73; CI no 45350 [518-47-8] $C_{20}H_{10}Na_2O_5$ (376.28).

Preparation—By heating resorcinol with phthalic anhydride at about 200°. After purifying, the phthalein is dissolved in the required amount of sodium hydroxide solution and evaporated to dryness.

Description—Orange-red, odorless powder; hygroscopic; aqueous solution is strongly fluorescent even in extreme dilution; the fluorescence disappears when the solution is made acid and reappears when the solution is again made alkaline.

Solubility—Freely soluble in water; sparingly soluble in alcohol.

Comments—Used as a sterile ophthalmic strip impregnated with drug, or as a 2% aqueous solution for the diagnosis of *corneal lesions*, pressure points on the surface of the cornea under contact lenses, and the detection of minute *foreign bodies* embedded in the cornea. A weak solution will not stain the normal cornea, but ulcers or injured epithelium and pressure points will become green and remain so for a time; foreign bodies will appear surrounded by a green ring; loss of substance in the conjunctiva is indicated by a yellow hue. It also reveals defects of the endothelium of the cornea, producing a deep coloration of the abnormal area.

It is particularly important that the preparation be sterile and that no accidental contamination of the solution occurs with *Pseudomonas aeruginosa* because this could cause blindness. Fluorescein is anionic and not compatible with preservatives such as benzalkonium chloride or substances known to be effective against *P aeruginosa,* such as polymyxin B sulfate. It is best used as a unit-dose package. When a sterile ophthalmic strip with fluorescein touches lacrimal fluid in the eye, it releases enough of the highly soluble drug to permit examination of the eye for lesions or injury.

Fluorescein Sodium Injection—[Fluorescite, Ful-Glo, Funduscein] *Comments:* A diagnostic aid in *ophthalmic angiography,* which includes examination of the fundus, evaluation of the iris' vasculature, distinction between viable and nonviable tissue, and observation of the aqueous flow. It is useful in the differential diagnosis of malignant and nonmalignant ocular tumors.

Adverse reactions include cardiac arrest, basilar artery ischemia, severe shock, and thrombophlebitis at the site of the injection. Transient nausea, vomiting, and allergic reactions have been reported in sensitive patients. A strong taste may develop following high dosage.

MEDICINAL AGENTS

Accu-Chek Active (*Roche Diagnostics*): alternate site testing; Accu-Chek Advantage (*Roche Diagnostics*): voice attachment available; Accu-Chek Compact (*Roche Diagnostics*): has a drum that holds 17 strips; Accu-Chek Complete (*Roche Diagnostics*); Free Style (*Therasense*): alternate site testing.

HEMOGLOBIN A1C TESTING

A1c Now: meter with test strip for measurement.

KETONE TESTING

Acetest : colometric urine test.
KetoStix: colometric urine test.
Precision Extra: meter reads blood ketone levels.

INFECTIOUS DISEASE TESTING

These tests require that a sample of capillary blood from a finger-stick be placed on a pad with reagents, and returned to a laboratory for analysis. Each test has a computer generated random number. The patient calls a toll-free phone number to speak with a trained professional to get the results, and counseling is available.

HIV

Home Access

HEPATITIS C

Hepatitis C Check

OVULATION TESTS

A test stick with monoclonal antibodies is either placed directly in the urine stream or dipped into a sample of urine in a container that *detect leutinizing hormone*. Capillary attraction moves the sample over the test area and a color is produced when the levels of leutinizing hormone reach levels that indicate that ovulation will occur. LH is released about 24 hours before ovulation. The tests come with multiple devices, usually 5 to 9 test sticks, because of the variation that occurs normally in the length of a woman's the menstrual cycle.

Clear Plan Easy Fertility Monitor is a new device that *detects both LH and estrone-3 glucuronide*, a metabolite of estrogen in the urine. It is an automated device programmed to predict fertility in stages ranging from low to high probability.

OVULATION TESTS

Answer 1 Step; Clearplan Easy; CVS brand; Eckerd brand; First Response; Target brand; Walgreen brand

PREGNANCY TESTING

A reagent stick with monoclonal antibodies *for detecting human chorionic gonadotropin (HCG)*, which is only secreted by the corpus luteum can be detected as early as 1 day after a missed menstrual period. The stick is placed in the urine stream or dipped in a same of urine and a positive test result produces a color.

PREGNANCY TESTS

Answer Quick & Easy; Clearblue Easy; Clear Choice; Confirm 1-step; e.p.t.; Quick Stick; First Response 1-Step

Comments—Some chain pharmacies also market their own brand name product as they do for ovulation tests above.

URINARY TESTING

BLOOD

EZ Detect for Hidden Blood in Urine

Comments—A colormetric, urine dipstick test. Users are advised to call their physician if the test is positive or if their symptoms persist after a negative test.

DRUGS OF ABUSE

Dr. Brown's Home Drug Testing System: mail sample; Parents' Alert: mail sample; Parents Home Drug Testing: in home result; QuickScreen A: in home result; American Medical Screening: a 10-drug test card for in home results.

Comments—Some OTC tests provide a result at the time of testing using a dipstick impregnated with reagent to produce a result. Other OTC products containing a random number require a urine sample be sent to a laboratory for analysis. A toll free phone number is provided for obtaining the results.

One OTC test, PDT-90, requires a sample of hair to be returned for analysis.

URINE TESTING FOR INFECTIONS

UTI: a nitrate to nitrite test; AZO Test Strips: a urinary nitrate to nitrite test combined with a dipstick that *detects leukocyte esterase*, an enzyme produced when leukocytes are release.

Comments—Patients using urinary test kits are advised to see their doctor if the test produces a positive result or if the result is negative but their symptoms persist.

Most bacteria responsible for urinary tract infections convert *urinary nitrates to nitrites*. A dipstick, colorometric test is used.

URINE TESTING FOR PROTEIN

Kidney Screen At Home

Comments—A colormetric, urine dipstick test that *detects albumin*. Users are advised to call their physician if the test is positive or if their symptoms persist after a negative test result.

REFERENCES

1. Roizen MF. *JAMA* 1994; 271:319.
2. Thrall JH. In:Swanson DP, Chilton HM, Thrall JH, eds. *Pharmaceuticals in Medical Imaging*. New York: Macmillan, 1990, Chap 8.
3. Singri N, Ahya SN, Levin ML. *JAMA* 2003; 289:747.
4. Nash K, Hafeez A, Hou S. *Am J Kidney Dis* 2002; 39:930.
5. Aspelin P, Aubry P, Fransson SG, et al. *N Engl J Med* 2003; 346:491.
6. Murray PR, Baron EJ, Jorgensen JH, et al, eds. *Manual of Clinical Microbiology*, 8th ed. Washington: ASM Press, 2003.
7. Truant AL, ed. *Commercial Methods in Clinical Microbiology*, Washington: ASM Press, 2003.
8. Grainger RG, Thomas AMK. In: Dawson P, Cosgrove DO, Grainger, RG, eds. *Textbook of Contrast Media*. Oxford: Isis Medical Media Ltd., 1999, Chap 1.
9. Freeman A. In: Dawson P, Cosgrove DO, Grainger, RG, eds. *Textbook of Contrast Media*. Oxford: Isis Medical Media Ltd., 1999, Chap 14.
10. Omnipaque Product Information. Princeton, NJ: Amersham Health, 2001.
11. GastroMARK Product Information. St. Louis: Mallinckrodt, 1997.
12. Teslascan Product Information. Princeton, NJ: Nycomed, 1997.
13. Definity Product Information. N. Billerica, MA: Bristol-Myers Squibb Medical Imaging, 2002.
14. Optison Product Information. Princeton, NJ: Amersham Health, 2003.

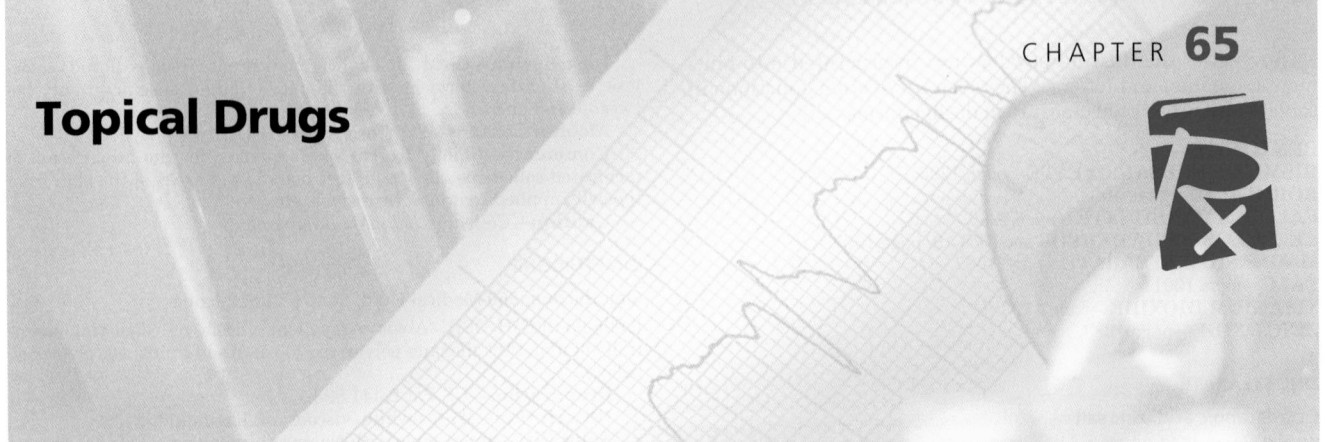

CHAPTER 65

Topical Drugs

Chemical agents may be applied to the skin and mucous membranes for localized effects within the skin or membrane. Many of these, such as antibiotics, antiseptics, corticosteroids, antineoplastics, and local anesthetics, belong to distinct pharmacological classes treated elsewhere in this text and are not discussed specifically in this chapter. However, transdermal delivery systems for compounds whose pharmacological activity is discussed elsewhere are outlined briefly from the delivery viewpoint in this chapter. The heterogeneous groups of agents that are not part of a pharmaceutical drug class but nonetheless have effects on epithelial surfaces and are mostly nonselective in action are the primary focus of this chapter.

Those locally acting topical agents that have limited chemical and pharmacological activity generally have a *physical* basis of action. Included in this group are protectives, adsorbents, demulcents, emollients, and cleansing agents. The relative inertness of many of these substances renders them of value as vehicles and excipients. Consequently, many agents in this group are also pharmaceutical necessities and may be treated in Chapter 55.

Topical agents that have general *chemical* reactivity include most astringents, irritants, rubefacients, vesicants, sclerosing agents, caustics, escharotics, many keratolytic (desquamating) agents, and a miscellaneous group of dermatologicals including hypopigmenting and antipruritic agents.

Although the skin (described in further detail in Chapter 37) and other membranes (see Chapter 44 concerning the eye and Chapter 59 concerning absorption across other membranes) differ considerably in structure and function, they exhibit similar absorption profiles for some chemical agents and similar responses to certain physical and pharmacological stimuli. Thus, many of the agents found in this chapter may be applied to other membranes. Nevertheless, it is obvious that many agents, for which there is either contraindication or no rationale for their application to the mucous membranes, may be applied only to the skin.

PROTECTIVES AND ADSORBENTS

In its broadest pharmacological sense a protective is any agent that isolates the exposed surface (skin or other membranes) from harmful or annoying stimuli. Substances that protect by mechanical or other physical means are considered to be protectives. While the surface action of adsorbents and demulcents may impart some protection, demulcents and emollients are placed in separate categories that reflect their primarily dermatological function.

The abridged category of protectives mainly comprises the dusting powders, adsorbents, mechanical protective agents, and plasters.

Dusting Powders

Certain relatively inert and insoluble substances are used to cover and protect epithelial surfaces, ulcers, and wounds. Usually these substances are very finely subdivided powders. They generally absorb moisture and, therefore, also act as cutaneous desiccants. The absorption of skin moisture decreases friction and also discourages certain bacterial growth.

The water-absorbent powders should not be administered to wet, raw surfaces because of the formation of cakes and adherent crusts. Starch and other carbohydrate powders may become doughy with absorption of aqueous-based fluids but also may ferment. Consequently, such powders often contain an antiseptic. Most impalpable powders are absorptive, to some extent. Whether absorption of substances, other than water, contributes to the protection of the skin is uncertain; however, absorption of fatty acids and perspiration constituents along with cutaneous drying, contributes to a deodorant action of such powders. It generally is held that the adsorptive capacity is important to the gastrointestinal (GI) protective action of chemically inert powders taken internally.

Chemically inert dusting powders are not entirely biologically inert, despite the name. When carried into pores or wounds or left upon skin or epithelial surfaces, dusting powders, eg, talc, may cause irritation, granulomas, fibrosis, or adhesions. Even without direct irritation or obstruction of the perspiration, dust can be troublesome.

Absorbable dusting powders (Biosorb, *Ezon*) are available for surgical gloves. This absorbable powder is mixed with 2% magnesium oxide and contains residual amounts of sodium sulfate and sodium chloride. This mixture produces no reaction in tissues and is absorbed completely within a short time. Starch also has drying and absorptive qualities (Fordustin powder; 90 and 24 g). These products, however, can be metabolized by *Candida* and thus can aggravate an infection.

A product containing detranomer (Debrisan) promotes debridement of secreting wounds, including venous stasis and decubitus ulcers, infected traumatic and surgical wounds, as well as infected burns. It consists of hydrophilic spherical beads (0.1–0.3 mm in diameter) of dextranomer. The beads are composed of a three-dimensional network of cross-linked dextran. This network selectively imbibes molecules on the basis of molecular mass (molecules <1000 daltons are imbibed; molecules 1000 to 5000 daltons experience decreased absorption with increasing molecular-weight and molecules >5000 daltons are not imbibed). Four milliliters of water are absorbed for each gram of dextranomer, and absorption is continuous so long as unsaturated beads are in proximity to the wound. This therapy is associated with the rapid and continuous exudate removal from wound surfaces, resulting in a marked reduction in inflammation, edema, and pain, as well as an increase in granuloma tissue formation and reduction in time for wound healing.

Several of the dusting powders are incorporated into ointments, creams, and lotions. They also serve other functions in tablets and other pharmaceutical dosage forms.

BENTONITE—page 1073.
BISMUTH, SUBSALICYLATE—page 1296.
BORIC ACID—page 1083.
CALCIUM CARBONATE—page 1296.
CELLULOSE, POWDERED—see RPS-19, page 1397.
MAGNESIUM STEARATE—page 1087.
TALC—page 1091.
TITANIUM DIOXIDE—page 1293.
ZINC OXIDE—page 1283.

ZINC STEARATE

Octadecanoic acid, zinc salt

Zinc stearate [557-05-1]. A compound of zinc with a mixture of solid organic acids obtained from fats, which consists chiefly of variable proportions of zinc stearate and zinc palmitate. It contains the equivalent of 12.5 to 14.0% of ZnO (81.38).

Preparation—An aqueous solution of zinc sulfate is added to a sodium stearate solution, and the precipitate is washed with water until free of sulfate and dried.

Description—Fine, white, bulky powder, free from grittiness, with a faint characteristic color; neutral to moistened litmus paper.

Solubility—Insoluble in water, alcohol, or ether; soluble in benzene.

Comments—In *water-repellent* ointments and as a *dusting powder* in dermatological practice for its desiccating, astringent, and *protective* effects. It has been removed from baby dusting powders, owing to accidental, fatal inhalations.

Mechanical and Chemical Protectives

Several materials may be administered to the skin to form an adherent, continuous film that may be either flexible or semi-rigid, depending on the materials and their formulations, as well as the manner in which they are applied. Such materials may serve several purposes including (1) providing occlusive protection from the external environment, (2) providing mechanical support, and/or (3) serving as vehicles for various medicaments.

The two principal classes of mechanical protectives are the collodions and plasters. Their use is decreasing with the increasing recognition of the importance of air exposure in maintaining a normally balanced cutaneous bacterial flora of low pathogenicity. Also, the mechanical protectives may be somewhat irritating because of interference with normal percutaneous water transport caused by certain oligomers, resins, and other components, especially in plasters. The cerates may be employed similarly to the plasters. Bandages, dressings, new vapor-permeable polymer membranes, and casts also afford mechanical protection and support (see Chapter 108 for additional information). A brief discussion of plasters is included in Chapter 44.

A number of insoluble and relatively inert powders that remain essentially unchanged chemically in the GI tract may possess surface properties that favor their absorption to the GI mucosa. Such materials may offer mechanical protection against abrasion and may even offer slight protection against toxins and chemical irritants. Many such protectives also are adsorbents (charcoal, bismuth compounds, kaolin) or astringents (zinc and bismuth compounds). They are discussed under those categories.

ALUMINUM HYDROXIDE GEL—page 1295.

COLLODION

Contains not less than 5.0%, by weight, of pyroxylin.

Pyroxylin	40 g
Ether	750 mL
Alcohol	250 mL
To make about	1000 mL

Add the alcohol and the ether to the pyroxylin contained in a suitable container, and stopper the container well. Shake the mixture occasionally until the pyroxylin is dissolved.

Description—Clear, or slightly opalescent, viscous liquid; colorless, or slightly yellowish, with the odor of ether; specific gravity between 0.765 and 0.775.

Alcohol Content—22% to 26% of C_2H_5OH.

Comments—Chiefly to seal small wounds, for the preparation of medicated collodions, and to protect nonaffected areas of the skin from topically applied irritants, corrosives, etc.

Caution—*Collodion is highly flammable.*

DIMETHICONE

Simethicone; 360 Medical Fluid; Sentry Dimethicone

[9006-65-9]$(C_2H_6OSi)_n$. A water-repellent silicone oil consisting essentially of dimethyl siloxane polymers (200 series of fluids; see *Silicones,* below).

Preparation—US Pat 2,441,098.

Description—Water-white, viscous, oil-like liquid.

Solubility—Immiscible with water or alcohol; miscible with chloroform or ether.

Comments—Exhibits skin-adherent and water-repellent properties. It is both a *protective* and an *emollient,* for which its Food and Drug Administration (FDA) classification is Category I. Applied to the skin, it forms a *protective* film that provides a barrier to ordinary soap and water and water-soluble irritants. The film may last several hours if the skin is exposed, mainly to aqueous media. The film provides a less effective barrier to synthetic detergents and lipid-soluble materials, such as organic solvents. It should not be applied except in contact dermatoses and dermatoses aggravated by substances that can be repelled by the silicone. It is useful in preventing irritation from ammonia produced by the urine of infants, but it may exacerbate preexisting irritation. The occlusive protection by the silicone is detrimental to inflamed, traumatized, abraded, or excoriated skin and to lesions requiring free drainage. However, applied adjacent to such lesions, it offers protection against irritating discharges and maceration. It practically is harmless and does not sensitize skin, but it does cause temporary irritation to the eyes. It may be incorporated into creams or lotions.

PETROLATUM GAUZE

Petrolated Gauze

Absorbent gauze saturated with white petrolatum. The weight of the petrolatum is 70–80% of the weight of the gauze. It is sterile.

Preparation—By adding, under aseptic conditions, molten, sterile, white petrolatum to dry, sterile, absorbent gauze, previously cut to size, in the ratio of 60 g petrolatum to each 20 g gauze.

Comments—A *protective* dressing; also as packing material for postoperative plugs, packs, rolls, and tampons, and as a wick, drain, or wraparound for tubing. It is claimed that there is no danger of tissue maceration and that no growth of granulation tissue through it occurs.

GELATIN SPONGE, ABSORBABLE—page 1337.
KAOLIN—page 1313.
LANOLIN—page 1078.
LANOLIN, ANHYDROUS—page 1077.
MINERAL OIL—page 1308.
MINERAL OIL EMULSION—see RPS-19, page 788.
MINERAL OIL, LIGHT—page 1087.
OLIVE OIL—see RPS-19, page 1400.
PEANUT OIL—page 1072.
PETROLATUM—page 1077.

SILICONES

Polyorganosiloxanes; Silastic; Silicone Rubber

Organosilicon polymers containing chains of alternating oxygen and silicon atoms with substituent organic groups, frequently methyl or phenyl, attached to each silicon atom.

Preparation—May be prepared synthetically by condensing alkylated or arylated *silanols*. Disubstituted *silanediols* [$R_2Si(OH)_2$] form linear polymers having the general formula.

$$HO-\underset{\underset{R}{|}}{\overset{\overset{R}{|}}{Si}}-O-\left[\underset{\underset{R}{|}}{\overset{\overset{R}{|}}{Si}}-O\right]_n-\underset{\underset{R}{|}}{\overset{\overset{R}{|}}{Si}}-OH$$

Cross-linked polymers result from condensation of mixtures of substituted silanediols and monosubstituted *silanetriols* [$RSi(OH)_3$], represented by the following partial formula where R is a hydrocarbon radical:

One method of preparation involves interaction of silicon tetrachloride with appropriate Grignard reagents to yield alkylated or arylated dichlorosilanes. After hydrolysis to the corresponding substituted silanols, dehydration procedures are used to effect condensation polymerization. The overall reaction, as it involves a disubstituted silanediol, may be represented as

$$SiCl_4 \xrightarrow{RMgX} R_2SiCl_2 \xrightarrow{HOH} R_2Si(OH)_2 \xrightarrow{-HOH} HO[Si(R)_2O]_nH$$

| Silicon tetrachloride | Disubstituted dichlorosilane | Disubstituted silanediol | Silicone linear polymer |

Description—Silicones with a wide range of properties may be produced by varying the molecular weight, tacticity, substituent R groups, R:Si ratios (whether linear, cyclic, or cross-linked polymers), and the degree of cross-linking. Physically, silicones vary from mobile liquids through low-viscosity liquids and semisolids to solids. Linear silicones (liquids to semisolids) have viscosities ranging from 0.65 to 1,000,000 centistokes. Higher-molecular-weight linear silicones form solids. Cross-linked silicones may exhibit gel-like to solid-like properties, depending on the degree of cross-linking and chemical structure of the repeat unit. In general, silicones are odorless, tasteless, water repellent, relatively inert chemically, stable under high and low temperatures, and efficient as antifoam agents.

Solubility—Unmodified silicones are generally insoluble in water, thus they frequently are termed *silicone oils*. However, a water-soluble sodium salt of a simple silicone, *sodium methyl siliconate* [$CH_3Si(OH)_2ONa$], has been marketed.

Comments—Preparations containing silicones have various dermatological uses (see *Dimethicone*) and are used as ingredients of bases for ointments and liniments. In the form of inhalation sprays, silicone preparations have been employed in the treatment of pulmonary edema nvolving frothing of fluid in the upper respiratory tract. They also are used orally as antiflatulent or gastric defoaming agents.

A silicone *bouncing putty* has found acceptance for use as a physical agent in treating conditions requiring finger exercise. The water-repellent properties of the silicones are employed in numerous applications in which drainage of aqueous fluids from surfaces is desirable.

Silicones exhibit low irritation as a result of their surface chemical, physical, and bulk mechanical properties. Consequently, silicone rubbers are component materials in various indwelling catheters and tubes designed for short-time use. Solid implants that incorporate silicone into their composition include nose, chin, and other types of prostheses used in plastic, reconstructive, and orthopedic procedures.

In addition to uses involving antifoaming, water-repellent, and non-irritating characteristics, silicone fluids also are employed to prevent adhesion between components or materials and as release agents. Examples of its usage as a release agent include release of rubber and plastics from molds, food from metal, ice from wings of aircraft and capsules and tablets from molds and dies in which they are fabricated.

Liquid silicones have been used to fill in hypoplastic body areas for cosmetic purposes, although these fluids tend to relocate because of flow under gravity and motion. While the use of silicone fluids in reconstructive breast surgery and similar applications is undergoing reassessment for safety concerns, solid materials continue to be well accepted in biomedical applications.

Higher-molecular-weight (solid) silicone rubbers are used to encapsulate steroid hormones and other drugs intended for chronic implantation. For example, Norplant *(Wyeth-Ayerst)* is a long- term contraceptive implant that incorporates levonorgestrel into silastic-based rods. The steroid is released slowly from the implant over an extended time period to provide approximately 5-yr continuous use.

Silicone-based materials are also an important class of contact lens materials. The silicone polymer is gas permeable, thus enabling oxygen to permeate the contact lens to the cornea. However, silicones are not hydrogels and do not absorb large amounts of water similar to hydrogel-based contact lenses. The materials exhibit minimal if any irritation as a result of surface chemical and physical properties and are comfortable to wear because of the gas permeation and mechanical properties.

ZINC CARBONATE

Smithsonite; Zincspar

[3486-35-9] CO_3Zn (125.38).

Description—White rhombohedroids.

Solubility—Soluble 10 ppm in water at 15°; soluble in dilute acids, alkalies, or solutions of ammonium salts.

Comments—Both for its lubricity and as a drying agent. As a skin protectant it falls into FDA Category I. It is included in commercial topical burn and sunburn products and extemporary protectants.

Occlusive Dressings

Occlusive dressings alter environmental aspects of certain types of wounds that may facilitate healing. While a moist wound environment may be beneficial, there are certain disadvantages. Moisture has been associated with enhanced rates of reepithelialization. Brief increases in the number of inflammatory cells within the wound site may break down cellular debris. While transient increases in bacterial counts have been observed with occlusive dressings, infection usually does not occur, in part as a result of the transitory increased inflammatory cell populations. Dermal and epidermal healing also may be aided by the low-pH and low-oxygen environment. Furthermore, such dressings provide physical protection.

Gas-permeable, synthetic, polymer-based dressings have been developed. These materials provide chemical and physical protection while maintaining a more acceptable microenvironment. Polyurethane-based films that are permeable to oxygen and water vapor include Op-site, Tegaderm, and Bioclusive. Duo-Derm *(Conva Tec)* is a hydrophobic polymer with embedded hydroactive particles that is oxygen- and water-vapor impermeable. Application depends on whether the dressing is self-adherent.

DEMULCENTS

Demulcents (L, *demulcere,* to smooth down) are protective agents that are employed primarily to alleviate irritation, particularly of mucous membranes or abraded tissues. They also often are applied to the skin. They generally are applied to the surface in viscid, sticky preparations that cover the area readily. They also may be medicated. The local action of chemical, mechanical, or bacterial irritants, thereby, is diminished, and pain, reflexes, spasm, or catarrh are attenuated. They also prevent drying of the affected surface. The demulcents may be applied to the skin (lotions, ointments, or wet dressings), GI tract (demulcent drinks or enemas), throat (lozenges or gargles), or corneal membranes (artificial tears and in wetting agents for contact lenses). When demulcents are applied as solid material (as in lozenges or powders), the liquid is provided by secreted or exuded fluids. Demulcents frequently are medicated. In such instances the demulcent may be an adjuvant, a corrective, or a pharmaceutical necessity. Many of the demulcents are also laxatives and are used as such, or they are used with laxatives or antacids for their demulcent and lubricating action.

A variety of chemical substances possess demulcent properties. Among these are the alginates, mucilages, gums, dextrins, starches, certain sugars, and polymeric polyhydric glycols. Mucus itself is a natural demulcent. Certain silicates that form silicic acid on exposure to air or gastric juice and glycerin, although the silicic acid has low molecular weight and relatively low binding power, frequently are placed among the demulcents. Also the colloidal hydrous oxides, hydroxides, and basic salts of several metals are claimed to be demulcent, but acceptable clinical proof of the claim has not been provided.

The hydrophilic colloidal properties of most demulcents enable them to function as emulsifiers and suspending agents in water-soluble ointments and suspensions. They also retard the absorption of many injections and, thus, may be employed in various depot preparations. Many of the demulcents mask the flavor of medicaments by means of at least three physical phenomena: (1) they apparently coat the taste receptors and render them less sensitive; (2) they incorporate many organic solutes into micelles and, thereby, diminish the free concentration of such solutes; and (3) they coat the surfaces of many particles in suspension. Because of the adhesiveness of the demulcents, they are employed widely as binding agents in tablets, lozenges, and similar dosage forms. Consequently, certain demulcents are discussed in Chapter 55.

ACACIA—pages 1070 and 1072.
AGAR—page 1073.

BENZOIN

Gum Benjamin; Benzoe

The balsamic resin obtained from *Styrax benzoin* Dryander or *Styrax paralleloneurus* Perkins, known in commerce as Sumatra Benzoin, or from *Styrax tonkinensis* (Pierre) Craib ex Hartwich, or other species of the Section *Anthostyrax* of the genus *Styrax,* known in commerce as Siam Benzoin (Fam *Styraceae*).

Sumatra benzoin yields not less than 75.0% of alcohol-soluble extractive, and Siam benzoin yields not less than 90.0% of alcohol-soluble extractive.

Constituents—Siam benzoin contains about 68% crystalline *coniferyl benzoate* [$C_{17}H_{16}O_4$]; up to 10% of an amorphous form of this compound is also present. Some *coniferyl alcohol* (*m-methoxy-p-hydroxycinnamyl alcohol,* mp 73° to 74°) occurs in the free state as well. Other compounds that have been isolated are *benzoic acid,* 11.7%; *d-iaresinolic acid,* 6%; *cinnamyl benzoate,* 2.3%; and *vanillin* 0.3%.

Sumatra benzoin has been reported to contain benzoic and cinnamic acid esters of the alcohol *benzoresinol* and probably also coniferyl alcohol, free *benzoic* and *cinnamic acids, styrene,* 2 to 3% *cinnamyl cinnamate* (also called *styracin*), 1% *phenylpropyl cinnamate,* 1% *vanillin,* a trace of *benzaldehyde,* a little *benzyl cinnamate,* and the alcohol *d-sumaresinol* $C_{30}H_{48}O_4$.

Description—*Sumatra Benzoin:* Blocks or lumps of varying size made up of compacted tears, with a reddish brown, reddish gray, or grayish brown resinous mass. *Siam Benzoin:* Compressed pebble-like tears of varying size and shape. Both varieties are yellowish to rusty brown externally and milky white on fracture; hard and brittle at ordinary temperatures but softened by heat; aromatic and balsamic odor; aromatic and slightly acrid taste.

Comments—A *protective* application for irritations of the skin. When mixed with glycerin and water, the tincture may be applied locally for *cutaneous ulcers, bedsores, cracked nipples,* and *fissures* of the lips and anus. For throat and bronchial inflammation, the tincture may be administered on sugar. The tincture and compound tincture sometimes are used in boiling water as steam inhalants for their *expectorant* and *soothing action* in acute laryngitis and croup. In combination with zinc oxide, it is used in baby ointments.

Compound Benzoin Tincture [Balsamum Equitis Sancti Victoris, Balsamum Commendatoris, Balsamum Catholicum, Balsamum Traumaticum, Balsamum Vulnerarium, Balsamum Persicum, Balsamum Suecium, Balsamum Friari, Balsamum Vervaini, Guttae Nader, Guttae Jesuitarium, Tinctura Balsamica, Balsam of the Holy Victorious Knight, Commander's Balsam, Friar's Balsam, Turlington's Drops, Persian Balsam, Swedish Balsam, Vervain Balsam, Turlington's Balsam of Life, Balsam de Maltha, Ward's Balsam, Jerusalem Balsam, Saint Victor's Balsam, Wade's Drops, Wound Elixir and Balsamic Tincture]

Preparation—With benzoin (in moderately coarse powder, 100 g), aloe (in moderately coarse powder, 20 g), storax (80 g), and tolu balsam (40 g), prepare a tincture (1000 mL) by Process M, using alcohol as the menstruum. *Alcohol Content:* 74% to 80% C_2H_5OH.

Comments—Especially valuable in acute *laryngitis,* also in croup, when added to hot water and the vapor inhaled. By adding a teaspoonful of the tincture to boiling water in an inhaler and inhaling the vapor, very effective results may be obtained. It also is used, on sugar, for throat and bronchial inflammation and as a local application, when mixed with glycerin and water, for *ulcers, bedsores, cracked nipples,* and *fissures* of the lips and anus.

CARBOMER METHYLCELLULOSE—see RPS-19, page 1396.
GELATIN—page 1074.
GLYCERIN—page 1081.
GLYCYRRHIZA—page 1064.
HYDROXYETHYL CELLULOSE—page 1074.
HYDROXYPROPYL CELLULOSE—page 1074.

HYDROXYPROPYL CELLULOSE INSERT

Lacrisert

Description—Sterile; translucent; rod-shaped.
Solubility—Soluble in water.
Comments—For administration into the inferior cul-de-sac of the eye. It is used when lacrimation is inadequate or to thicken tear film and prolong the tear-film breakup time, which usually is accelerated in patients with moderate to severe dry-eye states, including conjunctival hyperemia, corneal and conjunctival staining with rose bengal, exudation, itching, burning, foreign body sensation, smarting, photophobia, dryness, and blurred or cloudy vision.

HYDROXYPROPYL METHYLCELLULOSE—page 1074.

HYDROXYPROPYL METHYLCELLULOSE OPHTHALMIC SOLUTION

A sterile solution of hydroxypropyl methylcellulose, of a grade containing 19.0% to 30.0% methoxy and 4.0% to 12.0% hydroxypropoxy groups; may contain antimicrobial, buffering, and stabilizing agents.

Comments—A *wetting solution for contact lenses.* Its demulcent action decreases the irritant effect of the lens on the cornea. It also imparts viscous properties to the wetting solution, which assists the lens in staying in place. The demulcent effect also finds application in ophthalmic decongestants. *Artificial tear* formulations containing this drug may be used when lacrimation is inadequate. A 2.5% solution is used in gonioscopes.

METHYLCELLULOSE—page 1074.

METHYLCELLULOSE OPHTHALMIC SOLUTION

A sterile solution of methylcellulose; may contain antimicrobial, buffering, and stabilizing agents.

Comments—For the same purposes, and in the same manner, as *Hydroxypropyl Methylcellulose Ophthalmic Solution,* above.

PECTIN—page 1313.
POLYETHYLENE GLYCOLS—page 1079.
POLYVINYL ALCOHOL—page 1075.

POLYVINYL ALCOHOL OPHTHALMIC SOLUTION

VasoClear A

A sterile solution of polyvinyl alcohol, which may contain antimicrobial, buffering, and stabilizing agents and other demulcent substances. [9002-89-5] (Polyvinyl alcohol).

Preparation—By partial hydrolysis (*ca* 90%) of polyvinyl acetate.
Description—A white powder that is a linear polymer, —(CH_2—CHOH)$_n$—, where the value of n is between 500 and 5000; pH (1 in 25 aqueous solution) between 5 and 8.
Solubility—Soluble in water; insoluble in organic solvents.
Comments—A *wetting solution* for contact lenses. The polyvinyl alcohol has a demulcent action that helps protect the eye from irritation by the contact lens. It also is used in *artificial tears,* employed when there is insufficient lacrimation.

PROPYLENE GLYCOL—page 1082.
SODIUM ALGINATE—page 1073.
TRAGACANTH—page 1076.

EMOLLIENTS

Emollients (L, *emollier,* to soften) are bland, fatty, or oleaginous substances that may be applied locally, particularly to the skin but also to other mucous membranes. Skin usually appears *dry* because of a lack of moisture. Emollients or moisturizers increase the tissue moisture content, thereby rendering the skin softer and more pliable. Increased moisture content in the skin can be achieved by preventing water loss with an occlusive water-immiscible barrier, increasing the water-holding capacity of the skin with humectants, or altering the desquamation of the outermost skin layer, the streateum corneum.

The class of vehicles for emollients providing the range of the greatest moisturizing to the greatest drying effects on the skin include oleaginous bases, anhydrous absorption bases, W/O emulsions, O/W emulsions, the more-neutral, water-miscible compounds, and, finally, the more-drying gel and solution bases.

Emollients have certain disadvantages. It now is recognized that retention of perspiration below the emollient and exclusion of air render conditions favorable to the growth of anaerobic bacteria. Furthermore, rubbing and massaging during application aids in the spreading of cutaneous bacteria. Consequently, the use of emollients to cover burns and abrasions is diminishing. Some emollients (eg, lanolin, both the hydroxylated and acetylated forms; isopropyl myristate and palmitate; oleyl alcohol and sodium lauryl sulfate) are comedogenic. Other liquid emollients may be used for mild catharsis and for protection against GI corrosives; however, castor oil is hydrolyzed in the gut to the irritating ricinoleic acid and, hence, is employed as an emollient only externally. Orally administered liquid emollients may be aspirated into the trachea and lungs, especially by infants; in the debilitated, such aspiration induces *oil aspiration pneumonia.* This condition also may be induced by emollient nose drops.

The chief use of emollient or moisturizing substances beyond their therapeutic actions is to provide vehicles for lipid-soluble drugs (as in ointments and liniments); hence, many of them are described among the pharmaceutical necessities (Chapter 55). It is widely, but incorrectly, held that such vehicles facilitate the transport through the skin of their active ingredients. On the contrary, when the oil:water partition coefficient is greater than 1.0, the penetration is retarded, and the emollient vehicle prolongs the action of the active ingredient. Emollient substances also are employed in both cleansing and antiphlogistic creams and lotions. Compound ointment bases, creams, and other medicated applications are treated in Chapter 43. Only the simple emollients and important compounded ointments that are used frequently for their emollient actions are listed below.

Animal Fats and Oils

LANOLIN—page 1078.
MINERAL OIL—pages 1087 and 1308.
MINERAL OIL, LIGHT—page 1087.
PARAFFIN—page 1077.
PETROLATUM—page 1077.

RED PETROLATUM
Description—UV-absorbing qualities to 340 nm. It provides a water-protective action because of its petrolatum base.

Comments—Owing to its opacity, it is used as a *sunblock* in creams, ointments, and sticks. It also is used as a *sunshade* with zinc oxide in some formulations and for lip protection (20% petrolatum with 5% *p*-aminobenzoic acid (PABA)).

WHITE OINTMENT—page 1077.
WHITE PETROLATUM—page 1077.
YELLOW OINTMENT—page 1077.

Vegetable Oils

CASTOR OIL—page 1306.
COCOA BUTTER—page 1085.
COCONUT OIL—see RPS-18, page 1317.
CORN OIL—page 1071.
COTTONSEED OIL—page 1072.
OLIVE OIL—see RPS-19, page 1400.
PEANUT OIL—page 1072.
PERSIC OIL—see RPS-18, page 1323.
SESAME OIL—page 1072.

Waxes

CETYL ESTERS WAX—page 1077.
COLD CREAM—page 1078.
HYDROPHILIC OINTMENT—page 1078.
ROSE WATER OINTMENT—page 1078.

Other Emollients

CETYL ALCOHOL—page 1078.
GLYCERIN—pages 758, 1081 and 1423.
PETROLATUM, HYDROPHILIC—page 1078.
ISOPROPYL MYRISTATE—page 1086.

MYRISTYL ALCOHOL

Tetradecyl Alcohol

[112-72-1] $CH_3(C7H_2)_{12}CH_2OH$ (214.38).
Preparation—By reduction of fatty acid esters.
Description—White, crystalline alcohol; specific gravity 0.824; melts at 30°.
Solubility—Insoluble in water; soluble in ether; slightly soluble in alcohol.
Comments—An *emollient* in cold creams.

OLEYL ALCOHOL—page 1075.

SHARK LIVER OIL
The oil extracted from the livers of the *soupfin shark, Galeorhinus zyopterus* or *Hypoprion brevirostris,* both of which are rich in vitamins A and D.
Comments—An *emollient* and *protectant* (FDA classification Category I) used in burn and sunburn ointments.

ASTRINGENTS AND ANTIPERSPIRANTS

Astringents are locally applied, protein precipitants that have such a low cell penetrability that the action essentially is limited to the cell surface and the interstitial spaces. The permeability of the cell membrane is reduced, but the cells remain viable. The astringent action is accompanied by contraction and wrinkling of the tissue and by blanching. The cement substance of the capillary endothelium and the basement membrane is hardened, so that pathological transcapillary movement of plasma protein is inhibited, and local edema, inflammation, and exudation, thereby, are reduced. Mucus or other secretions also may be reduced, so that the affected area becomes drier.

Astringents are used therapeutically to arrest hemorrhage by coagulating the blood (*styptic* action) and to check diarrhea, reduce inflammation of mucous membranes, promote healing, toughen the skin, or decrease sweating.

The principal astringents are

1. Salts of the cations aluminum, zinc, manganese, iron, or bismuth.
2. Certain other salts that contain these metals (such as permanganates).
3. Tannins or related polyphenolic compounds.

Zinc sulfate (0.25%) is the only nonprescription astringent recommended. Acids, alcohols, phenols, and other substances that precipitate proteins may be astringent in the appropriate amount or concentration. However, such substances generally are not employed for their astringent effects, because they readily penetrate cells and promote tissue damage. Strongly hypertonic solutions dry the affected tissues and are often incorrectly called astringents, since protein precipitation also occurs. Many astringents are irritant or caustic in moderate to high concentrations. Consequently, strict attention must be paid to the appropriate concentration. Most astringents are also antiseptics, and many of them are discussed in Chapter 88.

Astringents also possess some *deodorant* properties by virtue of their interaction with odorous fatty acids liberated or produced by action of bacteria on lipids in sweat and by suppressing bacterial growth, partly because of a decrease in pH. The *antiperspirant* effect is the result of both the closure of the sweat ducts by protein precipitation to form a plug and peritubular irritation that promotes an increase in inward pressure on the tubule.

Antiperspirants and deodorants can be applied as aerosols, sprays, pads, sticks, and roll-on liquid, creams, and semisolids for the control of excessive perspiration and body odor. The general adult population secretes between 0.5 to 1.5 L of odorless perspiration a day. The unpleasant odor associated with perspiration is the result of chemical and bacterial

some sunscreens. It is included in some vulvovaginal deodorant preparations and in preparations for the treatment of hemorrhoids. It also is used in dental cements and temporary fillings. It is the essential ingredient in *Calamine*.

ZINC PYRITHIONE—see RPS-18, page 1173.
ZINC SULFATE—see RPS-19, page 1271.
ZINC UNDECYLENATE—see RPS-18, page 1237.

IRRITANTS, RUBEFACIENTS, AND VESICANTS

Irritants are drugs that act locally on the skin and mucous membranes to induce, based on irritant concentration, hyperemia, inflammation, and when the action is severe, vesication. Agents that induce only hyperemia are known as *rubefacients*. Rubefaction is produced by increased circulation to the injured area and is accompanied by a feeling of comfort, warmth, and sometimes itching and hyperesthesia. Appropriately low concentrations of directly applied or inhaled vapors of volatile aromatic irritants, such as camphor or menthol, induce a sensation of coolness rather than warmth. When the irritation is more severe, plasma escapes from the damaged capillaries and forms blisters (vesicles). Agents that induce blisters are known as *vesicants*. Most rubefacients also are vesicants in higher concentrations. Certain irritants may be relatively selective for various tissues or cell types, so that hypersecretion of the surface, seborrheic abscesses, paresthesia, or other effects may be noted in the absence of appreciable hyperemia.

Irritants have been used empirically for many centuries, probably even prehistorically. They may be employed for counterirritation, the mechanism of which is poorly understood. A moderate-to-severe pain may be obscured by a milder pain arising from areas of irritation appropriately placed to induce reflex stimulation of certain organs or systems, especially respiratory. Sensory and visible effects of irritation sometimes give patients the assurance that they are receiving effective medication. The rubefacient of choice is simply the applicant of heat, as drugs are much less efficient. Taken internally, many irritants exert either an emetic or laxative action. A few irritants, especially cantharides, on absorption into the bloodstream, irritate the urogenital tract and, consequently, have been dangerously employed as *aphrodisiacs*. Certain irritants also possess a healing action on wounds, possibly the result of local stimulation. Many condiments are irritants. In high concentrations, many irritants even can be corrosive.

ALCOHOL—pages 1080 and 1082.
ALCOHOL, RUBBING—see RPS-19, pages 1264 and 1510.

ANTHRALIN

1,8,9-Anthracenetriol; Dithranol; Dioxyanthranol; Cignolin; Anthra-Derm

1,8-Dihydroxyanthranol [480-22-8] $C_{14}H_{10}O_3$ (226.23).

Preparation—Anthraquinone is sulfonated to the 1,8-disulfonic acid, which is isolated from the reaction mixture and then heated with a calcium hydroxide–calcium chloride mixture to form 1,8-dihydroxy-9,10-anthraquinone, which is reduced with tin and HCl to anthralin.

Description—Yellowish brown, crystalline powder; odorless and tasteless; melts between 175° and 181°.

Solubility—Insoluble in water; slightly soluble in alcohol; soluble in chloroform; slightly soluble in ether.

Comments—Although long considered to be an irritant, its principal therapeutic action is the reduction of epidermal DNA synthesis and mitotic activity. It is used in the treatment of *psoriasis, alopecia areata, eczema,* and other *chronic dermatoses*. It usually is used in combination with ultraviolet light and a daily coal tar *bath*. To avoid harmful irritation, medicaments containing it should not be used on the face, scalp, genitalia, or intertriginous skin areas; they should not be applied to blistered,

raw, or oozing areas of the skin and should be kept from the eyes, since they may cause severe conjunctivitis, keratitis, or corneal opacity. Renal irritation, casts, and albuminuria may result when the drug is absorbed systemically. The hands should be washed immediately after applying medication. A reversible slight discoloration of the skin may occur.

BENZOIN TINCTURE, COMPOUND—page 1280.

CAMPHOR

2-Camphanone; 2-Bornanone; Gum Camphor; Laurel Camphor

[76-22-2] $C_{10}H_{16}O$ (152.24). A ketone obtained from *Cinnamomum camphora* (Linné) Nees et Ebermaier (Fam *Lauraceae*) (Natural Camphor) or produced synthetically (Synthetic Camphor).

Preparation—Natural crude camphor may be obtained by steam distilling chips of the camphor tree; the crude camphor so obtained is purified, usually by sublimation. One method of producing synthetic camphor starts with *pinene* [$C_{10}H_{16}$], a hydrocarbon obtained from turpentine oil. The pinene is saturated with hydrogen chloride at 0°, forming bornyl chloride [$C_{10}H_{17}Cl$]. On heating the bornyl chloride with sodium acetate and glacial acetic acid, it is converted into isobornyl acetate, which is hydrolyzed subsequently to isobornyl alcohol [$C_{10}H_{17}OH$] and oxidized with chromic acid to camphor. Synthetic camphor resembles natural camphor in most of its properties except that it is a racemic mixture and, therefore, lacks optical activity. When camphor is mixed in approximately molecular proportions with chloral hydrate, menthol, phenol, or thymol, liquefaction ensues; such mixtures are known as *eutectic mixtures*.

Description—Colorless or white crystals, granules, or crystalline masses or colorless to white, translucent, tough masses; a penetrating, characteristic odor, a pungent, aromatic taste and readily pulverizable in the presence of a little alcohol, ether, or chloroform; specific gravity about 0.99; melts between 174° and 179° and slowly volatilizes at ordinary temperature and in steam.

Solubility—1 g in about 800 mL water, 1 mL alcohol, about 0.5 mL chloroform, or 1 mL ether; freely soluble in carbon disulfide, solvent hexane, or fixed and volatile oils.

Incompatibilites—Forms a liquid or a soft mass when rubbed with *chloral hydrate, hydroquinone, menthol, phenol, phenyl salicylate, resorcinol, salicylic acid, thymol,* or other substances. It is precipitated from its alcoholic solution by the addition of water. It is precipitated from camphor water by the addition of soluble salts.

Comments—Locally, weakly *analgesic,* mildly *analgesic (antipruritic),* and *rubefacient* when rubbed on the skin. The spirit is applied locally to allay itching caused by insect stings. It also is used as a counterirritant in humans for *inflamed joints, sprains,* and *rheumatic* and other *inflammatory* conditions such as colds in the throat and chest. Although the patient may feel improved, the inflammation is not affected. However, reflexly induced local vasoconstriction may mediate a mild nasopharyngeal decongestant effect. When taken internally in small amounts it produces a feeling of warmth and comfort in the GI tract and, therefore, formerly was much used as a *carminative*. Systemically, it is a reflexly active *circulatory* and *respiratory stimulant*. However, its use as a stimulant is obsolete. It also possesses a slight *expectorant* action and is included in some cough-suppressant mixtures. Concentrations above 11% are not safe. Toxicity consists of nausea and vomiting, headache, feeling of warmth, confusion, delirium, convulsions, coma, or respiratory arrest. Camphor is a *pharmaceutical necessity* for *Salicylic Acid Collodion* and *Camphorated Opium Tincture*.

CANTHARIDIN

[56-25-7] $C_{10}H_{12}O_4$ (186.21). The active principle of *Cantharides*.

Preparation—*JACS* 1980; 102:6893.

Description—White platelets.

Solubility—1 g in 40 mL acetone, 65 mL chloroform, 560 mL ether, or 150 mL ethyl acetate; soluble in oils.

Comments—An *irritant* and *vesicant* on skin. As a result of its intradermal vesiculation, it also is employed to remove benign epithelial growths such as warts (particularly the periungual type), molluscum contagiosum, and thick hyperkeratotic lesions without leaving a scar. It usually is applied under occlusive bandages. The vesicle eventually breaks, becomes encrusted, and falls off in 1 to 2 weeks. It is not an aphrodisiac as folklore suggests.

CAPSICUM

The dried ripe fruit of *Capsicum frutescens* Linné, *Solonaceae*, which contains not less than 0.5% of capsaicin [(E)-N[4-hydroxy-3-methoxyphenyl]-8-methyl-6-nonaneamide [404-86-4] $C_{18}H_{27}NO_3$ (305.40), which is the active ingredient.

Comments—Its active ingredients are mildly irritant, causing erythema and a feeling of warmth without vesication. Its preparations are used as *counterirritants*.

COAL TAR

Pix Carbonis; Prepared Coal Tar BP; Pix Lithanthracis; Gas Tar

The tar obtained as a by-product during the destructive distillation of bituminous coal.

Description—Nearly black, viscous liquid, heavier than water, with a characteristic naphthalene-like odor and a sharp burning taste; on ignition it burns with a reddish, luminous, and very sooty flame, leaving not more than 2% of residue.

Solubility—Only slightly soluble in water, to which it imparts its characteristic odor and taste and a faintly alkaline reaction; partially dissolved by alcohol, acetone, methanol, solvent hexane, carbon disulfide, chloroform, or ether; to the extent of about 95% by benzene, and entirely by nitrobenzene with the exception of a small amount of suspended matter.

Comments—A *local irritant* used in the treatment of *chronic skin diseases*. Like anthralin, its primary action is to decrease the epidermal synthesis of DNA and, hence, to suppress hyperplasia. Occasionally, it may cause a rash, burning sensation, or other manifestations of excessive irritation or sensitization. Since photosensitization may occur, the treated area should be protected from sunlight. It should be kept away from the eyes and from raw, weeping, or blistered surfaces. Temporary discoloration of the skin may occur.

ICHTHAMMOL

Ammonium Ichthosulfonate; Sulfonated Bitumen; Ictiol; Ichthymall; Ichthyol

[8029-68-3]. It yields not less than 2.5% of ammonia and not less than 10% of total sulfur.

Preparation—By the destructive distillation of certain bituminous schists, sulfonating the distillate and neutralizing the product with ammonia.

Description—Reddish brown to brownish black, viscous fluid, with a strong, characteristic, empyreumatic odor.

Solubility—Miscible with water, glycerin fixed oils, or fats; partially soluble in alcohol or ether. *Incompatibilities:* Becomes granular in the presence of *acids* or under the influence of *heat*. In solution, it is precipitated by acids and *acid salts* as a dark, sticky mass; *alkalies* liberate ammonia; many *metallic salts* cause precipitation.

Constituents—It belongs to a class of preparations containing, as essential constituents, salts or compounds of a mixture of acids designated by the group name *sulfoichthyolic acid*, formed by sulfonation of the oil obtained in the destructive distillation of certain bituminous shales. Sulfoichthyolic acid is characterized by a high sulfur content, the sulfur existing largely in the form of sulfonates, sulfones, and sulfides.

Comments—A *mildly astringent irritant* and *local antibacterial agent* with moderate *emollient* and *demulcent* properties. It is used alone or in combination with other antiseptics for the treatment of skin disorders such as *insect stings and bites, erysipelas, psoriasis,* and *lupus erythematosus* and to produce healing in *chronic inflammations*. It also is used to treat *inflammation* and *boils* in the external ear canal. Medical opinion is divided as to whether this agent is useful. In higher concentrations, irritation is frequent and rashes may develop. It should be kept away from the eyes and other sensitive surfaces. It has been reported to cause hyperepithelialization, an action that would be counterproductive in the treatment of psoriasis.

JUNIPER TAR

Cade Oil

The empyreumatic volatile oil obtained from the woody portions of *Juniperus oxycedrus* Linné (Fam *Pinaceae*).

Description—Dark-brown, clear, thick liquid; tarry odor; faintly aromatic, bitter taste.

Solubility—Very slightly soluble in water; 1 volume in 9 volumes alcohol or 3 volumes ether, leaving a slight, flocculent residue; miscible with chloroform.

Comments—A mildly irritant oil that is employed as a *topical antipruritic* in several chronic dermatological disorders, such as *psoriasis, atopic dermatitis, pruritus, eczema,* and *seborrhea*. Since it is irritant to the conjunctiva and also may cause chemosis of the cornea, care should be taken to keep it out of the eyes. Systemic absorption may result in renal damage.

MENTHOL

Peppermint Camphor

[1490-04-6] $C_{10}H_{20}O$ (156.27). An alcohol obtained from diverse mint oils or prepared synthetically. It may be levorotatory [(−)-Menthol] from natural or synthetic sources, or racemic [(±)-Menthol)].

Preparation—It owes its odor chiefly to menthol, which is obtained from it by fractional distillation and allowing the proper fraction to crystallize or by chromatographic processes. Among numerous methods of synthesis of an optically inactive menthol, the most popular involves the catalytic hydrogenation of thymol (obtained from natural sources or synthesized from *m*-cresol or cresylic acid). The difficulty in the synthesis of (−)-menthol arises from the fact that menthol contains three asymmetric carbon atoms, and there are thus eight stereoisomers, designated as (−)- and (+)-menthol, (−)- and (+)-isomenthol, (−)- and (+)-neomenthol, and (−)- and (+)-neoisomenthol. To obtain a product meeting USP requirements, it is necessary to separate (−)-menthol from its stereoisomers, for which purpose fractional crystallization, distillation under reduced pressure, or esterification may be used. The other stereoisomers differ from the official (−)-menthol in physical properties and possibly to some extent in pharmacological action.

Description—Colorless, hexagonal, usually needle-like crystals or fused masses or a crystalline powder, with a pleasant, peppermint-like odor; (−)-menthol melts between 41° and 44°; (±)-menthol congeals at 27° to 28°.

Solubility—Very soluble in alcohol, chloroform, or ether; freely soluble in glacial acetic acid, mineral oil, or fixed and volatile oils; slightly soluble in water.

Identification—When mixed with about an equal weight of camphor, chloral hydrate, phenol, or thymol, it forms a *eutectic* mixture liquefying at room temperature.

Incompatibilities—Produces a liquid or soft mass when triturated with *camphor, phenol, chloral hydrate, resorcinol, thymol,* or numerous other substances. *Labeling:* The label on the container indicates whether it is levorotatory or racemic.

Comments—In low concentrations, it selectively stimulates the sensory nerve endings for cold and, hence, causes a *sensation of coolness*. Some *local analgesic* effects also accompany this effect. Higher concentrations not only stimulate sensory endings for heat and other pain, but also may cause some irritation. Consequently, there may first be a sensation of coolness, then a slight prickly and burning sensation. The *local analgesia* and *sensation of coolness* are employed in the treatment of insect bites and stings, itching (antipruritic effect), minor burns and sunburn, hemorrhoids, toothache, cankers, cold sores, and sore throat. The local analgesic effect also is the probable basis of the *antitussive* use, although the value of the drug as an antitussive remains unproved. Care must be taken to avoid the inhalation of irritant concentrations. The contribution of a placebo effect to some of these effects cannot be discounted. It is incorporated into *irritant* products used to treat acne vulgaris, dandruff, seborrhea, calluses, corns, warts, and athlete's foot and in vaginal preparations to lessen the sense of irritation. Whatever effects the rubbing of menthol-containing ointment on the chest possesses to relieve pulmonary congestion in colds and allergy are attributable to *counterirritation* and placebo effects. It also is contained in counterirritants for the treatment of muscle aches.

METHYL SALICYLATE—page 1065.

PERUVIAN BALSAM

Peru Balsam; Balsam of Peru; Indian Balsam; Black Balsam

Obtained from *Myroxylon pereirae* (Royle) Klotzsch (Fam *Leguminosae*). Contains from 60% to 64% of a volatile oil termed *cinnamein* and from 20% to 28% resin. Cinnamein is a mixture of compounds, among which the following have been identified: the esters *benzyl benzoate, benzyl cinnamate,* and *cinnamyl cinnamate (styracin)* and the alcohol *peruviol* (considered by some to be identical with the sesquiterpene alcohol *nerolidol,* $C_{15}H_{26}O$) as ester, free *cinnamic acid:* about 0.05% *vanillin;* and a trace of *coumarin*. The resin consists of benzoic and cinnamic acid.

Description—Dark brown, viscid liquid; transparent and appears reddish brown in thin layers; agreeable odor resembling vanilla; a bitter, acrid taste, with a persistent aftertaste and free from stringiness or stickiness. It does not harden on exposure to air; specific gravity, 1.150 to 1.170.

Solubility—Nearly insoluble in water; soluble in alcohol, chloroform, or glacial acetic acid, with not more than an opalescence; partly soluble in ether or solvent hexane.

Comments—A local *irritant* and *vulnerary*. It once was used as a dressing to promote growth of epithelial cells in the treatment of *indolent ulcers, wounds,* and certain *skin diseases,* eg, scabies. It presently is an ingredient in suppositories used in the treatment of hemorrhoids and anal pruritus. Allergic reactions to it occasionally occur. Ointments containing both this and sulfur present a problem in compounding, since the resinous part of the balsam tends to separate. This difficulty may be overcome by mixing the balsam with an equal amount of castor oil prior to incorporating it into the base or, alternatively, by mixing it with solid petroxolin—an ointment vehicle (oxygenated petroleum) consisting of liquid paraffin, oleic acid, and ammoniated alcohol.

PINE TAR

Pix Pini; Pix Liquida; Tar

The product obtained by the destructive distillation of the wood of *Pinus palustris* Miller or of other species of *Pinus* Linné (Fam *Pinaceae*). Usually obtained as a by-product in the manufacture of charcoal or acetic acid from wood. It is a complex mixture of phenolic bodies for the most part insoluble in water. Among these are *cresol, phlorol, guaiacol, pyrocatechol, caerulignol,* and *pyrogallol* ethers. Traces of *phenol* and *cresols* also are present as well as hydrocarbons of the paraffin and benzene series.

Description—Very viscid, blackish brown liquid; translucent in thin layers, but becomes granular and opaque with age; has an empyreumatic, terebinthinate odor, a sharp, empyreumatic taste, and is more dense than water; solution is acid to litmus.

Solubility—Miscible with alcohol, ether, chloroform, glacial acetic acid, or fixed and volatile oils; slightly soluble in water, the solution being pale yellowish to yellowish brown.

Comments—Externally as a mild *irritant* and *local antibacterial* agent in chronic *skin diseases,* especially eczema and psoriasis. Its volatile constituents are claimed to be *expectorant,* but their efficacy is unproven; its inhalations formerly were used for this purpose.

STORAX—page 1090.
TOLU BALSAM—page 1068.

SCLEROSING AGENTS

A number of irritant drugs are of sufficient activity to damage cells but are not so potent as to destroy large numbers of cells at the site of application. Such agents promote fibrosis and are used to strengthen supporting structures, close inguinal rings, etc. The intimal surface of blood vessels may break down under attack by such agents and thus initiate thrombosis, which may be an undesirable side effect. This action is the basis of the use of sclerosing agents in the reduction of varicose veins and hemorrhoids. They can be harmful when used improperly and sometimes even when used with caution.

MORRHUATE SODIUM INJECTION

Scleromate

A sterile solution of the sodium salts of the fatty acids of cod liver oil. It contains 50 mg of sodium morrhuate/mL. A suitable antimicrobial agent, not to exceed 0.5%, and ethyl or benzyl alcohol, not to exceed 3%, may be added.

Note—It may show a separation of solid matter on standing. Do not use the material if such solid does not dissolve completely upon warming.

Preparation—By heating cod liver oil with alcoholic sodium hydroxide until completely saponified. After dilution with water the alcohol is removed by distillation. Dilute H_2SO_4 then is added to the aqueous solution, and the liberated organic acids are separated or preferably extracted with a suitable immiscible solvent such as ether. Just-sufficient aqueous NaOH then is added to neutralize the acids. About 20 mg of benzyl alcohol/mL of the Injection usually is added to lessen the pain of injection.

Comments—Formerly, widely used as a *sclerosing* and *fibrosing* agent for obliterating *varicose veins.* Irritants of this type once were employed for closure of hernial rings, fibrosing of uncomplicated hemorrhoids, removal of condylomata acuminata, and in other conditions where the ultimate objective was production of fibrous tissue.

SODIUM TETRADECYL SULFATE

STS; Sotradecol

$$CH_3(CH_2)_3CH(CH_2)_2CHOSONa$$

[139-88-8] $C_{14}H_{29}NaO_4S$ (316.43).

Preparation—One method reacts the corresponding alcohol with $ClSO_3H$ and neutralizes the resulting hydrogen sulfate ester with Na_2CO_3.

Description—White, waxy, odorless solid.
Solubility—Soluble in water, alcohol, or ether.
Comments—A *sclerosing* agent similar in action to sodium morrhuate. It formerly was used widely as a buffered solution in the *obliteration of varicose veins and internal hemorrhoids.* For such purposes, the solution is injected directly into the vein. Injection outside of the vein may cause sloughing. For this reason, the substance is not used to close inguinal rings. The principal untoward effect is pain immediately upon injection, although brief; mild anaphylactoid and idiosyncratic responses rarely occur. Because the substance is an anionic surface-active agent, it also is used as a *wetting agent* to promote spreading of certain topical antiseptics.

CAUSTICS AND ESCHAROTICS

Any topical agent that causes destruction of tissues at the site of application is a *caustic* (or corrosive).

Caustics may be used to induce desquamation of cornified epithelium (*keratolytic* action) and, therefore, are used to destroy warts, condylomata, keratoses, certain moles, and hyperplastic tissues.

If the agent also precipitates the proteins of the cell and the inflammation exudate, there is formed a scab (or eschar), which later is organized into a scar; such an agent is an *escharotic* (or cauterizant). Most, but not all, caustics are also escharotic. Furthermore, certain caustics, especially the alkalies, redissolve precipitated proteins, partly by hydrolysis, so that no scab or only a soft scab forms; such agents penetrate deeply and generally are unsuitable for therapeutic use. Escharotics sometimes are employed to seal cutaneous and aphthous ulcers, wounds, etc. Since most escharotics are bactericidal, it formerly was thought that chemical cauterization effected sterilization; however, sterilization is not achieved always, especially by those agents that remain bound to the protein precipitate. The growth of certain bacteria even may be favored by the chemically induced necrosis and by the protection of the scab.

ACETIC ACID, GLACIAL—page 1083.
ALUM—page 1282.
ALUMINUM CHLORIDE—page 1282.

DICHLOROACETIC ACID

Bichloracetic Acid

$Cl_2CHCOOH$ [79-43-6] $C_2H_2Cl_2O_2$ (128.95).
Preparation—From chloral; *Chem Ind* 1960; 718.
Description—Pungent liquid; boils about 194°.
Solubility—Miscible with water, alcohol, or ether.
Comments—A *cauterizing agent.* It rapidly penetrates and cauterizes skin, keratins, etc. Its cauterizing ability compares with that of electrocautery or freezing. It is used on calluses, hard and soft corns, xanthoma palpebrarum, seborrheic keratoses, ingrown nails, cysts, and benign erosion of the cervix. See also *Trichloroacetic Acid.*

NITRIC ACID, CONCENTRATED

An aqueous solution containing 67% to 71% HNO_3.
Preparation—By oxidation of ammonia.
Description—Fuming liquid; very caustic; characteristic, highly irritating odor; boils at 120°; specific gravity about 1.41.
Solubility—Miscible with water.
Comments—A *cauterizing agent* for the immediate sterilization of dangerously infected wounds, such as the bite from a rabid animal; it does not penetrate too deeply and forms a firm eschar.

PHENOL—page 1087.

PODOFILOX

Furo[3',4':6,7]naphtho[2,3-d]-1,3-dioxol-6(5aH)-one, [5R-(5α,5aβ, 8aα,9α)]-5,8,8a,9-tetrahydro-9-hydroxy-5-(3,4,5-trimethoxyphenyl)-, Condylox

Podophyllotoxin [518-28-5] $C_{22}H_{22}O_8$ (414.41).

Found in the rhizomes of several species of plants, principally *Podophyllum peltatum* L *Berberidaceae, P emodi,* and *Juniperus virginiana* L *Coniferae.*

Preparation—See *JACS* 1981; 103:6208.

Description—Hydrated crystals; melts about 115° (dec) and about 184° after drying; a number of polymorphic forms exist.

Solubility—Very slightly soluble in water; soluble in alcohol, chloroform, or acetone.

Comments—Actions, uses, and adverse effects are those of *Podophyllum Resin* (below), except that the therapeutic index is greater. It is several times more potent.

PODOPHYLLUM

Mandrake; May Apple

The dried rhizome and roots of *Podophyllum peltatum* Linné (Fam *Berberidaceae*); it yields not less than 5% of podophyllum resin.

Constituents—From 3% to 6% resin along with up to 1% quercetin and podophyllotoxin and peltatin glucosides. At least 16 different compounds have been isolated and characterized. The aglycone *podophyllotoxin* [$C_{22}H_{22}O_8$] is the lactone of 1-hydroxy-2-(hydroxy-methyl)-6,7-methylenedioxy-4-(3',4',5'-trimethoxyphenyl)-1,2,3,4-tetrahydronaphthalene-3-carboxylic acid. Hydrolytic rupture of the lactone ring yields *podophyllic acid* [$C_{22}H_{24}O_9$], the 2,3-*trans* form of which is *podophyllinic acid,* while the 2,3-*cis* form is *picropodophyllinic acid.*

Although podophyllotoxin has been demonstrated to possess marked caustic, cathartic, and toxic properties, it is believed that not it, but an amorphous *resin,* called *podophylloresin,* is the chief cathartic principle of the drug. However, podophyllotoxin is safer and ultimately likely will replace the crude preparations.

Comments—See *Podophyllum Resin.*

PODOPHYLLUM RESIN

Comments—Supersedes *Podophyllum.* Certain glycosides and polynuclear lactones in the resin interact with tubulin and, thus, interfere with cell cycling and intracellular dynamics such as to cause the eventual death of affected cells. Applied topically, it is corrosive in the region of contact. It mainly is used in the treatment of *condyloma acuminatum* but also that of *juvenile papilloma of the larynx, multiple superficial epitheliomatoses* (basal cell and squamous cell carcinomas), *precancerous keratoses* (seborrheic, actinic, and radiation keratoses), *verrucae fibroids,* and *calluses.* Some pain usually occurs at the site of application; if it is excessive, the drug should be removed with ethyl or isopropyl alcohol. Resin on adjacent normal tissues also should be removed. Pain may be avoided somewhat by treating only a small area of surface at any one time. *It especially is irritating to the eyes and mucous membranes.* Treatment of large surfaces also may result in excessive absorption and systemic effects, such as nausea and vomiting, tachycardia, shallow respiration, leukopenia, thrombocytopenia, renal damage, paralytic ileus, lethargy, stupor, psychotic confusional states, and peripheral neuropathy, including flaccid paralysis. Systemic absorption is enhanced by occlusion. The drug is contraindicated in pregnancy and lactation.

POTASSIUM HYDROXIDE

Caustic Potash; Lye; Potash Lye

[1310-58-3] KOH (56.11); it contains not less than 85.0% K_2CO_3 (138.21).

Caution—Exercise great care in handling, as it rapidly destroys tissues. Do not handle it with bare hands.

Preparation—By electrolysis of a solution of potassium chloride in a diaphragm cell that does not allow liberated chlorine to react with it.

It is prepared in the form of sticks, pellets, flakes, or fused masses. Sticks or pellets are made by evaporating a solution of it to a fluid of oily consistency and then pouring the hot liquid into suitable molds in which it solidifies.

Description—White, or nearly white, fused masses, small pellets, flakes, sticks, and other forms; hard and brittle and shows a crystalline fracture; exposed to air it rapidly absorbs carbon dioxide and moisture and deliquesces; melts at about 360 to 380°; when dissolved in water or alcohol or when its solution is treated with an acid, much heat is generated; solutions, even when highly diluted, are strongly alkaline.

Solubility—1 g in 0.9 mL water, 3 mL alcohol, or 2.5 mL glycerin at 25°; very soluble in boiling alcohol.

Incompatibilities—Bases react with *acids* to form salts, liberate alkaloids from aqueous solutions of *alkaloidal salts,* and promote various hydrolysis reactions such as the decomposition of *chloral hydrate* into chloroform and a formate or the breakdown of *salol* into phenol and a salicylate. Only the alkali hydroxides are appreciably soluble in water. Nearly all common *metals* will be precipitated as hydroxides when solutions of their salts are added to solutions of the alkali hydroxides. Certain hydroxides, however, notably those of aluminum, zinc, arsenic, or lead, will dissolve in an excess of sodium or potassium hydroxide.

Comments—A *caustic,* principally in veterinary practice. The end of a stick of potassium hydroxide may be inserted into a section of rubber tubing or wrapped several times with tin foil to avoid cauterizing the fingers of the operator. It is used also as a *pharmaceutical necessity* in several pharmacopeial preparations.

SALICYLIC ACID—page 1288.

SILVER NITRATE

Nitric acid, silver(1+) salt; Argenti Nitras

Silver(1+) nitrate [7761-88-8] $AgNO_3$ (169.87).

Preparation—By the action of nitric acid on metallic silver.

Description—Colorless or white crystals; on exposure to light in the presence of organic matter, it becomes gray or grayish black; pH of solutions about 5.5.

Solubility—1 g in 0.4 mL water, 30 mL alcohol, about 250 mL acetone, slightly more than 0.1 mL boiling water or about 6.5 mL of boiling alcohol; slightly soluble in ether.

Incompatibilities—Easily reduced to metallic silver by most *reducing agents,* including *ferrous salts, arsenites, hypophosphites, tartrates, sugars, tannins, volatile oils,* and other *organic substances.* In neutral or alkaline solutions, precipitated by *chlorides, bromides, iodides, borax, hydroxides, carbonates, phosphates, sulfates, arsenites,* and *arsenates. Potassium permanganate, tannic acid,* and *soluble citrates and sulfates* may cause a precipitate if sufficiently concentrated. In acid solution, only the *chloride, bromide,* and *iodide* are insoluble. *Ammonia water* dissolves many of the insoluble silver salts through formation of the silver diamine complex, $Ag(NH_3)_2^+$.

Comments—Silver ions combine with proteins and cause denaturation and precipitation. As a result, silver ions have *astringent, caustic, bactericidal,* and *antiviral* properties. In low concentrations, silver-denatured protein is confined to the interstitial spaces and the surface of denuded, weeping areas, so that only astringent and antimicrobial effects occur; with higher concentrations, cell membranes are disrupted and caustic effects result. The corroded site will become covered with a scab of silver-protein precipitate.

It is used mainly in podiatry as a caustic to *destroy excessive granulation tissue,* such as *corns, calluses, granuloma pyogenicum,* and *plantar warts; reduce neurovascular helomas; remove papillomas; and cauterize small nerve endings* and *blood vessels.* As an astringent, it is used to treat *impetigo vulgaris* and *pruritus* as well as *indolent ulcers, wounds,* and *fissures.* It is used as a *styptic,* especially in dentistry.

As an antiseptic, it mainly is employed prophylactically against *ophthalmia neonatorum.* It formerly was applied regularly to burned surfaces because of its high efficacy against both staphylococci and pseudomonas. However, the precipitation of AgCl at the site of application and in dressing depletes plasma chloride and can cause serious electrolyte disturbances; consequently, the drug seldom is used in burn therapy today.

Excessive corrosion at the target site and corrosion from inadvertent application or leakage away from the intended site can occur. Dental cones or pieces of toughened silver nitrate that are accidentally ingested can cause death. Elemental silver from the bioreduction of silver ion may reside permanently at the site of application and cause a bluish-to-black discoloration called argyria. Locally injected sodium thiosulfate sometimes can remove the silver. Nitrate ion absorbed from large, denuded surfaces can cause methemoglobinemia. Only concentrations 0.5% or below should be applied to raw wounds, fresh cuts, or broken skin.

MEDICINAL AGENTS

TRICHLOROACETIC ACID

Tri-Chlor

[76-03-9] $C_2HCl_3O_2$ (163.39).

Preparation—Usually by oxidizing chloral hydrate with fuming nitric acid.

Description—Colorless, deliquescent crystals with a slight, characteristic odor; melts at about 58° and boils at 196° to 197°.

Solubility—1 g in about 0.1 mL water; soluble in alcohol or ether.

Comments—Precipitates proteins and used as a *caustic* on the skin or mucous membranes to destroy local lesions and for treatment of various dermatological disease. Its chief use is to destroy ordinary warts and juvenile flat warts. It is employed extensively as a precipitant of protein in the chemical analysis of body fluids and tissue extracts, as well as a *decalcifier* and *fixative* in microscopy.

Caution—Trichloroacetic Acid is highly corrosive to the skin.

KERATOLYTICS (DESQUAMATING AGENTS)

The epidermis consists of layers of flat cells, called *stratified squamous epithelial cells*. They are bound together by desmosomes and penetrating tonofibrils, both of which largely consist of keratin. The outer layer of the epidermis (cornified epithelium or stratum corneum) is composed of the collapsed ghosts of the squamous cells (keratinocytes or corneocytes) that are primarily tight networks of keratin and lipoprotein within a matrix of lipid multilayers. Unlike most cellular membranes, the lipids include fatty acids, neutral lipids, ceramides, etc, and are predominantly in the gel (solid-like) state. Certain fungi, especially the dermatophytes, use keratin and, therefore, reside in the stratum corneum in those places where the degree of hydration and the pH are sufficiently high. One way such mycoses may be suppressed is removal of the stratum corneum, a process called *desquamation*. Certain chemical substances, especially among phenols and sulfhydryl compounds, loosen the keratin and thus facilitate desquamation. These substances are called *keratolytics*. Aqueous maceration of the stratum corneum also favors desquamation. In addition to the treatment of epidermophytosis, keratolytics are used to thin hyperkeratotic areas. Most keratolytics are irritant. Irritants also can cause desquamation by causing damage to, and swelling of, the basal cells.

BENZOYL PEROXIDE

[94-36-0] $C_{14}H_{10}O_4$ (242.23); contains 65% to 82% of benzoyl peroxide; also contains about 26% of water for the purpose of reducing flammability and shock sensitivity.

Preparation—Benzoyl chloride is reacted with a cold solution of sodium peroxide.

Description—White, granular powder with a characteristic odor; melts about 104°; *may explode with heat.*

Solubility—Sparingly soluble in water or alcohol; soluble in acetone, chloroform, or ether.

Caution (for the drug entity, not the dosage forms)—It may explode at temperatures higher than 60° or cause fires in the presence of reducing substances. Store it in the original container, treated to reduce static charges. Do not transfer it to metal or glass containers fitted with friction tops. Do not return unused material to its original container, but destroy it by treatment with NaOH solution (1 in 10) until addition of a crystal of KI results in no release of free iodine.

Comments—Possesses *mild antibacterial* properties, especially against anaerobic bacteria. It is also mildly irritant, and it exerts moderate keratolytic and antiseborrheic actions. Its principal use is in the treatment of mild *acne vulgaris* (in which it is comedolytic) and *acne rosacea*, but it also is used in the treatment of decubital and stasis ulcers.

It causes stinging or burning sensations for a brief time after application; with continued use these effects mostly disappear. After 1 or 2 weeks of use there may be a sudden excess dryness of the skin and peeling. The drug must be kept away from the eyes and from inflamed, denuded, or highly sensitive skin, such as the circumoral areas, neck, and skin of children. It should not be used in conjunction with harsh abrasive skin cleansers. It can cause contact dermatitis. It can bleach hair and fabrics.

FLUOROURACIL—pages 1573 and 1680.

SALICYLIC ACID

Benzoic acid, 2-hydroxy-, *o*-Hydroxybenzoic Acid

Salicylic acid [69-72-7] $C_7H_6O_3$ (138.12).

Preparation—Mostly by the Kolbe-Schmidt process in which CO_2 is reacted with sodium phenolate under pressure at about 130° to form sodium salicylate, followed by treatment with mineral acid.

Description—White, fine, needle-like crystals or a fluffy, white, crystalline powder; the synthetic acid is white and odorless; sweetish, afterward acrid, taste; stable in the air; melts between 158° and 161°.

Solubility—1 g in 460 mL water, 3 mL alcohol, 45 mL chloroform, 3 mL ether, 135 mL benzene, or about 15 mL boiling water.

Comments—Used *externally* on the skin, where it exerts a slight *antiseptic* action and considerable *keratolytic* action. The latter property makes it a beneficial agent in the local treatment of certain forms of *eczematoid dermatitis*. It also is included in products for the treatment of *psoriasis,* for which the FDA classification is Category I. Tissue cells swell, soften, and ultimately desquamate. Salicylic Acid Plaster often is used for this purpose. The drug is especially useful in the treatment of *tinea pedis* (athlete's foot) and *tinea capitis* (ringworm of the scalp), since the fungus grows and thrives in the stratum corneum. Keratolysis both removes the infected horny layer and aids in penetration by antifungal drugs. It is combined with benzoic acid in an ointment long known as *Whitfield's Ointment* (see RPS-18, page 1235). It also is combined commonly with zinc oxide, sulfur, or sulfur and coal tar. It is incorporated into mixtures for the treatment of acne, dandruff, and seborrhea, insect bites, and stings and into soaps and vaginal douches, but efficacy remains to be established. In high concentrations it is *caustic* and may be used to remove *corns, calluses, warts,* and other growths.

Collodions or solutions of 17% or higher and other forms above 25% concentration should not be employed if the patient has diabetes mellitus, peripheral vascular disease, or inflammation or infection at the intended site of application. Continuous application of the drug to the skin can cause dermatitis. Systemic toxicity resulting from application to large areas of the skin has been reported. It is not employed internally as an analgesic because of its local irritating effect on the GI tract.

SULFUR, PRECIPITATED—page 1598.

TRETINOIN

Retinoic acid; Retin-A

All *trans*-Retinoic acid [302-79-4] $C_{20}H_{28}O_2$ (300.44).

Preparation—By oxidation of vitamin A aldehyde which may be obtained by oxidation of vitamin A. *Biochem J* 1964; 90:569.

Description—Yellow to light-orange crystals or crystalline powder with the odor of ensilage; should be stored in cold and protected from light and air; melts between 176° and 181°.

Solubility—Insoluble in water; slightly soluble in alcohol; slightly soluble in chloroform; 1 g in 10 mL boiling benzene.

Comments—It is retinoic acid, or so-called *vitamin A acid,* which is formed when the aldehyde group of retinene (retinal) is oxidized to a carboxyl group. It is not known whether retinoic acid has a physiological function, but some authorities consider it to be the form of vitamin A that acts in the skin. This view is supported by the fact that retinol and retinal have very little action on the skin but large systemic doses of vitamin A evoke prominent dermatological changes.

Topically, it causes inflammation, thickening of the epidermis (acanthosis), and local intercellular edema, which leads to some separation of the epidermal cells. Follicular epithelial cells become less adhesive, the stratum corneum loosens, and exfoliation may occur. High concentrations can cause vesiculation. These actions are used in the treatment of *acne vulgaris*. The loosened horny layer makes it easier for the comedo to rise up and discharge, and the inflammatory response mobilizes white cells that attack the bacteria in the follicle. In the early stages of treatment, the sudden surfacing of obscured preexisting comedones makes it appear that the acne has been exacerbated, but the new comedones do not coalesce into cysts or nodules, and scarring does not occur. The exaggerated stage may last for as long as 6 weeks, after which improvement comes rapidly. Shortly after discontinuation of treatment, relapses readily occur. Deep cystic nodular acne (acne conglobata) or severe cases usually are not improved by the drug.

Various hyperkeratotic conditions are reported to respond to it, responses being sometimes exceptionally dramatic. *Solar* and *follicular keratosis, lamellar ichthyosis, keratosis palmaris* and *plantaris,* and other hyperplastic dermatoses have been treated successfully with the drug. It also has been used in the treatment of some skin cancers. Recent reports indicate that it may somewhat rejuvenate sun-aged skin.

It is an antioxidant and free-radical scavenger. There is some evidence not only that topical applications may provide some protection from actinic and other radiation effects on the skin, including cancer, but that internally it may be protective against carcinogenesis from radiation and carcinogens. Systemically, it does not cause the toxic effects of large doses of vitamin A.

In concentrations of 0.05% to 0.1%, it causes a transient feeling of warmth or mild stinging, and erythema follows. Peeling of the skin may occur. Irritation and peeling are marked more when the concentration exceeds 0.1%. When peeling, crusting, or blistering occur, medication should be withheld until the skin recovers, or the concentration should be reduced. The drug should not be applied around the eyes, nose, or angles of the mouth, because the mucosae are much more sensitive than the skin to the irritant effects. It also may cause severe irritation on eczematous skin. It should not be applied along with, or closely following, other irritants or keratolytic drugs. Exposure to sunlight should be avoided if possible. Both hypo- and hyperpigmentation have been reported, but the conditions appear to be reversible and temporary.

TRICHLOROACETIC ACID—page 1288.

CLEANSING PREPARATIONS

The skin may be cleansed with detergents, solvents, or abrasives, singly or in combination. Among the detergents, the soaps have enjoyed the greatest official status, more through custom than through special merit. The nonsoap detergents became important not only as household hand cleansers, but in dermatological and surgical practice as well. However, because many nonsoap detergents do not decompose in sewage disposal plants, there has been a return to real soap. Some of the antiseptic *soaps* still contain synthetic detergents. Soap interferes with the action of many antiseptics, which is one reason synthetic detergents often are used in antiseptic cleansing preparations. However, synthetic detergents also interact with some antiseptics. Anionic nonsoap skin detergents rarely sensitize the skin and, thus, are prescribed when the user is allergic to soap.

Ordinary soaps tend to be alkaline, with pH ranging from 9.5 to 10.5. Superfatted soaps have a pH in the lower end of the range. Synthetic detergents usually have a pH $\leq$5.6. Neutral toilet bars contain synthetic detergents. Anionic surfactants and cationic detergents emulsify fats with water as well as assisting in the removal of foreign particulates from the skin, scalp, or hair.

Shampoos are liquid soaps or detergents used to clean the hair and scalp. Both soaps and shampoos often are used as vehicles for dermatological agents.

Many bar soaps contain either triclosan or triclocarban as antiseptics in concentrations that suppress bacterial production of body odors but that effectively are not antiseptic. A number of soaps and shampoos contain keratolytic and antiacne ingredients. Abrasive soaps contain particles of alumina, polyethylene, or sodium tetraborate decahydrate.

It commonly, but erroneously, is believed that soap has an antiseptic action. The promotion of either soap or synthetic detergents alone for the control of acne is unwarranted; antiseptic substances must be added to the cleansing material or be used separately. Quantitative studies of the cutaneous flora before and after cleansing with soap or with other anionic

detergents show a negligible antiseptic effect. However, the removal of loose epidermis lessens the likelihood that cutaneous bacteria will be transferred from the skin to other structures. Certain cationic detergents employed in dermatology are antiseptic. Detergents are treated under *Surface-Active Agents,* chapter 39.

The choice of organic solvents to cleanse the skin depends largely upon the nature of the material to be removed. In medical practice ethanol and isopropyl alcohol are the most frequently employed organic solvents. Cleansing creams act both as solvents and as detergents. Other soapless cleansers variously contain petrolatum, vegetable oils, lanolin, high-molecular-weight alcohols, various carbohydrate derivatives, oatmeal, and other ingredients.

ALCOHOL—pages 1080 and 1082.
ALCOHOL, RUBBING—see RPS-19, pages 1264 and 1510.
BENZALKONIUM CHLORIDE—page 1626.
HEXACHLOROPHENE CLEANSING EMULSION—page 1628.
ISOPROPYL RUBBING ALCOHOL—page 1629.
SELENIUM SULFIDE—page 1629.
SODIUM LAURYL SULFATE—page 1075.

TRANSDERMAL SYSTEMS

Transdermal systems are designed to employ the skin as either a rate-controlling barrier to drug absorption or a reservoir for drug absorption. The primary compounds delivered via transdermal systems include estradiol, page 1463; nitroglycerin, page 1359; nicotine, page 1371; clonidine, page 1270; fentanyl, page 1531; scopolamine, page 1408, and testosterone, page 1472.

These drugs are discussed elsewhere, since their pharmacological activity is not primarily skin-related. However, transdermal systems have been developed to deliver salicylic acid for localized therapy in the skin to remove warts (salicylic acid, page 1288).

The underlying principles of percutaneous absorption are discussed in further detail in Chapter 37, while the systems are discussed in Chapter 50. However, transdermal systems may give localized effects within skin because of increased hydration as a result of occlusion, drug metabolism or degradation within the skin, penetration enhancer–associated skin alterations, increased localized bacterial populations, etc.

MISCELLANEOUS DERMATOLOGICALS

Gargles, nasal washes, douches, enemata, etc, generally contain as basic ingredients substances described under other categories in this chapter.

Antiphlogistics include alcohol and several creams and lotions that cool the skin by evaporation. Many antiphlogistic preparations also contain an astringent and a local anesthetic or camphor or menthol.

Commonly employed *antipruritics* also depend to some extent upon local anesthetics and the soothing effect of cooling, although some emollients or demulcents may be included, especially depending upon the cause of the pruritus. The antipruritic properties of phenol preparations largely derive from superficial local anesthesia.

Vulnerary and *epithelizing* properties are attributed to numerous irritants and to several dyes; however, few reliable data exist to support most claims to vulnerary action.

Sunscreens contain aromatic compounds such as aminobenzoic acid, which efficiently absorb the harmful UV rays from the incident sunlight and transmit mainly the less harmful wavelengths, or titanium dioxide, which reflects sunlight from the surface of application. UV light in the spectral range of 290 to 320 nm causes suntan and sunburn; therefore, a sunscreen to prevent tan or burn should have a high molar absorptivity in this range. However, *photosensitization* (ie, the photoactivation of chemicals to make them toxic or allergenic) may occur with wavelengths as high as 500 nm; consequently, to protect recipients of certain drugs (tetracyclines, sulfonamides, erythromycin, promazine, chlorpromazine, promethazine, psoralens), sunscreens with a broader absorption spectrum are required. An adequately broad spectrum is usually achieved with combinations of sunscreens (eg, dioxybenzone and oxybenzone).

Melanizers are substances that promote the pigmentation of the skin. Most melanizers produce their effect by sensitizing the skin to UV light, so that the effect is principally the same as if the subject had been exposed for a long time to the sun.

This action is termed a *photodynamic action*. The term has been used loosely to include all instances of enhanced sensitivity to light, but in strict definition it is confined to photosensitization in which the participation of oxygen is required. In the photodynamic process, light of wavelengths too long to be ordinarily effective may be used, so that the activating spectrum may be shifted toward longer wavelengths.

Skin bleaches, or *demelanizers,* mostly contain hydroquinone derivatives.

Hair bleaches generally contain peroxides.

There is a large variety of *depilatories* on the market. Many of them are sulfhydryl compounds, especially thioglycollates, which reduce the disulfide bonds of keratin, thus softening the hair to the point where it can be separated easily from the epidermis. Some of the same compounds are used in lower concentrations in hairwaving preparations. There is one drug, minoxidil, an antihypertensive drug, which can *increase hair growth* and *treat baldness.*

Antiperspirants have been included among the astringents.

ALLANTOIN

Urea, (2,5-dioxo-4-imid-azolidinyl)-,

[97-59-6] $C_4H_6N_4O_3$ (158.12).

Preparation—By oxidation of uric acid.

Description—Colorless crystals; melts at 238°.

Solubility—1 g in 190 mL water or 500 mL alcohol; nearly insoluble in ether.

Comments—In World War I it was noticed that maggot-infested wounds seemed to heal better than uninfested wounds, an effect attributed to this drug produced by maggots. It is used topically as a *vulnerary* to stimulate tissue repair in suppurating wounds, resistant ulcers, acne, seborrhea, cold sores, hemorrhoids, and various dermatological infections and psoriasis. It frequently is combined with astringents, keratolytics, coal tar, antiseptics, and antifungal drugs. The silver salt has been used in the topical treatment of extensive burns.

AMINOBENZOIC ACID

Benzoic acid, 4-amino-, PABA

p-Aminobenzoic acid [150-13-0] $C_7H_7NO_2$ (137.14).

Preparation—*p*-Nitrotoluene is oxidized with permanganate to *p*-nitrobenzoic acid, and the nitro group then is reduced to an amino group with iron and hydrochloric acid.

Description—White or slightly yellow, odorless crystals or crystalline 8 powder; melts between 186° and 189°; discolors on exposure to air or light.

Solubility—Slightly soluble in water or chloroform; freely soluble in alcohol or solutions of alkali hydroxides and carbonates; sparingly soluble in ether.

Comments—A *sunscreen.* It absorbs UV light of wavelengths in the region of 260 to 313 nm; its molar absorptivity at 288.5 nm is 18,300. However, it does not absorb throughout the near UV range, so that drug-related photosensitivity and phototoxicity may not be prevented by it, but in combination with benzophenone it does protect against some drug-induced phototoxicities. Nevertheless, in the 260 to 313 nm range, it has the highest protection index of current sunscreen agents.

For animal species that do not use preformed folic acid, which contains the *p*-aminobenzoyl moiety, it is a B vitamin. However, man does not use it, and its promotion in vitamin preparations preys on the ignorance of the consumer. It or its potassium salt is promoted as an agent that softens or regresses fibrotic tissue in Peyronie's disease, scleroderma, dermatomyositis, morphea, and pemphigus. The claims for the antifibrotic actions are substantiated poorly, and the actions and uses are not mentioned in major works on pharmacology and therapeutics.

Topically, it is rarely allergenic to recipients, but phototoxicity and photoallergenicity occur. Systemic side effects include nausea, anorexia, fever, and rash.

CETYL ALCOHOL—page 1078.

CINOXATE

Propenoic acid, 3-(4-methoxyphenyl)-, 2-ethoxyethyl ester

[104-28-9] $C_{14}H_{18}O_4$ (250.29).

Preparation—Brit Pat 856,411.

Description—A viscous liquid; may have a slightly yellow tinge; boils about 185°.

Solubility—Practically insoluble in water; miscible with alcohol.

Comments—A *sunscreen* that absorbs UV light at 270 to 328 nm and has a relatively high molar absorptivity (19,400 at 306 nm) but is nonabsorbing throughout the entire offending range of UV light. Consequently, it is used principally in preparations intended to promote tanning rather than to protect against photosensitivity and phototoxicity.

DEXTRANOMER

For the complete monograph, see page 1290.

Comments—For *drying, cleansing,* and *debridement* of exudative *venous stasis ulcers; infected wounds* and *burns;* it is not useful for cleansing nonexudative wounds or lesions. The beads not only absorb water but also proteins, including fibrin/fibrinogen degradation products, and thus prevent encrustation. The beads are poured into the cleansed wound, which is circumscribed with petroleum jelly, and a compress is taped in place to retain the material. Changes may be made up to three or four times a day, as needed. The beads must be removed before skin grafting is attempted. Care must be taken to prevent cross-contamination from patient to patient. On the floor the beads are slippery and thus hazardous.

DIHYDROXYACETONE

Chromelin Complexion Blender

[96-26-4] $C_3H_6O_3$ (90.08).

Preparation—By oxidation of the secondary alcohol group of glycerin.

Description—Crystalline powder; fairly hygroscopic; characteristic odor; sweet taste; melts about 77°.

Solubility—*Dimer* (normal form): slowly soluble in 1 part water or 15 parts alcohol. *Monomer* (formed in solution): very soluble in water, alcohol, or ether.

Comments—Interacts with keratin in the stratum corneum to form a dark pigment that simulates the appearance of a suntan. It is incorporated in several *sunscreen* preparations. Since the sunscreen component is usually present in a concentration lower than optimal, such preparations may not provide protection to photosensitive persons. Also used to treat vitiligo.

DIOXYBENZONE

Methanone, (2-hydroxy-4-methoxyphenyl)(2-hydroxyphenyl)-, Solaquin

2,2′-Dihydroxy-4-methoxybenzophenone [131-53-3] $C_{14}H_{12}O_4$ (244.25).

Preparation—By a Friedel-Crafts reaction in which *o*-methoxy-benzoyl chloride is added gradually to a mixture of 1,3-dimethoxybenzene, chlorobenzene, and aluminum chloride. The reaction conditions are such that both methoxy groups ortho to the carbonyl bridge in the initial condensation product are demethylated. US Pat 2,853,521.

Description—Off-white to yellow powder; congeals not lower than 68°.

Solubility—Practically insoluble in water; freely soluble in alcohol or toluene.

Comments—A *sunscreen* of intermediate molar absorptivity (11,950 at 282 nm), but it absorbs throughout the UV spectrum and, hence, affords protection not only against sunburn but also against the photodynamic, photosensitizing, and phototoxic effects of drugs. At present, it is marketed in combination with the closely related *Oxybenzone*.

ETHYLHEXYL *P*-METHOXYCINNAMATE

Parsol MCX

Octyl methoxycinnamate [5466-77-3] $C_{18}H_{26}O_3$ (290.40).

Preparation—US Pat 4,713,473.

Description—High-boiling liquid.

Comments—A *sunscreen* with a narrow absorption band of 290 to 320 nm and a moderate molar absorptivity.

ETRETINATE

2,4,6,8-Nonanetetraenoic acid, 9-(4-methoxy-2,3,6-trimethylphenyl)-3,7-dimethyl-, ethyl ester *(all-E)*; Tegison

[54350-48-0] $C_{23}H_{30}O_3$ (354.49).

Preparation—One scheme involves the Wittig condensation of diphenyl 2,3,6-trimethyl-4-methoxybenzylphosphonium chloride and 8-oxo-3,7-dimethyl-2,4,6-octane-trienoic acid (all-*trans*) in the presence of butylene oxide; *Experientia* 1978; 34: 1113.

Description—Crystalline solid melting about 104°.

Solubility—Soluble in alcohol; insoluble in water.

Comments—Although not a topical drug, it is a retinoid closely related to tretinoin and is used only for its dermatological actions; consequently, it is included in this chapter. It is used in the treatment of recalcitrant *psoriasis,* especially the severe, pustular, erythrodermic type. It decreases scaling, erythema, and the thickness of lesions and causes epithelial and dermal cells to redifferentiate to normal cells. Sometimes, dramatic improvement occurs within 2 weeks and complete clearing in 1.5 to 4.5 months. However, relapses are frequent once treatment is discontinued and sometimes even during chronic maintenance. It can be used alone or in low-dose combination with PUVA (psoralen augmented UVA) therapy. The mechanism of action is unknown, but it is undoubtedly like that of vitamin A. Activity resides in the acid metabolite.

Adverse effects occur in more than 75% of recipients. They include chapped lips; peeling of the palms, soles, and fingertips; dryness of the mucous membranes; sore tongue; cheilitis; rhinorrhea; nosebleed; gingival bleeding; loss of hair; nail abnormalities; dry and irritated cornea, sclera, and conjunctiva (50%); epidermal fragility; easy sunburning; and other effects. Occasionally, pseudotumor cerebri, metastatic calcification of ligaments and tendons, and liver dysfunction or necrosis occur. In children and adolescents there may be premature closure of the epiphyses. Plasma cholesterol and triglycerides rise and high-density lipoprotein decreases. The drug is also teratogenic. Adverse effects are less with the low doses used in conjunction with PUVA therapy.

Absorption after oral administration is incomplete. It can be increased by whole milk and other lipid-containing foods. There is a rapid metabolism during which it is deesterified to the acid metabolite. A much slower degradation and conjugation follows, the metabolites being secreted into bile and urine. Nearly all of the circulating drug is bound to plasma lipoproteins, but the active metabolite is bound to albumin. Ultimately, it is taken up into fat, where it may be found even as long as 2 years after the last dose. The apparent elimination half-life is about 120 days. This persistence of drug in the body militates against the use of the drug in fertile women of child-bearing age, since the incidence of congenital defects is high even when conception occurs months after the drug is discontinued. The drug also is excreted into milk; effects in the nursing infant are not known.

HOMOSALATE

Benzoic acid, 2-hydroxy-, 3,3,5-trimethylcyclohexyl ester; ing of Coppertone

Homomenthyl salicylate [118-56-9] $C_{16}H_{22}O_3$ (262.36).

Preparation—US Pat 2,369,084.

Description—Colorless liquid boiling about 163° at 4 mm.

Comments—A liquid with relatively low molar absorptivity (6720 at 310 nm) and limited absorption in the near ultraviolet range (290–315 nm), so that it is used mainly to *promote tanning.* Photosensitive persons may not be protected from burns and phototoxicity.

HYDROGEN PEROXIDE SOLUTION—page 1628.

HYDROQUINONE

1,4-Benzenediol; *p*-Dihydroxybenzene; Hydroquinol; Quinol; Eldoquin and Eldopaque Forte

Hydroquinone [123-31-9] $C_6H_6O_2$ (110.11).

Preparation—Various processes are employed. One involves reacting a sulfuric acid solution of aniline with manganese dioxide and reducing the resulting *p*-benzoquinone with sodium bisulfite.

Description—Fine, white needles; darkens on exposure to air; melts between 172° and 174°.

Solubility—1 g in about 17 mL water, 4 mL alcohol, 51 mL chloroform, or 16.5 mL ether.

Comments—A *hypopigmenting* agent employed percutaneously to lighten localized areas of hyperpigmented skin, such as skin blemishes, lentigo, melasma, chloasma, freckles, etc. Its action is temporary, so that it is necessary to repeat the application at frequent intervals. It is a mild irritant, and erythema or rash may develop, which requires discontinuation of the drug. It should not be used near the eyes or in open cuts. It is contraindicated in the presence of sunburn, miliaria, or irritated skin. It is not to be used in children. Ingestion of 1 g results in tinnitus, nausea, vomiting, a sense of suffocation, shortness of breath, cyanosis, convulsions, delirium, and collapse. Death has occurred with ingestion of 5 g. Irritation of the GI tract occurs with oral ingestion. Dermatitis results from skin contact. Corneal staining and opacification have been noted in those exposed for prolonged periods to hydroquinone vapor at concentrations not sufficiently high for systemic effects.

HYDROXYUREA—page 1575 .

ISOTRETINOIN

13-*cis*-Retinoic Acid; Accutane

3,7-Dimethyl-9-(2,6,6-trimethyl-1-cyclohexen-1-yl)-2-*cis*-4-*trans*-6-*trans*-8-*trans*-nonatetraenoic acid [4759-48-2] $C_{20}H_{28}O_2$ (300.44). Differs from tretinoin (vitamin A) only in the configuration of the unsaturation at the α and β carbon atoms, which is *cis rather than trans*.

Comments—Although not a topical drug, it is a dermatological agent and, hence, is described here. Its primary action is to decrease the production of sebum, which lends itself to the treatment of severe *modular* and *cystic* acne (acne conglobata). The size of the sebaceous gland is decreased, and there is a change in the morphology and secretory capacity of the cells (dedifferentiation). Complete clearing of lesions is seen in about 90% of cases. A single course of treatment usually brings about long-lasting, sometimes permanent, remissions.

It also appears to diminish hyperkeratosis and has been reported to be effective in *rosacea,* gram-negative *folliculitis, lamellar ichthyosis, Darier's disease, pityriasis rubra pilaris,* and *keratocanthoma.*

Adverse effects include facial dermatitis, fragile skin, thinning and drying of the hair, reversible cheilitis, and dry skin, mouth, eyes, and conjunctivitis in 25 to 80% of recipients. Peeling of the palms and soles and sensitivity to sunburn occur in about 5% of users. Urethral inflammation also occurs frequently. Joint pains and exacerbation of rheumatoid arthritis also has been reported to occur in about 16% of patients. Sedimentation rate, serum triglyceride concentration and serum levels of alanine and aspartate transaminases transiently occur in about 25% of users. Vertebral hyperostosis has been noted with the current recommended dose regimen. It was noted originally in patients receiving isotretinoin for various keratinization disorders at higher dosages and for longer periods than those recommended for acne. In spite of the relatively high incidence of side effects, treatment rarely has to be discontinued.

After oral administration, peak blood concentrations occur within 1 to 4 hr. The compound is oxidized to 4-hydroxy-13-*cis*-retinoic acid, which then is glucuronidated and is secreted into the bile. The elimination half-life is 11 to 39 (mean 20) hr. Isotretinoin should not be given during pregnancy or nursing.

LISADIMATE

1,2,3-Propanetriol, 1-(4-aminobenzoate) ester; Escalol 106

Glyceryl *p*-aminobenzoate [136-44-7] $C_{10}H_{13}NO_4$ (211.21).

Preparation—By esterification of aminobenzoic acid with glycerin.

Description—Waxy semisolid or syrup.

Solubility—Insoluble in water, oils, or fats; soluble in alcohol, isopropyl alcohol, or propylene glycol.

Comments—A *sunscreen* that absorbs UV light at 264 to 315 nm and that has a relatively high molar absorptivity (17,197 at 295 nm) but a limited spectrum, therefore used primarily to promote tanning rather than to protect sensitive persons.

METHOXSALEN

7*H*-Furo[3,2-*g*][1]benzopyran-7-one, 9-methoxy-, Ammoidin; 9-Methoxypsoralen; Xanthotoxin; Oxsoralen

[298-81-7] $C_{12}H_8O_4$ (216.19).

Preparation—Occurs naturally in *Psorales coryfolia, Ammi majus, Ruta chalepensis,* and various other plants. It may be synthesized by methods described in *JACS* 1957; 79: 3491, and in US Pat 2,889,337.

Description—White to cream-colored, odorless, fluffy, needle-like crystals; melts between 143° and 148°.

Solubility—Practically insoluble in cold water, sparingly soluble in boiling water; freely soluble in chloroform; soluble in boiling alcohol, acetone, or acetic acid; soluble in aqueous alkalies with ring cleavage; reconstitution occurs on neutralization.

Comments—A *psoralen melanizer.* It increases the photodynamic pigmentation of skin; it does not induce pigmentation in the absence of UV light or melanocytes. It is used in the treatment of *vitiligo* and to *desensitize to sunlight.* Severe sunburning can occur with topical application; it is customary to protect the surrounding skin with a sunscreen. It also is used in PUVA treatment of *psoriasis, mycosis fungoides,* and *cutaneous T-cell lymphoma;* in these, irradiation activates it to cross-link DNA. It may have value in the PUVA treatment of *alopecia areata, inflammatory dermatoses, eczema,* and *lichen planus.* After oral administration GI upset and central nervous system toxicities, such as vertigo and excitement, also occur. Consequently, the drug should be used orally only under medical supervision. It is additive with other photosensitizing drugs and the furocumarin pigments in carrots, celery, figs, limes, mustard, parsley, and parsnips. It inhibits the metabolism of caffeine.

METHYL ANTHRANILATE

2-Aminobenzoic acid, methyl ester

[134-20-3] $C_8H_9NO_2$ (151.16).

Preparation—A constituent of several essential oils; also, by esterification of anthranilic acid with methyl alcohol.

Description—A crystalline substance; melts at 25°.

Solubility—Slightly soluble in water; freely soluble in alcohol or ether.

Comments—A *sunscreen,* with the lowest molar absorptivity of all sunscreens (941 at 315 nm); also, it does not absorb throughout the near UV range (absorption band, 290 to 320 nm) and, therefore, is used in combination with other sunscreens or light-protectives. It also is used as a perfume in ointments and cosmetics.

MONOBENZONE

Phenol, 4-(phenylmethoxy)-, Monobenzyl Ether of Hydroquinone; Benoquin

p-(Benzyloxy)phenol [103-16-2] $C_{13}H_{12}O_2$ (200.24).

Preparation—Prepared in various ways. One method involves condensing sodium *p*-nitrophenolate with benzyl chloride to produce benzyl *p*-nitrophenyl ether followed by (1) reduction of nitro to amino, (2) diazotization of amino, and (3) hydrolytic decomposition of the diazonium compound to the corresponding phenol.

Description—White, odorless, crystalline powder possessing very little taste; melts between 117° and 120°.

Solubility—1 g in >10,000 mL water, 14.5 mL alcohol, 29 mL chloroform, or 14 mL ether.

Comments—A *depigmenting agent* or *demelanizer.* It acts by interfering with the formation of melanin, which is the principal cutaneous pigment. It is recommended only for the final depigmentation in *vitiligo.* It is not recommended for treatment of lentigo, severe freckling, and other types of hyperpigmentation. It is not effective against pigmented moles or malignant melanoma. Its pigment-decreasing action is somewhat erratic. Irritation of varying degrees occurs in a considerable number of patients.

OXYBENZONE

Methanone, (2-hydroxy-4-methoxyphenyl)phenyl-,

2-Hydroxy-4-methoxybenzophenone [131-57-7] $C_{14}H_{12}O_3$ (228.25).

Preparation—Benzoic acid is condensed with resorcinol monomethyl ether by heating in the presence of $ZnCl_2$ or polyphosphoric acid (103% H_3PO_4 equivalent), and PCl_3. US Pat 3,073,866.

Description—White to off-white powder; congeals not lower than 62°.

Solubility—Practically insoluble in water; freely soluble in alcohol or toluene.

Comments—A *sunscreen* with a high molar absorptivity (20,381 at 290 nm), and it absorbs in both the long and short UV spectrum 270 to 350 nm. Therefore, it serves not only to prevent sunburn but also to protect against the photodynamic, photosensitizing, and phototoxic effects of various drugs. Contact with the eyes should be avoided. At present, it is marketed only in combination with other sunscreens.

PADIMATE A

Benzoic acid, 4-(dimethylamino)-, pentyl ester

[14779-78-3] $C_{14}H_{21}NO_2$ (235.33). A mixture of pentyl, isopentyl, and 2-methylbutyl esters of *p*-aminobenzoic acid.

Description—Yellow liquid; faint, aromatic odor.

Solubility—Practically insoluble in water or glycerin; soluble in alcohol, chloroform, isopropyl alcohol, or mineral oil.

Comments—A *sunscreen* of moderate molar absorptivity but relatively narrow UV absorption spectrum (290–315 nm) characteristic of other aminobenzoic acid derivatives.

PADIMATE O

Benzoic acid, 4-(dimethylamino)-, 2-ethylhexyl ester

[21245-02-3] $C_{17}H_{27}NO_2$ (277.41).

Preparation—By the esterification of *p*-dimethylaminobenzoic acid with 2-ethylhexanol in the presence of dry HCl. The product is liberated from the salt by neutralization with base.

Description—Light-yellow mobile liquid; faint, aromatic odor.

Solubility—Practically insoluble in water, alcohol, or mineral oil.

Comments—See Padimate A.

ROXADIMATE

Benzoic acid, 4-[bis-(2-hydroxypropyl)amino]-, ethyl ester; Amerscreen

[58882-17-0] $C_{15}H_{23}NO_4$ (281.35).

Comments—A *sunscreen* with a limited absorption spectrum (280 to 330 nm) characteristic of *p*-aminobenzoates but a relatively high molar absorptivity. It is used mainly in suntan products.

SODIUM FLUORIDE

Sodium fluoride [7681-49-4] NaF (41.99).

Preparation—By interaction of 40% HF with an equivalent quantity of NaOH or Na_2CO_3.

Description—White, odorless powder.

Solubility—1 g in 25 mL water; insoluble in alcohol.

Comments—A *dental caries prophylactic*. Fluoridation of municipal water supplies is considered a safe and practical public health measure; a concentration of about 1 ppm of fluoride in the water supply results in a 50% to 65% reduction in the incidence of dental caries in permanent teeth. Ingested fluoride is effective only while teeth are being formed. The fluoride is incorporated into tooth salts as fluoroapatite. Excessive intake during development of teeth may cause mottling; hence, mottling of newly erupted teeth is an indication to reduce fluoride intake. Where drinking water contains less than 0.7 ppm of fluoride, dietary supplements for children with unerupted teeth may provide some future protection.

Topical application results in changes only in the outer layers of enamel or exposed dentin. In children, repeated application of a 2% solution of the drug to cleaned teeth results in a 16% to 49% reduction of dental caries; adult teeth are protected to a lesser extent by topical application. Topical application also is used to *desensitize* teeth.

Orally administered, it produces new bone formation in some patients with osteoporosis, especially when calcium and vitamin D (and estrogens in women) are administered concomitantly to facilitate mineralization of the new bone. However, the bone may become brittle.

It removes calcium from tissues and also poisons certain enzymes. Large oral doses may cause nausea and vomiting, which usually can be prevented by taking the substance with food. Pastes, rinses, solutions, and gels for topical applications should not be swallowed.

SODIUM MONOFLUOROPHOSPHATE

Phosphorofluoridic acid, sodium salt

FPO(ONa)$_2$

Disodium phosphorofluoridate [10163-15-2] (143.95).

Preparation—Substantially pure drug is produced by fusing a mixture of sodium metaphosphate and sodium fluoride, in stoichiometric proportion, in a closed vessel from which moist air is excluded.

Description—White to slightly gray, odorless powder.

Solubility—Freely soluble in water.

Comments—Like *Sodium Fluoride*, above, it promotes the replacement of hydroxyapatite by fluoroapatite in the tooth salts and, hence, is used as a *dental prophylactic* against dental caries. It has the advantage over sodium fluoride in that the teeth do not require special preparation before application, it is effective when included in dentifrices, and in dentifrices there is no hazard with respect to local toxicity to the gingivae or systemic intoxication from ingestion.

STANNOUS FLUORIDE

Tin Difluoride; Fluoristan

Tin fluoride (SnF$_2$) [7783-47-3] (156.69); contains not less than 71.2% Sn$_2$$^+$ (stannous tin) and about 24% F$^-$ (fluoride).

Preparation—Stannous oxide is dissolved in 40% HF, and the solution is evaporated out of contact with air.

Description—White, crystalline powder with a bitter, salty taste; melts at about 213°.

Solubility—Freely soluble in water; practically insoluble in alcohol, ether, or chloroform.

Comments—Alters the composition and crystalline structure of the hydroxyapatite-like salts that make up the bulk of enamel and dentin, so that the tooth material is more resistant to acidic erosion and dental caries (decay). The substance is applied only topically, so that the tooth substance is only affected in the superficial layers, and it must be applied periodically. It is most effective when applied to the tooth surface after the teeth have been cleaned thoroughly by a dentist. However, there is good evidence that even when incorporated into toothpastes the drug has a retardant effect on the development of dental caries.

TITANIUM DIOXIDE

Titanic Anhydride

Titanium oxide (TiO$_2$) [13463-67-7] TiO$_2$ (79.88).

Preparation—By adding ammonia or an alkali carbonate to a solution of titanyl sulfate (TiOSO$_4$). Titanic acid Ti(OH)$_4$ or TiO(OH)$_2$ is precipitated and, after filtration and washing, is dried and ignited.

Description—White, amorphous, tasteless, odorless, infusible powder; density about 4; suspension in water (1 in 10) neutral to litmus.

Solubility—Insoluble in water, HCl, HNO$_3$, or dilute H$_2$SO$_4$.

Comments—Its powder has a very high reflectance at visible and UV wavelengths, and, hence, it serves as an excellent white pigment. In ointments or lotions it reflects a very high proportion of incident sunlight, hence, protecting the skin from sunburn and serving as a sunblock. It also is used in cosmetics and as a dusting powder. Topically, it is devoid of toxicity.

TRIOXSALEN

7*H*-Furo[3,2-*g*][1]benzopyran-7-one, 2,5,9-trimethyl-, 6-hydroxy-β,2,7-trimethyl-5-benzofuranacrylic acid, δ-lactone; Trisoralen

[3902-71-4] $C_{14}H_{12}O_3$ (228.25).

Caution—Avoid contact with the skin.

Preparation—2-Methylresorcinol is cyclized with ethyl acetoacetate with the aid of sulfuric acid to 7-hydroxy-4,8-dimethylcoumarin (I). Treatment with allyl bromide in the presence of potassium carbonate transforms I into the 7-allyloxy compound, which, on reacting with acetic anhydride in the presence of *N,N*-diethylaniline and anhydrous sodium acetate, rearranges and esterifies to give the 7-acetoxy-6-allyl compound (II). Bromination of II followed by reaction with sodium methoxide yields trioxsalen. US Pat 3,201,421.

Description—White to off-white, odorless, tasteless crystalline solid; stable in light, air, and heat; melts at about 230°.

Solubility—1 g in 1150 mL alcohol, 84 mL chloroform, or 43 mL methylenedichloride; practically insoluble in water.

Comments—Although not a topical drug, it closely relates to other drugs in this section. It facilitates the action of near UV light to induce melanin (skin pigment) formation. It is used to cause repigmentation in idiopathic *vitiligo* and to **enhance** pigmentation to *increase tolerance to sunlight* or for *cosmetic purposes*. The increased tolerance to sunlight does not occur until enhanced pigmentation has occurred, and the patient must be cautioned that severe sunburning with less than normal exposure can occur early during the course of treatment. The increase in dermal pigment occurs gradually over a period of several days of repeated exposure. Care must be taken to protect the eyes and lips during treatment. The manufacturer's recommended schedule of exposure should be used except at high altitudes, where exposure times should be appropriately reduced.

It is contraindicated in persons with photosensitizing diseases, such as infectious leukoderma, porphyria, or lupus erythematosus, and when photosensitizing drugs are being given. The drug sometimes may cause gastric irritation and emesis. Children under 12 should not take it.

ACKNOWLEDGMENTS–Kristine Knutson, PhD and Lynn K Pershing, PhD are acknowledged for their contributions in previous editions of this work.

MEDICINAL AGENTS

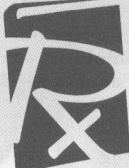

CHAPTER 66

Gastrointestinal and Liver Drugs

John E Hoover, BSc Pharm, RPh

The major categories of drugs included in this chapter areantacids, H_2-receptor antagonists, proton pump inhibitors, drugs that enhance mucosal resistance, digestants including pancreatic enzymes, laxatives, antidiarrheals, emetics, antiemetics, prokinetic agents, adsorbents, and miscellaneous drugs. A number of other drugs, used primarily for other indications but also used in the treatment of gastrointestinal (GI) diseases, are not included in this chapter. These include immunosuppressive drugs, anti-inflammatory drugs, immunostimulants and antibiotics.

DRUGS USED TO TREAT ACID PEPTIC DISEASES

Mucosal injury in the acid peptic diseases (ie, gastric ulcer, duodenal ulcer and gastroesophageal reflux disease (GERD)) is mediated by gastric acid. Hydrochloric acid is secreted by parietal cells in the body of the stomach. It is regulated by adjacent endocrine, paracrine, and neurocrine cells. The parietal cell has receptors for acetylcholine (neurocrine), gastrin (endocrine), histamine (paracrine), somatostatin (endocrine), and prostaglandin E_2 (paracrine). Acetylcholine and gastrin both activate calcium channels, albeit different channels. This leads to intracellular accumulation of calcium. Calcium, in turn, stimulates protein kinases that phosphorylate H^+K^+ ATPase, the proton pump. The physiological essence of the proton pump is to exchange extracellular K^+ for intracellular H^+. It is thus the final common pathway of acid secretion. Gastrin and acetylcholine are relatively weak stimuli of the parietal cell. They act primarily through the adjacent enterochromaffin-like (ECL) cell, causing the release of histamine. Histamine is the most potent stimulus of acid secretion and acts as the common mediator. It induces adenylate cyclase, which converts ATP to cyclic AMP (cAMP), which activates the protein kinases. This complex interaction accounts for the well-known phenomenon of potentiation, in which the effect of two or more stimuli is greater than the sum of their additive effects. The converse is also true; histamine antagonists inhibit acid secretion that is stimulated by gastrin and acetylcholine as well as histamine.

There are two types of acid secretion under physiological secretions: (1) meal stimulated, 90% of which is stimulated by gastrin, and (2) basal, which is mostly stimulated by acetylcholine. Meal-stimulated acid secretion is largely regulated by gastrin. Gastrin secretion is modulated by a negative feedback mechanism such that alkalization, ie, feeding, stimulates gastrin release and thus acid secretion, while acidification, ie, discontinuing eating, inhibits gastrin release and shuts down acid secretion. Food stimulates gastrin release by three mecha-

nisms: (1) gastric distention; (2) specific food constituents such as amino acids, protein hydrolysates, ethanol, and calcium; and (3) elevation of gastric pH. Acid is the major inhibitor of gastrin release and thus of acid secretion. Since ingestion of food increases gastric pH, gastrin release is disinhibited and acid secretion continues. As food intake stops, gastric pH falls, gastrin release is inhibited, and acid secretion returns to basal levels. It is in this way that eating regulates acid secretion. Acidification also causes adjacent D cells to release somatostatin, which appears to inhibit acid secretion by direct inhibition of adenyl cyclase in the parietal cell. The major effect of somatostatin, however, is inhibition of histamine release from the adjacent ECL cell.

Basal acid secretion exhibits a circadian rhythm in which gastric secretion is highest at night (approximately at midnight) and lowest in the early morning. This secretion is not paralleled by changes in circulating serum gastrin and is abolished by vagotomy. It appears, therefore, that basal secretion is largely controlled by the vagus nerve and its neurotransmitter, acetylcholine. The importance of basal secretion is twofold:

1. It accounts for the characteristic nighttime awakening with peptic ulcer pain.
2. It serves as the rationale for single nighttime dosing with H_2 receptor antagonists.

In addition to a stimulatory pathway of acid secretion, there is a closely related inhibitory system. This system is activated by prostaglandin E_2 (PGE_2), which appears to act on a membrane receptor that activates an inhibitory protein (GIP) that blocks the histamine activation of adenylate cyclase. An additional function of PGE_2 in the gastric mucosa is to increase bicarbonate and mucus secretion, which enhances mucosal resistance to injury. Thus, the combined effect of PGE_2 is to inhibit acid secretion and increase mucosal protection—yet another example of the constitutive or protective function of the prostaglandins. The inhibition of PGE_2 by nonsteroidal anti-inflammatory drugs (NSAIDs) is the underlying mechanism by which they cause injury. The other major inhibitor of acid secretion is somatostatin.

In general, ulcer disease occurs whenever there is an increase in acid secretion or a decrease in mucosal resistance. Conversely, acid peptic diseases can be treated by either decreasing acid or increasing mucosal resistance. Acid-mediated pain occurs when the gastric pH is below 2. Healing of the acid peptic diseases occurs when the mean 24-hr pH is kept above 3 to 4. The pH can be increased by either neutralizing acid (antacids) or inhibiting gastric secretion (H_2-receptor antagonists or proton pump inhibitors). Mucosal resistance can be increased with prostaglandin analogs.

DRUGS THAT DECREASE ACID

The exact mechanism of gastric acid secretion has yet to be elucidated. It is known that four endogenous substances—acetylcholine, the neurotransmitter of the vagus nerve; gastrin, a systemic hormone secreted by G cells in the antrum of the stomach; histamine, a paracrine hormone secreted by enterochromasin cells in the wall of the stomach; and calcium—all stimulate acid secretion. There are receptors for acetylcholine (muscarinic receptors), gastrin (gastrin receptors), and histamine (H_2-receptors). Calcium may both increase gastrin and act as a second messenger for gastrin and acetylcholine. Histamine probably activates adenylate cyclase, which converts cytosolic ATP to cAMP, which acts as a second messenger. There is some evidence that histamine may act as the common mediator of acid secretion, since it augments acetylcholine- and gastrin-stimulated secretion, and H_2-blockers inhibit both acetylcholine- and gastrin-stimulated secretion.

The final common pathway of acid secretion is the proton pump, Na^+/K^+ ATPase. The physiological essence of Na^+/K^+ ATPase is to exchange K^+ for H^+; H^+ is secreted against a profound concentration gradient of 2,000,000:1 or greater. This acid secretion is stimulated by the sight, smell, and ingestion of food. In addition to the stimulated acid secretion, there is a basal acid secretion that occurs independently of eating. An important feature of basal acid secretion is its diurnal variation, such that acid secretion is low during the day but relatively high at night—generally peaking between 10 PM and midnight. For this reason patients tend to wake up around midnight with dyspepsia and heartburn. It is at this time that gastric pH tends to drop to 1 or 2, since acid secretion is relatively high and is not neutralized by food.

During the day, the food that stimulates acid secretion also neutralizes it, keeping the gastric pH about 4 or 5. The diurnal variation in acid secretion forms the rationale for using H_2-receptor antagonists as a single evening dose in the treatment of gastric and duodenal ulcers.

As discussed above, PGE_2 acts both to inhibit acid secretion and increase mucosal protection. There are other inhibitors of acid secretion. Somatostatin and secretin are probably the most important under physiological conditions.

ANTACIDS

Antacids are drugs that react with hydrochloric acid to form salt and water. This neutralizes acid and, in so doing, raises gastric pH. The most widely used antacids are sodium bicarbonate, calcium carbonate, aluminum hydroxide, and magnesium hydroxide.

Antacids are used widely for the relief of heartburn and dyspepsia, as well as a large variety of nonspecific GI symptoms. The primary role of antacids in the management of acid peptic disorders is relief of pain. For the most part, they are safe, but in patients with compromised renal function, indiscriminate use can lead to alkalosis and other complications.

Antacids usually are used in combination. The differences in mixture account for the relative differences in neutralizing capacity and side effects. It is apparent that the more acid neutralized, the greater the efficacy of the antacid. For practical purposes, however, efficacy is obtained by increasing the gastric pH to 3.5 or greater. This is achieved readily with modern antacids, giving doses of 15 to 30 mL, 1 and 3 hr after meals. Such doses also heal ulcers in 4 to 8 weeks in approximately 80% of patients.

The mechanism of action of antacids is complex. A proposed mechanism is the prevention of back-diffusion of hydrogen ions across the GI mucosa. Fifty percent of the acid in a given amount of gastric juice with a pH of 1.3 can be neutralized by raising the pH to 1.6, 90% by raising the pH to 2.3, and 99% by raising the pH to 3.3. It generally is accepted that raising the gastric pH to approximately 4 prevents stress ulcer, which is thought to be mediated by acid back-diffusion. Another action of antacids is to prevent the conversion of gastric pepsinogen to pepsin, the active form. This is a proteolytic enzyme thought to mediate tissue injury in ulcer disease. Pepsinogens are inactivated irreversibly at pH 5 and inactivated at pH 7. It thus may be necessary to raise the pH to 5 to achieve the maximum benefit from antacids. Antacids also may enhance cytoprotection in the stomach. Finally, antacids may confer a therapeutic benefit by inactivating bile salts, which are thought to reflux from the duodenum into the stomach and play some role in acid peptic disease.

There are differences in the types of antacids in terms of their cation content, neutralizing capacity, duration of action, side effects, and cost. These must be considered when choosing an antacid for therapeutic use.

NEUTRALIZING CAPACITY—Antacids are compared quantitatively in terms of acid-neutralizing capacity (ANC), defined as the number of milliequivalents of hydrochloric acid required to maintain 1 mL of an antacid suspension at pH 3 for 2 hr *in vitro*. The rate of neutralization varies according to the degree of comminution, crystal form, precipitants used, and presence of reactive suspending agents. Consequently, the ANC and rate of neutralization of various antacids differ enormously. For example, 5 mL of aluminum hydroxide suspension (Amphojel) will neutralize 6.5 mEq of acid in 60 min, whereas a similar volume of aluminum hydroxide–magnesium hydroxide suspension (Delcid) will neutralize 42 mEq in the same period of time.

DOSING INTERVAL—An ideal antacid should be rapid in onset and provide a continuous buffering action. Antacids with a rapid onset include magnesium hydroxide, magnesium oxide, and calcium carbonate; those with an intermediate onset, magaldrate and magnesium carbonate; and those with a slow onset, magnesium trisilicate and the aluminum compounds. The duration of buffering action is determined largely by when the antacid is administered; if administered while food is in the stomach, the buffering action will last for 2 hr. An additional dose 3 hr after meals will extend the buffering time by 1 hr. Therefore, the ideal dosing interval is 1 and 3 hr after meals and at bedtime.

THE PATIENT—Certain patients by nature of their underlying disease may be at increased risk of antacid toxicity. For example, patients with heart failure may be at risk from excess sodium intake. Most available antacids are low in sodium and thus the presence of edema or heart failure precludes the use only of sodium bicarbonate. Patients with renal failure should not use magnesium-containing antacids, because of the possibility of hypermagnesemia, or sodium bicarbonate, which may cause systemic alkalosis. While patients with renal failure are sometimes given aluminum-containing antacids for their phosphate-lowering effect, there is increasing concern about aluminum neurotoxicity in such patients.

SIDE EFFECTS—A systemic antacid, such as sodium bicarbonate, is soluble and readily absorbed. It can cause electrolyte disturbances and alkalosis. The so-called nonsystemic antacids, such as aluminum-, calcium-, and magnesium-containing antacids, form relatively insoluble compounds in the GI tract. It is not true, however, that such compounds are not absorbed. Toxicity occurs as the result of systemic absorption of all of these antacids. Ingestion of large amounts of calcium carbonate can lead to hypercalcemia, alkalosis, and renal failure with so-called milk-alkali syndrome. Magnesium-containing antacids can cause both diarrhea and hypermagnesemia. Prolonged treatment with aluminum-containing antacids can cause phosphate depletion and, eventually, osteoporosis and osteomalacia as well as neurotoxicity. All of the toxicities of the nonsystemic antacid are more common and more serious in patients with renal failure.

ALUMINUM CARBONATE GEL, BASIC—see RPS-20, page 1221.

ALUMINUM HYDROXIDE GEL

Colloidal Aluminum Hydroxide; Amphojel; Alternagel

Aluminum Hydroxide [21645-51-2] $Al(OH)_3$ (78.00); a suspension each 100 g of that contains the equivalent of 3.6 to 4.4 g of aluminum oxide [Al_2O_3 = 101.96] in the form of aluminum hydroxide and hydrated oxide.

It may contain peppermint oil, glycerin, sorbitol, sucrose, saccharin, or other suitable flavors, and it may contain suitable antimicrobial agents.

Preparation—One process for the preparation of this type of aluminum hydroxide is as follows:

Dissolve 1000 g of $Na_2CO_3 \cdot 10H_2O$ in 400 mL of hot water and filter. Dissolve 800 g of ammonium alum in 2000 mL of hot water and filter into the carbonate solution with constant stirring. Then add 4000 mL of hot water and remove all gas. Dilute to 80,000 mL with cold water. Collect and wash the precipitate and suspend it in 2000 mL of purified water flavored with 0.01% peppermint oil and preserve with 0.1% of sodium benzoate. Homogenize the resulting gel.

The principal property desired is a very fine particle size to achieve large surface and thus maximum adsorption capacity.

Description—White, viscous suspension, from which small amounts of water may separate on standing; translucent in thin layers; affects both red and blue litmus paper slightly but is not reddened by phenolphthalein.

Incompatibilities—The use of Aluminum Hydroxide Gel and similar materials to reduce the GI problems accompanying use of tetracyclines has resulted in complexation with decreased absorption of the antibiotic.

Comments—Used primarily as an antacid in the management of *peptic ulcer, gastritis,* and *esophagitis.* It also is used as a skin protectant and mild astringent. It is a relatively weak antacid and does not elevate gastric pH sufficiently to inhibit pepsin activity. Aluminum hydroxide does not have significant demulcent properties. Although aluminum hydroxide is a nonsystemic antacid, significant amounts are absorbed in patients with renal failure. Aluminum hydroxide is excreted as the phosphate. This provides the basis not only for the occasional use of aluminum hydroxide for the treatment of *phosphate nephrolithiasis,* but also is the cause of the phosphate depletion syndrome sometimes observed after chronic administration. There is increasing concern that aluminum absorption may lead to dementation. The major advantage of aluminum hydroxide is that no systemic alkalosis is produced. Aluminum compounds decrease the absorption of certain drugs, such as tetracyclines. It also interferes with the defoaming action of simethicone. These compounds are also constipating.

BISMUTH SUBSALICYLATE

Basic Bismuth Subsalicylate; Pepto-Bismol

[14882-18-19] $C_7H_5BiO_4$ (362.11).

Solubility—Practicaly insoluble in water or alcohol; soluble in alkali; decomposed by hot water.

Comments—The principal ingredient in a popular over-the-counter (OTC) product employed for *indigestion, nausea,* and *diarrhea.* As an antidiarrheal agent it shows good activity versus *Salmonella* but less activity versus *Escherichia coli.* As an antiulcer drug, it seems to increase the rate of healing of peptic ulcers. It also reduces active intestinal secretion induced by *E coli* and *Vibrio cholerae.* This is thought to be due to antiprostaglandin activity by the subsalicylate component. It is used also as an antibiotic for the prophylaxis of traveller's diarrhea and amoebiasis. It also is used to treat the common form of gastritis and duodenal ulcer caused by *Helicobacter pylori.* In this circumstance, it is used in combination with an antibiotic (usually amoxicillin and/or metronidazole) and an H_2-blocker or proton pump inhibitor, but it is effective when given alone.

Bismuth subsalicylate has several properties aside from its effect on *H pylori* that may account for its efficacy in the treatment of ulcer disease. It forms a glycoprotein-bismuth complex with mucus that may create a protective barrier against acid peptic digestion. Furthermore, it may stimulate PGE_2, which in turn stimulates mucus and bicarbonate secretion. Finally, it may stimulate epidermal growth factor, which may enhance healing of ulcers.

Adverse Effects—Most ingested bismuth subsalicylate is excreted in feces as bismuth sulfide. However, small amounts are absorbed, and plasma levels are detectable. Encephalopathy has been reported with other bismuth salts. Its use is not recommended in patients with renal failure. The toxicity of long-term therapy is uncertain. Since this agent is a salicylate, it may cause ringing of the ears if taken with aspirin. Bismuth subsalicylate causes a temporary darkening of the stool and tongue. The darkening of the stool mimics melena and may mistakenly suggest GI bleeding.

CALCIUM CARBONATE

Mylanta; Titrilac

Calcium carbonate (1:1) [471-34-1] $CaCO_3$ (100.09).

Preparation—By double decomposition of calcium chloride and sodium carbonate in aqueous solution. Its density and fineness are gov-

erned by the concentration of the solutions; heavy and light forms are available on the market.

Description—Fine, white, microcrystalline powder, without odor or taste, and stable in air; aqueous suspension is practically neutral to litmus.

Solubility—Practically insoluble in water (its solubility in water is increased by the presence of any ammonium salt and by the presence of carbon dioxide; alkali hydroxide reduces its solubility); insoluble in alcohol; dissolves with effervescence in dilute acetic, hydrochloric, or nitric acids.

Comments—A rapidly acting *antacid.* It is used in the treatment of dyspepsia and heartburn and as an add-on treatment of gastritis, peptic ulcer disease, and esophagitis. Precipitated calcium carbonate also is employed in dentifrices and is a pharmaceutical necessity for Aluminum Subacetate Solution and antacid oral suspension dosage forms.

Adverse Effects—Although calcium carbonate is classified as a *nonsystemic* antacid, long-term therapy with large doses may cause systemic alkalosis and hypercalcemia (milk-alkali syndrome) in patients with renal failure. The salt reacts with hydrochloric acid in the stomach to form calcium chloride, which is largely (90%) insoluble. However, a proportion of the calcium (7–19%) is absorbed. Calcium is constipating. For this reason, calcium and magnesium antacids often are alternated in therapy or given in fixed combination.

Calcium-containing antacids cause *acid rebound*—an increase in acid secretion that occurs after the neutralizing effect occurs. Calcium-containing antacids are used for the prevention, not treatment, of osteoporosis. The goal of therapy is to maintain, rather than restore, bone mass. Large doses, ie, 1000 to 1500 mg, as elemental calcium daily are required in order to prevent or slow the progression of osteoperosis.

CALCIUM HYDROXIDE TOPICAL SOLUTION—page 1084.
CALCIUM PHOSPHATE, DIBASIC—page 1338.
DIHYDROXYALUMINUM SODIUM CARBONATE—see RPS-20, page 1221.

MAGNESIUM HYDROXIDE

Milk of Magnesia; Rolaids

[1309-42-8] $Mg(OH)_2$ (58.32).

Preparation—By precipitation using aqueous solutions of magnesium chloride or sulfate and sodium hydroxide. US Pat 3,127,241. A method for preparing it in various particle sizes is described in US Pat 3,232,708.

Description—White, very fine, bulky powder; slowly absorbs carbon dioxide on exposure to air.

Solubility—Practically insoluble in water or in alcohol; dissolves in dilute acids.

Comments—As a laxative and an antacid (although at usual doses it does not have enough neutralizing capacity to be defined as an antacid). Magnesium hydroxide is a mild cathartic that usually produces bowel movements in 1/2 to 6 hr. It probably acts by altering intestinal motility. It should not be used in patients with vomiting or abdominal pain.

It is not recommended, although frequently used as an antacid. As with other magnesium-containing compounds, it should not be used in patients with impaired renal function.

MAGNESIUM OXIDE

Magnesia; Light Magnesia; Calcined Magnesia; Heavy Magnesium Oxide; Heavy Magnesia; Heavy Calcined Magnesia; Uro-Mag and Mag-Ox 400

[1309-48-4] MgO (40.30)

Preparation—Light or heavy magnesium carbonate is exposed to red heat, whereupon CO_2 and H_2O are expelled, and light or heavy magnesium oxide is left. The density of the oxide also is influenced by the calcining temperature; high temperatures yielding more compact forms.

Description—Very bulky white powder, known as light magnesium oxide, or a relatively dense white powder, known as heavy magnesium oxide. Readily absorbs moisture and carbon dioxide when exposed to air.

Solubility—Practically insoluble in water to which, however, it imparts an alkaline reaction; insoluble in alcohol, soluble in dilute acids.

Comments—An effective, fairly long-acting, nonsystemic antacid. Since in water it is converted to the hydroxide, its biological properties are the same as those of the hydroxide. It is sometimes employed as a cathartic.

Light magnesia is preferable to heavy for administration in liquids, because being a finer powder, it suspends more readily.

Table 66-1. The Relative Onset and Duration of Action, Sodium Content, Acid Neutralizing Capacity (ANC), and Potential Adverse Effects of Common Single-Entity Antacids

ANTACID	ONSET OF ACTION	DURATION OF ACTION	SODIUM (MG/UNIT)	ANC[a]	ADVERSE EFFECTS[b]
Aluminum carbonate gel	Slow	Short	0.12	12	AFGI
Aluminum hydroxide gel	Slow	Prolonged	<2.5	16	AFGI
Calcium carbonate	Fast	Prolonged	<2.3	10	ABCEH
Magnesium carbonate	Intermediate	Prolonged	—	20/g	BD
Magnesium hydroxide	Fast	Short	0.12	14	BD
Magnesium oxide	Fast	Short	—	21	BD
Sodium bicarbonate	Fast	Short	88	12/g	CEJ

[a] ANC per capsule, tablet, or 5-mL suspension unless otherwise indicated.
[b] A, constipation; B, laxation; C, hypercalcemia; D, hypermagnesia; E, metabolic alkalosis; F, neurotoxicity in renal failure; G, osteomalacia and osteoporosis; H, renal calculi; I, phosphorus depletion; J, swelling of feet.

MAGNESIUM TRISILICATE

Hydrated Magnesium Silicate

Magnesium silicate hydrate [39365-87-2] $2MgO \cdot 3SiO_2 \cdot xH_2O$; *anhydrous* [14987-04-3] (260.86). A compound of magnesium oxide and silicon dioxide with varying proportions of water. It contains not less than 20% magnesium oxide [MgO = 40.30] and not less than 45% silicon dioxide [SiO$_2$ = 60.08].

Preparation—By precipitating a solution of sodium silicate of the proper composition [$Na_4Si_3O_8$, or having a ratio of Na_2O to SiO_2 of 1:1.5] with a solution of magnesium chloride or sulfate.

Description—Fine, white, odorless, tasteless powder, free from grittiness; its suspension is neutral or only slightly alkaline to litmus.

Solubility—Insoluble in water or alcohol; readily decomposed by mineral acids, with liberation of silicic acid.

Comments—A nonsystemic *antacid* and *adsorbent*. As an antacid, it has a slow onset of action and is relatively weak; as a single entity it does not meet current pH requirements for nonprescription antacids. It is available only in combination with other antacids. Approximately 5% of the magnesium and 7% of the silicate may be absorbed. Therefore, a number of cases of siliceous nephrolithiasis have been reported following chronic use. Large doses may cause diarrhea due to the action of the soluble magnesium salts on the GI tract.

SODIUM BICARBONATE

Carbonic acid monosodium salt; Baking Soda; Sodium Acid Carbonate; Brioschi; Neut

Monosodium carbonate [144-55-8] $NaHCO_3$ (84.01).

Preparation—May be produced by the ammonium-soda process, or *Solvay process*, as it is usually called. In this process, CO_2 is passed into a solution of common salt in ammonia water, sodium bicarbonate is precipitated, and ammonium chloride, being much more soluble, remains in solution. The ammonium chloride solution is heated with lime, whereby the ammonia is regenerated and returned to the process.

Description—White, crystalline powder; odorless and with a saline and slightly alkaline taste; solutions freshly prepared with cold water without shaking are alkaline to litmus paper; alkalinity increases as the solutions stand or are agitated or heated; stable in dry air, but slowly decomposes in moist air.

Solubility—1 g in 12 mL water; with hot water it is converted into carbonate; insoluble in alcohol.

Comments—Widely employed as an antacid, especially by the laity, despite its many disadvantages. Sodium bicarbonate reacts with HCl to produce CO_2, thus giving rise to epigastric distress and eructation. Although the onset of action is rapid, the duration of action is short. In the treatment of systemic acidosis, it is specific in that the salt is composed of the two ions essential to correct this condition.

It is used locally on the skin in the form of a moist paste or a solution. In this form, it is an effective antipruritic. The salt also is an ingredient of many effervescent mixtures, alkaline solutions, douches, etc.

Sodium bicarbonate is absorbed readily. Prolonged therapy with large doses will produce systemic alkalosis. Moreover, chronic therapy along with milk or calcium may precipitate the milk-alkali syndrome in patients with renal failure. Even moderate amounts may expand plasma volume, increase blood pressure, and lead to edema. Therefore, it may be hazardous in patients with renal insufficiency, hypertension, or cardiac failure.

ANTACID MIXTURES

Antacids are used commonly in combination in order to

1. Combine fast- and slow-reacting antacids to obtain a product with a rapid onset and relatively even, sustained action.

2. Lower the dose of each component and minimize the possibility of certain adverse effects.

3. Use one component to antagonize one or more side effects of another component (eg, laxation vs constipation).

The antacid substances listed in Table 66-1 are employed extensively in the preparation of antacid mixtures. Indeed, they are the principal ingredients in almost 100 OTC antacid preparations, including chewable tablets, suspensions, and gels. For example, examination of 78 antacid mixtures reveals that 72% are composed of aluminum hydroxide and magnesium hydroxide alone or with simethicone, 12% of aluminum hydroxide and either magnesium trisilicate or magnesium carbonate, 11% of magnesium oxide and/or calcium carbonate with simethicone, and 5% of magaldrate with simethicone. Simethicone is not an antacid. It is used in antacid combinations to defoam gastric juice to decrease the incidence of gastroesophageal reflux. It does not decrease the antacid requirement.

The acid neutralizing capacity (ANC) of the suspensions closely approximates that of the tablets, but in general their neutralizing capacity tends to be greater because tablets go into solution less well. Gaviscon is listed in Tables 66-2 and 66-3, although it is not used in peptic ulcer disease and the ANC of its regular preparation does not qualify it as an antacid. Its unique formulation produces a foam that floats on the stomach contents. When acid reflux occurs, the foam precedes the stomach contents into the esophagus and protects the mucosa from further irritation. Hence, it is formulated specifically for acid reflux.

H$_2$-RECEPTOR ANTAGONISTS

There are three types of histamine receptors. The second of these mediates acid secretion by the gastric parietal cells and is inhibited by the H$_2$-receptor blocking drugs (Black et al. *Nature* 1972; 236:385). The identification of this receptor and its modulation introduced an era of pharmacology and led to the awarding of the Nobel prize to Dr Black. The H$_2$-receptor antagonists are histamine analogs. They consist of ring structures with side chains. While the rings and the side chains differ among compounds, they all have in common a nitrogen either in the ring or immediately adjacent to the ring and a nitrogen on the side chain that is recognized by the receptor.

The H$_2$-receptor antagonists are designer drugs developed as the result of the intentional modification of the histamine structure in an effort to find analogs with a higher binding affinity than histamine for the H$_2$-receptor. Such compounds would displace histamine and thus act as competitive inhibitors. The first such substance was burimamide, but it was only effective when given intravenously. The next substance was metiamide, effective both orally and intravenously but abandoned because it caused agranulocytosis. Finally, in 1977, cimetidine was approved by the Food and Drug Administration (FDA). It quickly became the number-one-selling drug in the world. It contains a substituted imidazole ring like that in histamine. Subsequently, ranitidine, a substituted furan ring, and famotidine and nizatidine, substituted thiazoles, were approved.

The H$_2$-receptor antagonists are a remarkably safe group of drugs. The list of adverse reactions is long, but the incidence is low. Among the side effects associated with all four drugs are headache, dizziness, malaise, myalgia, nausea, diarrhea, constipation, rashes, pruritus, and impotence. It has been said that

Comments—A substituted furan derivative. It is an H_2-receptor antagonist indicated for the short-term treatment of duodenal ulcer and the management of hypersecretory conditions such as Zollinger-Ellison syndrome and systemic mastocytosis. The pharmacokinetic profile of ranitidine is similar to that of cimetidine. Oral absorption appears to be variable and decreased if given concurrently with antacids; bioavailability after an oral dose of 150 mg is approximately 50% (range 40–88%); 15% is bound to plasma protein; volume of distribution is 1.4 L/kg; 30% of the administered dose is excreted unchanged; elimination half-life ranges from 2.5 to 3 hr; serum concentrations vary from 36 to 94 ng/mL; and mean peak blood levels are 440 to 545 ng/mL. Ranitidine lacks a predictable dose/response relationship. For example, 75, 100, and 150 mg of ranitidine inhibit nocturnal gastric acid output by 95%, 96%, and 92%, respectively. Interactions with warfarin, benzodiazepines, fentanyl, metoprolol, nifedipine, and acetaminophen have been reported. Pharmacologic tolerance occurs rapidly with ranitidine. It loses 50% of its activity to suppress acid within 1 week.

Adverse reactions include headache, malaise, dizziness, constipation, nausea, abdominal pain, and rash. Decreased white blood cell and platelet counts also have been reported. Increases (up to five times the upper limit of normal) in serum aminotransferases and gammaglutamyl transpeptidase have been noted. Rare cases of hepatitis also have been reported. In normal volunteers, ALT was increased at least twice the pretreatment levels in 6 of 12 subjects given 100 mg four times a day, intravenously, for 7 days and in 4 of 24 subjects given 50 mg four times daily, intravenously, for 5 days. This dose-related effect, however, is not associated with hepatotoxicity. With respect to use in pregnancy and lactation, studies in rats and rabbits have revealed no evidence of impaired fertility or harm to the fetus. Nevertheless, it should not be used in pregnancy unless needed. Ranitidine is secreted in milk; therefore, it should not be used in nursing mothers unless absolutely necessary.

PROTON PUMP INHIBITORS

The final common pathway in gastric acid secretion is the *proton pump*—an H^+/K^+ ATPase. The physiological essence of this enzyme is the exchange of hydrogen ion for potassium ion. Thus, hydrogen is secreted by the parietal cell into the gastric lumen in exchange for potassium. The proton pump inhibitors lansoprazole and omeprazole belong to a new class of antisecretory drugs called substituted benzimidazoles. The prototype, omeprazole, is an irreversible inhibitors of the proton pump. It has a plasma half-life of 0.5 to 1 hr, but its duration of action is greater than 24 hr, reflecting the time required to generate new H^+/K^+ ATPase. The proton pump inhibitors should be taken prior to meals. This is because, in the resting state, the proton pump resides on the inner membrane of secretory vesicles within the parietal cell. When the cell is activated by eating (or by pharmacological stimulus), the inner membrane of the vesicle is externalized and becomes the outer; ie, the secretory membrane, of the secretory villus. The physiological importance of this is that the proton pump inhibitors are prodrugs that need to be protonated, and this can occur only when the proton pump is externalized and secreting acid. Thus, these drugs are more potent when taken prior to meals and when taken orally. They also are absorbed more effectively in the morning and thus should be dosed approximately 30 min prior to breakfast.

The proton pump inhibitors are used for the short-term treatment of acid peptic disease, gastroesophageal reflux, gastric ulcer, duodenal ulcer, and Zollinger-Ellison syndrome and

for maintenance treatment of GERD. The therapeutic advantages of the proton pump inhibitors over the H_2-receptor antagonists are a faster healing rate, a higher healing rate, and the ability to heal patients who have not been helped by H_2-receptor antagonist therapy.

There are numerous side effects of the proton pump inhibitors, but they occur infrequently. Headache, diarrhea, abdominal pain, dizziness, rash, and constipation are seen with about the same frequency as seen with H_2-blockers, ie, 1% to 5%. Of some concern with the use of proton pump inhibitors is an elevation of serum gastrin. The elevations are 1.5- to 4-fold—about twice that seen with H_2-blockers. Gastrin is a trophic hormone that causes enterochromaffin cells to proliferate in rats. These cells produce histamine and are the precursor to carcinoid tumors in rats. The effect in rats is almost certainly mediated through gastrin rather than from a carcinogenic effect of the drug itself, since the tumors do not occur after antrectomy, a situation that precludes an increase in serum gastrin. Human studies have shown only a slight increase in the enterochromaffin cell population with chronic use of proton pump inhibitors. Carcinoid tumors have not been reported in human subjects using omeprazole. Nevertheless, there is an increased incidence of carcinoid tumors in patients with pernicious anemia, a condition that also is associated with hypergastrinemia. The FDA initially warned against prolonged use of omeprazole. Long-term studies, however, support the view that omeprazole is safe and efficacious for long-term (10+ years) treatment of ulcer disease. Some of the properties of the proton pump inhibitors are shown in Tables 66-5 and 66-6.

ESOMEPRAZOLE MAGNESIUM

1H-Benzimidazole, 5-methoxy-2-[(S)-[(4-methoxy-3,5-dimethyl-2-pyridinyl)methyl]sulfinyl]-, magnesium salt, trihydrate; Nexium

[217087-09-7] $C_{34}H_{36}MgN_6O_6S_2 \cdot 3H_2O$ (767.17).

Preparation—see *Omeprazole*, page 1301.

Description—The *S*- enantiomer of *omeprazole*. The acidic form is a white to off-white crystalline powder from acetonitrile, melting about 156°. Mg salt is a white powder; $[\alpha]_D^{20} - 128.2$ c = 1, methanol).

Solubility—(Acidic form); freely soluble in ethanol or methanol; slightly soluble in acetone or 2-propanol; very slightly soluble in water. (Mg salt); slightly soluble in water. Stability is a function of pH; at pH 6.8 (phosphate buffer) the half-life is about 19 hrs at 25° and 8 hrs at 37°.

LANSOPRAZOLE

1H-Benzimidazole, 2-[[[3-methyl-4-(2,2,2-trifluoroethoxy)-2-pyridyl]methyl]sulfinyl-, Prevacid

[103577-45-3] $C_{16}H_{14}F_3N_3O_2S$ (369.36).

Table 66-6. Antisecretory Effects of Proton Pump Inhibitors

	LANSOPRAZOLE 30 MG			OMEPRAZOLE 20 MG	
	BASELINE	DAY 1	DAY 5	DAY 1	DAY 5
Mean 24-hr pH	21	3.6	4.9	2.5	4.6
Mean nighttime pH	1.9	2.6	3.8	2.2	3.0
% time pH > 3	18	51	72	30	60
% time pH > 4	12	41	66	19	51

Preparation—See US Pat 5,374,730 (1994).

Description—White to off-white, odorless crystals melting about 166° (180° decomposition).

Solubility—Freely soluble in DMF; soluble in methanol; slightly soluble in ethyl acetate, acetonitrile, or methylene chloride; very slightly soluble in ether; insoluble in water or hexane. Degrades in aqueous solution, and rate increases with decreasing pH. At 25°, $t_{1/2}$ = 0.5 hr at pH 5 and 18 hr at pH = 7.

Comments—A proton pump inhibitor. Like all proton pump inhibitors, it is a lipophilic weak base that is unstable in acid. It is administered as enteric-coated, acid-resistant granules that are released in the neutral-alkaline environment of the small intestine. The non-encapsulated granules can be suspended in apple juice or sprinkled in apple sauce to be taken orally or through a nasogastric tube. It is indicated for the short-term treatment of acute duodenal ulcer, gastric ulcer, and erosive esophagitis. It also is indicated for maintenance treatment of healed idiopathic duodenal ulcer, erosive esophagitis, and pathological hypersecretory states such as Zollinger-Ellison syndrome.

It is a prodrug that requires protonation for activation. Thus, it is most effective given 30 to 60 min prior to a meal. Peak concentration occurs at approximately 1.7 hr. The plasma elimination half-life is 1.5 hr, but because it is an irreversible inhibitor of the proton pump, its acid inhibitory effect is greater than 24 hr. On a molar basis, it is approximately 30% to 35% more potent than omeprazole, with the equivalent doses being lansoprazole 30 mg and omeprazole 40 mg.

Like other proton pump inhibitors, it is very effective in healing acid peptic disease with 4-week healing rates for duodenal ulcer of approximately 95%, 8-week healing rates for gastric ulcer of 95%, and 8-week healing rates for gastric ulcer of 95%, and 8-week healing rates for erosive esophagitis of 95%.

Adverse reactions occurring in more than 1% of patients include abdominal pain (1.8%), diarrhea (3.6%), and nausea (1.4%), but only diarrhea occurs with a higher frequency than with placebo. The initial concern about carcinoid tumors seen in male rats treated with high doses for prolonged periods has not been borne out in clinical studies. While there is an increase in serum gastrin levels and hyperplasia of enterochromaffin-like cells, dysplasia and carcinoids have not been seen in other animal species or man after several years of continuous treatment.

Lansoprazole is metabolized through the CYP3A and CYP2C19 isozymes. Studies have not shown significant interactions with commonly used drugs, except a 10% increase in theophylline clearance. This interaction appears to be of no clinical significance. Lansoprazole, however, should not be administered with ketoconazole, which requires low pH for absorption. The pregnancy category is B.

OMEPRAZOLE

1*H*-Benzimidazole, 5-methoxy-2-[[(4-methoxy-3,5-dimethyl-2-pyridinyl)-methyl]sulfinyl]-, Prilosec

[73590-58-6]$C_{17}H_{19}N_3O_3S$(345.42).

Preparation—US Pat 4,255,431.

Description—White crystals melting about 156°; pK$_a$ (pyridine-N) 4.0, (imidazole-N) 8.7.

Solubility—1 g in about 8000 mL water or 25 mL alcohol.

Comments—In the treatment of acid peptic disorders. It is approved for the short-term treatment of duodenal ulcer, severe or poorly responsive gastroesophageal reflux, and hypersecretory conditions such as Zollinger-Ellison syndrome, systemic mastocytosis, and multiple endocrine adenomas. It is also effective in the prevention of NSAID ulcers and their complications. While not approved for that use, it appears to be as effective as misoprostol and has fewer side effects. It is now thought that, with the exception of NSAID-induced and *H pylori*–induced ulcers, the acid peptic diseases are lifelong diseases that require a lifetime of therapy. Long-term studies have demonstrated efficacy in the prevention of recurrence of reflux esophagitis and duodenal ulcer. The current trend in practice is to use proton-pump inhibitors as both initial and maintenance therapy; the so-called black-box precaution for long-term use of omeprazole has been removed and it was never placed on lansoprazole, the subsequently approved proton pump inhibitor.

Omeprazole, because of its acid lability, is given as a delayed-release capsule. Absorption occurs in the small bowel, with peak plasma levels occurring at 0.5 to 3.5 hr. Peak plasma levels and area under the concentration-time curve (AUC) are approximately proportional to dose in the therapeutic range. Bioavailability is 30% to 40%. Plasma half-life is 0.5 to 1 hr with total body clearance of 500 to 600 mL/min. Protein-binding is approximately 95%. Two plasma metabolites have been identified: hydroxyomeprazole and its corresponding carboxylic acid. The metabolites have virtually no antisecretory activity. Most of the drug is eliminated as metabolites in the urine. Dosage adjustment is not needed for patients with impaired renal function.

The antisecretory effect of omeprazole occurs within 1 hr, with maximum effect occurring within 2 hr. Inhibition of secretion remains at about 50% at 24 hr and lasts approximately 72 hr. The prolonged effect, beyond that expected for a drug with a short half-life, is due to irreversible binding to the H$^+$/K$^+$ ATPase. The inhibition of acid secretion peaks in 3 to 4 days and lasts for 3 to 5 days after discontinuing treatment. Omeprazole, at therapeutic doses of 20 to 40 mg causes an 80% to 95% decrease in 24-hr intragastric acidity.

Duodenal ulcer healing occurs in 80% to 95% of patients at 4 weeks and greater than 95% at 8 weeks. Reflux esophagitis healing occurs in 8 weeks in approximately 80% of patients.

Adverse reactions reported to occur in more than 1% of patients include headache (6.9%), diarrhea (3.0%), abdominal pain (2.4%), nausea (2.2%), dizziness (1.5%), vomiting (1.5%), rash (1.5%), constipation (1.1%), asthenia (1.1%), and back pain (1.1%). The previous concern about the development of carcinoid tumors after long-term treatment is not justified after several years of clinical studies; in fact, such tumors have not been reported, other than in patients with Zollinger-Ellison syndrome and the multiple endocrine adenoma syndrome, Type C. These patients are predisposed to the development of gastric carcinoid tumors.

Omeprazole prolongs the elimination of diazepam, warfarin, and phenytoin. Clinical interactions have been seen with cyclosporine, disulfiram, and benzodiazepines. Omeprazole also inhibits the absorption of pH-dependent drugs such as ketoconazole and it should not be used during pregnancy.

PANTOPRAZOLE SODIUM

1*H*-Benzimidazole, 5-(difluoromethoxy)-2-[[(3,4-dimethoxy-2-pyridinyl)methyl]sulfinyl] -, sodium salt, hydrate(2.3); Protonix

[164579-32-2] $C_{16}H_{14}F_2N_3NaO_4S$.11/2H$_2$O (432.37).

Preparation—*J Med Chem*, 1992; 35: 1049 and US 4,758,579 (1986).

Description—(Acid form) weakly amphoteric, white to off-white solid melting about 136° (dec); pK$_{a1}$ 3.92, pK$_{a2}$ 8.19. (Salt) Off-white solid decomposing about 130°.

Solubility—(Salt) Freely soluble in water; slightly soluble in pH 7 phosphate buffer; insoluble in hydrocarbon solvents. Solution stability is pH dependent with degradation increasing with decreasing pH. At pH 5, $t_{1/2}$ is 2.8 hrs and 220 hrs at pH 7.8. The pH of the injection is 9 to 10.

RABEPRAZOLE SODIUM

1*H*-Benzimidazole, 2[[[4-(3-methoxypropoxy)-3-methyl-2-pyridinyl]methyl]sulfinyl]- , sodium salt; Pariprazole, Aciphex

[117976-90-6] $C_{18}H_{20}N_3NaO_3S$ (381.42).

Preparation—US Pat 5,045,552 (1991).

Description—(Acid form) White crystals from methylene chloride\ether melting about 100° (dec). Sodium salt occurs as white crystals from ether melting about 140° (dec). Stability is a function of pH, with rapid decomposition in acid medium.

Solubility—Very soluble in water or methanol; freely soluble in ethanol, chloroform or ethyl acetate; insoluble in ether or hexane.

DRUGS THAT ENHANCE MUCOSAL PROTECTION

MISOPROSTOL

Prost -13-en-1-oic acid, (11α, 13E)-(±)-11,16-dihydroxy-16-methyl-9-oxo-, methyl ester; Cytotec

[59122-46-2] $C_{22}H_{38}O_5$ (382.54).

Preparation—*J Med Chem* 1957; 20:1152.

Description—Pale yellow oil. It is a mixture of the (±)-*R* and (±)-*S* forms with reference to carbon atom no 16.

Solubility—1 g in 2500 mL of water or 100 mL of alcohol.

Comments—In the prevention of NSAID gastropathy. A prostaglandin E_1 analog, it differs from the naturally occurring compound in that it is more water soluble and has a longer half-life. It both inhibits gastric acid secretion and increases mucosal resistance. Its inhibition of acid secretion, however, may not be sufficient to cause a therapeutic effect. Misoprostol probably derives its therapeutic benefit in the GI tract by increasing mucus and bicarbonate secretion by the gastric epithelium by increasing epithelial regeneration and by enhancing mucosal blood flow, thus enhancing mucosal protection.

Misoprostol is used for the prevention of gastric injury by NSAIDs. Controlled studies demonstrate that doses of 100 μg four times a day, 200 μg four times a day, and 200 μg twice a day are effective in preventing gastric injury induced by NSAIDs and reducing the incidence of severe complications by approximately 50%. It is superior to H_2-blockers in preventing gastric ulcers but not duodenal ulcers. It is superior to sucralfate in preventing both gastric and duodenal ulcers and superior to H_2-receptor antagonists in preventing gastric ulcer.

It is not yet clear which patients should receive misoprostol routinely for prophylaxis of NSAID-induced injury or under what circumstances misoprostol is cost effective. The patients at greatest risk for NSAID injury are patients with a previous history of ulcer disease, the elderly, patients with concomitant debilitating disease, and patients on multiple drug therapy. It is becoming common practice to treat all such patients prophylactically.

Misoprostol is also effective in the treatment of gastric ulcer, duodenal ulcer, and stress ulcer but is not approved for these uses, presumably because it has more side effects and no therapeutic advantage over H_2-blockers or proton pump inhibitors. Side effects from misoprostol have, to some extent, limited its use. At a dosage of 200 μg four times a day, more than 30% of patients have diarrhea. This appears to be lower with 100 μg four times a day, which should be the initial dose. It has no effect on GI hormones (gastrin, motilin, somatostatin, and vasoactive intestinal peptide) and no effect on gastric motility.

Misoprostol, because it causes uterine contractions, is contraindicated in pregnancy. It is rapidly (T_{max}, 12 min) and extensively absorbed. It has a terminal half-life of 20 to 40 min, with 80% being recovered in the urine. Dosage adjustment is not needed in patients with renal impairment. There is no effect on hepatic mixed-function oxidase systems, and no drug interactions are known. Misoprostol does not inhibit the therapeutic benefit of NSAIDs in rheumatoid arthritis.

SUCRALFATE

α-D-Glucopyranoside, β-D-fructofuranosyl-, octakis(hydrogen sulfate), aluminum complex; Carafate

(*R* is $SO_3[Al_2(OH)_x(H_2O)_y]$)

[54182-58-0] $C_{12}H_mAl_{16}O_nS_8$ (*m* and *n* are approximately 54 and 75, respectively, giving an average molecular mass of about 2086 daltons).

Preparation—See US Pat 3,432,489.

Description—White powder; pK_a between 0.43 and 1.19.

Solubility—Practically insoluble in water; soluble in fixed alkali or acids.

Comments—Approved for short-term (8-week) therapy of duodenal ulcers and, at reduced dosage, for maintenance therapy of duodenal ulcer. Clinical reports indicate that 1 g four times a day for 4 weeks will heal 73% to 92% of duodenal ulcers. Antacids may be prescribed as needed for pain relief. Sucralfate is absorbed minimally from the GI tract. The mechanism by which sucralfate accelerates healing of duodenal ulcer remains to be defined fully. It reduces acid secretion by approximately 50%, and this is probably its most important effect. It also forms an ulcer-adherent complex with proteinaceous exudate at the ulcer site; this complex covers the ulcer site and protects it against further attack by acid, pepsin, and bile salts. Animal studies suggest that sucralfate also enhances local prostaglandin synthesis, which would increase mucosal protection by stimulating mucus and bicarbonate secretion. Whatever the mechanism, sucralfate is effective in healing ulcers. There are no known contraindications. Nevertheless, it should not be used during pregnancy or in nursing mothers unless clearly needed. Since sucralfate is an aluminum salt of a sulfated disaccharide, it may prevent absorption of tetracycline, phenytoin, H_2-blockers, warfarin, or digoxin if the drugs are given simultaneously; giving the drugs 2 hr apart minimizes these effects. Adverse effects occur in approximately 5% of patients; constipation is most common (2.2%). Other adverse effects include diarrhea, nausea, gastric discomfort, indigestion, dry mouth, rash, pruritus, back pain, dizziness, sleepiness, and vertigo.

PROKINETIC DRUGS

Prokinetic drugs enhance GI motility and are used in the treatment of gastroesophageal reflux disease (GERD), gastroparesis, and constipation. GI motility is regulated through a complex integration of the autonomic nervous system, the enteric nervous system, and GI hormones. Each organ, ie, the esophagus, stomach, small intestine, and colon, have both integrated physiological regulation as well as unique regulation for each organ. The features that are unique to each organ are poorly understood, and many of the specific receptors have not been identified. Thus, the drugs tend to have a broad range of activity, with the beneficial and adverse effects mimicking each other. It is important to realize that in disorders of gastric emptying, oral drug absorption may be impaired or delayed, and thus IV therapy may be needed to the initial treatment.

BETHANECHOL CHLORIDE

For the full monograph, see page 1390.

Comments—A parasympathemimetic that stimulates muscarinic receptors. It increases lower esophageal sphincter pressure and as such reduces nocturnal gastroesophageal reflux. It also increases contractions in the fundus and antrum of the stomach but does not trigger migratory motor activity. Thus, it does not enhance gastric emptying and is not a true prokinetic drug.

It is indicated for the treatment of acute postoperative and postpartum urinary retention in the absence of obstruction of the urinary tract.

CISAPRIDE

Benzamide, cis-4-amino-5-chloro-N-[1-[3-(4-fluorophenoxy)propyl]-3-methoxy-4-piperidinyl]-2-methoxy-, monohydrate; Propulsid

[81098-60-4] $C_{23}H_{29}ClFN_3O_4 \cdot H_2O$ (483.97).

Preparation—See US Pat 5,665,884 (1997).

Description—White to off-white powder melting about 110°.

Solubility—Practically insoluble in water; sparingly soluble in methanol or acetone.

Comments—It stimulates acetylcholine release from enteric nerves and acts as a direct smooth muscle stimulant. It also appears to be a serotonin 4 (5-HT$_4$) agonist and 5-HT$_3$ antagonist. It has effects along the entire GI tract. It increases lower esophageal sphincter pressure and also enhances esophageal peristalsis. It thus has a beneficial effect in GERD by increasing lower esophageal sphincter pressure and by increasing acid clearance from the esophagus.

Cisapride increases gastric liquid and solid emptying with a reduction of duodenogastric reflux. Thus, it has potential benefit in patients with disorders of gastric emptying such as diabetic gastroparesis.

It also has prokinetic effects on the jejunum and colon that account for its sometimes beneficial effect in patients with constipation but also its major side effect of diarrhea.

Cisapride is indicated for the symptomatic treatment of nocturnal heartburn but is used widely for gastroparesis, and constipation.

Peak plasma levels are achieved within 2 hr of the usual oral dose of 10 mg. The use of cisapride often is limited by the development of diarrhea, which occurs in 10% to 20% of patients. Tachyphylaxis occurs within a few months of continuous use.

Cisapride is metabolized by the CYP3A4 isoenzyme system. Drugs that inhibit this enzyme, such as fluconazole, ketoconazole, traconazole, miconazole, clarithromycin, and erythromycin elevate cisapride blood levels, which can lead to serious cardiac arrhythmias including ventricular tachycardia and torsades de pointes. Deaths have been reported. Pregnancy category is C. The FDA has restricted the use of cisapride due to cardiac effects.

ERYTHROMYCIN

For the full monograph, see page 1653.

Comments—While widely used as an antibiotic, it is apparent that low-dose erythromycin also has prokinetic activity. It is a motilin agonist causing premature migratory motor-complex activity when used at doses of 1 to 2 mg/kg. Interestingly, at high doses, it does not have significant prokinetic activity. Tachyphylaxis, a problem common to all prokinetic drugs, is a significant problem with erythromycin as well.

It has no approved indication for the treatment of gastroparesis but is used widely. It appears to be especially helpful when used IV for acute gastroparesis. It must not be used in conjunction with cisapride.

METOCLOPRAMIDE HYDROCHLORIDE

Benzamide, 4-amino-5-chloro-_N_-[2-(diethylamino)ethyl]-2-methoxy-monohydrochloride, monohydrate; Reglan

[54143-57-6]$C_{14}H_{22}ClN_3O_2 \cdot HCl \cdot H_2O$

Preparation—See _Arch Pharm_ 1980; 313:297.

Description—White crystals melting about 185° with decomposition.

Solubility—Soluble 1 g in about 0.7 mL of water, 3 mL of alcohol, or 55 mL of chloroform. A 10% aqueous solution has a pH of about 5.5.

Comments—A substituted benzamide with dopaminergic activity. Its prokinetic activities are limited to the proximal gut, and as such it is used for the prophylaxis of _vomiting_ associated with _cancer chemotherapy;_ relief of symptoms associated with _acute_ and _recurrent diabetic gastroparesis;_ it also is used as adjunctive therapy in patients with gastroesophageal reflux. When treating diabetic gastroparesis, it should be used IV until some gastric emptying is restored to ensure absorption.

In addition to its ability to stimulate the gut, it also has enteric cholinergic properties, apparently sensitizing intestinal smooth muscle to the action of acetylcholine rather than acting directly on cholinergic receptors. The drug is not effective in motion sickness. The use of metoclopramide is limited by two factors—a narrow therapeutic index and tachyphylaxis that usually occurs within 6 weeks.

DIGESTANTS

Bile Acids

Bile is composed of a variety of substances, but only the bile salts (salts of the native bile acids) are therapeutically important. When given by mouth the bile salts are absorbed from the intestine and reexcreted by the liver in the bile, thus, entering the same cyclic process (enterohepatic circulation) as endogenous bile salts. They are of little value in promoting the absorption of fats and fat-soluble vitamins from the GI tract but are useful in the dissolution of gallstones and in the treatment of primary biliary cirrhosis and, perhaps, steatohepatitis or fatty liver.

Bile, a viscid, bitter, alkaline (pH 7.8) fluid, isotonic with serum and yellowish brown to golden yellow in color, is excreted by adults at the rate of 500 to 1100 mL per 24 hr. The principal organic constituents are bile acids (as salts), bile pigments, cholesterol, lecithin, and mucin. The principal inorganic constituents are water, sodium, calcium, copper, iron, magnesium, potassium, bicarbonate, phosphate, and sulfate.

The bile acids, present as the sodium salts of a mixture of acids, are divided into two groups: primary (derived from cholesterol) and secondary (derived from primary bile acids). The bile salts are conjugated through peptide linkages to glycine or taurine. The primary bile salts are taurine or glycine conjugates of cholic acid and chenic acid; the secondary bile salts are taurine and glycine conjugates of deoxycholic and lithocholic acids.

The predominant bile acids represented in bile are cholic, chenic, deoxycholic, and lithocholic. The structural relationships among these and their parent molecule, 5b-cholanic acid, are shown below. The synthetic dehydrocholic acid is included for comparison.

These bile acids combine with phospholipid to solubilize cholesterol and fatty acid in the intestine as mixed micelles. In so doing, they solubilize lipids and promote the absorption of fats, cholesterol, and the fat-soluble vitamins. The major clinical use of bile acids, however, is the dissolution of cholesterol gallstones and the treatment of primary biliary cirrhosis.

URSODIOL

Cholan-24-oic acid, (3α,5β,7β)-3,7-dihydroxy-, Ursodeoxycholic Acid; Actigall; Urso

[128-13-2]$C_{24}H_{40}O_4$ (392.58).

Preparation—For the isolation, see _J Biochem (Japan)_ 1927; 7:505.

Description—Platelets, melting about 203°; p$K_a \approx 5$.

Solubility—Practically insoluble in water; freely soluble in alcohol; slightly soluble in chloroform; very slightly soluble in ether.

Comments—A naturally occurring bile acid that is found in small amounts in man and in large amounts in bear (hence the name _urso_). It is the 7β epimer of chenodeoxycholic acid—an important primary bile acid in man. It reduces the cholesterol saturation of bile by inhibiting HMG-CoA reductase, the rate-limiting enzyme in cholesterol synthesis. It is indicated for the dissolution of radiolucent (ie, cholesterol) gallstones and the treatment of primary biliary cirrhosis. It also is used in primary sclerosing cholangitis, chronic active hepatitis and nonalcoholic steatohepatitis (fatty liver), but without proved therapeutic benefit.

Ursodiol is 90% absorbed in the small bowel. Upon absorption, it enters the portal circulation and then is extracted by the liver, where it is conjugated with glycine or taurine and finally secreted into bile and ultimately back into the intestine. This intrahepatic recirculation of ursodiol ultimately results in some replacement of endogenous bile acids such that after about 3 weeks of therapy, ursodiol makes up about 60% of the total bile acid pool. Since the total bile acid pool also is increased, cholesterol more readily can be solubilized, and cholesterol gallstones are dissolved gradually. Once ursodiol is conjugated, little change occurs in the liver or intestine. Small amounts of 7-ketolithocholic acid or lithocholic acid are formed but mostly lost in the feces. This is helpful since larger amounts of lithocholic acid are hepatotoxic. There is also some deconjugation of ursodiol in the intestine. The resultant free ursodiol is reabsorbed and subsequently reconjugated in the liver.

Clinical trials with ursodiol in the treatment of primary biliary cirrhosis have shown a retardation of disease progression and delay in the need for liver transplantation.

Urosodiol reduces the amount of fat in the liver in patients with nonalcoholic steatohepatitis and by implication should reduce the progression of cirrhosis. That, however, has neither been proved nor is it known whether life expectancy is altered.

Clinical trials also have demonstrated that gallstone dissolution occurs in about 30% of patients with gallstones less than 20 mm in diameter treated for up to 2 yr. Patients with larger stones or with non-visualizing gallbladders on oral cholecystogram rarely dissolve their stones. However, patients with floating stones less than 0.5 cm in diameter have a greater than 50% chance of dissolution.

MALT EXTRACT—page 1076.

PANCREATIC ENZYMES

Pancreatic enzymes are approved for the treatment of malabsorption secondary to pancreatic insufficiency caused by chronic pancreatitis, pancreatectomy, and cystic fibrosis. They also have been advocated for the treatment of chronic pancreatitis and pancreatic fistulae. Pancreatic enzyme preparations consist of mixtures of lipase, amylase, and protease.

Lipase hydrolyzes dietary triglycerides at the alpha position, forming two molecules of fatty acid and a molecule of β-monoglyceride. In so doing, the large triglyceride molecule is converted into three smaller molecules that can be incorporated in mixed bile acid micelles for solubilization and transported in the intestine.

Amylase is an α-1,4-glucosidase that splits straight-chain polyglucosides (the amyloses in dietary starch) into maltose and maltotriose. These subsequently are cleaved into glucose by intestinal brush-border disaccharidase enzymes and absorbed.

Protease is a mixture of proteolytic enzymes—trypsin, chymotrypsin, and elastase—that cleaves peptide bonds in the center of proteins and polypeptides. The hydrolytic products of these enzymes are amino acids and oligopeptides. The amino acids are absorbed directly, while the oligopeptides are split further by brush-border enzymes or intracellular enzymes before being transported in the portal circulation to the liver.

The treatment of malabsorption is the usual indication for pancreatic enzymes. The major manifestation of pancreatic malabsorption is steatorrhea—a voluminous, malodorous stool that is light in color and laden with fat that is not being absorbed. Clinical steatorrhea does not occur until pancreatic lipase output is less than 10% of normal. Thus, the lipase content of the pancreatic enzyme replacement preparation is the critical factor in the treatment of steatorrhea. Approximately 28,000 U of lipase should be delivered during the 4-hr postprandial period.

Only a few preparations have sufficient lipase to be effective (Table 66-7 for enzyme contents). Because lipase is inhibited irreversibly below pH 4, the enzyme preparations either have to be enteric coated or need to be given with sodium bicarbonate supplementation to avoid inactivation. The new microsphere preparations, Creon, Entolase-HP, Pancrease MT16, and Zymase, appear to have the most bioavailability. The usual dose is 3 capsules prior to each meal. When using Viokase (8 tablets),

Cotazyme (6 capsules), or Ilozyme (4 capsules), adjuvant therapy with an H_2-receptor antagonist or proton pump inhibitor may be needed to ensure bioavailability. Dosing is generally 2 to 3 tablets or capsules with each meal but should be adjusted to alleviate steatorrhea.

The treatment of abdominal pain in patients with chronic pancreatitis is complex and controversial. Many of the patients have chronic pain syndrome with narcotic addiction.

An important component of pain management in these patients is withdrawal from pain medications that in themselves may be perpetuating the pain. Once this is done, correction of mechanical problems, ie, drainage of pseudocysts and the correction of duct stenosis, is essential. If pain persists, there is evidence that large doses of pancreatic enzymes will decrease pain in these patients. The rationale for this treatment is that *resting* the pancreas will allow it to heal.

Pancreatic enzymes inhibit cholecystokinin, which stimulates pancreatic secretion when food reaches the duodenum. Putting the pancreas to rest presumably eliminates the pain that occurs when the pancreas is actively secreting. The effective components of the pancreatic enzymes for relieving pain are the serine proteases (trypsin, chymotrypsin, and elastase). Patients with idiopathic chronic pancreatitis appear to respond better than patients with chronic alcoholic pancreatitis.

Finally, pancreatic enzymes also have been advocated for the treatment of pancreatic fistulae and for the reduction and frequency of attacks of acute recurrent pancreatitis. To date, there are no controlled studies to support this type of therapy.

LACTASE

Lactaid; Lactrase

Preparation—A β-D-galactosidase isolated from *Aspergillus oryzae* (caplets) or *Kluyveromyces lactis* (drops).

Comments—The enzyme lactase hydrolyzes lactose—the sugar found in milk—into two simple sugars: glucose and galactose. It is indicated for patients with symptomatic lactose deficiency manifested by abdominal cramps, bloating, flatulence, and diarrhea following the ingestion of dairy products. Its only known side effect is allergy. Diabetics should be aware that the glucose formed through degradation by lactase will be absorbed and, in effect, increase their sugar intake. Lactase drops are used for the treatment of milk prior to ingestion; adding 10 to 15 drops to a quart of milk reduces the lactose by 90% to 99%. Caplets are to be taken with meals that contain dairy products.

SACROSIDASE

β-Fructofuranosidase; Sucraid

[85897-35-4]

Table 66-7. Pancreatic Enzymes

NAME	FORMULATION	ENZYME CONTENT[a,b]
Cotazyme	Powder in capsules	L, 8000; P, 30,000; A, 30,000
Cotazyme S	Enteric-coated spheres in capsules	L, 8000; P, 30,000; A, 30,000
Creon 10	Enteric-coated microspheres in capsules	L, 8000; P, 13,000; A, 30,000
Creon 25	Enteric-coated microspheres in capsules	L, 25,000; P, 62,500; A, 74,700
Ku-zyme	Capsules	L, 1200; P, 6 mg; A, 30 mg
Pancrease	Enteric-coated microspheres in capsules	L, 4000; P, 25,000; A, 30,000
Pancrease MT 4	Enteric-coated microtablets in capsules	L, 4000; P, 12,000; A, 12,000
Pancrease MT 10	Enteric-coated microtablets in capsules	L, 10,000; P, 30,000; A, 30,000
Pancrease MT 16	Enteric-coated microtablets in capsules	L, 16,000; P, 48,000; A, 48,000
Viokase	Tablets	
Powder (1/4 tsp.)	L, 8000; P, 30,000; A, 30,000	

[a] L, lipase; P, protease; A, amylase.
[b] Expressed in USP units. USP units (*in vitro* test method) indicate digestive capacity such that 1000 units of lipase digests 3.5 g of fat, 1000 units of protease digests 1 g of protein, and 1000 units of amylase digests 1 g of starch.

Preparation—A β-D-fructofuranoside fructohydrolase obtained from baker's yeast (*Saccharomyces cerevisiae*).

Description—An enzyme of reported molecular weight between 97 and 140 kDa.

Comments—Sacrosidase is used in the treatment of congenital sucrase-isomaltase deficiency (CSID) as it hydrolyzes sucrose (in the gut) into its elements, glucose and fructose.

LAXATIVES

Laxatives are drugs that either accelerate fecal passage or decrease fecal consistency. They work by promoting one or more of the mechanisms that cause diarrhea.

Constipation has different meanings for different people but, in general, refers to stools that are too small, too infrequent, or too difficult to expel. Patients also may describe it as a sense of incomplete evacuation. None of these definitions is easy to quantify, and the normal range is wide. Normal stool weight is largely a function of diet. Thus, stools generated by the Western diet, which tends to be low in undigestible fiber, weigh 100 to 200 g a day, while stools in Africa tend to weigh 400 to 500 g a day. Similarly, the frequency of stools varies greatly and is largely a function of the diet. It is said that normal stool frequency varies from three stools a day to three a week. There are few studies to determine what really is normal, but in the Western world, it is believed that fewer than five stools a week is abnormal. Another definition is a change to lower frequency than usual for a particular individual.

Since constipation is a symptom rather than a disease, medical evaluation should be undertaken in patients who develop constipation. The wide availability and marketing of OTC laxatives have the potential to preclude appropriate diagnosis. The most common cause is irritable bowel syndrome, but constipation may be associated with neurogenic diseases, systemic diseases, and pharmacological causes. All of these may require primary treatment independent of symptomatic treatment with laxatives. Bowel disease, *per se,* other than irritable bowel syndrome usually does not cause constipation.

Laxatives are divided into several categories as a function of their mechanism of action.

Stimulant laxatives, such as bisacodyl, phenolphthalein, and senna, work by various mechanisms including inhibition of absorption, enhancement of secretion, and effects on motility. In general, these laxatives have the most toxicity and are less physiological in their actions.

Saline laxatives, such as magnesium citrate and sodium phosphate, exert an osmotic effect that increases the water content and volume of stool.

Hyperosmotic laxatives, such as lactulose, exert an osmotic effect, leading to water secretion into the intestine.

Bulk-forming laxatives consist of polysaccharides and cellulose derivatives that are undigestible (Table 66-8). Because they absorb water, they increase the bulk of stool and, in so doing, provide a physiological stimulus to defecation. They also may inhibit bile acid absorption, with subsequent effects on water absorption and secretion by the intestine.

Lubricant laxatives, such as mineral oil, allow easier passage of a stool because of an oil coating. They may also inhibit colonic reabsorption of water.

Emollient laxatives, such as docusate sodium, are surfactants that facilitate mixture of water and lipid soluble substances to soften stool. They also stimulate water secretion in the GI tract.

Patients who use laxatives should be reminded of the following points: laxatives are not for long-term use; if they are not effective after 1 week, a physician should be consulted. Laxative products that contain more than 15 mEq (345 mg) of sodium, more than 25 mEq (975 mg) of potassium, or more than 50 mEq (600 mg) of magnesium in the maximum daily dose should not be used if kidney disease is present. Phenolphthalein preparations should be discontinued if a rash appears. Saline laxatives should not be given orally to children under 6 or rectally to infants under 2 yr of age; mineral oil should not be given to children under 6 yr of age. Dioctyl sodium sulfosuccinate should not be used with mineral oil. To be effective, enemas and suppositories must be administered properly. *Laxatives should not be used to relieve GI symptoms of unknown cause.*

Although occasional use of a laxative is relatively harmless, depletion of fluids and electrolytes can result from their chronic use. Mineral oil should be given at bedtime to minimize its interference with the absorption of fat-soluble vitamins. In addition, aspiration of mineral oil may result in chronic pneumonitis; consequently, it is contraindicated in patients with disorders of gastric or esophageal emptying. Even the soft, bulk-forming laxatives have been reported to cause enteric obstruction in an occasional patient with inflammatory or neoplastic strictures of the gut.

Stimulant Laxatives

The *stimulant laxatives* have multiple actions on the intestine. These include stimulation of motor activity and effects on water reabsorption and secretion. What they have in common is the ability to increase the amount of water in the stool and the ability to decrease colonic transit time. The more commonly employed agents are the anthraquinone laxatives, *cascara sagrada* and *senna;* the diphenylmethane derivatives, *phenolphthalein* and *bisacodyl;* and *castor oil.*

The *anthraquinone-containing laxatives,* such as cascara and senna, are used widely. The active glycosides are absorbed in the small intestine, circulated through the portal system and into the general circulation and excreted in the bile, urine, saliva, colonic mucosa, and in the milk of lactating women. These glycosides stimulate Auerbach's plexus to increase peristalsis. They usually act within 6 to 12 hr of ingestion. The *diphenylmethane derivatives,* such as phenolphthalein and bisacodyl, have similar pharmacological actions; they stimulate sensory nerves in the colonic mucosa to initiate reflex peristalsis. Phenolphthalein is usually active within 6 to 8 hr after administration; bisacodyl results in a smooth, formed stool within 6 to 10 hr after oral administration and 15 to 60 min after rectal administration. *Castor oil* is classified as a stimulant laxative because lipolysis in the

Table 66-8. Composition and Dose of Some Bulk Laxatives

PRODUCT	ACTIVE INGREDIENT	AMOUNT OF FIBER (G/UNIT DOSE)	USUAL ADULT DOSE[a]
Citrucel Orange Flavor	Methylcellulose	2 g	1 tbs
Fiberall Powder	Polycarbophil	2.2 g	1 tsp
Fiberall Fiber Wafers	Psyllium	2.2 g	1 wafer
FiberCon	Polycarbophil	0.5 g	2 tablets
Hydrocil Instant	Psyllium	3.5 g	1 packet
Metamucil Regular	Psyllium	3.4 g	1 tsp
Metamucil Sugar Free Orange	Psyllium	3.4 g	1 packet
Perdiem Fiber	Psyllium	4 g	1 tsp
Serutan	Psyllium	2.5 g	1 tsp

[a] Teaspoonful and tablespoonful quantities are rounded unless otherwise stated.

other drugs. For the most part, they are safe. They are devoid of systemic side effects but may increase flatulence. Rare cases of intestinal and esophageal obstruction have been reported. It is important, therefore, to take these agents with large volumes of liquid, at least one glass with each dose. They are contraindicated in patients with known esophageal or intestinal obstruction. The dosing of these agents is highly variable and needs to be adjusted to the individual patient.

CARBOXYMETHYLCELLULOSE SODIUM—page 1073.
METHYLCELLULOSE—page 1074.

PSYLLIUM

Metamucil; Perdiem; Serutan

Description—Various preparations from the outer portions of the clean, dried, ripe seeds of *Plantago psyllium* Linné or *indica*. Known commercially as French Psyllium Seed. The seed are small, dark, odorless, and tasteless, and the ground hulls form a mucilaginous mass with water.

Comments—These are mild laxatives, mostly used in irritable bowel syndrome. They are pharmacologically inert but absorb water, thus increasing the bulk of the stool and producing a physiological stimulus for evacuation. They also are used in diarrheal states such as inflammatory bowel disease to increase the bulk and consistency of the stool. They are contraindicated in the presence of partial or complete obstruction anywhere in the GI tract.

POLYCARBOPHIL

Acrylic Acid-Divinyl Glycol Copolymer; Fiberall; Noveon

Polycarbophil [9003-97-8]; polyacrylic acid cross-linked with divinyl glycol.

Preparation—Acrylic acid and divinyl glycol (1,5-hexadiene-3,4-diol) are copolymerized in a hot salt slurry using azobis [methylpropionitrile] as the initiator. US Pat 3,202,577.

Description—White to creamy white granules with a slight, characteristic, esterlike odor; contains a maximum of 1.5% water.

Solubility—Swells but is insoluble in water; insoluble in most organic solvents.

Comments—A pharmacologically inert substance that has the capacity to bind free fecal water. Hence, it is used in diarrheal disorders to decrease the fluidity or looseness of stools. Orally adminstered, polycarbophil exerts its most marked hydrosorptive action only on reaching the slightly acid or alkaline medium of the small intestine and colon. Polycarbophil also is used as a bulk-forming laxative. This hydrophilic polyacrylic resin is indigestible and nonabsorbable and binds more water than other laxatives of this type. Polycarbophil is reported to have no effect on digestive enzymes, and is thus metabolically inactive. The only adverse effect noted is a sense of fullness and bloating in some patients; this can be minimized by giving smaller doses at shorter intervals. This compound contains calcium, which may interact with tetracycline. It is contraindicated in bowel obstruction or fecal impaction.

Lubricant Laxatives

The *lubricant laxatives* (mineral oil and vegetable oils) lubricate the intestinal tract, soften the fecal contents, and facilitate the passage of feces. The many untoward effects induced by mineral oil, such as *lipid pneumonitis, lipoid avitaminosis A,* foreign-body reactions in the intestinal mucosa, and anal leakage all argue against their use.

COTTONSEED OIL—page 1072.

MINERAL OIL

Liquid Paraffin; Liquid Petrolatum; White Mineral Oil; Heavy Liquid Petrolatum

A mixture of aliphatic hydrocarbons obtained from petroleum. It is indigestible and thus has limited absorption.

Preparation—After removing the lighter hydrocarbons from petroleum by distillation, the residue is again subjected to distillation at a temperature between 330° and 390°, and the distillate treated first with H_2SO_4, then with NaOH, and afterward decolorized by filtering through bone black, animal charcoal, or fuller's earth. The purified product is again chilled, to remove paraffin, and redistilled at a temperature above 330°. In some instances the H_2SO_4 treatment is omitted.

Description—Colorless, transparent, oily liquid, free or nearly free from fluorescence; tasteless and odorless when cold and develops not more than a faint odor or petroleum when heated; specific gravity between 0.860 and 0.905; kinematic viscosity not less than 38.1 centistokes at 37.8°.

Solubility—Insoluble in water or alcohol; miscible with most fixed oils, but not with caster oil; soluble in volatile oils.

Comments—Used internally as a *laxative.* When taken internally, mineral oil, by virtue of its ability to soften fecal contents and retard the absorption of water, is a mild laxative. It is probably harmless in occasional laxative doses but, if taken continuously in large amounts, may impair appetite, reduce the absorption of fat-soluble vitamins, and possibly be absorbed to an extent sufficient to cause recognizable changes in the liver and mesenteric lymph nodes. It should not be used when abdominal pain, nausea, or vomiting is present. The adverse effects, especially lipid pneumonia, argue against its use as a laxative, especially in children or the elderly.

Fecal Softeners

The fecal softeners represent the most recent approach to the management of constipation and fecal impaction. Substances included in this category are *surface-acting* or *wetting* agents, which are nonabsorbable and relatively nontoxic. Their action is attributed to their surface-active property; by lowering surface tension they permit the intestinal fluids to penetrate the fecal mass more readily and, thus, produce soft, easily passed stools. However, agents such as dioctyl sodium sulfosuccinate have been shown to increase mucosal cAMP and alter ion transport in a manner similar to that of the bile acids. Thus, cAMP-mediated active anion secretion may account for the increased accumulation of luminal fluid. The relative importance of these two mechanisms remains to be determined.

DOCUSATE CALCIUM

Butanedioic acid, sulfo-, 1,4-bis(2-ethylhexyl) ester, calcium salt; Bis(2-ethylhexyl) S-Calcium Sulfosuccinate; Dioctyl Calcium Sulfosuccinate; Surfak

[128-49-4] $C_{40}H_{74}CaO_{14}S_2$ (883.22).

Preparation—*Docusate Sodium* (below) is dissolved in 2-propanol and reacted with a methanolic solution of calcium chloride. US Pat 3,035,973.

Description—White, amorphous solid with the characteristic odor of octyl alcohol; free of the odor of other solvents.

Solubility—1 g in 3300 mL water, <1 mL alcohol, <1 mL chloroform, or <1 mL ether.

Comments—A *fecal-softening* agent useful in *preventing constipation* or in patients for whom laxative therapy is undesirable or contraindicated. It does not increase GI motility and, therefore, may be used in patients in whom cathartic medication is contraindicated. Except for occasional mild, transitory, cramping pains, dioctyl calcium sulfosuccinate is free from side effects and contraindications. It is used also as an emulsifying, wetting, and dispersing agent for external preparations.

DOCUSATE POTASSIUM—see RPS-20, page 1233.

DOCUSATE SODIUM

Butanedioic acid, sulfo-, 1,4-bis(2-ethylhexyl) ester, sodium salt; Dioctyl Sodium Sulfosuccinate; Colace

Sodium 1,4-bis(2-ethylhexyl) sulfosuccinate [577-11-7] $C_{20}H_{37}NaO_7S$ (444.56).

Preparation—Several patents have been issued covering the preparation of this compound. In general, maleic anhydride is treated with 2-ethylhexanol to produce dioctyl maleate, which then is reacted with sodium bisulfite under conditions conducive to saturation of the olefinic bond with simultaneous rearrangement of the bisulfite to the sulfonate structure.

Description—White, waxlike, plastic solid with a characteristic odor suggestive of octyl alcohol; usually available in the form of pellets.

Solubility—1 g slowly in about 70 mL water; freely soluble in alcohol or glycerin.

Comments—A surface-active agent used in the management of constipation and painful anorectal conditions. It is not a laxative but is used to soften the stools in such conditions as anal fissures and postoperative anal pain such as occurs after hemorrhoidectomy. It is also useful for constipation in geriatric, pediatric, and obstetric patients. However, 1 or 2 days of treatment may be necessary before an effect is observed. Although its action is attributed to its *detergent* or *wetting* properties, it does increase mucosal cAMP in a manner similar to that of bile acids, and this may increase fluid and electrolyte secretion into the intestine. As a pharmaceutical aid, it is used as an emulsifying, wetting, and dispersing agent in formulations for external use.

Laxative Combinations

There are many laxative products available to the public (OTC) that contain more than one type of laxative. For example, a product may contain both an emollient (stool softener) and a stimulant laxative. In general, combination products are more likely to cause adverse effects because of the multiple ingredients, especially when the separate ingredients are used in full dose. In addition, laxative combinations do not offer any advantage over products that contain only one type of laxative. The composition of some of the more commonly used laxative combinations, available in either capsule or tablet form, is shown in Table 66-9.

ANTIDIARRHEALS

Diarrhea is the manifestation of many illnesses. Its etiology includes infections (viral, bacterial, fungal, parasitic), irritable bowel syndrome, inflammatory bowel disease (ulcerative colitis, Crohn's disease and others), toxins (food poisoning and pseudomembranous colitis), drugs, surreptitious laxative abuse, neuroendocrine tumors, secretory tumors (villous adenoma), malabsorption syndromes (celiac sprue, lactase deficiency, motility disorders, diverticular disease, and ileostomy). Treatment should be directed to the underlying cause. Nevertheless, it is occasionally necessary to use antidiarrheals for convenience or for conditions for which there is no primary treatment, eg, ileorectal anastomosis and ileoanal pull-through surgery. The most commonly used antidiarrheals are anticholinergics, opioid narcotics, meperidine congeners (diphenoxylate), and loperamide.

DIPHENOXYLATE HYDROCHLORIDE

4-Piperidinecarboxylic acid 1-(3-cyano-3,3-diphenylpropyl)-4-phenyl-, ethyl ester, monohydrochloride; ing of Lomotil

Ethyl 1-(3-cyano-3,3-diphenylpropyl)-4-phenylisonipecotate monohydrochloride [3810-80-8] $C_{30}H_{32}N_2O_2 \cdot HCl$ (489.06).

Preparation—Ethyl 4-phenylisonipecotate (prepared as described under *Meperidine Hydrochloride* except omitting the final step of *N*-methylation), is condensed with 2,2-diphenyl-4-bromobutyronitrile by refluxing in toluene using either an excess of the ester or another suitable dehydrobrominating agent. US Pat 2,898,340. Combined with atropine subject.

Description—White, odorless, crystalline powder; pH (saturated solution) about 3.3; melts between 220° and 226°.

Solubility—Sparingly soluble in alcohol or acetone; slightly soluble in water or isopropyl alcohol; freely soluble in chloroform; practically insoluble in ether or solvent hexane.

Comments—A synthetic congener of meperidine that inhibits excessive GI propulsion by slowing intestinal motility. It is *effective as adjunctive therapy* in the management of diarrhea associated with gastroenteritis, irritable bowel, acute infections, food poisoning, and side effects of some drugs. It also is useful in the control of intestinal transit time in patients with ileostomies or colostomies and after ileoanal pull-through surgery.

Caution should be used in patients with ulcerative colitis and pseudomembranous colitis who are at increased risk of developing toxic megacolon. Also, it may prolong infectious diarrhea.

In high dosage (40–60 mg) it can produce morphine-like euphoria and prevent withdrawal symptoms in narcotic addicts, but in the recommended dosage range for antidiarrheal therapy no evidence for addiction liability has been reported. The available dosage forms contain a subtherapeutic dose of 0.025 mg of atropine sulfate and a 2.5-mg dose of the hydrochloride. Atropine sulfate decreases GI transit after accumulative dosage and also, because of side effects, discourages usage of excessive amounts, thereby minimizing abuse.

Side effects are usually minor and include nausea, sedation, vertigo, vomiting, pruritus, skin eruption, insomnia, and abdominal cramps. Numbness of the extremities, headache, blurring of vision, swelling of gums, and general malaise also have been reported. The drug is contraindicated in patients with cirrhosis or advanced liver disease and in children under 2 yr. Laboratory studies demonstrate that it inhibits microsomal enzymes. Therefore, it should be used with caution in patients on barbiturates, tranquilizers, and alcohol, because the activity of these drugs may be potentiated by diphenoxylate. Concurrent use with monoamine oxidase inhibitors (MAOIs) may, in theory, precipitate a hypertensive crisis.

LOPERAMIDE HYDROCHLORIDE

1-Piperidinebutanamide, 4-(4-chlorophenyl)-4-hydroxy-*N*,*N*-dimethyl-α, α-diphenyl-, monohydrochloride; Imodium

4-(*p*-Chlorophenyl)-4-hydroxy-*N*,*N*-dimethyl-α,α-diphenyl-1;piperidinebutyramide monohydrochloride [34552-83-5] $C_{29}H_{33}ClN_2O_2 \cdot HCl$ (513.51).

Preparation—4-Bromo-2,2-diphenylbutyric acid is converted in a series of reactions to dimethyl(tetrahydro-3,3-diphenyl-2-furylidene) ammonium bromide, which is reacted with *p*-chlorophenyl-4-piperidinol to produce loperamide. US Pat 3,714,159; *J Med Chem* 1973; 16:782.

Description—White to faintly yellow, amorphous or microcrystalline powder; melts about 222°.

Solubility—Slightly soluble in water; soluble in alcohol.

Comments—A synthetic agent used for the control and symptomatic relief of *acute nonspecific diarrhea* and *chronic diarrhea* associated with ileoanal pull-through surgery. It also is used for *reducing the volume of discharge* from ileostomies. Caution should be used in patients with ulcerative colitis, Crohn's colitis, and pseudomembranous colitis who are at increased risk for toxic megacolon. Also, loperamide may prolong the course of infectious diarrhea. Plasma levels are highest 5 hr after oral administration. The elimination half-life is 10.8 hr, with a range of 9.1 to 14.4 hr. Unchanged drug remains below 2 ng/mL after the intake of a 2-mg capsule. Most of the drug is excreted in the feces. The safe use of this agent during pregnancy, by nursing mothers, infants and children, has not been established. Adverse effects are minimal and usually self-limiting. Abdominal pain or discomfort, constipation, drowsiness, dizziness, dry mouth, nausea and vomiting, and tiredness have been reported. Hypersensitivity reactions have been reported. Loperamide should be discontinued if abdominal distention occurs or if other untoward symptoms develop in patients with ulcerative colitis.

EMETICS

An *emetic* is a drug that induces vomiting. They may act directly by stimulation of the *chemoreceptor trigger zone* located in the area postrema of the medulla oblongata, (eg, apomorphine, morphine, hydrogenated ergot alkaloids, and digitalis glycosides), or they may act reflexly by irritant action on the GI tract (eg, copper sulfate, mustard, sodium chloride, and zinc sulfate). They also may produce stimulation of the vagus (eg, veratrum). It should be remembered that a nasogastric tube is a safer and more efficient tool for emptying the stomach. Emetics should not be used in patients who are unconscious or semicomatose or in whom coma is expected imminently. They should not be used in patients with severe heart disease or advanced pregnancy. They are contraindicated in debilitated patients and in poisoning caused by corrosive or petroleum products.

EMETINE HYDROCHLORIDE—see RPS-20, page 1549.
SODIUM CHLORIDE—page 1341.

ANTIEMETICS

Nausea and vomiting are among the most frequent symptoms of both GI and systemic disease. They may be induced by drugs and frequently occur after surgery and radiation therapy, during pregnancy, with GI tumors, and as the result of certain types of motion in sensitive persons. Useful agents are found among the following six groups:

1. *Antipsychotics* (phenothiazines and butyrophenones) act at the chemoreceptor trigger zone (CTZ) to block dopaminergic emetic receptors excited by apomorphine.
2. *Antihistaminics* provide relief from motion sickness through an action on the vestibular apparatus.
3. *Anticholinergics* in combination with *d*-amphetamine and scopolamine are most effective against motion sickness (mechanism unknown).
4. *Cannabinoids* are especially useful in the emesis from cancer chemotherapy.
5. *5-HT$_3$-receptor antagonists* such as ondansetron block both peripheral and central 5-HT$_3$ receptors and are especially effective against the emetogenic effects of chemotherapy.
6. *Other agents,* such as trimethobenzamide and metoclopramide, block dopamine receptors in the CTZ, whereas diphenidol depresses the vestibular apparatus.

Centrally acting antiemetics, such as trimethobenzamide, the phenothiazines, and similar agents, should not be used for the treatment of uncomplicated vomiting in children because the extrapyramidal symptoms that often occur with these agents may be confused with the CNS signs of an undiagnosed primary disease responsible for the vomiting, eg, Reye's syndrome or other encephalopathy.

The phenothiazine antiemetics are capable of potentiating CNS depressants (eg, anesthetics, opiates, alcohol, etc).

Adverse reactions include

Phenothiazines (aliphatic)—Drowsiness, orthostatic hypotension, ocular changes, anticholinergic effects, extrapyramidal reactions (dystonia, akathisia, parkinsonian syndrome, dysarthria), hypersensitivity reactions, amenorrhea, reversal of epinephrine pressor effect, enhancement of CNS depressant drugs, gynecomastia, lactation, hyperglycemia, hypoglycemia, and glycosuria.
Antihistaminics—Drowsiness, lightheadedness, blurred vision, dryness of the mouth, and urinary retention.
Anticholinergics—Glycosuria, drowsiness, excitement or hallucinations, dryness of the mouth, mydriasis, blurred vision, and urinary retention.
Cannabinoids—Cardiac disorders, drug dependence, hypertension, mania, or depressive states or psychoses.
5-HT$_3$-receptor antagonists—Constipation, rash, and seizures.

Since drowsiness is common to most of these agents, patients should be cautioned not to drive or operate hazardous machinery while on these drugs.

Persistent vomiting results in loss of hydrochloric acid, alkalosis and dehydration, which in turn may precipitate further vomiting. Hence, a fluid electrolyte therapy may be necessary after vomiting has been present for some time.

APREPITANT

3*H*-1,2,4-Triazol-3-one, 5-[[(2*R*,3*S*)-2-[(1*R*)-1-[3,5-bis(trifluoromethyl)phenyl]ethoxy]-3-(4-fluorophenyl)-4-morpholinyl]methyl]-1,2-dihydro-, Emend

[170729-80-3] C$_{23}$H$_{21}$F$_7$N$_4$O$_3$. (534.43).
  Preparation—US Pat 5,719,147 (1998).
  Description—White to off-white crystals.
  Solubility—Practically insoluble in water, sparingly soluble in ethanol or 2-propanol; slightly soluble in acetonitrile.

CHLORPROMAZINE—page 1511.

DIMENHYDRINATE

1*H*-Purine-2,6-dione, 8-chloro-3,7-dihydro-1,3-dimethyl-, compd. with 2-(diphenylmethoxy)-*N,N*-dimethylethanamine (1:1); Dramamine

8-Chlorotheophylline, compound with 2-(diphenylmethoxy)-*N,N*-dimethylethylamine (1:1) [523-87-5] C$_{17}$H$_{21}$NO.C$_7$H$_7$ClN$_4$O$_2$ (469.97); contains 53–55.5% of diphenylhydramine (C$_{17}$H$_{21}$NO), and 44–47% of 8-chlorotheophylline (C$_7$H$_7$ClN$_4$O$_2$).
  Preparation—By interaction of diphenhydramine, a base, with 8-chlorotheophylline, an acid, in isopropyl alcohol.
  Description—White, crystalline, odorless powder; melts between 102° and 107°.
  Solubility—Slightly soluble in water; freely soluble in alcohol or chloroform; sparingly soluble in ether.
  Comments—An *antihistaminic* compound that is a combination of diphenhydramine (Benadryl) and 8-chlorotheophylline. The latter contributes little, if anything, to its action as an antiemetic or an antihistaminic agent. It is employed chiefly as an *antinauseant* in *motion sickness.* It also has been used with success in the management of the vertigo associated with Méniére's syndrome and radiation sickness. Mild sedation commonly attends it use. See this page. Because of its sedating properties, patients should be cautioned about driving or operating machinery.

DIPHENHYDRAMINE HYDROCHLORIDE—page 1545.
FLUPHENAZINE HYDROCHLORIDE—page 1512.

DOLASETRON MESYLATE

1*H*-Indole-3-carboxylic acid, (2α, 6α, 8α, 9aβ)-octahydro-3-oxo-2,6-methano-2*H*-quinolizin-8-yl ester, monomethanesulfonate salt; Anzemat

[115956-13-3] C$_{19}$H$_{20}$N$_2$O$_3$.CH$_4$O$_3$S (420.48).
  Preparation—US Pat 4,906,755 (1990) and Eur Pat Appl 266,730 (1988).
  Description—White to off-white crystalline solid melting about 278°.
  Solubility—Freely soluble in water and propylene glycol; slightly soluble in ethanol or normal saline.

DRONABINOL

6*H*-Dibenzo[*b,d*]pyran-1-ol, (6a*R-trans*)-6a,7,8,10a-tetrahydro-6,6,9-trimethyl-3-pentyl-, Delta-9-tetrahydrocannabinol; Marinol

[1972-08-3]C$_{21}$H$_{30}$O$_2$ (314.47)

Preparation—The Δ^1-3,4-*trans* isomer (Δ^9-THC) is the major active component of marijuana (hashish). For the isolation refer to *J Am Chem Soc* 1964; 86:1646; for synthesis, *ibid* 1974; 96:5860.

Description—Viscous, oily liquid; see *J Pharm Sci* 1973; 62:1601 for stability under various conditions of storage.

Solubility—Insoluble in water; soluble in 1 part of alcohol or acetone, 3 parts of glycerol; soluble in fixed oils. Stability of parental solutions; *J Pharm Sci* 1972; 61:1106.

Comments—Commonly known as delta 9-THC, it is an orally active cannabinol and one of the active ingredients of marijuana. As such, it may be habit forming. It is especially useful for cancer chemotherapy–induced nausea and vomiting. It is thought to act centrally. Following oral administration dronabinol has systemic bioavailability of 10% to 20%. Its onset of action is 0.5 to 1 hr, with a peak effect at 2 to 4 hr. The drug undergoes extensive first-pass metabolism. Numerous metabolites have been identified, including 11-hydroxytetrahydrocannabinol, which appears in the plasma in about the same concentration as the parent substance. Within 72 hr after oral administration, approximately 50% of the administered dose is excreted in the feces and 15% in the urine, either unchanged or as a metabolite.

Patients may experience mood changes, hallucinations, mental depression, nervousness, and tachycardia followed by bradycardia. Because of its effects on mental status, patients should be warned not to drive, operate machinery, or make judgment decisions. Thus, strict patient compliance to dosage prescribed must be emphasized, and the amount prescribed limited to that required for a single cycle of chemotherapy. Tachyphylaxis occurs to most of its effects but not its appetite-stimulating effect. Withdrawal symptoms consisting of irritability, insomnia, and restlessness occur within 12 hr of abrupt withdrawal.

GRANISETRON HYDROCHLORIDE

1H-Indazole-3-carboxamide, endo-1-methyl-N-(9-methyl-9-azabicyclo[3.3.1]non-3-yl-, Kytril

[107007-99-8] $C_{18}H_{24}N_4O.HCl$ (348.88).

Preparation—European Pat Appl. 200,444.

Description—White tufts melting about 291°.

Solubility—Very soluble in water or normal saline.

Comments—An injectable, selective 5-hydroxytryptamine (5-HT$_3$) receptor; 5-HT$_3$ receptors are located peripherally in vagal nerve terminals and centrally in the CTZ. It is indicated to control nausea and vomiting associated with cancer chemotherapy. It is effective in preventing emesis and nausea when used with cisplatin, carboplatin, and cyclophosphamide. It may also be co-administered with dexamethasone. Total clearance is reduced in patients with hepatic impairment due to metastasis, but dosage adjustment is not necessary.

Principal adverse effects are headache (14%), asthenia (5%), somnolence (4%), diarrhea (4%), and constipation (3%).

HYDROXYZINE HYDROCHLORIDE—pages 1491 and 1548.
HYDROXYZINE PAMOATE—page 1492.

MECLIZINE HYDROCHLORIDE

Piperazine, 1-[(4-chlorophenyl)phenylmethyl]-4-[(3-methylphenyl)methyl]-, dihydrochloride, monohydrate; Antivert; Bonine

[31884-77-2] $C_{25}H_{27}ClN_2.2HCl.H_2O$ (481.89); *anhydrous* [1104-22-9] (463.88).

Preparation—Meclizine is formed by condensing N-(m-methylbenzyl) piperazine with p-chlorobenzhydryl chloride in the presence of triethylamine. The purified base is dissolved in a suitable solvent and converted to the dihydrochloride by a stream of hydrogen chloride.

Description—White or slightly yellowish, crystalline powder; slight odor; tasteless; melts between 217° and 224°, with decomposition.

Solubility—Practically insoluble in water and ether; freely soluble in chloroform; slightly soluble in alcohol.

Comments—A long-acting antihistaminic effective in the prevention or treatment of *nausea, vomiting,* and *dizziness* associated with motion sickness. It may be effective in *vertigo* associated with diseases affecting the vestibular system. The antiemetic activity starts within 60 min and lasts for 8 to 24 hr. Like other antihistamines, it may cause drowsiness and other side effects, such as blurred vision, dryness of the mouth, and fatigue. Patients should be cautioned about driving and operating machinery. The action of a single dose can persist for 9 to 24 hr. Use of the drug in pregnancy or in women who may become pregnant is contraindicated. Because it has some anticholinergic activity, it should not be used in patients with asthma, glaucoma, or prostatic enlargement.

PERPHENAZINE—page 1514.

ONDANSETRON HYDROCHLORIDE

4H-Carbazol-4-one, (±)-1,2,3,9-tetrahydro-9-methyl-3- [(2-methyl-1H-imidazol-1-yl)methyl]-, monohydrochloride, dihydrate; Zofran

[103639-04-9] $C_{18}H_{19}N_3O.HCl.2H_2O$ (365.86).

Preparation—US Pat 4,695,578.

Description—White crystals melting about 180°; pK$_a$ 7.4.

Solubility—1 g dissolves in 3 mL of water.

Comments—A selective 5-HT$_3$-receptor antagonist. Such receptors are present in vagal nerve terminals and in the CTZ of the area postrema of the brain. It is not clear whether it acts peripherally, centrally, or both. Ondansetron is indicated for the prevention of nausea and vomiting associated with cancer chemotherapy. It appears that cytotoxic chemotherapy such as cisplatin is associated with release of serotonin from enterochromaffin cells in the small intestine. It is speculated that serotonin triggers vomiting through 5-HT$_3$ vagal receptors that activate the vomiting reflex.

Ondansetron is metabolized extensively; only 5% of unchanged compound is recovered in the urine. It initially undergoes hydroxylation of the indole ring, followed by glucuronidation or sulfation. The mean elimination half-life is approximately 4 to 5 hr but increases with age. Plasma protein binding is 70% to 75%.

Ondansetron is effective in reducing emesis in both cisplatin- and cyclophosphamide-based chemotherapy. Using a visual analog scale (0 to 100), global satisfaction is increased from 10.5 to 96 after single-day cisplatin therapy and from 52 to 100 after single-dose cyclophosphamide therapy.

The most common side effects of ondansetron are diarrhea (22%) and headache (16%). Other adverse reactions after multiple-day therapy include constipation, elevated liver enzymes, rash, bronchospasm, tachycardia, angina, hypokalemia, and seizures. Akathisia and dystonia, seen with metoclopramide, do not occur with ondansetron.

PALONOSETRON HYDROCHLORIDE

1H-benz[de]isoquinolin-1-one, (3aS)-2,3,3a,4,5,6-hexahydro-2-[(3S)-3-quinuclidinyl- , monohydrochloride; Aloxi

[135729-62-3] $C_{19}H_{24}N_2O.HCl$ (332.87).

Preparation—*J Med Chem,* 1993;36: 2645 and *Medicinal Research Rev,* 1997;17: 163

Description—White to off-white crystalline powder from 2-propanol/ether, melting above 270°; pK$_a$ 10.4.

Solubility—Freely soluble in water; soluble in propylene glycol; slightly soluble in ethanol or 2-propanol.

PROCHLORPERAZINE

10H-Phenothiazine, 2-chloro-10-[3-(4-methyl-1-piperazinyl)propyl]-, Chlorazine; Compro

[58-38-8]$C_{20}H_{24}ClN_3S$ (373.94).

Preparation—A toluene solution of 1-(3-chloropropyl)-4-methylpiperazine and 2-chlorophenothiazine is refluxed with sodamide for several hours. After filtering and distilling off the toluene, the prochlorperazine is obtained by short-path distillation under high vacuum.

Description—Clear, pale yellow, viscous liquid; sensitive to light.

Solubility—Very slightly soluble in water; freely soluble in alcohol, chloroform or ether.

Comments—A piperazine-type phenothiazine with actions, uses and limitations similar to those of *Prochlorperazine Maleate*. However, prochlorperazine, as the base, is administered rectally.

PROCHLORPERAZINE EDISYLATE

10H-Phenothiazine, 2-chloro-10-[3-(4-methyl-1-piperazinyl)propyl]-, 1,2-ethanedisulfonate (1:1); Prochlorperazine Ethanedisulfonate; Compro

[1257-78-9] $C_{20}H_{24}ClN_3S.C_2H_6O_6S_2$ (564.13).

For the structure of the base, see *Prochlorperazine*.

Preparation—*Prochlorperazine* is dissolved in a suitable solvent and treated with an equimolar portion of 1,2-ethanedisulfonic acid. The salt precipitates.

Description—White to very light yellow, odorless, crystalline powder; solutions are acid to litmus.

Solubility—1 g in about 2 mL water or about 1500 mL alcohol; insoluble in ether or chloroform.

Comments—Same actions and uses as Prochlorperazine Maleate except that it may be administered IM. Parenteral therapy usually is reserved for the treatment of severe nausea and vomiting, for the immediate control of acutely disturbed psychotics, or for patients who cannot or will not take oral medication. It should not be used in children with uncomplicated vomiting of unknown etiology. See *Prochlorperazine Maleate*.

PROCHLORPERAZINE MALEATE

10H-Phenothiazine, 2-chloro-10-[3-(4-methyl-1-piperazinyl)propyl]-, (Z)-2-butenedioate (1:2); Compro

[84-02-6] $C_{20}H_{24}ClN_3S.2C_4H_4O_4$ (606.09).

For the structure of the base, see *Prochlorperazine*.

Preparation—By the method described for *Prochlorperazine Edisylate* except that maleic acid is employed instead of ethanedisulfonic acid, and it is employed in double equimolar quantity in relation to the prochlorperazine base.

Description—White or pale yellow, practically odorless, crystalline powder; saturated solution is acid to litmus.

Solubility—Practically insoluble in water or alcohol; slightly soluble in warm chloroform.

Comments—An *antiemetic, antipsychotic,* and *tranquilizing agent*. It is an effective *antiemetic* in the control of mild or severe nausea and vomiting due to a variety of causes, such as early pregnancy, anesthesia, surgery, and radiation therapy. Safety in pregnancy has not been established. There are reports of prolonged jaundice, extrapyramidial signs, hyperreflexia or hyporeflexia in newborns whose mothers have received phenothiazines. Nevertheless, Compazine is used widely in pregnancy and has a long track record of safety. It, however, is not approved for this usage. It should not be used in children with uncomplicated vomiting of unknown etiology. The drug is also an *effective antipsychotic*. Beneficial results ascribed to its action include reduction in psychomotor agitation and excitement, diminished aggressiveness and destructiveness, mitigation of hallucinations and delusions, and a general calming effect. As a *tranquilizing agent*, it is possibly effective in mild mental disorders in which anxiety, tension, and agitation predominate.

Adverse reactions include *drowsiness, dizziness, amenorrhea, skin reactions, hypotension, cholestatic jaundice, neuromuscular (extrapyra-midal) reactions, motor restlessness, dystonias, pseudoparkinsonism, persistent tardive dyskinesia,* and *contact dermatitis*. Children with acute infections (chickenpox, CNS infections, measles, gastroenteritis) or dehydration are more susceptible to neuromuscular reactions, particularly dystonias; such patients should be kept under close supervision. This agent may mask signs of overdosage of toxic drugs or obscure diagnosis of conditions such as intestinal obstruction or brain tumor. Adverse drug reactions can be minimized by periodically evaluating the dosage employed by patients on long-term therapy.

PROMETHAZINE HYDROCHLORIDE—page 1545.
THIETHYLPERAZINE MALATE—see RPS-20, page 1237.
THIETHYLPERAZINE MALEATE—see RPS-20, page 1237.

TRIMETHOBENZAMIDE HYDROCHLORIDE

Benzamide, N-[[4-[2-(dimethylamino)ethoxy]phenyl]methyl]-3,4,5-trimethoxy-, monohydrochloride; Tigan

[554-92-7] $C_{21}H_{28}N_2O_3.HCl$ (424.92).

Preparation—4-[2-(Dimethylamino)ethoxy]benzylamine is condensed with 3,4,5-trimethoxybenzoyl chloride by refluxing in an inert solvent. The resulting trimethoxybenzamide may be converted to the hydrochloride by dissolving it in a suitable solvent and treating with HCl. The starting amine may be prepared in various ways, eg, by condensing sodium *p*-aminomethylphenoxide with 2-chloro-N,N-dimethylethylamine.

Description—White crystalline powder; slight phenolic odor; melts between 186° and 190°.

Solubility—1 g in 2 mL water, 59 mL alcohol, 67 mL chloroform, or 720 mL ether.

Comments—A dimethylaminoethanol derivative indicated for the control of *nausea* and *vomiting*. Its safety in pregnancy has not been established, but trimethobenzamide frequently is used in this situation. Its antiemetic potency is about 1/10 that of chlorpromazine when given subcutaneously and 1/4 that of the latter when given orally. Minor side effects that have been reported include drowsiness, vertigo, diarrhea, and local irritation. In patients with acute febrile illness, encephalitides, gastroenteritis, dehydration, and electrolyte imbalance (especially children and the elderly and debilitated), CNS reactions, such as opisthotonos, convulsions, coma, and extrapyramidal symptoms, have been reported, but it is not certain that these effects were in all cases due to use of the drug. Therefore, caution should be exercised when trimethobenzamide hydrochloride is used in these conditions. Drowsiness can occur, and patients should be cautioned about driving and operating machinery. The use of the injectable form of the drug in children, the suppositories in premature or newborn infants, and the use of the drug in patients hypersensitive to it are contraindicated. Also, suppositories should not be used in patients known to be sensitive to benzocaine or similar types of local anesthetics. Parkinson-like symptoms have been reported. Blood dyscrasias, blurred vision, coma, seizure, depression, diarrhea, drowsiness, muscle cramps, and jaundice also have been reported. A blanket warning on the label, relating to Reye's syndrome does not seem to be justified, but still should be considered.

ADSORBENTS

Adsorbents are chemically inert powders that have the ability to adsorb gases, toxins, and bacteria. The fine state of subdivision of these inert powders confers high adsorptive capacity upon them. However, in the complex milieu of the GI secretions, physical (van der Waals) adsorbents are more likely to be selective for surface-active substances such as bile salts than for bacterial toxins and other noxious substances. Consequently, only certain materials that possess chemical adsorptive properties lend themselves effectively to detoxification and to the adsorption of gases resulting from abnormal intestinal fermentation. Such substances are kaolin and activated charcoal. It is doubtful that either is an effective adsorbent in the lower GI tract, since passage through the upper tract saturates and deactivates these agents.

Many of the nonsystemic antacids may serve as internal protectives and adsorbents, especially after regeneration in the alkaline small intestine. Magnesium trisilicate is claimed to exert a protective action in the stomach by virtue of released silicic acid, which acts more as a demulcent than as a solid protective. *Antacids* commonly are combined with kaolin or other adsorbents.

BISMUTH SUBNITRATE—page 1083.

ACTIVATED CHARCOAL

Actidase; Charcoal Plus DS; Medicinal Charcoal

The residue from the destructive distillation of various organic materials, treated to increase its adsorptive power.

Preparation—Formerly, a product named *Carbo Ligni* or *Wood Charcoal* was produced by burning wood out of contact with air; the residue obtained consisted of nearly pure carbon. Charcoal made by this process was variable in its adsorptive powers, frequently being entirely devoid of such properties. It was found that the adsorptive powers of charcoal could be increased tremendously by treating it with various substances such as steam, air, carbon dioxide, oxygen, zinc chloride, sulfuric acid, phosphoric acid, or a combination of some of these substances, at temperatures ranging from 500 to 900°. This treatment is referred to as activation, the activating agent presumably removing substances previously adsorbed on the charcoal and, in some instances at least, breaking down the granules of carbon into smaller ones having a greater total surface area. It has been estimated that 1 mL of charcoal, finely divided, possesses a total surface of approximately 1000 m^2.

In addition to wood, many other substances are used as sources of charcoal, including sucrose, lactose, rice starch, coconut pericarp, bone, blood, various industrial wastes, etc. As many different activated charcoals are available for various purposes, one should be certain to use only the medicinal variety for medicinal purposes.

Description—Fine, black, odorless, and tasteless powder, free from gritty matter.

Solubility—Insoluble in water or the other known solvents.

Comments—Used for the acute treatment of poisoning—primarily as an emergency *antidote* in many forms of poisoning. It is the emergency treatment of choice for virtually all drugs and chemicals. Charcoal capsules also are used for the relief of flatulence and the discomfort of abdominal gas, but there is little evidence that it is effective for this purpose.

Industrially, it is used in large quantities in chemical and pharmaceutical manufacturing as a decolorizer.

KAOLIN

Light Kaolin; White Bole; China Clay; Kaolin-Pectin Suspension

A native hydrated aluminum silicate; powdered and freed from gritty particles by elutriation.

Preparation—Kaolin is distributed widely in nature. Most kaolin deposits, however, are contaminated with ferric oxide (hence the red color of ordinary clay) and some other impurities, such as calcium carbonate, magnesium carbonate, etc. To render kaolin suitable for pharmaceutical use, it has to be purified by treatment with hydrochloric acid or sulfuric acid, or both, then washed with water.

Kaolin of a high degree of purity, directly suitable for pharmaceutical use without acid purification, has been mined in the state of Georgia. England has large deposits of a fine grade of kaolin. The kaolin from these deposits is freed of coarse particles by elutriation or screening. Kaolin is essentially a colloid, and the *colloid kaolin* on the market differs only from ordinary kaolin in that it contains a larger percentage of fine particles and is prepared by special screening.

Description—Soft, white or yellowish white powder, or lumps; characteristic earthy or clay-like taste and, when moistened with water, becomes darker and develops a pronounced clay-like odor.

Solubility—Insoluble in water, cold diluted acids, or solutions of the alkali hydroxides.

Comments—Either alone or as *Kaolin Mixture with Pectin* (see below) it is used medicinally as an *adsorbent*. It is perhaps of value in the treatment of *diarrhea* caused by agents capable of being adsorbed; eg, the diarrhea of food poisoning or dysentery. Kaolin also has been used in the treatment of chronic ulcerative colitis, but it is doubtful whether any adsorptive capacity is retained by the time the preparation reaches the colon. Externally, kaolin has some use as a poultice, dusting powder, and an ingredient of toilet powders.

MAGNESIUM TRISILICATE—page 1297.

PECTIN

A purified carbohydrate product obtained from the dilute acid extract of the inner portion of the rind of citrus fruits or from apple pomace. It consists chiefly of partially methoxylated polygalacturonic acids.

Pectin yields not less than 6.7% of methoxy groups and not less than 74.0% of $C_6H_{10}O_7$ (galacturonic acid), calculated on the dried basis.

Pectin may be standardized to the convenient "150 jelly grade" by addition of dextrose or other sugars, and it may contain sodium citrate or other buffer salts. Such pectin is not suitable for medicinal use.

Description—Coarse or fine powder, yellowish white in color, almost odorless, and with a mucilaginous taste.

Solubility—Almost completely soluble in 20 parts of water at 25°, forming a viscous, opalescent, colloidal solution that flows readily and is acid to litmus; insoluble in alcohol or diluted alcohol and in other organic solvents; dissolves in water more readily if first moistened with alcohol, glycerin, or simple syrup or if first mixed with 3 or more parts of sucrose.

Incompatibilities—Precipitated from solution by an excess of *alcohol. Metals,* particularly the heavy metals, form insoluble derivatives. In the presence of *alkalies,* pectin undergoes progressive hydrolysis resulting in a demethylation followed by a splitting of the glycosidic linkages of the galacturonic acid units. *In cold acid solution* it is more stable; prolonged heating of such a solution causes hydrolysis. Liquefaction of pectin pastes may be due to a hydrolysis that accompanies growth of certain types of *mold.*

Comments—A protective used for the treatment of diarrhea in infants and children. The unchanged molecules of the polygalacturonic acids may have an adsorbent action in the intestine.

DRUGS USED FOR THE TREATMENT OF INFLAMMATORY BOWEL DISEASE

The major inflammatory diseases of the bowel are ulcerative colitis, which is confined to the colon, and Crohn's disease, which most often involves the terminal ileum and colon but can involve the entire GI tract. The etiologies are not known, but the injury in both diseases appears to be the consequence of an immune-mediated inflammatory reaction. Thus, therapy consists of anti-inflammatory agents (salicylates) and immunosuppressents (corticosteroids, azathioprine, methotrexate, cyclosporine, and monoclonal antibodies). The goals of therapy are to maintain nutrition, maintain a good quality of life, and prevent the development of cancer. There are two components to therapy—treatment of acute flareups and maintenance of remission.

CORTICOSTEROIDS—Corticosteroid therapy is used for acute flareups of moderate-to-severe Crohn's disease or ulcerative colitis. Dosing is generally started high (ie, prednisone 40 mg or equivalent per day) and tapered as the disease goes into clinical remission. At the same time, maintenance therapy is started with salicylates or immunosuppressents. Corticosteroids are ineffective in maintenance therapy and because of their side effects are contraindicated as maintenance therapy.

SALICYLATES—Sulfasalazine, the first of the salicylates, was developed in the 1930s for the treatment of rheumatoid arthritis. It subsequently was noted that patients with associated ulcerative colitis benefitted, and in the 1960s, placebo-controlled clinical trials confirmed that benefit. Later, it was noted that most of the severe adverse reactions to sulfasalazine occurred in slow acetylators of sulfapyridine and that 5- aminosalicylic acid (5-ASA) was the active moiety. Subsequently prodrugs and slow-release drugs consisting of 5-ASA and 4-ASA were developed that could deliver salicylate to the distal intestine. Olsalazine consists of two molecules of 5-ASA joined by an azo bond that is split by azo reductase liberated by colonic bacteria. Mesalamine is 5-amino-2-hydroxybenzoic acid that is enteric-coated to dissolve at approximately pH 6 to 7 in the small intestine and colon.

Despite considerable research, the mechanism of action of salicylates is only partially understood. Speculated actions include attenuation of various cytokines including interferon-γ and tumor necrosis factor, inhibition of chloride secretion, inhibition of HLA-DR expression, inhibition of adhesion molecules, inhibition of leukotriene B$_4$ synthesis, and scavenging of reactive oxygen species. Whatever the mechanism, salicylates are used widely for the initial treatment of mild disease and as the mainstay of maintenance therapy. Pentasa, because of its release throughout the GI tract, has theoretical advantages for the treatment of Crohn's disease involving the small intestine.

ALOSETRON HYDROCHLORIDE

1*H*-Pyrido[4,3-*b*]indol-1-one, 2,3,4,5-tetrahydro-5-methyl-2-[(5-methyl-1*H*-imidazol-4-yl)methy l]-, monohydrochloride; Lotronex

[122852-69-1] $C_{17}H_{18}N_4O \cdot HCl$ (330.82).

Preparation—EP306323 (1989) and US 5,360,800(1994).
Description—White to beige solid melting about 290°.
Solubility—(mg/mL of solvent); water (61); 0.1*N* HCl (43); pH 6 phosphate buffer (0.3); pH 8 phosphate buffer (0.1).

AMINOSALICYLIC ACID

Benzoic acid, 4-amino-2-hydroxy-, PAS; Paser

4-Aminosalicylic acid [65-49-6] $C_7H_7NO_3$ (153.14).

Caution—Under no circumstances use a solution if its color is darker than that of a freshly prepared solution.

Preparation—From *m*-aminophenol by a modification of the Kolbe-Schmitt reaction, which involves heating the phenol under pressure with a source of carbon dioxide such as ammonium carbonate or potassium bicarbonate.

Description—White, or nearly white, bulky powder: darkens on exposure to light and air; odorless, or has a slight acetous odor; melts between 135° and 140° with decomposition; pH (saturated aqueous solution) between 3 and 3.7.

Solubility—1 g in about 600 mL water and about 21 mL alcohol; slightly soluble in ether.

Comments—See *Aminosalicylate Sodium* for *antitubercular* actions, uses, adverse effects, and pharmacokinetics. It is also used to lower blood lipids; it can lower the low-density lipoproteins (and cholesterol) by 15% to 20% and the very-low-density lipoproteins (and tri glycerides) by 25%. It is used mainly in the treatment of *familial* hypercholesterolemia. The drug impairs absorption of cholesterol. The incidence of GI disturbances and of crystalluria is greater than with the sodium salt. A preparation of aminosalicylic acid stated to have much of its irritant impurities removed by recrystallization with ascorbic acid (PAS-C, *Hellwig*) is reported to induce a lesser incidence of GI side effects. Aminosalicylic acid can cause systemic acidosis in children. The urine should be alkalinized.

BALSALAZIDE DISODIUM

Benzoic acid, (*E*)-5-[[4-[[(2-carboxyethyl)amino]carbonyl]phenyl]a zo]-2-hydroxy-, disodium salt, dihydrate; Colazal

[150399-2-6] $C_{17}H_{13}N_3Na_2O_6 \cdot 2H_2O$ (437.32).

Preparation—US 4,412,992 (1983) and *Chem Abstr* 1978; 88: 69623x.

Description—(Acid) crystals from ethanol, melting about 255°; (salt, dihydrate) stable, odorless, non-hygroscopic, orange to yellow crystalline powder; melts above 350°.

Solubility—Freely soluble in water or normal saline; sparingly soluble in methanol or ethanol; practically insoluble in all other solvents.

MESALAMINE

Benzoic acid, 5-amino-2-hydroxy-, Asacol ; Canasa; Pentasa; Rowasa

[89-57-6] $C_7H_7NO_3$ (153.13).

Preparation—By reduction of *m*-nitrosalicylic acid with zinc dust or iron and HCl or by electrolytic reduction.

Description—Creamy white to off-white powder melting at about 280° (decomposition). Darkens on exposure to light.

Solubility—Soluble in dilute mineral acids and fixed bases; slightly soluble in water; more soluble in hot water.

Comments—*Asacol* and *Pentasa* are indicated for the treatment of mildly to moderately active ulcerative colitis and for the maintenance of remission of ulcerative colitis. The oral preparations are enteric-coated for slow release. Approximately 20% is absorbed, as is the case with suppositories and rectal suspensions. *Rowasa* suspension enema is indicated for treatment of mild to moderately active distal ulcerative colitis and proctitis. Suppositories are indicated for active ulcerative proctitis. Remission rates in mild-to-moderate ulcerative colitis vary from 30% to 65%. Numerous trials using mesalamine as maintenance therapy in ulcerative colitis have shown a 1-yr reduction in relapse from approximately 70% to 20%.

The mesalamines are less effective in Crohn's disease, but *Pentasa* has been shown to be effective at high dose (4 g/day) in ileal and ileal-colonic Crohn's disease.

The choice of salicylate depends on the anatomical extent of disease. *Pentasa*, which is released throughout the GI tract, is theoretically preferable for Crohn's disease involving the small bowel; however, none of the drugs has been shown to be effective in patients with proximal disease.

The most common side effects are diarrhea (2–3%), headache (2%), nausea (1–2%), abdominal pain (1–2%), and rash, but it is unusual to have to discontinue therapy because of adverse reactions.

OLSALAZINE SODIUM

Benzoic acid, 3,3′-azobis[6-hydroxy-, disodium salt; Dipentum

[6054-98-4] $C_{14}H_8N_2Na_2O_6$ (346.21).

Preparation—5-Nitrosalicylic acid is esterified with methanesulfonyl chloride, and the resultant sulfonated nitro compound is reduced with hydrogen and palladium to the amine, which is then diazotized and coupled with methyl salicylate under alkaline conditions. After acidification, this yields the dimethyl ester of the title compound with one hydroxyl group sulfonated. Boiling with sodium hydroxide and adjusting the pH to 6 affords the product.

Description—Yellow crystals melting about 240°.

Solubility—Soluble in water and DMSO; practically insoluble in ethanol, chloroform or ether.

Comments—Indicated for the maintenance of remission of ulcerative colitis in patients intolerant to sulfasalazine. Less than 1% of olsalazine is absorbed. The remaining 99% reaches the colon, where it is converted to mesalamine. It thus has the highest bioavailability of the salicylates, and one comparative study has shown it to be more effective than mesalamine. Its major side effect is diarrhea, which occurs in 3 to 5% of patients.

SULFASALAZINE

For the full monograph, see page 1633.

Comments—Poorly absorbed from the small intestine, so that the major portion of drug passes into the colon, where bacterial enzymes release both 5-aminosalicylic acid and sulfapyridine from the drug. It has a suppressive effect on *ulcerative colitis,* which is not defined precisely. The local antibacterial effect of sulfapyridine in decreasing anaerobic bacteria may not be significant because of systemic absorption. The 5-aminosalicylate inhibits arachidonic acid cascade, both cyclooxygenase and lipoxygenase pathways. Most important may be the inhibition of leukotriene B$_4$ production by PMNs.

Since some sulfapyridine is absorbed from the colon, this drug has the toxic potential of *Sulfapyridine*. Adverse effects mostly occur when plasma levels exceed 50 µg/mL of sulfapyridine. Heinz-body and acute hemolytic anemias occur, so that the hematological status of the patient must be monitored regularly. Folic acid absorption also is impaired by the drug. Toxic epidermal necrolysis has been reported. If the initial dose does not exceed 2 g/day, the toxic potential is said to be minimized without seriously compromising therapeutic action. It imparts a yellow color to alkaline urine. Iron compounds decrease its absorption, the therapeutic significance of which is unknown. There have been a few instances in which sulfasalazine exacerbated ulcerative colitis. Desensitization has been used when reinstitution is required in patients with hypersensitivity.

Relapses occur in about 33% of cases, so that continuous prophylactic use often is advocated. However, after a year of continuous successful suppression, the relapse rate is about the same as when no prophylaxis is used.

TEGASEROD MALEATE

Hydrazinecarboximidamide, 2-[(5-methoxy-1H-indol-3-yl)-methylene]-N-pentyl-, (2Z)-2-butenedioate salt (1:1); Zelnorm

[189188-57-6] $C_{16}H_{23}N_5O.C_4H_4O_4$ (417.46).

Preparation—US 5,510,353 (1996).

Description—Off-white to white crystalline powder. Base melts about 155°.

Solubility—Slightly soluble in ethanol; very slightly soluble in water.

IMMUNOSUPPRESSANTS—Azathioprine (page 1563) and its metabolite, 6-mercaptopurine (page 1579), have been demonstrated to be effective in the management of Crohn's disease. Patients usually are started on a low dose of 50 mg a day, gradually increased to 1.5 to 2.5 mg/kg a day or until the patient is slightly lymphopenic. The therapeutic effects are not seen until after 3 to 6 months. There has been some debate about the role that immunosuppressive therapy should play in Crohn's disease, but the trend has been to make it the mainstay of long-term treatment. There is some evidence that immunosuppressive therapy may be helpful in healing the fistulas of Crohn's disease.

The efficacy of azathioprine in the management of ulcerative colitis also has been demonstrated.

The limiting factor in the use of immunosuppressives is their toxicity, in that they commonly cause severe leukopenia. These drugs must be monitored very carefully and should be used only in compliant patients. Other toxicities include pancreatitis, allergic reactions, and infectious complications in 7% of patients. Neoplasms have been reported, but probably only histiocytic lymphoma of the brain is associated with the drug.

CYCLOSPORINE

For the full monograph, see page 1590.

Comments—There is increasing experience with both IV and oral cyclosporine in patients with severe Crohn's disease or ulcerative colitis. It initially is given IV at a dose of 4 mg/kg/day and then maintained at 5 to 8 mg/kg/day for 2 to 3 months, during which time immunosuppressive therapy with azathioprine or 6-mercaptopurine is started. Long-term use is precluded by nephrotoxicity.

INFLIXIMAB

Remicade

Description—A chimeric IgG1K monoclonal antibody with an approx mol wt of 149,000 Daltons. It is composed of human constant and murine variable regions.

Comments—It binds to human tumor necrosis factor alpha (TNFα), an inducer of proinflammatory cytokines such as IL-1 and IL-6. TNFα also enhances leukocyte migration, activates neutrophils, and induces acute phase reactants. Its activity is increased in Crohn's disease and correlates with disease activity. Treatment with this agent reduces infiltration of inflammatory cells and TNFα production in inflamed areas of intestine. It has been shown to reduce symptoms, reduce disease activity, and improve quality of life after a single IV dose in patients with Crohn's disease who have failed other therapy.

Infliximab is indicated for the treatment of moderate to severe Crohn's disease resistant to conventional therapy and in patients with enterocutaneous Crohn's fistulas.

It is given by IV infusion at 5 mg/kg. It has a terminal half-life of 9.5 days. The volume of distribution is increased by concomitant corticosteroid therapy. Up to two courses of therapy may be given at 2- and 4-month intervals.

It has been associated with hypersensitivity reactions including urticaria, dyspnea, and hypotension. Medications for treatment of hypersensitivity reactions should be on hand when infusing infliximab. Autoimmune reactions including a lupus-like syndrome with positive anti-dsDNA antibodies also may occur. Lymphomas have also been reported. Since Crohn's patients and patients on long-term immunosuppressive therapy are predisposed to develop lymphoma, the significance of the reported cases is uncertain. Adverse reactions occur in approximately 85% of patients and include headache, nausea, upper respiratory infections, abdominal pain, fever, rash, and vomiting—each occurring in more than 5% of patients.

METHOTREXATE

For the full monograph, see page 1580.

Comments—While not approved for the management of Crohn's disease or ulcerative colitis, it has been used and appears to be effective in inducing and maintaining remission in approximately 40% of patients. Like immunosuppressive therapy, it takes 3 to 6 months to obtain the full benefit. The major limiting factor in its use is its toxicity.

DRUGS USED FOR THE TREATMENT OF CHRONIC VIRAL HEPATITIS

Immunostimulation is used to treat chronic hepatitis B and C. Approximately 10% to 15% of patients who become infected with the hepatitis B virus develop chronic disease, manifested by chronic hepatitis, cirrhosis, and hepatocellular carcinoma. The reasons that patients develop chronic disease are uncertain. In some parts of the world, southeast Asia for example, almost 90% of infants born to hepatitis B–positive women will become chronically infected. When the disease is acquired at an older age, chronic disease is less likely to occur. Serum interferon levels are decreased in many patients with chronic hepatitis B. This may be secondary to the virus transfecting chromosome-9 at the site that codes for interferon. Interferon is antiviral because of two properties—it stimulates the synthesis of 2,5-A synthetase, which inhibits viral replication, and it induces the HLA major histocompatibility antigens on the hepatocyte surface so that they can become the target of cytotoxic T cells. The demonstration of interferon deficiency in chronic hepatitis B is the rationale for its use in that disease. It induces remission in about half the patients with a relapse rate of 2% to 3% a year. It is not known if it prevents hepatocellular carcinoma in such patients.

Approximately 85% of patients with hepatitis C become chronically infected. Approximately half of these patients will develop chronic hepatitis and cirrhosis. Once cirrhosis develops, hepatocellular carcinoma occurs at a rate of 2% to 3% a year. The mechanism of persistence probably relates to the development of mutants known as quasispecies that escape immune detection. Interferon trials for non-A, non-B hepatitis trials were started prior to the discovery of the hepatitis C virus. It was learned subsequently that most of the patients indeed had hepatitis C and that the drug induced remission in approximately 20% of these patients, with relapse occurring in about half of these patients by 1 yr. It subsequently has been learned that the standard pulse dosing of interferon at 3 MUs SQ tid induces mutations in the hepatitis C virus that may predispose to drug resistance. Thus, it is more common to treat patients with 3 MUs a day for 6 months to 1 yr.

INTERFERON ALFA-2B

Intron A

See also page 1577.

Comments—The alpha interferons are a family of proteins of MW 15,000 to 27,600 that are secreted by lymphocytes in response to viral infections. They bind to cellular proteins and exert a number of effects including induction of certain enzymes such as 2,5 A synthetase, which inhibits viral replication; inhibition of cell proliferation; and immune-modulating activity including expression of HLA major histocompatibility antigens that become the targets of cytotoxic T lymphocytes. Recent data indicate that interferons also may be anti- inflammatory, antifibrinogenic, and anticarcinogenic.

Interferon alfa at a dose of 5 MU a day is indicated for the treatment of chronic hepatitis B, which is continued for 6 months. There is frequently a flareup of the liver disease at 12 to 14 weeks, when the hepatitis e antigen converts to e antibody. This generally signals the end of viral replication and a positive response to treatment. Patients with decompensated liver disease manifested by ascites, encephalopathy, or coagulopathy should not be treated except under special, controlled circumstances, because of the high risk of fatal side effects, especially bacterial peritonitis with sepsis.

Side effects are common with interferon alfa-2b. Those seen in more than 10% of patients include fever (45%), headaches (45%), myalgias (40%), depression (40%), asthenia (20%), rigors (25%), fatigue (20%), arthralgias (20%), nausea (25%), diarrhea (15%), and alopecia (15%). Irritability, insomnia, abdominal pain, pruritus, retinitis, peripheral neuropathy, seizures, rash, and inflammation at the injection site also are seen. Thyroid dysfunction in the form of either hyper- or hypothyroidism occurs in approximately 1% of patients and has been irreversible in some. TSH monitoring prior to therapy and at 1 month is recommended, especially in women. Anemia, leukopenia, and thrombocytopenia occur in 10 to 30% of patients and may require dose modification or temporary discontinuance. Leukopenia is the rate limiting toxicity with interferon (IFN). CBCs are recommended at 2- to 4-week intervals to monitor patients. Despite the long list of side effects and their rather high frequency, therapy almost always can be completed. It should not, however, be used in patients with decompensated liver disease.

Indicated for the treatment of chronic hepatitis B and C, interferon alfa-2a and interferon alfacon-1 for the treatment of chronic hepatitis C. While the interferons are indicated for the treatment of patients 18 yr of age or older with compensated liver disease, it is now routine to treat all hepatitis C patients who are infected, including those with acute hepatitis C. Treatment of acute hepatitis C has reduced the rate of developing chronic disease from approximately 80% to 85% to 10% to 15%.

Initial studies for the treatment of chronic hepatitis C were done using SQ doses of 3 MU tiw for 3 to 6 months. Sustained remission rates of 15 to 20% were obtained. The pulse dosing initially used with alpha interferon was designed to reduce the toxicity. Pharmacokinetic data, however, show that serum levels are not sustained. Peak serum concentration occurs 3 to 12 hr after injection. The elimination half-life is 2 to 3 hr, and serum levels are undetectable after 16 hr. Hepatitis C replication rates are in the trillions a day, with viral half-life of approximately 5 hr. Thus, there is a pharmacokinetic/pharmacodynamic mismatch that ends up increasing the replication rate of the virus above baseline. It also was learned that such dosing increased the mutation rate, potentially leading to the formation of immune-evading quasispecies.

Subsequent studies have used 5 MU for 6 to 12 months and have doubled the sustained remission rate. It appears, however, that the optimum initial dose is 10 MU. Current studies using 10 MU a day for a few days followed by 5 MU a day for 6 to 12 months have shown promise of increasing the sustained remission rate even further. Furthermore, studies with pegelated interferon—a sustained-release form given once a week—have shown promise of even higher sustained remission rates with less toxicity.

RIBAVIRIN IN COMBINATION WITH INTERFERON ALFA-2B

Rebetron

Comments—A guanosine analog that has antiviral activity against respiratory syncytial virus but not hepatitis B or C virus. However, in combination with alpha interferon, it increases the sustained remission rate in chronic hepatitis C. It is packaged as interferon alfa-2b 3 million units/vial and ribavirin (Rebetol) capsule, 200 mg. It is indicated for the retreatment of chronic hepatitis C in both naive patients and those who have not responded to interferon therapy or who have relapsed after prior treatment with alpha interferon. In a large multicenter study, combination therapy for 24 weeks achieved a sustained virological response of 31%, compared with 6% for interferon alone (3 MU SC tiw).

DRUGS THAT DISSOLVE GALLSTONES

See *Bile, Bile Acids, and Bile Salts,* page 1303.

MISCELLANEOUS GASTROINTESTINAL DRUGS

Several drugs with diverse actions on the GI tract are included in this section. They range from the empirical carminative *peppermint spirit* to the novel gallstone dissolution agent *ursodiol* and the well-established *diphenoxylate hydrochloride–atropine sulfate* antidiarrheal combination. Carminatives are substances that were at one time used to relieve gaseous distention of the stomach or intestines. Many carminative volatile oils are used as flavoring agents.

ANISE OIL—page 1064.
CAMPHOR—page 1284.
CARDAMOM OIL—page 1064.
CARDAMOM SEED—page 1064.
CHLOROBUTANOL—page 1059.
CHLOROFORM—page 1085.

LACTULOSE

D-Fructose, 4-*O*-β-Dcnm-galactopyranosyl-, Cholac

4-*O*-β-D-Galactopyranosyl-D-fructofuranose [4618-18-2] $C_{12}H_{22}O_{11}$ (342.30).

Preparation—Lactulose (a disaccharide containing 1 molecule of galactose and 1 molecule of fructose) may be prepared by epimerization of lactose (a disaccharide containing 1 molecule of galactose and 1 molecule of glucose) in a lime water medium. *J Am Chem Soc* 130; 52:2101.

Description—White powder; melts at about 169°; levorotatory; reduces Fehling's solution; yields galactose and fructose on acid hydrolysis. The commercially available syrup is a pale yellow to yellow, viscous, sweet liquid; each 15 mL contains 10 g of lactulose (and less than 2.2 g galactose, less than 1.2 g lactose, and 1.2 g or less of other sugars).

Solubility—Very soluble in water; very slightly soluble in alcohol.

Comments—A disaccharide containing 1 molecule of galactose and 1 molecule of glucose. It is used to reduce blood ammonia levels in patients with portal-systemic encephalopathy. It improves the patients' mental state and EEG patterns but does not alter the course of the underlying liver disease. The action of lactulose, which is absorbed poorly after oral administration, depends on its breakdown by colonic bacteria to carbon dioxide, lactic acid, and small amounts of acetic and formic acids, which acidify the contents of the colon. The acidic environment converts ammonia to ammonium ion ($NH4^+$), which cannot be absorbed. It also favors diffusion of ammonia from blood into the colon. The osmotic laxative action of lactulose and/or its metabolites then expels the trapped ammonium ions from the colon. Therapy with lactulose is reported to reduce blood-ammonia levels by 25% to 50% and effect a favorable clinical response in about 75% of patients. Lactulose is poorly absorbed, with only 3% appearing in the urine in 24 hr.

Lactulose may produce gaseous distention with flatulence or belching and abdominal discomfort such as cramping in about 20% of patients. Excessive dosage produces diarrhea but some degree of diarrhea (2–4 loose stools per 24 hr) is needed for its maximum therapeutic effect. Nausea and vomiting have been reported infrequently.

Lactulose syrup contains some monosaccharides and should be used with caution in diabetics. Concomitant use of neomycin with lactulose may result in elimination of colonic bacteria that are essential for the required degradation of lactulose and thus prevent acidification of the colon. Other laxatives should not be used, especially during the initial phase of therapy, because loose stools falsely may suggest that lactulose dosage is adequate. Lactulose does not alter the course of the underlying liver disease, for which other therapy may be required. The safety of lactulose syrup during pregnancy and the effect on the mother and fetus have not been evaluated.

ORLISTAT

Leucine, *N*-formyl-, [2*S*-[2α(*R),3β]]-1-[(3-hexyl-4-oxo-2-ox etanyl)methyl]dodecyl ester; Xenical**

[96829-58-2] C$_{29}$H$_{53}$NO$_5$ (495.74).

Preparation—*J Biol Chem*, 1997; 272: 867 and *J Med Chem*, 2003;46:4209.

Description—The tetrahydro derivative of *lipstatin* which is isolated from the fermentation broth of *Streptomycin toxytricini*. White to off-white crystalline powder melting about 43°; [α]$^{20}_D$ − 32° (c = 1, CHCl$_3$).

Solubility—Practically insoluble in water; freely soluble in chloroform; very soluble in methanol or ethanol.

SIMETHICONE

Gas-X; Mylicon; Phazyme

Simethicone [8050-81-5]; a mixture of fully methylated linear siloxane polymers containing repeating units of the formula [M(CH$_3$)$_2$SiO]$_n$, stabilized with trimethylsiloxy end-blocking units of the formula [(CH$_3$)$_3$SiOM], and silicon dioxide.

Description—Translucent, gray, viscous fluid; specific gravity between 0.964 and 0.984; refractive index between 1.400 and 1.410; viscosity (25° ± 0.1°) not less than 300 centistokes.

Comments—An agent with defoaming action that is supposed to relieve gas in the GI tract. It is used as adjunctive therapy in conditions in which gas is a problem, such as *postoperative gaseous distention, air swallowing, functional dyspepsia, irritable colon,* and *diverticulosis.* It also is used in antacid combinations to defoam gastric juice, to decrease the tendency to gastroesophageal reflux; however, it does *not* decrease the antacid requirement. It has yet to be proved that simethicone has any therapeutic benefit. It is thought to be physiologically inert and devoid of toxicity.

CHAPTER 67

Blood, Fluids, Electrolytes, and Hematological Drugs

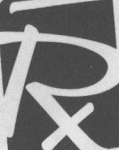

Blood is a unique tissue. As a tissue, it can be withdrawn from the body, and an extensive array of its parts can be separated for use in therapy. As a circulating body fluid, blood serves a vital set of physiological functions. A large number of drugs exert useful specific actions directed at maintaining or restoring these functions.

The reader is referred to Chapter 31 for a basic discussion of hematology and blood banking technology.

The responsibility for promulgating and administering federal regulations applicable to blood and blood products is that of the Food and Drug Administration (FDA), Bureau of Biologics. The applicable regulations are found in the *Code of Federal Regulations, 21 CFR 273.3*. Standards also are set by the American Association of Blood Banks and the World Health Organization (WHO).

WHOLE BLOOD AND BLOOD COMPONENTS

Blood serves many vital functions and also reflects the condition of other body tissues. Even though whole blood does not normally come into direct contact with noncirculating cells other than the vascular endothelium, electrolytes and many small organic compounds found in plasma freely exchange with both the lymph and the interstitial fluid. Thus, the composition of blood is an important indicator of cellular ion and metabolic status. Plasma is the vehicle for the transport of most nutrients to, and many wastes from, the tissues. Plasma transports drugs, often in combined, or bound, form; plasma is therefore an important factor in determining the effectiveness of drugs (Chapter 57). The proteins in plasma are involved importantly in the regulation of the hydration of the tissues by virtue of osmosis resulting from the impermeability of the vascular endothelium to most of the protein. Some of the plasma proteins are involved intimately in the clotting of blood and, therefore, in its conservation.

The erythrocytes are involved especially with oxygen and carbon dioxide transport. Leukocytes play major roles in the defense against infection (see Chapter 60), and platelets exert a variety of important functions in hemostasis and response to injury.

USES FOR BLOOD AND BLOOD COMPONENTS—
The many physiological functions of blood derive from the specific roles of its many parts; in addition to the formed elements there are more than 80 discrete proteins in plasma. When whole blood has been lost, as by hemorrhage, whole blood is required for replacement. However, the use of whole blood to overcome a deficiency of a single part constitutes a dissipation of the other useful parts.

In most instances, the administration of a single component in concentrated form elicits a far better response than the administration of that component as whole blood. Furthermore, by using the specific parts of the blood, the supply of blood can be used more economically; the net result is the use of the components of a single donation for several purposes.

The number of products now available is increasing but is still short of the number of known parts of blood. For example,

the red cells can be made available for the treatment of anemia, albumin for the treatment of shock, immune globulins for the prophylaxis of certain infectious diseases, granulocytes for granulocytopenia, and platelets for thrombocytopenia. These, and other important available blood components, are discussed in the following sections.

In the United States, the collection, processing, preservation, and distribution of blood and its separated components are performed by a wide variety of enterprises. For the purpose of this discussion, however, the important fact is where and how blood and its components are made available for the use of patients and the public at large. The main channels for dispensing blood services and blood products are

1. Blood centers and blood banks. These provide a wide array of services that reach the patient on prescription, usually through a hospital blood bank or transfusion service. The major services include the provision of whole blood, separated red cells, platelets, granulocytes, cryoprecipitated Factor VIII, single-donor plasma, and fresh frozen plasma. These usually are referred to as blood and blood components. They are distinguished by the fact that they are prepared locally in the blood center and dispensed in the form of individual units identified by the donor.
2. The pharmaceutical manufacturer and the pharmacy. This applies to the products of plasma fractionation, which are prepared by pharmaceutical manufacturers from large lots of pooled human plasma and are, therefore, subject to biological control regulations separate from those applying to simple units of blood and its components.
3. Public-health agencies and large blood centers. These may dispense directly to physicians or even to individual patients under certain circumstances.

TRANSMISSION OF INFECTION—The use of blood and its components is accompanied by some risk of transmission of serum hepatitis cytomegalovirus, human immunodeficiency viruses, Epstein-Barr virus, herpes simplex, infectious mononucleosis, syphilis, malaria, Chagas' disease, etc. This risk is different depending on which part of the blood is used and, also, on how it was prepared.

In the case of units of whole blood and blood components prepared and distributed by blood banks and blood centers, the degree of risk depends on the ability to detect the infectious agent in donor blood. Rapid progress is being made in this area. However, it probably will be some time, if ever, before the risk will reach zero; ie, before the absolute safety of donor blood can be assured. Still, the risk may be diminished or indeed eliminated by suitable processing treatments. Thus, immune globulin prepared by the ethanol-water fractionation procedure is free of virus even without specific viricidal treatment.

Human Albumin carries no risk of virus transmission, as a result of heating the solution to 60°C for 10 hr. Therefore, it is likely that any product that can be heated at 60°C for 10 hr will have a greatly diminished, if not zero, risk of viral transmission. Unfortunately, very few products can withstand such rigorous treatment, and other means have been sought to inactivate viruses, but with less than complete success. These include irradiation with ultraviolet light, cathode rays, and chemical treatment with various substances such as β-propiolactone. None of these methods, as presently used, can be relied on to inactivate completely all viruses that might be present, although they diminish the risk associated with use of the material.

In short, except for certain products such as albumin and immune globulin, which are known to be free of virus, most blood derivatives must be assumed to involve a risk of virus transmission, and this risk must be weighed against the medical consequences of withholding the product.

WHOLE BLOOD

Blood may be collected for human use only from persons who are certified by a physician as being free of transmissible disease, as far as can be determined from the donor's personal history, physical examination, etc. Unfortunately, in mass donations (eg, bloodmobiles) these examinations and certifications tend to be hasty and limited. The usual amount drawn is 500 mL. The blood is collected into an anticoagulant solution. A sample of blood is collected at the time of bleeding and subjected to serological and virological tests.

The use of the anticoagulant mixtures known as ACD and CPD extends the useful life of the red cells with the result that, following storage under proper conditions, the blood can be used with safety for a period of 21 days after collection. The addition of adenine to CPD solution (to make CPDA-1) increases the shelf life by another 14 days, thus enabling a useful storage time of 35 days. The use of these solutions has extended greatly the flexibility of hospital and community blood banks. However, with heparin the shelf life is much shorter, the official expiration time being 2 days.

If whole blood is used, it is handled carefully and stored in the cold without further processing or testing, except for occasional observation to detect evidence of hemolysis or contamination.

BLOOD COMPONENTS

Blood collection agencies—blood centers and blood banks—provide an array of blood services to the areas they serve. These include providing whole blood and several blood components prepared in the center from fresh donor blood. Blood components are made from single units of blood without opening or breaking the sterility of the plastic-bag system in which the blood originally was collected. These components thus are individualized with respect to the donor; if greater amounts are required than those available from one donor, multiple units are used. In addition to whole blood, components commonly available are CPD or CPDA-1 red blood cells, frozen red blood cells, saline-washed red blood cells, leukocyte-free red blood cells, granulocyte concentrate, platelet concentrate, cryoprecipitated antihemophilic factor, fresh frozen plasma, and liquid plasma.

WHOLE BLOOD

Blood that has been drawn from suitable human donors under rigid aseptic precautions. It contains citrate ion (acid citrate dextrose or citrate phosphate dextrose or citrate phosphate dextrose with adenine) or heparin as an anticoagulant. Preparations are designated ACD Whole Blood, CPD Whole Blood, CPDA-1 Whole Blood, or Heparinized Whole Blood according to the anticoagulant used. Whole blood from which the antihemophilic factor has been removed is designated Modified Whole Blood (see below).

Description—Deep-red, opaque liquid from which the corpuscles readily settle, on standing for 24 to 48 hr, leaving a clear, yellowish, or pinkish, supernatant layer. If the blood has been drawn soon after the donor has eaten, it may, on standing, acquire a layer of fatlike material near its surface. A deep-pink or red color in the plasma or a purplish tint at the surface of the cell portion usually indicates that the blood is unsatisfactory for use.

Comments—The natural replenisher for lost blood and hence indicated when there has been hemorrhage or traumatic blood loss of over 20% of the blood volume. When the blood loss is small, it is not essential that all of the lost blood be replaced, except in persons with high oxygen demand (eg, thyrotoxicosis, beri-beri) or in anemia. Consequently, some practitioners may replace only part of the lost blood and make up the remainder of the deficit with a saline, hetastarch, or dextran solution. In hemorrhagic shock, some medical opinion holds that the entire volume deficit should not be repaired by whole blood alone because of erythrocyte aggregation and sludging, and a dextran also sometimes is added concomitantly, to suppress not only erythrocyte aggregation but also platelet aggregation, since intravascular clotting sometimes is a complication. Adverse effects of whole blood include reactions from improperly matched blood, passive transfer of allergies, serum hepatitis and other infections, volume overload in improperly monitored administration, and increased viscosity of the circulating blood. Stored whole blood is nearly devoid of platelets and also may be deficient in Factors V and VII, so that clotting and coagulation defects may occur after massive transfusions.

WHOLE BLOOD MODIFIED

Single-donor whole blood from which antihemophilic factor (USP definition) or one or more other, nonerythrocyte components have been removed. Components and plasma may be removed either by sedimentation methods or by continuous separation devices; after selective separation, the plasma is reunited with the erythrocytes.

Comments—The uses are determined, in part, by the health of both the donor and recipient and the reason for removal of the component(s). If the reason for component-pheresis is to remove an adverse component, such as leukocytes in a leukemia or lymphocytes in an autoimmune disorder, the modified whole blood is returned autologously to the donor. If, instead, the donor is healthy and pheresis is conducted to provide a heterologous source of the component(s) for therapeutic purposes, the residual modified whole blood may be used for the same purposes as *Whole Blood*, provided that the volume to be transfused is small enough so as not to cause, by dilution, a clinically significant deficit of the corresponding component(s) in the recipient.

GRANULOCYTE CONCENTRATE

A single-donor concentrate of leukocytes obtained either by separation from sedimented whole blood or by pheresis with a continuous- or intermittent-flow centrifuge. The granulocytes (and entrained lymphocytes) are resuspended in the plasma of the recipient. The component should be used within 24 hr of collection.

Comments—Heterologously in patients with severe leukopenia, usually that which results from cancer chemotherapy or other adverse drug reactions.

LYMPHOCYTES FROZEN

A single-donor frozen concentrate of lymphocytes obtained by differential sedimentation from whole blood or from the removal of lymph from the thoracic duct. The cells are cooled at a rate of 3.5/min. DMSO is added to a 5% concentration when the temperature reaches 0°. Reconstitution requires careful thawing and repeated washout of DMSO. Viable cells are quantified from the uptake of radiothymidine into phytohemagglutinin-stimulated suspensions.

Comments—Investigationally in the treatment of neoplastic diseases, as exchange replacement for lymphocytes pheresed from the blood of patients afflicted with certain thymocyte-mediated autoimmune disorders, and as a diagnostic agent in specialized *in vitro* assessments of immune function.

SINGLE-DONOR PLASMA

Human Plasma

The liquid portion of a single unit of ACD, CPD-, or CPDA-1 whole blood, the separation of which was accomplished within the expiration time of the whole blood. It is stored at 1 to 6°; it may be stored for 5 days beyond the dating period of the whole blood from which it was separated (26 and 40 days if from CPD- or CPDA-1 whole blood, respectively). The ABO compatibility is that of the donor whole blood. One unit is 220 to 250 mL.

Description—Straw-colored transparent fluid that may sometimes exhibit a slight opalescence.

Comments—Mostly for *volume replenishment* in the treatment of *shock*, especially after severe burns, in which plasma protein loss is considerable. It is used occasionally as a source of the stable coagulation Factors II, VII, IX, and X, and thus can be used to treat hemophilia B. ABO compatibility is desirable but is not a prerequisite to use.

SINGLE-DONOR PLASMA FREEZE DRIED

Human Plasma Freeze-Dried

Single-donor plasma that has been cryodesiccated. If Fresh Frozen Plasma is the source of the cryodesiccate, the plasma may be designated an Antihemophilic Plasma. The expiration time of the reconstituted plasma is that of *Single-Donor Plasma*.

Comments—If the desiccate is made from *Fresh Frozen Plasma,* see the monograph; if made from Frozen Plasma, see *Single-Donor Plasma*.

SINGLE-DONOR PLASMA FRESH FROZEN

Human Plasma, Fresh Frozen; Antihemophilic Plasma

Single-donor human plasma frozen within 6 hr of collection and stored at a temperature of −20° or lower (preferably below −30°). The frozen plasma shall not be stored beyond 12 months. As a source of coagulation factors, the expiration time of thawed fresh frozen plasma is 24 hr; as a volume replenisher, the expiration time is that of Single-Donor Plasma. ABO compatibility is that of the donor whole blood. One unit is 200 to 250 mL.

Description—Light yellow to deep cream in color. When viewed microscopically, a reticulated structure without evidence of fusion may be seen.

Comments—Indicated especially for the treatment of *multiple coagulation factor deficiencies* (since the labile coagulation Factors V and XIII are preserved in fresh frozen plasma), such as those that occur in cases of massive transfusion with stored blood, after heparinization in disseminated intravascular coagulation, or in liver disease, and for *hemophilia*. The preparation also may be used as *Single-Donor Plasma* (above), although such use is unnecessarily expensive. It is the plasma of choice in patients with thrombotic thrombocytopenic purpura. It also is of value in patients with deficiencies of immunoglobulin and/or complement. Serum hepatitis virus is not killed by freezing.

SINGLE-DONOR PLASMA FROZEN

Human Plasma Frozen

Single-donor plasma that has been frozen within the expiration time of the liquid plasma but longer than 6 hr after removal from the donor. The expiration time of the thawed plasma is that of *Single-Donor Plasma*.

Comments—See *Single-Donor Plasma*.

PLATELET CONCENTRATE

Platelets taken from plasma obtained by whole-blood collection, by plasmapheresis or by plateletpheresis, from a single, suitable, human donor of whole blood; or from a plasmapheresis donor; or from a plateletpheresis donor. One unit of platelet concentrate consists of not less than 5.5×10^{10} platelets suspended in a specified volume of the original plasma. (See USP for collection procedure.)

Preserved platelets can be reinfused successfully into recipients suffering from platelet deficiency. Platelets obtained by plateletpheresis must be used within 24 hr of collection, because the open system allows bacterial contamination. Although the official expiration time is only 72 hr, it now is possible to store platelets for up to 120 hr, and it is likely that methods to preserve them for a longer period will be devised in the near future.

Comments—To arrest or prevent bleeding resulting from thrombocytopenia or thrombopathy. In platelet deficiency consequent to disseminated intravascular coagulation and thrombocytopenic purpura (in which a type of intravascular coagulation occurs), the platelets must be coadministered with heparin. When thrombocytopenia is caused by immune destruction, the administration of platelets mostly is futile because of rapid destruction of the added platelets. Likewise, in drug-induced thrombocytopenia, the effects of the platelets mostly are voided unless the drug is discontinued, preferably in advance. Platelets can be used in the priming of extracorporeal circuits, but they may be subjected to faster destruction in the circuit than endogenous platelets. The half-life of platelets is about 1 to 2 days.

RED BLOOD CELLS

Human Red Blood Cells; Red Cell Concentrate

Red cells of whole human blood, separated from plasma by centrifuging or subsidence during the dating period of the blood from which they are derived, but not later than 21 days after the blood is drawn if the anticoagulant solution is ACD or CPD solution; if acid citrate dextrose adenine solution has been used as anticoagulant, such preparation may be made within 35 days therefrom; if heparin is used, the expiration time is 48 hr. The expiration dates are valid only if the hematocrit does not exceed 80% and the seal is unbroken. Preparations are designated CPD Red Cells, CPDA-1 Red Cells, or Heparinized Red Cells, according to the anticoagulant used.

Description—Dark red when packed and may show a slight creamy layer on the surface and a small supernatant layer of yellow or opalescent plasma. Resuspended human blood cells is a dark-red fluid.

Comments—A *blood replenisher* in any condition in which the primary deficiency in the blood is of the erythrocytes. Thus, they are used in the emergency treatment of a number of the anemias that formerly were treated with whole-blood transfusions. They also may be returned to the donor by autologous transfusion after plasmapheresis or apheresis of other components. Human blood cells are not suitable alone as a replacement fluid in hemorrhage, but they may be employed in cases where chronic blood loss is not too great to decrease appreciably the plasma volume and plasma protein content. Each unit of concentrate preferably is mixed with 50 to 100 mL of 0.9% NaCl injection to decrease the viscosity. Lactated Ringer's injection is contraindicated because it provides enough calcium to initiate coagulation; dextrose injection is contraindicated because it causes hemolysis. The half-life is about 4 weeks but varies considerably depending on the recipient.

RED BLOOD CELLS FROZEN

Red Blood Cells (Human) Frozen; Red Cells Fresh Frozen

A preparation in which human red cells are suspended in a glycerol solution and frozen at temperatures ranging from −80 to −120°. There are two types of preparations: one that uses a low concentration of glycerol and rapid freezing and the other, which uses a high concentration of glycerol and slow freezing. The expiration time is 3 years. Before use, the suspension is thawed and the glycerol medium is replaced with a physiological solution. At this stage the preparation is designated Deglycerolized Red Cell Concentrate. The expiration time of the thawed preparation is 24 hr.

Comments—By freezing erythrocytes immediately or shortly after withdrawal, both ATP and 2,3-diphosphoglyceric acid (2,3-DPG) are preserved better than in the classical preparation and storage methods, and frozen erythrocytes have better oxygen-transport capacity. Therefore they especially are suited for use in newborn and premature infants and in older patients with excessive oxygen demands. Because of their single-donor origin they are used especially for autologous transfusions. They also are used when there is a rare blood requirement, in elective gynecological and cardiac surgery, hemodialysis, and kidney transplantation. They essentially are free of irregular antibodies and plasma proteins and hence are useful in patients with allergic, febrile reactions to saline-washed red cells or with nocturnal hemoglobinuria. Since there are few surviving leukocytes, the risk of graft-versus-host response is diminished. The freeze-thaw procedure removes senescent erythrocytes, thus leaving a younger population of cells with a longer survival time in the recipient. The postthaw washing procedure greatly decreases the risk of serum hepatitis and pyrogenic reactions to debris from leukocytes and platelets. Frozen red cells are very expensive.

RED BLOOD CELLS LEUKOCYTES REMOVED

Red Cell Concentrate, Leukocyte-Poor

A single-donor red cell concentrate that contains less than 25% of the original leukocytes. The expiration time is that of *Red Blood Cells* and is determined by the type of anticoagulant used. The hematocrit usually ranges from 0.7 to 0.8.

Comments—Mostly for autologous transfusion in leukemic individuals in whom a reduction in circulating leukocytes is imperative. May be used in heterologous erythrocyte replenishment if the original donor blood was normal (ie, donor blood served as a source of therapeutic leukocytes). Because the preparation has fewer pyrogenic leukocyte fragments than does Red Blood Cells, febrile reactions are less severe and less frequent.

RED BLOOD CELLS SALINE WASHED

Red Cell Concentrate, Washed

A single-donor red-cell concentrate in which most of the plasma, leukocytes, and platelets have been removed within 24 hr of transfusion by one or more washes with an isotonic saline solution. The hematocrit usually lies between 0.7 and 0.8.

Comments—Washing may be employed for five purposes: (1) to remove adverse components in specific disorders (eg, lymphocytes and/or immune globulins in certain autoimmune disorders, Rh factors in alloimmunity, anticoagulation factors in certain bleeding disorders, thyroid hormone in thyroid storm, etc; in such instances, the erythrocytes are to be reinfused into the donor; (2) to reduce the risk of blood-transmissible infections (not malaria); the erythrocytes are intended for heterologous transmission; (3) to remove citrate in citrated blood when the volume to be transfused is large and the intended recipient has a liver dysfunction in which citrate cannot be tolerated; (4) to decrease the intensity of heterologous transfusion reactions in emergency situations in which out-of-group (nonmatched) blood must be used; or (5) to decrease the incidence and severity of febrile transfusion reaction caused by fragments of leukocytes and platelets.

PLASMA EXPANDERS AND INTRAVENOUS FLUIDS

PROTEIN AND COLLOID SOLUTIONS

Hemorrhage and shock result in loss of blood volume, which, if carried beyond a certain critical point, leads to circulatory failure. Replacement of the plasma proteins or injection of a substance having similar osmotic properties will restore the blood volume at least temporarily, so that circulation of oxygen to the tissues may be maintained. Many substances have been employed for this purpose: *whole blood,* which in certain situations is ideal, but is not always immediately available; *plasma,* which is quite effective, but is unstable in the liquid form, relatively cumbersome in the dry form, involves injection of salt and water, which is in some cases undesirable, and, finally, cannot readily be rendered free of pathogenic viruses; *serum albumin,* the protein in the plasma that functions to control blood volume and polysaccharides, such as *dextrans* and *hetastarch.*

Physiologically, the most clearly established role of albumin appears to be its water-retaining (osmotic) capacity. It is due chiefly to plasma albumin that the water of the plasma, instead of diffusing into the tissues, is retained in the bloodstream, maintaining the volume of blood that is necessary for effective cardiac output and circulation. Albumin, although it comprises less than 60% of the plasma proteins, by virtue of having the lowest molecular weight of these proteins contributes 80% of their osmotic effect. Another highly important property of albumin is its capacity to bind various chemical substances, including certain ions, some hormones, and numerous drugs.

Methods have been devised for preparing human plasma albumin more than 99% pure. Unlike most plasma proteins, it is extraordinarily stable. It does not require desiccation or continuous refrigeration and, therefore, can be kept on hand as a 25% sterile solution, ready for instant use. Separation of the albumin leaves the remaining plasma proteins as by-products. It is possible to derive many specific pharmaceutical agents from one blood donation, enabling more efficient use of a given quantity of blood.

ALBUMIN HUMAN

Normal Human Serum Albumin; Albuminar; Albutein; Plasbumin; Buminate

Human albumin is a sterile, nonpyrogenic preparation of serum albumin, obtained by fractionating blood, plasma, serum, or placentas from healthy human donors and tested for absence of hepatitis B surface antigen. It is prepared by a process ensuring safety for intravenous use. The albumin content is not less than 96% of the total protein. The solution contains 5 or 25 g of albumin, respectively, corresponding to 100 or 500 mL of normal human plasma. It may contain sodium acetytryptophanate alone or with sodium caprylate as a stabilizing agent. The sodium content is not less than 130 mEq/L and not more than 160 mEq/L. No antimicrobial agent is added. It meets the requirements of tests for limit of heme, heat stability, and pH. Solutions are heated in final containers at 60° for 10 hr to kill any pathogenic organisms that may be present. The storage temperature is indicated on the label. The solution is not to be used if it is turbid or there is a sediment.

Description—Moderately viscous, clear, brownish fluid; practically odorless; may develop a slight granular or flaky deposit during storage. When dried, has a slight-yellow to deep-cream color.

Comments—Serves as an emergency agent for restoration of blood volume in the treatment of *shock* or *hemorrhage.* It especially is indicated when blood loss exceeds 20% of blood volume. If albumin is administered in hypertonic concentrations, it will abstract water from interstitial and intracellular fluids and increase blood volume by an amount more than the volume administered; in isotonic concentration it will expand blood volume only by an amount equal to the volume added. Each gram of albumin holds about 18 mL of water in the bloodstream. Because its action depends on the availability of tissue water, hypertonic albumin should not be used in severely dehydrated patients without simultaneous administration of saline or dextrose solutions.

It has been used in protein replacement therapy when serum protein levels are low because of excessive loss, as in extensive burns and nephrosis, certain skin diseases, and other conditions, or because of inadequate formation of proteins resulting from nutritional disturbances, cirrhosis, or other causes. However, the value of albumin in the therapy of chronic nephritis or cirrhosis is less impressive than in acute hypoalbuminemia. Hyperoncotic albumin solutions may be used to cause transient diuresis in edematous patients or in those undergoing renal dialysis. It also is used in the treatment of hyperbilirubinemia and erythroblastosis fetalis to increase the binding capacity for bilirubin.

Low salt content and the high stability of the single protein component present make *salt-poor* albumin the agent of choice in certain types of protein replacement therapy, bearing in mind the following limitations: Albumin does not, in any sense, replace red cells and, therefore, should not be used in hemorrhagic shock except as an emergency remedy. It lacks the other proteins contained in plasma, hence is not an adequate agent for treatment of deficiencies of specific plasma proteins (eg, fibrinogen, prothrombin) such as occur in acute hepatitis or burns. It does not replace lost fluids and therefore must be given with ample quantities of crystalloid solution when used in dehydrated patients, as noted above. Chills, fever, urticaria, and perturbations of respiration and blood pressure sometimes occur. Albumin is contraindicated in congestive heart failure. Large doses should not be given in severe anemia, in low cardiac reserve, and in the absence of hypoalbuminemia.

ANTIHEMOPHILIC FACTOR—page 1326.

PLASMA PROTEIN FRACTION

Human Plasma Protein Fraction; Plasmanate; Plasma Plex; Plasmatein; Protenate

A sterile solution of selected proteins derived from the blood plasma of healthy adult human donors. It contains 4.5 to 5.5 g of protein/100 mL, of which about 83 to 90% is albumin and the remainder is alpha and beta globulins. It contains no antimicrobial agent but may contain suitable stabilizers. The expiration time is 5 years if the storage temperature is 2° to 10°, 3 years if 11° through 29°, the time not to include 1 year of storage at the manufacturing plant at 5°.

Preparation—By a process similar to that by which albumin is made. The product resembles plasma from which certain unstable globulins have been removed, including gamma globulin and certain lipoproteins. The solution is treated by heating at 60° for 10 hr to reduce the risk of virus transmission. The solution is isotonic with normal plasma and is isotonic with respect to diffusible ions, the major ions being sodium and chloride.

Description—Transparent, nearly colorless or slightly brownish liquid; nearly odorless; may develop a slight granular or flaky deposit during storage.

Comments—Indicated, like albumin, as a substitute for plasma in treating nonhemorrhagic *shock.* It also is a convenient source of protein for intravenous nutrition. Because it does not contain any clotting factors, it is not a substitute for fresh plasma in treating hemorrhagic states. The plasma half-life is about 27 days.

Untoward effects are uncommon; they include nausea, vomiting, and increased salivation. Care must be exercised to prevent circulatory overload, especially in nonhypovolemic patients. Solutions of this fraction should not be mixed with other intravenous fluids, either in the bottle or in the tubing.

MEDICINAL AGENTS

DEXTROSE AND SODIUM CHLORIDE INJECTION

Sodium Chloride and Dextrose Injection

A sterile solution of dextrose and sodium chloride in water for injection. It contains 95 to 105% of the labeled amount of $C_6H_{12}O_6.H_2O$ and of NaCl. It contains no antimicrobial agents.

Preparation—This title may include a highly concentrated solution for use as a sclerosing agent or much weaker solutions to be used in a manner similar to the use of 5 or 10% dextrose solution. This may be a mixture of equal parts of isotonic sodium chloride solution and isotonic dextrose solution, or it may represent 5% dextrose in isotonic sodium chloride solution. Both of these should be prepared according to the suggestions given for the preparation of *Dextrose Injection*.

Description—Clear, colorless solution with a pH of 3.5 to 6.5, determined on a portion of injection diluted with water, if necessary, to a concentration of not more than 5% dextrose.

Comments—To provide dextrose as a nutrient (see above) in a medium that does not hydrate the tissues, or it may be employed as a source of isotonic sodium chloride, or both. When hypertonic solutions of dextrose are employed in cerebral edema or in hydrated states, isotonic sodium chloride in the injection prevents a delayed rebound hydration. Since dextrose, alone, cannot be given safely by the subcutaneous route (see *Dextrose Injection*), this is the preferred preparation.

FRUCTOSE INJECTION—page 1692.

ANTIBODIES AND ISOAGGLUTININS

Human plasma contains antibodies of various types, which are concentrated almost entirely in Fractions II and III. Some of these occur naturally, others arise as a result of infection or are stimulated by artificial immunization.

The serum of all human beings contains antibodies (agglutinins or isoagglutinins) that react with those principal blood-group factors (agglutinogens) that the individual does *not* possess (Table 67-1).

Thus, for example, 45% of the population of the *US* possesses the blood-group O factor in their red cells, and agglutinins against the A and B factors in the plasma. Should the whole blood or cells of a Group A individual be injected into a Group O patient, the anti-A agglutinins of the patient will clump the cells received and usually will destroy (lyse) them, causing a serious reaction in many cases, even if the volume of cells injected is as low as 50 mL.

The importance of establishing the blood group of anyone either giving or receiving whole blood is therefore obvious. This is done by mixing a specimen of the cells of the subject with the serum of a selected individual whose group is known; for example, if the cells of an untyped donor are clumped by the serum of a known Group B subject, but not by the serum of a known Group A subject, the donor evidently belongs to Group A.

In practice, anti-A isoagglutinins obtained from selected group B subjects, and anti-B isoagglutinins from similarly selected Group A subjects, have for years provided highly effective reagents for identification of the blood groups. It has been demonstrated that administration of small quantities of the specific blood-group substances A or B (which can be obtained from red blood cells or, in larger quantities, from other animal tissues) to individuals having the corresponding isoagglutinins will induce a tremendous rise in titer of the agglutinin. In this fashion, extremely potent blood-grouping sera have been prepared in ample quantities. It is also possible to produce blood-grouping sera as a by-product of ethanol fractionation of plasma.

In practice (see Chapter 31), it is customary not only to determine the blood group of a donor and recipient of a blood transfusion, but to *cross-match* the cells of the donor with the serum of the patient and *vice versa*, to detect any otherwise unpredictable incompatibility in the bloods of the two individuals. This extra precaution is invaluable, not only for the purpose indicated but also as a final check against mistaken identity of the specimens. Numerous other precautions are involved in correct blood grouping, so that it has become a highly specialized technique that should only be performed by a qualified technician.

THE Rh FACTOR—A much rarer antibody occurs in a small proportion of individuals as a result of injection of so-called *Rh-positive blood* or absorption of such blood across the placenta during pregnancy in gravid females. This *Rh factor* actually consists of at least nine different factors, any one or several of which may be present in the red cells of a given individual. Isoagglutinins reacting with these factors do not occur normally in humans, but appear only as a result of accidental *immunization* of individuals with a type of Rh factor which they do not possess. Actually, the blood of about 85% of Western Europeans or Americans contains one or two of the commonest of these factors, which also are the most potent as antigens. Therefore, in general practice it is customary and quite permissible to classify individuals simply as either *Rh-positive* or *Rh-negative*. The technique of Rh typing is essentially like that of blood grouping.

Like anti-A and anti-B blood-grouping serum, the principal source for Rh-typing serum is the blood of human donors who, by chance or intention, have become hyperimmunized to one of the Rh factors. One of the commonest sources is the blood of Rh-negative women who have borne several Rh-positive infants, absorbed their Rh factor, and thereby became sensitized. Another source is Rh-negative individuals who have been transfused with Rh-positive blood. Injection of small amounts of Rh substance in the latter individuals will induce very high antibody titers, rendering them suitable donors of hyperimmune serum for typing purposes. The danger of mismatched transfusion in such individuals is actually decreased, since they become extremely easy to identify.

BLOOD-GROUPING AND TYPING SERUMS

BLOOD-GROUP SPECIFIC SUBSTANCES A, B, AND AB

A sterile, isotonic solution of the polysaccharide–amino acid complexes that are capable of reducing the titer of the anti-A and anti-B isoagglutinins of group O blood. The blood-group specific substance A is prepared from hog gastric mucin, and the blood-group specific substances B and AB are prepared from the glandular portion of horse gastric mucosa. Blood-Group Specific Substances A, B and AB contains no preservative.

Description—Clear solution, which may have a slight odor due to the preservative; pH 6.0 to 6.8.

Comments—Added to group O blood as a *neutralizer of isoagglutinins*, and hence it makes the blood reasonably safe for transfusions into patients whose blood is of another group. It also may be used to condition plasma. However, conditioned plasma that contains immune anti-A and anti-B agglutinins may cause reactions. Furthermore, it must not be forgotten that blood from group O donors who previously have received conditioned group O blood may contain A and B isohemagglutinins. Such blood is dangerous to use in universal donation unless it is conditioned with blood group specific substances A and B.

Table 67-1. Blood-Group Factors

FACTORS PRESENT	BLOOD GROUPS (CELLS) FREQUENCY IN POPULATION	ISOAGGLUTININS (PLASMA)
O	45%	Anti-A and Anti-B
A	41%	Anti-B
B	10%	Anti-A
AB	4%	None

ANTI-A BLOOD-GROUPING SERUM

Derived from high-titered serums of humans, with or without stimulation by the injection of group-specific red cells or substances. It agglutinates human red cells containing A antigens; ie, blood groups A and AB (including subgroups A_1, A_2, A_3, A_1B, and A_2B). It may contain a suitable antibacterial preservative.

Description—Clear or slightly opalescent fluid unless artificially colored, when it has a blue or blue-green color. The dried product is light yellow to deep cream color, unless artificially colored as indicated for liquid serum, and microscopically has a honeycomb-like structure.

ANTI-B BLOOD-GROUPING SERUM

Derived from high-titered serums of humans, with or without stimulation by the injection of group-specific red cells or substances. It agglutinates human red cells containing B antigens; ie, blood groups B and AB (including subgroups A_1B and A_2B). It may contain a suitable antibacterial preservative.

Description—Clear or slightly opalescent fluid unless artificially colored, when it has a yellow color. The dried product is light yellow to deep cream color, unless artificially colored as indicated for liquid serum, and microscopically has a honeycomb-like structure.

ANTI-RH BLOOD-GROUPING SERUMS

Blood Grouping Serums Anti-D, Anti-C, Anti-E

Derived from the blood of humans who have developed specific Rh antibodies. Anti-Rh Blood-Grouping Serums are free from agglutinins for A or B antigens and from alloantibodies other than those for which claims are made in the labeling. They may contain suitable antimicrobial agents.

Two varieties of Anti-Rh Grouping Serums are recognized: (1) complete *(saline-agglutinating)* serums, which specifically agglutinate human red blood cells in saline TS, and (2) incomplete *(blocking)* serums, which agglutinate human red blood cells only in a medium containing protein or other macromolecular substances, which may be furnished in an accompanying diluent. Complete serums commonly are designated *For saline tube test,* and the incomplete serums are designated *For slide or modified (rapid) tube test.* In liquid form, the latter contain, as additives, the required micromolecular substances.

The left-hand column of Table 67-2 lists the designations of the most commonly used anti-Rh blood-grouping serums, and the right-hand column lists the blood factor(s) with which each serum specifically reacts. The designations used in an alternative system of nomenclature are indicated parenthetically.

Comments—As diagnostic agents.

IMMUNE GLOBULINS

Adult blood contains antibodies specific for various infectious agents to which the individual has built up a resistance. In pooled normal plasma used for fractionation some of these are in high enough concentration to have a protective action. This is usually true of measles and poliomyelitis antibodies. Antibodies from adult plasma will protect against the disease if given after exposure. In certain other conditions, it is possible to select individuals with already detectable antibody levels and, by injection of an appropriate vaccine, to raise their antibody level to very high titers, much as described above for blood grouping and Rh typing sera. This practice has been employed

Table 67-2.

SERUM	ANTIGEN(S) REACTING
Anti-D (Anti-Rh₀)	D (Rh₀)
Anti-C (Anti-rh`)	C (rh`)
Anti-E (Anti-rh``)	E (rh``)
Anti-CD (Anti-Rh₀`)	D (Rh₀), C (rh`)
Anti-DE (Anti-Rh₀``)	D (Rh₀), E (rh``)
Anti-CDE (Anti-Rh₀``)	D (Rh₀), C (rh`), E (rh``)
Anti-c (Anti-hr`)	c (hr`)
Anti-e (Anti-hr``)	e (hr``)

mainly in the production of pertussis hyperimmune globulin for the treatment or prophylaxis of whooping cough.

During the fractionation of plasma, most of the antibodies are concentrated into a single fraction (Fraction II); electrophoretically the proteins in this fraction are characterized as gamma globulins. Isolated immune globulins, dispensed as a 16% solution, represent a concentration of most antibodies approximately 25 times greater than that in plasma. As a result, they have been found useful in the prophylaxis of certain infectious diseases, including measles, infectious hepatitis (not to be confused with serum hepatitis), and poliomyelitis.

The usefulness derives from the immunity conferred by the *added* antibody. However, since the added antibody is metabolized slowly and therefore disappears, the immunity is passive, and lasts only so long as the concentration of antibody is above an effective level, usually from 1 to 2 months. Thereafter, the recipient once again becomes susceptible to infection. Alternatively, and particularly when exposure to infection can be ascertained with reasonable accuracy, as in measles, a modifying dose of antibodies may be administered.

While failing to prevent active infection, the added antibody lessens the severity of the disease, and patients respond to the infection by producing antibodies of their own. This production of antibodies persists for long periods thereafter, thus conferring long-lasting immunity.

Immune globulin is administered intramuscularly; it cannot be used intravenously. Reactions are uncommon and, when they do occur, chiefly are local and usually mild. Another source of gamma globulin is the blood from normal human placentas. Application of the methods of processing immune globulin from human blood, however, has made possible the preparation of a similar globulin from placentas.

Immune Globulin and immune globulins for *hepatitis B, pertussis, rabies, Rh₀(D), tetanus, cytomegalovirus, respiratory syncytial virus,* and *varicella-zoster* are described in Chapter 89.

IMMUNE SERA

Various biological products obtained from the blood of humans or animals and used for their prophylactic or therapeutic effects, eg, antitoxins, immune sera, and immune globulin, are discussed in Chapter 89.

AGENTS AFFECTING BLOOD COAGULATION

The clotting of blood is a very important process (see Chapter 31). It depends on the existence of a complex system of reactions involving plasma proteins, platelets, tissue factor, and calcium ion. This system normally is in a state of balance known as hemostasis, referring to the spontaneous arrest of bleeding. However, if a factor is defective or absent, as is the case in hemophilia, a hemorrhagic tendency exists that can lead to major hemorrhage under certain circumstances. In hemophilia, the defect is congenital. Other defects, often transient, may arise as the result of disease or malnutrition. Under certain circumstances, the reverse situation is encountered. Hypercoagu-

lability—an abnormal tendency for the blood to clot—can be very serious, leading to thrombosis.

BLOOD-CLOTTING PROTEINS

The inherited coagulation disorders associated with bleeding affect 1 in 10,000 to 15,000 persons, except von Willebrand's disease (VWD), which may affect up to 1% of the population. These diseases are usually the result of either qualitative or quantitative defects in a single plasma protein. In hemophilia

A, plasma levels of Factor VIII are decreased, and in hemophilia B, plasma levels of Factor IX are diminished. VWD is due to an abnormality in the Factor VIII–von Willebrand Factor (VWF) complex that is required for normal platelet adhesion. In its most common form, VWD is associated with mild, mucocutaneous bleeding such as bruising, epistaxis, and menorrhagia. There are also various acquired disorders that result in excessive bleeding, including vitamin K deficiency, liver disease, or circulating antibody inhibitors to Factor VIII that can occur with age, autoimmune disease, postpartum, or in previously transfused hemophilic patients. The principal treatment is replacement therapy of the deficient factor by use of blood products derived from normal people or animals or recombinant coagulation proteins. The activity of the various coagulation factors is expressed in units, referring to the activity found in 1 mL of fresh plasma pooled from normal donors.

ANTIHEMOPHILIC FACTOR

Humate P

A sterile, purified, lyophilized concentrate of human antihemophilic factor prepared from the Factor VIII–rich cryoprotein fraction of human venous plasma.

Preparation—Precipitated by glycine from a solution of AHF-rich first precipitate from pooled normal human plasma. After treatment to lower the content of glycine and inactive proteins, a solution of the active fraction is pasteurized by heating to 60°C for 10 hr in aqueous solution.

Description—White or grayish, to yellow, amorphous substance dried from the frozen state; colorless or opalescent when reconstituted with the diluent provided. One unit is the activity in 1 mL of pooled human plasma less than 1 hr old.

Comments—The coagulation defect in classical hemophilia (hemophilia A) is predominately a deficit of the coagulation Factor VIII, called antihemophilic factor (AHF). In severe hemorrhage in the patient with hemophilia A, it is used as a cryoprecipitate or concentrate, or in fresh plasma or whole blood, as required *to terminate hemorrhage* or to prevent hemorrhage in surgery or consequent to various procedures in which bleeding may occur. The concentrate generally is preferred to plasma or whole blood, since the AHF titers of blood and plasma are quite variable, but in VWD the cryoprecipitate (below) is more effective. Although the concentrate contains VWF, it lacks the high-molecular-weight multimeric forms found in plasma, and the cryoprecipitate product. The preparation is poorly effective in hemophilia B. AHF has a distribution half-life of 4 to 8 hr and an elimination half-life of 12 to 15 hr.

In the past, viral transmission of hepatitis and human immunodeficiency viruses (HIV) was substantial, as concentrated preparations were prepared from large plasma pools. Specific viral transmission has been reduced significantly, as the concentrates now are sterilized by solvent-detergent or heat treatment. The monoclonal antibody–prepared products have shown hepatitis safety and very low risk for HIV, whereas the recombinant products are considered very low to no risk for both hepatitis and HIV. Traces of ABO isohemagglutinins are present in glycine precipitates, so that large doses may sometimes cause severe hemolysis. In contrast, monoclonal antibody–purified products have reduced blood-group-specific antibodies significantly. In addition, an antibody inhibitor to Factor VIII occurs in approximately 10% of patients, secondary to previous transfusions. Patients with high-titer Factor VIII inhibitor are treated with Anti-inhibitor Coagulant Complex or animal-derived Factor VIII. Mild allergic reactions are frequent. Occasionally there may be chills, fever, erythema, urticaria, bronchospasm, headache, lethargy, somnolence, and backache. The concentrate is more expensive than the cryoprecipitate.

See Table 67-3.

CRYOPRECIPITATED ANTIHEMOPHILIC FACTOR

A sterile, frozen concentrate of antihemophilic factor prepared from the Factor VIII–rich cryoprotein fraction of a single unit of human venous plasma obtained from whole blood or by plasmapheresis. It can be kept for 1 year at −18° or below and is thawed at a temperature not to exceed 37° just before use.

Comments—See *Antihemophilic Factor*. The cryoprecipitated form is used when an autologous replacement is necessary. Also, cryopreservation maintains the potency better than liquid preservation. The cryoprecipitate contains other factors, including one that improves the bleeding time in patients with VWD. This factor is not present in marketed preparations of antihemophilic factor, and the cryoprecipitated preparation or fresh frozen plasma should be used instead. Since the cryoprecipitate is type-specific, it may be cross-matched to the patient's blood to avoid hemolysis.

ANTITHROMBIN III (HUMAN)

Thrombate III; AT nativ

[52014-67-2]

Antithrombin III (AT III) is an α_2-globulin of molecular weight about 60,000, found in blood, and a major endogenous coagulation inhibitor that inactivates various clotting cascade serine proteases including thrombin.

Preparation—Produced from pooled units of human plasma from normal donors by modifications and refinements of the cold ethanol method of Cohn (Cohn EJ, et al. *J Am Chem Soc* 1946; 68(3): 459.).

Table 67-3. Factor VIII Products

PRODUCT	PURIFICATION METHOD	PURITY
Human plasma–derived Factor VIII		
Alphanate (*Alpha Therapeutics*)	Solvent and detergent	High purity with VWF under evaluation
Hemofil M (*Baxter Healthcare*)	Monoclonal antibody plus solvent and detergent	High purity with reduced VWF
Trace amounts of murine protein		
Humate-P (*Centeon*)	Glycine precipitation; pasteurized	Some VWF
Koate-HP (*Cutter*)	Gel chromatography and solvent and detergent	High purity
Monoclate-P (*Centeon*)	Monoclonal antibody and heat treatment	High purity with reduced VWF
Trace amounts of murine protein		
Porcine plasma-derived Factor VIII		
Hyate: C (*Speywood*)	Cryoprecipitate fractionation	High purity with significant VWF
Recombinate Factor VIII		
Bioclate (*Centeon*)	Recombinant DNA product	Highest purity
Trace amounts of murine, hamster, and bovine protein		
Helixate (*Centeon*)	Recombinant DNA product	Highest purity
Trace amounts of murine and hamster protein		
Kogenate (*Bayer Biological*)	Recombinant DNA product	Highest purity
Trace amounts of murine and hamster protein		
Recombinate (*Baxter-Hyland*)	Recombinant DNA product	Highest purity
Trace amounts of murine, hamster, and bovine protein		

Description—Lyophilized powder consisting of a glycoprotein of molecular weight 58,000 that has a pH of 6.0 to 7.5 upon reconstitution.

Uses—Administered to patients with hereditary AT III deficiency prior to surgical or obstetrical procedures or when they suffer from thromboembolism. AT III is the major plasma inhibitor of thrombin because of its covalent binding with the active residue of thrombin forming an inactive complex. AT III also inactivates other components of the coagulation cascade including Factors IXa, Xa, XIa, and XIIa. The neutralization rate of these serine proteases is relatively slow but is greatly accelerated in the presence of heparin. The hereditary deficiency of AT III may result in spontaneous episodes of thrombosis and pulmonary embolism, and these risks are increased with age, surgery, pregnancy, or delivery. To either treat or prevent acute thrombotic events, the AT III level should be raised to normal and maintained at this level for 2 to 8 days, depending on the treatment indication as well as the patient's medical condition. In some situations such as hemorrhage or acute thrombosis, following surgery, or concomitant heparin therapy, the half-life of AT III may be decreased, so plasma levels should be monitored more frequently, and dosage or frequency of drug administration adjusted as necessary.

Dose—*Intravenous* administration of 1 U/kg raises the level of AT III by 1% to 2%, depending on the patient's condition. The loading dose should be determined on an individual basis, based on the pretherapy AT III level, to achieve the level found in normal plasma, using the following formula:

$$\text{Dosage units} = \frac{[\text{Desired AT III level (\%)} - \text{baseline AT III level (\%)}] \times \text{weight (kg)}}{1.4}$$

This formula is based on an expected incremental increase of 1.4% per IU/kg administered. As the increase varies among patients, it is essential to measure AT III levels preceding and 20 min postinfusion so that subsequent doses can be adjusted if necessary on the basis of the initial dose effect. Plasma levels of AT III should be monitored initially at least twice daily until the patient is stabilized and thereafter once every 24 hr with the goal of keeping plasma AT III levels above 80%. Levels should always be obtained before the next infusion of Thrombate III. Plasma levels between 80% and 120% usually are maintained by dosing every 24 hr with 60% of the initial loading dose. These recommendations are a general guideline for therapy, and adjustments in the maintenance dose and dosing intervals should be based on the actual AT III levels achieved. The suggested rate of infusion is 50 IU/min and should not exceed 100 IU/min.

ANTI-INHIBITOR COAGULANT COMPLEX

Autoplex; Feiba

A cryodesiccated complex of activated and precursor clotting factors and factors of the kinin-generating system that is prepared from pooled human plasma. It is standardized by its ability to restore normal clotting time to Factor VIII–deficient plasma. One correctional unit will correct the clotting time to 35 sec in the ellagic acid-APTT test. The complex is reconstituted with Sterile Water for Injection.

There should be no more than 2 U/mL of heparin and 0.02 *M* citrate after reconstitution.

Uses—As an alternative treatment for hemorrhagic diathesis in patients with titers of Factor VIII inhibitors above 5 Bethesda Units/mL only after the failure of conventional treatment. It is contraindicated when signs of fibrinolysis or disseminated intravascular coagulation exist. It may cause transient hypofibrogenemia in children, so fibrinogen levels should be monitored in young patients. Headache, flushing, tachycardia, and hypotension may result from too-rapid infusion. It is not free of the risk of serum hepatitis.

Dose—*Intravenous, initially* 25 to 100 U/kg, to be adjusted according to APTT 30 min after the end of infusion. The infusion rate should not exceed 10 mL/min.

FACTOR IX COMPLEX

Konyne

A preparation of pooled human plasma protein fraction containing clotting Factors II, VII, IX, and X and low levels of Factor VIII. The preparation is standardized in terms of Factor IX; the activity is one International unit (IU) of Factor IX, which is approximately equal to the level of Factor IX found in 1.0 mL of fresh normal plasma.

Preparation—See US Pat 3,717,708.

Description—White powder with a slight odor; fairly stable in light and air but unstable in heat. After reconstitution, solutions are stable up to 3 hr at room temperature; however, they should only be prepared immediately before use.

Solubility—Soluble in water.

Comments—Principally, as a source of Factor IX for the treatment of hemophilia B, a form of hemophilia separate and distinct from the more prevalent hemophilia A, or classic Factor VIII–deficient hemophilia. It can be used for the treatment of bleeding episodes in patients with hemophilia A (Factor VIII deficient) who have inhibitors to Factor VIII. Unlike earlier preparations, which were associated with a significant risk of posttransfusion hepatitis, the heat treatment employed in the preparation is thought to reduce the incidence of infectious transmission substantially. It also can be used in the treatment of congenital deficiencies of the other vitamin K–dependent coagulation factors, namely, Factors II, and X.

See Table 67-4.

Anticoagulants

Anticoagulants are substances or drugs that delay blood coagulation. They are of three general types.

Calcium Sequestering Agents—Calcium is essential to several steps in the clotting process; hence, its removal prevents clotting. The calcium-sequestering agents tie up calcium and other divalent cations; these agents are employed only in withdrawn blood. Thus, they find their most common use in anticoagulant solutions used by blood banks. These substances act rapidly, and their effect can be overcome rapidly by adding or

Table 67-4. Factor IX Products

PRODUCT	PURIFICATION METHOD	PURITY
Human Factor IX complexes		
Bebulin VH (*Immuno*)	2-step vapor heat treatment of 10 hr at 60° plus 1 hr at 80°	Hepatitis safety
Low Factor VII		
Konyne-80 Factor IX Complex (*Bayer Biologicals*)	Heat-treated for 72 hr at 80°	Low risk for HIV and hepatitis transmission
Low Factor VII		
Profilnine SD (*Alpha Therapeutics*)	Solvent and detergent (TNBP and polysorbate 80)	Reduced risk for HIV and hepatitis transmission
Low Factor VII		
Proplex T Factor IX Concentrate[a] (*Baxter-Biotech*)	Heat-treated for 144 hr at 60°	Risk for hepatitis and HIV seroconversion
Purified Factor IX products		
Alpha Nine SD (*Alpha Therapeutics*)	Affinity chromatography and solvent and detergent treatment	Hepatitis safety
Mononine (*Centeon*)	Monoclonal antibody and ultrafiltration	Hepatitis safety and low HIV risk
Trace amounts of murine protein		
Recombinant Factor IX		
BeneFIX (*Genetics Institute*)	Recombinant DNA product	Highest purity
Very low/no risk of viral transmission		

[a] Also indicated for Factor VII deficiency.

otherwise restoring calcium to normal. Thus, citrate-containing blood is, in effect, recalcified on transfusion back into the bloodstream.

Heparin and Heparin Substitutes—These agents combine with AT III. The complex then interacts with certain activated clotting factors, namely, Factors IX, X, XI, and XII, to prevent the conversion of prothrombin to thrombin. In high concentrations the complex interacts with thrombin and inhibits its effects to promote conversion of fibrinogen to fibrin. They inhibit the aggregation of platelets. They are fast-acting drugs. Heparin has the advantage of being a naturally occurring substance.

Prothrombopenic Anticoagulants (Oral Anticoagulants)—In this group dicumarol provides the prototype of action but not necessarily of structure. Prothrombopenic anticoagulants competitively inhibit vitamin K in the hepatic production of prothrombin (Factor II), the plasma content of prothrombin thus is reduced, and blood coagulation is impaired. These drugs also suppress formation of Factors VII, IX, and X, although the effect on prothrombin is the predominant one. Drugs in this category are slow because their effect is directed at inhibition of protein synthesis, and there is a latency determined by the long half-life (about 60 hr) of prothrombin. By the same token, their action is overcome only slowly by vitamin K.

The heparin and prothrombopenic anticoagulants generally are not employed for the same purpose, since chronic medication with heparin is expensive and entails the nuisance of parenteral administration. Rather, they may be complementary, heparin being employed acutely or initially, and prothrombopenic anticoagulants being employed for longer-term therapy. Anticoagulants should be used with extreme caution in disease states in which there is an increased risk of hemorrhage. These include severe uncontrolled hypertension, acute bacterial endocarditis, congenital or acquired bleeding disorders, active ulcerative disease, and stroke, periods shortly after brain, spinal, or ophthalmological surgery, and postoperative indwelling epidural catheter use.

The enzymes urokinase and streptokinase are not true anticoagulants, although their effects to increase the fibrinolytic activity of blood have the effect of retarding red thrombus formation.

PROTHROMBOPENIC ANTICOAGULANTS

ANISINDIONE

Miradon

[117-37-3] $C_{16}H_{12}O_3$ (252.27).

Preparation—By rearrangement of 3-(p-methoxybenzylidene) phthalide. US Pat 2,899,359.

Description—White or off-white, crystalline powder.

Solubility—Practically insoluble in water.

Comments—A prothrombopenic anticoagulant with actions and uses similar to those of *Dicumarol*. It is reserved for patients who cannot tolerate coumarins. Its onset of action is 24 to 72 hr, and duration of action is ordinarily 3 to 5 days. The effective dose and duration of action are affected by factors including dietary intake, bacterial synthesis of vitamin K, and concurrently administered drugs that affect the hepatic microsomal drug-metabolizing system. Agranulocytosis, dermatitis, and hepatitis have occurred in patients on this drug, so blood studies and liver function tests need to be performed periodically. If fever or dermatitis appears, the drug should be discontinued because of the possible danger of blood dyscrasias. As with other oral anticoagulants, the bleeding risk is increased and dose-related. Patients should be advised to have periodic coagulation testing. Overdoses can be antagonized with phytonadione (vitamin K₁) but there is a long delay before prothrombin levels return to a safe range. It may cause some orange discoloration of urine that may obscure onset of hematuria, an important sign of impending hemorrhage; the color disappears on acidification. Hemorrhagic complications, including hemorrhagic necrosis, and drug interactions are as for *Dicumarol*. The drug is contraindicated in pregnancy because of its teratogenic effects.

DICUMAROL

2H-1-Benzopyran-2-one, 3,3′-methylenebis[4-hydroxy-, Biscumarol; Bishydroxycoumarin; Dicumarol

3,3′-Methylenebis[4-hydroxycoumarin] [66-76-2] $C_{19}H_{12}O_6$ (336.30).

Preparation—Methyl acetylsalicylate is stirred with sodium, thus effecting ring closure through demethanolation to form the sodium derivative of 4-hydroxycoumarin. Treatment with HCl liberates 4-hydroxycoumarin, which readily forms methylenebishydroxycoumarin on heating with formaldehyde and water.

Description—White or creamy white, crystalline powder, with a faint, pleasant odor and a slightly bitter taste; melts at about 290°.

Solubility—Practically insoluble in water, alcohol, or ether; slightly soluble in chloroform; readily soluble in solutions of fixed alkali hydroxides.

Comments—A *prothrombopenic anticoagulant*. It depresses hepatic production of prothrombin, probably by competing with vitamin K, both for transportation into liver cells and at the major site of vitamin K–dependent synthesis of clotting factors; the resultant lowering of the blood level of prothrombin renders the blood less coagulable. The plasma levels of VII, IX, and X also are depressed; indeed, in some persons the major effect of dicumarol is upon these factors. Plasma levels of Factor VII are the first to fall, since it has a half-life of about 6 hr; the half-lives of Factors IX, X, and II (prothrombin) are 20, 40, and 60 hr, respectively.

It has advantages over heparin for ambulatory and prolonged anticoagulant therapy in that it is *orally effective*, has a longer duration of action (2–7 days; plasma half-life, about 8.2 hr at low doses, but up to 30 hr at high doses), and is considerably less expensive. It is unsuitable for short-term or emergency therapy in that the maximal effect of a full initial dose does not occur for 48 to 96 hr after administration, which reflects both the long half-life of prothrombin and the slow onset of the steady state. During the period of onset of action, heparin may be given. This drug or one of its congeners is employed for long-term therapy to a much greater extent than heparin. Patients must have their therapy monitored by frequent prothrombin tests, preferably with the International Normalized Ratio (INR), to avoid thrombosis or hemorrhage due to under- or overcoagulation. It may be used in the treatment of the following: *pulmonary embolism,* to prevent further embolism; primary acute and postoperative *thrombophlebitis* and *traumatic injuries to blood vessels,* to forestall *venous thrombosis* and to prevent *thromboemboli;* sudden *arterial occlusion from thrombosis or embolism;* prophylaxis of *postoperative venous thrombosis or embolism or vascular surgery,* and prophylaxis after mechanical prosthetic valves or tissue heart valves.

In the absence of specific contraindications, it frequently is used routinely in acute *coronary thrombosis* with myocardial infarction. It also is advocated in the treatment of chronic diseases that predispose to thrombi or emboli, such as congestive heart failure, persistent phlebitis migrans, recurrent thrombophlebitis, recurrent coronary thrombosis, and atrial fibrillation. However, the exact status of such long-term therapy is undetermined.

The aim of treatment is to maintain the blood prothrombin activity at a level of 15% to 25% of normal. The onset of action is 1 to 5 days; the duration is 2 to 10 days.

With the recommended dosage, the incidence of hemorrhage is 2% to 4%, and strict laboratory control is mandatory to prevent hemorrhagic diatheses. Bleeding is most common from the mucous membranes, skin, gastrointestinal tract, urogenital tract, and uterus. Stools should be monitored for occult blood loss and urine for hematuria. Hemorrhage can be arrested by vitamin K (which has a latency), fresh frozen plasma, whole blood, or Factor IX concentrate (which contains prothrombin along with other vitamin K–dependent coagulation factors).

Other side effects include anorexia, nausea, vomiting, and diarrhea. Rarely, there may be hypersensitivity reactions, such as purpura; alopecia; urticaria; necrosis of the skin, breast, and genitals; and purple coloration of the toes. Tissue necrosis has been associated with protein C deficiency and may be minimized by concurrent heparin therapy for the first 5 to 7 days of treatment. Protein C, a plasma glycoprotein, is a vitamin K–dependent factor that upon activation functions as an endogenous anticoagulant.

It has perhaps the most drug interactions of any commonly prescribed agent, as well as being affected by the nutritional and health status of the patient, all of which may lead to unpredictable results. Therefore, whenever a patient on this drug is subjected to a new drug regimen or an old drug is withdrawn, it is essential that the patient's prothrombin time be monitored and the dosage of dicumarol be adjusted if necessary.

Drug interactions occur in various ways. Mechanisms of antagonism and offending drugs are as follows (*italics* indicate the most-important clinical interactions):

Interference with absorption: *griseofulvin, cholestyramine,* clofibrate.

Stimulation of synthesis of clotting factors: *vitamin K,* glucocorticoids, estrogens.

Induction of hepatic enzymes: *barbiturates, ethchlorvynol, glutethimide, carbamazepine, griseofulvin,* meprobamate, phenytoin, rifampin.

Mechanisms of increasing the response to dicumarol, and the offending drugs are as follows:

Displacement from plasma protein: *aspirin, chloral hydrate* (as the trichloroacetate metabolite), *clofibrate,* diazoxide, ethacrynic acid, mefenamic acid, nalidixic acid, phenylbutazone and hydroxyphenylbutazone, long-acting sulfonamides.

Inhibition of hepatic metabolism: *chloramphenicol, clofibrate,* oral hypoglycemics, *cimetidine, disulfiram,* allopurinol, mercaptopurine, methylphenidate, nortriptyline.

Decrease in availability of vitamin K: *anabolic steroids, broad-spectrum antibiotics, clofibrate, cholestyramine, mineral oil,* D-thyroxine.

Inhibition of synthesis of clotting factors: acetaminophen, *anabolic steroids, glucagon,* mercaptopurine, *quinidine, salicylates.*

Increased catabolism of clotting factors: *anabolic steroids,* D-thyroxine.

Increased binding affinity to receptor enzyme: D-thyroxine.

Additivity of anticoagulant effects: *heparin, salicylates,* quinidine.

A complete table of interactions may be found in *USP DI.*

The drug is contraindicated if laboratory facilities are unavailable for determining prothrombin levels, and vitamin K, fresh blood, or plasma is not available. It also is contraindicated in any person with hemorrhagic tendencies, blood dyscrasias, peptic ulcer, ulcerative colitis, colitis, diverticulitis, subacute bacterial endocarditis, recent operations on the central nervous system (CNS), regional or lumbar block anesthesia, and severe renal or liver disease. Not only is it contraindicated in threatened abortion, but it should be withheld in pregnancy, since hemorrhage in the fetus can occur, and several teratogenic abnormalities including hydrocephaly, microcephaly, optic atrophy, other CNS defects, nasal hypoplasia, and chondrodysplasia punctata have been attributed to the drug. Patients with congestive heart failure are more sensitive to dicumarol than persons with normal cardiac function.

It is metabolized by the hepatic cytochrome P450 system. The half-life is 24 to 96 hr.

WARFARIN SODIUM

2H-1-Benzopyran-2-one, 4-hydroxy-3-(3-oxo-1-phenylbutyl)-, sodium salt; Coumadin; Panwarfin

3-(α-Acetonylbenzyl)-4-hydroxycoumarin sodium salt [129-06-6] $C_{19}H_{15}NaO_4$ (330.31); an amorphous solid or a crystalline clathrate. The clathrate consists principally of sodium warfarin, isopropyl alcohol, and water, the molecular proportions of which vary between 8:4:0 and 8:2:2.

Preparation—By addition of 4-hydroxycoumarin to benzalacetone under the catalytic influence of a mildly basic substance such as ammonia or piperidine. The reaction is a typical Michael *condensation.* Conversion to the sodium salt is effected by reacting purified warfarin with an equimolar portion of dilute NaOH solution at room temperature.

Description—White, odorless, amorphous or crystalline powder with a slightly bitter taste; discolored by light; pH (1 in 100 solution) 7.2 to 8.3.

Solubility—Very soluble in water, freely soluble in alcohol; very slightly soluble in chloroform or ether.

Comments—The most widely used *prothrombopenic anticoagulant* (see *Dicumarol*). Although usually it is administered orally, its chief distinction from other prothrombopenic drugs is the fact that it is water-soluble and may be administered intravenously. By the intravenous route its onset of action is 12 to 18 hr, and its duration is 5 to 6 days. It is metabolized by the hepatic cytochrome P-450 system. The plasma half-life is 41 to 57 hr, except about 27 hr in alcoholics and probably even less in persons using phenobarbital or other hepatic microsomal enzyme inducers.

The hemorrhagic complications, precautions, and drug interactions are those of *Dicumarol.* Influenza vaccine increases the response; this interaction probably occurs also with dicumarol and anisindione.

Dose—*Oral, intramuscular,* or *intravenous,* adults, 10 to 15 mg for 2 to 4 days, followed by a daily *maintenance* dose of 2 to 10 mg, according to the prothrombin time. A prothrombin time 1.2 to 1.5 times the control time is effective for anticoagulation yet is associated with an incidence of hemorrhage of only 4.3%.

NONPROTHROMBOPENIC ANTICOAGULANTS

ANTICOAGULANT CITRATE DEXTROSE SOLUTION MODIFIED

ACD Solution Modified

Each sterile 10 mL contains 80 mg citric acid, 224 mg anhydrous sodium citrate, and 120 mg anhydrous dextrose.

Comments—It is used with *Sodium Chromatic Cr 51 Injection* for the labeling of erythrocytes in *in vitro* and *in vivo* diagnostic tests.

ANTICOAGULANT CITRATE DEXTROSE SOLUTION

ACD Solution

A sterile solution of citric acid ($C_6H_8O_7$), sodium citrate ($C_6H_5Na_3O_7.2H_2O$), and dextrose ($C_6H_{12}O_6.H_2O$) in water for injection. It contains no antimicrobial agents.

Preparation—See the USP.

Comments—The citrate chelates calcium ions and thus acts as an anticoagulant. The ratio of citric acid to sodium citrate is such that the pH is optimal for storage of whole blood. The dextrose provides a substrate for glycolysis during storage, thus extending the lifetime of the erythrocytes. The expiration time of whole blood anticoagulated with ACD solution is 21 days. The sterile solution is employed mainly for the anticoagulation and preservation of whole blood for transfusion.

ANTICOAGULANT CITRATE PHOSPHATE DEXTROSE SOLUTION

CPD Solution

A sterile solution of citric acid ($C_6H_8O_7$), sodium citrate ($C_6H_5Na_3O_7.2H_2O$), sodium biphosphate ($NaH_2PO_4.H_2O$), and dextrose ($C_6H_{12}O_6.H_2O$) in water for injection. It contains no antimicrobial agents.

Preparation—See the USP.

Description—Clear, colorless, odorless liquid; pH 5.0 to 6.0.

Comments—Citrate ion chelates calcium, thus making calcium unavailable to the coagulation system. Citric acid, sodium citrate, and sodium biphosphate are in the proper proportions to buffer the solution at the optimal pH for the storage of blood and its components. Dextrose provides a substrate for glycolysis and increases both storage and posttransfusion lives of blood cells. The expiration time of whole blood with CPD solution is 21 days. The 2,3-diphosphoglycerate (2,3-DPG) content of erythrocytes stored in CPD solution is 120% of the original content at 7 days and 40% at 21 days. The preservation helps keep the oxygen affinity of hemoglobin low so that it can yield its oxygen readily to the tissues. Consequently, CPD is the preferred anticoagulant for blood to be used for exchange transfusion.

The sodium concentration is 284 mEq/L, and 17.8 mEq is thus added to each unit of whole blood.

ANTICOAGULANT SODIUM CITRATE SOLUTION

A sterile 4% solution of sodium citrate $C_6H_5Na_3O_7H_2O$ (294.10) in water for injection. It contains no antimicrobial agents.

Preparation—Dissolve 40 g sodium citrate in sufficient water for injection to make 1000 mL, and filter until clear. Place the solution in suitable containers, and sterilize.

Note—Anhydrous sodium citrate (35.1 g) may be used instead of the dihydrate.

Description—Clear, colorless solution possessing a slightly saline taste; pH 6.4 to 7.5.

Comments—Prevents clotting of blood by forming an undissociated calcium citrate chelate. The solution also prevents either crenation or swelling of the cells. The sterile solution is employed for preparation of blood for fractionation, for banked blood for transfusion, and for preparation of citrated human plasma.

EDETATE DISODIUM—page 1343.

ANTICOAGULANT CITRATE PHOSPHATE DEXTROSE ADENINE SOLUTION

CPDA-1 Solution; CPD-Adenine Solution

Comments—The addition of adenine to CPD solution increases the storage life of blood by 40%, that is, blood can now be stored for 35 days. However, CPDA-1 solution does not preserve 2,3-diphosphoglycerate as well as does CPD solution; there is 97% of the initial content at 7 days but only 10% at 21 days. Therefore, CPDA-1 whole blood should not be used in exchange transfusion.

Application—14 mL per 100 mL of whole blood.

DANAPROID SODIUM

Orgaran

Preparation—It is extracted from porcine mucosa and has an average molecular weight of approximately 5500.

Description—Danaproid consists of heparan sulfate (84%), dermatan sulfate (12%), and a small amount of chondroitin 4- and 6-sulfates (4%) as the sodium salts.

Comments—It is an antithrombotic that acts via antithrombin III to inhibit both Factor Xa and thrombin, with additional inhibitory effect on thrombin through heparin cofactor II. Its predominant inhibitory effect is exerted on Factor Xa with the anti-Xa and antithrombin ratio of >22. It has little effect on clotting tests (ie, the partial thromboplastin time [PTT] or prothrombin time [PT]) so they are not useful for monitoring therapy with this drug. It has only minor effects on platelet function and aggregability. It is indicated for the prophylaxis of postoperative deep venous thrombosis, which may lead to pulmonary embolism in patients undergoing elective hip replacement therapy. The drug is administered by subcutaneous injection. As with other anticoagulant agents, bleeding and hemorrhage are the major adverse events, and patients must be monitored carefully while on the medication. There is no evidence that protamine sulfate is able to reduce severe nonsurgical bleeding due to danaproid. In the event of serious bleeding the drug should be discontinued and transfusion of blood or blood products administered. As the agent includes sodium sulfite as a preservative, allergic type reactions including mild-to-severe asthmatic symptoms or anaphylaxis can occur with this drug. The sulfite sensitivity is more common in asthmatic than nonasthmatic patients.

FONDAPARINUX SODIUM

α-D-Glucopyranoside, methyl *O*-2-deoxy-6-*O*-sulfo-2-(sulfoamino)-α-D-gluco-pyranosyl-(1→4)-*O*-β-D-glucopyranuronosyl-(1→4)-*O*-2-deoxy-3,6-di-*O*-sulfo-2-(sulfoamino)-α-D-glucopyranosyl-(1→4)-*O*-2-*O*-sulfo-α-L-idopyranuronosyl-(1→4)-2-deoxy-2-(sulfoamino)-, 6-(hydrogen sulfate), decasodium salt; Arixtra

recommended dose, fondaparinux sodium does not affect fibrinolytic activity or bleeding time.

LOW-MOLECULAR-WEIGHT HEPARINS

Ardeparin, Dalteparin, Enoxaparin, Fragmin, Lovenox, Normiflo

There are several products consisting of a mixture of low-molecular-weight fragments of heparin obtained by the depolymerization of unfractionated porcine heparin. Ardeparin contains fragments of 5650 to 6350 daltons, Dalteparin contains fragments of 2000 to 9000 daltons, and Enoxaparin contains fragments of 2000 to 8000 daltons.

Comments—Standard heparin forms a ternary complex with AT III and thrombin, whereas the low-molecular-weight heparins form primarily binary complexes with AT III. This results in enhanced inhibition of Factor Xa, with less inhibitory effect on thrombin. As with heparin, these agents also inhibit thrombin by binding to heparin cofactor II. As small heparin molecules bound to AT III react only slightly with platelets, deep vein thrombosis can be prevented or retarded without as much risk of hemorrhage as with standard heparin.

Ardeparin is indicated for the prevention of deep vein thrombosis that may lead to pulmonary embolism in patients following knee replacement therapy. Dalteparin is indicated for the prophylaxis of deep venous thrombosis in patients undergoing abdominal surgery who are at risk for thromboembolic complications, ie, those over age 40, obese, having general anesthesia lasting more than 30 min, or those with a malignancy or previous history of thrombosis.

Enoxaparin is indicated for the prevention of deep venous thrombosis in patients undergoing hip or knee replacement therapy as well as for patients undergoing abdominal surgery who are at risk for thromboembolic complications. These agents have also been used (off-label) for systemic anticoagulation for both primary and secondary prophylaxis against thromboembolic events. These drugs are administered by subcutaneous injection only. The incidence of hemorrhagic complications is lower than with standard heparin; however, protamine sulfate is useful in treating patients who do experience hemorrhagic events. The concomitant use of antiplatelet agents or oral anticoagulants may increase the risk of hemorrhage.

[114870-03-0] $C_{31}H_{43}N_3Na_{10}O_{48}S_8$ (1728.08).

Preparation—US Pat 4,818,816 (1989) and *Mini Rev Med* 2004:4; 207–233.

Description—White, lyophilized powder; $[\alpha]^{23}_{D}$ +48° (c = 0.61, water).

Comments—The antithrombotic activity of fondaparinux sodium is the result of antithrombin III (ATIII)-mediated selective inhibition of Factor Xa. By selectively binding to ATIII, fondaparinux sodium potentiates (about 300 times) the innate neutralization of Factor Xa by ATIII. Neutralization of Factor Xa interrunpts the blood coagulation cascade and thus inhibits thrombin formation and thrombus development.

Fondaparinux sodium does not inactivate thrombin (activated Factor II) and has no known effect on platelet function. At the

These drugs should be administered with particular caution in patients who have a history of heparin-induced thrombocytopenia. In addition, there have been cases of epidural or spinal hematomas causing long-term or permanent paralysis with the use of low-molecular-weight heparins or heparinoids in patients undergoing spinal or dural anesthesia. The risk appears to be increased by repeated epidural or spinal puncture, by the use of indwelling epidural catheters, or by concomitant use of other drugs affecting hemostasis.

TINZAPARIN SODIUM

Tinzaparin sodium; Innohep, Logiparin

[9041-08-1].

n =1-25, R= H or SO₃Na
R' =H or SO₃Na or COMe
R" =H and R'''=CO₂Na or
R" =CO₂Na and R'''=H

Preparation—A low molecular weight heparin prepared by enzymatic depolymerization of porcine mucosal heparin with Flavobacterium heparinum. The reaction is followed using UV absorption (230-235 nm) and refractive index of a filtered portion of the medium to determine when the desired molecular weight is achieved.
US Pat 5,106,734 (1992).

Description—Average MW ranges from 5.5 to 7.5 kDa with 10% less than 2 kDa, 60% to 70% in the 2 to 8 kDa range and 22% to 36 % more than 8 kDa.

Comments-Tinzaparin sodium is a low molecular weight heparin with antithrombotic properties. Tinzaparin sodium inhibits reactions that lead to the clotting of blood including the formation of fibrin clots, both *in vivo* and *in vitro*. It acts as a potent co-inhibitor of several activated coagulation factors, especially Factors Xa and IIa (thrombin). The primary inhibitory activity is mediated through the plasma protease inhibitor, antithrombin.

Bleeding time is usually unaffected by tinzaparin sodium. Activated partial thromboplastin time (aPTT) is prolonged by therapeutic doses of tinzaparin sodium used in the treatment of deep vein thrombosis. Prothrombin time (PT) may be slightly prolonged with tinzaparin sodium treatment but usually remains within the normal range. Neither aPTT nor PT can be used for therapeutic monitoring of tinzaparin sodium.

Neither unfractionated heparin nor tinzaparin sodium have intrinsic fibrinolytic activity; therefore, they do not lyse existing clots. Tinzaparin sodium induces release of tissue factor pathway inhibitor, which may contribute to the antithrombotic effect. Heparin is also known to have a variety of actions that are independent of its anticoagulant effects. These include interactions with endothelial cell growth factors, inhibition of smooth muscle cell proliferation, activation of lipoprotein lipase, suppression of aldosterone secretion, and induction of platelet aggregation.

HEPARIN SODIUM

Heparin

A mixture of active glycosaminoglycans, having the property of prolonging the clotting time of blood. It usually is obtained from bovine or porcine lung tissue or intestinal mucosa. Potency: not less than 120 (when derived from lungs) and not less than 140 (when derived from other tissues) USP Heparin Units/mg.

Note—USP Heparin Units consistently are established on the basis of the USP assay, independently of International Units, and the respective units are not equivalent.

Preparation—Heparin is the body's natural anticoagulant, taking part in the physiological function of maintaining the fluidity of the blood. It is produced by the mast cells of Ehrlich, which are clustered in the perivascular connective tissue of the walls of major blood vessels and capillaries. Heparin is a polysulfuric ester of mucoitin. The molecular skeleton is constructed from acetylated glucosamine and glucuronic acid. The disaccharide unit is similar to that in *mucoitin sulfuric acid* and *hyaluronic acid*. Protein-free samples of heparin contain about 10% sulfur, present as ester sulfates. Original preparations of heparin contain mixtures consisting of mucoitin disulfuric and trisulfuric acids. The anticoagulant action is greater in preparations with the highest sulfuric content. Heparin in the final, therapeutic form is supplied in a solution made from the sodium salt, but in the steps of its purification the barium salts of heparin are prepared. Heparin, being a mixture of the several sulfuric esters, is not entirely homogeneous, and there is debate as to whether a truly crystalline or homogeneous preparation has been or ever can be prepared.

Description—White or pale-colored amorphous powder; odorless, or nearly so; hygroscopic. The molecular weight may vary from 6000 to 20,000, depending on the source and on the method used to determine the molecular weight. pH (1% solution) 5.0 to 7.5. It will not dialyze through a parchment membrane and only slightly through a collodion membrane. Heparin is resistant to all kinds of chemical agents, gives an insoluble precipitate with protamine and with toluidine blue, and interference with the sulfuric groups reduces its anticoagulant activity. It has a very low osmotic pressure in respect to its high degree of ionization. In contrast to the effect of oxalate, it has no osmotic influence on red blood cells. It may be stored for long periods without loss of activity.

Solubility—1 g in 20 mL of water; soluble in alcohol, acetone, and glacial acetic acid.

Comments—Its anticoagulant actions are described on page 1328. In addition, it releases lipoprotein lipase from the vascular endothelium, which has the effect of clearing chylomicrons and very-low-density lipoproteins from blood; only low doses are needed for this action. It has antiatherogenic activity, but only a few studies of its prophylactic efficacy have been made. It also has anti-inflammatory and antiallergy actions through its effects on the Hageman factor (XIIa), kallikreins, and other enzymes that have active groups containing or acting on substrates with lysine and/or arginine moieties.

It is employed clinically in conditions in which a rapid reduction in the coagulability of the blood is desired. It often is employed to initiate prolonged anticoagulant therapy to cover the latent period of onset of action of dicumarol-type anticoagulants. It also is used in lieu of dicumarol-type drugs in prolonged therapy when laboratory facilities are unavailable for determination of prothrombin time.

Some of the primary clinical applications are the treatment and prevention of *pulmonary embolism, prevention of mural thrombosis* after myocardial infarction, *initial treatment of deep-vein* and *proximal-vein thrombosis,* primary and postoperative *thrombophlebitis,* sudden *arterial occlusion* from thrombosis or embolism, prophylaxis of postoperative *venous thrombosis* or embolism, *prevention of cerebral thrombosis* during evolving stroke and after *vascular surgery.* For these purposes, low doses given subcutaneously are popular; however, recent reports indicate that blood levels are erratic, and monitoring is advisable. It is indicated for treatment of *diffuse intravascular coagulation* (DIC; consumptive coagulopathy) in patients with acute leukemia (only) and *immune thrombocytopenia* (in which vasculitis causes coagulopathy and consumption of platelets).

It sometimes is given during and after conversion of atrial fibrillation to prevent thrombosis from emboli and mural thrombi. It is recommended that myocardial infarction patients be treated with heparin for 24 to 72 hr following fibrinolytic therapy to reduce the risk of early reocclusion.

The indications for prolonged therapy are the same as with prothrombopenic anticoagulants (see *Dicumarol*), but usually this drug is used only during the early stages of treatment when the disorder is acute, to keep blood clotting suppressed until oral anticoagulants can be given and take effect. It also has special uses, such as prevention of clotting of blood samples or whole blood for transfusion; *prevention of clotting* during *blood transfusions, extracorporeal hemodialysis,* or *cardiopulmonary bypass;* and for the heparin tolerance test.

It is used in low concentrations in solutions for flushing intravenous catheters for intermittent injections; the residual heparin in the catheter keeps clots from occluding the catheter orifice. It also is used to prevent pleural and peritoneal *adhesions.* Sometimes it is used as an adjuvant to antineoplastic therapy to suppress formation of a fibrin network through which the neoplasm can spread.

Constant infusion appears to be more efficacious and safer than intermittent injection. Intramuscular injection often results in hematoma formation and should be avoided.

Hemorrhage is the principal toxic effect, usually the result of overdosage; protamine, with which it combines, may be employed for immediate control of hyperheparinemia. It must be administered cautiously when oral anticoagulants are in use or when there is thrombocytopenia, because of the enhanced risk of hemorrhage; it also interferes with laboratory tests for the effect of oral anticoagulants. The risk of hemorrhage also is increased by salicylates, dipyridamole, glyceryl guaiacolate, or other inhibitors of platelet adhesiveness.

Certain amine or ammonium compounds, especially bifunctional ones, interact with it directly and thus decrease the circulating levels in the blood; cimetidine, various antihistamines, quinine, and quinidine are examples. Even tetracyclines supposedly interact. Polymyxins and colistins are known to interact during simultaneous infusion but have not been reported to interact when administered separately.

Hypersensitivity and other adverse side effects may occur. Manifestations include bronchospasm (dyspnea, tightness in chest, wheezing), rash, urticaria, pruritus, chills, fever, vasospasm (chest pain, pain in extremities, priapism), neuropathy with paresthesias, and hair loss.

Thrombocytopenia occurs in up to 30% of patients, is often mild (platelet count remains $> 100,000/mm^3$), and may reverse or remain stable while heparin therapy continues. However, a more severe form of thrombocytopenia with platelet count $< 100,000/mm^3$ is accompanied by heparin resistance often leading to thromboembolism or DIC. Heparin therapy should be discontinued, and thromboembolic complications treated with lepirudin in such cases.

It is inactive orally and must be administered parenterally. Its plasma half-life is 1.3 to 1.6 hr.

POTASSIUM OXALATE

[583-52-8] $K_2C_2O_4.H_2O$ (183.23).

Description—Colorless crystals; effloresces in dry air.

Solubility—1 g in 3 mL water.

Comments—The oxalate anion of potassium oxalate combines with calcium ions to form the very insoluble calcium oxalate. Thus, when it is added to withdrawn (shed) blood it acts as an anticoagulant, for which purpose it may be employed in clinical laboratory procedures. Care must be exercised in its storage and use because it is highly toxic.

SODIUM CITRATE

1,2,3-Propanetricarboxylic acid, 2-hydroxy-, trisodium salt

$CH_2(COONa)C(OH)(COONa)CH_2COONa$

Trisodium citrate [68-04-2] $C_6H_5Na_3O_7$ (258.07) or trisodium citrate dihydrate [6132-04-3] (294.10).

MEDICINAL AGENTS

Preparation—Usually, by adding sodium carbonate to a solution of citric acid until effervescence ceases, evaporating, and granulating the product.

Description—Colorless crystals or a white, crystalline powder; cooling, saline taste; stable in air; the aqueous solution is slightly alkaline to litmus but should not be reddened by phenolphthalein.

Solubility—1 g in 1.5 mL water at 25° or in 0.6 mL boiling water; insoluble in alcohol.

Comments—The most important use is as an *anticoagulant* for blood or plasma that is to be fractionated or for blood that is to be stored. The anticoagulant effect is due to conversion of ionized calcium in the blood to a citrato-calcium chelate. It is an ingredient of *Anticoagulant Citrate Dextrose Solution, Anticoagulant Citrate Phosphate Dextrose Solution,* and *Sodium Citrate and Citric Acid Solution.*

It also is used as an *expectorant* and a systemic and urine *alkalinizer.* Saline expectorants are useful especially when it is desired to liquefy thick, tenacious sputum. In the body sodium citrate is oxidized to bicarbonate and excreted in urine. Thus, when given orally it is useful in acidosis, to overcome excessive urinary acidity and to assist in the dissolution of uric acid nephroliths.

It is a chelating agent and thus increases *urinary excretion of calcium* and *lead*. It has been employed in hypercalcemia and urolithiasis and to facilitate elimination of lead in poisoning due to the latter. As a *pharmaceutic aid,* sodium citrate may be used to prevent darkening when iron is included in preparations containing tannin.

SODIUM OXALATE

[62-76-0] $Na_2C_2O_4$ (134.01). The actions and uses of sodium oxalate are virtually identical to those of *Potassium Oxalate.*

THROMBOLYTIC AGENTS

The fibrinolytic system comprises a group of proteins that complexly interact to cause the lysis of thrombi and also to keep the fibrinolytic factors in check. Plasminogen plays a key role in the activation of fibrinolysis. It is a proenzyme that is converted to the active enzyme, plasmin, by interactions among circulating intrinsic factors (prekallikrein; kininogens; Factors XII, XIIIa, and plasminogen proactivator and the extrinsic factor; endothelial tissue, which releases plasminogen activator (tissue plasminogen activator, tPA). Fibrinolytic activity is kept in check by the inhibitors, C1-*in*activator, α_2-macroglobulin and α_2-antiplasmin. Once formed, plasmin cleaves fibrin into its split-products. However, it also can degrade Factors V, VIII, and XII and other proteins. The rates of formation and inactivation of plasmin normally are balanced, such that there is always a small amount of fibrin being formed to maintain normal vascular integrity and the remainder is lysed before clots form. Vascular injury and inflammation increase both fibrin deposition and fibrinolytic activity.

In the early 1960s, a bacterial product called streptokinase-streptodornase was discovered to activate plasminogen. Subsequently, the active component, streptokinase (SK) has been purified sufficiently to permit clinical use in the dissolution of thrombi. Interest has been high, especially with respect to the ability to dissolve coronary thrombi and restore coronary perfusion. Timing is very critical, because once the fibrin has *aged* (more than 4 hr), very little dissolution occurs. Originally, administration was via the intracoronary route, requiring the placement of a coronary catheter. However, SK and other thrombolytic agents now are administered primarily IV with efficacy similar to that with intracoronary delivery and fewer bleeding complications due to the invasive procedure. SK presently still confers a considerably high risk of hypersensitivity reactions.

A natural plasminogen activator, urokinase (UK) was isolated and purified for the same uses as SK. It is free of allergic potential but has a slightly lower potential for generalized fibrinolyisis and hemorrhage than SK. It is several times more expensive. There are fewer clinical data concerning the long-term efficacy of UK in treating myocardial infarction, as intracoronary administration is no longer common. More recently, several other plasminogen activators have been isolated, characterized, and modified. They are anisoylated plasminogen-streptokinase activator complex (APSAC) and tissue plasminogen activator (tPA). APSAC is an inactive complex of human plasminogen and SK that is gradually deacylated and thus activated after injection. It has efficacy similar to that of intracoronary SK in achiev-

ing reperfusion and may be slightly superior in preventing reocclusion. APSAC's major advantage over SK is its ease of administration due to the prolonged half-life.

Both recombinant forms of tPA theoretically have considerably lesser tendencies to produce hemorrhage, because they bind selectively to fibrin and not to circulating clotting factors. Thus, they are selective for the intended target, a previously formed clot. They are not free of bleeding risk, however, because they attack the many microclots that constantly are forming at the sites of endothelial breaks, and clinical opinion is divided over whether there is a significant advantage over SK and UK in this respect. In fact, target selectivity creates a bleeding problem, in that clots tend to form around the intravenous catheters used for infusion, so that heparin also is infused to prevent this effect. Furthermore, their short half-lives favor rethrombosis unless heparin is coadministered. Anistreplase and the recombinant tPA products are considerably more expensive than SK or UK.

With respect to the treatment of coronary occlusion, there is very little difference in the percentage of reopened coronary arteries and reperfusion (65–70%) or in the reocclusion frequencies (about 20%) if treatment is begun earlier than 4 hr after occlusion. It is thought by some that the very short lifetime of infused tPA limits the concentration at the target, a situation that might be correctable by higher rates of infusion. There appears to be some advantage with recombinant tPA at later times, for reasons not altogether clear.

ABCIXIMAB

Immunoglobulin G, ReoPro, Centocor

[143653-53-6]

Description—It is the Fab fragment of the chimeric human-murine monoclonal antibody 7E3 produced in mammalian cell culture. The 47,615-dalton Fab fragment is purified in a series of steps from the cell culture supernatant.

Comments—It binds to the platelet glycoprotein IIb/IIIa receptor, resulting in inhibition of platelet aggregation by preventing the binding of fibrinogen, VWF, and other adhesive molecules to this receptor. In addition it binds to the vitronectin receptor that mediates the procoagulant properties of platelets as well as the proliferative response of smooth muscle and endothelial cells. It is indicated as an adjunct to percutaneous coronary intervention for the prevention of cardiac ischemic complications in patients undergoing percutaneous coronary intervention. In addition, it is recommended for use in patients with unstable angina not responding to conventional therapy when percutaneous coronary intervention is planned within 24 hr. The safety and efficacy of abciximab have only been evaluated with concomitant administration of conventional therapy with heparin and aspirin. It has the risk of bleeding complications, which can be significantly reduced by the use of low-dose, weight-adjusted heparin, by early femoral sheath removal, by careful patient and access-site management, and by weight adjustment of the abciximab infusion dose. It is contraindicated in patients with significant bleeding risk including those with active internal bleeding, recent GI or GU bleeding, bleeding diathesis, recent major surgery or trauma, or severe, uncontrolled hypertension. In addition to bleeding, thrombocytopenia is a common occurrence and most often occurs within the first 24 hr of therapy. Platelet counts should be monitored prior to dosing, at 2 to 4 hr following dosing, and at 24 hr after dosing or prior to discharge, whichever is first. If thrombocytopenia is verified, the drug should be discontinued immediately.

ALTEPLASE (RECOMBINANT)

Activase

[105857-23-6] $C_{2736}H_{4174}N_{914}O_{824}S_{45}$ (59,050.00).

Purified glycoprotein of a single, continuous chain containing 527 amino acids, with three carbohydrate side chains. The biological potency is determined by an *in vitro* clot lysis assay expressed in International Units as tested against a WHO standard. See Chapter 49.

Preparation—Using the complimentary DNA (cDNA) for natural human tissue-type plasminogen activator obtained from a human melanoma cell line. The enzyme alteplase is secreted into the culture medium by an established mammalian cell line (Chinese hamster ovary cells) into which the DNA for alteplase has been inserted genetically. It is harvested, purified by chromatography, and lyophilized.

Description—White to off-white powder.

Comments—Indicated for thrombolysis in patients with acute myocardial infarction (MI), to improve ventricular function, reduce the incidence of congestive heart failure, and reduce mortality. It should be administered as soon as possible after the onset of symptoms. There is a standard and an accelerated dosing regimen, both of which also include concomitant administration of heparin and aspirin. The results of controlled studies comparing clinical outcomes with the two regiments are not currently available. The drug also is indicated for use in patients with acute massive pulmonary embolism when the diagnosis has been confirmed by objective means such as pulmonary angiography or lung scanning. Activase was approved in 1998 for the management of acute *ischemic* stroke in adults, for improving neurological recovery and reducing the incidence of disability. Treatment should only be initiated within 3 hr after the onset of stroke symptoms and after exclusion of intracranial hemorrhage by a cranial computerized tomography (CT) scan or other diagnostic imaging method sensitive to the presence of hemorrhage. Because of these stringent guidelines, there has been limited experience of therapeutic outcome in ischemic stroke patients treated with this drug. It is contraindicated if there is internal or external bleeding, arteriovenous malformation, aneurysm, severe hypertension, a history of cerebrovascular accident, recent (<2 months) trauma, or intracranial or spinal surgery. Adverse effects include nausea, vomiting, mild hypersensitivity reactions, fever, and bleeding. Part of the hemorrhage problem is the result of concomitant administration of heparin, which is given to prevent clots at the catheter tip and to decrease the reocclusion rate for MI patients. Alteplase is eliminated by the liver; the half-life is less than 5 min.

ANISTREPLASE

Eminase

[81669-57-0]

Preparation—By *p*-anisoylation of primary human lys-plasminogen SK complex (1:1) from Group C β-hemolytic streptococci.

Description—White to off-white powder.

Comments—Indicated for thrombolysis in patients exhibiting symptoms consistent with acute MI. Its comparison with SK is described above. Randomized, controlled studies comparing it with either placebo- or heparin-treated patients demonstrated that anistreplase significantly reduced mortality. As with other thrombolytics, it is contraindicated in patients with active internal bleeding, a history of cerebrovascular accident, recent intraspinal or intracranial surgery or trauma, severe hypertension, arteriovenous malformation, or aneurysm. Allergic type reactions including rash, bronchospasm, fever, angioedema, and anaphylaxis have been observed in patients receiving anistreplase and are similar in incidence to those with SK. Other reported adverse effects include facial flushing, nausea, vomiting, and muscle aches. The half-life of anistreplase is approximately 90 min, with a fibrinolytic activity duration of 4 to 6 hr after administration.

RETEPLASE

Retavase, 173-527-Plasminogen activator (human tissue type)

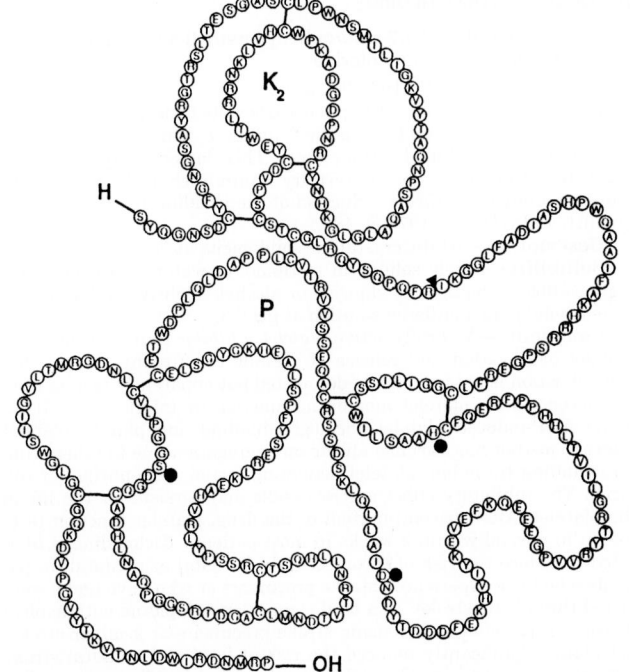

[133652-38-7]

Description—Nonglycosylated deletion mutant of tPA containing 355 of the 527 amino acids of native tPA; ie, amino acids 1–3 and 176–527. Occurs as a lyophilized powder.

Preparation—It is produced by recombinant DNA technology in *Esherichia coli,* and the protein is isolated as inactive inclusion bodies. It is converted into its active form by an *in vitro* folding process and purified by chromatography. Potency is expressed in units (U) using a reference standard that is specific for reteplase and is not comparable with units used for other thrombolytic agents.

Comments—It is indicated for use in the management of acute myocardial infarction in adults for the improvement of ventricular function, reduction of the incidence of congestive heart failure and reduction of mortality associated with myocardial infarction. The most common adverse reaction associated with reteplase administration is bleeding, and the drug is contraindicated in patients with significant bleeding risks. In addition, coronary thrombolysis may result in arrhythmias associated with reperfusion, and antiarrhythmic therapy should be readily available. Other adverse events include nausea and/or vomiting, hypotension, and fever. Reteplase is cleared primarily by the liver and kidney and has an effective half-life of 13 to 16 min.

STREPTOKINASE

Kabikinase; Streptase

[9002-01-1] Mol wt about 4700.

Preparation—A single-chain coenzyme obtained from cultures of the Group Cβ strain of *Streptococcus haemolyticus.* (*Methods Enzymol.* 1950; 19: 807.

Description—Hygroscopic white powder of friable solid.

Solubility—Freely soluble in water; unstable in concentrations of less than 10,000 IU/mL.

Comments—Indicated for the management of acute myocardial infarction (AMI) in adults, for the lysis of intracoronary thrombi; the improvement of ventricular function; the reduction of mortality associated with AMI, when administered by either the IV or the intracoronary route; as well as for the reduction of infarct size and congestive heart failure associated with AMI when administered by the IV route. Earlier administration is correlated with greater clinical benefit. It also is indicated for the lysis of objectively diagnosed pulmonary emboli, involving obstruction of blood flow to a lobe or multiple segments, with or without unstable hemodynamics. In addition, this drug is indicated for the lysis of objectively diagnosed, acute, extensive thrombi of the deep veins as well as arterial thrombi and emboli. Individuals with recent streptococcal infections may have significant amounts of circulating antistreptokinase antibodies; thus a loading dose sufficient to neutralize these antibodies is required. It is contraindicated in patients with a predisposition for bleeding. Fever and shivering occur in 1% to 4% of patients with other allergic manifestations including urticaria, itching, flushing, nausea, headache, and musculoskeletal pain, which is also relatively common. Anaphylactic reactions ranging in severity from minor breathing difficulties to bronchospasm, periorbital swelling, or angioedma have been observed more rarely but can require drug discontinuation. SK acts with plasminogen to form an *activator complex,* and the half-life of this complex is approximately 23 min. The complex is inactivated, in part, by antistreptococcal antibodies.

TENECTEPLASE

103-L-Asparagine-117-L-glutamine-296-L-alanine-297-L-alanine-298-L-alanine-299-L-alanineplasminogen activator (human tissue type); Arixtra, TNKase, Metalyse

SYQVICRDEK	TQMIYQQHQS	WLRPVLRSNR	VEYCWCNSGR
AQCHSVPVKS	CSEPRCFNGG	TCQQALYFSD	FVCQCPEGFA
GKCCEIDTRA	TCTEDQGISY	RGNWSTAESG	AECTNWQSSA
LAQKPYSGRR	PDAIRLGLGN	HNYCRNPDRD	SKPWCYVFKA
GKYSSEFCST	PACEGNSDC	YFGNGSAYRG	THSLTESGAS
CLPWNSMILI	GKVYTAQNPS	AQALGLGKHN	YCRNPDGDAK
PWCHVLKNRR	LTWEYCDVPS	CSTCGLRQYS	QPQFRIKGGL
FADIASHPWQ	AAIFAAAAAS	PGERFLCGGI	LISSCWILSA
AHCFQERFPP	HHLTVILGRT	YRVVPGEEEQ	KFEVEKYIVH
KEFDDDTYDN	DIALLQLKSD	SSRCAQESSV	VRTVCLPPAD
LQLPDWTECE	LSGYGKHEAL	SPFYSERLKE	AHVRLYPSSR
CTSQHLLNRT	VTDNMLCAGD	TRSGGPQANL	HDACQGDSGG
PLVCLNDGRM	TLVGIISWGL	GCGQKDVPGV	YTKVTNYLDW
IRDNMRP			

Recombinant (TNKase) thrombolytic [191588-94-0] $C_{2558}H_{3872}N_{738}O_{781}S_{40}$ (Mol wt about 65 kDa; polypeptide portion about 59kDa).

Preparation—(WO 93,24635) Tenecteplase is a tissue plasminogen activator (tPA) produced by a recombinant DNA procedure on a cell line from the ovaries of the Chinese hamster. It is a 527 amino acid glycoprotein formed by introducing the following modifications to the complementary DNA (cDNA) of natural human tPA:

In the kringle 1 domain; a. Substitution of threonine 103 with asparagine

b. Substitution of asparagine 117 with glutamine

In the protease domain; c. Substitution of amino acids 296 to 299 by tetra-alanine

The nutrient medium for the cell culture contains gentamycin (65 mg/L) but the antibiotic is not found in the final product at a limit of detection of 0.67 pg/vial.

Description—Sterile, white to off white, lyophilized powder.

Comments—Tenecteplase is a modified form of human tissue plasminogen activator (tPA) that binds to fibrin and converts plasminogen to plasmin. In the presence of fibrin, in vitro studies demonstrate that Tenecteplase conversion of plasminogen to plasmin is increased relative to its conversion in the absence of fibrin. This fibrin specificity decreases systemic activation of plasminogen and the resulting degradation of circulating fibrinogen as compared to a molecule lacking this property. Following administration of 30, 40, or 50 mg of TNKase, there are decreases in circulating fibrinogen (4-15%) and plasminogen (11-24%). The clinical significance of fibrin-specificity on safety (eg, bleeding) or efficacy has not been established. Biological potency is determined by an in vitro clot lysis assay and is expressed in Tenecteplase-specific units. The specific activity of Tenecteplase has been defined as 200 units/mg.

UROKINASE

Abbokinase

[9039-53-6]

Preparation—From human urine or tissue cultures of human kidney cells. (*Am J Physiol* 1952; 171: 768.

Description—A polypeptide chain of two active forms with molecular weights of 33,000 and 55,000; the principal component is the smaller of the two.

Solubility—Freely soluble in water.

Comments—Indicated for the lysis of acute massive pulmonary emboli and pulmonary emboli accompanied by unstable hemodynamics when the diagnosis has been confirmed by objective means such as pulmonary angiography or lung scanning. It has been reported to lyse acute thrombi obstructing coronary arteries associated with evolving transmural myocardial infarction (MI); however it has not been established that intracoronary administration during evolving MI results in salvage of myocardial tissue nor that it reduces mortality. The MI patients who might benefit from this therapy cannot be defined. As with other thrombolytics, it is contraindicated in conditions with a predisposition for bleeding. Relatively mild allergic reactions such as rash and bronchospasm have been reported. When administered intravenously it is cleared rapidly by the liver, with a plasma half-life of 20 min or less.

ANTIPLATELET DRUGS

Platelets play a key role in hemostasis and thrombus formation. Platelets adhere to thrombin, collagen, immunologically sensitized surfaces, and various other substances. At the site of vascular injury, collagen is exposed, thus causing platelet adhesion and the release of ADP, prostaglandins PGG_2 and PGH_2, TXA_2, and other substances. The growing platelet aggregate becomes a *white thrombus,* which may plug a small vascular break or grow sufficiently large to cause vascular occlusion. In a blood clot, adhesion to thrombin causes an aggregate known as the *white head* of a red thrombus, which by a self-regenerating process (since ADP and TXA_2 cause further aggregation) enlarges the thrombus. Serotonin, PGG_2, PGH_2, TXA_2, and platelet-derived growth factor (PDGF) cause local vasospasm, which helps arrest bleeding from ruptured capillaries.

Vascular endothelium generates prostacyclin (PGI_2), which suppresses platelet adherence and aggregation and thus is a protective substance that helps limit the progression of a white thrombus beyond the point of injury. PGI_2 is also a potent vasodilator.

Platelets adhering to the wall of a blood vessel promote atherogenesis. PDGF causes local smooth muscle cells to increase cholesterol synthesis, bind low-density lipoprotein (LDL), increase the rate of cell replication, and change into the foam cells characteristic of an atheroma. Platelets also are crucial to the process of thrombotic vascular occlusion once an atheroma has ruptured. Platelets also are involved in inflammation, bronchial asthma, eosinophilia, vascular tone, microcirculatory regulation, mitogenesis, and tissue growth and repair, but antiplatelet drugs have received little attention in these roles.

So-called antiplatelet drugs may suppress platelet adherence and aggregation and extend platelet viability by acting directly on mechanisms within the platelet (true antiplatelet activity) or indirectly, to decrease the availability of non-platelet-derived agonists that promote aggregation. Much interest has been on inhibitors of prostaglandin and thromboxane synthesis, especially of *aspirin.*

Aspirin irreversibly inhibits (by acetylation) the cyclooxygenase system that generates prostaglandins, prostacyclin, and TXA_2. The effect of decreasing TXA_2 is inhibition of platelet aggregation, but at first this is counterbalanced by a decrease in PGI_2. However, vascular endothelial cells continue to synthesize cyclooxygenase, whereas anuclear platelets do not. Therefore, within a few hours after the administration of aspirin, PGI_2 synthesis returns to normal, but TXA_2 synthesis does not. Furthermore, oral aspirin interacts with circulating platelets during absorption but with most endothelial cells only after passing through the liver, where first-pass metabolism greatly decreases the plasma concentration, and after dilution with nonhepatic blood; consequently, platelets are the more affected, and it is possible to suppress platelet aggregation with doses that have little effect on the generation of PGI_2. In addition, aspirin probably inhibits platelet function by additional mechanism(s) unrelated to TXA_2 inhibition.

Other nonsteroidal anti-inflammatory drugs (NSAIDs), such as other salicylates, hydroxychloroquin, indomethacin, etc, are not irreversible inhibitors of cyclooxygenase and are not as effective as antiplatelet drugs. Sulfinpyrazone is a weak inhibitor of cyclooxygenase and possibly may have another mechanism of action. Aspirin also has an action to suppress secretion of ADP-containing dense granules from platelets, which also contributes to antiplatelet activity.

TICLOPIDINE HYDROCHLORIDE

Thieno[3,2-e]pyridine, 5-[(2-chlorophenyl)methyl]-4,5,6,7-tetrahydro-, hydrochloride; Ticlid Hydrochloride

[53885-35-1] $C_{14}H_{14}ClNS.HCl$ (300.25).

Preparation—From 2-thiophenecarboxaldehyde plus 2-aminoacetaldehyde diethyl acetal to form the Schiff base, which is cyclized with acid to form pyrido[3,4-b]thiophene. This latter compound with α,2-dichlorotoluene yields the tertiary iminium chloride, which with sodium borohydride affects reduction of the pyridine ring to yield the product. (*J Med Chem* 1974; 9: 483.)

Description—White, crystalline solid; melts at 189°.

Solubility—Freely soluble in methanol or water to pH 3.6; sparingly soluble in methylene chloride or alcohol; slightly soluble in acetone; insoluble in a buffered solution at pH 6.3.

Comments—An orally active *platelet inhibitor* that prevents both platelet aggregation and release of granule constituents. Its mechanism of action is not completely delineated but apparently results from interference with platelet membrane function by inhibition of It. It inhibits ADP-induced platelet-fibrinogen binding and platelet-platelet interactions but has variable effects on aggregation due to other stimuli including thrombin, platelet-activating factor, epinephrine, or collagen. The inhibitory effect is irreversible and persists for the life of the platelet. After discontinuation of the drug, platelet function tests return to normal within 2 weeks in most patients. Ticlopidine is indicated to reduce the risk of thrombotic stroke (fatal or nonfatal) in patients who have experienced stroke precursors or who have had a completed thrombotic stroke. In a trial comparing ticlopidine with aspirin therapy in patients experiencing stroke precursors or a minor stroke, ticlopidine significantly reduced the risk of fatal and nonfatal stroke compared with aspirin. The risk reduction by ticlopidine was similar in women and men. Side effects were more frequent with ticlopidine than with aspirin, and GI symptoms were the most common complaint. Neutropenia is the most serious adverse effect of ticlopidine and occurred in 2.4% of patients. Consequently, patients *must* have their blood tested every 2 weeks for the first 3 months of therapy. Patients also should be advised to contact their physician immediately if they experience symptoms of infection such as fever, chills, or sore throat. The drug is metabolized extensively by the liver and is contraindicated in patients with severe liver impairment. In addition, it should not be given to patients who have a hematopoietic or hemostatic disorder or active pathological bleeding such as a bleeding peptic ulcer or intracranial bleeding.

Dose—*Oral, adults,* 250 mg twice a day taken with food.

Dosage Form—Tablets: 250 mg.

Other Antiplatelet Drugs

Other drugs work in other ways.

Dipyridamole inhibits platelet phosphodiesterase, thus increasing cyclic AMP levels, which suppresses platelet aggregation and dense-granule secretion. It also blocks the reuptake and metabolism of adenosine and potentiates the antiaggregating action of PGI_2.

Calcium channel blockers (page 1290) decrease intraplatelet calcium concentration and, hence, also suppress dense-granule secretion.

β-*Adrenergic blockers* prevent β-receptor operation of calcium channels.

α-Blockers prevent α-agonist-induced dense-granule secretion.

Anagrelide suppresses platelet response to all stimuli; its mechanism may be that of inhibiting a distinct pool of cAMP phosphodiesterase.

Other inhibitors of platelet function are dextrans, glyceryl guaiacolate (very active), penicillin, tricyclic antidepressants, glucocorticoids, clofibrate, pyridinol carbamate, PGE_1, glucagon, antiserotonin drugs, certain antihistamines, caffeine, theophylline, pentoxifyllin, general anesthetics, and ethanol in high concentration.

Clopidogrel Bisulfate—A thienopyridine derivative chemically related to ticlopidine that inhibits platelet aggregation by irreversibly modifying the platelet-ADP receptor. It is indicated for the reduction of atherosclerotic events including MI, stroke, and vascular death in patients with documented atherosclerosis. The major adverse effects include chest pain, flulike symptoms, abdominal pain, arthralgia, and purpura.

Eptifibatide—A cyclic heptapeptide that binds to the platelet glycoprotein IIb/IIIa receptor and thus inhibits platelet aggregation, similar to *Abciximab*. It is indicated for the treatment of patients with acute coronary syndromes including those to be managed medically as well as those undergoing percutaneous coronary intervention. In the clinical trials with this drug, it was shown to decrease the rate of a combined endpoint of death, new MI, or need for urgent intervention. Most patients were also receiving aspirin and heparin in these clinical trials. Experience in 1998 was limited to the treatment of large numbers of patients with this drug.

Tirofiban Hydrochloride—A nonpeptide antagonist of the platelet glycoprotein IIb/IIIa receptor, which reversibly inhibits platelet aggregation. It is indicated for use along with heparin in the treatment of acute coronary syndromes including those to be managed medically as well as those undergoing percutaneous coronary intervention. In this setting it has been shown to decrease the rate of a combined endpoint of death, new MI, or refractory ischemia/repeat cardiac procedure. Experience in 1998 was limited to the treatment of large numbers of patients with this drug.

No clinical use of antiplatelet drugs is without some controversy. In general, except for dextrans 70 and 75, antiplatelet drugs have not been found effective alone in preventing or limiting venous thrombosis and pulmonary embolism, but they probably improve the response to oral anticoagulants. In such a combination, aspirin increases the incidence and severity of GI hemorrhage, whereas dipyridamole does not. This deleterious effect of combination therapy is reduced if the dose of aspirin is lowered, ie, 325 mg a day or less. In addition, it is essential that coagulation and platelet function tests are monitored routinely, with anticoagulant doses adjusted accordingly.

Antiplatelet-anticoagulant drug combinations appear to be superior to oral anticoagulants alone in preventing thrombosis from prosthetic heart valves and other foreign surfaces. After hip surgery, aspirin alone (in men), aspirin-dipyridamole, and

hydroxychloroquin have been reported to be of value in preventing venous thrombosis and pulmonary embolism. Sulfinpyrazone decreases the incidence of systemic embolism in rheumatic mitral valve stenosis.

Aspirin is approved in the US to reduce the risk of death and/or nonfatal MI in patients with a previous infarction or unstable angina pectoris. One tablet is recommended immediately at the onset of symptoms of an MI. It also is approved to reduce the risk of stroke in persons experiencing transient ischemic attacks, although ticlopidine is perhaps superior. Completed strokes are not affected. Occlusive microvascular disorders in the fingers are resolved in 2 to 3 days and further prevented after treatment with aspirin. Microvascular occlusion after organ transplants also appears to be diminished by aspirin. In general, the combination of aspirin and dipyridamole is no more effective than aspirin alone.

There is much interest in the reputed ability of antiplatelet drugs to decrease the rate of MI. There have been two randomized trials examining whether aspirin has a protective effect in the primary prevention of vascular disease, with conflicting results. In a 5-year study, the US Physicians' Health Study, there was a 44% reduction (from approximately 0.4% to 0.2%/year) in the incidence of MI in men receiving aspirin (325 mg every other day) compared with placebo. This effect was only observed in men age 50 or over. Over the 5-year period the death rate from cardiovascular processes was similar in both placebo- and aspirin-treated groups. In contrast, in the British Doctors' Trial there was no difference in the rate of MI or cardiovascular death in the aspirin (500 mg/day) versus placebo group over a 6-year study period. In both of these studies there was a slight increase in the incidence of stroke and an increased risk of GI hemorrhage in the aspirin-treated cohort. The US Preventive Services Task Force recommends that "low-dose aspirin therapy may be considered for men aged 40 and over who are at a significantly increased risk of myocardial infarction and who lack contraindications to the drug." Aspirin therapy should be considered an adjunct approach in the management of cardiovascular disease. Reduction of significant risk factors including hypertension, high cholesterol levels, and smoking are the most effective treatment for patients at risk for MI and stroke. Of note, current epidemiological evidence suggests that aspirin is beneficial in women as well as men; however definitive recommendations must await the results of the ongoing Women's Health Study.

ANTICOAGULANT ANTAGONISTS

Anticoagulant therapy carries the risk of serious hemorrhage, so that there may be need to arrest the anticoagulant action. Prothrombopenic anticoagulants, as expected from their mode of action, are antagonized by vitamin K or its synthetic substitutes. Not all vitamin K preparations are equally effective, vitamin K_1 (phytonadione) being superior and menadione inferior. The efficacy of vitamin K preparations also varies according to the anticoagulant, but all agents of the dicumarol group may be antagonized by an appropriate dose of vitamin K_1. The antagonism is not manifested immediately, since normal coagulation is obtained only after the liver has had time to replenish the prothrombin and other vitamin K–dependent coagulation factors.

High doses of vitamin K_1 can antagonize oral anticoagulants, despite their being continually inhibited at their site of action, because high doses can activate a second latent enzyme not significantly productive with ordinary concentrations of vitamin K, which enzyme is not inhibited by the anticoagulants. Heparin is antagonized by various amines, ammonium compounds, and basic proteins that precipitate the polysulfate. Circulating heparinoid substances in the blood also can be assayed with such substances.

MENADIOL SODIUM DIPHOSPHATE—page 1700.
PHYTONADIONE—page 1700.

LEPIRUDIN

1-L-Leucine-2-L-threonine-63-desulfohirudin; *Hirudo medicinalis* **isoform HVI**

```
Leu-Thr-Tyr-Thr-Asp-Cys-Thr-Glu-Ser-Gly-Gln- Asn- Leu-Cys-Leu-
 1    2   3   4   5   6   7   8   9   10  11   12   13  14  15
Cys-Glu-Gly-Ser-Asn-Val-Cys-Gly- Gln-Gly-Asn-Lys-Cys-Ile-Leu-
 16  17  18  19  20  21  22  23   24  25  26  27  28  29  30
Gly- Ser-Asp-Gly-Glu- Lys-Asn-Gln-Cys-Val- Thr- Gly-Glu-Glu-Thr-
 31   32  33  34  35   36  37  38  39  40   41   42  43  44  45
Pro-Lys-Pro- Gln-Ser-His-Asn-Asp-Gly-Asp-Phe-Glu-Glu-Ile-Pro-
 46  47  48   49  50  51  52  53  54  55  56  57  58  59  60
Glu-Glu-Tyr-Leu-Gln
 61  62  63  64  65
```

[138068-37-8] $C_{287}H_{440}N_{80}O_{111}S_6$ (6979.56).

Description—Lepirudin is a recombinant hirudin composed of 65 amino acids and is produced in yeast. It differs from natural hirudin by the absence of a sulfate group on tyrosine at position 63 and the substitution of leucine for isoleucine at the amino terminus.

Comments—A direct inhibitor of thrombin, with one molecule of lepirudin combining with one molecule of thrombin. It has no effect on antithrombin III. It is indicated for anticoagulation in patients with heparin-induced thrombocytopenia (HIT) and associated thromboembolic disorders, to prevent further thromboembolic complications. The major adverse effect is bleeding, and intracranial bleeding has occurred in acute MI patients following concomitant thrombolytic therapy with alteplase or streptokinase. Other adverse events include allergic reations involving the skin and airways. The systemic clearance of lepirudin depends on the glomerular filtration rate, and dosage adjustment based on creatinine clearance is recommended. There is no specific antidote for lepirudin, and life-threatening bleeding requires immediate discontinuation of the drug as well as possible blood transfusion. Therapy is monitored using the PTT ratio, with a target range of 1.5 to 2.5, and current data suggest that higher ratios increase the bleeding risk without a significant increase in clinical efficacy.

PROTAMINE SULFATE

A purified mixture of simple protein principles obtained from the sperm or testes of suitable species of fish, which has the property of neutralizing heparin. Each milligram neutralizes not less than 80 USP Units of heparin activity derived from lung tissue and not less than 100 USP Units of heparin activity derived from intestinal mucosa.

Preparation—Frozen, ripe, salmon testes are ground, water-washed, centrifuged, and dehydrated by means of solvents and vacuum drying. The dried material then is extracted with 10% H_2SO_4, and after filtering, a protamine sulfate–rich fraction is precipitated from the filtrate with cold alcohol. This fraction is dissolved in hot water, and the protamine sulfate separates as an oil upon cooling. This protamine-rich oil is dissolved in hot water and fractionated again with cold alcohol. The resulting fraction is dehydrated by means of solvents and vacuum dried.

Description—Fine, white or faintly colored, amorphous or crystalline, hygroscopic powder.

Solubility—Sparingly soluble in water.

Comments—A *heparin antagonist*. Because it is a strongly basic macromolecule, it combines avidly with heparin, which is a polyanionic macromolecule. It combines with heparin in an approximately 1:1 ratio by weight regardless of the source of heparin; since the potency of heparin from different sources varies, the dose of protamine based on USP unitage also varies. It is injected slowly intravenously after suitable dilution with physiological salt solution, to counteract the effect of *overmedication with heparin*. The duration of the effect is about 2 hr.

Untoward effects are uncommon. They include abrupt hypotension, dyspnea, bradycardia, flushing, and a feeling of warmth. An overdose can itself exert an anticoagulant effect.

FIBRINOLYTIC INHIBITORS

AMINOCAPROIC ACID

Epsilon **Aminocaproic Acid; Aminocaproic Acid; Amicar**

$$H_2C(CH_2)_3CH_2COOH$$
$$\underset{NH_2}{|}$$

6-Aminohexanoic acid [60-32-2] $C_6H_{13}NO_2$ (131.17).

Preparation—The lactam group of the commercially available caprolactam (hexahydro-2*H*-azepin-2-one) is cleaved at the C-N linkage by heating an aqueous solution with calcium hydroxide. The calcium aminocaproate thus formed is reacted with sulfuric acid to free the official acid and precipitate the calcium. Various other methods of preparation are also available.

Description—Fine, white, crystalline powder; odorless, or nearly so; tasteless, stable in light and air; melts at about 205°.

Solubility—1 g in 3 mL water; slightly soluble in alcohol; practically insoluble in chloroform or ether.

Comments—A competitive inhibitor of plasminogen activators, which also expresses antiplasmin activity. It is used in the treatment of *procedures or disorders in which fibrinolysis is enhanced,* such as cardiac bypass, postcaval shunt, major thoracic surgery, prostatic postoperative hematuria, and also nonsurgical hematuria, leukemia, metastatic prostatic carcinoma, cirrhosis and other hepatic diseases, eclampsia, intrauterine fetal death, amniotic fluid embolism, and abruptio placentae. It also is used to correct excessive, treatment-induced fibrinolysis. It has been reported to be of use in angioedema and subarachnoid hemorrhage. The drug is of no value in hemorrhage due to thrombocytopenia, hyperheparinemia, or other coagulation defects or to vascular disruption.

It may cause itching, erythema, rash, diuresis, heartburn, nausea, and diarrhea. It also has an antiadrenergic effect similar to that of guanethidine, so that nasal stuffiness, conjunctival suffusion, and hypotension may occur. The drug may enhance thrombotic processes by suppression of reactive fibrinolysis, which tends to limit clot formation and favor clot resolution. Therefore, it should not be given unless there is unequivocal evidence that disseminated intravascular clotting is not the cause of elevated fibrinolytic activity. It is not known whether this drug can cause fetal harm, and it is currently in pregnancy Category C.

It is excreted by the kidney; in the presence of renal disease the dose should be reduced.

TRANEXAMIC ACID

Cyklokapron

[1197-18-8] $C_8H_{15}NO_2$ (157.21).

Preparation—*J Org Chem* 1959; 24: 115, and US Pat 3,499,925.

Description—White crystals; melts over 300°.

Solubility—1 g in about 6 mL water; very slightly soluble in alcohol or ether; 5% aqueous solution, pH 6.5 to 7.5.

Comments—Resembles aminocaproic acid in decreasing the activity of the fibrinolysis system, in part by inhibiting plasminogen; it is approved for use in hemophiliac patients to prevent hemorrhage and reduce the need for replacement of blood factors. Its most interesting use has been in the treatment of malignant ovarian tumors, to promote formation of a fibrin capsule to wall off and inhibit growth of the tumor. It also causes regression of ascites secondary to carcinoma. In these uses heparin was given concomitantly to prevent intravascular coagulation. It causes nausea, vomiting, diarrhea, occasional vertigo, and hypotension from rapid injection. It passes through the placental barrier. It is excreted rapidly in urine.

HEMOSTATICS AND STYPTICS

Many substances not especially related to the clotting mechanism are capable of promoting clotting. Upon contact with most surfaces, platelets adhere, aggregate, and release mediators that promote fibrin deposition. Spongy and gauzy materials, which provide a large surface area, thus are used to arrest bleeding; absorbable sponges may be left permanently at the site of bleeding. Fibrin, fibrinogen, and thrombin are also potent hemostatics. Astringents also initiate clotting by precipitating proteins and by labilizing platelets; mostly ferric salts are employed as styptics.

ALUM—page 1282.

MICROFIBRILLAR COLLAGEN

Avitene

A preparation of animal origin of the polypeptide substance occurring as the main constituent of skin, connective tissue, and the organic substance of bones.

Comments—Platelets adhere naturally to collagen and are stimulated to release substances that promote further aggregation. Microfibrillar collagen is used to arrest bleeding, especially during surgery except neurological, urological, and ophthalmological procedures. It usually stops capillary bleeding in 1 min, *brisk* bleeding in 4 to 5 min, and oozing from bone in 5 to 10 min. The collagen is absorbed in less than 84 days. It may cause mild, chronic inflammation at the site of application, probably as the result of slight contamination by bovine albumin. It does not interfere with regeneration of bone. It may interfere mechanically with the closure of incisions. Plugging of pores in cancellous bone diminishes the strength of methacrylate adhesives. Spillage on nonbleeding surfaces should be avoided because it may cause adhesions.

DESMOPRESSIN—page 1441.

ABSORBABLE GELATIN POWDER

Gelfoam

A fine, dry, heat-sterilized light powder prepared by milling absorbable gelatin sponge.

Comments—Sterile powder, saturated with sterile sodium chloride solution; is indicated in surgical procedures to control capillary, venous, and arteriolar bleeding when conventional procedures such as pressure or ligature are ineffective.

ABSORBABLE GELATIN SPONGE

Gelfoam

Gelatin in the form of a sterile, absorbable, water-insoluble sponge.

Description—Light, nearly white, nonelastic, tough, porous, hydrophilic solid; 10-mm cube weighing approximately 9 mg will take up approximately 45 times its weight of well-agitated oxalated whole blood; it is stable in dry heat at 150 for 4 hr.

Solubility—Insoluble in water, but absorbable in body fluids; completely digested by a solution of pepsin.

Comments—A *hemostatic* and *coagulant* used to control bleeding. It is moistened with sterile sodium chloride or thrombin solution and may then be left in place following closure of a surgical incision. It should not be used in the closure of skin incisions because of interference with the rejoining of edges. It is absorbed in 4 to 6 week.

THROMBIN

Thrombinair; Thrombogen; Thrombostat

A sterile protein substance prepared from prothrombin of bovine origin through interaction with added thromboplastin in the presence of calcium. It is capable, without the addition of other substances, of causing the clotting of whole blood, plasma, or a solution of fibrinogen. It may contain a suitable antibacterial agent.

Note: Solutions of thrombin should be used within a few hours after preparation, and are not to be injected.

Description—White or grayish, amorphous substance dried from the frozen state.

Comments—When concentrated, it has an extraordinarily potent hemostatic or clotting effect on blood. Its powerful coagulant action is employed in coagulating fibrinogen solution. It also is useful for local application to *cuts* or *injuries*. In surgery and in emergency, it is useful for local application in the control of minor oozing. For more extensive or inaccessible *hemorrhage,* a matrix must be applied to hold the thrombin in place and provide a structure for clot formation. Such a matrix is provided by various products, including fibrin foam, gelatin sponge, etc. It is ineffective in arterial bleeding.

ELECTROLYTES AND SYSTEMIC BUFFERS

The concentration of several of the electrolytes in plasma is critical for proper functioning of cells, especially those of the excitable tissues. The proper balance of the several ions is complex, depending not only on the concentration in the extracellular fluid (of which plasma is one compartment) but also on the intracellular concentration, the ratio across the cell membrane being an essential factor as well as the ratio of one ion type to another. Thus, plasma electrolyte concentrations provide only a crude clue to the electrolyte status of the patient, and balance or other ancillary studies are often necessary to determine the true electrolyte needs. Certain electrolytes, for example calcium and phosphate, serve also as structural elements in hard tissues (bone, teeth, etc) and may be employed for that purpose.

Several of the phosphates described in this section often are used to remove calcium from blood in hypercalcemia and to prevent and even dissolve calcific kidney stones rather than to add an electrolyte.

AMMONIUM CHLORIDE—page 1423.
CALCIUM CARBONATE—page 1296.

CALCIUM CHLORIDE

Calcium chloride, dihydrate [10035-04-8] $CaCl_2 \cdot 2H_2O$ (147.02); *anhydrous* [10043-52-4] (110.99).

Preparation—By saturating HCl with chalk or marble, then adding calcium hydroxide to alkalinity and boiling, which precipitates magnesium, iron, and other metals. After filtering, the filtrate is neutralized with HCl and evaporated until it contains about 24% water.

Description—White, hard, odorless fragments or granules; deliquescent.

Solubility—1 g in 0.7 mL of water or 4 mL of alcohol.

Comments—Provides calcium ions in the treatment of *hypocalcemic tetany*. It also relieves muscle spasms and pain from *black widow bites*. It is given during *exchange transfusions,* to repair the calcium deficit in citrated blood; however, calcium gluceptate is preferred for this use. It is *antispasmodic* to smooth muscle and effective in relieving

the abdominal pain and diarrhea of *intestinal tuberculosis* and *lead colic;* for this purpose it is given orally, a neutral salt being preferred. It stimulates cardiac automaticity and contractility and is used in *cardiac resuscitation.* Calcium is used in the management of *hypersensitivity reactions,* especially urticaria and angioneurotic edema, and of *insect bites* and *stings.*

It is a specific antidote in cases of *magnesium poisoning.* It is used in the treatment of *hyperkalemia,* since it antagonizes the cardiac effects of potassium.

As an *electrolyte replenisher* it is a pharmaceutical necessity for *Ringer's Injection, Lactated Ringer's Injection,* and *Ringer's Solution.*

Side effects result from too-rapid injection; these include vasodilation and a burning sensation in the skin. Overdosage can cause hypercalcemia, characterized by persistent nausea and vomiting, lethargy, weakness, coma, and sudden death. Because of the danger of overdosage, it is contraindicated in renal insufficiency, even if hypocalcemia exists. It should be given cautiously to the digitalized patient, and the electrocardiogram should be monitored. In general, plasma electrolyte concentrations should be monitored before and during use. Extravasation and intramuscular or subcutaneous injection can cause tissue necrosis. For this reason, less-irritant salts are preferred, especially in pediatrics.

CALCIUM CITRATE

1,2,3-Propanetricarboxylic acid, 2-hydroxy-, calcium salt (2:3), tetrahydrate; Citracal

$$\left[\begin{array}{c} CH_2COO- \\ | \\ HO-C-COO- \\ | \\ CH_2COO- \end{array} \right]_2 Ca_3 \cdot 4H_2C$$

[5785-44-4]

$C_{12}H_{10}Ca_3O_{14} \cdot 4H_2O$ (570.50).

Preparation—By treating citric acid obtained from citrus fruits, with lime.

Description—White, odorless, crystalline powder losing all of its water of crystallization at 120°.

Solubility—1 g in 1050 mL cold water; more soluble in hot water; insoluble in alcohol.

Comments—Most calcium compounds given orally as a source of calcium are soluble in gastric acid but are converted mostly to insoluble calcium carbonate in the duodenum, so that only a fraction of the calcium is available for absorption. Calcium carbonate, especially, depends greatly upon gastric acid to make some of the calcium bioavailable. Persons with achlorhydria, pyloroplasty, or other conditions in which a calcium compound is not in an acidic environment long enough to liberate or maintain much soluble calcium usually do not obtain adequate calcium absorption from calcium carbonate and certain other calcium compounds. In this drug, the calcium ion is chelated sufficiently firmly that a large proportion remains in the soluble form in the alkaline environment of the small intestine. In individuals with normal gastric acid secretion, 20% to 66% more calcium is bioavailable from the citrate than from the carbonate, and in persons with achlorhydria it is 100% more available. It is used to treat *hypocalcemia* and as a *supplement* to dietary calcium, especially in persons in whom there is a probability of developing or exacerbating osteoporosis.

CALCIUM GLUBIONATE

Calcium, (4-O-β-D-galactopyranosyl-D-gluconato-O¹)(D-gluconato-O1)-, monohydrate; Neo-Calglucon

[12569-38-9] $C_{18}H_{32}CaO_{19}.H_2O$ (610.53).

Comments—As a source of calcium, more as a dietary supplement than for the treatment of hypocalcemia.

CALCIUM GLUCEPTATE

D-*glycero*-D-*gulo*-Heptonic acid, calcium salt (2:1); Calcium Gluceptate

Calcium D-*glycero*-D-*gulo*-heptonate (1:2) [17140-60-2] $C_{14}H_{26}CaO_{16}$ (490.43); *hydrate* [56348-83-5] (508.45).

Preparation—From sodium glucoheptonate, US Pat 3,033,900.

Comments—To provide calcium ions when rapid availability is required. The clinical conditions in which calcium is required are stated under *Calcium Chloride*. This drug is even less irritating than *Calcium Gluconate,* so that it is preferred when intramuscular administration is required, as in neonatal tetany. Many authorities also prefer the gluceptate to the gluconate for intravenous injection, but once symptoms are controlled, maintenance usually is achieved with calcium gluconate given by intravenous infusion. The duration of action after intravenous administration is 2 to 3 hr and after intramuscular injection, 1 to 4 hr.

After rapid intravenous injection there may be tingling sensations and a chalky taste. The effects of overdoses, precautions, and drug interactions are those of *Calcium Chloride*. Mild local reactions may occur at the site of injection, but abscesses apparently do not occur.

CALCIUM GLUCONATE

D-Gluconic acid, calcium salt (2:1)

Calcium gluconate (1:2) [299-28-5] $C_{12}H_{22}CaO_{14}$ (430.38).

Preparation—D-Glucose is oxidized to gluconic acid in the presence of calcium carbonate. The oxidation may be effected by certain molds, eg, *Aspergillus niger,* or by bromine.

Description—White, crystalline granules or powder, without odor or taste; stable in air and does not lose its water on drying without un-

dergoing decomposition; solutions are neutral to litmus paper; decomposed by dilute mineral acids into gluconic acid and the calcium salt of the mineral acid used.

Solubility—1 g slowly in about 30 mL water or about 5 mL boiling water; insoluble in alcohol or many other organic solvents.

Comments—Its uses are those of *Calcium Chloride*. It is less irritating than calcium chloride and may be given orally or by intramuscular or intravenous injection. However, intramuscular injection may cause abscesses. It usually is considered to be the calcium salt of choice for intravenous use.

CALCIUM GLYCEROPHOSPHATE

Calphosan; Neurosin; Phos-Cal

$(HOCH_2)_2CHOPO_3Ca$

[27214-00-2] $C_3H_7CaO_6P$ (210.15). A mixture of the β-calcium salt (center hydroxyl of glycerol is phosphorylated) and the α-salt (end hydroxyl is phosphorylated). Since the α-salt enjoys a chiral center, it exists as two stereoisomers; only the racemic form is present in this salt.

Preparation—*J Chem Soc* 1914; 105: 1238.

Description—Odorless, tasteless powder; decomposes at about 170°.

Solubility—1 g in about 50 mL water at 20°; less soluble at higher temperatures.

Comments—The actions, uses and adverse effects are much like those of *Calcium Gluconate*. The effects of overdoses, drug interactions and precautions are those of *Calcium Chloride*. The salt is marketed only in combination with calcium lactate or calcium levulinate.

CALCIUM LACTATE

Propanoic acid, 2-hydroxy-, calcium salt (2:1), hydrate

Calcium lactate (1:2) hydrate [41372-22-9] $C_6H_{10}CaO_6.xH_2O$; *anhydrous* 814-80-2 (218.22); *pentahydrate* (308.30).

Preparation—By fermenting hydrolyzed starch with a suitable mold in the presence of calcium carbonate, and purifying until the product meets USP purity requirements. It also is obtained, now in decreasing quantities, by fermentation of the mother liquors resulting from the production of milk sugar.

Description—White, almost odorless powder or granules, somewhat efflorescent; it becomes anhydrous at 120°; aqueous solutions are prone to become moldy.

Solubility—1 g in about 20 mL of water; practically insoluble in alcohol.

Comments—An excellent source of calcium ion in the oral treatment of *calcium deficiency*. It causes less GI irritation than does calcium chloride. It is used in the prevention and retardation of *osteoporosis*. The bioavailability of calcium is not as gastric acid–dependent as is that of $CaCO_3$; consequently, the lactate is superior in many elderly patients.

CALCIUM LEVULINATE

Pentanoic acid, 4-oxo-, calcium salt (2:1)

$[CH_3COCH_2CH_2OOO-]_2Ca \cdot 2H_2O$

[5743-49-7] $C_{10}H_{14}CaO_6.2H_2O$ (306.33).

Preparation—From levulinic acid and calcium carbonate. The acid may be obtained from crude cellulose and as a by-product in the manufacture of furfural. (*Ind Eng Chem* 1956; 48: 1331.)

Description—White, crystalline or amorphous powder; faint odor suggestive of burnt sugar; bitter, salty taste.

Solubility—Freely soluble in water; slightly soluble in alcohol; insoluble in ether or chloroform.

Comments—Much like *Calcium Gluceptate* in that it is less irritating than calcium gluconate. The side effects also are essentially the same. The effects of overdoses, precautions, and drug interactions are those of *Calcium Chloride*. The salt is marketed only in combination with calcium glycerophosphate.

DIBASIC CALCIUM PHOSPHATE

Phosphoric acid, calcium salt (1:1); Dicalcium Orthophosphate

Calcium phosphate (1:1) anhydrous [7757-93-9] $CaHPO_4$ (136.06); *dihydrate* [7789-77-7] (172.09).

Preparation—A phosphate mineral, eg, *apatite*, or preferably ignited animal bone, is decomposed with H_2SO_4, resulting in the production of phosphoric acid and calcium sulfate. After filtering off the calcium sulfate, the proper quantity of calcium hydroxide is added to form dibasic calcium phosphate.

It also may be prepared from animal bones as described under the preparation of *Tribasic Calcium Phosphate,* using only sufficient calcium hydroxide to form the dibasic salt.

Description—White, odorless, tasteless powder; stable in air; aqueous suspension is neutral to litmus.

Solubility—Practically insoluble in water; readily soluble in diluted hydrochloric or nitric acids; insoluble in alcohol.

Comments—An excellent *source of calcium* and *phosphorus* during pregnancy, lactation, or mild-to-moderate *hypocalcemia* characterized by a low degree of tetany. Because of the phosphate content, it is contraindicated in hypoparathyroidism. If the tetany is severe, intravenous calcium medication is administered. See *Calcium Chloride, Calcium Gluconate, Calcium Gluceptate, Calcium Glycerophosphate,* or *Calcium Levulinate.*

TRIBASIC CALCIUM PHOSPHATE

Calcium Hydroxide Phosphate

$Ca_5(OH)(PO_4)_3$

[12167-74-7] $Ca_5HP_3O_{13}$ (502.32).

Preparation—Commercially from phosphate rock; also occurs naturally.

Description—Amorphous, odorless, tasteless powder.

Solubility—Insoluble in water, alcohol, or acetic acid; soluble in mineral acids.

Comments—Mainly for the prophylaxis and treatment of *hypocalcemia,* although it also serves as a source of phosphate.

POTASSIUM ACETATE

[127-08-2] $C_2H_3KO_2$ (98.14).

Preparation—Potassium bicarbonate or carbonate is reacted with acetic acid previously diluted with water, and the solution is evaporated to dryness.

Description—Colorless, monoclinic crystals or a white, crystalline powder; rapidly deliquesces in moist air; saline and slightly alkaline taste; aqueous solutions are alkaline to litmus, but do not affect phenolphthalein TS.

Solubility—1 g in about 0.5 mL water or about 3 mL alcohol.

Comments—Therapeutically, as a systemic and urinary *alkalinizer,* and for the effects of the *potassium ion.* Its value in hypokalemia is limited, since the condition frequently is associated with a hypochloremic alkalosis. Consequently, potassium chloride usually is preferred in hypokalemia. Acetate anion is metabolized to bicarbonate. When used orally as an alkalinizer the salt should be diluted liberally with water or fruit juice to avoid gastric distress. Indiscriminate use of this or other potassium salts may produce toxic manifestations of hyperkalemia (see *Potassium Chloride*).

POTASSIUM CHLORIDE

Potassium chloride [7447-40-7] KCl (74.55).

Preparation—Occurs in sea water and in many mineral springs. Formerly it largely was imported from Germany where it is mined at Stassfurt, occurring there as *carnallite* [KCl.MgCl$_2$.6H$_2$O] and as *sylvite* [KCl]. It now is obtained from the Searles Lake deposit in the Mojave Desert of southern California and from deposits of carnallite and sylvite in New Mexico and Texas. Another source is the Dead Sea, where considerable quantities are found as dissolved carnallite. This double salt, in aqueous solution, is treated with live steam, the two separate salts form, and the less-soluble salt, potassium chloride, crystallizes out as the solution cools. In the laboratory it may be prepared from potassium carbonate or bicarbonate and HCl.

Description—Colorless, elongated, prismatic, or cubical crystals, or as a white granular powder; odorless, saline taste and stable in air; pH (aqueous solution) about 7.

Solubility—1 g in 2.8 mL water at 25° or about 2 mL boiling water; insoluble in alcohol.

Comments—The salt most frequently employed when the action of potassium cation is desired. It is used when *hypokalemia* or *hypochloremic alkalosis* exists, as after prolonged diarrhea or vomiting or consequent to adrenal steroid therapy or treatment with certain diuretics, especially the thiazides. It is used when it is desired to elevate normal plasma potassium levels, as in the treatment of digitalis intoxication. It may be used as a diuretic. Potassium chloride is of value for the relief of the symptoms of *hypokalemic periodic paralysis,* a rare disease characterized by recurrent attacks of muscular weakness. An increase in the daily intake of potassium decreases the risk of stroke-associated mortality; an increment of 10 mEq a day results in an average decrement in mortality of 40%. Potassium salts have been found to relieve the symptoms of Méniére's disease.

Potassium chloride is an ingredient of *Lactated Potassic Saline Injection, Ringer's Solution, Lactated Ringer's Injection, Ringer's Injection* and various other parenteral and oral electrolyte combinations.

It is irritant to the GI tract, oral preparations may cause nausea, vomiting, epigastric distress, abdominal discomfort, and diarrhea. High, local concentrations in the GI tract can lead to ulceration. Esophageal ulceration may occur if there is dysphagia and gastric ulceration, especially if gastric emptying is delayed. Enteric coating lessens the incidence of such side effects but favors the development of small bowel lesions, especially when thiazides are used concurrently. In a wax matrix it has been promoted as a safe form, but esophageal, gastric, and small bowel ulcerations nevertheless occur occasionally. It is best to avoid solid forms; if they are used, they should be taken with one or more full glasses of water. Overdoses may cause paresthesias, generalized weakness, flaccid paralysis, listlessness, vertigo, mental confusion, hypotension, cardiac arrhythmias, and heart block. Death may ensue.

Signs of toxicity may occur even with apparently normal blood levels; consequently, the signs must be monitored frequently, and ambulatory patients must be apprised of premonitory symptoms. Most patients can be managed adequately and more safely with foods high in potassium and low in sodium (fruits, especially dried, and cereals).

It must be administered cautiously in the presence of heart or renal disease. It is contraindicated in untreated Addison's disease, heat cramps, adynamia episodica hereditaria, acute dehydration, and hyperkalemia from any cause.

POTASSIUM GLUCONATE

Kaon

[299-27-4] $C_6H_{11}KO_7$ (234.25).

Preparation—Glucose may be oxidized to gluconic acid by various processes, eg, electrolytic oxidation of an alkaline solution, reaction with hypobromites, or fermentation using *Aspergillus niger* or other microorganisms. Neutralization with potassium hydroxide provides the salt.

Description—White to yellowish white, crystalline powder or granules; odorless; slightly bitter taste; stable in air; solutions slightly alkaline to litmus.

Solubility—1 g in 3 mL water; practically insoluble in dehydrated alcohol, ether, or chloroform.

Comments—A *source of potassium* for management of *hypokalemic states,* such as occur consequent to adrenocorticosteroid therapy or use of thiazide diuretics, or for deliberate production of hyperkalemia, as for treatment of digitalis intoxication. The gluconate anion supposedly makes the compound better tolerated in the GI tract than is potassium chloride. It also is claimed that the potassium of the gluconate is absorbed high in the GI tract, above the location where mucosal lesions sometimes occur in combined thiazide-potassium therapy, whereas other salts are not absorbed so quickly. Such faulty suppositions and claims ignore the unavoidable chemical fact that irrespective of the salt used, potassium ion is only dissociable completely and hence is unaffected in its irritant actions and absorption by the anion in the compound.

Its sugar-coated tablets dissolve at a higher level than do enteric-coated tablets of potassium chloride but, by this very fact, are free to cause the irritation for which the chloride tablet was coated. The fact that it may cause nausea, vomiting, diarrhea, and abdominal discomfort shows that the gluconate has no advantage over non-enteric-coated potassium chloride tablets. A full glass of water taken with either greatly reduces the irritant effects of either salt. Hypochloremia is a frequent accompaniment of hypokalemia; in such instances the chloride definitely is preferred. Furthermore, since gluconate metabolizes to bicarbonate, it contributes to alkalosis, which also may be present in hypokalemia. Only in a hypokalemic, hyperchloremic acidosis (as in renal failure, dehydration, and occasional diabetic acidosis) is the drug rational; however, clinical experience indicates no obvious superiority over KCl. The use and toxicity of, and contraindications to, it are the same as for *Potassium Chloride.*

POTASSIUM MIXTURES

A number of potassium-containing products are mixtures of KCl and KHCO$_3$; KCl, KHCO$_3$, and K$_2$CO$_3$; KCl, KHCO$_3$, and citric acid; KCl, KHCO$_3$, and potassium citrate; KHCO$_3$ and citric acid; KCl and potassium gluconate; KHCO$_3$, potassium citrate, and potassium acetate; and potassium citrate and potassium gluconate. Those that combine KHCO$_3$ with citric acid are effervescent; some effervescent preparations contain betaine.HCl or lysine.HCl in lieu of, or in addition to, citric acid. Those that are not reconstituted for effervescence are intended for their alkalinizing effects in addition to their effects to repair potassium deficits. KHCO$_3$ and K$_2$CO$_3$ are directly alkalotic; potassium acetate, citrate, and gluconate all metabolize to KHCO$_3$. Since hy-

and sodium and for renal function at frequent intervals. Concurrent administration with thiazides may cause renal damage. Each milliliter of the injection described above represents 92 mg (4 mEq) of sodium, which should be taken into consideration in using the injection in patients on sodium restriction.

TROMETHAMINE

1,3-Propanediol, 2-amino-2-(hydroxymethyl)-, THAM

$$\begin{array}{c} CH_2OH \\ | \\ HOCH_2CCH_2OH \\ | \\ NH_2 \end{array}$$

2-Amino-2-(hydroxymethyl)-1,3-propanediol [77-86-1] $C_4H_{11}NO_3$ (121.14).

Preparation—Nitromethane is reacted additively with formaldehyde to yield tris(hydroxymethyl)nitromethane, and the nitro compound then is hydrogenated with the aid of Raney nickel. US Pat 2,174,242.

Description—White, crystalline powder with a slight, characteristic odor and a faint, sweet, soapy taste; stable in light and air; melts between 168 and 172°; pH (1 in 20 solution) 10.0 to 11.5.

Solubility—1 g in 1.8 mL water, 46 mL alcohol, or >10,000 mL chloroform.

Comments—For the prevention and correction of severe metabolic acidosis. It is a weak amine base with a pK_b of 7.8 at body temperature. This is close to plasma pH (7.4), so the compound is well-suited for the preparation of a buffer mixture for controlling extracellular pH.

Furthermore, at pH 7.4 it is 30% nonionized, and hence it gradually penetrates cells, where it also may buffer the intracellular contents. It can react with any proton donor, and the notion that it reacts primarily with carbonic acid or carbon dioxide is erroneous. By removing protons from hydronium ions, ionization of carbonic acid is shifted so as to decrease pCO_2 and to increase bicarbonate concentration. The excess bicarbonate then is excreted gradually in the kidney. This is an especially useful way to manage excessively high pCO_2 in *respiratory acidosis* (respiratory distress syndrome, asphyxia neonatorum, status asthmaticus, chronic respiratory insufficiency, drug intoxication, etc), in which pulmonary ventilation is inadequate. However, it equally is useful in the management of *metabolic acidosis* (drug intoxications, cardiac surgery, diabetic acidosis, etc), especially when the intracellular pH is low, since it readily penetrates cells.

It is used to prevent acidosis in cardiac bypass surgery, and it may be used in conjunction with other drugs in the treatment of cardiac arrest. The ionized drug is excreted by the kidney, so the effect is that of excretion of hydrogen ions. Elimination of the drug from the body is entirely by renal excretion. Excretion of tromethammonium ion is accompanied by osmotic diuresis, since clinical doses of the drug add considerably to the osmolarity of the glomerular filtrate. The drug should be used cautiously in renal disease. It also is used to buffer blood for transfusions, and it may be added to ACD blood as a buffer for storage purposes.

The principal untoward effects are related to its buffering action, namely that overdoses may cause alkalosis; respiration may be depressed because of the decrease in pCO_2 and increase in pH in plasma. Also, it is irritating locally because of its alkalinity; a slough may develop at a site of extravasation, and venospasm and thrombosis also may occur. The fact that about 70% remains in the extracellular space means that a sufficient amount of water must be given to prevent hyperosmolarity and hence to avoid tissue dehydration and the hemodynamic consequences of an increased blood volume.

Plasma hyperosmolarity, in general, causes hepatic and renal damage, and tromethamine is no exception. The hemorrhagic liver necrosis seen frequently in newborn infants treated with the drug may possibly have another origin, perhaps related to the route of administration (umbilical vein). The drug also causes hyperkalemia and hypoglycemia and may depress the respiratory center, especially in neonates and premature infants.

CATION-COMPLEXING AGENTS

The introduction of the arsenical war gas Lewisite and the proof by Carl Voegtlin that arsenicals combine with sulfhydryl groups led to the eventual development of dimercaprol (British antilewisite; BAL) in the 1940s. BAL has a high affinity constant because the two adjacent -SH groups enable the arsenic to attach to both sulfhydryl groups in a very stable five- membered ring structure. Such ring complexes were later called

chelates. BAL also was shown to chelate a number of heavy metals, and it monopolized the role as a heavy metal antidote for nearly two decades.

In 1962, edetate disodium was introduced into medicine. It chelates calcium (and to a lesser extent, magnesium) in addition to various heavy metals. This led to an era in which edetate was used widely to lower plasma calcium levels and to attempt the decalcification of ateriosclerotic and calcinosed organs, and later it became an important decorporant for lead. Despite a spate of even newer chelating compounds, these early drugs are still in use.

Selectivity is a major problem in chelation therapy. Monovalent cations cannot be chelated sufficiently strongly so that chelating agents can be used to decrease plasma concentrations. Certain crown ethers can sequester monovalent cations selectively, but at present, only oral cation-exchange resins are used clinically in the decorporation of monovalent ions. With polyvalent cations, selectivity is achieved through the types of reactive groups, internal dimensions, and steric relations in the reagent. Still, selectivity presently is inadequate. For example, chelating agents for calcium also decorporate zinc and other alkaline earth metals. With radionuclides, this problem is circumvented, in part, by using the zinc chelate as a reagent for the radionuclide. Development in this area has been slow, not only because of chemical limitations but also because of a small market and consequent meager investment incentives.

CELLULOSE SODIUM PHOSPHATE

Calcibind

[68444-58-6] An insoluble, nonabsorbable ion-exchange resin with a great affinity for calcium ions.

Preparation—US Pat 2,759,924.

Description—White to cream-colored powder; must be stored in tightly closed containers to minimize hydrolysis during storage. It contains about 34% inorganic phosphate and 11% sodium. Each gram exchanges approx 1.8 mmol of Ca.

Solubility—Practically insoluble in water, dilute acids, and organic solvents.

Comments—Exchanges sodium for calcium and other polyvalent cations. By the oral route it decreases the amount of calcium absorbed from the diet, supposedly without altering calcium balance. It is used to treat a type of absorptive hypercalciuria that occurs even on low-calcium diets. The effectiveness in suppressing nephrolith formation ranges from nil to much according to various reports. During treatment, hyperoxaluria and hypermagnesemia occur, both of which favor certain kinds of kidney stones. The drug is unpalatable and may cause GI discomfort. Acute arthralgias from drug-induced hyperparathyroidism have been reported. Every 15 g contains 25 to 50 mEq of sodium.

DEFEROXAMINE MESYLATE

Butanediamide, N'-[5-[[4-[[5-(acetylhydroxyamino)pentyl]amino]-1,4-dioxobutylhydroxyamino]pentyl]-N-(5-aminopentyl)-N-hydroxy-, monomethanesulfonate; Desferal Mesylate

$$H_2N(CH_2)_5\underset{OH}{N}\overset{O}{C}(CH_2)_2\overset{O}{C}NH(CH_2)_5\underset{OH}{N}\overset{O}{C}(CH_2)_2\overset{O}{C}NH(CH_2)_5\underset{OH}{N}\overset{O}{C}CH_3 \cdot CH_3SO_3H$$

[138-14-7] $C_{25}H_{48}N_6O_8CH_4O_3S$ (656.79).

Preparation—Isolated from cultures of *Streptomyces pilosus* by the method of Bickel *et al* (*Helv Chim Acta* 1960; 43: 2118) or synthesized by the method of Prelog and Walser (*Helv Chim Acta* 1962; 45: 631).

Description—White crystals; reconstituted solutions are stable for 2 weeks at room temperature.

Solubility—1 g in 5 mL water or 20 mL alcohol; practically insoluble in organic solvents.

Comments—A chelating agent that is selective for iron, but it does complex with aluminum. It is used for the treatment of *severe iron intoxication*, iron overload resulting from hemolysis (from drugs, thalassemia, sickle-cell anemia, frequent blood transfusions, etc.), or *iron storage disease*. It is used to treat *hemodialysis-related porphyria*. Stoichiometrically, 100 mg of deferoxamine sequesters 8.5 mg of ferric iron. Although it does not bind ferrous ion appreciably, it has, nevertheless, proved useful in the treatment of intoxication by ferrous and ferric salts, probably partly because some of the toxicity of ferrous salts is due to ferric ion resulting from oxidation of the divalent iron. Also, partly because complexation of the ferric ion favors further oxidation of ferrous ion and so promotes a diminution in the content of the divalent form. It can decorporate aluminum, and it has been used to manage aluminum accumulation in bone for patients on hemodialysis.

The drug is not absorbed orally and must be given parenterally. By intermittent or continuous subcutaneous infusion the drug is two to three times more effective than by intramuscular or intravenous injection. This can be achieved in ambulatory patients with an automatic syringe strapped to the waist. Ascorbic acid, 1 g twice a day, also greatly increases its efficacy.

Pain and induration may occur at the site of an intramuscular injection. Other untoward effects include erythema, flushing, diarrhea, blurring of vision, optic neuropathy, high-frequency hearing loss, abdominal discomfort, muscular spasms in the legs, itching, tachycardia, and fever. In long-term therapy, various allergic reactions, including anaphylaxis, have been reported. It is a growth factor for many bacteria and enhances virulence; *Yersinia* sepsis and mucormycosis have occurred in patients under treatment with the drug. Because of the side effects, it should not be used to treat mild iron intoxication. The drug is contraindicated in severe renal impairment. Long-term treatment has caused visual and hearing disturbances. The iron chelate (ferrioxamine) is excreted by the kidney and imparts a reddish color to the urine.

DIMERCAPROL

1-Propanol, 2,3-dimercapto-, British Anti-Lewisite; BAL in Oil

$$CH_2CHCH_2OH$$
$$\underset{SH}{|} \quad \underset{SH}{|}$$

[59-52-9] $C_3H_8OS_2$ (124.22) and not more than 1.5% 1,2,3-trimercaptopropane ($C_3H_8S_3$).

Preparation—A methanol solution of NaOH is saturated with hydrogen sulfide, resulting in the formation of sodium hydrogen sulfide (NaSH). 2,3-Dibromopropanol is added and the mixture heated at 40° under pressure. 2,3-Dibromopropanol is prepared by bromination of allyl alcohol.

Description—Colorless or almost colorless liquid; offensive, mercaptan-like odor; specific gravity, 1.242 to 1.244; boiling range, 66 to 68° (0.2 torr).

Solubility—1 g in about 20 mL water; soluble in alcohol, benzyl benzoate, or vegetable oils.

Comments—An *antidote*, in oil solution, in the treatment of *arsenic, gold,* or *mercury poisoning*. The drug may be of value in the treatment of antimony, thallium, or bismuth poisoning. It is used in the treatment of acute *lead encephalopathy* only in conjunction with *Edetate Calcium Disodium*. The thiol groups of dimercaprol compete with the physiologically essential-SH groups found in the tissues and thus remove the metal ions. The combination of heavy metal and dimercaprol is a stable compound that is excreted. It particularly is useful in hemorrhage encephalitis resulting from arsenotherapy, in arsenical or gold dermatitis, and, possibly, in postarsenical jaundice.

It usually causes hypertension and tachycardia, which lasts for about 2 hr. It often causes nausea, vomiting, headache, burning sensations in the mouth and throat, and a feeling of pressure in the throat, chest, and hands. It also may cause conjunctivitis, lacrimation, salivation and rhinorrhea, sweating, and abdominal pain. Sterile abscesses often occur at the site of injection. In children, fever frequently occurs; it appears after the third dose and remains throughout the course.

EDETATE CALCIUM DISODIUM

Calciate(2-), [[N,N'-1,2-ethanediylbis[N-(carboxymethyl)-glycinato-(4-)-N,N', O,O',O^N O^N -, disodium, hydrate (OC-6-21)-, Calcium Disodium Versenate

Disodium (ethylenedinitrilo)tetraacetato] calciate(2-) hydrate; calcium disodium ethylenediaminetetraacetate hydrate [23411-34-9] $C_{10}H_{12}$ $CaN_2Na_2O_8 \cdot xH_2O$; *anhydrous* [62-33-9] (374.27); a mixture of the dihyrate and trihydrate of calcium disodium ethylenediaminetetraacetate (predominantly the dihydrate).

Preparation—Among other ways, by boiling an aqueous solution of edetate disodium (below) with slightly more than an equimolar quantity of calcium carbonate until carbon dioxide no longer is evolved, filtering while hot, and crystallizing.

Description—White, crystalline granules or white, crystalline powder; odorless, slightly hygroscopic and a faint, saline taste; stable in air.

Solubility—Freely soluble in water.

Comments—Primarily in the diagnosis and treatment of *lead poisoning* but may be used for removing certain other heavy metals from the body. As a diagnostic agent, it causes a surge of lead into the urine, the magnitude of which reveals the extent of the body's burden of lead. Treatment is usually by intravenous infusion, but in lead encephalopathy the infusion fluid exacerbates the cerebral edema, so the drug is given, instead, by the intramuscular route in a hyperosmotic concentration. Since this agent already contains calcium it is useless as an anticoagulant or for treatment of hypercalcemia. Indeed, the purpose of calcium in the compound is to prevent the loss of calcium.

During infusion there may be transitory hypotension, inversion of the T-wave of the ECG, and prolongation of prothrombin time. Fever sometimes occurs 4 to 8 hr after an infusion. It is accompanied by malaise, fatigue, thirst, and chills. Myalgia, headache, vomiting, and increased urinary urgency often follow. Sneezing, nasal congestion, lacrimation, glycosuria, anemia, and dermatitis also occasionally occur. Edetate sometimes causes a usually reversible hydropic degeneration of the renal tubular epithelium, especially in the lower nephron. Some of the adverse effects are the result of decorporation of zinc.

It is eliminated entirely in the urine, with a half-life of 1 hr, except longer in renal insufficiency.

EDETATE DISODIUM

Glycine, N,N'-1,2-ethanediylbis[N-(carboxymethyl)-, disodium salt, dihydrate; Diso-Tate; Endrate; Edathamil; Disodium Versenate

$(HOOCCH_2)_2NCH_2CH_2N(CH_2COONa)_2 \cdot 2H_2O$

Disodium (ethylenedinitrilo)tetraacetate dihydrate [6381-92-6] $C_{10}H_{14}N_2Na_2O_8 \cdot 2H_2O$ (372.24); *anhydrous* [139-33-3] (336.21).

Preparation—(Ethylenedinitrilo)tetraacetic acid is dissolved in a hot solution containing two equivalents of NaOH, and the disodium salt is allowed to crystallize.

Description—White, crystalline powder.

Solubility—Soluble in water; pH (1 in 20 solution) 4.0 to 6.0.

Comments—To remove free calcium ions from solution, since it readily chelates calcium; thus, it may be used as an *anticoagulant* in the same manner as sodium citrate. Intravenously, it *temporarily lowers plasma calcium* concentration, but the effect is too brief to be of value in the treatment of hypercalcemia; constant infusion can yield a more sustained effect. It is employed occasionally to *terminate* abruptly *the effects of injected calcium* and to *antagonize digitalis toxicity,* or *suppress tachyarrhythmias*. The drug is not effective in the treatment of arteriosclerosis, since calcium is mobilized more easily from bone. It can dissolve precipitated calcium salts.

It may cause nausea, vomiting, diarrhea, transient circumoral paresthesias, numbness, headache, and a transient hypotension. Too-rapid an injection can cause death. Fever, anemia, exfoliative dermatitis, and other toxic effects on skin and mucous membranes occasionally occur. When given intravenously, it sometimes has a nephrotoxic action. Overdosage can result in damage to the reticuloendothelial system. Prolonged infusion may cause zinc and magnesium deficiencies. It is contraindicated in patients with impaired renal function with severe azotemia and should be used cautiously in the presence of liver impairment and hypokalemia.

PENICILLAMINE

D-Valine, 3-mercapto-, Cuprimine; Depen

β,β-Dimethylcysteine; D-3-Mercaptovaline [52-67-5] $C_5H_{11}NO_2S$ (149.21).

Preparation—By acid hydrolysis of penicillin. It is precipitated from the hydrolysis mixture as the mercuric salt, which is then collected, suspended in water, and treated with hydrogen sulfide to liberate the free acid. Purification involves only recrystallization from water. Penicillamine also is obtained by synthesis.

Description—Fine, white or practically white, crystalline powder; slight, characteristic odor and a slightly bitter taste; relatively stable in both light and air; melts at about 200° with decomposition; pH (1 in 100 solution) 4.5 to 5.5.

Solubility—Freely soluble in water; slightly soluble in alcohol; insoluble in chloroform or ether.

Comments—A chelating agent useful in the treatment of *Wilson's disease* and *biliary cirrhosis* (in which the serum and liver copper concentrations, respectively, are excessively high), and *lead, gold,* or *mercury poisoning*. It especially is useful in the long-term treatment of lead poisoning because of its oral efficacy, which the edetates lack. It also is useful in the treatment of *cystinuria* and *rheumatoid arthritis;* plasma cystine levels fall in the former during treatment but rise in the latter. The mechanism in rheumatoid arthritis is uncertain but has been attributed to a marked reduction in concentrations of IgM rheumatoid factor or to the scavenging of oxygen free radicals. The drug is investigational in the treatment of biliary cirrhosis.

Side effects most often appear shortly after therapy has begun. It may cause ecchymosis, hematuria dermatitis, eruptions of the mucous membranes, leukopenia, thrombocytopenia, agranulocytosis, fever, polyarthralgia, glomerulopathy, nephrosis, lymphadenopathy, and optic neuritis. Anorexia, nausea, epigastric pain, diarrhea, vomiting, stomatitis, peptic ulcer, and disorders of taste are also common effects. Some of these effects are the result of decorporation of zinc. Tinnitus and optic neuritis occur as the result of drug-induced pyridoxine deficiency; pyridoxine supplements are advised. Cholestatic jaundice, toxic hepatitis, lupus erythematosus, bronchiolitis, alveolitis, pemphigoid, myasthenia, and pancreatitis occur rarely. Blood counts must be made every 2 weeks during the first 6 months of therapy. Once therapy has begun, treatment should be continued on a daily basis, as even short interruptions have been followed by sensitivity reactions.

SODIUM POLYSTYRENE SULFONATE

Benzene, ethenyl-, homopolymer, sulfonated, sodium salt; Kayexalate

Styrene polymer sulfonated, sodium salt; a cation-exchange resin prepared in the sodium form. Each gram exchanges 2.8 to 3.5 mEq of potassium.

Description—Golden brown, fine powder; odorless and tasteless.

Solubility—Insoluble in water.

Comments—An ion-exchange resin used for the treatment of hyperkalemia resulting from acute renal failure. The resin is given orally by a stomach tube or as a high-retention enema. The sodium moiety of the resin is, in part, replaced by potassium, which subsequently is eliminated from the body when the resin is excreted in the feces or in the enema. The potassium-removing capacity of the resin is approximately 1/3 of that possible when measured under conditions in which potassium is the only cation present. The resin should be an adjunct to other therapeutic measures, such as restriction of electrolyte intake, control of acidosis, and high-caloric diet. Untoward effects include anorexia, nausea, vomiting, and constipation. Constipation and fecal impaction can be minimized by the administration of 70% sorbitol solution every 2 hr as needed to produce watery stools. Serum potassium levels should be determined daily to avoid hypokalemia.

The resin may cause gastric irritation, nausea, vomiting, and occasional diarrhea. Especially in elderly patients, large doses may cause fecal impaction. Since the resin can sequester calcium and magnesium, hypocalcemia, hypomagnesemia, or related effects may occur, and mineral metabolism should be monitored during prolonged treatment. The drug should be used with caution in patients with actual or impending cardiac failure; the absorption of the released (exchanged) sodium may be hazardous in such patients. It also may exaggerate the effects of digitalis.

SUCCIMER

Butanedioic acid, *(R,S)*-2,3-dimercapto-, Chemet

$$
\begin{array}{c}
COOH \\
| \\
H-C-SH \\
| \\
H-C-SH \\
| \\
COOH
\end{array}
$$

meso-2,3-Dimercaptosuccinic acid; DMSA; DIM-SA [304-55-2] $C_4H_6O_4S_2$ (182.21).

Preparation—*J Chem Soc* 1949; 71: 3109.

Description—White crystalline powder with an unpleasant mercaptan-like odor and taste; melts at about 193°.

Comments—Has a broader spectrum of chelating activity than does dimercaprol, owing to the presence of carboxyl groups in the molecule. However, it is selective for lead and is used in the treatment of lead intoxication. Its advantages are that it can be administered orally and that adverse effects are few and mild. Mild, transient elevation of plasma SGPT levels occurs. An increase in copper and zinc excretion has been noted, but no pathology attributed to loss of these metals has been observed. The drug probably will eventually replace dimercaprol in the treatment of lead and certain other heavy metal poisonings. Technetium-99 (^{99}Tc) DMSA is used for renal imaging. The compound is excreted in both the urine and bile.

TRIENTINE HYDROCHLORIDE

1,2-Ethanediamine, *N,N'*-bis(2-aminoethyl)-, dihydrochloride; Syprine (formerly Cuprid)

$H_2N(CH_2)_2NH(CH_2)_2NH(CH_2)_2NH_2 \cdot 2HCl$

Triethylenetetramine hydrochloride [38260-01-4] $C_6H_{18}N_4.2HCl$ (219.16).

Preparation—See *J Org Chem* 1944; 9: 125.

Description—White to pale-yellow hygroscopic crystals, melts about 117°.

Solubility—Freely soluble in water; slightly soluble in alcohol; insoluble in chloroform or ether.

Comments—A tetramine chelating agent that lacks sulfhydryl and oxygen-containing groups and hence has a low affinity for most of the transition and heavy metals, yet retains a high affinity for copper. The relative affinity for copper enables the drug to be used for the treatment of *Wilson's disease* without the side effects attributable to decorporation of zinc. It also presently does not appear to cause the hypersensitivity and immune disorders evoked by penicillamine. However, penicillamine-induced lupus erythematosus sometimes fails to remit or even recurs during treatment. It is approved only for the treatment of Wilson's disease in patients intolerant to penicillamine, but its low toxicity most certainly will result in the displacement of penicillamine in the treatment of this disease. The only significant adverse effect observed thus far is iron-deficiency anemia; that it is really the result of copper deficiency and not iron decorporation is demonstrated by the response of the anemia to copper.

HEMATOLOGICAL DRUGS AFFECTING BLOOD PRODUCTION

HEMATOPOIETICS

Hematopoietics are *antianemics* that aid in the production of red and white blood cells; *hematinics* are *antianemics* that increase the hemoglobin content of blood through erythropoiesis or through an increase in hemoglobin content of erythrocytes. The choice of a hematinic critically depends upon the nature of the anemia. The hypochromic anemias are nearly all iron-deficiency anemias in character and are treated with iron preparations. Occasionally, other accessory factors are indicated in the treatment of the hypochromic anemias. As long as 6 months of treatment may be required to replenish the body stores of iron and correct various anemias. For example, the anemia of nurslings may require copper to facilitate the mobilization of iron from the gut and tissues.

Ascorbic acid occasionally helps promote the antianemic action of iron. When given with iron salts, it promotes the absorption of iron, in part by reducing the less-well-absorbed ferric ion to the better-absorbed ferrous ion or maintaining the ferrous state of administered ferrous salts and in part by forming an absorbable complex with iron. However, ascorbic acid appears to have an additional but obscure role in hematopoiesis; it is included in a number of iron-containing products.

Cobalt and molybdenum probably also play a role in hematopoiesis, but deficiency syndromes in man are unknown, and the inclusion of these metals in hematinic preparations is irrational. The use of cobalt even may be dangerous. Although copper is known to have a hematopoietic function, a deficiency in man severe enough to impair erythropoiesis has never been demonstrated, although trientine can cause a copper-responsive anemia.

The macrocytic anemias all respond to cyanocobalamin, but the route of administration and accessory factors depend critically upon the particular anemia. In tropical sprue, the absorption of folic acid is impaired to a greater extent than that of vitamin B_{12}, so that folic acid usually elicits the greater hematopoietic response. For reasons stated elsewhere, the promiscuous use of folic and folinic acids should be condemned. In pyridoxine deficiency, protoporphyrin synthesis and hence erythropoiesis is impaired, and pyridoxine restores normal erythropoiesis.

Iron and Iron Compounds

Iron is used in medicine in the form of inorganic and simple organic ferrous compounds (ferrous sulfate, etc) and complex ferrous compounds.

Complex (nonionic) iron compounds do not respond to the ordinary tests for ferrous or ferric ions because the iron in them is part of a complex radical. The stabilities of these complex radicals differ widely. Some are converted to simple ionic iron by the action of dilute acids, while others resist treatment with strong acids or with alkalies. The complex iron compounds occurring naturally in animal and vegetable tissues (termed *food irons*) belong generally to the more resistant class, while the complex iron compounds produced artificially are as a rule decomposed rather readily. There is, however, no sharp distinction between the natural complex iron compounds and those products artificially produced, nor is there any good evidence that they differ in therapeutic action.

Comments—The principal use of iron is in the treatment of *hypochromic, iron-deficiency anemias,* that is, in anemias characterized by a deficiency of hemoglobin. The two most common causes of such anemias are nutritional (deficient intake, especially in infancy, in childhood, at puberty, during pregnancy, and late in menstrual life or at the menopause) and chronic blood loss (especially bleeding peptic ulcer, carcinoma of the colon or stomach, bleeding from the urinary tract, or excessive loss of blood during menstruation). Iron therapy is of no particular value in other forms of anemia, such as pernicious anemia, unless patients have entered an iron-deficiency stage of the disease.

Complex iron compounds generally are less prone to produce gastric distress than the simple ferrous compounds; they also are used less efficiently physiologically. Indeed, in some complexes the iron may be chelated so effectively as to escape use altogether.

Differences exist among the different iron preparations in their local irritant and astringent actions, which are absent in most of the complex iron compounds; for this reason the less-astringent and less-irritant ferrous salts are used rather than ferric salts. The irritation occurs mostly in the stomach and upper duodenum, where the pH is low. It can exacerbate peptic ulcer, regional enteritis, ulcerative colitis, and other GI disorders. Enteric coatings allow the preparations to pass into the more alkaline portions of the gut before release occurs. However, the absorption of iron from enteric-coated preparations is less than in uncoated ones, especially in persons with bowel hypermotility. In steatorrhea or in persons with partial gastrectomy, iron preparations often are absorbed poorly. Antacids also diminish absorption. Constipation consequent to local actions of iron may be countered by cathartics, properly individualized. Suitable diet (especially liver, kidney, and meat) is sometimes more effective than the iron preparations, presumably by the cooperation of other factors.

All of the iron preparations are capable of causing severe intoxication in overdoses, especially in children. Iron preparations are a common cause of lethal intoxication in children.

ASCORBIC ACID—pages 912 and 913.

FERROUS FUMARATE

2-Butenedioic acid, *(E)*-, iron(2+) salt

Iron(2+) fumarate [141-01-5] $C_4H_2FeO_4$ (169.90).

Preparation—Ferrous sulfate and sodium fumarate are metathesized in hot aqueous solution, whereupon the sparingly soluble, anhydrous ferrous fumarate precipitates.

Description—Reddish orange to red-brown, odorless powder; may contain soft lumps that produce a yellow streak when crushed.

Solubility—Slightly soluble in water; very slightly soluble in alcohol; its solubility in dilute HCl is limited by the separation of insoluble free fumaric acid.

Comments—In the clinical management of *iron-deficiency anemias*. Its efficacy is about the same as that of ferrous sulfate, but the untoward effects are somewhat less severe. The drug may sometimes be employed without difficulty in patients who cannot tolerate other preparations of iron. When side effects occur, they include anorexia, nausea, vomiting, cramping, and constipation or diarrhea. Like other iron preparations, this drug may exacerbate GI diseases, especially ulcerative ones. The effects generally subside as therapy is continued. The untoward effects are minimized if the dose is taken shortly after eating.

FERROUS GLUCONATE

D-Gluconic acid, iron(2+) salt (2:1), dihydrate

Iron(2+) gluconate (1:2) dihydrate [12389-15-0] $C_{12}H_{22}FeO_{14}.2H_2O$ (482.17); *anhydrous* [299-29-6] (446.14).

Preparation—By metathesis between hot solutions of calcium gluconate and ferrous sulfate whereby ferrous gluconate and insoluble calcium sulfate are formed. The mixture is filtered while hot to minimize the solubility of calcium sulfate, and the filtrate is evaporated to crystallization.

It also may be produced by heating freshly prepared ferrous carbonate with the proper quantity of gluconic acid in aqueous solution.

Description—Fine, yellowish gray or pale greenish yellow powder or granules, with a slight burnt-sugar-like odor; affected by light; the ferrous iron slowly oxidizes to ferric on exposure to air; aqueous solution is acid to litmus (color of the solution depends on pH—they are light yellow at pH 2, brown at pH 4.5, and green at pH 7); the iron rapidly oxidizes at higher pH.

Solubility—1 g in about 5 mL water with slight heating; practically insoluble in alcohol; it forms supersaturated solutions that are stable for a period of time; its solubility is increased by addition of citric acid or the citrate iron.

Comments—A *hematinic,* similar to other ferrous salts. Its side effects and toxicity are those of all iron compounds; it is claimed that it causes fewer side effects than ferrous sulfate (see under *Iron and Iron Compounds*). The elixir can cause staining of the teeth if taken undiluted.

FERROUS SULFATE

Sulfuric acid, iron(2+) salt (1:1), heptahydrate; Ferri Sulfas; Feosol

Iron(2+) sulfate (1:1) heptahydrate [7782-63-0] $FeSO_4.7H_2O$ (278.01); *anhydrous* [7720-78-7] (151.90).

Note—Do not use Ferrous Sulfate that is coated with brownish yellow basic ferric sulfate.

Preparation—By dissolving iron in diluted H_2SO_4. The resulting solution is filtered and concentrated, if necessary, to the point of crystallization of ferrous sulfate. Commercially, scrap iron is used in the process.

Description—Pale, bluish green crystals or granules; odorless, has a saline, styptic taste, and effloresces in dry air, becoming white; oxidizes readily in moist air to form brownish yellow basic ferric sulfate; pH (1 in 10 solution) about 3.7.

Solubility—1 g in 1.5 mL of water or 0.5 mL of boiling water; insoluble in alcohol.

Comments—One of the most commonly employed *hematinic preparations* used in iron-deficiency anemias (see under *Iron and Iron Compounds*). The drug is dispensed most commonly as capsules or tablets coated for protection from air and moisture. The salt sometimes is mixed with glucose or lactose to protect it from oxidation.

Its adverse effects are those of iron compounds in general, but they are rarely severe when the salt is taken in therapeutic doses; however, relatively small overdoses can cause serious intoxication in infants and children. The oral solution can cause staining of teeth if used undiluted.

About 20% of this drug is absorbed when taken orally. Timed-release and enteric-coated preparations tend to be absorbed more erratically and are not recommended. Magnesium and aluminum hydroxides, present in some preparations, make the iron unavailable for absorption.

IRON DEXTRAN INJECTION

InFeD

A sterile, colloidal solution of ferric hydroxide in complex with partially hydrolyzed dextran of low molecular weight, in water for injection. It may contain not more than 0.5% of phenol as a preservative.

Preparation—To an aqueous solution of partially depolymerized dextran (intrinsic viscosity 0.04–0.07) is added a solution of alkali and a solution of a ferric salt. The mixture is heated, then cooled to room temperature, clarified by centrifugation, and the solution dialyzed against running water. After concentrating to the required iron content, the solution is filtered, ampuled, and sterilized by autoclaving.

Description—Dark-brown, slightly viscous liquid; pH 5.2 to 6.

Comments—Because iron is strongly chelated by dextran, it is not locally irritating on intramuscular injection. Absorption is rapid from an intramuscular site. Thus the drug is used for intramuscular injection in patients with iron-deficiency anemias when oral therapy cannot be tolerated or does not evoke a therapeutic response. If the drug is administered to persons not in an iron-deficient state, hemosiderosis may occur. Absorption is very slow from a subcutaneous site, and a brown stain occurs that may remain for 1 to 2 years. Consequently, in injecting the drug, care must be taken to prevent leakage under the skin. Injections are given deeply into the upper-outer quadrant of the buttock by a special technique called a Z-track injection, which diminishes leakage to subcutaneous sites.

In the human the lymphatic system is well-developed, and the dose of the complex is relatively low, so that the danger of malignancy, as occurs in some animals, is very slight. However, it can cause fibrosis at the site of injection. Allergic reactions, even anaphylaxis, have occurred. Consequently, a test of 0.5 mL of the injection should be given prior to therapeutic administration. Headache, fever, nausea, vomiting, paresthesias, and regional lymphadenopathy are relatively common side effects. Hypotension, reactivation of quiescent arthritis, leukocytosis with fever, and sterile abscesses at an intramuscular injection site may occur. Phlebitis occasionally occurs after intravenous administration. The parenteral use of iron and carbohydrate has resulted in fatal anaphylactic-type reactions. Consequently, use of iron dextran should be reserved for patients with a clearly established iron deficiency not amenable to oral iron therapy.

POLYFEROSE

β-D-Fructofuranosyl α-D-glucopyranoside deriv, polymer, iron complex; Jefron

[9009-29-4] A chelate of iron with a polymerized derivative of sucrose, containing about 45% Fe.

Comments—For the treatment of iron-deficiency anemias. The complex is less astringent than ferrous salts and hence is more palatable in oral suspension.

Agents for Macrocytic Anemias

The macrocytic anemias are characterized by the presence of large, hypochromic erythrocytes. They include *pernicious anemia, the anemia of sprue, macrocytic tropical anemia, fish tapeworm anemia, achrestic anemia,* and anemias resulting from gastric carcinoma and resection or disease of the intestinal tract. In all of these, insufficient intake or absorption of *cyanocobalamin* (vitamin B_{12}) is the cause of the disorder, the vitamin being essential to normal hematopoiesis and to the integrity of the central nervous system. Early work on pernicious anemia established the need for a dietary factor, called the *extrinsic factor,* and a gastric and upper duodenal secretory factor, called the *intrinsic factor.*

It is now well-established that cyanocobalamin is the extrinsic factor; the vitamin is also the *antianemia component* of liver. The intrinsic factor is essential for the proper absorption of vitamins B_{12}. The intrinsic factor is absent in pernicious anemia; in this disease the secretion of hydrochloric acid and pepsin also is diminished or absent. Before the advent of cyanocobalamin (a vitamin B_{12}), various liver preparations were employed as sources of extrinsic factor, and stomach preparations as sources of the intrinsic factor. Since orally administered liver was not reliable, because it did not provide the

intrinsic factor, it was necessary to administer a stomach preparation at the same time or to administer the liver parenterally. Today, the preparation of choice is cyanocobalamin, which is cheaper and causes less discomfort at the site of injection than liver. Oral cyanocobalamin, of course, like liver, optimally requires a source of intrinsic factor.

For the patient with uncomplicated pernicious anemia in relapse, the initial dose of cyanocobalamin is 30 µg a day, parenterally, or every other day for 5 to 10 doses, followed by 15 to 30 µg once or twice a week until the blood picture is normal. For maintenance, 40 to 60 µg every 2 weeks or 80 to 100 µg once a month is usually adequate. If there is demonstrable neurological damage, it may be necessary to administer 1000 µg a week for several months before switching to the maintenance schedule. Therapy must be maintained for life, since the basic deficiency in GI physiology remains. Nevertheless, the patient may be kept in good health and may lead a fairly normal life.

Despite the superiority of cyanocobalamin, liver and stomach preparations still are available. The ingestion of 200 to 400 g of whole liver may be effective irregularly in inducing a remission in pernicious anemia. Concentrates for oral administration are made from such amounts of liver, but concentration results in some loss of activity. Extracts suitable for parenteral administration may be prepared from 10 to 15 g of liver. Similar effects may be produced by the ingestion of 30 to 40 g of desiccated stomach; however, the combinations of stomach and liver are required for optimal oral therapy.

Liver preparations for injection may be assayed microbiologically, employing *Lactobacillus leichmannii* ATCC 7830, the assay being expressed in terms of cyanocobalamin. However, since oral preparations rarely are effective, owing to the absence of the intrinsic factor, the assay must be made in the human pernicious anemia patient in relapse, and the assay is expressed in terms of oral units. This reflects the ridiculousness of using archaic and irregularly effective preparations when the active ingredient, cyanocobalamin, or derivatives, readily is available and is administered more easily and safely.

Megaloblastic anemia of infancy, megaloblastic anemia of pregnancy, achrestic anemia, and nutritional macrocytic anemia generally respond better to liver preparations than they do to cyanocobalamin, and deficiencies in *folic* and *folinic acid* intake or metabolism are implicated; thus, either of these two acids may evoke a dramatic response in such anemias. Ascorbic acid also occasionally may confer additional benefits. The metabolic functions of folic or folinic acid and vitamin B_{12} converge in certain respects. Thus, folic or folinic acid may induce a remission in the blood pathology in pernicious anemia, but it will not revert or delay the progression of the epithelial and neurological pathology, which may develop insidiously and emerge explosively and irreversibly. Therefore, folic or folinic acid therapy of pernicious anemia is to be condemned. *Equally offensive and irresponsible is the inclusion of these acids in liver or multivitamin-hematinic preparations* because, in allaying the blood pathology of undiagnosed pernicious anemia, they prevent detection of the disease until the neurological pathology has advanced to a dangerous state. Unfortified liver preparations also may contain enough folic acid to constitute the same danger. *In general, a hematinic should be employed only upon accurate diagnosis of the anemia and upon specific indication.* Multiple preparations are to be avoided.

HEMATOPOIETIC GROWTH FACTORS

The hematopoietic growth factors regulate the proliferation and differentiation of progenitor stem cells found in the bone marrow. They are glycoproteins that bind to specific cell surface receptors, resulting in a sequence of events culminating in hematopoiesis. Recombinant DNA technology has allowed the manufacture of sufficient quantities of these factors to enable clinical trials in patients. Erythropoietin, which stimulates red blood cell production was the first human hematopoietic growth factor to be isolated and studied. It improves the anemia associated with several clinical conditions. Several of the colony-stimulating factors also have been purified, molecularly cloned, and expressed as recombinant proteins. Clinical trials in progress are evaluating their effectiveness in treating patients for a variety of hematological disorders. Two of the colony-stimulating factors, granulocyte colony-stimulating factor (G-CSF) and granulocyte-macrophage colony-stimulating factor (GM-CSF) are efficacious in the management of bone marrow hypoplasia, particularly after myelosuppressive chemotherapy. They not only stimulate the progenitor cell target but also result in some functional activation of the mature cell. It is anticipated that future therapy will use additional hematopoietic growth factors in various conditions involving altered hematological status.

EPOETIN ALFA

1-165-Erythropoietin (human clone λHEPOFL 13 protein moiety), glycoform α; Epogen; Procrit

[113427-24-0] $C_{809}H_{1301}N_{229}O_{240}S_5$ (34,400 ± 400) A 165–amino acid glycoprotein produced by Chinese hamster ovary cells into which the human erythropoietin gene has been incorporated.

Comments—Erythropoietin, a naturally occurring glycoprotein, stimulates the division and differentiation of erythroid progenitors in the bone marrow, resulting in red blood cell production. The kidney is the major source of erythropoietin in adults. Epoetin alfa stimulates erythropoiesis in chronic renal failure (CRF) patients who are anemic because of impairment of their endogenous erythropoietin production. It is effective in both patients on dialysis and those not requiring regular dialysis. As it requires several days for erythroid progenitors to mature and be released into blood, a clinically significant increase in hematocrit generally is not observed before 2 weeks. The treatment goal is to increase hematocrit to 30% to 33% and eliminate the need for blood transfusions. The rate of hematocrit increase depends on several factors including availability of iron stores, baseline hematocrit, concurrent medical problems, and the dose administered. For reasons discussed below, a rapid increase in hematocrit (eg, >4 points in any 2-week period) is undesirable. Epoetin alfa also is indicated for treatment of anemias related to zidovudine (AZT) therapy in HIV-infected patients who have endogenous erythropoietin levels <500 mU/mL and are receiving <4200 mg a week of AZT. Patients with endogenous erythropoietin levels >500 mU/mL do not appear to have a clinically significant response with epoetin alfa.

Prior to and during therapy, the patient's iron stores should be evaluated; transferrin saturation should be at least 20%, and ferritin at least 100 ng/mL. Supplemental iron may be required to increase and maintain transferrin saturation to adequate levels. Epoetin alfa therapy has been associated with increased blood pressure in many CRF patients. Blood pressure should be controlled adequately prior to administration of the drug and must be monitored closely and controlled during therapy. During the time when hematocrit is increasing, approximately 25% of dialysis patients require initiation of, or increases in, antihypertensive medication. The dose of drug should be decreased in patients with an excessive rate of hematocrit rise (eg, >4 points in any 2-week period), as this rapid increase may exacerbate the hypertensive response. Epoetin alfa is contraindicated in patients with uncontrolled hypertension or known hypersensitivity to either mammalian cell–derived products or human albumin. During hemodialysis, patients on this drug may require increased anticoagulation with heparin to prevent clotting of the artificial kidney.

FILGRASTIM

Colony-stimulating factor (human clone 1034), N-L-methionyl-, Neupogen

[121181-53-1] $C_{845}H_{1339}N_{223}O_{243}S_9$ (18,000.00). A single chain of 175 amino acids, nonglycosylated, produced by recombinant DNA technology, expressed by *E coli*.

Comments—Granulocyte colony-stimulating factor (G-CSF) is an endogenous glycoprotein that acts primarily on hematopoietic cells regulating the production of neutrophils within the bone marrow. It is effective in accelerating the recovery of neutrophil counts following a variety of chemotherapy regimens. In addition to regulating the production of neutrophils, G-CSF also enhances neutrophil functional activity including enhanced phagocytic ability, priming of the cellular

metabolism associated with respiratory burst, and antibody-dependent killing. It is indicated to decrease the incidence of infection in patients with nonmyeloid malignancies receiving myelosuppressive anticancer drugs. Such patients experience a significant incidence of severe neutropenia with fever. Because of the potential sensitivity of rapidly dividing myeloid cells to cytotoxic agents, it should not be used 24 hr prior to, or within 24 hr after, chemotherapy. It is essential to obtain complete blood counts and platelet counts prior to the chemotherapy and twice a week during treatment with filgrastim. A transient increase in the neutrophil count typically occurs within the first 1 or 2 days following administration of filgrastim; however, for a sustained therapeutic effect it should be continued until the postchemotherapy nadir count reaches 10,000/mm³. Medullary bone pain of mild-to-moderate severity is the major adverse effect and occurs in approximately 24% of patients. It is most frequent in patients treated with higher doses (20–100 μg/kg/day) administered IV and is reported less in patients treated with lower SC doses (3 to 10 μg/kg/day). Although filgrastim is a growth factor that primarily stimulates neutrophils, it could potentially act as a growth factor for tumor cells, and caution should be used if this drug is administered in any malignancy with myeloid characteristics. It is contraindicated in patients with known hypersensitivity to *E coli*–derived proteins.

OPRELVEKIN

2-178-Interleukin 11 (human clone PXM/IL-11)

H- GPPPGPPRVS	PDPRAELDST	VLLTRSLLAD	TRQLAAQLRD
KFPADGDHNL	DSLPTLAMSA	GALGALQLPG	VLTRLRADLL
SYLRHVQWLR	RAGGSSLKTL	EPELGTLQAR	LDRLLRRLQL
LMSRLALPQP	PPDPPAPPLA	PPSSAWGGIR	AAHAILGGLH
LTLDWAVRGL	LLLKTRL-OH		

[145941-26-0] $C_{854}H_{1411}N_{253}O_{235}S_2$ (19,047.40).

Preparation—Oprelvekin is a nonglycosylated protein of approximately 19,000 daltons consisting of 177 amino acids which is produced by recombinant DNA technology in *E coli* bacteria. It differs from native IL-11, which is composed of 178 amino acids, only by lacking proline in the amino terminus.

Description—Interleukin eleven (IL-11) is a naturally occurring growth factor that stimulates the proliferation of hematopoietic stem cells and megakaryocyte progenitor cells as well as promoting megakaryocyte maturation resulting in increased platelet production.

Comments—It is indicated to increase platelet counts and decrease the need for platelet transfusion following chemotherapy in patients with nonmyeloid malignancies who are likely to develop thrombocytopenia. In clinical trials of patients undergoing chemotherapy for various malignancies who had previously required a platelet transfusion, oprelvekin was found to reduce platelet transfusions significantly compared with placebo administration. A trial in breast cancer patients who had not previously shown severe thrombocytopenia due to chemotherapy, demonstrated that 65% (26 of 40) of patients avoided platelet transfusion compared with 41% (15 of 37) in the placebo cohort following two dose–intensive chemotherapy with cyclophosphamide and doxorubicin. Oprelvekin has been administered safely using the recommended dosing schedule for up to 6 cycles following chemotherapy; however the efficacy and safety of more prolonged, chronic dosing is not established. Patients treated concurrently with G-CSF demonstrated no adverse effects on its activity by oprelvekin; little information is currently available regarding the combination of oprelvekin and GM-CSF. A complete blood count should be obtained prior to chemotherapy and at regular intervals during therapy with dosing continued until the postnadir platelet count is <50,000 cells/μL. Moderate decreases of 10 to 15% in hemoglobin, hematocrit, and red blood cell count commonly occur within a few days of drug initiation and are primarily due to an increase in plasma volume. Patients receiving this agent often experience mild-to-moderate fluid retention resulting in peripheral edema (~60%) and dyspnea with exertion (~50%). The fluid retention is reversible within several days following discontinuation of therapy. The drug should be used with caution in patients with congestive heart failure, and fluid balance should be monitored in these patients. Close monitoring of both fluid and electrolyte balance is also necessary in patients receiving chronic diuretic therapy. Transient atrial arrythmias occur in approximately 10% of patients treated with oprelvekin, and the drug should be used with caution in patients with a history of atrial arrthymias. No association of the agent with ventricular arrthymias has been found. Transient, mild visual blurring has been reported by patients taking oprelvekin, and the drug should be used with caution in patients with preexisting papilledema.

SARGRAMOSTIM

Colony-stimulating factor 2 (human clone pHG$_{25}$ protein moiety), 23-L-leucine-, rhu GM-CSF; Leukine; Prokine

[123774-72-1] $C_{639}H_{1002}N_{168}O_{196}S_8$ (15,500 to 19,500). A single chain of 127 amino acids, glycosylated, produced by recombinant DNA technology, expressed by *Saccharomyces cerevisiae*. There are three species having approx molecular weights of 19,500, 16,800, and 15,500, depending on the extent of glycosylation.

Description—White lyophilized powder.

Comments—Granulocyte-macrophage colony-stimulating factor (GM-CSF) is an endogenous multipotential hematopoietic growth factor that stimulates proliferation and differentiation of both early and late progenitor cells, resulting in increases in granulocytes and macrophages. It is indicated for accelerating myeloid engraftment in autologous bone marrow transplantation (BMT) in patients with non-Hodgkin's lymphoma, acute lymphoblastic leukemia, and Hodgkin's disease. It is effective in decreasing median duration of antibiotic therapy, reducing duration of infectious episodes, and shortening the median duration of hospitalization in these patients. It also is indicated for patients who have undergone allogeneic or autologous BMT in whom engraftment is delayed or has failed. In these patients, sargramostim is safe and effective in prolonging survival in both the presence or absence of infection. Hematological response to therapy should be assessed twice a week by CBC with differential. Sargramostim can induce WBC increases, and treatment should be interrupted or the dose reduced if excessive leukocytosis occurs (WBC > 50,000 cells/mm^3; absolute neutrophil count > 20,000 mm^3). It is contraindicated in patients with excessive (more than 10%) leukemic myeloid blasts in the bone marrow or peripheral blood or known hypersensitivity to yeast-derived products. Adverse effects include peripheral edema and a capillary leak syndrome, and it should be used with caution in patients with preexisting fluid retention, congestive heart failure, or pulmonary infiltrates. Because of the potential for promoting tumor growth, precaution is necessary when using this drug in any malignancy with myeloid characteristics.

ANTIHEMATOPOIETIC DRUGS

Polycythemia and erythrocytosis are conditions in which there is an increase in the number of circulating erythrocytes. The cause is usually the result of a deficient oxygenation of the arterial blood, and either condition may be corrected by management of the underlying primary disorder. However, in polycythemia rubra vera the condition is primary, and therapy thus is directed at the erythrocytes, either by their removal by venesection, their destruction by phenylhydrazines, or the suppression of their formation, by antihematopoietic drugs or by X-irradiation. Several of the antineoplastic drugs such as the nitrogen mustards, the antifolic acids, arsenicals, or radiophosphate may be employed. The *leukemias* result from excessive leukocytic hematopoietic activity of a neoplastic nature; either the bone marrow (myelogenous or granulocytic leukemia) or lymphatic tissue (lymphocytic leukemia) may be involved. In myelogenous leukemia there may be anemia because the erythropoietic cells are crowded out by leukopoietic cells.

MISCELLANEOUS DRUGS AFFECTING BLOOD

HEMIN

Ferrate(2−), chloro[7,12-diethenyl-3,8,13,17-tetramethyl-21*H*,23*H*-porphine-2,18-dipropanoato(4−)-*N*^{21},*N*^{22},*N*^{23},*N*^{24}]-, dihydrogen-, (*SP*-5-13).

Chlorohemin [16009-13-5] $C_{34}H_{32}ClFeN_4O_4$ (651.96).

Preparation—Usually from hemoglobin by treatment with a hot saline acetic acid solution. *Org Syn Coll*, vol III, 1955, p 442.

Description—Polychromatic crystals (usually brownish to blue) that do not melt above 300°.

Solubility—Freely soluble in dilute base through conversion to *hematin* by replacement of the chlorine atom by hydroxyl; sparingly soluble in alcohol; insoluble in water.

Comments—Inhibits the biosynthesis of porphyrin in juvenile erythrocytes and hence also indirectly decreases the rate of formation of porphyrins. It is used to ameliorate symptoms in *intermittent porphyria, porphyria variegata,* and hereditary *coproporphyria*. In some but not all patients pain, tachycardia, hypertension, mild-to-moderate neurological impairment, and abnormal mentation are abated. Neurological improvement is sometimes delayed weeks to months after treatment. Remissions are not permanent.

It is contraindicated in hypersensitivity to itself and in porphyria cutanea tarda. Excessive doses may cause renal failure. Phlebitis may occur in the injected vein. Coagulopathy and renal failure from an overdose have been reported. It may be antagonized by barbiturates, estrogens, and various steroid metabolites that induce aminolevulinate synthesis.

It is converted partially to bilirubin and partially excreted into the bile intact. Bilirubin metabolites and urobilinogen also appear in the urine.

METHYLENE BLUE

Phenothiazin-5-ium, 3,7-bis(dimethylamino)-, chloride, trihydrate; Methylthionine Chloride; Aniline Violet

C I Basic Blue 9 trihydrate [7220-79-3] $C_{16}H_{18}ClN_3S.3H_2O$ (373.90); *anhydrous* [61-73-4] (319.85).

Preparation—By treating a solution of *N*,*N*-dimethyl-*p*-phenylenediamine and *N*,*N*-dimethylaniline hydrochlorides with H_2S and $FeCl_3$ or another suitable oxidizing agent.

Description—Dark green crystals or a crystalline powder, with a bronze-like luster; odorless or with a slight odor; stable in air; solutions have a deep-blue color.

Solubility—1 g in 25 mL water or 65 mL alcohol; soluble in chloroform.

Comments—Readily reduced to leukomethylene blue, which, in turn, is readily reoxidized to methylene blue. Thus, it is useful as a reversible *oxidation-reduction* indicator. Its principal therapeutic use, in the *treatment of methemoglobinemia,* stems from this chemical property. It acts as an electron-acceptor in the transfer of electrons from reduced pyridine nucleotides (NADPH and NATPH) to methemoglobin, thus facilitating reduction of ferric to ferrous iron. Glucose 6-phosphate dehydrogenase is required; if this enzyme is absent, as it is in certain hemolysis-prone individuals, the drug is ineffective. If the dose is high, the oxidation potential favors the formation of methemoglobin from hemoglobin. This effect is used in the *treatment of cyanide poisoning.* The methemoglobin so formed complexes cyanide, which tends to spare the cytochrome system. However, other drugs are superior.

This drug formerly was employed as a urinary antibacterial agent, but this use is now obsolete. An outgrowth of this use is the belief that the drug is effective in the treatment of urolithiasis. Although a slight effect to retard crystal formation *in vitro* has been reported, no clinical benefits have been proven, and expert opinion holds the dye to be ineffective. Its use as an analgetic, antipyretic, and parasiticide has likewise been abandoned. The dye is used as a bacteriological stain.

It colors urine and feces green and the skin blue. It may cause bladder irritation, nausea, vomiting, and diarrhea. Large doses may cause vertigo, headache, confusion, sweating methemoglobinemia (paradoxical), and chest and abdominal pains. It can cause hemolysis in persons with glucose-6-phosphate dehydrogenase–deficient erythrocytes.

PENTOXIFYLLINE

1*H*-Purine-2,6-dione, 3,7-dihydro-3,7-dimethyl-1-(5-oxohexyl)-, Trental

1-(5-Oxohexyl)theobromine [6493-05-6] $C_{13}H_{18}N_4O_3$ (278.31).

Preparation—Ethyl acetoacetate and 1,3-dibromopropane are reacted to form the ethyl ester of 3*H*-dihydropyran-3-carboxylic acid, which is cleaved with HBr to form 6-bromo-2-hexanone. This latter compound, with theobromine, in the presence of base yields pentoxifylline.

Description—Bitter-tasting, colorless, odorless needles; melts about 105°.

Solubility—1 g in 13 mL water at 25° or in 5.5 mL at 37°; 1 g in 9 mL benzene.

Comments—Increases the ATP content of erythrocytes, which makes them both more deformable and less likely to aggregate. Consequently, they pass through precapillary sphincters and capillaries more easily, which improves blood flow through the microcirculation. It also stimulates the synthesis of prostacyclin by endothelial cells and inhibits phosphodiesterase activity (thus increasing cyclic AMP levels) in platelets; these two actions decrease the aggregation of platelets. It increases fibrinolytic activity and thus decreases fibrinogen concentration. These effects sum to decrease the viscosity of blood, which increases blood flow and decreases myocardial work. It is approved for the treatment of *intermittent claudication*. It is also investigational in the management of cerebrovascular insufficiency, transient ischemic attacks, stroke, diabetic angiopathy, sickle cell thalassemia and leg ulcers.

Adverse effects are dyspesia (2.8%), nausea (2.2%), vomiting (1.2%), bloating (0.6%), belching, flatus, anorexia, dry mouth, thirst, constipation, and cholecystitis; dizziness (1.9%), headache (1.2%), tremor (0.3%), anxiety and confusion; anginal pain (0.3%), hypotension and edema; blurred vision, conjunctivitis, and scotomata; dyspnea, flulike symptoms, laryngitis, nasal congestion and nose bleeds; brittle fingernails, pruritus, rash, and urticaria; earache, leukopenia, malaise, sialorrhea, bad taste, sore throat and swollen neck lymph glands, and change in weight; dysrhythmias, hepatitis and jaundice, hyperfibrinogenemia, pancytopenia, purpura, and thrombocytopenia are rare effects.

It is absorbed readily and first-pass metabolized by the oral route. Peak plasma levels occur in 2 to 4 hr. There are more than five metabolites, two of which probably have pharmacodynamic activity. The elimination half-life is only about 0.4 to 0.8 hr, but that of the major metabolites is 1 to 1.6 hr.

SODIUM NITRITE

Sodium nitrite [7632-00-0] $NaNO_2$ (69.00).

Preparation—By various methods, as by reduction of sodium nitrate with lead, a sulfite, or sulfur dioxide, or by absorption of NO obtained from catalytic oxidation of ammonia in sodium carbonate solution.

Description—White to slightly yellow, granular powder or white or nearly white, opaque, fused masses or sticks; deliquescent in air; solutions are alkaline to litmus.

Solubility—1 g in 1.5 mL water; sparingly soluble in alcohol.

Comments—Principally for treating *cyanide poisoning,* based on its causing methemoglobin, which complexes cyanide. In cyanide poisoning, it is injected intravenously in very large doses to produce methemoglobin, which combines with the highly lethal cyanide and renders it temporarily inactive as cyanmethemoglobin. Sodium thiosulfate then is injected intravenously to form the nontoxic thiocyanate. Nitrite ion relaxes smooth muscle, so sodium nitrite causes hypotension. Solutions are unstable and should be prepared directly before use.

ACKNOWLEDGMENTS—Karleen S Callahan, PhD is acknowledged for her efforts in previous editions of this work.

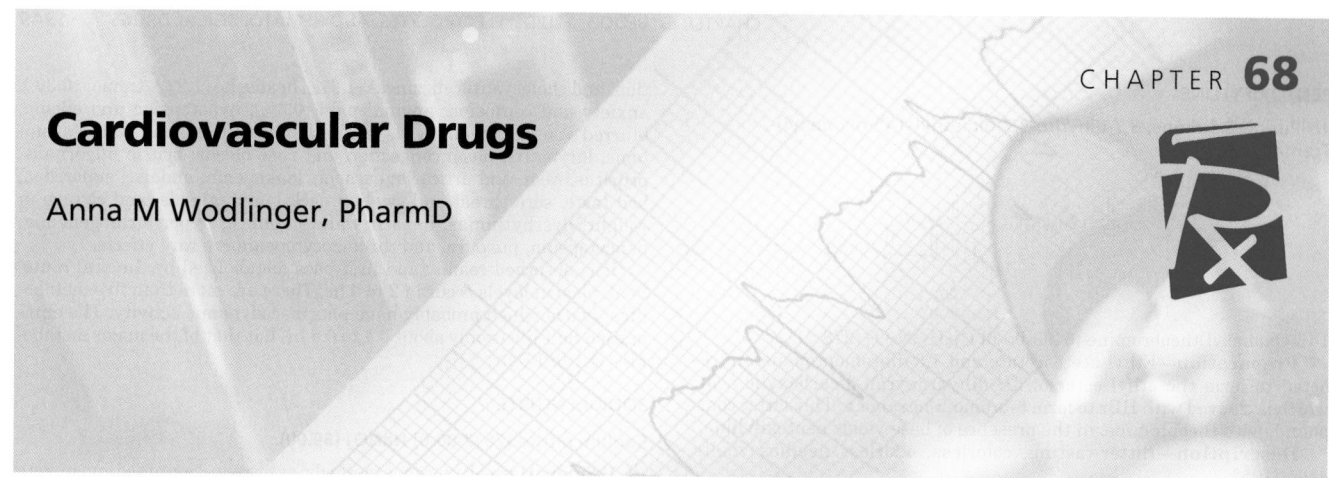

CHAPTER 68

Cardiovascular Drugs

Anna M Wodlinger, PharmD

The term *cardiovascular drug* refers to any medication that affects the heart, blood vessels, or the circulatory system. These drugs can be used alone or in combination with each other in the treatment of a variety of disease states such as hypertension, acute coronary syndromes, congestive heart failure (CHF), arrhythmias, and dyslipidemias. The majority of the drugs included in this category will be covered in this chapter, however some are discussed in more detail in other chapters and are referenced as such. The treatment of cardiovascular diseases is under constant study and recommendations may change. Several expert committees and associations publish guidelines periodically that provide specific treatment recommendations based on the most recent data available. I refer the reader to these publications for specific recommendations in the treatment of a particular cardiovascular disease state.

ANTIHYPERTENSIVE AND HYPOTENSIVE DRUGS

Hypertension is a disease characterized by an elevated blood pressure. The vast majority of patients with hypertension have primary (essential, idiopathic) hypertension in which the underlying cause is unknown. Secondary hypertension, in which there is an underlying cause such as renovascular disease or pheochromocytoma, affects a small percentage of patients. Malignant hypertension is a severe, progressive phase of primary hypertension. There are several drugs used in the treatment of hypertension, and no universal therapy for primary hypertension exists. Individual patients vary widely in response to antihypertensive drugs, and often more than one drug is necessary for effective treatment.

There are several factors that have been identified that contribute to the development of primary hypertension and several drugs target these processes. Some of these causes include abnormal central and autonomic nervous system response, abnormalities in renal or tissue autoregulatory processes, abnormality in the renin-angiotensin-aldosterone (RAS) system, vascular endothelium dysfunction, and dietary influences of sodium, calcium, and potassium.

Long-term studies have proven unequivocally that treatment of hypertension both decreases morbidity and prolongs life expectancy. Agents available for the treatment of hypertension include thiazide diuretics, β-adrenoreceptor-antagonists (β-antagonists), angiotensin converting enzyme (ACE) inhibitors, angiotensin receptor blockers (ARBs) or calcium channel blockers (CCBs) as single agents. If a single drug is not effective alone, two from different classes are used in combination. The choice of initial antihypertensive regimen or combination therapy should be made dependent upon the latest clinical data. Therapy should be specific for each patient, and drugs that have compelling indications in certain disease states (eg, ACE inhibitors in diabetes and CHF) should be used preferentially.

Currently, diuretics, ACE inhibitors, β-antagonists, calcium channel blockers, and angiotensin receptor blockers dominate the field. Drugs such as hydralazine, clonidine, and minoxidil are used as a tertiary drug for resistant cases. There has been a marked decline in use of guanethidine, reserpine, and methyldopa.

Diuretics

It long has been suspected that certain hypertensive persons have abnormal salt metabolism, and epidemiological and endemiological studies have established a relationship between salt intake and blood pressure. In the essential and malignant hypertensive individual with an expanded blood volume and high sodium burden, the rationale for use of diuretic drugs is almost self-evident. However, certain diuretic drugs even have been found to lower blood pressure of persons with essential hypertension in the absence of expanded blood volumes.

It is held widely that the vascular smooth muscles in such persons have high intracellular sodium content. When thiazide diuretics are given, the fall in blood pressure in the first week or two correlates with diuresis and the decrement in extracellular fluid volume (hence, in venous return, stroke volume, and systolic blood pressure). In this phase, heart rate is accelerated, and peripheral resistance may increase. The antihypertensive action passes into a phase in which the extracellular volume and heart rate return toward normal and peripheral resistance falls. Not all diuretics are alike in this effect, which suggests that something more than diuresis is involved. For example, loop diuretics do not lower vascular resistance, and blood pressure is lowered only because cardiac output is decreased. Spironolactone is a useful antihypertensive agent when aldosterone or 18-hydroxycorticosterone levels are high.

Homeostatic mechanisms increase plasma renin activity in response to excessive diuresis, which counterproductively increases plasma levels of the potent endogenous vasoconstrictor angiotensin II. If they were available, drugs that inhibit renin secretion would be rational agents to combine with diuretics.

At present, thiazide-like diuretics often are the first drugs to be used in the treatment of essential hypertension, customarily being used alone in mild essential hypertension; other drugs are added in moderate and severe essential hypertension. Loop diuretics should be used in congestive heart failure or in patients with renal impairment.

For the pharmacology of specific diuretics, see Chapter 75.

Peripheral Antiadrenergic Drugs

Regardless of whether there is a sympathetic component of essential or malignant hypertension, a reduction of whatever sympathetic activity exists can cause a lowering of blood pressure in four ways:

- A decrease in sympathetically (α-receptor)-mediated arteriolar constriction will decrease systemic peripheral resistance.
- A decrease in sympathetically (α₁-receptor)-mediated venous tone will increase venous capacitance and decrease venous return and, hence, cardiac output; however, this effect tends not to be sustained in the long run because of compensation by fluid retention.
- A decrease in sympathetically (β₁-receptor)-mediated cardiac contractility and heart rate will decrease cardiac output.
- A decrease in sympathetically (β₁-receptor)-modulated secretion of renin by the juxtaglomerular apparatus of the kidney will decrease the plasma levels of angiotensin II, a potent vasoconstrictor and sensitizer to sympathetic nervous activity and stimulant of the secretion of aldosterone, an antidiuretic hormone.

The exact mechanism by which β-antagonists are effective in the treatment of hypertension is unknown. Explanations include their ability to decrease cardiac output, renin secretion, and the release of norepinephrine at the adrenergic nerve terminals. They are effective alone and can be considered first-line therapy for the treatment of essential hypertension. They are also important adjuncts to diuretics, which increase renin secretion, and vasodilator drugs, which cause reflex sympathetic cardiac stimulation. Some β-antagonists, such as metoprolol, are selective for the β₁ receptor, and others, such as carvedilol and labetalol, are non-selective and affect both β₁ and β₂ receptors as well as α-receptors. The agents with both α- and β-adrenoreceptor blocking activity are useful in the treatment of essential hypertension, since blockade of one type of receptor cannot result in counteractive reflex activation of the other. Nonselective α-adrenoreceptor-antagonists, such as phenoxybenzamine and phentolamine, have antihypertensive actions, but reflex cardiac stimulation and increased renin secretion limit their efficacy and their role as antihypertensive agents is limited to the treatment of pheochromocytoma. The selective α₁-antagonists, such as prazosin, cause less of such counterproductive homeostatic adjustments and hence are more efficacious and can be used in the treatment of essential hypertension at low doses. However, at higher doses fluid and sodium retention occurs and concurrent diuretic therapy is necessary to maintain hypotensive effects. Drugs such as reserpine and guanethidine, which act on adrenergic nerve terminals to deplete norepinephrine or prevent release of norepinephrine, have limited use due to their side effect profiles.

The important antihypertensive α- and β-adrenoreceptor-blocking drugs and drugs that act on the adrenergic nerve terminals are described in Chapter 72.

DOXAZOSIN MESYLATE—page 1400.
PRAZOSIN HYDROCHLORIDE—page 1400.
TERAZOSIN HYDROCHLORIDE—page 1400.

Centrally Acting Antihypertensive Drugs

The drugs in this class stimulate α₂-receptors in the brain. The action of the α₂-receptor-agonists in the brain results in decreased sympathetic outflow to the blood vessels and heart and increased parasympathetic (vagal) outflow to the heart. This causes vasodilation, decreased heart rate, a decrease in renin release from the kidney, and blunted baroreceptor reflexes. It is also postulated that stimulation of presynaptic α₂-receptors peripherally contributes to the decrease in sympathetic tone. Only clonidine, guanabenz, guanfacine, methyldopa, and methyldopate are described in this section. There is no rationale for using more than one of these drugs at a time, and only clonidine is recommended for routine use.

Moderate doses of these drugs cause a high incidence of sedation, dry mouth, and mild-to-moderate orthostatic hypotension. Salt and water retention can occur with chronic use

and concurrent diuretic therapy may be necessary to maintain antihypertensive efficacy.

If the drugs are discontinued abruptly a compensatory increase in norepinephrine release may occur and a rebound hypertension could result. The occurrence of this is increased if the patient is receiving concurrent therapy with a β-antagonist due to unopposed α-receptor simulation.

CLONIDINE HYDROCHLORIDE

2-Imidazoline, 2-(2,6-dichlorophenylamino)-, hydrochloride; Catapres

[4205-91-8] $C_9H_9Cl_2N_3 \cdot HCl$ (266.56).

Preparation—Ammonium thiocyanate converts 2,6-dichloroaniline to the thiourea, which is treated with methyl iodide to yield the *S*-methylthiouronium salt. The latter compound, with ethylenediamine, closes the imidazoline ring to afford the product. See US Pat 3,202,660.

Description—White to off-white, odorless, bitter-tasting, crystalline powder; stable in light, air, and heat; does not exhibit polymorphism; melts about 300° with decomposition; pK_a 8.2.

Solubility—1 g in about 13 mL water (20°), about 25 mL alcohol, or about 5000 mL chloroform.

Comments—Available in a transdermal patch that delivers drug for 1 week.

GUANABENZ ACETATE

Hydrazine carboximidamide, 2-[(2,6-dichlorophenyl)methylene]-, monoacetate; Wytensin

[23256-50-0]$C_8H_8Cl_2N_4 \cdot C_2H_4O_2$ (291.14).

Preparation—Brit Pat 1,019,120.
Description—White solid; melts about 193° (dec).
Solubility—1 g in 90 mL water, 20 mL alcohol or 10 mL propylene glycol.

Comments—Efficacy is enhanced by diuretics. The half-life is 7 to 10 hr. It causes a mild, usually insignificant, postural or exercise hypotension.

GUANFACINE HYDROCHLORIDE

Benzeneacetamide, N-aminoiminomethyl)-2,6-dichloro-, monohydrochloride; Tenex

[29110-48-3] $C_9H_2Cl_2N_3O \cdot HCl$ (282.56).

Preparation—US Pat 3,632,645.
Description—White needles; melts about 215°.

Comments—Its longer half-life permits once-a-day dosing. Tolerance is common in the absence of a diuretic. Withdrawal hypertension may occur 2 to 7 days after discontinuation of treatment. Elimination is by both hepatic metabolism (60–70%) and renal excretion (30–40%); dosage is said not to require adjustments in renal failure. The elimination half-life is 14 to 17 hr.

METHYLDOPA

L-Tyrosine, 3-hydroxy-α-methyl-, sesquihydrate; Alpha-methyldopa; Aldomet

[41372-08-1] $C_{10}H_{13}NO_4 \cdot 1\frac{1}{2}H_2O$ (238.24); *anhydrous* [555-30-6] (211.22).

Preparation—The product of the reaction of 3,4-dimethoxyphenyl-lacetonitrile with sodium ethoxide is hydrolyzed with acid to give 3,4-dimethoxyphenylacetone. This is reacted with ammonium carbonate and potassium cyanide to form a substituted hydantoin intermediate, which, on alkaline hydrolysis, yields racemic methyldopa. The acetylated form of this racemate is resolved using (−)-α-methylbenzylamine. The isolated acetylated (−)-methyldopa salt is deacetylated with base and treated with mineral acid to liberate (−)-methyldopa. US Pat 2,868,818.

Description—White to yellowish white, odorless, fine powder, which may contain friable lumps; almost tasteless and relatively stable in both light and air; melts above 290° with decomposition; pK_a 2.2 (COOH), 10.6 (NH_2), 9.2 and 12 (ring OH).

Solubility—Sparingly soluble in water; very soluble in diluted hydrochloric acid; slightly soluble in alcohol; practically insoluble in ether.

Comments—Converted to methylnorepinephrine in the brain, which displaces norepinephrine from storage sites and is released as a *false transmitter* by nervous impulses in the adrenergic nerves. The metabolite α-methylnorepinephrine has potent a_2-agonist activity and probably acts to decrease blood pressure in the same way as clonidine. Its action begins in about 2 hr, becomes maximal in 6 to 8 hr, and lasts 18 to 24 hr. Used in hypertension in pregnancy.

METHYLDOPATE HYDROCHLORIDE

L-Tyrosine, 3-hydroxy-α-methyl-, ethyl ester, hydrochloride; Aldomet Ester Hydrochloride

[5208-79-4] $C_{12}H_{17}NO_4 \cdot HCl$ (275.73).

Preparation—By converting methyldopa to its ethyl ester and passing hydrogen chloride into a solution of the ester in a suitable organic solvent.

Description—White or practically white crystalline powder; odorless or practically odorless with a bitter taste; relatively stable both in light and air; melts about 160°; pH (1 in 100 solution) 3 to 5.

Solubility—Freely soluble in water, alcohol, or methanol; slightly soluble in chloroform; practically insoluble in ether.

Comments—Parenteral form for IV injection.

Antihypertensive Direct Vasodilators

Direct vasodilators act by several mechanisms, such as inhibition of cyclic nucleotide phosphodiesterase, adenosine mimicry, impairment of calcium and sodium influx in vascular smooth muscle, opening of potassium channels, release of nitric oxide (NO), stimulation of guanylate cyclase, and stimulation of dopamine receptors. Their usefulness in the treatment of hypertension depends a great deal on the selectivity of the drug for the resistance blood vessels, namely, the arterioles, which causes a lowering of blood pressure. If the capacitance veins also are dilated, venous return to the heart and hence cardiovascular adjustments to posture and exercise are impaired, and the patient may experience postural and exercise hypotensions, sometimes to the point of syncope. A slight degree of interference with venous return usually is considered to be desirable, especially in the treatment of severe hypertension, because it enables a greater lowering of blood pressure than arteriolar dilatation alone.

Some direct vasodilators can cause reflex palpitation and tachycardia and an increase in plasma renin activity that leads to fluid retention. Therefore, the long-term effectiveness of the drug is reduced unless combined with β-antagonists and/or diuretics to antagonize these effects.

DIAZOXIDE

2H-1,2,4-Benzothiadiazine, 7-chloro-3-methyl-, 1,1-dioxide; Hyperstat IV

[364-98-7] $C_8H_7ClN_2O_2S$ (230.67).

Preparation—One method reacts 2,4-dichloronitrobenzene with benzyl mercaptan and KOH and the 2-(benzylthio) group thus introduced is converted to —SO_2Cl with chlorine and aqueous acetic acid and thence to —SO_2NH_2 by reaction with NH_3. After reducing the NO_2 to NH_2 with Fe and NH_4Cl, cyclization is affected by condensation with ethyl orthoacetate. *Science* 133:2067, 1961. US Pats 2,986,573 and 3,345,365.

Description—White to cream-white crystals or crystalline powder; odorless; melts about 330°; pK_a 8.5.

Solubility—Practically insoluble to sparingly soluble in water.

Comments—A potent vasodilator, especially by the intravenous route. In therapeutic doses, vasodilation is primarily the result of arteriolar dilatation, so that orthostatic hypotension is usually minimal. The smooth muscle–relaxing effects result from hyperpolarization of vascular smooth muscle by activating ATPase-sensitive potassium channels. It can be used intravenously as a hypotensive drug in acute hypertensive crises. Increases in heart rate may occur following administration in response to blood pressure reduction.

Although it is a benzothiazide, it is not a diuretic but instead actually causes salt and water retention and consequent gain in weight. This action sometimes precipitates congestive heart failure, especially if renal function is impaired.

It should be used cautiously in persons with coronary or cerebral insufficiency and patients with impaired renal function. The drug is contraindicated if hypersensitivity to thiazides exists. Thiazide diuretics and other antihypertensive drugs increase the response to diazoxide, even when they fail to lower blood pressure themselves.

It is about 90% protein-bound, but rapid intravenous injection permits distribution to smooth muscle before it is bound to protein. Thus, a greater and longer-lasting fall in blood pressure accrues to faster rates of injection. The drug persists in blood longer than the hypotensive effect. The plasma half-life is 20 to 60 hr in persons with normal renal function, but the hypotensive effect lasts only 2 to 15 hr. Different populations may eliminate the drug differently, some mostly by renal tubular secretion and others mostly by biotransformation.

FENOLDOPAM MESYLATE

1H-3-Benzazepine-7,8-diol, 6-chloro-2,3,4,5-tetrahy-dro-1-(4-hydroxyphenyl)-, methanesulfonate (salt); Corlopam

[67227-57-0](salt), [67227-56-9] (base) $C_{17}H_{20}ClNO_6S$ (401.87).

Preparation—Reduction of 2-chloro-3,4-dimethoxyphenylacetonitrile with B_2H_6 in THF gives 2-chlorohomoveratryl amine. This latter compound with styrene oxide yields α-[[2-(2-chloro-3.4-dimethoxyphenyl)ethyl]aminomethyl]benzyl alcohol which is cyclized with a refluxing trifluoroacetic acid/sulfuric acid mixture to give 9-chloro-7,8-dimeth-oxy-5-(p-methoxyphenyl)-1,3,4,5-tetrahydro-3(2H)-benzazepine. Cleavage of the three ether groups to the corresponding phenols affords the base which is converted to the salt with methanesulfonic acid. *J Med Chem* 1980: 23; 973. Also US Pat 4,197,297 (1980).

Description—White to off-white crystals melting about 274° (dec).

Solubility—Sparingly soluble in water, methanol or ethanol; soluble in propylene glycol.

Comments—A dopamine receptor agonist that binds to the D_1-like receptor and also has moderate affinity for a_2-adrenoceptors. Vasodilator effects occur in the coronary and peripheral arteries and in the renal efferent and afferent arterioles. Fenoldopam is indicated for short-term, continuous intravenous management of hypertensive emergencies. Significant side effects include hypotension and tachycardia.

HYDRALAZINE HYDROCHLORIDE

Phthalazine, 1-hydrazino-, monohydrochloride; Apresoline

[304-20-1] $C_8H_8N_4 \cdot HCl$ (196.64).

Preparation—Phthalazone is converted to 1-chlorophthalazine by treatment with phosphorus oxychloride, condensed with hydrazine hydrate to form hydralazine and neutralized with HCl to produce the hydrochloride.

Description—White to off-white, crystalline powder; melts between 270° and 280° with decomposition; pK$_a$ 0.5, 7.3.

Solubility—1 g in 25 mL water, 500 mL alcohol; very slightly soluble in ether.

Comments—Causes vasodilation by stimulating guanylate cyclase in arteriolar smooth muscle; the stimulant appears to be nitric oxide (NO) from the local oxidation of the hydrazine moiety. NO is a natural, endothelium-derived relaxing factor.

It is one of the few drugs that cause substantial vasodilatation in the kidney, and it increases renal plasma flow even when the blood pressure drops considerably. Vasodilatation also is pronounced in the splanchnic, cerebral, and coronary vascular beds; it exerts only slight vasodilator actions in skin and skeletal muscle. The veins participate very little in the effect, so that postural hypotension is negligible. As the result of the fall in blood pressure, reflex tachycardia, palpitations, and increases in plasma renin activity occur, although the renin activity sometimes decreases in long-term treatment. The side effects of tachycardia and palpitations may precipitate attacks of angina pectoris.

Its principal serious toxic effects are syndromes resembling rheumatoid arthritis or lupus erythematosus, appearance of which necessitates withdrawal of the drug. This toxicity is more frequent in slow than in fast acetylators and is associated with chronic daily doses greater than 200 mg.

It is absorbed by the oral route. With low doses, first-pass metabolism limits bioavailability to 16% to 35%; food enhances the bioavailability. Elimination is by both ring hydroxylation and N-acetylation, and only 10% of hydralazine is excreted unchanged. Elimination is dose-dependent, and plasma levels increase disproportionately with dose. The half-life is 1.5 to 6 hr; the difference between slow and fast acetylators is usually minor. It accumulates in fat in vascular smooth muscle, where it has a longer life than in plasma.

MINOXIDIL

2,4-Pyrimidinediamine, 6-(1-piperidinyl)-, 3-oxide; Loniten; Rogaine

[38304-91-5] C$_9$H$_{15}$N$_5$O (209.25).

Preparation—US Pat 3,461,461.

Description—White to off-white, crystalline powder; pK$_a$ 4.6.

Solubility—1 g in about 500 mL water; 25 mL alcohol; practically insoluble in chloroform.

Comments—Dilates arterioles by opening potassium channels, which causes hyperpolarization and relaxation of smooth muscle. This lowers the total peripheral vascular resistance and hence the blood pressure. Dilatation of capacitance veins is only slight to moderate and therefore postural and exercise hypotensions are usually minimal.

Reflex tachycardia and palpitations occur, but they are less than that expected from the fall in blood pressure, which suggests cardioaccelerator-suppressant actions not yet elucidated. Plasma renin activity may be elevated as the result of reflex sympathetic activity or diminished by an unknown mechanism. Irrespective of the plasma renin activity, salt and water retention occurs sufficiently to cause considerable tolerance to the antihypertensive effects, and diuretics, even occasionally loop diuretics, are necessary to restore the antihypertensive effects.

Minoxidil is used as a last line of therapy to treat moderate to severe essential hypertension. It often is effective in hypertension refractory to all other therapy.

A side effect is excessive hair growth. Consequently, the drug is used topically to restore hair growth in androgenic alopecia and alopecia areata.

The drug is absorbed well by the oral route. The volume of distribution is 9 to 15 L/kg. It is concentrated in vascular tissue. Metabolism in the liver accounts for about 90% of elimination, and no modification of dose is required in renal failure or hemodialysis. The apparent half-life of about 4 hr appears to be a distribution parameter; the β-half-life is about 24 hr. The duration of action is 1 to 3 days.

SODIUM NITROPRUSSIDE

Ferrate(2-), pentakis(cyano-C)nitrosyl-, disodium, (OC-6-22)-dihydrate; Sodium Nitroferricyanide; Nipride; Nitropress

[13755-38-9] Na$_2$[Fe(CN)$_5$NO].2H$_2$O (297.95); *anhydrous* [14402-89-2] (261.92).

Preparation—Potassium ferrocyanide is dissolved in 50% HNO$_3$, and the solution is boiled for about 1 hr. After cooling and filtering to remove potassium nitrate, the solution is neutralized with Na$_2$CO$_3$ and evaporated to crystallization.

Description—Reddish brown, practically odorless, crystals or powder; freshly prepared solutions all have a faint brownish tint. Since nitroprusside ion forms colored compounds with many organic and inorganic substances, blue, green, red or any highly colored solutions should be discarded; aqueous solutions are photosensitive and should be protected from light.

Solubility—1 g in about 2.5 mL water; slightly soluble in alcohol.

Comments—A potent, directly acting peripheral vasodilator. It releases nitric oxide (NO), which is an endogenous, endothelium-derived relaxing factor. NO activates guanylyl cyclase in vascular smooth muscle to produce vasodilation. Its actions on arterioles decrease the total systemic vascular resistance, which is the main cause of the fall in blood pressure it evokes. Heart rate may be increased reflexly.

This drug has an immediate onset of effect and short duration of action so it is effective in treating hypertensive emergencies but must be given by continuous intravenous infusion. Side effects of this drug include significant hypotension and cyanide or thiocyanate toxicity.

Nitroprusside is broken down rapidly by reaction with hemoglobin to NO, cyanide ion, and cyanmethemoglobin, with a half-life of about 2 min. Cyanide is converted to thiocyanate by the enzyme rhodanese in the liver. Infants lack this enzyme, so the drug should not be used in neonates and probably also not in the treatment of toxemia of pregnancy. Conversion to thiocyanate requires endogenous thiosulfate, which can be depleted by high doses or prolonged administration, leading to toxic levels of cyanide. Thiocyanate is eliminated by the normal kidney, with a half-life of 3 days. Due to potential toxicities with accumulation of cyanide or thiocyanate high dosages and prolonged use, particularly in patients with renal or hepatic dysfunction, should be avoided.

Ganglionic Blocking Agents

The clinically available ganglionic blocking drugs compete with acetylcholine at postsynaptic nicotinic receptors. Since the ganglia of both the sympathetic and parasympathetic nervous systems are cholinergic, these drugs interrupt the outflow through both systems; thus, it is not possible to achieve a therapeutic block of autonomic outflow to a given locus without a number of undesirable side effects resulting from the blockade of other autonomic nerves. Blockade of sympathetic outflow to the blood vessels causes hypotension and increased blood flow.

Blockade of sympathetics to the heart may cause slowing, but the parasympathetic outflow also is blocked, so that acceleration can result in persons with predominantly parasympathetic tone. Orthostatic hypotension results from blockade of reflex adjustments to posture. Blockade of parasympathetic outflow results in dry mouth, mydriasis, cycloplegia (loss of ocular accommodation), diminished GI motility, and urinary retention.

The ganglionic blocking agents should be used cautiously when other hypotensive, antihypertensive, or anesthetic drugs are used concomitantly, because the hypotension may be exaggerated to such an extent that blood flow through the brain, heart, or kidney may be jeopardized. Overdose of the ganglionic blocking drug alone can have this effect. Because compensatory cardiovascular reflexes are suppressed by the ganglionic blocking drugs, pressor drugs given during ganglionic blockade may elicit dangerously enhanced responses.

Ganglionic blocking drugs are contraindicated when there is pyloric stenosis, cerebral arteriosclerosis, coronary insufficiency, recent myocardial infarction, or glaucoma. They should be used cautiously in elderly patients, patients with renal insufficiency, and those receiving neuromuscular blocking antibiotics. These drugs were used in the past to treat essential hypertension, but have been replaced by newer drugs

MECAMYLAMINE HYDROCHLORIDE

Bicyclo[2.2.1]heptan-2-amine, N,2,3,3-tetramethyl-, monohydrochloride; Inversine

[826-39-1] C$_{11}$H$_{21}$H.HCl (203.75).

Preparation—From camphene *J Am Chem Soc* 1946; 78:1514.

Description—White, crystalline powder; melts about 245° (dec); can be sterilized by autoclaving.

Solubility—1 g in 5 mL water, 12 mL alcohol, or 10 mL glycerol.

Comments—Differs from most other ganglionic blocking agents in that it is not a quaternary ammonium compound, so it is ionized poorly in the small intestine and thus is readily and completely absorbed. It is the only orally effective ganglionic blocker available. Its nonionic form permits it to pass into the CNS, so occasional bizarre central disturbances may occur. It has a low renal clearance and hence a long duration of action. It will produce a variety of unpleasant, unavoidable side effects that result from the interruption of both sympathetic and parasympathetic outflow. Orthostatic hypotension, blurring of vision, dry mouth, diarrhea followed by constipation, occasional paralytic ileus, nausea and vomiting, urinary retention, fatigue, sedation, and impotence are among these general side effects. Tremor and delusions or hallucinations may occur. It is absorbed readily from the gut. It penetrates the blood-brain barrier into the CNS and also into the fetus (hence, it should be avoided in pregnancy). Elimination is by renal tubular secretion. The duration of action is 6 to 12 hr.

TRIMETHAPHAN CAMSYLATE

Thieno[1′,2′:1,2]thienol[3,4-*d*]imidazol-5-ium, decahydro-2-oxo-1, 3-bis(phenylmethyl)-, salt with (+)-7,7-dimethyl-2-oxobicyclo[2.2.1]heptane-1-methanesulfonic acid (1:1); Arfonad

[68-91-7] $C_{32}H_{40}N_2O_5S_2$ (596.80).

Preparation—The bromide, prepared from an intermediate produced in the synthesis of biotin, is metathesized with silver *d*-camphor-10-sulfonate; the silver bromide is removed by filtration, and the camsylate is obtained by evaporating the filtrate.

Description—White crystals or crystalline powder; melts between 230° and 235° with decomposition.

Solubility—Freely soluble in water, alcohol, or chloroform; insoluble in ether.

Comments—Usually classified as a ganglionic blocking agent, but it only moderately blocks ganglia in the therapeutic dose range. Some of its hypotensive effects result from a direct peripheral vasodilator action. It has an extremely brief duration of action and must be administered via intravenous infusion. It can be used in the treatment of hypertensive emergencies, but other drugs are preferred. Adverse effects that are mostly the result of ganglionic blockade and necessitate a reduction in dosage include anorexia, nausea, vomiting, constipation, and possibility of paralytic ileus, mydriasis, cycloplegia, glaucomatous attack, dry mouth, anginal pain, tachycardia, postural hypotension, and urinary retention.

Drugs Affecting the Renin-Angiotensin System

Renin is a protease released by the kidney in response to reduced renal perfusion, hyponatremia, or sympathetic activity. It acts on the plasma α_2-globulin substrate, angiotensinogen, to yield the decapeptide, angiotensin I. Angiotensin I is hydrolyzed by a converting enzyme to yield the octapeptide angiotensin II. Angiotensin II may lose one amino acid residue to yield angiotensin III. Angiotensins II and III are destroyed by carboxypeptidases.

Angiotensin I is inactive in the cardiovascular system, although it may have some effect to contract the renal glomerular mesangium. Angiotensin II has several cardiovascular-renal actions.

It stimulates the zona glomerulosa of the adrenal cortex to secrete aldosterone. Aldosterone causes the renal retention of sodium (and hence of water) and the loss of potassium. The extracellular fluid volume and body burden of sodium are thus increased, which promotes an increase in blood pressure in many persons and edema in congestive heart failure. Angiotensin III also stimulates the adrenal secretion of aldosterone.

It is a very potent vasoconstrictor, which contributes to an elevation of blood pressure in most persons and to reduced cardiac output (from increased afterload), particularly in congestive heart failure.

It facilitates transmission in sympathetic ganglia, increases the release of norepinephrine at adrenergic nerve terminals, and increases the response of blood vessels and the heart to norepinephrine, thus amplifying sympathetic factors in the maintenance of elevated blood pressure.

It stimulates the release of ADH (vasopressin) from the neurohypophysis and thirst receptors, thus adding to volume and vasopressor factors in some conditions of hypertension and in congestive heart failure. Angiotensin II is also a putative neurotransmitter in the CNS.

The principal site of the angiotensin converting enzyme (ACE) is in the endothelial cells, but ACE also is found in many tissues including the kidney and lungs. ACE is the same enzyme as kininase II and therefore, inhibition of ACE not only decreases the amount of the vasoconstrictor, angiotensin II, but also increases the amount of bradykinin and other potent vasodilator peptides. The increased kinins may contribute to the hypotensive effects and side effects of ACE inhibitors.

ANGIOTENSIN CONVERTING ENZYME INHIBITORS

ACE inhibitors are used to treat mild-to-moderate essential and renovascular hypertension. These agents should be used as first line therapy in patients with compelling indications such as left ventricular dysfunction and/or diabetes mellitus. Alone or in combination, ACE inhibitors are becoming the drugs of choice in the first-line treatment of essential hypertension. Many drugs that lower blood pressure homeostatically increase renin release, hence increasing angiotensin II concentrations.

Centrally acting and β-antagonist antihypertensive drugs decrease sympathetically mediated, but not hemodynamically or intrarenally mediated, increases in angiotensin levels; ACE inhibitors suppress the production of angiotensin II that results from increased angiotensin levels from any cause. In combination with diuretics, they suppress the renin-angiotensin-aldosterone factor in diuretic-induced hypokalemia, thus attenuating the risk of hypokalemia. In fact, they may produce hyperkalemia, if there is concurrent renal failure or if potassium-sparing diuretics or potassium supplements are being taken. By preventing homeostatic rises in aldosterone levels and even by themselves causing a decrease in extracellular fluid volume, ACE inhibitors have a synergism with diuretics.

Except for captopril and lisinopril, all of the other ACE inhibitors listed below are esterified prodrugs, which are well absorbed from the GI tract and then deesterified to the much more active metabolite with a long duration of action. The suffix *-at* is added to the respective general name to denote the active metabolite (eg, enalaprilat, for IV administration). All of them except captopril are effective with single daily doses, although several are recommended to be administered twice daily when being used for the treatment of congestive heart failure.

Although ACE inhibitors, as a group, are relatively free of side effects or toxicities in most patients, they do occur and some can be life-threatening. Initial doses can produce first-dose hypotension, especially in patients currently taking diuretics or otherwise volume depleted. Reports of dizziness may be due to the expected but less severe reduction of blood pressure. Angioedema or angioneurotic edema occurs early in therapy in 0.1% to 0.2% of patients and is characterized by rapid swelling of tissues in the oral cavity, throat, and larynx, a life-threatening condition, which should be treated with epinephrine and/or a corticosteroid. This condition as well as the occurrence of a dry cough is thought to be due to inhibition of bradykinin metabolism by ACE.

Captopril contains a sulfhydryl group and has been reported to cause a rash in some patients. Neutropenia and hepatotoxicity are rare, but potentially serious side effects of ACE inhibitors; both are reversible if detected early. ACE inhibitors are definitely contraindicated in pregnancy, especially during the second and third trimesters when they are teratogenic; they should be discontinued as soon as pregnancy is detected.

BENAZEPRIL HYDROCHLORIDE

1H-1-Benzazepine-1-acetic acid, [S-(R*,R*)]-, 3-[[1-(ethoxycarbonyl)-3-phenylpropyl]-amino]-2,3,4,5-tetrahydro-2-oxo-, monohydrochloride, Lotensin

[86541-74-4] $C_{24}H_{28}N_2O_5 \cdot HCl$ (490.96).

Description—White to off-white crystalline powder.

Solubility—Greater than 1 g in 10 mL of water, ethanol, or methanol.

Comments—A prodrug rapidly absorbed and converted to the active ACE inhibitor benazeprilat, which has a half-life of 10 to 11 hr. It is approved for treating essential hypertension and may be effective for treating congestive heart failure.

CAPTOPRIL

L-Proline, 1-[(2S)-3-mercapto-2-methyl-1-oxopropyl]-, Capoten

[62571-86-2] $C_9H_{15}NO_3S$ (217.28).

Preparation—See *Science* 1977; 196:441.

Description—White crystals melting about 88° which resolidify and melt again about 105°; $pK_1 = 3.7$, $pK_2 = 9.8$.

Solubility—Freely soluble in water, alcohol, or chloroform.

Comments—The first orally effective ACE inhibitor to have been marketed. It is approved for use in the treatment of hypertension, heart failure, and left ventricular dysfunction post-myocardial infarction.

Rashes (erythematous, morbilliform, macropapular, edematous, urticarial) occur during the first 4 weeks of treatment in 4% to 10% of recipients. Approximately 7% to 10% of these manifest eosinophilia and antinuclear antibody, so that the rashes may have an immune origin. Eruptions do not occur until the dose exceeds 600 mg a day and may disappear even with continued treatment.

About 50% is eliminated in the urine, the remainder is metabolized. The half-life is less than 2 hr.

ENALAPRIL MALEATE

L-Proline, (S)-1-[N-[1-(ethoxycarbonyl)-3-phenylpropyl]-L-alanyl]-, (Z)-2-butenedioate (1:1); Vasotec

[76095-16-4] $C_{20}H_{28}N_2O_5 \cdot C_4H_4O_4$ (492.52).

Preparation—See *Nature* 1980; 288:280.

Description—White to off-white crystalline powder melting about 143°; pH (1% aqueous solution) about 2.5; pK_a 3.0, 5.4.

Solubility—Very soluble in water; soluble in ethanol; freely soluble in methanol.

Comments—A prodrug converted to the active ACE inhibitor enalaprilat. It is indicated for use in the treatment of hypertension, heart failure and asymptomatic left ventricular dysfunction.

About 60% is absorbed by the oral route. Peak plasma levels occur in 0.5 to 1 hr. In the body, about 40% is deesterified to enalaprilat, the active form of the drug (below). Enalaprilat and the remaining enalapril are eliminated in the urine. The half-life of enalapril is 1.3 hr, but that of enalaprilat is about 11 hr, thus providing a duration of action of over a day.

ENALAPRILAT

L-Proline, (S)-1-[N-[1-(carboxy)-3-phenylpropyl]-L-alanyl]-, dihydrate; Vasotec IV

[84680-54-6] $C_{18}H_{24}N_2O_5 \cdot 2H_2O$ (384.43).

Preparation—See *Enalapril Maleate*.

Description—White crystals melting about 150°.

Comments—The active form of enalapril (see above). It is water-soluble and hence is the parenteral form of enalapril. It is absorbed too slowly and erratically to be given orally.

FOSINOPRIL SODIUM

L-Proline, *trans*-4-cyclohexyl-1-[[[2-methyl-1-(1-oxopropoxy)propoxy] (4-phenylbutyl)phosphinyl]acetyl]-, sodium salt; Monopril

[88889-14-9] $C_{30}H_{45}NNaO_7P$ (585.65).

Preparation—See *J Med Chem* 1988; 31:1148.

Description—White to off-white crystalline powder.

Solubility—1 g in 10 mL water; soluble in methanol or ethanol.

Comments—A prodrug rapidly absorbed and hydrolyzed by esterases in the intestine and liver to the active ACE inhibitor fosinoprilat, which has a half-life of about 12 hr. It is approved for treating hypertension and heart failure. Total-body clearance is not reduced by renal impairment because it is conjugated to inactive glucuronide in the liver and excreted in the bile and urine.

LISINOPRIL

L-Proline, (S)-1-[N²-[1-(carboxy)-3-phenylpropyl]-L-lysyl]-, dihydrate; Prinivil

[83915-83-7] $C_{21}H_{31}N_3O_5 \cdot 2H_2O$ (441.52).

Preparation—US Pat 4,555,502.

Description—White crystals; pK_a 2.5, 4.0, 6.7, and 10.1.

Solubility—1 g in 10 mL water or 70 mL of methanol.

Comments—An ACE inhibitor approved for use in the treatment of hypertension, heart failure and acute myocardial infarction.

Only about 30% is absorbed by the oral route. Peak plasma levels occur in about 7 hr. Elimination is almost entirely by renal excretion; the dose must be adjusted in renal failure. The normal half-life is about 12 hr but is longer in elderly patients.

MOEXIPRIL HYDROCHLORIDE

3-Isoquinolinecarboxylic acid, (3S)-2-[(2S)-N-[(1S)-1-carboxy-3-phenyl-propyl]alanyl]-1,2,3,4-tetrahydro-6,7-dimethoxy-, hydrochloride; Univasc

[103775-14-0] $C_{25}H_{30}N_2O_7$ (470.53).

Description—Fine white to off-white powder.

Solubility—Soluble in water about 1 in 10 at 20°.

Comments–A prodrug converted to the active moexiprilat. Approved for the treatment of hypertension. Bioavailability is about 13% and is decreased by food.

PERINDOPRIL ERBUMINE

1H-Indole-2-carboxylic acid, [2S-[1[R*(R*)]],2α,3a,7aβ]]-1-[2-[[1-(ethoxycarbonyl)butyl]amino]-1-oxopropyl]octahydro-, compd with 2-methyl-2-propaneamine; Aceon; Procaptan

[82834-16-0] $C_{19}H_{32}N_2O_5.C_4H_{11}N$ (441.61).
Preparation—See US Pat 4,508,729 (1985).
Comments—Following absorption in the gut it releases perindoprilat in the liver. It is approved for the treatment of essential hypertension.

QUINAPRIL HYDROCHLORIDE

3-Isoquinolinecarboxylic acid, [3S-[2[R*(R*)]],3R*]-2-[2-[[1-(ethoxycarbonyl)-3-phenylpropyl]amino]-1-oxopropyl]-1,2,3,4-tetrahydro-, monohydrochloride, monohydrate; Accupril

[90243-99-5] $C_{25}H_{30}N_2O_5.HCl.H_2O$ (493.00).
Preparation—*J Med Chem* 1986; 29:1953.
Description—White crystals melting between 120 to 130° (dehydrated salt).
Comments—A prodrug rapidly absorbed and rapidly hydrolyzed to quinaprilat, which is active for 24 hr despite a plasma half-life of about 2 hr. It is approved for treating hypertension heart failure.

RAMIPRIL

Cyclopenta[b]pyrrole-2-carboxylic acid, [2S-[1[R*(R*)]],2α,3aβ,6aβ]]-1-[2-[[1-(ethoxycarbonyl)-3-phenylpropyl]amino]-1-oxopropyl]octahydro-, Altace

[87333-19-5] $C_{23}H_{32}N_2O_5$ (416.52).
Preparation—See *Arzneimittel-Forsch* 1984; 34:1399.
Description—Fine needles melting about 109°; pK_a (ramiprilat) 3.1, 5.6.
Solubility—Soluble in alcohol; very slightly soluble in water.
Comments—A prodrug rapidly absorbed and converted to ramiprilat, which has a half-life of 13 to 17 hr. It is approved for treating essential hypertension, heart failure post-myocardial infarction and for reducing the risk of myocardial infarction, stroke and death from cardiovascular causes in high risk patients. Dosage should be reduced in renal failure since 60% is excreted in the urine.

TRANDOLAPRIL

2-Indolinecarboxylic acid, (2S,3aR,7aS)-1-[(S)-N-[(S)-1-carboxy-3-phenylpropyl]alanyl]hexahydro-, Mavik; Odrik

[87679-37-6] $C_{24}H_{34}N_2O_5$ (430.54).

Preparation—See US Pat 4,933,361 (1990).
Description—Colorless crystals melting about 125°.
Solubility—Soluble in chloroform, methylene chloride, or methanol at greater than 100 mg/mL.
Comments—A prodrug of the nonsulfhydryl ACE, trandoliprat, which is formed by the hydrolysis of the ethyl ester. Approved for the treatment of hypertension and heart failure post-myocardial infarction.

ANGIOTENSIN II RECEPTOR ANTAGONISTS

The angiotensin II receptor blockers (ARBs) are a newer class of antihypertensive agents. They inhibit the effects of angiotensin II by directly blocking the angiotensin AT_1 receptor. The generation of angiotensin II can occur through mechanisms other than ACE activity and the AT_1 receptor is the site of action for angiotensin II that results in vasoconstriction, aldosterone, and ADH release, constriction of the efferent arteriole of the glomerulus and sympathetic activation. The ARBs inhibit the action of angiotensin II regardless of the pathway of generation; however, unlike the ACE inhibitors they do not block the breakdown of bradykinin. They are indicated for use in the treatment of hypertension and have also been studied in the treatment of heart failure and myocardial infarction. Their exact role in the treatment of heart failure and myocardial infarction has yet to be determined.

The side effects of the angiotensin II receptor antagonists are similar to those of the ACE inhibitors. However, the incidences of cough and angioedema are significantly lower, probably because of their lack of effect on bradykinin metabolism. They are contraindicated in pregnancy. Frank neutropenia or hepatotoxicity has not been reported, but caution should dictate until their use becomes more widespread.

CANDESARTAN CILEXETIL

(±)-1-H-Benzimidazole-7-carboxylic acid, 2-ethoxy-1-[[2′-(1H-tetrazol-5-yl)[1,1-biphenyl]-4-yl]methyl]-, 1-[[(cyclohexyloxy)carbonyl]oxy]ethyl ester; Atacand

[145040-37-5] $C_{33}H_{34}N_6O_6$ (610.67)
Preparation—See *J Med Chem* 1993; 36:2343; US Pat 5,196,444 (1993).
Description—Colorless crystals melting about 163° with decomposition.
Comments—Prodrug for the free acid which is formed by hydrolysis of the ethyl ester.

EPROSARTAN MESYLATE

2-Thiophenepropionic acid, (E)-α-[[2-butyl-1-[(4-carboxyphenyl)-methyl]-1H-imidazol-5-yl]methylene]-, monomethanesulfonate; Teveten

[44143-96-4] $C_{23}H_{24}N_2O_4S.CH_4O_3S$ (520.62).
Preparation—US Pat 5,185,351 (1993); *J Med Chem* 1991; 1514:34.

Methyl 4-(bromomethyl)benzoate and 5-chloro-2-propylimidazole are condensed using potassium carbonate in DMF to give the 1-(4-methoxycarbonyl)benzyl derivative of the imidazole (I). I, with the monomethyl ester of 2-thenylmalonate, in a solution of piperidine and pyridine in toluene forms the dimethyl ester of eprosartan, which is saponified to the diacid. The mesylate salt is obtained by reaction with methanesulfonic acid.

Description—Crystals from methanol. Free base melts about 260o.
Solubility—Insoluble in water; freely soluble in ethanol.

IRBESARTAN

Diazaspiro[4.4]non-1-en-4- one, 2-butyl-3-[[2′-(1H-tetrazol-5-yl)- [1,1-biphenyl]-4-yl]methyl]-, Avapro

[138402-11-6] $C_{25}H_{28}N_6O$ (428.53).
Preparation—US Pat 5,270,317 (1993); *J Med Chem* 1993; 36:3371.
A multi-step synthesis starting with butyl 2-[(4-methylamino)-phenyl] benzoate and 1-aminocyclopentane carboxylic acid.
Description—White to off-white crystals from ethanol; melts about 180°.
Log P (pH 10.1) 7.4.
Solubility—Slightly soluble in ethanol or methylene chloride; practically insoluble in water.

LOSARTAN POTASSIUM

1H-Imidazole-5-methanol, 2-butyl-4-chloro-1-[[2′(1H-tetrazol-5-yl)- [1,1-biphenyl]-4-yl]methyl]-, potassium salt; Cozaar

[124750-26-4] $C_{22}H_{22}ClKN_6O$ (461.01).
Preparation—See *J Med Chem* 1991; 34:2525; US Pat 5,138,069 (1992).
Description—White to off-white free-flowing crystalline powder melting at about 184°; pK_a approx 5.5 (free acid).
Solubility—Freely soluble in water; soluble in alcohol; slightly soluble in acetonitrile or 2-butanone.
Comments—Oxidation of the hydroxymethyl group on the 5- position of the imidazole ring yields the active metabolite.

OLMESARTAN

1H-Imidazole-5-carboxylic acid, 4-(1-hydroxy-1-methyl-ethyl)-2-propyl-1-[[(2′-(1H-tetrazol-5-yl) [1,1′-biphenyl]-4-yl]methyl]-, Benicar

[144689-24-7] $C_{24}H_{26}N_6O_3$ (446.50).
Preparation—US Pat 5,616,599 (1997); *J Med Chem* 1996; 39:323.
Description—White to light yellow crystals from ethanol melting about 180o (dec).
Solubility—Practically insoluble in water; sparingly soluble in methanol.
Comments—A Prodrug hydrolyzed to olmesartan during absorption from the gastrointestinal tract.

TELMISARTAN

[1,1′-Biphenyl]-2-carboxylic acid, 4′-[(1,4′-dimethyl-2′-propyl[2,6′-bi-1H-benzimidazol]-1′-yl)methyl]-, Micardis

[144701-48-4] $C_{33}H_{30}N_4O_2$ (514.62).
Preparation—EP 502,314 (1992); *Chem Abstr*; 1993;117: 251,352; also *J Med Chem* 1993;36: 4040.
Description—White solid melting about 262°.
Solubility—Practically insoluble in water or in aqueous solutions ranging from pH 3 - 9. Soluble in basic solutions above pH 10.

VALSARTAN

L-Valine, N-(1-oxopentyl)-N-[[2′-(1H-tetrazol-5-yl)[1,1′-biphenyl]-4-yl]methyl]-, Diovan

[137862-53-4] $C_{24}H_{29}N_5O_3$ (435.53).
Preparation—See US Pat 5,399,578 (1991).
Description—White crystals melting at about 117°.

PERIPHERAL VASODILATORS

Peripheral vasodilators are substances that dilate the arterioles and increase blood flow in the numerous systemic vascular beds, especially in the extremities. To the pharmacologist, the word peripheral may indicate that the action is directly on the arterioles, but to the clinician the word merely indicates the site of the final effect. Thus, centrally acting, reflexly acting, or ganglionic blocking drugs that reduce sympathetic tone to the periphery are peripheral vasodilators, clinically speaking. Consequently, all of the hypotensives listed in the previous section may be considered to be peripheral dilators. Some sympathomimetics with prominent β₂-receptor stimulant actions are employed for their peripheral vasodilator effects. The adrenergic blocking drugs also are used to improve flow through specific peripheral vascular beds (Table 68-1).

Table 68-1. Other Peripheral Vasodilators

DRUG	DESCRIPTION
Cyclandelate (Cyclospasmol)	Synthetic
Ethaverine HCl (Ethaquin, Ethatab)	Semisynthetic homolog of papaverine
Papaverine HCl	Nonopioid alkaloid in crude opium

Peripheral vasodilators are employed in the treatment of vasospastic disorders such as Raynaud's disease, causalgias and reflex dystrophy, vasospasm associated with arterial embolism and thrombophlebitis, immersion foot, trench foot, herpes zoster, decubitus ulcers, and degenerative arterial diseases such as thromboangiitis obliterans, arteriosclerosis obliterans, acrocyanosis, and diabetic gangrene. However, there is a great deal of justifiable skepticism about the value of peripheral vasodilators in most uses, since vasospastic ischemia usually is self-limiting because of autoregulatory factors that counteract the spasms. An organic obstruction cannot be corrected for by vasodilatation, since the obstruction is the principal resistance in the line. However, vasodilatation may (or may not) improve circulation in the ischemic area through collateral vessels. Papaverine, alone or in combination with phentolamine, has been used as an intracavernous injection for impotence.

DIPYRIDAMOLE—see RPS-18, page 844.
ISOXSUPRINE HYDROCHLORIDE—page 1384.
NYLIDRIN HYDROCHLORIDE—page 1384.
PHENTOLAMINE—page 1400.

ANTIANGINAL DRUGS

Drugs considered in this section are used primarily for the treatment of angina pectoris of several types: *classical* (exercise-induced or stable), *variant* (vasospastic or Prinzmetal's), and *unstable anginas.*

Three classes of drugs are the mainstays of angina therapy: the organonitrates, the calcium channel blockers, and the β-antagonists. Nitrates and calcium channel blockers dilate coronary arteries, which may contribute to their antianginal effects, particularly in vasospastic angina.

Organic nitrates dilate the capacitance veins (which decreases ventricular filling pressures) and the conducting arteries (which decreases arterial impedance). Both effects lead to a reduction in wall stress, the major determinant of myocardial oxygen demand, as a result of decreased ventricular volume and pressure and, hence, provide relief from anginal pain. There is also a decrease in cardiac output and total peripheral resistance, which may lower the blood pressure, eliciting reflex arteriolar constriction (which opposes the direct arteriolar dilating actions of the drug) and tachycardia, both of which are counterproductive.

The organonitrates also decrease pulmonary pressures. The result is a decrease in pulmonary congestion and edema in left heart failure, and hence, organonitrates can be used to relieve orthopnea and paroxysmal nocturnal dyspnea.

Organonitrates all have a common mechanism of action briefly summarized as follows. The nitrates are converted *in vivo* to nitric oxide (NO), which is an endothelium-derived relaxing factor (EDRF) endogenously generated by the oxidation of L-arginine. In turn, NO stimulates guanylate cyclase, thus causing smooth muscle relaxation. Sustained use of organic nitrates can produce tolerance to the nitrates. Therefore, many experts now recommend pulse or intermittent dosing (a 6- to 8-hour nitrate-free interval) rather than continuous nitrate administration, to reduce the likelihood of tolerance during chronic therapy. Sustained exposure to high doses of nitrates can result in a physical dependence that, upon abrupt discontinuation of drug, can be manifested as anginal attacks. They should be withdrawn gradually after continuous or chronic use.

Calcium entry blocking drugs act somewhat differently from the organonitrates in relieving angina. They are both coronary and peripheral arteriolar dilators, however their antianginal effect in exercise-induced and unstable anginas derives from the reduction in wall tension from a decrease in cardiac afterload. Coronary artery dilatation has some contribution, particularly in vasospastic angina. Effects on cardiac preload are negligible. Some calcium entry antagonists directly slow the heart; this effect decreases myocardial oxygen demand and blunts reflex responses to arteriolar dilatation. Prevention of calcium influx into ischemic myocardial cells also may have a direct effect to decrease myocardial oxygen demand by preserving myocardial ATP.

Other pharmacological approaches to the treatment of angina include the use of β-antagonists and various drugs that decrease the incidence and consequences of coronary artery disease.

Beta-antagonists increase exercise tolerance in angina because they improve blood flow to the vulnerable subendocardium, mostly by slowing the heart rate and increasing diastolic time, during which subendocardial perfusion mainly occurs. Also, a decrease in heart rate and contractility decreases myocardial oxygen demand. These drugs are discussed in Chapter 72.

The use of drugs to lower blood cholesterol and, hence, prevent coronary atherosclerosis are effective and are discussed later in this chapter.

Antiplatelet drugs prevent the formation of white thrombus that occurs following rupture of an atheromatous plaque. Aspirin and clopidogrel are effective as primary and secondary prevention of acute coronary syndromes that occurs from formation of thrombus in the coronary arteries.

ORGANONITRATES

Organonitrates are available in a variety of dosage forms listed below. For aborting an acute attack of angina, sublingual nitrates or lingual spray have a rapid onset of action and are effective for short periods. For chronic prophylaxis, sustained-release tablets or topical ointment provide antianginal effects for up to 8 hours and can be administered on a scheduled basis. Transdermal systems of nitroglycerin can provide sustained blood levels for up to 24 hr. Since tolerance can develop when used on a continuous basis, a 10- to 12-hour nitrate-free interval should occur in order to prevent tolerance.

AMYL NITRITE

Mixture of nitrous acid, 2-methylbutyl ester, and nitrous acid, 3-methylbutyl ester; Vaporole; Aspiroles

[8017-89-8] $C_5H_{11}NO_2$ (117.15).

Preparation—A good grade of commercial amyl alcohol (isoamyl alcohol) boiling above 125° is esterified with nitrous acid. The acid is generated in contact with the alcohol from sodium nitrite and dilute H_2SO_4.

Description—Clear, yellowish liquid with an ethereal, fruity odor and pungent, aromatic taste; boils about 96° but is volatile even at low temperatures and is flammable; slowly decomposes on exposure to air and light; moisture accelerates decomposition; specific gravity 0.870 and 0.876.

Solubility—Practically insoluble in water; miscible with alcohol, chloroform, or ether.

Comments—Although a nitrite, its actions are those of organonitrates (see the general statement). It causes more reflex arteriolar constriction than the nitrates. It is quite volatile and is inhaled to obtain a rapid effect (onset 0.5 min). In practice, however, amyl nitrite is employed rarely in the treatment of attacks of angina pectoris. An unusual, but at times life-saving, use for amyl nitrite is in the emergency treatment of cyanide poisoning, when nitrites are given to produce methemoglobin, which temporarily inactivates the toxic cyanide ion by combining with it to form cyanmethemoglobin. For this purpose, sodium nitrite is employed intravenously, but this drug may be inhaled while the solution of sodium nitrite is being prepared. It is administered by crushing a glass perle of this drug in a handkerchief and inhaling the liquid that volatilizes, or by dropping a small quantity on a handkerchief and inhaling the vapor. It has become a drug of abuse because of a rush (an acute vasodilatory episode) felt after inhalation. Abuse may cause methemoglobinemia, hemolytic anemia, and immunological disorders.

Caution—Amyl nitrite is very flammable. Do not use where it may be ignited.

ERYTHRITYL TETRANITRATE

(R*,S*)-1,2,3,4-Butanetetrol, tetranitrate; Tetranitrol; Cardilate

$$CH_2ONO_2$$
$$H-C-ONO_2$$
$$H-C-ONO_2$$
$$CH_2ONO_2$$

[7297-25-8] $C_4H_6N_4O_{12}$ (302.11); a dry mixture with lactose or other suitable inert excipients, to permit safe handling and compliance with federal ICC regulations pertaining to interstate shipment.

Caution: Undiluted erythrityl tetranitrate is a powerful explosive, and proper precautions must be taken in handling. It can be exploded by percussion or by excessive heat. Only extremely small quantities should be isolated.

Preparation—Erythritol is reacted with nitric acid in the presence of sulfuric acid under controlled temperature.

Description—White powder with a slight odor of nitric oxides and a bitter taste; unstable in light or heat.

Solubility—Soluble (undiluted) in acetone or alcohol; practically insoluble in water.

Comments—By the sublingual route, it has a relatively long duration of action (about 2 hr). By the oral route, the duration is longer, but quite variable. This agent should not be used as a chronic prophylactic therapy.

ISOSORBIDE DINITRATE

D-Glucitol, 1,4:3,6-dianhydro-, dinitrate; Isordil; Sorbitrate; Dilatrate-SR

$$CH_2$$
$$HCONO_2$$
$$CH \quad C$$
$$HC$$
$$O$$
$$HCONO_2$$
$$CH_2$$

[87-33-2] $C_6H_8N_2O_8$ (236.14).

Preparation—An aqueous syrup of 1,4:3,6-dianhydro-D-glucitol is added slowly to a cooled mixture of HNO_3 and H_2SO_4. After standing a few minutes, the mixture is poured into cold water, and the precipitated product is collected and recrystallized from ethanol.

Description—*Diluted* (with mannitol, lactose, or other inert ingredients): ivory-white, odorless powder. *Undiluted:* white, crystalline rosettes.

Solubility—*Undiluted:* very slightly soluble in water; very soluble in acetone; freely soluble in chloroform; sparingly soluble in alcohol.

Comments—The long-acting organonitrate of choice when chronic prophylaxis of angina is necessary. With sublingual and chewable tablet forms, the onset of effect is 2 to 5 min (absorption from the chewable tablet is also mainly from the mouth); with oral forms, the onset is about 30 min and duration is 4 to 6 hr; with sustained-release forms, the duration is 8 to 12 hr.

The most frequent complaint by users is headache. Oral bioavailability is approximately 22% because of high first-pass metabolism. Sublingual administration is said to increase bioavailability, but there is some disagreement on this point. However, sublingual and chewable tablet dosages are predicated on bioavailabilities at least twice the bioavailability with oral administration. The metabolites of isosorbide dinitrate are the 2- and 5-mononitrates, both of which have antianginal effects. The 5-mononitrate is the more active (see below). The half-life varies with the route of administration and ranges from 20 min (IV) to 4 hr (oral), probably because there is more mononitrate formed after oral administration; mononitrate inhibits the metabolism of the parent drug.

ISOSORBIDE MONONITRATE

D-Glucitol, 1:4,3:6-dianhydro-, 5-nitrate; ISMO

$$CH_2$$
$$HCOH$$
$$O-CH$$
$$HC-O$$
$$HCONO_2$$
$$CH_2$$

[16051-77-7] $C_6H_9NO_6$ (191.14).

Preparation—See *Acta Physiol Scand* 1948; 15:173.

Description—White powder melting about 90°.

Solubility—About 1 g in 20 mL alcohol or water.

Comments—A metabolite of isosorbide dinitrate (above). Its bioavailability is about 100%. The half-life is 4 to 6 hr. Advantages over isosorbide dinitrate include no first-pass metabolism, no active metabolites, and a significantly longer half-life.

NITROGLYCERIN

1,2,3-Propanetriol, trinitrate; Glyceryl Trinitrate, Glonoin, Trinitrin

$$CH_2ONO_2$$
$$H-C-ONO_2$$
$$CH_2ONO_2$$

Nitroglycerin [55-63-0] $C_3H_5N_3O_9$ (227.09).

Preparation—By nitrating glycerin with a mixture of nitric and sulfuric acids, called *nitration acid*. This acid usually consists of 3 parts of concentrated nitric acid and 5 parts of sulfuric acid.

Description—Practically colorless, odorless liquid with a sweet taste.

Packaging—Sufficiently volatile to require packaging of tablets in glass containers with tightly fitting metal screw caps and holding no more than 100 tablets in each container; only original unopened containers may be dispensed. Patients should keep the tablets in the original container, close it tightly after each use and avoid exposure to heat. Some manufacturers have added a *fixing* agent (polyethylene glycols) to the tablet preparation to minimize volatilization. Regardless, the unopened container *only* should be dispensed and under no circumstance should a label, absorbent cotton, or a desiccant be placed in the container.

Comments—The classical organonitrate once was the drug of choice for the treatment of angina pectoris. After oral administration, it is metabolized rapidly in the intestinal wall and liver, so systemic bioavailability is rather low. Consequently, oral doses are quite high, and plasma levels are erratic. The sustained-release forms are not recommended since oral bioavailability is so poor and tolerance is favored. Bioavailability is much greater by the buccal and sublingual routes. By the sublingual route, the vasodilator effects of the drug appear in 2 to 3 min and last about 20 min, but exercise tolerance may be increased for as long as an hour in some patients. Buccal tablets, if retained in the mouth, release nitroglycerin for 3 to 5 hr. Sustained-release oral capsules and tablets maintain plasma levels for 8 to 12 hr. A nitroglycerin ointment can provide therapeutic blood levels for 2 to 12 hr per application. Transdermal preparations may sustain plasma levels for 24 hr or longer. An intravenous formulation is available but has a short half-life of 1 to 5 minutes and, therefore, must be administered via continuous infusion.

Cerebral vasodilation may cause transient headaches. Paradoxical angina occurs when the dose is too large and blood pressure falls too low to sustain coronary flow. Dizziness, nausea, and other symptoms of hypotension also occur. High, repetitive doses can cause methemoglobinemia.

PENTAERYTHRITOL TETRANITRATE

1,3-Propanediol, 2,2-bis-[(nitrooxy)methyl]-, dinitrate, ester; Peritrate

$$CH_2-ONO_2$$
$$O_2NO-CH_2CCH_2-ONO_2$$
$$CH_2-ONO_2$$

[78-11-15] $C_5H_8N_4O_{12}$ (316.14).

Description—A dry mixture of pentaerythritol tetranitrate (prepared by nitration of pentaerythritol) with lactose or other suitable inert excipient to permit safe handling of the explosive undiluted substance; melts about 140°.

Solubility—Practically insoluble in water; sparingly soluble in polar organic solvents.

Comments—A so-called long-acting organonitrate, the long duration of which is mainly the result of prolonged release and absorption from oral dosage forms. Medical authorities state that the sustained-release forms are poorly effective. It is not absorbed sublingually. Since absorption by the oral route is erratic, efficacy is unpredictable.

VASOPRESSOR DRUGS

A number of drugs in several classes have vasoconstrictor or cardiostimulator activity and are necessary to elevate the blood pressure in certain conditions. These drugs are used in patients who require vasoconstrictive or inotropic support, primarily those with critically low blood pressure due to decreased cardiac output or systemic vasodilation, or both. Before initiating vasopressors treatment of underlying conditions, such as hypovolemic shock or sepsis, should be initiated. The most important of these drugs, the sympathomimetics, are alpha- and beta-receptors agonists and are discussed in detail in Chapter 70.

In the treatment of patients with cardiogenic shock, it is necessary to increase the cardiac output in order to maintain perfusion to vital organs. Dobutamine is an option in these patients because of its beta-agonist activities that result in positive inotropic activity. However, it may cause some afterload reduction resulting in hypotension and may cause arrhythmias. Dopamine has both alpha- and beta-agonist activity, depending on the dosage used, and will increase the cardiac output while not lowering afterload. For this reason, it is a better option in patients who require inotropic support but have low blood pressures.

DOBUTAMINE—page 1269.
DOPAMINE—page 1387.

CARDIAC GLYCOSIDES (DIGITALIS)

The primary action of digitalis on the heart is a direct cardiotonic action on the myocardium to increase the force of contraction. The increased contractility results from inhibition of the membrane sodium/potassium-activated ATPase, which inhibition ultimately increases the intracellular stores of calcium. In congestive heart failure, stroke volume may be increased, which more effectively empties the ventricles and lowers diastolic ventricular pressures and ultimately pulmonary and central venous pressures. Congestion thus is diminished.

Increased cardiac output improves renal blood flow and glomerular filtration and decreases juxtaglomerular renin secretion, so that the renal resorption of sodium and water is diminished. Hepatic blood flow also is increased, which increases the clearance of aldosterone. The result of this is a decrease in edema and an improvement in symptoms.

Slowing of the cardiac rate occurs only when the rate was originally rapid, as the result of compensatory sympathetic reflexes, consequent to failure. When the failure is abolished, there is no longer any need for the compensatory tachycardia, and consequently, the heart rate slows to normal. This slowing also has been attributed to a vagal action of digitalis. Digitalis does sensitize the sinoatrial node, atrium, and atrioventricular node to vagal impulses and increases vagal tone by actions in the CNS and on the baroreceptors. High doses also may slow the ventricle by a direct action on atrioventricular conduction.

The chief therapeutic use for digitalis is in the treatment of low-output congestive heart failure. When the failure is due to an acute toxic or infectious process, such as viral myocarditis, rather than to a chronic degenerative process such as arteriosclerosis or failure secondary to hypertensive heart disease, digitalis may give poor results. High-output failure in patients with anemia, hyperthyroidism, and thiamine deficiency is likewise not much benefited.

The action of digitalis to impair atrioventricular conduction is employed in the management of atrial flutter, atrial fibrillation, and paroxysmal supraventricular tachycardia (PSVT). The action sought is to decrease the ventricular rate toward a more optimal value, that is, a partial heart block to decrease the number of atrial impulses that pass through to the ventricles. In an occasional case of atrial flutter, the proper use of fairly large doses of digitalis may abolish the arrhythmia. In PSVT a properly selected dose can interrupt one segment of the reentrant pathway within the AV node, thus terminating the circus movement yet allowing orthograde conduction of normal impulses.

There are two glycoside products available. When absorbed in adequate amounts, the active digitalis principles produce identical effects on the myocardium, and their toxic effects are essentially the same, although there is some evidence that digitoxin gains better access to the CNS and causes more neurological side effects and CNS-initiated arrhythmias. They differ from each other largely in speed of onset of action, duration of cardiac effects, and the degree of absorption by the oral route. With some glycosides (eg, digoxin), bioavailability varies widely from product to product, which may require clinical or plasma-level monitoring.

Initial digitalization may be accomplished rapidly or slowly, depending on the urgency of the case. The vast majority of patients with congestive heart failure can be digitalized without a loading dose, so that about 5 half-lives are required to achieve a maintenance steady state.

In acute heart failure or symptomatic atrial tachyarrhythmias, loading may be desirable. The process of loading is known as rapid digitalization. It is not unusual to digitalize a patient in 12 or 24 hr by giving one-half of the calculated dose at once and the remainder in two or three divided doses at intervals of 6 hr. This principle is applied to other cardiac glycosides, and only the timing differs. Dosing should be individualized to the patients weight and renal function, and patients should be monitored closely to observe the developing effects of the drug and to prevent unpleasant or serious toxic effects from overdosage.

Intravenous administration can be utilized in patients who have severely symptomatic congestive heart failure or atrial tachyarrhythmias or who are unable to tolerate oral digitalis or who have GI disorders that preclude oral dosage.

Cardiac glycosides have a low margin of safety. They may cause nausea, vomiting, diarrhea, abdominal pain, headache, drowsiness, fatigue, malaise, backache, decreased libido, impotence, trigeminal neuralgia, white vision and other visual disturbances, convulsions, mental disturbances, eosinophilia, rashes, gynecomastia, and, rarely, thrombocytopenia.

Cardiac arrhythmias of all types are a sign of excessive plasma levels. Heart block and premature ventricular contractions (PVC) are the most frequent, ventricular tachycardia the most ominous. Toxic doses also can result in serious ventricular arrhythmias. Toxicity is more likely in the presence of hypokalemia, a common result of concomitant diuretic therapy for the cardiac edema.

Toxicity can be antagonized by digoxin immune Fab (see below), edetate disodium, potassium (especially if hypokalemia exists), lidocaine, phenytoin, or to a lesser extent, propranolol, quinidine, or procainamide.

DIGITOXIN

Card-20(22)-enolide, (3β,5β)-3-(*O*-2,6-dideoxy-β-D-*ribo*-hexopyra-nosyl-(1 → 4)-*O*-2,6-dideoxy-β-D-*ribo*-hexopyranosyl-(1 → 4)-2, 6-dideoxy-D-*ribo*-hexopyranosyl)oxy-14-hydroxy-,

[71-63-6] $C_{41}H_{64}H_{13}$ (764.95); a cardiotonic glycoside obtained from *Digitalis purpurea* Linné, *Digitalis lanata* Ehrh, and other suitable species of *Digitalis*.

The side chain consists of 3 molecules of digitoxose in glycosidic linkage. Removal of the side chain by hydrolysis yields the aglycone, digitoxigenin ($C_{23}H_{34}O_4$).

Description—White or pale buff, odorless, microcrystalline powder.

Solubility—Practically insoluble in water; 1 g in about 150 mL alcohol or 40 mL chloroform; very slightly soluble in ether.

Comments—This drug is currently not available in the United States. It is absorbed almost completely after oral administration. Action is maximal in 4 to 12 hr. After full digitalization, the duration of action is about 14 days. In plasma, about 97% is protein-bound. The volume of distribution is about 0.6 mL/g. Plasma concentrations of 15 to 25 ng/mL are considered to be therapeutic, and 35 to 40 ng/mL or more to be toxic. Hepatic metabolism accounts for 52% to 70% of elimination. The β-half-life ranges from 2.4 to 9.6 (av 7.6) days.

Caution—Handle digitoxin with exceptional care, since it is highly potent.

DIGOXIN

Card-20(22)-enolide, (3β,5β,12β)-3-[(*O*-2,6-dideoxy-β-D-*ribo*-hexopyranosyl-(1 → 4)-*O*-2,6-dideoxy-β-D-*ribo*-hexopyranosyl-(1 → 4)-2,6-dideoxy-β-D-*ribo*-hexopyranosyl)oxy]-12,14-dihydroxy-, Lanoxin, Digitek

[20830-75-5] $C_{41}H_{64}O_{14}$ (780.95); a cardiotonic glycoside obtained from the leaves of *Digitalis lanata Ehrh* (Fam *Scrophulariaceae*).

The side chain of digoxin consists of three molecules of digitoxose in glycosidic linkage. Hydrolytic cleavage yields the aglycone, digoxigenin ($C_{23}H_{34}O_5$).

Description—Clear to white crystals or a white crystalline powder; odorless; melts with decomposition above 235°.

Solubility—Practically insoluble in water or ether; slightly soluble in diluted alcohol or chloroform.

Comments—In plasma 20% to 30% is protein-bound. It has a high volume of distribution, with a volume of distribution of about 7 L/kg in normal adults and neonates and even larger in infants; in renal failure the volume of distribution is approximately 4-6 L/kg.

The therapeutic concentration in plasma is 0.5 to 2.0 ng/mL, although efficacy in heart failure has been observed with plasma concentrations ranging from 0.8 to 1.2 ng/mL. Concentrations above 2.0 ng/mL are considered toxic, although symptoms of toxicity may occur at lower concentrations when other conditions, such as hypokalemia and hypercalcemia, exist. In adults, renal excretion accounts for 60% to 90% of elimination. Biliary secretion and enterohepatic recirculation account for about 7% to 30%. The elimination half-life is 29 to 135 (usually 36–41) hours in normal adults. In renal failure, the β-half-life may be as long as 89 to 177 hours. By the oral route, about 50% to 85% is absorbed from solid dosage forms, but it is 90% to 100% absorbed from hydroalcoholic solutions in capsules.

DIGOXIN IMMUNE FAB (OVINE)

F(ab); Digibind

Comments—The toxicity and long half-life of digitalis glycosides led to the development of specific antidigoxin antibody fragments obtained from immunized sheep. The antibodies bind and inactivate molecules of digoxin or digitoxin, and the resulting complex is excreted in the urine. It takes 40 mg of Fab to bind about 0.6 mg of digoxin or digitoxin. Allergic reactions are rare (0.8%), but hypokalemic reactions can develop rapidly. It is administered intravenously, on the basis of the amount of drug ingested or serum digoxin concentration (see package insert for specific instructions).

PHOSPHODIESTERASE INHIBITORS

Cardiac glycosides had been the drugs of choice in the treatment of congestive heart failure for two centuries. Later, dopamine and dobutamine were introduced for their positive inotropic actions in the management of decompensated congestive heart failure. Dobutamine, initially, was the focus of attention because its vasodilator actions decrease the cardiac impedance (unload the left ventricle), which increases stroke output beyond that achieved by the positive inotropic action. The discovery of amrinone in 1977 has led to interest in drugs that combine positive inotropic with vasodilator actions. Such drugs are selective or nonselective phosphodiesterase inhibitors and have become known as inodilator drugs.

These drugs inhibit phosphodiesterase III and thus increase intracellular cAMP and calcium. In heart muscle the result is an increase in contractility, and in vascular smooth muscle the result is relaxation. Both effects contribute to improvement in cardiac output in congestive heart failure. Amrinone and milrinone are presently the only available inodilators, and their use is limited to decompensated heart failure that is refractory to other treatments.

AMRINONE

[3,4′-Bipyridin]-6(1*H*)-one, 5-amino-, amrinone, Inocor

[60719-84-8] $C_{10}H_9N_3O$ (187.20).

Preparation—US Pat 4,004,012.

Description—Pale-yellow crystals; melts about 295° with decomposition.

Solubility—At pH 4, 6, and 8 is 25, 0.9, and 0.7 mg/mL, respectively.

Comments—To avoid confusion with similarly sounding drugs, the name was changed from amrinone to inamrinone in 2000. Metabisulfite preservative in the preparation can cause hypersensitivity in certain individuals. Amrinone is not effective by the oral route even though it is absorbed. It has a volume of distribution of 1.2 L/kg. Over 70% is conjugated in the liver, the remainder is excreted in the urine. The half-life is about 3.6 hr in normal persons but 5 to 8 hr in subjects with heart failure. The duration of action is 30 to 120 min.

FLOSEQUINAN

4(1*H*)-Quinolone, 7-fluoro-1-methyl-3-(methylsulfinyl)-, Manoplax

[76568-02-0] $C_{11}H_{10}FNO_2S$ (239.26).

Preparation—US Pat 4,302,460.

Description—White crystals melting about 227°.

Comments—Not currently available in the United States. A fluoroquinolone derivative that produces both venous and arterial vasodilation and increases heart rate and contractility. Although its precise mechanism of action remains unknown, it appears to influence intracellular release of calcium by attenuating levels of inositol triphosphate or inhibiting protein kinase C. It is also a nonselective inhibitor of phosphodiesterases.

It is absorbed rapidly after oral administration and undergoes slow conversion to an equally active sulfone metabolite. Although the half-life of flosequinan is only about 1.7 hr, that of its active metabolite is 30 to 40 hr. Half-lives may be prolonged markedly in patients with congestive heart failure or with renal or hepatic impairment. The active and several inactive metabolites are excreted in the urine.

MILRINONE LACTATE

[3,4′-Bipyridine]-5-carbonitrile, 1,6-dihydro-2-methyl-6-oxo-, Primacor

[78415-72-2] $C_{12}H_9N_3O$ (211.22).

Preparation—US Pat 4,313,951.

Description—White crystals melting over 300°.

Comments—It is 20 to 30 times more potent than inamrinone as a positive inotropic agent and somewhat more potent as an arteriolar and venous dilator. It does not affect renal function significantly. In patients with congestive heart failure it improves cardiac index and decreases systemic vascular resistance. An oral form is not available. It has a volume of distribution of 0.4 L/kg and a mean half-life of 2.3 hr. It is excreted rapidly in the urine by active secretion.

ANTIARRHYTHMIC DRUGS

Cardiac arrhythmias may result from disturbances in the pacemaker function of the sinoatrial node, from alterations in conduction pathways and velocity, or from activation of pacemakers outside the sinus node and are often classified as tachyarrhythmias or bradyarrhythmias.

Autonomic drugs are often utilized to manage arrhythmias. Sinus tachycardia may be slowed by β_1-antagonists, and anticholinergics. β_1-agonists are used to revive an arrested heart and treat certain types of heart block.

Antiarrhythmic drugs have specific actions that alter cardiac conduction and are classified by their electrophysiological properties *in vitro*. The classification that follows is based on the classification of Vaughn-Williams. For simplicity, the most prominent effects at normal doses are used to determine placement in groups, but drugs may have properties that place them in more than one group. They may act differently in different parts of the heart, and in normal and diseased hearts the effects may be modified. Some drugs, such as digoxin or adenosine, are used in the treatment of arrhythmias; however, they are not included in the Vaughn-Williams classification.

Type I drugs are classified as sodium channel blockers. They inhibit the influx of sodium into the cardiac cell, thereby slowing conduction velocity. The action of the individual subclasses depends on the receptor binding and unbinding characteristics and the rate dependence properties.

Subtype IA drugs slow conduction velocity, prolong refractoriness, and decrease automaticity. They are typically effective for both supraventricular and ventricular arrhythmias.

Subtype IB drugs have minimal effects on conduction velocity but does shorten refractoriness and decreases automaticity. They are more effective in treating ventricular than supraventricular arrhythmias, particularly in ischemic tissue.

Subtype IC drugs decrease conduction velocity but have little effect on the refractory period. They are effective in the treatment of both supraventricular and ventricular arrhythmias; however, their use in patients with ischemic heart disease is limited secondary to the increased risk of proarrhythmias.

Type II drugs are the β-antagonists. These drugs are utilized in the treatment of arrhythmias, particularly tachyarrhythmias associated with high sympathetic tone. Their antiadrenergic properties make them particularly effective in the treatment of arrhythmias of the sinoatrial and atrioventricular node and in slowing the ventricular response in atrial tachyarrhythmias. These agents are discussed in detail in Chapter 72.

Type III drugs block the potassium channels thereby prolonging repolarization and increasing refractoriness. The individual properties of the drugs in this category are very different and several of them have multiple electrophysiologic actions.

Type IV drugs are the classical calcium entry blockers. These agents are similar to the Type II drugs in that they are particularly effective in the treatment of arrhythmias of the sinoatrial and atrioventricular node and in slowing the ventricular response in atrial tachyarrhythmias. They are discussed in more detail later in this chapter.

All antiarrhythmic drugs may cause new or worsened arrhythmias, a characteristic termed proarrhythmia. Although the incidence of proarrhythmias is higher with Type I and Type III drugs, both β-antagonists drugs (Type II) and calcium channel blocking drugs (Type IV) can be proarrhythmic, usually causing sinus bradycardia or AV block. These new arrhythmias are often difficult to distinguish from worsening of the original arrhythmia, which can lead to further or more aggressive treatment with the offending drug. A large clinical trial using several Type IC drugs in post–myocardial infarction patients found that there was a significant increase in mortality or nonfatal cardiac arrest in patients taking the drugs over those taking placebo.

ADENOSINE

9H-Purine, 6-amino-9-β-D-ribofuranosyl-, Adenocard

[58-61-7] $C_{10}H_{13}N_5O_4$ (267.24).

Preparation—Derived from yeast nucleic acids.

Description—White crystals melting at about 235°.

Solubility—Very soluble in water; solution may be sterilized by filtration or short-term autoclaving.

Comments—An antiarrhythmic drug approved for supraventricular tachycardia. It is given IV only and has a half-life less than 10 seconds. Major side effects are flushing and dyspnea.

AMIODARONE HYDROCHLORIDE

Methanone, (2-butyl-3-benzofuranyl)[4-[2-(diethylamino)ethoxy]-3,5-diiodophenyl]-, Cordarone

[1951-25-3] $C_{25}H_{29}I_2NO_3$ (645.32).

Preparation—US Pat 3,248,301.

Description—White to cream-colored, crystalline powder; melts about 156°; pK_a 6.56.

Solubility—Slightly soluble in water; soluble in alcohol; freely soluble in chloroform.

Comments—Type III antiarrhythmic drug used in atrial fibrillation and life- threatening recurrent ventricular arrhythmias that do not respond to other antiarrhythmic drugs. Its half-life is 25 to 100 days. Major side effects are serious pulmonary toxicity (about 10% fatal), complex CNS effects, proarrhythmia, hyper- and hypothyroidism, photosensitivity, drug deposits in the eye and skin, nausea, vomiting, and hepatic toxicity.

β-ANTAGONIST DRUGS—page 1400.

BRETYLIUM TOSYLATE

Benzenemethanaminium, 2-bromo-N-ethyl-N,N-dimethyl-, salt with 4-methylbenzenesulfonic acid (1:1); Darenthin; Bretylol

[61-75-6] $C_{18}H_{24}BrNO_3S$ (414.36).

Preparation—By interaction of *o*-bromobenzyl bromide and dimethylethylamine, the product being quaternized with *p*-toluenesulfonic acid.

Description—White, crystalline powder; melts about 98°.

Solubility—Freely soluble in water or alcohol.

Comments—Type III antiarrhythmic drug approved for life-threatening, ventricular arrhythmias that do not respond to first-line antiarrhythmic drugs and ventricular fibrillation. Intravenous use is limited to intensive-care units. A major side effect is hypotension (adrenergic neuron blocking mechanism).

DIGITALIS AND CARDIAC GLYCOSIDES—page 1360.

DISOPYRAMIDE PHOSPHATE

2-Pyridineacetamide, α-[2-[bis(1-methylethyl)amino]ethyl]-α-phenyl-, phosphate (1:1); Norpace

(CH₃)₂CH—NCH₂CH₂—C—CONH₂ • H₃PO₄
(CH₃)₂CH

[22059-60-5] $C_{21}H_{29}N_3O.H_3PO_4$ (437.47).

Preparation—One process for one synthesis of disopyramide converts 4-diisopropylamino-2-phenyl-2-(2-pyridyl)butyronitrile to the corresponding amide (disopyramide) by heating with concentrated H_2SO_4, followed by isolation and purification of the product (*CA 58*:12522c, 1963).

Description—White, crystalline powder; pK$_a$ 8:36.

Solubility—Freely soluble in water.

Comments—Subtype IA antiarrhythmic drug approved for life-threatening ventricular arrhythmias and may also be used in the treatment of paroxysmal supraventricular tachycardia. It has prominent antimuscarinic activity. Major side effects are proarrhythmia and typical antimuscarinic effects.

DOFETILIDE

Methanesulfonamide, N-[4-[2-[(methyl[2-[4-[(methylsulfonyl)amino]phenoxy]ethyl]amino]ethyl]phenyl]-, Dogmatyl, Dolasetron, Tikosyn

[115256-11-6] $C_{19}H_{27}N_3O_2S_2$ (441.58).

Preparation—By nucleophilic displacement of the halogen in 4-(2-bromoethoxy)methanesulfonanilide by *N*-methyl-*p*-nitrophenethylamine and potassium carbonate in acetonitrile, the tertiary amine precursor of the product is formed. The *p*-nitro group is catalytically reduced to the amine, which is then sulfonated with dimethyl sulfate in methylene chloride to afford the product. *J Med Chem* 1990: 33;1151. Also US Pat 4,959,366 (1990).

Description—White to off-white crystals from ethyl acetate/methanol melting about 149°. pK$_a$ 7.0, 9.0, 9.6. Log P (pH 7.4) 0.96.

Solubility: Very slightly soluble in water; soluble in acetone or 0.1 M HCl or NaOH.

Comments—A Type III antiarrhythmic agent approved for the treatment of atrial fibrillation/flutter. It is metabolized by CYP3A4 and also excreted unchanged in urine via both glomerular filtration and active tubular secretion and, therefore, has several drug interactions. Major side effects include proarrhythmias and QT prolongation.

FLECAINIDE ACETATE

Benzamide, N-(2-piperidinylmethyl)-2,5-bis(2,2,2-trifluorethoxy-, monoacetate; Tambocor

[54143-56-5] $C_{17}H_{20}F_6N_2O_3 \cdot C_2H_4O_2$ (474.40).

Preparation—See *J Med Chem* 1977; 20:821.

Description—White crystalline solid melting about 146°; pK$_a$ 9.3.

Solubility—1 g in about 21 mL water at 37° or 3.5 mL alcohol.

Comments—Subtype IC antiarrhythmic drug approved for atrial fibrillation/flutter, paroxysmal supraventricular tachycardia, and life-threatening ventricular arrhythmias. Major side effects include proarrhythmias, complex CNS effects, dizziness, dyspnea, headache, nausea, fatigue, and visual disturbances. Should be avoided in patients with structural heart disease.

IBUTILIDE FUMARATE

Methanesulfonamide, (±)-N-[4-[4-(ethylheptylamino)-1-hydroxybutyl]phenyl]-, (E)-2-butenedioate (2:1) salt; Covert

[122647-31-8] $(C_{20}H_{36}N_2O_3S)_2.C_4H_4O_4$ (885.23).

Preparation—See *J Med Chem* 1991; 34:308; US Pat 5,155,268.

Description—White to off-white powder melting about 118°.

Solubility—soluble (1 in 10) in water at pH 7 or below.

Comments—A Type III antiarrhythmic drug approved for atrial fibrillation/flutter. It is only available IV. A major side effect is proarrhythmia.

LIDOCAINE HYDROCHLORIDE

For the full monograph, see page 1481.

Comments—A Subtype IB antiarrhythmic drug approved for life-threatening ventricular arrhythmias. Most effective in arrhythmias associated with myocardial ischemia. Major side effects include seizures, dizziness, vertigo, nausea, parasthesia, rash, blood dyscrasias, and proarrhythmias.

MEXILETINE HYDROCHLORIDE

Ethylamine, 1-methyl-2-(2,6-xylyloxy)-, Mexitil

[31828-71-4] $C_{11}H_{17}NO$ (179.26).

Preparation—US Pat 3,659,019.

Description—White crystals; melts about 205°; pK$_a$ 8.4.

Solubility—1 g in 2 mL water or 3 mL alcohol.

Comments—A Subtype IB antiarrhythmic drug approved for used in the treatment of refractory life-threatening ventricular arrhythmias. Major side effects are proarrhythmias, complex CNS effects (including convulsions), nausea, vomiting, hepatoxicity, leukopenia, agranulocytosis, and rash.

MORICIZINE HYDROCHLORIDE

Carbamic acid, [10-[3-(4-morpholinyl)-1-oxopropyl]-10H-phenothiazin-2-yl]-, ethyl ester; Ethmozine

Ethyl 10-(3-morpholinopropionyl)phenothiazine-2-carbamate [31883-05-3] $C_{22}H_{25}N_3O_4S$ (427.52).

Preparation—US Pat 3,864,487.

Description—White crystals melting at about 190° (dec).

Solubility—Soluble in water or alcohol.

Comments—A Subtype IA antiarrhythmic drug approved for life-threatening ventricular arrhythmias. Major side effects are serious proarrhythmias, dizziness, and nausea.

PHENYTOIN SODIUM

For the full monograph, see page 1506.

Comments—A Subtype IB antiarrhythmic drug approved for ventricular arrhythmias and digitalis intoxication, but more often used as an antiepileptic agent. Major side effects are complex CNS effects, gingival hyperplasia, hirsutism, rash, blood dyscrasias, and proarrhythmias.

PROCAINAMIDE HYDROCHLORIDE

Benzamide, 4-amino-*N*-[2-(dimethylamino)ethyl]-, monohydrochloride; Procan; Pronestyl

$$NH_2—\bigcirc—CONHCH_2CH_2N(C_2H_5)_2 \cdot HCl$$

[614-39-1] $C_{13}H_{21}N_3O \cdot HCl$ (271.79).

Preparation—Among other ways, by condensing *p*-nitrobenzoyl chloride with β-diethylaminoethylamine and then reducing the nitro group to amino by any of the usual methods. The hydrochloride forms readily when a stream of hydrogen chloride is passed into a solution of the base in an appropriate organic solvent.

Description—White to tan, crystalline powder, odorless; pH (1 in 10 solution) 5 to 6.5; melts between 165° and 169°; pK_a 9.2.

Solubility—Very soluble in water; soluble in alcohol; slightly soluble in chloroform; very slightly soluble in ether.

Comments—A Subtype IA antiarrhythmic drug approved for life-threatening ventricular arrhythmias and also used for atrial fibrillation/flutter. It has less muscarinic effect than quinidine. Major side effects are proarrhythmias, lupus erythematosus syndrome, agranulocytosis, nausea, and diarrhea.

PROPAFENONE HYDROCHLORIDE

Propiophenone, 2'-[2-hydroxy-3-(propylamino)propoxy]-3-phenyl-, hydrochloride; Rythmol

[34183-22-7] $C_{21}H_{27}NO_3 \cdot HCl$ (377.91).

Preparation—Ger Pat 2,001,431.

Description—White crystals; pK_a 8.8.

Solubility—Soluble in hot water or alcohol; slightly soluble in cold water.

Comments—A Subtype IC antiarrhythmic drug approved for life-threatening ventricular arrhythmias and also used in the treatment of supraventricular arrhythmias. About 10% of patients are slow metabolizers with 3-fold increase in half-life. Major side effects are nausea, vomiting, unusual taste, dizziness, constipation, and blood dyscrasias.

QUINIDINE GLUCONATE

Cinchonan-9-ol, (9*S*)-6'-methoxy-, mono-D-gluconate (salt); Quinidine Monogluconate (salt); Quinaglute

[7054-25-3] $C_{20}H_{24}N_2O_2 \cdot C_6H_{12}O_7$ (520.58); the gluconate of an alkaloid that may be obtained from various species of *Cinchona* and their hybrids or from *Remijia pedunculata* Flückiger (Fam *Rubiaceae*) or prepared from quinine.

Description—White powder; odorless; very bitter taste.

Solubility—Freely soluble in water; slightly soluble in alcohol.

Comments—A Subtype IA antiarrhythmic drug approved for atrial fibrillation/flutter and ventricular tachycardia. It exerts antimuscarinic action on the heart and alpha-blockade on blood vessels. Major side effects are proarrhythmias, cinchonism, nausea, vomiting, diarrhea, quinidine syncope, and blood dyscrasias.

QUINIDINE POLYGALACTURONATE

Cardiaquin

A compound described as a polymer of quinidine and polygalacturonic acid and assigned the molecular formula $(C_{20}H_{24}N_2O_2 \cdot C_6H_{10}O_7 \cdot H_2O)_x$ [7681-28-9].

Preparation—From quinidine and polygalacturonic acid (from pectin); described in *Am J Pharm* 1958; 130:190; and US Pat 2,878,252.

Description—Creamy white, amorphous powder; melts about 180° with decomposition.

Solubility—Sparingly soluble in water.

Comments—See Quinidine Gluconate.

QUINIDINE SULFATE

Cinchonan-9-ol, (9*S*)-6'-methoxy-, sulfate (2:1) (salt), dihydrate

[6591-63-5] $(C_{20}H_{24}N_2O_2)_2 \cdot H_2SO_4 \cdot 2H_2O$ (782.95); anhydrous [50-54-4] (746.92); the sulfate of an alkaloid obtained from various species of *Cin*-

chona and their hybrids and from *Remijia pedunculata* Flückiger (Fam *Rubiaceae*) or prepared from quinine.

Quinidine is a stereoisomer of quinine and occurs in cinchona bark in amounts ranging from 0.3 to over 1%, although in some barks it may be practically absent. Quinidine of commerce usually is accompanied by up to 20% of *hydroquinidine* (which is quinidine with an ethyl group replacing the vinyl), which, however, is therapeutically as potent as quinidine and no more toxic.

Preparation—By treating quinine with a metallic alkoxide (Doering WE et al. *J Am Chem Soc* 1947; 69:1700; or by oxidizing quinine to quininone and then reducing the latter with sodium isopropoxide (Woodward RB et al. *J Am Chem Soc* 1945; 67:1428. It also may be obtained directly from the mother liquors remaining after removal of quinine from extracts of *Cinchona;* separation from cinchonine and other alkaloids is effected by special processes.

Description—Fine, needle-like, white crystals, frequently cohering in masses; very bitter taste; darkens on exposure to light; solutions neutral or alkaline to litmus; pK_{a1} 5.4; pK_{a2} 10.0.

Solubility—1 g in about 100 mL water, 10 mL alcohol, or 15 mL chloroform; insoluble in ether.

Comments—See Quinidine Gluconate.

SOTALOL HYDROCHLORIDE

For the full monograph, see page 1403.

Comments—A Type III antiarrhythmic drug approved for life-threatening ventricular arrhythmias and used in the treatment of atrial fibrillation/flutter. It is a β-antagonist with Type III actions. Major side effects include proarrhythmias, bradycardia and hypotension.

TOCAINIDE HYDROCHLORIDE

Propanamide, 2-amino-*N*-[2,6-dimethylphenyl)-, Tonocard

[35892-53-1] $C_{11}H_{16}N_2O \cdot HCl$ (228.72).

Preparation—*J Med Chem* 1979; 22:1171.

Description—White, crystalline powder; bitter taste; melts about 247°; pK_a 7.7.

Solubility—Freely soluble in water or alcohol.

Comments—A Subtype IB antiarrhythmic drug approved for life-threatening ventricular arrhythmias. Major side effects are proarrhythmias, dizziness, vertigo, paresthesia, rash, and blood dyscrasias.

CALCIUM CHANNEL BLOCKING DRUGS

Calcium channel blockers (CCBs) are a heterogeneous group of drugs consisting of four classes: the phenylalkylamines (verapamil), benzothiazepines (diltiazem), diarylaminopropylamine ethers (bepridil), and dihydropyridines (amlodipine, felodipine, nicardipine, nifedipine, nimodipine, and isradipine). Their main pharmacological effect is to block the voltage dependent, L-type calcium channels in the vascular smooth muscle and heart. The entry of calcium into cells is of fundamental importance for the normal functioning of the cardiovascular system, and the CCBs can affect this system in several ways. In vascular smooth muscle, calcium influx into cells is the excitation-contraction link that is necessary for smooth muscle contraction whenever smooth muscle is stimulated. The CCBs, by blocking the calcium channels in the arterial smooth muscle, result in peripheral vasodilation. The depolarization of the sinoatrial (SA) node and atrioventricular (AV) node in the heart is dependent on the inward movement of calcium ions through the slow channel. All CCBs reduce the inward current of calcium ions in the SA and AV node which has no effect on overall function, however diltiazem and verapamil delay the recovery of the channel which results in slowing of the SA node pacemaker rate and AV nodal conduction. In cardiac muscle the plateau phase of the action potential (Phase 2) is the result of inward calcium movement, which, in turn, couples the electrical excitation of these cells with muscle contraction. By blocking this process, the CCBs result in a negative inotropic effect. The reflex tachycardia that results from the significant peripheral vasodilation associated with the dihydropyridines is enough to overcome this negative inotropic effect. However, because of their effect on AV nodal conduction, verapamil and diltiazem prevent the tachycardic response and therefore the heart cannot overcome the negative inotropic effects of these drugs.

CCBs are utilized for the treatment of variant (vasospastic) and chronic stable angina pectoris. They are useful in the therapy of these diseases for three reasons: they directly dilate coronary arteries and increase myocardial blood flow, they decrease myocardial oxygen demand by peripheral arteriolar dilatation that decreases afterload, and they exert negative chronotopic (verapamil and diltiazem) and inotropic actions that also decrease oxygen demand.

Verapamil and diltiazem are utilized for the intravenous therapy of supraventricular tachyarrhythmias because of their significant depressant effects on SA nodal automaticity and AV nodal conduction. Oral verapamil and diltiazem can also be used for rate control in the treatment of chronic atrial flutter/fibrillation.

CCBs are utilized in the treatment of systemic hypertension because they are potent arteriolar vasodilators. They can be used as monotherapy or can be combined with other antihypertensive drugs. Newer formulations allow for once-daily or twice-daily dosing, and they are associated with minimal side effects. The CCBs, particularly diltiazem and verapamil because of their negative chronotropic and inotropic effects, should be used cautiously in patients with congestive heart failure. In those patients with CHF who are on appropriate therapy (ACE Inhibitors) that require additional afterload reduction, the dihydropyridine CCBs should be used preferentially to the non-dihydropyridines (verapamil and diltiazem).

Untoward effects of the CCBs are consequences of calcium entry blockade and are limited primarily to the cardiovascular system. Drug-induced vasodilatation leads to hypotension and to dizziness, lightheadedness, flushing, and headache. The non-dihydropyridines effects on decreased SA automaticity AV conduction can result in bradycardia and heart block. The use of these agents with β-antagonists, particularly, can induce heart block. Decreased myocardial contractility can result in congestive heart failure, particularly when these drugs are used with β-antagonists drugs. Peripheral edema caused by these drugs may be due to a combination of heart failure and peripheral vasodilatation, but direct effects to decrease sodium excretion have been noted with some CCBs.

Constipation sometimes is reported, particularly with verapamil and may be caused by mild excitation-contraction uncoupling in GI smooth muscle. Excitation-secretion coupling in exocrine and endocrine glands is another important role of calcium, but the effects of CCBs on glandular function have not proved to be important clinically, although nifedipine has been reported to decrease insulin secretion. In usual doses, CCBs do not appear to affect norepinephrine release from sympathetic nerve endings, although calcium is necessary for norepinephrine release. In contrast to the β-antagonists, CCBs do not increase airway resistance.

AMLODIPINE MALEATE

3,5-Pyridinedicarboxylic acid, 2-[(2-aminoethoxy)methyl]-4-(2-chlorophenyl)-1,4-dihydro-6-methyl-, 3-ethyl 5-methyl ester, (±)-, (Z)-2-butenedioate (1:1); Norvasc

[88150-47-4] $C_{20}H_{25}ClN_2O_5 \cdot C_4H_4O_4$ (524.96).

Preparation—J Med Chem 1986; 29:1696.
Description—White crystals melting about 180°; pK_a (base- NH_2) 9.0.
Comments—Approved for hypertension and angina (chronic stable or vasospastic). Its half-life is 34 hr.

BEPRIDIL HYDROCHLORIDE

β-[(2-methylpropoxy)methyl]-N-phenyl-N-(phenylmethyl)-, monohydrochloride, monohydrate; Vascor

[74764-40-2] $C_{24}H_{34}N_2O \cdot HCl \cdot H_2O$ (421.02).
Preparation—US Pat 3,962,238.
Description—White crystals melting about 91°.
Comments—Approved for chronic stable angina. Associated with proarrhythmias because of its Type I properties. Torsades de pointes has been reported rarely, and there have been some reports of agranulocytosis associated with its use.

DILTIAZEM HYDROCHLORIDE

Benzothiazepin-4(5H)-one, (+)-cis-3-(acetyloxy)-5-[2-(dimethylamino)ethyl]-2,3-dihydro-2-(4-methoxyphenyl)-, monohydrochloride; Cardizem; Dilacor XR, CartiaXT, Tiazac

[33286-22-5] $C_{22}H_{26}N_2O_4S \cdot HCl$ (450.98).
Preparation—Chem Pharm Bull 1971; 19:595.
Description—White crystals melting about 188°; pK_a 7.7.
Solubility—Freely soluble in water, alcohol, or chloroform; slightly soluble in dehydrated alcohol.
Comments—Indicated orally for the treatment of angina (chronic stable or due to coronary artery spasm) and hypertension or intravenously for atrial fibrillation/flutter or paroxysmal supraventricular tachycardia.

FELODIPINE

3,5-Pyridine dicarboxylic acid; (±)-4-(2,3-dichlorophenyl)-1,4-dihydro-2,6-dimethyl-, ethyl methyl ester; Plendil

[72509-76-3] $C_{18}H_{19}Cl_2NO_4$ (384.26).
Preparation—US Pat 4,264,611.
Description—White crystals melting about 145°.
Solubility—Practically insoluble in water, very soluble in alcohol.
Comments—Indicated for the treatment of hypertension.

ISRADIPINE

3,5-Pyridinedicarboxylic acid, (±)-4-(4-benzofurazanyl)-1,4-dihydro-2,6-dimethyl-, methyl 1-methylethyl ester; DynaCirc

[75695-93-1] $C_{19}H_{21}N_3O_5$ (371.39)

Preparation—US Pat 4,466,972.
Description—White crystals melting about 142°.
Solubility—Practically insoluble in water; very soluble in alcohol.
Comments—Indicated for the treatment of hypertension.

NICARDIPINE HYDROCHLORIDE

3,5-Pyridinedicarboxylic acid, 1,4-dihydro-2,6-dimethyl-4-
(3-nitrophenyl)-, methyl 2-[methyl(phenylmethyl)aminoethyl ester,
monohydrochloride; Cardene

[54527-84-3] $C_{26}H_{29}N_3O_6 \cdot HCl$ (515.99).

Preparation—*Chem Pharm Bull* 1979; 27:1426.
Description—White crystals melting about 180° (α-form) or about
169° (β-form); pK_a 7.2.
Comments—Indicated for oral use in the treatment of chronic
angina or hypertension. Also available parenterally for short-term
treatment of hypertension.

NIFEDIPINE

3,5-Pyridinecarboxylic acid, 1,4-dihydro-2,6-dimethyl-4-
(2-nitrophenyl)-, dimethyl ester; Adalat CC; Procardia

[21829-25-4] $C_{17}H_{18}N_2O_6$ (346.34).
Preparation—See US Pat 3,485,847.
Description—Yellow crystals melting about 174°.
Solubility—Practically insoluble in water; slightly soluble in alcohol; very soluble in chloroform or acetone; solutions are extremely light-sensitive.
Comments—Indicated for angina (vasospastic and chronic stable) and hypertension.

NIMODIPINE

3,5-Pyridinedicarboxylic acid, 1,4-dihydro-2,6-dimethyl-4-
(3-nitrophenyl)-, 2-methoxyethyl 1-methylethyl ester; Nimotop

[66085-59-4] $C_{21}H_{26}N_2O_7$ (418.45).
Preparation—US Pat 3,799,934.
Description—Yellow crystals melting at about 125°.
Solubility—Insoluble in water; soluble in alcohol.
Comments—Approved for *subarachnoid hemmorrhage* (the only CCB approved for this purpose). It causes high brain levels because of its high lipid solubility despite a short plasma half-life.

NISOLDIPINE

3,5-Pyridinecarboxylic acid, ($\pm$)-1,4-dihydro-2,6-dimethyl-4-
(2-nitrophenyl)-, methyl 2-methylpropyl ester; Sular

[63675-72-9] $C_{20}H_{24}N_2O_6$ (388.42).

Preparation—By the reaction of isobutyl 2-(*o*-nitrobenzylidene)-3-oxobutyrate and methyl 3-aminobutyrate in a Knoevenagel-type reaction. See US Pat 4,154,839 (1979).
Description—Yellow crystalline powder melting about 152°.
Solubility—Practically insoluble in water; soluble in ethanol.
Comments—Approved for hypertension.

VERAPAMIL HYDROCHLORIDE

Benzeneacetonitrile, α-[3-[[2-(3,4-dimethoxyphenyl)ethyl]-
methylamino]propyl]-3,4-dimethoxy-α-(1-methylethyl)-,
hydrochloride; Calan; Isoptin; Veralan

[52-53-9] $C_{27}H_{38}N_2O$ (454.61).
Preparation—See *Arzneimittel-Forsch* 1962; 12:563; and *Helv Chim Acta* 1975; 58:2050.
Description—White to off-white crystals melting about 140°; pH (7% w/w solution) about 4.2.
Solubility—1 g dissolves in about 15 mL water, 25 mL alcohol, or 2 mL chloroform; soluble in most polar organic solvents.
Comments—Approved orally for angina (vasospastic, chronic stable and unstable), atrial fibrillation/flutter and paroxysmal supraventricular tachycardia and hypertension. Also available parenterally for the management of supraventricular tachycardias and atrial fibrillation/flutter.

DRUGS AFFECTING BLOOD LIPIDS

Drugs that affect blood lipids are often classified as cardiovascular drugs because of the relation of blood lipids to atherosclerosis. Several studies, including the large epidemiological Framingham study, have found a positive correlation between elevated cholesterol levels and risk of coronary heart disease (CHD), and recent studies have shown inconclusively that lowering low-density lipoprotein (LDL) cholesterol is associated with a reduction in the risk of CHD. In addition to elevated total cholesterol (TC) and LDL levels, elevated triglycerides (TG) and/or low high-density lipoprotein (HDL) levels are independently associated with an increased risk of CHD. Studies have also demonstrated that raising HDL levels results in decreased risk of CHD.

Several drugs are available that lower TC, LDL, and TG levels and increase HDL levels. One source of cholesterol is from a diet with high cholesterol content. Consequently there are drugs, such as the recently approved ezetimibe, and plant derivatives that affect the absorption of cholesterol from the intestine in an attempt to decrease dietary absorption of cholesterol. These agents are used mainly for their LDL lowering effect. The bile acid sequestrants are utilized because of their ability to increase the catabolism of LDL cholesterol. In addition, the 3-hydroxy-3-methylglutaryl coenzyme A (HMG-CoA) reductase inhibitors (statins), which work by inhibiting the synthesis of cholesterol, are used primarily for their LDL lowering effect and also have some effect on lowering TG and raising HDL. Niacin inhibits the mobilization of free fatty acids from peripheral adipose tissue to the liver resulting in decreased TG synthesis and very-low density lipoprotein (VLDL) secretion that results in decreased TG and LDL levels. It also blocks the hepatic uptake of apolipoprotein A-I, a major component of HDL, resulting in increased HDL levels. Finally, the fibric acid derivatives (fibrates) increase lipoprotein lipase activity, inhibit the synthesis of triglyceride-containing very low density lipoprotein (VLDL), and increase synthesis of the major HDL apolipoproteins A-I and A-II. Their greatest effect is on lowering TG levels and increasing HDL. They also convert small, dense LDL particles to larger, more buoyant particles that are less atherogenic.

The statins, bile acid sequestrants, and fibrates have demonstrated a reduction in CHD risk and a reduction in overall mortality in dyslipidemic patients. Please refer to the latest report published by the National Cholesterol Education Program (NCEP) Expert Panel on Detection, Evaluation, and Treatment of High Blood Cholesterol in Adults (Adult Treatment Panel) for specific recommendations on the use of lipid lowering drugs.

CHOLESTYRAMINE RESIN

Cholybar; Questran

Cholestyramine [11041-12-6]; a strongly basic anion-exchange resin in the chloride form, consisting of styrene-divinylbenzene copolymer with quaternary ammonium functional groups. Each gram exchanges 1.8 to 2.2 g of sodium glycocholate, calculated on the dried basis.

Preparation—Polystyrene trimethylbenzylammonium chloride is copolymerized through cross-linkage with divinylbenzene.

Description—White to buff-colored, hygroscopic, fine powder; odorless or has not more than a slight amine-like odor; pH between 4 and 6 in a slurry (1 in 100).

Solubility—Very slightly soluble in water or alcohol; insoluble in chloroform or ether.

Comments—Binds weak acid anions with partial hydrophobic character. It binds bile acids in the intestine and, hence, prevents their absorption. The depletion of bile acids in the intestines not only decreases the absorption of dietary and enterohepatic cholesterol but also increases the synthesis of bile acids from cholesterol, which decreases the size of the systemic cholesterol pool. In familial hypercholesterolemia, the plasma concentration of LDL is decreased by 20% to 30%, which upregulates LDL-receptor populations in hepatocytes and vascular myocytes and thus accelerates LDL catabolism. The effect is even more pronounced in the presence of statins and niacin.

Side effects, attributable to depletion of intraintestinal bile acids, include constipation (20–50%), heartburn and dyspepsia, colic, belching, bloating, biliary stasis and lodged gallstones, steatorrhea and malabsorption syndrome (with doses > 24 g/day), and consequent hypovitaminoses A, D, and K. The bulkiness of the dose along with the decrease in bowel motility exacerbates constipation and favors impaction and may be the cause of nausea, vomiting, and GI bleeding from ulcers. Hypochloremic alkalosis sometimes occurs. In hypertriglyceridemias, the drug may elevate VLDLs and intermediate-density lipoproteins.

It binds numerous weakly acidic drugs and interferes with their absorption during concurrent oral administration.

COLESTIPOL HYDROCHLFORIDE

Tetraethylenepentamine polymer with 1-chloro-2,3-epoxypropane hydrochloride; Colestid

Copolymer of diethylenetriamine and 1-chloro-2,3-epoxypropane, hydrochloride [37296-80-3].

Preparation—Colestipol hydrochloride is a high-molecular-weight, highly cross-linked, basic anion-exchange copolymer of diethylenetriamine and 1-chloro-2,3-epoxypropane, with approximately one of five amine nitrogens protonated (chloride form). US Pat 3,692,895 and 3,803,237.

Description—White to pale-yellow beads; odorless; tasteless; hygroscopic.

Solubility—Insoluble in water, the beads swelling when placed in water or aqueous fluids.

Comments—An anion-exchange resin similar to Cholestyramine Resin (above) in its actions and uses, but there are differences in the anions for which it will exchange.

COLESEVELAM HYDROCHLORIDE

2-Propen-1-amine polymer with (choromethyl)oxirane, *N,N,N*-trimethyl-6-(2-propenylamino)1-hexanaminium chloride and *N*-2-propenyl-1-decanamine hydrochloride; WelChol

[182815-44-7] (HCl), [182815-43-6] (base).

$(C_3H_7N)_m(C_3H_5ClO)_n(C_{12}H_{27}N)_p \cdot xHCl$.

Preparation—US Pat 5,693,675 (1997).

Description—An alkylated cross-linked polymer.

Solubility—It is hydrophilic but insoluble in water.

Comments—Similar in action to the bile acid sequestrants it is a non-absorbed polymer that binds bile acids in the intestine, preventing their reabsorption. Unlike cholestyramine and colestipol, it is administered in tablet formulation and therefore is associated with less gastrointestinal discomfort and increased compliance.

EZETIMIBE

2-Azetidinone, [3*R*-[3α(*S**),4β]]-1-(4-fluorophenyl)-3-hydroxypropyl]-4-(4-hydroxyphenyl)-, Zetia

[163222-33-1] $C_{24}H_{21}F_2NO_2$ (409.43).

Preparation—An imine formed from 4-fluoroaniline and 4-(benzyloxy)benzaldehyde is treated with 4-(methoxycarbonyl)butanoyl chloride in heptane/tributyl amine which cyclizes to produce 1-(4-fluorophenyl)-3-(2-methoxycarbonyl)-4-(4-benzyloxyphenyl)-2-azetidinone. The racemic ester is resolved, hydrolyzed to the free acid, converted to the acyl chloride and reacted with 4-fluorphenylzinc bromide. The resulting ketone is reduced to the secondary alcohol, debenzylated and resolved on a chiral column to afford the product. US 5,767,115(1998); *J Med Chem* 1998; 41:973.

Description—White, crystalline solid melting about 165°.

$[\alpha]^{22}_D - 33.9$ (c = 3, MeOH).

Solubility—Freely soluble in methanol, ethanol, or acetone: practically insoluble in water.

Comments—This is a new class of lipid-lowering agents that inhibit the absorption of cholesterol from the intestine. Ezetimibe localizes and acts at the brush borders of the small intestine to inhibit the absorption of cholesterol, which leads to a decreased delivery of cholesterol to the liver. This reduction in hepatic cholesterol stores leads to an increase in cholesterol clearance from the blood. Ezetimibe has no effect on bile acid excretion or cholesterol synthesis. Side effects reported in clinical studies were minimal and similar to placebo.

FENOFIBRATE

Propionic acid, 2-[4-(4-chlorobenzoyl)phenoxy-, 1-methylethyl ester; Antara; Lofibra; Procetofene; TriCor

[49562-28-9] $C_{20}H_{21}ClO_4$ (360.84).

Preparation—One method involves the formation of the sodium salt of 4-chloro-4'-hydroxybenzophenone with sodium hydroxide in anhydrous acetone followed by nucleophilic reaction with α-chloroisobutyric acid to form the ether (Williamson method) and subsequent esterification with isopropyl alcohol to yield the product. See *Arzneimittel-Forsch* 1976; 26:885; US Pat 4,059,552 (1977).

Description—White crystals melting about 78°.

Solubility—Practically insoluble in water; slightly soluble in ethanol or methanol; soluble in ether, acetone, chloroform, or benzene.

Comments—A fibric acid derivative structurally similar to gemfibrozil. Mechanism of action is similar to gemfibrozil. Once-a-day dosing is an advantage.

GEMFIBROZIL

Pentanoic acid, 5-(2,5-dimethylphenoxy)-2,2-dimethyl-, Lopid

[25812-30-0] $C_{15}H_{22}O_3$ (250.34).

Preparation—See US Pat 3,674,836.

Description—White crystals melting about 61°.

Solubility—Practically insoluble in water or alcohol; slightly soluble in dilute alkali; pK$_a$ 4.7.

EPOPROSTENOL SODIUM

(5Z,9α,11α,13E,15S)-Prosta-5,13-dien-1-oic acid, 6,9-ep-oxy-11,15-dihydroxy-, sodium salt; Flolan

Prostacyclin, PGI$_2$, Prostaglandin I$_2$, Prostaglandin X.

Preparation—One method involves the conversion of arachidonic acid into prostenoids by prostaglandin G/H synthetase (PGHS).

Description—White to off-white powder. The injection has a pH of 10.2 - 10.8 and is unstable at lower pH.

Comments—Epoprostenol is a naturally occurring prostaglandin. Its actions include vasodilation of pulmonary and systemic arterial vasculature and inhibition of platelet aggregation. It is indicated for the treatment of primary pulmonary hypertension and pulmonary hypertension associated with the scleroderma spectrum of disease in NYHA Class III and Class IV patients failing to respond to conventional therapy. Epoprostenol has a short half-life (2.7 minutes) and must, therefore, be administered via continuous intravenous infusion. Dose-limiting adverse effects include flushing, jaw pain, nausea, headache, hypotension, and also include chest pain, anxiety, dizziness, bradycardia, dyspnea, abdominal pain, musculoskeletal pain, and tachycardia.

NESIRITIDE

Natriuretic factor-32; Natrecor

SPKMVQGSGC FGRKMDRISS SSGLGCKVLR RH

(Human brain clone λhBNP57) [124584-08-3] base;
[189032-40-4] citrate salt; C$_{143}$H$_{244}$N$_{50}$O$_{42}$S$_4$ (3464 daltons).

Preparation—From *E Coli* strain rhBNP.

Description—White to off-white lyophilized powder.

Comments—Nesiritide is a purified preparation of human B-type natriuretic peptide (hBNP). Human BNP has several actions including reducing systemic arterial pressures and the pulmonary capillary wedge pressure (PCWP). Nesiritide is indicated for the treatment of patients with acutely decompensated congestive heart failure who have dyspnea at rest or with minimal activity. Its use should be avoided in patients with systolic blood pressures less than 90 mm Hg. It is generally well tolerated with the most significant adverse effect being hypotension. It is currently only available intravenously and should be administered via continuous infusion.

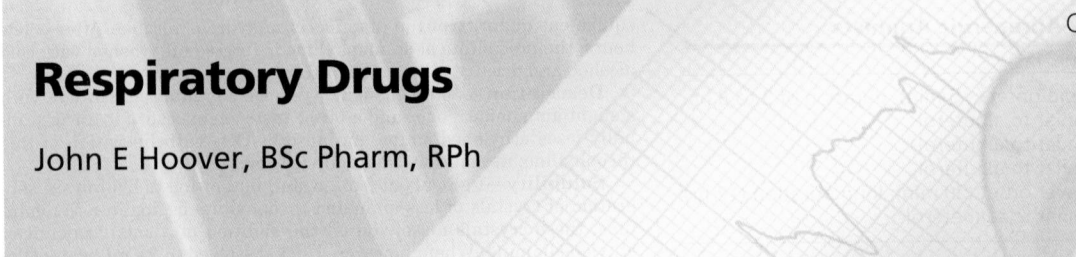

Respiratory Drugs

John E Hoover, BSc Pharm, RPh

The drugs used to treat asthma are the main group of respiratory drugs emphasized in this chapter because it is an extremely common respiratory disorder that afflicts 14 to 15 million people in the US. Asthma is now recognized to be an inflammatory illness that has bronchial hyperreactivity and bronchospasm that accounts for more than 100 million days of restricted activity and 470,000 hospital admissions annually. Clinical trials have shown the benefits of anti-inflammatory therapy for treatment of the underlying inflammatory component of this respiratory disorder and reserving bronchodilators primarily for symptomatic use. The drugs for asthma therapy include bronchodilators, corticosteroids, inhibitors of mediator release, leukotriene pathway inhibitors, and anticholinergic agents. Other important categories of respiratory drugs that are mentioned include antitussives, expectorants, and surfactant preparations.

Bronchodilators are used to open air passages and facilitate breathing as well as diminish bronchospasms by relaxing the smooth muscles of the bronchioles. They provide respiratory relief from conditions such as asthma, bronchitis, emphysema, or bronchiectasis. A number of pharmacologically different groups of drugs possess bronchodilator properties. *Sympathomimetic drugs,* such as metaproterenol, albuterol, terbutaline, isoetharine, pirbuterol, and salmetrol, exert a preferential effect on β_2-adrenergic receptors and mediate relaxation of the smooth muscle of the respiratory tract. The bronchial muscles are controlled by the autonomic nervous system with parasympathetic fibers predominating in number and effect. Stimulation of parasympathetic nerves causes calcium-dependent contraction of the bronchi and enhances the release of chemical mediators that induce bronchospasm. Consequently, *anticholinergic drugs* (eg, atropine) are useful for reducing bronchospasm (Table 69-1).

Corticosteroids (eg, beclomethasone dipropionate, dexamethasone, triamcinolone acetonide, flunisolide, and fluticasone) not only are effective anti-inflammatory agents, but also potentiate the bronchodilator effects of adrenergic drugs. These corticosteroids are not direct bronchodilators and are not effective for rapid relief of bronchospasm. Use of corticosteroid inhalers provides effective and localized anti-inflammatory activity within the bronchial airways, while having minimal systemic effects (Table 69-2).

Cromolyn sodium and nedocromil inhibit the release of mediators of inflammation from mast cells. These mediators include histamine, leukotrienes, platelet activating factor (PAF), prostaglandins, proteases, interleukins, and numerous cytokines. These diverse mediators are induced by specific antigens as well as nonspecific mechanisms (such as exercise) resulting in vasodilation, microvascular leakage, leukocyte chemotaxis, mucus secretion, and bronchoconstriction. The cells recruited during inflammation include eosinophils, T lymphocytes, basophils, and macrophages. Their mediators can cause epithelial disruption, bronchoconstriction, altered ciliary function, smooth muscle hypertrophy, mucus secretion, airway edema, and tissue damage. Early asthmatic reactions to allergen exposure are dominated by mediators released from mast cells, while delayed (2–8 hr) or late asthmatic reactions are related to mediators released from eosinophils.

Nedocromil and cromolyn block both early and late asthmatic responses induced by either episodic or continuous allergen inhalation or exercise. They control the symptoms of mild-to-moderate chronic asthma in 60% to 70% of patients in doses that induce few, if any, adverse effects. They are not recommended for acute asthma or status asthmaticus since they have no intrinsic bronchodilator activity. Cromolyn has local effects on the lungs and consequently is administered often in aerosol forms. It frequently is used in combination with corticosteroid and/or bronchodilator treatment.

Leukotriene pathway inhibitors include receptor antagonists and leukotriene synthesis inhibitors. Leukotrienes are endogenous mediators clearly involved in the inflammatory process associated with asthma and are recognized to have three main effects: increased vascular permeability, recruitment of inflammatory leukocytes (PMNs), and induction of bronchoconstriction. The first leukotriene synthesis inhibitor to be approved by the Food and Drug Administration (FDA) was zileuton, which inhibits 5-lipoxygenase and improves airway function and reduces asthma symptoms in mild-to-moderate asthma patients. Zafirlukast is the first leukotriene D4 receptor antagonist approved, but others are now under investigation that produce similar benefits without the increases in liver enzymes or drug interactions reported with zileuton and zafirlukast.

The *xanthine drugs,* especially theophylline, its soluble salts, and derivatives, are thought to be the most useful bronchodilators for moderate or severe reversible bronchospasm. Moreover, they also improve respiratory exchange by increasing diaphragmatic contractility. The mechanism for the therapeutic effect of theophylline on respiratory systems is not clear. However, the bronchodilator action may be due in part to increased cyclic adenosine monophosphate (cAMP) following competitive inhibition of phosphodiesterase, the enzyme that degrades cAMP. Other proposed mechanisms include mobilization of intracellular calcium in smooth muscle, inhibition of prostaglandin action, blockade of adenosine receptors, and inhibition of the release of histamine and leukotrienes from mast cells. This drug has several notable actions that influence other target organs such as cardiac muscle and the central nervous system (CNS) including

1. It competitively inhibits phosphodiesterase, which increases cAMP and the release of endogenous epinephrine.
2. It inhibits neural transmission at certain synapses, especially in the CNS, where adenosine, a structural analog, may be a neurotransmitter.
3. It antagonizes the action of PGE_2 and $PGF_{2\alpha}$.
4. It affects the mobilization of intracellular calcium.

Table 69-1. Inhaled β₂-Adrenergic Agonists

DRUG	COMMENTS
Albuterol	Rapid onset (<5 min), duration of 3 to 8 hr
Metaproterenol	Similar to albuterol
Pirbuterol	Similar to albuterol
Terbutaline	Similar to albuterol
Salmeterol	Slower onset (20 min), long duration (12 hr)
Fenoterol	Similar to salmeterol

It is important to note that theophylline induces learning and behavioral problems in about 5% of school children receiving the drug.

The effectiveness of the theophylline salts and derivatives in the treatment of bronchial asthma depends on their hepatic conversion to theophylline, which is the active constituent. Consequently, the dosage of theophylline, its salts, and dyphylline usually is expressed in terms of anhydrous theophylline base, despite the marked pharmacokinetic interpatient variability among these preparations. The approximate anhydrous theophylline content of some theophylline derivatives is theophylline monohydrate (91%), anhydrous aminophylline (86%), aminophylline dihydrate (79%), dyphylline (70%), and oxytriphylline (64%). Numerous sustained-action preparations of theophylline are also used to control nocturnal symptoms in asthma patients. A major variable with all of these products is the variability in pharmacokinetics, especially the hepatic metabolism of theophylline, which can be altered by an extensive list of other drugs. The adverse effects and potential toxicities of theophylline are dose-related, so it is often necessary to monitor serum levels in patients who receive chronic therapy. A summary of theophylline pharmacokinetics and associated adverse reactions is included in a monograph.

The anticholinergic drugs are discussed in Chapter ??, β₂ and other adrenergic drugs in Chapter ??, and corticosteroids in Chapter ??. The currently available inhaled β₂-adrenergic agonists used for treatment of asthma are shown in the cross references below.

ALBUTEROL—page 1382.

AMINOPHYLLINE

1*H*-Purine-2,6-dione, 3,7-dihydro-1,3-dimethyl-, compd with 1,2-ethanediamine (2:1)

Theophylline compound with ethylenediamine [317-34-0] $C_{16}H_{24}N_{10}O_4$ (420.43); *dihydrate* [49746-06-7] (456.46).

Preparation—By adding, with vigorous stirring, a weighted quantity of theophylline to a volume of solution containing the required

Table 69-2. Inhaled Corticosteroids

DRUG	COMMENTS
Beclomethasone dipropionate	High topical activity, active metabolite formed in lung fluids, low systemic bioavailability due to high lipophilicity
Budesonide	High topical activity, used as powder, rapid hepatic metabolism, limited systemic bioavailability
Flunisolide	Good topical activity, higher systemic bioavailability, short plasma half-life
Fluticasone propionate	Very high topical activity, very low systemic bioavailability
Triamcinolone acetonide	Good topical activity, short plasma half-life, limited systemic bioavailability

equivalent quantity of the diamine in anhydrous alcohol. After a few hours, the precipitate of aminophylline is filtered off, washed with cold alcohol, and dried at a low temperature.

Description—White or slightly yellowish granules or powder, with a slight ammoniacal odor and a bitter taste; on exposure to air it gradually loses ethylenediamine and absorbs CO_2 with liberation of free theophylline; its solution is alkaline to litmus.

Solubility—1 g in about 5 mL water, but, owing to hydrolysis, separation of crystals of less-aminated theophylline begins in a few minutes, these crystals dissolving on the addition of a small amount of ethylenediamine. When, however, 1 g is dissolved in 25 mL water, the solution remains clear; insoluble in alcohol or ether.

Incompatibilities—Aqueous solutions are alkaline and display the incompatibilities of the alkalies. *Acids* cause a precipitation of theophylline; even *carbon dioxide* of the air behaves thus.

Comments—Indicated for *bronchial asthma,* and for reversible bronchospasm associated with chronic bronchitis and emphysema. Aminophylline (injection, oral solution, enema) also is used as a respiratory stimulant in neonatal apnea and in Cheyne-Stokes respiration. It also is useful as a diuretic agent. Absorption from the GI tract after oral or rectal administration is incomplete, slow, and variable. Approximately 79% is converted to theophylline. Optimal serum therapeutic levels range from 10 to 20 μg/mL. It is most effective when given intravenously; if given slowly in dilute solution, the drug is relatively nontoxic, although nausea, vomiting, and anorexia may appear in some patients. The simultaneous administration of aluminum hydroxide decreases the incidence of this side effect. See *Theophylline.*

AROMATIC AMMONIA SPIRIT

Aromatic ammonia spirit contains, in each 100 mL, 1.7–2.1 g of total NH_3 (17.03), and ammonium carbonate corresponding to 3.5–4.5 g of $(NH_4)_2CO_3$ (96.09).

Description—A nearly colorless liquid when recently prepared, but gradually acquires a yellow color on standing. It has the taste of ammonia, has an aromatic and pungent odor, and is affected by light. Its specific gravity is about 0.90.

Comments—This preparation is given orally as a reflex respiratory stimulant. It should be well diluted with water.

ATROPINE—page 1408.
BITOLTEROL—page 1383.
CROMOLYN SODIUM—page 1547.

DOXAPRAM HYDROCHLORIDE

2-Pyrrolidinone, 1-ethyl-4-[2-(4-morpholinyl)ethyl]-3,3-diphenyl-, monohydrochloride, monohydrate; Dopram

1-Ethyl-4-(2-morpholinoethyl) -3,3-diphenyl -2- pyrrolidinone monohydrate [7081-53-0] $C_{24}H_{30}N_2O_2$·HCl·H_2O (432.99); anhydrous [113-07-5] (414.97).

Preparation—1-Ethyl-3-pyrrolidinol is reacted with thionyl chloride to form the 3-chloro compound which is condensed with diphenylacetonitrile in toluene solution with the aid of sodamide. The resulting α-(1-ethyl-3-pyrrolidinyl)diphenylacetonitrile is hydrolyzed with 70% H_2SO_4 to the corresponding acid. On treatment with thionyl chloride, the acid is converted into the acid chloride which immediately isomerizes to 4-(2-chloroethyl)-3,3-diphenyl-1-ethyl-2-pyrrolidinone. Condensation of this with morpholine in a dehydrohalogenating environment yields doxapram (base) which, on reaction with HCl, gives the official salt.

Description—White to off-white, odorless, crystalline powder; stable in light and air; melts at about 220°.

Solubility—1 g in 50 mL of water; soluble in chloroform; sparingly soluble in alcohol; practically insoluble in ether.

Comments—Doxapram hydrochloride has respiratory stimulant, pressor, and general CNS arousing properties. Respiratory stimulation is mediated principally through the central respiratory centers in the medulla. There may be some contribution through stimulation of peripheral carotid chemoreceptors.

Following a single intravenous injection of doxapram hydrochloride the onset of respiratory stimulation usually occurs in 20–40 seconds with peak effect at 1–2 minutes. The duration of effect may vary from 5–12 minutes. Continuous infusion is a means of controlling the effect and extending its duration.

The respiratory stimulant action is manifested by an increase in tidal volume associated with an increase in respiratory volume.

A pressor response with tachycardia is common following doxapram administration. The pressor response is due more to an increased cardiac output than to peripheral vasoconstriction. Following doxapram administration an increased release of catecholamines has been noted.

DYPHYLLINE

1-*H*-Purine-2,6-dione, 7-(2,3-dihydroxypropyl)-3,7-dihydro-1,3-dimethyl-, Dilor; Lufyllin

7-(2,3-Dihydroxypropyl)theophylline $C_{10}H_{14}N_4O_4$ (254.25).

Preparation—By interaction of 1-chloro-2,3-dihydroxypropane with theophylline dissolved in a sodium hydroxide or potassium hydroxide solution. US Pat 2,575,344 (see *CA* 1952; 46:1722i).

Description—White, crystalline powder; bitter taste; melts about 158°; pH (1 in 100 solution) 6.6 to 7.3; protect aqueous solutions from light.

Solubility—1 g in 3 mL water, 50 mL alcohol or 100 mL chloroform.

Comments—Indicated for relief of *bronchial asthma* and for reversible *bronchospasm* associated with *chronic bronchitis* and *emphysema*. It exhibits peripheral vasodilator and bronchodilator actions characteristic of theophylline. It also has some diuretic and myocardial stimulant effects, and is effective orally. Dyphylline is a derivative of theophylline and is not metabolized to theophylline *in vivo*. Following oral administration, dyphylline is 68% to 82% bioavailable. Peak plasma concentrations are reached in 1 hr; its half-life is 2 hr. The minimal therapeutic concentration is 12 μg/mL; 88% is excreted unchanged in the urine. Because of its somewhat shorter half-life, other theophylline derivatives usually are preferred for chronic bronchodilator therapy. Otherwise, its pharmacological profile, effective and toxic serum levels, contraindications, precautions, adverse reactions, and drug interactions are similar to those for theophylline.

EPHEDRINE—page 1385.
EPINEPHRINE—page 1386.
ETHYLNOREPINEPHRINE—page 1386.
ISOETHARINE—page 1383.
ISOPROTERENOL—page 1383.
METAPROTERENOL—page 1384.
NEDOCROMIL—page 1375.
OXTRIPHYLLINE—see RPS-20, page 1298.
PIRBUTEROL—page 1384.
SALMETROL—page 1385.
TERBUTALINE SULFATE—page 1385.

THEOPHYLLINE

1*H*-Purine-2,6-dione, 3,7-dihydro-1,3-dimethyl-, monohydrate or anhydrous; 1,3-Dimethylxanthine; Elixophyllin; Quibron

Theophylline monohydrate [5967-84-0] $C_7H_8N_4O_2.H_2O$ (198.18); *anhydrous* [58-55-9] (180.17).

Preparation—Present in tea but in too small an amount to make it an economical source. It has been made from caffeine but is produced more successfully by total synthesis.

Description—White, odorless, crystalline powder with a bitter taste; stable in air; melts between 270° and 274°; saturated aqueous solution is neutral or slightly acid to litmus; weaker as a base than caffeine or theobromine and scarcely forms salts even with the strong acids, but is more "acidic" than those and readily dissolves in ammonia water.

Solubility—1 g in about 120 mL water or 80 mL alcohol; more soluble in hot water; sparingly soluble in ether or chloroform; freely soluble in solutions of alkali hydroxides or ammonia.

Comments—Theophylline and its salts and derivatives are used as *bronchodilators* in the symptomatic treatment of *mild bronchial asthma* and *reversible bronchospasm,* which may occur in association with *chronic bronchitis, emphysema,* and *other obstructive pulmonary diseases*. The drug also suppresses exercise-induced asthma and, in doses that maintain therapeutic serum levels, prevents symptoms of chronic asthma. Theophylline is well absorbed after administration. Food has little effect on its availability, although absorption may be slower in the presence of food. Rectal suppositories are absorbed slowly and errati-

cally. The time required to reach peak plasma levels varies with the route and formulation used; following oral administration of liquids or uncoated tablets, peak plasma levels are reached in 2 hr. Average volume of distribution is 0.5 L/kg. Plasma or serum levels of about 10 to 20 μg/mL usually are needed to produce optimum bronchodilator response.

Theophylline is excreted by the kidneys. Less than 15% of the drug is excreted unchanged in the urine. Elimination kinetics vary greatly among individuals. The elimination half-life of theophylline averages about *7 to 9 hr in the adult nonsmoker, 4 to 5 hr in the adult smoker* (one or two packs per day), *3 to 5 hr in children,* and *20 to 30 hr in premature neonates*. The premature neonate excretes about 50% unchanged theophylline and may accumulate the caffeine metabolite. Theophylline, its salts, and dyphylline exert identical pharmacological actions.

Theophylline has less stimulatory effect on the CNS and skeletal muscles than caffeine but has a greater effect on coronary dilatation, smooth muscle relaxation, diuresis, and cardiac stimulation than caffeine. In general, it has relatively more pharmacological activity in all categories than theobromine.

Theophylline produces CNS stimulation and GI irritation following administration by any route. It and its salts and analogs are all somewhat irritating to gastric mucosa. The most common GI side effects (both locally and centrally mediated) include nausea, vomiting, epigastric pain, abdominal cramps, anorexia, and, rarely, diarrhea. Cardiovascular side effects include palpitation, sinus tachycardia, and increased pulse rate. These side effects are usually mild and transient. It also may produce transiently increased urinary frequency, dehydration, twitching of fingers and hands, and elevated SGOT levels. Hypersensitivity reactions characterized by urticaria, generalized pruritus, and angioneurotic edema have been reported with theophylline administration.

Drug interactions are common in patients on theophylline. Agents that *decrease* the effects of theophylline include cigarette and marijuana smoking, phenobarbital, and charcoal-broiled foods. Agents that *increase* the effects of theophylline include cimetidine, erythromycin, influenza virus vaccine, troleandomycin, allopurinol, and thiabendazole. Theophylline *increases* the effects of sympathomimetic drugs, digitalis, and oral anticoagulants. Theophylline *decreases* the effects of phenytoin and lithium carbonate. Concomitant administration of theophylline with β-adrenergic blocking agents may result in antagonistic effects; theophylline with reserpine or halothane may induce tachycardia or cardiac arrhythmias, respectively.

Theophylline toxicity is most likely to occur when plasma levels exceed 20 μg/mL and becomes progressively more severe at higher serum concentrations. Tachycardia, in the absence of hypoxia, fever, or administration of sympathomimetic drugs, may be an indication of theophylline toxicity. Anorexia, nausea and occasional vomiting, diarrhea, insomnia, irritability, restlessness, and headache commonly occur. Fatalities in adults have occurred during or following IV administration of large doses of theophylline in patients with renal, hepatic, or cardiovascular complications. In other patients, the rapidity of the injection, rather than the dose used, appears to be the more important factor precipitating acute hypotension, convulsions, coma, cardiac standstill, ventricular fibrillation, and death. There is no specific antidote for theophylline toxicity; therapy is usually supportive. Treatment includes stopping the drug, gastric lavage and/or emesis, and administration of antacids or demulcents and oxygen. Prompt restoration of fluid and electrolyte balance is essential. Other symptomatic procedures are instituted as necessary.

CORTICOSTEROIDS

In general, inhaled corticosteroids are used to treat persistent asthma and control the inflammatory component of this disease. However, oral corticosteroids may be used intensively for limited time periods to treat more severe, acute exacerbations when other measures, such as β2-selective agonists do not provide adequate relief. The long-term use of systemic corticosteroids may be necessary in some patients, which can cause adrenal insufficiency. Corticosteroid therapy for asthma is done often in combination with concurrent use of other asthma medication, such as inhaled β2-adrenergic agonists and/or sustained-action theophylline-related oral medication. Such combinations help to reduce the number of doses of corticosteroids required to provide adequate asthmatic control and decrease the chance of serious side effects. If done conservatively, inhaled glucocorticoids often are effective in relieving bronchial hyperreactivity associated with moderately severe asthma without significant suppression of adrenal function. However, oral inhalation of corticosteroids such as dexamethasone should not be used for the treatment of occasional mild attacks of asthma that are controlled adequately by treatments with β_2-selective sympathomimetics.

It should be remembered that corticosteroids are not bronchodilators and will not provide rapid relief from bronchospasm and thus should not be the primary treatment for status epilepticus or other acute episodes of asthma. The relative topical potency of inhaled corticosteroid agents is flunisolide = triamcinolone acetonide < beclomethasone dipropionate < budesonide < fluticasone propionate. The delivery systems used can affect the topical and systemic activity of inhaled corticosteroids. The factors that influence clinical efficacy and systemic toxicity of inhaled corticosteroids include topical activity, retention in bronchial fluids, and rapid inactivation when absorbed from the lungs. Increased lipophilicity can slow dissolution and prolong the residence in the lung, but complete pharmacokinetic studies have not compared all these parameters. Also, there is no clear evidence of greater efficacy of any inhaled corticosteroid when administered in equipotent dosages. The most common adverse effects associated with inhaled corticosteroids include a huskiness in the voice (dysphonia) and candidiasis. Rinsing the mouth after inhalation usually controls the potential for oral candidiasis. The higher doses of all inhaled corticosteroids can produce systemic effects that include hypothalamic-pituitary-adrenal axis suppression, bone resorption, carbohydrate and lipid metabolism changes, cataracts, skin thinning, and growth retardation. Some of the inhaled corticosteroids have less potential for such systemic effects because of their rapid hepatic metabolism upon systemic absorption, such as budesonide and beclomethasone dipropionate. These drugs are discussed in greater detail in Chapter ??. A summary of the currently available inhaled corticosteroids is shown below. The inhaled corticosteroids and some potent topical corticosteroids including dexamethasone are also available as either an aqueous spray or aerosol for intranasal administration and are used extensively for allergic rhinitis, without significant adverse effects in most patients. Some patients may experience mild nasopharyngeal irritation, dryness, and headache. Effects are not immediate, but regular use usually results in benefits within a few days.

OMALIZUMAB

Immunoglobulin G, anti-(human immunoglobulin E Fc region) (human-mouse monoclonal E25 clone pSVIE26 γ-chain), disulfide with human-mouse monoclonal E25 clone pSVIE26 -chain, dimmer; Xolair
[242138-07-4]

Preparation—From Chinese hamster ovary cell culture in a nutrient medium containing gentamycin (which is not detectable in the finished product).

Description—Sterile, white, lyophilized powder in a single dose vial. MW about 150 kDa.

Comments—Used to treat moderate-to-severe persistent allergic asthma not adequately controlled by inhalation corticosteroids. It inhibits the binding of IgE to the high-affinity IgE receptor (FcεRI) on the surface of mast cells and basophils. Reduction in surface-bound IgE on FcεRI-bearing cells limits the degree of release of mediators of the allergic response. Treatment with Xolair also reduces the number of FcεRI receptors on basophils in atopic patients.

LEUKOTRIENE PATHWAY ANTAGONISTS

The major differences in the new drugs designed to interfere with the formation or action of the bronchoconstrictor leukotrienes (LTC_4, LTD_4, and LTE_4) are their duration of action, frequency of side effects, and potential drug interactions. Zileuton inhibits the enzyme 5-lipoxygenase, which converts arachidonic acid to a leukotriene A that is a precursor to the proinflammatory leukotriene (LTB_4) that augments the migration of neutrophils and eosinophils as well as the potent bronchoconstrictor leukotrienes. Zafirlukast and montelukast are LTC_4 receptor antagonists that attenuate bronchoconstriction

resulting from the immediate and delayed release of this leukotriene in asthmatic patients exposed to allergens as well as other types of inhalation challenges. However, these drugs are not indicated for acute asthmatic attacks.

MONTELUKAST SODIUM

Cyclopropaneacetic acid, [R-(E)-1-[[[1-3-[2-(7-chloro-2-quinolinyl)ethenyl]-phenyl]-3-[2-(1-hydroxy-1-methylethyl)phenyl]propyl]thio]methyl]-, sodium salt; Singulair

[151767-02-1] $C_{35}H_{35}ClNNaO_3S$ (608.18)

Preparation—See *Drugs of the Future* 1997; 22:1103.

Comments—Approved for *oral prophylaxis* and *chronic treatment* of asthma in patients ≥ 6 yr of age. It is a selective leukotriene receptor antagonist of LTD_4 receptors. It is absorbed rapidly following oral administration, with mean bioavailability of 64% that is not influenced by food. It is extensively metabolized by CYP3A4 and CYP2C9 but does not inhibit these enzymes at therapeutic doses. The mean half-life is 2.7 to 5.5 hr. Adverse effects include some dyspepsia in a few patients. Phenobarbital can induce its metabolism.

ZAFIRLUKAST

Carbamic acid, [3-[[2-methoxy-4-[[[2-methylphenyl)sulfonyl]amino]carbonyl]phenyl]methyl]-1-methyl-1H-indol-5-yl]-, cyclopentyl ester; Accolate

Preparation—See US Pat 4,859,692; *J Med Chem* 1990; 33:1781.

Description—White solid melting about 139°.

Comments—Approved for *oral prophylaxis* and *chronic treatment* of asthma in patients ≥ 12 yr of age. It is a selective and competitive leukotriene receptor antagonist of LTD_4 receptors, which induce bronchoconstriction. It can attenuate the increase in bronchial hyperresponsiveness to inhaled histamine that follows inhaled allergan challenge. Pretreatment also attenuates early and late-phase reaction to inhaled allergens. It is absorbed rapidly following oral administration and is metabolized extensively, with a mean half-life of 10 hr. It inhibits the cytochrome P-450 isoenzymes 3A4 and 2C9. Food reduces bioavailability by 40%, so it should be taken 1 hr before or 2 hr after meals. Adverse effects include headache, dizziness, nausea, diarrhea, elevation of serum liver enzymes, and dyspepsia. Drug interactions due to inhibition of CYP2C9 and CYP3A4 include aspirin, erythromycin, terfenadine, theophylline, and warfarin.

ZILEUTON

Urea, (±)-N-(1-benzo[b]thien-2-ylethyl)-N-hydroxy-, Zyflo

[406-87-2] $C_{11}H_{12}N_2O_2S$ (236.29).

Preparation—In one procedure, 2-acetylbenzothiophene is converted to the oxime and reduced with BH_3/pyridine to form the corresponding hydroxylamine derivative. The latter is acylated and esterified with acetyl chloride in triethylamine; the ester cleaved with LiOH, then treated with HCl and phosgene to yield the N-hydroxyacyl chloride, which with ammonia is converted to the urea product. See US Pat 4,873,259 (1989).

Description—Crystals melting about 158°.

Comments—Approved for *oral prophylaxis* and *chronic treatment* of asthma in patients ≤12 yr of age. It is a specific inhibitor of 5-lipoxygenase, which results in the inhibition of leukotriene (LTB$_4$, LTC$_4$, LTD$_4$, LTE$_4$) formation. LTB$_4$ augments neutrophil and eosinophil migration as well as adhesion and activation of neutrophils. Increased inflammation, capillary permeability, edema, mucus secretion, and bronchoconstriction are produced by these leukotrienes. Zileuton is absorbed rapidly upon oral administration and can be taken with or without food. It is metabolized extensively by hepatic cytochrome P-450 enzymes (1A2, 2C9, and 3A4), with a mean half-life of 2.5 hr. Adverse reactions include hepatotoxicity, which requires monitoring of serum hepatic transaminases. Drug interactions are observed with several drugs undergoing hepatic metabolism such as propranolol, terfenadine, theophylline, and warfarin. Other adverse effects include dyspepsia and nausea in some patients.

OTHER INHALED DRUGS USED FOR ASTHMATIC PATIENTS (ANTICHOLINERGICS AND INHIBITORS OF MEDIATOR RELEASE)

The synthetic anticholinergic drug ipratropium bromide is a quaternary ammonium compound that acts like atropine to block muscarinic receptors. It is administered by inhalation to limit its systemic anticholinergic actions and to reduce bronchoconstriction due to parasympathetic tone that is present in some patients with chronic obstructive pulmonary disease (eg, chronic bronchitis and emphysema). The inhibitors of mediator release, cromolyn and nedocromil, are not used to treat acute bronchospasm but require several days to weeks before a decrease in the bronchospasm and congestive symptoms associated with the release of inflammatory mediators from mast cells, eosinophils, neutrophils, basophils, and alveolar macrophages that are involved in the inflammatory component of this disease. Combination therapy with these agents may help decrease the dose of inhaled or systemic corticosteroid therapy as well as decrease the frequency of use of inhaled β$_2$-selective agonists.

CROMOLYN SODIUM

Disodium salt of 1,3-bis(2-carboxychromon-5-yloxy)-2-hydroxy propane; C$_{23}$H$_{14}$Na$_2$O$_{11}$ (512.34)

For the full monograph see page 1547.

Comments—Prophylactic management of severe bronchial asthma by inhalation of nebulized solution, aerosol, or dry powder contained in capsules. Patients must have substantial bronchodilator-reversible component to their airway obstruction. Response to treatment generally occurs within the first 2 to 4 weeks. Therapy also may include prevention of exercise-induced bronchospasm or exposure to other known precipitating factors (eg, cold dry air, environmental pollutants, allergens). Nasal solution may be used to treat seasonal or perennial allergic rhinitis. Cromolyn inhibits the release of histamine and bronchoconstrictor leukotrienes from mast cells, which may involve effects on calcium channels, but its exact mechanism has not been defined. Only 7% to 8% of drug is absorbed from the lung after inhalation, and it is rapidly excreted unchanged in the urine and bile. When drug from the respiratory tract is swallowed, it is absorbed poorly from the GI tract. Adverse reactions with inhalation include dizziness, headache, cough, wheezing, nasal congestion, bad taste, and rash.

IPRATROPIUM BROMIDE

3-(3-hydroxy-1-oxo-2-phenylpropoxy)-8-methyl-(1-methylethyl)-bromide monohydrate; C$_{20}$H$_{30}$BrNO$_3$.H$_2$O (430.38)

For the full monograph, see page 1408.

Comments—As a *bronchodilator* by inhalation for maintenance of treatment of bronchospasm associated with chronic obstructive pulmonary disease (COPD), including chronic bronchitis and emphysema. It also is used as a nasal spray for symptomatic relief of rhinorrhea associated with allergic and nonallergic rhinitis in patients ≥12 yr of age. Ipratropium bromide is a synthetic quaternary anticholinergic ammonium compound that is chemically related to atropine. It has local effects when inhaled, and it is absorbed poorly into the systemic circulation from the nasal mucosa when used as an intranasal spray. About half the dose is swallowed and eliminated in the feces. The half-life is 3 to 4 hr. Adverse effects from inhalation are cough, mouth dryness, headache, dizziness, and nausea. Few systemic effects are observed in most patients. Use as a nasal spray induces epistaxis, nasal dryness, dry throat, and nasal congestion in some patients.

NEDOCROMIL SODIUM

4*H*-Pyrano[3,2-*g*]quinolone-2,8-dicarboxylic acid, 9-ethyl-6,9-dihydro-4,6-dioxo-10-propyl-, disodium salt; Tilade

[69049-74-7] C$_{19}$H$_{15}$NNa$_2$O$_7$ (415.31)

Preparation—See US Pat 4,474,787; *J Med Chem* 1985; 28:1832.

Description—Yellow powder.

Comments—Used as an inhaled aerosol in maintenance therapy for patients with mild-to-moderate bronchial asthma. It inhibits the activation and mediator release from a variety of inflammatory cell types associated with asthma including eosinophils, neutrophils, macrophages, mast cells, monocytes, and platelets. It inhibits release of mediators including histamine, leukotriene C$_4$, and prostaglandin D$_2$. These actions provide the basis for inhibition of the development of early and late bronchoconstrictor responses to inhaled antigen and other causes of bronchoconstriction such as exercise, cold air, and pollutants (eg, sulfur dioxide). Systemic bioavailability is low, and absorbed drug is excreted unchanged, with a mean half-life of 3.3 hr. The drug is well tolerated with few adverse reactions. Some patients experience unpleasant taste, upper respiratory tract infections, nausea, dyspepsia, and headache.

ANTITUSSIVES

Antitussives are substances that specifically inhibit or suppress the act of coughing. Such inhibition may be due to

1. Depression of the medullary center or associated higher centers.
2. Increased threshold of the peripheral reflexogenous zones.
3. Interruption of tussal impulses in the afferent limb of the cough reflex.
4. Inhibition of conduction along the motor pathways.
5. Removal of irritants by facilitating bronchial drainage and mucociliary activity.

The first four ways of inhibiting cough are believed to characterize the *antitussive* agents, whereas the last one is theoretically associated with *expectorant* agents.

Antitussives may be classified in various ways. For example, centrally acting antitussives either depress the CNS and inhibit the *cough center* in the medulla or raise the threshold for central noxious stimuli and diminish the cough reflex, whereas peripherally acting antitussives act principally within the respiratory tract. Another possible classification considers these drugs as *narcotic antitussives* or *nonnarcotic antitussives*. Agents that have addiction potential are identified, however, since the addiction liability of these substances is the same regardless of therapeutic use.

BENZONATATE

Benzoic acid, 4-(butylamino)-, 2,5,8,11,14,17,20,23,26-nonaoxaoctacosan-28-yl ester; Tessalon

Average: n = 8; [104-31-4] C$_{30}$H$_{43}$NO$_{11}$ (average, 603).

Benzonatate is a mixture of the *p*-butylaminobenzoate esters of the monomethyl ethers derived from a mixture of polyethylene glycols having the average composition of a nonaethylene glycol. The chemical name above is for the average compound.

Preparation—Ethyl *p*-(butylamino)benzoate is transesterified with a polyethylene glycol monomethyl ether fraction in a methanol solution of sodium methoxide. The crude ester is purified by extracting its benzene solution with sodium carbonate solution, the ester being retained in the benzene. US Pat 2,714,606.

Description—Pale yellow, clear, viscous liquid with a faint characteristic odor and a bitter taste followed by a sense of numbness.

Solubility—Freely soluble in chloroform, alcohol, or benzene; miscible with water in all proportions.

Comments—An *antitussive*. It is related to tetracaine and reduces the cough reflex at its source by anesthetizing the stretch receptors in the respiratory passages, lungs, and pleura. It begins to act within 15 to 20 min and its effect lasts for 3 to 8 hr. Although its antitussive potency essentially is the same as that of codeine when evaluated against experimentally induced cough in animals and man, it is somewhat less effective than codeine against cough associated with clinical illness. Benzonatate is tolerated well in therapeutic doses. Untoward effects reported to date include headache, mild dizziness, pruritus and skin eruptions, nasal congestion, constipation, nausea, GI upset, a sensation of burning of the eyes, and numbness or tightness in the chest. Hypersensitivity reactions have been reported. If the capsules are allowed to dissolve in the mouth, they exert a local anesthetic effect that is disagreeable to a few patients. Dependence, euphoria, respiratory depression, or constipation have not been reported. Overdosage can lead to CNS stimulation, resulting in restlessness, tremors, and, ultimately, seizures.

CODEINE—page 1527.
CODEINE PHOSPHATE—page 1527.
CODEINE SULFATE—page 1528.

DEXTROMETHORPHAN HYDROBROMIDE

(9α,13α,14α)-Morphinan, 3-methoxy-17-methyl-, hydrobromide, monohydrate

[6700-34-1] $C_{18}H_{25}NO \cdot HBr \cdot H_2O$ (370.33); *anhydrous* [125-69-9] (352.32).

Preparation—Dextromethorphan base (*d*-3-methoxy-*N*-methylmorphinan) is prepared from the corresponding *d*-3-hydroxy compound by methylation with phenyltrimethylammonium hydroxide. The procedure is analogous to that employed for the methylation of morphine to produce codeine. Treatment of the base with HBr yields the hydrobromide.

Description—Practically white crystals, or crystalline powder, with a faint odor; melts about 126° with decomposition, pH (1 in 100 solution) 5.2 to 6.5.

Solubility—1 g in about 65 mL water; freely soluble in alcohol or chloroform; insoluble in ether.

Comments—Dextromethorphan, the *d*-isomer of the codeine analog of levorphanol, is employed as an *antitussive agent*. It controls cough spasms by depressing the cough center in the medulla. Controlled studies in man indicate that it has a cough suppression potency approximately one-half that of codeine. The oral administration of 30 mg to an adult provides effective antitussive activity over an 8- to 12-hr period. Unlike codeine, it is devoid of analgesic properties and produces little or no depression of the CNS. Addiction does not usually occur even after the administration of rather large doses for prolonged periods. However, there have been reports of abuse of OTC dextromethorphan-containing cold and cough medicines, especially by teenagers. Animal studies suggest that this drug has some effects similar to those of phencyclidine (PCP), which may account for its abuse. Additional data are needed for better assessment of the potential for dextromethorphan dependence. High doses of this drug can cause ataxia, respiratory depression, and convulsions in children, while in adults high doses can alter sensory perception and cause ataxia, slurred speech, and dysphoria. The side effects include slight drowsiness and GI upset; these are less severe and less frequent than with codeine. Accidental poisoning in children is characterized by stupor and ataxia with rapid recovery after emesis. Dextromethorphan hydrobromide should not be given to patients on monoamine oxidase inhibitors.

DIPHENHYDRAMINE HYDROCHLORIDE—pages 1545 and 1548.
HYDROCODONE BITARTRATE—page 1528.
METHADONE HYDROCHLORIDE—page 1532.
MORPHINE SULFATE—page 1527.

EXPECTORANTS

Expectorants are drugs that have been proposed to be useful in loosening and liquefying mucous, in soothing irritated bronchial mucosa, and in making coughs more productive. Such agents are thought to affect the respiratory tract in two ways:

1. By decreasing the viscosity of the bronchial secretions and facilitating their elimination so that local irritants are removed and ineffectual coughing is alleviated or made more productive.
2. By increasing the amounts of respiratory tract fluid so that demulcent action is exerted on the dry mucosal lining, thus relieving the unproductive cough.

The FDA has proposed that orally administered expectorants available OTC be divided into three categories:

Category I—those generally recognized as safe and effective.
Category II—those not generally recognized as safe and effective.
Category III—those with insufficient data to classify as safe and effective.

The FDA has approved only guaifenesin for classification as a Category I expectorant. Thus, it is not surprising that many of the orally administered cough and cold combinations include guaifenesin as the expectorant. Even so, there is a lack of scientific evidence to demonstrate that guaifenesin is of value in the treatment of coughing. It should be remembered, however, that humidification of room air and adequate fluid intake (6–8 glasses of water a day) can effectively liquefy respiratory mucus and are useful therapeutic procedures.

ACETYLCYSTEINE

L-Cysteine, *N*-acetyl-, Mucomyst

N-Acetyl-L-cysteine [616-91-1] $C_5H_9NO_3S$ (163.19).

Preparation—By direct acetylation of L-cysteine.

Description—White, crystalline powder with a very slight acetic odor and a characteristic sour taste; stable in ordinary light; nonhygroscopic (oxidizes in moist air); stable at temperatures up to 120°; melts between 104° and 110°; pK$_a$ 3.24; pH (1 in 100 solution) 2 to 2.75.

Solubility—1 g in 5 mL water or 4 mL alcohol; practically insoluble in chloroform or ether.

Comments—To *reduce the viscosity of pulmonary secretions* and *facilitate their removal*. Hence, it is used as adjuvant therapy in bronchopulmonary disorders when mucolysis is desirable. It is thought the sulfhydryl group in the molecule *opens* the disulfide bonds in mucus and lowers the viscosity. The mucolytic activity of acetylcysteine is related to pH; significant mucolysis occurs between pH 6 and 9. Clinical studies indicate that after inhalation, onset of action is within 1 min, and time to peak effect is 5 to 10 min. Side effects are rare. However, bronchospasm, hemoptysis, and nausea and vomiting have been observed. Antimicrobial drugs, including ampicillin, tetracyclines, amphotericin B, and erythromycin lactobionate, should not be administered in acetylcysteine solution, since it inactivates antibiotics. Effectiveness of acetylcysteine as a mucolytic is difficult to assess and has been based on subjective observations; it may not be any greater than adequate humidification.

Acetylcysteine is used orally and parenterally as an antidote to prevent or minimize hepatotoxicity in acute acetaminophen overdosage. It also has been used with some success as an ophthalmic solution for the treatment of keratoconjunctivitis sicca (dry eye) and as an enema for the management of bowel obstruction due to meconium ileus.

AMMONIUM CHLORIDE—page 1423.
ANTIMONY POTASSIUM TARTRATE—page 1596.

CARBETAPENTANE TANNATE

ing of Tussizone-12, Rynatuss, Xiratuss, etc.

Preparation—Carbetapentane is dissolved in 2-propanol (water also has been used), heated to 65–70° to effect solution and a solution of tannic acid in the same solvent is added over a 60 min period while stirring. After cooling, the suspension is filtered, washed with solvent and vacuum dried. US Pat 5,663,415 (1997), US Pat 6,455,727 (2002).

Description—Light tan-colored powder; softens about 80 - 85°; purity is reported as approximately 95%.

Solubility—Slightly soluble in water or alcohol; insoluble in CH_2Cl_2.

Comments—For the symptomatic relief of cough associated with respiratory tract conditions such as the common cold, bronchial asthma, and acute and chronic bronchitis.

GLYCERIN—pages 758, 1081, and 1423.

GUAIFENESIN

1,2-Propanediol, 3-(2-methoxyphenoxy)-, Glyceryl Guaiacolate

3-(o-Methoxyphenoxy)-1,2-propanediol [93-14-1] $C_{10}H_{14}O_4$ (198.22).

Preparation—Guaiacol and 3-chloro-1,2-propanediol are condensed via dehydrochlorination by warming a mixture of the reactants with a base.

Description—White to slightly gray crystalline powder with a bitter taste; may have a slight characteristic odor; stable in light and heat and is nonhygroscopic; melts with a range of 3° between 78° and 82°; pH (1 in 100 solution) between 5 and 7.

Solubility—1 g in 60 to 70 mL water; soluble in alcohol, chloroform, glycerin, or propylene glycol; insoluble in petroleum ether.

Comments—Used for the *symptomatic relief of respiratory conditions* characterized by a dry, nonproductive cough and the presence of mucus in the respiratory tract. Subjective clinical studies suggest that the action of guaifenesin ameliorates dry unproductive cough by decreasing sputum viscosity and difficulty in expectoration and increasing sputum volume. However, experimentally, it only increases respiratory tract secretions, but only when given in doses larger than those used clinically. Adverse effects are infrequent and usually consist of nausea, gastric disturbance, and drowsiness. Guaifenesin may produce a false-positive test result for 5-hydroxyindoleacetic acid. It is an ingredient of many OTC proprietary expectorant formulations.

POTASSIUM IODIDE

Potassium iodide [7681-11-0] KI (166.00).

Preparation—Potassium iodide may be prepared by reacting iodine with a hot solution of potassium hydroxide, the iodate simultaneously formed being subsequently reduced to iodide by heating the dry reaction mixture with carbon.

Description—Hexahedral crystals, either transparent and colorless or somewhat opaque and white, or a white granular powder; slight hygroscopic in moist air; aqueous solution is neutral or slightly alkaline to litmus.

Solubility—1 g in 0.7 mL water, 22 mL alcohol, 2 mL glycerin, 75 mL acetone at 25°, or 0.5 mL boiling water; when dissolved in water heat is absorbed; 100 mL of a saturated aqueous solution at 25° contains 100 g of KI.

Comments—Used as an *expectorant* and when the action of iodide is desired. It is used as an expectorant to liquefy thick and tenacious sputum in chronic bronchitis, bronchiectasis, bronchial asthma, and pulmonary emphysema. It also is used as adjunctive treatment in cystic fibrosis, in chronic sinusitis, and after surgery to prevent atelectasis. However, the therapeutic value of potassium iodide as an expectorant has not been demonstrated convincingly. Although a substantial number of patients tolerate potassium iodide well, iodide-induced goiter and hypothyroidism have been observed. Consequently, alternative drugs that are safer and more effective should be considered when an expectorant action is desired.

Mild untoward reactions occur frequently with iodide medication. The syndrome is known as iodism. The symptoms include salivation, lacrimation, coryza, soreness of the teeth and gums, eruption of the skin, headaches, swollen salivary glands, and gastric irritation. The symptoms disappear when the drug is discontinued. Serious reactions occur very rarely. Concurrent use of potassium iodide with lithium and other antithyroid drugs may potentiate the hypothyroid and goitrogenic effects of these medications. Likewise, use with other potassium-containing medications and potassium-sparing diuretics may induce hyperkalemia and cardiac arrhythmias or cardiac arrest.

Potassium Iodide Solution—[Saturated Potassium Iodide Solution; Lugol's Solution] contains, in each 100 mL, 97 to 103 g of KI. *Preparation:* Dissolve potassium iodide (1000 g) in hot purified water (680 mL), cool to about 25°, and add sufficient purified water to make 1000 mL; filter, if necessary. *Note:* If the solution is not to be used within a short time, 500 mg of sodium thiosulfate should be added to each 1 L. *Description:* Clear, colorless, and odorless solution with a characteristic, strongly salty taste; neutral or slightly alkaline to litmus paper; specific gravity about 1.700. *Comment:* Iodide supplement and expectorant; see *Potassium Iodide.*

SODIUM CITRATE—page 1331.

TERPIN HYDRATE

Cyclohexanemethanol, 4-hydroxy-α,α-4-trimethyl-, monohydrate; Terpinum; Terpinol

p-Menthane-1,8-diol monohydrate [2451-01-6] $C_{10}H_{20}O_2.H_2O$ (190.28); *anhydrous* [80-53-5] (172.27).

Preparation—By hydration of the pinenes in turpentine oil (or pine oil) in the presence of a strong acid.

Description—Colorless, lustrous crystals, or as a white powder; slight odor, and efflorescent in dry air; a hot 1:100 aqueous solution is neutral to litmus; when dried over H_2SO_4 in a vacuum, it melts about 103°.

Solubility—1 g in about 200 mL water, 13 mL alcohol, 140 mL chloroform, or about 140 mL ether at 25°; 1 g in about 35 mL boiling water or about 3 mL boiling alcohol.

Comments—In *bronchitis* as an *expectorant.* Terpin hydrate elixir contains too little of the compound to be effective alone and is employed mainly as a vehicle for cough mixtures such as *Terpin Hydrate and Codeine Elixir* and *Terpin Hydrate and Dextromethorphan Elixir.*

Terpin Hydrate Elixir contains, in each 100 mL, 1.53 to 1.87 g of $C_{10}H_{20}O_2.H_2O$. *Preparation:* Dissolve terpin hydrate (17 g) in the alcohol (430 mL); add successively sweet orange peel tincture (20 mL), benzaldehyde (0.05 mL), glycerin (400 mL), syrup (100 mL), and purified water (qs) to make the product measure 1000 mL; mix well and filter, if necessary, until the product is clear. *Note*—The sweet orange peel tincture may be replaced by 1 mL orange oil dissolved in 15 mL alcohol. *Alcohol Content:* 39 to 44%. The high alcoholic content in this elixir is required for the solution of the terpin hydrate. *Incompatibilities:* Dilution of this elixir with water or liquids of low alcohol content causes precipitation of the terpin hydrate.

Terpin Hydrate and Codeine Elixir contains, in each 100 mL, 1.53 to 1.87 g of $C_{10}H_{20}O_2.H_2O$ (terpin hydrate), and 180 to 220 mg of $C_{18}H_{21}NO_3.H_2O$ (codeine). *Preparation:* Dissolve codeine (2 g) in terpin hydrate elixir (qs) to make the product measure 1000 mL. *Alcohol Content:* 39 to 44%. *Comments:* This elixir is an *expectorant* and *sedative* used to allay excessive coughing. Its value resides primarily in its content of codeine. *Caution*—This elixir is sometimes used by addicts, by whom it is known as *GI Gin,* for its alcohol and codeine content. In some states pharmacists are required to register and limit its sale. Its repeated sale to an individual should be noted and stopped.

Terpin Hydrate and Dextromethorphan Hydrobromide Elixir contains, in each 100 mL, 1.53 to 1.87 g of $C_{10}H_{20}O_2.H_2O$ (terpin hydrate), and 180 to 220 mg of $C_{18}H_{25}NO.HBr.H_2O$ (dextromethorphan hydrobromide). *Preparation:* Dissolve dextromethorphan hydrobromide (2 g) in terpin hydrate elixir (qs) to make the product measure 1000 mL. *Comments:* The same indications as *Terpin Hydrate and Codeine Elixir.* It is used in the control of coughs associated with the common cold, laryngitis, tracheitis and bronchitis. Dextromethorphan acts to elevate the threshold for coughing. Unlike codeine, it rarely produces drowsiness or GI disturbances.

TOLU BALSAM—page 1068.

Expectorant Combinations

The most frequent expectorant combinations include an antitussive with guaifenesin. However, expectorants also are found in combination with sympathomimetics, antihistamines, and analgesics in OTC cold and cough medicines. The benefit of such combinations in the treatment of coughing or other respiratory ailments is controversial.

SURFACTANT PREPARATIONS

Surfactant preparations are used as replacement therapy for the treatment of premature infants suffering from neonatal respiratory distress syndrome (also known as hyaline membrane disease). This pulmonary condition occurs in approximately 20% of the 250,000 premature babies born in the US each year and accounts for 5000 deaths annually. A substantial deficiency in the endogenous lung surfactant (of which beractant is the primary phospholipid) is the principal factor contributing to the pathology of respiratory distress syndrome. The lung surfactant preparations are used in combination with supplemental oxygen and mechanical ventilation to facilitate gas exchange for either prophylactic or rescue treatment of neonatal respiratory distress syndrome. The exogenous surfactants are either derived from animals or synthesized. The efficacy of lung surfactants has been demonstrated in double-blind, randomized studies in comparison to air placebo in premature infants with respiratory distress syndrome, particularly in infants with a birth weight exceeding 700 g. Studies suggest the exogenous lung surfactants are tolerated well, with few direct adverse effects.

BERACTANT

3,5,9-Trioxa-4-phosphapentacosan-1-aminium, *(R)*-4-hydroxy-*N,N,N*-trimethyl-10-oxo-7-[(1-oxohexadecyl)oxy]-, hydroxide, inner salt, 4-oxide; Survanta

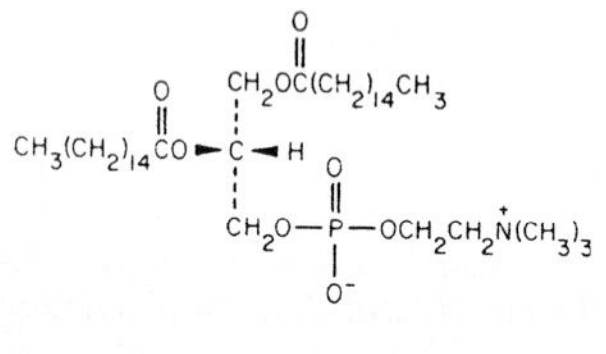

1,2-Dipalmitoyl-*sn*-glycero-3-phosphocholine [63-89-8] $C_{40}H_{80}NO_8P$ (734.05).

Comments—*Beractant* is a modified bovine extract consisting of phospholipids, neutral lipids, fatty acids, and surfactant-associated proteins beractant, palmitic acid, and tipalmitin are added to improve the surface-active properties. Exosurf is a synthetic lung surfactant composed of beractant, cetyl alcohol, and tyloxapol. The cetyl alcohol facilitates spreading and adsorption of beractant at the air-alveolar interface.

CALFACTANT

Calfactant; Infasurf

[183325-78-2]

Preparation—A natural surfactant extracted from the lungs of calves using a chloroform/methanol lavage.

Description—A sterile, non-pyrogenic lung surfactant; off-white suspension in 0.9% aqueous sodium chloride solution and contains 35 mg total phospholipids (including 26 mg phosphatidylcholine of which 16 mg is disaturated phosphatidylcholine) and 0.65 mg proteins including 0.26 mg of SP-B. It has a **pH** of 5.0-6.0.

Comments—Calfactant is indicated for the prevention of Respiratory Distress Syndrome (RDS) in premature infants at high risk for RDS and for the treatment ("rescue") of premature infants who develop RDS. It decreases the incidence of RDS, mortality due to RDS, and air leaks associated with RDS.

PORACTANT ALFA

Poractant Alfa; Curosurf

[129060-19-8]

Description—An extract of porcine lung containing not less than 90% of phospholipids, about 1% hydrophobic proteins (SP-B and SP-C) and about 90% of other lipids. The phospholipid component is composed of phosphatidyl choline and derivatives.

Comments—Poractant Alfa is used to treat or "rescue" premature babies with Respiratory Distress Syndrome (RDS). It reduces air trapped in the lining of the lungs (pneumothoraces) associated with RDS.

MISCELLANEOUS RESPIRATORY DRUGS

ALPHA-1 PROTEINASE INHIBITOR

Aralast, Prolastin, Zemaira

Alpha$_1$-PI, Alpha$_1$-antitrypsin

Preparation—From pooled human blood plasma by a cold ethanol fractionation. *Vox Sang* 1985; 48:333.

Description—White lyophilized powder. A single polypeptide chain of 394 amino acid molecules plus 3 carbohydrate molecules linked to asparagine residues. It is the major serine protease inhibitor in mammalian plasma.

Comments—Alpha-1 proteinase inhibitor is indicated for chronic augmentation therapy in patients having congenital deficiency of α1-PI with clinically evident emphysema. Clinical and biochemical studies have demonstrated that with such therapy, it is effective in maintaining target serum α1-PI trough levels and increasing α1-PI levels in epithelial lining fluid. Clinical data demonstrating the long-term effects of chronic augmentation or replacement therapy are not available. It is not indicated as therapy for lung disease patients in whom congenital α1-PI has not been established.

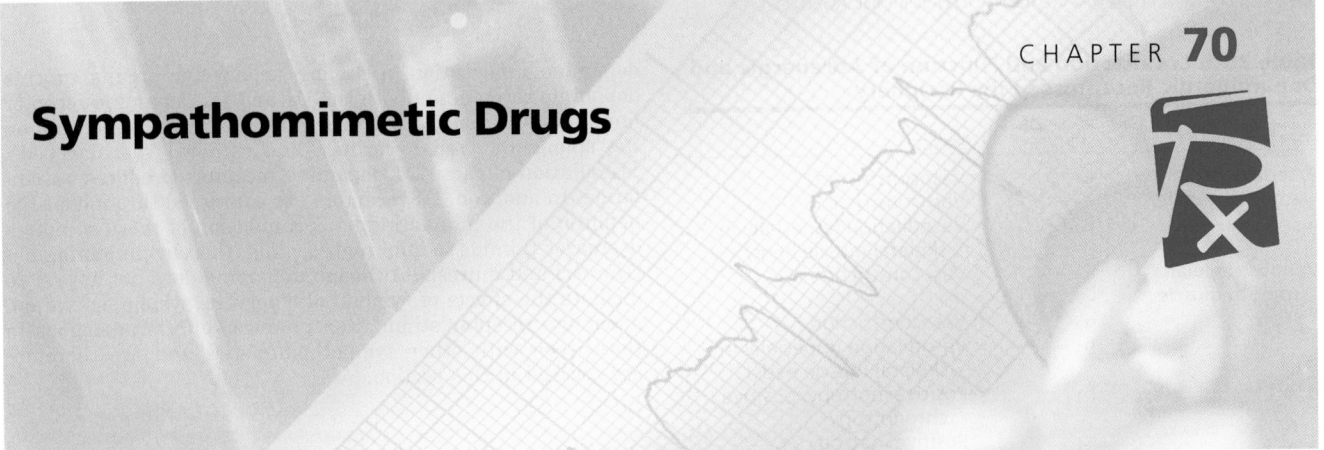

CHAPTER 70

Sympathomimetic Drugs

It is helpful to review briefly the autonomic nervous system (ANS) and the classification of drugs that act on or simulate components of that system. The ANS generally is defined as that aspect of the nervous system involved in the regulation of involuntary, visceral function. As such, the ANS is responsible for regulating the activity of cardiac muscle; the activity of smooth muscle of the viscera, blood vessels, and the eye; and the secretory activity of cells in the viscera, as well as sweat, salivary, and lacrimal glands. The ANS functions to maintain or restore homeostasis of vital physiological functions, such as cerebral blood flow, body temperature, visual accommodation, blood sugar, and body fluid composition.

There are two main efferent divisions to the ANS—the sympathetic (thoracolumbar) and the parasympathetic (craniosacral). Most organs or systems (effectors) receive innervation from both of these divisions. Generally, but not invariably, the two divisions exert opposite influences on a given effector.

The opposite effects exerted by the two divisions of the ANS arise largely because the chemical substances (neurotransmitter/neuromodulator) liberated by the postganglionic nerve terminals in the effector organs are not the same for the two divisions. Parasympathetic *post*ganglionic nerves liberate acetylcholine and, hence, are called *cholinergic*. This acetylcholine acts on muscarinic receptors in the effectors. Most sympathetic *post*ganglionic nerves liberate norepinephrine (noradrenaline), and thus are considered to be *noradrenergic*. The adrenal medulla, however, which is innervated by sympathetic preganglionic nerves, liberates both epinephrine (adrenaline/*adrenergic*) and norepinephrine, with epinephrine release predominating under many, but not all, conditions. These two catecholamines activate α- and β-adrenergic receptors. Although most *post*ganglionic sympathetic neurons are noradrenergic, it should be noted that sympathetic *post*ganglionic fibers to the sweat glands and a few fibers to the vascular beds of the mouth, face, and skeletal muscles are cholinergic.

In the sympathetic ganglia, *pre*ganglionic nerves of either division liberate acetylcholine (ie, are cholinergic). However, the acetylcholine released by the preganglionic neurons acts on nicotinic cholinergic receptors, rather than muscarinic receptors. Thus, the effects of acetylcholine release at these two sites (sympathetic ganglia versus effector organ) are not blocked by the same drugs. Somatic motor neurons also are cholinergic and are similar to autonomic preganglionic nerves in this regard. However, the nicotinic receptors at the neuromuscular junction also are pharmacologically distinguishable from those in the sympathetic ganglia.

Autonomic drugs are classified on the basis of their effects relative to activation of the ANS. Thus, *sympathomimetic drugs* are those whose effects mimic (hence *-mimetic*) the effects seen with activation of the sympathetic nervous system. Likewise, *parasympathomimetics* are drugs that mimic the effects of parasympathetic nervous system activation. Since the sympathetic nervous system liberates norepinephrine (noradrenaline) and epinephrine (adrenaline), sympathomimetics sometimes are referred to as adrenomimetics. Parasympathomimetics are referred to as cholinomimetics, since the parasympathetic system releases acetylcholine at the effector organ.

The effects of sympathetic nervous system activation and, therefore, the effects of sympathomimetic drugs are determined largely by the type and localization of the postsynaptic receptor to which the released neurotransmitter or exogenous sympathomimetic binds. Norepinephrine and epinephrine bind to two general families of receptors, the α- and β-adrenergic receptors. α-Adrenergic receptors have been further divided into α_1 and α_2 receptors on the basis of their pharmacology, and each of these subclasses can be divided further on the basis of their pharmacology and molecular biology. Thus, at least three distinct α_1 receptors have been identified, designated α_{1A}, α_{1B}, and α_{1D}. Similarly, molecular biological techniques have identified at least three distinct α_2 receptors, termed $\alpha_{2A\text{-}2C}$. The β receptors have been subdivided into β_1, β_2, and β_3 receptors on the basis of their pharmacological properties and molecular cloning as well. It should be noted, however, that despite the cloning of a number of α and β receptors, clinically available pharmacological agents at present only distinguish between the broad classes of α_1, α_2, β_1, and β_2 receptors. Therefore, in this chapter reference is not made to the subtypes of receptor within each broad classification.

α_1 Receptors increase phosphatidyl inositol hydrolysis, leading to the production of inositol trisphosphate (IP_3) and diacylglycerol (DAG). These second messengers lead to an increase in intracellular calcium concentrations. α_2 Receptors, on the other hand, are coupled negatively to adenylate cyclase through the $G_{i/o}$ signaling system, leading to a decrease in intracellular cyclic AMP (cAMP) levels. In addition, stimulation of α_2 receptors decreases the opening of voltage-sensitive calcium channels and increases the activity of voltage-sensitive potassium channels, both effects contributing to decreased cell excitability. All three types of β receptors are positively coupled to adenylate cyclase, leading to increased levels of cAMP and increased activity of protein kinase A in the cell.

Knowledge of the localization of the different adrenergic and dopaminergic receptors is critical for understanding the physiological effects of sympathomimetic drugs. The localization of the adrenergic and dopaminergic receptors in a number of effector organs important for the therapeutic usefulness of sympathomimetics and the effects of stimulation of those receptors are given in Table 70-1. The bold-face type indicates, where relevant, which receptor subtype dominates in determining function under normal conditions. It should be noted,

Table 70-1. Localization and Function of Adrenergic and Dopaminergic Receptors in the Periphery

EFFECTOR ORGAN	RECEPTOR SUBTYPE	EFFECT
Arterial vascular smooth muscle	α_1	Vasoconstriction
	α_2	Vasoconstriction
	β_2	Vasodilation (especially in skeletal muscle beds)
Venous vascular smooth muscle	α_1	Vasoconstriction
	α_2	Vasoconstriction
	β_2	Vasodilation (especially in skeletal muscle beds)
Heart	β_1	Positive inotropy, positive chronotropy
	α_1	Positive inotropy
Lungs	β_2	Relaxation of smooth muscle
Eye		
Radial muscle	α_1	Contraction (mydriasis)
Aqueous humor outflow	α_2	Decreased
Kidney	α_1	Decreased sodium and water excretion
		Decreased renin release
	β_1	Increased renin release
Gastrointestinal tract		
Motility	α_2	Decreased ACh release so decreased motility
Ion absorption	α_2	Increased Na^+ and Cl^- absorption
Pancreas	α_2	Decreased insulin release
Urinary bladder		
Detrusor muscle	β_2	Relaxation
Trigone muscle and sphincter	α_1	Contraction
Urethra	α_1	Contraction
Prostate gland	α_1	Contraction of smooth muscle
Uterus	α_1	Contraction
	β_2	Relaxation
Skeletal muscle	β_2	Increased K^+ uptake; increased glycogenolysis
Liver	β_2	Increased glycogenolysis; increased gluconeogenesis
	α_1	
Fat cells	β_3	Lipolysis; thermogenesis

however, that under pathological conditions, the relative contributions of the receptors may be altered. For example, whereas β_1 receptors predominate in regulating cardiac function under normal conditions, α_1-mediated effects become more prominent after chronic treatment with β-blockers, after myocardial ischemia, and in congestive heart failure. Knowledge of the localization of the different receptor subtypes and the effect of their stimulation on the effector organ allows prediction of many of the therapeutic indications and likely side effects of the sympathomimetic drugs. Because of this, the sympathomimetic drugs are classified largely relative to the receptor subtypes that they affect and are presented in this chapter in such a manner.

The role of dopamine in the sympathetic nervous system remains controversial. There is little evidence for dopamine nerves *per se* in the sympathetic nervous system. Although dopamine is the immediate biosynthetic precursor of norepinephrine and therefore is present in postganglionic sympathetic nerves, there is little support for the idea that dopamine is released as a neurotransmitter from those nerve terminals in response to sympathetic nervous system activation. Dopamine is thought to be synthesized, however, by cells in the proximal tubules of the kidney and might exert a paracrine function in that region. Despite the lack of

dopamine innervation, a number of effector organs express dopamine receptors of both the D1 and D2 dopamine-receptor families. For example, D1 dopamine receptors are located on the splanchnic, renal, cardiac, and cerebral vascular beds. Stimulation of these D1 dopamine receptors produces vasodilation. In addition, D1 receptors are expressed throughout the nephron of the human kidney. Stimulation of these receptors decreases tubular sodium reabsorption, thereby promoting natriuresis and diuresis. Although dopamine does not appear to mediate the effects of sympathetic nervous system activation, dopamine receptor stimulation produces effects analogous to those seen with other sympathomimetics and are therefore are covered in this section.

α_1 AGONISTS

Given the distribution of α_1 receptors outlined above and the effects of their stimulation, it follows that pure α_1 agonists often are used for their ability to produce vasoconstriction. Increases in total peripheral resistance achieved with systemic α_1 stimulation are useful in the management of hypotension associated with spinal shock or spinal anesthesia, situations in which there is a loss of sympathetic outflow to the vasculature. Although they can be used in the treatment of other types of shock once blood volume has been restored, their use in these situations is not recommended, as further vasoconstriction in vital organs that already are insufficiently perfused is undesirable.

Local administration of α_1 agonists is beneficial for the production of local vasoconstriction. Thus, local administration is often used in surgery to control local hemorrhage. This vasoconstriction is also of benefit when combined with a local anesthetic, as the vasoconstriction decreases absorption of the anesthetic, thereby prolonging its duration of action. When applied topically to the nasal mucosa or the eye, the local vasoconstriction produced promotes decongestion.

Stimulation of α_1 receptors in the eye produces mydriasis (pupillary dilation) due to contraction of the radial muscle of the iris. The α_1 agonists therefore are useful in producing mydriasis for ophthalmologic examinations.

As is the case for their clinical utility, most of the contraindications and side effects of the α_1 agonists arise from their marked ability to produce vasoconstriction. The resulting increase in blood pressure can precipitate cerebrovascular accidents (ie, stroke), coronary artery occlusion resulting in myocardial infarction, or aneurysm. Because the heart must work harder against the increased pressure, angina may result or heart failure may be exacerbated. For these reasons, the use of α_1 agonists in patients with *hypertension, coronary artery disease, arteriosclerosis, atherosclerosis, cardiac arrhythmias,* or a history of *myocardial infarction* is contraindicated except under strict medical supervision. They also are contraindicated in patients with *venous thrombosis* and *diabetes* because the vascular pathology that is or may be present in these patients can be exacerbated by the vasoconstriction produced. It should be noted that sufficient absorption of α_1 agonists can occur with topical administration to the conjunctiva or nasal mucosa to produce systemic hypertension.

Other peripheral side effects of the α_1 agonists arise from stimulation of α_1 receptors in other sites. Thus, stimulation of α_1 receptors in the urethra and sphincter of the bladder can lead to urinary retention. For this reason, α_1 agonists should be used cautiously in patients with *prostatic hypertrophy*. The mydriasis produced by stimulation of α_1 receptors in the radial muscle of the iris can lead to *photophobia*. Because rebound miosis can occur after the adrenergic effects wear off, α_1 agonists should be used cautiously when there is *retinal detachment*. In addition, the mydriasis produced by α_1 agonists may significantly increase intraocular pressure in patients with *angle-closure (narrow angle) glaucoma*.

MEPHENTERMINE SULFATE

Benzeneethanamine, *N*,α,α-trimethyl-, sulfate; Wyamine Sulfate

[1212-72-2] $(C_{11}H_{17}N)_2 \cdot H_2SO_4$ (424.60); *dihydrate* [6190-60-9] (460.63).

Preparation—By a seven-step synthesis starting with phenyl isopropyl ketone and conversion of the free base to the salt with sulfuric acid. US Pat 2,590,079.

Description—White, odorless crystals or a crystalline powder; solutions are acid to litmus, having a pH of about 6.

Solubility—1 g in 18 mL water, 220 mL alcohol, >1000 mL chloroform, or >10,000 mL ether.

Comments—Has indirect and direct actions.

METARAMINOL BITARTRATE

Benzenemethanol, [*R*-(*R**,*S**)]-α-(1-aminoethyl)-3-hydroxy-, [*R*-(*RI*,*R**)]-2-3-dihydroxybutanedioate (1:1) (salt) Aramine; Pressonex

(−)-α-(1-Aminoethyl)-*m*-hydroxybenzyl alcohol, tartrate (1:1) (salt) [33402-03-8] $C_9H_{13}NO_2 \cdot C_4H_6O_6$ (317.29).

Preparation—Among other methods, by reactions using *m*-hydroxybenzaldehyde and benzylamine as the principal reactants. The base is converted to the bitartrate with an equimolar quantity of tartaric acid.

Description—White, practically odorless, crystalline powder; melts between 171° and 175°; pH (1 in 20 solution) between 3.2 and 3.5.

Solubility—Freely soluble in water; 1 g in about 100 mL alcohol; practically insoluble in chloroform or ether.

Comments—A direct-acting α and β₁ agonist with little β₂ activity. It releases norepinephrine and is used mainly for maintaining blood pressure during spinal shock or spinal anesthesia.

METHOXAMINE HYDROCHLORIDE

Benzenemethanol, α-(1-Aminoethyl)-2,5-dimethoxy-, hydrochloride; Vasoxyl Hydrochloride

(±)-α-(1-Aminoethyl)-2,5-dimethoxybenzyl alcohol hydrochloride [61-16-5] $C_{11}H_{17}NO_3 \cdot HCl$ (247.72).

Preparation—Among other ways, from 2′,5′-dimethoxypropiophenone through reaction with nitrous acid to form the 2-isonitroso derivative followed by catalytic hydrogenation which reduces both the carbonyl function to carbinol and the isonitroso function to amino. The methoxamine, dissolved in a suitable organic solvent, is readily converted to the hydrochloride by a stream of hydrogen chloride.

Description—Colorless or white, plate-like crystals, or a white, crystalline powder; odorless or has only a slight odor; solutions are acid to litmus, having a pH of about 5; melts between 214° and 219°.

Solubility—1 g in about 2.5 mL water or 12 mL alcohol; almost insoluble in chloroform or ether.

Comments—A direct-acting α₁ agonist with a rapid and prolonged pressor action. It also has some β receptor–blocking properties. It is used mainly to support blood pressure during anesthesia.

NAPHAZOLINE HYDROCHLORIDE

1*H*-Imidazole, 4,5-dihydro-2-(1-naphthalenylmethyl)-, monohydrochloride; Privine Hydrochloride

2-(1-Naphthylmethyl)-2-imidazoline monohydrochloride [550-99-2] $C_{14}H_{14}N_2 \cdot HCl$ (246.74).

Preparation—In almost quantitative yields by heating 1-naphthalene-acetonitrile with ethylenediamine monohydrochloride at 175° to 200° for 1 hr. The 1-naphthaleneacetonitrile is made from naphthalene by chloromethylation with formaldehyde and HCl followed by treatment of the resulting 1-naphthylmethyl chloride with potassium cyanide.

Description—White, crystalline, odorless, bitter powder; melting range 253° to 258°, with decomposition; pH (1 in 100 solution) between 5 and 6.6.

Solubility—Freely soluble in water or alcohol; very slightly soluble in chloroform; practically insoluble in ether.

Comments—An OTC and Rx nasal and ocular decongestant used topically.

OXYMETAZOLINE HYDROCHLORIDE

Phenol, 3-[(4,5-dihydro-1*H*-imidazol-2-yl)methyl]-6-(1,1-dimethylethyl)-2,4-dimethyl-, monohydrochloride; Afrin; Neo-Synephrine; Visine

6-*tert*-Butyl-3-(2-imidazolin-2-ylmethyl)-2,4-dimethylphenol monohydrochloride [2315-02-8] $C_{16}H_{24}N_2O \cdot HCl$ (296.84).

Preparation—2,4-Dimethyl-6-*tert*-butylphenol is converted into the benzyl cyanide intermediate, which is reacted with ethylenediamine *p*-toluenenesulfonate whereby, through addition and deammoniation, the imidazoline ring is formed. The resulting oxymetazoline is converted to the salt through interaction with an equimolar quantity of hydrogen chloride. US Pat 3,147,275.

Description—White to nearly white, fine, crystalline powder; odorless; stable in light and heat, nonhygroscopic; melts about 300° with decomposition; pH (1 in 20 solution) between 4 and 6.5.

Solubility—1 g in 6.7 mL water, 3.6 mL alcohol or 860 mL chloroform; practically insoluble in ether.

Comments—An OTC drug used topically as a nasal and ocular decongestant. It causes less rebound congestion than *Naphazoline*.

PHENYLEPHRINE HYDROCHLORIDE

Benzenemethanol, 3-hydroxy-α-[(methylamino)methyl]-, hydrochloride

(−)-*m*-Hydroxy-α-[(methylamino)methyl]benzyl alcohol hydrochloride [61-76-7] $C_9H_{12}NO_2 \cdot HCl$ (203.67).

Preparation—*m*-Hydroxyphenacyl bromide is condensed with methylamine, and the carbonyl group then is reduced to a carbinol via catalytic hydrogenation. The phenylephrine so formed is dissolved in a suitable solvent and neutralized with HCl.

Description—White or nearly white crystals; odorless; bitter taste; melts between 140° and 145°.

Solubility—Freely soluble in water or alcohol.

Comments—Used to maintain blood pressure and as a nasal, scleroconjunctival, and uveal decongestant. It also is used as a mydriatic agent and to promote aqueous humor outflow in the treatment of open-angle glaucoma. Its vasoconstricting properties are used in conjunction with local or spinal anesthetics to prolong their duration of action. It is orally active.

TETRAHYDROZOLINE HYDROCHLORIDE

Imidazole, 4,5-dihydro-2-(1,2,3,4-tetrahydro-1-naphthalenyl)-, monohydrochloride; Collyrium Fresh; Murine; Soothe; Tyzine

[522-48-5] $C_{13}H_{16}N_2 \cdot HCl$ (236.74).

Preparation—Ethyl phenylacetate and methyl acrylate undergo a Michael condensation and cyclization using sodium ethoxide as catalyst, followed by acidification to form 4-keto-1,2,3,4-tetrahydro-1-naphthoic acid. The keto group is reduced by catalytic hydrogenation to methylene, and the resulting 1,2,3,4-tetrahydro-1-naphthoic acid is condensed with ethylenediamine in the presence of HCl.

Description—White crystals; odorless; melts with decomposition about 256°.

Solubility—1 g in 3.5 mL water or 7.5 mL alcohol; very slightly soluble in chloroform or ether.

Comments—An OTC drug used topically as a nasal and ocular decongestant. It causes systemic constriction.

XYLOMETAZOLINE HYDROCHLORIDE

1*H*-Imidazole, 2-[[4-(1,1-dimethylethyl)-2,6-dimethylphenyl]-methyl]-4,5-dihydro-, monohydrochloride; Otrivin Hydrochloride

2-(4-*tert*-Butyl-2,6-dimethylbenzyl)-2-imidazoline monohydrochloride [1218-35-5] $C_{16}H_{24}N_2 \cdot HCl$ (280.84).

Preparation—Using (4-*tert*-butyl-2,6-dimethylphenyl)acetonitrile as the participating nitrile, by the method described for *Naphazoline Hydrochloride,* page 1307.

Description—White, odorless, crystalline powder, melts above 300° with decomposition; pH (1 in 20 solution) between 5 and 6.6.

Solubility—1 g in about 30 mL water; freely soluble in alcohol; sparingly soluble in chloroform; practically insoluble in benzene or ether.

Comments—A nasal decongestant with possibly less reactive hyperemia.

α₂ AGONISTS

The α_2 agonists presented in this section are those used for their actions at peripheral α_2 receptors, thus mimicking the effects of sympathetic nervous system activation. These α_2 agonists are used peripherally in the treatment of open-angle glaucoma, as stimulation of α_2 receptors increases uveoscleral outflow and decreases the production of aqueous humor. Other α_2 agonists, such as clonidine and guanfacine, act on α_2 receptors in the central nervous system (CNS) to decrease sympathetic nervous system activity. Such drugs are reviewed in Chapter 68.

APRACLONIDINE HYDROCHLORIDE

1,4-benzenediamine,2,6-dichloro-*N₁*-2-imidazolidinylidene-, monohydrochloride; Iopidine

[73218-79-8] $C_9H_{10}Cl_2N_4 \cdot HCl$ (281.57)

Preparation—US Pat 4,517,199.

Description—White to off-white powder.

Solubility—1 g in 34 mL water, 74 mL ethanol, 13 mL methanol; practically insoluble in chloroform or nonpolar organic solvents, pH of a 1% soln is about 5.5.

Comments—Used to prevent increases in intraocular pressure following eye surgery including argon laser trabeculoplasty, iridotomy, capsulotomy, and cataract surgery. Its usefulness in the long-term management of glaucoma is limited by the development of tachyphylaxis and ocular allergy.

BRIMONIDINE TARTRATE

Quinoxalinamine, 5-bromo-*N*-(4,5-dihydro-1*H*-imidazol-2-yl)-, [*S*-(*R**,*R**)-2,3-dihydroxybutanedioate salt (1:1); Alphagan

[79570-19-7]) $C_{11}H_{10}BrN_5 \cdot C_4H_6O_6$ (442.23)

Preparation—See Ger 2,538,620 (1976).

Description—Yellow crystals melting about 207°.

Comments—The first selective α_2 agonist approved for long-term use in the treatment of open-angle glaucoma or ocular hypertension. It also is indicated for use in the prevention of increased intraocular pressure in patients undergoing argon laser trabeculoplasty. It is applied topically to the eye and has a peak effect 2 hr after instillation and a duration of action up to 12 hr. It is effective in the long-term management of patients with glaucoma who cannot tolerate a β-blocker or as add-on therapy. Although it has 1000-fold greater selectivity for α_2 over α_1 receptors, mydriasis, vasoconstriction, and eyelid retraction can occur because of α_1 stimulation. Adverse side effects are minimal and include dry mouth, eye redness or stinging (25%), and allergic reactions (10%). The effectiveness of brimonidine in decreasing intraocular pressure may decrease over time in some patients. Brimonidine is contraindicated in patients taking *monoamine oxidase inhibitors* (MAOIs).

β AGONISTS

The localization of β-receptors to the smooth muscle of the trachea and bronchi, as well as to uterine smooth muscle, underlies most of the clinical utility of the β agonists. Since the β receptors located on the smooth muscle in those effector organs are of the β_2 subtype, efforts have been focused on developing β_2-selective agonists. β agonists are used in the treatment of reversible obstructive pulmonary diseases such as asthma, emphysema, and bronchitis because they produce bronchodilation, inhibit the release of inflammatory mediators from mast cells, and increase ciliary motility. Their ability to cause relaxation of the uterine smooth muscle underlies their usefulness in the prevention of preterm labor and delivery. β_2 agonists also have been used to treat peripheral vascular disease, particularly intermittent claudication and thrombophlebitis, which has a predominate vasospastic component and occurs in vascular beds that contain β_2 receptors (eg, skeletal muscle). β agonists also are of some use in the emergency management of heart block, bradycardia, and torsades de pointes.

Selective β_2 receptor agonists have less tendency to produce cardiac stimulation than do nonselective β agonists that stimulate β_1 receptors in cardiac muscle. Thus, the incidence of adverse cardiac side effects such as tachycardia and more serious arrhythmias is lower, but not absent, in selective β_2 agonists. Patients with underlying cardiovascular disease and those on MAO inhibitors or tricyclic antidepressants are at greater risk for such cardiovascular side effects. β_1 agonists are therefore contraindicated in patients with *heart disease* or *cardiac arrhythmias.* They also are contraindicated in patients with *thyrotoxicosis,* as the heart in such patients is sensitized to the stimulatory effects of β receptor activation. β_2 receptor agonists also can precipitate tachycardia and arrhythmias because they can decrease blood pressure (by vasodilation), leading to reflex tachycardia. Consequently, they should be used with caution in patients with underlying cardiovascular disease as well. Other potential side effects of β agonists include skeletal muscle tremor (β_2), although tolerance to this effect usually develops; decreased arterial O_2 tension (β_1 and β_2); feelings of restlessness, anxiety, or apprehension; decreased plasma K^+ concentrations (β_2); and increased plasma glucose (β_2) and free fatty acid ($\beta_{1/3}$) concentrations. The decreased plasma K^+ concentration may be problematic for cardiac patients, especially those taking cardiac glycosides and diuretics, and the hyperglycemia may necessitate dietary or insulin changes in diabetic patients. All side effects are less likely when β agonists are administered by inhalation.

ALBUTEROL

1,3-Benzenedimethanol, α¹-[[(dimethylethyl)amino]methyl]-4-hydroxy-, Proventil; Ventolin

α¹-[(*tert*-Butylamino)methyl]-4-hydroxy-*m*-xylene-α,α-diol, [18559-94-9] $C_{13}H_{21}NO_3$ (239.31).

Preparation—*J Med Chem* 1970; 13:674.

Description—Off-white to white, crystalline powder; odorless; slightly bitter taste.

Solubility—1 g dissolves in 4 mL of water; slightly soluble in alcohol, chloroform or ether.

Comments—The prototypic β_2 selective agonist and the most widely used in the treatment of asthma and other forms of reversible obstructive pulmonary disease. It has weak β_1 agonist activity. It is administered via oral inhalation through a metered-dose inhaler or nebulizer (albuterol sulfate) or orally as a syrup or tablet (albuterol sulfate). Albuterol is the only metered-dose inhaler currently FDA approved for use in children age 4 yr and above. It often is administered nebulized in the emergency room for the treatment of acute exacerbations of asthma.

Although the oral administration of albuterol and other β_2 agonists has been used in the past to provide a more prolonged duration of action, this approach is being supplanted by the use of β_2 agonists that have long durations of action when administered by inhalation, as administration via inhalation decreases the incidence of systemic side effects.

BITOLTEROL MESYLATE

Benzoic acid, 4-methyl-, 4-[2-[(1,1-dimethylethyl)amino]-1-hydroxyethyl]-1,2-phenylene ester, methanesulfonate (salt); Tornalate

[30392-41]-7] $C_{28}H_{31}NO_5 \cdot CH_4O_3S$ (557.66)

Preparation—*J Med Chem* 1976; 19:834.

Description—Crystalline solid melting about 171°.

Comments.—A prodrug converted to colterol; a β_2-selective agonist. It is used as a bronchodilator with a long duration of action (5 to 8 hr).

FENOTEROL HYDROBROMIDE

1,3-benzenediol, 5-[1-hydroxy-2-[[2-(4-hydroxyphenyl)-1-methylethyl]amino]ethyl]-, hydrobromide salt; Berotec

[13392-18-2] (base) [1944-12-3] (HBr) $C_{17}H_{21}NO_4 \cdot HBr$ (397.26).

Preparation—3,5-Diacetoxyphenacyl bromide and 1-(*p*-methoxybenzyl)-2-propanamine react to form the fenoterol nucleus, wherein the three phenolic groups remain protected. Hydrolysis with acid removes the acetyl groups and demethylation of the methoxy group is accomplished with refluxing HBr to yield the product. US Pat 3,341,593 (1962).

Description—Crystals from methanol/ether melting about 222°.

FORMOTEROL FUMARATE

Formanilide, (±)-2'-hydroxy-5'-[(R*)-1-hydroxy-2-[[(R*)-p-meth-oxy-α-methylphenethyl]amino]ethyl]-, fumarate (2:1) salt; Foradil

[43229-80-7] $(C_{19}H_{24}N_2O_4)_2 \cdot C_4H_4O_4$ (804.88).

Preparation—*Pharm Chem Bull* 1977; 25: 1368 and US Pat 3,994,974.

Description—Crystals from 95% isopropyl alcohol melting about 139o; pK_{a1} 7.9, pK_{a2} 9.2; log P (octanol/water) 0.4 (pH 7.4).

Solubility—Readily soluble in water at physiological pH.

Comments—Formoterol fumarate is a long-acting selective beta₂-adrenergic receptor agonist (beta₂-agonist). Inhaled formoterol fumarate

acts locally in the lung as a bronchodilator. In vitro studies have shown that formoteral has more than 200-fold greater agonist activity at beta₂-receptors than at beta₁-receptors. Although beta₂-receptors are the predominant adrenergic receptors in bronchial smooth muscle and beta₁-receptors are the predominant receptors in the heart, there are also beta₂-receptors in the human heart comprising 10% to 50% of the total beta-adrenergic receptors. The precise function of these receptors has not been established, but they raise the possibility that even highly selective beta₂-receptors may have cardiac effects.

The pharmacologic effects of beta₂-adrenoceptor agonist drugs, including formoterol, are at least in part attributable to stimulation of intracellular adenyl cyclase, the enzyme that catalyzes the conversion of adenosine triphosphate (ATP) to cyclic 3', 5'-adenosine monophosphate (cyclic AMP). Increased cyclic AMP levels cause relaxation of bronchial smooth muscle and inhibition of release of mediators of immediate hypersensitivity from cells, especially from mast cells.

ISOETHARINE HYDROCHLORIDE

1,2-Benzenediol, 4-[1-hydroxy-2-[(1-methylethyl)amino]butyl]-, hydrochloride; *N*-isopropylethylnorepinephrine hydrochloride; Bronkosol; Arm-a-Med

3,4-Dihydroxy-α-[1-(isopropylamino)propyl]benzyl alcohol hydrochloride $C_{13}H_{21}NO_3 \cdot HCl$ [2576-92-1] (275.77).

Preparation—Synthesis of isoetharine and other 1-(3,4-dihydroxyphenyl)-2-monoalkyl-1-butanols, starting with 3,4-dihydroxybutyrophenone, is described in German Pat 638,650 (*CA* 1937; 31:3209⁴). The base is converted to the hydrochloride or the mesylate (below).

Description—White to off-white, crystalline solid; odorless; melts between 196° and 208° with decomposition.

Solubility—Soluble in water; sparingly soluble in alcohol; practically insoluble in ether.

Comments—A moderate α and β agonist used as a bronchodilator. It has a duration of action of 1 to 3 hr.

ISOETHARINE MESYLATE

1,2-Benzenediol, 4-[1-hydroxy-2-[(1-methylethyl)amino[butyl]-, methanesulfonate (salt); *N*-isopropylethylnorepinephrine methanesulfonate; Bronkometer

For the formula of isoetharine base, see *Isoetharine Hydrochloride*. 3,4-Dihydroxy-α-[1-(isopropylamino)propyl]benzyl alcohol methanesulfonate [7279-75-6] $C_{13}H_{21}NO_3 \cdot CH_4O_3S$ (335.41).

Preparation—See *Isoetharine Hydrochloride*.

Description—White to off-white, crystalline solid; odorless; slightly bitter, salty taste; melts about 165°.

Solubility—Freely soluble in water; soluble in alcohol; very slightly soluble in ether.

Comments—See *Isoetharine Hydrochloride*.

ISOPROTERENOL HYDROCHLORIDE

1,2-Benzenediol, 4-[1-hydroxy-2-[(1-methylethyl)amino]ethyl]-, hydrochloride; Isopropylarterenol Hydrochloride

3,4-Dihydroxy-α-[(isopropylamino)methyl]benzyl alcohol hydrochloride [51-30-9] $C_{11}H_{17}NO_3 \cdot HCl$ (247.72).

Preparation—By the synthetic procedure given for *Epinephrine* (page 1311), using isopropylamine in place of methylamine; the base is then converted to the hydrochloride without resolution.

Description—White to nearly white, odorless, crystalline powder, with a slightly bitter taste; gradually darkens on exposure to air and light; solutions become pink to brownish pink on standing exposed to air, and almost immediately so when rendered alkaline; pH (1% aqueous solution) about 5; melting range between 165° and 170°.

Solubility—1 g in 3 mL water or 50 mL alcohol; less soluble in dehydrated alcohol; insoluble in chloroform or ether.

Comments—A prototypic, nonselective β agonist used to stimulate heat rate in bradycardia, heart block, or *torsades de pointes*. Its use in

FENOLDAPAM MESYLATE

1H-3-Benzazepine-7,8-diol, 6-chloro-2,3,4,5-tetrahydro-1-(4-hydroxy-phenyl)-, methanesulfonate (salt); Corlopam

[67277-57-0] $C_{16}H_{16}ClNO_3 \cdot CH_4O_3S$ (401.86)

Preparation—Reduction of 3,4-dimethoxyphenylacetonitrile affords the corresponding amine, which is treated with 2-(4-methoxyphenyl)oxirane, opening the ethylene oxide ring through nucleophilic attack to form 2-[2-(3,4-dimethoxyphenylethylamino)]-1(4-methoxyphenyl)ethanol. With strong acid this latter compound yields the trimethoxylated benzazepine ring structure; this is demethylated with BBr$_3$ to the trihydroxy derivative, oxidized to the orthoquinone, and treated with 9N HCl to form the basic product.

Description—Melts about 274° with decomposition.

Comments—A selective D1 agonist used for the IV management of severe malignant hypertension in a hospital setting.

ACKNOWLEDGMENTS—The efforts of Kristen A Keefe, PhD in previous editions of this work are gratefully acknowledged.

CHAPTER 71

Cholinomimetic Drugs

Daniel J Canney, PhD

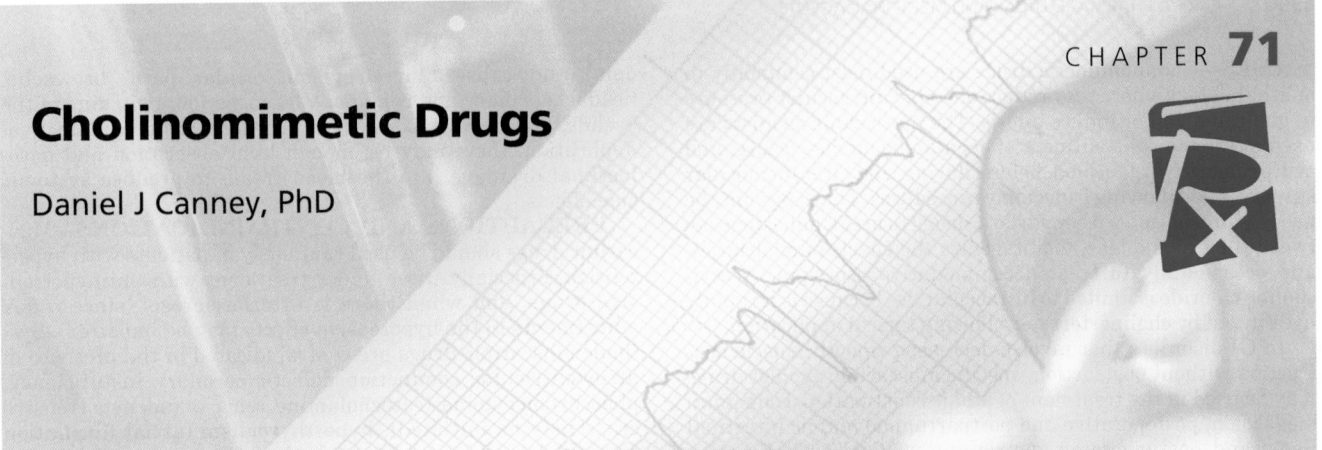

The autonomic nervous system (ANS) may be divided into two efferent portions called the sympathetic (thoracolumbar) and parasympathetic (craniosacral) divisions. The terms sympathetic and parasympathetic are anatomic terms that do not refer to the neurotransmitter being released at nerve terminals or the type of effects produced. The neurotransmitter of all preganglionic autonomic fibers, postganglionic parasympathetic fibers, and a few postganglionic sympathetic fibers (sweat glands) is acetylcholine (ACh). Most postganglionic sympathetic fibers use norepinephrine as the neurotransmitter. An historically important classification of autonomic nerves is dependent on the type of neurotransmitter released from nerve fibers. Hence, fibers that release ACh are cholinergic and include all autonomic preganglionic neurons, somatic nerve endings, parasympathetic postganglionic neurons, and certain neurons of the central nervous system. Those releasing norepinephrine are noradrenergic or adrenergic fibers and include most postganglionic sympathetic neurons and some neurons of the central nervous system.

The cholinergic neurotransmitter system is known to play an important role in both peripheral (PNS) and central nervous system (CNS) function. Cholinergic receptors are divided into nicotinic and muscarinic receptors based on the preferential binding of the alkaloids, nicotine or muscarine, respectively. Molecular biological studies, radio-ligand binding studies and functional assays have identified numerous subtypes of muscarinic and nicotinic receptors that exist in both the PNS and CNS. Acetylcholine binds nonselectively to each of these widely distributed receptors to elicit a large range of pharmacological actions. Cholinomimetic drugs may act at receptors in ganglia, neuromuscular junctions, in the central nervous system, and in parasympathetic neuroeffectors. By contrast, parasympathomimetic drugs are limited primarily to effects at the parasympathetic neuroeffectors innervated *via* muscarinic receptors. It is important to remember that selectivity for a particular receptor subtype is highly dependent on drug concentration. Thus, high concentrations of a muscarinic agonist can produce effects at receptors in the ganglia and/or the neuromuscular junction. Nonetheless, compounds that specifically target subtypes of muscarinic or nicotinic receptors may provide therapeutic agents that lack the side effect profiles of the currently available nonselective drugs.

Acetylcholine synthesis takes place in the cytoplasm of cholinergic neurons through the action of choline acetyltransferase. The newly synthesized ACh is transported into vesicles for storage. Following the release of ACh from the nerve terminal, it is rapidly hydrolyzed to choline and acetate by acetylcholinesterase. The enzyme is found in high concentrations in cholinergic neurons, surrounding neuromuscular junctions, and in other tissues. Butyrylcholinesterse (also known as serum esterase, pseudo-cholinsterase, cholinesterase) has a lower specificity for acetylcholine and is found in plasma, erythrocytes, liver, glia, and other tissues. Drugs that inhibit these enzymes prolong the life of ACh and elicit a variety of effects associated with muscarinic and nicotinic agonists. For this reason, acetylcholinesterase inhibitors generally are classified as cholinomimetics. These drugs have received considerable attention as therapeutic agents, insecticides, and as agents for chemical warfare. The discussion in this chapter will focus on those acetylcholinesterase inhibitors with therapeutic actions in the PNS and the CNS.

CHOLINOMIMETICS

The rapid destruction of systemically administered ACh by cholinesterases makes the endogenous neurotransmitter of limited clinical value. Clinically useful cholinomimetic drugs are either cholinergic agonists that are resistant to the hydrolytic action of cholinesterases, or agents that inhibit cholinesterases. Based on these mechanisms of action, cholinomimetic drugs may be classified as direct acting (agonists) and indirect acting agents (anticholinesterases). The cholinomimetic drugs are used for their effects at muscarinic receptors in the PNS and find utility in ophthalmologic, gastrointestinal, genitourinary, cardiovascular, and pulmonary practice. In addition to these uses, specific indirect acting drugs (anticholinesterases) are used for their CNS actions and in the treatment of Alzheimer's disease. Finally, nicotine is included as a cholinomimetic drug and is available as a smoking cessation aid.

The effects of drugs acting at muscarinic receptors in the periphery are varied. In the eye, stimulation of muscarinic receptors results in contraction of the ciliary muscle to produce accommodation while contraction of the iris sphincter muscle causes miosis. The prominent effects observed in the cardiovascular system are modified by important homeostatic reflexes and involve reduction of peripheral vascular resistance and changes in heart rate. In the gastrointestinal (GI) tract, muscarinic agonists increase the secretory activity of salivary and gastric glands and increase peristalsis activity. In the genitourinary tract muscarinic agonists promote urination due to contraction of the detrusor muscle and relaxation of the trigone sphincter. In the respiratory system, the bronchiolar smooth muscle is contracted, and the tracheobronchial glands are stimulated.

Widespread neuronal degeneration, neuritic plaques containing β-amyloid, and tau-rich neurofibrillary tangles are hallmark findings in Alzheimer's disease. The loss of markers for cholinergic neurotransmission has called attention to a cholinergic component in the disease. Presently, the only FDA-approved drugs for Alzheimer's disease are cholinomimetic drugs. The drugs are palliative and have no effect on the progression of the disease.

USES—Cholinomimetic drugs are used most commonly in ophthalmology where they reduce elevated intraocular pressure in glaucoma and/or induce miosis. The muscarinic agonists are used in the topical treatment of open-angle, angle-closure, and acute congestive glaucoma, before, during, and after intraocular surgery, and following iridectomy procedures. The drugs may be used in alternation with mydriatic drugs to break adhesions between the iris and lens, to antagonize the effects of mydriatics, and occasionally to treat accommodative esotripia. Acetylcholine chloride is limited to intraocular use because is it rapidly hydrolyzed by cholinesterases following topical application.

In GI disorders that involve decreased smooth muscle contraction without obstruction, specific muscarinic agonist drugs may be used in the treatment of atonic constipation, congenital megacolon, postoperative and postpartum adynamic intestinal ileus, and postvagotomy gastric atony. Pancreatic function tests may utilize muscarinic drugs to stimulate pancreatic secretions. Bethanechol has been used to increase the tone of the lower esophageal sphincter in the diagnosis (treatment) of reflux esophagitis. In the genitourinary tract, muscarinic agonists are useful in the treatment of postoperative and postpartum non-obstructive urinary retention and neurogenic atony of the urinary bladder with retention. The primary use of the drug in the cardiovascular field is in the diagnosis and possible arrest of paroxysmal atrial tachycardia. While therapeutic doses usually do not depress normal cardiac functioning, a conduction block in the aberrant conduction pathway within the atrioventricular node may be induced by the drugs. In pulmonary practice, the hypersensitivity of asthmatic patients to bronchiolar constriction induced by cholinomimetics makes methacholine useful in the diagnosis of asthma. Vasospastic peripheral vascular disorders such as Raynaud's disease and dermatitis congelationis (frost-bite) have been treated with these agents. However, superior drugs are available and cholinomimetic drugs are seldom used for this purpose. Lastly, muscarinic agonists are known to increase secretory activity in glands including the salivary and lacrimal glands and are used in the treatment of symptoms of dry mouth caused by radiotherapy for cancer of the head and neck, and symptoms associated with Sjogren's syndrome.

The cause of Alzheimer's disease is unknown, but abnormal processing of neuronal lipoproteins and marked changes in the level of many neurotransmitters including ACh have been implicated. A significant decrease in cholinergic neuronal activity is observed during the progression of the disease that is consistent with the observed deficits in memory and cognition. Based on these observations, drugs with cholinomimetic properties in the CNS are used in the treatment of Alzheimer's disease.

ADVERSE EFFECTS—Adverse effects produced by the cholinomimetics can be predicted based on the pharmacodynamic activity of the drugs. Thus, undesirable effects may include flushing, sweating (that may interfere with body temperature control), abdominal cramps, difficulty in visual accommodation, headache, and convulsions at high doses. Specific GI adverse effects include epigastric distress, belching, diarrhea, involuntary defecation, nausea and vomiting, and colic. In the genitourinary tract, there may be a feeling of tightness in the urinary bladder, urinary frequency, and enuresis. With regard to respiratory effects, bronchiolar constriction leading to bronchspasm and excessive salivary, nasopharyngeal, and bronchial secretions can result and lead to life-threatening blockade of the airway. In low doses, vasodilatation mainly may be confined to the skin (flush, burning sensation). Moderate to high doses may cause moderate-to-severe hypotension, leading to syncope and even shock. Excessive doses may cause severe bradycardia, even cardiac arrest, and atrioventricular conduction disturbances, especially heart block. Furthermore, reflex sympathoadrenal discharge coupled with direct muscarinic effects on conduction sets the stage for serious cardiac arrhythmias.

Topical muscarinic drugs applied to the conjunctiva or intraocularly may interfere with near vision (accommodative myopia) and cause blurred vision, ocular pain, browache, headache, ciliary and conjunctival congestion, twitching of the eyelids, and decreased vision in poor light. After conjunctival application, there may be enough local absorption and nasolacrimal drainage into the bloodstream to produce systemic side effects.

PRECAUTIONS AND CONTRAINDICATIONS—Muscarinic drugs should be used cautiously in patients with hypertension, especially those under treatment with antihypertensive drugs, and when there is arteriosclerosis (since reflex adjustments to the hypotensive effects may be impaired). Systemic muscarinic drugs are contraindicated in the presence of atrioventricular conduction defects, coronary insufficiency, pheochromocytoma (catecholamine release and hypertensive crisis may be initiated), hyperthyroidism (atrial fibrillation may result), asthma, and peptic ulcer. While systemic absorption following topical application in ophthalmology is rare, care must be exercised in patients with the conditions mentioned above. Digital compression of the nasolacrimal ducts following instillation of solutions into the conjunctival sac will minimize drainage and systemic absorption of the drugs.

The actions produced by cholinomimetic drugs are dose dependent, and at toxic levels nicotinic activity may be observed. In case of overdose, anticholinergic drugs may be useful to reverse and/or control some symptoms. The muscarinic actions of the drugs are antagonized by atropine (or other muscarinic antagonists) and the drug serves as an antidote in the treatment of overdose. The nicotinic actions in the PNS (ganglionic and neuromuscular stimulation) can be antagonized with ganglionic blocking drugs and neuromuscular blocking agents, respectively.

ACETYLCHOLINE CHLORIDE

Ethanaminium, 2-(acetyloxy)-*N,N,N*-trimethyl-, chloride; Miochol

$$CH_3CO(CH_2)_2N^+(CH_3)_3Cl^-$$

Choline chloride acetate [60-31-1] $C_7H_{16}ClNO_2$ (181.66).

Preparation—Trimethylamine is reacted with 2-chloroethyl acetate as described in *Bull Soc Chim France* 1914; 15(4):544.

Description—Hygroscopic, crystalline powder.

Solubility—Very soluble in cold water or alcohol; decomposed by hot water or alkalies; practically insoluble in ether.

Comments—Principally a topical ophthalmological drug to induce *miosis* during certain intraocular surgical procedures, such as cataract surgery (*after* the lens is delivered), iridectomy, penetrating keratoplasty, and other anterior segment surgery. It is given as an irrigant into the anterior chamber. When applied to the intact cornea, the poor absorption and rapid hydrolysis of ACh preclude its clinical use as a miotic agent.

There are no clinical uses for systemically administered ACh because it is rapidly hydrolyzed by acetylcholinesterase. When deaths due to huge doses have been reported, it is usually a hypoxic death from mucous plugs in the bronchial tree and/or a cardiac death due to arrhythmias.

BETHANECHOL CHLORIDE

1-Propanaminium, 2-[(aminocarbonyl)oxy]-*N,N,N*-trimethyl-, chloride; Duvoid; Urebeth; Urecholine Chloride

$$\left[\begin{array}{c} CH_3CHCH_2N^+(CH_3)_3 \\ | \\ OCONH_2 \end{array} \right] Cl^-$$

(2-Hydroxypropyl)trimethylammonium chloride carbamate [590-63-6] $C_7H_{17}ClN_2O_2$ (196.68).

Preparation—By treating propylene chlorohydrin with phosgene, reacting the condensation product (2-chloro-1-methylethyl chloroformate) with ammonia in ether solution, and heating the resulting urethan with trimethylamine.

Description—Colorless or white crystals or a white crystalline powder, usually having a slight, amine-like odor; slightly hygroscopic; pH (1% solution) between 5.5 and 6.5; exhibits polymorphism (one form melts about 211° and the other about 219°).

Solubility—1 g in 0.6 mL water or 13 mL alcohol; less soluble in dehydrated alcohol; insoluble in chloroform or ether.

Comments—A carbamate ester analog of ACh, bethanechol chloride is resistant to hydrolysis by the cholinesterases, and it has a relatively prolonged duration of action. The drug has minimal nicotinic activity and has somewhat stronger muscarinic activity for the GI and urinary tracts than for the cardiovascular system. Hence it is employed systemically only for the gastroenterological and genitourinary uses indicated in the general statement. See the general statement for adverse effects, precautions, and contraindications.

Bethanechol chloride is supplied for subcutaneous and for oral administration. It should be taken on an empty stomach. It should not be administered by the intravenous or intramuscular route as cholinergic crisis may result. Even with subcutaneous administration, adverse systemic effects may occur.

CARBACHOL

Ethanaminium, 2-[(aminocarbonyl)oxy]-*N,N,N*-trimethyl-, chloride; Miostat

$$[NH_2COOCH_2CH_2N^+(CH_3)_3]Cl^-$$

Choline chloride, carbamate [51-83-2] (182.65).

Preparation—By reaction of ethylene chlorohydrin with phosgene, the resulting chloroethyl chloroformate is treated with ammonia to produce chloroethyl urethan, which yields carbachol when reacted with aqueous trimethylamine.

Description—White or faintly yellow crystals or crystalline powder; odorless or with a slight amine-like odor; hygroscopic; melts between 200° and 204°; pK_a 4.8.

Solubility—1 g in about 1 mL water or 50 mL alcohol; practically insoluble in chloroform or ether.

Comments—A carbamate ester analog of ACh, carbachol is resistant to hydrolysis by the cholinesterases, and it has a relatively prolonged duration of action. It is a potent cholinergic agonist exhibiting both muscarinic and nicotinic activity. Currently, it is used in ophthalmology, mainly for the treatment of narrow-angle glaucoma and to induce miosis prior to ocular surgery. See the general statement for actions, adverse effects, and contraindications.

CEVIMELINE HYDROCHLORIDE

Spiro[1-azabicyclo[2.2.2]octane-3,5'-[1,3]oxathiolane], *cis*-2'-methyl-, hydrochloride, hydrate (2:1); Evoxac

$(\pm)$-*cis*-2'-Methylspiro[1,3-oxathiolane-5,3'-quinuclidine], hydrochloride, hemihydrate (2:1)

[153504-700-2]; free base [107233-08-9] $C_{10}H_{17}NOS.HCl.1/2H_2O$ (244.79).

Preparation—By reacting 3-hydroxy-3-mercaptomethylquinuclidine with acetaldehyde as described in Japanese Patent 2,804,797 (1986) and referenced in US Patent 5,340,821 (see also, *Drugs of the Future*, (2000), 25(6), 558–569).

Description—A white to off-white crystalline powder with a melting range of 201–203°. The pH of a 1% solution ranges from 4.6 to 5.6.

Solubility—Freely soluble in alcohol and chloroform, very soluble in water, and virtually insoluble in ether.

Comments—Muscarinic agonist that increases secretion of exocrine glands. Indicated for the treatment of symptoms of dry mouth associated with Sjogren's syndrome. The recommended dosage is 30 mg three times daily. Muscarinic agonists can increase secretion and increase tone of smooth muscle in the gastrointestinal and urinary tracts. The most commonly observed adverse effects (in order of frequency) included excessive salivation, nausea, rhinitis, diarrhea, and urinary frequency. The drug is contraindicated in patients with uncontrolled asthma, known hypersensitivity to cevimeline, and when miosis is undesirable (eg, acute iritis, narrow-angle glaucoma). The drug should be used with caution in patients with cardiovascular disease, pulmonary disease, and in other disorders where cholinomimetic effects may lead to complications. Cevimeline should be administered with caution in patients taking beta-adrenergic antagonists due to the possibility of conduction disturbances. The drug may interfere with the effects of antimuscarinic drugs when co-administered. (See the general statement for additional actions, adverse effects, and contraindications). Cevime-

line is metabolized by CYP2D6 and CYP3A4 and drugs that inhibit these enzymes may inhibit cevimeline metabolism. Use in caution in patients suspected of CYP2D6 deficiency. Exposure of CYP450 enzymes to cevimeline produced no inhibition in *in vitro* studies.

METHACHOLINE CHLORIDE

Propanaminium, 2-(acetyloxy)-*N,N,N*-trimethyl-, chloride; Provocholine

(2-Hydroxypropyl)trimethyl ammonium chloride acetate [62-51-1] $C_8H_{18}ClNO_2$ (195.69).

Preparation—From trimethylacetonylammonium chloride by reduction followed by acetylation. (US Pat 2,040,145).

Description—Highly deliquescent; faint, fishy odor; aqueous solutions are neutral and stable for only short periods even when refrigerated; alkaline excipients promote degradation.

Solubility—Freely soluble in water, alcohol, or chloroform.

Comments—The presence of a methyl group beta to the quaternary nitrogen of ACh results in decreased susceptibility to hydrolysis and selectivity for muscarinic receptors. However, weak nicotinic actions are manifested at the neuromuscular junction in myasthenic persons and at adrenal medullary tumors in pheochromocytoma. The drug is marketed only for the diagnosis of bronchial asthma. Persons with asthma are much more sensitive to the bronchoconstrictor actions than are normal persons. A positive test result is a 20% or greater decrease in the forced expiratory volume. However, there is a tendency toward false positives among nonasthmatic smokers and relatives of asthmatics; there is also a small percentage of false negatives. Hypertensives are excessively sensitive to the hypotensive effects, but persons with pheochromocytoma respond with an acute hypertension. Adverse effects of the inhaled drug are syncope and cardiac arrest, for which 0.5 to 1 mg of atropine is given. There is a rare incidence of vertigo, throat irritation, and itching. Methacholine is contraindicated in the presence of β-adrenoreceptor-blocking drugs. Cromolyn may attenuate the bronchoconstrictor response.

NICOTINE

Pyridine, 3-(1-methyl-2-pyrrolidinyl)-,

[54-11-5] $C_{11}H_{14}N_2$ (162-23). An alkaloid from *Nicotiana tabacum* or *N rustica*.

Preparation—Commercially, it is a byproduct of the tobacco industry where it occurs to the extent of 2–8%. It is extracted from waste tobacco with organic solvents and purified through the zinc chloride double salt.

Description—Poisonous, oily liquid; unpleasant tobacco-like odor; burning taste; strongly alkaline reaction; pK_1 6.16; pK_2 10.96 at 15°.

Solubility—Soluble in water, alcohol, chloroform, and most common organic solvents.

Comments—Nicotine is the prototype of cholinomimetics of the so-called nicotinic type. Because it was used by early investigators to determine both cholinomimetic agonist and antagonist actions at the ganglia, at the adrenal medulla, and at the neuromuscular junction, the cholinergic receptors at these sites are designated as the nicotinic subtypes. The action of nicotine in the body is characterized by a primary transient stimulation followed by a persistent depression of all sympathetic and parasympathetic ganglia. The actions are explained by a common mechanism, namely, that of depolarization of the postsynaptic membrane. During the onset of depolarization, nerve action potentials are generated. Once the postsynaptic membrane becomes fully depolarized, further action potentials cannot be initiated, since they require a polarized postsynaptic membrane at their outset. Thus, a block of synaptic transmission results from the persisting depolarization induced by nicotine. Even after the membrane potential is restored, the block may persist. The synaptic stimulatory and depressant effects of nicotine cannot be overcome by atropine.

Nicotine likewise stimulates then paralyzes skeletal muscles and thus induces a succinylcholine-like action, which is the major reason for the toxic effect of the alkaloid on respiration. However, nicotine is more active on ganglia than on skeletal muscles, whereas the reverse is true of succinylcholine. In addition to the above well-established actions, nicotine also first stimulates then depresses the central nervous system (CNS).

Cardiovascular effects of nicotine are hypertension (which may tend to shift to hypotension with time), a smearing of circadian cardiovascular rhythms, tachycardia, a positive inotropic effect (only a part of which can be explained by an effect on nicotinic receptors), and, in large doses, a variety of abnormal electrocardiographic effects. The relationship of these effects to the cardiomyopathy of smoking is unknown.

The CNS effects of nicotine probably are the most important to the initiation and maintenance of the smoking habit. Nicotine is a CNS stimulant that resembles psychomotor stimulants, and it may induce subtle, complex changes in behavior. Although it is often dysphoric in the naive user, it is euphorigenic in tobacco habitues. It increases alertness and attention and, consequently, may improve memory. It decreases irritability and appetite. Deep tendon reflexes and skeletal muscle tone are diminished, which may contribute to a feeling of relaxation. However, nicotine also may induce skeletal muscle tremor and even cause convulsions in large doses. Death may be either consequent to convulsions or respiratory arrest as the result of CNS depression and skeletal muscle paralysis. The adult lethal dose is 40 to 60 mg. Even low doses may cause nausea and vomiting by actions at the chemoreceptor trigger zone and the *vomiting center* in the medulla oblongata. The CNS actions result from a combination of the stimulation of nicotinic and dopaminergic receptors, blockade of some central cholinergic synapses, inhibition of choline acetylase, and release of acetylcholine, dopamine, norepinephrine, and serotonin. Nicotine also causes the release of several hormones, to which some effects are secondary.

Nicotine is metabolized to cotinine in the liver. The plasma half-life is about 2 hours. Nicotine, along with various other constituents of tobacco smoke, induces various hepatic microsomal enzymes in both phase 1 and phase 2 metabolism. Estrogen elimination is accelerated and may cause menopausal-like consequences. Nicotine also increases the elimination of hydrocortisone, which is counterbalanced by greater release of the hormone from the adrenal cortex because of enhanced ACTH release. The metabolism of caffeine, theophylline, imipramine, pentazocine, propranolol, propoxyphene, mexiletine, and numerous other drugs may be accelerated.

Nicotine delivery systems have been developed to be used as part of comprehensive behavioral smoking cessation programs. The systems are intended to help suppress withdrawal symptoms in chronic tobacco users who are trying to quit. The strategy attempts to substitute nicotine previously obtained from tobacco products with nicotine in the delivery systems. Specific quantities of nicotine are incorporated into the delivery device to permit tapering of the dose (over a period of weeks or months) until tobacco dependency subsides.

In nicotine *gum*, nicotine is complexed with a polyacrylic resin. Release from the resin is slow, so that euphorigenesis is less apparent. Nevertheless, nicotine dependence is maintained. Adverse effects from the nicotine content include (in decreasing order of incidence) nausea and vomiting, eructations, vertigo, sialorrhea, headache, and irritability. Effects from constant chewing are oropharyngeal soreness and jaw muscle ache. Each square contains 2 or 4 mg of nicotine; it should be chewed for 20 to 30 min, during which time about 90% of the nicotine is absorbed. Nicotine *transdermal systems* are attached to hairless, clean skin once a day and deliver a rapid initial release of nicotine followed by a slow release over the next 24 hours. A new patch must be applied every 24 hours to a different site to avoid skin irritation. Daily dosage (5–21 mg) is regulated and tapered by using patches of differing sizes (3.5–30 cm^2) and nicotine content. The most common adverse effect is a reversible erythema, pruritus, or burning at the site of patch. Hypersensitivity reactions occur in 2% of patients. A *nasal spray* is available in which each activation of the pump delivers a metered 50 μL spray containing 0.5 mg of nicotine. One dose is considered two sprays and delivers 1 mg of nicotine to the nasal mucosa. The maximum recommended duration of treatment is 3 months, and the maximum number of doses recommended in one day is 40. A nicotine *inhaler* has been developed that delivers 4 mg of nicotine from a cartridge (10 mg/cartridge) attached to a mouthpiece. Successful patients using this nicotine delivery system used 6 to 16 cartridges per day for a duration of 3 months and then were weaned off the inhaler over 6 to 12 weeks. The inhaler is not recommended for more than 6 months. Most recently a nicotine *lozenge* was introduced and is available as 2 mg and 4 mg strengths. The product is allowed to slowly dissolve to release nicotine in place of the usual tobacco product. Headache, insomnia, abnormal dreams, nervousness, insomnia, and GI complaints are relatively common with the nicotine systems. Serious toxicity can result from oral ingestion of patches or from application of multiple patches and overuse/misuse of the gum, lozenge, nasal spray or inhaled products (see effects of nicotine mentioned in the comment section above for additional effects).

PILOCARPINE

2(3*H*)-Furanone, (3*S*-*cis*)-3-ethyldihydro-4-[(1-methyl-1*H*-imidazol-5-yl) methyl]-, Ocusert

Pilocarpine monohydrochloride [92-13-7] $C_{11}H_{16}N_2O_2$ (208.25).

Preparation—The total alkaloids are extracted from the dried crushed leaves of *Pilocarpus microphyllus* or other suitable *Pilocarpus* species with alcohol containing a small amount of hydrochloric acid. The solvent is distilled, and the aqueous residue neutralized with ammonia and allowed to stand until the resins are all deposited. It is then filtered, and the filtrate is evaporated to a small bulk. Ammonia is added in excess, and the free alkaloids are extracted with chloroform. The solvent is removed by distillation, and the residue is allowed to crystallize.

Description—Colorless, translucent, odorless, faintly bitter crystals; hygroscopic and affected by light; solutions acid to litmus; melts within a range of 3° between 199° and 204°; pK$_{a1}$ 6.8, pK$_{a2}$ 1.3.

Solubility—Soluble in water, alcohol, or chloroform; sparingly soluble in ether.

Incompatibilities—See *Alkaloids*, Chapter 26. Since the free alkaloid is quite soluble in water, *alkalies* do not readily cause a precipitation when added to solutions of its salts. It reduces *silver nitrate*.

Comments—See *Pilocarpine Hydrochloride*.

PILOCARPINE HYDROCHLORIDE

2(3*H*)-Furanone, (3*S*-*cis*)-3-ethyldihydro-4-[(1-methyl-1*H*-imidazol-5-yl)methyl]-, monohydrochloride; Isopto Carpine, Salagen

Pilocarpine monohydrochloride [54-71-7] $C_{11}H_{16}N_2O_2 \cdot HCl$ (244.72)

Description—Colorless, translucent, odorless, faintly bitter crystals; hygroscopic and affected by light; solutions acid to litmus; melts within a range of 3° between 199° and 204°; pK$_{a1}$ 6.8, pK$_{a2}$ 1.3.

Solubility—1 g in 0.3 mL water, 3 mL alcohol, or 360 mL chloroform; insoluble in ether.

Incompatibilities—See *Alkaloids* (Chapter 26). Since the free alkaloid is quite soluble in water, *alkalies* do not readily cause a precipitation when added to solutions of its salts. It reduces *silver nitrate*.

Comments—A muscarinic agonist that is devoid of nicotinic activity but is nonselective with respect to muscarinic targets. Because it is a tertiary amine, it is reversibly protonated at physiological pH and penetrates membranes more effectively than do quaternary ammonium cholinomimetics. Consequently, it lends itself well to topical administration in ophthalmology (see below).

Pilocarpine is tolerated better than other miotics. It rarely causes irritation or hypersensitivity, and systemic responses following topical application are uncommon; however, absorption from solutions of high concentration may result in systemic side effects. Lens opacities may result from prolonged use. Ocular controlled-release systems may cause mechanical irritation of the conjunctiva and sometimes a slight increase in mucus secretion, which usually wanes during continued use.

The free base, pilocarpine, is employed in the ocular controlled-release system, since only the nonionized form can diffuse readily through the *hydrophobic* membrane. The hydrochloride or nitrate salt is employed to make solutions, gels, and tablets (see below); the less hygroscopic nitrate is the more convenient to handle pharmaceutically but offers no therapeutic advantage.

In narrow-angle glaucomatous patients who are responsive to pilocarpine and who can maintain the unit within the conjunctival sac, the ocular controlled-release system has the advantage of long duration; the system needs changing but once a week. Topically applied drops are suited better to the acute antagonism of antimuscarinic mydriatics. The salts also may be used in the management of both narrow-angle glaucoma and chronic simple glaucoma of the open-angle type.

Muscarinic agonists are known to increase secretory activity in glands including the salivary and lacrimal glands. Pilocarpine HCl is administered orally for the treatment of symptoms of dry mouth caused by radiotherapy for cancer of the head and neck, and symptoms associated with Sjogren's syndrome. The recommended dosage is 5 mg three times daily. See the adverse effects, contraindication sections for cholinomimetic drugs mentioned above for additional information.

PILOCARPINE NITRATE

2(3*H*)-Furanone, (3*S*-*cis*)-3-ethyldihydro-4-[(1-methyl-1*H*-imidazol-5-yl)methyl]-mononitrate; P.V. Carpine Liquifilm

Pilocarpine mononitrate [148-72-1] $C_{11}H_{16}N_2O_2 \cdot HNO_3$ (271.27).

Description—Shining, white crystals; stable in air but is affected by light; solutions are acid to litmus; melts within a range of 3° between 171° and 176°.

Solubility—1 g in 4 mL water or 75 mL alcohol; insoluble in chloroform or ether.

Incompatibilities—See *Pilocarpine Hydrochloride*.

Comments—See *Pilocarpine Hydrochloride*.

ANTICHOLINESTERASES

Cholinomimetic drugs may be classified as direct acting and indirect acting agents depending on their mechanism of action. The direct acting agents exert their effects by stimulating muscarinic and/or nicotinic receptors whereas indirect acting agents inhibit acetylcholinesterase. The activity of the indirect acting cholinomimetics is due primarily to inhibition of cholinesterase enzymes though several drugs have direct nicotinic actions. Drugs that inhibit acetylcholinesterase cause ACh to accumulate at cholinergic receptor sites and thereby facilitate cholinergic neurotransmission. The term *cholinesterase* is a generic term that includes all enzymes capable of hydrolyzing acetylcholine. There are two main categories of cholinesterase. The term *acetylcholinesterase* is applied to any or all of a family of serine-dependent isoenzymes that very selectively hydrolyze acetylcholine and hence are called true, or specific, cholinesterases; they are not truly specific, since other choline esters may be hydrolyzed at low velocities. Acetylcholinesterase is concentrated in the region of the motor endplate, at autonomic ganglia, in cholinergic neurons in and outside the CNS, and in erythrocytes. The term *butyrylcholinesterase* (also called cholinesterase, pseudocholinesterase, or nonspecific cholinesterase) is applied to a number of enzymes that may hydrolyze acetylcholine but for which butyrylcholine, not acetylcholine, is the optimal substrate. Butyrylcholinesterase is present in glial and satellite cells in the CNS and autonomic ganglia, in smooth muscle, exocrine glands, and various organs such as the liver, and plasma; its concentration in cholinergic neurons is usually insignificant.

The hydrolysis of the ACh molecule is carried out in several steps. Firstly, ACh binds to the catalytic site of the enzyme that includes an esteratic site and an anionic site. The next step involves attack by the hydroxyl group of an active-site serine on the acetate carbonyl of ACh. The resulting transition state is unstable and decomposes to produce free choline and the acetylated enzyme. The acetylated enzyme is hydrolyzed rapidly to regenerate the active enzyme and acetic acid. By changing the "acylating" group on the substrate (ACh) or on an enzyme inhibitor (eg, ester, carbamate, or phosphate), the rate of regeneration of the enzyme and hence the duration of inhibition can be controlled (see below).

Inhibition of acetylcholinesterase and butyrylcholinesterase has various consequences, depending on where the enzymes are inhibited. The function of the butyrylcholinesterase in plasma and the acetylcholinesterase in erythrocytes are poorly understood, and their inhibition has no known physiological consequences, but inhibition may cause moderate increases in the plasma half-life and concentration of acetylcholine and certain other hydrolyzable choline esters. Important effects accrue to inhibition at sites of cholinergic neuroeffector transmission. The preservation of acetylcholine at such sites prolongs and intensifies the cholinergic activity there. Thus, at the neuromuscular junction, anticholinesterases facilitate neuromuscular transmission, with an early increase in muscle strength (by recruiting subliminal junctions) and a late decrease in muscle strength, even paralysis, if many motor endplates remain depolarized by persisting levels of acetylcholine. Excessive muscular fasciculations and fibrillations also occur, which also decrease muscle strength, by causing asynchrony among motor units and fibers. At the autonomic ganglia, the predominant effect is to facilitate transmission, and the final result depends on the effector organ system innervated by the excited postganglionic nerves. In the case of the atria and the atrioventricular node, the activity in both adrenergic and cholinergic postganglionic nerves will be increased, so that the effects mediated by the parasympathetic nerves will be antagonized by those of the sympathetic nerves. However, in the parasympathetic innervation, acetylcholine is preserved by the anticholinesterase at two sites, the ganglia and the innervated heart cells, which amplifies the action, whereas, in the sympathetic innervation, transmission is facilitated only at the ganglia. Therefore, where there is dual and antagonistic innervation, as in the atria, atrioventricular node, pupil, stomach and intestines, urinary tract, etc, the parasympathetic effects predominate. Thus, bradycardia, partial heart block, miosis, increased gastric secretion and motility, and tendency to urination all result from significant anticholinesterase activity. The blood pressure may be elevated, because there is little cholinergic innervation of the vascular tree, and the facilitation in the sympathetic pathway is not antagonized at the vascular smooth muscle. Ciliary spasm may be intense, because there is a negligible antagonistic sympathetic innervation of the ciliary body. Facilitation in both sympathetic and parasympathetic pathways causes increased salivation and sweating (which is mostly cholinergic). Anticholinesterase action within the CNS may cause a mixture of stimulation and depression.

Most of the cholinesterase inhibitors fall into three chemical categories: (1) alcohols with quaternary ammonium groups (edrophonium), (2) carbamate esters of alcohols containing a tertiary or quaternary ammonium group (physostigmine; also bis-quaternary compounds), (3) and organic derivatives of phosphoric acid (echothiophate). *(Note: anticholinesterase drugs used to treat Alzheimer's disease do not fall into these categories.)* These drugs interact with the anionic sites and/or with the esteratic site of cholinesterase to inhibit the enzyme. The molecular details of the inhibition differ based on the chemical class of each drug. Thus, the quaternary amine containing alcohol, edrophonium, inhibits the enzyme through reversible electrostatic interactions. Interaction between the enzyme and the inhibitor does not involve covalent interactions, and consequently the duration of action is short-lived (minutes). The carbamate-containing group of drugs *(with the possible exception of bis-quaternary ammonium-containing compounds)* undergo hydrolysis by the enzyme as described for ACh. However, during the hydrolysis step, the carbamoylated enzyme (carbamate moiety rather than an acetate) is resistant to hydrolysis, and the regeneration of the active enzyme takes longer. Consequently, the duration of action of the drugs in this category is prolonged (hours). The organophosphate-type anticholinesterases result in a phosphorylated enzyme active site that is extremely stable to hydrolysis and may undergo additional reactions (aging) to further strengthen the bond. With these organophosphate-type drugs (like isofluorphate), the duration of action is dependent on the time for resynthesis of cholinesterase (weeks to months). The organophosphate-like agents are sometimes referred to as irreversible inhibitors due to their long duration of action.

The presence of a permanent positive charge on the quaternary amine containing carbamates limits their absorption from the lungs, skin, conjunctiva, and especially into the CNS. Amines like physostigmine (tertiary amine), however, are reversibly protonated at physiological pH. The drug is well absorbed from the eye, lungs, and other sites, can enter the CNS and is more toxic in overdose than the quaternary carbamates. The quaternary ammonium containing carbamates often may enhance neuromuscular function with only minimal-to-moderate autonomic side effects. The quaternary compounds have a nicotinic agonist activity, which, at the ganglia and neuromuscular junction, adds to the cholinomimetic effect. Due to this dual effect, these agents are often chosen to enhance neuromuscular function. Because of their confinement to the periphery, the quaternary agents also may be preferred for peripheral actions. The organophosphate-type anticholinesterases are lipophilic molecules that are absorbed through the skin, readily distribute throughout the body, and penetrate the blood-brain barrier to cause CNS effects. Their effects are long-lasting and consequently, overdoses are dangerous and include a significant CNS component. They generally do not enhance neuromuscular transmission without excessive effects on glands and smooth muscle.

USES—The anticholinesterases are applied topically to the eye in the treatment of primary *wide-angle glaucoma, accommodative convergent strabismus,* and *accommodative esotropia* and for the *emergency treatment of acute congestive glaucoma.* They also may be used to *treat marginal corneal ulcers.* In myasthenia gravis, topical application may be used to improve the function of the extraocular muscles and eyelids. The reversibly acting anticholinesterases may be alternated with mydriatics to *break adhesions between lens and iris.*

The quaternary ammonium anticholinesterases are used systemically to abolish muscular paralysis from competitive *neuromuscular blocking drugs,* to improve muscle function in *myasthenia gravis,* to treat *intestinal distention,* such as congenital *megacolon,* postoperative and postpartum *adynamic intestinal ileus, postvagotomy gastric atony,* and *functional urinary retention.* Edrophonium or neostigmine are used also in the differential *diagnosis of myasthenic crisis,* in which case they will improve muscle function; *cholinergic crisis,* in which case they will worsen function; and to diagnose *myotonia congenita.* Anticholinesterases, especially physostigmine, are used to treat atropine or tricyclic antidepressant poisoning.

Physostigmine, a blood-brain-barrier-penetrant amine anticholinesterase, is employed to *antagonize the toxic CNS effects of antimuscarinic drugs, tricyclic antidepressants,* and H_1-*antihistamines. An approach to protect against exposure to chemical warfare agents like the organophosphates involves pretreatment with reversible inhibitors (physostigmine). This prophylactic measure is used only when lethal exposue to chemical warefare agents is anticipated and very likely to occur.*

Alzheimer's disease is a neurodegenerative disorder that is characterized by the progressive loss of memory and cognitive functions (dementia). The cause of the disorder is unknown but abnormal processing of neuronal lipoproteins and marked changes in the functioning of many neurotransmitters (ACh, cholinergic, serotonin, glutamate, dopamine, norepinephrine, somatostatin) systems have been implicated. A significant decrease in cholinergic neuronal activity has been observed during the progression of Alzheimer's disease. Based on these observations, drugs that increase ACh levels (anticholinesterases) in the CNS are used in the treatment of Alzheimer's disease. If this purported mechanism of action is correct, these drugs will be beneficial only while cholinergic neurons are still intact (ie, early stages of the disease). There is no evidence that the cholinomimetic agents alter the progression of the disease.

ADVERSE EFFECTS AND INTOXICATION—Conjunctivally applied anticholinesterases locally may cause stinging, lacrimation, ocular pain and brow ache (from ciliary spasm), blurring of vision, blepharospasm, conjunctival and intraocular hyperemia, transient early rise in intraocular pressure, iridocyclitis, pigment cysts of the iris, anterior and posterior synechiae, and, rarely, retinal detachment. Atropine can antagonize some of these effects. Allergies also may occur. In addition, organophosphates may cause fibrinous iritis cataracts, especially in elderly patients (in 50% of cases chronically treated), and uveitis.

Adverse systemic effects, from systemic administration or systemic absorption after topical application, include excessive salivation, sweating, tracheobronchial secretion, lacrimation, bronchoconstriction, marked miosis, blurring of vision, nausea and vomiting, diarrhea, abdominal cramps and colic, involuntary defecation, pallor, hypertension or hypotension, bradycardia, and urinary frequency, urgency, and enuresis. These effects can be antagonized with sufficiently large doses of atropine. Laryngospasm, tremors, muscle fasciculations and twitching, weakness (even respiratory paralysis), potentiation of succinylcholine, and dizziness are nicotinic effects that cannot be antagonized with atropine. These effects usually occur only after quite large overdoses. Pralidoxime will antagonize these actions if

given early enough. Acute intoxication caused by large doses of physostigmine or organophosphates also induces CNS effects, such as confusion, ataxia, loss of reflexes, slurred speech, Cheyne-Stokes respiration, convulsions, coma, and respiratory and circulatory paralysis. Huge doses of atropine and pralidoxime, if used early, can suppress these effects. General supportive measures also are necessary in the management of both peripheral and central toxicity. Neuropathy associated with a latent demyelination of various nerve axons has been associated with chronic exposure to some organophosphates.

PRECAUTIONS AND CONTRAINDICATIONS—When systemic anticholinesterases are used, the margin between the first appearance of side effects and serious toxic effects is small. The first signs may be quite subtle. Furthermore, there is wide variation among patients and in the same patient from time to time, so each patient must be approached cautiously. Therefore, careful medical supervision is mandatory. Anticholinesterases should be used cautiously, or withheld, in patients with bronchial asthma, mechanical intestinal or urinary obstruction, peptic ulcer, vagotonia, bradycardia, hypotension, recent myocardial infarction, epilepsy, parkinsonism, or a known hypersensitivity to depolarizing neuromuscular blocking drugs and when cholinomimetics are to be used. Quinidine and quinine antagonize the neuromuscular effects of the anticholinesterases. They should not be applied topically to the eye when there is a history of retinal detachment, uveitis, or angleclosure glaucoma. Their potential systemic effects command the same precautions as for systemic anticholinesterases. Systemic anticholinesterases will antagonize ganglionic blocking drugs. The safety of the amine and quaternary ammonium agents in mother and fetus during pregnancy has not been established; systemic organophosphates are absolutely contraindicated.

AMBENONIUM CHLORIDE

Benzenemethanaminium, *N,N*'-[(1,2-dioxo-1,2-ethanediyl)bis-(imino-2,1-ethanediyl)]bis[2-chloro-*N,N*-diethyl]-, dichloride; Mysuran; Mytelase

[Oxalylbis(iminoethylene)]bis[(o-chlorobenzyl)diethylammonium] dichloride [115-79-0] $C_{28}H_{42}Cl_4N_4O_2$ (608.48); *tetrahydrate* [52022-31-8] (680.54).

Preparation—*N,N*-Diethylethylenediamine is reacted with ethyl oxalate to give *N,N*'-bis[2-(diethylamino)ethyl]oxamide which is doubly quaternized with 2-chlorobenzyl chloride. US Pat 3,096,373.

Description—White, odorless powder melting about 200°.

Solubility—1 g in 5 mL water, 20 mL alcohol, >1000 mL chloroform or >1000 mL ether.

Comments—A quaternary ammonium *anticholinesterase* drug with actions similar to those of neostigmine; ambenonium chloride is 2 to 4 times more potent, and its duration of action after oral administration (4 hr) may be slightly longer. It also is claimed to have a lower incidence of side effects than neostigmine, particularly of the GI tract. It is used in the treatment of *myasthenia gravis.* For side effects and precautions, see the general statement, above.

DEMECARIUM BROMIDE

Benzenaminium, 3,3'-[1,10-decanediylbis(methylimino)carbonyloxy]-bis[*N,N,N*-trimethyl-, dibromide; Humorsol

m-(Hydroxyphenyl)trimethylammonium bromide, decamethylenebis [methylcarbamate]

(2:1) [56-94-0] $C_{32}H_{52}Br_2N_4O_4$ (716.60).

Preparation—*N,N'*-Dimethyl-1,10-decamethylenediamine is added to molten 3-(dimethylamino)phenyl carbonate to produce 1,10-decamethylenebis {3-(dimethylenebis[3-(dimethylamino)phenyl]-N-methylcarbamate}. This ester, a viscous oil, is dissolved in ethanol and doubly quaternized with an acetone solution of methyl bromide. US Pat 2,789,981.

Description—White, or slightly yellow, slightly hygroscopic, crystalline powder; melts about 165° with decomposition; pH (1 in 100 solution) between 5 and 7.

Solubility—Freely soluble in water or alcohol; sparingly soluble in acetone; soluble in ether; aqueous solutions are stable and may be heat-sterilized.

Comments—A reversible anticholinesterase. It is used as a solution with a duration of action from 3 to 5 days.

ECHOTHIOPHATE IODIDE

Ethanaminium, 2-[(diethoxyphosphinyl)thio]-*N,N,N*-trimethyl iodide; Ecodide; Phospholine Iodide

(2-Mercaptoethyl)trimethylammonium iodide *S*-ester with *O,O*-diethyl phosphorothioate [513-10-0] $C_9H_{23}INO_3PS$ (383.22).

Preparation—β-(Dimethylamino)ethanol is reacted with sodium, and the resulting sodium alkoxide is condensed with *O,O*-diethyl phosphorochloridothioate [ClP(S)(OC$_2$H$_5$)$_2$] to yield *S*-[2-(dimethylamino)ethyl] *O,O*-diethyl phosphorothioate. This ester is quaternized with methyl iodide. US Pat 2,911,430.

Description—White, crystalline, hygroscopic solid with slight mercaptain-like odor; its solutions have a pH of about 4.

Solubility—1 g in 1 mL water, 3 mL methanol, or 25 mL dehydrated alcohol; practically insoluble in other organic solvents.

Comments—Due to a long duration of action, the drug may be considered an irreversible anticholinesterase. It is used as a solution with a duration of action from 3 to 7 days.

EDROPHONIUM CHLORIDE

Benzenaminium, *N*-ethyl-3-hydroxy-*N,N*-dimethyl-, chloride; Enlon-Plus; Tensilon

Ethyl (*m*-hydroxyphenyl) dimethylammonium chloride [116-38-1] $C_{10}H_{16}ClNO$ (201.70).

Preparation—*m*-Dimethylaminophenol is dissolved in a suitable organic solvent and quaternized with ethyl iodide. The dimethylethyl(3-hydroxyphenyl)ammonium iodide precipitates and is converted to the chloride in various ways, one of which involves treatment with moist silver oxide to form the quaternary base followed by neutralization with hydrochloric acid.

Description—White, odorless crystalline powder; 1 in 10 solution is practically colorless, pH (1 in 10 solution) between 4 and 5; melts between 165° and 170° with decomposition.

Solubility—1 g in 0.5 mL water or 5 mL alcohol; insoluble in chloroform or ether.

Comments—Inhibits cholinesterase primarily at the neuromuscular junction and very little at other sites. It also has some direct nicotinic stimulant actions at the neuromuscular junction but not at the autonomic ganglia. The duration of action of a single small dose is only about 5 min, but large doses may be effective for 1 to 2 hours. It is used to *abolish neuromuscular paralysis due to d-tubocurarine* or similarly acting motor endplate–stabilizing drugs. It also is used as a *diagnostic agent for myasthenia gravis* or to differentiate a myasthenic crisis from a cholinergic crisis. It may be used occasionally to treat *myasthenic crises*.

Transient blurring of vision, lacrimation, perspiration, and dizziness may accompany its use. It causes muscle fasciculations in the normal human. When it is used to differentiate myasthenic from cholinergic crisis, facilities for endotracheal intubation and artificial respiration must be available.

ISOFLUROPHATE

Phosphorofluoridic acid, bis(1-methylethyl) ester; DFP; Floropryl

Diisopropyl phosphorofluoridate [55-91-4] $C_6H_{14}FO_3P$ (184.15).

Preparation—Isopropyl alcohol is reacted with PCl$_3$ to form diisopropyl phosphite. Oxidation with chlorine gives diisopropyl phosphorochloridate, which metathesizes with NaF to yield the phosophorofluoridate.

Description—Clear, colorless, or faintly yellow liquid; boils about 183°; specific gravity about 1.05; vapor is extremely irritating to the eye and mucous membranes; in the presence of moisture, it decomposes with formation of hydrogen fluoride.

Solubility—Sparingly soluble in water; soluble in alcohol.

Comments—Due to a very long duration of action, this organophosphate may be considered an irreversible anticholinesterase. It is used as an ointment with a duration of action from 2 to 4 weeks.

NEOSTIGMINE BROMIDE

Benzenaminium, 3-[[(dimethylamino)carbonyl]oxy]-*N,N,N*-trimethyl-, bromide; Prostigmin Bromide

(*m*-Hydroxyphenyl)trimethylammonium bromide dimethylcarbamate [114-80-7] $C_{12}H_{19}BrN_2O_2$ (303.20).

Preparation—It may be prepared by reacting dimethylcarbamoylchloride [(CH$_3$)$_2$NCOCl] with potassium *m*-(dimethylamino)phenolate, then quaternizing with methyl bromide.

Description—White, crystalline powder; odorless and with a bitter taste; solutions are neutral to litmus; melts between 171° and 176° with decomposition.

Solubility—1 g in about 0.5 mL water; soluble in alcohol; practically insoluble in ether.

Comments—A quaternary ammonium anticholinesterase. It acts at the ester site of the enzyme to form the inactive dimethylcarbamoyl enzyme. Its effects are more prominent on certain structures than on others, being particularly effective on the bowel, urinary bladder, and skeletal muscle; the pupil, heart, blood pressure, and secretions are affected to a much lesser extent at doses that are ordinarily effective on the structures listed above. The duration of action by the oral route is 3 to 6 hours and by the intramuscular route, 2 to 4 hours.

Neostigmine can be employed for the genitourinary and neuromuscular uses indicated in the general statement. However, it is seldom used today to antagonize curare-like drugs or in the diagnosis of myasthenia gravis due to its long duration of action.

Orally, neostigmine is absorbed poorly; sometimes as little as 1%. Changes in bowel condition can alter absorption considerably, which may make management difficult. Neostigmine is administered parenterally as the methylsulfate and orally as the bromide salt.

NEOSTIGMINE METHYLSULFATE

Benzenaminium, 3-[[(dimethylamino)carbonyl]oxy]-*N,N,N*-trimethyl-, methyl sulfate; Prostigmin Methylsulfate

(*m*-Hydroxyphenyl)trimethylammonium methyl sulfate dimethylcarbamate [51-60-5] $C_{13}H_{22}N_2O_6S$ (334.39).

Preparation—It is made by the method outlined under *Neostigmine Bromide*, using dimethyl sulfate in place of methyl bromide.

Description—White, crystalline powder, odorless and has a bitter taste; solutions are neutral to litmus; melts between 144° and 149°.

Solubility—Very soluble in water; soluble in alcohol.

Comments—See *Neostigmine Bromide*.

PHYSOSTIGMINE SALICYLATE

Pyrrolo[2,3-*b*]indol-5-ol, (3a*S*-*cis*)-1,2,3,3a,8,8a-hexahydro-1,3a,8-trimethyl-, methylcarbamate (ester); mono-(2-hydroxybenzoate); Eserine Salicylate; Isopto-Eserine; Antilirium

Physostigmine monosalicylate [57-64-7] $C_{15}H_{21}N_3O_2 \cdot C_7H_6O_3$ (413.47).

Preparation—By extracting powdered *Physostigma* seeds with hot alcohol. After distilling off the alcohol, the residue is mixed with sodium carbonate and extracted with ether, from which solution the physostigmine is removed with dilute sulfuric acid. The free alkaloid may be obtained by alkalinizing the acid solution. The salicylate may be made by adding 2 parts of physostigmine to a solution of 1 part of salicylic acid in

35 parts of boiling distilled water and allowing the salt to crystallize on cooling.

Description—White or faintly yellow odorless powder or shining crystals; acquires a red tint when exposed to light and air; melts about 184°.

Solubility—1 g in 75 mL water, 16 mL alcohol, 6 mL chloroform, or about 250 mL ether.

Incompatibilities—Aqueous solutions tend to develop a red color on standing; a pink solution does not necessarily indicate complete ineffectiveness, but as the color deepens to red, the product rapidly loses its potency. Boric acid retards the change, but alkalies hasten decomposition. Alkali-free glass should be used. It is precipitated by the usual alkaloidal precipitants.

Comments—The oldest of the anticholinesterases. It combines with the enzyme at the esteratic site to yield the inactive methylcarbamoyl enzyme. It shares with neostigmine marked stimulatory actions on the bowel but causes more secretion of glands, more effect on blood pressure, more constriction of the pupil, and less action on skeletal muscle. Since it is a tertiary amine, it penetrates readily into the eye. Although its main use in medicine is topically in ophthalmology, for the purposes indicated in the general statement, there is some interest in its CNS uses. The salicylate is used for both its CNS and ophthalmological actions; the sulfate is used only in the eye. The duration of the ocular effects after topical application is 6 to 12 hours; the duration of systemic effects is less than 2 hours. The systemic bioavailability after oral administration is about 5 to 12%.

Physostigmine, a tertiary amine can penetrate the blood-brain-barrier and is employed to *antagonize the toxic CNS effects of antimuscarinic drugs, tricyclic antidepressants, and H_1-antihistamines.* An approach to protect against exposure to chemical warfare agents like the organophosphates involves pretreatment with reversible inhibitors like physostigmine. The rationale is to protect the enzyme by blocking it with a reversible agents rather than allowing the essentially irreversible inhibitors access to the enzyme. This prophylactic measure is used only when lethal exposure to chemical warfare agents is anticipated and very likely to occur.

The salicylate has the advantage of being less deliquescent than the sulfate. Addition of a small amount of boric acid to a solution of the salt is said to inhibit formation of the red decomposition product produced by alkalies, which frequently occurs in solutions of physostigmine salts dispensed on prescription. A solution that has developed a red color should not be used.

PYRIDOSTIGMINE BROMIDE

Pyridinium, 3-[[(dimethylamino)carbonyl]oxy]-1-methyl-, bromide; Mestinon; Regonal

3-Hydroxy-1-methylpyridinium bromide dimethylcarbamate [101-26-8] $C_9H_{13}BrN_2O_2$ (261.12).

Preparation—3-Pyridinol is condensed with dimethylcarbamoyl chloride in the presence of a suitable basic catalyst such as dimethylaniline, magnesium oxide, etc. The resulting ester, 3-pyridyl dimethylcarbamate, is isolated, dissolved in a suitable organic solvent, and quaternized with methyl bromide.

Description—White or practially white, crystalline, hygroscopic powder, with an agreeable, characteristic odor; melts between 154° and 157°.

Solubility—Freely soluble in water, alcohol, or chloroform; slightly soluble in hexane; practically insoluble in ether.

Comments—A quaternary ammonium anticholinesterase drug that is approximately one-fourth as potent as neostigmine at the neuromuscular junction and about one-eighth as potent on the bowel, genitourinary tract, and exocrine glands. Its duration of action by the oral route usually is somewhat longer and absorption is less erratic than with neostigmine, which are advantages. Because of its relative affinity for the neuromuscular junction, its principal use is in the treatment of *myasthenia gravis,* in which use it causes fewer side effects than does neostigmine. It is also superior to neostigmine in that the patient may be carried through the night without the necessity of interrupting sleep to take medication. However, in some patients, it provides less control of muscular weakness than does neostigmine. Pyridostigmine is administered orally except when the patient is to undergo surgery or childbirth or is in myasthenic crisis. Neonates born of myasthenic mothers also may be given parenteral pyridostigmine to improve respiration, swallowing, and suckling. The drug also is used to antagonize competitive neuromuscular-blocking drugs.

Anticholinesterases for Alzheimer's Disease

DONEPEZIL HYDROCHLORIDE

Inden-1-one, (±)-2,3-dihydro-5,6-dimethoxy-2-[[1-(phenylmethyl)-4-piperidinyl]methyl]-1*H*- hydrochloride; Aricept

(±)-2-[(1-Benzyl-4-piperidyl)methyl]-5,6-dimethoxy-1-indanone [120014-06-4 (base)] $C_{24}H_{29}NO_3$. HCl (415.96).

Preparation—In a crossed aldol reaction, 1-benzyl-4-piperidinecarboxaldehyde and 5,6-dimethoxy-2(1*H*)-indenone are reacted in the presence of butyl lithium with subsequent dehydration to form the alkene. Catalytic reduction yields the product. *Drugs of the Future* 1997; 22: 397.

Description—Donepezil hydrochloride is a white crystalline powder.

Solubility—Freely soluble in chloroform, soluble in water or glacial acetic acid, slightly soluble in ethanol or acetonitrile and practically insoluble in ethyl acetate or hexane.

Comments—A reversible cholinesterase inhibitor used to treat mild-to-moderate Alzheimer's disease. It is completely absorbed from the GI tract and has a half-life of about 70 hours. Clinical trials indicate modest improvement in cognitive function and activities of daily living; a minority of patients showed greater improvement. Muscarinic side effects and insomnia occur in some patients. Hepatic toxicity has not been reported. Cholinomimetics may have the potential to cause generalized convulsions. However, seizures may be a result of the neurological disorder and not the drugs. Donepezil may interfere with the effects of antimuscarinic drugs or other cholinomimetics (synergy) when co-administered. (See the general statement for additional actions, adverse effects, and contraindications). It is metabolized by CYP2D6 and CYP3A4 and drugs that inhibit or induce these enzymes may alter Donepezil metabolism. Use in caution in patients suspected of CYP2D6 deficiency. Exposure of CYP450 enzymes to donepezil produced no significant inhibition in *in vitro* studies. There is no evidence that the cholinomimetic agents alter the progression of the disease.

GALANTAMINE HYDROBROMIDE

6*H*-Benzofuro[3a,3,2-*ef*][2]benzazepin-6-ol, (4a*S*,6*R*,8a*S*)-4a,5,9,10,11,12-hexahydro-3-methoxy-11-methyl-, hydrobromide; Reminyl, Nivalin

Galanthamine Hydrobromide [1953-04-4] $C_{17}H_{21}NO_3$.HBr (368.27).

Preparation—It has been isolated from Caucasian snowdrop *Galanthus woronoyi.* Galanthamine may be isolated/derived from other plant sources including the bulbs of the daffodil, *Narcissus pseudonarcissus* (see US Pat 5,877,172). It may be synthesized by treating (-)narwedine with L-selectride in tetrahydrofurane followed by treatment with a 60% solution of HBr in ethanol. US Pat 6,407,229.

Description—White to off-white crystalline powder; melts about 245° (decomposition).

Solubility—Sparingly soluble in water, soluble in ethyl acetate, CHCl$_3$.

Comments—Tertiary alkaloid isolated from Caucasian snowdrop *Galanthus woronoyi* and other plant sources including the bulbs of the daffodil, *Narcissus pseudonarcissus.* The precise mechanism of action of the drug is unknown. It is a reversible competitive inhibitor of acetylcholinesterase and enhances cholinergic function in the CNS. In addition, it is postulated that the drug is a modulator of nicotinic receptors. These mechanisms may explain the clinical benefits of the drug. If this purported mechanism of action is correct the drug will be beneficial only while cholinergic neurons are still intact (ie, early stages of the disease). There is no evidence that the cholinomimetic agents alter the progression of the disease.

The drug is available as tablets (4 mg, 8 mg, and 12 mg dosages) and as an oral solution (4 mg/mL) supplied with a calibrated pipette. The dose should be titrated up starting with 4 mg twice daily (8 mg/day) and increased to 8 mg twice daily (16 mg/day) after 4 weeks. The recommended dosage range is 16–24 mg/day given twice daily. Dosage adjustments may be necessary in patients with hepatic renal impairment.

The most commonly observed adverse effects reported for the drug included nausea, vomiting, diarrhea, dizziness, and headache. The drug is contraindicated in patients with known hypersensitivity to galantamine. The drug should be used with caution in patients with cardiovascular disease, gastrointestinal conditions, pulmonary disease (asthma, COPD) and in other disorders where cholinomimetic effects may lead to complications. Cholinomimetics may have the potential to cause generalized convulsions. However, seizures may be a result of the neurological disorder and not the drugs. Galantamine may interfere with the effects of antimuscarinic drugs or other cholinomimetics (synergy) when co-administered. (See the general statement for additional actions, adverse effects, and contraindications). It is metabolized by CYP2D6 and CYP3A4 and drugs that inhibit or induce these enzymes may alter galantamine metabolism. Use in caution in patients suspected of CYP2D6 deficiency. Exposure of CYP450 enzymes to galantamine produced no significant inhibition in *in vitro* studies.

RIVASTIGMINE TARTRATE

Carbamic acid, *N*-ethyl-*N*-methyl-, 3-[1(*S*)-(dimethylamino)ethyl]phenyl ester, 2*R*,3*R*-dihydroxybutanedioate (1:1); Exelon

m-[(*S*)-1-(Dimethylamino)ethyl]phenyl ethylmethylcarbamate, hydrogen tartrate (1:1); [129101-54-8] $C_{14}H_{22}N_2O_2 \cdot C_4H_6O_6$ (400.42).

Preparation—Reaction of *N*-ethyl-*N*-methylcarbamoyl chloride and α-(*m*-hydroxy-phenylethyl)dimethylamine yields a racemic mixture of the product, which is resolved by heating with (+)- bis-[(*O,O*)-*p*-toluyl]tartaric acid in aqueous methanol. On cooling the solution is made alkaline and the *S*-enantiomer extracted with ether. US Pat 5,620,176 (1991).

Description—White to off-white crystals from ethanol melting about 124°. pK$_a$ 8.85, distribution coefficient 3.0 (octanol-phosphate buffer pH 7 at 37°); [α]$^{20}_D$ +4.7, c = 0, ethanol).

Solubility—Very soluble in water, soluble in ethanol and acetonitrile, slightly soluble in octanol, and very slightly soluble in ethyl acetate.

Comments—The precise mechanism of action of the drug is unknown. It is a reversible competitive inhibitor of acetylcholinesterase and enhances cholinergic function in the CNS. If this purported mechanism of action is correct the drug will be beneficial only while cholinergic neurons are still intact (ie, early stages of the disease). There is no evidence that the cholinomimetic agents alter the progression of the disease.

The drug is available as capsules containing rivastigmine tartrate equivalent to 1.5, 3.0, 4.5 and 6.0 mg and as an oral solution containing rivastigmine tartrate equivalent to 2.0 mg/mL of rivastigmine base for oral administration. The starting dose is 1.5 mg twice daily. The dose should be titrated up to the recommended dosage range (6–12 mg/day) based on how well it is tolerated. The drug should be taken with meals in the morning and evening. Dosage adjustments may not be necessary in patients with hepatic and renal impairment.

The most commonly observed adverse effects reported for the drug included nausea, vomiting, diarrhea, loss of appetite, dizziness and headache. The drug is contraindicated in patients with known hypersensitivity to rivastigmine, other carbamate derivatives or components of the formulation. The drug should be used with caution in patients with cardiovascular disease, gastrointestinal conditions, pulmonary disease (asthma, COPD) and in other disorders where cholinomimetic effects may lead to complications. Cholinomimetics may have the potential to cause generalized convulsions. However, seizures may be a result of the neurological disorder and not the drugs. Rivastigmine may interfere with the effects of antimuscarinic drugs or other cholinomimetics (synergy) when co-administered. (See the general statement for additional actions, adverse effects, and contraindications). The drug is metabolized primarily via cholinesterases. Based on in vitro and animal studies the CYP450 enzyme system is not a major route of metabolism and drug interactions related to the CYP450 enzymes have not been observed.

TACRINE HYDROCHLORIDE

Acridine, 9-amino-1,2,3,4-tetrahydro-, hydrochloride; Cognex

[1684-40-8] $C_{13}H_{14}N_2 \cdot HCl$ (234.73).

Preparation—By heating 9-chloro-1,2,3,4-tetrahydroacridine with ammonium carbonate in phenol at 130° followed by usual conversion to the hydrochloride. (See *J Soc Chem Ind* 1945; 64: 169.)

Description—Yellow needles melting about 284°; bitter taste; pH of 1.5% solution about 5.

Solubility—Soluble in water.

Comments—Tacrine or tetrahydroacridineamine (THA) possesses both an anticholinesterase action and an action to block potassium channels in cell membranes. The latter action causes prolonged action potentials, which, at cholinergic nerve endings, increase the release of acetylcholine. Thus, the two actions complement each other. Since the drug can penetrate the blood-brain barrier readily (in the nonionized form) and gain access to the CNS, it is of special interest as an anticholinesterase for actions in the CNS. The current focus is on its effects to improve learning, memory, and mood in patients with Alzheimer's type of senile dementia. AS with other agents used for Alzheimer's disease, the drug is only palliative and does not prevent the eventual degeneration of the affected nerve tracts. Typical muscarinic side effects occur in about 25–35% of recipients, but they are usually minimal and tolerated; they include belching, nausea, emesis, enuresis, abdominal discomfort, diarrhea, and sweating. Evidence of hepatic toxicity requires dosage reduction or discontinuation.

CHOLINESTERASE REACTIVATORS

Consumption of certain wild mushrooms, exposure to anticholinesterase insecticides, or exposure to organophosphate-like anticholinergics (chemical warfare agents) can result in acute cholinergic poisoning. This is a medical emergency that requires rapid treatment with appropriate supportive measures and anticholinergic medications. To ensure appropriate penetration into the CNS, tertiary amine-containing drugs (atropine) should be used to antagonize muscarinic effects. There is no effective way to antagonize the nicotinic effects of the drugs. However, there is class of compounds that can regenerate the active enzyme following exposure to the organophosphate-type inhibitors. As mentioned above, the phosphorylation of the enzyme active site by organophosphates is extremely stable to hydrolysis and may undergo additional reactions (aging) to further strengthen the bond. Several substances are capable of regenerating the active site by hydrolyzing the phosphorylated esteratic sites of cholinesterases poisoned by the drugs. The reactivators are site-directed nucleophiles designed with a cationic moiety to direct the molecule to the anioinic site of the enzyme. Once bound, the nucleophile (oxime) is in close proximity to the phosphorylated enzyme and a nucleophilic attach of the phosphorous by the oxime results. The oxime-phosphonate is split off to provide the free enzyme. Unfortunately, within a period of minutes to hours after poisoning with organophosphates, there is a change in the phosphorylated enzyme (*aging*, dealkylation of the alkyl phosphate moiety), so that the alkylphosphate-enzyme bond becomes too stable to be displaced by reactivators. The efficacy of reactivators may vary according to which organophosphate drug is involved because of the differences in electrophilicity of the phosphorus in the various phosphate radicals. Anticholinesterase agents have been reported that are refractory to displacement by cholinesterase reactivators. The CNS penetration of reactivators is a consideration in order to treat central effects of the drugs. Atropine also must be used concomitantly with reactivators for optimal therapy. The reactivators may be used prophylactically.

PRALIDOXIME CHLORIDE

Pyridinium, 2-[(hydroxyimino)methyl]-1-methyl-, chloride; 2-PAM Chloride; Protopam Chloride

2-Formyl-1-methylpyridinium chloride oxime [51-15-0] $C_7H_9ClN_2O$ (172.61).

Preparation—Picolinal is converted to its oxime, which is then quaternized with dimethyl sulfate. Metathesis of the resulting pralidoxime methosulfate with HCl yields the official chloride. US Pat 3,123,613.

Description—White to pale-yellow, crystalline powder; odorless; stable in air; melts between 215° and 225° with decomposition.

Solubility—Freely soluble in water.

Comments—A reactivator most effective in the regeneration of cholinesterase associated with neuromuscular junctions. The positively charged quaternary pyridine nitrogen prevents effective penetration into the CNS. The drug is used in the treatment of poisoning by organophosphate anticholinesterases; it has questionable value in poisoning by neostigmine or physostigmine. The therapeutic effect (remission) usually occurs within 1 hour. Pralidoxime also is given prophylactically to handlers of organophosphates and to those expected to come into contact with the organophosphate drugs used as chemical weapons. Pralidoxime does not enter the CNS and does not antagonize all anticholinesterase compounds; the manufacturer's package literature should be consulted to ascertain whether the drug will be effective. After a period of time, organophosphate-inhibited cholinesterase undergoes a change (aging) that makes reactivation difficult; with isoflurophate, this time is only about 1 hour. The plasma half-life of pralidoxime is about 2.5 hours. When pralidoxime is injected more rapidly than at the recommended rate, dizziness, nausea, headache, mild weakness, blurred vision, diplopia, or tachycardia may result.

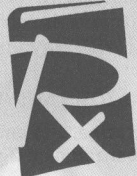

CHAPTER 72

Adrenergic Antagonists and Adrenergic Neuron Blocking Drugs

The term *blockade* is used to indicate interference with a response system such that the final effect is prevented. Thus, *adrenergic blockade* indicates interference with response systems involving the catecholamine neurotransmitters, epinephrine (adrenaline), norepinephrine (noradrenaline, levarterenol), and dopamine. Adrenergic blocking agents can be classified into two categories: adrenergic receptor (adrenoceptor) antagonists and adrenergic neuron blocking drugs. Adrenergic receptor antagonists are compounds that are devoid of intrinsic activity *per se* and instead exert effects by inhibiting the interaction of catecholamines or sympathomimetic agents with adrenergic receptors. In contrast, the term *adrenergic neuron blocking drugs* generally refers to those drugs that reduce delivery of catecholamines to the adrenergic receptors by disrupting catecholamine synthesis, storage, or release. Adrenergic blocking agents sometimes are called sympatholytics, because they abolish *(lyse)* the response to stimulation of the sympathetic nerves, or adrenolytics, because they abolish certain responses to epinephrine.

ADRENERGIC ANTAGONISTS

Based on their pharmacological properties, adrenoreceptors have been divided into three classes: alpha (α), beta (β), and dopamine. Whereas drugs that block peripheral dopamine receptors are of no established clinical importance, those that block central dopamine receptors are important psychopharmacological agents and are discussed in Chapter 82.

The α and β adrenoreceptors have been defined classically into four subclasses: α_1, α_2, β_1, and β_2. The respective pharmacological effects of activating these receptor subclasses is described in Chapter 70. Nonselective and selective antagonists targeting these subclasses are of considerable therapeutic importance and are described below. Recently, molecular biological studies have further identified at least three α_1 (α_{1A}, α_{1B}, α_{1D}) and three α_2 (α_{2A}, α_{2B}, α_{2C}) subtypes with specific regional distributions in the body. Moreover, an additional β subclass, β_3, has been identified in mammalian tissue. Although a few selective antagonists have been identified, therapeutic utility for selectively targeting these newly described adrenergic subclasses has yet to be demonstrated clinically.

α-ADRENERGIC RECEPTOR ANTAGONISTS

α-Adrenergic antagonists can bind reversibly (eg, phentolamine, prazosin) or irreversibly (eg, phenoxybenzamine) to their receptors. Blockade of α_1-adrenoreceptors causes readily apparent effects, whereas blockade of α_2-receptors generally causes subtle effects. Blockade of α_1-adrenergic impulses to the

arterioles decreases vascular resistance, thus tending to lower blood pressure and cause a pink, warm skin. α_1-Receptor blockade at the venules (capacitance vessels) increases venous capacitance and causes postural hypotension. These drugs decrease only that component of vascular resistance that is due to sympathetic activation.

Nonselective α-antagonists (eg, phentolamine, phenoxybenzamine) can cause palpitations and reflex tachycardia. These effects are partially attributable to activation of baroreflexes resulting from the hypotension produced by α_1-blockade. There also can be increased norepinephrine release from adrenergic nerve endings (transmitter *overflow*) as the result of concurrent block of α_2-adrenoreceptors, which subserve a negative-feedback function to decrease the release of transmitter. Consequently, tachycardia and palpitations may occur even when blood pressure falls very little. These reflex/overflow effects are counterproductive in the major uses of nonselective α-blocking drugs.

Other effects associated with α-receptor blockade include improved urine flow rates as a consequence of smooth muscle relaxation in the bladder neck and prostate. Miosis and nasal stuffiness also can occur after α-receptor antagonist administration.

Selective α_1-antagonists approved for use in the US include prazosin, terazosin, and doxazosin. Because these agents have little affinity for α_2-receptors, they do not increase catecholamine release and thereby do not cause excessive tachycardia. The most adverse side effect of α_1-blockade can be severe postural hypotension and syncope, especially early in treatment.

Selective α_2-antagonists include yohimbine and rauwolscine. Theoretically, such agents could be used to correct autonomic insufficiencies, since these agents increase norepinephrine release by blocking the inhibitory effects of norepinephrine at presynaptic α_2-receptors. Although there are presently no approved therapeutic indications for α_2-blockade, yohimbine has been used to treat diabetic neuropathy and impotence.

Some nonselective α-adrenoreceptor antagonists have been approved for use in the treatment of pheochromocytoma. The drugs may be used in advance of surgery to prevent hypertensive episodes caused by manipulation of the tumor or for the long-term treatment of an inoperable, metastatic pheochromocytoma. Other uses for nonselective α-antagonists have been reported, including treatment of:

1. Peripheral vascular disorders in which there is an adrenergically mediated vasospastic component, such as Raynaud's syndrome and frostbite.
2. Micturition disorders resulting from neurogenic bladder.

Theoretically, selective α_1-receptor antagonists should be useful in treating many of the same disorders as are the nonselective α-blockers, but α_1-antagonists are currently approved only for the treatment of hypertension and benign prostatic hyperplasia. However, these agents enjoy considerable use in the treatment of refractory heart failure and of vasospasm associated with Raynaud's disease.

DOXAZOSIN MESYLATE

Piperazine, 1-(4-amino-6,7-dimethoxy-2-quinazolinyl)-4-[(2,3-dihydro-1,4-benzodioxin-2-yl)carbonyl]-, monomethanesulfonate; Cardura

[77883-43-3] $C_{23}H_{25}N_5O_5 \cdot CH_4O_3S$ (547.58).

Preparation—See US Pat 4,188,390.

Description—Off-white powder; pK_a 6.93.

Solubility—Sparingly soluble in water and most common organic solvents.

Comments—A selective α_1-antagonist.

PHENOXYBENZAMINE HYDROCHLORIDE

Benzenemethanamine, N-(2-chloroethyl)-N-(1-methyl-2-phenoxyethyl)-, hydrochloride; Dibenzyline Hydrochloride

N-(2-Chloroethyl)-N-(1-methyl-2-phenoxyethyl)benzylamine hydrochloride [63-92-3] $C_{18}H_{22}ClNO \cdot HCl$ (340.29).

Preparation—One method starts with phenol undergoing addition to propylene oxide to give 1-phenoxy-2-propanol, which is reacted with thionyl chloride to yield 1-phenoxy-2-chloropropane. Refluxing the latter with excess ethanolamine gives N-(phenoxyisopropylamino) ethanol and additional refluxing of this with benzyl chloride in the presence of NaHCO$_3$ yields 2-[N-benzyl-N-(1-methyl-2-phenoxyethyl) amino]ethanol. Treatment with thionyl chloride and HCl in CHCl$_3$ completes the synthesis. US Pat 2,599,000.

Description—White, crystalline, odorless powder; melts between 136° and 141°.

Solubility—1 g in 25 mL water, 6 mL alcohol, 3 mL chloroform or >1000 mL ether.

Comments—An irreversible antagonist with nonselective actions.

PHENTOLAMINE MESYLATE

Phenol, 3-[[(4,5-dihydro-1H-imidazol-2-yl)methyl](4-methylphenyl)-amino]-, monomethanesulfonate (salt); Regitine Mesylate

[65-28-1] $C_{17}H_{19}N_3O.CH_4O_3S$ (377.46)

Preparation—m-(p-Toluidino)phenol is refluxed with 2-chloromethylimidazoline hydrochloride and the resulting phentolamine base treated with an equimolar portion of methanesulfonic acid.

Description—White or off-white, odorless, crystalline powder; solutions are acid to litmus, having a pH of about 5, and deteriorate slowly; melts about 178°.

Solubility—1 g in 1 mL water, 4 mL alcohol or 700 mL chloroform.

Comments—Phentolamine is a nonselective α-adrenoreceptor antagonist with an immediate onset and short duration of action. In addition to α-blocking activity, it has weak muscarinic activity in the gastrointestinal (GI) tract and weak-to-mild histaminergic activity in the stomach. These effects limit the dose that can be used; hence, α-blockade is usually incomplete. Its pharmacological effects are described in the general statement. This drug is approved therapy for treating individuals with a pheochromocytoma and the treatment or prevention of dermal necrosis and sloughing resulting from extravasation or intravenous administration of norepinephrine. Additional uses include the management of hypertensive crises caused by drug interactions with

monoamine oxidase inhibitors (MAOIs) or the abrupt withdrawal of clonidine. It is used as a diagnostic agent for pheochromocytoma, although determination of blood and/or urinary concentrations of catecholamines and/or their metabolites is a safer method. It has been combined with papaverine for intracavernous injection in impotence. The adverse effects are those of α-blockade (see the general statement), in addition to which there is weakness.

PRAZOSIN HYDROCHLORIDE

Piperazine, 1-(4-amino-6,7-dimethoxy-2-quinazolinyl)-4-(2-furanylcarbonyl)-, monohydrochloride; Minipress

1-(4-Amino-6,7-dimethoxy-2-quinazolinyl)-4-(2-furoyl)piperazine monohydrochloride [19237-84-4] $C_{19}H_{21}N_5O_4 \cdot HCl$ (419.87).

Preparation—4,5-Dimethoxyanthranilamide is treated with sodium cyanate to form the corresponding tetrahydroquinazoline-2,4-dione. The carbonyl groups are converted to chlorine and the heterocyclic ring aromatized using POCl$_3$ plus PCl$_5$. Subsequent treatment with ammonia replaces the chlorine atom adjacent to the benzenoid ring with an amino function, and the resulting monochloro derivative is condensed with 1-(2-furoyl)-piperazine to yield the product. See British Pat 1,156,973.

Description—White, crystalline powder; pK_a (in 1:1 water-ethanol solution) 6.5.

Solubility—Slightly soluble in water; very slightly soluble in alcohol.

Comments—A selective α_1-antagonist.

TERAZOSIN HYDROCHLORIDE

Piperazine, 1-(4-amino-6,7-dimethoxy-2-quinazolinyl-4-[(tetrahydro-2-furanyl)carbonyl], monohydrochloride, dihydrate; Hytrin

[70024-40-7] $C_{19}H_{25}N_5O_4 \cdot HCl \cdot 2H_2O$ (459.93)

Preparation—See *Prazosin Hydrochloride;* 1-(tetrahydrofuroyl) piperazine is condensed with the monochloroquinazoline.

Description—White crystalline powder.

Solubility—Freely soluble in water.

Comments—A selective α_1-antagonist.

β-ADRENERGIC RECEPTOR ANTAGONISTS

Most β-adrenergic receptor antagonists (β-*blockers*) reversibly and competitively inhibit the binding of norepinephrine to its receptors. Although most are pure antagonists, a few clinically relevant β-blockers have partial agonist activity. β-Blockers can be distinguished by several factors including relative affinity for the various β-receptor subtypes, duration of effect, local anesthetic activity, and lipid solubility.

Blockade of myocardial β$_1$-receptors causes bradycardia, suppression of some ectopic pacemakers, decreased force of myocardial contraction, and slowing of atrioventricular conduction. Impaired exercise tolerance can result. β-Blockers can decrease myocardial oxygen demand by preventing catecholamine-induced increases in heart rate and contractility. However, these agents can also increase myocardial oxygen demand by increasing end-diastolic pressure and the duration of systolic injection. Still, the net effect of β-receptor blockade on oxygen demand is usually advantageous. β-blockers are of value in the treatment of angina pectoris.

β-Antagonists are used for the management of both supraventricular and ventricular arrhythmias. These drugs also can be used to suppress tachycardia in thyrotoxicosis and pheochromocytoma. Many β-blockers act as sodium channel blockers and thereby as local anesthetics. This membrane-stabilizing activity was once considered to be responsible for the antiarrhythmic action of these agents, although it is now recognized that this effect is likely of little consequence, since the dose of β-blockers employed in treatment of arrhythmias is generally too low to exert this effect.

β-Antagonists are used in the treatment of essential hypertension. Although the precise mechanism for this effect has not been determined, it has been suggested that β-blockers decrease blood pressure by (1) a direct effect on the heart and blood vessels, (2) decreasing sympathetic outflow from the central nervous system (CNS), and/or (3) affecting the renin- angiotensin-aldosterone system. Although many β-blockers increase peripheral resistance acutely (probably by opposing β$_2$-mediated vasodilation), chronic therapy can result in a decreased peripheral resistance that contributes to the long-term hypotensive effects of the drug. β-Antagonists are especially useful in combination with antihypertensive vasodilators (ie, hydralazine, minoxidil) to prevent reflex tachycardia.

The rate of formation of intraocular fluid is decreased by β-antagonists; this effect is useful in the treatment of glaucoma. β-Blockers with significant local anesthetic activity generally are not used for this purpose, so as to prevent local anesthesia of the cornea. Betaxolol, carteolol, levobunalol, metipranolol, and timolol are applied topically in this disorder.

β-Antagonists have varied usefulness in the prophylaxis of migraine headache, diminishing pain in many instances but increasing it in others. Propranolol and timolol are approved for migraine treatment. The mechanism of action is presently unknown.

In the treatment of certain kinds of anxiety, such as stage fright and examination apprehension, β-antagonists are frequently effective. The efficacy is likely attributable to the prevention of the peripheral manifestations of sympathoadrenal discharge (ie, of tachycardia, palpitations, or muscle tremor) rather than to a central action. Their value in the treatment of pathological anxiety disorders is controversial, as they appear to have little effect on the underlying disorder.

Selective β$_1$-antagonists theoretically can be used for all the purposes listed under the nonselective blockers, although they have not been approved universally for these uses.

Not all β-antagonists penetrate into the CNS, nor do these drugs have similar CNS effects. Some, for example, block certain serotonin receptor subtypes. Central actions explain the increase in sleep disturbances, dizziness, and ataxia that can result from β-blocker administration. Drowsiness, lassitude, headache, vertigo, visual disturbances, depression, hallucinations, and mental confusion may also result from β-blocker administration. Tolerance to these effects is frequent. β-Blockers that are highly lipid soluble are more likely to penetrate the CNS.

Antagonism of β-receptors in the bronchioles causes an increase in airway resistance. This can cause bronchospasm in bronchial asthma, bronchitis, emphysema, and chronic obstructive pulmonary disease. Laryngospasm also may occur. In insulin overdosage, β$_2$-blockade may prevent the mobilization of glucose from the liver to offset hypoglycemia; furthermore, the prevention of reflex tachycardia deprives the patient of an early warning signal of impending insulin shock. β-Blockers can inhibit the lipolysis resulting from sympathetic nervous stimulation.

Other adverse effects of β-blockade include loss of libido in both men and women, impotence, increased very low-density and decreased high-density lipoproteins, occasional nausea and vomiting, mild diarrhea or constipation, and rare allergic responses, such as rashes, fever, and purpura.

Some β-antagonists also stimulate β-adrenoreceptors (ie, have intrinsic sympathomimetic activity, or ISA). For instance, carteolol and pindolol have appreciable partial agonist properties. Some authorities believe that partial agonist activity offers no advantage over full antagonist activity. Others contend

that partial agonist properties may be advantageous in patients prone to bradycardia.

ACEBUTOLOL HYDROCHLORIDE

Butaneamide, (±)-N-3-acetyl-4-[2-hydroxy-3-[(1-methylethyl)-amino[propoxy] phenyl-, hydrochloride; Sectral

(±)-3′-acetyl-4′[2-hydroxy-3-(isopropylamino)propoxy]butyranilide hydrochloride [34381-68-5] $C_{18}H_{28}N_2O_4$ · HCl (372.93)

Preparation—S Afr Pat 68 08,345.
Description—White to slightly off-white powder melting about 142°.
Solubility—Freely soluble in water; partially soluble in alcohol.
Comments—A β$_1$-selective drug with low lipid solubility.

ATENOLOL

Benzeneacetamide, 4-[2-hydroxy-3-[(1-methylethyl) amino]propoxy]-; Tenormin

2-[p-[2-Hydroxy-3-(isopropylamino)propoxy]phenyl]acetamide [29122-68-7] $C_{14}H_{22}N_2O_3$ (266.34)

Preparation—From p-hydroxyphenylacetamide, ethylene chlorohydrin and isopropylamine (US Pat 3,836,671).
Description—White crystals melting about 147°.
Comments—A β$_1$-selective drug with low lipid solubility.

BETAXOLOL HYDROCHLORIDE

2-Propanol, 1-[4-[2-(cyclopropylmethoxy)-ethyl]phenoxy]-3-[(1-methylethyl)amino]-, hydrochloride; Betoptic; Kerlone

[63659-19-8] $C_{18}H_{29}NO_3$ · HCl (343.89)

Preparation—The methyl ester of 2-(cyclopropylmethoxy)ethanesulfonic acid and p-benzyloxyphenol react to form 2-(cyclopropylmethoxy)ethoxyphenyl benzyl ether, which is debenzylated to yield the free phenol, treated with epichlorhydrin to form the glycidyl ether, followed by ring opening with isopropylamine to yield the product as the base. Treatment of the base in dry ether with HCl forms the salt. US Pat 4,252,984; Chem Abstr 87:13454.
Description—Crystals melting about 116°.
Comments—A β$_1$-selective drug with low lipid solubility. It is used to treat open-angle glaucoma.

BISOPROLOL FUMARATE

2-Propanol, (±)-1-[4-[[2-(1-methylethoxy)ethoxy]methyl]phenoxy]-3-[(1-methylethyl)amino]-, (E)-2-butenedioate (2:1) (salt); Zebeta

[104344-23-2] $(C_{18}H_{31}NO_4)_2$ · $C_4H_4O_2$ (766.97).

Preparation—Cyclization of 1-(isopropylamino)-3-phenoxy-2-propanol with $COCl_2$ forms a cyclic carbamate. Treatment with paraformaldehyde and HCl yields the p-chloromethyl derivative, which undergoes an S_N reaction with 2-isopropoxyethanol to form the ether.

Aqueous base opens the protective carbamate ring, yielding the product. See US Pat 4,258,062.

Description—White crystals melting about 100°; pK$_a$ (amine) 4.8.

Solubility—Very soluble in water; 1 g dissolves in 20 mL of alcohol.

Comments—A β$_1$-selective drug with low lipid solubility.

CARTEOLOL HYDROCHLORIDE

2(1H)-Quinolinone, 5-[3-[(1,1-dimethyl-ethyl)amino]-2-hydroxypropoxy]-3,4-dihydro-, monohydrochloride; Cartrol; Ocupress

[51781-21-6] C$_{16}$H$_{24}$N$_2$O$_3$ · HCl (328.84)

Preparation—It is synthesized from 3,4-dihydro-5-hydroxycarbostyril and epichlorhydrin to afford the 2,3-epoxypropyl ether. Opening the epoxide with t-butylamine yields the base, which is converted to the hydrochloride. See J Med Chem 1974; 17:529.

Description—White crystals melting about 278°.

Solubility—Soluble in water; slightly soluble in alcohol.

Comments—A nonselective drug with low lipid solubility. It is used to treat open-angle glaucoma.

CARVEDILOL

2-Propanol, (±)-1-(9H-carbazol-4-yloxy)-3-[[2-(2-methoxyphenoxy)ethyl]-amino]-, Coreg

[72956-09-3] C$_{24}$H$_{26}$O$_4$ (406.48).

Preparation—By condensation of 4-(2,3-epoxy-1-propyl)carbazole with 2-(2-methoxyphenoxy)ethyl amine. See US 4,503,067 (1985).

Description—Colorless crystals melting about 115°.

Comments—Has both nonselective β-antagonist and α-antagonist activity.

ESMOLOL HYDROCHLORIDE

Benzenepropanoic acid, (±)-4-[2-hydroxy-3-[(1-methylethyl)-amino]propoxy]-, methyl ester, hydrochloride; Brevibloc

[84057-94-3] C$_{16}$H$_{25}$NO$_4$ · HCl (331.84)

Preparation—J Med Chem 1982; 25: 1408.

Description—White crystals melting about 85°.

Comments—A β$_1$-selective drug with low lipid solubility. It has an ultrashort duration of action.

LABETALOL HYDROCHLORIDE

Benzamide, 2-hydroxy-5-[1-hydroxy-2-[(1-methyl-3-phenylpropyl)amino]ethyl]-, monohydrochloride; Normodyne; Trandate

5-[1-hydroxy-2-[(1-methyl-3-phenylpropyl)amino]ethyl]salicylamide monohydrochloride [32780-64-6] C$_{19}$H$_{24}$N$_2$O$_3$ · HCl (364.87).

Preparation—US Pat 4,012,444.

Description—White crystals.

Solubility—Soluble in water or ethanol; insoluble in ether or chloroform.

Comments—Has both nonselective β and selective α$_1$-antagonist activity.

LEVOBUNOLOL HYDROCHLORIDE

1(2H)-Naphthalenone, (−)-5-[3-[(1,1-dimethylethyl)-amino]-2-hydroxypropoxy]-3,4-dihydro-, hydrochloride; Betagan Liquifilm

[27912-14-7] C$_{17}$H$_{25}$NO$_3$ · HCl (327.85)

Preparation—See J Med Chem 1970; 13:684.

Description—White crystals melting about 210°.

Solubility—Soluble in water; slightly soluble in alcohol.

Comments—A nonselective drug used for open-angle glaucoma.

METIPRANOLOL HYDROCHLORIDE

Phenol, (±)-4-[2-hydroxy-3-[(1-methylethyl)amino]propoxy]-2,3,6-trimethyl-, 1-acetate, hydrochloride; MPR; OptiPranolol

[22664-55-7(base)] C$_{17}$H$_{27}$NO$_4$ (345.86).

Preparation—Czech Pat 128,471.

Description—White crystals melting about 106°.

Solubility—Slightly soluble in water.

Comments—A nonselective drug used for open-angle glaucoma.

METOPROLOL TARTRATE

2-Propanol, (±)-1-[4-(2-methoxyethyl)phenoxy]-3-[(1-methylethyl)amino]-, [R[(R*,R*)]]-2,3-dihydroxybutanedioate (2:1) (salt); Lopressor; Toprol XL

(±)-1-(Isopropylamino)-3-[p-(2-methoxyethyl)phenoxy]-2-propanol L-(±)-tartrate (2:1) (salt) [56392-17-7] (C$_{15}$H$_{25}$NO$_3$)$_2$ · C$_4$H$_6$O$_6$ (684.82).

Preparation—From 4-(2-methoxyethyl)phenol, 3-chloro-1,2-propanediol and isopropylamine (Swedish Pat 368,004).

Description—White, odorless powder; bitter taste; melts about 120°.

Solubility—Very soluble in water; soluble in alcohol or chloroform; insoluble in acetone or ether.

Comments—A β$_1$-selective drug with moderate lipid solubility.

NADOLOL

2,3-Naphthalenediol, cis-5-[3-[(1,1-dimethylethyl)amino]-2-hydroxypropoxy]-1,2,3,4-tetrahydro-, Corgard

1-(tert-Butylamino)-3-[(5,6,7,8-tetrahydro-cis-6,7-dihydroxy-1-naphthyl)oxy]-2-propanol [42200-33-9] C$_{17}$H$_{27}$O$_4$ (309.40).

Preparation—US Pat 3,935,267.

Description—White crystalline powder melting about 130°; pK$_a$ 9.68.

Solubility—Freely soluble in alcohol; slightly soluble in water or chloroform; insoluble in acetone or hydrocarbon solvents.

Comments—A nonselective drug with low lipid solubility.

PENBUTOLOL SULFATE

2-Propanol, (S)-1-(2-cyclopentylphenoxy)-3-[(1,1-dimethylethyl)amino]-, sulfate (2:1) (salt); Levatol

[38363-32-5] $C_{18}H_{29}NO_2)_2 \cdot H_2SO_4$ (680.94).

Preparation—See US Pat 3,551,493.

Description—White crystals melting about 217°.

Solubility—Soluble in water; slightly soluble in alcohol.

Comments—A nonselective drug with high lipid solubility. It has some agonist activity.

PINDOLOL

2-Propanol, 1-(1H-indol-4-yloxy)-3-[(1-methyl-ethyl)amino]-, Visken

[13523-86-9] $C_{14}H_{20}N_2O$ (248.32).

Preparation—Swiss Pat 472,404.

Description—Off-white, crystalline powder; almost odorless; melts about 172°.

Solubility—Practically insoluble in water; slightly soluble in anhydrous alcohol or chloroform.

Comments—A nonselective drug with moderate lipid solubility. It has partial agonist activity.

PROPRANOLOL HYDROCHLORIDE

2-Propanol, 1-[(1-methylethyl)amino]-3-(1-naphthalenyloxy)-, hydrochloride; Inderal

[318-98-9] $C_{16}H_{21}NO_2 \cdot HCl$ (295.81).

Preparation—α-Naphthol is reacted with epichlorohydrin in aqueous alkali to form 2,3-epoxypropyl α-naphthyl ether, and the epoxy ring is ruptured by reaction with isopropylamine. The base is converted to hydrochloride with HCl.

Description—White or almost white powder that is odorless, with a bitter taste; stable to heat, unstable in light, and nonhygroscopic; melts about 161°; pK_a 9.45.

Solubility—1 g in 20 mL water or 20 mL alcohol; slightly soluble in chloroform; practically insoluble in ether.

Comments—The prototype nonselective β-antagonist, with all the actions, uses, adverse effects, and contraindications characteristic of this class of drugs (see general statement), except that it is not used to treat glaucoma. The drug penetrates into the CNS and causes the central effects in the general statement. It has been reported to be of value in more than 20 noncardiovascular disorders, many of which are associated with the CNS. Its elimination $t_{1/2}$ is 4 to 6 hr.

SOTALOL HYDROCHLORIDE

Methanesulfonamide, N-[4-[1-hydroxy-2-[(1-methylethyl)-amino]ethyl]phenyl]-, monohydrochloride; Betapace

[959-24-0] $C_{12}H_{20}N_2O_3S \cdot HCl$ (308.82).

Preparation—One method involves the reaction of methanesulfonyl chloride with p-aminoacetophenone to form the sulfonamide, which is then brominated by a free radical procedure to yield the phenacyl bromide. A nucleophilic substitution of bromine by isopropyl amine affords the base which is converted to the salt. See J Med Chem 1967; 10:462.

Description—White crystals melting about 207°; pK_1 8.3, pK_2 9.8.

Solubility—Freely soluble in water; insoluble in alcohol.

Comments—A nonselective drug with low lipid solubility.

TIMOLOL MALEATE

2-Propanol, 1-[(1,1-dimethylethyl)amino]-3-[[4-(4-morpholinyl-1,2,5-thiadiazol-3-yl]oxy]-(S)-, (Z)-2-butenedioate (1:1) (salt); Blocadren, Timoptic

(−)-1-(tert-Butylamino)-3-[(4-morpholino-1,2,5-thiadiazol-3-yl)oxy]-2-propanol maleate (1:1) (salt) [26921-17-5] $C_{13}H_{24}N_4O_4 \cdot S \cdot C_4H_4O_4$ (432.49).

Preparation—J Med Chem 1972; 15:651.

Description—White crystals melting about 202°; pH (5% aqueous solution) about 4; stable in aqueous solution up to about pH 12.

Solubility—Freely soluble in water; soluble in alcohol; sparingly soluble in chloroform; practically insoluble in ether.

Comments—A nonselective drug with moderate lipid solubility. It is used for open-angle glaucoma.

ADRENERGIC NEURON BLOCKING DRUGS

The adrenergic neurotransmitter, norepinephrine, is synthesized in sympathetic adrenergic neurons. 3,4-Dihydroxyphenylalanine (DOPA), which is formed in the adrenergic neuron by the hydroxylation of tyrosine, is decarboxylated (by aromatic amino acid decarboxylase) to produce the catecholamine dopamine (3,4-dihydroxyphenylethylamine). Within the adrenergic neuron in the region of the nerve endings are granular organelles that contain the enzyme dopamine β-hydroxylase, which introduces the side-chain hydroxyl group onto dopamine to form norepinephrine. Norepinephrine is stored in the granular organelles. Nerve impulses cause the influx of calcium, which releases norepinephrine from the storage granules.

Adrenergic neuron blocking drugs reduce the delivery of catecholamines (eg, norepinephrine) to adrenergic receptors. As noted above, this can occur by disrupting catecholamine synthesis, storage, or release. The pharmacology of some such agents is described below.

GUANADREL SULFATE

Guanidine, (1,4-dioxaspiro[4.5]dec-2-ylmethyl)-, sulfate (2:1); Hylorel

[22195-34-2] $(C_{10}H_{19}N_3O_2)_2 \cdot H_2SO_4$ (524.63).

Preparation—US Pat 3,547,951.

Description—White solid melting about 235° with decomposition.

Solubility—1 g dissolves in about 13.5 mL water.

Comments—An adrenergic neuron blocking drug with a mechanism of action and hemodynamic properties like those of guanethidine, to which it is related chemically. Guanadrel inhibits vasoconstriction by inhibiting norepinephrine release in response to sympathetic nerve stimulation. The resulting antihypertensive effect is greater when standing than in the supine position. Orthostatic hypotension occurs frequently. Unlike guanethidine, it is used in the treatment of mild and moderate essential hypertension. Tricyclic antidepressants and other drugs that inhibit the amine reuptake into the adrenergic neurons prevent neuronal uptake of guanadrel and hence attenuate its effects. Frequent side effects include palpitations, shortness of breath, coughing, fatigue, headache, drowsiness, GI disturbances (diarrhea or constipation), edema, and excessive weight gain/loss.

GUANETHIDINE MONOSULFATE

Guanidine, [2-(hexahydro-1(2H)-azocinyl)ethyl-, sulfate (2:1); Ismelin Sulfate

$$\left[\raisebox{0.5em}{\begin{array}{c} N-CH_2CH_2-NH-C \begin{array}{c} NH \\ \\ NH_2 \end{array} \end{array}} \right]_2 \cdot H_2SO_4$$

[60-02-6] $(C_{10}H_{22}N_4)_2 \cdot H_2SO_4$ (494.69)

Preparation—Cycloheptanone oxime undergoes Beckmann rearrangement to form hexahydro-2(1H)-azoconone,—CH$_2$(CH$_2$)$_5$ CO—NH], which is then reduced to heptamethyleneimine [—CH$_2$(CH$_2$)$_6$—NH]. This is condensed with chloracetonitrile, and the resulting nitrile is hydrogenated to 1-(2-aminoethyl)-heptamethyleneimine. Condensation with 2-methyl-2-thiopseudourea [NH= C(SCH$_3$)NH$_2$] sulfate eliminates CH$_3$SH to produce crude guanethidine sulfate. See *Experientia* 1959; 15:267.

Description—White to off-white, crystalline powder.

Solubility—Sparingly soluble in water; slightly soluble in alcohol; practically insoluble in chloroform.

Comments—It is taken up into into noradrenergic nerve terminals via the same transporter responsible for uptake of the transmitter. Once inside, the drug is transported into, and concentrated within, vesicles, wherein it replaces norepinephrine. By replacing norepinephrine, guanethidine causes a gradual depletion of the catecholamine from the nerve terminal. Its onset of action is slow, requiring several hours to 2 or 3 days for its full effect, and its duration of action may be 4 or more days.

Guanethidine causes vasodilation and increases venous capacitance. The drug lowers blood pressure very effectively, especially when an individual is standing or exercising. Since blood pressure can fall to dangerously low levels in some patients, the drug usually is employed in submaximal doses and is combined with thiazides or hydralazine, to permit some adrenergic function. It usually is not employed to treat mild to moderate hypertension, only moderately severe to severe hypertension.

The most common untoward effects of guanethidine are those that obligatorily accrue because of the effects of sympathetic blockade. They include orthostatic hypotension with its attendant vertigo, weakness, lassitude, nausea and occasional syncope, bradycardia, dry mouth, diarrhea, urinary incontinence, and nocturia. Tricyclic antidepressants and other drugs that inhibit the amine reuptake into the adrenergic neurons prevent neuronal uptake of guanethidine and hence attenuate its effects. Guanethidine potentiates the pressor effects of norepinephrine and certain other directly acting α sympathomimetics by inhibiting uptake into the adrenergic nerve terminals and by causing supersensitivity of receptors. It also may cause release of catecholamines from pheochromocytomas and hence precipitate hypertensive crises. The drug is contraindicated in pheochromocytoma, in patients hypersensitive to the drug, and when MAOIs are in use.

METYROSINE

L-Tyrosine, (−)-α-methyl-, Demser

$$HO-\bigcirc-CH_2-\underset{NH_2}{\overset{CH_3}{\underset{|}{\overset{|}{C}}}}-COOH$$

[672-87-7] $C_{10}H_{13}NO_3$ (195.22).

Preparation—*J Org Chem* 1967; 32:4074.

Description—White, crystalline solid; melts about 310°.

Solubility—About 1 g in 1750 mL water.

Comments—Metyrosine inhibits the activity of the catecholaminergic neurons since it blocks tyrosine hydroxylase and thus suppresses the synthesis of catecholamines. This causes depletion of catecholamines in adrenergic neurons in both the sympathetic and central nervous systems and in the pheochrome cells in the adrenal medulla and accessory tissue. The drug is used to treat pheochromocytoma. Sedation is the most common side effect, but some tolerance occurs during the first week of treatment. Extrapyramidal dyskinesias occur in about 10% of recipients. Other adverse CNS effects include anxiety, confusion, depression, disorientation and hallucinations. GI side effects include di-

arrhea, nausea, vomiting, and abdominal pain. Other adverse effects are nasal stuffiness, impotence, dry mouth, headache, gynecomastia, galactorrhea, peripheral edema, urticaria, and eosinophilia. Metyrosine potentiates the extrapyramidal effects of phenothiazines and butyrophenones.

RESERPINE

Yohimban-16-carboxylic acid, (3β,16β,17α,18β,20α)-11,17-dimethoxy-18-[(3,4,5-trimethoxybenzoyl)oxy]-, methyl ester

[50-55-5] $C_{33}H_{40}N_2O_9$ (608.69)

Reserpine, one of more than 20 alkaloids in *Rauwolfia serpentina*, was first isolated in pure crystalline form by Müller *et al*, (*Experientia* 1952; 8: 338). Subsequently it was found also in other species of *Rauwolfia*. A procedure for its separation is described in US Pat 2,833,771 (1958). Although it has been synthesized (Woodward *et al*, *J Am Chem Soc* 1956; 78:2023), its production by this route is not economically feasible.

Description—White or pale-buff to slightly yellowish, odorless, crystalline powder; darkens slowly on exposure to light, but more rapidly when in solution; melts between 255° and 265° with decomposition.

Solubility—Insoluble in water; very slightly soluble in ether; 1 g in about 1800 mL alcohol or about 6 mL chloroform; slightly soluble in benzene; freely soluble in acetic acid.

Comments—Reserpine is an alkaloid derived from the roots of *Rauwolfia serpentina*. It acts to inhibit both neuronal and chromaffin granule transporters. As a consequence, catecholamine accumulation is blocked. Depletion is slower and less complete in the adrenal medulla than in other tissues. By preventing such storage, reserpine initially causes catecholamine release. This is followed by a profound depletion of transmitter that can persist for days to weeks. The effects of reserpine appear to be irreversible.

Reserpine was the first rauwolfia alkaloid to be recognized officially. It was used first for the symptomatic management of patients with anxiety or tension psychoneuroses or chronic psychoses involving anxiety, psychomotor hyperactivity, or compulsive aggressive behavior. It is a sedative and may cause mental depression. Extreme caution must be exercised when administering reserpine to patients with a history of depression, since reserpine can unmask or worsen this condition.

Because of the seriousness of side effects, reserpine is rarely used as an antianxiety or antipsychotic drug. Instead, reserpine is used in antihypertensive therapy. By depleting peripheral amines, reserpine lowers blood pressure. Central actions may also contribute to this antihypertensive effect. The drug is used chiefly in combination with thiazide diuretics for the management of mild-to-moderate essential hypertension.

Nasal congestion, scleroconjunctival congestion, drowsiness, bradycardia, nausea, vomiting, anorexia, weight gain, and diarrhea are frequently noted side effects. Dry mouth, headache, dizziness, dysuria, myalgia, and dull sensorium can also occur. Suicidal depression is the most serious untoward effect. Other serious reactions are orthostatic hypotension, fatigue, weakness, insomnia, nightmares, excitement, paradoxical anxiety, parkinsonian-like rigidity, glaucoma, angina-like symptoms, deafness, pruritus, rash, purpura, and optic atrophy.

The drug is absorbed poorly and erratically from the GI tract, which causes considerable differences in efficacy of oral doses. It characteristically has a long latency of onset and a prolonged duration of action. For example, with daily oral administration the effects of the drug usually are not fully manifest for several days to 2 weeks and may persist for as long as 4 weeks after oral medication is discontinued. Tolerance to the drug does not develop with continued administration.

ACKNOWLEDGMENTS—Annette E Fleckenstein, PhD is acknowledged for her efforts in previous editions of this work.

CHAPTER 73

Antimuscarinic and Antispasmodic Drugs

Daniel J Canney, PhD

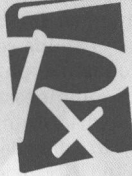

The preferential binding of the alkaloids nicotine and muscarine to cholinergic receptors has been used to classify them as nicotinic and muscarinic receptors, respectively. Further subtypes of muscarinic and nicotinic receptors have been identified in both the peripheral (PNS) and central nervous systems (CNS). Acetylcholine binds nonselectively to each of these widely distributed receptors to elicit a large range of pharmacological actions. Anticholinergic drugs or *cholinergic blocking drugs* may antagonize the effects of ACh at cholinergic receptors in ganglia, neuromuscular junctions, in the central nervous system or in parasympathetic neuroeffectors. By contrast, antimuscarinic drug actions are limited to antagonist effects at the parasympathetic neuroeffectors and certain central synapses innervated via muscarinic receptors. With the exception of certain quaternary ammonium antimuscarinics, these agents have little effect on nicotinic receptors. The quarternary ammonium-containing antimuscarinics have greater affinity for nicotinic receptors than other drugs in the class and may cause neuromuscular paralysis and/or ganglionic blockade even at therapeutic doses. In general, it is important to remember that the selectivity of drugs for a particular receptor subtype is highly dependent on the concentration (dose). Thus, at autonomic ganglia where ACh acts primarily at nicotinic receptors, antimuscarinic drugs may produce blockade at high doses. In the neuromuscular junction where receptors are almost exclusively nicotinic, antimuscarinic drugs may have slight effects at exceedingly high doses. Drugs that effectively target a specific subtype(s) of muscarinic or nicotinic receptor may provide therapeutic agents that lack the side effect profiles of nonselective drugs.

Atropine, the prototypic antimuscarinic agent, is an alkaloid isolated from the dried leaf and flowering or fruiting top of *Atropa belladonna* Linné. *Antimuscarinic* drugs are competitive antagonists that act on the cholinergic receptors at smooth muscle, secretory cells and certain central synapses. Other synonyms for the term antimuscarinic are *anticholinergic, cholinolytic, parasympatholytic,* and *parasympathetic blocking drugs*. Antagonist drugs that specifically target nicotinic receptors will be handled in the chapter on skeletal muscle relaxants.

ACTIONS AND SELECTIVITY—The effects of antimuscarinic drugs on the whole are predicted readily by considering the consequences of interruption of parasympathetic (and sympathetic cholinergic) nerve stimulation. Thus, the effects are decreased gastrointestinal (GI) motility, decreased gastric secretion, dry mouth, drying of the mucous membranes in general, mydriasis, loss of accommodation (with consequent tendency to increased intraocular pressure), urinary retention, decreased sweating and compensatory cutaneous flush, bronchial and biliary dilation, tachycardia (although effective block of the cardiac inhibitory nerves is difficult to achieve), etc. Some antimuscarinics have important actions in the CNS and are used in the treatment of Parkinson's disease (see below).

Current evidence suggests that there are at least five subtypes of muscarinic receptors that differ in their distribution and function. For example, the M1 subtype is distributed in the CNS, sympathetic postganglionic cell bodies, and at various presynaptic sites. The M2 receptors are found in smooth muscle organs, and the myocardium, and in the CNS while M3 are most commonly found on effector cell membranes of glandular and smooth muscle. Structure-activity relationship (SAR) studies indicate that each subtype differs in its structural requirements for blockage. Hence, subtype-selective muscarinic antagonists may provide therapeutic agents with more favorable side effect profiles than nonselective drugs.

Atropine is the prototypic antimuscarinic drug that guided early attempts to design additional drugs in the class. A close inspection of the molecule reveals a similarity to ACh that results in recognition and nonselective binding to muscarinic receptors. There are considerable differences in the effects elicited by currently available antimuscarinic drugs. These differences may be attributed to varying pharmacokinetic profiles (absorption, distribution, metabolism, excretion) and/or pharmacodynamic profiles (degree of receptor subtype selectivity). For example, scopolamine has excellent mydriatic and cycloplegic activity yet cannot block cardiac vagal activity in nontoxic doses, whereas its derivative methscopolamine is the most efficacious drug for the antagonism of vagally mediated cardiac effects. SAR studies indicate that numerous structural characteristics and functional groups may contribute to the different pharmacological and therapeutic profiles of the antimuscarinic drugs. One moiety of particular importance appears to be the amine group within the molecules. Hence drug with quaternary ammonium groups differ in important ways from the corresponding tertiary or secondary amine-containing drugs.

SOME DIFFERENCES BETWEEN QUATERNARY AND TERTIARY AMINE-CONTAINING ANTIMUSCARINICS—Quaternary ammonium groups in drug molecules carry a positive charge that makes the drug highly ionized. In general, these charged molecules do not penetrate cell membranes or the blood-brain barrier (BBB) very effectively. These properties result in erratic absorption from the GI and little to no CNS penetration. Similarly, the quaternary ammonium compounds poorly penetrate into the eye from the bloodstream or cornea and are less likely than the tertiary amines to cause mydriasis and cycloplegia. The quaternary compounds have a greater affinity for nicotinic receptors, so that some degree of ganglionic blockade may result from therapeutic doses of some quaternary ammonium antimuscarinic drugs. Some analogs also have a potential for neuromuscular paralysis, especially in drug interactions in persons with myasthenia gravis or when taken in toxic doses. The quaternary ammonium group seems to confer various degrees of selectivity for gastric secretory and, perhaps, other GI functions. The extent to which ganglionic blockade may be involved is not known. The quaternary ammonium-containing drugs tend to be excreted unchanged in the urine. In contrast, the tertiary (and secondary) amine containing antimuscarinic drugs are reversibly protonated at physiological pH and consequently can penetrate cell membranes and the BBB in the non-ionized form. Most topical mydriatic antimuscarinic drugs are tertiary amines. These drugs are may be useful for the treatment of CNS disorders and lead to CNS toxicities also. Lastly, the tertiary amine containing antimuscarinic drugs tend to undergo significant metabolic biotransformation in the liver.

USES—In gastroenterology, antimuscarinic drugs are used sometimes for their GI effects, although parasympathetic effects in the bowel are difficult to suppress completely (Table 73-1). In the *irritable colon syndrome* (spastic colon) they may provide some relief initially, but some refractoriness usually develops later. *Functional GI disorders (functional diarrhea, spastic constipation, cardiospasm, pylorospasm, neurogenic colon, general hypermotility)* may respond, as may mild-to-moderate, irritative or infectious disorders, such as *mild diarrhea;* however, severe infectious dysenteries, regional enteritis, and ulcerative colitis do not. *Acute enterocolitis, mucous colitis,* and *the splenic flexure syndrome* may respond erratically. *Diverticulitis* sometimes may be improved. Antimuscarinic drugs may be used in combination with meperidine in the relief of *biliary dyskinesia.* In these uses, belladonna alkaloids commonly are employed; although they are less expensive than nonsolanaceous antimuscarinic drugs, they also cause more intense side effects than many synthetic, especially quaternary ammonium, drugs (Table 73-2). Atropine is available in combination with diphenoxylate, a non-analgesic analog of meperidine, for the treatment of mild GI hypermotility (eg, traveler's diarrhea). Several antimuscarinic drugs are available for GI use in combination with barbiturates, benzodiazepines, and ergotamine. The therapeutic effectiveness of these combinations is questionable.

The levorotatory alkaloids of belladonna, homatropine hydrobromide, and hyoscyamine sulfate are of historical importance in the treatment of peptic ulcer disease. These agents were used extensively in spite of the fact that doses required to produce modest reduction of *gastric acid secretion* also produced significant, often intolerable, side effects. *Pirenzepine* (Gaotrozepine, *Boehringer Ingelheim*) is an M₁ selective antimuscarinic drug that effectively reduces acid secretion and

Table 73-2. Antimuscarinic/Antispasmodic Drugs Used for Effects on the Gastrointestinal Tract[a]

QUATERNARY AMINES DRUG (TRADE NAME)	TERTIARY AMINES DRUG (TRADE NAME)	ANTISPASMOTIC/MISC DRUG (TRADE NAME)
Clidinium bromide (Quarzan: in Librium)	L-alkaloids of belladonna (Various)	Dicyclomine hydrochloride (Bentyl)
Glycopyrrolate (Robinul)	Belladonna alkaloids (Various)	Oxybutynin chloride (Ditropan; Various)
Mepenzolate bromide (Cantil)	L-hyoscyamine hydrobromide, sulfate (Various)	
Methantheline bromide (Banthine)	Oxyphencyclimine hydrochloride (Daricon)	
Methscopalamine bromide (Pamine)	Scopolamine hydrobromide (Various)	Pirenzepine (M1 selective-not in USA)
Propantheline bromide (Pro-Banthine)		
Tridihexethyl chloride (Panthilon)		

[a] For further information, see RPS-18, Chap 46, page 907.

promotes ulcer healing with a low incidence of antimuscarinic side effects. Although available in many countries, it is not yet approved in the United States. The introduction of several highly effective, well tolerated classes of drugs (H₂ antagonists (eg, cimetidine) and the proton pump inhibitors *(eg, omeprazole)* led to the replacement of the antimuscarinic drugs in the treatment of peptic ulcer. In addition, recurrent ulcers are often associated with infections of the acid-stable bacteria, *Helicobacter pylori* (*H pylori*). Hence, therapy for recurrent ulcers involves regimens that include appropriate antibacterial therapy administered with an H₂ antagonist or a proton pump inhibitor.

In genitourinary practice, antimuscarinic drugs are used to relieve symptoms of bladder instability in patients with uninhibited and reflex neurogenic bladder that include *urinary frequency, urgency, leakage,* and *dysuria.* They also are used to control urinary incontinence and to control enuresis in children (Table 73-1).

In ophthalmology, antimuscarinic drugs are used topically to *dilate the pupil (cause mydriasis* to facilitate visualization of the optic fundus) and to *paralyze accommodation (cause cycloplegia* for refractive examination); some of these drugs (eg, homatropine) cannot effect a complete cycloplegia, so they are not all equivalent. Generally, short-acting topical antimuscarinic drugs (cyclopentolate, tropicamide, homatropine) are preferred for examination, so that interference with vision or intraocular tension will last for the shortest possible time. They are given in combination with phenylephrine to *promote maximal widening of the pupil* to allow greater surgical access and, after surgery, to *prevent adhesions* and, in alternation with miotics or with phenylephrine, to *break adhesions between the iris and lens* (synechiae). They also are used to *treat acute iritis, uveitis, iridiocyclitis, and keratitis.* Paradoxically, these drugs may be used to treat malignant (ciliary block) glaucoma; in this, the rationale is that relaxation of the ciliary muscle helps to push the lens/diaphragm posteriorly and reestablish an anterior direction of flow of intraocular fluid.

Antimuscarinic drugs, especially atropine, are used sometimes for *anesthetic premedication,* to *inhibit excessive salivary and bronchial secretions* (aspiration prophylaxis) and *prevent bronchospasm* and *laryngospasm.* The antisecretory effects also are sought in the treatment of *sialorrhea, acute coryza, hay fever,* and *rhinitis.* Several medications used to treat allergic rhinitis, for example, contain various belladonna alkaloids (eg, methscopalamine) in combination with antihistamines and de-

Table 73-1. Examples and Potential Uses of Products Containing Antimuscarinic Drugs

THERAPEUTIC USE	DRUG EXAMPLE
Antidiarrheals	Atropine sulfate (Various combinations)
Antispasmodic	Dicyclomine hydrochloride (Bentyl; Various)
Antivertigo (Motion sickness)	Scopalamine Transderm-Scop
Aspiration prophylaxis (inhibit secretions)	Atropine sulfate (Various)
Cardiology (bradycardia, cardiopulmonary resuscitaion)	Atropine sulfate (Various)
Ophthomology (Mydriasis, cycloplegia)	Tropicamide (Mydriacyl; various)
Overactive bladder	Tolterodine tartrate (Detrol) Oxybutynin hydrochloride (Ditropan; Various)
Parkinson's disease	Benztropine mesylate (Cogentin; Various)
Pulmonary (Asthma)	Ipratropium bromide (Atrovent and with albuterol)
Pulmonary (upper respiratory combinations)	Methscopalamine nitrate (Dallergy; Various)

congestants for this purpose. The therapeutic effectiveness and the adverse effects resulting from the combination of drugs is questionable, especially at the doses being administered.

The effects to antagonize parasympathetically mediated bronchospasm and bronchorrhea are employed also in the treatment of *bronchial asthma* and other chronic obstructive pulmonary diseases. When administered by inhalation, systemic side-effects are infrequent and often negligible. Ipratropium is available in aerosol form either alone or in combinations with sympathomimetic drugs for the treatment of asthma.

In cardiology and anesthesiology, antimuscarinic drugs (atropine) are used to prevent or suppress *vagally mediated bradyarrhythmias* (such as occur after coronary occlusion), *heart block,* or *cardiac syncope* due to hyperactive carotid sinuses.

Certain antimuscarinic drugs may be used for their CNS actions in the treatment of *parkinsonism* and to treat *extrapyramidal symptoms (pseudoparkinsonism)* associated with antipsychotic drugs (dopamine antagonists). Parkinson's disease is a chronic, progressive degenerative disorder involving areas of the brain that maintain posture and muscle tone, as well as, regulate voluntary motor activity. Patients have great difficulty translating the desire to move into the act of moving. Current drug therapy is based on the observation that dopaminergic neurons in certain brain areas are lost. It is hypothesized that the progressive loss of the inhibitory influence of dopamineric neurons and a relative increase in the influence of ACh leads to an imbalance that results in the symptoms. Current treatment options are palliative and include the use of drugs to increase dopaminergic neurotransmission or to decrease cholinergic neurotransmission in the CNS. Hence, centrally acting antimuscarinic drugs like benztropine (Cogentin), biperiden (Akineton), trihexyphenidyl, and procyclidine (Kemadrin) are used in the treatment of Parkinson's disease (see Chapter 74 under the discussion on *Antiparkinson Drugs*). These drugs are generally used in combination with other drugs and are especially useful in the treatment of tremor.

Antimuscarinic drugs (especially atropine) also are used as antidotes for central and peripheral muscarinic toxicity in *anticholinesterase intoxication and for* poisoning by *Amanita muscaria.* Atropine is available in combination with the cholinesterase reactivator, pralidoxime, for use by the military as a parenteral preparation to treat organophosphate poisoning. Scopolamine is highly effective against motion sickness and is sometimes used for its sedative and amnesic effects, but these effects are not typical of antimuscarinic drugs.

ADVERSE EFFECTS—With nearly all antimuscarinic drugs, *dry mouth* is the first and dry skin is the second most common side effect. *Thirst* and *difficulty in swallowing* occur when the mouth and esophagus become sufficiently dry; chronic dry mouth also fosters dental caries. Suppression of sweating causes reflexive *flushing* and *heat intolerance* and can result in heat exhaustion or heat stroke in a hot environment; it also contributes to the hyperthermia seen in intoxication. *Mydriasis* frequently occurs, especially with secondary and tertiary compounds; *photophobia* and *blurring of vision* are consequences of mydriasis. With the secondary and tertiary amines, *cycloplegia* (which exacerbates blurred vision) occurs approximately concomitantly with mydriasis, but usually higher doses are required with many quaternary ammonium antimuscarinic drugs. In susceptible persons, especially the elderly, cycloplegia may contribute to an *elevation of intraocular pressure.* Difficulty in urination and urinary retention may occur, especially in elderly males with prostate enlargement. Tachycardia is a common side effect. *Constipation,* even *bowel stasis,* may occur. Antimuscarinic drugs relax the lower esophageal sphincter and thus promote gastroesophageal reflux, heartburn, and reflux esophagitis. They are, therefore, contraindicated in these conditions.

At high therapeutic doses, the secondary and tertiary amine antimuscarinic drugs may cause *dizziness, restlessness, tremors, fatigue,* and *locomotor difficulties.* Serious systemic intoxication can occur even from topical ophthalmological application, especially in children, since both local absorption and nasolacrimal drainage into the gut can deliver considerable amounts to the circulation. In serious intoxication, *hyperpyrexia, flushing, nausea, vomiting, drowsiness, disorientation, stupor, hallucinations, leukocytosis, nonallergic rashes, circulatory or respiratory collapse,* and even *death,* in addition to all aforenamed effects, may occur. Children, especially *infants and children with Down's syndrome, spastic paralysis, or brain damage,* are more sensitive than adults to the toxic effects.

When barbiturates or benzodiazepines are included in an antimuscarinic product, adverse effects of these drugs must be anticipated. The possibility that chronic use will lead to dependence should be considered.

The quaternary ammonium drugs mostly have a low CNS component of toxicity but instead may *cause orthostatic hypotension* (from ganglionic blockade) and *neuromuscular paralysis.*

Hypersensitivity with a variety of manifestations, usually rash, may follow the use of any antimuscarinic drug, but it is more common with the solanaceous alkaloids.

Other drugs, such as phenothiazines, tricyclic antidepressants, certain antihistamines, meperidine, and others that have significant antimuscarinic activity, may intensify considerably the effects of antimuscarinic drugs. Drugs with neuromuscular paralyzant activity (neuromuscular blocking drugs, aminoglycosides, polymyxin, etc) and ganglionic blocking drugs will summate with quaternary ammonium antimuscarinic drugs. Aluminum and magnesium trisilicate–containing antacids have been shown to decrease the absorption of some antimuscarinic drugs.

PRECAUTIONS—If there is mydriasis and photophobia, *dark glasses* should be worn. The patient also should be warned that *driving or other vision-dependent capabilities* may be impaired. Appropriate dosage precautions must be taken with *infants, children, and persons with Down's syndrome, brain damage, spasticity, or light irides.* Elevated intraocular pressure, urinary difficulty and retention, and constipation are more probable in *elderly persons.* Men with *prostatic hypertrophy,* especially, should be monitored for urinary function. Antimuscarinics should be used cautiously in *toxic megacolon.* Because of the tachycardic effects of the drugs, care must be exercised when *tachycardia,* other *tachyarrhythmias, coronary heart disease, congestive heart disease,* or *hyperthyroidism preexist.* Persons with *hypertension* may experience both exaggerated orthostatic hypotension and tachycardia. Similarly, *autonomic neuropathy* requires caution. Persons with a history of *allergies* or *bronchial asthma* will show a higher than normal incidence of hypersensitivity reactions. Quaternary ammonium antimuscarinic drugs, especially, may cause neuromuscular paralysis (with fatal respiratory arrest) in persons with *myasthenia gravis.* Although these drugs sometimes are used in the treatment of *adhesions between lens and iris,* damage can occur, and expert precautions must be taken. When solutions of antimuscarinic drugs are applied topically to the eye, pressure should be applied just below the internal canthus of the eye to prevent nasolacrimal drainage.

Precautions are appropriate in *ulcerative colitis.* In *hiatus hernia or gastroesophageal reflux,* reflux and esophagitis are exacerbated by antimuscarinic drugs, because the lower esophageal sphincter is stimulated by cholinergic nerves. In a *hot environment,* the user is more susceptible to disruption of heat regulation. *Hepatic disease* for some and *renal disease* for other antimuscarinic drugs may decrease the rate of elimination. Cognizance should be taken of possible *drug interactions.* Lastly, until proven otherwise, it must be assumed that all antimuscarinic drugs can pass the placental barrier; the threat to the fetus *in utero* is unknown, but an infant born with an effective amount of drug aboard may have GI difficulties and problems in early nutrition.

CONTRAINDICATIONS—An antimuscarinic drug generally is contraindicated in *narrow-angle glaucoma, pyloric* or *intestinal obstruction, intestinal atony* of the elderly, *paralytic*

MEDICINAL AGENTS

ileus, achalasia of the esophagus, frank *bladder neck obstruction,* or when there is *hypersensitivity* to the drug or a closely related one. There are specific exceptions depending on the route employed and the degree of selectivity (profile of activity) of the drug used.

ATROPINE SULFATE

Benzeneacetic acid, *endo*-(±)-α-(hydroxymethyl)-, 8-methyl-8-azabicyclo[3.2.1]oct-3-yl ester, sulfate (2:1) (salt), monohydrate

1αH,5αH -Tropan-3α-ol (α)-tropate(ester) sulfate (2:1) (salt) monohydrate [5908-99-6] ($C_{17}H_{23}NO_3$)$_2$.H_2SO_4.H_2O (694.82); anhydrous [55-48-1] (676.82).

Caution—Atropine Sulfate is very poisonous.

Preparation—Atropine is dissolved in warm acetone, sufficient dilute sulfuric acid is added to form the 2:1 sulfate, and atropine sulfate is crystallized from the solution.

Description—Colorless crystals or a white, crystalline powder; odorless; effloresces in dry air; slowly affected by light; when previously dried at 120° for 4 hr, it melts not lower than 187°.

Solubility—1 g in 0.4 mL water, 5 mL alcohol, or about 2.5 mL glycerol.

Comments—Atropine is a tertiary amine antimuscarinic drug with all of the actions and most uses and adverse effects described in the general statement at the beginning of this chapter. The antimuscarinic activity mostly resides in the *l*-isomer (*l*-hyoscamine). By historical precedence, it has become the prototype and most widely used of antimuscarinic drugs.

Because atropine is obtained from species of *belladonna,* the word atropine often has been used as synonymous with belladonna. Actually, several genera of *Solanaceae* produce atropine and related alkaloids, so atropine and other related natural or semisynthetic congeners are sometimes called *solanaceous* alkaloids.

Atropine is absorbed rapidly and completely from the gut and is distributed rapidly throughout the body. Atropine is available in combination with diphenoxylate, a nonanalgesic analog of meperidine, for the treatment of mild GI hypermotility (eg, traveler's diarrhea). Following topical application atropine penetrates readily into the eye. It produces prolonged mydriasis and cycloplegia for more than 1 week. It is metabolized mainly in the liver. The plasma half-life of *l*-hyoscyamine is less than 4 hr. The half-life in the eye is long, and effects may last for 7 to 12 days after topical application to the eye. Intraocular inflammation, however, greatly shortens the half-life in the eye.

BELLADONNA

Deadly Nightshade Leaf; Belladonna Herb; Black Cherry Leaf; Dwale; Dwayberry Leaf

The dried leaf and flowering or fruiting top of *Atropa belladonna* Linné or of its variety *acuminata* Royle ex Lindley (Fam *Solanaceae*); it yields not less than 0.35% of the alkaloids of Belladonna Leaf USP.

Comments—Its actions are those of the principal alkaloids, hyoscamine and atropine (see the general statement).

LEVOROTATORY ALKALOIDS OF BELLADONNA

A synthetic mixture of the pure salts of the levorotatory alkaloids found in belladonna. The ratio of the salts is such that a single dose contains the approximate amount of each of the following: scopolamine hydrobromide, 0.006 mg; atropine sulfate, 0.02 mg and hyoscyamine sulfate, 0.1 mg.

Comments—See *Belladonna.*

HOMATROPINE HYDROBROMIDE

Benzeneacetic acid, (±)-α-hydroxy-, *endo*-8-methyl-8-azabicyclo[3.2.1]oct-3-yl ester hydrobromide

1αH,5αH-Tropan-3α-ol mandelate (ester) hydrobromide [51-56-9] $C_{16}H_{21}NO_3$.HBr (356.26); the hydrobromide of tropine mandelate.

Preparation—By heating *tropine* with *mandelic acid* in the presence of hydrochloric acid; ammonia is added, and the liberated homatropine extracted with chloroform; the solution is evaporated, hydrobromic acid added and the homatropine hydrobromide crystallized.

Description—White crystals, or a white crystalline powder; affected by light; melts between 214° and 217° with slight decomposition; aqueous solution is practically neutral or only faintly acid to litmus.

Solubility—1 g in 6 mL water, 40 mL alcohol or about 420 mL chloroform; insoluble in ether.

Comments—For ophthalmological use only. It has a duration of action from 0.5 to 2 days.

HYOSCYAMINE SULFATE

Benzeneacetic acid, α-(hydroxymethyl)-, [3(S)-endo]-8-methyl-8-azabicyclo[3.2.1]oct-3-yl ester, sulfate (2:1), dihydrate; Cystospaz

[6835-16-1] ($C_{17}H_{23}NO_3$)$_2$.$H_2SO_4$2H_2O (712.85); anhydrous [620-61-1] (676.82). The sulfate of an alkaloid usually obtained from species of *Hyoscyamus* Linné or other genera or Fam *Solanaceae*.

Caution—Hyoscyamine Sulfate is extremely poisonous.

Preparation—Isolated from the alkaloids of belladonna by resolution of atropine.

Description—White, odorless crystals or a crystalline powder; deliquescent; affected by light; when previously dried at 105° for 4 hr, does not melt below 200°; pH (1 in 100 solution) about 5.3.

Solubility—1 g in 0.5 mL water or 5 mL alcohol; practically insoluble in ether.

Comments—The levorotatory isomer of atropine. It is used as an *antispasmodic.*

IPRATROPIUM BROMIDE

(±)-(endo, syn)-8-Azoniabicyclo[3.2.1]octane, 3-(3-hydroxy-1-oxo-2-phenylpropoxy)-8-methyl-8-(1-methylethyl)-, bromide monohydrate; Atrovent

(8r)-3α-Hydroxy-8-isopropyl-1αH,5αH-tropanium bromide (±)-tropate monohydrate [66985-17-9]; anhydrous [22254-24-6] $C_{20}H_{30}BrNO_3$.H_2O (430.38).

Preparation—Atropine is quaternized with isopropyl bromide.

Description—White, crystalline substance with a bitter taste.

Solubility—Freely soluble in water or alcohol; insoluble in chloroform or ether.

Comments—A quaternary ammonium antimuscarinic drug used for the treatment of *bronchial asthma* and *chronic obstructive pulmonary disease,* for which it is given as an inhalant aerosol. It appears to be approximately equivalent to β$_2$-agonists in its efficacy against bronchial asthma, but the duration of action is longer. It appears to be more effective than β$_2$-agonists against chronic obstructive pulmonary disease. It seems to act mainly on the larger airways.

By inhalation, the incidence and severity of side effects is low, the most common effects being dry mouth, irritation in the throat, cough, and unpleasant taste. Other effects are quite rare and include blurring of vision, drowsiness, dizziness, *mild bradycardia,* and airway obstruction caused by sputum made viscous by diminished tracheobronchial secretions.

By inhalation, ipratropium causes bronchodilatation in doses 1/1000 those of oral or intravenous doses, which avoid most systemic side effects. Bronchodilatation occurs within a few minutes, peaks at 1 to 2 hr, and lasts 4 to 8 hr. About half the dose is eliminated in the feces. The half-life is 3 to 4 hr. Nasal sprays of ipratropium (0.03% and 0.06%) are now available for topical treatment of allergic rhinitis or rhinorrhea associated with the common cold, respectively.

SCOPOLAMINE HYDROBROMIDE

Benzeneacetic acid, [7(S)-(1α,2β,4β,5α,7β)]-α-(hydroxymethyl)-, 9-methyl-3-oxa-9-azatricyclo[3.3.1.0²,⁴]non-7-yl ester, hydrobromide, trihydrate; Transderm-Scop

6β,7β-Epoxy-1αH,5αH-tropan-3α-ol (-)-tropate(ester) hydrobromide trihydrate [6533-68-2] $C_{17}H_{21}NO_4$.HBr.3H_2O (438.31); anhydrous [114-49-8] (384.27).

Preparation—Scopolamine, an alkaloid occurring in several solanaceous plants, may be obtained from such plants by alkaloid extraction procedures followed by fractionation of the extract to remove other alkaloids, notable hyoscyamine.

Description—Colorless or white crystals or white, granular powder; odorless; slightly efflorescent in dry air; the anhydrous salt melts between 195° and 199°; pH (1 in 10 solution) between 4 and 5.5.

Solubility—1 g in 1.5 mL water or 20 mL alcohol; slightly soluble in chloroform; insoluble in ether.

Comments—It differs from other antimuscarinic drugs in that in therapeutic doses it is a sedative and tranquilizing depressant to the CNS. In its peripheral actions, it differs from atropine in that it is a stronger blocking agent for the iris, ciliary body, and salivary, bronchial, and sweat glands but is weaker in its action on the heart (in which it is incapable of exerting actions in tolerated doses), the intestinal tract, and the bronchial musculature. It is sometimes given as a *preanesthetic* medication for both its sedative-tranquilizing and antisecretory actions. It is effective as a prophylactic against *motion sickness,* for which slow-release transdermal dosage forms have been devised. Transdermal systems provide sustained release for 3 days. It also is used sometimes in other types of *vertigo.* It occasionally is used to suppress *delirium.* It is used as an *amnesic* agent in *obstetrics* (combined with morphine it was used formerly to produce *twilight sleep*). As a *mydriatic* and *cycloplegic,* it has a somewhat shorter duration (3–7 days), and intraocular pressure is affected less markedly than with atropine.

Except for drowsiness, its side effects are those of tertiary amine antimuscarinic drugs. Occasionally, with therapeutic doses a patient may experience excitement, restlessness, hallucinations, delirium or disorientation, confusion, memory loss, stupor, and, rarely, coma. Infants and young children are quite susceptible to the CNS toxicity. After a transdermal system has been in use for 3 or more days, removal sometimes causes a withdrawal syndrome consisting of dizziness, disequilibrium, nausea, vomiting, and headache. Rarely, there may be hypersensitivity, characterized by edema of the uvula, glottis, and lips. The toxic effects of overdoses, precautions, and contraindications are like those of tertiary amine antimuscarinic drugs.

TOLTERODINE TARTRATE

Phenol, (*R*)-2-[3-[bis(1-methylethyl)amino]-1-phenylpropyl]-4-methyl-, [*R*-(*R**,*R**)]-2,3-dihydroxybutanedioate (1:1) salt; Detrol, Detrol LA

bladder outflow obstruction and gastrointestinal obstructive disorders. The drug is extensively metabolized by CYP2D6 and potent inhibitors of the may lead to adverse effects. CYP3A4 inhibitors also may lead to elevated serum concentrations of the drug.

OPHTHALMOLOGICAL DRUGS

CYCLOPENTOLATE HYDROCHLORIDE

Benzeneacetic acid, α-(1-hydroxycyclopentyl)-, 2-(dimethylamino)ethyl ester, hydrochloride; AK-Pentolate; Cyclogyl

2-(Dimethylamino)ethyl 1-hydroxy-α-phenylcyclopentaneacetate hydrochloride [5870-29-1] $C_{17}H_{25}NO_3 \cdot HCl$ (327.85).

Preparation—The acid moiety of the ester, 1-hydroxy-α-phenylcyclopentaneacetic acid (I), may be prepared by adding sodium phenylacetate to an ethereal solution of isopropyl magnesium bromide; treatment of the resulting sodium phenylacetate magnesium bromide with an ethereal solution of cyclopentanone produces a Grignard addition product that on hydrolysis yields I. The ester is produced by metathesis

(+)-(*R*)-2-[1-[2-Diisopropylamino)ethyl]benzyl]-*p*-cresol L-tartrate (1:1) salt
[124937-52-6] $C_{22}H_{31}NO \cdot C_4H_6O_6$ (475.58).

Preparation—Crude 3-(2-methoxy-5-methylphenyl)3-phenyl-propionyl chloride is added dropwise to a stirred solution of diisopropylamine in dichloromethane at 0°. *N,N*-diisopropyl-3-(2-methoxy-5-methylphenyl)-3-phenylpropionamide is filtered, dried, and added to a stirred suspension of lithium aluminum hydride in dry ether and refluxed for 2 days. The compound was treated with BBr_3 to provide the free phenol. The amine was treated with a solution of L(+)-tartaric acid to provide the desired enantiomer. US Patent 5,382,600.

Description—White crystalline powder; pKa 9.87.

Solubility—Solubility in water is 12 mg/mL, soluble in methanol, slightly soluble in ethanol, and practically insoluble in toluene. The partition coefficient (octanol/water) is 1.83 at pH 7.3.

Comments—Competitive muscarinic antagonist with pronounced effects on bladder function. The drug is extensively metabolized by the liver following oral administration. The primary route of metabolism involved the oxidation of the 5-methyl group mediated by the CYP2D6. The 5-hydroxymethyl metabolite exhibits antimuscarinic activity similar to the parent drug and contributes significantly to the therapeutic effects of the drug. Certain individuals (7% of caucasian population) are devoid of the CYP2D6 enzyme. These patients are considered poor metabolizers and require dosage adjustments.

Immediate release tablets (1 mg and 2 mg) and extended release capsules (2 mg and 4mg) are available. The initial recommended dosage range for the immediate release product is 1–2 mg twice daily based on individual response and tolerability. The recommended dose for patients with impaired liver function and those taking CYP3A4 inhibitors is 1 mg twice daily.

The recommended dose for the extended release capsules is 2–4 mg once daily (taken with liquids and swallowed whole) based on individual response and tolerability. The recommended dose for patients with significantly impaired liver or renal function and those taking CYP3A4 inhibitors is 2 mg daily.

The drug is contraindicated in patients with known hypersensitivity to tolterodine or its ingredients and in patients with urinary retention, gastric retention, or uncontrolled narrow-angle glaucoma. Adverse effects include dry mouth, headache, constipation, abdominal pain, and abnormal vision. The drug should be used with caution in patients with

between the sodium salt of I and 2-dimethylaminoethyl chloride in isopropyl alcohol. After crystallization from acetone, the ester is converted to the hydrochloride with HCl.

Description—White, crystalline powder, which on standing develops a characteristic odor; melts between 137° and 141°; pH (1 in 100 solution) between 4.5 and 5.5.

Solubility—Very soluble in water; freely soluble in alcohol; insoluble in ether.

Comments—An *antimuscarinic* drug used primarily for its *ophthalmological* actions. After application to the cornea, cyclopegia is complete in 25 to 75 min; recovery is complete in 6 to 24 hr. The side effects and CNS toxicity are those of antimuscarinic drugs, but the duration of the effects is very short.

TROPICAMIDE

Benzeneacetamide, *N*-ethyl-α-(hydroxymethyl)-*N*-(4-pyridinylmethyl)-, Mydriacyl

N-Ethyl-2- phenyl - *N*- (4 - pyridylmethyl) hydracrylamide [1508-75-4 $C_{17}H_{20}N_2O_2$ (284.36).

Preparation—Tropic acid is esterified with acetyl chloride, and the resulting tropic acid acetate is converted to the corresponding acid chloride by reaction with thionyl chloride. Condensation of the acid chloride with 4-[(ethylamino)methyl] pyridine in the presence of an appropriate dehydrochlorinating agent yields the tropicamide acetate ester, which saponifies readily to tropicamide. US Pat 2,726,245.

Description—White or practically white, crystalline powder; odorless or has not more than a slight odor; melts between 96° and 100°.

Solubility—1 g in 500 mL water or 3 mL chloroform; freely soluble in alcohol or solutions of strong acids.

Comments—An *antimuscarinic* drug that is used to induce *mydriasis* and *cycloplegia* in ophthalmological practice. Applied topically to the eye, it has a short duration of action. The time to a maximal effect is usually 20 to 25 min. The duration of maximal effect is only about 15 to 20 min, but full recovery requires 5 to 6 hr. However, photophobia and other subjective indices of an effect may disappear as early as 2 hr after application. The drug, thus, has an obvious advantage over belladonna alkaloids in its shorter duration of action and over homatropine in its ability to induce cycloplegia. It is disadvantageous in that the ophthalmologist must time the examination to coincide with the time of maximal effect and has a brief time for examination or else it is necessary to repeat administration at 30-min intervals to obviate the timing problem.

Although tropicamide does not increase intraocular pressure in normal persons, it may do so in patients with glaucoma or those who have certain structural deformities of the anterior chamber of the eye. It should, thus, be used cautiously in such patients. If an antimuscarinic drug must be employed in such patients, tropicamide is indicated because of its brief duration of action.

Side effects can occur from passage of solutions through the nasolacrimal duct and subsequent absorption. Dry mouth and tachycardia have occurred. Although intoxication in children has not been reported, it must be kept in mind. Tropicamide usually stings transiently when applied.

ANTISPASMODIC DRUGS

The term *antispasmodic* is a general one that might be applied to the actions of many drugs with diverse mechanisms of action. Spasm may result from a local disorder in which cellular injury initiates the contractile process and local hormones or other excitatory or irritant substances are released (or local reflexes are activated) or it may be the result of hyperactivity in efferent excitatory autonomic nerves or electrolyte disturbances that favor increased neuronal and muscular activity. Therefore, according to the locus, cause, and mediators of a spastic condition, one or more of a number of classes of selective drugs may be employed, eg, neuromuscular blocking or centrally acting muscle relaxants for various spastic conditions of skeletal muscle, local anesthetics for some localized neurally mediated spasm, α-adrenoreceptor-blocking drugs or β$_2$-adrenoreceptor agonists for vasospasm, β$_2$-agonists for bronchial and uterine spasms, antimuscarinic drugs for ciliary spasm or spastic bowel, calcium for hypocalcemic tetany, calcium channel blockers for various smooth muscle spasms, etc. Thus, the term antispasmodic might apply to many different types of drugs.

The term antispasmodic should be reserved, however, for those drugs that relax smooth muscle nonselectively. Only flavoxate hydrochloride and oxybutinin chloride potentially influence all smooth muscle, regardless of the type of innervation and neurotransmitter affected. Calcium channel–blocking drugs are discussed elsewhere. The selective antagonists are treated in the appropriate chapters. Long before the selective competitive antagonistic actions of antimuscarinic drugs were known, some antimuscarinic preparations and drugs were known to relieve certain spastic conditions of the bowel. Therefore, the term antispasmodic came to connote antimuscarinic drugs that have important GI uses, and it has become common to include antispasmodics in chapters on antimuscarinic drugs.

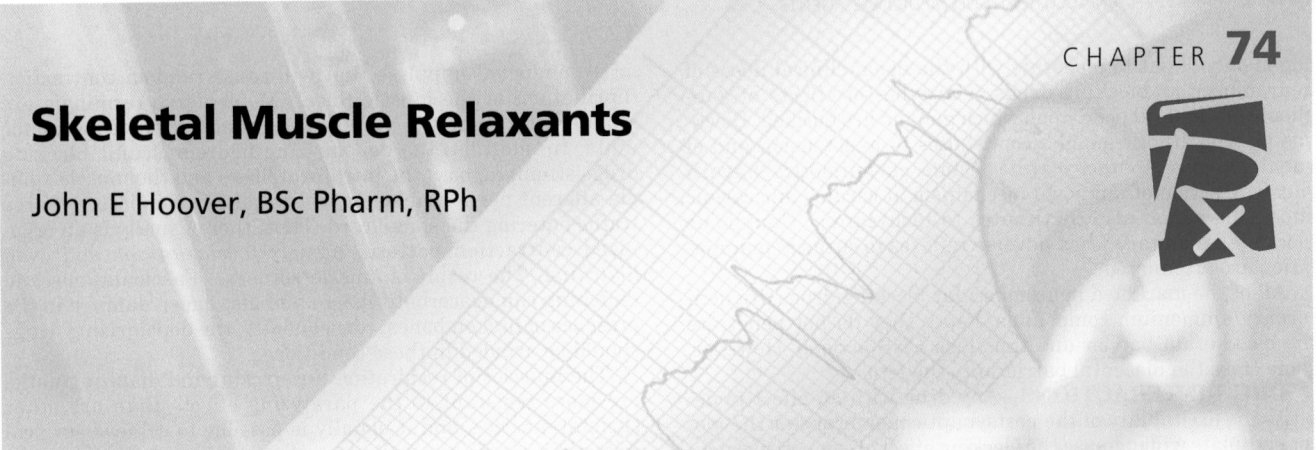

Skeletal Muscle Relaxants

John E Hoover, BSc Pharm, RPh

Skeletal muscle may be relaxed by blocking the effect of somatic motor nerve impulses, by depressing the appropriate neurons within the central nervous system (CNS) so that somatic motor nerve impulses fail to be generated, or by decreasing the availability of calcium ions to the myofibrillar contractile system. Interruption of certain afferent reflex pathways, as by local anesthesia, also may effect relaxation of circumscribed muscle groups; local anesthetic block of efferent somatic motor outflow also is employed sometimes to relieve localized skeletal muscle spasm. In this chapter only those drugs that act at the myoneural junction, the *neuromuscular blocking drugs,* and those drugs that act upon central neurons, the *centrally acting muscle relaxants,* are discussed.

NEUROMUSCULAR BLOCKING DRUGS

Neuromuscular blocking drugs prevent somatic motor nerve impulses from initiating contractile responses in the effector skeletal (striated) muscles and hence cause a paralysis of the muscles. There are two categories of such drugs: the *competitive (or stabilizing) paralyzants* and the *depolarizing paralyzants,* discussed separately.

USES—Competitive and depolarizing neuromuscular blocking drugs have the same major uses, in general. The pharmacokinetics and pattern of side effects, rather than their mechanism, determine the uses of any given agent. The principal use is to provide *adequate skeletal muscular relaxation* during *surgery, controlled respiration,* and *orthopedic manipulations.* The short-acting drugs are used to relax the laryngeal muscles during *endotracheal intubation* and *bronchoscopy.* Neuromuscular paralyzants may be employed to *decrease the severity of muscle contraction* during *electroconvulsive* treatment. Competitive neuromuscular paralyzants have been used in the management of *tetanus* and in *various spastic disorders,* but the results usually have been disappointing. Competitive blocking drugs may be used in the *diagnosis of myasthenia gravis;* the myasthenic patient is extremely sensitive to the paralyzant actions.

Competitive Neuromuscular Blocking Drugs

When impulses in the somatic motor nerves arrive in the nerve terminals in the motor end-plate region, they evoke the release of acetylcholine, which diffuses to the postsynaptic motor end-plate membrane. There, acetylcholine combines with nicotinic cholinergic receptors to activate them, which leads to the opening of transmembrane ion channels, ion flow, and consequent membrane depolarization. End-plate membrane depolarization is followed by depolarization of the muscle membrane and subsequent contraction. Any interruption of the above sequence of events leads to muscular paralysis.

The competitive neuromuscular blocking drugs combine with the nicotinic receptors and occupy them without activating them. Acetylcholine cannot activate the already occupied receptors, so motor nerve impulses cannot elicit contractions, and paralysis ensues. Some of them also lodge in the receptor-operated ionophore and, thus, decrease electrical activation of the postsynaptic membrane.

PHARMACOLOGICAL ANTAGONISM—The interaction of blocking drug and receptor is reversible and dynamic. Drug molecules combine, dissociate, recombine, etc, thus leaving receptor molecules transiently unoccupied. The probability that an acetylcholine molecule will find an unoccupied receptor is directly proportional to the concentration. If the concentration is elevated sufficiently, dissociated blocking drug molecules will find the receptors occupied with acetylcholine and will be prevented from recombining with the receptors to maintain blockade. Thus, a blockade can be overcome competitively. In practice, the acetylcholine concentration is raised by inhibiting acetylcholinesterase in the end-plate region. Neostigmine and edrophonium are the most commonly employed anticholinesterases for antagonizing competitive neuromuscular paralyzants. The anticholinesterases are discussed in Chapter 71.

SIDE EFFECTS AND PRECAUTIONS—The competitive neuromuscular blocking drugs are quite selective for the nonrespiratory muscles, so that it is possible to achieve surgical relaxation of the abdominal, limb, neck, or laryngeal muscles without significant loss of respiratory function. However, respiration often may be depressed to the point of danger, even apnea, so *these drugs should be used only when facilities for prolonged respiratory assistance are at hand and the trachea is intubated,* in case respiratory assistance is needed. In hypothermic procedures such as cardiopulmonary bypass surgery, blockade is less complete, so that larger than standard doses are required; excessive paralysis may ensue subsequently when body temperature is elevated.

The two other principal side effects are the release of histamine from mast cells and ganglionic blockade. The extent to which histamine release occurs varies among the several drugs; it is greatest with tubocurarine. The histamine released may cause vasodilation and consequent hypotension and reflex tachycardia, bronchospasm, urticaria, rash, and, rarely, even angioneurotic edema. *Histamine-releasing neuromuscular blocking drugs should be avoided in persons with a history of bronchial asthma, angioneurotic edema, or anaphylaxis.*

Ganglionic blockade may occur, because the postsynaptic ganglionic cholinergic receptors are nicotinic. However, these receptors have somewhat different structural requirements from those at the neuromuscular junction, so ganglionic blockade is only slight to moderate with the usual clinical doses of neuromuscular blocking drugs. The types of effects of ganglionic blockade depend upon which ganglia are blocked. Blockade of sympathetic ganglia contributes to hypotension and of vagal ganglia, to tachycardia. Some curimimetics have a *vagolytic* action of unknown mechanism at cardiac muscarinic sites; this action also contributes to tachycardia. Ganglionic blockade is salutary when adverse reflexes to surgical manipulation are attenuated.

All of the marketed neuromuscular blocking drugs are quaternary ammonium compounds, hence they do not penetrate the blood-brain barrier and thus lack CNS actions. However, some cross the placental barrier into the fetus.

DRUG INTERACTIONS—Any drug with an effect to depress the excitability of the postsynaptic membrane at the motor end-plate will increase the blocking effect of competitive neuromuscular blocking drugs. The anesthetic ethers, halothane, and propranolol, are among such drugs.

A number of antibiotics can cause neuromuscular paralysis in high doses and in therapeutic doses may increase neuromuscular blockade by the competitive blocking drugs. Some of these (gentamicin, kanamycin, neomycin, streptomycin, tobramycin, and paromomycin) apparently also act competitively on the nicotinic receptor and, hence, may be antagonized by anticholinesterases. Others (polymyxins, colistin, colistimethate, tetracyclines, lincomycin, and clindamycin) have a more obscure action and are not antagonized by anticholinesterases, although anticholinesterases will antagonize the neuromuscular blocking drug and relieve the exaggerated paralysis; calcium partially antagonizes these drugs. Local anesthetics (quinine, quinidine, ganglionic blocking drugs, and magnesium ion) also potentiate the neuromuscular blocking actions of the competitive blocking drugs.

Depolarizing Neuromuscular Blocking Drugs

The depolarizing neuromuscular blocking drugs are nicotinic agonists, which, like acetylcholine, interact with the postsynaptic nicotinic receptors to effect a depolarization of the membrane at the motor end-plate. Unlike acetylcholine their sojourn at the end-plate is long, so the postsynaptic membrane may remain depolarized. Since the muscle membrane and consequent contraction can be excited only by a fresh depolarization, the muscle remains paralyzed. That is to say, the trigger for the conducted muscle impulse is the transient fall in end-plate membrane potential and not the persisting depolarization.

Eventually, the motor end-plate membrane repolarizes despite the continuing presence of the drug (phase two block), owing to a shift in receptor conformation. Nevertheless, despite the fact that the membrane is poised for a new depolarization, motor nerve impulses and acetylcholine fail to elicit a response, because the nicotinic receptor is not in its appropriate configuration. During this phase, the neuromuscular blockade takes on some characteristics of competitive blockade and even may be antagonized partially by anticholinesterases. This second phase is erratic in onset among the various muscles, and blockade may be of a mixed type, thus complicating the treatment of overdoses. Furthermore, not all drug recipients respond alike. Electrolyte status, muscle condition, disease, genetic factors, the presence of other drugs, and temperature all affect the time of onset and extent of phase two block. Moreover, not all depolarizing drugs are identical in the pattern of blockade. Clinically, phase two is usually significant only when the drug dose is repeated or the drug is infused and blood levels sustained beyond the normal single-dose limit. Monitoring neuromuscular function by nerve stimulation to avoid overdose and/or conversion to phase two paralysis is advisable.

SIDE EFFECTS AND PRECAUTIONS—During the onset of the drug-induced depolarization, as the membrane potential depolarizes to the critical firing potential, there may

arise conducted impulses that will cause random contraction (fibrillation) of the muscle fibers. Motor nerve terminals are stimulated to generate axon reflexes that fire off entire motor units. In addition, the depolarizing neuromuscular blocking drugs stimulate both the intrafusal fibers and the muscle spindle afferent nerve endings, which results in facilitatory nerve traffic entering the spinal cord. Thus, there usually is an organized contraction pattern, namely *fasciculations* and even *twitching*. The result is muscle soreness. Fasciculations and twitching can exacerbate spasm and also cause damage in the presence of broken bones; consequently, the depolarizing drugs should be avoided in these conditions.

The muscles of respiration (intercostal and diaphragmatic) are more resistant to the paralyzing effects than are other skeletal muscles, and it usually is possible to achieve surgical relaxation of abdominal, limb, neck, or laryngeal muscles without significant loss of respiratory function. Nevertheless, respiration often may be depressed, sometimes to the point of apnea. This is likely especially after prolonged use, which favors considerable loss of potassium from the motor end-plate region. Consequently, *the depolarizing neuromuscular blocking drugs should be used only with tracheal intubation and when facilities for prolonged assisted respiration are at hand.* Care should be used when respiration already is depressed and also when the lithotomy or Trendelenburg positions are employed, especially in young children and the aged.

During the depolarizing phase of neuromuscular block, potassium is lost rapidly from the muscles, which may cause hyperkalemia. If a sufficient amount of the mobilized potassium is excreted, there may be a later hypokalemia. Various cardiac arrhythmias, even cardiac arrest, may result, especially if the patient is digitalized. Prolonged paralysis by these agents may lead to malignant hyperthermia.

The effects of depolarizing blocking drugs on autonomic ganglia and histamine stores are variable.

DRUG INTERACTIONS—Muscle paralysis with depolarizing neuromuscular blocking drugs is increased by hypothermia, hypokalemia, hypermagnesemia, polymyxin B, colistin, colistimethate, and aminoglycoside antibiotics (streptomycin, kanamycin, gentamicin, tobramycin, and neomycin).

ATRACURIUM BESYLATE

Isoquinolinium, 2,2′-[1,5-pentanediylbis[oxy(3-oxo-3,1-propanediyl)]]-bis[1-(3,4-dimethoxyphenyl)methyl]-1,2,3,4-tetrahydro-6,7-dimethoxy-2-methyl-, dibenzenesulfonate; Tracrium

[64228-81-5] $C_{65}H_{82}N_2O_{18}S_2$ (1243.49).

Preparation—Acryloyl chloride and 1,5-pentanediol are reacted to produce the diester, which then is treated with tetrahydropapaverine to yield the di-tertiary amine. This latter product, with methyliodide, forms the bis-quaternary iodide, which is converted to the besylate with benzenesulfonic acid. See US Pat 4,179,507.

Description—Off-white powder; melts at 87°. The molecule has the potential to conform to any of 16 different isomers, but due to its symmetry, only 10 exist. The drug entity consists of a mixture of several possible isomers, and the synthetic procedure results in the production of a consistent ratio of isomers, but in unequal amounts. The isomer that predominates (approximately in a 3:1 ratio) is that in which the quaternary methyl group and the dimethoxybenzyl group assume a *trans* configuration about the tetrahydroisoquinoline parent.

Solubility—1 g in 20 mL water.

Comments—A competitive neuromuscular paralyzant that is 2.5 times as potent as tubocurarine. Its effects are more predictable than are those of tubocurarine, especially with respect to repeated doses. Its duration of action is 33–50% of that of tubocurarine, 90% of recovery of muscle function occurring in 60 to 70 min. The drug thus lends itself to use in surgical procedures of short-to-intermediate duration. In therapeutic doses, side effects are minimal, but moderate degrees of histamine release and consequent sequelae occur occasionally.

Drug interactions and antagonism by anticholinesterases essentially are the same as with tubocurarine, but the potentiating effects of anesthetics are less marked.

It neither is metabolized appreciably in the liver nor excreted into the urine. Rather, the bridge between the isoquinoline moieties is ruptured spontaneously by Hoffman elimination and by hydrolysis in plasma. This unique elimination makes the effects and duration of action independent of liver and/or renal insufficiency. The elimination half-life is about 20 min.

CISATRACURIUM BESYLATE

Isoquinolinium, [1R-[1α,2α(1′R*,2′R*)]]-2,2′-[1,5-pentanediylbis[oxy(3-oxo-3,1-propanediyl)]bis[1-[3,4dimethoxyphenyl)methyl]-1,2,3,4-tetrahydro-6,7-dimethoxy-2-methyl-, dibenzenesulfonate; Nimbex

[96946-42-8] $C_{65}H_{82}N_2O_{18}S_2$ (12243.51).

Preparation—From racemic tetrahydropapaverine which is resolved to the *R*-form (**I**). A coupling compound (**II**) is made by forming the diacrylate estser of 1,5-pentanediol with 2-bromopropionic acid using p-toluenesulfonic acid and triethylamine. Two molecules of **I** are condensed with **II** at the piperidine nitrogen atoms using oxalic acid, to form the base. Benzenesulfonic acid converts the base to salt. Drugs of the Future 21:14, 1996. See also US Pat 4,179,507 (1979).

CURARE

Comments—A name applied to extracts principally of the bark and other parts of plants of certain species of *Chondodendron* or *Strychnos,* especially *Chondodendron tomentosum* and *Strychnos toxiferin,* prepared by South American Indians of the Upper Amazon and Orinoco basins for use as arrow poisons. The extracts contain neuromuscular paralyzant alkaloids and numerous other contaminants. The chondodendron alkaloids contain tertiary and quaternary benzylisoquinoline derivatives such as *d*-tubocurarine (see *Tubocurarine Chloride*), *curine,* and related compounds. The strychnos alkaloids contain β-carboline alkaloids such as the toxiferins and calabash *curarines*. None of the crude preparations currently is used in therapeutics. Only purified preparations or alkaloids from *Chondodendron tomentosum* are available commercially.

DANTROLENE SODIUM

2,4-Imidazolidinedione, 1-[[[5-(4-nitrophenyl)-2-furanyl]methylene]amino]-, sodium salt, hydrate (2:7); Dantrium

1-[[5-(*p*-Nitrophenyl)furfurylidene]amino]hydantoin sodium salt hydrate [24868-20-0] $C_{14}H_9N_4NaO_5.31/2H_2O$ (399.29).

Preparation—See *J Med Chem* 1967; 10:807, and US Pat 3,415,821.

Description—Orange powder; *free acid* melts about 280°; pK_a about 7.5.

Solubility—Slightly soluble in water; more soluble in alkali.

Comments—Differs from the classical neuromuscular blocking drugs in that its action is distal to the nicotinic receptors and neuromuscular junction. Instead, it suppresses excitation-contraction coupling by interfering with release of calcium from the sarcotubular reticulum. The muscle fibers still respond to nerve impulses; the contractile response is lessened but not abolished. Therefore, muscle weakness, rather than paralysis, is the result. Fast muscle fibers (white) are affected more than slow muscle fibers (red). Because the contractility of the intrafusal fibers in the muscle spindles also is decreased, spinal cord–mediated stretch reflexes are attenuated, which provides the primary explanation of its ability to relieve certain types of spasm. It is used

to treat *spasticity resulting from upper motor neuron* lesions, such as those with *spinal cord injury, stroke, multiple sclerosis,* and *cerebral palsy* but not spasticity resulting from musculoskeletal injury, lumbago, or rheumatoid disorders. It is possible that a direct effect on the motor neuron may be involved in this limited spectrum of activity, since the drug does exert some CNS-depressant actions. In fact, the drug is used to treat the *neuroleptic malignant syndrome*. Its effect on intracellular calcium also lends itself to the treatment of *malignant hyperthermia,* which can be triggered by general anesthesia and neuromuscular blocking drugs.

Interference with muscle function may cause weakness and fatigue, poor posture with consequent backache and myalgia, a feeling of suffocation, difficulties in swallowing, diplopia, and other visual disturbances. Effects on the CNS include drowsiness, dizziness, malaise, headache, nervousness, slurred speech, confusion, depression, and, rarely, convulsions. Other adverse effects include constipation, diarrhea, abdominal cramps, gastric irritation, GI bleeding, increased urinary frequency yet oliguria, lacrimation, sweating, disorders of taste, urticaria, acneiform rash, eczematoid dermatitis, pleural effusions and pericarditis, hepatitis, chills, and fever. It is contraindicated in liver and pulmonary disease, in situations in which alertness is essential, and when gross postural abnormalities result from its use. It may color the urine orange to red.

Orally, it is absorbed poorly but more or less consistently, so that blood levels are proportional to the dose. It is metabolized in the liver to several products. It is stated that the plasma half-life is 5 hr by the intravenous route but 9 hr by the oral route. The former is probably an approximation of the distribution (α) half-life and the latter of the elimination (β) half-life.

DOXACURIUM CHLORIDE

Isoquinolinium dichloride, 2,2′-[(1,4-dioxo-1,4-butanediyl)bis(oxy-3,1-propanediyl)] bis[1,2,3,4-tetrahydro-6,7,8-trimethoxy-2-methyl-1-[(3,4,5-tri-methoxyphenyl)methyl]-, Nuromax

[106819-53-8] $C_{56}H_{78}Cl_2N_2O_{16}$ (1106.15).

Comments—A long-acting, nondepolarizing, competitive, neuromuscular blocking drug whose action is reversed by anticholinesterases. Doxacurium is indicated as an adjunct to general anesthesia. Its time to onset following an intravenous dose is approximately 1.5 to 2 times longer than that of the intermediate-acting nondepolarizing agents atracurium and vecuronium and 4 to 5 times longer than that of the short-acting depolarizing agent succinylcholine. Time to 25% recovery is approximately 10 to 15 times longer than that of succinylcholine and 2 to 3 times longer than that of the intermediate agents. Doxacurium does not appear to cause histamine release. The major elimination pathway for doxacurium is through excretion of unchanged drug in the urine and bile. The duration of action of doxacurium is increased in patients with end-stage kidney and hepatic disease.

METOCURINE IODIDE—see RPS-20, page 1335.

MIVACURIUM CHLORIDE

Isoquinolinium, [R-[R*, R*-(E)]]-2,2′-[(1,8-dioxo-4-octene-1,8-diyl)bis(oxy-3,1-propanediyl)]bis-[1,2,3,4-tetrahydro-6,7-dimethoxy-2-methyl-1-[(3,4,5-trimethoxyphenyl)methyl]-, dichloride; Mivacron

[106861-44-3 (total racemate)] $C_{58}H_{80}Cl_2N_2O_{14}$ (1100.18).

Comments—A short-acting, nondepolarizing, competitive, neuromuscular blocking drug whose action is reversed by anticholinesterases. Its time to onset following a bolus dose is equivalent to the intermediate-acting nondepolarizing agents atracurium and vecuronium and two to three times longer than the short-acting depolarizing agent succinylcholine. Time to 25% recovery is approximately 2 times longer than with succinylcholine (16 versus 8 min, respectively) and two to three times shorter than with the intermediate agents (16 versus 25 to 45 min, respectively). For short-duration procedures not requiring rapid induction of anesthesia, mivacurium represents a viable alternative to succinylcholine. Bolus doses of mivacurium can cause histamine release that leads to cutaneous flushing of face and neck, increased heart rate, and hypotension. Like succinylcholine, mivacurium is metabolized rapidly by plasma cholinesterase. The duration of action of mivacurium is increased in patients with end-stage kidney and hepatic disease and patients with a deficiency of plasma cholinesterase.

PANCURONIUM BROMIDE—see RPS-20, page 1336.

ROCURONIUM BROMIDE

Pyrrolidinium, 1-(2β,3α,5α,16β,17β)-17-(acetyloxy)-3-hydroxy-2-(4-morpholinyl)androstan-16-yl]-1-(2-propenyl)-, bromide; Zemuron

1-Allyl-1-(3α,17β-dihydroxy-2β-morpholino-5α-andro-stan-16β-yl)pyrrolidinium bromide, 17-acetate [119302-91-9] $C_{32}H_{53}BrN_2O_4$ (609.69).

Preparation—US Pat 4,894,369 (1990).

Description—Crystals melting about 161–169°; $[\alpha]_D^{20}$ +18.7° (c = 1.03, CHCl$_3$); Octanol/water partition coefficient 0.5 at 20°.

Solubility—Soluble in water.

Comments—The injection is a nondepolarizing neuromuscular blocking agent with a rapid to intermediate onset depending on the dose and intermediate duration. It acts by competing for cholinergic receptors at the motor and end-plate. This action is antagonized by acetylcholinesterase inhibitors, such as neostigmine and edrophonium.

SUCCINYLCHOLINE CHLORIDE

Ethanaminium, 2,2'-[(1,4-dioxo-1,4-butanediyl)bis(oxy)]bis[N,N,N-trimethyl-, dichloride; Suxamethonium Chloride; Quelicin

Choline chloride succinate (2:1) *anhydrous* [71-27-2] $C_{14}H_{30}Cl_2N_2O_4$ (361.31); *dihydrate* [6101-15-1] (397.34); usually occurs as the dihydrate.

Preparation—It may be prepared by condensing succinyl chloride with β-dimethylaminoethanol and quaternizing the resulting ester with methyl chloride.

Description—White, odorless, crystalline powder; solutions are acid to litmus (pH of about 4); the dihydrate melts about 160°, the anhydrous about 190°; hygroscopic.

Solubility—1 g in about 1 mL water or about 350 mL alcohol; slightly soluble in chloroform; practically insoluble in ether.

Comments—A depolarizing neuromuscular blocking agent; see the introductory statement for actions, uses, side effects, precautions, and drug interactions. It usually has a very transient duration of action because of rapid hydrolysis of the drug by serum butyryl (pseudo)cholinesterases. The effects of a single injection usually last only a few minutes; consequently, it is of special use for muscle relaxation during brief manipulations. Prolonged muscular relaxation is achieved by continuous intravenous infusion, and the intensity of muscle paralysis is controlled readily by adjustment of the infusion rate. Alternatively, prolonged muscular relaxation may be achieved with periodic injections when the drug is given in combination with *hexafluorenium bromide* (above). Although a stabilizing phase of action can occur, its occurrence is erratic and usually results only from prolonged use.

It does not cause liberation of histamine, but hypersensitivity reactions sometimes occur. As the drug depolarizes the motor end-plate, axon reflex-conducted impulses and contractions of motor units (fasciculations) may occur. Muscle aching resulting from its transient stimulatory action is minimized by slow administration. Hyperkalemia, due to potassium loss from muscle, and myoglobinemia sometimes result from these stimulatory actions. Excessive salivation may occur; this is preventable by premedication with atropine or scopolamine. It may induce a bradycardia that can be suppressed by atropine or methscopolamine but not by scopolamine. It may cause cardiac arrhythmias in patients with myocardial damage. Among neuromuscular blocking drugs, it is unique in its effect to increase intraocular pressure; it is contraindicated in persons with glaucoma or retinal detachment and in persons with known hypersensitivity. Rarely, it may cause a severe (malignant) hyperthermia when an ether anesthetic or cyclopropane is used. No specific pharmacological antagonist of the skeletal muscle effects is available, but dantrolene can suppress malignant hyperthermia. Calcium channel–blocking drugs also are useful in this regard. Its actions may be prolonged in individuals with reduced plasma cholinesterase activity, such as results from a genetic defect or from liver disease or cachexia.

TIZANIDINE HYDROCHLORIDE

2,1,3-Benzothiadiazole-4-amine, 5-chloro-N-(4,5-dihydro-1H-imidazol-2-yl)-, monohydrochloride; Sirdalud; Zanaflex

5-Chloro-4-(2-imidazolin-2-ylamino)-2,1,3-benzothiadiazole monohydrochloride [51322-75-9] $C_9H_8ClN_5S\cdot HCl$ (290.18).

Preparation—4-Amino-5-chloro-2,1,3-benzothiadiazole is treated with thiophosgene to form the 4-thiocyanato derivative which is reacted with ethylene-diamine yielding the thiourea. Heating the latter compound in methanol evolves H$_2$S forming the imidazoleamino ring on the 4-position, which is the product.

Description—White to off-white odorless crystals from methanol melting about 222°.

Solubility—Slightly soluble in water or methanol; solubility decreases as pH increases.

Comments—An agonist at the α_2-adrenergic receptor sites and presumably reduces spasticity by increasing presynaptic inhibition of motor neurons. In animal models, it has no direct effect on skeletal muscle fibers or the neuromuscular junction, and no major effect on monosynaptic spinal reflexes. Its effects are greatest on polysynaptic pathways. The overall effect of these actions is thought to reduce facilitation of spinal motor neurons. Its imidazoline chemical structure is related to that of the antihypertensive drug clonidine and other α_2-adrenergic agonists.

TUBOCURARINE CHLORIDE

Tubocuraranium, 7',12'-dihydroxy-6,6'-dimethoxy-2,2',2'-trimethyl-, chloride, hydrochloride, pentahydrate; (+)-Tubocurarine Dichloride; d-Tubocurarine Chloride

(+)-Tubocurarine chloride hydrochloride pentahydrate [6989-98-6] $C_{37}H_{41}ClN_2O_6\cdot HCl\cdot 5H_2O$ (771.73); *anhydrous* [57-94-3] (681.65).

Preparation—Isolated from the stems and bark of the freshly gathered plant *Chondodendron tomentosum*, which is extracted with small portions of water.

Description—White or yellowish white to grayish white, odorless, crystalline powder; melts about 270°, with decomposition.

Solubility—1 g in 20 mL water or 45 mL alcohol; insoluble in chloroform or ether.

Comments—A competitive neuromuscular blocking agent; see the introductory statement for the actions, uses, side effects, and drug interactions.

It is not absorbed from the gut. After intravenous administration it rapidly disappears from the plasma, with a distribution half-life of about 12 min; however, its terminal plasma half-life is 1 to 3 hr. The duration of action of the first dose is 10 to 30 min, but a residual effect lasting several hours has been shown. Subsequent doses may have a longer action. It is both excreted into urine (43%) and degraded in the liver and kidneys, and either renal failure or hepatic failure can prolong the half-life.

VECURONIUM BROMIDE

Piperidinium, 1-[(2β,3α,5α,16β,17β)-3,17-bis(acetyloxy)-2-(1-piperidinyl)androstan-16-yl]-1-methyl-, bromide, diacetate

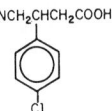

[50700-72-6] $C_{34}H_{57}BrN_2O_4$ (637.74).

Preparation—See *J Med Chem* 1973; 16:1116.
Description—White crystals; melts about 230°.
Solubility—Soluble in water.
Comments—It retains the competitive neuromuscular blocking activity of pancuronium but is devoid of some of the side effects and, consequently, has clinical advantages over pancuronium. It does not release histamine significantly, cause ganglionic blockade, or interfere with neuronal reuptake of norepinephrine, hence, has negligible cardiovascular side effects. The duration of action in adults is about 15 to 30 min for doses that cause less than 100% paralysis. Partial recovery sufficient to permit breathing may take even less time. Consequently, it may be used for relatively short surgical procedures and endotracheal intubation in adults. Recovery time is slightly longer in young children and more than twice as long in infants. When doses are repeated after only 25% of recovery of muscle function, accumulation apparently does not occur.

It is excreted mostly into the bile, and the degree of paralysis and duration of action are increased in liver failure. Ten to 25% is excreted into urine, and renal failure may prolong the duration of action by as much as 32%.

CENTRALLY ACTING MUSCLE RELAXANTS

The cell bodies of the somatic motor nerves lie within the spinal cord and, hence, within the CNS. The activity of motor neurons is affected not only by facilitatory and inhibitory modulation through feedback from contralateral and ipsilateral stretch and other receptors but also from centers in the brain. Spasticity can arise from musculoskeletal injury, which may cause aberrant afferent impulse traffic into the spinal cord, from injury to, or disease of, the motor nerves or related interneurons in the cord or sensory neurons in the sensory ganglia and from disorders in the brain that alter the flow of suprasegmental impulses to the motor neurons. Involuntary movement, such as is seen in palsies, chorea, or parkinsonism, mostly is the result of impairment of feedback control within the brain.

When the disorder is musculoskeletal or is within the spinal cord, the selectivity of drugs is relatively low, because the collective neurons involved in the reflex arcs are not sufficiently qualitatively different from the motor and sensory neurons in chemical sensitivity to permit a selective depression of the hyperactive influences on the motor neuron. However, some selectivity is achieved when interneurons are involved, simply because a small effect on each converging interneuron may summate to cause a moderate decrease in interneuronal input to the motor neuron. Because the interneurons are involved in the fine tuning of neuronal activity, their influences are balanced critically and hence are more susceptible to pharmacological action than the motor neuron itself. Consequently, most central relaxants are *interneuron depressants,* which, however, will manifest variable depressant actions throughout the CNS. Interestingly, many antianxiety and some sedative drugs possess muscle relaxant activity, probably because of the high

sensitivity of the critically balanced interneurons to perturbation.

In tolerated doses, the centrally acting muscle relaxants are erratic, owing to their limited selectivity. Orally, they are usually ineffective (the tolerated doses being much too low); intravenously, they have some established value in treating acute muscle spasms resulting from trauma or inflammation. Motor dysfunctions that accrue to spinal cord or brain disorders are affected little.

The central relaxant effects and uses of certain benzodiazepines, such as diazepam, differ from those of interneuron depressants.

BACLOFEN

Butanoic acid, 4-amino-3-(4-chlorophenyl)-, Lioresal

$$H_2NCH_2CHCH_2COOH$$

β-(Aminomethyl)-*p*-chlorohydrocinnamic acid [1134-47-0] $C_{10}H_{12}$ $ClNO_2$ (213.67).

Preparation—Synthesis by hydrogenation of β-cyano-*p*-chlorohydrocinnamic acid in acidified ethanol in the presence of platinic oxide catalyst is described in Swiss Pat 449,046 (*CA* 1968; 69:106273f).

Description—Crystalline powder; melts about 207° (190°?); pK_a 3.85, 9.25.

Solubility—Slightly soluble in water; poorly soluble in organic solvents.

Comments—Its muscle relaxant actions result from an action within the spinal cord, where both monosynaptic and polysynaptic reflexes are inhibited by the drug. It is an analog of γ-aminobutyric acid (GABA), an inhibitory neurotransmitter within the CNS. Part of the action of baclofen is likely attributable to its agonist properties at the $GABA_B$ receptor, which is coupled to a G-protein-activated K^+ channel. However, the precise mechanism of its muscle relaxant properties is unknown. Its sedative and ataxic actions are consistent with such an action in the brain.

It is used in the relief of painful spasticity in *multiple sclerosis,* for which it is more effective than diazepam. Some residual ambulatory function must be present; the drug will not make nonambulatory patients ambulatory. Although spasticity may be lessened, the gait and posture of some patients may be worsened, because of the unmasking of incoordination. It also may afford some relief in patients with *spinal cord disease* and *traumatic transverse myelopathies.* It is not as effective as carbamazepine in the treatment of neuralgias but is an important substitute when needed. It has been reported to be of value in tardive dyskinesia. It is useful in the management of *external urinary sphincter hypertonicity* and *detrussor–external sphincter dyssynergia.* It is not indicated in musculoskeletal spastic disorders.

Sedation is the most frequent adverse effect, although it is less frequent and severe than with diazepam. Its use in combination with other CNS depressants or ethanol should be avoided, if possible. Weakness may occur, but it is less handicapping than with dantrolene. Other common side effects include dizziness, insomnia, pruritus, and rashes. The drug is contraindicated when a hypersensitivity exists. Less frequent side effects include hypotension and mental confusion. Abrupt withdrawal has been reported to result in anxiety, tachycardia, and even visual hallucinations; therefore, dosage must be discontinued gradually. In patients with epilepsy, it may increase the frequency of seizures. Overdoses may cause seizures, coma, loss of brainstem reflexes and respiratory depression. It is teratogenic, and this risk must be considered in pregnancy. It also has been found to cause ovarian cysts and enlarged or hemorrhagic adrenal glands in experimental animals.

It is absorbed rapidly, orally; absorption time is approximately 2 hr. More than 80% of the drug is excreted in the urine. The elimination half-life is 3 to 4 hr.

CARISOPRODOL

1,3-propanediol, 2-methyl-2-propyl-, carbamate isopropylcarbamate; Carisprodate; Isobamate; Soma

$$(CH_3)_2CHNHCOOCH_2\overset{\overset{\displaystyle CH_3}{|}}{\underset{\underset{\displaystyle CH_2CH_2CH_3}{|}}{C}}CH_2OOCNH_2$$

[78-44-4] $C_{12}H_{24}N_2O_4$ (260.33).

vomiting are intolerable, they may be managed with non-phenothiazine-, non- pyridoxine-containing antiemetics. The second most common type of side effect is the appearance of abnormal involuntary movements, which usually start with the face and tongue and gradually move downward to involve the arms, hands, and trunk. These dyskinesias are most severe 1 to 2 hr after administration. These effects are not seen immediately but progress slowly over a year's time. Eventually, nearly 75% of patients will show some such movements; however, most patients accept such movements as the price of increased mobility. The involuntary movements can be decreased by lowering the dose or by use of haloperidol or pyridoxine, but these recourses also abolish the therapeutic response to this drug. Hypotension occurs in about 75%, and orthostatic hypotension in about 30% of recipients, but vertigo and syncope are uncommon. Cardiac arrhythmias occur occasionally. After 2 or 3 months, tolerance develops. Increased myocardial contractility, tachycardia, and atrial fibrillation may occur. Behavioral changes frequently accompany treatment. Increased CNS excitability, with nervousness, anxiety, insomnia, vivid dreams, tremor, and flushing occurs. Paranoid ideation, delusions, hallucinations (often olfactory), delirium, and loss of judgment sometimes occur. Easy sexual arousal and loss of sexual inhibitions are common; in part this is the result of the emergence of normal desire long suppressed by physical incapacity. Serum glutamic oxaloacetate transaminase and glutamic pyruvate transaminase may be elevated somewhat early during therapy, but they usually subside later. Transient granulocytopenia may occur; agranulocytosis no longer seems to be an adverse effect, since the dextro form was removed from the preparations. Dental caries is accelerated, and fillings often fall out, perhaps because the buffering effect of sialorrhea is diminished. Other miscellaneous side effects include increased pain when pain-producing pathology or headache exists, sweating, alopecia, cough, hoarseness, urinary frequency, incontinence or retention, nocturia, mydriasis, blurred vision, Horner's syndrome, fever, hot flashes, and loss or gain in weight. A mild natriuresis occurs, probably as the result of the action of dopamine formed in the kidney. Thrombocytopenia occurs rarely after long-term treatment.

Pyridoxine antagonizes levodopa, possibly by promoting premature decarboxylation (as a coenzyme to dopa decarboxylase) before levodopa has penetrated into the brain. Some antagonism occurs with even as little as a Recommended Dietary Allowance, so patients should not take multivitamin supplements containing pyridoxine. To what extent some of the side effects of the CNS are attributable to pyridoxine deficiency is not known. Carbidopa prevents antagonism by pyridoxine. Methyldopa and reserpine, which interfere with catecholamine synthesis and storage, exacerbate the parkinson syndrome and, hence, antagonize levodopa. Tricyclic antidepressants and MAOIs given concomitantly evoke hypertensive crises and may precipitate many of the adverse side effects of the CNS, because they increase the local concentrations of dopamine formed from levodopa. Such drugs should be discontinued 2 weeks prior to taking levodopa. Antacids decrease gastric emptying time and thereby promote absorption, thus increasing efficacy in some patients. Levodopa is synergized by antimuscarinics.

Levodopa is contraindicated when there is evidence of uncompensated endocrine, renal, hepatic, pulmonary, or cardiovascular disease; narrow-angle glaucoma; blood dyscrasia; or hypersensitivity to the drug. It should be used cautiously in diabetes, hyperthyroidism, wide-angle glaucoma, epilepsy, and hypotension or when antihypertensives are being used. The drug should be discontinued 24 hr prior to anesthesia. Levodopa is a precursor of melanin and may activate latent malignant melanoma; it should be withheld from persons with a history of malignant melanoma or suspicious skin lesions.

PERGOLIDE MESYLATE

Ergoline-, [8-(methylthio) methyl]-6-propyl-, methanesulfonate salt, Permax

[66104-23-2]C$_{19}$H$_{26}$S.CH$_4$O$_3$S(410.59).

Preparation—See US Pat 4,166,182.

Description—White solid; melts at 207°. Log P at 25° (CHC$_3$/water) 6.14 at pH 2.2; 119.6 at pH 4.

Solubility—Sparingly soluble in DMF or ethanol; slightly soluble in water, 0.01 N HCl, chloroform acetonitrile, methylene chloride, absolute alcohol; very slightly soluble in acetone; practically insoluble in dilute NaOH, HCl or ether.

Comments—Has actions and uses like those of bromocriptine and is indicated as an adjunct to levodopa/carbidopa for the management of Parkinson's disease. It has both D$_1$- and D$_2$-dopaminergic activity. Side effects include nausea and vomiting, postural hypotension, premature ventricular contractions, confusion and hallucinations, dyskinesias, elevated SGOT, sedation, hallucinations, xerostomia and, rarely, reversible pleural fibrosis. It is likely that other side effects like those of bromocriptine eventually will be reported. The duration of action exceeds 24 hr.

PRAMIPEXOLE DIHYDROCHLORIDE

2,6-Benzothiazolediamine, (S)-4,5,6,7-tetrahydro-N^6-propyl-, dihydrochloride; Mirapex

(S)-2-Amino-4,5,6,7-tetrahydro-6-(propylamino)benzothiazole, dihydrochloride monohydrate [104632-26-0 (free base)] C$_{10}$H$_{17}$N$_3$S.HCl.H$_2$O (302.27).

Preparation—Butanal and 2,6-diamino-4,5,6,7-tetrahydrobenzothiazole are heated in DMF and the imine reduced with sodium borohydride; water is added and acidified tp pH 1, extracted with ethyl acetate, which is discarded. The aqueous phase is made alkaline with potassium carbonate, extracted with ethyl acetate, dried, concentrated and the salt precipitated with ethereal HCl. *J Med Chem*, 1987; 30: 494. See also US Pat 4,886,812.

Description—White to off-white crystals from methanol; melts at 286–88°; [α]$_D^{20}$ -67.2° (c = 1, MeOH). **Note**: The bulk drug is stable but the tablets are susceptible to photo-degradation and should be protected from light.

Solubility—About 20% in water, 8% in methanol or 0.5% in ethanol. Insoluble in chlorinated hydrocarbons.

Comments—A nonergot dopamine agonist with high relative in vitro specificity and full intrinsic activity at the D$_2$ subfamily of dopamine receptors, binding with higher affinity to D$_3$ than to D$_2$ to D$_4$ receptor subtypes. The relevance of D$_3$ receptor binding in Parkinson's disease is unknown.

The precise mechanism of its action as a treatment for Parkinson's disease is unknown, although it is believed to be related to its ability to stimulate dopamine receptors in the striatum. This is supported by electrophysiologic studies in animals that have demonstrated that it influences striatal neuronal firing rates via activation of dopamine receptors in the striatum and the substantia nigra, the site of neurons that send projections to the striatum.

PROCYCLIDINE HYDROCHLORIDE

1-pyrrolidinepropanol, α-cyclohexyl-α-phenyl-, hydrochloride; Kemadrin

[1508-76-5] C$_{19}$H$_{29}$NO.HCl (323.91)

Preparation—From the cyclohexyl Grignard reagent and 3-(1-pyrrolidinyl)propiophenone; the resulting base then is converted to the hydrochloride.

Description—White, crystalline powder melts about 226°.

Solubility—About 1 g in 33 mL water; more soluble in alcohol.

Comments—An antimuscarinic drug used mostly as a substitute for trihexyphenidyl in the treatment of parkinsonism when the latter drug fails to control symptoms. Sometimes it is used in combination with other drugs. The side effects, precautions, and contraindications are those of trihexyphenidyl.

ROPINIROLE HYDROCHLORIDE

2(H)-Indol-2-one, 4-[2-(dipropylamino)ethyl]-1,3-dihydro-, monohydrochloride; Requip

[91374-20-8] $C_{16}H_{24}N_2O \cdot HCl$ (296.84).

Preparation—The acid chloride of 2-(2-methyl-3-nitrophenyl)acetic acid is prepared with thionyl chloride, then treated with dipropylamine to form the amide. The carbonyl group is reduced with borane in THF and then reacted with diethyl oxalate and sodium in alcohol in a Claisen-type reaction to produce the ethyl ester of 3-[[2-(dipropylamino)ethyl]-6-nitrophenyl]pyruvic acid. Hydrolysis and decarboxylation of the acid with peroxide and base removes the ethoxycarbonyl group and forms 2-[2-(dipropylamino)ethyl]-6-nitrophenylacetic acid. Cyclization to the product is effected by catalytic reduction of the nitro group, using palladium/hydrogen to give the amine, which through loss of water forms the lactam (indolone). Heating with HCl forms the title substance.

Description—White to pale yellowish green powder melting about 245°.

Solubility—About 130 mg/mL of water.

Comments—A dopamine receptor antagonist. This nonergot derivative displays high-affinity specificity for dopamine D_2 receptors.

It has been approved for the management of symptoms associated with mild-to-severe Parkinson's disease. The precise mechanism of action has not been elucidated clearly. Unlike levodopa, which is thought to act by elevating synaptic concentrations of dopamine, ropinirole is presumed to be effective by direct activation of postsynaptic dopamine receptors in the corpus striatum.

In several double-blind controlled trials, ropinirole was found to be effective in improving daily activities of patients with parkinsonian syndrome and reduce their motor manifestations such as bradykinesia, tremor, rigidity, and postural instability. In addition, it was reported to reduce the off-time of patients with advanced symptoms who were experiencing the deteriorating response to levodopa treatment.

Patients receiving dopamine agonists should be counseled to avoid rapid transitions in posture due to increased likelihood for development of orthostatic hypotension. Patients receiving ropirinole are also at increased risk for hallucinations. This particular adverse effect is greater in the geriatric population.

SELEGILINE HYDROCHLORIDE

Benzeneethanamine, N,α-dimethyl-N-2-propynyl-, hydrochloride; Deprenyl; L-Deprenyl; Eldepryl

[14611-52-0] $C_{13}H_{17}N \cdot HCl$ (223.78).

Preparation—By reacting propargyl bromide with L-(N,α-dimethyl)- phenethylamine and distilling the extracted oil. US Pat 3,496,195.

Description—Oil, boiling point 92° to 93° at 0.8 mm; η_D^{20} 1.518; $t\alpha_D$ −11.2. The HCl salt melts about 141°.

Solubility—Freely soluble in water, chloroform, or methanol.

Comments—An inhibitor of monoamine oxidase B, which enzyme is selective for dopamine over norepinephrine and epinephrine. As such, selegiline is an approved adjunct to levodopa for the treatment of parkinsonism. The drug decreases the effective dose of levodopa and smooths out dose-related fluctuations in efficacy, effects that should rouse only mild interest. However, recent reports indicate that it slows the progress of idiopathic parkinsonism and increases the lifespan of the afflicted. The drug is converted to amphetamine and methamphetamine in the body, which metabolites possibly account for some of the antiparkinson activity. Dyskinesias have been reported to occur in about one-third of users, but this high incidence of adverse effects is undoubtedly the result of fail-

ure to reduce the dose of levodopa to which the drug was added. Dry mouth, nausea, and dizziness occur in 10–20% of cases. Side effects of low incidence are postural hypotension, unpleasant taste, circumoral paresthesias, hallucinations, depression, and paranoia.

TOLCAPONE

Methanone, (3,4-dihydroxy-5-nitrophenyl)(4-methyphenyl)-; Tasmar

3,4-Dihydroxy-4′-methyl-5-nitrobenzophenone [134308-13-7] $C_{14}H_{11}NO_5$ (273.25).

Preparation—*Drugs of the Future* 16:719, 1991.

Description—Yellow, odorless, non-hygroscopic crystals from methylene chloride; melts about 147°.

TRIHEXYPHENIDYL HYDROCHLORIDE

1-Piperidinepropanol, α-cyclohexyl-α-phenyl-, hydrochloride; Artane; Benzhexol Hydrochloride

α-Cyclohexyl-α-phenyl-1-piperidinepropanol hydrochloride [52-49-3] $C_{20}H_{31}NO \cdot HCl$ (337.93).

Preparation—From a Mannich reaction of acetophenone, piperidine, and formaldehyde. The piperidinopropiophenone formed is treated as for *Procyclidine*.

Description—White or slightly off-white, crystalline powder; no more than a very faint odor; melts between 247° and 253° with slight decomposition.

Solubility—Slightly soluble in water; soluble in alcohol or chloroform.

Comments—Has weak *antimuscarinic* and *antispasmodic* activity. In the treatment of parkinsonism it is preferred to levodopa in patients with mild-to-moderate nonincapacitating symptoms, and most neurologists prefer to begin treatment of all patients with it. It is effective in all forms of the disease, although not uniformly. It is most effective against rigidity, but it also is useful in the relief of akinesia, tremor, sialorrhea, and oculogyria. Tolerance may develop, but not necessarily. It also is useful in the treatment of *drug-induced extrapyramidal dyskinesias*.

The adverse effects mostly derive from its antimuscarinic actions, but they are much less troublesome than with atropine. The most frequent are dry mouth, blurred vision, tachycardia, constipation, dry skin, nervousness, headache, sedation, and muscle weakness. Some of these effects subside after continued administration. Sometimes insomnia may occur. Urinary retention is infrequent, but it does occur. Occasionally, vomiting, severe tinnitus, vertigo, suppurative parotitis, or rash occur and may require discontinuation of medication. With large doses, inability to concentrate, impaired memory, disorientation, and confusion may occur, and if the dose is not reduced, they are followed by agitation, excitement, delirium, visual hallucinations, and psychoses. Elderly patients or persons with arteriosclerosis especially are susceptible to the adverse central effects. It should be used cautiously in persons with cardiovascular or liver pathology, glaucoma, bladder neck obstruction, prostatitis, hyperthyroidism, or arteriosclerosis and in elderly patients. Trihexyphenidyl may interact with CNS-active antihypertensive drugs, ethanol and other CNS depressants, tricyclic antidepressants, MAOIs, other antimuscarinic drugs, dopamine agonists, dopamine antagonists, phenothiazine, and procainamide. When it is used in combination with levodopa, bromocriptine, or amantadine, the doses of both drugs in combination may need reduction.

ACKNOWLEDGMENT—The author acknowledges the tremendous efforts of H Steve White, PhD in previous editions of this work.

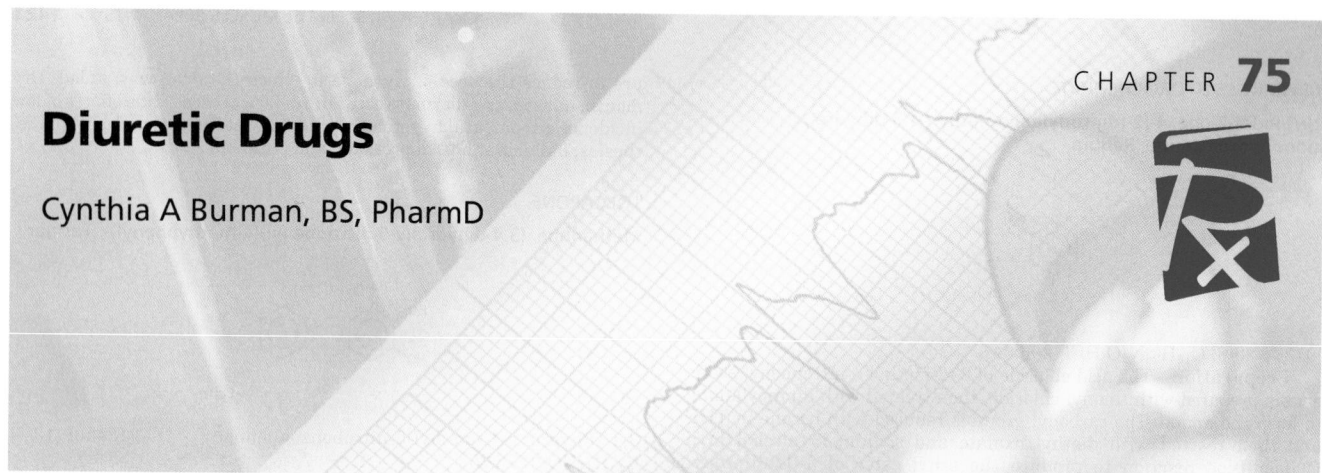

CHAPTER 75

Diuretic Drugs

Cynthia A Burman, BS, PharmD

Diuretics are drugs that reduce the volume of extracellular fluid, enhance the urinary excretion of sodium chloride, and, secondarily, increase the volume of urine excreted by the kidneys. They are used primarily to prevent and alleviate edema and ascites. These conditions occur in diseases of the heart, kidneys, and liver. Consequently, diuretics are used in the treatment of edema associated with chronic congestive heart failure, acute pulmonary edema, edema of pregnancy, brain edema, and cirrhosis associated with ascites. They also are used in hypertension, diabetes insipidus, renal calculi, hypercalcemia, acute and chronic renal failure, and the nephrotic syndrome.[1]

Some diuretics have highly specialized uses in glaucoma, hyperkalemia, bromide intoxication, anginal syndrome, epilepsy, migraine, and premenstrual depression, conditions in which edema is not present or at least not definitely established. In addition, diuretics sometimes are used to maintain adequate urine volume, as in the case of some severe traumatic injuries, or to reduce the concentration of a noxious agent in the urine, to minimize renal damage.

The formation of urine from the blood, in simplest terms, consists of glomerular filtration and selective tubular reabsorption and secretion. In healthy individuals, the filtration rate amounts to 180L/day.[1] As the glomerular filtrate passes through the tubules, substances essential to the blood and tissues—water, glucose, salts, and amino acids—are reabsorbed.

Other substances in the glomerular filtrate, such as urea, are not absorbed as readily by the tubules. Thus, it is thought that in the renal tubule there is a specific mechanism for the transport of each ionic species, the capacities of which are quite different. For example, the capacity of the renal tubule to reabsorb sulfate ion is limited. The tubular capacity for the reabsorption of phosphate is such that a sufficient amount is reabsorbed to maintain the normal extracellular level, and any excess is excreted. On the other hand, much larger amounts of bicarbonate ion and chloride ion can be reabsorbed.

Under normal circumstances the glomerular filtration rate is about 100 mL/min. About 99 mL of the fluid is returned to the blood, and only 1 mL is excreted as urine. It follows, therefore, that drugs may increase the rate of urine formation by:

1. Increasing glomerular filtration
2. Decreasing tubular reabsorption

Increasing glomerular filtration is not an efficient mechanism and usually causes only a moderate increase in urine formation. If, for example, the percentage of fluid reabsorbed by the renal tubules is assumed to remain constant, glomerular filtration rate would have to be increased twofold to double the urinary output. On the other hand, a 1% decrease in the tubular reabsorption of water, induced either by the administration of excessive quantities of electrolytes or nonelectrolytes (osmotic diuretics) or by agents that alter selective reabsorption of substances in the renal tubules, would double the urinary output.

Most diuretics block sodium and/or chloride reabsorption in the renal tubules.[2] This results in natriuresis and diuresis. However, the mechanism(s) by which diuretics block the reabsorption and the site of action varies; they may act at the proximal tubule, loop of Henle, distal tubule, collecting tubule, or combinations of these sites.

Osmotic diuretics are thought to produce diuresis by multiple mechanisms. Mannitol, the most widely used osmotic diuretic, is freely filtered at the glomerulus and is not reabsorbed by the renal tubules. Because of its osmotic action in the proximal tubule and thick ascending limb, mannitol prevents the reabsorption of water and impairs sodium and chloride reabsorption by lowering the concentration in the tubular fluid.[2] *Carbonic anhydrase inhibitors* act on the proximal convolution and possibly the collecting tubule to inhibit cytoplasmic and brush border carbonic anhydrase. This enzyme catalyzes the reaction $CO_2 + OH^- \rightarrow HCO_3^-$ The overall inhibition of carbonic anhydrase decreases bicarbonate reabsorption and passive forces favoring chloride reabsorption. The excess chloride (with accompanying sodium) subsequently is reabsorbed in the loop of Henle. The net effect is bicarbonate is excreted with both sodium and potassium, but the total diuretic effect is minimal.[2] After several days of continuous administration, a mild hyperchloremic acidosis develops, which decreases the diuretic effect.

Thiazide diuretics act mainly to block sodium and chloride reabsorption at the distal convoluted tubule, connecting tubule, and early collecting duct.[2] At sufficient concentrations thiazides have mild inhibitory activity toward carbonic anhydrase. The resulting natriuresis is accompanied by increased excretion of potassium (particularly in short-term treatment), bicarbonate, chloride, and water. However, glomerular filtration rate actually may be reduced by these drugs, causing a problem in patients with diminished renal reserve. The antihypertensive action of the thiazides may be attributable to:

A depletion of sodium and subsequent reduction in plasma volume
A decrease in peripheral resistance

Thiazides are useful in blunting the sodium retention that occurs with vasodilators.

Potassium-sparing diuretics interfere with sodium absorption in the distal tubules and collecting ducts, thereby promoting sodium excretion while conserving potassium. Aldosterone stimulates the exchange of sodium for potassium and hydrogen. Therefore, spironolactone, a competitive inhibitor of aldosterone, blocks sodium reabsorption through a different mechanism than triamterene and amiloride. Triamterene and amiloride interfere directly with electrolyte transport. These agents are not potent diuretics when used alone, but there main use is to correct potassium and/or magnesium deficiency.

Potassium-sparing diuretics are often with a thiazide diuretic. The onset of diuresis with combination therapy is much more rapid than with spironolactone alone (4 to 7 days).

Loop, or high-ceiling, diuretics act mainly on the medullary and cortical portions of the thick ascending loop of Henle and cause a peak diuresis far greater than that that occurs with other diuretics. At the thick ascending limb of the loop of Henle 20% to 30% of filtered sodium is reabsorbed and a maximally effective dose of a loop diuretic can cause excretion of 20% to 25% of filtered sodium.[3] The thick ascending limb is also important for urinary concentration ability. Loop diuretics reduce the osmotic gradient in the renal medulla that in turn impairs both the concentrating and diluting capacities of the kidney.[2] Although initially increasing renal blood flow, the reduction in extracellular fluid volume that is caused by the diuresis can result in a decrease in renal blood flow.

Contraindications and adverse effects resulting from diuretic therapy usually are due to electrolyte imbalance induced by these agents. Many commonly employed diuretics can produce acute and chronic sodium depletion, hypokalemia, hyperglycemia, and hyperuricemia, as well as alterations in chloride, magnesium, and calcium balance. Osmotic diuretics must be used with caution because they can produce a marked increase in vascular blood volume in patients with acute renal failure.[2] Hypersensitivity to diuretic agents sometimes occurs. Also, blood dyscrasias, pancreatitis (thiazides), decreased glucose tolerance (thiazides at doses higher than clinically useful), and ototoxicity (chronic high dose loop diuretics) occasionally are encountered during diuretic therapy.

Concurrent administration of diuretic agents and other drugs result in some of the most frequently encountered drug interactions. A common example is the prescribing of a cardiac glycoside and a diuretic; the diuretic-induced hypokalemia potentiates the cardiotoxicity of the glycoside. The adverse interaction can be minimized either by increasing potassium intake (potassium supplements, diet, or potassium-sparing diuretic) or by administering the diuretic intermittently (allows homeostatic mechanisms to correct imbalance). Other examples of adverse interactions include:

- More-intensive skeletal muscle blockade in patients on certain muscle relaxants and hypokalemia-inducing diuretics
- Orthostatic hypotension induced by concurrent administration of centrally acting antihypertensives and a diuretic
- Increased incidence of ototoxicity when patients on aminoglycoside antibiotics are given diuretics reported to cause ototoxicity (chronic high dose loop diuretics)
- Hyperkalemia when potassium salts are administered with potassium sparing diuretics
- Disruption of uricosuric therapy by administration of a diuretic that increases plasma uric acid levels (thiazides)
- An increased anticoagulant effect induced by displacement of warfarin from protein binding sites

Thoughtful management of these interactions will not only result in improved patient response, but also will spare the patient unnecessary inconvenience and expense.

Agents employed clinically as diuretics may be divided into two groups: (1) osmotic diuretics and (2) renal tubule–inhibiting diuretics. In this presentation a third category, miscellaneous renal agents, is provided for probenecid, an agent that is not a diuretic but inhibits renal tubule reabsorption of uric acid and blocks the renal excretion of a number of substances.

OSMOTIC DIURETICS

The capacity of the renal tubule to reabsorb various electrolytes and nonelectrolytes is limited and, as previously mentioned, varies for each ionic species. If large amounts of these substances are administered to an individual, their concentration in the body fluids and, subsequently, in the glomerular filtrate exceeds the reabsorption capacity of the tubule, and the excess

appears in the urine accompanied by an increased volume of water.

Traditionally, substances that increase urine formation in this manner are called osmotic diuretics. Osmotic agents may have multiple sites of action; nevertheless, their major component is a decrease in medullary solute content resulting in less water reabsorption from the thin descending limb of Henle and collecting duct and less sodium chloride reabsorption in the proximal tubule and thick ascending limb of Henle.

The major toxic effect of osmotic diuretics is related to the amount of solute administered and its effect on the volume and distribution of body fluids. For example, following its administration, mannitol is distributed throughout the extracellular fluid; consequently, the administration of hypertonic solutions sufficient to make a significant contribution to extracellular osmolarity will be accompanied by a significant expansion of extracellular fluid volume, largely at the expense of intracellular fluid volume. In edematous states accompanied by diminished cardiac reserve, the use of mannitol introduces a risk that far outweighs any advantages. Also, a variety of signs and symptoms suggestive of hypersensitivity reactions have accompanied the use of some osmotic diuretics.

This group of diuretics includes osmotic electrolytes (potassium and sodium salts), osmotic nonelectrolytes (urea, glycerin, and mannitol), and acid-forming salts (ammonium chloride). Osmotic diuretics are highly effective treatments for cerebral edema and are used primarily for this purpose.

AMMONIUM CHLORIDE

Muriate of Ammonia; Sal Ammoniac

Ammonium chloride [12125-02-9] NH_4Cl (53.49).

Preparation—By the following processes: (1) the ammoniacal liquid obtained from the destructive distillation of coal is neutralized with HCl and the crude product subsequently is purified, (2) the vapors of ammonia from synthetic processes are absorbed in HCl, and (3) as a byproduct in the Solvay process for sodium bicarbonate.

Description—Colorless crystals, or a white, fine or coarse crystalline powder; cool, saline taste; somewhat hygroscopic; when dissolved in water the temperature of the solution is lowered; pH (1 in 20 solution) between 4.6 and 6.

Solubility—1 g in 3 mL water, 100 mL alcohol, or 8 mL glycerin.

Comments—A *diuretic, systemic acidifier,* and *expectorant.* Ammonium chloride is a combination of a labile cation and a fixed anion. When the ammonium ion is converted to urea, the liberated hydrogen ion reacts with bicarbonate and other body buffers. The end result is that chloride ion displaces bicarbonate ion; the latter is converted to CO_2. Thus, the chloride load to the kidneys is increased, and an appreciable amount escapes reabsorption along with an equivalent amount of cation (predominantly sodium) and an isosmotic quantity of water. This is the basic mechanism by which ammonium chloride brings about a net loss of extracellular fluid and promotes the mobilization of edema fluid.

Ammonium chloride has limited value when used alone for its diuretic effects. It occasionally is combined with a xanthine for short-term relief from temporary water-related weight gain, bloating, or edema associated with menstrual periods.

The fact that ammonium chloride causes systemic acidosis makes the salt of some value in the treatment of alkalosis. It also renders the urine acidic and is prescribed for this purpose in conjunction with methenamine. In the rare instances when it is desired to produce an acidosis, ammonium chloride may be used. An example is in the treatment of lead poisoning when an acidosis is desired to hasten the excretion of lead or to treat alkalosis from excessive use of alkalinizing drugs.

GLYCERIN

1,2,3-Propanetriol; Glycerol; Ophthalgan; Osmoglyn

[56-81-5] $C_3H_8O_3$ (92.09)

Preparation—Obtained in the production of soaps and fatty acids through hydrolysis or by hydration of propylene.

Description—Syrupy liquid with a sweet warm taste; hygroscopic.

Solubility—Completely miscible with water or alcohol; insoluble in most nonpolar solvents.

Comments—*An oral osmotic agent for reducing intraocular pressure.*

GLUCOSE—pages 1885–1886
GLUCOSE, LIQUID—page 1886.

MANNITOL

Mannite; Manna Sugar; Osmitrol

D-Mannitol [69-65-8] $C_6H_{14}O_6$ (182.17).

Preparation—May be extracted from manna and other natural sources with hot alcohol or other selective solvents. Commercially, it is produced by catalytic or electrolytic reduction of certain monosaccharides such as mannose and glucose. Manufacture is somewhat complicated by the need for separation of stereoisomers.

Description—White, crystalline powder or free-flowing granules; odorless and with a sweetish taste; density about 1.52 at 20°; melts between 165° and 168°; pK_a (19°) 3.4.

Solubility—1 g in about 5.5 mL water; slightly soluble in pyridine; very slightly soluble in alcohol; soluble in alkaline solutions; practically insoluble in ether.

Comments—A *diuretic* and a *diagnostic agent for kidney function.* The intravenous administration of hypertonic solutions of mannitol is used to promote an *osmotic diuresis*. It is not absorbed significantly from the gastrointestinal (GI) tract, and if given orally, mannitol causes osmotic diarrhea.

Mannitol is a useful adjunct in the treatment of acute renal failure before irreversible renal failure becomes established. However, to be effective, there must be sufficient renal blood flow and glomerular filtration for mannitol to reach the kidneys. It also is used to reduce intracranial pressure, treat cerebral edema, reduce intraocular pressure when elevated pressure is not amenable to other therapy, and promote urinary excretion of toxic substances.

When administered parenterally, mannitol is distributed in the extracellular space. Only 7% to 10% is metabolized to glycogen, and the rest is excreted in the urine. Plasma half-life after a single IV dose is 15 min with normal renal function. In severe renal insufficiency, mannitol excretion is reduced greatly; retained mannitol may increase extracellular tonicity, expand extracellular fluid volume, and induce hyponatremia. It is superior to dextrose in that it is metabolized only slightly in the body and is reabsorbed only slightly by the renal tubule. Although it requires a larger volume, it produces fewer side effects than urea and is equally effective.

Side effects mostly are due to fluid and electrolyte imbalance. Significant accumulation of mannitol can occur because of rapid administration of large doses or inadequate renal output, leading to an expanded extracellular fluid volume. Isolated cases of adverse reactions (such as pulmonary congestion, fluid and electrolyte imbalances, acidosis, electrolyte loss, dryness of the mouth; thirst, osmotic nephrosis, marked diuresis, urinary retention, edema, headache, blurred vision, convulsions, nausea, vomiting, rhinitis, diarrhea, arm pain, thrombophlebitis, chills, dizziness, urticaria, dehydration, hypotension, hypertension, and anginal-like chest pains) have been reported during or following mannitol infusion.

Since only a negligible amount of mannitol, which appears in the glomerular filtrate, is reabsorbed by the renal tubule, it has been employed for the measurement of *glomerular filtration rate*.

Mannitol and Sodium Chloride Injection—A sterile solution of mannitol and sodium chloride in water for injection. It contains no bacteriostatic agents. pH between 4.5 and 7. *Uses*: See *Mannitol.*

ISOSORBIDE

D-Glucitol, 1,4:3,6-dianhydro-, Ismotic

[652-67-5] $C_6H_{14}O_4$ (146.14).

Preparation—By acid dehydration of sorbitol.

Description—White, crystals melting about 63°; usually supplied as an aqueous solution of approximately 75% concentration.

Solubility—Completely miscible with water; insoluble in most nonpolar organic solvents.

Comments—Used for short-term reduction of intraocular pressure.

UREA

Carbonyldiamide; Ureaphil

$CO(NH_2)_2$

Carbamide [57-13-6] CH_4N_2O (60.06).

Preparation—A product of the metabolism of proteins, it is excreted in human urine in average amounts of 30 g/day. In 1828, Wöhler obtained it on evaporating a solution containing potassium cyanate and ammonium sulfate, the ammonium cyanate first produced isomerizing to urea—reputedly the first synthesis of an organic compound from inorganic material.

A large-scale process for preparing urea is by heating calcium cyanamide with water under pressure:

$$CaNCN + 3H_2O \rightarrow CO(NH_2)_2 + Ca(OH)_2$$

Description—Colorless to white, prismatic crystals or a white, crystalline powder; almost odorless with a cooling, saline taste; may gradually develop a slight odor of ammonia, especially in the presence of moisture; melts between 132° and 135°; aqueous solutions are neutral to litmus but, on standing or heating, decompose into NH_3 and CO_2; pK_a (21°) 0.1.

Solubility—1 g in 1.5 mL water, 10 mL alcohol, 20 mL anhydrous alcohol, 6 mL methanol, or 2 mL glycerol; practically insoluble in chloroform or ether.

Comments—Used to reduce intracranial and intraocular pressure.

RENAL TUBULE–INHIBITING DIURETICS

The most powerful and consistently effective diuretics are those that depress tubular mechanisms responsible for the active reabsorptive transport of certain ions. Drugs that induce diuresis in this way may be divided into five groups: carbonic anhydrase inhibitors, benzothiadiazine and related derivatives, potassium-sparing diuretics, loop diuretics, and other renal tubular-inhibiting diuretics. The mechanisms, uses, and limitations of these several groups of diuretics are discussed in the introductory statement to the respective section.

DICHLORPHENAMIDE

1,3-Benzenedisulfonamide, 4,5-dichloro-, Daranide

4,5-Dichloro-*m*-benzenedisulfonamide [120-97-8] $C_6H_6Cl_2N_2O_4S_2$ (305.15).

Preparation—*o*-Chlorophenol is reacted with chlorosulfonic acid to produce 5-chloro-4-hydroxy-1,3-benzenedisulfonyl chloride, which is treated with PCl_5 to replace the 4-hydroxy with chlorine. Ammonolysis of the sulfonyl chloride yields the disulfonamide.

Description—White or nearly white, crystalline powder, with not more than a slight characteristic odor; melts between 236.5° and 240°.

Solubility—Very slightly soluble in water; freely soluble in 1 *N* NaOH; soluble in alcohol; slightly soluble in ether.

Comments—Used for primary, and the acute phase of secondary, glaucoma.

METHAZOLAMIDE

Acetamide, *N*-[5-(aminosulfonyl)-3-methyl-1,3,4-thiadiazol-2(3*H*)-ylidene]-,

N-(4-Methyl-2-sulfamoyl-Δ^2-1,3,4-thiadiazolin-5-ylidene)acetamide [554-57-4] $C_5H_8N_4O_3S_2$ (238.26).

Preparation—2-Acetamido-5-mercapto-1,3,4-thiadiazole, prepared as described under *Acetazolamide,* is treated with *p*-chlorobenzyl chloride to produce the *p*-chlorobenzylmercapto derivative, which, on treatment with methyl bromide in the presence of sodium methylate, undergoes methylation and rearrangement to yield the acetylimino thiadiazoline derivative. This is oxidized with chlorine water to the 2-sulfonyl chloride, which yields methazolamide on amidation with ammonia.

Description—White or faintly yellow, crystalline powder with a slight odor; melts about 213°; pKₐ 7.30.

Solubility—Weakly acidic; slightly soluble in water, alcohol or acetone; soluble in dimethylformamide.

Comments—Chemically related to *Acetazolamide*.

Carbonic Anhydrase Inhibitors

Carbonic anhydrase is an ubiquitous enzyme responsible for the catalytic reversible hydration of carbon dioxide and dehydration of carbonic acid, a process critical to the transport of carbon dioxide in the erythrocyte and its exchange in the parenchyma of the lungs. This enzyme also is found in the renal cortex, gastric mucosa, pancreas, eye, and central nervous system (CNS).

The renal tubular cells also contain substantial amounts of carbonic anhydrase, and the CO_2 produced metabolically in the cells of the renal tubule is converted immediately to carbonic acid by the enzyme. Urine is normally acidified by secretion of hydrogen ions derived from carbonic acid formed in the proximal tubular cells in exchange for sodium ions in the lumen of the tubule.

When carbonic anhydrase is inhibited, via adenyl cyclase stimulation, pH of the urine increases because the number of hydrogen ions available for exchange with sodium is decreased; the excess sodium ions retained in the tubule combine with bicarbonate and are excreted by the kidney with an increased volume of water and a loss of potassium. The diuretic effect is self-limiting when it is administered for longer than 48 hr, since the subsequent metabolic acidosis prevents further diuretic action by the carbonic anhydrase inhibitor.

Although carbonic anhydrase inhibitors were developed originally as diuretics, their major usefulness is in glaucoma. Inhibition of carbonic anhydrase in the ciliary body of the eye markedly reduces secretion of aqueous humor; oral or parenteral administration of carbonic anhydrase inhibitors decreases intraocular pressure in most patients with this ocular defect.

These agents also have been used in some cases of absence and generalized tonic-clonic epilepsy refractory to anticonvulsants. The anticonvulsant effects of the carbonic anhydrase inhibitors may be due to the metabolic acidosis caused by these agents.

Adverse reactions to carbonic anhydrase inhibitors are seldom serious and are reversed rapidly, since the drug is excreted rapidly. The most frequent adverse effects include paresthesia, particularly tingling in the extremities; loss of appetite; polyuria; some drowsiness; and confusion. During long-term systemic therapy, an acidotic state may supervene; this can be corrected by administration of bicarbonate. Transient myopia has been reported.

Other occasional reactions include urticaria, melena, flaccid paralysis, and convulsions. Drowsiness may impair ability to drive or perform other tasks requiring alertness; patients should be advised of this. Like other sulfonamide derivatives, the sulfonamide-type carbonic anhydrase agents may produce fever, rash, crystalluria, renal calculus, bone-marrow depression, thrombocytopenic purpura, hemolytic anemia, leukopenia, pancytopenia, and agranulocytosis. At the first signs of such reactions the drug should be discontinued and appropriate therapy instituted.

The safe use of these agents during pregnancy has not been established. These agents are contraindicated in patients with idiopathic renal hyperchloremic acidosis, renal failure, a known depletion of sodium and/or potassium, or Addison's disease and patients known to be sensitive to this class of drugs. Moreover, long-term therapy is contraindicated in patients with chronic, noncongestive, angle-closure glaucoma.

ACETAZOLAMIDE

Acetamide, *N*-[5-(aminosulfonyl)-1,3,4-thiadiazol-2-yl]-, Diamox

$$H_2NO_2S \underset{N-N}{\overset{S}{\diagup\!\!\diagdown}} NHCOCH_3$$

[59-66-5] $C_4H_6N_4O_3S_2$ (222.24).

Preparation—Hydrazine hydrate is reacted with a two-molar quantity of ammonium thiocyanate to produce 1,2-bis(thiocarbamoyl) hydrazine, which yields, through loss of ammonia and rearragement, 5-amino-2-mercapto-1,3,4-thiadiazole. This is acetylated and then oxidized to the 2-sulfonyl chloride with chlorine. The final step is amidation with ammonia.

Description—White to faintly yellowish white, crystalline, odorless powder; pKₐ: 7.2, 9.0.

Solubility—Very slightly soluble in water; sparingly soluble in hot water (90° to 100°); slightly soluble in alcohol.

Comments—A *carbonic anhydrase inhibitor* effective for adjunctive treatment of *edema due to congestive heart failure, drug-induced edema, absence* and other *centrencephalic epilepsies,* chronic simple (open-angle) *glaucoma,* secondary glaucoma and *preoperatively in acute angle-closure glaucoma* when it is desired to lower intraocular pressure prior to surgery.

It also is used in the prevention and amelioration of symptoms associated with acute mountain (high altitude) sickness. When used orally in tablet form to lower intraocular pressure, it has a rapid onset of action (1–1½ hr), reaches peak effect in 2 to 4 hr and the effect persists for 8 to 12 hr. When sustained-release capsules are employed, onset of action is approximately 2 hr, peak effect varies from 8 to 12 hr and the effects persist for 18 to 24 hr. It particularly is useful where careful following of blood electrolytes is not possible, as in outpatients. It has low toxicity. For additional information on adverse effects and precautions, see introductory statement.

ACETAZOLAMIDE SODIUM

Acetamide, *N*-[5-(aminosulfonyl)-1,3,4-thiadiazol-2-yl]-, monosodium salt; Diamox Sodium

[1424-27-7] $C_4H_5N_4NaO_3S_2$ (244.22); prepared from acetazolamide with the aid of NaOH. It is suitable for parenteral use. For the structure of the base, see *Acetazolamide*.

Preparation—Acetazolamide is dissolved in aqueous NaOH solution containing an equimolar quantity of NaOH, whereupon the acidic H of the—SO_2NH_2 group is replaced by Na. The solid sodium compound then may be produced by various drying or crystallization techniques.

Description—White solid, with the characteristic appearance of freeze-dried products; pH (freshly prepared solution, 1 in 10) between 9 and 10.

Comments—See *Acetazolamide*.

Benzothiadiazine and Related Diuretics

The benzothiadiazine diuretics occurred from efforts to develop more-potent carbonic anhydrase inhibitors. This resulted in the introduction of the prototype thiazide, chlorothiazide, in 1958, a widely used, reliable, well-tolerated, orally effective diuretic.

The thiazide diuretics increase urinary excretion of sodium and water by inhibiting sodium reabsorption on the distal convoluted tubule, connecting tubule, and early collecting duct. They also increase excretion of chloride, potassium, and, to a lesser extent, bicarbonate ions. The latter effect is due to their slight carbonic anhydrase–inhibitory action, although this action is usually of minor diuretic consequence. Because of their site of action, they interfere with the dilution, but not the concentration, of urine.

The thiazide drugs also decrease the glomerular filtration rate. This effect does not appear to contribute to the diuretic action of these drugs and may explain their diminished efficacy in the presence of impaired kidney function.

The thiazide drugs are frequently employed in the treatment of hypertension and can add to the effectiveness of other antihypertensive drugs and reverse the fluid retention caused by some of these agents. Although the precise mechanism of their antihypertensive action is unknown, it may be due to an altered sodium balance. Since the thiazides induce only a limited (10%) reduction in blood pressure, they are useful either in mild cases of hypertension or as adjunctive therapy to other drugs.

Thiazide diuretics are effective as adjunctive therapy in *edema* associated with *congestive heart failure, hepatic cirrhosis,* and *corticosteroid* and *estrogen therapy,* as well as edema due to *various forms of renal dysfunction (nephrotic syndrome, acute glomerulonephritis,* and *chronic renal failure)* if estimated creatinine clearance is > 40°mL/min. Thiazide diuretics also have been used successfully (alone or in combination with amiloride and/or allopurinol) to prevent the formation and recurrence of calcium stones in *hypercalciuric* and *normal calciuric patients.*

Thiazide diuretics are contraindicated in anuria, patients hypersensitive to these and other sulfonamide drugs and in otherwise healthy pregnant women with or without mild edema. Diuretics can decrease placental perfusion. Thiazides are excreted into breast milk; therefore, use by nursing mothers is not recommended. These drugs should be used with caution in patients with renal disease, since they may precipitate azotemia. They also should be used with caution in patients with impaired liver function, diabetes, gout, or a history of lupus erythematosus.

Adverse effects have been observed as follows: *GI* (anorexia, gastric irritation, nausea, vomiting, cramping, diarrhea, constipation, jaundice, pancreatitis, sialadenitis), *CNS* (dizziness, vertigo, paresthesias, headache, xanthopsia), *hematological* (leukopenia, agranulocytosis, thrombocytopenia, aplastic anemia), *cardiovascular* (orthostatic hypotension), *hypersensitivity* (purpura, photosensitivity, rash, urticaria, necrotizing angiitis, fever, respiratory distress, anaphylactic reactions), and *other* (hyperglycemia, glycosuria, hyperuricemia, muscle spasm, weakness, restlessness, transient blurred vision).

Periodic serum electrolyte determinations should be done on all patients to detect electrolyte imbalance such as hyponatremia, hypochloremic alkalosis, and hypokalemia. Finally, in higher doses, thiazides may increase total cholesterol, triglycerides, and low-density lipoproteins (LDLs).

Thiazides are involved in several clinically important drug interactions. They interact with adrenal corticosteroids to enhance hypokalemia, with vitamin D and calcium to induce hypercalcemia, with diazoxide to cause hyperglycemia, with indomethacin to decrease the natriuretic and/or antihypertensive effect, and with digitalis glycosides to produce digitalis toxicity. Moreover, the thiazides increase lithium levels and the neuromuscular blocking effect of tubocurarine but decrease the anticoagulant effect of the oral anticoagulants.

BENDROFLUMETHIAZIDE

2*H*-1,2,4-Benzothidiazine-7-sulfonamide, 3,4-dihydro-3-(phenylmethyl)-6-(trifluoromethyl)- 1,1-dioxide; Naturetin

[73-48-3] $C_{15}H_{14}F_3N_3O_4S_2$ (421.41).

Preparation—One method consists of cyclization of 4-amino-6-trifluoromethyl-*m*-benzenedisulfonamide through condensation with phenylacetaldehyde (*J Am Chem Soc* 1959; 81:4807).

Description—White to cream-colored, finely divided, crystalline powder that is odorless or has a slight, characteristic floral odor; melts about 220°. pK_a 8.5.

Solubility—1 g in 23 mL alcohol or 200 mL ether; practically insoluble in water, chloroform, or benzene.

Comments—A potent, orally effective thiazide diuretic.

BENZTHIAZIDE

2*H*-1,2,4-benzothiadiazine-7-sulfonamide, 6-chloro-3-[[(phenylmethyl)thio]methyl]- 1,1-dioxide; Aquatag, Proaqua; Exna; Hydrex

3-[(Benzylthio)methyl]-6-chloro-2*H*-1,2,4-benzothiadiazine-7-sulfonamide 1,1-dioxide [91-33-8] $C_{15}H_{14}ClN_3O_4S_3$ (431.93).

Preparation—4-Amino-6-chloro-*m*-benzenedisulfonamide is reacted with chloroacetic anhydride to give 2,3'-dichloro-4',6'-disulfamoylacetanilide, which is then condensed and cyclized with benzyl mercaptan in the presence of sodium hydroxide (US Pat 3,111,517).

Description—Fine, white, crystalline powder with both a characteristic odor and taste; stable in both light and air; melts about 240°.

Solubility—1 g in 41,000 mL water, 480 mL alcohol, 24,000 mL chloroform, or 2900 mL ether; soluble in alkaline solutions.

Comments—A diuretic and antihypertensive similar to the thiazides.

CHLORTHALIDONE

Benzenesulfonamide, 2-chloro-5-(2,3-dihydro-1-hydroxy-3-oxo-1*H*-isoindol-1-yl)-, Hygroton; Hylidone; Combipres

2-Chloro-5-(1-hydroxy-3-oxo-1-isoindolinyl)benzenesulfonamide [77-36-1] $C_{14}H_{11}ClN_2O_4S$ (338.76).

Preparation—3-Amino-4-chlorobenzophenone-2-carboxylic acid is diazotized, and the resulting diazonium chloride is reacted in the cold with sulfur dioxide in the presence of cupric chloride to form 4-chloro-2'-carboxybenzophenone-3-sulfonyl chloride (1). Heating 1 with thionyl chloride yields 3-chloro-3-(3'-chlorosulfonyl-4'-chlorophenyl)phthalide, which is reacted with ammonia. Removal of the solvent and treatment of the residue with HCl yields chlorthalidone (US Pat 3,055,904).

Description—White to yellowish white, crystalline powder; melts with decomposition above 215°; pK_a 9.4.

Solubility—Practically insoluble in water (12 mg/100 mL at 20°), chloroform, or ether; slightly soluble in alcohol; soluble in methanol. Soluble in alkali carbonates or basic solutions.

Comments—An orally effective nonthiazide diuretic.

CHLOROTHIAZIDE

2*H*-1,2,4-Benzothiadiazine-7-sulfonamide, 6-chloro-, 1,1-dioxide; Diachlor; Diuril

[58-94-6] $C_7H_6ClN_3O_4S_2$ (295.72).

Preparation—3-Chloroaniline is acylated with chlorosulfonic acid to produce the 4,6-disulfonyl chloride, which is amidated with ammonia to give the 4,6-disulfonamide. Heating the latter with formic acid results in cyclization through double condensation.

Description—White or practically white, odorless, crystalline powder; melts about 340°, with decomposition. pK_a 6.7, 9.5.

Solubility—Very slightly soluble in water (0.4 g/L at pH4, 0.65 g/L at pH 7); freely soluble in dimethylformamide or dimethyl sulfoxide; slightly soluble in methanol or pyridine; practically insoluble in ether, benzene, or chloroform. Soluble in alkaline solutions but decomposes on heating or standing.

Comments—The prototype benzothiadiazine diuretic, with the therapeutic indications, warnings, precautions, drug interactions, and adverse reactions described above. Diuretic effects are apparent within 2 hr after oral administration, reach peak activity in 4 hr, and persist for about 6 to 12 hr; after intravenous administration, effects are apparent in 15 min, reach a peak in 30 min, and persist for about 2 hr. Refractoriness to the drug is relatively uncommon, even after prolonged periods of continuous administration. For information on drug interactions of benzothiazides, see above.

CYCLOTHIAZIDE

2*H*-1,2,4-Benzothiadiazine-7-sulfonamide, 3-bicyclo[2.2.1]hept-5-en-2-yl-6-chloro-3,4-dihydro-, 1,1-dioxide; Anhydron

6-Chloro-3,4-dihydro-3-(5-norbornen-2-yl)-2*H*-1,2,4-benzothiadiazine-7-sulfonamide 1,1-dioxide [2259-96-3] $C_{14}H_{16}ClN_3O_4S_2$ (389.87).

Preparation—The process is analogous to that for *Chlorothiazide,* except that 5-norbornene-2-carboxaldehyde is employed in the cyclization step instead of formic acid (US Pat 3,275,625).

Description—White to nearly white, practically odorless powder; melts within a range of 4° between 217° and 225°.

Solubility—1 g in 70 mL alcohol or 30 mL methanol; practically insoluble in water, chloroform or ether.

Comments—An orally effective diuretic and antihypertensive.

HYDROCHLOROTHIAZIDE

2H-1,2,4-Benzothiadiazine-7-sulfonamide-, 6-chloro-3,4-dihydro-, 1, 1-dioxide

[58-93-5] $C_7H_8ClN_3O_4S_2$ (297.75).

Preparation—The process is identical with that for *Chlorothiazide*, except that formaldehyde is employed in the final cyclization step instead of formic acid.

Description—White, or practically white, odorless, crystalline powder; melts about 268° with decomposition; pK_{a1} 7.9; pK_{a2} 9.2.

Solubility—Slightly soluble in water; freely soluble in sodium hydroxide solution or dimethylformamide; sparingly soluble in methanol; insoluble in ether or chloroform.

Comments—A drug similar to *Chlorothiazide*.

HYDROFLUMETHIAZIDE

2H-1,2,4-Benzothiadiazine-7-sulfonamide, 3,4-dihydro, 6-(trifluoromethyl)-, 1,1-dioxide

[135-09-1] $C_8H_8F_3N_3O_4S_2$ (331.28).

Preparation—4-Amino-6-(trifluoromethyl)-*m*-benzenedisulfonamide is heated with formaldehyde in a sulfuric acid environment, thus effecting concomitant condensation and cyclization to hydroflumethiazide (US Pat 3,254,076).

Description—White to cream-colored, finely divided, crystalline powder; odorless; melts between 270° and 275°; pH (1 in 100 dispersion in water) between 4.5 and 7.5; pK_1 8.9, pK_2 10.7.

Solubility—1 g in >5000 mL water, 39 mL alcohol, >5000 mL chloroform, or 2500 mL ether.

Comments—A potent, oral thiazide diuretic.

INDAPAMIDE

Benzamide, 3-(aminosulfonyl)-4-chloro-N-(2,3-dihydro-2-methyl-1H-indol-1-yl)- Lozol

4-Chloro-N-(2-methyl-1-indolinyl)-3-sulfamoylbenzamide [26807-65-8] $C_{16}H_{16}ClN_3O_3S$ (365.84).

Preparation—*p*-Chlorotoluene is sulfonated and converted to the sulfonamide yielding 3-chloro-4-sulfamoylbenzoic acid. This acid is reacted with thionyl chloride to form the carbonyl chloride and treated with 2-methylindole (skatole) to give the product (US Pat 3,565,911).

Description—White to yellow orthogonal crystals melting about 161°; weak acid, $pK_a = 8.8$.

Solubility—Soluble in aqueous solutions of strong bases.

Comments—An oral diuretic and antihypertensive related to the indolines.

METHYCLOTHIAZIDE

2H-1,2,4-Benzothiadiazine-7-sulfonamide, 6-chloro-3-(chloromethyl)-3,4-dihydro-2-methyl-, 1,1-dioxide

[135-07-9] $C_9H_{11}Cl_2N_3O_4S_2$ (360.23).

Preparation—By a process analogous to that for *Chlorothiazide*, 4-amino-6-chloro-N^3-methyl-*m*-benzenedisulfonamide is cyclized through condensation with monochloroacetaldehyde or an acetal thereof (US Pat 3,163,644).

Description—White or practically white, crystalline powder; odorless or has a slight odor and is tasteless; chars slightly below 220° and decomposes at 220°; pK_a (extrapolated from water-acetone) 9.4.

Solubility—1 g in >10,000 mL water, 92.5 mL alcohol, >10,000 mL chloroform, or 2700 mL ether; freely soluble in acetone.

Comments—A thiazide diuretic.

METOLAZONE

6-Quinazolinesulfonamide, 7-chloro-1,2,3,4-tetrahydro-2-methyl-3-(2-methylphenyl)-4-oxo-, Diulo; Mykrox; Zaroxolyn

[17560-51-9] $C_{16}H_{16}ClN_3O_3S$ (365.83).

Preparation—5-Chloro-*o*-toluidine is converted through a series of reactions into *N*-(*o*-tolyl)-2-amino-4-chloro-5-sulfamoylbenzamide, which undergoes ring closure through reaction with acetaldehyde (US Pat 3,360,518; *J Med Chem* 1970; 13:886).

Description—Colorless, odorless, tasteless, crystalline powder; light-sensitive; pK_a 9.72; melts between 253° and 259°.

Solubility—Sparingly soluble in water or alcohol, more soluble in plasma, blood, alkali, and organic solvents.

Comments—A quinazoline-derived nonthiazide diuretic.

POLYTHIAZIDE

2H-1,2,4-Benzothiadiazine-7-sulfonamide, 6-chloro-3,4-dihydro-2-methyl-3-[[(2,2,2-trifluoroethyl)thio]methyl]-, 1,1-dioxide; Renese

[346-18-9] $C_{11}H_{13}ClF_3N_3O_4S_3$ (439.87).

Preparation—6-Amino-4-chloro-*N*′-methyl-*m*-benzenedisulfonamide is condensed with the dimethyl acetal of 2,2,2-trifluoroethylmercaptoacetaldehyde. The crude polythiazide, which precipitates when the reaction mixture is added to cold water, is recrystallized from 2-propanol (US Pat 3,009,911).

Description—White, crystalline powder with a characteristic odor; melts between 207° and 217°, with decomposition; pK_a 9.1.

Solubility—1 g in >1000 mL water, 150 mL alcohol, 175 mL chloroform or >1000 mL ether; soluble in acetone; soluble in aqueous alkali carbonates or hydroxides with increasing decomposition as pH increases.

Comments—A thiazide diuretic.

QUINETHAZONE

6-Quinazolinesulfonamide, 7-chloro-2-ethyl-1,2,3,4-tetrahydro-4-oxo

[73-49-4] $C_{10}H_{12}ClN_3O_3S$ (289.74).

Preparation—4′-Chloro-*o*-acetotoluidide is subjected to chlorosulfonation and subsequent amination to form 2-amino-4-chloro-5-sulfamoylbenzamide. Refluxing with an acidulated alcholic solution of the diethylacetal of propionaldehyde effects the required condensation cyclization to yield quinethazone (US Pat 2,976,289; *J Am Chem Soc* 1960; 82:2731).

Description—White to yellowish white, odorless, crystalline powder with a bitter taste; discolors in the presence of strong light and alkaline materials; melts between 250° and 252°.

Solubility—1 g in 500 mL alcohol; freely soluble in solutions of alkali hydroxides and carbonates; very slightly soluble in water.

Comments—A quinazoline derivative with 6-thiazide-like effect.

TRICHLORMETHIAZIDE

2H-1,2,4-Benzothiadiazine-7-sulfonamide, 6-chloro-3-(dichloromethyl)-3,4-dihydro-, 1,1-dioxide; Metahydrin; Naqua

[133-67-5] $C_8H_8Cl_3N_3O_4S_2$ (380.65).

Preparation—By reacting 4-amino-6-chloro-*m*-benzenedisulfonamide with dichloroacetaldehyde, or an acetal thereof, in a suitable condensation environment (US Pats 3,163,645 and 3,264,292).

Description—White, crystalline powder that is odorless or has a slight characteristic odor; light-sensitive, but stable in air and heat; melts about 274° with decomposition.

Solubility—1 g in 1100 mL water, 48 mL alcohol, 5000 mL chloroform, or 1400 mL ether.

Comments—An orally long-acting thiazide.

Potassium-Sparing Diuretics

The potassium-sparing diuretics include *spironolactone, triamterene,* and *amiloride.* The effects of these agents on urinary electrolyte composition are similar in that they cause a mild natruresis and decrease potassium and hydrogen ion excretion. Despite this similarity, these agents actually compose two groups with respect to mechanism of action.

Spironolactone, the prototype agent of the so-called *aldosterone antagonists,* is a specific competitive inhibitor of aldosterone at the receptor site level; hence, it is effective only when aldosterone is present. The other two potassium-sparing diuretics, triamterene and amiloride, exert their effect independent of the presence or absence of aldosterone.

Triamterene, on the peritubular side, inhibits the potential in the collecting duct and not on the distal tubule. Amiloride, on the other hand, inhibits the potential in both the collecting duct and the distal tubule. In addition, amiloride also decreases sodium transport in the proximal tubule. The potassium-sparing action common to all three of these agents is due to alteration of passive forces controlling movement of these ions.

The potassium-sparing agents are used in the management of *edema* associated with *congestive heart failure, hepatic cirrhosis with ascites, the nephrotic syndrome,* and *idiopathic edema* Because these diuretics have little antihypertensive action of their own they are used mainly in combination with other drugs in the management of hypertension and to correct hypokalemia often caused by other diuretic agents. Spironolactone also is used in *primary hyperaldosteronism.*

Potassium-sparing diuretics are contraindicated in patients with anuria, acute renal insufficiency, impaired renal function, or hyperkalemia. Adverse reactions include diarrhea, nausea, vomiting, weakness, headache, erythematous rash, and urticaria. Gynecomastia and carcinoma of the breast have been reported after spironolactone; however, no causal relationship between the latter and the drug has been established.

These drugs can cause life-threatening hyperkalemia in patients using potassium-containing *salt substitutes* or in those with renal impairment. Serum potassium levels should be monitored in diabetics, the elderly, and patients with renal failure.

AMILORIDE HYDROCHLORIDE

Pyrazinecarboxamide, 3,5-diamino-N-(aminoiminomethyl)-6-chloro-, monohydrochloride, dihydrate; Midamor

N-Amidino-3,5-diamino-6-chloropyrazinecarboxamide hydrochloride, dihydrate [2016-88-8] $C_6H_8ClN_7O \cdot HCl \cdot H_2O$ (302.12).

Preparation—Pyrazine-2,3-dicarboxamide is converted to 3-amino-2-carboxamide through a Hoffman degradation using one equivalent of NaOBr, the carboxamide forming the ethyl ester by ethanolysis, followed by reaction with sulfuryl chloride. This latter treatment forms the 5,6-dichloro derivative. As the 5-chloro is activated by the *p*- carboxyl it is readily converted to the amine with ammonia. Finally, the ester group is condensed with guanidine to yield the product (Belg Pat 639,386 [*CA* 1965; 62:14698f]).

Description—Odorless, pale yellowish-green powder melting about 240°; pK$_a$ 8.7.

Solubility—Soluble 1 g in 200 mL water or 350 mL alcohol; practically insoluble in chloroform or ether.

Comments—A potassium-conserving drug with natriuretic, diuretic, and antihypertensive activity. It is approved only for concurrent use with other thiazide diuretics or other kaliuretic-diuretic agents in the management of congestive heart failure or hypertension. It is used to restore normal serum potassium levels in patients who develop hypokalemia and in patients who would be exposed to a particular risk if hypokalemia were to develop.

Its effect on electrolyte excretion is first observed 2 hr after drug administration, reaches a peak between 6 and 10 hr, and lasts about 24 hr. Peak plasma levels are reached in 3 to 4 hr and plasma half-life varies from 6 to 9 hr. The drug is not metabolized by the liver and is excreted unchanged in the urine. It is contraindicated in patients with hyperkalemia or those taking potassium supplements or other potassium-sparing drugs, anuria, acute or chronic renal insufficiency, and diabetic nephropathy. It should be used with extreme care in patients with diabetes.

Amiloride usually is well-tolerated, and serious side effects are infrequent, although minor adverse effects occur in 20% of the users. Adverse effects include headache, nausea, anorexia, diarrhea, and vomiting (3–8%). Other adverse effects such as dizziness, encephalopathy, abdominal pain, constipation, weakness, muscle cramps, decreased libido, cough, and impotence occur less frequently. Amiloride alone has little effect on electrolytes other than potassium; however, electrolyte disturbances may occur when it is combined with other diuretics. Serum potassium levels should be monitored.

SPIRONOLACTONE

(7α, 17α)-Pregn-4-ene-21-carboxylic acid, 7-(acetylthio)-17-hydroxy-3-oxo γ-lactone; Aldactone

17-Hydroxy-7α-mercapto-3-oxo-17α-pregn-4-ene-21-carboxylic acid γ-lactone acetate [52-01-7] $C_{24}H_{32}O_4S$ (416.57).

Preparation—By treating dehydroepiandrosterone (prepared from cholesterol or sitosterol) with acetylene to form the 17α-ethynyl-17β-hydroxy derivative, which is carbonated to the 17α-propiolic acid. Reduction of the unsaturated acid in alkaline solution yields the saturated acid, which cyclizes to the lactone on acidification. Bromination to the 5,6-dibromo compound, followed by oxidation of the 3-hydroxyl group to the ketone, then dehydrobromination to the 7α-hydroxyl derivative, produces spironolactone when esterified with thiolacetic acid.

Description—Light, cream-colored to light tan, crystalline powder; faint to mild mercaptan-like odor; stable in air; melts between 198° and 207°, with decomposition.

Solubility—Practically insoluble in water; freely soluble in benzene and chloroform; soluble in alcohol; slightly soluble in fixed oils.

Comments—A synthetic steroid that acts as a competitive antagonist of the potent, endogeneous mineralocorticosteroid, aldosterone. It has a slower onset of action than triamterene or amiloride, but its natriuretic effect is slightly greater during long-term therapy.

It is indicated in the treatment of *essential hypertension, edema* associated with *congestive heart failure, hepatic cirrhosis* with ascites, the *nephrotic syndrome,* and *idiopathic edema, hypokalemia,* and in the diagnosis of *primary aldosteronism* By blocking the sodium-retaining effects of aldosterone on the distal convoluted tubule, it corrects one of the most important mechanisms responsible for the production of edema, but spironolactone is effective only in the presence of aldosterone.

Its onset of diuretic action is gradual (24–48 hr), reaches a peak in 48 to 72 hr, and lasts for 48 to 72 hr. It is a relatively weak diuretic and usually is employed as an adjunct to other diuretics, such as the thiazides. When used in this combined manner, it enhances the excretion of sodium and decreases the excretion of potassium.

Further increase in diuresis may be obtained by the use of a glucocorticoid with this drug in combination with another diuretic. It is metabolized rapidly after oral administration. The metabolites are excreted largely in the urine, but also in bile. The primary metabolite, canrenone, reaches peak plasma levels 2 to 4 hr after oral administration of the drug.

The half-life of canrenone, following multiple doses of the drug is 13 to 24 hr. Both this drug and canrenone are more than 90% bound to plasma proteins. It has been shown to be a tumorigen in chronic toxicity studies in rats; 500 mg/kg induced hepatocytomegaly, hyperplastic liver nodules, and hepatocellular carcinoma.

It is contraindicated in acute renal insufficiency, anuria, significant impairment of renal excretory function, and hyperkalemia. Patients on digoxin should be monitored closely. Concurrent use elevates digoxin plasma levels and may induce digoxin toxicity. Similarly, concurrent use with lithium increases the risk of lithium toxicity. Side effects include hyponatremia, hyperkalemia, and drowsiness. Other adverse effects include headache, diarrhea, rashes, urticaria, mental confusion, drug fever, ataxia, gynecomastia, decreased libido in the male, and mild androgenic effects, such as hirsutism, irregular menses, and deepening of the voice in the female.

TRIAMTERENE

2,4,7-Pteridinetriamine, 6-phenyl-, Dyrenium

2,4,7-Triamino-6-phenylpteridine [396-01-0] $C_{12}H_{11}N_7$ (253.27).

Preparation—5-Nitroso-2,4,6-triaminopyrimidine is refluxed with phenylacetonitrile in the presence of sodium methoxide (US Pat 3,081,230; *J Org Chem* 1963; 28:1191).

Description—Yellow, odorless, crystalline powder; stable to temperature and light; pK$_a$ 6.2.

Solubility—Practically insoluble in water, chloroform, or ether; very slightly soluble in alcohol.

Comments—Inhibits reabsorption of sodium ions in exchange for potassium and hydrogen ions at that segment of the distal tubule under the control of adrenal mineralocorticoids. The effect is unrelated to the level of aldosterone secretion. After oral administration, 30% to 70% is absorbed, and 50% to 67% is bound to plasma protein. Diuresis appears within 2 hr after administration, reaches a peak in 6 to 8 hr, and lasts for 12 to 16 hr.

It is metabolized primarily by the liver (hydroxytriamterene sulfate, an active metabolite), and about 3% to 5% is excreted unchanged in the urine. It also is used in combination with hydrochlorothiazide in treatment of edema associated with *congestive heart failure, cirrhosis,* and the *nephrotic syndrome.* It also is indicated in steroid-induced edema, idiopathic edema, edema due to secondary hyperaldosteronism, and in edematous patients unresponsive to other therapy. It directly inhibits the reabsorption of sodium and chloride independent of aldosterone.

Although it promotes the excretion of sodium and chloride, it is believed to conserve potassium by reducing the transport of this ion from the tubular cell to the tubular lumen.

It is contraindicated in patients with hyperkalemia or those taking potassium supplements or other potassium-sparing drugs, anuria, acute or chronic renal insufficiency, and diabetic nephropathy. Patients receiving long-term triamterene treatment should be monitored for electrolyte imbalances. Side effects are usually mild and include nausea, vomiting, GI disturbances, weakness, headache, dry mouth, and rash.

Loop Diuretics

The loop, or high-ceiling, diuretics, ethacrynic acid, furosemide, and bumetanide, are the most potent currently available diuretic agents. Although differences do exist between these agents, they are similar in that their most important action is in the medullary and cortical portions of the thick ascending limb of the loop of Henle. Loop diuretics inhibit active chloride, and possibly sodium, transport in the ascending thick limb of Henle.

The loop diuretics have a much greater diuretic effect than the thiazides and are effective even in the presence of elec-

trolyte and acid-base disturbances. Excess amounts of the potent diuretics can lead to serious water and electrolyte depletion; thus, careful medical monitoring is required. The time of onset and duration of action of the loop diuretics are shorter than those with the thiazides.

Despite their similar actions, there are some essential differences between the loop diuretics. Furosemide usually is preferred to ethacrynic acid for a number of reasons:

1. It has a broader dose-response curve.
2. It is less ototoxic.
3. It causes fewer gastrointestinal side effects.
4. It is more convenient for intravenous use.
5. It may be less likely to cause alkalosis.

Considerable controversy persists concerning the loop diuretic antihypertensive effectiveness compared with that of the thiazides. Studies have suggested that the loop diuretics are not more effective than the thiazides in the management of uncomplicated mild-to-moderate hypertension in most patients. There is little controversy relative to the superiority of the loop diuretics in hypertension associated with renal insufficiency. Moreover, the loop diuretics *increase* renal blood flow, whereas the thiazides tend to *decrease* renal blood flow and further compromise renal function.

Many of the adverse effects are similar for both the thiazides and loop diuretics, and the management of these effects are the same. However, because of the much greater potency of the loop diuretics, compared with the thiazides, close monitoring is warranted to avoid severe electrolyte imbalances.

BUMETANIDE

Benzoic acid, 3-(aminosulfonyl)-5-(butylamino)-4-phenoxy-, Bumex

3-(Butylamino)-4-phenoxy-5-sulfamoylbenzoic acid [28395-03-1] $C_{17}H_{20}N_2O_5S$ (364.41).

Preparation—3-Chloro-5-(chlorosulfonyl)benzoic acid is nitrated in the 3-position with nitric/sulfuric acid, treated with ammonia to form the sulfonamide, then with sodium phenoxide to form the phenyl ether (replacing the active ring halogen), the nitro group reduced with acid bisulfite to the amine and a butylamino group generated by reductive coupling of the ring amino group with butyraldehyde in the presence of Pd and H_2 This latter step also produces the butyl ester of the carboxylic acid function, which subsequently is saponified with base and the free acid generated with HCl (*J Med Chem* 1971; 14:432).

Description—White crystals melting about 230°; pK$_{a1}$ 0.3; pK$_{a2}$ 4.0; pK$_{a3}$ 10.

Solubility—1 gm in 30 mL alcohol or 10,000 mL water.

Comments—A metanilamide derivative that is a potent *loop diuretic* with efficacy and biochemical effects similar to those of furosemide. Orally, it is effective in patients with *chronic congestive heart failure, chronic renal failure, chronic hepatic disease,* and the *nephrotic syndrome.*

Orally, 1 mg is equivalent to 40 mg of furosemide. It is 95% protein bound and the volume of distribution is 12 to 35 L. Approximately 45% of an oral dose is excreted unchanged. The half-life is 1 to 1.5 hrs and is prolonged in patients with renal failure. Onset of diuresis is observed within 30 to 60 mins following oral administration, reaches a peak in 1 to 2 hr and persists for 4 to 6 hrs. Diuresis starts within minutes following intravenous administration and reaches maximum levels in 15 to 30 mins. It inhibits both chloride and sodium reabsorption in the ascending limb of the loop of Henle; it is somewhat more chloruretic than natriuretic.

Bumetanide causes dilation of renal vasculature and increases renal blood flow. Since fluid and electrolyte changes are similar to those for furosemide, the same precautions apply (see this page). It also may cause azotemia, hyperuricemia, and rarely, impaired glucose tolerance.

Nausea, dizziness, muscle cramps, hypotension, and headache have been reported. Thrombocytopenia has occurred rarely. Reported drug interactions are similar to those for furosemide.

ETHACRYNIC ACID

Acetic acid, [2,3-dichloro-4-(2-methylene-1-oxobutyl)phenoxy]-, Edecrin

[2,3-Dichloro-4-(2-methylenebutyryl)phenoxy]acetic acid [58-54-8] $C_{13}H_{12}Cl_2O_4$ (303.14).

Caution—Use care in handling, since it irritates the skin, eyes, and mucous membranes.

Preparation—2,3-Dichlorophenoxyacetic acid is subjected to a Friedel-Crafts reaction with butyryl chloride to form the 4-butyryl derivative. This undergoes a Mannich reaction with formaldehyde and dimethylamine, the product decomposing thermally to introduce the methylene group (*J Med Pharm Chem* 1962; 5:660).

Description—White or practically white, crystalline powder that is odorless or practically odorless and has a bitter taste; relatively stable in light and at room temperature; nonhygroscopic; melts between 121° and 125°; pK_a 3.5.

Solubility—1 g in 1.6 mL alcohol, 3.5 mL ether, or 6 mL chloroform; very slightly soluble in water.

Comments—An aryloxyacetic acid derivative that is a potent, short-acting diuretic. Maximum water and sodium diuresis is similar to that with furosemide but greatly exceeds that with the thiazides. It is useful especially in patients who require an agent with greater diuretic potential than those commonly employed. It is also useful in patients with a documented sulfa allergy. It is used in the treatment of *edema* caused by *congestive heart failure, cirrhosis of the liver,* and *renal disease,* including the nephrotic syndrome.

It also is recommended for the short-term management of ascites due to malignancy, idiopathic edema, and lymphedema. In addition, it is useful for the short-term management of hospitalized pediatric patients with congenital heart disease or the nephrotic syndrome. It has also been used as adjunctive therapy for acute pulmonary edema. It exerts its action on the cortical ascending (thick) loop of Henle and on the proximal and distal tubule, where it affects both the concentrating and diluting mechanisms of the kidney.

It causes the excretion of virtually an isoosmotic urine by preventing sodium reabsorption from the loop of Henle. Initially chloride excretion exceeds that of sodium. With prolonged administration, chloride excretion declines. Ethacrynic acid is almost 100% bioavailable following oral administration. After oral administration, diuresis begins within 30 mins, reaches a peak in 2 hrs, and persists for 6 to 8 hrs. After intravenous administration, diuresis begins within 5 mins, reaches a peak in 15 to 30 mins, and lasts about 2 hrs. Approximately 95% of the drug is bound to plasma proteins. Plasma half-life is about 1 hr. It can be used with additive effect with diuretics having different sites of action.

Adverse reactions include anorexia, malaise, abdominal discomfort, dysphagia, nausea, vomiting, diarrhea, hyperuricemia, and acute gout have been reported. Blood dyscrasias (agranulocytosis, severe neutropenia, and thrombocytopenia) have been reported rarely. Patients should have determinations of blood urea nitrogen, serum carbon dioxide, and electrolytes and white blood cell counts made frequently.

ETHACRYNATE SODIUM

Acetic acid, [2,3-dichloro-4-(2-methylene-1-oxobutyl)phenoxy]-, sodium salt; Edecrin Sodium

Sodium [2,3-dichloro-4-(2-methylenebutyryl)phenoxy]acetate [6500-81-8] $C_{13}H_{11}Cl_2NaO_4$ (325.12).

Preparation—A sterile, cryodesiccated powder prepared by the neutralization of ethacrynic acid with NaOH.

Comments—See *Ethacrynic Acid.*

FUROSEMIDE

Benzoic acid, 5-(aminosulfonyl)-4-chloro-2-[(2-furanylmethyl)amino]-, Lasix

4-Chloro-*N*-furfuryl-5-sulfamoylanthranilic acid [54-31-9] $C_{12}H_{11}ClN_2O_5S$ (330.74).

Preparation—2,4-Dichlorobenzoic acid is heated with chlorosulfonic acid, and the resulting 5-chlorosulfonyl derivative is reacted with concentrated ammonia to convert it to the 5-sulfamoyl analogue (I). Refluxing I with furfurylamine in large excess or in the presence of sodium bicarbonate yields crude furosemide, which is recrystallized from aqueous ethanol (US Pat 3,058,882).

Description—Fine, white to off-white, crystalline powder; odorless and practically tasteless; unstable in light but stable in air; melts between 203° and 205° with decomposition; pK_a 3.9 (acid).

Solubility—Practically insoluble in water; freely soluble in acetone or solutions of alkali hydroxides; sparingly soluble in alcohol; slightly soluble in ether; very slightly soluble in chloroform.

Comments—A *diuretic* chemically related to the sulfonamide diuretics. It is characterized by high efficacy, rapid onset of action, comparatively short duration of action, and a tenfold ratio between minimum and maximum diuretic dose. Moreover, it is slightly more potent than the organomercurial agents, is orally effective, and its diuretic action is independent of alterations in body acid-base balance. It acts not only on the proximal and distal tubules but also on the ascending limb of the loop of Henle.

It is indicated for the treatment of *edema* associated with *congestive heart failure, cirrhosis of the liver,* and *renal disease,* including the *nephrotic syndrome.* It is indicated particularly when a greater diuretic potential is needed than that produced by commonly employed diuretic agents. It is thought to decrease peripheral resistance in hypertensive patients and dilate the veins in patients with congestive heart failure (*TIPS* 1987; 8:254).

It is given by both oral and parenteral routes of administration; parenteral administration should be reserved for those cases in which oral therapy is not practical. Orally, the diuretic effect begins within 1 hr, reaches a peak in 1 or 2 hr and persists for 6 to 8 hr. Administered intravenously, the diuretic effect begins within 5 mins, reaches a peak in 30 min, and persists for 2 hrs.

Clinical pharmacokinetic studies carried out after a single intravenous dose of 0.5, 1.0, or 1.5 mg/kg indicate that peak diuresis occurs between 20 and 60 min after injection. Apparent volume of distribution of the drug averages 11.4% of the body weight and is independent of the dose. Mean plasma half-life in these studies was 29.5 min, with a clearance rate of 162 mL/min.

Renal excretion was found to be the main route of elimination and averaged 92% of the administered dose, with a mean renal clearance of 149 mL/min. Since this exceeds the glomerular filtration rate, it is thought that tubular secretion of this drug occurs, despite the fact that 95% of it is bound to plasma protein. The bioavailability of furosemide is considerably less than with other loop diuretics.

Like the other diuretics, furosemide is known to be involved in a number of drug interactions. It increases the toxicity of lithium, digitalis, anticoagulants, and theophylline. It decreases the arterial responsiveness of norepinephrine and antagonizes the skeletal muscle relaxant effects of tubocurarine and may potentiate the action of succinylcholine. Concomitant administration of indomethacin may reduce the natriuretic and antihypertensive effects of the drug. This effect also may occur with other nonsteroidal anti-inflammatory drugs such as ibuprofen or naproxen. Metolazone acts synergistically with this to stimulate profound diuresis in patients resistant to it.

It is contraindicated in anuria, in hepatic coma, and in patients known to be sensitive to the drug. Adverse effects that may result from therapy include reduction of renal, cerebral, and cardiac blood flow; potassium loss with resultant cardiac and neuromuscular abnormalities; elevation of blood uric acid and blood sugar levels; allergic reactions; rare cases of exfoliative dermatitis; pruritus; and blood dyscrasias (thrombocytopenia and leukopenia). Paresthesia, blurring of vision, postural hypotension, nausea, vomiting, or diarrhea may occur. In addition, cases of reversible deafness and tinnitus have been reported. Ototoxicity is associated with rapid injection, severe renal impairment, with doses several times the usual dose, and with concurrent use with other ototoxic drugs.

Diuresis induced by the drug also has been accompanied by weakness, fatigue, light-headedness or dizziness, muscle cramps, thirst, and urinary frequency. Excessive therapy can lead to profound diuresis with water and electrolyte depletion. Patients on this drug should be tested at frequent intervals for blood urea nitrogen, sodium, potassium, chloride, and carbon dioxide concentrations. The drug should not be used in cirrhotic patients, unless they do not respond to other therapy.

Other Renal Tubule–Inhibiting Diuretics

THEOBROMINE—see RPS-19, page 1050.

MISCELLANEOUS RENAL AGENT

PROBENECID

Benzoic acid, 4-[(dipropylamino)sulfonyl]-, Benemid

$$(CH_3CH_2CH_2)_2NSO_2—\langle\bigcirc\rangle—COOH$$

[57-66-9] $C_{13}H_{19}NO_4S$ (285.36).

Preparation—Oxidation of the methyl group of *p*-toluenesulfonyl chloride produces *p*-carboxybenzenesulfonic acid. This acid is then converted into the corresponding sulfonyl chloride by treatment with chlorosulfonic acid, which is condensed with di-*n*-propylamine (US Pat 2,608,507).

Description—White or nearly white, fine, crystalline powder; practically odorless; melts between 198° and 200°; pK_a 5.8.

Solubility—Soluble in alcohol, chloroform, or acetone; practically insoluble in water. Soluble in dilute aqueous alkali.

Comments—An agent that blocks both renal and CSF transport of weak acids. With respect to the inward renal transport, it is an effective *uricosuric* agent for the treatment of gout and gouty arthritis. It inhibits tubular reabsorption of urate at the proximal convoluted tubule, thus increasing urinary excretion of uric acid and decreasing serum uric acid levels. With regard to outward renal transport probenecid blocks secretion of weak organic acids at the proximal and distal tubules and is effective as an adjuvant therapy with penicillin G, O, or V, or with ampicillin, methicillin, oxacillin, cloxacillin, or nafcillin for elevation and prolongation of penicillin plasma levels by whatever route the antibiotic is given.

It inhibits the renal excretion and may increase the plasma levels of methotrexate, sulfonamides, sulfonylureas, naproxen, indomethacin, rifampin, aminosalicylic acid, dapsone, clofibrate, or pantothenic acid. Patients concurrently taking any of these agents should be monitored closely and the dosage regimen adjusted appropriately.

It is absorbed rapidly and completely after oral administration. Plasma levels of 100 to 200 µg/mL are necessary for an adequate uricosuric effect, whereas plasma levels of only 40 to 60 µg/mL produce maximal inhibition of penicillin excretion. Plasma levels of 25 µg/mL are reached 30 min after a single 1-g oral dose; plasma levels reach a peak in 2 to 4 hr and remain above 30 µg/mL for 8 hr. Following a single 2-g oral dose, peak plasma levels of 150 to 200 µg/mL are reached in 4 hr, and levels of 50 µg/mL are sustained for 8 hr; the plasma half-life ranges from 4 to 17 hr. At a plasma concentration of 14 µg/mL, about 17% of the drug is bound to plasma protein.

It is contraindicated in hypersensitive individuals, children under 2 years, and persons with known blood dyscrasias or uric acid stones. Therapy should not be started until an acute gouty attack has subsided. Exacerbation of gout following therapy may occur; in such cases, colchicine or other appropriate therapy is advisable. The drug should not be given with methotrexate, since plasma levels of the latter agent have been reported to be increased. Use of salicylates also is contraindicated because these substances antagonize the drug's uricosuric action. Patients who require a mild analgesic should be advised to use acetaminophen rather than salicylates. Probenecid is devoid of analgesic activity.

It is tolerated well, but an occasional patient may experience headache, anorexia, nausea, vomiting, urinary frequency, hypersensitivity reactions, sore gums, flushing, dizziness, and anemia. In gouty patients, exacerbation of gout and uric acid stones with or without hematuria, renal colic, and costovertebral pain have been observed. Nephrotic syndrome, hepatic necrosis, and aplastic anemia occur rarely. Hemolytic anemia, which in some cases could be related to genetic deficiencies of red blood cell glucose 6-phosphate dehydrogenase, has been reported.

REFERENCES

1. *Am J Med Sci* 2000; 319:51.
2. *Am J Med Sci* 2000; 319:38
3. *Kidney Int* 1979; 16:187.

MEDICINAL AGENTS

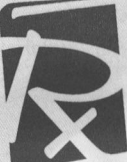

CHAPTER 76

Uterine and Antimigraine Drugs

John E Hoover, BSc Pharm, RPh

OXYTOCICS

Drugs that stimulate the smooth muscle of the uterus are known as oxytocics. Three chemical types of oxytocics are principally used clinically: (1) the oxytocic fraction (oxytocin) of the posterior pituitary extract, (2) certain ergot alkaloids (ergonovine), and (3) certain prostaglandins (dinoprostone). However, a number of other agents possess mild to intense oxytocic actions. Some of these (eg, hydrastis and quinine) have been used formerly but are now archaic. The main clinical uses of the oxytocics include (1) induction of abortion, (2) evacuation of the uterus in situations of incomplete abortions, (3) induction and augmentation of labor, and (4) involution of the uterus to normal during puerperium.

The response of the uterus to oxytocics depends on estrogenic and progestational hormonal influences. Progesterone hyperpolarizes the uterine smooth muscle and, thus, diminishes its responsiveness and coordination, while estrogen increases myometrial excitability. Consequently, and fortunately, during the first two terms of pregnancy, oxytocics generally are incapable of inducing labor. Late in the third term, as the progesterone levels decline and the estrogen influence increases, uterine responsiveness rises sharply in advance of pelvic relaxation, cervical dilatation, and the coordination of uterine contractions necessary for proper delivery of the fetus. The premature induction of labor by oxytocics can result in harm to both mother and infant and may result in stillbirth if premature separation of the placenta, placental vasoconstriction, or umbilical strangulation occur. Therefore, only under rare circumstances should oxytocics be used to induce labor; indeed, they generally are withheld during labor until the cervix is dilated and presentation of the fetus has occurred (ie, until the third stage of labor). The oxytocic then is given to hasten the delivery of the placenta and to diminish uterine bleeding by contractile compression of the blood sinuses and vasoconstriction. Oxytocics also may be employed during the puerperium to aid in the involution of the uterus to normal. Oxytocin promotes and facilitates the normal phasic contractions that are characteristic of normal delivery. The ergot alkaloids induce prolonged contractions or contracture, which may be detrimental to safe delivery, and hence, they are employed mainly in the third stage of labor to diminish bleeding. Prostaglandins, notably PGE_2 and PGF_2, promote normal-type phasic contractions. However, the effects of the prostaglandins are not so dependent on the estrogen-progesterone balance as those of oxytocin, so prostaglandins can induce labor considerably in advance of term and, hence, can be used to induce abortion.

CARBOPROST TROMETHAMINE

Prosta-5,13-dien-1-oic acid (5Z,9α,11α,13E,15S)-9,11,15-trihydroxy-15-methyl-, compound with 2-amino-2-(hydroxymethyl)-1,3-propanediol (1:1); Hemabate

(15S)-15-Methylprostaglandin $F_α$ tromethamine [58551-69-2] $C_{21}H_{36}O_5 \cdot C_4H_{11}NO_3$ (489.65).

Preparation—By a series of complex alterations on a prostaglandin precursor. See US Pat 3,728,382.

Comments—Dinoprost-like, with a longer duration of action.

DIHYDROERGOTAMINE MESYLATE

Ergotaman-3′,6′,18-trione, (5′α)-9,10-dihydro-12′-dihydroxy-2′-methyl-5′-(phenylmethyl)-, monomethanesulfonate (salt); DHE 45; Migranal

Dihydroergotamine monomethanesulfonate [6190-39-2] $C_{33}H_{37}N_5O_5 \cdot CH_4O_3S$ (679.79).

Preparation—Dihydroergotamine, prepared by catalytic hydrogenation of ergotamine, is reacted with an equimolar portion of methanesulfonic acid in a suitable solvent.

Description—White, yellowish, or faintly red powder; pH (1 in 1000 solution) between 4.4 and 5.4.

Solubility—1 g in 125 mL water, 90 mL alcohol, 175 mL chloroform, or 2600 mL ether.

Comments—A smooth muscle stimulant with somewhat weaker actions than ergotamine.

DINOPROSTONE

Prosta-5,13-dien-1-oic acid, (5Z,11α,13E,15S)-11,15-dihydroxy-9-oxo-, Cervidil; PGE₂; Prepidil; Prostin E₂

Prostaglandin E_2 [363-24-6] $C_{20}H_{32}O_5$ (352.47).

Preparation—The limited availability of the prostaglandins from natural sources has spurred efforts to synthesize them, and total synthesis of prostaglandins F_2 (dinoprost) and E_2 (dinoprostone) has been achieved. The complex syntheses are described in articles in *J Am Chem Soc* 1969; 91:5675; 1586, 1970; 92:397; 1972; 94:2123, 4342.

Description—Colorless crystals or white to off-white crystalline solid; melts between 66° and 68°.

Solubility—1 g in about 1000 mL water; soluble in alcohol.

Comments—It is one of a family of over 30 natural, partially cyclic, alkenoic acids, called prostaglandins, derived from arachidonic acid. They are involved in the regulation of endocrine, reproductive, secretory, digestive, nervous, cardiovascular, respiratory, renal, and hemostatic systems. Certain prostaglandins are involved in the cyclical changes in uterine tone and activity and the changes consequent to pregnancy. Furthermore, prostaglandins in semen stimulate the myometrium and fallopian tubes in a way that facilitates the transport of sperm to the ovum. Not all prostaglandins have the same actions; some are vasodilators and others vasoconstrictors, etc. Some prostaglandins, eg, prostaglandins E_2 (PGE$_2$, dinoprostone), are oxytocic and also induce cervical softening. Unlike oxytocin, they are oxytocic even in the second trimester of pregnancy and, hence, can be used as an early abortifacient. Dinoprostone is used to terminate pregnancy from the 12th week through the second trimester (80–90% effective), to evacuate the uterus in intrauterine fetal death or missed abortion up to 28 weeks after conception, and to manage benign hydatidiform mole. It also is used to induce labor in midtrimester and later, contract the postpartum uterus and, hence, decrease hemorrhage and ripen the cervix prior to curettage or abortion procedures.

Endovaginally, it may be absorbed sufficiently into the bloodstream to cause systemic side effects; some of the effects attributed to the drug possibly may be the result of hormonal changes and of release of substances from the fetoplacental unit or hydatidiform mole consequent to sloughing and movement or to movement itself. Adverse effects include the following: nausea and vomiting (67%), transient fever (50%; PGE$_2$ is the mediator of pyrogens), diarrhea (40%), headache (10%), chills and shivering (10%), hypotension (10%), backache, arthralgia, flushing, vertigo, vaginal pain, chest pain, dyspnea, endometritis, faintness, syncope, vulvovaginitis, asthenia, muscle cramps and myalgia, tightness in the chest, breast tenderness, blurred vision, cough, rash, stiff neck, dehydration, tremor, paresthesias, impaired hearing, urinary retention, pharyngitis, laryngitis, sweating, wheezing, tachycardia, skin discoloration, vaginismus, tension, and convulsions (rare). Also, it is not fetotoxic, and near the end of the second trimester a live fetus may be presented. Caution should be exercised when there is asthma or chronic obstructive pulmonary disease, hypotension, hypertension, other cardiovascular disease, renal or hepatic disease, anemia, jaundice, diabetes, a past history of epilepsy, endocervical disease, vaginitis, or cervicitis. It is contraindicated in acute pelvic inflammatory disease and when there is hypersensitivity to the drug.

ERGONOVINE MALEATE

Ergoline-8-carboxamide, [8β(S)]-9,10-didehydro-N-(2-hydroxy-1-methylethyl)-6-methyl-, (Z)-2-butenedioate (1:1) (salt); Ergometrine Maleate

9,10-Didehydro-N-[(S)-2-hydroxy-1-methylethyl]-6-methyl-ergoline-8β-carboxamine maleate (1:1) (salt) [129-51-1] $C_{19}H_{23}N_3O_2 \cdot C_4H_4O_4$ (441.48).

Preparation—May be prepared from the natural alkaloid ergonovine by dissolving the latter in a suitable solvent and reacting it with an equimolar portion of maleic acid.

Ergonovine alkaloid also is prepared synthetically from isolysergic acid obtained by alkaline hydrolysis of ergot alkaloids. One of the methods of synthesis involves the following steps: (1) conversion of the acid to its methyl ester by reaction with diazomethane; (2) hydrazinolysis of the ester to lysergic acid hydrazide; (3) condensation of the hydrazide with nitrous acid to form the azide; (4) metathesis of the azide with D-2-amino-1-propanol to form the amide; and (5) isomerization of the amide to the normal form by treatment with acetic or phosphoric acid.

Description—White to grayish white or faintly yellow, odorless, microcrystalline powder; affected by light.

Solubility—1 g in about 36 mL water or about 120 mL alcohol; insoluble in ether or chloroform.

Comments—Ergonovine is the most valued of the ergot alkaloids for obstetrical use. It is a powerful uterine stimulant and is active after either oral or parenteral administration. It is less toxic than the other natural alkaloids of ergot and is much less prone to cause gangrene. It is given after the delivery of the placenta for the purpose of inducing prolonged, nonphasic contractions of the uterus, to reduce postpartum bleeding. It also may be administered during the puerperium to promote involution of the uterus. In incomplete abortion, it may be used to accelerate the expulsion of the uterine contents. It constricts the cerebral vessels and, hence, is used in the treatment of migraine headache, but it is inferior for this purpose and not recommended. It constricts coronary arteries; in variant angina pectoris the arteries respond to otherwise ineffective doses, so low doses may be used in the diagnosis of variant angina pectoris.

It may cause nausea and vomiting, especially when given intravenously. Like other oxytocics, occasionally it evokes severe hypertensive episodes, especially in hypertensive or toxemic patients or when regional anesthetics containing vasoconstrictors have been used. Such hypertensive episodes can be suppressed by chlorpromazine. Hypersensitivity, including anaphylactic shock, has been reported.

It is contraindicated before the fetus has been presented and should not be used to induce or augment labor. In addition, ergonovine should not be used in persons with known allergy to ergot alkaloids, in uterine sepsis, toxemia of pregnancy, peripheral vascular disease, coronary insufficiency, or kidney or liver disease. It should be used cautiously if there is cardiac disease or hypertension. The actions are antagonized by hypocalcemia, and calcium gluconate can be used judiciously to improve the response.

When used properly, there is little problem with adverse side effects; however, high doses administered by the IV route can cause nausea and vomiting, headaches, tinnitus, dyspnea, muscle cramps, nasal congestion, diarrhea, and a foul taste.

METHYLERGONOVINE MALEATE

Ergoline-8-carboxamide, [8β(S)]-9,10-didehydro-N-[1-(hydroxymethyl)propyl]-6-methyl-, (Z)-2-butenedioate (1:1) (salt); Methergine; Methylergometrine Maleate

9,10-Didehydro-N-[(S)-1-(hydroxymethyl)propyl]-6-methyl-ergoline-8β-carboxamide maleate (1:1) (salt) [7054-07-1] [57432-61-8] $C_{20}H_{25}N_3O_2 \cdot C_4H_4O_4$ (455.51).

Preparation—Synthesized by the method described above for ergonovine except that in step (4), D-2-amino-1-butanol is employed. The base, dissolved in a suitable solvent, yields the maleate by reaction with an equimolar quantity of maleic acid.

Description—White to pinkish tan, microcrystalline powder; odorless and a bitter taste; must be protected from light and heat; pH (1 in 5000 solution) between 4.4 and 5.2.

Solubility—1 g in 100 mL water, 175 mL alcohol, 1900 mL chloroform, or 8400 mL ether.

Comments—Has actions similar to those of ergonovine.

MIFEPRISTONE

11β,17β-Estra-4,9-dien-3-one, 11-[4-(diethylamino)phenyl]-17-hydroxy-17-(1-propynyl)-; Mifeprex

[84371-65-3] $C_{29}H_{35}NO_2$ (429.59).

Preparation—In a multi-step synthesis from 3,3-ethylenendioxy)estra-5(10),9(11)-diene-17-one.[1,2]

Description—Yellow powder melting about 150°; $[\alpha]_D^{20} = 139°$ (c = 0.5, CHCl$_3$)[1]; melting range[3] 191–196°.

Solubility—Very soluble in methanol, chloroform, or acetone, poorly soluble in water, hexane, or isopropyl ether.

Comments—Its antiprogestational activity results from competition interaction with progesterone at progesterone-receptor sites. Based on studies with various oral doses in several animal species (mouse, rat, rabbit, and monkey), the compound inhibits the activity of endogenous or exogenous progesterone. The termination of pregnancy results.

OXYTOCIN

Alpha-Hypophamine; Pitocin

H-Cys-Tyr-Ile-Glu(NH$_2$)-Asp(NH$_2$)-Cys-Pro-Leu-Gly-NH$_2$
   1   2   3   4   5   6   7   8   9

[50-56-6] $C_{43}H_{66}N_{12}O_{12}S_2$ (1007.19).

Preparation—Obtained from the posterior lobe of the pituitary of healthy hogs or cattle; from either source it has the same amino acid

1. *Drugs of the Future* 1994; 9:755.
2. US Pat 4,386,085 (1982).
3. Danco Labs LLC, FDA label information.

USP Units in gelatin medium possess the approximate clinical efficacy of 40 USP Units of aqueous solution by intermittent intramuscular injection.

Description—White or practically white, soluble, amorphous solid with the characteristic appearance of substances prepared by freeze-drying; pH (of the liquid form or after reconstitution from the solid state) between 3 and 7.

Comments—Stimulates the adrenal gland to produce hydrocortisone, desoxycorticosterone, and androgens. It is used as a diagnostic drug to assess the functional capacity of the adrenal gland. After injection, a rise in plasma cortisol or urinary 17-hydroxycorticosterone indicates a functional gland. This is at present the most important clinical use of this agent. This drug has been promoted as a therapeutic agent in a wide variety of glucocorticoid-responsive disorders. In general, with the exception of primary adrenal insufficiency, it is effective in all of the conditions for which glucocorticoids are found useful, but it is ineffective when applied locally. The continued administration of large amounts of the hormone may result in one or more of the manifestations of Cushing's syndrome, may exacerbate the symptoms of latent or frank diabetes, and, because of its anti-inflammatory action, may mask symptoms of infection. The need for adequate medical supervision during its use, therefore, cannot be overemphasized. They occur frequently when the dosage exceeds 40 Units a day.

Abrupt cessation of corticotrin injections may be followed by withdrawal effects that take the form of symptoms of adrenal insufficiency. These result from pituitary inhibition that occurs during treatment with corticotrin and may be minimized or eliminated by gradually reducing the amount injected. Corticotrin causes some side effects not caused by glucocorticoids, namely, hypersensitivity, salt and water retention, and androgenic effects (acne, hirsutism, and amenorrhea) in women. It is contraindicated if there is osteoporosis, systemic mycosis, corneal herpes, or scleroderma.

ENTACAPONE—page 1419.

GONADORELIN ACETATE

Luteinizing hormone–releasing factor acetate (salt) hydrate; LH-RH; Lutrepulse

$$5\text{-oxoPro-His-Trp-Ser-Tyr-Gly-Leu-Arg-Pro-Gly-NH}_2 \cdot x C_2H_4O_2 \cdot y H_2O$$

[52699-48-6] $C_{55}H_{75}N_{17}O_{13} \cdot xC_2H_4O_2 \cdot yH_2O$

Preparation—By synthesis or from the hypothalamus, *Science* 1973; 179:34.

Description—Faint-yellow powder.

Solubility—1 g in 25 mL water, 50 mL methanol, or 25 mL 1% acetic acid.

Comments—Identical to natural GnRH. Gonadorelin is used in the treatment of primary hypothalamic amenorrhea. Gonadorelin hydrochloride (Factrel, *Ayerst*) is a related preparation and is used as a diagnostic agent to determine whether hypogonadism is the result of a defect in anterior pituitary release of LH or in hypothalamic release of LH-RH. If gonadorelin evokes a rise in LH levels, the disturbance is in the hypothalamus; if it does not, the disturbance is in the anterior pituitary. Administered in pulsatile fashion, it evokes secretion of both FSH and LH. However, if plasma levels remain high for periods longer than a few hours, preceptor down-regulation occurs. LH receptors are affected more than FSH receptors. By careful selection of dose regimen it is thus possible to increase or decrease male or female fertility, in the latter instance without marked changes in estrogen secretion.

Local swelling, itching, or pain and occasional rash at the injection site may occur after subcutaneous injection. Headache, nausea, lightheadedness, abdominal discomfort, and rare flushing may occur. It does not cause multiple births.

LEUPROLIDE—page 1577.
LEVODOPA/CARBIDOPA—pages 1418 and 1419.

MENOTROPINS

Pergonal

Menotropins [9002-68-6]; an extract of postmenopausal urine containing the follicle-stimulating hormone (FSH) and luteinizing hormone (LH) in a 1:1 ratio.

Comments—Has the gonadotropic activities of FSH and LH It is used to induce ovulation in women with infertility consequent to insufficient endogenous production of gonadotropins. HCG is given following menotropins. Clinical experience is that about 75% of anovulatory women ovulate after treatment, and 25% become pregnant after two courses of treatment. Multiple gestation occurs in about 15% to 30% of completed pregnancies. The hyperstimulation syndrome occurs in 1% to 2% of cases.

It also is used concomitantly with HCG for >3 months to induce spermatogenesis in men with hypogonadotropic hypogonadism.

Side effects include ovarian enlargement, flatulence, abdominal discomfort, oliguria, weight gain, ascites, pleural effusion, hypotension, and hypercoagulability; these are all evidence of hyperstimulation. Other adverse reactions include arterial thromboembolism, hypersensitivity, and febrile reactions. Birth defects occurred in 5 of 287 pregnancies. Occasionally, ovarian rupture and intraperitoneal hemorrhage occur, and surgery is required.

NAFARELIN ACETATE

Luteinizing hormone-releasing factor (pig), 6-[3-(2-naphthadenyl)-D-alanine, acetate (salt), hydrate; Synarel

H-5-oxo-L-Pro-L-His-L-Trp-L-Ser-L-Tyr—N---C---C—
L-Leu-L-Arg-L-Pro-Gly—NH$_2$ • xCH$_3$COOH • yH$_2$O

[86620-42-0] $C_{66}H_{83}N_{17}O_{13} \cdot xC_2H_4O_2 \cdot yH_2O$.

Preparation—US Pat 4,234,571.

Comments—An agonist for LH-RH receptors. However, the duration of action is too long for pulsatile dosing, so the effect of repetitive administration is that of down-regulation of LH-RH receptors. It has been found to be effective in the treatment of endometriosis and central precocious puberty. In women, adverse effects are those of hypoestrogenemia, namely, hot flashes, vaginal dryness, decreased libido, and a moderate decrease in trabecular bone mineralization in the spine in about 67% of patients. In men, weight gain, hot flashes, decreased libido, and decreased drive and initiative occur. These effects disappear after discontinuation of the drug. It is absorbed rapidly by the intranasal but not sublingual route. Intranasal bioavailability is about 21%. The drug is metabolized to at least six metabolites. The half-life is about 2 hr.

OCTREOTIDE

L-Cysteinamide, [R-(R*,R*)]-D-phenylalanyl-L-cysteinyl-L-phenyl-alanyl-D-tryptophyl-L-threonyl-N-[2-hydroxy-1-(hydroxy-methyl)propyl]-, cyclic (2 → 7)-disulfide; Sandostatin, Sandostatin LAR

S————————S
H—D-Phe-Cys-Phe-D-Trp-Lys-Thr-Cys-Thr-ol

[83150-76-9] $C_{49}H_{66}N_{10}O_{10}S_2$ (1019.24).

Preparation—US Pat 4,395,403.

Comments—An analog of somatostatin that differs in that it inhibits growth hormone secretion in lower doses than affect insulin secretion, it is long acting (2-hr half-life), there is no rebound hypersecretion after discontinuation, and it is orally effective. It is approved for symptomatic treatment of carcinoid tumors and profuse diarrhea associated with vasoactive intestinal peptide tumors (lipomas, vipomas). In light of octreotide's short half-life a depot injection (Sandostatin LAR) was formulated for chronic use of carcinoid tumors and vipomas and can be administered every 4 weeks. However, patients should be stabilized on subcutaneous octreotide for 2 weeks prior to switching to the long-acting intramuscular depot injection.

The drug is tolerated well. During the first few days of treatment there are flatulence, loose stools, diarrhea, and abdominal pains. A mild steatorrhea occurs in some patients and may persist during treatment or disappear in a few days. Malabsorption does not occur. There may be a moderate decrease in postprandial glucose tolerance, but no complications have been recorded.

PERGOLIDE MESYLATE—page 1420.
PRAMIPEXOLE—page 1420.
ROPINIROLE—page 1421.

SOMATREM AND SOMATROPIN

N-L-Methionylsomatotropin (human); Protropin
[82030-87-3] $C_{995}H_{1537}N_{263}O_{301}S_8$ (22,256.21)

SOMATROPIN

Genotropin, Humatrope, Nutropin

Growth hormone, human; somatotropin (human) [12629-01-5] $C_{990}H_{1528}N_{262}O_{300}S_7$ (21,500.00)

Preparation—A single polypeptide chain of 191 amino acids once obtained from the anterior lobe of the human pituitary gland. See US Pat 3,118,815.

Comments—Both somatrem and somatropin products are from recombinant DNA–directed syntheses. Somatropin is identical to human pituitary–derived somatropin. Somatrem (Protropin) is identical to natural growth hormone except it contains an additional methionine on the *N*-terminus of the molecule. However, the effects and potencies are identical; therefore, both peptides are considered together. Somatropin from pituitary extracts was discontinued because of reports that its use was sometimes the cause of Creutzfeldt-Jakob disease. For description, actions, and uses see *Growth Hormone.*

Intramuscular administration of the hormone is preferred to subcutaneous injection because the hormone causes lipodystrophy or lipoatrophy at the cutaneous injection site. Pain and swelling usually occur on injection, so sites should be rotated. Hypercalciuria occurs frequently but usually regresses in 2 to 3 months. Hyperglycemia and frank diabetes mellitus due to insulin resistance may occur. Myalgia and early morning headaches are relatively frequent. Antibodies to the hormone may be found in 30% to 40% of recipients given somatrem, but patients rarely fail to respond to therapy. Approximately 2% of patients receiving somatropin developed antibodies, but growth responses have not been limited in such patients. Occasionally, somatotropin causes hypothyroidism. If the epiphyses are closed, the hormone should not be used because continued stimulation of growth of the phalanges and jawbone, but not other bones, can cause abnormal body proportions. Available products are exceedingly expensive.

THE POSTERIOR PITUITARY (NEUROHYPOPHYSIS)

The posterior pituitary contains two peptide hormones, oxytocin and vasopressin. Neither is made in the posterior pituitary, but rather they are synthesized in neurons in the hypothalamus. Oxytocin is synthesized in the paraventricular nucleus, and vasopressin in the supraoptic nucleus. The axons of the hormone-secreting nerve cells pass from the hypothalamus to the internal infundibular zone of the posterior pituitary (hence the name neurohypophysis). The hormones flow down the axons as granules or vesicles composed of a hormone and a carrier protein called neurophysin. Their release at the nerve terminals is effected by nerve impulses. Thus, the control of release is actually in the appropriate hypothalamic nuclei.

Human and most mammalian vasopressin is Cys-Tyr-Phe-Gln-Asn-Cys-Pro-Arg-GlyNH$_2$, called arginine vasopressin. An exception is pigs whose vasopressin called lypressin contains lysine at position 8. Vasopressin possesses antidiuretic hormone (ADH) and vasopressor activities. The ADH activity decreases urine flow by increasing the resorption of water from the distal convoluted tubules and collecting ducts of the kidney. The effect is a decrease in the osmolarity of the extracellular fluid.

When there is a defect in the hypothalamic-pituitary secretion of ADH, diabetes insipidus results in a watery diuresis. Vasopressin is used mainly for its antidiuretic effects in this disease rather than for its vasoconstrictor actions, from which the name vasopressin is derived. However, not only does vasopressin stimulate vascular smooth muscle, but also it increases bowel motility, and it has been used to treat bowel stasis and to expel gas postsurgically. The vasoconstrictor and bowel spastic actions have special usefulness in arresting hemorrhage from peptic ulcers. The smooth muscle stimulant effects occur with higher doses than are necessary to affect renal function. Vasopressin also has weak oxytocic activity. Vasopressin has a brief half-life (less than 20 min).

Oxytocin stimulates the contraction of smooth muscle in the uterus and alveoli of the lactating breast. At coitus, uterine stimulation by oxytocin causes peristaltic activity that assists the migration of spermatozoa. During parturition, the hormone enhances the uterine contractions. The uses of oxytocin in labor and breast engorgement are described in Chapter 76. Neither vasopressin nor oxytocin survives the acid and enzymes of the gastrointestinal (GI) tract, so they must be given parenterally or intranasally.

Each of the octapeptides has been synthesized. Oxytocin has the structure

Oxytocin

The structure of vasopressin from human, monkey, dog, cat, ox, camel, rabbit, and rat pituitaries is identical with that of oxytocin, except that the isoleucine and leucine residues are replaced by residues of phenylalanine and arginine, respectively. The successful synthesis of the naturally occurring posterior lobe hormones has provided the impetus for the synthesis of a number of analogs of both oxytocin and vasopressin. Thus, substances in which one or more of the amino acids of the native hormones have been replaced by others or that contain fewer or additional amino acid residues have been prepared, and their pharmacological properties explored. One of these was the compound vasotocin, containing the pentapeptide ring of oxytocin and the tripeptide side chain of vasopressin. This substance possesses the biological properties of both neurohypophyseal hormones, although in lesser degree. Synthetic analogs of oxytocin and vasopressin, in which one or more of the amino acids of the native hormones have been replaced, are named by using numbers to denote the alterations represented in the synthetic. A synthetic vasopressin in which the moiety at position 8 is arginine is named simply 8-arginine vasopressin.

DESMOPRESSIN ACETATE

Vasopressin, 1-(3-mercaptopropionic acid)-8-D-arginine, monoacetate (salt), trihydrate; DDVAP; Stimate

[62357-86-2] C$_{48}$H$_{68}$N$_{14}$O$_{14}$S$_2$·3H$_2$O (1183.22).

Preparation—A synthetic analog of 8-arginine vasopressin in which the amino group has been removed from the *N*-terminal cysteine and L-arginine at position 8 has been replaced by the D-enantiomer. *Helv Chim Acta* 1966; 49:695.

Description—White fluffy powder; pK$_a$ (gly-NH$_2$) 4.8.

Solubility—Soluble in alcohol or water.

Comments—Used in the treatment of central *(neurogenic)* diabetes insipidus. It also is used to test the ability of the kidney to concentrate urine. Since the hormone can raise the plasma levels of Factor VIII (antihemophilic factor), it is sometimes used to treat Factor VIII bleeding disorders and to increase Factor VIII levels prior to surgery. It may be used alone or as an adjunct for some refractory cases of primary nocturnal enuresis.

Headache, mild hypertension, nasal congestion, mild abdominal cramping, water intoxication, and vulval pain sometimes occur. Chlorpropamide and clofibrate potentiate, and glyburide inhibits, antidiuretic action.

VASOPRESSIN

Beta-Hypophamine; Pitressin

$$\text{Lys}-\text{Tyr}-\text{Phe}-\text{Glu}-\text{Asp}-\text{Cys}-\text{Pro}-\overset{*}{\text{Arg}}-\text{Gly}-\text{NH}_2$$
$$1 \quad\;\; 2 \quad\;\; 3 \quad\;\; 4 \quad\;\; 5 \quad\;\; 6 \quad\;\; 7 \quad\;\; 8 \quad\;\; 9$$

(* in pig vasopressin, Arg is Lys)

8-L-Lysine (or arginine) vasopressin: Lysine form-[50-57-7] $C_{46}H_{65}N_{13}O_{12}S_2$ (1056.22); Arginine form-[113-79-1] $C_{46}H_{65}N_{15}O_{12}S_2$ (1084.23).

Comments—Its actions are discussed on page ____. It is employed for its antidiuretic effect in central diabetes insipidus and to dispel gas shadows in bowel roentgenography and pyelography. It should not be used as a pressor agent.

Untoward effects related to overdosage include water intoxication (with headache, nausea and vomiting, confusion, lethargy, coma, and convulsions), especially when patients drink excessive amounts of water or are given intravenous fluids, and stimulation of vascular, uterine, and intestinal smooth muscle, which may result in pallor, hypertension, coronary constriction (with anginal chest pain, electrocardiographic changes, and occasional myocardial infarction), uterine cramps, menorrhagia, and nausea, vomiting, diarrhea, and abdominal cramps. Hypersensitivity occasionally occurs; manifestations include urticaria, neurodermatitis, flushing, fever, wheezing, dyspnea, and rare anaphylactic shock. Large doses are oxytocic and also cause milk ejection. Alcohol, heparin, demeclocycline, lithium, and large doses of epinephrine antagonize it; carbamazepine, chlorpropamide, clofibrate, glucocorticoids, and urea potentiate it.

The plasma half-life is 10 to 20 min. However, the effect of an intramuscular injection lasts from 2 to 8 hr. From 10% to 15% is excreted unchanged. Vasopressin tannate is also available as a longer-acting preparation.

THE ADRENOCORTICAL STEROIDS

The steroid hormone products of the adrenal cortex are grouped into two classes: the corticosteroids (glucocorticoids and mineralocorticoids), which have 21 carbons, and the androgens, which have 19. Adrenal corticosteroids differ in their relative glucocorticoid (carbohydrate-regulating) and mineralocorticoid (electrolyte-regulating) activities. In humans hydrocortisone (cortisol) is the main glucocorticoid and aldosterone is the main mineralocorticoid. The cortex, or outer portion, of the adrenal gland is one of the endocrine structures most vital for normal metabolic function. While it is possible for life to continue in the complete absence of adrenal cortical function, serious metabolic derangements ensue, and the capacity of the organism to respond to physiological or environmental stress is lost completely.

PHYSIOLOGICAL ACTIONS—Adrenocortical steroids have diverse effects that include alterations in carbohydrate, protein, and lipid metabolism; maintenance of fluid and electrolyte balance; and preservation of normal function of the cardiovascular system, the immune system, the kidney, skeletal muscle, the endocrine system, and the nervous system. One of the major pharmacological uses of this class of drugs is based on their anti-inflammatory and immunosuppressive actions. A protective role for cortisol is apparent in the physiological response to severe stress that can increase daily production over 10-fold. Furthermore, many immune mediators associated with the inflammatory response can lead to decreased vascular tone and cardiovascular collapse if unopposed by adrenal corticosteroids. The relative or complete absence of adrenocortical function, known as Addison's disease, is accompanied by loss of sodium chloride and water, retention of potassium, lowering of blood-glucose and liver-glycogen levels, increased sensitivity to insulin, nitrogen retention, and lymphocytosis. The disturbances in electrolyte metabolism are the cause of morbidity and mortality in most cases of severe adrenal insufficiency. All of these disorders may be corrected by administration of adrenal cortical extract or the pure adrenal cortical steroids now available.

In its biosynthesis of the steroid hormones, the adrenal cortex uses cholesterol, which is present in large amounts in the gland; during periods of secretory activity it also consumes large quantities of ascorbic acid, which is likewise present in high concentration. The synthesis and secretion of the gluco-

corticoids (essentially hydrocortisone) takes place in the zona fasciculata. Corticotropin (ACTH) is the primary stimulus to hydrocortisone secretion. ACTH is released in response to the hypothalamic hormone CRH (see page ____). Glucocorticoid secretion, then, is regulated through suprahypothalamic and hypothalamic nuclei, which integrate responses to sensory, emotional, and chemical inputs, including the glucocorticoids themselves, and the basophilic cells of the adenohypophysis, release from which is suppressed by circulating glucocorticoids. Physical (injury, surgery, etc.) and emotional stress and hypoglycemia increase secretion. Synthesis in the zona fasciculata can be altered by drugs that inhibit specific enzymes involved. CRH, ACTH, and glucocorticoid release follows a circadian rhythm such that blood concentrations of hydrocortisone are highest between 6 and 8 AM and lowest around midnight.

The synthesis and release of the mineralocorticoid aldosterone takes place in the zona glomerulosa. ACTH has only a slight effect on secretion. Rather, angiotensins II and III are the primary stimulants, although hyperkalemia is also an important stimulus. The production of the angiotensins is under renal, CNS, and sympathetic nervous system control. In the kidney, the macula densa around the juxtaglomerular distal tubules monitors Na^+ and Cl^- concentrations and luminal osmolarity. Low Na^+ concentration and osmolarity or high Cl^- causes signals to be sent to the juxtaglomerular (JG) cells in the afferent arterioles, which then release renin. Renin secretion also is increased by low blood pressure at the JG cells and by sympathetic impulses, which work through β_1-adrenoreceptors. Renin then cleaves angiotensin I from angiotensinogen, both locally and in the blood. Angiotensin I is converted to angiotensin II by a converting enzyme (CE or kininase II), mainly in the lung. (Angiotensin III is a metabolite of II.) Thus, a variety of electrolyte, emotional, cardiovascular, and drug factors can affect aldosterone secretion indirectly.

STRUCTURE-ACTIVITY RELATIONSHIP—Clinical experience has indicated that the anti-inflammatory activity of adrenal cortical steroids in man correlates well with their glucocorticoid activity. The undesirable side effects of sodium retention and edema are associated with mineralocorticoid activity. Synthetic steroids possessing higher glucocorticoid and lower mineralocorticoid activity than cortisone or cortisol have been prepared and marketed. A comparison of some commonly used systemic corticosteroids is included in Table 77-2.

All adrenal corticoids require the 3-keto group and 4,5 unsaturation. Additional unsaturation in Ring A enhances the anti-inflammatory properties while at the same time reducing the sodium-retaining effect. The presence of oxygen at position 11 is necessary for significant glucocorticoid activity; the 11β-hydroxy group is more potent than the 11-keto group; the 11-keto group is converted to the active β-hydroxy group in the body. The 17α-hydroxy group also is important to glucocorticoid activity. Introduction of either a methyl or hydroxyl group at position 16 markedly reduces mineralocorticoid activity but only slightly decreases glucocorticoid and anti-inflammatory activity. The 9α-fluoro group enhances both glucocorticoid and mineralocorticoid activities, but the effects of substituents at the 6 and 16 positions override this effect.

BIOLOGICAL ACTIVITY—The glucocorticoids appear to affect all cells, although not all in the same way. Clinical interest primarily focuses on their anti-inflammatory and immunosuppressant effects. They prevent release of various lytic enzymes that extend tissue damage during inflammation and generate leukotactic substances. Glucocorticoids decrease phagocytosis by macrophages. Anti-inflammatory effects include the retardation of the migration of polymorphonuclear leukocytes, suppression of repair and granulation, reduction in the erythrocyte sedimentation rate, decreased fibrinogenesis, and diminished elaboration of C-reactive protein. Glucocorticoids suppress the production of cytokines (eg, IL-1, IL-6, interferon gamma, TNF-alpha, and others) by inflammatory cells (eg, monocytes, macrophages, and lymphocytes) that recruit eosinophils. They also decrease lipid eicosanoid and prostaglandin production by inhibiting the

Table 77-2. Major Adrenal Corticosteroids[a]

DRUG	RELATIVE ACTIVITY			DOSAGE FORM
	ANTI-INFLAM	TOPICAL	NA + RET	
Short- to medium-acting glucocorticoids				
Hydrocortisone (Cortisol)	1	1	1	Oral, Inj, Top
Cortisone	0.8	0	0.8	Oral, Inj, Top
Prednisone	4	0	0.3	Oral
Prednisolone	5	4	0.3	Oral, Inj, Top
Methylprednisolone	5	5	0	Oral, Inj, Top
Intermediate-acting glucocorticoids				
Triamcinolone	5	5–100	0	Oral, Inj, Top
Fluprednisolone	15	7	0	Oral
Long-acting glucocorticoids				
Betamethasone	25–40	10	0	Oral, Inj, Top
Dexamethasone	30	10–40	0	Oral, Inj, Top
Mineralocorticoids				
Fludrocortisone	10	10	250	Oral, Inj, Top
Desoxycorticosterone acetate	0	0	20	Inj, pellets

[a]Legend: Relative activity, potency relative to hydrocortisone; anti-inflammatory, anti-inflam; sodium retention, Na + Ret; Injection, Inj; topical, Top.

production of cytokines that induce cyclooxygenase-II in inflammatory cells. The immunosuppressant effects may be partly the result of the suppression of phagocytosis, gene expression of cytokines and a decrease in the number of eosinophils and lymphocytes, suppression of delayed hypersensitivity reactions, decrease in tissue reaction to antigen-antibody interactions, and reduction in plasma immunoglobulins.

Effects on carbohydrate, fat, and protein metabolism are responsible for both beneficial and untoward effects. These hormones increase hepatic gluconeogenesis and glycogen deposition, both lipolysis and lipogenesis (but increase fat deposition at only a few specialized sites), and protein catabolism in various tissues (especially skeletal muscle).

In addition to the above-mentioned changes brought about by glucocorticoids are the so-called permissive effects. In these, the steroids do not themselves cause change but physiological amounts are required for certain organs or structures to respond to stimuli. For example, neither the kidney can respond to a water load nor the arterioles to epinephrine in the absence of adequate levels of glucocorticoids.

Once a glucocorticoid hormone has permeated a cell membrane, it combines with a cytosolic glucocorticoid receptor that is inactive because it is bound to some specific proteins, including some heat shock proteins that prevent them from reaching the nucleus and binding to DNA. The glucocorticoid-receptor complex undergoes conformational changes that allow dissociation from the heat shock proteins and other immunomodulatory proteins, then it is translocated to the cell nucleus, where it attaches to glucocorticoid receptor elements in the DNA. The result is an enhancement or reduction of the gene transcription that leads to an increased or decreased synthesis of certain proteins. Other transcription factors also interact at the same DNA binding sites. The protein produced is determined, in part, by the glucocorticoid receptor, of which there is more than one kind within the cell. There are estimated to be from 10 to 100 glucocorticoid target genes per cell, but not all of them are expressed in every cell. Tissue selectivity for different steroid hormones seems to be considerably determined by steroid-metabolizing enzymes that differentially alter intracellular steroids that upon transport to the nucleus bind to specific hormone response elements in the DNA.

Mineralocorticoids act on the distal tubules and collecting ducts of the kidney to increase the expression of genes that encode for proteins that enhance reabsorption of Na^+ from the tubular fluid. The effects on electrolytes are associated with an increase in the number of open Na^+ and K^+ channels in the luminal membrane tubular cells, and they increase the activity of basolateral membrane Na^+/K^+-activated ATPase. The net result is a return of Na^+ to the systemic circulation in exchange for K^+. Similar electrolyte effects are promoted by mineralocor-

ticoids in other tissues (eg, colon, salivary glands, and sweat glands).

Glucocorticoids also inhibit membrane lipid peroxidation, which possibly contributes to the salutary effects in brain edema; the effect appears to be one of decreasing the activity of membrane-bound, superoxide radical-generating mixed-function enzymes. Possibly related is an action to block phospholipase-A2, which prevents the release of arachidonic acid from membrane phospholipids and its subsequent conversion to eicosanoids. This inhibitory effect results from the production of an inhibitory protein, lipocortin, in leukocytes.

The primary effects of mineralocorticoids are on cortical collecting tubule cells in the kidney to increase sodium reabsorption and potassium secretion. Thus, elevated aldosterone titers cause sodium retention and potassium depletion with accompanying volume expansion and weight gain, hypertension, and metabolic alkalosis.

SIDE EFFECTS—Certain side effects may appear during the first week of treatment with glucocorticoids; they include euphoria and a rare paradoxical suicidal depression, psychoses (especially with high doses), hypertension (rare), anorexia, occasional hyperglycemia, colonic ulceration (rare), increased susceptibility to infections (especially viral infections, fungal infections, tuberculosis), and acne. After 7 to 10 days of treatment, the pituitary release of ACTH is suppressed, and the adrenal secretion of cortisol is temporarily inadequate once glucocorticoid administration ceases. In the case of a medical emergency, the depressed pituitary-adrenal response may make the patient unable to respond to stress. Additional exogenous corticosteroid is given in a dosage and for a duration appropriate for the severity of the stress. Consequently, patients on high-dose or long-term treatment should carry identification stating that they are under treatment with corticosteroids. Withdrawal of corticosteroids should be slow.

From the first week through the first year of therapy, additional side effects may appear, namely, fat redistribution to the nape of the neck *(buffalo hump)* and lower abdomen, diabetes mellitus and hyperglycemia, *moon face* and other edematous states, and renal potassium loss (from mineralocorticoid activity), alkalosis, additional infections (including tuberculosis), papilledema, glaucoma, posterior subcapsular cataracts, diplopia, 6th nerve palsies, osteoporosis, myopathy, ecchymoses and purpura, and cutaneous striae. After prolonged suppression of the anterior pituitary secretion of ACTH, there may be a permanent defect in pituitary-adrenal function. Continuous or repetitive use of glucocorticoids may cause painless joint destruction, especially if the drug is given intra-articularly. After prolonged glucocorticoid therapy, additional untoward effects include bone fractures and vertebral collapse (from marked osteoporosis), hyperlipidemia, and possible premature atherosclerosis.

MEDICINAL AGENTS

Adverse effects of glucocorticoids applied to the skin include stinging or burning sensations, itching, irritation, dryness, scaliness, vasoconstriction, folliculitis, acne, bacterial or yeast infections, hypopigmentation, atrophy, and striae. Systemic effects also can occur, especially if occlusive dressings are used. Topical ophthalmological glucocorticoids not only may cause serious exacerbations of viral, fungal, and bacterial infections of the eye but also glaucoma. From all of the above, it can be seen that glucocorticoids are drugs that have numerous and potentially serious side effects.

Because the mineralocorticoids are used mainly in physiological doses for replacement therapy, untoward effects are usually infrequent and mild. Sodium and water retention (with *moon face*), potassium loss, alkalosis, and hypertension can occur with excessive doses.

DRUG INTERACTIONS—Glucocorticoids decrease the hypoglycemic activity of insulin and oral hypoglycemics, so that a change in dose of the antidiabetic drugs may be necessitated. In high doses, glucocorticoids also decrease the response to somatotropin. The usual doses of mineralocorticoids and large doses of some glucocorticoids cause hypokalemia and may exaggerate the hypokalemic effects of thiazide and high-ceiling diuretics. In combination with amphotericin B they also may cause hypokalemia. Glucocorticoids appear to enhance the ulcerogenic effects of nonsteroidal anti-inflammatory drugs (NSAIDs). They decrease the plasma levels of salicylates, and salicylism may occur on discontinuing steroids. Glucocorticoids may increase or decrease the effects of prothrombopenic anticoagulants. Estrogens, phenobarbital, phenytoin, and rifampin increase the metabolic clearance of adrenal corticosteroids and hence necessitate dose adjustments.

PRECAUTIONS AND CONTRAINDICATIONS—Both glucocorticoids and mineralocorticoids must be used cautiously in congestive heart failure, hypertension, liver failure, renal failure, or nephrolithiasis. When glucocorticoids are used in persons with emotional instability or psychotic tendencies, hyperlipidemia, diabetes mellitus, hypothyroidism, myasthenia gravis, osteoporosis, peptic ulcer, ulcerative colitis, chronic infections (especially tuberculosis or a positive test), or a history of herpetic infections, patients should be monitored frequently for untoward effects. Topical application to the eye is absolutely contraindicated in the presence of ophthalmological infections.

PHARMACOKINETICS—Most corticosteroids are absorbed rapidly and completely from the GI tract. Some corticosteroids (hydrocortisone and some inhaled congeners including beclomethasone and budesonide) are rapidly inactivated by metabolism as they pass through the liver. Thus, some corticosteroids must be given parenterally for systemic effects. Esterification with large hydrophobic organic acids decreases solubility and therefore slows systemic absorption from sites of injection. Esterification with water-soluble acids, such as phosphoric or succinic, increases the rate of absorption from injection sites and even may permit intravenous administration. All of the glucocorticoids are absorbed from the skin, but some slowly enough that metabolic destruction can limit systemic accumulation. Many glucocorticoids also are metabolized in the skin. Fluorination at the 9-position and various substituents at the 17-position make glucocorticoids resistant to local destruction and hence make these derivatives more likely to cause systemic effects.

In the plasma, corticosteroids are bound to both corticosteroid-binding globulin (CBG, transcortin, α_1-macroglobulin) and albumin, which serve as transport vehicles. The extent of binding varies among the steroids. Various drugs and diseases can affect the concentration of transport proteins and their capacities. Corticoids cross the placental barrier and may cause congenital malformations. They also appear in breast milk and may suppress growth of the infant. The action of a steroid-receptor complex at the genes long outlasts significant plasma concentrations of the steroid, so that the plasma half-life has little relevance to a dosage regimen. Instead, a parameter known as the biological half-life is the primary determinant of dosage intervals.

THERAPEUTIC USES—The adrenal corticosteroids are used for replacement therapy in adrenal insufficiency (eg, Addison's disease and congenital adrenal hyperplasia). In this use, toxic effects are infrequent, since the aim is to approximate the equivalent of physiological body concentrations. Both mineralocorticoids and glucocorticoids may be required. Glucocorticoids additionally are used to treat rheumatic, inflammatory, allergic, neoplastic, and other disorders; the effects are palliative only and do not eradicate the underlying disorders. It is necessary to use supraphysiological doses, so some untoward effects are unavoidable.

The anti-inflammatory actions of the glucocorticoids are employed in the treatment of noninfectious acute ocular inflammation and certain infectious inflammations, especially in combination with antibiotics. Glucocorticoids are of value in decreasing some cerebral edemas (eg, vasogenic). Their value in the treatment of bacterial meningitis probably accrues to decreased permeability of the blood-brain barrier plus inhibition of cytokine production, especially tumor necrosis factor (TNF-alpha).

In serious acute allergic disorders, systemic glucocorticoids may be indicated; they should not be used chronically in allergic disorders, except in acute flare-ups. However, potent topical corticosteroids are now regularly used by inhalation for chronic treatment of bronchial asthma and intranasally for chronic noninfectious rhinitis (see *Respiratory Drugs* in Chapter 69). Similarly, acute bronchial asthma, status asthmaticus, and some chronic obstructive pulmonary disease may require systemic glucocorticoids. These drugs suppress allergic and inflammatory manifestations of trichinosis.

Topical or systemic glucocorticoids often markedly improve certain skin diseases, such as pruritus, psoriasis, dermatitis herpetiformis, and eczema; pemphigus, erythema multiforme, exfoliative dermatitis, and mycosis fungoides usually require systemic treatment, which may be life-saving.

Probably the most widely known application of the anti-inflammatory actions of the glucocorticoids is in the treatment of the arthritic and rheumatic disorders. Immunosuppressant actions also may play a role in the treatment of such disorders. These disorders are systemic lupus erythematosus, polyarteritis nodosa, temporal arteritis, Wegener's granulomatosis, polymyositis, and polymyalgia rheumatica. Glucocorticoids may be indicated in severe cases of rheumatoid arthritis unresponsive to other treatment, Still's disease, mixed connective tissue disease, drug-induced lupoid syndromes, and psoriatic arthropathy.

Rheumatic or arthritic conditions in which glucocorticoids may or may not provide temporary relief but are not justified chronically because of a high toxicity/benefit ratio are osteoarthritis, systemic ankylosing spondylitis, gout fibrositis, and Reiter's syndrome. Even though the nephrotic syndrome is not inflammatory, it may respond to treatment, perhaps as the result of immunosuppression. Ulcerative colitis sometimes may respond dramatically. The beneficial effects in myasthenia gravis are probably immunosuppressant. Chronic multiple sclerosis does not respond, but acute relapses may. The incidence and severity of the respiratory distress syndrome in premature infants can be decreased by glucocorticoid treatment.

Glucocorticoids may be palliative in acute leukemia and also in chronic lymphocytic leukemia, and they are components of certain curative antineoplastic combinations. They suppress the associated autoimmune hemolytic anemia and the nonhemolytic anemia, granulocytopenia, and thrombocytopenia that result from encroachment on the bone marrow. The effects are only temporary, and the patient eventually becomes refractory to steroid therapy. Hodgkin's disease, lymphosarcoma, and multiple myeloma also may be suppressed temporarily.

In the treatment of endotoxin shock, massive doses of glucocorticoids suppress the vasculotoxic effects of the toxin. In all kinds of shock, massive doses decrease peripheral resistance, stimulate the heart, and decrease the amount of circulating myocardial depressant factor. To be optimally effective they must be given as boluses.

MODALITIES AND REGIMENS OF CORTICOS-
TEROID THERAPY—*Replacement Therapy*—Treatment of primary and secondary adrenal insufficiency requires replacement of both glucocorticoids and mineralocorticoids in sufficient doses to relieve the signs and symptoms of insufficiency. However, when the patient experiences an additional stress, supplements of glucocorticoids may be required. The dose and dose-interval vary from patient to patient, but the doses are small, and complications are infrequent and minimal; the most difficult challenge is in the adjustment of dosage in response to changes in stress.

CHRONIC LOW-DOSE SYSTEMIC THERAPY OF DISEASE—In mild inflammatory or collagen disorders, low doses of glucocorticoids often are sufficient to be palliative, and low-dose regimens are preferable, since adverse effects usually are of low intensity, provided that the therapeutic endpoint is only amelioration and not elimination of the morbidity. Although low-dose therapy may cause some suppression of pituitary-adrenal function, the suppression is readily reversible, and some reserve exists in the system. However, abrupt withdrawal of the drug may be followed not only by a return to the previous condition but also an acute exacerbation of the disease. Pituitary-adrenal suppression and consequent acute flare-up after withdrawal may be lessened by avoiding round-the-clock administration and, instead, giving the drug between 6 and 9 AM, so that plasma levels and, hence, pituitary-adrenal suppression are at a minimum during the early morning sleeping hours, when pituitary adrenal function is at its diurnal peak. Moreover, the selection of a steroid with a short biological half-life allows some drug-free time during the day, during which pituitary-adrenal recovery can occur.

CHRONIC HIGH-DOSE SYSTEMIC THERAPY—In serious chronic inflammatory or immunological disorders or in glucocorticoid-responsive neoplasia, large doses of glucocorticoids may be given for long periods of time. Consequently, side effects are frequent, and pituitary-adrenal suppression may be severe. The suppression may continue for weeks to months after cessation of treatment, so withdrawal must be tapered slowly to allow the pituitary-adrenal system to recover.

Abrupt withdrawal will result in adrenal insufficiency, which may be life-threatening, as well as an acute recrudescence of the original disorder. Pituitary-adrenal suppression and systemic side effects may be less severe if the dose is given in the morning, so that nocturnal pituitary-adrenal activity is less inhibited. Another device to minimize such adverse systemic effects is use of alternate-day therapy. Thus, twice the usual daily dose is given, but only every other day, which permits the hypothalamic-pituitary segment of the pituitary-adrenal negative feedback system and various undiseased target organs time to recover partially between doses. Only glucocorticoids with an intermediate duration of action (12–36 hr) should be used for alternate drug therapy.

INTENSIVE SHORT-TERM SYSTEMIC THERAPY—Massive doses of glucocorticoids may be required in certain acute conditions, such as bacteremic shock or status asthmaticus. The short duration of such treatment, sometimes no longer than 48 hr, is not enough to give rise to pituitary-adrenal suppression, serious immunosuppression, or opportunistic infections, although in septic shock, suprainfections may occur. Psychosis, GI bleeding, and hyperosmolar diabetic coma can occur in such short-term use.

LOCAL TREATMENT (TOPICAL APPLICATION)—Topical efficacy depends on the inherent glucocorticoid activity (or potency) of the steroid, the concentration in the preparation, permeability coefficient, the vehicle and excipients, and local metabolic processes. Except for serious conditions, low-potency glucocorticoids are preferred by many authorities, because adverse effects on the skin appear to be less severe than with high-potency agents, even if the latter are used at appropriately lower concentrations. Only hydrocortisone and its acetate are available for nonprescription topical use.

Drugs with a high lipid-water distribution coefficient penetrate well from absorbable or nonoleaginous vehicles and tend to remain longer in the skin than water-soluble agents, exerting a more extended local action but lesser systemic side effects, especially if the drug is metabolized rapidly systemically. However, it is desirable that the agents be metabolized in the skin, so that less is delivered to the systemic circulation. Steroids that have the 17-OH group substituted and/or that are fluorinated are metabolized poorly locally and hence may have a significant potential for systemic effects; for this reason, special caution is urged when such compounds are used in children.

Occlusive dressings may be used, especially for low-potency, poorly penetrant steroids. The stratum corneum under the dressing becomes macerated and more permeable. However, such dressings increase absorption into the bloodstream and hence favor systemic effects. The relative potency of several of the most commonly used topical corticosteroids are summarized in Table 77-3.

LOCAL TREATMENT (LOCAL INJECTION)—To achieve high, rapidly acting local concentrations of a glucocorticoid, it sometimes is injected as a very soluble derivative that rapidly generates the parent steroid. However, such soluble

Table 77-3. Potency Ranking of Some Commonly Used Topical Corticosteroids[a]

Super-potent
Group I
  Betamethasone dipropionate ointment or cream 0.05%
  Clobetasol propionate ointment or cream 0.05%
  Diflorasone diacetate ointment 0.05%
Potent
Group II
  Amcinonide ointment 0.1%
  Betamethasone dipropionate ointment 0.05%
  Desoximetasone cream, gel or ointment 0.25%
  Diflorasone diacetate ointment 0.05%
  Fluocinonide cream, gel or ointment 0.05%
  Halcinonide cream 0.1%
Group III
  Betamethasone benzoate gel 0.025%
  Betamethasone dipropionate cream 0.05%
  Betamethasone valerate ointment 0.1%
  Diflorasone diacetate cream 0.05%
  Mometasone furoate cream or ointment 0.1%
  Triamcinolone acetonide cream or ointment 0.5%
Mid-strength
Group IV
  Desoximetasone cream 0.05%
  Fluocinolone acetonide cream 0.2% or ointment 0.025%
  Flurandrenolide ointment 0.05%
  Hydrocortisone valerate ointment 0.2%
  Triamcinolone acetonide cream or ointment 0.1%
Group V
  Betamethasone benzoate cream 0.025%
  Betamethasone diproprionate lotion 0.02%
  Betamethasone valerate cream or lotion 0.1%
  Fluocinolone acetonide cream 0.025%
  Flurandrenolide cream 0.05%
  Hydrocortisone butyrate cream 0.1%
  Hydrocortisone valerate cream 0.2%
  Triamcinolone acetonide cream or lotion 0.1%
Mild
Group VI
  Alclometasone dipropionate cream or ointment 0.05%
  Desonide cream 0.05%
  Fluocinolone acetonide solution 0.01%

[a]Legend: Relative potency, Group I > II > III > IV > V > VI; topical activity of corticosteroids may vary considerably depending upon the vehicle, site of application, disease, individual patient, and whether or not an occlusive dressing is used. Approximate relative activity is based on vasoconstrictor assay and/or clinical effectiveness in psoriasis (preparations in each group are approximately equivalent).

forms also rapidly leave the region of injection. For this reason, insoluble derivatives may be included or injected alone, so that a sustained action in parallel with slow dissolution may be effected.

INHALATION AND INTRANASAL TREATMENT—Inhalers and nasal sprays are now available with glucocorticoids that possess high topical activity and low systemic bioavailability. These corticosteroids (beclomethasone, budesonide, fluticasone, and fluocinolide) have either low systemic absorption and/or high first-pass hepatic metabolism. These drugs are discussed in Chapter 69.

INHIBITORS OF BIOSYNTHESIS—Several drugs that interfere with the biosynthesis of adrenocorticoids are used clinically as *antiadrenal* drugs. Their mechanisms of action vary. Mitotane causes adrenocortical atrophy and a consequent decrease in the biosynthesis of all products of adrenocortical cells. Aminoglutethimide blocks the conversion of cholesterol to pregnenolone, and trilostane the dehydrogenation of the 3β-hydroxyl group of pregnenolone; hence, they both interrupt the biosynthesis of all active adrenal-derived steroids, including androgens and estrogens.

Mitotane blocks 11β-hydroxylation and hence the biosynthesis of aldosterone, cortisone, and hydroxycortisone. Mitotane and aminoglutethimide, especially, are used in the treatment of adrenal tumors, and aminoglutethimide also to suppress the production of androgens and estrogens in carcinoma of the breast. These two drugs are discussed in Chapter 86. Since blocking 11-hydroxylation leads to the homeostatic overflow of ACTH and the 11-deoxy precursors of cortisone and hydrocortisone, metyrapone is used diagnostically to ascertain the source of excess hydrocortisone in suspected adrenal carcinoma or autonomous adenoma by monitoring plasma ACTH and 11-deoxycorticoids. Metyrapone and trilostane are used in the management of Cushing's syndrome.

BECLOMETHASONE DIPROPIONATE

Pregna-1,4-diene-3,20-dione, (11β,16β)-9-chloro-11-hydroxy-16-methyl-17,21-bis(1-oxopropoxy)-, Beclovent; Beconase; Vanceril; Vancenase

[5534-09-8] $C_{26}H_{37}ClO_7$ (521.05).

Preparation—Synthesis of beclomethasone, a 9-chloro-16β-methyl derivative of prednisolone, and esters of beclomethasone, from steroid intermediates is described in British Pats 901,093 and 912,378 (*CA* 1963; 58:3488c and 1963; 59:14082b).

Description—White to cream-white powder; odorless.

Solubility—Very slightly soluble in water; very soluble in chloroform; freely soluble in alcohol or acetone.

Comments—Has 500 times the topical anti-inflammatory activity of dexamethasone but is less active as a systemic glucocorticoid and is almost inactive by the oral route. The low systemic activity is the result of rapid deesterification and further metabolism in the liver. Also, it has a high lipid, but low water, solubility, so that it not only is absorbed well topically but also tends to remain at the site of application. Thus, it may be administered by oral inhalation with usually negligible systemic side effects. It is indicated for treatment of bronchial asthma. As long as 2 to 4 weeks may be required for the onset of a beneficial effect. It is also employed in the treatment of noninfectious rhinitis.

The most common side effects of the inhaled drug are dry mouth, hoarseness, sore throat, and pharyngeal or tracheal candidiasis. Usually, the effects on pituitary-adrenal function are negligible, but suppression of plasma cortisol levels occurs in a few percent of adult patients who receive higher doses. Adverse effects of intranasal administration include epistaxis, nasal irritation, sneezing, and nasopharyngeal candidiasis. Hypersensitivity or other adverse effects of the propellants (CHF_3 and CH_2F_2) and oleic acid (a dispersing agent)

may occur; hypersensitivity absolutely contraindicates use of the aerosol. The plasma half-life is about 0.5 hr based on intravenous administration.

BETAMETHASONE

Prena-1,4-diene-3,20-dione, (11β,16β)-9-fluoro-11,17,21-trihydroxy-16-methyl-, Celestone

[378-44-9] $C_{22}H_{29}FO_5$ (392.47).

Preparation—Betamethasone is prepared from 16-dehydropregnenolone (see *Progesterone*, page 1468) by treatment with methylmagnesium iodide to insert the 16β-methyl group, catalytic reduction of the remaining double bond, enol acylation at position 20, and reaction with peracetic acid followed by hydrolysis to the 16β-methyl-17α-hydroxy compound. Bromination and acetoxylation give the 3β-hydroxy-21- acetoxy derivative, which is oxidized to the 3-oxo compound with chromic acid. Dibromination at positions 1 and 4 followed by dehydrobromination with dimethylformamide to the 1,4-diene, then incubation with *Pestalotia foedans* (or a similar organism) results in the 11α-hydroxy derivative. Esterification at the 11-position with ethyl chloroformate, elimination of the ester function with acetic acid to form the 1,4,9(11)-triene, treatment with *N*-bromoacetamide and perchloric acid gives the 9α-bromo-11β-hydroxy compound. Abstraction of HBr with potassium acetate affords the 9β,11β,-epoxy derivative, which by treatment with HF in a halogenated hydrocarbon yields the 9α-fluoro-11β-hydroxy analog, betamethasone.

Description—White to practically white, odorless, crystalline powder; melts about 240° with some decomposition.

Solubility—1 g in 5300 mL water, 65 mL alcohol or 325 mL chloroform; very slightly soluble in ether.

Comments—An extremely potent glucocorticoid with actions, uses, and side effects typical of this class of steroids (see the introduction to this section). Its activity is 20 to 30 times that of cortisol. However, it only rarely induces sodium and water retention and potassium loss such as accompany treatment with cortisone and many other adrenal corticoids; on occasion, it even may increase sodium excretion and induce diuresis. In the usual doses, the incidence of characteristic adrenal corticoid untoward effects such as anorexia, protracted weight loss, vertigo, headache, and muscle weakness is quite low. The plasma half-life is about 6.5 hr, and the biological half-life, 36 to 54 hr. The volume of distribution is 1.8 L/kg.

BUDESONIDE

Pregna-1,4-diene-3,20-dione, [11β,16α(17R)]-16,17-butylidenebis(oxy)-11β,21-dihydroxy-, and 11β,16α(17S)]-isomer; Pulmicort; Rhinocort

and

"

[51333-22-3] [51372-29-3] [51372-28-2] $C_{25}H_{34}O_6$ (430.54).

Preparation—11β, 16α,17,21-Tetrahydroxypregna-1,4-diene-3,20-dione is converted to the 16,17-acetal with butyraldehyde. US Pat 3,929,768 (1973); *Arzneimittel-Forsch* 1979; 29:1607.

Description—Off-white crystals melting about 225° (decompn.). A mixture of *R* and *S* isomers (40–51% *S*-isomer), but not necessarily a racemic mixture.

Solubility—Practically insoluble in water or hydrocarbon solvents; sparingly soluble in alcohol; freely soluble in chloroform. Partition coefficient (octanol/water) at pH 4 is 1.6×10^3.

Comments—It is orally inhaled for maintenance treatment of asthma as well as intranasally for treatment of allergic rhinitis. The onset of action is within 24 hr, which is relatively rapid for an inhaled corticosteroid, but maximum benefit may not be achieved for 1 to 2 weeks or longer. The oral availability of inhaled drug is low (~10%) primarily because of extensive first-pass metabolism in the liver (half-life, 2 hr). It has higher topical activity than beclomethasone propionate. The most common side effects of the inhaled drug are dry mouth, hoarseness, sore throat, and pharyngeal or tracheal candidiasis.

DEXAMETHASONE

(11β-16α)-Pregna-1,4-diene-3,20-dione, 9-fluoro-11,17,21-trihydroxy-16-methyl-, Decadron

[50-02-2] $C_{22}H_{29}FO_5$ (392.47).

Preparation—In a manner quite similar to that for *Betamethasone*, the difference being that the 16-methyl group is inserted in the α-configuration.

Description—White to practically white, odorless, crystalline powder; stable in air; melts about 250° with some decomposition.

Solubility—1 g in 42 mL alcohol or 165 mL chloroform; sparingly soluble in acetone, dioxane, or methanol; very slightly soluble in ether; practically insoluble in water.

Comments—Possesses glucocorticoid activity, for which it is used clinically (see the introduction to this section). It especially is used as an anti-inflammatory and antiallergic drug. Topically, it is employed in the treatment of glucocorticoid-responsive dermatoses. Systemically, it decreases the incidence and severity of hearing loss consequent to bacterial meningitis. Its systemic glucocorticoid potency is about 25 times that of cortisone. It is capable of inducing all the usual side effects of adrenal corticoids, except that the mineralocorticoid-like side effects are less pronounced than with cortisone acetate.

Its effect to suppress pituitary-adrenocortical function is used for differential diagnostic purposes in Cushing's syndrome. The plasma half-life is 3 to 4 hr, and the biological half-life is 36 to 54 hr. The volume of distribution is 0.75 L/kg. It binds linearly to albumin but does not bind to transcortin.

FLUDROCORTISONE ACETATE

(11β)-Pregn-4-ene-3,20-dione, 21-(acetyloxy)-9-fluoro-11,17-dihydroxy-, Florinef Acetate

[514-36-3] $C_{23}H_{31}FO_6$ (422.49).

Preparation—One method starts with *Hydrocortisone Acetate*, which is first dehydrated to the 4,9-diene. The 9α-fluoro and 11β-hydroxy groups are inserted by a method similar to that used for *Betamethasone*.

Description—Fine, white to pale-yellow powder that is odorless or practically odorless; hygroscopic; melts about 225° with some decomposition.

Solubility—Insoluble in water; soluble 1 g in 50 mL alcohol, 50 mL chloroform, or 250 mL ether.

Comments—A potent mineralocorticoid with considerable glucocorticoid activity. Its uses and side effects are those of mineralocorticoids, except that when used for replacement therapy in adrenal insufficiency it may not always be necessary to use a glucocorticoid concurrently, although usually hydrocortisone or cortisone are administered also. As with the doses used for replacement therapy, glucocorticoid side effects of the drug alone are mild and infrequent. The plasma half-life is about 3.5 hr, and the biological half-life is 18 to 36 hr.

FLUNISOLIDE

Pregna-1,4-diene-3,20-dione, (6α,11β,16α)-6-fluoro-11,21-dihydroxy-16,17-[(1-methylethylidene)bis(oxy)]-, hemihydrate; AeroBid; Nasalide, Nasarel

[77326-96-6] $C_{24}H_{31}FO_6 \cdot 1/2H_2O$ (443.51).

Preparation—See US Pat 3,124,571.

Description—White to creamy white crystalline powder melting about 245°.

Solubility—Soluble in acetone; sparingly soluble in chloroform; slightly soluble in methanol; practically insoluble in water.

Comments—A topical glucocorticoid for the treatment of noninfectious rhinitis and bronchial asthma. It has a high lipid/water- distribution coefficient, which favors both absorption into nasal and pulmonary tissue and retention at the site of application. By inhalation, about 40% is absorbed, which is considerably more than is absorbed of beclomethasone. The plasma half-life is about 1.8 hr, so absorbed steroid is destroyed rapidly enough so that pituitary-adrenocortical suppression does not occur with recommended doses. Dry mouth, hoarseness, sore throat, and pharyngeal, laryngeal, or tracheal candidiasis sometimes occur after continuous use. Occasional coughing, wheezing, and chest tightness are attributable to the vehicle and/or propellant.

FLUTICASONE PROPIONATE

Androsta-1,4-diene-17-carbothioic acid, (6α,11β,17α)-6,8-difluoro-11-hydroxy-16-methyl-3-oxo-17-(1-oxopropoxy)-, S-fluoromethyl ester; Cutivate; Flonase; Flovent

[80474-14-2] $C_{25}H_{31}F_3O_5S$ (500.57).

Preparation—US 4,335,121(1981); Neth Appl 8,100,707 (1981)

Description—White to off-white crystals melting about 272° (decomposition).

Solubility—Practically insoluble in water; freely soluble in DMSO or DMF; slightly soluble in ethyl alcohol or methanol.

Comments—It is similar to other potent inhaled corticosteroids that are useful in the maintenance treatment of chronic asthma and intranasally to treat allergic rhinitis. About 30% of the inhaled dose is absorbed from airways and is systemically available, with an elimination half-life of about 14 hr. The most common side effects include oral candidiasis and hoarseness. Higher doses of inhaled fluticasone can suppress the hypothalamic-pituitary-adrenal axis.

HYDROCORTISONE

(11β)-Pregn-4-ene-3,20-dione, 11,17,21-trihydroxy-, Compound F; Reichstein's "Substance M"; Cortef, Hydrocortone, Hytone

Cortisol [50-23-7] $C_{21}H_{30}O_5$ (362.47).

Preparation—The most attractive commercial synthesis involves the oxidation of 17α-21-dihydroxypregn-4-ene-3,20-dione, which is readily obtainable from diosgenin. Microbiological hydroxylation at the 11β-position is effected on the diacetate of the above compound employing organisms of the *Rhizopus, Aspergillus,* or *Streptomyces* species. Saponification then yields hydrocortisone.

Description—White to practically white, odorless, crystalline powder; melts about 215°, with decomposition.

Solubility—1 g in 40 mL alcohol; very slightly soluble in water or ether; slightly soluble in chloroform.

Comments—The principal natural glucocorticoid in man and thus the prototype of all glucocorticoids (for actions, uses, and side effects of glucocorticoids, see the introduction to this section). Systemic side effects can result from topical application. Allergic bronchospasm after use in asthmatics has been reported. The plasma half-life is 1.5 to 3 hr, and the biological half-life is 8 to 12 hr. The volume of distribution is 0.3 to 0.5 L/kg, varying with the dose.

METHYLPREDNISOLONE

(6αa,11β)-Pregna-1,4-diene-3,20-dione, 11,17,21-trihydroxy-6-methyl-, Medrol;

[83-43-2] $C_{22}H_{30}O_5$ (374.48).

Preparation—*Progesterone* is converted to the 6α-methyl derivative in the same manner as indicated in the synthesis of *Medroxyprogesterone Acetate*. Incubation of the 6α-methyl compound with an ascomycetes, such as *Pestalotia*, forms the 11α-hydroxy derivative, which is oxidized to the 3,11-diketo compound with chromic acid. Further treatment with ethyl oxalate followed by bromination, rearrangement with sodium methoxide, and debromination with zinc dust gives the methyl ester of the 4,17(20)-diene-21-carboxylate. With pyrrolidine, lithium aluminum hydride reduction, and treatment with alkali, the 11β,21-dihydroxy-4,17(20)-diene is formed, which is converted to the 21-acetate and then oxidatively hydroxylated to 6α-methylhydrocortisone acetate. Saponification, followed by dehydrogenation with *Septomyxa affinis* gives the 1,4,17(20)-triene, which is again converted to the 21- acetate, oxidatively hydroxylated to yield the 17α-hydroxy derivative, and saponified to give methylprednisolone.

Description—White to practically white, odorless, crystalline powder; melts about 240° with some decomposition.

Solubility—1 g in 10,000 mL water, 100 mL alcohol, 800 mL chloroform, or 800 mL ether.

Comments—A glucocorticoid with actions, uses, and side effects typical of drugs of this class (see the introduction to this section). It induces considerably less retention of sodium and water than the parent prednisolone. Because it possesses only weak mineralocorticoid activity, it is not employed in the management of acute adrenal insufficiency. The plasma half-life is 3 to 4 hr, and the biological half-life is 18 to 36 hr. The volume of distribution is 0.7 L/kg. The drug does not bind to transcortin.

PREDNISOLONE

(11β)-Pregna-1,4-diene-3,20-dione, 11,17,21-trihydroxy-, Prelone

[50-24-8] $C_{21}H_{28}O_5$ (360.45); *sesquihydrate* [52438-85-4] (387.47); anhydrous or contains one and one-half molecules of water of hydration.

Preparation—From hydrocortisone by a microbiological process using *Corynebacterium simplex*, which selectively dehydrogenates cortisol at the 1 and 2 positions.

Description—White to practically white, odorless, crystalline powder; melts about 235° with some decomposition.

Solubility—1 g in 30 mL alcohol or 180 mL chloroform; very slightly soluble in water.

Comments—A glucocorticoid with the actions, uses, and side effects typical of drugs of this class (see the introduction to this section). It is four times as potent as, but relatively somewhat weaker than, hydrocortisone as a mineralocorticoid, although sodium retention and potassium depletion can occur. The plasma half-life is said to be about

3 hr, and the biological half-life is 18 to 36 hr. However, the pharmacokinetics are dose-dependent because of nonlinear protein binding. With high doses the plasma half-life may approach 1.7 hr. Except for its higher solubility, it may be considered equivalent to prednisone; it is the biologically active metabolite of *Prednisone*.

PREDNISONE

Pregna-1,4-diene-3,11,20-trione, 17,21-dihydroxy-, Deltasone, Orasone

[53-05-2] $C_{21}H_{26}O_5$ (358.43).

Preparation—As described for *Prednisolone* except that cortisone is used instead of hydrocortisone.

Description—White to practically white, odorless, crystalline powder; melts about 230°, with some decomposition.

Solubility—1 g in 150 mL alcohol or 200 mL chloroform; very slightly soluble in water.

Comments—The active form of the drug is its metabolite, prednisolone. It has three to five times the glucocorticoid activity of hydrocortisone but somewhat less of mineralocorticoid activity, although sodium retention and potassium depletion may occur. It cannot be used alone for replacement therapy in adrenal insufficiency. It is the glucocorticoid predominantly used in cancer chemotherapy, always in combination with other drugs. In pediatrics it is used widely to treat nephrosis, rheumatic carditis, leukemias, other tumors, and tuberculosis. The plasma half-life is 3 to 5 hr, but the biological half-life is 12 to 36 hr.

TRIAMCINOLONE

(11β,16α)-Pregna-1,4-diene-3,20-dione, 9-fluoro-11,16,17,21-tetrahydroxy-, Aristocort; Kenacort

[124-94-7] $C_{21}H_{27}FO_6$ (394.44).

Preparation—From hydrocortisone acetate via the 3,20-bisketal by treatment with thionyl chloride, refluxing with potassium hydroxide and acetylation to give 21-acetoxy-4,9,11(16)-pregnatriene-3,20-dione. Oxidation with osmium tetroxide to the 16α,17α-dihydroxy derivative and subsequent insertion of the 9α-fluoro and 11β-hydroxy groups as indicated for *Betamethasone* (page 1444) gives a product lacking only a double bond at the 1-position. This latter step is accomplished by incubation with *Nocardia corallina*, followed by saponification of the acetate to yield triamcinolone. Alternatively, the compound can be made from *Fludrocortisone* by enzymatically inserting the 16α-hydroxyl group and dehydrogenating as above at the 1,2-position.

Description—Fine, white or practically white, crystalline powder with not more than a slight odor; its polymorphic forms and/or solvates melt between 248 and 250°, 260 and 263°, or 269 and 271°.

Solubility—1 g in about 5000 mL water, 70 mL propylene glycol, or less than 20 mL dimethyl sulfoxide; slightly soluble in alcohol or chloroform.

Comments—A glucocorticoid with actions, uses, and side effects typical of drugs of this class (see the introduction to this section). It is 7 to 13 times more potent than hydrocortisone. It has been claimed that therapeutic doses of this drug are nearly devoid of mineralocorticoid and other side effects of hydrocortisone, but the mineralocorticoid actions vary from patient to patient. It appears that the drug may induce natriuresis, negative sodium balance with weight loss in most patients (along with headache, dizziness, and fatigue), and sodium retention with weight gain, moon face, etc. in others. Nearly every side effect seen with hydrocortisone has been observed with this drug, but the relative frequencies are lower; however, it does not increase appetite and thus differs from other glucocorticoids. By the oral route, more of it survives the first pass through the liver than does hydrocortisone, and blood levels are somewhat more predictable. The plasma half-life is about 5 hr, and the biological half-life is 18 to 36 hr. The volume of distribution is 1.4 to 2.1 L/kg, depending upon the dose.

THE PANCREATIC HORMONES

The larger portion of the pancreas consists of glandular tissue that contains acinar cells that secrete digestive enzymes. However, there also are isolated groups of pancreatic cells called the islet of Langerhans that are composed of four cell types, each of which produces a distinct polypeptide hormone: insulin in the beta (β) cell, glucagon in the alpha (α) cell, somatostatin in the delta (δ) cell, and pancreatic polypeptide in the PP or F cell. β cells make up 60% to 80% of the islet. Dysregulation of certain pancreatic cell function can lead to a disorder known as diabetes mellitus.

Diabetes mellitus is a group of metabolic diseases characterized by hyperglycemia resulting from defects in insulin secretion, action or both. This condition affects approximately 17 million persons in the United States. Diabetes mellitus can be divided into 3 major types, Type 1, Type 2, and gestational diabetes.

Type 1 diabetes mellitus, (formerly known as juvenile diabetes or insulin dependent diabetes mellitus(IDDM) comprises about 10% of the diabetic population. It typically occurs during childhood and has an abrupt onset. Type 1 diabetes mellitus results from an autoimmune attack on the beta-cells of the pancreas and often times follows some environmental triggers such as certain viruses. There also may be some genetic component. Type 1 diabetes mellitus is associated with certain HLA phenotypes with detectable serum antibodies to islet cells. There is an absolute deficiency of insulin secretion from the β-cells of the pancreas and patients must be treated with exogenous insulin to sustain life.

Type 2 diabetes mellitus, formally known as non-insulin dependent diabetes mellitus (NIDDM), makes up approximately 90% of all cases of diabetes mellitus. Historically it was thought to occur mainly in adults greater than 40 years of age, however, the incidence has been increasing in younger patients due to physical inactivity and obesity. The onset is gradual and is often diagnosed at a routine physical examination with the patient unaware of any signs and symptoms. Type 2 diabetes mellitus may result from a deficiency of insulin secretion from the β-cells of the pancreas, peripheral insulin resistance, and/or persistent hepatic glucose production. There is a strong correlation to heredity and many Type 2 patients have central upper body obesity. Treatment of Type 2 diabetes mellitus can be accomplished by using diet and exercise, and if need be, using oral antidiabetic medication(s) or even insulin.

Typical signs and symptoms of diabetes mellitus are polyuria, polydipsia, and polyphagia. The increase in plasma glucose causes a marked glucosuria and an osmotic diuresis, resulting in dehydration. Hyperglycemia may also cause blurred vision, fatigue, nausea, and lead to increase incidence of various fungal and bacterial infections.

Complications of diabetes mellitus can be classified as acute and chronic. Hypoglycemia is an acute complication that occurs if there is excess insulin. The blood glucose concentration falls below a patient specific range and manifests by episodes of sweating, hunger, incoherence, palpitations, convulsions, coma and death. Severe cases of hypoglycemia can be treated with glucagon, which will increase blood glucose. Hyperglycemic crisis is an acute complication that occurs when the blood glucose concentration rises above a patient specific range. Type 1 patients are at risk for diabetic ketoacidosis, and Type 2 patients are at risk for hyperglycemic hyperosmolar non-ketotic syndrome.

Chronic complications can be classified as microvascular and macrovascular. Cardiovascular, cerebrovascular, and peripheral vascular diseases are examples of macrovascular complications all occurring at higher rates in the diabetic population. Examples of microvascular complications include peripheral and autonomic neuropathies, retinopathy, where it is the leading cause of blindness in the United States, and nephropathy, where it is responsible for 50% of all cases of dialysis. The results of the Diabetes Complications and Control Trial (DCCT) established that intensive treatment of diabetic patients can prevent or slow the progression of chronic complications.

Recent research and evidence has described a constellation of disorders comprising the metabolic syndrome (or Syndrome X). Hypertension, dyslipidemia, obesity and diabetes mellitus are the components of the metabolic syndrome and should be treated as a whole in order to prevent serious consequences to the cardiovascular system.

INSULIN—Insulin, a hormone secreted by the pancreas, was discovered more than 75 years ago and was initially extracted from beef and pork sources. These products were associated with immunologically mediated sequelae such as lipodystrophy and hypersensitivity reactions. The purity of animal derived insulins was improved over subsequent years. Finally Human insulin was introduced. This form of insulin is the most widely used insulin in therapeutic practice today. Current insulin preparations are available from two different species including pig, and human. Beef insulin, formally available in the United States has been removed from the market due to concerns regarding the transmission of Bovine Spongiform Encephalopathy (BSE) also known as "Mad Cow Disease." Human insulin is produced by recombinant DNA technology by inserting human genes into *Escherichia coli*. The recombinant products have the same physiological properties as insulin from beef or pork but are much less likely to cause allergic reactions and refractoriness.

Insulin is a protein containing 51 amino acids; it consists of A and B chains (containing 21 and 30 amino acids) linked by disulfide bonds. The 2 chains are produced along with C-peptide from a single proinsulin molecule. C-peptide can be measured clinically as an indicator of endogenous insulin production in diabetic patients It has a molecular weight of 6000. In aqueous solution, insulin polymerizes to form macromolecules of molecular weight 12,000 or 36,000, depending on pH and concentration. The isoelectric point of insulin is 5.3.

The physicochemical properties of human and porcine insulins differ slightly because of substitutions in a couple of amino acids. Porcine insulin differs from human insulin by only one carboxy-terminal amino acid of the B chain. The human insulin analogue Lispro inverts the amino acids at positions 28 (proline) with position 29 (lysine). Insulin Aspart differs from human insulin by the substitution of aspartic acid at amino acid position 28. The changes of amino acids in Insulin Lispro and Aspart result in quicker onset of action and activity that more closely mimics normal physiologic insulin secretion in response to meals.

Regular insulin is a clear solution that has the FDA indication to be administered subcutaneously, intramuscularly or intravenously. (Please note that this is currently the only insulin that can be administered IV). Lispro and Aspart are clear solutions that have been studied by the intravenous route, however do not have the indication for such use and should therefore be administered subcutaneously. Glargine is also clear solution, but must be given by the subcutaneous route because it depends on precipitation in order to exert its long-acting effect. All other currently available insulins are suspensions because regular insulin has been complexed with protamine (NPH) or Zinc (Lente and UltraLente) to extend their actions. These solutions should never be given intravenously.

PHYSIOLOGY AND ACTIONS—Insulin is the hormone that facilitates the uptake of glucose into skeletal muscle and adipose tissue by increasing the number of glucose transporters (specifically the GLUT1 and GLUT4 subtypes) that facilitate glucose diffusion in these target cells. In response to insulin, vesicles containing GLUT-4 move to the plasma membrane, where they dock, forming complexes. The vesicles fuse with the plasma membrane, increasing the number of GLUT-4 molecules in the membrane and thus the rate of glucose transport into cells. Insulin also decreases hepatic gluconeogenesis and increases glycogenesis. As previously stated, when the supply of, or response to, insulin is inadequate, a disease known as diabetes mellitus occurs.

Although attention focuses on the intervention of insulin in glucose metabolism, it also has independent actions to stimulate lipogenesis and promote the synthesis of many proteins important for cell growth and differentiation. Other actions include the suppression of synthesis of some proteins that regulate catabolic states that promote hepatic gluconeogenesis.

Insulin binds to the α-subunit of the insulin receptors. This evokes tyrosine kinase activity in the β-subunit and autophosphorylation of the receptor and also the translocation of glucose transporters to the plasma membrane. Phosphatidyl-inositol system coupling also occurs; inositol phosphates mediate recruitment of intracellular calcium, and inositol phosphate glycans and diacylglycerol mediate the activation of receptor-contained threonine and serine kinases and gene transcription. Furthermore, phosphodiesterase activity is increased, which decreases cAMP, and guanylate cyclase activity is increased. Inward potassium and magnesium transports are stimulated. Intracellular enzyme activities are altered variously by phosphorylation, dephosphorylation, and changes in protein synthesis. Overall, protein, lipid, and DNA syntheses are increased, and cell growth is promoted. Down-regulation of the insulin receptors begins within minutes of receptor activation and becomes maximal within a few hours.

In Type 1 diabetes mellitus, insulin injections must be spaced throughout the day, usually being given before meals. During the night, when no insulin is available, the blood sugar rises and is usually at its highest point before the morning dose. This erratic behavior of the level of blood sugar can be controlled more adequately by the use of insoluble insulins, which are absorbed more slowly and thus can exert a continuous, even action over a period as long as 24 hr (see below). Several different types of continuous infusion pumps for insulin are available that are easy to program for pulse injections at times of increased insulin demand. Devices for the nasal inhalation of insulin, and dry-powder for oral inhalation of insulin are under investigation but none are currently on the market.

The major insulin preparations are summarized in Table 77-4. The different insulin preparations are categorized according to their onset and duration of action.

PREPARATIONS—*Crystalline Zinc Insulin*—By addition of appropriate amounts of zinc salts, insulin may be crystallized. This achieves a superior degree of purification in order to minimize possible allergic sensitivity reactions to earlier insulin products. The speed and duration of action of the zinc insulins depends on the crystal size. The microcrystalline form (regular insulin) dissolves promptly and hence, by the subcutaneous route, has an onset of action of 0.5 hours, a peak of 2 to 4 hours, and duration of action of 4 to 6 hours.

Zinc insulins of larger crystal size have slow-release properties that depend on crystal size. Thus Insulin Zinc Suspension (Lente) has a duration of 12 to 18 hours, and Extended Insulin Zinc Suspension (UltraLente) has a duration of 18 to 36 hours.

Crystalline Protamine Zinc Insulin—*Insulin or zinc insulin may be combined with protamine to yield complexes of larger molecular weight.*

Neutral Protamine Hagedorn insulin (NPH) is injected as a suspension. It goes into solution slowly, and this limits the rate of absorption. It has a duration of action of about 12 to 16 hours.

Proinsulin—This is the single-chain protein precursor of insulin. The removal of the C-peptide moiety leaves insulin. When administered exogenously, its metabolic effects differ somewhat from those of insulin in that it mostly suppresses hepatic glucose output and has only a slight action to stimulate peripheral glucose uptake. Therefore, it has a much lower probability of causing severe hypoglycemia. The locus of action especially lends itself to the treatment of Type 2 diabetes mellitus. The pharmacokinetics permit once-a-day dosage. A recombinant human product is undergoing clinical trials.

Glucagon (Hyperglycemic Factor; Hgf)—In addition to insulin, the pancreas also produces a substance that exerts an effect on blood sugar opposite to that of insulin. This HGF, or glucagon, is produced by the α-cells of the Islets of Langerhans. It plays an important role in the physiological regulation of blood sugar, and defects in the control of glucagon secretion are a factor in certain types of diabetes mellitus.

Somatostatin (Gh-Rif)—Somatostatin also is produced in the pancreas, where it inhibits release of both insulin and glucagon; it is involved in the physiological regulation of the secretion of these hormones. In diabetes mellitus, the persistence of glucagon output contributes to hyperglycemia and ketoacidosis; administration of somatostatin improves the metabolic condition by suppressing glucagon blood levels. Unfortunately, the half-life of somatostatin is very short, so that longer-lived congeners with separate activities to treat diabetes, acromegaly, peptic ulcer, and other disorders are being developed.

GLUCAGON

Glucagon (pig)

H - His - Ser - Glu(NH₂) - Gly - Thr - Phe - Thr - Ser - Asp - Tyr - Ser - Lys - Tyr - Leu - Asp - Ser -
 1   2   3   4   5   6   7   8   9   10   11   12   13   14   15   16

Arg - Arg - Ala - Glu(NH₂) - Asp - Phe - Val - Glu(NH₂) - Trp - Leu - Met - Asp(NH₂) - Thr - OH
 17   18   19   20   21   22   23   24   25   26   27   28   29

Glucagon [16941-32-5] $C_{153}H_{225}N_{43}O_{49}S$ (3482.78); a polypeptide occurring in the pancreas glands of domestic mammals used for food by man, which has the property of increasing the blood glucose concentration. It is employed as the hydrochloride.

Description—Fine, white or faintly colored, crystalline powder; practically odorless and tasteless.

Solubility—Soluble in dilute alkali or acid solutions; insoluble in most organic solvents.

Comments—Stimulates the hepatic adenylate cyclase system and hence promotes the breakdown of liver glycogen. The end result is the release of glucose and an elevation of blood glucose. Stimulation of adenylate cyclase in the heart causes positive inotropy and in intestinal muscle, relaxation. After parenteral injection the glucose response is quite prompt. The action lasts but 45 to 90 minutes. It is used primarily to terminate hypoglycemic coma, such as may occur from an overdose of insulin. It is dubious that it offers any compelling advantage over intravenous dextrose for this purpose, except when it is difficult to give an intravenous infusion. Its value in idiopathic hypoglycemia, islet cell car-

Table 77-4. Summary of Major Insulin Preparations

TYPE OF INSULIN	ONSET (HOURS)	PEAK (HOURS)	DURATION (HOURS)	APPEARANCE
Rapid-acting				
Aspart	<¼	1–2	2–4	Clear
Lispro	<½	1–3	2–4	Clear
Short-acting				
Regular	<½–1	2–4	4–6	Clear
Intermediate-acting				
Lente	1–2	6–14	12–18	Cloudy
NPH	1–2	6–14	10–16	Cloudy
Long-acting				
Glargine	1–2	2–20	20–24+	Clear
Ultralente	4–10	8–30	18–36+	Cloudy

cinoma, and glycogen storage disease has not yet been determined fully. However, it can be used to diagnose glycogen storage disease and to determine pancreatic β-cell secretory reserve; in the latter test, the amount of C-peptide that appears in the plasma quantifies the reserve. It must be used cautiously in islet cell carcinoma, because it stimulates the release of insulin and may cause hypoglycemia. Even in the diabetic patient it may cause rebound hypoglycemia, mostly, however, because of the persistence of insulin levels from the overdose for which glucagon was administered. It is used as an adjunct in hypotonic radiography of the GI tract, to relax the smooth muscle. Side effects include dizziness, nausea, vomiting, hypotension, and rebound hypoglycemia, especially after intravenous administration. Occasional allergy causes dyspnea or rash.

INSULIN INJECTION

Rapid-Acting Insulins

INSULIN ASPART

Insulin Aspart; NovoLog

```
Gly- Ile- Val- Glu- Gln- Cys- Cys- Thr- Ser- Ile- Cys- Ser- Leu- Tyr- Gln- Leu-
 1    2    3    4    5    6    7    8    9   10   11   12   13   14   15   16
Glu- Asn- Tyr- Cys- Asn
 17   18   19   20   21
Phe- Val- Asn- Gln- His- Leu- Cys- Gly- Ser- His- Leu- Val- Glu- Ala- Leu- Tyr-
 1    2    3    4    5    6    7    8    9   10   11   12   13   14   15   16
Leu- Val- Cys- Gly- Glu- Arg- Gly- Phe- Phe- Tyr- Thr- Asp- Lys- Thr
 17   18   19   20   21   22   23   24   25   26   27   28   29   30
```

28^{B}-L-Aspartic acid-insulin (human) [11609423-6] $C_{256}H_{381}N_{65}O_{79}S_{6}$ (5825.54).

Preparation—Using a recombiant technology utilizing Brewer's yeast (*Saccharomyces cerevisiae*).

Description—It is homologous with human insulin with the exception of a single substitution of proline by aspartic acid in position B28.

Comments—A rapid-acting insulin that can be injected 5 to 10 minutes prior to a meal. It has an onset within 15 minutes as well as a much shorter peak (0.5–1.5 hr) and duration (2–4 hr) than regular insulin injection. It is therefore associated with greater reductions in postprandial blood glucose concentrations. Because of its short duration of action, it is most commonly used in regimens that contain an intermediate-acting or long-acting insulin.

INSULIN LISPRO

Insulin(human), 28B-L-lysine-29B-L-proline-, Humalog

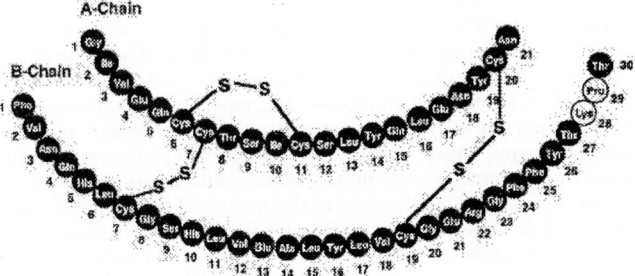

[133107-64-9]

Preparation—US Pat 5,514,646 (1966).

Description—A Lys(B28), Pro(B29) human insulin analog created when the amino acids at positions 28 and 29 on the insulin B-chain are reversed. This type of analog is less prone to dimerization or self association to higher molecular weight forms, thus possessing a more rapid onset of activity while retaining the biological activity of native human insulin.

Comments—A rapid-acting insulin that can be injected immediately prior to a meal. It has an onset of action within 15 minutes. It has a much shorter peak (0.5–1.5 hours) and duration (2–4 hours) than regular insulin injection. It is therefore associated with greater reductions in postprandial blood glucose concentrations. Because of its short dura-

tion of action, it is most commonly used in regimens that contain an intermediate-acting or long-acting insulin.

Short-Acting Insulins

REGULAR INSULIN

Humulin R and Novolin R

A sterile, acidified or neutral solution of insulin. The solution has a potency of 100, or 500 USP Insulin Units in each mL.

Description—When containing in each mL not more than 100 USP Units, it is a colorless or almost colorless liquid; that containing 500 Units may be straw-colored; substantially free from turbidity and from insoluble matter; contains from 0.1% to 0.25% (w/v) of either phenol or cresol and 1.4% to 1.8% (w/v) of glycerin; pH, determined potentiometrically, between 2.5 and 3.5 for acidified injection, and 7.0 and 7.8 for neutral injection.

Comments—Regular insulin is a short-acting insulin that is injected prior to a meal. It has an onset of action of about 30 to 60 minutes. It has a relatively short peak (3–4 hours) and duration (6–8 hours). It is commonly used in regimens that contain an intermediate-acting or long-acting insulin in order to attain better control of blood glucose concentrations. It is an insulin that may be administered by the intravenous route (IV).

Intermediate-Acting Insulins

ISOPHANE INSULIN SUSPENSION (NEUTRAL PROTAMINE HAGEDORN)

Humulin N and Novolin N

NPH Insulin

A sterile suspension of zinc-insulin crystals and protamine sulfate in buffered water for injection, combined in a manner such that the solid phase of the suspension consists of crystals composed of insulin, protamine, and zinc. The protamine sulfate is prepared from the sperm or from the mature testes of fish belonging to the genera *Oncorhynchus* Suckley or *Salmo* Linné (Fam *Salmonidae*).

Each mL is prepared from sufficient insulin to provide 100 USP Insulin Units of insulin activity.

Description—White suspension of rod-shaped crystals approximately 30 μm in length and free from large aggregates of crystals following moderate agitation; contains either (1) 1.4% to 1.8% (w/v) glycerin, 0.15% to 0.17% (w/v) metacresol, and 0.06% to 0.07% (w/v) phenol or (2) 1.4% to 1.8% (w/v) glycerin and 0.20% to 0.25% (w/v) phenol; contains 0.15% to 0.25% (w/v) dibasic sodium phosphate; contains also 0.01 to 0.04 mg of zinc and 0.3 to 0.6 mg of protamine for each 100 USP Insulin Units; when examined microscopically, the insoluble matter in the suspension is crystalline and contains not more than traces of amorphous material; pH between 7.1 and 7.4, determined potentiometrically.

Comments—An intermediate-acting insulin that is typically injected twice daily. It has an onset of action of 1 to 2 hours, a peak of 6 to 14 hours and a duration of action of approximately 10 to 16 hours. There may be occasional hypersensitivity to the protamine component. It is never given intravenously.

INSULIN ZINC SUSPENSION

Lente

A sterile suspension of insulin in buffered water for injection, modified by the addition of zinc chloride in a manner such that the solid phase of the suspension consists of a mixture of crystalline and amorphous insulin in a ratio of approximately 7 parts of crystals to 3 parts of amorphous material. Each mL is prepared from sufficient insulin to provide 100 USP Insulin Units of insulin activity.

Description—Almost colorless suspension of a mixture of characteristic crystals predominantly 10 to 40 μm in maximum dimension and many particles that have no uniform shape and do not exceed 2 μm in maximum dimensions; contains 0.15% to 0.17% (w/v) sodium acetate, 0.65% to 0.75% (w/v) sodium chloride, and 0.09% to 0.11% (w/v) methylparaben; contains also, for each 100 USP Insulin Units, 0.12 to 0.25 mg of zinc of which 20% to 65% is in the supernatant liquid; pH between 7.2 and 7.5.

Comments—An intermediate-acting insulin that is typically injected twice daily. It has an onset of action of 1 to 2 hours, a peak of 6 to 14 hours and a duration of action of approximately 10 to 16 hours. It is never given intravenously.

A theoretical advantage of Lente insulin is its freedom from foreign proteins, such as protamine, to which certain patients are sensitive (however the most commonly used intermediate-acting insulin remains NPH).

Long-Acting Insulins

INSULIN GLARGINE

Insulin (human), 21ᴬ-glycine-30ᴮa-L-arginine-30ᴮb-L-arginine-, Lantus

```
Gly-Ile-Val-Glu-Gln-Cys- Cys-Thr-Ser-Ile-Cys-Ser-Leu-Tyr-Gln-Leu-
 1   2   3   4   5   6    7   8   9   10  11  12  13  14  15  16
Glu-Asn-Tyr-Cys-Gly
 17  18  19  20  21
Phe-Val- Asn-Gln-His-Leu-Cys-Gly-Ser- His- Leu-Val-Glu-Ala- Leu-Tyr-
 1   2    3   4   5   6   7   8   9    10   11  12  13  14   15  16
Leu-Val-Cys-Gly- Glu- Arg- Gly- Phe-Phe- Tyr-Thr-Pro- Lys-Thr-Arg-Arg
 17  18  19  20   21   22   23   24  25   26  27  28   29  30  31  32
```

[160336-95-1] $C_{267}H_{404}N_{72}O_{78}S_6$ (6062.89).

Preparation—By a recombinant DNA procedure using a non-pathogenic strain of *E coli* (K_{12}).

Description—Differs from human insulin in that asparagine, at position A21 is replaced by glycine.

Comments—A long-acting insulin that has a pKa of 4.0. When administered by the subcutaneous route, the clear solution precipitates, releases slowly, and thus provides a sustained duration of action. It has an onset of action of approximately 2 hours, is lacking an appreciable peak of action, and has a duration of action of 24 hours. It is the only true 24-hour insulin available. This insulin most closely mimics the human bodies' production of a basal insulin concentration throughout the day. It is a clear solution, but must never be given IV. It must be administered subcutaneously. It must never be administered in the same syringe as other insulins.

EXTENDED INSULIN ZINC SUSPENSION

Ultra-Lente

A sterile suspension of insulin in buffered water for injection, modified by the addition of zinc chloride in a manner such that the solid phase of the suspension is predominantly crystalline. In its preparation, sufficient insulin is used to provide 100 USP Insulin Units for each mL of the suspension.

Description—Almost colorless suspension of a mixture of characteristic crystals the maximum dimension of which is predominantly 10 to 40 μm; contains, for each 100 USP Units of insulin, 0.12 to 0.25 mg of zinc (of which 20–65% is in the supernatant liquid) and not more than 0.70 mg of nitrogen; contains also 0.15% to 0.17% (w/v) sodium acetate, 0.65% to 0.75% (w/v) sodium chloride, and 0.09% to 0.11% (w/v) methylparaben; pH, between 7.2 and 7.5.

Comments—The crystals in this form are of sufficient size to have a slow rate of dissolution. It is a long-acting insulin with an onset of action of 4 to 8 hr, a peak at 10 to 30 hr, and duration usually in excess of 36 hr (Although this has been very variable in clinical practice). A theoretical advantage is that it is free of protamine and other foreign proteins so the incidence of allergic reactions is possibly minimized.

COMBINATION INSULIN PRODUCTS

Insulin 70/30: 70% NPH and 30% Regular (Humulin 70/30, Novolin 70/30)

Insulin 50/50: 50% NPH and 50% Regular (Humulin 50/50)

Insulin 75/25: 75% Insulin Lispro Protamine (Intermediate-acting) and 25% Lispro (Humalog Mix 75/25)

ORAL ANTIDIABETIC DRUGS

As discussed previously, patients with Type 2 diabetes mellitus have a defect in insulin secretion from the pancreas, inappropriate hepatic glucose production, tissue insulin resistance, or a combination of any of these as a major cause of the glucose dysregulation. In Type 2 diabetic patients, as the fasting plasma glucose concentration rises, insulin secretion from the pancreas decreases progressively. Also the rate of basal hepatic glucose output is excessive. Defects in insulin receptor function and glucose transport contribute to tissue insulin resistance. Drugs that improve insulin secretion, decrease hepatic glucose production and improve insulin sensitivity at the tissue receptors are therefore effective in treating type 2 diabetes mellitus.

Sulfonylureas

The sulfonylurea drugs have been available in the United States since 1954 and have been the mainstay of oral antidia-

betic therapy for many years. They are classified as either first-generation (Acetohexamide, Chlorpropamide, Tolbutamide, and Tolazamide) or second-generation (Glyburide, Glipizide, and Glimeperide) based on their pharmacokinetic profiles. Second generation sulfonylureas tend to be prescribed more frequently based on their tolerability and dosing schedule.

The sulfonylureas exert their blood glucose lowering actions by stimulating insulin release from β- cells in the pancreatic islets. They bind to the sulfonylurea receptor found on the surface of the pancreatic β-cells. This interaction leads to a closure of voltage dependent potassium adenosinetriphosphate channels, which leads to decreased potassium influx and β-cell membrane depolarization. This depolarization opens a voltage-gated calcium channel that results in calcium influx and the secretion of insulin. Some functional β-cells must be present for an effect on blood glucose. Although this is the primary mechanism of action, the possibility that sulfonylureas decrease hepatic glucose production as well as a decrease in tissue insulin resistance has arisen. Typical reduction in fasting plasma glucose is 50–60 mg/dl, and decrease in HgA1c by 1% to 2%.

There are two types of drug failure with regard to the sulfonylurea agents. First is primary failure, which is when the patient does not respond to a properly titrated course of therapy. Secondary failure describes a tolerance that may develop during chronic treatment such that a blood glucose lowering response in not seen. It also could be due to a failure to follow diet and exercise regimens or certain stressful situations that worsen the appearance of glycemic control.

In the past there were concerns about the adverse cardiac effects from the use of sulfonylureas. The results of the UKPDS trial showed that there was no link between the use of sulfonylureas and increased incidence of coronary artery disease in patients with Type 2 diabetes mellitus, which refutes the results from an earlier study by the University Group Diabetes Program.

α-Glucosidase Inhibitors

Dietary carbohydrates require enzymatic degradation by α-glucosidase to monosaccharides within the gastrointestinal tract in order to be able to be absorbed. The α-glucosidase inhibitors (Acarbose and Miglitol) are a unique class of drugs that act on this enzyme in the brush border of the proximal small intestine epithelium. By competitively inhibiting the enzyme α-glucosidase, these agents result in a delay of intestinal carbohydrate absorption. These agents should be taken at the beginning of each meal in order to exert their pharmacologic actions. They seem to be useful when there is consistent postprandial hyperglycemic episodes. Typical reduction in postprandial plasma glucose is 25-50 mg/dl, and decrease in HgA1c by 0.5% to 1%.

The widespread use of these agents is limited because of the occurrence of gastrointestinal side effects such as abdominal pain, flatulence, and diarrhea. Increase liver enzymes have been reported with high doses of Acarbose. When used as monotherapy, these agents do not cause hypoglycemia, however the incidence rises when combined with insulin or other insulin secretagogues. Because of the nature of the mechanism of action, it is imperative to treat episodes of hypoglycemia with a source of sucrose as opposed to more complex carbohydrates.

Biguanides

Metformin, a biguanide that has been in clinical use for more than 40 years, was introduced in the United States in 1995. It is chemically related to an earlier Biguanide, Phenformin, which was removed from the market in the 1970s due to an association with lactic acidosis. Metformin, however, differs structurally from Phenformin and rarely causes lactic acidosis in diabetic patients. The decrease incidence of lactic acidosis has to due in part by the strict contraindications to its use. All of the following are contraindications to the use of metformin: serum creatinine in males ≥1.5 mg/dl and females ≥1.4 mg/dl, abnormal creatinine clearance, active liver disease, active alcoholics, conditions that may cause significant hypoxemia, patients with CHF requiring pharmacologic therapy, and concurrent use of IV contrast dyes for imaging tests (Metformin must be discontinued before the test and not restarted until 48 hours after the test as long as renal function seems adequate).

Metformin exerts its blood glucose lowering effect primarily by the inhibition of basal hepatic glucose production. In addition, metformin may lower blood glucose secondarily by increasing tissue sensitivity to insulin. Typical reduction in fasting plasma glucose is 50 to 70 mg/dl, and decrease in HgA1c by 1.5% to 2%.

Since metformin lacks any insulin secretagogue activity, it does not cause hypoglycemia when used as monotherapy. Based on the results of the UKPDS trial in which metformin showed significant improvement in glucose control in overweight diabetic patients, it should be considered the drug of choice in obese Type 2 diabetic patients unless contraindicated.

Meglitinides

The meglitinides, Repaglinide and Nateglinide, are structurally different from the sulfonylureas; however, they exert their blood glucose lowering action by the same mechanism. They bind to a different portion of the sulfonylurea receptor found on the surface of the pancreatic β-cells. This interaction leads to a closure of voltage-dependent potassium adenosinetriphosphate channels, which leads to decreased potassium influx and β-cell membrane depolarization. This depolarization opens a voltage-gated calcium channel that results in calcium influx and the secretion of insulin. They are insulin secretagogues, like the sulfonylureas, but result in a much more rapid, and short-lived release of insulin. These agents are particularly useful in patients who demonstrate consistent postprandial hyperglycemia. Typical reduction in fasting plasma glucose is 50–60 mg/dl, and decrease in HgA1c by 1% to 2%.

Thiazolidinediones

The thiazolidinediones, Pioglitazone and Rosiglitazone, are chemically related to Troglitazone, which was removed from the market because of rare idiosyncratic hepatocellular injury. Pioglitazone and Rosiglitazone have a unique mechanism of action, binding to a novel receptor known as the peroxisome proliferator activated receptor γ (PPARγ). When activated, the receptor binds with response elements on DNA, altering transcription of a variety of genes that regulate carbohydrate and lipid metabolism. The primary effect is decreasing tissue insulin resistance thereby stimulating glucose uptake by peripheral tissues. Secondarily, thiazolidinediones may decrease hepatic glucose production, and this may aid in the overall blood glucose reduction. These agents do not stimulate the β-cells of the pancreas to secrete insulin; however, they may enhance the responsiveness and efficacy of the β-cells. Historically not thought of as first line therapy for Type 2 diabetic patients, preliminary data suggest that these agents may actually prolong β-cell survival, and should be considered earlier in therapy. Typical reduction in fasting plasma glucose is 50–60 mg/dl, and decrease in HgA1c by 1% to 2%.

Pioglitazone and Rosiglitazone appear to be safer with regard to hepatic injury, possibly due to the strict guidelines for monitoring liver function in these patients. Patients who are prescribed Pioglitazone or Rosiglitazone need to have baseline LFTs performed, and repeated monitoring every 2 months for the first year of therapy, then quarterly thereafter. If at any time the LFTs are >2.5 times the upper limit of normal, these medications should be discontinued. Other side effects include edema, weight gain, and certain lipid abnormalities. Due to the edema that may occur when using Thiazolidinediones, there is a precaution for use in patients with congestive heart failure.

ACARBOSE

Glucose, O-4,6-dideoxy-4-[[[1S-(1α,4α,5β,6α)]-4,5,6-trihydroxy-3-(hydroxymethyl)-2-cyclohexen-1-yl]amino]-α-D-glucopyranosyl-(1→4)-O-α-D-glucopyranosyl-(1→4)-, Precose

[56180-94-0] $C_{25}H_{43}NO_{18}$ (645.61).

Preparation—An oligosaccharide obtained through fermentation processes involving *Actinoplanes utahensis*. US Pat 4,062,950(1975); *Carbohydrate Res* 1989; 189:309.

Description—Amorphous powder.

Solubility—Soluble in water; pK_a is 5.1.

Comments—Acarbose is an oral antidiabetic agent in the α-glucosidase class that is used to treat Type 2 diabetes mellitus. It is indicated as monotherapy or in combination with sulfonylureas. It is not bound to plasma proteins. It is primarily metabolized within the GI tract by intestinal bacteria. The metabolites are excreted in the urine. Side effects include gastrointestinal disturbances and rash. Since Acarbose is not an insulin secretagogue, there is no risk for hypoglycemia when used as monotherapy, however the risk increases when used in combination with other insulin secretagogues.

Acarbose is dosed initially at 25 mg three times a day and the maintenance dose is 50 mg three times a day (if patient weighs <60 kg) or 100 mg three times a day (if patient weighs >60 kg). Drug interactions are mainly with drugs that may bind Acarbose in the GI tract (Example: digestive enzymes and charcoal).

ACETOHEXAMIDE

Benzensulfonamide, 4-acetyl-N-[[cyclohexylamino]carbonyl]-, Dymelor

[968-81-0] $C_{15}H_{20}N_2O_4S$ (324.39).

Preparation—p-Acetylbenzenesulfonamide in acetone is treated with anhydrous potassium carbonate and the resulting potassium salt of the sulfonamideis reacted with cyclohexyl isocyanate. After removal of the solvent, the residual potassium salt of acetohexamide is acidified to precipitate the product. US Pat 3,320,312 (1967).

Description—White, practically odorless, crystalline powder melting about 183°.

Solubility—1 g in 230 mL of alcohol or 210 mL of chloroform; practically insoluble in water or ether.

Comments—A first generation sulfonylurea oral hypoglycemic agent that stimulates the β-cells of the pancreas to secrete insulin. It is indication to treat Type 2 diabetes mellitus as monotherapy or in combination with other oral anti-diabetic agents (Metformin, Thiazolidinediones, or α-glucosidase inhibitors), except the meglitinides. It is extensively bound to plasma proteins. It is metabolized in the liver to an inactive metabolite and is excreted through the kidneys. Side effects include hypoglycemia, weight gain, gastrointestinal disturbances, skin rash, and insulin resistance.

Acetohexamide is dosed 250 to 1500 mg once daily. See Table 77-5 for a list of possible drug interactions.

CHLORPROPAMIDE

Benzenesulfonamide, 4-chloro-N-[(propylamino)carbonyl]-, Diabinese

1-[(p-Chlorophenyl)sulfonyl]-3-propylurea [94-20-2] $C_{10}H_{13}Cl$-N_2O_3S (276.74).

Preparation—p-Chlorobenzenesulfonamide undergoes addition to propyl isocyanate by warming a solution of equimolar quantities of the two reactants.

Description—White, crystalline powder, with a slight odor; melts between 125° and 129°.

Solubility—Practically insoluble in water; soluble in alcohol; sparingly soluble in chloroform.

Comments—A first generation sulfonylurea oral hypoglycemic agent that stimulates the β-cells of the pancreas to secrete insulin.

It is indicated to treat Type 2 diabetes mellitus as monotherapy or in combination with other oral anti-diabetic agents (metformin, thiazolidinediones, or α-glucosidase inhibitors), except the meglitinides. Chlorpropamide is highly bound to plasma proteins, is metabolized 80% hepatically, and cleared renally. It has a long half-life (25–60 hr) and duration of action (about 24–48 hr).

Side effects include hypoglycemia, weight gain, gastrointestinal disturbances, skin rash and insulin resistance. In addition, chlorpropamide may increase the endogenous release of vasopressin (ADH) and thus causes water retention with resultant hyponatremia and hypoosmolality with symptoms similar to SIADH and should be avoided in the elderly who are at increased risk. There have been reports of a disulfiram reaction when taking concomitantly with alcohol. Chlorpropamide is dosed 250 mg to 500 mg once daily. See Table 77-5 for a list of possible drug interactions.

GLIMEPERIDE

Urea, 1-[[p-[2-(3-ethyl-4-methyl-2-oxo-3-pyrroline-1-carboxamido)ethyl]phenyl]sulfonyl]-3-(4-methylcyclohexyl)-, Amaryl

[93479-97-1] $C_{24}H_{34}N_4O_5S$ (490.62).

Preparation—US Pat 4,379,785 (1983).

Description—White to yellowish-white crystalline, practically odorless powder melting about 207°.

Comments—A second-generation sulfonylurea oral hypoglycemic agent that stimulates the β-cells of the pancreas to secrete insulin.

It is indicated to treat Type 2 diabetes mellitus as monotherapy or in combination with other oral anti-diabetic agents (metformin, thiazolidinediones, or α-glucosidase inhibitors), except the meglitinides.

Glimeperide is highly protein bound, but principally nonionic which may make for less propensity to be displaced from proteins by other highly protein bound drugs. It is metabolized hepatically and cleared renally. It has a half-life of 9 hours and duration of action of about 24 hours.

Side effects include hypoglycemia, weight gain, gastrointestinal disturbances, skin rash, and insulin resistance.

Glimeperide is dosed 1 to 8 mg once daily. See Table 77-5 for a list of possible drug interactions.

GLIPIZIDE

Pyrazinecarboxamide, N-[2-[4-[[[(cyclohexyl-amino)carbonyl]amino]sulfonyl]phenyl]ethyl]-5-methyl-, Glucotrol, Glucotrol XL

[29094-61-9] $C_{21}H_{27}N_5O_4S$ (445.54).

Preparation—By the condensation of 4-[2-(5-methyl-2-pyrazine-carboxamido)ethyl]benzenesulfonamide and cyclohexyl isocyanate; *Arzneimittel-Forsch* 1971; 21:200.

Description—White, odorless powder; pKa 5.9; melts about 205°.

Solubility—Insoluble in water or polar solvents; freely soluble in dimethylformamide or fixed alkalies.

Comments—A second- generation sulfonylurea oral hypoglycemic agent that stimulates the β-cells of the pancreas to secrete insulin.

Table 77-5. Drug Interactions with Sulfonylureas

ADDED DRUG	MECHANISM
Highly protein bound drugs	Displacement of sulfonylureas
β-Blockers	Increase blood glucose
Corticosteroids	concentrations
Diazoxide	
Nicotinic acid	
Sympathomimetics	
Thiazide diuretics	
Charcoal	Decrease absorption

*This list is not all-inclusive. See Facts and Comparisons for a comprehensive list of medications that could possibly interact with sulfonylureas.

It is indicated to treat Type 2 diabetes mellitus as monotherapy or in combination with other oral anti-diabetic agents (Metformin, Thiazolidinediones, or α-glucosidase inhibitors), except the meglitinides..

Glipizide is highly protein bound, but principally nonionic which may make for less propensity to be displaced from proteins by other highly protein bound drugs. It is metabolized hepatically and cleared renally. It has a half-life of 2 to 4 hours and duration of action of about 12 to 24 hours.

Food delays the absorbtion but not affect the peak concentrations of Glipizide.

Side effects include hypoglycemia, weight gain, gastrointestinal disturbances, skin rash, and insulin resistance.

Glipizide is dosed 5 to 40 mg once daily. It is available in an extended-release formulation. See Table 77-5 for a list of possible drug interactions.

GLYBURIDE

Benzamide, 5-chloro-N-[2-[4-[[[(cyclohexyl-amino)carbonyl]amino]sulfonyl]phenyl]ethyl]-2-methoxy-, DiaBeta; Glynase Pres Tab; Micronase

Glybenclamide [10238-21-8] $C_{23}H_{28}ClN_3S$ (494.00).

Preparation—See *Arzneimittel-Forsch* 1966; 16:640; *CA* 66: 65289h.

Description—White to off-white crystalline powder; melts about 170°; pKa 5.3.

Solubility—Sparingly soluble in water or ether; 1 g dissolves in 330 mL of alcohol or 36 mL of chloroform.

Comments—A second-generation sulfonylurea oral hypoglycemic agent that stimulates the β-cells of the pancreas to secrete insulin.

It is indicated to treat Type 2 diabetes mellitus as monotherapy or in combination with other oral anti-diabetic agents (metformin, thiazolidinediones, or α-glucosidase inhibitors), except the meglitinides.

Glyburide is about 97% is bound to plasma albumin as a weak-acid anion and, hence, is susceptible to displacement by many weak acid drugs. It is metabolized hepatically and eliminated in both the urine and feces equally. The half-life is approximately 5 hr, and the duration of action is 12 to 24 hours.

Side effects include hypoglycemia, weight gain, gastrointestinal disturbances, skin rash, and insulin resistance. In addition, glyburide has been associated with a disulfiram reaction if taken concomitantly with alcohol, cholestatic jaundice, and eosinophilia.

Glyburide is dosed 2.5 mg to 20 mg once daily. It is available in a micronized formulation that is dosed 1.5 mg to 12 mg once daily. See Table 77-5 for a list of possible drug interactions.

METFORMIN HYDROCHLORIDE

Imidodicarbonimidic diamide, N,N-dimethyl-, monohydrochloride; Glucophage;Glucophage XR; Metiguanide

[657-24-9] $C_4H_{11}N_5 \cdot HCl$ (165.67).

Preparation—By the reaction of dimethylamine hydrochloride with dicyandiamide to yield the base; *J Am Chem Soc* 1959; 81:2220, 3728.

Description—White crystals melting about 230°

Solubility—Soluble in water or alcohol; practically insoluble in ether or chloroform.

Comments—An oral antidiabetic agent of the Biguanide class that is used in the management of Type 2 diabetes mellitus. It is indicated as monotherapy or as an adjunct to diet or other oral antidiabetic agents (sulfonylureas, thiazolidinediones, α-glucosidase inhibitors or meglitinides) and insulin. In Type 2 diabetic patients, metformin may decrease insulin requirements. Metformin does not bind to plasma proteins to any appreciable extent. It is not metabolized by the liver and is excreted primarily by the kidneys through the process of glomerular filtration and proximal tubular secretion.

Side effects include gastrointestinal disturbances that can happen in up to 30% of patients started on metformin and are a primary reason for patients not continuing therapy. This can be minimized by taking metformin after a meal and by slow careful dose titration. Since metformin is not an insulin secretagogue, there is no risk for hypoglycemia when used as monotherapy. This is not true when metformin is used in combination with insulin or other insulin secretagogues. Other side effects include vitamin b-12 deficiency (clinical implications are unknown), minor rash, and the rare complication of lactic acidosis. (Please see contraindications in the Biguanide description section). Unlike certain other oral antidiabetic medications, metformin has neutral or even beneficial effects on serum lipids. In studies, metformin was shown to reduce triglycerides and LDL-cholesterol levels.

Metformin is dosed 500 mg to 1000 mg twice daily. Maximum dose is 2550 mg daily. Blood glucose lowering as well as an improvement in HgA1c levels are not seen until a dose of 1000 to 1500 mg a day are achieved. It is available as an extended-release product. Metformin is available in combination products with glyburide (Glucovance), glipizide (Metaglip) and Rosiglitazone (Avandamet) which have been shown to be very effective in reducing blood glucose concentrations.

MIGLITOL

Piperidinetriol, 1-(2-hydroxyethyl)-2-(hydroxymethyl)-[2R-(2α,3β,4α,5β)]-, Glyset

[72432-03-2] $C_8H_{17}NO_5$ (207.22).

Preparation—One method involves the of nojirimycin, a natural product obtainable from the leaves of the mulberry tree (*M elba, M bombycis, or M nigra*).

Nojirimycin retains the configuration of D-glucose with the ether linkage replaced by a secondary amino group. The hydrogen atom on carbon-1 is removed by regioselective oxidation with *Gluconobacter oxydans* to form 1-deoxynojirimycin. The amine hydrogen atom is replaced by a hydroxyethyl group to form the product.

US Pat 4,639,436(1987) and www.wiley-vch.de/books/biotech/pdf/v08b_regi.pdf.

Description—Crystals from ethanol melting about 114°.

Solubility—Soluble in water; pKa 5.9.

Comments—Miglitol is an oral antidiabetic agent in the α-glucosidase class that is used to treat Type 2 diabetes mellitus. It is indicated as monotherapy or in combination with sulfonylureas. It is not bound to plasma proteins, is not metabolized, and is excreted unchanged in the urine. Side effects include gastrointestinal disturbances and rash. Since miglitol is not an insulin secretagogue, there is no risk for hypoglycemia when used as monotherapy, however the risk increases when used in combination with other insulin secretagogues.

Miglitol is dosed initially at 25 mg three times a day and a maintenance dose of 50 mg to 100 mg three times a day. Drug interactions are mainly with drugs that may bind Miglitol in the GI tract (Example: digestive enzymes and charcoal).

NATEGLINIDE

D-Phenylalanine, N-[[trans-4-(1-methylethyl)cyclohexyl]carbonyl]-, Starlix

[105816-04-4] $C_{19}H_{27}NO_3$ (317.42).

Preparation—4-Isopropylbenzoic acid is catalytically reduced to the cyclohexyl derivative yielding a mixture of both *cis* and *trans* isomers. The cyclohexanecarboxylic acid is converted to the acyl chloride and then the methyl ester. At this point the racemic mixture is resolved using chiral HPLC and the trans-ester saponified to the acid, converted back to the acyl halide, which then is coupled with phenylalanine to form the product. US Pat 4,816,484 (1989) and *J Med Chem* 1989; 32:1436.

Description—White crystals from methanol melting about 130°. [α]$^{20}_D$ −9.4°, (c=1, methanol).

Solubility—Freely soluble in methanol, ethanol or chloroform; soluble in ether;

Comments—Nateglinide is an oral antidiabetic agent of the meglitinide class that is used to treat Type 2 diabetes mellitus. It is approved for use as monotherapy, or in combination with Metformin

It is extensively protein bound (98%). It is metabolized by the cytochrome P450 2C9 and 3A4 and is primarily excreted through both urine and feces.

Side effects include hypoglycemia, upper respiratory tract infection, and gastrointestinal disturbances. Nateglinide is dosed as 60 mg to 120 mg three times a day. Drug interactions involving the CYP 450 system are lacking.

PIOGLITAZONE

(±)-2,4-Thiazolidinone, 5-[[4[2-(5-ethyl-2-pyridinyl)ethoxy]phenyl]methyl]-, monohydrochloride; Actos

[112529-15-4] $C_{19}H_{20}N_2O_3S$·HCl (392.90). US Pat 4,687,777 (1987).

Description—White, odorless crystalline powder melting about 193°.

Solubility—Soluble in DMF; slightly soluble in absolute ethanol; very slightly soluble in acetone or acetonitrile; practically insoluble in water; insoluble in ether.

Comments—Pioglitazone is an oral antidiabetic agent of the Thiazolidinediones class that is used to treat Type 2 diabetes mellitus. It is indicated as monotherapy or in combination with insulin or other oral antidiabetic agents (sulfonylureas, metformin, meglitinides, α-glucosidase inhibitors).

It is highly protein bound (>99%). It is metabolized by cytochrome P450 2C8, 3A4, and 1A1. It is excreted through both the urine and feces.

Side effects include headache, edema, and weight gain, and increased liver function tests. Pioglitazone appears safer than Troglitazone with respect to hepatic injury. (Please see LFT monitoring parameters in the Thiazolidinedione description section). Since Pioglitazone is not an insulin secretagogue, there is no risk for hypoglycemia when used as monotherapy. The risk is greater when used in combination with other insulin secretagogues. Pioglitazone may have a neutral or beneficial effect on lipids. In studies, Pioglitazone decreased triglycerides and LDL-cholesterol levels.

Pioglitazone is dosed as 15 to 45 mg once daily. The maximum benefit of Pioglitazone may take from 8 to 12 weeks. Since Pioglitazone is metabolized by CYP450 3A4, combining medications that inhibit or induce this pathway should be done cautiously. Pioglitazone has the possibly of decreasing the effect of oral contraceptives.

REPAGLINIDE

p-Toluic acid, (+)-2-ethoxy-α-[[(S)-α-isobutyl-o-piperidinobenzyl]carbamoyl]-, Prandin

[135062-02-1] $C_{27}H_{36}N_2O_4$ (452.59).

Preparation—See Int Pat Appl WO 93 00,337 (1993).

Description—White powder melting about 129°.

Comments—Repaglinide is an oral antidiabetic agent in the meglitinide class used in the treatment of Type 2 diabetes mellitus. It is indicated as monotherapy or in combination with metformin. It is bound to plasma proteins > 98%. It is metabolized by cytochrome P450 3A4 and is excreted through the feces and urine. Side effects include hypoglycemia, upper respiratory tract infection and gastrointestinal disturbances.

Repaglinide is dosed as 0.5 mg to 4 mg taken with meals. Since Repaglinide is metabolized by CYP450 3A4, combining medications that inhibit or induce this pathway should be done cautiously.

ROSIGLITAZONE MALEATE

2,4-Thiazolidinedione, (±)-5-[[4-[2-(methyl-2-pyridylamino)-ethoxy)phenylmethyl]-, maleate salt (1:); Avandia

[155141-29-0] [122320-73-4](base) $C_{18}H_{19}N_3O_3S$·$C_4H_4O_4$ (473.50).

Preparation—*J Med Chem* 1994; 37:3977 and US Pat 5,002,953 (1991).

Description—(Base) Crystals from methanol melting about 154°; (maleate) white to off-white solid melting about 122°. pK$_{a1}$6.1; pK$_{a2}$ 6.8.

Solubility—Readily soluble in methanol or aqueous solutions buffered to pH 2.3–2.5. Solubility decreases with increase in pH.

Comments—Rosiglitazone is an oral antidiabetic agent of the Thiazolidindione class that is used to treat Type 2 diabetes mellitus. It is indicated as monotherapy or in combination with insulin or other oral antidiabetic agents (sulfonylureas, metformin, meglitinides, α-glucosidase inhibitors). When added to regimens containing insulin, rosiglitazone may decrease the insulin requirements. It is highly protein bound (>99%). It is metabolized by cytochrome P450 2C8 and 2C9 and is excreted through both the urine and feces.

Side effects include headache, edema, and weight gain, and increased liver function tests. Rosiglitazone appears safer than troglitazone with respect to hepatic injury. (Please see LFT monitoring parameters in the thiazolinidione description section.) Since rosiglitazone is not an insulin secretagogue, there is no risk for hypoglycemia when used as monotherapy. The risk is greater when used in combination with other insulin secretagogues. Rosiglitazone is available in a combination product with metformin (Avandamet).

Rosiglitazone is dosed as 4 to 8 mg once daily. The maximum benefit of rosiglitazone may take from 8 to 12 weeks. There are no significant drug interactions seen with rosiglitazone

TOLAZAMIDE

Benzenesulfonamide, N-[[(hexahydro-1H-azepin-1-yl)amino]carbonyl]-4-methyl-, Tolinase

CH$_3$—◯—SO$_2$NHCONH—N◯

[1156-19-0] C$_{14}$H$_{21}$N$_3$O$_3$S (311.40).

Preparation—Methyl p-toluenesulfonylcarbamate undergoes an ammonolysis type of reaction with 1-aminohexamethylenetetramine. US 3,063,903 (1962).

Description—White to off-white crystalline powder; odorless or slight odor; melts between 161° and 169°.

Solubility—Very slightly soluble in water; freely soluble in chloroform; soluble in acetone; slightly soluble in alcohol.

Comments—A first generation sulfonylurea oral hypoglycemic agent that stimulates the β-cells of the pancreas to secrete insulin. It is indication to treat Type 2 diabetes mellitus as monotherapy or in combination with other oral anti-diabetic agents (metformin, thiazolidinediones, or α-glucosidase inhibitors), except the meglitinides. It is extensively bound to plasma proteins. It is metabolized in the liver to an inactive metabolite and is excreted through the kidneys. Side effects include hypoglycemia, weight gain, gastrointestinal disturbances, skin rash, and insulin resistance.

Tolazamide is dosed as 100 to 1000 mg daily. See Table 77-5 for a list of possible drug interactions.

TOLBUTAMIDE

Benzenesulfonamide, N-[(butylamino)carbonyl]-4-methyl-, Orinase

CH$_3$—◯—SO$_2$—NHCONH(CH$_2$)$_3$CH$_3$

1-Butyl-3-(p-tolylsulfonyl)urea [64-77-1] C$_{12}$H$_{18}$N$_2$O$_3$S (270.35).

Preparation—Toluene is treated with chlorosulfonic acid and the resulting p-toluenesulfonyl chloride is converted into p-toluenesulfonamide by interaction with ammonia. Condensation of the sulfonamide with ethyl chloroformate in the presence of pyridine or another suitable basic catalyst produces ethyl N-p-toluenesulfonylcarbamate. Aminolysis with butylamine in ethylene glycol monomethyl ether solutions yields tolbutamide.

Description—White, or practically white, crystalline powder; slightly bitter and practically odorless; melting range is 126° to 132°.

Solubility—Practically insoluble in water, soluble in alcohol or chloroform.

Comments—A first generation sulfonylurea oral hypoglycemic agent that stimulates the β-cells of the pancreas to secrete insulin. It is indication to treat Type 2 diabetes mellitus as monotherapy or in combination with other oral anti-diabetic agents (metformin, thiazolidinediones, or α-glucosidase inhibitors), except the meglitinides. It is extensively bound to plasma proteins. It is metabolized in the liver to an inactive metabolite and is excreted through the kidneys. Side effects include hypoglycemia, weight gain, gastrointestinal disturbances, skin rash and insulin resistance.

Tolbutamide is dosed as 500 to 3000 mg once daily. See Table 77-5 for a list of possible drug interactions.

COMBINATION ORAL ANTIDIABETIC AGENTS

GLUCOVANCE—(Glyburide and Metformin)
METAGLIP—(Metformin and Glipizide)
AVANDAMET—(Rosiglitazone and Metformin)

THE PARATHYROID HORMONE AND CALCITONIN

Spontaneous atrophy or injury (as at thyroidectomy) of the parathyroid glands is followed by a decrease in the concentration of serum calcium and an increase in serum phosphorus. These changes can be reversed by the parenteral administration of suitably prepared extracts of the parathyroids of domestic animals. The active principle of the parathyroid gland is a protein of molecular weight 9500. Active amino-terminal and carboxyl-terminal fragments of lower molecular weight (3800 and 6900, respectively) are found in plasma. These products possess 1/4 to 1/2 the specific calcium-mobilizing activity of parathyroid hormone (PTH).

Various cancers produce an active peptide homologous to the amino end of PTH, which is called parathyroid hormone–like peptide (PTH-LH) and causes hypercalcemia, bone destruction, and pain. PTH-LH also is found in lactating mammary tissue and plays a role in the mobilization of calcium to milk.

Secretion of PTH is stimulated by a fall in the free Ca^{2+} concentration of the plasma. The hormone then acts to restore Ca^{2+} concentration by (1) increasing reabsorption of calcium and the excretion of phosphate and decreasing the absorption of bicarbonate by the kidney; (2) increasing resorption of bone, with release of Ca^{2+}; and (3) increasing absorption of calcium and phosphate from the GI tract. The GI effects are mediated by 1α,25-dihydroxycholecalciferol (calcitriol), a metabolite of vitamin D$_3$ that may be considered a hormone; PTH is a trophin for renal synthesis of calcitriol. The metabolite also promotes the action of vitamin D$_3$ on bone. Vitamin D$_2$ (calciferol) and dihydrotachysterol can simulate the hypercalcemic effect of PTH; these compounds, moreover, are active orally. Overdosage with any of these compounds can lead to dangerously high calcium concentrations in the blood, with attendant complications, such as calcification of kidneys and blood vessels.

The thyroid gland produces a hormone, thyrocalcitonin, that reduces serum calcium concentration. A small amount of calcitonin also is produced in the parathyroid gland as well as the thymus, but the main source is the thyroid gland. The biological function of calcitonin is to prevent excessive hypercalcemia from parathyroid hormone activity. It has an effect to decrease osteoclastic activity, thus inhibiting the movement of bone salts from bone to the blood. It decreases the renal tubular secretion of calcium and probably inhibits calcium pumping in many types of cells. It also increases renal excretion of phosphate. It has very little effect on the absorption of calcium from the intestine. It plays a role in the homeostasis of blood calcium. When plasma calcium levels are elevated, thyrocalcitonin is released in increased quantities. Thus it tends to oppose parathyroid hormone but at different cell targets. The molecular weight of monomeric thyrocalcitonin is 3500. It is a polypeptide of 32 amino acid units. Despite only a 50% homology between human and salmon calcitonins, their biochemical actions are the same. However, salmon calcitonin is allergenic.

CALCITONIN

Calcitonin; Calcimar; Miacalcin

Cys-Ser-Asn-Leu-Ser-Thr-Cys-Val-Leu-Gly-Lys-Leu-Ser-Gln-Glu-Leu-His-
1   2   3   4   5   6   7   8   9   10 11 12 13 14 15 16 17

Lys-Leu-Gln-Thr-Tyr-Pro-Arg-Thr-Asn-Thr-Gly-Ser-Gly-Thr-Pro-NH$_2$
18 19 20 21 22 23 24 25 26 27 28 29 30 31 32

[47931-85-1] C$_{145}$H$_{240}$O$_{48}$S$_2$ (3431.88).

A polypeptide hormone secreted by the parafollicular cells of the thyroid gland in mammals and by the ultimobranchial gland of birds and fish, isolated from various of these sources, all apparently containing 32 amino acid residues but differing in the linear sequence. Human and salmon calcitonin differ at 18 positions. Both human and salmon calcitonins are available as synthetic products. The source of the product is indicated in the labeling.

Description—White, fluffy powder; lyophilized.

Solubility—Very soluble in water; slightly soluble in alcohol; insoluble in chloroform or ether.

Comments—Does not have much effect on normal plasma calcium, and patients with calcitonin-producing tumors of the thyroid medulla often do not manifest disturbances of calcium metabolism. It appears to act only in hypercalcemia, such as that caused by hyperparathyroidism, various carcinomas, and multiple myeloma. It normalizes plasma calcium and causes a favorable change in bone structure in Paget's disease; 3 to 12 months of treatment may be required to restore plasma electrolyte, alkaline phosphatase, and hydroxyproline to normal. Human calcitonin is less potent than salmon calcitonin because it is more rapidly degraded. Used alone against osteoporosis the hormone has a variable effect that may be related to the formation of antibodies. In combination with calcitriol and calcium it may be effective against senile and postmenopausal osteoporosis.

Side effects are mild nausea, vomiting, diarrhea, facial flushing, and malaise. Rashes may occur with salmon calcitonin. Inflammation and pain at the injection site sometimes occur. Diuresis at the onset of treatment often occurs.

The half-life of human calcitonin is about 1 hr; that of salmon calcitonin is considerably longer, but the exact figure is unknown. The duration of action is 6 to 8 hr.

AGENTS AFFECTING BONE MINERALIZATION

The two hormones that serve as the principal regulators of calcium and phosphate homeostasis in bone and the extracellular fluid are PTH and vitamin D, which acts as a prohormone because it must be metabolized to the biologically active calciferol and calcitriol. Other hormones that are considered secondary regulators include calcitonin, prolactin, growth hormone, insulin, thyroid hormone, and sex hormones. However, the most important agents used therapeutically are calcitonin, glucocorticoids, estrogen, and the bisphosphonates (nonhormonal analogs of pyrophosphate). Bone undergoes a continuous remodeling process involving resorption and formation, so alterations in the balance of controlling factors can lead to increased resorption, resulting in osteoporosis.

The principal effects of calcitonin are to lower serum calcium by effects on bone and kidney. Calcitonin inhibits osteoclastic bone resorption and reduces renal reabsorption of calcium and phosphate plus other ions, namely sodium, potassium, and magnesium. Prolonged use of glucocorticoids inhibit collagen synthesis in bone and antagonize vitamin D actions on intestinal calcium absorption and renal excretion; the result is an increased incidence of osteoporosis in adults and stunted growth in children. Estrogens can prevent accelerated bone loss during the immediate postmenopausal period and transiently increase bone in these patients. Estrogen receptors are present in bone and have some direct effects on bone remodeling that involves the osteoclasts that resorb bone and osteoblasts that are responsible for bone formation but are influenced by osteoclasts.

Treatment of postmenopausal osteoporosis is an important area of new drug development because estrogen replacement therapy is associated with increased cardiovascular problems as well as the potential increased risk of endometrial and breast cancer in some patients. Parenteral salmon calcitonin causes nausea, flushing, and formation of antibodies that may lead to resistance to the drug. A potential improvement is the availability of salmon calcitonin as a nasal spray that has little toxicity other than nasal irritation, but it appears to be less potent than the bisphosphonates.

New-drug developments include the selective estrogen- receptor modulators (SERMs) such as raloxifene plus new-generation bisphosphonates (alendronate) and slow-release formations of fluoride. Raloxifene represents a new class of synthetic estrogen analogs that have selectivity for the signal transduction that occurs at estrogen receptors; raloxifene has an agonist

effect on bone and an antagonist effect on both the breast and the uterus. Alendronate has improved efficacy over etidronate for increasing bone mass and decreasing bone fractures in patients with osteoporosis. Unlike bisphosphonates and calcitonin, which decrease bone resorption, sodium fluoride stimulates osteoblast proliferation and increases bone formation. However, too much fluoride can increase bone fragility. Slow-release sodium fluoride has been successful in maintaining serum fluoride concentrations in the therapeutic range associated with increased formation of normal bone, and clinical trials have demonstrated increased bone mass in women with severe postmenopausal osteoporosis. Plain sodium fluoride can cause moderately serious GI effects, including bleeding, but the slow-release form has only minor GI toxicity.

BISPHOSPHONATES—This group of agents are analogs of pyrophosphate in which the P-O-P bond is replaced by a non-hydrolyzable P-C-P bond. The bisphosphonates have the ability to retard formation and dissolution of hydroxyapatite crystals within bone and other sites, although the exact mechanism by which they selectively inhibit bone resorption is unclear. The first bisphosphonate available for clinical use was etidronate, but several new analogs are now available including pamidronate, alendronate, tiludronate, and risedronate. The limitations of etidronate include the lack of efficacy in increasing bone mass and reducing fractures in patients with osteoporosis for more than 2 years, plus it has potential toxicity of a mineralization defect called osteomalacia with higher doses. Alendronate is absorbed poorly and must be given on an empty stomach but has a greater efficacy in increasing bone density and reducing fractures over at least 5 years of continuous therapy. Pamidronate can cause an acute flulike illness and must be given by the intravenous route because it causes gastric irritation. The bisphosphonates are useful in treating hypercalcemia associated with malignancy, osteoporosis, and syndromes of ectopic calcification. They also are used to manage Paget's disease, which is a localized disease characterized by uncontrolled osteoclastic bone resorption with secondary increases in bone formation. Tiludronate and risedronate are available for oral treatment of Paget's disease. A summary of the comparative features of bisphosphonates is included in Table 77-6.

Other agents used to treat hypercalcemia include gallium nitrate and plicamycin, which have toxicity problems. Gallium nitrate inhibits bone resorption but has potential nephrotoxicity. Therapy with plicamycin is associated with sudden thrombocytopenia followed by hemorrhage as well as hepatic and renal toxicity. Chronic hypercalcemia of sarcoidosis, vitamin D intoxication, and certain cancers may be treated with glucocorticoids.

ALENDRONATE SODIUM

Phosphonic acid, (4-amino-1-hydroxybutylidene)bis-, monosodium salt, trihydrate; Fosamax; Onclast

[121268-17-5] $C_4H_{12}NNaO_7P_2.3H_2O$ (325.12).

Preparation—Orthophosphorous acid is heated with 4-aminobutyric acid in an atmosphere of nitrogen and phosphorous trichloride is added to the melt. Finally, water is added, the solution is decolorized with charcoal, and diluted with methanol to precipitate the free acid which is treated with one equivalent of sodium hydroxide. US Pat 4,705,651 (1987).

Description—(Acid) White crystalline, nonhygroscopic powder melting about 234° (decomposition). pK_1 2.27; pK_2 8.73; pK_3 10.5; pK_4 11.6 (in 0.1M KCl).

Solubility—(salt) Very soluble in water.

Comments—The first oral bisphophonate to be approved for the treatment and prevention of osteoporosis in postmenopausal women. It is more potent than etidronate and also is used to treat Paget's disease. Alendronate is a highly selective inhibitor of bone resorption (100–500

Table 77-6. Major Features of Bisphosphonates

BISPHOSPHONATES	COMMENTS
Etidronate	Less potent inhibitor of bone resorption; causes mineralization defects
Pamidronate	Only IV administration; causes acute flulike illness
Alendronate	Useful in treatment of osteoporosis; may cause esophageal ulcers
Tiludronate	Similar to etidronate but does not cause mineralization defects
Risedronate	More potent inhibitor than etidronate of bone resorption; may cause flulike syndrome and arthralgia

× more potent), while etidronate has the disadvantage of secondarily reducing bone formation that is coupled to resorption. The drug should be taken at least 30 min before food, beverage, or other medication. The mean oral bioavailability is 0.7%, which can be decreased by food. It is not metabolized and is eliminated from the systemic circulation by renal excretion. Several GI adverse effects may occur that include flatulence, acid regurgitation, dysphagia, and gastritis. Other effects include headache, musculoskeletal pain, and rash. Upper GI side effects including esophagitis and gastritis may be increased with higher doses used to treat Paget's disease.

CALCITRIOL

(1α,3β,5Z,7E)-9,10-Secocholesta-5,7,10(19)-triene-1,3,25-triol; Dihydrotachysterol; DHT; Calcijex; Rocaltrol; Topitrol

[3222-06-3] $C_{27}H_{44}O_3$ (416.65).

Preparation—Stereospecific synthesis from *d*-carvone in Lednicer D, Mitscher LA. *The Organic Chemistry of Drugs,* vol 3. New York: Wiley, 1984, pp 103–106; Baggiolini et al. *J Am Chem Soc* 1982; 104:2945.

Description—White crystals melting about 114°. Sensitive to air and light.

DIHYDROTACHYSTEROL

9,10-Secoergosta-5,7,22-trien-3-ol, (3β,5E,7E,10α,22E)-, Dihydrotachysterol; DHT

9,10-Secoergosta-5,7,22-trien-3β-ol [67-96-9] $C_{28}H_{46}O$ (398.67).

Preparation—Calciferol (activated ergosterol) is dissolved in a suitable organic solvent and subjected to catalytic hydrogenation until the proper amount of hydrogen has reacted.

Description—Colorless or white crystals, or a white, crystalline powder; odorless; melts between 123.5° and 129° for one form, or about 113° for the other form.

Solubility—Practically insoluble in water; soluble in alcohol; freely soluble in ether or chloroform; sparingly soluble in vegetable oils.

Comments—Chemically closely related to vitamin D_2 (calciferol) and consequently classified frequently as a D vitamin. However, it possesses very weak antirachitic activity, being only about 1/400 as potent as calciferol in this respect, mainly because its effects on calcium absorption from the intestine are quite weak. But it has potent calcemic activity (ie, raises plasma calcium concentration) and is similar to parathyroid hormone in this action. Consequently, it long has been used in lieu of parathyroid hormone in the treatment of idiopathic and postoperative tetanies, hypocalcemia, and hypoparathyroidism. The drug should not be used in the presence of renal insufficiency or hyperphosphatemia. Extreme care must be used to prevent overdosage.

Adverse effects result mainly from hypercalcemia. They include anorexia, nausea, vomiting, diarrhea, languor, osteoporosis, weight loss, metastatic calcification, renal damage, anemia, band keratitis, and convulsions. In severe hypercalcemia there may be headache, vertigo, tinnitus, abdominal cramps, polyuria, thirst, ataxia, albuminuria, and xanthemia.

ETIDRONATE DISODIUM

Phosphonic acid, (1-hydroxyethylidene)bis-, disodium salt; Didronel

$C_2H_6Na_2O_7P_2$ (249.99).

Preparation—Etidronic acid may be prepared in various ways, as by passing gaseous phosphorus trichloride into acetic acid at about 75°, by reaction of the same substances in a lower aliphatic tertiary amine such as tributylamine, or by reaction of an anhydrous mixture of phosphorous acid, acetic anhydride, and acetic acid.

Description—White powder.

Solubility—Very soluble in water.

Comments—This first-generation bisphosphonate is approved for treatment of Paget's disease but is a less potent inhibitor of bone resorption than new analogs. It is adsorbed onto hydroxyapatite (bone crystal), where it interferes with resorption of the crystals in osteoclasia and, in higher concentration, with osteoblastosis. In Paget's disease (osteitis deformans), for which it mainly is used, it slows the rate of turnover of bone, decreases excessive osteoclastic and osteoblastic cellular activities, and diminishes hydroxyproline levels in blood and urine and brings the elevated serum alkaline phosphate down toward normal. Usually several months of treatment are required to effect a considerable improvement. It also is used in the prophylaxis or slowing of heterotopic ossification (eg, after hip replacement or vertebral injury) and to suppress hypercalcemia of malignancy.

In high doses or after prolonged use, increased bone pain, decreased mineralization, and increased bone fractures may occur as the result of inhibition of osteoid formation. Even with the usual dosage, there may be occasional nausea, vomiting, diarrhea, and abdominal cramps, which can be lessened by dividing the dose into two or more portions.

It is 50% absorbed by the oral route. Various constituents in food and antacids, especially calcium, impair absorption. The distribution half-life is 5 to 7 hr; the elimination half-life is about 24 hr. The drug is eliminated entirely by renal excretion. Therefore, it should be used cautiously in renal failure. Urine hydroxyproline levels and serum alkaline phosphatase activity should be monitored periodically during treatment.

GALLIUM NITRATE

Nitric acid, gallium salt, nonahydrate: Ganite

$Ga(NO_3).9H_2O$[135886-70-3] $GaN_3O_9 \cdot 9H_2O$ (417.87).

Preparation—By dissolution of gallium metal or gallium oxide in nitric acid.

Description—White, deliquescent crystals; decomposes about 110°; forms Ga_2O_3 at 200°.

Solubility—Very soluble in water; soluble in anhydrous alcohol.

Comments—To treat cancer-related hypercalcemia unresponsive to adequate hydration. It inhibits calcium resorption from bone, possibly by reducing increased bone turnover. The precise mechanism has not been determined. The plasma half-life is 72 to 115 hr with a prolonged intravenous infusion, and the major route of elimination is renal excretion.

Adverse effects include nephrotoxicity, transient hypophosphatemia, anemia, and leukopenia. It should not be used with other nephrotoxic drugs.

THE THYROID HORMONES

The thyroid gland modulates the energy metabolism and certain nonenergetic metabolic functions of the body. In the absence of the thyroid gland the basal metabolic rate is less than 55% of normal, and growth and development are impaired. In the presence of a hyperactive gland the metabolic rate may be up to 160% of normal; the excitability of irritable tissues is increased, and tachycardia, nervousness, etc. result. Thyroid *hormone* is used clinically mainly to replenish the corporal hormone supply in conditions of thyroid insufficiency (hypothyroidism), such as may result from a natural thyroid or pituitary pathology or from thyroid surgery. The *hormone* rarely is administered to increase the metabolic rate and organic activity above normal, and such iatrogenic hyperthyroidism may indeed be dangerous.

The mediator by which the thyroid gland stimulates the tissues to a higher activity and rate of metabolism is called the thyroid hormone, but there are actually four active substances, all iodinated thyronines, released by the gland. Thyroxine (L-3,5,3′,5′-tetraiodothyronine, or T_4 is found in the greatest amount in blood (about 75% of the thyroid hormone content of the plasma), and the moderately less active L-3,3′-diiodothyronine is present in the next greatest amount (25%). L-3,5,3′-Triiodothyronine (liothyronine, or T_3, which is 3 to 10 times as active as thyroxine, and L-3,3′,5′-triiodothyronine make up less than 3% of the plasma thyroid hormone content. But since the triiodothyronines disappear more rapidly from blood than thyroxine, they probably constitute a somewhat larger proportion of the glandular secretion; in the thyroid gland they account for about 1/5 of the hormone content and as much as 40% of its hormone activity. Furthermore, in the tissues, some thyroxine is converted to liothyronine and perhaps as much as 1/2 to 2/3 of the body liothyronine is derived from thyroxine. Liothyronine regulates TRH release in the hypothalamus and is probably the principal hormone involved in the long negative-feedback-loop regulation of TSH (thyroid-stimulating hormone, or thyrotropin) release.

The thyroid gland concentrates iodide ion from the plasma and converts it to free iodine, which then reacts with tyrosine moieties within the substance of the gland eventually to produce the thyroid hormones. The glandular accumulation of iodine and the conversion to the intermediate 3,5- diiodotyrosine are under the control of the thyrotropic hormone. Iodine deficiency results in a compensatory increase in the size of the thyroid gland in a usually fruitless homeostatic attempt to manufacture more hormone. Iodine administration corrects this type of goiter and permits the normal production of the thyroid hormones. The incorporation of sodium iodide into table salt helps protect against iodine-deficiency thyroid disorders. In children under 14 years, iodine supplementation corrects endemic cretinism.

In the colloid of the thyroid gland these thyronine derivatives are bound to a globulin, thyroglobulin, which formerly was thought to be the thyroid hormone. About 90% of the thyroid hormone content of the gland is in the thyroglobulin complex. The molecular weight of thyroglobulin is 650,000. Before thyroxine and liothyronine can be released into the bloodstream, the thyroglobulin must be assimilated by the thyroid follicular cells, within which the globulin is split by proteases to release the hormones. In the blood, the hormones are bound mainly to an albumin; the complex is dissociable, so the hormones are free to pass into the body cells.

The thyroid hormones interact with nuclear receptors to increase RNA polymerase and also to increase the number of initiation sites for the polymerase. The result is an increase in transcription for a number of proteins, and the synthesis thereof is increased. Thyroid hormone also has a regulatory action on tRNA. The synthesized proteins in turn regulate various enzymes and enzyme complexes, so that oxidative phosphorylation in the mitochondria may become partially uncoupled, membrane ATPase activity is increased, adenylate cyclase activity is enhanced, etc. There also are some direct actions on cellular functions, such as stimulation of autocrine growth factors and amino acid transport systems and inhibition of some zinc-dependent dehydrogenases, prostaglandin dehydrogenases, etc. The uses and adverse effects of the thyroid hormones are indicated in the monograph on *Thyroid*. Thyroid hormones lower plasma lipid concentrations. However, because of their effect to increase the metabolic rate, they are not used clinically to lower blood lipids. The lipid-lowering action is possessed also by the dextro isomers of thyroid hormones, but the dextro forms have only a very weak effect on the metabolic rate. Consequently, dextrothyroxine is employed to lower blood lipids.

Table 77-7. Thyroid Hormone Products

PREPARATION	COMPOSITION (RATIO OF T_4/T_3)	COMMENTS
Crude hormone		
Thyroid	2–5	Powdered extract from domestic animals
Thyroglobulin	2.5	Extracted from hog thyroid glands
Thyroid strong	3.1	Desiccated thyroid with higher iodine content, 50% stronger than thyroid
Synthetic hormone		
Levothyroxine	Pure T_4	Longer half-life (6–7 days)
Liothyronine	Pure T_3	Short half-life (<2 days), potency 4× > T4
Liotrix	4	Mixture of pure T4 and T3

A summary of the thyroid hormone products is shown in Table 77-7.

LEVOTHYROXINE SODIUM

l-Tyrosine, *O*-(4-hydroxy-3,5-diiodophenyl)-3,5-diiodo-, monosodium salt, hydrate; Levothroid; Levoxyl, Synthroid, Unithroid

Monosodium L-thyroxine hydrate [25416-65-3] $C_{15}H_{10}I_4NNaO_4 \cdot xH_2O$; *anhydrous* [55-03-8] (798.86); the sodium salt of the levo isomer of thyroxine, an active physiological principle obtained from the thyroid gland of domesticated animals used for food by man, or prepared synthetically. It contains 61.6% to 65.5% of iodine, corresponding to 97% to 103% of levothyroxine sodium.

Preparation—L-Thyroxine is dissolved in dilute NaOH solution, and the resulting sodium salt is precipitated by saturating the solution with NaCl.

Thyroxine may be prepared from thyroid glands or by synthesis. Preparation from the glands (fresh or desiccated) involves extraction with dilute sodium hydroxide followed by acidification with hydrochloric acid, whereupon a very crude form of thyroxine is precipitated. Purification involves repeated solubilization by means of sodium hydroxide and reprecipitation with acid, these operations being conducted under increasingly refined conditions and with the aid of auxiliary operations designed to enhance the purity of the final precipitate of thyroxine.

The key compound in the synthesis of thyroxine is 3,5-diiodo-4- (*p*-methoxyphenoxy)nitrobenzene (I), which is readily formed by condensing *p*-methoxyphenol with 3,4,5-triiodonitrobenzene under the influence of anhydrous potassium carbonate. A series of subsequent operations involves (a) reduction of nitro to amino; (b) replacement of amino by cyano by treatment with cuprous cyanide and butyl nitrite;

(c) hydration of cyano to carboxyl, and (d) reduction of carboxyl to formyl. The resulting aldehyde may be converted into thyroxine in various ways. One involves condensation with 2-phenyl-2-oxazolin-5-one to produce II, which is then simultaneously hydrogenated, demethylated, and reductively cleaved by hydrogen iodide in the presence of phospho-

MEDICINAL AGENTS

rus and acetic anhydride to give the DL-form of 3-[4-(4-hydroxyphenoxy)-3,5-diiodophenyl]alanine (III), which is resolved, and the isolated L-enantiomorph is iodinated with ammoniacal potassium triiodide solution at the 3,5-positions on the phenoxy ring to give levothyroxine. Neutralization of this acid with NaOH yields the salt.

Description—Light yellow to buff-colored, odorless, tasteless, hygroscopic powder; stable in dry air but may assume a slight pink color upon exposure to light; pH (saturated solution) about 8.9.

Solubility—1 g in about 700 mL water or about 300 mL alcohol; insoluble in acetone, chloroform, or ether; soluble in solutions of alkali hydroxides.

Comments—Has the actions, uses, side effects, and limitations of thyroid. The sodium salt lends itself to intravenous administration in the treatment of myxedemic coma, although the more rapidly acting liothyronine is preferred. Approximately 50% of an oral dose is absorbed. The plasma half-life is about 9 to 10 days in hypothyroid, 6 to 7 days in euthyroid and 3 to 4 days in hyperthyroid persons, but the time for the intensity of its effect to fall to 1/2 of its initial value is 9 to 12 days, and some residual effects may be apparent for several weeks after the last dose. Although the *l*-form is twice as active as the racemic mixture, it offers no particular therapeutic advantage over the *dl*-form, and it has the disadvantage of being more expensive.

LIOTHYRONINE SODIUM

L-Tyrosine, *O*-(4-hydroxy-3-iodophenyl)-3-5-diiodo-, monosodium salt; Cytomel, Triostat, Liothyronine Sodium

Monosodium L-3-[4-(4-hydroxy-3-iodophenoxy)-3,5-diiodophenyl]alanine [55-06-1] $C_{15}H_{11}I_3NNaO_4$ (672.96).

Preparation—3,5-Diiodo-L-thyronine, the L-enantiomorph of compound (III) in the thyroxine synthesis described under *Levothyroxine Sodium*, is dissolved in methanol and iodinated only at the 3-position by treatment with ammonia and iodine at room temperature. The liothyronine (acid) is then liberated by acidifying the reaction mixture. It is purified and neutralized with NaOH to give the salt.

Description—Light-tan, odorless, crystalline powder.

Solubility—Very slightly soluble in water; slightly soluble in alcohol; practically insoluble in most other organic solvents.

Comments—Four times more potent than *Levothyroxine Sodium*. The actions and uses are those of *Thyroid* and *Levothyroxine Sodium*. It also has been used to reduce goiter, but it is less effective than Levothyroxine in suppressing TSH release. Because of the lesser pituitary suppression and the wide fluctuation in plasma levels, which negate monitoring, it is not the agent of choice for maintenance, especially after ablative radioiodine treatment. It is the treatment of choice to treat myxedemic coma, because of the rapid onset of action. It may be used to suppress goiter preparatory to surgery.

It has a rapid onset of action. The peak effect occurs in 1 to 3 days, and the offset of action is about 3 days. The prompt onset and rapid offset (compared with levothyroxine) are considered to be an advantage over thyroid or levothyroxine. The time for the intensity of its effect to fall to 1/2 of its initial value is 4 to 10 days. Liothyronine is absorbed erratically from the GI tract, and 30 to 40% may be recovered from the stools. Liothyronine is only loosely bound to plasma proteins and hence does not elevate the plasma protein-bound iodine (PBI) significantly. It crosses the blood-brain barrier and hence is not recommended for use in children.

THYROID

Desiccated Thyroid, Armour Thyroid, Thyroid USP

The cleaned, dried, and powdered thyroid gland previously deprived of connective tissue and fat. It is obtained from domesticated animals that are used for food by man.

Thyroid contains 0.17% to 0.23% of iodine (I) in thyroid combination and is free from iodine in inorganic or any form of combination other than that peculiar to the thyroid gland. A desiccated thyroid of a higher iodine content may be brought to this standard by admixture with a desiccated thyroid of a lower iodine content with lactose, sodium chloride, starch, sucrose, or dextrose.

Description—Yellowish to buff-colored, amorphous powder, with a slight characteristic, meat-like odor and a saline taste.

Comments—Essential for normal metabolism and development. The congenital absence of thyroid hormone results in a condition known as cretinism. In childhood or adult life, absence of thyroid hormone causes myxedema. These conditions are characterized by an abnormally low basal metabolic rate. The primary therapeutic use is in their treatment.

These preparations may be used to suppress the secretion of thyrotropin in simple nonendemic goiter (hence decreases thyroid size) and

chronic lymphocytic thyroiditis (Hashimoto's disease). These hormones do not decrease hyperthyroid exophthalmus. The use of them in the diagnosis of hyperthyroidism is outlined under *Liothyronine Sodium*.

In the absence of hypothyroidism, these hormones do not improve skin conditions, mental depression, fatigue, lethargy, obesity, irritability, nervousness, menstrual irregularities, and other endocrine and reproductive disorders, and there is danger that untoward effects may be produced.

Untoward effects of overdoses of these hormones include tachycardia, arrhythmias, angina pectoris, hypertension, insomnia, nervousness, hyperkinesis, tremors, diaphoresis, hot skin, GI disturbances, and hypoadrenocorticism. Even with physiological doses, it may be advisable to administer glucocorticoids concurrently. It may cause allergic reactions.

It has a very slow onset of action. A given dose does not exert its maximum effect for several days and will continue to have some degree of action for 2 to 3 months. Therefore, caution must be exercised in judging the dose, in that cumulative effects must be anticipated.

ANTITHYROID DRUGS

A number of linear and heterocyclic derivatives of thiourea inhibit the production of thyroid hormone by the thyroid gland. The mechanism of action is that of preventing iodination of tyrosine and the coupling between iodotyrosines. They also inhibit the conversion of thyroxine to liothyronine in the periphery. The decline in thyroid hormone output and the resultant lowering of plasma levels of the thyroid hormones is sensed in the hypothalamus, which through the long-loop feedback and intermediation of the thyrotropin-releasing factor stimulates the adenohypophysis to produce more thyrotropic hormone. Consequently, the thyroid gland is stimulated to enlarge, even though the enlarged gland cannot produce more thyroid hormone. Because of the thyroid enlargement consequent to the use of the thiourea class of antithyroid compounds, such compounds are called goitrogens. The goitrogens are employed in the control of hyperthyroidism. An enlarged thyroid gland is very vascular and friable, which makes surgery difficult. Therefore, iodine (or a thyroid hormone), which reduces the size of the gland, is added to the regimen preparatory to thyroid surgery. Antithyroid drugs also decrease T-lymphocyte cytotoxicity and restore normal suppressor-cell activity and are thought thus to decrease thyroid autoimmunity in Grave's disease.

Several other classes of compounds also are antithyroid agents. Compounds such as thiocyanates and perchlorates competitively inhibit the iodine uptake mechanism. Large doses of iodine inhibit the enzyme tyrosine iodinase and thus interfere with the production of thyroid hormone. Therefore, iodine also may be used in the treatment of hyperthyroidism. Curiously, this action of iodine is not goitrogenic; in fact, iodine opposes the goitrogenic effects of certain antithyroid drugs. Radioiodine I-131 (^{131}I) is antithyroid by virtue of tissue destruction caused by radiation. Thyroid hormones are antigoitrogenic by the long-loop homeostatic feedback mechanism to reduce the hypothalamic release of thyrotropin-releasing factor.

METHIMAZOLE

2*H*-Imidazole-2-thione, 1,3-dihydro-1-methyl-, Tapazole

1-Methylimidazole-2-thiol [60-56-0] $C_4H_6N_2S$ (114.16).

Preparation—One method consists of cyclizing (methylamino)acetaldehyde diethyl acetal with thiocyanic acid via de-ethanolation. Details are provided in *J Am Chem Soc* 1949; 71:4000.

Description—White to pale buff, crystalline powder, with a faint characteristic odor; solutions are practically neutral to litmus; melting range 144 to 147°.

Solubility—1 g in 5 mL water, 5 mL alcohol, 4.5 mL chloroform, or 125 mL ether.

Comments—An antithyroid drug for the preparation of the hyperthyroid patient for surgery and for the total treatment of hyperthyroidism. It is approximately 10 times as potent as propylthiouracil and is more prompt in eliciting an antithyroid response. The drug also exhibits a more prolonged action than propylthiouracil; a single dose of 5 mg may inhibit the synthesis of thyroid hormone for 24 hr. The plasma half-life is 6 to 8.5 hr in hyperthyroid, but 8 to 18 hr in hypothyroid, patients; therefore, as the drug lowers the metabolic rate, its own metabolism is slowed, and accumulation will occur unless the dose is adjusted.

Approximately 6% of patients taking the drug experience some untoward effect. Thus, the incidence of untoward reactions is somewhat higher than with propylthiouracil but considerably lower than with other antithyroid drugs. Cross-sensitization to other thiouracils can occur. Three times as much of this drug crosses the placental barrier as propylthiouracil.

POTASSIUM IODIDE—page 1377.

PROPYLTHIOURACIL

4(1*H*)-Pyrimidinone, 2,3-dihydro-6-propyl-2-thioxo-, Propacil

6-Propyl-2-thiouracil [51-52-5] $C_7H_{10}N_2OS$ (170.23).

Preparation—By condensation of ethyl 3-oxocaproate with thiourea (*J Am Chem Soc* 1945; 67:2197).

Description—White, powdery, crystalline substance; starch-like in appearance and to the touch; bitter taste; melts about 220°.

Solubility—Slightly soluble in water; sparingly soluble in alcohol; slightly soluble in chloroform or ether; soluble in ammonia or alkali hydroxides.

Comments—Since the drug does not interfere with the release or use of stored thyroid hormone, the period that elapses between the beginning of medication and the manifestations of its antithyroid action depends upon the quantity of thyroid hormone stored in the gland. The marked hyperplasia of the thyroid gland that follows its administration is a result of a compensatory increase of thyrotropin release consequent to a reduction in the thyroid hormone titer of the blood. In the preparation of the hyperthyroid patient for surgery, when treatment with the drug has brought the basal metabolic rate to normal (euthyroidism) or nearly so, iodine is administered to reduce the marked vascularity and friability of the gland. In the total (medical) treatment of hyperthyroidism, the duration of treatment usually ranges from 6 months to 3 years, after which thyroid function may remain normal. However, at least half of patients so treated may be expected to have a recurrence 6 to 12 months after cessation of medication.

The most serious toxic actions are granulocytopenia, leukopenia, drug fever, and dermatitis. Joint pains and urticaria may occur. Cross-sensitivity to other thiouracils may occur. A small percentage of patients experience nausea, abdominal discomfort, headache, drowsiness, vertigo, paresthesias, and loss of taste sense. The overall incidence of untoward reactions to propylthiouracil is approximately 4%; the incidence of agranulocytosis approaches 0.5%. The drug passes the placental barrier and may affect the fetus, so that during pregnancy the lowest possible dose should be used. It also is secreted into milk, and the drug should be withheld from nursing mothers.

Only about 75% is absorbed by the oral route. There is considerable confusion about the elimination half-life, probably because redistribution has been confused with elimination and because of analytical difficulties. The elimination half-life is probably about 3 to 5 hr in hyperthyroid, 6 to 8 hr in euthyroid, and 24 to 34 hr in hypothyroid, persons; thus since the drug decreases the metabolic rate, the dose should be adjusted accordingly, to avoid accumulation.

THE GONADAL HORMONES AND INHIBITORS

Three main classes of steroid hormones are produced by gonadal tissues: estrogenic, progestational, and androgenic hormones. The ovary is the primary site for synthesis and secretion of estrogenic and progestational hormones in women. At puberty, the ovary begins a 30- to 40-year period of cyclic function called the menstrual cycle that is regulated by the pulsatile production of hypothalamic gonadotropin-releasing hormone (GnRH) that stimulates the release of follicle-stimulating hormone (FSH) and luteinizing hormone (LH) from the anterior pituitary. In men and postmenopausal women, the principal source of estrogen is adipose tissue stroma, where the level of estrogens is regulated in part by the availability of androgenic precursors secreted from the adrenal cortex.

The most important androgenic hormone produced by the testes in men is testosterone, although the adrenal cortex also produces some androgenic hormones in both men and women. FSH and LH also regulate testosterone production by specific cells in the testis that control spermatogenesis and the development of primary and secondary sexual characteristics in men.

STRUCTURE—The natural estrogens are all steroids (see Chapter 26) containing 18 carbon atoms, oxygenated at carbons 3 and 17. Ring A of all the estrogens is aromatic and is formed from either androstenedione or testosterone precursors by a monooxygenase enzyme complex called aromatase that uses NADPH and molecular oxygen as cosubstrates.

Progesterone, the hormone of the corpus luteum, is a 21-carbon-atom steroid possessing, like adrenal cortical steroids, an α,β-unsaturated ketone component in Ring A. It differs from the latter in that its C17 does not carry a hydroxyl group.

The natural androgenic steroids are 19-carbon-atom compounds. They are characterized by a partly or completely saturated ring A and by either a hydroxyl or a keto group at C3 and C17. As with all other classes of steroids, stereoisomerism is of fundamental importance with the sex hormones; and the α- and β-configuration conventions are applied in drawing the structural formulas.

The Ovarian Hormones

The ovaries serve the dual purpose of secreting the female hormones and producing the ova that, after the menarche, are liberated normally at the rate of one every 4 weeks. The menstrual cycle can be described in terms of the development of both the ovarian follicles and changes in the endometrial lining of the uterus. The proliferative and secretory phases of the endometrial changes coincide with the follicular and luteal stages of the ovarian follicles, respectively. Estrogen predominates during endometrial proliferation and maturation of an ovarian follicle that is released at the time of ovulation. Both estrogen and progesterone are produced by the ruptured follicle that becomes the corpus luteum, which secretes estrogen and progesterone. Progesterone levels are greatest during the secretory phase of the endometrium and the luteal phase of the corpus luteum. Estrogen levels fall at the time of menstruation and are associated with bleeding and sloughing of the highly vascularized endometrium; if the released ovum or corpus luteum is not sustained by successful fertilization it regresses. During pregnancy the placenta produces large quantities of estrogen. The ovaries also secrete small amounts of androgens, adrenal steroids, and the nonsteroidal hormone relaxin (see below).

The ovarian production of hormones is regulated by the gonadotropic hormones of the anterior pituitary. However, the control of pituitary gonadotropin production is, in turn, modulated by the estrogens and progesterone, which in low plasma concentrations appear to stimulate, and at high concentrations inhibit, the production of FSH, LH, and LRH. Thus, a complex positive and negative feedback system subserves the cyclic phenomena of ovulation and menstruation. The exact details in this concert are not known completely for humans. It is known that in women ovulation can be prevented by estrogens as the result of suppression of FSH production. However, estrogen alone is not satisfactory for oral contraception, owing to what is termed *breakthrough* bleeding, except when high doses of estrogen are used. In large doses, progesterone also inhibits ovulation, presumably because of suppression of the pulsatile secretion of the hypothalamic GnRH. Furthermore, progesterone can favor infertility by antagonism of some estrogen actions, by maintaining the endometrium in a hypoproliferative and hyposecretory state that is unfavorable to implantation of the fertilized ovum. It now is known that some progestins have an antifertility effect at doses well below those necessary to suppress endometrial proliferation and secretion.

Intermenstrual bleeding occurs during continuous treatment with many progestins, and it was found desirable to add estrogens. Estrogen not only helped normalize cyclic bleeding but also contributed to the contraceptive effect. Progestins alone can be used for contraception, but their mechanism does not totally depend upon inhibition of ovulation that occurs in 70% to 80% of cycles by slowing the frequency of the GnRH pulse generator and blunting the LH surge. A thickening of the cervical mucus to decrease sperm penetration and endometrial changes that impair implantation are thought to contribute to their efficacy. Progestins alone avoid the drawbacks of estrogens, namely nausea, vomiting, headache, a tendency to venous thrombosis, and other untoward effects, but they are slightly less effective contraceptives than are the estrogens.

The luteinized granulosa cells of the corpus luteum also produce relaxin, a peptide with a tertiary structure similar to that of insulin and some growth factors. There are two chains linked through disulfide bonds. The molecular weight is about 6000. It relaxes the estrogen-primed symphysis pubis and increases the viscous pliability of the cervix, thus assisting the birth canal to prepare for parturition. It also increases glycogen synthesis and water uptake by the myometrium and decreases uterine contractility, which suggests a role during gestation. During the menstrual cycle, blood levels are high just following the LH surge and during menstruation. Much of its physiology remains to be learned. Relaxin also is found in the placenta and uterus.

Another relaxing peptide, lututrin, is produced in the ovary. Very little is known of its physiological functions. Relaxin and lututrin have been used to treat dysmenorrhea, premature labor, cervical dystocia, and scleroderma, but efficacy never has been proved.

NATURAL ESTROGENIC HORMONES AND CONGENERS

Natural estrogenic hormones are secreted by the ovarian follicles. They stimulate or regulate the growth and development of the uterus, the vaginal mucous membrane, and other structures such as mammary glands, subcutaneous fat, axillary and pubic hair, and certain elements in the skin. These latter comprise the secondary female sex characteristics. Therefore the estrogens also are called female sex hormones. Of the estrogens the most potent occurring naturally are β-estradiol and its two principal metabolic products, estrone and estriol, which also are estrogenic. Several other products of metabolic change occur in smaller amounts, but these are not offered as single substances for therapy. Estrogens are secreted throughout the period of activity of the ovaries, but at varying rates at different times of the menstrual cycle.

The naturally occurring estrogens can be prepared synthetically, but at greater cost than by extraction from natural materials or by simple chemical processing of natural estrogens as they occur in urine. An interesting improvement of the natural estrogen has been the synthetic modification of β- estradiol, the most potent natural estrogen, by the addition of a side chain, producing ethinyl estradiol. This has a very high activity when administered orally.

USES—Estrogens are used as substitution therapy when menopausal symptoms occur after cessation of ovarian function, following ovariectomy or x-ray or radium therapy, or in the natural menopause (also called the climacteric). There is general agreement that low-dose estrogen treatment will ameliorate the symptoms of vasomotor instability (hot flashes), prevent or reverse urogenital atrophy in menopausal women.

The beneficial effects of estrogen therapy on irritability, depression, anxiety, and insomnia are more unpredictable. Estrogen administration can alter high-density lipoproteins (HDLs) and low-density lipoproteins (LDLs), which improves the relative lipoprotein profile. However, any potential benefits of estrogen replacement therapy must be weighed against serious cardiovascular and breast cancer risk (see *Side Effects* below).

At this time estrogen replacement therapy can only be recommended for short-term management of menopausal symptoms.

Estrogens are used in young women in whom there is failure of steroidogenesis; treatment brings about acceleration of delayed development of the uterus, the appearance of secondary sex characteristics, and subtle biochemical and behavioral changes. Applied locally, the estrogens are useful in the treatment of atrophic or senile vaginitis, vulvovaginitis, or cervicitis resulting from hypoestrogenesis but not from other causes.

A number of menstrual irregularities may be treated with estrogens. Some of these, such as amenorrhea, may be the result of an asynchrony in the release of hypothalamic release factors and pituitary gonadotropin release. Estrogens used cyclically may regularize some of these conditions. They are of value in symptoms of premenstrual tension such as headache and electrolyte imbalance. In endometriosis, estrogens are effective for only a short time, endometrial hyperplasia eventually resulting. In dysmenorrhea and dysfunctional uterine bleeding, combined treatment with estrogens and progestogens is used, and normal withdrawal bleeding may follow the abrupt cessation of treatment.

Estrogens also are used to treat acne vulgaris and hirsutism. They may be used in the induction of parturition and in the postpartum period to reduce breast engorgement.

There is a choice of compounds for estrogenic therapy. A comparison of some major features of estrogenic agents is included in Table 77-8. Estrone is employed commonly by intramuscular injection, but considerable activity is lost if the oral route is used. Ethinyl estradiol is the most active of all oral estrogens, and its oral activity is nearly equal to its parenteral activity. Conjugated estrogens retain much of their activity on oral administration and are used extensively by this route. Estrogens also can be given by topical, intravaginal or with transdermal systems.

Synthetic or Nonsteroidal Estrogens

The best known is diethylstilbestrol, which possesses most of the therapeutic and untoward actions of the natural estrogenic hormones. Since nonsteroidal estrogens lose little activity after oral administration, they have advantages over the natural estrogens, but the comparative toxicities are not clear. Attempts to explain why such nonsteroidal compounds are estrogenically potent have been intriguing. There is a spatial resemblance between them and the true hormone estradiol. Others have focused attention on the closeness of the dimensions of the synthetics (especially length, width, and distance between OH groups) and those of estradiol. The synthetic estrogens combine with the same cytoplasmic receptors as natural estrogens and presumably also with the same nuclear receptor.

Table 77-8. Major Features of Estrogens

ESTROGENS	COMMENTS
Natural estrogens	
Estradiol	Low oral bioavailability due to extensive first-pass hepatic metabolism; oral, IM, topical, and transdermal forms
Conjugated estrogens	
Esterified estrogens	Mixture of sulfate esters of estrogenic substances from pregnant mares; predominantly estrone and equilin; used orally or topically
Synthetic estrogens	
Ethinyl estradiol	Slower metabolism; half-life = 13–27 hr
Mestranol	Metabolized to ethinyl estradiol
Nonsteroidal estrogens	
Diethylstilbesterol	Good oral absorption; slow inactivation

Synthetic estrogens have a greater bioavailability than natural ones. Regarding the latter it must be recalled that the oral doses of natural estrogens, with the possible exception of ethinyl estradiol (a derivative of a natural estrogen), may have to be five or more times that of the parenteral doses to secure similar results. This is the result of first-pass metabolism, excretion into bile, and destruction in the intestines. One disadvantage of some synthetic estrogenic compounds is that nausea follows the use of even the minimum effective dose in some women. It is most distressing in the first 2 weeks of use, after which tolerance develops. In such women the synthetic materials must be replaced by natural products. Whether the synthetic estrogens are more toxic than natural estrogens is not established unequivocally, but diethylstilbestrol differs significantly from natural compounds (see the introduction to this section and *Diethylstilbestrol*).

SIDE EFFECTS—Nausea and vomiting are frequent side effects of estrogens. These effects appear to be mainly of CNS origin. Estrogens may cause fluid retention and breast tenderness. They also may cause breast engorgement, in part by promoting the proliferation of the secretory acini and ducts. Headache and dizziness are more frequent with high doses and severe migraine may occur even with low doses. Malaise, irritability, and depression occasionally occur with small doses and frequently with large doses. The effect on libido is erratic, being increased in some and decreased in others.

Estrogens effect changes in the concentration of some of the clotting factors in blood, and therapeutic doses of semisynthetic and synthetic estrogens increase the incidence of thrombophlebitis and thromboembolism in both the superficial and deep veins. Pulmonary embolism, cerebral embolism with stroke, and mesenteric vascular occlusion occur. Coronary thrombosis also seems to be increased among users of estrogens.

Estrogens alter hepatic function, which may alter results of various tests of liver function as well as various synthetic and biotransformation processes. Effects of estrogen alone to decrease glucose tolerance are now believed to be related to their combined effects with progestins. 17-Alkyl derivatives, especially, occasionally cause cholestatic jaundice. The composition of the bile is altered, and there is a slightly increased incidence of gallstones after long-term use.

Acute porphyria may be precipitated. Changes in the concentration of blood proteins may occur; thyroxine- and glucocorticoid-binding proteins are increased, which may alter endocrine relationships. Aldosterone secretion is increased, which not only accounts for sodium retention but also for an abnormal incidence of hypertension among users of estrogens. Estrogen-induced hypertension is reversible.

Estrogens may induce changes in the skin, such as dermatitis, increased pigmentation (in combination with progestins, causes chloasma), a tendency to vaginal candidiasis, and spider angiomas. Photosensitization may occur, and protective measures are advisable. Although estrogens may improve acne, they only do so after a temporary worsening of the condition. Estrogens may cause a loss of scalp hair in some users and hypertrichosis in others. Allergic reactions include rashes, erythema multiforme, erythema nodosum, and cholestatic jaundice.

Recent data have shown the relationship of estrogen therapy to an increased risk of breast cancer for premenopausal women. Estrogens increase the risk of endometrial carcinoma by 4.5 to 13.9 times, and the incidence appears to depend on duration and dose. When diethylstilbestrol is taken during pregnancy, there is an increased likelihood of vaginal adenocarcinoma in the daughter after maturity; whether natural and semisynthetic estrogens are similarly fetotoxic is not known. There also is an increased likelihood of functional abnormalities in the reproductive tracts in both female and male offspring.

Hypercalcemia may occur, especially in men taking large doses for prostatic carcinoma.

In women, chronic use may cause spotting or breakthrough vaginal bleeding; after discontinuation, withdrawal bleeding usually occurs.

A discussion of the role of estrogens in the adverse effects of oral contraceptives is included under *Oral Contraceptives, Adverse Effects*.

PHARMACOKINETICS—Naturally occurring estrogens are not effective orally because they are destroyed almost totally in a single pass through the liver (first-pass effect). Oral effectiveness can be improved by administration of conjugated or esterified estrogens, by use of synthetic estrogens that are metabolized more slowly, or, in the case of estradiol, by preparation of the drug in a micronized form that is absorbed into the thoracic duct rather than into the portal circulation.

Estrogens are absorbed rapidly from intramuscular sites, mucous membranes, skin, and other sites of therapeutic application. The half-life of estradiol is 40 to 50 min, but other estrogens persist much longer. Estrogens circulate in both free and conjugated forms. These are bound in varying amounts to albumin and to a specific sex hormone–binding globulin (SSHBG).

Estrogens are excreted primarily in the conjugated form in urine. Some free estrogen is secreted in bile, from which some is excreted in feces and most returns to the systemic circulation by the enterohepatic route. Estrogens are excreted in breast milk, so their use in nursing mothers is not recommended.

DRUG INTERACTIONS—Drugs that induce the hepatic microsomal mixed oxygenase system (eg, phenobarbital, phenytoin, and rifampin) will accelerate estrogen metabolism.

Estrogens antagonize oral anticoagulants and also interfere with tests of coagulation. They also interfere with tests of thyroid function.

ESTRADIOL

(17β)-Estra-1,3,5(10)-triene-3,17-diol, 17-Beta-estradiol; Estrace

Dihydrotheelin; [50-28-2] $C_{18}H_{24}O_2$ (273.39).

Preparation—Has been isolated from ovarian follicular fluid and from placental tissue and is the most potent of the natural estrogens. It is usually prepared through reduction of the 17-keto group of *Estrone*.

It is curious that the urine of stallions and of the males of other *Equidae* contains 3 to 5 times as much estradiol as that of the female of the species.

Description—White or creamy white, small crystals or a crystalline powder; odorless and stable in air; hygroscopic; melts about 175°.

Solubility—1 g in 28 mL alcohol, 435 mL chloroform, or 150 mL ether; practically insoluble in water.

Comments—A natural estrogen used for replacement mainly in the postmenopause but also in ovarian hypofunction and after ovariectomy. It has a high presystemic elimination rate, hence a low bioavailability by the oral route. However, a micronized preparation (*Estrace*) is absorbed rapidly enough to flood the pertinent liver enzyme sufficiently to make oral administration feasible. Transdermal systems also are used effectively for replacement. Intravaginal estradiol (cream and ring) work topically in atrophic vaginitis, but the action to correct kraurosis vulvae is probably partly systemic. Estradiol is considerably converted to estrone in the body. The half-life is about 1 hr. Employ the lowest effective dose for the shortest duration to control menopausal symptoms.

DIETHYLSTILBESTROL

Phenol, (E)-4,4'-(1,2-diethyl-1,2-ethenediyl)bis-, DES

α,α'-Diethyl-(*E*)-4,4'-stilbenediol [56-53-1] $C_{18}H_{20}O_2$ (268.35).

Preparation—A synthetic estrogen first synthesized by Dodds et al in 1938. As to be expected, the compound exists in two geometric isomeric forms. The *cis*-isomer(*Z*), which has less than one-tenth the activity of the *trans*(*E*) and does not form readily, is unstable and tends to revert to the *trans*-isomer; hence the official product is *trans*- diethylstilbestrol.

Several methods of synthesis have been devised. That of Kharasch and Kleiman (*Medicinal Chemistry*, vol II, New York: Wiley, 1956) uses anethole hydrobromide as the starting material and is most convenient.

Description—White, odorless, crystalline powder; melts within a range of 4°, between 169° and 175°.

Solubility—Practically insoluble in water; soluble in alcohol, ether, chloroform, fatty oils, or dilute alkali hydroxides.

Comments—It is absorbed well orally. The rate of inactivation is slow. It can be administered orally in single daily doses, even with large doses.

Nausea and vomiting appear to be caused, in part, by local actions of the drug. Enteric coatings on tablets slow the rate of release and lessen the incidence and intensity of such local effects. It is advised to start with smaller doses for patients who tend to develop disagreeable symptoms such as nausea. It is contraindicated in pregnancy because of the danger of inducing a latent vaginal carcinoma in female offspring and structural abnormalities in the genitourinary tract in male offspring.

CONJUGATED ESTROGENS

Premarin

A mixture containing the sodium salts of the sulfate esters of the estrogenic substances, principally estrone and equilin, that are of the type excreted by pregnant mares. Conjugated estrogens contains 50% to 65% of sodium estrone sulfate, and 20% to 35% of sodium equilin sulfate, calculated on the basis of the total estrogens content.

Preparation—The urine of pregnant mares is subjected to a solvent extraction process. US Pats 2,565,115 and 2,720,483.

Description—Buff-colored powder; odorless or with a slight, characteristic odor.

Solubiltiy—Soluble in water.

Comments—Most commonly prescribed estrogen product, however it has fallen out of favor due to recent clinical trial data demonstrating increased risk of stroke, DVT/PE, CHD events and breast cancer. At this time therapy can only be recommended for short-term management of menopausal symptoms. Employ the lowest effective dose for the shortest duration as needed to control menopausal symptoms.

ESTROPIPATE

Estra-1,3,5(10)-triene-17-one, 3-(sulfooxy)-, compd with piperazine (1:1); Ogen; Ortho-Est

Piperazine estrone sulfate [7280-37-7] $C_{18}H_{22}O_5S.C_4H_{10}N_2$ (436.56).

Preparation—Estrone is treated with sulfur trioxide in DMF and excess piperazine is added which precipitates the product. US Pat 3,525,738 (1970), *Anal Profiles of Drug Subst* 5:375.

Description—Yellowish-white odorless, tasteless, crystalline powder melting about 190°, resolidifying and decomposing about 245°; racemic form melts about 251°.

$$[\alpha]^{20}_D = +87.8° \ (c = 1, 0.4\% \ NaOH).$$

Solubility—1 g in > 2000 mL water, alcohol, chloroform or ether.

Comments—Approved for the treatment of moderate-to-severe vasomotor menopausal symptoms. At this time therapy can only be recommended for short-term management of menopausal symptoms. Employ the lowest effective dose for the shortest duration as needed to control menopausal symptoms.

ETHINYL ESTRADIOL

(17α)-19-Norpregna-1,3,5(10)-trien-20-yne-3,17-diol, 17-Ethynylestradiol

[57-63-6] $C_{20}H_{24}O_2$ (296.41).

Preparation—By the Nef reaction, or a modification thereof, whereby estrone is caused to react with sodium acetylide in liquid am-

monia. Hydrolysis of the sodoxy addition complex yields the desired carbinol. It also may be prepared by a typical Grignard reaction from estrone and ethynyl magnesium bromide.

Description—White to creamy white, odorless, crystalline powder; melting range 180° to 186°; also exists in a polymorphic modification melting between 142° and 146°.

Solubility—Insoluble in water; soluble in alcohol, chloroform, or ether.

Comments—Has the actions, uses, and limitations of the other estrogens. It has an anovulatory effect at relatively low doses; it is the most widely used estrogen in oral contraceptive combinations. The ethinyl radical delays the decomposition of the estradiol molecule that occurs during absorption by the oral route. It is one of the most potent oral estrogens known.

MESTRANOL

(17α)-19-Norpregna-1,3,5(10)-trien-20-yn-17-ol, 3-methoxy-,

[72-33-3] $C_{21}H_{26}O_2$ (310.44).

Preparation—Estrone is converted to its 3-methoxy analog by reaction with methyl sulfate. The ethynyl group may then be introduced at position 17 either through reaction with sodium acetylide in liquid ammonia followed by hydrolysis of the sodoxy compound, or through grignardization with ethynyl bromide. US Pat 2,666,769.

Description—White to creamy white, odorless, crystalline powder; melts within a range of 4° between 146° and 154°.

Solubility—Freely soluble in chloroform; sparingly soluble in ether; slightly soluble in alcohol; insoluble in water.

Comments—This drug was incorporated with norethynodrel in the historically famous oral contraceptive, Norethynodrel with Mestranol, and it is now combined with several progestins in oral contraceptives. When suppression of the pituitary release of gonadotropins occurs with these preparations, it is likely that inhibition is more attributable to this drug than to the progestin. However, oral contraceptive preparations containing mestranol do not suppress ovulation in a large fraction of users, and the oral contraceptive effect cannot thus be correctly attributed to an anovulatory effect of the estrogen. It is an effective estrogen for the usual uses of estrogens, but it is not marketed as a single entity.

ANTIESTROGENS AND AROMATASE INHIBITORS

In a broad sense, antiestrogens are substances that suppress the effects of estrogens, regardless of mechanism. Androgens and progestins would thus qualify as incomplete antiestrogens, since they are antagonists to estrogens in some of their effects. With the advent of competitive antagonists of estrogens, the term *antiestrogen* has become restricted in use to apply only to such drugs. A number of estrogens have been found that reduce the intensity of response to other estrogens, behaving as agonists at some target organs and antagonists at other sites. Raloxifene is the first drug available in the new class of drugs called selective estrogen receptor modulators (SERMs). Raloxifene acts similarly to estrogen on bone, where it decreases bone resorption and increases bone mineral density; it also has estrogen-like effects on lipid (decrease in total and LDL cholesterol) metabolism. It is approved for prevention and treatment of postmenopausal osteoporosis. Raloxifene does not increase the incidence of uterine or breast tumors, which is consistent with the selective ability to act as an agonist at some but not all estrogen target tissues. Raloxifene is considered a second generation SERM. Studies with several estrogen target tissues have shown that some estrogenic drugs can promote selective gene transcription by activation of different estrogen-receptor elements upon transport of the drug-receptor complex to its nuclear binding site on DNA.

Tamoxifen is considered a first generation SERM because while it acts as an antagonist in bone, it demonstrated partial agonist activity in the uterus. The latter could be responsible for the increased incidence of uterine malignancies. Tamoxifen is indicated for primary and adjuvant therapy of breast cancer.

A closely related compound, clomiphene, has an even stronger antiestrogenic action in the hypothalamus but is sufficiently weak in the periphery so as not to interfere with the peripheral effects of endogenously released estrogens. By blocking the effects of endogenous estrogen to suppress adenohypophyseal release of gonadotropins, antiestrogens allow the anterior pituitary to produce more gonadotropins than normally. The ovaries are thus stimulated to a greater extent, and follicular development and maturation are enhanced. In cases of infertility resulting from failure to ovulate this effect may result in ovulation and the development of fertility.

Another approach to suppress the effects of endogenous estrogens is to decrease their synthesis. A new class of drugs for this purpose are the aromatase inhibitors. Aromatase is an enzyme complex that converts androgen precursors into estrogens. Inhibition of this enzyme complex decrease estrogen synthesis making these agents useful for the treatment of advanced breast cancer.

ANASTROZOLE

1,3-Benzenediacetonitrile, α,α,α′,α′-tetra-methyl-5-(1H-1,2,4-triazol-1-ylmethyl)-, Arimidex

[120511-73-1] $C_{17}H_{19}N_5$ (293.37).

Preparation—A mixture of 3,5-bis(bromomethyl)toluene, tetrabutylammonium bromide, dichloromethane and water is heated, then extracted with ethyl acetate and the extract evaporated to give 2,2′-(5-methyl-1,3-phenylene)diacetonitrile. To this latter compound is added iodomethane in DMF followed by sodium hydride in mineral oil to yield 2,2′-(5-bromomethyl-1,3-phenylene)diacetonitrile which is coupled with the sodio derivative of triazole using NBS and benzoyl peroxide to form the product, after suitable purification. US Pat 4,935,437 (1980).

Description—Crystals from ethyl acetate/cyclohexane melting about 81°.

Solubility—About 0.5 mg/mL at 25°; freely soluble in methanol, acetone, ethanol or THF; very soluble in acetonitrile.

Comments—It is indicated as first-line treatment of postmenopausal woman with hormone receptor positive or hormone receptor unknown advanced or metastatic breast cancer. It is also indicated for treatment of advanced breast cancer following tamoxifen therapy.

CLOMIPHENE CITRATE

Ethanamine, 2-[4-(2-chloro-1,2-diphenylethenyl)phenoxy]-N,N-diethyl-, 2-hydroxy-1,2,3-propanetricarboxylate (1:1); Clomid; Milophene; Serophene

2-[p-(2-Chloro-1,2-diphenylvinyl)phenoxy]triethylamine citrate (1:1) [50-41-9] $C_{26}H_{28}ClNO.C_6H_8O_7$ (598.09).

Preparation—4-Hydroxybenzophenone is condensed with 2-(diethylamino)ethyl chloride in toluene in the presence of alkali. The 4-[2-(diethylamino)ethoxy]benzophenone thus formed is grignardized with benzyl chloride, and the tertiary carbinol thus produced is dehydrated to give 2-[p-(1,2-diphenylvinyl)phenoxy]triethylamine. This compound is chlorinated to yield clomiphene and then reacted with an equimolar quantity of citric acid. Clomiphene citrate is a mixture of (E)- and (Z)-geometric isomers containing 30.0 to 50.0% of the latter isomer.

Description—White to pale yellow powder, essentially odorless; not appreciably hygroscopic; melts about 118° with decomposition.

Solubility—Sparingly soluble in alcohol; slightly soluble in water or chloroform; insoluble in ether.

Comments—An antiestrogenic drug used to induce ovulation (increase fertility) in anovulatory and oligoovulatory women who have adequate endogenous estrogens and in whom the hypothalamic–anterior pituitary has a latent capacity to function. It blocks the negative feedback action of endogenous estrogens by blocking cytosolic estrogen receptors in the hypothalamus and diminishing their number. The result is an increase in the secretion of GnRH and, hence, in gonadotropins (FSH and LH). However, its effect is uneven, since it seems to be most effective in the late follicular, and not in the luteal, phase of the estrous cycle. The elevated LH levels bring about ovulation; sometimes more than one ovum is released, which may result in multiple pregnancies. In properly selected patients, 80% may be induced to ovulate, and successful pregnancy is achieved in 30% to 40%. The probability of multiple pregnancy is increased to eight times normal. This is about the same order of success as with human chorionic gonadotropin (HCG).

In addition to multiple pregnancy, the major side effect is cystic enlargement of the ovaries. Increased cyclic ovarian pain, breast enlargement, and hot flashes that resemble those of the menopause also occur. Nausea is frequent. Blurred vision and scintillating scotoma may occur, and they require discontinuation of the treatment.

EXEMESTANE

Androsta-1,4-diene-3,17-dione, 6-methylene-, Aromasin

[107868-30-4] $C_{20}H_{24}O_2$ (296.41).

Preparation—One method involves the 1,2-dehydrogenation of 6-methylene-andros-4-ene-3,17-dione with selenium dioxide or dichlorodicyanobenzoquinone. US Pat 4,808,616 (1989).

Description—White to slightly yellow powder melting about 190°.

Solubility—Freely soluble in dimethylformamide (DMF); soluble in methanol; practically insoluble in water.

Comments—It is indicated for the treatment of advanced breast cancer following tamoxifen therapy.

LETROZOLE

Benzonitrile, 4,4′-(1H-1,2,4-triazol-1-ylmethylene)bis-, Femara

[112809-51-5] $C_{17}H_{11}N_5$ (285.31)

Preparation—Imidazole and 4-(bromomethyl)benzonitrile in dichloromethane are stirred at room temperature, diluted with water, the organic layer separated and the solvent removed to form 4-[(1H-imidazole-1-yl)methyl]benzonitrile. This latter compound is treated with potassium t-butoxide and 4-fluorobenzonitrile in DMF to yield the product. US Pat 4,978,672 (1990).

Description—Practically odorless, white to off-white powder melting about 185°.

Solubility—Freely soluble in dichloromethane; slightly soluble in ethanol; practically insoluble in water.

Comments—It is indicated as first-line treatment of postmenopausal woman with hormone receptor positive or hormone receptor unknown advanced or metastatic breast cancer. It is also indicated for treatment of advanced breast cancer following anti-estrogen therapy.

RALOXIFENE HYDROCHLORIDE

Methanone, [6-hydroxy-2-(4-hydroxyphenyl)benzo[b]thien-3-yl]-[4-[2-(1-piperidinyl)ethoxy]phenyl]-, hydrochloride; Evista

[82640-04-8] $C_{28}H_{27}NO_4S.HCl$ (510.05).

Preparation—Condensation of α-bromo-p-methoxyacetophenone with m-methoxythiophenol using polyphosphoric acid yields α-(m-methoxyphenylthio)-p-methoxy-acetophenone, which is cyclized by a Friedel-Crafts-type reaction to form 2-(p-methoxyphenyl)-6-methoxy-benzothiazole. The methoxyphenyl group apparently shifts from the theoretical 3- to the 2-position on the thiazole ring. The two methyl ether groups are removed and the resulting phenols reacted with methanesufonyl chloride to form the sulfonate ester (I). Methyl paraben is alkylated with 1-(2-chloroethyl)piperidine to yield the piperidinoethyl ether; the ester is hydrolyzed to the acid and converted to the acyl halide (II). Compound I is then acylated with II (Friedel-Crafts), which attaches the carbonyl group to the 3-position of the thiazole ring, and finally the sulfonate esters are hydrolyzed to the free base of the title compound. *J Med Chem* 1984; 27:1057.

Description—Off-white to pale yellow crystals melting about 258°.

Solubility—Very soluble in water.

Comments—A selective estrogen receptor modulator (SERM) that is used in the prevention and treatment of osteoporosis in postmenopausal patients. It has estrogen-like effects on bone (in bone mineral density and decreases bone resorption) and on lipid (decrease in total and LDL cholesterol) metabolism; in addition, it is an estrogen antagonist and lacks estrogen-like effects in uterine and breast tissues.

Raloxifene is absorbed rapidly after oral administration, with about 60% of dose absorbed. However, absolute bioavailability is only 2% because the drug undergoes extensive first-pass metabolism in the liver to glucuronide conjugates and enterohepatic cycling that prolongs the elimination half-life to 27.7 hr. Cholestyramine may decrease absorption and enterohepatic cycling. The drug is >95% bound to plasma proteins and may be displaced by other drugs such as clofibrate, ibuprofen, and naproxen.

The most common side effects are hot flashes and leg cramps that seem to be dose-related. Other side effects may be observed such as insomnia, rash, and weight gain. The risk of developing venous thromboembolism seems to be similar to that with estrogen replacement therapy.

TAMOXIFEN CITRATE

(Z)-2-[4-(1,2-diphenyl-1-butenyl)phenoxy]-N,N-dimethyl-, Nolvadex

(Z)-2- [p - (1,2-Diphenyl-1-butenyl)phenoxy]-N,N-dimethylethylamine citrate (1:1) [54965-24-1] $C_{26}H_{29}NO.C_6H_8O_7$ (563.65).

Preparation—4-β-Dimethylaminoethoxy-α-ethyldesoxybenzoin by reaction with phenylmagnesium bromide or phenyl lithium is converted to 1-(4-β-dimethylaminoethoxyphenyl)-1,2-diphenyl butanol, which on dehydration yields a mixture of tamoxifen and its cis-isomer that may be separated with petroleum ether; tamoxifen is converted to the 1:1 citrate for dispensing use. See *Nature* 1966; 212:733; *CA* 1967; 67:90515g.

Description—White, crystalline powder; melts about 140°.

Comments—A nonsteroidal antiestrogen for palliative therapy of breast cancer in postmenopausal women. The drug competes with estrogens for cytosol estrogen receptors and thus blocks estrogen effects in the target tissue. Tumors with negative receptor assays do not respond to it. Adverse effects frequently reported are hot flashes, nausea, and vomiting. The drug also can cause vaginal bleeding and discharge, rashes, transient leukopenia, and thrombocytopenia. Increased bone and tumor pain may occur. Infrequent side effects are anorexia and hypercalcemia. There is an increased risk of uterine cancer. A few patients have developed retinal abnormalities.

The oral bioavailability is 25% to 100%. The half-life of a single dose is 18 hr, but it is only 7 hr at steady state.

PROGESTINS AND ANTAGONISTS

Progesterone is the primary progestational substance produced by ovarian cells of the corpus luteum. It has a physiological action that is unique and distinct from that of estrogen. Progestins (progesterone and its derivatives) transform the proliferative endometrium into secretory endometrium. This alteration is part of the change that is essential to provide for the implantation of a fertilized ovum and for the continuing development of the placenta. This endometrial alteration requires the cooperation of an estrogen; in the absence of an estrogen, a progestin that is devoid of estrogenic activity will exert an atrophic effect on the endometrium.

Progestins also cause an increase in the viscosity of cervical secretions, which impedes the movement of sperm. Progestins in high doses suppress the pituitary release of luteinizing hormone and the hypothalamic release of GnRH, thus preventing ovulation.

Progestins also decrease uterine motility, which may contribute to a contraceptive effect. In addition, they antagonize the endometrial actions of estrogens, especially the natural estrogens. Progestins have the ability to stimulate development of the glandular portions of the mammae. They also exert some effects upon the capacity of tissues to retain water in the intercellular spaces. They also have a thermogenic action.

Progesterone is biotransformed in vivo, beginning with 5-α and 5-β reductions, to several active metabolites that affect the CNS in multiple ways and that may be responsible for some of the effects of progesterone described above. The metabolites decrease brain electrical activity, inhibit calcium entry into nerve terminals and norepinephrine release, and modify behavior. They also participate in the control of gonadotropin secretion. The metabolites appear to function both by modifying gene expression or by altering membrane permeability.

Progestins may be used cyclically in the treatment of infertility in which the uterus is not receptive to implantation; the progestin sustains the secretory endometrium during the third and fourth weeks of the menstrual cycle. They are used cyclically with estrogens in the treatment of secondary amenorrhea and dysfunctional uterine bleeding. They also may be used to lessen premenstrual tension, although they cause salt and water retention, which is a factor in this disorder.

The effect to suppress the release of LH and GnRH is used to prevent ovulation, not only with some oral contraceptives but also in the treatment of primary dysmenorrhea and endometriosis. In sexual infantilism in the female, progestins may be combined with estrogens to bring about genital development and maturation. Progestins may decrease breast size in mastodynia. In preeclampsia and toxemia of pregnancy due to hormonal imbalance, progestins plus estrogens may improve the condition, even though both types of hormone can cause salt and water retention, and estrogens can cause hypertension. They may be used in large doses as adjunctive treatment in endometrial carcinoma. They have been used in the past to prevent habitual abortion or treat threatened abortion.

The use of these agents during the first 4 months of pregnancy is not recommended because there is evidence that the fetus may be harmed; progestins may increase the risk of heart defects and deformed arms and legs in their children.

Untoward effects of progestins include nausea, vomiting, diarrhea, edema and weight gain, headache, fatigue, hirsutism, urticaria, ulcerative stomatitis, pruritus vulvae, and a tendency to galactorrhea and vaginal candidal infections. Some are locally irritating. Some have mild androgenic activity that may result in masculinization, especially in the female fetus. Others have a weak estrogenic component of activity. Some have both estrogenic and androgenic actions.

Progestins increase the cutaneous pigmenting effect of estrogens, thus favoring chloasma (melasma) when used in combination. It is probable that they increase the intensity of adverse effects of estrogens, especially headache and hypertension. There may be breakthrough bleeding when continuous high doses are used that suppress menstruation, yet there also may be decreased menstrual flow in many patients.

SUBCLASSES OF PROGESTINS—These agents can be grouped into three general categories, based on their structure: progesterone derivatives, 17α-ethinyl testosterone derivatives, and 19-nortestosterone derivatives. The most important differences between these synthetic agents are pharmacological changes in their activity profile. Table 77-9 provides a summary of several progestins that have been compared using various endpoints and target tissues, some of which may not apply to humans. In general, the 21-carbon compounds that are

Table 77-9. Major Features of Progestins

PROGESTINS	ACTIVITY PROFILE			
	PROGESTIN	ESTROGEN	ANTIESTROGEN	ANDROGEN
Progesterone and derivatives				
Progesterone	+ + + +	0	+	0
Hydroxyprogesterone	+ + +	+	0	+
Megestrol acetate	+ + +	0	0	+
17α-Ethinyl testosterone derivatives				
Dimethisterone	+	0	+	0
19-Nortestosterone derivatives				
L-Norgestrel	+ + +	0	+ +	+ + +
Desogestrel	+ + +	0/+	+ + +	0/+
Norgestimate	+ + +	0	+ + +	0
Ethynodiol diacetate	+ +	+	+	+ +
Norethindrone acetate	+	+	+ + +	+ +
Norethindrone	+	+	+	+ +
Norethynodrel	+	+ + +	0	0

derivatives of progesterone closely reproduce the pharmacological actions of the natural hormone progesterone. The greatest variability in pharmacological actions of progestins is demonstrated by the 19-nortestosterone derivatives that vary in their relative androgenic (masculinizing effects), estrogenic, antiestrogenic, and progestational effects.

Most oral contraceptives contain both an estrogen and a progestogen. Certain progestins may be used alone.

PROGESTERONE ANTAGONISTS

In addition to the widespread use of progestins in oral contraceptive agents, drugs that are classified as progesterone antagonists are receiving considerable attention in reproductive pharmacology. Since progesterone is essential for nidation and maintenance of early pregnancy, blockade of progesterone receptors or interference with progesterone synthesis prevents pregnancy and/or causes abortion early in gestation. Two such agents have been studied in some detail in experimental animals and humans.

Mifepristone (RU486) combines with progesterone receptors and acts as a progesterone antagonist. The drug is an abortifacient and acts as a contraceptive. The exact clinical status of mifepristone as an abortifacient remains to be established, but the potential availability of methods to produce safe, noninvasive abortions raises significant medical, social, and legal questions.

LEVONORGESTREL

(17α)-(−)-18,19-Dinorpregn-4-en-20-yn-3-one, 13-ethyl-17-hydroxy-,

[797-63-7] $C_{21}H_{28}O_2$ (312.45). This compound is the (−)-isomer of norgestrel, but the D-configurational isomer. A former designation as the *d*-enantiomer is incorrect.

Preparation—Refer to *Experiential* 1963; 19:394 for the (±)-form and US Pat 3,413,314 for both enantiomers.

Description—White crystals melting about 240°.

Solubility—Practically insoluble in water; soluble in chloroform; slightly soluble in ether or dioxane; sparingly soluble in ether.

Comments—The levo-isomer of norgestrel (see RPS-19, page 1097). It is the active form of norgestrel, hence it is twice as potent on a weight basis as norgestrel. Otherwise, the pharmacological properties of norgestrel and this drug are the same. It is used alone in subdermal implants and in combinations with ethinyl estradiol as an oral contraceptive.

MEDROXYPROGESTERONE ACETATE

(6α)-Pregn-4-ene-3,20-dione, 17-(acetyloxy)-6-methyl-, Cycrin, Depo-Provera, Provera

17-Hydroxy-6α-methylpregn-4-ene-3,20-dione acetate [71-58-9] $C_{24}H_{34}O_4$ (386.53).

Preparation—From 17α-hydroxyprogesterone by first forming the 3,21-bisethylene acetal with ethylene glycol, then treating with peracetic acid to give a mixture of the 5α,6α- and 5β,6β-epoxides. With methyl magnesium iodide the α-epoxide isomer yields the 5α-hydroxy-6β-methyl derivative, which dehydrates and epimerizes with hydrogen chloride in chloroform to the Δ⁴-6α-methyl compound, medroxyprogesterone. Acylation with acetic anhydride and *p*-toluenesulfonic acid in acetic acid gives medroxyprogesterone acetate.

Description—White to off-white, odorless, crystalline powder; melts at about 205°; stable in air.

Solubility—Insoluble in water; freely soluble in chloroform; soluble in acetone or dioxane; sparingly soluble in alcohol or methanol; slightly soluble in ether.

Comments—Actions, uses, and side effects of the progestins in general. Its oral efficacy is an advantage over progesterone. The drug is teratogenic during the first 4 months of pregnancy and hence should not be used for threatened abortion. The long duration of action of intramuscular drug makes it popular in some countries. It is effective as a contraceptive when given IM at the recommended dose to women every 3 months. There is a black box warning stating "prolonged use may increase the loss of significant bone mineral density. Bone loss is greater with increasing duration of use and may not be completely reversible. Depo-Provera Contraceptive should be used as a long-term birth control method (eg, longer than 2 years) only if other birth control methods are inadequate. Gonadotropin secretion is inhibited, which prevents follicular maturation and ovulation and results in endometrial thinning. It has been found to be beneficial in some cases of sleep apnea. Aqueous suspensions administered intramuscularly have a duration of action of weeks to months.

NORETHINDRONE

(17α)-19-Norpregn-4-en-20-yn-3-one, 17-hydroxy-,; Micronor; Nor-Q.D.; Norlutin

[68-22-4] $C_{20}H_{26}O_2$ (298.42).

Preparation—The methyl ether of estrone is reacted with lithium metal in liquid ammonia to reduce ring A to the 4-ene state and the reduced compound is oxidized with chromic acid in aqueous acetic acid to form estr-4-ene-3,17-dione (I). To prevent the 3-keto group from participating in the ensuing ethynylation reaction, I is reacted with ethyl orthoformate in the presence of pyridine hydrochloride to form the 3-ethoxy-3,5-diene compound (II). Acetylene is passed into a solution of II in toluene, previously admixed with a solution of sodium in *tert*-amyl alcohol, to form the 17-ethynyl-17-hydroxy compound. Hydrolysis at the 3-ethoxy linkage by heating with dilute HCl is accompanied by rearrangement of the 3-hydroxy-3,5-diene compound to the 3-oxo-4-ene state. US Pat 2,744,122.

Description—White to creamy white, odorless, crystalline powder; melts about 205°; stable in air.

Solubility—Practically insoluble in water; sparingly soluble in alcohol; soluble in chloroform or dioxane; slightly soluble in ether.

Comments—In addition to its progestational actions, it has weak estrogenic actions, owing to biotransformation to an estrogenic metabolite. Among the progestational drugs, it ranks high in ability to postpone menstruation, and it is used for this purpose for both medical and social reasons. In high doses it prevents ovulation by suppressing pituitary gonadotropin output. In lower doses it suppresses the endometrium and decreases the fluidity of the cervical mucus. Consequently, the steroid is an important oral contraceptive. As an oral contraceptive, it is used alone or combined with an estrogen, especially *Mestranol* and *Ethinyl Estradiol;* when used alone, the pregnancy rate is about three times that when used in combination with an estrogen.

In some women with Type V hyperlipoproteinemia, it markedly decreases the concentrations of VLDL and chylomicrons; however, it also lowers HDL and hence is used only when the condition is refractory to other drugs. The drug has weak androgenic properties and may cause deepening of the voice, hirsutism, and acne, and it may cause masculinization of the fetus.

PROGESTERONE

Pregn-4-ene-3,20-dione; Prometrium, Crinone

Progesterone [57-83-0] $C_{21}H_{30}O_2$ (314.47).

Preparation—From animal ovaries, synthesized from stigmasterol, or better from diosgenin (extracted from *Dioscorea mexicana,* a Mexican yam). The latter synthesis involves acetolysis, chromic acid oxidation, cleavage of the ketoester diacetate with boiling acetic acid to 16-dehydropregnenolone acetate, which on catalytic reduction yields pregnenolone acetate. Saponification of the acetate ester to the 3β-alcohol followed by Oppenauer oxidation affords progesterone. Progesterone in pure form was first isolated, from corpus luteum, in 1934 by Butenandt.

Description—White or creamy white, crystalline powder; odorless and stable in air; melts about 128°; a polymorphic modification melts about 121°.

Solubility—Practically insoluble in water; soluble in alcohol, acetone, or dioxane; sparingly soluble in vegetable oils.

Comments—Its plasma half-life is only about 5 min, so it is extremely difficult to achieve effective blood levels with any convenient dosage schedules. It can be given intramuscularly as a suspension or solution in oil and intravaginally. Recently a Micronized progesterone formulation is available for oral administration.

One intrauterine contraceptive device (Progestasert, *Alza*) contains 38 mg of progesterone in silicone oil. The hormone is said to enhance the contraceptive effectiveness of the device by a local effect on the endometrium and by effects on sperm motility, capacitation, and metabolism. Progesterone is released at an average rate of 65 µg daily for 1 year, at which time the device is replaced. The device increases the risk of pelvic inflammation and actinomycotic infections.

HORMONAL CONTRACEPTIVES

MECHANISMS—The various mechanisms whereby hormonal contraceptives can prevent conception are complex. The mechanisms involved vary with the particular agent(s) in a preparation, the dose(s), and whether a cyclic or continuous schedule is used. It is probable that several mechanisms operate simultaneously with some preparations.

SUPPRESSION OF GONADOTROPIC OUTPUT—During the menstrual cycle, there are two periods of elevated FSH secretion, a sharp peak just preceding ovulation and a long wave beginning just before menstruation. In sufficient doses, estrogens can suppress both phases by feedback actions on both the hypothalamus and the anterior hypophysis; FSH and LH output is desynchronized at the early peak, ovulation may be prevented, and the estrogen-progestin priming of the uterus is defective. Estrogens also suppress the hypophyseal output of LH. Progestins also can suppress the LH peak (by an action at the hypothalamus, only), but their action is weak, owing to their antiestrogenic effects, which oppose the suppressant actions of endogenous and exogenous estrogen. Very high doses of progestins are necessary to suppress LH output, unless the progestin is combined with an estrogen. A progestin alone desynchronizes the FSH and LH output, thus sometimes preventing ovulation; long-term use of a combination of progestin and estrogen depresses the output of both gonadotropins and more consistently prevents ovulation.

OVARIAN EFFECTS—Estrogens and progestins decrease the ovarian response to their respective gonadotropins. The result may be a failure to ovulate or, if ovulation does occur, a smaller, hyposecreting corpus luteum, the latter especially when a progestin is in the contraceptive preparation.

TUBAL EFFECTS—In some species progestins and in others estrogens accelerate the ciliary and peristaltic egg transport in the fallopian tubes and increase secretions. Consequently, the ovum arrives in the uterus before the endometrium is prepared for nidation. The tubal effects of these hormones in women may involve a tubal action.

EFFECTS ON THE ENDOMETRIUM—Long-acting injectable progestins in appropriate doses cause endometrial atrophy. Oral preparations vary according to the drug and the dose, some permitting a normal endometrium and others causing regression. In combination with estrogens, progestins effect a decrease in tortuosity and secretion of the endometrial glands with thinning of the endometrium after several cycles of use.

EFFECTS ON THE CERVIX—Estrogens favor a thin and watery secretion, while progestins promote more-viscous cervical secretions that impede the mobility of sperm. In the combination contraceptives, the progestins predominate.

EFFECTS ON CAPACITANCE—Capacitance is the ability of the sperm to penetrate into the ovum. Progestins are thought to decrease capacitance, by an unknown mechanism, probably involving prostaglandins. It is speculated that the low-dose, continuously administered progestin contraceptives are effective by the anticapacitant action.

TYPES OF PREPARATIONS—The first oral contraceptives to be marketed were progestin-estrogen combinations. In some preparations, called *monophasic* combinations, the progestin and estrogen are present in fixed amounts, so that blood levels rise and fall together, in contrast to the levels in the normal menstrual cycle, in which one estrogen peak appears 11 days in advance of the combined estrogen-progesterone peak. With the combined preparations, an artificial menstrual cycle is induced by using the contraceptive for only 20 to 21 days of every 28; if they were to be used continuously instead, no regular menses would occur, but breakthrough bleeding would occur eventually.

The artificial menses caused by the cyclic use of combination contraceptives usually is not normal but oligemic. During the 7 to 8 days in which no hormones are taken, some products provide placebo or iron tablets in lieu of the combination; in these products, the pills are packaged to be taken serially by number. Over the years since combinations appeared on the market, the estrogen content has been decreased considerably in several products because of the possible adverse effects of the estrogen component.

Attempts to develop more nearly physiological regimens have led to the so-called *biphasic* and *triphasic* combinations.

In the former, the progestin dose is increased during the last 11 days of the medication cycle; in the latter, the progestin/estrogen ratio is changed 3 times during the cycle by altering the doses of either progestin or estrogen or both.

Continuous progestin-only oral products do not contain any estrogen and furthermore contain the progestin in amounts smaller (the so-called *mini-pill*) than those used in combination products. The dose is small enough not to prevent ovulation and menstruation in most users, yet to act sufficiently on the uterus, cervix, or capacitance to prevent conception. However, the efficacy is lower than that of combination or sequential products. A progesterone-containing IUD and continuous- progestin injectable products, repository forms of progestins, also are available.

Emergencyl have been used, to prevent pregnancy in girls or women who are caught without contraceptive preparation; these preparations, however, are not for routine use. They are effective if taken within 72 hr after coitus.

EFFICACY AND FAILURES—The efficacy of an oral contraceptive depends on the type and the dose of hormonal ingredients. The combined type, which contains relatively high doses of estrogens, is nearly 100% effective when taken correctly; failures probably can be attributed to the negligence of the user. There appears to be a finite, though small, probability of ovulation and hence of later conception if a single pill is missed, because of the rebound oversecretion of the gonadotropins. If one pill is skipped, the user should take it immediately upon discovery of the skip and take the rest on their schedule; if two or more are missed, she should additionally use other methods of contraception until her next cycle. Lowering the estrogen content in combination preparations decreases the side effects but increases the risk of pregnancy. The long-acting combinations have a relatively high failure rate. The continuous low-dose oral progestin products have a failure rate several times that of combination products.

ADVERSE EFFECTS—The adverse effects vary in incidence and severity according to the type of preparation. Most side effects are from the estrogens in combination contraceptives, but progestins also cause adverse effects. The estrogen-progestin ratio is important to the type and incidence of side effects. A summary of the dose-related side effects of oral contraceptives is shown in Table 77-10.

Oligomenorrhea, or low menstural flow, occurs in 20% to 80% of users of combination and some continuous progestin contraceptives, and amenorrhea occurs in some. The greatest offenders are the 19-nortestosterone derivatives. Spotting and breakthrough bleeding that is unpredictable or irregular in onset may also occur; sometimes such bleeding is more voluminous than in regular menstruation.

Other side effects can occur such as tiredness, weakness, malaise, changes in libido, dizziness, and nonspecific headaches. An increase in the incidence of migraine headaches is especially notable in some patients; the estrogen component

appears to be responsible. Weight gain occurs with some but not all preparations; salt and water retention is caused mostly by estrogen components, whereas anabolic effects are caused by higher doses of the 19-nortestosterone-derived progestins (not the 17α-hydroxyprogesterones).

Chloasma occurs in about 4% of users of combination contraceptives during the first year and 37% by the fifth year; it is attributable to the combined action of the two active components. Milk flow in lactating women may be decreased by an average of 50% when combination preparations are used. Estrogen-containing contraceptives also cause an uncommon choreiform movement.

Serious side effects of oral contraceptives are multiple. A reversible hypertension is observed in approximately 15% of users of estrogen-containing contraceptives. The prevalence of hypertension increases with duration of use and is greater in older women. Incidence of thromboembolic disorders, including stroke and myocardial infarction, is higher in women using oral contraceptives; the relative risk may be several times greater in users than in control populations. Further, the risk increases sharply in women over 35 years who are smokers.

Contraceptive use also has been associated with increased evidence of benign liver tumors. The relative risk of liver tumors appears to rise with duration of use of the drugs. In one study, mestranol-containing preparations were implicated almost exclusively, thus indicating that the type of synthetic estrogen might be important. The risk of gallbladder disease is increased twofold in contraceptive users. Fetal abnormalities may result if the mother continues to take the pill after becoming pregnant. Neuroocular lesions have been associated with use of oral contraceptives. Some other possible complications of contraceptive use include breast cancer (pill use actually protects against the development of benign breast lesions) and cancer of the uterus, cervix, and vagina. Any of the other side effects of estrogens or progestins given above also may be caused by these drugs.

Irregular bleeding is initially a problem for some women with depot progestin administration. However, after 1 year most women are completely amenorrheic. Patients taking oral contraceptives must be informed of their effectiveness and risks.

MALE CONTRACEPTIVES

Since 1980 there has been considerable effort to develop male contraceptives. In China, gossypol, a polyphenol-aldehyde isolated from cottonseed oil, has been under investigation since the mid-1950s. It is an inhibitor of human sperm acrosin and an LDD isoenzyme known as LDH-C. It also interferes with epididymal function and elicits structural alterations. A clinical trial in over 4000 healthy men found gossypol to be 99.9% effective as a contraceptive. However, it causes hypokalemia and other untoward effects and has a narrow margin of safety. Its effects are irreversible in 10 to 20% of users. Investigations of related compounds are in progress.

The inhibitory effect of testosterone and other androgens on hypothalamic release factor signalling and anterior pituitary secretion of gonadotropins results in decreased spermatogenesis, and aspermia may result from prolonged, vigorous use. Because of the adverse effects, however, (see the introduction under *The Testicular Hormones*), this approach has limited promise. Low-dose androgen-progestin combinations, which suppress anterior pituitary release of LH/FSH with less intense androgenic side effects, are being investigated also.

A more encouraging approach is the use of analogs of GnRH, such as goserelin, nafarelin, buserelin, and leuprolide, which cause a down-regulation of pituitary release hormone receptors during continuous administration. Both steroidogen-

Table 77-10. Summary of Dose-Related Side Effects of Oral Contraceptives

Estrogen excess	Progestin excess
Nausea	Increased appetite
Cervicomyxorrhea	Weight gain
Melasma	Tiredness, fatigue
Migraine headache	Hypomenorrhea
Hypertension	Acne, oily skin
Breast tenderness	Hair loss
Edema	Depression
Estrogen deficiency	*Progestin deficiency*
Early or midcycle breakthrough bleeding	Late breakthrough bleeding
Increased spotting	Amenorrhea
Hypomenorrhea	Hypermenorrhea

esis and spermatogenesis are diminished reversibly. Decreased libido occurs, so to be acceptable to many men, use must be supplemented with androgens. The Sertoli cell peptide, inhibin, and related proteins, which inhibit the anterior pituitary release of FSH, are under active investigation but are not ready for clinical trials. They, too, probably will decrease libido and hence may not be acceptable to a large percentage of potential users.

Perhaps the most promising but nascent developments are vaccines against one or more spermatic proteins. The sperm lactic dehydrogenase, LDH-C4, and possibly various protamines are presently investigational targets for monoclonal and other antibodies. The first vaccines for human use are likely to be against LDH-C4. The effects of vaccines, are not likely to be readily reversible, although some memory immune cells have relatively short lifetimes.

THE TESTICULAR HORMONE (TESTOSTERONE)

The testis has a dual function, to produce the germ cell (the sperm) and supply the male hormone (testosterone). Two clearly defined groups of cells are found in the testes; the one group in the seminiferous tubules produces the sperm, while the other, clustered in between the tubules, consists of interstitial cells (Leydig cells). The spermatogenic tissue produces an exocrine secretion and probably also androgens needed for spermatogenesis.

The interstitial cells are the seat of production of a steroid hormone, testosterone. However, it is mainly the metabolite dihydrotestosterone that stimulates and maintains the secondary sex organs; these are the penis, prostate gland, seminal vesicles, vas deferens, and scrotum. It also exerts sustaining effects on the spermatogenic cells, and it stimulates the development of bone, muscle, nerves, skin and hair growth, and emotional responses to produce the characteristic adult masculine traits. Testosterone, itself, regulates the anterior pituitary release of LH. This group of combined actions of this hormone is termed androgenic actions. Testosterone also antagonizes a number of the effects of estrogens and sometimes is employed clinically for this purpose. This is especially important in the suppression of metastatic carcinoma of the breast. Since it promotes development of the clitoris, which is an anatomical homolog of the penis, androgens may increase the libido of women.

The naturally occurring androgens (androsterone and testosterone) are derivatives of androstane. Testosterone and its esters (testosterone propionate) and derivatives (methyltestosterone) are the most commonly used androgenic steroids. In addition to their androgenic properties, however, these compounds exert widespread anabolic effects and promote the retention of calcium. In attempts to dissociate the virilizing and anabolic properties (for use in women) a number of compounds with high anabolic:androgenic ratios have been prepared. However, it has not been possible yet to abolish completely the androgenic effects. A summary of the comparative actions of androgens and anabolic agents is shown in Table 77-11.

USES—For replacement therapy in men who have climacteric symptoms or in men or youths with hypogonadism (eunuchism, Klinefelter's syndrome). They have been employed to facilitate development of adult masculine characteristics when the adolescent process has been delayed. In cryptorchidism they may be used adjunctively with gonadotropins. They also are very useful in therapy of patients with hypopituitarism and with Addison's disease. They are of value in the treatment of frigidity and occasionally in impotence. The use of androgens for relief of impotence not associated with evidence of testicular underactivity (psychic causes) is known to be futile in most cases.

Table 77-11. Major Features of Androgens and Anabolic Steroids

ANDROGEN/ANABOLIC ACTIVITY		COMMENTS
Androgens		
Testosterone	1:1	Given IM/transdermally; inactive orally
Methyltestosterone	1:1	Orally active; short half-life (2.5 hr)
Fluoxymesterone	1:2	Orally active; long half-life (10 hr)
Danazol	—	Weak androgen; orally active
Anabolic steroids		
Oxymetholone	1:3	Orally active
Oxandrolone	1:3–1:13	Orally active
Nandrolone phenpropionate	1:3–1:6	Given IM
Stanozolol	1:3–1:6	Orally active

Low doses of androgens have been used in pituitary dwarfism to accelerate growth, but care must be exercised not to arrest growth by epiphyseal closure. They also are used sometimes to promote hematopoiesis. In doses that are 10 to 200 times larger than normal, anabolic steroids increase athletic performance and aggressiveness. Their use has been condemned by the American College of Sports Medicine. Because of their potential for some serious adverse effects and their potential abuse these drugs are highly publicized for their inherent risks. Female performance is improved, but at the expense of virilization and acne vulgaris.

With estrogens, androgen therapy may be efficacious in the treatment of the menopause. The anabolic effects are possibly of some benefit in the postclimacteric person, and they may retard osteoporosis, although many authorities do not believe that any lasting benefit is achieved. They also help relieve vasomotor instability in postmenopausal women in whom estrogens alone do not relieve symptoms. In functional dysmenorrhea androgens may give relief through an antiestrogenic action, although they also are combined often with estrogens to treat this disorder. They may be used to treat endometriosis. They also may be used in the treatment of postpartum breast engorgement and for suppression of lactation.

Testosterone and related compounds find widespread application in the palliative treatment of cancer of the breast in women. Its use in men with prostatic cancer, however, is contraindicated.

SIDE EFFECTS—Androgens cause hirsutism, deepening or hoarseness of the voice, precocious puberty and epiphyseal closure in immature males, increased libido (in both male and female), priapism, oligospermia and testicular atrophy (from negative feedback on LH and FSH production), enlargement of the clitoris in the female, flushing, decreased ejaculatory volume and sperm population, gynecomastia (from conversion to estrogens), hypersensitivity, acne, weight gain, edema, and hypercalcemia. Prolonged use increases aggressivenessWhile paranoia-like and other psychotic behavior has been reported. Biliary stasis and jaundice occur. There have been a few cases reported of hepatoma following long-term therapy. The 17α-methylated androgens are more prone to disturb liver function (peliosis hepatis, cholestasis, and hepatic failure) than are the nonsubstituted drugs. Blood lipid changes associated with increased risk of atherosclerosis are seen, including decreased HDL and sometimes increased LDL. Hypercalcemia requires discontinuation of therapy, and edema requires diuretic therapy.

Except in the treatment of breast cancer, a reduction in dosage is indicated upon virilization in women. The administration of androgens to patients on anticoagulant therapy may increase the effect of anticoagulants and, thus, may require an adjustment of the dose of the latter. Likewise, dosage of insulin or oral hypoglycemic agents may require adjustment when anabolic androgens are administered to diabetic patients.

DANAZOL

(17α)-Pregna-2,4-dien-20-yno[2,3-d]isoxazol-17-ol, Chronogyn; Danocrine

[17230-88-5] $C_{22}H_{27}NO_2$ (337.46).

Preparation—Danazol is a derivative of ethisterone (17α-ethynyltestosterone) in which an isoxazole ring is fused to the 2,3-position of the steroid nucleus. Methods for preparing such steroidal heterocycles have been described by Manson et al. *J Med Chem* 1963; 6:1; also in US Pat 3,135,743.

Description—Pale yellow, crystalline powder; melts about 225°.

Solubility—Practically insoluble in water; sparingly soluble in alcohol.

Comments—An *impeded* androgen (ie, weak androgenic activity). It binds to androgen, glucocorticoid, and progesterone receptors, but it evokes no glucocorticoid, progestational, or estrogenic effects except that it suppresses the release of LH and FSH, even in women. It suppresses ovarian steroidogenesis, induces the hepatic metabolism of progesterone, and binds to α-macroglobulin, causing partial displacement of other steroids. It is used in the treatment of endometriosis in patients who do not respond to or cannot tolerate other drug therapy and in the management of fibrocystic breast disease and periareolar abscesses. It may prevent attacks of hereditary angioedema. It increases platelet populations in idiopathic and immune thrombocytopenias. However, it also can cause thrombocytopenia. It relieves migraine in some persons.

Androgenic side effects include deepening of the voice in women, acne, edema, mild hirsutism, decrease in breast size, oiliness of the skin and hair, weight gain, and clitoral hypertrophy. Hypoestrogenic manifestations include amenorrhea; vasomotor instability; vaginitis with itching, burning, and vaginal bleeding; and emotional lability. It also may cause muscle cramps, asthenia, rhabdomyolysis, testicular atrophy, and rare hematuria. It has an adverse effect on plasma lipids. In doses over 400 mg a day, it may cause hepatic injury, including carcinoma. It has been reported to lower serum levothyroxine levels.

FLUOXYMESTERONE

(11β,17β)-Androst-4-en-3-one, 9-fluoro-11,7-dihydroxy-17-methyl-, Halotestin

[76-43-7] $C_{20}H_{29}FO_3$ (336.45).

Preparation—From 17-methyltestosterone first by introduction of a hydroxyl group at position 11 through oxidation with a microorganism (such as *Pestalotia* or *Aspergillus*), followed by dehydration, epoxidation, and treatment with HF, as for *Betamethasone.*.

Description—White or practically white, odorless, crystalline powder; melts about 240° with some decomposition.

Solubility—Practically insoluble in water; sparingly soluble in alcohol; slightly soluble in chloroform.

Comments—The same actions, uses, and limitations as the androgens (page 1390).It is approximately five times more potent than testosterone and is orally effective. Nevertheless, it is less effective than testosterone in hypogonadism and is seldom used to initiate treatment but rather for maintenance. In addition to the side effects of testosterone, this drug may cause occasional cholestatic jaundice, gynecomastia, oligospermia after prolonged use, and hypersensitivity. It sometimes is combined with an estrogen for treatment of postmenopausal osteoporosis. The half-life is about 10 hr.

METHYLTESTOSTERONE

(17β)-Androst-4-en-3-one, 17-hydroxy-17-methyl-, Android; Methitest

[58-18-4] $C_{20}H_{30}O_2$ (302.46).

Preparation—From dehydroepiandrosterone (prepared from cholesterol) by subjecting it to a Grignard reaction with CH_3MgI followed by an Oppenauer oxidation. The first reaction creates the tertiary carbinol structure at C_{17}, while the second oxidizes the secondary carbinol group at position 3 to carbonyl and causes a rearrangement of the double bond from the 5,6- to the 4,5-position.

Description—White or creamy white crystals or a crystalline powder; odorless; stable in air, but slightly hygroscopic; affected by light; melts about 165°

Solubility—Practically insoluble in water; soluble in alcohol, methanol, ether, or other organic solvents; sparingly soluble in vegetable oils.

Comments—The same actions, uses, and limitations as the androgens. It is effective orally. In addition to the side effects caused by testosterone, it may cause oligospermia, hypersensitivity with dermatological manifestations, and a rare type of cholestatic jaundice.

It is metabolized rapidly by the liver and undergoes first-pass metabolism. By the buccal route, potency is twice that by the oral route. The half-life is about 2.5 hr.

OXANDROLONE

(5α,17β)-2-Oxaandrostan-3-one, 17-hydroxy-17-methyl-, Oxandrin

17β-Hydroxy-17-methyl-2-oxa-5α-androstan-3-one [53-39-4] $C_{19}H_{30}O_3$ (306.44).

Preparation—Methyldihydrotestosterone is converted into the corresponding 1,2-dehydro compound by bromination followed by dehydrobromination. Ring A is then ruptured through ozonization and subsequent hydrolysis to yield the aldehyde-acid (I). Reduction of the formyl group in I yields the expected hydroxy acid implied in the partial structure (II) which is lactonized to oxandrolone.

(I)   (II)

Description—White, odorless, crystalline powder; stable in air but darkens when exposed to light; melts about 225°.

Solubility—1 g in 5200 mL water, 57 mL alcohol, <5 mL chloroform, 860 mL ether, or 69 mL acetone.

Comments—Although strictly speaking not a steroid, its configuration is that of a 17-methyl androgenic steroid. Its anabolic actions are strong relative to its androgenic actions. Consequently, it is used in the treatment of chronic wasting diseases, conditions in which negative nitrogen balance exists. The drug may cause virilization in children or women, especially if the recommended doses are exceeded. The potential toxicity is that of the androgens, but the incidence and severity are less than with testosterone. It may affect liver function tests adversely, and the possibility of cholestatic jaundice must be kept in mind. Leukopenia also has been reported. It is contraindicated in prostatic cancer, breast cancer in some women, pregnancy, nephrosis, and premature and newborn infants. It is also available as an IND for treatment of constitutional delay of growth and puberty.

OXYMETHOLONE

(5α,17β)-Androstan-3-one, 17-hydroxy-2-(hydroxymethylene)-17-methyl-, Anadrol

[434-07-1] $C_{21}H_{32}O_3$ (332.48).

Preparation—17β-Hydroxy-17-methylandrostan-3-one (17-methyldihydrotestosterone) is reacted with ethyl formate and sodium hydroxide by stirring the mixture under nitrogen for several hours, thus forming the 2-(sodoxymethylene) derivative. Treatment of the washed sodium compound with cold dilute hydrochloric acid liberates the oxymetholone, which may be purified by recrystallization from ethyl acetate. *J Am Chem Soc* 1959; 81:427.

Description—White to creamy white crystals or crystalline powder; odorless and stable in air; tautomeric in nature and can exist as either tautomer or as a mixture of both, the exact composition depending on solvent and rate of crystallization; melts about 175°.

Solubility—1 g in >10,000 mL water, 40 mL alcohol, 5 mL chloroform, 82 mL ether, or 14 mL dioxane.

Comments—An androgenic steroid with relatively greater anabolic activity than androgenic activity. Consequently, it is employed mainly to promote nitrogen anabolism and weight gain in cachexia and debilitating diseases and after serious infections, burns, trauma, or surgery. It may be used for its erythropoietic effects in the treatment of hypoplastic and aplastic anemias. Side effects include nausea, vomiting, anorexia, burning of the tongue, increased or decreased libido, acne, suppression of gonadotropin secretion, virilization (especially in women and children), gynecomastia in males, oligospermia, sodium retention and edema, abnormal liver function tests, cholestatic jaundice, decrease in several clotting factors, and hemorrhagic diathesis in the presence of anticoagulants.

STANOZOLOL

(5α,17β)-2'H-Androst-2-enol[3,2-c]pyrazol-17-ol, 17-methyl-, Winstrol

[10418-03-8] $C_{21}H_{32}N_2O$ (328.50).

Preparation—17-Methyl-5α-androstan-17β-ol-3-one is converted into its 2-formyl derivative, which is then condensed with hydrazine hydrate. US Pat 3,030,358.

Description—Nearly colorless, odorless, crystalline powder; exists in two forms: *needles,* melting about 155°, and *prisms,* melting about 235°.

Solubility—1 g in >1000 mL water, 41 mL alcohol, 74 mL chloroform, or 370 mL ether.

Comments—An androgen with relatively strong anabolic and weak androgenic activity. Consequently, it is employed mainly to promote nitrogen anabolism and weight gain in cachexia and debilitating diseases and after serious infections, burns, trauma, or surgery. It may have an erythropoietic effect in hypoplastic and aplastic anemias. It also is used in the prophylaxis of hereditary angioedema, which is now the only approved use.

Side effects include increased or decreased libido, virilization (especially in women and children), sodium retention and edema, hypercalcemia, insomnia, restlessness, chills, hemorrhage in patients on anticoagulants, acne, and hepatic dysfunction. Potentially, any of the side effects of testosterone may occur. However, these rarely occur during the usual 5-day course.

TESTOSTERONE

(17β)-Androst-4-en-3-one, 17-hydroxy-,

17β-Hydroxyandrost-4-en-3-one [58-22-0] $C_{19}H_{28}O_2$ (288.43).

Preparation—First isolated in crystalline form by Laquer in 1935 who obtained it from animal testes. Although small amounts of testosterone may be extracted from testicular material, the synthetic commercial supply is derived from cholesterol. The key intermediate in the synthesis is dehydroepiandrosterone, which can be treated further, by either chemical or microbiological processes, to yield testosterone. US Pat 2,236,574.

Description—White or slightly creamy white crystals or crystalline powder; odorless; stable in air; melts about 155°.

Solubility—Practically insoluble in water; 1 g in about 6 mL of dehydrated alcohol, 1 mL chloroform, or 100 mL ether; soluble in vegetable oils.

Comments—See the introduction to this section, page. It is not effective orally because it is destroyed in the liver on absorption. Its plasma half-life is 10 to 20 min. However, two different transdermal preparations are now available to use as replacement therapy for primary or secondary hypogonadism in men. One is placed on scrotal skin *(Testoderm)* and provides a maximum serum concentration within 2 to 4 hr and returns to baseline within 2 hr after removal. Daily applications of transdermal systems are applied at 10 PM and left in place for 22 to 24 hr. The nonscrotal transdermal preparation *(Androderm)* is applied at two sites (on back, abdomen, upper arms, or thighs) and should never be applied to the scrotum because it is a higher-dose preparation. Side effects from transdermal preparations include local irritation at sites of application. It is also available as a topical gel and implantable pellets.

ANDROGEN HORMONE INHIBITORS AND ANTIANDROGENS

Drugs may be used to suppress the effects of androgens by inhibition of gonadotropin production or by inhibition of enzymes involved in the production of androgen or their precursors. Analogs of the hypothalamic gonadotropin-releasing hormone, GnRH, can be given in a continuous release preparation to inhibit pituitary LH and suppress production of testosterone in the testis. Although testosterone levels fall after a month of therapy with GnRH analogs, an initial increase in testosterone occurs. Inhibitors of the 17-hydroxylation of progesterone or pregnenolone can lead to decreased levels of androgen precursors. More-specific inhibition of androgenic effects can achieved by inhibition of the 5α-reductase enzyme that converts testosterone to dihydrotestosterone, the active androgenic hormone in specific tissues such as prostate, seminal vesicles, epididymis, and skin. Other drugs are classified as antiandrogens if they can specifically block testosterone receptors. The most important drugs currently available as androgen hormone inhibitors and antiandrogens are shown in Table 77-12.

The subcutaneous injection of leuprolide or other GnRH analogs (goserelin, nafarelin, and buserelin) has been used successfully in the treatment of prostatic carcinoma. The combination of a GnRH analog with finasteride, an inhibitor of 5α-reductase, can inhibit the initial stimulation of testosterone

Table 77-12. Features of Androgen Hormone Inhibitors and Antiandrogens

	COMMENTS
Androgen Hormone Inhibitor	
Finasteride	Inhibits 5α-reductase in prostate
Leuprolide acetate	GnRH agonist injected SC; inhibits gonadotropin secretion resulting in decreased gonadal testosterone production
Goserelin	GnRH agonist similar to leuprolide in action
Antiandrogens	
Cyproterone acetate	Antagonist at androgen receptors
Flutamide	Competitive antagonist at androgen receptors

production and provide a more effective inhibition of androgenic activity. Finasteride is used in the treatment of benign prostate hypertrophy and male pattern baldness.

The antiandrogens or testosterone receptor antagonists are used in the treatment of conditions associated with androgen excess such as hirsutism, excessive libido, and prostate cancer. Flutamide is a potent nonsteroidal antiandrogen that competitively blocks nuclear androgen receptors in prostate tissue. It is used in the treatment of prostatic carcinoma.

Other drugs are under development in the area of androgen suppression and antagonism or receptors that should improve the efficacy and reduce the side effects of these agents. Common adverse effects of these agents in men are gynecomastia, decreased libido, and infertility.

DUTASTERIDE

Androst-1-ene-17-carboxamide, (5α,17β)-N-[2,5-bis(trifluoromethyl)phenyl]-3-oxo-4-aza-, Avodart

[164656-23-9] $C_{27}H_{30}F_6N_2O_2$ (528.54).

Preparation—By a multi-step synthesis from diosgenin. See *J Med Chem* 1995; 38:3189, WO95 07927 and *Ann Rep Sankyo Res Lab* 2000; 52:1-14.

Description—White to pale yellow crystals melting about 245°.

Solubility—(mg/mL) ethanol (44); methanol (64); PEG 400 (3); insoluble in water.

Comments—It is indicated for the treatment of symptomatic benign prostatic hyperplasia in men with an enlarged prostate to reduce symptoms.

FINASTERIDE

4-Azaandrost-1-ene-17-carboxamide, (5α-17β)-N-(1,1-dimethyl-ethyl)-3-oxo-, Proscar

[98319-26-7] $C_{23}H_{36}N_2O_2$ (372.55).

Preparation—*J Am Chem Soc* 1988; 110:3319.

Description—White to off-white crystals; melts about 257°.

Solubility—Very slightly soluble in water or dilute acid or base; freely soluble in alcohol or chloroform.

Comments—An androgen hormone inhibitor that acts by competitive inhibition of steroid 5-reductase, which converts testosterone to potent 5-dihydrotestosterone (DHT) in the prostate gland, liver, and skin. DHT induces its effects by binding to androgen receptors in cell nuclei of organs containing this enzyme. It is used to treat symptomatic benign prostatic hyperplasia. A lower-dose preparation is used to treat male pattern baldness. The drug generally is tolerated well, with reports of impotence (3.7%), decreased libido (3.3%), and decreased volume of ejaculation (2.8%).

FLUTAMIDE

For the full monograph, see page 1573.

Comments—An orally active and potent competitive inhibitor of nuclear androgen receptors in target tissues such as the prostate, seminal vesicles, and adrenal cortex. It is used in the treatment of prostatic cancer that is clinically localized and is given in combination with a GnRH analog (eg, goserelin and leuprolide acetate). Its pharmacological activity is substantially due to the principal metabolite, 2-hydroxyflutamide. Approximately half of the drug is eliminated in the urine within 72 hr, and the hydroxylated metabolite has a half-life that varies with the dose from 6 to 22 hr. A high incidence of gynecomastia and some GI discomfort are observed. Some cases of severe hepatotoxicity were reported. Periodic liver function tests should be performed.

MEDICINAL AGENTS

CHAPTER 78

General Anesthetics

Michael R Borenstein, PhD

General anesthetics are a remarkably diverse group of chemical agents with the common property of inducing a profound but reversible central nervous system (CNS) depression resulting in loss of consciousness. The mechanism of action of these drugs has not been fully elucidated and may represent a number of non-specific pharmacologic processes as diverse as their structures. No one particular cellular target can explain the myriad of brain functions affected by, nor has any pharmacologic antagonist to general anesthetics been discovered. Thus, it is safe to assume that a number of physicochemical events are involved in the production of general anesthesia. Included among these may be effects at cell membranes and proteins, as well as enzyme and receptor systems.

The ideal anesthetic agent should possess the following characteristics: rapid and pleasant induction and withdrawal from anesthesia, skeletal muscle relaxation, analgesia, high potency, a large therapeutic index, non-flammability, and chemically inertness with regard to anesthetic delivery devices. In practice it is common to employ a variety of drugs since no one agent meets all these criteria.

The route of administration of general anesthetics is via inhalation or intravenous injection. This chapter reviews the volatile compounds in clinical use, as well as a number of parenterally administered agents that produce loss of consciousness and some degree of analgesia or muscle relaxation. There are a number of drugs discussed elsewhere that often play an adjunct role in general anesthesia these include opioids, muscle relaxants, and benzodiazepines.

A general note of caution with regard to general anesthetic administration and the recent increased use of natural products has been issued by the American Society of Anesthesiologists. It is recommend that patients stop taking herbal medications at least 2 to 3 weeks before surgery in order to decrease the risk of adverse effects resulting from an enhancement or prolongation of anesthetic effects. This is particularly important in those patients using St. John's Wort, *Hypericum perforatum.*

INHALATION ANESTHETICS

In 1846 William Morton reported the first use of diethyl ether as a volatile inhaled agent to produce surgical anesthesia. This was followed by the introduction of chloroform, nitrous oxide, and the halogenated hydrocarbons in the 1950s. Although neither diethyl ether or chloroform are in widespread clinical use today, they served as the structural templates for synthetic manipulations that have produced today's potent congeners. The volatile anesthetics in common clinical use are either halogen-substituted ethers or extensively halogenated alkanes. In addition, there are inorganic gases with relatively weak anesthetic

activity that must be administered in combination with opiates, muscle relaxants, or other agents in order to produce acceptable surgical anesthesia.

Inhalation anesthetics are produced from volatile liquids or gases. Thus, they require the use of specialized delivery systems employing various combinations of vaporizers, absorbers, and flowmeters to deliver a constant and precisely controlled amount of drug to the respiratory system of the patient. Rapid metabolism and pulmonary excretion aid in the reversal of the anesthetic state. There are several physicochemical parameters that describe the efficacy of volatile anesthetics. The minimal alveolar concentration (MAC) is a measure of anesthetic potency as reflected in the concentration of anesthetic agent in the alveoli required to produce immobility in 50% of adult patients subjected to a noxious stimulus, typically a surgical incision. As the concentration of anesthetic in the lungs increases, a concomitant rise in blood concentration will follow. The blood solubility of anesthetics is reflected in the blood/gas partition coefficient and determines how rapidly surgical anesthesia is attained. MAC and partition coefficient values are inversely related to potency and time to onset of anesthesia, respectively.

Modern inhalation anesthetics are conveniently divided into potent carbon-based drugs and relatively weak anesthetics such as nitrous oxide and the still experimental xenon. The difference lies in the fact that the potent inhalation agents provide the entire anesthetic requirement in the presence of an adequate amount of oxygen. The inorganic anesthetics must be administered in an appropriate combination with opioids, muscle relaxants, or hypnotic adjuvants.

HALOGENATED ALKANES

HALOTHANE

Ethane, 2-bromo-2-chloro-1,1,1-trifluoro-, Fluothane

2-Bromo-2-chloro-1,1,1-trifluoroethane [151-67-7] $C_2HBrClF_3$ (197.38); contains 0.008% to 0.012% thymol, by weight, as a stabilizer.

Preparation—Commercially available 2-chloro-1,1,1-trifluoroethane is subjected to direct bromination, and halothane is isolated from the reaction product by fractional distillation.

Description—Colorless, mobile, nonflammable, heavy liquid; characteristic odor resembling that of chloroform; sweet taste and produces a burning sensation; distills between 49° and 51°; specific gravity between 1.872 and 1.877 at 20°.

Solubility—Slightly soluble in water; miscible with alcohol, chloroform, ether, or fixed oils.

Comments—Introduced into clinical practice in 1956, it is the only volatile anesthetic to contain a bromine atom that may contribute to its potency. It has an intermediate solubility (blood/gas partition coefficient, 2.5) and low MAC (0.7%). Halothane causes dose-dependent vasodilation, myocardial depression, and decreases in sympathetic tone. Like the other potent inhalation anesthetics, halothane provides muscle relaxation and in addition has a low incidence of nausea and vomiting.

Halothane is subject to oxidative degradation to hydrochloric and hydrobromic acid, as well as phosgene. For this reason it is stored in amber-colored bottles with the preservative thymol. It is reactive with most metals except titanium, nickel, or chromium. As a myocardial depressant, halothane decreases cardiac output to 80% of normal at 1 MAC and 70% of normal at 2 MAC. The drug also sensitizes the myocardium to the dysrhythmic actions of epinephrine more than the ether-based anesthetics. This effect is accentuated by hypercarbia. Like all other potent inhalation anesthetics, halothane decreases the normal ventilatory responses to hypoventilation and hypoxemia.

A relatively large amount of the administered dose of halothane is metabolized. This has been associated with its hepatotoxicity and led to the development of the newer ether anesthetics (see below).

HALOGENATED ETHERS

Fluorinated derivatives of diethyl ether were developed in an attempt to improve upon the adverse effect profile of halothane. As a class, they are nonflammable, stable, and nonarrhythmogenic. They differ in their degree of metabolism and effects on respiration, circulation, or the CNS.

DESFLURANE

Ethane, (±)-2-(difluoromethoxy)-1,1,2,2-tetrafluoro-, Suprane

[57041-67-5] $C_3H_2F_6O$ (168.04)

Description—Extremely volatile; nonflammable and not explosive at clinical concentrations.

Solubility—Insoluble in water; soluble in organic solvents.

Comments—Approved for clinical use in the US in 1993. It is minimally metabolized (0.02%) and has a low solubility (blood/gas partition coefficient, 0.42), leading to a rapid onset and recovery and extensive use in the outpatient surgical procedure environment. Its low boiling point necessitated the development of a heated vaporizer to ensure consistent drug delivery. Desflurane is less potent (MAC, 6.0%) than the other ethers.

Dose-related decreases in blood pressure and cardiac output are similar to isoflurane. Increases in heart rate and blood pressure have been noted upon introduction of the agent because of stimulation of the sympathetic nervous system following the production of carbon monoxide. These effects may be minimized by the use of new carbon monoxide absorbents. Desflurane is the most pungent of the inhalation anesthetics, causing breath-holding and coughing, and is not recommended for inhalation induction of general anesthesia in children. Desflurane either increases or does not change intracranial pressure (ICP) in patients with space-occupying tumors. It causes cerebral vasodilation and dose-dependent decreases in the cerebral metabolic rate of oxygen consumption ($CMRO_2$) similar to isoflurane and sevoflurane.

ENFLURANE

Ethane, 2-chloro-1-(difluoromethoxy)-1,1,2-trifluoro-, Ethrane

2-Chloro-1,1,2-trifluoroethyl difluoromethyl ether [13838-16-9] $C_3H_2ClF_5O$ (184.49).

Preparation—May be synthesized by a series of reactions starting with trifluorochloroethylene. US Pats 3,469,011 and 3,527,813.

Description—Clear, colorless, volatile liquid; pleasant hydrocarbon like odor; boils at 56.6°; nonflammable.

Solubility—Soluble in water to the extent of 0.275%, and water-soluble in enflurane to the extent of 0.13%; miscible with organic solvents.

Comments—Introduced in 1973, it has intermediate blood solubility (blood/gas partition coefficient, 1.9; MAC, 1.7) and excellent muscle relaxant properties. Approximately 2–10% is hepatically metabolized to produce fluoride but at low enough levels to preclude nephrotoxicity. An increase in metabolism is seen in the obese patient and those taking isoniazid or other hydrazine compounds. Enflurane produces spiking discharges on the electroencephalogram (EEG) at high doses. Its use is avoided in epileptics, patients at risk for nephrotoxicity, and those with a history of malignant hyperthermia.

ISOFLURANE

Ethane, 2-chloro-2-(difluoromethoxy)-1,1,1-trifluor-, Forane, AErrane [Veterinary]

1-Chloro-2,2,2-trifluoroethyl difluoromethyl ether [26675-46-7] $C_3H_2ClF_5O$ (184.49).

Preparation—Trifluoroethanol is methylated with dimethyl sulfate to form the methyl ether, which is then chlorinated to the dichloromethyl ether, $CF_3CHClOCHCl_2$. This latter compound, on treatment with $HF/SbCl_5$ forms the product. See *J Med Chem* 1971; 14:517.

Description—Low-boiling liquid (48.5°) with a slight odor; nonflammable.

Solubility—Miscible with most organic solvents including fats or oils; practically insoluble in water.

Comments—Similar to its isomer enflurane it was approved for use in the US in 1979. Its has a good safety record, acceptable physical properties (blood/gas partition coefficient, 1.5; MAC, 1.15), and a low rate of metabolism (0.2%). Its irritating pungent odor requires the use of intravenous induction agents. It can cause uterine relaxation and is contraindicated in patients with a history of malignant hyperthermia.

SEVOFLURANE

Propane, 1,1,1,3,3,3-hexafluoro-2-(fluoromethoxy)-, Ultane

[28523-86-6] $C_4H_3F_7O$ (200.06)

Description—Nonflammable, highly volatile.

Solubility—Insoluble in water.

Comments—Approved for clinical use in the US in 1995. It has a low solubility (blood/gas partition coefficient, 0.69) that is slightly higher than that of nitrous oxide and desflurane and an intermediate potency (MAC, 2.05%). Three to 5% of the drug is metabolized in the body, with a by-product being inorganic fluoride. Although fluoride toxicity (high-output renal failure) was a concern with this agent, it has not been seen in a clinical context. Sevoflurane is also subject to degradation by the basic environment present in the carbon dioxide absorbent in the gas delivery system. The breakdown products include pentafluoroisopropenyl fluoromethyl ether (PIFE) also know as Compound A, a substance associated with renal injury in rats and non-human primates. Clinical conditions including low fresh gas flows through the vaporizer and pre-existing renal failure in the patient are relative contraindications to using this agent. Thus far, renal injury due solely to sevoflurane has not been reported.

Dose-related decreases in blood pressure and cardiac output are similar to those seen with isoflurane. Sevoflurane is the least pungent of the potent inhaled agents and is used commonly for inhalation induction of anesthesia in children. It is a potent bronchodilator and can be used to treat acute bronchoconstriction. It is similar to isoflurane in its effect on cerebral hemodynamics, decreasing ICP with hyperventilation, decreasing $CMRO_2$, and preserving the response of the cerebral vasculature to carbon dioxide. The physical properties of sevoflurane allow a smooth, rapid inhalation induction and a quick emergence from anesthesia. The addition of nitrous oxide to sevoflurane during induction decreases induction time and decreases excitatory phenomena such as movement.

INORGANIC GASES

Only one agent is currently approved for use in the US; however, clinical trials of the inert gas Xenon indicate promise as an effective anesthetic with a reduced cardiovascular adverse effect profile.

NITROUS OXIDE

Dinitrogen Monoxide; Laughing Gas

Nitrogen oxide (N_2O) [10024-97-2]; contains not less than 99.0%, by volume, of N_2O (44.01). The remainder is chiefly nitrogen.

Preparation—Usually by heating ammonium nitrate to about 170° to produce nitrous oxide and water. Nitrous oxide is furnished in compressed form in metallic cylinders.

Description—Colorless gas, without appreciable odor or taste; specific gravity 1.53; 1 L, at a pressure of 760 torr at 0°, weighs about 1.97 g.

Solubility—1 volume dissolves in about 1.4 volumes of water at 20° under normal pressure; freely soluble in alcohol; soluble in ether or oils.

Comments—The narcosis-producing effects of nitrous oxide (N_2O) were described by Sir Humphry Davy in 1799. It is a powerful analgesic and a weak anesthetic (MAC, 105%) with a rapid onset and recovery (blood/gas partition coefficient, 0.47) available as a compressed gas. It is often used in combination with other anesthetics as part of a *balanced technique* or as an adjunct to potent inhalation agents to decrease the concentration necessary to achieve MAC. Nitrous oxide is considered to be nonflammable but will support combustion. It has been suggested that nitrous oxide causes ordination of the cobalt atom in vitamin B_{12} resulting in an inhibition of methionine synthetase activity, leading to megaloblastic anemia after prolonged (days) administration. The same mechanism is presumably responsible for the nitrous oxide induced increases in total homocysteine plasma levels which are associated with an increase in perioperative myocardial ischemia.

Nitrous oxide has a minimal effect on respiration, although hypoxic drive is blunted. Cardiac output is maintained with increasing dose, presumably through mild sympathetic stimulation. In clinical situations where there are enclosed air-containing spaces, such as inner ear surgery, abdominal surgery, sitting craniotomy, or pneumothorax, nitrous oxide will diffuse into the space 35 times faster than nitrogen diffuses out, resulting in expansion of the air-containing spaces. There is evidence that nitrous oxide may increase postoperative nausea and vomiting. It has wide utility in dental procedures where full anesthesia is not essential. Recent reports have indicated that the use of nitrous oxide during general anesthesia in gas-filled eyes may have disastrous visual results caused by gas expansion and elevated intraocular pressure.

INTRAVENOUS ANESTHETICS

The parenteral route for the administration of general anesthetics offers the advantage of less cumbersome delivery systems when compared to the inhalation route. A major disadvantage is the lack of control regarding the time course for the anesthetic effect. Inhalation anesthetics are dosed in response to the hemodynamic parameters of the patient, and adequate levels can be monitored with end-tidal measurement of the respiratory gas. A similar monitor of the dose-effect ratio is not currently available for intravenous anesthetics, so a rough dose estimate must be made on the basis of the population pharmacodynamics and pharmacokinetics. Wide variations exist between patients and clinical situations, making accurate titration of intravenous agents difficult.

Interestingly, the precise pharmacologic targets for these agents have been more fully defined than those for the inhalation anesthetics, nevertheless actions at single sites do not account for the profound anesthesia produced by these compounds. The inhibitory GABA receptor appears to be a primary mediator for the activity of many of these agents but the opioid, NMDA, serotonin, or muscarinic receptors may also be involved.

Similar to the inhalation agents, there is no ideal intravenous anesthetic and combinations of both are common. Intravenous drugs have found a particularly useful role in the in-

duction of general anesthesia, which is often maintained by the addition of inhalation anesthetics or other adjuvant agents including opioids and benzodiazepines.

Barbiturates

The ultra short-acting barbiturates produce rapid unconsciousness but lack analgesic or muscle relaxant activity and are therefore typically used as induction agents or for short procedures. There are two classes of barbiturates used in anesthesia, thiobarbiturates such as thiopental, and oxybarbiturates such as methohexital. The drugs differ in potency, metabolism, and clinical use, as reviewed below. Common to all barbiturates is the proscription in patients with latent or clinical porphyria. Induction of cytochrome enzyme systems predisposes such patients to a possibly fatal episode.

METHOHEXITAL SODIUM

2,4,6(1*H*,3*H*,5*H*)-Pyrimidinetrione, (±)-1-methyl-5-(1-methyl-2-pentynyl)-5-(2-propenyl)-, monosodium salt; Brevital Sodium

Sodium 5-allyl-1-methyl-5-(1-methyl-2-pentynyl)barbiturate [309-36-4] $C_{14}H_{17}N_2NaO_3$ (284.29).

Preparation—1-Butynyl magnesium bromide is treated with acetaldehyde, and the resulting alcohol is treated with PCl_5 to produce 2-chloro-3-pentyne. Condensation with ethyl cyanoacetate in the presence of sodium ethylate yields ethyl 1-methyl-2-pentynylcyanoacetate which, on similar further condensation with allyl bromide, yields ethyl (1-methyl-2-pentynyl)allylcyanoacetate. Reaction with *N*-methylurea yields the iminobarbituric acid, which, on acid-catalyzed hydrolysis, forms methohexital. Neutralization with sodium hydroxide produces the sodium salt.

The two diastereoisomers of the barbituric acid have been designated as α- and β-forms in the literature. The α-form is the one used medicinally (the β-form causes undesirable side effects) and is formed almost exclusively by the above process. The malonic ester synthesis described under *Barbital* (RPS-18, p 1067) is not used because it yields mainly the unwanted β-form.

Description—White to off-white hygroscopic powder; essentially odorless; solutions are alkaline to litmus.

Solubility—Soluble in water.

Comments—Used primarily for short, mildly painful procedures and induction of general anesthesia. An induction dose of 1 mg/kg reliably produces unconsciousness in 30 sec; the pharmacological effect terminates with rapid redistribution from the brain to peripheral sites. Recovery from methohexital is more rapid, and there is less myocardial depression than with thiopental. Intravenous injection may be painful, and tremor, coughing, and hiccups occur occasionally. Methohexital has been used to elicit spiking discharges on the EEG in patients undergoing testing for seizure activity. In the anesthetic realm, it has been used during closed reduction of fractures, electroconvulsive therapy, cardioversion, and testing of automatic defibrillators.

Methohexital is metabolized only in the liver, causing induction of cytochrome enzymes. Intravenous injection may result in anaphylaxis (1/30,000), and seizures are reported after a continuous infusion (1/3).

THIOPENTAL SODIUM

4,6-(1*H*,5*H*)-Pyrimidinedione, 5-ethyldihydro-5-(1-methylbutyl)-2-thioxo-, monosodium salt; Thiopentone Sodium; Pentothal Sodium

Sodium 5-ethyl-5-(1-methylbutyl)-2-thiobarbiturate [71-73-8] $C_{11}H_{17}N_2NaO_2S$ (264.32).

Preparation—In the same manner as *Amobarbital* (RPS-20, p 1415), using 2-bromopentane as the alkyl halide and the ethyl 1-methyl-butylmalonate is condensed with thiourea [$CS(NH_2)_2$].

Description—White to off-white, crystalline powder or a yellowish white to pale greenish yellow hygroscopic powder; may have a disagreeable odor; aqueous solution is alkaline to litmus; solutions decompose on standing and, on boiling, precipitation occurs. Carbon dioxide also causes precipitation in the solution.

Solubility—Soluble in water or alcohol; insoluble in absolute ether, benzene, or solvent hexane.

Incompatibilities—Thiopental precipitates in acid solutions.

Comments—Used for induction of general anesthesia, brain protection therapy, and as an anticonvulsant. It is not used for short procedures requiring unconsciousness and amnesia because recovery occurs faster with methohexital or propofol. A single induction dose (3–5 mg/kg) will cause unconsciousness in 30 to 40 sec, and its action is terminated by redistribution of drug away from the brain. Pain at the injection site is less common than with methohexital or propofol. There is a transient decrease in blood pressure (20%) and a compensatory increase in heart rate on injection. Hypovolemic patients are at risk for major hemodynamic sequelae because of the vasodilation caused by thiopental. Intra-arterial injection leads to arterial thrombosis and necrosis of the involved limb.

Thiopental is metabolized mainly in the liver, although the kidney and muscle tissue may participate. Intravenous injection has been associated with anaphylaxis and porphyria attacks in susceptible individuals.

Thiopental has been used to treat acute increases in ICP and as a brain protectant during surgical procedures in which there is risk of ischemia due to lack of blood flow. Monitoring of the EEG is helpful in determining the thiopental dose needed to cause burst suppression. Although the mechanism of this effect is not certain, it is thought that decreasing oxygen consumption or free radical scavenging is involved.

Nonbarbiturates

ETOMIDATE

1*H*-Imidazole-5-carboxylic acid, (±)-1-(1-phenylethyl)-, ethyl ester, Amidate

(+)-Ethyl (1-(α-methylbenzyl)imidazole-5-carboxylate [33125-97-2] $C_{14}H_{16}N_2O_2$ (244.99).

Preparation—From a-methylbenzyl amine and ethyl chloroacetate in 8 steps.

Description—White or yellow crystals or amorphous; melts about 67°.

Solubility—Insoluble in water; soluble in common polar organic solvents.

Comments—A hypnotic agent used for induction of general anesthesia. Intravenous injection of this water-soluble agent at 0.3 mg/kg leads to a rapid loss of consciousness within one arm-to-brain circulation time. Etomidate is known for its cardiovascular stability and quick emergence after a single dose because of rapid redistribution. Adverse reactions include pain on injection, respiratory depression (less than the barbiturates), and myoclonus. Myoclonic activity results from a disinhibition of subcortical structures and is not associated with seizure activity on EEG. Adrenocortical suppression has been reported for induction doses and is more common after an intravenous infusion of etomidate. This effect is due to an inhibition of 11-β-hydroxylase activity lasting 4 to 8 hr after an induction dose. The clinical significance of this finding remains unclear but suggests the choice of other agents in the critical care setting where adrenocortical dysfunction may lead to mortality.

Metabolism of etomidate takes place in the liver. Recovery from etomidate anesthesia is associated with a greater incidence of nausea and vomiting, and emergence delirium has been noted after long infusions.

Etomidate is an alternative to barbiturate induction in patients with unstable cardiovascular systems, in hypovolemic patients, and as a supplement to other anesthetic agents in a balanced technique. Although it decreases ICP, $CMRO_2$, and EEG activity as thiopental does, its efficacy as a brain protectant has been questioned recently.

KETAMINE HYDROCHLORIDE

Cyclohexanone, 2-(2-chlorophenyl)-2-(methylamino)-, hydrochloride; Ketaject, Ketalar

(±)-2-(*o*-Chlorophenyl)-2-(methylamino)cyclohexanone hydrochloride [1867-66-9] Base [6740-88-1] $C_{13}H_{16}ClNO \cdot HCl$ (274.19).

Preparation The product resulting from a Grignard reaction involving *o*-chlorobenzonitrile and bromocyclopentane is treated in the presence of strong alkali to form the epoxy compound (I). Reaction of this (I) with methylamine yields the imine (II), which rearranges on heating in the presence of hydrochloric acid. Belgian Pat 634,208.

I II

Description—White, crystalline powder with a characteristic odor; solutions are acid to litmus; melts between 258° and 261° with decomposition; pH (1 in 10 solution) between 3.5 and 4.1.

Solubility—1 g in 5 mL water, 14 mL alcohol, 60 mL chloroform, or 60 mL absolute alcohol.

Comments—Unique as an intravenous anesthetic in that it provides anesthetic, sedative, amnesiac, and analgesic action. Induction doses (1–2 mg/kg) produce surgical anesthesia within 30 sec. Patients maintain ventilation and cardiovascular function. Ketamine produces a state of *dissociative anesthesia;* patients may appear awake and be non-communicative yet experience intense analgesia and amnesia. Some protective reflexes (gag, laryngeal tone, spontaneous ventilation) remain intact.

Intravenous injection is not painful, and the action of the drug is terminated by redistribution. Ketamine is metabolized by the liver (CYP3A4 predominates). Tolerance to the drug may develop after repeated dosing. Cardiovascular effects resemble sympathetic stimulation (increases in heart rate, cardiac output, blood pressure), possibly through direct interaction with the sympathetic nervous system. *In vitro,* ketamine is a myocardial depressant. Thus, patients with depleted catecholamine stores (trauma, critical illness) may experience cardiovascular collapse upon induction with ketamine. Emergence delirium (1% of patients) is characterized by visual and auditory hallucinations that may continue up to 24 hr after administration. This effect is attenuated by coadministration of benzodiazepines or other anesthetic agents. Patients receiving ketamine should not be released from care until recovery is complete and should be accompanied by a responsible adult.

Ketamine is used as an intravenous induction agent in adults and as an intramuscular injection in difficult-to-manage children (4 mg/kg). It is used for short painful procedures (ie, burn wound dressing, emergency induction for c-section). It may also be given by mouth. Ketamine is a bronchodilator and so is useful for asthmatic patients but should be avoided in clinical situations with cardiovascular and neurosurgical concerns.

PROPOFOL

Phenol, 2,6-diisopropyl-, Diprivan

[2078-54-8] $C_{12}H_{18}O$ (178.27)

Preparation—See *J Org Chem* 21:712, 1956.

Description—Oily liquid; melts about 19°, pK_a 11.

Solubility—Slightly soluble in water; very soluble in alcohol.

Comments—Propofol has a rapid onset (within one arm-brain circulation time), and its pharmacological action is terminated by redistribution. Pain on injection is common unless the drug is injected into a large vein or preceded by injection of a local anesthetic or potent opioid. Rapid recovery is facilitated by a short initial distribution half-life (2–8 min), with clearance by glucuronide and sulfate conjugation and possibly extrahepatic site metabolism with less than 0.3% excreted unchanged.

An induction dose (1.5–2.5 mg/kg) leads to a greater decrease in blood pressure than with thiopental, through vasodilation and a direct myocardial depressant effect. There is little or no change in heart rate or cardiac output. Dose-dependent respiratory depression occurs in 25 to 35% of patients after an initial dose; it is also a bronchodilator and decreases the normal response to hypoxia and hypercarbia. Propofol decreases $CMRO_2$ and ICP and is reported to have brain-protectant qualities. Substantial decreases in blood pressure leading to clinically significant decreases in cerebral perfusion pressure limits it application in neuroanesthesia. Side effects include precipitation of excitatory motor activity (myoclonus and opisthotonus) and antiemetic properties. It is not a trigger for malignant hyperthermia (MH) and is the agent of choice in patients susceptible to MH. Propofol is contraindicated in critically ill pediatric patients where it has been shown to produce a "propofol syndrome" consisting of metabolic acidosis and cardiac failure.

Propofol is used as an induction agent for general anesthesia and as a maintenance hypnotic under constant intravenous infusions. It has found utility in the outpatient surgical environment. Patients tend to awake quickly from a propofol-based anesthetic with, at times, a feeling of euphoria. There is a significant amnestic effect at high doses.

BIBLIOGRAPHY

Badner NH, Freeman D, Spence JD. *Anesthesia & Analgesia* 2001; 93(6):1507.

Barash PG, Cullen BF, Stoelting RK. *Clinical Anesthesia,* ed 3. Philadelphia: JB Lippincott, 1996.

Cheng MA, Theard MA, Tempelhoff R. *Crit Care Clin* 1997; 13(1):185.

Eger EI 2nd. *Anesthesiology* 1994; 80(4):906.

Farnsworth S, Johnson J. *Am J Anesth* 1995; 12:139.

Gillman MA, Lichtigfeld FJ. *Int J Neurosci* 1998; 93(1–2):55.

Goa KL, Noble S, Spencer CM. *Paediatric Drugs* 1999; 1(2):127–53, 1999

Hijazi Y, Boulieu R. *Drug Metabolism & Disposition* 2002; 30(7):853.

Katzung BG. *Basic & Clinical Pharmacology,* ed 8. New York: Lange Medical Books/McGraw-Hill, 2001.

Krasowski MD, et al. *Mol Pharmacol* 1998; 53(3):530.

Ries CR, Scoates PJ, Puil E. *Can J Anaesth* 1994; 41(5Pt1):414.

Roberts RG, Redman JW. *Anaesthesia* 2002; 57(4):413.

Rosow CE. *J Clin Anesth* 1997; 9(6 Suppl): 27S.

Rossaint R, Reyle-Hahn M, Schulte AM et al. *Anesthesiology* 2003; 98(1):6.

Seaberg RR, Freeman WR, Goldbaum MH, et al. *Anesthesiology* 2002; 297(5):1309.

Stoelting RK. *Pharmacology and Physiology in Anesthetic Practice,* ed 3. Philadelphia: Lippincott, 1998.

Sullivan RL. *ASA Newsletter* 1999; 11(63).

Tempelhoff R. *J Neurosurg Anesthesiol* 1997; 9(1):6971.

Umbrain V, Shi L, Camu F. *Acta Anaesthesiologica Belgica* 2002; 53(3):187.

Williams DA, Lemke TL. *Foye's Principles of Medicinal Chemistry,* ed 5. Baltimore: Lippincott Williams & Wilkins, 2002.

Wooltorton E. *CMAJ* 2002; 167(5):507.

Yaksh TL, Lynch C, Zapol WM, et al. *Anesthesia: Biologic Foundations*, Philadelphia: Lippincott-Raven, 1998.

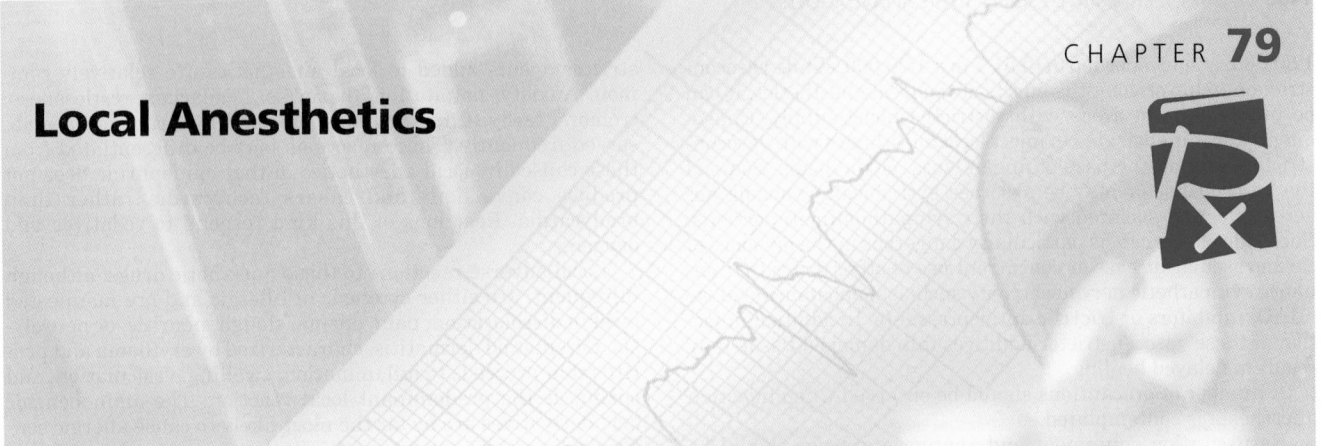

CHAPTER 79

Local Anesthetics

Local anesthetics reversibly block impulse conduction in any part of the nervous system and in all nerves, including sensory, motor, and autonomic types. They often are used to produce a transient loss of sensation in a circumscribed area of the body without causing a general loss of consciousness. This action can be used to block pain sensation—or sympathetic vasoconstrictor impulses—to specific areas of the body. Hence, local anesthetics are used to prevent pain in surgical procedures, dental manipulations, injury, and disease. The synthetic local anesthetic agents may be divided into two groups: the slightly soluble compounds and the soluble compounds. The slightly soluble local anesthetics are used only for surface (topical) application, since their slow absorption renders them safe for use on ulcers, wounds, and mucous surfaces. The anesthesia that they induce is not as complete as that induced by soluble compounds, but the duration is longer. Many soluble anesthetics also may be used for topical anesthesia. On the other hand, only soluble local anesthetics of relatively low toxicity should be injected.

Local anesthesia induced by injectable agents is designated according to the technique or anatomical site of the injection. Infiltration anesthesia refers to injection directly into the area that is painful or is to be subjected to surgical trauma. Field block is accomplished by administering the local anesthetic to a region of the nerve proximal to the site to be anesthetized. Peripheral nerve block, commonly called regional anesthesia, places the anesthetic agent in direct contact with the nerve or nerve plexus. Paravertebral nerve block places the anesthetic agent in direct contact with the nerve as it exits the intervertebral foramina. Epidural and caudal blocks are similar; caudal block is an epidural block in the caudal region. Subarachnoid block, commonly called spinal anesthesia, but more correctly spinal analgesia, requires that the anesthetic be placed within the subarachnoid space so that the anesthetic agent mixes with spinal fluid.

The use of a hyperbaric (heavy) solution or hypobaric (light) solution and proper positioning of the patient on the operating table permits manipulation of anesthesia for various body areas.

Local anesthetics prevent both the generation and the conduction of the nerve impulse. The excitable membrane of nerve axons maintains a transmembrane potential of -90 to -60 mV. During excitation, the sodium channels open, and a fast inward sodium current quickly depolarizes the membrane toward the sodium equilibrium potential ($+40$ mV). As a result of depolarization, the sodium channels close (inactivate), and potassium channels open. The outward flow of potassium repolarizes the membrane toward the potassium equilibrium potential (-95 mV); repolarization returns the sodium channels to the rested state. The transmembrane ionic gradients are maintained by the sodium pump.

When increasing concentrations of a local anesthetic are applied to a nerve fiber, the threshold for excitation increases, the impulse conduction slows, the rate of rise of the action potential declines, the action potential amplitude decreases, and, finally, the ability to generate an action potential is abolished. All these effects result from the binding of the local anesthetic to sodium channels, which in turn blocks the transient permeability to sodium. If the sodium current is blocked over a critical portion of nerve, propagation of an impulse over the blocked area is no longer possible.

When infiltration, conduction, or regional techniques are employed, both nerve fibers and nerve endings are anesthetized. The ease with which a nerve fiber may be anesthetized is related to its type and size. Although there are exceptions, large myelinated nerves usually require a higher concentration of anesthetic solution and more time to be blocked than small nonmyelinated fibers. Accordingly, small nerve fibers concerned with vasoconstriction, temperature, and surface pain are anesthetized most easily, whereas large fibers associated with the sensation of touch, pressure, deep pain, and the sensations from joints and tendons are anesthetized with more difficulty. In spinal anesthesia, it is probable that both sensory and motor nerve fibers are anesthetized. In surface (topical) anesthesia, the sensory nerve endings are the chief nerve structures affected.

The nerve-blocking action of the local anesthetics is pH sensitive. Because these drugs generally are marketed as water-soluble salts, the injected solutions are mildly acidic. To block nerve activity, the local anesthetic must become deprotonated and diffuse through cellular membranes to reach its intracellular site of action. However, because the cationic species is the form of the local anesthetic that interacts preferentially with the sodium channels, molecules that have crossed the membranes must be protonated again to be effective. Changes in extracellular pH can disrupt the balance between protonated and deprotonated forms and interfere with local anesthetic activity. This can occur in areas of tissue damage or inflammation or following multiple administrations of the acidic local anesthetic solutions.

The duration of action of a local anesthetic is proportional to the time during which it is in actual contact with nervous tissues. Consequently, procedures that help localize the drug at the nerve prolong anesthesia. Cocaine itself constricts blood vessels, prevents its own absorption, and has a duration of action longer than most local anesthetics. A vasoconstrictor drug, such as epinephrine, norepinephrine, or levonordefrin, is included frequently in local anesthetic solutions. The presence of one of these drugs in the local anesthetic solution retards absorption of the local anesthetic solution, thereby reducing its systemic toxicity, increasing its duration of action, and increasing its efficiency by decreasing the volume of solution required. The pressor potency relative to epinephrine (shown in parentheses), maximal total dose, and usual concentration are as follows: epinephrine (1), 0.2 mg, 1:50,000 to 1:200,000; norepinephrine (0.6), 0.34 mg,

1:30,000; and levonordefrin (0.5), 1 mg, 1:20,000. While vasoconstriction helps prolong the effects of the local anesthetics, it can be problematic in areas with restricted blood supply. Consequently, it is inadvisable to inject local anesthetics with vasoconstrictors around the base of fingers, toes, or the penis. Some of the vasoconstrictor may be absorbed systemically, causing adverse effects associated with their sympathomimetic actions. Such side effects can be particularly dangerous in the presence of cardiovascular disease or concurrent use of other drugs that enhance sympathetic nervous activity such as monoamine oxidase (MAO) inhibitors or tricyclic antidepressants. In addition, injection of these vasoconstrictor additives into damaged tissue may result in delayed healing.

A number of precautions should be observed when injection anesthesia is contemplated.

Resuscitation equipment and appropriate drugs should be immediately available.

The safe use of these agents in pregnancy, with respect to adverse effects on fetal development, has not been established.

Local anesthetic procedures should be used with caution when there is inflammation and/or sepsis in the region of the proposed injection.

Local anesthetics containing epinephrine should be used with extreme caution in patients on MAO inhibitors, tricyclic antidepressants, phenothiazines, etc, as either severe hypertension or hypotension may occur.

Vasopressor agents used in caudal or other epidural blocks should be used with extreme caution in patients on oxytocic drugs, since the resulting interaction may produce severe persistent hypertension and/or rupture of cerebral blood vessels.

Serious, dose-related cardiac arrhythmias may occur if local anesthetics containing a vasoconstrictor such as epinephrine are employed in patients during or following the administration of chloroform, halothane, cyclopropane, trichloroethylene, or other inhalation anesthetics.

Factors that must be given careful consideration prior to concurrent use of general and local anesthetics include the effect of both agents on the myocardium, the concentration and volume of the vasoconstrictor, and the elapsed time since injection.

Adverse reactions to local anesthetics may be divided into two groups: systemic and local adverse reactions. In general, these reactions are qualitatively similar for all local anesthetic agents.

Systemic adverse reactions usually are associated with high blood levels of the drug and result from overdosage, rapid systemic absorption, or inadvertent intravenous injection. Because local anesthetics can affect all excitable membranes, the reactions usually involve the central nervous and cardiovascular systems.

The initial CNS reactions are excitatory and/or depressant and may be characterized by nervousness, agitation, dizziness, blurred vision, and tremors, followed by drowsiness, convulsions, unconsciousness, and possibly respiratory arrest. Other systemic effects may include nausea, vomiting, chills, pupil contraction, or tinnitus. The excitatory reactions may be very brief or absent, in which case the first manifestation of toxicity may be drowsiness, merging into unconsciousness and respiratory arrest.

Cardiovascular reactions usually require high systemic concentrations, are depressant, and may be characterized by hypotension, cardiovascular collapse, bradycardia, and possibly cardiac arrest. Treatment of a patient with toxic manifestations includes reassurance, maintaining a patent airway, and supporting ventilation using oxygen and assisted or controlled respiration. Should circulatory depression occur, vasopressors, such as ephedrine or metaraminol, and IV fluids may be used. Should a convulsion persist despite oxygen therapy, diazepam given IV is usually the treatment of choice.

Allergic reactions are characterized by cutaneous lesions, urticaria, edema, or anaphylactoid reactions. Untoward reactions from overdosage with epinephrine and other vasoconstrictor agents added to local anesthetics are relatively common. Anxiety, palpitation, dizziness, headaches, restlessness, tremors, tachycardia, anginal pain, and hypertension are observed frequently. These reactions may be differentiated from those caused by local anesthetics in that epinephrine does not produce convulsions and causes tachycardia rather than bradycardia. Reactions of this kind respond to sedatives and oxygen.

Local adverse reactions to these anesthetic drugs, although infrequent, are either cytotoxic or allergic and are manifested by skin discoloration, pain, edema, slough, neuritis, or neurolysis. Eczematoid dermatitis, characterized by erythema and pruritus that proceeds to inflammation, swelling, vesiculation, and oozing, is the predominant local reaction. The aminobenzoic acid derivatives are by far the most likely to cause allergic sensitivity reactions; cross-sensitivity between members of this group often is reported. If a patient is allergic or does not tolerate a particular local anesthetic, it is advisable to use a drug from a different chemical family. Unfortunately, tests for sensitivity such as skin, conjunctival, and patch tests are not reliable for predicting the possibility of allergic reactions.

All local anesthetics are toxic, and the tolerance of patients varies. Safe dosage, therefore, is limited for each drug and must be individualized. The choice of drug, concentration, rate and site of injection, and age and emotional and physical status of the patient are a few factors that must be considered. In general, the smallest amount of the least toxic drug that will serve the purpose should be used, if reactions are to be avoided. In some patients, premedication with diazepam may be advisable to minimize the incidence of toxic reactions. Many local anesthetics occasionally give rise to dermatitis. When this is severe, the use of the anesthetic should be discontinued.

The interested reader is referred to the following reviews on the subject: Courtney KR. Structural elements that determine local anesthetics activity. In *Handbook of Experimental Pharmacology*, vol 81, Strichartz GR, ed. Berlin: Springer-Verlag, 1987, p 53, and McLeskey CH. Rational use of local anesthetics. *NC Med J* 1982; 43:496.

INJECTION ANESTHETICS

Injectable local anesthetic drugs can be divided conveniently into two groups: esters and nonesters. The esters are primarily of the *para*-aminobenzoic acid type and include chlorpromazine, procaine, propoxycaine, and tetracaine. The nonesters are anilides (amides or nonesters) that include lidocaine, mepivacaine, bupivacaine, etidocaine, and prilocaine. This classification is particularly important from the point of view of possible allergic reactions as well as biotransformation. Thus, local anesthetics with an ester linkage (aromatic acid + amino alcohol) such as procaine and those with an amide linkage (aromatic amine + amino acid) such as lidocaine differ significantly in hypersensitivity, metabolism, and duration of action. Hypersensitivity seems to occur most prominently in response to local anesthetics of the ester-type and frequently extends to chemically related compounds. Allergic reactions to the amide type are extremely rare, and substitution of such amide-type, compounds to avoid allergic responses is usually possible.

The metabolic fate of local anesthetics is of great practical importance because their toxicity depends largely on the balance between their rate of absorption and their rate of destruction. The ester-type local anesthetic appears to be hydrolyzed by both liver esterase and plasma esterase. Metabolic degradation by plasma esterase is particularly important in man; human plasma esterase can hydrolyze local anesthetics 4 to 20 times faster than can animal plasma esterases. Consequently, very little of the ester-type agent is available for hydrolysis by liver esterase. Spinal fluid contains little or no esterase; hence, anesthesia produced by intrathecal injection of an ester-type local anesthetic will persist until the local anesthetic agent is absorbed into the blood.

On the other hand, amide-type local anesthetics are degraded by hepatic microsomes; the initial reactions involve *N*-dealkylation and subsequent hydrolysis. Consequently, the amide-type local anesthetics usually have a longer duration of action than the ester type.

Considerable pharmacokinetic data have been accumulated on the amide-type local anesthetics, particularly lidocaine, mepivacaine, bupivacaine, and etidocaine (the data are presented in the respective monographs). Comparatively little such information is available on the older ester-type agents; for the most part their rapid metabolism has hindered most attempts to measure their blood concentrations after less than heroic doses in man. Consequently, most studies with the latter agents deal with potency, toxicity, time for onset, and duration of action. The descriptive phrase *short-acting* suggests a duration of 45 to 75 min, medium-acting, 90 to 150 min, and long-acting, 180 min or longer.

With the exception of solutions for use in spinal anesthesia, local anesthetic solutions should be isotonic to avoid edema, local irritation, and inflammation at the site of injection. Solutions for spinal anesthesia may be isobaric, hypobaric, or hyperbaric, depending on the desired level of anesthesia. The total maximal dosages employed with injection anesthetics vary markedly, depending on the technique used and the patient's age, weight, and physical condition. In general, the physician should administer the smallest volume of the most dilute solution that is effective. For adverse effects and special warnings in the use of these agents, refer to the introductory statement.

BUPIVACAINE HYDROCHLORIDE

2-Piperidinecarboxamide, 1-butyl-*N*-(2,6-dimethylphenyl)-, hydrochloride; Marcaine Hydrochloride; Sensorcaine

1-Butyl-2′,6′-pipecoloxylidide monohydrochloride [14252-80-3] $C_{18}H_{28}N_2O \cdot HCl \cdot H_2O$ (342.91).

Preparation—Similar to that of *Mepivacaine Hydrochloride*, except that butyl bromide instead of dimethyl sulfate is used for alkylation. *J Med Chem* 1971; 14:891.

Description—White, crystalline powder; odorless; melts with decomposition about 250°. pK$_a$ 8.05.

Solubility—1 g in 25 mL water or 8 mL alcohol; slightly soluble in chloroform.

Comments—For local infiltration (0.25% soln), lumbar epidural (0.25%, 0.5%, and 0.75% soln), caudal block (0.25% and 0.5%), peripheral nerve block (0.25% and 0.5% soln), retrobulbar block (0.75% soln), sympathetic block (0.25% soln), and dental block (0.5% soln). It is not used for obstetrical paracervical block or topical anesthesia. The onset of action after local injection is rapid (5 min); however, onset may be delayed as long as 20 min when used for brachial plexus or peridural anesthesia. The duration of peripheral nerve blocks produced may be up to 7 hr, whereas the duration of peridural anesthesia is about 4 hr. Epidural block with 0.75% solution induces complete motor block; hence, abdominal operations requiring complete muscle relaxation may be done. It also has been noted that a period of analgesia persists after the return of sensation; during this time the need for analgesics is reduced. It has a t$_{1/2}$ of 2.7 hr, V$_d$ of 1.04, and a partition coefficient of 130; 84% to 95% of the drug is bound to plasma protein. Consequently, it has a low degree of placental transmission of parenteral local anesthetic and may cause the least fetal depression.

After injection for caudal, epidural, or peripheral nerve block in humans, peak blood levels of approximately 1.2 µg/mL are reached in 30 to 45 min, followed by a decline to insignificant levels within 3 to 6 hr. Like other local anesthetics with an amide structure, it is not detoxified by plasma esterases but is detoxified in the liver, via conjugation with glucuronic acid.

Contraindications, general warnings, precautions, and adverse reactions are similar to those of other amide-type local anesthetics (see *Lidocaine*, page 1484. It is not recommended for children under 12 yr, and the solution for spinal anesthesia should not be used in children under 18 yr. The safe use in pregnancy, with respect to adverse effects on fetal development, has not been established.

CHLOROPROCAINE HYDROCHLORIDE

Benzoic acid, 4-amino-2-chloro-, 2-(diethylamino)ethyl ester, monohydrochloride; Nesacaine, Nesacaine-MPF

2-(Diethylamino)ethyl 4-amino-2-chlorobenzoate monohydrochloride [3858-89-7] $C_{13}H_{19}ClN_2O_2 \cdot HCl$ (307.22).

Preparation—2-Chloro-4-nitrobenzoic acid is reacted with thionyl chloride, and the resulting acid chloride is condensed with 2-(diethylamino)ethanol. Reduction of the nitro ester with iron and acidulated water yields chloroprocaine base, which may be converted into the hydrochloride by dissolving in a suitable solvent and introducing hydrogen chloride.

Description—White, crystalline powder; odorless and stable in air; solutions acid to litmus; exhibits local anesthetic properties when placed on the tongue; melts about 175°.

Solubility—1 g in about 20 mL water or about 100 mL alcohol; very slightly soluble in chloroform; practically insoluble in ether. Aqueous solutions are acid to litmus and if discolored, should not be used.

Comments—Infiltration and nerve block (mandibular, infraorbital, or brachial plexus anesthesia, 2% soln; digital, 1%; pudendal, 2%; and paracervical block, 1% soln). Caudal and epidural block, 2 or 3% solution. It is not effective topically. Its onset of action is about 6 to 12 min, and anesthesia lasts from 30 to 60 min; with the addition of epinephrine 1:200,000, duration is increased to 60 to 90 min. For adverse reactions see the introductory statement.

ETIDOCAINE HYDROCHLORIDE

Butanamide, (±)-*N*-(2,6-dimethylphenyl)-2-(ethylpropylamino)-, monohydrochloride; Duranest

(±)-2-(Ethylpropylamino)-2′-6′-butyroxylidide monohydrochloride [3667-18-0 (free base)] $C_{17}H_{28}N_2O \cdot HCl$ (312.88).

Preparation—Etidocaine is synthesized by the interaction of 2,6-xylidine, 2-bromobutyric acid, and ethyl *n*-propylamine. German Pat 2,162,744 (*CA 77:* 101244c, 1972).

Description—White, crystalline powder; pK$_a$ 7.74 (etidocaine).

Solubility—Soluble in water; freely soluble in alcohol.

Comments—It has a rapid onset (3–5 min) and a prolonged duration of action (5–10 hr). The duration of sensory analgesia is 1.5 to 2 times longer than that of lidocaine; duration in excess of 9 hr is not infrequent in peripheral nerve blocks. It also produces a significant degree of motor blockade and abdominal muscle relaxation when used for peridural analgesia. Because of its tendency to block voluntary expulsive muscles, etidocaine should not be used in vaginal deliveries. This drug also should not be used for spinal anesthesia.

Contraindications, warnings for use, precautions, and adverse reactions are similar to those for lidocaine. Its safe use in pregnancy, with respect to adverse effects of fetal development, has not been established. The use of this agent in children under 14 years has not been investigated.

LIDOCAINE—page 1484.

LIDOCAINE HYDROCHLORIDE

Acetamide, 2-(diethylamino)-*N*-(2,6-dimethylphenyl)-, monohydrochloride, monohydrate; Lignocaine

2-(Diethylamino)-2′,6′-acetoxylidide monohydrochloride [6108-05-0] $C_{14}H_{22}N_2O \cdot HCl \cdot H_2O$ (288.82); *anhydrous* [73-78-9] $C_{14}H_{22}N_2O \cdot HCl$ (270.80).

For the structure of the base, see *Lidocaine*, page 1484.

Description—White, odorless, crystalline powder; slightly bitter taste; melts about 76°. pK$_a$ 7.86 (base).

Solubility—1 g in 0.7 mL water or 1.5 mL alcohol; pH (0.5% solu), 5.0 to 7.0; solutions may be sterilized by autoclaving.

Comments—A widely employed amide-type local anesthetic and antiarrhythmic drug. As a local anesthetic, it is employed for infiltration and field block anesthesia in a concentration of 0.5%; for periph-

MEDICINAL AGENTS

eral nerve block in concentrations of 0.5% and 1%; for paravertebral nerve block in a concentration of 0.5% to 1.5%; for epidural or caudal anesthesia in a concentration of 1.5% with 7.5% dextrose; and in subarachnoid block (spinal analgesia) in a concentration of 5% made hyperbaric with 7.5% dextrose. It also is used topically on mucous membranes as a 1% to 4% aqueous solution, 2% jelly, 2.5% and 5% ointment, and 2.0% viscous. It is also used in the form of suppositories for temporary relief of pain associated with inoperative, irritated, or inflamed anorectal conditions.

Some of its injections contain epinephrine to delay absorption, prolong its action, and reduce its toxic effects. Because it is also effective without a vasoconstrictor, it appears to be the anesthetic of choice for use in those individuals who are sensitive to epinephrine and its congeners. In addition, it is so dissimilar in chemical structure to procaine and related anesthetics that it is the agent of choice in individuals sensitive to procaine.

Its local anesthetic action is more rapid in onset, more intense, and of longer duration than that of procaine. It also is more potent than procaine. Because of its local vasodilating action, epinephrine often is combined with lidocaine. When used alone, anesthesia after perineural injection lasts 60 to 75 min; with epinephrine, anesthesia lasts 2 hr or more. This drug and procaine are approximately equally toxic when administered extravascularly in 0.5% solutions; when higher concentrations are used, this is 1 1/2 times as toxic as procaine. By the intravenous route, it is twice as toxic as procaine.

As an antiarrhythmic agent it is administered intravenously for the management of ventricular arrhythmias occurring during cardiac manipulation, such as cardiac surgery, and life-threatening arrhythmias that are ventricular in origin, such as occur during acute myocardial infarction. For this purpose it usually is given in a dose of 50 to 100 mg intravenously at a rate of 25 to 50 mg/min. If the initial injection does not produce the desired clinical response, a second dose (1/3–1/2 the initial dose) may be given after 5 min.

No more than 200 to 300 mg of lidocaine should be administered during a 1-hr period. Smaller doses should be used in cardiac failure, a reduced cardiac output from any cause, and in patients over 60 years. It exhibits a biphasic half-life. The distribution phase ($t_{1/2}$: 7 to 8 min) accounts for the short duration of action after intravenous administration (10–20 min). The terminal elimination half-life is 1 to 2 hr.

Therapeutic antiarrhythmic plasma levels range from 1.5 to 5.5 µg/mL; subjective toxic effect levels range from 3 to 5 µg/mL; and objective adverse manifestations such as muscular irritability, convulsions, and coma appear at plasma levels of 6 to 10 µg/mL. Thus, there is considerable overlap between therapeutic levels and subjective toxic effect levels. Moreover, toxicity may be significantly altered by the coadministration of other drugs. For example, coadministration with propranolol impairs the clearance of lidocaine and enhances toxicity; concomitant intravenous administration of phenytoin and lidocaine may induce excessive cardiac depression; and additive neurological effects may be produced during concurrent administration of procainamide and lidocaine.

It should be emphasized that after administration as a local anesthetic agent, systemic absorption may result in blood concentrations in the usual therapeutic antiarrhythmic, or even toxic, ranges. Plasma levels vary according to the site at which the local anesthetic is injected: subcutaneous, 1.2 µg/mL/100 mg; epidural, 1.1 µg/mL/100 mg; and subcutaneous (abdominal), 0.5 µg/mL/100 mg. Thus, the epidural injection of 25 mL of a 1.5% solution (375 mg) has the potential for producing a plasma level of 4.13 µg/mL, a value well within the range that induces subjective toxic effects (3 to 5 µg/mL) and approaching that which results in objective adverse manifestations (6–10 µg/mL).

After absorption, it partitions extensively into body tissues. Studies in monkeys indicate that it has a high affinity for spleen (tissue to plasma coefficient 3.5), lung (3.1), kidney (2.8), adipose tissue (2.0), brain (1.2), heart (0.96), and musculoskeletal tissues (0.6). Because of the avidity with which tissues take up the drug, only about 6% of a given dose is found in the blood at steady state. It then redistributes to muscle and adipose tissue, and these tissues become the major storage reservoirs. For more detailed pharmacokinetic data, the interested reader is referred to the excellent review by Benowitz and Meister (*Clin Pharmacokinet* 1978; 3:177).

This drug is a weak base with a pKa of 7.86, $t_{1/2}$ of 1.6 hr, and V_d of 1.3 L/kg; 60% to 80% is bound to plasma protein. Maximal excretion in an acid urine is only 10%. The major portion of this agent is metabolized by the liver microsomal system. Two major metabolites have been identified: monoethylglycinexylidide and glycinexylidide. Animal experiments indicate that both metabolites have antiarrhythmic and convulsant activities; the former has potency similar to this drug itself, while the latter is only 10% to 26% as potent. Both metabolites, after further biotransformation in the liver, are excreted in the urine.

Some adverse CNS effects frequently are observed during therapy. These commonly include drowsiness, dizziness, paresthesia, and euphoria. Typical symptoms with higher doses include confusion, agitation, dysarthria, vertigo, visual disturbances, tinnitus, and nausea. Sweating, muscle tremor, or fasciculations also may occur. Manifestations of severe toxicity include psychosis, seizures, respiratory depression, and coma. Seizures that persist after the administration of oxygen may be controlled by intravenous administration of 2.5-mg increments of diazepam. Caution must be exercised, since overdosage may occur if sufficient time is not allowed for the anticonvulsant action of the individual doses to become apparent. Diazepam has been recommended for prophylaxis of convulsions during local anesthetic therapy.

MEPIVACAINE HYDROCHLORIDE

2-Piperidinecarboxamide, *N*-(2,6-dimethylphenyl)-1-methyl-, monohydrochloride; Carbocaine; Polocaine

1-Methyl-2',6'-pipecoloxylidide monohydrochloride [1722-62-9] $C_{15}H_{22}N_2O \cdot HCl$ (282.81).

Preparation—Picolinic acid (2-pyridinecarboxylic acid) is condensed with 2,6-xylidine to 2',6'-picolinoxylidide, which is reacted with dimethyl sulfate in xylene solution. Reduction of the pyridine ring followed by treatment with HCl yields the product. *Acta Chem Scand* 1957; 11:1183.

Description—White, odorless, crystalline solid; melts with decomposition about 258°; pH (1 in 50 solution) about 4.5; pKa 7.73 ± 0.08.

Solubility—Freely soluble in water or methanol; very slightly soluble in chloroform; practically insoluble in ether.

Comments—An amide anesthetic employed for nerve block (1 or 2% soln), paracervical block in obstetrics (1% soln), caudal and epidural block (1, 1.5, or 2% soln), infiltration (1% soln), therapeutic block (1 or 2% soln), and dental procedures (1, 2, or 3% soln). It is not effective topically, except in large doses; therefore it should not be used for this purpose. It has a $t_{1/2}$ of 1.9 hr, a V_d of 1.2 L/kg, and a partition coefficient of 12.1. Approximately 60% to 80% of that in blood is bound to serum proteins.

When used in obstetrics, maternal plasma concentrations vary from 2.9 to 6.9 µg/mL, whereas the umbilical vein concentration varies from 1.9 to 4.9 µg/mL; thus, the fetus is exposed to only 60% to 70% of that in maternal plasma. It has an action similar to that of lidocaine hydrochloride; however, its onset is faster, and its duration of action is somewhat longer.

Anesthesia develops in 3 to 5 min and lasts 2 to 2 1/2 hr. It may be used for many purposes without epinephrine. Thus, it particularly is indicated in circumstances in which epinephrine is contraindicated. The systemic effects are similar to those produced by other local anesthetics. For additional information, see the introductory statement.

PRILOCAINE HYDROCHLORIDE

Propanamide, *N*-(2-methylphenyl)-2-(propylamino)-, monohydrochloride; Citanest

2-(Propylamino)-*o*-propionotoluidide monohydrochloride [1786-81-8] $C_{13}H_{20}N_2O \cdot HCl$ (256.77).

Preparation—*o*-Toluidine is condensed with 2-bromopropionyl bromide, and the resulting 2-bromo-*o*-propionotoluidide is condensed with propylamine to yield prilocaine (base). An acetone solution of the base treated with hydrogen chloride yields the official salt. Brit Pat 839,943.

Description—White, odorless, crystalline powder; initially an acid and then bitter taste, stable in light and air; melts about 167°; pKa 7.89.

Solubility—1 g in 3.5 mL water, 4.2 mL alcohol or 175 mL chloroform; practically insoluble in ether.

Comments—An amide-type local anesthetic chemically related to lidocaine and mepivacaine. For the most part, it is used for dental procedures and administered either by infiltration or nerve block. An initial dose of 40 to 80 mg (1–2 mL of a 4% solution) is usually sufficient, with a maximum dose of 600 mg (8 mg/kg). Onset of action after infiltration averages 1 or 2 min; duration of action is 60 min or longer. For major nerve blocks (epidural), the onset of analgesia is approximately 2 min longer than that for lidocaine; whereas the duration of action is 30 to 60 min longer. Approximately 55% is bound to plasma protein. After 600 mg of the drug, peak plasma levels are reached in 20 min, at which time plasma levels average 4 μg/mL; the same dose with epinephrine also peaks at 20 min, but the plasma level is only 2 μg/mL. Consequently, this drug generally is used without epinephrine. Hence, this local anesthetic is particularly useful for patients who cannot tolerate vasopressor agents, eg, patients with hypertension, diabetes, thyrotoxicosis, or other cardiovascular disorders.

Like other amide-type local anesthetics, prilocaine is not metabolized by plasma esterases; it is metabolized by both the liver and the kidney and excreted by the kidney. One of its metabolites is *o*-toluidine, a substance known to induce methemoglobinemia. Methemoglobin levels up to 15% and cyanosis have been reported following doses of 600 mg or more. Other clinical symptoms of methemoglobinemia, such as tachycardia, fatigue, headache, lightheadedness, and dizziness, may occur at higher doses. Except for methemoglobinemia, its side effects are similar to those observed with other local anesthetics. When methemoglobinemia occurs, it can be reversed by intravenous injection of methylene blue, 1 to 2 mg/kg of a 1% solution administered over a 5-min period. As with other local anesthetics, prilocaine is contraindicated in the presence of shock, severe cardiovascular disease, or heart block. For other adverse effects, see the introductory statement.

PROCAINE HYDROCHLORIDE

Benzoic acid, 4-amino-, 2-(dimethylamino)ethyl ester, monohydrochloride; Novocain

2-(Diethylamino)ethyl *p*-aminobenzoate monohydrochloride [51-05-8] $C_{13}H_{20}N_2O_2 \cdot$ HCl (272.77).

Preparation—2-(Diethylamino)ethanol is made by reacting ethylene chlorohydrin or bromohydrin with diethylamine. The diethylaminoethanol is then heated with *p*-nitrobenzoyl chloride, forming diethylaminoethyl *p*-nitrobenzoate. The NO$_2$ group is reduced with iron or tin and HCl. US Pat 812,554.

Description—Small, white, odorless crystals or a white crystalline powder; melts about 157°; pK$_a$ 8.7 (base).

Solubility—1 g in 1 mL of water or 15 mL of alcohol; slightly soluble in chloroform; practically insoluble in ether.

Comments—An ester-type local anesthetic. It is used for infiltration (0.25–0.5% soln), peripheral nerve block (0.5–2% soln), and spinal anesthesia (10% soln). It is ineffective when applied topically. The drug has a slower onset of action than lidocaine or prilocaine; its duration of action is short, about 1 hr.

It produces vasodilation, and thus vasoconstrictor drugs such as norepinephrine or levonordefrin may be required to retard absorption, prolong duration of action, and maintain homeostasis. Following absorption, it is hydrolyzed rapidly by esterases in both the plasma and liver (see the introductory statement). Since spinal fluid contains little or no esterase, when given by this route of administration it remains active until it is absorbed into the general circulation.

The products of metabolic degradation include *para*-aminobenzoic acid and diethylaminoethanol; the former inhibits the action of sulfonamides. Therefore, it and other ester-type local anesthetics should not be used in any condition in which therapy with sulfonamide is being employed. This drug and its congeners also interfere with the laboratory determination of sulfonamide concentration in biological fluids. Local anesthetics other than derivatives of *para*-aminobenzoic acid should be used in all circumstances when sulfonamide therapy has been instituted. The IV use of procaine is contraindicated in patients receiving digitalis, anticholinesterase drugs, or succinyl choline. For adverse effects, see the introductory statement.

TETRACAINE—page 1485.

TETRACAINE HYDROCHLORIDE

Benzoic acid, 4-(butylamino)-, 2-(dimethylamino)ethyl ester, monohydrochloride; Amethocaine Hydrochloride; Pontocaine Hydrochloride

2-(Dimethylamino)ethyl *p*-(butylamino)benzoate monohydrochloride [136-47-0] $C_{15}H_{24}N_2O_2 \cdot$ HCl (300.83).

For the structure of the base see page 1485.

Preparation—By dissolving tetracaine (base) in a solvent such as benzene and passing hydrogen chloride into the solution, whereupon the salt precipitates. For the preparation of the base, see *Tetracaine.*

Description—Fine, white, crystalline, odorless powder; slightly bitter taste followed by a sense of numbness; solutions neutral to litmus; melts about 148°; two polymorphic modifications melt about 134° and 139°, respectively; mixtures of these may melt between 134° and 147°; pK$_a$ 8.39. Protect solutions from light.

Solubility—Very soluble in water; soluble in alcohol; insoluble in ether or benzene.

Comments—An ester-type local anesthetic used topically on the eye and in the nose or throat and by infiltration for subarachnoid block (spinal analgesia). When used in the eye, it does not dilate the pupil, paralyze accommodation, or increase intraocular pressure. It is particularly suitable for spinal anesthesia, especially for surgical procedures requiring 2 to 3 hr. Although it is an ester-type local anesthetic, it is only slowly hydrolyzed by plasma and liver esterases. It has a delayed onset of action, often as long as 15 min, but a long duration of action; spinal anesthesia may last as long as 3 hr. Since its *para*-aminobenzoic acid metabolite may antagonize the activity of aminosalicylic acid and sulfonamides, it should not be used in patients receiving these drugs. For information on cautions, contraindications, and adverse effects, see the introductory statement.

TOPICAL ANESTHETICS

The salts and base forms of the esters and amides included in this section are used to produce topical (surface) anesthesia. The salts do not penetrate intact skin, but both forms penetrate abraded or raw, granulated skin surfaces. The base forms relieve pruritus, burning, and surface pain on intact skin but penetrate only to a limited degree. Wounds, ulcers, and burns preferably are treated with preparations that are relatively insoluble in tissue fluids. Mucous membranes of the nose, mouth, pharynx, larynx, trachea, bronchi, and urethra are anesthetized readily by both salt and base forms. Consequently, these agents are used prior to inserting intratracheal catheters, pharyngeal and nasal airways, nasogastric and endoscopic tubes, urinary catheters, laryngoscopes, proctoscopes, sigmoidoscopes, and vaginal specula. Many of these agents also are used in the eye for such procedures as tonometry and gonioscopy, for removal of foreign bodies from the cornea, or for short operative procedures on the cornea or conjunctiva. For precautions, warnings, and adverse effects, see the introductory statement.

BENZOCAINE

Benzoic acid, 4-amino-, ethyl ester; Benzocaine; Anesthesin

Ethyl *p*-aminobenzoate [94-09-7] $C_9H_{11}NO_2$ (165.19).

Preparation—*p*-Nitrobenzoic acid, obtained by nitration of toluene and oxidation of the resulting *p*-nitrotoluene, is converted into the ethyl ester by heating with alcohol and sulfuric acid. The resulting ethyl *p*-nitrobenzoate is reduced with tin and hydrochloric acid.

Description—Small, white, odorless crystals or a white crystalline powder; melts within a 2° range between 88° and 92°; pK$_a$ 2.5.

Solubility—1 g in about 2500 mL water, 5 mL alcohol, 2 mL chloroform, 4 mL ether, or 30 to 50 mL expressed almond oil or olive oil; soluble in dilute mineral acids.

Comments—An insoluble local anesthetic. It usually is employed as an ointment to relieve pain associated with ulcers, wounds, and mucous surfaces. It also is used as a lubricant and anesthetic on intratracheal catheters, pharyngeal and nasal airways, nasogastric and endoscopic tubes, etc. It is included in proprietary creams, lozenges, ointments, powders, sprays, and suppositories to relieve pain of damaged skin surfaces and inflamed mucous membranes, particularly those in the anorectal area. It also is used as an otic preparation for the temporary relief of ear pain. Benzocaine commonly is combined with antitussives, such as dextromethorphan, in cold medications. It acts only as long as it is in contact with the skin or mucosal surface. Peak effect occurs within 1 min after application and lasts for 36 to 60 min. For adverse reactions, see the introductory statement in this chapter.

CHLOROBUTANOL—page 1059.

COCAINE

8-Azabicyclo[3.2.1]octane-2-carboxylic acid, [1R-(exo,exo)]-3-(benzoyloxy)-8-methyl-, methyl ester

Methyl 3β-hydroxy-1αH,5αH-tropane-2β-carboxylate benzoate (ester) [50-36-2] $C_{17}H_{21}NO_4$ (303.36); an alkaloid obtained from the leaves of *Erythroxylon coca* Lamarck and other species of *Erythroxylon* Linné (Fam *Erythroxylaceae*) or by synthesis from ecgonine or its derivatives.

History—Isolated by Gaedken in 1844 from Brazilian coca leaves, which for many years was the only source of cocaine. At present the alkaloid is obtained principally from Java coca leaves. Brazilian coca leaves contain from 0.5 to 1% methylbenzoylecgonine or cocaine, whereas the Java leaves contain very little cocaine as such. However, there are present in the latter such derivatives as benzoylecgonine, cinnamoylecgonine, methylecgonine, etc, to the extent of 1.5 to 2%, all of which are converted to cocaine in the manufacturing process.

Preparation—By moistening ground coca leaves with sodium carbonate solution, percolating with benzene or other solvents such as petroleum benzin, shaking the liquid with diluted sulfuric acid, and adding to the separated acid solution an excess of sodium carbonate. The precipitated alkaloids are removed with ether, and after drying with sodium carbonate, the solution is filtered and ether distilled off. The residue is dissolved in methyl alcohol and the solution heated with sulfuric acid or with alcoholic hydrogen chloride. This treatment splits off any acids from ecgonine and esterifies the carboxyl group. After dilution with water the organic acids that have been liberated are removed with chloroform. The aqueous solution is concentrated, neutralized and cooled with ice, whereupon methylecgonine sulfate crystallizes. This is benzoylated by heating with benzoyl chloride or benzoic anhydride to about 150°. On adding water and sodium hydroxide methylbenzoylecgonine or cocaine is precipitated. The cocaine is extracted with ether and the solution concentrated to crystallization. For the purification of cocaine recrystallization from a mixture of acetone and benzene generally is preferred.

Total synthesis of cocaine was achieved by Willstäter *et al, Ann* 1923; 434:111.

Description—Colorless to white crystals, or a white, crystalline powder; odorless; melts at about 97°; solution (in diluted HCl) levorotatory; saturated solution alkaline to litmus.

Solubility—1 g in about 600 mL water, 7 mL alcohol, 1 mL chloroform, 3.5 mL ether, about 12 mL olive oil, or 80 to 100 mL liquid petrolatum; very soluble in warm alcohol.

Comments—The first local anesthetic to be discovered. While it is considered too toxic for any anesthetic procedure requiring injection, it is still employed topically in a 1 or 2% solution for anesthesia of the ear, nose, throat, rectum, and vagina because of its intense vasoconstrictive action. When in solution as the hydrochloride salt it is used for local anesthesia of mucous membranes. For topical application (ear, nose, throat, or bronchoscopy) concentrations of 4 to 10% are employed. Besides its local anesthetic properties, cocaine enhances catecholamine systems by interfering with uptake of their transmitters into neuronal terminals. Peak effect is reached within 2 to 5 min and lasts from 1/2 to 2 hr. Toxic symptoms occur frequently because it is absorbed readily and dosage often is not monitored carefully. CNS effects include euphoria and cortical stimulation manifested by excitement and restlessness.

Stimulation of the lower motor centers causes hypertension, tachycardia, and tachypnea. Repeated use results in psychic dependence and tolerance, the euphoric effects of which are almost indistinguishable from those induced by amphetamines. Indeed, knowledgeable human subjects cannot distinguish between the subjective effects induced by the intravenous injection of 8 to 10 mg of the drug and those induced by 10 mg of dextroamphetamine. The drug is abused by intranasal, parenteral, or inhalation administration because of its CNS-stimulating effects. It is listed under Schedule II of the Controlled Substances Act. Severe toxic effects have been reported with doses as low as 20 mg, while the fatal dose is approximately 1.2 g. For adverse reactions, see the introductory statement.

DIBUCAINE

4-Quinolinecarboxamide, 2-butoxy-N-[2-(diethylamino)ethyl]-, Nupercainal

2-Butoxy-N-[2-(diethylamino)ethyl]cinchoninamide [85-79-0] $C_{20}H_{29}N_3O_2$ (343.47).

Preparation—May be synthesized by the following sequence of reactions: (1) Acetylation of isatin (obtained by oxidation of indigo) to N-acetylisatin, (2) rearrangement of 2-hydroxycinchoninic acid by treatment with alkali, (3) formation of 2-chlorocinchoninoyl chloride by reaction with phosphorous pentachloride; (4) conversion to 2-chloro-N-[2-(diethylamino)ethyl]cinchoninamide with *asym*-diethylethylenediamine, and (5) heating with sodium butoxide. US Pat 1,825,623.

Description—White to off-white powder; slightly characteristic odor; somewhat hygroscopic; darkens on exposure to light; melts about 63°.

Solubility—1 g is soluble in 4600 mL water, in less than 1 mL of alcohol or chloroform, or in 1.4 mL ether.

Comments—Topically, for the temporary relief of pain and itching associated with burns, sunburn, insect bites, or minor skin irritation. Ointment or suppositories are used topically for the relief of the pain and itching of hemorrhoids. Its toxicity caused it to be removed from the US market as an injectable local anesthetic.

DYCLONINE HYDROCHLORIDE

1-Propanone, 1-(4-butoxyphenyl)-3-(1-piperidinyl)-, Dyclone

4'-Butoxy-3-piperidinopropiophenone hydrochloride [536-43-6] $C_{18}H_{27}NO_2 \cdot HCl$ (325.88).

Preparation—p-Hydroxyacetophenone is reacted with butyl bromide in a basic environment to produce the butoxy compound, which is reacted with piperidine hydrochloride and formaldehyde in an organic solvent under acidic conditions. US Pat 2,771,391 and 2,868,689.

Description—White crystals or white, crystalline powder; may have a slight odor; melts about 175°; pH (1 in 100 solution) 4 to 7.

Solubility—1 g in 60 mL water, 24 mL alcohol, or 2.3 mL chloroform. Insoluble in ether or hexane.

Comments—To anesthetize accessible mucous membranes (eg, the mouth, pharynx, larynx, trachea, esophagus, and urethra) prior to various endoscopic procedures. The 0.5% solution also may be used to block the gag reflex and to relieve pain associated with oral or anogenital lesions. Dyclonine-containing lozenges are used to relieve minor sore throat or mouth discomfort. It is contraindicated in cystoscopic procedures following intravenous pyelography; the drug precipitates iodine and interferes with visualization. When instilled into the conjunctival sac, it induces anesthesia without miosis or mydriasis. It also has antimicrobial properties. The clinical significance of this property has not been determined. Because of irritating properties, dyclonine should not be injected. For adverse effects, see the introductory statement.

ETHYL CHLORIDE—see RPS-19, page 1141.

LIDOCAINE

Acetamide, 2-(diethylamino)-N-(2,6-dimethylphenyl)-, Xylocaine

2-(Diethylamino)-2',6'-acetoxylidide [137-58-6] $C_{14}H_{22}N_2O$ (234.34).

Preparation—By chloroacetylation of 2,6-xylidine and condensation of the resulting chloroacetoxylidide and diethylamine.

Description—White or slightly yellow, crystalline powder; characteristic odor; stable in air; melts about 67°; pK_a 7.86.

Solubility—Very soluble in alcohol or chloroform; freely soluble in benzene or ether; practically insoluble in water; dissolves in oils.

Comments—A local anesthetic used as an ointment topically on mucous membranes on minor burns, abrasions, and anorectal lesions; also used as an anesthetic lubricant for endotracheal intubation. See *Lidocaine Hydrochloride.*

LIDOCAINE HYDROCHLORIDE—pages 1481 and 1482.

PRAMOXINE HYDROCHLORIDE

Morpholine, 4-[3-(4-butoxyphenoxy(propyl]-, hydrochloride; Tronothane; Proctofoam; Prax

CH₃CH₂CH₂CH₂O—⟨benzene⟩—OCH₂CH₂CH₂—N⟨O⟩ · HCl

4-[3-(*p*-Butoxyphenoxy)propyl]morpholine hydrochloride [637-58-1] $C_{17}H_{27}NO_3 \cdot HCl$ (329.87).

Preparation—An acqueous mixture of 4-(3-chloropropyl)morpholine and *p*-butoxyphenol is refluxed until condensation is complete. The reaction mixture is cooled, and the base is extracted with benzene. After evaporation of the benzene, the purified base is converted to the hydrochloride with HCl. *J Am Chem Soc* 1951; 73:2281.

Description—White to nearly white, crystalline powder; numbing taste; may have a light aromatic odor; pH (1 in 100 solution) about 4.5; melts about 182°.

Solubility—1 g in about 35 mL chloroform; freely soluble in alcohol and water; very slightly soluble in ether.

Comments—A surface anesthetic that has low indices of sensitization and toxicity and is unrelated structurally to either ester- or amide-type agents. Consequently, it may be useful in patients sensitive to these classes of drugs. Local anesthesia develops in 3 to 5 min; its potency is comparable to that of benzocaine and is not sufficient to abolish the gag reflex. It is applied locally in a 1% concentration for relief from discomfort and pain in hemorrhoids and rectal surgery, episiotomies, anogenital pruritus, itching dermatoses, and minor burns. It is too irritating to be used in the eye. For adverse effects, see the introductory statement.

PROPARACAINE HYDROCHLORIDE

Benzoic acid, 3-amino-4-propoxy-, 2-(diethylamino)ethyl ester, monohydrochloride; Alcaine; Ak-Taine; Ophthaine; Ophthetic

CH₃CH₂CH₂O—⟨benzene, NH₂⟩—COOCH₂CH₂N(C₂H₅)₂ · HCl

2-(Diethylamino)ethyl 3-amino-4-propoxybenzoate monohydrochloride [5875-06-9] $C_{16}H_{26}N_2O_3 \cdot HCl$ (330.85).

Preparation—*p*-Hydroxybenzoic acid is reacted with *n*-propyl chloride in alkaline solution and the resulting *p*-propoxybenzoic acid is nitrated to the 3-nitro compound. Treatment with thionyl chloride yields the acid chloride, which is coupled with 2-(diethylamino)ethanol. The resulting nitro ester is reduced to the base, which reacts with an equimolar quantity of HCl to form the hydrochloride. *J Am Chem Soc* 1952; 74:592.

Description—White to off-white, or faintly buff-colored, crystalline powder; odorless; on heating or exposure to air the compound tends to discolor; solutions exposed to air slowly discolor and finally become dark, with some loss of potency; crystals melt within 2° range between 178 and 185°; pK$_a$ 3.2.

Solubility—1 g in about 30 mL water or 30 mL warm alcohol or methanol; insoluble in ether or benzene. Solutions are neutral to litmus.

Comments—An effective ester-type surface anesthetic with a potency about equal to that of tetracaine. It is a useful anesthetic in ophthalmology and induces little or no initial irritation. Its onset of action is rapid; surface anesthesia of sufficient intensity to permit tonometry can generally be obtained within about 20 sec after the instillation of 1 or 2 drops of a 0.5% solution. The duration of such anesthesia is about 15 min. It is useful for most ocular procedures that require topical anesthesia such as cataract extraction, tonometry, removal of foreign bodies and sutures, gonioscopy, conjunctival scraping for diagnosis, and short operative procedures involving the cornea and conjunctiva. Although it is too toxic for use as an injection anesthetic, its ophthalmic use has been relatively free from side effects or untoward reactions. For adverse effects, see the introductory statement.

TETRACAINE

Benzoic acid, 4-(butylamino)-, 2-(dimethylamino)ethyl ester; Pontocaine

CH₃(CH₂)₃NH—⟨benzene⟩—COOCH₂CH₂N(CH₃)₂

2-(Dimethylamino)ethyl *p*-(butylamino)benzoate [194-24-6] $C_{15}H_{24}N_2O_2$ (264.37).

Preparation—Ethyl *p*-aminobenzoate is butylated by refluxing with *n*-butyl bromide and ethanol in the presence of sodium carbonate. The resulting ethyl *p*-butylaminobenzoate is transesterified by heating with 2-(dimethylamino)ethanol in the presence of sodium ethoxide such that the liberated ethanol is distilled continously from the reaction mixture. US Pat 1,889,645.

Description—White, or light yellow, waxy solid; melts about 43°.

Solubility—1 g in 1000 mL water, 5 mL alcohol, 2 mL chloroform, or 2 mL ether.

Comments—See *Tetracaine Hydrochloride,* page 1483.

ACKNOWLEDGMENTS—H Steve White, PhD is acknowledged for his efforts in previous editions of this work.

CHAPTER 80

Antianxiety Agents and Hypnotic Drugs

Laura A Mandos, BS, PharmD

Antianxiety agents that were defined in the past as primarily sedatives are the most commonly used psychotropic medications.[1] The term *sedative* refers to a quieting effect accompanied by relaxation and rest but not necessarily sleep.[2] The term *hypnotic* refers to the production of sleep.[2] Hypnotic drugs are used to produce drowsiness and help the onset and maintenance of sleep. Since most of the current drugs have both sedative and hypnotic actions, the distinction is artificial. A small dose of a drug may act as a sedative, whereas a large dose of the same drug may act as a hypnotic. In this respect, the benzodiazepines have several clear advantages to the older classes of sedative-hypnotic drugs such as the barbiturates: a greater dose margin between anxiolysis and sedation, less abuse potential, a wider therapeutic index, and less tendency to produce tolerance and dependence.[3] Other antianxiety agents can also have an anxiolytic effect without the sedative actions associated with the benzodiazepines. Examples of the nonsedating antianxiety agents include the azapirone buspirone, the selective serotonin reuptake inhibitor antidepressant paroxetine, and the selective serotonin/norepinephrine reuptake inhibitor antidepressant venlafaxine.[4–6] Tricyclic antidepressants that have both serotonergic and noradrenergic effects have also been studied in the treatment of generalized anxiety disorder.[7] Imipramine has been found to be at least as effective as benzodiazepines in the treatment of generalized anxiety disorder.[7] The adverse effect profile of imipramine makes the drug less tolerable than the newer antidepressants. A more in-depth discussion of imipramine, paroxetine, and venlafaxine will be covered in a different chapter. Agents used as sedatives and hypnotics include a large number of compounds of diverse chemical structure and pharmacological properties, which, with the exception of the benzodiazepines (eg, diazepam), buspirone, and the aforementioned antidepressants, have in common the ability to induce a nonselective, reversible depression of the central nervous system (CNS). Thus, inorganic salts (bromide), chloral derivatives (chloral hydrate), acetylenic alcohols (ethchlorvynol), cyclic ethers (paraldehyde), carbamic acid esters of glycols (meprobamate), diureides (barbiturates), piperidinedione derivatives (glutethimide), and some miscellaneous aromatic tertiary alkylamines such as antihistaminics (diphenhydramine) and parasympatholytics (scopolamine) all exhibit pronounced sedative and hypnotic effects. The antihistamines (diphenhydramine) and parasympatholytics (scopolamine) that exhibit sedative and hypnotic effects will be discussed elsewhere.

For convenience, the antianxiety agents will be divided into two categories: benzodiazepines and nonbenzodiazepine anxiolytics. The hypnotic agents will also be divided into two categories: the barbiturates and nonbarbiturate hypnotics. The hypnotic benzodiazepines will be included in this section.

In addition to their use as anxiolytics and hypnotics, the medications discussed in this chapter are also administered as muscle relaxants, preanesthetic medications, anticonvulsants, and therapeutic aids in psychiatry.

As *antianxiety agents,* they are used in the management of anxiety disorders such a generalized anxiety disorder and panic attacks. Anxiety may manifest as a transient situational response to stress, a secondary reaction to a medical condition, or as a primary anxiety disorder. Generalized anxiety disorder (GAD) is a prevalent condition that frequently presents in primary care settings as fluctuating levels of worry associated with insomnia and symptoms of being easily fatigued, feeling irritable or on edge, poor concentration, and skeletal muscle tension. In the general population, GAD is reported to have a lifetime prevalence of 4% to 6%.[8] To meet the DSMIV-TR GAD criteria, patients suffering from generalized anxiety must have been ill on more days than not for a minimum of 6 months. Those who suffer from briefer episodes of generalized anxiety are placed in the residual diagnostic category of anxiety disorder NOS (not otherwise specified).[9] A panic attack is a discrete period of intense fear or discomfort in the absence of real danger that is accompanied by at least four of 13 somatic or cognitive symptoms. Symptoms include palpitations, sweating, trembling or shaking, the sensation of smothering or shortness of breath, feeling of choking, chest pain or discomfort, nausea or abdominal distress, dizziness or lightheadedness, derealization or depersonalization, fear of losing control or "going crazy", fear of dying, paresthesias, and chills or hot flushes.[9] The attack has a sudden onset and builds to a peak rapidly often with a feeling of impending doom. Panic attacks can be unexpected or situationally cued. Regardless of presentation, generalized anxiety disorder and panic attacks can be extremely debilitating and disabling.

Insomnia is a ubiquitous disorder of insufficient sleep or unsatisfying sleep. Insomnia may present as difficulty falling asleep, difficulty staying asleep, or feeling nonrefreshed from sleep. Insomnia can be a primary disorder, a comorbid disorder with a psychiatric, medical or other sleep condition, or an adverse effect of a medication.[10] Insomnia may also be classified by duration: transient meaning two to three nights, short-term meaning less than 3 weeks, or long-term meaning greater than 3 weeks of difficulty sleeping.[11] It should be remembered that not all patients with insomnia require hypnotic drug therapy. Assessment of insomnia should begin with a history obtained from the patient and bed partner and continue with a physical examination. Questioning should be directed at determining predisposing factors, precipitating events, lifestyle, and use of caffeine, alcohol, and drugs (prescription, nonprescription, and illicit). Many patients will respond to nonpharmacologic therapy. Common recommendations include: regular daytime exercise; avoiding large meals at night, avoiding caffeine, tobacco, and alcohol; reducing evening fluid intake; limiting the use of the bedroom to sleep and sex; maintaining a consistent wake-up time; avoiding or limiting daytime napping; and avoiding bright lights, noise, and temperature extremes.[11] Nonspecific hypnotic therapy should be employed only when specific causes of the insomnia *cannot* be identified and eliminated.

To induce sleep, hypnotic agents are selected on the basis of the characteristics of the insomnia. Some patients have difficulty only in falling asleep and, once asleep, need no drug assistance; a rapidly acting hypnotic drug with a short duration of action will suffice for these patients. Other patients fall asleep readily, but experience one or more periods of wakefulness during the night; a hypnotic drug with a longer duration of action usually is indicated in such cases. Still other patients have trouble falling and staying asleep; a rapidly acting hypnotic drug that exerts an effect throughout part or most of the night is required for such patients. In all cases, however, consideration should be given to what the patient does on the day following a night of drug-induced sleep. Persons who must be alert the following day usually will object to drugs that leave residual sedation, whereas hospitalized patients or individuals with no place to go and nothing to do actually may benefit from the sedative aftereffects the next day.

A number of the sedative-hypnotic drugs have *anticonvulsant* properties. Several benzodiazepines have excellent anticonvulsant actions, and some are used to treat epilepsy. Clonazepam is used alone or as an adjunct in the management of absence (petit mal), petit mal variant, and especially akinetic and myoclonic seizures. Diazepam is used as adjunctive therapy in status epilepticus and severe recurrent seizures as well as treatment of acute seizures resulting from drug overdoses or exposure to toxins.

All barbiturates exhibit anticonvulsant activity, but only phenobarbital, mephobarbital, and metharbital are sufficiently selective to be clinically useful *antiepileptics*. Phenobarbital is useful in the management of generalized tonic-clonic seizures and as adjunctive therapy in complex partial (temporal lobe) seizures.

Sedative and hypnotic agents frequently are used as *preanesthetic medication* and as *adjunctive therapy* in psychiatry. Benzodiazepines and barbiturates are used commonly to allay anxiety and apprehension prior to surgery or other medical and dental procedures. In psychiatry, barbiturates with a short half-life have been used in *narcoanalysis* and *narcotherapy*. Sedative and hypnotic drugs also are employed in the treatment of dependence on CNS depressants. Chlordiazepoxide, diazepam, lorazepam, and oxazepam have all been used to manage symptoms associated with acute alcohol withdrawal.[12]

A number of the sedative-hypnotic drugs cross the placental barrier. Consequently, their chronic use during pregnancy may cause withdrawal effects in the newborn infant. Moreover, many of these substances are excreted in breast milk. Their chronic use during breastfeeding may cause sedation in the nursing infant.

Drowsiness is a side effect common to sedative-hypnotic agents. Patients taking such substances should be cautioned about operating hazardous machinery or operating a motor vehicle while taking such medication. Concurrent use of sedative-hypnotic drugs with alcohol, other CNS depressants, monoamine oxidase (MAO) inhibitors, or tricyclic antidepressants should be avoided. More-detailed information with respect to adverse effects and drug interactions is provided in the introductory statement to each section and in the individual monographs.

Prolonged overdosage with most of these drugs can result in habituation and dependence liability. However, the *dependence risk* varies markedly among the various agents. For example, the dependence risk with benzodiazepines is very low and has been estimated to be as few as one case per 5 million patient-months *at risk* for all recorded cases and one case per 50 million months in therapeutic use. Even though it is likely that in the past problems with benzodiazepines have been underesti-

mated, there is no question that these agents are considerably safer than most other sedative and hypnotic drugs, such as barbiturates. Accordingly, alprazolam, lorazepam, clonazepam, and other benzodiazepines are listed in *Schedule IV* under the *Controlled Substances Act*.

On the other hand, the dependence risk with amobarbital, pentobarbital, and related substances is very high, with severe abuse potential. Consequently, these agents are listed in *Schedule II* under the *Controlled Substances Act*.

Finally, the marketing of buspirone and the antidepressants paroxetine and venlafaxine as anxiolytic agents provide another therapeutic option for treatment of anxiety in patients with a high risk of dependence. Buspirone, paroxetine, and venlafaxine lack significant abuse potential.

BENZODIAZEPINES

Despite the fact that modern guidelines for treating anxiety disorders has evolved from recommending the benzodiazepines to recommending serotonergic agents as first-line therapy, diazepam, lorazepam, alprazolam, and clonazepam remain in the top 200 most frequently prescribed medications in the US.[13,14] In 2002, alprazolam was the only benzodiazepine in the top 20 most frequently prescribed generic drugs.[14] These findings demonstrate the great popularity enjoyed by the benzodiazepines despite public perception that benzodiazepine use has diminished over the last decade.

The benzodiazepines are not general depressants of the CNS like the barbiturates, ethanol, and various other sedative-hypnotic agents and general anesthetics. There are marked differences among the various agents in selectivity, pharmacological profile, clinical usefulness, and pharmacokinetic properties (Table 80-1). Moreover, they do not induce a true "anesthetic effect," since awareness is still present and total muscular relaxation is not obtained even after large doses. Anterograde amnesia may take place, and this creates the illusion that anesthesia has occurred. True surgical anesthesia can be obtained only when benzodiazepines are combined with other drugs that depress the CNS.

Acting through its gamma-aminobutyric acid A (GABA$_A$) receptor, the amino acid neurotransmitter GABA is the major inhibitory neurotransmitter in the brain. GABA$_A$ receptors are ligand-gated channels, meaning the neurotransmitter-binding site and an effector ion channel is part of the same macromolecular complex. Benzodiazepines produce their effects by binding to a specific site on the GABA$_A$ receptor. The pharmacologic effects of benzodiazepines can be explained by an increase of GABA inhibitory impulses mediated via the benzodiazepine receptor. They do so by allosterically regulating the receptor (changing its conformation) so that it has a greater affinity for GABA.[15] The pharmacology of the GABA$_A$ receptor is complex; GABA$_A$ receptors are the primary site of action not only of the benzodiazepines but also of the barbiturates and some of the intoxicating effects of ethanol. Benzodiazepines and barbiturates act at separate binding sites on the receptor to potentiate the effects of GABA. In addition, each drug increases the affinity of the receptor for each other.[16] The cellular mechanisms, pharmacokinetics, basic pharmacology, and clinical pharmacology of the benzodiazepines have been reviewed by MacDonald and Olsen.[17]

The benzodiazepines are used in the symptomatic relief of anxiety and tension states resulting from a stressful environment or emotional factors. They also are useful in psychoneurotic states characterized by tension, anxiety, apprehension, fatigue, depression symptoms, or agitation, and the benzodiazepine alprazolam has been approved for treatment of panic attacks. Chlordiazepoxide, lorazepam, oxazepam, and diazepam also are useful in acute alcohol withdrawal to provide symptomatic relief from acute agitation, tremors, and impending delirium tremens and hallucinosis.

Table 80-1. Benzodiazepine Anxiolytics

AVAILABLE PREPARATIONS	ORAL DOSAGE EQUIVALENCY (MG)	TIME TO PEAK PLASMA LEVEL (H)	PROTEIN BINDING (%)	ELIMINATION HALF-LIFE (H) PARENT COMPARED	ACTIVE METABOLITE	METABOLIC PATHWAY
Alprazolam (Xanax and generics)	0.5	1–2	80	12–15	One	Oxidation
Chlordiazepoxide (Librium and generics)	10	1–4	96	5–30	Four	N-dealkylation Oxidation
Clonazepam (Klonopin and generics)	0.25	1–4	85	30–40	None	Nitroreduction
Clorazepate (Tranxene and generics)	7.5	1–2	97	Prodrug	Two	Oxidation
Diazepam (Valium and generics)	5	0.5–2	98	20–80	Two	Oxidation
Lorazepam (Ativan and generics)	1	2–4	85	10–20	None	Conjugation
Oxazepam (Serax and generics)	15	2–4	97	5–20	None	Conjugation

Data from Kirkwood CE, Melton ST. Anxiety Disorders. In: DiPiro JT, Talbert RL, Yee GC, et al., eds. *Pharmacotherapy: A Pathophysiologic Approach, Fifth Edition.* New York: McGraw Hill, 2002. and Arana GW and Rosenbaum JF. *Handbook of Psychiatric Drug Therapy,* 4th ed. Philadelphia: Lippincott Williams and Wilkins, 2000.

Clonazepam is useful alone or as an adjunct in the management of several types of epileptic seizures. Diazepam is used as an adjunct therapy to endoscopic procedures, in the management of acute skeletal muscle spasm, and, by parenteral injection, in status epilepticus, to control convulsions resulting from overdosage with local anesthetics and other severe recurrent convulsive seizures. The benzodiazepines also are useful adjunct therapy in the management of apprehension and anxiety that precedes or accompanies surgical procedures and disease states.

Benzodiazepines are similar in mechanism of action as well as side effect profile. They differ in terms of potency and pharmacokinetic parameters (see Table 80-1).[18,19] After oral administration, the time to peak plasma level varies from 1 to 4 hours, depending on the formulation given. Protein binding varies from 80% with alprazolam to 98% with diazepam. The extent to which benzodiazepines interact with other protein-bound drugs is not known; the absence of reports of such adverse interactions suggests that such competition is not of clinical significance.

The benzodiazepines are metabolized by hepatic microsomal enzymes to form demethylated, hydroxylated, and oxidized products that pharmacologically active. The active metabolites are then conjugated with glucuronic acid and the resulting glucuronides are inactive. The glucuronides are more water-soluble than the parent compound and are readily excreted in the urine. Clorazepate, chlordiazepoxide, diazepam, and flurazepam are transformed to active metabolites, primarily to *N*-demethylated products with a longer half-life than the parent drug. This metabolite may be particularly significant in the elderly, newborns, or those with severe liver disease. Lorazepam, oxazepam, and temazepam are conjugated with glucuronic acid to form inactive metabolites and are a safer choice of medication in the elderly or patient with impaired hepatic function.[19] Benzodiazepines cross the placental barrier and are excreted in human milk.

Patients on these drugs should be warned about potential effects induced by the concomitant use of alcohol or other CNS depressants such as other antianxiety and hypnotic drugs, tricyclic antidepressants, opiate analgesics, antipsychotics, and antihistamines, including nonprescription sleep aids and cold remedies. They also should be warned not to operate a motor vehicle or hazardous machinery while on these drugs.

Side effects most commonly reported after the use of benzodiazepines include drowsiness, fatigue, confusion, dizziness, weakness, ataxia, syncope, venous thrombosis, and phlebitis at the site of the injection. Other, less frequent side effects include anterograde amnesia, blurred vision, diplopia, and nystagmus;

urticaria and rash; hiccups; changes in salivation; constipation; changes in appetite; bizarre behavior; antisocial acts; neutropenia; and jaundice. Paradoxical reactions such as acute hyperexcited states, anxiety, hallucinations, increased muscle spasticity, insomnia, rage, and sleep disturbances also have been reported; should these occur the drug should be discontinued. Since significant amounts of benzodiazepines are found in maternal and cord blood, these agents are not recommended for obstetrical use. The safe use of benzodiazepines in children under 12 years has not been established.

Physical and *psychological dependence* may occur, especially following prolonged use, although dependence also can occur with short-term, high-dose treatment. Symptoms of benzodiazepine dependence can resemble those associated with barbiturate or alcohol dependence and include slurred speech, ataxia, and drowsiness. Abrupt discontinuation of long-term benzodiazepine treatment can result in severe withdrawal symptoms as with other CNS depressants. To prevent such consequences, these drugs should be withdrawn gradually. Individuals known to be addictive-prone or those whose history suggests they modify drug dosage on their own initiative should not be given the drug. Withdrawal symptoms resemble those resulting from barbiturate withdrawal. The benzodiazepines are listed in *Schedule IV* under the *Controlled Substances Act.*

ALPRAZOLAM

4*H*-[1,2,4]Triazolo[4,3-*a*][1,4]benzodiazepine, 8-chloro-1-methyl-6-phenyl-, Xanax

[28981-97-7] $C_{17}H_{13}ClN_4$ (308.77).

Preparation—See *J Med Chem* 1977; 20:1694.
Description—White crystals; melts about 228°.
Solubility—Practically insoluble in water; soluble in methanol or ethanol.
Comments—For the management of anxiety disorders or the short-term relief of the symptoms of anxiety. It also is indicated for the adjunctive treatment of anxiety associated with mental depression. Alprazolam also has been found to be effective in the short-term (4- to 10-week) treatment of panic disorder with or without agoraphobia. Although not evaluated in well-controlled studies, the drug has been used effectively for 8 months or longer. In many patients, discontinuation of alprazolam results in a relapse of panic attacks and anxiety. After oral

administration peak plasma levels are reached in 1 to 2 hr, and half-life is 12 to 15 hr. Thus, it has a short to medium half-life compared with other benzodiazepines. Accumulation is minimal during multiple dosage, and steady-state plasma concentration usually is attained within 2 to 3 days. Elimination is rapid following discontinuation of therapy. Therefore, chronic therapy should not be terminated abruptly. Medical problems and adverse effects are similar to those for other benzodiazepines. See the introductory statement.

CHLORDIAZEPOXIDE

3*H*-1,4-Benzodiazepin-2-amine, 7-chloro-*N*-methyl-5-phenyl-, 4-oxide; Libritabs; Menrium

7-Chloro-2-(methylamino)-5-phenyl-3*H*-1,4-benzodiazepine 4-oxide [58-25-3] $C_{16}H_{14}ClN_3O$ (299.76).

Preparation—For the preparation of chlordiazepoxide, see *Chlordiazepoxide Hydrochloride,* below.

Description—Yellow, practically odorless, crystalline powder; sensitive to sunlight; melts about 242°; pK_a 4.6.

Solubility—1 g in >10,000 mL water, 50 mL alcohol, 6250 mL chloroform, or 130 mL ether.

Comments—See *Chlordiazepoxide Hydrochloride.*

CHLORDIAZEPOXIDE HYDROCHLORIDE

3*H*-1,4-Benzodiazepin-2-amine, 7-chloro-*N*-methyl-5-phenyl-, 4-oxide, monohydrochloride; Librium

[438-41-5] $C_{16}H_{14}ClN_3O \cdot HCl$ (336.22).

For the structure of the base, see above.

Preparation—By condensation cyclization of 2-amino-5-chlorobenzophenone oxime with chloroacetyl chloride to form 6-chloro-2-chloromethyl-4-phenylquinazoline 3-oxide, which subsequently is reacted with methylamine in methanol solution. US Pat 2,893,992.

Description—White or nearly white, crystalline powder; odorless; sensitive to sunlight; melts about 215° with decomposition.

Solubility—1 g in 10 mL water or 40 mL alcohol.

Comments—Indicated for the relief of anxiety and tension, withdrawal symptoms of acute alcoholism, preoperative apprehension and anxiety, and adjunct therapy in various disease states in which anxiety and tension are prominent features. Its efficacy for long-term use (ie, for longer than 4 months) has not been established; therefore, the need for continued therapy with the drug should be reevaluated periodically. It has a pK_a of 4.6 and a half-life of 8 to 20 hr. During chronic administration, accumulation occurs, not only of the parent substance but also of three active metabolites (desmethylchlordiazepoxide, demoxepam, and desoxydemoxepam). Demoxepam has a half-life of 37 (range, 28–63) hr and desoxydemoxepam of 44 (range, 39–61) hr. These metabolites probably contribute to the overall activity of this drug, since they are pharmacologically active in animals. Steady-state plasma levels of chlordiazepoxide, desmethylchlordiazepoxide, and demoxepam average 0.75, 0.54, and 0.36 µg/mL, respectively. It is excreted in the urine; 1–2% is excreted unchanged, and 3–6% as a conjugate.

As with other benzodiazepines, this drug requires the same warnings and precautions regarding its use in patients with known hypersensitivity, elderly and excessively depressed individuals, pregnant and lactating mothers, patients with known renal and hepatic impairment, patients on other CNS-depressant drugs, and patients with a history of either drug addiction or indiscriminate alteration of drug dosage.

Chlordiazepoxide is also available commercially in anxiolytic products, combined with anticholinergic (clidinium) and anti depressant (amitriptyline) agents. The therapeutic value of these fixed combinations has not been established.

Adverse reactions include drowsiness, ataxia, confusion, skin eruptions, edema, menstrual irregularities, nausea and constipation, extrapyramidal symptoms, and decreased libido in some patients; blood dyscrasias (agranulocytosis), jaundice, and hepatic dysfunction have occasionally been reported. Paradoxical reactions of rage, excitement, stimulation, hostility, and depersonalization have sometimes followed administration to severely disturbed patients. Rashes, nausea, headache, and decreased tolerance to alcohol also have been reported. The chronic administration of large doses of chlordiazepoxide hydrochloride may result in the development of tolerance and physical dependence.

CLONAZEPAM—page 1503.

CLORAZEPATE DIPOTASSIUM

1*H*-1,4-Benzodiazepine-3-carboxylic acid, 7-chloro-2,3-dihydro-2-oxo-5-phenyl-, potassium salt, compound with potassium hydroxide (1:1); Tranxene

[57109-90-7] $C_{16}H_{11}ClK_2N_2O_4$ (408.92).

Preparation—2-Amino-5-chlorobenzonitrile is treated with phenylmagnesium bromide, and the resulting ketimine is condensed via deamination with diethyl aminomalonate. The diester is then saponified with KOH in aqueous methanol, and the resulting dipotassium dicarboxylate cyclizes via isomerization. US Pat 3,516,988.

Description—Fine, light-yellow, practically odorless, crystalline powder; slightly burning taste; sensitive to light, moisture, and excessive heat; aqueous solutions are unstable (clear, light-yellow, and alkaline to litmus).

Solubility—Very soluble in water; very slightly soluble in alcohol; insoluble in chloroform, ether, benzene, or acetone.

Comments—For the symptomatic relief of anxiety associated with neurosis, psychoneuroses with symptoms of anxiety, acute alcohol withdrawal, and other conditions in which anxiety is a prominent feature and as adjunctive therapy in the management of partial seizures. This substance is hydrolyzed in the stomach to desmethyldiazepam, a metabolic precursor of oxazepam and also a metabolite of both chlordiazepoxide and diazepam. The metabolite is absorbed rapidly (1–2 hr); the volume of distribution is 0.93 to 1.47 L/kg, and the half-life ranges from 50 to 100 hr. Desmethyldiazepam accumulates for about 7 days and then reaches a steady state. Consequently, clorazepate can be given once a day as well as in divided doses.

It requires the same warnings and precautions regarding use with other drugs, in hypersensitive individuals, during pregnancy and in young children, in elderly and excessively depressed patients, in patients with impaired renal or hepatic function, and in patients with a history of drug addiction as other benzodiazepines. Drowsiness is the most common adverse effect. Less-common untoward reactions include dizziness, various gastrointestinal (GI) complaints, nervousness, blurred vision, dry mouth, headache, and mental confusion. Other adverse reactions include insomnia, transient rashes, fatigue, ataxia, genitourinary complaints, irritability, diplopia, depression, and slurred speech. Hypotension, decreased hematocrit, and abnormal liver and kidney function also have been reported.

DIAZEPAM

2H-1,4-Benzodiazepin-2-one, 7-chloro-1,3-dihydro-1-methyl-5-phenyl, Valium; Zetran; Diazepam Solution

[439-14-5] $C_{16}H_{13}ClN_2O$ (284.74).

Preparation—2-(Methylamino)-5-chlorobenzophenone in ethereal solution is reacted with bromoacetyl bromide to form 2-(2-bromo-*N*-methylacetamido)-5-chlorobenzophenone. The latter is then reacted with ammonia in methanol solution, whereby the bromine is replaced by amino followed by cyclization through a dehydration involving the hydrogens of the amino group and the oxygen of the starting phenone. The crude diazepam may be purified by recrystallization from ether. US Pat 3,136,815.

Description—Off-white to yellow, practically odorless, crystalline powder; stable in the air; melts about 133°; pK_a 3.7, 3.2.

Solubility—1 g in 333 mL water, 16 mL alcohol, 2 mL chloroform, or 39 mL ether.

Comments—A benzodiazepine indicated for the symptomatic relief of tension and anxiety, acute alcohol withdrawal, and adjunctive therapy in skeletal muscle spasms and preferred by many clinicians for the management of status epilepticus. It is used preoperatively because of its ability to relieve anxiety, sedate, and cause light anesthesia and anterograde amnesia. It is absorbed well after single oral doses (pK$_a$ 3.3), leading to rapid onset of clinical effects. Initially these effects may be transient due to extensive distribution to body tissues.

After distribution is complete, elimination is slow, with a half-life of 20 to 50 hr. Effective plasma levels vary from 0.2 to 0.5 µg/mL. With chronic administration, the drug and its major active metabolite, desmethyldiazepam, accumulate and reach a steady state in about 7 days. Consequently, it may take this long to achieve maximal sedative and antianxiety effects, at which time the patient can usually be maintained by giving the drug once or twice a day. Patients on the drug should be cautioned not to drive an automobile or to operate dangerous machinery until a few days after the drug has been discontinued.

LORAZEPAM

2H-1,4-Benzodiazepin-2-one, 7-chloro-5-(2-chlorophenyl)-1,3-dihydro-3-hydroxy-; Ativan

[846-49-1] C$_{15}$H$_{10}$Cl$_2$N$_2$O$_2$ (321.16).

Preparation—Syntheses of a number of substituted 1,4-benzodiazepin-2-ones, including lorazepam, have been described by Bell et al (*J Med Chem* 1968; 11:457; see also *J Org Chem* 1962; 27:1691). It differs from oxazepam in having a 5-*o*-chlorophenyl substituent in place of the 5-phenyl.

Description—White to off-white powder; no characteristic odor; melts about 173° with decomposition; pK$_a$ 1.3, 11.5.

Solubility—Practically insoluble in water; slightly soluble in alcohol or chloroform.

Comments—A benzodiazepine used orally for anxiety and transient situational stress. Its effectiveness for long-term use (more than 4 months) has not been assessed. It is used parenterally for *preanesthetic* medication, producing sedation and decreased ability to recall events related to the surgery. It is absorbed rapidly after oral administration; peak plasma levels after a 2-mg dose are about 20 ng/mL, and maximal clinical effects occur within 2 hr after administration. Its mean plasma half-life is about 12 hr, whereas that of its conjugated metabolite, lorazepam glucuronide, is about 18 hr. Approximately 85% is bound to plasma proteins. There is no evidence of its accumulation on administration for up to 6 months.

Adverse reactions, if they occur, usually appear at the beginning of therapy and disappear on continued medication or on decreasing the dose. Sedation is the most frequent adverse reaction (15.9%) and may persist up to 6 to 8 hours following an injection. Other common side effects include dizziness (6.9%), weakness (4.2%), and unsteadiness (3.4%). Less-frequent adverse effects are disorientation, depression, nausea, headache, sleep disturbance, agitation, dermatological symptoms, eye function disturbance, GI symptoms, and autonomic manifestations. The incidence of sedation and unsteadiness usually increases with age.

It requires the same warnings and precautions regarding use with other drugs, in hypersensitive individuals, during pregnancy and in young children, in elderly and excessively depressed patients, in patients with impaired renal or hepatic function, and in patients with a history of drug addiction that other benzodiazepines require.

MIDAZOLAM HYDROCHLORIDE

4H-Imidazo[1,5-a][1,4]benzodiazepine, 8-chloro-6-(2-fluorophenyl)-1-methyl-, monohydrochloride; Versed

[59467-96-8]C$_{18}$H$_{13}$ClF$_3$N.HCl (362.23); [59467-70-8] (335.76) (base).

Preparation—One method starts with 2-amino-4-chloro-2'-fluorobenzophenone in eight steps. See *J Org Chem* 1978; 43:936 and 4480.

Description—Colorless crystals melting about 159°; pK$_a$ 6.2.

Solubility—Soluble in water.

Comments—An imidazobenzodiazepine, short-acting CNS depressant. The sedative potency of midazolam is likely two to four times that of diazepam. It is administered intramuscularly for preoperative sedation and perioperative amnesia. The oral syrup carries the same indications. Because of its relatively rapid onset and short duration, it is considered by some clinicians to be the best benzodiazepine for preoperative use with short surgical procedures. Midazolam also is administered by the intravenous route, often combined with a narcotic, for conscious sedation associated with minor surgical or dental procedures or for short diagnostic or endoscopic procedures. It has been used IV as part of balanced anesthesia (eg, nitrous oxide and oxygen). It also has been administered orally for preoperative sedation and short-term management of insomnia. Midazolam is absorbed rapidly from IM injection sites, and pharmacological effects are apparent within 5 to 15 min and maximal in 20 to 60 min. The duration of action of this drug is 1 to 6 hr. Following IV injection, onset of sedation and amnesic effect is usually within 1 to 5 min. After oral dosing, midazolam is absorbed rapidly from the GI tract and achieves maximum plasma concentration within 1 hr; however, up to 60% is altered with first-pass hepatic metabolism to 1-hydroxymethylmidazolam or 4-hydroxymidazolam. Approximately 95% of midazolam is bound to plasma proteins, and it is excreted principally as a conjugated metabolite in the urine.

Midazolam can cause serious respiratory depression or arrest, especially with high doses, when given IV for conscious sedation. Consequently, it should only be given IV in hospital or ambulatory-care facilities that are equipped to provide respiratory and cardiac monitoring and render resuscitative care if necessary. Patients with chronic obstructive pulmonary disease (COPD) are particularly sensitive to midazolam-induced respiratory depression. There also have been rare reports of hypotensive responses to this drug that required treatment, although changes in blood pressure and heart rate frequently occur after parenteral administration of midazolam. Adverse responses to this drug, which are similar to the side effects of other benzodiazepines, include excessive sedation, drowsiness, prolonged emergence from anesthesia, euphoria, dysphoria, confusion, agitation, sleep disturbance, weakness, lethargy, slurred speech, nausea and vomiting, blurred vision, and visual disturbances. Some local tenderness following parenteral administration of midazolam has been reported but appears to be less than with other benzodiazepines.

Similar cautions should be used for midazolam as used for other benzodiazepines. Midazolam is a potent drug, and dosing should be individualized for the patient. It should not be administered during pregnancy. Midazolam will potentiate the action of other CNS depressants.

OXAZEPAM

2H-1,4-Benzodiazepin-2-one, 7-chloro-1,3-dihydro-3-hydroxy-5-phenyl-, Serax

[604-75-1] C$_{15}$H$_{11}$ClN$_2$O$_2$ (286.72).

Preparation—2-Amino-5-chlorobenzophenone is acylated with chloroacetyl chloride, and the product is refluxed with sodium iodide to form the iodoacetamido compound (I). Reaction of I with hydroxylamine effects dehydration and dehydrohalogenation to form the benzodiazepine derivative (II). Treatment of II with acetic anhydride causes rearrangement to oxazepam, which is simultaneously esterified to acetate. Saponification liberates oxazepam.

Description—Creamy white to pale-yellow powder; practically odorless; bitter taste; stable in light and non-hygroscopic; melting point indefinite; pH (1 in 50 suspension) 4.8 to 7.0.

Solubility—1 g in >10,000 mL water, 220 mL alcohol, 270 mL chloroform, or 2200 mL ether.

Comments—A congener of chlordiazepoxide and diazepam; it is a mild sedative useful in the management and control of anxiety, tension, agitation, irritability, and related symptoms, particularly in elderly patients. Also, it is useful for the control of acute tremulousness, inebriation, or anxiety associated with alcohol withdrawal. Unlike diazepam, this drug is absorbed slowly after oral administration (1–4 hr) and has a simple, one-step elimination pathway without active intermediate metabolites. Its half-life is short (5–15 hr), there is little accumulation, and full therapeutic effect can be expected with the first few doses. However, several daily doses may be necessary to reach a clinical steady state. Excessive and prolonged use may result in the development of physical dependence on the drug. Withdrawal symptoms following abrupt discontinuance of oxazepam are similar to those seen with barbiturates.

As with other sedative agents, patients on this drug should be cautioned against driving automobiles or operating dangerous machinery. Other warnings, contraindications, and precautions are similar to those for other benzodiazepines. Untoward effects include transient mild drowsiness, dizziness, vertigo, headache, and, rarely, syncope. Mild paradoxical reactions such as excitement and excessive stimulation also have been recorded.

Other side effects that have been observed include rashes, nausea, lethargy, edema, slurred speech, tremor, and altered libido. More severe reactions include leukopenia and jaundice. Fortunately, the latter reactions only occasionally are observed. Patients on the drug should be observed carefully for the appearance of other untoward effects characteristic of benzodiazepine drugs.

Benzodiazepine Combinations

Some examples of benzodiazepine combinations (with milligrams/unit provided) are as follows:

Chlordiazepoxide with Amitryptyline Hydrochloride [Limbritol, Limbritol DS *(Roche)*]—5 or 10 mg with 12.5 or 25 mg, respectively.
Chlordiazepoxide Hydrochloride with Clidinium Bromide [CDP Plus *(Gold Line)*; Clindex *(Rugby)*; Clindibrax *(Pharmaceutical Basics)*; Clinoxide *(Geneva Generics, Halsey)*; Librax *(Roche)*; Lidox *(Major)*; Lidoxide *(Interstate)*]—5 mg with 2.5 mg, respectively.

NONBENZODIAZEPINE ANXIOLYTIC AGENTS

An anxiolytic drug that is structurally and pharmacologically distinct from the benzodiazepines and barbiturates is the arylpiperazine derivative, buspirone. This drug is distinguished from the other sedatives because it relieves anxiety without causing drowsiness or impairing psychomotor function and appears to lack abuse potential. Hydroxyzine is a piperazine derivative chemically unrelated to the benzodiazepines, barbiturates, or meprobamate. Hydroxyzine has demonstrated clinical efficacy in the management of neuroses and in emotional disturbances manifested by anxiety, tension, agitation, or apprehension.

BUSPIRONE HYDROCHLORIDE

Azaspiro[4,5]decane-7,9-dione, 8-[4-[4-(2-pyrimidinyl)-1-piperazinylbutyl-, monohydrochloride; BuSpar

[33386-08-2] $C_{21}H_{31}N_5O_2 \cdot HCl$ (421.97).

Preparation—Piperazine and 2-chloropyrimidine are reacted to form 2-(1-piperazinyl)pyrimidine (I). Treatment of I with γ-chlorobutyronitrile N-alkylates the free piperazinyl nitrogen atom to yield II. With spirocyclopentane-1, 3′-glutaric anhydride, the free base of buspirone is produced, which is then converted to the hydrochloride; *J Med Chem* 1969; 12:876, and *ibid,* 1972; 15:477.

Description—White, crystalline solid melting about 200°; pK_a 1.22 and 7.32.

Solubility—1 g in 1 mL water, 50 mL alcohol.
Comments—An antianxiety agent that is unrelated either chemically or pharmacologically to the benzodiazepines, barbiturates, or other sedative/anxiolytic drugs. It is used in the management of anxiety disorders, the short-term relief of the symptoms of anxiety, or phobic neurosis. Although its long-term effectiveness as an anxiolytic has not been proven, there are reports of use in patients for 6 to 12 months without apparent loss of clinical benefit. The antianxiety effects of buspirone in general have been found to be comparable to that of the benzodiazepines, with some exceptions, while causing fewer adverse CNS side effects, such as sedation, psychomotor impairment, or dependence. Buspirone has been used successfully as an anxiolytic in patients who experience disinhibition or aggressive behavior when taking benzodiazepines. The mechanism of its anxiolytic effect is not known, but appears to be different from that of the benzodiazepines and barbiturates and likely involves multiple transmitter systems, particularly those of a serotonergic nature. It is absorbed rapidly and undergoes extensive first-pass metabolism. However, buspirone tends to have a slow onset of antianxiety action, which can cause patients to be discouraged during initial therapy. Peak plasma levels of 1 to 6 mg/mL usually occur within 40 to 90 min; approximately 95% is bound to plasma protein; 29–63% is excreted in the urine, and 18–38% in the feces. Elimination half-life of the unchanged drug is about 2 to 3 hr.

Even though it appears that this drug has no abuse potential and does not induce either tolerance or psychological dependence, patients on the drug should be monitored closely. Although animal studies suggest that the drug does not cause fetal damage, use during pregnancy should be limited to those clearly in need of the medication. Since it is excreted in breast milk, administration to nursing women is not recommended. Safety and efficacy in children under 18 years has not been established.

Common adverse effects include dizziness, nausea, headache, nervousness, drowsiness, lightheadedness, excitement, and mood changes. Chest pain, tachycardia, syncopy, hypo- and hypertension, sore throat, blurred vision, rashes, leukopenia, and shortness of breath also have been observed. Patients should notify their physician if any abnormal chronic muscle movements occur. Although buspirone generally does not impair psychomotor function at usual therapeutic doses, there is enough individual variation that patients should be warned that their ability to perform mental or motor tasks may be impaired.

DOXEPIN HYDROCHLORIDE—page 1520. See *Psychopharmacologic Agents* chapter.

HYDROXYZINE HYDROCHLORIDE

Ethanol, 2-[2-[4-[(4-chlorophenyl)methyl]-1-piperazinyl]ethoxy]-, dihydrochloride; Atarax

[2192-20-3] $C_{21}H_{27}ClN_2O_2 \cdot 2HCl$ (447.83).
Preparation—By condensing *p*-chlorobenzhydryl chloride (I) with N-[2-(2-hydroxyethoxy)ethyl]piperazine (II). Conversion to the hydrochloride may be effected by dissolving the base in a double molar quantity of hydrochloric acid and evaporating the solution to dryness.

It may be synthesized by treating benzaldehyde with *p*-chlorophenylmagnesium bromide and reacting the resulting *p*-chlorobenzhydrol with a suitable halogenating agent. II may be synthesized by interaction of piperazine and ethylene oxide.

Description—White, odorless powder; melts with decomposition about 200°.

Solubility—1 g in 1 mL of water, 4.5 mL of alcohol, 13 mL of chloroform or >1000 mL of ether.

Comments—A piperazine derivative used for the management of neuroses and emotional disturbances characterized by anxiety, tension, agitation, apprehension, or confusion. This includes its use in anxiety and apprehension associated with organic diseases, alcoholism, allergic conditions, pre- and postoperative conditions, and cardiac conditions. Hydroxyzine also is used to control motion sickness, and nausea and vomiting of various causes. It is contraindicated in early pregnancy and in patients who have shown a previous hypersensitivity to it. Like most other sedatives it should be used with caution, with proper dose adjustment in patients on other CNS-depressant drugs. Therefore, when used as preanesthetic medication with other agents, such as meperidine and a barbiturate, the dosage should be adjusted on an individual basis. Because of its anticholinergic action, the effects of hydroxyzine may be additive with those of atropine and other belladonna alkaloids. Since the drug may cause drowsiness, the patient should be warned not to drive a car or operate hazardous machinery while on the drug.

Adverse reactions are relatively mild and include drowsiness and dryness of the mouth. Less frequent side effects are dizziness, ataxia, agitation, and anxiety. Involuntary motor activities, including rare instances of tremor and convulsions, have been reported. Because of marked local irritation and possible tissue necrosis, hydroxyzine should not be administered by subcutaneous, intra-arterial, or IV injection. Clinical studies substantiate the absence of toxic effects on the liver or blood. *The potentiating effect of this drug must be taken into consideration when it is used in conjunction with CNS-depressants such as narcotics and barbiturates.*

HYDROXYZINE PAMOATE

Ethanol, 2-[2-[4-[(4-chlorophenyl)phenylmethyl]-1-piperazinyl]ethoxy]-, compd with 4,4′-methylenebis[3-hydroxy-2-naphthalenecarboxylic acid] (1:1); Vistaril

[10246-75-0] $C_{21}H_{27}ClN_2O_2 \cdot C_{23}H_{16}O_6$ (763.29).

Preparation—Hydroxyzine, prepared as described under *Hydroxyzine Hydrochloride*, is reacted with an equimolar portion of 4,4′-methylenebis[3-hydroxy-2-naphthoic acid].

Description—Light-yellow, practically odorless, powder.

Solubility—1 g in >1000 mL water, 700 mL alcohol, >1000 mL chloroform, >1000 mL ether, or 10 mL dimethylformamide.

Comments—See *Hydroxyzine Hydrochloride.*

IMIPRAMINE HYDROCHLORIDE—see *Psychopharmacologic Agents* chapter.

MEPROBAMATE

1,3-Propanediol, 2-methyl-2-propyl-, dicarbamate

[57-53-4] $C_9H_{18}N_2O_4$ (218.25).

Preparation—2-Methyl-2-*n*-propyl-1,3-propanediol, in toluene solution, is condensed at about 0° with phosgene in the presence of dimethylaniline to yield the chloroformate diester, which is then subjected to ammonolysis to form the dicarbamate ester.

Description—White powder; characteristic odor and a bitter taste; melts within a range of 2° between 103° and 107°.

Solubility—Slightly soluble in water; freely soluble in alcohol or acetone; sparingly soluble in ether.

Comments—A propanediol derivative chemically related to mephenesin, indicated for the management of *anxiety disorders* or for the short-term relief of the *symptoms of anxiety*. Anxiety or tension associated with the stress of everyday life usually does not require treatment with an anxiolytic. It is contraindicated in patients with acute, intermittent porphyria and in patients allergic to meprobamate or related agents, such as carisoprodol, mebutamate, or carbromal. Much like the barbiturates, physical and psychological dependence is known to occur after chronic use of high doses. Sudden withdrawal of the drug after prolonged, excessive use should be avoided to minimize withdrawal effects. Withdrawal symptoms usually appear 12 to 48 hr after discontinuation of meprobamate and usually cease within the next 12 to 48 hr. The drug should not be prescribed for patients with a history of drug abuse or those known to increase the dosage of drugs on their own initiative. Patients should be warned not to attempt potentially hazardous tasks or take other CNS-depressant drugs while on this drug. The drug should be used with caution in elderly or debilitated patients, epileptic patients, patients with compromised hepatic or renal function, and patients with suicidal tendencies. It is capable of producing a variety of side effects and untoward reactions. Briefly, these include *CNS:* drowsiness, ataxia, dizziness, slurred speech, headache, vertigo, weakness, paresthesias, impaired visual accommodation, euphoria, overstimulation, and para-

doxical excitement; *GI:* nausea, vomiting, and diarrhea; *cardiovascular:* palpitation, arrhythmias, syncope, and hypotensive crises; *allergic or idiosyncratic:* a variety of reactions including various skin, blood, and hypersensitivity reactions (also, Stevens- Johnson syndrome and bullous dermatitis) have been observed: *hematological:* agranulocytosis, aplastic anemia, and rare cases of thrombocytopenic purpura have been reported. Exacerbation of porphyric symptoms also has been observed.

Plasma half-life ranges from 6 to 17 hr (average 10 hr). Therapeutic blood levels range from 0.5 to 2.0 mg%; levels of 3 to 10 mg% usually correlate with mild-to-moderate symptoms of overdosage, ie, stupor or slight coma; and levels of 10 to 20 mg%, with deeper coma requiring intensive therapy, with some fatalities occurring. At levels above 20 mg% more fatalities than survivors can be expected. It is evident, therefore, that the drug should be employed with the same discretion as other CNS-depressant agents and with due cognizance of the possibility of untoward effects.

PAROXETINE HYDROCHLORIDE—see *Psychopharmacologic Agents* chapter.
VENLAFAXINE HYDROCHLORIDE—see *Psychopharmacologic Agents* chapter.

BARBITURATES

The introduction of barbital in 1903 and phenobarbital in 1912 initiated the barbiturate era. For over half a century they reigned as the preeminent sedative-hypnotic agents. Although several so-called nonbarbiturates attempted to displace the barbiturates from time to time, it was not until chlordiazepoxide was marketed in 1961 that their position was challenged seriously. The benzodiazepine hypnotics and several of the non-benzodiazepine hypnotics (zolpidem, zaleplon) have replaced the use of barbiturates as hypnotics. Barbiturates are rapidly tolerated, have a high risk of abuse and dependence, and a narrow margin of safety, and significant drug interactions.[20] Because of the safety considerations, the barbiturates have few indications as hypnotics.

The development of clinical pharmacokinetic data on hypnotic drugs revealed that the traditional classification of barbiturates into long-, intermediate-, and short-acting compounds bears little relation to the rate of elimination of these agents in man. Moreover, these data indicate that onset (rate of absorption) and duration of action (rate of elimination) are essential factors to be considered in their use. In general, barbiturate salts are absorbed rapidly, in contrast to the free acids. Liver disease tends to decrease the elimination rate of these substances, whereas renal insufficiency may give rise to accumulation of polar metabolites. For these reasons and for ready reference, the elimination half-lives, apparent volumes of distribution, and clearance values of barbiturates are summarized in each monograph.

Although traditionally used as nonspecific CNS depressants for daytime sedation and short-term treatment of insomnia, the barbiturates generally have been replaced by the benzodiazepines for these purposes. However, they are still given for preoperative medication to allay anxiety and facilitate induction of anesthesia. The anticonvulsant barbiturates, such as phenobarbital, mephobarbital, and metharbital, are still useful alternatives for the long-term management of generalized tonic-clonic and cortical focal seizures and are given intravenously for the management of acute convulsive episodes, such as status epilepticus, eclampsia, meningitis, tetanus, and toxic reactions to strychnine or local anesthetics. The barbiturates also are administered rectally to infants and children when oral or parenteral therapy may be undesirable.

Elixirs of certain barbiturates are still available for use as somnifacients and sedatives for children, despite the availability of more effective agents. They also are used in the relief of colic, excitation, and restlessness due to illness. Sedative doses may be administered as frequently as 3 to 4 times a day in cases of pylorospasm, whooping cough, nausea, and vomiting of functional origin, etc.

Barbiturates are contraindicated in patients with a history of porphyria. They should be used with caution in patients with impaired hepatic or renal function and in debilitated patients with depressed respiration. They also are contraindicated in persons with known previous addiction to the sedative/hypnotic drugs. Moreover, they should not be used in women of child-bearing age, since their safe use in pregnancy has not been established. Patients on barbiturates should avoid alcoholic beverages as well as other CNS depressants and refrain from driving an automobile or operating hazardous machinery while receiving such drugs.

Drug interactions are relatively common in patients taking barbiturates in combination with other drugs. For this reason patients on these drugs should be monitored closely. The most common problems relate to the ability of barbiturates (especially phenobarbital) to induce the hepatic microsomal enzyme system and increase the rate of metabolism of coumarin anticoagulants, tricyclic antidepressants, oral contraceptives, corticosteroids, digitoxin, phenytoin, phenothiazines, doxycycline, and other agents. Accordingly, the effectiveness of these agents may be decreased when given to a patient already on a barbiturate, and contrariwise, patients on both a barbiturate and one of these agents may experience adverse effects if the barbiturate is discontinued during chronic therapy, ie, a patient on coumarin may hemorrhage if the barbiturate is stopped and the anticoagulant dosage is not readjusted.

Barbiturates (especially phenobarbital) may competitively inhibit the metabolism of some drugs, such as phenytoin. Barbiturates have been shown to decrease the GI absorption of dicumarol and griseofulvin. Some barbiturates potentiate the adverse effects of tricyclic antidepressants by competing for the same hydroxylating enzymes. MAO inhibitors, valproic acid, chloramphenicol, and acute alcoholic intoxication inhibit the metabolism of barbiturates. Chronic alcoholic intoxication, on the other hand, increases the metabolism of barbiturates. Concomitant use of ether or curare-like drugs may produce additive respiratory depression. It also has been suggested that sulfisoxazole competes with thiopental for plasma-protein binding sites and decreases the amount of the latter necessary for anesthesia. Finally, additive depressant effects may occur with concomitant use of barbiturates and other CNS-depressant drugs.

Adverse reactions to barbiturates include:

CNS: somnolence, agitation, confusion, hyperkinesia, ataxia, nightmares, lethargy, paradoxical excitement, nervousness, hallucinations, insomnia, anxiety, and dizziness.
Respiratory: apnea, hypoventilation, respiratory depression, bronchospasm, and circulatory collapse.
Cardiovascular: bradycardia, hypotension, and syncope.
Hypersensitivity: rashes, angioneurotic edema, fever, serum sickness, morbiliform rash, urticaria, exfoliative dermatitis, and Steven-Johnson syndrome.
Other: physical and psychological dependence, headache, blood dyscrasias, myalgia, neuralgia, and arthritic pain.

For these and other reasons mentioned in this section, their indiscriminate use should be avoided.

Accidental and suicidal deaths from acute barbiturate poisoning are encountered, but the incidence has decreased with their diminished use. Treatment varies with the degree of intoxication. In general, emergency measures in acute poisoning are directed toward maintenance of respiration and cardiac function, followed by gastric decontamination. The latter is accomplished by gastric lavage, administration of activated charcoal (20–25 g in a child, 50 g in an adult) by gastric lavage tube, and a saline cathartic to clear the gut. In severe intoxication, measures to enhance elimination of absorbed barbiturate may be necessary, such as diuresis, urine alkalinization, dialysis, and hemoperfusion. The prognosis in barbiturate poisoning, with adequate medical care, is very good; mortality is less than 1%.

Continual use of barbiturates can result in tolerance, which encourages an increase in dosages. Tolerance to the effects of barbiturates on mood, sedation, and hypnosis is greater than tolerance to respiratory depression; consequently, with tolerance comes a decrease in the therapeutic index.

Serious withdrawal symptoms, including convulsions and psychoses, may occur when a barbiturate is withheld from dependent patients. In some chronically intoxicated individuals, even though they have no previous history of epilepsy, major convulsive seizures follow the sudden withdrawal of barbiturate. It is advisable to reduce the dose of barbiturate gradually in both epileptic and nonepileptic patients when cessation of chronic barbiturate medication is contemplated. It also should be emphasized that barbiturate therapy is contraindicated in patients with a history of drug addiction.

AMOBARBITAL

2,4,6(1*H*,3*H*,5*H*)-Pyrimidinetrione, 5-ethyl-5-(3-methylbutyl)-, Amylobarbitone; Amytal

5-Ethyl-5-isopentylbarbituric acid [57-43-2] $C_{11}H_{18}N_2O_3$ (226.27).

Preparation—A typical method starts with monochloroacetic acid, which is treated with sodium cyanide to form cyanoacetic acid; the latter is reacted with hydrochloric acid in the presence of alcohol, yielding the diethyl ester of malonic acid. This ester, in absolute alcohol solution, is treated with the theoretical quantity of metallic sodium to replace one hydrogen of the CH_2 group, then a slight excess of the theoretical amount of an ethylating agent, such as ethyl bromide, is added. The second hydrogen is replaced similarly, using isopentyl bromide as the alkylating agent. The diethyl ester of ethyl isopentyl malonic acid thus obtained is heated in an alcoholic solution, in the presence of sodium, with urea. Sodium amobarbital is formed, from which amobarbital is liberated with HCl. The alkylation of the CH_2 group of the malonic ester, whether the alkyls are both the same as in barbital or different, as in amobarbital, may be done in two stages, introducing one alkyl group at a time.

Description—White, crystalline, odorless, bitter powder; pH (saturated solution) about 5.6; melts within a 3° range between 156° and 161°.

Solubility—1 g in about 1300 mL of water, 5 mL of alcohol, about 17 mL of chloroform, or 6 mL of ether; soluble in solutions of fixed alkali hydroxides and carbonates.

Comments—A *sedative* and *hypnotic*. It may be used in any condition that requires sedation, ranging from relief of anxiety and tension to hypnotic doses for preanesthetic medication. Because of tolerance, its use as a hypnotic is limited to 2 weeks. See the introductory statement on *Barbiturates*. It is a *Schedule II* drug under the *Controlled Substances Act*.

AMOBARBITAL SODIUM

2,4,6(1*H*,3*H*,5*H*)-Pyrimidinetrione, 5-ethyl-5-(3-methylbutyl)-, monosodium salt; Amylobarbitone Sodium; Amytal Sodium

Sodium 5-ethyl-5-isopentylbarbiturate [64-43-7] $C_{11}H_{17}N_2NaO_3$ (248.26).

Preparation—By reacting amobarbital with a solution containing a chemically equivalent quantity of sodium hydroxide or sodium carbonate, evaporating to dryness, and crystallizing the residue from a solution in a suitable solvent such as alcohol.

Description—White, friable, hygroscopic, odorless, granular powder with a bitter taste; pH (1 in 20 solution) 9.6 to 10.4.

Solubility—Very soluble in water; soluble in alcohol; practically insoluble in ether or chloroform.

Comments—A *hypnotic* and *sedative*. It is indicated for sedation and relief of anxiety, preanesthetic medication, and the control of acute convulsive disorders. The onset of action varies from 45 to 60 min, half-life is approximately 25 hr, and duration of action is 6 to 8 hr. See the introductory statement on *Barbiturates*. It is a *Schedule II* drug under the *Controlled Substances Act*.

BUTABARBITAL SODIUM

2,4,6(1H,3H,5H)-Pyrimidinetrione, 5-ethyl-5-(1-methylpropyl)-, monosodium salt; Butisol Sodium

Sodium 5-sec-butyl-5-ethylbarbiturate [143-81-7] $C_{10}H_{15}N_2NaO_3$ (234.23).

Preparation—By preparing butarbital using a method similar to that for *Amobarbital,* using ethyl bromide and *sec*-butyl bromide as the alkylating agents. Then treating an alcoholic solution of butabarbital with an equimolar quantity of NaOH and removing the solvent by evaporation.

Description—White, bitter powder; pH (1 in 10 solution) 9.5 to 10.2.

Solubility—1 g in 2 mL of water, 7 mL of alcohol, 7000 mL of chloroform, or >10,000 mL of ether.

Comments—A *sedative* and *hypnotic.* Used for short-term treatment of insomnia. Because of tolerance, barbiturates lose efficacy after 2 weeks of use. See the introductory statement on *Barbiturates.* It is a *Schedule III* drug under the *Controlled Substances Act.*

MEPHOBARBITAL

2,4,6(1H,3H,5H)-Pyrimidinetrione, 5-ethyl-1-methyl-5-phenyl-, Prominal; Phemitone; Mebaral

5-Ethyl-1-methyl-5-phenylbarbituric acid [115-38-8] $C_{13}H_{14}N_2O_3$ (246.27).

Preparation—The diethyl ester of ethylphenylmalonic acid is prepared by the general method described under *Amobarbital* and is then condensed with *N*-methylurea in the presence of sodium ethylate. The resulting sodium mephobarbital is treated with HCl, whereupon mephobarbital crystallizes.

The *N*-methylurea is prepared as follows. Methylamine is passed into a mixture of sulfuric acid and absolute alcohol until the mixture is alkaline. Potassium cyanate then is added, and the mixture is refluxed overnight, whereupon the monomethyl ammonium cyanate produced initially by metathesis rearranges (Wöhler) to *N*-methylurea.

Description—White, crystalline powder; odorless; bitter taste; saturated solution acid to litmus; melts about 178°; pK$_a$ 8.8.

Solubility—1 g in >1000 mL water, >1000 mL alcohol, 50 mL chloroform, or >1000 mL ether; soluble in solutions of fixed alkali hydroxides or carbonates.

Comments—A barbiturate with strong *sedative* and *anticonvulsant* actions but a relatively mild *hypnotic* action. Hence, it is used for relief of anxiety, tension, and apprehension and as an antiepileptic in the management of generalized tonic-clonic (grand mal) and absence (petit mal) seizures. See also the introductory statement on *Barbiturates.*

METHOHEXITAL SODIUM—page 1476.

PENTOBARBITAL

2,4,6(1H,3H,5H)-Pyrimidinetrione, 5-ethyl-5-(1-methylbutyl)-, Nembutal

5-Ethyl-5-(1-methylbutyl)barbituric acid [76-74-4] $C_{11}H_{18}N_2O_3$ (226.27).

Preparation—By the general method described under *Amobarbital,* using ethyl bromide and 1-methylbutyl bromide as alkylating agents.

Description—White to practically white, fine powder; practically odorless; melts about 130°.

Solubility—1 g in >2000 mL water, 4.5 mL alcohol, 4 mL chloroform, or 10 mL ether.

Comments—see *Pentobarbital Sodium.* It is a *Schedule II* drug under the *Controlled Substances Act.*

PENTOBARBITAL SODIUM

2,4,6(1H,3H,5H)-Pyrimidinetrione, 5-ethyl-5-(1-methylbutyl)-, monosodium salt; Pentobarbitone Sodium; Soluble Pentobarbital; Nembutal Sodium

Sodium 5-ethyl-5-(1-methylbutyl)barbiturate [57-33-0] $C_{11}H_{17}N_2$ NaO$_3$ (248.26).

Preparation—By the process given for *Amobarbital,* using 2-bromopentane instead of ethyl bromide to react with one of the hydrogens in the CH$_2$ of the malonyl group. It then is converted into the soluble sodium salt by the addition of the required amount of NaOH.

Description—White, odorless, crystalline granules or a white powder with a slightly bitter taste; pH (1 in 10 solution) 10.0 to 10.5 when used in parenterals; otherwise, 9.7 to 10.2; solutions decompose on standing, heat accelerating the decomposition; pK$_{a1}$ 8.17; pK$_{a2}$ 12.67.

Solubility—Very soluble in water; freely soluble in alcohol; practically insoluble in ether.

Comments—Used as a *sedative* or *hypnotic* for the short-term (up to 2 weeks) management of insomnia and as preanesthetic medication. It also is indicated, in anesthetic doses administered intravenously, for control of certain convulsive syndromes. This barbiturate is thought to reduce cerebral blood flow and thereby decrease edema and/or intracranial pressure. See also the introductory statement on *Barbiturates.* It is a *Schedule II* drug under the *Controlled Substances Act.*

PHENOBARBITAL

2,4,6(1H,3H,5H)-Pyrimidinetrione, 5-ethyl-5-phenyl-, Phenylethylmalonylurea; Phenobarbitone; Luminal

5-Ethyl-5-phenylbarbituric acid [50-06-6] $C_{12}H_{12}N_2O_3$ (232.24).

Preparation—Benzyl chloride is converted into phenylacetic ester (ethyl phenylacetate) by treating with sodium cyanide and then hydrolyzing with acid in the presence of alcohol. The ester is condensed in the presence of alcohol and metallic sodium with ethyl oxalate, forming diethyl sodium phenyloxaloacetate. HCl is added to liberate diethyl phenyloxaloacetate, which on being distilled at 180° splits off carbon monoxide and forms phenylmalonic ester [$C_6H_5CH(COOC_2H_5)_2$]. The hydrogen of the CH in the phenylmalonic ester is then ethylated, and the resulting ethylphenylmalonic ester condensed with urea as described under *Amobarbital.*

Description—White, odorless, glistening, small crystals or a white crystalline powder, which may exhibit polymorphism; stable in air; pH (saturated solution) about 5; melts about 176°; pK$_a$ 7.6.

Solubility—1 g in about 1000 mL water, 10 mL alcohol, about 40 mL chloroform, or 15 mL ether.

Comments—This classical barbiturate is a *sedative, hypnotic,* and *antiepileptic* drug. In appropriate doses it is used in neuroses and related tension states when mild, prolonged sedation is indicated, as in hypertension, coronary artery disease, functional GI disorders and preoperative apprehension. In addition, it has specific usefulness in the symptomatic therapy of *epilepsy.* It is especially useful in patients with generalized tonic-clonic seizures (grand mal) and complex partial (psychomotor) seizures. Effective doses usually produce a degree of drowsiness or sluggishness. Phenobarbital also has been found to be effective in the treatment and prevention of hyperbilirubinemia in neonates. Approximately 80% of an oral dose is absorbed, and peak plasma levels are reached in 16 to 18 hr. Because of its slow onset of action, phenobarbital generally is not used orally to treat insomnia, but is used to help withdraw people who are physically dependent on other CNS depressants. The apparent volume of distribution is 0.7 to 1 L/kg. Therapeutic plasma levels range from 10 to 30 μg/mL. About 45 to 50% of the drug is bound to plasma protein. Apparent plasma half-life varies from 50 to 120 hr in adults and 40 to 70 hr in children. Approximately 65% of the drug is metabolized (largely to the inactive *p*-hydroxyphenyl derivative), and 35% is excreted by the kidney unchanged. Plasma clearance is slow and approximates 0.004 L/kg/hr. With the exception of metharbital and mephobarbital, this is the only barbiturate effective in epilepsy. See the introductory statement on *Barbiturates*.

PHENOBARBITAL SODIUM

2,4,6(1*H*,3*H*,5*H*)-Pyrimidinetrione, 5-ethyl-5-phenyl-, monosodium salt; Sodium Phenobarbital; Soluble Phenobarbital; Phenobarbitone Sodium; Luminal Sodium

Sodium 5-ethyl-5-phenylbarbiturate [57-30-7] $C_{12}H_{11}N_2NaO_3$ (254.22).

Preparation—By dissolving phenobarbital in an alcohol solution of an equivalent quantity of NaOH and evaporating at low temperature.

Description—Flaky crystals or white, crystalline granules, or white powder; odorless; bitter taste; hygroscopic; solutions alkaline to phenolphthalein and decompose on standing; pH (1 in 10 solution) 9.2 to 10.2.

Solubility—Very soluble in water; soluble in alcohol; practically insoluble in ether or chloroform.

Comments—Because it is soluble in water, it may be administered parenterally. It is given by slow intravenous injection for control of acute convulsive syndromes. For additional information see *Phenobarbital* and the introductory statement on *Barbiturates*.

Note: Doses should be reduced significantly in elderly or debilitated patients. No barbiturate should be given parenterally without full knowledge of its particular characteristics, dosage, and recommended rate of administration. Because of potentially severe respiratory depression, phenobarbital sodium should not be administered at a rate that exceeds 60 mg/min.

SECOBARBITAL

2,4,6(1*H*,3*H*,5*H*)-Pyrimidinetrione, 5-(1-methylbutyl)-5-(2-propenyl)-, Seconal

5-Allyl-5-(1-methylbutyl)barbituric acid [76-73-3] $C_{12}H_{18}N_2O_3$ (238.29).

Preparation—By the general method described under *Amobarbital*, using allyl bromide and 1-methylbutyl bromide as alkylating agents at the 5-position.

Description—White, amorphous or crystalline, odorless powder; slightly bitter taste; pH (saturated solution) about 5.6; melts about 98°.

Solubility—Very slightly soluble in water; freely soluble in alcohol, ether, or solutions of alkali hydroxides; soluble in chloroform.

Comments—A *sedative* and *hypnotic*. See also *Secobarbital Sodium* and the introductory statement on *Barbiturates*. It is a *Schedule II* drug under the *Controlled Substances Act*.

SECOBARBITAL SODIUM

2,4,6(1*H*,3*H*,5*H*)-Pyrimidinetrione, 5-(1-methylbutyl)-5-(2-propenyl)-, monosodium salt; Quinalbarbitone Sodium; Seconal Sodium

Sodium 5-allyl-5-(1-methylbutyl)barbiturate [309-43-3] $C_{12}H_{17}N_2NaO_3$ (260.27).

Preparation—By treatment of secobarbital with a chemically equivalent portion of NaOH as described under *Phenobarbital Sodium*.

Description—White, odorless, hygroscopic powder; bitter taste; pH (1 in 20 solution) 9.7 to 10.5; solutions decompose on standing, heat accelerating the decomposition.

Solubility—Very soluble in water; soluble in alcohol; practically insoluble in ether.

Comments—A short-acting barbiturate widely used *sedative* and *hypnotic*. The drug also is used, in anesthetic doses intravenously, for the control of certain acute convulsive conditions, such as those associated with tetanus, status epilepticus, and toxic reactions to strychnine and local anesthetics. Within 2 hr after oral administration, 90% is absorbed from the GI tract. The effect after a hypnotic dose occurs in 15 to 30 min with oral or rectal administration and persists for 1 to 4 hr. The elimination half-life is about 30 hr. Secobarbital has been used rectally in children to induce anesthesia. See the introductory statement on *Barbiturates*. It is a *Schedule II* drug under the *Controlled Substances Act*.

THIOPENTAL SODIUM—page 1476.

Barbiturate Combinations

Some examples of barbiturate combinations (with milligrams/unit provided) are as follows:

Butalbital, Acetaminophen and Caffeine [Fioricet *(Sandoz)*]—50, 325, and 40 mg, respectively.
Butalbarbital, Aspirin and Caffeine [Fiorinal *(Sandoz)*]—50, 325, and 40 mg, respectively.

NONBARBITURATE HYPNOTICS

Benzodiazepine Hypnotics

Benzodiazepines markedly influence CNS activity of humans in both the awake and sleep state. In the waking human electroencephalogram (EEG), alpha activity is decreased, fast activity (primarily beta) is increased, and the energy content of the EEG is decreased.

With respect to sleep, the benzodiazepines decrease sleep latency and decrease the number of awakenings and the time spent in Stage 0 (wakefulness). They also increase the awakening threshold. The time spent in Stage 1 (descending drowsiness) is decreased by flurazepam, and lorazepam, but increased by chlordiazepoxide, diazepam, and oxazepam. The time spent in Stage 2 (major fraction of non–rapid eye movement (REM) sleep) is increased by all benzodiazepines. The time spent in Stages 3 and 4 (slow wave sleep) usually is decreased; however, a few agents may increase these stages. Because of suppression of Stage 4 sleep, diazepam has been used to prevent night terrors in adults. Please refer to Table 80-2 for a discussion of the pharmacokinetic parameters of the benzodiazepine hypnotics.[21, 22]

The benzodiazepines increase the latency to REM sleep, decrease REM sleep time, and increase the number of REM cycles. Total sleep time is increased by the benzodiazepines. The greatest increase is observed in subjects with the shortest baseline sleep time. In such individuals, total sleep time may increase threefold.

ESTAZOLAM

4*H*-[1,2,4]Triazolo [4,3-*a*][1,4]benzodiazepine, 8-chloro-6-phenyl-, ProSom

[29975-16-4] $C_{16}H_{11}ClN_4$ (294.74).

Table 80-2. Benzodiazepine Hypnotics

AVAILABLE PREPARATIONS	ORAL DOSAGE EQUIVALENCY (MG)	TIME TO PEAK PLASMA LEVEL (H)	PROTEIN BINDING (%)	ELIMINATION HALF-LIFE (H) PARENT COMPARED	ACTIVE METABOLITE	METABOLIC PATHWAY
Estazolam (ProSom and generics)	2	2	93	12–15	One	Oxidation
Flurazepam (Dalmane and generics)	30	1	97	8	Three	Oxidation N-dealkylation
Quazepam (Doral)	15	2	>95	39	Two	Oxidation N-dealkylation
Temazepam (Restoril and generics)	30	1.5	98	10–15	None	Glucuronidation
Triazolam (Halcion and generics)	0.25	1	90	2	One	Oxidation

Data from Curtis JL, Germaine DM. Sleep Disorders. In: DiPiro JT, Talbert RL, Yee GC, et al, eds. *Pharmacotherapy: A Pathophysiologic Approach*, 5th ed. New York: McGraw Hill, 2002., Arana GW and Rosenbaum JF. *Handbook of Psychiatric Drug Therapy, Fourth Edition*. Philadelphia: Lippincott Williams and Wilkins, 2000, and http://www.efactsweb.com. Accessed June 25, 2003.

Preparation—From 7-chloro-1,3-dihydro-5-phenyl-2*H*-benzo-[1,4]-diazepin-2-thione and formylhydrazine in boiling *n*-butyl alcohol; see *J Org Chem* 1964; 29:231, and *J Med Chem* 1971;14:1078.

Description—White crystals; melts at about 230°.

Comments—A triazolobenzodiazepine derivative that structurally resembles alprazolam and triazolam. Estazolam has an intermediate half-life: the peak plasma concentration is reached 1.5 to 2 hr after oral administration. It undergoes hepatic microsomal oxidation and has an elimination half-life of 2 to 15 hr. Some clinicians believe that triazolobenzodiazepines, such as estazolam, cause more serious toxicity and withdrawal reactions than other benzodiazepines. The adverse effects of estazolam are like those of other benzodiazepines and include sedation, drowsiness, dizziness, incoordination, and possible recall impairment. Sudden discontinuation can cause significant transient rebound insomnia. Because use of benzodiazepines during pregnancy can result in fetal damage, estazolam should not be administered to pregnant women. Since the elimination of this drug may be slowed in geriatric patients, the doses of estazolam should be individualized carefully for this age group.

FLURAZEPAM HYDROCHLORIDE

2*H*-1,4-Benzodiazepin-2-one, 7-chloro-1-[2-(diethylamino)ethyl]-5-(2-fluorophenyl)-1,3-dihydro-, dihydrochloride; Dalmane

[1172-18-5] $C_{21}H_{23}ClFN_3O \cdot 2HCl$ (460.81).

Preparation—Aqueous CrO_3 is added dropwise to an acetic acid solution of 2-aminomethyl-5-chloro-1-2-(diethylamino)ethyl-3- (*o*-fluorophenyl)indole dihydrochloride, and the mixture is stirred overnight. US Pat 3,567,710.

Description—Off-white to yellow, crystalline powder; slight odor to odorless; melts with decomposition about 212°; moderately hygroscopic; pK_a 1.9, 8.2.

Solubility—1 g in 2 mL water; 4 mL alcohol; slightly soluble in chloroform.

Comments—A benzodiazepine widely used in short-term treatment (up to 4 weeks) of all types of insomnia such as difficulty in falling asleep, frequent nocturnal awakenings, and/or early morning awakening. It also is used in acute and chronic medical situations in which restful sleep is desirable. It is absorbed rapidly from the GI tract and rapidly metabolized by the liver. Following a single oral dose, peak plasma concentrations ranging from 0.5 to 4.0 ng/mL are reached in 60 min. After 7 to 10 days of treatment the major metabolite, N^1-desalkylflurazepam, reaches steady-state levels 5- to 6-fold higher than the 24-hr levels observed on day 1. The parent compound disappears rapidly from the blood; *N*-desalkylflurazepam remains active and has a half-life that ranges from 47 to 100 hr. The major urinary metabolite is conjugated N^1-hydroxyethylflurazepam and accounts for 22–55% of the dose.

This drug is excreted primarily in the urine. Less than 1% is excreted in the urine as N^1-desalkylflurazepam. The onset of sleep ranges from 15 to 45 min. Maximum effectiveness may not be achieved for 3 or 4 nights. Thus, the metabolite is responsible for the clinical effect as well as the residual effects that persist after the drug is discontinued. It requires the same warnings and precautions regarding use with other drug therapy, in hypersensitive individuals, during pregnancy, in children under 12 years, in elderly and excessively depressed patients, in patients with impaired renal or hepatic function, and in patients with a history of drug addiction that other benzodiazepines require.

Adverse reactions include dizziness, drowsiness, lightheadedness, ataxia and falling (especially in elderly or debilitated persons), and severe sedation. The last usually is due to drug intolerance or overdosage. Other reported side effects include headache, heartburn, upset stomach, nausea, vomiting, diarrhea, constipation, GI pain, nervousness, talkativeness, apprehension, irritability, weakness, palpitation, chest pains, body and joint pain, and genitourinary complaints. Less frequently, sweating, flushes, blurred vision, difficulty in focusing, burning eyes, faintness, hypotension, shortness of breath, pruritus, rash, dry mouth, bitter taste, excessive salivation, anorexia, euphoria, depression, slurred speech, confusion, restlessness, hallucinations, and paradoxical reactions (excitement, stimulation, and hyperactivity) have been observed.

QUAZEPAM

2*H*-1,4-Benzodiazepine-2-thione, 7-chloro-5-(2-fluorophenyl)-1,3-dihydro-1-(2,2,2-trifluorethyl)-, Doral

[36735-22-5] $C_{17}H_{11}ClF_4N_2S$ (386.79).

Preparation—It is synthesized in a manner similar to that for midazolam; *J Med Chem* 1974; 16:1354.

Comments—A benzodiazepine with a relatively long elimination half-life (39.3 hr). It is used for the short-term (up to 4 weeks) management of insomnia. Its two principal metabolites (2-oxoquazepam and N-desalkylflurazepam) are pharmacologically active with long elimination ($t_{1/2s}$, 40.2 and 69.5 hr). These long half-lives likely account for the drowsiness and hangover effects that persist for 2 to 3 days following discontinuation of therapy. However, because of its slow elimination, this drug is unlikely to cause significant withdrawal such as hyperexcitability or rebound insomnia. Adverse effects, drug interactions, and precautions appear to be similar to those of other benzodiazepines.

TEMAZEPAM

2*H*-1,4-Benzodiazepin-2-one, 7-chloro-1,3-dihydro-3-hydroxy-1-methyl-5-phenyl-, Restoril

[846-50-4] $C_{16}H_{13}ClN_2O_2$ (300.74).

Preparation—The synthesis is similar to that of oxazepam, using 2-(methylamino)-5-chlorobenzhydrol as the starting material. See *J Org Chem* 1962; 27:1691.

Description—White crystals melting about 120°.

Solubility—Very slightly soluble in water; sparingly soluble in alcohol; pK_a 1.6.

Comments—A hypnotic drug indicated for the short-term (up to 5 weeks) relief of *insomnia* associated with difficulty falling asleep, frequent nocturnal awakenings, and/or early morning awakenings. Oral bioavailability is relatively slow (mean times to peak concentration, 2 to 3 hr); 96% is bound to plasma proteins. Volume distribution ranges from 1.4 to 1.5 L/kg, and clearance from 1.10 to 1.36 mL/kg/min. The elimination half-life varies from 3 to 38 hr (mean, 14.7 hr). It is conjugated with glucuronic acid and excreted in the urine. Since metabolic enzyme induction does not appear to occur after 5 to 7 days of administration, tolerance to repeated use is not troublesome.

Adverse effects are usually mild and diminish with continued administration. Those observed most frequently include morning drowsiness, dizziness, lethargy, confusion, and GI disturbances (anorexia, diarrhea). Other, less-frequent adverse effects include vertigo, dryness of the mouth, paresthesias, tachycardia, panic reactions, nystagmus, paradoxical excitement, and hallucinations. Precautions and possible drug interactions are the same as those for other benzodiazepines. Dysmorphogenic changes in rib formation have been observed in two animal species given 50 to 100 times the human therapeutic dose. Use during pregnancy should be avoided if possible.

TRIAZOLAM

4*H*-1,2,4-Triazolo[4,3-*a*][1,4]benzodiazepine, 8-chloro-6-(2-chlorophenyl)-1-methyl-, Halcion

[28911-01-5] $C_{17}H_{12}Cl_2N_4$ (343.21).

Preparation—Ethyl α-aminoacetate and 2-amino-2′,4-dichlorobenzophenone are reacted in pyridine, which upon elimination of the elements of water and ethanol yields 7-chloro-5-(2-chlorophenyl)benzodiazepin-2-one. The latter, with P_2S_5 forms the 2-thiono derivative, which when treated with acetyl hydrazide gives the 2-acetamidoimino compound (I). Upon heating I over 200°, water is eliminated to form the triazole ring of triazolam. See Ger Pat 2,533,924.

Description—Tan crystals from isopropyl alcohol; melts about 235°.

Solubility—Very slightly soluble in water; slightly soluble in alcohol.

Comments—In the short-term management (up to 6 weeks) of insomnia characterized by difficulty in falling asleep, frequent nocturnal awakenings, and/or early morning awakenings. It is absorbed rapidly after oral administration; approximately 90% is bound to plasma proteins. Time to peak concentration is 1 hr. Volume distribution ranges from 0.8 to 1.3 L/kg. The elimination half-life is 2.0 (1.7–5.2) hr. The metabolites have little if any hypnotic activity. Common adverse effects include drowsiness, dizziness, and headache. Hallucinations and marked confusion also have been reported. Some reports suggest that anterograde amnesia and other side effects, such as confusion, bizarre behavior, agitation, and hallucinations may occur more often with triazolam than with most of the other benzodiazepines. Thus, patients using this drug should be monitored and treatment discontinued if such symptoms appear. Prescribers should be alert to the usual drug interactions common to benzodiazepines. The safe use of this drug during pregnancy or lactation has not been established.

MISCELLANEOUS HYPNOTICS

In addition to the benzodiazepines and barbiturates discussed in the previous two sections, there are a number of other agents that possess hypnotic properties. These are derived from several heterogeneous structures, including alcohols (ethchlorvynol), chloral hydrate, cyclic ether (paraldehyde), piperidinediones (glutethimide, methyprylon), imidazopyridines (zolpidem) and pyrazolopyrimidines (zaleplon). In addition to their hypnotic properties, several of these substances possess anticonvulsant, antispasmodic, local anesthetic, and weak antihistaminic properties. Zolpidem is an imidazopyridine agent that is an agonist at the benzodiazepine omega$_1$ receptor component of the GABA$_A$ receptor.[23] Zolpidem has shown weaker anxiolytic, anticonvulsant, and myorelaxant effects than benzodiazepines.[24] Today, zolpidem is the most commonly prescribed hypnotic, and it ranked 38th out of the top 200 most commonly prescribed medications in 2002.[14] Zaleplon, like zolpidem, acts as a selective agonist at the benzodiazepine omega$_1$ receptor subunit of the GABA$_A$ receptor complex in the brain.[25]

The older hypnotics, including ethchlorvynol, chloral hydrate, methprylon, glutethimide, and paraldehyde, do not differ qualitatively from the barbiturates in their desirable and undesirable effects. Hence, patients should be cautioned about concomitant use of alcohol or other CNS depressants and warned about operating a motor vehicle or hazardous machinery while on such drugs. It should be remembered that safe and effective use of many of these agents during pregnancy and in pediatric patients has not been established. Also, many of these agents will produce physical dependence and habituation when taken chronically in excessive doses. For this reason, glutethimide is listed in *Schedule II* under the *Controlled Substances Act*. Other substances in this section have lower abuse potential and are listed in *Schedule IV*. Nevertheless, they all should be used with caution in patients with a previous history of drug dependence. Again, due to safety considerations, use of these agents has largely been replaced by the hypnotic benzodiazepines and the nonbenzodiazepines zolpidem and zaleplon.

CHLORAL HYDRATE

1,1-Ethanediol, 2,2,2-trichloro-, Chloral

$CCl_3CH(OH)_2$ Chloral hydrate [302-17-0] $C_2H_3Cl_3O_2$ (165.40).

Preparation—By hydration of trichloroacetaldehyde (chloral) obtained by action of chlorine on alcohol.

Description—Colorless, transparent, or white crystals; aromatic, penetrating, and slightly acrid odor; slightly bitter, caustic taste. Melts about 55°; slowly volatilizes in air.

Solubility—1 g in 0.25 mL water, 1.3 mL alcohol, 2 mL chloroform, or 1.5 mL ether; very soluble in olive oil.

Comments—Principally for the short-term (2-week) treatment of insomnia. It is used preoperatively to allay anxiety and to induce sedation and/or sleep. It is used postoperatively as an adjunct to opiates and other analgesics to control pain. It also has been used to produce sleep prior to EEG evaluations. It is also effective in reducing anxiety associated with the withdrawal of alcohol and other drugs such as opiates and barbiturates.

Following oral administration, chloral hydrate is converted rapidly to trichloroethanol (TCE), which is largely responsible for its hypnotic action. Other metabolites are trichloroacetic acid (TCA) and trichloroethanolglucuronide (TCEG). Peak plasma levels of TCE and TCEG are reached in 20 to 60 min; plasma half-lives are 8.0 (7.0–9.5) hr and 6.7 (6.0–8.0) hr for TCE and TCEG, respectively. The half-life for TCA is 4 days. These data suggest that this drug has desirable properties, since the half-life of its active metabolite is short. The formation of TCA is a matter of concern, since its effect on the patient is unknown. It must be used with caution in patients receiving oral anticoagulants because TCA displaces warfarin from plasma protein binding sites; it is likely that dicumarol is affected similarly. Also, concomitant administration of alcohol and chloral hydrate should be avoided; significant potentiation may occur.

Gastric irritation occurs in some patients. Paradoxical excitement is observed rarely. The continued use of large doses causes peripheral vasodilation, hypotension, ventilatory depression, arrhythmias, and myocardial depression. Overdosage produces symptoms similar to those caused by barbiturate overdosages and may result in coma. Patients with serious heart, kidney, or liver disease should not be given this drug. If gastritis is present, the drug may be administered by rectum in olive oil as a retention enema. The acute toxic oral dose for adults is approximately 10 g; death has been reported after as little as 4 g, and individuals have survived after ingesting 30 g.

For oral use, it is sometimes given in a flavored syrup. As alkali causes decomposition of chloral hydrate, it is important that the vehicle not be alkaline.

ETHCHLORVYNOL

1-Penten-4-yn-3-ol, 1-chloro-3-ethyl-, Placidyl

$$HC \equiv C - \overset{\overset{\displaystyle OH}{|}}{\underset{\underset{\displaystyle CH_2CH_3}{|}}{C}} - CH = CHC^-$$

[113-18-8] C_7H_9ClO (144.60).

Preparation—By reacting ethyl chlorovinyl ketone (I) with lithium acetylide under Grignard reaction conditions. The alkoxide addition complex reacts readily with dilute acid to form crude ethchlorvynol, which is extracted with a suitable water-immiscible organic solvent such as ether and is subsequently purified by distillation. Compound I may be prepared in good yield by addition of propionyl chloride to acetylene at a temperature of about 40° in the presence of zinc chloride. US Pat 2,746,900.

Description—Colorless to yellow liquid with a characteristic pungent odor; darkens on exposure to light and air; specific gravity 1.068 to 1.071; refractive index 1.476 to 1.480; boils about 170°.

Solubility—Immiscible with water; miscible with most organic solvents.

Comments—A mild hypnotic that induces sleep within 15 min to 1 hr and has a duration of action of approximately 5 hr. Elimination half-life varies from 10 to 25 hr. Its effect is less profound and not as predictable as that obtained with benzodiazepines. It is indicated as short-term (up to 1 week) hypnotic therapy in insomnia. This drug is thought to have little effect on REM sleep; hence, REM rebound is not a major problem. It has been reported to increase the metabolism of coumarin anticoagulants by enzyme induction; patients on oral anticoagulants should be monitored closely when this drug is started or stopped. It is contraindicated in patients with porphyria and those with known hypersensitivity to the drug.

Patients should be cautioned about concomitant use of alcohol, barbiturates, other CNS depressants, or MAO inhibitors, since such combinations may produce exaggerated depressant effects. Also, they should be warned against operating a motor vehicle or hazardous machinery while on the drug. The excessive chronic use of large doses has been reported to cause psychic and physical dependence, tolerance, and withdrawal symptoms much like that caused by chronic use of barbiturates or alcohol and including severe convulsions when the drug is discontinued. It should not be used in patients with a history of drug abuse, mental depression, or suicidal tendencies, and the drug should be withdrawn gradually from patients taking excessive quantities. The drug is metabolized primarily by the liver, although the kidneys appear to contribute also.

Side effects, such as nausea, mental confusion, headache, and dermatitis, have been observed in some patients. In addition, hypotension, blurring of vision, dizziness, facial numbness, and allergic reactions have been reported. There have been rare reports of cholestatic jaundice and a few instances of thrombocytopenia. The safe and effective use of this agent during pregnancy and in pediatric patients has not been established.

GLUTETHIMIDE

2,6-Piperidinedione, 3-ethyl-3-phenyl-, Doriden

2-Ethyl-2-phenylglutarimide [77-21-4] $C_{13}H_{15}NO_2$ (217.27).

Preparation—Benzyl cyanide in toluene solution is treated with ethyl chloride in the presence of sodamide to yield α-ethylbenzyl cyanide. This is then caused to undergo addition (Michael condensation) to methyl acrylate under the catalytic influence of piperidine, thus forming methyl 4-cyano-4-phenylhexanoate (I). After purifying by low-pressure distillation, I is cyclized in acid medium. The cyclization may be represented as involving hydration of the cyanide group to amide and saponification of the ester, followed by dehydration between the amide and carboxyl groups.

Description—White, crystalline powder; saturated solution slightly acid; melts about 88°.

Solubility—Freely soluble in ethyl acetate, acetone, ether, or chloroform; soluble in alcohol or methanol; practically insoluble in water.

Comments—A hypnotic used to induce sleep in all types of insomnia. Overdosage is less likely to depress respiration but more likely to cause hypotension than most barbiturates. The onset of ac-

tion begins about 30 min after the administration of a hypnotic dose and generally lasts from 4 to 8 hr. Oral absorption is variable, with peak plasma level times between 1 and 6 hr. Elimination half-life varies from 5 to 22 hr, with an average value of 11.6 hr. It is contraindicated in hypersensitive patients, and patients should be warned about the concomitant use of alcohol and other CNS-depressant drugs. Patients also should be cautioned about engaging in activities that require alertness until 4 or 5 hr have elapsed following ingestion of the drug. It induces liver microsomal enzymes; therefore, therapy in patients on coumarin anticoagulants may require adjustment of the coumarin dose during and upon cessation of such therapy.

Adverse reactions include a generalized rash (in this case the drug should be withdrawn); occasionally, a purpuric or urticarial rash; exfoliative dermatitis has been observed rarely; nausea, hangover, paradoxical excitation, and blurred vision have occurred. Some of these side effects may be due to the anticholinergic activity of this drug. Porphyria or blood dyscrasias (thrombocytopenic purpura, aplastic anemia, or leukopenia) also have been reported. Habituation and physical dependence, like that which occurs with the barbiturates, may result from the prolonged administration of excessive doses. It is currently a *Schedule II* drug under the *Controlled Substances Act*. The drug should be used with caution in patients with a history of drug abuse.

PARALDEHYDE

1,3,5-Trioxane, 2,4,6-trimethyl-, Paracetaldehyde; Paral

2,4,6-Trimethyl-*s*-trioxane [123-63-7] $C_6H_{12}O_3$ (132.16); a trimer of acetaldehyde.

Caution—*It is subject to oxidation to form acetic acid. It may contain a suitable stabilizer.*

Preparation—By treating acetaldehyde with small quantities of sulfur dioxide, hydrochloric acid, carbonyl chloride, or zinc chloride; almost complete conversion occurs, and by freezing the liquid and then distilling the crystallized material, if necessary, the pure compound is produced.

Description—Colorless, transparent liquid; a disagreeable taste and a strong, characteristic, but not unpleasant or pungent odor; specific gravity about 0.99; does not congeal below 11° and distills at 120° to 126°; in contact with air it slowly oxidizes to acetic acid.

Solubility—1 mL in about 10 mL water or about 17 mL boiling water; miscible with alcohol, chloroform, ether, or volatile oils.

Incompatibilities—*Acids* convert it into acetaldehyde, which is prone to oxidation.

Comments—One of the oldest *sedatives* and *hypnotics*. It is absorbed rapidly after oral administration and produces sleep within 10 to 15 min after a 4- to 8-mL dose. It is detoxified by the liver (70–80%) and 11%–28% is excreted by the lungs. A negligible amount is excreted in the urine. Its chief disadvantage is that, being in part excreted through the lungs, it imparts an odor to the exhaled air, causes irritation, and thus should not be used in patients with asthma or other pulmonary diseases. Also, it has an unpleasant taste and may irritate the throat and gastric mucosa unless dispensed in suitable vehicles and should not be used in patients with gastroenteritis. It is poorly soluble in water; hence, it usually is prescribed in combination with alcoholic liquors, elixirs, etc. The drug also can be taken in milk, fruit juices, or iced tea or with cracked ice. Finally, it can be administered as a rectal retention enema in olive oil. It is effective in status epilepticus but should be reserved for patients who do not respond to phenobarbital. It occasionally is employed as an *obstetrical analgetic*, in which case large doses are administered, usually by rectum.

PROMETHAZINE HYDROCHLORIDE—page 1545.
PYRILAMINE MALEATE—see RPS-19, page 1227.
SCOPOLAMINE HYDROBROMIDE—page 1408.

ZALEPLON

Acetamide, N-[3-(3-cyanopyrazolo[1,5-a]pyrimidin-7-yl)phenyl]-N-ethyl-; Sonata

3′-(3-Cyanopyrazolo[1,5-a]pyrimidin-7-yl)-N-ethylacetamide [151319-34-5] $C_{17}H_{15}N_5O$. (305.34).

Preparation—The condensation of *m*-acetylacetanilide with N-(dimethoxy-methyl)dimethylamine forms 3-[3-(dimethylaminoacrylyl) derivative (I). Alkylation of I with ethyl iodide and sodium hydride ethylates the amido nitrogen and the pyrazolopyrimidine ring is closed with 3-aminopyrazine-4-carbonitrile in hot acetic acid. US Pat 4,626,538.

Description—Off-white powder; melts about 186°. Over the range of pH 1 to 7, log P (octanol-water partition coefficient) is 1.23.

Solubility—Practically insoluble in water; sparingly soluble in ethanol or propylene glycol.

Comments—A nonbenzodiazepine hypnotic from the pyrazolopyrimidine class. While zaleplon has a chemical structure that is unrelated to benzodiazepines or barbiturates, it acts as a selective agonist at the benzodiazepine omega$_1$ receptor subtype on the GABA$_A$ receptor complex in the brain.[25] Subunit modulation of the GABA-BZ receptor is hypothesized to be responsible for its hypnotic properties. It is rapidly and almost completely absorbed following oral administration. Zaleplon has an absolute bioavailability of 30% because of extensive first-pass metabolism.[26] Peak plasma concentrations are attained within 1 hour of administration with a mean elimination half-life of one hour. Because of its rapid onset of action, zaleplon should only be ingested immediately prior to going to bed or after the patient has gone to bed. Metabolism of zaleplon is primarily by oxidation via the enzyme aldehyde oxidase to 5-oxo-zaleplon, an inactive metabolite. Zaleplon is also metabolized to desethylzaleplon via the cytochrome P4504A4 system, which is a minor metabolic pathway.[25] Total protein binding is about 60%, independent of concentrations between 10 to 1000 ng/mL. A high fat/heavy meal will delay the t_{max} of zaleplon by approximately 2 hours and decrease the C_{max} by approximately 35% with no change in the AUC or elimination half-life.[26] For faster sleep onset it should not be administered with, or immediately following, a meal. Like other hypnotics, zaleplon may produce additive CNS depressant effects when coadministered with other psychotropic medications, antihistamines, ethanol, and other drugs that produce CNS depression.[26] The most common side effects are headache, drowsiness, dizziness, and lightheadedness.[25] There are no studies of zaleplon in pregnant women so its use is not recommended in this population.

ZOLPIDEM TARTRATE

Imadazolo[1,2-a]pyridine-3-acetamide, N,N,6-trimethyl-2-(4-methyl-phenyl)-, [R-(R*,R*)]-2,3-dihydroxybutanedioate; Ambien

[99294-93-6] $(C_{19}H_{21}N_3O)_2 \cdot C_4H_4O_6$ (764.88).

Preparation—The condensation of *p*-(bromomethyl)benzophenone and 5-methyl-2-pyridineamine yields 2-(p-tolyl)-6-methylimidazolo[1,2-a]pyridine. This latter compound, with dimethylamine and formaldehyde, in a classic Mannich reaction, adds the dimethylamino group on position-3, which is quaternized with methyl iodide, and the quaternary group is replaced with a nitrile, followed by conversion of the CN to the N,N-dimethylamide; the title compound. US Pat 4,382,938 (1983). *Drugs of the Future* 1987; 12:777.

Description—White to off-white crystals melting about 196°; pK$_a$ 6.2 (for the base).

Solubility—(Salt) Soluble 23 mg/mL in water.

Comments—Zolpidem is an imidazopyridine agent that is an agonist at the benzodiazepine omega$_1$ receptor component of the GABA$_A$ receptor.[23] Three subtypes of the omega receptor have been identified, and zolpidem in vitro binds to the omega$_1$ receptor preferentially. This selective binding may explain the relative absence of myorelaxant and anticonvulsant effects as well as the preservation of deep sleep (stages 3 and 4) in human.[27] It is absorbed rapidly in the GI tract; with a mean

elimination half-life of 2.6 (range 1.4–3.8) hr. Total protein binding is about 93%, independent of concentration between 40 and 790 ng/mL. When taken with food the mean AUC and C_{max} were decreased by 15 and 25%, respectively, and mean T_{max} was prolonged by 60% (from 1.4 to 2.2 hr) with no change in $t_{1/2}$. For faster sleep onset it should not be administered with, or immediately following, a meal. The most common side effects are drowsiness, dizziness, and diarrhea.[24] Zolpidem may produce additive CNS depressant effects when combined with other psychotropic agents, antihistamines, or alcohol. These combinations should be avoided.

There have been no well controlled studies examining the effects of zolpidem in pregnant women. Use during pregnancy only if clearly needed.[27] The use of zolpidem in nursing mothers is not indicated.

BENZODIAZEPINE ANTAGONIST

Because of the widespread use and the growing abuse of the benzodiazepines, attempts have been made to develop selective benzodiazepine antagonists to treat suspected benzodiazepine overdoses. These efforts have met with some success, and the Food and Drug Administration (FDA) has approved the use of flumazenil (Mazicon) as an adjunct to conventional therapy for overdosing with the benzodiazepines.

FLUMAZENIL

4H-Imidazo[1,5-a][1,4]benzodiazepine-3-carboxylic acid, 8-fluoro-5,6-dihydro-5-methyl-6-oxo-, ethyl ester; Romazicon

[78755-81-4] $C_{15}H_{14}FN_3O_3$ (303.29).

Preparation—Sarcosine and 6-fluorisatoic anhydride are condensed to 7-fluoro-5-methylbenzo[1,4]diazepin-2,5-dione. The dione, with ethyl α-isonitriloacetate forms a Schiff base through nucleophilic reaction with the amido hydrogen atom. A Claisen condensation closes the imidazole ring between positions 1 and 2 on the diazepine ring to yield the product. US Pat 4,316,839.

Description—White crystals melting about 202°.

Solubility—Insoluble in water; slightly soluble in aqueous acid.

Comments—An imidazobenzodiazepine that binds directly to the benzodiazepine (BDZ) recognition site on the GABA/BDZ receptor complex. It acts as a selective competitive antagonist to block the CNS actions of the benzodiazepines. Flumazenil only blocks the psychomotor, cognitive, and memory impairment caused by the benzodiazepines and has no effect on the actions of other CNS depressants (eg, ethanol, barbiturates, or general anesthetics). The effects are dose-dependent, with approximately 0.1 to 0.2 mg of flumazenil causing partial antagonism, and 0.4 to 1.0 mg producing complete blockade of benzodiazepine effects. After IV administration, the reversal of BDZ effects occurs within 1 to 2 min, with peak inhibition at 6 to 10 min. However, because of extensive first-pass elimination, oral administration results in low plasma drug concentration and is not recommended. Extensive and rapid ($t_{1/2}$ = 0.7–1.3 hr) hepatic metabolism results in no active metabolites. Despite a rapid clearance (31–78 L/hr), flumazenil can block benzodiazepine effects up to 6 hr. This drug was found to improve psychomotor performance, coordination, short-term memory loss, and subjective feelings of pain and drowsiness within 30 min of administration to patients pretreated with midazolam.

Flumazenil is to be used as an adjunct to, not a substitute for, proper airway and circulatory management in the case of BDZ overdosing. Although large IV doses produce no serious side effects in healthy volunteers, in BDZ-dependent patients this BDZ antagonist can provoke severe withdrawal effects such as anxiety, panic attacks, hot flashes, tremors, and seizures. Consequently, flumazenil generally is not to be used in patients with BDZ-dependence. Deaths have resulted from using this drug in patients with serious underlying diseases or in patients who overdosed on BZs in combination with large amounts of nonbenzo-

MEDICINAL AGENTS

diazepine drugs (eg, tricyclic antidepressants). In such cases, the flumazenil blocks the protective action of the BZs and unmasks the toxic effects of the other drugs. In the absence of BZs, it causes no serious adverse effects.

Besides the treatment of BZD overdoses, flumazenil has been used to reverse the sedative effects of BDZ used for general anesthesia. It has been suggested that this drug is able to reverse hepatic encephalopathy in some patients with acute and chronic liver failure. However, its effects are short-lasting.

Flumazenil should be titrated to the desired pharmacological effect by administering a series of small infusions (not a single large bolus) through a freely flowing IV tube in a large vein.

REFERENCES

1. Schatzberg AF, Cole JO, DeBattista C. *Manual of Clinical Psychopharmacology,* 4th ed. Washington, DC: American Psychiatric Publishing, 2003.
2. Friel JP, ed. *Dorland's Medical Dictionary,* 26th ed. Philadelphia: WB Saunders, 1981.
3. Sellers EM, Schneiderman JF, Romach MK, et al. *J Clin Psychopharmacology* 1992; 12:79.
4. Ballenger JG. *Biol Psychiatry* 1999; 46:1579
5. Rocca P, Fonzo V, Scotta M, et al. *Acta Psychiatr Scanda* 1997; 95:444.
6. Rickels K, Pollack MH, Sheehan DV, et al. *Am J Psychiatry* 2000; 157:968.
7. Rickels K, Downing R, Schweizer E, et al. *Arch Gen Psychiatry* 1993; 50:884.
8. Robins LE, Reiger DM, eds. *Psychiatric Disorders in America: The Epidemiologic Catchment Area Study.* New York: The Free Press, 1991.
9. American Psychiatric Association. *Diagnostic and Statistical Manual of Mental Disorders, Fourth Edition, Text Revision.* Washington, DC: American Psychiatric Association, 2000.
10. Schneck CH, Mahowald MW, Sack RL. *JAMA* 2003; 289:2475.
11. Holbrook AM, Crowther R, Lotter A, et al. *Can Med Assoc J* 2000; 162:210.
12. Kosten TR, O'Connor PG. *N Engl J Med* 2003; 348:1786.
13. Stahl SM. *J Clin Psychiatry* 2002; 63:756.
14. *Pharmacy Drug Cards,* 18th ed. Lawrence: Sigler and Flanders, Inc., 2002.
15. Moller HJ. *J Clin Psychopharmacology* 1999; 19:[suppl 2]2S.
16. Pritchett DB, Sontheimer H, Shivers B, et al. *Nature* 1989; 338:582.
17. MacDonald RL, Olsen RW. *Annu Rev Neuroscience* 1994; 17:569.
18. Kirkwood CK, Melton ST. In: DiPiro JT, Talbert RL, Yee GC, et al, eds. *Pharmacotherapy: A Pathophysiologic Approach,* 5th ed. New York: McGraw-Hill, 2002, Chap 71.
19. Arana GW, Rosenbaum JF. *Handbook of Psychiatric Drug Therapy,* 4th ed. Philadelphia: Lippincott Williams and Wilkins, 2000.
20. Neylan TC, Reynolds CF, Kupfer DJ. In: Hales RE, Yudofsky SC, Talbott JA, eds. *Textbook of Psychiatry,* 3rd ed. Washington, DC: American Psychiatric Press, 1999, Chap 24.
21. Curtis JL, Germaine SM. In: DiPiro JT, Talbert RL, Yee GC, et al, eds. *Pharmacotherapy: A Pathophysiologic Approach,* 5th ed. New York: McGraw-Hill, 2002, Chap 73.
22. Drug Facts and Comparisons. [resource on World Wide Web] URL: http://www.efactsweb.com. Accessed June 25, 2003.
23. Holm KJ, Goa KL. *Drugs* 2000; 59:865.
24. Langtry HD, Benfield P. *Drugs* 1990; 40:291.
25. Dooley M, Plosker GL. *Drugs* 2000; 60:413.
26. Drug Facts and Comparisons. [resource on World Wide Web] URL: http://www.efactsweb.com. Accessed August 25, 2003.
27. Drug Facts and Comparisons. [resource on World Wide Web] URL: http://www.efactsweb.com. Accessed August 27, 2003.

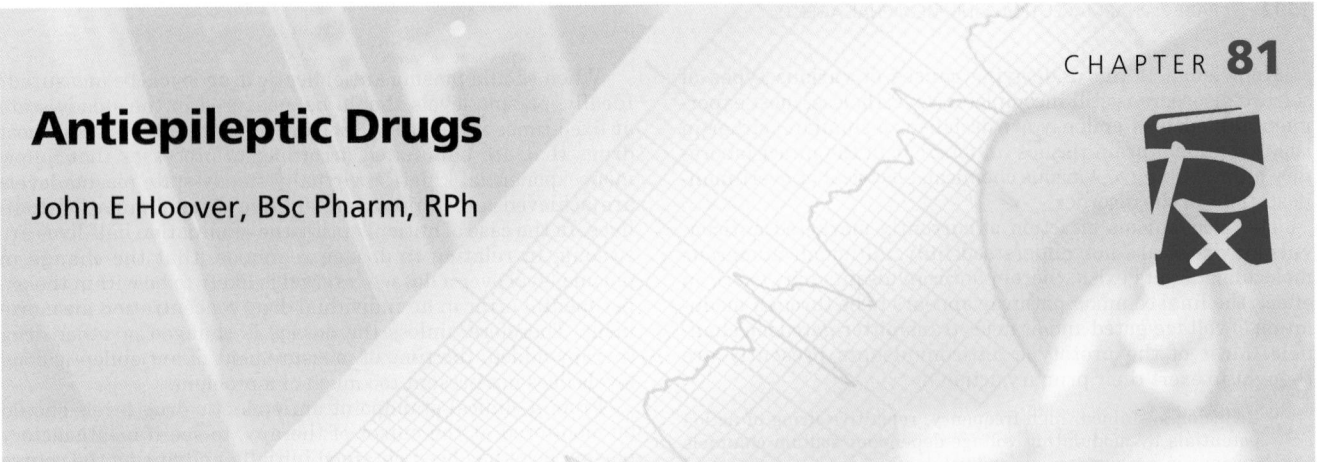

CHAPTER 81

Antiepileptic Drugs

John E Hoover, BSc Pharm, RPh

Epilepsy may be defined as a paroxysmal, self-sustaining, and self-limiting cerebral dysrhythmia characterized by an abnormal and excessive EEG discharge and a loss of consciousness. It may or may not be associated with body movements or hyperactivity of the autonomic nervous system. The epileptic attack is initiated by an abnormal focus of electric discharge, originating either in the grey matter or in the other part of the brain. The discharge spreads to other parts of the CNS and results in convulsions and other manifestations of the disorder.

There are many conditions that result in seizures. These include the entire range of neurological diseases from infection to neoplasm to head injuries. Contrary to popular opinion, hereditary factors are involved in only a few subtypes of seizures. The antiepileptic drugs described in this chapter also are used in patients who have febrile seizures or who have seizures as a result of an acute illness such as meningitis, even though the term epilepsy is not applied to such patients unless they later develop chronic seizures. Seizures also may result from an acute toxic or metabolic disorder; in such cases appropriate therapy is directed to the specific abnormality, such as hypocalcemia. In most cases of epilepsy, the choice of medication is dictated by the seizure classification.

Based on a modification of the International Classification (*Epilepsia* 1981; 22:489), epileptic seizures may be divided into two groups:

I. *Partial Seizures* (Focal Seizures).
    A. Partial seizures with elementary symptomatology (cortical focal). Generally without impairment of consciousness. Includes seizures confined to a single limb or muscle group (Jacksonian motor epilepsy), those who have sensory or somatosensory symptoms (Jacksonian sensory epilepsy) and those who have other limited symptoms, depending on the particular cortical area involved.
    B. Partial seizures with complex symptomatology (temporal lobe, psychomotor seizures). Generally with impairment of consciousness. Attacks of confused behavior with a wide variety of clinical manifestations, associated with bizarre generalized EEG activity during the seizure and temporal lobe abnormalities during the interictal period.
    C. Partial seizures secondarily generalized.
II. *Generalized Seizures* (bilaterally, symmetrical seizures). Includes absences (*petit mal*), characterized by brief, abrupt loss of consciousness associated with synchronous, 3-per-second spike-and-wave pattern in the EEG, usually with symmetrical clonic motor activity (eyelid blinking or jerking of entire body). *Bilateral massive epileptic myclonus,* isolated clonic jerks with brief burst of multiple spikes in EEG; *infantile spasms,* motor spasms with bizarre diffuse changes in the interseizure EEG, ie, hypsarrhythmia and progressive mental retardation; *clonic seizures,* rhythmic clonic contraction of all muscles, loss of consciousness and autonomic manifestations; *tonic seizures,* opisthotonos, loss of consciousness, and autonomic manifestations; *tonic-clonic seizures* (grand mal), characterized by a sequence of maximal tonic spasms of all body musculature followed by synchronous clonic jerking and profound depression of all central functions; *atonic seizures,* loss of postural tone with sagging of the head or falling; *akinetic seizures,* impaired consciousness and complete muscle relaxation, secondary to excessive inhibitory discharge.

The limitation of this type of description is that it is confined to describing individual seizure types and does not take into account a description of the numerous epileptic syndromes which continue to be described. To satisfy the need for a more accurate description of a seizure disorder, the International Classification of Epilepsies and Epileptic Syndromes was proposed to supplement the above classification. An epileptic syndrome is characterized by a variety of signs and symptoms. A particular syndrome will attempt to incorporate a number of items, including type of seizure, etiology, anatomy, precipitating factors, age of onset, severity, chronicity, diurnal and circadian cycling and often prognosis (*Epilepsia* 1989; 30(4):389).

A number of specific childhood epileptic syndromes have been recognized and classified by age. The notable examples include Early Myoclonic Encephalopathy; Lennox-Gastaut Syndrome; Absence Epilepsy Syndromes such as typical absence, juvenile absence and juvenile myoclonic epilepsy; and Progressive Myoclonic Epilepsy. One major advantage of this classification is that it recognizes that a simple partial seizure can progress to a complex partial seizure, and then to a secondary generalized seizure. In so doing, this classification does not require that a seizure be classified into one specific seizure category (*Univ Rep Epilepsy* 1992; 1(1):1).

One approach to the treatment of seizure disorders employs the use of antiepileptic drugs. The many medical therapies of antiquity have been replaced by a rational therapeutic approach which had its origin in the beginning of the 19th century. It has progressed from the use of bromides in 1857 and phenobarbital in 1912 to the modern era marked by introduction of diphenylhydantoin (phenytoin) in 1938. The clinical efficacy of the latter established the fact that chemicals effective in epilepsy need not be hypnotics and stimulated the laboratory search for other effective anticonvulsant agents. As a result, a number of anticonvulsant barbiturates, benzodiazepines, deoxybarbiturates, dipropylacetic acid derivatives, hydantoins, oxazolidinediones, and succinimides have been introduced in the last 50 years. Since 1993, five new drugs have been approved for the adjunctive treatment of partial seizures (ie, felbamate, gabapentin, lamotrigine, topiramate, and tiagabine). Of these five, serious idiosyncratic adverse effects have been identified for felbamate which include aplastic anemia and hepatic failure. As a result of these advances in drug therapy, it generally is stated that 50% of all individuals who have epileptic disorders can be satisfactorily controlled with available drugs and that the incidence of seizures can be reduced in another 25% of epileptic persons.

Knowledge of the underlying causes of various types of seizure disorders is still incomplete. Nevertheless, most experimental models of epilepsy are designed to simulate, either in isolated animal brain tissues (*in vitro*) or in the intact laboratory animal (*in vivo*), various chemical, electrical or overt manifestations of the disorder.

The mechanisms of action of currently marketed anticonvulsant drugs are not understood fully. Although numerous molecular targets exist wherein anticonvulsants may exert an effect, the final common pathway appears to be through modulation of voltage-gated and/or neurotransmitter-gated ion channels. Most of the prototype anticonvulsants presently are thought to exert their primary action by

- Reducing sustained, high-frequency, repetitive firing of action potentials by modulating voltage-dependent sodium channels (phenytoin, carbamazepine, and valproate).
- Enhancing GABA-mediated inhibitory neurotransmission via a receptor-gated chloride channel (benzodiazepines).
- Modulating neurotransmitter release and neuronal bursting through an effect on voltage-gated and receptor-gated calcium channels (ethosuximide, dimethadione, and valproate (*Epilepsia* 1989; 30 (4):389).

In addition, newer anticonvulsant substances still under preclinical development have been found to open potassium channels (*Brain Res* 1989; 495:189; *Eur J Pharmacol* 1989;167:181). Another promising area currently being pursued involves identifying novel therapies that are aimed at either reducing excitation by blocking specific excitatory amino-acid receptors and those aimed at enhancing inhibition by blocking high-affinity uptake of neuronally released GABA. It is anticipated that the increased appreciation of the processes underlying the initiation, propagation, and amelioration of seizure activity will lead to the introduction of mechanistically novel drugs in the not-too-distant future.

No one anticonvulsant drug is effective equally in all types of epilepsy. Hence, antiepileptic therapy must be individualized and drug therapy selected on the basis of seizure type, epileptic syndrome, and patient response. In generalized tonic-clonic seizures (*grand mal*) and simple and complex partial (focal, psychomotor), the drugs of choice are phenytoin, carbamazepine, or valproate; in generalized absence seizures (*petit mal*), ethosuximide and valproate with clonazepam as an alternate; for myoclonic epilepsy, valproate. It should be noted that valproate is effective in all of the above.

Status epilepticus, a succession of tonic-clonic seizures without intervening return of consciousness, requires prompt intravenous medication. The objective of treatment is suppression of the seizures, but all of the drugs used to treat this medical emergency can be lethal if they are given too rapidly or in overdosage. Intravenous diazepam is preferred by many clinicians, but since it is short-acting, maintenance must be started promptly. Some clinicians prefer intravenous phenytoin, especially in patients already on this drug. Phenobarbital is an effective alternative for the management of this disorder. If these drugs do not suppress the continuous seizure activity, general anesthesia may be used as an emergency treatment.

Until the 1970s, antiepileptic polytherapy was the most widely accepted practice in the treatment of epilepsy. Now, monotherapy is considered the superior therapeutic practice in the management of this disorder. This change was encouraged by refinements in diagnosis and the availability of broadspectrum antiepileptics such as valproic acid. Successful monotherapy involves three basic principles.

- Careful diagnosis of the specific type of seizures
- Accurate selection of the most suitable antiepileptic drug for the patient's seizures
- Appropriate drug use and monitoring

Monotherapy has been shown to improve seizure control and reduce the risk of idiosyncratic reactions, dose-related adverse effects, and complex drug interactions. Monotherapy also encourages better patient compliance and is cost effective.

When should plasma antiepileptic drug levels be measured? Ideally, plasma levels should be measured in the steady state at fixed times in relation to the drug dosage interval. For most drugs that are eliminated according to processes that follow monoexponential kinetics, virtually steady-state plasma levels are achieved after approximately five drug-elimination half-lives. In the case of antiepileptics, the elimination half-lives are so long, in relation to dosage regimens, that the change in plasma level over a dosage interval is likely to be within the experimental error in an individual drug concentration measurement. Therefore, unless the dosage is changed or other drug therapy added, the time of measurement of antiepileptic drug levels does not present too much of a problem.

From a clinical standpoint antiepileptic drug levels should be monitored at the outset of therapy, to see if a satisfactory plasma level has been obtained initially and during the course of therapy. The latter is especially important if the seizures are not controlled, intercurrent illness develops, antiepileptic drug dosage is changed, dosage of any other drug is changed or symptoms occur that appear to be caused by the drug. It also is important to monitor the epileptic patient during pregnancy, since antiepileptic drug levels tend to fall during pregnancy and rise again during puerperium. Such monitoring increases the changes of controlling epilepsy in patients and decreases the risk of their being overdosed in the process.

Behavioral disturbances and cognitive effects have been observed in patients on antiepileptic drug therapy (*Pediatrics* 1985; 76:644). Phenobarbital is associated with hyperactivity, fussiness, lethargy, disobedience, and stubbornness; phenytoin with unsteadiness, involuntary movements, tiredness, and alterations of emotional state; carbamazepine with sleep disorders, agitation, irritability, and emotional liability; clonazepam with irritability, aggression, hyperactivity, disobedience, and antisocial activities; and valproic acid with drowsiness. In addition, some have been shown to induce deficits in neuropsychological tests and impair attention and short-term memory. Physicians and parents should be alert for such behavioral and cognitive changes. Of the newer antiepileptic drugs, topiramate has the greatest liability for inducing cognitive impairment. However, this effect can be markedly reduced or even eliminated by initiating therapy at low doses and after a slow-titration rate.

Antiepileptic drugs may add to or potentiate the action of other CNS depressants, including other anticonvulsants and alcohol. A number of drugs, when concurrently administered with various antiepileptic agents, have been reported to alter the patient's response either to the antiepileptics or the other drugs.

Whether or not the effects are clinically significant cannot be stated categorically; they must be evaluated by careful observation of the individual patients, with monitoring of blood plasma levels of the concurrently administered drugs after which dosage adjustments of the interacting drugs may be necessary. For these reasons patients on antiepileptic medication should not take other drugs, either OTC or prescription, without the knowledge and approval of the physician responsible for their seizure therapy.

As tricyclic antidepressants may precipitate seizures, patients being treated with anticonvulsants should be observed closely for decreased seizure control if tricyclic antidepressant therapy is commenced; if necessary, the dosage of the anticonvulsant should be adjusted.

Children of epileptic mothers who receive anticonvulsant medication during the early months of pregnancy have an increased incidence of birth defects. The risk is approximately 7% as compared with 2% or 3% in the general population. Data are more extensive with respect to phenytoin, phenobarbital, and trimethadione. More recent observations indicate that valproate may be associated with spinal defects in the fetus.

Although systematic or anecdotal reports suggest a possible similar association with the use of all known anticonvulsant drugs, therapeutic abortion should be considered when trimethadione has been used during pregnancy. The great majority of mothers on anticonvulsant medication, however, deliver normal infants. It also is important to note that anticonvulsant drugs should not be discontinued in patients in whom the drug is administered to prevent generalized tonic-clonic seizures because of the strong possibility of precipitating status epilepticus with an attendant hypoxia and threat to life. In individual cases where the severity and frequency of the seizure disorder are such that the removal of medication does not pose a serious threat to the patient, discontinuation of the drug may be considered prior to and during pregnancy, although it cannot be said with any confidence that even seizures do not pose some hazard to the developing embryo or fetus. The prescribing physician will wish to weigh the risk/benefit of these considerations in treating or counseling epileptic women of childbearing age.

Antiepileptic agents have several uses in the nonepileptic patient. They have been used to soften the seizures in patients undergoing electroshock therapy, control convulsions occurring in dementia paralytica and tetanus, and lessen muscular rigidity in certain cases of cerebral palsy. Phenytoin administered intravenously has been reported to be effective in suppressing - recurrent cardiac arrhythmias. In addition, phenytoin, trimethadione, and phenacemide have been employed for the treatment of disturbed nonepileptic psychotic patients, particularly in catatonic excitement states, and in the management of children who have behavioral disorders. The latter use is especially intriguing and warrants careful clinical study. In addition, a number of the established as well as the newer generation antiepileptic drugs are sometimes employed in the management of bipolar disorder, aggression, and certain forms of chronic pain.

ACETAZOLAMIDE—page 1425.

CARBAMAZEPINE

5H-Dibenz[b, f]azepine-5-carboxamide; Tegretol

[298-46-4]$C_{15}H_{12}N_2O$ (236.27).

Preparation—5H-Dibenz[b, f]azepine, which may be prepared by thermal deammoniation of 2-(o-aminostyryl) aniline hydrochloride, is condensed with carbamoyl chloride by refluxing in an inert solvent in the presence of sodamide. US Pat 2,948,718.

Description—White to off-white powder; melts within a range of 3° between 187 and 193°.

Solubility—Practically insoluble in water; soluble in alcohol or in acetone.

Comments—Considered the drug of choice for complex partial seizures (temporal lobe, psychotomotor). It is preferred by many physicians for generalized tonic-clonic seizures (grand mal) and simple partial (focal, Jacksonian) seizures, particularly in patients who have not responded to other less-toxic anticonvulsants. It sometimes is effective in patients who have mixed seizure patterns which include the above, or other partial or generalized seizures. It is also useful in treatment of pain associated with true trigeminal neuralgia. Beneficial results also have been reported in glossopharyngeal neuralgia. Carbamazepine also has been used with some benefit for the management of acute mania, maintenance therapy of bipolar affective disorder and for the management of aggression and alcohol withdrawal syndrome (*Am Pharm* 1993; NS33(2): 47). The drug has a neutral pK_a; from 60% to 73% of the drug is bound to plasma protein, volume distribution usually is between 0.8 to 1.4L/kg; and half-life varies from 10 to 25 hr in adults and 8.5 to 19 hr in children. Therapeutic plasma levels range from 4 to 12 µg/mL. It should not be used in combination with other drugs; for example, troleandomycin, erythromycin, cimetidine, isoniazid, and propoxyphene inhibit the metabolism of carbamazepine and elevate the plasma concentration of this agent. The steady-state plasma concentration of carbamazepine is reduced by the concomitant administration of felbamate (see brainstem). In contrast, felbamate increases the concentration of carbamazepines-active metabolites. On the other hand, carbamazepine decreases the plasma levels of clonazepam, diazepam, ethosuximide, phenytoin, phenobarbital, primidone, and valproic acid.

To minimize adverse effects, initial dosage and daily increments should be limited to 200 mg. Adverse are encountered in approximately 50% of patients who have serum levels from 8.5 to 10 µg/mL, but few occur with concentrations less than 5 µg/mL. Diplopia, dizziness,

drowsiness, and ataxia occur with concentrations greater than 6 µg/mL; nystagmus may occur at serum levels below the therapeutic range. Other reactions include anorexia and nausea, rash (including the Stevens-Johnson syndrome), and edema. More-serious adverse effects include aplastic anemia, agranulocytosis, thrombocytopenia, and transient leukopenia. Therefore, all patients should be subjected to a complete blood test before being placed on the drug; additional blood tests should be done at weekly intervals during the first month of therapy, every 2 weeks during the 2nd and 3rd month, and at monthly intervals as long as the patient is on the drug. Patients should be made aware of the early toxic signs and symptoms of hematological problems such as fever, sore throat, ulcers in the mouth, easy bruising, and petechial or purpuric hemorrhage. If any blood abnormality is observed, the drug should either not be used or stopped if the patient is already on the drug. If adverse effects are of such severity that the drug must be withdrawn, the physician must be aware that abrupt discontinuation of any anticonvulsant drug in a responsive patient may lead to increased seizure incidence or even status epilepticy.

The safe use of the drug in pregnancy, lactation and in women of childbearing age has not been established. See the introductory statement.

CLONAZEPAM

2H-1,4-Benzodiazepin-2-one, 5-(2-chlorophenyl)-1,3-dihydro-7-nitro-, Klonopin

[1622-61-3] $C_{15}H_{10}CIN_3O_3$ (315.72).

Preparation—o-Chlorobenzoyl chloride is reacted with p-nitroaniline to form 2-amino-5-nitro-2′-chlorozophenone, and this is condensed with bromacetyl to form 2-bromoacetamido-5-nitro-2′-chlorobenzophenone, then with ammonia to form the corresponding acetamido compound. The acetamido compound is converted to its hydrochloride with anhydrous HCl in methanol, dissolved in boiling methanol, and cyclized to clonazepam with pyridine as the catalyst.

Description—Light-yellow, crystalline powder; faint odor; melts at approximately 238°; pK_a 1.5 (deprotonation of nitrogen in 4 position), 10.5 (deprotonation of nitrogen in 1 position).

Solubility—Practically insoluble in water; slightly soluble in alcohol; sparingly soluble in chloroform; slightly soluble in ether.

Comments—One of the drugs of choice for the management of myoclonic epilepsy. It also is useful alone or as an adjunct in the management of several types of generalized seizures such as absence (petit mal) attacks not responsible to either valproate or ethosuximide, the Lennox–Gestaut syndrome (petit mal variant) and akinetic seizures. Approximately 87% of the drug is bound to plasma protein; volume distribution is 3.2 L/kg and its half-life varies from 19 to 46 hr in adults and from 13 to 33 hr in children. Therapeutic plasma levels range from 20 to 80 ng/mL.

As with diazepam, which it resembles, tolerance develops in approximately 30% of patients as shown by a loss of anticonvulsant activity; adjustment of dosage may reestablish efficacy. Consequently, the drug should be withdrawn gradually during simultaneous substitution of another anticonvulsant. When used in patients who have mixed seizure types, it may increase the incidence or precipitate the onset of generalized tonic-clonic seizures (grand mal). This may require the use of either increased dosage or addition of other antiepileptic medication. Like other benzodiazepines, it is characterized in laboratory animals by its remarkable ability to antagonize pentylenetetrazole-induced seizures; it also has a taming effect in aggressive primates and induces muscle weakness and hypnosis.

Its depressant effects may be potentiated by alcohol, narcotics, barbiturates, nonbarbiturate hypnotics, antianxiety agents, the phenothiazines, thioxanthene, and butyrophenone classes of antipsychotic agents, monoamine oxidase inhibitors and the tricyclic antidepressants, as well as by other anticonvulsant drugs. Phenobarbital or phenytoin may decrease steady-state plasma levels of this drug by enzyme induction. Its concomitant use with valproate may produce absence status.

The most frequently occurring side effects are referable to CNS depression; drowsiness occurs in approximately 50% of patients and ataxia in approximately 30%. Other adverse reactions, listed by systems are

- *Neurological:* abnormal eye movements, aphonia, choreiform movements, coma, diplopia, dysarthria, dysdiadochokinesis, *glassy-eyed* appearance, headache, hemiparesis, hypotonia, nystagmus, respiratory depression, slurred speech, tremor and vertigo.

- *Psychiatric:* confusion, depression, forgetfulness, hallucinations, hysteria, increased libido, insomnia, psychosis, and suicidal tendencies.
- *Respiratory:* chest congestion, rhinorrhea, shortness of breath, and hypersecretion in upper respiratory passages.
- *Cardiovascular:* palpitations.
- *Dermatological:* hair loss, hirsutism, skin rash, and ankle and facial edema.
- *Gastrointestinal:* anorexia, coated tongue, constipation, diarrhea, dry mouth, encopresis, gastritis, hepatomegaly, increased appetite, nausea and sore gums.
- *Genitourinary:* dysuria, enuresis, nocturia, and urinary retention.
- *Musculoskeletal:* muscle weakness and pains.
- *Miscellaneous:* dehydration, general deterioration, fever, lymphadenopathy, and weight loss or gain.
- *Hematopoietic:* anemia, leukopenia, thrombocytopenia, and eosinophilia.

Its safe use in pregnancy, in lactation, and in women of childbearing age has not been established. See the introductory statement.

DIAZEPAM—page 1489.

DIVALPROEX SODIUM

Pentanoic acid, 2-propyl-, sodium salt (2:1); Depakote

Sodium hydrogen bis(2-propylvalerate)[76584-70-8] $C_{16}H_{31}NaO_4$ (310.41).

Preparation—Neutralization of a solution of valproic acid (page ??) with 1/2 equivalent of sodium hydroxide and the solvent removed yields the product.

Comments—An antiepileptic agent that dissociates in the GI tract into two molecules of valproate. Hence, it has the same indications, adverse reactions, and contraindications as valproate. It differs from valproate, however, in that it is available in tablet form. See *Valproate Sodium*, page 1508.

ETHOSUXIMIDE

2,5-Pyrrolidinedione, 3-ethyl-3-methyl-, Zarontin

2-Ethyl-2-methylsuccinimide [77-67-8]$C_7H_{11}NO_2$ (141.17).

Preparation—Methyl ethyl ketone is condensed with ethyl cyanoacetate to yield ethyl 2-cyano-3-methyl-2-pentenoate, which, in ethanolic solution, adds hydrogen cyanide to form ethyl 2,3-dicyano-3-methylpentanoate. Proton-catalyzed saponification of the latter ester is accompanied by decarboxylation to produce 2-methyl-2-ethylsuccinonitrile. This, on heating with aqueous ammonia, cyclizes to ethosuximide. US Pat 2,993,835.

Description—White to off-white crystalline powder or waxy solid; characteristic odor; stable in light, air and heat at 37°; melts at approximately 50°; pKa 9.5.

Solubility—Soluble in alcohol or ether; freely soluble in water or chloroform; very slightly soluble in solvent hexane.

Comments—The drug of choice for control of uncomplicated absence seizures (*petit mal*). It suppresses the paroxysmal 3 cycles/s spike and the wave activity associated with lapses of consciousness characteristic of this disorder. It should not be used alone in mixed seizure types since it may increase the incidence of generalized tonic-clonic seizures in such patients. It is absorbed completely after oral administration. The drug is not bound to plasma protein; volume distribution is 0.7 L/kg; its half-life is approximately 60 hr in adults and 30 hr in children. It is excreted slowly in the urine; approximately 20% is excreted unchanged and as much as 50% as the hydroxylated metabolite or its glucuronide or as both. Therapeutic plasma levels range from 40 to 100 μg/mL. Maximal serum concentrations are usually achieved within 5 days after oral surgery is begun.

Adverse effects involve the GI, hemopoietic, nervous, and integumentary systems. GI symptoms occur frequently and include anorexia, nausea, vomiting, cramps, epigastric distress, and abdominal pain; blood disturbances such as leukopenia, agranulocytosis, pancytopenia, aplastic anemia, and eosinophilia have occurred; neurologic and sensory reactions observed include drowsiness, headache, dizziness, euphoria, hyperactivity, and ataxia; skin manifestations include urticaria, Stevens–Johnson syndrome, lupus erythematosus, and pruritic erythematous rashes; other reactions reported include myopia, vaginal bleeding, gum hypertrophy, and hirsutism. Periodic blood and urine tests should be made on patients who are taking the drug. It should be with extreme caution in patients known to have liver or renal disease. Its safe use in pregnancy, lactation, and women of childbearing age has not been established. See the introductory statement.

ETHOTOIN

Imidazolidin-2,4-dione, 3-ethyl-5-phenyl-, Peganone

[86-35-1]$C_{11}H_{12}N_2O_2$ (204.23).

Preparation—From mandelonitrile and urea to form *N*-(α-cyanobenzyl) urea that cyclizes with HCl to yield the imino derivative of hydantoin. Hydrolysis of the imine followed by ethylation with C_2H_5I forms ethotoin. See *Ber*, 1888; 21:2320.

Descriptions—White, crystalline powder; melts about 94°.

Solubility—Sparingly soluble in water; freely soluble in alcohol.

Comments—Used for the management of generalized tonic-clonic and complex partial seizures. With plasma levels less than 8 μg/mL, the half-life ranges from 3 to 9 hr. Therapeutic plasma levels range from 15 to 50 μg/mL. It is contraindicated in patients who have hepatic and hematological disorders. Untoward effects include nausea, vomiting, fatigue, dizziness, headache, diplopia, nystagmus, skin rash, numbness, fever, diarrhea, and chest pain. Ataxia and gum hyperplasia have occurred rarely; lymphadenopathy has been reported in some patients. See the introductory statement on the use of antiepileptics during pregnancy.

FELBAMATE

1, 3-Propanediol, 2-phenyl-, bis(carbamate) ester; Felbatol

[25451-15-4] $C_{11}H_{14}N_2O_4$ (238.24).

Comments—The first new drug approved for the management of epilepsy since 1978. It represents the first new chemical entity to emerge from the National Institute for Neurological Disorders and Stroke's comprehensive Anticonvulsant Drug Development Program. Felbamate is approved for the add-on treatment of partial seizures in patients 14 years of age and older. It also has been approved for the adjunctive therapy of partial and generalized seizures associated with Lennox–Gastaut syndrome, which is characterized by a mixture of several seizure types and usually is uncontrolled with other available anticonvulsants.

In laboratory animal models of epilepsy, it is effective against seizures induced by maximal electroshock, pentylenetetrazol, or picrotoxin. This unique profile is broader than that of phenytoin, carbamazepine, or ethosuximide, and slightly narrower than that of valproate; this suggests that felbamate has the ability to limit the spread of seizure activity and to raise seizure threshold. Its mechanism of action has yet to be clearly established. However, felbamate has been shown to inhibit high-frequency repetitive firing of spinal cord neurons and to modulate the strychnine-insensitive glycine recognition site of the NMDA receptor-ionophore complex. Felbamate is a weak inhibitor at the benzodiazepine recognition site of the GABA_A receptor and the GABA_A-receptor. It is devoid of any activity at the MK-801 binding site of the NMDA-preferring receptor.

Felbamate is well absorbed after oral administration. Absorption of the tablet formulation does not appear to be affected by food. Approximately 40% to 50% of the absorbed dose is excreted in the urine unchanged. An additional 40% appears as unidentified metabolites and conjugates. It is approximately 22% to 25% bound to protein and displays a terminal half-life of 20 to 23 hrs. The C_{max} and AUC are proportional to dose after single and multiple doses over a range of 100 to 800 mg and single doses of 1200 to 3600 mg.

Felbamate is reported to produce only mild dose-related side effects. The most common adverse reactions seen in adults receiving felbamate monotherapy include anorexia, vomiting, insomnia, nausea, and headache. The most commonly reported side effects in pediatric patients during adjunctive therapy are anorexia, vomiting, headache, and somnolence.

Unfortunately, felbamate use has been associated with an increased risk of aplastic anemia and acute hepatic failure. Recognition of this liability has clearly curtailed felbamate use since 1994. Now, both physicians and patients are required to sign an informed consent form prior to felbamate's being dispensed.

The addition of felbamate to other anticonvulsant drugs affects the steady-state plasma concentrations of the coadministered drug. It has been shown in clinical trials to increase the plasma concentration of phenytoin or valproate, decrease the plasma concentration of carbamazepine, and increase the concentration of the active metabolite of carbamazepine. Phenytoin and carbamazepine have been shown to increase the clearance of felbamate and to reduce its steady-state concentration. The available data suggest that there is no significant effect of valproate on the clearance of felbamate. These interactions necessitate careful titration of felbamate and scheduled dosage reduction of concomitant antiseizure drugs when it is administered concurrently with other antiseizure drugs. The safety and efficacy of felbamate during pregnancy has not been established and the drug should only be used during pregnancy if clearly needed.

GABAPENTIN

Cyclohexaneacetic acid, 1-(aminomethyl)-, Neurontin

[60142-96-3] $C_9H_{17}NO_2$ (171.24).

Preparation—Cyclohesane-1,1-diacetic acid is monoesterified with methanol and the ester reacted with ethyl chloroformate in the presence of triethylamine followed by reaction with sodium azide to yield the 1-isocyanatomethyl derivative of the monoester. This latter compound is converted to the 1-(aminomethyl) product and the lactam, through the cyclization of the ester and the free amine. The mixture is refluxed with dilute HCl to give the product. US Pat 4,024,175 (1977).

Description—White crystals melting about 164°–167°; HCl melts about 70° · pK_{A1} 3.68; pK_{A2} 10.7.

Solubility—Greater than 100 mg/mL in water at pH 7.4.

Comments—Approved as adjunctive therapy for the management of partial seizures in adults. Although the precise mechanism of action of gabapentin remains unknown, several molecular mechanisms have been proposed. These include an ability to limit sustained repetitive firing of action potentials with prolonged exposure. This effect suggests an action at the voltage-sensitive sodium channel. Furthermore, gabapentin has been found to increase brain GABA levels in epilepsy patients. Last, gabapentin may modify neurotransmitter release through an interaction with the a2d auxiliary subunit of the voltage-sensitive calcium channel.

Side effects are fairly mild but may include dizziness and aggressiveness at higher therapeutic doses. In some patients, gabapentin may produce significant weight gain. Gabapentin is not significantly metabolized in humans; nor does it induce liver enzymes. Gabapentin, which is excreted unchanged by the kidneys, is the only new antiepileptic drug to be introduced into the US market since 1993. As such, it displays minimal potential for drug–drug interactions. One major disadvantage of gabapentin is its short half-life (approximately 4–6 hrs), which necessitates multiple daily dosing (3–4 times a day).

Gabapentin has been endorsed as an effective drug for the management of neuropathic pain. However, its use for this indication is currently relegated as off-label.

LAMOTRIGINE

1,2,4-Triazine-3,5-diamine, 6-(2,3-dichlorophenyl)-, Lamictal

[84057-84-1] $C_9H_7Cl_2N_5$ (256.09).

Preparation—Reaction of 2,3-dichlorobenzoyl chloride with cyanide ion forms the benzoylcyanide derivative that is then treated with aminoguanidine to form a Schiff base through loss of water between the carbonyl group and the one primary amine function of the guanidine. Ring closure by addition of the lone free primary amino group remaining on the guanidine moiety to the nitrile function is accomplished by base catalysis and yields the product. US Pat 4,602,017 (1986).

Description—White crystals melting about 217°.

Comments—Approved for the adjunctive management of partial seizures in adults. In addition, anecdotal evidence suggests that lamotrigine is effective against a broad spectrum of seizure disorders, including generalized absence seizures. In addition to its anticonvulsant effects, lamotrigine appears to be effective in the management of bipolar disorder; however, this use is currently unapproved by the FDA. Lamotrigine, like phenytoin and carbamazepine, appears to exert its anticonvulsant effect through its ability to inhibit voltage-sensitive sodium channels in a voltage- and use-dependent manner.

Lamotrigine use does not affect the metabolism of other antiepileptic drugs; however, the metabolism of lamotrigine can be modified by the addition of other drugs. This latter effect is particularly problematic when lamotrigine is administered in conjunction with valproic acid.

Lamotrigine is generally well tolerated in both normal and epilepsy patients. However, the incidence of a severe life-threatening rash with lamotrigine use had led the FDA to issue a *black box* warning in 1997. There appears to be a greater risk in children (1:100) as opposed to adults (1:1000). The risk of rash is lower with slower titration rates. Patients should be counseled to contact their physician at the first sign of rash. The incidence of rash appears to be greater with concomitant use of valproic acid. This is most likely related to the ability of valproic acid to increase lamotrigine plasma levels by modification of the metabolism of lamotrigine. For example, the half-life of lamotrigine is increased from 24 to 59 hrs by concomitant administration of valproic acid.

LEVETIRACETAM

1- Pyrrolidineacetamide, (S)-α-ethyl-2-oxo-, Keppra

[102767-28-2] $C_8H_{14}N_2O_2$ (170.21).

Preparation—Butyrolactam and 2-oxobutyric acid are condensed by dehydration using refluxing toluene with a Dean-Stark trap to form 2- (2-oxopyrrolidino)-2-butenoic acid (Z to E ratio - 80:1). Recrystallization from acetone improves the Z to E ratio to 149:1. The unsaturated acid is converted to the acyl chloride with PCl_5 then to the amide with dry NH_3. Asymmetric hydrogenation of the unsaturation using Rh-(Et,Et)DUPHOS catalyst is 97% stereoselective and yields primarily the S- product. US Pat 4,997,955(1991) and US Pat 6,713,635(2004).

Description—White to off white powder from acetone, with a bitter taste; melts about 119°.

Solubility—In (g/100 mL) of solvent: water(104), $CHCl_3$ (65.3), methanol(53.6), ethanol(16.5), acetonitrile(5.7); practically insoluble in hexane.

Comments—The precise mechanism(s) by which levetiracetam exerts its antiepileptic effect is unknown and does not appear to derive from any interaction with known mechanisms involved in inhibitory and excitatory neurotransmission. The antiepileptic activity of levetiracetam was assessed in a number of animal models of epileptic seizures. Levetiracetam did not inhibit single seizures induced by maximal stimulation with electrical current of different chemoconvulsants and showed only minimal activity in submaximal stimulation and in threshold tests. Protection was observed, however, against secondarily generalized activity from focal seizures induced by pilocarpine and kainic acid, two chemoconvulsants that induce seizures that mimic some features of human complex partial seizures with secondary generalization.

MEPHENYTOIN—see RPS-20, page 1425.

METHSUXIMIDE

2,5-Pyrrolidinedione, 1,3-dimethyl-3-phenyl-, Celontin

N,2-Dimethyl-2-phenylsuccinimide [77-41-8]$C_{12}H_{12}NO_2$ (203.24).

Preparation—2-Methyl-2-phenylsuccinic acid is dissolved in excess 40% methylamine. The water and excess urine are distilled off, and the residue of the di(methylamine) salt of the acid is pyrolyzed at 250° until no more distillate is formed. The residue of crude methsuximide may be purified by vacuum ditilation. US Pat 2,643,257.

Description—White to grayish white, crystalline powder; odorless or not more than a slight odor; melts about 53°.

Comments—Similar in spectrum to *Ethosuximide* (ie, absence seizures). It does not worsen or increase generalized tonic-clonic seizures.

OXCARBAZEPINE

5*H*-Dibenz[*b,f*]azepine-5-carboxamide, 10,11-dihydro-10-oxo-, Trileptal

[28721-07-5] $C_{15}H_{12}N_2O_2$ (252.27).

Preparation—10-Methoxy-5*H*-dibenz[*b,f*]azepine is treated with phosgene to form the 5-carbonyl chloride which is converted to the amide with ammonia, then refluxed with 2*N* HCl to yield the 10-oxo-10,11-dihydro derivative which is oxcarbazepine. US Pat 3,642,775(1972).

Description—White to faint orange crystals from ethanol, melting about 215°.

Solubility—Slightly soluble in chloroform, methylene chloride, acetone or methanol; practically insoluble in ethanol, ether or water.

Comments—The pharmacological activity of oxcarbazepine is primarily exerted through the 10-monohydroxy metabolite (MHD) of oxcarbazepine. The precise mechanism by which oxcarbazepine and MHD exert their antiseizure effect is unknown; however, in vitro electrophysiological studies indicate that they produce blockade of voltage-sensitive sodium channels, resulting in stabilization of hyperexcited neural membranes, inhibition of repetitive neuronal firing, and diminution of propagation of synaptic impulses. These actions are thought to be important in the prevention of seizure spread in the intact brain. In addition, increased potassium conductance and modulation of high-voltage activated calcium channels may contribute to the anticonvulsant effects of the drug. No significant interactions of oxcarbazepine or MHD with brain neurotransmitter or modulator receptor sites have been demonstrated.

PARAMETHADIONE—see RPS-20, page 1426.
PHENACEMIDE—see RPS-20, page 1426.
PHENSUXIMIDE—see RPS-20, page 1426.

PHENYTOIN

2,4-Imidazolidinedione, 5,5-diphenyl-, Diphenylhydantoin; Dilantin

5,5-Diphenylhydantoin [57-41-0] $C_{15}H_{12}N_2O_2$ (252.27). See *Phenytoin Sodium* for the formula.

Preparation—Phenytoin sodium, prepared as described below yields the base on acidification of its aqueous solution.

Description—White powder, odorless; melts about 295°.

Solubility—Practically insoluble in water; slightly soluble in cold alcohol, chloroform, or ether.

Comments—See *Phenytoin Sodium*.

PHENYTOIN SODIUM

2,4-Imidazolidinedione, 5,5-diphenyl-, monosodium salt; Diphenylhydantoin Sodium Salt; Diphenylhydantoin Sodium; Soluble Phenytoin; Dilantin Sodium

5,5-Diphenylhydantoin sodium salt [630-93-3] $C_{15}H_{11}N_2NaO_2$ (274.25).

Preparation—By treating benzaldehyde with a solution of sodium cyanide, 2 mol of benzaldehyde are condensed (benzoin condensation) into 1 mol of benzoin, which is oxidized to benzil with nitric acid or cupric sulfate. The benzil is then heated with urea and in the presence of sodium ethoxide or isopropoxide, forming phenytoin sodium.

Description—White, odorless powder; somewhat hygroscopic and on exposure to air, gradually absorbs carbon dioxide with the liberation of the base. pK_a 8.32.

Comments—One of the drugs of choice for the management of generalized tonic-clonic (grand mal) seizures, complex partial (temporal lobe; psychomotor) seizures, and simple partial (focal, Jacksonian) seizures. It is not recommended for the management of pure absence (petit mal) epilepsy. Parenterally, it is used for the control of status epilepticus of the generalized tonic-clonic (grand mal) type and in the management of seizures occurring during neurosurgery. Intravenous phenytoin sodium may be useful in the treatment of paroxysmal atrial tachycardia, ventricular tachycardia, and digitalis-induced cardiac arrhythmias. Oral phenytoin sodium also may afford benefit in the treatment of behavioral disorders and, in large doses, the management of trigeminal neuralgia. It is much less effective in the latter than carbamazepine. Approximately 87% to 93% of the drug is bound to plasma protein, volume distribution ranges from 0.5 to 0.8 L/kg, and half-life is approximately 22 hrs in adults and 18 to 22 hrs in children. Therapeutic plasma levels range from 10 to 20 µg/mL in adults and 5 to 20 µg/mL in children. Toxic levels range from 30 to 50 µg/mL, and lethal levels are approximately 100 µg/mL.

It acts on the motor cortex where it stabilizes the neuronal membrane and inhibits the spread of the seizure discharge. Present evidence suggests that it limits sustained high-frequency repetitive firing by blocking Na^+-channels in a use- and frequency-dependent manner. It also enhances calcium binding to phospholipids in neuronal membranes. These effects result in a more stable membrane configuration.

These observations are in harmony with the fact that its most easily demonstrated properties are its ability to limit the development of maximal seizure activity and to reduce the spread of the seizure process from the active focus. Both features are undoubtedly related to its clinical usefulness.

There are two distinct forms of Phenytoin Sodium Capsules: the rapid-release type (Prompt Phenytoin Sodium Capsules) and the slow-dissolution type (Extended Phenytoin Sodium Capsules). The former have a dissolution rate of not less than 85% in 30 min and are used for 3- or 4-times/day dosing, whereas the latter has a slow dissolution rate of 15% to 35% in 30 min, 45% to 65% in 1 hr, and not less than 85% in 2 hr and may be used for once/day dosing. Studies comparing doses of 100 mg three times a day of Prompt Phenytoin Sodium Capsules with a single, daily dose of 300 mg of Extended Phenytoin Sodium Capsules (Dilantin Kapseals, *Parke-Davis*) indicate that absorption, peak plasma levels, biological half-life, difference between peak and minimum values, and urinary recovery are equivalent. *Because of the differences in dissolution rates among various brands, physicians should be cautioned to keep patients on one manufacturer's product.*

Its metabolism may be altered significantly by concomitant use of other drugs. Drugs that increase the serum levels include chloramphenicol, dicumarol, tolbutamide, isoniazid, phenylbutazone, acute alcohol intake, salicylates, chlordiazepoxide, phenothiazines, felbamate, diazepam, estrogens, ethosuximide, halothane, methylphenidate, sulfonamides, cimetidine, and trazodone. Drugs that *decrease* the serum levels include carbamazepine, chronic alcohol abuse, reserpine, and preparations containing calcium. Drugs that *either increase or decrease* the serum levels include phenobarbital, valproic acid, and valproate sodium.

This is a fairly safe anticonvulsant, although many adverse effects have been observed. Nystagmus may appear with serum concentrations of 8 to 20 µg/mL and is nearly always present at higher levels. At concentrations greater than 30 µg/mL, ataxia and dysarthria commonly occur. Gingival hyperplasia and hirsutism are often intolerable, particularly in the young. A morbilliform rash may occur, usually in the first 10 days of treatment, and it rarely progresses to exfoliate dermatitis or the Stevens-Johnson syndrome; the drug should be stopped if a rash appears. There also are reports of peripheral neuropathy, a lupus erythematous syndrome, hepatitis, lymphadenopathy, megaloblastic anemia and rickets, and osteomalacia because of interference with vitamin D metabolism. Serum folic acid and vitamin K levels also may be depressed, and bleeding disorders have been reported in infants born to mothers taking the drug. Overdosage causes an acute cerebellar syndrome, delirium, and rarely, coma.

It is contraindicated in patients who have a history of sensitivity to hydantoins. Abrupt withdrawal of this medication may precipitate status epilepticus; when the dosage needs to be reduced or when substitution of another antiepileptic appears desirable, such alteration in therapy should be done gradually. Recent reports suggest an association between the use of anticonvulsant drugs by women who have epilepsy and an increased incidence of birth defects in children born to these women. The prescribing physician should weigh the benefit and risk potential of antiepileptic agents when treating or counseling epileptic women of childbearing age. See the introductory statement.

PRIMIDONE

4,6-(1*H*,5*H*)-Pyrimidinedione, 5-ethyldihydro-5-phenyl-, Mysoline

[125-33-7] $C_{12}H_{14}N_2O_2$ (218.25).

Preparation—A solution of ethylphenylmalonamide (I) in a large molecular excess of formamide (II) is refluxed for 2 hr. The cyclization may be viewed as being brought about by a Cannizzaro type of disproportionation of II followed by a deammoniation and a dehydration between I and the highly reactive methanolamine resulting from the disproportionation.

Description—White, odorless; crystalline powder; slightly bitter taste; melts about 281°.

Solubility—1 g in 2000 mL water or 200 mL alcohol; slightly soluble in most organic solvents.

Comments—Either alone or in combination with other antiepileptics, used as alternate therapy in the control of generalized tonic-clonic seizures (grand mal), complex partial seizures (temporal lobe; psychomotor), and focal epileptic seizures. It is metabolized to phenylethylmalonamide (PEMA) and phenobarbital. Phenobarbital formation ranges from 15% to 25%. The plasma half-life of PEMA is 24 to 48 hr, whereas that of phenobarbital is 48 to 120 hr. Both substances tend to accumulate during chronic medication.

PEMA is an active antiepileptic but is less potent and less toxic than phenobarbital. From 0% to 30% of this drug is bound to plasma protein, volume distribution averages 0.6 L/kg and plasma half-life in adults range from 9 hr in combination therapy to 15 hr in monotherapy; in children, half-life varies from 6 to 8 hr. Therapeutic plasma concentrations range from 6 to 12 µg/mL for this drug and from 15 to 45 µg/mL for pheobarbital. Few interactions with other drugs have been reported, but those for phenobarbital also apply. The ratio of phenobarbital to this unmetabolized drug in serum is significantly higher in epileptic patients treated with a combination of this drug and phenytoin than in patients on this drug alone. It decreases the prothrombin response to dicumarol and warfarin. Also, concurrent treatment with valproate increases the plasma level of phenobarbital in patients on this drug.

The most frequent side effects include ataxia and vertigo; these tend to disappear with continued or reduced therapy. Occasionally, nausea, anorexia, vomiting, fatigue, irritability, emotional disturbances, diplopia, nystagmus, drowsiness, and morbilliform rashes occur. Megaloblastic anemia may occur as a rare idiosyncrasy; this anemia responds to folic acid, 15 mg a day, without the medicine's being discontinued.

TIAGABINE HYDROCHLORIDE

3-Piperidinecarboxylic acid, 1-[4,4-(bis-(3-methyl-2-thienyl)-3-butenyl]-, hydrochloride; Gabitril

[145821-59-6] $C_{20}H_{25}NO_2S_2$.HCl (412.02).

Preparation—Cyclopropyl magnesium bromide and 2,2′-dithienyl ketone yield an oil that is treated with aqueous HBr to yield 4,4′-bis(2-thienyl)-1-bromobutene-3, which is refluxed with ethyl nipecotate and potassium carbonate in acetone and purified by column chromatography to form tiagabine methyl ester. The ester is saponified with alcoholic base to yield the acid which is converted to the hydrochloride. US Pat 5,010,090 (1991); *J Med Chem* 1993; 36:1776.

Description—Off-white crystals melting about 192° (decompn); base melts about 64°. pK$_{a1}$ 3.3; pK$_{a2}$ 9.4.

Solubility—Approximatley 30 mg/mL in water; insol in hydrocarbon solvents.

Comments—Approved for the adjunctive treatment of partial seizures in adults. Tiagabine was introduced into the US market in 1997 and was derived from a mechanistic-based drug discovery program that targeted the GABA-uptake carrier in the CNS. By selectively blocking GABA reuptake into both neurons and glial, tiagabine enhances GABA-mediated neurotransmission within the CNS. It is through this effect that tiagabine is thought to exert its anticonvulsant action.

Tiagabine is highly protein bound and extensively metabolized by the hepatic P-450 drug-metabolizing enzyme system. Both of these properties of tiagabine are likely to contribute to numerous drug–drug interaction and should be considered when tiagabine is added to the therapeutic regimen of patients who have epilepsy. The short half-life (7–9 hr) of tiagabine may necessitate multiple daily dosing (three to four times a day). Tiagabine does not appear to induce the metabolism of other antiepileptic drugs. For example, in patients being concomitantly treated with an enzyme-inducing antiepileptic drug (eg, phenytoin, carbamazepine, and phenobarbital), the half-life of tiagabine can be reduced from 7–9 to 4–7 hr.

Because an increase in seizure frequency has been reported after the discontinuation of therapy, the dosage should be reduced slowly.

The most commonly reported side effects associated with tiagabine use include somnolence, dizziness, and cognitive effects.

TOPIRAMATE

β-D-Fructopyranose, 2,3:4,5-bis-O-(1-methylethylidene)-, sulfamate; Topamax

[97240-79-4] $C_{12}H_{21}NO_8S$ (339.37).

Preparation—Fructose and acetone form the diacetonide (acetal) with the hydroxyl group in the C-1 position remaining free. The hydroxyl hydrogen is treated with NaH to form the alkoxide and then with sulfamoyl chloride to yield the product. US Pat 4,513,006 (1985); *J Med Chem*, 1987; 30: 880.

Description—White crystals that melt about 126°.

Comments—Topiramate was approved for the adjunctive treatment of partial seizures in 1996. Anecdotal reports suggest that the anticonvulsant profile of topiramate also includes efficacy against generalized seizures, including absence and myoclonic seizures. Topiramate has been reported to possess multiple mechanisms of action. For example, it appears to inhibit voltage-sensitive sodium channels, block non–NMDA-evoked glutamate currents, enhance GABA-evoked chloride currents, and inhibit carbonic anhydrase.

In clinical trials, the most troublesome adverse effects associated with topiramate use were CNS related. These included somnolence, fatigue, and certain troublesome cognitive side effects such as psychomotor slowing and word-finding difficulties. The cognitive effects associated with topiramate use were later shown to be lessened when the titration rate was decreased. There appears to be greater incidence of renal stones associated with topiramate use; however, this effect is reduced by maintenance of adequate hydration and probably is related to the carbonic inhibitory properties of topiramate. Last, a significant percentage of patients experienced weight loss.

TRIMETHADIONE

2,4-Oxazolidinedione, 3,5,5,-trimethyl-,Tridione

[127-48-0] $C_6H_9NO_3$ (143.14).

Preparation—By a series of reaction beginning with acetone and involving the following steps: conversion with HCN to acetone cyanhydrin, hydrolysis, and esterification with alcohol to ethyl dimethylgylcolae, condensation with urea to 5,5-dimethyloxazolidine-2,4-dione and methylation with dimethyl sulfate to trimethadione.

Description—White, crystalline granules; slight, camphor-like odor; melts about 46°.

Solubility—Soluble in water; freely soluble in alcohol, ether, or chloroform.

Comments—An alternate for the treatment of refractory generalized absence seizures. A frequent and troublesome adverse effect is hemeralopia.

VALPROATE SODIUM

Pentanoic acid, 2-propyl-, sodium salt; Depakene

$$CH_3CH_2CH_2CHCOONa$$
$$|$$
$$CH_3CH_2CH_2$$

Sodium 2-propylpentanoate; sodium 2-propylvalerate [1069-66-5] $C_8H_{15}NaO_2$ (166.20).

Preparation—Valproic acid may be synthesized from 4-heptanol by successive conversions to 4-bromoheptane with HBr, to 4-cyanoheptane with HCN and to 2-proplpentanoic (valproic) acid by alkaline hydrolysis of the 4-cyanoheptane.

Description—White, crystalline powder; odorless; saline taste; pK_a 4.95.

Solubility—Soluble in water or in alcohol.

Comments—It is unique both in its experimental and clinical profile of anticonvulsant action. It is effective in nontoxic doses against tonic seizures induced by either electroshock or strychnine, as well as against minimal-threshold seizures induced by either pentylenetetrazol, bicuculline, or picrotoxin. Clinical efficacy confirms this broad spectrum of antiepileptic activity. It is one of the drugs of choice in the management of simple absence seizures. Similarly, atypical absence seizures and myoclonic epilepsies respond well and, since there has never been an entirely satisfactory drug for these types of childhood epilepsy, this is an important advance. It also is effective in generalized tonic-clonic. In some refractory patients it has been used effectively in the management of partial seizures with complex symptomatology (psychomotor or temporal lobe seizures) or myoclonic and akinetic seizures. Like carbamazepine, valproate has been used with some success in the management of bipolar disorder and in the treatment of aggression or violence (*Am Pharm* 1993; NS33 (2): 47).

Approximately 90% to 95% is bound to plasma protein, volume distribution ranges from 0.1 to 0.5 L/kg (mean 0.2 L/kg), and half-life varies from 6 to 17 hr in adults and 4 to 14 hr in children. Therapeutic plasma levels range from 50 to 100 µg/mL; levels greater than 100 µg/mL are potentially toxic. More than ten metabolites have been identified in human blood and urine. Only 0.5% to 20% is excreted unchanged in the urine. Of the several metabolites, only 2-propyl-2-pentenoic acid (2–2-en-VPA) has been shown to accumulate in the brain. The 2–VPA metabolite is approximately 1.3 times more potent than the parent drug and may contribute significantly to the anticonvulsant effect of chronically administered valproate.

The precise mechanism of its anticonvulsant action is still unknown. It has been postulated that its administration inhibits GABA-transaminase and thus increases the concentration of cerebral GABA. However, other saturated straight-chain fatty acids (propionic, butyric, and pentanoic) that lack anticonvulsant properties are more potent inhibitors of GABA-transaminase than is valproic acid. It has been also reported that there is a strong correlation between the anticonvulsant potency of valproate and other branched-chain fatty acids and their ability to reduce the concentration of cerebral aspartate.

It may decrease binding to serum proteins or block hepatic metabolism of phenobarbital. Administration of the drug to patients in a steady state while on phenobarbital (or primidone, which is metabolized to phenobarbital) can increase the plasma levels of phenobarbital from 35% to 200%, causing excessive somnolence. Present evidence indicates this is caused by an immediate decrease in the rate of elimination of phenobarbital. This drug interacts unpredictably with phenytoin; it has been associated not only with lowered serum phenytoin levels and increased seizure frequency, but also with increased free phenytoin levels and phenytoin toxicity. Valproate also has been found to increase the clearness of felbamate significantly and to reduce its plasma concentration correspondingly. Conversely, phenobarbital, primidone, phenytoin, and other drugs may induce enzymes that metabolize this drug and reduce its half-life. In contrast, felbamate has been shown to increase the plasma concentration of valproate when the two drugs are administered concurrently.

More than 40 cases of fatal hepatic failure have been reported in patients on this therapy. The risk of hepatic failure is drastically less in patients on monotherapy (*ca* 1/37,000) compared with those on polytherapy (*ca* 1/6500). Moreover, the incidence is much greater in children younger than 2 yr and who are on polytherapy (monotherapy, 1.42/10,000; polytherapy, *ca* 1/500).

The most commonly observed side effects in patients on monotherapy (valproate) are weight gain (11%), sedation (10%), nausea (6%), headache (3%), tremor (3%), hair loss (1%), and dizziness (1%). Other rarely observed untoward effects include skin rashes, enuresis, insomnia, anxiety, fatigue, and paresthesias. Teratogenic effects have been reported in animals. Moreover, its use by women who have epilepsy during the first trimester (3 months) of pregnancy has been reported by the Centers for Disease Control, United States Public Health Service (USPHS), to be associated with increased risk (1.2%) of spina bifida in their infants (*MMWR* 1982; 31). Although the majority of women who have epilepsy and who are taking this drug will give birth to nonaffected babies, it is recommended that they consider prenatal testing for neural tube defects.

ZONISAMIDE

2-Benzisoxazole-3-methanesulfonamide; Zonegran

[68291-97-4] $C_8H_8O_3S$ (212.23).

Preparation—A mixture of 3-bromoethyl-1,2-benzisoxazole with sodium sulfite in methanol/water is stirred at 50° for 4 hrs, vacuum distilled and crystallized to yield 3-(1,2-benzisoxazolyl)methanesulfonic acid, converted to the acid chloride with $POCl_3$ and then treated with ammonia to form the amide which is zonisamide. *J Med Chem* 1974; 22:180.

Description—White needles from ethyl acetate melting about 163°; pK_a 12.2.

Solubility—Sparingly soluble in water (0.8 mg/mL), chloroform or hexane; soluble in methanol, ethanol, ethyl acetate or acetic acid.

Comments—The precise mechanism through which zonisamide exerts its antiseizure activity is unknown. It demonstrated anticonvulsive activity in several experimental models. The effects may be produced through action at sodium and calcium channels. In vitro pharmacological studies suggest that zonisamide blocks sodium channels and reduces voltage-dependent, transient inward currents (T-type Ca^{2+} currents, consequently stabilizing neuronal membranes and suppressing neuronal hypersynchronization. In vitro binding studies have demonstrated that zonisamide binds to the GABA/benzodiazepine receptor ionophore complex in an allosteric fashion which does not produce changes in chloride flux. Other in vitro studies have demonstrated that zonisamide suppresses synaptically driven electrical activity without affecting postsynaptic GABA or glutamate responses or neuronal or glial uptake of [^{3}H]-GABA. Thus, zonisamide does not appear to potentiate the synaptic activity of GABA. In vivo microdialysis studies demonstrated that zonisamide facilitates both dopaminergic and serotonergic neurotransmission. Zonisamide also has weak carbonic anhydrase inhibiting activity, but this pharmacologic effect is not thought to be a major contributing factor in the antiseizure activity of zonisamide.

OTHER ANTIEPILEPTIC DRUGS

Several other established antiepileptic drugs are available for management of seizure disorders; however, these have been relegated to late-stage treatment primarily because of the development of less toxic and more efficacious agents.

CHAPTER 82

Psychopharmacologic Agents

Joel Shuster, PharmD, BCPP

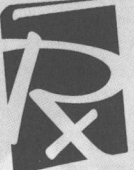

Many conditions that afflict people are related to mental function. Some of these are transient with symptoms that are moderately uncomfortable but that are not incapacitating. Often, these symptoms are responses to events in our lives, but in some cases there is not an identified precipitating cause. On the other end of the spectrum are severe mental disorders that prevent an individual from functioning appropriately in society. It is estimated that approximately 20% of people will suffer sometime during their life from a mental condition that affects their ability to function with normal efficiency. Although some of the conditions related to mental function can be resolved through counseling and nondrug therapy, management of others requires pharmacological intervention. Although pharmacotherapy does not cure mental disorders in the same sense that antibiotics cure infectious diseases, the available drugs do control most symptomatic manifestations and behavioral problems, facilitate the patient's tendency toward remission, and improve his or her capacity for social, occupational, and familial adjustment.

Drugs that alter the mind and behavior have attracted the attention of man since the beginning of recorded history. Without the benefits of science and medicine, mankind has sought emotional comfort or novelty through the use of drugs for a venerable period of time. To cite two examples, alcohol and opium have been used for this purpose since antiquity. However, it was the inadvertent discovery of the unusual psychotomimetic properties of lysergic acid diethylamide in 1943 and the subsequent demonstration that these effects were similar to those induced by mescaline that marked the beginning of psychopharmacology. Additional interest in this new science was created with the introduction of chlorpromazine for the empiric treatment of mental disorders. The successful clinical use of this agent not only led to the realization that behavior can be studied objectively in laboratory animals but also resulted in the discovery of a host of new drugs that stimulate, sedate, or otherwise change behavior.

More than 1500 compounds classified as psychoactive or psychotropic drugs have been described, and approximately 20% of all prescriptions written in the US are for medications intended to alter mental processes and behavior. Those agents employed in the treatment of psychotic illnesses and depressant disorders are the focus of this chapter. Antianxiety drugs are not discussed here because the spectrum of effects of these agents includes sedative-hypnotic actions. These drugs are covered in Chapter 80 with the conventional sedative and hypnotic agents.

ANTIPSYCHOTIC AGENTS

One of the major uses of the antipsychotic drugs is treatment of schizophrenia. Manifestations of the disease include two types of symptoms: positive and negative. Positive symptoms tend to be exaggerations of normal functioning. For example, a distortion of perceptions may be manifest as an auditory hallucination, and a distortion of thought process may be manifest as delusions. Negative symptoms involve loss of normal functioning and include blunted affect, asociality, reduced ability to relate to others, lack of motivation and drive, narrowing of ideation, and poverty of speech. The spectrum of symptoms varies widely between afflicted persons. To aid in diagnosis and treatment, psychiatrists have classified schizophrenia into various types: disorganized (hebephrenic), paranoid, catatonic, undifferentiated, and residual. Symptoms usually manifest during the early years of adulthood, and approximately 1% of people are affected across all cultures and ethnic groups. Oftentimes, the symptoms are debilitating relative to the ability to function in society. The illness is chronic, and less than 20% of patients recover fully from a single episode of psychosis. Rates of employment among people who have schizophrenia rarely exceed 20%, and schizophrenia accounts for approximately 10% of all suicides.

The cause of schizophrenia is unknown, although it is almost certainly the result of flawed neurochemistry. The fact that major symptoms do not manifest until young adulthood suggests that abnormalities in brain development might be involved. Imaging techniques show alterations in patterns of activity in a variety of brain regions, with the prefrontal cortex and the thalamic areas being particularly affected. Because an underlying morphological or structural deficit likely is the cause of schizophrenia, pharmacotherapy cannot cure but can only hope to normalize the balance between various brain circuits.

The first successful pharmacological treatment of schizophrenia was introduced in 1952 with the advent of the use of chlorpromazine (which was originally marketed as a new antihistamine) to treat psychotic illness. Over the years, other antipsychotic drugs with similar efficacy have become available. These drugs are now grouped together under the title "typical" antipsychotics or neuroleptics. They are mainly effective against the positive symptoms of schizophrenia and often cause both short- and long-term movement disorders. Thus, in schizophrenic patients, the typical antipsychotics reduce or eliminate the positive symptoms of hallucinations, delusions, and thought disorganization in a majority of patients. The widespread use of these moderately safe compounds has greatly reduced the number of chronic patients residing in public mental hospitals, shortened the duration of hospitalization for acute episodes, and shifted the focus of treatment of mental disorders from institutional care to community-based ambulatory treatment programs. This clinical efficacy is accompanied by significant adverse effects. Depending on the agent used, adverse effects include sedation, dry mouth, sexual dysfunction, akathisia, bradykinesia, rigidity, and sometimes tardive dyskinesia. Although these drugs are a major advance in the treatment of schizophrenia, as many as 33% of those treated do not respond to therapy, and as many as 40% of those whose symptoms are alleviated by drug therapy discontinue their medication because of adverse effects. In addition to their use to treat schizophrenia, several of these drugs are also effective antiemetic and antinausea agents.

A new type of antipsychotic medication became available with the introduction of clozapine in 1990. After its success, other medications with similar clinical profiles have been developed. These *atypical* or *novel* antipsychotic agents are effective against both the positive and the negative symptoms of schizophrenia and seldom cause movement disorders. Although the atypical agents are more expensive than the typical drugs, recent evaluations of the total costs of treatment show that the atypical drugs are economically superior. This is because the increased efficacy and higher rate of compliance result in fewer hospital admissions and other emergency interventions.

Although pharmacotherapy normalizes many aspects of thinking and emotion, the antipsychotic drugs alone do not allow most patients to function fully in society. Intensive training in social and job-related skills is often required.

The mechanism of action of the antipsychotic agents is complex, and many details remain to be established. However, evaluation of properties shared by effective antipsychotic agents provides clues to their mechanism of action. All of the typical antipsychotic agents block postsynaptic dopaminergic receptors (in the basal ganglia, hypothalamus, limbic system, brainstem, and medulla) and act as competitive antagonists of dopamine centrally and peripherally. The clinically observed potency of the drugs in this class is directly correlated with the affinity for binding to the D2 family of dopaminergic receptors. This observation coupled with the fact that drugs increase dopaminergic activity (levodopa, amphetamine, cocaine, apomorphine) aggravate schizophrenia or produce it in some nonpsychotic individuals led to the hypothesis that excessive activity of dopaminergic systems may be a cause of schizophrenia. However, the dopamine hypothesis of schizophrenia does not account for all of the pathology of the disease. For example, many patients do not respond to treatment with drugs that block dopaminergic receptors, the degree of dopaminergic receptor block shown in positron emission tomography (PET) scans does not correlate with clinical responses, and the atypical agents show little dopaminergic receptor antagonism. Some of the atypical antipsychotic drugs have a high affinity for the serotonin 5-HT2 receptor, making it likely that a combination of interference with some subset of dopaminergic and serotonergic neurotransmission is required for clinical effectiveness. However, the situation may be even more complex, as some studies suggest a correlation of clinical efficacy with α-adrenoceptor blocking potency.

Relating to mechanism of action of antipsychotic drugs, schizophrenic patients often require weeks of treatment to attain therapeutic benefit, and many patients experience an increase in clinical efficacy with long duration of treatment. These and other observations suggest that it is the response of brain systems to long-term effects of the antipsychotic drugs that accounts for their therapeutic effectiveness. One experimental model supporting this concept shows that chronic treatment of animals with any active antipsychotic drug results eventually in the loss of ability (called depolarization block) of these drugs to increase ventral-tegmental area dopaminergic cell firing.

The effective antipsychotic drugs vary significantly in selectivity and potency for the three known subtypes of receptor within the dopaminergic D2 family, and all, to some degree, are competitive antagonists of other neurotransmitters. This variation in activity at a variety of receptors accounts for differences in adverse effects of the drugs. The extrapyramidal toxicity appears to be related to antagonism of the dopaminergic D2 family of receptors in the caudate-putamen brain areas. The extrapyramidal toxicity also is related inversely to the central anticholinergic properties of the drugs. Many of the various peripheral effects, including the cardiovascular effects of some of these agents, are attributable to anticholinergic properties and peripheral α-adrenergic blockade.

A drug with significantly different action is lithium carbonate. Its major use is in the treatment of bipolar (manic depressant) affective disorder. In addition, it is sometimes used as an adjunct with other antipsychotic drugs in the treatment of a variety of psychotic disorders.

Typical Antipsychotics

Several different typical antipsychotics are available. Structurally, they can be divided into five groups: phenothiazines, thioxanthenes, butyrophenones, dihydroindolone derivatives, and dibenzoxazepines. The numerous phenothiazines and related congeners have qualitatively similar clinical efficacy, but their potency and side effects are influenced significantly by their chemical structure. For example, congeners with an aliphatic side chain, such as chlorpromazine, are fairly low in potency and high in sedative effects. Conversely, congeners with a piperazine constituent are more potent and have less sedative effects but more prominent extrapyramidal toxicity. A thioxanthene is a phenothiazine in which the nitrogen at the 10 position is replaced by a carbon atom with a double bond to the side chain. Thus phenothiazines and thioxanthenes are closely related chemically and have many biological effects in common.

Experimentally, the phenothiazines suppress or abolish conditioned avoidance responses in trained rats, prevent morphine-induced mania in cats, and reduce the toxicity of amphetamine in aggregated mice. Many of these compounds also suppress vomiting from apomorphine, irradiation, and motion sickness but, in laboratory animals, do not affect the emesis from morphine, veratrum alkaloids, digitalis, and copper sulfate. In addition, they decrease spontaneous motor activity, lower electroshock seizure threshold, and cause skeletal muscle relaxation. The phenothiazines also exhibit weak adrenolytic, hypotensive, antispasmodic, hypothermic, and antihistaminic effects.

In general, the typical antipsychotic drugs are highly lipid soluble and protein bound (92–99%). Consequently, they tend to have large volumes of distribution (usually more than 7 L/kg); bioavailability after oral administration is variable and low (25–35%). Plasma half-life tends to be short, ranging from 10 to 20 hr, but the duration of the antipsychotic action is much longer. Metabolites may be found in the urine weeks after the last dose of drug. This suggests that large amounts of the drug are sequestered in the tissues.

The phenothiazines are indicated for the management of psychotic disorders, control of nausea and vomiting, control of manic depression, relief of intractable hiccups and acute intermittent porphyria, and as an adjunct in the treatment of tetanus. The thioxanthenes (chlorprothixene and thiothixene) are used for the management of the symptoms of psychotic disorders. Butyrophenone (haloperidol) also is employed for the management of symptoms of psychoses, including schizophrenia, the manic phase of manic depressive illness or psychotic reactions associated with organic brain syndrome or mental retardation. Dibenzoxazepine (loxapine succinate) is indicated for the management of schizophrenia.

Many of the contraindications to the use of these drugs are similar. For example, they are contraindicated in comatose patients who have received large amounts of central nervous system (CNS)-depressant drugs (alcohol, barbiturates, narcotics, etc.), in patients who have Parkinson's disease and in patients who have a known history of hypersensitivity to these agents. It is not known whether there is cross sensitivity between the phenothiazines and the thioxanthenes, but this possibility should be kept in mind.

The safe use of many of these agents during pregnancy has not been established with respect to possible adverse effects on fetal development. The safe use of thioxanthenes in children has not been established. It is recommended that these agents not be used in children younger than 12 years of age. Geriatric or debilitated patients usually require a lower initial dose of these agents; the dose then is increased as needed and tolerated. Both phenothiazines and thioxanthenes have an anticholinergic effect; hence, they should be used with extreme caution in patients who have a history of glaucoma or prostatic hypertrophy. All agents in these groups tend to impair the mental and the physical ability required for operating a motor vehicle or complex hazardous machinery. Patients should be warned accordingly.

Phenothiazines and thioxanthenes may significantly affect the actions of other drugs (see Chapter 102 for additional information concerning specific drug interactions). They may increase, prolong, or intensify the action of CNS depressants (anesthetics, alcohol, barbiturates, narcotics, etc); therefore, appropriate adjustments in dosage of narcotics and barbiturates should be made when such agents are to be administered concomitantly. These agents also lower convulsive threshold; hence, they should be used with extreme caution in patients who have a history of epilepsy. They also should be cautiously used in patients receiving atropine and related drugs because of the possible additive anticholinergic effect. Because these agents have antiemetic properties, they may mask signs of drug overdosage and obscure symptoms of brain tumor or intestinal obstruction. These agents also should be used with extreme caution in patients who have cardiovascular disease, chronic respiratory disorders, impaired liver function, or a history of gastric ulcer; the aggravation of a preexisting ulcer has been reported.

Although not all the adverse reactions listed herein have occurred after administration of either phenothiazines or thioxanthenes, the chemical and the pharmacological similarities of the two groups suggest that all of the known side effects and toxicities associated with these agents should be kept in mind. CNS effects include drowsiness, particularly during the first or the second week of therapy; and extrapyramidal reactions (EPS or EPRs) may be fairly common. Extrapyramidal effects are usually of three types: (1) Parkinsonian-like syndrome, (2) dystonia and dyskinesia, including torticollis, tics, and other involuntary muscle movements, and (3) akathisia, shown by restlessness and an urge to move about. Hyperreflexia has been reported in the newborn when phenothiazines are used during pregnancy. *Grand mal* seizures, catatonic-like states, psychotic symptoms, and cerebral edema also have been reported. Cardiovascular effects include postural hypotension, tachycardia, bradycardia, faintness, dizziness, and cardiac arrest. Hematological effects, including agranulocytosis, eosinophilia, leukopenia, hemolytic anemia, thrombocytopenic purpura, and pancytopenia have been reported. Liver jaundice has been observed but is usually reversible. Allergic reactions of urticaria or dermatitis also occur in approximately 5% of patients. Photosensitivity, resulting in an increased propensity to sunburn, occurs in some patients. Antipsychotic drugs exert endocrine effects: these agents block ovulation, suppress the menstrual cycle, and cause infertility and pseudopregnancy, lactation, and breast engorgement in females. They reduce urinary levels of gonadotropins, estrogens, and progestins. In males, gynecomastia or changes in libido have been observed. Cholesterol levels also are increased significantly. Other reported reactions include dry mouth, nasal congestion, constipation, myosis, mydriasis, urinary retention, increased appetite, weight gain, peripheral edema, fever, and suppression of cough reflex. The last may enhance the potential of aspiration or asphyxia. Prolonged therapy with antipsychotic drugs at high doses may cause pigmentation of exposed skin areas; ocular changes consisting of lenticular and corneal opacities, epithelial keratopathies, and pigmentary retinopathy; impaired vision (Table 82-1). See also Chapter 61.

CHLORPROMAZINE HYDROCHLORIDE

10*H*-Phenothiazine-10-propanamine, 2-chloro-*N*,*N*-dimethyl-, monohydrochloride; Thorazine Hydrochloride

2-Chloro-10-[3-(dimethylamino)propyl]phenothiazine monohydrochloride [69-09-0] $C_{17}H_{19}ClN_2S \cdot HCl$ (355.32)

Table 82-1. Table of Typical Antipsychotic Drugs

GENERIC NAME	TRADE NAME	COMMENTS
Chlorpromazine	Thorazine	A phenothiazine with low clinical potency, medium extrapyramidal toxicity, high sedative effect, and high hypotensive action
Droperidol	Inapsine	A butyrophenone with low clinical potency, medium extrapyramidal toxicity, and high sedative effect—only approved for sedation and treatment of nausea and vomiting; high hypotensive action
Fluphenazine	Permitil, Prolixin	A phenothiazine with high clinical potency, high extrapyramidal toxicity, low sedative effect, and low hypotensive action
Haloperidol	Haldol	A butyrophenone with high clinical potency, high extrapyramidal toxicity, low sedative effect, and low hypotensive action
Loxapine	Loxitane	A dibenzoxazepine with medium clinical potency, medium extrapyramidal toxicity, low sedative effect, and low hypotensive action
Mesoridazine	Serentil	A phenothiazine with medium clinical potency, low extrapyramidal toxicity, high sedative effect, and medium hypotensive action
Molindone	Moban	A dihydroindolone with medium clinical potency, low extrapyramidal toxicity, medium sedative effect, and no hypotensive action
Perphenazine	Trilafon	A phenothiazine with high clinical potency, medium extrapyramidal toxicity, medium sedative effect, and low hypotensive action
Pimozide	Orap	High clinical potency, high extrapyramidal toxicity, low sedative effect, and low hypotensive action
Prochlorperazine	Compazine	A phenothiazine used for treatment of nausea and vomiting
Promazine	Sparine	A phenothiazine with low clinical potency, medium extrapyramidal toxicity, high sedative effect, and high hypotensive action
Thioridazine	Mellaril	A phenothiazine with low clinical potency, low extrapyramidal toxicity, high sedative effect medium, and hypotensive action
Thiothixene	Navane	A thioxanthene with high clinical potency, medium extrapyramidal toxicity, medium sedative effect, and medium hypotensive action
Trifluoperazine	Stelazine	A phenothiazine with high clinical potency, high extrapyramidal toxicity, low sedative effect, and low hypotensive action

MEDICINAL AGENTS

Description—White or slightly creamy white, odorless, crystalline powder; darkens on prolonged exposure to light; melts about 196°.

Solubility—1 g in 1 mL of water, 1.5 mL of alcohol, or 1.5 mL of chloroform; insoluble in ether or in benzene.

Comments—A *phenothiazine* with low clinical potency, medium extrapyramidal toxicity, high sedative effect, and high hypotensive action.

DROPERIDOL

2H-Benzimidazol-2-one, 1-[1-[4-(4-fluorophenyl)-4-oxobutyl]-1,2,3,6-tetrahydro-4-pyridinyl-1,3-dihydro-, Inapsine

1-[1-[3-(p-Flurorbenzoyl)propyl]-1,2,3,6-tetrahydro-4-pyridyl]]-2- benzimidazolinone [548-73-2] $C_{22}H_{22}FN_3O_2$ (379.43).

Preparation—4-Chloro-4'-flurobutyrophenone is prepared from γ-butyrolactone and reacted with 1-(1,2,3,6-tetrahydro-4-pyridyl)-2-benzimidazolinone in the presence of a suitable condensing agent. US Pat 3,161,645.

Description—White to light tan, amorphous or microcrystalline powder; odorless and tasteless (*Note:* Because this compound is extremely potent, no taste test is recommended.); sensitive to light, air, and heat; hygroscopic; melts at approximately 146° after being dried in a vacuum at 70° for 4 hr, pKa 7.6.

Solubility—1 g in 10,000 mL of water, 140 mL of alcohol, 4 mL of chloroform, or 500 mL of ether.

Comments—A *butyrophenone* with low clinical potency, medium extrapyramidal toxicity, high sedative effect, and high hypotensive action. It is approved only for sedation and treatment of nausea and vomiting.

FLUPHENAZINE DECANOATE

1-Piperazineethanol, 4-[3-[2-(trifluoromethyl)-10H-phenothizin-10-yl]-propyl]-, decanoate (ester); Prolixin Decanoate

[30909-31-4] $C_{32}H_{44}F_3N_3O_2S$ (591.77).

Preparation—Fluphenazine (see *Fluphenazine Hydrochloride*) is esterified with decanoyl chloride in the presence of pyridine. US Pats 3,194,733 and 3,394,131.

Description—Pale yellow to yellowish orange viscous liquid with a characteristic odor; light sensitive; melts about 31°.

Solubility—Insoluble in water; soluble in alcohol, acetone, benzene, or ether.

Comments—See *Fluphenazine Hydrochloride*.

FLUPHENAZINE ENANTHATE

Prolixin Enanthate

[2746-81-8] $C_{29}H_{38}F_3N_3O_2S$ (549.69).

Preparation—Fluphenazine is esterified through reaction with enanthoyl chloride in the presence of pyridine. For the preparation of fluphenazine, see *Fluphenazine Hydrochloride*. US Pat 3,058,979.

Description—Pale yellow to yellow-orange, clear to slightly turbid, viscous liquid with a characteristic odor; *not recommended to be tasted*; unstable in strong light, but stable in air at room temperature.

Solubility—1 g in <1 mL of alcohol, <1 mL of chloroform, or 2 mL of ether; insoluble in water.

Comments—See *Fluphenazine Hydrochloride*.

FLUPHENAZINE HYDROCHLORIDE

Permitil; Prolixin

[146-56-5] $C_{22}H_{26}F_3N_3OS.2HCl$ (510.44).

Preparation—Fluphenazine may be prepared by condensing 2-(trifluoromethyl)-10-(3-chloropropyl)phenothiazine with 1-piperazineethanol in toluene with the aid of sodamide. Reaction of the purified base with a double molar quantity of hydrogen chloride yields the official salt. The starting phenothiazine compound may be prepared by heating 3-(trifluoromethyl)diphenylamine with sulfur and condensing the resulting 2-(trifluoromethyl)phenothiazine with 1-bromo-3-chloro-propane. US Pat 3,058,979.

Description—White or nearly white, odorless, crystalline powder; melts within a 5° range above 225°.

Solubility—1 g in 1.4 mL of water or 6.7 mL of alcohol; slightly soluble in chloroform; practically insoluble in ether.

Comments—A *phenothiazine* with high clinical potency and extrapyramidal toxicity, low sedative effect, and low hypotensive action.

HALOPERIDOL

1-Butanone, 4-[2-(chlorophenyl)-4-hydroxy-1-piperidinyl]-1-(4-fluorophenyl)-, Haldol

4-[4-(p-Chlorophenyl)-4-hydroxypiperidino-4'-fluorobutyrophenone [52-86-8]

$C_{21}H_{23}ClFNO2$ (375.87).

Preparation—4-(p-Chlorophenyl)-4-piperidinol is condensed with 4-chloro-4'-fluorobutyrophenone in a toluene solution. The haloperidol thus formed is isolated and recrystallized from a solvent such as disopropyl ether. The starting substituted piperidinol may be prepared from p-chloro-α-methylstyrene by the method described by Schmidle and Mansfield (*J Am Chem Soc* 1956; 78:1702).

Description—White to faintly yellowish, odorless, amorphous, or microcrystalline powder; light sensitive and nonhygroscopic; saturated solution is neutral to litmus; melts about 150°; pKa 8.2 to 8.3.

Solubility—1 g in >10,000 mL of water, 60 mL of alcohol, 15 mL of chloroform, or 200 mL of ether.

Comments—A butyrophenone that is indicated for the management of symptoms of psychotic disorders and the control of tics and vocal utterances of Tourette's Disorder. Haloperidol is effective for the treatment of severe behavior problems in children who have combative, explosive hyperexcitability. Haloperidol is effective in the short-term treatment of hyperactive children who show excessive motor activity with accompanying conduct disorders consisting of some or all of the following symptoms: impulsivity, difficulty sustaining attention, aggressiveness, mood lability, and poor frustration tolerance. Haloperidol should be reserved for use in managing behavioral problems of children who fail to respond to psychotherapy or other medications.

The bioavailability of haloperidol has been reported to be approximately 60% via the oral route. The half-life of elimination ranges from 12 to 38 hr after oral administration of the drug but is reduced to 10 to 19 hr after intravenous administration. Therapeutic plasma levels usually range from 3 to 10 ng/mL, but some patients require significantly higher levels before adequate antipsychotic effects are observed.

Haloperidol is contraindicated in severe toxic CNS depression or comatose states from any cause and in individuals who are hypersensitive to this drug or who have Parkinson's disease. Potential adverse effects from the use of haloperidol include tardive dyskinesia (potentially irreversible, involuntary, dyskinetic movements—rhythmical involuntary movements of tongue, face, mouth or jaw), neuroleptic malignant syndrome (hyperpyrexia, muscle rigidity, altered mental status, autonomic instability), extrapyramidal symptoms (Parkinson-like symptoms, akathisia, dystonia). Care should be exercised when antihypertensive agents, general anesthetics, hypnotics, alcohol, analgesics, and other CNS depressants are used concomitantly with this drug, because it may potentiate their actions. There is considerable variation from patient to patient in the amount of medication required for treatment.

HALOPERIDOL DECANOATE

Decanoic acid, 4-(4-chlorophenyl)-1-[4-(4-fluorophenyl)-4-oxo-butyl]-4-piperidinyl ester; Haldol Decanoate

[74050-97-8] $C_{31}H_{41}ClFNO_3$ (530.13).

Preparation—The alcohol moiety of the ester is obtained by the condensation of 4-(p-chloro-4'-fluorobutyrophenone and 4-(p-chlorophenyl)-4-piperidinol in toluene solution which is esterified with decanoyl chloride. *JACS* 1956; 78:1702 and Eur Pat Appl 260,070.

Description—Log P 3.98.

Solubility—Almost insoluble in water (0.01 mg/mL), but is soluble in most organic solvents. The IM injection is in sesame oil.

LITHIUM CARBONATE

Carbonic acid, dilithium salt; Eskalith

Dilithium carbonate [554-13-2] Li_2CO_3 (73.89).

Preparation—Lithium chloride is metathesized with sodium carbonate in aqueous solution.

Description—White, light, granular powder; melts about 62°.

Solubility—1 g in 78 mL of cold water or 140 mL of boiling water; slightly soluble in alcohol; dissolved by dilute acids.

Comments—Indicated for the treatment of *bipolar disorder*, both for treatment of acute mania and for prophylaxis against recurrences. Other psychiatric conditions that may be benefited include recurrent severe depressions without manic episodes, schizoaffective psychosis, episodic alcoholism, periodic antisocial behavior, and periodic schizophrenic illness. Bipolar affective (manic depressive) is a very serious psychiatric disorder characterized by wide fluctuations in mood. Patients who have cyclic attacks of mania have many symptoms that resemble paranoid schizophrenia (grandiosity, bellicosity, paranoid thoughts, and over activity). These are interspersed with periods of fairly normal mood and behavior and periods of depression. Maintenance therapy with lithium prevents or diminishes the intensity of subsequent episodes of mania in those manic-depressive patients. The overall success rate for achieving remission from the manic phase of bipolar disorder is reported to be 60% to 80%.

Neither the cause of bipolar disorder nor the mechanism of action of lithium is known. The best-defined pharmacological effect of lithium is alteration of second messenger pathways involving inositol phosphate compounds. Lithium blocks several enzymes involved in recycling of inositol compounds, eventually leading to a depletion of phosphatidylinositol-4,5-bisphosphate, the membrane precursor of inositol-based second messengers and diacylglycerol. Lithium also inhibits second messenger systems involving adenylyl cyclase, alters sodium transport in nerve and muscle cells, and affects a shift toward interneuronal metabolism of catecholamines and serotonin.

Lithium carbonate is completely absorbed 6 to 8 hours after oral administration. Its plasma half-life is approximately 24 hr. It is excreted by the kidneys, and approximately 80% of filtered lithium is reabsorbed by a carrier in the renal tubules. Lithium competes for this carrier with sodium, and therefore sodium depletion decreases renal excretion of lithium, resulting in lithium accumulation. The lithium ion is distributed in total body water but is concentrated in various tissues to different degrees. After a steady state has been reached, approximately 40% is contained in cerebrospinal fluid, and renal clearance is somewhat constant. Serum levels should be maintained between 0.7 and 1.3 mEq/L. Adverse effects are noted at levels higher than 1.5 mEq/L, and serious toxicity is common when concentrations exceed 2.0 mEq/L. Because toxicity develops at serum levels little higher than effective therapeutic levels, frequent monitoring and dosage adjustments are mandatory for successful therapy.

Nausea, vomiting, and diarrhea are presumptive evidence of toxicity and indicate the dose should be reduced. The most common untoward effects are slight tremor and polyuria; these ordinarily do not require a reduction in dosages. CNS effects, such as slurred speech, blurred vision, confusion, and lethargy, require immediate withdrawal of the drug and the administration of sodium chloride (at least 4 g extra a day) to facilitate the excretion of lithium. Adverse cardiovascular

effects include arrhythmias and hypotension. Goiter, hypothyroidism, and diabetes insipidus also have been observed. Lithium should not be used in patients who have cardiovascular or renal disease. Lithium must be used with caution during pregnancy as it can cause cardiac and other birth defects. The drug should not be used in children younger than 12 yr.

LOXAPINE SUCCINATE

Dibenz[*b,f*][1,4]oxapine, 2-chloro-11-(4-methyl-1-piperazinyl)-, butanedioate (salt); Loxitane

[27833-64-3] $C_{18}H_{18}ClN_3$.$C_4H_6O_4$ (445.90).

Preparation—A method of synthesis of loxapine starting with anthone oxime is described in US Pat 3,412,193. Other procedures are summarized in *CA* 1965; 63:11592h.

Description—White to off-white, crystalline powder; pK_a 6.6 (loxapine).

Solubility—Slightly soluble in water or alcohol.

Comments—A *dibenzoxazepine* with medium clinical potency and extrapyramidal toxicity, low sedative effect, and low hypotensive action.

MESORIDAZINE BESYLATE

10*H*-Phenothiazine, 10-[2-(1-methyl-2-piperidinyl)ethyl]-2-(methylsulfinyl)-, monobenzenesulfonate; Serentil

[32672-69-8] $C_{21}H_{26}N_2OS_2$.$C_6H_6O_3S$ (544.74).

Preparation—Nitrophenide [bis(3-nitrophenyl)disulfide)] is converted by a series of reactions into 2-(methylthio)phenothiazine. Oxidation with H_2O_2 yields the corresponding sulfinyl compound that is reacted with 1-methyl-2-(2-chloroethyl)piperidine in the presence of a suitable condensing agent and the mesoridazine thus formed is converted, with benzenesulfonic acid, to the besylate salt. US Pat 3,084,161.

Description—White to pale yellow, crystalline powder with a faint odor; melts about 178°.

Solubility—1 g in 1 mL of water, 11 mL of alcohol, 3 mL of chloroform, or 6300 mL of ether.

Comments—A *phenothiazine* with medium clinical potency, low extrapyramidal toxicity, high sedative effect, and medium hypotensive action.

MOLINDONE HYDROCHLORIDE

4*H*-Indol-4-one, 3-ethyl-1,4,6,7-tetrahydro-2-methyl-5-(4-morpholinylmethyl)-, monohydrochloride; Moban

[15622-68-8] $C_{16}H_{24}N_2O_2$.HCl (312.84).

Preparation—From 4-(morpholinyl)-1,3-cyclohexanedione and 2-oximino-3-pentanone in acetic acid by refluxing with powdered zinc yields the base that may be converted to the hydrochloride by usual procedures. See Belg Pat 670,798; *CA* 1966; 65,7148f.

Description—White crystals; melts about 180°.

Solubility—Freely soluble in water or alcohol.

Comments—A *dihydroindolone* with medium clinical potency, low extrapyramidal toxicity, medium sedative effect, and no hypotensive action.

PERPHENAZINE

1-Piperazineethanol, 4-[3-(2-chloro-10H-phenothiazin-10-yl)propyl]-, Trilafon

[58-39-9] $C_{21}H_{26}ClN_3OS$ (403.97).

Preparation—A toluene solution of 2-chloro-10-(3-chloropropyl) phenothiazine and 1-piperazineethanol is refluxed with sodamide and the resulting perphenazine purified by means of vacuum distillation. US Pat 2,766,235.

Description—White to creamy white, light-sensitive powder; almost odorless and has a bitter taste; melts about 97°.

Solubility—1 g in 7 mL of alcohol or 13 mL of acetone; practically insoluble in water; freely soluble in chloroform.

Comments—A *phenothiazine* with high clinical potency, medium extrapyramidal toxicity, medium sedative effect, and low hypotensive action.

PIMOZIDE

2H-Benzimidazol-2-one, 1-[1-[4,4-bis(fluorophenyl)butyl]-4-piperindinyl]-1,3-dihydro-, Orap

[2062-78-4] $C_{28}H_{29}F_2N_3O$ (461.55).

Preparation—The ethyl ester of 1-benzyl-4-oxo-3-piperidinecarboxylic acid and *o*-phenylenediamine are condensed, with the loss of the elements of water and ethanol, to yield I. With hydrogen and Pd catalyst, the benzyl group is removed from I, and the unsaturation is reduced to give II, 1(2H)-(4-piperidinyl)benzimidazol-2-one. The other necessary intermediate is formed from a Grignard reaction between *p*-fluoro-phenylmagnesium bromide and ethyl cyclohexyl-propanecarboxylate to give 4,4′-difluorophenyl)-4-chloro-1-butene. Catalytic reduction of the 1,1-bis(4-fluorophenyl)-4-chloro-1-butene. Catalytic reduction of the double bond followed by condensation with II in the presence of Na_2CO_3 yields pimozide.

(I)   (II)

Description—Crystals; melts about 216°; pKa, 7.32.

Solubility—Practically soluble in water; 1 g in 140 mL of alcohol, 5 mL of chloroform, or 500 mL of ether; slightly soluble in dilute aqueous acid solution.

Comments—Has high clinical potency, high extrapyramidal toxicity, low sedative effect, and low hypotensive action.

PROCHLORPERAZINE

For the full monograph, see page 1312.

Comments—A *phenothiazine* used for treating nausea and vomiting.

PROMAZINE HYDROCLORIDE

10H-Phenothiazine-10-propanamine, N,N-dimethyl-, monohydrochloride; Sparine; Prozine

10-[3-Dimethylamino)propyl]phenothiazine monohydrochloride [53-60-1] $C_{17}H_{20}N_2S.HCl$ (320.88).

Preparation—Phenothiazine is dissolved in an inert solvent and condensed with 3-chloro-*N,N*-dimethylproplyamine in the presence of sodium hydride to yield promazine. After purification, it is dissolved in an organic solvent and reacted with an equimolar quantity of HCl.

Description—White to slightly yellow, practically odorless, crystalline powder; oxidizes upon prolonged exposure to air and acquires a blue or pink color; melts within a 3° range between 172° and 182°

Solubility—1 g in 3 mL of water; free soluble in chloroform.

Comments—A *phenothiazine* with low clinical potency, medium extrapyramidal toxicity, high sedative effect, and high hypotensive action.

THIORIDAZINE

10H-Phenothiazine, 10-[2-(1-methyl-2-piperdinyl)ethyl]-2-(methylthio)-, Mellaril-S

[50-52-2] $C_{21}H_{26}N_2S_2$ (370.57).

Preparation—2-(Methlythio)phenothiazine, which may be prepared by reacting 2-chlorophenothiazine with (methylthio)sodium, is condensed with 2-(1-methyl-1-piperidyl)ethyl chloride with the aid of a dehydrochlorinating agent such as sodamide. US Pat 3,239,514.

Description—Crystals; melts about 73°; pKa 9.5 (methylamino group).

Solubility—1 g in 6 mL of alcohol; practically insoluble in water.

Comments—See *Thioridazine Hydrochloride.*

THIORIDAZINE HYDROCHLORIDE

10H-Phenothiazine, 10-[2-(1-methyl-2-piperdinyl)ethyl]-2-(methylthio)-, Mellaril

[130-61-0] $C_{21}H_{26}N_2S_2 \cdot HCl$ (407.03).

For the structure and preparation of the base, see *Thioridazine.*

Description—White to slightly yellow, granular powder with a faint odor and a very bitter taste; stable in moderate heat, nonhygroscopic and darkens on exposure to light; melts within a range of 3° between 157° and 163°; pH (1 in 100 solution) between 4.2 and 5.2.

Solubility—1 g in 9 mL of alcohol or in 10 mL of water; freely soluble in chloroform or methanol; slightly soluble in benzene; insoluble in ether.

Comments—A *phenothiazine* with low clinical potency, low extrapyramidal toxicity, high sedative effect, and medium hypotensive action.

THIOTHIXENE

(Z)-9H-Thioxanthene-2-sulfonamide, N,N-dimethyl-9-[3-(4-methyl-1-piperazinyl)propylidene]-, Navane

[5591-45-7 and 3313-26-6(Z)] $C_{23}H_{29}N_3O_2S_2$ (443.62).

Preparation—2-Chlorobenzoic acid is converted into its 5-dimethylsulfamoyl derivative by successive reaction with chlorosulfonic acid and dimethylamine. The chlorine is then replaced with the phenylthio group by treatment with benezenethiol in the presence of alkali, and the resulting 2-phenylthio derivative is cyclized with polyphosphoric acid to form N, N-dimethyl-9-oxothioxanthene-2-sulfonamide. Reaction of this compound with [3-(4-methyl-1-piperidyl)-propylidene]triphenylphosphorane replaces the oxo oxygen with the appropriately substituted propylidene group to yield thiothixene. US Pat number 3,310,553.

Description—White to tan, crystalline powder; practically odorless; very bitter taste; unstable in light; melts about 150° (*cis* or *Z* isomer).

Solubility—Practically insoluble in water; 1 g in 110 mL of anydrous alcohol, 2 mL of chloroform, or 120 mL of ether; slightly soluble in methanol or acetone.

Comments—A *thioxanthene* with high clinical potency, medium extrapyramidal toxicity, medium sedative effect, and medium hypotensive action.

THIOTHIXENE HYDROCHLORIDE

(Z)-9H-Thioxanthene-2-sulfonamide, N,N-dimethyl-9-[3[3-(4-methyl-1-piperazinyl)propylidene]-, dihydrochloride, dihydrate, Navane Hydrochloride

[22189-31-7 and 49746-09-0(Z)] $C_{23}H_{29}N_3O_2S_2.2HCl.2H_2O$ (552.57); *anhydrous* [49746-04-5] (516.54). For the structure of the base, see *Thiothixene*.

Preparation—*Thiothixene* is reacted with aqueous HCl, and the hydrochloride is crystallized there from.

Description—White, or nearly white, crystalline powder; slight odor; affected by light.

Solubility—1 g in 8 mL of water, 270 mL of anhydrous alcohol, or 280 mL of chloroform; practically insoluble in benzene, acetone, or ether.

Comments—See *Thiothixene*.

TRIFLUOPERAZINE HYDROCHLORIDE

10H-Phenothiazine, 10-[3-(4-methyl-1-piperazinyl)propyl]-2-(trifluoromethyl)-, dihydrochloride; Stelazine

[440-17-5] $C_{21}H_{24}F_3N_3S.2HCl$ (480.42).

Preparation—By the process described for *Triflupromazine Hydrochloride*, except that 1-(3-chloropropyl)-4-methylpiperazine is used as the condensing amine in place of (3-chloropropyl)dimethylamine. US Pat 2,921,069.

Description—White to pale yellow, crystalline powder; practically odorless; bitter taste; melts about 242° with decomposition. pK_a 8.1 (piperazine).

Solubility—1 g in 3.5 mL of water, 11 mL of alcohol, or 100 mL of chloroform; insoluble in ether; protect aqueous solutions from light.

Comments—A *phenothiazine* with high clinical potency, high extrapyramidal toxicity, low sedative effect, and low hypotensive action.

Atypical or Novel Antipsychotics

Antipsychotics are classified as atypical based on three important clinical observations. Atypical antipsychotic agents are effective against the negative symptoms of schizophrenia (as well as the positive symptoms), often effective in patients refractory to treatment with typical antipsychotics, and seldom induce motor-related adverse effects. These agents have significant activity on central serotonergic tracts, especially $5HT_2$ receptors. Other serotonin receptors may be affected. Clozapine, the first of these agents to appear, was approved for use in the US in 1989. The major limitation to use of clozapine has been that it induces agranulocytosis in approximately 1% of those receiving it. Thus, patients being treated with clozapine need to have routine blood analyses performed. Other agents have become available that do not induce agranulocytosis and that appear to have an efficacy similar to that of clozapine. They also have a reduced adverse effect spectrum compared with typical antipsychotics. Treatment with all of these atypical or novel antipsychotic agents is associated with improved efficacy and better rates of compliance than is treatment with the typical antipsychotics. The absence of motor-related adverse effects appears to correlate with lower affinity for the D2-specific receptor within the family of dopaminergic D2 receptors. Risperidone, and to a lesser degree olanzapine, do elicit motor disorders at higher doses; hence these do not fit into the class of atypical antipsychotics as completely as the other agents. The newest agents, quetiapine, ziprasidone, and aripiprazole have very low EPS potential. Many of these agents have a propensity to cause lipid abnormalities and/or glucose intolerance (or the development of diabetes mellitus) (Table 82-2).

ARIPIPRAZOLE

2(1H)-Quinolinone, 7-[4-[4-(2,3-dichlorophenyl)-1-piperazinyl]butoxy]-3,4-dihydro-, Abilify

[129722-12-9] $C_{23}H_{27}Cl_2N_3O_2$ (448.39).

Preparation—7-Hydroxy-3,4-dihydro-2(1H)-quinolinone is refluxed with 1,4-dibromobutane plus K_2CO_3 in DMF to form the 7-(4-bromobutoxy) derivative which iscondensed with 1-(3,4-dichlorophenyl)piperazine to yield the product. *J Med Chem* 1998; 41:658. Also US Pat 5,006,528 (1991).

Description—White, crystalline powder from ethanol melting about 139°.

Comments—Classed as an *atypical antipsychotic*, this agent may have a unique mechanism of action in that it may modulate dopamine activity in a different manner than other atypical antipsychotic agents. Adverse effects include gastrointestinal effects and hypotension early in therapy, but the drug is very well tolerated. Weight gain is less than with most other agents.

CLOZAPINE

5H-Dibenzo[b,e][1,4]diazepine, 8-chloro-11-(4-methyl-1-piperazinyl)-, Clozaril

[5786-21-0] $C_{18}H_{19}ClN_4$ (326.83).

Table 82-2. Atypical Antipsychotic Drugs

GENERIC NAME	TRADE NAME	COMMENTS
Aripiprazole	Abilify	Adverse effects are moderate and include sedation and orthostatic hypotension.
Clozapine	Clozaril	Adverse effects include sedation, orthostatic hypotension, weight gain. Must monitor WBC count for possible agranulocytosis. Monitor blood sugar.
Olanzapine	Zyprexa	Adverse effects include orthostatic hypotension, sedation, weight gain and mild antimuscarinic effects. Higher doses may produce extrapyramidal effects. Monitor blood sugar.
Quetiapine	Seroquel	Adverse effects include dizziness, somnolence, agitation, and weight gain
Risperidone	Risperdal	Adverse effects include nasal congestion, orthostatic hypotension, insomnia, and possible extrapyramidal symptoms. Monitor blood sugar.
Ziprasidone	Geodon	Adverse effects are moderate and include sedation and hypotension.

Preparation—Clozapine may be prepared by means of intramolecular condensation of 2-amino-4-chlorodiphenylamine-2'-carboxylic acid 4-methylpiperazide in the presence of phosphorous oxychloride and *N*, *N*-dimethylformamide. The desired product is extracted with benzene, extracted from the organic solution with dilute acetic acid, and then precipitated by addition of concentrated ammonia water. Neth Pat 293,201.

Description—Yellow, tasteless crystals; melts between 183° and 184°.

Solubility—Slightly soluble in water; soluble in ether.

Comments—A *dibenzodiazepine-derived atypical antipsychotic* indicated for the management of symptoms of schizophrenia. In several trials, clozapine has been effective in patients refractory to treatment with typical antipsychotic drugs. In addition to its antipsychotic actions, clozapine may also help reduce aggressive and hostile behavior and the risk of suicide. It has also been used in the treatment of L-dopa–induced psychotic symptoms in patients who have Parkinson's disease.

Although clozapine does not produce the extrapyramidal symptoms and other motor irregularities associated with typical antipsychotic drugs, it does have significant adverse effects. These include drowsiness, headaches, disturbed sleep, dizziness, fever (5%), changes in blood pressure (less than 10%), tachycardia (25%), cardiac arrhythmias, dry mouth or hypersalivation (50–80%), nasal congestion, pallor, bowel irregularities, nausea or vomiting, respiratory irregularities and rash (2%), and seizures (3-5%). The most serious problem is agranulocytosis, which occurs in 0.5% to 1.5% of patients taking the drug. More than 95% of incidents of agranulocytosis occur within the first 6 months of therapy. Patients taking clozapine should be monitored closely with weekly white blood cell (WBC) assessments for the first 6 months. After 6 months of therapy the WBC must be measured every 2 weeks. Another adverse effect is a rebound psychosis from discontinuance of drug therapy. May cause weight gain and an increased tendency for glucose intolerance (de novo diabetes mellitus).

OLANZAPINE

10*H*-Thieno[2,3-*b*][1,5]benzodiazepine, 2-methyl-4-(4-methyl-1-piperazinyl)-, Zyprexa

[132539-06-1] $C_{17}H_{20}N_4S$ (312.43).

Preparation—A mixture of sulfur, propanol, DMF, and trimethylamine are heated during the addition of malononitrile to produce 2-amino-5-methylthiophene-3-carbonitrile. Reaction of this compound with 2-fluoronitrobenzene and sodium hydride forms 2-(2-nitroanilino)-5-methylthiophene-3-carbonitrile, which is subsequently treated with anhydrous stannous chloride to close the diazepine ring. The diazepine with 1-methylpiperazine in DMSO yields the product (base).

Description—Yellow crystals.

Solubility—Practically insoluble in water.

Comments—An *atypical antipsychotic*. Its adverse effects include orthostatic hypotension, sedation, and mild antimuscarinic activity. Higher doses may produce extrapyramidal effects. May cause weight gain and an increased tendency for glucose intolerance (de novo diabetes mellitus).

QUETIAPINE FUMARATE

Ethanol, 2-[2-(4-dibenzo[*b*,*f*][1,4[-thizaepin-11-yl-1-piperazinyl)ethoxy]-, (*E*)-2-butanedioate (2:1) salt; Seroquel

[111974-72-2] $(C_{21}H_{25}N_3O_2S_2)_2 \cdot C_4H_4O_4$ (833.11).

Preparation—The cyclic amide, dibenzo[*b*,*f*][1,4]thiazepin-11-one is converted to the 11-chloro derivative with phosphorus oxychloride. Nucleophilic displacement of the halogen by 2-[2-(piperazin-1yl)ethoxy]ethanol yields the product (base). The salt is prepared by mixing saturated solutions of the base and fumaric acid in ethanol. *Drugs of the Future* 1986; 21:483–489.

Description—White crystals that melt about 129°; base, 172°; HCl, 218°

Comments—An *atypical antipsychotic*. Its adverse effects include dizziness, somnolence, and weight gain.

RISPERIDONE

4*H*-Pyrido[1,2-*a*]pyrimidin-4-one, 3-[2-[4-(6-fluoro-1,2-benzisoxazol-3-yl)-1-piperidinyl]ethyl]-6,7,8,9-tetrahydro-2-methyl-, Risperdal

[106266-06-2] $C_{23}H_{27}FN_4O_2$ (410.49).

Preparation—A Friedel-Crafs condensation of 1-acetylpiperidone-4-carbonyl chloride and 2,4-difluorobenzene, followed by hydrolysis of the *N*-acetyl group yields 4-(2,4-difluorobenzoyl)piperidone and the benzoyl carbonyl is converted to the oxime. With alkali, the fluorine atom in the 2-position is displaced through ring closure to form the isoxazole moiety. The secondary amine of the piperidine ring is alkylated with 3-(2-chloroethyl)pyrido[1,2-*a*]pyrimidin-4-one to yield the product.

Description—Off-white crystals that melt about 170°.

Solubility—Practically insoluble in water; freely soluble in methylene chloride; soluble in methanol and 0.1 *M* HCl.

Comments—An *atypical antipsychotic* and *neuroleptic*. Its adverse effects include nasal congestion, orthostatic hypotension, insomnia, and possible extrapyramidal symptoms (EPS). Causes more EPS (at higher doses) than other atypical agents. May cause weight gain and an increased tendency for glucose intolerance (de novo diabetes mellitus).

ZIPRASIDONE HYDROCHLORIDE

2*H*-Indol-2-one, 5-[2-[4-(1,2-benzisothiazol-3-yl)-1-piperazin-yl]ethyl]-6-chloro-1,3-dihydro-, monohydrochloride, monohydrate; Geodon, Zeldox

[13898-67-9] $C_{21}H_{21}ClN_4OS \cdot HCl \cdot H_2O$ (467.42).

Preparation—By refluxing 5-(2-chloroethyl)oxindole and *N*-(1, 2-benzisothiazol-3-yl)piperazine with sodium carbonate and sodium iodide in methyl isobutyl ketone, followed by evaporation of the solvent and chromatography on silica gel with 4% methanol in methylene chloride. The salt is formed from the amine by addition of ether saturated with HCl gas. US Pat 4,831,031 (1989).

Description—White to faint pink powder. Hemihydrate melts above 300°.

Comments—An *atypical antipsychotic*, this agent must be given with food twice daily for maximum effect. Adverse effects include somnolence and minor QT_c prolongation. Currently, this is the only atypical antipsychotic available in a parenteral (IM) formulation.

Antidepressants

Antidepressants relieve the symptoms of depressive disorders. Depression is a common ailment, which afflicts approximately 5% to 6% of the population. It estimated that 10% to 15% of people experience depression sometime during their lifetime. The diagnosis of depression excludes behaviors resulting from normal bereavement, physical conditions, and drug use. Depression varies significantly in intensity and in the clinical symptoms manifested. Patients who have depression experience symptoms of depressed mood or loss of interest or pleasure in normal activities. They commonly complain of fatigue, decreased productivity, changes in appetite or weight, insomnia or somnolence, difficulty concentrating, and anhedonia. For such patients, nearly 75% experience clinically significant improvement with antidepressant drug treatment, and approximately 50% experience complete recovery. Treatment is characterized by a long interval (weeks to months) from the time that the patient begins taking medication to the time that improvement in symptoms occurs.

Many antidepressants are also indicated or used effectively for a variety of psychiatric disorders including generalized anxiety disorder (GAD), post-traumatic stress disorder (PTSD), obsessive-compulsive disorder (OCD), social anxiety disorder, and eating disorders.

Several effective antidepressants are currently available. These drugs vary significantly in chemical and pharmacological properties. One convenient way of characterizing the drugs is to combine the chemical and the pharmacological criteria and group the drugs into four major categories: tricyclic (based on three rings in the chemical structure), selective serotonin reuptake inhibitors (SSRIs) (based on pharmacological action), monoamine oxidase inhibitors (MAOIs) (based on pharmacological effect), and heterocyclics (whatever does not fit into the other three categories).

Generally, when tested in a broad population of patients, all of the antidepressants have equal efficacy. However, the drugs have significantly different spectra of adverse effects. Thus, the choice of drug is often made on the basis of least potential adverse effects. The SSRIs and some of the agents from the heterocyclic group show significantly less incidence of adverse effects than the tricyclic agents or the MAOIs. Clinical trials indicate equal efficacy of antidepressants when tested across a wide population. Recent research indicates that some patients who are refractory to treatment with most antidepressant drugs may still respond to one of the other antidepressant drugs. Because standard criteria are not available for determining what agent is effective in the nonresponding group, several agents may need to be tried.

The SSRIs (citalopram, escitalopram, fluoxetine, fluvoxamine, paroxetine, and sertraline) are currently the most commonly used antidepressant drugs. Generally, these have a low incidence of adverse effects, especially when compared with the tricyclic antidepressants and the MAOIs. Some adverse effects associated with the SSRIs are related to their ability to increase synaptic levels of serotonin. Because the GI tract utilizes more serotonin than any other body organ, the most common adverse effects are GI disturbances. Other adverse effects include headache, incoordination, sleep disturbance, sexual dysfunction, and tremor. Sexual dysfunction is becoming increasingly recognized with this class of agents. Anorgasmia is the most common effect, but loss of libido and erectile dysfunction are also seen. Some of these effects are transient and disappear with continued use of the drug. In some patients, a potentially fatal "serotonin syndrome" can occur. Symptoms of the serotonin syndrome include agitation, diaphoresis, diarrhea, fever, hyperreflexia, incoordination, mental status changes, myoclonus, shivering, and tremor. The syndrome is usually associated with a defect in serotonin metabolism accompanied by the stimulation of release of serotonin from its storage sites. MAO inhibitors have caused many of these reactions and are contraindicated in combination with SSRIs. Meperidine has also been implicated. The syndrome has been precipitated by the concomitant use of St. John's Wort. Nonprescription cold remedies and diet pills contain agents that release serotonin (dextromethorphan, sympathomimetics) may precipitate the syndrome in patients taking SSRIs. Other prescription drugs that affect serotonin levels such as the newer migraine agents and antiemetics may also precipitate such a reaction. The syndrome is reversible when the stimulus for serotonin release is removed, and it can be treated acutely with serotonin antagonists such as cyproheptadine or propranolol. Dantrolene may be used for hyperthermia.

The heterocyclic group (amoxapine, bupropion, maprotiline, mirtazapine, nefazodone, trazodone, and venlafaxine) of antidepressants (sometimes termed miscellaneous antidepressants) have little in common other than clinical efficacy. These drugs have a different spectrum of adverse effects from the SSRI group and can often be taken by patients who do not tolerate the SSRIs. The drugs in the heterocyclic group have a much lower incidence of adverse effects than the tricyclic or the MAOI antidepressants.

The tricyclic antidepressant compounds (amitriptyline, clomipramine, desipramine, doxepin, imipramine, nortriptyline, protriptyline, and trimipramine) generally have antianxiety and sedative properties. Some tricyclic antidepressants (imipramine and, to a lesser extent, amitriptyline and nortriptyline) are also helpful in alleviating enuresis in children and adolescents. The tricyclic antidepressant drugs induce a wide variety of adverse effects. Because all of these drugs have antagonist activity at muscarinic receptors, many adverse effects are related to this action. The most common include dryness of the mouth, constipation, blurred vision, and drowsiness. Other adverse effects associated with tricyclic antidepressants are excessive perspiration and weight gain. Occasionally, manic episodes, tremors, heart block, tachycardia and other arrhythmias, rashes, and facial sweating are observed. Cholestatic jaundice, bone-marrow depression, epileptiform seizures, peripheral neuropathy, and photosensitization occur rarely. Urinary retention, especially in men, also has been reported. Doses must be increased very slowly to allow patient to accommodate to adverse effects.

The MAOIs (isocarboxazid, phenelzine, and tranylcypromine) are used for symptomatic relief of severe reactive or endogenous depression in hospitalized or closely supervised patients who have not responded to other antidepressant therapy. They must be used with caution because they are more toxic than the other antidepressant drugs. The untoward reactions produced by MAOIs include postural hypotension. In addition, certain foods and drugs when combined with a MAOI can produce a hypertensive crisis characterized by headache, palpitation, nausea and vomiting, and, occasionally, subarachnoid or intracranial hemorrhage. This reaction may be induced by the ingestion of certain kinds of sharp cheese, yeast extracts, broad beans, chicken livers, pickled herring, and chocolate. Other adverse reactions include restlessness, insomnia, dry mouth, nausea, dizziness, constipation, and anorexia; occasionally, patients may experience flushing, urinary retention, tremors, impotence, and paresthesias; and rarely, patients might develop skin rash, hepatitis, tinnitus, muscle spasms, and mania.

The mechanism by which antidepressant drugs exert their effects is complex. Certain conclusions emerge from a comparison of pharmacology of active agents. All antidepressant drugs affect norepinephrine and serotonin synapses in the brain. However, the nature of the acute effects on synaptic transmission and the selectivity for one of these two neurotransmitter systems varies significantly. The MAOIs increase amount of monoamine neurotransmitters available by interfering with their metabolism. Several of the tricyclic drugs and the SSRI class block uptake of neurotransmitters from the synapse into the presynaptic terminal. Drugs that selectively block uptake of either serotonin or norepinephrine are effective antidepressants. Further, there seems little evidence to distinguish between effectiveness of these two types of antidepressants. Drugs that block the uptake of norepinephrine or serotonin selectively are equally effective as drugs that block the uptake of both neurotransmitters. Several antidepressant drugs are antagonists at the serotonin 5-HT2A receptor, and this antagonism has been postulated to reduce anxiety. As all of the antidepressant drugs necessitate 3 to 4 weeks or more of therapy before clinical benefit is observed, it would appear that neuronal adaptations to the presence of the drugs correlate with efficacy. All of the compounds that enhance norepinephrine neurotransmission induce a delayed down regulation of β-adrenergic receptors and a decreased ability to increase levels of cyclic adenosine monophosphate (cAMP) by activation of β-adrenergic receptors. Such observations suggest that clinical effectiveness may be produced through adaptations in second-messenger systems stimulated by norepinephrine. All of the compounds that enhance serotonergic neurotransmission appear to alter the balance between effects mediated by presynaptic and postsynaptic serotonin receptors, such that an increase in serotonergic transmission is observed.

Patients taking antidepressants should avoid all other medications, including over-the-counter (OTC) preparations, unless specifically approved by their physician. They should be advised not to use alcoholic beverages and to limit the amount of caffeine-containing beverages while on these medications. Special precautions should be taken when antidepressants are used with other medications. The tricyclic compounds may decrease the effect of anticonvulsant medication, necessitating dosage adjustment. Many tricyclic agents potentiate the effects of antihistaminics, antimuscarinics, and other CNS depressants; block the antihypertensive effects of clonidine and guanethidine; alter blood glucose levels; and decrease the effectiveness of hypoglycemic medication. Their effectiveness is reduced by concurrent use of estrogens. Their concurrent use with MAOIs should be avoided as a hyperpyretic crisis, severe convulsions, and death may occur. A minimum of 14 days should elapse between the discontinuance of MAOIs and the initiation of tricyclic antidepressant therapy and vice versa. Likewise, concurrent use of tricyclic antidepressants with sympathomimetics may result in severe hypertension or hyperpyrexia; these agents may enhance the possibility of cardiac arrhythmias in patients on thyroid medication. The tricyclic compounds are contraindicated in patients who have congestive heart failure, angina pectoris, and paroxysmal tachycardia. Also, they should be used with caution in patients who have urinary retention, glaucoma, diabetes, impaired liver function, asthma, and a history of convulsive seizures.

MAOIs potentiate the effects of many other drugs (barbiturates, insulin, procaine, adrenergic agents, methyldopa, thiazide diuretics, anti-Parkinson agents, phenothiazines, and morphine analgesics); thus, a reduced dosage of each agent is necessary if the drugs are used concomitantly. The MAOIs should not be administered with or immediately after other MAOIs or other antidepressants. Such combinations can produce a hypertensive crisis, fever, significant sweating, excitation, delirium, tremor, twitching, convulsions, chorea, and circulatory collapse. At least 14 days should elapse between discontinuing an MAOI and the institution of another antidepressant or MAOI. A similar period should elapse before patients on MAOIs undergo elective surgery. The MAOIs should not be used in patients who have cerebrovascular defects or in patients who have cardiovascular disease, hypertension, or pheochromocytoma.

The safe use of tricyclic compounds or MAOIs during pregnancy or lactation has not been established. These agents should not be used in children younger than 12 years for the same reason. Also, geriatric, adolescent, and black patients on tricyclic compounds usually require reduced dosage; this is thought to be related to slower drug metabolism. Antidepressant drugs are toxic agents and should be employed only with a full knowledge of their precautions and potential adverse effects (Table 82-3).

AMITRIPTYLINE HYDROCHLORIDE

1-Propanamine, 3-(10,11-dihydro-5*H*-dibenzo[*a,d*]cyclohepten-5-ylidene)-*N,N*-di-methyl-, hydrochloride; Elavil

[549-18-8] $C_{20}H_{23}N.HCl$ (313.87).

Table 82-3. Antidepressant Drugs

GENERIC NAME	TRADE NAME	COMMENTS
Amitriptyline	Elavil	A tricyclic with high sedation, intense antimuscarinic effects, high hypotension, and weight gain
Amoxapine	Asendin	A heterocyclic with moderate sedation and moderate antimuscarinic effects
Bupropion	Wellbutrin	A heterocyclic with no sedation, no antimuscarinic effects
Citalopram	Celexa	An SSRI with low sedation, no antimuscarinic effects
Clomipramine	Anafranil	A tricyclic with high sedation, intense antimuscarinic effects, high hypotension, and weight gain
Desipramine	Norpramin, Pertofrane	A tricyclic with low sedation, low antimuscarinic effects
Doxepin	Sinequan	A tricyclic with high sedation, intense antimuscarinic effects, moderate hypotension, and weight gain
Duloxetine Hydrochloride	Cymbalta	An SSRI with low sedation, no antimuscarinic effects
Escitalopram	Lexapro	An SSRI with low sedation, no antimuscarinic effects. Active s-enantiomer of citalopram
Fluoxetine	Prozac	An SSRI with no sedation, no antimuscarinic effects
Fluvoxamine	Luvox	An SSRI: only approved in US for obsessive-compulsive disorder
Imipramine	Tofranil	A tricyclic with moderate sedation, moderate antimuscarinic effects, high hypotension, and weight gain
Isocarboxazid	Marplan	An MAOI with low sedation, low antimuscarinic effects, and weight gain
Maprotiline	Ludiomil	A heterocyclic with moderate sedation and moderate antimuscarinic effects
Mirtazapine	Remeron	A heterocyclic with high sedation, no antimuscarinic effects
Nefazodone	Serzone	A heterocyclic with low sedation, low antimuscarinic effects; black box warning for possible hepatotoxicity
Nortriptyline Hydrochloride	Aventyl, Pamelor	A tricyclic with moderate sedation and moderate antimuscarinic effects
Paroxetine	Paxil	A SSRI with low sedation, no antimuscarinic effects
Phenelzine Sulfate	Nardil	An MAOI with low sedation, low antimuscarinic effects, and weight gain
Protriptyline Hydrochloride	Vivactil	A tricyclic with no sedation, moderate antimuscarinic effects
Sertraline	Zoloft	A SSRI with low sedation, no antimuscarinic effects
Tranylcypromine	Parnate	A MAOI with low sedation, low antimuscarinic effects
Trazodone Hydrochloride	Desyrel	A heterocyclic with high sedation, no antimuscarinic effects
Trimipramine	Surmontil	A tricyclic with high sedation, high antimuscarinic effects, high hypotension, and weight gain
Venlafaxine	Effexor	A heterocyclic with no sedation and no antimuscarinic effects

Preparation—Phthalic anhydride is reacted with phenylacetic acid to form 3-benzylidenephthalide, which is hydrogenated to 2-phenethylbenzoic acid. Conversion to the acid chloride followed by intramolecular dehydrochlorination yields the ketone (5H-dibenzo[a,d]cyclohepten-5-one), which is grignardized with 3-(dimethylamino)propyl chloride. Dehydration of the resulting tertiary carbinol gives amitriptyline, which is dissolved in a suitable solvent and converted to the hydrochloride by a stream of HCl. US Pat 3,205,264.

Description—White or practically white, odorless or practically odorless, crystalline powder or small crystals; melts about 197°; pH (1 in 100 solution) 5 to 6; pKₐ 9.4.

Solubility—1 g in in 1 mL water, 1.5 mL alcohol, 1.2 mL chloroform, or 1 mL methanol; insoluble in ether.

Comments—A *tricyclic* used for the relief of symptoms of depression. Endogenous depression is more amenable to amitriptyline therapy than are other depressive states. It is useful in the management of depression accompanied by anxiety. It is also useful in temporarily alleviating enuresis in children and adolescents.

Amitriptyline is contraindicated in patients who have shown previous hypersensitivity to it. It should not be given concomitantly with MAOIs. Hyperpyretic crises, severe convulsions, and deaths have occurred in patients receiving tricyclic antidepressant and MAO-inhibiting drugs simultaneously. When a MAOI is replaced with amitriptyline, a minimum of 14 days withdrawal should be allowed before initiation of the new therapy. Amitriptyline is not recommended for use during the acute recovery phase after myocardial infarction.

Amitriptyline is absorbed rapidly after either oral or parenteral administration; (31–61% is bioavailable); peak plasma levels occur within 2 to 12 hr; 96% is bound to plasma proteins. The plasma half-life ranges from 31 to 46 hr; volume of distribution is 5 to 10 L/kg; therapeutic plasma levels range from 80 to 200 ng/mL. It is metabolized in the liver by P-450 2D6. At least one active metabolite, nortriptyline, has been identified. Approximately 25% to 50% is excreted in the urine as inactive metabolites within 24 hr; small amounts are excreted in the feces via the bile.

Adverse effects associated with amitriptyline include drowsiness, xerostomia, tremor, fatigue, weakness, blurring of vision, constipation, urinary retention, edema, tachycardia, and orthostatic hypotension. Most untoward effects can be controlled by a reduction in dosage. Patients taking large doses over an extended period should be watched closely for possible changes in liver and hematopoietic functions.

AMOXAPINE

Dibenz[b,f][1,4]oxazepine, 2-chloro-11-(1-piperazinyl)-, Asendin

[14028-44-5] C₁₇H₁₆ClN₃O (313.79).

Preparation—See *Helv Chim Acta* 1967; 50:245.

Description—White crystals; melting about 175°.

Solubility—Practically insoluble in water; freely soluble in chloroform; sparingly soluble in acetone or methanol.

Comments—A *heterocyclic* with moderate sedative and antimuscarinic effects.

BUPROPION HYDROCHLORIDE

1-Propanone, 1-(3-chlorophenyl)-2-[(1-dimethylethyl)amino]-, hydrochloride; Wellbutrin, Zyban

[31677-93-7] C₁₃H₁₈ClNO.HCl

Preparation—*m*-Chlorobenzonitirile is reacted with ethyl Grignard reagent in ether to produce *m*-chlorobenzyl ethyl ketone, which is brominated in dichloromethane. The product is reacted with tertiary butyl amine in acetronitrile to yield bupropion base. Treatment of an ethereal solution of the base with dry HCl yields the salt. Ger Offen 2,059,618.

Description—White solid; melting about 233° to 234°.

Solubility—1 g in 3.5 mL water or 5 mL ethanol.

Comments—A *heterocyclic* with no sedative or antimuscarinic effects. Also used as an aid in smoking cessation

CITALOPRAM HYDROBROMIDE

5-Isobenzofurancarbonitrile, 1-[3-(dimethylamino)propyl]-1-(4-fluorophenyl)-1,3-dihydro-, monohydrobromide; Celexa

1-[3-(Dimethyamino)propyl]-1-(p-fluorophenyl)-5-phthalan- carbonitrile monohydrobromide [59729-33-8] C₂₀H₂₁FN₂O.HBr (405.30).

Preparation—A multi-step synthesis involving the interaction of the Grignard reagent from *p*-bromochlorobenzene and 5-bromophthalide to form 4'-chloro-4-bromo-2-(hydroxymethyl)benzophenone (I). I, with another Grignard, 3-dimethylaminopropyl-magnesium chloride, yields α-(3-dimethylaminopropyl)-α-(p-chlorophenyl-α-4-bromo-2-hydroxymethyl)benzyl alcohol, which is cyclized with hot phosphoric acid to give the 5-bromophthalan. Conversion of the bromine atom to 5-cyano with copper cyanide affords the product. US Pat 6,455,710(2002); *Eur J Med Chem Ther* 1977;12:289.

Description—Crystals from 2-propanol melting about 182°.

Solubility—Sparingly soluble in water; soluble in ethanol.

Comments—An *SSRI*, indicated for treatment of depression.

CLOMIPRAMINE HYDROCHLORIDE

5H-Dibenz[b,f]azepine-5-propanamine, 3-chloro-10,11-dihydro-N,N-dimethyl-, monohydrochloride; Anafranil

[17321-77-6] C₁₉H₂₁ClN₂.HCl (351.32).

Preparation—3,9-Dichloroacridine is refluxed with P₂O₅ in dry xylene to form 3-chloro-5H-dibenz[b,f]azepine, which is catalytically reduced using PtO₂ in ethanol at room temperature giving 3-chloro-10,11-dihydro-5H-dibenz[b,f]azepine. Treatment of the latter compound with sodamide in toluene followed by reaction of the sodio salt with 3-chloro-N,N-dimethylpropylamine gives the free amine which is converted to the hydrochloride. *J Org Chem* 1961; 26:135.

Description—Crystals from methanol/ether melting about 190°. Log P, 3.3; pKₐ 3.6–4.6.

Solubility—Ethanol, 1 in 5; water, 1 in 8. Freely soluble in methanol or methylene chloride. Insoluble in ether or benzene.

Comments—A *tricyclic*, with high sedative and intense antimuscarinic effects, causing hypotension and weight gain. Initially indicated only for obsessive-compulsive disorder.

DESIPRAMINE HYDROCHLORIDE

5H-Dibenz[b,f]azepine-5-propanamine, 10,11-dihydro-N-methyl-, monohydrochloride; Norpramin; Pertofrane

[58-28-6] C₁₈H₂₂N₂.HCl (302.85).

Preparation—Pyrolysis of the methanesulfonate of 4,4'-diaminobibenzyl results in cyclization with formation of 10,11-dihydro-5H-dibenz[b,f]azepine. This is condensed with N-(3-chloropropyl)-N-methylbenzylamine in the presence of alkali to form N-benzylated desipramine, which, after debenzylation through reductive cleavage, is reacted with an equimolar quantity of HCl. Brit Pat 908,788; US Pat 3,454,698.

Description—White to off-white, crystalline powder; odorless; bitter taste; unstable after long exposure to light, heat, and air; melts within a 5° range between 208° and 218°; pKₐ 10.2 (methylamino).

Solubility—1 g in 12 mL of water, 14 mL of alcohol, 3.5 mL of chloroform, or >10,000 mL of ether.

Comments—A *tricyclic* with low sedative and antimuscarinic effects. Active metabolite of imipramine.

DOXEPIN HYDROCHLORIDE

1-Propanamine, 3-(dibenz[b,e]oxepin-11(6H)-ylidene)-N,N-dimethyl-, hydrochloride; Adapin; Sinequan

[1229-29-4; 4698-39(E); 251127-31-5(Z)] $C_{19}H_{21}NO.HCl$ (315.84). Doxepin hydrochloride, an (E) and (Z) geometric isomer mixture, contains the equivalent of not less than 85.0% and not more than 92.0% of $C_{19}H_{21}NO$ (doxepin), calculated on the dried basis. It contains not less than 12.0% and not more than 16.0% of the (Z)-isomer and not less than 72.0% and not more than 78.0% of the (E)-isomer.

Preparation—6,11-Dihydrodibenz[b,e]oxepin-11-one is prepared from ethyl 2-(bromomethyl)benzoate and phenol to produce 2-(phenoxymethyl)benzoic acid, which is converted to 6,11-dihydrobenzo[b,e]oxepin-11-one by cyclization with polyphosphoric acid. This latter compound is transformed to 11-[3-(dimethylamino)propyl]-6H-dibenz[b,e]oxepin-11-ol through Grignard reaction with 3-(dimethylamino)propyl chloride. Dehydration of the alcohol with mineral acid yields the base that is reacted with HCl.

Description—White, odorless, bitter, crystalline substance; decomposes slowly in light, nonhygroscopic up to 75% RH, and relatively stable in heat; melts about 188°; pK$_a$ 8.

Solubility—1 g in 1 mL water, 2 mL alcohol, or 10 mL chloroform.

Comments—A *tricyclic* with high sedative and intense antimuscarinic effects, causing moderate hypotension and weight gain.

ESCITALOPRAM OXALATE

S-(+)-5-Isobenzofurancarbonitrile, 1-[3-(dimethylamino)propyl]-1-(4-fluorophenyl)-1,3-dihydro-, oxalate (salt; 1:1); Lexapro

[219861-08-2] $C_{20}H_{21}FN_2O.C_2H_2O_4$ (414.43).

Preparation—Escitalopram is the (S)-isomer of the racemic citalopram. The isomer is produced by resolution of the enantiomer and conversion to the oxalate salt. US Pat 6,455,710.

Description—White to off-white powder.

Solubility—Freely soluble in methanol or DMSO. Soluble in normal saline, sparingly soluble in water or ethanol, slightly soluble in ethyl acetate.

Comments—An *SSRI*, it is the active S-enantiomer of citalopram (see above). Dosage is half that of citalopram. No advantage over citalopram.

FLUOXETINE HYDROCHLORIDE

Propylamine, (±)-3-(p-trifluoromethylphenoxy)-N-methyl-3-phenyl-, Prozac, Serafem

[56296-78-7] $C_{17}H_{18}F_3NO.HCl$ (345.79, hydrochloride salt).

Preparation—β-(Dimethylamino)propiophenone is reduced by diborane to the corresponding secondary alcohol. The hydroxyl group is substituted by chlorine using hydrochloric acid in chloroform. The product is reacted with sodium 4-trifluoromethylphenoxide in a Williamson synthesis to produce the dimethyl analog of the desired compound. Mono-demethylation is accomplished by successive reaction with BrCN and KOH. German Pat 2,500,110.

Description—Off-white crystalline solid.

Solubility—1 g in 70 mL of water.

Comments—An *SSRI* indicated for treatment of depression, obsessive-compulsive disorder, and bulimia nervosa. Besides its use in the treatment of major depression, fluoxetine also has been used in patients who have bipolar disorder, obesity, and panic attacks.

Although fluoxetine has a wide margin of safety, it can have undesirable actions on nervous and GI systems that cause discontinuance in 15% of patients. These effects include anxiety, nervousness, insomnia, dizziness, headaches, and nausea. Significant weight loss may occur. Fluoxetine is contraindicated in patients known to be allergic to it. Fluoxetine should not be used in combinations with an MAOI or within 14 days of discontinuing therapy with an MAOI. Fluoxetine forms an active metabolite norfluoxetine, which has a half-life of approximately 7 to 9 days. Therefore, after stopping fluoxetine, allow at least a 5-week interval before starting an MAOI.

Fluoxetine is well absorbed from the GI tract (60–80%), and peak plasma levels occur 4 to 8 hr after administration. The elimination half-life of fluoxetine is approximately 2 to 3 days (range of 1–9 days), and the half-life of its active metabolite, norfluoxetine, is 7 to 9 days (range of 3–15 days); thus, adverse effects may disappear slowly after discontinuing the drug. Fluoxetine is metabolized principally in the liver, and blood levels are increased in patients who have liver dysfunction.

FLUVOXAMINE MALEATE

1-Pentanone, E-5-methoxy-1-[4-(trifluoromethyl)phenyl]-, O-(2-aminoethyl) oxime; Luvox

[54739-18-3] $C_{15}H_{21}F_3N_2O_2.C_4H_4O_4$ (434.41).

Preparation—A Friedel Crafts reaction of α,α,α-trifluorotoluene and 5-methoxyvaleryl chloride forms 1-(4-trifluoromethylphenyl)-5-methoxyvalerophenone, which with 2-aminoxyethyl amine hydrochloride yields the oxime product. US Pat 4,058,225 (1978).

Description—White to off-white, odorless crystals that melt about 121°.

Solubility—Sparingly soluble in water; freely soluble in ethanol or chloroform; practically insoluble in ether.

Comments—An *SSRI* approved in the US only for obsessive-compulsive disorder.

IMIPRAMINE HYDROCHLORIDE

5H-Dibenzo(b,f)azepine-5-propanamine, 10,11-dihydro-N,N-dimethyl-, mono-hydrochloride; Tofranil, Janamine

[113-52-0] $C_{19}H_{24}N_2.HCl$ (316.87).

Preparation—Dimerization of o-nitrotoluene is affected with sodium ethoxide and an oxidizing agent to produce 1,2-bis(o-nitrophenyl)ethane. This compound is reduced to the corresponding diamine, 2-(o-aminophenethyl)aniline hydrochloride, which is condensed with 3-chloro-N,N-dimethylpropylamine by refluxing in benzene solution with the aid of sodamide. The basic constituents are then extracted with aqueous HCl and the extract is rendered alkaline and extracted with ether. After drying, the solvent is evaporated and the residue is vacuum distilled to yield the base. Treatment with alcoholic HCl produces the hydrochloride. US Pat 2,553,736.

Description—White to off-white, odorless crystalline powder; melts about 172°; pK$_a$ 9.4.

Solubility—1 g in approximately 5 mL of water, approximately 10 mL of alcohol, or approximately 15 mL of acetone; insoluble in ether or benzene.

Comments—A *tricyclic* with moderate sedative and antimuscarinic effects, causing hypotension and weight gain.

IMIPRAMINE PAMOATE

5-[3-(Dimethylamino)propyl]-10,11,-dihydro-dH-dibenz[b,f]-azepine compound (2:1) with 4,4-methylene-bis][3-hydroxy-2-naphthoic acid]; Tofranil-PM

For the structure and preparation of the base, see *Imipramine Hydrochloride*.

[10075-24-8] $(C_{19}H_{24}N_2)_2.C_{23}H_{16}O_6$ (949.20).

Description—Yellow powder; tasteless; odorless.

Solubility—Insoluble in water; soluble in alcohol, ether, or chloroform.

Comments—See *Imipramine Hydrochloride*.

ISOCARBOXAZID

3-Isoxazolecarboxylic acid, 5-methyl-, 2-(phenylmethyl)hydrazide; Marplan

[59-63-2] $C_{12}H_{13}N_3O_2$ (231.26).

Preparation—Acetonylacetone is reacted with nitric acid to form 5-methyl-3-is-oxazolecarboxylic acid, which is converted to the ethyl ester. The ester, with hydrazine hydrate, forms the acid hydrazide, which is condensed with benzaldehyde to yield the 2-benzylidenehydrazide. This latter compound is reduced with $LiAlH_4$ to the product. *J Med Pharm Chem* 1960; 2:133. *Anal Profiles of Drug Subst* v 2, p 295-314.

Description—White to off-white crystalline powder from methanol; slight characteristic odor; stable in dry air; melts about 106°; pK_a 10.4. Octanol/water partition coefficient, 30.

Solubility—Sparingly soluble in hot water; very soluble in ethanol, glycerol or propylene glycol.

Comments—An *MAOI* with low sedative effects. Was off the market for a few years and was then reintroduced in 1998. No advantages over phenelzine or tranylcypromine.

MAPROTILINE HYDROCHLORIDE

9,10-Ethananthracene-9(10*H*)-propanamine, *N*-methyl-, hydrochloride; Ludiomil

[10347-8] $C_{20}H_{23}N \cdot HCl$ (313.87).

Preparation—Refer to *Helv Chim Acta* 1969; 52:1385.

Description—White crystals; melting about 230°; pK_a 10.5.

Comments—A *heterocyclic* with moderate sedative and antimuscarinic effects.

MIRTAZAPINE

Pyrazino[2,1-*a*]pyrido[2,3-*c*][2]benzazepine, (±)1,2,3,4,10, 14*b*-hexahydro-2-methyl-, Remeron

[61337-67-5] $C_{17}H_{19}N_3$ (265.36).

Preparation—The reaction of 2-chloropyridine-3-carbonitrile and 3-phenyl-1-methylpiperazine forms 2-(4-methyl-2-phenylpieridin-1-yl)nicotrinonitrile. Hydrolysis of the nitrile to the acid followed by reduction with diborane converts the carboxyl to a carbinol. Concentrated sulfuric acid closes the azepine ring and yields the product.

Description—White to off-white crystals that melting about 116°.

Solubility—Slightly soluble in water.

Comments—A *heterocyclic* with high sedative and no antimuscarinic effect.

NEFAZODONE HYDROCHLORIDE

3*H*-1,2,4-Triazol-3-one, 2-[3-[4-(3-chlorophenyl)-1-piperazinyl]]-propyl]-5-ethyl-2,4-dihydro-4-(2-phenoxyethyl)-, monohydrochloride; Serzone

[82752-99-6]$C_{25}H_{32}ClN_5O_2 \cdot HCl$ (506.48).

Preparation—Heating phenol and 2-ethyloxazoline yields *N*-(2-phenoxyethyl)propionamide, which with phosgene forms the imidoyl chloride derivative. This latter compound with ethyl hydrazinocarboxylate, yields I. *J Hetero Chem* 1985; 22:11211. US Pat 4,338,317 (1982).

(I)

Compound I undergoes base-catalyzed intramolecular rearrangement to form the triazole moiety of the drug. The secondary amine fragment of the triazole is alkylated with 1-(3-chlorophenyl)-4-(3-chloropropyl)piperazine to form the product (base).

Description—White, nonhygroscopic crystals that melt about 187° (slow cooling); polymorph, which melts about 182° (rapid cooling) from 2-propanol; m 177° from ethanol. See US Pat 4,338,317 (1982).

Solubility—Freely soluble in chloroform; soluble in propylene glycol; slightly soluble in water or polyethylene glycols.

Comments—A *heterocyclic* with low sedative and antimuscarinic effects. Has black box warning for possible hepatotoxicity.

NORTRIPTYLINE HYDROCHLORIDE

1-Propanimine, 3-(10,11-dihydro-5*H*-dibenzo[*a,d*]cyclohepten-5-ylidene)-*N*-methyl-, hydrochloride; Aventyl; Pamelor

[894-71-3] $C_{19}H_{21}N \cdot HCl$ (299.84).

Preparation—10,11-Dihydro-5*H*-dibenzo[*a,d*] cyclohepten-5-one, which may be prepared as described under *Cyproheptadine Hydrochloride*, is reacted with an alkali metal derivative of *N*-methyl-2-propynylamine and the product hydrolyzed to form the carbinol. The acetylenic bond is then saturated by hydrogenation and the resulting carbinol dehydrated to yield nortriptyline (base). Reaction of the base with hydrogen chloride produces the hydrochloride.

Description—White to off-white powder; slight, characteristic odor; melts within a range of 3° between 215° and 220°. pK_a is 9.73.

Solubility—1 g in 90 mL water, 30 mL alcohol, 20 mL chloroform, or 10 mL methanol.

Comments—A *tricyclic* with moderate sedative and antimuscarinic effects. Active metabolite of amitriptyline.

PAROXETINE

Piperidine, (3*S-trans*)-3-[(1,3-benzodioxol-5-yloxy)methyl]-4-(4-fluorophenyl)-, Paxil (as the hydrochloride)

[61869-08-7] $C_{19}H_{20}FNO_3 \cdot HCl$ (365.87).

Preparation—A Grignard reaction between 4-fluorophenylmagnesium bromide and methyl 1,2,5,6-tetrahydronicotinate produces methyl 4-(4-fluorophenyl)nipecotate. This ester is reduced with LiAlH$_4$ and the resulting carbinol condensed with 3,4-methylenedioxybenzyl alcohol in the presence of cyclohexylcarbodiimide to yield the product, an ether (base). US Pat 4,721,723 (1988) and US Pat 4,007,196 (1977).

Description—Off-white powder that melts about 120° to 134°; HCl. ½H$_2$O, 131°; maleate, 138°; [α]$_D$ - 87° (c = 5, ethanol).

Solubility—Soluble 5.4 mg/mL in water.

Comments—An *SSRI* with low sedative and no antimuscarinic effects. More drug interactions than most SSRIs. Also indicated for social anxiety disorder, GAD, OCD, PTSD, and panic disorder.

PHENELZINE SULFATE

Hydrazine, (2-phenylethyl)-, sulfate (1:1); Nardil

Phenethylhydrazine sulfate (1:1) [156-51-4] $C_8H_{12}N_2.H_2SO_4$ (234.27).

Preparation—Phenethyl alcohol is reacted with thionyl chloride to give phenethyl chloride, which is then added to hydrazine hydrate to yield phenethylhydrazine hydrochloride. Reaction with sodium hydroxide liberates the base, which is then reacted sulfuric acid to form the sulfate. US Pat 3,314,855.

Description—White to yellowish-white powder; characteristic odor; subject to oxidation and must be protected from heat and light; melts about 166°; pH (1 in 100 solution) 1.4 to 1.9.

Solubility—1 g in about 7 mL water; practically insoluble in alcohol, chloroform, or ether.

Comments—An MAOI with low sedative and antimuscarinic effects, causing weight gain.

PROTRIPTYLINE HYDROCHLORIDE

5H-Dibenzo[a,d]cycloheptene-5-propanamine, N-methyl-, hydrochloride; Vivactil

[1225-55-4] $C_{19}H_{21}N.HCl$ (299.84).

Preparation—5H-Dibenzo[a,d]cyclohepten-5-one, prepared as described under *Cyproheptadine Hydrochloride* (page 1547), is reduced to the corresponding carbinol that is then converted to the 5-chloromethyl compound (I). Reaction with HCl gives the hydrochloride.

Description—White to yellowish powder; odorless or has not more than a slight odor; a bitter taste; reasonably stable in light, air, and heat under the usual prevailing temperature conditions; melts about 168°; pH (1 in 100 solution) 5 to 6.5.

Solubility—1 g in 2 mL water, 4 mL alcohol, 2.3 mL chloroform, or 2 mL methanol; practically insoluble in ether.

Comments—A *tricyclic* with no sedative and moderate antimuscarinic effects.

SERTRALINE HYDROCHLORIDE

Naphthalenamine, (1S-cis)-4-(3,4-dichlorophenyl)-1,2,3,4-tetrahydro-N-methyl-, hydrochloride, Zoloft

[79559-97-0] $C_{17}H_{17}Cl_2N.HCl$ (342.70).

Preparation—4-(3,4-Dichlorophenyl)-3,4-dihydro-1(2H)-naphthalenone, methylamine, and titanium tetrachloride are reacted to form a Schiff base, which then is reduced with sodium borohydride to produce a mixture of geometric isomers. The *cis* and *trans* isomers are separated by use of chromatography on silica gel. The purified base is dissolved in ether and converted to the salt with HCl gas in ether. *J Med Chem* 1984; 27:1508.

Comments—An *SSRI* with low sedative and antimuscarinic effects. Also indicated for OCD, PTSD, panic disorder, and pre-menstrual dysphoric disorder.

TRANYLCYPROMINE SULFATE

Cyclopropanamine, trans-(±)-2-phenyl-, sulfate (2:1); Parnate

[13492-01-8] $(C_9H_{11}N)_2.H_2SO_4$ (364.46).

Preparation—Styrene is reacted with ethyl diazoacetate to form ethyl 2-phenylcyclopropanecarboxylate. Saponification of this ester

with sodium hydroxide and subsequent acidification yields a mixture of the *cis* and the *trans* forms of the corresponding acid, and the *trans* form is isolated by fractional crystallization from water. The *trans* acid is then subjected to the Curtius reaction, whereby carboxyl is transformed successively through the acyl chloride, acyl azide, and isocyanate states to yield finally the base. Reaction with a 1/2 equimolar quantity of H_2SO_4 gives the sulfate. US Pat 2,997,422.

Description—White, crystalline powder; odorless or a faint, cinnamaldehyde-like odor; slightly acid taste; stable in light, heat, and air; melts with decomposition at 218°; pK_a 8.2.

Solubility—1 g in 25 mL of water; slightly soluble in alcohol or ether; practically insoluble in chloroform.

Comments—An *MAOI* with low sedative and antimuscarinic effects.

TRAZODONE HYDROCHLORIDE

1,2,4-Triazolo[4,3-a]pyridin-3(2H)-one, 2-[3-[4-(3-chlorophenyl)-1-piperazinyl]propyl]-, monohydrochloride; Desyrel

[25332-39-2] $C_{19}H_{22}ClN_5O.HCl$ (408.33).

Preparation—Semicarbazide and 2-chloropyridine are condensed with loss of water and ammonia to form 1,2,4-triazolo[4,3-a]pyridin-3(2H)-one, which on treatment with 1-(3-chlorophenyl)4,3-chlorophenyl)piperazine (I) and sodamide, yields trazodone. I is prepared form 1-(3-chlorophenyl)piperazine with 1-bromo-3-chloropropane. See US Pat 3,381,009.

Description—White crystals; melts about 90°; pK_a (in 50% ethanol) 6.14.

Solubility—Sparingly soluble in water or alcohol; soluble in chloroform.

Comments—A *heterocyclic* with high sedative and no antimuscarinic effects.

TRIMIPRAMINE MALEATE

5H-Dibenz[b,f]azepine-5-propanamine, 10,11-dihydro-N,N,β-trimethyl-, (Z)-2-butenedioate (1:1); Surmontil

[521-78-8] $C_{20}H_{26}N_2.C_4H_4O_6$ (410.51).

Preparation—As per imipramine, page 1520, except that the side chain is attached with 3-(dimethylamino)-2-methylpropylchloride. See *Compt Rend* 1961; 252:2117.

Description—White crystals; bitter taste; slight numbing characteristic; melts about 143°; pK_a 7.72 (dimethylamino).

Solubility—Slightly soluble in water or in alcohol; freely soluble in chloroform.

Comments—A *tricyclic* with high sedative, antimuscarinic, and hypotensive effects, causing weight gain.

VENLAFAXINE HYDROCHLORIDE

Cyclohexanol, (±)-1-[2-(dimethylamino)-1-(4-methoxyphenyl)ethyl-, hydrochloride; Effexor

[99300-78-4] $C_{17}H_{27}NO_2.HCl$ (313.87).

Preparation—Under basic conditions an aldol-type condensation of the anion nucleophile of 4-methoxyphenylacetonitrile and cyclohexanone yield 2-(2-hydroxycyclohexyl)-2-(4-methyoxyphenyl)acetonitrile. Reduction of the nitrile to the primary amine followed by N-methylation gives the product (base). *J Med Chem* 1990; 33:2899. US Pat 4,535,186 (1985).

Description—Off-white crystals that melt about 217°; (+)-form, 102° to 104° from ethanol; (−) form, 241° from methanol or ether. Octanol-0.2 M NaCl partition coefficient, 0.543.

Solubility—Soluble at 572 mg/mL in 0.2 M NaCl.

Comments—A *heterocyclic* with no antimuscarinic effects. May cause increase in blood pressure of 5-7 mm Hg. Also indicated for GAD.

DULOXETINE HYDROCHLORIDE

2-Thiophenepropaneamine, (*S*)-*N*-methyl-γ-(1-naphthyloxy)-, hydrochloride; Cymbalta

136434-34-9] $C_{18}H_{19}NOS.HCl$ (333.88).

Preparation—*Tetr Lett* 1990; 31:1990 and US Pat 5,023,269 (1991).

Description—White solid, pK_a (66% DMF/water)9.6.

Solubility—Slightly soluble in water.

BIBLIOGRAPHY

ANTIPSYCHOTICS

Bristow MF, Hirsch SR. Pitfalls and problems of the long term use of neuroleptic drugs in schizophrenia. *Drug Safety* 1993; 8:136.
Carpenter WT Jr, Buchanan RW. Schizophrenia. *N Engl J Med* 1994; 330:681.
Deutch AY, Moghaddam B, Innis RB, et al. Mechanisms of action of atypical antipsychotic drugs: Implications for novel therapeutic strategies for schizophrenia. *Schizophrenia Res* 1991; 42:121.
Ereshefsky L, Tran-Johnson TK, Watanabe MD. Pathophysiologic basis for schizophrenia and the efficacy of antipsychotics. *Clin Pharm* 1990; 9:682.
Kapur S, Remington G. Atypical antipsychotic agents: New directions and new challenges in schizophrenia treatment. *Annu Rev Med* 2001; 52:503.

Keith SJ. Pharmacologic advances in the treatment of schizophrenia. *N Engl J Med* 1997; 337:851.
Levinson DF. Pharmacologic treatment of schizophrenia. *Clin Ther* 1991; 13:326.
Littrell RA, Schneiderhan M. The neurobiology of schizophrenia. *Pharmacotherapy* 1996; 16:153S.
McGavin JK, Goa KL. Aripiprazole. *CNS Drugs* 2002; 16:779.
Reynolds GP. Developments in the drug treatment of schizophrenia. *Trends Pharmacol Sci* 1992; 13:118.
Ryan PM. Epidemiology, etiology, diagnosis, and treatment of schizophrenia. *Am J Hosp Pharm* 1991; 48:1271.

ANTIDEPRESSANTS

Blier P, de Montigny C. Current advances and trends in the treatment of depression. *Trends Pharmacol Sci* 1994; 15:220.
Brown TM, Skop BP, Mareth TR: Pathophysiology and management of the serotonin syndrome. *Ann Pharmacother* 1996; 30:527.
Caldecott-Hazard S, Schneider LS. Clinical and biochemical aspects of depressive disorders: III. Treatment and controversies. *Synapse* 1992; 10:141.
Cohen LJ. Rational drug use in the treatment of depression. *Pharmacotherapy* 1997; 17:45.
Frazer A. Antidepressants. *J Clin Psychiatry* 1997; 58(suppl 6):9.
Gardier AM, Malagié I, Trillat AC, et al. Role of 5-HT$_{1A}$ autoreceptors in the mechanism of action of serotoninergic antidepressant drugs: Recent findings from in vivo microdialysis studies. *Fund Clin Pharmacol* 1996; 10:16.
de Jonghe F, Swinkels JA. The safety of antidepressants. *Drugs* 1992; 43(suppl 2):40.
Kasper S, Fuger J, Moller JJ. Comparative efficacy of antidepressants. *Drugs* 1992; 43(suppl 2):11.
Keller MB. Citalopram therapy for depression: A review of 10 years of European experience and data from U.S. clinical trials. *J Clin Psychiatry* 2000; 61:896.
Keck PE, Nelson EB, McElroy SL. Advances in the pharmacologic treatment
DJ, Glue P. Clinical pharmacology of anxiolytics and antidepressants: A psychopharmacological perspective. *Pharm Ther* 1989; 44:309.
Schatzberg AF. Recent developments in the acute somatic treatment of major depression. *J Clin Psychiatry* 1992; 53(suppl 3):20.
Scott MA, Shelton PS, Gattis W. Therapeutic options for treating major depression, and the role of venlafaxine. *Pharmacotherapy* 1996; 16:352.
Waugh J. Goa KL. Escitalopram: A review of its use in the management of major depressive and anxiety disorders. *CNS Drugs* 2003; 17:343f

MEDICINAL AGENTS

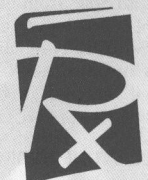

CHAPTER 83

Analgesic, Antipyretic, and Anti-Inflammatory Drugs

Robert B Raffa, PhD

Analgesics are agents that relieve pain without significantly disturbing consciousness or altering other afferent input (sensory modalities). Hence, many drugs that are used to relieve pain are not truly analgesics. For example, general anesthetics reduce pain, but interfere with consciousness; local anesthetics reduce pain by blocking peripheral nerve fibers that carry other sensory input; antispasmodics indirectly relieve certain kinds of pain by relaxing smooth muscle; and adrenal corticoids relieve pain associated with rheumatoid arthritis by their anti-inflammatory action. These drugs are considered elsewhere in this text. Antipyretics are drugs that reduce elevated body temperature (fever) to normal levels. Certain analgesics and antipyretics also possess anti-inflammatory properties; such substances are used in the treatment of arthritis and other inflammatory conditions. The drugs considered in this chapter have demonstrated analgesic action (or antagonism), with or without antipyretic or anti-inflammatory action. The drugs include opioid (morphine-like) agonists and antagonists, mixed-action agents, traditional NSAIDs (non-steroidal anti-inflammatory drugs), COX-2 inhibitors, and acetaminophen.

Pain serves several useful purposes. It warns of present or potential tissue damage and activates reflex or conscious withdrawal of the affected tissue from the source of injury, and it elicits a natural tendency to protect the injured site in order to prevent further injury. However, persistent pain adversely affects a patient's quality of life, can lead to pain hypersensitivity due to an increase in excitability of spinal cord neurons ('central sensitization'), and can delay recovery. Analgesics can inhibit the sensation of pain or alter the perception of pain. Modulation of the affective component of pain can improve a patient's quality of life even in the presence of a continuing sensation of pain. Since pain often originates from multiple sources, it involves multiple types of pain and multiple pain transmission pathways. Because of the multifaceted nature of some pain, treatment can often benefit from, or require, a combination of pharmacologic and non-pharmacologic approaches. The optimal pharmacologic treatment of pain requires classification of the type of pain and not merely of the severity of pain. Hence, an understanding of the differences in the mechanisms of action of the commonly available analgesics is helpful for the judicious selection of the optimal agent. A particularly important aspect of the treatment of pain is that a variety of chemical signals can be involved. Inflammatory pain may be an additional component of the overall pain profile. For example, pain caused by an inflammatory condition might best be treated with a 'weaker' anti-inflammatory drug, such as a cyclooxygenase inhibitor, rather than with a 'stronger'–but not anti-inflammatory–opioid analgesic.

At the site of an injury, tissues are damaged and cells release chemical mediators that trigger a pain signal. The released substances, such as histamine, bradykinin, and postaglandins, are either inherently painful or amplify the pain signal transmitted by other chemical mediators. The pain signal is transmitted from the site of injury to the central nervous system (CNS) via primary afferent sensory neurons. The anatomy of neurons influences the characteristics of the pain signal. For example, primary afferents of the Aδ type are highly myelinated and transmit their action potential rapidly–giving rise to a 'sharp' and localized type of pain. In contrast, C-fiber afferents are less heavily myelinated, slower conducting, and give rise to a more 'dull', diffuse, or vague type of pain. The cell bodies of afferent neurons, which comprise the DRG (dorsal root ganglion), can be damaged, giving rise to aberrant or false pain signaling (perhaps one explanation of 'phantom' pain). The signal enters the CNS through the dorsal horn of the spinal cord; many of the primary afferent fibers synapse in the *substantia gelatinosa* and adjacent layers, where neurotransmitters and neuromodulators are located within synapses between primary and secondary neurons. Substance P and glutamate are considered to be important mediators of the pain signal at this level. The secondary fibers decussate within the spinal cord and travel to the brain in ascending pathways such as the lateral spinothalamic tract. Within thalamic and associated nuclei, an affective component is superimposed upon the pain sensation. For example, an awareness of the magnitude of the discomfort and an emotional overlay is added to the pain sensation and memory of previously experienced pain is recruited. Higher CNS centers, including the cerebral cortex, contribute an additional affective component to the pain signal. Individual, cultural, and religious differences in pain response or interpretation are partly explained by this level of processing of the pain signal. In addition to these ascending pathways that carry the signal to higher CNS centers for processing, evaluation, and response, descending pathways modulate transmission of the incoming pain signal. Several neurotransmitter systems are involved in this descending modulation, including the endogenous opioid system (endorphins, enkephalins), norepinephrine from the *locus cœruleus*, and 5-hydroxytryptamine (serotonin) from the *raphe* nuclei. These pathways can be activated subconsciously or consciously, possibly accounting for the large placebo effect observed in clinical trials.

From the above considerations, it is clear that the mechanism(s) of action of a particular analgesic will determine the types of pain that the drug can be expected to treat. Although there are many analgesics available either by prescription or over-the-counter (OTC), there are relatively few categories from which to choose based upon the pharmacologic mechanism of action. The major categories of current analgesic pharmacotherapy are: (1) opioids; (2) mixed-action analgesics; (3) traditional NSAIDs and the newer selective cyclooxygenase-2 (COX-2) inhibitors; (4) acetaminophen, which is not an NSAID; (5) adjuvants (drugs not thought of as primarily analgesic, but are helpful in certain situations); and (6) combinations of these.

Table 83-1. Profile of the Analgesic Categories Most Commonly Used to Treat Pain

Opioids
  Maximum single-agent analgesic efficacy.
  Not anti-inflammatory
  MOA: 7-TM GPCR receptors (μ, δ, and κ)
  PK: good absorption; moderate onset; hepatic metabolism; renal excretion
  AEs: constipation; respiratory depression; abuse potential
NSAIDs
  Good analgesic efficacy (less than opioids)
  Anti-inflammatory
  MOA: inhibition of COX-1 and COX-2
  PK: good absorption; rapid onset; hepatic metabolism; renal excretion
  AEs: GI bleeding (potentially fatal); retention of Na^+/H_2O
COX-2 inhibitors
  Analgesic efficacy equivalent to traditional NSAIDs
  Ant-iinflammatory
  MOA: selective inhibition of COX-2
  PK: good absorption; rapid onset; hepatic metabolism; renal excretion
  AEs: to be established (possible cardiovascular, renal)
Acetaminophen
  Efficacy equivalent to traditional NSAIDs and COX-2 inhibitors
  Not anti-inflammatory
  MOA: not known (central)
  PK: good absorption; rapid onset; hepatic metabolism; renal excretion
  AEs: hepatotoxicity in overdose or compromised liver

MOA = mechanism of action; PK = pharmacokinetics; AE = adverse effects; 7-TM GPCR = 7-transmembrane spanning G protein-coupled receptors.

The characteristics of the major classes of currently available analgesics can be summarized as shown in Table 83-1.

OPIOID ANALGESICS

The analgesic properties of opium ('juice' of *Papaver somniferum*) and derivatives has been known for centuries. Morphine (after Morpheus, the Greek god of dreams) was isolated by Sertürner in 1806. Opioid receptors were discovered in the early 1970s by three groups: Pert & Snyder (*Science* 179:1011, 1973); Simon et al. (*PNAS* 70:1947, 1973); and Terenius (*Acta Pharmacol Toxicol* 32:317, 1973). Based on the assumption that the body would not have receptors for opioid drugs unless it produces an endogenous opioid-like substance, Hughes and Kosterlitz at the University of Aberdeen in Scotland isolated and identified such material, which they called *enkephalins*, from pig brain (*Nature* 258:577, 1975). Two of the identified brain peptides have the structure tyrosine-glycine-glycine-phenylalanine-X, differing only in the *N*-terminal amino acid (Met-enkephalin when X = methionine and Leu-enkephalin when X = leucine). The enkephalins are now known to be members of a family of endogenous opioids, which also includes endorphins (contracted from endogenous and morphine) and dynorphins. *Opiates* are drugs derived from opium and include, for example, morphine and codeine. *Opioids* is a general term referring to natural, synthetic, or endogenous morphine-related substances. *Narcotics* ('stupor') are drugs of certain legal status, the term has lost any pharmacologic specificity. Opioid analgesics fundamentally mimic the action of endogenous opioids.

It is now known that opioid analgesics produce their effects by binding to (affinity) and activation of (intrinsic activity; efficacy) the opioid receptors. There are three major types of opioid receptors, which are termed μ, δ, and κ. Each has been cloned and each is a 7-TM GPCR (7-transmembrane G protein-coupled receptor). Most of the currently used opioid analgesics act pri-

marily at μ receptors; some have an admixture of activity at the other types. Opioid receptors are located pre- and post-synaptically along the pain transmission pathways. High densities of receptors are found in the dorsal horn of the spinal cord and higher CNS centers. Opioid receptors in the brainstem are responsible for the respiratory depressant effects produced by opioid analgesics. Constipation results from activation of opioid receptors in the CNS and in the GI tract. Opioid receptors in higher CNS centers probably account for the effect of opioids on the affect component of pain. The cellular actions of opioid agonist analgesics involve enhancement of neuronal K^+ efflux and inhibition of Ca^{2+} influx. Enhanced K^+ efflux increases the transmembrane potential, which hyperpolarizes neurons and makes them less likely to respond to a pain stimulus. Because Ca^{2+} entry is necessary for vesicle merging with neuronal membranes and the subsequent release of neurotransmitters into the synapse, inhibition of Ca^{2+} entry by opioid analgesics decreases neurotransmitter release from neurons located along the pain transmission pathway.

The available opioid analgesics are derivatives of a relatively small number of chemical groups (eg, phenanthrenes, phenylheptylamines, phenylpiperidines, morphinans, and benzomorphans). Pharmacologically, opioids differ in their affinity for opioid receptors and in their intrinsic activity; some have high efficacy (eg, morphine); others moderate efficacy (eg, codeine); whereas others have zero efficacy, ie, are antagonists (eg, naloxone). Some opioid derivatives exhibit mixed agonist-antagonist activity (eg, nalbuphine).

Morphine is the prototype of the opioid analgesics, all of which have similar actions and overlapping clinical usefulness. They are used in the management of almost all types of moderate to severe pain, to inhibit cough and treat gastrointestinal (GI) and urinary tract disorders. They depress respiration at high doses, increase nonpropulsive intestinal spasms, decrease the propulsive motility of the small and the large intestines, and diminish biliary, pancreatic, and intestinal secretions. The consequences of these actions are periods of slight atony, causing a delay in the passage of bowel contents and an increase in stool viscosity. Constipation at analgesic doses is not uncommon. Also, they cause nausea and vomiting in some individuals and may induce cutaneous pruritus. These and other actions of morphine and related compounds tend to limit their usefulness. If these agents are given for long periods, tolerance to the analgesic effect develops so that the dose must be periodically increased to obtain equivalent pain relief.

The opioid analgesics generally are *contraindicated* in patients who have myxedema, Addison's disease, and hepatic cirrhosis. Such patients are especially sensitive to these agents. Consequently, respiratory depression, stupor, and even coma may result from relatively small doses of the opioids. Because opioids decrease ventilation, which causes hypercapnia and progresses to cerebrovascular dilatation and increased intracranial pressure, they should be used with caution in head injuries, cerebral edema, and delirium tremens. These agents also should be used with caution in patients who have cardiac arrhythmias, chronic ulcerative colitis, and impaired kidney function. Moreover, opioid analgesics cross the placental barrier; hence, newborn infants whose mothers have been administered such analgesics during labor should be observed closely for signs of respiratory depression and be treated for opioid overdosage if necessary. Individuals sensitive to a particular opioid agent, or group of agents, should avoid these drugs.

The analgesic and depressant effects of these agents provide the basis for many interactions with other drugs. Alcohol, antihistamines, muscle relaxants, antipsychotics, tricyclic antidepressants, or sedative-hypnotics may interact with opioids to intensify their overlapping actions, such as respiratory depression and anticholinergic effects. Particular caution is necessary if monoamine oxidase inhibitors (MAOIs) are administered concurrently with opioid analgesics because of intensification of action (use of meperidine in patients treated with MAOIs has produced severe and occasionally fatal reactions). Doses of the opioid analgesics should be adjusted to avoid these enhanced reactions.

Tolerance and physical dependence develop, which, combined with euphoria, can contribute to excess use or abuse by susceptible/predisposed individuals. For these reasons, it is important that morphine and its derivatives be taken only as directed by the physician (never in a greater dose, more often, or longer than prescribed) and never be used for pain when some other type of analgesic is satisfactory. Because drowsiness and decreased alertness are not uncommon, the patient taking any opioid analgesics usually should avoid tasks that require intact reflexes, coordination, and mental alertness. Many of the drugs described in this section come under the control of the *Comprehensive Drug Abuse Prevention and Control Act of 1970*. This law, commonly referred to as the *Controlled Substances Act*, is designed to regulate the distribution of all drugs with abuse potential as designated by the Drug Enforcement Administration, Department of Justice. The actual abuse by pain patients has been documented to be quite low and many patients unnecessarily go undertreated for their pain.

OPIUM

Gum Opium; Crude Opium; Raw Opium; Thebaicum; Meconium

The air-dried milky exudate obtained by incision of unripe capsules of *Papaver somniferum* Linné or its variety *album* De Candolie (Fam *Papveraceae*). It yields not less than 9.5% of anyhydrous morphine.

History—As a medicinal drug, it has been known and cultivated for many centuries, but it was not until the investigations of Sertüner, published in the early 1800s, that it was known that the drug contained certain definite principles now called *alkaloids*.

Dioscorides, in the 2nd century, was the first writer to discuss opium and its uses at length. He gave the recipe for a preparation called *diacodion*, which is the prototype of the formerly official syrup of poppies. Paracelsus used opium extensively in the 15th century and referred to it as the "stone of immortality." Van Helmont, early in the 17th century, used opium so freely that he was referred to as Doctor Opiatus. Sydenham, a little later in the same century, praised opium as the most valuable gift of God to man.

The principal opium exporting countries have been Turkey, Iran, Yugoslavia, and India. The Turkish and Yugoslavian products are nearly alike in their physical properties: color, odor, and consistency. Iranian and Indian opiums, although closely resembling each other, differ from the former in physical properties—they are darker and have a somewhat different odor and consistency. There also is a significant difference between the two groups in the amounts of the principal opium alkaloids.

Constituents—It owes its activity to the opioid alkaloids; 25 have been found in the various kinds of opiums, and several more have been suspected, but their existence has not been confirmed. Three acids occur combined with the alkaloids—*viz*, meconic, lactic, and sulfuric acids. Also present are *meconin* [$C_{10}H_{10}O_4$], pectin, glucose, mucilage, caoutchoue, wax and odorous, fatty, and coloring matters.

Description—More or less rounded, oval, brick-shaped or elongated, somewhat flattened masses, usually approximately 8 to 15 cm in diameter and weighing approximately 300 g to 2 kg each. Externally, it is pale olive-brown or olive-gray, having a coarse surface and covered with a thin coating consisting of fragments of poppy leaves and, at times, with fruits of a species of *Rumex* adhering from the packing. It is more or less plastic when fresh, becoming hard or tough on storage. Internally, it is reddish brown and coarsely granular. It has a very characteristic odor and a bitter taste.

Comments—It owes its chief pharmacological effects to its morphine content, other alkaloids not being present in sufficient amount to modify significantly the morphine type of action. Thus, it has many of the same uses as morphine, but the latter drug nearly always is preferred, inasmuch as it can be administered in a variety of ways. The average adult dose of opium is 60 mg, taken orally. This is the equivalent of 6 mg of morphine. Like morphine, this drug has *analgetic* and other *opioid* effects. It acts as an *antiperistaltic* agent by causing spasm of the bowel musculature and preventing propulsive movements. Traditionally, it is used for *diarrheas* and *dysenteries* rather than morphine. It produces *sedation* and *sleep*. It also controls *cough* and *dyspnea*. Thus, it has a variety of therapeutic uses in medicine and surgery.

Caution—Opium, and all opium derivatives and related synthetic compounds, are listed in Schedule II *of the Controlled Substances Act* (Chapter 111). It should not be dispensed except upon the presentation of a physician's prescription. See *Morphine.*

Powdered Opium is opium dried at a temperature not exceeding 70° and reduced to a fine powder and yields 10.0–10.5% of anhydrous morphine. It may contain any of the diluents, permitted for powdered extracts under *Extracts.*.

Description—Light brown to moderate yellowish brown, consisting chiefly of yellowish-brown to yellow, more or less irregular and granular fragments of latex, varying from 15 to 150 μm in diameter; a few fragments of strongly lignified, thick-walled, 4- to 5-sided or narrowly elongated, epidermal cells of the poppy capsule; few fragments of tissues of poppy leaves, poppy capsules, and, occasionally, *Rumex* fruits. In addition, there are the microscopic characteristics of the diluent if any has been used in the preparation of the powder.

Comments—A pharmaceutical necessity for *Paregoric*. See *Opium* and *Morphine.*

Paregoric [Camphorated Opium Tincture USP XVI; Paregoric Elixir; Tinctura Opii Benzoica; Tinctura Thebaica Benzoica] yields, from each 100 mL, 35 to 45 mg of anhydrous morphine.

Preparation—Macerate powdered opium (4.3 g), anise oil (3.8 mL), benzoic acid (3.8 g), and camphor (3.8 g) for 5 days, with occasional agitation, in a mixture of diluted alcohol (900 mL) and glycerin (38 mL). Then filter, and pass enough diluted alcohol through the filter to obtain 950 mL of total filtrate. Assay a portion of this filtrate as directed in the USP, and dilute the remainder with a sufficient quantity of diluted alcohol containing, in each 100 mL, 0.4 mL of anise oil, 400 mg of benzoic acid, 400 mg of camphor, and 4 mL of glycerin, to produce a solution containing, in each 100 mL, 40 mg of anhydrous morphine.

History—This preparation was originated about 1715 by Professor LeMort of the University of Leyden. It was official in the 1721 edition of the London Pharmacopaeia as *Elixir Asthmaticum*, which was changed to *Elixir Paregoricum*, meaning soothing elixir, in 1746. It also has been known as *Tinctura Camphorae Composita* and *Tinctura Opii Benzoica*, and the formula has changed in minor details many times since its introduction into medicine. *Alcohol Content: 44–46%.*

Comments—An *antidiarrheal agent* and mild *anodyne* in cough, nausea, and *abdominal pains*. It should never be used to quiet restless infants, as a habit may be induced. It contains 0.4% opium. Paregoric is listed in *Schedule III* of the *Controlled Substances Act*; hence, it only can be obtained on a prescription order (either oral or written) of a licensed practitioner.

MORPHINE

History—Morphine was the first alkaloid discovered. In the 17th and 18th centuries, many attempts were made to separate from opium the active ingredient. Preparations thought to represent these active principles but were really extracts, were employed in medicine under the name of *Magisterium Opii*. Bucholz was the first to endeavor to obtain a crystalline product from opium. About 1800 learned apothecaries of the time devoted their attention to the separation of the suspected active drug. One of these apothecaries, Derosne, succeeded in isolating narcotine in 1803, and the following year Seguin read a paper to the Institute of France describing the isolation of a substance that is now recognized as morphine. He did not publish his paper, however, until 1814 and in 1806, Frierich William Adam Sertüner, an apothecary of Einbeck, Germany, announced the separation of a basic crystalline substance that existed in opium in combination with a special acid. He later published, in 1817, the results of further investigation in which he named the substance *morphium* and described it as a *vegetable alkali*. Liebig, in 1831, assigned to it the formula $C_{34}H_{36}N_2O_6$, which was later modified by Laurent to the present formula, $C_{17}H_{19}NO_3$ (285.33).

It was only after almost 100 years of intensive research that the correct structural formula, which adequately explains the chemical transformations of morphine, could be proposed. Final confirmation of this structure came with the successful total synthesis of morphine in 1952.

Preparation—Several processes are in use. In all or nearly all of them the morphine and most of the other opium alkaloids are extracted from the opium with water alone or with slightly acidulated water. In one of the processes, the extract, after concentration, is neutralized, a solution of calcium chloride added, and the mixture filtered and further concentrated. Crude morphine hydrochloride crystallizes and is purified by precipitation with ammonia and recrystallized as the sulfate or hydrochloride. In another process the concentrated water extract is mixed with alcohol and made alkaline with ammonia. The morphine, being but slightly soluble in dilute alcohol, separates, whereas the greater part of the other alkaloids remain in solution. The crude morphine so obtained is purified by repeated crystallization as the sulfate or hydrochloride and reprecipitation if necessary in the presence of alcohol.

Description—*Monohydrate:* colorless or white, shining, rhombic prisms, fine needles or a crystalline powder; darkens on exposure to air; a saturated aqueous solution is alkaline to litmus; melts with decomposition at approximately 255°.

Solubility—*Monohydrate:* 1 g in approximately 5000 mL water (1100 mL boiling water), 210 mL alcohol (98 mL boiling alcohol), 1220 mL chloroform, 6500 mL ether, or 100 mL lime water; insoluble in benzene; readily soluble in solutions of fixed alkali or alkaline earth hydroxides from which it is reprecipitated by ammonium chloride or sulfate.

Comments—An *analgesic, adjunct to anesthesia, antitussive, and nonspecific antidiarrheal agent.* It is a strong analgesic, altering the psychological response to pain and suppressing anxiety and apprehension. It is the drug of choice for the treatment of pain associated with myocardial infarction and for dyspnea associated with acute left ventricular failure and pulmonary edema. It is used in small to moderate doses to relieve constant dull pain and in moderate to large doses to alleviate intermittent, sharp pain of traumatic or visceral origin. Although effects may begin earlier, maximal analgesic effect occurs approximately 20 min after intravenous injection, 50 to 90 min after subcutaneous injection, and 30 to 60 min after intramuscular injection. Analgesia persists for approximately 4 hr, but, in some patients, it may be as short as 2.5 hr or as long as 7 hr.

Although its role as a *preanesthetic* medication is still being elucidated, it generally is agreed that it is of particular value when pain is present preoperatively, in selected types of cardiac surgery, and in poor-risk patients in general. It is an effective *antitussive* agent, but because of its erratic absorption after oral administration and its dependence liability, it should be used as an antitussive agent only when cough is associated with severe pain and cannot be controlled by antitussives having less potential for abuse. This drug and other opioids, such as paregoric, are the most effective and prompt-acting *nonspecific antidiarrheal* agents. They act by enhancing tone in long segments of the longitudinal muscle and inhibiting propulsive contraction of both circular and longitudinal muscle. They are used to treat acute, self-limited diarrhea.

When administered orally, it is absorbed rapidly but incompletely and metabolized equally rapidly to the glucuronide. Thus, the plasma levels after this route are usually only 1/5 to 1/3 those obtained after parenteral injection. The half-life of morphine in plasma or serum during the first 6 hr is between 2 and 3 hr; the serum half-life, between 6 and 48 hr after intravenous administration, ranges from 10 to 44 hr. Approximately 35% of the drug is bound, primarily to the albumin fraction. After parenteral administration 70–80% is excreted during the first 48 hr with 60% as conjugated morphine. After oral administration, approximately only 60% of a given dose is excreted; this probably reflects the incomplete absorption from the GI tract.

Overt symptoms of *overdosage* include coma, pinpoint pupils, and depressed respiration. Shock, decreased body temperature, and pulmonary edema may occur. Treatment includes establishing a patent airway and ventilating the patient. If significant respiratory depression occurs, a suitable opioid antagonist, such as naloxone, should be administered. Other supportive measures should be applied as indicated. Morphine is a *Schedule II* drug under the *Controlled Substances Act.*

MORPHINE SULFATE

Morphinan-3,6-diol, (5α,6α)-7,8-didehydro-4,5-epoxy-17-methyl-, sulfate (2:1) (salt), pentahydrate

[6211-15-0] $(C_{17}H_{19}NO_3)_2 \cdot H_2SO_4 \cdot 5H_2O$ (758.83); *anhydrous* [64-31-3] (668.76).

Description—White, feathery, silky crystals, as cubical masses of crystals, or as a white crystalline powder; odorless and when exposed to air gradually loses water of hydration; darkens on prolonged exposure to light.

Solubility—1 g in 16 mL water, 570 mL alcohol, 1 mL water at 80° or approximately 240 mL alcohol at 60°; insoluble in chloroform or ether.

Comments—See *Morphine* and *Morphine Sulfate Injection.*

MORPHINE SULFATE INJECTION

A sterile solution of morphine sulfate in water for injection. It may contain suitable antimicrobial agents.

Preparation—Solutions of morphine sulfate at a pH above 7 decompose quickly even at room temperature. At a pH of less than 5.5, no change is reported in a 1% solution heated for 1 hr. The pH should be between 2.5 and 6.0. Sterilization should be conducted with a minimum of heat.

Comments—Indicated for the relief of severe pain. It is effective in the control of postoperative pain as well as for relieving preoperative apprehension. Its most important actions are on the brain, especially its higher functions. An initial transitory stimulation is followed by depression of the brain, its higher functions, and its medullary centers. The reflexes and spinal functions usually are stimulated. It affects perception in such a way that the patient is more tolerant to discomfort and pain. In addition it appears to interfere with pain conduction. It depresses the respiratory center, stimulates the vomiting center, depresses the cough reflex, constricts the pupils, increases the tone of the GI and genitourinary tracts, and produces mild vasodilation.

It is contraindicated in bronchial asthma, respiratory depression, or idiosyncrasy to the drug. Overdoses may cause respiratory depression, coma, and death. The drug should be used with caution in extreme ages (infants and elderly) as well as in the debilitated patient, or in patients who have increased intracranial pressure, toxic psychoses, myxedema, or prostatic hypertrophy. Untoward reactions may include allergic reactions, nausea, vomiting, constipation, urinary retention, depression, delirium, and convulsions. Morphine Sulfate Injection is a *Schedule II* drug under the *Controlled Substances Act.*

CODEINE

Morphinan-6-ol, (5α,6α)-7,8-didehydro-4,5-epoxy-3-methoxy-17-methyl-, monohydrate; Methylmorphine

[6059-47-8] $C_{18}H_{21}NO_3 \cdot H_2O$ (317.38); *anhydrous* [76-57-3] (299.37).

History—Isolated from opium by the French chemist Robiquet in 1832, who gave it a name derived from the Greek word meaning poppy 'capsules'.

Preparation—Although some codeine is obtained from opium directly, the quantity is not sufficient to meet the extensive use of this alkaloid as a valuable medicinal agent. Much more codeine is used than morphine. This need is met by making it by partial synthesis from morphine. The process involves methylating the phenolic OH of the latter with phenyltrimethylammonium hydroxide. Dry morphine is dissolved in a solution of potassium hydroxide in absolute alcohol, the methylating agent added, and the solution heated. After cooling, water is added, the solution acidified with sulfuric acid, the dimethylaniline product separated, and the alcohol removed by distillation. Treatment with caustic soda solution precipitates the codeine, while any unreacted morphine is held in solution by the sodium hydroxide. The crude codeine is purified by crystallization as the sulfate.

Description—Colorless or white crystals, or a white, crystalline powder; effloresces slowly in dry air and is affected by light; when rendered anhydrous by drying at 80°, it melts within a 2° range between 154° and 158°; sublimes (anhydrous) under reduced pressure; pH (saturated aqueous solution) approximately 9.8.

Solubility—1 g in 120 mL water, 2 mL alcohol, about 0.5 mL chloroform, 50 mL ether, or about 20 mL benzene. When heated in an amount of water insufficient for complete solution, it melts to oily drops that crystallize on cooling.

Incompatibilities—Precipitated from its aqueous solution by most *alkaloidal precipitants* but not by sodium, potassium or ammonium carbonate, or sodium bicarbonate. Aqueous solutions are sufficiently alkaline to precipitate other less soluble alkaloids from solutions of their salts. Ammonia may be liberated from *ammonium salts.*

Comments—May be viewed as morphine with less ceiling efficacy, which fails to produce proportionately greater analgesia as the dose is increased. Indeed, large amounts of codeine may cause excitement. Average doses are *sedative, analgetic,* and *antitussive.* When administered by the oral route 30 to 60 mg is equivalent in analgesic effectiveness to approximately 650 mg of aspirin; subcutaneously, 60 mg is somewhat less effective than 10 mg of morphine. Because of different mechanisms of action, codeine plus salicylates or acetaminophen produces enhanced analgesic action.

Codeine is useful for inducing sleep in the presence of mild pain. It is absorbed rapidly after either oral or parenteral administration; onset of action occurs in 15 to 30 min, and analgesia is maintained for 4 to 6 hr. Codeine is metabolized mainly in the liver where it undergoes *O*-demethylation, *N*-demethylation and partial conjugation with glucuronic acid. The drug is excreted largely in the urine as narcodeine and free and conjugated morphine. Like morphine, this drug also produces cortical and respiratory depression, but serious degrees of either are practically unknown. It is less apt than morphine to cause nausea, vomiting, constipation, and miosis. Both tolerance and addiction occur, however, and the same precautions should be observed in its use as for morphine. *Naloxone* is a specific antagonist in cases of acute intoxication.

This drug, like morphine, is employed as an *analgetic, sedative, hypnotic, antiperistaltic,* and *antitussive* agent. It commonly is given in combination with aspirin, acetaminophen, or other agents. Administered alone, codeine is a *Schedule II* drug under the *Controlled Substances Act. In combination with aspirin-like drugs, it is classified as Schedule III.*

CODEINE PHOSPHATE

Morphinan-6-ol, (5α,6α)-7,8-didehydro-4,5-epoxy-3-methoxy-17-methyl-, phosphate (1:1) (salt), hemihydrate

[41444-62-6] $C_{18}H_{21}NO_3 \cdot H_3PO_4 \cdot 1/2H_2O$ (406.37); *anhydrous* [52-28-8] (397.36).

Preparation—By dissolving codeine in an equimolecular quantity of aqueous phosphoric acid, adding alcohol, and allowing the salt to crystallize from solution.

Description—Fine, white, needle-shaped crystals or a white, crystalline powder; odorless; readily loses water of hydration on exposure to air and is affected by light; solutions are acid to litmus and levorotatory.

Solubility—1 g in 2.5 mL water, 325 mL alcohol, 0.5 mL water at 80°, or 125 mL boiling alcohol.

Comments—See *Codeine, Morphine,* and *general statement.* Being more soluble then codeine sulfate, the phosphate is preferred to the sulfate.

CODEINE SULFATE

Morphinan-6-ol, (5α,6α)-7,8-didehydro-4,5-epoxy-3-methoxy-17-methyl-, sulfate (2:1) (salt), trihydrate

[6854-40-6] $(C_{18}H_{21}NO_3)_2.H_2SO_4.3H_2O$ (750.86); *anhydrous* [1420-53-7] (698.81).

Preparation—By crystallization from a solution of codeine in diluted H_2SO_4.

Description—White crystals, usually needle-like or a white, crystalline powder; effloresces in dry air and is affected by light; aqueous solution is practically neutral or only slightly acid to litmus.

Solubility—1 g in 30 mL water, 1300 mL alcohol, or approximately 6.5 mL water at 80°; insoluble in chloroform or ether.

Incompatibilities—See the *Alkaloids.* It reacts with *phenobarbital sodium* to produce free alkaloid and phenobarbital, both of which may precipitate unless the vehicle contains a moderate proportion of alcohol.

Comments—See *Codeine, Morphine,* and the introductory statement.

Semisynthetic Opioid Analgesics

In the effort to obtain an agent with the advantages of morphine or codeine without their disadvantages, chemists have modified the structure of these natural alkaloids of opium. Some of these modifications, eg, hydrocodone, hydromorphone, or nalorphine result from making minor chemical alterations in the natural alkaloids, the characteristic nucleus remaining intact. For pharmacological convenience, all of these agents are classified here as semisynthetic opioids. In general, the pharmacological properties exhibited by these agents differ quantitatively from those of the parent substance, but qualitatively they are similar. The several semisynthetic agents employed clinically are described below.

HYDROCODONE BITARTRATE

Morphinan-6-one, (5α)-4,5-epoxy-3-methoxy-17-methyl-, [R-(R,*R*)]-2,3-dihydroxybutanedioate (1:1), hydrate (2:5); Dihydrocodeinone Bitartrate

[34195-34-1] [6190-38-1] $C_{18}H_{21}NO_3.C_4H_6O_6.2$ 1/2H_2O (494.50); *anhydrous* [143-71-5] (449.46).

Preparation—This synthetic alkaloid, 7,8-dihydrocodeinone, is prepared either by catalytic rearrangement of codeine or by controlled hydrolysis and oxidation of dihydrothebaine.

Description—Fine white crystals or a fine white crystalline powder; affected by light; pH (1 in 50 solution) 3.2 to 3.8.

Solubility—1 g in 16 mL water; slightly soluble in alcohol; insoluble in ether or chloroform.

Comments—For the relief of moderate to severe pain and for the symptomatic relief of cough. It is an opioid that is somewhat more sedating and addictive than codeine, and is a *Schedule III* drug under the *Controlled Substances Act. It frequently is combined with other drugs such as aspirin-like analgesics, antihistamines, expectorants, and sympathomimetics.*

HYDROMORPHONE HYDROCHLORIDE

Morphinan-6-one-, (5α)-4,5-epoxy-3-hydroxy-17-methyl-, hydrochloride, Dihydromorphinone Hydrochloride; Dilaudid Hydrochloride

[71-68-1] $C_{17}H_{19}NO_3.HCl$ (321.80).

Hydromorphone hydrochloride is 7,8-dihydromorphinone hydrochloride.

Preparation—By electrolytic reduction of morphine or by oxidation of dihydromorphine and then reacting with HCl. US patent 2,649,454.

Description—Fine, white, odorless, crystalline powder, affected by light; aqueous solution is practically neutral or only slightly acid to litmus.

Solubility—1 g in about 3 mL water; sparingly soluble in alcohol; practically soluble in ether.

Incompatibilities—Reactions characteristic of alkaloids are generally applicable to this substance.

Comments—A semisynthetic *analgetic,* chemically and pharmacologically similar to morphine, indicated for the relief of moderate to severe pain of myocardial infarction, cancer, trauma (soft tissue and bone), biliary and renal colic, burns, and postoperative pain. It also is used occasionally for its antitussive effects. It is one-fifth as potent orally as intramuscularly; the peak effect occurs later, and the duration of analgesia is longer after oral administration. After parenteral administration, analgesic action is apparent within 15 to 30 min and lasts for 4 to 5 hr. After oral administration, onset of analgesia is approximately 30 min. Slower absorption and hence longer relief from pain can be obtained from its use in suppository form. It has less tendency to cause sleep than morphine when given in equivalent analgesic doses, and thus relief from pain can be obtained without sleep or stupefaction. It is contraindicated in bronchial asthma, respiratory depression, or idiosyncrasy to the drug. It is claimed that the drug causes less constipation and vomiting than morphine; also, it produces less euphoria. However, tolerance and addiction do occur with the drug, and it must be used with the same precautions as for morphine. It can be given by mouth, by rectum in suppository form, or injected subcutaneously or intravenously (in emergency). The high-dose injection (10 mg/mL) should be used only in patients who are tolerant to the opioids and require large doses of these drugs for relief.

Caution—This drug, being a morphine derivative, is a *Schedule II* drug under the *Controlled Substances Act. Naloxone* is a specific antagonist in cases of acute intoxication.

LEVORPHANOL TARTRATE

Morphinan-3-ol, 17-methyl-, [R-(R*,R*)]-2,3-dihydroxybutanedioate (1:1) (salt), dihydrate; Levo-Dromoran

17-Methylmorphinan-3-ol tartrate (1:1) (salt) dihydrate [5985-38-6] $C_{17}H_{23}NO.C_4H_6O_6.2H_2O$ (443.49); *anhydrous* [125-72-4] (407.46).

Preparation—5,6,7,8-Tetrahydro-2-methylisoquinolinium bromide (I) is metathesized with *p*-methoxybenzyl magnesium bromide (II), and the product rearranges at the expense of the 1,2-double bond to form 1-(*p*-methoxybenzyl)-2-methyl-1,2,5,6,7,8-hexahydroisoquinoline (III). III may be redrawn as shown below to display the ensuing reactions more clearly. A solution of the hydrochloride of III is then hydrogenated at the 3,4-positions with the aid of platinized charcoal, and subsequent treatment with ammonia liberates the *dl*-1,2,3,4,5,6,7,8-octahydro compound (IV), which may be resolved into its (+)- and (−)-enantiomers by the usual procedures. The final step in the preparation of the base involves heating the (−)-enantiomer with phosphoric acid at 150° whereby cyclization between the isoquinoline residue and the benzene ring occurs at the expense of the remaining double bond of the isoquinoline. During the treatment with phosphoric acid, the methoxy group simultaneously is converted to hydroxy, thus producing levorphanol (V).

The tartrate may be produced by dissolution of the base in aqueous tartaric acid solution and crystallizing.

Description—Practically white, odorless, crystalline powder; melts about 115° (anhydrous, about 207°).

Solubility—1 g in 50 mL water or 120 mL alcohol; insoluble in chloroform and ether.

Comments—A potent synthetic analgesic related chemically and pharmacologically to morphine. It produces analgesia at least equal to that of morphine and greater than that of meperidine with much smaller doses than either. It also is longer acting than either of the above; from 6 to 8 hr of pain relief can be achieved after either oral or parenteral administration. Its margin of safety is essentially the same as that of morphine, but it is less likely to produce nausea, vomiting, and constipation. It is indicated whenever an opioid analgesic is required; it is effective for moderate to severe pain and is used parenterally for preoperative sedation as well as an adjunct to nitrous oxide-oxygen anesthesia. The drug is contraindicated in acute alcoholism, bronchial asthma, increased intracranial pressure, respiratory depression, and anoxia. Other precautions and adverse reactions are similar to those induced by other opioid analgesics. It is an opioid with addiction liability similar to that of morphine; therefore, the same precautions should be observed when prescribing this drug as for morphine. The drug is a *Schedule II* drug under the *Controlled Substances Act*.

OXYCODONE HYDROCHLORIDE

4,5-Epoxy-14-hydroxy-3-methoxy-17-methylmorphinan-6-one Hydrochloride; Dihydrodihydroxycodeinone Hydrochloride; OxyContin

[124-90-3] $C_{18}H_{21}NO_4 \cdot HCl$ (351.83).

Preparation—From thebaine, also obtained from opium. Thebaine is the 3,6-dimethoxy-$\Delta^{6,8}$-diene that on oxidation with H_2O_2 inserts an OH at position 14 and a hemiacetal at 6. Hydrolysis of the hemiacetal forms the ketone at position 6; see Manske, *Chemistry of the Morphine Alkaloids*, Oxford Press, 1954. The hydrochloride is prepared from the base by the usual means.

Description—Odorless, white, crystalline powder; saline, bitter taste; melts with decomposition between 274° and 278°.

Solubility—1 g in 10 mL water or 60 mL alcohol.

Comments—For the relief of moderate to moderately severe pain. Like codeine and methadone, it retains one half of its analgesic activity after oral administration. It often is used to relieve postoperative, posttextractional, and postpartum pain. Although oxycodone has less analgesic capability than morphine, it possesses comparable addiction potential and is a *Schedule II* drug under the *Controlled Substances Act*. *It frequently is used in combination with aspirin or acetaminophen.*

OXYMORPHONE HYDROCHLORIDE

(5α)-Morphinan-6-one, 4,5-epoxy-3,14-dihydroxy-17-methyl-, hydrochloride; Numorphan

[357-07-3] $C_{17}H_{19}NO_4 \cdot HCl$ (337.80).

Preparation—Thebaine is dissolved in aqueous formic acid and treated with 30% hydrogen peroxide, after which neutralization with aqueous ammonia yields 14-hydroxycodeinone. This then is dissolved in acetic acid and hydrogenated with the aid of palladium-charcoal catalyst to form 14-hydroxy-7,8-dihydrocodeinone (oxycodone). In the form of its hydrochloride, this compound is demethylated by means of heating with pyridine hydrochloride to yield crude oxymorphone hydrochloride, which then is purified. US Pat 2,806,033.

Description—White, acicular crystals or as a white or slightly off-white powder; odorless; darkens on prolonged exposure to light; pH (aqueous solutions) approximately 5.

Solubility—1 g in 4 mL water, 100 mL alcohol, >1000 mL chloroform or >1000 mL ether.

Comments—A semisynthetic opioid analgesic with actions, uses, and side effects similar to those of hydromorphone and morphine, except it possesses no significant antitussive activity. After parenteral administration, 1 mg of this drug is approximately equivalent in analgesic activity to 10 mg of morphine. Onset of action is rapid; initial effects usually are seen within 5 to 10 min, duration of action is approximately 3 to 6 hr. It satisfactorily controls postoperative pain, the more severe pain of advanced neoplastic diseases, and other types of pain that ordinarily can be controlled by morphine. It also is used parenterally for preoperative medication as well as a supplement to anesthesia. Except that it is somewhat less constipating, the overall incidence and severity of side effects are similar to those of morphine. Its addiction liability is approximately the same as morphine. It is a *Schedule II* drug under the *Controlled Substances Act*.

Opioid Antagonists

Although *N*-allylnorcodeine was observed in 1915 to prevent or abolish morphine- and heroin-induced respiratory depression, more than 25 yr elapsed before it was demonstrated that *N*-allylnormorphine (nalorphine; no longer available in the US) had even more pronounced morphine-antagonizing properties. Even then the clinical significance of this antagonizing effect was not explored until 1951. Two years later it was shown that nalorphine would precipitate acute abstinence syndromes in postaddicts who had been given morphine, methadone, or heroin for brief periods. It also was shown that nonaddicted subjects given large doses of nalorphine exhibited dysphoria and anxiety rather than euphoria. Subsequently, it was noted that, although nalorphine antagonized the analgesic effects of morphine, it was a potent analgesic when given to patients who have postoperative pain.

Except for meperidine, the substitution of an allyl group for the *N*-methyl group in most of the opioids (eg, morphine, levorphanol, methadone, oxymorphone, and phenazocine) results in drugs with varying levels of opioid antagonistic effect. It should be emphasized that this is not restricted to allyl substitution, because the substitution of other groups (methallyl, propyl, isobutyl, propargyl, or cyclopropargylmethyl) for the *N*-methyl group of opioid analgesics also produces substances that are antagonists.

The term *antagonist*, as used in this section, includes naloxone and naltrexone, which are antagonists with little or no agonist actions. These competitive opioid antagonists are effective in the management of *severe respiratory depression* induced by opioid drugs and of *asphyxia neonatorum* caused by administration of these drugs to the expectant mother and for the *diagnosis or treatment of opioid addiction*.

NALOXONE HYDROCHLORIDE

(5α)-Morphinan-6-one, 4,5-epoxy-3,14-dihydroxy-17-(2-propenyl)-, hydrochloride, Narcan

[357-08-4] $C_{19}H_{21}NO_4 \cdot HCl$ (363.84); *dihydrate* [51481-60-8] (399.87).

Preparation—*Oxymorphone* is demethylated and the resulting 4,5α-epoxy-3,14-dihydroxymorphinan-6-one is *N*-allylated by reaction in ethanol with allyl bromide in the presence of $NaHCO_3$. The resulting naloxone is reacted with ethanolic HCl. US Pat 3,254,088.

Description—White to slightly off-white powder; aqueous solutions are acidic; melts about 203°.

Solubility—Soluble in water; slightly soluble in alcohol; practically insoluble in chloroform or ether.

Incompatibilities—Long-chain or high-molecular-weight anions (forms relatively insoluble salts) and with alkaline solutions (base precipitates if concentration is high enough); however, the injection is compatible with bulk IV solutions that are slightly alkaline. Also, oxygen, oxidizing agents, bisulfites, or metabisulfites.

Comments—A synthetic opioid antagonist essentially devoid of opioid agonist properties. Hence, it does not possess morphine-like properties, such as respiratory depression, psychotomimetic effects, and pupillary constriction, characteristic of other opioid antagonists. Available evidence suggests that it antagonizes these opioid effects by competing for the same receptor sites. It is the drug of choice for management of respiratory depression induced by natural and synthetic opioid analgesics, including depression induced by the partial agonist pentazocine. It also is indicated for diagnosis of acute opioid overdosage. It is not effective against nonopioid respiratory depression. Naloxone has been used to detect opioid abuse and can precipitate severe opioid withdrawal symptoms in physically dependent patients. The use of this drug may diminish opioid-dependent euphoria and help reduce the desire for these drugs.

The drug rapidly disappears from serum in man. After an intravenous dose, naloxone is distributed rapidly in the body. The onset of activity generally is apparent within 2 to 5 min; the onset of action is only slightly less rapid when administered by the subcutaneous or intramuscular routes. The mean half-life in adults ranges from 30 to 81 min (means of 64 and 12 min); the mean half-life in neonates is 3.1 and 0.5 hr. It is metabolized in the liver, primarily by glucuronide conjugation, and excreted in the urine. This short duration of action necessitates multiple dosing. Hence, considerable research effort has been directed toward the development of antagonists with a much longer duration of action (see Naltrexone following). Safe and effective use in children younger than 12 yr and in pregnant women has not been established. Adverse effects are said to be rare and usually consist of nausea and vomiting. It is *unscheduled* under the *Controlled Substances Act.*

NALTREXONE HYDROCHLORIDE

Morphinan-6-one, (5α)-17-(cyclopropylmethyl)-4,5-epoxy-3,14-dihydroxy-, Trexan

[16676-29-2] $C_{19}H_{21}NO_4$·HCl (377.87).

Preparation—From normorphine by oxidation at the allylic positions C6 and C14; hydrogenation of the C7-8 double bond and *N*-alkylation with cyclopropylmethyl halide. US Pat 3,332,950.

Description—White crystals; melts about 275°.

Solubility—1 g in approximately 1 mL water.

Comments—Naltrexone generally has little or no agonist activity. Its opioid antagonist activity is reported to be 2 to 9 times that of naloxone and 17 times that of nalorphan. Consequently, it is used as an adjunct to the maintenance of the opioid-free state in detoxified, formerly opioid-dependent, individuals. It also has been used in the treatment of postconcussional syndrome unresponsive to other treatments. It is absorbed rapidly and almost completely after oral administration, but undergoes extensive first-pass metabolism in the liver. Only 5–20% of an orally administered dose reaches systemic circulation unchanged. The major metabolite is 6β-naltrexol; this also is a pure antagonist and may contribute to the opioid receptor blockade. Mean elimination half-lives for naltrexone and 6β-naltrexol are 3.9 and 12.9 hr, respectively; pharmacological effects are apparent for 24 and 72 hr and appear to be independent of dose. The drug does not accumulate after chronic administration but is excreted primarily in the urine. Adverse effects most frequently observed (10%) include anxiety, nervousness, headache, low energy, abdominal cramps, nausea, vomiting, and joint and muscle pain. Liver test abnormalities and lymphocytosis have been reported. Patients should wear some identification indicating they are taking this drug.

SYNTHETIC OPIOID AGONIST/ANTAGONIST

The undesirable side effects of morphine and addiction potential stimulated the search for synthetic drugs that would be as analgesic as morphine but have fewer undesirable effects and less addiction potential. Although the ideal analgesic agent has yet to be developed, currently available synthetic agents have valuable analgesic and pharmacological properties that are described in this section.

ALFENTANIL HYDROCHLORIDE

Propanamide, *N*-[1-[2-(4-ethyl-4,5-dihydro-5-oxo-1*H*-tetrazol-1-yl)ethyl]-4-(methoxymethyl)-4-piperidinyl]-*N*-phenyl-, monohydrochloride, monohydrate; Alfenta

[70879-28-6] $C_{21}H_{32}N_6O_3$·HCl (471.00).

Preparation—See *J Med Chem* 1986; 29:2290.

Description—White crystals; melts at 138°.

Comments—A potent synthetic opioid analgesic related to fentanyl but with a more rapid onset of action and a shorter duration of opioid ef-

fects. The brief duration (30–60 min after 50 mg/kg intravenous) is advantageous for short surgical procedures but requires frequent injection or continuous infusion for longer operations. Because it is less lipid-soluble than fentanyl, it is less likely to accumulate with prolonged or repeated administration.

Adverse effects include muscular rigidity (chest wall, trunk, and extremities), hypotension and bradycardia, respiratory depression, nausea, vomiting, and dizziness. Large doses over a long period also may prolong postoperative awakening and respiratory depression. It is a *Schedule II* drug under the *Controlled Substances Act.*

BUPRENORPHINE HYDROCHLORIDE

6,14-Ethenomorphinan-7-methanol, 17-(cyclopropylmethy)-α-(1,1-dimethylethyl)-4,5-epoxy-18,19-dihydro-3-hydroxy-6-methoxy-α-methyl-, hydrochloride; Buprenex

Preparation—From thebaine; US Pat 3,433,791.

Description—White crystalline powder; aqueous solutions are weakly acidic.

Solubility—Slightly soluble in water.

Comments—A semisynthetic centrally acting opioid analgesic derived from thebaine, it is used for the relief of moderate to severe pain particularly associated with postoperative discomfort. It is approximately 30 times as potent as morphine and exerts its analgesic effect by binding to CNS opioid receptors. It is classified as a partial agonist and exhibits antagonist effects in higher doses. Onset of analgesia occurs within 15 min after intramuscular injection, peaks at 1 hr and persists for up to 6 hr. Approximately 96% is bound to plasma protein and metabolized by the liver. Terminal half-life is 2 to 3 hr. The drug is excreted in the feces as free buprenorphine. Chronic use may produce psychological dependence and may infrequently produce limited physical dependence. Adverse effects related to the *CNS* include sedation (66%), dizziness (5–10%), headache (1–5%), confusion, slurred speech, depression, and hallucinations; *cardiovascular* adverse effects are hypotension or hypertension, tachycardia or bradycardia; *GI* adverse effects are nausea and vomiting, dry mouth, dyspepsia, or flatulence; *respiratory* adverse effects are hypoventilation, dyspnea, or cyanosis; *ophthalmological* adverse effects are miosis, blurred vision, diplopia, or conjunctivitis; *other adverse effects* include pruritus, urinary retention, flushing, chills or coldness, and tinnitus. Safety and efficacy in children has not been established.

Buprenorphine has recently been approved for use in the treatment of opioid abuse.

BUTORPHANOL TARTRATE

(−)-Morphinan-3,14-diol, 17-(cyclobutylmethyl)-, [R(R*,R*)]-2,3-dihydroxybutanedioate (1:1) salt; Stadol

(−)-17-(Cyclobutylmethyl)morphinan-3,14-diol tartrate (1:1) salt [58786-99-5] $C_{21}H_{29}NO_2$·$C_4H_6O_6$ (477.55).

Preparation—Total synthesis of *N*-substituted 3,14-dihydroxymorphinans, including butorphanol, from 7-methoxy-1-tetralone, has been reported by Monkovic et al (*J Am Chem Soc* 1973; 95:7910).

Description—White, crystalline powder; melts about 219°.

Solubility—Soluble in water.

Comments—A potent analgesic with both opioid agonist and antagonist effects. Analgesic potency is 3.5 to 7 times that of morphine, 30 to 40 times that of meperidine, 15 to 20 times that of pentazocine, and 1/40 the antagonist potency of naloxone. It is indicated for moderate to severe postsurgical pain to supplement balanced anesthesia and to relieve postpartum pain. After intramuscular injection, analgesia begins within 10 min, reaches peak activity in 30 to 60 min and persists for 3 to 4 hr. After intravenous administration, peak activity is reached within a few minutes. A 2-mg intramuscular dose is equivalent in analgesic effect to 10 mg of morphine. Although completely absorbed from the GI tract after oral administration, it undergoes approximately 80% first-pass metabolism. Adverse effects observed are similar to those observed after morphine, including dizziness, lightheadedness, and nausea. Transient but disturbing psychotomimetic reactions have been reported after doses of 2 to 4 mg. Two mg depresses the respiration to the same extent as 10 mg of morphine; slow, shallow respiration has been reported in patients taking recommended doses of the drug. The respiratory depression and other effects can be reversed by naloxone. Like pentazocine, the drug increases arterial resistance and the work of the heart; consequently, it is contraindicated in patients who have acute myocardial infarction. It is known to cause euphoria, and tolerance to the analgesic effect has been reported in animals. It also can precipitate withdrawal in opioid-dependent patients. It is a *Schedule IV* drug under the *Controlled Substances Act.*

DEZOCINE

(−)(5α,11α,13S*)-5,11-Methanobenzocyclodecen-3-ol, 13-amino-5,6,7,8,9,10,11,12-octahydro-5-methyl-, Dalgan

[53648-55-8] $C_{16}H_{23}NO$ (245.37).

Preparation—1-Methyl-7-methoxy-2-tetralone is treated with $Br(CH_2)_5Br$ and NaH to insert a pentamethylene bridge between positions 1 and 3 of the tetralone molecule. Reductive amination of the carbonyl group with NH_2OH and Ni/H_2 followed by demethylation of the 7-methoxy group with HBr affords the product; *J Med Chem* 1973; 16:595.

Comments—A synthetic opioid agonist-antagonist structurally similar to pentazocine. Its analgesic and pharmacokinetic properties are similar to morphine. Its adverse effects are like those of other opioid analgesics and include nausea, vomiting, sedation, and respiratory depression. Dizziness, anxiety, disorientation, hallucinations, and sweating also have been reported. Dezocine is not recommended for use in patients physically dependent on opioids. Extreme caution should be exercised if dezocine is used in combination with other CNS-depressant drugs due to an increased risk to the patient. Although it is likely that because of its opioid agonist-antagonist properties, dezocine has less abuse potential than some of the other opioid analgesics, it probably does have some potential for dependence, particularly in patients who have a history of opioid drug abuse. Dezocine is metabolized extensively in the liver by glucuronide conjugation and excreted in the urine.

FENTANYL CITRATE

Propanamide, N-phenyl-N-[1-(2-phenylethyl)-4-piperidinyl]-, 2-hydroxy-1,2,3-propanetricarboxylate (1:1); Sublimaze; ing of Innovar

N-(1-Phenethyl-4-piperidyl)propionanilide citrate (1:1) [990-73-8] $C_{22}H_{28}N_2O.C_6H_8O_7$ (528.60).

Preparation—One method consists of condensing propionyl chloride with *N*-(4-piperidyl)aniline, then treating the resulting *N*-(4-piperidyl)propionanilide with phenethyl chloride, aiding each condensation by the presence of a suitable dehydrochlorinating agent. Reaction of the base with an equimolar portion of citric acid yields the (1:1) citrate. US Pat 3,164,600.

Description—White, crystalline powder or glistening crystals; odorless and tasteless (*Note:* because this compound is extremely potent, no taste test is recommended); stable in air; melts at 147° to 152°; pKa 8.3.

Solubility—1 g in approximately 40 mL of water, 140 mL of alcohol or 350 mL of chloroform.

Comments—A potent opioid analgesic with rapid onset and short duration of action when administered parenterally. Administration of the base via a transdermal patch has a much slower onset (8–12 hr) and

a longer duration of action (>72 hr) and often is used to manage chronic pain that necessitates an opioid analgesic. It has a profile of pharmacological action similar to morphine, except that it does not cause emesis or release histamine. Equianalgesia can be obtained with a dose 1/150 that of morphine. After intravenous injection, peak analgesia appears within 3 to 5 min and lasts 30 to 60 min. Fentanyl produces signs and symptoms typical of opioid analgesics, such as miosis, euphoria, and respiratory depression. It is used primarily as an analgesic for the control of pain associated with all types of surgery. It also can be used as a supplement to all agents commonly employed for general and regional anesthesia. It also is an ingredient in *Fentanyl Citrate and Droperidol Injection*, see RPS-18, page 1045.

It is contraindicated in children 2 yr and younger, in asthmatic patients, and in patients who have a history of myasthenia gravis. Other depressant drugs, such as barbiturates, major tranquilizers, tricyclic antidepressants, opioids, and general anesthetics have an additive or potentiating effect on the drug. Its safe use in pregnancy has not been established. It crosses the placental barrier; use during labor may lead to respiratory depression in the newborn infant. It should be used with caution in patients who have liver and kidney disease. Adverse reactions include respiratory depression, apnea, muscular rigidity, and hypotension. Less frequently, nausea and vomiting may occur. Infrequently, dizziness, visual disturbance, itching, euphoria, and spasms of the sphincter of Oddi have been observed. It is a *Schedule II* drug under the *Controlled Substances Act.*

MEPERIDINE HYDROCHLORIDE

4-Piperidinecarboxylic acid, 1-methyl-4-phenyl-, ethyl ester, hydrochloride; Pethidine Hydrochloride; Dolantin, Dolantol, Eudolat, Isonipecaine; Demerol Hydrochloride

Ethyl 1-methyl-4-phenylisonipecotate hydrochloride [50-13-5] $C_{15}H_{21}NO_2.HCl$ (283.80).

Preparation—One of several methods in which benzyl chloride, diethanolamine, and benzyl cyanide are used in the following principal steps:

Removal of the *N*-benzyl group is accomplished by catalytic hydrogenation in acetic acid solution in which a palladium catalyst is used. The addition of formaldehyde to the reduction mixture followed by further catalytic hydrogenation leads to meperidine. The free base is converted to the hydrochloride by neutralization with HCl.

Description—Fine, white, crystalline, odorless powder; stable in air at ordinary temperatures; pH (1 in 20 solution) approximately 5; melts between 186° and 189°; pKa 7.7 to 8.15.

Solubility—Very soluble in water; soluble in alcohol; sparingly soluble in ether.

Comments—A synthetic opioid analgesic with multiple actions qualitatively similar to those of morphine; the most prominent of these actions are on the CNS and on organs composed of smooth muscle. It acts principally to induce analgesia and sedation. It is indicated for preoperative use, relief of moderate to severe pain, support anesthesia, and obstetrical analgesia. It crosses the placental barrier; use during labor may lead to respiratory depression in the newborn infant. Available evidence suggests it produces less smooth muscle spasm, constipation, and depression of cough reflex than equianalgesic doses of morphine. In a 60- to 80-mg parenteral dose, it essentially is equal in analgesic effectiveness to 10 mg of morphine; the onset of action is slightly more rapid, and the duration of action is somewhat shorter than morphine.

It is significantly less effective by the oral than by the parenteral route. After intravenous administration of meperidine in healthy adults, the volume distribution at steady state was 269 L; plasma clearance was 1.06 L/min; and elimination half-life was 3.6 hr. Evidence exists that the disposition of meperidine varies between day and night, with elimination half-life shorter and plasma clearance greater at night. It is contraindicated in patients on MAO inhibitors; it inconsistently has precipitated severe, and occasionally fatal, reactions within 14 days in patients who have received such medication. The drug should be used with caution and in reduced dosage in patients on other opioid analgesics, general anesthetics, phenothiazines, sedatives, tricyclic antidepressants, and other CNS depressants. Major adverse reactions include respiratory depression, circulatory depression, respiratory arrest, shock, and cardiac arrest. The most frequent untoward effects include dizziness, sedation, nausea, vomiting, and sweating. Other adverse reactions include euphoria, weakness, headache, agitation, tremor, seizures, transient hallucinations, and disorientation. Some of the CNS toxicity may be due to the neurotoxic metabolite, normeperidine. Because of concern about the incidence and severity of the CNS adverse effects, many clinicians recommend its short-term use only in otherwise healthy adults who are unable to receive other agents. Other effects involving the GI tract, cardiovascular system, and genitourinary tract are similar to morphine. Analgesia is possible with doses that do not cause stupefaction, a decided advantage over morphine. Pain usually is relieved within 20 min to 1 hr, analgesia lasting from 2 to 5 hr. Naloxone is a specific antagonist in cases of acute intoxication It is a *Schedule II* drug under the *Controlled Substances Act.*

METHADONE HYDROCHLORIDE

3-Heptanone, 6-(dimethylamino)-4,4-diphenyl-, hydrochloride; Dolophine Hydrochloride

Amidone Hydrochloride; [1095-90-5] $C_{21}H_{27}NO.HCl$ (345.91).

Preparation—Diphenylacetonitrile is condensed with 2-chloro-1-dimethylaminopropane in the presence of sodamide, yielding 4-(dimethylamino)-2,2-diphenylvaleronitrile and an unwanted isomeric nitrile in approximately equal amounts. The isomers are separated and the former is subjected to Grignard addition with ethyl magnesium bromide. Subsequent hydrolysis in the presence of hydrochloric acid yields methadone hydrochloride.

Description—Colorless crystals or a white, crystalline, odorless powder; pH (1 in 100 solution) 4.5 to 6.5; optically inactive (the official salt is a racemic mixture of which only the levo form has analgetic activity).

Solubility—1 g in 13 mL water, 8 mL alcohol, or 3 mL chloroform; practically insoluble in ether or glycerin.

Comments—A synthetic *opioid analgesic* with multiple actions quantitatively similar to morphine, the most prominent of which involve the CNS and organs composed of smooth muscle. The principal actions of therapeutic value are those of *analgesia, sedation,* and *detoxification* or *temporary maintenance* in opioid addiction. It also has

significant *antitussive* properties but is no longer approved for this use in the US. It is rapidly but probably incompletely absorbed after oral administration, because only 52% of a given dose appears in the urine. Mean plasma levels of 182 and 420 ng/mL have been reported in patients maintained on a daily oral dose of 40 and 80 mg, respectively, 71–87% of which is in bound form. The half-life is approximately 25 hr, with a range of 13 to 47 hr. A parenteral dose of 8 to10 mg is approximately equivalent in analgesic effectiveness to 10 mg of morphine; onset and duration of action of the two drugs are similar.

It is approximately half as potent orally as parenterally. It is indicated for the relief of moderate to severe pain, for detoxification treatment of opioid addiction, and for temporary, or sometimes long-term, maintenance treatment of opioid addiction. If it is administered for heroin treatment for longer than 3 wk, the procedure passes from treatment of the acute withdrawal syndrome (detoxification) to maintenance therapy; the latter use can be undertaken *only* in approved programs, unless the addict is hospitalized for conditions other than addiction. Its abstinence syndrome qualitatively is similar to that of morphine; however, the onset is slower, the course more prolonged, and the symptoms less severe. It can produce drug dependence of the morphine type; therefore, it should be prescribed and administered with the same degree of caution as morphine.

It is contraindicated in patients known to be sensitive to it. The drug should be used with caution and in reduced dosage in patients on other opioid analgesics, general anesthetics, phenothiazine, and other tranquilizers, sedative-hypnotics, tricyclic antidepressants, MAOIs, and CNS depressants as respiratory depression; hypotension, profound sedation, or coma may result. Patients on a maintenance program are given methadone only as an oral liquid form and should not be given pentazocine or rifampin because these drugs may induce withdrawal symptoms. The safe use of the drug in pregnancy has not been established. It is not recommended for obstetrical analgesia, because its long duration may induce respiratory depression in the newborn. Adverse reactions are similar to those for other opioid analgesics (see especially *Meperidine*). It is widely employed in the withdrawal management of patients addicted to morphine, heroin, and related opioid drugs. *Naloxone* is an effective antagonist in cases of acute intoxication. It is a *Schedule II* drug under the *Controlled Substances Act.*

NALBUPHINE HYDROCHLORIDE

(5α,6α)-Morphinan-3,6,14-triol, 17-(cyclobutylmethyl)-4,5-epoxy-, hydrochloride, Nubain

[23277-43-2] $C_{21}H_{27}NO_4.HCl$ (393.91)

Preparation—Refer to US Pat 3,393,197.

Description—*Base:* white crystals; melts about 230°.

Comments—For the relief of moderate to severe pain. It also may be used for preoperative analgesia, as a supplement to surgical anesthesia and for obstetrical analgesia during labor. It is related chemically to oxymorphone and to the opioid antagonist naloxone. It possesses both agonist and antagonist properties. Thus, it resembles pentazocine pharmacologically. Its analgesic potency when administered parenterally, on a milligram basis, is approximately the same as that of morphine and approximately three to four times greater than that of pentazocine; its antagonistic potency is approximately 10 times greater than that of pentazocine. The onset of action occurs within 2 to 3 min after intravenous administration and within 15 min after intramuscular or subcutaneous administration; it is metabolized in the liver; its plasma half-life is 5 hr and the duration of effect is 3 to 6 hr. Adverse reactions are the same as those for morphine and other potent analgesics. Those most frequently observed include sedation (36%), sweaty or clammy skin (9%), nausea and vomiting (6%), dizziness and vertigo (5%), dry mouth (4%), and headache (3%). Respiratory depression may occur with usual doses of nalbuphine, but it is not dose related; however, it plateaus with a cumulative intravenous dose of approximately 30 mg. The abrupt withdrawal after prolonged administration causes opioid-like abstinence symptoms that are milder than those of morphine but more intense than those of pentazocine. Although it possesses opioid antagonist activity, evidence exists that in nondependent patients it does not antagonize an opioid analgesic administered just before, concurrently, or just after an injection of the drug. Therefore, patients receiving opioid analgesics, general anesthetics, phenothiazines, other sedatives, hypnotics, or CNS depressants concomitantly may exhibit additive effects. Thus, the dose of one or both agents should be reduced. Clinical experience to support use in children younger than 18 yr is presently unavailable.

PENTAZOCINE

2,6-Methano-3-benzazocin-8-ol, (2α,6α,11R*)-1,2,3,4,5,6-hexahydro-6,11-dimethyl-3-(3-methyl-2-butenyl)-, Talwin

[359-83-1] $C_{19}H_{27}NO$ (285.43).

Preparation—1,2,3,4,5,6-Hexahydro-6,11-dimethyl-2,6-methano-3-benzazocin-8-ol (I) is condensed with 1-bromo-3-methyl-2-butene by refluxing in N,N-dimethylformamide in the presence of sodium bicarbonate. The reaction mixture is filtered, and the crude pentazocine is isolated by means of a suitable solvent extraction process and finally crystallized from aqueous methanol. US patent 3,250,678.

Compound I may be prepared by the following sequence of reactions: 3,4-dimethylpyridine methiodide is converted to 1,3,4-trimethyl-2-(p-methoxybenzyl)-1,2-dihydropyridine with p-methoxybenzylmagnesium chloride, reduced to 1,3,4-trimethyl-2-(p-methoxybenzyl)-1,2,5,6-tetrahydropyridine with sodium borohydride, cyclized (with H_3PO_4 or HBr) to 1,2,3,4,5,6-hexahydro-3,6,11-trimethyl-2,6-methano-3-benzazocin-8-ol, esterified with acetic anhydride and reacted with cyanogen bromide to form 3-cyano-1,2,3,4,5,6-hexahydro-6,11-dimethyl-2,6-methano-3-benzazocin-8-ol acetate, and hydrolyzed with dilute HCl to compound I.

Description—White to pale tan, crystalline powder; odorless; slightly bitter taste; stable in light, heat (ambient room temperature), and air; melts between 147° and 158°; pKa approximately 8.95.

Solubility—1 g in >1000 mL of water, 11 mL of alcohol, 2 mL of chloroform or 42 mL of ether.

Comments—A synthetic analgesic agent. When administered orally in a 50-mg dose, it appears to be equivalent in analgesic effectiveness to 60 mg of codeine. When given in usual parenteral doses, it is as effective in relieving moderate to severe pain as usual parenteral doses of morphine, meperidine, butorphanol, or nalbuphine. Significant analgesia occurs within 15 to 30 min after oral administration, 15 to 20 min after intramuscular injection, and 2 to 3 min after intravenous administration. Duration of action is usually 3 hr or longer. Half-life after intramuscular administration is 2.1 hr. Onset, duration of action, and degree of pain relief are related both to dose and to the severity of pain. It weakly (approximately 1/50 that of nalorphine) antagonizes the analgesic effect of morphine and meperidine. It also produces incomplete reversal of the cardiovascular, respiratory, and behavioral depression induced by morphine and meperidine. It also has some sedative properties. It is indicated for the control of moderate to severe pain. It is contraindicated in patients hypersensitive to it. It should be used with caution in patients who have head injuries and increased intracranial pressure. Except during labor, its use during pregnancy has not been established. Because of limited experience in children younger than 12 yr, its use in this age group is not recommended. Patients on the drug should be warned not to drive an automobile, operate machinery, or expose themselves to hazards. Although some patients on therapeutic doses exhibit acute CNS manifestations (hallucinations, disorientation, and confusion), such instances are rare and usually clear spontaneously.

GI (nausea, vomiting, diarrhea, infrequent constipation, and abdominal distress), CNS (dizziness, lightheadedness, sedation, euphoria, headache, disturbed dreams, insomnia, syncope, visual blurring, and hallucinations), autonomic (sweating, flushing, and chills), allergic (rash, urticaria, and edema of the face), and cardiovascular (hypotension and tachycardia) adverse effects have been reported. Respiratory depression has also been included among these adverse effects.

Pentazocine has been reported to cause psychological and physical dependence after both oral and parenteral use. This is more common in patients who have a history of drug abuse. It has been abused in combination with the antihistamine, tripelennamine, by parenteral injection. This combination is reported to cause effects similar to those of heroin. It is a *Schedule IV* drug under the *Controlled Substances Act*.

PROPOXYPHENE HYDROCHLORIDE

Benzeneethanol, [S-(R*,S*)]-α-[2-(dimethylamino)-1-methylethyl]-α-phenyl-, propanoate (ester), hydrochloride; Darvon

[1639-60-7] $C_{22}H_{29}NO_2$·HCl (375.94).

Preparation—The Mannich base formed by condensation of propiophenone and dimethylamine with formaldehyde is grignardized with benzyl magnesium chloride to produce a mixture of the racemates of the two diastereoisomers (designated commercially as α and β) of the alcohol. The desired α-*dl* form is isolated by fractional crystallization and resolved by means of *d*-camphorsulfonic acid. The desired α-*d* enantiomorph is propionylated with propionic acid in the presence of trimethylamine to form propoxyphene, which adds an equivalent of HCl in forming the hydrochloride.

Description—White, crystalline powder; odorless; bitter taste; melts within a 3° range between 163.5° and 168.5°.

Solubility—Freely soluble in water; soluble in alcohol, chloroform, or acetone; practically insoluble in benzene or ether.

Comments—A mild analgesic structurally related to the opioid analgesic methadone. Although its pharmacological properties resemble those of the opioids as a group, it does not compare with them in analgesic potency. Well-controlled studies indicate that the milligram potency of propoxyphene is approximately one-third to two-thirds that of codeine. It appears that its effectiveness in a dose of 32 mg is questionable, and in a dose of 65 mg it is not more, and usually less, effective than the same dose of codeine or 650 mg of aspirin. It has no anti-inflammatory or antipyretic action and little antitussive activity, despite the fact its levo isomer is used for this purpose. It is indicated for the control of *mild-to-moderate* pain. It is absorbed completely after oral administration; however, first-pass elimination of 30% to 70% significantly reduces its bioavailability. The apparent volume of distribution is 700 to 800 L; oral clearance is 1.3 to 3.6 L/min; and half-life is 6 to 12 hr. The major metabolite, norpropoxyphene, has a half-life of 30 to 36 hr. It is contraindicated in patients hypersensitive to it and to aspirin, phenacetin, or caffeine. The drug should not be used during pregnancy unless in the physician's judgment the potential benefits exceed the potential hazards. The most frequent adverse effects are dizziness, sedation, nausea, and vomiting. Other adverse reactions include constipation, abdominal pain, skin rashes, lightheadedness, headache, weakness, euphoria, dysphoria, and minor visual disturbances. The chronic ingestion of 800 mg/day has caused toxic psychoses and convulsions. The depressant effects of propoxyphene may be experienced with those of other depressant drugs, such as alcohol, tranquilizers and sedative-hypnotics. Moreover, deaths have been reported in patients on excessive doses, either alone or in combination with other CNS depressant drugs. Because both psychological and physical dependence have been induced with this agent, it should be prescribed with the same degree of caution as codeine. Drowsiness or dizziness may occur, which may impair ability to drive or perform other tasks requiring alertness. It is not recommended for children.

PROPOXYPHENE NAPSYLATE

Benzeneethanol, [S-(R*,S*)]-α-[2-(dimethylamino)-1-methylethyl]-α-phenyl-, propanoate (ester), compound with 2-naphthalenesulfonic acid (1:1) monohydrate; Darvon-N

[26570-10-5] $C_{22}H_{29}NO_2$·$C_{10}H_8O_3S$ · H_2O (565.72); *anhydrous* [17140-78-2] (547.71).

For the structure of the base, see *Propoxyphene Hydrochloride*.

Preparation—*Propoxyphene* is reacted with an equimolar quantity of aqueous 2-naphthalenesulfonic acid and the salt is crystallized therefrom.

Description—White, bitter, crystalline powder; essentially no odor; melts within a 4° range between 155° and 165°.

Solubility—1 g in 10,000 mL water, 15 mL alcohol, or 10 mL chloroform; soluble in ether.

Comments—Actions, uses, and precautions are the same as *Propoxyphene Hydrochloride*, except that, because of its larger molecular weight, a dose of 100 mg is needed instead of the 65-mg dose of the hydrochloride. This compound permits more stable liquid and tablet dosage forms because of its very slight solubility in water.

SUFENTANIL

Propanamide, N-[4-(methoxymethyl)-1-[2-(thienyl)ethyl]-4-piperidinyl]-N-phenyl-, 2-hydroxy-1,2,3-propanetricarboxylate (1:1); Sufenta

[60561-17-3] $C_{22}H_{30}N_2S.C_6H_8O_7$ (578.68).

Preparation—*Arzneimittel-Forsch* 26:1521, 1976.

Description—White crystals; melts about 97°.

Comments—A strong opioid analgesic. Its analgesic potency is 5 to 12 times that of fentanyl on a weight basis. High doses can cause amnesia and a loss of consciousness. It is used for balanced anesthesia in general surgery as an adjunct to nitrous oxide and oxygen. It also may be used for induction of surgical anesthesia and as the sole anesthetic agent with a muscle relaxant and oxygen for cardiovascular and neurosurgical procedures. Given intravenously it is metabolized rapidly (elimination half-life, 2.4 hr). The volume of distribution is 2.5 L/kg; 92.5% is bound to plasma protein; plasma clearance is 0.8 L/min. The most common adverse effects include respiratory depression and skeletal muscle rigidity. The rapid intravenous administration of sufentanil may induce a general increase in muscle tone, including chest-wall spasm. Other adverse effects include bradycardia, hypotension, and hypertension. After low doses recovery time is approximately the same as that for fentanyl. Sufentanil is a *Schedule II* drug under the Federal *Controlled Substances Act*.

Mixed-Action

TRAMADOL HYDROCHLORIDE

Cyclohexanol, (±)-*cis*-2-[dimethylaminomethyl]-1-(3-methoxyphenyl)-, hydrochloride; Ultram; Zydol

[22204-88-2]$C_{16}H_{25}NO_2$.HCl (299.84).

Preparation—See US Pat 3,652,589 (1965).

Description—White crystals that melt at approximately 180°

Solubility—Soluble in water.

Comments—It exerts analgesic effect partly by activating the μ opioid receptor, but it is neither an opium derivative nor a semisynthetic derivative. It also inhibits the neuronal reuptake of norepinephrine and serotonin, which is thought to contribute to its analgesic effects. The pain-relieving action of tramadol is only partially blocked by naloxone. It is effective against moderate to moderately severe postoperative, gynecologica, obstetric, cancer, and other pain. Tramadol's principal metabolite is 6 times more potent as an analgesic and has 200 greater affinity for the μ receptor. Although tramadol shares pharmacological and adverse effects of other opioid agonists, such as drowsiness, dry mouth, nausea, and pruritus, the abuse potential appears to be low. Consequently, tramadol is not subject to regulation by the Federal *Controlled Substances Act* of 1970 and is not a scheduled substance. Tramadol causes minor tolerance and withdrawal. In addition, respiratory depression is significantly less than with morphine. The onset of analgesia with this drug occurs within 1 hr and peaks at 2 to 4 hr. Usually the duration of the pain relief is 3 to 6 hr. Seizures have occurred in patients using tramadol.

ANALGESICS, ANTIPYRETICS, AND ANTI-INFLAMMATORIES

Drugs of the analgesic, antipyretic, and anti-inflammatory class include a heterogeneous group of compounds that, unlike those presented in the preceding section, are without significant addiction liability and, therefore, are not subject to regulation under the *Controlled Substances Act*. Many of these agents affect pain, fever, and inflammation and are referred to as the nonsteroidal anti-inflammatory drugs (NSAIDs). Consequently, they are used widely for minor aches and pains, headaches, the general feeling of malaise that accompanies febrile illnesses, and to alleviate symptoms of rheumatic fever, arthritis, gout, and other musculoskeletal disturbances. Acetaminophen is not an NSAID, because it lacks significant anti-inflammatory action, but it has uses similar to the NSAIDs. Several agents (eg, allopurinol, colchicine, probenecid) have pain-relieving properties in various conditions (eg, gout, arthritis); however, because they are of no value in other types of pain, they cannot be classed as true analgesic drugs and are not discussed in this section.

Nonsteroidal Anti-inflammatory Drugs

The principal mechanism of action for all NSAIDs appears to be inhibition of prostaglandin synthesis by blocking the activity of the precursor enzyme, cyclooxygenase (COX). Their actions on prostaglandins likely account for many of the side effects of the NSAIDs. Although, in general, there is little difference between the efficacy of different NSAIDs, some patients may respond to one agent better than another. This is difficult to predict and often necessitates trial and error to find the most suitable drug.

The discovery that NSAIDs inhibit prostaglandin biosynthesis was made by John Vane and coworkers in the early 1970s. Tissue injury activates an enhanced conversion of arachidonic acid to prostaglandins *via* the COX pathway, which is so-named because COX enzymes catalyze the conversion. Because some prostaglandins amplify pain signals, inhibition of COX results in analgesia. NSAIDs have good analgesic efficacy, but less than that of opioids; a relatively rapid onset; well-known adverse effects, including potentially fatal gastrointestinal bleeding and disturbance of salt and water balance. They also have a relatively well-defined mechanism of action. All of the effects of NSAIDs–analgesic, antiinflammatory, antipyretic, and antiplatelet–are believed to be due, directly or indirectly, to inhibition of the biosynthesis of prostanoids, such as PGE_2, which induce inflammation and sensitize nociceptors. Inhibition of other routes of arachidonic acid metabolism, such as the lipoxygenase pathway, does not produce a strong analgesic effect. From x-ray crystallographic studies, it appears that most traditional NSAIDs bind to the polar amino acid arginine at position 120 (Arg^{120}) of cyclooxygenase enzymes. There are at least 2 COX isozymes (COX-1 and COX-2). Because COX-1 and COX-2 isozymes both have an arginine in position 120, the traditional NSAIDs inhibit the catalytic activity of both COX isoforms (ie, they are nonselective COX inhibitors).

The clinical usefulness of NSAIDs is restricted by several adverse effects. Phenylbutazone has been implicated in hepatic necrosis and granulomatous hepatitis; and sulindac, indomethacin, ibuprofen, and naproxen has been implicated in hepatitis and cholestatic hepatitis. Transient increases in serum aminotransferases, especially alanine aminotransferase, have been reported. All of these drugs, including aspirin, because of their inhibition of prostaglandins, can interfere with regulation of glomerular filtration and renal sodium and water excretion. Thus, the NSAIDs can cause fluid retention and decrease sodium excretion, followed by hyperkalemia, oliguria and anuria. Moreover, all of these drugs can adversely affect the stomach and may even cause peptic ulceration. Other side effects include diarrhea with meclofenamate; tinnitus with aspirin; headache with indomethacin, and upper abdominal pain with ketoprofen, meclofenamate, and tolmetin. The ranking of NSAIDs according to toxicity shows indomethacin, tolmetin, and melofenamate to be the most toxic with coated or buffered aspirin and ibuprofen the least. Blood dyscrasias associated with NSAIDs are rare, but death has been attributed to the use of these drugs (estimates range to over 10,000 per year in the United States). All of them can interfere with platelet function and may cause bleeding in patients taking anticoagulants. In addition, agranulocytosis or aplastic anemia have been reported in patients on indomethacin, ibuprofen, fenoprofen, naproxen, tolmetin, and piroxicam. Phenylbutazone has caused agranulocytosis and aplastic anemia, especially in the elderly, and may cause leukemia.

Other adverse effects attributed to these drugs include dermatitis and allergic reactions as well as CNS effects, such as sedation, agitation, headaches, and tinnitus. Patients taking these drugs for long periods should have periodic white cell counts and determinations of serum creatinine levels and hepatic enzyme activities.

Salicylate-like Nonsteroidal Anti-inflammatory Drugs

The salicylate group of analgesics and antipyretics are commonly employed. Indeed, these are consumed at a rate in excess of 10,000 tons annually. In general, salicylates are contraindicated in hypersensitive individuals and in those who have GI disturbances, particularly hemorrhaging ulcers. They also should be used with caution in patients on anticoagulant therapy and avoided in patients on uricosurics. The salicylates interact with a wide variety of agents, some of which are important clinically, whereas others are largely of theoretical interest. Nevertheless, the well-informed pharmacist should be knowledgeable of the potential interactions between salicylate drugs:

Antidiabetic agents (increased hypoglycemia)
Oral anticoagulants (displacement of anticoagulants from protein binding sites, increased anticoagulant effect)
Uricosuric agents (relative effect of large and small doses of salicylates)
Antiarthritic drugs (may lower plasma concentrations of these agents)
Alcohol (which enhances GI bleeding)
Tetracycline (may complex with buffering agent in some aspirin products)

ASPIRIN

Benzoic acid, 2-(acetyloxy)-,

Acetylsalicylic acid [50-78-2] $C_9H_8O_4$ (180.16).

Preparation—Salicylic acid is acetylated directly with acetic anhydride and the crude material purified by recrystallization from benzene or various other nonaqueous solvents. A granulated form of aspirin, either white or colored, also is available commercially for compression into tablets.

Description—White crystals, commonly tabular or needle-like, or a white, crystalline powder; odorless or a faint odor; stable in dry air (in moist air it gradually hydrolyzes into salicylic and acetic acids, the odor of the latter becoming noticeable); melts about 135°, but the exact melting temperature varies with the conditions of the test; an alcoholic solution is not colored violet by ferric chloride (distinction from salicylic acid).

Solubility—1 g in approximately 300 mL water, 5 mL alcohol, 17 mL chloroform, or approximately 10 to 15 mL of ether; less soluble in absolute ether; dissolves with decomposition in aqueous solutions of alkali hydroxides or carbonates.

Incompatibilities—Can form a damp to pasty mass when triturated with *acetanilid, acetophenetidin, antipyrine, aminopyrine, methenamine, phenol,* or *salol.* Powders containing aspirin with an alkali salt such as *sodium bicarbonate* may become gummy on contact with atmospheric moisture owing to a partial solution and subsequent hydrolysis of the aspirin. Hydrolysis likewise occurs in admixture with salts containing water of crystallization. Solutions of alkali acetates and citrates, as well as alkalies themselves, dissolve this drug, but the resulting solutions hydrolyze rapidly to form salts of acetic and salicylic acids. Sugar and glycerin have been shown to hinder the decomposition. It very slowly liberates hydroidic acid from *potassium* or *sodium iodide.* Subsequent oxidation by the air produces free iodine.

Comments—Of the salicylate drugs, aspirin (acetylsalicylic acid) is the most frequently used. All commercially available salicylates have similar pharmacological properties, so aspirin is discussed as the prototype for this group. Aspirin is employed as an antipyretic and analgetic

in a variety of conditions. It is indicated for the relief of pain from simple headache, discomfort, and fever associated with the common cold and minor muscular aches and pains. When drug therapy is indicated for the reduction of a fever, it is one of the most effective and safest drugs.

Epidemiological evidence has suggested the possibility of an association between the use of aspirin in the treatment of fever in children who have varicella (chickenpox), a common cold, or influenza virus infections and the subsequent development of Reyes syndrome. The current opinion is that aspirin should not be prescribed under usual circumstances for children who have upper respiratory, viral infections. If control of fever, aches, and pains are necessary, alternative measures should be employed.

In gout and in acute rheumatic fever, the salicylates, including aspirin, have a fairly specific action. In gout, large doses must be given often, and the results are somewhat less drastic than with phenylbutazone or allopurinol. In acute rheumatic fever, full doses are given every hour until salicylism occurs (ringing in ears, dizziness); thereafter, it is given every 4 hr for days or weeks. In neither of the above-mentioned conditions are the salicylates a cure, and other forms of treatment are employed simultaneously. After oral administration, peak plasma levels are reached within 1 to 2 hr, and fairly constant levels are maintained for 4 to 6 hr.

Plasma half-life after oral administration of 1 g of aspirin ranges from 4.7 to 9 hr, with an average of 6 hr. With toxic doses (10–20 g) the half-life may be increased to 22 hr. A direct correlation between plasma levels and clinical effectiveness has not been established, but analgesia usually is achieved at plasma levels of 15 to 30 mg/100 mL, anti-inflammatory activity at 20 to 40 mg/100 mL, and some symptoms of salicylism at 35 mg/100 mL. It is bound poorly to plasma protein; nevertheless, with therapeutic doses, from 50% to 80% is bound to plasma proteins.

Adverse effects from usual doses of the drug are infrequent; most common are GI disturbances (dyspepsia, nausea, vomiting, and occult bleeding). Prolonged administration of large doses (3.6 g/day) results in occult bleeding and may result in anemia. Massive GI hemorrhage can occur and, although its relation to peptic ulcer is uncertain, a nonsalicylate analgesic may be preferred in high-risk patients.

As evidenced by substantial fecal blood loss, alcohol increases the gastric bleeding caused by aspirin in many patients. Concomitant use of the drug and corticosteroids or pyrazolone derivatives (phenylbutazone) may increase the risk of GI ulceration. Its use with fenoprofen, ibuprofen, indomethacin, or naproxen may cause a lowering of plasma concentrations and thus reduce the effectiveness of the latter drugs. It displaces highly bound coumarin-type anticoagulants from protein-binding sites and thus increases the concentrations and effects of the anticoagulants.

The hypoglycemic action of oral sulfonylureas may be increased by concurrent administration of the drug. The uricosuric activity of probenecid and sulfinpyrazone are inhibited when either drug is administered simultaneously with aspirin. Buffered aspirin formulations that contain calcium, magnesium, or aluminum may form complexes with tetracycline from which absorption of the antibiotic is impaired.

Salicylates account for many accidental poisonings that may result from promiscuous use of large doses of these agents by the laity. To avoid accidental poisoning of children, this drug and other salicylate drugs should be kept out of their reach; also, caution in use of these drugs in children who have fever and dehydration is necessary because they are particularly prone to intoxication from relatively small doses of the drugs. In addition, some few people manifest idiosyncrasy in the form of an allergic sensitivity to salicylates, especially this drug, and may suffer from serious, if not fatal, asthma after ingestion of a single 300-mg dose. Consequently, it should be used with great care in patients who have asthma, nasal polyps, or allergies.

It crosses the placental barrier and is excreted into breast milk. As use of aspirin before delivery may have inhibited platelet aggregation and diminished factor XII plasma levels in newborn infants, it has been suggested that no salicylate be ingested during the last month of pregnancy. Chronic high-dose therapy has been reported to increase the length of gestation and to prolong labor.

Several studies indicate that low doses of aspirin reduce the risk of myocardial infarction, stroke, and perhaps colon cancer.

Nonsalicylate Nonsteroidal Anti-Inflammatory Drugs

This group of NSAIDs include derivatives from propionic, acetic, and anthranilic acids, as well as oxicam. Little distinguishes the clinical profile of these NSAIDs from the others.

BROMFENAC SODIUM

Benezenacetic acid, 2-amino-3-(4-bromobenzoyl)-, monosodium salt, sesquihydrate; Duract

[12638-5-3] $C_{15}H_{11}BrNNaO_3.1\ 1/2H_2O$ (338.17).

Preparation—From 2-amino-4′-bromobenzophenone and ethyl 2-(methylthio)acetate in the presence of t-butyl hypochlorite to form 3-(methylthio)-6-(p-bromobenzoyl)-2(1H)-indoline through the sulfonium ion intermediate, followed by rearrangement. The methylthio group is removed by catalytic reduction (Raney nickel) with subsequent hydrolysis of the resulting amide to yield the free acid. See *J Med Chem*1984; 27:137.

Description—Orange crystals melting about 285° with decomposition.

Solubility—Soluble in water, alcohol, or dilute aqueous alkali; insoluble in organic solvents or dilute aqueous acid.

DICLOFENAC SODIUM

Benzeneacetic acid, 2-[(2,6-dichlorophenyl)amino]-, monosodium salt; Voltaren

[15307-79-6] (salt); [15307-86-5] (free acid) $C_{14}H_{10}Cl_2NNaO_2$ (318.13).

Preparation—Oxalyl chloride and 2,6-dichlorodiphenylamine are condensed to form the N, N-diphenyloxanilyl chloride that cyclizes under Friedel-Crafts conditions to yield 1-(2,6-diphenyl)isatin. Wolff-Kishner reduction of the 3-oxo group gives the lactam, which on hydrolysis affords the free acid. Neutralization with NaOH produces the salt; US Pat 3,558,690.

Description—White crystals; melts about 284°; pK$_a$ 4.0.

Solubility—Soluble in water; insoluble in organic solvents.

Comments—A pharmacological activity much like the other NSAIDs. As with other drugs in this group, diclofenac is thought to exert many of its effects as a result of its ability to inhibit prostaglandin synthesis.

Diclofenac is used as an anti-inflammatory, analgesic, and occasionally an antipyretic. Its anti-inflammatory action is similar to other NSAIDs with a potency, on weight basis, that is approximately 2.5 times that of indomethacin. On a weight basis, its analgesic potency is 8 to 16 times that of ibuprofen. It is used in the symptomatic relief of acute and chronic rheumatoid arthritis, osteoarthritis, and ankylosing spondylitis. It also has been used to relieve mild-to-moderate postoperative pain associated with dental, orthopedic, or postpartum procedures. It is also effective in relieving some cancer-related visceral pains. Diclofenac doses of 75 to 100 mg/day are equally effective in relieving pain as 0.9 to 2.7 g of aspirin or 1.2 g of ibuprofen. It is also effective in relieving some of the discomforts associated with dysmenorrhea.

Most of the adverse effects of diclofenac are similar to those of other NSAIDs and occur in several systems. The GI effects can include irritation, bleeding, ulceration, and eventually wall perforation. Such effects usually are associated with chronic, high-dose treatments. However, with usual therapeutic doses, diclofenac is less likely to cause serious GI problems than aspirin or naproxen. Diclofenac can cause headaches and dizziness in 3–9% and 1–3%, respectively, of patients. Use of this drug has been associated with renal impairment in less than 1% of patients. Severe hepatic reactions occur rarely, whereas 1–3% of patients may experience a rash or pruritus when using the drug. Tinnitus has been reported in 1–3% of patients using this drug, and fluid retention occurs in 3–9%. Because of its anticlotting actions, Diclofenac should be used with caution in patients who would be put at risk by prolonging bleeding time.

DIFLUNISAL

[1,1′-Biphenyl]-3-carboxylic acid, 2′,4′-difluoro-4-hydroxy-, Dolobid

[22494-42-4] $C_{13}H_8F_2O_3$ (250.20).

Preparation—Refer to US Pat 3,714,226.

Description—White crystals; melts at approximately 210°.

Solubility—Sparingly soluble in water; soluble in most organic solvents or dilute aqueous bases.

Comments—A prostaglandin inhibitor, nonsteroidal analgesic, and anti-inflammatory drug used in the management of mild-to-moderate pain and osteoarthritis. It also has measurable, but not clinically useful, antipyretic activity. Double-blind studies indicate that a 500-mg dose of the drug is more effective in the control of postoperative episiotomy pain than 600 mg of aspirin; in postoperative oral surgery 500 to 1000 mg of the drug was more potent than 600 mg of acetaminophen alone and comparable with 600 mg of acetaminophen with 60 mg of codeine, and more effective than 100 mg of propoxyphene napsylate. Moreover, it had a longer duration of action. After oral administration, peak plasma levels occur within 2 to 3 hr. Approximately 99% is bound to plasma proteins. Plasma half-life is 8 to 12 hr. Approximately 90% of the drug is excreted in the urine as two soluble glucuronide conjugates. Although it is a derivative of salicylic acid, it is not metabolized to salicylic acid.

The drug is contraindicated in patients in whom acute asthmatic attacks, urticaria, or rhinitis are precipitated by aspirin. It prolongs the clotting time in patients on anticoagulant therapy, significantly increases plasma levels of hydrochlorathiazide and acetaminophen, decreases the hyperuricemic effect of furosemide, and significantly decreases the urinary excretion of naproxen and its glucuronide metabolite. The most prominent side effects include nausea, dyspepsia, GI pain, and diarrhea; dizziness, headache, and rash also have been reported in 3–9% of patients. It appears to cause less GI bleeding than aspirin. Aspirin or acetaminophen should not be taken with this drug, except on professional advice.

ETODOLAC

Pyrano[3,4-b]indole-1-acetic acid, 1,8-diethyl-1,3,4,9-tetrahydro-, Lodine

[41340-25-4] $C_{17}H_{21}NO_3$ (287.36).

Preparation—See *J Med Chem* 19:391, 1976.

Description—White crystals; melts about 147°; pK$_a$ 4.65.

Solubility—1 g in 10 mL water or 4 mL alcohol.

Comments—An *NSAID* used for osteoarthritis and rheumatoid arthritis.

FENOPROFEN CALCIUM

Benzeneacetic acid, (±)-α-methyl-3-phenoxy-, calcium salt (2:1), dihydrate; Nalfon

(±)-Calcium m-phenoxyhydratropate dihydrate [53746-45-5] $C_{30}H_{26}CaO_6.2H_2O$ (558.64); *anhydrous* [34597-40-5] (522.61).

Preparation—From p-phenoxyacetophenone by reduction of the phenone carbonyl group to the secondary alcohol; replacing the OH with Br using PBr$_3$; nucleophilic substitution of Br by CN followed by hydrolysis to the acid, which is converted to the calcium salt. *J Med Chem* 19:391, 1976.

Description—White, crystalline powder; pK$_a$ 4.5 (fenoprofen).

Solubility—Slightly soluble in water; sparingly soluble in alcohol.

Comments—An *NSAID* propionic acid derivative like *Ibuprofen*.

FLURBIPROFEN

(±)-[1,1′-Biphenyl]-4-acetic acid, 2-fluoro-α-methyl-, Ansaid

[5104-49-4] $C_{15}H_{13}FO_2$ (255.26)

Preparation—The Willgerodt reaction on 3-fluoro-4-phenylacetophenone yields the corresponding phenylacetic acid ester, which, with $NaOC_2H_5$ and ethyl carbonate, forms the substituted malonic ester. The ester is methylated by the classical method, hydrolyzed, and decarboxylated to the product; US Pat 3,755,427.

Description—White to slightly yellow powder; melts about 110°.

Solubility—Slightly soluble in water; soluble in dilute alkali; freely soluble in alcohol.

Comments—An *NSAID* used topically in ophthalmology to prevent miosis during ocular surgery.

IBUPROFEN

Benzeneacetic acid, (±)-α-methyl-4-(2-methylpropyl)-, Rufen, Nuprin, Advil, Haltran, Motrin, Medipren

(±)-*p*-Isobutylhydratropic acid; (±)-2-(*p*-isobutylphenyl)propionic acid [15687-27-1] $C_{13}H_{18}O_2$ (206.28).

Preparation—Isobutylbenzene is acetylated in the *para* position by a Friedel-Crafts procedure on acetophenone, which is treated with HCN to yield the cyanohydrin. Heating with HI and red P hydrolyzes the nitrile to the acid and simultaneously reduces the hydroxyl group; *J Org Chem* 43:2936, 1978.

Description—White to off-white, crystalline powder; slight characteristic odor and taste; melts about 75°; apparent pK_a 5.2.

Solubility—Slightly soluble in water; soluble in alcohol or other organic solvents.

Comments—An *NSAID* that possesses *analgesic* and *antipyretic* activities. In mild-to-moderate pain, 200 mg appears to be as effective as 650 mg of aspirin. When used to relieve dysmenorrhea, it is as effective as mefenamic acid and more effective than aspirin or propoxyphene. Like other NSAIDs its mechanism of action likely relates to its inhibition of prostaglandin synthesis. Evidence that it does have a salutary effect in the treatment of chronic rheumatoid arthritis and osteoarthritis is shown by a reduction of joint swelling, decrease in pain, decrease in duration of morning stiffness, and improved functional capacity as indicated by an increase in grip strength, a delay in the time to onset of fatigue, and a decrease in the time to walk 50 ft.

The drug is absorbed rapidly after oral administration, and peak plasma serum levels generally are attained within 1 to 2 hr after oral administration. With single doses from 200 to 800 mg, a dose–response relation exists between the amount of drug administered and the integrated area under the serum drug concentration versus time curve. It is metabolized rapidly and eliminated in the urine; excretion virtually is complete 24 hr after the last dose of drug. The serum half-life is 1.8 to 2.0 hr.

It is indicated for relief of symptoms of rheumatoid arthritis and osteoarthritis. It also is indicated for the relief of mild-to-moderate pain, for the treatment of primary dysmenorrhea, and as an antipyretic. It is contraindicated in individuals sensitive to the drug or in individuals who have the syndrome of nasal polyps, angioedema, and bronchospastic reactivity to aspirin or other NSAIDs. Peptic ulceration and GI bleeding have been reported. Consequently, it should be given under close supervision to patients who have a history of upper GI tract disease. Blurred or diminished vision, scotomata, and other changes in color vision have been noted; should such occur, the drug should be discontinued and the patient given an ophthalmological examination.

Patients should be cautioned to report signs or symptoms of GI ulceration or bleeding, blurred vision or other eye symptoms, skin rash, weight gain, or edema to their physicians. This drug, like aspirin and other NSAIDs, can inhibit platelet function and prolong bleeding time, but the effects are reversible and not as long lasting as those of aspirin. Nevertheless, it should be administered with caution to patients on anticoagulants. It is not recommended for use in pregnant women or nursing mothers.

Adverse reactions with an incidence greater than 1% may be categorized as *GI* (4–16%) (eg, nausea, epigastric pain, heartburn, diarrhea, abdominal distress, nausea and vomiting, indigestion, constipation and abdominal cramps, or pain), *CNS* [eg, dizziness (3–9%), headache, nervousness, and tinnitus], *dermatologic* [eg, rash (3–9%) and pruritus], and *metabolic* (eg, decreased appetite, edema, and fluid retention).

Adverse effects with an incidence of less than 1% include *GI* (gastric or duodenal ulcer with bleeding or perforation), *dermatologic* (vesiculobullous eruptions, urticaria, and erythema multiforme), *CNS*

(depression or insomnia), *special senses* [amblyopia (blurred or diminished vision, scotomata, or other changes in vision)], *hematologic* (leukopenia and decreases in hemoglobin and hematocrit), and *cardiovascular* (congestive heart failure in patients who have marginal cardiac function and elevated blood pressure). Other reactions have been reported but under circumstances in which a causal relation could not be established.

INDOMETHACIN

1*H*-Indole-3-acetic acid, 1-(4-chlorobenzoyl)-5-methoxy-2-methyl-, Indocin, Indocin SR

[53-86-1] $C_{19}H_{16}ClNO_4$ (357.79).

Preparation—*p*-Anisidine is diazotized and the diazonium compound reduced with sodium sulfite. The resulting *p*-methoxyphenylhydrazine undergoes the Fisher indole synthesis with methyl levulinate. The steps involved include formation of the hydrazone (I), rearrangement of I to the enamine compound II, and cyclization of II through loss of ammonia to form III. III is then hydrolyzed to the acid, which is re-esterified by means of the anhydride to give the *tert*-butyl ester. Acylation with *p*-chlorobenzoyl chloride followed by debutylation yields indomethacin. US Pat 3,161,654.

Description—Pale-yellow to yellow-tan, crystalline powder; odorless or a slight odor; slightly bitter taste; light sensitive, stable in air and stable in heat under the usual prevailing temperature conditions; one polymorphic form melts about 155°, the other about 162°.

Solubility—1 g in 50 mL alcohol, 30 mL chloroform, or 40 mL ether; practically soluble in water.

Comments—A nonsteroidal drug with anti-inflammatory, antipyretic, and analgesic properties. *It is not a simple analgesic and, because of its potential serious untoward effects, should not be used for trivial or minor problems.* It is indicated for the treatment of *rheumatoid arthritis, ankylosing (rheumatoid) spondylitis, osteoarthritis, bursitis, tendinitis, gouty arthritis,* and *patent ductus arteriosus in premature neonates.* The drug is absorbed rapidly after oral administration; peak plasma levels are reached in 2 hr; 97% of the drug is protein bound. It has a half-life of 2.6 to 11.2 hr; 10–20% of the drug is excreted unchanged in the urine. Because it is a potent drug and has a potential to cause severe adverse effects, it should be considered carefully for an active disease unresponsive to adequate trial with salicylates and other established measures, such as appropriate rest. The drug is contraindicated in children, pregnant women, and nursing mothers, patients who have GI problems, and patients who are allergic to aspirin.

The incidence of untoward effects has been reported to vary from a few percent to 75% of patients. Most frequent untoward actions include *GI* (single or multiple ulcerations, hemorrhage, GI bleeding, increased pain in ulcerative colitis, gastritis, nausea, vomiting, and epigastric distress), *eye reactions* (corneal deposits, retinal disturbances, and blurring of vision), *hepatic* [toxic hepatitis and jaundice (some fatalities have been reported)], *hematologic* (aplastic anemia, hemolytic anemia, depression of the bone marrow, agranulocytosis, leukopenia, and thrombocytopenia purpura), *hypersensitivity* [acute respiratory (including asthma and dyspnea), angiitis, pruritus, urticaria, skin rashes, etc.], *ear* [deafness (rarely) and tinnitus], *CNS* (psychotic disturbances, depersonalization, depression, mental confusion, coma, convulsions, peripheral neuropathy, drowsiness, lightheadedness, dizziness, and headache); *cardiovascular renal* (edema, hypertension, hematuria), *dermatologic* (loss of hair and erythema nodosum), *miscellaneous* (vaginal bleeding, hyperglycemia, glycosuria, ulcerative stomatitis, and epistaxis). Both the incidence and the severity of side effects appear to be dose related.

The high potential for dose-related adverse reactions (see above) makes it imperative that the smallest effective dosage be determined for each patient. GI reactions may be reduced if the patient takes the drug with food, immediately after meals, or with antacids. The occurrence of ocular or hematological disturbances in some patients on prolonged therapy with the drug indicates the need for periodic ophthalmological examination and appropriate blood tests. Whether the drug has any effect on anticoagulants is uncertain, but concurrent administration may be hazardous because of increased risk of GI bleeding.

It may aggravate psychiatric disturbances, epilepsy, and parkinsonism; it should be used with considerable caution in patients who have these conditions. Patients should be warned that ability to drive or perform other activities requiring alertness might be affected adversely. The drug should be discontinued if any of the untoward effects listed above occurs, pending consultation with the physician.

KETOPROFEN

Benzeneacetic acid, 3-benzoyl-α-methyl-, Orudis

[22071-15-4] $C_{16}H_{14}O_3$ (254.28).

Preparation—The diazonium salt prepared from 2-(*p*-aminophenyl)propionic acid is converted to the mercaptan (**I**) with potassium ethyl xanthate followed by hydrolysis. **I**, with *o*-iodobenzoic acid yields the corresponding diphenyl sulfide. The carboxyl group *ortho* to the sulfur atom cyclizes with the adjacent ring to form a thioxanthone configuration followed by desulfurization to reopen the ring and reform the benzophenone product; *Farmaco Ed Sci* 35:684, 1980.

Description—White to off-white, odorless, crystalline, nonhygroscopic powder; melts about 95°.

Solubility—Practically insoluble in water; soluble in fixed bases; freely soluble in alcohol, chloroform, acetone, or ether.

Comments—An *NSAID* propionic derivative like *Ibuprofen*, but lower doses are needed and available.

MECLOFENAMATE SODIUM

Benzoic acid, 2-[(2,6-dichloro-3-methylphenyl)amino]-, monosodium salt, monohydrate

Monosodium *N*-(2,6-dichloro-*m*-tolyl)anthranilate monohydrate [6385-02-0] $C_{14}H_{10}Cl_2NNaO_2 \cdot H_2O$ (336.15).

Preparation—By the Ullman condensation of *o*-iodobenzoic acid and 2,6-dichloro-*m*-toluidine in the presence of copper-bronze, *J Med Chem* 11:1009, 1968.

Description—White crystals; melts about 290°; a saturated solution in water (1 g in 65 mL) is slightly turbid; pH approximately 7.5.

Comments—An *NSAID* related to *Mefenamic Acid*.

MEFENAMIC ACID

Benzoic acid, 2-[(2,3-dimethylphenyl)amino]-, Ponstel

N-(2,3-Xylyl)anthranilic acid [61-68-7] $C_{15}H_{15}NO_2$ (241.29).

Preparation—*o*-Chlorobenzoic acid is condensed with 2,3-xylidine with the aid of potassium carbonate, and the resulting potassium salt is treated with mineral acid to liberate the desired acid. *J Med Chem* 11:111, 1968.

Description—White to off-white, crystalline powder; odorless; little initial taste, but a bitter aftertaste; darkens on prolonged exposure to light, nonhygroscopic; stable up to 45°; decarboxylates at temperature above its melting point (at 300°, 100% is decarboxylated in 3 min); melts about 230°.

Solubility—1 g in 220 mL of alcohol; insoluble in water; sparingly soluble in chloroform or ether.

Comments—An analgesic drug used for the relief of moderately severe pain when *therapy will not exceed 1 wk* and for the treatment of *primary dysmenorrhea*. It also is indicated for the relief of pain resulting from postoperative pain. It is contraindicated in patients who have ulceration of the upper or lower intestinal tract, children younger than 14 yr, women during pregnancy, or patients known to be hypersensitive to the drug. Untoward effects include diarrhea, which may be severe and indicates the drug should be stopped; autoimmune hemolytic anemia; thrombocytopenic purpura; leukopenia; pancytopenia; agranulocytosis; and bone-marrow hypoplasia.

Minor reactions include drowsiness, GI discomfort, dizziness, headache, vomiting, urticaria, rash, eosinophilia, blurred vision, insomnia, and perspiration. Rarely, palpitations, facial edema, dyspnea, eye pain, ear pain, dysuria, hematuria, reversible loss of color vision, and increased insulin need in diabetic patients. Mild renal and hepatic toxicity also have been reported. As with all drugs, physicians would be well advised to consider its use only in cases that either cannot tolerate or do not respond to less-toxic agents.

MELOXICAM

2*H*-1,2-Benzothiazine-3-carboxamide, 4-hydroxy-2-methyl-*N*-(5-methyl-2-thiazolyl-, 1,1-dioxide; Mobic

[71125-38-7] $C_{14}H_{13}N_3O_4S_2$ (351.41).

Preparation—The imide of 2-carboxybenzenesulfonic acid and methyl chloroacetate are reacted in a modified Hinsberg reaction to yield the *N*-methoxy-carbonylmethyl derivative, which is isomerized by sodium methoxide in a mixture of toluene and *tert*-butyl alcohol to form the benzothiazine ring. Refluxing this latter compound with methyl iodide in methanol affords the *N*-methyl derivative (**I**). Compound **I** is refluxed with 2-amino-5-methylthiazole in xylene, with the reaction being driven by removal of the methanol formed using a molecular sieve in a Soxhlet apparatus. On cooling the product crystallizes. US Pat 4,233,299.

Description—Yellow solid melting about 254°. Log P approx. 0.1 (octanol/pH 7.4 buffer); pK$_a$ 1.1 and 4.2.

Solubility—Practically insoluble in water; more soluble at high or low pH; very slightly soluble in methanol.

Comments—A nonsteroidal anti-inflammatory drug (NSAID) that exhibits anti-inflammatory, analgesic, and antipyretic activities. Might have greater selectivity for COX-2. Clinical trials have demonstrated pain relief in osteoarthritis. Peak plasma levels occur about 4 to 5 hr after oral administration. It is ~99% bound to plasma protein. It is almost completely metabolized to four inactive metabolites (predominantly through P450 2C9 and 3A4) and eliminated in the urine and feces. The major metabolite is 5'-carboxy meloxicam. Half-life is about 15 to 20 hr. Patients with severe hepatic impairment have not been studied; it is not recommended in patients with advanced kidney disease.

It is contraindicated in patients with known hypersensitivity to it or demonstrated allergic-type reactions to NSAIDs. It has not been evaluated in persons under 18 yrs old.

NABUMETONE

2-Butanone, 4-(6-methoxy-2-naphthalenyl)-, Relafen

4-(6-Methoxy-2-naphthyl)-2-butanone; [42924-53-8] $C_{15}H_{16}O_2$ (228.29).

Preparation—Acetone and 6-methoxynaphthalenecarboxaldehyde are reacted in aldol fashion to form 5-(6-methoxy-2-naphthyl)-3-buten-2-one, which is reduced catalytically to nabumetone. See *J Med Chem* 21:1260, 1978.

Description—White crystals; melts about 80°.

Solubility—Practically insoluble in water; sparingly soluble in alcohol.

Comments—An *NSAID* with a metabolite similar to *naproxen*.

NAPROXEN

2-Naphthaleneacetic acid, (+)-6-methoxy-α-methyl-, Equiproxen (Veterinary), Naprosyn

[22204-53-1] $C_{14}H_{14}O_3$ (230.26).

Preparation—6-Methoxynaphthalene is acetylated in the 2- position and the acetyl group is then converted to—$CH(CH_3)COOH$ by a sequence of reactions—Willgerodt-Kindler, esterification, alkylation and hydrolysis—yielding DL-naproxen (*CA 71*:91162j, 1969). Resolution of the racemate may be effected through precipitation of the more potent D-enantiomer as the cinchonidine salt (*J Med Chem 13*:203, 1970).

Description—White to off-white, crystalline powder; bitter taste; melts about 155°; apparent pK_a 4.15.

Solubility—Practically insoluble in water at pH 2; freely soluble in water at pH 8 or above; sparingly soluble in alcohol.

Comments—A propionic acid derivative that has anti-inflammatory, analgesic, and antipyretic activities. It is commercially available both as the acid and the sodium salt and is sold OTC. It is indicated for relief of symptoms of rheumatoid arthritis, both of acute flares and long-term management of the disease. Symptomatic improvement, when use of the drug is indicated, usually begins within 2 wk but a longer trial period may be necessary. It is comparable to aspirin in controlling disease symptoms, but with lesser frequency and severity of nervous system and milder GI adverse effects. It is used to relieve mild-to-moderate postoperative pain as well as postpartum pain, primary dysmenorrhea, orthopedic pain, headache, and visceral pain associated with cancer. Its analgesic effects are comparable with those of aspirin or indomethacin with usual doses.

It appears to be absorbed completely from the GI tract after oral administration. Peak plasma levels (approximately 55 mg/mL) are reached in 2 to 4 hr after a 500-mg dose, and steady-state levels are attained after 4 or 5 doses at 12-hr intervals. More than 99% is bound to serum albumin. The mean plasma half-life is approximately 13 hr. Approximately 95% of a dose is excreted in the urine, principally as conjugates of naproxen and its inactive metabolite 6-demethylnaproxen. The adverse effects, precautions, contraindications and drug interactions are essentially the same as for *Fenoprofen Calcium*.

NAPROXEN SODIUM

2-Naphthaleneacetic acid, 6-methoxy-α-methyl-, sodium salt; Anaprox

[26159-34-2] $C_{14}H_{13}NaO_3$ (252.24).

Comments—See *Naproxen*, above.

OXYPHENBUTAZONE

3,5-Pyrazolidinedione, 4-butyl-1-(4-hydroxyphenyl)-2-phenyl-, monohydrate

4-Butyl-1-(*p*-hydroxyphenyl)-2-phenyl-3,5-pyrazolidinedione monohydrate [7081-38-1] $C_{19}H_{20}N_2O_3 \cdot H_2O$ (342.39); *anhydrous* [129-20-4] (324.38).

Preparation—Diethyl butylmalonate is condensed with *p*-benzyloxyhydrazobenzene, with the aid of a solution of sodium ethoxide in anhydrous ethanol, to form 1-(*p*-benzyloxy)-2-phenyl-4-butyl-3,5- pyrazolidinedione (I). Completion of the reaction is effected by the addition of xylene and by heating of the mixture to about 140° for several hours, thus removing the alcohol released by the cyclizing condensation. Debenzylation of I is effected by Raney nickel hydrogenation at ambient temperature and pressure. Recrystallization of the initial product is from ether/petroleum ether. US Pat 2,745,783.

Description—White to yellowish white, odorless, crystalline powder; melts over a wide range between 85° and 100°.

Solubility—1 g in >10,000 mL water, 1.5 mL alcohol, 4 mL chloroform, 15 mL ether.

Comments—An *NSAID* propionic acid derivative.

PHENYLBUTAZONE

3,5-Pyrazolidinedione, 4-butyl-1,2-diphenyl-, Butazolidin

[50-33-9] $C_{19}H_{20}N_2O_2$ (308.38).

Preparation—Butylmalonyl chloride is condensed with hydrazobenzene in ether solution at 0° with the aid of pyridine. After extraction of the pyridine with aqueous HCl, the phenylbutazone is extracted with aqueous Na_2CO_3 and then precipitated by addition of HCl. US Pat 2,562,830.

Description—White to off-white, odorless, crystalline powder; melts about 105°.

Solubility—1 g in approximately 20 mL alcohol; slightly soluble in water; freely soluble in acetone or ether.

Comments—A synthetic pyrazolone derivative chemically related to aminopyrine and that has anti-inflammatory, antipyretic, analgesic, and mild uricosuric properties. Like other NSAIDs, these pharmacological effects likely relate to inhibition of prostaglandin synthesis caused by this drug. It is indicated for the symptomatic relief of *gout, rheumatoid arthritis, rheumatoid spondylitis, osteoarthritis, psoriatic arthritis, acute superficial thrombophlebitis,* and *painful shoulder*. Its anti-inflammatory and analgesic actions are comparable with that of usual doses of indomethacin, ibuprofen, or tolmetin. Because of the risk of agranulocytosis and aplastic anemia, it should be used only after other nonsteroidal and anti-inflammatory drugs have proved unsatisfactory; it is not recommended for use as a simple analgesic or antipyretic.

Therapy should not be started until the patient has been subjected to a complete physical and laboratory examination, including a hemogram and urinalysis, and has been adequately warned of potential adverse effects. In particular, it is contraindicated in patients who have severe renal, hepatic, or cardiac disease and should not be prescribed for those not available for frequent observation. Patients should be warned not to exceed the recommended dosage and to immediately report any fever, sore throat, or lesions in the mouth (symptoms of blood dyscrasia), dyspepsia, epigastric pain, symptoms of anemia, unusual bleeding, bruising, black or tarry stools (symptoms of intestinal lesions), and significant weight gain or anemia.

The goal of therapy should be *short-term* relief of *severe* symptoms to a level tolerable with the smallest possible drug dosage. If a favorable response is not observed within 1 wk, the drug should be discontinued. The drug is contraindicated in patients who have GI problems, have a history of drug allergy, and in children younger than 14 yr. It also is contraindicated in patients on other concurrent therapy, such as potent chemotherapeutic drugs and anticoagulant medication.

It is absorbed rapidly after oral administration and highly bound to plasma protein. Phenylbutazone's time to peak serum concentration is approximately 2.5 hr; however, the usual time for onset of antigout activity varies from 1 to 4 days and that for antirheumatic activity 3 to 7 days. Therapeutic serum concentrations average approximately 43 mg/mL; elimination half-life is approximately 84 hr. The drug (1%) and its major metabolite (oxyphenbutazone, 2%) are excreted by the kidneys.

It produces untoward effects in approximately 40% of patients; approximately 15% have to discontinue the drug because of toxic effects. Consequently, the drug should be employed only in those patients who fail to respond adequately to less hazardous substances. The most frequently encountered untoward effects are water retention, nausea, rash, epigastric pain, vertigo, and stomatitis. Other less frequent but more severe effects include hepatitis, hypertension, transient psychosis, moderate leukopenia, agranulocytosis, and thrombocytopenia. CNS stimulation, visual symptoms, anemia, lethargy, constipation, diarrhea, GI hemorrhage, fever, and cardiac arrhythmias also have been observed.

Numerous drug interactions have been reported. Some of these interactions may be due to microsomal induction caused by phenylbutazone and its metabolite, oxyphenylbutazone. Generally, it should not be administered to patients taking anticoagulants, anti-inflammatory agents, bone-marrow depressants, digitoxin, hypoglycemics, methotrexate, phenytoin, or sulfonamides.

MEDICINAL AGENTS

Because it is a potent drug and misuse can lead to serious results, physicians are well advised to familiarize themselves with its GI, acid-base balance, hepatic, dermatological, allergic, renal, cardiovascular, ocular, metabolic, and endocrine effects before prescribing this drug. It should be used with caution in pregnant women, nursing mothers, elderly patients, and patients known to have other illnesses. This drug should be taken with milk or with meals to minimize gastric irritation.

PIROXICAM

2H-1,2-Benzothiazine-3-carboxamide, 4-hydroxy-2-methyl-N-pyridinyl-, 1,1-dioxide; Feldene

[36322-90-4] $C_{15}H_{13}N_3O_4S$ (331.35).

Preparation—See *J Med Chem* 14:1171, 1971 and *Ibid* 15:848, 1972.

Description—White crystals; melts about 200° a saturated solution in dioxane:water (2:1) has a pKₐ of approximately 6.3.

Solubility—Slightly soluble in water.

Comments—An *NSAID* structurally unrelated, but pharmacologically similar, to other NSAIDs.

SULINDAC

1H-Indene-3-acetic acid, (Z)-5-fluoro-2-methyl-1-[[4-(methylsulfinyl)phenyl] methylene]-, Clinoril

[38194-50-2] $C_{20}H_{17}FO_3S$ (356.41).

Preparation—The reaction of *p*-fluorobenzyl chloride with methylmalonic ester in the classic malonic ester synthetic route yields 3-(p-fluorophenyl)-2-methylpropanoic acid. Cyclization with polyphosphoric acid gives 6-fluoro-2-methylindanone which is reduced by means of a Reformatsky reaction to the alcohol, dehydrated to the indene, condensed with *p*-(methylthio)benzaldehyde to the 3-benzylidene derivative, the ester hydrolyzed and the thio group oxidized to the sulfoxide; *J Org Chem* 42:1914, 1977.

Description—Yellow crystals; melts at about 183° with decomposition; pKₐ 4.5.

Solubility—Practically insoluble in water; sparingly soluble in alcohol.

Comments—An *NSAID* structurally related to *Indomethacin*.

TOLMETIN SODIUM

1H-Pyrrole-2-acetic acid, 1-methyl-5-(4-methylbenzoyl)-, sodium salt, dihydrate; Tolectin, Tolectin DS

[64490-92-2] $C_{15}H_{14}NNaO_3.2H_2O$ (315.31).

Preparation—The corresponding acetonitrile is obtained by a Friedel-Crafts reaction between 1-methylpyrrole-2-acetonitrile and *p*-methylbenzoyl chloride; after separation from the 4-aroyl isomer, produced simultaneously, by fractional crystallization or adsorption chromatography, the acetonitrile is converted to tolmetin by saponification and subsequently to its sodium salt (*J Med Chem* 14:646, 1971).

Description—Light yellow, crystalline powder; pKₐ 3.5 (free acid).

Solubility—Freely soluble in water; slightly soluble in alcohol.

Comments—A nonsteroidal compound that has anti-inflammatory, analgesic, and antipyretic activities. Its mode of action is unknown, although inhibition of prostaglandin synthesis likely contributes to its anti-inflammatory action. In patients who have rheumatoid arthritis, various manifestations of its anti-inflammatory and analgesic actions are observed, but there is no evidence of alteration of the progressive course of the underlying disease.

The drug is absorbed rapidly and almost completely with peak plasma levels being reached within 30 to 60 min after an oral therapeutic dose. It is bound approximately 99% to plasma proteins; the mean plasma half-life is approximately 1 hr. Essentially, all of a dose is excreted in the urine within 24 hr, either as an inactive oxidative metabolite or as conjugates of tolmetin.

The drug is indicated for the relief of signs and symptoms of rheumatoid arthritis, both for acute flares and for long-term management of the disease. Safety and effectiveness in patients who are incapacitated, largely or wholly bedridden, or confined to a wheelchair, with little capacity for self-care have not been established. The drug is comparable with aspirin and with indomethacin in controlling disease activity; however, the frequency of the milder GI adverse effects is reported to be less than in aspirin-treated patients and the incidence of CNS adverse effects less than in indomethacin-treated patients. Concomitant administration of this drug and aspirin is not recommended because there does not appear to be any greater benefit from the combination over that achieved with aspirin alone and the potential for adverse reactions is increased.

It is contraindicated in patients demonstrated to be hypersensitive to the drug and also in those in whom aspirin and other NSAIDs induce symptoms of asthma, rhinitis, or urticaria. In patients who have active rheumatoid arthritis who also have an active peptic ulcer, treatment with nonulcerogenic drugs should be attempted; if it must be given, the patient should be observed closely for signs of ulcer perforation or severe GI bleeding. Because it is eliminated primarily by the kidneys, patients who have impaired renal function should be monitored closely and dosage reduced or discontinued if necessary. Because it prolongs bleeding time, patients who may be affected adversely should be observed carefully when treated with the drug. Patients who have compromised cardiac function should be treated with caution because the drug causes some retention of water and sodium, with a resultant mild peripheral edema.

The most frequent adverse reactions are GI in nature and include, in descending order of frequency, epigastric or abdominal pain or discomfort (approximately 1 of 6 patients), nausea, vomiting, indigestion, heartburn, constipation, and dyspepsia. The most common nervous system reactions are headache (1 of 15 patients), followed by dizziness and lightheadedness, tension and nervousness, and drowsiness. Tinnitus occurs in 1 of 40 patients. Mild edema is observed in approximately 1 of 50 patients. Rash, including maculopapular eruptions or urticaria, develops in 1 of 30 patients and pruritus in approximately 1 of 50 patients. Small and transient decreases in hemoglobin and hematocrit, not associated with GI bleeding, occur infrequently as also do a few cases of granulocytopenia.

Safe use in children younger than 2 yr has not been established, although the drug has been used safely and effectively in children older than 2 yr. Use of the drug in pregnancy is not recommended, and because it is secreted in human milk, its use by nursing mothers also is not recommended.

Selective COX-2 Inhibitors

Whereas traditional NSAIDs block COX-1 and COX-2 isozymes non-selectively, the 'COX-2 inhibitors' inhibit COX-2 more selectively. The (simplified) concept is that COX-2 is induced during inflammation and pain and is not needed for protection of the GI mucosa, raising hopes that targeted therapy would have minimal impact on mucosal integrity and would reduce inflammation and relieve pain without producing GI bleeding. The ability to selectively inhibit the COX-2 isozyme is related to the difference in amino acids at position 523 of COX-1 and COX-2–isoleucine in COX-1, but valine in COX-2. The smaller valine forms a binding pocket in the channel leading to the catalytic site of the enzyme, which is believed to be a primary site of attachment of the selective COX-2 inhibitors.

The analgesic efficacy of the selective COX-2 inhibitors (the coxibs) is approximately equivalent to that of the traditional NSAIDs, and both have a relatively rapid onset of action. The adverse effects of COX-2 inhibition have yet to be fully characterized and are still somewhat controversial. It is unclear whether the adverse effects are specific to the individual agents currently marketed or will be observed with all COX-2 inhibitors (ie, are attributable to the mechanism of this class of agents).

Like other NSAIDs, the selective COX-2 inhibitors can cause renal toxicity (mainly edema and worsening of hypertension) and may decrease the antihypertensive effects of ACE inhibitors and diuretics. Unresolved at this time is the extent of sparing of GI ulcerations (with or without aspirin) and possible prothrombotic action that might increase cardiovascular risks.

CELECOXIB

Benzenesulfonamide, 4-[5-(4-methylphenyl)-3-(trifluoro-methyl)-1H-pyrazol-1-yl]-; Celebrex

p-[5-*p*-tolyl-3-(trifluoromethyl)pyrazol-1-yl]benzenesulfonamide [169590-42-5] $C_{17}H_{14}F_3N_3O_2S$ (381.38).

Preparation—Methyl trifluoroacetate and 4-methylbenzophenone are refluxed with sodium methoxide in methanol to yield 1-(*p*-tolyl)-4,4,4-trifluoro-1,3-butanedione. This latter compound is heated with *p*-hydrazinobenzenesulfonamide, closing the pyrazole ring forming the product. *Drugs of the Future* 1997; 22:71.

Description—Pale yellow crystals melting about 158°; pK$_a$ 9.7.

Solubility—Sparingly soluble in water.

Comments—A nonsteroidal anti-inflammatory drug (NSAID) that exhibits anti-inflammatory, analgesic, and antipyretic activities. Its mode of action is due to inhibition of prostaglandin synthesis, primarily via inhibition of COX-2. Peak plasma levels occur about 3 hr after oral administration. It is ~97% bound to plasma protein. Its elimination is predominantly by hepatic metabolism and elimination in the urine and feces. The primary metabolites are the carboxylic acid and glucuronide. Half-life is about 11 hr. Dose should be reduced in patients with hepatic impairment and is not recommended in patients with severe renal insufficiency.

Clinical trials have demonstrated pain relief in osteo- and rheumatoid-arthritis and in acute analgesic models of post-oral surgery, post-orthopedic surgery, and primary dysmenorrhea.

It is contraindicated in patients with known hypersensitivity to it or demonstrated allergic-type reactions to sulfonamides or NSAIDs. Significant interactions may occur when administered together with drugs that inhibit P450 2C9; potentially with fluconazole, lithium, furosemide, or ACE inhibitors. It has not been evaluated in persons under 18 yrs old. Because of its lack of platelet inhibiting effects, it is not a substitute for aspirin for cardiovascular prophylaxis.

ROFECOXIB

2(5H)-Furanone, 4-[p-(methylsulfonyl)phenyl]-3-phenyl-

[162011-90-7] C17H14O4S (314.36).

Preparation—One method involves the Friedel-Crafts condensation of acetyl chloride and methylmercatobenzene to form 4-(methylthio)acetophenone which is then oxidized using hydrogen peroxide catalyzed by sodium tungstate yielding the sulfone(I). Bromination of I yields the phenacyl bromide derivative which, with sodium phenylacetate, undergoes nucleophilic displacement of bromine to produce the 4-(methylsulfonyl)phenacyl ester of phenylacetic acid. Heating this ester with diisopropylamine forms the 2(5H)-furanone ring, which is the product. *Drugs of the Future* 1287: 23, 1998.

Description—White to light yellow powder.

Solubility—Sparingly soluble in acetone; slightly soluble in methanol or isopropyl acetate; very slightly soluble in 1-octanol.

Comments—A nonsteroidal anti-inflammatory drug (NSAID) that exhibits anti-inflammatory, analgesic, and antipyretic activities. Its mode of action is due to inhibition of prostaglandin synthesis, primarily via inhibition of COX-2. The median time to peak plasma levels is 2 to 3 hr (range 2–9 hr) after oral administration. It is ~87% bound to plasma protein. Its metabolism is primarily mediated through reduction by cy-

tosolic enzymes and elimination in the urine (~70–75%) and feces. The major metabolites are the *cis*- and *trans*-dihydro derivatives. The effective half-life (based on steady-state levels) is approximately 17 hr. Dose should be adjusted in patients with hepatic impairment and is not recommended in patients with advanced renal disease.

Clinical trials have demonstrated pain relief in osteo- and rheumatoid-arthritis and in acute analgesic models of post-oral surgery, post-orthopedic surgery, and primary dysmenorrhea.

It is contraindicated in patients with known hypersensitivity to it or demonstrated allergic-type reactions to sulfonamides or NSAIDs. It has not been evaluated in persons under 18 yrs old. Because of its lack of platelet inhibiting effects, it is not a substitute for aspirin for cardiovascular prophylaxis.

Note: Vioxx has been withdrawn from the market in October 2004.

VALDECOXIB

Benzenesulfonamide, 4-(5-methyl-3-phenyl-4-isooxazolyl-; Bextra

[181695-72-7] $C_{16}H_{14}N_2O_3S$ (314.36).

Preparation—One method involves conversion of benzyl phenyl ketone to the oxime which is deprotonated with butyl lithium and the product condensed with ethyl acetate to yield 3,4-diphenyl-5-methyl-4,5-dihydroisoxazolin-5-ol (I). Treatment of I with chloroformic acid followed by aqueous ammonia gives the product. *J Med Chem* 2000; 775: 43.

Description—Melts about 173°; pK$_a$ 9.8.

Solubility—Insoluble in water; as with most sulfonamides it is more soluble in aqueous solution at high pH; soluble in most organic solvents.

Comments—A nonsteroidal anti-inflammatory drug (NSAID) that exhibits anti-inflammatory, analgesic, and antipyretic activities. Its mode of action is due to inhibition of prostaglandin synthesis, primarily via inhibition of COX-2. Peak plasma levels occur about 3 hr after oral administration. It is ~98% bound to plasma protein. It undergoes extensive hepatic metabolism involving P450 isozymes (3A4 and 2C9) and non-P450 dependent pathways (eg, glucuronidation). Less than 5% is excreted unchanged in the urine. The mean half-life is about 8 to 11 hr and increases with age. It is not recommended in patients with severe hepatic impairment or advanced renal disease.

Clinical trials have demonstrated pain relief in osteo- and rheumatoid-arthritis and in primary dysmenorrhea.

It is contraindicated in patients with known hypersensitivity to it or demonstrated allergic-type reactions to sulfonamides or NSAIDs. It has not been evaluated in persons under 18 yrs old. Because of its lack of platelet inhibiting effects, it is not a substitute for aspirin for cardiovascular prophylaxis.

Acetaminophen

Acetamide, N-(4-hydroxyphenyl)-, N-Acetyl-p-aminophenol; p-Acetamidophenol

4′-Hydroxyacetanilide [103-90-2] $C_8H_9NO_2$ (151.16).

Preparation—*p*-Nitrophenol is reduced and the resulting *p*-aminophenol is acetylated by means of heating with a mixture of acetic anhydride and glacial acetic acid. The crude product may be purified by recrystallization from an ethanol–water mixture.

Description—White, odorless, crystalline powder; slightly bitter taste; melts about 170°; pH (saturated solution) 5.3 to 6.5; pK$_a$ 9.51.

Solubility—1 g in 70 mL water, 20 mL boiling water, 10 mL alcohol, 50 mL chloroform, 40 mL glycerin; slightly soluble in ether.

Comments—The analgesic efficacy of acetaminophen is essentially equivalent to that of NSAIDDs, but acetaminophen is not anti-inflammatory. The mechanism of action of acetaminophen is unknown, but the prevailing evidence suggests that involves a central component. Several possible actions have been proposed on the basis of *in vitro* studies. The oldest proposal is that acetaminophen inhibits COX-1, but rather than in the periphery. Another proposal is that acetaminophen inhibits a specific type of COX activity or under select conditions. Other reports suggest that descending modulatory mechanisms are involved, possibility involving 5-HT or endogenous opioid pathways. Taken together, the findings suggest that acetaminophen has a direct action at the level of the spinal cord and in addition stimulates a supraspinal system that modulates neurotransmitters at the level of the spinal cord. This dual mechanism may explain why it has previously been so difficult to elucidate the basis for the analgesic effect of acetaminophen. It is effective in the treatment of a wide variety of arthritic and rheumatic conditions involving musculoskeletal pain as well as the headache pain, dysmenorrhea, myalgias, and neuralgias. It also is useful in diseases accompanied by pain, discomfort, and fever, such as the common cold and other viral infections. It is useful particularly as an analgesic-antipyretic in patients who experience untoward reactions to aspirin. It rarely induces untoward effects in therapeutic doses and usually is well tolerated by aspirin-sensitive patients. Rarely, a sensitivity reaction may occur; in this case the drug should be stopped. Acetaminophen frequently is combined with other drugs, such as caffeine, aspirin, and opiates, such as codeine and oxycodone. It lacks the anti-inflammatory action of the salicylates; hence, it is of only limited usefulness in inflammatory rheumatic disorders and is often not considered an NSAID agent. Unlike aspirin, acetaminophen does not antagonize the effects of uricosuric agents. Although large doses have been reported to potentiate anticoagulants, therapeutic doses have no effect on prothrombin time.

Absorption of the drug after oral administration is rapid and peak plasma levels are reached in 30 to 120 min. The therapeutic half-life is approximately 3 hr. Approximately 2% is excreted unchanged in the urine; the glucuronide and the sulfate conjugates are nontoxic and account for approximately 95% of the drug. A much smaller amount, estimated to be 3%, is oxidized via the hepatic cytochrome P-450 system to a chemically reactive intermediate that combines with liver glutathione to form a nontoxic substance. However, after massive single doses of the drug, the supply of liver glutathione is exhausted and the excess reactive arylating intermediate covalently binds to vital hepatocellular macromolecules, leading to necrosis. Hepatic necrosis and death have been observed after overdosage; hepatic damage is likely if an adult takes more than 10 to 15 g in a single dose or if a 2-year-old child takes more than 3 g.

Both *in vivo* and *in vitro* studies have shown that agents that stimulate metabolism, such as phenobarbital, phenytoin, and alcohol, potentiate acetaminophen-induced hepatotoxicity. The best indicator of potential liver injury is the half-life of its elimination. A half-life longer than 4 hr is associated uniformly with liver injury. Also, plasma levels greater than 300 mg/mL at 4 hr postingestion are consistent with liver injury, whereas levels less than 120mg/mL at 4 hr postingestion usually are not.

Treatment of overdosage includes administration of acetylcysteine to help conjugate the hepatotoxic metabolite plus symptomatic and supportive care. The label on its dosage forms carries the following (or equivalent) statement: *Warning—Do not use more than 10 days unless directed by a physician. Keep this medication out of reach of children.*

OTHER DRUGS TO RELIEVE PAIN (ADJUVANTS)

Certain drugs, although not classified as analgesics, are helpful in treating certain types of pain. Such drugs may be used alone or in concert with standard analgesics. Examples include an-

Table 83-2. Possible Mechanism(s) of Action of Some Adjuvants Used for Pain

ADJUVANT	POSSIBLE MECHANISM(S) OF ACTION
Antidepressants	Enhancement of descending modulatory pathways by inhibition of neuronal reuptake of norepinephrine and 5-HT. SSRI's are generally less effective than are non-selective agents.
α_2-adrenoceptor agonists	Potentiation of endogenous or exogenous opioid action at the level of the spinal cord.
Corticosteroids	Interruption of the inflammatory cascade by inhibition of cytokine production.
Anticonvulsants	Interruption of ectopic foci by action on ion channels.
GABA-related	Hyperpolarization of neurons by enhancement of Cl^- influx.
Calcitonin	Potentiation of amine reuptake; direct binding to CNS sites; release of endogenous opioids; decrease of Ca^{2+}.

GABA = γ-amino butyric acid; SSRI = selective serotonin reuptake inhibitor.

tidepressants, α_2-adrenoceptor agonists, corticosteroids, anticonvulsants, agents related to γ-amino butyric acid (GABA), and calcitonin. In addition, muscle relaxants and benzodiazepines can relieve some musculoskeletal pains. The little that is known about the mechanisms by which these agents work to relieve pain is summarized in Table 83-2.

COMBINATIONS OF ANALGESICS

Analgesic combinations offer a potential benefit over individual agents, including increased compliance and reduced side-effects (if the same level of analgesia can be achieved with the lower doses of each component in the combination). Combining analgesics that have different mechanisms of action offers the additional potential advantage of being able to treat a broader spectrum of pain. Such an approach has been recommended by the World Health Organization (WHO). However, not all analgesic combinations lead to an improved clinical outcome. Therefore, each combination (and dose-ratio) must be evaluated independently. In addition, caution must be exercised to ensure that the maximum daily dose of either component of the combination is not exceeded. This is particularly important when one or both components are available separately OTC.

CHAPTER 84

Histamine and Antihistaminic Drugs

John E Hoover, BSc Pharm, RPh

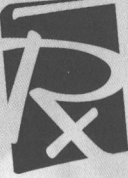

Histamine is a physiologically active, endogenous substance (autocoid) that is produced within the body by the decarboxylation of the amino acid, histidine, and then stored in mast cells and basophils where it is protected from ubiquitous destructive enzymes, such as histaminase. It binds to and activates histamine H_1- and H_2-receptors in various sites in the body. H_3-receptors, which may be involved in the control of histamine synthesis, also have been described.

The action of histamine on the cells depends to some extent on the function of the cell as well as on the ratio of its H_1- and H_2-receptors. The cardiovascular effects of histamine include direct and indirect microvascular dilation (involving H_1- and H_2-receptors) and increased vascular permeability (probably involving H_1-receptors); as a result, intracutaneous injection of histamine produces a *triple response* characterized by local reddening, a bright halo or flare, and wheal formation. Histamine also binds to and activates specific receptors in the nose, eyes, respiratory tract, and skin, causing characteristic allergic signs and symptoms. Activation of H_1-receptors (H_1-antagonists) block these actions.

Historically, the term antihistamine has been used to describe drugs that act as H_1-receptor antagonists. Activation of H_2-receptors stimulates gastric acid secretion; drugs that antagonize H_2-receptors (eg, cimetidine/nizatidine, ranitidine, or famotidine) are referred to as H_2-receptors antagonists (see Chapter 66). The H_2-antagonists inhibit gastric secretion stimulated not only by histamine, but also by insulin, pentagastrin, food, or physiological vagal reflex.

Another amine, 5-hydroxytryptamine, also is distributed widely in animals and is present in some plants. This substance, discovered independently by three groups of workers, is also known as enteramine and serotonin. It is found in largest amounts in the brain, blood, spleen, stomach, intestine, lungs, and skin. It has been suggested that 5-hydroxytryptamine may be involved in the regulation of vascular tone, motor, and secretory activity of the gastrointestinal (GI) tract and kidney function. Serotonin also functions as a neurotransmitter in the brain, and drugs that prevent its reuptake (eg, fluoxetine) possess antidepressant activity. These observations and the demonstration that tumors of the argentaffin cells of the intestinal mucosa (argentaffinomas or carcinoids) secrete large amounts of 5-hydroxytryptamine have stimulated the search for 5-hydroxytryptamine antagonists. The pharmacological actions of 5-hydroxytryptamine are varied and complex. Liberation of excessive amounts in man, as in argentaffin cell tumors, produces episodic flushing, tachycardia, and hypertension followed by cyanosis, diarrhea, asthma, and pulmonary stenosis. 5-Hydroxytryptamine an-

tagonists have been employed in the management of this malignancy, as well as certain skin diseases and psychoses. Several of the antihistamines described below possess both antihistaminergic and antiserotonergic activity. However, there are several clinically useful serotonin antagonists (granisetron hydrochloride, methysergide maleate, and ondansetron hydrochloride) that have been introduced into the clinical arena in recent years for the management of nausea or vomiting associated with carcinoid syndrome (granisetron, methysergide, and ondansetron) and vascular headache (methysergide). The remainder of this chapter is focused primarily on the role of histamine and uses of H_1-receptor antagonists.

HISTAMINE PHOSPHATE

1H-Imidazole-4-ethanamine, phosphate (1:2)

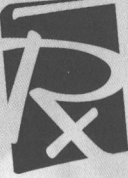

4-(2-Aminoethyl)imidazole phosphate (1:2) [51-74-1] $C_5H_9N_3 \cdot 2H_3PO_4$ (307.14).

Preparation—Histamine occurs in small amounts in ergot. It is among the products of bacterial decomposition of histidine, and this constitutes one of the methods for its production. It also is produced synthetically from imidazolylpropionic acid by several methods.

Description—Long prismatic crystals; colorless; odorless stable in air but affected by light; aqueous solutions are acid to litmus; when dried at 105° for 2 hr, melts at approximately 140°; pH (4.1% aq soln, iso-osmotic with serum) about 5.

Solubility—1 g in approximately 4 mL of water; slightly soluble in alcohol.

Pharmacology—Although many tissues contain a lethal amount of histamine in a bound or inactive form, no effect is produced until it is released in free form into body fluids as a result of certain stimuli. Because it is destroyed in the intestinal tract by the enzyme histaminase, it is ineffective when taken orally. After injection, it constricts certain smooth muscles such as the bronchi, uterus, and intestines and dilates the capillary bed. Characteristically, increased capillary permeability accompanies the dilation, and there is seepage of fluid, plasma, proteins, and even some cellular elements of the blood into extracellular spaces. Dilation of the capillaries and arterioles produces flushing of the face, fall in blood pressure, and increase in skin temperature.

It stimulates all types of glandular secretions—gastric, duodenal, salivary, and lacrimal. An important effect in man is the stimulation of the gastric glands, which increases the hydrochloric acid of the stomach. This effect of histamine was the basis of a diagnostic test that had been used in the past to differentiate between nonspecific hypochlorhydria and that caused by pernicious anemia. The preferred agent for this purpose is pentagastrin.

One highly characteristic effect of this agent is the *triple response* induced by the intracutaneous injection of small amounts of this agent.

It consists of

1. a local reddening at the site of the injection,
2. a wheal or patch of localized edema that obscures the original red spot, and
3. the scarlet flare that surrounds the wheal.

The initial red spot is due mostly to local capillary dilatation, and the wheal develops from arteriolar dilation and increased capillary permeability. The flare is a local phenomenon produced by an axon reflex involving peripheral sensory nerves. Because the flare does not appear in the presence of atrophy or degeneration of the nerve, this reaction has been used as a diagnostic test to distinguish between real and pseudoanesthesia.

When injected intravenously, it provokes an increased output of epinephrine from the adrenal medulla as indicated by a secondary rise in blood pressure. In the past, clinical use was made of this action on the adrenals by the use of it as a test agent in the diagnosis of pheochromocytoma. This test is now considered obsolete because of its hazardous nature and because chemical assays are now available for detecting and quantitating the levels of catecholamines and their metabolites in patients suspected of having pheochromocytoma.

Comments—Used primarily as a positive control in evaluation of allergenic skin testing. It has a few other minor diagnostic applications. Because the *flare* that results from intracutaneous injection of this agent is mediated by an axon reflex, this approach has been used as a test for the integrity of sensory nerves; the wheal that results has been used as a test for circulatory competency.

Adverse reactions are observed even after small doses, such as those employed in gastric analysis [0.01 mg/kg subcutaneously (SC)]. These include flushing, dizziness, headache, bronchial constriction, dyspnea, visual disturbances, faintness, syncope, urticaria, asthma, significant hypertension or hypotension, palpitation, tachycardia, nervousness, abdominal cramps, diarrhea, vomiting, metallic taste, allergic manifestations, or collapse with convulsions. The hypotension usually is postural and requires no treatment other than the patient's assuming a recumbent position. If treatment is required, epinephrine (0.3 mg SC) is an effective physiological antagonist.

ANTIHISTAMINES

All clinically available antihistamines antagonize histamine to approximately the same extent, regardless of their chemical class (ethanolamines, ethylenediamines, alkylamines, phenothiazines, or piperidines). They all induce some degree of sedation and anticholinergic activity. Only the ethanolamines and phenothiazines possess antiemetic properties. The clinical and pharmacological differences, therefore, are related chiefly to variations in adverse effects and to nonhistamine antagonizing actions, such as their atropine-like effects, central nervous system (CNS) effects (depression, stimulation, antiemetic, antitremor, and motion sickness), and local anesthetic properties. A knowledge of these factors is essential for proper drug selection.

All currently available antihistamines (H_1-receptor antagonists) act by competitively antagonizing the effects of histamine at receptor sites; they do not block the release of histamine and, hence, offer only palliative relief of allergic symptoms. After oral administration, effects are apparent within 15 to 30 min, are maximal within 1 hr, and persist for 4 to 6 hr. The liver is the principal site of metabolism; the agents are excreted in urine as unidentified metabolites.

Clinically, indications for the use of the various antihistaminic drugs vary considerably. The majority of these agents are *effective* for *perennial* and *seasonal allergic rhinitis, vasomotor rhinitis, allergic conjunctivitis, urticaria and angioedema, allergic reactions to blood and plasma, and dermographism* and as adjuncts to conventional therapy in *anaphylactic reactions.* A few antihistamines probably are effective in mild, local *allergic reactions to insect bites; physical allergy;* and minor *drug* and *serum* reactions characterized by *pruritus.* Selected antihistamines (eg, diphenhydramine hydrochloride) reduce rigidity and tremors in *paralysis agitans* (Parkinson's disease) and in *drug-induced extrapyramidal symptoms.* Some antihistamines (eg, buclizine, cyclizine, dimenhydrinate, diphenhydramine, meclizine) are also effective

in the *active and prophylactic* management of *motion sickness.* More sedative agents (eg, diphenhydramine, doxylamine, promethazine) sometimes are used in *insomnia* and in *insomnia* predominant in certain medical disorders. Certain antihistamines, such as chlorpheniramine, doxylamine succinate, and pyrilamine maleate, are used in proprietary medication advertised as daytime sedatives and sleep aids. Methapyrilene, formerly used in virtually all nonprescription sleep aids in the US, was removed from these products in 1979 because of its possible carcinogenic properties.

The phenothiazine antihistamines possess other useful clinical properties not shared by conventional antihistamines. For example, promethazine hydrochloride is useful for *preoperative, postoperative,* and *obstetric sedation;* prevention and control of *nausea* and *vomiting* associated with certain types of anesthesia and surgery; and as *adjunctive therapy* to meperidine or other analgesics for the *control of postoperative pain.*

The usefulness of antihistamines in various other clinical conditions (eg, bronchial asthma, atopic dermatitis, neurodermatitis, allergic eczema, various contact and chemotoxic dermatitides, and generalized pruritus) and for cardiac arrhythmias, spasmolysis in GI allergies, prophylaxis of drug reactions, etc. must await further clinical investigation before a final assessment can be made. It is generally agreed that *most* antihistamines are *ineffective* in migraine and histamine headache; for prevention or reduction of the sequelae of pain, edema, and hemorrhage in oral surgery; and for potentiation of narcotic analgesic drugs, as antiemetics in postoperative patients and as antitussives or for treatment of nocturnal leg cramps, leg cramps of pregnancy, and functional dysmenorrhea.

The most common side effect of antihistamines is sedation, evidenced principally by drowsiness, plus a diminished alertness and ability to concentrate. Less-common effects—unless large doses are used—include dryness of the mouth, blurred vision, vertigo, and GI distress (see also above). The sedative effect of some antihistamines may be so intense as to impair driving ability and performance of duties that necessitate mental alertness. Other side effects elicited by these drugs include nausea, headache, and restiveness. Dermatological complications and skin eruptions have followed local application or oral administration of antihistamines. In a few individuals, certain antihistamines produce signs of central excitation such as insomnia and nervousness. Concurrent use of antihistamines and certain other CNS-active drugs should be avoided because the depressant effects of alcoholic beverages and other drugs that depress the CNS (tranquilizers, hypnotics, sedatives, antianxiety agents, depressants, analgesics, etc.) are increased by antihistamines. Patients being treated with monoamine oxidase inhibitors (MAOIs), or who have been treated with such drugs within the preceding 2 weeks, should not be given antihistamines.

Because of their drying effect on mucous membranes, antihistamines may exacerbate wheezing and therefore should not be used during an asthmatic attack. Because of the anticholinergic action of antihistamines, their use in the following diseases may be contraindicated or subject to great caution: narrow-angle glaucoma, prostatic hypertrophy, stenosing peptic ulcer, pyloroduodenal obstruction, bladder-neck obstruction, increased intraocular pressure, history of bronchial asthma, hyperthyroidism, cardiovascular disease, or hypertension. Antihistamines should not be given to premature or newborn infants and may be denied by the physician for patients breastfeeding infants.

These brief observations call attention to the enormous number of clinical conditions for which antihistaminic drugs have been suggested. They also point up the fact that these drugs vary from *effective* to *ineffective* in these conditions.

When considering the multiplicity of available antihistamines, their numerous untoward reactions, and their propensity to induce sedation of variable intensity, one can appreciate the complex therapeutic problem that confronts both the patient and the physician in the selection of an antihistamine for a particular patient with a histamine-related clinical condition. Three monographs that highlight prototype antihistamines of the alkylamine (chlorpheniramine), ethanolamine (diphenhydramine), and phenothiazine (promethazine) classes of antihistamines are presented below.

CHLORPHENIRAMINE MALEATE

2-Pyridinepropanamine, γ-(4-chlorophenyl)-N,N-dimethyl-, (Z)-2-butenedioate (1:1); Chlor-Trimeton

2-[p-Chloro-α-[2-(dimethylamino)ethyl]benzyl]pyridine maleate (1:1) [113-92-8] $C_{16}H_{19}ClN_2 \cdot C_4H_4O_4$ (390.87).

Preparation—By condensing 2-[p-chloro-α-(2-chloroethyl)benzyl]pyridine with dimethylamine in the presence of sodamide. Treatment of the base with an equimolar portion of maleic acid results in the formation of the maleate.

Description—White, crystalline powder; odorless; solutions are acid to litmus (pH 4 to 5); melts about 130° to 135°; pK_a 9.2.

Solubility—1 g in 4 mL water, 10 mL alcohol, or 10 mL chloroform; slightly soluble in ether or benzene.

Comments—An alkylamine antihistamine that is a common ingredient in over-the-counter (OTC) antitussive formulation. It has a mild sedative action and slight anticholinergic activity. It is probably effective in allergic and vasomotor rhinitis, allergic conjunctivitis, mild urticaria and angioedema, allergic reactions to blood and plasma in sensitive patients, and dermographism and as adjunct therapy in anaphylactic shock. It is used widely as an ingredient in proprietary antitussive formulations. It undergoes significant first-pass metabolism (40–55%). Peak plasma levels of 5.9 and 11 ng/mL are achieved in 2 to 6 hr. It has a low incidence of side effects; these side effects are similar to those induced by other antihistamines. See the introductory statement.

CHLORPHENIRAMINE TANNATE

ing of Tussizone-12, Rynatuss, Xiratuss, etc.

Preparation—US Pat 5,663,415 (1997); US Pat 6,455,727 (2002); see also *Carbetapentane tannate*.

Description—Tan solid of undetermined purity.

Comments—See Chlorpheniramine Maleate.

DIPHENHYDRAMINE HYDROCHLORIDE

Ethanamine, 2-(diphenylmethoxy)-N,N-dimethyl-, hydrochloride; Benadryl Hydrochloride

2-(Diphenylmethoxy)-N, N-dimethylethylamine hydrochloride [147-24-0] $C_{17}H_{21}NO \cdot HCl$ (291.82).

Preparation—By heating diphenylbromomethane, β-dimethylaminoethanol and sodium carbonate in toluene. After the toluene is distilled off, the purified diphenhydramine is converted to the hydrochloride with hydrogen chloride.

Description—White, crystalline powder; slowly darkens on exposure to light; solutions are practically neutral to litmus; melts about 167° to 172°.

Solubility—1 g in 1 mL water, 2 mL alcohol, 2 mL chloroform, or 50 mL acetone; slightly soluble in benzene or ether.

Comments—A potent ethanolamine antihistamine that possesses significant anticholinergic (drying), antitussive, antiemetic, and sedative effects. It is effective for use in perennial and seasonal allergic rhinitis; vasomotor rhinitis; allergic conjunctivitis caused by inhalant allergens and foods; mild, uncomplicated allergic skin manifestations of urticaria and angioedema; alleviation and prevention of allergic reactions to blood or plasma in patients who have a known history of such reactions; dermographism; therapy for anaphylactic reactions adjunctive to epinephrine and other standard measures after the acute manifestations have been controlled; parkinsonism (including drug induced) in the elderly unable to tolerate more potent agents; mild cases of parkinsonism (including drug induced) in other age groups; other

cases of parkinsonism (including drug induced) in combination with centrally acting anticholinergic agents and active and prophylactic treatment of motion sickness. It also has significant antitussive activity; the syrup is used as a cough suppressant for the control of cough due to colds or allergy.

It is probably effective for use in mild, local allergic reactions to insect bites; physical allergy; minor drug and serum reactions characterized by pruritus; and intractable insomnia and insomnia dominant in certain medical disorders. Other suggested uses require further investigation. Although it is well absorbed after oral administration, first-pass metabolism is so extensive that only 40–60% reaches systemic circulation unchanged. Peak plasma concentrations are attained in 1 to 4 hr; 80–85% is bound to plasma protein; and elimination half- life ranges from 2.4 to 9.3 hr.

Patients, observed while on this drug, have shown numerous side effects such as drowsiness, confusion, restlessness, nausea, vomiting, diarrhea, blurring of vision, diplopia, difficulty in urination, constipation, nasal stuffiness, vertigo, palpitation, headache, and insomnia. Other side effects observed were urticaria, drug rash, photosensitivity, hemolytic anemia, hypotension, epigastric distress, anaphylactic shock, tightness of the chest and wheezing, thickening of bronchial secretions, dryness of the mouth, nose and throat and tingling, and heaviness and weakness of the hands.

Dimenhydrinate (Dramamine) contains approximately 50% diphenhydramine. The former agent is capable of masking symptoms of ototoxicity; therefore, dimenhydrinate and diphenhydramine should be used with caution in patients receiving aminoglycoside antibiotics (streptomycin, neomycin, or kanamycin) or other ototoxic drugs.

Because it has an atropine-like action, it should be used with caution in patients who have asthma. Likewise, patients should be cautioned about taking this drug with other depressant substances, because of the additive effect. Persons also should be advised not to operate a motor vehicle, fly an airplane, or operate hazardous machinery while on this drug. The incidence of side effects is approximately 30–60%.

PROMETHAZINE HYDROCHLORIDE

10H-Phenothiazine-10-ethanamine, N,N,α-trimethyl-, monohydrochloride; Phenergan

10-[2- (Dimethylamino)propyl]phenothiazine monohydrochloride [58-33-3] $C_{17}H_{20}N_2S \cdot HCl$ (320.88).

Preparation—By reacting phenothiazine with 1-chloro-2-(dimethylamino)propane hydrochloride in the presence of sodamide and sodium hydroxide in xylene. The base is extracted, purified, and converted to the hydrochloride.

Description—White to faint yellow, crystalline powder; practically odorless; slowly oxidized, particularly when moistened, on prolonged exposure to air, becoming blue in color; pH (1 in 20 solution) 4.0 to 5.0; melts within a 3° range between 215° and 225°; pK_a 9.1.

Solubility—Soluble in water, hot dehydrated alcohol, or chloroform; practically insoluble in ether, acetone, or ethyl acetate.

Comments—A phenothiazine antihistamine with significant sedation and antiemetic actions. It has significant anticholinergic activity. It has marked potency and prolonged duration of action. It is effective for use in perennial and seasonal allergic rhinitis; vasomotor rhinitis; allergic conjunctivitis caused by inhalant allergens and foods; mild, uncomplicated allergic skin manifestations of urticaria and angioedema; alleviation and prevention of allergic reactions to blood or plasma in patients who have a known history of such reactions; dermographism; therapy for anaphylactic reactions adjunctive to epinephrine and other standard measures after the acute manifestations have been controlled; preoperative, postoperative, or obstetric sedation; prevention and control of nausea and vomiting associated with certain types of anesthesia and surgery; therapy adjunctive to meperidine or other analgesics for control of postoperative pain; sedation in both children and adults as well as relief of apprehension and production of light sleep from which the patient can easily be aroused; active and prophylactic treatment of motion sickness; and antiemetic action in postoperative patients.

It is well absorbed, and peak effects occur within 20 min after oral, rectal, or intramucular (IM) administration; 76% to 80% is bound to plasma proteins; the duration of antihistaminic effect may persist for 12 hr or longer. The drug is excreted slowly in the urine and feces, primarily as inactive sulfoxides and glucuronides.

Untoward reactions include dryness of the mouth, blurring of vision, and, rarely, dizziness. Rare cases of leukopenia and one case of agranulocytosis have been reported. Minor increases in blood pressure and occasional mild hypotension have been documented. The appearance of photosensitivity may contraindicate further treatment. Excessive doses in adults have resulted in deep coma, sedation, and, rarely, convulsions; in children such doses have resulted in hyperexcitability and nightmares. See the introductory statement.

ANTIHISTAMINE COMBINATIONS

Typically, most antihistamine combinations include an antihistamine, a decongestant (eg, phenylephrine, or pseudoephadrine), a cough suppressant (eg, dextromethorphan, codeine, or hydrocodone), and an analgesic (eg, acetaminophen or aspirin). Because there are literally dozens of OTC and prescription antihistamine combinations available, it is recommended that the reader refer to a current *Facts and Comparisons Drug Information* or *Physicians' Desk Reference* (for both prescription and nonprescription drugs) for a listing of the available products, dosage, and suppliers.

INHIBITORS OF HISTAMINE RELEASE

The antihistamines described in the previous section antagonize, in varying degrees, most but not all pharmacological effects of histamine. They appear to accomplish this by occupying the *receptor sites* on the effector cell to the exclusion of the agonist, histamine, without initiating a response. Typically, they are competitive antagonists and do not prevent the release of histamine in response to injury, drugs, or antigens. However, a more recently developed drug, cromolyn sodium, can prevent the release of histamine from mast cells that have been sensitized by specific antigens.

ASTEMIZOLE—see RPS-20, page 1467.

ACRIVASTINE

2-Propenoic acid, (*E,E*)-3-[6-[1-(4-methylphenyl)-3-(1-pyrrolidin-yl)-1-propenyl]-2-pyridinyl]-, ing of Semprex-D

[87848-99-5] $C_{22}H_{24}N_2O_2$ (348.44).

Preparation—A multistep procedure starting with 2-bromo-6-(p-toluoyl)pyridine, ethyl acrylate and triphenylphosphine with a Pd(II)acetate catalyst, under pressure to form a triphenyl-2-pyrrolidinoethylphosphonium bromide. This latter compound with butyl lithium, hot sulfuric acid and an elaborate clean-up procedure affords the product. US Pat 4,501,893(1985).

Description—Odorless white to cream-colored crystalline powder from 2-propanol.

Solubility—Soluble in chloroform and ethanol; slightly soluble in water.

Comments—Acrivastine, a structural analog of triprolidine hydrochloride, exhibits H₁-antihistamine activity in isolated tissues, animals, and humans, and has sedative effects in humans. The propionic acid derivative of acrivastine is a metabolite in several animal species (as well as man) and also exhibits H₁-antihistaminic activity. Pseudoephedrine hydrochloride is an indirect sympathomimetic agent. It releases norepinephrine from adrenergic nerves. *In vitro* tests and *in vivo* studies in animals of acrivastine and pseudoephedrine in combination failed to demonstrate evidence of any beneficial or deleterious pharmacologic interaction between the two agents.

AZATADINE MALEATE

5*H*-Benzo[5,6]cyclohepta[1,2-*b*]pyridine, 6,11-dihydro-11-(1-methyl-4-piperidinylidene)-, (*Z*)-2-butenedioate (1:2); ing of Trinalis

6,11-Dihydro-11-(1-methyl-4-piperidylidene)-5*H*-benzo[5,6]-cyclohepta[1,2-*b*]pyridine maleate (1:2) [3978-86-7] $C_{20}H_{22}N_2$ $2C_4H_4O_4$ (522.55).

Preparation—Azatadine is a chemical relative of cyproheptadine, differing from the latter in that a pyridine ring replaces one of the benzene rings of cyproheptadine and in the saturation of the cycloheptane ring of the latter compound. It may be prepared by dehydrating the condensation product formed in the presence of sodium and liquid ammonia from 4-chloro-*N*-methylpiperidine and 5,6-dihydro-11*H*-benzo-[5,6]cyclohepta[1,2-*b*]pyridine-11-one. Treatment of the base with a bimolar quantity of maleic acid forms the maleate salt. US Pat 3,326,924.

Description—White to off-white powder; non-hygroscopic; melts at approximately 153°; pKₐ 8.4.

Solubility—1 g in 30 mL of water or 30 mL of alcohol.

Comments—An antihistamine structurally related to cyproheptadine with antiserotonin activity, mild to marked sedative action, and slight anticholinergic activity.

AZELASTINE HYDROCHLORIDE

1(2*H*)-Phthalazinone, (±)-4-[(4-chlorophenyl)methyl]-2-(hexahydro-1-methyl 1*H*-azepin-4-yl)-, monohydrochloride; Astelin; Optvar

[100643-71-8] $C_{22}H_{24}ClN_3 \cdot HCl$ (418.37).

Preparation—US Pat 3,813,384 (1974)

Description—A racemic mixture of white crystals melting about 225°–229° with a bitter taste; pH of a saturated aqueous solution between 5.0 and 5.4.

Solubility—Sparingly soluble in water, methanol, or propylene glycol; slightly soluble in ethanol, octanol, or glycerine.

Comments—A relatively selective histamine H₁ antagonist and an inhibitor of the release of histamine and other mediators from cells (eg, mast cells) involved in the allergic response. Based on in vitro studies using human cell lines, inhibition of other mediators involved in allergic reactions (eg, leukotrienes and PAF) has been demonstrated with this drug. Decreased chemotaxis and activation of eosinophils also has been demonstrated.

BROMPHENIRAMINE MALEATE

2-Pyridinepropanamine, γ-(4-bromophenyl-*N,N*-dimethyl-, (*Z*)-butenedioate (1:1); ing of Dimetapp

2-[*p*-Bromo-α-[2-(dimethylamino)ethyl]benzyl]pyridine maleate (1:1) [980-71-2] $C_{16}H_{19}BrN_2 \cdot C_4H_4O_4$ (435.32).

Preparation—α-(*p*-Bromophenyl)-2-pyridineacetonitrile is converted to its sodium derivative with sodium amide and condensed with 2-chloro-*N*, *N*-dimethylethylamine. The resulting nitrile is hydrolyzed to the corresponding acid, which is decarboxylated by treatment with H₂SO₄. The base, obtained on alkalinization, is solvent extracted and reacted with maleic acid.

Description—White, crystalline powder; odorless; melts about 130° to 135°; pH (1 in 100 solution) 4.0 to 5.0; pKₐ 3.9, 9.1.

Solubility—1 g in 5 mL water, 15 mL alcohol or 15 mL chloroform; slightly soluble in ether or benzene.

Comments—A mildly sedative bromine analog of chlorpheniramine with slight anticholinergic activity. It is an alkylamine derivative.

CARBINOXAMINE MALEATE

Ethanamine, 2-[(4-chlorophenyl)-2-pyridinylmethoxy]-N,N-dimethyl-, (Z)-2-butenedioate (1:1); ing of Rondec

2-[p-Chloro-α-[2-(dimethylamino)ethoxy]benzyl]pyridine maleate (1:1) [3505-38-2] $C_{16}H_{19}ClN_2O \cdot C_4H_4O_4$ (406.87).

Preparation—Picolinaldehyde and p-chlorophenylmagnesium bromide undergo a Grignard reaction to produce p-chloro-α-(2-pyridyl)benzyl alcohol. This is converted into its sodium alkoxide derivative with sodamide; β-Dimethylaminoethyl chloride is added to form carbinoxamine and the base converted into the maleate by reaction with maleic acid.

Description—White, crystalline powder; odorless; melts about 116° to 121°; pH (1 in 100 solution) 4.6 to 5.1; pK_a 8.7.

Solubility—1 g in <1 mL of water, 1.5 mL alcohol, 1.5 mL chloroform or 8300 mL ether.

Comments—An ethanolamine antiemetic with significant sedation and significant anticholinergic activity. It is useful for treating motion sickness.

CETIRIZINE HYDROCHLORIDE

Acetic acid, [2-[4-[(4-chlorophenyl)phenylmethyl]-1-piperazinyl]-ethoxy-, dihydrochloride; Zyrtec

[83881-52-1] $C_{21}H_{25}ClN_2O_3 \cdot 2HCl$ (461.82).

Preparation—Piperazine is condensed with 1 mol of 4-chlorobenzhydryl bromide under slightly alkaline conditions, and then the free secondary amine on the ring is further alkylated with 2-(2-chloroethoxy)acetamide to yield the amide of cetirizine that is hydrolyzed to the free acid. US Pat 4,525,358 (1985).

Description—Crystals that melt about 112° (base); dihydrochloride melts about 225°.

Solubility—Soluble in water.

Comments—A long-acting carboxylic acid metabolite of hydroxyzine with negligible anticholinergic activity. It is a piperazine derivative.

CLEMASTINE FUMARATE

Pyrrolidine, [R-(R*,R*)]-2-[2-[1-(2-[2-[1-(4-chlorophenyl)-1-phenylethoxy]ethyl]-1-methyl-, (E)-2-butenedioate (1:1); Tavist

(+)-(2R)-2-[2-[(R)-p-Chloro-α-methyl-α-phenylbenzyl)oxy]ethyl]-1-methylpyrrolidine fumarate (1:1) [14976-57-9] $C_{21}H_{26}ClNO \cdot C_4H_4O_4$ (459.97).

Preparation—Various benzhydryl ethers that have histamine-inhibiting action, clemastine being one, may be prepared by heating a mixture of the appropriate benzhydryl bromide and N-methyl-2-piperidylethanol in the presence of sodium carbonate. Details of the process, as well as of an alternate synthesis, are described in British patent 942,152 (see CA 60: 9250g, 1964).

Description—White to faintly yellow, crystalline powder; practically odorless; melts 176° to 181° with decomposition.

Solubility—Slightly soluble in water, chloroform, or ether; slightly soluble in alcohol.

Comments—A long-acting ethanolamine antihistamine with slight anticholinergic activity. It has sedative and anticholinergic side effects.

CROMOLYN SODIUM

4H-1-Benzopyran-2-carboxylic acid, 5,5′-[(2-hydroxy-1,3-propanediyl)-bis[4-oxo-, disodium salt; DSCG; Sodium Chromoglycate; Crolom; Gastrocrom, Intal, Nasalcrom, Opticrom

[15826-37-6] $C_{23}H_{14}Na_2O_{11}$ (512.34).

Preparation—2,6-Dihydroxyacetophenone is reacted with epichlorohydrin in the presence of a basic catalyst to yield the diether, 2′, 2″-[(2-hydroxytrimethylene)dioxy]bis[6′-hydroxyacetophenone]. Reaction with diethyl oxalate affects dehydration and deethanolation of each hydroxyacetophenone portion, thus introducing the fused oxopyrancarboxylate groups as ethyl esters. This diester is then saponified with NaOH. US Pat 3,419,578.

Description—White, crystalline powder; odorless; tasteless but with a slightly bitter aftertaste; hygroscopic; pK_a believed by analogy with similar monochromes to be approximately 1.5 to 2; melts about 261°; does not exhibit polymorphism.

Solubility—1 g in 20 mL of water; insoluble in alcohol or chloroform.

Comments—An antiasthmatic, antiallergic, and mast-cell stabilizer used in the management of severe bronchial asthma; the prevention of exercise-induced and acute bronchospasm and allergic rhinitis; the treatment of allergic ocular disorders, such as vernal keratoconjunctivitis, vernal conjunctivitis, giant papillary conjunctivitis, vernal keratitis, and allergic keratoconjunctivitis; and in the management of mastocytosis. Animal studies show that it inhibits the degranulation of sensitized mast cells that occurs after exposure to specific antigens. Thus, it inhibits the release of histamine and SRS-A (slow-reacting substance of anaphylaxis) from the mast cell. It has no vasoconstrictor, antihistaminic, or anti-inflammatory activity.

It is absorbed poorly from the GI tract, lung (7–8%), or eye (0.03%). The systemically absorbed drug is excreted unchanged in the bile and the urine. Adverse reactions from the use of capsule and aerosol preparations include lacrimation, swollen parotid glands, nausea, dysuria, dizziness, headache, rash, urticaria, angioedema, joint swelling and pain; adverse reactions from the use of a nebulizer or nasal solutions are cough, nasal congestion, sneezing, nasal itching, epistaxis, postnasal drip, headache, and abdominal pain; and adverse reactions from ocular solutions include stinging or burning on instillation, puffy eyes, eye irritation, and styes. It is contraindicated in patients hypersensitive to cromolyn or any component of the product.

CYPROHEPTADINE HYDROCHLORIDE

Piperidine, 4-(5H-dibenzo[a,d]cyclohepten-5-ylidene)-1-methyl-, hydrochloride, sesquihydrate; Periactin

4-(5H-Dibenzo[a,d]cyclohepten-5-ylidene)-1-methylpiperidine hydrochloride sesquihydrate [41354-29-4] $C_{21}H_{21}N \cdot HCl \cdot 1 1/2H_2O$ (350.89); *anhydrous* [969-33-5] (323.86).

Preparation—Phthalic anhydride is reacted with phenylacetic acid to form 3-benzylidenephthalide that, on isomerization and hydrogenation, gives 2-phenethylbenzoic acid. This is converted to its acid chloride, which then undergoes condensation to close the 7-membered ring and gives 10,11-dihydro-5H-dibenzo[a,d] cyclohepten-5-one. Bromination at the 10 position followed by dehydrobromination introduces the 10,11 double bond. Grignardization of this ketone with 4-chloro-1-methylpiperidine followed by dehydration of the resulting carbinol yields cyproheptadine (base), which, on reacting with an equimolar quantity of hydrogen chloride, forms the hydrochloride. US Pat 3,014,911.

Description—White to slightly yellow, crystalline powder; odorless or practically odorless; slightly bitter taste; relatively stable in light, stable at room temperature; nonhygroscopic; sesquihydrate is stable in air; anhydrous form melts about 250° and sesquihydrate melts about 162°.

Solubility—1 g in 275 mL of water, 35 mL of alcohol, or 26 mL of chloroform; practically insoluble in ether.

Comments—An antihistamine with slight anticholinergic activity. It has mild sedative and antiserotonin activity.

DESLORATADINE

5*H*-Benzo[5,6]cyclohepta[1.2-*b*]pyridine, 8-chloro-6,11-dihydro-11-(4-piperidinylidene)-; Clarinex

[00643-71-8] $C_{19}H_{19}ClN_2$ (310.80).

Preparation—A multi-step synthesis starting with either 3-methylnicotinonitrile or ethyl nicotinate and 3-chlorophenyllactonitrile. *Drugs of the Future* 2000; 25:339-346.

Description—Crystals, melting about 152°.

Solubility—Slightly soluble in water; very soluble in ethanol or propylene glycol.

Comments—A long-acting tricyclic histamine antagonist with selective histamine H_1 receptor e antagonist activity. Receptor binding data indicate that a concentration of 2–3 ng/mL (7 nanomolar), it shows significant interaction with the huma histamine H_1 receptor. It inhibited release from human mast cells in vitro.

DEXBROMPHENIRAMINE MALEATE

2-Pyridinepropanamine,(*S*)-γ-(4-bromophenyl)-*N*,*N*-dimethyl-, (*Z*)-2-butanedioate (1:1); ing of Drixoral

(+)-2-[*p*-Bromo-α-[2-dimethylamino)ethyl]benzyl]pyridine maleate (1:1). [2391-03-9] $C_{16}H_{19}BrN_2 \cdot C_4H_4O_4$ (435.32).

Preparation—As for *chlorpheniramide*, using the *p*-bromo derivative, rather than chloro. The racemic mixture produced is resolved to yield the product. See US Pats 2,676,964 and 3,061,517.

Description—White, crystalline powder; odorless; pH (1 in 100 solution) approximately 5; melts about 103° to 113°.

Solubility—1 g in 1.2 mL water, 2.5 mL alcohol, 2 mL chloroform, or 3000 mL ether.

Comments—The *d*-isomer of brompheniramine with slight anticholinergic activity. It is an alkylamine derivative.

DEXCHLORPHENIRAMINE MALEATE

2-Pyridinepropanamine, (*S*)-γ-(4-chlorophenyl)-*N*,*N*-dimethyl-, (*Z*)-2-butenedioate (1:1)

(+)-2-[*p*-Chloro-α-[2-(dimethylamino)ethyl]benzyl]pyridine maleate (1:1) [2438-32-6] $C_{16}H_{19}ClN_2 \cdot C_4H_4O_4$ (390.87).

Preparation—Racemic chlorpheniramine (see *Chlorpheniramine Maleate*) is resolved with the aid of (+)-phenylsuccinic acid. The (+)-enantiomorph of the base then is liberated from its (+)-phenylsuccinate salt by treatment with sodium hydroxide and reacted with an equimolar portion of maleic acid.

Description—White, crystalline powder; odorless; melts at 110 to 115°; pH (1 in 100 solution) 4.0 to 5.0.

Solubility—1 g in 1.1 mL water, 2 mL alcohol, 1.7 mL chloroform, or 2500 mL ether.

Comments—The *d*-isomer of chlorpheniramine with twice the potency and a wide margin of safety. It has minimal anticholinergic activity. It is an alkylamine derivative.

DIMENHYDRINATE

For the full monograph, see page 1310.

Comments—An ethanolamine antihistamine causing significant sedation. It is an antinauseant in motion sickness and vertigo associated with Meniere's syndrome. It has significant anticholinergic activity.

DIPHENHYDRAMINE HYDROCHLORIDE

Ethanamine, 2-(diphenylmethoxy)-*N*,*N*-dimethyl-, hydrochloride; Benadryl Hydrochloride

2-(Diphenylmethoxy)-*N*,*N*-dimethylethylamine hydrochloride [147-24-0] $C_{17}H_{21}NO \cdot HCl$ (291.82).

Preparation—By heating diphenylbromomethane, β-dimethyl-amino-ethanol, and sodium carbonate in toluene. After distilling off the toluene, the purified diphenhydramine is converted to the hydrochloride with hydrogen chloride.

Description—White, crystalline powder; slowly darkens on exposure to light; solutions are practically neutral to litmus; melts 167° to 172°.

Solubility—1 g in 1 mL water, 2 mL alcohol, 2 mL chloroform, or 50 mL acetone; slightly soluble in benzene or ether.

Comments—An ethanolamine antihistamine with significant anticholinergic activity.

DOXYLAMINE SUCCINATE—see RPS-20, page 1469.

EMEDASTINE DIFUMARATE

1*H*-Benzimidazole, 1-(2-ethoxyethyl)-2-(hexahydro-4-methyl-1*H*-1,4diazepin-1-yl)-, (*E*)-2-butenedioate (1:2); Emadine

[87233-62-3] $C_{17}H_{26}N_4O \cdot 2C_4H_4O_4$ (534.57).

Preparation—1-Chloro-2-ethoxyethane and 2-chlorobenzimidazole are heated and stirred at 120° for 2 hrs. The mixture is made alkaline, extracted with ethyl acetate, dried, concentrated, and chromatographed to purify. The solvent is removed, the residue dissolved in hot ethanol, and fumaric acid added to yield the crystalline difumarate.

Description—Melts about 142°.

Solubility—Soluble in water.

Comments—A relatively selective, histamine H_1 receptor antagonist. In vitro examinations of emedastne's affinity for histamine receptors demonstrate relative selectivity for the H_1 histamine receptor. In vivo studies have shown concentration-dependent inhibition of histamine-stimulated vascular permeability in the conjunctiva following topical ocular administration. It appears to be devoid of effects on adrenergic, dopaminergic, and serotonin receptors.

FEXOFENADINE HYDROCHLORIDE

Benzeneacetic acid, (±)-4-[1-hydroxy-4-[4-hydroxydiphenylmethyl)-1-piperdinyl]butyl]-α,α-dimethyl-, hydrochloride; Allegra

[138452-21-8] $C_{32}H_{39}NO_4 \cdot HCl$ (538.13).

Preparation—One method involves reduction of 2-methyl-2-phenylpropanoic acid with LiAlH$_4$, esterification of the resulting alcohol with acetic anhydride to form the acetate, **I**. A Friedel-Crafts reaction of **I** with 4-chlorobutyryl chloride yields the *p*-(4-chlorobutyryl) derivative, **II**. *N*-Alkylation by **II** of α,α-diphenyl-4-piperidinemethanol in the presence of $KHCO_3$, followed by reduction of the carbonyl group to a secondary alcohol with $NaBH_4$ gives the methyl ester of fexofenadine. Hydrolysis with base affords the product, which is converted to the hydrochloride. *Arzneimittel-Forsch.* 1982; 32:1185.

Description—White crystals that melt about 143°.

Solubility—Freely soluble in ethanol or methanol; slightly soluble in chloroform or water; insoluble in hydrocarbon solvents.

Comments—An active metabolite of terfenadine without the cardiotoxic and drug-interaction potential. It has no anticholinergic activity. It is a piperidine derivative.

HYDROXYZINE HYDROCHLORIDE

For the full monograph, see page 1491.

Comments—A piperazine antihistamine with significant sedation often used as a preanesthetic. It has no anticholinergic activity.

KETOTIFEN FUMARATE

10*H*-Benzo[4,5]cyclohepta[1,2-*b*]thiophene-10-one, 4,9-dihydro-4-(1-methyl-4-piperidinylidene)-, (*E*)-2-butenedioate (1:1); Zaditor

[34580-14-8] $C_{19}H_{19}NOS.C_4H_4O_4$ (425.51).

Preparation—A multi-step procedure starting with 9,10-dihydro-4*H*-benzo[4,5]cyclohepta[1,2-*b*]thiophen-4-one. *Helv chim Acta* 1976; 59:866. See also US Pat 3,682,930 (1971).

Description—Crystals from ethyl acetate. Melting point: base, 152–3°; fumarate, about 153°.

LORATADINE

1-Piperidinecarboxylic acid, 4-(8-chloro-5,6-dihydro-11*H*-benzo[5,6]-cyclohepta [1,2-*b*]pyridin-11-ylidene)-, Alavert; Claritin

[79794-75-5] $C_{22}H_{23}ClN_2O_2$ (382.89).

Preparation—*J Med Chem* 1972; 15:750. US Pat 4,282,233 (1981).

Description—Crystals that melt about 135°.

Comments—A long-acting, nonsedating tricyclic antihistamsine. It has no anticholinergic activity.

MECLIZINE HYDROCHLORIDE

For the full monograph, see page 1311.

Comments—A piperazine antihistamine with slight sedation. Its major use is for prophylactic treatment of motion sickness. It has no antichloinergic activity.

OLOPATADINE HYDROCHLORIDE

Dibenz[*b,e*]oxepin-2-acetic acid, *Z*-11-[3-(dimethylamino)-propylidene-6,11-dihydro-, hydrochloride; Patanol

[140462-76-6] $C_{21}H_{23}NO_3.HCl$ (373.88).

Preparation—By condensation of the sodium salt of methyl *p*-hydroxyphenyl acetate with phthalide to form the *o*-carboxyphenyl methyl ether. The ring is closed with trifluoroacetic anhydride and BF_3 in ether to yield the methyl ester of 10-oxobenz[*b,e*]oxapinacetic acid. Treatment with 3-dimethylaminopropyl triphenyl phosphonium bromide and hydrolysis of the ester which is formed, yields the product. *Drugs of the Future* 1993; 18:794.

Description—White crystals, soluble in water. Melts about 248° (dec).

Solubility—Soluble in water.

Comments—An inhibitor of the release of histamine from the mast cell and a relatively selective histamine H_1 antagonist that inhibits the *in vivo* and *in vitro* type 1 immediate hypersensivity reaction including inhibition of histamine-induced effects on human conjunctival epithelial cells. It is devoid of effects on a-adrenergic, dopamine, and muscarinic type 1 and 2 receptors. Following topical ocular administration in humans, it was shown to have low systemic exposure.

PHENINDAMINE TARTRATE

1*H*-Indeno[2,1-*c*]pyridine-, 2,3,4,9-tetrahydro-3-methyl-9-phenyl-, [*R*-(*R**,*R**)]-2,3dihydroxybutanedioate salt (1:1); Nolahist; Nolamine

[569-59-5] $C_{19}H_{19}N.C_4H_6O_6$ (411.46).

Preparation—Methylamine HCl, acetophenone and paraformaldehyde are refluxed in alcohol to form 3,3′-methyliminobispropiophenone HCl. Ring closure is achieved by heating with HBr to yield 2,3-dihydro-1-methyl-9-phenyl-1*H*-indeno[2,1-*c*]pyridine hydrobromide. Catalytic hydrogenation and treatment with alkali forms the base which is converted to the tartrate. US Pat 2,470,109 (1949).

Description—Creamy white powder; faint odor. Melts about 161° and on continued slow heating solidifies about 163° and melts again about 168° with decomposition.

Solubility—1 g in about 40 mL of water or 350 mL of alcohol; practically insoluble in chloroform, ether or benzene. Aqueous solutions are acid to litmus.

TRIPELENNAMINE CITRATE

1,2-Ethanediamine,*N,N*-dimethyl-N′-(phenylmethyl)-*N*′-2-pyridinyl-, 2-hydroxy-1,2,3-propanetricarboxylate (1:1); PBZ; Pyribenzamine

2-[Benzyl[2-(dimethylamino)ethyl]amino]pyridine citrate (1:1) [6138-56-3] $C_{16}H_{21}N_3 \cdot C_6H_8O_7$ (447.49).

Preparation—Tripelennamine is reacted with an equimolar portion of citric acid in a suitable volatile solvent. For the preparation of the base, see *Tripelennamine Hydrochloride*.

Description—White, crystalline powder; solutions are acid to litmus; melts about 107°.

Solubility—1 g in approximately 1 mL of water; freely soluble in alcohol; slightly soluble in ether; practically insoluble in chloroform or benzene.

Comments—An antihistamine said to be more palatable by the oral route of administration than the hydrochloride. Otherwise, its actions and uses are the same. See *Tripelennamine Hydrochloride*.

TRIPELENNAMINE HYDROCHLORIDE

1,2-Ethanediamine, *N,N*-dimethyl-*N*′-(phenylmethyl)-*N*′-2-pyridinyl-, monohydrochloride; PBZ; Pyribenzamine

2-[Benzyl[2-(dimethylamino)ethyl]amino]pyridine monohydrochloride [154-69-8] $C_{16}H_{21}N_3.HCl$ (291.82). For the structure of the base, see *Tripelennamine Citrate*.

Preparation—As follows: 2-aminopyridine, prepared by the action of sodamide on pyridine, is reacted with β-dimethylaminoethyl chloride in the presence of sodamide, and the resulting 2-[2-(dimethylamino)ethylamino]pyridine is condensed with benzyl bromide in the presence of sodamide. The hydrochloride is formed from the base by treatment with hydrogen chloride in an organic solvent.

Description—White, crystalline powder; slowly darkens on exposure to light; solutions practically neutral to litmus; melts at 188° to 192°.

Solubility—1 g in 1 mL water, 6 mL alcohol, 6 mL chloroform, or about 350 mL acetone; insoluble in benzene, ether or ethyl acetate.

Comments—An ethylenediamine antihistamine with moderate sedation. It has slight anticholinergic activity.

TRIPROLIDINE HYDROCHLORIDE

Pyridine, *E*-2-[1-(4-methylphenyl)-3-(1-pyrrolidinyl)-1-propenyl]-monohydrochloride, monohydrate; ing of Actifed

[6138-79-0] $C_{19}H_{22}N_2 \cdot HCl \cdot H_2O$ (332.87); *anhydrous* [550-70-9] (314.86).

Preparation—4′-Methylacetophenone is reacted with formaldehyde and pyrrolidine to form 3-(1-pyrrolidinyl)-4′-methylpropiophenone. Reaction with 2-pyridylsodium and subsequent hydrolysis produces the tertiary carbinol, α-[2-(1-pyrrolidinyl)ethyl]-α-*p*-tolyl-2-pyridinemethanol, which is dehydrated with sulfuric acid to introduce the propenyl double bond. Alkalinization liberates triprolidine, which is purified and reacted with an equimolar portion of HCl. US Pats 2,712,020 and 2,712,023.

Description—White, crystalline powder; no more than a slight, but unpleasant, odor; bitter taste; solutions are alkaline to litmus; melts about 115°; light sensitive; non-hygroscopic; stable to reasonable heat; pK$_a$ 3.6, 9.3.

Solubility—1 g in 2.1 mL water, 1.8 mL alcohol, 1 mL chloroform, or 2000 mL of ether.

Comments—A propylamine antihistamine with a rapid onset and long duration of action found in OTC cold and sinus preparations. It has no anticholinergic activity.

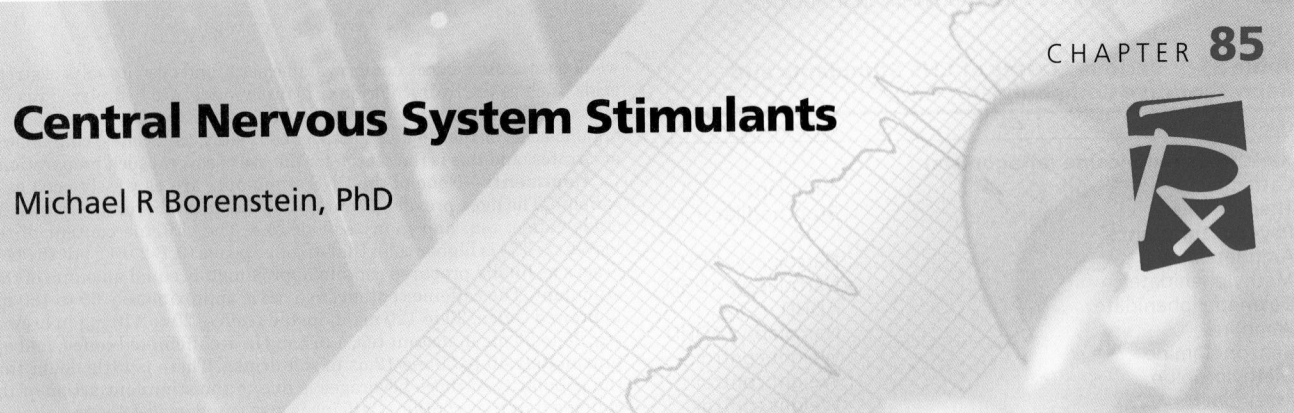

CHAPTER 85

Central Nervous System Stimulants

Michael R Borenstein, PhD

Central nervous system (CNS) stimulants are substances that increase excitability within various regions of the brain or the spinal cord. The prominent effects produced by many of these drugs are arousal and increased motor function that result in subjective feelings of increased mental alertness, decreased fatigue, improved concentration, increased energy and motivation, and an elevation in mood. Excessive CNS excitation produced by these drugs can lead to dose-dependent adverse effects such as extreme nervousness, agitation, anxiety, and seizures.

Excitability of the CNS reflects an intricate balance between excitatory and inhibitory activity within the brain. Stimulants of the CNS directly or indirectly enhance excitatory activity or block inhibitory components. The excitatory transmitters, glutamate and aspartate, are important neurotransmitters at excitatory synapses where their actions are mediated through N-methyl-D-aspartate (NMDA) or non-NMDA (kainate or AMPA/quisqualate) receptors. In contrast, gamma-aminobutyric acid (GABA) and glycine are prominent inhibitory neurotransmitters. The neuromodulator, adenosine, also plays an important role in CNS excitation in that it can exert a depressant action, owing to its ability to decrease impulse-generated transmitter release and to limit excitation of postsynaptic elements by direct hyperpolarization of the neuronal membrane. Many CNS stimulants produce excitation through their antagonism at GABA, glycine, or adenosine receptors. The indirect-acting sympathomimetics, produce pronounced CNS stimulation by enhancing the actions of endogenous catecholamines because of their ability to increase release or prevent the uptake of endogenous catecholamines (Table 85-1).

The CNS stimulants are a diverse group of pharmacological agents. Many are used therapeutically and are prescription drugs (eg, the psychostimulant amphetamine). Others, such as the xanthine derivative, caffeine, are found predominately in nonprescription preparations or in common beverages. See Table 85-1 for classification of the CNS stimulants.

The xanthine derivatives (caffeine and theophylline) are mild CNS stimulants. Indeed, the ability of caffeine to increase alertness is one reason for the high consumption of caffeine-containing beverages. Of this class, only caffeine is used therapeutically for its stimulant effects. It is available in nonprescription preparations for use in promoting wakefulness. It is also found as an adjunct in various analgesic drug preparations, including prescription and nonprescription drugs, although its efficacy in the treatment of pain is not well established.

The indirect acting sympathomimetics (eg, methylphenidate and the amphetamines) are more potent CNS stimulants than caffeine but have limited therapeutic use. They are used in the treatment of attention deficit hyperactivity disorder (ADHD), narcolepsy, and obesity. However, because these CNS stimu-

lants convey a sense of self-confidence, well-being, and euphoria, they are highly addictive and some are widely abused (eg, amphetamines, especially methamphetamine). Because of their abuse potential, the search continues to find alternative therapies for the potent CNS stimulants in these disorders. As relates to weight loss therapy, the amphetamines have limited usefulness because of the development of tolerance to their anorexic actions. Research in the area of obesity has revealed the role of various hormones and neuropeptides in lipid metabolism and satiety. It is likely that in the future, alternative therapeutics will be developed as more efficacious agents in the treatment of obesity.

CNS stimulation can be an adverse effect of some drugs at therapeutic doses. Common examples include sympathomimetic amines, nicotine, serotonin reuptake inhibitors, MAO inhibitors and various alkaloids. A number of agents are stimulant only at toxic doses. These include local anesthetics and salicylates. Only those drugs that have central stimulation as a predominant action are described in this section.

XANTHINE DERIVATIVES

Xanthine derivatives include caffeine, theophylline, theobromine, and several related synthetic derivatives, all of which have similar pharmacological properties but differ considerably in the intensity of their actions in various structures. For example, the stimulant effects of caffeine and theophylline on the CNS and on skeletal muscle are much greater than those of theobromine. However, theophylline surpasses caffeine in its diuretic, cardiac, and smooth muscular actions. Therefore, in the therapeutic application of these drugs for a specific effect, side effects can be minimized and the desired effect intensified by careful selection of the xanthine employed. For example, theophylline, but not caffeine, is used in the treatment of asthma because of its greater action on smooth muscle and its ability to alleviate bronchoconstriction. Because the principal therapeutic application of caffeine is as a CNS stimulant, its actions are discussed in this section. The principal therapeutic use of theophylline and related compounds is as a bronchodilator in the management of asthma; these drugs are discussed in Chapter 69.

AMINOPHYLLINE—page 1372.

CAFFEINE

1*H*-Purine-2,6-dione, 3,7-dihydro-1,3,7-trimethyl-, Theine: Nō Dōz; Tirent; Vivarin; Dexitac; Quick Pep

1,3,7-Trimethylxanthine [58-08-2] $C_8H_{10}N_4O_2$ (194.19); *monohydrate* [5743-12-4] (212.21).

Preparation—Caffeine may be isolated from tea or coffee by boiling with water in the presence of lime or magnesium oxide, which

Table 85-1. Various Classes of CNS Stimulants and Representative Compounds

CLASS/COMPOUND	PRIMARY USE
Xanthines (adenosine antagonists)	
Caffeine	Stimulant
Theophylline	Bronchodilator
Psychostimulants[a]	
Amphetamine	Narcolepsy, ADHD
Methylphenidate	Narcolepsy, ADHD
Dexmethylphenidate	ADHD
Pemoline	Narcolepsy, ADHD
Benzphetamine	Weight control
Diethylpropion	Weight control
Mazindol	Weight control
Phendimetrazine	Weight control
Phentermine	Weight control
Sibutramine	Weight control
Cocaine	Drug of abuse
Methamphetamine	Drug of abuse
Modafinil[c]	Narcolepsy

[a] Increase aminergic activity by releasing monoamines or blocking their reuptake.
[b] Stimulates medullary respiratory centers.
[c] Mechanism unclear, possible adrenergic α-1B agonist.

serves to precipitate the tannins and some of the coloring matter. After filtration, the crude caffeine that separates is recrystallized from hot water after treatment with decolorizing charcoal. A source of the commercial supply is tea dust or sweepings. Increasing quantities of caffeine are now obtained as a byproduct in the manufacture of "decaffeinized coffee." It is also produced by methylation of theobromine (partial synthesis) and by total synthesis from urea or dimethylurea by variations of Traube's classic process (*Ber* 33:3052, 1900). The essential steps of a synthesis of theophylline and caffeine from urea are shown below:

Theophylline

Description—White powder or white, glistening needles, usually matted: odorless and has a bitter taste; pH (1% solution) 6.9; the hydrate is efflorescent in air and loses all its moisture at 80°; when rendered anhydrous by drying, it melts between 235° and 237.5°; pK$_a$ 13.9.

Solubility—1 g of anhydrous caffeine dissolves in approximately 50 mL water, 6 mL of water at 80°, 75 mL alcohol, approximately 25 mL alcohol at 60°, approximately 6 mL chloroform, or 600 mL ether. Being a

weak base, caffeine does not form stable salts, and even its salts of strong acids, such as the hydrochloride or hydrobromide, are hydrolyzed readily by water. The solubility of caffeine in water is increased by the presence of organic acids or their alkali salts, eg, benzoates, salicylates, cinnamates, or citrates, and this is the reason for the use of several such preparations.

Comments—None of the CNS stimulants are as widely used as is caffeine. The most prevalent sources of caffeine are beverages, which include coffee, tea, and many soft drinks. The caffeine content of tea leaves (2–3%) is higher than that of coffee beans (0.7–2.0%), but the beverages as finally prepared contain approximately equal amounts of this stimulant. The caffeine content (in 5 oz) is approximately 60 to 180 mg in brewed coffee, 30 to 120 mg in instant coffee, 20 to 110 mg in brewed tea, 25 to 50 mg in instant tea, 1 to 5 mg in decaffeinated coffee, and approximately 40 to 50 mg/12 oz in soft drinks. There is little doubt that the popularity of these beverages is due to the stimulant action of the caffeine that they contain. Caffeine is also found in oral nonprescription and prescription drugs.

Pharmacokinetics—Caffeine is absorbed readily after oral administration. After the oral administration of 100 mg of caffeine (amount contained in a cup of coffee), peak plasma levels of approximately 1.5 to 1.8 µg/mL are reached after 15 to 20 min. Plasma concentrations >20 µg/mL commonly produce adverse reactions. The lethal concentration is >100 µg/mL. Caffeine is distributed rapidly throughout all body tissues, readily crossing the placenta and the blood–brain barrier. Approximately 17% of the drug is bound to plasma proteins. Plasma half-life is 3 to 4 hr in adults; in preterm infants the half-life may be >100 hr. The longer half-life in infants is because of a much slower rate of metabolism because of the immaturity of the P-450-metabolizing systems. Therefore, if caffeine is used therapeutically in neonates (eg, in the treatment of prolonged apnea in preterm infants), dosing intervals need to be adjusted accordingly and its plasma concentration needs to be closely monitored. Caffeine is metabolized rapidly by the liver to 1-methyluric acid, 1-methylxanthine, and 7-methylxanthine. Less than 10% is excreted unchanged by the kidneys.

Pharmacology—Several mechanisms have been proposed for caffeine's stimulant actions. For many years it was thought that the stimulant action of caffeine was caused by its inhibition of the enzyme phosphodiesterase in the brain and the resulting accumulation and actions of cyclic 3′,5′-adenosine monophosphate (c-AMP). However, several compounds that are more potent than caffeine in inhibiting phosphodiesterase activity lack CNS-stimulant actions. Moreover, the concentration of caffeine needed to inhibit phosphodiesterase activity is 100 times greater than blood levels achieved after caffeine consumption. The more likely mechanism for the stimulant actions of caffeine is its blockade of adenosine receptors. Adenosine exerts prominent presynaptic and postsynaptic inhibition of neuronal activity. Blockade of this inhibition by caffeine would result in increased excitatory activity of neurons.

System Effects—Caffeine exerts effects on many systems. For example, in one double-blind clinical study, oral administration of 250 mg of the drug to nine healthy young noncoffee drinkers who had no coffee, tea, or cola in the previous 3 wk increased plasma renin activity (57%); plasma norepinephrine (75%); and plasma epinephrine by (207%); urinary normetanephrine and metanephrine were increased 52% and 100%, respectively; mean blood pressure increased 14/10 Torr within 1 hr; heart rate first decreased and then increased; and respiratory rate increased 20%.

- *CNS:* Caffeine stimulates all levels of the CNS. In oral doses of 100 to 200 mg, it stimulates the cerebral cortex, producing a more rapid and clear flow of thought, wakefulness, or arousal in fatigued patients, as well as improved psychomotor coordination. However, tasks requiring finite muscular coordination or timing may be adversely affected. Its cortical effects are milder and of shorter duration than those of the amphetamines. In larger doses, caffeine stimulates medullary vagal, vasomotor, and respiratory centers, inducing bradycardia, vasoconstriction, and an increased respiratory rate.

- *Cardiovascular:* In the heart, caffeine has a positive inotropic effect on the myocardium and a positive chronotropic effect on the sinoatrial node, causing a transient increase in heart rate, force of contraction, cardiac output, and work of the heart. In doses in excess of 250 mg, the centrally mediated vagal effects of caffeine may be masked by increased sinus rates; tachycardia, extrasystoles, or other ventricular arrhythmias may result. In the vasculature, caffeine, in normally ingested amounts, produces vasoconstriction of blood vessels, presumably by blocking adenosine receptors located in the smooth muscle of the vasculature. It is thought that the vasoconstriction of the cerebral blood vessels by caffeine contributes to its ability to relieve headaches. In the peripheral vasculature, caffeine ingestion results in increased vascular resistance and a slight increase in blood pressure, probably because of the action of caffeine on the smooth muscle of the vessels and on catecholamine release.

- *Skeletal Muscle:* Caffeine stimulates voluntary skeletal muscle, increasing the force of muscle contraction and decreasing muscular fatigue.
- *Gastrointestinal (GI):* Caffeine stimulation of parietal cells increases gastric acid secretion.
- *Renal:* Caffeine induces a mild diuresis by increasing renal blood flow and glomerular filtration rate and by decreasing proximal tubular reabsorption of sodium and water.
- *Metabolism:* Caffeine increases glycogenolysis and lipolysis, although the increases in blood glucose and plasma lipids usually are not of physiological consequence in healthy humans.

Adverse Effects—Dose-related adverse effects of caffeine include nervousness, anxiety, tremulousness, irritability, headache, excitation, restlessness, insomnia, tinnitus, GI irritation, nausea, vomiting, tachycardia, palpitations, and extrasystoles. Miscellaneous effects include hypersensitivity, urticaria, hyperglycemia, and diuresis.

Toxicity—Large doses are usually associated with GI pain, muscle twitching, facial flushing, dizziness, dyspnea, mild delirium, diuresis, dehydration, nausea, vomiting, and fever. More serious symptoms include cardiac arrhythmias and convulsions. The acute lethal dose of caffeine in adults appears to be approximately 5 to 10 g. Caffeine may aggravate diarrhea in patients who have irritable bowel, or it may exacerbate duodenal ulcers. Safety for pregnancy has not been established, but moderate intake does not appear to be harmful to the fetus.

Tolerance—Prolonged, high intake may produce tolerance to the diuretic, cardiovascular, and CNS system effects as well as physical dependence. Abrupt discontinuation of the stimulant may produce withdrawal symptoms of fatigue, headache, anxiety, nausea, vomiting, irritability, impaired psychomotor function, restlessness, lethargy, and less commonly, yawning and rhinorrhea. A typical symptom is headache that results from a rebound vasodilation of the brain vasculature upon withdrawal from caffeine. Symptoms appear within 24 hr after the last ingestion of caffeine, peak within 48 hr, and may persist for as long as 1 wk.

Drug Interactions—Caffeine and other xanthines may modify the effects of other drugs. These drugs can enhance the cardiac inotropic effects of beta-adrenergic stimulating agents and decrease the effect of benzodiazepines. Because caffeine ingestion results in reduced liver blood flow, the metabolism and elimination of drugs that are eliminated primarily by hepatic metabolism may be slowed.

Laboratory Tests—The ingestion of caffeine can cause a slight increase in urine levels of vanillylmandelic acid, catecholamines, and 5-hydroxyindoleacetic acid. Because high urine levels of vanillylmandelic acid or catecholamines may result in a false-positive diagnosis of pheochromocytoma or neuroblastoma, caffeine intake should be avoided during these tests.

Uses—Nonprescription caffeine preparations are used orally as a mild CNS stimulant to aid in staying awake and to restore mental alertness. Caffeine is the only stimulant approved by the Food and Drug Administration (FDA) for nonprescription use. Caffeine also is found in nonprescription drugs containing analgesics (acetaminophen, aspirin) for the treatment of mild pain, for relief from vascular headaches such as migraine and cluster headaches, and for the treatment of menstrual pain and discomfort (usual caffeine content of 30 to 65 mg/tablet). It is also a component in various cold remedies. Although the efficacy of caffeine in the analgesic preparations is controversial, results from some clinical studies indicate that the adjunct use of caffeine with analgesics may lower the amount of analgesic needed for pain relief. Caffeine is also used in combination with ergotamine in prescription drugs for migraine headaches, presumably because of its actions on extracranial vasculature and trigeminal afferents. Caffeine is used to treat preterm apnea in infants. However, the combination of caffeine with sodium benzoate is contraindicated for use in these infants because the benzoate can cause metabolic disturbances and bilirubinemia.

CAFFEINE, CITRATED

Xanthine, 1,3,5-trimethyl-, citrate salt; Cafcit

[69-22-7] Caffeine citrate

Preparation—Fifty grams each of caffeine and citric acid are dissolved in 100 mL of hot distilled water, the solution evaporated to dryness with constant stirring. It is usually prepared simply by dry-mixing equal quantities of each component.

Description—White, odorless powder; slightly bitter, acid taste; acid reaction. Solutions are adjusted to pH 4.7.

Solubility—1 g in approximately 4 mL warm water; the caffeine gradually precipitating on diluting the solution with an equal volume of water but redissolving on further dilution with sufficient water.

Incompatibilities—Neutralization of the citric acid by *alkalies* or *alkaline salts* causes precipitation of caffeine if in sufficient concentration. The alkali salts of organic acids may release either caffeine or the

free organic acid. Generally, it displays the incompatibilities of the citric acid that it contains.

Comments—Approved by the FDA in 1999 as a solution for intravenous injection and oral administration for the short-term treatment of apnea of prematurity (AOP) in infants between 28 and <33 weeks gestational age.

Pharmacology—The mechanism of action of caffeine in AOP is not known but may be related to its following effects: stimulation of the respiratory center, increased minute ventilation, decreased threshold to hypercapnia, increased response to hypercapnia, increased skeletal muscle tone, decreased diaphragmatic fatigue, increased metabolic rate, and increased oxygen consumption.

Pharmacokinetics—Peak plasma levels of caffeine are reached 30 minutes to 2 hours following oral administration of 10 mg of caffeine base/kg to preterm neonates. The elimination of caffeine is much slower in infants compared to adults. Mean half-life in neonates is 3 to 4 days, and 86% is excreted unchanged.

Adverse Effects—Published long-term follow-up studies have not shown caffeine to adversely effect neurologic development or growth. Necrotizing enterocolitis, feeding intolerance, and the development of rash were the most commonly reported events, but the potential exist for CNS stimulation, cardiovascular and gastrointestinal effects, as well as alterations in metabolism and renal effects.

CAFFEINE AND SODIUM BENZOATE INJECTION

A sterile solution of caffeine and sodium benzoate in water for injection; contains an amount of anhydrous caffeine ($C_8H_{10}N_4O_2$) equivalent to 45% to 52%, and an amount of sodium benzoate ($C_7H_5NaO_2$) equivalent to 47.5% to 55.5%, of the labeled amounts of caffeine and sodium benzoate.

Description—pH between 6.5 and 8.5.

Comments—see *Caffeine* page 1551.

DYPHYLLINE—page 1373.
OXTRIPHYLLINE—page 1383.
THEOPHYLLINE—page 1373.
THEOPHYLLINE, EPHEDRINE HYDROCHLORIDE, AND PHENOBARBITAL—see RPS-19, page 973.

PSYCHOSTIMULANTS

Most of the compounds included under this heading are indirect-acting sympathomimetic drugs and are more potent central stimulants than the xanthine derivatives. These compounds do not stimulate monoaminergic receptors directly, but rather they increase the actions of endogenous monoamines. This is because of their ability to inhibit the uptake of the catecholamine from the synaptic cleft after release (eg, cocaine, methylphenidate, mazindol, or sibutramine) or to cause catecholamine release (amphetamine and congeners). The actions of diethylpropion and phentermine are primarily on adrenergic neurotransmission, pemoline on dopaminergic neurotransmission, and those of mazindol and sibutramine increase adrenergic, dopaminergic, and serotonergic activity. Because of their propensity to produce euphoria, many of these drugs are widely abused and are controlled substances. Given the abuse liability and dependence potential of many of these compounds, the therapeutic use of these drugs needs to be monitored closely. Other compounds in this category (eg, cocaine, methamphetamine) have limited therapeutic use but are some of the most widely abused drugs in the world.

Many drugs in this class are used in the treatment of ADHD in children and adults. This is a disorder characterized by a variety of symptoms, including an unacceptable degree of hyperactivity, inability to concentrate, short attention span, difficulty in learning, emotional lability, and compulsiveness. Paradoxically, CNS stimulants can be beneficial in the treatment of this disorder although the mechanisms by which they provide benefit is unknown. Although their use remains controversial, there is a patient group with severe, persistent hyperactivity, and a short attention span that benefit from treatment with these agents. Drug treatment is not indicated for all children who have this disorder; stimulants are not indicated for the child who exhibits symptoms secondary to environmental factors or primary psychiatric disorders. Consequently, these should be ruled out and remedial psychological, educational, and social resources should be used before drug therapy is instituted. In the adult population, cardiovascular effects of these stimulants often preclude their use. The psychostimulants most frequently used for this purpose are amphetamine and methylphenidate; pemoline is also used but is not the first choice of drug for treatment.

Narcolepsy is another condition that requires long-term treatment. This disorder, characterized by sleep attacks, cataplexy (loss of muscle tone), hypnagogic hallucinations, sleep paralysis, and nocturnal sleep disruption, may result from an impairment in catecholamine neurotransmission. The psychostimulants are effective in preventing the daytime symptoms (sleep attacks and cataplexy), although they can also interfere with nighttime sleep. In the US, the drugs approved for use for narcolepsy are amphetamine, methylphenidate, pemoline, and modafinil.

Obesity is the only other condition for which the psychostimulants are approved for use. Amphetamine and its analogs have significant anorexic effects. The mechanisms by which these drugs reduce appetite are not fully established, but it is thought that stimulation of satiety centers in the hypothalamus and limbic areas is involved. However, tolerance readily develops to this action within a few weeks. Because of the development of tolerance, the production of undesirable side effects, and the high abuse potential of the amphetamines, many in the medical field believe that the use of these drugs for weight reduction purposes is inappropriate. Others would argue that their use is appropriate when all other approaches have failed and if drug use is carefully monitored. The drugs primarily used as appetite suppressants are benzphetamine, diethylpropion, mazindol, methamphetamine, sibutramine, phendimetrazine, and phentermine. Although these drugs may differ in potency and some of their adverse effects, their qualitative pharmacological effects are similar.

The psychostimulants can improve psychomotor performance and enhance wakefulness, although it is questionable whether concentration in complex learning situations or judgment is improved. Their effects are thought to be mediated through cortical stimulation and possibly through stimulation of the reticular activating system. For the amphetamines, the (S), (+), or dextro- isomers are somewhat more potent than the (R), (−), or levo- isomers (eg, amphetamine isomer effects differ by 3- to 4-fold) in elicitation of CNS responses the dextro enantiomer of methylphenidate is also the more potent isomer. The alerting effect of the psychostimulants, their anorectic effect, and their locomotor-stimulating action are likely mediated by enhancement of the actions of norepinephrine and dopamine in various brain regions. Euphoric effects are likely related to actions on dopamine within the limbic system. That the CNS-stimulating effects of these compounds are mediated through the catecholamines is suggested by animal studies findings that the inhibition of catecholamine synthesis prevents the behavioral activation produced by the drugs.

Adverse effects of the psychostimulant drugs are generally extensions of their therapeutic actions but may differ somewhat with the individual agents owing to their differences in potency and the specificity of their pharmacological action. In general, adverse effects include nervousness, insomnia, anorexia, nausea, palpitations, headache, dyskinesias, blood pressure and pulse changes, tachycardia, angina, cardiac arrhythmias, abdominal pain, weight loss, and hypersensitivity reactions. Acute CNS toxicity with these agents can produce restlessness, dizziness, tremor, hyperactive reflexes, talkativeness, irritability, weakness, insomnia, and fever. Larger doses can produce confusion, increased libido, anxiety, panic states, hallucinations, psychotic behavior, and seizures. Some of these effects may also be caused by the ability of these drugs to enhance the actions of 5-hydroxytryptamine (5-HT) from serotonergic neurons. In addition, there may be pronounced cardiovascular and GI effects. Symptoms of overdose may include vomiting, agitation, tremors, hyperreflexia, muscle twitching, convulsions (may be followed by coma), euphoria, confusion, hallucinations, delirium, sweating, hyperpyrexia, tachycardia, palpitations, cardiac arrhythmias, hypertension, mydriasis,

and dryness of the mucous membranes. Tolerance, psychological dependence, abnormal behavior, and physical dependence can occur with the psychostimulants. Characteristics of high-dose use that may emerge include severe dermatoses, significant insomnia, irritability, hyperactivity, personality changes, disorganized thought, poor concentration, compulsivity, hallucinations, and possibly, a severe psychotic state resembling paranoid schizophrenia.

Severe *drug interactions* may occur between the psychostimulants and other drugs, especially those that also have actions on monoaminergic neurons. For example the psychostimulants and selective serotonin-reuptake inhibitors (eg, fluoxetine, paroxetine, sertraline, or fluvoxamine) may result in a group of symptoms (termed *serotonin syndrome*) which include excitation, hypomania, restlessness, loss of consciousness, confusion, disorientation, anxiety, agitation, motor weakness, myoclonus, tremor, hemiballismus, hyperreflexia, ataxia, dysarthria, hyperthermia, shivering, diaphoresis, emesis, and tachycardia. Similarly, the use of psychostimulants in patients being treated with monoamine oxidase inhibitors (MAOIs) is contraindicated. Because of their cardiovascular effects, stimulants are contraindicated in patients who have a history of coronary heart disease, chronic heart failure, arrhythmias, stroke, or glaucoma. In addition, the psychostimulants need to be used cautiously in patients being treated with other drugs that affect cardiovascular function, including nonprescription drugs containing phenylpropanolamine, ephedrine, or pseudoephedrine. The use of psychostimulants is not recommended for patients taking antidepressants, lithium, sumatriptan, tryptophan, or dihydroergotamine. In general, psychostimulants are contraindicated in patients who have agitation, cardiovascular disorders, hypertension, hyperthyroidism, glaucoma, hypersensitivities to the drugs, motor tics, a diagnosis of or family history of Tourette's syndrome, a history of epilepsy or abnormal EEGs, or a history of drug abuse because their use could exacerbate the symptoms associated with these disorders or disease states. The safe use of the psychostimulants in children younger than 6 yrs. of age has not been established. See Chapter 70 for additional discussion of the amphetamines, contraindications for use, and drug interactions.

Cocaine is also a potent sympathomimetic CNS stimulant with actions similar to those of the amphetamines but with a much shorter duration of action. In contrast to the amphetamines, which cause monoamine release, cocaine's actions are thought to be mediated primarily by its blockade of the reuptake of released monoamines. Cocaine has local anesthetic actions; however, its use for this purpose is limited, having been replaced by synthetic local anesthetics that have little CNS stimulation. The importance of cocaine lies in its abuse potential; it is currently one of the most widely abused drugs in the United States.

AMPHETAMINE SULFATE—see RPS-19, page 986.
BENZPHETAMINE HYDROCHLORIDE—see RPS-19, page 987.
COCAINE—page 1484.
DEXTROAMPHETAMINE SULFATE—see RPS-19, page 987.
DIETHYLPROPION—see RPS-19, page 987.
MAZINDOL—see RPS-19, page 992.
METHAMPHETAMINE—see RPS-19, page 994.

METHYLPHENIDATE HYDROCHLORIDE

2-Piperidineacetic acid, (R*,R*)-(±)-α-phenyl-, methyl ester, hydrochloride, Ritalin; Concerta

[298-59-9] $C_{14}H_{19}NO_2 \cdot HCl$ (269.77).

Preparation—2-Chloropyridine is condensed with phenylacetonitrile and the resulting α-phenyl-2-pyridineacetonitrile is hydrated to its corresponding amide. The pyridine ring then is hydrogenated catalytically and the amide converted to its corresponding carboxylic acid. Esterification with methanol, with the aid of HCl, yields the final product.

Description—White, odorless, fine, crystalline powder; melts about 75°; solutions are acid to litmus, pKa 8.9.

Solubility—Freely soluble in water or methanol; soluble in alcohol; slightly soluble in chloroform or acetone.

Comments—A mild *CNS stimulant* with a potency intermediate to caffeine and amphetamine. It is effective as adjunctive therapy to other remedial measures (psychological, educational, and social) in the management of ADHD. It is also effective in the treatment of narcolepsy and possibly effective in mild depression and in apathetic or withdrawn senile behavior. Methylphenidate also shares the abuse potential of the amphetamines. The drug should not be used to alleviate normal fatigue.

Pharmacokinetics—Methylphenidate is readily absorbed from the GI tract. Peak blood levels are reached in 1 to 3 hr, and the plasma half-life ranges from 1 to 3 hr. The pharmacological effects persist from 4 to 6 hr after oral administration of conventional tablets and approximately 8 hr for extended-release preparations. Approximately 80% of an oral dose is metabolized to ritalinic acid and excreted in the urine.

Pharmacology—Its pharmacological properties are essentially the same as those of the amphetamines. Its actions appear to be mediated by blockade of norepinephrine and dopamine into the presynaptic neuron and increase the release of these monoamines into the extraneuronal.

See the general statement for effects, adverse effects, and contraindications for use of methylphenidate. Additional adverse reactions reported with methylphenidate use include leukopenia and anemia, and a few cases of scalp hair loss have been reported with methylphenidate.

Drug Interactions—In addition to above discussion of drug interactions, human studies indicate methylphenidate may inhibit metabolism of coumarin anticoagulants, anticonvulsants, and tricyclic antidepressants. Dosage of these agents may require downward adjustment when given concomitantly with this drug.

DEXMETHYLPHENIDATE HYDROCHLORIDE

2-Piperidineacetic acid, (R*,R*)-(+)-α-phenyl-, methyl ester, hydrochloride, Focalin

[40431-64-9] $C_{14}H_{19}NO_2.HCl$ (269.77).

Preparation—See US Pat 6,162,919 (1998).

Description—The *d-threo* isomer of methylphenidate, which is a racemic mixture of the d-threo and l-threo isomers. White to off white powder; solutions are acid to litmus.

Solubility—Freely soluble in water or methanol; soluble in alcohol; slightly soluble in chloroform or acetone.

Comments—Dexmethylphenidate was approved by the FDA in 2001 for treatment of ADHD in children greater than 6 years of age. It is the d-threo enantiomer (the more pharmacologically active enantiomer) of racemic methylphenidate hydrochloride. It is not approved for use in narcolepsy.

Pharmacokinetics—Dexmethylphenidate is readily absorbed following oral administration, reaching a maximum concentration 1 to 1.5 hours post dose. The mean plasma elimination half-life is approximately 2.2 hours.

Pharmacology—See methylphenidate.

Drug Interactions—See methylphenidate

PEMOLINE

4(5H)-Oxazolone, 2-amino-5-phenyl-, Cylert

[2152-34-3] $C_9H_8N_2O_2$ (176.17).

Preparation—Ethyl mandelate, $C_6H_5CH(OH)COOC_2H_5$, is reacted with guanidine, $HN=C(NH_2)_2$, in boiling alcoholic solution. US Pat 2,832,753.

Description—White, crystalline powder; odorless and tasteless; melts about 256° with decomposition.

Solubility—Practically insoluble in water, chloroform, dilute HCl, or ether; slightly soluble in alcohol or propylene glycol.

Comments—A CNS stimulant that is structurally different from the amphetamines and methylphenidate. It has less abuse potential than the amphetamines and is classified as a *Schedule IV* drug (amphetamines are *Schedule II* drugs). Although laboratory studies indicate that pemoline may act through dopaminergic mechanisms, the mechanism and site of action in man are not known. It is used in the treatment of narcolepsy and as adjunctive therapy in children who have attention deficit disorder; however, its efficacy is less than that of amphetamine or methylphenidate. It also has less sympathomimetic effects than the amphetamines. Pemoline has been used in the treatment of fatigue, mental depression, chronic schizophrenia, and as a mild stimulant in geriatric patients; however, clinical benefits from such use are minimal. It should not be used for the prevention or the treatment of normal fatigue.

Pharmacokinetics—Peak serum levels of the drug are reached 2 to 4 hr after ingestion of a single oral dose; the serum half-life is approximately 12 hr, and a steady-state level is reached in 2 to 3 days of multiple dosage. Approximately 50% of the drug is bound to serum proteins. Approximately 75% of an oral dose is excreted in the urine within 24 hr, approximately 43% is excreted unchanged, and 22% is excreted as pemoline conjugates.

Adverse Effects and Toxicity—In addition to adverse effects common to the psychostimulants, pemoline use can produce dyskinetic movements of the tongue, lips, face, and extremities as well as abnormal oculogyric function (nystagmus and oculogyric crises). Pemoline has been associated with life-threatening hepatic failure and, for this reason, it is not recommended as the first choice of drug in treatment.

SIBUTRAMINE HYDROCHLORIDE

(±)-Cyclobutanemethanamine, 1-(4-chlorophenyl)-N,N-dimethyl-α-(2-methylpropyl)-, hydrochloride, monohydrate; Meridia; Reductil

[125494-59-9] $C_{17}H_{26}ClN.HCl.2H_2O$ (334.33).

Preparation—See US Pat 4,929,629 (1987).

Description—White crystals melting about 193° to 196°.

Solubility—Moderately soluble in water.

Comments—An appetite-suppressant drug that was approved by the FDA in 1997. It can be considered a prodrug because its pharmacological activity actually resides in two of its desmethylated metabolites (formed from CYP-3A4 metabolism of the parent drug). The pharmacological effects of the active sibutramine metabolites block the uptake of all three monoamines but with a slightly greater potency on norepinephrine and dopamine uptake than on serotonin uptake.

Pharmacokinetics—The drug is rapidly absorbed after oral administration. Sibutramine undergoes extensive first-pass metabolism (half-life is approximately 1 hr). Concentrations of the active metabolites peak at 3 to 4 hr and have half-lives of 14 to 16 hr. These metabolites are further metabolized by hydroxylation and conjugation to inactive substances and excreted in the urine.

Adverse Effects and Contraindication—Similar to other psychostimulants.

MODAFINIL

Acetamide, 2-[(diphenylmethyl)sulfinyl]-, Provigil

[68693-11-8] $C_{15}H_{15}NO_2S$ (273.35).

Preparation—See US Pat 4,177,290 (1978).

Description—White crystals melting about 164° to 166°.

Comments—Modafinil is a psychostimulant with a mechanism of action distinct from other agents in this class. It is approved for use in the US for the treatment of the symptoms of daytime sleepiness in narcolepsy and other sleep disorders. Modafinil is a drug that possesses alerting properties (eugeroic), although its precise mechanism of action is not known. Psychometric, psychobiological tests, and electroencephalogram (EEG) profiles show changes that are viewed as improvements in vigilance. There is some suggestion that modafinil may be somewhat less effective than amphetamine or methylphenidate. However, unlike the amphetamines, modafinil does not reduce Stage 2 rapid eye movement (REM) sleep or alter heart rate or blood pressure.

Pharmacology—The exact mechanism of antinarcoleptic action is unknown. Limited studies have indicated that it may increase glutaminergic transmission in the thalamus and hypothalamus or have an agonist effect at central alpha 1-B adrenergic receptors.

Pharmacokinetics—Peak plasma concentrations are reached 2 to 3 hr after oral administration of the drug. Plasma half-life is 8 to 10 hr.

Adverse Effects—Dose-related adverse effects include dry mouth, dry eyes, nausea, inner tension, sleep disturbances, sweating, headache, dizziness, hot flashes, and gastralgia. Other effects include tachycardia, hypersalivation, anorexia, anxiety, choking, dysphoria, bad temper, hypertension, excitation, fatigue, sexual hyperactivity, weight gain, euphoria, and motor excitation.

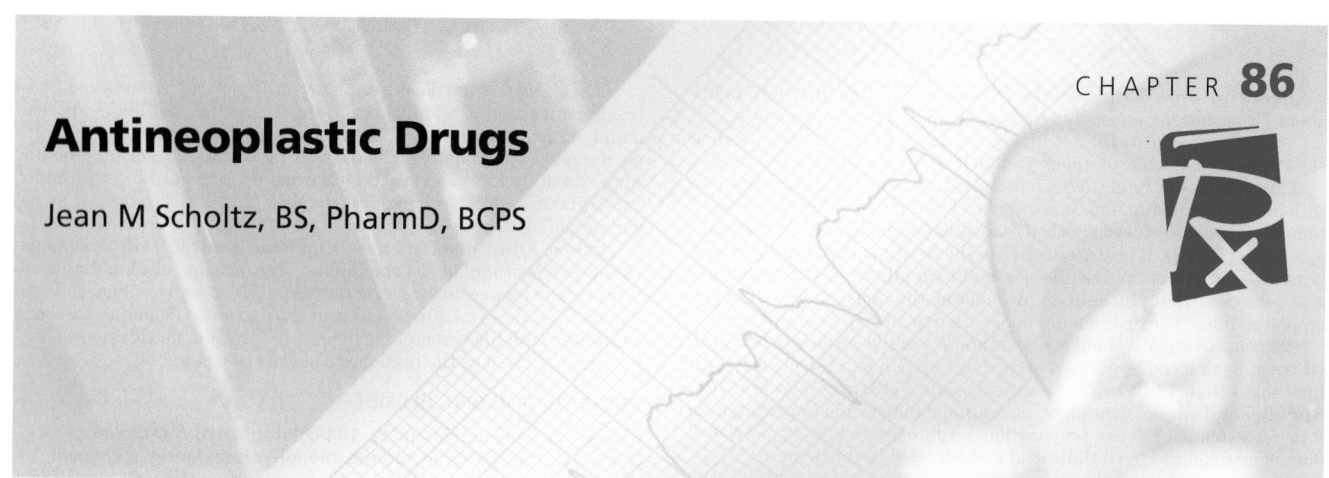

CHAPTER 86

Antineoplastic Drugs

Jean M Scholtz, BS, PharmD, BCPS

Before the 1940s the principal nonsurgical treatment of neoplasms was radiograph and radium therapy, although certain arsenicals and urethane were also in use. During the 1940s, there were three main developments: radioisotopes, nitrogen mustards, and antifolic acid agents. The use of sex hormones for the treatment of certain types of neoplasms and of adrenal corticoids and adrenocorticotropic hormone (ACTH) for the treatment of leukemia also developed considerably during these years.

Much excitement was generated by these early developments in antineoplastic therapy, but it was later tempered by the realization not only that the drugs were not curative but also that, for the most part, life-expectancy was negligibly increased, the drugs being mainly palliative. Subsequently, there has been a great proliferation in both the number and the classes of anticancer drugs and in the theory of cell kinetics and cancer at the molecular level. Recent progress in the understanding of oncogenes and tumor-suppressor, and their role in pathogenesis of cancer have led to the development of new classes of drugs. Long-term cures and disease-free remissions continue to be achieved with various combinations of these drugs, with more research being performed in the chemoprevention arena.

Tumor Growth and Kinetics

The principal difference between mature normal tissues and tumors is not in the rate of cell replication but in that the rate of proliferation for most normal tissues equals the rate of cell death, whereas in neoplasms, proliferation exceeds the death rate. Proliferation in normal tissue responds to subtle signals that indicate when proliferation is needed for repair, regeneration or growth, and development. Neoplasms seem to lack such an autoregulation of proliferation, and the cell-replication rate appears to depend mostly on an intrinsic rate modulated by the adequacy of the vascular supply.

EXPONENTIAL GROWTH AND DOUBLING TIMES— In the early stages, the growth of a tumor is approximately constant. The doubling time is the mean (*average*) interval between successive mitoses. It is characteristic of the particular type of tumor cell. Doubling time varies significantly among various kinds of tumors. In Burkitt's tumor, it is approximately 24 hours; in acute leukemia, 2 weeks; in breast cancer, 3 months; and in multiple myeloma, 6 to 12 months. Contrary to common belief, these doubling times are within the range of those for normal tissues. For example, white-cell precursors divide approximately every 12 hours and mucosal cells of the rectum every 24 hours.

A tumor becomes detectable when the number of cells reaches approximately 10^9 to 10^{10} cells. This requires 30 to 33 doubling times. The neoplasm becomes lethal when the population reaches approximately 5×10^{11} to 5×10^{12} cells, after 39 to 42 doubling times.

PHASES OF THE CELL CYCLE—Some drugs can exert a lethal action only when a cell is in a particular stage of activity and growth. Therefore, a knowledge of cell kinetics will be useful. After mitosis and cell division, the new daughter cells are in a resting state, terms phase G_0 (G for gap). The length of time spent in G_0 depends on both the type of cell and the autoregulatory factors. In some tissues, such as bone marrow, gastrointestinal (GI) mucosa, and skin, G_0 is prolonged only moderately during maturation and aging, whereas with others, such as nerve and skeletal muscle cells, G_0 becomes essentially infinitely long well in advance of maturity. In solid tumors, G_0 is longer when the cell mass is large than when small, because the vascular supply cannot keep pace with the rate of growth. Ultimately, the cell enters a postresting phase, called G_1. In this phase, metabolism appears to be normal, but the cell is committed to divide. After a latency period, the cell enters the S-phase, in which DNA synthesis is activated, in preparation for mitosis. The cell then enters another phase, G_2, the premitotic phase, in which DNA synthesis is essentially at rest but protein synthesis and other metabolic activities are increased and the cell volume grows. Finally, the cell undergoes mitosis (phase M) and cellular fission.

The cell cycle can be thought of as existing in two superstages: G_0 as one, and all of $G_1 + S + G_2 + M$ as the other, the latter comprising all phases committed to cellular division. The entity $(G_1 + S + G_2 + M)/(G_0 + G_1 + S + G_2 + M)$ is known as the growth fraction. In tumors, it usually lies between 0.2 and 0.7. Although the growth fraction tends to be greater in the more rapidly proliferating tissues and tumors, this is not always the case. The proliferation of normal cells is tightly controlled by proto-oncogenes and tumor-suppressor genes. These provide stimulatory and inhibitory signals, respectively, which regulate the cell cycle. The evolution of cells through the cell cycle is a tightly-regulated process. Various proteins, called cyclins, along with enzymes called cyclin-dependent kinases (CDKs), regulate movement of cells through the cell cycle. Various gene mutations, such as loss or mutation of tumor suppressor gene p53, result in excessive cell proliferation. Apoptosis and senescence (aging) are other mechanisms that control excessive cell division. Research is ongoing to discover genes, proteins, and receptors involved in the growth of cancer cells, and strategies or agents to alter their effects on the cell cycle and cell growth.

Chemotherapeutic Intervention

PHASE SPECIFICITY—Antineoplastic drugs are of two general categories: (1) those that can act on the cell throughout its cycle (such drugs are said to be phase nonspecific) and (2) those that act preferentially during one or more of the nonresting phases (these drugs tend to be ineffective if delivered to the cell during the wrong phase). Even phase-nonspecific drugs have greater activity during the growth phases. The particular phase during which a drug acts depends on the lethal mechanism. Those that combine irreversibly with DNA can do so at any time and hence are phase nonspecific. However, more DNA is exposed during the growth phases than during G_0, so that even these drugs have some phase selectivity. Drugs that interfere with DNA synthesis are specific to the S phase; those that block protein synthesis are specific mainly to phases S and G2; and those that inhibit microtubule assembly are specific mainly to M.

TUMOR SELECTIVITY AND RESPONSE—Especially for phase-specific drugs, the probability of a lethal action on a tumor cell (or normal cell) is directly proportional to the percent of time spent in the vulnerable phase. It follows that the percent of time spent in the vulnerable phase is an important determinant of the susceptibility of tumors of different cell types. Even without reference to any particular growth phase, the generality that those tumors with a large growth fraction are more susceptible to chemotherapy than those with a low fraction is an important precept. Examples of tumors with high growth fractions that respond well to chemotherapy are acute leukemia in children, Burkitt's lymphoma, choriocarcinoma, chronic myelogenous leukemia (these last three now are considered curable), lymphocytic leukemia, Hodgkin's disease, Wilms' tumor, and breast cancer. Examples of neoplasms that respond poorly are malignant melanoma, carcinoma of the GI tract, bronchogenic carcinoma, and tumors of the uterus and cervix.

Because growth fractions are higher in small, recent tumors, it follows that efficacy is enhanced by early treatment. Different cell types spend different proportions of time in one as opposed to another phase (ie, more in G_2 than S, etc.). Therefore, the most effective drug would be expected to be of a type that is specific to the phase of longest duration. In part, this may account for the differences in efficacy among drugs of different mechanisms and phase specificity.

There has been interest in and investigation of the possibility of *synchronizing* tumor cells so that all cells are in the same phase of the cycle. If the cells were synchronized and the host cells were not, then the tumor could be made more vulnerable to appropriate drugs given at the proper time, and the therapeutic index could be increased. Synchronization is attempted by a holding *pulse* of a mitostatic or some other drug that holds the cells in a given phase until the out-of-phase cells also come into that phase. Discontinuation of the synchronizing drug simultaneously releases the cells to resume their cycle, all starting from the same phase. In combination chemotherapy, drugs often are administered in sequence, rather than simultaneously; the first-given drug sometimes serves as a synchronizing drug.

DETERMINANTS OF SENSITIVITY AND SELECTIVITY—In addition to the growth fraction or vulnerable phase time of a tumor, other factors also determine the selectivity of drugs for certain cell types. The demand for nutrients varies among tumor types but also differs between tumor cells and normal cells. For example, many tumors require more asparagine than normal cells, so that if the plasma asparagine is destroyed enzymatically (see *Asparaginase,* page 1562, the tumor cells are selectively *starved* to death.

Some drugs are metabolized in the peripheral cells as well as in the liver, and the different cell types differ in their ability to metabolize these drugs. For example, with bleomycin, there is evidence to suggest that the drug is metabolized less in susceptible tumor cells than in other cells, thus permitting higher local concentrations. Several drugs are converted to active metabolites by the target cells (*lethal synthesis*), and differences in the rates of conversion may contribute to selectivity.

Differences in penetrance account for some differences among drugs; lipid-soluble antineoplastic drugs are more effective than water-soluble ones for neoplasms in the central nervous system (CNS). With some drugs, active transport into tumor cells is greater than into normal cells; with other drugs, there are differences in outward transport. An unassessed factor in selectivity is that of effects on the immune system. There

are not only tumor-cell-attacking *killer* T cells but also suppressor T cells and blocking factors from B cells that protect certain neoplastic cells from immune attack. According to which immune cells are the most suppressed, some antineoplastic drugs might antagonize the immune response to neoplastic cells, and other drugs augment it.

REQUIREMENTS FOR "KILL"—A remission usually can be achieved with a kill of 90% to 99% of the neoplastic cells. A kill of 99% would leave at least 10^7 to 10^8 surviving cells to carry on tumor growth, and the remission would last only 3 to 4 doubling times. With those neoplasms against which the immune system is ineffective, a 100% kill is necessary to effect a true cure, because it has been shown experimentally that a single implanted neoplastic cell can develop into a tumor. However, a true cure may not always be necessary. For example, with a tumor, the doubling time of which is 12 months, a kill of 99.99% (which would leave perhaps 10^6 surviving cells) would require approximately 13 years for the tumor cell population to recover to the number extant at the time of treatment.

A second course of an appropriate chemotherapy might add another 13 years, which, with middle-aged or elderly patients, might be beyond the normal life expectancy. However, with a rapidly doubling tumor such as Burkitt's tumor, the survival time in the untreated patient is measured in days, not years; even if all but a single cell were killed by an antineoplastic drug, survival would be prolonged less than 2 months; therefore, either a complete kill or sustained or frequently repeated courses are imperative. Fortunately, 50% to 60% of Burkitt's tumor cells are in the S phase and are thus highly susceptible to drugs that are S-phase specific.

COMBINATION CHEMOTHERAPY—One way of increasing the percent of kill is to combine two or more antineoplastic drugs. Radiation also is a modality that often can be combined effectively with drugs. There are four criteria to optimize such combinations:

1. Each component drug must have some efficacy by itself.
2. Each component drug should have a different mechanism of cytotoxic activity and, preferably, phase specificity.
3. Each component drug should have a different spectrum of toxicity than the other components, in order to avoid overwhelming toxicity of a given type.
4. The mechanism of resistance to each component should be different to that of the other components.

LOG CELL-KILL PRINCIPLE—Antineoplastic drugs may be characterized by their log cell-kill index, that is, by the negative log of the fraction of the tumor cell population that survives a single course of treatment. Thus a drug that kills 99.99% of the tumor cell population, ie, leaves 0.0001 (or $1/10^4$) of the population, is known as a 4-log drug; a second drug that kills 99.9% is known as a 3-log drug. The log cell-kill index is a tenuous number, but it is useful in predicting the effects of combinations that meet criteria 1 and 2. The predicted effect of a combination is obtained by addition of the indices of the component drugs. Theoretically, a 4-log drug plus a 3-log drug should provide a 7-log combination, that is, kills 99.99999% or leaves $1/10^7$ of the population. A third drug that kills 99% (2-log drug) would further reduce the remaining population to $1/10^9$, which comes close to complete eradication of a tumor caught early.

DRUG RESISTANCE—Some tumor populations appear to be heterogeneous by the time the tumor is discovered, some of the cells being resistant to certain drugs at the outset of treatment. This is well established for adrenal, colon, jejunal, kidney, and liver carcinomas. As many as four different cancer cell types have been identified in a single tumor. Differences among some of these cell types do not represent different genes necessarily but rather, sometimes, differences in the number of copies of a single gene. Resistance in cancer cells can occur de novo or develop during treatment as a result of cell mutation. The resistant daughter cells then can proliferate in the environment of the drug. Whatever the cause, resistance often terminates the usefulness of an antineoplastic drug.

Various mechanisms of resistance have been identified, and include the following:

1. Improved proficiency in the repair of potentially lethal DNA damage
2. Loss of a transport system essential for the permeation of the drug into the tumor cell, as happens with methotrexate.
3. Increases or decreases in the amounts or binding affinity of target enzymes necessary for the intratumor *lethal synthesis* of an essential active metabolite (DHFR, topoisomerase II)
4. An increase in outward active transport or efflux of the drug, so that effective intracellular concentrations cannot be achieved or maintained (multidrug or pleiotropic drug-resistance)
5. Overexpression of metallothionine (resistance to platinum-containing and certain alkylating antineoplastics)
6. Antibody formation (eg, interferons)
7. Membrane changes that confer resistance to natural killer (NK) cells
8. Increased glutathione synthesis in cancer cells treated with anthracyclinedione cells

Lipophilic anticancer drugs such as the vinca alkaloids, certain alkylaminoanthraquinones actinomycin-D, colchicine, verapamil, and probably other drugs are transported outwardly by an adenosine-triphosphate-(ATP-)–dependent pump, known as *P*-glycoprotein. This is produced excessively by some tumor cells, and accounts for the primary mechanism of multiple drug resistance. Various drugs, such as verapamil, cyclosporine, and quinidine, compete for this pump, thereby inhibiting P-glycoprotein. However, the concentrations of these agents required to inhibit P-glycoprotein results in excessive toxicity, and thus their use continues to be examined. Studies with new more potent agents are being performed.

TOXICITY—Neoplastic cells have compositions and activities very much like those of the host cells. This has made it impossible thus far to design antineoplastic drugs that also do not attack normal cells. Every antineoplastic drug has a therapeutic index less than 1.0. This may be changing with some of the new *targeted therapies,* although many of these new therapeutic agents lack significant cytotoxicity when used independently. The principles that apply to antitumor efficacy also apply to the toxicity. Thus the tissues most affected are those with high growth fractions, and the integrity of the highly proliferative tissues can be disturbed considerably. Consequently, the bone marrow, lymphoblasts, mucous membranes, skin, and gonads are affected to a greater extent than other cells. Because the myelogenous leukocyte turnover is faster and the growth fraction is greater than those of erythrocytes, *bone-marrow depression* usually causes a more severe neutropenia and thrombocytopenia than anemia. Bone-marrow depression is a major adverse effect of antineoplastic drugs.

Suppression of proliferation of mucosal cells causes mucositis, characterized by aphthous and gastrointestinal ulceration or mucositis. Arrest of the proliferation of the cutaneous epithelial cells may cause alopecia, scaliness of the skin, sometimes even desquamation. Some drugs that lack significant dermatological actions may nevertheless recall cutaneous toxicities induced by previous drugs or radiation.

Aspermia may result from actions on the seminiferous tubules and amenorrhea from actions on the ovaries (where the growth fraction but not the turnover rate is high). The immune cells have a rapid turnover and are highly susceptible to certain cytotoxic agents. *Immunosuppression* makes the patient more vulnerable to *infection*; it is noteworthy that 50% of cancer patients die of intercurrent infections rather than from the terminal phases of the neoplastic disease.

Immunosuppression probably enhances the growth of certain neoplasms. Because they interfere with genetic mechanisms, certain antineoplastic drugs are mutagenic and carcinogenic, and the patient is subjected to the risk of future neoplasia. The incidences of acute leukemia and bone sarcoma are considerably higher in persons who have been treated with antineoplastic drugs than in the general population. Theoretical considerations predict that all neoplastic drugs are teratogenic, and teratogenic activity has been shown with some.

There are also other toxicities related to antineoplastic actions. For example, massive cell destruction results in the release of large quantities of purine from the nucleic acids of the dead cells; these purine bases are metabolized to uric acid. Hyperuricemia, renal damage consequent to hyperuricuria and also some neurological damage may result. Hence, it is common to give allopurinol along with antineoplastic drugs. Massive destruction of certain leukemic cells may also cause an acute hypotensive crisis that sometimes is called *anaphylaxis* despite its not being a true allergic response. For reasons not understood, treatment of breast cancer is thrombogenic in approximately 7% of cases, irrespective of the drug used.

Some of the local adverse effects also are related to the antineoplastic mechanisms. Extravasation, or leakage of the drug out of the vein, may present high concentrations to the cells in the local area, leading to vesication, ulceration, sloughing, or tissue necrosis. Other drugs may cause phlebitis, or pain and irritation, along the vein during or following administration. Gastrointestinal toxicity may cause nausea, vomiting, diarrhea, cramping, or constipation.

Other toxicities may not be seen immediately, but weeks or months after chemotherapy is initiated. These include pulmonary fibrosis, cardiac toxicity, liver and renal toxicity. The specific toxicities are discussed under the specific agents listed below. A few of these may be minimized or prevented by using various antidotes including amofostine, dexrazoxane, and mesna.

PRECAUTIONS AND CONTRAINDICATIONS—With all drugs that cause bone-marrow depression, it is essential to monitor the blood cell count, which may serve both as a guide to adequate dosage and as a precaution against overdoses. The minimum advisable leukocyte and platelet count varies somewhat among the drugs but is usually 3000 to 4000 leukocytes and 20,000 to 100,000 platelets. When the count falls below these limits, the drug dosage should be reduced or the drug discontinued until there is recovery. It usually is not advisable to begin treatment with a bone-marrow depressant drug within 4 weeks of the administration of another bone-marrow depressant drug or radiation therapy. The use of colony stimulating factors, which stimulate the bone marrow to produce granulocytes, have greatly improved the morbidity and delays in treatment due to chemotherapy-induced bone marrow suppression. In most malignancies, chemotherapy cannot be administered if the blood cell count is < 2500 leucocytes.

Antineoplastic drugs are teratogenic, and should not be used during pregnancy unless the risk-benefit ratio has been discussed. Because most antineoplastic drugs can be found in breast milk, infants must not be nursed during antineoplastic therapy. Studies have shown that improper handling during mixing or administration of anticancer drugs may result in urine mutagenicity and chromosomal damage, and although controversial, are thought to be due to exposure to cytotoxic agents. They are fetotoxic in pregnant nurses that handle such drugs. All antineoplastic agents must be handled with proper attention to aseptic techniques during preparation and administration, as well as proper disposable.

CLASSES AND MECHANISMS OF DRUGS—Antineoplastic drugs may be conveniently grouped into several categories. Some of the categories are based on chemical and mechanistic properties and others on the origins of natural products.

Alkylating Agents—The subgroups of the alkylating agents include: nitrogen mustards, nitrosoureas, methylhydrazines, ethylenimines, platinum analogues, and alkylsulfonates. The nitrogen mustards are all bis(β-chloroethyl)amines. The mustards are important drugs in treatment regimens; cyclophosphamide, the most useful alkylating agent, is a member of this class.

The ethylenimines contain three ethylenimine groups per molecule, and the alkylsulfonates are bismethylsulfonates. Thus these compounds are all polyfunctional alkylating agents, a fact that relates importantly to the mechanism of action. The alkylating groups react with nucleophilic centers in many different kinds of molecules; guanine is the most reactive target in DNA. However, their bifunctional or trifunctional character allows them to cross-link double-stranded DNA, thus preventing the strands from separating for replication. The platinum analogs are alkylating-like agents in which the chloride atoms are lost intracellularly resulting in a reactive electrophile. This covalently binds to DNA forming intra- and inter- strand crosslinks.

Nitrosoureas—These usually are classified as alkylating agents. Carmustine is bifunctional and may be able to cross-link double-stranded DNA. Lomustine contains a single β-chloroethyl group but can cross-link DNA by use of the nitroso group as a second electrophilic group. Streptozocin lacks a bifunctional alkylating moiety. Carbamoylation of the nucleoside bases in nucleic acids has been suggested as a possible mechanism of action. However, the nitroso group is also a free radical and an ion generator, which could confer radiomimetic properties.

Methylhydrazines—Procarbazine and dacarbazine sometimes are classified as alkylating agents, because an *alkylating* moiety is liberated within the target cell. However, like other hydrazines, they generate free hydroxyl radicals and ions and thus also are considered radiomimetic.

Antimetabolites—There are three subcategories of antimetabolites: purine analogs, pyrimidine analogs, and folinic acid analogs. The purine analogs are incorporated into DNA as the deoxyribotides and into RNA as the ribotides, where they interfere with coding and replication. They also act like the natural purine bases in inhibiting synthesis of purine bases by acting through the allosteric feedback systems (pseudofeedback). The pyrimidine analogs inhibit enzymes in the biosynthetic pathways for pyrimidine ribotides and deoxyribotides; thymidylate synthetase, orotic acid decarboxylase, aspartate carbamoyltransferase, dihydroorotase, and DNA polymerase are inhibited. Methotrexate and trimetrexate bind very tightly to dihydrofolate reductase and thereby prevent the conversion of dihydrofolate (folinate) to tetrahydrofolate.

Antibiotics and Natural Products—This is a miscellaneous group of drugs with respect to mechanism of action. Mitomycin appears to be an alkylating agent, the anthracyclines and epipodophyllotoxins act therapeutically by inhibiting topoisomerase II, and the vinca alkaloids and taxols interfere with microspindle function. Dactinomycin binds to DNA and inhibits DNA synthesis, and mithramycin inhibits DNA-dependent RNA polymerase. Bleomycin both acts as an antimetabolite of thymidine and causes fragmentation of DNA.

Steroid Hormones—The steroid hormones are transported to the cell nucleus, where they attach to chromatin and usually stimulate transcription and, hence, protein synthesis. However, the glucocorticoids suppress mitosis in lymphocytes, and fibroblasts and appear to inhibit transcription. This so-called lympholytic effect is employed in the chemotherapy of the lymphocytic leukemias and in immunosuppression.

The estrogens, progestins, and androgens also probably inhibit transcription and prevent mitosis in those cell types that are derived from normal cells that are suppressed by these hormones in the natural hormonal physiology. Thus, the normal prostate gland is suppressed by estrogens, apparently by a comparative antagonism of androgens, and estrogens are used to treat cancer of the prostate gland, etc. Similarly, androgens exert an antiestrogen effect on certain breast tumors; only tumors of a cell type that contain estrogen receptors are responsive. Antiestrogens also are used to suppress such tumors. Estrogens also suppress the growth of some breast tumors, but the mechanism of the effect is understood poorly. Luteinizing hormone releasing hormone (LHRH) analogs act centrally to inhibit androgen and estrogen synthesis. Progestins behave as antiestrogens in the endometrium and, hence, may be employed in the chemotherapy of endometrial carcinoma.

Monoclonal Antibodies—These agents directly target receptors that are overexpressed in tumor cells. Rituximab is directed against CD20 on B lymphocytes, thus binding to the antigen and activating complement dependent cytoxicity. Gemtuzumab is directed against CD33, which is expressed on leukemic blasts.

Miscellaneous—Porfimer is a photosensitizing agent used in the photodynamic therapy. Isotretinoin is a differentiating agent useful in the treatment of leukemias.

KINETICS AND REGIMENS—With drugs with phase-specific actions, the temporal window of vulnerability is the duration of the vulnerable phase of the cell cycle. With rapidly proliferating cells, this may be only a few hours for any given cell. If the cell cycles are synchronized, only a brief exposure to the drug may be needed to accomplish a high degree of cell kill; the optimal drug would be one with a half-life such that it does not persist in the body beyond the time necessary to act upon the tumor cells, so that there would be the least necessary exposure of normal cells to the drug. However, the synchronization of cell cycles is yet in its infancy, and most regimens attack a tumor cell population that randomly is in various phases of the cell cycle. In this case, it is optimal to keep the drug in the body for slightly longer than the duration of the entire cell cycle.

In the case of Burkitt's lymphoma, with a doubling time of 24 hours, exposure to drug should be approximately a day to effect the greatest tumor cell kill. Unfortunately, white-cell stem cells have a doubling time of only 12 hours and GI cells approximately 24 hours, so that it is not possible to expose Burkitt's lymphoma cells for the duration of an entire cell cycle without causing a life-threatening kill of certain kinds of normal cells. The clinical problem, then, is to devise a regimen that is more sparing of normal cells yet causes an adequate remission, though not complete elimination of the tumor. This is possible, despite the shorter cell cycles of certain normal cells, because the normal cells spend more time in G_0 than do Burkitt's lymphoma cells. Problems of this kind usually are resolved by repeating courses of submaximal tumor-killing doses.

It is much more difficult to devise an effective yet safe regimen for the treatment of tumors with long doubling times, because the tumor doubling time may be many times longer than the hematopoietic stem, immune, and mucosal cells. Long, multicourse combination treatments are the rule. Most are quite empirical with respect to kinetic considerations. In these, because the duration of a course is inevitably longer than the elimination lifetime of the drugs in use, a regimen needs maintenance dosing or constant infusion. One example of this is the prolonged, low-dose infusions of 5-fluorouracil over several months.

Site-directed administration of antineoplastic drugs by intra-arterial infusion is advantageous to intravenous administration only if the concentration of drug in the blood in systemic circulation is substantially lower than that infused into the artery. This is thought to occur when a high rate of systemic clearance of the drug exists, so that toxic amounts of the drug do not accumulate. However, experience with intra-arterial fluorouracil, a drug with a half-life of less than 20 minutes, has been disappointing. It has been explained that the local extraction ratio of fluorouracil during prolonged intra-arterial infusion is sufficiently low that there is not a sufficiently selective uptake into the target to gain much advantage by local infusion.

In contrast, the nitrosourea, carmustine has a high extraction ratio by the intracarotid arterial route and, consequently, is advantageous by this route (for CNS tumors), even though there is considerable local toxicity. Similarly, diaziquone has a high local extraction ratio and is advantageous by the intra-arterial route. The local clearance of an intra-arterially infused drug of low extraction ratio may be increased by decreasing the rate of blood flow with a vasoconstrictor. Although most regimens are largely empirical, improvisation, or failure to follow the regimen as recommended, is a common cause of early relapse, especially in pediatrics.

Circadian rhythms may not only affect the metabolism of many drugs but also the susceptibility of the patient to the toxic effects of antineoplastic drugs. Many studies have been performed, and the effects shown. However, the data does not warrant clinical changes in anticancer regimens at this time based on circadian kinetics.

As among drugs in general, various antineoplastic drugs are involved in pharmacokinetic drug interactions. For example, cisplatin and daunorubicin induce the hepatic enzymes for the metabolism of carbamazepine, phenytoin, and valproate. Verapamil competes for the active transport of lipophilic anticancer drugs out of cells. Some of these interactions are due to biochemical modulation. Methotrexate and leucovorin cause this effect. Sequential methotrexate, followed by 5-fluorouracil, results in increased activation of 5-fluorouracil to the active moiety, FUTP, leading to increased cell kill due to increased concentrations in RNA. The combination of leucovorin with 5-fluorouracil causes increased cell death by providing an exogenous source of reduced folate, thus increasing the binding of FdUMP to thymidylate synthetase.

IMMUNOACTIVE DRUGS

The immune system is quite complex. Several types of cells are involved. These are cells, the ancestral line of which has derived from bone marrow stem cells. Some of the descendants of the stem cells migrate to sites elsewhere in the body, where they become small lymphocytes. There are two general types of lymphocytes involved in the immune responses: the B cells and the T cells. The B lymphocytes get the designation B from the fact that in birds they derive from stem-cell clones in the bursa of Fabricus; in man, the location of analogous clones may be in the intestinal mucosal Peyer's patches. The T cells get their designation from the fact that they are derived from stem cells cloned in the thymus gland. Undifferentiated lymphocytes take up residence in lymph tissue in the spleen, tonsils, intestines, and other sites.

B and T cells respond to antigen by cellular transformation, proliferation, and differentiation. Proliferation increases the population of immunocompetent cells and differentiation creates cells with various roles to play in the immune response. Both B and T cells differentiate into what broadly may be termed effector cells and memory cells. The memory cells revert to an inactive state (G_0) but respond to later immune challenge by accelerated proliferation, differentiation, and activity. During their residence in the bursa equivalent, the future effector B cells become programmed to respond to an antigen by transformation into plasma cells, which produce antibodies (immunoglobulins I_A, I_D, I_E, I_G, and I_M), the role of which is to combine with circulating antigens. The immunity conferred by B cells is known as humoral immunity.

Hypersensitivity mediated through the humoral immune system is called immediate hypersensitivity, because the response is rapid. T cells become programmed in the thymus to respond in various ways to antigen that has become fixed to cell surfaces or engulfed by macrophages. The cytotoxic T cell (effector cell, *killer* cell), with the aid of complement, attacks and lyses those cells to which the offending antigen is attached. There are different cytotoxic T cells for different antigens. There are also helper T cells, which promote B-cell activity, and suppressor T cells, which restrain both the cytotoxic T cells and the B cells. Helper and suppressor B cells also exist. T-cell-mediated immunity is known as cell-mediated immunity. This is the immune response involved in graft rejection, autoimmunity, and delayed hypersensitivity.

The priming of lymphocytes in response to antigen is known as the primary response. The final effector response is known as the secondary, or efferent, response.

There are other bone-marrow, stem-cell-derived cells, such as macrophages and K cells, that participate in the immune response. In the primary response, the macrophages engulf antigens, process them, and present the processed antigen to helper T lymphocytes, which initiate the recruitment of other lymphocytes. Thus the macrophages are an integral part of the afferent limb of the primary response. They also appear to be involved in the efferent response; they fix and alter antigen prior to its recognition by the T cells. Details of the immune system may be found in Chapter 89.

OTHER IMMUNOMODULATORS—Because immunosuppression is a common adverse effect of antineoplastic drugs and also because many immunosuppressive drugs have come from among the antineoplastics, it is common to believe that antineoplastic cytotoxicity automatically suppresses the immune system. However, the immune system has helper, suppressor, and killer components, so that the net effect depends on which components are affected most. IL-2 (interleukin-2) is used for its direct stimulation of T lymphocytes. Indeed, there is thought to be immunostimulatory components to the actions of some antineoplastic drugs.

Conversely, the situation is analogous with the so-called immunostimulants, because the net effect on any given immune response depends on which of the sundry participating cells are stimulated most. For example, levamisole is called an immunostimulant, but it either can augment or suppress an immune response depending on factors such the type of response, dose, and timing. T-lymphocyte function is augmented more than B-lymphocyte function. The drug tends to normalize a disturbed immune system. A similar bifunctionalism exists among the various cytokines. Interferons, for example, stimulate some immune cells and suppress others. Diethyl dithiocarbamate, however, is nearly a pure immunostimulant; it induces the recruitment of T lymphocytes and promotes cytotoxicity. Every vaccine is an immunostimulant and often selective. However, some, such as staphage lysate, cause rather general immunostimulation and may be used to confer varying degrees of immunity to various nonbacterial invaders.

It is now known that certain autonomic and CNS transmitters and neuromodulators also have influences on the immune system. Enkephalins and endorphins stimulate B-lymphocyte proliferation and antibody production and promote T-lymphocyte and natural killer-cell cytotoxicity. Opioid drugs mimic some of the immunomodulatory actions of the peptides. It is believed that these peptides are part of a neuroendocrine-immune system loop. Histamine stimulates suppressor T lymphocytes and thus tends to limit immune responses. The action is mediated through H_2-receptors. Consequently, H_2-antagonists, such as cimetidine and ranitidine, tend to augment the efferent immune response. Various immune cells also possess alpha- and beta-adrenoreceptors, through which immune functions can be affected by circulation of epinephrine and sympathetically released norepinephrine and their antagonists. The overall effect of alpha-agonism is immunosuppression but that of beta-agonism varies according to the immune status under various conditions.

ANTINEOPLASTIC DRUGS

ABARELIX

D-Alaninamide, *N*-acetyl-3-(2-naphthalenyl)-D-alanyl-4-chloro-D-phenylalanyl-3-(3-pyridinyl)-D-alanyl-L-seryl-*N*-methyl-L-tyrosyl-D-asparaginyl-L-leucyl-*N* [6]-(1-methylethyl)-L-lysyl-L-prolyl-, Plenaxis

[183552-38-7] $C_{72}H_{95}ClN_{14}O_{14}$ (1416.08).

Preparation—A synthetic decapeptide initially manufactured as an acetate-water complex, then converted into a carboxymethylcellulose complex to prepare the drug product. The reconstituted injection (with normal saline) has a pH of 5 ± 1.

Description—White to off-white powder.

Comments—Acts by directly suppressing luteinizing hormone and follicle stimulating hormone secretion and thereby reducing the secretion of testosterone by the testes. Used for palliative treatment of men with advanced symptomatic *prostate cancer*. May prolong QTc interval, therefore may interact with Class I and III antiarrythmic agents. It is highly protein bound (96–99%). The most common side effects experienced in clinical trials were serious allergic reactions (including loss of consciousness), hot flashes, sleep disturbances, pain, including back pain, breast enlargement or pain, and constipation.

ALDESLEUKIN

Interleukin-2 Recombinant; Proleukin

2-133-Interleukin 2 (human reduced) [110942-02-4] $C_{690}H_{1115}N_{177}O_{203}S_6$ (15,600).

Preparation—A continuous chain of 133 amino acid residues; a product of recombinant DNA technology with genetically engineered *E coli* strains containing an analog of the human IL-2 gene.

Comments—Identical to a cytokine, IL-2, secreted by activated helper T lymphocytes that is a colony-stimulating factor for active T lymphocytes, immature thymocytes, natural killer (NK) cells, antigen-activated B lymphocytes, and probably other cells of the immune system. The ability to stimulate proliferation of cytotoxic T lymphocytes and NK cells has led to clinical trials against several kinds of cancer. It is approved for *metastatic renal cancer and metastatic melanoma*. Treatment consists of the administration of IL-2 alone, prior to, or along with, autologous lymphokine-activated killer (LAK) cells; the IL-2 for the purpose of encouraging the proliferation of LAK cells. At present, the combination has been found effective in some cases of *colorectal carcinoma* and *Hodgkin's disease*, but treatment of other cancers is under active investigation. It is also under investigation as an anti-infective agent; it is in Phase II trials for use in AIDS.

Common adverse effects attributable to IL-2 are nausea, vomiting, diarrhea, fever, malaise, pruritus, severe anemia, hyperbilirubinemia, and elevated plasma creatinine. Less-common effects are elevated capillary permeability with pulmonary edema, fluid retention, hypotension, cardiac dysrhythmias, thrombocytopenia, and disorientation, even coma. Approximately 20% of patients treated with IL-2 and LAK cells develop hypothyroidism. It is contraindicated in patients with an abnormal thallium stress test or abnormal pulmonary function tests and those with organ allografts. Treatment is prohibitively expensive. The peptide nature of IL-2 requires parenteral administration. The half-life is less than 1 hr, and is administered by a 15-minute infusion every 8 hours for a maximum of 14 doses. Following 9 days of rest, the schedule may be repeated as tolerated for a maximum of 28 doses per course with a 7-week break between each course of treatment.

ALEMTUZUMAB

Immunoglobulin G 1 (human-rat monoclonalCAMPATH-1H 1-chain anti-human antigen CD52), disulfidewith human-rat monoclonal CAMPATH-1H light chain, dimer; CamPath

[CAS-216503-57-0]

Preparation—It is produced in a mammalian cell (Chinese hamster ovary) suspension culture in a medium containing neomycin. Neomycin is not detectable in the final product. A recombinant DNA-derived humanized monoclonal antibody (Campath-1H) that is directed against the 21–28 kD cell surface glycoprotein, CD52. that is expressed on the surface of normal and malignant B and T lymphocytes, NK cells, monocytes, macrophages, and tissues of the male reproductive system. The Campath-1H antibody is an IgG1 kappa with human variable framework and constant regions, and complementarity-determining regions from a murine (rat) monoclonal antibody (Campath-1G). The Campath-1H antibody has an approximate molecular weight of 150 kDa. US Pat 5,846,534 (1998).

Description—Campath is a sterile, clear, colorless, isotonic solution for injection; pH 6.8–7.4.

Comments—A recombinant DNA-derived human monoclonal antibody that is indicated for the treatment of *B-cell chronic leukemia* in patients who have failed fludarabine therapy. It acts against the 21–28 kD by binding to cell surface glycoprotein, CD52, that is expressed on the surface of normal and malignant B and T lymphocytes. This agent causes myelosuppression, which may result in severe, and sometimes fatal, pancytopenia or serious opportunistic and bacterial infections. Other side effects include nausea and vomiting, rash, and pneumonia. Gradual dose escalation is recommended to reduce the incidence of

infusion-related reactions, including hypotension, rigors, fever, shortness of breath, bronchospasm, chills, and/or rash. The average half-life is about 12 days, and it is administered by intravenous infusion over a two hour period three times weekly.

ALTRETAMINE

1,3,5-Triazine-2,4,6-triamine, *N,N,N',N',N'',N''*-hexamethyl-, Hexamethylmelamine; Hexalen

[645-05-6] $C_9H_{18}N_6$ (210.28).

Preparation—*J Am Chem Soc* 73:2984, 1951.

Description—White needles; melts about 173°.

Solubility—Practically insoluble in water; increasingly soluble at pH less than 3.

Comments—A Group C oral alkylating agent related to triethylenemelamine, an early alkylating agent. It is one of several secondary drugs for treatment of *ovarian tumors*. It is approved as a single agent for *refractory ovarian cancer*. It also has proved useful in the treatment of both *Hodgkin's* and *non-Hodgkin's lymphomas, oat-cell bronchogenic carcinoma*, and *breast tumor*. Nausea and vomiting are the main acute adverse effects. Delayed toxicity includes bone-marrow depression, CNS depression, peripheral neuritis, ataxia, hallucinations, psychoses, pruritus, and dermatitis. The drug is metabolized in the liver. The terminal half-life is 4.7 to 10.2 hr, which may increase with concomitant cimetidine therapy. Phenobarbital may decrease the half-life, and severe hypotension may occur with concomitant MAO inhibitor agents.

AMIFOSTINE

Ethanethiol, (*S*)-2-[(3-aminopropyl)amino]-, dihydrogen phosphate (ester); Ethiotos; Ethyol

[20537-88-6] $C_5H_{15}N_2O_3PS$ (214.21).

Preparation—1,3-Propanediamine is monoalkylated with 2-chloroethanol to form 2-[3-(aminopropyl)amino]ethanol and the free OH converted to Br by use of HBr. Treating the resulting alkyl bromide with sodium thiophosphate (Na₃PO₃S), followed by acidification affords the product. *J Med Chem* 1969; 12:236. US Pat 3,892,824 (1973).

Description—White crystalline solid melting about 161° (dec).

Solubility—Freely soluble in water; $pK_{a1} < 2.0$; pK_{a2} 4.2; pK_{a3} 9.0; pK_{a4} 11.7.

Comments—Approved for reduction of renal toxicity caused by repeated administration of cisplatin. It is a thiophosphate prodrug that once dephosphorylized provides a reduced thiol. It is indicated to reduce cumulative renal toxicity associated with repeated doses of cisplatin for the treatment of advanced ovarian cancer or non-small cell lung cancer. It also reduces the incidence of xerostomia in patients with head and neck cancer undergoing post-operative radiation treatments involving the parotid gland. It has been used to treat myelodysplasia and may protect against cisplatin and paclitaxel induced neurotoxicity.

It is rapidly metabolized and after only 6 min, less than 10% remains in the plasma. The thiol metabolite is distributed rapidly throughout the body. Approximately 62% of treated patients experienced hypotension, 19% experienced severe nausea and vomiting. Administration should be interrupted if systolic blood pressure drops significantly. Antiemetics should be coadministered, including a 5HT3 receptor antagonist. Hypersensitivity reactions also were reported.

AMINOGLUTETHIMIDE

2,6-Piperidinedione, 3-(4-aminophenyl)-3-ethyl-, Cytadren

2-(*p*-Aminophenyl)-2-ethylglutaramide [125-84-8]$C_{13}H_{16}N_2O_2$ (232.28).

Preparation—By a procedure similar to *Glutethimide* with nitration of the α-ethylbenzyl cyanide to the *p*-nitro derivative. This then, is reduced to the amine after ring closure. US Pat 2,848,455.

Description—White crystals; melts about 150°.

Solubility—Slightly soluble in water; freely soluble in many organic solvents.

Comments—Inhibits the first step in adrenalcorticoid biosynthesis by inhibiting the conversion of cholesterol to Δ5-pregrenolone. It also inhibits the aromatase that converts androstenedione to estrone and estradiol, thus eliminating the adrenal source, the only source of estrogens in postmenopausal and oophorectomized women. It is approved for *suppression of adrenalcorticoid production* in selected Cushing's syndrome patients. Treatment with aminoglutethimide is preferred to adrenalectomy in postmenopausal women who have *estrogen receptor-positive breast carcinoma.* Hydrocortisone is administered concomitantly to suppress the counterproductive, counterregulatory increase in ACTH release that accrues to the drug-induced lowering of plasma hydrocortisone. The regimen, however, causes more adverse effects than does tamoxifen and hence is a second-choice treatment. It also is useful in the management of certain cases of *Cushing's syndrome and prostate cancer.*

Early adverse effects include lethargy (40% of recipients), ataxia (10% of recipients), nausea, vomiting, and anorexia, and morbilliform rash; tolerance to this effects develops in 1 to 6 wk. Delayed adverse effects mostly relate to mineralocorticoid insufficiency and include orthostatic hypotension (10% of recipients; symptoms are dizziness and weakness) so that mineralocorticoids may require supplementation. Occasional adverse effects include pruritus, myalgia, headache, masculinization and hirsuitism in women, precocious sexual development in boys, hypothyroidism with goiters after long-term use, leukopenia, thrombocytopenia, granulocytopenia, and pancytopenia. Alkaline phosphatase and serum glutamic oxaloacetic transaminase (SGOT) activities in serum frequently occur, and cholestatic jaundice occurs rarely. Aminoglutethimide induces the metabolism of dexamethasone, thus that particular glucocorticoid should not be used concomitantly. It also enhances the clearance of digitoxin, theophylline, and warfarin.

Aminoglutethimide is well absorbed orally. Initially, approximately 50% is excreted in the urine unchanged, but induction of liver metabolism diminishes the importance of renal elimination. The elimination half-life is initially approximately 13 hr but decreases to approximately 7 hr after 1 to 2 wk.

ANASTRAZOLE

1,3-Benzenediacetonitrile, α,α,α',α'-tetramethyl-5-(1*H*-1,2,4-triazol-1-ylmethyl)-, Arimidex

[120511-73-1] C$_{17}$H$_{19}$N$_5$ (293.37).

Preparation—A mixture of α,α'-dibromomesitylene, tetra-(*t*-butyl) ammonium bromide, and KCN in methylene chloride or methylene chloride/water is heated to produce 5-methyl-1,3-phenylenebisacetonitrile. Refluxing this latter compound with methyl iodide and NaH in DMF yields the α,α-dimethyl derivative of both nitrile side chains. Further treatment with NBS and benzoyl peroxide brominates the free aryl methyl group, and reaction with sodiated 1,2,4-triazole forms the product. US Pat 4,935,437 (1990).

Description—Off-white crystals melting about 82°.

Solubility—Freely soluble in methanol, ethanol, acetone, or tetrahydrofuran (THF); soluble in acetonitrile; soluble in 0.5 mg/mL water.

Comments—Approved for use in postmenopausal women with hormone receptor positive or hormone receptor unknown locally advanced or metastatic breast cancer or those who have advanced breast cancer with disease progression after tamoxifen therapy. It is a potent non-steroidal inhibitor of aromatase, and, as such, inhibits conversion of androstenedione to estrone. It significantly reduces levels of circulating estradiol up to 80% after daily dosing with no detectable effect on adrenal corticosteroids of aldosterone. In clinical trials it proved similar in efficacy to megosterol in objective response and stabilization of disease in postmenopausal (primarily ER-positive) women who had progressing breast cancer, evidencing progression after tamoxifen therapy. ER-negative breast cancer rarely responds to anastrozole.

It is well absorbed when taken orally with or without food. Approximately 85% of the dose can be recovered from the urine and the feces. Approximaely 85% of the dose is eliminated by means of hepatic

metabolism and another 11% by means of renal excretion. The major circulating metabolite has no pharmacological activity. It has a terminal half-life of approximately 50 hr, concordantly steady-state levels are reached after 7 days of dosing.

Hepatic function is important for its clearance; clearance was reduced as much as 30% in patients who have cirrhosis of the liver. Vaginal bleeding occurs infrequently in the first weeks after the switch to therapy with this drug.

ARSENIC TRIOXIDE

Arsenic trioxide; Trisenox

Arsenous acid, arsenous oxide [13276-53-3] As$_4$O$_6$ (395.68).

Preparation—Occurs naturally in the mineral claudetite.

Description—Odorless, transparent crystals or white powder. Melts about 315° (with sublimation) and boils about 465°. Sp gr 3.74.

Solubility—Reported from 1.2 to 3.7 g/100 mL, at 20° in various references.

Comments—Used for remission, induction, and consolidation of the acute promyelocytic (M3) subtype of acute myeloid (myelogenous, nonlymphocytic) leukemia (AML, ANLL) with the t(15:17) chromosomal translocation that is refractory to retinoid and anthracycline therapy or has relapsed despite such therapy. Extensively metabolized via reduction by arsenate reductase and methylation (mainly in the liver) by methyltransferases, widely distributed throughout the body, and eliminated principally by metabolism and urinary excretion. Acts by inducing differentiation through degradation of the chimeric PML/RAR-alpha protein, and also induces apoptosis through a mitochondrion-dependent process, resulting in subsequent release of cytochrome C with caspase activation. The main toxicities are fatigue, electrocardiographic changes with QT prolongation, arrhythmias, and a syndrome characterized by fever, dyspnea, skin rash, fluid retention, and weight gain. Should be used caution in patients receiving drugs that may prolong the QT interval or those that may cause electrolyte abnormalities.

ASPARAGINASE

L-Asparagine amidohydrolase; E.C. 3.5.1.1.; Elspar

L-Asparaginase [9015-68-3], an enzyme of molecular weight 133,000 ± 5000, believed to consist of four equivalent subunits.

Preparation—L-Asparaginase, an enzyme that catalyzes hydrolysis of L-asparagine to l-aspartate and ammonia, occurs in many species. Isolated in pure form from several sources, it usually is obtained from *E coli* or *Erwinia caratovora,* which produces also an asparaginase devoid of antileukemic activity, that is removed on purification of the enzyme. See Mashburn and Wriston, *Arch Biochem Biophys* 105:450, 1964.

Description—White, crystalline powder.

Solubility—Freely soluble in water; practically insoluble in chloroform or in methanol.

Comments—Protein synthesis in several normal as well as malignant cell types depends partly on exogenous asparagine, and, in a few cells, such as lymphoblasts and certain other leukemic cells, essentially is dependent totally. The enzymatic destruction of asparagine by asparaginase injected into plasma deprives the dependent cells of the essential asparagine and, thus, not only arrests their growth but also might even result in some cell death and tumor regression. It is approved for use in *acute lymphocytic leukemia.*

Currently, it is used mainly in chemotherapy of acute lymphocytic leukemia, T-cell leukemias, and lymphomas in sequential combinations with other drugs. When it is administered immediately after a course of vincristine and a glucocorticoid (usually prednisone or dexamethasone) for the induction of the first remission in children, the median duration of remission is more than doubled. Addition of doxorubicin and intrathecal cytarabine further prolongs survival. Some studies indicate a small increase in the incidence of complete remissions. The enzyme also is useful for induction of remission in children who have relapsed acute lymphocytic leukemia. It is not recommended for maintenance. Asparaginase protects some tissues and cancers from some antimetabolites (eg, methotrexate, cytarabine), probably by preventing DNA synthesis. Such interactions, especially with methotrexate, should be anticipated. In patients allergic to asparaginase, pegaspargase, a polyethylene-glycol (PEG) conjugated l-asparaginase preparation is available. Also, Erwinia asparaginase is an orphan drug for use in patients allergic to asparaginase from *E coli.*

Sixty to 90% of recipients of asparaginase show laboratory evidence of an impairment of liver function, such that plasma fibrinogen and other clotting factors may be diminished, and most patients have a considerable elevation of blood ammonia. Effects on the pancreas also are common; insulin production is diminished; there may be hyperglycemia; serum amylase activity may increase; and acute pancreatitis, sometimes hemorrhagic, may occur in as many as 5% of recipients. There also are actions on the CNS to cause impairment of the sensorium, mental depression, and rare coma. Nausea, vomiting, chills, and fever also occur frequently. Hypersensitivity reactions, ranging from mild rash to anaphylaxis and death, occur in 5% to 20% of recipients, so that sensitivity testing before administration is necessary and desensitization may be necessary before a second course is administered. *Erwinia* (Porton) asparaginase is less sensitizing than that from *E. coli.* Both enzymes also have immunosuppressant activity.

It must be administered parenterally. The rate of clearance varies considerably between preparations. Its half-life is approximately 16 hr.

AZACITIDINE

1,3,5-Triazin-2(1*H*)-one, 4-amino-1-β-D-ribofuranosyl-, Mylosar, Vidaza

[320-67-2] $C_8H_{12}N_4O_5$ (244.20).

Preparation—A ring analog of cytidine, obtained by synthesis or produced microbiologically. US Pat 3,350,388.

Description—White powder that melts about 229°.

Solubility—1 g in 25 mL water or 1000 mL alcohol. Reconstituted intravenous solutions are not stable for more than a few hours.

Comments—A pyrimidine nucleoside analog of cytidine, this antimetabolite is used to treat patients with various myelodysplastic syndromes subtypes including refractory anemias with sideroblasts or excess blasts and chronic myelomonocytic leukemia. It causes acute nausea, vomiting, diarrhea, and fever. Delayed toxicity, which is not dose-related, includes prolonged leukopenia, thrombocytopenia, and hepatotoxicity. The mortality rate has been reported to be approximately 6%. It should not be used in patients with severe hepatic impairment. It is administered subcutaneously once daily for seven days at 4-week intervals. Metabolites are excreted primarily by the kidneys, and dosage adjustments are required with impaired renal function.

AZATHIOPRINE

1*H*-Purine, 6-[(1-methyl-4-nitro-1*H*-imidazol-5-yl)thiol]-, Imuran

6-[(1-Methyl-4-nitroimidazol-5-yl)thio]purine [446-86-6] $C_9H_7N_7O_2S$ (277.26).

Preparation—*N,N*'-Dimethyloxaldiamide is reacted with phosphorus pentachloride to give 5-chloro-1-methylimidazole. This is nitrated, and the resulting 5-chloro-1-methyl-4-nitroimidazole condensed with purine-6-thiol (mercaptopurine) in an appropriate dehydrohalogenating environment. US Pat 3,056,785.

Description—Yellow, matted powder that is odorless and has a slightly bitter taste; light sensitive, nonhygroscopic, and stable to reasonable temperatures; decomposes at approximately 245°.

Solubility—Insoluble in water; slightly soluble in alcohol or chloroform; soluble in dilute solutions of alkali hydroxides (unstable); sparingly soluble in dilute mineral acids.

Comments—Approved for prevention of renal transplant rejection. It is a derivative of *Mercaptopurine* into which it largely is converted in the body, but not all of its actions are those of mercaptopurine. It is used only as an *immunosuppressive* drug. It suppresses T-lymphocyte and monocyte (hence macrophage) production more than B-lymphocyte production. It probably has been used more than any other immunosuppressive drug in *kidney transplantations.* Currently, approximately one-half of kidney transplants survive for longer than 3 yr when azathioprine is used, but other measures also contribute to this rate of success. It also is used in other organ transplantations.

Azathioprine works in the afferent and not the efferent immune phase and hence does not suppress ongoing graft rejection. It appears to bring about a satisfactory response in a high percentage of patients who have *ulcerative colitis, regional enteritis, polymyositis,* or *refractory idiopathic thrombocytopenic purpura* but induces considerable toxicity. In *rheumatoid arthritis,* it is used when conventional therapy fails. It is almost as effective as gold, penicillamine, or cyclophosphamide and less toxic than penicillamine or cyclophosphamide. It may improve metabolic control in recent-onset diabetes mellitus. It is usually of little benefit in *systemic lupus erythematosus.*

Nausea and vomiting are frequent. Other toxicity or intercurrent infection (see the introductory statement) occurs in approximately one-third of patients under immunosuppressive treatment with the drug. Bone-marrow depression is the most frequent, occurring in approximately 11% of patients; leukopenia (28 to more than 50%, as much as 16% serious), thrombocytopenia, and, to a lesser extent, anemia or pancytopenia are manifested.

In antiarthritic doses, infections are not increased, and other adverse effects are less frequent and less severe. Pancreatitis, alopecia, arthralgia, skin rashes, serum sickness, stomatitis, esophagitis, steatorrhea, retinopathy, peritoneal hemorrhage, and pulmonary edema also may occur in a small percentage of cases. Occasionally, hepatic damage, with elevation of the plasma content of liver enzymes and jaundice, is seen, but damage seems slight and seems to disappear during the course of treatment. However, in the presence of liver dysfunction the drug should be withheld. Although the incidence is rare, an increase in reticulum cell sarcoma and lymphoma has been noted in transplant patients receiving azathioprine; it is unclear whether this is from immunosuppression or from the successfully sustained transplant. However, the drug is carcinogenic in experimental animals.

Although it is degraded rapidly in the liver, it is important that the kidney regulates the plasma concentration of the effective metabolites, so that toxicity is greatly increased in the presence of allopurinol or renal impairment, unless the dosage is properly adjusted. It should not be used during pregnancy if possible.

It is metabolized rapidly to 6-MP, so that its useful half-life is that of 6-MP. Because allopurinol inhibits the metabolism of 6-MP, the dosage of this drug must be reduced to approximately one-third of the usual dose when allopurinol is used concurrently. Hepatic insufficiency diminishes efficacy.

BCG VACCINE

TICE BCG; TheraCys, BCG Live (intravesical)

Preparation—TICE is an attenuated live culture preparation of the Bacillus of Calmette and Guerin (BCG) strain *Mycobacterium.* The culture is grown on a medium containing glycerin, asparagine, citric acid, potassium phosphate, magnesium sulfate, and iron ammonium citrate. Prior to freeze-drying lactose is added. Each 10^8 colony-forming units (CFU) is equivalent to approximately 50 mg net weight.

TheraCys is a freeze-dried suspension of the same bacterium grown on Sauton medium (potato and glycerin based). Each approx 10^9 CFU weighs approximately 80 mg.

See, Guerin C, *The History of BCG in BCG Vaccines: Tuberculosis-Cancer,* Rosenthal SR, ed. Littleton, MA: PSG, 1980.

Comments—Approved for treatment of primary cancer of the urinary bladder. TICE BCG is freeze dried and (attenuated), whereas TheraCys is live, but both are used by intravenous instillation into the urinary bladder. The exact mechanism is unknown, but BCG instillation elicits an inflammatory response with leukocytic infiltration into the bladder. This is associated with an eradication or reduction of superficial carcinoma lesions. In clinical trials approximately 50% of patients treated with TICE BCG showed complete responses and appeared disease-free; approximately 75% showed positive response. In patients who have *in situ* carcinoma and are treated with TheraCys, approximately 71% showed good clinical response. Following bladder instillation, the drug is retained for 2 hours and then voided. Bladder irritability occurs in 50% of patients in the following 24 to 72 hours.

BCG should not be given to patients who have compromised immune systems or who are receiving immunosuppressants, antimicrobial agents, or radiation therapy. Deaths have occurred owing to systemic infections, and therapy should be interrupted if patients show high or persistent fever and malaise.

BEVACIZUMAB

Immunoglobulin G1 (human mouse monoclonal rhuMAb-VEGF γ-chain anti-human vascular endothelial growth factor), disulfide with human-mouse monoclonal rhuMAb-VEGF light chain dimer; Avastin

[216974-75-3] $C_{6638}H_{10160}N_{1720}O_{2109}S_{44}$ (149,214.2).

Preparation—Produced in a Chinese Hamster Ovary mammalian cell expression system in a nutrient medium containing gentamycin.

Description—Clear to slightly opalescent, colorless to pale brown in the sterile, IV infusion; pH 6.2.

Comments—recombinant humanized monoclonal IgG1 antibody that binds to and inhibits a natural protein called human vascular endothelial growth factor (VEGF) which plays a role in the formation and maintenance of tumor blood vessels. This monoclonal antibody belongs to a new class of drugs called angiogenesis inhibitors, and is believed to work by targeting and inhibiting the function of a natural protein called "vascular endothelial growth factor" (VEGF) that stimulates new blood vessel formation or angiogenesis. When this binding occurs, the tumor cannot stimulate the growth of blood vessels, thus denying tumors blood, oxygen, and other nutrients needed for growth. Indicated in combination with intravenous 5-fluorouracil—based chemotherapy for first-line treatment of patients with metastatic carcinoma of the colon or rectum.

Common side effects include hypertension, tiredness, blood clots, diarrhea, leukopenia, headache, anorexia, stomatitis, constipation, upper respiratory infection, epistaxis, dyspnea, exfoliative dermatitis, and proteinuria. Serious, but uncommon side effects include gastrointestinal perforation (sometimes leading to intra-abdominal infections), impaired wound healing, and internal bleeding.

BEXAROTENE

Benzoic acid, 4-[1-(5,6,7,8-tetrahydro-3,5,5,8,8-pentamethyl-2-naphthalenyl)ethenyl]-, Targretin

[153539-49-0] $C_{24}H_{28}O_2$ (348.48).

Preparation—US Pat 5,466,861(1995).

Description—White to off-white powder from methylene chloride melting about 231°.

Solubility—Insoluble in water; soluble in ethanol or vegetable oils.

Comments—a synthetic retinoid analog, is an antineoplastic agent that selectively binds with and activates retinoid X receptor (RXR) subtypes (RXR$_\alpha$, RXR$_\beta$, and RXR$_\gamma$). Bexarotene is an oral orphan drug for the treatment of skin manifestations of cutaneous T-cell lymphoma (CTCL) in patients who are refractory to at least one prior systemic therapy. Metabolized through oxidation by the cytochrome P-450 (CYP) 3A4 isoenzyme and primarily eliminated by biliary excretion with a terminal half-life of 7 hrs. Plasma concentrations after a 300-mg dose increased by approximately 48% after a meal containing fat compared with a glucose solution. Adverse reactions include skin rash, dry skin, flu-like symptoms, anemia, fever, hyperlipemia, hypothyroidism, leukopenia, peripheral edema, photosensitivity, and increased liver function tests. Drug interactions may occur with protein bound drugs, gemfibrozil, hormonal contraceptives, tamoxifen, oral hypoglycemic agents, or inhibitors or inducers of the cytochrome P-450 system.

BICALUTAMIDE

Propanamide, (±)-N-[4-cyano-3-(trifluoromethyl)phenyl]-3-[4-(fluorophenyl)sulfonyl]-2-hydroxy-2-methyl-, Casodex

[90357-06-5] $C_{18}H_{14}N_2O_4S$ (430.38).

Preparation—Thiophenol is reacted with methyl 2,3-epoxy-2-methylpropanoate and NaH in THF to yield the methyl ester of 2-hydroxy-2-methyl-3-(phenylthio)propionic acid (I). Saponification of I, to form the acid, followed by treatment with thionyl chloride, and the acyl chloride reacted with 4-amino-3-(trifluoromethyl)benzonitrile, produces the corresponding amide. Oxidation of the thio ether linkage with 3-chloroperbenzoic acid gives the title compound.

Description—White to off-white crystals that melt about 192°. It is a racemic mixture and the S-isomer is essentially inactive; pK$_a \sim$ 12.

Solubility—Soluble in 5 mg/mL water; soluble in acetone or in THF; slightly soluble in chloroform or anhydrous alcohol; sparingly soluble in methanol.

Comments—Approved for use in advanced prostate cancer in combination with LHRH analogs. It is a nonsteroidal antiandrogen that acts by inhibiting androgen uptake or nuclear binding target tissues.

When 50 mg of this drug was given once a day, it proved no different from flutamide 250 mg tid in patients who had either leuprolide or goserelin depot or implants. Time to treatment failure was no different.

Bicalutamide is well absorbed orally with or without meals. The active (R) isomer is inactivated largely by oxidation followed by glucuronidation. The (S) isomer is cleared rapidly, and does not contribute significantly to steady-state plasma levels. Peak levels are reached approximately 3 hr after a single dose and exhibit a half-life of 5.8 days. Mean steady-state plasma concentration in cancer patients is 8.9 mcg/mL. Renal and hepatic function impairment did not affect the affect the drug's elimination.

Elevations in plasma testosterone and estradiol levels are noted when bicalutamide is used as a single agent. Gynecomastia and breast pain were reported in approximately 38% of treated patients. The most frequent adverse reaction was hot flashes reported in 49% of patients. Diarrhea was also reported. It can displace coumarin anticoagulants from plasma protein binding sites, thus caution should be exercised when treatment is started in patient being treated with anticoagulants. Patients should be monitored for possible increases in liver enzymes, as rare cases of death due to hepatotoxicity have occurred.

BLEOMYCIN SULFATE

Blenoxane

(Main component: Bleomycin A_2, in which **R** is $(CH_3)_2S^+CH_2CH_2CH_2$—)

Bleomycin Sulfate (salt) [9041-93-4].

A mixture of the sulfate salts of a group of related basic glycopeptide antibiotics, notably bleomycin A_2 and bleomycin B_2, obtained from cultures of Streptomyces verticillus; bleomycin A_2 is the main component of the bleomycin used clinically.

Preparation—For the purification and separation of the bleomycins see Umezawa et al. *J Antibiot* 1966; 19:200, 210, also Takita. *J Antibiot* 1968; 21:79, and 1969; 22:237.

Description—Cream-colored, hygroscopic powder.

Solubility—Soluble in water; sparingly soluble in alcohol.

Comments—Causes fragmentation of DNA and also inhibits incorporation of thymidine into DNA. It stops the progression of cells through the G_2 and the M phases of the cell cycle. Despite these actions, it has little effect on bone marrow, a circumstance that gives it a special usefulness in drug combinations. Its selectivity appears to be related to distribution. It is approved as palliative treatment of *lymphomas, testicular carcinoma,* and *squamous cell carcinoma.* A component of all three preferred combinations is used for the treatment of *testicular carcinoma* and of two for cervical cancer. It is included in one of two preferred combinations to treat *squamous cell carcinoma of the head and neck.* It also has been used successfully in the treatment of squamous cell carcinomas of the skin, penis, and vulva. It is in two of five preferred for *Hodgkin's disease.* It is a component of four of seven preferred combinations to treat diffuse lymphocytic lymphoma. It has shown efficacy against reticulum cell sarcoma, lymphosarcoma, chloriocarcinoma, teratocarcinoma, and AIDS related Kaposi's sarcoma. It is also sometimes used intrapleurally for sclerotherapy in the management of malignant pleural effusions and is also effective against *common warts.*

It is toxic, and 10% to 40% of patients develop a pneumonitis that progresses to pulmonary fibrosis: 1% of bleomycin-treated patients die of pulmonary complications. The effect is most likely to occur in elderly patients or those who have received a total of 400 Units. The drug must be used extremely cautiously in the presence of pulmonary disease. Acute hyperpyrexia and cardiorespiratory collapse also occur, especially in patients who have lymphomas; for this reason, patients who have lymphomas are given two test doses of 5 U or less and are observed for a day before treatment is begun. Anticalmodulin drugs (eg, trifluperazine) enhance lethal toxicity. Bleomycin commonly causes nausea, vomiting, chills, and fever, and in half the patients, it causes erythema and hyperkeratosis, which sometimes progresses to vesication. Other occasional adverse effects are cutaneous desquamation, hyperesthesia, confusion, vertigo, pruritus, tenderness, alopecia, and aphthous ulcers. Cutaneous toxicity is most likely to occur when the total cumulative dose exceeds 150 U.

It is absorbed poorly orally and also is inactivated in the gut and the liver. Consequently, it must be administered parenterally. Higher concentrations are reached in certain neoplasms (carcinomas more than sarcomas), lungs, and skin than in other tissues, which accounts for the selectivity and the loci of toxicities. In the tissues, the drug appears to be deaminated and, possibly, also hydrolyzed by peptidases. The enzymatic destruction is less in those tissues in which the higher concentrations are reached. Sixty to 70% is excreted in the urine. In patients who have normal renal function, the elimination half-life is approximately 2 hr; in renal failure the half-life may be as long as 21 hr. Care must be exercised in the presence of renal impairment.

BORTEZOMIB

Boronic acid, [(1R)-3-methyl-1-[[(2S)-1-oxo-3-phenyl-2-[(pyrazinylcarbonyl)amino]propyl]amino]butyl]-, Velcade

[179324-69-7] $C_{19}H_{25}BN_4O_4$ (328.24).

Preparation—The pinanediol ester of leucineboronic acid is coupled with an *N*-Boc protected amino acid in the presence of TBTU (*O*-(benzotriazol-1-yl)-*N,N,N',N'*-tetramethyluronium tetrafluoroborate). Deprotection and *N*-acetyl-ation yields the dipeptideboronic ester. *Biorg Med Chem Lett,* 1998; 8:336 and US Pat 4,499,087 (1985) in *Chem Abstr* 1985; 103:71709.

Description—The pure drug substance exists in the cyclic anhydride form as a trimeric boroxine. The injectable exists as a mannitol boronic ester which, after reconstitution, is in equilibrium with the monoboronic acid, the hydrolysis product.

Solubility—In water; 3.3 to 3.8 mg/mL in a pH range of 2 to 6.5.

Comments—reversible inhibitor of the chymotrypsin-like activity of the 26S proteasome (large protein complex that degrades ubiquitinated proteins). The ubiquitin-proteasome pathway are essential in regulating the intracellular concentration of specific proteins, thereby maintaining homeostasis within cells. Inhibition of the 26S proteasome prevents this targeted proteolysis which can affect multiple signaling cascades within the cell. This disruption of normal homeostatic mechanisms can lead to cell death. Indicated for multiple myeloma in patients who have received at least two prior chemotherapy regimens and experienced disease progression. Adverse effects may be severe and life-threatening, and include peripheral neuropathy (paresthesias and/or loss of reflexes), asthenia, hypotension, diarrhea, constipation, vomiting, thrombocytopenia, neutropenia, or fever.

In vitro studies with human liver microsomes and human cDNA-expressed cytochrome P450 isozymes indicate that bortezomib is primarily oxidatively metabolized via cytochrome P450 enzymes, 3A4, 2D6, 2C19, 2C9, and 1A2. The major metabolic pathway is deboronation to form two deboronated metabolites that subsequently undergo hydroxylation to several metabolites. Deboronated-bortezomib metabolites are inactive as 26S proteasome inhibitors.

BROMOCRIPTINE—page 1418.

BUSULFAN

1,4-Butanediol, dimethanesulfonate; Tetramethylene Dimethanesulfonate; Myleran
$CH_3SO_2O(CH_2)_4OSO_2CH_3$

1,5-Butanediol dimethanesulfonate [55-98-1] $C_6H_{14}O_6S_2$ (246.29).

Preparation—By esterifying 1,4-butanediol with methanesulfonyl chloride in the presence of pyridine.

Description—White, crystalline powder; melting about 116°.

Solubility—Slightly soluble in water; slightly soluble in alcohol; 1 g in approximately 45 mL acetone.

Comments—An alkylating agent that is efficacious as an *antineoplastic* drug in certain cases. It is phase nonspecific. Its principal distinction is that in the usual doses it exerts little action on rapidly proliferative tissues other than bone marrow. With low doses, granulocytopoiesis can be suppressed selectively without affecting erythropoiesis. Thus, it is approved for the palliative treatment of *chronic granulocytic* (myelogenous, myeloid, myelocytic) *leukemia;* for this type of leukemia, it is one of two drugs of choice. It is not to be used in terminal or acute phases of the disease. It is also quite effective in the treatment of *polycythemia vera* and *primary thrombocytosis*. Because it has little effect on lymphopoiesis, it is of no value in lymphocytic leukemia, Hodgkin's disease, or malignant lymphoma. It is useless against solid tumors, but is used in high dosages for pretransplant conditioning regimens in patients undergoing autologous or allogeneic bone marrow transplantation for acute or chronic leukemias.

Its principal toxicity is pancytopenia and long-lasting thrombocytopenia. Lymphocytopenia is uncommon. A complete differential blood count (including thrombocytes) once a week is mandatory. Nausea, vomiting, diarrhea, impotence, amenorrhea, sterility, and fetal malformation occasionally occur. Granulocyte destruction results in a high rate of excretion of urates, the precipitation of which may cause renal damage; cotreatment with allopurinol may avoid such damage. It also sometimes causes cheilosis, glossitis, interstitial pulmonary fibrosis, anhidrosis, skin pigmentation (which may be the result of adrenalcortical hypofunction), alopecia, and gynecomastia.

It is not immunosuppressive. It is rapidly and completely absorbed, and metabolized in the liver mainly by glutathione conjugation (spontaneous and glutathione *S*-transferase-mediated). The glutathione conjugate is then further metabolized in the liver by oxidation with an elimination half-life is 2 to 3 hr.

CAPECITABINE

Carbamic acid, [1-(5-deoxy-β-D-ribofuranosyl)-5-fluoro-1,2-di-hydro-2-oxo-4-pyrimidinyl]-, pentyl ester; Xeloda

[154361-50-9] $C_{15}H_{22}FN_3O_6$ (359.35).

Preparation—5'-Deoxy-5-fluorocytidine is acetylated with acetic anhydride to form the 2',3'-diacetate, which on treatment with *n*-pentyl chloroformate yields the N^4-propxycarbonyl derivative. The esters are saponified using dilute NaOH to give the product. US Pat 5,472,949 (1995).

Description—Off-white crystalline powder or crystals from ethyl acetate, melting about 110–120°. It is the prodrug of doxifluridine and is designed to be metabolized in the body to 5-fluorouracil.

Solubility—Water; 26 mg/mL at 20°.

Comments—A fluoropyrimidine carbamate prodrug indicated for the treatment of metastatic breast cancer and colorectal cancer. It undergoes extensive metabolism in the liver by the enzyme carboxylesterase to an intermediate, 5'-deoxy-5-fluorocytidine, which is converted to 5'-deoxy-5-fluorouridine by the enzyme cytidine deaminase. The 5'-deoxy-5-fluorouridine metabolite is then hydrolyzed by thymidine phosphorylase to fluorouracil in the tumor. Peak plasma levels are achieved in about 1.5 hours, and peak fluorouracil levels are reached at 2 hours after oral administration and oral bioavailability is about 70% to 80%.

The main toxicities consist of diarrhea, hand-and-foot syndrome, myelosuppression, nausea, and vomiting. Myelosuppression, nausea and vomiting, and mucositis occur at a significantly less incidence than that seen with intravenous fluorouracil. Its toxicity may be increased with concomitant administration of leucovorin. Drug interactions may occur resulting in increased phenytoin levels or increased bleeding with warfarin.

CARBOPLATIN

Platinum, diammine [1,1-cyclobutanedicarboxylato(2-)-O,O']-, CBDCA, Paraplatin

[41575-94-4] $C_6H_{12}N_2O_4Pt$ (371.25).

Preparation—Silver sulfate is reacted with *cis*-diammine platinum diiodide to yield the diaquodiammine platinum sulfate. Interaction with barium 1,1-cyclobutanedicarboxylate precipitates $BaSO_4$, and forms the product. *Inorg Chem Acta* 1980; 46:L15.

Description—White crystals.

Solubility—1 g in approximately 10 mL water or 1000 mL alcohol.

Comments—Its *antineoplastic* activity results from binding to DNA and inhibiting DNA synthesis. Specifically, bidentate dicarboxylate ligands of carboplatin are displaced by water (aquation), forming positively charged platinum complexes that react with nucleophilic sites on DNA. Cisplatin has the same mechanism of action providing the same clinical antitumor spectrum. Carboplatin and cisplatin are activated by an initial aquation reaction, carboplatin is a more stable compound and is activated more slowly than cisplatin Carboplatin produces predominantly DNA intrastrand cross-links from the formation of adducts between the activated platinum complexes of the drug and the N-7 atom on guanine. Interstrand cross-linking within the DNA helix also occurs which are stable bonds that do not dissociate easily. Higher concentrations of carboplatin than cisplatin are required to produce equivalent levels of DNA binding

Carboplatin is less nephrotoxic and ototoxic compared to cisplatin. It is approved as palliative relief for *ovarian cancer*. It is presently an alternative drug for treatment of *small-cell* and *non–small-cell lung cancer, ovarian, head and neck, Wilms' tumor, brain, bladder* and *testicular carcinomas*. Immediate adverse effects are nausea and vomiting. Delayed toxicity includes myelosuppression with sometimes pronounced thrombocytopenia, renal, and otic toxicities. The drug is not effective orally. In plasma, less than 10% is protein bound. The elimination half-life is 3 to 7 hr. Dosage adjustments are required based on renal function.

CARMUSTINE

Urea, N,N'-bis(2-chloroethyl)-N-nitroso-, BiCNU

1,3-Bis(2-chloroethyl)-1-nitrosourea [154-93-8] $C_5H_9Cl_2N_3O_2$ (214.05).

Preparation—Like other cytotoxic nitrosoureas, it may be synthesized by nitrosation with sodium nitrite of the appropriate substituted urea—in this case 1,3-bis(2-chloroethyl)urea—in a cold, acid medium (eg, formic acid). Methods of synthesis of nitrosoureas have been published by Johnston et al. *J Med Chem* 1963; 6:669.

Description—White or light yellow powder; melts, with decomposition to an oily liquid about 30°.

Solubility—Slightly soluble in water; freely soluble in alcohol; highly soluble in lipids; decomposes rapidly in acid or aqueous solutions with a pH greater than 7.

Comments—Although this is an alkylating drug, it also carbamoylates amino and other groups. Its cytotoxic effect is likely due to its ability to cross-link cellular DNA. Synthesis of DNA and RNA is inhibited. It is phase nonspecific. Carmustine is approved for intravenous use in *brain tumors, multiple myeloma, Hodgkin's disease,* and *non-Hodgkin's lymphomas*. The drug is used mainly in the treatment of *brain glioblastoma* (for which it shares drug-of-choice status with its congener lomustine), *Hodgkin's disease* and other *lymphomas;* it is a component of a first-choice combination for *myeloma*. It has been reported to have a high efficacy against *Burkitt's tumor*. Although it has activity against various other carcinomas, including melanoma and renal cell carcinoma, it is not among the usual choices for such diseases. It usually is given in combination with radiotherapy in the treatment of brain tumors and with vincristine, procarbazine, and glucocorticoids (eg, prednisone) in the treatment of the various lymphomas and multiple myeloma. An intracranial carmustine wafer implant is available as an adjunct to surgery in palliative treatment of recurrent glioblastoma multiforme in patients for whom surgical resection is indicated. It is

also effective topically for the palliative treatment of cutaneous T-cell lymphoma (mycosis fungoides).

Within 2 hr after administration and lasting for 4 to 6 hr, nausea and vomiting occur frequently and usually severely. Rapid intravenous infusion causes intense flushing and conjunctival suffusion with a similar time course. There may be a burning sensation but rarely thrombosis at the site of injection. Delayed bone-marrow toxicity occurs; also, thrombocytopenia that reaches a nadir in approximately 4 wk and a less severe leukepenia in approximately 6 wk occur, each lasting 2 to 7 wk; mild anemia may occur. With repeated doses, bone-marrow depression is cumulative. Leukocyte and platelet counts and signs of intercurrent infections should be monitored carefully throughout treatment. Severe dyspnea and a sometimes fatal interstitial pulmonary fibrosis occasionally occur. There also may be a mild, reversible hepatotoxicity in approximately 25% of recipients. Other adverse effects include slight nephrotoxocity [with a transient elevation of blood urea nitrogen (BUN)] to severe nephrotoxicity and renal failure, and with large cumulative doses, vertigo and ataxia occur. There is an increased risk of nonlymphocytic leukemia.

By the oral route, it is metabolized almost completely as it passes through the liver; consequently, it must be given intravenously. After intravenous administration, its plasma half-life is short, reported variously as from 3 to 30 min. Because the drug is highly lipid soluble, it readily passes the blood-brain barrier, and concentrations of metabolites in the cerebrospinal fluid range from approximately 50% to 115% of those in plasma.

CETUXIMAB

Immunoglobulin G1, anti-(human epidermal growth factor receptor) (human-mouse monoclonal C225γ-chain), disulfide with human-mouse monoclonal C225 K-chain, dimer; Erbitux

[205923-56-4] Molecular weight is approximately 170,000 daltons.

Preparation—Produced in mammalian (murine myeloma) cell cultures. Also US 6,645,990 and US Pat Appl 0040096890 (2004).

Description—White, amorphous particulate.

Comments—Recombinant, human/mouse chimeric monoclonal antibody that targets a natural protein called "epidermal growth factor receptor" (EGFR) on the surface of cancer cells, thus interfering with their growth. This binding to EGFR blocks phosphorylation and activation of receptor-associated kinases, resulting in inhibition of cell growth, induction of apoptosis, and decreased matrix metalloproteinase and vascular endothelial growth factor production. In vitro assays and in vivo animal studies have shown that only the growth and survival of tumor cells that over-express the EGFR are inhibited. Approved as a single agent is indicated for the treatment of EGFR-expressing, metastatic colorectal carcinoma in patients who are intolerant to irinotecan-based chemotherapy, or in combination with irinotecan, for the treatment of EGFR-expressing, metastatic colorectal carcinoma in patients who are refractory to irinotecan-based chemotherapy.

Common side effects include acne-like rash, dry skin, tiredness or weakness, fever, constipation, and abdominal pain. Severe infusion reactions occurred in approximately 3% of patients, rarely with fatal outcome (<1 in 1000). Approximately 90% of severe infusion reactions were associated with the first infusion. Severe infusion reactions are characterized by rapid onset of airway obstruction (bronchospasm, stridor, hoarseness), urticaria, and hypotension. Other less common but more serious events are interstitial lung disease, pulmonary emboli, and sepsis. Studies have shown a mean half-life was 114 hours (range, 75–188 hours).

CHLORAMBUCIL

Benzenebutanoic acid, 4-[bis(2-chloroethyl)amino]-, Leukeran

4-[*p*-[Bis(2-chloroethyl)amino]phenyl]butyric acid [305-03-3] $C_{14}H_{19}Cl_2NO_2$ (304.22).

Preparation—4-Phenylbutyric acid is nitrated and the resulting p-nitric acid is esterified with isopropyl alcohol. The nitro ester then is hydrogenated to the aminoester. Reaction with ethylene oxide converts the—NH_2 into—$N(CH_2CH_2OH)_2$, which then is converted into—$N(CH_2CH_2Cl)_2$ by treatment with $POCl_3$. Hydrolysis of the ester yields the acid, chlorambucil.

Description—Off-white, slightly granular powder.

Solubility—Slightly soluble in water; soluble in dilute alkali; 1 g in 2 mL acetone.

Comments—An alkylating agent effective by the oral route. It is approved for and is the agent of choice in the treatment of *chronic lymphocytic leukemia.* It also is effective in the treatment of *Waldenstrom's macroglobulinemia, multiple myeloma, lymphosarcoma, giant-cell follicular lymphoma,* and, to a lesser degree, in *choriocarcinoma, Hodgkin's disease,* and *ovarian and testicular tumors.* As an immunosuppressant it is considered of value in the treatment of the nephrotic syndrome and vasculitis associated with *systemic lupus erythematosus, Wegner's granulomatosis, idiopathic membranous nephropathy,* and *Behçet's disease.*

It is the slowest-acting and least toxic of currently used nitrogen mustards. Its toxicity is manifested mainly as bone-marrow depression, although in therapeutic doses it generally is moderate and reversible. Most patients have some neutropenia after the third week of treatment until approximately 10 days after discontinuation of treatment. Slowly progressing lymphopenia also occurs, but it repairs itself quickly after treatment. Thrombocytopenia and anemia also occur sometimes. When the total accumulated dose exceeds 6.5 mg/kg the incidence of severe bone-marrow damage becomes high, and even irreversible toxicity may occur. It is mandatory that hemoglobin, leukocyte and platelet counts be monitored closely. It is contraindicated for 4 wk after radiotherapy or other drugs that depress bone marrow. If possible, it should be avoided during the first trimester of pregnancy.

It is adsorbed well by the oral route. It is degraded extensively in the body. The elimination half-life is approximately 1.5 hr.

CHLOROQUINE PHOSPHATE—page 1666.

CISPLATIN

Platinum, diamminedichloro-, (*SP*-4-2), Platinol

cis-Diamminedichloroplatinum [15663-27-1]Cl$_2$H$_6$N$_2$Pt (300.06).

Preparation—A solution of potassium tetrachloroplatinate(II), which is prepared by reduction of the hexachloroplatinate(II) salt with hydrazine, is neutralized with ammonium chloride and ammonium hydroxide. The cis-isomer precipitates (*Inorg Synth* 1963, 7:239).

Description—White, lyophilized powder; melts about 207°.

Solubility—1 g in approximately 1000 mL of water or normal saline; 1 g in approximately 42 mL of dimethylformamide.

Comments—Cross-links DNA and hence acts like alkylating antineoplastic agents. It is approved as palliative relief for metastatic testicular and ovarian tumors and for advanced bladder cancer. It is used in various first-choice combinations for the treatment of metastatic carcinomas of the testes, ovary, prostate, and cervix; squamous cell carcinoma of the head and neck; small-oat-cell and non-small-cell cancer of the lung; advanced cancer of the bladder, medulloblastoma, and retinoblastoma that has proved refractory to surgery or radiation. It also is used alone in the treatment of bladder cancer.

Acute toxicity includes severe nausea, vomiting, and anorexia, which occurs in almost all recipients but can be controlled largely with antiemetics. Occasional anaphylactoid reactions occur. Delayed toxicity includes ototoxicity (tinnitus or hearing loss in approximately 30% of patients), which requires audiometric monitoring. Nephrotoxicity, which requires monitoring of serum creatinine, urate, and BUN and avoidance of other nephrotoxic drugs, is a serious side effect in all patients and is controlled by forced diuresis (administration of mannitol and saline) and hydration prior to and following administration. Use of prophylactic amifostine, a phosphorylated sulfhydryl compound, decreases the incidence and severity of nephrotoxicity and is administered immediately prior to cisplatin administration. Bone-marrow depression occurs in 25% to 30% of recipients, typically at the higher dosages. Peripheral neuropathies, loss of taste, and convulsions are other side effects experienced. In studies of patients with advanced ovarian cancer, the incidence and severity of cisplatin-induced neurotoxicity appeared to be reduced in patients who received prophylactic amifostine. Electrolyte deficits, perhaps from hemodilution by fluids, have been reported, and consist primarily of hypomagnesemia, hypokalemia, and hypocalcemia. It combines tightly with various proteins, which stimulates the immune system to produce various antibodies; the adverse effect of such immune stimulation are not known.

It is not absorbed orally and must be given intravenously. Intra-arterial and peritoneal administration has shown to be effective in select patients. Approximately 90% is bound to plasma proteins. It does not cross the blood-brain barrier. Elimination is mainly renal, partly by tubular secretion; excretion is nonlinear. It is contraindicated in patients with poor renal function. The distribution half-life of the unbound drug is 25 to 49 min and the elimination half-life of total platinum is normally 58 to 73 hr but may be as long as 240 hr in anuria. However, platinum can be identified in tissues, especially liver, kidney, testes, and intestine, for prolonged periods of time. Sodium thiosulfate decomposes the drug and complexes platinum and thus protects against renal damage and certain other toxicity.

CLADRIBINE

Adenosine, 2-chloro-2'-deoxy-, Leustatin

[4291-63-8] C$_{10}$H$_{12}$ClN$_5$O$_3$ (285.69).

Preparation—By condensing 2,6-dichloropurine with 1-chloro-2-deoxy-3,5-di-*O*-(*p*-tolyl)-α-D-*erythro*-pentofuranose in acetonitrile, the product(s) purified and separated by chromatography and the 7- substituted isomer heated with ammonia-saturated methanol, whereby the free chloro group is replaced by amino, to give the product.

Description—White crystals melting about 212°; solidifies and does not remelt below 300°.

Solubility—Soluble in water and DMF.

Comments—Approved for use in hairy-cell leukemia and is used in the treatment of chronic lymphocytic leukemia and low-grade non-Hodgkin's lymphoma. It is a synthetic antimetabolite that passively crosses the plasma membrane and is activated by deoxycytidine kinase to 2-CdAMP. It is both incorporated into DNA and inhibits DNA single-strand-break repair. Poly adenosine diphosphate-(ADP-) ribosylation of the damaged DNA depletes cellular NAD and ATP and disrupts cell cycling. In clinical trials, 92% of previously untreated patients and 84% of previously treated patients displayed positive clinical responses to a single course of 0.09 mg/kg/day administered for 7 consecutive days.

It is usually administered by continuous intravenous infusion. It has a terminal half-life of elimination of approximately 5.4 hr. It is cleared mainly by the kidney. In patients who have normal renal function, no accumulation of the drug is seen after the normal 7-day course of therapy. Severe neutropenia is seen in approximately 70% of treated patients starting therapy. This is frequently accompanied by fever or infection. Severe anemia appeared in approximately 12% of patients. Headache and rash are also common side effects. A prolonged bone-marrow hypocellularity has been noted in 34% of treated patients. This condition may last for as long as 3 yr, although its significance is unknown. At high doses, it may cause severe, irreversible neurotoxicity, acute nephrotoxicity, and severe bone marrow suppression.

CYCLOPHOSPHAMIDE

2*H*-1,3,2-Oxazaphosphorin-2-amine, *N,N*-bis(2-chloroethyl)-tetrahydro-, 2-oxide, monohydrate; Cytoxan; Neosar

[6055-19-2] C$_7$H$_{15}$Cl$_2$N$_2$O$_2$P.H$_2$O (279.10); anhydrous [50-18-0] (261.09).

Preparation—3-Amino-1-propanol is condensed with *N,N*-bis(2-chloroethyl)phosphoramidic dichloride [(ClCH$_2$CH$_2$CH$_2$)$_2$N—POCl$_2$] in dioxane solution under the catalytic influence of triethylamine. The condensation is double, involving both the hydroxyl and the amino groups, thus effecting the cyclization.

Description—White, crystalline powder; liquefies on loss of its water of crystallization.

Solubility—1 g in approximately 25 mL water; soluble in alcohol.

Comments—An alkylating agent. Unlike other β-chloroethylamino alkylators, it does not cyclize readily to the active ethyleneimonium form until activated by hepatic enzymes. The liver is protected by the further metabolism of activated metabolites to inactive end products. Thus, the substance is stable in the GI tract, tolerated well, and effective by the oral and parenteral routes; it does not cause local vesication, necrosis, phlebitis, or even pain.

Cyclophosphamide is approved for *Stage III and IV, malignant lymphomas, multiple myeloma, leukemias, mycosis fungoides, neuroblastoma, retinoblastoma,* and *carcinoma of the breast.* Alone or in combination, it is the drug of choice for treatment of Burkitt's and non-Hodgkin's lymphomas. It is a component of various first-choice combinations for treatment of Hodgkin's disease, follicular lymphoma, diffuse histiocytic lymphoma, multiple myeloma, squamous cell, and large-cell anaplastic carcinomas, and adenocarcinoma of the lung, small- (oat-) cell lung cancer, soft-tissue sarcomas, embryonal rhabdomyosarcoma, osteogenic sarcoma, retinoblastoma, neuroblastoma, pediatric solid tumors, Ewing's sarcoma, breast tumor, ovarian tumors, and testicular tumors. In combination, it shares alternative drug status with various other drugs for chemotherapy of acute lymphocytic leukemia, testicular cancer, Wilms' tumor, glioblastoma, cervical cancer, head and neck squamous cell carcinoma, islet cell carcinoma, Kaposi's sarcoma, and chronic lymphocytic leukemia. Active metabolites appear in cerebrospinal fluid but in insufficient quantities to treat meningeal leukemia. It is used in high dosages in combination with busulfan as a conditioning regimen prior to allogeneic hematopoietic progenitor cell transplantation in leukemias.

It is an immunosuppressive drug. It has been shown to be of value in the treatment of rheumatoid arthritis, Wegner's granulomatosis, hemophilia A with factor VIII destruction, idiopathic thrombocytopenic purpura (alone or in combination), erythroid aplasia, childhood nephrotic syndrome, pemphigus and vulgaris and dermatomyositis (in combination). It appears to be erratic against systemic lupus erythematosus. It possibly may be efficacious in the management of uveitis. In combination with radiation treatment, it improves the survival of bone marrow and probably of heart transplants. The long-term toxicities of cyclophosphamide should be considered if the drug is to be used as other than a cancer chemotherapeutic agent.

Alopecia occurs in approximately 50% of patients receiving maximal prolonged treatment. Leukopenia is the inevitable side effect and is used as an index of dosage. Other side effects include sterile hemorrhagic cystitis in 20% of those receiving treatment, anorexia, nausea, and vomiting (regardless of route of administration), anaphylactoid reactions, fever, hemolytic-uremic reaction, pulmonary infiltrates and fibrosis, mucosal ulcerations, dizziness, occasional thrombocytopenia, hypoprothrombinemia, nail ridging, cutaneous pigmentation, water intoxication, aspermia in males (3–6 months or longer in onset), anovulation in 30% to 50% of females, and occasional hepatic dysfunction. Bladder telangiectasis and abnormal urinary cytology occur; in long-term use, bladder fibrosis and transitional cell carcinoma occasionally occur. Sodium 2-mercaptoethanesulfonate (Mesna), a synthetic sulfhydryl compound, interacts with acrolein and other metabolites to decrease the incidence and severity of hemorrhagic cystitis. The blood count should be monitored closely during induction and at least weekly thereafter. Cyclophosphamide is relatively platelet sparing; cyclophosphamide is carcinogenic.

It is absorbed orally. It is distributed to the tissues with a volume of distribution greater than the total body water. The drug is metabolized by the hepatic microsomal system to alkylating metabolites that, in turn, are converted to phosphoramide mustard and acrolein. High doses rapidly induce the metabolism of the drug. The plasma half-life is 4 to 6 hr. Although the clinical significance has not been clearly elucidated, caution should be used with concomitant therapy with drugs which induce liver microsomal enzymes, as this may result in an increased pharmacologic effect and toxicity of cyclophosphamide because of increased conversion to active metabolites.

CYCLOSPORINE

For the full monograph, see page 1590.

Comments—Suppresses helper T lymphocytes without significantly affecting suppressor T or B lymphocytes. Thus, it is a selective immunosuppressive drug without the cytotoxicity characteristic of most other immunosuppressive drugs. Because it works only in the primary (afferent) immune phase, it must be administered before exposure to the attacking antigen. It has a modest effect to suppress some humoral immunity.

It is the most efficacious immunosuppressive and is approved for prevention of graft rejection in allogenic transplantation of kidney, liver, or heart. It is less successful in pancreatic, lung, or bone-marrow transplantation. It also is used in the management of severe aplastic anemia, some cases of myasthenia gravis, childhood diabetes (Type I) of recent onset, Graves' disease, Crohn's disease, multiple sclerosis, pemphigus and pemphigoid, dermatomyositis, polymyositis, atopic dermatitis, severe psoriasis, Behçet's disease, uveitis, biliary cirrhosis, and pulmonary sarcoidosis. It usually is employed in combination with a glucocorticoid. Although combination with other immunosuppressives

usually is avoided, in bone-marrow transplantation it commonly is combined with methotrexate.

Nephrotoxicity is a common, serious adverse effect, occurring with an incidence of approximately 25% in renal and 40% in heart transplantations. In renal transplantation, nephrotoxicity is difficult to distinguish from graft rejection. Nonsteroidal anti-inflammatory drugs (NSAIDs), aminoglycosides, trimethoprim, or sulfamethoxozole favor nephrotoxicity. Hepatotoxicity occurs in 4 to 7% of cases. Hypertension occurs in approximately 26% of cases. Benign breast tumors and lymphoproliferative disorders may occur; the latter usually remit after the drug is discontinued.

CNS toxicity includes headache, parethesias (50%), lethargy, weakness, loquaciousness, sleep disorders, confusion, depression, blurred vision, tremors (12%), ataxia, quadraplegia, coma, hallucinations, mania, and convulsions. Severe CNS effects have been associated with low plasma cholesterol, hypomagnesemia, hypokalemia, high-dose methylprednisolone, aluminum overload (from dialysis), and hypertension.

Hirsutism occurs with an incidence of 21% and acne with an incidence of 6%. Gum hyperplasia and diarrhea occur in 3% to 4% of cases. Leukopenia, anemia, and thromboembolism occur rarely. Insulin-dependent diabetes may result from cyclosporine-glucocorticoid combination. Rare anaphylactoid reactions occur during intravenous infusion; polyoxyethylated castor oil in the injection is the usual culprit. There is a danger of severe infection, especially when other immunosuppressives or verapamil are used concurrently. It is teratogenic. It also is exceedingly expensive, which leads some authorities to doubt the cost-effectiveness of the drug. The systemic bioavailability by the oral route averages 27% but varies greatly; the intravenous dose is approximately 1/3 the oral dose. Plasma levels peak in approximately 3.5 hr. In plasma, approximately 90% is protein bound. The pharmacokinetics are multicompartmental. The volume of distribution is 1 to 13 (av 4) L/kg; it is concentration dependent. Nearly all of the drug is metabolized by cytochrome P-450 III in the liver; 94% of the metabolites are excreted into the bile, and 6% are excreted into the urine. The elimination half-life is 10 to 27 hr; there is a circadian periodicity to the elimination rate, the rate being faster in the morning. In infants and children, the volume of distribution and clearance are greater than in adults. Androgens, cimetidine, danazol, erythromycin, ketoconazole, and miconazole each slows the elimination rate and increases plasma levels. Trough plasma levels should be monitored as should be renal function, because many treatment failures result from low concentrations.

CYTARABINE

2(1*H*)-Pyrimidinone, 4-amino-1-β-D-arabinofuranosyl- Cytosine Arabinoside; Cytarabine; Cytosar-U; DepoCyt; Alexan; Arabitin; Aracytin; Aracytine; Citarabina; Iretin; Laracit; Novumtrax; Udicil; Udicil CS

1-β-D-Arabinofuranosylcytosine [147-94-4] $C_9H_{13}N_3O_5$ (243.22).

Preparation—Cytidine is reacted with fuming HNO_3 and the resulting cytidine 2′,3′,5′-trinitrate is boiled in alcohol containing dilute alkali hydroxide to form the inverted 2′-hydroxy compound. Remaining nitrate groups are removed by means of saponification. *CA* 1971; 75:130077q.

Description—White to off-white, odorless, crystalline powder; nonhygroscopic and stable at 40°; melts about 216°.

Solubility—1 g in 5 mL water, 500 mL alcohol, 1000 mL chloroform, or 300 mL methanol.

Comments—A pyrimidine nucleoside antimetabolite that is cytotoxic to a number of cell types. Incorporation of the nucleotidase into DNA inhibits polymerization by termination of strand synthesis. It is S-phase specific. It is approved for use in *acute lymphocytic leukemia*. It is a component of first-choice combinations to treat both *acute* and *chronic myeloblastic leukemias* and *non-Hodgkin's* and *Burkitt's lymphomas*. By the intraventricular route, it is the first alternate to methotrexate to treat *leukemic metastases in the CNS* and also other meningeal soft-tissue metastases. With other drugs it shares alternative-drug status for treatment of *acute lymphocytic leukemia* and *diffuse histiocytic lymphoma*. There does not appear to be cross refractoriness to mercaptopurine, methotrexate, or prednisone. By constant intravenous infusion, or with frequent low doses, it is also effective in the treatment of *preleukemic syndromes*.

This drug is not absorbed sufficiently orally to be maximally effective by this route. Oral bioavailability is less than 0.2. However, it does penetrate into the cerebrospinal fluid and reaches a concentration of as much as 40% of that in plasma. Conversely, intrathecal administration can result in systemic toxicity. In the body, 90% is destroyed by deamination; the plasma elimination half-life is 1 to 3 hr. The elimination half-life in the cerebrospinal fluid is approximately 3.5 hr. Because detoxification takes place throughout the body, the drug may be given in the presence of renal impairment, but the dose should be reduced in hepatic failure.

The primary adverse effects are leukopenia (66%), thrombocytopenia (62%), and, less frequently, anemia and megaloblastosis, which are actually closely related to the therapeutic response and hence, are essentially unavoidable. Bone-marrow depression is more severe when the drug is given in high-dose regimens (15 times the usual dose) and by continuous intravenous infusion than by single injection. However, there are indications that with low rates of infusion an antineoplastic effect can be achieved without serious immunosuppression.

Other side effects are nausea, vomiting (especially after intravenous administration), diarrhea, aphthous ulceration, abdominal pain and bowel necrosis, esophagitis, chest pain, thrombophlebitis at the site of injection, neuritis, arthalgias, flushing, rash, alopecia, sepsis, and teratogenicity. Liver damage may occur. It should be given cautiously and in reduced doses to patients who have liver impairment or bone-marrow depression. It must not be given in combination with methotrexate. Leukocyte and platelet counts should be made daily during the initial course of treatment and at regular intervals during maintenance. High-dose treatment may cause serious neurotoxicity (in peripheral nerves, mood, ideation, memory, cerebellum, and seizures) and skin and ocular toxicities.

DACARBAZINE

1*H*-Imidazole-4-carboxamide, 5-(3,3-dimethyl-l-triazenyl)-, DIC; DTIC-Dome

5-(3,3-Dimethyl-l-triazeno)imidazole-4-carboxamide [4342-03-4] $C_6H_{10}N_6O$ (182.18).

Preparation—5-Diazoimidazole-4-carboxamide, obtained by reaction between 5-aminoimidazole-4-carboxamide and sodium nitrite in acid solution, is reacted with an anhydrous solution of dimethylamine in methanol at 5 to produce dacarbazine (Shealy et al. *J Org Chem* 1962; 17:2150).

Description—Colorless to ivory-colored microcrystalline powder; sensitive to light and heat; reported to melt at 205° and decompose explosively at 250° to 255°; pKa 4.42.

Solubility—Slightly soluble in water or alcohol.

Comments—It is converted in the body to an alkylating metabolite that primarily impairs DNA. It is approved for the treatment of *metastatic malignant melanoma*. The objective response rate is approximately only 20%. It is also a component of first-choice combinations for *Hodgkin's lymphoma* [adriamycin, bleomycin, vinblastine, dacarbazine (ABVD)], and is useful in some adult soft-tissue tumors. With several drugs it shares alternative status for *islet-cell carcinoma* and *neuroblastoma*.

The most serious adverse effect is bone-marrow depression, which occasionally is fatal; leukocytes and platelets are the most affected, anemia being mild, when it occurs. Careful monitoring of leukocytes, platelets, and erythrocytes is required. If there is preexisting bone-marrow depression, or if another bone-marrow suppressant drug is in use or has been used within 4 wk, the dose must be reduced. Anorexia, nausea, and vomiting lasting 1 to 12 hr occur in more than 90% of recipients of the drug, thus aggressive antiemetic therapy is required. A flu-like syndrome accompanied by fever as high as 39° can occur; myalgia and malaise sometimes occurs approximately 1 wk after large doses and may continue for 1 to 3 wk. Facial flushing, facial paresthesias, and alopecia also have been observed. Abnormalities in liver or renal function have been reported, and the drug should be used cautiously in patients who have liver or renal damage. Extravasation of dacarbazine may cause pain and local necrosis. The drug is mutagenic and teratogenic.

It is eliminated with a terminal half-life of 5 hr. Dacarbazine requires initial activation by the cytochrome P450 system of the liver through an *N*-demethylation reaction. Approximately 50% of an intravenous dose is metabolized in the liver; by the oral route, little remains unchanged, thus making the intravenous route necessary. Approxi-

mately 40% of the drug appears unchanged in the urine within 6 hr. The unmetabolized drug is excreted in the urine by tubular secretion. The volume of distribution is larger than total body water.

DACTINOMYCIN

2-bis[Cyclo(N-methyl-L-valyl-sarcosyl-L-prolyl-D-valyl-L-threonyl)]-1,9 dimethyl-4,6 3H-phenoxazinone; Dactinomycin; Meractinomycin; Cosmegen; Actinomycin-D; Lyovac; Ac-De; Dacmozen

Actinomycin D [50-76-0]; $C_{62}H_{86}N_{12}O_{16}$ (1255.43).

Caution—Handle with exceptional care, to prevent inhaling particles of it and exposing the skin to it.

Preparation—Elaborated during the culture of *Streptomyces parvulus*. After extracting from the fermentation broth, it is purified through chromatographic and crystallization processes. US Pat 2,378,876.

Description—Bright-red crystalline powder; light sensitive and should be protected appropriately; should be protected from excessive heat and moisture; melts about 246° with the decomposition; contains in each milligram an amount of antibiotic activity of not less than 900 µg of dactinomycin.

Solubility—1 g in approximately 8 mL alcohol, 25 mL water (at 10°), 1000 mL water (at 37°), or approximately 1666 mL ether.

Comments—An antineoplastic drug that inhibits DNA-dependent RNA polymerase, approved for use in *Wilms' tumor, rhabdomyosarcoma, Ewing's sarcoma*, and *carcinoma of the testis and the uterus*. It is a component of first-choice combinations for treatment of *choriocarcinoma, embryonal rhabdomyosarcoma*, and *Wilms' tumor*. Tumors that fail to respond to systemic treatment sometimes respond to local perfusion. Dactinomycin potentiates radiotherapy (*radiation recall*) and is a secondary immunosuppressive.

Nausea and vomiting are usual and occur within the first few hours after administration of dactinomycin and require antiemetic therapy. Anorexia, abdominal pain, diarrhea, proctitis, and GI ulceration follow. The patient also may experience malaise, fatigue, lethargy, myalgia, and fever. Cheilitis, ulcerative stomatitis, pharyngitis, esophagitis, and proctitis are common. Because agranulocytosis, leukopenia, pancytopenia, thrombocytopenia, and anemia frequently occur, and *must be monitored closely*. Cutaneous eruptions, alopecia, hyperpigmentation, and erythema also occur. Anaphylaxis has been reported. Side effects appear to be reversible. The drug is toxic locally, and phlebitis and cellulitis may occur at the site of injection; extravasation may cause serious local tissue damage. Venous thrombosis also may result from local effects.

Half of the dose is excreted intact into the bile and 10% into the urine; the half-life is approximately 36 hr. The drug does not pass the blood–brain barrier.

DAUNORUBICIN HYDROCHLORIDE

5,12-Naphthacenedione, (8S-*cis*)-8-acetyl-10-[(3-amino-2,3,6-trideoxy-α-L-*lyxo*-hexanopyranosyl)oxy]-7,8,9,10-tetrahydro-6,8,11-trihydroxy-10-methoxy-, hydrochloride; Cerubidine; Daunomycin HCl; Daunoblastin; Daunoblastina; Rubilem; Trixilem

[23541-50-6] $C_{27}H_{29}NO_{10} \cdot HCl$ (563.99).

Preparation—An antibiotic produced by *S peuceticus* or *S coeruleorubidus*.

Description—Red needles decomposing about 190°; pH (aqueous solution containing 5 mg/mL) 4.5 to 6.5.

Comments—Intercalates into DNA, inhibits topoisomerase II, produces oxygen radicals, and inhibits DNA synthesis. It can prevent cell division in doses that do not interfere with nucleic acid synthesis.

It is approved for use in acute *nonlymphocytic leukemia* in adults and for *acute lymphocytic leukemia* in adults and in children. In combination with other drugs it is included in the first-choice chemotherapy of *acute myelocytic leukemia* in adults (for induction of remission), *acute lymphocytic leukemia,* and the *acute phase of chronic myelocytic leukemia.* The drug is not given as a single agent.

Acutely, it causes nausea, vomiting and fever; rarely, it causes convulsions, cardiac dysrhythmias, S-T depression, and pulmonary edema; occasionally, it is fatal. Phlebitis at the site of injection or tissue necrosis from extravasation may occur. It also colors the urine red for 1 to 2 days. Delayed toxicity includes frequent bone-marrow depression (with leukopenia and thrombocytopenia), which may be severe, and a dose-limiting, irreversible congestive heart failure (CHF). Other toxicities include stomatitis and aphthous ulceration, anorexia, hemorrhagic mucositis enterocolitis, abdominal pain, fever, rashes, usually reversible alopecia (80% of recipients), renal tubular damage, and hematuria. Cardiotoxicity also may be delayed. Rhythm disturbances are not related to cumulative dose, but a late CHF is frequent when the cumulative dose exceeds 550 mg/m^2. The onset of failure may occur as long as 1 to 6 months after discontinuation of treatment. Daunorubicin is teratogenic, mutagenic, and carcinogenic. Monitoring of blood-cell counts, renal function, and electrocardiogram (ECG) is required.

Oral absorption is poor, and it must be given intravenously. The half-life of distribution is 45 min and of elimination, approximately 19 hr. The half-life of its active metabolite, daunorubicinol, is approximately 27 hr. Daunorubicin is metabolized mostly in the liver and also secreted into the bile (ca 40%). Dosage must be reduced in liver or renal insufficiencies.

DAUNORUBICIN CITRATE LIPOSOMAL

DaunoXome

Preparation—See *Stealth Liposomes*, D Lasic & F Martin, CRC Press, Boca Raton, FL, 1995.

Description—*Daunorubicin*, as the citrate salt, encapsulated in liposomes.

Comments—A liposomal preparation formulated to maximize the delivery and selectivity of daunorubicin to solid tumors *in situ*. Indicated as a first line cytotoxic therapy for advanced HIV-associated Kaposi's sarcoma. While in the circulation, the liposome formulation protects the drug from chemical and enzymatic degradation, minimizes protein binding, and generally decreases uptake by normal (non-reticuloendothelial system) tissues. Increased cytotoxicity may also be due to increased permeability of the tumor neovasculature to some particles in the size range of daunorubicin citrate liposome. Once within the tumor environment, daunorubicin is released over time enabling it to exert its antineoplastic activity. Liposomal encapsulation substantially affects the functional properties relative to those of the unencapsulated drug.

Primary toxicities of daunorubicin citrate liposome are myelosuppression, mainly of the granulocytes (which may be severe), and cardiac toxicity, which is usually cardiomyopathy associated with a decrease of the left ventricular ejection fraction (LVEF). Measurement of LVEF should be performed at total cumulative doses of 320 mg/m^2, 480 mg/m^2 and every 240 mg/m^2 thereafter. A triad of back pain, flushing, and chest tightness has been reported in 13.8% of the patients (16/116) treated in the randomized clinical trial and in 2.7% of treatment cycles (27/994). Dosage should be reduced in patients with impaired hepatic function. Pharmacokinetics of liposomal daunorubicin differs significantly from conventional daunorubicin hydrochloride. The liposomal form has has smaller steady-state volume of distribution 6.4 L and clearance of 17 ml/min. These differences result in a higher daunorubicin exposure (in terms of plasma AUC) from the liposomal form. The apparent elimination half-life of daunorubicin citrate liposome is 4.4 hours.

DEXRAZOXANE

2,6-Piperazinedione, (S)-4,4'-(1-methyl-1,2-ethanediyl)bis-, Zinecard, Razoxin

[24584-09-6] C$_{11}$H$_{16}$N$_4$O$_4$ (268.27).

Preparation—The *S*-isomer of propane-1,2-diamine is treated with excess chloroacetic acid to yield the tetra-carboxymethyl derivative, which is cyclized with formamide at each pair of acetic acid fragments to form a bis-imide (2,6-piperazinedione), the title product. US Pat 3,941,791 (1976).

Description—White crystals that melt at approximately 194°. Octanol-water partition coefficient 0.025; pK$_a$ 2.1.

Solubility—In milligrams per milliliter: water, 10 to 12; 0.1 *N* HCl, 35 to 43; 0.1 *N* NaOH, 25 to 34; 10% alcohol, 6.7 to 10; methanol, 1; 0.1 *M* citrate buffer pH 4, 9.7 to 14.5; 0.1 *M* borate buffer pH 9, 8.7 to 13. Practically insoluble in nonpolar organic solvents. If the pH is greater than 7, it rapidly degrades.

Comments—Approved for reduction of the incidence or severity of cardiomyopathy associated with doxorubicin use in women who have breast cancer and whose total doxorubicin dose has reached 300 mg/m^2. It is a cyclic ethylenediamine tetra-acetic acid (EDTA) derivative that penetrates cell membranes. Intracellularly, the ring opens and it chelated iron, thereby interfering with the free-radical generation that contributes to doxorubicin cardiomyopathy.

Peak plasma concentrations are reached 15 to 30 min after a 15-min infusion of a 500-mg/m^2 dose. It is not bound to plasma proteins, and approximately 42% of the above dose is cleared in the urine. When started with the seventh course of 5-FU, adriamycin, cyclophosphamide (FAC) therapy in patients continuing the therapy, it reduced the incidence of CHF from 22% to 3%. In other studies, it was shown to reduce loss of cardiac function and the risk of heart attack.

It may add to the myelosuppressive action of anticancer regimens. Evidence also exists that this drug will reduce the efficacy of FAC therapy if used too early. It should be used only in patients who have received a cumulative dose of 300 mg/m^2. The recommended dosage ratio of dexrazoxane:doxorubicin is 10:1 (eg, 500 mg/m$_2$ dexrazoxane:50 mg/m$_2$ doxorubicin) given by slow IV push or IV infusion. Proper administration is required for maximum protective effect. After completing the infusion of dexrazoxane, and prior to a total elapsed time of 30 minutes (from the beginning of the dexrazoxane infusion), the IV injection of doxorubicin should be given.

DOCETAXEL

(2R,3S)-N-Carboxy-3-phenylisoserine, N-tert-butyl ester, 13-ester with 5β,20-epoxy-1,2α,4,7β,10β,13α-hexahydroxytax-11-en-9-one 4-acetate-2-benzoate; Taxotere; Daxotel; Dexotel; Oncodocel

[114977-28-5] C$_{43}$H$_{53}$NO$_{14}$ (807.89).

Preparation—Complex synthesis with a precursor obtained from the needles of the yew plant. US Pat 4,814,470 (1989); *J Org Chem* 1991; 56:6939.

Description—White to off-white powder that melts about 232°.

Solubility—Practically insoluble in water; highly lipophilic.

Comments—Active as a single agent for treatment of locally advanced or metastatic breast cancer after failing anthracycline-based therapy or in locally advanced or metastatic non-small lung cancer failing platinum-based chemotherapy. It induced clinical response in approximately 45% of patients who had advanced breast cancer and who progressed after anthracycline treatment with approximately 2% complete responses. Also approved combined with cisplatin as first-line therapy for unresectable, locally advanced or metastatic non-small cell lung cancer and in combination with prednisone for hormone refractory metastatic prostate cancer. It promotes the inappropriate assembly of microtubules and prevents their disassembly. Cells experiencing this, arrest in mitosis.

After a 1-hr infusion, its distribution is characterized by three compartments with half-lives of 4 min, 36 min, and 11.1 hr. In the blood, it is approximately 94% protein bound. Approximately 80% of an administered dose is excreted after 1 wk, with approximately 75% appearing in the feces. The excreted drug is primarily the major metabolite that is produced by cytochrome P-450 oxidation of the tertbutyl ester group. In patients who have moderate hepatic impairment, total clearance of the drug reduced 27%, increasing the AUC 38%.

Neutropenia is the major toxicity and occurs in virtually every patient. Deaths due to sepsis are the most common drug-related lethality, as high as 11% in patients who have abnormal liver function. Frequent monitoring of blood counts is essential so that doses can be adjusted. The drug should not be administered to patients who have neutrophil counts less than 1500/mm^3. Deaths due to thrombocytopenia and bleeding were seen in patients who had severe liver function impairment. Pain, paresthesia, and asthenia are reported frequently, and nausea and vomiting is mild to moderate. Hypersensivity reactions (characterized by hypotension and/or bronchospasm, or generalized rash/erythema) and severe fluid retention may occur; therefore, all patients require a 3 to 5-day dexamethasone regimen beginning one day prior to initiation of therapy.

DOXORUBICIN HYDROCHLORIDE

5,12-Naphthacenedione, (8S-cis)-10-[(3-amino-2,3,6-trideoxy-α-L-lyxo-hexopyransoyl)oxy]-7,8,9,10-tetrahydro-6,8,11-trihydroxy-8-(hydroxyacetyl)-1-methoxy-, hydrochloride; Hydroxydaunorubicin Hydrochloride; Adriamycin; Rubex; Doxorubicin

14-Hydroxydaunorubicin hydrochloride [25316-40-9] $C_{27}H_{29}NO_{11}$.HCl (579.99).

Preparation—An anthracycline antibiotic isolated from cultures of *Streptomyces peucetius var caesius* (US Pat 3,590,028). It differs from *Daunorubicin* only in having a hydroxyacetyl group in place of the acetyl group in daunorubicin, in position 8.

Description—Red-orange, crystalline powder; almost odorless; hygroscopic; melts about 205° with decomposition; pKa 8.22.

Solubility—1 g dissolves in approximately 10 mL water or approximately 2000 mL alcohol.

Comments—Approved for use in *acute lymphoblastic* and *myeloblastic leukemias; Hodgkin's* and *non-Hodgkin's lymphomas; Wilms' tumor; neuroblastoma; sarcomas,* and *breast, ovarian, transitional cell, bronchogenic, gastric,* and *thyroid carcinomas.* It has the widest anti neoplastic spectrum and usefulness of the antineoplastic drugs. It intercalates the base pairs of the DNA double helix, thus inhibiting nucleic acid synthesis, inhibiting topoisomerase II and produceing oxygen radicals. Administered alone, it is the drug of first choice for the treatment of *thyroid adenoma* and *primary hepatocellular carcinoma.* It is a component of 31 first-choice combinations for the treatment of *ovarian, endometrial,* and *breast tumors; bronchogenic oat-cell carcinoma, non-small-cell lung carcinoma; gastric adenocarcinoma; retinoblastoma; neuroblastoma; mycosis fungoides; pancreatic carcinoma; prostatic carcinoma; bladder carcinoma; myeloma; diffuse histiocytic lymphoma; Wilms' tumor; Hodgkin's disease; adrenal tumors; osteogenic sarcoma; soft-tissue sarcoma; Ewing's sarcoma; rhabdomyosarcoma;* and *acute lymhocytic leukemia.* It is an alternative drug for the treatment of *islet cell, cervical, testicular,* and *adrenocortical cancer.* It is also an immunosuppressant, but its status remains to be determined. Tumor resistance to this drug may be suppressed by verapamil.

There is a high incidence of bone-marrow depression, which manifests itself mainly as a neutropenia that is most severe 10 to 14 days after treatment and lasts approximately 7 days; a white-cell count as low as 1000/mm^3 is to be expected. Monitoring of leukocytes and erythrocytes and signs of intercurrent infection is mandatory. Other frequent adverse effects are nausea and vomiting and reversible alopecia. Stomatitis and esophagitis may occur 5 to 10 days after treatment. Anorexia and diarrhea occur occasionally. Rarely, there may be hypersensitivity (fever, chills, urticaria), hyperpigmentation of the nails, lacrimation, conjunctivitis, and recurrence of skin reactions caused by previous radiotherapy. Hyperuricemia from rapid lysis of neoplastic cells may occur.

A serious toxicity is acute left-ventricular irreversible cardiomyopathy, which may be treated with digitalis. An early change in ECG patterns is not prodromal of the more serious CHF. This cardiotoxicity is most likely to occur with patients in whom the cumulated dose is 550 mg/m^2. Prior radiotherapy to the chest, concomitant cyclophasphamide therapy, or hyperthermia may cause the cardiomyopathy to occur with a total dose as low as 400 mg/m^2. Antineoplastic activity has been dissociated from cardiotoxicity in certain chemical congeners that may eventually replace this drug. Toxicity appears to result from oxidant

and free-radical metabolites. Certain antioxidants, such as dexrazoxane (ICRF-187), protect against cardiotoxicity.

It is locally toxic and causes venous streaking, and extravasation results in pain, cellulitis, and sloughing. Its natural color may cause the urine and other body secretions to be red. It may potentiate hemorrhagic cystitis caused by cyclophosphamide, mucositis by radiotherapy, hepatotoxicity by 6-MP and the bone-marrow depressant actions of other antineoplastic drugs.

It is absorbed poorly and must be administered intravenously. The pharmacokinetics are multicompartmental. Distribution phases have half-lives of 12 min and 3.3 hr. The elimination half-life is approximately 30 hr. Forty to 50% is secreted into the bile. Most of the remainder is metabolized in the liver, partly to an active metabolite (doxorubicinol), but a few percent is excreted into the urine. In the presence of liver impairment, the dose should be reduced.

DOXORUBICIN HYDROCHLORIDE LIPOSOMAL

Doxil

Preparation—See *Stealth Liposomes,* D Lasic & F Martin, CRC Press, Boca Raton, FL, 1995.

Description—*Doxorubicin hydrochloride* encapsulated in liposomes.

Comments—A liposomal coated core of doxorubicin coated with a polyethylene glycol derivative. The polymer coating masks recognition by the reticuloendothelial cells, resulting in increased blood circulation time and half-life. Active for AIDS-related Kaposi's sarcoma in patients with disease that has progressed on prior therapy or who are intolerant to therapy. Also indicated for treatment of metastatic ovarian cancer refractory to paclitaxel and platinum-based therapy.

Adverse reactions are similar to doxorubicin. Dose limiting effect is severe myelosuppression. Palmar-plantar erythrodysesthesia is cumulative and consists of painful red palms and soles progressing to ulceration if doses are not reduced. Acute infusion-related reactions (flushing, shortness of breath, facial swelling, headache, chills, back pain, tightness in the chest or throat, and/or hypotension) have occurred in up to 10% of treated patients. Cardiomyopathy may be lessened, but not eliminated. Dosage must be reduced with impaired hepatic function.

EPIRUBICIN HYDROCHLORIDE

5,12-Naphthacenedione, 10-[3-amino-2,3,6-trideoxy-α-L-ara-bino-exopyranosyl)oxy]-7,8,9,10-tetrahydro-6,8,11-trihydroxy-8-(hydroxyacetyl)-1-methoxy-, hydrochloride; Ellence, Pharmorubicin

[56390-09-1] $C_{27}H_{29}NO_{11}$.HCl (579.98).

Preparation—*J Med Chem,* 1977; 18:703 and US Pat 4,058,519 (1977).

Description—Orange-red solid melting about 185° (dec). [α]$^{20}_D$ + 274° (c = 0.01, methanol). It is the 4'-epimer of doxorubicin.

Solubility—Solutions are light sensitive.

Comments—Anthracycline agent that forms a complex with DNA by intercalation between base pairs triggering DNA cleavage by topoisomerase II, thus causing inhibition of DNA and protein synthesis. Indicated as a component of adjuvant therapy in patients with evidence of axillary node tumor involvement following resection of primary breast cancer. Also shown to be effective in the treatment of small cell lung cancer, non-small cell lung cancer, non-Hodgkin's lymphoma, Hodgkin's disease, gastric cancer, bladder cancer, ovarian cancer, prostatic cancer, and primary hepatocelluar carcinoma.

Extensively and rapidly metabolized by the liver; dosage adjustments required with liver or severe renal impairment. Primary dose limiting toxicity consists of dose-dependent, reversible leukopenia and/or neutropenia, with nadir reached 10 to 14 days from drug administration. Other adverse effects include acute (sinus tachycardia and/or ECG abnormalities) or delayed cardiotoxicity (decreased left ventricular ejection fraction and/or signs and symptoms of congestive heart failure). Life-threatening cardiotoxicity is dependent on the cumulative dose of epirubicin, and usually occurs late in therapy or within 2 to 3 months after completion of treatment. The estimated risk of epirubicin-treated patients developing clinically evident CHF was 0.9% at a cumulative dose of 550 mg/m^2, 1.6% at 700 mg/m^2, and 3.3% at 900 mg/m^2. The risk increases steeply after 900 mg/m^2. Other adverse effects include hair loss, nausea, vomiting, diarrhea, mouth sores.

ESTRAMUSTINE PHOSPHATE SODIUM

Estra-1,3,5(10)-triene-3,17-diol(17β), 3-[bis(2-chloroethyl)carbamate] 17-, (dihydrogen phosphate), disodium salt; Emcyt; Estracyte

[52205-73-9] $C_{23}H_{30}Cl_2NNa_2O_6P$ (564.35).

Preparation—A compound of estradiol with a nitrogen mustard moiety.

Description—Off-white powder.

Solubility—Freely soluble in water or in methanol; slightly soluble in chloroform or in anhydrous ethanol; pH of 0.5% solution, 8.5 to 10.

Comments—An alkylating agent that is approved for metastatic and/or progressive cancer of the prostate, but is also active for advanced breast cancer. It causes nausea and vomiting, delayed bone-marrow depression, mild gynecomastia, perianal anesthesia, thrombophlebitis, occasional myocardial infarction, hypertension, hypoglycemia, and hepatotoxicity. It is nearly 75% absorbed orally and metabolized in the liver. It is excreted in the urine, bile, and feces with a prolonged half-life of about 20–24 hr.

ETOPOSIDE

Vepesid, VP16

9-[(4,6-O-Ethylidene-β-D-glucopyranosyl)oxy]-5,8,8a,9-tetrahydro-5-(4-hydroxy-3,5-dimethoxyphenyl)furo[3',4':6,7]-naphtho[2,3-d]-1,3-dioxol-6(5aH)-one [33419-42-0] $C_{29}H_{32}O_{13}$ (588.56).

Preparation—A semisynthetic derivative of podophyllotoxin. See *J Med Chem* 1971, 14:936.

Description—White to yellow-brown powder; melts about 221°.

Solubility—Soluble in methanol or in chloroform; slightly soluble in ethanol; sparingly soluble in water or in ether.

Comments—Damages DNA, most likely by means of topoisomerase II cleavage, and arrests the cell cycle primarily in phase G$_2$, although it has some action in late S and M. It is approved for *refractory testicular tumors* and *small-cell lung cancer*. Alone, it is one of two drugs of choice for the treatment of *Kaposi's sarcoma* and one of three for *non-Hodgkin's lymphoma*. It also is a component of first-choice combinations to treat *oat-cell bronchogenic carcinoma* and *refractory disseminated germ-cell tumors*. It is an alternative drug for use against *acute lymphocytic leukemia, acute myelocytic leukemia, Hodgkin's disease, Wilms' tumor, choriocarcinoma, diffuse histiocytic lymphoma, Ewing's sarcoma, hepatocellular carcinoma, neuroblastoma, non-Hodgkin's lymphoma,* and *non-small cell bronchogenic carcinoma.*

Acute adverse effects of mild nausea and vomiting, chills and fever; postural hypotension, tachycardia, palpitations, and bronchospasm occur during and after rapid intravenous infusion. Delayed toxicity includes leukopenia (60–90%), thrombocytopenia (28–41%), anemia (≤ 33%), diarrhea, fever, alopecia, rash, stomatitis, Stevens-Johnson syndrome, various other allergic responses, hepatotoxicity (3%), and peripheral neuropathy. It increases the hypoprothrombopenic affects of warfarin.

Oral absorption is 25% to 75%. In plasma, approximately 94% is protein bound, and the concentration in the cerebrospinal fluid is less than

10% of that in plasma. Distribution is slow; the initial half-life being approximately 1.5 hr. Approximately 35% is excreted unchanged in the urine and approximately 6% into bile. A hydroxyacid metabolite is excreted in the bile, and the sulfate and glucuronide metabolites are excreted in urine. The elimination half-life is 4 to 11 hr. Dosage reduction is required for elevated bilirubin or liver impairment.

ETRETINATE—page 1291.

EXEMESTANE

Androsta-1,4-diene-3,17-dione, 6-methylene-, Aromasin

[107868-30-4] $C_{20}H_{24}O_2$ (296.41).

Preparation—US Pat 3,622,841 (1987).

Description—White to slightly yellow crystalline powder melting about 190°.

Solubility—Freely soluble in DMF; soluble in methanol; practically insoluble in water.

Comments—irreversible, selective aromatase inhibitor that acts as false substrate for aromatase converting reactive alkylating intermediates that bind covalently to the substrate binding site of the enzyme thus inactivating it. Used in the treatment of advanced breast cancer in postmenopausal women whose disease has progressed following tamoxifen therapy.

Exemestane selectively inhibits the conversion of androgens to estrogens and does not affect synthesis of adrenal corticosteroid, aldosterone, or thyroid hormone. Adverse effects include hot flushes (flashes), nausea, fatigue, increased sweating, increased appetite, excessive weight gain, and increases in liver function tests.

FLOXURIDINE

Uridine, 2'-deoxy-5-fluoro-, FUDR

[50-91-9] $C_9H_{11}FN_2O_5$ (246.19).

Preparation—*J Am Chem Soc* 1959; 81:4112.

Description—White to off-white, odorless solid; melts about 151°.

Solubility—1 g in 3 mL water, 12 mL alcohol, or more than 10,000 mL chloroform or ether; pH of 2% solution, 4.0 to 5.5.

Comments—In the body it is converted into a false nucleotide that interferes with the synthesis of DNA. It also is converted to fluorouracil, so that it potentially has all the actions and uses of Fluorouracil. It is approved for *GI adenocarcinoma with metastasis to the liver*. However, currently, its use is restricted to regional intraarterial infusion of carcinomas that are judged incurable by surgery or other chemotherapy, mainly *colorectal cancer metastatic to the liver* and *hepatocellular carcinoma*. In these uses, it does not appear to be superior to fluorouracil.

The most frequent adverse effects are nausea, vomiting, diarrhea, enteritis, localized erythema along the course of infused artery, leukopenia, and elevation in serum transaminase, alkaline phosphatase, bilirubin, and lactic dehydrogenase. Other effects are abdominal cramps, anorexia, duodenal ulcer, duodenitis, gastroenteritis, pharyngitis, glossitis, gastritis, alopecia, dermatitis, hyperpigmentation, edema, peeling of the skin, pruritus, various rashes and skin ulceration, abscesses, ataxia, blurred vision, convulsions, depression, hemiplegia, hiccoughs, lethargy, nystagmus, malaise, pain, vertigo, asthenia, dysuria, fever, hypoadrenalism, thrombocytopenia, prothrombinopenia, hypoproteinemia, and aberrations in the sedimentation rate and BSP test.

It is contraindicated in patients who have cachexia, potentially serious infections, or bone-marrow depression. The drug is metabolized mainly in the body, but some is excreted unchanged in the urine.

FLUDARABINE PHOSPHATE

9*H*-Purin-6-amine, 2-fluoro-9-(5-*O*-phosphono-β-D-arabinofuranosyl)-, Fludara

[75607-67-9] $C_{10}H_{13}FN_5O_7P$ (365.21).
Preparation—US Pat 4,357,324.
Description—White powder.
Solubility—Soluble in water.
Comments—Supplied as the monophosphate but is rapidly dephosphorylated *in vivo* to yield the free nucleoside that is actively transported into susceptible cells. Once rephosphorylated and part of the nucleotide pool of the cell, fludarabine is a potent inhibitor of DNA and RNA synthesis, by inhibition of many enzymes involved in nucleic acid synthesis. The synthesis of DNA appears to be inhibited at lower intracellular concentrations of fludarabine nucleotides. Fludarabine is approved for use in *chronic lymphocytic leukemia* that has proved refractory to at least one alkylating agent. It also has activity against *Hodgkin's* and *non-Hodgkin's lymphomas, mycosis fungoides,* and *macroglobulinemia.* Fludarabine, administered IV, has a short initial half-live of approximately 80 min. The most severe adverse effects involve a CNS syndrome and suppression of the hematopoietic system. The CNS syndrome includes a delayed blindness, coma, and death that appear at high doses. This syndrome is rare in patients receiving the recommended dose for chronic lymphocytic leukemia. Severe bone-marrow suppression results in decreased counts of neutrophil (< 500/μl in 59% of patients), hematocrit, and platelets in 50 to 60% of patients. The myelosuppression may be cumulative. It also is reported to cause pulmonary dysfunction, skin rashes, and pruritus.

FLUOROURACIL

2,4(1*H*,3*H*)-Pyrimidinedione, 5-fluoro-, 5-FU; Adrucil; Efudex; Fluoroplex

5-Fluorouracil [51-21-8] $C_4H_3FN_2O_2$ (130.08).
Preparation—Potassium fluoroacetate is reacted with methyl bromide to form methyl fluoroacetate that is then subjected to a Claisen condensation with methyl formate and sodium ethoxide to produce the potassium enolate of the methyl ester of α-fluoromalonaldehydic acid (I). Cyclization of I is affected through condensation under anhydrous conditions with *S*-benzylisothiourea. The resulting 2-(benzylthio) compound is hydrolyzed readily in the presence of acid to form fluorouracil. US Pat 2,802,005.
Description—White to practically white, practically odorless, crystalline powder; stable when exposed to air; decomposes about 282°.
Solubility—1 g in 80 mL water, 170 mL alcohol, or 55 mL methanol; practically insoluble in chloroform, ether, or benzene; solubility in aqueous solutions increases with increasing pH.
Comments—A congener of uracil that acts both as a surrogate and as an antimetabolite of that nucleotide. Its metabolite, 5-fluorodeoxyuridine-5'-monophosphate (FUMP), blocks the synthesis of thymidylic acid and hence of deoxyribonucleic acid; it also is incorporated into RNA. Uracil is used preferentially by neoplastic tissue; thus the antimetabolite has some degree of selectivity for the neoplasm. It is approved for palliative treatment of *cancer of the colon, rectum, stomach, breast,* and *pancreas.* It is not curative, but it may bring approximately regression of a number of neoplasms. It is the antineoplastic of choice of the treatment of *colorectal cancer.*

In combination with other drugs it provides chemotherapy of first choice in the treatment of *breast cancer, islet-cell tumors, squamous cell carcinoma* of the *head* and *neck, non-small-cell carcinoma* of the *lung, pancreatic* and *gastric carcinomas, primary hepatocellular carcinoma, testicular* and *prostatic carcinomas,* and *bladder tumors.* It shares alternative-drug status for the treatment of *endometrial carcinoma; squamous cell tumors of the head, neck,* and *cervix;* and *ovarian tumors.* It

may be useful in the treatment of *neoplasms of the gallbladder* and, to a lesser extent, those of the esophagus, larynx, thyroid, and pharynx. Remissions of as long as 4 yr have been noted in a few instances, although the average is a few months.

The drug also is used topically in the treatment of precancerous dermatoses, especially *actinic keratosis,* for which it is the treatment of choice if the lesions are multiple. Even lesions that are not clinically discernible respond. For this reason, the drug is applied to the entire affected area. Healing continues for 1 to 2 months after treatment. The drug does not affect nonkeratotic lesions. It is a secondary (efferent) immunosuppressive agent and therefore has not been used in organ transplantation.

The drug is toxic, approximately two-thirds of patients showing signs of toxicity; the mortality rate is approximately 3% when treatment is initiated by daily doses. When the drug is administered by intravenous bolus, leukopenia is the principal adverse effect, usually occurring between day 7 and day 14, with a nadir at days 21 to 25. Leucocytes readily recover if the dose is lowered promptly. Thrombocytopenia is less frequent, with a nadir occurring between day 7 and day 17. Aphthous ulceration may occur or the appearance of diarrhea are signs that therapy should be discontinued temporarily. Other toxic effects include vomiting, nausea, GI ulceration (the dose-limiting effect of constant infusion), alopecia, dermatitis, hyperpigmentation, pharyngitis, esophagitis, cerebellar ataxia (sometimes irreversible), and epistaxis. Lassitude and asthenia, lasting from 12 to 35 hr after an injection, may occur; severe CNS depression may occur in patients who have familial pyrimidinemia. When the drug is administered as a continuous low-dose protracted infusion, the dose-limiting toxicity is hand-foot syndrome, which involves painful and erythematous desquamation of the palms and soles. Topically, it may induce photosensitization and always erythema, scaling, fissuring, tenderness, and usually erosion, ulceration, necrosis, and re-epithelialization as the result of the therapeutic action, although some persons appear to be resistant to this effect. The antineoplastic effect as well as the toxicities are potentiated by concomitant administration with leucovorin (folinic acid).

By the oral route, there is poor absorption and variable first-pass elimination of the drug by the gut and liver, so that intravenous administration is required. At least 60% is metabolized to CO_2, but more than 15% is excreted into the urine. The drug enters the cerebrospinal fluid and effusions. The plasma half-life is approximately 10 min, but the active metabolite, FUMP, may be detectable for days.

FLUOXYMESTERONE—page 1471.

FLUTAMIDE

Propaneamide, 2-methyl-*N*-[4-fluoro-3-(trifluoromethyl)phenyl]-, Eulexin

[13311-84-7] $C_{11}H_{11}F_3N_2O_3$ (276.21).
Preparation—See *J Med Chem* 1967; 10:93.
Description—Yellow crystals melting about 110°.
Solubility—Practically insoluble in water.
Comments—Approved for use in Stage D or metastatic prostate cancer in combination with LHRH analogs. It is a nonsteroidal antiandrogen that acts by inhibiting androgen uptake or nuclear binding at target tissues. When used with goserelin or leuprolide an radiation, in patients who have fairly advanced prostate cancer (StageB2-C), this drug significantly lowered local failure rate against radiation alone and with hormonal therapy reduced distant metastasis from 36% to 16%; it also increased disease-free survival time in patients receiving complete hormone therapy to 4.4 yr versus 2.6 yr for those receiving radiation alone.

It is absorbed rapidly and completely when taken orally; it is also metabolized rapidly. The major plasma metabolite is the pharmacologically active alpha hydroxylate, which accounts for 23% of the dose 1 hr after administration. The half-life of this metabolite is approximately 6 hr in normal healthy volunteers, approximately 9 hr at steady state in the elderly. The drug itself accounts for approximately only 2.5% of the drug in plasma 1 hr after administration. Both flutamide and the alpha hydroxylate are >90% plasma protein bound. In patients who have renal impairment, the half-life of the major metabolite was slightly prolonged.

Hepatotoxicity has been noted with the use of flutamide, and hepatic function should be monitored. Treatment should be discontinued if serum transaminase levels exceed 2 or 3 times the normal upper limit. Likewise, methemoglobinemia, hemolytic anemia, and cholestatic jaundice have been noted. Malignant breast neoplasms and gynecomastia have occurred in male patients taking drug. Urine discoloration and photosensitivity also occur with drug intake.

FULVESTRANT

Estra-1,3,5(10)-triene-3,17-diol, (7α,17β)-7-[9-[(4,4,5,5,5-penta-fluoropentyl)sulfinyl]nonyl]-, Faslodex

129453-61-8] $C_{32}H_{47}F_5O_3S$ (606.77).

Preparation—*J Med Chem*, 1991; 34:1624-30.

Description—White powder.

Comments—an estrogen antagonist without known agonist effects that competitively binds to and downregulates estrogen receptors in human breast cancer cells. It inhibits the growth of tamoxifen-resistant as well as estrogen-sensitive human breast cancer (MCF-7) cell lines in vitro and in vivo. It does not appear to exhibit peripheral steroidal effects as there are no changes in concentrations of follicle-stimulating hormone (FSH) and luteinizing hormone (LH) in post-menopausal women receiving 250 mg of fulvestrant IM monthly. Peak plasma concentrations of fulvestrant are attained approximately 7 days after IM administration and persist for at least 1 month. Steady-state plasma fulvestrant concentrations usually are achieved within 3 to 6 months after administration of once-monthly IM injections. The drug is approximately 99% bound to plasma proteins and is extensively metabolized in the liver with an elimination half-life of about 40 days. Metabolism of fulvestrant appears to involve a combination of various biotransformation pathways (eg, oxidation, aromatic hydroxylation, conjugation), but it does not appear to substantially inhibit any of the major cytochrome P-450 (CYP) isoenzymes, including 1A2, 2C9, 2C19, 2D6, and 3A4 in vitro. Main side effects include gastrointestinal effects, headache, back pain, vasodilation (hot flushes), and pharyngitis.

GEFITINIB

Quinazolinamine, N-(3-chloro-4-fluorophenyl)-7-meth-oxy-6-[3-(4-morpholinyl)propoxy]-, Iressa

[184475-35-2] $C_{22}H_{24}ClFN_4O_3$ (446.91).

Preparation—*J Med Chem* 2002; 45:3772 and *J Med Chem* 1999; 42:1803.

Description—White to off-white powder; pK_{a1} 5.4; pK_{a2} 7.2.

Solubility—Freely soluble in glacial acetic acid or DMSO; soluble in pyridine; sparingly soluble in THF; slightly in methanol, anhydrous alcohol, 2-propanol or acetonitrile.

Solubility—Sparingly soluble at pH1, almost insoluble above pH 7, with solubility dropping sharply between pH 4 and pH 6. In nonaqueous solvents, gefitinib is freely soluble in glacial acetic acid and dimethyl-sulphoxide, soluble in pyridine, sparingly soluble in tetrahydrofuran, and slightly soluble in methanol, ethanol (99.5%), ethyl acetate, propan-2-ol and acetonitrile.

Comments—An inhibitor of epidermal growth factor receptor (EGFR) tyrosine kinase . Effective orally as monotherapy in patients with locally advanced or metastatic non-small cell lung cancer in patients failing platinum-based and docetaxel regimens. Inhibits the intracellular phosphorylation of numerous tyrosine kinases associated with transmembrane cell surface receptors, including the tyrosine kinases associated with the EGFR (which are expressed on cell surfaces on normal cells and cancer cells). Activation of EGFR tyrosine kinase appears to initiate a cascade of intracellular signaling events leading to cell proliferation and influencing processes critical to cell survival and tumor progression (eg, angiogenesis, apoptosis, metastasis); however, the precise mechanism of antineoplastic activity of gefitinib has not been fully elucidated. Undergoes extensive hepatic metabolism, mainly by CYP3A4. If used concomitantly with potent cytochrome P-450 (CYP) isoenzyme 3A4 inducers (eg, rifampin, phenytoin), the dosage of gefitinib must be increased.

Adverse effects occurring in 5% or more of patients receiving gefitinib (250 mg once daily) during clinical trials include diarrhea, rash, acne, dry skin, nausea, vomiting, pruritus, anorexia, and asthenia. Gefitinib-associated pulmonary toxicity has been described as interstitial pneumonia, pneumonitis, and alveolitis at an incidence of 1%.

GEMCITABINE HYDROCHLORIDE

Cytidine, 2′-deoxy-2′,2′-difluoro-, monohydrochloride; Gemzar

[122111-03-9] $C_9H_{11}F_2N_3O_4 \cdot HCl$ (299.66).

Preparation—The acetonide of 2,3-dihydroxypropanal (chiron—from mannitol) undergoes a Reformatsky reaction with ethyl 2,2-di-bromo-2-fluoroacetate to yield the classic alcohol product, which is then benzylated to protect the generated OH group. Treatment with acid removes the acetonide group and the resulting diol forms a lactone with the γ-OH function. The free OH is benzylated (protection) and the lactone carbonyl reduced to form a mixture of isomers of 3,3-difluoro-4,5-di(ben-zyloxy)-2-furanol and the free OH is converted to a mesyl ester (I) with methanesulfonyl chloride and base. Cysteine is reacted with trimethylsi-lyl chloride to silylate the hydroxyl and amino groups (II). Compound I reacts with II, accompanied by loss of the mesyl group and, after removal of the benzyloxy groups with ammonia, yields the title compound.

Description—White to off-white powder that melts about 290° (dec).

Solubility—Soluble in water; slightly soluble in methanol; practically insoluble in ethanol or in polar organic solvents.

Comments—Indicated as first-line treatment for Stage II or above adenocarcinoma of the pancreas or in patients previously treated with 5-FU. Also active for colon cancer and in combination with cisplatin for the first-line treatment of inoperable, locally advanced or metastatic non-small cell lung cancer. After uptake into the cellular phosphoneu-cleotide pool, its triphosphate salt serves as a substrate for DNA polymerase but results in inhibition of DNA strand elongation. Clinical trials have shown that this drug yielded significant improvement over 5-FU for previously untreated pancreatic cancer, both with respect to time to disease progression and survival. The volume of distribution increases with duration of infusion, indicating that shorter infusions do not reach maximal distribution. It is eliminated by the kidneys, with no drug accumulating after weekly dosing.

Nausea and vomiting are relatively common adverse reactions, although myelosuppression is dose-limiting toxicity. Approximately 19% of patients required red-blood-cell (RBC) transfusions, and 16% suffered mild hemorrhage. Dyspnea was reported in 235 of the patients.

GEMTUZUMAB OZOGAMICIN

Mylotarg

n, average loading of calicheamicin derivative on antibody (hP67.6), is 2 to 3 moles/mole

[220578-59-6]

Preparation—Isolated from the fermentation of *Micromonospora echinospora* ssp. *calichensis.*

Description—A recombinant humanized IgG4 kappa antibody conjugated with a cytotoxic antitumor antibiotic, calicheamicin. Drug product is light sensitive and solutions should be protected from UV light. The drug product is a sterile, white, preservative-free lyophilized powder.

Comments—Recombinant DNA-derived humanized anti-CD33 monoclonal antibody. Effective for the treatment of patients with CD33-positive acute myeloid leukemia (AML) in first relapse who are 60 years of age or older and who are not considered candidates for other cytotoxic chemotherapy. The antibody component is an IgG$_4$ kappa immunoglobulin that is conjugated with the cytotoxic antitumor antibiotic calicheamicin. It binds specifically to antigen CD33, a sialic acid-dependent adhesion protein that is expressed on leukemic blasts in more than 80% of patients with acute myeloid leukemia (AML). Following binding, a complex is formed that is internalized by the myeloid cell. Calicheamicin is released (presumably via hydrolysis) within the lysosomes of the myeloid cell and binds to DNA in the minor groove, resulting in double strand breaks and cell death.

Severe myelosuppression (neutropenia, thrombocytopenia, anemia) occurs in all patients, with a median recovery pf neutrophils occurring 40.5 days after the first dose. Severe hypersensitivity reactions, including infrequently fatal anaphylaxis, have occurred. Acute infusion reactions, including shaking chills, fever, nausea, vomiting, headache, hypotension, hypertension, hypoxia, dyspnea, hyperglycemia, and anaphylaxis, may occur during the first 24 hours after administration. Severe adverse pulmonary events, including dyspnea, pulmonary infiltrates, pleural effusions, noncardiogenic pulmonary edema, pulmonary insufficiency and hypoxia, and acute respiratory distress syndrome, have occurred as sequelae of infusion reactions and infrequently were fatal. Severe hepatotoxicity, including hepatic veno-occlusive disease (VOD) and hepatic failure, has occurred and sometimes resulted in death.

GOLD AU—See page 367.

GOSERELIN ACETATE

Luteinizing hormone-releasing factor (pig) 6-[*O*-(1,1-dimethylethyl)-D-serine]-10-deglycinamide-, 2-(aminocarbonyl)hydrazide, acetate salt; Zoladex

$$\text{H}-5\,\text{oxoPro}-\text{His}-\text{Trp}-\text{Ser}-\text{Tyr}-\text{D-Ser}(t-\text{Bu})-\text{Leu}-\text{Arg}-\text{Pro}-\overset{\displaystyle O}{\overset{\|}{\text{NH}-\text{NH}-\text{C}}}-\text{NH}_2 \cdot \text{CH}_3\text{COOH}$$
$$123456789$$

[65807-02-5 (goserelin)] $C_{59}H_{84}N_{18}O_{14} \cdot C_2H_4O_2$ (1329.48).

Preparation—*J Med Chem* 1978; 21:1018.

Description—White to off-white powder.

Solubility—Soluble in water, dilute acids, or bases; aqueous solution pH approximately 6.0.

Comments—A synthetic LHRH (GnRH) analog that acts as a potent inhibitor of pituitary gonadotropin secretion. Proliferation of prostatic cells and usually prostatic neoplastic cells are simulated by dihydrotestosterone generated locally from circulating testosterone (80%); hence it is directly under the control of LH-RH/FSH/RH. Like the natural releasing hormone, treatment with this drug initially causes an acceleration of the growth of prostatic tumors; however, it later causes a decline in tumor growth rate, as a result of down regulation (densensitization) of LH-RH/FSH-RH receptors in the anterior hypophysis and androgen receptors in prostatic tumor cells. It is approved for palliative treatment of *prostatic carcinoma;* however, it is active against *estrogen receptor positive breast cancer.*

Recipients often experience an exacerbation of the cancer during the first few weeks of treatment. This results in temporarily increased bone destruction and pain in approximately 8% of cases; hypercalcemia, renal insufficiency, and urinary obstruction may occur. The concurrent use of the antiandrogen and flutamide, prevents these flareups. As downregulation develops and androgen-estrogen blood levels decline to castration levels, approximately 60% of the patients have hot flashes that gradually recede. In male patients, loss of libido and sexual dysfunction are common. Plasma levels of phosphatase and appropriate sex hormone should be monitored; hormone levels reach castration values in approximately 2 wk; and phosphatase returns to baseline levels in 4 wk.

HYDROXYPROGESTERONE CAPROATED—see RPS-19, page 1095.

HYDROXYUREA

Hydroxycarbamide; Mylocel

[127-07-1] $CH_4N_2O_2$ (76.05).

Preparation—By interaction of hydroxylamine hydrochloride and potassium cyanide.

Description—White powder; odorless; essentially tasteless; melts about 135°.

Solubility—Freely soluble in water.

Comments—Inhibits synthesis of DNA but not of RNA. It is lethal to cells in the S phase and also holds cells in the G$_1$ phase in which they are more sensitive to irradiation. It shares first-choice status with busulfan for the treatment of the *chronic phase* of *chronic myelocytic leukemia.* The value of either drug as a backup drug for the other may be limited by cross resistance. It sometimes is combined with radiation to treat squamous cell carcinoma of the head and neck or used alone to treat inoperable ovarian carcinoma or malignant melanoma in which it has erratic palliative actions; superior chemotherapy is retiring it from such uses. Hydroxyurea is also approved for the treatment of adult patients with sickle cell disease. The drug reduces the number of painful crises, the frequency of acute chest syndrome and hospitalization, and the need for blood transfusion

As an *immunosuppressant,* it may be used in the treatment of *psoriasis.* It appears to improve the condition of the patient in a high percentage of cases, but the quality of the response may not be as good as with some other drugs. Adverse effects include severe bone barrow suppression (leukopenia, thrombocytopenia, anemia), maculopapular rash, elevation of hepatic enzymes, and gastrointestinal toxicity (nausea, vomiting, diarrhea, mucositis).

IDARUBICIN HYDROCHLORIDE

5,12-Naphthacenedione, (7S-cis)-9-acetyl-7-[(3-amino-2,3,6-trideoxy-α-L-*lyxo*-hexopyranosyl)oxy]-7,8,9,10-tetrahydroxy-, hydrochloride; Idamycin; Zavedos

[57852-57-0] $C_{26}H_{27}NO_9 \cdot HCl$ (533.96).

Preparation—See US Pat 4,046,879 (1977).

Description—Orange crystals that melt about 184° (or 173°).

Comments—Approved for use with other approved drugs for the treatment of acute myelogenous leukemia (AML) in adults. Clinical trials showed it to be superior to daunorubicin when used with cytarabine in the induction and the duration of remissions in previously untreated AML. It is also active for the blast phase of chronic myelogenous leukemia and acute lymphocytic leukemia. It is a highly lipophilic synthetic anthracycline. Its cellular uptake is increased over other anthracyclines, although it shares the topoisomerase II cellular target. It exhibits high levels of tissue binding and undergoes extensive extrahepatic metabolism. Elimination is primarily by means of biliary and secondarily by means of renal excretion of the biologically active major metabolite idarubicinol (13-dehydroidarubicin). It is thought to penetrate into the cerebrospinal fluid, and both idarubicin and idarubicinol are approximately 95° bound to plasma proteins.

The terminal half-life of elimination for idarubicin varies widely, but averages approximately 22 hr. The half-life for elimination of idarubicinol is longer than 45 hr; thus it accumulates to higher levels than idarubicin and may contribute significantly to the therapeutic effect. Patients who have moderate levels of hepatic dysfunction exhibit elevated levels of circulating drug, so care must be taken in treating such patients. The drug should not be administered if bilirubin levels are higher than 5 mg/dL.

Myelosuppression is the major toxicity resulting from idarubicin administration; care should be taken when the drug is administered to patients who have low WBC counts or who previously have received radiation therapy. Bleeding and infection have followed therapy. Caution must be taken during administration to avoid extravasation as this agent is a tissue vesicant. Cardiotoxicity resembling CHF is common, and is the primary dose-limiting toxicity. Although difficult to predict, cardiotoxicity is associated with a decrease in left ventricular end volume. Administration necessitates close monitoring of the patient for blood counts and cardiac, renal, and hepatic function.

IFOSFAMIDE

2H-1,3,2-Oxazaphosphorin-2-amine, N,3-bis(2-chloroethyl)-tetrahydro-, 2-oxide; Ifex

[3778-73-2] $C_7H_{15}Cl_2N_2O_2P$ (261.09).

Preparation—Reaction of 3-(chloromethylamino)-1-propanol with $POCl_3$ yields the N-(2-chloroethyl)-P-chlorooxaphosphorane oxide, which with 2-chloroethylamine yields the product. US Pat 3,732,340.

Description—White crystals that melt about 40°.

Solubility—Soluble in water.

Comments—An alkylating agent isomeric with cyclophosphamide. It is a component of a first-choice combination for the treatment of adult soft-tissue sarcomas and *testicular cancer*. It is an alternative drug for the treatment of *acute lymphocytic leukemia, acute myelocytic leukemia, breast carcinoma, Burkitt's lymphoma, colorectal carcinoma, diffuse histiocytic lymphoma, bone and soft tissue sarcoma, melanoma, non-small-cell lung carcinoma, oat-cell carcinoma, pancreatic carcinoma, testicular carcinoma, ovarian carcinoma,* and *Wilms' tumor.* Nausea and vomiting occur acutely. Delayed toxicity includes bone-marrow depression, hemorrhagic cystitis, alopecia, and a usually temporary sterility. It is converted slowly to an active metabolite, the half-life being approximately 15 hr. The active metabolites are rapidly bound to proteins. The volume of distribution is larger than that of total body water. To avoid bladder toxicity, it must be given with extensive hydration and a cytotoxic protector, such as mesna. Neurologic toxicity (lethargy, ataxia, stupor, somnolence, disorientation, seizures) occurs at a higher incidence in patients receiving high doses or with impaired renal function.

IMATINIB MESYLATE

p-Toluidide, α-(4-methyl)-1-piperazinyl-3'-[[4-(3-pyridyl)-2-pyrimidinyl]amino]-p-tolu-p-toluidide; Gleevec

[152459-95-5] $C_{29}H_{31}N_7O.CH_4SO_3$ (589.71).

Preparation—*Tetr Lett*, 2001; 3: 2273 and US Pat 5,521,184 (1996).

Description—(Salt) White to off-white to brownish or yellow tinged crystalline powder; α-form melts about 226°, β-form melts about 217°. (Base) Melts about 211°; pK_{a1} 8.07, pK_{a2} 3.73, pK_{a3} 2.56, pK_{a4} 1.52.

Solubility—(Salt) Very soluble in water or aqueous buffers ≤ pH 5.5: soluble 100g/L at pH 4 and 49 mg/L at pH 7. Soluble to some extent in DMSO, methanol or ethanol; insoluble in 1-octanol, acetone or acetonitrile.

Comments—Protein-tyrosine kinase inhibitor that inhibits the Bcr-Abl tyrosine kinase, the constitutive abnormal tyrosine kinase created by the Philadelphia chromosome abnormality in chronic myeloid leukemia (CML). It inhibits proliferation and induces apoptosis in Bcr-Abl positive cell lines as well as fresh leukemic cells from Philadelphia chromosome positive chronic myeloid leukemia. Also an inhibitor of the receptor tyrosine kinases for platelet-derived growth factor (PDGF) and stem cell factor (SCF), c-kit, and inhibits PDGF- and SCF-mediated cellular events. In vitro, inhibits proliferation and induces apoptosis in gastrointestinal stromal tumor (GIST) cells, which express an activating c-kit mutation. Indicated for the treatment of newly diagnosed adult patients with Philadelphia chromosome positive CML in chronic phase, patients with Philadelphia chromosome positive CML in blast crisis, accelerated phase, or in chronic phase after failure of interferon-alpha therapy and pediatric patients with Ph$^+$ chronic phase CML whose dis-

ease has recurred after stem cell transplant or who are resistant to interferon alpha therapy. Also indicated for the treatment of patients with Kit (CD117) positive unresectable and/or metastatic malignant gastrointestinal stromal tumors.

Well absorbed after oral administration (oral bioavailability 98%) with C_{max} achieved within 2 to 4 hours post-dose. Hepatic metabolism, primarily by CYP3A4, with elimination half-lives of imatinib and major active metabolite, the N-desmethyl derivative, are approximately 18 and 40 hours, respectively. Binding to plasma proteins in vitro approximately 95%, mostly to albumin and α_1-acid glycoprotein. Dosage adjustments are required with liver dysfunction. Altered metabolism may occur when administered with cytochrome P-450 (CYP) isoenzyme 3A4 (CYP3A4) inhibitors (eg, clarithromycin, erythromycin, itraconazole, ketoconazole) and inducers (eg, carbamazepine, dexamethasone, phenobarbital, phenytoin, rifampin, St John's wort). Imatinib appears to inhibit CYP3A4, thus may increase plasma CYP3A4-substrate concentrations when used with CYP3A4 substrates (eg, cyclosporine, pimozide, triazolo-benzodiazepines, dihydropyridine calcium-channel blockers, certain HMG-CoA reductase inhibitors). Also appears to inhibit CYP2C9 resulting in increased anticoagulant effect and inhibits CYP2D6.

Main toxicities associated with this drug include fluid retention/edema which could be severe resulting in pleural effusion, pericardial effusion, pulmonary edema, ascites, and superficial edema (ie, rapid weight gain, anasarca). Also hematologic effects (Grade 3 or 4 neutropenia, anemia, or thrombocytopenia occurred in up to 30–40% of patients), increases in liver enzymes (Grade 3 or 4 hyperbilirubinemia occurred in up to 4% of patients), nausea, vomiting, muscle cramps, diarrhea, rash, myalgias, headache, and hypokalemia may occur.

INTERFERON ALFA-2A, RECOMBINANT

Comments—Identical to one of the human alpha-interferons. Interferons and other cytokines are discussed in Chapter 60. It increases class I histocompatibility molecules on lymphocytes, enhances the production of ILs-1 and -2 (which mediate much of the toxic and therapeutic effects), modulates antibody responses, and enhances NK cell activity. It also inhibits tumor-cell growth by its ability to inhibit protein synthesis. It also is antiproliferative and thus can be immunosuppressive. The action on NK cells is the most important for its *antineoplastic* action. It is approved for use in *hairy-cell leukemia* and *AIDS-related Kaposi's sarcoma*. It shares first-choice status for the treatment of *hairy-cell leukemia* and *Kaposi's sarcoma* and is the drug of choice for treatment of *renal cell carcinoma*. It also is an alternative drug for use against *chronic myelocytic leukemia multiple myeloma* (21% respond), *melanoma* (13–23% respond), and *advanced cutaneous T-cell lymphomas*. Preliminary trials also show promising efficacy against ovarian carcinoma, non-Hodgkin's lymphoma, and metastatic carcinoid tumor.

It has *antiviral* activity, especially against RNA viruses. It has been shown to be effective in the treatment of varicella in immunocompromised children, non-A and non-B hepatitis, genital warts, and lymphoproliferative disorders caused by Epstein-Barr virus and in the prevention of cytomegalovirus, rhinoviral colds, and even possibly opportunistic bacterial infections in renal and other transplant recipients. Other investigations are in progress.

It enhances the targeting of monoclonal antibody-tethered cytotoxic drugs to cancer cells.

Toxicity varies directly with the dose and the rate of absorption. Antiviral effects, without toxicity, can be achieved with 3×10^5 IU. No adverse effects accrue to intranasal doses of 2.5×10^7 IU.

Antibodies to rIFN-αA develop, which may cause refractoriness to occur.

The following adverse effects with antineoplastic doses have incidences of 75% through 98% (in order of decreasing incidence): fever (IL-1-mediated), fatigue, elevated SGOT, and myalgias; 50% through 74%: headache, leukopenia, chills, neutropenia, and hypocalcemia; 25% through 49%: proteinuria, elevated alkaline phosphatase, anorexia, thrombocytopenia, nausea, hyperglycemia, hyperbilirubinemia, diarrhea, and proteinuria; 10% through 24%: dizziness, rash, hyperphosphatemia, oropharyngeal inflammation, hyperuricemia, weight loss, pruritus, dry skin, and azotemia; 5% through 9%: anemia, emesis, confusion, arthralgia, sweating, alopecia, paresthesias, numbness, lethargy, and hypotension; less than 5%: lethargy, nervousness, night sweats, conjunctivitis, sleep disturbances, edema, dysrhythmias and chest pain, decreased libido, impotence, etc. Interstitial nephritis and renal failure rarely occur. Many of the adverse effects diminish after several days of continued treatment. Interferons are expensive.

It is not absorbed orally. By the intravenous route, it entirely disappears within 4 hr, but by the intramuscular or subcutaneous route disapperance takes 6 to 7 hr.

INTERFERON ALFA-2B, RECOMBINANT

Comments—It is approved for use in *hairy-cell leukemia, AIDS-related Kaposi's sarcoma, chronic myelogenous leukemia, melanoma, condylomata acuminata,* and *chronic hepatitis*. Its actions are nearly those of rIFN-αA, and the uses are presently the same, except that it appears to be somewhat less effective against melanoma, and antibody formation is less. Neither alpha interferon has been studied in a sufficient number of cases to ascertain whether adverse effects differ substantially; they seem to be qualitatively the same but perhaps of slightly lower incidence and severity with rIFN-α-2.

IRINOTECAN HYDROCHLORIDE TRIHYDRATE

[1,4′-Bipiperidine]-1′-carboxylic acid, 4,11-diethyl-3,4,12,14-tetra-hydro-4-hydroxy-3,14-dioxo-1H-pyrano[3′,4′:6,7]indolizino-[1,2-b]quinolin-9-yl ester, monohydrochloride, trihydrate; Camptosar; CPT-11

[136572-09-3] $C_{33}H_{38}N_4O_6 \cdot HCl \cdot 3H_2O$ (677.20).

Preparation—A semisynthetic derivative of camptothecin, an alkaloid derived from plants (eg, *Camptotheca acuminata*). US Pat 4,604,463 (1986).

Description—Pale yellow needles that melt about 257°.

Solubility—Slightly soluble in water or organic solvents; pH of a 2% aq solution is 4.

Comments—Indicated in as first-line therapy in combination with 5-fluorouracil/leucovorin of metastatic carcinoma of the colon or the rectum or for metastatic carcinoma of the colon or the rectum in patients failing 5-FU therapy. It is a prodrug that is converted to the active metabolite, SN-38, in vivo. This conversion is attributed primarily to carboxylesterase enzymes located in the liver and is linear with dose. The activating enzymes do not appear to be saturable or inducible. SN-38 is a potent inhibitor of topoisomerase I. It causes the enzyme to freeze at a step in catalysis where it exists as a covalent adduct to a nicked strand of the DNA helix. Cancer-cell resistance to SN-38 may arise from lowered levels of topoisomerase I or from specific topoisomerase I mutations.

SN-38 is inactivated largely by glucuronidation. Urinary excretion of irinotecan accounts for approximately 15% of the dose. Very little SN-38 is eliminated via the kidney, but 3% of the dose appears in the urine as the SN-38-glucuronide. Cumulative urinary and biliary excretion over 48 hr ranges from 25% to 50%. After IV infusion, drug levels in plasma drop in a multiexponential manner with a terminal half-life of approximately 6 hr. The terminal half-life for SN-38 is approximately 10 hr. Maximal concentrations of SN-38 are generally seen 1 hr after a 90-min infusion of the drug. After a 125-mg/m² infusion. Maximal plasma concentrations of irinotecan equal approximately 1660 ng/mL, whereas maximal SN-38 concentrations equal approximately 26 ng/mL.

This drug can induce early and late forms of diarrhea, which must be treated promptly. The early form is transient and is cholinergic in derivation. The later form of diarrhea, due to cytotoxic effects on gut lining, can be prolonged and can result in dehydration or electrolyte imbalance. Severe myelosuppression and death due to sepsis have followed its administration. Therapy should be discontinued temporarily if neutropenic fever occurs or if the neutrophil count drops to less than 500/mm³ or if total WBC count drops to less than 2000/mm³. Patients previously receiving pelvic or abdominal irradiation are at particular risk for myelosuppression. This drug may harm the fetus and may be excreted in breast milk.

LETROZOLE

Benzonitrile, 4,4′-(1H-1,2,4-triazol-1-ylmethylene)bis-, Femara

[112809-51-5] $C_{17}H_{11}N_5$ (285.31).

Preparation—A mixture of α-bromo-*p*-tolunitrile and 1,2,4-triazole in chloroform and acetonitrile is stirred to give 1-(*p*-cyanotolyl)-1,2,4-triazole which is then treated with α-fluoro-*p*-tolunitrile and potassium *t*-butoxide to yield the product. US Pat 4,978,672 (1990) and US Pat 5,473,078 (1995).

Description—White to yellowish-white, practically odorless, crystalline powder melting about 185°.

Solubility—Freely soluble in methylene dichloride; slightly soluble in ethanol; practically insoluble in water.

Comments—Approved for first-line treatment of hormone receptor-positive or hormone receptor-unknown locally advanced or metastatic breast cancer in postmenopausal women as well as use in postmenopausal women who have breast cancer that has progressed after antiestrogen therapy. It is a nonsteroidal inhibitor of aromatase. It binds the heme portion of the P-450 subunit of the enzyme and reduces the production of estrogen in all tissues. Treatment with this drug significantly lowers serum estrone and estradiol. It is effective as ovarectomy at raising serum luteinizing hormone (LH) while not increasing follicle-stimulating hormone (FSH). It causes regression of estrogen-stimulated neoplasia.

It is rapidly and completely absorbed from the GI tract. Its absorption is unaffected by coadministration wit food. Plateau blood levels are reached after 2 wk daily dosing with 25-mg tablets. It has a large volume of distribution and displays a terminal half-life for elimination of approximately 2 days. The major pathway for elimination is by means of metabolism to an inactive carbinol metabolite and the renal clearance of the glucuronide conjugate of the carbinol. Approximately 90% of the drug appears in the urine, approximately 75% of it as the conjugated metabolite. Cytochrome P-450 enzymes are likely responsible for the metabolism, and the drug is known to inhibit some of these enzymes. Renal dysfunction was not found to affect circulating drug levels, while moderate hepatic dysfunction increased levels of circulating drug 37%.

In clinical studies, approximately 3% of patients discontinued therapy for reasons other than cancer progression. A minor incidence of thromboembolism and vaginal bleeding was observed. Patients receiving the drug did not require replacement corticoid therapy. The most frequently reported adverse experiences were bone pain, hot flushes, back pain, nausea, arthralgia and dyspnea.

LEUCOVORIN CALCIUM—page 1705.

LEUPROLIDE ACETATE

6-D-Leucine-9-(N-ethyl-L-prolinamide)-10-deglycinamide-, monoacetate salt; Lupron

Leuprorelin; LH releasing factor (pig). [74381-53-6] $C_{59}H_{84}N_{16}O_{12} \cdot C_2H_4O_2$ (1269.47).

Comments—An analog of the gonadotropin-releasing hormone, LH-RH/FSH-RH. Proliferation of prostatic and usually of prostatic neoplastic cells is stimulated by dihydrotestosterone generated locally from circulating testosterone (80%); hence it is indirectly under the control of LH-RH/FSH-RH. Like the natural releasing hormone, treatment with this drug initially causes an acceleration of the growth of prostatic tumors; however, it later causes a decline in tumor growth rate, as the result of downregulation (densensitization) of LH-RH/FSH-RH receptors in the anterior hypophysis and androgen receptors in prostatic tumor cells. It is approved for use only for palliative treatment of *prostatic carcinoma* when orchiectomy or estrogen therapy is rejected by the patient; however, it is analogously active against estrogen receptor-positive breast cancer. Metabolism and elimination have not been fully elucidated to date, but studies show an elimination half-life of about 3 hours following IV administration.

Recipients often experience an exacerbation of the cancer during the first few weeks of treatment. This results in temporarily increased bone destruction and pain in 3% to 10% of cases, and hypercalcemia and urinary obstruction may occur. The concurrent use of the antiandrogen, flutamide, prevents these flareups. As downregulation develops and androgen-estrogen blood levels decline to castration levels, approximately half of the patients have hot flashes which gradually recede. In male patients there is commonly loss of libido, impotence, and gynecomastia. Nausea and vomiting, edema, changes in bone density and thrombophlebitis are uncommon complications. Plasma levels of phosphatase and appropriate sex hormone should be monitored; hormone levels reach castration values in approximately 2 wk and phosphatase to baseline levels in 4 wk.

MEDICINAL AGENTS

LEVAMISOLE HYDROCHLORIDE

Imidazo[2,1-*b*]thiazole, (*S*)-2,3,5,6-tetrahydro-6-phenyl-, monohydrochloride; Ergamisol

[16595-8-5] $C_{11}H_{12}N_2S.HCl$ (240.75).

Preparation—US Pat 3,274,209 or 3,579,530.

Description—White to cream-colored crystals.

Solubility—1 g in 2 mL water or 5 mL methanol; practically insoluble in ether.

Comments—A drug that predominantly stimulates, but also suppresses, immune responses to a variety of antigens, depending on dose and timing of administration. It acts upon T lymphocytes, B lymphocytes, monocytes, macrophages, and neutrophils to modify their proliferation, mobility, and factor-release. It does not act on killer or NK cells. An increase in monocyte chemotaxis is thought to be the most important action. Its effects on T lymphocytes are more pronounced than those on B lymphocytes. Clinical interest focuses on the immune stimulatory effects, especially in the treatment of cancer. Indicated as adjuvant treatment in combination with fluorouracil after surgical resection in patients with Dukes' stage C colon cancer. It is most ineffective in the induction of tumor regression, although it may be occasionally effective against breast carcinoma, ovarian carcinoma, and AML. It is most useful for the *stabilization of remission in breast carcinoma, bronchogenic carcinomas, squamous cell sarcomas of the head and neck, gastric carcinoma, leukemias, and myeloma.* It has been reported to be effective in the management of certain immune disorders, namely, erythema multiforme, lupus erythematosis, and *rheumatoid arthritis,* against which it seems to be as effective as penicillamine. There also are reports of anti-infectious activity against aphthous stomatitis, chronic brucellosis, leprosy, and staphylococcal infections. Adverse effects are usually mild and infrequent. They include vertigo (especially with ethanol), nausea, vomiting, headache, fever, dermatitis, and granulocytopenia. It readily is absorbed orally. It is metabolized nearly entirely in the liver. The elimination half-life is approximately 4 hr.

LOMUSTINE

Urea, *N*-(2-chloroethyl)-*N*′-cyclohexyl-*N*-nitroso-, CCNU; CeeNU

1-(2-Chloroethyl)-3-cyclohexyl-1-nitrosourea [13010-47-4] $C_9H_{16}ClN_3O_2$ (233.70).

Preparation—This drug, a cytotoxic nitrosourea, may be prepared by nitrosation of its substituted urea moiety (see preparation of *Carmustine*), page ___.

Description—Yellow powder.

Solubility—Practically insoluble in water, soluble in alcohol; highly soluble in lipids.

Comments—It has been approved for use in *brain cancer* and *Hodgkin's disease.* A chemical congener of *Carmustine* and has similar mechanisms of action and shares some of the same uses. Like carmustine, it reaches high concentrations in the cerebrospinal fluid and hence shares with carmustine a first-choice status for the treatment of *glioblastoma.* It has alternative drug status for treatment of *Hodgkin's* and *diffuse histiocytic lymphomas, multiple myeloma, non-small-cell lung cancer,* and *renal carcinoma.* It also is used in *bone-marrow transplantation* in Hodgkin's disease.

The adverse effects are similar to those of carmustine except that there may be rare interstitial pulmonary fibrosis (may occur at any dosage, but typically with cumulative doses exceeding 1100 mg/m²). Nausea and vomiting occur later (3–6 hr) and last longer (24 hr). Thrombocytopenia and leukopenia reach nadirs in 4 and 6 weeks, respectively, and last 1 to 2 wk. Stomatitis, alopecia, anemia, and mild, transient hepatotoxicity occasionally occur. Dysarthria, ataxia, lethargy, and disorientation have been reported. Monitoring of leukocyte counts is required. When other myelosuppressive drugs are in use or have been used within the previous 4 wk, the dose of lomustine should be reduced.

Lomustine is absorbed well orally and survives the first pass through the liver to be effective by the oral route. It is distributed among the tissues with a volume of distribution greater than total body water. In the cerebrospinal fluid, the concentration of metabolites reaches 150% of that in plasma. Biotransformation occurs throughout the body; the half-life is approximately 15 min; the half-lives of metabolites are 48 hr. The dosage is 100–130 mg/M² as a single oral dose every 6 weeks.

LYMPHOCYTE IMMUNE ANTI-THYMOCYTE GLOBULIN (EQUINE)

Atgam

A preparation of equine immunoglobulin containing antibodies (primarily IgG) prepared from the hyperimmune serum of horses immunized with human thymus lymphocytes.

Description—Transparent to slightly opalescent (pink) aqueous solution of the protein.

Comments—Attacks T lymphocytes but not B lymphocytes. Its approved use is the *prevention of allograft rejection* in renal transplantation. Efficacy is enhanced and adverse effects are attenuated when the globulin is used in combination with other immunosuppressive agents. The globulin also has been reported to be of value in the treatment of T-cell leukemias, graft-versus-host disease, and selected cases of aplastic anemia. Frequent adverse effects include chills, fever, urticaria, pruritus, generalized rashes, leukopenia, and thrombocytopenia. Less frequently experienced adverse effects are nausea, vomiting, stomatitis, diarrhea, hypotension, chest pain, back pain, night sweats, pain at the injection site, and peripheral thrombophlebitis. Rarely there may be tachycardia, myalgias, pulmonary edema, serum sickness, anaphylaxis, laryngospasm, local and systemic infections, and activation of herpes simplex infections. Prior to use, a skin test for sensitivity to horse serum is advisable. The half-life 3 to 9 days.

MECHLORETHAMINE HYDROCHLORIDE

Ethanamine, 2-chloro-*N*-(2-chloroethyl)-*N*-methyl-, hydrochloride; Nitrogen Mustard: HN2; Mustargen

$$CH_3N(CH_2CH_2Cl)_2 \cdot HCl$$

2,2′-Dichloro-*N*-methyldiethylamine hydrochloride [55-86-7] $C_5H_{11}Cl_2N.HCl$ (192.52).

History—The medical uses for nitrogen mustards were discovered as a result of chemical warfare research on vesicant agents during World War II. After noting that these agents brought about dissolution of lymphoid tissue, L Goodman, A Gilman, and T Dougherty were prompted to study the effect of nitrogen mustards on transplanted lymphosarcoma in mice. The first clinical trial with these agents was conducted in 1942.

Preparation—Among other ways, the base may be synthesized by reacting methylamine with a double equimolar portion of ethylene oxide to produce *N*-methyldiethanolamine, which then is reacted with thionly chloride. After purification, the base then may be converted conveniently to the hydrochloride by dissolving it in a suitable organic solvent and passing HCl into the solution.

Description—White, crystalline, hygroscopic powder that melts about 109°; pH (1:500 aqueous solution) 3 to 5.

Solubility—Soluble in water; soluble in alcohol.

Comments—The prototype of a series of alkylating agents called the nitrogen mustards. The β-chloroethyl groups lose chloride ions to generate carbonium and azaridium (ethylenimonium) ions, which are extremely reactive and alkylate many biologically important chemical groups. In DNA they alkylate guanine groups; if one *arm* alkylates one guanine moiety and the second arm another guanine on the opposing strand of double-stranded DNA, the DNA becomes irreversibly crosslinked. This inhibits mitosis and also may cause chromosomal breakage. Relatively undifferentiated germinal cells are nonproliferative and hypertrophied during exposure to the drug, but the more differentiated germinal cells disintegrate. Certain neoplastic growths, particularly of the lymph nodes and bone marrow, are somewhat more sensitive to the drug than are the normal more slowly proliferating tissues. It is approved for use in *Hodgkin's disease, lymphosarcoma, chronic lymphocytic* and *myelocytic leukemia, polycythemia vera, mycosis fungoides,* and *bronchogenic carcinoma.*

Although this was the drug that ushered in the era of cancer chemotherapy, it is still used today. The combinations known as MOPP (mechlorethamine, vincristine, procarbazine, prednisone) and MOP (MOPP without prednisone) offer options for treatment of *Hodgkin's disease.* It is also a component of first-choice combinations to treat *medulloblastoma* and *diffuse histiocytic lymphoma.* Mechlorethamine's only other therapeutic status of note is as the drug of choice in the topical treatment of mycosis fungoides and intrapleural, intrapericardial, or intraperitoneal palliative treatment of effusions resulting from metastatic carcinomas. In *polycythemia vera,* remissions of several months to 2 yr have been achieved. All of the above diseases eventually develop resistance to nitrogen mustards.

It is an immunosuppressive drug, but the requirement for intravenous administration and its high toxicity have discouraged its use. In the treatment of *"malignant" rheumatoid arthritis* it effects a good initial response in nearly all patients; maintenance is carried on with cyclophosphamide or other immunosuppressive drugs. It also has been reported to improve the condition of a high percentage of patients who have *ulcerative colitis.*

Nausea and vomiting commonly occur within 30 to 180 min after administration, but sedative and antiemetic agents greatly diminish the incidence of such untoward actions originating centrally. Diarrhea also occurs frequently. Bone-marrow depression may result in lymphocytopenia followed by leukopenia and occasionally thrombocytopenia and thus in bleeding tendencies. Serious and potentially lethal hematological responses mainly occur when the total accumulated dose in a course of therapy exceeds 0.4 mg (400 µg)/kg. Skin eruptions are noted rarely, but herpes zoster (shingles) commonly occurs, especially in the treatment of malignant lymphoma. Sometimes temporary menstrual irregularities occur in females. In patients who have large tumor masses which involute rapidly with treatment, there may be hyperuricemia, and adequate fluid intake and allopurinol are needed to prevent crystalluria and kidney damage. Alopecia, metallic taste, headache, drowsiness, asthenia, tinnitus, and deafness sometimes occur.

It is teratogenic and carcinogenic and should not be used during the first trimester of pregnancy. Several local reactions to mechlorethamine, as well as rapid chemical breakdown of the drug, require that therapy be limited to the intravenous route; even so, extravasation may cause tender local induration and tissue necrosis, and irritation from within the lumen of the vessel may cause phlebothrombosis or thrombophlebitis, especially if the infusion rate is too rapid or the concentration of solution is too high. Extravasation should be treated with 1/6 *M* sodium thiosulfate solution.

MEDROXYPROGESTERONE ACETATE—page 1467.

MELPHALAN

L-Phenylalanine, 4-[bis(2-chloroethyl)amino]-, Alkeran, L-PAM, Phenylalanine mustard; L-sarcolysin

$$(ClCH_2CH_2)_2N \!-\!\!\bigcirc\!\!-\! CH_2 \!-\!-\! \underset{\underset{H}{|}}{\overset{\overset{NH_2}{|}}{C}} \!-\! COOH$$

[148-82-3] $C_{13}H_{18}Cl_2N_2O_2$ (305.20).

Preparation—L-3-Phenylalanine is nitrated and the *p*-nitro compound is reduced to L-3-(*p*-aminophenyl)alanine. This is reacted with ethylene oxide to form the corresponding bis(2-hydroxy-ethyl)-amino compound that then is treated with phosphoryl chloride to yield the drug.

Description—Off-white to buff powder having a faint odor; sensitive to light, heat, and moisture; melts about 180° with decomposition.

Solubility—Practically insoluble in water, chloroform, or ether; slightly soluble in alcohol; soluble in dilute mineral acids.

Comments—An alkylating agent of the bischloroethylamine type. Cytotoxicity appears to be related to the extent of its interstrand crosslinking with DNA, probably by binding at the N^7 position of guanine. It is approved for use in *multiple myeloma* and *nonresectable epithelial carcinoma of the ovary.* In combination with prednisone either it or cyclophosphamide is the drug of choice for treatment of *multiple myeloma.* Seventy to 80% of patients show subjective improvement; 33% to 50% show objective improvement for periods from 6 months to 2 yr; and life expectancy may be increased even when no objective signs of improvement are obtained. It is a component of the combination of choice against *ovarian carcinoma.* It is used occasionally in the *treatment of tumors of the testis, osteogenic sarcoma, non-small cell lung cancer,* and *chronic granulocytic leukemia.*

Adverse effects include mild nausea and vomiting after large doses, bone-marrow depression with anemia, neutropenia, thrombocytopenia, and occasional azotemia. Aphthous ulceration, GI hemorrhage, skin eruptions, and bronchopulmonary dyplasia also occur occasionally. Regular blood-cell counts are required. It should be given cautiously if the patient has been receiving radiation or other cancer chemotherapy. It is contraindicated in thrombocytopenia, anemia, and leukopenia and during the first trimester of pregnancy. In the presence of impaired renal function the drug should be used cautiously. IV melphalan may cause anaphylaxis, diaphoresis, hypotension, tachycardia, bronchospasm, dyspnea, and cardiac arrest.

It is absorbed well by the oral route, being as efficacious as by the intravenous route. It is transformed into active metabolites in probably all tissues. The elimination half-life is approximately 1 to 3 hr. Following IV administration, drug plasma concentrations declined rapidly in a biexponential manner with distribution phase and terminal elimination phase half-lives of approximately 10 and 75 minutes, respectively. Estimates of average total body clearance varied among studies, but typical values of approximately 7–9 ml/min/kg (250–325 ml/min/m²) were ob-

served with mean (±SD) peak melphalan plasma concentrations in myeloma patients given IV melphalan at doses of 10 or 20 mg/m² were 1.2 ± 0.4 and 2.8 ± 1.9 ug/ml, respectively. The steady-state volume of distribution of melphalan is 0.5 L/kg, with plasma protein binding ranging from 60% to 90%.

MERCAPTOPURINE

6*H*-Purine-6-thione, 1,7-dihydro-, monohydrate; Purinethol; 6-MP

Purine-6-thiol monohydrate (tautomer) [6112-76-1] $C_5H_4N_4S.H_2O$ (170.19); *anhydrous* [50-44-2] (152.17).

Preparation—Thiourea and ethyl cyanoacetate are reacted in the presence of sodium methylate to give 2-thiol-4-amino-6-hydroxypyrimidine (I) that then is converted to the 5-nitroso derivative (II) by treatment with sodium nitrite and acetic acid. Reduction of II with sodium hydrosulfite yields the corresponding diamino compound (III) which then is desulfurized by hydrogenolysis in the presence of Raney nickel to yield 4,5-diamino-6-hydroxypyrimidine (IV). The imidazole ring closure then is effected by double condensation of IV with formic acid (V), and the resulting hypoxanthine is thiolated with P_2S_5.

Description—Yellow, crystalline powder; odorless or practically odorless; melts with decomposition at temperatures above 308°.

Solubility—Insoluble in water, acetone, or ether; soluble in hot alcohol or in dilute aqueous alkali; slightly soluble in diluted H_2SO_4.

Comments—It is converted to 6-thioinosinic acid, which acts as an antimetabolite to inhibit synthesis of adenine and guanine and also to prevent conversion of purine bases into nucleotides. It also mimics inosinic acid in exerting a negative feedback suppression of the synthesis of inosinic acid. Some mercaptopurine also is converted to thioguanine, which is incorporated into both DNA and RNA to generate defective nucleic acids. Thus nucleic acid synthesis and functions are impaired several ways. Cell mitosis is inhibited.

In combination with methotrexate it provides a combination of first choice in the *maintenance chemotherapy of acute lymphocytic leukemia* (this is its approved use). It is an alternative drug for the treatment of *stable chronic myelocytic leukemia;* the remission rate is approximately 80% if the disease is caught early, but cures are not achieved. Induction sometimes is accomplished with busulfan and maintenance with mercaptopurine. There is no cross resistance between this drug and nonpurine antineoplastic drugs.

It is mostly a secondary (efferent) *immunosuppressive* drug that is capable of eliciting a high percentage of favorable responses in *ulcerative colitis* and *psoriatic arthritis.* It also is moderately effective in the treatment of *systemic lupus erythematosus, dermatomyositis,* and *polymyositis.* However, it probably will not become the drug of choice for any of these disorders. Immunosuppression predisposes to intercurrent infections.

Bone-marrow depression occurs during treatment. Leukopenia and thrombocytopenia (with hemorrhage) are common and may be severe, but anemia is rare. Frequent monitoring of the blood-cell population is mandatory. Nausea, vomiting, and anorexia may occur; they signal onset of GI toxicity, which may take the form of mucositis and ulceration. Oral, pharyngeal, and esophageal mucositis may also occur, with thrushlike stomatitis or aphthous ulceration. Diarrhea and spruelike symptoms occasionally occur. There also may be jaundice in 10% to 40% of patients who have acute leukemia due to hepatic injury which can occur with any dosage, but seems to occur when doses of more than 2.5 mg/kg/day. The histologic pattern of mercaptopurine hepatotoxicity includes features of both intrahepatic cholestasis and parenchymal cell necrosis. In patients who have high WBC counts or massive disease, cellular destruction leads to hyperuricemia and sometimes to tubular clogging with urate crystals and consequent oliguria, thus necessitating use of allopurinol.

The systemic bioavailability by the oral route ranges from 5% to 37%, owing to first-pass metabolism in the intestinal mucosa and liver. Both oxidation by xanthine oxidase and *S*-methylation occur. The xanthine oxidase inhibitor, allopurinol, considerably increases plasma levels from oral, but not from intravenous, drug, so that only approximately one-third of the usual oral dose should be given in the presence of allopurinol. Approximately 20% of the drug in plasma is protein bound, and the volume of distribution is larger than the extracellular space; however, the access to cerebrospinal fluid is slight. The half-life averages 47 min in adults and 21 min in children. Inhibition of the anticoagulant effect of warfarin, when given with mercaptopurine, has been reported.

MESNA

Ethanesulfonic acid, monosodium salt; Mesnex

$$Na^+ \left[HS-CH_2-CH_2-SO_3 \right]^-$$

[19767-45-4] $C_2H_5NaO_3S_2$ (164.17).

Preparation—Reaction of sodium vinylsulfonate with NaSH or H_2S, in an anti-Markovnikov addition yields the product.

Description—White crystalline powder with a "rotten egg" odor.

Solubility—Freely soluble in water; sparingly soluble in organic solvents.

Comments—Approved for prevention of ifosfamide-induced hemorrhagic cystitis. It is a mercaptan which scavenges and inactivates reactive molecules such as acrolein produced by ifosfamide activation. In clinical trials, patients treated with ifosfamide and traditional protective strategies (diuretics and alkalinization of urine) suffered approximately 20% hematuria. Those treated with this drug suffered none. It is eliminated rapidly by the kidneys. Approximately 33% of a dose appears in the urine within 24 hr, the largest fraction within the first 4 hr. The half-life ranges from 1.2–8.3 hours following oral administration of the drug, with a volume of distribution of approximately 0.65 L/kg.

It should not be used in patients hypersensitive to thiol-containing agents. Adverse reactions include nausea, vomiting, and diarrhea. The drug may cause a false positive test for urinary ketones.

METHOTREXATE

L-Glutamic acid, *N*-[4-[[(2,4-diamino-6-pteridinyl)methyl]methylamino]benzoyl]-, Folex: Methotrexate; Mexate

4-Amino-10-methylfolic acid; [59-05-2]; a mixture of 4-amino-10-methylfolic acid and closely related compounds and contains not less than 85.0% of $C_{20}H_{22}N_8O_5$ (454.44).

Preparation—2,3-Dibromopropionaldehyde (I) is condensed in an aqueous medium with 2,4,5,6-tetraminopyrimidine (II). The condensation is multiple, consisting of (a) dehydrobromination, involving a hydrogen of the 5-amino group and the 2-bromine; (b) dehydration, involving two hydrogens of the 6-amino group and the oxygen in II; and (c) dehydrogenation, involving the remaining hydrogen of the 5-amino group and the 2-hydrogen of II. The dehydrogenation in step (c) is brought approximately by another molecule of II that, by effecting the dehydrogenation, is reduced to 2,3-dibromo-1-propanol. The overall effect of these condensations is the cyclization of I with II to produce 6-bromomethyl-2,4-diaminopteridine (III). Further condensation (dehydrobromination involving the bromine in III and the hydrogen of the methylamino group in *N*-[*p*-(methylamino)benzoyl]glutamic acid) yields the crude drug, which is purified.

Description—Orange-brown, crystalline powder.

Solubility—Practically insoluble in water, alcohol, chloroform, or ether; freely soluble in dilute solutions of alkali hydroxides or carbonates; slightly soluble in dilute hydrochloric acid.

Comments—Inhibits dihydrofolate reductase, and thus prevents conversion of deoxyuridylate to thymidylate and blocks the synthesis of new DNA needed for cellular replication. Methotrexate is approved for use, and is the drug of choice, in *trophoblastic tumors* such as choriocarcinoma, *hydatidiform mole*, and *chorioadenoma destruens*. It also is approved for *prophylaxis of and treatment of meningeal leukemias* and for *breast cancer* and *nonmetastatic osteosarcoma*. It sometimes is combined with dactinomycin in these uses. When given intrathecally, it is the drug of choice for *CNS prophylaxis in acute lymphocytic leukemia*. In combination with other drugs it provides the therapy of choice. It is a component of first-choice combinations for induction and maintenance in *acute lymphocytic leukemia, diffuse histiocytic leukemia, cervical cancer, medulloblastoma, osteogenic sarcoma, breast cancer, non-Hodgkin's lymphomas, Burkitt's lymphoma, bladder carcinoma, squamous cell carcinoma of the head and neck, oat-cell* and *non-small-cell lung cancers*. It is an alternative drug for treatment of *adult soft-tissue sarcoma, follicular lymphoma, embryonal rhabdomyosarcoma,* and *colorectal carcinoma*. It also is used sequentially with fluorouracil in the treatment of node-negative breast cancer.

It may be given by intra-arterial infusion into the affected region in the treatment of a variety of carcinomata of the head, neck, pelvis, and limbs; the local concentrations achieved may be high enough to be effective and yet low enough in the rest of the body not to be toxic. The endocellular transport competitor, folinic acid (leucovorin), is also often given systematically to prevent generalized toxicity.

It is a secondary (efferent) immunosuppressive drug. It is one of a few drugs used to treat *Reiter's syndrome,* although results range from poor to good. It is employed to treat *psoriasis* refractory to other drugs; with methotrexate, approximately 50% of affected joints and 65% of skin lesions improve. It is used successfully to treat severe, progressive, refractory *rheumatoid arthritis* and glucocorticoid-dependent asthma. It has provided improvement in *dermatomyositis* and *polymyositis* (40–100% improvement), *Wegner's granulomatosis, pemphigus vulgaris, pityriasis rubra pilaris, bullous pemphigoid,* and *thrombocytopenic purpura,* but other drugs appear to be equal or superior.

The toxic effects are extensions of its antimetabolite effects; sometimes toxicity occurs first. They include bone-marrow hypoplasia with leukopenia, thrombocytopenia (with hemorrhage), and anemia. Depression of cellular proliferation along the GI tract results in diarrhea, ulcerative stomatitis, hemorrhagic enteritis, and perforation. Alopecia also may occur. Dosage schedules in which methotrexate is given chronically daily may cause liver damage. The drug must not be used when there is preexisting liver damage or bone-marrow depression, or during pregnancy. Daily blood counts and triweekly creatinine determinations are mandatory. The toxicity and therapeutic effects may be antagonized by leucovorin (leucovorin or thymidine *rescue*); if the leucovorin is given after an appropriate delay, it can prevent the toxic but not the therapeutic effect on certain tumors or the immune system. The drug is concentrated in the urine, and precipitation may cause renal failure; alkalinization and high water intake help protect the kidneys. Nitrous oxide, often used in pediatric oncology units, increases its cytotoxicity and probably its efficacy.

In doses less than 30 mg/m², it is absorbed well by the oral route; but approximately 1/3 of an oral dose is metabolized by intestinal bacteria, and antibiotics affect the amount absorbed. In doses greater than 80 mg/m², the amount absorbed is reduced further by 30 to 50%. Only approximately 50% of the drug is bound to plasma protein, but it does not gain much access to the cerebrospinal fluid because it is strongly ionized and outwardly transported at the choroid plexus; consequently, it must be administered intrathecally for use in the CNS. In the usual doses, it actively is transported into all tissues, but it is transported preferentially into responsive neoplastic cells. Intensification of therapy, alternating with or followed by leucovorin rescue, may achieve sufficient plasma levels (1 μM) to effect meningeal leukemias and lymphomas without intrathecal administration. Plasma clearance is triexponential, with a distribution half-life of approximately 45 min, a second phase of approximately 3.5 hr (possibly an enterohepatic component, because 10% of the drug is secreted into bile), and an elimination half-life of 6 to 69 hr. Renal tubular secretion accounts for approximately 80% of elimination, and probenecid, salicylate, and other NSAIDs, etc, interfere with excretion. Because methotrexate is partly bound to serum proteins, its toxicity may be increased as a result of displacement by certain drugs such as salicylates, sulfonamides, sulfonylureas, phenytoin, phenylbutazone, tetracyclines, chloramphenicol, and aminobenzoic acid. The dose must be adjusted in renal failure.

MITOMYCIN

Azirino[2′,3′:3,4]pyrrolo[1,2-a]indole-4,7-dione, [1aR-(1aα,8β,8aα, 8bα)]-6-amino-8-[[(aminocarbonyl)oxy]methyl]-1,1a,2,8,8a,8b-hexahydro-8a-methoxy-5-methyl-, Mitocin-C; Mutamycin

Mitomycin C [50-07-7] $C_{15}H_{18}N_4O_5$ (334.33).

Preparation—One of three closely related entities isolated from the antibiotic complex produced by *Streptomyces caespitosus*, an organism from Japanese soil.

Description—Blue-violet, crystalline powder.

Solubility—Soluble in water and in common organic solvents.

Comments—Inhibits DNA synthesis by cross-linking double-stranded DNA through guanine and cytosine. It is approved for palliative treatment of *disseminated adenocarcinoma of the stomach and the pancreas that have failed other treatments*. It is a component of second-line combinations for the treatment of *cervical, gastric,* and *pancreatic carcinomas* and *non-small-cell bronchogenic carcinoma*. It is instilled into the bladder in *papilloma*. It is an alternative drug for use against *head* and *neck squamous cell carcinoma, bladder carcinoma,* and *osteogenic sarcoma.* Acute adverse effects occur in approximately 14% of patients; they include nausea, vomiting, anorexia, fever, local irritation, and cellulites or tissue necrosis from extravasation at the site of injection. Delayed toxicity includes cumulative, frequently irreversible, bone-marrow depression (64% of recipients), stomatitis, alopecia, and renal impairment (20% of recipients). Pulmonary toxicity with hemoptysis, dyspnea, coughing, and pneumonia and hemolytic uremic syndrome occur infrequently, but may be severe.

MITOTANE

Benzene, 1-chloro-2[2,2-dichloro-1-(4-chlorophenyl)ethyl]-, *o,p'*-DDD; Lysodren

1,1-Dichloro-2-(*o*-chlorophenyl)-2-(*p*-chlorophenyl)ethane [53-19-0] $C_{14}H_{10}Cl_4$ (320.05).

Preparation—Chlorobenzene is condensed with 2,2-dichloro-1- (*o*-chlorophenyl)ethanol with the aid of H_2SO_4.

Description—White, tasteless, crystalline powder; slight aromatic odor; stable in light, air, and heat; melts about 78°.

Solubility—Practically insoluble in water; soluble in alcohol, ether, solvent hexane, or fixed oils or fats.

Comments—Because it is toxic to the adrenal cortex, it is approved for the treatment of *inoperable adrenal cortical carcinoma.* Nearly 50% of patients respond to treatment. It also is used to treat *Cushing's syndrome* and *Leydig carcinoma of the testicle.* Causes focal degeneration in the zona fasciculata and reticularis of the adrenal cortex with resultant atrophy and usually causes only minimal degeneration in the zona glomerulosa (site of aldosterone biosynthesis). Adverse effects of adrenal insufficiency may necessitate adrenal steroid replacement; these effects include anorexia, nausea, vomiting (in 80%), diarrhea, lethargy, somnolence (25%), dizziness (15%), headache, confusion, asthenia, tremors, ataxia, speech difficulties, neuropathies, dermatitis (15%), hypersensitivity, flushing, hyperpyrexia, postural hypotension, alopecia, pigmentation, leukopenia, thrombocytopenia, hyperbilirubinemia, albuminuria, hemorrhagic cystitis, elevated serum transaminase, blurred vision, diplopia, lens opacities, and retinopathy. The drug should be used with caution in the presence of liver damage, bone-marrow depression, dermatitis, or neuropathy. It is metabolized in the liver and reported to increase the metabolism of warfarin through induction of hepatic microsomal enzymes.

MITOXANTRONE HYDROCHLORIDE

9,10-Anthracenedione, 1,4-dihydroxy-5,8-bis-[[2-[(2-hydroxyethyl)amino]ethyl]amino]-, dihydrochloride; Novantrone

Mitozantrone [70476-82-3] $C_{22}H_{28}N_4O_6 \cdot 2HCl$ (517.41).

Preparation—*J Med Chem* 1978, 21:291.

Description—Blue-black solid; hygroscopic; melts about 161°; pKa 5.99, 8.13.

Solubility—Sparingly soluble in water; slightly soluble in methanol.

Comments—An alkylaminoanthraquinone antineoplastic drug related to doxorubicin. It is approved for the treatment of *acute nonlymphocytic leukemia* when combined with other agents and in combination with a corticosteroid in the palliative treatment of advanced, symptomatic (ie, painful) *hormone-refractory prostate cancer.* It is also indicated for reducing neurologic disability and/or the frequency of clinical relapses in patients with secondary (chronic) progressive, progressive relapsing, or worsening relapsing-remitting multiple sclerosis (ie, patients whose neurologic status is significantly abnormal between relapses), but not for treatment of patients with primary progressive multiple sclerosis. It is an alternative drug for the treatment of *acute lymphoblastic leukemia, chronic myelogenous leukemia, ovarian* and *breast carcinoma.* Immediate adverse effects include nausea, vomiting, and phlebitis. Tissue necrosis and sloughing result from extravasation. Delayed adverse effects include myelosuppression and cardiac, renal, and hepatic toxicities. The *N*-substitution on the aminosugar decreases

the cardiotoxicity. The drug is not absorbed orally. It is eliminated mostly in the bile and has a half-life of 20 to 36 hr.

Myocardial toxicity, manifested in its most severe form by potentially fatal congestive heart failure (CHF), may occur either during therapy with mitoxantrone or months to years after termination of therapy. In cancer patients, the risk of symptomatic CHF was estimated to be 2.6% for patients receiving up to a cumulative dose of 140 mg/m^2. Cardiovascular disease, prior or concomitant radiotherapy to the mediastinal/pericardial area, previous therapy with other anthracyclines or anthracenediones, or concomitant use of other cardiotoxic drugs may increase the risk of cardiac toxicity.

NILUTAMIDE

2,4-Imidazolidindione, 5,5-dimethyl-3-[4-nitro-3-(trifluoromethyl)phenyl]-, Nilandron; Anandron

[63612-50-0] $C_{12}H_{10}F_3N_3O_4$ (317.23).

Preparation—By reaction of 5,5-dimethylhydantoin with 5-chloro-2-nitro-α,α,α-trifluorotoluene in diphenyl ether or diglyme at 200° with CuO, Cu_2O, or NaOH as the condensing agent. US Pat 5,166,358 (1992).

Description—Microcrystalline, off-white powder that melts about 154°.

Solubility—Freely soluble in ethyl acetate, acetone, chloroform, ethanol, methylene chloride, or methanol; slightly soluble in water (<0.1% at 25°).

Comments—Approved for use in metastatic prostate cancer (Stage D) in combination with castration. It is a nonsteroidal antiandrogen that interacts with the testosterone receptor and prevents its response or nuclear binding at target tissues. It is absorbed rapidly and completely after oral administration. After a detectable distribution phase, it is metabolized extensively, less than 2% is excreted unchanged in the urine within 5 days. Several metabolites have been identified, one with 25% to 50% of the activity of the parent drug. The majority of the administered doses (62%) appears in the urine within 120 hr of administration. The average half-life is approximately 45 hr after a single dose. During multiple dosing (3 × 50 mg twice a day), steady-state levels were reached in 2 to 4 wk. It is bound by plasma proteins. Severe hepatic impairment is a contraindication for this drug.

Interstitial pneumonitis had been reported in 2% of patients receiving the drug. Signs of pneumonitis most often appeared within the first 3 months of treatment. Serum increases in hepatic enzymes led to discontinuation of the drug in 1% of patients. The drug should be discontinued if liver serum enzyme levels increase to 2- or 3-fold the normal upper limit. As many as half the patients report a delay in adapting to the dark; wearing tinted glasses seems to help in this respect. It inhibits several P-450 enzymes and care should be taken to monitor coadministered drugs that necessitate liver metabolism.

OXALIPLATIN

Platinum, [*SP*-4-2-(1*R-trans*)]-(1,2-cyclohexanediamine-*N,N'*)[ethanedioato(2-)-*O,O'*]-, Eloxatin

[61825-94-3] $C_8H_{14}N_2O_4Pt$ (397.30).

Preparation—*J Med Chem*, 1978; 21:1315.

Description—Colorless plates.

Solubility—6 mg/mL in water; very slightly soluble in methanol and practically insoluble in ethanol or acetone.

Comments—undergoes nonenzymatic conversion forming several transient reactive species, including monoaquo and diaquo DACH platinum, which covalently bind with macromolecules. Both inter- and intra-strand Pt-DNA cross-links are formed. Crosslinks are formed between the *N7* positions of two adjacent guanines (GG), adjacent adenine-guanines (AG), and guanines separated by an intervening nucleotide (GNG). These crosslinks inhibit DNA replication and transcription. It is indicated in combination with fluorouracil and leucovorin, for the treatment of metastatic cancer of the colon or rectum in patients whose disease has recurred or progressed during or within 6 months following first-line therapy with the combination regimen of fluorouracil, leucovorin, and irinotecan. It also has shown activity in ovarian cancer, germ-cell cancer, and cervical cancer.

Pharmacokinetics of oxaliplatin are triexponential with short initial α and β distribution phases (0.28 hour and 16.3 hours, respectively) and a long terminal γ phase (273 hours). Approximately 80% of oxaliplatin is bound to plasma proteins, and it undergoes extensive biotransformation, and has a very large volume of distribution. Over 5 days, approximately 50% will be excreted in the urine, and only 5% will be excreted in the feces. The dose-limiting toxicity of oxaliplatin is a peripheral neuropathy that is often triggered by exposure to cold, and manifests as paresthesias and/or dysesthesias in the upper and lower extremities, mouth, and throat. The peripheral neuropathy is cumulative; 75% of patients receiving a cumulative dose of 1560 mg/m^2 experience some neurotoxicity. Hematologic toxicity is mild to moderate, and nausea is well controlled with antiemetics. Anaphylactic-like reactions to oxaliplatin have been reported.

PACLITAXEL

5β,20-Epoxy-1,2α,4,7β,10β,13α-hexahydroxytax-11-en-9-one 4,10-diacetate 2-benzoate 13-ester with (2R,3S)-N-benzoyl-3-phenylisoserine; FK + 506; Taxol; Anzatax; Biotax; Bristaxol; Ifaxol; Intaxel; Medixel; Onxol; Parexel; Paxene; Praxel

[33069-62-4] $C_{47}H_{51}NO_{14}$ (853.92).

Preparation—Extracted from the bark of the Pacific yew tree (*Taxus brevifolia, Taxaceae*).

Description—White needles that melt about 215° with decomposition.

Solubility—Highly lipophilic and insoluble in water

Comments—Inhibits mitosis by stabilizing mitotic spindles by preventing depolymerization and promoting their formation. This causes inhibition of the normal dynamic reorganization of the microtubule network that is essential for interphase and mitotic cellular functions. May induce cell death by triggering apoptosis. Taxol is approved as first-line and subsequent therapy for use in *ovarian cancer* and as adjuvant treatment of *node-positive or metastatic breast cancer given sequentially to doxorubicin-containing regimen*. It is also indicated in combination with cisplatin as first line treatment for non-small cell lung cancer in patients who cannot tolerate surgery and/or radiation therapy and for second-line treatment of AIDS-related Kaposi's sarcoma. It has shown activity in malignant melanoma, gastric cancer, and acute leukemia.

Following IV administration, paclitaxel is widely distributed into body fluids and tissues with the mean apparent volume of distribution at steady state ranging from 227–688 L/m^2 with 88% to 98% bound to plasma proteins. The average distribution half-life ($t_{1/2\alpha}$) is 0.27 to 0.34 hours, and an average elimination half-life ($t_{1/2\beta}$) is 2.33 to 5.8 hours, depending on infusion time. It is extensively metabolized in the liver to its major metabolite, 6α-hydroxypaclitaxel, which is mediated by cytochrome P-450 isoenzyme CYP2C8.

Bone marrow suppression (primarily neutropenia), peripheral neuropathies (62% incidence consisting of numbness, tingling, and pain in hands and feet), and mucositis are dose-dependent and the dose-limiting toxicities. Anaphylaxis and severe hypersensitivity reactions consisting of dyspnea and hypotension requiring treatment, angioedema, and generalized urticaria have occurred in 2% to 4% of patients in clinical trials. All patients must be pretreated with corticosteroids, diphenhydramine, and H$_2$ antagonists. Severe cardiac changes (bradycardia, hypotension, chest pain, tachycardia, complete AV block) have been documented in <1% of patients during therapy. The drug is an irritant and potentially a vesicant. It also causes alopecia, facial flushing, and elevations in liver enzymes.

PEGASPARGASE

(Monomethoxypolyethylene glycol succinimidyl)$_{74}$-L-asparaginase; Oncaspar

[130167-69-0].

Preparation—See US Pat 4,179,337 (1979).

Description—The reaction product of L-asparaginase (derived from *E coli*) with succinic anhydride and esters with polyethylene glycol monomethyl ether. Its molecular weight is about 5000.

Comments—Approved for patients who have acute lymphoblastic leukemia who require, but who have developed hypersensitivity to, L-asparaginase. It generally is used in combination with other drugs. It is the enzyme L-asparaginase, obtained from *E coli*, that has been modified covalently by the addition of methoxypolyethylene glycol (mol wt 5000 daltons). Rapid depletion of asparagine by the administration of pegaspargase kills leukemia cells hat rely on exogenous sources of asparagine for growth. In asparaginase-hypersensitive patients, 93% of whom had relapsed from previous therapy, 50% evidenced reinduction after multiple injections of pegasparagase, 36% showing complete remissions.

The half-life of this drug in the blood is 3 to 6 days, with the volume of distribution approximating plasma volume. L-asparaginase is detectable in the blood 15 days after an administration of pegaspargase. Adverse reactions were relatively minor with elevations of liver enzymes, thrombosis, hyperglycemia, and pancreatitis being reported in less than 5% of patients. Allergic reactions, including rash and bronchospasm, were reported in greater than 5% of patients. Pegaspargase was administered intravenously and intramuscularly to 48 and 126 patients respectively. The incidence of hypersensitivity reactions when pegaspargase was administered intramuscularly was 30% in patients who were previously hypersensitive to native L-asparaginase and 11% in non-hypersensitive patients. The incidence of hypersensitivity reactions when pegaspargase was administered intravenously was 60% in patients who were previously hypersensitive to native L-asparaginase and 12% in non-hypersensitive patients.

PENTOSTATIN

Imidazo[4,5-d][1,3]diazepin-8-ol, (R)-3-(2-deoxy-β-D-*erythro*-pentofuranosyl)-3,6,7,8-tetrahydro-, Nipent, 2′-deoxycoformycin (DCF)

[63677-95-2] $C_{11}H_{16}N_4O_4$ (268.27).

Preparation—*J Org Chem* 1982, 47, 3457. Usually isolated from *Streptomyces antibioticus*.

Description—White crystals that melt about 223°; pKa 5.2.

Comments—Inhibits adenosine deaminase, thus leading to an accumulation of 2′-deoxyATP. Inhibition of cell proliferation results. Lymphocytes are especially sensitive to this drug. It is approved for use in *α-interferon refractory hairy-cell leukemia*. It is an alternative drug for use against chronic *lymphocytic leukemia, mycosis fungoides, acute lymphoblastic leukemia*. Adverse effects include myelosuppression sometimes with severe lymphopenia, conjuctivitis, panserositis, lethargy, coma, pulmonary toxicity, hyperuricemia and immunosuppression; various infections may occur, herpes simplex infections being the most common.

PLICAMYCIN

Aureolic acid; Mithramycin; Mithracin

[18378-89-7] $C_{52}H_{76}O_{24}$ (1085.16).

Preparation—Produced by cultures of *Streptomyces argillaceus, S plicatus,* and *S tanashiensis.*

Description—Yellow, crystalline powder; odorless; hygroscopic; melts about 182°.

Solubility—Slightly soluble in water, slightly soluble in alcohol; freely soluble in ethyl acetate.

Comments—An antibiotic elaborated during culture of certain strains of *Streptomyces.* A yellow, crystalline powder; odorless; hygroscopic; slightly soluble in water; slightly soluble in alcohol. It has various uses: Binds to guanine-rich DNA and thus inhibits DNA-dependent RNA polymerase. It acts mainly during the S phase. It is approved for and used to treat *carcinoma* of the *testes,* but use has been replaced by other more effective agents. It also is an alternative drug for *blast phase* of *chronic myelogenous leukemia,* especially in combination with hydroxyurea. Because it suppresses osteoclast activity, it often is used to treat *malignant hypercalcemia* (neoplasms that cause dissolution of bone salts) unresponsive to conventional treatment and *Paget's disease* of the bone..

It is toxic, and drug-induced mortality ranges from 0.09% to 0.7%, depending on dose. Death results from hemorrhagic diatheses resulting from hypoprothrombinemia,, thrombocytopenia, increased clotting and bleeding times, and abnormal clot retraction. The hemorrhagic episode usually begins with nosebleed, but it may begin with hematemesis. The most common untoward effects are nausea, vomiting, diarrhea, anorexia, and stomatitis. Less frequently there occur fever, facial flushing, rash, phlebitis, malaise, headache, drowsiness, asthenia, lethargy, depression, hepatic dysfunction, renal insufficiency, hypocalciuria, hypokalemia, hypophosphatemia, and leukopenia. The hemorrhagic syndrome occurs in approximately 5% of patients who receive no more than 30 µg/kg/day for no more than 10 doses, whereas it is approximately 12% for higher doses. It is locally toxic and can cause necrosis and sloughing if extravasated.

PORFIMER SODIUM

Polymorphin oligomer containing ester and ether linkages; Photofrin

[87806-31-1].

Preparation—See US Pat 4,649,151 (1987).

Description—The purified product as a mixture of oligomers formed by ester and ether linkages to as many as eight porphyrin units with aggregates of a combined molecular weight of approximately 10^5.

Solubility—The reconstituted product should be protected from heat and light and used immediately. **DO NOT MIX** with other drugs in the same solution.

Comments—Approved for photodynamic therapy of obstructive esophageal cancer and for the treatment of microinvasive endobronchial NSCLC in patients for whom surgery and radiotherapy are not indicated. It is injected intravenously after which 40 to 70 hr are allowed for clearance. It is retained in a few tissues, notably spleen, liver, and skin, and tumor. Laser light at 630-nm wavelength then is used to irradiate the esophagus. The drug that is present is excited by the light to initiate the production of reactive oxygen species. These are tissues damaging on their own but, in addition, they induce necrosis in the tumor by means of ischemia mediated by the production of thromboxane A2 and vascular occlusion. In a clinical trial of 17 patients who have obstructive esophageal cancer, 93% showed objective response after therapy, and 65% received clinically important benefit.

After a 2-mg/kg dose the half-life for elimination was 250 hr. It is approximately 90% protein bound in the serum. Patients treated with this drug are photosensitive and should take care to remain protected from sunlight and bright indoor light for a minimum of 30 days. Serious side effects were noted in less than 5% of patients and were primarily related to inflammation at the illumination site.

PREDNISONE—page 1448.

PROCARBAZINE HYDROCHLORIDE

Benzamide, *N*-(1-methylethyl)-4-[(2-methylhydrazino)methyl]-, monohydrochloride; Matulane

N-Isopropyl-α-(2-methylhydrazino)-*p*-toluamide monohydrochloride [366-70-1] C12H19N3O.HCl (257.76).

Preparation—1,2-Bis(carbobenzoxy)-1-methylhydrazine is reacted with 4-(bromoethyl)benzoic acid methyl ester ultimately to yield 4-[[2-methyl-1,2-di(carbobenzoxy)hydrazino]methyl]benzoic acid. Thionyl chloride is used to obtain the acid chloride which is reacted with isopropylamine to give the *N*-isopropylamide compound. Treatment with 33% HBr in glacial acetic acid removes the protecting carbobenzoxy groups, and thus resulting hydrobromide may be converted to the hydrochloride by the usual process. US Pat 3,520,926.

Description—White to pale yellow, crystalline powder; slight odor and a bitter taste; solutions are acid to litmus; stable in light, slowly oxidized in air, and stable at room temperature (in the presence of oxygen, oxidation is accelerated by increased temperature); melts about 223° with decomposition; pK$_a$ (at room temperature) 6.8.

Solubility—1 g in 7 mL water or 100 mL alcohol; slightly soluble in chloroform; insoluble in ether.

Comments—Unstable in aqueous solutions, it breaks down to form the methylazoxy derivative, the active form of the drug. It generates hydrogen peroxide, hydroxyl, and methyl-free radicals, the latter being thought to alkylate DNA, resulting in degradation and chromosomal breaks; DNA synthesis, and hence protein synthesis, is impaired. It is approved as part of a combination therapy for *Hodgkin's disease.* The most important use of procarbazine is as a component of several combinations of choice for *Hodgkin's disease, nonHodgkin's lymphoma, mycosis fungoides, multiple myeloma,* and *medulloblastoma.* It is an alternative drug to treat non-small-cell *bronchogenic carcinoma;* it is rarely used alone. Cross resistance with other agents or radiation apparently does not occur.

Untoward reactions include frequent leukopenia, thrombocytopenia, anemia, less frequent nausea, and vomiting; rare reactions are anorexia, dry mouth, stomatitis, dysphagia, diarrhea, constipation, myalgia and arthralgia, chills and fever, sweating, fatigue, asthenia, lethargy, and drowsiness. Ascites, edema, effusions, cough, intercurrent infections, epistaxis, hemorrhaging, melena, pruritus, allergic dermatitis, allergic pneumonitis, flushing, alopecia, pigmentation, herpes, jaundice, headache, vertigo, depression, paresthesias, neuropathies, insomnia, nightmares, ataxia, confusion, coma, tremors, and convulsions may occur. Rarely, there may be hoarseness, hypotension, tachycardia, syncope, hemolysis, nystagmus, photophobia, photosensitivity, retinal hemorrhage, diplopia, papilledema, impaired hearing, and slurred speech. It is mutagenic, teratogenic, and carcinogenic in experimental animals. Thus, it must be regarded as a dangerous drug.

CNS depressants should not be given at the same time, except under supervision. Because the drug is a monoamine oxidase inhibitor, tricyclic antidepressants, various sympathomimetics and tyramine-containing foods should be avoided. Because it has disulfiram-like activity, patients should be warned against ingestion of alcoholic beverages. Caution must be exercised in the presence of liver damage, respiratory disorders, renal impairment, or bone-marrow depression.

It is absorbed almost completely by the oral route. It penetrates readily into the cerebrospinal fluid. Peak plasma and cerebrospinal fluid levels occur approximately 60 min after an oral dose. It is metabolized rapidly and auto-oxidized, with an elimination half-life of only approximately 7 min. Almost none is excreted unchanged.

SODIUM IODIDE I 131—See Chapter 29
SODIUM PHOSPHATE P 32—See Chapter 29.

STREPTOZOCIN

D-Glucopyranose, 2-deoxy-2[[(methylnitrosoamino)carbonyl]amino]-, Streptozocin; Zanosar

[18883-66-4] C8H15N3O7 (265.22).

Preparation—A nitrosourea antibiotic isolated from *Streptomyces achromogenes* fermentation broth; also synthesized; *J Am Chem Soc* 1969; 52:2555.

Description—Plates or prisms; melts about 115° with decomposition.

Solubility—Soluble in water or in alcohol.

Comments—It is approved for and has become the drug of first choice (in combination with fluorouracil) for treatment of *islet-cell carcinoma*. It also is used with fluorouracil and mitomycin for *pancreatic carcinoma*. It is an alternative drug for use against *malignant carcinoid tumors, non-small cell lung cancer, squamous cell carcinoma of the oral cavity,* and *hepatomae*. Acute adverse effects include severe nausea and vomiting, proteinuria, local pain at the site of administration, and chills. Renal damage is the principal delayed toxicity, but hepatotoxicity also occurs. Bone-marrow depression occurs in approximately 20% of recipients. The drug is mainly metabolized; its half-life is approximately 15 min. Dosage adjustments are recommended with decreased renal function.

TAMOXIFEN CITRATE

(Z)-2-[4-(1,2-diphenyl-1-butenyl)phenoxy]-N,N-dimethyl-, Nolvadex

(Z)-2- [p - (1,2-Diphenyl-1-butenyl)phenoxy]-*N,N*-dimethylethylamine citrate (1:1) [54965-24-1] $C_{26}H_{29}NO.C_6H_8O_7$ (563.65).

Preparation—4-β-Dimethylaminoethoxy-α-ethyldesoxybenzoin by reaction with phenylmagnesium bromide or phenyl lithium is converted to 1-(4-β-dimethylaminoethoxyphenyl)-1,2-diphenyl butanol, which on dehydration yields a mixture of tamoxifen and its cis-isomer that may be separated with petroleum ether; tamoxifen is converted to the 1:1 citrate for dispensing use. See *Nature* 1966; 212:733; *CA* 1967; 67:90515g.

Description—White, crystalline powder; melts about 140°.

Comments—A nonsteroidal antiestrogen approved for palliative therapy of breast cancer in men and postmenopausal women. It is also effective as adjuvant therapy in axillary node-negative or node-positive breast cancer following total mastectomy, axillary dissection, and breast irradiation. The drug competes with estrogens for cytosol estrogen receptors and thus blocks estrogen effects in the target tissue. Tumors with negative receptor assays do not respond to it. Adverse effects frequently reported are hot flashes, nausea, and vomiting. The drug also can cause weight gain, vaginal bleeding and discharge, rashes, transient leukopenia, increased hepatic enzymes, and thrombocytopenia. Increased bone and tumor pain may occur. Infrequent side effects are deep vein thrombosis and hypercalcemia.

The oral bioavailability is 25% to 100%. The half-life of a single dose is 18 hr, but it is only 7 hr at steady state.

TEMOZOLOMIDE

Imidazo[5,1-d]-as-tetrazine-8-carboxamide, 3,4-dihydro-3-methyl-4-oxo-,Temodar

[85622-93-1] $C_6H_6N_6O2$ (194.15).

Preparation—The dimethyl ester of 4-aminopyrazole-3,5-dicarboxylic acid is diazotized with sodium nitrite and HCl and the diazonium salt treated with methylamine to yield the product. *J Med Chem* 1995; 38:1496

Description—White to light tan powder melting about 180°. It is the prodrug for *dacarbazine* which is formed by hydrolysis of the amide group (carbonyl and adjacent *N*-atom bearing the methyl group) in the tetrazine ring. The molecule is stable below pH 5 but rapidly transforms to *dacarbazine* at pH >7; $[\alpha]^{20}_D$ +43 ± 2°, c = 1, water).

Solubility—(mg/mL) Water (3), ethanol(1), DMSO(22–25),

Comments—Undergoes rapid non-enzymatic conversion at physiologic pH to the reactive ompound, 3-methyl-(triazen-1-yl)imidazole-4-carboxamide(MTIC), whick alkylates DNA. Alkylation (methylation) occurs mainly at the O^6 and N^7 positions of guanine. Indicated for the treatment of adults with refractory anaplastic astrocytoma who have experienced disease progression on a drug regimen containing a nitrosourea and procarbazine. Completely absorbed after oral administration; food reduces the rate and extent of absorption. Rapidly eliminated with a mean elimination half-life of 1.8 hours and mean apparent volume of distribution of 0.4 L/kg (%CV=13%). It is weakly bound to human plasma proteins, with an overall clearance of about 5.5 L/h/m². Most frequently occurring adverse effects were nausea and vomiting, fatigue, headache, and dose-limiting myelosuppression (thrombocytopenia and neutropenia).

TENIPOSIDE

Furo[3′,4′:6,7]naphtho[2,3-d]-1,3-dioxol-6(5aH)-one, [5R-[5α,5aβ,8aα,9β(R*)]]-5,8,8a,9-tetrahydro-5-(4-hydroxy-3,5-dimethoxyphenyl)-9-[[4,6-O-(2-thienylmethylene)-β-D-glucopyranosyl]oxy]-, VM-26; Vumon

[29767-20-2] $C_{32}H_{32}O_{13}S$ (656.66).

Preparation—A semisynthetic derivative of podophyllotoxin.

Description—White crystals that melt about 245°.

Comments—A drug related to podophyllotoxin and similar to etoposide in antieoplastic activity. It arrests the cell cycle in late S and G_2 phases. It is approved for use in *relapsed or refractory acute lymphocytic leukemia in children*. It is an alternative drug for the treatment of *cutaneous T-cell lymphoma, Kaposi's sarcoma,* and *small cell lung brain metastases*. The principal adverse effects (leukopenia, thrombocytopenia, etc) result from myelosuppression, but hypotension, thrombophlebitis, and anaphylaxis also occur. The drug is not absorbed orally. In plasma it is almost completely protein bound. It is eliminated mainly by hepatic metabolism, with a half-life of 8 to 24 hr.

TESTOLACTONE—see RPS-19, page 1104.
TESTOSTERONE PROPIONATE—see RPS-19, page 1105.

THIOGUANINE

6H-Purine-6-thione, 2-amino-1,7-dihydro-, Tabloid

2-Aminopurine-6(1*H*)-thione [154-42-7] $C_5H_5N_5S$ (167.19); *hemihydrate* [50322-14-0] (176.20).

Preparation—By thionation of guanine with phosphorus pentasulfide. US Pat 2,884,667.

Description—Pale yellow, crystalline powder, odorless or practically odorless.

Solubility—Insoluble in water, alcohol, or chloroform; freely soluble in dilute solutions of alkali hydroxides.

Comments—An antimetabolite of guanine which is converted into 6-thioguanine-ribose-phosphate; this not only is incorporated into DNA and RNA but also interferes with guanine synthesis. It acts mainly in the S phase of the cell cycle, but cell replication ultimately is prevented. It also promotes differentiation of some cancer cells. Its actions are very similar to those of mercaptopurine, some of which is converted to thioguanine and cross resistance occurs between the two drugs; however, its actions and uses are not identical. It is approved for *acute non-lymphocytic leukemia*. With other drugs, thioguanine is a component of combinations that are treatments of choice for *AMLs* and the *acute phase of chronic granulocytic leukemia*. It is an alternative drug for use against *acute lymphocytic leukemia*. It sometimes is used in the stable phase of *chronic myelocytic leukemia*. It also is a potent *immunosuppressive drug,* but its status has yet to be settled. It has been used especially in the treatment of *nephrosis* and *collagen-vascular disorders*.

Its adverse effects are virtually the same as those for mercaptopurine (see page 1497), except that the incidence of GI toxicity is less and there is no adverse interaction with allopurinol.

It is metabolized nearly completely in the body; the 6-thiol group is methylated and the 8-amino group removed to yield 6-methyl-mercaptopurine. Xanthine oxidase is not involved.

THIOTEPA

Aziridine, 1,1′,1,″-phosphinothioylidynetris-,
Triethylenephosphoramide; Thioplex

[52-24-4] $C_6H_{12}N_3PS$ (189.2).

Preparation—By condensing ethylenimine with thiophosphorylchloride ($PSCl_3$) in the presence of triethylamine as the acid receptor.

Description—Fine, white, crystalline flakes; faint odor; melts about 54°.

Solubility—1 g in 13 mL water, 8.3 mL alcohol, 1.9 mL chloroform, or 4.1 mL ether.

Comments—An alkylating agent. However, it has a much lower chemical reactivity than the β-chloroethylamines and hence has a low degree of local irritancy and lacks the vesicant properties. For this reason it currently is used mainly for local application, where appropriate. It is approved for use in *adenocarcinoma of the breast and ovary*. Local instillation into the urinary bladder for *papillary carcinoma* is sometimes effective. It also may be instilled into other cavities (ie, intrathecally) to control serous infusions consequent to certain neoplasms. It occasionally may be infiltered directly into tumors, especially obstructive lesions. Given systemically, its bone-marrow toxicity is unpredictable, so that such use is dangerous; consequently, it is nearing obsolescence for systemic treatment. The neoplasm for which it is still a possible desperation choice is *embryonal rhabdomyosarcoma*.

Local adverse effects include local pain, weeping, and occasional perforation through the lesion. The most serious systemic adverse effect is bone-marrow depression, characterized by neutropenia, thrombocytopenia, and usually low-grade anemia. It is mandatory to monitor the blood-cell counts. The effects may not appear for 5 to 30 days, which complicates management. Anorexia, nausea, and vomiting are not as common as with other alkylating agents. Headache, dizziness, fever, and tightness in the throat may occur. Hyperuricemia may result from massive cell destruction, and crystalluria and oliguria are possible. Hypersensitivity is uncommon, but hives, skin rash, and even anaphylaxis can occur. Depression of spermatogenesis and ovarian function have been reported. Systemic side effects from local instillation can occur. It is excreted mostly unchanged, so that the dose should be reduced in renal failure. It is contraindicated if there is previous bone-marrow depression or pregnancy.

TOPOTECAN HYDROCHLORIDE

1*H*-Pyrano[3′,4′:6,7]indolizino[1,2-*b*]quinoline-3,14(4*H*,12*H*)-dione, 10-[(dimethylamino)methyl]-4-ethyl-4,9-dihydroxy-, monohydrochloride; Hycamtin

[119413-54-6] $C_{23}H_{23}N_3O_5$.HCl (457.92).

Preparation—Semisynthetic derivative of camptothecin derived from *Camptotheca acuminata*. *J Med Chem* 1991; 34:98.

Description—Light yellow to greenish-yellow crystals that melt about 215° (dec).

Solubility—Soluble 1 mg/mL in water.

Comments—Indicated in metastatic ovarian cancer that has failed at least one round of alternative therapy. It is a potent inhibitor of topoisomerase I. It causes the enzyme to freeze at a step in catalysis where it exists as a covalent adduct to a nicked strand of the DNA helix. Can-

cer-cell resistance to this drug may arise from lowered levels of topoisomerase I or from specific topoisomerase I mutations.

It undergoes reversible hydrolysis of the lactose moiety to yield a pharmacologically inactive ring-opened form. Liver metabolism plays only a minor role in inactivation of the drug. Approximately 30% of the drug is excreted in the urine; thus renal clearance is important. It exhibits multiexponential elimination from the plasma with a terminal half-life of approximately 2.5 hr. Approximately 35% is bound to plasma proteins. It is given by IV infusion over 30 minutes for 5 days every 21 days.

Bone-marrow suppression is its dose-limiting toxicity, most commonly neutropenia. The drug should not be administered if baseline neutrophil counts are less than 1500/mm³ or platelet counts less than 100,000/mm³. Neutropenia is most common during the first course of treatment, approximately a 60% frequency, but occurs during all courses at approximately a 40% frequency. The nadir of the neutrophil count is approximately 11 days. Thrombocytopenia occurs in approximately 25% of patients. Anemia occurs in approximately 40% of patients, with the nadir in RBC count at approximately day 15. It may harm the fetus and may appear in breast milk. Nausea and vomiting and total alopecia are noted in approximately 50% of patients.

TRETINOIN

Vesanoid

See page 1288 for full monograph.

Comments—Approved for induction of remission in patients who have acute promyelocytic leukemia displaying the t(15;17) translocation and who are refractory or who have relapsed from anthracycline therapy. It is a transretinoic acid related to vitamin A. It induces differentiation of promyelocytic cell and can induce complete remissions. Administered daily for as long as 90 days, it induced complete remissions in 50% to 80% of relapsed patients. It induces leukocytosis in approximately 40% of patients.

A single 45-mg/m² oral dose yields peak blood concentrations in approximately 1.5 hr; it is >95% bound to plasma proteins, largely albumin. Approximately 65% of a dose appears in the urine within 72 hr; approximately 30% appears in the feces within for 6 days. Cytochrome P-450 is involved in the metabolic activation of this drug, and several metabolites have been identified. This metabolism in inducible, and blood levels decrease by approximately one third after a 1-wk continuous treatment. Ketoconazole pretreatment led to a 72% increase in tretinoin AUC.

Almost all patients experience adverse reactions characteristic of high-dose vitamin A ingestion. Fever, headache, skin dryness, bone pain, malaise, chest discomfort, edema, DIC, etc. It can induce benign intracranial hypertension. Symptoms include headache, nausea, and visual disturbances. GI hemorrhage, pain, diarrhea, and constipation have been reported.

URACIL MUSTARD

2,4(1*H*, 3*H*)-Pyrimidinedione, 5-[bis(2-chloroethyl)amino-, Uramustine; Uracil Mustard

5-[Bis(2-chlorethyl)amino]uracil [66-75-1] $C_8H_{11}Cl_2N_3O_2$ (252.10).

Preparation—Using 5-aminouracil, ethylene oxide and thionyl chloride as reactants.

Description—Off-white, crystalline powder; odorless; melts about 200° with decomposition. Unstable in high humidity or aqueous vehicles.

Solubility—1 g in more than 1000 mL water or in 50 mL alcohol.

Comments—An alkylating agent of the nitrogen-mustard-type. It is essentially an obsolete drug, having been displaced by the more efficacious and less toxic chlorambucil. However, this drug still may have a special use in the treatment of *primary thrombocytosis*. Other neoplasms for which the drug is used occasionally are non-Hodgkin's lymphomas, chronic lymphocytic leukemia, chronic myelocytic leukemia, mycosis fungoides, and polycythemia vera. The most common untoward effects are nausea, vomiting, and diarrhea. Pruritus, dermatitis, and partial alopecia do occur, but less frequently than with cyclophosphamide. Nervousness, irritability, depression, amenorrhea, and oligospermia occur infrequently. Bone-marrow depression with leukopenia, thrombocytopenia, and even anemia may occur, and the blood counts must be monitored twice a week during the first month of treatment. The bone-marrow damage may become irreversible when the cumulative dose approaches 1 mg/kg. Rapid involution of tumors may cause hyperuricemia and consequent nephropathy and renal failure, so that plasma uric acid levels should be determined regularly and the patients should drink a lot of water.

VALRUBICIN

Pentanoic acid, (2S-cis)-2-[1,2,3,4,6,11-hexahydro-2,5,12-tri-hydroxy-7-methoxy-6,11-dioxo-4-[[2,3,6-trideoxy-3-[(trifluoro-acetyl)amino]-α-L-lyxo-hexopyranosyl]oxy]-2-naphtha-cenyl]-2-oxoethyl ester; Valstar

[56124-62-0] $C_{34}H_{36}F_3NO_{13}$ (723.65).

Preparation—US Pat 4,035,566 (1977).

Description—Orange or orange-red powder; highly lipophilic.

Solubility—Soluble in methylene chloride, ethanol, methanol or acetone; relatively insoluble in water.

Comments—indicated intravesically for the treatment of BCG-refractory carcinoma *in situ* (CIS) of the urinary bladder in patients who are not candidates for immediate cystectomy because of unacceptable morbidity or mortality. Principal toxicity is local bladder irritation, which occurs during or shortly after instillation in most patients receiving the drug and usually resolves within 1 to 7 days. The most common local bladder symptoms reported are urinary frequency, urinary urgency, and dysuria, which occur in 61%, 57%, and 56% of patients, respectively. Bladder spasm, hematuria, and bladder pain have been reported in 31%, 29%, and 28% of patients, respectively. It must not be administered intravenously.

VINBLASTINE SULFATE

Vincaleukoblastine, sulfate (1:1) (salt); Velban

(R is CH₃)

[143-67-9] $C_{46}H_{58}N_4O_9 \cdot H_2SO_4$ (909.06).

Preparation—By extracting the leaves, bark, or stems of *Vinca rosea* with aqueous or aqueous-alcoholic sulfuric acid, isolating the alkaloid from the extract by the usual precipitation and solvent techniques and purifying by chromatography on aluminum oxide. Conversion to the (1:1) sulfate may be effected by dissolution of the alkaloid in an equimolar quantity of dilute H_2SO_4 and either evaporating to dryness or precipitating with a suitable organic solvent. US Pat 3,097,137.

Description—White to slightly yellow, amorphous or crystalline powder; odorless; hygroscopic.

Solubility—Freely soluble in water.

Comments—Interferes with the assembly of the microtubules, by combining with tubulin; the result is mitotic arrest in metaphase. However, there is also evidence that vinblastine exerts its antineoplastic effect by interfering with glutamate and aspartate metabolism. The antineoplastic spectrum and toxicity are much different than for vincristine, which also interacts with tubulin. It is approved for use in *advanced Hodgkin's disease, lymphocytic* and *histiocytic lymphoma, mycosis fungoides, testicular cancer,* and *Kaposi's sarcoma.* This drug is a compo-

nent of first-choice combinations for the treatment of *testicular carcinoma, Hodgkin's disease,* and *bladder cancer.* It is an alternative drug for *choriocarcinoma, squamous cell carcinoma* of the head and neck, *renal-cell carcinoma, neuroblastoma, breast tumors, cervical carcinoma, Kaposi's sarcoma, melanoma,* and *mycosis fungoides.* It also has been used to treat lymphosarcoma, lymphocytic lymphoma, reticulum-cell sarcoma, and Letterer-Siwe's disease. This drug is subject to pleiotropic drug resistance.

Nausea, vomiting, headache, and paresthesias occur within 4 to 6 hr and last from 2 to 10 hr. Severe bronchospasm may occur, especially if mitomycin has been given. Diarrhea, constipation, adynamic ileus, anorexia, and stomatitis also may occur and are premonitory of neurotoxic effects, such as severe headache, malaise, mental depression, paresthesias, and loss of deep tendon reflexes. Neurotoxicity occurs in 5% to 20% of cases, more frequently at higher doses. CNS damage occasionally is permanent when excessive doses have been used. Blindness and death have been reported. Alopecia occurs in approximately 30 to 60% of users, but it generally is reversible. Mild bone-marrow depression with leukopenia occurs in a high percentage of patients and may require discontinuation of the drug. The thrombocytes are less affected, unless other thrombocytogenic drugs also are being given or recently have been given. Anemia is rare. The blood-cell count must be determined weekly. The drug is toxic locally, and extravasation should be avoided. It may cause phlebitis at the site of injection. Inappropriate secretion of ADH may occur. It is teratogenic in animals, and probably should not be used during the first trimester of pregnancy.

In plasma it is approximately 75% protein bound. It manifests three-compartment kinetics, the second phase having a half-life of 1 to 1.5 hr and an elimination half-life of 18 to 40 hr. It is metabolized largely by the liver and doses should be reduced by 50% in patients who have impaired liver function.

VINCRISTINE SULFATE

Vincaleukoblastine, 22-oxo-, sulfate (1:1) (salt); Oncovin; Vincasar PFS

Leurocristine sulfate (1:1) (salt) [2068-78-2] $C_{46}H_{56}N_4O_{10} \cdot H_2SO_4$ (923.04).

The structure is the same as for *Vinblastine Sulfate,* except that R is CHO, an aldehyde.

Preparation—With suitable modifications in the chromatographic part of the process, vincristine sulfate may be prepared as described above for *Vinblastine Sulfate.* US Pat 3,205,220.

Description—White to slightly yellow, amorphous or crystalline powder: odorless; hygroscopic.

Solubility—Freely soluble in water.

Comments—Combines with the protein tubulin and prevents assembly of microtubules, thus disrupting various cellular processes, including spindle formation and mitosis. Synthesis of RNA and proteins also is suppressed. It is approved for use in *Hodgkin's lymphomas, rhabdomyocsarcoma, neuroblastoma,* and *Wilms' tumor.* The alkaloid is the second most widely used of the antineoplastic drugs. It is especially useful in the treatment of hematological malignancies. It is a component in 27 first-choice combinations for the treatment of *acute lymphocytic leukemia,* the *acute phase of chronic myelocytic leukemia, Hodgkin's disease, non-Hodgkin's lymphoma, Burkitt's lymphoma, diffuse histiocytic lymphoma, follicular lymphoma, cervical carcinoma, oat-cell bronchogenic carcinoma, Wilms' tumor, medulloblastoma, soft-tissue sarcomas, Ewing's sarcoma,* and *embryonal rhabdomyosarcoma.* It is an alternative drug for treatment of *breast carcinoma, cervical carcinoma, testicular carcinoma, glioblastoma, neuroblastoma,* and *chronic lymphocytic leukemia.* Some authorities prefer to use this drug only to induce remissions and not for maintenance, because chronic use often results in neurotoxicity. Cross resistance to other drugs occurs by means of pleiotropic drug resistance.

It differs from most other antineoplastics in that bone-marrow depression frequently does not occur; this is one reason why vincristine is used in combinations. However, leukopenia can occur, and WBC counts should be made before each dose. Treatment usually is limited by the neurotoxic effects. Adverse effects usually begin with nausea, vomiting, constipation, abdominal cramps, and weight loss; these effects readily are reversible. Severe bronchospasm may occur, especially if mitomycin has been given. The drug also may cause slowly reversible reactions, such as alopecia and peripheral neuropathy, Serious neuropathic effects may occur; they include loss of deep tendon reflexes, neuritic pain, numbness of extremities, headache, ataxia, and visual defects; paresis or paralysis and atrophy of certain extensor muscles may occur late; paralysis of cranial nerves 2, 3, 6, and 7 may occur. Neuropathies may persist for several months. Severe hypertension, agitation, or mental depression also may occur transiently. The drug is toxic locally, and extravasation should be avoided. It is best given into the tubing of a running intravenous solution.

It is cleared rapidly from the blood. It manifests three-compartment kinetics, with half-lives of 0.08, 2.3, and 85 hr. Seventy percent is secreted into the bile. In obstructive jaundice or impaired liver function the toxicity is greater, and the dose should be reduced by 50%. Approximately 12% is excreted in urine. It does not penetrate into the brain, hence it cannot be used for CNS leukemias. Caution must be taken never to administer this agent intrathecally as it will result in death of the patient.

VINORELBINE

Didehydrodeoxynorvincaleukoblastine; Navelbine

$C_{45}H_{54}N_4O_8.2C_4H_6O_6$

Preparation—White to yellow or light brown amorphous powder

Description—Large dimeric asymmetric compound composed of a dihydroindole nucleus (vindoline), which is the major alkaloid present in the periwinkle (*Catharanthus roseus* [Apocynaceae]), and an indole nucleus (catharanthine), which is present in low concentrations in the plant.

Solubility—aqueous solubility of the drug exceeds 1000 mg/mL in distilled water; pH of approximately 3.5.

Comments—Vinorelbine is a semisynthetic vinca alkaloid whose mechanism of action is identical to that of vinblastine and vincristine (ie, inhibits cell mitosis in the M phase through inhibition of tubulin polymerization) resulting in inhibition of microtubule assembly and cellular metaphase arrest. Indicated for the treatment of unresectable, advanced non-small cell lung cancer (NSCLC) as a single agent or for Stage III or IV NSCLC in combination with cisplatin for first-line treatment. Also active for metastatic breast cancer, Hodgkin's disease, and advanced ovarian cancer. Myelosuppression with neutropenia is the dose-limiting toxicity, but nausea and vomiting, transient elevations in liver function tests, mild to moderate peripheral neuropathy (paresthesias, loss of deep tendon reflexes, myalgias) and SIADH are also reported. Dosage must be adjusted for hepatic insufficiency. Caution must be used to avoid extravasation as it is a vesicant.

Extensively metabolized in the liver by the cytochrome P-450 (CYP3A) isoenzymes to two metabolites, vinorelbine *N*-oxide and deacetylvinorelbine. Deacetylvinorelbine, the primary metabolite, has been shown to possess antitumor activity similar to the parent drug. Concurrent administration of drugs that effect CYP3A isoenzyme may effect the metabolism of this agent and cause increased toxicities. A steady-state volume of distribution of 25.4–40.1 L/kg has been reported and mean terminal elimination half-life of 27.7–43.6 hours and a mean plasma clearance of 0.97–1.26 L/hour per kg have been reported.

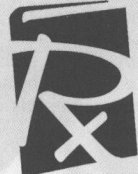

CHAPTER **87**

Immunoactive Drugs

Daniele K Gelone, PharmD

The immune system is a highly orchestrated specialized series of responses the immune system is quite complex. Several types of cells are involved. These are cells, the ancestral line of which has derived from bone marrow stem cells. Some of the descendants of the stem cells migrate to sites elsewhere in the body, where they become small lymphocytes. There are two general types of lymphocytes involved in the immune responses: the B cells and the T cells. The B lymphocytes get the designation B from the fact that in birds they derive from stem-cell clones in the bursa of Fabricus; in man, the location of analogous clones may be in the intestinal mucosal Peyer's patches. The T cells get their designation from the fact that they are derived from stem cells cloned in the thymus gland. Undifferentiated lymphocytes take up residence in lymph tissue in the spleen, tonsils, intestines, and other sites.

B and T cells respond to antigen by cellular transformation, proliferation, and differentiation. Proliferation increases the population of immunocompetent cells and differentiation creates cells with various roles to play in the immune response. Both B and T cells differentiate into what broadly may be termed effector cells and memory cells. The memory cells revert to an inactive state (G_0) but respond to later immune challenge by accelerated proliferation, differentiation, and activity. During their residence in the bursa equivalent, the future effector B cells become programmed to respond to an antigen by transformation into plasma cells, which produce antibodies (immunoglobulins I_A, I_D, I_E, I_G, and I_M), the role of which is to combine with circulating antigens. The immunity conferred by B cells is known as humoral immunity.

Hypersensitivity mediated through the humoral immune system is called immediate hypersensitivity, because the response is rapid. T cells become programmed in the thymus to respond in various ways to antigen that has become fixed to cell surfaces or engulfed by macrophages. The cytotoxic T cell (effector cell, *killer* cell), with the aid of complement, attacks and lyses those cells to which the offending antigen is attached. There are different cytotoxic T cells for different antigens. There are also helper T cells, which promote B-cell activity, and suppressor T cells, which restrain both the cytotoxic T cells and the B cells. Helper and suppressor B cells also exist. T-cell-mediated immunity is known as cell-mediated immunity. This is the immune response involved in graft rejection, autoimmunity, and delayed hypersensitivity.

The priming of lymphocytes in response to antigen is known as the primary response. The final effector response is known as the secondary, or efferent, response.

There are other bone-marrow, stem-cell-derived cells, such as macrophages and K cells that participate in the immune response. In the primary response, the macrophages phagocytose antigens, process them, and present the processed antigen to helper T lymphocytes, which initiate the recruitment of other lymphocytes. Thus the macrophages are an integral part of the afferent limb of the primary response. They also appear to be involved in the efferent response; they fix and alter antigen prior to its recognition by the T cells.

IMMUNOACTIVE AGENTS—An immunoactive drug is one that can attenuate the expression of at least one type of immune response. The numerous cell types involved in the immune system afford an equal number of places of immunosuppressive drugs to intervene. It is conceivable that a T cell responsive to one antigen may be affected more than is another T cell specific to another antigen, or that suppressor T cells might be affected more than cytoxic or helper T cells.

AZATHIOPRINE

1*H*-Purine, 6-[(1-methyl-4-nitro-1*H*-imidazol-5-yl)thiol]-, Imuran

6-[(1-Methyl-4-nitroimidazol-5-yl)thio]purine [446-86-6] $C_9H_7N_7O_2S$ (277.26).

Preparation—*N,N'*-Dimethyloxaldiamide is reacted with phosphorus pentachloride to give 5-chloro-1-methylimidazole. This is nitrated, and the resulting 5-chloro-1-methyl-4-nitroimidazole condensed with purine-6-thiol (mercaptopurine) in an appropriate dehydrohalogenating environment. US Pat 3,056,785.

Description—Yellow, matted powder that is odorless and has a slightly bitter taste; light sensitive, nonhygroscopic, and stable to reasonable temperatures; decomposes at approximately 245°.

Solubility—Insoluble in water; slightly soluble in alcohol or chloroform; soluble in dilute solutions of alkali hydroxides (unstable); sparingly soluble in dilute mineral acids.

Comments—Approved for prevention of renal transplant rejection. Azathioprine (AZA) is an imidazole derivative of the antimetabolite 6-mercaptopurine, which was developed in the 1950s. It is a pro-drug of 6-mercaptopurine (6-MP) and classified as an antimetabolite agent. It has been utilized by solid organ transplant clinicians for nearly 30 years. It was also commonly used in the treatment of a variety of autoimmune diseases like rheumatoid arthritis and certain malignancies, such as leukemia. After the introduction of cyclosporine, the role of AZA was consigned to that of an adjunctive agent. Although it had significantly impacted medical practice, resulting in the awarding of the Nobel prize, it has now been largely replaced at most transplant centers with newer more effective and better tolerated immunoactive agents (eg, mycophenolate mofetil or sirolimus).

AZA is rapidly converted in the liver and RBCs into 6-MP, which is then metabolized to an inactive metabolite, 6-thiouric acid. The active metabolite (6-MP) is incorporated into the cellular DNA inhibiting purine nucleotide synthesis and interfering with the synthesis and metabolism RNA. This effectively inhibits gene replication and resultant T cell activation. It suppresses T lymphocyte and monocyte (hence macrophage) production more than B lymphocyte production. AZA works in the afferent and not the efferent immune phase and hence does not suppress ongoing graft rejection.

After oral administration, AZA is rapidly and incompletely absorbed. It is distributed quickly and widely throughout all body fluids. The bioavailability of AZA is ~15% with ~40% detected as 6-MP. Despite having relatively short plasma half-lives (~50 and 75 minutes, respectively), the affect on purine inhibition and subsequent T activation is significant and persists much longer than either AZA or 6-MP. Clinical experience has indicated that once daily dosing is adequate as dosing regimens greater than twice daily administration have failed to improve therapeutic results. Clinicians have often employed a milligram-per-milligram conversion between the oral and intravenous doses for the sake of simplicity. However, given the bioavailability, some recommend reducing the intravenous dose to one half the oral dose. Acute toxicity is seen more frequently after intravenous administration, particularly with long courses of therapy, and is most likely caused by greater bioavailability. Full doses may be appropriate in patients' whose complete blood count is normal.

The parent compound and its metabolites are excreted primarily in the urine; however, dosage adjustments are not recommended in renal failure as the kinetics of the active compounds are unaltered. Dosage adjustments may be necessary in patients experiencing oliguria or tubular necrosis immediately status post cadaveric renal transplant.

Myelosuppression, manifested as leukopenia, megaloblastic anemia, or thrombocytopenia, is the major dose-limiting adverse event associated with azathioprine occurring in ~11% of patients. It appears approximately 2 weeks post initiation of the agent. Dosage adjustments should be based according to complete blood counts, white blood cells >3500/mm^3, and platelets. Nausea, vomiting, and diarrhea are frequent and may occur acutely. Occasionally, hepatotoxicity may occur and is reflected by abnormal liver function tests, including elevated bilirubin or transaminases, but damage seems slight and seems to disappear during the course of treatment. However, in the presence of liver dysfunction the drug should be withheld. Other toxicity or intercurrent infection occurs in approximately one-third of patients under immunosuppressive treatment with the drug.

In antiarthritic doses, infections are not increased, and other adverse effects are less frequent and less severe. Pancreatitis, alopecia, arthralgia, skin rashes, serum sickness, stomatitis, esophagitis, steatorrhea, retinopathy, peritoneal hemorrhage, and pulmonary edema also may occur in a small percentage of cases. Although the incidence is rare, an increase in reticulum cell sarcoma and lymphoma has been noted in transplant patients receiving azathioprine. The incidence of adverse effects is less when azathioprine is used in combination regimens, which allows clinicians to reduce doses of the agents. All immunosuppressants increase the risk of infections as well as certain types of cancer, including post-transplant lymphoproliferative disease.

It should be noted that a clinically significant drug-drug interaction exists between allupurinol and aziothioprine. Allupurinol, a xanthine-oxidase inhibitor, impairs the degradation of 6-MP resulting in significantly increased plasma concentrations of 6-MP. If not appropriately recognized and managed, concomitant use of these agents may result in a life-threatening pancytopenia. Thus, azathioprine therapy is considered a contraindication to allopurinol use. If necessary, allopurinol should be used with extreme caution and requires dose reductions of 60% to 80% to azathioprine, followed by more frequent monitoring of complete blood counts. Mycophenolate mofetil is preferred as an alternate to azathioprine as it does not interact with allopurinol.

Therapeutic drug monitoring of azathiorpine or 6-MP is not performed. In organ transplantation doses are based on milligram per kilogram basis. Most protocols employ initial doses ranging from 1mg/kg to 3mg/kg of body weight administered as a single daily dose. Doses are typically adjusted thereafter according to complete blood counts. Doses should reduced or discontinued in the face of hepatotoxicity or cytopenia

CYCLOPHOSPHAMIDE

2H-1,3,2-Oxazaphosphorin-2-amine, N,N-bis(2-chloroethyl)-tetrahydro-, 2-oxide, monohydrate; Cytoxan; Neosar

[6055-19-2] $C_7H_{15}Cl_2N_2O_2P.H_2O$ (279.10); anhydrous [50-18-0] (261.09).

Caution: Great care should be taken to prevent inhaling its particles and exposing the skin to it.

Preparation—3-Amino-1-propanol is condensed with N,N-bis(2-chloroethyl)phosphoramidic dichloride [(ClCH$_2$CH$_2$CH$_2$)$_2$N–POCl$_2$] in dioxane solution under the catalytic influence of triethylamine. The condensation is double, involving both the hydroxyl and the amino groups, thus effecting the cyclization.

Description—White, crystalline powder; liquefies on loss of its water of crystallization.

Solubility—1 g in approximately 25 mL water; soluble in alcohol.

Comments—An alkylating agent. Unlike other β-chloroethylamino alkylators, it does not cyclize readily to the active ethyleneimonium form until activated by hepatic enzymes. The liver is protected by the further metabolism of activated metabolites to inactive end products. Thus, the substance is stable in the GI tract, tolerated well, and effective by the oral and parenteral routes; it does not cause local vesication, necrosis, phlebitis, or even pain.

Cyclophosphamide is approved for Stage III and IV, malignant lymphomas, multiple myeloma, leukemias, mycosis fungoides, neuroblastoma, retinoblastoma, nephritic syndrome, and carcinoma of the breast. Its use in solid organ transplantation has been limited to rare instances. In prior years, it was employed as an alternative in patients experiencing leukopenia or hepatotoxicity with azathioprine use. In more recent years, it has been relegated to rare use in solid organ transplantation recipients undergoing rejection episodes characterized as severe, refractory, or extended episodes that are resistant to conventional/standard therapies.

It has been shown to be of value in the treatment of rheumatoid arthritis, Wegner's granulomatosis, hemophilia A with factor VIII destruction, idiopathic thrombocytopenic purpura (alone or in combination), erythroid aplasia, childhood nephrotic syndrome, pemphigus and vulgaris, dermatomyositis, or systemic lupus erythematosus. The long-term toxicities of cyclophosphamide should be considered if the drug is to be used as other than a cancer chemotherapeutic agent.

Cyclophosphamide is one of the most potent immunosuppressive agents, inhibiting both humoral and cell-mediated immunity. It is a prodrug. The drug is metabolized by the hepatic microsomal system to alkylating metabolites, adolphosphamide and 4-hydroxycyclophosphamide, that, in turn, are converted to phosphoramide mustard and acrolein, which are thought to be responsible for its cytotoxic effects.

After oral administration, cyclophosphamide is well absorbed yielding >75% bioavailabilty. Cyclophosphamide and its metabolites are distributed throughout the body. It is distributed to the tissues with a volume of distribution greater than the total body water. It is undergoes extensive metabolism in the liver through the cytochrome p450 mixed function oxidase enzymes with up to ~30% of the drug excreted unchanged in the urine. High doses rapidly induce the metabolism of the drug.

Approximately 25% of the drug is protein bound. The half-life of cyclophosphamide following oral and intravenous administration range from ~1 to 6.8 hours and ~4 to 16 hours, respectively. Renal or hepatic dysfunction does not require dosage alterations. However, dosage adjustments may be necessary in patients undergoing hemodialysis as ~72% of cyclophophamide is removed after 6-hour hemodialysis treatment.

Cyclophosphamide causes dose dependent bone marrow suppression. Leukopenia is the inevitable side effect and is used as an index of dosage. Clinicians should monitor white blood counts (avoidance of WBC <3500/mm^3) with expected nadir typically occurring within 2 weeks after therapy initiation. Dosages should be adjusted to achieve WBC between 4000 and 6000/mm^3. Anemia and thrombocytopenia may occur, although less frequently than leukopenia. Alopecia occurs in approximately 50% of patients receiving maximal prolonged treatment. Other side effects include sterile hemorrhagic cystitis in 20% of those receiving treatment, anorexia, nausea and vomiting (regardless of route of administration), anaphylactoid reactions, fever, hemolytic-uremic reaction, pulmonary infiltrates and fibrosis, mucosal ulcerations, dizziness, occasional, hypoprothrombinemia, nail ridging, cutaneous pigmentation, water intoxication, aspermia in males (3–6 months or longer in onset), anovulation in 30% to 50% of females, and occasional hepatic dysfunction. Bladder telangiectasis and abnormal urinary cytology occur; in long-term use, bladder fibrosis and transitional cell carcinoma occasionally occur. 2-Mercaptoethanesulfonate (Mesna) protects the bladder from this acrolein metabolite. The blood count should be monitored closely during induction and at least weekly thereafter. Cyclophosphamide is relatively platelet-sparing; cyclophosphamide is carcinogenic. All immunosuppressants increase the risk of infections as well as certain types of cancer, including post-transplant lymphoproliferative disease.

CYCLOSPORINE

Cyclosporine; Sandimmune, Gengraf, Neoral

[59865-13-3] $C_{62}H_{111}N_{11}O_{12}$ (1202.63).

Preparation—US Pat 4,117,118 (1978).

Description—A fungal metabolite first isolated from cultures of *Trichoderma polysporum* and *Cylindrocarpon ilucidivum*. White, prismatic needles from acetone melting about 150°. $[\alpha]^{23}_D$ -244° (c = 0.6, chloroform); -189° (c = 0.5, methanol).

Solubility—Insoluble in water or alcohol.

Comments—Suppresses helper T lymphocytes without significantly affecting suppressor T or B lymphocytes. Thus, it is a selective immunosuppressive drug without the cytotoxicity characteristic of most other immunosuppressive drugs. Because it works only in the primary (afferent) immune phase, it must be administered before exposure to the attacking antigen. It has a modest effect to suppress some humoral immunity.

Cyclosporine is a nonpolar, cyclic polypeptide antibiotic consisting of 11 amino acids of fungal origin. The unique cyclic structure of the drug is responsible for its immunosuppressive effects. It gained widespread clinical use in the early 1980s and significantly improved 1-yr graft survival rates, which in turn revolutionized transplant clinical practice and ushered in the modern era of selective immunosuppressive therapy. For most centers, kidney transplant 1-yr graft survival rates improved from 50% to 90% the world over; however, longer-term graft survival rates of that period were not impacted to the same degree with the initiation of CSA. Over the past two decades, CSA has become a mainstay of therapy at many transplant centers today. It is usually employed in combination with other immunoactive agents allowing clinicians the opportunity to reduce doses and minimize side effects associated with each agent. Typically cyclosporine is used in triple combination maintenance regimens, which includes steroids and an additional immunosuppressive agent with distinct mechanism of action.

It is a very effective immunosuppressive and is approved for organ transplant rejection, prevention of cardiac, kidney, or liver transplant rejection, rheumatoid arthritis, and severe recalcitrant psoriasis. It is less successful in pancreatic, lung, or bone-marrow transplantation. It has also been employed in graft-versus-host disease and its prevention.

Cyclosporine is a calcineurin phosphatase inhibitor, which inhibits T cell activation and proliferation, including production of interleukins from CD4 cells while sparing CD8 cells, B cells, macrophages, and granulocytes. The exact mechanism of immunosuppressive action of cyclosporine is not fully understood but appears to mainly involve inhibition of lymphocytic proliferation and function.

Following oral administration, cyclosporine is incompletely and variably absorbed. It exhibits considerable inter- and intra-individual variation, bioavailability ranging from 2% to 89%, depending on numerous variables including organ transplant type, individual patient, post-transplantation time, bile flow (micellar absorption of the drug involving bile), GI state (eg, decreased with diarrhea), and the formulation administered. Several oral preparations (Sandimmune, Neoral) are commercially available and corresponding bioavailability varies with each. Following oral administration with Sandimmune cyclosporine, oral bioavailabilty ranges from 10% to 90%, with overall absorption of ~30%. Oral absorption of Sandimmune is highly dependent on bile, which results in enhanced variability among patients experiencing diarrhea, diabetic gastroparesis, biliary diversion, or malabsorption. Currently, the Neoral formulation of cyclosporine has now largely replaced Sandimmune in clinical practice. Neoral imparts a much improved bioavailability ranging from 30% to 45%, less dependence on bile for absorption, more consistent oral absorption and less variable pharmacokinetic profile. However, some patients may still be maintained on the Sandimmune formulation. It should be noted that the oil-based Sandimmune formulation is not bioequivalent to the microemulsion Neoral formulation or its AB-rated generic equivalents.

Plasma levels peak in approximately 3.5 hr. In plasma, approximately 90% is protein bound, ~58% bound to red blood cells and ~33% bound primarily to lipoproteins. The pharmacokinetics are multicompartmental. The volume of distribution is 1 to 13 (average, 4) L/kg; it is concentration-dependent. Nearly all the drug is metabolized by cy-

tochrome P-450 III in the liver and gut; 94% of the metabolites are excreted into the bile, and 6% are eliminated into the urine. The pharmacokinetic inter-/intra-patient variabilities exhibited by the CSA formulations may also be caused by inherent polymorphisms expressed by metabolic enzymes (cyp3A4) and or p-glycoprotein countertransport proteins. In infants and children, the volume of distribution and clearance are greater than in adults. Thus, pediatric and African-American patients may require increased dosages. Additionally, elderly patients or those experiencing liver dysfunction may require longer intervals between dosage administration. The elimination half-life is 10 to 27 hr; there is a circadian periodicity to the elimination rate, the rate being faster in the morning.

Nephrotoxicity is a common, serious adverse effect, which may be related to renal vasoconstrictive or tubular toxicity associated with the agent. Cyclosporine causes both acute and chronic renal insufficiency. Concomitant use with other potentially nephrotoxic agents, such as nonsteroidal anti-inflammatory drugs (NSAIDs), aminoglycosides, trimethoprim, or sulfamethoxozole may increase patients susceptibility to nephrotoxicity. Other adverse effects include hypertension, hyperlipidemia, glucose intolerance, bruising, nausea, vomiting, hepatotoxicity, electrolyte imbalances manifested as hypomagnesemia, hyperuricemia or hypokalemia, headaches, or diarrhea. Neurotoxicity manifests as parasthesias, tremors, convulsions, or encephalopathy. Hemolytic-uremic syndrome with microangiopathic anemia and thrombocytopenia has been reported with CSA use and requires discontinuation of the agent. Several unique side effects of CSA include gingival hyperplasia, acne, hirsutism, increased appetite, and pancreatitis. Leukopenia, anemia, and thromboembolism occur rarely. All immunosuppressants increase the risk of infections as well as certain types of cancer, including post-transplant lymphoproliferative disease. It is teratogenic.

It should also be noted that CSA is subject to many clinically significant drug-drug interactions secondary to inhibition, induction, or competitive metabolism through the cytochrome p450 3A4 isozyme system. Therefore, the addition of any new agent should be screened for drug interactions (decreased or increased metabolism; potentiation of side effects) potential prior to implementation. Decreased cyclosporine plasma concentrations have occurred with concomitant phenobarbital, phenytoin, carbamazepine, rifampin, naficillin, Saint John's Wort, or rifabutin use. Increased cyclosporine plasma concentrations have occurred with concomitant amiodarone, fluconazole, itraconazole, ketoconazole, diltiazem, nicardipine, verapimil, erythromycin, cimetidine, clarithromycin, danazol, grapefruit juice, miconazole, metoclopramide, or bromocriptine.

Dosage guidelines vary according to disease, organ transplant type, time post-transplant, concomitant immunosuppression, and transplant center. Initial oral dosages may range from 3 to 15mg/kg/day given as divided dose every 12 hours. The intravenous dose is approximately 1/3 the oral dose. Thereafter, dosages are adjusted to achieve specific goal trough levels. Goal trough concentrations vary according to disease, concomitant immunosuppression, organ transplant type, time post-transplant, transplant center, and assay type. Therapeutic drug monitoring is routinely performed. Whole blood assay therapeutic range is 100 to 400 mcg/L. Plasma assay therapeutic range 50 to 200 mcg/L.

TACROLIMUS HYDRATE

Prograf, FK506

[109581-93-3] $C_{44}H_{69}NO_{12} \cdot H_2O$ (822.05).

Preparation—Obtained from *Streptomyces tsukubaensis*.

Description—Colorless prisms that melt about 128°.

Solubility—Soluble in methanol, ethanol, acetone, ethyl acetate, chloroform, or ether; sparingly soluble in hexane or ligroin; practically insoluble in water.

Comments—Tacrolimus is approved for prophylaxis and treatment of kidney and liver transplant rejection. It has also been useful in the prevention of rejection in heart and lung transplantation. It is a macrolide lactone antibiotic compound, which is structurally related to sirolimus. First approved for use in the liver transplant population, it has since gained in popularity and is used in the majority (>50%) of centers. Tacrolimus, a calcineurin phosphatase inhibitor, shares a similar mechanism of action to that of CSA. However, it binds specifically to its own cytoplasmic immunophilin, FK-binding protein, thereby forming a complex that inhibits calcium-sensitive phosphatase calcineurin. It inhibits T-cell activation and, as such, broadly suppresses the immune system. Based on in vitro concentrations, it is purported to be significantly more potent (10–100 times greater) than cyclosporine.

Tacrolimus is available as both intravenous and oral preparations. Absorption from the gut is variable and erratic, with approximately 20% to 25% bioavailability from 1- or 5-mg capsules, and peak blood concentrations were achieved 1.5 to 3.5 hr after ingestion. Unlike cyclosporine, its absorption is independent of bile secretion. Tacrolimus is widely distributed throughout the blood. It is highly protein bound with a terminal half-life for elimination of 11.7 hr in liver transplant patients; ~19 hours in renal transplant patients. Like CSA, tacrolimus is metabolized through the liver and gut (cytochrome p450 3A4 isoenzyme system) and is subject to similar clinically significant drug-drug interactions (see above). It is primarily excreted in bile with minimal renal elimination. It is also subject to inter-/intra-patient pharmacokinetic variability, which may be caused by polymorphisms expressed by metabolic enzymes (cyp3A4) and or p-glycoprotein countertransport proteins. As with CSA, the addition of any new agent should be screened for drug interactions (decreased or increased metabolism; potentiation of side effects) potential prior to implementation.

The most common side effects are headache, fever, tremor, hypertension, abdominal pain, diarrhea, nausea, renal dysfunction, and insomnia. Overall, the incidence of adverse reactions was comparable with cyclosporine-based immunosuppressive therapy. However, alopecia, glucose intolerance and neurotoxicity seem to occur more frequently with tacrolimus.

Dosage guidelines vary according to disease, organ transplant type, time post-transplant, concomitant immunosuppression, and transplant center. Initial oral dosage may range from 0.1 to 0.3 mg/kg per day administered as a divided dose every 12 hours. The intravenous dose may range from 0.05 to 0.10 mg/kg/day as a continuous infusion. Some centers may recommend lower initial doses. Thereafter, dosages are adjusted to achieve specific goal trough levels. Goal trough concentrations vary according to disease, concomitant immunosuppression, organ transplant type, time post-transplant, transplant center, and assay type. Therapeutic drug monitoring is routinely performed. Whole blood assay therapeutic range is 5 to 20 mcg/L. Plasma assay therapeutic range is 0.1 to 0.5 mcg/L.

LYMPHOCYTE IMMUNE ANTI-THYMOCYTE GLOBULIN (EQUINE)

Atgam

A preparation of equine immunoglobulin containing antibodies (primarily IgG) prepared from the hyperimmune serum of horses immunized with human thymus lymphocytes.

Description—Transparent to slightly opalescent (pink) aqueous solution of the protein.

Comments—Historically, Atgam, one of the first commercially available polyclonal antibody agents, has played an important role in transplantation. Antithymocyte globulin equine (ATG [equine]) (Atgam) is used for the treatment of acute rejection in renal allograft recipients. It has also been used to prevent renal, cardiac, and lung transplant rejection. The globulin also has been reported to be of value in the treatment of T-cell leukemias, graft-versus-host disease, and selected cases of aplastic anemia. Typically it is used as an adjunctive to other immunosuppressive therapy. Polyclonal agents are usually administrated in combination with other immunosuppressive agents as induction or sequential therapy or in the treatment of acute rejection. Induction or sequential therapy is used to induce acceptance of the newly transplanted organ or provide an increased overall immunosuppressive effect for a short period of time when acute rejection is most likely, typically the first 3 months post-transplantation. The term *sequential therapy* is used as most induction or sequential therapy agents, such as Atgam or Thymoglobulin, are administered for short courses (up to 14 days immediately post-transplant dependent on the agent used) while providing prolonged levels of immunosuppression secondary to exceptionally long half-lives and effect. The agents used in combination with sequential or induction agents are deemed maintenance agents, such as cyclosporine, mycophenolate mofetil, and corticosteroids, as patients are required to take these agents for the lifetime of the graft. Although polyclonal agents have been highly effective, they are also costly and potent immunosuppressive agents, and not without considerable long-term effects. Therefore, over the past decade, clinicians have tried to optimize results through judicious use of these agents in patient populations with the greatest need and greatest potential for gain. Currently, most transplant protocols utilize polyclonal antibody preparations in high immunologic risk patients. Patients characterized as high immunologic risk may include patients with elevated pre-transplant panel reactive antibodies, African-American recipients, re-transplants, and cases of delayed graft function.

Atgam has now been largely replaced by its successor, Thymoglobulin, at most transplant centers as clinical trial data has proven it superior in both the treatment and prevention of rejection.

Atgam attacks T lymphocytes but not B lymphocytes. Efficacy is enhanced, and adverse effects are attenuated when the globulin is used in combination with other immunosuppressive agents. After administration of the antithymocyte agent, profound depletion of peripheral blood lymphocytes ensues and is mediated by several pathways including cells coated with antibodies undergo complement-mediated cell lysis of lymphocytes, clearance by the reticuloendothelial system or T lymphocyte proliferation may also be affected. Additionally, its immunosuppressive effect continues long after therapy discontinuation. This is demonstrated by the blunted proliferative response of lymphocytes that return to circulation and continued suppression of the CD4 subset, which may be effected for several years.

Atgam is administered intravenously in a dose of 10 to 20 mg/kg/day for a course of 7 to 14 days. However, most centers use shorter courses of therapy for induction regimens. Atgam exhibits an extended half-life ranging from 3 to 9 days. But, large inter-patient variations have been reported. The first dose is administered over a 6-hour infusion; subsequent doses may be administered over shorter infusion times (4 hours). Anaphylactic reactions and allergic reactions are possible, and prophylactic regimens are commonly employed. Prior to use, a skin test for sensitivity to horse serum is advisable. Patients are premedicated with acetaminophen, diphenhydramine, and methylprednisolone 1 hour prior to administration to ameliorate side effects.

Frequent adverse effects include chills, fever, urticaria, pruritus, generalized rashes, leukopenia, diarrhea, arthralgias, headache, and thrombocytopenia. Dosage adjustments may be necessary in the face of leukopenia or thrombocytopenia. Complete blood counts should be monitoring daily while on therapy. Less frequently experienced adverse effects are stomatitis, hypotension, chest pain, back pain, night sweats, pain at the injection site, and peripheral thrombophlebitis. Rarely there may be tachycardia, myalgias, pulmonary edema, serum sickness, anaphylaxis, malignancies, laryngospasm, local and systemic infections, and activation of herpes simplex infections. All immunosuppressants increase the risk of infections as well certain cancers, including post-transplant lymphoproliferative disease. It is important to ensure that patients receive appropriate antiviral prophylaxis while receiving Atgam or any other potent immunosuppressive regime.

LYMPHOCYTE IMMUNE ANTI-THYMOCYTE GLOBULIN (RABBIT)

Thymoglobulin

A preparation of rabbit immunoglobulin containing antibodies (primarily IgG) prepared from the hyperimmune serum of rabbit immunized with human thymus lymphocytes.

Thymoglobulin, a polyclonal anti-thymocyte globulin, is derived by inoculating rabbits with human thymocytes, purifying the resulting solution from unwanted materials, yielding a solution specific for lymphocytes. Approved in 1999, it is the second commercially available polyclonal antibody preparation available on the market. Since its introduction, it has become the preferred polyclonal agent used to treat and prevent rejection in solid organ transplant recipients. It has also been useful in treating graft-versus-host disease, steroid-resistant rejection, and aplastic anemia. Thymoglobulin is used in clinical practice in the same manner as Atgam; as either an induction or sequential therapy (see above for full description) or as treament for rejection. It has, however, replaced Atgam secondary to superior results including: improved rates of graft survival, less severe rejection, fewer rejection episodes, greater reversed rejection episodes, and fewer recurrent rejection episodes.

Thymoglobulin exerts its immunosuppressive action similarly to Atgam (see above). After its administration, a profound decrease in circulating lymphocytes occurs. The usual dose of thymoglobulin is 1.5 to

2.5mg/kg per day administered intravenously (first dose over 6-hour continuous infusion, subsequent doses over 4-hour continuous infusion) for a duration of 5 to 14 days. However, many centers may use modified protocols with lower doses or alternate day dosing schedules. Again, shorter courses of therapy are commonly used for induction regimens. It has a half-life of ~30 days; inter-patient variation exists. As with Atgam and OKT3, premedication regimens (acetaminophen, diphenhydramine, and methylprednisolone) should be administered 1 hour prior to Thymoglobulin administration to offset known side effects. Allergies are possible, however, skin tests are not necessary prior to Thymoglobulin use. However, patients possible allergy to rabbits should be ascertained prior to administration.

Thymoglobulin has similar side effect profile to Atgam. These include leukopenia (occurs more frequently with thymoglobulin), fever, chills, nausea, diarrhea, headaches, and arthralgias. Dosage adjustments may be necessary in the face of leukopenia or thrombocytopenia. Complete blood counts should be monitored daily while on therapy. All immunosuppressants increase the risk of infections as well certain cancers, including post-transplant lymphoproliferative disease. It is important to ensure that patients receive appropriate antiviral prophylaxis while receiving Thymoglobulin or any other potent immunosuppressive regime.

MUROMONAB-CD3

Orthoclone OKT3

A murine monoclonal antibody (anti-CD3), $IgG_{2\alpha}$, of two chains having molecular weights of approximately 50,000 and 25,000.

Preparation—Mouse myeloma is fused into lymphocytes from immunized animals producing a hybridoma, which then secretes antigen-specific antibodies to the T3 antigen of T lymphocytes.

Comments—OKT3, or muromonab-CD3, approved in the mid-1980s, was the first monoclonal antibody preparation approved for therapeutic use in humans. Muromonab-CD3 is a murine IG2 monoclonal antibody that targets the ε chain of CD3. Initially it was commonly used to treat rejection and eventually to prevent it. OKT3 has been proven useful in both the prevention and treatment of rejection. In renal graft rejections, the success rate has been reported to be as much as 94%. Despite that, it has now been relegated to a secondary role as newer polyclonal antibody agents are preferable first-line options, given their similar efficacy and reduced toxicity profiles. Currently, OKT3 is reserved to treat severe rejection episodes or steroid resistant rejection episodes. When employed, it is used in combination with triple-drug immunosuppressive maintenance regimen.

OKT3 is a potent immunoactive agent with several pathways thought responsible for its effect. Anti-CD3 blocks cell signals that induce proliferation of cytotoxic lymphocytes and also causes the removal of T lymphocytes from the circulation, returning only after several days after administration. The mechanisms involved include T cell opsonization and their clearance by mononuclear phagocytic cells, complement mediated cell lysis, modulation of TCR-CD3 complex off the T cell surface, and steric hindrance. During therapy, CD3 positive cells are depleted while other T-cells (CD2, CD4, and CD8) reappear. T cells containing CD3 and other surface markers reappear ~2 days after discontinuation of therapy. It has a half-life of ~18 hours. However, short-term treatment with OKT3 or polyclonal antibody preparations has been associated with persistent immunosuppressive effects. It is administered intravenously as a bolus (over 1 minute) and various regimens exist. A typical regimen used is 5mg/day for 10 to 14 days. However, doses as low a 2 mg/day have proven effective as induction therapy.

OKT3 has many significant adverse drug reactions. The most dangerous of which is "cytokine release syndrome," which is characterized by flu-like symptoms, high fever, chills, arthralgias, headache, chest pain, tacchycardia, wheezing, nausea, and diarrhea. Some patients may experience more severe reactions including hypotension, rapidly developing pulmonary edema (dyspnea may be seen clinically), seizures, encephalopathy, aseptic meningitis or renal insufficiency. Cytokine release syndrome results from muromonab-CD3-activated T cells and monocytes releasing IL-1, IL6, and tumor necrosis factor. Adverse reactions occur most frequently following the initial dosage administration or upon dose increases. Most adverse effects persist only during the first 2 days of treatment. Rarely occurring side effects include anaphylaxis and coagulopathies such as thrombocytopenia or graft thrombosis. The severity of these reactions may be blunted with the use of premedications including methylprednisolone, acetaminophen, or diphenhydramine. Premedications are administered 1 hour prior to the administration of muromonab-CD3. Additionally, ensure that patients are within 3% of his/her dry body weight as another preventive measure. All immunosuppressants increase the risk of infections as well as certain types of cancer, including post-transplant lymphoproliferative disease. It has been implicated with higher rates of post-transplant lymphoproliferative disease when used in combination with triple-drug regimens or in patients receiving cumulative doses totaling >75mg of OKT3 (administered over greater than a 2-week period). Therefore, doses exceeding these specific parameters are not recommended. However, many clinicians conclude it is not specifically due to this specific agent but rather to the overall net immunosuppressive effect. Various opportunistic infections have occurred, herpes simplex and cytomegalovirus infections being the most common. Therefore, it is important to ensure that patients receive appropriate antiviral prophylaxis while receiving OKT3 or any other potent immunosuppressive regime.

MYCOPHENOLATE MOFETIL

4-Hexenoic acid, (*E*)-6-(1,3-dihydro-4-hydroxy-6-methoxy-7-methyl-3-oxo-5-isobenzofuranyl)-4-methyl-, 2-(4-morpholinyl)ethyl ester (and hydrochloride); CellCept (base); CellCept IV (hydrochloride)

(Base) [115007-34-6] $C_{23}H_{31}NO_7$ (433.49). (HCl) [116680-01-4] $C_{23}H_{31}NO_7 \cdot HCl$ (469.96).

Preparation—*J Am Chem Soc*, 1986; 108:806.

Description—(Base) White to off-white crystalline powder. Apparent Log P (pH 7.4 buffer) is 238. pK_a 5.6 (morpholino group) and 8.5 (phenolic OH).

Solubility—(Base) In water 43 μg/mL at pH 7.4; 4.27 mg/mL at pH 3.6; in DMSO 50 mg/mL. Freely soluble in acetone; soluble in methanol and sparingly soluble in ethanol. (HCl) 65.8 mg/mL in 5% dextrose.

Comments—Approved for prophylaxis of organ rejection in renal, cardiac, and liver transplant patients. It has also been used to treat a wide-variety of autoimmune diseases, diffuse proliferative nephritis, prevention of lung or pancreas transplant rejection, psoriasis, and refractory uveitis. Mycophenolic acid, the active metabolite of mycophenolate mofetil, was originally discovered in 1896. Mycophenolate mofetil was developed as an alternative to azathioprine for maintenance immunoactive agent, specifically designed to improve potency and selectivity for immune tissue throughout the body. The morpholinoethyl ester derivative of MPA, mycophenolate mofetil, was pursued because of its improved bioavailability. Safety and efficacy of the agent were proven in three pivotal trials. Clinically, mycophenolate mofetil (used as part of triple-drug regimens) has resulted in significantly improved acute rejection rates, morbidity, and mortality. Hence, it has successfully replaced AZA in the large majority of transplant programs. It is also thought to have improved chronic rejection rates as well. Generally, it is used in triple-drug combination regimens with cyclosporine or tacrolimus or sirolimus and steroids. However, it has also been useful in the development of novel transplant immunoactive regimens including steroid-sparing regimens and treatment for acute rejection (in addition to other therapy).

On metabolism to its active metabolite MPA, it inhibits *de novo* guanine–purine biosynthesis and thereby suppresses lymphocyte production. It is absorbed rapidly and completely from the GI tract and undergoes virtually complete metabolism of MPA, which itself may be metabolized further to an inactive glucuronide. MPA is 97% bound to albumin in the blood. Coingestion of food decreased blood levels by 40%. Oral bioavailability, based on MPA blood levels, is approximately 94%. More than 94% appears in the urine, the majority of which is the MPA glucuronide (MPAG). However, enterohepatic recirculation of the inactive metabolite, MPAG may occur. Concomitant agents such as cyclosporine (results in lower serum [MPA]), antibiotics, bile acid sequestrants, or other disease states may alter this process. Patients experiencing renal dysfunction are susceptible to accumulation of MPA. This is thought to be due to the reconversion through beta-glucuronidation of MPAG to MPA. The half-life of MPA in the blood is approximately 17.9 hr. Both the parent compound (~99%) and MPA (~82%) are highly protein bound to albumin. Use caution when administering mycophenolate mofetil in patients experiencing uremia, hyperbilirubinemia, hypoalbuminemia, or those receiving other highly protein bound agents.

Mycophenolate mofetil (MMF) is available as both an intravenous and oral preparations. The majority of transplant recipients are well enough immediately post-transplant to receive the oral formulation. Typical oral dosage is 1g administered orally twice a day. Doses may vary (500 mg up to 1.5 g administered orally twice a day) dependent on concomitant immunosuppresion, organ transplant type, or immunologic risk. Doses greater than 3g/day have been associated with higher rates of side effects, particularly GI disturbances. Therapeutic drug monitoring is not the standard of care at most centers; however, MPA levels may be performed for cause.

Mycophenolate mofetil is well tolerated. The most commonly occurring side effects are GI intolerances; diarrhea (~30%), constipation, nausea, dyspepsia, and vomiting. Other common adverse reactions include leukopenia, anemia, thrombocytopenia, or leukocytosis. Dosage adjustments may be necessary with hematologic and GI side effects (change schedule to QID). Dosage reductions, in face of GI intolerances, are associated with increased risks of acute rejection. Thus, every attempt should be made to maintain patients on full-dose therapy. All immunosuppressants increase the risk of infections as well as certain types of cancer, including post-transplant lymphoproliferative disease.

MYCOPHENOLIC ACID

4-Hexenoic acid, (*E*)-6-(1,3-dihydro-4-hydroxy-6-methoxy-7-methyl-3-oxo-5-isobenzofuranyl)-4-methyl-, Myfortic

[24280-93-1] $C_{17}H_{20}O_6$ (329.34).

Preparation—*J Am Chem Soc* 1986; 108:806. Total synthesis, *Tetrahedron*, 2003; 59:1989–1994.

Description—Produced by *Penicillium brevi-compactum* and related organisms. Needles from water melting about 141°.

Solubility—Practically insoluble in water; freely soluble in alcohol; moderately soluble in ether or chloroform; sparingly soluble in hydrocarbon solvents.

Comments—Introduced onto the market in 2004, Myfortic is the enteric-coated formulation designed to deliver the active component, mycophenolic acid. It is the second product commercially available. Myfortic was designed to overcome the GI adverse events associated with its predecessor, MMF. Additionally, they sought to improve clinical effectiveness by enhancing adherence to full-dose regimens, as GI intolerances (previous experience with MMF) led to dose reductions or discontinuations, which increased risk of rejection. Clinical trials have proven Myfortic equally safe and effective to MMF. Both agents have comparable side effect profiles (see above). The most commonly occurring side effects were diarrhea and leukopenia. Despite its enteric coating, it did not correlate clinically to improved GI tolerability. Considering the data available to date, Myfortic does not impart any clinical advantage over mycophenolate mofetil.

Typically dosage is 720 mg twice daily with or without food. Compared with MMF 1000 mg twice daily, the Myfortic regimen provides equimolar amounts of MPA. Myfortic therapy should be initiated within 24 hours post-transplant in de novo transplant recipients. Dose adjustments are not necessary in the elderly or in patients with delayed graft function. Patients with severe chronic renal insufficiency (glomerular filtration rate of <10 mL/min), however, should be monitored for signs of MPA toxicities. A pharmacokinetic analysis demonstrated that mycophenolate sodium achieved higher serum MPA concentrations compared with MMF equal doses. This did not result in improved efficacy, but rather suggests that relative to overall exposure, tolerability may be improved. Additionally, it may allow patients to achieve higher therapeutic MPA concentrations. Following mycophenolic acid administration, mean absolute bioavailability of MPA is 71%; peak plasma concentration is achieved in 1.5 to 2 hours.

SIROLIMUS

Rapamycin; Rapamune

[53123-88-9] $C_{51}H_{79}NO_{13}$ (914.17).

Preparation—Produced by *Streptomyces hygroscopicus*. *J Antibiot*, 1975; 28:721 and US Pat 5,100,899 (1992).

Description—White to off-white powder melting at 181°.

Solubility: Insoluble in water; freely soluble in benzyl alcohol, chloroform, acetone and acetonitrile. Soluble in DMSO.

Comments—Sirolimus, or rapamycin, is a new immunoactive agent approved in 1999 for use in kidney transplantation. It is a macrocyclic triene antibiotic derived from *Streptomyces hygroscopicus* from soil samples collected on Easter Island (Rapa Nui) in 1968. Originally pursued for its potential as an antifungal agent, sirolimus' immunosuppressive activities were later recognized and studied following the discovery of tacrolimus' immunosuppressive prowess. It is a macrolide antibiotic, which is structurally similar to tacrolimus. But sirolimus demonstrates a novel mechanism of action and distinct side effect profile. Like the calineurin phosphostase inhibitors, sirolimus is also an immunophilin binding agent. Sirolimus engages immunophilin forming the rapamycin-FK binding protein (FKBP) complex. Unlike the calcineurin inhibitors, rapamycin-FKBP complexes do not inhibit calcineurin phosphatase or cytokine transcription but rather binds a kinase enzyme, the mammalian target of rapamycin (mTOR). mTOR inhibition prevents cytokine mediated cell proliferation between phase G1 and S and results in T- and B- cell inhibition. Since its introduction, it has provided clinicians with another effective alternative maintenance agent. Additionally, it has been instrumental in the development of novel immunosuppressive regimens, including steroid sparing protocols and calcineurin inhibitor sparing regimens. Sirolimus is available as an oral solution or in tablets. Following oral administration, it is poorly absorbed. Bioavailability is reported at ~15%. The half-life is between ~57 and 62 hours but has been reported to be reduced in the pediatric population. Like, CSA and tacrolimus, sirolimus is subject to variable pharmacokinetics. Sirolimus' distribution is relatively similar to tacrolimus, approximately 95% is bound to red blood cells with 3% in plasma. Up to 40% in the plasma fraction are associated with lipoproteins, and the remaining amount (60%) is free unbound drug. Sirolimus is very lipophilic and has a large volume of distribution. It is metabolized through the liver and gut (p450 3A4) into multiple metabolites. Additionally, like CSA and tacrolimus, it is also susceptible to drug interactions mediated by the cytochrome p450 3A4 isoenzyme system as well as p-glycoprotein. It is eliminated largely in feces (~90%) with minimal excretion in the urine (2%).

It should also be noted that sirolimus is subject to many clinically significant drug-drug interactions secondary to inhibition, induction, or competitive metabolism through the cytochrome p450 3A4 isozyme system. Therefore, the addition of any new agent should be screened for drug interactions (decreased or increased metabolism; potentiation of side effects) potential prior to implementation. Increased sirolimus levels have been reported with concomitant fluconazole, itraconazole, ketoconazole, clotrimazole, diltiazem, nicardipine, verapimil, erythromycin, cimetidine, clarithromycin, danazol, grapefruit juice, miconazole, metoclopramide or bromocriptine. Decreased sirolimus levels have been reported with phenobarbital, phenytoin, carbamazepine, rifampin, or rifabutin use. Additionally, concomitant cyclosporine use increases overall sirolimus exposure (AUC increased by 230%). Upon 4-hour separation between the two agents, the magnitude of the effect was greatly diminished (AUC sirolimus increased by 80%). Thus, clinicians have targeted lower cyclosporine trough concentrations and/or lowered doses. The aforementioned interaction does not occur with concomitant tacrolimus therapy. The magnitude of some the interactions can be severe; ketoconazole increase sirolimus levels by 990%; rifampin reduces sirolimus concentrations by ~90%. Therefore, these combinations should be avoided.

Dosage guidelines vary according to disease, organ transplant type, time post-transplant, concomitant immunosuppression, and transplant center. Initial loading dosages are typical and range from 6 to 15 mg administered orally once per day; maintenance oral doses range from 2 to 5 mg administered orally once per day. Thereafter, dosages are adjusted to achieve specific goal trough levels. Target trough concentrations vary according to disease, concomitant immunosuppression, organ transplant type, time post-transplant, transplant center, and assay type. Therapeutic drug monitoring is routinely performed. Whole blood assay therapeutic range is 3–36 ng/mL.

Sirolimus is has several unique and dose-dependent adverse events, the most notable being hyperlipidemia, manifested as hypertriglyceridemia or hypercholesterolemia. This side effect is more severe when sirolimus is used in combination with cyclosporine. Thus, it is imperative to appropriately recognize and treat it with non-pharmacologic measures and 3-hydroxy-3-methylglutaryl coenzyme A reductase inhibitors (HMG-CoA reductase inhibitors). Patients who receive both sirolimus and an HMG CoA reductase inhibitor are more susceptible to myopathy or rhabdomyolysis as both are substrates of the p450 system. Additionally, although sirolimus does not cause nephrotoxicity alone, it does, however, potentiate cyclosporine-induced nephrotoxicity when they are coadministered. Other side effects include bone marrow suppression such as leukopenia, anemia, or thrombocytopenia; liver dysfunction; GI intolerance such as nausea, vomiting, dyspepsia and diarrhea; delayed wound healing (particularly with high doses); electrolyte disturbances; skin ulcers; lymphocytes. All of the above side effects are dose dependent.

DACLIZUMAB

Humanized anti-TAC monoclonal antibody comprised of four subunits, two heavy chains and two light chains; Zenapax

```
            MATURE HUMANIZED HEAVY CHAIN

H    QVQLVQSGAE    VKKPGSSVKV    SCKASGYTFT    SYRMHWVRQA
     PGQGLEWIGY    INPSTGYTEY    NQKFKDKATI    TADESTNTAY
     MELSSLRSED    TAVYYCARGG    GVFDYWGQGT    LVTVSSASTK
     GPSVFPLAPS    SKSTSGGTAA    LGCLVKDYFP    EPVTVSWNSG
     ALTSGVHTFP    AVLQSSGLYS    LSSVVTVPSS    SLGTQTYICN
     VNHKPSNTKV    DKKVEPKSCD    KTHTCPPCPA    PELLGGPSVF
     LFPPKPKDTL    MISRTPEVTC    VVVDVSHEDP    EVKFNWYVDG
     VEVHNAKTKP    REEQYNSTYR    VVSVLTVLHQ    DWLNGKEYKC
     KVSNKALPAP    IEKTISKAKG    QPREPQVYTL    PPSRDELTKN
     QVSLTCLVKG    FYPSDIAVEW    ESNGQPENNY    KTTPPVLDSD
     GSFFLYSKLT    VDKSRWQQGN    VFSCSVMHEA    LHNHYTQKSL
     SLSPGK-OH
```

```
            MATURE HUMANIZED LIGHT CHAIN

H    DIQMTQSPST    LSASVGDRVT    ITCSASSSIS    YMHWYQQKPG
     KAPKLLIYTT    SNLASGVPAR    FSGSGSGTEF    TLTISSLQPD
     DFATYYCHQR    STYPLTFGQG    TKVEVKRTVA    APSVFIFPPS
     DEQLKSGTAS    VVCLLNNFYP    REAKVQWKVD    NALQSGNSQE
     SVTEQDSKDS    TYSLSSTLTL    SKADYEKHKV    YACEVTHQGL
     SSPVTKSFNR    GEC-OH
```

```
        LOCATION OF DISULFIDE BRIDGES
```

Type	Location		Description
bridge	Cys-22	-Cys-96	disulfide bridge
bridge	Cys-143	-Cys-199	disulfide bridge
bridge	Cys-219	-Cys-213	disulfide bridge
bridge	Cys-225	-Cys-225	disulfide bridge
bridge	Cys-228	-Cys-228	disulfide bridge
bridge	Cys-260	-Cys-320	disulfide bridge
bridge	Cys-366	-Cys-424	disulfide bridge
bridge	Cys-22	-Cys-96	disulfide bridge
bridge	Cys-143	-Cys-199	disulfide bridge
bridge	Cys-219	-Cys-213	disulfide bridge
bridge	Cys-366	-Cys-320	disulfide bridge
bridge	Cys-366	-Cys-424	disulfide bridge
bridge	Cys-23	-Cys-87	disulfide bridge
bridge	Cys-133	-Cys-193	disulfide bridge
bridge	Cys-23	-Cys-87	disulfide bridge
bridge	Cys-133	-Cys-193	disulfide bridge

[152923-56-3] Daclizimab [$C_{6394}H_{9888}N_{1696}O_{2012}S_{44}$ (protein moiety) MW ca 144 to kDa, as predicted from DNA sequencing.

Preparation—US Pat 5,530,101 (1996).

Description—A composite of 90% human and 10% murine antibody sequences. The human elements are from human IgG1 and the Eu myeloma antibody. Murine sequences are from the complimentarity-determining regions of a murine anti-TAC subunit.

Solubility—The product, as the concentrate, contains 25 mg in 5 mL of pH 6.9 buffer.

Daclizumab, an IL-2 receptor antagonist, is one of the newest monoclonal antibody preparations available on the market. It is a monoclonal antibody composed of human and murine antibody sequences. It contains primarily human components (90%) with smaller proportion being murine (10%) in nature. Currently, IL-2 receptor antagonists are used primarily as induction agents in immunosuppressive protocols. Compared with polyclonal antibody induction therapy, IL-2 receptor antagonists did not provide adequate rejection prophylaxis among high immunologic risk renal transplant recipients when used in combination with triple-drug maintenance immunosuppression regimens. Consequently, they are no longer favored in that population and have been relegated to use among lower risk patients. Those regimens have been proven safe and effective in adult and pediatric patients in reducing acute rejection. Additionally, they have been increasingly used in novel immunosuppressive regimens such as calcineurin-free or sparing regimens and steroid-free or withdrawal regimens.

IL-2 receptor antibodies specifically bind to the alpha-subunit of the interleukin-2 receptor (CD-25) located on the surface of activated T lymphocytes. It interferes with IL-2 driven proliferation and differentiation. This usually results in diminished T cell responses that yields prolonged immunosuppressive action (at least 6 weeks). Daclizumab has an exceptionally long half-life; ranging from 11 to 38 days.

The above mechanisms may explain the prolonged immunosuppressive action demonstrated by the IL-2 receptor antagonists.

Daclizumab is administered intravenously over 15 minutes. The recommended dose is 1mg/kg/day within 24 hours of surgery followed by equal doses administered every 14 days for up to five doses. This dosing regime is possible because of its extended half-life. Many centers may use alternate protocols requiring fewer doses.

Daclizumab has a relatively mild side effect profile. Unlike OKT3 or polyclonal antibody agents, it is not associated with first dose effects or cytokine release syndrome. In clinical trials, it has demonstrated side effects similar to those reported among patients receiving placebo; including infection and malignancy. Hypersensitivity may occur. No significant drug interactions are reported for daclizumab.

BASILIXIMAB

Immunoglobulin G1, anti-(human interleukin 2 receptor) (human-mouse monoclonal CHI621 γ1-chain), dusulfide with human-mouse monoclonal CHI621 light chain, dimer; Simulect

[179045-86-4] Immunosuppressant monoclonal antibody.

Preparation—A glycoprotein produced by recombinant DNA technology and obtained from fermentation media of an established mouse myeloma cell line. EP 449,769 (1991).

Description—Approximate MW 144 kDa.

Solubility—Soluble in water.

Basiliximab is an anti-CD25 monoclonal antibody preparation. Like daclizumab, it is considered an IL2 receptor antagonist. It is a chimeric antibody composed of 75% human and 25% murine components. Therefore, basiliximab does not have the same affinity for the IL-2 receptor when compared to daclizumab. Compared to older monoclonal antibodies such as OKT3, daclizumab and basiliximab demonstrate low immunogenic potential as well as improved side-effect profiles. Clinical applications of basiliximab are similar to that of daclizumab (see above). It also demonstrates the same mechanism of action as described for daclizumab (see above).

It is administered intravenously as a single 20-mg dose on the day of transplant surgery and on the 4th day post-transplantation. Unlike OKT3 or polyclonal antibody agents, it is not associated with first dose effects or cytokine release syndrome. Basiliximab is well tolerated. In clinical trials, it has demonstrated side effects similar to those reported among patients receiving placebo, including infection and malignancy. Hypersensitivity may occur. No significant drug interactions are reported for basilximab.

Parasiticides

Steven P Gelone, PharmD

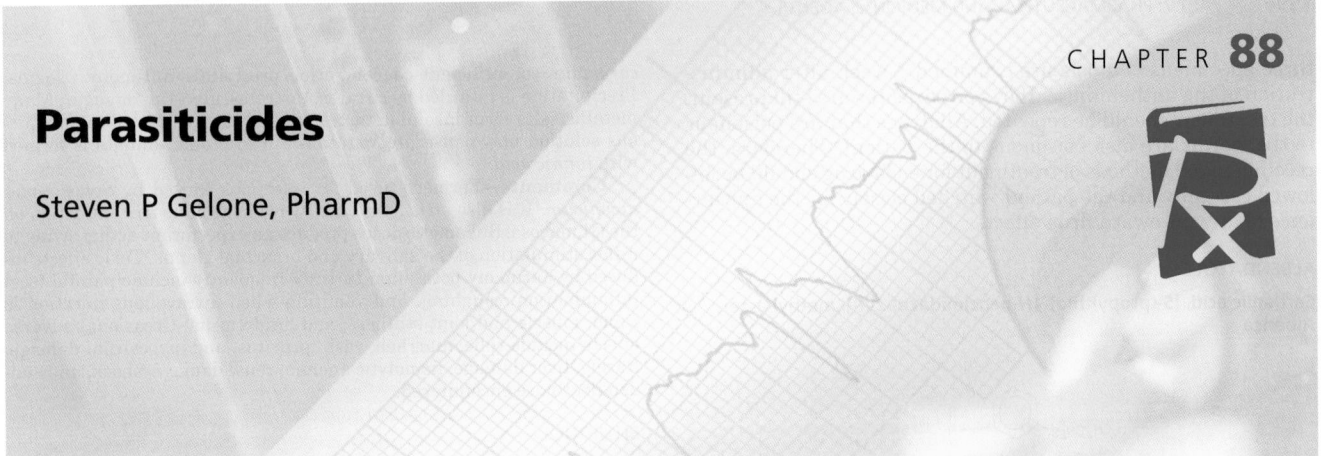

Parasitic infections are now a worldwide problem. Increased travel, use of immunosuppressants, and the spread of AIDS has led to a greater prevalence of parasitic infections (*Med Lett Drugs Ther* April 2002). Consequently, the subject is an important part of pharmacology. In its broadest aspects, it includes the problem of eradication of all organisms that live within or upon man. However, the discussion in this chapter is limited to the anthelmintics and those agents that are applied directly to the skin of the human host in the treatment of pediculosis and scabies.

ANTI-INFECTIVES

The term *anthelmintic* frequently is restricted to drugs acting locally to expel parasites from the GI tract. However, there are several types of worms that penetrate other tissues; drugs that act on these parasitic infections are also known as anthelmintics. Furthermore, drugs that kill worms are referred to commonly as vermicides; those that affect the worm in such a manner that peristaltic activity or catharsis expels it from the intestinal tract are referred to as vermifuges. This arbitrary division serves no useful purpose because many anthelmintics manifest both actions, according to the dose employed. Therefore, the anthelmintics are defined more properly as drugs used to combat any type of helminthiasis.

The worm parasites of man belong to two phyla: *Nemathelminthes* (roundworms) and *Platyhelminthes* (flat worms).

The roundworms include the hookworm, roundworm, whipworm, pinworm, *Strongyloides stercoralis, Trichinella spiralis,* and *Wuchereria bancrofti.*

There are two common varieties of hookworm: *Necator americanus,* the American variety, and *Ancylostoma duodenale,* the European variety. They are cylindrical worms, 1 to 2 cm long, with two pairs of hooks near the mouth. They attach themselves to the mucosa of the duodenum and derive their nourishment by sucking blood from the surrounding blood vessels.

The common roundworm, *Ascaris lumbricoides,* is the most prevalent of human helminths. It may be 7 to 23 cm in length, 3 to 6 mm in diameter, grayish to reddish in color, and inhabits the upper part of the small intestine; therefore, it is vomited up occasionally.

The whipworm, *Trichuris trichiura,* is approximately 5 cm long and resembles a whip. It inhabits the cecum principally, but is found also in the lower part of the ileum and the appendix.

The pinworm or threadworm, *Enterobius vermicularis,* is 1.5 to 3 mm long. It inhabits the small intestine, cecum, and colon.

S stercoralis is only approximately 2 mm long. It inhabits the duodenum chiefly, but may be found in the stomach, biliary passages, pancreatic ducts, and various parts of the intestinal tract.

Infection with *T spiralis* causes trichinosis, a condition that results from eating incompletely cooked pork infested with the larvae of the worm. When such meat is eaten, the cysts dissolve, the parasites mature, and a new crop of larvae develops that penetrate the intestinal mucosa and eventually lodge in the muscles.

The most important filarial worm is *W bancrofti,* which is transmitted by the bite of the mosquito. Symptoms result from the blocking of the lymphatic ducts with the adult worms.

The flatworms are of two types: segmented (cestodes) and nonsegmented (trematodes). The cestodes include the tapeworms, and the trematodes include the flukes.

Four common varieties of parasitic tapeworms are found in man; *Taenia saginata* (beef tapeworm), *Taenia solium* (pork tapeworm), *Diphyllobothrium latum* (fish tapeworm), and *Hymenolepis nana* (dwarf tapeworm). Except for the dwarf tapeworm, they are from 2 to 10 m in length and may contain 3000 to 4000 segments, each segment being capable of producing hundreds of eggs. The dwarf tapeworm is only 6 to 12 mm in length, but it consists of 150 to 200 segments. The larval stage of all tapeworms is spent in the muscles of the intermediate host, and human infection occurs through eating imperfectly cooked meat and fish.

Three varieties of blood fluke inhabit the blood stream of man, causing schistosomiasis: *S haematobium, S mansoni, S mekongi,* and *S japonicum.* These parasites cause epigastric distress, abdominal pain, anorexia, diarrhea with blood and mucus in the stools, enlarged and tender liver, pyrexia, and ascites. The intermediate host is either a freshwater snail or a freshwater mollusk. Transmission is by way of contaminated water.

Parasitic worms are harmful to the human host for several reasons. They deprive the host of food, injure organs or obstruct ducts, may elaborate substances toxic to the host, and may provide a portal of entry for other organisms. It is desirable, therefore, to eradicate the parasites as soon as they have been discovered. Nevertheless, the need for treatment must be weighed carefully against the toxicity of the drug; the mere presence of a parasite does not necessarily demand that it must be treated.

Proper choice of the anthelmintic is important, as most drugs are more effective against some species than others, and virtually all antiparasitic drugs induce some adverse effects. The drug selected should offer the best combination of effectiveness and relative safety. There is an excellent review (*Med Lett Drugs Ther* April 2002) of the choice of drugs for parasitic infections.

Many of the newer drugs require little or no change in the patient's normal routine. When the patient has a tapeworm infestation, a thorough examination of the stools produced by the second purgation is necessary. Unless the head of the worm has been expelled and identified, the worm regenerates. Usually three specimens of stools are examined 1 week after administration of the anthelmintic. If ova or parasites are still present, the treatment should be repeated. All drugs that are poisonous to the worms are also poisonous to the patient. Therefore, the recommended methods of treatment for each drug should be followed carefully and the patient watched closely for the appearance of any untoward drug effects.

ALBENDAZOLE

Carbamic acid, [5-(propylthio)-1H-benzimidazol-2yl-], methyl ester; Albenza

[54965-21-8] $C_{12}H_{15}N_3O_2S$ (265.34).

Preparation—Etherification of 4-mercaptoacetanilide with *n*-propyl bromide yields 2-nitro-4-(propylthio)acetanilide, which is hydrolyzed to the amine, reduced to the diamine with stannous chloride, then converted to the benzimidazole structure with *S*-methylthiourea, and finally acylated at the 2-amino group with methyl choloformate. *J Med Chem* 1971;14:580. US Pat 3,915,986 (1975).

Description—Colorless crystals melting about 209° (decompn).

Solubility—Insoluble in water; soluble in dimethyl sulfoxide (DMSO), acetic acid, strong acids, or bases; can be regenerated from these solutions by neutralization if not heated or kept for too long a time.

Comments—A synthetic, benzimidazole-derivative anthelmintic that is used for the treatment of parenchymal neurocysticercosis resulting from active lesions produced by the larval form of *T solium* (pork tapeworm) and the treatment of cystic hydatid disease of the liver, lung, and peritoneum, produced by the larval form of the dog tapeworm (*Echinococcus granulosus*).

The precise mechanism of action is not clear; however, it appears to exert its primary anhelmintic effice by binding to the free β-tubulin in parasite cells, thereby producing a selective inhibition of parasite micotubule polymerization, and inhibition of micotubule-dependent glucose uptake. Inhibition of parasite β-tubulin occurs at lower concentrations of albendazole than those that are needed to inhibit human microtubule polymerization.

When employed in the treatment of neurocysticercosis, corticosteroids are often administered in conjunction with albendazole to reduce the frequency and severity of adverse nervous system effects. When employed for the treatment of cystic hydatid disease, it is most often used perioperatively to reduce the risk of intraoperative dissemination of daughter cysts.

Albendazole is administered orally with food. Bioavailability is increased by the presence of fat. For example, in the presence of 40 g of fat, the plasma concentrations of albendazole are approximately 5 times that observed in fasting patients. It is contraindicated during pregnancy because of potential risk to the fetus. In addition, liver function tests are recommended prior to each course of treatment and at 2-week intervals during treatment. Should clinically important increases in liver function test results be observed, its use should be discontinued.

ANTIMONY POTASSIUM TARTRATE

Antimonate(2-), bis[μ-[2,3-dihydroxybutanedioato(4-)-O¹, O², O³, O⁴]]-di-,dipotassium, trihydrate, stereoisomer

Tartar Emetic [28300-74-5] $C_8H_4K_2Sb_2O_{12}.3H_2O$ (667.85); anhydrous [11071-15-1] (613.81).

Preparation—By dissolving a mixture of 10 parts of potassium bitartrate with 8 parts of antimony trioxide [Sb_2O_3] in 75 parts of boiling water, filtering the solution while hot and allowing it to crystallize.

Description—Colorless, odorless, transparent crystals or a white powder; the crystals effloresce on exposure to air; solutions are acid to litmus.

Solubility—1 g dissolves in 12 mL water, approximately 15 mL glycerin or approximately 3 mL boiling water; insoluble in alcohol.

Incompatibilities—*Mineral acids,* when added to aqueous solutions of antimony potassium tartrate, precipitate basic salts of antimony, with possibly some potassium bitartrate. *Alkali hydroxides* and

carbonates of sufficient concentration precipitate antimony trioxide. Precipitation is retarded by citrates, tartrates, glycerin, or sugar. Many metallic salts form insoluble tartrates. Addition of *alcohol* to an aqueous solution may cause precipitation. An insoluble tannate is formed with *tannic acid.*

Comments—Formerly used for infections caused by *Schistosoma japonicum.* It is also an *emetic,* chiefly by virtue of its irritant action on the GI mucosa. Subemetic doses produce an expectorant action owing to reflex stimulation of the salivary and bronchial glands. Toxic effects induced by antimony potassium tartrate frequently include painful local inflammation, coughing, and vomiting when intravenous injection is rapid, muscle and joint stiffness, and bradycardia. Occasional adverse effects include colic, diarrhea, rash, pruritus, and myocardial damage. Rarely, liver damage, hemolytic anemia, renal damage, shock, and sudden death are encountered.

BITHIONOL

Phenol, 2,2′-Thiobis(4,6-dichloro-,

[97-18-7] $C_{12}H_6Cl_4O_2S$ (356.05).

Preparation—By reaction of 2,4-dichlorophenol and sulfur chloride.

Description—White or off-white, crystalline powder; melts about 188°.

Solubility—Practically insoluble in water; freely soluble in alcohol or ether; soluble in solutions of alkali hydroxides.

Comments—The drug of choice for infections caused by *Fasciola hepatica* (sheep liver fluke) and, alternative drug for those caused by *Paragonimus westermani* (lung fluke). Untoward reactions are frequent and include photosensitivity skin reactions, vomiting, diarrhea, abdominal pain, and urticaria. Available from the Parasitic Disease Drug Service, CDC, Atlanta, GA 30333.

DIETHYLCARBAMAZINE CITRATE

1-Piperazinecarboxamide, N,N-diethyl-4-methyl-, 2-hydroxy-1,2,3-propanetricarboxylate; Hetrazan

N,N-Diethyl-4-methyl-1piperazinecarboxamide citrate (1:1) [1642-54-2] $C_{10}H_{21}N_3O.C_6H_8O_7$ (391.42).

Preparation—By acylating piperazine with diethylcarbamoyl chloride, and then methylating at the N^4-position by treatment with formaldehyde and formic acid. Treatment of the purified base with an equimolar portion of citric acid yields the official citrate.

Description—White, crystalline powder; odorless, or has a slight odor; slightly hygroscopic; melts between 134° and 139°.

Solubility—Very soluble in water; sparingly soluble in alcohol; practically insoluble in acetone, chloroform, or ether.

Comments—The drug of choice for treating filariasis infections (*W bancrofti, Brugia malayi, Mansonella ozzardi, Loa loa,* and *tropical eosinophilia*). In adequate dosage it clears the blood rapidly of the microfilariae and appears to be curative. The drug should be administered with special caution in Loa loa, because it can provoke an encephalopathy. Antihistamines or corticosteroids may be needed to control the allergic reactions caused by the disintegration of microfilariae.

Untoward reactions are frequent but not serious; they include severe allergic or febrile reactions, owing to the filarial infection, and GI disturbances. Rarely, encephalopathy and loss of vision are encountered.

Note—Available only from the manufacturer.

EMETINE HYDROCHLORIDE—page 1310.

MEBENDAZOLE

Carbamic acid, (5-benzoyl-1H-benzimidazol-2-yl)-, methyl ester; Vermox

Methyl 5-benzoyl-2-benzimidazolecarbamate [31431-39-7] $C_{16}H_{13}N_3O_3$ (295.30).

Preparation—Synthesis of mebendazole and related anthelmintic benzimidazolecarbamates is described in German Pat 2,029,637 (corresponding to US Pat 3,657,267). See *CA* 74:100047s, 1971.

Description—White to slightly yellow powder; melts about 290°.

Solubility—Practically insoluble in water, alcohol, ether, or chloroform.

Comments—The anthelmintic of choice in hookworm (*Ancylostoma duodenale* and *Necator americanus*), pinworm (*Enterobius vermicularis*), roundworm (*Ascaris lumbricoides*), whipworm (*T trichiura*), and guinea worm (*Dracunculus medinensis*); in filariasis (*Mansonella perstans*); and as an alternative drug for *Visceral Larva Migrans*. It also is used as an adjunct to steroids for the treatment of trichinosis (*T spiralis*). It blocks the glucose uptake by susceptible helminths, thereby depleting glycogen stored within the parasite. The glycogen depletion results in a decreased formation of adenosine triphosphate (ATP); the latter is required for survival and reproduction of the helminth. Side effects are usually mild and transient; abdominal pain and diarrhea have occurred in cases of massive infection and expulsion of worms. Leukopenia is rare but has been reported. The drug is contraindicated in pregnancy and in persons who have shown hypersensitivity to it.

METRONIDAZOLE—page 1669.

OXAMNIQUINE

6-Quinolinemethanol, 1,2,3,4-tetrahydro-2-[[(1-methylethyl)amino]methyl]-7-nitro-, Vansil

[21738-42-1] $C_{14}H_{21}N_3O_3$ (279.34).

Preparation—From 6-(methoxymethyl)quinaldinic acid to form the acyl chloride, which with diethylamine yields the amide. Reduction of the amide with lithium aluminum hydride and Raney nickel produces the diethylaminomethyl derivative. Nitration of the latter compound in the 7-position followed by demethylation of the 6-position yields oxamniquine (US Pat 3,821,228).

Description—A light, orange, crystalline powder melting about 151°.

Solubility—Soluble in 3300 in water; soluble in acetone, chloroform, or methanol.

Comments—An alternate drug for infection caused by *Schistosoma mansoni*, including the acute and the chronic phase with hepatosplenic involvement. It significantly reduces the egg load of *S mansoni*. Contraindicated in pregnancy. Adverse effects observed include occasional headache, fever, dizziness, somnolence, nausea, diarrhea, rash, insomnia, and electrocardiogram (ECG) changes. Convulsions and neuropsychiatric disturbances also have been observed, but are rare.

PIPERAZINE

[110-85-0] $C_4H_{10}N_2$ (86.14).

Preparation—By catalytic deamination of diethylenetriamine and of ethylenediamine. US Pat 2,267,686.

Description—White to slightly off-white lumps or flakes having an ammoniacal odor; melts between 109° and 113°; boils between 145° and 146°; in water it crystallizes with $6H_2O$ in colorless crystals called *piperazine hydrate,* melting at 44° and boiling between 125° and 130°. Soluble in water or alcohol; insoluble in ether. Incompatible with salts of heavy metals, alkaloidal salts or with acetanilid, phenacetin, or nitrites.

Comments—*Piperazine and several of its salts—the adipate, calcium edetate, citrate, phosphate,* and *tartrate*—have been used as anthelmintics for treatment of roundworm and pinworm infections. When administered orally, therapeutic doses have little or no pharmacological effects on the host. Adverse effects are transient, usually mild and disappear when the drug is discontinued. Occasionally, patients may complain of nausea, vomiting, mild diarrhea, abdominal cramps, headache, and dizziness.

More serious adverse effects such as seizures and respiratory depression are rare and occur after large doses. Piperazine should be used with caution in patients who have severe malnutrition oranemia. It is contraindicated in patients who have impaired renal or hepatic function

or seizure disorders and in those patients who are hypersensitive to piperazine. Although piperazine has been used, without adverse effects, in pregnant women, its safe use in pregnancy has not been established clearly.

PRAZIQUANTEL

4H-Pyrazino[2,1-a]isoquinolin-4-one, 2-(cyclohexylcarbonyl)-1,2,3,6,7,11b-hexahydro-, Biltricide

[55268-74-1] $C_{19}H_{24}N_2O_2$ (312.41).

Preparation—Aminomethyltetrahydroisoquinoline, cyclohexane carbonyl chloride, acetonitrile, and aqueous hydrochloric acid are refluxed in the presence of pyridine to first form the cyclohexanecarbamoylmethyl derivative that cyclizes to form the product (US Pat 4,001,411).

Description—A hygroscopic solid with a bitter taste, melting about 137°.

Solubility—Freely soluble in chloroform; soluble in ethanol; very slightly soluble in water.

Comments—The drug of choice for infections caused by *S japonicum, S mekongi, S haematobium,* and *S mansoni.* It is also an investigational drug of choice for tapeworm infestations and numerous fluke infections. It increases the permeability of the worm's cell membrane to calcium ions; this causes massive contraction and paralysis of its musculature and disintegration of its tegumental layer. Adverse effects include sedation, abdominal discomfort, fever, sweating, nausea, eosinophilia, headache, and dizziness.

PYRANTEL PAMOATE

(E)-1,4,5,6-tetrahydro-1-methyl-2-[2-(2-thienyl)ethenyl]-, compd with 4,4′-methylenebis[3-hydroxy-2-naphthalenecarboxylic acid] (1:1); Antiminth

[22204-24-6] $C_{11}H_{14}N_2S.C_{23}H_{16}O_6$ (594.68).

Preparation—Thiophene is converted to 2-thiophenecarboxaldehyde (I) via a Vilsmeier-Haack reaction. *N*-Methyl-1,3-propanediamine is condensed with acetonitrile to yield 1,4,5,6-tetrahydro- 1,2-dimethylpyrimidine, which is then coupled with I in the presence of methyl formate to yield pyrantel (base). The pyrantel is isolated as the tartrate and metathesized with a soluble alkali-metal pamoate.

Description—Yellow to tan powder that is tasteless and free of characteristic odor; decomposes slowly in light; nonhygroscopic in air under ordinary conditions; relatively stable in heat; melts with decomposition between 247° and 261°.

Solubility—Insoluble in water; very slightly soluble in alcohol.

Comments—One of the anthelmintics of choice in the treatment of *ascariasis* (common roundworm infection) and *enterobiasis* (pinworm) infection. It is also an investigational drug for the treatment of hookworm, moniliformis, and trichostrongylus infections. Side effects occur only occasionally and are relatively mild; GI disturbances, headache, dizziness, rash, and fever have been reported.

QUINACRINE HYDROCHLORIDE—page 1667.
SURAMIN SODIUM—see RPS-19, page 1326.

THIABENDAZOLE

1H-Benzimidazole, 2-(4-thiazolyl)-, Mintezol; Thibenzole

2-(4-Thiazolyl)benzimidazole [148-79-8] $C_{10}H_7N_3S$ (201.25).

Preparation—Ethyl pyruvate is brominated, and the resulting 2-bromo ester is reacted with thioformamide whereby cyclization occurs with formation of ethyl 4-thiazolecarboxylate. This ester is saponified and condensed with o-phenylenediamine to introduce the benzimidazole moiety. US Pat 3,017,415.

Description—White to practically white, odorless or practically odorless, tasteless powder; stable in light and nonhygroscopic; melts between 296° and 303°; pK_a 4.7.

Solubility—Practically insoluble in water; slightly soluble in acetone or alcohol; very slightly soluble in chloroform or ether.

Comments—The anthelmintic of choice in *S stercoralis,* cutaneous larva migrans (creeping eruption), *Angiostrongylus costaricensis.* It also is recommended as an alternate drug in the treatment of *Capillaris philippensis, D medinensis* (guinea worm) infections, and visceral larva migrans. No special diet or purgation is needed with this drug. Side effects usually include nausea, vomiting, vertigo, headache, and weakness. Leukopenia, crystalluria, rash, disturbance of color vision and hallucinations also have been reported. In rare instances, shock, tinnitus and Stevens–Johnson syndrome have been observed. Because from one third to one half of patients usually are incapacitated for several hours after receiving the drug, it should be given on days when the patient does not have to go to school or work. Patients on the drug should be cautioned not to engage in activities requiring mental alertness.

PEDICULICIDES AND SCABICIDES

Pediculicides are compounds effective in the treatment of pediculosis. Pediculosis in man is caused by three species of sucking lice known as *Pediculus humanus* variety *capitis* (the head louse), *P humanus* variety *corporis* (the body louse) and *Phthirius pubis* (the crab louse). These parasitic, wingless insects thrive where personal hygiene is neglected. The eggs (nits) of the body louse are attached to the fibers of clothing while those of the other two species are attached to hairs by a chitin-like cement. Cutting the hair short or shaving the area is helpful in destroying the eggs. The period of development from egg to adult is approximately 2 to 4 weeks. To be effective completely, an antipedicular agent must kill both parasites and eggs. Should the latter fail to be destroyed, repeated applications of the agent may be necessary to destroy the newly hatched lice.

Scabicides are compounds that are effective against *Sarcoptes scabiei,* the animal parasite that causes scabies in man. The parasite, a mite, thrives where personal hygiene is neglected. After copulation takes place on the surface of the skin, the female mite excavates a sinuous inward-sloping burrow in the corneous layer of the skin. The eggs are laid in the burrow and, after hatching, the larvae and nymphs may exit. For this infestation to be eradicated, an antiscabious agent must kill both parasites and eggs. If the eggs are not destroyed, repeated applications of the antiscabious agent may be necessary. The life cycle from egg to adult parasite is from 8 to 15 days. Sulfur ointment has been a time-honored scabicide. Except for alternate use in scabies (*S scabies*), it now has been replaced by more effective agents. Because many agents possess both antipedicular and anti-scabious properties, the pediculicides and scabicides are listed together.

CROTAMITON

2-Butenamide, *N*-ethyl-*N*-(2-methylphenyl)-, Eurax

CH$_3$CH=CHCONCH$_2$CH$_3$

N-Ethyl-*o*-crotonotoluidide [483-63-6] C$_{13}$H$_{17}$NO (203.28).

Preparation—By condensation of a crotonyl halide, ester, salt, or a derivative thereof with *N*-ethyl-*o*-toluidine.

Description—Colorless to slightly yellowish oil; faint aminelike odor.

Solubility—Practically insoluble in water; miscible with alcohol.

Comments—A scabicidal and antipruritic agent, effective in eradicating scabies infestations and useful for symptomatic treatment of pruritic skin. Allergic sensitivity or primary irritation reactions may occur in some patients. It should not be applied to acutely inflamed skin, raw, weeping surfaces, or in the eyes or mouth. In scabies, it is recommended that crotamiton be thoroughly massaged into the skin of the entire body, from the chin down; a second application 24 hours later is advised to assure complete eradication of mites. A cleansing bath should be taken 48

hours after the last application. In pruritus the cream is massaged gently into affected areas until absorbed; repeated as needed.

LINDANE

Cyclohexane, (1α,2α,3β,4α,5α,6β)-1,2,3,4,5,6-hexachloro-, Gamma Benzene Hexachloride; Gammexane; BHC; 666;

γ-1,2,3,4,5,6-Hexachlorocyclohexane [58-89-9] C$_6$H$_6$Cl$_6$ (290.83).

Gamma benzene hexachloride, as this compound was formerly officially called, is one of the nine theoretical stereoisomeric forms of 1,2,3,4,5,6-hexachlorocyclohexane. It has been shown to have the conformation

and, in terms of equatorial-axial notation, becomes *1e,2e,3e,4a,5a,6a*-hexachlorocyclohexane.

Preparation—By the chlorination of benzene in the presence of light. The reaction product is a mixture of stereoisomers containing from 10% to 15% of the insecticidally active gamma isomer that may be separated by solvent extraction processes.

Description—White, crystalline powder; slight, musty odor.

Solubility—Practically insoluble in water; slightly soluble in ethylene glycol; 1 g in 20 mL dehydrated alcohol, 3.5 mL chloroform or 40 mL ether.

Comments—Widely used as an *ectoparasiticide* and *ovicide.* It is an alternative drug for the treatment of *Sarcoptes scabiei* (scabies), *P capitis* (head lice) and *P pubis* (crab lice). As a *scabicide,* it is employed in a 1% concentration in a vanishing cream or lotion. The mixture is applied in a thin layer over the entire cutaneous surface from the neck down. One ounce usually is sufficient for an adult. Leave it on for at least 12 hr; remove it by thorough washing. One application is usually curative; retreatment is indicated only if living mites can be demonstrated. The shampoo is used for the treatment of *P pubis* and *capitis.* Approximately 1 oz (for short hair) and 2 oz (for long hair) is worked thoroughly into the hair and allowed to remain in place for 4 min; small quantities of water are added then until a lather forms; the hair is rinsed thoroughly, toweled briskly and any nits removed with nit comb or tweezers.

Adverse effects include occasional eczematous skin rash and conjunctivitis; rarely, convulsions and aplastic anemia have been observed.

MALATHION—page 1732.

PRECIPITATED SULFUR

Precipitated Sulphur; Lac Sulfuris; Milk of Sulfur

Sulfur [7704-34-9] S (32.06).

Preparation—To a slurry of 1 part of lime and 10 parts of water, 2 parts of sublimed sulfur are added, thoroughly mixed and the mixture boiled with frequent agitation until all of the sulfur is dissolved:

$$12S + 3Ca(OH)_2 \rightarrow 2CaS_5 + CaS_2O_3 + 3H_2O$$

After cooling, the clear liquid is decanted through a filter, and a slight excess of HCl, calculated from the quantity of lime used, is added to the filtrate. The acid decomposes the calcium pentasulfide and the thiosulfate with the precipitation of sulfur:

$$2CaS_5 + CaS_2O_3 + 6HCl \rightarrow 3CaCl_2 + 12S + 3H_2O$$

Description—Very fine, pale yellow, amorphous or microcrystalline powder; odorless and tasteless.

Solubility—Practically insoluble in water; very slightly soluble in alcohol; slightly soluble in olive oil. Distinguished from other forms of sulfur by more rapid solubility in carbon disulfide: on shaking 1 g of precipitated sulfur with 5 mL carbon disulfide, it should dissolve quickly except for a small amount of insoluble matter usually present.

Incompatibilities—Sufficiently hydrophobic that it sometimes causes trouble in lotions, where it tends to float on the surface. Among substances that have been shown to promote the wetting of sulfur, and thus aid its dispersion, are triethanolamine oleate and benzoin tincture. Trituration of the sulfur with a few drops of alcohol, glycerin, or a dilute solution of a wetting agent is also of some service.

Comments—An active parasiticide; a 10% sulfur paste or ointment is used as an alternative treatment for *S scabiei* (mites). Sulfur also is actively keratolytic and, in the form of full-strength ointment or in combination with other keratolytic agents such as salicylic acid, it is used in the treatment of skin disorders such as *psoriasis, seborrhea, eczema-dermatitis* and *lupus erythematosus*. The percentage of sulfur in an ointment should be reduced in the event that a patient's skin shows intolerance. Prolonged use of sulfur may result in a characteristic dermatitis venenata.

PYRETHRINS WITH PIPERONYL BUTOXIDE

RID; A-200 Pyrinate

Preparation—Pyrethrins are the insecticidal extracts of the pyrethrum flower and are usually synthesized from pyrethrolone [(Z)(+)-4-hydroxy-3-methyl-2-(2,4-pentadienyl)-2-cyclopentene-1-one, $C_{11}H_{14}O$] and chrysanthemic acid [2,2-dimethyl-3-(2-methyl-1 propenyl)cyclo-propanecarboxylic acid, $C_{10}H_{17}O_2$] to yield a mixture of pyrethrins I and II. Piperonyl butoxide, [5-[[2-(2-butoxyethoxy)ethoxy]methyl]-6-propyl-1,3-benzodioxazole, $C_{19}H_{30}O_5$] has a synergistic effect on pyrethrins and rotenone, another floral insecticide.

Comments—This combination (pyrethrins 0.3%, piperonyl butoxide 3.0%) is an alternative treatment for *P humanis, P capitis,* and *P pubis*. It is contraindicated in individuals sensitive to the ingredients or ragweed, harmful if swallowed or inhaled, and may be irritating to the eyes and mucous membranes. Discontinue use and notify a physician if irritation or skin rash occurs. Usually it is applied topically only once and after 5 to 7 days later if needed to kill hatching progeny.

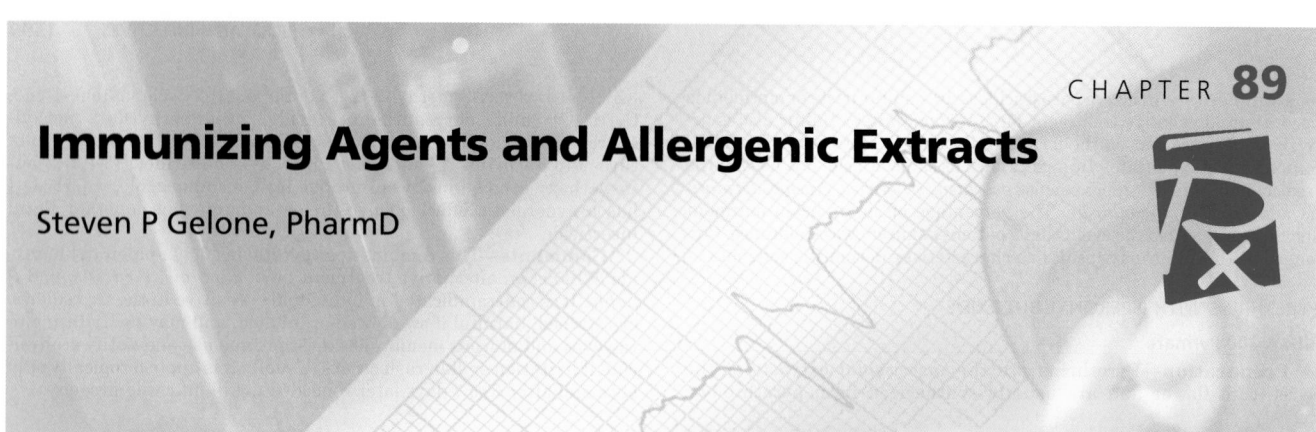

CHAPTER 89

Immunizing Agents and Allergenic Extracts

Steven P Gelone, PharmD

Immunizing agents and allergenic extracts are two of the main groups of drugs that are classified as *biologics* by the Food and Drug Administration (FDA). The properties of these agents are sufficiently unique that they are under the control of a separate division of the FDA; ie, the *Center for Biologics Evaluation and Research* (CBER) rather than the *Center for Drug Evaluation and Research* (CDER). This is perhaps one of the things that has confused many laymen and professionals alike into thinking that biologicals are not drugs. To the contrary, they were the first group of drugs to fall under Federal Control and were originally defined in the Public Health Service Act of 1902. More importantly, the biologics as a group and, more specifically the active immunizing agents, have likely prevented more morbidity and mortality than all other drugs combined. *Vaccina vaccine* must be considered the most effective drug to date since it has totally eradicated smallpox from our world. A similar success for the *poliomyelitis virus vaccines* appears imminent.

Characteristics of Biologics

Biologics (Table 89-1) are drugs in every sense of the word but they have unique characteristics that are helpful to review before considering the specific groups and individual agents. To be sure, none of the characteristics listed below is completely unique to biologics but, considered together, they describe what make these drugs special when compared to what are called *conventional drugs* for the purpose of this discussion.

1. Biologics are *natural products*. Virtually all of the drugs in this group are derived from once living organisms including man, higher animals, plants, and microorganisms. Although there may ultimately be a few exceptions to this rule, even the so-called *synthetic proteins* today are produced in living systems.
2. Biologics are relatively *crude products* by contemporary pharmaceutical standards. Most of these products contain cells, tissues, or even entire organisms. Even the relatively *pure* products that contain no biological structural elements are often mixtures of chemicals with varying degrees of activity.
3. The active constituents of biologics are *macromolecules,* proteins and/or, less commonly, polysaccharides. This is a particularly important consideration with respect to formulation, administration, and pharmacokinetics.
4. Most biologics are *standardized by bioassay*. The doses of very few of these products can be expressed in the conventional units of mass of active constituent but rather are usually expressed in units of biological activity that are characteristic to the individual agent.
5. Biologics are *immunogenic*. Conventional drugs with low molecular weights can induce immune responses by acting as haptens, but this is a relatively uncommon occurrence with most drugs. Biologics virtually always contain complete immunogens (proteins and polysaccharides) that are highly immunogenic by themselves. Even the increasingly common *human* or *humanized pro-*

teins are rarely completely identical to their natural analogs and are usually more immunogenic than conventional drugs. There is nothing more central to understanding biologics than knowledge of the principles of immunology.
6. Biologics have some very *unique hazards*. Adverse toxic, idiosyncratic and, as noted above, allergic reactions can occur with biologics as with other drugs. But some biologics consist of living microorganisms that actually infect the patient and, on occasion, may even be transmitted to others. Some biologics carry a significant risk of microbial contamination because of their source. Certainly any product containing cells carries some risk of carrying an unknown biological contaminant. Those vaccines that are used for mass immunization have a very unique ability to alter the epidemiological patterns of disease that may have both advantages and disadvantages within a community.

IMMUNIZING AGENTS

Immunizing agents are among the oldest of modern drugs and can be dated to the beginning of immunology in 1798 when Edward Jenner introduced his vaccine for smallpox. The active immunizing agents are also, from virtually all perspectives, the most successful and powerful drugs yet developed. First, their main action is to *prevent* rather than to treat disease; most of the commonly used agents are highly effective and several have been singularly successful as noted earlier. Second, in spite of a number of real and potential hazards, they have generally proven to be remarkably *safe* in actual practice. Finally, and very importantly, active immunizing agents are generally available at a relatively *low cost*.

Passive immunizing agents date to the early part of the 20th century following the discovery of antibodies. Various antitoxins derived from animals held an important place in therapy prior to the development of antibiotics but these products, in contrast to the vaccines, had a number of problems with respect to both efficacy and safety and for a number of years their utility was quite limited. Presently, antibody preparations are rapidly gaining prominence in therapeutics largely because of the following developments: availability of human immune globulins; development of intravenous dosage forms; monoclonal antibody (MAb) technology; and the ability to prepare humanized MAbs.

Immunity

Immunity in the broadest sense may be defined simply as inborn or acquired resistance to disease and necessarily involves all of what may collectively be called the *host defenses* (Fig 89-1). It is common practice to restrict immunity and related terms to specific defenses and use *resistance* to denote those that are nonspecific. This is not fixed, however, and one will see the

Table 89-1. Biologicals[a]

Active Immunizing Agents (Vaccines)
Allergenic Extracts
Biological Response Modifiers (Cytokines)
Blood and Blood Derivatives
Cellular Therapies
Diagnostic Products
  In vitro antibodies and antigens
  ***In vivo* diagnostic skin test antigens**
Enzymes and Venoms
Passive Immunizing Agents (Antibody Products)

[a] Products considered in this chapter are indicated in bold type. Consult *Establishments and Products Licensed under Section 351 of the Public Health Services Act* at the FDA Web site [http://www.fda.gov] for a complete list of currently licensed biologics.

terms used in a variety of different contexts. What is most important to understand is that much of the terminology of immunology is context-based, and the observer must be careful in trying to apply rigid definitions.

Immunizing agents are broadly classified on the basis of the type of immunity that they induce and knowing the properties of the different types of immunity is fundamental to the understanding of immunizing agents and their applications. *Active immunity* is a form of acquired immunity that develops in an individual in response to an immunogen. This may be naturally acquired by exposure to an infectious disease or artificially acquired by receiving active immunizing agents *(vaccines)*. The term *vaccination* is used as a synonym for active immunization. There is a lag time of several days after first exposure to an immunogen and protective levels of immunity are typically not achieved for 1 to 2 weeks. Because of the phenomenon of *immunologic memory*, second and subsequent exposures to the same immunogen usually result in faster and stronger responses. However, it is important to recognize that immunologic memory is not infinite and will wane in the absence of periodic *booster doses* of the immunogen.

Passive immunity involves the transfer of the effectors of immunity, usually the specialized molecules called immunoglobulins or antibodies, from an immune individual to another. This occurs naturally by the active transport across the placental barrier of IgG antibodies from mother to fetus and, to a lesser extent, by the transfer of sIgA antibodies in the mother's milk. Passive immunizing agents include those derived from humans *(homologous)* or other higher animals *(heterologous)*. The onset of passive immunity is much quicker, but the duration is much shorter because there is no active immune response to the immunogen and thus no memory. Immunoglobulins, especially if derived from foreign sources, are highly immunogenic proteins and may elicit an active immune response that is the basis for *serum sickness* and other allergic reactions.

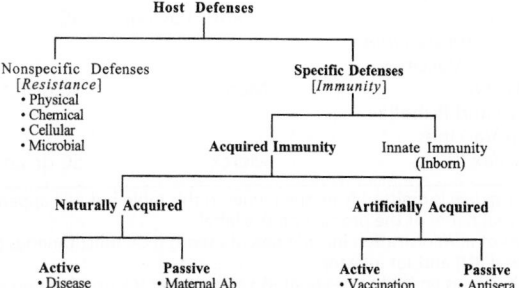

Figure 89-1. The host defenses.

ACTIVE IMMUNIZING AGENTS

Active immunizing agents are immunogenic drugs that are usually administered to a patient prior to their being exposed to a disease with the intention of providing long-term, even permanent, protection against the disease. Often there is the secondary goal of preventing the patient from serving as a reservoir and thereby transmitter of the disease. Active immunization can conceivably and, perhaps, one day will be used for a variety of conditions ranging from cancer to drug abuse. But all of the currently available active immunizing agents (Tables 89-2–89-5) are employed in the control of infectious disease and the discussion of these agents is restricted to this perspective.

Types of Products

Vaccine may be defined as pharmaceutical suspension or solution of an immunogenic substance or compound(s) that is intended to induce active immunity. In the past it was common to limit the term to products that contained whole microorganisms, but today the term may be applied to all active immunizing agents and the process of active immunization is called *vaccination*.

The majority of vaccines still consist of entire microorganisms that may be either *inactivated* (killed) or *live attenuated*. Attenuated refers to strains of organisms that have a reduced disease-causing capacity but that retain the major immunogenic characteristics of the so-called *wild* strains that circulate in the community. It can be seen that viruses comprise most of the live attenuated vaccines while most of the bacterial vaccines contain killed bacteria or their components. It is important to understand that the live vaccines contain less immunogen than the killed and must actually cause an infection and replicate within the patient in order to induce a protective immune response. In evaluating a vaccine, the first two things that should be looked at are (1) the identity of the immunogen(s), ie, the disease(s) protected against, and (2) whether the product contains live or inactivated immunogen.

Toxoids are protein toxins that have been modified (eg, by treatment with formalin) to reduce the toxicity without significantly altering the immunogenicity. Two of the oldest and best known active immunizing agents are diphtheria toxoid and tetanus toxoid that protect against the bacteria exotoxins elaborated by *Corynebacterium diphtheriae* and *Clostridium tetani*, respectively.

Better methods of producing and purifying macromolecules in recent years have led to significant advances in the production of vaccines containing more highly purified compounds that represent important *virulence factors* of the microorganisms. The antiphagocytic capsular polysaccharides of *Hemophilus influenzae* type b, *Streptococcus pneumoniae*, and *Neisseria meningitidis* have been used to prepare effective vaccines against these important bacterial pathogens. The hepatitis B virus vaccine is the first to be produced by recombinant technology and contains a synthetic protein that has immunogenic epitopes of the hepatitis B surface antigen. Several acellular pertussis vaccines have been licensed and are expected ultimately to replace the killed whole cell vaccine of *Bordetella pertussis*.

The products described above are formulated as aqueous suspensions or lyophilized powders for reconstitution. In some cases the antigen has been *adsorbed* on an *adjuvant* (eg, alum or aluminum hydroxide) that enhance the immune response, probably by delaying absorption and prolonging the period of immunogenic stimulation. The diphtheria and tetanus toxoids and pertussis vaccine (DTP) are adsorbed in the vast majority of the products in which they occur, and this is so noted on the label; products containing no adjuvants are commonly referred to as *fluid* preparations.

Table 89-2. Bacterial Vaccines[a]

VACCINE	DISTRIBUTOR	ADMINISTRATION[b]
Live Attenuated Vaccines		
Bacillus Calmette Guérin (BCG) Vaccine		PC
Mycobax	Aventis Pasteur	
Tice BCG	Organon Technika	Intravesical
Typhoid Vaccine, Live, Oral		
Vivotif Berna	Berna Products	Oral
Inactivated Vaccines		
Anthrax VaccineAdsorbed	BioPort Corporation	SC
Cholera Vaccine	Wyeth	ID, SC, IM
Hemophilus Influenza Type B		IM
Conjugate Vaccines		
ActHIB (Tetanus toxoid conjugate)	Aventis Pasteur	
HibTITER (Diphtheria CRM$_{197}$ conjugate)	Wyeth	
PedvaxHIB (Meningococcal Protein Conjugate)	Merck	
Lyme Disease Vaccine *LYMErix*	Merck	
Meningococcal Polysaccharide Vaccine, Groups A, C, Y, and W-135		SC or Jet
Menomune-A/C/Y/W-135	Aventis Pasteur	
Pertussis Vaccine, Adsorbed	Michigan Biologic Products Inst	IM
Pneumococcal Conjugate Vaccine, 7-Valent *Prevnar*	Wyeth	
Pneumococcal Vaccine, 23-Valent		SC or IM
Pneumovax-23	Merck	
Pnu-Imune-23	Wyeth	
Tetanus Toxoid, Adsorbed	Aventis Pasteur	
Massachusettes Public Health Biologic Lab	IM or Jet	
Te Anatoxal Berna	Berna Products	
Typhoid Vi Capsular Polysaccharide Vaccine		IM
Typhim Vi	Aventis Pasteur	
Typhoid Vaccines, Inactivated	Wyeth	SC
Typhoid Vaccine, live-oral	Berna Biothech, Ltd.	

[a] The terms *live* and *inactivated* (*Killed*) are omitted from some of the names in this table but will appear in the official name of the product on the label.
[b] Routes of administration include intradermal (ID), intramuscular (IM), percutaneous (PC), subcutaneous (SC) and Jet injector.

Table 89-3. Combined Bacterial Vaccines[a]

VACCINE	DISTRIBUTOR
Diphtheria and Tetanus Toxoids and Whole-Cell Pertussis Vaccine (DTwP)	Aventis Pasteur
Tri-Immunol	Wyeth–Lederle
Diphtheria and Tetanus Toxoids and Acellular Pertussis Vaccine (DTaP)	
Acel-Imune	Wyeth–Lederle
Infanrix	GSK
Tripedia	Aventis Pasteur
Diphtheria and Tetanus Toxoids, Adsorbed, for Pediatric	
Use (DT)	Biocine Sclavo
Aventis Pasteur	
Wyeth	
Diphtheria and Tetanus Toxoids, Adsorbed, for Adult	
Use (Td)	Biocine Sclavo
Aventis Pasteur	
Massachussettes Public Health Biologic Lab	
HIB Conjugate Vaccine and Hepatitis B Virus Vaccine	
Comvax	Merck

[a] The term *inactivated* (*Killed*) is omitted from some of the names in this table but will appear in the official name of the product on the label. All products in this table are administered by the intramuscular route except for the Mixed Respiratory Vaccine that is administered subcutaneously. Hepatitis B is a virus not a bacterial vaccine.

Table 89-4. Live Attenuated Virus Vaccines[a]

VACCINE	DISTRIBUTOR	ADMINISTRATION[b]
Influenza Virus Vaccine		
FluMist	MedImmune	IN
Measles Virus Vaccine		
Attenuvax	Merck	SC or Jet
Mumps Virus Vaccine		
Mumpsvax	Merck	SC or Jet
Poliovirus Vaccine, Oral Trivalent		
Poliovax	Aventis Pasteur	
Rubella Virus Vaccine		
Meruvax II	Merck	SC or Jet
Smallpox Vaccine		
Dryvax	Wyeth/DoD	PC
Varicella Virus Vaccine		
Varivax	Merck	SC
Yellow Fever Virus Vaccine[c]		
YF-Vax	Aventis Pasteur	SC
Combination Vaccines		
MMR Virus Vaccines		
M-M-R II	Merck	SC or Jet
Measles and Rubella Virus Vaccines		
M-R Vax II	Merck	SC or Jet

[a] The term *live* is omitted from the names in this table but will appear in the official name of the product on the label.
[b] Routes of administration include percutaneous (PC), subcutaneous (SC), intranasal (IN) and Jet injector.
[c] Distribution is limited to designated Yellow Fever Vaccination Centers authorized by state health departments to issue yellow fever certificates of vaccination.

Table 89-5. Inactivated Virus Vaccines[a]

VACCINE	DISTRIBUTOR	ADMINISTRATION[b]
Hepatitis A Vaccine		
Havrix	GSK	IM or Jet
Vaqta	Merck	
Hepatitis B Vaccine		
Engerix-B	GSK	IM
Recombivax-HB	Merck	
Hepatitis A and Hepatitis B combination vaccine		
Twinrix	GSK	IM
Influenza Virus Vaccines, Trivalent Types A & B		IM or Jet
Fluvirin (Purified surface antigen)	Evans Vaccines	
Fluzone (Subvirion or whole-virion)	Aventis Pasteur	
Japanese Encephalitis Vaccine		
JE-Vax	Aventis Pasteur	SC
Poliovirus Vaccine, Inactivated		
Ipol	Aventis Pasteur	SC
Rabies Virus Vaccine	Bioport	IM
Imovax Rabies (Human diploid cell)	Aventis Pasteur	IM or ID
RabAvert (Purified chicken embryo cell)	Chiron Behring GmbH and Co	IM

[a] The term *inactivated* (*Killed*) is omitted from some of the names in this table but will appear in the official name of the product on the label.
[b] Routes of administration include intradermal (ID), intramuscular (IM), subcutaneous (SC) and Jet injector.

A *simple vaccine* is one that protects against a single disease whereas a *combined vaccine* is, as the name implies, a combination product that protects against two or more diseases (cp, Tables 89-3 and 89-4). This should not be confused with the *valency* of a vaccine that refers to the number of strains of an organism causing a single disease.

Virtually all of the information described above is found in the official name of the product (Tables 89-2–89-5). This name provides a guide to most of the important information that one needs to know about any vaccine.

Storage, Handling, and Administration

It is common practice to assume that when a vaccine is administered that the patient is immunized and generally no measures are taken to confirm this (eg, serological confirmation of antibody formation). The validity of this assumption depends in large measure upon the vaccine being properly stored, handled, and administered. Anyone administering vaccines, and this is increasingly including the pharmacist, should be familiar with the *General Recommendations on Immunization* published by CDC.[3]

The immunogens in vaccines are susceptible to alteration or inactivation by heat, freezing, and extremes of pH and care should be taken to store and reconstitute the products within the labeled limits. Most vaccines should be stored at refrigerator temperatures (2–8 °C) but a few are frozen (eg, varicella vaccine) and some for *field use* may not require refrigeration. Unless designed to do so, vaccines should never be mixed with each other or with other drugs.

The route of administration can have a profound effect on the quantity and quality of the immune response. The majority of vaccines are still administered by a parenteral route (Tables 89-2–89-5). Adjuvant products and killed bacterial vaccines are usually administered by intramuscular injection; subcutaneous injection usually provides an immune response but often results in a painful sterile cyst at the injection site. Live virus vaccines are usually administered by subcutaneous injection. A few vaccines are administered by intradermal injection (eg, typhoid, some rabies vaccines) and multiple puncture techniques (eg, BCG, vaccinia). Jet injectors may be used with some products to expedite the vaccination of large numbers of people. Vaccines should never be administered intravascularly since this is both less effective and results in more adverse reactions.

The quantity of immunogen in a vaccine is determined by a bioassay and expressed in units that are nearly always unique to that immunogen; a notable exception is those vaccines that contain purified microbial components that are expressed in mcg. Parenteral vaccines are typically administered in volumes of 0.1 to 1 mL with 0.5 mL being the most common. It should be noted that the products from different manufacturers do not always contain completely identical immunogens and some may have different dosage regimens (cp, *Hemophilus influenzae* type b vaccines). When multiple vaccines are available, the best practice is to complete an immunization series with the same vaccine. However, in those cases where this is not possible, it is generally better to use a different vaccine than to not vaccinate.

A distinction needs to be made between the multiple doses in a *primary immunization series* and *booster* doses of a vaccine. Primary immunization series are designed to assure that most if not all of those vaccinated will elicit a positive immune response. For example, if the efficacy of a single dose of a vaccine is 80%, a primary series of 3 doses would be expected to immunize most of the vaccinees. Primary series are especially important in pediatric immunizations since very young children may fail to respond because of underdeveloped immune systems (< 2 years of age) and/or interference by maternal antibodies (< 6 months of age).

A true *booster* dose of a vaccine is intended to enhance immunity in an immunized individual. In this respect, it is important to recognize that immunologic memory is not infinite in duration in spite of the apparent *life long immunity* imparted by either vaccination or having a disease. Immunity may be boosted following primary immunization by exposure to the natural disease, exposure to cross-reacting antigens or nonspecific activation during another immune response by the so-called *bystander effect*. The first of these is probably most important, and it follows that any mass immunization program that reduces the prevalence of a disease also reduces the opportunity for *natural boosters*. Most of the mass immunization procedures have not been in effect long enough to completely evaluate if this is a problem, but it's clear from the experience with diphtheria immunization that immunity can wane with age in the absence of booster doses of vaccine.

Efficacy

The effectiveness of a vaccine can be measured in several ways. Serological responses, such as the appearance of *neutralizing antibody* in the serum, are most easily measured and are often used as an indication of immunity. However, in many diseases cell-mediated immunity or local mucosal immunity are more

Table 89-6. Routine Pediatric Immunization

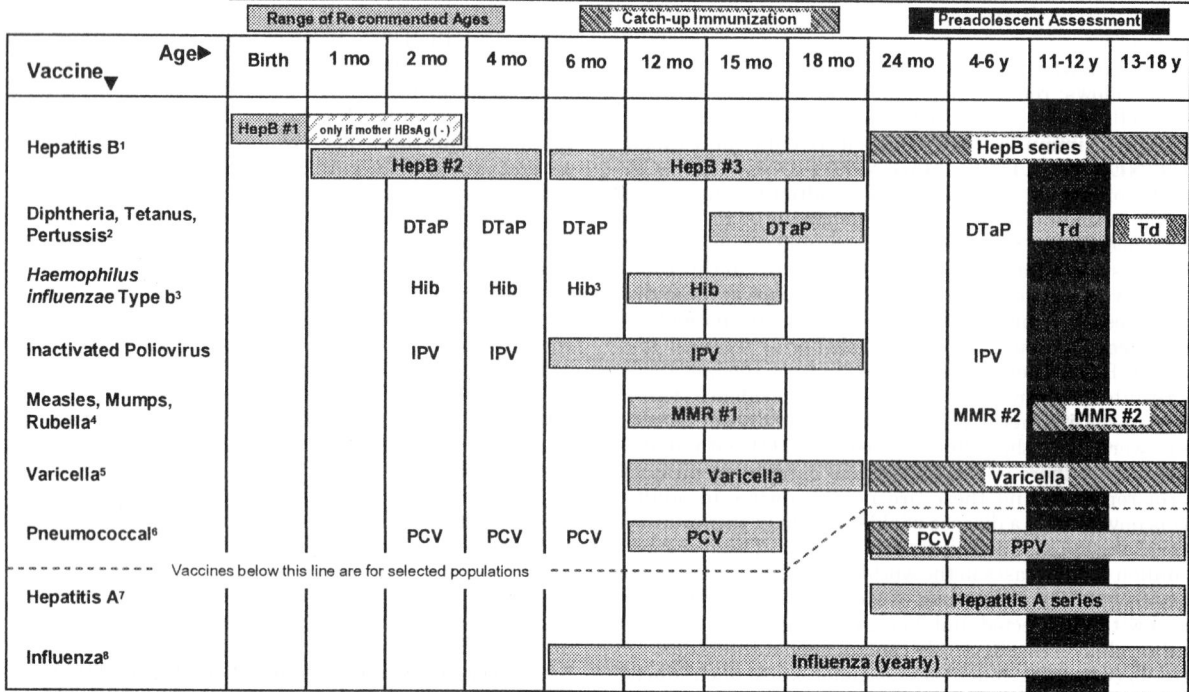

Recommended Childhood and Adolescent Immunization Schedule — United States, January – June 2004

Vaccine ▼ Age ►	Birth	1 mo	2 mo	4 mo	6 mo	12 mo	15 mo	18 mo	24 mo	4-6 y	11-12 y	13-18 y
Hepatitis B[1]	HepB #1	only if mother HBsAg (–)									HepB series	
		HepB #2				HepB #3						
Diphtheria, Tetanus, Pertussis[2]			DTaP	DTaP	DTaP		DTaP			DTaP	Td	Td
Haemophilus influenzae **Type b[3]**			Hib	Hib	Hib[3]	Hib						
Inactivated Poliovirus			IPV	IPV		IPV				IPV		
Measles, Mumps, Rubella[4]						MMR #1				MMR #2	MMR #2	
Varicella[5]						Varicella				Varicella		
Pneumococcal[6]			PCV	PCV	PCV	PCV				PCV	PPV	
Vaccines below this line are for selected populations												
Hepatitis A[7]										Hepatitis A series		
Influenza[8]						Influenza (yearly)						

Column group headers: Range of Recommended Ages | Catch-up Immunization | Preadolescent Assessment

This schedule indicates the recommended ages for routine administration of currently licensed childhood vaccines, as of December 1, 2003, for children through age 18 years. Any dose not given at the recommended age should be given at any subsequent visit when indicated and feasible. ▨ Indicates age groups that warrant special effort to administer those vaccines not previously given. Additional vaccines may be licensed and recommended during the year. Licensed combination vaccines may be used whenever any components of the combination are indicated and the vaccine's other components are not contraindicated. Providers should consult the manufacturers' package inserts for detailed recommendations. Clinically significant adverse events that follow immunization should be reported to the Vaccine Adverse Event Reporting System (VAERS). Guidance about how to obtain and complete a VAERS form can be found on the Internet: http://www.vaers.org/ or by calling 1-800-822-7967.

1. Hepatitis B (HepB) vaccine. All infants should receive the first dose of hepatitis B vaccine soon after birth and before hospital discharge; the first dose may also be given by age 2 months if the infant's mother is hepatitis B surface antigen (HBsAg) negative. Only monovalent HepB can be used for the birth dose. Monovalent or combination vaccine containing HepB may be used to complete the series. Four doses of vaccine may be administered when a birth dose is given. The second dose should be given at least 4 weeks after the first dose, except for combination vaccines which cannot be administered before age 6 weeks. The third dose should be given at least 16 weeks after the first dose and at least 8 weeks after the second dose. The last dose in the vaccination series (third or fourth dose) should not be administered before age 24 weeks.

Infants born to HBsAg-positive mothers should receive HepB and 0.5 mL of Hepatitis B Immune Globulin (HBIG) within 12 hours of birth at separate sites. The second dose is recommended at age 1 to 2 months. The last dose in the immunization series should not be administered before age 24 weeks. These infants should be tested for HBsAg and antibody to HBsAg (anti-HBs) at age 9 to 15 months.

Infants born to mothers whose HBsAg status is unknown should receive the first dose of the HepB series within 12 hours of birth. Maternal blood should be drawn as soon as possible to determine the mother's HBsAg status; if the HBsAg test is positive, the infant should receive HBIG as soon as possible (no later than age 1 week). The second dose is recommended at age 1 to 2 months. The last dose in the immunization series should not be administered before age 24 weeks.

2. Diphtheria and tetanus toxoids and acellular pertussis (DTaP) vaccine. The fourth dose of DTaP may be administered as early as age 12 months, provided 6 months have elapsed since the third dose and the child is unlikely to return at age 15 to 18 months. The final dose in the series should be given at age >4 years. **Tetanus and diphtheria toxoids (Td)** is recommended at age 11 to 12 years if at least 5 years have elapsed since the last dose of tetanus and diphtheria toxoid-containing vaccine. Subsequent routine Td boosters are recommended every 10 years.

3. *Haemophilus influenzae* type b (Hib) conjugate vaccine. Three Hib conjugate vaccines are licensed for infant use. If PRP-OMP (PedvaxHIB or ComVax [Merck]) is administered at ages 2 and 4 months, a dose at age 6 months is not required. DTaP/Hib combination products should not be used for primary immunization in infants at ages 2, 4 or 6 months but can be used as boosters following any Hib vaccine. The final dose in the series should be given at age >12 months.

4. Measles, mumps, and rubella vaccine (MMR). The second dose of MMR is recommended routinely at age 4 to 6 years but may be administered during any visit, provided at least 4 weeks have elapsed since the first dose and both doses are administered beginning at or after age 12 months. Those who have not previously received the second dose should complete the schedule by the 11- to 12-year-old visit.

5. Varicella vaccine. Varicella vaccine is recommended at any visit at or after age 12 months for susceptible children (i.e., those who lack a reliable history of chickenpox). Susceptible persons age >13 years should receive 2 doses, given at least 4 weeks apart.

6. Pneumococcal vaccine. The heptavalent **pneumococcal conjugate vaccine (PCV)** is recommended for all children age 2 to 23 months. It is also recommended for certain children age 24 to 59 months. The final dose in the series should be given at age >12 months. **Pneumococcal polysaccharide vaccine (PPV)** is recommended in addition to PCV for certain high-risk groups. See *MMWR* 2000;49(RR-9):1-38.

7. Hepatitis A vaccine. Hepatitis A vaccine is recommended for children and adolescents in selected states and regions and for certain high-risk groups; consult your local public health authority. Children and adolescents in these states, regions, and high-risk groups who have not been immunized against hepatitis A can begin the hepatitis A immunization series during any visit. The 2 doses in the series should be administered at least 6 months apart. See *MMWR* 1999;48(RR-12):1-37.

8. Influenza vaccine. Influenza vaccine is recommended annually for children age >6 months with certain risk factors (including but not limited to children with asthma, cardiac disease, sickle cell disease, human immunodeficiency virus infection, and diabetes; and household members of persons in high-risk groups [see *MMWR* 2003;52(RR-8):1-36]) and can be administered to all others wishing to obtain immunity. In addition, healthy children age 6 to 23 months are encouraged to receive influenza vaccine if feasible, because children in this age group are at substantially increased risk of influenza-related hospitalizations. For healthy persons age 5 to 49 years, the intranasally administered live-attenuated influenza vaccine (LAIV) is an acceptable alternative to the intramuscular trivalent inactivated influenza vaccine (TIV). See *MMWR* 2003;52(RR-13):1-8. Children receiving TIV should be administered a dosage appropriate for their age (0.25 mL if age 6 to 35 months or 0.5 mL if age >3 years). Children age <8 years who are receiving influenza vaccine for the first time should receive 2 doses (separated by at least 4 weeks for TIV and at least 6 weeks for LAIV).

For additional information about vaccines, including precautions and contraindications for immunization and vaccine shortages, please visit the National Immunization Program Web site at www.cdc.gov/nip/ or call the National Immunization Information Hotline at 800-232-2522 (English) or 800-232-0233 (Spanish).

Approved by the Advisory Committee on Immunization Practices (www.cdc.gov/nip/acip), the American Academy of Pediatrics (www.aap.org), and the American Academy of Family Physicians (www.aafp.org).

Table 89-6. (continued)

Recommended Childhood and Adolescent Immunization Schedule
United States   July–December 2004

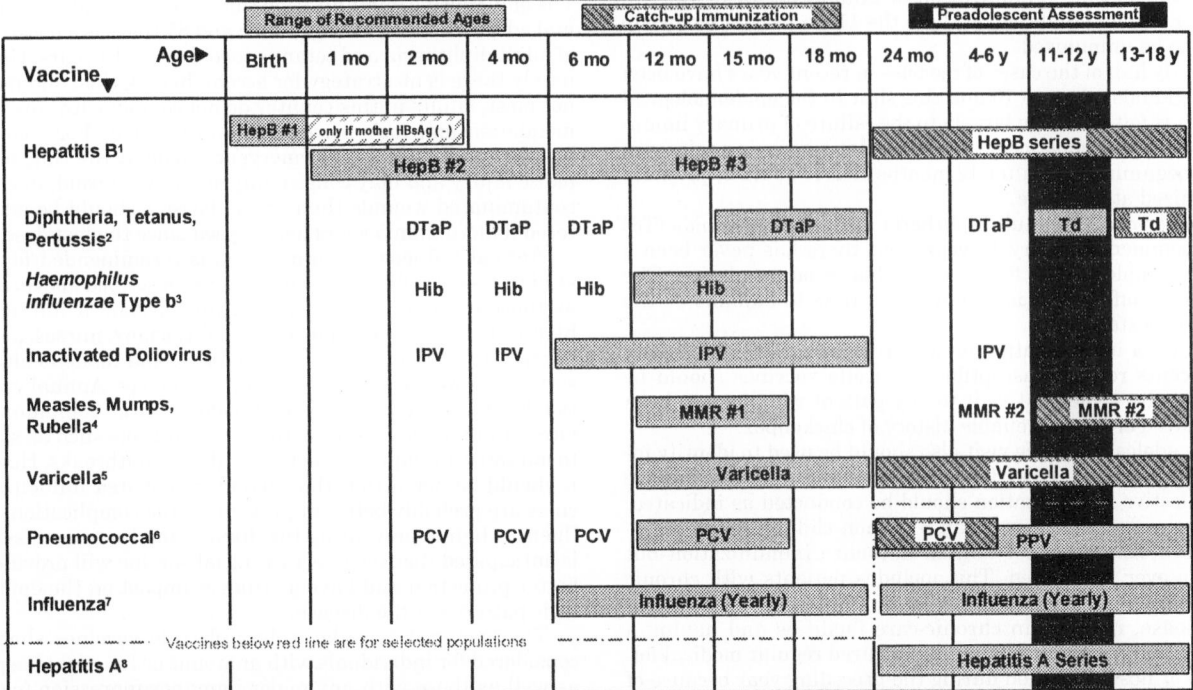

This schedule indicates the recommended ages for routine administration of currently licensed childhood vaccines, as of April 1, 2004, for children through age 18 years. Any dose not given at the recommended age should be given at any subsequent visit when indicated and feasible. ▨Indicates age groups that warrant special effort to administer those vaccines not previously given. Additional vaccines may be licensed and recommended during the year. Licensed combination vaccines may be used whenever any components of the combination are indicated and the vaccine's other components are not contraindicated. Providers should consult the manufacturers' package inserts for detailed recommendations. Clinically significant adverse events that follow immunization should be reported to the Vaccine Adverse Event Reporting System (VAERS). Guidance about how to obtain and complete a VAERS form can be found on the Internet: www.vaers.org or by calling 800-822-7967.

1. Hepatitis B (HepB) vaccine. All infants should receive the first dose of hepatitis B vaccine soon after birth and before hospital discharge; the first dose may also be given by age 2 months if the infant's mother is hepatitis B surface antigen (HBsAg) negative. Only monovalent HepB can be used for the birth dose. Monovalent or combination vaccine containing HepB may be used to complete the series. Four doses of vaccine may be administered when a birth dose is given. The second dose should be given at least 4 weeks after the first dose, except for combination vaccines which cannot be administered before age 6 weeks. The third dose should be given at least 16 weeks after the first dose and at least 8 weeks after the second dose. The last dose in the vaccination series (third or fourth dose) should not be administered before age 24 weeks.

Infants born to HBsAg-positive mothers should receive HepB and 0.5 mL of Hepatitis B Immune Globulin (HBIG) within 12 hours of birth at separate sites. The second dose is recommended at age 1–2 months. The last dose in the immunization series should not be administered before age 24 weeks. These infants should be tested for HBsAg and antibody to HBsAg (anti-HBs) at age 9–15 months.

Infants born to mothers whose HBsAg status is unknown should receive the first dose of the HepB series within 12 hours of birth. Maternal blood should be drawn as soon as possible to determine the mother's HBsAg status; if the HBsAg test is positive, the infant should receive HBIG as soon as possible (no later than age 1 week). The second dose is recommended at age 1–2 months. The last dose in the immunization series should not be administered before age 24 weeks.

2. Diphtheria and tetanus toxoids and acellular pertussis (DTaP) vaccine. The fourth dose of DTaP may be administered as early as age 12 months, provided 6 months have elapsed since the third dose and the child is unlikely to return at age 15–18 months. The final dose in the series should be given at age ≥4 years. **Tetanus and diphtheria toxoids (Td)** is recommended at age 11–12 years if at least 5 years have elapsed since the last dose of tetanus and diphtheria toxoid-containing vaccine. Subsequent routine Td boosters are recommended every 10 years.

3. *Haemophilus influenzae* type b (Hib) conjugate vaccine. Three Hib conjugate vaccines are licensed for infant use. If PRP-OMP (PedvaxHIB or ComVax [Merck]) is administered at ages 2 and 4 months, a dose at age 6 months is not required. DTaP/Hib combination products should not be used for primary immunization in infants at ages 2, 4 or 6 months but can be used as boosters following any Hib vaccine. The final dose in the series should be given at age ≥12 months.

4. Measles, mumps, and rubella vaccine (MMR). The second dose of MMR is recommended routinely at age 4–6 years but may be administered during any visit, provided at least 4 weeks have elapsed since the first dose and both doses are administered beginning at or after age 12 months. Those who have not previously received the second dose should complete the schedule by the visit at age 11–12 years.

5. Varicella vaccine. Varicella vaccine is recommended at any visit at or after age 12 months for susceptible children (i.e., those who lack a reliable history of chickenpox). Susceptible persons age ≥13 years should receive 2 doses, given at least 4 weeks apart.

6. Pneumococcal vaccine. The heptavalent **pneumococcal conjugate vaccine (PCV)** is recommended for all children age 2–23 months. It is also recommended for certain children age 24–59 months. The final dose in the series should be given at age >12 months. **Pneumococcal polysaccharide vaccine (PPV)** is recommended in addition to PCV for certain high-risk groups. See *MMWR* 2000;49(RR-9):1-35.

7. Influenza vaccine. Influenza vaccine is recommended annually for children aged ≥6 months with certain risk factors (including but not limited to asthma, cardiac disease, sickle cell disease, HIV, and diabetes), healthcare workers, and other persons (including household members) in close contact with persons in groups at high risk (see *MMWR* 2004;53;[RR-6]:1-40) and can be administered to all others wishing to obtain immunity. In addition, healthy children aged 6–23 months and close contacts of healthy children aged 0–23 months are recommended to receive influenza vaccine, because children in this age group are at substantially increased risk for influenza-related hospitalizations. For healthy persons aged 5–49 years, the intranasally administered live, attenuated influenza vaccine (LAIV) is an acceptable alternative to the intramuscular trivalent inactivated influenza vaccine (TIV). See *MMWR* 2004;53;[RR-6]:1-40. Children receiving TIV should be administered a dosage appropriate for their age (0.25 mL if 6–35 months or 0.5 mL if ≥3 years). Children aged ≤8 years who are receiving influenza vaccine for the first time should receive 2 doses (separated by at least 4 weeks for TIV and at least 6 weeks for LAIV).

8. Hepatitis A vaccine. Hepatitis A vaccine is recommended for children and adolescents in selected states and regions and for certain high-risk groups; consult your local public health authority. Children and adolescents in these states, regions, and high-risk groups who have not been immunized against hepatitis A can begin the hepatitis A immunization series during any visit. The 2 doses in the series should be administered at least 6 months apart. See *MMWR* 1999;48(RR-12):1-37.

For additional information about vaccines, including precautions and contraindications for immunization and vaccine shortages, please visit the National Immunization Program Web site at www.cdc.gov/nip/ or call the National Immunization Information Hotline at 800-232-2522 (English) or 800-232-0233 (Spanish).

Approved by the Advisory Committee on Immunization Practices (www.cdc.gov/nip/acip), the American Academy of Pediatrics (www.aap.org), and the American Academy of Family Physicians (www.aafp.org).

MEDICINAL AGENTS

Most persons in this country infected with hepatitis B virus acquired their infection as an adolescent or young adult; the virus is transmitted primarily through sexual contact, intravenous drug use, household contacts, or occupational exposure. Since the routine immunization of infants began in 1991, a number of individuals currently in the 11- to 12-year old group needs to be immunized.

Nearly half of the cases of measles in recent years have been in individuals over age 10 and this shift in the epidemiological pattern is felt to be due largely to the failure of primary immunization. Those adolescents who have not received two doses of MMR beginning at or after 12 months of age should be properly immunized at this time.

Booster doses of adult diphtheria and tetanus toxoids (Td) are recommended every 10 years, but there has never been a strategy implemented for effecting this recommendation. The adolescent office visit is a convenient time to administer the first Td booster.

Varicella immunization became routine in 1995 and many adolescents remain susceptible. Varicella vaccines should be given at the adolescent visit to any patient who has not been immunized or has no reliable history of chickenpox.

The adolescent office visit also should be used to identify individuals who are at risk for other vaccine-preventable disease and selective immunization should be conducted as indicated. It is estimated that more than 8 million children and adolescents are candidates for annual influenza immunization but few are ever vaccinated. This includes patients with chronic pulmonary disease (eg, asthma, cystic fibrosis) or cardiovascular disease; residing in chronic-care facilities and having a chronic medical condition; having required regular medical follow-up or hospitalization during the preceding year because of chronic metabolic disease (eg, diabetes), renal disease, hemoglobulinopathy, or immunosuppression; or receiving long-term aspirin therapy and at a risk of developing Reye's syndrome after influenza infection (up to 18 years of age).

It is estimated that 340,000 persons from 2 to 18 years of age have chronic illnesses that increase the risk of pneumococcal disease and should be vaccinated with the 23-valent vaccine. This includes those with anatomic or functional asplenia including sickle cell disease, nephrotic syndrome, cerebrospinal fluid leaks, or conditions associated with immunosuppression.

Hepatitis A virus infections occur in about 140,000 persons a year in the US and the highest rates of disease are in those 5 to 14 years of age. Hepatitis A vaccine should be administered to adolescents who plan to travel of work in areas where the disease is prevalent; human immune globulin may be used for short term prophylaxis when protection is needed faster than the vaccine can provide. Vaccination may be considered for adolescents who reside in communities that experience periodic outbreaks of hepatitis A. Adolescents should definitely be vaccinated if they have chronic liver disease, are receiving clotting factors, use illegal drugs of any kind or are males who have sex with males.

There are other selective immunizations that may be occasionally indicated in adolescents and many of these are described under adult immunizations.

IMMUNIZATION OF ADULTS UNDER AGE 65—The first thing to consider about the immune state of an adult patient is whether or not they have completed the recommended pediatric immunizations. Pertussis vaccine is not recommended for adults but the other nine vaccines are commonly indicated under different circumstances if there is not evidence of immunity; ie, reliable history of having the disease or positive serological test. When a patient is found to be susceptible to any of these nine diseases, their history should be reviewed vis-a-vis the recommendations for the appropriate vaccine(s) to determine if vaccination is indicated. Three circumstances where it is particularly important that the pediatric immunizations are up-to-date are the following:

1. Women of child-bearing age who may become pregnant since the immunity (ie, IgG) that they transfer to the fetus depends on their immune status.

2. Individuals with chronic diseases since they may be more susceptible to the disease or its adverse effects.
3. Individuals who travel internationally since some of these diseases remain prevalent in other parts of the world.

The only routine immunization that is recommended for all normal adults between the ages of 18 and 65 years is a booster dose of adult diphtheria and tetanus toxoid every 10 years. Unfortunately there is no strategy for accomplishing this, and many, if not most, adults in this country do not comply with this recommendation and may not even be aware of it. For some, this booster is received in the emergency room at the time of traumatic injury and may consist only of tetanus toxoid; in cases of contaminated wounds the tetanus booster should be administered if more than 5 years has elapsed since the last dose.

Annual influenza immunization is recommended for those at high-risk of influenza complications (described above) as well as those capable of nosocomial transmission of influenza to high-risk patients; ie, pharmacists, physicians, nurses, and others who provide in-patient, out-patient, and home health-care services as well as nonprofessional caregivers. Annual vaccination is also wise for those who provide essential community services, and individuals in institutional settings such as schools, to minimize disruption of activities during outbreaks. However, it should be noted that the current inactivated influenza vaccines are probably better at preventing the complications of influenza than of preventing the disease and its transmission. It is anticipated that the live, intranasal vaccine will provide both better protection and have a stronger impact on the epidemiologic patterns of the disease.

The bacterial capsular polysaccharide vaccines should be considered for individuals with anatomic or functional asplenia as well as those with any major immunosuppression (eg, HIV infection, organ transplant, some cancers). Pneumococcal vaccine should be administered to other high-risk individuals including those with cardiovascular or pulmonary disease, chronic hepatic or renal disorders, and diabetes mellitus. Meningococcal vaccine is recommended for some travelers and some closed populations where outbreaks may occur.

International travel is very common today for business, travel, and hobby, and all travelers should review the current recommendations of CDC[7] well in advance of any trip. Most travelers to developed areas of the world need only to have their routine immunizations up-to-date. The only disease for which an *International Certificate of Vaccination* may still be required is yellow fever. Travelers to underdeveloped countries or the back country of developed countries may find other vaccines recommended; hepatitis A vaccine is most likely but cholera, plague, and typhoid vaccines may occasionally be suggested.

Hepatitis B immunization is essential for health-care workers with exposure to human blood and tissues, and there are a number of other vaccinations that are recommended for those in high-risk occupations. Laboratory and field workers exposed to *Yersinia pestis* or wild rodents and fleas should receive plague vaccine. Military recruits will receive adenovirus, hepatitis A, and meningococcal vaccines and sometimes others.

The majority of vaccines are administered prior to exposure to the infectious organism but in diseases with long incubation periods postexposure active immunization, with or without concurrent passive immunization, may be effective. Postexposure active immunization is routinely used to prevent rabies in individuals exposed through the bites of infected animals while the usual pre-exposure immunization is recommended only for those who have occupational exposure. Both hepatitis A and hepatitis B have sufficiently long incubation periods to warrant postexposure vaccination when needed.

BCG vaccine is one of the most widely used worldwide but is very rarely recommended in this country. It appears to be effective in preventing serious miliary and meningeal tuberculosis, but its efficacy in preventing common pulmonary tuberculosis is questionable. It is recommended only in extremely high-risk individuals where other controls are impractical. It should be mentioned that BCG vaccine is commonly used to treat bladder cancer by direct instillation into the bladder. This is sometimes called nonspecific immunotherapy, but the precise mechanism is unknown; the vaccine does promote a local inflammatory response that may be responsible for the anti-tumor effects.

IMMUNIZATION OF ADULTS AGE 65 AND OVER— Older age is often thought of as being synonymous with declining immunity, although there is little objective evidence to indicate that most older persons suffer from major immunodeficiency. There is an increasing incidence and severity of chronic diseases that often increase the risk and complications of a number of infectious diseases. The elderly may respond poorer to some vaccines, but this does not appear to be a general problem. Although applicable throughout life, an important principle in preparing for old age is to effect immunization while still healthy whenever possible. The routine pediatric and selective immunizations described earlier are an important factor contributing to the increasing number of persons reaching old age. Evaluation of immune status and appropriate vaccination at age 65 is important to the quality of the later years.

Every individual should continue to receive adult diphtheria and tetanus toxoid boosters every 10 years and, if this has not been done, it is important to update these vaccinations at age 65. Unfortunately many older Americans are susceptible to these diseases as reflected in the epidemiological pattern of tetanus.

All individuals age 65 and over should receive annual influenza immunization and a single dose of pneumococcal vaccine. Those who received pneumococcal vaccine prior to age 65 should receive a booster dose if it has been 5 or more years since the first dose. Those at highest risk of fatal pneumococcal disease (eg, asplenia) also should receive a booster dose at 5 years after the initial dose.

Pharmacists and other health professionals should encourage individuals of all ages to receive appropriate immunization. Although the immunization rates for children in this country are generally good, the immunization rates for both healthy and chronically ill adults of all ages are relatively poor.

Adverse Reactions

The vaccines that are routinely used today are generally very safe as well as highly effective. There are, as with any drugs, risks of vaccination that range from common, minor, and inconvenient to rare, serious, and life-threatening. There are also some misconceptions on the part of both lay persons and professionals that may unnecessarily prevent or delay vaccination. As with most drugs, the acute hazards are much better understood than the chronic, and there are some potential risks associated with vaccines that should always be kept in mind. Pharmacists and others who administer vaccines will find the CDC publication on the risks of vaccination[8] helpful.

The most common adverse effects of vaccines are mild toxic and/or allergic reactions although, as with most adverse drug reactions, the mechanism usually remains unconfirmed. Both of these tend to be more common with the inactivated products than with live vaccines since they usually contain more antigen and require booster doses. It is not surprising, for example, that products containing whole, killed, gram-negative bacteria such as the cholera, plague, and killed typhoid vaccines frequently cause minor inflammation at the site of injection as well as mild systemic febrile responses. Reactions such as this occurring shortly after injection, and especially after the first dose, are almost certainly direct toxic reactions.

That vaccines may cause allergic reactions is also quite predictable considering their immunogenic character. This is an uncommon problem with the live virus vaccines that are administered locally and/or boosted less frequently. The too-frequent administration of tetanus toxoid, which was formerly very commonly done in emergency rooms, is associated with lo-

cal and systemic immune complex reactions. These Arthus-type skin reactions or any of the systemic symptoms of serum sickness are expected to occur within several hours of administration, especially following booster vaccination with an inactivated product.

IgE-mediated or anaphylactic sensitivity is more cause for concern and may take the form of urticaria (hives), angioedema, wheezing or even life-threatening shock. These reactions usually occur soon (0–60 minutes) after administration and, if due to the vaccine antigen, will generally occur after a booster dose. Reactions to components of the production medium (eg, eggs), antibiotics (eg, neomycin) or preservatives (eg, thimerosol) are very rare today but are likely to occur on the first dose in previously sensitized persons who are strongly allergic. Anaphylactic sensitivity to a vaccine or component is generally a contraindication to vaccination but there are some protocols for immunizing sensitive individuals.[3]

Inactivated vaccines pose very little infectious hazard if they are manufactured properly. That accidents may happen is best illustrated by the so-called *Cutter incident* in 1955 when improperly inactivated polio virus in IPV caused disease in a number of vaccinees.

Live vaccines are unique among pharmaceutical products in that infection of the patient receiving the product is intentional. There are several obvious as well as some subtle hazards associated with these products.

Live vaccines generally are contraindicated in pregnancy but the risk, at least with the current vaccines, is largely theoretical and occasionally the benefits merit vaccinating a pregnant woman who is at serious risk of disease. Rubella has, of course, been of particular concern and there is some evidence that the vaccine virus may be transmitted to the fetus; there have been many pregnant women inadvertently immunized with rubella vaccine but never a confirmed case of vaccine-associated congenital rubella. The medicolegal aspects of vaccinating a pregnant woman also must be considered, particularly in light of the relatively high incidence of miscarriages and birth defects during usual pregnancies.

Severely immunocompromised individuals can be safely administered inactivated vaccines, although the immune response may be poor, but should generally not receive live vaccines that have the potential to cause serious disease in such individuals. Serious immunosuppression can result from congenital immunodeficiency, HIV infection, malignancy (eg, leukemia, lymphoma, generalized malignancy), chemotherapy, and/or immunosuppressive therapy. The decisions in this area can be difficult, and there may or may not be data available to guide the clinician. For example, immunization of HIV-positive patients with MMR has caused no problems to date, and it is generally recommended that it be given to asymptomatic patients and considered even for those with symptoms. The immunosuppressive effects of corticosteroids are poorly defined but most steroid therapy is *not* a contraindication for live vaccines including the following: short-term therapy of less than 2 weeks; low to moderate dose therapy including physiologic maintenance doses (replacement therapy); long-term alternate day therapy; and topically or locally administered steroids including aerosols and intra-articular injections. The best practice is, whenever possible, to vaccinate prior to the immunosuppression.

Live vaccines also may pose a threat to the unvaccinated contacts of recent vaccinees. Poliovirus may be transmitted and cause disease especially in household contacts; vaccinees living with immunosuppressed individuals should only receive IPV. Varicella vaccine may cause chickenpox or shingle-type rashes in immunosuppressed individuals (eg, leukemia patients), and they may transmit the virus to susceptible contacts. Although vaccinees may shed measles, mumps, and rubella viruses after vaccination, there is no evidence of transmission of the viruses following MMR.

In addition to the real risks of vaccines, there are several potential problems that merit mention. Mass active immunization changes the epidemiological pattern of a disease and can

MEDICINAL AGENTS

have several consequences. What were formerly childhood diseases may in the unvaccinated be deferred until later in life where some are more serious; this has been the concern of some with mumps immunization particularly if the immunity is not as long as desired. On a longer term, the absence of a disease from a community for generations may result in a population even more susceptible than it was prior to immunization; apathy in immunization coupled with reintroduction of the disease could prove devastating to a community.

The viruses for vaccines are much like other drugs in the fact that much more is understood about their acute adverse effects than the chronic. The possibility of the virus causing an inapparent chronic or integrated infection as well as the potential for such things as oncogenesis and tetratogenesis cannot be completely ignored. The requirement that viruses be grown in living cells also increases the risk for inadvertent contamination with unknown organisms. These esoteric concerns are far outweighed by the benefits of vaccination, but their existence emphasizes two important points: first, active immunization should not be considered for trivial conditions and second, continuous diligence and study is required of all immunizing agents and procedures.

Contraindications

The contraindications given above are associated with adverse reactions to vaccination while those described below are generally related to achieving a poor immune response.

Active immunization should generally not be conducted in infants under 1 or 2 years of age unless there is a special risk and/or an effective procedure has been established. Maternal antibodies can persist for 6 or more months in a neonate, and it takes several years for the immune system to develop completely; infants usually respond poorly to any immunizing agent relative to older individuals, and there may be a risk of vaccine-induced illness if live vaccines are administered too early. Those pediatric immunizations recommended before 1 year of age all require completion of a primary series of doses to assure effectiveness. When other vaccines must be given early, revaccination at a later age is virtually always indicated.

Serious febrile illness is a contraindication to active immunization, especially with live virus vaccines, but there can be much confusion about this. Most acute febrile illnesses are caused by viruses that induce interferon and can interfere with virus replication and the response to the vaccine. The administration of any vaccine to a seriously ill individual can confound the evaluation of the illness and/or any reaction to the product. These factors must be weighed against the urgency for the vaccination. All vaccines can be administered to individuals with minor illnesses such as common diarrhea and mild upper respiratory disease with or without fever. These conditions are so common in children that failure to do so may seriously interfere with the vaccination program.

Live vaccines are contraindicated for varying periods after administration of immunoglobulin containing preparations because specific antibodies can interfere with the immune response; this is usually not a problem with killed vaccines that contain sufficient immunogen to overcome any inhibition. The products that can interfere with immunization include all human immune globulin preparations, whole blood, and several blood components (eg, packed RBCs, plasma/platelet products).

The effect of immune globulin on virus vaccines varies considerably with the vaccine. For example, OPV and yellow fever vaccines can be administered without regard to immune globulin administration. It has generally been recommended to wait 6 weeks to 3 months before administering most live vaccines such as MMR. But this interval is not sufficient for measles vaccine when high doses of intravenous immune globulin are administered and vaccination may have to be delayed for up to 11 months.[5] As always, the recommended intervals have to be

viewed with respect to the urgency of vaccination in the individual case.

National Childhood Vaccine Injury Act

The National Childhood Vaccine Injury Act (NVICA) became effective March 21, 1988 and has two main objectives: (1) to avoid future crises that may interrupt the National Immunization Program and (2) to provide financial compensation for patients who suffer vaccine-related injuries. The act requires that the providers of vaccinations keep certain permanent records of covered vaccinations as well as to report on certain adverse events. A surcharge is placed on the price of covered vaccines to fund the program, and compensation is paid to persons who suffer specified injuries from receiving these drugs. The covered vaccines currently include all of the routine pediatric immunizations (Table 89-6). The details of the record-keeping and reporting requirements as well as the current list of covered vaccines may be found at the CDC Web site.

Immunization Records

Proper documentation of immunizations is important from several respects. It helps ensure that those in need of vaccination receive it without the need for serologic testing and helps prevent overvaccinating, which increases the risks of hypersensitivity reactions. A comprehensive vaccination record should include not just the history of vaccinations but also ancillary information such as documentation of having had a disease or serologic testing for immunity. The NVICA specifies the records to be maintained by the provider.[2]

Official immunization cards have been adopted by every state to facilitate the assessment of immunization status by schools and child-care centers. A permanent immunization record card should be established for each newborn infant and maintained by the parents. Some states are developing computerized immunization record systems, and there is even consideration of a national immunization registry.

PASSIVE IMMUNIZING AGENTS

Passive immunization in the broadest sense involves the administration of any specific immune effector, antibody or effector T cell. In practice it has been restricted to the use of antibodies since effector T cells are limited in number, difficult to harvest and, perhaps most importantly, MHC-restricted and not usually effective when transferred from one individual to another. There have, however, been recent attempts to harvest the T cells of the individual patient, expand their number *in vitro* with colony-stimulating factors, and reintroduce the cells into the patient. The currently employed passive immunizing agents are all derived from immunoglobulins, and the majority of these consist mainly of IgG isotypes (see Chapter 60).

Human serum was used as early as 1907 for the prevention of measles and later for mumps and pertussis. Animal-derived antitoxins were used extensively prior to World War II to treat diphtheria, tetanus, scarlet fever, and other diseases with mixed results. Intramuscular human immune globulin (IGIM) became available after the war and was first used to treat a form of agammaglobulinemia (Bruton's disease) in 1952. Intravenous human immune globulin (IGIV) was developed over the 1980s and represents a major advance in passive immunizing agents. The first MAbs (digoxin immune Fab and muromonab CD3) were licensed in 1986, but only as the 20th century closes is this technology beginning to have a major impact on clinical medicine.

The antibody-containing products available in the US as of January 2000 are listed in Tables 89-7–89-9. Depending on how one defines passive immunization, it can be correctly argued that not all of these are passive immunizing agents. The emphasis at this point will be on those products that are used to

Table 89-7. Routine Adult Vaccine Recommendations

Recommended Adult Immunization Schedule, United States, 2003-2004 by Age Group

	For all persons in this group	Catch-up on childhood vaccinations	For persons with medical / exposure indications

Age Group ▶ / Vaccine ▼	19-49 Years	50-64 Years	65 Years and Older
Tetanus, Diphtheria (Td)*	1 dose booster every 10 years [1]		
Influenza	1 dose annually [2]	1 dose annually [2]	
Pneumococcal (polysaccharide)	1 dose [3,4]		1 dose [3,4]
Hepatitis B*	3 doses (0, 1-2, 4-6 months) [5]		
Hepatitis A	2 doses (0, 6-12 months) [6]		
Measles, Mumps, Rubella (MMR)*	1 dose if measles, mumps, or rubella vaccination history is unreliable; 2 doses for persons with occupational or other indications [7]		
Varicella*	2 doses (0, 4-8 weeks) for persons who are susceptible [8]		
Meningococcal (polysaccharide)	1 dose [9]		

See Footnotes for Recommended Adult Immunization Schedule, by Age Group and Medical Conditions, United States, 2003-2004 on back cover

*Covered by the Vaccine Injury Compensation Program. For information on how to file a claim call 800-338-2382. Please also visit www.hrsa.gov/osp/vicp To file a claim for vaccine injury contact: U.S. Court of Federal Claims, 717 Madison Place, N.W., Washington D.C. 20005, 202-219-9657.

This schedule indicates the recommended age groups for routine administration of currently licensed vaccines for persons 19 years of age and older. Licensed combination vaccines may be used whenever any components of the combination are indicated and the vaccine's other components are not contraindicated. Providers should consult the manufacturers' package inserts for detailed recommendations.

Report all clinically significant post-vaccination reactions to the Vaccine Adverse Event Reporting System (VAERS). Reporting forms and instructions on filing a VAERS report are available by calling 800-822-7967 or from the VAERS website at www.vaers.org.

For additional information about the vaccines listed above and contraindications for immunization, visit the National Immunization Program Website at www.cdc.gov/nip or call the National Immunization Hotline at 800-232-2522 (English) or 800-232-0233 (Spanish).

Approved by the Advisory Committee on Immunization Practices (ACIP), and accepted by the American College of Obstetricians and Gynecologists (ACOG) and the American Academy of Family Physicians (AAFP)

impart passive immunity for infectious and toxic diseases, but, as will be seen, the difference between these and the other antibody products is not always clear. All of the products are listed in the tables to assist the reader in making comparisons, but some of the products are described in greater detail in other chapters under their respective therapeutic categories.

Types of Products

When considering immunoglobulin-containing products, it is useful to think in terms of three dichotomies: human or animal, intramuscular or intravenous, polyclonal or monoclonal.

Human immune globulin products are derived from pooled plasma obtained from 1000 or more donors. The antibody content of all of these products is primarily IgG (90–98% depending on the product), and the four isotypes are generally within the range of their natural distribution: IgG_1 (60–70%), IgG_2 (23–29%), IgG_3 (4–8%) and IgG_4 (2–6%). The other isotypes are largely removed since they usually contribute little to the activity of the products and may give rise to adverse reactions. The composition of the products is very similar for both the so-called *normal* immune globulin preparations (IGIM, IGIV) as well as the specific or *hyperimmune* globulin products (eg, hepatitis B immune globulin). The former are standardized by assaying for several common antibodies (eg, measles, diphtheria, poliovirus, and often others), while the specific immune globulins also are assayed for the labeled antibody; the latter products are obtained from the pooled plasma of individuals having high titers of the labeled antibody such as recent vaccinees.

Heterologous antibody products (Table 89-8) must have their source displayed on the label, and this is nearly always equine. The horse was chosen because it has a large blood volume and is rarely used as a food animal in this country, which lessens the chance for sensitization. MAbs are often derived from sheep (ovine) or mice (murine). There is little functional difference between human and animal antibodies, but there is sufficient structural difference that allergy is a major problem with heterologous sera. *Serum sickness* is a systemic immune complex disease that occurs 5 to 14 days after administration of foreign antibodies; this active immune response also serves to clear the antibodies and heterologous products thus have a shorter duration of action than the homologous. Subsequent administration of a heterologous serum will result in an even faster and stronger reaction and may even be accompanied by IgE-mediated anaphylactic reactions. It is apparent that heterologous products are severely limited and has been a major factor in delaying the development of products containing MAbs; there are technical difficulties in producing human MAbs by hybridoma technology (Chapter 60). Technological advances in preparing *chimeric* (human-animal) and *humanized* MAbs has led to a number of products at the end of the millennium, and many more can be expected early in the 21st century.

Table 89-7. (continued)

Recommended Adult Immunization Schedule, United States, 2003-2004 by Medical Conditions

| | For all persons in this group | Catch-up on childhood vaccinations | | For persons with medical / exposure indications | Contraindicated |

Medical Conditions ▼ / Vaccine ▶	Tetanus-Diphtheria (Td)*,1	Influenza 2	Pneumo-coccal (polysacch-aride) 3,4	Hepatitis B*,5	Hepatitis A6	Measles, Mumps, Rubella (MMR) *,7	Varicella*,8
Pregnancy		A					
Diabetes, heart disease, chronic pulmonary disease, chronic liver disease, including chronic alcoholism		B	C		D		
Congenital Immunodeficiency, leukemia, lymphoma, generalized malignancy, therapy with alkylating agents, antimetabolites, radiation or large amounts of corticosteroids			E				F
Renal failure / end stage renal disease, recipients of hemodialysis or clotting factor concentrates			E	G			
Asplenia including elective splenectomy and terminal complement component deficiencies		H	E, I, J				
HIV infection			E, K			L	

See Special Notes for Medical Conditions below —also see Footnote for Recommended Adult Immunization Schedule, by Age Group and Medical Conditions, United States, 2003-2004 on back cover

Special Notes for Medical Conditions

A. For women without chronic diseases/conditions, vaccinate if pregnancy will be at 2nd or 3rd trimester during influenza season. For women with chronic diseases/conditions, vaccinate at any time during the pregnancy.

B. Although chronic liver disease and alcoholism are not indicator conditions for influenza vaccination, give 1 dose annually if the patient is age 50 years or older, has other indications for influenza vaccine, or if the patient requests vaccination.

C. Asthma is an indicator condition for influenza but not for pneumococcal vaccination.

D. For all persons with chronic liver disease.

E. For persons < 65 years, revaccinate once after 5 years or more have elapsed since initial vaccination.

F. Persons with impaired humoral immunity but intact cellular immunity may be vaccinated. MMWR 1999; 48 (RR-06): 1-5.

G. Hemodialysis patients: Use special formulation of vaccine (40 ug/mL) or two 1.0 mL, 20 ug doses given at one site. Vaccinate early in the course of renal disease. Assess antibody titers to hep B surface antigen (anti-HBs) levels annually. Administer additional doses if anti-HBs levels decline to <10 milliinternational units (mIU)/ mL.

H. There are no data specifically on risk of severe or complicated influenza infections among persons with asplenia. However, influenza is a risk factor for secondary bacterial infections that may cause severe disease in asplenics.

I. Administer meningococcal vaccine and consider Hib vaccine.

J. Elective splenectomy: vaccinate at least 2 weeks before surgery.

K. Vaccinate as close to diagnosis as possible when CD4 cell counts are highest.

L. Withhold MMR or other measles containing vaccines from HIV-infected persons with evidence of severe immunosuppression. MMWR 1998; 47 (RR-8):21-22; MMWR 2002; 51 (RR-02): 22-24.

Intramuscular human immune globulin (IGIM) is the prototype for the specific immune globulins that are administered by this route. A major limitation of these products is that, even with painful injections at several sites, the desired blood levels of IgG are not always attainable. Care must be taken not to inject these products intravascularly, for they contain immunoglobulin aggregates that can activate the complement system and cause serious anaphylactic reactions.

Intravenous human immune globulin (IGIV) is the prototype for the specific immune globulins that are administered by this route. Intravenous preparations are treated to prevent aggregation of the immunoglobulins, and there are virtually no limitations with respect to attainable blood levels. The first of these products marketed in the early 1980s were of questionable activity because of alteration of the Fc portion of the IgG molecules; ie, loss of the complement-activating and opsonizing activities required for antibacterial effects. The current products are evaluated for these *secondary* antibody activities. Later some of the products were associated with transmission of hepatitis C, but virus inactivation is now required in the manufacture of all immune globulins; the *P* in some of the product names represents *pasteurization* and *S/D* stands for surfactant/detergent, which are processes used to inactivate viruses.

IGIM and IGIV are polyclonal antibody preparations containing perhaps 10^7 different antibody specificities. These products are extremely broad spectrum when compared to MAbs but of relatively low activity for each specificity. MAbs are specific

for essentially a single epitope (assuming no cross reactivity) and are highly concentrated when compared to the polyclonal products. This level of specificity is desirable when the drug is targeting a specific receptor in the body such as a tumor antigen (eg, rituximab), physiologically active molecule such as tumor necrosis factor (eg, infliximab), or drug (eg, digoxin immune Fab) but is likely a disadvantage when the goal is to neutralize an infectious organism. *Immunologic redundancy* with polyclonal antibodies specific for different epitopes, and of multiple isotypes, is probably more effective against pathogens. It also should be recalled that all of the epitopes in an MAb are highly concentrated and some of these may be foreign and cause allergic reactions; eg, idiotopes, allotypic markers (Gm, Km).

Immune Globulin Intramuscular

The IGIM products are aqueous solutions containing 15% to 18% protein of which more than 90% is IgG and each lot represents the pooled plasma of more than 1000 donors. They are standardized for antibody to measles, diphtheria, and poliovirus to assure reasonable uniformity of product but contain antibodies specific for numerous bacteria, viruses, and fungi.

The main indications of IGIM is for IgG-replacement therapy in disorders where there is a deficiency of IgG antibodies and for the passive prevention or modification of hepatitis A and measles in susceptible persons when given shortly after ex-

Table 89-8. Human Immune Globulins

IMMUNE GLOBULIN	DISTRIBUTOR
Immune Globulin Intramuscular (IGIM)	
BayGam	Bayer
Gammar-P.I.M.	Centeon LLC
Immune Globulin Intravenous (IGIV)	
Gammar-P.I.V.	Aventis Biologicals
Gamimune N	Bayer
Gammagard S/D	Hyland Immuno HealthCare
Iveegam	Immuno-Hyland
Polygam S/D	American Red Cross
Sandoglobulin	Novartis
Venoglobulin-I and *Venoglobulin-S*	Alpha Therapeutics
Anti-Infective Immune Globulins	
Cytomegalovirus Immune Globulin Intravenous	
CytoGam	MedImmune
Hepatitis B Immune Globulin	
BayHep B	Bayer
Nabi-HB	North American Biologicals.
Rabies Immune Globulin	
BayRab	Bayer
Imogam Rabies	Pasteur–Mérieux Connaught
Respiratory Syncytial Virus Immune Globulin, Intravenous	
RespiGam	Medimmune and Wyeth–Lederle
Tetanus Immune Globulin	
BayTet	Massachusetts Public Health Biologics Lab
Vaccinia Immune Globulin	Bayer
	Centers for Disease Control and Prevention
	Massachusetts Public Health Biologics Lab
Varicella-Zoster Immune Globulin	
Immunosuppressive Immune Globulins	
Rh$_O$ (D) Immune Globulin	
BayRho-D	Bayer
Gamulin Rh and *Mini-Gamulin Rh*	Centeon LLC
Rh$_O$GAM and *MICRh$_O$GAM*	Ortho Diagnostics
Rh$_O$ (D) Immune Globulin Intravenous	
WinRho SDF	North American

posure; passive immunization for measles is particularly important in household contacts less than 1 year of age since they are particularly prone to measles complications and have not yet been vaccinated. IGIM is not standardized for hepatitis B, and the specific immune globulin should be used in this case. IGIM can be used for the prevention of varicella in immunocompromised patients if varicella-zoster immune globulin is not available. It also has been used to prevent fetal damage in women who are exposed to rubella during the first trimester of pregnancy and who do not want a therapeutic abortion, but it is of questionable value for this purpose. The ACIP recommends immune globulin (IM or IV) administration to symptomatic HIV-positive and other severely immunocompromised patients who are exposed to measles, regardless of their immunization status.

Immune globulins are probably effective in preventing or modifying infections by encapsulated bacteria and their complement-activating and opsonizing activities are most important in this respect. Antibody is more effective in preventing virus, fungal and other intracellular infections than in the resolution of established infection where cell-mediated immunity is much more important.

In treating immunodeficiency diseases the goal is to maintain IgG levels at about 200 mg/dL, which may require IGIM doses of 1mL/kg or more; lower doses are generally indicated for the other uses. Injection is preferably in the upper, outer quadrant of the gluteal region and doses of more than 10 mL should be divided and injected at several sites to reduce discomfort. The IgG titers peak within 2 to 5 days, and the serum half-life of IgG is usually about 20 to 25 days, but this can vary considerably.

There are few adverse reactions associated with IGIM except for local pain and tenderness at the injection site. Serious anaphylactic reactions occur occasionally and, as with all immune globulin products, are most often associated with selective IgA deficiency. This is the most common selective immunoglobulin deficiency, but the true incidence is not known and estimates range from 1:700 to 1:2,500.

IGIM is reported to be 80% to 95% effective in preventing hepatitis A depending upon the degree of exposure and time of treatment. It is probably much less effective in completely preventing the other virus diseases but is believed to lessen the in-

Table 89-9. Heterologous Antisera

ANTISERUM	DISTRIBUTOR
Antitoxins	
Botulism Antitoxin Types A, B, and E (Equine)	CDC[a]
Botulism Antitoxin Monovalent Type E (Equine)	CDC[a]
Diphtheria Antitoxin (Equine)	CDC[a]
Antivenins	
Crotalidae Antivenin Polyvalent (Equine)	Wyeth–Ayerst
Micrurus fulvius Antivenin (Equine)	Wyeth–Ayerst
Latrodectus Mactans Antivenin (Equine)	Merck
Sculpturatus centruroides Antivenin (Caprine)	Arizona State University
Immunosuppressive	
Anti-thymocyte Globulin (Equine)	
ATGAM	Upjohn

[a] Centers for Disease Control and Prevention.

cidence of severe disease and complications. IGIM helps in controlling infections in antibody deficiency disorders, but serious immunodeficiency disease involves multiple problems that are not addressed by IGIM.

The fundamental properties of the specific immune globulins for hepatitis B, rabies, tetanus, vaccinia, and varicella-zoster are very similar to those of IGIM.

Immune Globulin Intravenous

The IGIV products are aqueous solutions or lyophilized powders that are reconstituted to provide 5% or 10% protein solutions except for Sandoglobulin, which is prepared as 3, 6, 9, or 12% solutions. The IgG content ranges from greater than 90% to 99% depending upon the specific product and is nearly all monomeric (>92% to 99%). Each lot represents the pooled plasma of from more than 1000 to 50,000 donors. Most of the powders can be stored at room temperature and the solutions at 2–8°, but there are some differences in the way that individual products are stored and reconstituted so that pharmacists should become familiar with the properties of the individual products used. Some of the products have less IgA and may be able to be used in some IgA-sensitive patients. There is much variation in the reported mean serum half-life (23–40 days) of the products, but this also varies considerably between patients. The individual products also vary in the approved labeled indications but, for most purposes, they are considered to be therapeutically equivalent and will be discussed as such below.

IGIV is especially useful in those conditions where rapid and/or high levels of antibody are desired and cannot be achieved with IGIM or in patients where IGIM is contraindicated because of such things as limited muscle mass or bleeding tendencies. The indications and uses of IGIV are somewhat paradoxical in that these products are employed both as anti-infectives and as immunosuppressive agents. Note however that the dose levels in the first case are similar to those for IGIM with the goal being to maintain baseline serum levels of IgG of at least 200 mg/dL; the dose levels of IGIV when used as an immunosuppressive generally exceed those that can be easily attained with IGIM. Several days is required for the serum levels of IgG to equilibrate since IgG is extensively redistributed to extravascular spaces.

IGIV is indicated for the treatment of primary immunodeficiency disease in much the same way as IGIM (see above). It also is indicated for the prevention of bacterial infections in patients with B cell chronic lymphocytic leukemia, the most common form of adult leukemia, and in children with AIDS. Doses in the range of 100 to 400 mg/kg every 3 to 4 weeks will usually maintain the IgG serum levels at the desired 200 mg/dL.

IGIV also is indicated for immune thrombocytopenia purpurea (ITP), Kawasaki disease, and bone marrow transplant patients. IGIV is presumably acting as an immunosuppressive in these conditions, but the reader should be aware that neither the detailed mechanisms of these diseases nor of IGIV are completely understood at this time.

Both the anti-infective and immunosuppressive activities of IGIV are important in bone marrow transplantation where it is effective in reducing the incidence and severity of both infections and *graft-versus-host disease*. Doses of 500 mg/kg are administered 7 and 2 days prior to transplantation, or at the beginning of conditioning therapy, and are continued weekly after transplantation for about 13 weeks.

In Kawasaki disease, IGIV plus aspirin therapy reduces the incidence of coronary artery abnormalities significantly more than aspirin therapy alone. Several different dosing schedules are used including a single dose of 2 g/kg within 10 days of onset of the disease or 400 mg/kg on four consecutive days.

The efficacy of IGIV in ITP depends on the age of the patient and form of the disease and, while often helpful in restoring platelet levels, is difficult to predict; acute childhood ITP probably responds best, but this is also the form with the highest rate of spontaneous remission. A wide variety of dosage regimens have been used to attain the goal of a platelet count of 30,000 to 50,000 cells/mm^3; one example is induction therapy of 400 to 2000 mg/kg for 1 to 7 consecutive days and, if required, maintenance therapy of 400 to 2000 mg/kg every 2 weeks.

The mechanism of the immunosuppressive activity of IGIV is not well understood but likely involves multiple mechanisms of varying importance depending upon the condition.[9] For example, ITP involves *antibody-dependent cell-mediated cytotoxicity* in which the antibody-coated platelets are lysed, primarily in the spleen, by effector cells such as macrophages that have Fc receptors for the autoantibodies. One theory is that antibodies in the IGIV, after forming immune complexes with their complementary antigens, compete for the Fc binding sites with the antibody-coated platelets; the efficacy of Rh$_o$(D) immune globulin intravenous in treating ITP in Rh-positive patients is notable in this respect. Another possibility is that the IGIV contains anti-idiotypic antibodies specific for the anti-platelet antibodies. It also may be speculated that immune complexes suppress the immune response by binding to Fc receptors and inhibiting B cell responsiveness, which appears to be a mechanism of feedback inhibition of antibody production. Note however that the mechanism of action of the immunosuppressive antibodies used in the management of allograft rejection (anti-thymocyte globulin, muromonab CD3 and daclizumab) is likely quite different than that of IGIV; these antibodies all inhibit specific receptors on lymphocytes and thereby suppress ongoing immune responses.

There are many off-label uses of IGIV, and an expert panel has reviewed and made recommendations on 53 of these.[10] The majority of the diseases are known or suspected to be immunologically mediated diseases (eg, autoimmune). Lassister's[11] evaluation of the studies of IGIV in the management of neonatal sepsis contains an excellent review of the factors to be considered in fetal and neonatal immunity.

The adverse reactions of IGIV tend to be mild and transient. Mild fever, chills, arthralgia, myalgia, and many other minor symptoms are most likely to occur when there are large time intervals (greater than 8 weeks) between treatment and a build up of what may be called the *antigen load*; the administered antibodies react with their complementary antigens that have accumulated since the last dose of IGIV and the immune complexes formed may cause the mild reactions until they are cleared. Such reactions can be controlled, in part, by using slower initial infusion rates. More serious anaphylactic reactions are rare and usually associated with IgA deficiency.

Cytomegalovirus immune globulin and respiratory syncytial virus immune globulin are both intravenous preparations that share the essential properties of IGIV except that their use is restricted to the conditions for which they are named.

Other Antibody Products

The heterologous antisera currently available are all, with the exception of anti-thymocyte globulin, used to treat intoxications by venomous animals or bacterial exotoxins. Each of these products have limited and specific indications that are well described in the product literature. Patients should always be skin-tested for anaphylactic sensitivity prior to receiving heterologous products; it is also notable that most of these products are administered by slow IV infusion since the onset of activity with IM administration is too slow to deal effectively with a serious intoxication. It is of interest to compare these products with digoxin immune Fab that is an immunoantidote derived from MAb technology. It too is a heterologous product, but it demonstrates the potential to develop humanized MAbs (or Fab fragments) for the safer and more effective management of intoxications of many types.

The MAb products marketed as of April 2004 are listed in Table 89-10. The six therapeutic categories represented by the

Table 89-10. Monoclonal Antibodies[a]

ANTIBODY	DISTRIBUTOR
Anticoagulant Antibodies	
Abciximab (Chimeric)*	
ReoPro	Lilly
Anti-Infective Antibodies	
Palivizumab (Humanized)	
Synagis	Medimmune and Ross Products
Antiinflammatory Antibodies	
Infliximab (Chimeric)	
Remicade	Centocor
Antineoplastic Antibodies	
Rituximab (Chimeric)	
Rituxan	IDEC and Genentech
Tratuzumab (Humanized)	
Herceptin	Genentech
Immunoantidote Antibodies	
Digoxin Immune Fab (Ovine)*	
Digibind	Glaxo–Wellcome
Digidote	Boehringer Mannheim
Immunosuppressive Antibodies	
Daclizumab (Chimeric)	
Zenapax	Hoffmann–LaRoche
Muromonab-CD3 (Murine)	
Orthoclone-OKT3	IDEC and Genentech

[a] Includes Fab fragments (*) derived from monoclonal antibodies but does not include the radioisotope-conjugated MAbs and fragments licensed for diagnostic purposes as of January 2000.

eight current products only partially reflect the potential of MAbs as therapeutic agents. Conceivably every known therapeutic class could ultimately be represented, possibly along with some that are currently unknown.

The MAb that is definitely a passive immunizing agent is palivizumab. This antibody is specific for an epitope in the F protein of the respiratory syncytial virus (RSV). The F protein on the surface of RSV is necessary for the virus to infect cells and, as expressed on the surface of the infected cells, is responsible for the cell fusion that results in syncytia. Palivizumab exhibits both *virus-neutralizing* and *fusion inhibitory activity*. It is indicated, as is RSV immune globulin intravenous (Table 89-7), for the prevention of serious lower respiratory tract disease caused by RSV in high-risk infants. This product may, more than any of the others, best reflect the future of passive immunization.

ALLERGENIC EXTRACTS

Allergenic extracts comprise a large group of products that are unique compared to other biologics and conventional pharmaceuticals. A specific license is required for their manufacture, and they are available mainly from specialty companies. In spite of nearly 90 years of clinical use for the diagnosis and treatment of allergy, allergenic extracts are relatively crude drugs by contemporary standards. Their composition is heterogeneous and ill-defined, their mechanism of action is understood poorly, and to date there are no totally reliable standards of potency. Allergenic extracts are administered (or dispensed) primarily in the allergist's office, and with few exceptions, these drugs do not enter conventional pharmaceutical distribution systems.

Common allergies are estimated to affect 10% to 30% of the population, and allergenic extracts, despite their shortcomings, are mainstays in the control of these diseases. Every pharmacist should have a fundamental understanding of allergenic extracts, and some clinical, institutional, and industrial specialists require expertise. In recent years allergy research has intensified, but an unfortunately small number of pharmaceutical scientists have entered the field.

Because of the complexity and large number of allergenic extracts, only the fundamental terminology, principles, properties, and types of products are included in this chapter. As noted earlier, the *diagnostic skin antigens* for infectious diseases are included in this discussion of allergenic extracts (*delayed hypersensitivity tests*) since they are most closely related to these products in both composition and use (Table 89-11).

ALLERGY

Allergy (*hypersensitivity*) may be defined as an *untoward immunological reaction* to an environmental immunogen called the *allergen*. The phenomenon is not a simple cause-effect rela-

Table 89-11. Mechanisms and Manifestations of Allergy[a]

	TYPE I[b]	TYPE II	TYPE III	TYPE IV
Names	IgE-Mediated Immediate Hypersensitivity	Cytotoxic	Immune Complex Arthus-type	Cell-Mediated Delayed Hypersensitivity Tuberculin-type
Immune Effectors	IgE	IgG	IgG, IgM	CD4+ T Cells CD8+ T Cells
Major cells involved in inflammation	Mast Cell Basophil	Macrophage (Antibody-dependent cell-mediated cytotoxicity) or, less commonly,	Neutrophil	Macrophage
Mediators	Histamine		Cytokines	
Leukotrienes	Complement-mediated lysis	Lysozomal enzymes		
Onset in sensitized individual	0–30 minutes	Immediate (but symptoms inapparent)	2–24 hours	6–24 hours
Manifestations Allergic asthma Atopic dermatitis Gastroenteropathy	Allergic rhinitis			
	Hemolytic anemia Neutropenia Thrombocytoenia	Vasculitis		
Serum Sickness Glomerulonephritis Arthus-type rash	Allergic contact dermatitis Hypersensitivity pneumonitis			

[a] Based upon the classification of Coombs and Gell.[12]
[b] The characteristics of *late phase reactions* are not represented in this table.

tionship, however, for exposure to an allergen results in disease only in a small portion of the population. The occurrence of allergic disease is determined by the characteristics of the individual as well as those of the allergen and the conditions of exposure. Disease occurs only in those previously sensitized by exposure to the allergen and the ability to become sensitized is, at least sometimes, genetically determined (see *Atopy*). Sensitization also may vary with the age of the individual, nature of the allergen, route and degree of exposure and many other factors.

The immunological processes involved in allergy result in inflammation and tissue damage but otherwise do not differ fundamentally from those seen in the normal immune response (Chapter 60). The classification system of Coombs and Gell (Table 89-1) that considers four basic mechanisms of immunologically mediated disease remains a very useful frame of reference for allergic disease

Most of the common allergies are *IgE-mediated* and allergenic extracts are most useful in the diagnosis (*immediate sensitivity tests*), and to a lesser extent immunotherapy, of these conditions. *Cytotoxic allergy* and *immune complex disease* are more prominent in autoimmune and alloimmune diseases (Chapter 60) and are not as important in the present context. Many environmental allergens, including the well-known poison ivy, produce allergic contact dermatitis and this cell-mediated immunity is the basis for *delayed hypersensitivity tests*.

Atopy

Atopy is the inherited tendency to develop IgE-mediated allergy to common inhaled and ingested allergens. The atopic diseases include the common *allergic rhinitis* (hay fever) and *allergic asthma*, *atopic dermatitis*, and, less commonly, *allergic gastroenteropathy*. Allergenic extracts are most useful in the management of the first two conditions.

The etiology of atopy is poorly understood. The atopic individual frequently has a family history of allergy and typically is allergic to multiple allergens. Serum IgE usually is elevated, and eosinophilia is usually present in the blood and tissues. The shock tissues are hyperresponsive, and this may involve autonomic imbalance such as a β-adrenergic deficit (or cholinergic excess) in the case of asthma. The nature of the allergen and the route of exposure via mucous membranes undoubtedly play important roles.

The IgE-mediated conditions *urticaria-angioedema* and *anaphylaxis* are nonatopic diseases in that there is no genetic predisposition, and the shock tissues not hyperirritible. The allergens are most often ingested or injected, and the most common offenders are foods and drugs. Sensitivity testing and immunotherapy are of limited value in these nonatopic conditions with the notable exception of *Hymenoptera (stinging insect) sensitivity*.

The manifestations of both atopic and nonatopic IgE-mediated disease are what are often considered to be the *typically allergic symptoms*. It is important for the pharmacist to understand that allergy can be manifest by other symptoms and, especially, that rhinitis, asthma, urticaria, and anaphylaxis can result by nonimmunological mechanisms.

Allergens

Allergens are the inciting agents of allergy. It is common to speak of substances such as pollens, danders, dusts, etc, as allergens when, in fact, the true allergens are found in the individual compounds within these substances. As in other immunological reactions, the specificity resides in small fragments within the molecules called *epitopes*.

The chemical identity of most allergens is unknown, but the tools of molecular biology are being employed for both the elucidation of structure and synthesis of recombinant allergens. When isolated, individual allergens are named by the system of the International Union of Immunological Societies.[13]

The first three letters of the genus are followed by the first letter of the species and then a Roman numeral; eg, *Amb a I* is antigen E of short ragweed (*Ambrosia artemisifiolia*). Baldo has reviewed the structural characteristics of both environmental and drug allergens.[14]

Most known allergens are proteins or glycoproteins and do not appear to differ much from other immunogens except perhaps being somewhat smaller (mol wt 10,000-70,000). Most allergenic substances contain multiple allergens that vary in their allergenic potency, ie, *major* and *minor* allergens. Allergens from related sources often are similar chemically and *cross-allergenicity* is common between biologically related substances. The number and diversity of potential allergens in the environment is great, which provides a major complication in the control of allergy.

A variety of low-molecular-weight chemicals may serve as allergenic *haptens* (partial immunogens) and induce allergy after combining covalently with a suitable protein carrier. While this is an important process in drug allergy, most common environmental allergens appear to be complete immunogens. A notable exception is the case of common allergic contact dermatitis caused by a variety of plants, drugs, clothing additives, and other substances. The plants most responsible for contact dermatitis in North America belong to the Anacardiaceae family, primarily the genus *Toxicodendron* (Rhus), and include poison ivy, oak, and sumac. The allergic components of these plants, called urushiols, are found in the oleoresin fraction and are derivatives of pentadecylcatechol or heptadecylcatechol. Many plants of the *Compositae* family, which includes the ragweeds, also cause contact dermatitis, and the allergens have been identified as sesquiterpenoid lactones.

The chemical differences between the common atopic and contactant allergens are of significance in the preparation of allergenic extracts. The plant oleoresins containing the contactants usually are removed during the defatting process and are not present in the aqueous allergenic extracts. The ether-soluble fraction, on the other hand, can be used for the preparation of patch-testing materials.

Diagnosis of Allergy

The diagnosis of an allergic disease requires first the determination of allergic etiology and second the identification of the specific allergen(s). Understanding the fundamental principles in the diagnosis of allergy is important to pharmacists, particularly in the community setting, where they are called upon for the initial evaluation of reactions to both drugs and environmental substances. In such cases important decisions must be made whether to refer the patient to a physician or emergency facility, recommend OTC therapy or to take another course of action.

Physical diagnosis, while important, is not sufficient to establish allergic etiology since the symptoms of allergic diseases can result from other causes. Important in this respect are the *intrinsic* (nonallergic) diseases of asthma, rhinitis, and urticaria that should be distinguished from the *extrinsic* (allergic) diseases. This distinction between allergy and intrinsic diseases is not always clear, and some clinical conditions likely involve both. It is important, however, since a number of drug idiosyncrasies are associated with intrinsic disease and may be mistaken for allergy.

A *detailed history* is perhaps the most important step both in determining whether the condition is an allergy as well as suggesting possible allergens. This should include consideration of the patient's symptoms in relation to familial, seasonal, home environment, occupational, medication, and related personal factors.

Clinical laboratory tests are assuming greater importance in the diagnosis of allergy. Diagnostic testing services are available to measure total serum IgE and immunogen-specific IgE for many allergens. These tests can be used in conjunction with sensitivity tests and in those with dermographia, very young patients or others where skin testing may be unreliable. Determination of IgG, IgA, and IgM may be helpful in differentiating various autoimmune, infectious, or other diseases that may mimic allergies. These and related tests also may be used to monitor immunotherapy.

Sensitivity testing with allergenic extracts is still the principal method of determining specific allergic etiology. Sensitivity testing has been used since the early part of the century for the diagnosis of allergy. A variety of different test methods may be employed, but all involve the administration of a small amount of allergen to the patient who is observed for reactions suggestive of allergy. While simple in principle, both the administration and interpretation of sensitivity tests require a great deal of expertise and should be conducted only by qualified individuals. Also, since sensitivity testing is a costly, discomforting, and time-consuming procedure, it is impractical to test the patient for all possible allergens. A detailed history provides the main basis for selection of the specific tests to be performed.

Immediate Sensitivity Tests

These tests, as the name implies, are used to detect IgE-mediated allergy, and there are two general types of test procedures.

CUTANEOUS TESTS—These are the simplest of the immediate sensitivity tests and somewhat safer than intradermal tests. The back as well as the arms can be used for testing that enables 50 or more allergens to be evaluated in a single office visit. Cutaneous tests also are less sensitive, which some feel is an advantage that provides better correlation with clinical allergy. Allergists often employ a cutaneous test for preliminary screening followed by intradermal tests for more complete evaluation of the allergens to which the patient is sensitive. The skin is abraded with a sharp needle (*prick test*) or scarifier (*scratch test*) either before or after application of a drop of a relatively concentrated (1:00 to 1:10 *w/v*) allergenic extract. The test sites, grading of reactions, and precautions are similar to those described for the intradermal tests.

INTRADERMAL TESTS—These are the most sensitive of the immediate sensitivity tests and are accomplished by injecting relatively dilute (1:1000 to 1:100 *w/v*) allergenic extracts directly into the skin on the volar surface of the lower or upper arm. The back should not be used because of the difficulty in dealing with systemic reactions. Multiple extracts can be tested at one time using sites 2 to 3 inches apart and marked with an appropriate code. The tests are inspected after 15 minutes or again at 30 minutes if the characteristic wheal and flare reactions are not developed fully. The tests are graded from 0 to 4+ depending upon the size of the wheal. Generalized allergic reactions are relatively uncommon, but a rubber tourniquet and epinephrine (1:1000) should always be available when these tests are performed.

Histamine controls are used to eliminate false-negative reactions by confirming the wheal/flare reaction of the skin and quality of the technique. Diluent controls are used to detect the rare individual with *dermographia* that gives positive tests to the skin trauma. Although a single concentration of allergenic extract often is used for testing, more information can be obtained by a *threshold dilution titration* using a 10-fold dilution series.

Other types of immediate sensitivity tests using allergenic extracts such as *provocation tests* and *passive transfer tests* are employed less commonly and are described in standard references on allergy.

EFFECT OF DRUGS ON SENSITIVITY TESTS—Antihistamines (H$_1$-antagonists) and other drugs with antihistaminic activity such as the tricyclic antidepressants suppress the immediate skin-test reactions. Long-acting agents may suppress the reaction for as long as 6 weeks. H$_2$-antagonists do not suppress the immediate skin-test reactions alone but may act synergistically with the H$_1$-antagonists. Oral and parenteral β$_2$-adrenergic agonists have been reported to decrease

the allergen induced wheal, and potent topical corticosteroids may suppress skin reactivity locally. Inhaled β$_2$-adrenergic agonists, methylxanthines, and cromolyn do not interfere with skin testing. Oral corticosteroids and nonsteroidal anti-inflammatory agents have little effect on immediate skin tests. It is recommended that tricyclic antidepressants, chlorpromazine, and hydroxyzine be discontinued for at least 5 days before testing, and that the short-acting antihistamines be discontinued for at least 24 hours. Beta-blocking agents can increase the immediate skin test reaction significantly and patients on these drugs may be less responsive to the beta-agonists needed to treat a systemic reaction to an allergenic extract. The optimal time for skin testing is when the patient has recently taken no drugs that may potentially interfere, and in all cases it is important to administer a positive control (ie, histamine).

Treatment of Allergy

The types, causes, and contributing factors of allergy are numerous. Therapy is thus complex and variable but can be divided into three main types.

Environmental controls are designed to eliminate or at least minimize exposure to the allergen.[15] The avoidance of an allergen is relatively simple and effective in some instances but most allergens cannot be eliminated totally from the environment. However, minimizing exposure to the allergen always enhances the effectiveness of other therapeutic measures and should always be accomplished as much as possible.

Symptomatic drug therapy is required in the control of most common allergies. The many drugs used for this purpose include the antihistamines and leukotriene antagonists, corticosteroids, and sympathomimetics.

Specific *immunotherapy* may be employed for certain allergies as described below.

Immunotherapy

The immunotherapy of allergy is accomplished by administration of gradually increasing doses of allergen over a period of months or years with the anticipation of the patient developing increasing tolerance to the allergen. This is called commonly *desensitization* or *hyposensitization,* but these terms tend to imply unconfirmed mechanisms and may be confused with other clinical procedures. For example, different *desensitization* procedures have been used in drug allergy (eg, penicillin, sulfonilamide, insulin, etc) but these are short-term procedures that likely involve different mechanisms.

Immunotherapy was first used for hay fever in England in 1911 and is still used nearly exclusively in the treatment of IgE-mediated allergy. There have been many attempts to desensitize against the cell-mediated *Rhus* contact dermatitis (poison ivy and oak), but they have met with little success and the products marketed for this purpose remain controversial.

The precise mechanism of immunotherapy remains unknown, but a variety of both humoral and cellular immunological changes have been observed over the course of allergen administration.[16] Clinical improvement in some patients correlates well with the level of IgG *blocking antibodies* that, as suggested by the name, may bind the allergen and prevent its interaction with the mast cell-bound IgE. This is undoubtedly too simple an explanation, and it appears that the parenteral exposure to allergen (most disease involves mucosal exposure) alters the factors that regulate the production of allergen specific IgE.

The efficacy of immunotherapy is difficult to judge. There have been many controlled clinical trials, but most of these have considered allergic rhinitis and asthma caused by common aeroallergens (eg, ragweed pollens, common grass, and tree pollens). Immunotherapy commonly is recommended and is considered to be effective for these conditions when properly employed. The treatment of hay fever and asthma due to other aeroallergens (eg, molds) is based mainly upon experience with the common allergens but is common and likely effective in skilled hands. Hymenoptera insect venom therapy is highly effective and recommended for any patient who has experienced systemic anaphylaxis following a sting. Immunotherapy is not recommended for food allergies that are best treated by elimination diets or for dander allergies except in rare instances where avoidance is impossible (eg, veterinarians).

The variety of regimens and techniques used in the immunotherapy of allergy are described in standard reference works on allergy. The optimum duration of therapy is uncertain but usually continues until the patient is symptom-free for at least 1 year. The average course of therapy may require 3 to 5 years. Success often is relative but some patients remain free of symptoms for extended periods. In others there is sufficient reduction of symptoms that symptomatic therapy alone can be employed but some patients require resumption of immunotherapy.

Immunotherapy is not without risk.[17] Most patients develop some swelling and redness at the injection site, but reactions that persist for more than 24 hours are a signal to proceed cautiously. Particularly uncomfortable local reactions may be treated with oral antihistamines and cold compresses. The possibility of serious generalized allergic reactions always is present. Patients should remain in the physician's office for at least 20 minutes after each course of immunotherapy or longer if they are in one of the following high-risk groups: unstable asthma, seasonal exacerbation, high degree of hypersensitivity, receiving beta-blockers or *rush immunotherapy* (ie, more rapid dose escalation than with conventional therapy). During pregnancy there is no evidence of major adverse effects of allergenic extracts on the fetus, but uterine contractions may occur as part of a generalized allergic reaction. It generally is recommended that immunotherapy not be started during pregnancy and that slight reduction of the maintenance dose be considered for those who become pregnant during therapy.

It should be remembered that the most successful therapy of allergy is achieved by avoidance of the allergen(s) and that all other forms of therapy are essentially adjunctive. Immunotherapy should not be continued indefinitely in the absence of clinical improvement. Treatment failures may result from improper selection of allergens, development of new sensitivities, improper use of environmental controls, and various problems associated with the allergenic extracts that are discussed in the next section.

ALLERGENIC EXTRACTS

Allergenic extracts are concentrated solutions or suspensions of allergens used for the diagnosis and treatment of allergic diseases. Most are injectable products administered in the physician's office, and for many years they were prepared by the individual users. Commercial extracts gradually replaced extemporaneous preparation as a number of small specialty companies began marketing allergenic extracts several decades ago. More recently, many of the familiar names in allergy products have merged into the larger pharmaceutical companies, and today several of the manufacturers of allergenic extracts are multinational corporations. There are more than 900 different diagnostic allergenic extracts and about 600 therapeutic extracts currently licensed by the FDA. Because of the great number of allergenic extracts on the market only the general characteristics of the products are described here. Additional information on these and related products may be obtained from the licensed manufacturers listed in Table 89-12.

Handling

Allergenic extracts usually are designated as being *aqueous* or *glycerinated* products. Normal saline or similar isotonic electrolyte solution is the diluent for the former while the latter contain 50% glycerin in the diluent. The preparations normally are buffered to pH 8 and contain phenol (0.4%) as a preserva-

Table 89-12. Licensed Manufacturers of Allergenic Extracts[a]

ALK Laboratories, Inc.
Allergologisk Laboratorium A/S
ALO Laboratories, Inc.
Allergy Laboratories, Inc.
Allermed Laboratories, Inc.
Antigen Laboratories, Inc.
Center Laboratories, Inc[b]
Greer Laboratories, Inc
Hollister-Steir Labs[b]
Nelco Laboratories, Inc

[a] *Establishments and Products Licensed under Section 351 of the Public Health Services Act,* available at the FDA Web site [http://www.fda.gov].
[b] Aqueous and alum precipitated extracts.

tive. The preparation of allergenic extracts is described in earlier editions of this book and more detailed information on their production is available from the manufacturers and FDA.

The most common measures of allergenic potency are by *weight/volume* (*w/v*) and the *protein nitrogen unit* (PNU) (Table 89-13). Weight/volume is the weight of allergenic substance extracted per volume of extracting fluid. For example, a 1:50 extract is prepared by extracting 1 g of substance with 50 mL of solvent and decimal dilutions of this extract provide 1:500, 1:5000, etc concentrations. One protein nitrogen unit represents 0.01 mcg of total protein nitrogen in the product.

A typical allergenic substance contains multiple allergenic molecules and epitopes of varying potency, and there is significant chemical and biological variation with different lots of the substance. Neither the *w/v* concentration nor the PNU are directly related to allergenic potency nor can the two units be reliably compared with each other. One must understand well this variation that occurs between the lots of the same product and between similar products produced by different manufacturers in order to safely and effectively employ allergenic extracts in the clinic.

The FDA has licensed *standardized allergenic extracts* (Tables 89-14–89-18) since 1983 that are bioassayed against FDA reference standards. The potency of these products are expressed in terms of *allergy units* (AU) or *bioequivalent allergy units* (BAL). The potency between lots is definitely more consistent than with conventional extracts, but variation may still occur and the same general principles of use still apply.

The absence of a completely reliable method of standardization along with the extreme variation between patients dictates that the appropriate dosage for immunotherapy must be determined clinically. The initial dilution of extract, starting dose, and progression of dosage is determined by a skilled clinician on the basis of the patient's history and sensitivity tests. Some things to keep in mind are that dilute extracts tend to lose activity more rapidly and that care must be exercised when changing to a new lot since it may be significantly more potent.

Table 89-13. Units of Potency for Allergenic Extracts

UNIT	DESCRIPTION
Weight/Volume (*w/v*)	Allergenic substance (g) per volume (mL) of extracting fluid
Protein Nitrogen Unit (PNU)	1 mg protein N 5 100,000 PNU
Allergy Unit (AU)	Bioassay compared to reference standard
Bioequivalent Allergy Unit (BAU)	Bioassay compared to reference standard

Table 89-14. Pollen Extracts

Trees

Acacia	Elderberry	Orange
Alder, grey	Elm, American	Osage orange
Almond	Eucalyptus	Palo verde
Apple	Fir	Peach
Apricot	Hackberry	Pear
Arbor vitae	Hazelnut	Pecan
Ash	Hemlock	Pepper tree
Aspen	Hickory	Pine
Bayberry	Hop-hornbeam	Plum
Beech	Ironwood	Poplar
Birch, spring	Juniper	Privet
Birch, white	Locust	Redwood
Bottle brush	Maple	Russian olive
Box elder	Melaleuca	Spruce
Carob tree	Mesquite	Sweet gum
Cedar	Mock orange	Sycamore
Cherry	Mulberry	Tamarack
Chestnut	Oak, white	Tree of heaven
Cottonwood	Olive	Walnut
Cypress		Willow

Grasses

Bahia		**Redtop**[a]
Barley	Corn	
Beach	**Fescue, meadow**[a]	**Rye grass, perennial**[a]
Bent	Grama	Salt
Bermuda grass[a]	Johnson	Sorghum
Bluegrass, Kentucky[a]	Koeler's	Sudan
Brome	Oats	
Orchard grass[a]	**Sweet vernal grass**[a]	**Timothy grass**[a]
Bunch	Quack	Velvetgrass
Canarygrass		Wheat

Weeds and garden plants

Alfalfa	Fireweed	Poppy
Amaranth	Gladiolus	Povertyweed
Aster	Goldenrod	Quailbush
Balsam root		
Bassia	Greasewood	
Hemp	**Ragweed, giant**[a]	
Beach bur		
Broomweed	Honeysuckle	
Hops		
	Ragweed, short[a]	
Burrow brush		
Careless weed	Iodine Bush	
Jerusalem oak	**Ragweed, western**[a]	
Castor bean	Kochia	Rose
Chamise	Lamb's quarters	Russian thistle
Clover	Lily	Sagebrush
Cocklebur	Marigold	Saltbrush
Coreopsis	Marshelder	Scale
Cosmos	Mexican tea	Scotch broom
Daffodil	Mugworta	Sea blight
Dahlia	Mustard	Sheep sorrel
Daisy	Nettle	Snapdragon
Dandelion	Pickleweed	Sugar beet
Dock	Pigweed	Sunflower
Dog fennel	Plantain, English	Western waterhemp
		Winter fat
		Wormseed
		Wormwood

[a] Standardized extract for which FDA reference standard is available. The FDA discontinued licensing of the 8 nonstandardized grass extracts July 1998.

Scratch test extracts are glycerinated products supplied in 1 to 5 mL dropper vials. They are relatively concentrated solutions, usually in strengths of 1:5 to 1:20 depending on the allergen. *Intradermal test extracts* are aqueous solutions supplied in 1 to 5 mL multiple dose vials and are more dilute (1:500 to 1:5000). *Therapeutic extracts* are supplied in multiple-dose vials in a variety of sizes (5–100 mL) and dilutions (1:10 to 1:100). Since these extracts are diluted before use, most companies provide a variety of dilution vials that contain a volume of diluent that facilitates preparation of 10-fold dilutions. *Adjuvant extracts* of several types have been used for many years but only alum-adsorbed extracts are available

Table 89-15. Dust Extracts

House dusts		
House	Mattress	Upholstery
Dust mites		
D farniae[a]	**D pteronyssinus**[a]	**Mite mix**[a]
Other dusts[b]		
Cedar and red cedar	Cotton gin	Oak
Grain, elevator	Padauk	Wood dusts

[a] Standardized extract for which FDA reference standard is available.
[b] See also Table 89-16.

commercially (Table 89-12). *Autogenous extracts* sometimes are prepared from allergenic substances collected from the individual patient's environment. Standard and custom diagnostic and therapeutic sets and mixtures also are available as are a variety of auxiliary supplies used in allergy practice.

Prescriptions for therapeutic allergenic extracts may contain up to a dozen or more allergens, although many clinicians prefer to use multiple extracts if more than 4 to 5 allergens are to be included. These prescriptions are labeled according to clinician preference on the basis of the total allergen content or the concentration of the greatest single allergen present. The prescriptions are usually prepared in the allergist's office or obtained through the manufacturers' prescription service. A few pharmacists offer this specialized service.

It is vitally important that allergenic extracts be handled and stored properly. They tend to show reduced potency within a matter of weeks or months after their preparation, but there have been few detailed studies on the stability of these products. Both high temperatures and freezing usually have deleterious effects, and the latter may cause agglomeration of adjuvant extracts. Some extracts contain proteolytic enzymes that may contribute to decomposition of the allergens. Both glycerinated and lyophilized products are more stable than aqueous extracts. Very dilute extracts tend to lose potency by adsorption to the surfaces of containers and syringes and thus usually are prepared close to the time use. All allergenic extracts should be refrigerated at 2° to 8° and freezing should be avoided. Care must be exercised in changing to new lots or different dilutions of extracts because of possible variations in potency. It generally is recommended that quantities of extract sufficient to last the patient for 1 year be prepared to avoid frequent changes in extracts.

Role of the Pharmacist

Few pharmacists are called on today to prepare allergenic extracts or to dispense prescriptions for these products. Some pharmacies, particularly in hospitals, may stock allergenic extracts and related supplies for allergists. Actually, the training of a pharmacist is suited uniquely to many of the services required in the allergy clinic, and it is unfortunate that more pharmacists have not become involved in this area.[18]

Table 89-16. Fungal Extracts

Alternaria	Fusarium	Phoma
Aspergillus	Gelasinospora	Pullularia
Botrytis	Geotrichum	Rhizopus
Candida	Gliocladium	Rhodotorula
Cephalosporium	Helminthosporum	Rusts
Cephalothecium	Hormodendrum	Saccharomyces
Chaetomium	Microsporium	Smuts
Cladosporium	Mucor	Spondylocladium
Cryptococcus	Mycogone	Stemphylium
Curvularia	Nigraspora	Trichoderma
Epicoccum	Paecilomyces	Trichophyton
Epidermophyton	Penicillium	Verticillium

Table 89-17. Miscellaneous Inhalant Extracts

Mammalian epidermals		
Camel	Dog	Horse
Cat hair[a]	Gerbil	Mohair
Cat pelt[a]	Goat	Monkey
Chinchilla	Guinea pig	Mouse
Cow	Hamster	Rabbit
Deer	Hog	Wool (sheep)
Feathers		
Canary	Duck	Pigeon
Chicken	Goose	Turkey
	Parakeet	
Miscellaneous inhalants		
Acacia	Hemp fiber	Lycopodium
Algae	Henna	Orris root
Castor bean	Flaxseed	Pyrethrum
Cotton linters	Guar gum	Silk, raw
Cottonseed	Jute	Sisal
Derris root	Karaya gum	Tobacco leaf
Fern spores	Kapok	Tragacanth
Grain dusts	Leather	Wood dusts

[a] Standardized extract for which FDA reference standard is available.

In a few institutions allergenic extracts are provided by the pharmacist on a prescription order. Some patients require only a single extract, but even in these cases appropriate dilutions must be prepared. More frequently, patients are allergic to multiple allergens, and complex extract mixtures are required. The basic techniques and facilities required for this service are essentially the same as those used in a typical IV-additive program, but the pharmacist should have some additional training and experience in handling allergenic extracts.[18]

In addition to assuming responsibility for the preparation and control of allergenic extracts, the pharmacist also may provide a variety of patient-oriented services in the allergy clinic.[19] These services include obtaining patient histories, performing allergy testing procedures, and patient consultation. Common allergic diseases are found in up to 30% of the population, and patients with these ailments obtain a variety of drugs and medical supplies from community pharmacies. Thus, there are many opportunities for pharmacists to be of service to the allergy patient in traditional practice sites as well as the allergy clinic. To accomplish this effectively, pharmacists must have a fundamental understanding of allergy and the products used in the control of allergic diseases.

PRODUCTS

This section contains a summary of the principal allergenic extracts available today. It is impractical to provide an individual monograph for each product, and they have been grouped according to the type of allergenic substance (eg, pollens or dusts). This type of classification is used in the manufacturers' literature and also has merit when considering both the product characteristics and clinical allergy. These are described briefly for each group with emphasis on the following: clinical significance of the allergen group, most-common offenders of the group, and general usefulness and limitations of the extracts.

The lists of allergenic extracts are not intended to be comprehensive but rather to illustrate the scope of the problem in each case. Only one name, usually the common one, is given for each extract, while in practice a number of both common and scientific names may be used. Similarly, individual extracts usually are derived from a single species of plant, animal, or microorganism, but only the genus is given in the list; however, extracts of most of the common allergenic species are commercially available. Extracts containing allergens from more than one source are designated as mixtures and, while many are commercially available, only a few are

Table 89-18. Insect Extracts[a]

Stinging Insect-Whole Body

Ant, black	Ant, carpenter	Ant, fire
Ant, red	Ant mix (black/red)	

Stinging Insect-Venom Protein

Honey bee[a]	**Wasp**[a]	**White-faced hornet**[a]
Yellow hornet[a]	**Yellow jacket**[a]	**Mixed vespid**[a]

Inhalant Allergy to Insects

Aphid	Deerfly	**Mites, dust**[a]
Black fly	Fruit fly	Mosquito
Butterfly	Honey bee, whole body	Moth
Caddis fly	Horse fly	Mushroom fly
Cicada/locust	House fly	Screwworm fly
Cricket	Leafhopper	Sow bugs
Cockroach	May fly	Spider
Daphnia	Mexican bean weevil	Water flea

[a] Standardized extracts. The potency of insect venom extract is expressed in mg.

listed. Not all manufacturers produce all of the extracts, and it should be recognized that different companies may employ significantly different source materials and processes in preparing products of the same name. The products from different manufacturers cannot be considered to be equivalent in all respects.

Most of the products listed are provided as diagnostic extracts for both scratch and intradermal testing, but therapeutic extracts may or may not be routinely available. Similarly, the availability of both lyophilized and adjuvant products is limited. Many of the extracts also are available in diagnostic test sets. These are not listed but include various regional, pollen, food, mold, pediatric, titration, and other test sets. Manufacturing services for custom therapeutic mixtures and autogenous extracts are also available. The individual manufacturers should be contacted for more specific information on their products and services.

Pollen Extracts

Pollens (Table 89-14) are the most common group of atopic allergens and, in fact, hay fever is sometimes called *pollinosis*. Pollens are produced only by seed-bearing plants and not by algae, fungi, mosses, or ferns. Not all pollens are of equal clinical significance for there is variation in both allergenicity and degree of exposure. Allergy usually results from *anemophilous* (wind-borne) rather than *entomophilous* (insect-borne) pollens. Conifers such as the pines are copious pollen producers but the pollens, with few exceptions, are less allergenic than others.

Pollen allergy is largely a problem of temperate climates. In Arctic and alpine regions where summers are short, plants generally reproduce vegetatively (asexually), and most subarctic plants are conifers. In the tropics there tends to be a proliferation of species with a small number of individual plants so that the degree of exposure to a specific pollen is minimized. Anemophilous plants also tend to be less common in regions of extremely high humidity.

Seasonal and geographical variation is more pronounced with pollen allergy than other types. Pollen seasons vary with both the plant and locale, but the following generalizations can be made: trees from late winter to spring, grasses from spring to early summer, and weeds from late summer to fall. Pollen allergy is a significant problem in most parts of North America, but the allergens vary somewhat with the region and are determined best by consulting one of the published guides. Perhaps 100 of the approximately 300 pollens represented in commercial extracts are fairly common offenders.

Allergenic extracts prepared from some of the common pollens (eg, ragweed, several grasses, and trees) have been among the most widely studied. Controlled studies generally have shown these products to be reliable for both diagnosis and therapy when properly prepared and employed. Many of the products listed have not been studied extensively, but their reliability often is assumed based on extrapolation of the data on the common pollens.

Dust Extracts

House dust is the most common atopic allergen, and the dust mite (*Dermatophagoides* spp) is by far the most important allergenic constituent. Although house dust may contain a wide variety of other allergens that may be important in individual cases, the dust mite is definitely the number one offender.

The dust mite appears to be distributed virtually universally and usually is found in furnishings stuffed with vegetable fibers (eg, cotton) used by humans. In contrast to the cockroach, another important arthropod allergen, dust mites are not associated with poor hygiene.

House-dust sensitivity differs from pollen allergy in several respects and is suspected particularly when the patient's history includes one or more of the following factors: perennial symptoms that worsen when the patient remains indoors, increased nocturnal symptoms, increased symptoms when performing household chores, and increased symptoms associated with turning on heating or air conditioning systems.

House dust is a ubiquitous allergen, and its total elimination is virtually impossible; however, it is important that the patient maintain as dust-free an environment as possible, particularly in the bedroom. Instructions for the preparation of dust-free rooms and products to minimize the circulation of dust and kill mites are available.

The reliability of sensitivity testing for the diagnosis of house dust allergy has improved greatly with the introduction of standardized dust mite extracts (Table 89-15). These products are also effective for immunotherapy, however, it is still important to employ stringent environmental controls in the management of house dust allergy.[15]

Relatively little information is available on other dust extracts. These are generally less-common allergens, and many are associated with occupational allergies. Some of these are implicated as a cause of extrinsic allergic alveolitis described under *Fungal Extracts*.

Fungal Extracts

The fungi are a large group of organisms that may be involved in many types of diseases, including intoxications, infections and allergy (Table 89-16). Most fungi are saprophytes and compared to bacteria are relatively uncommon causes of infectious disease. Mycotoxins are of great concern in several areas of health including as possible contaminants of allergenic extracts. A number of fungi have been implicated increasingly as important causes of several types of allergic disease.

Molds are one of the major causes of atopic allergy. Allergic asthma and rhinitis, as well as various cutaneous reactions, can be precipitated by inhalation of mold spores or mycelial fragments in sensitive individuals. Fungi are ubiquitous and may be found in the home on textiles, leather goods, upholstered furniture, food, and plants. Damp, warm places such as basements and closets tend to favor mold growth, which is often encountered as common *mildew*, which most often is *Aspergillus* or *Penicillium* spp. Fungal allergy resulting from indoor exposure tends to be perennial; that from outdoor exposure shows more distinctive seasonal and geographical patterns but these are less pronounced than in pollen allergy. Fungal allergy is generally more difficult to evaluate because of taxonomic confusion, biologic complexity, and less predictable seasonal and geographical patterns than with pollens.

Sensitivity testing for fungal allergens appears to be generally reliable. It also is useful at times to identify the specific fungi in the patient's environment and fungal identification services are available. Therapy should include efforts to create a mold-free environment, but this is difficult to accomplish completely. Several studies indicate that immunotherapy may be of value for some patients. One problem is that the allergenic extracts are prepared variously from mycelium, medium, or both, and too little is known about the fungal allergens to know the most-appropriate method of preparation.

Fungi, along with a variety of organic dusts, have been found to be important causes of another respiratory allergy, *extrinsic allergic alveolitis* (hypersensitivity pneumonitis). Many names related to either the allergen or affected individuals have been applied to this condition; eg, farmer's lung, mushroom-workers disease, wood-dust asthma, etc. The disease shows no relationship to atopy but usually can be related to recent high-level exposures to the offending inhalant.

Extrinsic allergic alveolitis results primarily from a cell-mediated reaction to allergens in the lung but may involve some immune complex disease in the early stages. Diagnosis is based mainly on a detailed personal history. Both cell-mediated and immune complex allergy may provide cutaneous reactions on allergen challenge, but they differ in time-course and appearance from the immediate skin test reactions. The products listed in Table 89-16 are not useful in the diagnosis of extrinsic allergic alveolitis and effective therapy depends mainly on avoidance of the allergen.

Miscellaneous Inhalant Extracts

Atopic allergies may be caused by a variety of inhalant allergens other than pollens, dusts, and molds. The epidermals from domestic animals (cat, dog, horse) are the best-known, but the variety of inhalant allergens is remarkable. Exposure of an average individual to some of the substances listed below might appear unlikely, but this is not necessarily the case. Probably few people recognize that camel hair may be found in imported textiles and rugs, that the plant gums acacia, karaya, and tragacanth are present in hundreds of food, cosmetic, and drug products, and that pyrethrum is an active constituent of many household insecticides. Many of these substances are also ingestant (see *Food Extracts*) and contactant (see *Patch-Testing Materials*) as well as inhalant allergens.

Sensitivity testing with many of the extracts listed in Table 89-17 is fairly common but based largely on experience with common aeroallergen extracts. Little information is available on the use of most of these products for immunotherapy. Several cat allergens have been characterized and standardized extracts are available. Avoidance of the allergen remains the preferred method of control and usually can be achieved, although at times only with great effort.

Insect Allergy

Insect allergy is a term rather loosely applied to describe allergy from both insects and arthropods such as spiders and mites. Allergy may result from inhalation of body emanations but most often occurs following a sting or bite.

Allergy to stinging insects of the order *Hymenoptera* is of greatest clinical significance and has been studied most widely. The honeybee is the most common offender, but the bumblebee, wasp, hornet, and yellow jacket also may cause reactions. Hymenoptera sensitivity is estimated to result in 40 deaths annually in this country and the incidence of serious allergy is estimated at 1 to 10:100,000. Allergy with few exceptions involves IgE-mediated reactions and may be manifest as urticaria, angioedema, asthma, or systemic anaphylaxis. Death usually results from cardiovascular collapse and/or respiratory failure and typically occurs within 1 hour following the sting.

Serious reactions may occur in individuals without a history of sensitization, but they are more common in those who have previously exhibited a systemic reaction following a sting. It is of the utmost importance that sensitive individuals be aware of their problem and understand preventive measures and emergency procedures. *Emergency kits* are available for the treatment of *Hymenoptera* sensitivity in the field. These and the services that can be rendered by the community pharmacist are discussed by Sadik.[20]

Diagnosis of insect allergy usually is self-evident, but problems may arise in identifying the insect. Cross-sensitivity among *Hymenoptera* is common but by no means absolute, and species-specific allergens are important.

Sensitivity testing and immunotherapy commonly are recommended and employed for allergy to the stinging insects. The venom extracts (Table 89-18) have been shown to be highly effective when properly employed. These products are standardized somewhat differently than the other standardized extracts. The venoms are assayed for several known components (ie, hyaluronidase, antigen 5, phospholipase A), as well as total protein nitrogen. The quantity and potency of the products are expressed in mcg rather than allergy units.

Fire-ant allergy is being reported with increasing frequency. The fire ant has now spread over 13 southern states and is particularly a problem along the Gulf coast. It is a member of the *Hymenoptera* and causes similar allergic reactions, but its allergens appear to differ considerably from those of other stinging insects. Skin-testing with whole-body extracts appears to be reliable for the determination of sensitivity and reports on immunotherapy are encouraging.

Allergic reactions have been attributed to many biting insects including the mosquito, chigger, flea, louse, bedbug, kissing bug, and many flies. The majority of the reactions have been localized, with both the immediate- and delayed-types reported. The pathogenesis of most of these sensitivities remains to be verified, but since many appear to be cell-mediated reactions, it is not surprising that the limited information on sensitivity testing and immunotherapy is contradictory.

Allergic rhinitis and asthma can develop after inhalation of scales, hairs, or other emanations of various insects. This is analogous to the allergy seen with common inhalants but most often is seen in individuals who by reason of occupation or hobby are exposed to large numbers of insects. The cockroach has been increasingly implicated as an important cause of allergic asthma especially in central city areas. The caddis fly, mayfly, and aphid occur in large numbers in some locales and have been implicated frequently. Allergenic extracts for a number of these have proven to be effective for skin-test diagnosis and may be of value for immunotherapy (Table 89-18).

Food Extracts

Various food products are the most common ingestant allergens. Food allergy may seem simple but, in fact, is an extremely complex clinical entity. One problem stems from the tendency of many to attribute virtually any GI disturbance of unknown etiology to *food allergy*. GI disturbance may arise from many causes, including enzyme deficiencies (lactose intolerance), intoxications, infections, and others. Also, food allergy may and often is manifest outside the GI tract. The indiscriminate use of the term *food allergy* is to be condemned strongly.

Food allergens (Table 89-19) may cause atopic (asthma, rhinitis, gastroenteropathy) and nonatopic (urticaria-an-gioedema, anaphylaxis) symptoms, but both are IgE-mediated. Food allergy is usually not life-threatening, but some individuals may suffer serious exacerbation of asthma or, on rare occasions, systemic anaphylaxis. Strongly allergic individuals must be trained on how to deal with serious reactions and some should carry emergency kits with epinephrine to deal with inadvertent exposures.

Relatively few foods are responsible for the majority of reactions (peanuts, milk, nuts, fish, shellfish, eggs, and soy are the most common offenders) but many others may cause food allergy.[21] Food allergy may occur at any age but is probably most common in childhood and may be related to an underdeveloped GI system. Patients commonly appear to *outgrow* some food allergy (eg, cow's milk), but this is probably not the case with most foods.

Only a few food allergens have been characterized, but it is possible that many are not present in fresh foods but are the products of food processing or digestion. The diagnosis of food allergy depends heavily upon a detailed history along with the use of carefully designed elimination and challenge test diets. Skin testing is useful in the hands of experienced clinicians but requires some modified techniques.[21]

The therapy of food allergy is often even more difficult than the diagnosis. Elimination of the offending food(s) is about the only effective therapy, but it is often difficult to design a nutritious and palatable diet when multiple and/or common allergens are involved (eg, milk, eggs, peanuts). Immunotherapy is very difficult to assess for reasons noted above and therapeutic food extracts are not generally recommended.

It is notable that, of all of the allergies to environmental substances, food allergy is the most similar to that of drug allergy.[22] Ingestants (ie, foods and drugs) and injectants (ie, drugs and *Hymenoptera* stings) are the major cause of the nonatopic, IgE-mediated urticaria(hives), angioedema and anaphylaxis.

Table 89-19. Food Extracts[a]

Meat		
Beef	Goat	Rabbit
Chicken	Goose	Turkey
Deer	Lamb	
Duck	Pork	
Dairy		
Casein	Egg, whole	Milk, cow
	Egg, white	Milk, goat
	Egg, yolk	
Fish		
Bass	Halibut	Sardine
Bluefish	Herring	Scallop
Carp	Lobster	Shrimp
Clam	Mackerel	Smelt
Codfish	Oyster	Swordfish
Crab	Pike	Trout
Flounder	Red Snapper	Tuna
Haddock	Salmon	Whitefish
Nuts		
Almond	Chestnut	Peanut
Brazil	Coconut	Pecan
Cashew	English Walnut	Pistachio
	Filbert	
Grains		
Barley	Corn	Rye
Buckwheat	Oat	Wheat
	Rice	
Fruits		
Apple	Cranberry	Peach
Apricot	Date	Pear
Avocado	Fig	Pineapple
Banana	Grape	Plum
Blackberry	Grapefruit	Raspberry
Blueberry	Honeydew	Strawberry
Carrot	Lemon	Tangerine
Cantaloupe	Lime	Watermelon
Cherry	Orange	
Vegetables		
Artichoke	Celery	Pea
Asparagus	Cucumber	Potatoes
Beans	Eggplant	Pumpkin
Beet	Green Pepper	Radish
Broccoli	Lentil	Rhubarb
Brussell Sprouts	Lettuce	Spinach
Cabbage	Mushroom	Squash
Carrot	Olives	Tomato
Cauliflower	Onion	Turnip
Spices		
Allspice	Garlic	Peppermint
Bay Leaf	Licorice	Poppy Seed
Caraway Seed	Mustard Seed	Sage
Cinnamon	Nutmeg	Sesame
Clove	Oregano	Spearmint
Dill	Paprika	Thyme
Ginger	Pepper, Black	Vanilla

[a] This is not a comprehensive list and the absence of a food does not imply that it is never allergenic.

Veterinary Allergenic Products

Veterinary allergy is an emerging field, and pharmacists involved in animal health can expect increasing activity in this area. The general principles of immunology and allergy noted earlier apply for the most part to animals as well. Veterinary biologics are controlled by the US Department of Agriculture (USDA) as described earlier. Greer Laboratories markets a line of veterinary allergenic extracts and supplies. Most of the currently available products are marketed primarily for dogs.

It is estimated that as many as 20% of the dogs in the US have allergies. *Flea allergic dermatitis* is the most common canine allergy, and its control requires the complete eradication of fleas from the environment. Immunotherapy is rarely successful.

Atopy is the second most common allergic condition in dogs and, as in humans, is associated with inhaled pollens, molds, house dust, and other aeroallergens. *Canine allergic inhalant dermatitis* is a common form of atopy and is manifest by pruritus (scratching, foot licking, face rubbing) and sometimes sneezing, rhinitis, and conjunctivitis. Immunotherapy is often successful in the management of atopy.

Food allergy and *contact dermatitis* are also common in dogs; immunotherapy is of no value in the treatment of these conditions. It is apparent that the problems of canine allergy are quite analogous to those of human allergy.

DELAYED HYPERSENSITIVITY TESTS

Delayed hypersensitivity tests are used to detect the presence or absence of cell-mediated allergy and, as their name indicates, the time-course of a positive reaction varies considerably from those of the immediate hypersensitivity tests discussed above. Cell-mediated responses begin in a sensitized individual as early as 5 to 6 hours after exposure to the immunogen, and a maximum response is usually observed within 96 hours.

Table 89-20. Patch-Testing Allergens

American College of Dermatology
  Standard-Tray Allergens[a]

Balsam of Peru	Imidazolidinyl urea
Benzocaine	Lanolin alcohol
Black rubber mix	Mercaptobenzothiazole
p-tert-Butylphenolformaldehyde	Mercapto mix
Carba mix	Neomycin sulfate
Cinnamic aldehyde	Nickel sulfate anhydrous
Colophony	*p*-Phenylenediamine
Epoxy resin	Potassium dichromate
Ethylenediamine dihydrochloride	Quaternium-15
Formaldehyde	Thiuram mix

Commercial Patch Test Products

Standard-Tray Allergens	Hermal Laboratories
(in reclosable syringes)	
T.R.U.E. Test[b]	GSK

[a] For a description of the individual standard-tray allergens, consult Marks and DeLeo.[3]
[b] *T.R.U.E.* stands for *thin-layer rapid use epicutaneous test* and consists of two unit dose patches, each with 12 allergens, for administration to the upper back.

There are two main types of clinically useful delayed hypersensitivity tests: the *patch test* used to evaluate allergic contact dermatitis (Table 89-20) and diagnostic skin antigens used to evaluate several infectious diseases and the status of cell-mediated immunity (Table 89-21).

Patch-Testing

Contact dermatitis is a term that has been used in two main ways: first, to describe any rash resulting from a substance touching the skin and second, as a synonym for *allergic contact dermatitis*. The latter is used in present context and refers to eczematous lesions resulting from cell-mediated hypersensitivity reactions analogous to tuberculin sensitivity.

Table 89-21. Diagnostic Skin Antigens

VACCINE	DISTRIBUTOR
Candida albicans Skin Test Antigen	
Candin	ALK
Coccidioidin	
BioCox (Coccidioidin Mycelial Derivative)	Iatric
Spherulin (Coccidioidin Spherule Derivative)	ALK
Histoplasmin	
Generic (Mycelial Derivative)	Pfizer
Histolyn-CYL (Controlled Yeast Lysate)	ALK
Multiple Skin-Test Antigen Device	
Multitest CMI	Aventis Pasteur
Mumps Skin Test Antigen	
MSTA	Aventis Pasteur
Tetanus Toxoid Fluid	Aventis Pasteur
Wyeth	
Trichophyton	
Dermatophytin	Bayer
Tuberculin, Old (OT), Multiple Puncture Device	
Mono-Vac Test (OT)	Aventis Pasteur
Tuberculin, Tine Test OT	Wyeth
Tuberculin, Purified Protein Derivative (PPD)	
Multiple Puncture Device	
Aplitest	Pfizer
Sclavo Test-PPD	Biocine Sclavo
Tuberculin, Tine Test PPD	Wyeth
Tuberculin, Purified Protein Derivative (PPD)	
Intradermal Solution	
Aplisol	Pfizer
Tubersol Diagnostic Antigen	Aventis Pasteur

Similar clinical manifestations may occur by other mechanisms: primary irritant dermatitis, from direct chemical irritation; photocontact (phototoxic) dermatitis, which requires light to generate the irritant; and photoallergic dermatitis, which requires light to generate the allergen. These are not necessarily independent, for a number of contact allergens also may be irritants, but allergic reactions generally occur with lower concentrations of the offending agent. A variety of other conditions also must be differentiated from contact dermatitis (eg, atopic dermatitis, dermatomycoses), and virtually any disease of the skin may result in increased response to both contact irritants and allergens.

The best known and most common contact dermatitis in North American is *rhus dermatitis* (poison ivy, poison oak, and poison sumac[23]), but the scope of the problem is much greater than this. It is estimated that at least 35 million Americans are affected by contact dermatitis with the incidence and causes varying in different populations. The overall socioeconomic impact is great for it is a leading cause of industrial illness. The 20 American Academy of Dermatology standard-tray allergens (Table 89-20) are among the most common causes of allergic contact dermatitis and illustrate some of the complexity of the problem. Particularly notable are the drugs and drug additives that laymen may not recognize as constituents of drug products. The pharmacist can assist the sensitive patient with both drug product selection and avoidance.

The diagnosis of contact dermatitis depends mainly on a detailed history and complete physical examination. The area of the body affected is suggestive of the contactant and other factors (eg, light, dermatophytes). The patch test is presently the only practical way to demonstrate contact sensitivity and is used for the following purposes: to verify clinically diagnosed contact sensitivity; to determine the specific allergens including those that may not have been clinically suspected; as a predictive test to determine what the patient can safely tolerate; and to exclude contact dermatitis in puzzling clinical situations.

Patch testing usually involves application of the test substance to a piece of cloth or soft paper placed on the outer arm or upper back, covered with an impermeable substance and taped in place. After 24 to 48 hours, the patch is removed and the test site examined for presence of the characteristic rash. Patients receiving anti-inflammatory steroids or immunosuppressive therapy and those with other significant deficiency of cell-mediated immunity may be expected to have a reduced skin-test response. The monograph of Marks and DeLeo[24] is an excellent introduction to patch testing and includes a description of each of the allergens included in the American Academy of Dermatology standard tray.

The therapy of contact dermatitis involves, most importantly, avoidance of the contactant. Cool compresses and topical steroids are the mainstays of therapy, but systemic steroids may be employed for serious cases. Other topical medications should be avoided since they may contain irritants or sensitizers.

There have been a number of attempts at both oral and parenteral immunotherapy for poison ivy and several reports of success over the years; however, both forms of therapy have the potential of precipitating serious reactions in highly sensitive individuals and immunotherapy is not generally applicable in the management of contact dermatitis. Avoidance of the allergen is definitely the preferred and generally effective method of control.

Diagnostic Skin Test Antigens

Dermal reactivity in the form of delayed hypersensitivity develops in the course of many infectious diseases. Much study over the years has shown that this dermal sensitivity not only indicates that the patient is or has been infected with the microorganism in question, but also reflects the patency of cell-mediated immunity. Delayed hypersensitivity testing is of major value in the management of tuberculosis and is of some utility for the evaluation of several systemic mycoses (coccidiomycoses, histoplasmosis). These and other skin test antigens (Table 89-21) also are used to evaluate the status of cell-mediated immunity.

Tuberculin testing is an important procedure in the management of tuberculosis in this country. High-risk populations are screened to identify those who may be infected and benefit from chemoprophylaxis as well as those who have clinical disease and require therapy. Two forms of tuberculin products (Table 89-21) are available: old tuberculin (OT) and purified protein derivative (PPD). Both of these are available in multiple puncture devices (*tine test*) for transcutaneous administration; these products can be stored at room temperature and are particularly useful for the rapid mass screening of large groups. PPD solutions for intradermal administration (*Mantoux test*) are more sensitive, must be refrigerated and are used for definitive tuberculin testing of individuals.

Tuberculin tests are read 48 to 96 hours after administration and a positive reaction consists of induration of 2 mm or greater in diameter, or the presence of any vesiculation at the site of application. A positive test indicates only that the individual is hypersensitive to tuberculin, which implies past or present infection with *Mycobacterium tuberculosis*. A positive tuberculin test is an indication for additional diagnostic testing (eg, chest x-ray) to determine if prophylactic or therapeutic measures are required.

The other skin test antigens listed in Table 89-21 are very similar to the tuberculin test in principle and application. They have not, however, proven to be as useful in the evaluation of infection for a number of reasons including the problem of frequent cross-reactivity with immunogens from other organisms giving rise to false positive reactions.

A number of drugs can interfere with delayed hypersensitivity tests. Dermal reactivity may be depressed in patients taking corticosteroids or other immunosuppressive agents as well as those recently vaccinated with live virus vaccines (eg, measles, mumps, rubella, and polio viruses). Tuberculin testing can be administered simultaneously with these vaccines, but otherwise it should be deferred until 4 to 6 after vaccination. Persons immunized with BCG vaccine often convert to tuberculin positive and the interpretation of the test results is more complicated in these patients.

Delayed hypersensitivity may be suppressed in patients with a variety of conditions including acquired and congenital immune deficiencies, autoimmune disease, infections (bacterial, fungal, mycobacterial, virus), malignancy, malnutrition, and others. The absence of a dermal reactivity in a patient who has been sensitized to the immunogen in question is called *anergy*.

The usual method for assessing the competence of cell-mediated immunity is to employ a battery of 4 to 6 common immunogens referred to as an *anergy-test panel*. The panel is selected with the expectation that the patient will show a positive delayed hypersensitivity response to at least 2 to 4 immunogens if not anergic. This testing is of little value in evaluating primary immune deficiency during the first year of life since a failure to react may simply represent lack of exposure to the immunogens.

REFERENCES

1. Stites DP, Terr AI, Parslow TG, eds. *Medical Immunology*, 9th ed. Los Altos, CA: Appleton & Lange, 1997.
2. Grabenstein JD. *ImmunoFacts: Vaccines and Immunologic Drugs.* St. Louis: Facts & Comparisons, 1999.
3. *MMWR* 1994; 43(RR-1):1, 1994.
4. *MMWR* 1997; 46(RR-3):1.
5. *MMWR* 1998; 47(RR-8):1.
6. *MMWR* 1996; 45(RR-13):1.
7. *Health Information for International Travel, 1996-97.* Washington, DC: USGPO, 1996.
8. *MMWR* 1996; 45(RR-12):1.
9. Kaveri S, et al. *Multiple Sclerosis* 1997; 3:121.
10. Ratko TA, et al. *JAMA* 1995; 273:1865.
11. Lassiter HA. *Adv Pediatr* 1992; 39: 71.
12. Coombs RRA, Gell PGH. In Gell PGH, Coombs RRA, Lachmann PJ, eds. *Clinical Aspects of Immunology.* London: Blackwell, 1975.
13. *Bull WHO* 1994; 72:797.
14. Baldo BA. *Curr Opin Immunol* 1991; 3:841.
15. Evans R. *J Allergy Clin Immunol* 1991; 90: 462.
16. Creticos PS. *Immunol Clin North Am* 1992; 12:13.
17. Turkeltaub PC. *FDA Med Bull* 1994; 24:7.
18. Grabenstein JD. *Hosp Pharm* 1992; 27:145.
19. Hunter RB, Osterberger DJ. *Am J Hosp Pharm* 1975; 32:392.
20. Sadik F. *Handbook of Nonprescription Drugs*, 11th ed. Washington DC: APhA, 1996.
21. Sachs MI, Yunginger JW: *Immunol Allergy Clin North Am* 1991; 11:743.
22. VanArsdel PP: *Immunol Allergy Clin North Am* 1991; 11:461.
23. Wormser H. In *Handbook of Nonprescription Drugs*, 11th ed Washington DC: APhA, 1996.
24. Marks JG, DeLeo VA: *Patch Testing for Contact and Occupational Dermatology*. St Louis: Mosby Year Book, St Louis, 1992.

BIBLIOGRAPHY

Baldo BA: Structural features of allergens large and small with emphasis on recombinant allergens. *Curr Opin Immunol* 1991; 3:841.
Concepts in Immunology and Immunotherapeutics, 3rd ed. Bethesda, MD: ASHP, 1997.
Evans R. Environmental control and immunotherapy for allergic disease. *J Allergy Clin Immunol* 1991; 90:462.
Grabenstein JD. Drug-interactions involving immunologic agents: I. Vaccine-vaccine, vaccine-immunoglobulin, and vaccine-drug interactions. *DICP-Ann Pharmacother* 1990; 24:67.
Grabenstein JD. Drug-interactions involving immunologic agents: II. Immunodiagnostic and other immunologic drug interactions. *DICP-Ann Pharmacother* 1990; 24:186.
Grabenstein JD. Allergen extract compounding by pharmacists. *Hosp Pharm* 1992; 27:145.
Grabenstein JD. *ImmunoFacts: Vaccines and Immunologic Drugs.*, St Louis: Facts & Comparisons, 1999. [Updated biannually]
Hunter RB, Osterberger DJ. Role of the pharmacist in an allergy clinic. *Am J Hosp Pharm* 1975; 32:392.
IUIS/WHO Allergen Nomenclature Committee. Allergen nomenclature. *Bull WHO* 1994; 72:797.
Ratko TA, et al. Recommendations for off-label use of intravenously administered immunoglobulin preparations. *JAMA* 1995; 273:1865.
Stites DP, Terr AI, Parslow TG, eds: *Medical Immunology*, 9th ed. Los Altos, CA: Appleton & Lange, 1997.
VanArsdel PP. Drug allergy. *Immunol Allergy Clin North Am* 1991; 11:461.

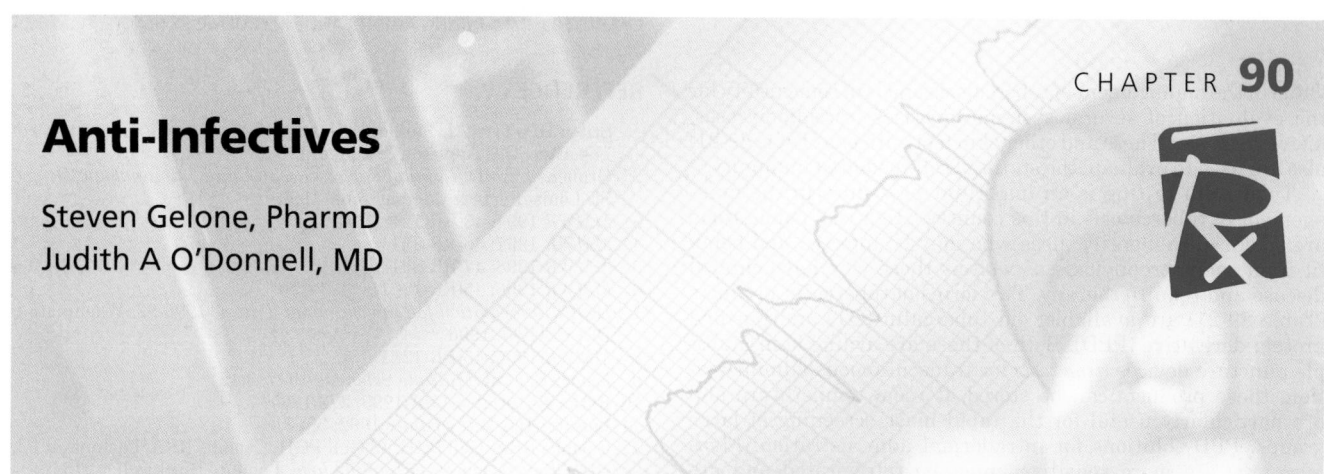

CHAPTER 90

Anti-Infectives

Steven Gelone, PharmD
Judith A O'Donnell, MD

The distinction between the terms *antibiotic* and *antimicrobial agent* has little meaning today. The term antibiotic traditionally refers to a substance produced by a microorganism. However, most agents are produced by chemical synthesis, or various moieties are attached to the basic core structure of an antibiotic after microbial fermentation.

The pathogenic microorganisms that can invade the human body and cause disease include a number of bacteria, viruses, fungi, and parasites. The major pharmacological approaches to treat these infections will be covered under the following headings: antiseptics and disinfectants, systemic antimicrobials, antimycobacterials, antifungals, and antivirals. Only the major antimicrobial drugs will be discussed in each section of this chapter to emphasize the general characteristics of specific drug families and their major subclasses. Common features will be summarized, and unique uses or problems will be highlighted for important drugs within each class.

ANTISEPTICS, DISINFECTANTS AND SPERMICIDES

The terms *antiseptic* and *disinfectant* refer to an agent that kills microbes upon contact. Drugs in this category are not taken internally and are not used to treat disease. These agents are used to prevent infection by destroying microorganisms on foreign surfaces and skin. Antiseptics are applied to living tissues and inhibit microorganism growth but this degerming action is only temporary. Presurgical scrubs reduce the normal and pathogenic flora on the skin if used appropriately, but bacterial multiplication resumes in minutes to hours.

The agents in this class are very diverse groups of chemicals and have a variety of mechanisms of action that include: highly reactive oxidizing and alkylating agents (ie, general protoplasmic poisons); protein denaturing agents that damage microbial cell walls or cytoplasmic membranes; lower surface tension; inhibit essential enzymes; and other examples of nonselective actions. The effectiveness of antiseptics and disinfectants is influenced by concentration, temperature, and time of exposure.

Many of these agents are poorly effective in the presence of serum or other organic media, or else they are excessively damaging to the tissues. Tissue damage, of course, is not of concern when such agents are employed for the disinfection of inanimate objects; on the other hand, corrosiveness, staining, and other effects then become important considerations. The best and most effective antiseptics are iodine and chlorhexidine in combination with alcohol.

Notable problems of commonly used preparations are listed in each monograph. Cationic detergents are very poor antiseptics or disinfectants due to their inactivation by soap and organic tissue components. It commonly is believed that antiseptics are nonselective and that they have a continuous spectrum of activity. Although this is essentially true, certain significant absolute exceptions exist, and the relative susceptibilities of the numerous microorganisms must be considered in antiseptic use. For example, hexachlorophene is effective primarily against gram-positive organisms, and cationic antiseptics are not effective against sporulating organisms. Certain bacteria are even capable of growing in 70% ethanol.

No really satisfactory classification of antiseptics exists. The most widely used scheme is the chemical classification. Nevertheless, the drugs listed below are not arranged according to chemical type. However, it will be noted that the major chemical categories represented are oxidizing agents (including the halogens and halogen-releasing compounds), phenols and related compounds, compounds of heavy metals (especially of mercury), surface-active agents (especially the cationic detergents) and scattered representatives from the alcohols and glycols, aldehydes, and acids. Locally effective antibiotics are discussed with the antibiotics.

It should be kept in mind that systemic antimicrobial drugs are often superior to topical ones. This is because topical agents usually do not penetrate into infected sites as well as systemic agents do. Nevertheless, topical drugs are often efficacious, simply by limiting surface infections so that tissue defenses can clean up below without continual reinfection from superficial foci. Furthermore, some superficial disorders do not seem to respond to safe systemic agents, or, if they do, there may be cogent reasons for withholding systemic drugs, for example, to avoid sensitizing the patient or creating resistant microorganisms. Therefore, there is still an important place for topical antiseptics. However, topical antiseptics can damage tissue defenses, so that sometimes they may exacerbate lesions. Such occasions are not always predictable, and they evidently depend in part on the condition of the patient and the activity of the immunological response to infection. A summary of the activities of antiseptics is shown in Table 90-1.

ACETIC ACID, DILUTED—page 1083.
ACRISORCIN—see RPS-17, page 1226.

ALCOHOL

For the full monograph, see RPS-20, page 1038.

Comments—An *antiseptic* with the following susceptibilities: gram–positive and gram–negative bacteria, highly susceptible; spores, resistant; lipophilic viruses, susceptible; hydrophilic viruses, variable; and fungi, no data.

ALUMINUM ACETATE TOPICAL SOLUTION—page 1282.
BACITRACIN—page 1653.

BENZALKONIUM CHLORIDE

**Ammonium, alkyldimethyl(phenylmethyl)-, chloride;
Zephiran Chloride**

Alkylbenzyldimethylammonium chloride [8001-54-5]; a mixture of alkylbenzyldimethylammonium chlorides of the general formula

Table 90-1. Activities of Antiseptics

CHEMICAL	CLASS/AGENTS GM+	GM−	ACTIVITY	BACTERIA SPORES	VIRUSES LIPOPHILIC	FUNGI HYDROPHILIC	USE
Alcohols							
Ethanol	HS	HS	R	S	V	—	Antiseptic
Isopropanol							
Aldehydes	S	HS	S	S	MS	S	Disinfectant
Formaldehyde							
Glutaraldehyde							
Chlorhexidine gluconate	HS	MS	R	V	R	—	Antiseptic
Chlorine sodium	HS	HS	S	S	S	MS	Disinfectant, irrigant
hypochlorite							
Hexachlorophene	S	R	R	R	R	R	Soap, shampoo
Iodine	HS	HS	S	S	R	S	Antiseptic
Povidone-iodine							
Phenols	HS	HS	R	R	R	—	Disinfectant
Oxidizing agents	HS	HS	S	V	V	S	Disinfectant, irrigant
Hydrogen peroxide							
Quaternary	HS	HS	R	S	R	—	Disinfectant
Ammonium (Benzalkonium							
chloride Cetylpyridinum							
chloride Benzethonium							
chloride)							

Key: HS = highly susceptible, MS = moderately susceptible, S = susceptible, R = resistant, V = variable, —no data.

$[C_6H_5CH_2N(CH_3)_2R]Cl$, in which R represents a mixture of alkyls, including all or some of the group beginning with n-C_8H_{17} and extending through higher homologs, with n-$C_{12}H_{25}$, n-$C_{14}H_{29}$ and n-$C_{16}H_{33}$ comprising the major portion. On the anhydrous basis, the content of n-$C_{12}H_{25}$ homolog is not less than 40%, and the content of the n-$C_{14}H_{29}$ homolog is not less than 20%, of the total alkylbenzyldimethylammonium chloride content. The amounts of the n-$C_{12}H_{25}$ and n-$C_{14}H_{29}$ homolog components comprise together not less than 70% of the total alkylbenzyldimethylammonium chloride content.

Preparation—By treating a solution of N-alkyl-N-methylbenzylamine in a suitable organic solvent with methyl chloride, the solvent being so chosen that the quaternary compound precipitates as it is formed.

Description—White or yellowish white, thick gel or gelatinous pieces; aromatic odor and a very bitter taste; solutions are alkaline to litmus and foam strongly when shaken.

Solubility—Very soluble in water and alcohol; 1 g of the anhydrous form dissolves in approximately 6 mL benzene and in approximately 100 mL ether.

Incompatibilities—Like other cationic surface-active agents, benzalkonium chloride is incompatible with *soap* and other *anionic agents*. The large organic ions of the two agents are oppositely charged and, in sufficient concentration, can precipitate from solution. *Nitric acid* and *nitrates* cause precipitation.

Comments—A *bacteriostatic* in low and bactericidal in high concentrations. Gram–positive bacteria are more sensitive than gram–negative bacteria. The antiseptic has a slow action. It requires 7 min for the bacterial count on the skin to be decreased by a mere 50%, while only 36 sec is required by 70% ethanol; to effect a 90% reduction, 25 min is required for this compared to 2 min for the 70% ethanol.

It is used for application to skin and mucous membranes. It is used widely in OTC ophthalmic solutions and as applications to contact lenses. It also is used for the sterilization of inanimate articles, such as surgical instruments. Its solutions have low surface tension and possess detergent and emulsifying actions. It has relatively low systemic toxicity. It does not destroy bacterial spores, it is ineffective against some viruses, it is inactivated by soap and other anionic surface–active agents, and when applied to the skin, it has a tendency to form a film under which bacteria remain viable. Organic matter from tissue inactivates the drug, so that it has limited efficacy in the disinfection of wounds. The drug can cause irritation and damage the epidermis, and it also can cause allergies.

BENZETHONIUM CHLORIDE

Benzenemethanaminium,N,N-dimethyl-N-[2-[2[4-(1,1,3,3-tetramethylbutyl)phenoxy]ethoxy]ethyl]-, chloride

Benzyldimethyl[2-[2-[p-(1,1,3,3-tetramethylbutyl)phenoxy]-ethoxy]ethyl]ammonium chloride. [121-54-0] $C_{27}H_{42}ClNO_2$ (448.09).

Preparation—From p-diisobutylphenol with dichlorodiethyl ether, dimethylamine and benzyl chloride.

Description—White crystals; mild odor; very bitter taste; melts at approximately 160°; aqueous solution (1%) slightly alkaline, and foams strongly when shaken.

Solubility—1 g in 0.6 mL water, 0.6 mL alcohol, 1 mL chloroform or 6000 mL ether.

Comments—A *disinfectant* with the following susceptibilities: gram–positive and gram–negative bacteria, highly susceptible; spores, resistant; lipophilic viruses, susceptible; hydrophilic viruses, resistant; and fungi, no data.

BENZOIC ACID—see RPS-19, page 1327.
BENZYL ALCOHOL—see RPS-19, page 1151.
BORIC ACID—page 1083.
BUTYLPARABEN—see RPS-18, page 1170.

CHLORHEXIDINE GLUCONATE

D-Gluconic acid, compd with N,N''-bis(4-chlorophenyl)-3,12-diimino-2,4,11,13-tetraazatetradecanediimidamide (2:1); Hibiclens, Hibistat

1,1′-Hexamethylenebis[5-(p-chlorophenyl)biguanide] di-D-gluconate [18472-51-0] $C_{22}H_{30}Cl_2N_{10}\cdot2C_6H_{12}O_7$ (897.77).

Preparation—Chlorhexidine base may be prepared by refluxing a mixture of hexamethylenebis [dicyandiamide], [NCNHC(:NH)-NH-(CH$_2$)$_3$]$_2$, and p-chloroaniline hydrochloride in 2-ethoxyethanol at 130° to 140° for 2 hours (Rose, Swain. *CA* 1956; 50: 1082h). The digluconate, diacetate, and dihydrochloride salts may be obtained by neutralizing the base with the respective acids.

Description—Colorless to pale-yellow solution. Usually available in 5% or 20% aqueous solution. pH (5% aqueous solution) 5.5 to 7.

Solubility—Very soluble in water; 1 g in 5 mL alcohol or 3 mL acetone.

Comments—*Bactericidal* to both gram-positive and gram-negative bacteria, although it is not as potent against the latter. It disrupts the plasma membrane of the bacterial cell, and cellular contents are lost.

In a 4% aqueous solution as a surgical scrub, it decreases the cutaneous bacterial population more than either hexachlorophene or povidone-iodine. It is slightly less effective than povidone-iodine if the skin is contaminated with certain *gram-negative bacteria*. A 1% aqueous solution has erratic antiseptic effects, but a 0.5% solution in 95% ethanol is more effective than a 4% aqueous solution. Chlorhexidine solutions leave a residue on the skin that gives a persistent antibacterial effect lasting 1 or 2 days. Its actions are not affected by blood, pus, or soaps.

It is used for the preoperative preparation of both surgeon and patient, for the treatment of superficial skin infections, burns, acne vulgaris, the irrigation of wounds, and surgical infections. It can be used in the hospital nursery to bathe neonates for prophylaxis against staphylococcal and streptococcal infections.

It is absorbed negligibly from the skin and mucous membranes; it has low systemic toxicity. However, serious injury may occur when it enters open wounds of the eye, and deafness may occur if it enters the middle ear through a perforated eardrum. A few cases of sensitization have been reported.

ETHYLENE OXIDE

Oxirane

Ethylene oxide [75-21-8] C_2H_4O (44.05).

Preparation—Ethylene is catalytically oxidized with air at high temperature.

Description—Colorless, flammable gas; liquid at less than 12°.

Solubility—Soluble in water, alcohol, or ether.

Comments—An *alkylating agent* that has a very broad germicidal spectrum, including spores and viruses. Since it is reactive at room temperature, it may be used for the disinfection and sterilization of heat-labile objects, such as certain catheters and endoscopes in the hospital. Because it is applied as a gas, it is advantageous for the sterilization of objects that would be harmed by immersion in aqueous or other media.

Inhalation of the gas causes nausea, vomiting, and neurologic disorders, and severe exposures can cause death. Consequently, sterilization must be done only in appropriate chambers or rooms. Chemical burns can result from the wearing of ethylene oxide-sterilized clothing, shoes, or gloves that have been aired inadequately after sterilization; thrombophlebitis or hemolysis can result from the use of catheters, and tracheitis from endotracheal tubes that have retained a residue of the gas. Polyvinyl tubing and bags are especially dangerous because of the formation of chlorohydrin. Therefore, after exposure, these items should be aired for 5 days at room temperature or 8 hr at 120°. The gas also is used as a fumigant.

The gas is highly explosive at concentrations above 3%, so that it needs to be mixed with CO_2 or fluorocarbons before use.

The gas kills vegetative bacteria very rapidly, but desiccated microorganisms and spores are killed only slowly, so that a 3-hr exposure at 30° is advised. The optimal humidity for action is 30% to 40%.

ETHYLPARABEN—see RPS-18, page 1171.

FORMALDEHYDE

Comments—A *disinfectant* with the following susceptibilities: gram-positive bacteria, susceptible; gram-negative bacteria, highly susceptible; spores, susceptible; lipophilic viruses, susceptible; hydrophilic viruses, moderately susceptible; and fungi, susceptible.

GLUTARAL

Pentanedial; Glutaraldehyde; Glutaric Dialdehyde; Cidex

$OCH(CH_2)_3CHO$ [111-30-8] $C_5H_8O_2$ (100.12).

Preparation—The 1:1 Diels-Alder adduct of acrolein and a vinyl alkyl ether is hydrolyzed, forming glutaral and an alkanol.

Description—Colorless liquid; pungent odor; boils about 188° with decomposition; stable in light; oxidizes in air; polymerizes on heating. *Glutaral Concentrate* is a 50% (w/w) solution in water.

Solubility—Soluble in water and in alcohol.

Comments—A *disinfectant* with the following susceptibilities: gram-positive bacteria, susceptible; gram-negative bacteria, highly susceptible; spores, susceptible; lipophilic viruses, susceptible; hydrophilic viruses, moderately susceptible; and fungi, susceptible.

HEXACHLOROPHENE

Phenol, 2,2'-methylenebis[3,4,6-trichloro-, G-11; AT-7;

[70-30-4] $C_{13}H_6Cl_6O_2$ (406.91).

Preparation—By the Baeyer condensation reaction involving two molecules of 2,4,5-trichlorophenol, and one molecule of formaldehyde. Sulfuric acid is employed as the dehydrant.

Description—White to light tan, crystalline powder; odorless or only slightly phenolic odor; melting range 161° to 167°; incompatible with benzalkonium chloride; pK_a 5.7.

Solubility—Insoluble in water; freely soluble in acetone, alcohol and ether; soluble in chloroform and dilute solutions of fixed alkali hydroxides.

Comments—An effective *bacteriostatic antiseptic* against gram-positive bacteria but it has low activity against gram-negative organisms. On the skin the bacterial population initially will decrease by only 30% to 50% but within 1 hr the decrease will exceed 90%. When washes are repeated 2 or more times a day, the decrease will reach 95% to 99% in 3 or 4 days from a persisting residuum of the drug in the skin. This reservoir can be removed by ethanol, isopropyl alcohol and soap and water washes or other detergents. The drug is effective whether applied as a tincture, detergent emulsion or soap; the tincture is the most effective and a 0.23% tincture foam has been reported to be more effective than a 3% soap. In soaps, one hydroxyl group is neutralized, which moderately decreases activity.

Preparations containing this are used widely as antiseptic scrubs by physicians, dentists, food handlers and others. The incidence and severity of pyogenic skin infections are reduced by routine use.

In infants, it can cause myelinopathy and spongiform encephalomalacia following topical application; for this reason, it is no longer used in hospital nurseries to bathe infants. Avoid contact with eyes and do not use on burns or mucous membranes. By the oral route it can cause nausea, vomiting and abdominal cramps with associated water and electrolyte derangements. Topically, the drug can cause dermatitis and sensitization. It is teratogenic.

HYDROGEN PEROXIDE SOLUTION

Hydrogen Dioxide

[7722-84-1] H_2O_2 (34.01).

Preparation—Hydrogen peroxide: by many methods, one of the most important ones involving electrolysis of sulfuric acid in a solution containing sulfate, whereby persulfate is formed, which is hydrolyzed to hydrogen peroxide. Solutions containing as much as 90% H_2O_2 in each 100 mL.

Description—Clear liquid; colorless; odorless or having an odor resembling that of ozone; usually deteriorates on standing or on protracted agitation; decomposes rapidly when in contact with many oxidizing or reducing substances; when rapidly heated, it may decompose suddenly.

Comments—A *germicide* active by virtue of the release of nascent oxygen; it is short acting because the release occurs rapidly. It is the substance released by activated neutrophils, and it is an effective *microbicide* when applied in close contact with most microorganisms. However, the ubiquitous enzyme catalase often destroys it before it reaches organisms in wounds. Effervescence helps cleanse wounds mechanically.

IODINE

Iodine

[7553-56-2] I (126.90).

Preparation—From the iodide in the ashes of seaweed by chlorination, from the iodate in chile saltpeter by reduction with sulfite ion, or from the iodide in oil well brines by oxidation with chlorine or nitrite ion.

Description—Heavy, grayish black plates or granules, a metallic luster; characteristic odor; specific gravity approximately 4.9; melts at approximately 114° but volatilizes even at room temperature.

Solubility—1 g in 3000 mL water, 13 mL alcohol, 80 mL glycerin; freely soluble in chloroform, carbon tetrachloride, ether, and glacial acetic acid; soluble in solutions of iodides by the formation of I_{3^-}.

Incompatibilities—Oxidizes *hypophosphites, sulfites*, the lower valence forms of some *metals* and *other reducing agents*, the iodine being reduced to an iodide. *Thiosulfates* (hyposulfites) also react with free iodine. It reacts with *fixed oils* to form addition compounds, and with *volatile oils* to form various derivatives. The reaction with *turpentine oil* is violent. An explosive iodide of nitrogen may be formed with *ammonia water* or *ammoniated mercury*. *Alkali hydroxides* and *carbonates* react with iodine to form iodides and iodates. Many *alkaloids* are precipitated from aqueous solutions of their salts. In *alcoholic solution* iodine slowly forms hydrogen iodide if alkali iodide is absent.

Comments—One of the best all-around *antiseptics*. It is active against bacteria, fungi, spores, yeasts, protozoa and viruses. Although it is available in high concentration in various complexes (with iodide ion, poloxamer, povidone, etc, called iodophores) or tinctures, its solubility in water is only 0.033% (1:3,000). The advantage of iodophores or concentrates is that they provide a reservoir (called available iodine) from which to replenish iodine that is depleted in combining with microbial components and organic materials resulting in a sustained action. Iodine can complex loosely with amino and heterocyclic groups in tissues constituents that serve as repository iodine. Ethanol and other organic solvents in tinctures act superadditively with free iodine.

Most bacteria are killed within 10 sec by a 1% solution, 1 min by 1:20,000 (0.05%) and 10 min by 1:500,000 (0.0002%). A 0.15% solution may kill wet bacterial spores, amebic cysts, and enteric viruses in about 15 min, but dry spores may require hours, even with 1:3000. On the skin, a 1% tincture will kill 90% of the bacteria in 90 sec.

Its tinctures and solutions are used widely by the lay public for the *disinfection of cuts and abrasions*. The 2% solution is the best-available OTC preparation for this purpose because it lacks the irritancy of tinctures and hypertonicity of the strong solution. Solutions are effective even in strengths as low as 0.1%, which is sometimes used for *wound irrigation*. The tincture is the best preparation for *presurgical preparation of the intact skin*. It may be used to purify drinking water. However, *Giardia* is less sensitive than bacteria and amebae and requires higher concentrations and longer incubations.

It has a high therapeutic index among antiseptics. Tinctures sting and also cause local damage. The strong tincture, especially, can cause burns, even on intact skin; it was this toxicity that gave iodine a bad reputation.

ISOPROPYL ALCOHOL

2-Propanol

$CH_3CH(OH)CH_3$ [67-63-0] C_3H_8O (60.10).

Preparation—Most of the isopropyl alcohol prepared commercially is obtained by treating propylene with H_2SO_4 followed by hydrolysis. The olefin is obtained in the cracking of petroleum.

Some of the alcohol also is obtained by the reduction of acetone through high-pressure hydrogenation.

Description—Transparent, colorless, mobile, volatile liquid; characteristic odor; slightly bitter taste; specific gravity 0.783 to 0.787; distilling range 81° to 83°; refractive index 1.376 to 1.378 at 20°.

Solubility—Miscible with water, alcohol, ether, and chloroform.

Comments—For the *disinfection* of hypodermic syringes and needles and, as the rubbing alcohol, a skin antiseptic. It is superior to ethyl alcohol in regard to its *antiseptic* properties. All concentrations greater than 70% are effective skin disinfectants. It does promote bleeding at an injection site, which may make reading of allergic tests difficult. It cannot be relied on to destroy the spores of organisms such as *Clostridium tetani*, *Clostridium welchii*, or *Bacillus anthracis*. It has a greater effect than ethanol to dry and irritate the skin. It is not potable and should not be given by mouth. It is recognized as a rubefacient, although it is used more widely as an antiseptic.

METHYLENE BLUE—page 1348.
METHYLPARABEN—see RPS-18, page 1172.

NITROFURAZONE

Hydrazinecarboxamide, 2-[(5-nitro-2-furanyl)methylene]-, Furacin; Amifur

5-Nitro-2-furaldehyde semicarbazone [59-87-0] $C_6H_6N_4O_4$ (198.14).

Preparation—By condensing 5-nitro-2-furaldehyde with semicarbazide hydrochloride in the presence of sodium acetate.

Description—Odorless, lemon-yellow, crystalline powder; nearly tasteless, but develops a bitter aftertaste; darkens slowly on exposure to light; melts at approximately 236° with decomposition; pH (saturated solution) 5 to 7.5.

Solubility—1 g in 4200 mL water, 590 mL alcohol, 350 mL propylene glycol, and polyethylene glycol mixtures as much as 1%; practically insoluble in chloroform and ether.

Comments—A *local antibacterial* agent with a broad spectrum of activity.

Most bacteria of surface infections of the skin or mucosal surfaces are sensitive to the drug. It is applied topically in the treatment of mixed, superficial infections of the skin. It finds use, especially, in the treatment of 2nd- and 3rd-degree burns and in skin grafting in which there are complications from bacterial infections that are refractory to the usual drugs of choice but in which bacterial sensitivity to the drug is demonstrable. It has not yet been shown to be useful in the treatment of minor burns, wounds, or cutaneous ulcers that are infected. It retains its antibacterial activity in blood, serum, and pus; phagocytosis is not inhibited, and nitrofurazone does not interfere with healing. However, it is a slowly acting drug, and at least 24 hr are required for it to take effect properly. Therefore, no treatment should be less than 2 or 3 days in duration.

Approximately 1% of patients become sensitized to the drug, sometimes within 5 days of initiation of treatment. The systemic toxicity is low.

PHENOL—page 1087.
PHENYLETHYL ALCOHOL—page 1066.
PHENYLMERCURIC ACETATE—see RPS-18, page 1172.
PHENYLMERCURIC NITRATE—page 1059.
PINE TAR—page 1286.
POLYMYXIN B SULFATE—page 1654.
POTASSIUM PERMANGANATE—see RPS-19, page 1270.

POVIDONE-IODINE

2-Pyrrolidinone, 1-ethenyl-, homopolymer, compd with iodine

1-Vinyl-2-pyrrolidinone polymer compd with iodine [25655-41-8]; contains 9–12% of available iodine.

Preparation—Povidone having an average molecular weight of 40,000 is heated with elemental iodine in the presence of a little water whereby a small amount of the iodine enters into loose organic union with the polymer to form a compound which contains approximately 10% of available iodine.

Description—Yellowish-brown, amorphous powder; slight, characteristic odor; aqueous solution is acid to litmus.

Solubility—Soluble in water or alcohol; practically insoluble in chloroform, carbon tetrachloride, ether, solvent hexane or acetone.

Comments—Kills both gram-positive and gram-negative bacteria, fungi, viruses, protozoa, and yeasts. The povidone component increases the solubility of iodine and provides a slow-release form of iodine. The affinity of povidone for iodine is greater than that of iodide, so that the concentration of free iodine is less than 1 ppm. Consequently the immediate bactericidal action of povidone-iodine is only moderate compared to that of iodine solutions. Although it takes 6 to 8 hr for the skin bacterial population to return to normal, which is longer than with iodine solutions, the effective duration of action for surgical purposes is only about 1 hr.

It is claimed that it stings less than iodine preparations. This is not true; it is iodine tincture that stings, and tinctures of this drug also sting. Iodine solutions are more effective in wound irrigation. It stains the skin and clothing less than iodine solutions and is also less of an irritant under occlusive dressings.

Its antiseptic preparations are indicated clinically for the prevention and treatment of surface infections as well as to degerm the skin prior to injection and hyperalimentation procedures; for seborrhea; for disinfection of wounds, burns, lacerations, and abrasions; for preoperative and postoperative scrubbing and washing of hospital operating-room personnel and for preoperative skin preparation of patients. It has no clear advantage over iodine solutions or tinctures.

PROPYLENE OXIDE—see RPS-18, page 1173.
PROPYLPARABEN—see RPS-18, page 1173.
PYRITHIONE ZINC—see RPS-18, page 1173.
SALICYLIC ACID—page 1288.

SELENIUM SULFIDE

Selenium Disulfide, Selsun; Exsel; Selsun Blue

Selenium sulfide (SeS_2) [7488-56-4] SeS_2 (143.08); contains 52.0 to 55.5% of selenium.

Preparation—Among other ways, by adding an aqueous solution of selenious acid to an aqueous solution containing a stoichiometric excess of hydrogen sulfide.

Description—Reddish brown to bright-orange powder; not more than a faint odor.

Solubility—Practically insoluble in water or organic solvents.

Comments—An *antibacterial, antifungal*, and *mildly keratolytic* agent used in the local treatment of seborrheic dermatitis of the scalp. It is effective in the treatment of tinea versicolor. It is also useful in the management of acne vulgaris and juvenilis and atopic eczema, but it has not been approved for these uses. Some authorities attribute its antiseborrheic efficacy to cytostatic actions. It induces inflammation of the mucous membranes and exposed tissues, so that care should be exercised in the application of the compound. It also causes *rebound* oiliness of the scalp. It should not be allowed to get into the eyes.

Occasionally, it causes loss of hair. Although it has considerably lower toxicity than selenites and some other selenium compounds and is available OTC, care nevertheless should be taken to keep preparations away from the mouth.

SILVER NITRATE—page 1287.
MILD SILVER PROTEIN—see RPS-18, page 1173.

SILVER SULFADIAZINE

Benzenesulfonamide, 4-amino-N-2-pyrimidinyl-, monosilver (1+) salt; Silvadene; SSD

N^1-2-Pyrimidinylsulfanilamide monosilver(1+) salt [22199-08-2] $C_{10}H_9AgN_4O_2S$ (357.13).

Description—A white powder.

Solubility—Practically insoluble in water.

Comments—Combines in one compound the *antibacterial* properties of silver ion and sulfadiazine; it is especially effective against *Ps aeruginosa.* It is indicated for topical use as an adjunct for prevention and treatment of wound sepsis in patients with second-and third-degree burns. It can penetrate the eschar. Although some sulfadiazine is absorbed, it is rarely sufficient to cause crystalluria. However, bacterial resistance to sulfonamides can occur. The drug does not cause pain at the site of application. Hypersensitivity may occur. Silver inactivates proteolytic enzymes used for debridement.

SODIUM BENZOATE—see RPS-19, page 1271.

SODIUM HYPOCHLORITE SOLUTION

Antiformin, Dakin's Solution, Hyclorite

An aqueous solution containing 4.0 to 6.0% *w/w* of sodium hypochlorite [7681-52-9] NaClO (74.44).

Preparation—By electrolysis of a solution of sodium chloride in a cell permitting reaction of chlorine with sodium hydroxide; an equivalent quantity of sodium chloride is produced simultaneously.

Description—Clear, pale greenish yellow liquid; slight odor of chlorine; affected by light.

Comments—A *disinfectant* and *irrigant* with the following susceptibilities: gram-positive and gram-negative bacteria, highly susceptible; spores, susceptible; lipophilic and hydrophilic viruses, susceptible; and fungi, moderately susceptible.

SYSTEMIC ANTIBACTERIAL DRUGS

Systemic antibacterial agents can be bactericidal (kill microbes) or bacteriostatic (growth inhibition) but also rely on host defenses to aid in eliminating bacterial pathogens. A given agent may be bactericidal under some conditions but be only bacteriostatic at other times, depending on the concentration of drug and type of bacteria. For a neutropenic patient a bactericidal agent would be necessary to maximize the potential for successful treatment.

The antibacterial agents can be classified into specific classes as well as divided into five major groups according to their primary mechanism of action or cellular biochemical pathway that is inhibited. The antibiotics and systemic antibacterial agents will be grouped into the following categories: inhibition of bacterial cell wall synthesis (penicillins, cephalosporins, carbapenems, and vancomycin), damage to cytoplasmic membrane (polymyxins), modification of synthesis or metabolism of nucleic acids (quinolones, rifampin and nitrofurantoin), inhibition of protein synthesis (aminoglycosides, tetracyclines, chloramphenicol, erythromycin, and clindamycin) and folate-inhibitors or modification of energy metabolism (sulfonamides and trimethoprim).

Factors to consider when selecting systemic antimicrobial agents for therapy in patients should include identification of likely or specific microorganism, antimicrobial susceptibility, bactericidal versus bacteriostatic, and host status (ie, allergy history, age, pharmacokinetic factors, renal and hepatic function, pregnancy status, genetic or metabolic abnormalities, anatomical site of infection and host defenses, especially neutrophil function). The systemic antibacterial drugs will be described according to their major chemical families because similarities of antibiotics within each class are extensive. The major differences of unique members within each subclass will be emphasized.

Sulfonamides

The sulfonamides and trimethoprim act by inhibiting folic acid synthesis that most bacteria must synthesize whereas humans can rely on dietary sources. Sulfonamides were the first antimicrobial agents, but their clinical use has been greatly restricted as a result of the development of resistant bacteria, their significant side effects, and the availability of other drugs. The sulfonamides are no longer the preferred drugs for treat-

Table 90-2. Sulfonamides

DRUG	COMMENTS
Sulfisoxazole	Highly soluble, short half-life
Sulfmethoxazole	Highly soluble, intermed. half-life
Sulfadiazine	Best tissue levels, intermed. half-life
Sulfathalidine	Not absorbed orally, used only for ulcerative colitis
Sulfacetamide	Only used topically, ophthalmic

ment of urinary tract infections (UTIs) but are still effective for some infections. Some examples include the treatment of initial, uncomplicated UTIs, nocardiosis, and topical treatment of burn areas. The trimethoprim-sulfamethoxazole combination has many therapeutic applications that expand the usefulness of sulfonamides to treat some urinary, respiratory and GI infections, pneumocystis, toxoplasmosis, and prevention of bacterial peritonitis (Table 90-2).

HISTORY—The compound *p*-aminobenzenesulfonamide, now known as *sulfanilamide*, was first synthesized in 1908, but it was many years before its therapeutic value was discovered. In 1932 a German firm prepared a red dye, 4-(4′-sulfamylphenylazo)-m-phenylenediamine or, p′-sulfamylchrysoidine, and in 1935 Domagk reported remarkable curative effects of this compound and named it *Prontosil.*

In the same year, a group of French investigators found that the antibacterial property of the drug resided in the *p*-aminobenzenesulfonamide portion of the molecule. In 1937 Ewins and Phillips of England synthesized sulfapyridine, which was the first sulfonamide used with great success in combating pneumonia. Then followed sulfathiazole, sulfadiazine, and a large number of other sulfonamides.

All the official, and generally all the therapeutically useful, antimicrobial sulfonamides are characterized by the structure.

ANTIMICROBIAL PROPERTIES—The sulfonamides originally possessed a wide antimicrobial spectrum that included all gram-positive cocci, except enterococcus, all gram-positive bacilli, nearly all *Enterobacteriaceae* and gram-negative cocci, *H influenzae, Bordetella pertussis, Pasteurella,* some *Pseudomonas, Chlamydia* (psittacosis, *Trachoma, Lymphogranuloma venereum*), *Actinomycetes, Nocardia,* and some *Toxoplasma* and malaria. However, resistance to the drugs has limited the spectrum greatly.

In most circumstances, these agents exert only a bacteriostatic action, and ultimate elimination of the invading microorganisms depends upon the cellular and humoral defense mechanisms of the host. However, bactericidal concentrations of these agents sometimes are attained in the urinary and intestinal tracts, where the concentration of drug may be quite high.

The mechanism of the antimicrobial action of the sulfonamides has been analyzed extensively. The sulfonamides compete with *p*-aminobenzoic acid and prevent its normal cellular use, particularly its incorporation into folic acid (pteroylglutamic acid, PGA). Thus, sulfonamide-sensitive organisms are primarily those that synthesize their own folic acid. Organisms able to use preformed folic or tetrahydrofolic acid or the tetrahydrofolate-dependent pyrimidines and thymidine are not affected by these agents generally. This mechanism is of importance as an example of the general concepts of biological antagonism and antimetabolites. The efficacy of sulfonamides generally is enhanced when the drugs are used in combination with trimethoprim that inhibits conversion of dihydrofolate to tetrahydrofolic acid and thence to folinic acid.

Microorganisms initially sensitive to the sulfonamides may become resistant to these drugs. The clinical importance of such acquired bacterial resistance is attested by the fact that the majority of the strains of *N gonorrhoeae* now isolated from patients with gonococcal urethritis are resistant to these agents, whereas the sulfonamides were once the agents of choice against such organisms. *Enterobacteriaceae*, especially, have become resistant.

Certain combinations of the sulfonamides with various antibiotics minimize the development of bacterial resistance and achieve chemotherapeutic results not attainable with either agent alone. Specific examples of valid combinations of the sulfonamides with other chemotherapeutic agents are indicated below.

ABSORPTION, DISTRIBUTION, AND EXCRETION— Sulfonamides in which the para-amino group is free are absorbed readily into the blood stream, mostly via the small intestine. Although only a small amount may remain unabsorbed, the local concentration in the bowel may be high enough to exert a prominent antibacterial action on some of the bowel flora. Absorption from the skin and vagina is erratic. Once into the bloodstream, sulfonamides bind to serum albumin to varying degrees, ranging from less than 10% to more than 90%, depending on the particular drug. Protein binding limits penetrance into the tissues, and glomerular filtration is a determinant of the rate of excretion.

Concentrations in tissue fluids usually range from about 50% to 80% of those in the plasma. Highly polar sulfonamides do not penetrate tissues well, but they are excreted rapidly.

Thus, sulfisoxazole is mainly extracellular in distribution and is of limited usefulness in systemic infections; because it is filtered rapidly in the renal glomerulus and resorbed poorly by the renal tubules (being lipid-insoluble), high concentrations are reached in the urine, which makes it effective in the treatment of UTIs. Nevertheless, when the UTI is extraluminal, more widely distributed sulfonamides, such as sulfadiazine, may be more effective.

Sulfonamides are acetylated in the liver to an extent of 30% to 85% depending on the sulfonamide and the patient. The fraction of the acetylate conjugate in the urine varies accordingly. Crystallization of sulfonamide, conjugate, or both may occur in the urine, depending on the solubility properties of each form of the drug at the pH of the urine and on the volume of urine. In general, both parent and acetylated sulfonamides are more soluble in alkaline than acid urine.

TOXICITY—Untoward effects during therapy with sulfonamides represent the major limitation to their clinical use. The most frequently observed side effects are crystalluria and related renal damage, hematuria being noted in approximately 2% of patients receiving sulfadiazine or other pyrimidine congeners. GI side effects include nausea, vomiting, abdominal pain, diarrhea, anorexia, stomatitis and rare pancreatitis. Of the neurologic effects, headache, vertigo, and insomnia are the most frequent, but tinnitus, psychic depression, ataxia, hallucinations, peripheral and optic neuritis, acute myopia, and convulsions occasionally occur. This incidence is less when adjuvant alkali and fluid therapy is instituted or when sulfonamide mixtures or the more soluble congeners are employed.

Hypersensitivity reactions, such as drug fever, dermatitis, hepatitis, polyarteritis nodosa, lupoid syndrome, pulmonary eosinophilia, and rare myocarditis, occur in about 2% of patients receiving most present-day sulfonamides. The incidence of hypersensitivity reactions is higher in patients receiving sulfapyridine. Agranulocytosis, aplastic anemia, leucopenia, and thrombocytopenia have been noted during sulfonamide therapy, but the incidence is low when sulfadiazine and the other newer congeners are employed.

Hemolytic anemia may occur; persons whose erythrocytes are deficient in glucose 6-phosphate dehydrogenase (G6PD) are especially susceptible. Sulfonamide-induced hepatocellular jaundice is now rare. Long-acting sulfonamides that may cause exudative erythema multiforme (Stevens-Johnson syndrome) are no longer available in the US.

CNS effects are observed infrequently during current sulfonamide therapy, and cyanosis, acid-base disturbances, and other miscellaneous toxic effects, formerly common during therapy with sulfanilamide, sulfathiazole, or sulfapyridine, are observed only rarely during the administration of sulfadiazine.

Sulfonamides displace bilirubin from plasma proteins and hence can cause kernicterus in the newborn. It is not recommended that sulfonamides be administered to infants younger than 2 mo. Consequently, sulfonamides should be avoided in pregnant women near term and in newborn or premature infants. Some sulfonamides have been shown to be teratogenic in rats. If at all possible, then, sulfonamides should be avoided in pregnancy.

Because the sulfonamides may cause serious untoward effects, they should be administered only when bacteriological diagnosis indicates that these agents can be expected to be superior to drugs of other classes. Constant medical surveillance, preferably daily, is necessary, and periodic blood counts and urinalysis are mandatory.

COMMENTS—Sulfonamide therapy alone has a minor place in the chemotherapy of infectious diseases. Major advantages of sulfonamides are their low cost and ease of administration; major disadvantages are their untoward effects and limited efficacy. The combination, trimethoprim-sulfamethoxazole is the treatment of choice for infections caused by *Shigella, Nocardia, Ps maltophila, Ps cepacia, Yersinia enterocolitica, Aeromonas hydrophila* and *Pneumocystis carinii*. Sulfonamides share alternate-drug status with other drugs in the treatment of infections caused by *H influenzae* (if not life-threatening), *Mycobacterium fortuitum, Chlamydia trachomatis*, lymphogranuloma venereum, and meningococcal meningitis.

Sulfonamides sometimes are combined with penicillin or erythromycin in the treatment of otitis media and may be combined with pyrimethamine in toxoplasmosis. Many strains of meningococcus are more sensitive to sulfonamides, but the occurrence of resistant strains has made penicillin G the drug of first choice. They are of use in some UTIs caused by *E coli, Salmonella, Shigella, Staphylococcus, Klebsiella-Enterobacter, Pr mirabilis,* and *Pr vulgaris*.

Sulfonamides are given with pyrimethamine to treat toxoplasmosis in immunosuppressed patients. In regions in which there is a problem of resistance of malarial parasites to the usual antimalarials, sulfonamides may be given in combination with trimethoprim, quinine, pyrimethamine, or other antimalarials. The beneficial effect of sulfasalazine in ulcerative colitis is understood poorly.

TYPES AND CHOICE OF PREPARATIONS—The antimicrobial spectrum of all sulfonamides is essentially the same. However, on the basis of solubility and degree of absorption from the GI tract, the sulfonamides can be divided into two broad classes, namely, those employed for systemic chemotherapy and those intended only for intestinal chemotherapy.

Oral administration of the sulfonamides is preferred. However, when medication cannot be taken by mouth, the soluble sodium or diolamine salts may be given parenterally. Topical chemotherapy rarely is effective, except in the most superficial infections, and may be dangerous because of sensitization. A possible exception is topical use of sulfacetamide sodium in trachoma and inclusion conjunctivitis, for which both topical and systemic treatments are used. A summary of the sulfonamides is presented in Table 90-2.

MIXTURES—Sulfonamide mixtures are designed to minimize the incidence of crystalluria and related renal injury associated with systemic use of sulfonamides. Since the solubility of a particular sulfonamide is not influenced by the presence of others in the same solution, a higher total concentration of sulfonamide can be attained in the urine without precipitation after administration of a mixture than is possible if a single sulfonamide is given.

There is no clinical necessity for less soluble triple sulfonamides because preparations that are more water-soluble are available.

INCOMPATIBILITIES—The sodium derivatives are soluble in water, invariably imparting to the solution a marked alkalinity. Hence, such solutions are incompatible with all acidic substances and with precipitable amines.

Local anesthetics related to para-aminobenzoic acid antagonize the action of the sulfonamides. Ethyl aminobenzoate, procaine, isocaine, butacaine, and tetracaine are related in this way.

PHTHALYLSUFATHIAZOLE

Benzoic acid, 2-[[[4-[(2-thiazolylamino)sulfonyl]phenyl]-amino]-carbonyl]-, Sulfathaladine

[85-73-4] $C_{17}H_{13}N_3O_3S_2$ (403.43).

Preparation—US Pat 2,324,015 (1943).

Description—Foams about 244° to 250° then melts about 272° to 277° dec.

Solubility—Slightly soluble in alcohol, very slightly soluble in ether, very soluble in fixed bases and acids, practically insoluble in water.

Comments—A sulfonamide which is not absorbed orally and is used only for ulcerative colitis.

SULFACETAMIDE

Acetamid, N^1-sulfanilyl-; ing of Sultrin, Trysul

[144-80-9] $C_8H_{10}N_2O_3S$ (214.24).

Preparation—By reacting sulfanilamide with acetic anhydride, followed by controlled alkaline hydrolysis to remove the N^1-acetyl group and subsequent acidification to a pH of approximately 4.

Description—White, crystalline powder; melts about 183°; pK_a 1.78.

Solubility—1 g in approximately 140 mL water; soluble in alcohol; insoluble in ether.

Comments—Employed topically in combination with sulfabenzamide and sulfathiazole for the treatment of vaginitis caused by *Gardnerella (Hemophilus) vaginalis*.

SULFACETAMIDE SODIUM

Acetamide, N-(4-aminophenyl)sulfonyl-, monosodium salt, monohydrate; Soluble Sulfacetamide

N-Sulfanilylacetamide monosodium salt monohydrate [6209-17-2] $C_8H_9N_2NaO_3S \cdot H_2O$ (254.24); *anhydrous* [127-56-0] (236.22).

Preparation—By reacting sulfanilamide with acetic anhydride, followed by controlled alkaline hydrolysis to remove the N^1-acetyl group and subsequent acidification to a pH of approximately 4 to form sulfacetamide which is dissolved in the required quantity of NaOH solution and the solution is evaporated to dryness or precipitated with alcohol.

Description—White, crystalline powder; odorless; bitter taste; pH (1 in 20 solution) between 8 and 9.5.

Solubility—1 g in 2.5 mL water; sparingly soluble in alcohol; practically insoluble in benzene, chloroform, or ether.

Comments—Its *antibacterial* spectrum is similar to that of the other sulfonamides, but it is less potent, owing to poor penetration into both tissues and bacteria. Employed in high concentration by local application, it is of benefit in various ophthalmologic infections, especially those caused by pyogenic cocci, gonococcus, *E coli*, and Koch-Weeks' bacillus.

Trachoma also may respond well sometimes. Since the drug is nonirritating even in high concentration, it can be employed in sufficient concentration to achieve penetration of the ocular tissues.

SULFADIAZINE

Benzenesulfonamide, 4-amino-*N*-(2-pyrimidinyl)-,

N^1-2-Pyrimidinylsulfanilamide [68-35-9] $C_{10}H_{10}N_4O_2S$ (250.27).

Preparation—By combining *p*-acetamidobenzenesulfonyl chloride with 2-aminopyrimidine in the presence of a mild alkaline agent, then splitting off the acetyl group by hydrolyzing with acid or alkali.

Description—White or slightly yellow powder; odorless or nearly so; stable in air, but slowly darkens on exposure to light; melts between 251° and 254°.

Solubility—1 g in approximately 13,000 mL water; sparingly soluble in alcohol and acetone; 1 g in approximately 620 mL human serum at 37; freely soluble in dilute mineral acids, solutions of potassium and sodium hydroxides or ammonia TS.

Comments—The therapeutic uses have been described in the general statement. Sulfadiazine is bound to plasma proteins to the extent of 40% to 50%, and concentrations of the drug in the CSF vary from 50% to 80% of those in the plasma; this is a good tissue concentration, as antibacterial agents go. Thus, it is the sulfonamide of choice for CNS infections susceptible to sulfonamides and for which superior agents are not available; nocardiosis is an example, as is antibiotic-resistant meningococcal meningitis. It readily enters cells, and the volume of distribution is slightly greater than total body water. The tissue-penetrating properties have proven to be of importance in combating UTIs, so that in some such infections it may be superior to the more soluble sulfonamides.

SULFADOXINE

Sulfanilamide, N^1-(5,6-Dimethoxy-4-pyrimidinyl)-, Fanasil, Fanzil

[2447-57-6] $C_{12}H_{14}N_4O_4S$ (310.34).

Preparation—By the general method for N^1-substituted sulfanilamides using 4-amino-5,6-dimethoxypyrimidine for the condensation with the sulfonyl chloride.

Description—White, to creamy white, crystalline powder; melts about 192°.

Solubility—Very slightly soluble in water; slightly soluble in alcohol.

Comments—Has antimicrobial activity similar to that of *Sulfadiazine*. Its principal use, however, is in the prophylaxis or suppression of malaria caused by chloroquine-resistant *P falciparum*. It is used only in combination with pyrimethamine, in a fixed-dose formulation.

SULFAMETHOXAZOLE

Benzenesulfonamide, 4-amino-*N*-(5-methyl-3-isoxazolyl)-, Gantanol

N^1-(5-Methyl-3-isoxazolyl)sulfanilamide [723-46-6] $C_{10}H_{11}N_3O_3S$ (253.28).

Preparation—By the general method for N^1-substituted sulfanilamides using 3-amino-5-methylisoxazole as the coupling amine. The latter may be prepared by heating ethyl 5-methylisoxazole-3-carbamate with aqueous sodium hydroxide. US Pat 2,888,455.

Description—White to off-white, crystalline powder; practically odorless; stable in air; melts about 172°.

Solubility—1 g in 3400 mL water, 50 mL alcohol, 1000 mL chloroform, or 1000 mL ether.

Comments—Chemically, closely related to *Sulfisoxazole*; has high aqueous solubility and low tissue penetrance, with the volume of distribution being considerably less than the extracellular space. It is bound to plasma proteins to the extent of about 68%. Thus, it is best suited to treatment of UTIs caused by susceptible organisms. It is the sulfonamide most used around the world in combination with trimethoprim or pyrimethamine for the treatment of various systemic infections.

SULFAMETHOXAZOLE AND TRIMETHOPRIM

Co-Trimoxazole, TMP-SMZ, Bactrim, Septra

Comments—Sulfamethoxazole and trimethoprim inhibit sequential steps in the formation of tetrahydrofolic acid. Thus, the inhibition is magnified by the independent actions at two consecutive metabolic steps, and bacteriostasis may be altered to that of bactericidal. The incidence of resistance is low but has been increasing with widespread use of the drug. The double blockade also widens the antibacterial spectrum from that of either agent alone.

The predominant use is in the treatment of UTIs, especially recurrent, chronic, or complicated infections not considered controllable by single drugs. With these limitations of use, the rate of development of resistant strains in a community can be retarded. UTIs caused by *E coli, Klebsiella-Enterobacter,* and *Proteus* spp are the ones mostly treated. The combination provides the treatment or prophylaxis of choice for pneumonitis caused by *Pneumocystis carinii* and enterocolitis caused by *Isospora* in immunocompromised patients. However, tissue distribution of sulfamethoxazole is poor, and the pharmacokinetics of the mixture is not optimal for treatment of systemic infections. Trimethoprim enters the CSF and tissues more readily than does sulfamethoxazole, so that the ratio is less than 20:1 at these sites.

In the presence of the sulfonamide, trimethoprim is bound poorly by plasma proteins, so that it filters rapidly into the urine, and less than 40% is metabolized. Consequently, the urine concentration may be 100 times that in plasma, whereas the sulfamethoxazole concentration may be only 3 times higher, thus departing from the supposedly optimal 20:1 ratio. The half-life of trimethoprim is about 9 hr. Impairment of renal function increases the half-life of each drug, the greater effect being on that of sulfamethoxazole.

SULFASALAZINE

Benzoic acid, 2-hydroxy-5-[[4-[(2-pyridinylamino)sulfonyl]phenyl]azo]-, Salicylazosulfapyridine; Azulfidine

[599-79-1] $C_{18}H_{14}N_4O_5S$ (398.39).

Preparation—N^1-2-Pyridylsulfanilamide is diazotized and coupled with salicylic acid.

Description—Light brownish yellow to bright yellow, fine powder; practically tasteless and odorless; melts about 255° with decomposition.

Solubility—1 g in >10,000 mL water, 2900 mL alcohol, >10,000 mL chloroform, or >10,000 mL ether.

Comments—Poorly absorbed from the small intestine, so that the major portion of drug passes into the colon where bacterial enzymes release both 5-aminosalicylic acid and sulfapyridine from the drug. It has a suppressive effect on *ulcerative colitis*, that is not defined precisely. The local antibacterial effect of sulfapyridine in decreasing anaerobic bacteria may not be significant due to systemic absorption. The 5-aminosalicylate inhibits arachidonic acid cascade, both cyclooxygenase and lipoxygenase pathways. Most important may be the inhibition of leukotriene B_4 production by PMNs.

Since some sulfapyridine is absorbed from the colon, this drug has the toxic potential of *Sulfapyridine*.

SULFISOXAZOLE

Benzenesulfonamide, 4-amino-N-(3,4-dimethyl-5-isoxazolyl)-, Gantrisin

N^1-(3,4-Dimethyl-5-isoxazolyl)sulfanilamide [127-69-5] $C_{11}H_{13}N_3O_3S$ (267.30).

Preparation—By the general method for N^1-substituted sulfanilamides using 3,4-dimethyl-5-aminoisoxazole for the condensation with the sulfonyl chloride.

Description—White to slightly yellowish crystalline powder; odorless; melts about 199°.

Solubility—1 g in approximately 6700 mL water; soluble in diluted hydrochloric acid.

Comments—The *antibacterial* properties and therapeutic uses resemble those of sulfadiazine. However, it does not penetrate cells and pass barriers as well as most sulfonamides. Consequently, it is not always effective against systemic infections that are sensitive to other sulfonamides. UTIs caused by sulfonamide-susceptible bacteria respond favorably. However, in genitourinary tract infections in which penetration into the involved tissues is required, it may not be as effective as sulfadiazine. It is secreted into prostatic fluid, but it is not known whether it is secreted into other genitourinary fluids. The extent of protein binding in plasma is 86%. It is metabolized primarily by acetylation and oxidation in the liver. Both it and the conjugate are excreted rapidly by the kidney and reach high concentrations in the urine. The half-life is about 6 hr. Since both the free and acetylated forms are highly soluble, even in acidic urine, adjuvant alkali therapy is not necessary and fluids need not be forced. The incidence of renal toxicity is lower than that caused by sulfadiazine or sulfonamide mixtures. With this excep-

tion, untoward effects during its therapy are similar to those caused by other sulfonamides (see the general statement).

Antibiotics

Antibiotic substances are technically chemical compounds produced by living cells and that inhibit, in very low concentrations, the growth of microorganisms although the term has come to refer to all systemic drugs used to treat bacterial infections. Although antibiotics have been isolated from tissues of higher plants and animals, the term generally has come to refer to inhibitory substances of microbial origin.

The historical development of the field of antibiotics began with the discovery by Chain, Florey, and associates at Oxford University who discovered the favorable therapeutic and pharmacological properties of extracts of cultures of the mold *Penicillium notatum,* found to produce penicillin by Fleming in 1929. The introduction of various acids, amines, or amides into the medium in which the mold is developing leads to the production of biosynthetic penicillins. Dozens of biosynthetic penicillins have been prepared in this manner in an attempt to obtain compounds superior to penicillin G with respect to various physical, microbiological, or pharmacological properties. In 1958 methods were devised for preparing the penicillin nucleus, thus making it possible to biosynthesize penicillins that could not be formed in a more normal medium. The resulting compounds were often more acid-stable, more penicillinase-resistant, or had a wider antibacterial spectrum.

The wide use of antibiotics in animal nutrition and disease has resulted in the sensitization of a relatively large number of the susceptible people, many of whom have serious reactions upon contact with these drugs. Such agricultural use also contributes to the pool of antibiotic-resistant bacteria in a community.

In this chapter penicillin is considered in detail because it is the historical prototype. It was the first antibiotic to be produced commercially and still assumes a position of major importance in this field.

DETECTION AND ISOLATION OF ANTIBIOTIC-PRODUCING ORGANISMS

The detection of productive organisms is based on the ability of cultures of the candidate organism to inhibit certain concomitantly cultured test bacteria under controlled conditions in vitro. A number of different test organisms are used, because no one organism is representative of the antibiotic susceptibilities or organisms in general. Thus, the use of a certain strain of *S aureus* as the test organism will detect all antibiotics inhibitory to that organism, but the antibiotic may or may not also be effective against *E coli,* for example, or even against various other strains of *S aureus.* To ensure securing a valid antibacterial spectrum, a number of species and types of strains must be used in the testing.

Antibiotic-producing organisms can be obtained by testing pure cultures of organisms available in culture collections or isolated from natural sources, and "screening," or selection through suitable techniques from the vast heterogeneous mixed population of the soil or other natural habitations of microorganisms. In the first case, the practice consists simply of adding to broth or agar cultures, seeded with the test organism, suitable quantities or culture filtrates of the cultures being examined, incubating and inspecting for inhibition of the test organism. The screening method involves plating out in serial dilution an aqueous extract of soil or other natural substrate using a medium, usually agar, previously seeded with the test organism. During incubation the various organisms of the soil population develop, and those forming antibiotic substances are distinguished by a clear zone or halo around the colony, indicative of inhibition of the test organism which, in the region beyond the clear zone, grows abundantly in the form of a marked turbidity throughout the agar.

Many modifications of this principle are employed. Thus, the use of different media, pH, temperature, and substrates will expose, for screening, different types of soil organisms. These conditions must be compatible with the growth of the particular test organism employed. Theoretically, the best chance for detecting the largest possible number of antagonists lies in the preincubation of the agar cultures containing the soil dilutions, but without the test bacteria. This is followed by a secondary incubation after the test organism is applied to the plate by streaking or spraying. In this manner slow-growing soil organisms are given the opportunity to develop and manifest antibiotic-producing ability.

Once detected, the antagonist is isolated in pure culture and identified, and the optimal conditions for production of the antibiotic substance produced by it are investigated. The composition of the medium is important. Different organic and inorganic nitrogenous substances are tested, with and without various carbohydrates, minerals, heavy metals, etc.

Once a favorable medium is established, other known strains of the antagonist, obtained either from stock-culture collections or isolated from nature, are compared for the character and amount of the antibiotic produced, and the highest yielding strain selected for further work. The antibacterial spectrum is obtained, ie, the relative effectiveness of the antibiotic in inhibiting the growth of a large variety of gram-positive and gram-negative bacteria, rickettsiae, viruses, and fungi, especially those that are pathogenic. This indicates those infections in which it may be useful chemotherapeutically.

Several concentrates or isolates of the antibiotic, not necessarily pure, then are examined for toxicity in mice. Only low-toxicity preparations and, in particular, those in which toxicity is inversely proportional to the antibacterial potency are of interest. Toxicity and pharmacological data are obtained in animals and, if favorable, in clinical trials on human beings. If the clinical trials show the antibiotic to be a promising therapeutic agent, attention is turned to large-scale manufacture. Chemical studies of the structure of the pure compound will indicate the feasibility of chemical synthesis. Generally, antibiotics are complex substances whose synthesis may be extremely difficult, or at least uneconomical, compared with microbiologic production. This is the case now with most of the successful antibiotics, such as penicillin, streptomycin or chlortetracycline.

The gradual increase in numbers of strains of microorganisms resistant to antibiotics, especially the staphylococci, and the numbers of individuals developing sensitivity to them make it extremely desirable that screening programs for the isolation and development of new agents be continued.

PRODUCTION

The development and operation of the large-scale commercial production of antibiotic substances may be exemplified by a description of the manufacture of penicillin. In general, the approach and methods employed are typical. Two types of processes for the microbiological production of antibiotics are:

The surface process, in which the antibiotic-producing organism grows in the form of a pad on the surface of a liquid medium in trays or bottles, or on the surface of a finely divided moist solid substrate such as wood shavings or wheat bran.

The submerged process, in which the organism develops in a liquid medium, maintained continuously under mechanical agitation and aeration, so that the organism develops uniformly and homogeneously in the form of a suspension of single cells, or small aggregates or colonies, throughout all portions of the culture liquid.

The penicillin is excreted into the culture fluid. The molds used industrially today are derived from *Penicillium chrysogenum*.

In the submerged process, growth is accelerated greatly and the handling of large quantities greatly facilitated. It is considerably more efficient than the surface processes, and hence is the only feasible method for large-scale commercial production. Stationary, closed tanks, known as fermenters, of 5000- to 30,000-gal capacity, are used in penicillin manufacture. Most of these are equipped with vertical single-shaft propeller or turbine-type agitators and with a mechanical means of comminuting and distributing sterile air, introduced for maximum dispersal effect in the region of the agitator. The tanks have a detachable manhole on the top, sight glasses, and outlets to valve-closed sampling lines and accessory feed chambers, enabling inoculation by hand if necessary, particularly in small seed tanks, and the addition whenever necessary of other (sterile) materials, such as antifoam agents, during the fermentation. All outlets from the tank are exposed continuously to flowing steam to minimize chances of contamination. The culture medium is sterilized by high-pressure steam and subsequently cooled. Temperature control during growth of the mold is maintained automatically at 23° to 25°. The compressed air, which is introduced into the fermenters, is sterilized by filtration through steam-sterilized cartridges of suitable size and filled, for example, with glass wool.

Inoculum for large tanks is obtained by building up the amount of growth successively through a series of seed tanks, from tank to tank, and transferring under air pressure through sterile pipe lines. Generally, this massive inoculum amounts to 5% to 10% of the main batch and, consequently, seed tanks are approximately 1/10 the volume of the next larger tank. The first and smallest seed tank is inoculated with a laboratory-prepared culture, consisting either of spores or of a small flask of submerged growth obtained on a laboratory-, rotary-, or reciprocal-type shaking machine.

The stock or master culture of the penicillin-producing mold is dry and cold-preserved in the form of spores. Continuous vegetative transfer of the mold on artificial media leads to loss of penicillin-producing power (physiological degeneration). Hence, the number of intermediate transfers between master culture and the final batch is kept at a minimum.

A Typical Production Medium	
Corn-steep liquor (solids)	2 to 5%
Crude lactose	2 to 3%
Calcium carbonate	0.5 to 1%

The culture medium used for commercial production of penicillin generally contains natural nitrogenous material, nitrate, α-aminoadipic acid, cottonseed meal, or corn-steep liquor, which is a by-product of the corn-milling industry, lactose, side-chain precursor, surface-active agent, and mineral salts (including sulfate). The penicillin potency is followed by assay every 3 to 6 hours and, at the time when the potency stops rising, the batch is harvested. Maximum activity generally is reached in 50 to 90 hours. Because of the instability of penicillin at ordinary temperatures, the batch is cooled to 5° and the mycelium filtered off by pressure filtration.

The penicillin is extracted and concentrated by charcoal adsorption or solvent extraction.

IMPROVEMENTS IN PRODUCTION—The greatest advancements in the production of penicillin have been the use of the submerged or tank method of production, the use of corn-steep liquor, and the progressive improvement in the penicillin-producing capacity of the mold.

The earliest widely used strain in tank production was *Penicillium notatum*, No 832, which yielded 50 to 60 units/mL. Later, a strain of *Penicillium chrysogenum*, No 1951B25, with maximum yields of 250 units/mL, was discovered. Spores of this organism, exposed to x-ray irradiation and tested from single spore isolates, led to selection of a mutant strain X1612 producing approximately 500 units/mL. Strain X1612 was subjected to ultraviolet irradiation and strain Q176, yielding penicillin potencies of more than double that of X1612, was obtained. This strain has been used widely in commercial production, but industry has even improved on it. Some variant strains produce several thousand units/mL. The improvement in strains suit-able for the surface production of penicillin followed a similar path although these were obtained by testing single spore isolates from parent cultures. A strain excellent in submerged culture is not necessarily good for surface culture, and *vice versa*. Surface culture methods are no longer used for commercial production of any of the presently useful antibiotics.

A large number of different fungi are now known to produce penicillin. More than 20 different species of *Aspergillus* and *Penicillia* produce penicillin, as do the dermatophyte *Trichophyton mentagrophytes* and a thermophilic fungus, *Malbranchea pulchella*.

CONTROL

Federal control of antibiotics dates back to an amendment of the 1938 Food, Drug and Cosmetic Act (Section 507) under which the FDA was required to pretest all forms of penicillin and its preparations before releasing them for sale. This certification covered potency, demonstration of nontoxicity and moisture content (the presence of excess moisture makes penicillin less stable). When intended for parenteral use, it also was tested for freedom from pyrogens, for sterility, clarity, and pH of its solutions.

This amendment included the provision that when it was found by the Federal Security Administrator (now Secretary HHS) that the pretesting of penicillin or its preparations was no longer necessary to insure safety and efficacy of such drugs, they could be exempted from the pretesting requirement.

Under this provision of the Act the Federal Security Agency, FDA Division, finding that certain new, highly purified forms of penicillin no longer required pretesting, issued a notice in the *Federal Register* of April 13, 1949, exempting Crystalline Penicillin G Potassium and Crystalline Penicillin G Sodium from this provision.

In March 1947, the Congress of the US placed streptomycin under the certification system and in July 1949 included chlortetracycline, chloramphenicol, and bacitracin. Because these amendments include all derivatives as well, both dihydrostreptomycin and tetracycline, as well as pyrrolidinomethyl tetracycline and demeclocycline, were certifiable drugs.

In May 1963, the Drug Amendments passed by Congress in 1962 became effective and superseded all previous rulings. These now provide that all antibiotics used in humans are subject to certification. Furthermore, those certifiable prior to passage of these latest amendments, ie, chlortetracycline, bacitracin, streptomycin, penicillin, and chloramphenicol, also must be certified for veterinary use.

CLASSES AND AGENTS

Antibiotics are classified by various schemes, the two most important being according to mechanism of action and according to chemical relationship. The antibiotic monographs that follow will be arranged according to chemical relationships.

Beta-Lactam Antibiotics

PENICILLINS

HISTORY—During an inspection of some culture plates in the laboratory of St Mary's Hospital London, in 1928, Professor Alexander Fleming observed the lysis of staphylococcus organisms by a contaminating mold. Upon subculturing the mold he found in the broth a powerful, but nontoxic, antibacterial substance. He gave it the name "penicillin" from the organism *Penicillium notatum*, which caused the generation of the antibiotic.

CHEMISTRY—The name "penicillin" now designates a number of antibiotic substances produced by the growth of various *Penicillium* species or by other means. The better known natural penicillins are listed in Table 90-3. Penicillins F, G, and X were referred to formerly as I, II, and III, respectively.

The parent compound is (2*S*-*cis*)-4-thia-1-azabicyclo[3.2.0] hepatane-2-carboxylic acid (I). The 3,3-dimethyl-7-oxo deriva-

tive of I is known commonly by the trivial name penicillanic acid (II) and the penicillins are α-carboxamido derivatives of it (III):

Penicillins are named variously in the literature as derivatives of I, II, or III above. Nomenclature by I is purely systematic, whereas that by II or III is trivial. As derivatives of II, it is merely necessary to identify the specific α-carboxyamido group; as derivatives of III, only the R of the α-carboxamido group is identified.

The introduction of various acids, amines, or amides into the medium in which the mold is developing leads to the production of biosynthetic penicillins which differ only in R. Dozens of biosynthetic *penicillins* have been prepared in this manner in an attempt to obtain compounds superior to penicillin G with respect to various physical, microbiological, or pharmacological properties. In 1958 methods were devised for preparing the penicillin nucleus, thus making it possible to biosynthesize penicillins that could not be formed in a more normal medium. The resulting compounds were often more acid-stable, more penicillinase-resistant, or had a wider antibacterial spectrum.

Table 90-3. Penicillins

CLASS	COMMENTS
Natural Penicillins (best streptococcal and narrow spectrum)	
Penicillin G	Best narrow spectrum (streptococci), IV, IM
Penicillin V	Same spectrum as Pen G, oral only
Penicillinase-resistant Penicillins (antistaphylococcal)	
Cloxacillin	Oral
Dicloxacillin	Preferred oral
Methicillin	IV, interstitial nephritis may occur
Nafcillin	Preferred IV drug for Staph.
Oxacillin	Oral
Aminopenicillins (improved gram-neg, *H influenzae*, *Enterococcus*, *Shigella*, *Salmonella*)	
Amoxacillin	Good oral absorption,
Ampicillin	Preferred IV drug, incomplete oral absorp., diarrhea, rash
Bacampicillin	Oral prodrug converted to ampicillin
Extended-spectrum (antipseudomonal) penicillins	
Carbenicillin	IV, high sodium, oral prodrug available
Ticarcillin	IV, similar to carbenicillin but less sodium
Mezlocillin	IV, similar to piperacillin
Piperacillin	Preferred IV, best gram-neg. spectrum
Beta-Lactamase Combinations (expand spectrum to staph., beta-lactamase producers)	
Clavulanalate-Amoxacillin	Oral, more diarrhea than amoxacillin
Sulbactam-Ampicillin	IV, active vs. staph. and beta-lactamase-producing *H influenzae* and *Strep pneum*
Clavulanate-Ticarcillin	IV, active vs. more gram-neg. bacilli
Tazobactam-Piperacillin	IV, active vs. more gram-neg. bacilli

Much of the penicillin of commerce is pure crystalline G. It occurs in fermentation liquors together with variable amounts of K and F penicillins and smaller amounts of others, and is separated from the other penicillins during purification. Commercial practice suppresses, to a certain extent, the natural tendency of the mold to form penicillins other than the desired G by the incorporation of a precursor of G, namely phenylacetic acid, phenylacetamide, phenylethylamine, or other substance containing the phenylacetyl radical, which is built directly into the penicillin G molecule. Penicillin G has the additional advantage of being much easier to crystallize than K or F.

As seen in figures I, II, and III, penicillins are acids. The potassium salt predominates in use, with the sodium salt next. These salts are very soluble in water. The acid moiety can be used to combine penicillins with various bases, such as procaine or benzathine, to create insoluble salts, for repository use, or for the purpose of decreasing solubility so as to make the compound more resistant to gastric acid.

Penicillin in solution is very unstable at pH 5 or less and at 8 or more. Solutions of penicillin begin to deteriorate upon standing a few days, even in the cold. Certain penicillins are more resistant to acid hydrolysis and thus lend themselves better to oral administration.

CLASSIFICATION AND SPECTRUM—Penicillins formerly were classified according to pseudohistorical divisions, by "generation," similar to the classification of the cephalosporins. However, it is more useful to classify them according to a mixture of chemical and antimicrobial designations. The categories are *penicillin G, acid-stable penicillins, penicillinase-resistant penicillins, amino penicillins, extended-spectrum penicillins,* and *amdinopenicillins.* There is a great deal of overlap in the properties among the categories. For example, two of the penicillinase-resistant, all of the amino penicillins and one extended-spectrum penicillin are sufficiently acid-stable to be orally effective; amino penicillins, extended-spectrum penicillins, and amdinocillin are all resistant to certain β-lactamases (which often are called penicillinases indiscriminately) and variably resistant to Class II β-lactamases, to which the term, penicillinase, is becoming restricted. All penicillins are bacteriostatic at low and bactericidal at high concentrations. Their antimicrobial spectra differ according to the pattern of β-lactamase resistance, the ability to penetrate the outer membrane of gram-negative bacteria and selectivities for the various bacterial transpeptidases (penicillin binding proteins; PBPs).

Although penicillin G is destroyed largely by gastric acid, its low oral bioavailability can be compensated by increased dosage. Penicillin V is the only marketed member of the acid-stable class. These two drugs/classes have nearly identical antimicrobial spectra, except that sensitivities to penicillin-V are not high enough for a number of gram-negative infections to be treated by the oral route. The spectrum is *narrow* and mostly limited to gram-positive bacteria, gram-negative cocci, and a few miscellaneous bacteria. They are especially active against gram-positive bacteria, particularly *Strep pyogenes,* most *pneumococci, Cl tetani* and *perfringens, Coryn diphtheriae, B anthracis, Bacteroides, Eubacterium, Fusobacterium, Listeria monocytogenes, Peptococcus,* and *Peptostreptococcus.*

Although *Staph aureus* and *epidermidis* were originally mostly sensitive, they are now over 90% resistant in hospital populations and 50% in the community. *Strep viridans* is variably sensitive. *Strep faecalis* (enterococcus) is usually resistant. The gram-negative cocci, *N meningitidis* and *N gonorrhoeae,* are mostly sensitive, although resistance is increasing rapidly. Activity against the gram-negative bacilli is usually too low to be of clinical significance, but over 80% of strains of *E coli, Enterobacter,* most *Prot mirabilis* and some *Salmonella* and *Shigella* are sufficiently sensitive to respond in the urinary tract, where drug concentrations are high. Concentrations are also high in the bile, and these penicillins may be used to treat biliary tract infections caused by some enterobacteria and enterococci. These drugs are also active against *Actinomycetes, Leptospira, Providencia, Spirillum minus, Streptobacillus moniliformis,* and *Treponema pallidum.*

Resistance of gram-positive and a number of gram-negative bacteria to penicillins G and V results from the bacterial elaboration of so-called penicillinase. This kind of resistance was obviated by the development of penicillins, which penicillinase cannot destroy. The first member of the penicillinase-resistant class was *methicillin,* to which *cloxacillin, dicloxacillin, nafcillin,* and *oxacillin* were added. These drugs have approximately the same spectrum of activity as the former two drugs, except increased activity against most staphylococci (especially), enterococci, gonococci, and meningococci.

The *amino penicillins* include *ampicillin, amoxacillin, becampicillin, cyclicillin,* and *epicillin.* Each has an amino group adjacent to the carbonyl of the *N*-acyl substituent. Efficacy is increased against enterococcus, meningococcus, and several gram-negative bacilli, such as community-acquired *E coli, H influenzae, Pr mirabilis,* various *Salmonella* and *Shigella.* However, there is less activity against most gram-positive bacteria, *N gonorrhoeae, B anthracis, Bacteroides, Clostridium, Corynebacterium, Enterobacter, Eubacterium, Listeria, Peptococcus, Peptostreptococcus, Providencia, Streptobacillus, Actinomyces,* and *Treponema*; consequently, this group also has been called *shifted-spectrum penicillins.* There are important differences among the spectra of the various members, ampicillin having the broadest spectrum but amoxacillin being the only one to be effective against *Strep viridans.* Only ampicillin has clinically significant activity against *Salmonella* and *Shigella.*

The *extended-spectrum* (antipseudomonal) *penicillins* include *azlocillin, carbenicillin, indanylcarbenicillin, mezlocillin, piperacillin,* and *ticarcillin.* There is increased activity against *Acinetobacter, Citrobacter, E coli, Enterobacter, H influenzae, Klebsiella, Morganella morganii, Pr mirabilis* and *vulgaris, Providencia rettgeri* and *stuartii, Ps aeruginosa, Bacteroides, Clostridium, Eubacterium, Fusobacterium, Peptococcus, Peptostreptococcus,* and *Veillonella.* They are even less active than amino penicillins against most gram-positive bacteria, *Actinomycetes* and *Treponema,* and they are not used to treat infections by these pathogens. There are considerable differences among the members. Neither azlocillin nor mezlocillin is active against staphylococci; azlocillin is inactive against *Pseudomonas* or *Neisseria* and *carbenicillin* is inactive against *Eubacterium.* Only piperacillin is active against *Strep viridans* and azlocillin and mezlocillin against *Providencia stuartii.*

Amdinocillin is the only marketed member of the class by the same name. It has a very limited spectrum. No infections by gram-positive or anaerobic bacteria are treatable. Among the gram-negative bacteria only *Citrobacter, Enterobacter, E coli, Klebsiella, Salmonella, Serratia,* and *Shigella* are sensitive enough so that this drug is used alone to treat infections by them. In combination with other β-lactams, it may be used against *Prot mirabilis, Morganella morganii,* and *Providencia.*

RESISTANCE—The penicillin resistance of many gram-positive and gram-negative bacteria is owing to their elaboration of penicillin-destroying enzymes called *beta-lactamases.* They are produced by large numbers of bacteria and actinomycetes and convert penicillin into inactive *penicilloic acid* by liberation of a second carboxyl group. The enzymes from staphylococci, enterococci, meningococci, gonococci, and various other bacteria were the first-known beta-lactamases and were called *penicillinases.* Penicillinases are Group II beta-lactamases, acidic proteins which are resistant to mercuric ions. Although they are inducible, the capacity for induction is determined by a plasmid-located gene.

Resistance of bacteria to penicillin cannot be explained entirely on penicillinase production because many resistant organisms produce little or no penicillinase. Nonpenicillinase-mediated resistance is called *methicillin resistance.* It is caused by an alteration in the target transpeptidase (penicillin-binding protein I). With some bacteria, eg, *Staph aureus,* resistance develops very fast clinically, but some microorganisms, eg, *T pallidum,* never become resistant. Resistance by staphylococci currently is a major hospital problem.

More resistant bacteria dwell in hospital personnel than in the community at large, because such personnel are close to patients under treatment. Acquired resistance is the result of the selection of natural penicillin-resistant strains that ordinarily are held in check by the sensitive parent strain. Resistant genes may be acquired by mutation, transduction by viruses, transformation, and conjugative transfer of resistant-gene-containing plasmids.

MECHANISM—Penicillin is known to interfere with the synthesis of peptidoglycans, which are part of the cell-wall material. Consequently, the growing protoplast cannot form a protective cell wall. Several wall enzymes are reversibly inhibited, the most important being a D, D-carboxypeptidase, which also functions as a transpeptidase. Conditions favoring rapid growth of bacteria are best for the inhibitory action of penicillin, owing to the fact that the cell must be producing cell wall-lysing enzymes during the time transpeptidases are inhibited in order for cell-wall lysis to occur. Under favorable conditions, penicillin exerts a direct bactericidal action, and successful penicillin therapy may be relatively independent of immunity mechanisms of the host.

POTENCY—The potency of penicillin is expressed in units/mg. *One International Unit is equivalent to the activity of 0.6 μg of pure crystalline sodium penicillin G* to which, by international conference, a potency of 1667 units/mg has been assigned. See Table 90-3. Because of the large doses now used, it is common to speak in terms of megaunits, ie, 1 megaunit equals 10^6 Units.

ASSAY—See *Biological Testing.*

COMMENTS—Although penicillin G is the original penicillin, it remains the drug of choice for the treatment of almost all infections caused by nonpenicillinase-producing, nonmethicillin-resistant gram-positive bacteria, the integrity of which depends upon cell walls. Thus, it is the drug of choice against infections by gram-positive, nonpenicillinase-producing cocci, such as *Staph aureus* or *epidermidis, Strep bovis,* Group B, *pyogenes, viridans, faecalis* (enterococcus; in combination with gentamycin, for serious infections, only) or *pneumoniae* (pneumococcus), *Peptococcus* or *Peptostreptococcus* and gram-positive bacilli, such as *B anthracis* or *Cl perfringens* or *tetani.* It is thus also the drug of choice against infections by nonpenicillinase-producing strains of the gram-negative coccus, *N meningitidis,* the gram-negative bacillus *Bacteroides fragilis* (especially oropharyngeal strains), *Fusobacterium, Leptotrichia buccalis, Pasteurella multicida, Spirillum minus,* or *Streptobacillus moniliformis,* the actinomycete, *Actinomyces israelii,* or the spirochete, *Leptospira* or *Treponema pallidum.*

It is an alternative drug to treat infections by *Coryn, diphtheriae, Vibrio vulnificus,* or *Borrelia burgdorferi.* Penicillin V shares with penicillin G first choice status in the treatment of lesser staphylococcal infections and streptococcal (pneumococcal) pneumonia.

Penicillinase-resistant penicillins are drugs of choice only for the treatment of infections by penicillinase-producing staphylococci. They also can be used as penicillinase inhibitors, to combine with penicillin G; however, clavulanate, sulbactam, and tazobactam are preempting that use.

An aminopenicillin is the drug of choice for the treatment of infections by *Strep* Group B (ampicillin; shares status with penicillin G), *Branhamella* catarrhalis (amoxacillin), *E coli* (ampicillin, combined with an aminoglycoside), *Prot mirabilis, Salmonella* (except *typhi*), *Eikenella corrodens* (with or without clavulanate or sulbactam), mild-to-moderate infections by *H influenzae* (with or without clavulanate or sulbactam), or *Listeria monocytogenes* (with or without gentamycin).

It is an alternate drug for the treatment of infections by penicillinase-producing *Staphylococcus* (with clavulanate), *Bordetella pertussis, E coli* (with clavulanate, sulbactam, or tazobactam), *Gardnerella vaginalis, H influenzae* (serious infections; initially in combination with chloramphenicol), *Kl pneumoniae* (with clavulanate or sulbactam), *Morganella morganii, Prot vulgaris* (with clavulanate or sulbactam), *Pasteurella multicida* (with clavulanate or sulbactam), *Salmonella typhi,* or *Shigella.*

An extended-spectrum (antipseudomonal) penicillin is the drug of choice only for the treatment of infections by sensitive *Ps aeruginosa.* It is an alternate drug for the treatment of infections by penicillinase-producing *Staphylococcus, Acinetobacter, Bacteroides fragilis* (gastrointestinal strains), *Enterobacter, Kl pneumoniae* (with clavulanate or sulbactam), *Morganella morganii* (with clavulanate or sulbactam), *Prot mirabilis* or *vulgaris* (with clavulanate or sulbactam), *Providencia rettgeri* or *stuartii* (with clavulanate or sulbactam), *Ps aeruginosa* (urinary tract infections), or *Serratia.*

A penicillin is employed sometimes in *combination* with other agents. The results of such therapy are often, but not invariably, superior to those obtainable with a penicillin alone. When it is administered with the tetracyclines, chloramphenicol, or the sulfonamides, antagonism may be noted if the microorganism is highly susceptible to a penicillin when it is administered alone. Nevertheless, it often is used in combination with chloramphenicol in the treatment of bacterial meningitis caused by *H influenzae.*

The number of bacteria and the quantity of pus appear to have only a minor influence upon the antibacterial action of penicillin, except when the organism produces an appropriate β-lactamase.

ADVERSE EFFECTS—Penicillin is practically nontoxic. However, hypersensitivity reactions occur in several percent of patients, depending on the type of preparation employed and the route of administration. The most-common manifestation of this allergic response is a skin rash. Nondermatological manifestations of allergy include serum sickness, angioedema, nephropathy, rare hemolytic anemia, Arthus reaction, rare pericarditis, enteropathy, hepatotoxicity, and anaphylaxis. Neutropenia, which occasionally results from high-dose therapy, does not appear to involve an immune process.

Side effects of oral administration of penicillins are nausea, vomiting, epigastric distress, diarrhea, and black "hairy" tongue.

Like other antibiotics, penicillin markedly can alter the normal bacterial flora of man. As a result, superimposed infection by a penicillin-resistant microorganism may develop during the course of treatment, and appropriate chemotherapy should be instituted as soon as possible. Overgrowth (suprainfection) even occurs in the bowel, because penicillin is secreted into the bile, which keeps the intestinal levels high. Coagulation disorders also may occur as the result of the suppression of enteric bacteria that synthesize vitamin K.

Very high concentrations of penicillin are neurotoxic, and nerve damage has resulted from intramuscular administration. Crystalline penicillin has an irritating effect when applied directly to the central nervous system. Symptoms after intrathecal administration include listlessness, headache, nausea, vomiting, respiratory difficulty, cyanosis, fall in blood pressure, thready pulse, muscular twitching, and convulsions. These are reduced or eliminated by lowering dosage.

With sodium and potassium salts, the effect of the cation load must be considered. Lastly, untoward effects sometimes result from the rapid bactericidal effects, because of the release of endotoxins and other bacterial cell components.

ABSORPTION, DISTRIBUTION, AND EXCRETION—Penicillin G in the form of its sodium or potassium salt is absorbed rapidly from subcutaneous and intramuscular sites. The intramuscular route is preferred. Penicillin G is given intravenously by continuous infusion only when it is imperative to maintain very high blood concentrations such as in the treatment of subacute *bacterial endocarditis.* The rate of absorption from intramuscular sites of injection may be slowed markedly by the use of repository (depot) preparations consisting of relatively insoluble salts of penicillin in a suitable vehicle. For example, therapeutic blood levels (for some purposes) persist 12 to 24 hours after a single 300,000-unit dose of *Procaine Penicillin in Aqueous Suspension,* 24 to 48 hours after *Procaine Penicillin in Oil,* and 1 wk or more after 1.2 million units of *Benzathine Penicillin G.* However, the slower the absorption, the lower the peak plasma level, and some uses are precluded.

The absorption of penicillin G from the gastrointestinal tract is incomplete and irregular, but some acid-stable penicillins are absorbed well. To obtain the same blood concentrations as by the intramuscular route, 3 to 5 times the parenteral dose of penicillin G must be employed. Penicillin G should be ingested when the stomach is empty because penicillin binds to food substances. Although hydrochloric acid in the gastric juice destroys penicillin G, buffer agents have not proved to be necessary for successful oral medication, because the dose can be raised to compensate. Oral penicillin G therapy should never be relied upon alone in severe infections.

Penicillins are distributed in the extracellular water, but they penetrate cells poorly. Tissue concentrations are approximately ¼ the plasma concentration *at equilibrium*. Plasma levels fall so fast that there is not enough time for the build-up of high concentrations in many tissues. Diffusion of penicillins into CSF is minimal unless the meninges are inflamed. The preferred route of administration for treatment of bacterial meningitis is IV supplemented by IM injection. It usually is not recommended to use intrathecal administration of penicillins because of the irritative effect of even low doses of penicillin on the CNS. Local instillation may be used in various body cavities to supplement systemic administration.

Penicillins are secreted mostly into the urine, partly by glomerular filtration but mostly by tubular secretion (80%). Substances that interfere with renal tubular excretion of penicillin (see *Probenecid*) serve to enhance and prolong the effective blood levels of the antibiotic. Probenecid can block completely the renal tubular secretion of penicillin, which slows excretion; it also decreases removal from the CSF. Phenylbutazone also interferes with excretion to a degree comparable to probenecid; sulfinpyrazone, aspirin, indomethacin, and some sulfonamides also moderately interfere with the excretion of penicillin. The normal plasma half-time of penicillin G is approximately 45 minutes, but in persons over 65 years it is almost twice as long. In oliguria, it may be 7 to 10 hours. The penicillins are summarized in Table 90-3.

AMOXICILLIN

[2S-[2α,5α,6β(S*)]]-4-Thia-1-azabicyclo[3.2.0]heptane-2-carboxylic acid, 6-[[amino(4-hydroxyphenyl)acetyl]amino] 3,3-dimethyl-7-oxo-, trihydrate

D(−)-α-Amino-*p*-hydroxybenzylpenicillin; [61336-70-7] $C_{16}H_{19}N_3O_5S \cdot 3H_2O$ (419.45); *anhydrous* [26787-78-0] (365.30).

Preparation—By acylation of 6-aminopenicillanic acid with D-(−)-2-(*p*-hydroxyphenyl)glycine.

Description—Fine, white to off-white, crystalline powder; bitter taste; high humidity and temperature over 37°adversely affect stability.

Solubility—1 g in 370 mL water or 2000 mL alcohol.

Comments—Amoxicillin, the *p*-hydroxy analog of ampicillin, has an antibacterial spectrum similar to that of *Ampicillin*, except that it is less active against *Streptococcus*, *N meningitidis*, *Clostridium*, *Salmonella*, and *Shigella*. Like ampicillin, it is destroyed by β-lactamases. However, it is more acid-stable than ampicillin, and absorption is not affected appreciably by food; it cannot be given parenterally. It is the drug of choice for infections caused by *Enterococcus faecalis* (enterococcus), *Branhamella catarrhalis,* or *Bacteroides fragilis* (mild to moderate infections). It is an alternate drug for infections by penicillinase-producing *Staphylococcus* (combined with clavulanate), *N gonorrhoeae* (with probenecid), *E coli* (with clavulanate), or *Pasteurella multicida* (with clavulanate). It cannot be given parenterally for severe infections. The toxicity is that of ampicillin, but there is less diarrhea and rash.

By the oral route, 75% to 90% is absorbed. In plasma, it is 17% protein-bound. The volume of distribution is 0.31 mL/g. From 50% to 72% is eliminated by renal tubular secretion. The half-life is about 1 hr when renal function is normal and 8 to 16 hr in renal failure.

AMPICILLIN

[2S-[2α,5α,6β(S*)]]-4-Thia-1-azabicyclo[3.2.0]heptane-2-carboxylic acid, 6-[(aminophenylacetyl)amino]-3,3-dimethyl-7-oxo-,

[69-53-4] $C_{16}H_{19}N_3O_4S$ (349.40); *trihydrate* [7177-48-2] (403.45). Potency: 900 to 1050 μg of $C_{16}H_{19}N_3O_4S$/mg, calculated on the anhydrous basis.

Preparation—6-Aminopenicillanic acid is acylated with D-glycine. US Pat 2,985,648.

Description—White, crystalline powder; practically odorless; occurs as the trihydrate, which is stable at room temperature.

Solubility—1 g in approximately 90 mL water or 250 mL absolute alcohol; practically insoluble in ether or chloroform.

Comments—The *first aminopenicillin* (see the general statement). Its in vitro spectrum against gram-positive cocci is similar to but generally somewhat less effective than that of penicillin G, except that it is somewhat more effective against *Enterococcus faecalis* (enterococcus). It is ½₀ as effective against *Strep pyogenes*.

It is poorly effective against penicillinase-producing organisms. It is the drug of choice for treatment of infections due to sensitive strains of Strep Group B, *Enterococcus faecalis* (combined with gentamycin), *Listeria monocytogenes* (with or without gentamycin), *E coli* (with or without gentamycin) and *Prot mirabilis*, and *Salmonella* (not *typhi*). It is an alternative drug against *Kl pneumoniae* (with sulbactam), indole-positive *Proteus* (*M morganii*, *Pr vulgaris* and *Providencia rettgeri*; with sulbactam), *Salmonella typhi*, *Shigella*, *Gardnerella vaginalis*, *H influenzae* (serious infections; initially combined with chloramphenicol) or *Nocardia*. Some of these readily acquire resistance by elaboration of penicillinase, so it is given often in combination with sulbactam.

It causes allergic reactions typical of other penicillins. It is 5 times as allergenic as penicillin G. The incidence of rashes is about 7%, but most of these are not allergenic; they are especially prevalent in patients with infectious mononucleosis. Patients allergic to penicillin G are often also allergic to ampicillin. The drug also may cause nausea and vomiting, diarrhea, glossitis, and stomatitis. It is acid-resistant and is 30% to 50% absorbed by the oral route.

AMPICILLIN SODIUM

[2S-[2α,5α,6β(S*)]]-4-Thia-1-azabicyclo[3.2.0]heptane-2-carboxylic acid, 6-(aminophenylacetyl)amino]-3,3-dimethyl-7-oxo-, monosodium salt

[69-52-3] $C_{16}H_{18}N_3NaO_4S$ (371.39). Potency: not less than 845 μg of ampicillin/mg, on the anhydrous basis.

Preparation—*Ampicillin* is dissolved in a suitable organic solvent and precipitated as the sodium salt by the addition of sodium acetate.

Description—White to off-white, crystalline powder; hygroscopic; pK_{a1} 2.66; pK_{a2} 7.24.

Solubility—Very soluble in water, isotonic NaCl or dextrose solutions.

Comments—Has the actions and uses of *Ampicillin*, and is the form in which ampicillin is employed for intramuscular and intravenous administration.

AZLOCILLIN SODIUM—see RPS-18, page 1187.

BACAMPICILLIN HYDROCHLORIDE

4-Thia-1-azabicyclo[3.2.0]heptane-2-carboxylic acid,[2S-[2α,5α,6β(S*)]]-,-6-[(aminophenylacetyl)amino]-3,3-dimethyl-7-oxo-, 1-[(ethoxycarbonyl)oxy]ethyl] ester, monohydrochloride,

[37661-08-8]$C_{21}H_{27}N_4O_7S \cdot HCl$ (501.98).

Preparation—US Pat 3,939,270.

Description—White crystals; melts about 175°; pH (2% aqueous solution) 3 to 4.5.

Solubility—1 g in approximately 15 mL water, 7 mL alcohol or 10 mL chloroform.

Comments—An *aminopenicillin* with improved gram-negative activity against *H influenzae*, *Enterococcus*, *Shigella*, and *Salmonella*. It is an oral prodrug converted to *Ampicillin*.

CARBENICILLIN DISODIUM

[2S-(2α,5α,6β)-4-Thia-1-azabicyclo[3.2.0]heptane-2-carboxylic acid, 6- [(carboxyphenylacetyl)amino]-3,3-dimethyl-7-oxo-, disodium salt; Geopen, Pyopen

(α-Carboxybenzyl)penicillin Disodium [4800-94-6] $C_{17}H_{16}N_2Na_2O_6S$ (422.36). Potency: the equivalent of not less than 770 μg of carbenicillin/mg, calculated on the anhydrous basis.

Preparation—One method consists of hydrolyzing esters of the type

(R = alkyl, aryl, or benzyl) with the aid of a suitable esterase, such as α-chymotrypsin or pancreatin, and extracting the acid and reacting it with aqueous $NaHCO_3$. *Chem Abstr* 1970; 72:41674a. The starting esters may be prepared by acylating 6-aminopenicillanic acid with monoesters of phenylmalonic acid. US Pats 3,282,926 and 3,492,291.

Description—White to off-white, crystalline powder; bitter taste; hygroscopic; odorless, pH (1% solution, *w/v*) 8.0. pK_{a1} 2.76; pK_{a2} 3.5.

Solubility—1 g in 1.2 mL water or 25 mL alcohol; practically insoluble in chloroform or ether.

Comments—An *extended-spectrum (antipseudomonal) penicillin.* It is given IV with high sodium. An oral prodrug (indanyl sodium) is available.

CLOXACILLIN SODIUM

[2S-(2α,5α,6β)]-4-Thia-1-azabicyclo[3.2.0]heptane-2-carboxylic acid, 6-[[[3-(2-chlorophenyl)-5-methyl-4-isoxazolyl]carbonyl]amino]-3,3-dimethyl-7-oxo-, monosodium salt, monohydrate; Cloxacillin Sodium Monohydrate, Tegopen, Cloxapen

[7081-44-9] $C_{19}H_{17}ClN_3NaO_5S·H_2O$ (475.88); *anhydrous* [642-78-4] (457.86). Potency: the equivalent of not less than 825 μg of cloxacillin/mg.

Preparation—6-Aminopenicillanic acid is acylated with 3-(*o*-chlorophenyl)-5-methyl-4-isoxazolecarboxylic acid and the resulting cloxacillin is purified by recrystallization and converted to the sodium salt.

Description—White, odorless, crystalline powder having a bitter taste; stable in light and only slightly hygroscopic; decomposes about 173°; pH (1 in 100 solution) 7.5; pK_a (COOH) 2.7.

Solubility—Freely soluble in water; soluble in alcohol; slightly soluble in chloroform.

Comments—A *penicillinase-resistant penicillin (antistaphylococcal)* administered orally.

DICLOXACILLIN SODIUM

[2S-(2α,5α,6β)]-4-Thia-1-azabicyclo[3.2.0]heptane-2-carboxylic acid, 6-[[[3-(2,6-dichlorophenyl)-5-methyl-4-isoxazolyl]carbonyl]amino]-3,3-dimethyl-7-oxo-, monosodium salt, monohydrate; Dynapen, Pathocil, Dycill

[13412-64-1] $C_{19}H_{16}Cl_2N_3NaO_5S·H_2O$ (510.32); *anhydrous* [343-55-5] (492.31). Potency: the equivalent of not less than 850 μg of dicloxacillin/mg.

Preparation—6-Aminopenicillanic acid is acylated with 3-(2,6-dichlorophenyl)-5-methyl-4-isoxazolecarboxylic acid and the resulting dicloxacillin (acid) is purified by recrystallization and converted to the sodium salt.

Description—White to off-white, crystalline powder; faint, characteristic odor; melts about 225° with decomposition; pK_a 2.67.

Solubility—Freely soluble in water; soluble in alcohol.

Comments—An oral *penicillinase-resistant penicillin* (see the general statement). As with all penicillinase-resistant penicillins, it is not as effective as penicillin G except against those organisms whose resistance depends on penicillinase production. Therefore, its use should be limited to the treatment of susceptible penicillinase-producing strains of *Staph aureus* or *epidermidis*.

The toxicity is the same as that of penicillins in general (see the general statement). Nausea and diarrhea sometimes occur, but they usually do not necessitate discontinuation of the drug. Rare hepatotoxicity has been observed. In persons with a low sodium tolerance, the sodium content must be taken into account.

By the oral route the amount absorbed is 37% to 50%. It is bound to plasma proteins to the extent of 90% to 97%, the highest among the penicillins. The volume of distribution is only 0.1 mL/g. Approximately 60% is excreted into the urine. Its half-life in plasma is 0.5 to 1.5 hr in normal patients but is 1 to 3 hr in renal insufficiency.

METHICILLIN SODIUM

4-Thia-l-azabicyclo[3.2.0]heptane-2-carboxylic acid, [2S-(2α,5α,6β)] 6-[(2,6-dimethoxybenzoyl)amino]-3,3-dimethyl-7-oxo-, monosodium salt, monohydrate

[7246-14-2]$C_{17}H_{19}N_2NaO_6S·H_2O$ [132-92-3](anhydrous);[61-32-5](methicillin, acid) (420.41).

Preparation—Fermentation-produced 6-aminopenicillanic acid is condensed with 2,6-dimethoxybenzoyl chloride in a suitable organic solvent and the resulting methicillin is precipitated as the sodium salt by the addition of sodium acetate.

Description—Fine, white, crystalline powder; odorless, or a slight odor.

Solubility—Freely soluble in water; slightly soluble in chloroform; insoluble in other.

Comments—A *penicillinase-resistant penicillin (antistaphylococcal).* It is given IV. Interstitial nephritis may occur.

MEZLOCILLIN SODIUM

[2S-[2α,5α,6β(S*)]]-4-Thia-1-azabicyclo[3.2.0]heptane-2-carboxylic acid, 3,3-dimethyl-6-[[[[3-(methylsulfonyl)-2-oxo-1-imidazolidinyl]carbonyl]amino]phenylacetyl]amino]-7-oxo-, monosodium salt; Mezlin

[51841-65-3] $C_{21}H_{24}NaN_5O_8S_2$ (561.56).

Preparation—Ger Pat 2,318,955.

Description—Yellowish-white powder; pK_a 2.7.

Solubility—Very soluble in water; soluble in DMF or methanol; very slightly soluble in alcohol or acetone.

Comments—An *extended-spectrum (antipseudomonal) penicillin.* It is given IV and is similar to *Piperacillin.*

NAFCILLIN SODIUM

[2S-(2α,5α,6β)]-4-Thia-1-azabicyclo[3.2.0]heptane-2-carboxylic acid, 6-[[(2-ethoxy-1-naphthalenyl)carbonyl]amino]-3,3-dimethyl-7-oxo-, monosodium salt, monohydrate; Unipen, Nafcil, Nallpen

[7177-50-6] $C_{21}H_{21}N_2NaO_5S \cdot H_2O$ (454.47); *anhydrous* [985-16-0] (436.46). Potency: equivalent to not less than 820 µg of nafcillin/mg.

Preparation—6-Aminopenicillanic acid is acylated by treatment with 2-ethoxy-1-naphthoyl chloride in an anhydrous organic solvent containing triethylamine. An aqueous extract of this product is admixed with a water-immiscible solvent and nafcillin is precipitated by the addition of sulfuric acid. Nafcillin sodium is precipitated by mixing ethanolic solutions of the acid and sodium ethylhexanoate. US Pat 3,157,639.

Description—White to yellowish white powder; not more than a slight characteristic odor.

Solubility—Freely soluble in water or chloroform; soluble in alcohol.

Comments—A *penicillinase-resistant penicillin*, the use of which is restricted to the treatment of infections caused by penicillinase-producing cocci (mostly staphylococci). After oral administration, serum levels are low and unpredictable, therefore the oral route is not recommended.

It is destroyed partly by gastric acid, and about 36% is absorbed from the gut, somewhat erratically. For serious infections, initial therapy should be by parenteral administration. About 90% is bound to protein in plasma. The volume of distribution is 0.26 to 0.44 mL/g. Only about 10% is eliminated unchanged in the urine. Nafcillin is excreted primarily by the liver with 60% of dose metabolized and 10% secreted unchanged in the bile. The half-life is 0.5 to 1 hr, except 1.2 to 1.5 hr in renal failure.

Untoward reactions are similar to those shown by other penicillins. It causes occasional nausea and diarrhea. It is irritating and may cause pain and an increase in serum transaminase activity after IM injection. Thrombophlebitis can occur with IV injection.

Cross-sensitivity between it and other penicillins may occur. It is preferred in adults because of the association of interstitial nephritis with methicillin. The sodium content must be considered when the drug is used in persons with a low sodium tolerance.

OXACILLIN SODIUM

[2S-(2α,5α,6β)]-4-Thia-1-azabicyclo[3.2.0]heptane-2-carboxylic acid, 3,3-dimethyl-6-[[(5-methyl-3-phenyl-4-isoxazolyl)carbonyl]-amino]-7-oxo-, monosodium salt, monohydrate; Bactocill, Prostaphlin

[7240-38-2] $C_{19}H_{18}N_3NaO_5S \cdot H_2O$ (441.43); *anhydrous* [1173-88-2] (423.42). Potency: equivalent to 815 to 950 µg of oxacillin $(C_{19}H_{19}N_3O_5S)$/mg.

Preparation—Fermentation-produced 6-aminopenicillanic acid is condensed with 5-methyl-3-phenyl-4-isoxazolyl chloride in a suitable organic solvent and the resulting oxacillin is precipitated as the sodium salt by the addition of sodium acetate.

Description—Fine, white, crystalline powder; odorless or a slight odor.

Solubility—Freely soluble in water; slightly soluble in absolute alcohol, chloroform; insoluble in ether.

Comments—A *penicillinase-resistant penicillin (antistaphylococcal)* given orally.

PENICILLIN G BENZATHINE

[2S-(2α,5α,6β)]-4-Thia-1-azabicyclo[3.2.0]heptane-2-carboxylic acid, 3,3-dimethyl-7-oxo-6-[(phenylacetyl)amino]-, compd with N,N'-bis-(phenylmethyl)-1,2-ethanediamine (2:1), tetrahydrate; Bicillin, Permapen

[41372-02-5] $C_{16}H_{20}N_2 \cdot 2C_{16}H_{18}N_2O_4S \cdot 4H_2O$ (981.19); *anhydrous* [1538-09-6] (909.13). Potency: 1090 to 1272 Penicillin Units/mg. One mg of Penicillin G Benzathine represents 1211 Penicillin G Units.

Preparation—Precipitates on mixing aqueous solutions containing N,N-dibenzylethylenediamine diacetate and sodium penicillin G in the required molar proportion.

Description—White, odorless, crystalline powder; pH (saturated solution) 5 to 7.5.

Solubility—1 g in approximately 5000 mL water and approximately 65 mL alcohol.

Comments—Low water-solubility; hence, on IM injection, it is released slowly and yields prolonged blood levels of penicillin, generally for 1 to 4 wk. Its antibacterial activity is that of the penicillin G moiety (see the general statement), except that its long duration of action makes it especially suitable for *prophylaxis of rheumatic fever*. However, by the IM route the blood levels are quite low and are not suitable for most of the uses of the drug. For example, 1.2 million units will yield an average plasma level of only 0.15 unit/mL on the 1st day, and by the 14th day it will have fallen to 0.03 unit/mL. CSF concentrations are negligible. With concurrent probenecid the levels will be somewhat higher. Consequently, it is indicated only for the *prophylaxis* and *treatment* of *infections* caused by highly susceptible *group A streptococcus, syphilis* and *yaws*.

PENICILLIN G POTASSIUM

[2S-(2α,5α,6β)]-4-Thia-1-azabicyclo[3.2.0]heptane-2-carboxylic acid, 3,3-dimethyl-7-oxo-6-[(phenylacetyl)amino]-, monopotassium salt; Benzylpenicillin Potassium

[113-98-4] $C_{16}H_{17}KN_2O_4S$ (372.48). Penicillin G Potassium has a potency of not less than 1440 and not more than 1680 Penicillin G Units/mg.

Preparation—From 6-aminopenicillanic acid and phenylacetyl chloride in an inert organic solvent; the sodium salt is precipitated with sodium acetate.

Description—Colorless or white crystals, or a white, crystalline powder; odorless or practically so; moderately hygroscopic; decomposed by prolonged exposure to temperatures of approximately 100°, moisture accelerating decomposition; not appreciably affected by air or light; solutions deteriorate at room temperature, but solutions stored lower than 15° remain stable for several days; rapidly inactivated by acids and alkalies, and also by oxidizing agents; pH (aqueous solution, 30 mg/mL) 5 and 7.5; pK$_a$ (acid) 2.8.

Solubility—Very soluble in water, normal saline, or dextrose solutions; soluble in alcohol (but is inactivated by this solvent), glycerin or many other alcohols.

Comments—See the uses of penicillins in the general statement. The potassium salt has no advantage over the sodium salt except when high doses are used in patients on sodium restriction. The potassium salt also avoids the hypokalemic alkalosis that sometimes occurs during treatment with high doses of penicillins. The possibility of potassium intoxication from massive doses in oliguric patients should be kept in mind. The bioavailability by the oral route is 15% to 33%. In plasma 50% to 65% is protein-bound. The volume of distribution is 0.47 mL/g. Renal elimination is 60% to 90% of the total, the remainder being mostly biliary. The half-life is 0.5 to 0.7 hr, except 2.5 to 10 hr in renal failure or after probenecid.

PENICILLIN G PROCAINE

[2S-(2α,5α,6β)]-4-Thia-1-azabicyclo[3.2.0]heptane-2-carboxylic acid, 3,3-dimethyl-7-oxo-6-[(phenylacetyl)amino]-, compd with 2-(diethylamino)ethyl 4-aminobenzoate (1:1), monohydrate

[6130-64-9] $C_{16}H_{18}N_2O_4S \cdot C_{13}H_{20}N_2O_2 \cdot H_2O$ (588.72); *anhydrous* [54-35-3] (570.70). Potency: 900 to 1050 Penicillin Units/mg. One mg represents 1009 Penicillin G units.

Preparation—An aqueous solution of sodium (or potassium) penicillin G undergoes metathesis with an equimolar quantity of procaine hydrochloride.

Description—White, fine crystals or a white, very fine, microcrystalline powder; odorless or practically so; not appreciably affected by air or light; pH (saturated solution) 7.5; rapidly inactivated by acids and by alkali hydroxides, also by oxidizing agents.

Solubility—1 g in 250 mL water, approximately 30 mL alcohol, or approximately 60 mL chloroform.

Comments—Upon IM injection it slowly releases the penicillin G and provides prolonged duration of effective blood levels. An IM dose of 300,000 units yields a peak plasma concentration of 1.5 units/mL at 1 to

3 hr, and the level is about 0.2 unit/mL at 24 hr and 0.05 unit/mL at 48 hr. Because of the relatively low peak blood levels, the drug is indicated only for *mild* to *moderately severe infections* by very susceptible organisms. For its uses and toxicity see the general statement. Allergies can occur due to the procaine component but other toxic effects of procaine are very rare. IV injection should never be used.

PENICILLIN V POTASSIUM

[2*S*-(2α,5α,6β)]-4-Thia-1-azabicyclo[3.2.0]heptane-2-carboxylic acid, 3,3-dimethyl-7-oxo-6-[(phenoxyacetyl)amino]-, monopotassium salt; Penicillin Potassium Phenoxymethyl

[132-98-9] $C_{16}H_{17}KN_2O_5S$ (388.48). Penicillin V Potassium has a potency of not less than 1380 and not more than 1610 Penicillin V units/mg.

Preparation—As for *Penicillin G*, using phenoxyacetyl chloride.

Description—White, odorless, crystalline powder; pH (aqueous solution, 30 mg/mL) 7.5; pK_a 2.73.

Solubility—Very soluble in water; 1 g in approximately 150 mL alcohol.

Comments—The antibacterial spectrum is essentially that of penicillin G against gram-positive bacteria, but this is less potent and effective against gram-negative bacteria. Consequently, it shares the same uses (see the general statement), except that in severe acute infections parenteral penicillin G is mandatory. It is inactivated less by gastric juice than is penicillin G. Penicillin V is the *preferred oral penicillin* for *less serious infections* because serum levels are 2 to 5 times higher than comparable doses of penicillin G and there is less individual variability in absorption. Like penicillin G, it may cause allergic reactions, and it frequently shows cross-sensitivity to the other penicillins. Its other toxicities are also those of penicillin G. The oral bioavailability is about 60% at best. It is 75% to 80% bound to plasma proteins. The volume of distribution is 0.73 mL/g, which is considerably larger than that of penicillin G. Only 20% to 40% is excreted unchanged in the urine. The half-life is about 0.5 to 1 hr.

PIPERACILLIN SODIUM

[2*S*-[2α,5α,6β(*S**)]]-4-Thia-1-azabicyclo[3.2.0]heptane-2-carboxylic acid, 6-[[[[(4-ethyl-2,3-dioxo-1-piperazinyl)carbonyl]amino]-phenylacetyl]amino]-3,3-dimethyl-7-oxo-, monosodium salt; Pipracil

[59703-84-3] $C_{23}H_{26}N_5NaO_7S$ (539.54). Potency: the equivalent of not less than 863 µg piperacillin/mg.

Preparation—US Pat 4,087,424.

Description—White crystals.

Solubility—1 g in approximately 1.5 mL water or methanol; 5 mL of ethyl alcohol.

Comments—An *extended-spectrum penicillin* with antibacterial activities characteristic of its class (see the general statement). It is the most active penicillin against *Ps aeruginosa*, with a potency nearly that of gentamicin. It is one of five drugs of choice for use against infections caused by *Ps aeruginosa*. It is more potent against *Klebsiella* and several other enteric bacilli than is carbenicillin or ticarcillin. It is an alternative drug for use against infections by *Acinetobacter, Bacteroides fragilis* (GI strains), *Enterobacter, E coli, Kl pneumoniae, Morganella morganii, Pr mirabilis* or *vulgaris, Providencia rettgeri* or *stuartii, Ps aeruginosa* (UTIs) or *Serratia*. It has a low efficacy against penicillinase- and other β-lactamase-producing bacteria. Resistance can develop rapidly to piperacillin during use, so that it should be administered only in combination with an aminoglycoside or penicillinase inhibitor (tazobactam) when used against *Ps aeruginosa* and other hard-to-suppress bacilli.

The oral bioavailability is too low and erratic to be of use. In plasma, 16% to 22% is protein-bound. The volume of distribution is about 0.18 to 0.30 mL/g. Renal excretion accounts for 60% to 80% of elimination. The half-life is 0.5 hr, except 0.6 to 1.2 hr in renal failure.

TICARCILLIN DISODIUM

[2*S*-[2α,5α,6β(*S**)]]-4-Thia-1-azabicyclo[3.2.0]heptane-2-carboxylic acid, 6-[(carboxy-3-thienylacetyl)amino]-3,3-dimethyl-7-oxo-, disodium salt; Ticar

[4697-14-7] $C_{15}H_{14}N_2Na_2O_6S_2$ (428.38). Potency: equivalent to not less than 800 µg of ticarcillin ($C_{15}H_{16}N_2O_6S_2$)/mg, calculated on the anhydrous basis.

Preparation—Belgian Pat 646,991. 2-(3-Thienyl)malonic acid, monobenzyl ester is converted to the acid chloride which is condensed with 6-aminopenicillanic acid, followed by hydrogenation to convert the ester to the free acid.

Description—White to pale-yellow powder; hygroscopic; unstable in acid medium; pK_a (acid form) 2.44, 3.64; acid solutions are unstable.

Solubility—1 g in 10 mL water or 66 mL ethanol; pH of a concentrated solution (>100 g/100 mL) approximately 7.0.

Comments—An *extended-spectrum penicillin* almost identical to *Carbenicillin* in its antibacterial spectrum and potency, except that it is twice as active against *Ps aeruginosa*. Resistance develops rapidly. With many infections, resistance is obviated by adding clavulanate. Also, for gram-negative infections, it is often combined with gentamicin or tobramycin to enhance activity and delay resistance.

The adverse effects are those of penicillins in general (see the general statement), and cross-sensitivity to penicillin occurs. Sodium overload and hypokalemia can occur, especially with high doses. In renal failure, high doses may inhibit platelet aggregation, and hemorrhagic phenomena may result.

It is not absorbed orally. In plasma, 55% to 65% is protein-bound. The volume of distribution is 0.22 mL/g. It is 86% eliminated by renal excretion. The half-life is 0.5 to 1 hr, except 15 hr in renal failure.

Beta-Lactamase Combinations

CLAVULINATE-AMOXICILLIN—A combination given orally. It has a broader spectrum of activity than amoxicillin (including anaerobic organisms) but causes more diarrhea than amoxicillin.

CLAVULANATE-TICARCILLIN—A combination given IV. It is active versus more gram-negative bacilli and anaerobes.

SULBACTAM-AMPICILLIN—A combination given IV. It is active versus *Staphylococcus* and beta-lactamase producing *H influenzae* and *Strep pneumoniae* and anaerobes.

TAZOBACTAM-PIPERACILLIN—A combination given IV. It is active versus more gram-negative bacilli and anaerobes.

CEPHALOSPORINS

The cephalosporins are a group of antibiotics closely related to the penicillins. The cephalosporanic acid moiety characteristic of cephalosporins is an analog of the penicillanic acid moiety characteristic of penicillins; cephalosporanic acid contains a dihydrometathiazine ring, while penicillanic acid contains a tetrahydrothiazole (thiazolidine) ring. Both have a beta-lactam ring. The 7-aminocephalosporanic acid derivatives are much more acid-stable than the corresponding 6-aminopenicillanic acid compounds. Cephamycins are cephalosporins that possess a 7-methoxy group that enhances beta-lactamase resistance. Cephamycins may induce beta-lactamase production.

The cephalosporins have a mechanism of action very similar to that of the penicillins, namely, they bind to one or more penicillin-binding proteins (PBPs) that are transpeptidases and inhibit the cross-linking of the peptidoglycan units in the bacterial cell wall. The intrinsic activity of a cephalosporin depends in part on resistance to beta-lactamases, affinity to PBPs and their ability to reach these targets that are extracellular for gram-positive bacteria and periplasmic for gram-negative bacteria. See Table 90-4.

Currently, the cephalosporins are classified into four generations based on their gram-negative spectrum and stability in

Table 90-4. Cephalosporins

CLASS	COMMENTS
First generation (Staph, some enteric gram-neg. bacilli)	
Cefadroxil	Oral, intermediate acting
Cefazolin	IM, IV, intermed. duration, less painful
Cephalexin	Oral, short acting
Cephalothin	IM, IV, short acting, weakest spectrum
Cephapirin	IM, IV, short acting
Cephradine	IM, IV, oral, short acting
Second generation (more active vs gram-neg, some active vs _H influenzae_ & anaerobes)	
Cefaclor	Oral, short acting, active vs _H influenzae_
Cefamandole	IM, IV, short acting
Cefmetazole	IV, short acting, good vs. anaerobes
Cefonicid	IM, IV, intermed-long acting
Ceforanid	IM, IV, intermed acting
Cefotetan	IM, IV, intermed-long acting, good vs anaerobes
Cefoxitin	IM, IV, short acting, good vs anaerobes
Cefprozil	Oral, short acting
Cefuroxime	IM, IV, oral, beta-lactamase resist., active vs _H influenzae_, good csf levels
Loracarbef	Oral, short acting, active vs _H influenzae_
Third generation (best gram-neg. spectrum, beta-lactamase resistant, poor vs staph.)	
Cefixime	Oral, intermed-long acting
Cefpodoxime	Oral, intermed acting, similar to cefixime
Cefoperazone	IM, IV, intermed acting, good vs _Pseud_
Cefotaxime	IM, IV, shortest acting, metab, good csf
Ceftazidime	IM, IV, short acting, good vs _Pseud_
Ceftizoxime	IM, IV, short acting, good csf levels
Ceftriaxone	IM, IV, long acting, good vs gonococci
Ceftibuten	Oral, similar to cefixime
Cefdinir	Oral, similar to cefixime
Fourth Generation	
Cefepime	IV, better vs staph and strep than 3rd gen

the presence of beta-lactamases. However, this classification scheme is becoming less reliable because newer agents have led to more exceptions and less precise criteria for differences in antibacterial spectrum.

The _first-generation cephalosporins_ (cefazolin, cephalothin, cephapirin, cephradine, cephalexin, and cefadroxil) have the highest activity against gram-positive and the lowest against gram-negative bacteria. In summary, they are effective against the following antibacterial spectrum: good activity against most staphylococci (even penicillinase-producers, but not methicillin-resistant staphylococci) plus most common streptococci (_Strep pyogenes, viridans_ and _pneumoniae_), but not enterococci; moderately active against certain gram-negative bacteria, such as _N gonorrhoeae_ and _meningitidis_, many _E coli_, some _H influenzae_, and non-hospital-acquired _Klebsiella_ and _Pr mirabilis_ and some _Salmonella_ and _Shigella_.

The _second-generation cephalosporins_ (cefuroxime, cefamandole, cefmetazole, cefonicid, cefoxitin, cefotetan, cefaclor, cefprozil, and loracarbef) are more active against gram-negative and less active against gram-positive bacteria than are first-generation members. Notable differences include the increased activity against most _H influenzae_ and the efficacy of some cephalosporins (cefoxitin, cefotetan, cefmetazole) against some more resistant hospital-acquired infections due to anaerobic bacteria (_Bacteroides fragilis_) and indole-positive _Proteus_. Like the first-generation, members of this group are inactive against _Ps aeruginosa_.

The _third-generation cephalosporins_ (cefotaxime, ceftizoxime, ceftriaxone, cefpodoxime, ceftibuten, moxalactam, ceftazidime, cefoperazone, and cefixime) are considerably less active than first-generation drugs against gram-positive bacteria (especially staphylococci) but have a much expanded spectrum of activity against gram-negative organisms and have more resistance to gram-negative beta-lactamases. They are

quite active against gram-negative anaerobes and are frequently active against _Enterobacteriaceae_ (_E coli, Enterobacter, K pneumoniae_). Of special interest is the activity some members of this group (ceftazidime and cefoperazone) that have high activity against _Pseudomonas_ but possess a weaker overall gram-negative spectrum.

The current _fourth-generation cephalosporin_ classification (cefepime) is based on an improved gram-positive spectrum while retaining the expanded gram-negative activity of third-generation cephalosporins.

RESISTANCE—As with the penicillins, one common mechanism of resistance is that of elaboration of a beta-lactamase. Although some cephalosporins are inactivated by penicillinase-types of beta-lactamase, many beta-lactamases are selective for cephalosporins and are called cephalosporinase types. Other resistance mechanisms include failure to bind to PBPs as occurs with methicillin-resistant strains of staphylococci.

INDICATIONS—The cephalosporins are effective in a wide variety of infections because they have a broad spectrum and high therapeutic/toxic ratio. The first- and second-generation cephalosporins are used frequently for prophylaxis during certain surgical procedures to reduce the risk of postoperative wound infections. Cefazolin is preferred over other first-generation analogs because it has a higher serum concentration and longer elimination half-life; also it is less painful upon IM administration. Cefoxitin, cefotetan, and cefmetazole are cephamycins that are preferred for intra-abdominal surgery because of their beta-lactamase resistance and activity against _Bacteroides fragilis_. A number of second- and third-generation cephalosporins are effective alternatives as prophylactic agents for various surgical procedures.

Cephalosporins are generally not the first drug of choice for any bacterial infections because of the availability of equally effective and less expensive alternatives. First-generation cephalosporins are preferred alternatives to antistaphylococcal penicillins or penicillin G for serious staphylococcal and/or streptococcal infection except enterococcal infections or meningitis. The non-cephamycin second-generation cephalosporins such as cefuroxime have similar antimicrobial spectra and may be used as alternatives to treat most serious infections caused by staphylococci and aerobic gram-negative bacilli. Only the third-generation cephalosporins are approved for treatment of meningitis caused by enteric gram-negative bacilli. Cefuroxime may be used to treat meningitis caused by _H influenzae_, although a third-generation cephalosporin is still the preferred choice.

Cefotaxime, ceftizoxime, and ceftriaxone are third-generationcephalosporins that are effective against serious hospital-acquired infections caused by enteric gram-negative bacilli, such as _Enterobacter_, indole-positive _Proteus, Providencia stuartii_, and _Serratia_. Against _H influenzae_, cefotaxime and ceftriaxone are preferred for parenteral therapy, although cefuroxime is an alternative.

Ceftriaxone is the drug of choice for treatment of gonorrhea, and any cephalosporin may be preferred over an extended-spectrum penicillin against _Kl pneumoniae_. The cephalosporins are also alternatives to penicillins to treat infections caused by _Branhamella catarrhalis_ and less serious infections of streptococci, staphylococci, _H influenzae_, _N meningitides_, and _E coli_.

Several oral cephalosporins have increased activity against _H influenzae_ including cefaclor, cefuroxime axetil, cefixime, cefprozil, and cefpodoxime proxetil. Ceftazidime and cefoperazone are preferred in the treatment of infections caused by _Ps aeruginosa, cepacia_, or _maltophilia_. Third-generation cephalosporins such as cefotaxime and ceftizoxime are expensive alternatives against indole-positive _Proteus, Providencia,_ and nontyphoid _Salmonella_.

ADVERSE EFFECTS—Hypersensitivity occurs in about 5% to 10% of recipients of cephalosporins; manifestations are eosinophilia, drug fever, maculopapular rash, urticaria, serum sickness, angioneurotic edema, anaphylaxis, positive Coombs test associated with rare hemolytic anemia and infrequent transient hepatic abnormalities (increased SGOT, SGPT and total bilirubin), thrombocytopenia, neutropenia, and interstitial nephritis. There is an appreciable incidence of cross-sensitization with penicillin; when previously manifested, penicillin sensitivity has not been serious. A cephalosporin, especially cefazolin, may be administered cautiously after sensitivity testing, but only if necessary; skin tests often give false negatives. If the previous reaction to penicillin was severe, such as with anaphylaxis or angioneurotic edema, or if the patient reacts to penicillin minor determinants, a cephalosporin usually is discouraged.

Other adverse effects of cephalosporins include pain, induration, sterile abscess, and sloughing at the site of IM injection, thrombophlebitis after IV administration, nausea, vomiting, glossitis, diarrhea, loose stools, abdominal pain and heartburn, especially with oral administration, sodium load, and water retention with sodium salts, antibiotic-associated colitis (especially with poorly absorbed members) and a false-positive urine test for glucose (Benedict, Fehling, and Clinitest, but not Tes-Tape). Present cephalosporins are not significantly nephrotoxic alone but may increase considerably the nephrotoxicity of an aminoglycoside.

Cephalosporins should not be used in combination with other antibiotics that cause nephrotoxicity or ototoxicity. High-ceiling diuretics (eg, furosemide and ethacrynic acid) also enhance nephrotoxicity and make certain cephalosporins ototoxic. The acquisition costs of some cephalosporins is very high. Suprainfections by gram-negative bacteria and *Candida* may occur. There may be occasional hypoprothrombinemia and disulfiram-like reaction with alcohol; those drugs with *N*-methylthiotetrazole side chains seem to be the serious offenders that include cefamandole, cefoperazone, cefotetan, and cefmetazole.

PHARMACOKINETICS—Cephalosporins vary considerably in their peroral bioavailability (15–86%), protein binding (14–96%) and half-lives (0.5–6.5 hr). Elimination is mainly by glomerular filtration and tubular secretion (except for cefoperazone) and some biliary secretion (and reabsorption), except that most of cephaloglycin and some of cefotaxime, cephalothin, cephapirin, and cephacetrile are deacetylated and subsequently further transformed; consequently, renal failure may greatly increase the half-lives of most cephalosporins. Cephalosporins vary in their penetrance into tissues. Only cefuroxime and third-generation cephalosporins achieve therapeutic concentrations in CSF, and then only in inflammation of the meninges. The first- and second-generation cephalosporins should not be used for meningitis.

Cephalosporins cross the placental barrier and reach plasma concentration in the fetus in about 10% of maternal concentrations; effects on the fetus are unknown, but it is advisable to avoid treatment of pregnant women with cephalosporins if possible. A summary of the cephalosporins is included in Table 90-5.

CEFACLOR

5-Thia-1-azabicyclo[4.2.0]oct-2-ene-2-carboxylic acid, [6R-[6α,7β(R*)]]-7-[(aminophenylacetyl)amino]-3-chloro-8-oxo-, monohydrate; Ceclor

[70356-03-05] $C_{15}H_{14}ClN_3O_4S\cdot H_2O$ (385.82)]. Cefaclor is a semisynthetic cephalosporin related to cephalexin.

Preparation—See *J Med Chem* 1975; 18:403.

Description—White crystalline solid; aqueous solutions are most stable at pH of approximately 3.5, which is the pH of a 2% solution.

Solubility—Soluble in water (1 in 100); practically insoluble in most organic solvents.

Comments—A *second-generation cephalosporin* with typical antibacterial activities and adverse effects (see the general statement). It

Table 90-5. Carbapenems

DRUG	COMMENTS
Imipenem	IV, metabolized by renal enzymes
Carbapenem	IV, not metabolized by renal enzymes

was the first orally efficacious member of its group. It is approved for use in the treatment of *upper respiratory tract infections, pharyngitis,* and *tonsillitis* caused by *Strep pyogenes*; lower respiratory tract infections caused by *Strep pneumoniae, pyogenes,* and *H influenzae*; otitis media caused by *Strep pneumoniae or pyogenes*, staphylococci and *H influenzae*; cutaneous infections caused by *Staph aureus* and *Strep pyrogens*; and UTIs caused by *E coli, Pr mirabilis, Klebsiella* spp, and coagulase-negative staphylococci. In plasma, 25% is bound to protein. The volume of distribution is 0.24 to 0.36 mL/g. About 60% to 85% is excreted unchanged into the urine. The half-life is 0.6 to 0.9 hr, except longer in renal failure.

CEFAMANDOLE NAFATE

5-Thia-1-azabicyclo[4.2.0]oct-2-ene-2-carboxylic acid, [6R-[6α,7β(R*)]]-7-[[(formyloxy)phenylacetyl]amino]-3-[[(1-methyl-1H-tetrazol-5-yl)-thio]methyl]-8-oxo-, monosodium salt, Mandol

[42540-40-9] [34444-01-4(acid)] $C_{19}H_{17}N_6NaO_6S_2$ (512.49).

Preparation—US Pat 3,641,021.

Description—White crystals; melts about 190° with decomposition; pK_a 2.8.

Solubility—Soluble in water or methanol; insoluble in nonpolar solvents.

Comments—A *second-generation cephalosporin* given IM and IV. It is short-acting.

CEFAZOLIN SODIUM

5-Thia-1-azabicyclo[4.2.0]oct-2-ene-2-carboxylic acid, 3-[[(5-methyl-(6R-trans)-1,3,4-thiadiazol-2-yl)thio]methyl]-8-oxo-7-[[(1H-tetrazol-1-yl)acetyl]-amino]-, monosodium salt; Ancef, Kefzol

[27164-46-1] $C_{14}H_{13}N_8NaO_4S_3$ (476.48). Potency: not less than 850 μg and not more than 1050 μg of cefazolin ($C_{14}H_{14}N_8O_4S_3$)/mg, calculated on the anhydrous basis.

Preparation—The sodium salt of 7-aminocephalosporanic acid is acylated with 1*H*-tetrazole-1-acetyl chloride and the acetoxy group is then displaced by reaction with 5-methyl-1,3,4-thiadiazole-2-thiol; the resulting cefazolin is converted to the sodium salt.

Description—White to off-white, crystalline powder.

Solubility—Freely soluble in water, saline TS or dextrose solutions; very slightly soluble in alcohol; practically insoluble in chloroform or ether.

Comments—A *first-generation cephalosporins* given IV or IM. Some gram-negative organisms and penicillinase-producing staphylococci resistant to both penicillin G and ampicillin are sensitive to cefazolin. Gram-negative activity essentially limited to *E coli, Klebsiella* and *Pr mirabilis*.

The drug can be used to treat infections of the respiratory tract, skin, soft tissues, bones, joints, and urinary tract and endocarditis and septicemia caused by susceptible organisms. Among UTIs, cystitis responds much better than pyelonephritis. It is the preferred cephalosporin for most surgical prophylaxis, because of its (relatively) long half-life.

The adverse effects are those of cephalosporins in general (see the general statement). It causes some pain at the site of injection and occasional phlebitis. Oral, genital, and vaginal candidiasis and anal pruritus occur. It causes a transient increase in blood urea nitrogen yet seems to have negligible nephrotoxicity.

It is not absorbed orally. It is bound to the extent of 70% to 85% by plasma proteins and has a low volume of distribution of only 0.10 to 0.14 mL/g. From 95% is excreted into urine. The half-life is 1.5 to 2 hr in normal persons but 3 to 42 hr in renal failure.

CEFDINIR

5-Thia-1-azabicyclo[4.2.0]oct-2-ene-2-carboxylic acid, [6R-[6α,7β(Z)]]-7-[[2-amino-4-thiazolyl) (hydroxyimino)acetyl]amino]-3-ethenyl-8-oxo-, Omnicef

[91832-40-5] $C_{14}H_{13}N_5O_5S_2$ (395.42).
Preparation—US Pat 4,559,334(1985).
Description—White to slightly brownish yellow powder melting about 170° (dec); pK_a 9.7.
Solubility—Slightly soluble in dilute HCl; sparingly soluble in 0.1M phosphate buffer.
Comments—A third generation cephalosporin given orally. It has a similar action as *Cefixime*.

CEFEPIME HYDROCHLORIDE

Pyrrolidinium, [6R-[6α,7β(Z)]]-1-[[7-(2-amino-4-thiazolyl) (methoxyimino)acetyl]amino]-2-carboxy-8-oxo-5-thia-1-azabicyclo[4.2.0]oct-2-ene-3-yl]methyl]-1-methyl-, hydroxide, inner salt hydrochloride; Maxipime

[88040-23-7] $C_{19}H_{24}N_6O_5S_2$·HCl (527.08).
Preparation—US Pat 4,406,899 (1983).
Description—Colorless solid melting about 150° (dec) (base). White to pale yellow powder (HCl); the commercial product is the hydrochloride dihydrate.
Solubility—Very soluble in water (hydrochloride).
Comments—A *fourth-generation cephalosporin* that retains an extended gram-negative spectrum against gram-negative aerobic bacilli covered by cefotaxime and ceftazidime including some strains resistant to these third-generation cephalosporins. It has improved activity against *Strep pneumoniae* and *Staph aureus* compared to the third-generation cephalosporins. Its activity against *P aeruginosa* is clinically relevant and it has become one of the agents of choice (often in combination with another anti- Pseudomonal drug) to treat this difficult pathogen.

The drug may be given IV or IM for treatment of UTIs, pneumonias, and skin infections. It is eliminated like most cephalosporins by renal excretion and has a half-life of 2 hr. Its adverse effects resemble the other cephalosporins.

CEFIXIME

5-Thia-1-azabicyclo[4.2.0]oct-2-ene-2-carboxylic acid, [6R-[6α,7β(Z)]]-7-[[(2-amino-4-thiazolyl)][(carboxymethoxy)imino]acetyl]amino]-3-ethenyl-8-oxo-, Suprax

[79350-37-1] $C_{16}H_{15}N_5O_7S_2$ (453.44).
Preparation—US Pat 4,098,888.
Description—Off-white crystals; melts over 250°; distinguished from the *E*-trihydrate which melts about 220° with decomposition; pK_a (acid) 2.5.
Solubility—1 g in 125 mL water or 2000 mL alcohol.

Comments—An oral *third-generation cephalosporin* with excellent activity against most *E coli* and *Klebsiella, H influenzae, Branhamella catarrhalis, N gonorrhoeae* and *meningitidis*, including β-lactamase-producing strains. It is active against common streptococci but staphylococci are resistant. It is used for respiratory infections, otitis media, and uncomplicated UTIs, but its therapeutic role remains to be defined.

It is absorbed slowly and incompletely from the GI tract and has a bioavailability of 40% to 50%. The oral suspension produces peak concentrations that are 25% to 50% higher than equivalent doses of tablet formulations. Food does not affect the amount of cefixime absorbed but delays absorption. Approximately 65% to 70% is bound to plasma protein. Renal excretion is the main route of elimination although biliary excretion is greater than 10%. The serum half-life is 3 to 4 hr but is prolonged with renal impairment.

The most common adverse reactions are gastrointestinal, primarily diarrhea. Other GI side effects may occur such as nausea, dyspepsia, and flatulence. Dizziness, headache, genital pruritus, and hypersensitivity reactions may occur.

CEFMETAZOLE SODIUM

5-Thia-1-azabicyclo[4.2.0]oct-2-ene-2-carboxylic acid, (6R-cis)-7-[[[(cyanomethyl)thio]acetyl]amino]-7-methoxy-3-[[(1-methyl-1H-tetrazol-5-yl)thio]methyl]-8-oxo-, monosodium salt, Zefazone

[56796-39-5], [5796-20-4 (acid)] $C_{15}H_{16}N_7NaO_5S_3$ (493.51).
Preparation—*J Antibiot* 1976; 29:554.
Description—White solid.
Solubility—Very soluble in water or methanol; soluble in acetone.
Comments—A *second-generation cephalosporin* given IV. It is short-acting and has good activity versus anaerobes.

CEFONICID SODIUM

5-Thia-1-azabicyclo[4.2.0]oct-2-ene-2-carboxylic acid, [6R-[6α,7β(R*)]-7-[(hydroxyphenylacetyl)amino]-8-oxo-3-[[[1-(sulfomethyl)-1H-tetrazol-5-yl]thio]methyl]-, disodium salt, Monocid

[61270-78-8] $C_{18}H_{16}N_6Na_2O_8S_3$ (586.52).
Preparation—Ger Pat 2,611,270; *CA* 1977; 86:2985t.
Description—pH (5% solution) 3.5 to 6.5.
Comments—A *second-generation cephalosporin* given IM and IV. It is intermediate-acting.

CEFOPERAZONE SODIUM

5-Thia-1-azabicyclo[4.2.0]oct-2-ene-2-carboxylic acid, [6R-[6α,7β(R*)]]-7-[[[(4-ethyl-2,3-dioxo-1-piperazinyl)carbonyl]amino]-(4-hydroxyphenyl)acetyl]amino]-3-[[(1-methyl-1H-tetrazol-5-yl)-thio]methyl]-8-oxo, monosodium salt, Cefobid

[62893-20-3] $C_{25}H_{26}N_9NaO_8S_2$ (667.65).
Preparation—See Belg Pat 837,682; *CA* 1977; 87:6002v.
Description—White powder; melts about 170°; pH (25% aqueous solution), 4.5 to 6.5; unstable in alkaline solution.

Comments—A *third-generation cephalosporin* given IM and IV. It is intermediate-acting and has good activity versus *Pseudomonas*.

CEFOTAXIME SODIUM

5-Thia-1-azabicyclo[4.2.0]oct-2-ene-2-carboxylic acid, [6*R*-[6α,7β(*Z*)]]-3-[(acetyloxy)methyl]-7-[[(2-amino-4-thiazolyl)-(methoxyimino)acetyl]amino]-8-oxo-, monosodium salt, Claforan

[64485-93-4] $C_{16}H_{16}N_5NaO_7S_2$ (477.44).

Preparation—*Chem Pharm Bull* 1980; 28:2629.

Description—White to off-white solid; pH (10% solution) approximately 5.5; pK$_a$ (acid) 3.75.

Solubility—Freely soluble in water; practically insoluble in most organic solvents.

Comments—A *third-generation cephalosporin*, given IV or IM, with an antibacterial spectrum characteristic of its class (see the general statement). Against many gram-negative bacilli it is equal to the aminoglycosides, except against *Ps aeruginosa*, *Acinetobacter* and some *Enterobacter*. It is more active against multiple-drug-resistant gram-negative bacilli than are moxalactam ceftazidime and cefoperazone. It is highly resistant to β-lactamases. Against *S aureus*, it is less active than first-or second-generation cephalosporins. It is a preferred third-generation cephalosporin for gram-negative meningitis and other serious gram-negative bacillary infections outside the CNS. It is used for surgical prophylaxis. When appropriate, it may be combined with an aminoglycoside. It has no unique toxicity (see the general statement). It is very expensive.

The drug is absorbed poorly by the oral route. In plasma, 38% is protein-bound. The volume of distribution is 0.25 to 0.39 mL/g. It penetrates into the CSF. About 85% is eliminated in the urine and 8% in the feces. The half-life is 1 to 1.2 hr, except 3 to 12 hr in renal failure. It is 30% to 50% metabolized to an active β-lactamase-stable metabolite.

CEFOTETAN DISODIUM

5-Thia-1-azabicyclo[4.2.0]oct-2-ene-2-carboxylic acid, [6*R*-6α,7α)]-7-[[[4-(2-amino-1-carboxy-2-oxoethylidene)-1,3-dithietan-2-yl]carbonyl]amino]-7-methoxy-3-[[(1-methyl-1*H*-tetrazol-5-yl)-thio]methyl]-8-oxo-, disodium salt; Cefotan

[74356-00-6] $C_{17}H_{15}N_7Na_2O_8S_4$ (619.57).

Preparation—See *Chem Pharm Bull* 1980; 28:2629.

Description—White to pale yellow powder; pH (freshly reconstituted solution) approximately 5.5; pK$_a$ 2.1, 3.3.

Solubility—Very soluble in water (the color varies from colorless to yellow depending on the concentration).

Comments—A *second-generation cephalosporin* given IM and IV. It is intermediate-acting and has good activity versus anaerobes.

CEFOXITIN SODIUM

(6*R*-cis)-5-Thia-1-azabicyclo[4.2.0]oct-2-ene-2-carboxylic acid, 3- [[(aminocarbonyl)oxy]methyl]-7-methoxy-8-oxo-7-[(2-thienylacetyl)amino]-, sodium salt; Mefoxin

[33564-30-6] $C_{16}H_{16}N_3NaO_7S_2$ (449.43).

Preparation—A semi-synthetic, broad spectrum cepha antibiotic derived from cephamycin C, which is produced by *S lactamdurans*. See *J Am Chem Soc* 1972; 94:1410.

Description—Crystals melting about 150°; pK$_a$ 2.2 (acid).

Solubility—Very soluble in water; soluble in methanol; sparing soluble in ethanol or acetone.

Comments—A *second-generation cephalosporin*. It is not the drug of choice for any infection, but it is an alternative drug for intra-abdominal infections, colorectal surgery, or appendectomy and ruptured viscus because it is active against most enteric anaerobes including *Bacteroides fragilis*. It is approved for use in the treatment of bone and joint infections caused by *S aureus*, gynecological and intra-abdominal infections by *Bacteroides* spp, and other common enteric anaerobes and gram-negative bacilli; lower respiratory tract infections by *Bacteroides* spp, *E coli*, *H influenzae*, *Klebsiella* spp, *S aureus*, or *Streptococcus* spp (except enterococci); septicemia by *Bacteroides* spp, *E coli*, *Klebsiella* spp, *S aureus*, or *Strep pneumoniae*; skin infections by *Bacteroides* spp, *E coli*, *Klebsiella* spp, *S aureus* or *epidermidis*, or *Streptococcus* spp (except enterococci) or UTIs by *E coli*, *Klebsiella* spp, or indole-positive *Proteus*, and for perioperative prophylaxis. It is absorbed poorly by the oral route. Elimination is essentially renal. The half-life is 40 to 60 min, except 13 to 22 hr in renal failure.

CEFPODOXIME PROXETIL

5-Thia-1-azabicyclo[4.2.0]oct-2-ene-2-carboxylic acid, [6*R*-[6α,7β(*Z*)]]-7-[[(2-amino-4-thiazolyl)(methoxyimino)acetyl]amino]-3-(methoxy-methyl)-8-oxo-, 1-[[(1-methylethoxy)-carbonyl]oxy]ethyl ester, Vantin

[87239-81-4], [80210-62-4 (acid)] $C_{21}H_{27}N_5O_9S_2$ (557.59).

Preparation—*J Antibiot* 1987; 40:370. The ester is the prodrug of the metabolite, cefpodoxime, with the free carboxyl group at position 4 of the thiazine ring.

Comments—A *third generation cephalosporin* given orally. It is intermediate-acting. It is similar to *Cefixime*.

CEFPROZIL

5-Thia-1-azabicyclo[4.2.0]oct-2-ene-2-carboxylic acid, [6*R*-[6α,7β(*R**)]]-, 7-[[amino(4-hydroxyphenyl)acetyl]amino]-8-oxo-3-(1-propenyl)-, Cefzil

[92665-29-7] $C_{18}H_{19}N_3O_5S$ (389.43).

Comments—A *second-generation cephalosporin* given orally. It is short-acting.

CEFRADROXIL

[6*R*-[6α,7β(*R**)]]-5-Thia-1-azabicyclo[4.2.0]oct-2-ene-2-carboxylic acid, 7-[[amino-(4-hydroxyphenyl)acetyl]amino]-3-methyl-8-oxo-, monohydrate; Duricef

[66592-87-8] $C_{16}H_{17}N_3O_5S \cdot H_2O$ (381.42).

Preparation—US Pat 4,504,657 (1985); German Pat 2,163,514 (1973).

Description—White to yellow-white crystals melting about 197° (dec).

Solubility—Soluble in water; stable in acid solution.

Comments—A *first-generation cephalosporin* given orally. It is intermediate-acting and effective against *Staphylococcus* and some enteric gram-negative bacilli.

CEFTAZIDIME

Pyridinium, [6R-[6α,7β(Z)]]-1-[[7-[[(2-amino-4-thiazolyl)-[(1-carboxy- 1-methylethoxy)imino]acetyl]amino]-2-carboxy-8-oxo-5-thia-1-azabicyclo[4.2.0]oct-2-ene-3-yl]-methyl]-, hydroxide, inner salt pentahydrate; Fortaz,Tazicef,Tazidime

[78439-06-2] $C_{22}H_{22}N_6O_7S_2$·$5H_2O$ (636.67).

Preparation—See Ger Pat 2,921,316; *CA 92*: 198413c, 1980.

Description—Ivory-colored powder; pK$_a$ 1.8, 2.7, 4.1.

Comments—A *third-generation cephalosporin* given IV or IM. It is a broad-spectrum antibiotic. It is of special interest because of its high activity against *Pseudomonas* and *Enterobacteriaceae* but not enterococci. It is resistant to penicillinases. It is an alternative drug for the treatment of hospital-acquired gram-negative infections. It may be combined with amikacin in the treatment of infections in immunocompromised patients when *Ps aeruginosa* is a potential causative organism.

It is approved for use in the treatment of bone and joint infections, CNS infections, gynecological infections, lower respiratory tract infections, septicemia, skin and UTIs.

The adverse effects are those of the cephalosporins in general.

It is absorbed poorly by the oral route. It is 80% to 90% eliminated in the urine. The half-life in normal persons is about 2 hr but longer in renal failure.

CEFTIBUTEN

5-Thia-1-azabicyclo[4.2.0]oct-2-ene-2-carboxylic acid, [6R-[6α,7β(Z)]]-7-[[2-(2-amino-4-thiazolyl)-4-carboxy-1-oxo-2-butenyl]amino]-8-oxo-, dihydrate; Cedax

[97519-39-6] $C_{15}H_{14}N_4O_6S_2$·$2H_2O$ (410.43).

Preparation—US Pat 4,634,697 (1987).

Description—The commercial product is the dehydrate.

Comments—A *third generation cephalosporin* given orally with activity similar to *Cefixime*.

CEFTIZOXIME SODIUM

[6R-[6α,7β,(Z)]]-5-Thia-1-azabicyclo[4.2.0]-oct-2-ene-2-carboxylic acid, 7-[[(2,3-dihydro-2-imino-4-thiazolyl)(methoxyimino)acetyl]amino]-8-oxo-, monosodium salt; Cefizox

[68401-82-1] $C_{13}H_{12}N_5NaO_5S_2$ (405.38).

Preparation—See US Pat 4,166,155.

Comments—A *third-generation cephalosporin* given IV with antibacterial activity typical of this class (see the general statement). It is about as active as cefotaxime and more active than cefoperazone against gram-negative enteric bacilli but is less active than cefoperazone against *Ps aeruginosa*. It has unreliable activity against anaerobes. It is not active against enterococci. It is approved for the treatment of bone and joint infections, gonorrhea, intra-abdominal infections, lower respiratory tract infections, meningitis, septicemia, skin infections, or UTIs. In serious infections caused by gram-negative bacilli, it usually is combined with an aminoglycoside.

Its adverse effects are those of cephalosporins in general. The drug is not effective orally. IM and IV doses of 1 g yield respective concentrations of 36 and 80 to 90μg/mL 30 min after administration. Only 30% is protein-bound in plasma. About 80% is eliminated in the urine. The half-life is about 1.7 hr but much longer in renal failure.

CEFTRIAXONE SODIUM

[6R-[6α,7β(Z)]]-5-Thia-1-azabicyclo[4.2.0]-oct-2-ene-2-carboxylic acid, 7-[[(2-amino-4-thiazolyl)(methoxyimino)acetyl]amino]-8-oxo-3-[[(1,2,5,6-tetrahydro-2-methyl-5,6-dioxo-1-2,4-triazin-3-yl)-thio]methyl]-, disodium salt; Rocephin

[74578-69-1] $C_{18}H_{16}N_8Na_2O_7S_3$ (598.53).

Preparation—See Brit Pat 2,022,090; *CA 1980*; 93:95289h.

Description—White to yellowish orange crystalline powder (hemiheptahydrate); melts over 155° with decomposition; pK$_a$ ≈ 3 (COOH); 3.2 (NH$_3$ $^+$); 4.1 (enolic OH); solution color varies from light yellow to amber depending on concentration and length of storage; pH (1% solution) approximately 6.7).

Solubility—Readily soluble in water (approximately 40g/100 mL at 25°); sparingly soluble in methanol; very slightly soluble in alcohol.

Comments—A *third-generation cephalosporin* that is the drug of choice for uncomplicated and disseminated gonococcal infections. It is an effective alternative for meningitis in infants caused by *H influenzae, N meningitides,* and *Strep pneumoniae.* It is effective against gram-negative bacillary meningitis and other serious gram-negative infections, including complications associated with Lyme disease. It is not used for enterococci. It is approved for the treatment of bone and joint infections, intra-abdominal infections; lower respiratory tract infections, pelvic infections, skin and urinary tract infections. It also is indicated for perioperative prophylaxis, for which it is as effective as cefazolin.

The side effects are those of the cephalosporins. Some patients show symptoms of cholecystitis.

It is not orally effective. Redistribution time is about 2 hr. In plasma, 83% to 96% is protein-bound. Elimination is 40% to 65% renal. The elimination half-life is 6 to 9 hr, except up to 34 hr in renal failure; the long half-life is an important advantage of the drug that permits a single daily administration.

CEFUROXIME SODIUM

5-Thia-1-azabicyclo[4.2.0]oct-2-ene-2-carboxylic acid, (6R,7R)-7-[2-(2-furyl)glyoxylamido]-3-(hydroxymethyl)-8-oxo-, 7-(Z)-mono (O-methyloxime) carbamate (ester); Kefurox, Zinacef,

[56238-63-2] $C_{16}H_{15}N_4NaO_8S$ (446.37).

Preparation—See US Pat 3,974,153.

Description—Off-white to white powder; unbuffered aqueous solutions are stable for approximately 12 hr at room temperature; approximately 15% decomposition occurs after 24 hr. Suspensions for IM use and solutions for IV infusion are usually stable for 48 hr if stored between 2° and 10°. May become yellowish on standing; pK$_a$ (acid) 2.5.

Solubility—1 g in 5 mL of water; slightly soluble in alcohol. A 10% aqueous solution has a pH of approximately 7.

Comments—A *second-generation cephalosporin* with antibacterial activity typical of that class (see the general statement). Its activity against *H influenzae* and ability to penetrate into the CSF make it particularly useful for treating meningitis caused by that organism; it also is approved to treat meningitis caused by *Strep pneumoniae, N meningitidis* and *Staph aureus.* It has excellent activity against all gonococci, hence is used to treat gonorrhea. It may be used to treat lower respiratory tract infections caused by *H influenzae and parainfluenzae, Klebsiella* spp, *E coli, Strep pneumoniae* and *pyogenes,* and *Staph aureus.* It is approved for use against UTIs caused by *E coli* and *Klebsiella,* a more limited approval than for other second-generation drugs. It also is approved for bone infections, septicemias, and surgical prophylaxis. The adverse effects are those of cephalosporins in general (see the general statement). Pain at the injection site is usually slight. However, supra infections caused by *Pseudomonas* and *Candida* may occur more frequently than with first- and other second-generation cephalosporins.

It is absorbed poorly by the oral route. However, the axetil ester is available for oral therapy of otitis media, pneumonia, and UTIs.

In plasma, 33% is protein-bound. The volume of distribution is 0.19 mL/g. It penetrates into CSF. More than 85% is eliminated in the urine; the half-life is 1.3 to 1.7 hr but may be as much as 24 hr in renal failure.

The axetil amide of cefuroxime is more lipid-soluble than the sodium salt, so that it is better absorbed by the oral route. Oral bioavailability without food is 36% compared to 50% fasting. It is approved for the treatment of otitis media caused by *Branhamella catarrhalis, H influenzae,* and *Strep pneumoniae* or *pyogenes;* pharyngitis and tonsilitis by *Strep pyogenes;* lower respiratory tract infections by *H influenzae* or *parainfluenzae* and *Strep pneumoniae;* skin infections by *Staph aureus* and *Strep pyogenes;* and UTIs by *E coli* and *Kl pneumoniae.*

CEPHALEXIN

5-Thia-1-azabicyclo[4.2.0]oct-2-ene-2-carboxylic acid, [6R-[6α,7β(R*)]]-7-[(aminophenylacetyl)amino]-3-methyl-8-oxo-, monohydrate; Keflex

[23325-78-2] $C_{16}H_{17}N_3O_4S \cdot H_2O$ (365.40).

Preparation—*J Med Chem* 1969; 12:310.

Description—White crystals; pK_a 5.2, 7.3; pH (0.5% solution) approximately 4.5.

Solubility—1 g in 100 mL water; soluble in dilute aqueous alkaline solutions; very slightly soluble to practically insoluble in organic solvents.

Comments—An *oral first-generation cephalosporin* with antimicrobial activity and adverse effects characteristic of that class (see the general statement). It is approved for use against respiratory infections by pneumococcus and Group A beta-hemolytic streptococci; otitis media by *H influenzae, Branhamella catarrhalis,* pneumococcus, staphylococci and streptococci; bone and joint infections by *Pr mirabilis* and staphylococci; skin and soft tissue infections by staphylococci and streptococci; and UTIs by *E coli, Klebsiella,* and *Pr mirabilis.* It is effective orally.

Elimination is by renal excretion with a half-life of 0.9 hr, except 5 to 30 hr in renal failure.

CEPHALOTHIN SODIUM

5-Thia-1-azabicyclo[4.2.0]oct-2-ene-2-carboxylic acid, (6R-trans)-3-[(acetyloxy)methyl]-8-oxo-7-[(2-thienylacetyl)amino]-, monosodium salt, Keflin, Leutral

[58-71-9] $C_{16}H_{15}N_2NaO_6S_2$ (418.41).

Preparation—7-Aminocephalosporanic acid is *N*-acetylated with 2-thiopheneacetyl chloride in a dehydrochlorinating environment. The starting acid may be prepared from the natural antibiotic, cephalosporin C, by either proton-catalyzed or enzymatic hydrolysis. The cephalothin thus prepared may be converted into its sodium salt by interaction with sodium acetate in a suitable organic solvent.

Description—White to off-white, crystalline powder; practically odorless; moderately hygroscopic; decomposes on heating; pK_a 2.2.

Solubility—Freely soluble in water, normal saline or dextrose solution; slightly soluble in alcohol; insoluble in most organic solvents.

Comments—A *first-generation cephalosporin* given IM and IV. It is short-acting and has the weakest spectrum of its class.

CEPHAPIRIN SODIUM

5-Thia-1-azabicyclo[4.2.0]oct-2-ene-2-carboxylic acid, [6R-trans]-3-[(acetyloxy)methyl]-8-oxo-7-[[(4-pyridylthio)acetyl]amino]-, monosodium salt; Cefadyl

[24356-60-3]$C_{17}H_{16}N_3NaO_6S_2$ (445.46).

Preparation—From 7-aminocephalosporanic acid by bromomethylation of the amino group to form the bromacetamide and then displac-

ing the bromine with 4-mercapto-pyridine to produce the thioether. Treatment with sodium bicarbonate gives the salt. US Pat 3,578,661 (1970); *J Med Chem* 1973; 16:1413.

Description—Soluble in water.

Solubility—Soluble in water.

Comments—A short-acting *first-generation cephalosporin* given IM or IV.

CEPHRADINE

5-Thia-1-azabicyclo[4.2.0]oct-2-ene-2-carboxylic acid, [6R-[6α,7β- (R*)]]-7-[(amino-1,4-cyclohexadien-1-ylacetyl]amino]-3-methyl-8-oxo-, Velosef

[31828-50-9 (non-stoichiometric hydrate)] [38821-53-3 (anhydrous)] $C_{16}H_{19}N_3O_4S$ (anhydrous)(349.40).

Preparation—From cephalosporanic acid. US Pat 3,485,819 (1969); *J Med Chem* 1971; 14:117.

Description—Colorless crystals (monohydrate) melting about 141°; pK_{a1} −2.63, pK_{a2} −7.27.

Solubility—Slightly soluble in acetone or alcohol; soluble in propylene glycol.

Comments—A short-acting first generation cephalosporin given IM or IV. The dosage form contains a non-stoichiometric hydrate containing up to 16% water and products must indicate by the labeling on the package and each label of a bulk shipment, eg, "Each capsule contains X mg of cephradine as the dihydrate."

LORACARBEF

1-Azabicyclo[4.2.0]oct-2-ene-2-carboxylic acid, [6R-[6α,7β(R*)]]-7-[(aminophenylacetyl)amino]-3-chloro-8-oxo-, monohydrate, Lorabid

[124750-99-8] $C_{16}H_{16}ClN_3O_4 \cdot H_2O$ (367.79).

Preparation—US Pat 4,708,956 (1987).

Description—White solid melting about 210°.

Solubility—Slightly soluble in water.

Comments—An oral *second-generation cephalosporin* with good beta-lactamase resistance. It is actually a carbacephem that has an antibacterial spectrum similar to cefaclor, cefprozil, or cefuroxime axetil. It is an alternative agent for upper and lower respiratory tract infections due to *Strep pneumoniae, H influenzae,* or *Branhamella catarrhalis.* It also may be used for uncomplicated UTIs caused by *E coli* or *Staph saprophyticus.*

It has a serum half-life of 1 hr and is eliminated almost entirely by renal excretion. Protein binding is 25%. The most common adverse effect is diarrhea, but limited experience with this beta-lactam antibiotic suggests that one consider its potential for allergic reactions including anaphylaxis. Patients allergic to penicillin may also be allergic to loracarbef.

Carbapenems and Monobactams

Carbapenems (imipenem and meropenem) are penicillin-related antibiotics in which the sulfur atom in the A ring of penicillanic acid has been replaced by carbon. A double bond in the A ring helps the planarity of the ring to approximate that of penicillanic acid. The carbapenems bind to penicillin-binding Proteins 1 and 2 and thus have antibacterial actions similar to those of the penicillins. However, they also bind to binding-Protein 7, which enables them to kill nongrowing bacteria, a property that undoubtedly will be found to be important in the treatment of infections with large populations of dormant cells (endocarditis, meningitis, ophthalmitis, osteomyelitis, etc). Carbapenems induce beta-lactamases but are resistant to them, which accounts for their efficacy against more than 90% of gram-negative species of bacteria.

Some important advantages of carbapenems include better activity against many highly penicillin-resistant strains of *Strep pneumoniae* and gram-negative aerobes, especially *Enterobacter*. They are not active against methicillin-resistant strains of staphylococci and *Enterococcus*. They also penetrate body tissues and fluids well including the CSF. They are eliminated by the kidney that can inactivate imipenem. Consequently, imipenem is only available with cilistatin, an inhibitor of renal dehydropeptidases. Patients allergic to penicillin may be sensitive to carbapenems. Other common side effects of these parenteral drugs are nausea, vomiting, skin rashes, and reactions at infusion sites. Excessive blood levels in patients with renal failure may lead to seizures, which are less frequently observed with meropenem (Table 90-5).

Monobactams (aztreonam) are natural or synthetic analogs of a monocyclic beta-lactam antibiotic isolated from certain soil bacteria. They bind only to penicillin-binding Protein 3, so that their activity is limited to aerobic gram-negative organisms; gram-positive and anaerobic organisms are insensitive. β-4-Alkyl groups confer resistance to most β-lactamases. Monobactams do not induce β-lactamases.

AZTREONAM

Propanoic acid, [2S,2α,3β(Z)]]- 2-[[[1-(2-amino-4-thiazolyl)-2-[(2-methyl-4-oxo-1-sulfo-3-azetidinyl)amino]-2-oxoethylidene]amino]-oxy]-2-methyl-, Azactam

[78110-38-0] $C_{13}H_{17}N_5O_8S_2$ (435.43).

Preparation—Neth Pat Appl 81 00571; *CA* 1982; 96:181062x.

Description—White powder; decomposes about 227°; pK$_a$ −0.5, 2.6, 3.7.

Solubility—Very soluble in water; slightly soluble in methanol; soluble in DMF; practically insoluble in nonpolar solvents.

Comments—A monobactam with antibacterial activity against most *Enterobacteriaceae* comparable to that of the extended-spectrum penicillins or third-generation cephalosporins. However, it is not active against *Acinetobacter* and is variably active against *Ps aeruginosa*. Against β-lactamase-producing, nonenteric gram-negative bacilli, such as *H influenzae* and *N gonorrhoeae*, it is as effective as third-generation cephalosporins. This drug and aminoglycosides mutually enhance antibacterial efficacy. In bacteremias, intra-abdominal infections, pneumonias, skin and soft-tissue infections and UTIs, efficacy ranges from 80% to 90%. Gram-positive organisms are not sensitive.

It causes the adverse effects characteristic of penicillins and cephalosporins except that coagulation defects do not occur. However, it does not cause cross-sensitization with penicillins or cephalosporins.

Oral bioavailability is low. In plasma, 56% is protein-bound. The volume of distribution is 0.18 mL/kg. The drug crosses the placental barrier and also is excreted in milk. Renal tubular secretion accounts for about 67% of elimination; 7% is converted to a metabolite and excreted and over 1% is secreted into bile. The half-life is 1.7 hr in healthy adults but longer in renal failure or if given with probenecid.

ERTAPENEM SODIUM

1-Azabicyclo[3.2.0]hept-2-ene-2-carboxylic acid, [4R-[3(3S*,5S*),4α,5β, 6β(R*)]]-3-[[5-[[(3-carboxyphenyl)amino]carbonyl]-3-pyrrolidinyl]thio-6-(1-hydroxyethyl)-4-methyl-7-oxo-, monosodium salt; Invanz

[153832-38-3] $C_{22}H_{24}N_3NaO_7S$ (497.50).

Preparation—US Pat 5,952,323 (1009) and *Albany Molecular Research Tech Report*, 7(66):21-28.

Description—White to off-white hygroscopic, crystalline powder

Solubility—Soluble in water or 0.9% saline; practically insoluble in ethanol; insoluble in isopropyl acetate and THF.

Comments—A carbapenem anti-infective with enhamced stability against beta-lactamase enzymes. Not clinically active against *P aeruginosa* or *A baumannii*. Clinically useful in the treatment of mixed infections and respiratory tract infections in patients at high-risk for poor outcomes. Adverse effects are similar to other beta-lactam anti-infectives.

IMIPENEM

1-Azabicyclo[3.2.0]hept-2-ene-2-carboxylic acid, [5R-[5α,6α (R*)]]-6-(1-hydroxyethyl)-3-[[2-[(iminomethyl)amino]ethyl]thio]-7-oxo-, monohydrate; ing of Primaxin

Imipemide[74431-23-5] $C_{12}H_{17}N_3O_4S \cdot H_2O$ (317.36).

Preparation—*J Med Chem* 1979; 22:1435. A crystalline derivative of thienamycin, produced by *S cuttleya*.

Description—White solid; nonhygroscopic; pK$_a$ 3.2, 9.9.

Solubility—1g in 1000 mL water or 2000 mL methanol; practically insoluble in ethanol, DMF or DMSO.

Comments—A *carbapenem*. It binds to bacterial penicillin-binding Proteins 1 and 2 and thus interferes with cell-wall synthesis, so that elongation and lysis occur. It is not destroyed by β-lactamases except those from *Ps maltophila* and occasional strains of *Bacteroides fragilis*. It has a broader antibacterial spectrum than any other β-lactam. It includes all cocci (except methicillin-resistant staphylococci and enterococci), *Enterobacteriaciae, Haemophilus, Ps aeruginosa*, and most anaerobes, including *Bacteroides fragilis*. It surpasses cephalosporins against staphylococci, equals penicillin G against streptococci, equals third-generation cephalosporins against most aerobic gram-negative bacilli and is comparable to ceftazidime against *Ps aeruginosa*. It is comparable to clindamycin or metronidazole against anaerobes. It is particularly useful for treatment of mixed bacterial infections. It should not be used alone for serious infections due to *Ps aeruginosa* because resistance may occur.

The adverse effects are those of other β-lactams. Nausea and vomiting occur with an incidence of 4%, diarrhea 3%, and hypersensitivity 3%. A reported incidence of seizures in 1.5% of recipients of imipenem-cilastatin requires confirmation; high doses, neurological disorders, and renal failure are said to contribute. The incidence of suprainfections is about 4%.

The induction of β-lactamases jeopardizes other β-lactam therapy. There is acquired resistance in up to 60% of strains of Pseudomonas. The oral bioavailability is low. Inflamed meninges are penetrated by the drug. Elimination is primarily renal, but the renal tubular cells inactivate the drug. The dehydropeptidase inhibitor, cilastatin, prevents inactivation, and enables tubular reabsorption; when it is coadministered, renal excretion of it is about 70%. It is marketed only in combination with cilastatin. Elimination half-life of both imipenem and cilastatin is 1 hr but is increased with decreased renal function.

MEROPENEM

1-Azabicyclo[3.2.0]hept-2-ene-2-carboxylic acid, [4R-[3(3S*,5S*)-4α,5β,6β(R*)]]-3-[[5-(dimethylamino)carbonyl]-3-pyrrolidino]thio]-6-(1-hydroxyethyl)-4-methyl-7-oxo-, trihydrate; Merrem

[119478-56-7] $C_{17}H_{25}N_3O_5S \cdot 3H_2O$ (437.52).

Preparation—US Pat 4,943,569 (1990).

Description—White to pale yellow crystalline powder. Solutions vary from colorless to yellow, depending on the concentration.

Solubility—Sparingly soluble in water; soluble in 5% monobasic sodium phosphate solution; very slightly soluble in alcohol; practically insoluble in acetone or ether.

Comments—A *carbapenem* similar to imipenem with slightly different affinity for specific PBPs (primary targets include PBPs 2 and 3)

depending on the strain of gram-negative bacteria. It has a similar distribution to imipenem. However, it is not degraded by renal dehydropeptidases. It has the same side effects as imipenem but is less likely to cause seizures. Because of this decreased potential, meropenem is the primary carbapenem used in the treatment of central nervous system infections.

Beta-Lactamase Inhibitors

Enzymes that open the β-lactam rings of penicillins, cephalosporins, and related compounds at the β-lactam bond are known as β-lactamases. There are several classes; classification is based upon general substrate selectivity and inhibition, the acidity or basicity of the enzyme protein, and the intra- and extracellular location of the enzyme. Those that are excreted mainly from the bacterium and the genes for which are located on plasmids are called penicillinases. They are Type II β-lactamases. They are mainly responsible for the penicillin-resistance of gram-positive bacteria, gram-negative cocci, and a number of gram-negative bacilli.

Penicillinase-resistant penicillins bind to the penicillinases but dissociation of the drug-enzyme complex is relatively rapid. They have been supplanted by clavulanate, sulbactam, and tazobactam. These newer inhibitors are β-lactams that acylate the enzyme by forming a double bond and consequently dissociate very slowly. They greatly increase the potency of the penicillins against certain bacteria and thus enhance efficacy. The combinations currently available in the US include clavulanate with amoxacillin and ticarcillin, sulbactam with ampicillin, and tazobactam with piperacillin.

CLAVULANATE POTASSIUM

[2R-(2α,3Z,5α)]-4-Oxa-1-azabicyclo[3.2.0]heptane-2-carboxylic acid, 3-(2-hydroxyethylidene)-7-oxo-, monopotassium salt; ing of Augmentum and Timentin

[61177-45-5] $C_8H_8KNO_5$ (237.25).

Preparation—A β-lactamase inhibitor, produced by *S clavuligerus*. It is the first reported naturally occurring fused β-lactam containing oxygen. *J Antibiot* 1976; 29:668.

Description—White powder; bitter-tasting.

Solubility—1 g in 2.5 mL alcohol or in less than 1 mL water.

Comments—The sulfur at Position 1 of the β-lactam ring has been replaced by oxygen and there is an ethylidene moiety at Position 2, which greatly enhances reactivity with the classic exopenicillinases of *Staph aureus* and *epidermidis* and the gram-negative β-lactamases of the Richmond Types II and III (*Haemophilus, Niesseria, E coli, Salmonella,* and *Shigella*), IV (*Bacteroides, Klebsiella,* and *Legionella*) and V. These are all plasmid-mediated enzymes; chromosomally mediated enzymes are not inhibited. It reacts irreversibly with some but not all β-lactamases. It is not presently available in a single-entity product but is marketed only in combination with amoxicillin and ticarcillin (see the separate monographs for use in particular infections).

It is absorbed well by the oral route but is also suitable for parenteral administration. In plasma, about 30% is protein-bound. About 25% to 50% is eliminated by renal tubular secretion, which is inhibited by probenicid; some is metabolized. The half-life is about 1 hr.

SULBACTAM SODIUM

(2S-cis)-4-Thia-1-azabicyclo[3.2.0]heptane-2-carboxylic acid, 3, 3-dimethyl-7-oxo-4,4-dioxide, sodium salt; ing of Unasyn

[69388-84-7] $C_8H_{10}NNaO_5S$ (255.22).

Preparation—6-aminopenicillanic is diazotized to form the unstable diazo derivative, which is immediately converted to the 6,6-dibromo compound if the reaction is carried out in the presence of bromine. Cat-

alytic hydrogenolysis of the bromine atoms forms the product. *J Org Chem* 1982; 47:3344.

Comments—A greater activity against Type I β-lactamases than clavulanate, but does not penetrate the cell walls of gram-negative bacteria as well. It extends the antibacterial spectrum of ampicillin to include β-lactamase-producing strains of *Acinetobacter, Bacteroides,* and other anaerobes, *Branhamella, Enterobacter, E coli, Klebsiella, Neisseria, Proteus,* and *Staphylococcus*. It has weak antibacterial activity of its own. It is important to note it does possess moderate antimicrobial activity against *Acinetobacter* sp that may be clinically relevant.

It is absorbed by the oral route but is also suitable for parenteral administration. The volume of distribution is about 0.27 mL/g.

Elimination is mostly by renal tubular secretion; however, it does not interfere significantly with the elimination of ampicillin, the only β-lactam antibiotics with which it is combined. It also is secreted into milk. The plasma half-life is about 1 hr. It is not currently available in a single-entity product.

TAZOBACTAM SODIUM

4-Thia-1-azabicyclo[3.2.0]-heptane-2-carboxylic acid, (2α,3α,5α)-3-methyl-7-oxo-3-(1H-1,2,3-triazol-1-ylmethyl)-, 4,4-dioxide, sodium salt; Ing of Zosyn

[89785-84-2] $C_{10}H_{11}N_4NaO_4S$ (322.27)

Preparation—*Microbiol Lett* 1997; 57:805.

Solubility—(Acid) Moderately soluble in water (5.5 mg/mL); solubility increases with increase in pH; partially soluble in methanol, acetone, ethanol; slightly soluble in ethyl acetate, ether or chloroform; insoluble in hydrocarbon solvents. (Salt) Soluble in water.

Comments—Enhanced activity against Type I beta-lactamse enzymes. It extends the spectrum of activity of piperacillin to include beta-lactamase producing strains of *Acinetobacter, Bacteroides* and other anaerobes, *Moraxella, Enterobacter, E coli, Klebsiella, Neisseria, Proteus, Pseudomonas,* and *Staphylococcus*. It has weak antibacterial activity of its own.

AMINOGLYCOSIDES

The aminoglycosides each contain one or more aminosugars, such as glucosamine or neosamine, linked by glycoside linkages to a basic (amino or guanidino) 6-membered carbon ring (eg, streptidine or streptamine).

ANTIBACTERIAL SPECTRUM—The major spectrum of activity of aminoglycosides include aerobic gram-negative bacilli and *Staph aureus*. Only gentamicin, tobramycin, amikacin, and netilmicin are reliable against most hospital-acquired infections due to aerobic gram-negative bacteria. Other aminoglycosides have distinct limitations and disadvantages that restrict their uses. It is easier to state what organisms are not affected: anaerobes (*Bacteroides, Clostridium, Entameba histolytica, Trichomonas vaginalis*), *Rickettsia*, fungi, *Trypanosoma* and viruses (Table 90-6).

MECHANISM—The aminoglycosides combine with bacterial (not mammalian) ribosomes to arrest protein synthesis. The initiation complex can be formed, but cannot pass into, subsequent stages of protein synthesis. The binding is quite firm, so that inhibition is severe enough that a bactericidal effect can result. The drugs also appear to interfere with the binding of aminoacetyl-t-RNA, which prevents chain elongation. They fur-

Table 90-6. Aminoglycosides

DRUG	COMMENTS
Amikacin	More resistant to bacterial enzymes, active vs some gentamicin resistance strains
Gentamicin	Least expensive
Netilmicin	Similar to gentamicin spectrum
Tobramycin	Similar to gentamicin spectrum
Streptomycin	Used mainly for TB

ther appear to cause misreading of some RNA codons, such that inappropriate proteins can be formed when protein synthesis is not prevented completely.

Toxicity in the human is unrelated and, instead, results from blockade of N-type calcium channels and inhibition of lysosomal phospholipase and sphingomyelinase.

RESISTANCE—Resistance to aminoglycosides develops very rapidly with some bacteria, sometimes as a single-step high resistance. With meningococcus, *Hemophilus* and some other bacteria, even dependence on the drug can occur.

Although resistance to one amino glycoside often confers resistance to others, there are important exceptions that may determine the choice of amino glycoside for the treatment of certain infections. Both acquired and natural resistance often resulting from bacterial elaboration of amino glycoside-destructive enzymes; nine such enzymes have been identified. Because of the rapid acquisition of resistance, it is common to employ aminoglycosides only in combination with other antibacterial drugs when the organism is one that rapidly develops high resistance.

COMMENTS—Aminoglycosides have been a very important class of antibiotics to treat infections caused by gram-negative bacilli. Treatment of most nosocomial gram-negative bacillary infections with third-generation cephalosporins, carbapenems, and new fluoroquinolones have made the aminoglycosides alternative drugs unless resistant strains are suspected in immunosuppressed patients.

TOXICITY—Most of the toxic actions are common among all aminoglycosides, although there are important quantitative differences in incidence and severity. Hypersensitivity, mostly manifested as rashes but sometimes as drug fever and blood dyscrasias, occurs in 5% to 10% of recipients. Eosinophilia is relatively common. A history of sensitization contraindicates use. Cross-sensitization occurs. Vestibular and auditory function may be impaired; in the early stages it may be reversible, but often it becomes irreversible if medication is not stopped. Headaches, dizziness, and nausea and vomiting during movement are early signs of impairment of vestibular function. Loss of auditory perception of high-frequency sound signals onset of auditory toxicity. Aminoglycosides vary with respect to whether auditory or vestibular function is most affected. High-ceiling diuretics increase risk of ototoxicity. Nephrotoxicity, manifested by albuminuria, hematuria, cylindruria, azotemia, tubular necrosis, and renal failure, is common to all aminoglycosides, although there are marked differences in incidence and severity. Aminoglycosides should not be used in combination with other nephrotoxic substances. Neuromuscular blockade also occurs with high doses, as the result of both postjunctional and prejunctional inhibitory actions, probably because of interference with movement of calcium into nerve terminals and motor endplate. Low plasma-calcium predisposes to the blockade. Aminoglycosides greatly will increase neuromuscular paralysis induced by curare-like drugs and ether anesthetics. Supra infections (*overgrowth*), most often candidal, may occur during prolonged use, as the result of interference with the normal microbial flora.

Therapeutic drug monitoring may be used to determine appropriate drug intervals and renal function must be monitored. Signs and symptoms of toxicity should be monitored. The use of single daily dosing of aminoglycosides may be used if renal function is not compromised. Aminoglycosides have a post-antibiotic effect and the rate of killing is concentration-dependent so that the total daily dose may be given once daily. This approach allows plasma levels to be below the threshold for MIC and decrease drug accumulation in sites that cause toxicities.

PHARMACOKINETICS—At the pH of the lower small bowel, aminoglycosides are polycationic and, hence, are absorbed poorly from the gut. For the same reason, they are confined mostly to the extracellular space and penetrate cells poorly. The distribution coefficients (Δ') range from 0.19 to 0.28 mL/g. Aminoglycosides penetrate the blood-brain barrier only slightly, unless the meninges are inflamed. Binding to plasma protein is low and ranges from 0% to 34%. The drugs are excreted mostly into urine, the amount ranging from 60% to 100%. The average clinically significant half-lives are about 2 to

3 hr, but there is a much slower phase of elimination that relates to the gradual release of tissue-bound drug; there is greater variation among recipients than there is among the drugs. Renal failure greatly prolongs the half-life. Half-lives in the inner ear are 4 to 5 times those in plasma; the half-lives in the renal cortex range from 25 to 700 hr. These facts help explain the predisposition to vestibular, auditory and renal toxicities.

AMIKACIN SULFATE

D-Streptamine, (S)-O-3-amino-3-deoxy-α-D-glucopyranosyl-(1 → 6)-O-[-6- amino-6-deoxy-α-D-glucopyranosyl-(1 → 4)]-N¹-(4-amino-2-hydroxy-1-oxobutyl)-2-deoxy-, sulfate (1:2) salt; Amikin

[39831-55-5] $C_{22}H_{43}N_5O_{23}\cdot 2H_2SO_4$ (781.78).

Preparation—Amikacin, the 1-L-(−)-4-amino-2-hydroxybutyryl derivative of kanamycin, is obtained by acylation of the C-1 amino group of the 2-deoxystreptamine moiety of kanamycin with L-(−)-4-amino-2-hydroxybutyric acid. German Pat 2,234,315, corresponding to US Pat 3,781,268 (*CA* 1973; 78:136615x).

Description—Amikacin base: white to off-white flocculent powder, which is converted to the sulfate salt in preparing injection dosage forms; melts (base) at approximately 203°, (sulfate) about 225° with decomp; pK_a (base) 8.1.

Solubility—Amikacin base: freely soluble in water; insoluble in alcohol.

Comments—The N-(4-amino-2-hydroxy-1-oxobutyl) group protects the amino glycoside from all but one of the nine amino glycoside-inactivating enzymes and acetyltransferase. In one study, more than 80% of strains of bacteria resistant to one or more aminoglycosides were sensitive in vitro to this drug. The greatest differences are shown with *Ps aeruginosa* and to a lesser extent with various *Enterobacteriaceae*.

Amikacin is considered the drug of choice for empirical therapy of infections caused by gram-negative bacilli in hospitals where bacterial strains are common that are resistant to gentamicin or tobramycin. Development of resistance to amikacin has not occurred where hospitals have used it as the primary amino glycoside. Septicemia, and serious infections of burns, urinary tract, respiratory tract and various soft tissues, meningitis, peritonitis, osteomyelitis, omphalitis in neonates, and serious surgical infections are indications for use.

The toxicity is that of the aminoglycosides in general (see the general statement). Tremors, paresthesias, arthralgia, and hypotension also occur. Plasma levels should be monitored where possible, and auditory tests and examination of the urine are mandatory. The effect on the fetus is unknown, and use in pregnancy should be avoided, if possible.

The absorption, distribution, and elimination is that of aminoglycosides in general (see the general statement). The drug is eliminated totally unchanged in the urine. The half-life is 2 to 3 hr in adults with normal renal function but up to 30 hr in renal failure; in neonates it is 4 to 8 hr.

GENTAMICIN SULFATE

Gentamicin, sulfate

Gentamycins sulfate [1405-41-0]; the sulfate salt of the antibiotic substances produced by the growth of *Micromonospora purpurea*. Potency: not less than 590 μg of gentamicin/mg, on the anhydrous basis.

Gentamicin is a mixture of gentamicin C_1, gentamicin C_2 and gentamicin C_{1A}. Gentamicin C_{1A} is O-3-deoxy-4-C-methyl-3-(methylamino)-β-L-arabinopyronosyl-(1 → 6)-O-[2,6-diamino-2,3,4,6-tetradeoxy-α-D-*erythro*-hexopyranosyl-(1 → 4)-2-deoxy-D-streptamine.

Preparation—Recovered from a fermentation broth produced when submerged cultures of two subspecies of *Micromonospora purpurea* are grown in a yeast extract-cerelose medium. US Pat 3,136,704.

Description—White to buff powder; odorless; stable in light, air and heat; melts with decomposition between 220° and 240°.

Solubility—Soluble in water; insoluble in alcohol, acetone, or benzene.

Comments—Currently the most important amino glycoside for use in the treatment of infections caused by most aerobic gram-negative bacteria and many strains of staphylococci. It has broad-spectrum antibacterial activity. The action against *Pseudomonas* is of especial interest, since species of that genus resistant to other antibiotics have become an important cause of surgical infections. They also almost always invade burned skin and, furthermore, cause some serious UTIs. However, because of systemic toxicity, present systemic use is limited mainly to life-threatening infections caused by *Pseudomonas, Klebsiella-Enterobacter-Serratia, Citrobacter*, and *Proteus*. In these infections it may be combined with an appropriate cephalosporin or penicillin.

It is used topically in the treatment of impetigo, infected bed sores, burns and nasal staphylococcal carrier state, pyodermata, and in infections of the external eye.

The absorption, distribution, elimination, and toxicity are those of aminoglycosides in general (see the general statement).

NEOMYCIN SULFATE

Fradiomycin Sulfate, Mycifradin Sulfate

Neomycin sulfate [1405-10-3]; the sulfate of an antibacterial substance produced by the growth of *Streptomyces fradiae* Waksman (Fam. *Streptomycetaceae*). Potency: equivalent to not less than 600 μg of neomycin/mg, calculated on the dried basis.

Neomycin consists almost entirely of a pair of $C_{23}H_{46}N_6O_{13}$ epimers designated as neomycin B and neomycin C, and the ratio of B to C has been observed to vary widely among different production lots. The total structure and the common names of the component parts of neomycin C are shown below. One g of salt should contain no less than 600 mg of the base.

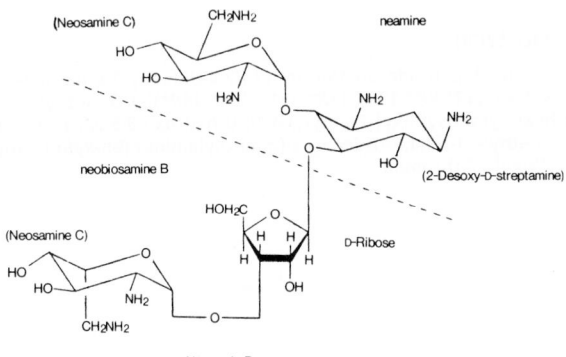

Systematically, it is O-2,6-diamino-2,6-dideoxy-α-D-gluco-pyranosyl-(1 → 3)-O-β-D-ribofuranosyl-(1 → 5)-O-[2,6-diamino-2,6-dideoxy-α-D-gluco-pyranosyl-(1 → 4)-2-deoxy-d-streptamine. Neomycin B is identical except that the α-D-glucopyranosyl residue in the neobiosamine moiety is β-L-idopyranosyl.

Description—White to slightly yellow powder or cryodesiccated solid; odorless or practically odorless; hygroscopic; pH (aqueous solution 33 mg/mL) between 5 and 7.5.

Solubility—1 g in approximately 1 mL water; very slightly soluble in alcohol; practically insoluble in acetone, chloroform or ether.

Comments—Used topically in a wide variety of local infections caused by common aerobic gram-negative bacteria in the *Enterobacteriaceae* family plus gram-positive cocci (*Staph* and *Enterococcus* but not streptococci). Some examples include infected dermatoses, burns, wounds, ulcers, impetigo, furunculosis, otitis externa, conjunctivitis and sty, as well as for irrigation of the bladder and urethra during catheterization, as prophylaxis. It mostly is combined with other antibiotics, especially polymyxin B sulfate, bacitracin zinc and gramicidin.

Orally, the drug is used to produce intestinal antisepsis prior to large bowel surgery, for the treatment of gastroenteritis caused by toxigenic *E coli* and to suppress ammonia-producing bowel flora in the management of hepatic coma. Because of rapid overgrowth of nonsusceptible bacteria, including staphylococci, oral therapy should not be continued for longer than 72 hr.

Although the orally administered drug rarely causes systemic toxic effects, it frequently produces loose stools, nausea, vomiting, and malabsorption syndromes. Applied topically, the drug is tolerated well, relatively nonirritating and has a low index of sensitivity. However, contact dermatitis occasionally occurs. Injected parenterally, it causes serious nephrotoxic, ototoxic, and neurotoxic effects. Because of the potential toxicity, parenteral injection and prolonged oral administration are avoided if possible.

NETILMICIN SULFATE

D-Streptamine, O-3-deoxy-4-C-methyl-3-(methylamino)-β-L-arabino-pyranosyl-(1 → 6)-O-[2,6-diamino-2,3,4,5-tetradeoxy-α-D-*glycero*-hex-4- enopyranosyl-(1 → 4)]-2-deoxy-N^1-ethyl-, sulfate (2:5) (salt), pentahydrate; Netromycin

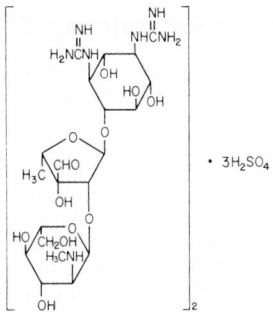

[56391-57-2] $(C_{21}H_{41}N_5O_7)_2$·5H$_2$O (1441.54); contains not less than 595 μg of netilmicin base calculated on the dried basis.

Preparation—A semi-synthetic derivative of sisomicin formed by ethylation of the amino group in the 1-position of the 2-deoxystreptamine ring; see *Chem Commun* 1976; 206.

Description—Off-white powder, p (1 in 25 solution) between 3.5 and 5.5; pK$_a$ 8.1.

Solubility—Very soluble in water.

Comments—An *aminoglycoside* with a spectrum similar to *Gentamicin.*

PAROMOMYCIN—page 1668.

STREPTOMYCIN SULFATE

D-Streptamine, O-2-deoxy-2-(methylamino)-α-L-glucopyranosyl-(1 → 2)-O-5-deoxy-3-C-formyl-α-L-lyxofuranosyl-(1 → 4)-N,N'-bis(aminoiminomethyl)-, sulfate (2:3) (salt)

Streptomycin sulfate (2:3) (salt) [3810-74-0] $(C_{21}H_{39}N_7O_{12})_2$·3H$_2SO_4$ (1457.38). Potency: equivalent to 650 to 850 μg of streptomycin $(C_{21}H_{39}N_7O_{12})$/mg.

Streptomycin is an organic base, consisting of N-methyl-*l*-glucosamine and streptidine linked through the carbohydrate streptose. The overall structure is portrayed above.

Preparation—Isolated from soil by Waksman and his colleagues of Rutgers University in 1943.

Streptomycin is produced in organic or synthetic media, in surface or submerged cultures of an actinomycete, *Streptomyces griseus*, a mold-like organism with filaments (mycelium) of bacterial thickness.

Commercially, streptomycin is manufactured much like penicillin, microbiologically in tank fermenters with aeration and agitation.

Description—White or practically white powder; odorless or has not more than a faint odor; hygroscopic; but stable toward air and light; pH (1 in 5 solution) between 4.5 and 7.0.

Solubility—Freely soluble in water; slightly soluble in alcohol; practically insoluble in chloroform.

Comments—Bacteriostatic in low concentrations and bactericidal in high concentrations to a large number of gram-negative and gram-positive bacteria. *Brucella, H ducreyi, Yersinia pestis, Francisella tu-*

larensis, many strains of *Mycobacterium tuberculosis* are sensitive to concentrations that are usually achievable in man.

The only infections in which it alone is the drug of choice are tularemia and bubonic plague. In combination with a tetracycline it is used in the treatment of brucellosis and infections caused by *Pseudomonas mallei*. It is an alternate choice drug in the treatment of chancroid, rat-bite fevers (*Spirillum* and *Streptobacillus*) and tuberculosis; in tuberculosis, however, it is never used alone, because of the rapidity of development of resistance.

The toxicity is that of aminoglycosides in general (see the general statement). In addition, malaise and myalgia may occur. Vestibular disturbances are more frequent than loss of hearing.

The absorption, distribution, and elimination are those of aminoglycosides in general.

TOBRAMYCIN

D-Streptamine, *O*-3-amino-3-deoxy-α-D-glucopyranosyl- (1 → 6)-*O*-[2,6-diamino-2,3,6-trideoxy-α-D-*ribo*-hexopyranosyl-(1 → 4)]-2-deoxy-, Tobrex, Nebcin (sulfate)

[32986-56-4] $C_{18}H_{37}N_5O_9$ (467.52). Potency: not less than 900 µg of $C_{18}H_{37}N_5O_9$ /mg, calculated on the anhydrous basis.

Preparation—An antibiotic entity separated from an antibiotic complex produced by *Streptomyces tenebrarius*. In its injection dosage form tobramycin is present as a sulfate.

Description—White or off-white, hygroscopic powder; hygroscopic; pK_a 6.7, 8.3, 9.9.

Solubility—1 g in 1.5 mL water; slightly soluble in alcohol; practically insoluble in chloroform or ether; a 1 in 10 aqueous solution, pH between 9 and 11.

Comments—An *aminoglycoside* with a spectrum similar to *Gentamicin*.

Aminoglycoside-Containing Combinations

Some examples of aminoglycoside-containing combinations (with content/mL or g provided) are as follows:

NEOMYCIN SULFATE AND POLYMYXIN B SULFATE—[Neosporin G.U. Irrigant]—40 mg and 200,000 Units, respectively; G.U. irrigant. [Neosporin, Startol]—3.5 and 10,000 Units, respectively; cream, ophthalmic ointment.—3.5 mg and 16,250 units, respectively; ophthalmic solution.

NEOMYCIN SULFATE, POLYMYXIN B SULFATE AND BACITRACIN ZINC—[Neosporin and Neosporin Ophthalmic, Triple Antibiotic, Mycitracin Triple Antibiotic and Mycitracin Ophthalmic,]—3.5 or 5 mg, 5000 Units and 400 or 500 Units, respectively; ointment and ophthalmic ointment.

NEOMYCIN SULFATE, POLYMYXIN B SULFATE AND GRAMICIDIN—[AK-Spore, Neocidin, Neosporin Ophthalmic]—1.75 mg, 10,000 units and 0.025 mg, respectively; ophthalmic solution.

Macrolides

The macrolides are hydroxylated macrocyclic lactones containing 12 to 20 carbon atoms in the primary ring. There are 37 known members of this class but only erythromycin and its derivatives have been used widely. New macrolides, clarithromycin, dirithromycin and azithromycin were approved in 1991. These are chemically similar to the 14-membered-ring macrolide, erythromycin. Azithromycin is a 15-membered-ring macrolide.

The macrolides are active against gram-positive and gram-negative aerobic bacteria and atypical organisms including chlamydiae, mycoplasmae, legionellae, rickettsiae, and spirochetes. Erythromycin is the prototypical macrolide and has been used in treating a wide variety of infections over the years. However, its use has been diminished by its gastrointestinal intolerance. The newer macrolides are better tolerated, have a broader spectrum of activity (*H influenzae*, *Mycobacterium avium*), and possess longer half-lives

The mechanism of action of the macrolides is inhibition of bacterial protein synthesis by binding to the 50s subunit of the bacterial ribosome. The complex has a relatively low affinity constant that some protein synthesiscan occur, so that these drugs are mainly bacteriostatic in therapeutic concentrations. Macrolides bind equally to ribosomes from gram-positive and gram-negative bacteria; the much greater effect on gram-positive organisms is the result of greater permeation of the cell membrane.

The macrolides in general are considered safe agents. Gastrointestinal effects such as abdominal pain, nausea, and vomiting are most common. The newer macrolides cause fewer GI side effects. Hepatotoxicity related to the macrolides is rare but may be serious. It is also less common with the newer agents. Extremely high doses of IV erythromycin and oral clarithromycin have been associated with ototoxicity. Phlebitis may occur with the intravenous administration of the macrolides.

The macrolides are separated into groups based on clinical significance of drug interactions. It is postulated that structural features of the compounds contribute to their interacting potential. Group 1 includes the prototype, erythromycin, a documented inhibitor of the cytochrome P450 enzyme system. It has been shown to prolong the half-life of an extensive list of agents including cyclosporine, theophylline, rifampin, and the HMG-CoA reductase inhibitors. These interactions are also likely to occur in Group 2 which includes clarithromycin. The newer marcolides in Group 3, azithromycin and Dirithromycin, do not form CYP 450 complexes so the possibility of interactions is low (Table 90-7).

AZITHROMYCIN

Oxa-6-azacyclopentadecan-15-one, 13-[(2,6-dideoxy-3-*C*-methyl-[2*R*-(2*R**,3*S**,4*R**,5*R**,8*R**,10*R**,11*R**,12*S**,13*S**,14*R**)]-3-*O*-methyl-α-L-*ribo*-hexopyranosyl)oxy]-2-ethyl-3,4,10-trihydroxy-3,5,6,8,10,12,14-heptamethyl-11-[[3,4,6-trideoxy-3-(dimethylamino)-β-D-*xylo*-hexopyr anosyl]oxy]-, Zithromax

[83905-01-5] $C_{38}H_{72}N_2O_{12}$ (749.00).

Preparation—A semisynthetic macrolide similar to erythromycin A; US Pat 4,517,359.

Description—White crystals; melts about 114°.

Comments—A new alternative macrolide to erythromycin that has a similar spectrum of activity. It is active against staphylococci and

Table 90-7. Macrolides

DRUG	COMMENTS
Azithromycin	Expanded spectrum, less GI effects, does not affect CYP enzymes, long half-life
Clarithromycin	Improved spectrum over erythromycin,less GI effects, inhibits CYP enzymes
Erythromycin	Frequent GI effects, inhibits CYP enzymes

streptococci but is more active than erythromycin against *H influenzae* and some aerobic gram-negative bacilli. Azithromycin suspension should be taken at least 1 hr before or 2 hr after a meal but tablets (as the dihydrate) are unaffected by food. It has a half-life of approximately 50 hours, which is much longer than any other macrolide. Only 6% is recovered from the urine; hepatic metabolism and biliary excretion account for most of its clearance.

Side effects most frequently reported are diarrhea, nausea, and abdominal pain, but these are less than those observed with erythromycin. Antacids containing aluminum or magnesium affect absorption. In addition, this new macrolide does not form complexes with the CYP 450 system so the possibility of interactions is low. Azithromycin is most commonly used in the treatment of respiratory tract infections (sinusitis, bronchitis, pneumonia) as well as for the prophylaxis of Mycobacterium avium infections in AIDS patients.

CLARITHROMYCIN

Erythromycin, 6-*O*-methyl; Biaxin

[81103-11-9] $C_{38}H_{69}NO_{13}$ (747.96). For the structure of *Erythromycin base,* see next monograph.

Preparation—US Pat 4,331,802.

Description—Crystals; colorless; melts about 220° with decomposition.

Comments—An alternative to erythromycin that is two- to fourfold times more active than erythromycin against most streptococci and staphylococci. It has moderate activity against *H influenzae* and *N gonorrhoeae* and is also active against the atypical organisms as well as mycobacteria. Clarithromycin is well absorbed from the GI tract with or without food. Bioavailability is approximately 50%. It is metabolized in the liver, and 30% to 40% of the dose is recovered in the urine. It is 65% to 70% bound to plasma proteins but penetrates well into tissues and cells, including macrophages and polymorphonuclear leukocytes. It may increase serum concentrations of theophylline or carbamazepine. Diarrhea, nausea, vomiting, dyspepsia, and metallic taste may occur but seem to be less frequent than reported with erythromycin.

Clarithromycin is an alternative to erythromycin that has a more convenient twice daily dosage regimen for the treatment of upper and lower respiratory tract infections. It is also a first-line agent used in combination with ethambutol for the treatment of *Mycobacterium avium* infection in AIDS patients.

DIRITHROMYCIN

Comments—Prodrug converted to erythromycylamine during intestinal absorption. The bioavailability of the oral formulation is 10%. Dirithromycin is enteric-coated to protect contents from gastric acid. The protein binding of dirithromycin ranges from 15% to 30%. The agent is primarily eliminated in the bile and undergoes little hepatic metabolism. The mean half-life is estimated to be approximately 8 hours. Rapid distribution of dirithromycin into tissues results in significantly higher concentrations in tissue than in serum. As a result, dirithromycin is not recommended for use in the treatment of known or suspected bacteremias due to inadequate serum levels to provide sufficient coverage of the bloodstream.

ERYTHROMYCIN

(3*R**,4*S**,5*S**,6*R**,7*R**,9*R**,11*R**,12*R**,13*S**, 14*R**)-4-[(2,6-Di-deoxy-3-*C*-methyl-3-*O*-methyl-α-ʟ-*ribo*-hexopyranosyl) oxy]-14-ethyl-7,12,13-trihydroxy-3,5,7,9,11,13-hexamethyl-6-[[3,4,6-trideoxy-3-(dimethylamino)-β-ᴅ-*xylo*-hexopyranosyl]oxy]oxacyclotetradecane-2, 10-dione; Ilotycin; E-Mycin

[114-07-8] $C_{37}H_{67}NO_{13}$ (733.94). Potency: not less than 850 μg of $C_{37}H_{67}NO_{13}$/mg, calculated on the anhydrous basis.

Preparation—Elaborated during the growth of a strain of *Streptomyces erythreus.* US Pat 2,823,203.

Description—White or slightly yellow crystals or powder; odorless or practically odorless; slightly hygroscopic; pK_a 8.7.

Solubility—1 g in approximately 1000 mL of water; soluble in alcohol, chloroform, or ether.

Comments—The prototypical macrolide with activity against gram-positive, gram-negative, and the atypical organisms (*Mycoplasma, Chlamydia, Legionella*).

Nausea, vomiting, and occasionally, diarrhea and stomatitis may occur, particularly with large doses. Hypersensitivity, skin eruptions, fever, and eosinophilia occasionally occur. The drug antagonizes lincomycin and chloramphenicol. Hepatic dysfunction, with or without jaundice, occurs in some patients receiving oral erythromycin products (especially the estolate).

It is absorbed variably after oral administration. Food interferes with absorption. The antibiotic is destroyed by gastric acid so enteric-coated preparations of the free base and acid-resistant salts or esters are used. It is 73% bound to plasma proteins. The volume of distribution is 0.72 mL/g. The plasma half-life is 1.2 to 2 hr but may be prolonged up to 5 to 6 hr in renal insufficiency.

The antibiotic does not diffuse readily into CSF, but attains antibacterial concentrations in peritoneal and pleural fluids. Only 2% of oral and 20% of parenteral erythromycin is excreted in active form by the kidney. The antibiotic is concentrated in the liver and excreted in active form in the bile. Erythromycin increases the plasma levels of theophylline, caffeine, alfentanil, carbamazepine, cyclosporine, digoxin, warfarin, and bilirubin.

Polypeptides

The polypeptide antibiotics (bacitracin and polymyxin B) are restricted to topical use because of their systemic toxicity. They differ from each other in their mechanism of action and antibacterial spectrum. Bacitracin is mainly effective against gram-negative bacteria and inhibits cell wall synthesis by interfering with the transfer of peptidoglycan subunits to the cell wall. Polymyxin are active against gram-negative bacteria by virtue of their cationic detergent-like disruption of bacterial cytoplasmic membranes.

BACITRACIN

Ayfivin; Penitracin; Topitracin; Zutracin

Bacitracin [1405-87-4]; polypeptide produced by the growth of the *licheniformis* group of *Bacillus subtilis* (Fam *Bacillaceae*). It has a potency of not less than 40 USP Units of bacitracin/mg. (The USP Unit of Bacitracin is the bacitracin activity exhibited by the weight of USP Bacitracin Reference Standard indicated on the label of the Standard. The USP unit and that defined by the FDA are equivalent.) Sterile bacitracin has a potency of not less than 50 Units/mg.

Bacitracin is a mixture of at least nine polypeptides, principally bacitracin A, $C_{66}H_{103}N_{17}O_{16}S$ (1411). The structure of bacitracin A has been shown to be

in which the detailed structure at the upper right represents a cyclic condensation moiety derived from cysteine and isoleucine.

Preparation—Several methods for isolation and purification of this antibiotic have been published. For details of certain of these multistep procedures see US Pats 2,498,165, 2,828,246, and 2,915,432.

Description—White to pale-buff powder; odorless or has a slight odor; hygroscopic; solutions rapidly deteriorate at room temperature; precipitated from its solutions and is inactivated by salts of many of the heavy metals; solutions retain their potency for several weeks if kept in a refrigerator.

Solubility—Freely soluble in water; soluble in alcohol; insoluble in chloroform or ether.

Comments—Effective mainly against gram-positive bacteria. It is limited largely in its use to infections that can be treated by topical application or local infiltration. The high incidence of nephrotoxicity (albuminuria, cylindruria, azotemia, accumulation of drug) that follows its parenteral administration precludes systemic use except in life-endangering staphylococcal infections (pneumonia, empyema) in infants in which other antibiotics have proved to be ineffective or in the treatment of antibiotic-associated (pseudomembranous) enterocolitis caused by *Cl difficile*.

It is effective topically in the treatment of the following cutaneous bacterial infections where the pathogen is bacitracin-sensitive:impetigo contagiosa, folliculitis, pyoderma, ecthyma, furunculosis, decubitus ulcer, infectious eczematoid dermatitis, scabies, and dermatophytosis. The drug is used in the treatment of ophthalmological conditions. The zinc salt often is preferred for topical therapy and is the form most often incorporated into combinations. It usually is combined with neomycin and polymyxin B sulfate. Development of bacterial resistance is much less frequent and slower for bacitracin than for penicillin, and for most organisms it is essentially nil.

In addition to renal damage, toxic effects of parenteral use include pain, induration and petechiae at the site of injection, skin rash, malaise, anorexia, nausea, and vomiting. In a few instances tinnitus and a peculiar taste may be noted. Topical application is usually not irritating and rarely induces allergic reactions.

POLYMYXIN B SULFATE

Polymyxin B, sulfate; Aerosporin

Polymyxin B sulfate [1405-20-5]; the sulfate salt of a substance produced by the growth of *Bacillus polymyxa* (Prazmowski) Migula (Fam *Bacillaceae*). It has a potency of not less than 6000 Units of polymyxin B/mg, calculated on the anhydrous basis.

Preparation—The filtered broth from the fermentation step is treated with a certified dye and the polymyxin B-dye salt complex thus precipitated is collected by filtration, washed with water and treated with an alcoholic solution of a lower aliphatic amine sulfate. The polymyxin B sulfate thus formed is filtered off, purified and lyophilized.

There are several polymyxins each of which is an *N*-monoacylated decapeptide with seven of the amino acid residues in cyclic union. Polymyxin B is a mixture of polymyxin B_1 ($C_{56}H_{98}N_{16}O_{13}$) and polymyxin B_2 ($C_{55}H_{96}N_{16}O_{13}$) the only difference being in the composition of the *N*-acyl group:

$$
\begin{array}{c}
O \\
\parallel \\
\text{Dbu-Thr-Dbu-C-R} \\
|
\end{array}
$$

$$\boxed{\text{Dbu-Dbu-Thr-Dbu-Dbu-DPhe-Leu}}$$

(Dbu = 2,4-diaminobutyric acid)
Polymyxin B_1 R = (+)-5-methylheptyl
Polymyxin B_2 R = 5-methylhexyl

The close relationship between these polymyxins and the colistins (see preceding article) is readily apparent.

Description—White to buff-colored powder; odorless or a faint odor; solutions are slightly acid or are neutral to litmus (pH 5 to 7.5); pK_a 8 to 9.

Solubility—Freely soluble in water; slightly soluble in alcohol.

Comments—In vitro and in vivo antimicrobial spectrum of activity is restricted to gram-negative bacteria, including *Aerobacter, Acinetobacter, Escherichia, Haemophilus, Klebsiella, Pasteurella, Pseudomonas, Salmonella, Shigella*, most *Vibrio* and *Yersinia*; all strains of *Pr providencia* and most of *Serratio marcescens* are unaffected by the antibiotic. In particular, it possesses activity against many multiply resistant strains of Acinetobacter and Pseudomonas species. All gram-positive bacteria are resistant.

The drug is used topically for the treatment or the prevention and treatment of external ocular infections caused by susceptible microorganisms, especially *Ps aeruginosa*. In topical therapy, it often is combined with neomycin, gramicidin, and bacitracin. It also is included in glucocorticoid ophthalmological topical preparations.

When given parenterally, it adversely can affect the nervous system and the kidney. Substances such as soap, which antagonize cationic surface-active agents, impair the action of the antibiotic.

VANCOMYCIN—page 1662.

Tetracyclines

The tetracyclines are all very much alike with respect to their antimicrobial spectra and the untoward effects they elicit. They differ mainly in their absorption, duration of action and suitability for parenteral administration (Table 90-8).

Table 90-8. Tetracyclines

DRUG	COMMENTS
Chlortetracycline	Short acting, incomplete oral abs
Demeclocycline	Intermed. acting, more phototoxicity
Doxycycline	Long acting, good oral abs, biliary excretion
Minocycline	Long acting, good oral abs, dizziness, and vertigo, metabolized
Methacycline	Intermed acting
Oxytetracycline	Short acting, incomplete oral abs
Tetracycline	Short acting, incomplete oral abs

ANTIMICROBIAL ACTIONS—The tetracyclines are broad-spectrum antibiotics. They are mainly bacteriostatic. They bind to the bacterial 30s ribosomes and prevent t-RNA from combining with m-RNA. Thus, protein synthesis is inhibited. The drugs have activities against both gram-positive and gram-negative bacteria, mycobacteria, *Mycoplasma*, treponemas, leptospira, rickettsia, actinomycetes, *Coxiella*, *Chlamydiae*, and plasmodia. The susceptible gram-positive bacteria are variable.

Although resistance to the tetracyclines is not acquired as rapidly as to penicillin, it nevertheless does occur readily. Among the gram-positive bacteria up to 44% of *Strep pyogenes* are resistant and 74% of *Enterococcus fecalis*. The incidence of resistance among hospital strains of *Staph aureus* may run from 30% to 50% but may increase to as high as 75% after several days of treatment. Highly resistant gonococci have become prevalent; however, topical tetracycline is comparable with silver nitrate in the prophylaxis of ophthalmia neonatorum and does not cause chemical conjunctivitis.

Various streptococci and pneumococci also become resistant. The incidence of resistance among various gram-negative bacteria is also very high, especially among the *Enterobacteriaceae*, which in the intestine can pass resistance-controlling genes from one species, even genus, to another (infectious drug resistance). Resistance to one tetracycline usually confers resistance to all others, except that some tetracycline-resistant strains of streptococci and *E coli* may retain sensitivity to minocycline. Cross-resistance between penicillin and tetracyclines or between other classes of antibiotics and tetracyclines is uncommon, except in infectious drug resistance, in which the acquired episome or plasmid contains more than one gene for resistance to other drugs.

COMMENTS—A tetracycline alone is the drug of choice in the treatment of cholera, relapsing fever, granuloma inguinale and infections caused by rickettsia, *Borrelia, Mycobacterium fortuitum* and *marinum,* and *Chlamydia psittaci* and *trachomatis* (except pneumonia and inclusion conjunctivitis). With erythromycin it shares first-choice status for the treatment of *Mycoplasma pneumonia* (primary atypical pneumonia). A tetracycline is a component of first-choice combinations for the treatment of brucellosis, glanders and infections by *Ps pseudomallei*. It is an alternative drug for the treatment of actinomycosis, anthrax, chancroid, melioidosis, plague, rat-bite fevers, syphilis, and yaws. However, in the treatment of acne, tetracyclines maintain a favored but challengeable status; if there is inflammation with pustules and cysts, an antibiotic may be indicated.

Doxycycline has been shown to prevent travelers' diarrhea caused by enterotoxigenic *E coli*. In UTIs, other drugs usually are preferred, unless sensitivity testing especially indicates tetracyclines. However, tetracyclines are used in nongonococcal urethritis and in prostatitis (often a mycoplasma). In UTIs and urethritis, the urine should be acidified to favor antibacterial action. In the treatment of the meningococcal carrier state, minocycline, but not other tetracyclines, appears to be effective.

In combination with quinine, a tetracycline is an alternative drug for the treatment chloroquine-resistant *Plasmodium falciparum* malaria.

Tetracyclines are used as an alternative to silver nitrate in the prevention of neonatal ocular prophylaxis of chlamydial and gonococcal conjunctivitis, but studies have shown them to be inferior.

ADVERSE EFFECTS—The tetracyclines cause a number of untoward effects. GI toxicity is common with oral use; it is probably the combined effect of local irritation and alteration of the intestinal flora. Manifestations are heartburn, epigastric distress, nausea, vomiting, diarrhea and rare esophageal ulceration in persons with esophageal obstruction or spastic disease.

The broad-spectrum antibacterial activity of the tetracyclines causes marked alterations in the floral ecology, so that microorganisms formerly held in check overgrow to cause superinfections. This occurs most frequently in the bowel but it also may occur readily in the mouth, lungs, vagina, and occasionally elsewhere. The most common superinfection is candidiasis, but overgrowth from staphylococci, enterococci, *Proteus, Pseudomonas,* or *Cl difficile* (cause of antibiotic-associated colitis) occurs. Staphylococcal enteric superinfections are frequently fatal.

Various hypersensitivity reactions, especially urticaria, asthma or facial edema, occur, but they are uncommon. Phototoxicity can occur with all tetracyclines, but it is most frequent with demeclocycline.

Hepatotoxicity, which is sometimes fatal, occasionally results when the daily dose in adults exceeds 1 g/day, especially if the tetracycline is given intravenously; pregnancy and renal failure predispose to this toxicity. Tetracyclines also may increase the risk of hepatic damage by other hepatotoxic drugs.

Although tetracyclines probably do not affect normal kidney function, they aggravate preexisting renal insufficiency, which can lead to extreme azotemia, but without oliguria. Doxycycline appears to be free of this effect. Old preparations that have undergone decomposition on the shelf are serious offenders in causing nephrotoxicity. Minocycline can cause vestibular toxicity.

Tetracyclines pigment developing teeth and reversibly impair bone growth through complexation with the bone salts and fixation to matrix proteins. The implication is that tetracyclines should be avoided in children up to 8 yr of age, in whom the cosmetically important permanent teeth have not erupted. It also should be avoided in pregnancy.

IV tetracyclines may cause thrombophlebitis, caused mainly by the acid required to effect solution. IM injections cause local pain, unless a local anesthetic is included.

ABSORPTION, DISTRIBUTION, AND ELIMINATION—The extent of GI absorption is 58% to 100%. Doxycycline and minocycline are absorbed the best. Tetracyclines complex with bivalent and trivalent metal ions, so that their absorption is greatly impaired by calcium-, magnesium- and aluminum-containing antacids and by iron preparations. Food, especially milk products or other high-calcium foods, also interferes with oral absorption of tetracyclines, although a minimal effect occurs with doxycycline and minocycline. Phosphate appears to improve absorption, in part by removing calcium.

All tetracyclines are bound to plasma proteins, to an extent ranging from 35% to 91%. Volumes of distribution range from 0.14 to 1.79 mL/g. Half-lives vary from 6 to 17 hr in normal persons but 12 to 108 hr in renal failure. Doxycycline and minocycline are longer acting, the most lipophilic and pentrate tissues more efficiently. Therapeutic concentrations of minocycline are achieved in saliva and tears to eradicate the meningococcal carrier state. Renal excretion is the principal mode of elimination, except that minocycline is excreted mostly in the bile and doxycycline is more than 50% metabolized and/or excreted into the colon. The tetracyclines penetrate well into the tissues and body fluids, but penetration into the CSF is low by the oral route. All tetracyclines are excreted somewhat into the bile and not resorbed completely in the intestine, so that even IV doses are capable of altering the bowel flora.

DEMECLOCYCLINE HYDROCHLORIDE

2-Naphthacenecarboxamide, [4S-(4α,4aα,5aα,6β,12aα)]-7-chloro-4-(dimethylamino)-1,4,4a,5,5a,6,11,12a-octahydro-3,6,10,12,12a-pentahydroxy-1,11-dioxo-, monohydrochloride; Declomycin

7-Chloro-6-demethyltetracycline hydrochloride [64-73-3] $C_{21}H_{21}ClN_2O_8 \cdot HCl$ (501.32). Potency: not less than 900 μg of $C_{21}H_{21}$-$ClN_2O_8 \cdot HCl/mg$, calculated on the anhydrous basis.

Preparation—An appropriate mutant strain of *Streptomyces aureofaciens* is grown in an appropriate liquid nutrient medium under controlled conditions of temperature, pH, and aeration. The harvested broth is acidified and filtered, and the antibiotic is isolated from the filtrate, either by solvent extraction or by chemical precipitation, and converted into the hydrochloride.

Description—Yellow, crystalline powder; odorless; bitter taste; pH (1 in 100 solution) approximately 2.5; pK$_a$ 3.3, 7.2, 9.3.

Solubility—1 g in approximately 60 mL water, 200 mL ethanol, or 50 mL methanol; sparingly soluble in solutions of alkali hydroxides or carbonates; practically insoluble in chloroform.

Comments—A *tetracycline*. It is intermediate-acting and causes more phototoxicity than other members of its class.

DOXYCYCLINE

2-Naphthacenecarboxamide, [4S-(4α,4aα,5α,5aα,6α,12aα)]-4-(dimethyl-amino)-1,4,4a,5,5a,6,11,12a-octahydro-3,5,10,12,12a-pentahydroxy-6-methyl-1,11-dioxo-, monohydrate; Vibramycin

[1086-28-1] $C_{22}H_{24}N_2O_8 \cdot H_2O$ (462.46); anhydrous [564-25-0] (444.44). Potency: 880 to 980 μg of $C_{22}H_{24}N_2O_8$ /mg.

Preparation—6-Deoxy-6-demethyl-6-methylene-5-oxytetracycline (see *Methacycline*) is dissolved or suspended in an inert liquid such as methanol and hydrogenated under the influence of catalytic amounts of noble metals such as rhodium or palladium to give a mixture of the 6α- and 6β-methyl epimers. The desired epimer is then isolated by chromatographic processes. US Pat 3,200,149.

Description—Yellow, crystalline powder; bitter taste; pK$_a$ 3.4, 7.7, 9.7.

Solubility—Very slightly soluble in water; freely soluble in dilute acid or alkali hydroxide solutions; sparingly soluble in alcohol; practically insoluble in chloroform or ether.

Comments—The actions and uses generally are the same as other tetracyclines (see the general statement). Against gram-positive bacteria it is about twice as potent as tetracycline, except that it is up to 10 times as potent against *Strep viridans*. Furthermore, strains of *Enterococcus fecalis* that are resistant to other tetracyclines may be sensitive to the drug.

Against gram-negative bacteria it is as potent to twice as potent as tetracycline. It is the drug of first choice for prophylaxis of *travelers' diarrhea*, commonly caused by enterotoxigenic *E coli*. It is the best of the tetracyclines against anaerobes.

It is absorbed more completely (90–100%) after oral administration than other tetracyclines, and its absorption does not appear to be inhibited by foods. Plasma-protein binding is about 93%. It has a volume of distribution of 0.75 mL/g. It readily penetrates cells, body fluids and cavities. Elimination is about 65% by hepatic metabolism and 35% by biliary/renal excretion. The rate of excretion is slow and the half-life is the longest of the tetracyclines, namely, 12 to 22 hr. Renal insufficiency has little influence on plasma levels or duration of action.

The toxicity is that of tetracyclines in general, but there is a three-fold greater incidence of GI effects and more frequent skin rashes than with other tetracyclines. Photosensitization occurs much more frequently than with shorter-acting tetracyclines. It complexes calcium to a lesser extent than other tetracyclines not affected by food or dairy products.

MINOCYCLINE HYDROCHLORIDE

2-Naphthacenecarboxamide, [4S-(4α,4aα,5aα,12aα)]-4,7-bis(dimethyl-amino)-1,4,4a,5,5a,6,11,12a-octahydro-3,10,12,12a-tetrahydroxy-1,11-dioxo-, monohydrochloride; Minocin

7-Dimethylamino-6-demethyl-6-deoxytetracycline [13614-98-7] $C_{23}H_{27}$ N_3O_7·HCl (493.94). Potency: equivalent to not less than 785 µg of minocycline ($C_{23}H_{27}N_3O_7$)/mg.

Preparation—6-Demethyltetracycline, dissolved in tetrahydrofuran containing methanesulfonic acid, is reacted with dibenzyl azodicarboxylate to form 7-[1,2-bis(carbobenzoxy)hydrazino]-6-demethyltetracycline. Palladium-catalyzed hydrogenation in the presence of formaldehyde yields minocycline which reacts with an equimolar quantity of HCl to form the monohydrochloride. US Pats 3,148,212 and 3,226,436.

Description—Yellow, crystalline powder; odorless; slightly bitter taste; slightly hygroscopic; stable in air when protected from light and moisture (strong light and/or moist air causes it to darken); potency in solution affected primarily caused by epimerization; pH (1 in 100 solution) between 3.5 and 4.5; pK_{a1} 2.8; pK_{a2} 5; pK_{a3} 7.8; pK_{a4} 9.3.

Solubility—1 g in approximately 60 mL water and approximately 70 mL alcohol; soluble in solutions of alkali hydroxides or carbonates; practically insoluble in chloroform or ether.

Comments—The actions and uses are essentially the same as those of the tetracyclines in general (see the general statement). Against most gram-positive organisms it appears to be generally two to four times as potent as tetracycline, but it shares an equally low potency against *Enterococcus fecalis*. Against *Strep viridans* it is about eight times as potent. Against gram-negative bacteria it is generally two to four times as potent as tetracycline. It is especially effective against *Mycobacterium marinum*, and it is now the drug of choice for treating infections caused by that bacterium. It differs from other tetracyclines in that bacterial resistance to the drug is of a lower order and incidence; this is especially true of staphylococci, in which cross-resistance has been reported to be as low as 4%.

The incidence and severity of the usual side effects of tetracyclines, effects like phototoxicity and GI upsets, are less than with other tetracyclines. However, nausea and vomiting are frequent, as the result of ototoxicity and CNS effects.

It is 90% to 100% absorbed by the oral route. Its absorption is diminished slightly by food and milk and markedly by nonsystemic antacids and iron preparations. It is 70% to 75% protein-bound in plasma. The volume of distribution is 0.14 to 0.7 mL/g. The half-life is 11 to 17 hr. Only 10% is reported to be excreted unchanged, but the half-life has been reported to be greatly prolonged in renal failure.

OXYTETRACYCLINE

2-Naphthacenecarboxamide, [4S-(4α,4aα,5aα,5aα,6β,12aα)]-4-(dimethylamino)-1,4,4a,5,5a,6,11,12a-octahydro-3,5,6,10,12,12a-hexahydroxy-6-methyl-1,11-dioxo-, dihydrate; Terramycin

[6153-64-6] $C_{22}H_{24}N_2O_9$·2H_2O (496.47); *anhydrous* [79-57-2] (460.44). Potency: not less than 832 mg of $C_{22}H_{24}N_2O_9$/mg.

Preparation—By the growth of a selected strain of *Streptomyces rimosus* on a medium consisting of water, proteins, and nutrient salts.

Description—Pale yellow to tan, odorless, crystalline powder; stable in air, but exposure to strong sunlight causes it to darken; deteriorates in solutions of pH less than 2, and is rapidly destroyed by alkali hydroxide solutions; saturated solution is nearly neutral to litmus, having a pH of approximately 6.5.

Solubility—1 g in 4150 mL water, 100 mL alcohol, >10,000 mL chloroform, 6250 mL ether; freely soluble in diluted hydrochloric acid or alkaline solutions.

Comments—A *tetracycline*. It is short-acting with incomplete oral absorption.

TETRACYCLINE

2-Naphthacenecarboxamide, [4S-(4α,4aα,5aα,6β,12aα)]-4-(dimethylamino)-1,4,4a,5,5a,6,11,12a-octahydro-3,6,10,12,12a-pentahydroxy-6-methyl-1,11-dioxo-,

[60-54-8] $C_{22}H_{24}N_2O_8$ (444.44). Potency: equivalent to not less than 975 µg of tetracycline hydrochloride ($C_{22}H_{24}N_2O_8$·HCl)/mg, calculated on the anhydrous basis.

Preparation—By removal of chlorine from chlortetracycline by hydrogenation. Also obtained from a *Streptomyces* species cultured in an appropriate nutrient medium.

Description—Yellow, crystalline powder; odorless; stable in air, but exposure to strong sunlight causes it to darken; potency is affected in solutions of pH less than 2, and is destroyed rapidly by alkali hydroxide solutions; more soluble than chlortetracycline and within the physiological and moderately alkaline range of pH is more stable; its solutions darken more rapidly than chlortetracycline but less than oxytetracycline; pH (aqueous suspension, 10 mg/mL) between 3.0 and 7.0; pK_a 3.3, 7.7, 7.9.

Solubility—1 g in approximately 2500 mL water and approximately 50 mL alcohol; freely soluble in dilute HCl or alkali hydroxide solutions; practically insoluble in chloroform or ether.

Comments—The antibiotic spectrum, actions, toxicity, absorption, fate and excretion, doses and uses essentially the same as those of the tetracyclines in general (see the general statement). It has been reported to be useful in the treatment of toxoplasmosis; it is not known whether this use can be extended to all tetracyclines. The GI side effects are less than those from chlortetracycline and oxytetracycline but more than from demeclocycline. About 77% of an oral dose is absorbed. In the plasma 25% to 55% is bound to proteins. The volume of distribution is 1.5 mL/g.

About 60% is eliminated by renal excretion. The plasma half-life is 6 to 11 hr in patients with normal renal function; in oliguria it may be as long as 2 to 4 days, and dosage must be adjusted accordingly.

FLUOROQUINOLONES

The quinolone antibacterial drugs have been in use since 1964 when nalidixic acid was released. Oxolinic acid and cinoxacin were introduced later but have fallen into disuse because of their limited antibacterial spectra and rapid development of resistance The introduction of 6-fluoro and 7-(1-piperazinyl) groups to the existing structure has expanded the spectrum, increased potency, and may prevent the development of plasmid-mediated resistance. Since 1990, the fluoroquinolones have become a dominant class of antimicrobial agents. The fluoroquinolones are bactericidal agents. They are strong inhibitors of DNA gyrase (topoisomerase II) and topoisomerase IV. These enzymes are critical to the process of supercoiling DNA. Without such enzymatic activity, DNA replication cannot occur.

In general, the fluoroquinolones possess activity against gram-positive, gram-negative, and the atypical organisms. The older fluoroquinolones (ciprofloxacin, norfloxacin, ofloxacin) are highly active against gram-negative pathogens including *Pseudomonas aeruginosa* but their activity against streptococci and staphylococci is limited. Ciprofloxacin remains the fluoroquinolone with the most potent in vitro activity against *Pseudomonas aeruginosa*. The newer fluoroquinolones (levofloxacin, gatifloxacin, moxifloxacin, trovafloxacin) have enhanced activity against the gram-positive pathogens (*S aureus*, *S pneumoniae*) while maintaining similar gram-negative activity with the exception of *Pseudomonas aeruginosa*. Moxifloxacin is unique in that it possesses anti-anaerobic activity but lacks sufficient activity against *Pseudomonas aeruginosa*. Trovafloxacin has the broadest spectrum and best overall activity including better activity against anaerobes. Resistance to one fluoroquinolone usually confers resistance to all other quinolones but not to other classes of antimicrobial drugs.

Adverse effects are usually mild and transient. They include GI disturbances (nausea, vomiting, diarrhea, dyspepsia, flatulence, constipation, heartburn, abdominal discomfort); CNS symptoms (ranging from headache and dizziness to seizures); mild or moderate rash and/or pruritus (photosensitivity, especially severe with sparfloxacin); arthropathy in growing children; increased likelihood of tendon ruptures (especially Achilles in adults); and arthralgias. Prolongation of QT interval occurs with some new fluoroquinolones. Some fluoroquinolones prolong the half-life of theophylline. Erosion of cartilage has been documented in young animals so the fluoroquinolones are not recommended for use in children under 18 years old or pregnant or nursing women. However, the agents have been used safely in the childhood population of patients with cystic fibrosis without sequelae.

Fluoroquinolones are all effective orally but also may be administered parenterally. They have large volumes of distribution and reach therapeutic concentrations in most tissues. They have long half-lives and may be administered only once or twice a day (Table 90-9).

Fluoroquinolones are used to treat upper and lower respiratory infections, gonorrhea, bacterial gastroenteritis, skin and soft tissue infections including osteomyelitis and both uncomplicated and complicated UTIs,.

CIPROFLOXACIN HYDROCHLORIDE

3-Quinolinecarboxylic acid, 1-cyclopropyl-6-fluoro-1,4-dihydro-4-oxo-7-(1-piperazinyl)-, monohydrochloride, monohydrate; Ciloxan, Cipro

[8693-32-0] $C_{17}H_{18}FN_3O_3 \cdot HCl \cdot H_2O$ (385.82).

Preparation—From 3-chloro-4-fluoroaniline by condensation with diethyl ethoxymethylenemalonate to form the imine which is thermally cyclized to ethyl 7-chloro-6-fluoro-4-hydroxyquinoline-3-carboxylate. *N*-alkylation with cyclopropyl iodide followed by nucleophilic displacement of the 7-chloro group by *N*-methylpiperazine and hydrolysis of the ester affords the product. *J Med Chem* 1976;19:1138.

Description—Pale-yellow crystals; amphoteric; pK_a 6, 8.8.

Solubility—1 g in 25 mL water.

Comments—It is approved for use in the treatment of bone and joint infections, infectious diarrhea, lower respiratory tract infections, and urinary tract infections. For hospital-acquired infections, ciprofloxacin remains the preferred agent because it possesses the best activity against Pseudomonas aeruginosa. Ciprofloxacin is also recommended for meningococcal prophylaxis.

The oral bioavailability is about 70% to 80%. Urinary excretion accounts for the elimination of 40% to 50% of an oral dose. Twenty to 35% is eliminated in the feces. There is hepatic biotransformation of four known metabolites, which accounts for 15% of a dose. The half-life is about 4 hr.

Table 90-9. Fluroquinolones

DRUGS	COMMENTS
Classical Fluoroquinolones	
Ciprofloxacin	Intermed. spectrum, good distribution
Norfloxacin	Incomplete oral absorption, limited spectrum
Ofloxacin	Intermed. spectrum
Levofloxacin	More active than ofloxacin, long acting
Enoxacin	Limited spectrum
Lomefloxacin	Intermed. spectrum, phototoxicity
Pefloxacin phototoxicity	Intermed. spectrum, long acting,
Newest Fluoroquinolones	
Sparfloxacin	Expanded spectrum, long acting, serious phototoxicity problems
Grepafloxacin	Expanded spectrum, long acting
Trovafloxacin	Expanded spectrum, no effect on drug metabolizing enzymes

ENOXACIN

1,8-Naphthyridine-3-carboxylic acid, 1-ethyl-6-fluoro-1,4-dihydro-4-oxo-7-(1-piperazinyl)-, Penetrex

[74011-58-8] $C_{15}H_{17}FN_4O_3$ (320.32).

Preparation—The active 2-chloro group of 2,6-dichloro-3-nitropyridine is nucleophilically displaced by *N*-carbethoxypiperazine; then the 6-chloro atom is displaced with ammonia and the resulting amined acylated to the acetamide. The nitro group is reduced, diazotized, and treated with HBF_4 to yield the fluoro derivative. The balance of the synthesis is analogous to that for *ciprofloxacin*; *J Med Chem* 1984; 27:292.

Description—White crystals; bitter taste; melts at approximately 222°.

Solubility—1 g in 3330 mL water.

Comments—A *limited-spectrum fluoroquinolone*.

GATIFLOXACIN

3-Quinolinecarboxylic acid, (±)-1-Cyclopropyl-6-fluoro-1,4-di-hydro-8-methoxy-7-(3-methyl-1-piperazinyl)-4-oxo-, sesquihydrate; Tequin

[160738-57-8](anhydrous) $C_{19}H_{22}FN_3O_4 \cdot \frac{1}{2}H_2O$ (402.42).

Preparation—A 10-step synthesis starting with 2,4,5-trifluoro-3-hydroxybenzoic acid. *J Med Chem* 1995; 38:4478.

Description—White to pale yellow crystalline powder melting about 160°.

Solubility—Aqueous solubility is pH dependent with maximum (40-60 mg/mL) at pH 2-5.

Comments—An 8-methoxyfluoroquinolone with enhanced activity against gram-positive organisms (especially S. pneumonia). Not clinically active against *P aeruginosa*. Clinically useful in the treatment of upper and lower respiratory tract infections. It is available both orally and parenterally.

LEVOFLOXACIN

7*H*-Pyrido[1,2,3-*de*]-1,4-benzoxazine-6-carboxylic acid, (*S*)-9-fluoro-2,3-dihydro-3-methyl-10-(4-methyl-1-piperazinyl)-7-oxo-, hemihydrate; Levaquin; Cravit

[138199-71-0] $C_{18}H_{20}FN_3O_4 \cdot \frac{1}{2}H_2O$ (369.93).

Preparation—US Pat 4,382,892 (1983); Lednicer D, et al. *Org Chem of Drug Syn*, vol 4, New York: Wiley, 1990, p 141.

Description—White to light yellow needles melting about 226° (dec). It is the (−) isomer; the racemic form is *ofloxacin*. Forms stable coordination complexes with metal ions (eg, Al > Cu > Zn > Mg > Ca in order if decreasing stability).

Solubility—Essentially constant from pH 0.6 to 5.8 (100 mg/mL). Above pH 5.8 solubility increases rapidly and at pH 6.7 it reaches a max of 272 mg/mL. Above pH 6.7 solubility decreases to a min of 50 mg/mL at pH 6.9.

Comments—The more active *levo* isomer of ofloxacin (a racemic mixture of D,L-isomers) that has improved activity against gram-positive pathogens (in particular against S. pneumoniae) compared to ciprofloxacin. It is well absorbed after oral administration and more than 80% of dose is excreted in urine. Its side effects are similar to other fluoroquinolones. Useful in the treatment of urinary tract infections, lower respiratory tract infections.

LOMEFLOXACIN HYDROCHLORIDE

3-Quinolinecarboxylic acid, ($\pm$)-1-ethyl-6,8-difluoro-1,4-dihydro-7-(3-methyl-1-piperazinyl)-4-oxo-, monohydrochloride; Maxaquin

[98079-52-8] $C_{17}H_{19}F_2N_3O_3\cdot HCl$ (387.81).

Preparation—By a method analogous to that for *Enoxacin*; US Pat 4,528,287.

Description—Colorless needles; melts about 295° with decomposition.

Solubility—Soluble in water.

Comments—Another limited-spectrum fluoroquinolone that is similar in antibacterial activity to enoxacin. It is approved only for treatment of UTIs and bronchitis caused by *H influenzae* or *Branhamella catarrhalis*. It covers gram-negative organisms frequently associated with UTIs but does not have the activity to cover the same bacterial infections which respond to ciprofloxacin and ofloxacin.

MOXIFLOXACIN HYDROCHLORIDE

3-Quinolinecarboxylic acid, (4aS-cis)-1-cyclopropyl-6-fluoro-1,4-dihydro-8-methoxy-7-(octahydro-6H-pyrrolo[3,4-b]pyridin-6-yl)-4-oxo-, monohydrochloride; Avelox, Vigamox

[186826-86-8] $C_{21}H_{24}FN_3O_4\cdot HCl$ (437.89).

Preparation—US Pats 4,254,135 (1981) and 4,990,517 (1991).

Description—Slightly yellow to yellow crystals melting about 325°. $[\alpha]^{25}_D$ -256° (c = 0.5, water).

Comments—An 8-methoxy fluoroquinolone with enhanced activity against gram-positive organisms (in particular *S pneumoniae*) and moderate anti-anaerobic activity. Not clinically active against *P aeruginosa*. Clinically useful for the treatment of upper and lower respiratory tract infections. It is available both orally and parenterally.

NORFLOXACIN

3-Quinolinecarboxylic acid, 1-ethyl-6-fluoro-1,4-dihydro-4-oxo-7-(1-piperazinyl)-, Chibroxin, Noroxin

[70458-96-7] $C_{16}H_{18}FN_3O_3$ (319.34).

Preparation—Similar to *Ciprofloxacin*, see *J Med Chem* 1980; 23:1358.

Description—White to pale-yellow crystalline powder; melts about 221°; hygroscopic and forms a hemihydrate in air; pK$_a$ 6.3, 8.8.

Solubility—Very slightly soluble in water, methanol or alcohol; freely soluble in glacial acetic acid.

Comments—A *limited-spectrum fluoroquinolone*. It has incomplete oral absorption.

OFLOXACIN

7H-Pyridol[1,2,3-de]-1,4-benzoxazine-6-carboxylic acid, ($\pm$)-9-fluoro-2,3-dihydro-3-methyl-10-(4-methyl-1-piperazinyl)-7-oxo-, Floxin

[82419-36-1] $C_{18}H_{20}FN_3O_4$ (361.38). The carbon atom to which the methyl group is attached, in the oxazine ring, is chiral and the clinically used substance is a racemic mixture, whereas the (+) form has twice the activity of the (−) form.

Preparation—By a method analogous to that for *Ciprofloxacin*; US Pat 4,382,892.

Description—Colorless needles; melts about 255° with decomposition; pK$_a$ 7.9.

Solubility—Poorly soluble in water or ethanol.

Comments—An *intermediate-spectrum fluoroquinolone*.

PEFLOXACIN

3-Quinolinecarboxylic acid, 1-ethyl-6-fluoro-1,4-di-hydro-7-(4-methyl-1-piperazinyl)-4-oxo-,

Preparation—US Pat 4,292,317 (1981); Lednicer D, et al. *Org Chem of Drug Syn*, vol 4, p 141. New York: Wiley, 1990.

Description—White crystals melting about 271° (dec). It is the *N*-methyl analog of norfloxacin.

Solubility—Slightly soluble in water; soluble in fixed acids or alkalies.

Comments—An intermediate spectrum, long acting fluoroquinolone; causes.

SPARFLOXACIN

3-Quinolinecarboxylic acid, cis-5-amino-1-cyclopropyl-7-(3,5-dimethyl-1-piperazinyl)-6,8-difluoro-1,4-dihydro-4-oxo-, Zagam

[110871-86-8] $C_{19}H_{22}F_2N_4O_3$ (392.41).

Preparation—US Pat 4,795,751 (1989); *J Med Chem* 1990; 33:1645.

Description—Yellow crystalline powder melting about 268°(dec); pK$_{a1}$ −6.25; pK$_{a2}$ −9.30.

Solubility—Sparingly soluble in glacial acetic acid or chloroform; very slightly soluble in alcohol; practically insoluble in water or ether. Soluble in dilute mineral acids or fixed bases (ca 0.1 *N*).

Comments—It is a newer fluoroquinolone with improved activity against *Strep pneumoniae* and other lower respiratory pathogens covered by grepafloxacin. It is more active against *Mycoplasma* than other fluoroquinolones. It has excellent oral bioavailability (92%) and is metabolized mainly by hepatic glucuronidation rather than cytochrome P450-mediated pathways. Consequently, it does not affect the clearance of other drugs (like theophylline, cimetidine, digoxin, warfarin and cyclosporine) that occurs with some fluoroquinolones. It has a half-life of approximately 20 hr. Its side effects are similar to other fluoroquinolones except that photosensitivity is much more severe.

TROVAFLOXACIN

1,8-Naphthyridine-3-carboxylic acid, (1α,5α,6α)-7-(6-amino-3-azabicyclo[3.1.0]hex-3-yl)-1-(2,4-diflourophenyl)-6-fluoro-1,4-dihydro-4-oxo-, monomethanesulfonate; Trovan

[147059-75-4] $C_{20}H_{15}F_3N_4O_3\cdot CH_4O_3S$ (512.47).

Preparation—US Pat 5,164,402 (1992).

Description—White to off-white powder.

Comments—It is a newer fluoroquinolone that is similar to the antibacterial spectrum of grepafloxacin that involves a better activity against some respiratory pathogens than the older fluoroquinolones such as ciprofloxacin. It is more active against *Strep pneumoniae* (including penicillin-resistant strains), *Staph aureus* (including methicillin-resistant strains), Enterococcus faecalis, and most important respiratory tract pathogens (*H influenzae, Moraxella, Legionella, Neisseria*). It is highly active against *Chlamydia, Mycoplasma*, and *Ureaplasma*, plus covers important anaerobes such as *Bacteroides fragilis* and the gram-negative *Enterobacteriaciae*, including *Ps aeruginosa*. Its use has been very limited secondary to serious adverse events.

ALATROFLOXACIN MESYLATE

L-Alaninamide, (1α,5α,6α)- L-alanyl-*N*-[3-[6-carboxy-8-(2,4-difluorophenyl)-3-fluoro-5,8-dihydro-5-oxo-1,8-naphthyridin-2-yl]-3-azabicyclo[3.1.0]hex-6-yl-, monomethanesulfonate; Trovan (Tablets only)

[157605-25-9] $C_{26}H_{25}F_3N_6O_5 \cdot CH_4O_3S$ (654.63).

Preparation—US Pat 5,164,402 (1992) and *J Chem Soc Perkin Trans* 2000; 1:1615.

Description—White to light yellow powder. *Alatrofloxacin* is *Trovaloxacin* with the L-alanyl-L-alanine side chain appended to the amino group on the 3-member ring of the azabicyclohexyl moiety.

Comments—The intravenous form of trovafloxacin.

MISCELLANEOUS ANTIBACTERIAL AGENTS

These antibacterial agents are principally second-line drugs because of emerging resistance, concerns with toxicity, or special activity against selected organisms. Chloramphenicol has the potential for causing aplastic anemia but is an alternative for treatment of life-threatening infections such as bacterial meningitis or rickettsial infections. Clindamycin is a unique licosamide antibiotic that is useful for anaerobic infections but is only bacteriostatic against streptococci and staphylococci. It also covers some parasitic infections such as pneumocystis and toxoplasmosis that occur in immunosuppressed patients. Spectinomycin is only used to treat gonococcal infections in patients unable to receive first-line drugs. Rifampin is important for prophylaxis of meningococcal disease and *H influenzae* meningitis plus some cases of *Mycobacterium avium* infections in AIDS patients. Vancomycin is a very specialized glycopeptide antibiotic for serious hospital infections caused by staphylococci (especially methicillin-resistant strains) and enterococci. Consequently, vancomycin should be reserved for those conditions where it is often the only effective drug available for such infections.

AMPHOTERICIN B—page 1670.

CHLORAMPHENICOL

Acetamide, [*R*-(*R**,*R**)]-2,2-dichloro-*N*-[2-hydroxy-1-(hydroxymethyl)-2-(4-nitrophenyl)ethyl-, Chloromycetin

D-*threo*- (−)-2,2-Dichloro-*N*-[β-hydroxy-α-(hydroxymethyl)-*p*-nitrophenethyl]acetamide [56-75-7] $C_{11}H_{12}Cl_2N_2O_5$ (323.13). Potency: not less than 900 μg of $C_{11}H_{12}Cl_2N_2O_5$/mg.

Preparation—Chloramphenicol is believed to be the first naturally occurring compound known to contain a nitro group or to be a derivative of dichloroacetic acid. Its stereochemical configuration is analogous to that of (−)-norpseudoephedrine, and is the only one of the four related stereoisomers that has antibiotic activity.

Chloramphenicol can be obtained from the filtrate of a *Streptomyces venezuelae* culture by extraction with ethyl acetate. If the charcoal extract is rich in chloramphenicol, the latter can be crystallized from the ethyl acetate by diluting with many volumes of kerosene.

Several synthetic methods of preparation are known. One of the better known commences with *p*-nitroacetophenone and, after converting it into *p*-nitro-2-aminoacetophenone, proceeds through the following steps: (a) acetylation of the—NH_2 group, (b) reaction with HCHO to introduce the terminal—CH_2OH group, (c) reduction with aluminum isopropoxide to give a mixture of the racemates of the *threo* and *erythro* forms of *p*-$NO_2PhCH(OH)CH(NH_2)CH_2OH$, (d) isolation of the *threo* racemate and resolution of it using *d*-camphorsulfonic acid, and (e) condensing the (−) enantiomorph with methyl dichloroacetate.

Description—Fine, white to grayish white or yellowish white, needle-like crystals or elongated plates; odorless; intensely bitter taste; pH (saturated solution) between 4.5 and 7.5; reasonably stable in neutral or moderately acid solutions but rapidly destroyed in alkaline solutions; melts between 149° and 153°; pK_a 5.5.

Solubility—1 g in approximately 400 mL water; freely soluble in alcohol; slightly soluble in ether or chloroform.

Comments—A wide spectrum of antibacterial activity. The drug is effective in rickettsial diseases including epidemic, murine and scrub typhus, Rocky Mountain spotted fever, rickettsial pox and Q fever; chlamydial diseases including the psittacosis-lymphogranuloma group and many gram-positive and gram-negative bacterial infections including the anaerobes (especially *Bacteroides fragilis*). Because of serious toxic reactions, the systemic use of the drug should be limited only to very serious infections that cannot be managed by other drugs. It is still the drug of choice for typhoid fever.

It is used topically for superficial conjunctival infections and blepharitis caused by *E coli, H influenzae, Moraxella lacunata, Staph aureus*, and *Strep hemolyticus*. Bone-marrow injury is the major toxic effect. Thrombocytopenia, granulocytopenia, and aplastic anemia are the most serious hematopoietic disturbances observed and have resulted in a number of fatalities.

In neonates it may cause the *Gray syndrome*, a fatal cyanosis (40% of cases) with symptoms of vomiting, abdominal distention, and loose, green stools, owing to the inability of the infant to metabolize the drug in consequence of glucuronyl transferase deficiency. Optic atrophy and blindness occur in a small number of cases, mainly in children on prolonged therapy.

Minor untoward effects such as transient mild euphoria, skin rash, and GI disturbances have been observed; the drug is contraindicated in patients with a history of previous sensitization.

Occasional untoward effects include glossitis, stomatitis, and pharyngitis. Its use, as with other antibiotics, may result in an overgrowth of microorganisms not susceptible to the drug. Oral anticoagulants, oral hypoglycemics, phenytoin, and perhaps acetaminophen inhibit its metabolism and increase the risk of intoxication; appropriate dose adjustments should be made. Rifampin decreases plasma concentrations.

The drug is absorbed rapidly from the GI tract, with a bioavailability of about 90%. Sixty percent of the drug in blood is bound to serum albumin. The volume of distribution is about 0.7 mL/g. From 85% to 95% is biotransformed in the liver. The half-life is 1.5 to 5 hr, except over 24 hr in neonates 1 to 2 days old and 10 hr in infants 10 to 16 days old. Because of considerable variability, plasma levels must be monitored. Also, the clearance increases with continuous use, and dose adjustments are necessary. When there is impaired hepatic function, and sometimes of renal function as well, the dosage must be reduced, according to determined plasma concentrations. It can cross the placental barrier and intoxicate the fetus, so that the drug should be avoided in pregnancy, if possible.

CLINDAMYCIN HYDROCHLORIDE

L-*threo*-α-D-*galacto*-Octopyranoside, methyl (2*S*-*trans*)-7-chloro-6,7,8-trideoxy-6-[[(1-methyl-4-propyl-2-pyrrolidinyl)carbonyl]-amino]-1-thio-, monohydrochloride; Cleocin Hydrochloride

(*) Indicates site of esterification to form the palmitate or phosphate derivatives.

[21462-39-5] $C_{18}H_{33}ClN_2O_5S \cdot HCl$ (461.44). Potency: equivalent to not less than 800 μg of clindamycin/mg.

Preparation—Lincomycin is treated with a solution of Rydon reagent prepared from triphenylphosphine, acetonitrile, and chlorine. The base is ultimately reacted with HCl. *CA* 1970; 73:15185*v*.

Description—White or practically white, crystalline powder; strong, characteristic taste; odorless or has a faint mercaptan-like odor; stable in air and light; pK$_a$ 7.72; melts about 142°.

Solubility—1 g in 2 mL water or 200 mL ethanol.

Comments—An antibacterial spectrum very much like that of *Lincomycin*, from which it is derived. However, among staphylococci and several streptococci it may be as much as 20 times more potent. It is also more potent against certain gram-negative organisms, but not against gram-negative cocci; with the recommended doses the plasma levels usually are not high enough to be effective against gram-negative bacteria. It is especially useful in the treatment of several infections caused by anaerobes; it is the drug of choice for treatment of GI infections caused by *Bacteroides fragilis*. It is important as an alternate drug for treating infections caused by penicillin-resistant *Staph aureus*. It also is used for treatment of respiratory tract infections and pharyngitis or tonsillitis caused by *Strep pyogenes*. It is perhaps the best drug for the topical treatment of acne vulgaris (used as the phosphate).

It may cause abdominal pain, nausea, vomiting, diarrhea and loose stools, which may occasionally contain blood and mucus. Incidence of benign diarrhea is about 10% to 20%. Incidence of antibiotic-associated (pseudomembranous) colitis is estimated to be 1:10,000. Allergic rashes and urticaria occur with an incidence of about 10%.

By the oral route, bioavailability is about 90% with low doses. The presence of food in the stomach and intestines does not appear to interfere with absorption. In plasma it is 60% to 95% protein-bound. Its volume of distribution is about 0.66 mL/g. It is distributed widely in most tissues, body fluids and bone.

However, high enough concentrations are not achieved in CSF to be used to treat meningitis. Most of it is eliminated in the liver, only about 10% being excreted in the urine. The half-life is 2.4 to 3 hr, except 3.5 to 5 hr in anuria and 7 to 14 hr in liver disease. Hepatic failure can be expected to reduce the dose requirement more than renal failure.

FOSFOMYCIN TROMETHAMINE

Phosphonic acid, (2R-cis)-(3-methyloxiranyl)-, compd with 2-amino-2-(hydroxymethyl)-1,3-propanediol (1:1); Monurol

[78964-85-9] C$_3$H$_7$O$_4$P·C$_4$H$_{11}$NO$_3$ (259.20).

Preparation—The thermal rearrangement of di-*tert*-butyl 2-propynyl phosphite yields the ester, di-*tert*-butyl propadienyl phosphonate. Selective hydrogenation followed by acid-catalyzed cleavage of the *t*-butyl groups forms *cis*-propenylphosphonic acid. Treatment of the acid with hydrogen peroxide and sodium tungstate gives the epoxide, which is resolved to the 2*R-cis* compound. Final reaction with 2-amino-2-(hydroxymethyl)-1,2-propanediol yields the salt. *J Org Chem* 1970; 35:3510 and US Pat 3,914,231 (1969).

Description—(Acid) White granular solid melting about 133°. [α]$^{28}_{405}$ -2.6° (c = 5, water); + 18.7° (c = 3, DMF).

Comments—A single dose treatment option for uncomplicated urinary tract infections in women. A less effective treatment alternative than fluorquinolones for this condition, but a viable choice in patients who have a contraindication to fluoroquinolone therapy. Adverse events commonly are gastrointestinal in nature.

Oxazolidinones

The oxazolidinones are a totally synthetic antibiotic class first investigated in the late 1980s as antidepressant agents. Serendipitously, these agents were discovered to have excellent antibacterial activity. The main reason for their development has been the increase and spread of resistance in gram-positive pathogens. The first agent in this class, l inezolid, was approved by the FDA in April 2000.

The oxazolidinones are protein-synthesis inhibiting compounds that most commonly produces a bacteriostatic effect. They bind to the 50S ribosome at a unique site and disrupt protein synthesis. The principal activity of the class is against gram-positive aerobic organisms including staphylococci, streptococci, and enterococci. In particular, activity against resistant pathogens such as methicillin-resistant staphylococci, penicillin-resistant streptococci, and vancomycin-resistant enterococci, is excellent.

LINEZOLID

Acetamide, (S)-N-[[3-[3-fluoro-4-(4-morpholinyl)phenyl]-2-oxo-5-oxazolidinyl]methyl]-, Zyvox

[165800-03-3] C$_{16}$H$_{20}$FN$_3$O$_4$ (337.35).

Preparation—Several multi-step methods starting with *p*-acetylphenyliso-thiocyanate. US Pat 5,688,792 (1997) ; *Tetrahedron Letters* 1999; 40:4855 and *Albany Molecular Research, Tech Reports* 9(17):14-18.

Description—White crystals from ethyl acetate melting about 182°; [α]$^{20}_D$ − 9° (c = 0.919, chloroform).

Comments—The only oxazolidinone commercially available to date. Both intravenous and oral formulations are commercially available. The bioavailability of the oral formulation is 100%. Linezolid is predominately eliminated by nonrenal mechanisms. Its metabolism does not involve the cytochrome P450 system. Two inactive metabolites are the major by-products of this conversion to water-soluble products that are excreted by the kidney.

In general, linezolid is well tolerated. The most common adverse effects are diarrhea, nausea, taste perversion, and vomiting. Thrombocytopenia has been reported in up to 4% of patients in clinical trials and has been associated with more than 2 weeks duration of therapy. Linezolid also possesses weak monoamine oxidase inhibitory activity. Therefore, the potential for drug interactions with sympathomimetic agents or foods rich in tyramine does exist.

Linezolid has proven useful in the treatment of a variety of infections caused by resistant gram-positive pathogens such as MRSA and VRE.

Streptogramins

The streptogramin antibiotics are naturally occurring products that have been in clinical use in Europe fpr more than 30 years as oral agents to treat mild to moderate infections. A semisynthetic derivative, quniupristin/dalfopristin, is the first injectable streptogramin antibiotic.

The streptogramins inhibit protein synthesis by binding to the 50S ribosome. The interaction of quinupristin and dalfopristin is synergistic. Either compound alone is bacteriostatic whereas the combination results in a bactericidal effect. The streptogramins are bactericidal against most organisms with the exception of enterococcus.

The principal activity of the streptogramins is against gram-positive aerobic organisms including staphylococci, streptococci, and enterococci. In particular, activity against resistant pathogens such as methicillin-resistant staphylococci, penicillin-resistant streptococci, and vancomycin-resistant *E faecium*, is excellent. Quinupristin/dalfopristin is not active against *Enterococcus faecalis*.

DALFOPRISTIN

Virginiamycin M$_1$, (26R, 27S)- 26-[[2-(diethylamino)ethyl]sulfonyl]-26,27-dihydro-, Ing of Synercid, which is approx 30% *Quinupristin* and 70% *Dalfopristin*

[112362-50-2] C$_{34}$H$_{50}$N$_4$O$_9$S (690.85).

Preparation—US Pat 4,669,669 (1987).

Description—White to slightly yellow hygroscopic powder melting about 150°. A synthetic polyunsaturated macrolactone type II *Streptogramin* derived from pristinamycin.

QUINUPRISTIN

Virginiamycin S₁, (S)-4-[4-(dimethylamino)-N-methyl-L-phenyl-alanine]-5-[5-[(1-azabicyclo[2.2.0]oct-3-ylthio)methyl]-4-oxo-L-2-piperidinecarboxylic acid]-, Ing of Synercid

[120138-50-3] $C_{53}H_{67}N_9O_{10}S$ (1022.23).

Preparation—US Pat 4,798,703 (1987).

Description—White crystals from methanol.

Comments—The only streptogramin commercially available in the United States. Quinupristin/dalfopristin is not absorbed from the gastrointestinal tract. After intravenous administration, both compounds have a serum half-life of approximately 1 hour. Clearance of both agents is through the liver. Although the cytochrome P450 system is not involved in the metabolism, CYP3A4 is significantly inhibited by quinupristin/dalfopristin, potentially increasing the levels of agents such as cyclosporine, warfarin, and the azoles. The most common adverse effects are infusion related. Infusion site reactions including pain, inflammation, edema and thrombophlebitis have been reported in as many as 75% of patients who received the drug through a peripheral IV catheter. Arthralgias and myalgias have also been reported which may be severe and require discontinuation of therapy. The most common laboratory abnormality is hyperbilirubinemia.

Quinupristin/dalfopristin has been used primarily in the treatment of resistant gram-positive infections including methicillin-resistant staphylococci, penicillin-resistant pneumococci and vancomycin-resistant E. faecium.

SPECTINOMYCIN HYDROCHLORIDE

4H-Pyrano[2,3-b][1,4]benzodioxin-4-one, [2R-(2α,4aβ,5aβ,6β,7β,8β,9α,9aα,10aβ)]-decahydro-4a,7,9-trihydroxy-2-methyl-6,8-bis(methyl-amino)-, dihydrochloride, pentahydrate; Trobicin

[22189-32-8]; $C_{14}H_{24}N_2O_7 \cdot 2HCl \cdot 5H_2O$ (495.35); *anhydrous* [21736-83-4] (405.27). Potency: equivalent to not less than 603 μg spectinomycin/mg.

Preparation—By growth of the soil microorganism *Streptomyces spectabilis*. Reaction with a double equimolar quantity of HCl yields the hydrochloride. *Antibiot Chemother* 1961; 11:118 and 661, US Pat 3,234,092.

Description—White, odorless, crystalline powder; slightly bitter taste; stable in light; nonhygroscopic; stable in air at room temperature; pKₐ 6.88, 8.84.

Solubility—1 g in approximately 7 mL water; practically insoluble in alcohol, chloroform or ether.

Comments—A wide-spectrum antibiotic with moderate activity against both gram-positive and gram-negative bacteria. However, it is employed clinically for only one purpose, namely, to treat

or prevent acute gonorrhea when the organism is resistant to penicillin, or when the patient is allergic to penicillin. It is not as effective as ceftriaxone. Resistance sometimes develops. It is not effective in eradicating pharyngeal gonococcal infections in more than 50% of patients.

Orally, the drug is absorbed poorly and must be given intramuscularly. The distribution coefficient is 0.12 mL/g. About 75% is excreted into urine unchanged. Plasma half-life is approximately 1 to 3 hr.

Untoward effects caused include frequent pain at the site of injection and infrequent headache, nausea, vomiting, insomnia, chills, fever, mild pruritus, and urticaria. It does not eradicate *Treponema* or *Chlamydia trachomatis*, which are common sexually transmitted pathogens.

TRIMETHOPRIM

2,4-Pyrimidinediamine, 5-[(3,4,5-trimethoxyphenyl)methyl]-, Proloprim, Trimpex

2,4-Diamino-5-(3,4,5-trimethoxybenzyl)pyrimidine [738-70-5] $C_{14}H_{18}N_4O_3$ (290.32).

Preparation—By interaction of a-(ethoxymethyl)-3,4,5-trimethoxycinnamonitrile and guanidine, the former prepared by condensing 3,4,5-trimethoxybenzaldehyde with β-ethoxypropionitrile. US Pat 3,049,544.

Description—White to cream-colored crystals or crystalline powder; odorless; bitter taste; melts about 199°; pKₐ approximately 6.6.

Solubility—Very slightly soluble in water; 1 g in approximately 285 mL absolute alcohol or 53 mL chloroform.

Comments—A congener of pyrimethamine and it similarly inhibits dihydrofolate reductase, although it is considerably less potent. It was introduced as an antimalarial drug (mostly against *Plasmodium falci-parum*) and is still used somewhat for that purpose, usually in combination with an appropriate sulfonamide. However, its most important use is as an antibacterial agent. Bacterial dihydrofolate reductases are generally more susceptible than are the plasmodial ones. Therefore, the drug is effective against all bacteria that must synthesize their own folinic acid (leucovorin). This gives it a wide spectrum of activity that includes *Strep pyogenes, viridans* and *pneumoniae, Staph aureus* and *epidermidis, H influenzae, Klebsiella-Enterobacter-Serratia, E coli*, various *Shigella* and *Salmonella, Bordetella pertussis, Vibrio cholerae, Pneumocystis carinii, Toxoplasma gondii*, and *Plasmodia*. It is not effective against *Ps aeruginosa* but is against *Ps cepaciae* and *pseudomallei*. Many of these same organisms must also synthesize their own folic acid. Sulfonamides and dapsone block the incorporation of *p*-aminobenzoate into folate, thus inhibiting a crucial biosynthetic step just previous to that where this drug acts. Therefore, the combination of this drug and sulfonamides or dapsone is supposedly more effective than either drug alone, although clinical confirmation of significant synergism is lacking. Nevertheless, it is widely used in combination with sulfamethoxazole. It alone is approved for the same uses as the above combination. It would seem prudent to use the combination for UTIs, even though the cost is greater, but the pharmacokinetics are such that sulfamethoxazole in the present formulation adds little to this drug alone for systemic infections. The combination of dapsone and trimethoprim is used in the treatment of leprosy and infections by *Mycobacterium avium*.

Mammalian dihydrofolate reductase is about 1:10,000 to 1:50,000 as sensitive to it as the bacterial enzymes, so that there is little interference with folate metabolism in man. The toxicity is low. It includes occasional nausea and vomiting, diarrhea, malaise, immunosuppression and, rarely, rash, leucopenia, and thrombocytopenia. It increases bone-marrow suppression and immunosuppression by antineoplastics. It is potentially teratogenic.

By the oral route, it is well absorbed and reaches a peak in 2 to 3 hr. About 45% is protein-bound in plasma. The volume of distribution is about 1.8 mL/g. The concentration in CSF reaches 30% to 50% of that in plasma. It is excreted mainly into the urine. The half-life is 9 to 12 hr in normal adults, but may be increased 2- to 3-fold when the creatinine clearance falls below 10 mL/min. It is considerably shorter in infants and children. The drug decreases the renal clearance of procainamide and acecainide. Rifampin accelerates its elimination.

VANCOMYCIN HYDROCHLORIDE

Vancomycin, hydrochloride; Lyphocin; Vancocin, Vancoled

Vancomycin hydrochloride [1404-93-9] is a substance produced by growth of *Streptomyces orientalis* (Fam *Streptomycetaceae*). Potency: equivalent to not less than 900 µg of vancomycin/mg, calculated on the anhydrous basis.

Preparation—Vancomycin is produced by the submerged fermentation process. After purification the base is converted to the soluble hydrochloride with HCl. See *Antibiot Ann* 1955–1956; 606. US Pat 3,067,099.

Description—Tan to brown, free-flowing powder; odorless; bitter taste.

Solubility—Freely soluble in water; insoluble in ether or chloroform.

Comments—A glycopeptide highly active against gram-positive cocci, *Neisseria* and *Clostridia*. It inhibits synthesis of peptidoglycan in cell-wall formation. It is one of the drugs of choice in the treatment of antibiotic-associated colitis and other infections caused by *Cl difficile*. The rapid emergence of methicillin-resistant staphylococci makes this drug valuable in the treatment of severe staphylococcal infections. Development of resistance to vancomycin is uncommon, but has been seen in Enterococci and rarely in Staphylococci. There is no cross-resistance to other antibiotics. Streptococcal (especially *Strep vividans* and *bovis*), enterococcal and pneumococcal infections also are treated with the drug. It is used only in combination with an aminoglycoside in treating enterococcal endocarditis.

It is absorbed poorly from the GI tract, so that it may be used orally against staphylococcal and enterococcal enteritis and antibiotic-associated enterocolitis. In plasma, 55% is protein-bound. It poorly enters the CSF with uninflammed meninges. The volume of distribution is 0.7 L/kg. The distribution half-life is 0.5 hr. The elimination half-life is 4 to 6 hr in adults.

Since the drug is 70% eliminated by excretion in urine, the half-life in anuric patients ranges from 3 to 10 days and doses must be appropriately adjusted.

It is irritating to tissue and may cause thrombophlebitis, or pain at the site of injection and necrosis occurs if extravasated; also chills, fever, occasional urticaria and maculopapular rashes with hypotension (red man's syndrome), nephrotoxicity and ototoxicity and, rarely, thrombocytopenia and neutropenia. True allergy is very rare.

ANTIMYCOBACTERIAL DRUGS

Drugs used in the treatment of tuberculosis, *Mycobacterium avium* and leprosy can be grouped together because all involve slow growing microorganisms that cause chronic diseases. Therapeutic problems are also similar and consist of prolonged therapy regimens with drug toxicity, microbial resistance and the challenges of patient compliance.

The first-line drugs for tuberculosis include isoniazid, rifampin, ethambutol, pyrazinamide, and streptomycin. Excellent responses can now be obtained with a 6-month regimen: isoniazid, rifampin, and pyrazinamide for the first 2 mo, followed by isoniazid and rifampin for the remaining 4 mo. Isoniazid is the only drug approved for prophylaxis of tuberculosis. Hepatoxicity is observed with chronic use of isoniazid, rifampin, and pyrazinamide. The first new drug approved in the

last 25 yr for tuberculosis is rifapentine, a cyclopentyl derivative of rifampin. It has a longer half-life (16 hr vs 3 hr) and shares some of the same problems as observed with rifampin including potential hepatoxicity, drug interactions, and red-orange discoloration of secretions. In areas where resistance occurs therapy involves up to four drugs for as long as 24 mo. Second-line drugs for tuberculosis are more toxic but may be required with resistance problems. These drugs include some fluoroquinolones (ofloxacin and ciprofloxacin), cycloserine, ethionamide, aminosalicylic acid, aminoglycosides (amikacin, kanamycin), clofazimine, and capreomycin.

Mycobacterium avium complex infection as well as tuberculosis are increased because of the high numbers of AIDS patients that coexist in the large inner city populations and homeless shelters. Antimicrobial drugs used to treat *Mycobacterium avium* complex include rifabutin, the new macrolides (clarithromycin and azithromycin), the fluoroquinolones, and combination regimens of ethambutol (or other tuberculosis drugs) with clarithromycin (or azithromycin).

The drugs most frequently used to treat leprosy are dapsone, clofazimine, and rifampin for 6 mo to 2 yr depending on the type of disease. All of these drugs have some serious toxicities that can develop with the prolonged therapeutic regimens required. Therefore, patient compliance must be well supervised and patients should be informed of the need to discuss side effects of their treatment.

CLOFAZIMINE

2-Phenazinamine, *N*,5-bis(4-chlorophenyl)-3,5-dihydro-3-[(1-methylethyl)imino]-, Lamprene

3-(*p*-Chloroanilino)-10-(*p*-chlorophenyl)- 2,10-dihydro- 2 -(isopropylimino)phenazine; [2030-63-9] $C_{27}H_{22}Cl_2N_4$ (473.40).

Preparation—*J Chem Soc* 1958; 859.

Description—Dark-red crystals; melts about 210°.

Solubility—Practically insoluble in water; soluble in alcohol, acetone, ethyl acetate, chloroform, or benzene.

Comments—In combination with other drugs, used for the treatment of leprosy and infections caused by *Mycobacterium avium* in AIDS patients. It is not significantly active against other bacteria. It binds to mycobacterial DNA and interferes with growth. It is bactericidal, but as long as 50 days may be required before killing is evident. Nausea, vomiting, diarrhea, abdominal pain, and eosinophilic enteritis may occur. Crystalline deposits of the drug in the viscera may cause GI bleeding and/or obstruction. Antimuscarinic actions cause dry skin and dryness, burning, itching, and irritation of the eyes. The drug also causes long-persisting, rufous discoloration of the skin, cornea, conjunctiva, and body fluids. The oral-systemic bioavailability is about 50%. The drug has a predilection for adipocytes, reticuloendothelial cells, and other macrophages, in which crystals may accumulate. During maintenance, the elimination half-life is about 70 days.

DAPSONE

Benzenamine 4,4'-sulfonylbis-, DDS

4,4'-Sulfonyldianiline [80-08-0] $C_{12}H_{12}N_2O_2S$ (248.30).

Preparation—Benzene is condensed with sulfuric acid to yield phenyl sulfone [$(C_6H_5)_2SO_2$] which is then nitrated by standard procedures to yield the 4,4'-dinitro derivative. Reduction with tin and HCl or with various other appropriate reductants yields dapsone.

Description—White or creamy white, crystalline powder; odorless; slightly bitter taste; melts between 175° and 181°.

Solubility—Very slightly soluble in water; freely soluble in alcohol; soluble in dilute mineral acids.

Comments—Has an antibacterial spectrum and mechanism of action similar to those of sulfanilamide (see *Sulfonamides*), of which it originally was studied as a congener. Limited success against tuberculosis has been achieved with it, but it is far surpassed by other agents. However, in combination with rifampin, it is the drug of choice in the chemotherapy of leprosy. Most of the sulfones used in the treatment of this disease owe both their activity and toxicity to dapsone released from the molecule. For this reason, the drug is the preferred sulfone, since it is cheaper than and equally efficacious to the others. However, resistance is becoming common. Combined with trimethoprim, it is as effective as trimethoprim-sulfametoxazole in the treatment of *Pneumocystis carinii pneumonia*. It is also useful as a suppressant in the treatment of dermatitis herpetiformis and relapsing polychondritis.

It is absorbed by the oral route. Absorption is more efficient with low than with high doses. It is eliminated in the liver by acetylation. There are slow and fast acetylators among patients. The half-life is 10 to 50 hr, and at least 8 days are required to reach plateau concentrations.

It may cause hemolytic anemia in glucose 6-phosphate dehydrogenase-deficient persons, methemoglobinemia, GI upset, headache, nervousness, giddiness, tachycardia, motor neuropathy, blurred vision, paresthesias and pruritus, hematuria, liver damage, and jaundice or rash that may become exfoliative. The dermatitis frequently occurs during the 5th week of therapy, followed by *Hypermelanosis*. Lepra reactions (erythema nodosum-like) may occur from a flooding of the body with endotoxins released from killed organisms. Careful initial grading of dose and rest periods avoids much of the toxicity.

ETHAMBUTOL HYDROCHLORIDE

[R-(R*,R*)]-1-Butanol, 2,2′-(1,2-ethanediyldiimino)bis-, dihydrochloride; Myambutol

$$CH_3CH_2-\underset{\underset{H}{|}}{\overset{\overset{CH_2OH}{|}}{C}}-NHCH_2CH_2NH-\underset{\underset{CH_2OH}{|}}{\overset{\overset{H}{|}}{C}}-CH_2CH_3 \quad \cdot \; 2HCl$$

(+)-2,2′-(Ethylenediimino)di-1-butanol dihydrochloride [1070-11-7] $C_{10}H_{24}N_2O_2 \cdot 2HCl$ (277.23).

Preparation—(±)-2-Aminobutanol is resolved via its tartrate and the (+)-enantiomorph is condensed with 1,2-dichloroethane in an appropriate dehydrochlorinating environment. The ethambutol thus formed is dissolved in a suitable solvent and reacted with HCl. US Pat 3,297,707.

Description—White, crystalline powder; essentially odorless; a bitter taste; stable in light and heat but is hygroscopic when exposed to high relative humidities; melts between 198° and 202°; pKa 6.3, 9.5.

Solubility—1 g in 1 mL water or 4 mL alcohol; slightly soluble in ether or chloroform.

Comments—A tuberculostatic drug that is effective against tubercle bacilli resistant to isoniazid or streptomycin. It acts only on proliferating cells, apparently by interfering with synthesis of RNA. When used alone in the treatment of tuberculosis, the drug may clear the sputum of mycobacteria within 3 mo in the majority of patients, but bacterial resistance occurs in 35% of cases, and relapses frequently occur. In combination with isoniazid or other tuberculostatic drugs, relapses are uncommon. It should be used as a companion drug to isoniazid. The ethambutol-isoniazid rifampin combinations are now the most frequently used for patients exposed to drug-resistant organisms.

It occasionally causes optic neuritis, with blurred vision and diminished visual acuity to green light; the effect relates to the duration of use of the drug. Although these effects disappear on discontinuation, the drug should be discontinued at the first indication of a loss in visual acuity. Eye tests should be made before and at monthly intervals after the onset of therapy.

Other untoward effects include dermatitis, pruritus, anorexia, nausea, vomiting, abdominal pain, pyrosis, fever, headache, vertigo, malaise, mental confusion, disorientation, hallucinations, paresthesias, elevated serum urate levels (and gout), and abnormal liver function.

Multivitamins should be given concurrently. Leukopenia and anaphylaxis are rare occurrences.

The oral bioavailability is 75% to 80%. It is distributed well into most tissues and fluids but poorly in CSF. The volume of distribution is 1.6 mL/g. Over 80% is eliminated in the urine. The half-life is 3 to 4 hr but up to 8 hr in renal failure.

ISONIAZID

4-Pyridinecarboxylic acid, hydrazide; Isonicotinylhydrazine; INH

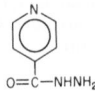

Isonicotinic acid hydrazide [54-85-3] $C_6H_7N_3O$ (137.14).

Preparation—By heating isonicotinic acid or its ethyl ester with anhydrous hydrazine. Isonicotinic acid may be synthesized by various oxidative processes starting with 4-methylpyridine.

Description—Colorless or white crystals, or a white, crystalline powder; odorless; slowly affected by exposure to air and light; solutions are practically neutral to litmus; melts between 170° and 173°; pKa 1.8, 3.5, 9.5; pH (1 in 100 solution) 5.5 to 6.5.

Solubility—1 g in approximately 8 mL water and approximately 50 mL alcohol; slightly soluble in chloroform and ether.

Comments—The most potent and selective of the known tuberculostatic antibacterial agents. It is tuberculocidal to growing bacteria and regarded as the most effective agent in the therapy of tuberculosis. The fact that it gains access to all organs and to all body fluids, including CSF, renders the drug of special value in treating tuberculous meningitis and other extrapulmonary forms of the disease. The drug is never used alone because of the rapid emergence of resistance. Used in combination with other antitubercular drugs, it enhances the clinical response, permits lower doses of the other active agent(s) to be used and retards emergence of resistant tubercle bacilli. It is the central drug around which various combinations are formulated. The first-choice combination contains isoniazid and rifampin, with or without pyrazinamide. It also is used as a prophylactic.

Untoward effects are relatively few except in persons who are slow acetylators, when the dose must be lowered. The effects may include restlessness, insomnia, muscle twitching, hyperreflexia, paresthesia, and even convulsions, toxic encephalopathy, optic neuritis, atrophy, and psychoses. These neurologic disorders result from competition of the drug with pyridoxine; pyridoxine administration suppresses the neurological disorders without antagonizing the antitubercular action. Other signs of pyridoxine deficiency may occur. The drug also may cause nausea, vomiting, epigastric distress, agranulocytosis, hemolytic or aplastic anemia, thrombocytopenia, eosinophilia, fever, various rashes and dermatoses, and rheumatoid and lupoid syndromes. Hepatitis, with jaundice, is uncommon in patients under 35 yr but occurs in about 2% of recipients over 50 yr, but 10% to 20% will show elevations in SGOT and SGPT. The hepatic, hematologic, and dermatologic effects are probably all allergic.

It is mostly acetylated by the liver; the rate varies considerably. In fast acetylators, the half-life is 1 to 1 1/2 hr; in slow ones, it is 2 to 5 hr.

IM injections cause local irritation.

PYRAZINAMIDE

Pyrazine carboxamide

[98-96-4] $C_5H_5N_3O$ (123.11).

Preparation—By thermal decarboxylation of 2,3-pyrazinedicarboxylic acid to form the monocarboxylic acid, which is esterified with methanol and then subjected to controlled ammonolysis. *J Am Chem Soc* 1952; 74:3617.

Description—White to practically white, crystalline powder; sublimes about 60°; melts about 190°; pKa 0.5.

Solubility—1 g in 67 mL water, 75 mL methanol, 175 mL absolute ethanol, 135 mL chloroform, 1000 mL ether, or 110 mL alcohol.

Comments—An antituberculosis drug used for initial treatment in combination with isoniazid and rifampin. It generally is administered with isoniazid, which it potentiates. However, it is quite toxic and should be held in reserve until other therapy fails. It may cause fever, anorexia, malaise and hepatic damage, with or without jaundice, and death can occur. All patients intended to be treated with this drug should have prior liver function tests, which tests also must be repeated periodically during therapy. All patients should be hospitalized during treatment. It may cause retention of uric acid.

RIFABUTIN

(9S,12E,14S,15R,16S,17R,18R,19R,20S,21S,22E,24Z)-6,16,18,20-tetrahydroxy-1'-isobutyl-14-methoxy-7,9,15,17,19,21,25-hepta-methylspiro[9,4-(epoxypentadeca[1,11,13]trienimino)-2H-furo[2',3':7,8]naphth[1,2-d]imidazole-2,4'-piperidine]-5,10,26-(3H, 9H)-trione-16-acetate; Mycobutin

[72559-06-9] $C_{46}H_{62}N_4O_{11}$ (847.02).

Comments—A semisynthetic ansamycin antibiotic that has antimycobacterial activity. It inhibits DNA-dependent RNA polymerase in susceptible strains of bacteria. It is indicated for prevention of disseminated *Mycobacterium avium* complex (MAC) disease in patients with advanced HIV infection.

It should not be administered to patients with active tuberculosis because single-agent therapy is likely to lead to development of tuberculosis that is resistant both to rifabutin and rifampin. Adverse reactions primarily may include rash (4%), GI intolerance (3%), and neutropenia (2%). Other reactions may include flu-like syndrome, hepatitis hemolysis, arthralgia, parathesia, aphasia, confusion, and nonspecific T-wave changes on ECG.

Oral doses are absorbed readily from the GI tract and slowly eliminated with a half-life of 16 to 69 hr. It has a high volume of distribution and good tissue uptake due to its lipophilicity. About 30% of dose is excreted in the feces, and 53% is excreted in urine primarily as metabolites.

RIFAMPIN

Rifamycin, 3-[[(4-methyl-1-piperazinyl)imino]methyl]-, Rifampicin, Rifadin, Rimactane

[13292-46-1] $C_{43}H_{58}N_4O_{12}$ (822.95). Potency: not less than 900 μg of $C_{43}H_{58}N_4O_{12}$/mg.

Preparation—Rifamycin SV, which may be prepared by the method of Sensi et al (US Pat 3,313,804), is converted to the 8-carboxaldehyde derivative, known also as 3-formylrifamycin SV, and this is condensed with 1-amino-4-methylpiperazine to form a Schiff base, which is rifampin.

Description—Red-brown, crystalline powder; odorless; unstable in light, heat, air, and moisture; melts between 183° and 188° with decomposition; pK_a 1.7, 7.9.

Solubility—1 g in approximately 762 mL water; freely soluble in chloroform; soluble in ethyl acetate or methanol.

Comments—A broad-spectrum antibiotic effective against most gram-positive bacteria, especially *Staph pyogenes, Strep pyogenes, viridans,* and *pneumoniae,* and variably active against gram-negative organisms, especially *H influenzae,* meningococci and gonococci. Both *Mycobacterium tuberculosis* and *Mycobacterium leprae* are very susceptible to the drug. Its clinical use is mainly in the treatment of tuberculosis. The rate of development of resistance of the mycobacterium is low. Nevertheless, it always is used in combination with other antitubercular drugs. It also appears to be an excellent drug for prophylaxis of meningococcal meningitis and pneumonia from *H influenzae* Type B and treatment of meningococcal carrier state. It may cause heartburn, epigastric distress, gas, cramps, diarrhea, anorexia, and nausea and vomiting. Headache, drowsiness, and fatigue commonly occur. Inability to concentrate, confusion, muscular weakness, ataxia, pain in the extremities, visual disturbances, and generalized numbness are other

CNS side effects. Jaundice and other manifestations of hepatotoxicity have occurred. It is teratogenic in laboratory animals and should therefore be withheld in pregnancy.

It induces the hepatic drug-metabolizing enzyme system and accelerates the metabolism of digitoxin, methadone, phenytoin, beta blockers, verapamil, theophylline, chloramphenicol, oral contraceptives and estrogens, oral anticoagulants, barbiturates, tolbutamide, and itself.

It is 100% absorbed after oral administration, but food in the stomach delays absorption of the drug. The drug is distributed widely in the body, even into CSF. In plasma 98% is protein-bound. The volume of distribution is 0.9 mL/g. About 85% of the drug is eliminated by biotransformation in the liver. An active metabolite is secreted into bile, where it is therapeutically effective. The risk of hepatotoxicity is increased when it is used with isoniazid. It imparts a reddish-orange color to urine, stools, sweat, saliva, and tears. Soft contact lenses may be stained permanently.

MISCELLANEOUS SYSTEMIC URINARY TRACT ANTISEPTICS

These drugs are used for chronic suppressive therapy of UTIs. The primary agents in this group are methenamine and nitrofurantoin. Both drugs are given orally for recurrent urinary tract pathogens and require an acidic urine for efficacy. They are not first-line agents to treat an initial UTI.

METHENAMINE

1,3,5,7-Tetraazatricyclo[3.3.1.1³,⁷]decane; Aminoform; Cystamin, Cystogen, Hexamine, Uritone, Urised

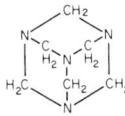

Hexamethylenetetramine [100-97-0] $C_6H_{12}N_4$ (140.19).

Although a cyclic tetramine, the therapeutic action of this compound depends exclusively on its ability to liberate formaldehyde under suitable environmental conditions.

Preparation—By adding a moderate excess of ammonia water to formaldehyde solution, and evaporating to dryness.

Description—Colorless, lustrous crystals or a white crystalline powder; practically odorless; aqueous solution is alkaline to litmus; sublimes about 260°; when ignited it burns with a smokeless flame.

Solubility—1 g in 1.5 mL water, 12.5 mL alcohol, 10 mL chloroform or 320 mL ether.

Incompatibilities—Alkaline in reaction and forms salts with weak acids. *Strong acids* and concentrated solutions of organic acids decompose it with liberation of formaldehyde. With prolonged contact, weak acids also decompose it, as do acidic vehicles.

It liquefies, in some cases with decomposition, when rubbed with *aspirin, antipyrine, benzoic acid, lithium carbonate, menthol, phenol, potassium acetate, sodium benzoate, sodium salicylate,* etc.

Ammonium salts and *alkalies* darken it. In capsules, it may combine slowly with the gelatin, rendering it insoluble.

Comments—A urinary tract anti-infective, provided it is acting in an acid medium. It is excreted rapidly and thus reaches effective antiseptic concentrations in the urine. The drug depends for its action on the liberation of free formaldehyde. This occurs to the extent of 20% of theoretical at pH 5, 6% at pH 6, and almost not at all at pH 7.6.

Consequently, precaution must be taken to maintain an acid urine (pH 6 or below) during medication with it. This usually is accomplished by administration of sodium biphosphate, mandelic acid, hippuric acid, ascorbic acid, or cranberry juice. Ammonium chloride should not be used, since NH_4^+ drives the equilibrium to the left. At a pH of 6, a daily dose of 2 g will yield an average 24-hr urine concentration of about 18 to 60 μg/mL, which is about 40 times the minimum to inhibit the growth of most bacteria that cause UTIs. However, it will not prevent growth of *Candida albicans.* It is improbable that products that provide only 40.8 to 81.6 mg/dose can provide a high enough concentration of formaldehyde, since the urine contains substances that bind some of the formaldehyde.

It is of particular value in the treatment of *E coli* infections of the urinary tract. It also is especially useful in patients with renal insufficiency. Because of its low systemic toxicity, failure to excrete the drug causes no harmful consequences, unless renal insufficiency is severe.

Approximately 10% to 30% is converted to formaldehyde in the acid stomach contents unless enteric capsules are employed. Even with enteric coatings, nausea, vomiting, diarrhea, and other GI distress often occur when the dose exceeds 500 mg 4 times a day. Take with food to minimize GI upset. Formaldehyde liberated from the compound presumably is the cause of the distress. Other untoward effects are occasional pruritus and skin rashes and bladder irritation, painful and frequent urination, and hematuria in persons who have taken the drug longer than 3 to 4 wk. Dyspnea, lipoid pneumonitis, and headache occur rarely. In persons with acidosis or renal failure, the acid salts usually given concomitantly may be detrimental. The drug should not be used if hepatic insufficiency exists.

NITROFURANTOIN

2,4-Imidazolidenedione, 1-[[(5-nitro-2-furanyl) methylene]amino]-, Furadantin, Macrodantin

1-[(-5-Nitrofurfurylidene)amino]hydantoin [67-20-9] $C_8H_6N_4O_5$ (238.16).

Caution—It is discolored by alkali and by exposure to light, and is decomposed upon contact with metals other than stainless steel or aluminum.

Preparation—5-Nitro-2-furaldehyde (1) readily undergoes condensation with 1-aminohydantoin (II) to yield nitrofurantoin. I is synthesized by direct nitration of "2-furfural diacetate" [2-furanmethanediol diacetate (III)], prepared by the addition reaction between 2-furaldehyde and acetic anhydride] followed by saponification to regenerate the formyl group which, had it not been so protected, would have been oxidized to carboxyl during the nitration. II may be synthesized by effecting the addition of cyanic acid to hydrazinoacetic acid (IV) to produce the 3-carbamoyl derivative (V) which cyclizes by dehydration to II.

Description—Lemon-yellow crystals or fine powder; odorless; bitter aftertaste; pk_a 7.2.

Solubility—Very slightly soluble in water or alcohol.

Comments—Effective against a majority of urinary tract pathogens, including certain strains of *E coli, Enterobacter, Klebsiella, Proteus* spp, *Staph aureus,* and *Strep faecalis.* It is also effective against many staphylococci, clostridia, and *B subtilis.* It is indicated for the treatment of infections of the urinary tract caused by the above bacteria: pyelonephritis, cystis, and pyelitis. An acid urine favors activity. It is not the drug of first choice in the treatment of any acute infection, and it rarely is used. In chronic bacteriuria, it is a second- or third-choice agent. However, as a prophylactic in the prevention of recurrences it is effective, being slightly superior to methenamine mandelate but inferior to sulfamethizole. It is not indicated for treatment of associated perinephric or renal cortical abscesses, prostatitis, or other genitourinary tract infections, since in these the blood level is more important than urine concentration. The microcrystalline form is absorbed rapidly and completely; the macrocrystalline form is more slowly and less completely absorbed. About 67% is metabolized in the body, and 33% is excreted into the urine unchanged. The half-life is only 0.3 hr; slow absorption helps to sustain urine levels. Dose adjustment must be made in renal failure. Overall, the side effects are high (10% or more). Nausea, vomiting, and diarrhea occur in an appreciable number of patients. Reduction in dosage, or administration with food or milk, lessens the incidence; it is claimed that use of "macrocrystalline" product diminishes the incidence and intensity of GI upsets without affecting potency. Absorption is delayed, but bioavailability is not diminished. GI effects also occur in some patients receiving the drug intravenously. Hypersensitivity reactions with dermatological manifestations also occur. Headache, vertigo, drowsiness, malaise, muscular aches, nystagmus, and polyneuropathy occasionally occur.

Neuropathies appear to be more likely to occur if there is renal insufficiency; they appear to be caused by metabolites. Hemolytic anemia, megaloblastic anemia, granulocytopenia, leukopenia, esoinophilia, and maculopapular rashes occur occasionally. It also causes infrequent cholestatic jaundice and hepatocellular damage. Pneumonitis and pulmonary fibrosis can occur, especially in elderly patients. Occasionally, there is transient alopecia. Superinfections may occur. The drug is mutagenic in the Ames test.

PHENAZOPYRIDINE HYDROCHLORIDE

2,6-Pyridinediamine, 3-(phenylazo)-, monohydrochloride; Pyridium

2,6-Diamino-3-(phenylazo)pyridine monohydrochloride [136-40-3] $C_{11}H_{11}N_5 \cdot HCl$ (249.70).

Preparation—Aniline is diazotized with sodium nitrite and excess HCl, and the resulting benzenediazonium chloride is coupled with 2,6-diaminopyridine.

Description—Light or dark red to dark violet, crystalline powder; odorless or has a slight odor; melts about 235° with decomposition.

Solubility—1 g in <10 mL water, 59 mL alcohol, 331 mL chloroform, >5000 mL ether, or 100 mL glycerin.

Comments—A drug used for symptomatic relief of pain, burning, urgency, frequency, and other discomforts arising from irritation of lower urinary tract mucosa caused by infection, trauma, surgery, endoscopic procedures or passage of catheters. When taken systemically, it is excreted quickly into the urine, so that a high local concentration is reached. Thus, the drug either may be administered orally or instilled locally.

However, a considerable proportion of the drug is converted metabolically to an inactive form, so that large oral doses are required to exert a therapeutic effect. The relief of discomfort is attributable mostly to a local anesthetic action rather than to an antibacterial action. Treatment should not continue beyond 2 days because there is no evidence it provides greater benefit than sulfonamides alone. GI irritation, jaundice, hemolytic anemia, and methemoglobinemia have been reported. After oral administration, the color of the urine may be orange red to dark red, if the urine is acidic. Large doses and prolonged treatment can give rise to renal stones of the drug. It is contraindicated in renal insufficiency, severe hepatitis, and pyelonephritis of pregnancy, and it should be used cautiously in the presence of GI disturbances. It often is combined with sulfonamides or methenamine salts.

ANTIMALARIALS

Malaria is caused by several species of the protozoan *Plasmodium*, of which *Plasmodium vivax*, and *Plasmodium falciparum* are the most common. The most serious infections involve *Plasmodium falciparum*, which causes a higher incidence of complications and deaths. They all have complex life cycles involving both the anopheles mosquito and the erythrocyte of the human host. In *Plasmodium vivax*, a persisting tissue phase continues to infect the blood at intervals for many years. Thus, the ideal antimalarial not only should eradicate the microzoan from the blood (ie, to *suppress* the clinical attack) but from the tissues as well, to effect a *radical cure*. The several antimalarials differ in their point of interruption of the cycle of the parasite and in the type of malaria affected. In addition, parasite resistance (especially *Plasmodium falciparum*) to these drugs is an important therapeutic problem.

The 4-aminoquinolines (amodiaquine, chloroquine, and hydroxychloroquine) and quinacrine cause similar adverse effects. GI side effects such as nausea, vomiting, diarrhea, and sialorrhea are common; they can be diminished by administering the drugs with meals and milk.

Oropharyngeal and dermatologic side effects may occur, especially during protracted therapy. They include pigmentation of the skin, nailbeds, and palate (especially quinacrine), bleaching of hair, pruritus, and lichenoid and pleomorphic skin eruptions. They may precipitate severe attacks of psoriasis in patients with that disease. The drugs should not be coadministered with phenylbutazone or gold salts, which have similar dermatotoxicities. There is cross-sensitization among all the 4-aminoquinolines. The drugs may cause neurologic disturbances, such as fatigue, lassitude, neuromyopathy, polyneuritis, toxic psychosis, and ototoxicity with vertigo and/or decreased auditory sensitivity. The knee and ankle reflexes should be monitored periodically. Ocular disorders, such as corneal opacities, keratopathy, and retinopathy (the drugs are concentrated in the retina) occur, especially during long-term treatment. Periodic ophthalmologic examinations are advised. The drugs are contraindicated if retinal or visual field disease is present.

The 4-aminoquinolines are concentrated in the liver and may cause hepatotoxicity, and they may precipitate attacks of porphyria; they must be used cautiously in persons with liver disease or who are under medication with other potentially hepatotoxic drugs (gold salts, erythromycin estolate, indomethacin, phenylbutazone, certain anabolic steroids, etc).

Hematologic disorders occasionally caused by the 4-aminoquinolines include leukopenia, pancytopenia, and agranulocytosis; periodic white-blood-cell counts are necessary. The drugs may depress the electrocardiographic T-wave.

The drugs pass the placental barrier and can cause cochleovestibular paresis in the fetus; they should be withheld in pregnancy, although chloroquine has been given safely in low doses for chemoprophylaxis.

CHLOROQUINE PHOSPHATE

1,4-Pentanediamine, N^4-(7-chloro-4-quinolinyl)-N^1,N^1-diethyl-, phosphate (1:2); Aralen Phosphate

7-Chloro-4-[[4-(diethylamino)-1-methylbutyl]amino]quinoline phosphate (1:2) [50-63-5] $C_{18}H_{26}ClN_3 \cdot 2H_3PO_4$ (515.87).

Preparation—By addition of concentrated phosphoric acid to a hot ethanolic solution of chloroquine base.

Description—White, crystalline powder; odorless; bitter taste; slowly discolors on exposure to light; pH (aqueous solution) approximately 4.5; is dimorphic; one form melts about 193° to 195° (usual form) or 210° to 215° (other polymorphic form); pK_{a1} 7; pK_{a2} 9.2.

Solubility—Freely soluble in water; practically insoluble in alcohol, chloroform, or ether.

Comments—An *antimalarial* that causes dysfunction of the acid phagosomes in plasmodia and also in human leukocytes and macrophages. It is used both for control of acute attacks of vivax malaria and for suppression against all plasmodia except chloroquine-resistant *Plasmodium falciparum*. The drug is neither a prophylactic nor a radical curative agent in vivax malaria. In regions where *Plasmodium falciparum* is generally sensitive to chloroquine, it is markedly effective in terminating acute attacks of nonresistant falciparum malaria and usually brings about complete cure in this type of malaria. However, in some regions a high incidence of resistance (up to 90%) exists, so that other drugs, such as quinine or quinidine, alone or in combination with pyrimethamine, sulfadiazine, or tetracycline, may have preference. Resistant strains of *Plasmodium vivax* also occur.

It is the drug of choice for the oral treatment of all malaria except that caused by resistant *Plasmodium falciparum*; the hydrochloride is second to quinine or quinidine for parenteral treatment.

Although not useful in intestinal amebiasis, it is an effective agent in the treatment of extraintestinal amebiasis, especially amebic hepatitis. It is not used alone but rather in combination with dihydroemetine or emetine. The combination is only the treatment of second choice, behind metronidazole-diiodohydroxyquin. Since chloroquine is well tolerated, it has been recommended that it be employed routinely even in cases of amebiasis without demonstrable hepatic involvement. Like quinacrine, it also may be of value in chronic discoid lupus erythematosus and rheumatoid arthritis. It is quite effective in the treatment of photoallergic reactions.

The adverse effects are those of the 4-aminoquinolines (see the general statement). The incidence is low, except for the GI side effects of the oral forms.

The drug is absorbed almost completely from the GI tract and usually is administered orally. It (as the hydrochloride) is given intramuscularly when necessary to resort to parenteral administration. Tissues bind the drug, although not quite to the same degree as quinacrine. It is degraded in tissues to unknown products. The drug is slowly excreted in the urine with an initial half-life of 1 wk, changing to 17 days after 4 wk, then ultimately becoming months.

DAPSONE—page 1662.

MEFLOQUINE HYDROCHLORIDE

4-Quinolinemethanol, (*R**, *S**)-(±)-α-2-piperidinyl-2,8-bis(trifluoromethyl)-, hydrochloride; Lariam

[51773-92-3] $C_{17}H_{16}F_6N_2O \cdot HCl$ (414.78).

Preparation—*J Med Chem* 1971; 14:926.

Description—White powder; bitter taste; melts about 260° with decomposition; the secondary alcohol group is chiral, but the racemate is used clinically; pK_a 8.6.

Solubility—1 g in 6 mL water or 250 mL alcohol.

Comments—Can eliminate fever and parasitemia and cause a radical cure in infections caused by *Plasmodium falciparum* and can suppress infections caused by *Plasmodium vivax*; with *Plasmodium vivax*, infections usually recur at a later time. Its mechanism is unknown. Resistance develops rapidly (the WHO is investigating combinations to delay resistance) and it is absorbed well orally. In plasma, it is extensively bound to plasma proteins and is concentrated in the liver and lungs. It is eliminated mainly in the feces, mostly after biliary secretion. The half-life is about 13 to 24 days.

PRIMAQUINE PHOSPHATE

1,4-Pentanediamine, N^4-(6-methoxy-8-quinolinyl)-, phosphate (1:2)

8-[(4-Amino-1-methylbutyl)amino]-6-methoxyquinoline phosphate (1:2) [63-45-6] $C_{15}H_{21}N_3O \cdot 2H_3PO_4$ (455.34).

Preparation—2-Chloropentylamine is condensed with 8-amino-6-methoxyquinoline, and the resulting primaquine base is reacted with a double molar quantity of phosphoric acid.

Description—Orange-red, crystalline powder; odorless; bitter taste; solutions are acid to litmus; melts about 200°.

Solubility—1 g in approximately 15 mL water; insoluble in chloroform or ether.

Comments—An *antimalarial* that is very important for the radical cure (ie, prevention of relapse) of relapsing vivax or ovale malaria; it is not employed for suppressive therapy or for control of the acute clinical attacks of the disease. It often is administered in combination with chloroquine. The incidence of serious untoward effects is low. Administration of the drug with milk, food, or antacids lessens GI adverse effects of abdominal cramps and epigastric distress; however, aluminum-containing antacids interfere with absorption. Mild hemolytic anemia, cyanosis (methemoglobinemia), and leukocytosis also may be observed. At higher dose levels these symptoms are accentuated, and leukopenia may be noted. Impairment of liver function has not been noted, even in patients with infectious hepatitis. Persons with tendencies toward granulocytopenia (eg, lupus erythematosus or rheumatoid diseases) should not take it because the blood dyscrasia may be precipitated. Other hemolyzing drugs should not be administered concurrently.

Untoward effects in non-Caucasians are similar, but the incidence and degree of anemia and intravascular hemolysis are greater especially in patients whose erythrocytes are deficient in glucose 6-phosphate dehydrogenase. Bone-marrow depressant drugs (eg, antineoplastics, colchicine, gold salts, penicillamine, phenylbutazone, hydroxyphenylbutazone, or quinacrine) given concurrently can cause excessive bone-marrow depression.

PYRIMETHAMINE

2,4-Pyrimidinediamine, 5-(4-chlorophenyl)-6-ethyl-, Daraprim

2,4-Diamino-5-(*p*-chlorophenyl)-6-ethylpyrimidine [58-14-0] $C_{12}H_{13}ClN_4$ (248.71).

Preparation—Ethyl propionate is condensed with *p*-chlorophenylacetonitrile in the presence of sodium methylate. The resulting α-propionyl-*p*-chlorophenylacetonitrile is reacted with isoamyl alcohol to form the hemiacetal which undergoes dehydration to α-(*p*-chlorophenyl)-β-ethyl-β-isoamyloxylacrylonitrile (I). I is reacted with guanidine whereupon cyclization occurs because of (*a*) the liberation of isoamyl alcohol by condensation involving the imino hydrogen of guanidine and the isoamyloxy group of I, and (*b*) an addition reaction involving an amino group of guanidine and the nitrile group of I.

Description—White, crystalline powder; odorless; melting range 238 to 242°; pK$_a$ 7.3.

Solubility—Practically insoluble in water; 1 g in approximately 200 mL alcohol or 125 mL chloroform.

Comments—Inhibits dihydrofolate reductase in plasmodia; thus the developing parasite cannot synthesize and use nucleic acid precursors needed for growth. Its action in preventing the development of the erythrocytic phase of the parasite is slow, so that it is of little value in suppression of acute attacks, except as an adjunct to quinine; rather it is used mainly as a suppressive prophylactic for the prevention of clinical attacks by *Plasmodium falciparum* in regions where the organism is resistant to chloroquine, in which use it is combined with sulfadoxine. It also renders the parasites incapable of sporulating in the mosquito, so that the life cycle of the parasite is broken. In some regions, treatment with the drug is successful in up to 90% of cases; addition of quinine increases the success rate to about 95%. Combination of the drug and trisulfapyrimidines is the treatment of choice for toxoplasmosis.

The toxicity is low. Anorexia and vomiting are common with large doses. Skin rashes are rare. In high doses it may cause megaloblastic anemia and, less commonly, leukopenia, thrombocytopenia and pancytopenia as the result of antagonism of folic acid. Atrophic pharyngitis and esophagitis occasionally results. CNS signs of folate deficiency may occur. Because of the intensive dose regimen for toxoplasmosis, semiweekly blood-cell and platelet counts should be made. The hematopoietic toxicity can be reversed by leucovorin. The antifolate actions are damaging to the fetus, so that the drug should be avoided in pregnancy, if possible, or be coadministered with leucovorin.

QUINACRINE HYDROCHLORIDE

1.4-Pentanediamine, *N*⁴-(6-chloro-2-methoxy-9-acridinyl)-*N*¹,*N*¹-diethyl-, dihydrochloride, dihydrate, Atabrine Hydrochloride

6-Chloro-9-[[4-(diethylamino)-1-methylbutyl]amino]-2-methoxyacridine dihydrochloride dihydrate, [6151-30-0] C$_{23}$H$_{30}$ClN$_3$O·2HCl·2H$_2$O (508.91).

Preparation—2,4-Dichlorobenzoic acid is condensed in alkaline solution with *p*-anisidine, and the product, on treatment with phosphorus oxychloride, is cyclized to methoxydichloroacridine. This is heated with 2-amino-5-(diethylamino)pentane in phenol solution and the reaction mixture is added to acetone containing hydrochloric acid. Quinacrine is precipitated as the dihydrochloride while the phenol is held in solution by the acetone.

Description—Bright-yellow, crystalline powder; odorless; bitter; pH (1 in 100 solution) approximately 4.5; melts about 250° with decomposition.

Solubility—1 g in approximately 35 mL water; soluble in alcohol; almost insoluble in chloroform.

Comments—Now generally considered an alternative choice for giardiasis for patients who do not tolerate metronidazole. It is obsolete for treating of malaria. A small percentage of patients treated with it exhibit untoward effects. These are essentially the same as those caused by the 4-aminoquinolines (see the general statement), of which quinacrine can be considered to be an analog. The GI irritancy is higher than with the 4-aminoquinolines, and it is common to give sodium bicarbonate concomitantly. Children do not tolerate it well, and patients with psoriasis should not receive quinacrine because it may exacerbate the condition. Toxic psychosis has been reported in 1.5% of adults who take it. It is absorbed readily from the GI tract and from IM and intracavitary sites of injection. It is excreted very slowly in the urine and accumulates in tissue on chronic administration. It usually is administered orally; each dose is given with water after a meal. If the oral route cannot be employed, IM injection is preferred over the IV injection.

QUINIDINE GLUCONATE—see page 1364.

QUININE SULFATE

(8α,9*R*)-Cinchonan-9-ol, 6′-methoxy-, sulfate (2:1) (salt), dihydrate

Quinine sulfate (2:1) (salt) dihydrate [6119-70-6]
(C$_{20}$H$_{24}$N$_2$O$_2$)$_2$·H$_2$SO$_4$·2H$_2$O (782.95); *anhydrous* [804-63-7] (746.92); the sulfate of an alkaloid obtained from the bark of *Cinchona officinalis Linné* (*C ledgeriana* Moens) (Fam *Rubiaceae*) or other species of *Cinchona*.

Contains not more than 10.0% of dihydroquinine.

Preparation—The crude sulfate, obtained when quinine is isolated from the bark of *Cinchona* sp, is recrystallized once or twice from hot water slightly acidified with sulfuric acid.

Description—White, fine, needle-like crystals; usually lusterless, making a light and readily compressible mass; odorless; persistent, bitter taste; when exposed to light, it acquires a brown tint; pK$_a$ 4.1, 8.5.

Solubility—1 g in approximately 500 mL water, 120 mL alcohol, 35 mL water at 100°, or approximately 10 mL alcohol at 80°; slightly soluble in chloroform or ether.

Comments—The *original antimalarial drug*. It only affects the erythrocytic form of the plasmodia and hence is used only as a suppressive in the management of acute attacks of vivax, malariae or ovale malaria. It may cure up to 50% of infections caused by falciparum plasmodia, but some strains are resistant. The drug may be combined with pyrimethamine and a sulfonamide, but it appears to be antagonized by chloroquine. The quinine-pyrimethamine-sulfadiazine (or sulfadoxine) combination is presently the treatment of choice for infections caused by chloroquine-resistant *Plasmodium falciparum*; an alternative is quinine with tetracycline. In severe infections, IV dihydrochloride or quinidine gluconate is the drug of choice. The combination, clindamycin-quinine, is the treatment of choice for babesiosis.

It has an effect to suppress neuromuscular transmission. In the symptomatic treatment of a rare myopathy known as myotonia congenita, or Thomsen's disease, it exerts a neuromuscular depressant action. It occasionally benefits patients with spasmodic torticollis (torsion spasm) and also persons with nocturnal leg cramps. It is a frequent constituent of bitter tonics and stomachic preparations.

A syndrome of toxic effects known as *cinchonism*, follows the repeated use of full therapeutic doses. Mild cinchonism is characterized by tinnitus, headache, nausea, and slight disturbance of vision. In severe cinchonism the skin is hot and flushed, rashes are frequent, and the CNS is involved; headache, fever, vomiting, apprehension, excitement, confusion, delirium, and syncope are common. The emesis is due to a central action of the drug as well as to its local irritant action on the intestinal mucosa. In a few cases, renal damage, photosensitivity, and hypoprothrombinemia may occur. Agranulocytosis has been observed rarely. Transient ventricular tachycardia is noted in rare instances after massive acute overdosage. Although it generally exerts vasodilator actions, retinal vasoconstriction, leading to loss of vision, has been described; and these effects mostly have followed rapid IV injections or large overdoses. It is absorbed readily from the GI tract. It is only moderately concentrated in tissues and undergoes degradation particularly in the liver. The drug and its degradation products are excreted rapidly in the urine, and for this reason the drug must be given every 6 hr in order to maintain relatively constant plasma levels. The half-life is 5 to 16 hr.

An alkaline urine prolongs the half-life. See the USP DI for the various pharmacokinetic drug interactions. The drug is given after meals to minimize gastric irritation. IM and SC injections are painful and frequently are followed by local tissue injury. The IV route is used rarely and only in emergencies.

SULFADIAZINE—page 1632.
SULFADOXINE—page 1632.

AMEBICIDES

Endemic amebiasis is relatively rare in the US but it still has a prevalence of 2% to 4% in some areas. Most infections are essentially asymptomatic, but the number of severe infections is still large. Amebic infections generally remain confined to the intestines, where they may give rise to dysentery, but in an appreciable fraction of cases the amebae may locate elsewhere, especially in the liver. The chemotherapy of amebiasis thus must provide drugs to treat both the intestinal and extraintestinal forms of the disease. In addition, the ideal amebicide also is capable of eliminating amebic cysts from the intestine. No safe drug exists that will eradicate all of motile forms, cysts, and extraintestinal amebas, but judicious combined therapy can eliminate the parasite from all sites. Metronidazole acts on amebae within the lumen and wall of the intestine as well as other organs. Diloxanide, iodoquinol, and paromomycin are oral luminal amebicides. Emetine and chloroquine are tissue amebicides.

The most commonly reported intestinal protozoal infection in the US is giardiasis, caused by the flagellated protozoan, *Giardia lamblia*. Most individuals are asymptomatic. However, these organisms cause a diarrhea that can be transient or persistent. Infection results from ingestion of cysts from fecal contamination of water, especially from lakes and streams in back country areas where various mammalian species can serve as reservoirs. Cysts change into motile trophozoites in the upper intestine where disease may be produced. Chemotherapy with metronidazole or quinacrine usually is successful.

EMETINE HYDROCHLORIDE

Emetan, 6',7',10,11-tetramethoxy-, dihydrochloride

[316-42-7] $C_{29}H_{40}N_2O_4 \cdot 2HCl$ (553.57); the hydrochloride of an alkaloid obtained from ipecac, or prepared by methylation of cephaeline, or prepared synthetically.

Description—White or slightly yellowish, crystalline powder; odorless; affected by light; pK_a 7.4, 8.3.

Solubility—1 g in 8 mL water or 12 mL alcohol.

Comments—Eradicates *Entameba histolytica* from both intestinal and extraintestinal sites. It is an alternative drug for severe intestinal amebiasis or amebic hepatitis; it ranks only as an alternative when other drugs fail. It is concentrated in the liver, hence its value in amebic hepatitis; it is also of considerable value in the treatment of amebic abscesses in other locations. Occasionally, the drug may be life-saving. It rapidly relieves symptoms of intestinal amebiasis by destroying motile amebas, but the percentage of cures is below 15%, since cysts are affected little; other agents are not only safer but superior. It may be used initially to control quickly severe intestinal amebiasis; the drug then is followed by treatment with other agents. It has no place in the therapy of mild ambulatory or chronic cases.

The incidence of toxic effects is very high, both by local and systemic administration. Thus, the IV route is contraindicated. Large doses produce acute lesions in the heart, liver, kidney, and intestines, and the dose is now restricted. Nevertheless, deaths still sometimes occur, often because of repeated courses of treatment at close intervals; the drug has a probable half-life on the order of weeks to months. Diarrhea, nausea, and vomiting are frequent, as are also skeletal muscle weakness, stiffness, and aching. Sensory disturbances also occur. By far the most important toxic effects are cardiovascular; they include hypotension, precordial pain, dyspnea, tachycardia, and long-persisting electrocardiographic changes; electrocardiographic and blood-pressure recordings at daily intervals are necessary. It is contraindicated in patients with organic disease of the heart or kidney, unless there is no therapeutic alternative, in pregnancy, and when there has been a previous course of therapy within 6 wk.

A course of the drug should not continue for more than 5 days. The patient should be kept in bed, and carefully watched for toxic effects. Do not give the drug IV. Dehydroemetine is available in US but only from the CDC.

IODOQUINOL

8-Quinolinol, 5,7-diiodo-, Diiodohydroxyquinoline; Diodohydroxyquin; Yodoxin

[83-73-8] $C_9H_5I_2NO$ (396.95).

Preparation—8-Quinolinol is iodinated by treatment with iodine monochloride or with a solution of iodine in potassium iodide.

Description—Light yellowish to tan, microcrystalline powder; wetted by water with difficulty; odorless or nearly so; stable in air; melts about 210° with decomposition.

Solubility—Practically insoluble in water; sparingly soluble in alcohol or ether.

Comments—The drug of choice for the treatment of asymptomatic intestinal amebiasis (cyst carrier state) caused by *Entameba histolytica*. In symptomatic intestinal disease, it follows initial treatment with metronidazole or dehydroemetine. In hepatic abscess, it follows metronidazole or emetine. Bed rest is not required. It is the drug of choice in the treatment of infections caused by *Dientameba fragilis*. It is a second-choice drug in the treatment of balantidial dysentery.

It has caused subacute myelo-optic neuropathy when doses larger than recommended for amebiasis were given for 3 wk, so long term therapy should be avoided. Iodine toxicoderma, chills, fever, mild to severe dermatitis, irritation, abdominal discomfort, diarrhea, and headache occur. The drug may cause goiter. It also can interfere with certain thyroid tests, and protein-bound iodine may remain elevated for as long as 6 mo after termination of a course of treatment. Systemic toxicity can result from topical, especially intravaginal, application. Because of GI irritation, it should be taken after meals.

METRONIDAZOLE—page 1669.

PAROMOMYCIN SULFATE

D-Streptamine, *O*-2-amino-2-deoxy-α-D-glucopyranosyl-(1 → 4)-*O*-[*O*-2,6-diamino-2,6-dideoxy-β-L-idopyranosyl-1(1 → 3)-β-D-ribofuranosyl-(1 → 5)]-2-deoxy-, sulfate (salt); Humatin

[1263-89-4];[7542-37-2;59-04-1 (paramomycin)] $C_{23}H_{45}N_5O_{14} \cdot xH_2SO_4$; the sulfate of an antibiotic substance or substances produced by the growth of *Streptomyces rimosus* var *paromomycinus*, or a mixture of two or more such salts. Potency: equivalent to not less than 675 µg of paromomycin ($C_{23}H_{45}N_5O_{14}$)/mg, calculated on the anhydrous basis.

Preparation—Paromomycin is isolated from fermentation broths by ion-exchange adsorption.

Description—Off-white to light-yellow, amorphous powder; odorless or practically so; hygroscopic.

Solubility—1 g in <1 mL water; >10,000 mL alcohol, chloroform, or ether.

Comments—Effective against most clinically significant gram-negative bacteria, especially various species of *Shigella* and *Salmonella* and strains of *E coli*. It is not effective against *Ps aeruginosa*. Among the gram-positive organisms, only staphylococci are sufficiently sensitive to be of clinical significance. It has been used to treat gastroenteritis or bacterial dysentery caused by these organisms, but resistance develops rapidly, the relapse rate is high and other antibiotics are more successful. It also has been used to reduce the bacterial content of the intestine prior to surgery on the bowel or to rid the bowel of nitrogen-forming bacteria in patients with hepatic coma.

Its principal and approved use (US) is in the treatment of asymptomatic intestinal amebiasis, for which it is an alternative drug. It alters the ecology of the intestinal flora in such a way that growth of intestinal amebas is discouraged and it also helps to prevent secondary infections that may follow or facilitate amebic invasion of the intestinal walls. It is of no value in treating hepatic or other extraintestinal abscesses. It also is used to treat infections caused by *Dientamoeba fragilis*. It is an obsolete drug for the treatment of tapeworm infestations.

It often causes GI hypermotility, nausea, diarrhea, and abdominal cramps, which generally appear on the 2nd or 3rd day of treatment and when the daily dose exceeds 2 g. Occasionally, the drug may cause headache, vertigo, vomiting, abdominal pain, or skin rash.

Overgrowth of enteric staphylococci and other pathogenic bacteria rarely occurs, but may if treatment is prolonged. Malabsorption syndromes have not been reported. There is mutual cross-resistance to kanamycin and neomycin, and often to streptomycin. Although it is absorbed poorly from the gut, there is potential nephrotoxicity, especially in the presence of renal disease.

MISCELLANEOUS ANTIPROTOZOAL DRUGS

Among the protozoal infections that are endemic to the US are trichomoniasis, amebiasis, giardiasis, and malaria. Other protozoal infections, uncommon in the US, nevertheless constitute serious public health and agricultural problems within the possessions and elsewhere. The amebicides and antimalarials are useful in the treatment of a number of other protozoal infections. The antimalarials and amebicides have been treated in separate sections.

Two important protozoal infections that occur in immunocomprimised patients (especially AIDS) are pneumocystis and toxoplasmosis. The intracellular protozoa *Toxoplasma gondii* is responsible for congenital infections (usually ocular) or encephalitis that are treated with trimethoprim-sulfamethoxazole or pyrimethamine-sulfadoxine. Alternative regimens include spiramycin, clindamycin, trimetrexate and atovaquone. The incidence of pneumonias due to *Pneumocystis carinii* (PCP) are increasing in AIDS patients and drug-induced immunosuppressed patients because more physicians are aware of this life-threatening risk to such patient populations. Therapy for PCP includes trimethoprim-sulfamethoxazole in most cases. However, some patients intolerant to this regimen are treated with pentamidine isethionate or atovaquone.

ANTIMONY POTASSIUM TARTRATE—page 1596.

ATOVAQUONE

1,4-Naphthalenedione, *trans*-2-[4-(4-chlorophenyl)cyclohexyl]-3-hydroxy-, Mepron

[95233-18-4]$C_{22}H_{19}ClO_3$ (366.85).

Preparation—A mixture of acetyl chloride, anhydrous $AlCl_3$, cyclohexene, and chlorobenzene is heated in CS_2 to form 4-(*p*-chlorophenyl)cyclohexyl methyl ketone. The haloform reaction with hypobromite yields 4-(*p*-chlorophenyl)cyclohexanecarboxylic acid. This latter compound with 2-chloro-1,4-naphthoquinone boiled in an aqueous solution containing silver nitrate, CH_3CN and ammonium persulfate yields the title compound with the ring hydroxyl replaced by Cl. The halogen is replaced with OH by boiling with aqueous alkali to yield the product. US Pats 5,053,532 and 4,981,874 (both 1991).

Description—Yellow crystals melting about 218°.

Solubility—Practically insoluble in water.

Comments—An analog of ubiquinone with antiprotozoal activity against *Pneumocystis carinii, Plasmodium* spp, and *Toxplasma gondii*. Its mechanism of action is not fully elucidated but antiprotozoal activity may be explained by an ability to inhibit selectively mitchondrial electron transport that results in inhibition of *de novo* pyrimidine synthesis.

It is highly lipophilic with low aqueous solubility. Bioavailability is increased significantly with food, but especially by fat. It has a half-life of 2.9 days and is believed to be excreted in the bile and to undergo enterohepatic cycling with almost all of the drug eliminated in the feces. It is highly protein-bound (>99.9%).

It is indicated for acute oral treatment of mild to moderate *Pneumocystis carinii* pneumonia (PCP) in patients who are intolerant to trimethoprim-sulfamethoxazole. It has not been evaluated adequately as a chronic suppressive agent to prevent PCP in patients at high risk for it.

Adverse effects in one study of 203 patients have included rash (23%), nausea (21%), diarrhea (19%), headache (16%), vomiting (14%), fever (14%), insomnia (10%), asthenia (8%), pruritus (5%), oral monilial (5%), abdominal pain (4%), constipation (3%), and dizziness (3%).

IODOQUINOL—page 1668.

METRONIDAZOLE

1*H*-Imidazole-1-ethanol, 2-methyl-5-nitro-, Flagyl

2-Methyl-5-nitroimidazole-1-ethanol [443-48-1] $C_6H_9N_3O_3$ (171.16).

Preparation—2-Methyl-5-nitroimidazole is condensed with ethylene chlorohydrin by heating with a large excess of the chlorohydrin. After removing the surplus chlorohydrin, the residue is extracted with water and the extract is alkalinized and extracted with chloroform. Evaporation of the chloroform yields crude metronidazole which is recrystallized from ethyl acetate. US Pat 2,944,061.

Description—White to pale-yellow, crystals or crystalline powder; odorless; stable in air, but darkens on exposure to light; melts between 159° and 163°; pK_a 2.62.

Solubility—Sparingly soluble in water, alcohol or chloroform; slightly soluble in ether.

Comments—Bactericidal to anaerobic and microaerophilic microorganisms, including *Bacteroides, Clostridium* sp, *Endolimax nana, Entameba histolytica, Fusobacterium vincentii, Gardnerella vaginalis, Giardia lamblia, Peptococcus, Peptostreptococcus,* and *Trichomonas vaginalis*. These organisms reduce the nitro group and generate metabolites that inhibit DNA synthesis. It long has been the drug of choice for the treatment of trichomoniasis and more recently in combination with iodoquinol for the treatment of symptomatic amebiasis (except in brain). Because it is absorbed well orally, concentrations in the lower bowel sometimes are not high enough to eradicate amebas, so that it is combined with iodoquinol to make a first-choice combination. It is also the drug of choice for the treatment of Dracunculus (guinea worm) infestations. It is the alternative drug to treat giardiasis (although some authorities consider it the drug of first choice), balantidiasis, blastocystisis, and infections by *Entameba polecki*. It is used widely for the treatment and prophylaxis of infections caused by anerobic bacteria; it is a drug of choice against GI strains of *Bacteroides fragilis* and vaginal infections by *Gardnerella vaginalis*. It has been used successfully in the treatment of antibiotic-associated pseudomembranous colitis, for which it may be given orally or intravenously. It also has been reported to be of value in Crohn's disease. The drug sensitizes hypoxic tumor cells to radiation and has been employed as an adjunct to radiation therapy.

The most common untoward effects are nausea, diarrhea, anorexia, epigastric distress, and abdominal cramps. Unpleasant taste, vomiting, furry tongue, and stomatitis are fairly frequent. Urticaria, pruritus, flushing, dysuria, cystitis, dry mouth, dry vulva and vagina, feeling of pelvic pressure, vaginal burning, rash, vertigo, headache, numbness, paresthesias, and insomnia occur occasionally. Incoordination and ataxia are rare. Sudden overgrowth of monilia sometimes occurs. The urine sometimes turns a dark color. During treatment the patient should refrain from drinking alcoholic beverages, since the drug has a mild effect similar to *Disulfiram*. Neutropenia occurs, so that a blood count should be made, especially before a second course of the drug. In patients with blood dyscrasias great care must be exercised. It should not be used in patients with diseases of the CNS. The drug has been found to be carcinogenic in mice and rats, and mutagenic. Substances mutagenic in the Ames test have been found in the urine of recipients. It has been used in pregnancy without consequence, but it is advisable to withhold it during pregnancy, if possible.

It is usually about 80% absorbed by the oral route, but in some patients absorption is low. Bowel surgery decreases presystemic elimination. Feces contain 6% to 20% of an oral dose. Although metabolism is performed by target anaerobes and microaerophiles, the principal route of elimination is hepatic oxidation and glucuronidation. About 20% of unchanged drug and all of the hepatic metabolites are excreted into the urine. The half-life is about 6 to 12 hr. The drug inhibits the oxidation of warfarin.

PENTAMIDINE ISETHIONATE

4,4′-(Pentamethylenedioxy)dibenzamidine, bis(2-hydroxyethanesulfonate; Pentam 300, NebuPent

[140-64-7] $C_{19}H_{24}N_4O_2 \cdot 2C_2H_6O_4S$ (592.68).

Preparation—*J Chem Soc* 1942; 103.

Description—Crystals; hygroscopic; melts about 180°.

Solubility—Soluble in water; slightly soluble in alcohol; insoluble in ether or chloroform; pK_a 11.4 (base).

Comments—The alternate drug to suramin for treatment of the hemolymphatic stage of African sleeping sickness (trypanosomiasis) caused by *T brucci gambiense* and *T brucei rhodesiense*. It is the alternate drug for the treatment and the drug of choice for prophylaxis of infections caused by *Pneumocystis carinii*; some reports indicate an efficacy equal to that of trimethoprim-sulfamethoxazole and comparable toxicity in patients with AIDS. It is also an alternative drug for the treatment of kala azar and visceral leishmaniasis. It concentrates in some organs and is eliminated mainly by the kidney. It has a half-life of 6.4 hr and 9.4 hr after 1 IM or IV administration, respectively. Frequent adverse effects include pain and swelling at the site of injection, hypotension, vomiting, blood dyscrasias, and renal damage. Occasional effects are diabetes, hypoglycemia, shock, and liver damage. Herxheimer reactions are rare. Too-rapid injection causes hypotension.

SULFADOXINE—page 1632.
TRIMETREXATE—see RPS-19, page 1262.

ANTIFUNGAL DRUGS

Human fungal infections have increased in recent years because more patients are now at risk for these pathogens. The increased exposure is explained by more frequent surgeries, the use of broad spectrum antimicrobials, immunosuppressive drug therapy for cancer and organ transplantation patients and the HIV epidemic. The antifungal drugs are grouped into the following categories: drugs for systemic mycoses, oral drugs for mucocutaneous infections and topical drugs for mucocutaneous infections (Table 87-10).

The major drugs for systemic mycoses include amphotericin B (a polyene macrolide), flucytosine (a pyrimidine analog), and the relatively nontoxic, orally-active azoles (ketoconazole, itraconazole, and fluconazole). These azoles are synthetic compounds that possess either an imidazole or triazole group. The major attributes of the lipophilic amphotericin B are its broad fungicidal activity and potential for serious nephrotoxicity. Flucytosine has a very restricted spectrum and causes bone marrow suppression and transient hepatoxicity. In contrast, the azoles have a broad antifungal spectrum and cause only relatively minor GI upset. Ketoconazole inhibits adrenal and gonadal steroid hormone synthesis and some hepatic metabolizing enzymes. However, itraconazole and fluconazole have much less potential for the inhibition of hepatic metabolism of other drugs.

Amphotericin B is relatively selective for fungal membranes because it binds to ergosterol, the predominant sterol in these microbes, whereas the main sterol in bacteria and human cells is cholesterol. Upon binding to ergosterol, amphotericin B alters the permeability of fungal cells resulting in pores allowing

Table 90-10. Antifungals

DRUG	COMMENTS
Drugs for Systemic Mycoses	
Amphotericin B	IV only, broad spectrum, nephrotoxicity
Flucytosine	Narrow spectrum, bone marrow suppression
Fluconazole	IV or oral, good oral abs and distribution, long acting
Ketoconazole	Oral abs good unless reduced gastric acid, limited distribution, inhibits CYP3A4
Itraconazole	Very lipophilic, so food improves p oral abs, metabolized, inhibits CYP3A4
Oral Drugs for Cutaneous Mycoses	
Griseofulvin	Food improves oral abs, fungistatic
Terbinafine	Good oral abs., fungicidal, shorter therapy
Topical Drugs for Cutaneous Mycoses	
Clotrimazole	High efficacy vs dermatophytes
Miconazole	Best efficacy vs dermatophytes
Ciclopirox	High efficacy vs dermatophytes
Tolnaftate	Good efficacy vs dermatophytes
Haloprogin	Good efficacy vs dermatophytes
Undecylenic acid	Lower efficacy vs dermatophytes

leakage of intracellular ions and macromolecules. Resistance occurs if ergosterol binding is impaired.

Flucytosine is converted to 5-fluorouracil and then a monophosphate and triphosphate inside the fungal cell where it inhibits DNA and RNA synthesis. Human cells are unable to convert the parent drug to its active metabolites.

The antifungal activity of azole drugs is based on their inhibition of fungal cytochrome P450 enzymes that participate in ergosterol sytnesis. Ketoconazole (an imidazole) is less selective and inhibits adrenal and gonadal cytochrome P450 enzymes (causing gynecomastia, infertility, and menstrual irregularities) as well as hepatic enzymes involved in drug metabolism. Itraconazole and fluconazole (both triazoles) have less interaction with hepatic microsomal enzymes.

The other major differences in these systemic antifungal drugs involve their pharmacokinetics. Amphotericin B is given by IV infusion and must be formulated as a colloidal suspension because of its low water solubility. Reactions due to IV infusion include fever, chills, headache, and hypotension. New liposomal formulations are now available to reduce the renal toxicity by decreasing its accumulation in renal cell membranes and increase delivery at other sites such as liver, spleen, lymph nodes, and lung.

The distribution of flucytosine is very extensive including the CSF in contrast to amphotericin B that must be given intrathecally to treat fungal meningitis. Flucytosine is eliminated by renal excretion, while amphotericin is mainly metabolized. The azoles vary in their water solubility and route of administration. Fluconazole is the most water soluble and best orally absorbed. It also has good CSF levels and is eliminated by renal excretion. Both ketoconazole and itraconazole have low water solubility, variable oral absorption, low CSF levels and undergo metabolism.

AMPHOTERICIN B

Fungizone

$[1R - (1R*,3S*,5R*,6R*,9R*,11R*,15S*,16R*,17R*,18S*,19E,21E,23E, 25E,27E,29E,31E,33R*,35S,36S*,37S*)]$-33-[(3-Amino-3,6-dideoxy-β-D-mannopyranosyl)oxy]-1,3,5,6,9,11,17,37-octahydroxy-15,16,18-trimethyl-13-oxo-14,39-dioxabicyclo[33.3.1]nonatriaconta-19,21,23,25,27, 29,31-heptaene-36-carboxylic acid [1397-89-3] $C_{47}H_{73}NO_{17}$ (924.09); a substance produced by the growth of *Streptomyces nodosus*. Potency: not less than 750 μg of amphotericin B/mg.

Preparation—By the growth of selected strains of *Streptomyces nodosus* in an appropriate medium under controlled conditions of temperature, pH, and aeration. After extracting from the medium, the crude product is purified by treatment with various solvents at controlled acidity.

Description—Yellow to orange powder; odorless or practically so; pK_a (acid) 5.7, (amine) 10.0.

Solubility—Insoluble in water, anhydrous alcohol or ether; aqueous solubility can be increased to approximately 50 mg/mL by complexation with sodium desoxycholate.

Comments—The widest spectrum of antifungal activity of any systemic antifungal drug. By the IV route it is an extremely useful drug for therapy of systemic fungus diseases, especially coccidioidomycosis, cryptococcosis, systemic moniliasis, histoplasmosis, aspergillosis, rhodotorulosis, sporotrichosis, phycomycosis (mucormycosis), and North American blastomycosis. It also is used topically in the treatment of superficial monilial infections and by nasal spray in the prophylaxis of aspergillosis in immunocompromised patients.

It is absorbed very poorly from the GI tract. It is highly bound predominantly to β-lipoproteins and is excreted slowly by the kidneys but neither renal failure nor hemodialysis has a consistent effect on plasma levels. The initial half-life is 24 hr, is followed by a terminal half-life of about 15 days.

It may induce chills and fever, nausea and vomiting, diarrhea, abdominal *cramps*, hemorrhagic gastroenteritis, dyspepsia, headache, vertigo, pain in the vein injected, thrombophlebitis, muscle and joint pains, anemia, purpura, hypertension, hypotension, cardiac arrest, ventricular fibrillation, skin rashes, hypokalemia, hypomagnesemia, renal damage, blood dyscrasias, loss of hearing, and other untoward effects. When given intrathecally it may cause grand mal convulsions, radiculitis, arachnoiditis, paralysis of the extremities, urinary retention, and other difficulties.

ANTHRALIN—page 1284.
BUTYLPARABEN—page 1627.

CASPOFUNGIN ACETATE

1-[(4*R*,5*S*)-5-[(2-Aminoethyl)amino]-*N*²-(10,12-dimethyl-1-oxo-tetradecyl)-4-hydroxy-L-ornithine]-5-[(3*R*)-3-hydroxy-L-ornithine]pneumocandin B₀, diacetate (salt); Cancidas

[179463-17-3] $C_{52}H_{88}N_{10}O_{15}\cdot 2C_2H_4O_2$ (1213.42).

Preparation—Synthesized from a fermentation product of *Glarea lozoyensis.*

US Pat 5,378,804 (1995).

Description—White to off white hygroscopic powder. Saturated solution has pH of about 6.6.

Solubility—Freely soluble in water or methanol; slightly soluble in ethanol.

Comments—A polypeptide antifungal related to pneumocandin B0. It is a glucan synthesis inhibitor of the echinocandin structural class. It is available as a parenteral agent for intravenous injection. This agent is very active against *Candida* species (including azole-resistant strains) and possesses moderate to good activity against *Aspergillus* species. Adverse effects are uncommon but have included histamine release associated with infusion of caspofungin as well as altered liver function tests. Of note, drug intereactions with cyclosporine may occur, and patients should be closely monitored.

CLOTRIMAZOLE

1*H*-Imidazole, 1-[(2-chlorophenyl)diphenylmethyl]-, Gyne-Lotrimin, Lotrimin, Mycelex, Mycelex-G

1-(*o*-Chloro-α,α-diphenylbenzyl)imidazole [23593-75-1] $C_{22}H_{17}ClN_2$ (344.84).

Preparation—From the reaction between imidazole and 2-chlorotriphenylmethyl chloride using trimethylamine as a proton receptor.

Description—White, to pale-yellow, crystalline powder; melts about 147° with decomposition weakly basic; hydrolyses on heating with aqueous acid.

Solubility—Slightly soluble in water; soluble in alcohol or chloroform; slightly soluble in ether.

Comments—A broad-spectrum antifungal agent that inhibits growth of pathogenic dermatophytes. It exhibits fungicidal activity in vitro against isolates of *Trichophyton rubrum* and *mentagrophytes, Epidermophyton floccosum, Microsporum canis,* and *Candida albicans.*

It shares with econazole and miconazole first-choice status for topical treatment of tinea pedis, tinea cruris, and tinea corporis due to any of the aforementioned organisms, candidiasis due to *Candida albicans.* It is effective for the topical treatment of vulvovaginal and oropharyngeal candidiasis.

Adverse effects from topical use include erythema; stinging, blistering and peeling of the skin; pruritus and urticaria.

FLUCONAZOLE

1*H*-1,2,4-Triazole-1-ethanol, α-(2,4-difluorophenyl)-α-(1*H*-1,2,4-triazol-l-ylmethyl), Diflucan

[86386-73-4] $C_{13}H_{12}F_2N_6O$ (306.27).

Preparation—US Pat 4,404,216.

Description—White crystals; melts about 139°.

Comments—A highly selective inhibitor of fungal cytochrome P-450 and sterol C-14 α-demethylation that results in inhibition of ergosterol synthesis. It is a broad-spectrum bistriazole antifungal agent that is primarily fungistatic with activity against *Cryptococcus neoformans* and *Candida* spp. In common with other azole antifungal drugs, most fungi are more susceptible in vivo. It is approved for systemic candidiasis, oropharyngeal and esophageal candidiasis, and cryptococcal meningitis.

The bioavailability of oral fluconazole is over 90% compared with IV administration. The volume of distribution is 0.8 g/L and reaches concentrations in the CSF that are 80% of that in serum of patients with meningitis. Plasma protein binding is 11%, and fluconazole is cleared primarily by renal excretion with 80% of the dose unchanged and 11% as metabolites in the urine. The plasma half-life is about 30 hr. Fluconazole may alter cytochrome P-450 pathways of metabolismof several drugs including phenytoin, cyclosporine, warfarin, and sulfonylureas.

The most common adverse effects of fluconazole are nausea, vomiting, bloating, and abdominal discomfort. Elevated hepatic aminotransferase activity and allergic rashes may occur.

FLUCYTOSINE

Cytosine, 5-fluoro-, 5-FC; Ancobon

[2022-85-7] $C_4H_4FN_3O$ (129.09).

Preparation—5-Fluorouracil is reacted with POCl₃ to form 2,4-dichloro-5-fluoropyrimidine which is reacted with NH₃ to produce 2-chloro-4-amino-5-fluoropyrimidine. Heating the latter in concentrated HCl yields flucytosine. US Pat 3,368,938.

Description—White to off-white, crystalline powder; odorless or has a slight odor; melts about 295° with decomposition; stable in light; nonhygroscopic; stable for at least 3 months at 45°; pKₐ 2.9, 10.7.

Solubility—1 g in approximately 83 mL water or approximately 12 mL 0.1 *N* HCl; slightly soluble in alcohol; practically insoluble in chloroform or ether.

Comments—Converted in the fungus to 5-fluorouracil, which is incorporated into RNA, which interferes with normal protein synthesis. Certain fungal organisms are more sensitive to interference from the drug than are human cells, so that the drug is useful in the treatment of some fungal infections. Most clinical isolates of *Cryptococcus* and 40 to 92% of *Candida* are sensitive to the drug. It is the drug of choice to treat chromomycosis and of second choice to treat systemic candidiasis. It may be combined with amphotericin B for first-choice treatment of aspergillosis or cryptococcosis, especially with meningitis.

Nausea, vomiting, diarrhea, and rash rather commonly are caused by the drug. Bone-marrow depression, manifested by anemia, leucopenia, and thrombocytopenia, occur in about 10% of patients; there have been a few fatalities.

Sedation, confusion, hallucinations, headache, and vertigo occur infrequently. Mild azotemia and an increase in liver enzymes in the plasma are rather common effects. Monitor hepatic function and hematopoietic system during therapy.

About 90% is absorbed orally. It is distributed well among all the tissues, including the CNS. About 80% to 90% is excreted unchanged in the urine with a half-life 0.5 to 1 hr, except 4 to 6 hr in renal failure. The dose needs to be adjusted if renal function is abnormal.

FORMALDEHYDE—page 1628.
GENTIAN VIOLET—see RPS-18, page 1171.

HALOPROGIN

Benzene, 1,2,4-trichloro-5-[(3-iodo-2-propynyl)oxy]-, ing of Halotex

[777-11-7] $C_9H_4Cl_3IO$ (361.39).

Preparation—CA 1963; 58:14635g.
Description—White or pale-yellow, crystalline powder; melts about 114°; decomposes at 190°.
Solubility—Very slightly soluble in water; soluble in alcohol.
Comments—A *topical antifungal* with good efficacy versus dermatophytes, used for cutaneous mycoses.

ICHTHAMMOL—page 1285.
IODINE—pages 1628 and 1716.

ITRACONAZOLE

3H-1,2,4-Triazol-3-one, (±)-4-[4-[4-[4-[[2-(2,4-dichlorophenyl)-2-(1H-1,2,4-triazol-1-ylmethyl)-1,3-dioxolan-4-yl]methoxy]-phenyl]-1-piperazinyl]phenyl]-2,4-dihydro-2-(1-methylpropyl)-, Sporanox

[84625-61-6] $C_{35}H_{38}Cl_2N_8O_4$ (705.65).

Preparation—J Med Chem 1984; 27:894. The racemate is used clinically.
Description—White crystals; melting about 166°; pKa approximately 3.5.
Solubility—1 g in 10,000 mL water or 1000 mL of alcohol; more soluble in acidulated polyethylene glycols.
Comments—A triazole antifungal agent with a mechanism of action and broad spectrum similar to fluconazole. It also inhibits chitin synthesis in both yeast-budding and hyphal growth of fungi. It is used to treat fungal infections in immunocompromised and nonimmunocompromised patients who have cryptococcosis, blastomycosis, histoplasmosis and aspergillosis. Unlabeled uses include superficial mycoses, systemic mycoses and subcutaneous mycoses.

Bioavailability is 55% and food enhances oral absorption. It is 99.8% protein bound and is eliminated in urine and bile after extensive hepatic metabolism. The half-life is 20 to 30 hr. Negligible levels reach CSF.

Adverse effects include nausea, epigastric pain, edema, and hypokalemia. Reversible alterations in liver function have been reported in a few cases. Some interactions with drugs metabolized by P450 pathways have been observed in some patients.

KETOCONAZOLE

Piperazine, cis-1-acetyl-4-[4-[[2-(2,4-dichlorophenyl)-2-(1H-imidazol-1-ylmethyl)-1,3-dioxolan-4-yl]methoxy]phenyl]-, Nizarol

[65277-42-1] $C_{26}H_{28}Cl_2N_4O_4$ (531.44).
Preparation—J Med Chem 1979; 22:1003.
Description—White crystals melting about 146°.
Comments—Blocks the fungal synthesis of ergosterol, which is essential to the integrity of the cell membranes of nearly all the pathogenic fungi. Consequently, it has a broad spectrum of antifungal activity. It or amphotericin B is the drug of choice for the treatment of

blastomycosis, coccidiodosis, histoplasmosis, and paracoccidiodosis. It is an alternative drug for candidiasis and chromoblastomycosis. Successful treatment sometimes requires months.

Nausea and vomiting are the most frequent (3–10%) side effects; these can be avoided by taking the drug with food. Pruritus is the next most frequent (1.5%) and abdominal cramps, third (1.2%). Other effects are pruritus, sleepiness, headache, diarrhea, photophobia, fever, thrombocytopenia, gynecomastia, impotence, and oligospermia (from low testosterone levels). A disulfiram-like reaction to alcohol occurs. Most adverse effects are transient and all are reversible, except that three cases of liver necrosis have been fatal. Monitoring of liver function is mandatory. In rats, it is teratogenic; thus, it should not be used during pregnancy. It inhibits certain cytochrome P-450 enzymes; plasma levels of cyclosporine, estradiol, hydrocortisone, methylprednisolone, rifampin, and theophylline can be increased. Cimetidine inhibits and rifampin induces the metabolism of the drug. Ketoconazole inhibits steroid C17-20 lyase and thus decreases the biosynthesis of adrenalcorticoids, androgens, and estrogens. This is the basis of its uses to treat Cushing's syndrome, precocious puberty, and prostatic carcinoma.

It is absorbed well by the oral route. In plasma, 95% to 99% is protein-bound. The principal route of elimination is hepatic metabolism and biliary secretion of the metabolites, less than 4% being renal excretion. There are a number of metabolites. Enterohepatic circulation complicates the pharmacokinetics. During the first 10 hr (alpha-phase), the half-life is 1.4 to 3.3 hr; thereafter (beta-phase), it is 6 to 10 hr.

VORICONAZOLE

4-Pyrimidineethanol, (αR,βS)-α-(2,4-difluorophenyl)-5-fluoro-β-methyl-α-(1H-1,2,4-triazol-1-ylmethyl)-, Vfend

[137234-62-9] $C_{16}H_{14}F_3N_5O$ (349.32).

Preparation—A Friedel-Crafts reaction between 1,3-difluorobenzene and chloroacetyl chloride yields 2,4-difluorophenacyl chloride. This latter compound with

1H-1,2,4-triazole forms the1-phenacyl derivative (I). Also, 4-chloro-5-fluoro-6-ethylpyrimidine, with NBS and AIBN forms the 1-bromoethyl product(II). Compounds I and II, with Zn/I₂, couples to form the variconazole nucleus in the *RS/SR* configuration of the alkyl side chain, in a 12:1 ratio. The compound is dechlorinated and resolved to yield the product. *Albany Molecular Research Tech Reports* 2003; 8(80):6-9.

Description—White to light yellow powder melting about 127°. $[\alpha]^{25}_D$ -62° (c = 1, methanol).

Comments—Triazole antifungal with enhanced activity against Aspergillus species. Clinically considered to be one of the treatments of choice for infections caused by this species. Also active against most "azole-resistant Candida species". Available both orally and parenterally. Adverse reactions area similar to itraconazole with a noted addition of transient visual disturbances. A potent inhibitor of cytochrome P450 enzymes. Caution should be exercised in patients receiving "narrow index" medications concomitantly with voriconazole.

SYSTEMIC DRUGS FOR MUCOCUTANEOUS INFECTIONS

Systemic treatment of dermatophyte infections of skin, hair, and nails has been restricted for many years to the fungistatic drug, griseofulvin. Its action involves deposition in newly formed skin and nail beds where it binds to keratin protecting these sites from new infection. It is given orally for prolonged periods with numerous side effects (headaches, nausea, hepatoxicity, skin rashes, and photosensitivity).

More recently, terbinafine (an allylamine) and itraconazole (an azole) have become available as oral fungicidal drugs for dermatophytes. Terbinafine is especially useful for antifungal therapy of nail beds (onychomycosis) because it is more effective over a shorter time period. It inhibits the fungal enzyme squalene epoxidase leading to the accumulation of the toxic sterol, squalene. Adverse effects are much less but involve some cases of GI upset and headache. Itraconazole is the azole of choice for treatment of dermatophytoses and onychomycosis.

GRISEOFULVIN

Spiro[benzofuran-2(3H),1′-[2]cyclohexene]-3,4-dione, 7-chloro-2,4,6-trimethoxy-6-methyl-, (1′S-trans)-,

[126-07-8] $C_{17}H_{17}ClO_6$ (352.77); a substance produced by the growth of *Penicillium griseofulvum* or by other means. It has a potency equivalent to not less than 900 μg of $C_{17}H_{17}ClO_6$/mg.

Preparation—By the submerged process using selected strains of *Penicillium patulum*.

Description—White to creamy white, powder, in which particles of the order of 4 μm in diameter predominate; odorless.

Solubility—Soluble in chloroform; sparingly soluble in alcohol; slightly soluble in water.

Comments—An effective agent in the treatment of superficial fungus infections. It is fungistatic and not fungicidal. Administered systemically, the drug is highly effective in the management of tinea capitis, tinea corporis, tinea unguium (onychomycosis) and the chronic form of tinea pedis caused by the dermatophytes, *Microsporon, Trichophyton,* and *Epidermophyton*.

Since it does not kill but only arrests reproduction of the organism, it is necessary to continue medication long enough for the entire epidermis to be shed and replaced in order to remove reinfecting organisms. It is deposited in the keratin precursor cells and is carried outwards into the epidermis as normal skin growth proceeds. This also makes for a long latency from the time medication is begun until evidence of improvement occurs.

Serious untoward reactions are infrequent, but skin eruptions, leukopenia, granulocytopenia, and allergic reactions such as serum sickness or angioneurotic edema are among the serious side effects reported. It also may cause nausea, vomiting, epigastric distress, and diarrhea; these often may be avoided by giving the drug with or shortly following a meal. Headache is also relatively frequent. Infrequently, phototoxicity, proteinuria, lassitude and fatigue occur and, rarely, there is mental confusion and motor incoordination. It is advisable to monitor kidney, blood, and liver functions. Ingestion of alcohol during treatment with the drug causes tachycardia and flushing.

The oral bioavailability depends upon particle size; the smaller the crystal size, the more complete the absorption. The percent absorbed from the microsize preparations is 25% to 70%; from the ultramicrosize preparations it is almost complete. Absorption is greater if the drug is administered with a high-fat meal. The principal route of elimination may be transepidermal loss, although a considerable hepatic metabolism and biliary secretion probably also occur. The half-life is 24 to 36 hr. It induces the hepatic microsomal system, and the metabolism of warfarin, mexiletine and oral contraceptives is increased, thus necessitating dosage adjustments.

TERBINAFINE HYDROCHLORIDE

1-Naphthalenemethaneamine, (E)-N-(6,6-dimethyl-2-hepten-4-ynyl)-N-methyl-, monohydrochloride; Lamasil

[78628-80-5] $C_{21}H_{25}N·HCl$ (327.90).

Preparation—*J Med Chem* 1984; 27:1539; Lednicer D, et al. *Org Chem of Drug Syn*, vol 4, Wiley, NY, 1990, p 55.

Description—White to off-white crystalline powder.

Solubility—Freely soluble in methanol and methylene chloride; soluble in alcohol; slightly soluble in water.

Comments—The *first allylamine* available for systemic use in the treatment of all dermatophytes (*Trichophyton, Epidermophyton*, and *Microspora*). It is also available for topical therapy of dermatophytes in-

cluding *tinea* infections. It selectively inhibits fungal squalene epoxidase causing a fungicidal action due to the intracellular accumulation of the toxic sterol, squalene; it also exerts a fungistatic action by depletion of ergosterol. One tablet daily for 12 wk achieves a 90% cure rate for onychomycosis that is more effective than griseofulvin or itraconazole. It does not seem to affect the cytochrome P450 metabolism of other drugs. The most common adverse effects are headache, diarrhea, dyspepsia, and abdominal pain. Taste disturbances do occur and may persist for several weeks after discontinuing the drug.

TOPICAL DRUGS FOR MUCOCUTANEOUS INFECTIONS

Nystatin is a topical polyene macrolide analog of amphotericin B with a similar mode of action but too toxic for parenteral use. It is active against most *Candida* spp and may be used for oropharyngeal thrush, vaginal candidiasis, and intestinal candidiasis. However, the most frequently used topical antifungal therapy today for oral thrush and dermatophytic infections are the azoles, clotrimazole and miconazole. Other azoles also available for topical use include econazole, oxiconazole, and sulconazole. The allylamines available of topical treatment of tinea infections are terbinafine and naftifine.

BUTENAFINE HYDROCHLORIDE

1-Naphthalenemethaneamine, N-[[4-(1,1-dimethylethyl) phenyl]methyl]-N-methyl-, hydrochloride; Mentax

[101827-46-7] $C_{23}H_{27}N·HCl$ (353.94).

Preparation—N-Methyl-1-naphthylmethaneamine is treated with *p-tert*-butylamine in DMF. Sodium carbonate is added and, after prolonged stirring, butenafine base separates, is filtered and converted to the hydrochloride by usual methods.

Description—White, odorless crystalline powder from methanol/acetic acid melting about 200°.

Solubility—Freely soluble in methanol, ethanol, chloroform or methylene chloride; slightly soluble in water.

Comments—Butenafine inhibits ergosterol biosynthesis by blocking squalene epoxidation. Butenafine appears as an alternative for treatment of various dermatophytosis, such as tinea pedis, tinea cruris, tinea corporis, and onychomycosis. Its rapid and persistent antifungal activity is attractive. Butenafine is available for topical administration in 1% cream formulation. The most striking feature of butenafine is its superior fungicidal activity against this group of fungi when compared to that of terbinafine, naftifine, tolnaftate, and clotrimazole. It is active also against *Candida albicans,* and this activity is superior to that of terbinafine and naftifine. Butenafine also generates low MICs for Cryptococcus neoformans and *Aspergillus* spp as well. Butenafine appears as an alternative for treatment of various dermatophytosis, such as tinea pedis, tinea cruris, tinea corporis, and onychomycosis. Its rapid and persistent antifungal activity is attractive.

CLOTRIMAZOLE—page 1671.

ECONAZOLE NITRATE

1H-Imidazole, (±)-1-[2-[(4-chlorophenyl)methoxy]-2-(2,4-dichlorophenyl)ethyl]-, mononitrate, Spectrazole

(±)-1-[2,4-Dichloro-β-[(p-chlorobenzyl)oxy]phenethyl]imidazole mononitrate [68797-31-9] $C_{18}H_{15}Cl_3N_2O·HNO_3$ (440.70).

Preparation—2,4-Dichloroacetophenone is further chlorinated to the phenacyl chloride and this compound treated with imidazole with loss of HCl to yield 1-(1*H*)-(2,4-dichlorophenacyl)imidazole (I). Reduction of the ketone group of I with sodium borohydride forms the secondary alcohol (II). With sodium hydride, the alcoholate of II is produced, which on reaction with *p*-chlorobenzyl chloride produces econazole base. See *J Med Chem* 1969; 12:784.

Description—White crystals; melts at approximately 162°; pK$_a$ 6.6.

Solubility—Very slightly soluble in water or most organic solvents.

Comments—Antifungal activity against the dermatophytes (*Epidermophyton floccosum, Microsporon auduoni, cani,s* and *gypseum, and Trichophyton rubrum, mentagrophytes,* and *tonsurans*), *Pityrosporon obiculare* (*Malasserzia furfur*) and *Candida albicans.* It is employed in the treatment of *cutaneous Candidiasis,* and *tineas corporis, cruris, pedis,* and *versicolor* (*pityriasis versicolor*). Its efficacy is comparable to that of miconazole or clotrimazole. It readily penetrates into the stratum corneum, where effective concentrations persist for as long as several days. In approximately 3% of recipients, local erythemia, burning sensation, stinging, and itching occur.

MERCURIC OXIDE, YELLOW—see RPS-18, page 1172.
MERCURY, AMMONIATED—see RPS-18, page 1172.

MICONAZOLE

1*H*-Imidazole, 1-[2-(2,4-dichlorophenyl)-2-[(2,4-dichlorophenyl)methoxy]ethyl]-, Micatin, Monistat

1-[2,4-Dichloro-β-[(2,4-dichlorobenzyl)oxy]phenethyl]imidazole [22916-47-8] C$_{18}$H$_{14}$Cl$_4$N$_2$O (416.12).

Preparation—2,4-Dichlorophenacyl bromide is used to alkylate imidazole followed by reduction of the ketone group to a secondary alcohol which is converted to the alkoxide. Williamson alkylation with α,*p*,-dichlorotoluene yields the product. *J Med Chem* 1969; 12:784.

Comments—Fungicidal to various species of *Aspergillus, Blastomyces, Candida, Cladosporium, Coccidioides, Epidermophyton, Histoplasma, Microsporon, Paracoccidioides,* and *Trichophyton.* It inhibits ergosterol synthesis, which disrupts fungal cell membranes. The drug readily penetrates into the stratum corneum and remains there in high concentration for as long as 4 days, which probably contributes to its efficacy against the dermatophytoses. In tinea pedis (athlete's foot) a mycological cure rate of 96% has been reported with the nitrate salt, which considerably exceeds that of any other drugs except clotrimazole and econazole.

Topically, for vulvovaginal candidiasis, the reported cure rate varies from 80% to 95%, considerably superior to that with nystatin (65%) and amphotericin B (75%). Often pruritus is relieved after a single application. It is also effective against some vaginal infections caused by *Trichophyton glabratus.* The free base is useful in the topical treatment of various ophthalmic mycoses. The base has been used successfully in the systemic treatment of several deep or systemic mycoses, especially those of candidiasis and cryptococcosis.

Burning, itching, and maceration sometimes occurs after application of the nitrate to the skin, as happens frequently with effective antifungal drugs. Intravaginally, burning, itching, pelvic discomfort, urticaria, and headache occur in 6% to 7% of users, especially during the first few days of treatment. Experimental and clinical studies suggest that the drug is safe for use in pregnancy, but systemic use during pregnancy should probably be avoided, if possible. Orally, it appears to be tolerated well, but nausea, vomiting, and diarrhea occur. No evidence of renal or hepatic toxicity has been observed.

IV administration may cause phlebitis, hypercholesterolemia, and hypertriglyceridemia (caused by the vehicle), hyponatremia (from ADH secretion), nausea, vomiting, diarrhea, anorexia, and infrequent allergic and immune reactions, such as fever, chills, pruritus, rashes, thrombocytopenia, anaphylaxis, and anemia. Wheezing and tachypnea and sinoatrial and ventricular tachycardias occur, which can be avoided by slower rates of infusion. Intrathecally, it may cause some meningeal irritation, but the route appears to be safe.

From topical sites, only trace amounts of the drug appear in the blood or urine. Slightly less than 50% of an oral dose is absorbed. In plasma, about 93% is bound to proteins. Less than 1% of an oral dose appears unchanged in urine. The drug manifests three-compartment pharmacokinetics. The terminal (elimination, β) half-life is about 1 day. Systemically, it inhibits the metabolism of warfarin.

NYSTATIN

Nystatin [1400-61-9] is a substance produced by the growth of *Streptomyces noursei* Brown, et al (Fam *Streptomycetaceae*). It contains not less than 4400 Units of nystatin activity/mg. Nystatin is a mixture of 4 different tetraenes, nystatin A, (principally) and nystatin A$_2$, A$_3$ and polyfungin B. Nystatin A$_1$ [34786-70-4] C$_{47}$H$_{75}$NO$_{17}$ is closely related to *Amphotericin B.* Each is a macrocyclic lactone containing a ketal ring, an *all-trans* tetraene system and a mycosamine (3-amino-3-deoxyrhamnose) moiety.

Description—Yellow to light-tan hygroscopic powder; odor suggestive of cereals; hygroscopic; affected by long exposure to light, heat or air; pK$_a$ 4.5, 8.64; gradually decomposes at temperatures higher than 160° without melting.

Solubility—(mg/mL, at approximately 30) Water, 4; alcohol 1.2; methanol 11.2; chloroform, 0.48; or ethylene glycol, 8.75.

Comments—Active *in vitro* against a number of yeasts and molds, but its clinical usefulness is limited to the treatment of *candidiasis.* The antibiotic is absorbed poorly from the gastrointestinal tract; consequently it is not effective against systemic infections, but is effective against *intestinal candidiasis.* It may prevent emergence of candidal suprainfections resulting from oral therapy with broad-spectrum antibiotics, although such suprainfections are so infrequent that routine "prophylactic" use of nystatin is not worthwhile. It does *not* prevent diarrhea from oral broad-spectrum antibiotics. It has been employed with variable success in the treatment of oral "thrush" (moniliasis). It is used alone to treat vulvovaginal candidiasis. For use on the skin, it may be combined with neomycin, gramicidin and triamcinolone acetonide. It is not the drug of first or second choice in any use. It is relatively nontoxic, but nausea, vomiting and diarrhea may occur with oral therapy.

OXICONAZOLE NITRATE

Ethanone, (*Z*)-1-(2,4-dichlorophenyl)-2-(1*H*-imidazol-1-yl)-*O*-[(2,4-dichlorophenyl)methyl]oxime, mononitrate; Oxistat

[64211-46-7]C$_{18}$H$_{13}$Cl$_4$N$_3$O·HNO$_3$ (492.15).

Preparation—An exothermic reaction occurs upon mixing 2,4-dichlorophenacyl chloride and imidazole in acetonitrile. The product, 2,4-dichlorophenacylimidazole, is refluxed with hydroxylamine HCl in pyridine to form the oxime, which is heated with 2,4-dichlorobenzyl chloride in ethanolic pyridine to yield the base of the title compound. US Pat 4,124,767 (1978).

Description—White crystals melting about 138°.

Solubility—Soluble in methanol; sparingly soluble in alcohol, chloroform, or acetone; very slightly soluble in water.

Comments—An antifungal agent used for the topical treatment of *tinea pitryasis versicolor* and for *tinea pedis, tinea cruris* and *tinea corporis* due to *Trichophyton rubrum*, *T mentagrophytes,* or *Epidermophyton floccosum.*

SULCONAZOLE NITRATE

1*H*-Imidazole, (±)-1-[2-[[(4-chlorophenyl)methyl]thio]-2-(2,4-dichlorophenyl)ethyl]-, mononitrate; Exelderm

[61318-91-0] C$_{18}$H$_{15}$Cl$_3$N$_2$S·HNO$_3$ (460.77).

Preparation—US Pat 4,038,409 (1977); Lednicer D, et al. *Org Chem of Drug Syn*, vol 3, NY, Wiley, 1984, p 133.

Description—White to off-white crystals melting about 130°.

Solubility—Freely soluble in pyridine; slightly soluble in alcohol, acetone, or chloroform; very slightly soluble in water.

Comments—Used for various *tinea* conditions (athlete's foot), such as *T corporis*, *T pedis*, or *T cruris*; action is similar to *oxiconazole*.

POTASSIUM IODIDE—page 1377.
POTASSIUM PERMANGANATE—see RPS-19, page 1270.
PROPYLPARABEN—see RPS-18, page 1173.
SALICYLIC ACID—page 1288.
SODIUM BENZOATE—see RPS-19, page 1271.
SODIUM HYPOCHLORITE SOLUTION—page 1630.

ANTIVIRAL DRUGS

Viruses cause much of the morbidity and mortality in populations worldwide, but the number of drugs available are still quite limited. Antiviral drug development has become a very active area in the last decade, especially with the challenges of the AIDS epidemic. The need to develop more selective inhibitors of viral function has increased the number of antiviral drugs in clinical trials for the human immunodeficiency virus (HIV) and should lead to important advantages in the next decade.

Viruses cannot replicate independently because they use the energy-generating, DNA or RNA replicating, and protein synthesizing pathways of the host cells to replicate. Viral replication can be targeted at several steps:

1. Adsorption to and penetration into susceptible host cells
2. Uncoating of viral nucleic acid
3. Synthesis of early, regulatory proteins (eg, nucleic acid polymerase)
4. Synthesis of RNA or DNA
5. Synthesis of late structural proteins
6. Assembly of viral particles
7. Release of infectious virions from the cell

Replication of the virus peaks after or before manifestation of clinical symptoms, so early initiation of therapy or prevention of infection is important for optimal clinical efficacy. Some good examples of successful early therapy or prevention include acyclovir to treat varicella-zoster infections and amantidine prophylaxis against influenzae A. The development of many pyrimidine and purine nucleoside analogs have lead to new compounds that selectively inhibit viral DNA synthesis. The selectivity of drugs for the HIV retrovirus was derived from reverse transcriptase inhibitors that block transcription of the HIV RNA genome into DNA and protein synthesis. More recently, protease inhibitors have been developed that prevent the synthesis of late protein and packaging of the virion.

The major antiviral drugs will be discussed under the following categories: inhibitors of viral uncoating, inhibitors of viral nucleic acid synthesis, reverse transcriptase inhibitors, protease inhibitors and immunostimulants (Table 90-11).

Amantadine and rimantidine are orally active inhibitors of viral uncoating that are effective for prophylaxis of influenzae A. These antiviral drugs are tricyclic amines that differ only in their pharmacokinetics. Renal excretion predominates for amantadine while rimantidine is extensively metabolized.

Acyclovir and other closely related guanosine analogs (ganciclovir, valacyclovir, and famciclovir) are the most important group of antiherpes drugs that act by inhibition of viral nucleic acid synthesis. These nucleoside antivirals have to be monophosphorylated by viral thymidine kinase and then are further phoshorylated to triphosphates that inhibit virus growth in three ways. First, the acyclovir triphosphate acts as a competitive inhibitor of DNA polymerases, while the human enzyme is much less susceptible than the viral enzyme; second, it can be a chain terminator; and third, it can produce irreversible binding between DNA polymerase and the interrupted chain causing permanent inactivation.

Foscarnet, a phosphonoformic acid, inhibits DNA polymerases, RNA polymerases, and reverse transcriptases. It is used primarily for AIDS patients with CMV retinitis but can be used against CMV herpes viruses resistant to acyclovir.

Table 90-11. Antiviral Drugs

DRUG	COMMENTS
Nucleic Acid Synthesis Inhibitiors	
Purine Analogs	
Acyclovir	Antiherpes (IV, oral, or topical), CNS effects
Cidofovir	For CMV, nephrotoxicity
Famciclovir	Prodrug of penciclovir
Ganciclovir	For CMV, bone marrow suppression
Penciclovir	Topical antiherpes, similar to acyclovir
Ribovarin	For RSV, potential embryotoxicity
Valacyclovir	Prodrug of acyclovir, better oral absorption
Pyrimidine Analogs	
Fluorouracil	Topical for warts
Idoxuridine	Topical for herpes simplex
Trifluridine	Topical for herpes simplex
Nonnucleosides	
Foscarnet	For CMV, acyclovir-resistant herpes, nephrotoxicity
HIV Reverse Transcriptase Inhibitors	
Pyrimidine Nucleosides	
Lamivudine	Well tolerated
Stavudine	Peripheral neuropathy
Zalcitabine	Peripheral neuropathy
Zidovudine	Anemia, neutropenia, GI effects, CNS effects
Purine Nucleosides	
Didanosine	Peripheral neuropathy, pancreatitis, GI effects
Nonnucleosides	
Nevirapine	Rash, fever, nausea, headache
Delavirdine	Rash
HIV Protease Inhibitors	
Indinavir	Good bioavailability, kidney stones, inhibits CYP3A4
Nelfinavir	Less side effects, some dirrhea
Ritonavir	Good bioavailability, more side effects, many drug interactions (CYP3A4 related)
Saquinavir	Lower bioavailability, less side effects, CYP3A4 related drug interactions
Inhibitors of Influenza Viral Penetration or Uncoating	
Amantidine	Renal excretion, more CNS toxicities
Rimantidine	Metabolized, similar toxicity as amantidine

Ribovarin is a synthetic purine nucleoside analog that is phosphorylated by host cell adenosine kinase resulting in a monophosphate that inhibits cellular inosine monophosphate formation. The net result is depletion of guanosine triphosphate and inhibition of viral protein synthesis plus suppression of initiation or elongation of viral mRNA.

The family of nucleoside reverse transcriptase inhibitors includes zidovudine (azidodeoxythymidine) several dideoxynucleosides (didanosine, zalcitabine, lamuvidine, and stavudine) that are competitive inhibitors of the HIV enzyme that converts viral RNA into DNA and act as DNA chain terminators upon phosphorylation to the triphosphate nucleotide derivatives. These nucleoside antivirals also inhibit mammalian DNA polymerases but require higher concentrations than those effective on HIV reverse transcriptase. Resistance to these compounds occurs from mutations in reverse transcriptase, so they need to be used in combination with each other or the HIV protease inhibitors. Two reverse transcriptase inhibitors are usually combined with a protease inhibitor to decrease the development of resistance. Nevirapine and delavirdine are nonnucleoside inhibitors of reverse transcriptase that also disrupts the catalytic site of this enzyme.

Idoxuridine and trifluridine are pyrimidine analogs that are incorporated into viral DNA resulting in inhibition of DNA synthesis. They are only used topically for herpes simplex infections of the cornea because of their toxicity problems. Fluorouracil, another pyrimidine nucleoside, acts by blocking production of thymidylate and interrupts normal cellular RNA and DNA synthesis. Consequently, it is also restricted to topical therapy of warts.

The protease inhibitors (saquinavir, ritonavir, indinavir, and nelfinavir) are peptide analogs that inhibit the HIV-1-specific protein cleaving enzyme necessary for the production of infectious HIV virions and act synergistically with reverse transcriptase inhibitors. It is important to use them in combination HIV therapy because resistance occurs if they are used alone or intermittently. Two reverse transcriptase inhibitors may be used in combination with one protease inhibitor or alternatively two protease inhibitors may be used with a reverse transcriptase inhibitor. The success of individual combination regimens has been variable but the overall success of combination therapy has been able to decrease viral replication, improve the immunologic status (ie, increase CD4$^+$ cell counts), delay complications and prolong life.

Interferons and immunoglobulins are examples of endogenous compounds that stimulate immune responses to virus infections. Interferons are glycoproteins produced by lymphocytes, macrophages, fibroblasts, and other cells. The three distinct immunologic and chemical classes of interferons are alpha, beta, and gamma. They act by inhibiting viral protein synthesis or assembly or by stimulating the immune system. Interferons have specific intracellular actions that result in several effects including inhibition of viral penetration, uncoating, translation of viral proteins plus assembly and release of virus. Immunoglobulins can be used to prevent some viral infections by using antibody preparations with high titers of specific binding to viruses (especially, hepatitis B and rabies).

The limitations of specific oral antiviral drugs are determined by the profile of adverse effects. Amantidine and rimantidine cause GI upset and CNS effects. Acyclovir and its related analogs (valacyclovir and famciclovir) cause CNS effects and decreased renal function. Other specific problems may occur with some analogs such as ganciclovir that causes bone marrow suppression. The nucleoside reverse transcriptase inhibitors have individual differences in their adverse effect profiles, but the most notable side effects include bone marrow suppression (zidovudine, lamivudine), neuropathy (didanosine, zalcitabine, stavudine) and pancreatitis (didanosine). The protease inhibitors vary in their inhibition of cytochrome P450 metabolism (notably CYP3A isoenzyme), but all possess some potential for drug interactions.

ABACAVIR SULFATE

2-Cyclopentene-1-methanol, (1S-cis)-4-[2-amino-6-(cyclopropyl-amino)-9H-purin-9-yl-, sulfate; Ziagen

[188062-50-2] $(C_{14}H_{18}N_6O)_2 \cdot H_2SO_4$ (670.74).

Preparation—2-Amino-4,6-dichloropyrimidine is coupled with *syn*-5-amino-3-cyclopentenemethanol to yield a secondary amine (I) by displacement of one chlorine atom, while retaining the *cis*-configuration. Treatment of I with *p*-chlorobenzenediazonium chloride forms an azo linkage on the sole unsubstituted position of the pyrimidine ring. The azo group is then reduced with zinc and acid to yield the free diamine (II).

I   II   III

Compound II, with ethyl orthoformate and acid forms a 5-membered imidazole ring involving the adjacent primary and secondary amino groups (III). Finally, the halogen atom on the pyrimidine ring is replaced by cyclopropylamino using cyclopropyl amine in alcohol affording the product. US Pat 6,294,540 (1991), US Pat 5,034,394 (1992), US Pat 6,294,540 (2001).

Description—(Base) White to off-white crystals from acetonitrile melting about 165°; $\alpha^{20}/_D$ -59.7° (c = 0.15, methanol); log P 1.22(0.1M sodium phosphate); pK_a 5.01. (Salt) log P 1.20, pH 7.1-7.3 buffer at 25°.

Solubility—(Salt) 77 mg/mL in water at 25°.

Comments—A nucleoside analogue used as part of combination therapy for the treatment of HIV infection. It is the most potent nucleoside analogue. Generally a well-tolerated antiretroviral. Adverse reactions include: Hypersensivity Reaction-fever, rash, fatigue, malaise, GI symptoms, and arthralgia (noted in 2-3% of patients). Mandatory d/c with hypersensivity rxn. Do not rechallenge. Rare cases of lactic acidosis +/- hepatomegaly w/ steatosis. Rare:Tubular injury

ACYCLOVIR

6H-Purin-6-one, 2-amino-1,9-dihydro-9-[(2-hydroxyethoxy)methyl]-, Zovirax

9-[(2-Hydroxyethoxy)methyl]guanine [59277-89-3] $C_8H_{11}N_5O_3$ (225.21).

Preparation—Guanine is alkylated with 2-(chloromethoxy)ethylbenzoate and the resulting ester hydrolyzed to the product; See Ger Pat 2,539,963.

Description—White crystals melting about 257°.

Solubility—In water, 1.3 mg/mL.

Comments—Activity against *Herpes simplex viruses* (HSV) 1 and 2, varicella-zoster, Epstein-Barr viruses and cytomegalovirus. Inside an infected cell, it is changed into the triphosphate, which then is incorporated into DNA; this terminates elongation of the DNA and prevents viral replication. The sodium salt is approved in the US for the oral treatment of recurrent mucosal and cutaneous infections caused by HSV-1 and HSV-2 in immunocompromised adults and children and for severe initial herpes genitalis infections in immunocompetent patients. However, the drug has been employed effectively in the treatment of HSV encephalitis and neonatal infections and in the treatment of chicken pox, cytomegalovirus, and varicella-zoster infections. The drug also is approved for the topical treatment of nonfulminating HSV-1 and HSV-2 infection (except in the eye), but it is only moderately effective, especially against genital herpes in women. It does not eradicate latent herpes. It is somewhat unpredictable as a topical prophylactic against recurrent infections by HSV-1 and HSV-2. Resistance of herpes simplex and cytomegaloviruses occurs and is a source of concern.

The most frequent adverse effect of systemic treatment is irritation at the site of injection (9%). The drug may crystallize in the urine, cause hematuria, and impair renal function if fluid intake is inadequate, glomerular filtration rate is low, the dosage interval is too short, or the drug is given as a bolus. Metabolic encephalopathy (1%) with hallucinations, confusion, tremors and seizures, bone-marrow depression, and alterations in hepatic function also may result from parenteral therapy. Untoward effects from oral administration are more frequent with long-term than with short-term therapy. In the short term, there may be nausea and vomiting (2.7%), headache (0.6%), diarrhea, dizziness, fatigue, skin rash, sore throat (all 0.3%), anorexia, edema, lymphadenopathy (especially inguinal), and leg pain. In the long term there may be headache (1.9%), diarrhea (2.4%), nausea and vomiting (2.7%), arthralgia, vertigo (both 3.6%), insomnia, fatigue, irritability, depression, rash, acne, alopecia, fever, palpitations, sore throat, muscle cramps,and lymphadenopathy. The drug is mutagenic and should be avoided in pregnancy, if possible. Topically, adverse effects occur in about 30% of recipients and consist of local stinging, burning or pain (28%), itching (4%), vulvitis (0.3%), and rash (0.3%).

In plasma, only 9% to 33% is protein-bound. Renal excretion after IV and oral use accounts for 62% to 91% and 9% to 20%, respectively. The half-life is about 2.5 hr but may be as long as 19.5 hr in renal failure.

ADEFOVIR DIPIVOXIL

Propanoic acid, 2,2-dimethyl-, [[[2-(6-amino-9*H***-purin-9-yl)-ethoxy]methyl]phosphinylidene]bis(oxymethylene) ester; Hepsera, Preveon**

[142340-99-6] $C_{20}H_{32}N_5O_8P$ (501.47).

Preparation—*J Med Chem* 1996; 39:4958 and US Pat 6,451,340 (2002).

Description—White to off-white crystals melting over 250°. Log P (phosphate buffer, pH 7) 1.91; pK_{a1} 2.0; pK_{a2} 6.8.

Solubility—In water; 19 mg/mL at pH 2.0 and 0.4 mg/mL at pH 7.2.

Comments—A nucleoride analougue used for the treatment of chronic hepatitis B, including patients with clinical evidence of lamivudine-resistant hepatitis B with either compensated or decompensated liver function. Most experts would recommend use in combination with lamivudine. Adverse reactions: Generally well tolerated. Occasional: Increase in creatinine (with underlying renal insufficiency); asthenia, abd pain; h/a; fever; n/v/d; exacerbation of hepatitis (with discontinuation of therapy); pruritus; rash; cough. Rare: nephrotoxicity, lactic acidosis.

AMANTIDINE HYDROCHLORIDE

Tricyclo[3.3.1.1^{3,7}]decan-1-amine, hydrochloride; Symmetrel, Symadine

1-Adamantanamine hydrochloride [665-66-7] $C_{10}H_{17}N \cdot HCl$ (187.71).

Preparation—Adamantane is halogenated, with chlorine or bromine in the presence of $AlCl_3$, at the bridgehead carbon atom to yield a reactive tertiary halide, incapable of dehydrohalogenation. Therefore, even with a weak base, such as CH_3CN, it undergoes an S_N1 reaction to the acetamido derivative. Hydrolysis affords the product, which is converted to the salt. *J Med Chem* 1963; 6:760.

Description—White crystals; decompose over 360°; pK_a 10.4, (amino group).

Solubility—1 g in 3 mL water or 5 mL alcohol.

Comments—A *narrow-spectrum antiviral* active against all influenzae A virus strains, some C virus strains, but not effective against B strains. It is approved for chemoprophylaxis and treatment of respiratory tract illness caused by influenzae A virus strains, when immunization is contraindicated or not feasible. It is indicated especially for high-risk patients because of underlying disease (eg, cardiovascular, pulmonary, metabolic, neuromuscular, or immunodeficiency disease), close-household or hospital-ward contacts of index cases, immunocompromised patients, and health-care and community-services personnel.

Amantidine is well tolerated by most patients, but CNS side effects are most common and include difficulty in thinking, confusion, lightheadedness, hallucinations, anxiety, and insomnia. These side effects are reversible upon discontinuation of the drug. More severe adverse effects such as mental depression and psychoses may occur with doses exceeding 200 mg daily. Less common side effects include anorexia, nausea, vomiting, and orthostatic hypotension. The peripheral and central effects of anticholinergic drugs are increased by concomitant use of amantidine.

Oral absorption is rapid and complete. It is not metabolized and 90% of the dose is excreted unchanged in the urine. The half-life is about 20 hr, and it reaches levels in the cerebral spinal fluid that are 60% of the plasma concentration. The dose must be reduced with renal insufficiency and in the elderly who have decreased renal function.

AMPRENAVIR

[3*S***-[3***R*****(1***R*****,2***S*****)]]-3-[[(4-Aminophenyl)sulfonyl](2-methyl-propyl)amino]-2-hydroxy-1-(phenylmethyl)propyl]tetrahydro-3-furanyl carbamate; Agenerase**

[161814-49-9] $C_{25}H_{35}N_3O_6S$ (505.63).

Preparation—US Pat 5,585,397 (1996).

Description—White to cream-colored solid.

Solubility—0.04 mg/mL in water at 25°; soluble in methanol, ethanol, chloroform, DMSO, acetonitrile, and methylene chloride; insoluble in hydrocarbon solvents.

Comments—A protease inhibitor used as part of combination therapy to treat HIV-infection. First once a day PI approved when used with ritonavir. Adverse reactions include: GI intolerance most common (N/V/D); oral paresthesias; headache; rash (in 11% of patients); lipodystrophy syndrome; hyperglycemia; increased triglycerides and/or cholesterol; transaminase elevation. TOXICITY FROM PROPYLENE GLYCOL IN THE ORAL SOLUTION. Co-administration contraindicated with: Terfenadine, astemizole, cisapride, ergot alkaloid, rifampin, bepridil, midazolam and triazolam. Dose modification needed with: Rifabutin, HMG-Coa reductase inhibitors, sildenafil,Dual-protease or NNRTI combination.

ATAZANAVIR SULFATE

2,5,6,10,13-Pentaazatetradecanedioic acid, (3*S***,8***S***,9***S***,12***S***)-3,12-(bis(1,1-dimethylethyl)-8-hydroxy-4,11-dioxo-9-(phenylmethyl)-6-[[4-(2-pyridinyl)phenyl]methyl]-, dimethyl ester, sulfate (1:1) salt; Reyataz**

[229975-97-7] $C_{38}H_{52}N_6O_7 \cdot H_2SO_4$ (802.94).

Preparation—US Pat 5,849,911(1998).

Description—White to pale yellow crystalline powder.

Solubility—Slightly soluble in water; pH of water-saturated solution about 2 at 25°.

Comments—A protease inhibitor used as part of combination therapy for the treatment of HIV-infection. A benefit in terms of lipid profile is consistently shown. This may offer a distinct advantage to patients with established CV disease risks, high lipid levels at baseline or high levels post-therapy with other PIs. Adverse reactions include: Common: Reversible benign hyperbilirubinemia (grade 3-4 occurring in 35-47% of patients), jaundice, and scleral icterus. Occasional: nausea, vomiting, abdominal pain, lipodystrophy, rash, h/a, and mild transaminase elevation (unrelated to UGT 1A1 inhibition). Contraindicated: Rifampin, irinotecan, ergot Alkaloid, cisapride, St. John's Wort, midazolam, triazolam, bepridil, pimozide, simvastatin, lovastatin, indinavir, and all proton pump-inhibitors.

CYTARABINE—page 1568.

CIDOFOVIR

Phosphonic acid, (*S*)-[[2-(4-amino-2-oxo-1(2*H*)-pyrimidin-yl)-1-(hydroxymethyl)ethoxy]methyl]-, dihydrate; Vistide

[149394-66-1] $C_8H_{14}N_3O_6P \cdot 2H_2O$ (315.22).

Preparation—From guanine; US Pat 5,142,051 (1992).

Description—White powder melting about 260°; log P (octanol/pH 7.1 buffer) −3.3.

Solubility—Approximately 170 mg/mL at pH 6–8.

Comments—A nucleic acid synthesis inhibitor (purine analog) used for cytomegalovirus (CMV). It causes nephrotoxicity.

DELAVIRDINE MESYLATE

Piperazine, 1-[3-[(1-methylethyl)amino]-2-pyridin-yl]-4-[[5-[(methylsulfonyl)amino-1*H*-indol-2-yl]carbonyl]-, monomethanesulfonate; Rescriptor

[147221-93-0] $C_{22}H_{28}N_6O_3S \cdot CH_4O_3S$ (552.68).

Preparation—US Pat 5,691,372 (1997); *J Med Chem* 1993; 36:1505.

Description—White to tan crystals melting about 227° (base).

Solubility—(Base) Approximately 2.9 µg/mL at pH 1, 295 µg/mL at pH 2 and 0.81 µg/mL at pH 7.4.

Comments—An HIV reverse transcriptase inhibitor (non-nucleoside). It causes rash.

DIDANOSINE

Inosine, 2′,3′-dideoxy-, ddL; Videx

[69655-05-6] $C_{10}H_{12}N_4O_3$ (236.23).

Preparation—*Nucleosides Nucleotides* 1988; 7:147.

Description—White solid; melts about 160° to 163°.

Comments—A nucleoside analog that is incorporated into retroviral DNA contributing to chain termination and inhibition of viral replication. The active metabolite, dideoxyadenosine triphosphate, is a reverse transcriptase inhibitor that is active against the human immunodeficiency virus (HIV) infected T cell and monocyte/macrophage cell cultures.

The approved indication is treatment of adult and pediatric patients with advanced HIV infection who have received prolonged prior *zidovudine* therapy or who have demonstrated intolerance or significant clinical or immunological deterioration during zidovudine therapy.

The major clinical toxicities of didanosine are pancreatitis (9%) and peripheral neuropathy (34%). Several other adverse effects are observed frequently including diarrhea (25%), asthenia (25%), insomnia (25%), nausea and vomiting (25%), rash/pruritus (24%), abdominal pain (21%), CNS depression (19%), constipation (16%), stomatitis (14%), myalgia (13%), arthritis (11%), taste loss/perversion (10%), pain (10%), dry mouth (9%), alopecia (8%), and dizziness (7%).

The average bioavailability of didanosine is reported to be 33% after a single dose. The elimination half-life is 1.6 hr and renal clearance is about 50%. There is no evidence of accumulation after either IV or oral dosing.

EFAVIRENZ

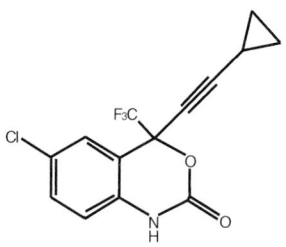

2*H*-3,1-Benzoxazin-2-one, (*S*)-6-chloro-4-(cyclopropylethynyl)-1,4-dihydro-4-(trifluoromethyl)-, Sustiva

[154598-52-4] $C_{14}H_9ClF_3NO_2$ (315.67).

Preparation—US Pat 5,519,021 (1996).

Description—White to slightly pink crystalline powder melting about 179°.

Solubility—Freely soluble in dilute HCl; practically insoluble in water; soluble 6.06 mg/mL in ethanol.

Comment—A non-nucleoside reverse transcriptase inhibitor used as part of combination therapy for the treatment of HIV-infection. Adverse events include: Morbilliform rash in (15-27% of patients with 1-2% requiring discontinuation); one case of Steven Johnson Syndrome reported; CNS effects (confusion, depersonalization, abnormal dreams) usually seen on day 1 (in up to 52% of patients); resolves in 2 to 4 weeks. Co-administration contraindicated with: Ergot alkaloid, midazolam, triazolam, terfenadine, astemizole, cisapride. Dose modification needed with: Saquinavir, amprenavir, indinavir, ethinyl estradiol, and rifabutin.

EMTRICITABINE

2-(1*H*)-Pyrimidinone,)2*R-cis*)-4-amino-5-fluoro-1-[2-(hydroxymethyl)-1,3oxathiolan-5-yl]-, Emtriva, Coviracil

[143491-57-0] $C_8H_{10}FN_3O_3S$ (247.24).

Preparation—A synthetic nucleoside of cytosine. *J Med Chem*, 1993; 36:181.

Description—White to off-white powder from methanol-ether melting about 138°.

Log P −0.43; pK_a 2.65; $[\alpha]_{25}^D$ -133.6° c = 0.23, methanol).

Solubility—112 mg/mL in water at 25°.

Comments—A once-daily nucleoside reverse transcriptase inhibitor used as part of combination therapt for the treatment of HIV-infection. Like lamivudine, possesses activity against the hepatitis-B virus. Adverse reactions include: Common: Generally well tolerated. Mild asymptomatic skin hyperpigmentation on the palm and/or soles. Asymptomatic and transient CPK elevation. Occasional: Headache, diarrhea, nausea, asthenia, and rash that required discontinuation in approx. 1% of patients. Emtricitabine is not a substrate, inhibitor, or inducer of any CYP450 isoforms, likelihood of clinically significant drug interactions are low.

ENFUVIRTIDE

Enfuvirtide; Fuzeon

[159519-65-0] $C_{204}H_{301}N_{51}O_{64}$ (4491.93).

Preparation—US Pat 6,333,395 (2001).

Description—White to off-white solid. A segment of the trans-membrane envelope glycoprotein (gp41) of human immunodeficiency virus, type (HIV-1).

Solubility—Practically insoluble in water. Solubility increases in buffered solutions; in pH 7.5 buffer, 0.85–1.42 g/mL.

Comments—The first "fusion inhibitor" used in combination for the treatment of HIV-infection. It is administered subcutaneously. It is most commonly used in patients who have been previously treated with a variety of other antiretroviral agents. A clear advantage of enfuvirtide is the lack of cross-resistance with currently available antiretrovirals, however, as with other antiretrovirals and as seen in clinical trials, salvage therapy with enfuvirtide is only as good as the background regimen with which it is combined. Adverse reactions include: Common ADR: local site reaction (grade 3 or 4) including pain (9%), erythema (32%), pruritus (4%), induration (57%), and nodules or cysts (26%)(with 3% requiring d/c).Occ: Eosinophilia; Bacterial pneumonia (in 4.68 events vs. 0.61 events per 100 pts-years.

FAMCICLOVIR

1,3-Propanediol, 2-[2-(2-amino-9H-purin-9-yl)ethyl]-, diacetate (ester); Famvir

[104227-87-4] $C_{14}H_{19}N_5O_4$ (321.34).

Preparation—One method involves first the formation of 5-(2-hydroxy- ethyl)-2,2-dimethyl-1,3-dioxolane(**I**) by the reaction of tri-ethylethane-1,1,2-tricarboxylate with THF and lithium aluminum hydride to form an oil which reacts with 2,2-dimethoxypropane in the presence of *p*-toluenesulfonic acid to yield **I**. The OH group is replaced by bromine using CBr$_4$ and trimethyl phosphine. The bromo derivative is combined with 2-amino-6-chloropurine to alkylate in the 7-position. The dioxalane ring is opened by warming with dilute HCl and the resulting diol esterified with acetic anhydride using 4-(dimethylamino)pyridine as the acid scavenger. US Pat 5,075,445 (1991); *J Med Chem* 1989; 32:1738.

Description—White to pale yellow platelets melting about 103° Non-hygroscopic below 80% relative humidity. Partition coefficient; octanol/water(pH 4) P = 1.09; octanol/pH 7.4 phosphate buffer P = 2.08.

Solubility—In water at 25° it initially is freely soluble (up to 25%) but forms a sparingly soluble monohydrate (about 3% soluble) which precipitates. Freely soluble in methanol or acetone; sparingly soluble in alcohol or 2-propanol.

Comments—An purine analog which is an inhibitor of nucleic acid synthesis; a prodrug of *penciclovir*.

FOSCARNET SODIUM

Phosphinecarboxylic acid, dihydroxy-, oxide, trisodium salt; Foscavir

Phosphonoformic acid, trisodium salt [63585-09-1] CNa_3O_5P (191.95).

Preparation—*Ber* 1924; 57B:1023.

Description—White crystals (usually as the hexahydrate); melts above 250°; pK$_a$ 7.27, 3.41, 0.49.

Solubility—Soluble in water; insoluble in alcohol.

Comments—An antiviral agent that acts at the pyrophosphate-binding site and inhibits viral DNA polymerases and reverse transcriptases at concentrations that do not affect cellular DNA polymerases. It does not require activation (phosphorylation) by a kinase. All known *herpes* viruses are inhibited in vitro including cytomegalovirus (CMV), *herpes simplex* 1 and 2 (HSV-1, HSV-2), human *herpes* virus 6 (HHV-6), *Epstein-Barr* virus (EBV) and *varicella zoster* virus (VZV). The only approved indication is the treatment of CMV retinitis in patients with AIDS.

The major toxicity is renal impairment that occurs in 33% of all patients, so everyone receiving it should be monitored for renal function. The other frequent adverse reactions include fever (65%), nausea (47%), anemia (33%), diarrhea (30%), vomiting or headache (26%), and seizures (10%). Electrolyte abnormalities must be monitored because of the propensity of foscarnet to chelate divalent cations. The drug is only administered by controlled IV infusion to decrease the incidence of toxicity as a result of excessive plasma levels.

Approximately 80% to 90% of IV foscarnet is excreted unchanged in the urine. Plasma half-life of foscarnet increases as renal function is impaired, but initial half-lives of 2 to 8 hr have been reported for patients with normal renal function. The safety and efficacy of foscarnet in children has not been studied because it is deposited in teeth and bone, and deposition is greater in young and growing animals. Development of tooth enamel is adversely affected in studies of animals.

FOMIVIRSEN SODIUM

Deoxyribonucleic acid, d(P-thio)G-C-G-T-T-T-G-C-T-C-T-T-C-T-T-C-T-T-G-C-G), eicosasodium salt; Vitravene

[160369-77-7] $C_{204}H_{243}N_{63}O_{114}P_{20}S_{20}$ (7122.04).

Preparation—One method involves a recombinant M 13 phage containing a negative stranded viral DNA or recombinant DNA vector containing the double-stranded viral DNA which may be produced by growing *E coli* harboring these vectors. Vectors containing the viral genes are isolated and subjected to restriction endonuclease for excision of the viral genes. The viral gene and vector DNA mixture is separated by chromatography. The DNA molecules so obtained are shortened by partial digestion or ultrasonics. The chain length of the viral DNA fragments are adjusted to between 9 and 100 nucleotides using gel electrophoresis or sephadex chromatography. The double-stranded DNA is then converted to isolate the negative strand using affinity chromatography.

Description—White to off-white hygroscopic, amorphous, powder. The IV preparation has an osmolality of 290 mOsm/L at pH 8.7.

Comments—An antisense phosphorothioate oligonucleotide inhibits CMV by binding to complementary sequences on messenger RNA transcribed from the major immediate-early transcriptional unit of the virus. Used as an intraveitreal injection for the treatment of cytomegalovirus retinitis.Active against strains of CMV that are resistant to ganciclovir, cidofovir, and foscarnet. Adverse reactions include: Ocular inflamation (iritis and vitritis) in 15% to 25%-usually respond to topical steroid. Increased intraocular pressure-transient (19%), but should be monitored.

FOSAMPRENAVIR CALCIUM

Carbamic acid, [(1S,2R)-3-[[(4-aminophenyl)sulfonyl](2-methyl-propyl)amino]-1-(phenylmethyl)-2-(phosphonooxy)propyl]-, C-[(3S)-tetrahydro-3-furanyl] ester, monocalcium salt; Lexiva

[226700-80-7] $C_{25}H_{34}CaN_3O_9PS$ (623.67).

Preparation—*J Med Chem* 2003; 46:4124.

Description—White to cream-colored solid. A prodrug of amprenavir to which it is converted in vivo by cellular phosphatases.

Solubility—About 0.31 mg/mL in water at 25°.

Comments—Fosamprenavir is a prodrug of amprenavir developed to overcome the high (16) pill burden associated with amprenavir. Adverse reactions include: Common: Rash 12% to 33% (severe in <1%). Severe GI intolerance in up to 5% to 10%. Occasional: Elevated triglyceride(less common without RTV) and LDL, insulin resistance, hepatitis. Do not co-administer: Ergot Alkaloid, Midazolam, Triazolam, Terfenadine, Astemizole, Cisapride, Pimozide, Flecainide, propafenone.

FLUOROURACIL

For the full monograph, see page 1573.

Comments—A *nucleic acid synthesis inhibitor* (pyrimidine analog) used topically for warts.

GANCICLOVIR SODIUM

6*H*-Purin-6-one, 2-amino-1,9-dihydro-9-[[2-hydroxyl-1-(hydroxymethyl)ethoxy]methyl]-, Cytovene

9-[[2-Hydroxyl-1-(hydroxymethyl)ethoxy]methyl]guanine [82410-32-0] $C_9H_{13}N_5O_4$ (255.23).

Preparation—US Pat 4,355,032; *J Med Chem* 1983; 26:759.

Description—White powder.

Solubility—1 g in 250 mL water.

Comments—An antiviral drug active against cytomegalovirus (CMV), *herpes simplex* virus-1 and -2 (HSV-1, HSV-2), *Epstein-Barr* virus and *viricella zoster* virus. It is approved for treatment of CMV retinitis in immunocompromised patients, including those with AIDS and prevention of CMV disease in transplant patients at risk for CMV disease. Upon entry into host cells, CMV induce kinases that phosphorylate ganciclovir to its active triphosphate form that is believed to inhibit viral DNA synthesis by competitive inhibition of viral DNA, resulting in termination of viral DNA elongation.

The major clinical toxicities of ganciclovir include granulocytopenia (40%) and thrombocytopenia (20%). In animal studies it is carcinogenic, teratogenic, and causes aspermatogenesis. Other adverse effects that have led to its withdrawal or interrupted its use in clinical trials are headache (17%), confusion (6%), abnormal thoughts or dreams, ataxia, dizziness, nervousness, parasthesia, psychosis, somnolence, tremor, arrhythmia, hypertension, rash, pruritus, alopecia, urticaria, nausea, vomiting, anorexia, diarrhea, abdominal pain, sepsis, fever, chills, edema, malaise, and dyspnea. Retinal detachment has occurred before and after initial treatment of CMV retinitis, so ophthalmological evaluations are advised. Renal toxicity may occur in heart allograft recipients, so renal function should be monitored during therapy.

Ganciclovir is given by IV infusion. Phlebitis and pain at the site of injection occur. The high pH (11) of solution may result in severe tissue irritation if given SC or IM. It is eliminated unmetabolized by renal excretion that accounts for 90% of the administered dose. The plasma half-life with normal renal function is about 3 hr but is increased to more than 10 hr with severe renal impairment. There is limited evidence to suggest that ganciclovir crosses the blood-brain barrier in adequate concentrations.

IDOXURIDINE

Uridine, 2′-deoxy-5-iodo-, IDU; Herplex; Stoxil

2′-Deoxy-5-iodouridine [54-42-2] $C_9H_{11}IN_2O_5$ (354.10).

Preparation—By refluxing a solution of deoxyuridine in aqueous mineral acid in the presence of iodine. Brit Pat 1,024,156. For the preparation of deoxyuridine, see *J Chem Soc* 1958:3035.

Description—White, crystalline powder; practically odorless; turns black 171°; pH (0.1% aqueous solution) about 6; a 0.1% solution in distilled water and preserved with 1:50,000 thimerosal is stable at room temperature for over a year; pKa 8.25.

Solubility—Slightly soluble in water or alcohol; practically insoluble in chloroform or ether; 1g in 2.5 mL DMSO.

Comments—A *nucleic acid synthesis inhibitor* (pyrimidine analog) used topically for herpes simplex.

INDINAVIR SULFATE

D-*erythro*-Pentanamide, [1(1*S*,2*R*,5(*S*)]-2,3,5-trideoxy-*N*-(2,3-dihydro-2-hydroxy-1*H*-inden-1-yl)-5-[2-[[(1,1-dimethylethyl)amino]carbonyl]-4-(3-pyridinylmethyl)-1-piperazinyl]-2-(phenylmethyl)-, sulfate(1:1 salt), monohydrate; Crixivan

[157810-81-6] $C_{36}H_{47}N_5O_4 \cdot H_2SO_4$ (711.88).

Preparation—US Pat 5,413,999 (1995).

Description—White to off-white hygroscopic powder; (as the monoethanolate) melts at 152°(dec). Loses ethanol on exposure to moist air and forms the hydrate.

Solubility—Very soluble in water or methanol.

Comments—A synthetic peptide analog that is a specific inhibitor of HIV-1 and -2 proteases that are essential enzymes for production of mature infectious virions. It has excellent oral bioavailability but must be consumed on an empty stomach. Resistance is mediated by expression of multiple and variable protease amino acid substitutions. Cross-resistance commonly occurs for indinavir, saquinavir, and ritonavir. Combination therapy with nucleoside reverse transcriptase inhibitors is used to decrease resistance. Adequate water consumption is important to prevent kidney stones (nephrolithiasis). Other side effects include thrombocytopenia, nausea, vomiting, diarrhea, hemolytic anemia, hepatitis, and irritability. Inhibition of cytochrome P450 enzymes (notably CYP3A4) results in numerous drug interactions. Increased serum levels of antihistamines, cispride, benzodiazepines, and riftabutin occur because they are metabolized by CYP3A4 and results in an increase in their potential toxicity. Serum levels of indinavir may be increased by antifungal azoles and decreased by riftabutin and rifampin.

INTERFERONS—see also Chapter 29.

INTERFERON ALFA

(available as 2a, 2b or 2c)

Comments—This glycopeptide is produced by genetic engineering techniques based on the human sequence. It affects many stages of viral infections but primarily inhibits viral protein translation. It is used for therapy of hepatitis B and C. The drug is administered by SC or IM injection. It is rapidly inactivated, but the effects outlast the plasma concentration. Toxicities include flu-like syndrome, bone marrow suppression, and neurotoxicity. Drug interactions can result from its ability to reduce hepatic cytochrome P450-mediated metabolism.

LAMIVUDINE

2(1*H*)-Pyrimidinone, (2*R-cis*)-4-amino-1-[2-(hydroxy-methyl)-1,3-oxathiolan-5-yl]-, Epivir; 3TC

[134678-17-4] $C_8H_{11}N_3O_3S$ (229.26).

Preparation—*J Org Chem* 1992; 55:2217.

Description—White to off-white powder melting about 161°.

Solubility—About 70 mg/mL in water at 20°.

Comments—An HIV reverse transcriptase inhibitor (pyrimidine nucleoside) which is well tolerated.

LOPINAVIR

1(2H)-Pyrimidineacetamide, [1S-[1R*(R*),3R*,4R*]]-N-[4-[[2,6-dimethylphenoxy)acetyl]amino]-3-hydroxy-5-phenyl-1-(phenylmethyl)pentyl]tetrahydro-α-(1-methylethyl)-2-oxo-, Ing of Kaletra (in combination with *Ritonavir*).

[192725-17-0] $C_{37}H_{48}N_4O_5$ (628.81).

Preparation—US Pat 5,914,332 (1999).

Description—White to light tan powder from ethyl acetate; melts about 126°.

Solubility—Freely soluble in methanol and ethanol; soluble in 2-propanol; practically insoluble in water.

Comments—A protease inhibitor that is formulated as a combination product along with ritonavir. Very potent and currently among the first-line treatment options for HIV-infection. Adverse reactions include: Frequent: Diarrhea in 13.8% to 23.8% of patients. Occasional: Nausea, vomiting, abdominal pain, asthenia, headache, and rash have also been reported. Like other protease inhibitors, class adverse events such as hyperlipidemia, fat redistribution, and hyperglycemia. Contraindicated: Flecainide, propafenone, astemizole, terfenadine, dihydroergotamine, ergonovine, ergotamine, methylergonovine, cisapride, pimozide, midazolam, triazolam, Rifampin, hypericum perforatum (St John's wort), lovastatin, and simvastatin.

NEVIRAPINE

6H-Dipyrido[3,2-b:2',3'-e][1,4]diazepin-6-one, 11-cyclopropyl-5,11-dihydro-4-methyl-, Viramune

[129618-40-2] $C_{15}H_{14}N_4O$ (266.30).

Preparation—US Pat 5,075,455 (1991); *J Med Chem* 1991; 34:2331.

Description—White crystals melting about 248°; pK < 3.

Solubility—Slightly soluble in water at pH7; very soluble at pH < 3.

Comments—An HIV reverse transcriptase inhibitor (pyrimidine nucleoside). It causes rash fever, nausea and headache.

OSELTAMIVIR PHOSPHATE

1-Cyclohexene-1-carboxylic acid, [3R-(3α,4β,5α)]-4-(acetyl- amino)-5-amino-3-(1-ethylpropoxy)-, ethyl ester, phosphate salt (1:1); Tamiflu

[204255-11-8] $C_{16}H_{28}N_2O_4 \cdot H_3PO_4$ (410.40).

Preparation—A multi-step synthesis beginning with either (-)shikimic acid or (−)quinic acid. Shikimic acid is obtained from star anise by fermentation using genetically engineered *E coli*. Quinic acid is derived from cinchona bark. US Pat 5,763,483(1998); *J Org Chem* 1981; 46:2381 and *Albany Molecular Research Tech Reports* 2000; 4(39):7-9.

Description—White, crystalline solid. Oseltamivir is a pro-drug requiring the hydrolysis of the ethyl ester to form the free acid, which is the active principle.$pK_a = 7.7$ (base).

Comments—An oral neuramidase inhibitor that is active against influenza A and B. Treatment must be started within 48 hours of the onset of symptoms. Adverse reactions include nausea, vomiting, diarrhea.

PEGINTERFERON ALFA-2A

Interferon αA (human leucocyte), mono(N^2, N^6-dicarboxyl-L-lysyl) derivative, diester with α-methyl-ω-hydroxypoly(oxy-1,2-ethanediyl)-, Pegasys

[198153-51-4]

Preparation—By pegylation of the interferon with polyethylene glycol (PEG). Many protein drugs suffer rapid enzyme degradation and clearance from the body. The optimal mass of a PEG required to retard renal and cellular clearance of protein molecules is estimated to be between 40 and 60 kDa. Pegylation of IFN alfa-2a has optimized pharmacological activity and minimized adverse effects. *J Adv Drug Deliv Rev*, 2002; 54: 571 and http://www.americanpeptide.com/corp/PEGylation.pdf

PEGASYS, peginterferon alfa-2a, is a covalent conjugate of recombinant alfa-2a interferon (approximate molecular weight [MW] 20,000 daltons) with a single branched bis-monomethoxy polyethylene glycol (PEG) chain (approximate MW 40,000 daltons). The PEG moiety is linked at a single site to the interferon alfa moiety via a stable amide bond to lysine. Peginterferon alfa-2a has an approximate molecular weight of 60,000 daltons. Interferon alfa-2a is produced using recombinant DNA technology in which a cloned human leukocyte interferon gene is inserted into and expressed in *Escherichia coli*.

Solubility—The drug product contains approximately 1.3 mL of solution containing 180 μg of drug..

Comments—Pegylated formulation of interferon alpha-2a or 2-b. Results in improved pharmacokinetic profile offering patients a once-weekly dosing schedule with greater efficacy, less side effects, and better patient adherence. Used as monotherapy or combination therapy (most commonly) for the treatment of chronic hepatitis C vius infection. Adverse reactions include: Common: Flu-like symptoms, headache, dizziness, fatigue, fever, rigor, injection site inflamation, depression (29%), insomnia, alopecia, GI (abdominal pain, anorexia, n/v/d). Occasional: thrombocytopenia, neutropenia, hypo- and hyperthyroidism, LFTs elevation.

PENCICLOVIR

6H-Purin-6-one, 2-amino-1,9-dihydro-9-[4-hydroxy-3-(hydroxy-methyl)butyl]-, Denavir

[39809-25-1] $C_{10}H_{15}N_5O_3$ (253.25).

Preparation—US Pat 5,075,445 (1991); *J Med Chem* 1987; 30:1636.

Description—White to pale yellow non-hygroscopic crystals melting at approximately 275° (monohydrate); log P (octanol/water, pH 7.5) 1.62.

Solubility—Approximately 1.7 mg/mL in water at 20°; 0.2 mg/mL in methanol; 1.3 mg/mL in propylene glycol; or 10mg/ml in pH 2 buffer.

Comments—A nucleic acid synthesis inhibitor (purine analog) similar to *acyclovir* and used topically for *herpes*.

RIBAVIRIN

1*H*-1,2,4-Triazole-3-carboxamide, 1-β-D-ribofuranosyl-, Virazole

Tribavirin; [36791-04-5] $C_8H_{12}N_4O_5$ (244.21).

Preparation—*J Med Chem* 1972; 15:1150.

Description—Colorless, crystalline powder existing in two polymorphic forms: melts about 167° (from aqueous ethanol) and melts about 175° (from ethanol).

Solubility—142 mg/mL in water at 25°; slightly soluble in alcohol.

Comments—A nucleoside analog with significant activity against influenza B, respiratory syncytial virus (RSV), and herpes simplex virus. It also has lesser activity against a wide variety of other viruses, such as those of herpes, varicella, Lassa fever, infectious hepatitis, dengue fever, measles, and AIDS. It is converted to metabolites that inhibit the 5′ capping of viral mRNA, so that ultimately viral protein synthesis of both DNA and RNA viruses are affected. It is approved for use only in the treatment of severe upper respiratory infections caused by RSV in infants and children. If the duration of the infection is judged to be less than that of a full course of treatment, the drug is contraindicated. It has been used successfully as an aerosol in the treatment of influenza A and B. Varying success has been achieved against infectious hepatitis, measles, Lassa fever, and Asian hemorrhagic fever.

IV or oral doses of more than 1 g a day suppress erythropoiesis, characterized mostly by normocytic anemia and reticulocytosis. The effect is reversible. There is also occasional hypotension, cardiac arrest, or digitalis intoxication. Adverse effects of the inhalation aerosol include occasional rash and conjunctivitis. In chronic obstructive pulmonary disease, pulmonary function often deteriorates. It antagonizes the effect of zidovudine on human immunodeficiency virus replication. It is contraindicated in pregnancy and during breast-feeding.

Systemic absorption occurs after aerosol administration, but bioavailability is unknown. It is highly accumulated in erythrocytes but is not bound to plasma proteins. In the cells, the drug is degraded by deribosylation and amide hydrolysis and the product is mono-, di-, and triphosphorylated.

The triphosphate is thought to be the active metabolite. It is formed more in lung and liver than in other tissues, hence the drug is most effective against infections in these organs. It does not pass the blood-brain barrier. Drug and known metabolites are excreted in the urine (50%) and feces (15%). The plasma half-life is 9.5 hr, while the half-life in erythrocytes is about 40 days.

RIMANTADINE HYDROCHLORIDE

Tricyclo[3.3.1³,⁷]decane-1-methaneamine-, α-methyl-, hydrochloride; Flumadine

[1501-84-4] $C_{12}H_{21}N \cdot HCl$ (215.77).

Preparation—From 1-bromoadamantane by addition of vinyl bromide, using $AlCl_3$ catalyst, to yield the 1-(2,2-dibromoethyl) derivative which undergoes classical dehydrohalogenation by heating with alkali to form the corresponding acetylene. The ketone is formed from the triple bond using mercury-catalyzed hydration with aqueous sulfuric acid. The carbonyl group is converted to the oxime which is the reduced with $LiAlH_4$ to form the product. US Pat 3,352,912 (1967).

Description—White to off-white crystals melting about 376° (sealed tube).

Solubility—Freely soluble in water (50 mg/mL at 20°).

Comments—An inhibitor of influenza viral penetration or *uncoating*. When metabolized it exhibits toxicity similar to *amantidine*.

NELFINAVIR MESYLATE

3-Isoquinolinecarboxamide, [3*S*-[2(2*S,3*S**),3α,4aβ,8aβ]]-*N*-(1,1-dimethylethyl)decahydro-2-[2-hydroxy-3-[(3-hydroxy-2-methylbenzoyl)amino]-4-(phenylthio)butyl]-, monomethanesulfonate (salt); Viracept**

[159989-65-8] $C_{32}H_{45}N_3O_4S \cdot CH_4O_3S$ (663.91).

Preparation—*Drugs of the Future* 1997; 22:371–377.

Description—White to off-white amorphous powder.

Solubility—Slightly soluble in water at pH ≥ 4; freely soluble in methanol, ethanol, isopropyl alcohol, or propylene glycol.

Comments—Similar to other peptide analogs that inhibit HIV-1 specific cleaving enzyme. It is used in combination with reverse transcriptase inhibitors to prevent resistance. Resistance to other protease inhibitors may not lead to cross-resistance with nelfinavir. Oral absorption is moderate and may be increased if drug is taken with a meal. It is similar in its adverse effects and drug interactions due to inhibition of CYP3A enzymes. The most common side effect is diarrhea.

RITONAVIR

2,4,7,12-Tetraazatridecan-13-oic acid, [5*S*-(5*R,8*R**,10*R**,11*R**)]-10-hydroxy-2-methyl-5-(1-methylethyl)-1-[2-(1-methylethyl)-4-thiazolyl]-3,6-dioxo-8,11-bis(phenylmethyl)-5-thiazolylmethyl ester; Norvir, Ing of Kaletra**

[155213-67-5] $C_{37}H_{48}N_6O_5S_2$ (720.96).

Preparation—PCT Int Pat Appl 94 14,436(1994); *Drugs of the Future* 1996; 21:700-705.

Description—White to light tan powder with a bitter metallic taste.

Solubility—Freely soluble in methanol or ethanol; soluble in isopropyl alcohol; practically insoluble in water.

Comments—A synthetic peptide analog and inhibitor of HIV-1 and -2 proteases. It has high oral bioavailability (60–80%) and is taken with meals. Used as part of combination therapy to treat HIV-infection. Most commonly used to increase the serum levels of other antiretroviral agents due to its ability to potently inhibit cytochrome P450 enzymes. Commercially available alone or in a combination product along with lopinavir. Adverse reactions include: Severe GI intolerance (N/V/D; abdominal pain, common with 600 mg bid dosing); taste perversion; asthenia; circumoral and peripheral paresthesias; lipodystrophy syndrome; hyperglycemia; increased triglycerides and/or cholesterol; transaminase elevation. Co-administration contraindicated with: Terfenadine, astemizole, cisapride, ergot alkaloid, midazolam, triazolam, propafenone, quinidine, flecainide, amiodarone, bepridil, pimozide, simvastatin, lovastatin.

SAQUINAVIR MESYLATE

Butanediamide, [3*S*-[2(1*R(*R**),2*S**),3α,4aβ,8aβ]]-*N*¹-[3-[3-[[(1,1-dimethylethyl)amino]carbonyl]octahydro-2(1*H*)-isoquinolinyl]-2-hydroxy-1-(phenylmethyl)propyl]-2-[(2-quinolinylcarbonyl)amino]-, monomethanesulfonate; Invirase**

[127779-20-8] $C_{38}H_{50}N_6O_5 \cdot CH_4O_3S$ (766.96).

Preparation—US Pat 5,196,438 (1993); *J Org Chem* 1994; 59:3656.
Description—White to off-white fine powder.
Solubility—Water; 2.22 mg/mL at 25°.
Comments—A synthetic peptide analog and inhibitor of HIV-1 and -2 proteases. It is used in combination with reverse transcriptase inhibitors, but is has less cross-resistance with other protease inhibitors. It has poor oral bioavailability (4%) and should be taken within 2 hr of a full meal for enhanced absorption. Adverse effects include GI disturbances and rhinitis. Potential drug interactions occur with drugs metabolized by CYP3A4.

STAVUDINE

Thymidine, 2′,3′-didehydro-3′-deoxy-, Zerit; d4t

[3056-17-5] $C_{10}H_{12}N_2O_4$ (224.22).
Preparation—US Pat 5,130,421 (1992).
Description—White to off-white crystals melting about 166° (174°). Octanol-water partition coefficient 0.144 at 23°.
Solubility—At 23°; water, 83 mg/mL, propylene glycol 30 mg/mL.
Comments—An HIV reverse transcriptase inhibitor (pyrimidine nucleoside). It causes peripheral neuropathy.

SURAMIN—see RPS-19, page 1326.

TENOFOVIR DISOPROXIL FUMARATE

2,4,6,8-Tetraoxa-5-phosphanonanedioic acid, (*R*)-5-[[2-(6-amino-9*H*-purin-9-yl)-1-methylethoxy]methyl]-, bis(1-methylethyl) ester, 5-oxide, (*E*)-2-butenedioate (1:1); Viread

[202138-50-9] $C_{19}H_{30}N_5O_{10}P·C_4H_4O_4$ (635.51).
Preparation—One method involves a 9 step synthesis beginning with D- (+)-isobutyl lactate. *Tetrahedron Lett* 1998; 39:1853 and US Pat 5,922,695 (1999).
Description—White to off white crystalline powder. Log P, 1.25 (pH 6.5 phosphate buffer at 25°).
Solubility—13.4 mg/mL, water at 25°.
Comments—A nucleotide analog used as part of combination therapy for the treatment of HIV-infection. Advantages includes: once daily administration, good side effect profile, active against hep B, active against strains that are often resistant to nucleosides. Adverse reactions include: Nausea and vomiting. Asymptomatic elevation of CPK and transaminase levels in 10% [AAC 2001;45:2733]. Neutropenia in 7% and increased amylase in 6%.

TRIFLURIDINE

Thymidine, α,α,α-trifluoro-, Viroptic

2′-Deoxy-5-(trifluoromethyl)uridine [70-00-8] $C_{10}H_{11}F_3N_2O_5$ (296.20).

Preparation—*J Am Chem Soc* 1962; 84:3597.
Description—White crystals; melts about 188°.
Comments—A *nucleic acid synthesis inhibitor* (pyrimidine analog) used topically for herpes simplex.

VALACYCLOVIR HYDROCHLORIDE

L -Valine, 2-[(2-amino-1,6-dihydro-6-oxo-9*H*-purin-9-yl)-methoxy]ethyl ester, monohydrochloride; Valtrex

[124832-27-5] $C_{13}H_{20}N_6O_4·HCl$ (360.80).
Preparation—US Pat 4,957,924 (1990).
Description—White to off-white crystals, pK_{a1} 1.90, pK_{a2} 7.47, pK_{a3} 9.43.
Solubility—174 mg/mL in water at 25°.
Comments—A nucleic acid synthesis inhibitor (purine analog). A prodrug of *acyclovir* but with better oral absorption.

VALGANCICLOVIR HYDROCHLORIDE

L-Valine, ester with 9-[[2-hydroxy-1-(hydroxymethyl)ethoxy]-methyl]guanine, monohydrochloride; Valcyte

[175865-59-5] $C_{14}H_{22}N_6O_5·HCl$ (390.82).
Preparation—*Org Biomol Chem*, 2004, 2(8):1164.
Description—The L-valyl ester (prodrug) of *ganciclovir* (page XXXX). White to off-white crystalline powder. Melting about 175°. Log P 0.009 (1-octanol/pH 6.9 buffer); pKa 7.6.
Solubility—10.4 mg/mL (95% ethanol); 30 mg/mL (acetone).
Comments—The valine-prodrug of ganciclovir. Has a 10-fold improvement in absorption over oral ganciclovir. The AUC of oral valganciclovir 900 mg is comparable to 5 mg/kg IV ganciclovir. Oral valganciclovir is equivalent to IV ganciclovir for the treatment of CMV retinitis in HIV-positive patients. Adverse reactions include: Frequent: diarrhea, nausea, vomiting, neutropenia and anemia (comparable to IV ganciclovir). Occasional: thrombocytopenia, headache, fever, rash, confusion, abnormal LFTs. Contraindicated if ANC<500/mm3, Plt <25,000/ml or hemoglobin <8g/dl. Myelosuppressive drugs (ie, zidovudine)-increased risk of hematologic toxicity. Didanosine- potential increase in didanosine serum level. Probenecid-potential increase in ganciclovir serum level (monitor for ganciclovir toxicity).

ZALCITABINE

Cytidine, 2′,3′-dideoxy-, ddC, Hivid

[7481-89-2] $C_9H_{13}N_3O_3$ (211.22).
Preparation—*Chem Pharm Bull* 1974; 22:128.
Description—White crystals; melts about 216°.
Comments—Antiviral activity against human immunodeficiency virus (HIV) is mediated by its conversion within infected cells to the active nucleoside triphosphate metabolite that inhibits HIV reverse transcriptase and viral DNA synthesis. It is approved for combination therapy with *zidovudine* in advanced HIV infection (CD4 cell

count\H300/mm³) who have demonstrated significant clinical or immunological deterioration.

The major clinical toxicities of *zalcitabine* are peripheral neuropathy (17–31%) and pancreatitis (<1%). It may exacerbate hepatic dysfunction and a greater risk of toxicity may occur in patients with renal impairment. Infrequent cases of esophageal ulcers have been attributed to zalcitabine therapy. Other adverse effects include oral ulcers, nausea, dysphagia, anorexia, abdominal pain, vomiting, diarrhea, rash, pruritus, headache, dizziness, myalgia, arthralgia, fatigue, pharyngitis, fever, rigors, chest pain, and weight decrease. The mean oral bioavailability is >80%, but food decreases the extent and rate of absorption. Renal excretion is the major route of excretion with little if any degree of hepatic metabolism. The half-life is 1 to 3 hr, but impaired renal function prolongs elimination.

ZANAMIVIR

D-*Glycero*-D-*galacto*-Non-2-enonic acid, 5-(acetylamino)-4-[(aminoiminomethyl)amino]-2,6-anhydro-3,4,5-trideoxy-, Relenza

[139110-80-8] $C_{12}H_{20}N_4O_7$ (332.32).

Preparation—From (-)shikimic or (-)quinic acid; *J Am Chem Soc* 1997; 119:681.

Description—White to off white powder; $[\alpha]^{20}_D$ + 40.9° (c = 0.9, water)

Solubility—18 mg/mL in water at 20°.

Comments—An aerosolized neuramidase inhibitor anti-infuenza agent with activity against influenza A and B. Effective for treatment only if treatment is started within 48 hours of onset of symptoms. Adverse reactions include: Occasional: bronchospasm (caution in patients with COPD or asthma); cough. Rare: headache; diarrhea; nausea; vomiting; dizziness; increase in liver enzyme and CPK; lymphopenia and neutropenia.

ZIDOVUDINE

Thymidine, 3′-azido-3′-deoxy-, AZT; Retrovir

Azidothymidine; [30516-87-1] $C_{10}H_{13}N_5O_4$ (267.24).

Preparation—*Tetrahedron Letters* 1988; 29:5349.

Description—White needles; from petroleum ether melts about 110°; from water, melts about 121°; pK_a 9.68.

Solubility—1 g in 40 mL water or 15 mL alcohol.

Comments—Incorporated into retroviral DNA by reverse-transcriptase to make a nonsense sequence that terminates DNA chain synthesis. The reverse-transcriptase is 100 times more susceptible to the drug than mammalian DNA polymerase. It has activity against human immunodeficiency virus; consequently, it is used for the treatment of AIDS and AIDS-related complex (ARC). It increases the survival and improves the quality of life of patients with complications, such as severe weight loss, fever, pneumocystosis, herpes zoster, herpes or thrush. Because it crosses the blood-brain barrier, it has a favorable effect on the neurological symptoms of AIDS. During prolonged therapy resistance may occur.

It causes severe anemia from bone-marrow depression in patients with AIDS; 25% of infected persons without AIDS develop anemia. It causes granulocytopenia and/or thrombocytopenia in about 5% of AIDS patients. However, it may increase platelet count if the count is depressed as the result of the disease. Nausea (46%), headaches (42%), GI pain (20%), rash (17%), fever (16%), diarrhea (12%), anorexia (11%), myalgia (8%), somnolence (8%), malaise (8%), vomiting, dizziness, paresthesias (each 6%), insomnia, dyspnea, sweating (all 5%), and macrocytosis occur. Polymyositis sometimes occurs. It is weakly mutagenic and should be withheld in pregnancy, if possible. In vitro antagonism of AZT inhibition of HIV-1 by ribovarin has been demonstrated, so those agents should not be used simultaneously. Drugs that inhibit hepatic glucuronidation, such as acetaminophen, aspirin, indomethacin, probenecid, pyrimethamine, and trimethoprim decrease elimination and increase toxicity.

Oral bioavailability is 52% to 75%. CSF levels are nearly the same as in plasma. The drug is metabolized rapidly in liver with a half-life of 0.8 to 1.9 hr. Only 14% of intact drug is eliminated in urine.

CHAPTER 91

Enzymes

Michael R Franklin, PhD

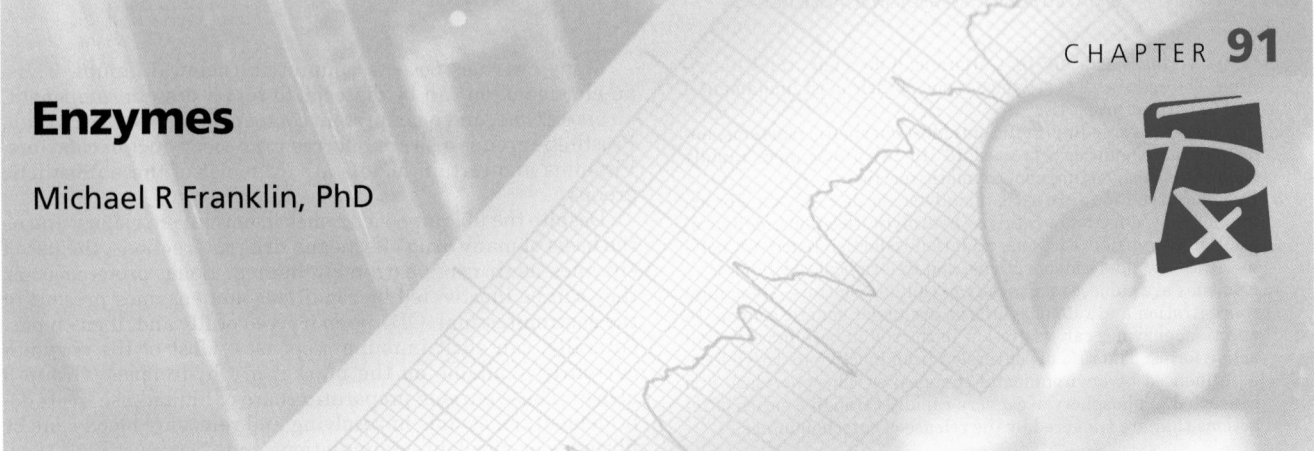

The functions of all living organisms depend on chemical reactions. For example, conversion of sugar to carbon dioxide and water with the release of energy proceeds through a series of chemical reactions, each of which requires a biological catalyst for the reaction to occur. Enzymes are proteins that serve as biological catalysts. Without these enzymes conditions for reaction would be required that would be incompatible with the life of the cell. Thus, enzymes play a vital role in the function of the normal cell.

The importance of enzymes in normal body function is illustrated dramatically in conditions when an enzyme is nonfunctional as a result of a disease state or a congenital abnormality. Patients with these *inborn errors of metabolism* are strikingly abnormal. Phenylketonuric infants who are born without the enzyme phenylalanine hydroxylase (which is responsible for the conversion of phenylalanine to tyrosine) develop motor disturbances; light coloration of the skin, hair, and eyes; and in early childhood (if not in infancy), remain mentally retarded.

Since most chemical reactions in the body require the action of an enzyme, these biological catalysts often serve as the focal point for the regulation of body function. Increased enzyme activity accelerates the formation of a given product that may be essential for a particular function. The synthesis of norepinephrine illustrates this principle well. Heart rate will increase when norepinephrine is released from the sympathetic nerves. Norepinephrine is synthesized through a series of enzymatic reactions of which the rate-limiting, and therefore the most important, regulating enzyme is tyrosine hydroxylase. Increased tyrosine hydroxylase activity brings about conversion of more tyrosine to dihydroxyphenylalanine (DOPA), which is converted by dopa decarboxylase to dopamine. Dopamine is converted to norepinephrine by the enzymatic activity of dopamine-β-hydroxylase. The formation of norepinephrine can be regulated by a number of factors, including a feedback mechanism. Increased levels of norepinephrine inhibit the enzyme tyrosine hydroxylase so that less norepinephrine is synthesized. Thus, levels of norepinephrine can control the amount of norepinephrine synthesized.

The actions of a considerable number of drugs representing a wide variety of pharmacological agents depend on an enzyme-drug interaction. Notable examples demonstrating this diversity include the following:

The hydrolysis of acetylcholine by cholinesterase is blocked in a competitive manner by physostigmine and in a noncompetitive manner by diisopropyl fluorophosphate, organophosphate insecticides, and several chemical warfare agents.

The oxidation of norepinephrine and serotonin by monoamine oxidase (MAO) is inhibited by the antidepressant phenelzine.

The oxidation of acetaldehyde to acetate by aldehyde dehydrogenase is inhibited by disulfiram.

The oxidation of arachidonic acid to prostaglandins by cyclooxygenase is inhibited by, and is the common mode of action of, nonsteroidal anti-inflammatory drugs such as aspirin and indomethacin.

The hydrolysis of one of the cellular mediators of hormonal action, cyclic 3′,5′-adenosine monophosphate, by phosphodiesterase is inhibited by methylated xanthines, such as caffeine and theophylline.

The 11β-hydroxylation reaction in the synthesis of cortisol, corticosterone and aldosterone is inhibited by metyrapone.

The thyroid peroxidase responsible for the synthesis of thyroxine is inhibited by propylthiouracil and methimazole.

The conversion of xanthine to uric acid by xanthine oxidase is inhibited by allopurinol, which is used therefore in the treatment of gout.

The bacterial synthesis of the essential vitamin folic acid is competitively inhibited by the sulfonamide antibiotics.

The cancer chemotherapeutic agent fluorouracil is converted to a compound that inhibits the enzyme thymidylate synthetase, which is needed for DNA synthesis.

These examples illustrate the importance of drug-enzyme interactions in the pharmacological actions of therapeutic agents. The actions of drugs of the future also undoubtedly will depend on drug-enzyme interaction. Indeed, the pharmacological action of many drugs currently being prescribed by the physician probably will be found to involve such interplay. Since enzymes are involved so intricately in regulation of function, it is only logical to suppose that drugs may increase or decrease function by stimulating or depressing enzyme activity, respectively. A knowledge of enzymes and their properties, therefore, becomes increasingly important to the pharmacist, to understand the action of drugs.

In addition to the action, the pharmacokinetics, drug interactions, and toxicities of many drugs depend on enzyme activity. The enzymes responsible for these phenomena are those generally termed drug-metabolizing enzymes and are located predominately in the liver. Contrary to most others, these enzymes typified by cytochrome P-450 and UDP-glucuronosyl transferase exhibit broad substrate specificity. The ability to metabolize a wide variety of drugs to more-readily excretable products carries with it the potential for mutual competition when several drugs are administered simultaneously, thus altering the pharmacokinetics from that seen if a single drug is given. Toxicities arise from the two-phase nature of drug metabolism, the introduction of a reactive site suitable for conjugation and masking of that site with an endogenous polar molecule to form an excretable water-soluble conjugate. Failure to mask a reactive site allows it to interact with cell macromolecules (proteins, DNA, membranes) to produce cell damage, carcinogenesis, or cell death.

PROPERTIES—Four properties of enzymes make them specialized catalysts.

1. Most enzymes will catalyze only a specific range of reactions, and in many cases only one reaction will be catalyzed by a given enzyme. Some enzymes have a low degree of specificity; eg, pepsin hydrolyzes almost all soluble native proteins, but the hydrolysis is limited to certain very specific peptide linkages. On the other hand, urease is a highly specific enzyme; its only known substrate is urea. Almost all enzymes show a high degree of spatial speci-

ficity. Arginase acts only on L-arginine; it does not attack D-arginine. The specificity of enzymes is one of their most fundamental and important properties.

2. Enzymes are exceedingly efficient. Most enzymatic reactions, under optimal conditions, proceed 10^8 to 10^{11} times more rapidly than the corresponding nonenzymatic reactions.

3. Enzymes as a group are exceptionally versatile catalysts. For example, they effectively catalyze hydrolytic reactions, dehydrations, acyl transfer reactions, oxidation-reduction reactions, polymerizations, aldol condensations, and free-radical reactions.

4. Enzymes are subject to a variety of cellular controls. Their final concentration and rate of synthesis are under genetic control. In addition, enzymes can be present in the cell in both inactive and active forms. The rate of conversion from inactive to active form is influenced by environmental changes; eg, phosphorylase *b* is converted to phosphorylase *a* very rapidly through a series of reactions that are triggered by the release of catecholamines.

NOMENCLATURE—Enzymes usually are named in terms of the reactions that are catalyzed. Usually, the suffix *-ase* is added to the name of the substrate upon which the enzyme acts, ie, the enzyme that attacks urea is urease, and arginine is acted upon by arginase. Enzymes also are classified according to the reaction they catalyze, eg, reductases and dehydrogenases. Some older names that are unrelated to the function of the enzyme remain in usage, eg, renin, trypsin, and pepsin.

The Commission on Enzymes of the International Union of Biochemistry has established a complete but rather complex system of classification and nomenclature. According to this classification enzymes are divided into six general groups:

1. *Oxidoreductases*—catalyzing oxidation-reduction reactions.
2. *Transferases*—catalyzing transfer of a chemical group from one molecule to another.
3. *Hydrolases*—catalyzing hydrolytic reactions.
4. *Lyases*—catalyzing the addition of groups to double bonds or *vice versa*.
5. *Isomerases*—catalyzing intramolecular rearrangements.
6. *Ligases* (also known as synthetases)—catalyzing the condensation of two molecules, coupled with the cleavage of a pyrophosphate bond of ATP or similar triphosphate.

In this system every enzyme is coded in a four-number system according to the type of reaction catalyzed, type of isomerization, type of bond hydrolyzed, etc.

Many enzymes possess nonprotein chemical groups. Thus, an enzyme often can be dissociated into a protein component, an *apoenzyme,* and a nonprotein component, a *prosthetic group*. Prosthetic groups also are referred to as coenzymes or cofactors. Vitamins and certain metals are examples of these prosthetic groups.

Despite the ubiquity of enzymes in normal physiology and as the basis of many drug effects and drug interactions, the use of enzymes as drugs is extremely limited. Being proteinaceous, they can be inactivated by conditions and enzymes present in the gastrointestinal (GI) lumen if given orally and, if given parenterally, can elicit immune responses. Most of the enzymes currently available on the market are hydrolases (Group 3 above). These enzyme preparations are of limited use in (1) debridement, ie, as aids in resolving and removing blood clots or fibrinous or purulent accumulations and (2) replacement therapy to correct certain GI deficiencies (Table 91-1).

ALTEPLASE—page 1332.
ASPARAGINASE—page 1562.

COLLAGENASE

Santyl

A product of *Clostridium histolyticum,* which breaks down native and denatured collagen in necrotic (not in healthy) tissue at physiological pH and temperature. It is a fermentation-produced enzyme complex.

Description—Fine, brown, amorphous powder; heat-labile.
Solubility—Soluble in water or alcohol.
Comments—Collagen constitutes about 75% of the dry weight of the skin and is the main constituent of necrotic debris and of the eschar that covers the surface of an ulcer; hence, collagenase is indicated for debridement of severely burned areas and dermal ulcers. Its effectiveness in the treatment of other necrotic skin lesions requires further investigation. The enzyme is compatible with antibiotics such as polymyxin B sulfate, neomycin, or bacitracin. It is adversely affected by heavy metal antiseptics, detergents, and hexachlorophene, so that these agents must be removed before using the enzyme.

DEOXYRIBONUCLEASE RECOMBINANT

Pulmozyme

Dornase alpha is a purified solution of recombinant human deoxyribonuclease I produced in genetically engineered Chinese hamster ovary cells. It is sensitive to light and heat.

Table 91-1. Pancreatic Enzymes: Dose and Dosage Forms

TRADE NAME	LIPASE[a]	PROTEASE[a]	AMYLASE[a]	DOSE
Pancrease-MT Capsules				In units of lipase activity: *children, 6 mo to 1 yr,* 2000 Units/meal; *1 to 6 yr,* 4000 to 8000 Units/meal; *7 to 12 yr,* 4000 to 12,000 Units/meal; *adults,* 4000 to 16,000 Units/meal
MT4	4	12	12	
Pancrease	5	25	20	
MT10	10	30	30	
MT16	16	48	48	
MT20	20	44	56	
Ultrase MT Capsules				
MT12	12	39	39	
MT20	20	65	65	
MT24	24	78	78	
Ilozyme	11	30	30	
Cotazyme	5	20	20	
Cotazyme-S	8	30	30	1 to 3 capsules prior to each meal or snack
8X Pancreatin Tablets	22.5	180	180	1 or 2 tablets with each meal; 1 tablet with a snack
Creon Capsules	8	13	30	Same as above
Creon 10	10	38	33	1 to 3 capsules with each meal
Creon 20	20	75	66	
Ku-Zyme-HP Capsules	8	30	30	
VioKase				
Tablets	8	30	30	Same as above
Powder	16.8	70	70	For *cystic fibrosis,* 1/4 tsp (0.7 g) with meals
Zymase Capsules	12	24	24	1 or 2 capsules with each meal

[a] In thousands of USP Units/dosage unit.

Comments—Deoxyribonuclease selectively cleaves DNA, which is present at high concentrations in the secretions of cystic fibrosis patients following release from leukocytes that accumulate in response to infection. Its action reduces the viscoelasticity of the secretion.

HYALURONIDASE FOR INJECTION

Wydase

A sterile, dry, soluble, enzyme product prepared from mammalian (bovine) testes and capable of hydrolyzing mucopolysaccharides of the hyaluronic acid type; its potency is not less than the labeled potency in Hyaluronidase Units and it contains not more than 0.25 µg of tyrosine for each Hyaluronidase Unit. It may contain a suitable stabilizer.

Description—White, odorless, amorphous solid or a nearly colorless glass-like solid; it is destroyed by heat; its solutions are colorless.

Comments—Intercellular cement, which binds together the parenchymal cells of organs; appears to be a gel of highly polymerized polysaccharide, hyaluronic acid. The latter is present in all organs but is most abundant in tissues of mesenchymal origin (eg, connective tissue and blood vessels); the testis is the richest source of hyaluronidase in mammals. Hyaluronidase hydrolyzes hyaluronic acid by splitting the glucosaminidic bond between carbon-1 of the glucosamine moiety and carbon-4 of glucuronic acid. Hyaluronidase accelerates the subcutaneous spread of both particulate matter and solutions by depolymerizing the hyaluronic acid. This results in a larger area of distribution of drugs in the tissue spaces and facilitates their absorption.

The chief clinical use of hyaluronidase is to facilitate administration of fluids by hypodermoclysis. It has been used as an adjunct in subcutaneous urography to improve resorption of radiopaque agents and to enhance absorption of drugs in tissue spaces, transudates, and various edemas. Its use with local anesthetics is not recommended. Hyaluronidase should not be used in infected areas because of the danger of spreading the infection.

LACTASE

Lactaid

A β-D-galactosidase derived from *Kluyveromyces lactis* yeast.

Comments—Added to, or ingested with, milk to convert the disaccharide lactose into glucose and galactose for patients suffering from lactase insufficiency (lactose intolerance).

MALT EXTRACT—page 1076.

PANCREATIC ENZYMES

A substance containing enzymes, principally amylase, protease, and lipase, obtained from the pancreas of the hog, *Sus scrofa* Linné var. *domesticus* Gray (Fam *Suidae*) or of the ox, *Bos taurus* Linné (Fam *Bovidae*).

Pancreatin contains, in each milligram, not less than 2 Units of lipase activity, not less than 25 Units of amylase activity and not less than 25 Units of protease activity. Pancreatin of a higher digestive power may be labeled with a whole-number multiple of the three minimum activities or may be diluted by admixture with lactose or with sucrose containing not more than 3.25% of starch or with pancreatin of lower digestive power.

Pancrelipase contains, in each milligram, not less than 24 Units of lipase activity, not less than 100 Units of amylase activity, and not less than 100 Units of protease activity.

Description—Cream-colored, amorphous powders, with a faint, characteristic, but not offensive, odor. They hydrolyze fats to glycerol and fatty acids, change protein into proteoses and derived substances, and convert starch into dextrins and sugars. Their greatest activities are in neutral or slightly alkaline media; more than traces of mineral acids or large amounts of alkali hydroxides render them inert. An excess of alkali carbonate also inhibits their action.

Solubility—Slowly and incompletely soluble in water; insoluble in alcohol.

Incompatibilities—*Mineral acids* or excess *alkali hydroxides* or carbonates render it inert. They are precipitated by *strong alcoholic solutions* and by many *metallic salts*.

Comments—In the treatment of patients with cystic fibrosis (mucoviscidosis), chronic pancreatitis, partial or complete surgical pancreatectomy, and other conditions associated with exocrine pancreatic insufficiency. The administration of pancreatin decreases the nitrogen and fat content of the stool. The use of pancreatin except in pancreatic insufficiency is of no known value. The efficacy of pancreatin in the treatment of gaseous distention has not been demonstrated. When treating pancreatic insufficiency, a high-caloric diet that is high in protein and low in fat is recommended. A significant amount of the enzyme activity can be lost by peptic digestion during passage through the stomach. The efficacy of pancreatin is enhanced by simultaneous administration of cimetidine, which increases intragastric pH. Dietary and enzyme regimens are best based on repeated clinical evaluation and, in

hospitalized patients, periodic measurements of fecal fat and nitrogen loss. Since the underlying pancreatic deficiency is unchanged, replacement pancreatin therapy is permanent. At high doses, pancreatin can cause nausea, abdominal cramps, and diarrhea. The enzyme dust is irritating to the nasal membrane, so inhalation should be avoided.

PAPAIN

Panafil

A proteolytic enzyme from the fruit of the tropical melon tree, *Carica papaya*. It exhibits broad-spectrum specificity over a wide pH range, including peptides, amides, esters, and thioesters, all being susceptible to papain-catalyzed hydrolysis. Nonviable protein is susceptible, but it is harmless to viable tissue.

Comments—In the debridement of necrotic tissue.

SUTILAINS

Travase

A substance, containing proteolytic enzymes, derived from the bacterium *Bacillus subtilis*. Elaborated by fermentation with *B subtilis* and purified by filtration, salt and solvent precipitation, and lyophilization. Potency not less than 2,500,000 Casein Units of proteolytic activity/g.

Description—Cream-colored odorless powder; *do not taste* (irritating to oral membranes); stable in light, hygroscopic, and decomposes in solvents.

Solubility—1 g in 100 mL of water; insoluble in alcohol or other organic solvents.

Comments—An adjunct to established methods of wound care for biochemical debridement of the following lesions: 2nd- and 3rd-degree burns; decubitus ulcers; incisional, traumatic, and pyrogenic wounds; and ulcers secondary to peripheral vascular disease. The enzyme digests denatured proteins found in necrotic tissues, and a moist environment is essential to optimal enzyme activity. Detergents and antiseptics may render the substrate refractory, and heavy-metal antibacterials may denature the enzyme. It is contraindicated for wounds communicating with body cavities or those containing exposed nerves or nervous tissue, for fungating neoplastic ulcers, and in wounds in women of childbearing potential. It should not be allowed to come in contact with the eyes. If this should occur inadvertently, the eyes should be rinsed immediately with copious amounts of water (preferably sterile water).

CRYSTALLIZED TRYPSIN

Granulex

A proteolytic enzyme crystallized from an extract of the pancreas of the ox, *Bos taurus* Linné (Fam *Bovidae*); its potency is not less than 25,000 Trypsin Units/mg.

Description—White to yellowish white, odorless or amorphous powder.

Solubility—An amount equivalent to 500,000 Units is soluble in 10 mL water or saline TS; pH (1% soln) 3 to 5.5; max activity at pH 8.

Comments—Promotes proteolysis of a variety of protein substrates, including clotted blood, purulent exudates (pus), and necrotic tissue, but not living tissue. Especially in the presence of blood its duration of action is limited because of the presence of inhibiting substrates. Solutions also have been inhaled to liquefy viscous sputum.

OTHER ENZYMES

Fibrinolysin and Deoxyribonuclease [Elase]—A mixture of fibrinolysin of bovine plasma and deoxyribonuclease obtained from bovine pancreas. These two enzymes function together when used topically to lyse fibrin and liquefy pus, thus aiding in the removal of necrotic material from both the skin and certain body cavities. It is used as a debriding agent in surgical wounds, ulcerative lesions, and 2nd and 3rd degree burns and is used intravaginally in severe cervicitis and vaginitis. It is not suitable for parenteral use and is not to be used in thromboembolic diseases. The commercial product named above is supplied as a lyophilized powder (25 units of fibrinolysin and 15,000 units of deoxyribonuclease), from which a solution for topical use may be prepared, and in ointment form (30 units of fibrinolysin and 20,000 units of deoxyribonuclease). It also is available combined with 1% chloramphenicol, but systemic toxicities with the antibiotic have been reported.

DIGESTIVE AIDS

Numerous preparations, both prescription and OTC, are available as aids for digestion, particularly for conditions in which deficiencies of natural digestive enzymes exist. They contain some or all of the following categories of enzymes: amylolytic, proteolytic, cellulytic, and lipolytic. In addition, the preparations often include bile salts or bile extracts. α-D-Galactosidase is used to reduce gassiness or bloating following ingestion of grains, cereals, nuts, seeds, or vegetables containing raffinose, verbascose, and stachyose.

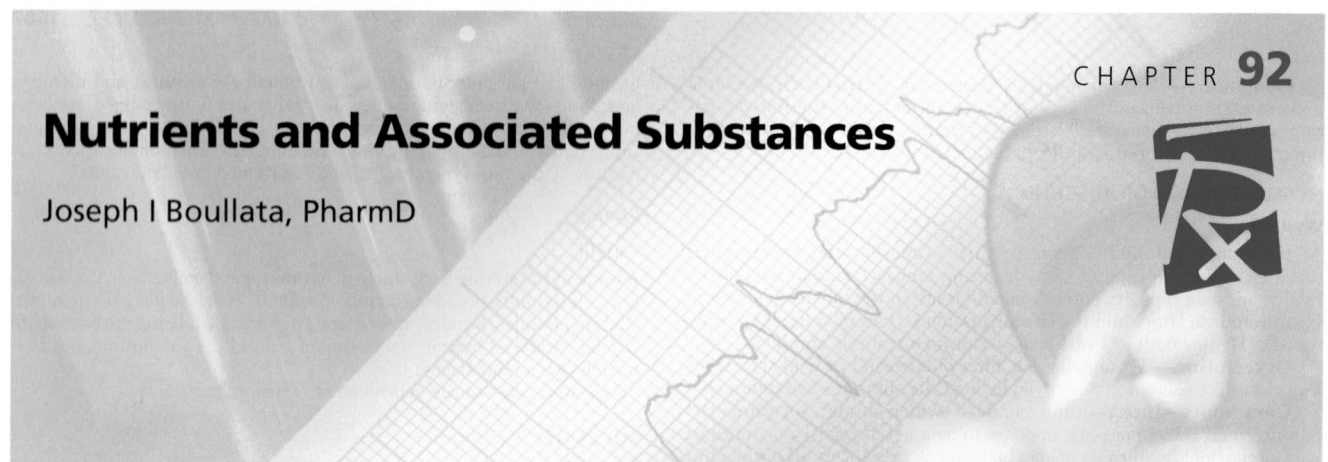

CHAPTER 92

Nutrients and Associated Substances

Joseph I Boullata, PharmD

Food, containing nutrients and associated substances, has been at the forefront of the preventive aspects of healthcare for over a century. In recent years more attention has been given to the specific aspects of the diet that not only prevent deficiencies but also can be used to prevent chronic disease, augment growth and development, and possibly treat select disorders of health.

From a pharmaceutical point of view nutrients and the associated substances typically found in the healthy diet may be consumed through a number of dosage delivery systems. This begins with conventional foods, fresh and processed. Besides providing traditional nutrients, some foods may contain other active ingredients (naturally or through manipulation) that may enhance health (ie, "pharmafoods," "functional foods," or "designer foods"). Nutrients may also be administered as dietary supplements. These products may contain nutrients or associated substances as the sole ingredient, but more often are included in multi-ingredient products. The latter sometimes combine nutrients with botanical and other non-nutrient ingredients in a dietary supplement product. Meal replacement formulas and medical foods intended for patients unable to consume adequate nourishment orally are additional delivery vehicles for nutrients. Some nutrients are found as drug products—in oral and parenteral dosage forms. These nutrient-containing products are often intended for specific disorders. Parenteral nutrients can be combined to form a parenteral nutrient admixture used to support patients unable to otherwise take or assimilate nutrients through the gastrointestinal tract. The analogy to medicines does not end with delivery systems.

Nutrients and associated substances found in foods are physiologically active substances. The chemical structure and structure-activity relationships of individual nutrients are no different than any other natural or synthetic drug. In fact the kinetic behavior of some nutrients is more complex than that of many drugs. Nutrient bioavailability can vary greatly with the delivery vehicle and dosage form. Additionally nutrient absorption, distribution, and elimination will vary with an individual's nutritional status. Pharmacists can be involved to varying degrees in helping consumers and patients alike with preventive strategies as well as therapies involving nutrients.

There exists a nutrition continuum from health to disease, across the life cycle, in which pharmacists have become involved based on their knowledge set and clinical opportunity. Together, as found in foods, nutrients and associated substances are critical to growth and development, as well as health maintenance. Issues relating to nutrients or to an individual's nutritional status is prominent in the management of many diseases, both acute and chronic. In the absence of the anatomic or physiologic ability to consume food products, some patients require enteral or parenteral nutrient formulations to therapeutically maintain or improve their metabolic status

lasting from several days to the remainder of their lives. A vast amount of confusion and nonscientific information surrounds the relationship of foods, as specially formulated food products, to health and prevention or cure of various disease conditions. However, food behaviors of increasing numbers of people are influenced by misrepresentations and false claims made for *health* foods, fad diets, and miracle cures by individuals and groups who profit from sale of such foods or ideas. Particularly in the field of nutrition, where misinformation may endanger the health of individuals, consumers must be provided opportunity to learn to make sound decisions regarding their health and nutritional status. Pharmacists can be involved in educating patients on various aspects of nutrition, screening patients for poor nutritional status, suggesting referral for more specific needs, and managing therapeutic regimens in patients requiring dietary supplementation or nutrition support. Furthermore, depending on the setting, pharmacists may be involved in clinical or basic research that involves nutrients. They may also be involved with local or national organizations whether nonprofit or corporate. Pharmacy has a vital role to play directly when it comes to nutrition in support of patient care.

NUTRIENTS

Many materials involved in human metabolism either cannot be synthesized by the body or in quantities insufficient to meet needs. These essential substrates, nutrients, need to be delivered exogenously—ideally through a healthy diet. Nutritional status is considered optimal when nutrient requirements are balanced by nutrient intake, while body composition and function is maintained. The nutrients have been reasonably well classified as either macronutrients or micronutrients. While macronutrients are required in gram quantities daily, the micronutrients are generally required in milligram quantities or less daily. Macronutrients include protein, carbohydrate, lipid, and water. The three carbon-based nutrients flow through common routes of intermediary metabolism and contribute to the energy needs of the body, with most reactions occurring in an environment containing water. Indeed, more than 50% of body weight is made up of water. When completely metabolized, protein, carbohydrate, and fat yield 4, 4, and 9 kcal of energy per gram of nutrient, respectively. Besides roles in energy metabolism, macronutrients provide structural and transport roles within the body, and individual amino acids and fatty acids have specific physiologic roles. Evidence is also growing that the amount and form of carbohydrate and fat have profound effects on development of degenerative diseases.

Although micronutrients provide no calories toward energy needs, this group of nutrients, which includes vitamins and minerals, are physiologically important in regulating metabolism through roles as co-enzymes and co-factors, free radical scavenging, intracellular signaling, and gene expression. Other components of food are rapidly being recognized for their importance to health, although not currently classified as nutrients. These other compounds found in food include substances such as carotenoids, flavonoids, and other phenolic derivatives. Most of these substances are found in foods of plant origin and are secondary metabolites of plant physiology intended to protect plants from their environments. Some of these substances may have roles in human health. Nutrients and associated substances are included for their roles in health, essentially no different than any other substance adopted into clinical practice that is covered in this section of the book. The current emphasis in practice should be on the overall health effects of food consumption, rather than solely on individual nutrients or associated substances. This does however require knowledge of the individual substances.

Dietary Guidelines and Nutrient Standards

The specifics of a number of nutrients and associated substances, including those found as pharmaceutical preparations, will be discussed in sections below. An appreciation for dosing strategies will be needed. The optimum human diet should meet all nutrient needs through the consumption of a wide variety of food. It should also help maintain appropriate body mass, or growth and development in children and pregnant women. The optimum diet should also prevent illness caused by deficiency or excess nutrient intake. Healthy eating patterns are those that follow the principles of adequacy, balance, and moderation by using all available guidelines related to achieving the optimum diet. Most people do not follow healthy eating patterns. It is not necessary to follow strict meal plans on a daily basis or fad diets that cannot be adhered to long-term to achieve a healthy eating pattern, but merely follow or work toward the general guidelines available.

Guidelines for nutrient intake are based on a number of science-based as well as public policy-driven initiatives. In the US this includes several qualitative and quantitative guidelines. The Healthy People 2010 is a governmental report comprising close to 500 national objectives organized into 28 focus areas, for improving health. Included in the report are about 40 objectives relating to nutrition, with one focus area dedicated to nutrition. It provides outcome targets for the year 2010 for each objective (eg, 75% of people should meet calcium requirements, currently less than 50% do). The government also provides a set of 10 general dietary guidelines for Americans as well as specific guidelines on apportioning calorie, cholesterol, and sodium intake. These guidelines on the percent of calories to be derived from various macronutrients and cholesterol and sodium intake have become similar to nutrition guidelines prepared by various non-governmental organizations (eg, American Heart Association, American Diabetic Association, American Cancer Society) to prevent or manage chronic disease. Beyond the guidelines exist some specific food guides (eg, food guide pyramid) to more easily help consumers in food selection for maintaining health.

All of the aforementioned guidelines, while updated regularly and helpful to the public in terms of making food choices consistent with a healthy eating pattern, are qualitative when it comes to intake of specific nutrients. Nutrient-specific standards are also available. The Dietary Reference Intakes (DRIs) are prepared by expert panels through the Institute of Medicine's Food and Nutrition Board to provide nutrient dosing standards based on the available evidence. These serve as the benchmark for nutritional adequacy in the US and Canada—with similar provisions in many other countries—and are a more complete set of standards that replace the periodic revision of the recommended dietary allowances that began in the 1940s. The dosing levels provided in the DRI reports are intended for healthy persons as part of the normal diet to reduce the risk of chronic disease and developmental disorders, as well as to prevent nutrient deficiencies. The DRIs encompass four types of

reference values and 12 life-stage groups as data permits. The reference values include the recommended dietary allowances (RDAs) for each nutrient with adequate supporting data, or the adequate intake (AI) levels in the absence of sufficient data.

In contrast to these nutrient dosing standards, the Food and Drug Administration (FDA) sets nutrient labeling standards for foods to help consumers see how a food fits into an overall healthy eating plan. This includes use of a Daily Value (DV) for a number of nutrients, a term that encompasses two types of reference values–the Daily Reference Values (DRV) for macronutrients, cholesterol, sodium, and potassium, and the Reference Daily Intake (RDI) levels for other micronutrients. In many, but not all cases, the DV levels are the same as the highest RDA or AI level. The DV replaced the term US Recommended Daily Allowance (US RDA) in use since 1974, which itself replaced the Minimum Daily Requirements established by the FDA in 1940. Besides the labeling standards for food, health claims for food products are also under the purview of the FDA. Regarding dietary supplement products, although standards for labeling and claims exist, no review of safety, efficacy, or product quality is currently required as it is for medications. Products are labeled with *Nutrition Facts* if they are regulated as food but with *Supplement Facts* if they are regulated less closely as dietary supplements.

Nutrient Therapy

Poor nutritional status (ie, malnutrition) refers to nutrient intake not in balance with nutrient requirements. It is more common than appreciated, often present alongside a variety of clinical disorders. It can refer to undernutrition, obesity, specific nutrient imbalances, and altered states of metabolism. Poor nutritional status contributes to poor patient outcome and should therefore be regularly evaluated by health care providers. The plan to manage malnourished patients and those at risk for malnutrition will differ based on the patient and the setting. Patient-related factors that can affect nutrient needs include the following:

- Interference with food consumption (eg, impaired appetite, gastrointestinal (GI) disease, traumatic neurological disorders interfering with self-feeding, neuropsychiatric disorders, disease of soft or hard oral tissue, alcoholism, pregnancy anorexia and vomiting, food allergy, adverse drug effects, and disease requiring a restricted diet).
- Interference with absorption (eg, absence of normal digestive secretions, intestinal hypermotility, reduction of effective absorbing surface, impairment of intrinsic mechanism of absorption, and drugs preventing absorption.)
- Interference with utilization or storage (eg, impaired liver function, hypothyroidism, neoplasm of GI tract, and drug therapy or radiation).
- Increased destruction of tissues and/or function (eg, severe trauma, achlorhydria in the GI tract, heavy metals, and other metabolic antagonists).
- Increased excretion or loss of nutrients (eg, lactation, burns, glycosuria and albuminuria, acute chronic blood loss, and drug-induced).
- Increased nutrient requirements (eg, increased physical activity, periods of rapid growth, pregnancy and lactation, fever, hyperthyroidism, and drug therapy).

The approach to the patient requiring nutritional intervention may include education, referral to a dietitian or other health care provider, or a therapeutic regimen. Regimens can include diet therapy under the care of a dietitian, as well as nutrient therapy as dietary supplements, medical foods, drugs, or specialized nutrition support.

Nutrition Support

For patients who are otherwise unable to maintain or improve their nutritional status through an oral diet, specialized nutrition support regimens may be required. The route of adminis-

MEDICINAL AGENTS

tration will depend in large part on the status of the GI tract. Enteral nutrition (ie, tube feeding) is used if the GI tract is functional and safe access exists. When enteral feeding is impractical or contraindicated, the alternative is intravenous feeding known as *parenteral nutrition (PN),* sometimes referred to as *total parenteral nutrition*, and previously referred to as *intravenous* or *parenteral hyperalimentation.* Such feeding provides essential macronutrients and micronutrients in a sufficiently concentrated form that does not exceed normal daily fluid requirements. These necessarily hypertonic admixtures are infused at a constant rate throughout the entire day into a large-diameter *central* vein where rapid dilution by high blood-flow minimizes vascular damage and the risk of phlebitis or thrombosis that is likely to occur on injection into a peripheral vein. Ambulatory patients may receive the infusion for only part of the day. The infusion is generally through a catheter whose distal end is in the superior vena cava.

A critical component in PN is a nitrogen source available for repletion and/or maintenance of lean body mass and proteins essential for wound healing, tissue repair, and growth. Solutions of mixed crystalline L-amino acids serve as the nitrogen source. Crystalline L-amino acids appear to be more efficiently metabolized and better tolerated in the body than were the peptides of protein hydrolysates used years ago. Also, individual amino acids may be readily and reproducibly formulated to meet specific requirements of patients (eg, pre-

mature infants). So that amino acids may be used for protein synthesis and to achieve positive nitrogen balance and weight gain in debilitated patients it is necessary to provide a nonprotein calorie source. Both concentrated dextrose solutions (50%, 70%) and intravenous lipid emulsions (10%, 20%, 30%) are available as caloric sources. The hydrated dextrose product provides 3.4 kcal/g, while the lipid emulsions provide 9 kcal/g plus the additional calories from the glycerol used to make the product isotonic. The lipid emulsion is also a source of essential fatty acids. Occassionally, based on PN stability or clinical circumstances, the lipid emulsion is not included in the admixture. If administered separately the 10% and 20% emulsion products may be administered through central or peripheral veins. If an intravenous emulsion is not used at all, large amounts of dextrose are required to achieve caloric balance and this may increase the risk of adverse effects from the dextrose.

In addition to amino acids, dextrose, and lipids, PN admixtures will contain vitamins, minerals, and electrolytes (often added to meet individual patient requirements). The final, patient-specific admixture is compounded using aseptic technique, under laminar airflow conditions and usually dispensed in an appropriate single, daily container. The preparation of the admixture is expected to follow accepted guidelines and standards of practice for dosing, labeling, and compounding with particular attention to stability and compatibility.

PROTEINS AND AMINO ACIDS

Proteins serve a structural role in all cells of the body and function as enzymes, hormones, and membrane transporters. The fundamental units of any protein are the amino acids. Protein and amino acids are consumed in the human diet. Some amino acids are considered indispensable (essential) in that they cannot be synthesized endogenously, and therefore are required in the diet (Table 92-1). The remaining amino acids are dispensable (non-essential) although many of them become indispensable under certain physiologic or pathologic conditions and are referred to as conditionally indispensable (conditionally essential) amino acids (see Table 92-1). The recommended protein requirement for healthy individuals across the life stages is provided in Table 92-2. Specific dosing requirements for individual amino acids are being generated as well. In recent years certain free amino acids have been prescribed for a variety of medical conditions for which neither drug nor food approval have been obtained. Regulations on the food-additive use are limited to providing protein requirements. Therefore, these uses of single amino acids are without approved status. Consumption of high levels of single amino acids has been associated with severe metabolic and medical consequences. For patients unable to consume food orally, a source of amino acids can be provided enterally or parenterally.

Commercially available amino acid injections used in preparing PN vary in the amount of protein (3.5–15 g/100 mL), nitrogen (0.55–2.37 g/100 mL), indispensable and dispensable amino acids, pH (4.5–7), osmolarity (357–1388 mOsm/L), and electrolyte content. These synthetic, crystalline L-amino acids replaced use of protein hydrolysates. A number of amino acids are either too poorly soluble and/or unstable to be included in amino acid products (eg, cysteine, glutamine).

CHEMISTRY—The USP has provided monographs of standards and tests for each of the crystalline amino acids used in amino acid dosage forms. For comparative purposes the formulas and chemical names of the L-amino acids are given in Chapter 26 and other chemical data are provided in Table 92-3.

Each of the amino acids is synthesized readily, by a variety of methods, but always as a DL-mixture. Resolution to obtain the L-form in most cases is conveniently accomplished.

The articles that follow describe a few amino acids that are used for certain nonnutritional purposes as well as components of nutritional formulations.

ARGININE HYDROCHLORIDE

R-Gene 10

L-Arginine monohydrochloride [1119-34-2] $C_6H_{14}N_4O_2$.HCl (210.66). For the structural formula of arginine, see Chapter 26.

Preparation—Arginine is present in the hydrolysis products of many proteins; for a method of separating it from gelatin hydrolysate. See *J Biol Chem* 1940; 132: 325. It is converted to the hydrochloride by reaction with HCl.

Description—White crystals or crystalline powder; practically odorless.

Solubility—Soluble in water; slightly soluble in hot alcohol.

Comments—Arginine has been variously used in clinical practice. Intravenous administration in the symptomatic management of severe encephalopathies associated with ammoniacal azotemia, on the theory that arginine combines with ammonia to form asparagine, has not been of value in significantly reducing blood ammonia levels or in improving the clinical status of patients, and use of the amino acid for this purpose is no longer approved by the FDA. Oral administration to patients with cystic fibrosis to correct malabsorption and steatorrhea and by inhalation as a mucolytic have not been effective. It is used as a nutritional supplement in conditions in which its dibasic amino character or possible blood ammonia–reducing power is useful. As a precursor of nitric oxide, its clinical use should be approached with caution.

Table 92-1. Amino Acids

INDISPENSABLE	CONDITIONALLLY INDISPENSABLE	DISPENSABLE
Histidine	Arginine	Alanine
Isoleucine	Cysteine	Aspartate
Leucine	Glutamine	Asparagine
Lysine	Glycine	Glutamate
Methionine	Proline	Serine
Phenylalanine	Tyrosine	
Threonine		
Tryptophan		
Valine		

Table 92-2. Dietary Reference Intakes—Macronutrients

LIFE STAGE GROUP	Protein (g/kg/d)	Carbohydrate (g/d)	Fat (g/d)	Energy (kcal/d)	Fiber (g/d)
Infants					
0–6 months	1.52*	60*	31*	520-570	ND[1]
7–12 months	1.5	95*	30*	676-743	ND
Children					
1–3 years	1.1	130	ND[1]	992-1046	19*
4–8 years	0.95	130	ND	1642-1742	25*
Males					
9–13 years	0.95	130	ND	2279	31*
14–18 years	0.85	130	ND	3152	38*
19–30 years	0.8	130	ND	$3067 - x$[2]	38*
31–50 years	0.8	130	ND	$3067 - x$	38*
51–70 years	0.8	130	ND	$3067 - x$	30*
>70 years	0.8	130	ND	$3067 - x$	30*
Females	0.95	130	ND	2071	26*
9–13 years	0.85	130	ND	2368	36*
14–18 years	0.8	130	ND	$2403 - y$[3]	25*
19–30 years	0.8	130	ND	$2403 - y$	25*
31–50 years	0.8	130	ND	$2403 - y$	21*
51–70 years	0.8	130	ND	$2403 - y$	21*
>70 years					
Pregnancy					
≤18 years		175	ND	2368-2820	28*
19–30 years		175	ND	2403-2855	28*
31–50 years		175	ND	2403-2855	28*
Lactation					
≤18 years		210	ND	2698-2768	29*
19–30 years		210	ND	2733-2803	29*
31–50 years		210	ND	2733-2803	29*

* Adequate Intake Level, otherwise values represent Recommended Dietary Allowances:
[1] Not determined or not described in the current recommendations.
[2] $x = 10$ kcal/d for each year above 19 years is subtracted from 3067 kcal/d.
[3] $y = 7$ kcal/d for each year above 19 years is subtracted from 2403 kcal/d.

Table 92-3. L-Amino Acids

AMINO ACID[a]	MOLECULAR FORMULA	MOLECULAR WEIGHT	SOLUBILITY IN WATER	pK VALUES
L-Alanine 56-41-7	$C_3H_7NO_2$	89.09	1 g in 6 mL	pK$_1$ 3.34 pK$_2$ 8.17
L-Arginine 74-79-3	$C_6H_{14}N_4O_2$	174.20	1 g in 5 mL	pK$_1$ 2.18 pK$_2$ 9.09 pK$_3$ 13.2
L-Aspartic acid 56-84-8	$C_4H_7NO_4$	133.10	1 g in 200 mL	pK$_1$ 1.88 pK$_2$ 3.65 pK$_3$ 9.60
L-Cysteine 52-90-4	$C_3H_7NO_2S$	121.16	Freely soluble	pK$_1$ 1.71 pK$_2$ 8.33 pK$_3$ 10.78
L-Cystine 56-89-3	$C_6H_{12}N_2O_4S_2$	240.30	1 g in 9 L	pK$_1$ 1 pK$_2$ 2.1 pK$_3$ 8.02 pK$_4$ 8.71
L-Glutamic acid 56-86-0	$C_5H_9NO_4$	147.13	1 g in 115 mL	pK$_1$ 2.19 pK$_2$ 4.25 pK$_3$ 9.67
L-Glutamine 56-85-9	$C_5H_{10}N_2O_3$	146.15	1 g in 31 mL	pK$_1$ 2.17 pK$_2$ 9.13
L-Glycine	$C_2H_5NO_2$	75.07	1 g in 4 mL	pK$_1$ 2.34 pK$_2$ 9.6
L-Histidine 71-00-1	$C_6H_9N_3O_2$	155.16	1 g in 24 mL	pK$_1$ 1.78 pK$_2$ 5.97 pK$_3$ 8.97
L-Hydroxyproline	$C_5H_9NO_3$	131.13	1 g in 3 mL (α-form)	pK$_1$ 1.82 pK$_2$ 9.65
L-Isoleucine[b] 73-32-5	$C_6H_{13}NO_2$	131.17	1 g in 25 mL	pK$_1$ 2.36 pK$_2$ 9.68
L-Leucine[b] 61-90-5	$C_6H_{13}NO_2$	131.17	1 g in 42 mL	K$_a$ 2.5×10^{-10} K$_b$ 2.3×10^{-2}
L-Lysine[b] 56-87-1	$C_6H_{14}N_2O_2$	146.19	Freely soluble	pK$_1$ 2.20 pK$_2$ 8.90 pK$_3$ 10.28

(continues)

Table 92-3. (continued)

AMINO ACID[a]	MOLECULAR FORMULA	MOLECULAR WEIGHT	SOLUBILITY IN WATER	PK VALUES
L-Methionine[b] 63-68-3	$C_5H_{11}NO_2S$	149.21	Soluble	pK$_1$ 2.12 pK$_2$ 9.28
L-Phenylalanine[b] 63-91-2	$C_9H_{11}NO_2$	165.19	1 g in 34 mL	pK$_1$ 2.16 pK$_2$ 9.18
L-Proline 147-85-3	$C_5H_9NO_2$	115.13	1 g in 0.7 mL	pK$_1$ 1.99 pK$_2$ 10.60
L-Serine 56-45-1	$C_3H_7NO_3$	105.09	1 g in 20 mL	pK$_1$ 2.19 pK$_2$ 9.21
L-Taurine 107-35-7	$C_2H_7NO_3S$	125.14	1 g in 16 mL	pK$_1$ 1.50 pK$_2$ 8.74
L-Threonine[b] 72-19-5	$C_4H_9NO_3$	119.12	Freely soluble	pK$_1$ 2.15 pK$_2$ 9.12
L-Tryptophan[b] 73-22-3	$C_{11}H_{12}N_2O_2$	204.22	1 g in 88 mL	pK$_1$ 2.38 pK$_2$ 9.39
L-Tyrosine 60-18-4	$C_9H_{11}NO_3$	181.19	1 g in 2.2 L	pK$_1$ 2.20 pK$_1$ 9.11 pK$_2$ 10.07
L-Valine[b] 72-18-4	$C_5H_{11}NO_2$	117.15	1 g in 12 mL	pK$_1$ 2.32 pK$_2$ 9.62

[a] The number below the name of each amino acid is its *Chemical Abstracts Service* (CAS) Registry Number. For structures and nomenclature see Chapter 26.
[b] Indispensable amino acids.

It stimulates pituitary release of growth hormone and prolactin and pancreatic release of glucagon and insulin, and arginine hydrochloride is used diagnostically to evaluate pituitary growth hormone reserve and detect deficiency of the hormone in various conditions. It is administered by intravenous infusion, and blood samples are taken at 30-min intervals after beginning infusion, for 2.5 hr; the plasma growth hormone levels in these samples and in others taken 30 min before and at the start of infusion are determined and diagnostically evaluated.

GLYCINE

Aminoacetic Acid; Glycocoll

NH$_2$CH$_2$COOH [56-40-6] C$_2$H$_5$NO$_2$ (75.07).

Preparation—Aminoacetic acid is a constituent of many proteins. It may be synthesized by many processes; industrially it is prepared by interaction of ammonia with chloroacetic acid.

Description—White, odorless, crystalline powder, with a sweetish taste; solution is acid to litmus; pK$_a$ 9.78.

Solubility—1 g in 4 mL water or 1254 mL alcohol; very slightly soluble in ether.

Comments—As an irrigating fluid in transurethral resection of the prostate. The acid also is used in an antacid preparation, as a complex salt. However, its limited buffering capacity does not warrant the expense of such a preparation. It is used primarily in admixture with other amino acids in PN formulations.

CARBOHYDRATES

Carbohydrates include simple pentoses and hexoses, as well as disaccharides and polymers of the simpler molecules. In the form of D-glucose (dextrose) carbohydrates provide cellular energy. Specific carbohydrates have alternative physiologic roles beyond energy (eg, ribose in nucleic acids). The chemistry of the sugars is discussed in Chapter 26. As part of a healthy eating pattern carbohydrates should make up about 45% to 65% of energy intake. The recommended dietary intake is provide in Table 92-2. For patients unable to consume food orally, a source of carbohydrate can be provided enterally or parenterally. In the section below are listed only those sugars that are used in medicine as aliments. Some of the carbohydrates also have important uses as pharmaceutical necessities, in parenteral fluids, as diuretics, as osmotic filler for injection of other drugs, etc; consequently, the monographs of certain nutrient carbohydrates may be found elsewhere in this volume.

DEXTROSE—page 1085.
DEXTROSE INJECTION—page 1323.
DEXTROSE AND SODIUM CHLORIDE INJECTION—page 1324.

FRUCTOSE

D(−)-Fructose; Levulose

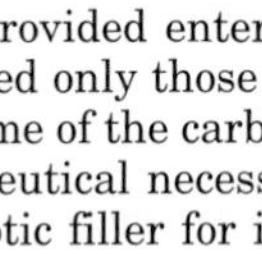

D(−)-Fructose; Levulose

β-D-Fructopyranose

D-Fructose [57-48-7] C$_6$H$_{12}$O$_6$ (180.16); a sugar usually obtained by the inversion of aqueous solutions of sucrose and subsequent separation of fructose from glucose.

Preparation—Sucrose is inverted by treatment with dilute acid at moderate temperature, and the fructose is separated by precipitation of the lime-fructose complex. Fructose is released from the complex with carbon dioxide, which precipitates the calcium as carbonate. After filtering, the fructose solution is purified with activated carbon and ion-exchange resins and evaporated to dryness.

Description—Colorless crystals or a white, crystalline or granular powder, which is odorless and has a sweet taste; specific rotation, −89 to −91°.

Solubility—1 g in about 15 mL alcohol or about 14 mL methanol; freely soluble in water.

Comments—A ketohexose used parenterally as a carbohydrate nutrient. It is converted to liver glycogen and metabolized more rapidly than dextrose, without requiring insulin, and thus may be used in diabetic patients. It is indicated in patients requiring fluid replacement and caloric feeding but contraindicated in hypoglycemia, for which dextrose should be used. It also is contraindicated in patients with hereditary fructose intolerance.

LACTOSE—page 1087.
LIQUID GLUCOSE—page 1086.
SUCROSE—page 1067.
SYRUP—page 1071.

OTHER SUGARS

Invert Sugar

[8013-17-0]—An equimolar mixture of glucose and fructose, produced by hydrolysis of sucrose. Forms clear, colorless solutions with a pH of 3.5 to 6. *Comments:* Instead of dextrose, for parenteral administration of carbohydrate. While it has the same caloric value as dextrose (4 kcal/g), invert sugar is utilized more rapidly and may be administered intravenously twice as fast as dextrose.

LIPIDS AND FATTY ACIDS

Dietary fat provides much of the energy required and is more calorically dense than carbohydrate. Dietary lipids contain predominantly triglycerides, which are made up of 3 fatty acids on a glycerol backbone. There are about 3 dozen fatty acids found in nature that vary in terms of carbon chain length and in degree of saturation. Some fatty acids contribute to increasing chronic disease risk while others may reduce it. Only two fatty acids are considered to be essential—linoleic acid, and α-linolenic acid. As part of a healthy eating pattern, lipids should make up about 20% to 35% of energy intake. The amounts of saturated and trans fatty acids should be limited in preference for unsaturated fatty acids. The ideal amount of monounsaturated, ω-6 or ω-3 polyunsaturated fatty acids required for health continue to be investigated. Besides energy provision, fatty acids play a role in transport, membrane structure and integrity, serving as eicosanoid precursors and in intracellular signaling and gene expression.

In recent years, it has been shown that the digestion and absorption of short- and medium-chain triglycerides (MCTs) are different from those of the long-chain triglycerides that are characteristic of most food fat. The hydrolysis and absorption of MCTs are faster than those of long-chain triglycerides, and it is possible for MCTs to be absorbed directly into the intestinal mucosa without first being hydrolyzed, making it possible to absorb MCTs in the absence of pancreatic juice and bile. MCTs only yield about 7 kcal/g. Coconut oil contains more medium-chain fatty acids than other fats and oils and is used as a source for fractionation and preparation of MCTs. MCTs are commercially available as relatively pure 8-carbon or 10-carbon triglycerides and as a 4:1 mixture. MCTs have been found to be useful in conjunction with the usual therapy in the treatment of diseases such as pancreatic insufficiency, cancer of the pancreas, cystic fibrosis of the pancreas, obstruction of the bile duct, cer-

tain abnormalities in the lymphatic system, regional enteritis, and postoperative cases involving the removal of much of the stomach or small intestine. The most consistent beneficial effects reported from the use of MCTs are a decrease in the fecal loss of fat and less diarrhea. There is commercial interest in continuing to develop triglycerides that contain mixtures of long-chain, medium-chain, and even short-chain fatty acids on the same glycerol backbone (ie, structured triglycerides).

For patients unable to consume food orally, a source of fatty acids can be provided enterally or parenterally.

Intravenous fat emulsions typically contain safflower and/or soybean oil, egg yolk phospholipids, glycerin, and water for injection. The fat particles containing long-chain triglycerides are less than 0.5 μm in diameter, similar in size to naturally occurring chylomicrons. These emulsions are available in 10%, 20%, and 30% products and provide the essential fatty acids. Dosing does not usually exceed 1 g/kg daily. Although not yet available on the US market, intravenous lipid emulsions containing physical mixtures of long-chain and medium-chain triglycerides are available elsewhere. Additionally, use of structured triglycerides for intravenous use continues to be investigated.

Intravenous Fat Emulsion [Liposyn; Intralipid]—*Description:* Water emulsions of 10%, 20%, and 30% using safflower and/or soybean oil; osmolarity of 258–310 mOsm/L; pH 6–9; particle size less than 0.5 μm in diameter. *Comments:* As source of calories and essential fatty acids, usually for patients requiring parenteral nutrition for more than 5 days. The predominant fatty acids in these products are linoleic acid (50–66%) and oleic acid (18–26%), with lesser quantities of several other fatty acids including linolenic acid (4–11%).

CORN OIL—page 1071.
OLIVE OIL—see RPS-19, page 1400.
PEANUT OIL—page 1072.

WATER

Human water requirements are individualized to maintain fluid balance and daily solute load. For the average adult consuming a typical diet and maintaining a moderate activity level a daily dose of 30–40 mL/kg is considered adequate. Recently published DRIs for water and the electrolytes suggest adult AI levels for water of 2.7 L (women) and 3.7 L (men) from foods as well as beverages. While water is most appropriately administered orally with a diet, or through an enteral access device along with an enteral nutrient formulation, some patients require intravenous administration. Options to deliver water intravenously must necessarily take

into consideration physiologic issues. Administration of hypotonic fluid into the vascular space will decrease serum osmolality leading to lysis of cells if severe. For this reason sterile water for injection can only be administered as part of an admixture with an estimated osmolarity closer to the physiologic range. Very specific clinical exceptions exist for the use of hypertonic admixtures. Dextrose-containing intravenous fluid may be used to deliver water (ie, electrolyte-free water).

WATER FOR INJECTION—pages 809 and 1070.
DEXTROSE IN WATER INJECTION—page 1323.

VITAMINS

Vitamins are organic compounds required for normal human growth, development, and maintenance that are unable to be synthesized by anabolic processes. Those with adequate data supporting dietary recommendations are listed in Table 92-4 (fat-soluble) and Table 92-5 (water-soluble). These compounds are effective in small amounts, do not furnish energy, and are not used as building units for the structure of the organism, but are essential for transformation of energy and for regula-

tion of the metabolism of structural units. In addition to protein, carbohydrates, fats, mineral salts, and water, it is essential that the food contain small amounts of these organic substances. If any one of these compounds is lacking in the diet, biochemical alterations result in changes in tissue/organ structure/function that subsequently results in clinical manifestations known as deficiency diseases.

Table 92-4. Dietary Reference Intakes — Fat-Soluble Vitamins

LIFE STAGE GROUP	Vitamin A (μg/d)[1]	Vitamin D (μg/d)[2]	Vitamin E (mg/d)[3]	Vitamin K (μg/d)
Infants				
0-6 months	400*	5*	4*	2*
7-12 months	500*	5*	6*	2.5*
Children				
1-3 years	300	5*	6	30*
4-8 years	400	5*	7	55*
Males				
9-13 years	600	5*	11	60*
14-18 years	900	5*	15	75*
19-30 years	900	5*	15	90*
31-50 years	900	5*	15	90*
51-70 years	900	10*	15	90*
>70 years	900	15*	15	90*
Females				
9-13 years	600	5*	11	60*
14-18 years	700	5*	15	75*
19-30 years	700	5*	15	90*
31-50 years	700	5*	15	90*
51-70 years	700	10*	15	90*
>70 years	700	15*	15	90*
Pregnancy				
≤18 years	750	5*	15	75*
19-30 years	770	5*	15	90*
1531-50 years	770	5*	15	90*
Lactation				
≤18 years	1200	5*	19	75*
19-30 years	1300	5*	19	90*
31-50 years	1300	5*	19	90*

* Adequate Intake Level, otherwise values represent Recommended Dietary Allowances:
[1] As retinol activity equivalents (RAE), 1 μg RAE = 1 μg all-trans retinol or 12 μg β-carotene or 24 μg α-carotene or β-cryptoxanthin
[2] As cholecalciferol, 1 μg = 40 IU vitamin D
[3] As α-tocopherol, including RRR-α-tocopherol and the 2R-stereoisomeric forms, but not the 2S-stereoisomeric forms of α-tocopherol

Table 92-5. Dietary Reference Intakes—Water-Soluble Vitamins

LIFE STAGE GROUP	Thiamine (mg/d)	Riboflavin (mg/d)	Niacin (mg/d)[1]	Vitamin B6 (mg/d)	Folate (μg/d)[2]	Vitamin B12 (μg/d)	Pantothenic Acid (mg/d)	Biotin (μg/d)	Choline (mg/d)	Vitamin C (mg/d)
Infants										
0-6 months	0.2*	0.3*	2*	0.1*	65*	0.4*	1.7*	5*	125*	40*
7-12 months	0.3*	0.4*	4*	0.3*	80*	0.5*	1.8*	6*	150*	50*
Children										
1-3 years	0.5	0.5	6	0.5	150	0.9	2*	8*	200*	15
4-8 years	0.6	0.6	8	0.6	200	1.2	3	12	250*	25
Males										
9-13 years	0.9	0.9	12	1	300	1.8	4*	20*	375*	45
14-18 years	1.2	1.3	16	1.3	400	2.4	5*	25*	550*	75
19-30 years	1.2	1.3	16	1.3	400	2.4	5*	30*	550*	90
31-50 years	1.2	1.3	16	1.3	400	2.4	5*	30*	550*	90
51-70 years	1.2	1.3	16	1.3	400	2.4	5*	30*	550*	90
>70 years	1.2	1.3	16	1.3	400	2.4	5*	30*	550*	90
Females										
9-13 years	0.9	0.9	12	1	300	1.8	4*	20*	375*	45
14-18 years	1	1	14	1.2	400	2.4	5*	25*	400*	65
19-30 years	1.1	1.1	14	1.3	400	2.4	5*	30*	425*	75
31-50 years	1.1	1.1	14	1.3	400	2.4	5*	30*	425*	75
51-70 years	1.1	1.1	14	1.5	400	2.4	5*	30*	425*	75
>70 years	1.1	1.1	14	1.5	400	2.4	5*	30*	425*	75
Pregnancy										
≤18 years	1.4	1.4	18	1.9	600	2.6	6*	30*	450*	80
19-30 years	1.4	1.4	18	1.9	600	2.6	6*	30*	450*	85
31-50 years	1.4	1.4	18	1.9	600	2.6	6*	30*	450*	85
Lactation										
18 years	1.4	1.6	17	2	500	2.8	7*	35*	550*	115
19-30 years	1.4	1.6	17	2	500	2.8	7*	35*	550*	120
31-50 years	1.4	1.6	17	2	500	2.8	7*	35*	550*	120

* Adequate Intake Level, otherwise values represent Recommended Dietary Allowances
[1] As niacin equivalents, 1 mg niacin = 60 mg tryptophan
[2] As dietary folate equivalents (DFE), 1 μg DFE = 1 μg food folate = 0.6 μg folic acid consumed with food = 0.5 μg folic acid supplement taken on an empty stomach

Vitamins are unlike each other in chemical composition and function. They are alike only in that they cannot be synthesized at all or at least not at an adequate rate in human tissues. The functions they serve fall into two categories, the maintenance of normal structure and of normal metabolic functions.

It is convenient in a discussion of this subject to divide these nutritional substances into two groups, the *fat-soluble* and the *water-soluble factors*, although a more clinical distinction is needed (eg, therapeutic index). Vitamins A, D, E, and K fall into the fat-soluble group, since they can be extracted with fat solvents and are found in the fat fractions of tissues. The water-soluble vitamins include ascorbic acid and the B group of vitamins, which consists of some 10 or more well-defined compounds. The characterization of vitamins as essential metabolic factors with discrete chemical structures required their isolation in pure form from natural sources and subsequent laboratory synthesis. Commercial chemical or microbiological syntheses, some from relatively simple compounds, are the source of most of the vitamins now used in pharmaceutical preparations, dietary supplements, and fortified foods.

Vitamin activity or potency has been measured by three principal types of methods: biological, microbiological, and chemical assays.

The status of vitamin methods of assay is now such that manufacturers of vitamin preparations find it possible to state with precision the potency of their products, and tables of vitamin content of foods are, for most vitamins, quite complete. Methods of assay are described briefly in the individual vitamin sections.

In the interest of improvement and uniformity of expressing the results of such assays, the World Health Organization (WHO) of the United Nations has sponsored the preparation and distribution of Standards. The USP provides such reference standards for the US. As a rule, an International Standard is no longer provided once the substance responsible for its characteristic activity has been isolated, identified, and made readily available. Availability of the vitamins in pure form encouraged transition from the use of International Units to the use of weight in expressing amounts present in vitamin products, although the FDA has yet to implement this for labeling provisions.

The Fat-Soluble Vitamins

VITAMIN A

Vitamin A was the first fat-soluble vitamin discovered. Animal nutritionists observed growth failures in calves born of cows maintained on wheat or oats alone, whereas whole corn plants supported growth and development of the animals. The vitamin was found to be related to chlorophyll and carotenoid-containing plants. Later study revealed that the vitamin is essential for the maintenance of normal tissue structure and for other important physiological functions such as vision and reproduction.

Chemistry and Assay—Vitamin A is represented primarily by the cyclic polyene alcohol vitamin A_1 (retinol) with an empirical formula of $C_{20}H_{30}O$ and whose four conjugated double bonds in the side chain are in the *trans* arrangement.

Vitamin A (Retinol) (Vitamin A_1)

Other naturally occurring forms have low biological activity and no commercial significance.

Vitamin A_1 is a pale yellow crystalline compound, is soluble in lipid solvents, and has a UV absorption maximum at 328 nm. The vitamin is not readily destroyed by heat but is oxidized easily and is less stable in acid than in alkaline solution. The esters of vitamin A_1 with the fatty acids acetic and palmitic are commercially important, since they are considerably more stable than the alcohol.

An additional source of vitamin A is the carotenoid pigments, the yellow-colored compounds in all chlorophyll-containing plants. At least 10 different carotenoids exhibit provitamin A activity, but only α- and β-carotene and cryptoxanthin are important in animal nutrition, β-carotene being the most important.

β-Carotene

Theoretically one molecule of β-carotene should yield two molecules of vitamin A_1; however, the availability of carotene in foods as sources of vitamin A for humans is low and extremely variable. This utilization efficiency of carotene is generally considered to be 1/12 for humans; that is, 1 μg of β-carotene would have the same biological activity as 0.083 μg of retinol. This conservatively takes into account the decremental effects on carotene utilization of absorption, transport, and tissue conversion to the active vitamin. The conversion of the provitamin to vitamin A occurs primarily in the walls of the small intestine and perhaps to a lesser degree in the liver; conversion is linked to body stores of vitamin A. Like vitamin A_1, the carotenes are soluble in fat solvents, in crystalline form appear deep orange or copper-colored, and have characteristic absorption spectra.

Total synthesis of vitamin A_1 and β-carotene is achieved commercially, vitamin A usually being prepared as the acetate. Concentration of vitamin A from animal fats and fish liver oil is still important. The principal steps in the process are molecular distillation, saponification and crystallization of the distillate, and acylation to the desired ester.

The USP Unit for vitamin A is identical to the International Unit and equals the biological activity of 0.3 μg of the all-trans isomer of retinol. The USP Reference Standard for vitamin A is a 3.7% solution of crystalline vitamin A acetate in cottonseed oil and peanut oil.

Vitamin A can be assayed by direct measurement of its ultraviolet absorption by photometric evaluation of the color reaction with antimony trichloride in chloroform (the Carr-Price reaction), by high-pressure liquid chromatographic separation and ultraviolet and visible spectrometry, or by a biological method based on the resumption of growth of rats when the vitamin activity is added to a vitamin A–deficient diet.

Metabolic Functions—Vitamin A and its metabolites can serve as ligands for several binding proteins and receptors important for transport and effect. Of the known functions of vitamin A in the body, its role in the visual process is established best. The retina of man contains two distinct photoreceptor systems. The rods, which are the structural components of one system, are especially sensitive to light of low intensity. A specific vitamin A aldehyde is essential for the formation of rhodopsin (the high-molecular-weight glycoprotein part of the visual pigment within the rods) and the normal functioning of the retina. By virtue of this relation to the visual process, vitamin A alcohol has been named retinol, and the aldehyde form named retinal. A vitamin A–deficient person has impaired dark adaptation (*night-blindness*).

Vitamin A also participates in the maintenance of the integrity of the epithelial membranes such that normal structures may be substituted by stratified keratinizing epithelium in the eyes, paraocular glands, and respiratory, alimentary, and genitourinary tracts under the stresses of a deficiency. The basal cells do not lose their function under such conditions, however, and are able to be restored to normal when sufficient vitamin A is absorbed. Abnormalities of nerve and connective tissue and of bones are further consequences of a dietary deficiency of the vitamin. In severe deficiency the affected epithelial and connective tissue may become the site of infections because of the cells' reduced resistance to bacterial invasion. This gave rise to the notion that administration of vitamin A was useful in the treatment of skin infections. Both topical and oral vitamin A, and especially vitamin A acid (*trans*-retinoic acid, tretinoin), are prescribed by some physicians to treat acne vulgaris; however, *trans*-retinoic acid has been shown to be equally effective, with less harmful side effects than oral isotretinoin (*cis*-retinoic acid).

There is a growing body of epidemiological data that suggest that foods that are a good source of vitamin A and carotenoids are protective against a variety of epithelial cancers. This association simply may be a result of a chronic vitamin A deficiency, since vitamin A is required for normal cell differentiation of stem cells in epithelial tissue. Also, there is the possibility that the observed protective effect could have been due to other undetected carotenoids, other vitamins, or compounds present in these foods. Some, but not all, animal studies show a positive effect for vitamin A and synthetic retinoids against epithelial cancers of the skin, lung, bladder, and breast.

The common severe deficiency symptoms are increased susceptibility to microbial infections, xerophthalmia and other eye disorders, loss of appetite and weight, and sterility, conditions that require a long time for their development. Although the recommended dietary allowance is no more than 900 µg/day, in a deficiency much greater amounts are indicated. For example, a therapeutic single oral dose range is from 7.5–30 mg for older children and non-pregnant adults.

If large doses of vitamin A are ingested for long periods of time, manifestations of toxicity develop. In the absence of a deficiency, chronic administration of 7.5–15 mg of vitamin A daily induces pathological changes in bone and periosteal tissues, skin and mucous membranes, and liver and changes in behavior. Doses as low as 5.5 mg of a water-dispersed vitamin A preparation daily for 1 to 3 months are reported to be toxic for infants 3 to 6 months of age. Vitamin A toxicity has occurred in infants who were given liver daily for a period of 3 months. Animal studies show that levels as low as four times the requirements increase the incidence of birth defects. Epidemiological studies in humans have indicated that levels as low as 4.5 mg during the first trimester of pregnancy may increase the risk of birth defects.

Dietary Requirement and Food Sources—The current dietary intake requirements for vitamin A for all life-stages can be found in Table 92-4.

About 1/2 of the vitamin A activity in the average American diet comes from β-carotene and related compounds. The other 1/2 is provided by the vitamin itself present in foods of animal origin. Not all of the carotene present in the food eaten is converted into vitamin A. Some passes through the digestive tract and is excreted as such. Of that absorbed, only the amounts necessary to meet requirements are converted to vitamin A. The rest is stored in the body or excreted. Intake of large amounts of carotene frequently causes a yellow-orange color to the skin, which is considered to be harmless. The richest sources of carotene are yellow and green (leafy) vegetables and yellow fruits. Preformed vitamin A_1 is supplied primarily from the fat of dairy products and egg yolk, but other important sources in some diets are liver, kidney, and fish. Federal regulations provide for the optional addition of 4.5 mg of vitamin A per pound of margarine. Almost all margarine is so fortified. There are also provisions for marketing vitamins A- and D–fortified nonfat dry milk containing 150 µg vitamin A and 2.5 µg vitamin D/8 fl oz reconstituted.

VITAMIN A PREPARATIONS

Contains a suitable form of retinol ($C_{20}H_{30}O$; vitamin A alcohol). It may consist of retinol or esters of retinol formed from edible fatty acids, principally acetic and palmitic acids. It may be diluted with edible oils, or it may be incorporated in solid, edible carriers or excipients, and it may contain suitable antimicrobial agents, dispersants, and antioxidants.

Note—In stating the potency and dosage of vitamin A dosage forms µg of retinol is preferred. It was customary to use either the International Unit (IU) or the equivalent USP Unit, where one USP Unit (or International Unit) of vitamin A is defined as the specific biological activity of 0.3 µg of the all-*trans* isomer of retinol.

Description—Yellow to red, oily liquid that may solidify upon refrigeration; in solid form, it has the appearance of any diluent that has been added; may be nearly odorless or may have a fish odor but has no rancid odor or taste; unstable to air and light.

Solubility—In liquid form, insoluble in water or glycerin; soluble in absolute alcohol or vegetable oils; very soluble in ether or chloroform. In solid form, may be dispersible in water.

Comments—The only valid therapeutic uses are in the treatment of vitamin A *deficiency* or in the *prophylaxis* of deficiency in persons with a known dietary deficiency, a high requirement, or an absorption defect. Large doses produce toxicity (see the general statement), symptoms of which may not be evident for 6 months or longer. Daily doses larger than 7500 µg should not be prescribed unless severe deficiency exists.

Vitamin A Acetate [Retinol Acetate; $C_{22}H_{32}O_2$]—Light-yellow to red oil with a slight fishy odor; light and oxygen cause deterioration; tasteless. Soluble in lipid solvents; insoluble in water. *Comments:* A form of vitamin A; 0.344 µg is equivalent to 1 USP Unit or to 0.6 µg of β-carotene.

Vitamin A Palmitate [Retinol Palmitate; $C_{36}H_{60}O_2$]—Light-yellow to red oil; odorless in the pure state but otherwise has a slight fishy odor; unstable in light and air. Soluble in oils and lipid solvents; insoluble in water. *Comments:* A form of vitamin A.

TRETINOIN—pages 1288 and 1585.

VITAMIN D

Vitamin D is the antirachitic vitamin effective in promoting calcification of the bony structures of man. It sometimes is known popularly as the *sunshine* vitamin because it is formed by the action of the sun's ultraviolet rays on precursor sterols in the skin. Exposure to sunlight, therefore, has a powerful antirachitic effect. The term *rachitic* denotes the condition of a person affected with the deficiency disease rickets, in which bone is poorly mineralized and unable to support the weight of the body.

Chemistry and Assay—The two immediate biological precursors (provitamins) of the vitamins D are the steroid alcohols ergosterol (ergosta-5,7,22E-trien-3β-ol) and 7-dehydrocholesterol (cholesta-5,7-dien-3β-ol). Under the influence of UV light, each undergoes scission of the 9(10) bond of the steroid nucleus with the simultaneous creation of a 10(19) double bond yielding, respectively, vitamin D_2 (ergocalciferol) and vitamin D_3 (cholecalciferol).

Vitamin D_2 (Ergocalciferol)
Vitamin D_3 (Cholecalciferol):
same except C_{17} side chain is

Pure vitamins D_2 and D_3 are white, odorless crystals that are soluble in fat solvents such as ether, alcohol, or chloroform but insoluble in water. The compounds have characteristic absorption spectra, useful in their identification. Both forms of the vitamin are stable to oxidation by air and to moderate heat in neutral and alkaline solutions. Upon alkaline saponification of fats, the vitamin appears in the nonsaponifiable fraction. It withstands autoclaving temperatures of 120° in the absence of air but at this temperature is subject to oxidation, and it is destroyed completely by heating at 170°. Vitamin D is stable over long periods of storage in oil solution but is quite unstable in the presence of mineral salts, such as tricalcium phosphate, when compounded in tablet form. It may be stabilized by dispersion in gelatin or a similar protective coating.

The international standard for vitamin D is a crystalline preparation of pure vitamin D_3 assigned a potency of 40 million units/g or 40 units/µg. The USP adopted an equivalent standard of vitamin D_3 with the same assigned potency. The USP unit for vitamin D, therefore, is equivalent to the IU, and USP reference standards exist for both cholecalciferol and ergocalciferol.

The provitamins D are found in both plant and animal tissue; 7-dehydrocholesterol is found principally in animal skin and ergosterol in relatively large amounts in yeasts, although it was first isolated from ergot. The vitamin D that is absorbed through the intestinal wall from dietary sources or that is formed in the skin from 7-dehydrocholesterol enters the circulatory system and excesses are stored. Vitamin D is stored predominantly in the adipose tissue and muscle of man. The liver oils, particularly of fish, are the most potent natural sources of the vitamin. The vitamin D of commerce now is synthesized principally from readily available, structurally related compounds, such as cholesterol, which often are obtained as packing house by-products.

There are three methods for quantitative physicochemical assay of vitamin D. For years, the biological assay based on the curative effects of the vitamin on experimental rickets in young rats has been used to measure the total biological activity of the vitamin in complex materials of low potency. Minimal amounts of the vitamin are needed by the rat; therefore, the rachitic condition is produced by using an extremely low-calcium, low-phosphorus diet. Now the preferred method for minimal amounts is high-pressure liquid chromatography for separation and UV spectrometry. For relatively concentrated solutions of vitamin D in alcohol (but not in oil), UV spectrometric determination is made at the wavelength of maximum absorption. Antimony trichloride reacts with various vitamins D in a Carr-Price reaction to yield a yellow color whose intensity is proportional to the vitamin D present. The reaction is satisfactory only for concentrated preparations; cholesterol and vitamin A interfere only when present in amounts in excess of certain limits.

Metabolic Functions—Both vitamin D_2 (ergocalciferol) and vitamin D_3 (cholecalciferol) are biologically inactive molecules. After absorption, they are converted, primarily in the liver, to 25-hydroxy(OH) D_2 and D_3 (25-OH D_3), respectively, and are the most predominant forms found in the blood. Both of these compounds appear to facilitate phosphate resorption in the renal tubule; however, their most important function is as a precursor of 1,25-$(OH)_2$ calciferol, which is formed in the kidney. This compound is a true hormone, referred to as calcitriol, and is excreted in response to specific stimuli from an organ distal to its target organ. Calcitriol is transported in the blood bound to a protein. There is a rapid turnover of 1,25-$(OH)_2$ calciferol, which depends on vitamin D status (greater turnover if body stores and plasma levels are low). Normal plasma values range from 18 to 60 pg/mL in children and 15 to 45 pg/mL in adults. It is likely that some forms of vitamin D–resistant rickets can be explained by possible genetic inability of the body to produce adequate amounts of either 25-OH calciferol or 1,25—$(OH)_2$ calciferol. Conversely, some children may have an enhanced capacity to convert vitamin D to the more active metabolites and, thereby, manifest a hyperreactivity to amounts of the ingested vitamin very slightly in excess of recommended dietary allowances.

Vitamin D, through the action of these active metabolites on molecular targets via vitamin D receptors, aids in the absorption of calcium from the intestinal tract and the resorption of phosphate in the renal tubule. Vitamin D is necessary for normal growth in children, probably having a direct effect on the osteoblast cells that influence calcification of cartilage in the growing areas of bone. 1,25—$(OH)_2$ calciferol also plays an essential management role in the regulation of various genes important to cell proliferation and lymphokine expression in systems not involved in mineral homeostasis.

A deficiency of vitamin D leads to inadequate absorption of calcium and phosphorus from the intestinal tract and retention of these minerals in the kidney and thence to faulty mineralization of bone structures. The inability of the soft bones to withstand the stress of weight results in skeletal malformations. Early rickets is difficult to diagnose, but fully developed cases in infants and children present characteristic signs. These include delayed closure of the fontanelles and softening of the skull; soft fragile bones with bowing of the legs and spinal curvature; enlargement of wrist, knee, and ankle joints; poorly developed muscles; and restlessness and nervous irritability. A form of *adult rickets* called osteomalacia similarly may occur. It, too, represents a failure of the process of calcification caused by simple vitamin D lack and calcium or phosphorus inadequacy.

With adequate calcium-phosphorus intake, adult osteomalacia and uncomplicated rickets can be cured by the ordinary daily intake of 10 µg of vitamin D. Larger doses (about 40 µg or more daily) are more rapidly effective, the first evidence of improvement—a rise in serum phosphorus—occurring in about 10 days.

Vitamin D has a serious toxic potential. There is a wide range of susceptibility to the toxic effects of vitamin D. Most adults will require more than 1250 µg of vitamin D/day to produce intoxication. However, levels as low as 375 µg/kg for 2 weeks have produced acute toxicity in adults. Long-term consumption of as little as 25 µg/kg may lead to hypercalcemia and attendant complications, such as metastatic calcification and renal calculi in adults, provided there are high levels of calcium in the diet. As little as 50 µg can inhibit linear growth of normal children. In advanced stages, demineralization of bones occurs, and multiple fractures may result from very slight trauma. Chronic excessive intake will result in liver accumulation, and detoxification will take many months. Classic features of vitamin D intoxication are hypercalcaemia, hyperphosphatemia, and impaired renal function. Painful joints and muscle weakness also may occur, which impair mobility.

Dietary Requirement and Food Sources—Requirements for vitamin D vary with the amount of exposure to UV light. Some individuals can obtain their entire requirements by skin irradiation, but age, skin pigment, and other conditions can effect the need for dietary supplies. Current recommendations are included in Table 92-4 and assume limited sun exposure.

Vitamin D is not found naturally in many food sources. Egg yolks, which are the best food source, vary in content from winter to summer depending most upon the content of the vitamin in the hen's diet. Unfortified dairy products contain some vitamin D, but again the potency varies with the season. Varieties of fish, whose muscle tissues contain substantial quantities of oil and fat, may supply an appreciable part of the dietary requirement. The livers of a number of fish, or the oils extracted from the livers, are extremely rich in vitamin D. Addition of vitamin D to appropriate foods has been an important factor in the prevention of any significant incidence of rickets in this country, although deficits of this vitamin do continue to be reported.

The major sources of vitamin D in the diets of most Americans are those foods that have been fortified. Vitamin D–fortified whole milk, nonfat dry milk, and evaporated milk containing 400 IU/qt (or reconstituted quart in the case of nonfat dry milk and evaporated milk) are particularly effective because of their use in infant feeding during the stage of growth most susceptible to rachitic changes. Fortification is accomplished by addition of vitamin D concentrates, mainly in the form of vitamin D_3. Fortification of other foods, such as processed cereals and margarine, is practiced to a limited degree.

VITAMIN D PREPARATIONS

CHOLECALCIFEROL

(3β)-9,10-Secocholesta-5,7,10(19)-trien-3-ol, Vitamin D_3; Activated 7-Dehydrocholesterol

9,10-Secocholesta-5,7,10(19)-trien-3β-ol [67-97-0] $C_{27}H_{44}O$ (384.64); an antirachitic vitamin obtained from natural sources or prepared synthetically.

Description—White, odorless crystals; affected by air and light; melts between 84 and 88°.

Solubility—Insoluble in water; soluble in alcohol, chloroform, or fatty oils.

Comments—The only valid therapeutic (as opposed to dietary) uses are in the *treatment* of vitamin D *deficiency* or in the *prophylaxis* of deficiency in persons with a known deficiency, a high requirement or an absorption defect. However, the substance may be employed to treat *hypocalcemic tetany* and *hypoparathyroidism*. Also, there is a growing medical opinion that it facilitates the prophylaxis of osteoporosis by calcium in postmenopausal women. It should not be employed in the presence of renal insufficiency or hyperphosphatemia.

COD LIVER OIL

Oleum Morrhuae; Oleum Jecoris Aselli; Oleum Gadi

The partially destearinated fixed oil obtained from fresh livers of *Gadus morrhua* Linné and other species of the Family *Gadidae;* contains in each gram not less than 255 µg (850 USP Units) of vitamin A and not less than 2.125 µg (85 USP Units) of vitamin D.

It may be flavored by the addition of not more than 1% of a suitable flavoring substance or a mixture of such substances.

Preparation—The highest grade of this medicinal oil is manufactured from fresh cod livers from healthy fish, removed from the fish within a few hours after they are caught. The oil is separated from the livers by heating with low-pressure steam. When livers of high quality are used and the manufacturing procedure is carried out under carefully controlled sanitary conditions the resulting crude oil is a light yellow color and has good flavor and odor. Such an oil requires no purification or chemical refining.

Due, however, to long-established trade demands, it is necessary to remove the cod liver stearin so that the oil will remain clear at temperatures above freezing. To accomplish this, the oil is chilled to precipitate the stearin, which is removed by pressure filtration. To preserve the natural vitamin content of the oil it should be stored out of contact with air and light, preferably in a cold place.

Constituents—Consists chiefly of unsaturated glycerides but contains *palmitin* and *stearin,* as well as traces of *chlorine, bromine, phosphorus,* and *sulfur.* American cod liver oils may contain as much as 3 ppm of arsenic, but there is little evidence as to how completely it may be assimilated. American cod liver oils are rich in *iodine*—one sample was found to contain nearly 15,000 parts of iodine/billion parts of oil.

The vitamins of this oil occur in the unsaponifiable fraction. Since some persons object to taking oils, tablets and capsules containing the unsaponifiable fraction of the oil are manufactured. In general the procedure consists of saponifying the oil, separating the unsaponifiable portion, and extracting it with suitable solvents. The extract is diluted with corn oil and filled with capsules or mixed with solid materials and manufactured into tablets. The vitamin potency of these preparations can be adjusted to the patient's requirements, but obviously they do not supply the constituents present in the saponifiable portion of the oil from which they were prepared.

Description—Thin, oily liquid, with a characteristic, slightly fishy, but not rancid, odor and a fishy taste; specific gravity, 0.918 to 0.927.

Solubility—Slightly soluble in alcohol; freely soluble in ether, chloroform, carbon disulfide, or ethyl acetate.

Comments—A source of vitamins A and D. The vitamins are present in such proportion that an oral dose of 5 mL can provide a significant portion of the daily requirements for children or adults of both of these dietary essentials. It has been employed in the prophylaxis of rickets in infants.

DIHYDROTACHYSTEROL—page 1458.

ERGOCALCIFEROL

(3β,5Z,7E,22E)-9,10-Secoergosta-5,7,10(19),22-tetraen-3-ol, Calciferol; Vitamin D_2

[50-14-6] $C_{28}H_{44}O$ (396.65). It is obtained by exposing ergosterol to UV light for the proper length of time. Insufficient irradiation results in the production of products with little or no antirachitic activity, and prolonged exposure causes the production of toxic products.

high requirement, and the criterion of activity (blood *prothrombin time*) is readily measurable, but species differences in biological activity are known to occur.

Metabolic Functions, Dietary Requirement, and Food Sources—Vitamin K is necessary for the formation of prothrombinogen and other blood-clotting factors in the liver. During clotting, circulating prothrombin is required for the production of thrombin; in turn, the thrombin converts fibrinogen to fibrin, the network of which constitutes the clot. It is obvious from this description that interference with formation of prothrombin will reduce the clotting tendency of the blood. In a severe deficiency of the vitamin, a condition of hypoprothrombinemia occurs, and blood-clotting time may be prolonged greatly or even indefinitely. Internal or external hemorrhages may ensue, either spontaneously or following injury or surgery. Other vitamin K-dependent proteins, including osteocalcin and matrix gla protein, have been identified in bone.

A group of substances termed vitamin K antagonists are characterized by their property to decrease plasma prothrombin levels and their usefulness in medicine as anticoagulants. Representative of this group is dicumarol, originally isolated from spoiled sweet clover hay, in which it is formed by bacterial action on coumarin. An important use of vitamin K is in the treatment of hypoprothrombinemia consequent to prothrombopenic anticoagulant therapy. Vitamin K_1 is the preferred form. Large doses of salicylates also antagonize vitamin K.

Optimal absorption of vitamins K requires the presence of bile or bile salts in the intestine. Menadione, the synthetic water-soluble analog, is absorbed easily in the absence of bile. The average diet apparently contains adequate amounts of vitamin K_1, since few if any malnourished humans have presented findings of dietary lack of vitamin K uncomplicated by intestinal disease, which prevents absorption. Current dietary recommendations are listed in Table 92-4.

The premature infant appears to be particularly sensitive to a lack of the vitamin and to an excess in the case of menadione. Because of this potential toxicity, the inclusion of menadione in OTC dietary supplements for the pregnant women is prohibited. Vitamin K_1 does not exhibit this toxicity and is the preferred form. For newborn infants and especially those born prematurely (and anoxic), a single dose of 1 mg of vitamin K_1, immediately after birth, is often a routine measure to prevent hemorrhagic disease. Vitamin K_1 may be administered to the mother 12 to 24 hr prior to the expected delivery or at the first sign of labor, especially if the mother has been receiving prothrombopenic anticoagulants. Requirements normally decrease after the neonatal period; however, it is important to ensure that adequate amounts of vitamin K_1 are present in infant formulas, since these are likely to be the sole nutriment during this period. Milk-substitute formulas containing less than 4 µg/100 kcal are required to have vitamin K_1 added to attain the level of 4 µg/100 kcal required by infant formula regulations.

Although extensive measurements of dietary intakes and food content of vitamin K_1 have not been made, primarily because suitable analytical methods have not been developed, most diets contain sufficient amounts as evident by adequate body stores for a very high proportion of the population. The green, leafy vegetables, tomatoes, cauliflower, egg yolk, soybean oil, and liver of all kinds are good sources. Since it is insoluble in water, there is no loss in ordinary cooking. The human may use to a limited extent vitamin K synthesized by certain enteric bacteria.

VITAMIN K PREPARATIONS

MENADIOL SODIUM DIPHOSPHATE

1,4-Naphthalenediol, 2-methyl-, bis(dihydrogen phosphate), tetrasodium salt, hexahydrate; Kappadione; Synkavite

2-Methyl-1,4-naphthalenediol bis(dihydrogen phosphate) tetrasodium salt, hexahydrate [6700-42-1] $C_{11}H_8Na_4O_8P_2$·6H$_2$O (530.18); *anhydrous* [131-13-5] (422.09).

Preparation—Reduction of menadione to the diol compound by treatment with zinc in the presence of acid, followed by double esterification with HI, metathesis of the resulting 1,4-diiodo compound with AgH$_2$PO$_4$, and neutralization of the bis(dihydrogen phosphate) ester thus formed with NaOH.

Description—White to pink powder, with a characteristic odor; hygroscopic; solutions are neutral or slightly alkaline to litmus, pH about 8.

Solubility—Very soluble in water; insoluble in alcohol.

Comments—See *Phytonadione*. In the body it is converted to menadione, and consequently, it has the same uses and limitations, except that it is water-soluble and does not require the presence of bile salts for its absorption; therefore, it is especially useful in the presence of biliary obstruction.

PHYTONADIONE

R-[*R**,*R**(*E*)]]-1,4-Naphthalenedione, 2-methyl-3-(3,7,11,15-tetramethyl-2-hexadecenyl)-, 2-Methyl-3-phytyl-1,4-naphthoquinone; Vitamin K_1; Mephyton

Phylloquinone [84-80-0] $C_{31}H_{46}O_2$ (450.70). It is a mixture of *cis*- and *trans*-isomers; it contains not more than 20.0% of the *cis*-isomer.

Description—Clear, yellow to amber, very viscous, odorless or nearly odorless liquid; specific gravity about 0.967; stable in air but decomposes on exposure to sunlight; solution (1 in 20) in alcohol is neutral to litmus; refractive index, 1.523 to 1.526 at 25°.

Solubility—Insoluble in water; soluble in dehydrated alcohol, benzene, chloroform, ether, or vegetable oils.

Comments—The natural product, vitamin K_1. For the metabolic functions of vitamin K, see the general statement.

It has a more prompt and prolonged action than menadiol and other synthetic analogs of vitamin K, and it is more reliable in restoring prothrombin to the blood in conditions of *hypoprothrombinemia. Hypoprothrombinemia in the newborn* may be prevented or treated by the administration of phytonadione to the mother shortly before parturition or by giving the infant a single dose shortly after birth. In *hypoprothrombinemia consequent to prothrombopenic anticoagulant therapy,* an adequate intravenous injection usually will stop hemorrhage within 3 to 4 hr and restore the plasma prothrombin level to normal in 12 to 24 hr. In hypoprothrombinemia resulting from liver disease it may have limited value, especially if the disease is hepatocellular; in *biliary obstruction or fistula,* in which only the absorption of vitamin K is impaired, hypoprothrombinemia responds promptly to parenteral phytonadione. In other enteric diseases in which absorption is defective—as in *sprue, regional enteritis, enterocolitis, ulcerative colitis, dysentery, extensive bowel resection, and other causes of intestinal failure*—it will correct hypoprothrombinemia if given parenterally.

It must be emphasized that it cannot be used to check bleeding irrespective of its origin. It is of no benefit in diseases of the blood-forming organs, thrombocytopenic purpura, hemophilia, etc.

The Water-Soluble Vitamins

Except for ascorbic acid, all the vitamins in this category belong to the B-group of vitamins. Some still retain their original individual designations, such as B_6, and B_{12}, whereas comparable names for other vitamins have become obsolete.

In 1930, when it was clear that vitamin B was of multiple nature, the term vitamin B complex was coined to refer to the group of water-soluble animal growth factors found in relatively high concentrations in such products as liver, yeast, and rice bran. This was a convenient term to use in the early scientific literature, but it was not intended to be a specific name for pharmaceutical preparations that contain varying proportions of the B vitamins. The term was intended to apply to a group of vitamins whose identity was still being sought, rather than to a group of compounds whose identity had been established. Since the nature of the *complex* has been characterized, the term vitamin B complex is no longer appropriate.

Ascorbic Acid (Vitamin C)

Vitamin C, or ascorbic acid (antiscorbutic vitamin), is necessary for the prevention and cure of the deficiency disease scurvy.

Scurvy has been recognized since the Middle Ages and was found widespread in northern Europe and among the crews of sailing ships. During the 18th century it was learned that when fresh fruit was made available aboard sailing vessels, scurvy was avoided. In 1907 Holst and Frolich observed a scurvy-like syndrome in guinea pigs that was similar to human scurvy and cured it by feeding citrus juices. This gave an experimental means for the rapid development of our knowledge of vitamin C, to which many workers have contributed.

Chemistry and Assay—Ascorbic acid is a white, crystalline compound structurally related to the monosaccharides. It exists in nature in both a reduced and the oxidized form, dehydroascorbic acid. These substances are in a state of reversible equilibrium in biological systems, and both have the same biological activity.

L-Ascorbic Acid   **Dehydroascorbic Acid**

Ascorbic acid is stable in the dry state but is easily oxidized in aqueous solution in the presence of air. Oxidation is accelerated by heat, light, alkalies, oxidative enzymes, and traces of copper and iron. Because of its relative instability, ascorbic acid is readily lost during cooking if simple precautions to avoid aeration are not taken. Also, because of its high aqueous solubility, the vitamin is lost to a considerable extent when large amounts of cooking water are discarded. Progressive loss of vitamin C in fresh fruits and vegetables occurs during storage.

Solutions of ascorbic acid are strongly reducing, and the vitamin is oxidized easily. In animal tissues the greater part of the vitamin is in the reduced form, but as scurvy develops, the ratio of oxidized to reduced form rises. This property of reversible oxidation-reduction is the most likely basis for the role of the vitamin in biochemical reactions.

The article of commerce is produced exclusively by synthesis. Sorbitol, a hexose occurring in several fruits but commercially obtained by hydrogenating dextrose, is the raw material for production of ascorbic acid. Amounts of ascorbic acid are expressed in terms of weight, as milligrams. The USP provides a Reference Standard of L-ascorbic acid for assay purposes. The practical methods of ascorbic acid assay are based on its powerful reducing properties, which enable determination by oxidimetric titration. The three most-used reagents for this titration are chloramine-T, 2,6-dichlorophenolindophenol, and iodine. Another practical assay is based on the conversion of ascorbic acid to oxalic acid 2-nitrophenylhydrazide by treatment with diazotized 2-nitroaniline. This yields a colored compound that is measured photometrically. Still another is the photometric assay of total ascorbic acid (ascorbic acid plus dehydroascorbic acid) by conversion of the vitamin to its 2,4-dinitrophenylhydrazone.

Metabolic Function, Dietary Requirement, and Food Sources—Vitamin C is known to be essential for the formation of intercellular collagen. In scorbutic tissues the amorphous ground substance and the fibroblasts in the area between the cells appear normal but without the matrix of collagen fibers. These bundles of collagenous material appear within a few hours after the administration of ascorbic acid. This points to the relationship of the vitamin in maintenance of tooth structures, matrix of bone, and the walls of capillaries. In scurvy, these are the tissues found to be faulty.

The picture of clinical scurvy in humans is one that can be related to the general breakdown of intercellular collagen substance. Bleeding is common, particularly at sites of pressure. The occurrence of petechiae, pinpoint hemorrhages that occur in the skin under reduced pressure, has been used as a diagnosis of scurvy. This is an indication of weakness or fragility of the walls of capillaries. Bones become brittle and cease to grow, and normal structures are replaced by connective tissue that contains calcified cartilage. Anemia is a common occurrence in scurvy, caused by an impairment of hematopoiesis. Also, vitamin C has been shown to change iron absorption. Tooth enamel, cementum, and particularly dentin change in structure, and the gums about the teeth become spongy and bleed easily. Keratoconjunctivitis sicca, xerostomia, salivary gland enlargement, xerosis, hyperpigmentation, ichthyosis, neuropathies, and mental depression may occur, even when the full-blown picture of scurvy is absent.

Vitamin C is essential for the healing of bone fractures. Such fractures heal slowly in a patient deficient in vitamin C. Wound-healing also is impaired.

There is evidence to indicate that the vitamin functions in the metabolism of tyrosine. There is an abnormal excretion of homogentisic, p-hydroxyphenylpyruvic, and p-hydroxyphenyllactic acids in scorbutic guinea pigs following administration of tyrosine, which, of course, is corrected with ascorbic acid. The excretion of tyrosyl derivatives in humans on a low–vitamin C diet given 20 g of tyrosine daily also is affected by ascorbic acid administration. In some newborns, the occurrence of tyrosinemia possibly accruing to high protein intakes suggests that this relationship be taken into consideration in evaluating the ascorbic acid requirement for the infant.

An intake of 10 to 20 mg a day of ascorbic acid is sufficient to protect an adult from classical scurvy, and 45 mg a day will maintain an adequate body pool of 1500 mg. The current dietary recommendations are provided in Table 92-5. Smokers likely require an additional 35 mg daily. The vitamin C requirements are increased following trauma, during infections, and during periods of vigorous physical activity; in such circumstances the requirement may be 100 to 200 mg a day.

The regular ingestion of 1 g or more of ascorbic acid a day has been suggested as a means of shortening the illness period and alleviating the symptoms of the *common cold* and other disorders but is not fully supported by the evidence.

A number of epidemiological studies show a protective association between the consumption of foods that contain vitamin C and cancers of the esophagus, stomach, and cervix. Animal studies testing precursors of known carcinogens showed a reduced number of tumors when the animals were given vitamin C. Biochemical studies suggest that vitamin C blocks the formation of active carcinogens from precursors. There is also the hypothesis that vitamin C has an effect as a free radial scavenger. Although vitamin C in large amounts may have some pharmacological effects, these are not related to the normal functioning of the vitamin at nutritional levels. There is no evidence that levels exceeding the recommended amount have any additional benefit, and contrary to those who advocate the use of megadose quantities (gram quantities), such practices can be harmful to some individuals.

The prolonged ingestion of supplements of ascorbic acid in excess of about 2 g a day (the upper tolerable intake level) is not without potential danger. GI disturbances (nausea followed by diarrhea), kidney or bladder stone formation (resulting from an increased excretion of oxalate, urate, and calcium), prenatal conditioning of the fetus to deficiency symptoms, interference with simple tests for glycosuria, and interference with the anticoagulant effect of heparin are clinical problems that may occur.

For therapeutic purposes in treatment of adult scurvy, 1000 mg of ascorbic acid a day, in divided doses, for 1 week is recommended, then 500 mg until all signs disappear. It also is used in the treatment of idiopathic methemoglobinemia to reduce the ferric iron in heme to the ferrous state.

Ascorbic acid facilitates the absorption of dietary iron by keeping the iron in the reduced form. A few microcytic anemias respond to ascorbic acid treatment, which may be in part due to improved absorption of iron.

Vitamin C is found in all living plant cells, is synthesized during the germination of seeds, and is concentrated relatively in the rapidly growing parts of the plant. It is present in all animal tissues as well, but only guinea pigs, primates, a few exotic animal species and humans are unable to meet body needs by synthesis and must rely upon a dietary source.

Although vitamin C appears to be present in all living tissues, our best sources of supply are fresh fruits such as citrus fruits, strawberries, and melons and green vegetables such as lettuce and cabbage. An average serving of potatoes contains enough vitamin C when first harvested to meet the adult RDA, but contains only half that amount by the following spring. It is a common practice, and a sound one, to rely to a large extent on citrus fruits and juices as important vitamin C carriers, particularly in infant feeding. An ounce of orange or lemon juice a day is sufficient to prevent scurvy in humans on an otherwise low–vitamin C diet.

It is fairly common practice to add ascorbic acid to foods for technical purposes; eg, as an antioxidant to protect natural flavors and colors.

VITAMIN C PREPARATIONS

L-Ascorbic acid [50-81-7] $C_6H_8O_6$ (176.13).

Preparation—The article in commerce is produced exclusively by synthesis. Sorbitol, a hexose sugar, occurring in several fruits but commercially obtained by hydrogenating dextrose in the presence of a Cu-Cr catalyst, is the raw material for the production of ascorbic acid. The D-sorbitol in aqueous solution is converted by the action of the organism *Acetobacter suboxydans* to L-sorbose, which is a ketose. The L-sorbose then is condensed with acetone by means of sulfuric acid to form diacetone sorbose. The object of the acetonation is to protect the hydroxyl group from oxidation in the subsequent steps. The diacetone sorbose, after suitable purification, is oxidized by potassium permanganate and then hydrolyzed, forming 2 keto-L-gulonic acid. This acid is esterified with methanol, and an intermediate sodio compound is formed with sodium methoxide. Hydrolysis with aqueous HCl removes the methyl group and sodium and lactonizes it to form ascorbic acid. The process is illustrated as follows:

CHO — D-Glucose → (H₂) CH₂OH — D-Sorbitol → (A Sub-oxydans) CH₂OH — L-Sorbose

$$\text{D-Glucose} \xrightarrow{H_2} \text{D-Sorbitol} \xrightarrow{A\ Sub\text{-}oxydans} \text{L-Sorbose}$$

Diacetone L-Sorbose

2-Keto-L-gulonic Acid

$$\text{2-Keto-L-gulonic Acid} \xrightarrow[\text{then } CH_3ONa]{CH_3OH + HCl} \xrightarrow{HCl} \text{L-Ascorbic Acid}$$

Description—White or slightly yellow crystals or powder; odorless and on exposure to light gradually darkens; in the dry state, reasonably stable in air, but in solution rapidly deteriorates in the presence of air; melts at about 190°; specific rotation (1 in 10 aqueous solution) between +20.5 and +21.5°; aqueous solution has the acidic properties of a monobasic acid, and it forms salts with metallic ions. pK_a 4.2 and 11.6.

Solubility—1 g in about 3 mL water or 40 mL alcohol; insoluble in chloroform, ether, or benzene.

Incompatibilities—Stable in the dry state but in solution oxidizes rapidly in the presence of air. The reaction is accelerated by *alkalies and certain metals,* especially *copper;* it is retarded by acids. Aqueous solutions are strongly acidic, with a pH of 2 to 3.

Comments—It is sometimes given orally with iron salts in the treatment of iron-deficiency anemia; it functions to keep the iron in the ferrous state and hence to improve absorption. Apart from coadministration of vitamin C and iron preparations, a few cases of hypochromic anemia improve upon increasing the intake of vitamin. For additional information, see the general statement on *Ascorbic Acid.*

It also is used as a urinary-acidifier to enhance the effectiveness of methenamide by lowering the pH of the urine and thus aiding in the formation of formaldehyde.

The effect of megadoses (10 or more times the RDA) has not been proved, and large overdoses should be discouraged.

Numerous, unapproved uses for ascorbic acid have been claimed, such as in the prevention and treatment of cancer, for infections of the gingiva, hemorrhagic states, mental depression, dental caries, acne, collagen disorders, ulcers of the skin, hay fever, and the common cold.

No more than the RDA should be given to the pregnant woman; the metabolism of the fetus adapts to high levels of the vitamin, and scurvy may develop after birth when the intake drops to normal levels.

SODIUM ASCORBATE

L-Ascorbic acid, monosodium salt; Cevalin

Monosodium L-ascorbate [134-03-2] $C_6H_7NaO_6$ (198.11).

Description—White or very faintly yellow crystals, or crystalline powder; odorless or practically odorless; relatively stable in air; on exposure to light it gradually darkens; pH (1 in 10 solution) between 7.5 and 8.

Solubility—1 g in 1.3 mL of water; very slightly soluble in alcohol; insoluble in chloroform or ether.

Comments—A pharmaceutical necessity for *Decavitamin Capsules* and *Decavitamin Tablets.* It also is used as an antioxidant in fruit and vegetable canning and in the processing of meat.

THE B VITAMINS

The *water-soluble B* of McCollum, or the *antiberiberi vitamine* of Funk, has now been differentiated into at least 11 separate and distinct chemical entities. It has been established that 8 of these are required in human nutrition. They are thiamine, riboflavin, niacin, folic acid, pyridoxine, vitamin B_{12}, biotin, pantothenic acid, and choline. When the dietary intake of methionine is adequate, choline can be synthesized endogenously; therefore, the human requirement is relative to the methionine intake, similar to the relationship between niacin and tryptophan. *p*-Aminobenzoic acid, and inositol have an essential part in cellular metabolism in plants and animals, but this alone does not constitute presumptive evidence of their importance in human nutrition. It can be stated categorically that the human does not require either an exogenous or endogenous source of *p*-aminobenzoic acid. Although inositol deficiency has not been demonstrated in humans, it may be an important nutrient in infant nutrition. Mammalian milk contains inositol, and since milk is the sole item of the diet of infants during this critical growth period, it is appropriate to include it in non-milk-based formulas, a practice that has existed since the early 1960s.

There is no one natural source of the B vitamins as a group that is necessarily superior to another source. No natural source contains all the water-soluble factors in the proportions that are needed in human nutrition, and the therapeutic value of any vitamin-containing material depends on the needs of the individual to whom it is being administered. Nevertheless, multiple deficiencies of B vitamins often coexist. Furthermore, the repair of one B-vitamin deficiency may increase the need for another; thus, the administration of thiamine in clinical or subclinical beriberi increases the need for riboflavin. Consequently, there is some justification for multivitamin therapy with those five B vitamins for which clinical deficiencies occur (thiamine, niacin, riboflavin, folic acid, and vitamin B_{12}). Human deficiencies in biotin and pantothenic acid have only been produced experimentally, and pyridoxine deficiency has occurred in infants fed an unfortified formula.

Biotin

cis-Hexahydro-2-oxothieno[3,4-d]imidazole-4-valeric acid

Before this nutritional factor was identified as a discrete chemical substance, it variously was called vitamin H, anti-egg-white injury factor, coenzyme R, Bios II, and others. Its discovery was an outgrowth of studies on the *toxicity* of large amounts of unheated egg white as the sole source of protein for rats.

Chemistry and Assay—Biotin is a colorless, crystalline, monocarboxylic acid, only slightly soluble in water or alcohol (its salts are quite soluble). Water solutions are stable at 100°, and the dry substance is both thermostable and photostable. Biotin is unstable, however, in strong acids and alkaline solutions and in oxidizing agents. The vitamin is optically active, and the natural isomer, which alone possesses biological activity, is the D-form (rings are *cis*-fused and the isomer is designated (+)-biotin).

HOOC(CH₂)₄— **Biotin**

Although biotin with the above structure is the compound present in food sources, the sulfur atom can be replaced with an oxygen atom without reduction in its metabolic activity. Biotin occurs in animal and plant tissues primarily in combined forms that are liberated by enzymatic hydrolysis during digestion. One of the simplest such complexes is biocytin, ε-*N*-biotinyl-L-lysine. The amount of the vitamin in a product is expressed solely in terms of the weight of the chemically pure substance, the free monocarboxylic acid.

Only microbiological methods are feasible for the quantitative assay of biotin because of their sensitivity to the low concentrations usually encountered. After simple aqueous or acid extraction combined with heating, a microbiological assay using growth of the test organisms *Allescheria boydii* or *Lactobacillus arabinosus* as the criterion is carried out.

Metabolic Functions, Dietary Requirement, and Food Sources—Attempts to induce deficiency in man by inclusion of large amounts (200 g) of dried unheated egg white for several days in the diet have resulted in the appearance of vague symptoms such as change in skin color and dermatoses, slight change in lingual papillae of the tongue, muscle pains, loss of appetite, sleeplessness, and extreme lassitude. Raw egg white contains a protein, avidin, which combines with biotin and prevents absorption of the vitamin from the intestine. Rapid relief from such symptoms was observed with administration of biotin. This condition is difficult to produce in human subjects, and since a frank and specific deficiency disease is not discernible, there is uncertainty as to the exact nature of the deficiency syndrome as well as the need for a dietary source of biotin in human nutrition. Intestinal synthesis is undoubtedly an important factor in the supply of biotin to the body.

Biotin functions in carbon dioxide fixation reactions in intermediary metabolism, transferring the carboxyl group to acceptor molecules. It similarly acts also in decarboxylation reactions. For its part in these vital enzymatic steps, in catalyzing deamination of amino acids and in oleic acid synthesis, biotin is essential in human metabolism and presumed to be a dietary essential in the absence of adequate microbial synthesis in the intestine.

Diets providing a daily intake of 150 to 300 μg of biotin are considered adequate. The current dietary requirements are found in Table 92-5. These amounts are readily met and exceeded when milk, meat, and eggs are frequent items of the diet.

Choline

Although it is synthesized in the human body, choline plays an important role both as a structural component of tissues and in biological methylation reactions. Dietary deficiency of it leads to gross pathology in several species of animals.

Chemistry—Choline is (β-hydroxyethyl)trimethylammonium hydroxide. Since it is completely dissociated, it is comparable to alkali hydroxides as a base. Consequently, it does not exist as a base at body pH but rather as a salt; the anion is that present in its immediate biological environment. The β-(hydroxyethyl)trimethylammonium cation is the biologically important moiety. The cation is incorporated into phospholipids, such as lecithin and sphingomyelin, and acetylcholine, a substance released at cholinergic nerve junctions during transmission of nerve impulses. Acid hydrolysis of phospholipids yields the free choline salt, which is very soluble in water and to a lesser extent in ethanol. Assay for choline is accomplished with a microbiological method using a mutant strain of *Neurospora*.

$$\left[\text{HOCH}_2\text{CH}_2\!-\!\overset{\displaystyle \text{CH}_3}{\underset{\displaystyle \text{CH}_3}{\overset{|}{\underset{|}{\text{N}}}}}{}^{+}\!\!-\!\text{CH}_3 \right] \text{OH}^-$$

Choline

Metabolic Functions, Dietary Requirement, and Food Sources—Besides its vital function as a precursor of acetylcholine, which is important in the sequence of nerve-muscle stimulations, choline is an important contributor of methyl groups needed for the *in vivo* synthesis of metabolites and perhaps some hormones. The biogenesis of choline appears to be universal in nature and is the result of the three-step transfer of methyl groups to an acceptor, which may be either free aminoethanol or phosphatidyl aminoethanol. Such transfers require methionine as a methyl donor (actually, *S*-adenosylmethionine). Choline is indirectly a source of methyl groups; it is first oxidized to betaine, which then may transfer a methyl group to homocysteine to form methionine. By thus regenerating methionine lost in transmethylation reactions, exogenous choline can spare the amino acid for use in protein synthesis. Methionine is an essential amino acid.

Choline has the property of preventing the deposition of excess fat or of causing the removal of excess fat from the liver of experimental animals fed high-fat diets and, because of this, it is often classified as a *lipotropic agent*. The lipotropic action probably relates to the incorporation of choline into phosphatidylcholine (lecithin), which, in turn, is incorporated into phospholipids and lipoproteins. The lipotropic action is independent of the function of choline as a reservoir of methyl groups.

There is presumptive evidence from nutritional and metabolic studies and teleological considerations that choline is important, if not essential, for the infant. It is appropriate to ensure, therefore, that choline is present in infant formulas at least to the level found in human milk. This is about 90 mg/L. Most infant formulas contain about 1 1/2 times this amount. It is equally appropriate to include choline in chemically defined diets to be used as the sole source of nutrients for critically ill patients.

An average mixed diet consumed by man in the US has been estimated to contain 500 to 900 mg of choline a day, an amount known to be adequate when compared with animal requirements. Current requirements for choline are listed in Table 92-5. Foods that supply large amounts of choline are liver, kidney, brain, muscle meats, fish, nuts, beans, peas, and eggs. Moderate amounts exist in cereals, milk, and a number of vegetables.

CHOLINE PREPARATIONS

Choline Bitartrate [(2-Hydroxyethyl)trimethylammonium Bitartrate; [87-67-2] $C_9H_{19}NO_7$ (253.25)]—*Preparation:* See *Choline Chloride,* below. *Description and Solubility:* A white, hygroscopic, crystalline powder with an acidic taste; odorless or may have a faint trimethylamine-like odor. Freely soluble in water, slightly soluble in alcohol, and insoluble in benzene, chloroform, or ether. *Comments:* As a nutrient or dietary supplement.

Choline Chloride [(2-Hydroxyethyl)trimethylammonium chloride; [67-48-1] $C_5H_{14}ClNO$ (139.62)]—*Preparation:* For the preparation of choline, see *Choline Dihydrogen Citrate. Description and Solubility:* White, deliquescent crystals; a 10% aqueous solution has a pH of about 4.7. Very soluble in water or alcohol. *Comments:* The salt is used to reduce fatty infiltration of the liver and thus supposedly to prevent degeneration and cirrhosis. Such infiltration may occur after exposure to certain chemical intoxicants, such as carbon tetrachloride, chloroform, and various other halogenated hydrocarbons (including several general anesthetics), divinyl ether, etc. Moderate-to-severe ethanol intoxication and habitual ingestion of ethanol also predispose to fatty infiltration of the liver. Patients who are acutely ill and cannot eat or persons on a high-fat diet frequently develop fatty livers, for which this vitamin may be given. In none of these conditions has there been clearly demonstrable efficacy. Furthermore, a high-protein diet, especially one that includes eggs, meat, liver, and milk, not only provides some of this vitamin but also methionine, which promotes the endogenous synthesis of *Choline*. Once cirrhosis occurs, it is probably too late for any possible benefits. There is no evidence that it is helpful in infectious hepatitis. For the above reasons, there is no longer any official preparation of it. Since the anion is irrelevant to the metabolic effects, the chloride is neither superior nor inferior to other salts. Its value in patients requiring long-term parenteral nutrition is being evaluated.

Choline Dihydrogen Citrate [(2-Hydroxyethyl)trimethylammonium Dihydrogen Citrate; [77-91-8] $C_{11}H_{21}NO_8$ (295.29)]—*Preparation:* By treating aqueous trimethylamine with ethylene oxide. Conversion to the dihydrogen citrate is conveniently effected by dissolving the base in a suitable solvent such as ethanol and treating with an equimolar portion of citric acid. *Description and Solubility:* Colorless, translucent crystals, or a white, granular to fine, crystalline powder; odorless or may have a faint trimethylamine odor and has an acidic taste; hygroscopic when exposed to air; melts between 103 and 107.5°; 1 g dissolves in 1 mL water or 42 mL alcohol; very slightly soluble in ether, chloroform, or benzene. *Comments:* See *Choline Chloride,* above.

Folic Acid

The vitamin derives its name from the Latin word *folium,* leaf. It was first isolated from spinach leaves where it is now known to occur in relatively minute amounts compared with other food sources. Several apparently unrelated factors had been isolated in various laboratories before realization that they had in common the same parent compound, pteroyl-L-glutamic acid: Factor U (a chick growth factor), vitamin M (a factor for monkeys), vitamin B_c (a chick antianemia factor), liver and yeast *L casei* factors (bacterial growth factors), and others., Folates found in nature may contain numerous glutamate residues and may exist in a number of reduced forms, but folic acid refers specifically to pteroyl-mono-glutamate. The term folate is used to describe all the aforementioned compounds. However, the USP continues to call pteroylglutamic acid by the descriptor folic acid, and medical and biochemical practice usually does the same.

Chemistry and Assay—Pteroylglutamic acid crystallizes from cold water, in which it is only slightly soluble, as yellow spear-shaped platelets. It is readily destroyed by boiling in acid solution, and its solutions will deteriorate in sunlight. It is insoluble in alcohol or the usual organic solvents but readily dissolves in dilute solutions of alkali hydroxides and carbonates. The characteristic UV absorption spectrum of pteroylglutamic acid in dilute NaOH is used to aid in identification and measurement of the compound.

A series of compounds with several molecules of glutamic acid attached to the first glutamic acid radical in peptide linkage have been synthesized. Compounds with one, two, three, and seven glutamic acid groups have been isolated. The latter three are known as conjugates. Some animals and man can utilize them as a source of pteroylglutamic acid, presumably because appropriate digestive enzymes can hydrolyze them. Microorganisms can use them to only a variable and limited extent unless they are first hydrolyzed to the free form with liver, kidney, or pancreatic enzymes, called conjugases.

The functional form of this vitamin group is basically the 5,6,7,8-tetrahydrofolic acid in which a formyl group (-CHO), when present, is attached at either or both the N^5 or N^{10} positions. The hydrogenated N^5-formyl compound, formerly called *folinic acid,* or leucovorin, is available, as is the monosodium salt of folic acid, as a discrete pharmaceutical preparation. It properly is termed 5-formyltetrahydrofolic acid. These compounds similarly serve as standards during assay of the vitamin. A USP Reference Standard Folic Acid is available. Separately, the three moieties that make up the folic acid molecule (pteroic acid, *p*-aminobenzoic acid, and glutamic acid) have no vitamin activity.

The quantitative assay of folate in natural products is mainly by biological or microbiological methods. In the chick assay, the birds are placed on a folic acid–free diet until they became anemic, after which folic acid supplements and the test material are administered. The degree of recovery is related to the quantity of reference folic acid fed. The two organisms most used in the microbiological method are *Lactobacillus casei* and *Streptococcus faecalis.* The method is based on the fact that pteroylglutamic acid is a required growth factor for each; however, the assay is complicated when biological material is analyzed, because naturally occurring folic acid derivatives do not all have the same biological activity for the two organisms.

Folic acid can be determined by either of two physicochemical methods, provided the compound is present in relatively pure form. One method is the spectrophotometric measurement of the extinction maxima of the UV absorption curve; the other is the spectrometric measurement after oxidative fission of folic acid to 4-aminobenzoylglutamic acid followed by diazotization and coupling to give an azo dye. Folic acid also can be determined with high-pressure liquid chromatography.

Metabolic Functions—Folic acid is one of the important hematopoietic agents necessary for proper regeneration of the blood-forming elements and their functioning. Although the mechanism whereby folic acid performs this vital role is not understood, much is known about the involvement of folic acid as a coenzyme in intermediary metabolic reactions in which one-carbon units are transferred. These reactions are important in interconversions of various amino acids and in purine and pyrimidine synthesis. This role is in contrast to that of choline in furnishing and transferring so-called labile methyl groups in transmethylation reactions. The biosynthesis of purines and pyrimidines is linked ultimately with that of nucleotides and ribo- and deoxyribonucleic acids, functional elements of all cells.

The concept of antivitamins or vitamin antagonists is exemplified in a particular aspect of folic acid metabolism. By virtue of its structural similarity, sulfanilamide competes with *p*-aminobenzoic acid in the biological synthesis of folic acid. The organism is thus deprived of needed folic acid. Sulfonamides act, therefore, as growth inhibitors of certain pathogenic organisms, a competitive antagonism that is responsible for the antibacterial action of sulfa drugs. Since mammals use preformed folic acid, sulfonamides do not disrupt the host metabolism.

Numerous analogs of pteroylglutamic acid have been prepared that exhibit potent antifolic acid activity. Several compounds, notably aminopterin (4-aminopteroylglutamic acid) and methotrexate (4-amino-N^{10}-methylpteroylglutamic acid), compete with folic acid in nucleic acid synthesis and have been used in the treatment of various cancers, psoriasis, and certain immune disorders. The antimicrobial drugs trimethoprim and pyrimethamine also are antifolate drugs.

Dietary Requirement and Food Sources—Folic acid deficiency results in megaloblastic anemia, glossitis, diarrhea, and weight loss. A deficiency is best diagnosed by reduced levels of folic acid in the serum or red blood cells. The condition of megaloblastic anemia arising as a result of dietary folate deficiency occurs most frequently after the age of 65, in persons suffering from malabsorption syndromes, in women during the last trimester of pregnancy, and in infants receiving unfortified proprietary formulas or goat's milk. In the treatment of megaloblastic or macrocytic anemia, folic acid should be administered as the sole therapy only when the possibility of pernicious anemia and other primary diseases of the small bowel has been excluded absolutely, a restriction necessitated by the vitamin's ability to mask other diagnostic signs of these conditions.

In recent years folic acid has been linked as a possible agent in lowering the risk of rare but serious defects in fetal development of the brain and spinal cord, including spina bifida and anencephaly. These conditions generally are referred to as neural tube defects (NTDs). In some interventional and observational studies in which women of childbearing age were given folic acid supplements, lower levels of NTDs were observed than with placebo controls. It should be noted that these studies were accomplished in areas where the pretreatment rates of NTDs were near or above 2 per 1000 live births, and supplemental levels of folic acid were between 0.4 and 4 mg/day. Also, data obtained for populations in which folic acid intakes were exceedingly low showed no relationship with the rates of NTDs, and therefore, the condition does not appear to be caused by classic folic acid deficiency. Furthermore, research with animals has not shown any increase in NTDs with folic acid–deficient diets.

No mechanism for the observed relationship of folic acid consumption and NTD rates in humans has been proposed. The US Public Health Service has recommended that all women who are capable of becoming pregnant should consume 0.4 mg of folic acid per day throughout their childbearing years for the purpose of reducing their risk of an NTD pregnancy.

The current dietary recommendations for folate intake levels are provided in Table 92-5. Note that they are described in units of dietary folate equivalents (DFE), where 1 µg DFE = 1 µg food folate = 0.6 µg folic acid consumed with food = 0.5 µg folic acid supplement taken on an empty stomach based on differing bioavailability.

A balanced American diet for adults contains approximately 0.2 to 0.6 mg of total folic acid activity, and the intestinal microflora also provide some absorbable amounts of the vitamin. Since 1998 grain products in the US have been fortified with 140 µg folic acid per 100 g of grain. Other food sources of folic acid are liver, kidney, dry beans, asparagus, mushrooms, broccoli, and collards, as well as spinach, peanuts, lima beans, cabbage, sweet corn, chard, turnip greens, lettuce, and milk.

FOLIC ACID PREPARATIONS

L-Glutamic acid, N-[4-[[(2-amino-1,4-dihydro-4-oxo-6-pteridinyl)-methyl]amino]benzoyl]-, PGA; Folacin; Pteroylglutamic Acid; Folvite

N-[*p*-[[(2-Amino-4-hydroxy-6-pteridinyl)methyl]amino]benzoyl]-L-glutamic acid [59-30-3] $C_{19}H_{19}N_7O_6$ (441.40).

Preparation—Commercial syntheses use different processes. In one of these, 2,3-dibromopropionaldehyde, dissolved in a water-miscible organic solvent (alcohol, dioxane), is added to a solution of equal molecular quantities of 2,4,5-triamino-6-hydroxypyrimidine and *p*-aminobenzoylglutamic acid, maintaining a pH of about 4 by the controlled action of alkali as the reaction progresses. The scheme of the reaction is analogous to that described for *Methotrexate,* the only difference being the starting pyrimidine compound.

Description—Yellow or yellowish orange, odorless, crystalline powder.

Solubility—Very slightly soluble in water; insoluble in alcohol, chloroform, or ether; readily dissolves in dilute solutions of alkali hydroxides or carbonates and is soluble in hot diluted hydrochloric or sulfuric acid, forming very pale yellow solutions.

Comments—The only valid therapeutic use is in the treatment of a deficiency of the vitamin or prophylactically in instances in which the folate requirement is increased, as in pregnancy. *Megaloblastic anemias* in which folic acid deficiency occurs may result from malabsorption syndromes, such as *sprue, idiopathic steatorrhea, celiac disease, intestinal reticulosis, regional jejunitis, jejunal diverticulosis, blind loop syndrome, and gastroenterostomy* and from antacid use in the elderly. Megaloblastic anemia of infancy is generally the result of generalized malnutrition, as is nutritional megaloblastic anemia. In all of the above-named megaloblastic anemias vitamin B12 deficiency often coexists, and folic acid, alone, may be inadequate. Pernicious anemia should be ruled out, lest the vitamin mask the disease (see below). In the megaloblastic anemias of nutrient deficiency, a low serum folic acid level is likely. However, in megaloblastic anemias consequent to treatment with pyrimethamine, phenytoin and related substances, or methotrexate, the serum folic acid levels may be normal; the signs of deficiency result from the antimetabolite effects of the drugs, and they may be overcome competitively by increasing its intake. It is not effective in the treatment of aplastic anemia, leukemia, anemias of infection and nephritis, and general reduction in bone marrow activity of unknown origin.

The vitamin usually is absorbed readily from the GI tract and from parenteral sites of administration. The portion of administered folic acid that is excreted in the urine varies directly with the dose; only a small fraction appears in the urine following the oral ingestion of 0.1 mg, but up to 90% may be excreted by the kidney when a single dose of 15 mg is ingested. The fate of the unrecovered vitamin is unknown. The indications for parenteral use are rare. A solution in water for injection, prepared with the aid of sodium hydroxide or sodium carbonate, is the preferred form for injection.

It is capable of bringing about an incomplete and temporary hematopoietic response in pernicious anemia, which may cause the clinician to overlook the basic disorder. But it does not affect the progressive neurological lesions of the disease, which may appear explosively and in an irreversible stage. Doses that will correct a deficiency but do not generally cause a remission in pernicious anemia are on the order of 0.1 to 0.4 mg.

Infants fed on a goat milk formula should have a 50 μg a day supplement of folic acid.

For additional information concerning folic acid see the general statement on *Folic Acid.*

LEUCOVORIN CALCIUM

L-Glutamic acid, *N*-[[(2-amino-5-formyl-1,4,5,6,7,8-hexahydro-4-oxo-6-pteridinyl)methyl]amino]benzoyl]-, calcium salt (1:1), pentahydrate; Folmic Acid; Citrovorum Factor

Calcium *N*-[*p*-[[(2-amino-5-formyl-5,6,7,8-tetrahydro-4-hydroxy-6-pteridinyl)methyl]amino]benzoyl]-L-glutamate (1:1) pentahydrate [6035-45-6] $C_{20}H_{21}CaN_7O_7 \cdot 5H_2O$ (601.58); *anhydrous* [1492-18-8] (511.51).

Preparation—Folic acid simultaneously is hydrogenated and formylated in 90 to 100% formic acid under the influence of platinum oxide catalyst at low temperature and atmospheric pressure to yield leucovorin. Conversion to the calcium salt may be accomplished by dissolving the leucovorin in NaOH solution, treating with CaCl₂, and precipitating with ethanol.

Description—Yellowish white or yellow, odorless powder; pK_a 3.8, 4.8, and 10.4.

Solubility—Very soluble in water; practically insoluble in alcohol.

Comments—Leucovorin is folinic acid. The calcium salt is a convenient pharmaceutical form that is preferred for intramuscular injection. Consequently, its uses and limitations in the *treatment of the megaloblastic anemias* are the same as those for folic acid. However, it is superior to folic acid in *counteracting the excessive effects of the folic acid antagonists (methotrexate)*, since the antagonists competitively antagonize the conversion of folic acid to leucovorin and not the leucovorin itself and also since leucovorin is an excellent competitor for the inward transport system.

Sodium Folate [Monosodium Folate [6484-89-5] $C_{19}H_{18}N_7NaO_6$ (463.38); Folvite Sodium]—*Preparation:* Folic Acid is reacted with NaHCO₃. *Description and Solubility:* Clear, mobile liquid with a yellow or orange-yellow color; pH between 8.5 and 11. *Comments:* Has the actions of *Folic Acid*; however, the salt is preferred for parenteral use.

INOSITOL

Inositol is hexahydroxycyclohexane (1,2,3,4,5,6-cyclohexanehexol; *i*-inositol; *myo*-inositol; *meso*-inositol). Actually, there are nine stereoisomeric cyclohexanols, all of which now are referred to commonly as inositols. Several occur in nature; the isomer described above is by far the most prevalent and is the only one that is biologically active.

Inositol

Inositol occurs normally in nearly all plant and animal cells, either free or combined, suggesting that it is an essential cell constituent. In animal tissues it occurs as a constituent of phospholipids. In plants it usually is found as *phytic acid,* the hexaphosphate ester of inositol. There has as yet been no demonstration of need for inositol in human nutrition. In fact, large amounts of phytic acid in the diet interfere with the absorption of minerals, especially calcium, zinc, and iron.

Although inositol possesses weak lipotropic activity, it is not as effective as methionine or choline. There is no known valid therapeutic use of the compound. It may, however, be important to ensure its presence, at levels customarily found in human milk, in foods that are fed to infants and critically ill patients as the sole item of the diet. Inositol is measured by a microbiological assay.

Niacin (Nicotinic Acid or Nicotinamide)

Nicotinic acid (niacin) and nicotinamide (niacinamide) have identical properties as vitamins. Both compounds had been known for approximately 20 years before their biological significance was realized. In 1867 nicotinic acid was synthesized by the oxidation of nicotine with nitric acid. But it was not until 1937 that it was isolated from biological sources and found to be effective in the cure of black tongue in dogs and, later, pellagra in humans. The vitamin has none of the pharmacological properties of nicotine, however. In the 1940s the term *niacin* was adopted as a synonym for food labeling purposes to avoid association with the nicotine of tobacco. The term *niacin* is used generically to include both nicotinic acid and nicotinamide.

Chemistry and Assay—Nicotinic acid is pyridine-3-carboxylic acid. The structures of nicotinic acid and nicotinamide are shown below.

Nicotinic Acid   Nicotinamide

Niacin, the most stable of the vitamins, is not destroyed by heating in acid or alkaline solution. It withstands mild oxidation and retains its biological activity during the processing of food and the preparation and storage of pharmaceuticals. It is readily soluble in water or alcohol but insoluble in ether or chloroform. Niacinamide, on the other hand, may be extracted from water solution with ether. The amide is hydrolyzed readily to the free acid by heating in acid or alkaline solution.

The usual commercial synthesis of nicotinic acid used in foods and drugs is by the oxidation of quinoline with potassium permanganate or manganese dioxide, and monodecarboxylation of the purified quinolinic acid with controlled heating. Nicotinamide usually is prepared by esterifying nicotinic acid with methanol followed by ammonolysis.

The activity of both forms of the vitamin is expressed in milligrams of the chemically pure substance. Because they have identical biological activity and their molecular weights are nearly identical, they are equivalent on a weight basis. Reference Standard Niacin and also Niacinamide Reference Standard are available from the USP.

Niacin may be determined in food, drugs, and biological materials by microbiological assay or by chemical methods. No animal biological method exists. The chemical determination involves reaction of the pyridine ring with cyanogen bromide and coupling of the fission product with an aromatic amine. The yellow polymethine dye that is formed is measured in a spectrometer at 436 nm. In natural products niacin occurs mainly in combined form as a coenzyme and must be liberated by acid hydrolysis before assay.

The microbiological assays employ *Lactobacillus arabinosus* as the test organism. A quantitative discrimination between nicotinic acid and nicotinamide in a sample is possible by assaying with both this organism, which uses both forms, and *Leuconostoc mesenteroides,* which can use only nicotinic acid.

Metabolic Functions—In the body niacin is converted to nicotinamide, which is an essential constituent of coenzymes I and II that occur in a wide variety of enzyme systems involved in the anaerobic oxidation of carbohydrates. The coenzyme serves as a hydrogen acceptor in the oxidation of the substrate. These enzymes are present in all living cells and take part in many reactions of biological oxidation.

Nicotinamide adenine dinucleotide (NAD) is the inner salt of the 5′-ester of 3-carbamoyl-1-D-ribofuranosylpyridinium hydroxide with adenosine 5′-pyrophosphate and has the structure shown below. Nicotinamide adenine dinucleotide phosphate (NADP) differs only in that the adenosine moiety is esterified at its 2′-position with phosphoric acid.

NAD

These coenzymes are synthesized in the body and take part in the metabolism of all living cells. Since they are of such widespread and vital importance, it is not difficult to see why serious disturbance of metabolic processes occurs when the supply of niacin to the cell is interrupted.

The observations of numerous nutritionists that the daily requirement for niacin is influenced by the amount and kind of dietary protein led to the discovery that the amino acid tryptophan functions as a potential precursor of niacin. The efficiency of the conversion indicates that 60 mg of dietary tryptophan is equivalent to 1 mg of niacin. This relationship has given rise to the use of the term *niacin equivalent,* which is defined for the purpose of estimating the adequacy of diets in this vitamin as 1 mg of niacin or 60 mg of dietary tryptophan.

Niacin is absorbed readily from the intestinal tract, and large doses may be given orally or parenterally, with equal effect. Niacin, as nicotinic acid, is prescribed widely by physicians in gram amounts for the purpose of lowering blood cholesterol levels. The mechanism for this action is not fully understood; however, the effect is known to occur as a result of decreased cholesterol synthesis in the liver. Only the nicotinic acid form of the vitamin provides the effects. The use of such high doses of nicotinic acid can have serious side effects, including impairment of liver function. Nicotinic acid at these levels should be used only in conjunction with appropriate monitoring of normal liver function.

The principal excretory product of niacin in the urine is *N*-methylnicotinamide, a fluorescent compound formed in the liver. On a normal diet approximately one-fourth of the niacinamide ingested is excreted as *N*-methylnicotinamide. With increased levels of niacin intake the percentage of ingested niacin excreted as the fluorescent substance is decreased.

Dietary Requirement and Food Sources—Pellagra, which means rough skin, is the primary deficiency disease due to lack of sufficient niacin in the diet, and it appears only after months of dietary deprivation. The condition involves the GI tract, the skin, and the nervous system. Loss of weight, anorexia, weakness, insomnia, headache, and diarrhea are common and appear without obvious cause. Other early symptoms may include abdominal pain, nervousness, and mental confusion.

Typical manifestations of pellagra in a well-advanced stage are diarrhea, dermatitis, and dementia. GI difficulties vary in severity, and absence of gastric secretion is a common finding. In the more advanced state, diarrhea is severe. Dermatitis has a characteristic appearance and occurs at those sites subject to exposure or irritation. The skin lesions are usually bilaterally symmetrical and appear first as erythematous patches, changing to brown pigmented areas, followed by desquamation and thickening. Glossitis is common; it is characterized by swelling and redness at the margins and tip of the tongue. Because of inflammation and superficial desquamation, the tongue, gums, and lips appear scarlet and smooth. Mental symptoms vary in occurrence and intensity; they include irritability, mental depression, and emotional instability. A confused mental state with hallucinations, mania, and delirium is seen in advanced stages of the disease. Pellagra is a complex deficiency, and symptoms of riboflavin, thiamine, and folate deficiency frequently complicate the clinical picture.

Treatment of the disease requires immediate change to a nutritionally adequate diet and the administration of niacin or niacinamide. When neurological symptoms are present, use of thiamine and riboflavin may be necessary as well. Recovery from the acute condition is dramatic in most instances and occurs within 24 to 48 hr. Small doses given frequently during the day have been found to be more effective than a single large daily dose. Niacinamide is prefer-

able to niacin because it does not produce vasodilation in the skin with sensations of itching, burning, or tingling. With severe nausea and diarrhea, intravenous injection of niacinamide is of additional advantage.

In considering dietary requirement and the foods that contribute to it, one must consider the content of preformed niacin and the niacin available by conversion from tryptophan, an essential amino acid present in all good-quality proteins. The minimum requirement to prevent pellagra is the equivalent of about 4.4 mg of niacin/1000 kcal/day. The recommended dietary allowance is provided in Table 92-5. Most diets consumed in the US supply from 500 to 1000 mg or more of tryptophan a day and 8 to 17 mg of preformed niacin, equivalent to 16 to 33 mg of niacin.

Poultry, meats, and fish constitute the most important single food group source of niacin. Organ meats are somewhat superior to muscle tissue. Potatoes, legumes, and some green leafy vegetables contain moderate amounts of preformed niacin, as do whole grains. An important public-health nutrition practice, begun in the 1940s, is the nutrient enrichment of cereal products: wheat flour, farina, corn products, rice, macaroni and noodle products, and bread. Niacin, thiamine, riboflavin, and iron are mandatory ingredients in products that are labeled *enriched*. The level of enrichment for niacin is such that a significant proportion of the daily requirement is obtainable from a generous serving of these foods.

NIACIN PREPARATIONS

3-Pyridinecarboxylic acid; Nicotinic Acid

Nicotinic acid [59-67-6] $C_6H_5NO_2$ (123.11).

Preparation—Niacin may be variously prepared, as by oxidation of nicotine with nitric acid or potassium permanganate, by oxidation of quinoline, or synthesis from pyridine.

Description—White crystals or crystalline powder; odorless or with a slight odor; melts at about 235°; pK$_a$ 4.85.

Solubility—1 g in about 60 mL water; freely soluble in boiling water, boiling alcohol, or also solutions of alkali hydroxides or carbonates; practically insoluble in ether.

Comments—Chiefly in the treatment of pellagra, a disease common among the poor in subtropical countries because of diet deficiency. It also has been found useful in conjunction with thiamine and riboflavin in the treatment of nutritional deficiency in chronic alcoholism.

In doses of 20 mg or more in humans, niacin elicits a vasodilator effect that occurs a few minutes after oral ingestion or immediately after intravenous injection and lasts for a few minutes to an hour. Symptoms of flushing, itching, burning, or tingling occur, along with an increased skin temperature and increased motility and gastric secretion. Nicotinyl alcohol also shares this vasodilator property, and at one time both nicotinic acid and the alcohol popularly were used in the treatment of peripheral vascular disease and senility (as a cerebral vasodilator). These uses are obsolete and now are but an annoying side effect of large doses. The vasodilator effect of the oral drug is lessened if it is given with a meal.

Larger doses lower blood cholesterol, phospholipids, triglycerides, and free fatty acids, and the drug is used in the treatment of hypercholesterolemia, mostly in combination with cholestyramine, colestipol, or clofibrate. Nicotinamide does not possess the hypolipemic or the vasodilator property.

Large doses, especially those over 3 g a day, cause abnormalities in liver function, including jaundice. The risk may be greater with SR products.

Niacin is absorbed well orally, and the oral and parenteral doses are the same. With large doses, a considerable amount is excreted into the urine, so it is advisable to give several small doses during the day rather than one large one.

For additional information see the general statement on *Niacin*.

NIACINAMIDE

3-Pyridinecarboxamide; Nicotinamide; Nicotinic Acid Amide

Nicotinamide [98-92-0] $C_6H_6N_2O$ (122.13).

Preparation—From niacin by various methods, as by reaction with thionyl chloride followed by treatment with ammonia, or by interaction of ammonia gas with molten niacin.

Description—White, crystalline powder; odorless or nearly so, and with a bitter taste; solutions are neutral to litmus paper; melts between 128 and 131°.

Solubility—1 g in 1.5 mL water, 5.5 mL alcohol, or 10 mL glycerin.

Comments—This drug lacks the vasodilator, GI, hepatic, and hypolipemic actions of niacin. Consequently, it is preferred to niacin in the treatment of deficiency.

Pantothenic Acid

Knowledge of the identity and importance of pantothenic acid grew principally from experimental studies on microorganisms and chicks. Because of its wide distribution in nature it was named *pantothenic* (Greek, *pantothen*, from all sides). The terms vitamin B₃ and chick antidermatitis factor once were applied to variously purified concentrates of the factor, but they are now obsolete. No known therapeutic value exists for pantothenic acid, except perhaps in the treatment of frank or suspected cases of combined nutritional deficiencies.

Chemistry and Assay—Pantothenic acid is optically active (chiral). Maximum vitamin activity resides only in the D-form, and it is readily available as either the sodium or calcium salt, which are crystalline substances. Another commercially available form used in liquid preparations is D-pantothenyl alcohol (panthenol). Chemically, pantothenic acid is a composite structure of β-alanine and 2,4-dihydroxy-3,3-dimethylbutyric acid γ-lactone, connected in peptide linkage.

D-Pantothenic Acid

The free acid is fairly stable in neutral solution but sensitive to acids, bases, and heat. The salts are somewhat more stable, but even these are destroyed by autoclaving.

Pantothenic acid, its salts and alcohol, can be assayed by both chemical and microbiological methods. A chick growth method has been used, but it is time-consuming and has been replaced since suitable methods are available for releasing the bound vitamin (a protein enzyme) from its first combination in plant and animal tissue. The first step in chemical assay is acid or alkaline hydrolysis. This cleaves the molecule at the peptide linkage into an alanine part and a pantoic acid part. These fission products then can be determined photometrically by suitable color reactions. In addition both gas-liquid chromatography and high-pressure liquid chromatographic methods now exist. *Saccharomyces carlsbergensis* and *Lactobacillus plantarum* are used for the microbiological assay of pantothenic acid and its salts. There is available a USP Reference Standard Calcium Pantothenate.

Metabolic Functions, Dietary Requirement, and Food Sources—Pantothenic acid is of the highest biological importance because of its incorporation into coenzyme A (CoA), which is involved in many vital enzymatic reactions transferring a two-carbon compound (the acetyl group) in intermediary metabolism. It is involved in the release of energy from carbohydrate, in the degradation and metabolism of fatty acids, and in the synthesis of such compounds as sterols and steroid hormones, porphyrins, and acetylcholine. CoA is composed of one mole each of adenine, ribose, and β-mercaptoethylamine and three moles of phosphate for each mole of pantothenate.

Many microorganisms depend on the same metabolic pathways for their growth and reproduction as do animal species and humans and thus also require pantothenic acid. Some have the ability to synthesize pantothenic acid at a life-sustaining rate from proper precursors. Synthesis by the bacterial flora of the intestine in humans appears to be an important source of the vitamin and is the probable explanation, in part, of why pantothenic acid deficiency in humans is seldom encountered. A deficiency syndrome has been experimentally induced in human volunteers by the oral administration of a pantothenic acid antagonist, ω-methylpantothenic acid, imposed on a pantothenic acid–deficient diet. It has been impossible so far to induce an isolated deficiency of the vitamin in less than at least 9 months on anything resembling a natural diet alone, because of the occurrence of significant amounts of pantothenic acid in such a wide variety of foods.

The symptoms that appear to be specific for a lack of available pantothenic acid from the studies using the antivitamin are neuromuscular disorders (paresthesias of the hands and feet and cramping of the legs and impairment of motor coordination), loss of normal eosinopenic response to adrenal corticotrophic hormone (ACTH), heightened sensitivity to a test dose of insulin, and, in concert with pyridoxine, a loss of antibody production. Fatigue, malaise, headache, sleep disturbances, nausea, abdominal cramps, epigastric distress, occasional vomiting, and an increase in flatus were subjective observations of the pantothenic acid–deficient human volunteers.

Usual diets of adult Americans furnish about 10 to 15 mg of pantothenic acid a day, with a probable range of 6 to 20 mg. The recommended daily intake of pantothenic acid is found in Table 92-5. Human milk contains about 2 mg/L; cow's milk, about 3.5 mg/L. Liver and other organ meats and eggs are particularly good sources. Broccoli, cauliflower, white and sweet potatoes, tomatoes, and molasses are quite high in pantothenic acid. Muscle tissue of beef, pork, lamb, and chicken also is a good source.

PANTOTHENIC ACID PREPARATIONS

CALCIUM PANTOTHENATE

β-Alanine, *(R)-N*-(2,4-dihydroxy-3,3-dimethyl-1-oxobutyl)-, calcium salt (2:1); Dextro Calcium Pantothenate

Calcium D-pantothenate (1:2) [137-08-6] $C_{18}H_{32}CaN_2O_{10}$ (476.54); the calcium salt of the dextrorotatory isomer of pantothenic acid.

Preparation—Several syntheses are available. In one, isobutyraldehyde is converted to the lactone of 2,4-dihydroxy-3,3-dimethylbutyric acid, the D-enantiomer of which, obtained by resolution, is combined with β-alanine to form D-pantothenic acid and then converted to the calcium salt.

Description—Slightly hygroscopic, white powder; odorless, has a bitter taste and is stable in air; unstable to heat both in the dry state and in acid or alkaline solution; most stable at pH 5.5 to 6.5, and its solutions may be autoclaved at this pH for a short time without appreciable loss; solutions are neutral or slightly alkaline to litmus, with a pH of 7 to 9; specific rotation (calculated on the dried basis and in a 5% solution) +25 to +27.5°.

Solubility—1 g in about 3 mL water; soluble in glycerin; practically insoluble in alcohol, chloroform, or ether.

Comments—See the general statement on *Pantothenic Acid*. Since a deficiency of pantothenic acid alone is virtually unknown, the primary indication for use is a general nutritional deficiency. Clinical cases have been too few to supply creditable data on dosage.

Pyridoxine (Vitamin B₆)

Vitamin B₆ does not denote a single substance but is rather a collective term for a group of naturally occurring pyridines that are metabolically and functionally interrelated; namely, pyridoxine, pyridoxal, and pyridoxamine. They are interconvertible *in vivo* in their phosphorylated form. There is no information on the relative biological activity of the three compounds in humans, and since pyridoxine is the most stable, it probably contributes the most vitamin activity to the diet.

Chemistry and Assay—Pyridoxine as the free base has a bitter taste and is readily soluble in water, alcohol, or acetone. It crystallizes as the hydrochloride and is prepared in this form for commercial use. Pyridoxine is one of the more stable vitamins and in the alcohol form withstands heating in acid or alkaline solution. Pyridoxal and pyridoxamine are less stable, however, and are known to undergo destruction in the more severe heat treatments sometimes used in food processing. Under most conditions of processing and storage of foods and pharmaceutical preparations, the vitamin is retained well.

The structures of the three active forms of the vitamin and the phosphorylated form of one of them, pyridoxal phosphate, are shown below.

Pyridoxine   **Pyridoxal**

Pyridoxamine

Pyridoxal Phosphate

The biological activity of the vitamin is expressed in milligrams of the chemically pure substance, usually pyridoxine hydrochloride, for which a USP Reference Standard is available. Chicks and rats have been used for the biological assay of vitamin B₆ by placing the animals on a deficient basal diet that, when supplemented with known amounts of the test vitamin, supports a degree of growth related to the amount present. It is necessary to measure the three forms of vitamin B_6 to determine accurately the total biological activity. This can be accomplished with a high-pressure liquid chromatographic method. Microbiological assays also can discriminate between the individual vitamin B_6 components. A very useful technique employed in this type of assay is the preliminary separation of the different vitamin forms by a column chromatographic procedure using an ion exchanger. The column eluates then are analyzed by procedures suited to the vitamin form present in the eluates. The organisms most commonly used are *Saccharomyces carlsbergensis*, *Lactobacillus casei*, and *Streptococcus faecalis*.

Metabolic Functions, Dietary Requirement, and Food Source—Vitamin B_6 in the form of pyridoxal phosphate or pyridoxamine phosphate functions in carbohydrate, fat, and protein metabolism; its major functions are most closely related to protein and amino acid metabolism. The vitamin is a part of the molecular configuration of many enzymes (a coenzyme), notably glycogen phosphorylase, various transaminases, decarboxylases, and deaminases. The latter three are essential for the anabolism and catabolism of proteins.

The biological activity of vitamin B_6 seems to be a function of the molecule as a whole, since small changes in structure render it inactive. Deoxypyridoxine, a derivative of the vitamin in which one of the methanol groups is reduced to a methyl group, has potent antivitamin activity, but it is of limited experimental use in man because of its toxicity. The antivitamin isonicotinic acid hydrazide (isoniazid) has been used widely in the treatment of tuberculosis. It is chemically related to pyridoxine and acts also as an antagonist, thus requiring physicians to be alert to the pyridoxine nutriture of patients so treated. A similar antagonism is possible during treatment of hypertension with the drug hydralazine.

No classic syndrome of pyridoxine deficiency exists, probably because it is distributed widely in nature and unique or unusual dietary habits have not so far produced an uncomplicated deficiency. That it is essential for the growth of animals and human infants is well-established. Other manifestations of deficiency in humans are probably an acrodynia-like syndrome characterized by edema and loss of hair, nerve degeneration resulting in behavioral changes, and, in infants, convulsive seizures. The latter symptom was shown to result when infants were fed a proprietary milk-based formula, unsupplemented with pyridoxine, in which the natural vitamin content was destroyed inadvertently during sterilization. In this instance, marked changes in electroencephalogram patterns of the infants were produced, and they returned to normal minutes after pyridoxine administration.

In infants, although daily requirements of the vitamin are met by consumption of adequate quantities of normal breast milk, the protein–vitamin B_6 relationship is critical. General experience with proprietary formulas suggests that metabolic requirements are satisfied if the vitamin is present in amounts of 0.015 mg/g of protein, or 0.04 mg/100 kcal. The recommended dietary allowances are provided in Table 92-5.

The best food sources of vitamin B_6 are muscle meats, liver, green vegetables, and whole-grain cereals. The bran from the cereal grains has especially large amounts. Nuts, corn, eggs, and milk are also good sources.

If large doses of vitamin B_6 are ingested for long periods of time, peripheral neuropathies develop. In most observations these involve levels in excess of 250 mg a day.

VITAMIN B₆ PREPARATIONS

PYRIDOXINE HYDROCHLORIDE

3,4-Pyridinedimethanol, 5-hydroxy-6-methyl-, hydrochloride; Vitamin B₆ Hydrochloride

Pyridoxol hydrochloride [58-56-0] $C_8H_{11}NO_3 \cdot HCl$ (205.64).

Preparation—Several processes are available. One may be viewed as a cyclizing dehydration of ethyl glycinate (I), ethyl pyruvate (II), and 1,4-diethoxy-2-butanone (III) followed by saponification and decarboxylation at position 2 and cleavage of the three ethoxy groups with HI or another suitable reagent. Reaction of the base with HCl yields the hydrochloride. US Pats 2,904,551, 3,024,244, and 3,024,245.

Description—Colorless or white crystals or a white, crystalline powder; stable in air and slowly affected by sunlight; solutions are acid to litmus, with a pH of about 3; melting range 202 to 206°, with some decomposition.

Solubility—1 g in 5 mL water or 115 mL alcohol; insoluble in chloroform or ether.

Comments—Deficiency in adults is extremely difficult to induce, and the therapeutic need for this vitamin, alone, in the adult is of rare occurrence. However, it is justified to give it along with other B vitamins when there is evidence of a *multiple B-vitamin deficiency*. It may be used prophylactically to prevent, or to treat, peripheral neuritis in *patients treated with isoniazid*. It has been claimed that the vitamin controls the *nausea and vomiting of pregnancy* or of *radiation sickness*, but unequivocal proof has never been presented. In infants with *convulsive seizures due to pyridoxine dependency*, administration of the vitamin promptly corrects the condition (see the general statement on *Pyridoxine*). It has been claimed to be medically effective in treating the carpaltunnel syndrome; however, more data are required to substantiate this claim. Extremely high doses (600 to 3000 mg per day) have been administered to schizophrenics, autistic children, and children exhibiting hyperkinesis. However, clear evidence of benefit has not been established. Caution needs to be exercised with these levels of administration because of reports of severe sensory-nervous-system dysfunction after daily consumption of 2 to 5 g. It may be effective in correcting hypochromic or megaloblastic anemia in patients with adequate levels of iron who have not responded to other hematopoietic agents. Since it antagonizes levodopa, patients with Parkinson's disease treated with the latter drug should not take multivitamin supplements containing pyridoxine.

Riboflavin

Riboflavin was formerly known as vitamin B_2 or G and lactoflavin. It owes its discovery as one of the components of the B-vitamin group to its characteristic fluorescence and pigmenting quality in such common foods as milk and egg yolk. Isolation and characterization of the yellow protein enzyme originally from yeast led to studies on the essential nature of the flavin pigment part of the enzyme in human metabolism, growth, and health.

Chemistry and Assay—Riboflavin is a yellow to orange-yellow, crystalline powder with a slight odor. When dry, it is not appreciably affected by diffused light.

In alkaline solution it is readily soluble but quite unstable to heat and to light, forming lumiflavin, a fluorescent degradation product that is without biological activity. Riboflavin is more stable to heat in acid solution, particularly from pH 1 to 6.5, but upon irradiation forms lumichrome, also biologically inactive. Photodegradation occurs in the skin, and infants with kernicterus who are treated with UV light may become riboflavin-deficient. Riboflavin is adsorbed readily from acid or neutral solution on such agents as frankonite, fuller's earth, and certain zeolites and eluted with acetone or pyridine solutions. Adsorbates have been used in pharmaceutical preparations, but from some of these the vitamin has been found to be unavailable to the human because of difficulty of elution in the intestinal tract.

Solutions of riboflavin have a characteristic yellow-green fluorescence that has a maximum absorption at 565 nm in the acid pH range. This property is made use of in the chemical determination of riboflavin. It is reduced rapidly by hydrosulfite, or by hydrogen in the presence of zinc in acid solution, to the leuco form, which is colorless and nonfluorescent. The leucoriboflavin is reoxidized easily by shaking in air. This oxidation-reduction property (see below) is the probable basis for the biological importance of riboflavin in the respiratory enzyme systems.

One gram dissolves in 3000 to about 20,000 mL of water, the variations in the solubility being due to differences in the internal crystalline structure of the riboflavin; it is more soluble in isotonic sodium chloride or alkaline solution than in water and less soluble in alcohol. It is insoluble in most lipid solvents. Derivatives such as the phosphate or acetate have been prepared for use in pharmaceutical preparations when higher concentrations are desired.

Riboflavin   **Leucoriboflavin**

The activity of riboflavin is expressed in milligrams of the chemically pure substance, and a USP Reference Standard Riboflavin is available for assay purposes. In early work, the riboflavin content of substances was measured by a rat growth bioassay method, but this has been replaced by both physicochemical and microbiological methods.

Chemical determinations are based on colorimetric and fluorometric procedures. Straightforward measurement of the intrinsic yellow color of riboflavin is often sufficient for assaying pharmaceutical preparations. The fluorometric method is more sensitive and free of interferences and is therefore more suited to the assay of the vitamin in foods. It depends upon the extraction of the vitamin with dilute acid, filtration, treatment of the filtrate with permanganate and hydrogen peroxide to destroy interfering pigments, and measurement of the fluorescence. Assays also can be accomplished using high-pressure liquid chromatography and a fluorometric detector.

Lactobacillus casei is used as the test organism for microbiological assay of riboflavin. It is determined by measurement of the growth stimulation of the organism or by alkaline titration of the acid produced during incubation.

Metabolic Functions—Riboflavin plays its physiological role as the prosthetic group of a number of enzyme systems that are involved in the oxidation of carbohydrates and amino acids. It functions in combination with a specific protein, either as a mononucleotide containing phosphoric acid (FMN) or as a dinucleotide combined through phosphoric acid with adenine (FAD).

Flavin-adenine dinucleotide (FAD)

The specificity of each of the enzymes is determined by the protein in the complex. By a process of oxidation-reduction, riboflavin in the system either gains or loses hydrogen. The substrate, either carbohydrate or amino acid, may be oxidized by a removal of hydrogen. The first hydrogen acceptor in the chain of events is NAD or NADP, the di- or trinucleotide containing nicotinic acid and adenine. The oxidized riboflavin system then serves as hydrogen acceptor for the coenzyme system and in turn is oxidized by the cytochrome system. The hydrogen finally is passed on to the oxygen to complete the oxidative cycle. A number of flavoprotein enzymes have been identified, each of which is specific for a given substrate.

There is evidence that some of the flavin enzymes contain metallic constituents. These metalloflavoproteins may contain iron, copper, or molybdenum. Succinic dehydrogenase, for example, contains iron, and xanthine oxidase contains molybdenum as well as iron.

After phosphorylation, riboflavin is absorbed from the intestinal tract and excreted in the urine. A human adult on an ordinary diet excretes from 0.5 to 1.5 mg in 24 hr, depending on the content of the diet. Of a 10-mg dose taken by mouth, 50% to 70% is excreted within 24 hr. In riboflavin deficiency there is little or none found in the urine. Measure of excretion has been used as a diagnostic sign of deficiency. Riboflavin, like thiamine, is stored to a limited extent, and constant dietary supply is needed to maintain normal body levels. Liver, kidney, and heart tissues contain relatively large amounts of riboflavin because of their high enzyme content.

Dietary Requirement and Food Sources—Symptoms of human ariboflavinosis include cheilosis (reddening of the lips and the appearance of fissures at the corners of the mouth), characteristic changes in color of the mucous membranes, inflammation of the tongue, and denuding of the lips. Lesions of a seborrheic nature also have been observed as a result of riboflavin deficiency. Ocular manifestations that appear in man are characterized chiefly by corneal vascularization, in which the cornea is extensively invaded by small capillaries. This usually is accompanied by sensations of itching, burning, and roughness of the eyelid and lacrimation, photophobia, and visual fatigue. Some of these conditions may, of course, arise from other causes and do not necessarily indicate riboflavin deficiency.

Riboflavin deficiency in humans has not been found to be widespread in any part of the world, but is undoubtedly a complicating factor in other deficiency diseases such as pellagra. For therapeutic purposes, doses of 1 to 10 mg a day have been given. Rapid disappearance of symptoms of ariboflavinosis occurs with 10-mg doses, and some question the need for administering amounts larger than this.

Studies dealing with the quantitative riboflavin requirement of the human indicate that it is related to body size, metabolic rate, and rate of growth. The parameter used to express these most closely is metabolic body size, represented as kilograms of body weight taken to the 3/4 power. The recommended daily dietary allowance of the Food and Nutrition Board for riboflavin is listed in Table 92-5. In general, the minimum requirement for riboflavin is about 0.3 mg for adults and 0.8 mg for infants on a 1000-kcal-intake basis. From a physiological point of view, an intake of more than 0.5 to 0.6 mg/1000 kcal may be of little extra value in normal adult persons.

Riboflavin is widely distributed in nature, in both plants and animals, as an essential constituent of all living cells, and therefore is found widely distributed in small amounts in foods. It is quite stable during the processing of food, except when there is excessive exposure to light. Because of its water solubility, there is moderate loss of riboflavin in cooking when the cooking water is discarded. This loss, however, is generally smaller than that of thiamine, niacin, or ascorbic acid.

Foods that make important contributions of riboflavin to the diet are liver and other organ tissues, milk, and eggs. Vegetables and fruits furnish a small but constant supply.

Many species of microorganisms are capable of synthesizing riboflavin, and because of the extensive bacterial growth in the human intestinal tract, this may form an important and constant source of supply of riboflavin and may account for the limited occurrence of deficiency in humans, although this has yet to be well studied.

When it was recognized that cereal products would be a good vehicle to use to improve the content of riboflavin in many diets, its mandatory addition as an enriching ingredient was adopted. In concert with thiamine, niacin, and iron, riboflavin is present in nutritionally significant amounts in enriched wheat flour, farina, corn products, bread, macaroni, and noodle products. Because of certain cooking habits and the apparent unacceptability of the unnatural yellow color, the enrichment of rice with riboflavin has been resisted.

RIBOFLAVIN PREPARATIONS

Lactoflavin; Vitamin B$_2$

Riboflavin [83-88-5] $C_{17}H_{20}N_4O_6$ (376.37).

Preparation—Mostly by synthesis. In one method, 1-(6-amino-3,4-xylidino)-1-deoxy-D-ribitol (I) is condensed with alloxan (II) in acetic acid with boric acid as a catalyst. Among other ways, I may be prepared by condensing D-ribitol with 4,5-dimethylphenylenediamine. US Patent 2,807,611.

Description—Yellow to orange-yellow, crystalline powder with a slight odor; melts at about 280°; saturated solution is neutral to litmus; when dry not appreciably affected by diffused light, but when in solution, light induces quite rapid deterioration, especially in the presence of alkalies.

Solubility—Very slightly soluble in water, alcohol, or isotonic sodium chloride solution; very soluble in dilute solutions of alkalies; insoluble in ether or chloroform.

Comments—To treat ariboflavinosis (riboflavin deficiency) and also to supplement other B vitamins in the treatment of pellagra and beriberi (see the general statement on *Riboflavin*).

Thiamine

Concentrates of thiamine, often termed vitamin B$_1$, were given the latter name by early workers in this country who recognized that at least two accessory dietary factors were needed for normal growth of laboratory rats, one in butter fat and the other in *milk sugar*. The names they suggested for these factors were fat-soluble vitamin A and water-soluble vitamin B. It was shown subsequently by a number of investigators that the latter consisted of a group of substances rather than a single compound, but vitamin B$_1$ was finally the first pure compound of the group to be laboriously isolated from rice polishings. In the pioneer studies on this substance it was found that a thiamine concentrate prevented polyneuritis in chickens, which later was found to be caused by the ab-

Vitamin B$_{12}$ (cyanocobalamin) in an atmosphere of hydrogen with a platinum catalyst is reduced to a red crystalline compound with slightly changed UV-absorption maxima, and a reduced stability to heat. Vitamin B$_{12a}$ results from such reduction. Vitamin B$_{12b}$, another reduced form, occurs in natural sources.

Commercially, vitamin B$_{12}$ is obtained from fermentation by *Streptomyces griseus*. The vitamin is precipitated from aqueous solutions saturated with ammonium sulfate by 1-butanol. Purification is achieved by chromatography, using bentonite or aluminum silicate as the adsorbent. Sharply defined red bands are formed during the development of the chromatograms, indicating the location of the vitamin. The red band is separated mechanically and eluted with water. The concentrated water solution on addition of acetone gives the crystalline vitamin, which can be purified further by recrystallization from aqueous acetone.

The USP provides a Reference Standard Cyanocobalamin for use in assay of the vitamin. A physicochemical method for determining vitamin B$_{12}$ involves measurement of light absorbance at certain specific wavelengths characteristic for cyanocobalamin. This method is only applicable to relatively concentrated solutions of the compound, such as pharmaceutical preparations. Vitamin B$_{12}$ also can be determined with high-performance liquid chromatography.

Vitamin B$_{12}$ is one of the most active biological factors known; its activity for bacteria is measured in terms of millimicrograms. Because of this sensitivity of some bacteria to such low levels of the vitamin and the fact that foods contain exceptionally low concentrations of the vitamin, microbiological methods (using *Lactobacillus leichmannii, Ochramonas malhamensis,* and *Euglenia gracilis*) were widely used until newer radioligand binding assays were introduced.

Metabolic Functions, Dietary Requirement, and Food Sources—The vitamin is essential for the normal functioning of all cells, but particularly for cells of the bone marrow, the nervous system, and the GI tract. It appears to facilitate reduction reactions and participate in the transfer of methyl groups. Evidence exists that vitamin B$_{12}$ is involved in protein, carbohydrate, and fat metabolism, but its chief importance in mammalian tissues seems to be, together with folic acid, in the anabolism of deoxyribonucleic acid in all cells. Coenzyme forms of vitamin B$_{12}$, in which the vitamin is linked to adenine and a sugar, which catalyze specific reactions in intermediary metabolism, have been isolated from bacterial cultures and probably have similar vitamin roles in mammalian cells.

The biochemical fault in pernicious anemia, a condition caused by a prolonged deficiency of vitamin B$_{12}$, is a failure of elaboration of the intrinsic factor, normally secreted by the parietal cells of the stomach mucosa. This intrinsic factor, which is essential for the absorption of the vitamin through the intestinal wall, forms a complex with vitamin B$_{12}$. Intrinsic factor is a glycoprotein of 45,000 daltons.

Vitamin B$_{12}$ is a requisite for normal blood formation, and certain macrocytic anemias respond to its administration. In pernicious anemia, unless accompanied by intrinsic factor, the vitamin is not absorbed orally in effective amounts and must be administered parenterally in microgram quantities. Vitamin B$_{12}$ deficits not associated with intrinsic factor pathology may be managed orally. Preparations containing vitamin B$_{12}$ and intrinsic factor concentrate are now available for oral use and have been shown for short-term use at least to be equivalent in value to the injections. Clinical studies indicate that if milligram amounts of the vitamin are administered orally in the absence of intrinsic factor, enough of the vitamin passes through the intestinal wall to be effective in maintaining the pernicious anemia patient. However, the injectable form of vitamin B$_{12}$ continues to be the drug of choice because of the desirability of regular attention of a physician to the condition of the patient.

The evidence indicating that vitamin B$_{12}$ is the antipernicious anemia factor is complete. In treating pernicious anemia, vitamin B$_{12}$ administered intramuscularly produces a maximal reticulocyte response in 4 to 9 days and a restoration of red- and white-cell counts in 4 to 6 weeks. The change in bone marrow from a megaloblastic to a normoblastic state is dramatic and occurs within a few hours after the injection of as little as 1 μg of the vitamin. Vitamin B$_{12}$ is considered to be the extrinsic factor of Castle, the absorption of which from the intestinal tract is facilitated by the intrinsic factor present in normal gastric juice. The biochemical defect in pernicious anemia, then, is a failure of elaboration of the intrinsic factor. Because of this relationship, vitamin B$_{12}$ given orally is much less effective in the pernicious anemia patient and entirely ineffective if there is complete absence of intrinsic factor.

The vitamin is effective in preventing the occurrence of neurological changes common to pernicious anemia. These symptoms are observed more frequently among the elderly because absorption of vitamin B$_{12}$ has been shown to decrease among this population. However, it is not uncommon to identify women with neurological changes caused by vitamin B$_{12}$ deficiency in their mid-thirties to late thirties. Acute symptoms of combined-system disease have been found to disappear rather promptly after B$_{12}$ administration, but recovery appears to depend more

on the chronicity of the disease than on the extent of neurological involvement, and conditions of long standing are less apt to show recovery. Osteoblast activity probably also depends upon vitamin B$_{12}$.

A simple nutritional concept of pernicious anemia that seems valid is that of essentially an uncomplicated deficiency of vitamin B$_{12}$ conditioned by the lack of intrinsic factor and, hence, the inability to absorb the vitamin from ingested food. This validation rests on several types of evidence; particularly convincing is the comparison of the clinical development of vitamin B$_{12}$ deficiency in vegans, in patients who had total gastrectomy (resulting in removal of intrinsic factor and interference with absorption of the vitamin), and the relapse following withholding of therapy from previously adequately treated patients with pernicious anemia. Simple experimental dietary deficiency of vitamin B$_{12}$ has not yet been produced in the adult human under conditions of careful continuous observation. It seems probable that the requirements for parenterally administered (or absorbed) vitamin B$_{12}$ by the patient with pernicious anemia or gastrectomy are similar to the requirements of the normal subject. The recommended daily dietary allowance of the Food and Nutrition Board is provided in Table 92-5.

Vitamin B$_{12}$ occurs in meat and dairy products but is not present to any measurable extent in plants or cereal grains. It is probable that indigenous bacteria in plant foods synthesize sufficient vitamin B$_{12}$ to meet the requirement of those individuals whose dietary habits preclude the use of animal food sources.

VITAMIN B$_{12}$ PREPARATIONS

CYANOCOBALAMIN

α-5,6-Dimethylbenzimidazolylcobamide cyanide; Vitamin B$_{12}$

Vitamin B$_{12}$ [68-19-9] C$_{63}$H$_{88}$CoN$_{14}$O$_{14}$P (1355.38).

Preparation—Vitamin B$_{12}$ can be isolated from aqueous liver extracts and from *Streptomyces griseus* fermentation. Commercially, it is obtained from the latter source.

Description—Dark red, hygroscopic crystals or amorphous or crystalline powder; when the anhydrous compound is exposed to air it may absorb about 12% water.

Solubility—1 g in 80 mL water; soluble in alcohol; insoluble in acetone, chloroform, or ether.

Comments—This and other forms of vitamin B$_{12}$ are used to treat various megaloblastic anemias, especially *pernicious anemia* and other anemias in which the secretion of the intrinsic factor is impaired, as in *gastric cancer, gastric atrophy, total* or even *subtotal gastrectomy*. It also may be used to treat the megaloblastic anemias of *tropical sprue, idiopathic steatorrhea, gluten-induced enteropathy, regional ileitis, ileal resection, malignancies, granulomas, strictures or other structural disorders of the ileum* in which vitamin B$_{12}$ absorption is impaired; in most of these folic acid deficiency is even more severe, and combined therapy is indicated. Its deficiencies untreated for periods of more than 3 months may result in permanent degenerative spinal cord lesions. The megaloblastic anemia associated with *fish tapeworm infestation* also responds to the vitamin. The megaloblastic anemias of pregnancy, infancy, alcoholism, and poverty usually are due to folic acid deficiency and only infrequently respond to it. The vitamin is *not useful* in the treatment of infectious hepatitis, multiple sclerosis, trigeminal neuralgia, anorexia, miscellaneous neuropathies, thyrotoxicosis, retarded growth, aging, and various psychiatric disorders, and claims to the contrary and promotion therefore represent misuse without support from clinical trials. It should not be administered intravenously and is contraindicated in patients who are sensitive to it or cobalt. Patients with Leber's disease have been found to suffer severe and rapid opticatrophy when treated with it. Either cyanocobalamin or hydroxocobalamin may be used for a loading dose in the Schilling test for malabsorption of the vitamin in diseases that affect the lower bowel, such as *sprue*.

A nasal spray has been developed that is said to provide significant absorption in the nasal mucosa and may supplant the parenteral dosage forms.

In addition to intrinsic factor, GI absorption requires an alkaline pH. In the presence of pancreatic disease it may be necessary to administer the oral vitamin with bicarbonate or give the vitamin parenterally.

For additional information about cyanocobalamin see the general statement on *Vitamin B12*.

HYDROXOCOBALAMIN

Cobinamide, dihydroxide, dihydrogen phosphate (ester), mono(inner salt), 3′-ester with 5,6-dimethyl-1-α-D-ribofuranosyl-1H-benzimidazole; Vitamin B$_{12a}$

Cobinamide dihydroxide dihydrogen phosphate (ester), mono(inner salt), 3′-ester with 5,6-dimethyl-1-α-D-ribofuranosylbenzimidazole

[13422-51-0] $C_{62}H_{89}CoN_{13}O_{15}P$ (1346.37); an analog of *Cyanocobalamin* in which a hydroxyl radical has replaced the cyano radical.

Preparation—Cyanocobalamin in solution is hydrogenated at room temperature with the aid of Raney nickel. The solution then is exposed to air and diluted with acetone. Oxidation takes place, and upon standing, the hydroxocobalamin crystallizes.

Description—Dark red crystals or red crystalline powder; odorless or has no more than a slight acetone odor; anhydrous form is very hygroscopic; pH (2 in 100 solution) between 8 and 10.

Solubility—1 g in 50 mL water, 100 mL alcohol, 10,000 mL chloroform, or 10,000 mL ether. It is preferable to make aqueous solutions in acetate buffer at a pH between 3.5 and 4.5 in which 1 g dissolves in about 100 mL water.

Comments—See *Cyanocobalamin*.

MULTIVITAMIN PREPARATIONS

In the preceding text and in various monographs, attention was called in several instances to the fact that it is desirable at times to administer more than one vitamin for what appear to be the symptoms of a single deficiency. The quotation "In the shadow of pellagra walks beriberi" has considerable substance in fact. Diets deficient in niacin are frequently also deficient in thiamine and certain other B vitamins of similar dietary source. The same relationship holds frequently for folate and vitamin B_{12}. Malabsorption syndromes affect the assimilation of several vitamins. Furthermore, the repair of a deficiency of one vitamin may increase the requirement for another; for example, repletion of thiamine increases the need for riboflavin. Diseases in which there is increased metabolism, such as thyrotoxicosis, increase the need for more of the vitamins, as do periods of hard physical work, stress, pregnancy, and lactation. Therefore, multivitamin therapy is often rational. Multivitamin therapy also is recommended for individuals who are on restricted diets for weight control or lack vitality, those who are debilitated, and those working in hazardous environments. Use of multivitamin supplements for infants and preschool children should be done on the advice of a pediatrician. For patients unable to consume an oral diet, injectable multivitamin products containing 13 vitamins are available to be administered diluted in parenteral fluid or in parenteral nutrition admixtures.

OTHER PREPARATIONS

Levocarnitine, L-Carnitine [L-(3-Carboxy-2-hydroxypropyl)trimethylammonium hydroxide inner salt; [461-06-3] Vitamin B_7; $C_7H_{15}NO_3$ (161.20); Carnitor]—*Preparation:* It may be isolated from meat extracts or prepared synthetically. *Description and Solubility:* White, very hygroscopic solid melting at about 197°. Readily soluble in water or hot alcohol; practically insoluble in most organic solvents. *Comments:* Required in mammalian energy metabolism and has been shown to facilitate long-chain fatty acid entry into cellular mitochondria, therefore providing the substrate for β-oxidation and subsequent production of energy. It is synthesized in the liver from lysine. Deficiency may occur from impaired hepatic synthesis or transport from liver to muscle. Carnitine deficiency may lead to elevated triglyceride and free fatty acid concentrations, diminished ketogenesis, and lipid infiltration of muscle and liver.

Betaine (anhydrous) {107-43-7]1-Carboxy-*N,N,N*-trimethylmethanaminium inner salt; trimethyl glycine; $C_5H_{11}NO_2$ (117.15) Cystadane. *Description and Solubility*—White, granular, hygroscopic powder; very soluble in water, soluble in methanol and in ethanol, sparingly soluble in ether. *Comments*—A methyl group donor used in the management of inborn errors of metabolism that result in homocystinuria. The orphan drug product is administered as a solution prepared from an anhydrous powder form.

MINERALS

Minerals can be further differentiated as macro-minerals and micro-minerals. The micro-minerals are also referred to as trace elements and will be presented in the next section. Macro-minerals are found in larger quantities in the human body and as such have higher requirements for intake. Those with adequate data supporting dietary recommendations are listed in Table 92-6. Dietary and supplementary intake of minerals is often in a salt form. These minerals can be found in dissociated ionic form in physiologic fluids in which case they are referred to as electrolytes. These electrolytes can each be administered intravenously as part of an admixture to maintain or replete total body stores of the electrolyte when the gastrointestinal route cannot be used.

SODIUM—(See *Blood, Fluids, Electrolytes, and Hematologic Drugs*).
POTASSIUM—(See *Blood, Fluids, Electrolytes, and Hematologic Drugs*).
CALCIUM—(See *Blood, Fluids, Electrolytes, and Hematologic Drugs*).
PHOSPHATE—(See *Blood, Fluids, Electrolytes, and Hematologic Drugs*).
MAGNESIUM—(See *Gastrointestinal Drugs*).

TRACE ELEMENTS

The trace elements, or micro-minerals, are inorganic nutrients found in small quantities in the human body and have intake requirements in the mg or μg range. The essentiality of several trace elements was established for humans during the 1930s. Those with adequate data supporting dietary recommendations are listed in Table 92-6. Fourteen elements now are thought to be essential, although dietary requirements have been established for only nine (Table 92-6). Some elements, notably manganese and chromium, can exist in several oxidation states; however, only one or two are compatible with a biological environment and function. Evidence to support required functions in humans is still incomplete for nickel, silicon, tin, and vanadium. There also is some evidence that boron may be essential. Although based on limited data, dietary intake of the remaining trace elements is about 15-160 μg cobalt, 100-150 μg nickel, 1.5-3.5 mg tin, and 10-20 μg vanadium.

Information on trace-element distribution in foods is presented in Table 92-7. This is an attempt to indicate important sources of the elements or the level, particularly if low, in important foods. This table is of rather limited usefulness because it is based on so little information. At present, too little is known about the effect of agricultural practices and manufacturing processes on trace-element content.

Our understanding of trace-element function in humans is less complete than that of vitamins. Study of a deficiency syndrome in animals often precedes recognition of deficiency or metabolic problems in humans, particularly as related to a disease. Notable exceptions have been reports of deficiency in patients receiving parenteral nutrition not providing a particular element. For this reason, deficiency syndromes in animals are described for each element known to be essential.

Similarly, our knowledge of trace-element toxicity in humans is limited, and we must rely on animal data. Two problems must be considered. One is the effect of long-term supplementation with a *moderate* excess above requirement. It is important to consider not only the amount of a single trace element, but also the balance among all required elements. This area requires periodic review as knowledge increases. The other toxicity problem relates to short-term intake of multiple recommended doses, either accidentally or purposefully. This must be regarded as undesirable, depending on the excess intake level. It is well known to be very serious in the case of infants swallowing capsules containing ferrous sulfate.

Inorganic elements are very different from the various organic nutrients in that they cannot be destroyed or converted

Table 92-6. Dietary Reference Intakes – Minerals

LIFE STAGE GROUP	Ca (mg/d)	P (mg/d)	Mg (mg/d)	F (mg/d)	Se (µg/d)	Cr (µg/d)	Cu (µg/d)	I (µg/d)	Fe (mg/d)	Mn (mg/d)	Mb (µg/d)	Zn (mg/d)
Infants												
0-6 months	210*	100*	30*	0.01*	15*	0.2*	200*	110*	0.27*	0.003*	2*	2*
7-12 months	270*	275*	75*	0.5*	20*	5.5*	220*	130*	11	0.6*	3*	3
Children												
1-3 years	500*	460	80	0.7*	20	11*	340	90	7	1.2*	17	3
4-8 years	800*	500	130	1*	30	15*	440	90	10	1.5*	22	5
Males												
9-13 years	1300*	1250	240	2*	40	25*	700	120	8	1.9*	34	8
14-18 years	1300*	1250	410	3*	55	35*	890	150	11	2.2*	43	11
19-30 years	1000*	700	400	4*	55	35*	900	150	8	2.3*	45	11
31-50 years	1000*	700	420	4*	55	35*	900	150	8	2.3*	45	11
51-70 years	1200*	700	420	4*	55	30*	900	150	8	2.3*	45	11
>70 years	1200*	700	420	4*	55	30*	900	150	8	2.3*	45	11
Females												
9-13 years	1300*	1250	240	2*	40	21*	700	120	8	1.6*	34	8
14-18 years	1300*	1250	360	3*	55	24*	890	150	15	1.6*	43	9
19-30 years	1000*	700	310	3*	55	25*	900	150	18	1.8*	45	8
31-50 years	1000*	700	320	3*	55	25*	900	150	18	1.8*	45	8
51-70 years	1200*	700	320	3*	55	20*	900	150	8	1.8*	45	8
>70 years	1200*	700	320	3*	55	20*	900	150	8	1.8*	45	8
Pregnancy												
≤18 years	1300*	1250	400	3*	60	29*	1000	220	27	2*	50	13
19-30 years	1000*	700	350	3*	60	30*	1000	220	27	2*	50	11
31-50 years	1000*	700	360	3*	60	30*	1000	220	27	2*	50	11
Lactation												
>18 years	1300*	1250	360	3*	70	44*	1300	290	10	2.6*	50	14
19-30 years	1000*	700	310	3*	70	45*	1300	290	9	2.6*	50	12
31-50 years	1000*	700	320	3*	70	45*	1300	290	9	2.6*	50	12

* Adequate Intake Level, otherwise values represent Recommended Dietary Allowances.

Table 92-7. Distribution of Essential Trace Elements in Foods[a]

	FOOD SOURCE AND CONTENT	
ELEMENT	AVERAGE TO HIGH	LOW
Chromium	Dried brewers' yeast, bran and germ of cereal grains, molasses, liver Refined cereals, refined sugar	
Cobalt	Leafy vegetables	Milk, refined cereals
Copper	Liver, kidney, shellfish, nuts, dry legumes, whole-grain cereals	Milk, muscle meat, eggs, fruit, vegetables
Fluorine[b]	Seafish, red meat, eggs, tea	Milk
Iodine[b]	Seafish, shellfish, iodized salt, milk	
Iron	Liver, kidney, shellfish, muscle meats, poultry, heart, egg yolk, dried legumes, cane molasses, nuts	Milk, refined sugar
Manganese	Whole-grain cereals, dried legumes, tubers, fruits, nonleafy vegetables Milk, poultry, fish	
Molybdenum	Liver, kidney, dried legumes, whole-grain cereals, leafy vegetables Fruits, root and stem vegetables, muscle meats, milk	
Nickel	Whole-grain cereals, vegetables	Muscle meats, fats, eggs, milk
Selenium	Liver, kidney	
Silicon	Whole-grain cereals, chicken skin, beer	Animal foods
Tin[d]	Cereals, muscle meats Milk	
Vanadium[b]	Liver, muscle meats, fish, bread, some cereal grains, nuts, a few root vegetables, oils from corn and soybeans	Milk, most vegetables
Zinc	Meat, egg yolk, whole-grain cereals, oysters, fowl, milk Fruits, fish, vegetables	

[a] Bioavailability is not taken into consideration; see text for individual elements.
[b] Most foods are highly variable.
[c] Selenium content is markedly affected by available selenium during growth of the plant or animal food. Cooking losses can occur.
[d] The tin content is markedly increased by exposure to tin-plated containers.

into another substance by the metabolic processes. In most cases the trace elements are bound to an organic ligand. This is the means for effecting elemental transport and function and minimizing toxicity. The binding may be very loose or very firm. Many of the elements are part of metalloenzymes. Nucleic acids also bind metal ions in a consistent pattern. Other mechanisms of function are described for individual elements below.

Many pairs or groups of essential elements may have chemical properties that are closely similar. This can result in competition for binding sites that may alter transport, storage, excretion, and function. In other words setting the stage for mineral-mineral interactions.

There are many elements in biological systems that have no known essential function but that have some chemical properties similar to those of required elements. These elements can become a health threat when they are present in sufficient quantity to replace a required element or to bind excessively to some organic ligand and cause a physiological aberration. Modern industrial technology has effected translocation of large quantities of many minerals from their native stores in the ground to the air, the water, and ultimately the food supply. Three elements that have caused concern and some isolated severe problems for humans are mercury, cadmium, and lead. The nutritional status of an exposed person can modify the severity of adverse response to a toxic level of an element. A deficiency of certain nutrients can result in a more severe adverse effect, while a moderate excess of other nutrients can afford some protection. The possibility must be kept in mind that elements now regarded only as toxic may at some future time have an essential function described for them at a very low level of intake.

Analysis of trace elements can be accomplished by both chemical and physical techniques. Current techniques such as induction coupled plasma, atomic absorption spectrometry, and neutron activation analysis provide rapid, accurate, and low-cost measurements.

CHROMIUM

Function and Deficiency Syndrome—For biological activity, chromium must be trivalent. The most active form of chromium is that which is incorporated into a low-molecular-weight organic molecule that occurs in many foods. Its structure is not known yet. This compound has been designated GTF (glucose tolerance factor). From a variety of biochemical studies, it appears that the presence of insulin is required for all functions of chromium. GTF is the only one of many compounds tested that passed through the rat placenta into the fetus.

The principal defect in chromium deficiency is an impairment of glucose utilization downstream from the insulin receptor; however, disturbances in protein and lipid metabolism also have been observed. In the young animal, growth rate may be reduced. Corneal lesions have been observed in rats deficient in both chromium and protein; no lesions have been seen with either single deficiency.

Impaired glucose utilization occurs in many middle-aged and elderly human beings. In experimental studies, significant numbers of such persons have shown improvement in their glucose utilization after treatment with chromium. There also have been improvements in diabetic children and infants with kwashiorkor.

Metabolism and Bioavailability—Chromium is transported by transferrin in the plasma and competes with iron for binding sites. The main excretory route is through the urine; however, some chromium is excreted in the bile and by the small intestine. The newborn animal has large stores of chromium that decline with age.

Toxicity—In animals, a wide margin of safety separates toxicity from the nutritional requirement of chromium (III). Hexavalent chromium is considered to be toxic.

COBALT

Function, Metabolism, and Deficiency Syndrome—The only known essential function of cobalt is as a component of vitamin B_{12}.

Cobalt salts are absorbed poorly. Excretion is via the bile and through the intestinal wall. Cobalt is widely distributed in the body, with the highest concentrations in the liver, kidney, and bone.

Toxicity—High levels of cobalt can produce a polycythemia in many species, an effect that is unrelated to vitamin B_{12}. Cobalt usually is considered relatively nontoxic; however, severe cardiac failure and some deaths in humans have resulted from consumption of large amounts of

beer containing 1.2 to 1.5 ppm of cobalt. The element was added to the beer to promote optimal foam stabilization.

COPPER

Function and Deficiency Syndrome—Several copper-containing metalloproteins have been isolated from animal tissues, including tyrosinase, ascorbic acid oxidase, laccase, cytochrome oxidase, urate oxidase, monoamine oxidase, δ-aminolevulinic acid dehydrase, and dopamine-β-hydroxylase. Copper functions in the absorption and utilization of iron, electron transport, connective tissue metabolism, phospholipid formation, purine metabolism, and development of the nervous system. Ferroxidase I (ceruloplasmin), a copper-containing enzyme, effects the oxidation of Fe (II) to Fe (III), a required step for mobilization of stored iron. There is evidence that a copper-containing enzyme is responsible for the oxidative deamination of the epsilon amino group of lysine to produce desmosine and isodesmosine, the cross-links of elastin. In copper-deficient animals the arterial elastin is weaker, and dissecting aneurysms may occur.

The most common defect observed in copper-deficient animals is anemia. Other abnormalities include growth depression, skeletal defects, demyelination and degeneration of the nervous system, ataxia, defects in pigmentation and structure of hair or wool, reproductive failure, and cardiovascular lesions, including dissecting aneurysms. Copper deficiency occurs very infrequently in human beings. Deficiency has been observed in some patients receiving nutrition support regimens deficient in copper.

Metabolism and Bioavailability—Copper is absorbed from the small intestine. Most of the copper in the plasma is in ceruloplasmin; however, significant amounts are loosely bound to albumin, and this fraction is important in transport. The plasma copper level increases in acute infections, in pregnancy, and in women taking oral contraceptives. Small amounts of copper are excreted in the urine, but the major excretory pathway is via bile and feces.

Copper is present in high concentrations in the brain, liver, heart, and kidney, with the highest levels occurring at birth. It is important that pregnant women receive adequate copper during pregnancy, so that the infant will have adequate stores of copper at birth.

The chemical form of copper in food is largely unknown. A variety of salts of copper have been used in animal studies and may vary in bioavailability. These salts include the sulfate, nitrate, chloride, carbonate, hydroxide, iodide, glutamate, glycerophosphate, aspartate, citrate, nucleinate, and pyrophosphate. Elemental copper, copper sulfide and oxide are utilized poorly. The absorption of copper can be decreased by large amounts of phytic acid, ascorbic acid, calcium, and zinc.

Toxicity—Wilson's disease, a genetic disease in humans, leads to excess copper accumulation in the brain, liver, and kidney, which results in mental and neurological abnormalities. The disease is treated by administration of a chelating agent, penicillamine (β,β-dimethylcysteine), which removes excess copper from the tissues and results in its excretion.

FLUORINE

Function and Deficiency Syndrome—The most important relationship of fluoride to health is that of preventing dental caries. Fluoride has been shown to enter the hydroxyapatite of teeth to form a more perfect crystal that resists acid attack more effectively. In areas where the fluoride content of the drinking water is unusually high, osteoporosis and calcification of the aorta of elderly persons are less than in control population groups not receiving high fluoride. In these areas the effective fluoride concentration is high enough to cause mottling of the tooth enamel in young children.

Metabolism and Bioavailability—The absorption of fluoride from the GI tract is rapid and complete. Even the water-insoluble forms are absorbed fairly well. Fluoride can cross membranes easily, and it passes readily from the plasma into the tissues; however, the mammary gland and the placenta offer some resistance to transport. Excess fluoride is excreted in the urine.

Bones typically have high concentrations of fluoride, which gradually increase throughout life to about age 55 years. Fluoride supplementation increases bone density but is reported to increase brittleness. Of the soft tissues, the kidney is highest in fluoride. Calcium and aluminum can decrease the absorption of fluoride, and sodium chloride can depress the skeletal uptake of fluoride.

Toxicity—Toxic doses of fluoride cause loss of appetite and body weight, muscular weakness, clonic convulsions, pulmonary congestion, and respiratory and cardiac failure.

Chronic exposure to fluoride most often comes through consumption of drinking water, usually from deep wells drilled through or near fluoride-containing rocks. Levels of fluoride around 2 ppm or higher produce a permanent brownish mottling of tooth enamel when the exposure is during the time of tooth formation.

IODINE

Function, Metabolism, and Deficiency Syndrome—The only known function of iodine is for the production of the thyroid hormones, which regulate cellular oxidation.

The absorption of iodide can occur at all levels of the GI tract. Iodinated amino acids can be absorbed as such but less efficiently than iodide. Excretion of iodine is primarily via the urine, and the amount is a reasonably good indicator of thyroid status. Iodine in saliva is reabsorbed.

The iodine-deficiency disease is goiter. In iodine-deficient young, growth is depressed and sexual development is delayed, the skin and hair are typically rough, and the hair becomes thin. Cretinism, feeble-mindedness and deaf-mutism occur in a severe deficiency. There is reproductive failure in the female and decreased fertility in the male.

Goiter has been observed in human beings in many areas of the world, with incidence in women and children usually higher than in the adult male. As a public-health measure, use of iodized salt has markedly reduced the incidence of goiter. Goitrogens, including those found in food, also can cause goiter.

IRON

Function and Deficiency Syndrome—Iron is an essential component of several important metalloproteins. These include hemoglobin, myoglobin and many oxidation-reduction enzymes. In iron deficiency, there may be reduced concentrations of some of the iron-containing enzymes, such as cytochrome c in liver, kidney, and skeletal muscle and succinic dehydrogenase in the kidney and heart.

Hypochromic microcytic anemia is the characteristic end result of iron deficiency. Depending on the severity, the anemia is accompanied by listlessness and tiredness, palpitation on exertion, sore tongue, angular stomatitis, dysphagia, and koilonychia.

Metabolism—Iron is absorbed from the small intestine by a complex but incompletely understood mechanism. Heme iron is more readily absorbed than non-heme iron. The proportion of dietary iron absorbed is greater in iron-deficient anemic individuals. Iron is transported via the blood, in which it is bound to transferrin, a β_1-globulin.

The iron from deteriorated red blood cells is reused. Under normal circumstances, the loss of iron from the body is very small, about 1 mg a day for men and an additional average daily loss of 0.5 mg a day by menstruating women. Iron is stored in the bone marrow, intestinal wall, liver, and spleen, with the latter organs containing the largest amounts.

Bioavailability—The recognition of anemia as a major public-health problem for menstruating women and young children throughout the world has focused on the need for more-extensive and better fortification of foods. This has stimulated a great deal of research on the availability of iron from foods and inorganic sources. Iron compounds that are utilized readily by experimental animals and humans are ferric ammonium citrate, ferrous sulfate, ferrous gluconate, ferrous fumarate, and ferrous ammonium sulfate. Average to poor sources of iron are reduced iron, ferric chloride, and ferric pyrophosphate. Very poor sources are ferric oxide, ferrous carbonate, sodium iron pyrophosphate, and ferric orthophosphate. The availability of iron from foods can vary also.

Several dietary components can affect the availability of iron from many sources. Phytic acid and antacids can decrease iron absorption. The availability of dietary iron is increased by a variety of reducing compounds such as ascorbic acid and molecules with sulfhydryl groups, as well as histidine and lysine. The smaller the particle size of elemental iron, the greater is the intestinal absorption and use. Heme iron is absorbed as such. High intakes of zinc, copper, manganese, and cadmium can decrease the absorption of iron. Many additional studies are needed to evaluate adequately the availability of iron as influenced by composition of the diet and method of food preparation beyond single test meals.

Toxicity—Because iron absorption is regulated by the body, moderate excess above the RDA was considered harmless. Some individuals have a metabolic defect such that their iron absorption is not carefully controlled, and even a normal iron intake can lead to excess tissue accumulation. A disease known as hemochromatosis results. It usually can be controlled by phlebotomy at periodic intervals; however death can result if the disease is not treated. Epidemiological data suggest that continued high intake of iron may raise the risk for chronic disease occurrence, especially in susceptible individuals, particularly those diseases that are increased with free radical formations. Deaths have occurred, however, in children who swallowed capsules or tablets containing a readily available source of iron, such as ferrous sulfate. Acute effects include vomiting, hematemesis, hepatic damage, tachycardia, and peripheral vascular collapse.

MANGANESE

Function and Deficiency Syndrome—Manganese is required for the synthesis of mucopolysaccharides of cartilage and for the conversion of mevalonic acid to squalene. Glucose utilization is impaired in manganese deficiency. Pyruvate carboxylase is a manganese metalloenzyme. It also participates in superoxide dismutase.

Manganese deficiency has been produced experimentally in many animals. Characteristics of the deficiency include growth depression of the young animal, skeletal abnormalities (ranging from mild rarefaction to crippling deformities), mortality of the young, perosis (slipping of the Achilles tendon and accompanying joint deformity) in birds, depressed reproduction of both males and females, nutritional chondrodystrophy of the chick embryo, and ataxia in newborn mammals, with head retraction, tremor, abnormal otoliths, and semicircular canals in the ears. Newborn manganese-deficient guinea pigs have aplasia or marked hypoplasia of the pancreas. Manganese deficiency has not been well recognized in humans.

Metabolism and Bioavailability—The homeostatic mechanism for regulating the concentration of manganese in the body is very precise. Manganese is absorbed from the small intestine and then is transported via the blood in the trivalent form bound to a β_1-globulin, transmanganin. Manganese is excreted in the bile and through the intestinal wall. The latter constitutes the principal mechanism for regulating the amounts of manganese in the tissues. With a high manganese intake, the element also is excreted in the pancreatic juice. The amount excreted in the urine is very small.

High levels of manganese occur in bone, liver, kidney, pancreas, and the pituitary, whereas the concentration in the skeletal muscle is very low. The manganese in bone cannot be mobilized to meet a need. The stores of manganese, in the order of their importance, are found in the liver, skin, and skeletal muscle. There is not a special store in the newborn.

Bioavailability of manganese from various salts (oxide, carbonate, sulfate, and chloride) has not been well evaluated. High dietary intakes of calcium and phosphorus can decrease manganese absorption.

Toxicity—Miners exposed to manganese oxide dust for long periods of time develop psychiatric abnormalities that resemble schizophrenia. This is followed by crippling neurological disorders similar to those found in Parkinson's disease.

MOLYBDENUM

Function, Metabolism, and Deficiency Syndrome—Xanthine oxidase is an important molybdenum-containing enzyme. Due to a variety of indirect evidence and the importance of xanthine oxidase, molybdenum is considered to be an essential trace mineral for humans, required in very small amounts.

Molybdenum supplied by water-soluble salts is absorbed readily. The element crosses the mammary gland easily. Excretion is into both urine and feces. The liver and kidney have the highest soft-tissue concentrations of molybdenum. Changes in level of dietary intake can be reflected in the concentrations in liver, kidney, skin, bones, and hair. The newborn does not have special stores of the element. Sulfate can affect the absorption, tissue distribution, and excretion of molybdenum. The content of molybdenum in erythrocytes decreases in many types of anemia. Adverse effects due to simple deficiency of molybdenum in healthy humans and in experimental animals have not been observed.

Toxicity—The tolerance of animals to high intakes of molybdenum varies with species, age, and the level of numerous other dietary components. The toxicity is decreased by copper, inorganic sulfate, and the sulfur amino acids.

NICKEL

Evidence that nickel is an essential element is based on abnormalities produced in chicks and rats fed diets containing 3 to 4 ppb of nickel. Lipid metabolism was affected. Rats maintained through successive generations on the nickel-deficient diet had increased fetal mortality.

Absorption of nickel is small from ordinary diets. Excretion is primarily through the feces; however, significant amounts can be lost in sweat. Phytate can form a very stable complex with nickel, so it is possible that phytate may decrease absorption of nickel. Further studies are required to establish clearly the essentiality of nickel and its significance to human health.

A low level of toxicity has been established for nickel in rats, mice, monkeys, and chicks.

SELENIUM

Function and Deficiency Syndrome—Selenium is an essential component of several enzymes including glutathione peroxidase. This provides a link between the antioxidant properties of vitamin E and the biological function of selenium in preventing most of the same selenium-deficiency problems. Animal studies have indicated that selenium may be useful as a chemoprevention agent, but studies in humans have not been accomplished. Experimentally, selenium has been shown to provide protection to pulmonary oxygen toxicity similar to that observed for vitamin E.

Depending on species, age, and specific diet composition, a deficiency of selenium can lead to one or more of the following abnormalities: growth depression, muscular dystrophy, degeneration of the myocardium, neurological lesions, liver necrosis, pancreatic fibrosis, exudative diathesis, ceroid-pigment deposition in adipose tissue, and death. Deficiency occurs in domestic animals with intakes below 0.02 to 0.05 ppm. Deficiency in humans has been demonstrated in China, where extremely low intake causes a cardiomyopathy in children (Keshan disease Other geographic areas with low selenium soil content also exist. Most deficiency syndromes responsive to selenium also respond favorably to vitamin E. An exception is pancreatic fibrosis, which occurs only in selenium deficiency.

Metabolism—Selenium is absorbed from the duodenum. It can be metabolized to a variety of compounds and lost from the body via the bile, pancreatic and intestinal secretions, and ultimately through the feces, urine, and expired air. Selenium can replace sulfur in the normal sulfur amino acids, and selenite also can bind to sulfur amino acids. It also is incorporated into selenonucleosides and may be involved in genetic translation. The highest tissue concentrations of selenium occur in the kidney, pancreas, pituitary, and liver.

Toxicity—Acute selenium toxicity is characterized by abdominal pain, excess salivation, grating of the teeth, paralysis, and blindness. Eventually, disturbed respiration leads to death.

Selenium is one of the most toxic of the essential nutrients, and the quantitative separation of required and chronic toxic levels is not very large. The source of selenium has a significant impact on the level that will cause toxicity to develop. Organic compounds containing selenium enhance absorption and, therefore, are toxic at lower levels. For domestic animals, the requirement is about 0.1 to 0.2 ppm, and 3 to 4 ppm in the diet are beginning levels for chronic toxicity. Intakes above 500 μg for long periods of time are considered to present a risk of toxicity in man. The upper tolerable intake level set by the Food and Nutrition Board is 400 μg daily for adults. A reported carcinogenicity for selenium is an elusive association that has not been clarified finally.

SILICON

With highly purified diets it has been possible to produce a deficiency of silicon in chicks and rats. The deficiency affected growth rate, bones, and integumental tissues. The primary biochemical lesion in the deficient animals was an effect on the cartilage matrix.

Silicon (as silicates) is absorbed easily from the intestinal tract and excreted readily in the urine, in part as SiO_2. Silicon is distributed widely in soil, plants, and animal tissues. It is relatively nontoxic; however, siliceous kidney stones have been reported in persons who live in regions with water high in silicate concentration or who chronically ingest magnesium trisilicate antacids.

TIN

Through rigid exclusion of environmental and dietary tin, it has been possible to produce growth retardation responsive to this element in rats. A maximal growth effect was obtained with 1 ppm of tin in the diet, a level similar to that found in many foods.

Tin is absorbed poorly and most of that in the diet is excreted in the feces. Tin has a low order of toxicity.

VANADIUM

Chicks and rats fed a diet containing less than 10 ppb of vanadium had slow growth, defective bones, and altered lipid metabolism. At low doses the element may influence glycemic control. Vanadium is a rather toxic element. The addition of 25 to 50 ppm of vanadium to the diet of rats causes diarrhea and mortality.

ZINC

Function and Deficiency Syndrome—Zinc is known to occur in many important metalloenzymes. These include carbonic anhydrase,

carboxypeptidases A and B, alcohol dehydrogenase, glutamic dehydrogenase, D-glyceraldehyde-3-phosphate dehydrogenase, lactic dehydrogenase, malic dehydrogenase, alkaline phosphatase, aldolase, and others. Impaired synthesis of nucleic acids and proteins has been observed in zinc deficiency. There is some evidence that zinc may be involved in the secretion of insulin and in the function of the hormone. It appears to be a modulator of neurohumoral transmission.

Zinc is required for growth of every animal species studied; therefore, growth depression of young animals is invariably observed if the zinc deprivation is severe enough. Other characteristics of deficiency include skin lesions, alopecia, abnormal feathering in birds, deformed and poorly mineralized bones, hyperkeratinization of the esophagus, reduced numbers of circulating lymphocytes, impaired reproduction in males and females, fetal abnormalities, and decreased learning ability. Persons with impaired taste acuity and discrimination and delayed healing of wounds and burns have responded favorably to therapeutic doses of zinc in some cases.

Nutritional dwarfism has been studied extensively in the Middle East. The syndrome includes delayed sexual development, reduced height and weight, hepatosplenomegaly, spoon nails, and usually anemia. Although the subjects were deficient to some degree in several nutrients, zinc was required to correct the hypogonadism and growth depression. The syndrome occurs in both males and females. Indolent ulcers and delayed wound healing in patients with low plasma zinc levels have been reported, and both systemic and topical administration of zinc compounds are followed by accelerated healing. There is limited evidence that some young children and elderly persons in the United States do not receive adequate zinc.

Metabolism and Bioavailability—Zinc can bind readily to sulfhydryl groups, amino groups, and imidazole groups of proteins, amino acids, and other organic molecules.

Zinc is absorbed primarily from the duodenum. It binds to all proteins of the plasma; however, it is bound most loosely to albumin, and this may be important for transport to and from tissues. The concentration of zinc in plasma decreases rapidly when a low-zinc diet is fed, and it is reduced in pregnancy and in women taking oral contraceptives. The principal route of excretion is via the feces. Small amounts of zinc are excreted daily in the urine; these increase when there is tissue catabolism such as occurs in burns and in fasting. Significant losses of zinc also can occur in the sweat.

Zinc is present in all tissues, with very high concentrations in the prostate and choroid of the eye. Generally, tissue concentrations are not affected greatly by zinc deficiency. The stores of zinc in the body are thought to be small.

Zinc bioavailability may vary with the wide variety of inorganic salts as well as metallic zinc. Phytic acid can markedly decrease absorption of zinc, particularly in the presence of large amounts of calcium. Consumption of whole-wheat bread, which contains phytic acid, has been shown to be primarily responsible for the zinc-deficiency dwarfism observed in the Middle East. The toxic effects of cadmium are probably partially related to interference with the normal physiological pathways and functions of zinc.

Toxicity—The taste threshold for a soluble salt of zinc in water is 15 ppm of zinc, whereas 40 ppm have a very definite taste. A dose of 225 to 450 mg of zinc has an emetic effect in an adult man. Acute toxicity of zinc is characterized by dehydration, electrolytic imbalance, stomach pain, lethargy, dizziness, muscular incoordination, and renal failure. High zinc intakes are known to lower copper absorption; therefore zinc supplements should be taken only with adequate intakes of copper. Zinc has been used successfully to treat Wilson's disease.

ZINC SULFATE—see RPS-19, page 1271.

ASSOCIATED DIETARY SUBSTANCES

A large number of substances, predominantly from plant sources (ie, phytochemicals), are found in the human diet. An understanding of these compounds and their potential impact on health and disease risk are only beginning to be described. Whether they will constitute a new class or classes of nutrients will depend on the essentiality to health of each individual class. Those undergoing the most scrutiny include the carotenoids, flavonoids and phenolic acids, as well as phytosterols, organosulfurics, indoles and isothiocyanates, lignans, stilbenes, terpenes, and tannins. Recent food composition

databases contain estimates of carotenoid and flavonoid content of foods commonly consumed.

CAROTENOIDS

There are an estimated 600 or more different carotenoids found naturally, of which several dozen are consumed in the human diet, a number of which can be routinely assayed in humans. Circulating concentrations of carotenoids are biological mark-

Table 92-8. Common Dietary Phenolic Compounds

CLASS	COMPOUNDS	FOOD SOURCES
Flavonoids		
• Flavones	Apigenin, luteolin	Parsley, peppers
• Flavonols	Kaempferol, quercetin	Apples, onions
• Flavanones	Hesperetin, naringenin	Citrus fruit, prunes
• Flavanols	Catechins, theaflavins	Cocoa, tea
• Anthocyanidins	Cyanidin, malvidin	Cherries, grapes
• Isoflavones	Daidzein, genistein	Soybeans, legumes
Phenolic acids	Caffeic acid, curcumin, ferulic acid	Apples, tomato, turmeric, wheat bran
Organosulfurics	Allylic sulfides, glucosinolates	Garlic, onions, leeks, cruciferous vegetables
Indoles	Indole-3-carbinol	Cruciferous vegetables
Lignan	Enterodiol, enterolactone	Grains, flax meal
Stilbenes	Resveratrol	Wine, grapes, peanuts
Triterpenes	Limonin, nomilin	Citrus fruit, spices

ers for fruit and vegetable consumption; and increased intakes are associated with lower risk of chronic disease. Most naturally occurring carotenoids exist in the all-trans configuration, and they serve to protect plants against photosensitization, but may possess antioxidant and other health-related activity. While a small number of them are known to be precursors to retinol (vitamin A), most are not. The carotenoids α-carotene, β-carotene, and β-cryptoxanthin are known to be pro-vitamin-A compounds that may be partially converted to retinol at the gastrointestinal mucosa. This is the only currently recognized nutrient function of carotenoids in humans. Other widely recognized carotenoids include lycopene, lutein, and zeaxanthin. Data on the absorption, metabolism, and excretion of carotenoids continue to be generated. Carotenoid bioavailability varies considerably with the food matrix it is part of and compounds it is administered with, as well as with the specific carotenoid. Lipoproteins serve as the route of transport for carotenoids. The recent DRIs provided no quantitative recommendations for carotenoid intake because data is insufficient to establish requirements; beyond consuming a wide variety of fruits and vegetables. It is known that the average dietary intake of carotenoids includes about 8 mg of lycopene, 2 mg of β-carotene, 1.7 mg of lutein and zeaxanthin, 400 μg of α-carotene, and about 100 μg of β-cryptoxanthin daily. Several carotenoids have been included in dietary supplement products. A valid method for assaying β-carotene and other carotenoids found in these products is currently being explored.

FLAVONOIDS

A large number of phenolic compounds are consumed in the human diet. These range from simple phenolic molecules (ie, phenolic acids) to high molecular weight, highly polymerized polyphenols (ie, tannins). These phytochemicals have been classified into groups that include flavonoids, and phenolic acids (Table 92-8). The flavonoids, once referred to as "vitamin P," are the largest class of polyphenols containing several thousand compounds, and are further broken down into a number of subclasses. The most common subclasses of flavonoids are the flavones, flavonols, flavanones, flavanols, anthocyanidins, and the isoflavones. Except for the flavanols, which exist in free form or as gallic esters, most of the other compounds exist in glycosylated forms. Flavonoids in plants are produced as a result of stressors that include climate, ultraviolet radiation, herbivores, and pathogens. These secondary metabolites are involved in plant communication and defense. As such the flavonoid content

of foods can be quite variable depending on conditions of development and growth. Antioxidant, free-radical scavenging, enzyme inhibiting and other activities of the flavonoids are being explored. Select flavonoids have been added as ingredients to dietary supplement products, although the data do not currently support this pharmacological use of individual flavonoids.

ACKNOWLEDGMENTS—The author acknowledges the tremendous efforts of Ernestine Vanderveen, PhD and John E Vanderveen, PhD in previous editions of this work.

REFERENCES

1. AOAC. Official Methods of Analysis of AOAC International., 17th ed. Washington, DC: AOAC International, 2002.
2. Bendich A, Deckelbaum RJ, eds. *Preventive Nutrition*, 2nd ed. Totowa, NJ: Humana Press, 2001.
3. Institute of Medicine, Food and Nutrition Board. *Dietary reference intakes: calcium, phosphorus, magnesium, vitamin D, and fluoride.* Washington, DC: National Academy Press, 1997.
4. Institute of Medicine, Food and Nutrition Board. *Dietary reference intakes: thiamin, riboflavin, niacin, vitamin B6, folate, vitamin B12, pantothenic acid, biotin, and choline.* Washington, DC: National Academy Press, 1998.
5. Institute of Medicine, Food and Nutrition Board. *Dietary reference intakes: vitamin C, vitamin E, selenium, and carotenoids.* Washington, DC: National Academy Press, 2000.
6. Institute of Medicine, Food and Nutrition Board. *Dietary reference intakes: vitamin A, vitamin K, arsenic, boron, chromium, copper, iodine, iron, manganese, molybdenum, nickel, silicon, vanadium, and zinc.* Washington, DC: National Academy Press, 2001.
7. Institute of Medicine, Food and Nutrition Board. *Dietary reference intakes: macronutrients and energy.* Washington, DC: National Academy Press, 2002.
8. Institute of Medicine, Food and Nutrition Board. *Dietary reference intakes: water, potassium, sodium, chloride, and sulfate.* Washington DC: National Academy Press, 2004.
9. Nutrient Data Laboratory. *Food composition database.* www.nal.usda.gov/fnic/foodcomp, 2003.
10. Shils ME, Olson JA, Shike M, Ross AC, eds. *Modern Nutrition in Health and Disease*, 9th ed. Philadelphia: Lippincott Williams & Wilkins, 1999.
11. Sikorski ZE, ed. *Chemical and Functional Properties of Food Components*, 2nd ed. Boca Raton, FL: CRC Press, 2002.
12. Stipanuk MH, ed. *Biochemical and Physiological Aspects of Human Nutrition.* Philadelphia: WB Saunders, 2000.
13. United States Pharmacopeial Convention. United States Pharmacopoeia / National Formulary, Edition 26/21. Rockville, MD: United States Pharmacopoeial Convention, 2003.
14. Yeo IB. *Food in Health and Disease.* Philadelphia: Lea Brothers & Co., 1894.

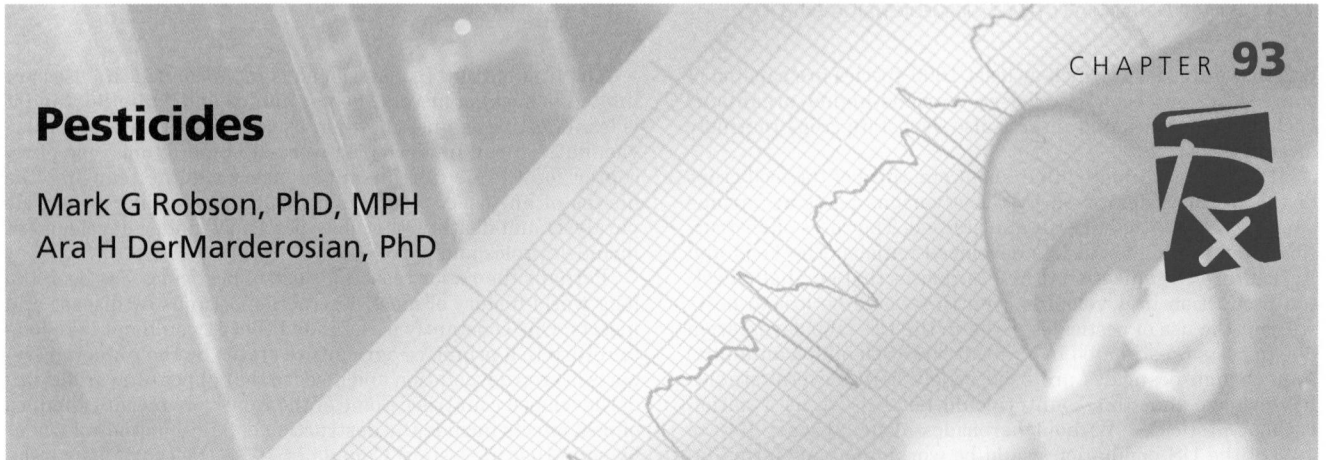

Pesticides

Mark G Robson, PhD, MPH

Ara H DerMarderosian, PhD

Pesticides may be defined simply as chemical agents used to control pests. In its broadest sense it includes insecticides, rodenticides, fungicides, and herbicides. These substances represent big business, with the US once being the largest producer in the world.

For the US, the Environmental Protection Agency (EPA) reports that pesticide use has remained stable, with year-to-year variations resulting from changes in acreages planted and weather conditions. In the most recent report, *Pesticide Industry Sales and Usage—1998 and 1999 Market Estimates,* released in August 2002, the EPA reported that the use of herbicides to control weeds has increased slightly over the previous 3 years. An average of $4200 per farm was expended in 1995 on pesticides. Conventional pesticides account for 27% of all pesticides used annually in the US and total an estimated 1.2 billion pounds. Wood preservatives account for 16% of all pesticides used and total about 0.72 billion pounds; speciality biocides, such as those used to control bacterial growth in cooling towers, are about 6% and total 0.26 billion pounds; and chlorine/hypochlorites, used in water-purifying plants and swimming pools represent 51% of all pesticides used and total 2.32 billion pounds.

The specific results of the National Home and Garden survey revealed that

In households without children under 5 years old, about 75% had at least one pesticide stored less than 4 feet off the ground and not locked in a cabinet (ie, within reach of children).

In homes with children under 5 years of age, about 47% stored at least one pesticide within reach of children. Overall, an estimated 85% of all households have at least one pesticide in storage and around the home.

Most families have between one and five pesticide products stored, and slightly over 27% of single family households have over six products stored.

Some 76% of all households used pesticides in their homes themselves, while about 20% hired a commercial applicator to treat such pests as roaches, fleas, or ants (termites are not included in these estimates).

Less than 25% could recall receiving written notification about the pesticides used in their home or any safety precautions to follow.

About 15% of households had pesticides applied in or around their homes by someone outside the household. Only half of these people recall receiving written information regarding the pesticides used and safety precautions to be followed.

In the households that dispose of concentrated pesticides, 67% use regular trash, 16% use special collections, and 17% give it away or pour it down the toilet or sink, on the street, in the gutter or sewer, or on the ground.

Some 44% of all households identified at least one insect that was considered a major problem.

Some 25% of all households were treated for cockroaches in 1990. It appears that cockroaches are the most common pest problem for households living in multifamily dwellings. For households in single-family dwellings, ants are the most common problem.

The most difficult pest to control was identified as fleas.

One of the most interesting reports on this scientific random sampling was an amazing response rate of 85%. The executive summaries of this 400-page National Home and Garden Pesticide Use Survey are available and may be obtained from the Communications Branch of EPA's Pesticide Programs (telephone: 703-305-5017).

Pharmacies throughout the US stock a myriad of consumer pesticide products used for these purposes. This represents an important area in which pharmacists can exercise their knowledge and skills, particularly for proper use, handling, and disposal of pesticides.

The EPA published the *Status of Pesticides in Registration and Special Review* (Rainbow report) that contains a general management directory, a chemical review manager directory, and a general information section that covers purpose, timing, comments, additional information, and electronic access (see EPA website, www.epa.gov, for the latest information).

Chapter 2 is entitled *Special Review* and is organized so that the first section explains the special review process including the criteria that EPA uses to initiate a special review, the steps it takes to conduct a Special Review, and the risk-reduction alternatives to the conventional Special Review process.

The following section gives an *At a Glance* summary of the dates when Special Review decision documents were published in the *Federal Register*.

The third section provides a comprehensive reference list of all chemicals that have been or are currently in the Special Review program. The various chemicals are listed in alphabetical order.

The final section lists the chemicals in identical sequence and additionally, gives the details of Special Review criteria met or exceeded as well as the outcomes of the reviews. The entire report is 377 pages long and lists almost 1500 compounds.

Further, the EPA lists numerous solvents, surfactants, stabilizers, and similar substances. Various economic, political, and toxicological considerations that crop up routinely in the pesticide business preclude any more-accurate figures within a given year.

For those who question the use of pesticides at all it is important to know something about what damage pests can do on a worldwide basis. First it should be understood that plants are the world's major source of food. These plants are susceptible to 80,000 to 100,000 diseases caused by everything from viruses to bacteria, fungi, algae, and even other higher plants. Food plants have to compete with some 30,000 different species of weeds worldwide, of which at least 1800 species are capable of causing serious economic losses. Various higher organisms such as nematodes and insects also devastate crops routinely around the world.

It has been estimated that about one-third of the food crops of the world is destroyed by these various pests at various stages, *viz*, growth, harvest, and storage. The rates of destruction often are higher in less developed nations. The Food and Agriculture Organization (FAO) estimates that one-half of cotton production in developing countries would be lost to pests without the use of pesticides. Even in the US, crop devastation due to pests is estimated to be about 30% ($20 billion annually) even though pesticides are used widely here. Several studies have shown that this country could not survive as a nation without pesticides. Without herbicides alone, at least 10% to 12% of the US population would be working on our farms instead of the current 3%.

Another important consideration of recent origin is the concept of minimum or reduced tillage. In this relatively new farming practice, herbicides help promote energy savings and soil conservation by reducing plowing and cultivation drastically. Now, farmers till only enough to plant new crops. Previous crop debris and weeds are left on the soil, and insects and weeds are controlled chemically rather than mechanically through unnecessary plowing. This method of control requires some 80% less energy.

There have been many who have argued for the return of what is called *organic* farming. Generally, organic farmers prefer to avoid the use of synthetic chemical products at all. They prefer naturally occurring chemicals such as rock phosphate and limestone and the manure of domestic animals. Also, leguminous plants are used as a nitrogen source as well as other plants that contain natural pesticidal compounds. While these are laudable practices, they generally result in higher prices because of the costs of these less available materials and the higher costs involved in the more labor-intensive practices of organic farming. In addition, more land with lower yielding capability would have to be farmed to make up for the lower efficiency of organic farming.

From a scientific point of view all natural materials are not necessarily organic, and organic substances are not necessarily natural. All things on earth are made up of chemicals, and plants do not really differentiate between what is made by man or nature. However, organic farming practices are sensible for the smaller farmer who wishes to avoid excess use of unnecessary chemicals and does not mind the use of extra labor practices to save money on materials.

According to a study by the Natural Resources Defense Council entitled "Harvest of Hope," alternative farming techniques could reduce pesticide applications 25% to 80% on nine crops grown in California and Iowa. The study showed that over 580 million pounds of pesticide-active ingredients were sold in California in 1987, and 57 million pounds of herbicide per year were used by Iowa farmers.

The study further stated that many ill effects have resulted from use of all of these, including pesticide contamination of the food supply, farm worker illness, ecosystem degradation, and water pollution. The council study calls on the federal government to redirect its agricultural research to make development of alternative farming systems a priority and to adopt alternative farming systems, including crop rotations, without incurring financial penalties. In addition, it promotes the concept that federal and state governments should levy fees on fertilizers and pesticides to help finance alternative agricultural research. At the same time that alternative ways of controlling pests are being sought, there are efforts to develop new chemicals with greater specificity to a particular pest and less toxicity to nontarget species. Proponents claim that having different chemical pesticides on hand with varying mechanisms of action allows rotation of these to limit development of resistance.

The first of this type developed is *imidacloprid*. Its uses are limited to sucking insects such as aphids and whiteflies, and it is less effective against chewing insects (worms, caterpillar larvae, butterflies). Imidacloprid works to bind to one type of receptor for the neurotransmitter acetylcholine, causing the nerves of an insect to fire uncontrollably, leading to muscle paralysis and death. Other new pesticides under development include fiproles and pyrroles.

Perhaps the major reason for use of pesticides has been the long world history of mass destruction of crops by disease and insects. One constantly is reminded that it would not take long to return to a primitive agriculture status by the numerous reports of crop devastation and disease that appear in various underdeveloped countries. Some of the relatively recent examples of pest effects include the destruction of 3 million tons of wheat by stem rust in western Canada in 1954, the continuous problem of arthropod-borne encephalitides that caused an average of 205 human cases in the US annually between 1964 and 1973, and the reduction of the annual death rate of malaria through the use of pesticides. The death rate in 1939 was 6 million, compared with 1996 estimates of 1.5 to 2.7 million. There are at least 24 common diseases (eg, encephalitis, typhus, anthrax, and dysentery) still of concern to man that are transmitted by a myriad of insects, ticks, or mites.

As with all substances used by modern man, pesticides offer a risk-benefit ratio that must be assessed for each application. A modern, concerned society should always advocate very specific, carefully planned usage of pesticides, well-integrated with other control practices. This approach has become quite popular today and is referred to as Integrated Pest Management (IPM). It consists of determining a workable combination of the best parts of all possible control procedures and applying them to a specific problem. The concept is to keep pests at a controllable level within the confines of sound ecological principles so that economic injury to plants or man is avoided. Overall, while mistakes have been made (eg, DDT), pesticides have contributed significantly to the increased productivity of the US farmer.

According to the American Crop Protection Association, less than 2% of Americans are farmers, compared with 30% in 1920. According to the US Department of Agriculture, in 1950 one farmer in the US fed 27 people; in 1970, 73; and in 1992, 129.

In recent years, there is a new trend in pesticide chemistry and application technology. For example, a 1-lb bottle of a new rice herbicide can control 10 acres of weeds; 5 years ago this area would have required 20 lb of pesticide.

EPA requires a new pesticide product to undergo rigorous registration requirements. Up to 120 safety, health, and environmental tests are required for registration. Typically it takes 10 years for a product to move from discovery to market, with an average cost of $35 to 50 million.

PESTICIDES AND LAW

In the US, numerous federal laws protect the user of pesticides as well as the consumers. Many of these laws are quite old and have been amended from time to time for obvious reasons. Since they are all complex and change with time, a brief summary is presented here so the pharmacist will be aware of who is responsible for which laws and what the current status of pesticide registration is.

The Federal Insecticide, Fungicide and Rodenticide Act (FIFRA) as amended (EPA, Oct 1996) is administered by the EPA. These new amendments require a substantial acceleration of the reregistration process for previously registered (licensed) pesticides and authorize the collection of fees to support reregistration activities. This law also changes EPA's responsibilities and funding requirements for the storage and disposal of suspended and cancelled pesticides and the indemnification of holders of remaining stocks of such canceled pesticides. Hence, under FIFRA, all pesticides have to be registered with the EPA before they may be sold or distributed in commerce in the US.

This agency establishes an overall risk-benefit standard for pesticide registration, requiring that pesticides show efficacy when employed according to label instructions and show no unreasonable risk of adverse effects on human health or the environment. Laws require that EPA take into account the economic, social, and environmental costs and benefits of pesticide uses.

Because FIFRA was originally enacted in 1947, there has been developed since literally thousands of pesticides registered for use. However, over time, the standards of use obviously have changed and evolved in tandem with general advances in science and public policy. Specifically, for example, test-data requirements for pesticides have become increasingly stringent in the light of modern advances in analytical chemistry and toxicology. So now, more than ever, companies that hold pesticide registrations are responsible for providing all test data needed to satisfy EPA's registration requirements. To be sure all of these things are done, FIFRA requires the review and *reregistration* of all existing pesticides.

The Food Quality Protection Act of 1996 (PL 104-170) amends both the Federal Food, Drug, and Cosmetic (FD&C) Act and FIFRA to provide a comprehensive and protective regulatory scheme for pesticides.

Highlights of the new laws are
FD&C ACT PROVISIONS
Health-Based Safety Standard for Pesticide Residues in Food—Establishes a strong, health-based safety standard for pesticide residues in all foods. It uses "a reasonable certainty of no harm" as the general safety standard, the same approach used in the Administration's 1994 bill.

1. Eliminates longstanding problems posed by multiple standards for pesticides in raw and processed foods with a single health-based standard.
2. Requires the EPA to consider all non-occupational sources of exposure, including drinking water, and exposure to other pesticides with a common mechanism of toxicity when setting tolerances.

Special Provisions for Infants and Children—Incorporates language virtually identical to the Administration's 1994 bill to implement key recommendations of the National Academy of Sciences report, "Pesticides in the Diets of Infants and Children."

1. Requires an explicit determination that tolerances are safe for children.
2. Includes an additional safety factor of up to 10-fold, if necessary, to account for uncertainty in data relative to children.
3. Requires consideration of children's special sensitivity and exposure to pesticide chemicals.

Limitations on Benefits Considerations—Places specific limits on benefits considerations, unlike previous law, which contained an open-ended provision for the consideration of pesticide benefits when setting tolerances.

1. Applies only to non-threshold effects of pesticides (eg, carcinogenic effects); benefits cannot be taken into account for reproductive or other threshold effects.
2. Limits further by three *backstops* on the level of risk that could be offset by benefits considerations: a limitation (1) on the acceptable risk in any 1 year, which greatly reduces the risks; (2) on the lifetime risk, which would allow the EPA to remove tolerances after specific phaseout periods; and (3) on not allowing benefits to be used to override the health-based standard for children.

Tolerance Reevaluation—Requires that all existing tolerances be reviewed within 10 years to make sure they meet the requirements of the new health-based safety standard.
Endocrine Disruptors—Incorporates provisions for endocrine testing and also provides new authority to require that chemical manufacturers provide data on their products, including data on potential endocrine effects.
Enforcement—Includes enhanced enforcement of pesticide residue standards by allowing the FDA to impose civil penalties for tolerance violations.
Right-to-Know—Requires distribution of a brochure in grocery stores on the health effects of pesticides, how to avoid risks, and which foods have tolerances for pesticide residues based on benefits consider-

ations. Specifically recognizes a state's right to require warnings or labeling of food that has been treated with pesticides, such as California's Proposition 65.
Uniformity of Tolerances—Prohibits states from setting tolerance levels that differ from national levels unless the state petitions the EPA for an exception, based on state-specific situations. National uniformity, however, would not apply to tolerances that included benefits considerations.

FEDERAL INSECTICIDE, FUNGICIDE, AND RODENTICIDE ACT PROVISIONS (FIFRA)
Pesticide Reregistration Program—Reauthorizes and increases (from $14 to 16 million per year) user fees necessary to complete the review of older pesticides to ensure that they meet current standards. Requires tolerances to be reassessed as part of the reregistration program.
Pesticide Registration Renewal—Requires the EPA to review pesticide registrations periodically, with a goal of establishing a 15-year cycle, to ensure that all pesticides meet updated safety standards.
Registration of Safer Pesticides—Expedites review of safer pesticides to help them reach the market sooner and replace older and potentially more risky chemicals.
Minor-Use Pesticides—

1. Establishes minor-use programs within the EPA and USDA to foster coordination on minor-use regulations and policy and provides for a revolving grant fund to support development of data necessary to register minor-use pesticides.
2. Encourages minor-use registrations through extensions for submitting pesticide residue data, extensions for exclusive use of data, and flexibility to waive certain data requirements and requires the EPA to expedite review of minor-use applications. These incentives are coupled with safeguards to protect the environment.

Antimicrobial Pesticides—Establishes new requirements to expedite the review and registration of antimicrobial pesticides and ends regulatory overlap in jurisdiction over liquid chemical sterilants. Office of Prevention, Pesticides and Toxic Substances (7506C) (August 1996)

Readers are advised to write or call the Special Review and Reregistration Div (H-7508W), Office of Pesticide Programs, US EPA, Washington, DC 20460; telephone: 703-308-8000.

For similar reasons it has not been possible to provide the exact status of every pesticide mentioned in this chapter. For completeness, however, the longstanding status and general properties of many *classically* used pesticides have been retained.
THE ENVIRONMENTAL PROTECTION AGENCY RESPONSIBILITIES. Interpret its laws and implement its provisions.

Established, by regulation, 10 categories of certification for commercial applicators. These include (1) agricultural pest control (plant and animal); (2) forest pest control; (3) ornamental and turf pest control; (4) seed treatment; (5) aquatic pest control; (6) right-of-way pest control; (7) industrial, institutional, structural, and health-related pest control; (8) public health pest control; (9) regulatory pest control; and (10) demonstration and research pest control.

Set general standards of knowledge for all categories of certified commercial applicators of pesticides. In each state, the certification is carried out by an appropriate regulatory agency, usually the state department of agriculture. Pesticide applicators are trained through the various cooperative extension services of the state.

The US Food and Drug Administration, Center for Food Safety and Applied Nutrition has published and put on its web sites (FDA/CFSAN Pesticides, Metals, and Industrial Chemicals; http://www.cfsan.fda.gov/~lrd/pestadd.html) several pesticide-related topics including various guidance articles, certain residue monitoring reports, and at least five technical references of the past 2 to 3 years. Other related web sites (http://www.cfsan.fda.gov/~dms/pes93rep.html and http://www.cfsan.fda.gov/~dms/pesrpts.html) provide over 30 pages on the FDA Pesticide Program residue monitoring from 1993 to 2001 These cover the FDA monitoring program, regulatory monitoring, analytical methods, FDA–state cooperation, animal feeds, international activities, incidence level monitoring, total diet studies, and results and discussions.

STATE REGULATION

Since these vary considerably for each state there is little room to include them in this chapter. For the most part, these laws are similar to the federal regulations. Refer to local state agricultural agencies for specific information.

MEDICINAL AGENTS

Pesticides and the Law

At the international level, the World Health Organization (WHO) and the Food and Agriculture Organization (FAO) of the United Nations continue to press for wider use of certain pesticides to help raise the level of efficiency in agriculture. Recent WHO literature relates international concern on safe use of pesticides and pesticide residues in food.

Interest in pesticides extends beyond their use simply to increase crop yields, specifically to their use in the control of pests as vectors of disease. For example, it is well-known that insects such as chiggers, itch mites, and ticks transport disease to humans directly or via foodstuffs, and that mosquitos, tsetse flies, rat fleas, and others are capable of directly injecting disease organisms into the bloodstream. Pest control also enters into areas where livestock must be protected against predatory animals such as coyotes, wolves, and bobcats.

It should be stated at the outset that the various pesticides discussed in this chapter are subject to numerous constraints under new and continually changing rulings. For this reason it is suggested that reference be made directly to the EPA for definitive information on specific pesticides and their registered uses. Each state also publishes its own set of pesticide recommendations.

Last updated in August 1997, the EPA has published a list of banned and severely restricted pesticides.

A *banned* pesticide is a pesticide for which all registered uses have been prohibited by final government action or for which all requests for registration or equivalent action for all uses have, for health or environmental reasons, not been granted.

BANNED PESTICIDES

1. Aldrin	23. EDB
2. Benzene hexachloride [BHC]	24. Endrin
	25. EPN
3. 2,3,4,5-Bis(2-butylene) tetrahydro2-furaldehyde [Repellent-11]	26. Ethyl hexyleneglycol [6–12]
	27. Hexachlorobenzene [HCB]
4. Bromoxynil butyrate	28. Lead arsenate
5. Cadmium compounds	29. Leptophos
6. Calcium arsenate	30. Mercurous chloride
7. Captafol	31. Mercuric chloride
8. Carbon tetrachloride	32. Mevinphos
9. Chloranil	33. Mirex
10. Chlordane	34. Monocrotophos
11. Chlordimeform	35. Nitrofen (TOK)
12. Chlorinated camphene [Toxaphene]	36. OMPA (octamethyl-pyrophosphoramide)
13. Chlorobenzilate	37. Phenylmercury acetate [PMA]
14. Chloromethoxypropyl-mercuric acetate [CPMA]	38. Phenylmercuric oleate [PMO]
15. Copper arsenate	
16. Cyhexatin	39. Potassium 2,4,5-trichloro-phenate [2,4,5-TCP]
17. DBCP	40. Pyriminil [Vacor]
18. Decachlorooctahydro-1,3,4-metheno-2*H*-cyclo-buta(cd) pentalen-2-one [chlordecone]	41. Safrole
	42. Silvex
	43. Sodium arsenite
	44. TDE
19. DDT	45. Terpene polychlorinates [Strobane]
20. Dieldrin	46. Thallium sulfate
21. Dinoseb and salts	47. 2,4,5-Trichlorophenoxy-acetic acid [2,4,5-T]
22. Di(phenylmercury) dodecenylsuccinate [PMDS]	48. Vinyl chloride

A *severely restricted* pesticide is a pesticide for which virtually all registered uses have been prohibited by final government regulatory action but for which certain specific registered use or uses remain authorized.

SEVERELY RESTRICTED PESTICIDES

1. Arsenic trioxide	4. Heptachlor
2. Carbofuran	5. Sodium arsenate
3. Daminozide	6. Tributyltin compounds

Although it is difficult to classify all pesticides chemically or biologically, it is useful to list some of the major categories, with a few examples in each class. Some of the examples provided are considered restricted-use pesticides.

Insecticides

Stomach Poison or Protective Insecticides—Chlorinated hydrocarbons (methoxychlor); miscellaneous (carbaryl).

Contact Insecticides—Botanicals (pyrethrum, rotenone); organic phosphorus compounds (parathion, malathion); miscellaneous (carbaryl).

Fumigants—Gaseous materials used in tightly closed spaces such as warehouses, ship holds, mills, grain elevators, boxcars, and vaults and in the soil; these include methyl bromide and paradichlorobenzene.

Acaricides (Miticides)—Phosphate insecticides.

Fungicides—Chemicals and formulations used to control fungi and bacteria on living and nonliving plants and plant parts, as well as on or in all materials and surfaces but *excluding* all uses on living humans or animals and all uses on or in processed foods, beverages, or pharmaceuticals. A *localized fungicide* is dodine; examples of *complete fungicides* are benomyl and thiabendazole.

Nematicides—Chemicals and formulations used to control nematodes (roundworms) inhabiting soil and water that are associated with damage to plants or plant parts. A *postplanting nematicide* is VC-13; a *systemic nematicide* is aldicarb.

Herbicides

Selective—Dalapon, siduron, 2,4-D.
Nonselective—Bromacil.
Contact—Cacodylic acid, paraquat.
Translocated—2,4-DB, MCPA.

Plant Regulators—All preparations intended to alter the behavior or products of plants through physiological action, such as gibberellic acid and maleic hydrazide.

Defoliants and Desiccants—Preparations intended to cause leaves or foliage of plants to drop prematurely and usually used to aid harvesting of certain crops such as cotton. Endothall, arsenic acid, and sodium chlorate are in this class.

Rodenticides—Strychnine, zinc phosphide, warfarin, chlorophacinone.

Sex Pheromones—Chemical substances produced and released by one sex of an insect (usually the female) that elicit a sexual response in an individual of the opposite sex. *cis*-7,8-Epoxy-2-methyloctadecane (Disparlure) is a gypsy moth lure.

Juvenile Hormones (Insect Growth Regulators)—A relatively new type of pest control agent that regulates insect growth. Isopropyl-11-methoxy-3,7,11-trimethyldodeca-2,4-dienoate (generic name, methoprene; brand name, Altosid) is used to arrest mosquito development at the pupal stage.

Attractants—These are insect sexual pheromones that are used to attract specific pests to traps where they may be destroyed. Examples include boll weevil sex attractant and muscalure (Z-9-tricosene), a sex and aggregation pheromone for the common fly *(Musca domestica)*.

Many of the chemical names given to pesticides are contractions of longer systematic nomenclature that usually serve as nonproprietary names. As with drugs, many proprietary names are featured. Many pesticides are put into proprietary formulations that include the active ingredients often coupled with some adjuvant such as abscission agents, acidifying agents, buffering agents, antifoaming agents, antitranspirants, colors and dyes, compatibility agents, crop oil concentrates, surfactants, deposition agents, dispersants, drift control agents, foam-markers, gustatory/feeding stimulants, harvest aids, spreaders, penetrants, wetting agents, stickers, extenders, adhesive agents, and suspension and gelling agents.

According to the major purpose for which pesticides are used, they may be classified as

Acaricides—Control ticks or mites.

Algicides—Destroy algae and other aquatic vegetation.

Antiseptics—Protect objects from damage by microorganisms.
Arboricides—Defoliate and/or destroy trees or shrubby vegetation.
Bactericides—Control bacterial infection in plants.
Fungicides—Control fungal infection in plants.
Herbicides—Control weeds or undesirable species of plants.
Insecticides—Control harmful insects. Several specific terms named for the insect group have been coined; eg, aphicides—agents that control aphids.
Larvicides—Control larval stages of insects.
Limacides or Molluscicides—Control mollusks, including gastropods.
Nematicides—Control roundworms (nematodes).
Predacides—Control predatory mammals or birds.
Zoocides—Control rodents (rodenticides).

GENERAL SUGGESTIONS TO PHARMACISTS

The pharmacy is a logical source to obtain pesticide and pest-control information. However, pharmacists who desire to handle pesticides and build a permanent patronage should acquaint themselves with the common pest problems, with chemicals recommended, and how such materials should be used. In particular, they should be acquainted with the classification of pesticides since they will be handling and selling the *general-use* type and not the *restricted-use* group.

Pharmacists should keep abreast of new laws that influence the ways in which chemicals may be used legally. Particular attention should be placed on becoming familiar with the Pesticide Chemicals Amendment to the FD&C Act dealing with the safety determination needed on the residue of pesticides on raw agricultural commodities. This amendment is known commonly as the *Miller Bill* and was passed in 1954.

The pharmacist should study the Chemical Additives Amendment to that same Act passed in 1958 and fully effective in 1960. An annual updating of federal and state pesticide legislation may be obtained through the most recent edition of the *Farm Chemicals Handbook,* published by Meister Publ Co, 37733 Euclid Ave, Willoughby, OH 44094. This reference features a buyer's guide, application equipment, fertilizer, tradenames and dictionary, and a pesticide dictionary. Particularly noteworthy in this edition is description of crop chemicals, toxicity class, and handling and storage cautions. The current regulatory file is an important new supplement and incorporates information on regulatory action at both the federal and state level in the US affecting pesticides. Further information is included on the Endangered Species Act, Superfund Amendment and Reauthorization Act (SARA), the OSHA Hazard Communication Standard, and California's Proposition 65.

The following are some websites that the authors consider beneficial. The authors and the publisher make no claims as to the accuracy and quality of this information.

http://www.igc.apc.org/panna—The Pesticide Action Network North America Regional Center (PANNA) is a nonprofit organization working to advance ecological alternatives to pesticides. This website provides many links to various sources of information on pesticides.

http://chemfinder.camsoft.com—The CambridgeSoft Corp is a distributor of information supplied by third parties. The ChemFinder webserver will search by CAS number, molecular weight, formula, or name. It will search by chemical name or tradename and provides links to other websites for more information about the specific chemical searched.

http://www.cdpr.ca.gov—The California Environmental Protection Agency, Dept of Pesticide Regulations, provides access to general consumer fact sheets for safe pesticide handling and precautions. It also provides pesticide-related links and database resources.

http://pmep.cce.cornell.edu—The Pesticide Management Education Program at Cornell Univ promotes the safe use of pesticides and provides information such as chemical information on active ingredients and external links to other websites. Chemical information is sorted by type, eg, herbicides, then alphabetically. It does not have a search engine for chemical or tradename.

http://www.epa.gov/pesticides—The US EPA, Office of Pesticide Programs, offers a broad range of information.

http://ace.ace.orst.edu/info/extoxnet—EXTOXNET, the Extension Toxicology Network, is a cooperative effort of the Univ of California-Davis, Oregon State Univ, Michigan State Univ, and Cornell Univ. The *Global Search and Browse* page will search by chemical and tradename and yields detailed information about the specific pesticide searched.

http://hammock.ifas.ufl.edu—The Florida Agricultural Information Retrieval System (Univ of Florida) website has information on pesticide poisoning, listed under the heading *Pesticide Management Topics.* It provides several vehicles for searching for the pesticide of interest and includes signs/symptoms of poisoning as well as treatment methods.

http://atsdr1.atsdr.cdc.gov:8080—The Agency for Toxic Substances and Disease Registry (DHHS) lists ToxFAQs for Hazardous Substance Fact Sheets. The number of pesticides is limited.

http://www.acpa.org—The American Crop Protection Assoc provides scientific and regulatory information in the form of downloadable files. Other information on agriculture industry issues is available. This website does not allow searching by chemical or tradename. Information is focused on agricultural applications.

http://www.state.XX.us—To search for state and local information about pesticides, enter the two-letter state abbreviation for *XX.* This provides access to the state's homepage that links to state government health, environment, and agricultural departments. The quality of information and hyperlinks vary.

The entomologist and plant physiologist of the state agricultural experiment station and the county agent of the state's cooperative extension service should be consulted for identification of insects and up-to-date information about plant diseases. Publications on weed, insect, and plant disease control may be obtained from the state experiment station. Also, the Office of Information, USDA, Washington, DC, supplies on request a publications list from which those needed for a personal reference library may be selected for ordering. To learn about applicator certification, contact the local state department of agriculture.

Meetings of insecticide dealers, held annually in many states, also can be important sources of knowledge of new developments in the field of insecticides. Information about the scheduling of such meetings may be obtained from the local county agricultural agent. Each year the cooperative extension service in each state publishes recommendations on pesticides.

Since there are many dependable sources of pesticides, pharmacists generally will find it advantageous to stock packaged materials for their sales. To aid in contacting wholesalers, the guide known as ENTOMA, prepared and distributed by the Entomological Society of America, 4603 Calvert Rd, College Park, MD 20740, is invaluable.

Guidance on methods of rodent and predatory animal control may be obtained from the US Fish and Wildlife Service, Dept of the Interior, Washington, DC 20240.

Authority for promulgating regulations establishing tolerances for pesticide chemicals in or on raw agricultural commodities or exempting any pesticide chemical from the necessity of such a tolerance is vested in the administrator of the EPA, according to the Miller Amendment (Sec 408) of the FD&C Act. It should be emphasized that both FEPCA and state laws require that pesticides be used according to label directions. Failure to do so can result in civil and criminal penalties.

Since garden insecticides are of fair importance in suburban areas, pharmacists should be aware of the numerous inexpensive publications that are available from the Superintendent of Documents, US Government Printing Office, Washington, DC 20402. These include discussion of such topics as diseases and pests of garden and ornamental plants.

Finally, it has been noted that pharmacists frequently are consulted on venereal diseases, which have increased dramatically in recent years. Beyond the usual recommendation to consult a physician, the pharmacist may be of direct service in recommending agents for body lice infestation.

CONTROL OF INSECTS

Insects may be controlled through proper application of chemicals by means of suitable techniques.

CLASSIFICATION OF INSECT CONTROL CHEMICALS

Insect control chemicals may be classified as insecticides, fumigants, repellents, or attractants.

INSECTICIDES—Insecticides often are classified according to the type of action that results in destruction of the insect. Three broad categories, namely stomach poisons, contact insecticides, and fumigants, are recognized generally. Among older insecticides such classification was rather distinct. However, with the new synthetic organic compounds, a single material often produces insecticidal action in several ways. Certain materials often are selected and used, however, in such a manner as to accomplish control primarily by stomach, contact, or fumigating action.

Stomach Poisons—For control of insects by this method it usually is necessary to apply the insecticide to the food that they consume. Stomach poisons are used widely to control leaf-feeding insects or other pests of plants that will result in consumption of the surface-contaminated material. Stomach poisons also are used in specially prepared baits for controlling a variety of insects. With the rapid advances in employing systemic insecticides it is now feasible to destroy by stomach action certain insects that feed on plant juices or blood and tissues of animals, which in the past were considered vulnerable only to contact insecticides.

Systemic insecticides are those chemicals that move in plants and animals from one location where applied to another location where the insect may be feeding. Some of the more widely used systemic insecticides include *O,O*-diethyl-*O*(and *S*)-2-(ethylthio)ethylphosphorothioates), *Meta Systox R,* and *dimethoate,* (*O,O*-dimethyl *S*-methylcarbamoylmethyl- phosphorodithioate). Stomach poisons include a variety of organic *arsenicals, fluosilicates, rotenone,* various *chlorinated hydrocarbons,* and the *organic phosphates* and *carbamates.*

Contact Insecticides—Most of the insecticides in use today depend largely on contact action to destroy insects. *Pyrethrum, rotenone, oil emulsions, nicotine,* and *soaps* have been used for this purpose for many years. The chlorinated hydrocarbon insecticides (eg, lindane), the organic phosphates (eg, malathion), and the carbamates (eg, carbaryl) have been employed extensively for many years. Some have restricted use for specific purposes as stated in the EPA's banned and severely restricted pesticide list of Aug 1997. Contact insecticides are employed against chewing as well as sucking insects.

Often insecticides appear on the market with added compounds called synergists, which may enhance the effects of the insecticides considerably. Some, like piperonyl butoxide, help block metabolic degradation of the insecticide by the insect.

Fumigants—These are gases or vapors used for the control of insects, usually in enclosed spaces. The fumigants include *ethylene dichloride, methyl bromide, chloropicrin,* and many others. A number of the *chlorinated hydrocarbon* and *organic phosphorus* insecticides have sufficiently high vapor toxicity to cause marked fumigating action against insects, particularly in enclosed spaces and in soils, but many of these, like lindane, have been cancelled for use in vaporizers.

REPELLENTS—A variety of insect control chemicals possess repellent action. *Citronella* and *creosote* are examples of older materials. *Ethohexadiol* and *diethyltoluamide* are examples of materials more recently developed. Such materials often cause insects to avoid contact with treated surfaces. Repellency in a strict sense might vary greatly in mode of action. Some insecticides, such as pyrethrum, have little or no repellent action except on contact. However, the action of *pyrethrum* is so rapid that the spraying of animals may cause flies and mosquitos to leave after alighting and before biting.

ATTRACTANTS—The use of attractants to lure insects to poisons or traps has been employed as a means of control for many years. The attractants employed are usually favorite foods for the particular insect involved, such as *molasses, sugar,* or *milk* for houseflies; *sugar* or *grease* for ants; *bran* for cutworms; *bananas* for cockroaches; decaying *meats* for blowflies; and *protein hydrolysate materials* for tropical fruit flies such as the Mediterranean fruit fly. In some cases specific chemicals prove highly attractive. Notable examples are *methyl eugenol* for attracting males of the Oriental fruitfly, a serious pest of fruits in some tropical areas, and many synthetic substitutes such as 10-dodecadienol, the codling moth sex attractant, and *cis*-7,8-epoxy-2-methyloctadecane *(Disparlure),* the gypsy moth sex attractant.

A new trap for Japanese beetles, now on the market, combines a controlled-release strip containing a furanone sex attractant and a eugenol odor attractant.

QUALIFICATIONS OF SUPPLIERS OF INSECTICIDES

Mere stocking of insecticides is not enough to establish a professionally recognized and economically successful enterprise as a supplier of insecticides, for three basic services must be provided in addition to physical supplies. These services, principally of information, are

Recognition of the type of insect causing the damage, from examination of either the insect or the injury it produces.

Recommendation of a remedy, based on knowledge of the action of various insecticides or other insect-control chemicals and of the life history, habits, and structure of the insect responsible.

Familiarity with methods of application of the remedy, for which the user is largely responsible but who may need instruction in such methods.

Pharmacists will find the following specific information useful in developing the aforementioned services:

An understanding of the relative importance of different insects and the relation of the cost of treatment to the increase in value resulting therefrom to the product injured is necessary. Not infrequently, the cost will exceed the damage that might be done. If the value of the product is small, the insect may not cause appreciable loss, even though it may be conspicuously evident. Again, the damage may have been done before its recognition, and the delayed treatment will not affect the insect or aid in preventing the damage.

A knowledge of the life history and habits of the common insects is desirable, as all insect control methods are based on a knowledge of these things.

The ability to recognize the common insects is a great aid, as it is the first step in providing suitable control. The county agents, federal entomologists, and the members of the staff of the respective state agricultural experiment stations are usually available to aid in the identification of insect pests.

A knowledge of how insecticides kill, of the relation of types of mouthparts to the kind of insecticide to use, and when and how the material should be applied is useful.

A knowledge of the usual insect problems of a community will enable the supplier to carry in stock the insecticides likely to be needed. This will eliminate surplus stock and will provide the materials that so often fill emergency needs.

A knowledge of the toxicity of an insecticide to warm-blooded animals, persistence of residues on plants or in animal tissues, hazard of the materials to bees or fish and wildlife is important so that advice can be given on precautions that should be taken in the use of certain chemicals. A wide variety of chemicals is in use today. They vary in their toxicity and hazards to different organisms. The degree of danger is governed not only by the inherent toxicity to higher animals and beneficial organisms in a lower category but also by the manner of use and extent of exposure. A highly toxic material properly applied in small amounts may be less hazardous than a material low in toxicity that is applied in larger amounts.

The variety of insect control chemicals is clearly apparent by mentioning some of the materials in wide use today. They include some organic arsenicals, nicotine compounds, a few chlorinated hydrocarbon insecticides (methoxychlor, lindane), and the insecticides grouped as *organic phosphates,* which at present include *parathion, malathion, dipterex, diazinon, dursban, imidan,* and the newer carbamates, which include *Sevin* (carbaryl, 1-naphthyl-*N*-methylcarbamate) and others. Several pamphlets are available from the EPA that deal with pesticide disposal, pesticide dust-avoidance respirators, and diagnosis and treatment of poisoning by pesticides. These should be kept on hand for reference by pharmacists providing poison control information on pesticides.

It is important to follow the recommendations for each locality. An insecticide effective in one region may not be in others.

It is essential to understand the labels on tradenamed preparations and follow the directions very carefully.

A knowledge of the essentials of a good insecticide, its effect on insects, and its availability and cost, is important.

Those manufacturing and offering preparations such as insecticides and rodenticides for sale on the open market must familiarize themselves with the various regulations of the individual states where the products are being manufactured or are to be sold. If such products are shipped in interstate commerce, these preparations also must comply with the various federal regulations, especially the FEPCA of 1972 and subsequent EPA amendments.

Many states require dealers in pesticides to be licensed. Some require the dealer to pass a written test to obtain the license. The test usually focuses on pesticide laws and regulations.

MOUTHPARTS AND THEIR RELATIONSHIP TO INSECT CONTROL—In general, pests have two kinds of mouthparts: chewing and sucking. An understanding of the mouthparts and how they relate to the use of different chemical insecticides often will aid in recommending a satisfactory insecticide treatment.

Chewing insects include the *grasshoppers, cockroaches, crickets, bird lice, beetles, slugs,* and *caterpillars.* Such insects have mandibles or jaws that enable them to cut off solid tissue and take it into their stomachs. Consequently, an insecticide can be used that kills when taken into the stomach with food eaten by the insect. Most of the newer insecticides, however, are active both as contact and stomach poisons.

Sucking insects include *plant bugs, leafhoppers, scale insects, aphids, fleas, mosquitos, flies,* and *sucking lice* on animals. Such an insect punctures the plant or animal but does not take any of the surface tissue into its stomach; consequently, stomach poisons that have no contact action will be ineffective when applied to the surface.

Recently, however, a variety of compounds has been found that are absorbed through the roots, stems, or leaves and transported to various parts of the plant where the chemical is available to sucking or chewing insects that feed inside or on the plant or fruit. These compounds are referred to as systemics. Insecticides having systemic action offer great promise for controlling insects, and a number of such compounds now are being employed on both plants and animals.

Plants that have been attacked by chewing pests frequently are recognized by the appearance of the eaten areas. Some plant feeders eat the entire tissue, as do *potato beetles;* others eat holes in leaves, as do *flea beetles;* while some chewing insects skeletonize the leaves, as do *slugs* and the *Mexican bean beetle.*

Sucking insects injure plants in different ways, and it is often difficult to determine the kind of insect responsible for the damage unless specimens are available. Sucking insects or mites may remove the sap and cause the plant to "stand still," wilt, or drop its foliage; or they may deform the plant, causing the leaves or shoots to curl and become deformed. Some sucking insects, such as the *potato leafhopper,* the *tarnished plant bug,* and *plant lice (aphids),* inject toxic secretions at the time of feeding, causing the death of plant cells,

while others, such as *plant lice, leafhoppers,* and *striped cucumber beetles,* may injure plants directly by feeding as well as through the transmission of plant diseases. Sucking insects also may affect animals by removing the blood, injecting toxic secretions, causing swelling and irritation, or carrying disease organisms.

LIFE HISTORY AND HABITS OF INSECTS—In general, there are two types of metamorphosis or development among insects: incomplete and complete. Those with incomplete metamorphosis, such as aphids, grasshoppers, plant bugs, and scale insects, have only three stages in development: the *egg* or *embryo,* the *nymph,* and the *adult* or *imago.* Insects with complete metamorphosis, such as beetles, butterflies, moths, flies, bees, ants, and wasps, have four stages in development. In this type, the larva hatching from the egg has no resemblance to the adult, there being also an intermediate resting stage known as the *pupa,* during which remarkable changes in structure take place.

The interrelation of insects, where they hibernate, when they are actively feeding, where they lay their eggs, if they have natural enemies that feed on destructive pests, all have an important bearing on controls. The ant is essential to the life of the corn root aphid, and cultural practices that eliminate the ant likewise will eliminate the aphid; the fact that *Anopheles* mosquitos often rest in homes and other sheltered areas explains the great success of residual sprays such as malathion and baytex for controlling malaria, which such mosquitos transmit; a knowledge of the preferred oviposition sites for grasshoppers permits surveys of egg abundance or abundance of newly hatched nymphs to forecast impending outbreaks of grasshoppers.

METHODS OF INSECT CONTROL

For convenience, insect controls can be grouped as follows.

NATURAL CONTROLS—Those that are usually present and that normally tend to hold insects in check.

Natural Enemies—Parasitic and predacious insects. Every insect is more or less hindered in its increase by other insects as well as by predacious birds, mammals, and other animal life. Although insect-eating birds and certain mammals are important, the insect parasites, predators, and insect diseases are usually the most important factors in natural insect control. In fact, it is probable that outbreaks of insects, such as the army worm, often are due not so much to favorable conditions for the pests as to unfavorable conditions for the insect parasites and predators that normally hold them in check. The use of a specific insecticide against a major pest on a crop might lead to a serious outbreak of a secondary pest because of the destruction of natural enemies that normally keep it in check, particularly if the pesticide chosen was largely ineffective against the secondary pest. Such an upset in the balance between destructive and useful insects is a problem of increasing concern in developing insect control chemicals.

Weather and Topographic Influences—Summer and winter temperatures, rainfall, soil, and atmospheric humidity plus all similar natural factors have their effect on insects and their hosts. No definite statement can be made concerning the effect of these factors on all insects. A severe winter may be harmful to some insects such as those that winter in an exposed condition; on the other hand, such conditions may have little effect on insects that are well-protected. Similarly, a severe winter may weaken trees and make them more susceptible to insect attack, or it may kill the fruit buds and deprive fruit-infesting insects of their food. However, it should be remembered that insects have a high reproductive capacity, and the seasonal conditions, especially spring and early summer conditions, may aid insects in becoming destructively abundant, even though they pass the winter few in numbers. On the other hand, an insect overwintering in large numbers may not be important the following season if the weather is not favorable for increase.

In tropical, temperate, and frigid climates there are to be found insect pests peculiar to these areas because of their adaptation to prevailing weather and topographic influences. Topographic features, such as mountain ranges, act as rather effective barriers to insect migration. However, the great increase in the amount and speed of national and international travel and commerce during the last few decades has provided greater opportunities for hitchhiking insect species to overcome such barriers.

tion for such a problem is to destroy the source of the infestation rather than to use insecticides repeatedly.

A homeowner might be alarmed, and rightly so, when an infestation of fleas is detected in the home. In most modern dwellings the odds are great that the source of the fleas is the cat or dog that has not had proper care. The householder can minimize the danger of flying pests such as mosquitos and flies getting into the premises by maintaining screen doors and windows in proper condition and by closing any openings into the home. Poorly cared-for garbage containers can be responsible for serious fly problems by attracting adult flies and by providing places for fly breeding. A few tin cans or tire casings that catch rainwater can provide the moisture essential for mosquito breeding on the premises.

The four general control measures for the prevention of insect and mite damage without chemicals are physical, mechanical, cultural, and biological.

Physical control simply involves direct action by hand, eg, removal of insect nests or egg masses.

Mechanical control involves the use of equipment specifically designed to control insects, eg, applying sticky bands around tree trunks to trap tent caterpillars and frequent hosing of foliage to prevent red spider mites and mealybugs from taking hold.

Cultural control is based on knowledge of the life history and habit pattern of insects and controlling these in various ways, eg, cultivating the soil when many insects are in the pupal stage, breeding insect-resistant plants or interplanting. Interplanting marigolds, which discourage nematode growth, with tomatoes is an example.

Biological control involves, eg, the use of the praying mantis, which devours insects.

It is recognized, however, that in spite of proper precautions, every homeowner is likely to be faced with insect problems that must be solved by applying insect-control chemicals. In some cases, however, the solution is not simple. It may require knowledge of the habits of the pest, a thorough survey of the problem, and know-how to control the pest involved. Often, it is not practical for the owner to attempt to do the job himself. In such circumstances the services of a licensed pest control operator (listed in the yellow pages of telephone directories) should be sought. The National Pest Control Association is in a position to advise on qualified pest-control firms in almost every city. County agents and entomologists in state experiment stations and with the federal government are prepared to give advice and furnish publications that will be helpful in many cases.

For insect control in living quarters, in food-handling establishments, and on the person, the factor of safety in handling and applying toxic chemicals must be considered fully. Fortunately, a number of efficient insecticides have low levels of hazard to man and animals, although no insecticide can be considered completely harmless. The petroleum oil solvent most commonly used as the carrier in household sprays is in itself sufficiently hazardous to cause toxic effects if the operator is careless in use and permits overexposure to it.

Foods and food utensils should not be left uncovered while insecticides are being used. All food preparation surfaces, utensils, and food serving areas should be cleaned thoroughly before the next use, to avoid contamination by pesticide residues. Care is needed in handling and applying pesticides to avoid excessive inhalation or skin contact. All poisons should be stored so that they are inaccessible to children and unauthorized people or where they cannot be mistaken for food. It also must be kept in mind that many preparations containing petroleum oil are flammable, or the vapors are explosive.

While stressing necessary precautions, it must be kept in mind that the proper use of insecticides should not be discouraged. Many pests in and around homes are capable of transmitting diseases, and experience has shown that the disease hazard may be far greater than that of the chemicals needed to control the insects responsible for propagating an epidemic.

ANTS—Several species of ants are pests in the home or around the premises. In the past, poison baits of various kinds were used to destroy them. Such methods are still effective un-

der certain conditions, but the use of newer sprays or dusts provides more effective and more rapid results.

Efforts should be made to locate the colony and destroy it if possible, although inside buildings the colony often cannot be found or may be inaccessible for treatment. The use of dusts and suitable sprays applied to the point of runoff on runways and other surfaces where ants have been seen, and along baseboards, borders of floors, window frames, doorsills, and similar places usually will give satisfactory control, although followup treatments may be necessary. In general, the procedure for poisoning ants is similar to that for controlling roaches.

For ant control on lawns or in gardens, the best procedure is to locate the ant colony and apply Baygon, Dursban, Ficam, or one of the other pyrethrin derivatives. Baygon, a carbamate insecticide, and Dursban, an organic phosphate insecticide, have become popular for this use. These currently are formulated at higher concentrations for use by professional applicators only. The material may be applied with a sprinkling can, sprayer, or any other convenient method, being sure to follow product labels, particularly on those allowed for lawn use only. A concentration of 0.25% of these insecticides is suggested for treating individual mounds. The amount to apply varies with the size of the colony. A quart may be sufficient for small colonies and up to 3 gal may be necessary for large fire ant colonies 1 ft high and 2 to 3 ft in diameter at the base. The surface of the mound or soil should be disturbed by raking, and the material poured on and around the nest.

Children and pets should not be permitted to play on the lawns until the area has been watered or rained on and allowed to dry. It is advised that the insecticide be washed off vegetation, into the ground, by sprinkling; this will not reduce the efficacy of the treatment.

Chlorpyrifos *(Dursban)*, and synergized pyrethrum sprays, may be employed for ant control in homes.

Bedbugs are controlled effectively by thorough spraying of the bed frame, springs, and edges and ticking of mattresses with 1% to 3% malathion by a professional applicator. Cracks, crevices, and surfaces behind objects near a wall also should be treated. Bedbugs stay well hidden in such places. Spraying the bed and other hiding places to the point of running off of the solution will provide long-lasting control. The treated mattress should be aired well before use.

Chiggers or red bugs cause severe annoyance to many people. These mites are most common in southern and midwestern areas. Some individuals are particularly susceptible to chigger bites, especially if they have not previously been exposed to them.

The insect repellents dimethyl phthalate, dimethyl carbate, diethyltoluamide, 2-ethyl-1,3-hexanediol, and benzyl benzoate, when applied to clothing, are excellent in preventing attack by chiggers. The repellents may be applied by hand to socks, inside cuffs of trousers and sleeves, and on the edges of any other openings in the clothing. Additional application of the repellent to the skin on the legs and forearms and base of neck will increase the probability of complete protection. Chiggers seldom attack the exposed portion of the body and are killed or repelled while crawling over treated clothing or exposed skin.

Clothing may be made repellent by light spraying, by drawing the mouth of the bottle along the parts of cloth to be treated (eg, cuffs and fly), or by complete impregnation of the cloth.

Although the repellents are highly effective in providing protection against chigger attack, persons often become exposed in areas where they do not expect chiggers to be present. After chiggers attack, there is no known treatment of the bites that will destroy the toxic substance that causes the irritation, although certain local anesthetics such as benzocaine will provide relief for several hours. A thorough, soapy bath as soon as chigger irritation is noted, which may be within a few hours after exposure, will reveal those attached and thus allow removal and subsequent reduction of irritation.

COCKROACHES—The German, American, and brown-banded are the most common cockroach species found in homes and industrial establishments. Although the efficacy of different insecticides varies with the species, those in common use can be employed effectively in most instances. The German roach accounts for 98% of the problem in the US.

Most aerosol formulas contain pyrethrum, allethrin, or resmethrin. Although intended primarily for flying insects, the aerosols can be used fairly effectively for roach control if applied in considerable amounts directly into the hiding places or released in high concentration in closed rooms. A thorough spray or dust treatment is considered more effective and longer-lasting. Many purchasers of aerosols expect roach control in the home by a light treatment. Such treatment, although satisfactory for flies, mosquitos, and similar pests, is inadequate for good roach control.

Boric acid and *borax* in finely powdered form, applied to hiding places and runways, are used for roach control, although they are less effective and slower to produce results than most other insecticides. The materials also are used in tablet form mixed with food baits that the roaches must eat. When well-distributed in office buildings or rooms where there is little food for roaches, they often provide satisfactory control.

Dursban (chlorpyrifos) sprays and dusts are widely used insecticides for roach control. The sprays, either oil-based or prepared from an emulsifiable concentrate, should contain about 2% and dusts about 5% of the insecticide as described on the label.

During the day, roaches usually remain well hidden in cracks and crevices and behind objects. It is important to know where the roaches hide and where they run. The coarse, wet insecticide sprays are applied into these runways and hiding places. A few puffs of a mist spray will not provide satisfactory control. A paint brush may be used to apply the solution instead of a sprayer, if label directions allow it. A dust should be blown directly into hiding places and placed along runways. Dursban *O,O*-diethyl-*O*-(3,5,6-trichloro-2-pyridyl)phosphorothionate may be recommended as a first-use agent.

Ficam (2,2-dimethyl-1,3-benzodioxol-4-yl), or bendiocarb (generic name), also is useful and is popular as a highly effective broad-spectrum carbamate insecticide for control of at least six species of cockroach.

Pyrethrum sprays or dusts usually will provide satisfactory roach control. It is necessary, however, to treat with pyrethrum often to obtain and maintain control. The use of synergists with this insecticide has made it more effective.

When chlorinated hydrocarbon resistance is encountered in roaches, malathion as a 1 to 2% spray has proved to be an effective substitute. *Diazinon O,O*-diethyl-*O*-(2-isopropyl-4-methyl-6-pyrimidinyl)phosphorothioate also has proved useful when roach resistance has been a problem. The residual life of malathion is generally less than that obtained with methoxychlor prior to the appearance of insecticide-resistant strains.

Fleas often are pests in homes and even in lawns in some areas. Infestations usually are associated with the presence of cats, dogs, rats, or other animals. To prevent recurrence of fleas, the source of the trouble should be treated. For dogs, powders containing 1% lindane, pyrethrum, or rotenone are used per label directions. For cats, only rotenone or pyrethrum insecticides are recommended, because these animals are very susceptible to the toxic effects of chlorinated hydrocarbons. If the source of the fleas is rats, the host animals should be eliminated by following suitable rodent-control measures.

Actual flea control in homes is usually not difficult. Bedding where dogs sleep should be removed, and the area thoroughly cleaned. Ordinary household sprays containing pyrethrum also may be used, although several repeat treatments may be required. Certain volatile organophosphate insecticides are the active ingredients of *flea collars* for dogs and cats. A new insect growth regulator, *methoprene,* is giving effective indoor flea control. This agent interferes with the life cycle of insects undergoing complete metamorphosis.

Finally, attention must be given to the pesticide label precautions. Some dogs and many cats are allergic to collars. Malathion and Sevin (carbaryl) are excellent materials for the control of fleas in the home or in infested yards.

FLIES—For most homes or industrial establishments flies can be eliminated by using ordinary household sprays or aerosols. The most common ones consist of deodorized kerosene, about 0.1% pyrethrins or allethrin, and 0.75% of a synergist such as piperonyl butoxide or sulfoxide. Many variations in percentages of such insecticides are included in different formulations. Aerosol formulas often contain 0.25% to 0.6% pyrethrins or allethrin, 0.8% to 1% synergist, and 1% to 2% methoxychlor. The method of using the sprays or aerosols generally is known and usually well-described on the labels.

If flies are a serious problem on the premises, other methods of control must be followed. Recently, the use of poison baits has become more widespread.

Malathion and Diazinon sprays as residual treatments outdoors around homes, in livestock buildings (including inside dairy barns), and similar places have come into use. When used according to label directions, these materials often provide good fly control up to several weeks after application. Flytraps (paper) and mechanical devices for trapping are still available and popular.

ITCH MITE—Many preparations have been employed for controlling the itch mite, or scabies. One of the most successful was the NBIN emulsion employed for head-louse control. It is important to treat all portions of the body and to delay a bath for about 12 hr after treatment. A second treatment may be needed after 1 week, although one thorough treatment will usually eliminate the infestation.

LICE—Three kinds of lice attack man: the *body louse, head louse,* and *crab (pubic) louse*. In the US, head louse and pubic louse infestations are more common than those of the body louse.

Body louse infestations can be controlled by regular changes of clothing and sterilization of all wearing apparel and bedding. Synergized pyrethrum dusts are also highly effective for body louse control. It also has been found that allethrin is about as effective as pyrethrins in such formulations. The material most commonly used today for head and body louse treatment is synergized pyrethrum (eg, the OTC product RID).

Head louse infestations are controlled readily with benzyl benzoate followed by a thorough shampoo the next morning. Weekly treatments may be needed. Since eggs are not destroyed easily, treatments should be repeated. One treatment applied to the hair on the head before bedtime will kill all motile stages of the lice, which may be brushed or washed out of the hair in the morning.

Crab louse infestations are controlled effectively with any of the preparations discussed under head louse. It is important that all hairy portions of the body be treated.

Mosquitos that occasionally enter homes can be killed easily with the type of space sprays and aerosols discussed in connection with fly control. Mosquitos often breed in areas several miles from the places where they are serious nuisances. Community mosquito control programs are the only real solution to this problem. The problem of achieving satisfactory mosquito control in a community is usually so complex and extensive that the help and advice of specialists are necessary.

Persons exposed to mosquitos, biting gnats, and flies outdoors in connection with work or recreation can obtain relief by applying skin repellents. The most common individual repellents available on the market are *diethyltoluamide, dimethyl phthalate, ethohexadiol,* and *dimethyl carbamate.* Various combinations of these also are available. All of these materials used as directed on container labels will provide transient relief from insect attack.

In some circumstances treatment of the exposed skin alone is inadequate because the mosquitos also may bite through clothing. The application of repellents to clothing by impregnation, by light spraying, or by hand will prevent the attack. The same repellent materials intended for skin application may be used. Most of the repellents are plasticizers. They should not be applied to rayons and similar synthetic clothing.

MOTHS AND CARPET BEETLES—Every homeowner is likely to encounter damage due to clothes moths or carpet beetles, often called *buffalo* moths. The damage caused by these insects to woolens and other items such as furs, materials made of animal hair, or feathers is very great.

For many years the fumigants naphthalene and para-dichlorobenzene were the chief means of control. It takes a high concentration of vapor to kill clothes moths or carpet beetles, however. Many pounds of these fumigants are needed to eliminate infestations in closets that are not tight or where the doors are opened too often to permit sufficient concentration of vapor. In using these fumigants add crystals, flakes, or balls at the rate of 1 lb/100 ft^3, and make closets tight by sealing cracks and edges of doors. Since the gas is considerably heavier than air, the fumigant should be placed high in the closet. For protecting clothing, furs, etc in trunks and other storage spaces for long periods, about 1 lb suffices for an average-size trunk.

Moth infestations are destroyed and woolen items effectively protected against subsequent infestations by treating with paradichlorobenzene, naphthalene, or DDVP (dichlorvos).

SILVERFISH—For the control of silverfish, use carefully applied residual insecticide sprays and dusts such as bendiocarb, diazinon, propoxur, and silica gel. Silverfish may be found in many places in the home—basement, attic, around books, and behind wall paper. They feed on the starchy material used as glues or for sizing paper.

Ticks are serious pests in some areas. If the infested areas must be used, it is possible to kill the ticks by following the procedures suggested for area chigger control. Protection of individuals from tick attack, however, is fairly effective if clothing is thoroughly impregnated with certain repellents. Emulsions of dimethyl phthalate and diethyltoluamide may be used for such treatment.

Insecticides, Fumigants, and Repellents

The number of insecticides and repellents currently in use has increased greatly during the past 30 years. New synthetic compounds have come into use for many pests for which practical chemical control methods were unknown, and in some cases have largely replaced certain inorganic compounds and insecticides of plant origin. However, some of the more recently developed chemicals are being replaced by even newer materials because of development of resistance by various insects to insecticides. This is a problem of major significance in insect control. The housefly, for example, became resistant to DDT and other chlorinated hydrocarbon insecticides within 5 to 10 years after they came into extensive use.

Organic phosphorus insecticides were developed as substitutes, but within a few years evidence of resistance to them became apparent. A wide variety of insects affecting man, livestock, fruits, vegetables, and cotton are resistant to one or more of the newer insecticides. Currently, the resistant strains still are restricted generally to certain localities. However, authorities in insect control generally are agreed that such local resistance problems are likely to become more widespread with continued use of the materials. The use of piperonyl butoxide as a mixed-function oxidase inhibitor and an inducer of cytochrome P-450 has led to the reduction of resistance to many insecticides by many insects.

The more widely employed insect control chemicals and their areas of use are discussed briefly. The extensive literature on the many insecticides may be consulted for further details, and the US Dept of Agriculture, state experiment stations, the US Public Health Service, and manufacturers of specific insecticides are prepared to provide more-detailed information. The EPA should be consulted for the latest information about a particular pesticide, since its status may change at any time. A chart for emergency treatment of acute pesticide poisoning is available from the US Navy Disease Vector Ecology and Control Center, Jacksonville, FL 32212.

COMMON INSECTICIDES

Allethrin (*dl*-2-allyl-4-hydroxy-3-methyl-2-cyclopenten-1-one esterified with a mixture of *cis* and *trans dl*-chrysanthemum monocarboxylic acids)—This synthetic pyrethrin-like compound has been developed as the result of basic studies on the complex composition of the active principles in pyrethrum insecticides. It has many of the desirable features of pyrethrum—high insecticidal activity with low toxicity to warm-blooded animals. In general, allethrin is effective against the same insects as pyrethrum. For some species such as the *housefly* and the *body louse* it is equally effective, but against others it is less effective than pyrethrum. At present it can be produced commercially at a cost somewhat lower than the cost of the pyrethrins (principal active ingredients in pyrethrum). This advantage in practical use is offset, however, because the insecticidal activity of allethrin is not increased to the same degree as that of the pyrethrins when combined with synergists available at present.

The development of allethrin is of great significance however. It is now used in household sprays and aerosols as a substitute for pyrethrins or to supplement the pyrethrins. The Dept of Defense uses the insecticide in sprays and aerosols supplied to troops. Research has shown that allethrin is highly efficient for the control of lice affecting man. The availability of allethrin ensures a supply of a pyrethrum-like insecticide in the event our source of supply of pyrethrum is cut off or greatly reduced as during World War II.

Arsenicals—These are among the older insecticides and are still employed to a very limited extent. Many compounds, such as lead arsenate and calcium arsenate, have been canceled voluntarily for use by the manufacturers. Due to the development and availability of many new insecticides equally effective and often less hazardous to plants and animals, the arsenicals have been replaced largely by other insecticides.

Lime-Sulfur (Calcium Polysulfides)—Originally used as a *sheep dip* for the control of *mites* and *ticks*, lime-sulfur in liquid and dry form is now better known as a dormant spray for the control of *scale insects* and as a summer spray for the control of certain *plant diseases*. For the methods of using the lime-sulfur liquid concentrate, follow the recommendations on the container. It generally is used to control apple scab and powdery skin irritation mildews.

Oil Sprays—Oils made from petroleum are among the insecticides that have been used for many years, chiefly as contact insecticides for *scale insects* and *mites* attacking plants. They are very important today. Oils will destroy other insects however, including *aphids, thrips, and leafhoppers,* and *eggs* of certain *Lepidopterous* spp. There are two classes of oils used as insecticides: the *dormant oils* and *summer oils*. The dormant oils are applied to hardier trees during the dormant period. The summer oils are used on fruit and vegetable crops during the growing season. The chief differences between the two types are the degree of refinement and their heaviness or viscosity, which determine in part the degree of phytotoxicity. The oils are applied as emulsions that permit dilution with water and more-uniform distribution on the plants. The concentration of oil in the finished spray for citrus usually is 1.66% to 2.0%. Small amounts of insecticides such as parathion added to the oil sprays increase their efficacy against various insects.

Pyrethrum—Pyrethrum flowers, the first widely used insecticide, possess unusually fast contact action against many insects, causing paralysis in a few minutes. Their low mammalian toxicity and rapid toxic action against many pests are features that are not present in the newer materials.

The active substances, pyrethrins I and II, occur in the oleoresin secretion of certain floral parts (achenes) of the closed or partially open flowers. A maximum of about 1.4% pyrethrins has been adopted by the foremost manufacturers of pyrethrum insecticides.

Formerly, pyrethrum insecticides were prepared as dusts by using the finely ground flowers or were prepared and used as liquids by extracting the active ingredients from the flowers with special fractions of light petroleum oil, preferably odorless kerosene. Today, manufacturers extract and concentrate the active ingredients in products containing about 20% pyrethrins. This concentrate is used to prepare the various preparations employed by the public including dusts, petroleum oil solutions, emulsion concentrates, wettable powders, and aerosol formulations.

Pyrethrum still is used as an ingredient in most household sprays and aerosols, chiefly for its *knockdown* effects against insects. It also is used in dusts and liquid preparations for controlling a variety of garden pests and *fleas, lice,* and *ticks* on pets.

The continued prominent place of pyrethrum as an insecticide has been maintained chiefly because of the development of chemicals that, when combined with pyrethrum, have the remarkable property of increasing the insecticidal activity of the insecticide even though the material added alone has little or no insecticidal properties. This cooperative potentiation is known as *synergism*.

These compounds include piperonyl butoxide, sulfoxide, and others and are called *synergists*. The development of these synergists has increased the range of activity of pyrethrins and at the same time permits reduction in the cost of formulas containing it.

Synergized pyrethrum combinations, although not so long-lasting as the chlorinated hydrocarbon insecticides, are used chiefly in household sprays and aerosols for *flies, mosquitos,* and other *household pests,* in liquid and dust preparations for controlling *external parasites* on pets, as sprays for flies on dairy cattle, and as dusts and sprays for controlling certain *vegetable pests.* Synergized pyrethrum powders and liquids were employed extensively for a time in controlling *lice* attacking man during World War II. Some preparations include pyrelline, pyrenone, and pyrocide. Most of these contain pyrethrins in varying concentrations and other materials such as piperonyl butoxide, rotenone, or ryania. Many pyrethroid synthetics have been found effective and now are registered for use. These include newer allethrin derivatives, resmethrin products, and S-bioallethrin.

Rotenone—This is a useful botanical insecticide and represents the chief chemical constituent of derris (*D elliptica* and *D chinensis*) and cube roots (species of *Lonchocarpus*) and other sources. Rotenone ($C_{23}H_{22}O_6$) is commercially available as such or in the form of derris and cube roots, sold with assayed rotenone content, usually 5%.

It is classified incorrectly as a nontoxic insecticide. It can cause skin irritation. Its use for louse control on humans is not recommended, since irritation often is produced, especially in the groin region. On internal administration in moderately large doses, especially in the presence of fatty foods, it is very toxic to higher animals. In general, however, rotenone insecticides are considered low in hazard. The relatively small amounts applied and rapid loss of toxic action results in minor residues on food crops. Rotenone is used mainly to kill unwanted fish in a pond prior to restocking.

Its paralyzing action on insects is slower than that of pyrethrum but more certain, with usually no recoveries. As a dry, crystalline powder, it is odorless and relatively stable. It is soluble in alcohol, oils, chloroform, and carbon tetrachloride (used in the extraction from the crude drug and its quantitative determination). It is slightly soluble in water, but aqueous sprays, particularly in the presence of alkaline soaps, quickly deteriorate and must be prepared fresh before use.

Its dusts at concentrations of 0.75% to 1.0% still are used to control pests such as the *Mexican bean beetle, cabbage worms, leaf hoppers,* and other insects attacking a variety of vegetables. It is especially useful for application to vegetables near the time for harvest, when certain of the effective newer insecticides cannot be used because of potentially excessive residues.

It also is used for controlling insect parasites of animals. It is effective for controlling *cattle grubs* and is employed also for *lice, fleas,* and *ticks* on pets and livestock.

Sulfur is used widely in insecticide preparations. It formerly was used for controlling such insects as *plant mites, fleahoppers* on cotton, *lice* on livestock, and *chiggers*. The new insecticides available today are far more efficient than sulfur for most insects. However, it is still one of the more effective insecticides for certain species of plant mites. Sulfur also is used in combination with many other insecticide dusts as a diluent. It serves a useful purpose in such combinations in controlling or preventing a buildup of mites and for the control of *plant diseases*. It is employed as a spray made from wettable sulfur or is used in wettable powder preparations containing other insecticides.

Other Materials—A number of other insecticides that have been used as pesticides, but for limited purposes, include *pentachlorophenol* ($C_6C_{15}OH$), widely used as a wood preservative to control termites, other wood-infesting insects, and wood rots (it is under investigation for dioxin contamination and the health ramifications of this contaminant); *Ryania,* a plant product containing alkaloids, used to some extent for controlling corn borers and codling moths on apples; and *sabadilla,* another plant product, which is effective for controlling squash bugs, lygus bugs, and harlequin bugs.

Also of interest in the biopesticide group are the avermectins. These are macrocyclic lactones isolated from the soil organism *Streptomyces avermitilis*. Known by the common name abamectin, it is considered an insecticide as well as a miticide.

Another interesting modern pesticide of biological origin is *neem*. This is a general name given the plant and its products. It is a subtropical shade tree *(Azadirachta indica)* native to the arid regions of India, Pakistan, and parts of Africa. Its most important constituent is a limonoid compound named azadirachtin. The tree has been known for centuries as being free of insects, disease, and nematodes. All parts of the tree, especially the seeds, are resistant. The bark, leaves, and fruit have been used in traditional medicinal remedies, and various extracts have been long used as insect repellents and antifeedants in Asia.

In June 1993 the Clinton administration announced an effort to encourage farmers to reduce their use of pesticides. This was due partly to a National Academy of Sciences report that said that pesticides may have a greater effect on children and that studies should be expanded to determine the possible dangers to children, who may consume more pesticides relative to their body weight.

Leaders in biotechnology are expanding efforts to circumvent the use of pesticides and hope to replace 10% to 20% of the current chemical pesticides in use. Already, biotechnology is being used to develop

squash plants that are immune to a killer virus by activating the plant's natural defenses. In a similar way, hybrid corn, using genes from rare species, may allow resistance to corn borer worm.

Opponents are concerned that biotechnology raises ethical questions about tinkering with nature. Of course, this approach will take time and money to see if it will be successful. Until then, the older advice of shopping for fresh vegetables frequently, serving a variety of fruits, and washing and peeling vegetables should be continued to minimize pesticide residue consumption.

CHLORINATED HYDROCARBON INSECTICIDES

The advances in insect control since about 1940 have been phenomenal because of the development and extensive use of a variety of chemical compounds broadly classified as synthetic chlorinated hydrocarbons. The use of this class of insecticides began with DDT, which was employed first in Switzerland, but within a decade a number of new similar insecticides of comparable, or in some instances greater, insecticidal activity came into use. These materials, although effective against similar pests in many instances, vary in their usefulness for controlling insects.

Insect species vary in their susceptibility to the different compounds. In addition, a factor of great significance that limits the practical use of many insecticides is the hazard associated with their use. Some of the insecticides possess long residual action—which may be of great advantage in controlling certain pests—but which is an objectionable feature when applied to food plants consumed by man and animals. Some of the materials are stored in fat or are excreted in milk of animals when the residues are consumed on forage treated for insect control or when the insecticides are applied to the animals for controlling pests. Such residues of some insecticides may persist for months, while others are eliminated within a few days or weeks.

Because of the persistence in the environment, DDT, aldrin, and dieldrin have been canceled by the EPA. Although their uses have been banned or severely restricted, approximately 1 million households still have products containing chlordane, 150,000 households have products containing DDT, and 70,000 have heptachlor.

Obviously, it is not possible in this chapter to discuss in detail the many uses for the various chlorinated hydrocarbon insecticides. The formulation to use, amount to apply, method and time of application, precautions that must be observed in avoiding harmful residues on the harvested crop, and many other aspects must be considered. Discussion is limited to those products whose use is currently approved by the EPA.

Lindane [γ-1,2,3,4,5,6-hexachlorocyclohexane]—This insecticide is used in household sprays and dusts on livestock and other animals and for controlling some pests on fruits and vegetables. When lice resistant to 10% DDT powder appeared in Korea the Dept of Defense substituted a 1% lindane dust to control this insect attacking man. The acute oral toxicity of lindane to animals is somewhat higher than that of DDT, but when absorbed through the skin it is more toxic than DDT. Lindane possesses high insecticidal activity in vapor form. This property has resulted in certain restricted use for the compound in devices that generate vapors with the aid of heat. Lindane has been canceled for use in vaporizers, canceled for indoor use in smoke fumigation devices, and a host of new restrictions were developed for limited use on commercial and homeowner ornamentals, such as hardwood logs and lumber, dog dips, moth sprays, seed treatments, flea collars, etc.

Methoxychlor [1,1,1-trichloro-2,2-bis(*p*-methoxyphenyl)ethane]— This has chemical and physical properties similar to those of DDT. The chief advantage of this over other chlorinated hydrocarbon insecticides is its low hazard to animals. It is satisfactory for controlling *flies* and other *household pests,* including *clothes moths* and *flies* and *lice* on livestock, *Mexican bean beetles,* and a variety of other insects attacking fruit, vegetable, and forage crops. It is available in 25 to 50% concentrations in various application forms.

It is one of the few chlorinated hydrocarbon insecticides that is not readily stored in animal fat or excreted in milk when consumed as residues on forage crops. For this reason it is used for controlling various insects on livestock feeds and forage. It also was used as a spray for controlling flies and lice on dairy cows but is no longer used thus because small amounts of the insecticide occur in milk.

MITICIDES. A variety of synthetic organic insecticides is used for controlling mites on plants, in addition to older insecticides such as sulfur and the organic phosphates discussed in the next section. Among the compounds used are *Ovex* (p-chlorophenyl p-chlorobenzenesulfonate) and *Kelthane* (1,1-bis(p-chlorophenyl)-2,2,2-trichloroethanol), used extensively on fruits and vegetables. These miticides may be used as dusts or sprays, and they often are combined with other insecticide applications or in insecticide-fungicide formulations.

ORGANIC PHOSPHORUS COMPOUNDS

A large variety of organic compounds of phosphorus possesses high insecticidal activity. They often are referred to as organophosphorus compounds. Some of these compounds also have unusually high potency as miticides, and many are also extremely toxic to man and other warm-blooded animals because of their action as irreversible inhibitors of cholinesterase.

A number of human fatalities in the US and other parts of the world have occurred as a result of exposure to phosphate insecticides, and many other persons have suffered ill effects. It is important, therefore, that the more toxic of these insecticides be handled with extreme caution and strictly in accordance with recommendations outlined by the manufacturer and federal and state agencies.

The reputation of the organic phosphorus insecticides is such that to the uninformed, most compounds in this class are regarded as dangerous to use. This is a misconception. The mammalian toxicity of some of the compounds is of a low order, and they can be handled with no more danger than that associated with the use of a number of the synthetic chlorinated hydrocarbon insecticides that are employed without serious toxic reactions.

The organophosphorus compounds will control a wide range of pests and disease carriers. Certain of these compounds possess systemic action, a characteristic that offers great promise for controlling important insect pests of crops as well as livestock.

The organic phosphorus insecticides are used extensively, in many instances replacing in part, at least, some of the chlorinated hydrocarbons and older insecticides such as rotenone. This trend is due to several factors. Resistance to the chlorinated hydrocarbons by a number of pests has necessitated substitute materials possessing a different mode of insecticidal action. Several of the organic phosphorus compounds do not accumulate in meat and milk as readily as do certain chlorinated hydrocarbon insecticides when consumed as residues on forage crops.

The phosphorus insecticides have not been in use as long as the older materials, and relatively few insects have become resistant to them. There is no assurance, however, that many pests will not in time become resistant to the phosphorus materials. A number of species of mites on plants became resistant within a few years, and as already mentioned, the house fly also has developed resistance to certain organic phosphorus compounds. There is some evidence, however, that in some insect species, resistance to the phosphorus insecticides does not develop to the high level of the chlorinated hydrocarbons.

Organic phosphorus insecticides generally destroy a wide range of insect species. Consequently, their use often kills many parasites, predators, and pollinating insects, as well as the destructive pests.

The more widely used organic phosphorus insecticides are described briefly, and some of their more important uses are given.

Ciodrin [3-hydroxycrotonic acid α-methylbenzyl ester dimethyl phosphate; Crotoxyphos]—An insecticide for control of animal parasites and for premises use.

Diazinon [O,O-diethyl O-(2-isopropyl-4-methyl-6-pyrimidinyl)-phosphorothioate; Spectracide *Knox Out*]—An amber-colored liquid with a somewhat objectionable odor in its technical form; it is an excellent insecticide. It is less toxic than parathion but more so than malathion to warm-blooded animals. It is highly toxic to flies as a contact and residual spray as well as a stomach poison and is in use for

controlling these insects both as sprays and in poison baits. It also is effective against aphids, mites, leafhoppers, the codling moth, fruitflies, cabbage worms, mosquitos, roaches, and other insects. Some resistant strains of houseflies have been reported. It also is used as a bait to control scavenger yellowjackets in 11 contiguous Western states.

Dibrom [1,2-dibromo-2,2-dichloroethyl dimethylphosphate; Naled]—A broad-spectrum insecticide for both plant protection and premises use. Not approved for use in grain bins.

Dipterex [O,O-dimethyl-2,2,2-trichloro-1-hydroxyethylphosphonate; trichlorofon]—A white, crystalline solid; soluble in water. The material is used in poison baits for controlling flies and for controlling many different species of insects. Its toxicity to warm-blooded animals is reported to be of a low order.

Guthion [O,O-dimethyl S-(4-oxo-3H-1,2,3-benzotriazine-3-methyl) phosphorodithionate; azinphosmethyl]—A crystalline material relatively insoluble in water. It has a wide spectrum of activity as a contact insecticide for the control of insect pests. It is generally more persistent on plants than other commonly used organophosphorus insecticides. The material is employed as a dust or spray.

Although the toxicity of Guthion is somewhat lower than that of parathion, it is in the class of highly toxic materials and must be handled with extreme caution. It is finding wide use for controlling cotton insects, particularly the boll weevil, which has become resistant to chlorinated hydrocarbon insecticides. It is also highly effective for the control of fruit pests such as the plum curculio, codling moth, stink bugs, aphids, and mites. This has proven useful in integrated fruit-pest control.

Malathion—This phosphorus compound, S-(1,2-dicarbethoxyethyl)-O,O-dimethyldithiophosphate, as produced commercially, is a light-amber liquid, with a sulfur-like odor. It is relatively low in toxicity to most warm-blooded animals and is active against a wide range of insects, although in general it is less effective than parathion or TEPP. The much lower toxicity to warm-blooded animals and rapid loss of residues on plants make it an acceptable insecticide for many uses.

It is used extensively for controlling insects on vegetables, fruits, and cereal and forage crops as well as for controlling insects affecting man and animals. The residues disappear in a few days to 2 weeks, thus permitting application near the harvest period. The compound is available commercially as emulsifiable concentrates, wettable powders, dusts, and for ultra-low-volume spraying. In the US Malathion ULV concentrate is the only grade registered for use on stored grain, recommended for use inside homes, and accepted for use on humans. Over 25 commercial products are marketed in the US that contain this ingredient.

Methyl Parathion—Closely related to parathion, with insecticidal and toxic properties somewhat similar to it. It is employed for controlling mites, aphids, thrips, and other insects, including such pests as the boll weevil. All applications are classified by the EPA as restricted use.

Parathion [O,O-diethyl O-p-nitrophenyl phosphorothioate]—This insecticide is a pale yellow liquid and is highly active against most insects. Its use is restricted because of its high toxicity to humans and animals. Parathion products are available commercially as dusts and as emulsifiable and wettable powder concentrates for mixing sprays. As of December 31, 1991, parathion was voluntarily canceled for use on over 80 crops in the US.

Phorate [O,O-diethyl S-(ethylthio)methyl phosphorodithioate; Thimet]—A liquid material with an objectionable odor. It is relatively insoluble in water. It is one of the more toxic of the organophosphorus insecticides and must be handled with extreme caution. It is primarily systemic in action and is absorbed readily by the roots of plants when applied to the seeds or when added to the soil. It has had limited use for controlling aphids, spider mites, thrips, leafhoppers, and certain other insects on cotton and sugar beets. It is now classed as an RUP by the EPA.

Phosphamidon [2-chloro-2-diethylcarbamoyl-1-methylvinyl dimethyl phosphate]—An organic phosphate, a water-miscible oil, used as a systemic insecticide, with strong stomach action, in small grains, cotton, and other field crops.

CARBAMATE INSECTICIDES

These insecticides, like the organic phosphorus insecticides, inhibit insect cholinesterases. Their mode of action is sufficiently different, however, for them to be considered a separate class of insecticides. The carbamates of interest as insecticides include

Carbaryl [1-naphthyl N-methylcarbamate; *Sevin*]—Occurring as crystals, it is slightly soluble in water and highly effective against a wide range of insects, including the *codling moth, Mexican bean beetle, cabbage worms, gypsy moth, boll weevil* and *pink bollworm*. It is not highly effective against most insects of medical importance or against mites affecting plants. Although the carbamate insecticides are considered to be of moderate to low toxicity to higher animals, carbaryl is highly toxic to the honey bee. It has the greatest range of controlled pests of any insecticide; vegetables, fruits, field crops, ornamentals, and pets. It is classed as a broad-spectrum insecticide.

NEWER METHODS OF INSECT CONTROL

Extensive research continues on new methods of insect control that reduce or avoid the dangers of toxic insecticide residues. Three experimental procedures that illustrate how such control may be achieved are

1. The use of irradiation to destroy the breeding capacity of the insect. Certain insects breed only once, and when the female of such a species is mated with a sterile mate, that female will not produce fertile eggs. Advantage has been taken of this biological fact in controlling the screw worm—a serious pest of cattle in the Southern US. In this operation males are irradiated with controlled doses of radioactive cobalt and then are released in tremendous numbers in the areas to be protected. Preliminary results have been so promising that this procedure is being considered for use against other species of insects with the same biological characteristics.
2. Distribution of the spores of organisms that are pathogenic for certain insect species only. Spores of *Bacillus thuringiensis, Berliner,* var *Kurstaki* have been shown to have value in controlling a small number of insect species and are now commercially available as Bactur, Thuricide, and others. The toxin is referred to as deltaendotoxin. Another is *Bacillus popilliae dutky,* also referred to as Milky Disease Spores.
3. The use of certain of the silica aerogels that act on soft-bodied insects by desiccation. Since the silica aerogels are exceedingly low in toxicity to humans, residues may be insignificant.

Pheromones are potentially important for monitoring insect populations. They are chemical substances produced and released by one sex of an insect (usually the female) that elicit a sexual response in an individual of the opposite sex. The specificity of pheromones makes them valuable for detecting and estimating insect populations before an infestation can enlarge or spread. There are at least 90 different pheromones currently available, eg, the boll weevil *(Grandlure),* coddling moth *(Codlelure),* house fly *(Muscalure),* and Mediterranean fruit fly *(Trimedlure).*

Insect population suppression also can be achieved by using large numbers of attractant-baited traps (mass-trapping), by disruption of normal communication between sexes *(confusion technique),* and by using a mixture of pheromone and a chemical sterilant.

FUMIGANTS

Fumigants have been, and still are being, used extensively for controlling a wide range of insects. Homes, industrial establishments, ships, and other structures may be fumigated to control household or structural pests. Large amounts of fumigants are employed to control pests in grains and woolens, in soil, and in living plants or plant products such as nursery stock, fruits, and vegetables.

The most common fumigants and their uses are discussed briefly below.

Aluminum Phosphide—A pelletized source of phosphine plus fire retardant. It is used widely in grain fumigation. It is available as *Phostoxin, Alphos, Celphine,* and others.

Carbon Disulfide [CS2]—This is one of the older fumigants. A colorless to slightly yellow liquid with a disagreeable odor. The vapor is about 2.6 times as heavy as air. Its chief disadvantage is its extreme explosiveness. It also is toxic to animals, and lengthy exposure must be avoided. It is not registered for use in fumigating stored beans, cowpeas, or peas. Fumigants are employed most extensively in grain fumigation. *Caution*—It can be toxic on inhalation. It is no longer allowed for home use and is not registered for use in fumigating dry beans, peanuts, or peas.

Chloropicrin, (Trichloronitromethane [CCl₃NO₂])—A colorless liquid that causes intense irritation of the eyes and throat and induces vomiting. It is used chiefly as a *soil fumigant.* It may be injected

in the soil in combination with xylene, carbon tetrachloride, or ethylene dichloride to help distribute the gas. It also is used in combination with certain other fumigants for *treating stored products* by sprinkling or spraying the infested materials. Since the gas is only slowly volatilized, thorough airing after use is required. Several products are on the market, eg, *Acquinite.* It is now classed as an RUP by the EPA.

Methyl Bromide (CH₃Br)—A colorless and usually odorless gas at ordinary temperatures, approximately three times as heavy as air. The gas is nonflammable and sometimes is used as a fire extinguisher. It is highly toxic to humans and the absence of odor and slow toxic action are characteristics that increase its hazard. It is among the most widely used fumigants. It destroys a wide range of pests. It is not highly toxic to most plants and leaves no objectionable odor in food. Since the chemical is a gas at ordinary temperatures, it is applied from containers into which it has been compressed as a liquid. It readily vaporizes at temperatures ordinarily encountered in fumigating. It usually is formulated with a small amount of chloropicrin to recognize the presence of this colorless and odorless gas.

Some important uses are for *fumigating warehouses, ships, railroad cars, residences, grains, living plants* shipped under quarantine regulations, *tobacco,* and many other products. The fumigant also is used to destroy *soil pests.* During World War II it was used successfully to *fumigate clothing of refugees and prisoners of war* to control *body lice.* Currently, all applications are classified by the EPA as RUPs. Only the registrant is authorized to refill cylinders.

INSECT REPELLENTS

Repellents are substances used to protect humans, animals, and plants from insects by making the hosts objectionable or unattractive by disguising the characteristic odor of the hosts.

During World War II, troops on many fronts in tropical and semitropical regions employed repellents effectively in the preventive campaign to keep away mosquitos and other annoying and disease-carrying insect pests. The problem here was to use compounds that not only had effective staying and nonirritating properties when applied to the skin of man and animals, but also were without pronounced and penetrating odors that would give the enemy information about patrolling or combat activities and locations of hideouts. During and since World War II more than 10,000 chemicals have been tested for use as insect repellents.

Perhaps the best all-purpose repellent developed since World War II is *diethyltoluamide,* which in various tests has been shown to be the most effective agent against a wide variety of insects.

Repellents, single- or multi-ingredient, generally are compounded in solution, emulsion, cream, or semisolid stick application forms. Most will provide relief from attack from mosquitos, biting flies, and gnats for periods of 30 min to 2 hr or longer.

The volatile oils of citronella, cedarwood, eucalyptus, pennyroyal, bergamot, cassia, clove, wintergreen, and lavender are, to some degree, repellent to mosquitos and other annoying insects but are not nearly as effective as the aforementioned chemicals.

Individuals who are allergic or sensitive to repellents may show various skin reactions, such as burning, itching, and swelling. Most repellents cause smarting when applied to broken skin or mucous membranes, hence care should be exercised when applying them around the eyes or other sensitive areas.

A brief chemical and physical description of the principal repellents follows.

Avitrol [4-Aminopyridine]—An avian repellent. It controls several species of birds, eg, blackbirds, crows, gulls, pigeons, sparrows, starlings, and other birds in and around structures and agriculture (eg, field corn and sunflowers). The odor causes the birds to signal vocal and physical distress that acts as an area repellent to the flock.

n-**Butyl phthalate [1,2-benzenedicarboxylic acid dibutyl ester; C₁₆H₂₂O₄]**—An oily liquid used as an insect repellent for impregnation of clothing.

Diethyltoluamide [*N,N*-diethyl-*m*-toluamide; *N,N*-diethyl-3-methylbenzamide; (*Delphene,* Deet); C₁₂H₂₇NO]—A colorless liquid with a faint, pleasant odor; practically insoluble in water, miscible with alcohol. This is a repellent for mosquitos, biting flies, gnats, chiggers, ticks, fleas, and certain other biting insects. Safe for use on human skin.

Pentachloronitrobenzene [PCNB, Terraclor]—A nitrobenzene compound used as a soil fungicide effective against many soil pathogens that attack vegetables, turf, and ornamentals. It also is used as foliar spray on young lettuce, cabbage, and cauliflower as well as on fruit trees.

Sulfur—For a long time one of the standard fungicide materials and still used widely to control a wide variety of plant diseases. It is sold as a dry powder ground to varying degrees of fineness, as a paste, or fused with clay (bentonite) and subsequently ground. Many special brands are available, and each manufacturer claims special virtues for his particular product. They all depend for their effectiveness on its inherent toxic property in affecting the growth processes of various fungi. The directions on the packages are a guide to their use. It is one of the cheapest fungicide materials and probably will continue to be used extensively as spray or dust for many years to come.

Combined with lime and water and heated for a considerable period, it forms complex *polysulfides*. This reaction product, called lime-sulfur, was described above under *Lime-Sulfur Solution*. If it is added to slaking stone lime and the only heat supplied is that of the stone lime combining with water, another type of spray called *self-boiled lime-sulfur* results. Properly prepared self-boiled lime-sulfur has a very low calcium polysulfide content and produces very little injury; it can be used with safety on peaches during the growing season, whereas lime-sulfur used at that time would cause excessive injury to the trees.

Yellow Cuprous Oxide—This material, containing 47% metallic copper, is sold under the tradename *Yellow Cuprocide* and may be used as a spray or dust. It is effective against celery blight, *Alternaria* blight of tomato, early and late blights of potato, anthracnose, downy mildew, and other leaf diseases of cucurbits, and is recommended for a variety of vegetable crops whenever a copper spray is needed.

Zineb [Zinc ethylenebisdithiocarbamate]—Exceptionally effective in the control of potato and tomato late blight in Florida. It has not been much superior to copper compounds in the more northern tomato-growing sections. It is less injurious to the tomato and potato plants than copper compounds, a factor of considerable importance in the South where numerous spray applications are required during the long growing season.

It also has been used on cucumbers, muskmelons, and watermelons for downy mildew and anthracnose control, especially in Florida. The lack of injury on these plants is a specially valuable feature of this compound, since cucumbers and melons are extremely susceptible to copper injury. For the same reason this compound has proved of value for the control of cabbage and cauliflower diseases and also has many uses on fruits. It sometimes is used to control fire blight on apple and pear trees. It also has been applied as a dust containing 8 to 10% of the fungicide.

Ziram [Zinc dimethyldithiocarbamate]—A white powder that does not leave an objectionable residue. It has found extensive use in the control of vegetable diseases (celery leaf blight, downy mildew of cucurbits, bean anthracnose, cabbage downy mildew, and squash black rot). It also has been used for peach brown rot control but is apt to produce leaf injury and fruit russet when used on apples, sour cherries, pears, and several other fruits. It is not an effective material for the control of potato or tomato late blight.

Relatively crude, denatured forms of streptomycin and oxytetracycline are being used to control many bacterial diseases of plants. Cycloheximide is used to control cherry leaf spot and dollar spot of turf.

ANTIBIOTICS

Streptomycin—Marketed as the sulfate or nitrate under the tradenames *Agri-Mycin 17* and *Phytomycin*. It is formulated as a dry, wettable powder (sulfate) and liquid (nitrate). Its salts are very soluble in water. It has general use as an antibacterial against fire blight of apples and pears and similar infections on ornamentals, including woody and herbaceous plants. It persists on plant surfaces for up to 4 months but is considered of low general toxicity. It can produce allergenic reactions such as rashes, conjunctivitis, and bronchial asthma. This agent should not be applied following Bordeaux mixture, and it is incompatible with lime-sulfur, pyrethrane, and aldrin.

Other animal and plant diseases can be controlled with aureomycin and terramycin.

CONTROL OF WEEDS AND PLANTS

Approximately $7.5 billion/year is spent in the US on agricultural pesticides. Herbicides account for about two-thirds of the agricultural expenditures for pesticides. Since 1990 herbicide use has remained relatively stable at 325 to 350 million pounds of active ingredient. High-activity compounds based on new chemistry have been developed that permit significantly lower application rates, employing new modes of action and lower environmental hazards.

Many herbicides are used for weed control, and others are being evaluated experimentally to determine their usefulness. Only those of current general interest and usefulness are described below.

Available information on the degree of toxicity of herbicides is listed in the descriptions of chemicals used for weed control. The symbol LD_{50} (lethal dose that kills 50% of the experimental animals) precedes each number that indicates relative oral toxicity. For example, the single acute oral dose for calcium cyanamide, $LD_{50} = 1400$ mg/kg, indicates a relatively low oral toxicity. The larger the LD_{50} number, the less poisonous the herbicide.

All LD values listed in this guide are based on a single dose of material orally administered to animals, followed by observation of the treated animals for a definite period of time. However, these findings do not indicate the possible hazards that may arise from skin contact or inhalation of the substance or substances indicated. Likewise, these data do not accurately predict the toxicity of a formulation that may differ depending on the solvent or diluent employed.

Herbicides are materials used mainly for the control of weeds and are used in five general ways:

Preplanting, which means that the herbicides are applied after the soil has been prepared but before seeding of the desired plant.

Preemergence or *contract,* which means that nonresidual dosages of herbicide are used after seeding but before emergence of the crop seedlings.

Preemergence or *residual,* which means that the herbicide is applied at the time of seedling or just prior to crop emergence, so that it kills weed seeds and germinating seedlings.

Postemergence, which refers to herbicide application after emergence of a crop.

Sterilant or *nonselective,* which means that sufficient herbicide is used to effect a complete kill of all treated plant life.

INORGANIC HERBICIDES. The major examples in this class are ammonium sulfamate and copper sulfate.

Copper Sulfate (Pentahydrate) [Basicap]—A blue, water-soluble crystalline material, widely used as a fungicide. However, it is used also as a herbicide, specifically for the control of algae and pond weeds in impounded potable waters. It also is used in irrigation water conveyance systems, root control in sewers, and in rice patties to control algae. *Signal Word:* Danger. *Toxicity Class:* I. *Toxicity:* Acute oral LD_{50}, 470 mg/kg; 1 mg/m^3 for all copper dusts or mists. Toxic to fish.

Antidote/Treatment: See a physician. May be corrosive to mucous membranes, eyes, skin, and gastrointestinal (GI) tract if swallowed. For oral poisoning, give two glasses of milk of magnesia, water, or milk to dilute the chemical, then induce vomiting. This should be repeated until vomitus is clear. *Handling and Storage Cautions:* Avoid direct contact. Do not use excessive amounts in ponds, streams, or lakes as a herbicide. Protective equipment and clothing should be worn during handling. *Formulation:* Numerous crystal forms and sizes, solutions, and powders are available from several manufacturers.

PETROLEUM OILS (90-PAR, VOLCK OILS, WHITE OILS, REFINED GRADES). These long have been used as insecticides, insecticide solvents, and insecticide adjuvants to increase their efficacy. Some are used as herbicides by themselves. They are applied as contact herbicides, being used for general or selective weed control. Petroleum products used as herbicides include Stoddart solvent (petroleum distillate between gasoline and kerosene, known also as mineral spirits) and diesel oil. These should be used with caution and are placed in *Toxicity Class III*. Various physical and chemical properties of the oils are important in determining their final use, eg, sulfonation percentage (indicates degree of refinement), volability, density, and viscosity.

ORGANIC ARSENICALS. This group includes monosodium methanearsonate (MSMA), disodium methanearsonate (DSMA), and cacodylic acid.

Cacodylic Acid [Hydroxydimethylarsine oxide; dimethylarsinic acid]—A nonselective herbicide, cotton defoliant, and silvicide (tree killer) for forestry use. *Toxicity Class:* III; use with caution. *Toxicity:* Acute oral LD_{50} (rat), 700 mg/kg. It also is used in a number of combination products.

Disodium Methanearsonate (DSMA)—Marketed under a variety of tradenames (eg, *Ansor DSMA Liquid, Arsinyl*) and used as a selective postemergence herbicide for cotton and as a directed spray on weeds such as Johnson grass, cocklebur, dallisgrass, watergrass, nutgrass, and goosegrass, particularly in noncrop areas. *Toxicity and Caution:* Similar to MSMA.

Monosodium Methanearsonate (MSMA) *[Ansar, Arsonate Liquid]*—A white, crystalline solid (mp, 132 to 139°C). It is a herbicide used for postemergent control of Johnson grass and other grassy weeds along the banks of ditches, storage yards, rights-of-way, and other noncrop locations; preplant in cotton; bearing citrus (except in Florida); nonbearing orchards; and crabgrass and certain broadleaf control in turf; and as a tree killer. *Toxicity Class:* III; it should be used with caution. *Toxicity:* Acute oral LD$_{50}$ (rat), 700 mg/kg; Arsonate Liquid (51% MSMA); acute oral LD$_{50}$ (rat) 1738 mg/kg; acute dermal LD$_{50}$ (rabbit) 2500 mg/kg; acute inhalation LD$_{50}$ (rat) 20 mg/L. It is mildy irritating to skin and eyes (rabbit). *Antidote/Treatment:* If swallowed, induce vomiting; drink lots of water.

PHENOXY-ALIPHATIC ACIDS. This group incudes many socalled plant hormones and related substances such as 2,4-D, 2,4-DB and MCPA.

2,4-D [(2,4-dichlorophenoxy) acetic acid; *Weed-B-Gon]*—Selective herbicide whose application is for grasses, wheat, barley, oats, sorghum, corn, sugarcane, and rice (Philippines) and noncrop areas for postemergent control of weeds such as Canada thistle, dandelion, annual mustards, ragweed, and lambs-quarters. Certain formulations are registered for pine release, water hyacinth control, and prevention of seed formation, and others for control of wild radish and other broadleaf weeds in cereals. For specific cautions, see the labels of different formulations. The dimethylamine salt form: *Toxicity Class:* I (eyes); EC:III (oral). *Toxicity:* Acute LD$_{50}$ (rat), 375 mg/kg, 700 mg/kg (isopropyl); 666 to 805 mg/kg (sodium salts). At the usual application rates (usually quite dilute), it has no adverse effect on soil microorganisms. Since this compound is active at low concentrations, spray equipment contaminated with it must be cleaned scrupulously before use for any other material. Avoid contamination in irrigation water. When using its preparations, plastic gloves, goggles, aprons, and dust masks are recommended. There are hundreds of commercial formulations and combinations of this agent on the market.

SUBSTITUTED AMINES. The substituted amine herbicides include alachlor, naptalam and propanil.

Alachlor [Chimichlor; 2-chloro-2′,6′-diethyl-N-(methoxymethyl) acetanilide]—A preemergence herbicide used to control most annual grasses and certain broadleaf weeds in corn, dry beans, peanuts, and soybeans. Leaves no carryovers residue in soil.

Naptalam [sodium 2-[(1-naphthalenylamino)carbonyl]benzoate]—A herbicide for numerous broadleaf weeds on cucurbits and nursery stock.

Propanil [Prop Job; N-(3,4-dichlorophenyl)propionamide]—A postemergence, contact-type herbicide with no residual effect against numerous grasses and broad-leaved weeds in rice.

NITROANILINES. These herbicides include benefin and triflaralin.

Benefin [Benfluralin, N-Butyl-N-ethyl-α,α,α,-trifluoro-2,6-dinitro-p-toluidine; Balan, Quilan]—Selective preemergence herbicides to control annual grasses and broadleaf weeds in seeded alfalfa, direct-seeded lettuce, peanuts, tobacco, and established turf. It may be applied and soil incorporated as much as 10 weeks prior to planting; however, it will not control established weeds. The caution signal word varies with the formulation used. *Toxicity:* Acute oral LD$_{50}$ (rat): over 10,000 mg/kg.

The pure compound is a yellow-orange, crystalline solid that is readily soluble in organic solvents. It has a flashpoint of 25.5° (78°F). These characteristics dictate caution in handling and storage. It should not be frozen, or stored above 4.5° (40°F), particularly near heat or open flame. It is corrosive and has caused severe eye irritation in lab animals. Certain individuals may show skin-sensitization reactions to it. It can be harmful if swallowed, inhaled, or absorbed through the skin. In case of contact, the eyes and skin should be flushed immediately with plenty of water. Protective clothing is recommended during usage. Several formulations and combination products are marketed.

SUBSTITUTED UREAS. These herbicides include baturon, diuron, linuron, and monuron.

Diuron; 3-(3,4-Dichlorophenyl)-1,1-dimethylurea; N′-(3,4-dichlorophenyl)-N,N-dimethylurea; Cekiuron, Unidron]—Used at low rates as a selective herbicide to control germinating broadleaf grass weeds in numerous crops such as sugarcane, pineapple, alfalfa, grapes, cotton, and peppermint. At higher rates of application it can be used as a general weed killer. As a soil sterilant, it is more persistent and preferred over monuron on lighter soil and/or in areas of heavy rainfall. *Toxicity Class:* III. *Toxicity:* Acute oral LD$_{50}$ (rat), 3400 mg/kg. *Handling and Storage Cautions:* Similar to those for other herbicides. It is

used commonly as a flowable, wettable powder in formulations, and numerous combination products exist.

CARBAMATES

Propham [Isopropyl carbanilate; IPC]—Used primarily as a preemergence and postemergence herbicide. It prevents cell division and acts on meristematic tissue. Major uses include control of weeds in alfalfa, ladino clover, flax, lettuce, safflower, lentils, and peas and on fallow land. *Toxicity Class:* III. *Toxicity:* Generally low toxicity to wildlife and fish; acute oral LD$_{50}$ (rat), 5000 mg/kg. It is available in flowable suspensions, wettable powders, and various combination products.

THIOCARBAMATES. These include pebulate, diallate, and EPTC (S-Ethyldipropylthiocarbamate; Alirox).

Pebulate [S-Propyl butylethylthiocarbamate; R-2061]—A preplant selective herbicide for the control of both grassy and broadleaf weeds. It has been used for selective weed control in sugar beets, tobacco, and tomatoes. The signal word is *caution. Toxicity Class:* III. *Toxicity:* Acute oral LD$_{50}$ (rat), 921 to 1900 mg/kg; acute dermal LD$_{50}$ (rabbit) >4640 mg/kg. Formulations include emulsifiable concentrate (6 lb/gal) and granules (10%).

HETEROCYCLIC NITROGEN COMPOUNDS. These herbicides include amitrole, pyrazon, and picloram.

Amitrole [1H-1,2,4-triazol-3-amine; Amerol, Simazol]—Used mainly as a nonselective systemic herbicide for control of annual grasses, broadleaf weeds, perennial broadleaf weeds, poison ivy, and certain aquatic weeds in marshes and drainage ditches. All applications are classified by the EPA as restricted use. It is restricted to noncropland use. The signal word is caution. *Toxicity Class:* III. *Toxicity:* Acute oral LD$_{50}$ (male albino rat), up to 10,000 mg/kg caused no death or symptoms of systemic activity. It has an indefinite shelf-life and should be stored at room temperature. It is available in liquid and solid powder formulations as well as pressurized-container products. Numerous combination products are also available.

TRIAZINES. These herbicides include atrazine, simazine, propazine, prometone, and cyanazine. The EPA currently is conducting a special review of triazine herbicides. In 1995 the manufacturers of cyanazine voluntarily withdrew its registration rather than proceed with the special review. Cyanazine, which is identified as a carcinogenic material, is the third most-used herbicide on corn and cotton and is commonly used on sorghum and other crops to control grasses and broadleaf weeds. The manufacturer agreed to stop selling products containing cyanazine in 1999.

Atrazine [2-Chloro-4-ethylamino-6-isopropylamino-1,3,5 triazine]—A selective herbicide used in season-long weed control in corn, sorghum, and certain other crops. It also is used at higher rates of application for nonselective weed control in noncropped areas. *Toxicity Class:* III. *Toxicity:* Acute oral LD$_{50}$ (rat), 1780 mg/kg. It is listed as harmful if swallowed, and contact with eyes and skin should be avoided. Another caution listing states "do not contaminate food, feed or water supplies with the product." The shelf-life is given as 3 years under environmental conditions, provided that the product is stored in its unopened and undamaged original containers, in shaded, possibly well-aired, fresh, and dry storehouse conditions and kept away from sources of heat, free flames, or spark-generating equipment. Formulations include dry flowable powders, flowable liquids, and wettable powders. Numerous combination products are on the market.

URACILS. These herbicides are bromacil and terbacil.

Bromacil [5-Bromo-3-sec-butyl-6-methyluracil]—A weed and brush herbicide in noncrop areas, especially for perennial grasses. It also has been used in selective weed control in pineapple and citrus growing. The dry formulations are water-soluble. *Toxicity Class:* III (dry); II (liquid). *Toxicity:* Acute oral LD$_{50}$ (rat), 5200 mg/kg. *Handling and Storage Cautions:* There are several because of its irritant and combustible qualities. Protective clothing is advised for proper handling. The formulations include granular powder, liquid, water-soluble liquid, and wettable powder. Several combination products are available, particularly with various contact and hormone weed killers.

ALIPHATIC ACIDS. These herbicides include *dalapon* and *TCA* (trichloroacetic acid).

Dalapon [2,2-Dichloropropionic acid]—A selective herbicide and growth regulator used for quackgrass, bermudagrass and other perennial and annual grasses as well as cattails and rushes. This herbicide is used commonly as a preplant treatment to control established perennial grasses in cropland, noncropland areas, and irrigation ditch banks in 17 Western states. It acts by being translocated to the roots of most species, where it acts as a growth regulator. *Toxicity Class:* II. *Toxicity:* Acute oral LD$_{50}$ (female rats), 970 mg/kg (tech ai); 7570 mg/kg (sodium salt). The acid is not used directly, and commercial products usually contain 85% sodium salt or mixed sodium and magnesium salts. *Handling and Storage Cautions:* There are several, including the avoidance of skin and eye contact because of irritancy and the avoidance of contamination of water, food, or feed through storage or disposal. It is formulated mainly as a water-soluble powder and in several combination products.

ARYLALIPHATIC ACIDS. The herbicides that belong to this class include dicamba, fenac, 2,3,6-TBA (trichlorobenzoic acid) and DCPA (Dacthal; dimethyl tetrachloroterephthalate).

Dicamba [2-Methoxy-3,6-dichlorobenzoic acid; 3,6-dichloro-*o*-anisic acid]—A herbicide. *Toxicity Class:* II. *Toxicity:* Acute oral LD_{50} (rat), 1707 mg/kg; acute dermal LD_{50} (rabbit), 2000 mg/kg. Formulations of a flowable liquid potassium product (Marksman) and the dimethylamine salt (4 lb/gal) are available. Several combination products are marketed.

PHENOL DERIVATIVES

DNOC [4,6-Dinitro-*o*-cresol; 2-methyl-4,6-dinitrophenol]—Insecticide, fungicide, herbicide, and defoliant properties. It has use as a dormant spray for killing insect eggs and in apple scab control. The triethanolamine salt has promise as a complete dormant apple spray for light infestations of mite and aphid eggs as well as other pests. The sodium salt has been used as a weed killer and on apple and peach trees to thin fruit. The signal word is *Danger. Caution:* Very phytotoxic. *Toxicity Class:* III; I. *Toxicity:* Acute oral LD_{50} (rat), 20 to 50 mg/kg. It should be stored in cool, well-ventilated areas away from heat and foodstuffs. Formulations include the ammonium salt (50%), flakes (98 to 100% free acid), and a flowable, wettable powder.

SUBSTITUTED NITRILES. These herbicides include dichlobenil and bromoxynil.

Dichlobenil [2,6-Dichlorobenzonitrile; Casoron]—For selective weed control in cranberry bogs, ornamentals, nurseries, fruit orchards, vineyards, forest plantations, and public green areas and for total weed control (such as industrial sites, railway lines, etc, under asphalt). It also is used to control aquatic weeds in nonflowing water. It has been recommended for selective weed control in woody perennial crops and for total weed control on industrial sites, car parks, roadsides, railways, and related areas. *Toxicity Class:* III. *Toxicity:* Acute oral LD_{50} (rat), 3160 mg/kg; acute dermal LD_{50} (rabbit), 1350 mg/kg. It is toxic to germinating seeds. It should not be stored with propagative structures such as seeds, bulbs, tubers, or nursery stock or with food or feed products. It is available as granules and wettable powder and in several combinations.

BIPYRIDYLIUMS. These herbicides include diquat and paraquat.

Paraquat [1,1′-Dimethyl-4,4′-bipyridinium ion (present as the dichloride salt); Herboxone]—A contact herbicide used in the desiccation of seed crops and for noncrop and industrial weed control in bearing and nonbearing fruit orchards, shade trees, and ornamentals. Other uses include defoliation and desiccation of cotton; a harvest aid in soybeans, sugarcane, sunflowers; pasture renovation; and eradication of weeds in coffee plantations and similar situations. Some or all applications may be classified by the EPA as RUP. The signal words are *danger* and *poison. Toxicity Class:* I. *Toxicity:* Acute oral LD_{50} (rat), 150 mg ion/kg. It can kill if swallowed. Use only with protective clothing, and wash thoroughly after using. Various formulations include soluble dichloride concentrate and various liquid and granular forms. Several combination products are available.

MISCELLANEOUS HERBICIDES. Herbicides in this miscellaneous group include endothall and bensulide.

Endothall [7-Oxabicyclo [2.2.1] heptane-2,3-dicarboxylic acid]; Accelerate]—A pre- and postemergence herbicide, defoliant, desiccant, aquatic algicide and growth regulator. *Toxicity Class:* I. *Toxicity:* Acute oral LD_{50} (rat), 51 mg/kg.

Bensulide [S-(*O,O*-Diisopropyl phosphorodithioate) ester of *N*-(2-mercaptoethyl)benzenesulfonamide; Bensumec, Exporsan, Prefar]—For preemergence control of annual grasses and crop use in carrots, cucumbers, peppers, and tomatoes, among others. *Toxicity Class:* III. *Toxicity:* Acute oral LD_{50} (rat), 271 to 1470 mg/kg. Various formulations and combination products exist.

PLANT REGULATORS

A plant-growth regulator is a preparation that in minute amounts alters the behavior of ornamental or crop plants or the products thereof through physiological (hormone) action rather than physical action. It may act to accelerate or retard growth, prolong or break a dormant condition, promote rooting, or act in other ways. A classification of plant-growth regulators usually includes auxins—2,4-D, MCPB, BNOA; gibberillins; cytokinins—kinetin; ethylene generators—ethylene ethephon; inhibitors—benzoic acid, MH; and retardants—A-Rest.

Gibberellic acid is used extensively as seeds to aid in uniform germination and growth and on grapes to increase size. 2-Methyl-4-chlorophenoxyacetic acid (MCPA) and a number of related chemicals are used to thin blossoms, stop the premature drop of fruits or vegetables before harvest, increase the uniformity of ripening, and a wide variety of other purposes. For ex-ample, when applied properly, 2,4-D will increase the red color in potatoes, and other chemicals will produce pineapples of more uniform shape than untreated ones. This field of chemical usage is expanding and appears to have a future limited only by the necessity to prove that the uses are safe, from both the toxicological and nutritional viewpoints. Also, 2,4-D is used on tomatoes to cause all fruits to ripen at the same time for machine harvesting.

The identification of vegetable-growth inhibitors may yield improved storage methods for crops. Growth inhibitors for onions and cabbage have been identified, but further studies are necessary to determine their ultimate value. Other growth regulators of potential value include

Ethrel [2-Chloroethylphosphonic acid], which functions by releasing ethylene in plant tissues; it can increase appearance of fruit on pineapple.

Captan [*N*-(trichloromethylthio)-4-cyclohexene-1,2-dicarboximide], which is registered for use in increasing the fruit set of both oranges and tangelos.

Ripenthol, which contains endothall (7-oxabicyclo[2.2.1]heptane-2,3-dicarboxylic acid) and can delay sucrose breakdown in mature sugarcane, giving planters a longer harvest period; this has increased yields of sugar in sugarcane.

DESICCANTS AND DEFOLIANTS

Desiccants and defoliants become increasingly important as mechanical harvesting gains popularity. In the same way that removal of weeds by use of herbicides just before the combines are put into the fields to harvest wheat prevents clogging of the machines with weed debris, the removal of cotton leaves by chemical treatment aids mechanical harvesting of cotton and other leafy crops. Arsenic acid, pentachlorophenol, and more complex chemicals such as S,S,S-tributylphosphorotrithionate and S,S,S-tributylphosphorotrithioite and others are being used for this purpose. Requests for information concerning developments in this field should be addressed to the USDA, state experiment stations, or manufacturers of specific products. Questions on the legal status of pesticides should be sent to Director, Pesticides Regulation Div, Environmental Protection Agency (EPA), Washington, DC 20460.

Acknowledgment is made of helpful comments and suggestions by Drs M Lee, R Taylor, and D MacIver and information provided by Susan Lawrence, Chief, Public Response and Program Resources Branch, Field Operations Div, Office of Pesticide Programs, EPA.

BIBLIOGRAPHY

Agricultural Resources and Environmental Indicators. USDA, Economic Research Service, 1996–97.

Biological effects of pesticides in mammalian systems. *Ann NY Acad Sci* 1969; 160(art 1): 1.

Brooks GT. *Chlorinated Insecticides*, vol I, *Technology and Application.* Cleveland OH: Chem Rubber Press, 1974; vol II, *Biological and Environmental Aspects*, 1975.

Citizens Guide to Pesticides. Washington, DC: EPA, Office of Pesticide Programs, Sep 1987.

40 CFR 150-189 (as of July 1, 1987), Protection of Environment. USGPO, 1987.

De Ong ER, *et al. Insect Disease and Weed Control.* New York: Chem Publ, 1972.

Djerassi C, *et al.* Insect control of the future: operational and policy aspects. *Science* 1974; 186: 596.

Edwards CA. *Persistent Pesticides in the Environment.* Cleveland, OH: Chem Rubber Press, 1970.

EPA Pesticides Industry Sales and Usage 1990 and 1991 Market Estimates (H-7503Q), Fall 1992.

Eto M. *Organophosphorus Pesticides: Organic and Biological Chemistry.* Cleveland, OH: Chem Rubber Press, 1974.

Farm Chemicals Handbook, ed 8. Willoughby, OH: Meister Publ, 1998.

The Federal Insecticide, Fungicide, and Rodenticide Act (as amended) (540/09-012). Washington, DC: EPA, Oct 1988.

Hassall K. *The Chemistry of Pesticides*. Deerfield Beach, FL: Verlag Chemie, 1982.

Herbicide Handbook, ed 5. Champaign, IL: Weed Sci Soc Am, 1983.

Jacbson M. *Pesticides of the Future*. New York: Dekker, 1975.

Klingman GC, Ashton FM, Noordhoff LJ. *Weed Science: Principles and Practices*. New York: Wiley, 1975.

Matsumura F, ed. *Environmental Toxicology of Pesticides*. New York: Academic, 1972.

Melnikov NN. *Chemistry of Pesticides*. New York: Springer-Verlag, 1971.

Morgan DP. *Recognition and Management of Pesticide Poisonings* (EPA-540/9-80), ed. 3. Washington, DC, Jan 1982.

National Home and Garden Pesticide Use Survey, Final Report, vol 1: Executive Summary, Results, and Recommendations. Research Triangle Park, NC: RTI, Mar 1992.

Pesticide Fact Handbook (EPA regulatory status of 550 tradenamed pesticides). Park Ridge, NJ: Noyes Data Corp, 1988; vol 2 (430 tradenamed pesticides), 1990.

Regulating Pesticides in Food. Washington, DC: Natl Acad Press, 1987.

Sherma J. Pesticides. *Anal Chem* 1987; 59: 18R.

Stevens-White R, ed. *Pesticides in the Environment,* vol 1, pt 1. New York: Dekker, 1071; vol 1, pt 2, 1971.

Storck WJ. Pesticides growth slow. *Chem Eng News* 1987; (Nov 16): 35.

Street JC, ed. *Pesticide Symposia* (Toxicology). Miami: Halos & Assoc, 1970.

Ware GW. *Pesticides. Theory and Application*. San Francisco: WH Freeman, 1983.

Wiswesser WJ, ed. *Pesticide Index,* ed 5. College Park, MD: Entomol Soc Am, 1976.

MEDICINAL AGENTS

PART **8**

Pharmacy Practice

Nicholas G Popovich, PhD
Professor and Head
Department of Pharmacy Administration
University of Illinois at Chicago
College of Pharmacy
Chicago, IL

Fundamentals of Pharmacy Practice

Nicholas G Popovich, PhD
Professor and Head
Department of Pharmacy Administration
University of Illinois at Chicago
College of Pharmacy
Chicago, IL

CHAPTER 94

Application of Ethical Principles to Practice Dilemmas

Amy Marie Haddad, PhD

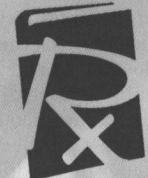

The growing sophistication and complexity of contemporary health care practice presents many ethical challenges including: protecting privacy and confidentiality in an environment of easily accessible information and perplexing regulations, maternal-fetal conflicts, threats to the rights of human subjects in research, genetic engineering and screening, and delivery of treatment and services in a highly fragmented system to name only some of the more problematic issues. As pharmacy practice becomes more complex and increasingly patient-oriented, pharmacists have to deal with the aforementioned broader ethical issues shared by all health professionals and those unique to or more commonly encountered in pharmacy practice. New and difficult questions face pharmacists. Is it ever right to use controversial drugs such as cannabis or heroin in treating terminally ill patients? How does one reduce or eradicate the undertreatment of pain? Whose responsibility is it to manage an impaired colleague? What is the best system to lower the number of medication errors? When, if ever, should a pharmacist participate in assisted suicide? How will changing state and federal laws and new court decisions impact the delivery and quality of pharmaceutical care?

"Because ethical dilemmas are commonplace in pharmacy practice, pharmacists must develop a working knowledge of formal and systematic ethical analysis, as well as learn to distinguish ethical issues from social, psychological, political, and legal issues."[1] Moreover, the difficulty of the ethical issues mentioned thus far suggests that a collaborative approach to resolving them would be preferable to individuals struggling alone. Pharmacists must be able to work with others on the health care team to find a justifiable resolution. To collaborate with others and work effectively, there must be a systematic approach to working through an ethical dilemma. The purpose of this chapter is to define applied ethics and its application to pharmacy practice with emphasis on the use of normative models of ethical decision-making to resolve practice dilemmas. A process for ethical decision-making is explained and applied to clinical cases that refer to issues encountered on an individual, institutional, and societal level. Resources to help in the resolution of ethical dilemmas are also noted.

APPLIED ETHICS AND HEALTH CARE

The application of the ideas and concepts of ethics to issues in health care began in the late 1960s with questions about the allocation of the new technologies of hemodialysis, vital organ transplantation, and the treatment of human research subjects. Normative ethics is that branch of ethical inquiry that considers ethical questions whose answers have a relatively direct bearing on practice.[2] The results of such ethical inquiry have immediate application for actions or policies. Hence, the term "applied" ethics, in this case is applied to pharmacy practice. To arrive at a clearer understanding of ethics in general, it helps to have a baseline of key terms. Three terms underlie all the discussion in this chapter: (1) ethics, (2) values, and (3) dilemmas.

Ethics

Ethics is a careful, systematic inquiry into the nature of morality, guidelines, or standards that give meaning and direction to the human community. Simply put, ethics is the study of good and evil, of right and wrong. But, ethics is much more than that. Ethics is concerned with the duties and obligations one has to others and to him- or herself. Ethics is also concerned with the rights of individuals and how those rights are recognized and respected. The systematic nature of ethics helps illuminate what one ought to do, who one should be as a human being, and what and whom one should nurture and sustain in life.

Values

Values are an important part of ethics. One uses values to help explain how and why things are important to us. "Values are not to be confused with concrete goods. They are ideas, images, and notions. Values attract us. One aspires after the good they articulate. One expects to find our own good in relation to what they offer."[3] When one looks at the goodness or badness of an action, one must also look at the values attached to the action. Values are the internal motivators for our actions. Evidence of values is observed in human behavior. True values elicit deeply held positive or negative attachments. Basic values and a value system are developed in childhood and result from such influencing factors as family, teachers, friends, religious traditions, and culture. People of different religious faiths or of no faith ascribe to many values and principles one acts upon on a daily basis. Values also have their roots in professions. Some traditional values of the pharmacy profession are compassion, faithfulness, and fairness. With the introduction of pharmaceutical care as a standard for pharmacy practice, the values of patience, responsiveness, and kindness have been added to the list of traditional values.[4]

Usually, values remain unchanged after one reaches adulthood unless they are challenged by great spiritual or emotional distress. Of course, values can also change when it becomes apparent that an old value system doesn't work anymore. Whatever their origin or evolution, the resulting personal and professional values can profoundly affect the ethical decisions that pharmacists make.

Dilemmas

An individual has a dilemma when, wanting to make a good choice realizes that no matter what is done, a choice will result in loss or harm. Simply put, a dilemma is choosing among equally unappealing alternatives. "A difficult problem becomes a 'dilemma' when one is quite sure that one will be making a big mistake regardless of what path one choose. It is instructive to consider moral dilemmas in this context. The anxiety one experiences as one faces each unpalatable alternative informs us about the nature of moral dilemmas. It seems that any decision one makes will violate one or another value which one holds dear."[5] In particular, moral dilemmas in pharmacy can arise in several ways. They can arise when the right thing to do, such as telling the truth, conflicts with obligations like loyalty to a peer or protecting the patient from harm. They can also arise when what is best for the patient runs counter to patient self-determination or one's own well being–one's health, obligations to family or one's employer, and so on. To resolve a dilemma effectively, one must have a method for reviewing the facts, generating alternatives, and choosing the "best" alternative given the circumstances of the dilemma.

A PROCESS FOR APPROACHING AND RESOLVING ETHICAL DILEMMAS

A method to resolve ethical dilemmas should closely resemble the methods of work-up for drug-related or medical problems. In both cases, the pharmacist needs to know how to collect information, analyze it, and use the findings in ways compatible with standards of pharmacy practice. For example, when a patient asks the pharmacist for help in treating a rash that covers his arms and trunk, the pharmacist begins the assessment process with a careful history including questions about medications, dietary changes, allergies, what treatments have been tried, what has worked, and use of new products such as lotion or laundry detergents. Depending on the clinical setting, the pharmacist may conduct a physical inspection of the rash noting its appearance. When the collected data are analyzed, a clinical judgment designed to best help the patient is made. In resolving ethical dilemmas, a similar stepwise process is followed.

The following is a suggestion for such an approach that takes into account the impact of the decision on the patient, family, and health care team. There are five steps in this proposed model. The five steps are (1) gather clinical and situational information; (2) identify values of the people involved and legal implications; (3) identify the ethical problem or problems in terms of principles; (4) seek a justifiable resolution; (5) anticipate arguments to the proposed resolution and respond.[6] By following the stepwise process, one is able to recognize and remedy faulty thinking, avoid simplistic decisions or snap judgments, clarify conflicts between values and principles, explain *why* a choice is right or wrong, and guide us to the right choice in ambiguous or confusing situations.

Gather Clinical and Situational Information

Clinical facts include diagnosis, prognosis, what treatments, including drugs have been attempted, the success or failure of such treatments, and other pertinent data that would affect a decision. Once the clinical facts are clearly outlined, one can then look at the specific context of those facts.

Situational or contextual facts include information about the individuals involved in the case, their relationships, as well as their authority and stake in the outcome. The context of an ethical problem has direct bearing on how the problem is perceived and what resolutions are possible. For example, two patients may share the same diagnoses and prognoses but differ greatly in their cultural backgrounds, religious beliefs, or where they live any of which can impact ethical choices.

Identify Values

It is important to gather information about the values that the individuals involved in a case have. These include values toward quality of life, honesty and responsibility to others, among others. By identifying basic values, it is easier to determine the nature of the conflict in the case. Because patients' wishes generally take priority over other parties, their beliefs, wishes and values should be considered first. Also, it is important to ascertain the validity of the information on which a patient bases his or her values. If the patient doesn't have sound clinical information, that information should be provided in clear, understandable terms. Sometimes, merely by clarifying values and correcting misinformation, an ethical problem can be resolved or avoided entirely.

Identify the Ethical Problem

Most problematic situations in pharmacy practice contain more than one ethical problem. Often there is a conflict between two moral goods, such as the pharmacist's duty to do good for the patient by providing appropriate drug therapy and counseling and the patient's right to self-determination that can result in noncompliance. The four principles approach to biomedical ethics proposed by Beauchamp and Childress, provides a comprehensive framework for ethical analysis.[7] Besides the four basic principles of respect for autonomy (self-determination or freedom of choice), nonmaleficence (the duty not to harm), beneficence (the duty to do good), and justice, the derivative principles of truth telling, fidelity, and avoidance of killing are also addressed as they all play a central role in health care.

AUTONOMY, SELF-DETERMINATION AND FREEDOM OF CHOICE—Respect for persons and an individual's autonomy are foundational principles in most ethical traditions. The principle of respect for autonomy states that human beings have a moral dignity that should be respected. And, individuals should be able to exercise freedom in decisions that affect their lives with undue interference from others. To make sound decisions about one's life plans, one needs good information. So the doctrine of informed consent is derived from the basic principle of respect of autonomy. Pharmacists address the issue of autonomy when they contemplate whether to advise a patient that he or she needs additional medical attention for his or her condition in the case of an inappropriate prescription.

BENEFICENCE AND NONMALEFICENCE—Because pharmacists are in professional practice to care for others, it is almost automatic in the provision of care to assume the principle of beneficence, that is, to help or assist patients. A closely related principle is nonmaleficence, which requires the avoidance of harm in all cases. Specifically, the principle of beneficence applies to actions in pharmacy practice that prevent harm, remove harm, and the provision of benefit. In the delivery of pharmaceutical care, beneficence requires respect for the wishes and choices of patients and their families. Moreover, the principle of nonmaleficence requires that pharmacists deliver safe and quality care. For example, when a pharmacist is confronted with a prescription that will not be harmful but probably will not help the patient, he or she is dealing with weighing the benefits and harms of therapy.

JUSTICE—The principle of justice addresses the fair distribution of burdens and benefits. Allocating health care resources is an increasing problem in all areas of health care delivery. Pharmacy practice is no exception and perhaps one of the most problematic areas of health care because of the high cost of drug products. Pharmacists not only deal with the societal issue of fair drug costs, but with the more personal, direct meanings of justice, for example, whether to treat patients differently depending on their ability to pay.

Justice embodies the ethical ideal of fairness. Implicit in the idea of fairness is the conflict between interests to which the ethical principle provides resolution. Justice gives us the rules and standards by which to mediate these claims that human beings make against each other on a daily basis. Justice requires that the pharmacist examine the fairness with which care is delivered in relationship to other competing demands. Consider this scenario, three patients arrive at a pharmacy at the same time, all equally sick and in need of the pharmacist's attention. When resources are limited, in this case the pharmacist's time, a decision must be made on some principle of justice to "break the tie" so to speak. The pharmacist could decide to spend his or her time where it would do the most good. Or, the pharmacist could decide to address the needs of the patient who holds the lengthiest relationship with the pharmacy, in a sense rewarding the patient's loyalty. This latter understanding of justice is referred to as "merit." In sum, determining the distribution of health care resources, whether it is a pharmacist's time or dollars, is one of the most complicated and painful areas of conflict in health care today.

TRUTHTELLING, HONESTY AND INTEGRITY—Regard for self-determination requires that health professionals be honest with their patients. Patients need accurate and understandable information to make good decisions. "Traditional ethics holds that it is simply wrong morally to lie to people, even if it is expedient to do so, even if greater good will come from the lie. According to this view, lying to people is morally wrong in that it shows lack of respect for them."[8] Pharmacists face the question of honesty when they are asked to withhold information from patients on the request of the physician or family member. Even if the reason for the request is to protect the patient from unnecessary harm, withholding the truth deprives the patient of his or her autonomy. Truth telling is one of the two cornerstones of trust between patient and pharmacist. Promise-keeping is the other.

PROMISE-KEEPING, COVENANT, OR FIDELITY—The principle of fidelity requires that promises, once made, should be kept. Our faithfulness in our relations with others ought to be respected and held in high esteem. When a pharmacist enters a relationship with a patient, there is an implicit agreement in the form of a promise or in the language of pharmaceutical care, a "covenant." It is important to explore the idea of covenant in pharmacy practice because it is a departure from the traditional relationship between patient and health professional that is based on a contractual model. Implicit in the covenantal relationship is the invitation for the patient to trust the pharmacist. Rather than a mere contract, which is external to a relationship, a covenant is internal to both parties. Covenants have a growing nature to them that extends rather than limits the relationship. This understanding of covenant requires that the pharmacist "be there" for the patient. So, when a pharmacist wonders whether to sell ineffective but heavily promoted nonprescription drug products or herbal remedies, the principle of fidelity asserts itself. What would this action do to the trust that patients place in the pharmacist?

AVOIDANCE OF KILLING—More and more, pharmacists will find themselves in positions where they will be parties to patient suicides or requests for active killing through lethal prescriptions. Although the principle of nonmaleficence counts strongly against taking the life of another human being, the seriousness and irreversible nature of killing requires a separate principle. Not all behavior that shortens an individual's life should be considered killing. For example, the use of opioids to manage pain in the terminally ill may hasten death, but the motive is not to kill the patient. Rather the intent in such situations is to manage pain even though an earlier death is a foreseen result. Many moral and religious traditions condemn active killing even for reasons of mercy. "If killing is always a wrong-making characteristic, then avoidance of killing can be thought of as another moral principle that must hold beneficence and nonmaleficence in check."[9]

Principles can be a means to determine if an ethical dilemma exists in a particular situation. By asking the following series of questions, one can quickly determine whether any of the principles previously mentioned are at work in a case. If the answer to any one of the questions is "yes," an ethical problem is present.

1. Is this unfair? To whom?
2. Does this break a promise?
3. Will this be harmful? To whom?
4. Will this threaten future or existing relationships?
5. Will I be compromising someone's rights (including my own)?
6. Will this benefit the patient from the patient's perspective?
7. Is this disrespectful? To whom?[10]

Seek a Justifiable Resolution

At this point, one can begin to explore possible courses of action. If the case is one of high urgency, there is little time to explore a variety of options. In those cases, it is best to comply with previously established policies or guidelines rather than responding rashly and emotionally. Principles can be action guides to moral behavior, in addition to helping one determine the source of the moral problem. Although it is likely that there will be conflicts between moral principles in a dilemma, it is a good place to begin to determine the morally correct thing to do. If there is time to reflect on various courses of action, it helps to consult with colleagues to determine the best course of action.

Anticipate Arguments and Respond

After determining the best course of action, it is prudent to critically look at one's choice by asking what others would think of the alternative. "Moral or practical reasoning entails defending judgments in a certain way. The goal in a moral justification is to be clear, to use all relevant information, and to give cogent reasons for one's views."[11]

APPLICATION TO COMPLEX CASES

Components of the five-step process of approaching ethical decisions is applied to three cases dealing with pharmacists involved in some aspect of clinical practice. The cases differ in that they explore three different levels of ethical importance. The first case explores personal, direct involvement with a patient and a colleague. The second case moves to an institutional level in which the pharmacist must attend not only to the needs of a particular patient but other patients with similar diagnoses, the values and concerns of co-workers, and the institution's reputation in the community. The third case explores societal implications of a decision at the institutional level as well as inequities in access to health care resources.

CASE ONE: PROTECTING THE REPUTATION OF A PEER AND PATIENT WELL-BEING—Jane Wagner, a 40-year-old freelance writer with a history of depression, left the community mental health center after her appointment and went straight to the nearest pharmacy to have her prescription filled before her long drive home. Ms. Wagner lived in the foothills of a mountain range. The closest town to her home was Maple River, 50 miles away, where Ms. Wagner did her shopping and visited the clinic. Ms. Wagner handed her prescription to Tara Sadler, PharmD, at the Maple River Pharmacy and told Dr. Sadler that she had some errands to run and would return for the prescription later. Dr. Sadler was the only pharmacist on duty with the help of one technician. Even though Maple River wasn't a large town, the pharmacy was exceptionally busy on this Friday afternoon. All Ms. Sadler had time for was to dispense prescriptions. Dr. Sadler barely had time to fill Ms. Wagner's prescription before she returned to the pharmacy to pick it up.

About 2 hours later, Ms. Wagner called the pharmacy and asked to speak to Dr. Sadler.

"I just opened my prescription and the pills are a different color than the ones I got the last time. These are blue and the last ones were pink. Are you sure these are right? I just drove 50 miles to get home and I sure don't want to turn around and drive another 100 miles round trip to get the right drug," Ms. Wagner stated.

Dr. Sadler quickly checked her records and noted that she must have dispensed 30-mg tablets rather than the 20-mg tablets prescribed BID. But, the written record showed that she dispensed the 20-mg tablets.

"Are you sure they're blue?" Dr. Sadler asked.

"Of course," Ms. Wagner responded. "I'm not color-blind!!"

Dr. Sadler responded, "Well, those pills will be okay. You're right, they are a different color from your last ones, but if you break them in half, they will be close enough to your old prescription. I think it will be just fine and it will save you a trip back into town. Just break them in half at the line down the middle."

Dr. Sadler hung up and returned to the rest of the prescriptions that were waiting for her. She reasoned that 15mg was close enough to 20mg Ms. Wagner was supposed to receive and wouldn't make that much difference.

One month later, Ms. Wagner visits Maple River Pharmacy for a refill on her prescription. John Winchester, PharmD, the manager of the pharmacy, notes that Ms. Wagner is right on time for her refill. Dr. Winchester asks Ms. Wagner how she is doing.

Ms. Wagner states, "I'm doing fine. By the way, I want you to fill this prescription with those blue tablets rather than the pink ones. I've been breaking the pills in half and taking a half in the morning and a half in the evening. I'm doing well on this dose."

Dr. Winchester was confused. "I don't understand. Who told you to break the pills in half?"

"The other pharmacist." Ms. Wagner replied.

After verifying that the prescription refill was for 20mg BID and that Dr. Sadler had filled the prescription a month ago, Dr. Winchester called Dr. Sadler at home to help resolve the situation. Dr. Sadler stated, "I won't admit to an error because I never saw the prescription after it left the pharmacy. The patient called and said the tablets were blue. I remember I checked the records and it said that I dispensed the 20-mg tablets. Since I didn't see the pills, its her word against mine."

Dr. Winchester is not happy with Dr. Sadler's attitude, but decides to refill the prescription as written until he can figure out where the true problem lies. When Ms. Wagner gets her prescription, she opens the bag, looks in the bottle and states, "These aren't blue. I told you I want the same prescription I got the last time. I'm not leaving until you fill this the right way." Dr. Winchester wonders what is the right thing to do.

Case One is fundamentally concerned with ethical issues on an individual level. "This realm also deals with weighing and balancing the values/goods/loyalties that stand in tension between two or more individuals."[12] For example, one must weigh Ms. Wagner's right to the most effective medication for her condition and Dr. Winchester's responsibility to dispense prescriptions as written.

Before the ethical problem or problems can be named in this case, it helps to gather information that is not in the case or that would help in understanding the different perspectives of those involved. The clinical or technical facts of the case are fairly clear. Ms. Wagner claims that she received blue (30-mg tablets) rather than the pink (20-mg) tablets she was supposed to receive. Dr. Sadler instructed Ms. Wagner to take half the blue tablet (15-mg) BID assuring her that it would be close enough to her prescribed dose. One month later when Ms. Wagner comes for a refill, Dr. Winchester discovers that Ms. Wagner claims she got 30mg tablets rather than the 20mg tablets ordered. Dr. Winchester checks with Dr. Sadler who denies making an error or instructing Ms. Wagner to take half a tablet twice a day. Ms. Wagner will not accept the correctly filled prescription and demands the "blue pills."

Other clinical or technical facts that are relevant in this case are: Ms. Wagner has a history of depression that requires medication; she lives in a rural, isolated area; she is functional enough to receive mental health services from a community mental health center; she pays attention to her prescriptions and the effect of the drug; she claims to be doing well on the 30-mg/day dose.

There are clinical facts that one does not know. For example, it would be important to know what drug is involved, its efficacy, dosing, and so on. It would also help to know Ms. Wagner's drug history, particularly, with antidepressants. What has worked for her before? Is one month long enough to know if this is the proper dose for Ms. Wagner? She seems to be compliant, but it would be important to know if this is a pattern or not.

The situational facts of the case include who is immediately involved in the case, their relationships, and perspectives. Situational information also includes attention to the context of a case such as time constraints or other environmental factors that could influence a decision. There is a sense of urgency in this case because Ms. Wagner is literally standing in the pharmacy waiting for an answer. Dr. Winchester has some time, but not a lot to come to a resolution. One knows that Dr. Winchester is the manager of the pharmacy so that places added responsibility on him. Dr. Sadler is not a manager, but a staff pharmacist so she is subordinate in the organization to Dr. Winchester. Because of the way the case is written in the third person voice, the reader of the case has more facts than Dr. Winchester. For example, one knows that Dr. Sadler did tell the patient to split the tablets in half even though she denies it. There is no information about any relationship between Ms. Wagner and the pharmacists at Maple River Pharmacy beyond that she is a customer. One does not know if she is a routine patient at the pharmacy or not. An important person in the case who remains unnamed is the prescriber who could be a physician's assistant, nurse practitioner, or physician. Regardless, the prescriber wrote a prescription for a drug at a specific dose. She or he presumes that the prescription was filled as written. There is no description of the relationship between the pharmacy and the mental health center nor the relationship between Dr. Winchester and the staff at the mental health center. We know Maple River is not a "large" town, but just how big a town is it? The size of the community can profoundly impact the relationships between health care institutions in the community and between individual health professionals. All these relationships play a part in formulating possible resolutions to the ethical problems posed by the case.

The relevant human values in the case can be discerned from the actions of the parties involved. Ms. Wagner appears to be an assertive patient with a history of mental illness that responds well to drug therapy if one is to accept her self-assessment about the medication's effects. In a way, Ms. Wagner is demanding respect from the pharmacists who care for her.

Dr. Sadler, at least when one first meets her in the case, is overworked. She tries to cover-up an error. She decides that she perhaps no real harm would come to the patient by "prescribing" a 30-mg/day dose. Later, she is unwilling to admit her mistake. Whether she denies wrongdoing because she is afraid of the repercussions or prideful, it is hard to say.

Dr. Winchester appears to want to do the right thing. He seems cautious. At first, he shows loyalty to his colleague and employee when he tries to sort out just what happened with Ms. Wagner's previous prescription. It seems that he values patient well-being. Although one does not have any information to gauge how he feels about the present situation, it is likely that he is feeling a sense of unfairness or anger at being placed in the center of a dilemma that he did not create. The case is a dilemma because whatever choice Dr. Winchester makes, there will be bad feelings and other harms.

The legal implications of the case include that Dr. Sadler prescribed 15-mg BID rather than the 20-mg BID that was ordered. One will assume that Dr. Sadler practices in a state that does not allow pharmacist prescribing. Even if Dr. Sadler could prescribe, one would expect that she would discuss a change in the medication with the original prescriber.

The ethical problem in the case can be posed as a question: How should Dr. Winchester fulfill his duty of beneficence to his patient, Ms. Wagner, and protect the reputation of his colleague, Dr. Sadler from unnecessary damage from the patient's and prescriber's perspectives? Moreover, Dr. Winchester has an obligation of honesty to the patient and prescriber that is in conflict with loyalty to a colleague.

Dr. Sadler did not fulfill her responsibility to the patient to dispense the medication as prescribed. Ms. Wagner has a right to properly dispensed medication. The judgment Dr. Sadler made about the safety and efficacy of the drug, that is, ". . . it will be close enough to your old prescription" could have resulted in harm to the patient. Dr. Sadler is not honest with the patient or her colleague, Dr. Winchester. Dr. Winchester is caught between his duty to do good and prevent harm to the patient. He also has a basic obligation to be loyal to his colleagues.

A duty also exists to the prescriber to dispense the medication as ordered. Ms. Wagner's autonomy is threatened because of lack of accurate information. Dr. Sadler's irresponsible behavior could reflect badly on Maple River Pharmacy and the pharmacy profession as a whole.

There are at least six actions that Dr. Winchester could take. First, he could fill the prescription as Ms. Wagner has requested. On one level this would be supported by beneficence because Ms. Wagner sees this as a good (ie, she claims that she is doing well on this dose). Second, Dr. Winchester could call the prescriber and explain that there was a prescription error, but the patient reports doing well on 15-mg BID. Dr. Winchester could do this without telling Ms. Wagner about the error. This action is supported by beneficence regarding the dose that Ms. Wagner wants, but suppresses the truth and limits patient autonomy because Ms. Wagner doesn't have all the information. Also, the prescriber may tell Ms. Wagner about the error during a later visit that could affect her trust in the pharmacy. Truth telling to the prescriber is supported by the principle of veracity. But, Dr. Winchester's honesty could be met by anger or mistrust by the prescriber.

Third, Dr. Winchester could follow the same actions as in alternative #2 but this time tell the patient about Dr. Sadler's error. This action would fulfill all the principles mentioned in alternative #2, but also includes veracity to the patient. Like the prescriber, Ms. Wagner could be angry or mistrustful because of learning about Dr. Sadler's error and the way she chose to remedy it.

Fourth, Dr. Winchester could stall. He could tell Ms. Wagner that he needs to speak to the prescriber to straighten out some confusion with the prescription. This is dishonest to a degree because he is not telling Ms. Wagner the truth. This alternative, at a minimum, would inconvenience the patient by making her wait or return at a later time for her prescription. One knows that she lives 50 miles from the pharmacy and the extra driving is time consuming.

Fifth, Dr. Winchester could call Dr. Sadler and demand that she come into the pharmacy and resolve the problem because she created it in the first place. This alternative is not supported by any of the ethical principles mentioned thus far. Dr. Winchester cannot shift responsibility this easily. He knows about the mix-up, and he has attempted to refill Ms. Wagner's prescription as written. Dr. Sadler could resolve the problem by dispensing the wrong dose again. Then, it might be clearer to Dr. Winchester what to do with his colleague.

Sixth, Dr. Winchester could bring all the parties involved together and resolve the problem through a discussion. This action is supported by autonomy and veracity. Practically speaking, this may not be possible. Also, this action could result in bad feelings and disrespect among parties, for example, the prescriber may not trust the pharmacy in the future or the patient could be angry and accusatory.

The best option, based on available facts and the values of the parties involved, is the third one of informing the prescriber and Ms. Wagner about the error. Also, Dr. Winchester should bring in Dr. Sadler to discuss her moral standards about personal responsibility, patient welfare, and obligations to peers. This alternative, although fraught with unpleasantness, places the welfare of the patient first (care-orientation), honors patient autonomy and veracity, and honors veracity with the prescriber. Dr. Winchester's willingness to be honest with the prescriber could result in getting the best therapy for the patient. Even if therapy weren't changed in the way Ms. Wagner would like, future medication adjustments would be made on facts rather than fallacies. Dr. Winchester would need the virtue of courage because revealing Dr. Sadler's actions does expose the profession to criticism for incompetence and deception. But, by being honest, it also shows a willingness to correct errors and assume responsibility.

An objection to this action could be that Dr. Winchester is somehow being disloyal to a colleague and is, perhaps, harming the reputation of the profession unnecessarily. A response to this objection would be based on the primacy of patient welfare and the trust relationships between all parties involved in patient care.

In brief, the first case deals with questions about individual good and relationships between a specific patient and two pharmacists. The second case moves the ethical analysis to the level of the organization or institution in which pharmacists work, in this case a hospital. Just as individuals have relationships, commitments, and claims, so do organizations. Hospitals not only have responsibilities to patients and families, they also have responsibilities to employees and the community at large.

CASE TWO: INCOMPETENT PATIENTS AND LIFE-SUSTAINING TREATMENT—Julian Russell is a 25-year-old man with a history of severe mental retardation (microcephaly) secondary to prematurity. He has been a resident of a custodial care center for most of his life. Besides profound mental incapacity, he has spasticity, severe scoliosis, and multiple contractures. He also has significant ocular myopathy, is nonverbal, and does not respond to verbal or tactile stimuli. He does respond to painful stimulation with grimacing and physical withdrawal.

Mr. Russell was admitted with a principle diagnosis of anemia secondary to Grade III-IV esophagitis. Diagnostic tests led to a thoracotomy and surgical repair. Following surgery, Mr. Russell was placed in the intensive care unit (ICU). Twenty-four hours postoperatively, he experienced severe respiratory distress. Chest x-rays showed a right upper lobe infiltrate, so he was intubated and placed on a ventilator for 3 weeks. To prevent him from extubating himself, which he repeatedly attempted, he was placed in full restraints. Tube feedings began during this period by a Dobhoff tube. When he was finally transferred to a general floor 1 month after surgery, the main concern was to encourage him to take food by mouth with supplementation from the tube feeding for 12 hours at night. Although Mr. Russell ate well before his hospitalization, he now refused most oral feedings. He continued to require restraints because he attempted to remove the feeding tube at every opportunity. The attending physician is contemplating ordering the placement of a percutaneous endoscopic gastrostomy (PEG).

Mr. Russell's father is his legal guardian and only living family member. The senior Mr. Russell has been consulted by telephone for every surgical permit. At no time during the hospitalization did the senior Mr. Russell visit his son. The father told the physician at the outset of Julian's hospitalization, "I agree to whatever you think is best for my son."

Before the attending physician decides about further surgery, he requests a consultation from the institution's ethics committee (IEC). Christine Gibbs, PharmD is a member of the ethics committee and works on the critical care units at the hospital. She is familiar with Mr. Russell's case. The nursing staff expressed much concern about the continued use of restraints and were equally worried about sedating Mr. Russell. Dr. Gibbs was personally concerned about the treatment of patients like Mr. Russell who were never competent.

This case is fundamentally concerned with ethical issues on an institutional basis although Mr. Russell's case is the genesis for these institutional concerns. When Dr. Gibbs worries about "the treatment of patients like Mr. Russell," she moves the focus to the institution as a whole considering the good of "never competent" patients overall. The concerns expressed by the nursing staff can also be viewed on an institutional level by considering the affect of working in such an environment (ie, one that restrains helpless patients or forces unwanted treatment on patients over time).

Gathering clinical facts in Mr. Russell's case about his medical condition is the most important first step in determining what is the right thing to do in his case, and by extension, cases like his. Understanding his medical status is key to resolving the ethical questions his case raises. For decisions involving withholding or withdrawing of treatment, the following questions are relevant:

- What is the patient's present medical status? Are there other contributing medical conditions?
- What is the diagnosis? Prognosis?
- How reliable are these?
- Are there other medical tests that could help clarify the situation?
- What is the life expectancy and general condition if treatment(s) is (are) given?
- Is treatment overall expected to benefit the patient?
- What are the goals of treatment?

The diagnosis, prognosis, and goals of treatment may point to the most appropriate alternative for treatment and eliminate some alternatives as well. For example, in Mr. Russell's case, an underlying condition such as impaired respiratory function due to pulmonary edema, pneumonia, or ineffective breathing, may keep him dependent on the ventilator. Such clinical information is essential to answering questions about further treatment.

All treatment options need to be considered in light of the goals of treatment and future quality of life of the patient. Medical goals differ depending on the clinical facts of the case. For example, if the main treatment goal is to make Mr. Russell comfortable and decrease his agitation, then inserting the PEG tube will be seen in a different light. Even if a treatment can achieve a limited goal such as maintenance of nutrition and hydration in a less uncomfortable manner, this should be examined in light of long-range goals for the patient.

Sometimes clinical facts point to a clear course of action. Only one right thing can be done if a patient presents with severe chest pain in the emergency department because he can't find his nitroglycerin prescription. The ethically correct course of action dictates the treatment of a reversible, acute condition. In a complex, chronic case, like Mr. Russell's, patient benefit is decidedly less clear. Would it benefit Mr. Russell in the long run to continue to provide artificially administered nutrition and hydration? What about continuing ventilator support? These types of questions regarding withholding or withdrawing life-sustaining treatment are always difficult, but if a patient's preferences are known it helps diminish doubts about the right course of action. Mr. Russell's case is complicated by the situational facts, particularly involving his incapacity to participate in decisions about his treatment.

As a rule, most ethicists agree that competent patients have the right to make decisions about their own care, including the right to refuse life-sustaining treatment such as a ventilator, artificial food and fluids, or medications. In this case, Mr. Russell is not presently competent nor has he ever been so. That fact cuts out the possibility of previously expressed medical preferences in the form of a living will or durable power of attorney for health care decisions. In the case of never competent patients, the pharmacist and other members of the health care team must do their best to determine what is best for the patient by consulting with others who have prior knowledge of the patient and his life. In short, the health care team and the IEC in such circumstances are seeking to base decisions on withholding or continuing treatment on the judgment of persons who know the patient best. The patient's father probably never heard his son express any medical preferences, but he would most likely be a sympathetic surrogate decision-maker for him. Also, it is likely that the senior Mr. Russell would be serving his son's best interest. But, this would only be true if he fully understood his son's present condition, the goals of treatment, and probability of reaching agreed upon goals.

It is not clear that Mr. Russell fulfills the previously stated criteria for being a morally valid surrogate. From the little one can gather about the senior Mr. Russell's acceptance of the role of decision maker, he has delegated his autonomy to the physician. In other words, the physician has Mr. Russell's permission to act in his son's best interest. But, the physician still has doubts and has decided to consult the IEC.

Situational facts of the case also include the views of other caregivers. When an ethics committee is asked to consider a case, it is good to invite the primary caregivers to be present for the discussion. Because the primary physician instigated the meeting with the IEC, the other caregivers who might be asked to attend are the nurses, the social worker, therapists from occupational, physical or respiratory therapy, and perhaps the chaplain. It is important to use this forum for discussion of the views of these "others" involved in Mr. Russell's care so that their feelings can be expressed and areas of disagreement or conflicts of values, such as comfort *versus* sustaining biological life, can be resolved.

One can determine the ethical problem(s) in the case by using the series of questions previously listed, for example, "Is this unfair? To whom?" In a complex case such as this, it is possible that more than one question could be answered in the affirmative, thus showing that more than one ethical principle is involved. First, could the treatment to date and future treatment decisions such as the placement of the PEG be considered fair? The concept of fairness is integral to an understanding of justice. Justice requires that patients should be treated as equals unless there is a compelling reason to treat individuals differently. Mr. Russell seems to have received the same treatment anyone with his medical condition would receive. The decision-making process surrounding withholding or withdrawing treatment is fair in that this is the standard applied to all "never competent" patients. Health professionals use the "best interest" standard, the generally agreed upon standard in law and ethics, to determine what is best for a patient who never expressed any views on end-of-life treatment. Furthermore, Mr. Russell's case has been brought to an IEC to assure that the patient's care receives impartial, thoughtful consideration.

As for the next question regarding promise keeping, an implicit promise of providing quality care is made to all patients who receive care in a hospital. It does not appear that this promise has been broken or compromised in any way. If the treatment team decides to withhold the PEG or withdraw the ventilator, it needs to be certain to keep the basic promise of caring for Mr. Russell and not abandon him. Specifically, the pharmacist should attend to measures to keep Mr. Russell comfortable and calm.

The third question, "Will this be harmful? To whom?" is pivotal. All treatments and procedures, particularly those that are invasive and painful will be construed as harmful and frightening from Mr. Russell's perspective because he is incapable of assigning meaning to the experiences. The very act of restraining an agitated, confused patient can cause physical and emotional harms. The harms of surgery, continual restraints, and dependence on a ventilator must be weighed against the potential benefits to be gained for Mr. Russell. Because he cannot make sense of the experience and cannot speak, the health care team must rely on the nonverbal messages his struggle sends as well as a judgment about objective best interest. Because the answer to the question regarding harm is "yes," it is clear that the case does contain ethical issues. The principles of non-maleficence and beneficence are in conflict. Perspectives about what benefit means in light of Mr. Russell's present state can vary between members of the health care team. And, there are harms to other individuals besides Mr. Russell that should be considered. The nursing staff could be psychologically harmed if it believes it is causing harm to Mr. Russell out of proportion to benefit. Therapists who work with Mr. Russell may see their work as futile at a minimum or harmful to the patient because it causes discomfort to the patient and little to no benefit. Once the key ethical issues are identified, one can move to determining alternative courses of action.

Some possible alternatives that the IEC could explore are (1) continue all reasonable measures of life-sustaining treatment including drugs, surgery, ventilator support, among others, even if it requires physical or chemical restraints; (2) continue with ventilator support and comfort measures to decrease pain and anxiety, but do not place the PEG, offer fluids or ice chips by mouth, and the like; (3) discontinue all life-sustaining measures and offer comfort measures only perhaps including terminal sedation when the ventilator is withdrawn. Terminal or total sedation is pharmacologically induced reduction of patient awareness to obviate symptoms of intractable pain or, in this case, overwhelming distress that often accompanies disconnection from a ventilator.[13]

All health care treatments are morally required or not based on considerations of their benefits and burdens. "If the benefits exceed the burdens, then the treatment is acceptable; if they do not, then it makes no sense to require it. This notion of the relative amount of benefits and burdens is now generally referred to as the criterion of proportionality."[14] The ethics committee should review these alternatives and others to determine if the burdens equal or exceed the benefits for each alternative. The IEC can then advise the attending physician which alternative brings about the most benefit.

Before leaving this case, it is important to explore the institutional implications, that is, the individual (patients, staff members) good within the institution and the common good of the society within which the institution exists. "For health care institutions not only provide health services, they are also a powerful cultural force and agent. By their presence, their promotional efforts, their budgets and their services health care institutions have a significant influence on what the general population thinks, hopes and demands in terms of health care. Hospitals not only respond to but also create demand in the general public about what to expect of a hospital by way of service, convenience, and opulence."[15]

Thus, the IEC needs to focus on individual patients and their needs, and the overall well-being of the whole and its public position on complex issues such as end-of-life care. The IEC must consider the impact of policies and guidelines on the internal workings of the hospital while also promoting the common good of society in such areas as respect for persons, support of the dying, and avoidance of futile treatment, to name a few. The final case deals with the societal realm of ethics as well as institutional ethical concerns.

CASE THREE: RESTRICTIONS ON OUTPATIENT PRESCRIPTIONS—The Good Shepherd Hospital, a private, not-for-profit, religiously based institution, adopted a policy based on its mission statement that any person "in the community" who experiences a medical emergency or is in labor can and will be treated in the emergency department (ED) regardless of ability to pay. This policy was extended to the hospital's inpatient pharmacy as well. The inpatient pharmacy dispensed the prescriptions of the "outpatients" in the ED because technically ED patients are "inpatients" of the hospital while they are being treated. Also, it seemed more practical to have prescriptions dispensed at the inpatient pharmacy because most pharmacies in the area were closed in the middle of the night and some prescriptions needed to be dispensed immediately.

ED patients who came to the inpatient pharmacy and presented their prescriptions had their insurance billed if they belong to a drug card plan. For patients without insurance, their bills were marked "self-pay." This practice went on for a while until the Director of Pharmacy Services, Natalie Norita, PharmD began to review accounts left unpaid by patients. What she found were patient accounts from the community who had unpaid balances in the thousands of dollars. For example, one patient had an outstanding debt of $8,000. Many patients with unpaid accounts were repeat patients in the ED who continued to use the inpatient pharmacy to get their prescriptions. Second, Dr. Norita was concerned that Good Shepherd might be attracting patients to their ED because of the "self-pay" policy. She suspected that word had gotten out that Good Shepherd would dispense prescriptions for free if a patient was treated in the ED. Third, there were several cases in which patients returned to the inpatient pharmacy shortly after receiving a prescription for a narcotic analgesic claiming that they had "dropped" their medication on the sidewalk and needed more.

Dr. Norita decided that drastic measures were in order because pressure was being placed on all units of the hospital to be more efficient and stop loss. The pharmacy could not continue losing money in this way. Dr. Norita posted the new policy in the inpatient pharmacy— no prescriptions for outpatients would be dispensed. There would be no exceptions even if the patient had insurance or the ability to pay. The policy was in place for less than a week when Dr. Norita heard from the ED physicians who complained, "How can we provide adequate care to patients when they can't get the prescriptions that we write filled at the hospital?" The nursing staff joined those who were unhappy with the new policy. The head of nursing stated, "The Code of Ethics for nurses states that we are to serve all patients regardless of economic status. I think the policy puts the nursing staff in conflict with the Code. Also, I don't think it is a good idea to inconvenience everyone merely because of the bad actions of a few." Dr. Norita wasn't really certain that her "no prescriptions" policy was the answer to the problems with bad debt in the ED, but it was a start. It appeared that the policy needed more work and perhaps input from others who would be affected by it.

The situation at Good Shepherd Hospital in the pharmacy department is a complicated one as Dr. Norita is discovering. There is a lot of information that is missing and would help in developing an ethical policy. Whatever policy is developed will have implications for the community that Good Shepherd serves. Questions at the societal level of ethics take on a broader perspective than those encountered at the institutional and individual levels. Clinical questions now look at groups of patients and their collective well-being. First, how does the pharmacy director define "emergency?" What is meant by "treatment?" Is sufficient treatment a few doses of a drug to get the patient through a couple of days or is it, for example, a full course of antibiotic drug therapy?

Situational data concerns relationships between groups and organizations within the community. For example, is Good Shepherd the only hospital in the community who is willing to care for indigent patients? Are unpaid accounts or bad debt basically different from those involving patients who request refills on lost or "dropped" medications? How many patients does this really involve? Is it possible to determine which patients have the ability to pay, which patients might be eligible for welfare and which patients' care will need to written off as unrecoverable debt? What is the overall institutional position on care for indigent patients?

Dr. Norita has a responsibility as Director of Pharmacy to the hospital as a whole, to the staff pharmacists who work for her, to other health professionals who work there, and last, but assuredly not least, patients. In an attempt to reduce loss and perhaps to be absolutely fair, Dr. Norita decided no prescriptions for outpatients would be dispensed. Although Dr. Norita is treating everyone equally, it may not be in everyone's best interest for her to do so. Under this absolute policy, children who are diagnosed with otitis media would not receive appropriate medications from the inpatient pharmacy. Perhaps Dr. Norita believed that the policy would stop patients from "abusing" the inpatient pharmacy and didn't anticipate the impact it would have on "deserving" patients with true medical emergencies.

The basic ethical problem in the case can be posed in the form of a question: How can Good Shepherd Hospital fulfill its mission to serve "all patients" and stay fiscally sound? What would be a reasonable balance between these competing goods?

Because the problem includes institutional and societal concerns, it makes sense that the deliberations about the policy would be best conducted with an interdisciplinary committee that would represent the different constituencies affected by the policy. At whatever level the deliberations take place, Dr. Norita should be involved to present the pharmacy perspective.

An IEC might be the place to start such a discussion, but it is not the only committee or group that can discuss such an issue. In fact, most ethics committees have dealt narrowly with patient care issues "at the bedside" and not institutional or organizational ethical issues. "Organizational ethics may be defined as the study of the ethical issues associated with the systems, structures and processes that shape the encounter between health care providers and patients."[16] The senior administrative team of Good Shepherd, rather than the ethics committee, is the proper group to address the larger questions that Dr. Norita's policy raises because they are the ones who make staffing and budget determinations. A reasonable argument could be made that senior management teams act as ethics committees when they are making value-based decisions that impact the organization as a whole and the community the organization serves. If Good Shepherd wants to survive as an institution, it must balance the need to increase contribution to margin (revenue minus variable costs) to better cover fixed costs, provide indigent care, and meet other community service responsibilities.[17] Decisions made at this level of an organization have far-reaching implications and affect a broader constituency. The basic ethical principles that are action guides for moral decisions on an individual level can be used to resolve societal level problems, but must be reconstructed and, perhaps, prioritized differently. For example, the good of one patient is conceptually and practically different from the good of many patients, as in the third case where one considers all patients who cannot pay for their medications. In reaching a resolution to Dr. Norita's problem in pharmacy, one must remember that Dr. Norita's problem doesn't exist in isolation. The optimum resolution will take into account the connection between balancing the pharmacy's budget, the institution's mission, and implications for the individuals the hospital serves.

CONTRIBUTION OF ETHICS TO CLINICAL PRACTICE

Sometimes, even when the normative model for decision-making is followed to the letter, it is not possible to arrive at a resolution. At this point, one might believe that a resolution could be reached if only there were more information or if there were a better model for making such decisions. However, even with the best models and information, it may not be possible to resolve a problem because of the limits of human knowledge and understanding. Further, it is the nature of ethical dilemmas to involve tragedy and loss. A morally correct way of dealing with dilemmas is to share them *as* dilemmas with those involved. Face the fact that serious matters are at issue. Do not allow secondary inference that there is no right answer to detract from the seriousness of the situation and the benefits of systematically working toward a solution.[18]

Besides decision-making models, there are other sources for moral guidance such as family and peers, laws and regulations (although the law sometimes diverges from ethics), professional codes of ethics, and religious beliefs. Further, there are resources within organizations such as policies and guidelines that have been thoughtfully written with ethical norms in mind. Colleagues in specialty areas of pharmacy practice could work together to establish mutually held values about complex ethical issues that are encountered in daily practice.

As noted in case two, IECs are becoming more common in hospitals and long-term care facilities. Pharmacists should not only seek out the advice and guidance of an IEC when problems seem beyond resolution; they should also offer to serve on such committees and bring their expertise regarding drugs and proper use of medications to the overall treatment plan. Unfortunately, the perspective and assistance of pharmacists is often missing from the committee's membership. Although IECs do not make the decision for the individuals involved in the ethical problem, they do offer a safe environment in which to discuss contentious issues and guidelines that affirm the values of the institution so that sound decisions can be reached.

REFERENCES

1. Veatch R. *Am J Hosp Pharm* 1989; 46:109.
2. Solomon WD. In: Reich WT, ed. *The Encyclopedia of Bioethics,* 2nd ed. New York: Macmillan, 1995, p 736.
3. Ogletree TW. In: Reich WT, ed. *The Encyclopedia of Bioethics,* 2nd ed. New York: Macmillan, 1995, p 2515.
4. Buerki RA, Vottero LD. Ethics and pharmaceutical care. In: Knowlton C, Penn R, eds. *Pharmaceutical Care,* 2nd ed. Bethesda: American Society of Health Systems Pharmacists, 2003, p 305.
5. Hundert EM. A model for ethical problem solving in medicine, with practical applications. *Am J Psychiatr* 1987; 144:839.
6. Haddad AM, Kapp MB. *Ethical and Legal Issues in Home Health Care,* Norwalk, CT: Appleton and Lange, 1991.
7. Beauchamp TL, Childress JF. *Principles of Biomedical Ethics,* 5th ed. New York: Oxford University Press, 2001.
8. Veatch R, Haddad AM. *Case Studies in Pharmacy Ethics.* New York: Oxford University Press, 1999, p 97.
9. Veatch R. *A Theory of Medical Ethics.* New York: Basic Books, 1981, p 227f.
10. Chater R, Dockter D, Haddad A, et al. *American Pharmacy* 1993; NS33(4):80.
11. Kopelman LM. *Ethics and Health Care* 2002; 5(1):5.
12. Glaser JW. *Three Realms of Ethics,* Kansas City, MO: Sheed and Ward, 1994, p 12.
13. Fine PG. *Journal of Hospice and Palliative Nursing* 2001; 3(3):81.
14. Congregation for the Doctrine of The Faith. Declaration on Euthanasia. Rome: *The Sacred Congregation for the Doctrine of the Faith,* May 5, 1980.
15. Glaser JW. *The Three Realms of Ethics.* Kansas City, MO: Sheed and Ward, 1994, p 14.
16. Hooyman T. In: Haddad A, Middleton C, Hooyman T, eds. *Ethics Committee Resource Manual.* Denver: Catholic Health Initiatives, 2002, p 24.
17. Dexter F, Blake JT, Penning DH, et al. *Anesthesiology-Analgesia* 2002; 94(1):138–142.
18. Erde EL. In: Mongale J, Thomasma DC, eds. *Health Care Ethics: Critical Issues for the 21st Century.* Gaithersburg, MD: Aspen Publishers, 1998, p537.

BIBLIOGRAPHY

Brannigan MC, Boss JA, eds. *Healthcare Ethics in a Diverse Society.* Mountain View, CA: Mayfield, 2001.

Fletcher JA, Quist N, Jonsen AR, eds. *Ethics Consultation in Health Care.* Ann Arbor, MI: Health Administration Press, 1989.

Haddad AM, Buerki RA, eds. *Ethical Dimensions of Pharmaceutical Care.* Binghamton, NY: Pharmaceutical Products Press, 1996.

Ross JW, Glaser JW, Rasinski-Gregory D, et al, eds. *Health Care Ethics Committees: The Next Generation.* Chicago: American Hospital Association, 1993.

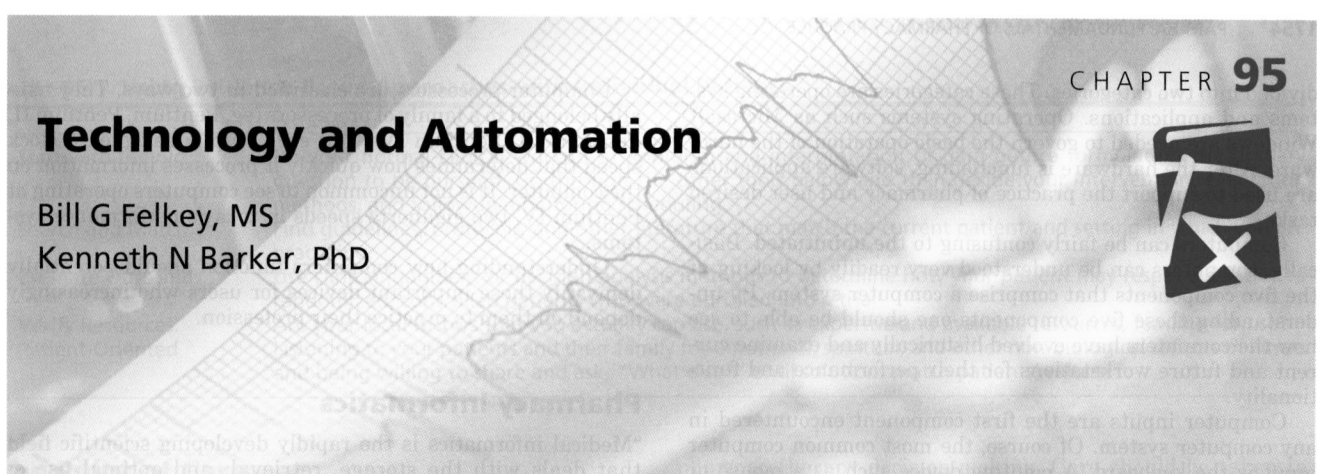

CHAPTER 95

Technology and Automation

Bill G Felkey, MS

Kenneth N Barker, PhD

The American Heritage Dictionary defines a system as, "A group of interacting, interrelated, or interdependent elements forming a complex whole; a condition of harmonious, orderly interaction."[1] Providing contemporary pharmacy services involves a sufficiently complex process that it most certainly necessitates a systems approach. Pharmacy is, of course, a subsystem of a larger, comprehensive health-care system. In this chapter, the authors will attempt to focus on a systems approach in utilizing technology to support a practice of pharmacy and describe the complex interactions that occur in a pharmacy practice between people and technologies. These interactions focus primarily on the welfare of patients and are performed by pharmacists and their associates who share a common vision because they are involved in the pursuit of rendering appropriate pharmaceutical care.[2]

It is impossible to imagine any scenario for the future of pharmacy that does not involve the use of many forms of technology and automation. This assumption holds true regardless of the practice setting selected. Consider that technology has two primary purposes. Both of the purposes of technology involve the work of humans. One purpose for technology is to replace completely the work done by humans. Technology usually excels at replacing work that is repetitive and work that is often found to be tedious by humans. Ideally, technology should be considered for selection and implementation when it can free a human being to be redeployed into a work process that requires the abstract, judgmental, and higher-level cognitive processes at which humans excel.[3]

The second role of technology involves the enhancement of human work. With over 6000 articles being published every week in the biomedical literature, it is impossible for any human to "keep up" with the dynamic field health care represents. Evidence-based medicine experts estimate that in even the narrowest specialty approximately 14 articles per day would need to be read from the literature to maintain one's professional competency at the highest level. Information technology can present the highest quality, empirically derived, evidence-based information that reduces a pharmacist's uncertainty while making decisions. Information technology helps to overcome the limits of human memory and helps reduce the use of conjecture (opinion-based) decision-making.[4]

Another example of a performance enhancing technology can be found in the use of bar codes. In community pharmacies, hospitals, and nursing homes, bar codes can be scanned in the dispensing process and at the point-of-administration to assure that the right drug is being given to the right patient in the right form by the right route in the right strength at the right time. Use of bar codes in health-care are proving to significantly reduce accidents and errors.[5]

Generally, one can assert that, over time, technology continues to weigh less while it does more. The ubiquitous nature of the Internet, microcomputers, and personal digital assistants (PDAs) makes technology touch everyone to an increasing amount in our everyday work and existence. Do you know anyone who receives more voicemail than e-mail? Are you aware that the new definition of the Internet involves every computer, cell phone, PDA, and pager in the world now potentially being able to communicate with one another? Where will it end? It is difficult to imagine all of the permutations and possibilities.

Health care as a discipline tends to lag behind other areas and industries with regard to its adoption and diffusion of technological innovation. In fact, health care had been described as one of the few remaining predigital industries. The authors believe the banking and financial industry is the best example to follow when determining how health care will continue to evolve. Granted there are differences, but trust is needed in both systems and technologies. If people are willing to trust their money to banking technologies, it might follow that they will become more comfortable trusting the management of their health-care information to technology. Most pharmacists state that they are less than 10% paperless in their practices. The authors can imagine no scenario where the digitization of transactions will not increase over time.[6]

Compare the adoption of "cash cards," a.k.a. ATM cards and imagine that a similar card for health care would serve as the means for caregivers to gain access to patients' medical records. There are several technologies that provide this kind of access. Everything from biometric fingerprint or retina scanning to smart cards is being examined. No true standard has emerged as of yet. In fact, some people say (tongue in cheek), that the nice thing about information technology standards is that there are so many to pick from. The authors do not believe the smart card is the future unless it can totally reduce the thickness of one's wallet by serving all identity functions for all health, business, travel, entertainment, and other related transactions of daily living.[7] Getting all of the businesses represented to agree on a single standard would certainly be a prodigious task.

Understanding Computers

Computers constitute a core technology in support of the practice of pharmacy. When anyone thinks about technology or automation, it is likely that computers are involved in almost every circumstance. Our watches, automobiles, entertainment systems, and even kitchen appliances are getting "smarter" through the incorporation of computers into their design. Computers are data processors. Simply stated, computers receive input, they process that input, and they produce outputs. The hardware components of the computer are controlled by software systems. Software that constitutes a set of instructions used to tell computer hardware how to operate can be further

Table 95-2. CPOE Attributes and Functions

CPOE must be selected and implemented with the following in mind:
- Access to the system is simple where the application sign-on and sign-off is achieved through a combination of password, biometrics, or proximity devices.
- Access to needed decision support information is available from any patient care setting, pharmacy, physician's office, or home.
- Mobility is maintained through a combination of mobile and stationary devices that are readily available and located at various point of care locations based on the workflow of the specific patient care area.
- Navigation is from a main screen with direct links to screens designed for patient data review, ordering, and information compendia. Moving forward and back to the main screen is clear and easy.
- Patient data to support the ordering process is readily available electronically. Prerequisites for most forms of decision support are allergies, height, weight, current medications, laboratory values, radiology results, and medical problem list.
- The maximum amount of relevant information is available on each screen. (Content beats aesthetic design every time.)
- System response is fast, and there is virtually no down time.[18]

The possession of Internet connectivity in pharmacies is high, but the use of Internet connectivity at the point of care is lagging behind the front and back office operations of pharmacy. A major movement toward application service providers (ASP) that essentially offer subscription based access via the Internet to remote servers externally is likely to be the information technology architecture utilized by most physicians and pharmacists in the future. While currently there are many concerns about mission critical information being stored and secured externally, adoption of this architecture is increasing.

Grover et al. looked at how patients desired better access to health services and not surprisingly found that they wanted more than was there. "Patients were especially interested in getting e-mail reminders. They wanted online booking of appointments in real time and wished to receive updates about new advances in treatment. Patients were also interested in virtual visits for simple and chronic medical problems and for following chronic conditions through virtual means. We concluded that computer-using patients desire Internet services to augment their medical care."[22]

Telepharmacy

Telehealth is the use of communication and information technology to deliver health, health-care services, and information over large and small distances.[23] While most people think of telehealth in relation to surgeries performed between countries using remote robotic control, telehealth can be delivered in the same room in which a practitioner is standing. Consider that a diabetes educator can delegate the initial education of the newly diagnosed patient with diabetes to a technology that is a multimedia program. This program can deliver age-specific, gender-specific, race-specific, and diagnosis-specific education in an interactive format that allows the patient to comprehend and retain the educational material as effectively as a one-to-one interaction with a human educator.

As long as the content provided by the technology is maintained to be accurate, complete, reliable, and relevant one can allow technology to totally replace the repetitive work of educating a newly diagnosed patient with diabetes. What is left for the practitioner is the more complex customization and troubleshooting that is needed by these patients. By delegating to the technology, the practitioner is able to be in two places at the same time in a literal sense.

Telepharmacy involves bringing care to patients when it is not feasible to have patients brought to the care setting. Many clinics, upon diagnosis, would like to dispense prescriptions and other medical supplies to patients, but the clinic volume of prescribing activity may not be significantly high enough to justify the placement of a pharmacist in the clinic. Some clinics are connecting, using telecommunication technology dispensing devices, to a remotely located pharmacist who is able to control the verification and dispensing process without physically being in the clinic.

Using video conferencing, pharmacists are able to provide real-time patient counseling and manage a medication use sys-

tem via remote control. Telepharmacy operations are proving to be a cost-effective method to render high-quality pharmacy services in underserved regions and can be a much-preferred alternative to physician/nurse/clerk dispensing options. Organizations such as the Veterans Administration are reporting early successes for many of their telehealth initiatives. Outside of closed system uses of this technology, reimbursement is a barrier to the implementation of the technology. Currently, real-time, live consultation over telecommunication technologies is the only practice interventions/consultation being reimbursed by the payers who recognize the value of these services. "Despite the slow growth of interactive and noninteractive telemedicine, technological development continues, and many new applications are under study. Remote patient monitoring programs, especially those based on store-and-forward technologies, are appealing because they are relatively inexpensive, increasingly convenient for patients and providers, and have the potential to cut the costs of care while improving outcomes. Medicare and other insurer reluctance to cover telemedicine has slowed its dissemination, but recent years have seen progressive, though limited, steps to extend reimbursement."[24]

Outcomes Measurement

"Outcome measures are used to monitor the effects of interventions in clinical practice or in formal clinical trials. They may also be used to assess changes within populations either spontaneously or as a result of public-health measures. They are used to monitor the course of illness as part of a management plan or, for larger groups, to identify changes brought about, for instance, by migration or immunization."[25]

Currently, outcomes are divided into four categories. The first category, therapeutic outcomes, requires the measurement of objective clinical results following the appraisal and intervention steps in the work-up of patients in a clinical setting. For example, patients are diagnosed with hypertension and will receive a prescription to treat this condition. The desired therapeutic outcome in the case of a normal adult would be a 120 systolic over a diastolic of 80 mm Hg. Technology is readily available to assist in the measurement of therapeutic outcomes. These technologies can enter measurements directly into a medical record or even a patient's specific web page.

The second outcome category, financial outcomes, measures the cost to achieve a therapeutic outcome. In the example of a patient with hypertension, the most cost-effective financial outcome could come from a lifestyle change on the part of the patient. Many patients' blood pressure will respond to positive changes in their diet and exercise. If a medication is required, a simple potassium sparing diuretic that achieves the therapeutic objective would have a favorable financial outcome when compared with a prescribed combination of calcium channel blocker and ACE inhibitor interventions. The selection of interventions that are effective and contain health-care costs can be assisted by care management algorithms' practice guidelines, and decision support software that prompts practitioners through the intervention selection process.

The third outcome category, quality of life (QOL), measures how health-care impacts patients' activities for daily living and physical and emotional performance in their work, home life, or recreation. It may be possible to achieve a therapeutic outcome at a cost that would meet the objectives for financial outcomes in the treatment of hypertension, but do this at the expense of patients' quality of life. For example, a male can be well-controlled with regard to his blood pressure when he is in his 30s through the use of a beta blocker. Upon entering his 40s, however, the same medication could cause him to experience fatigue and even impotence. Thus, a therapeutic and financial objective would be met but results in a negative quality of life impact. Some health-care systems administer QOL scales to patients to assess this outcome.

The fourth outcome category, satisfaction with the health-care system, has been measured in increasing numbers as managed care organizations seek to measure quality in the provision of health services. A "report card" called the Health Employer Data and Information Set (HEDIS) is given to patients to provide feedback to health systems and the employers who are paying for health services. Satisfaction can be determined by patients through factors such as how long it takes to get an appointment with a primary care physician and how they are treated during their appointments.

Technology can be employed to support the measurement of therapeutic outcomes. Technology can direct the achievement of a desired financial outcome. QOL can be assessed by technology and the results can be fed back into the healthcare system. Patient satisfaction can be measured and addressed using technological means. What is required is a systems approach throughout the delivery of care to assure maximum efficacy and the avoidance of negative outcomes.

Technology and HIPAA

"Medical records contain intimate information about a person's physical and mental health, behaviors, and relationships. Intrusions into privacy can result in loss of trust, with an unwillingness to confide in health care professionals. Unauthorized disclosures of intimate information can cause embarrassment, stigma, and discrimination."[26] Many pharmacists are greatly concerned that the legislation called Health Insurance Portability and Accountability Act (HIPAA) will make technological innovation more difficult. The new laws require that identifiable or protected patient information be held confidentially and the regulations impose severe penalties for security breaches. The authors know of at least 14 different methods to secure electronically held information. In many ways, it is more secure than paper records.

The regulations of HIPAA also provide that patients should have better access to their own medical records. In most US states, patients own the information contained in their medical records. Unfortunately, they do not feel as if they all miss information. Some US companies are creating a collaborative medical record that allows patients, through the World Wide Web, to become partners or coproducers in their own healthcare by allowing access to their medical records. The patient can also elect to allow access to their medical record by trusted relatives and other agents. In this way, an adult child can "look in" on his parents or grandparents health status.

Other technologies such as prescriber order entry are actually complementing HIPAA regulations and provide additional incentives for moving toward electronic medical record implementation. The portability aspect of the regulations can also be made possible through technology support. An Internet standard called extensible markup language (XML) allows the use of health information that is stored on the World Wide Web to be able to "move" between systems because the information on the web page is field tagged so that it can be portable between systems. Technology standards will again facilitate many processes and are necessary for rapid improvement.

Documentation of Interventions

There is a saying in health care, "If it wasn't documented, you didn't do it!" The authors believe that the documentation component of health care has been one of the reasons that pharmacy has struggled with obtaining provider status in Medicare regulations and other private sector circumstances. The ideal documentation system would allow documentation to take place as a natural byproduct of the rendering of patient care.

"Coding systems are important tools for the documentation of drug-related problems and following interventions. They should be suitable for scientific studies and for the broader implementation of Pharmaceutical Care in the pharmacy. A suitable coding system must be easy to use in a daily routine. To facilitate later computer aided use, it should be preferably structured like a decision tree and consist of three parts: the classification of drug-related problems; the intervention taken to solve the problem; and the degree to which the problem was solved."[27] Table 95-3 describes other documentation attributes and principles.

For example, if a drug reference is accessed at the point of care to determine what alternative dosing strategy should be

---

Table 95-3. Essential Documentation Principles

The following list contains the principles and summarizes what the systems, policies and practices should provide to accomplish them.
- Unique patient identification. Provide unique identification of each patient when recording or accessing information; provide—within and across organizations.
- Accuracy. Promote accuracy throughout information capture and report generation and during transfer among systems.
- Completeness. Identify minimum set of information required to completely describe incident, observation or intent; provide means to ensure that recorded information meets legal, regulatory, institutional policy or other requirements for specific reports.
- Timeliness. Require and facilitate healthcare documentation during or immediately after event so memory is accurate and information is immediately available for subsequent care.
- Interoperability across documentation systems. Provide highest realistically achievable level of interoperability; enable authorized practitioners to capture, share, and report information from any system, whether paper or electronic.
- Retrievability. Support achievement of worldwide consensus on information structuring—requiring use of standardized titles, formats, templates, macros, terminology, abbreviations and coding; enable authorized data searches, indexing and mining.
- Authentication and accountability. Uniquely identify persons, devices, systems that create or generate information and that take responsibility for its accuracy, timeliness; require that all information be attributable to its source (person or device); require that unsigned documents be readily recognizable as such; require review of documents before authentication.
- Auditability. Allow users to examine basic information elements, such as data fields; audit access and disclosure of protected health information; alert users of errors, inappropriate changes, potential security breaches; promote use of performance metrics as part of audit capacity.
- Confidentiality and security. Demonstrate adherence to related legislation, regulations, guidelines, and policies throughout the documentation process; alert users to potential confidentially and security breaches.[28]

used for a medication, an intervention communication and documentation application would automatically grab the medication name (and any patient information that was active) and populate those fields in the intervention and documentation program.

Some pharmaceutical care software packages manage the entire process and integrate clinical "to do's" into a pharmacist's calendar. For example, if a pharmacist is doing an appraisal with a pediatric patient diagnosed with asthma, the software will prompt the appropriate questions to ask. If a drug-related problem is identified, the software will prompt the appropriate options for intervention. If an intervention is initiated, the software will require that an evaluation of the intervention be performed at an appropriate interval. Once the evaluation is performed the software will schedule the patient for monitoring and follow-up intervals. All of these functions are integrated into the time management features of the software so that a pharmacist must respond or be "nagged" until the clinically appropriate action is taken.

The Role of Automation

Automation in general means that the machines that are used to perform work are controlled by a computer. The scope here is limited to machines used in pharmacy practice sites for work that includes the storage, packaging, compounding, dispensing, and distribution of medications. It includes collecting, controlling, and maintaining transaction information during such work, but excludes drug delivery systems such as infusion pumps.

The potential benefits of automated pharmacy are substantial. Automated systems can outperform humans in tasks that require tedious repetition, tiresome movement, intense concentration, immense memory retention, and meticulous record keeping. This describes many (though not all) of the tasks in the distribution process. Automated pharmacy systems are replacing many labor-intensive tasks already, thereby saving pharmacist, technician, and nursing time.

Of particular importance to the profession is the potential value of automation as an enabler for the re-engineering of pharmacy practice and for freeing pharmacists for the practice of pharmaceutical care. Automated pharmacy systems can reduce medication errors, improve documentation, increase authorized access to both medications and information, and enhance security. Turnover of personnel and on-the-job stress may be reduced when pharmacists are freed from "count and pour" dispensing. These potential benefits can be summarized in terms of increased productivity, accuracy, drug use control, and improved patient care.

Automated work systems are desirable because they are capable of achieving efficiency and accuracy far superior to that achievable in any other way, in appropriate applications. Identifying those applications where automation can and should be applied in pharmacy is still underway at this time. It is clear that factors such as proper training and the redesign of the physical environment to accommodate such automation are important. Automation to reduce medication errors may actually increase costs. Efforts are underway to show that error reduction actually reduces costs related to corrective actions and liability, which in turn offsets the cost of the automation.

Automated pharmacy systems (ie, pharmacy work systems incorporating one or more automated processes) are in widespread use throughout pharmacy practice. Their primary use today is for the functions of counting, packaging, and labeling dosage forms for pharmacists to dispense and/or administer to patients while electronically documenting the process.

Automated pharmacy systems may be centralized, pharmacy-based devices, or decentralized devices on nursing units, in long-term care facilities, and in other health care facilities. Currently, there are two types of pharmacy-based automated pharmacy systems: systems that repackage medications from bulk, and robotic systems that utilize "overwrapping" of unit-dose medications.

Decentralized automated pharmacy systems store and dispense drugs and supplies in locations outside the pharmacy, and may be interfaced to a central pharmacy computer to maintain centralized control over the drug storage and distribution processes. Some devices are used to dispense multiple-dose packages, while others dispense unit-doses. Some systems package the doses, while others dispense only prepackaged medications.

Community pharmacies have used technology to improve the efficiency of the drug distribution process since the 1970s; the first such system simply counted tablets. Today, automated pharmacy systems are available that automate the entire dispensing process. There are automated medication dispensing devices that serve different segments of the community pharmacy market based on prescription volume.

Prescription processing begins when an order is inputted into the pharmacy computer system and sent to the automated pharmacy system computer, which then initiates printing of bar-coded labels and receipts, selecting the prescription bottle, labeling of the container, filling, and capping. A video image of the drug inside the bottle is obtained before capping. After the bottle-specific bar code is scanned by the pharmacist, the video image for that medication is displayed to allow for a final check by the pharmacist. The technology allows for pricing of the prescription, adjusting the inventory, and documenting the transaction.

Mail service pharmacies use "assembly line," automated, drug distribution systems to dispense prescriptions. These are checked by a pharmacist and mailed with patient information directly to the patient. Mail service pharmacy has taken advantage of the economies of scale offered by automation, and is attractive for serving some patients with chronic diseases who are taking maintenance medication and need to have the prescription delivered to their homes.

Large, fully automated mail service pharmacies integrate the patient medication database with "assembly line," automated drug distribution systems to dispense thousands of prescriptions per day. In the Veterans Affairs (VA) system, consolidated mail outpatient pharmacies (CMOPs) located across the country use automation to fill 8,000 to 10,000 prescriptions in a 10-hour day. This has freed pharmacists to spend more time on direct patient care.[29]

Medication orders are entered into patient databases at the local VA medical center and are electronically transmitted to the CMOP where they are automatically processed. All items to be dispensed to one patient are placed in a bar-coded tote bin. A technician scans the tote's bar code and a computer screen indicates which items are needed. The tote is placed on a conveyor belt, where prepackaged items, loaded into racks mounted over the conveyor belt, are automatically dispensed onto an area of the belt that the computer has designated for the individual order. The items are then transported to a chute and deposited into the appropriate tote. The tote travels to the final dispensing area, where machines automatically dispense oral solids into plastic vials. The automated bottle filler scans the tote to determine what medication is to be dispensed. A label containing the patient and medication information is printed and applied to the vial, and the vial is filled and capped. Before releasing the vial, the computer verifies the tablet count, cap integrity, and label placement. When the order is complete, a pharmacist checks the items and sends the tote to technicians who prepare the medications for mailing.[29]

Hospitals and institutional long-term care pharmacies employ various centralized automated pharmacy systems, which are integrated with the pharmacy information system, for repackaging and labeling of solid oral medications. These automated pharmacy systems count, package, and label medication in patient-, date-, and time-specific single unit-dose, multidose, or patient "med pak" packaging (all medications for a particular administration time are packaged together).

Bulk medications are identified by humans and manually loaded into an individual, medication-specific canister that is calibrated, according to the size and shape of the specific drug product, and that will only fit into its assigned location. Some systems incorporate bar-code labeling on the canister, which can be scanned against the bulk medication supply to ensure accuracy. With information downloaded from the pharmacy information system, the automated pharmacy system packages medication in unit-dose packets, labels the packet with the required information, and dispenses the medications in the order in which they appear on the fill list. Integrated robotic systems that read bar-coded over-wrapped unit-dose packages are used to prepare patient medication cassettes and have the ability to return unused medications to stock. These systems are not limited solely to oral solid mediations; injectables, suppositories, and liquid unit-dose containers can all be handled·

A comprehensive and electronically sophisticated automated pharmacy system counts, packages, and labels patient-specific medications in unit-of-use envelopes at the time of mediation administration, and also sorts the envelopes by patient in the order in which the medications are to be administered. It can be used centrally in the pharmacy or in decentralized patient care areas. Nursing unit-based, decentralized systems feature "ATM-like" dispensing cabinets, which offer secure, computer-controlled access to medications and related supplies. When linked with the pharmacy computer system, as soon as a pharmacy-verified order is activated, the nurse may request a dose from the automated pharmacy system. Mobile systems offer the ability to move the dispensing cabinets from bedside to bedside, and enter and review orders from a terminal mounted on the cabinet. An important optional feature permits bar-code checking and the reading of the dose being administered at the patient's bedside.

Today, integrated drug distribution systems are being planned to meet the needs of an entire community by providing seamless distribution to primary care clinics, hospitals, long-term care facilities, and private homes. Automated pharmacy systems are making it possible for large health care systems to provide just-in-time deliveries of doses to refill drug distribution machines in an area-wide system of health care delivery sites.

The central fill concept allows a group of pharmacies to operate a central, high-volume dispensing facility. Once filled, the prescriptions are delivered to the patient's local pharmacy.[30] Telepharmacy is the provision of medications and pharmaceutical care by remote control from a distance. The Veterans Health Care System and others have demonstrated that such systems can provide pharmacy services to sites where the demand is too small to justify employment of a pharmacist in that location.[31]

In community pharmacy, the use of some form of automated dispensing automation differs widely. Among chain pharmacies, the percentage utilizing automated counting devices is high; among independent pharmacies, it is only about one in five.[32] In hospital pharmacies, automation is used to support centralized unit dose dispensing in 9.4% of hospitals, decentralized drug storage and distribution in 49.2%, IV production and manufacturing in 27.5%, and for transportation systems in 29.4%. Use of automation is more common in larger hospitals and systems, and those affiliated with a medical school.[33]

In pharmacy, the application of bar-code systems has received considerable attention for a long time, because of the recognition that pharmacy practice must store, process, and distribute a type of product (eg, dosage forms) which have numerous and a challenging variety of forms, storage, labeling, security, and patient safety requirements. The need for product identification by machines at the manufacturing, wholesaling, and ambulatory pharmacy level is similar to that for the processing of many other types of products (eg, canned foods) and the National Drug Code system maintained by the FDA has served well for this purpose.

In community pharmacy practice, the benefits of bar coding appear so evident and achievable that three major organizations,

the American Pharmaceutical Association, the National Association of Chair Drug Stores, and the National Community Pharmacists Associations joined in recommending the use of bar-code verification in all pharmacy practices within 3–5 years.[34]

In hospital pharmacy practice, though the benefits of the bar coding of drug products at the unit dose level are very attractive in theory, as a practical matter the complexity involved has thwarted years of attempts to achieve this goal. The problems have included such practical matters as the small size of unit dose packaging, the unwillingness of the pharmaceutical industry to offer larger packages, the difficulty in achievement a standardized approach, and the unwillingness of hospitals to pay the extra premium at which such packaging has been offered or can be achieved by in-house packaging operation.

The technology of product recognition by machines has advanced such that alternatives to bar-code systems are becoming available. Though the barriers to achievement are being narrowed to cost alone, that may not be inconsiderable. For example, the added cost of nursing time required for involvement in the bar-code reading process has been projected to have a negative effect on nursing productivity nationally.[35] In a report on pharmacy manpower in 2002, Knapp estimated that by the year 2020, the need for pharmacists would exceed the supply by 157,000. Though today automated systems prepare only 125,000 of the 3 billion prescriptions dispensed annually, Knapp assumed that by 2020 the use of automation and information technology plus supportive personnel will achieve an improvement in productivity by a factor of *five*. One of the assumptions was that a properly designed automated system would *not* require a personal final check by a pharmacist of every filled order, currently a requirement in many states.[36] Nevertheless, the projected shortfall accompanied by rising salaries makes further automation of the dispensing function appear essential.

Automation and Patient Safety

Patients are threatened by adverse drug events, and there is evidence that many can be prevented by pharmacy automation. The death rate associated with medication errors in hospitals was estimated in 1999 to be about 7,000 per year.[37] The relative frequency of medication errors was studied in 2002 in 36 hospitals and skilled nursing facilities in Georgia and Colorado, using three different methods to detect and confirm each error: direct observation of the nurses as they administered the doses, chart review, and incident report review. Medication errors were common: almost one of every five doses were in error in the typical facility. The percentage rated potentially harmful was 7%, or more than 40 per day in a typical 300 patient facility.[38]

The death rate from ambulatory patient errors has been difficult to estimate. Although the patients are not as ill, there are many more of them. The relative frequency of medication errors in ambulatory pharmacies was estimated in 2003 in a study involving the observation of pharmacists filling prescriptions in 50 pharmacies in six major cities. Prescriptions containing one or more errors occurred at a rate of 1.7%, or about four per day in a pharmacy dispensing 250 prescriptions daily. The percentage rated potentially harmful was 7%. Based on these findings, among the approximately 3 billion prescriptions filled annually are an estimated 51.5 million prescriptions that contain one or more errors, of which 3.3 million are potentially dangerous.[39] The need for the improvement in the quality of the drug dispensing and administration processes, in institutional and community pharmacies, is clear and compelling.

In hospitals, the first measure of the impact of automation on medication errors was reported in 1969. A patient-profile linked dispensing envelope system delivered each unit dose to the patients' bedside at the time for administration, in an envelope labeled with the complete physicians order. In a prospective, controlled clinical trial, data were collected by direct observation of the nurses and pharmacists at work, involving 192 8-hour work shifts observed for the old system and 64 work shifts for the new (automated) system. The error rate declined from 13% to 1.9%.[40]

In 1975, a similar system achieved an error rate reduction from 7.35% to 1.61% (omission errors were not counted).[41] Barker et al. reported a prospective controlled clinical trial in 1984 in which a bedside unit-dose dispensing machine system controlled by a pharmacy computer reduced the error rate from 15.9% to 10.6% on a medical-surgical nursing unit. The design involved a crossover design during the 2-week study period.[40]

In 1995, two studies focused on a nursing unit-based automated device. When used for narcotics and selected first-dose medications and not integrated with the patient's medication profile, the error rate for all doses retrieved from the Pyxis device as detected by observation was 16.3%, compared to 5.4% for doses retrieved from a medication drawer.[43]

The same year, Borel and Rascati compared medication error rates before and 2 months after implementation of Pyxis integrated with the patient profiles and found that the error rate declined from 16.9% down to 10.4%.[44] In community pharmacy, in 1993 Maliekal evaluated an automated dispensing system in an ambulatory pharmacy, by pulling 270 prescriptions off the line, and comparing the count delivered with that called for by the label. Thirty-eight discrepancies were discovered; 22 overfills, 14 underfills, and two could not be classified.[45]

Current studies underway at Auburn University have demonstrated that in a prospective controlled clinical trial an automated prescription filling system (ie, ScriptPro) reduced the rate of dispensing errors among the prescriptions to which it was applied from 2.8% down to 2.1% in a community pharmacy, and from 0.3% down to zero in a chain pharmacy. Each pharmacy was observed for 2 weeks before and after the implementation of the automated system.[46]

Automation may contribute to human errors when it engenders complacency. In a hospital study, the observers reported that typically nurses administered drugs from an automated device without checking them, whereas those taken from the patient's medication drawer were typically checked.[43] It must be recognized that automation is only one component of a human-machine system, and the education and training required for the human part must not be neglected.

Features shown desirable for reducing errors in automated pharmacy systems, as supported by research to date, are outlined below:

1. Controls are comprehensive—Controls extend all the way from the point of order-entry to the point of dispensing or administration, and are integrated with the pharmacy or facility information system.
2. *Electronic identification (eg, bar coding)*—All components including the drug, patient, and person dispensing are identified.
3. *Access to medications is limited and controlled*—Medications are accessible only when needed, and only by authorized personnel.
4. *Dispensing/administration is captured*—Documentation is automatic and complete.
5. *Drug use information is provided*—Access must be immediate.
6. *Labeling machine prints and affixes a label*
7. Controls are not easily compromised—System overrides are signaled visibly and/or audibly at the time of the event, and electronically documented.[47]

Although there are no *national* standards for automated pharmacy systems, most State Boards of Pharmacy have, or are in the process of writing, regulations for the use of automated systems. Model regulations for automated pharmacy systems have been adopted for incorporation into the National Association of Boards of Pharmacy Model State Pharmacy Act and Model Rules.[48]

The American Society of Health-Systems Pharmacists has published Guidelines on the Safe Use of Automated Storage and Distribution Devices.[49] The Joint Commission of the Accreditation of Healthcare Organizations has published standards for automated medication distribution systems.[50]

Pharmacists contribute to positive medication outcomes by assuring that each patient receives safe, appropriate, and effective drug therapy through the provision of pharmaceutical care, which is the responsible provision of drug therapy for the purpose of achieving defined therapeutic outcomes that improve a patient's quality of life while minimizing patient risk.[49] The provision of pharmaceutical care extends the pharmacist's responsibility beyond the delivery of the drug product to include the outcomes of drug therapy. Within the broad concept of pharmaceutical care, the public must be assured that pharmacists will retain their crucial role in the medication use process—specifically the pharmacist's review and evaluation of all prescriptions or medication orders before dispensing or administration, and control of the distribution of every dose dispensed or administered to every individual patient—even as the dispensing process becomes increasingly automated.

Although control of medication distribution will be increasingly exercised through automated systems, the ultimate responsibility for these systems must remain with the pharmacist, the drug use expert who best understands the purpose of these systems and their limitations. The exercise of control over an automated pharmacy system will require that the pharmacist implement standards developed by the profession for the performance of the system, and provide a mechanism for identifying deviations from those standards and a responsive system for taking action to correct any deviations when they occur. Thus, in each of the automated pharmacy systems evolving, the focus of the pharmacist should be on the control system—its performance standards and contribution to the achievement of pharmaceutical care outcomes. Pharmacists must obtain the needed education and training to implement and monitor these control systems effectively.

As the use of automation increases, the complexity of drug distribution systems will be such that the pharmacist will no longer be able to comprehend all aspects of these systems, nor should the pharmacist be expected to do so. The crucial new skills for the pharmacist will encompass: (1) how to operate automated pharmacy systems to produce the outcomes desired, (2) how to recognize when a system failure occurs or is imminent, (3) how to compensate to protect patient safety when failures occur, and (4) how to get failures corrected expeditiously.

A *White Paper on Automation in Pharmacy* describes automation including quality, safety, manpower and professional issues, and model regulations for State Boards of Pharmacy.[48]

The Systems Approach

The authors began this chapter by defining the word *system*. They continued throughout the chapter looking at subsystems and focal points for the use of technology in pharmacy practice. The authors propose that all of the pieces of the technology puzzle are truly in place and are readily available for implementation into all pharmacy practice settings.

Taking any technology topic to a search engine such as www.google.com will yield hundreds and potentially thousands of "hits" for consideration. Technology vendors are fully aware of the marketing potential for their products and services via the World Wide Web. The authors believe pharmacists will increase their efficiency and effectiveness through the appropriate selection of technology.

To maximize operational effectiveness in pharmacy practice, it is necessary to approach any pharmacy operation with a goal of integration of work systems in mind. It is usually possible to build an interface between any two devices such as a pharmacy management system and an automated dispensing robot. A simple interface between two devices is called a "point-to-point" interface. Multiple interfaces can exist in any pharmacy operation. The authors promote a systems approach that seeks to integrate the entire operation through the interconnection of all work systems.

For example, consider a retail pharmacy operation. The operation can be divided into the following functional areas: intake; processing and exceptions; fulfillment; quality assurance; front store; counseling; delivery; knowledge management; and external connectivity. Specific technologies exist within each functional area. For example, integration within the intake area might involve electronic prescribing, interactive voice response systems, a fax server, predictive fulfillment applications, and customer relations management software.

The authors recommend that a careful examination of opportunities for integration takes place for the entire operation. One goal should be to take work out of the system that would normally be performed by costly personnel. Error reduction is another primary goal. Providing value added services and features and benefits from association with the pharmacy operation is another desired goal. While it is possible to achieve some benefits from piecemeal enhancements to a pharmacy operation, the authors are confident that a combination of technology, training, and facilities designed will maximize results.

Emerging Technologies

"The imperatives of improving documentation, reducing error, and empowering patients will continue to motivate use of information technology in health care."[51] There are so many exciting and emerging technologies to investigate that we usually find it more interesting to look at the technological "low hanging fruit" than we do future implications of genomics and nanotechnologies. There are a number of futurists who predict that disruptive technologies must be anticipated because they will heavily impact organizations on both strategic and tactical levels. One nonprofit organization that looks 2–5 years into the future is the HealthTech Center (www.healthtech.org). This organization envisions a bulging pipeline of new clinical technologies that excites consumers and drives and integrates change in health-care systems.

HealthTech predicts that less invasive surgeries and therapies will take place as care increasingly moves to ambulatory and home care settings. It reports that patients and caregivers will see more real-time access to health data. Further, it also predicts that work for shortages will be softened by technology deployment.

Another corporation HEALTHvision (www.healthvision. com) predicts the future containing technology offered through subscription services via the Internet to caregivers. This corporation anticipates the complete electronic prescription pad to be a near future reality. It also anticipates that patient access to a shared medical record will occur in increasing numbers. Finally, HEALTHvision sees a proliferation of health device monitoring at home and the realization of health demographic and clinical information availability on the Internet.

At Auburn University, the authors investigate technologies such as continuous speech recognition. While many believe that this technology is not ready for prime time, these authors use it on a daily basis. They are tracking literally thousands of innovations that include clinician-tailored software, PDA programming for patient health-care uses, the use of digital pens in health-care, and all modes of wireless communication.

Surveys performed in 2003 are still demonstrating that the establishment of wireless networks in health-care systems remains a top priority for implementation. A combination of cellular, WiFi (802.11b), Bluetooth, 3G, and infrared technologies are rapidly proliferating to assure real-time access to needed information.[52] A Danish implementation of a wireless healthcare network successfully used existing capability with wireless phones to move clinical information to the point of care. "The Wireless Application Protocol (WAP) technology implemented in newer mobile phones has built-in facilities for handling much of the information processing needed in clinical work."[53]

Currently, the authors are tracking over 160 technologies to impact patient compliance to drug therapies. This is believed to be a natural outreach activity for the pharmacist wishing to move beyond a product focused, traditional practice.

REFERENCES

1. *The American Heritage Dictionary of the English Language*, 4th ed. Boston: Houghton Mifflin, 2000 from www.dictionary.com. Accessed March 28, 2003.
2. Cipolle RJ, Strand LM, Morley PC. *Pharmaceutical Care Practice*. New York: McGraw Hill, 1998.
3. Felkey BG, Barker, KN. *Am J Health-Syst Pharm* 1995; 52:537.
4. Felkey BG. *Int Pharm J* 1995; 9: 108
5. Knowlton CH, Penna RP. *Pharmaceutical Care*. Bethesda: ASHP, 2003.
6. Felkey BG, Barker KN. *J Am Pharm Assoc* 1996; 36:309.
7. Felkey BG. *Am J Health-Syst Pharm* 1997; 54:274.
8. Blois MS, Shortliffe EH. *Medical Informatics: Computer Applications in Health Care*. Boston: Addison-Wesley, 1990.
9. Felkey BG, Buring SM. *J Am Pharm Assoc* 2000; 40:546.
10. Felkey BG. *Am J Health-Syst Pharm* 1997; 54:1505.
11. Davidoff F. *Mt Sinai J Med* 1999; 66:75.
12. The Evidence-Based Medicine Working Group. *JAMA* 1992; 268: 2420.
13. Rosenberg W, Donald A. *Br Med J* 1995; 310:1122.
14. Sackett DL. *Br Med J* 1996; 312:71.
15. Schattner A. *QJM* 2003; 96:1.
16. Ferren AL. *J Healthcare Info Mgmt* 2002; 16:66.
17. Bates DW, Kuperman G, Teich JM. *Qual Man Health Care* 1994; 4:18.
18. Stablein D, Drazen E. *Healthcare Informatics* 2003; 20:96
19. Taylor H. Available at: http://www.harrisinteractive.com/ harris_poll/index.asp?PID=104. Accessed March 25, 2003.
20. Eysenbach G, Powell J, Kuss O, et al. *JAMA* 2002; 287:2691.
21. Felkey BG, Fox BI. *J Am Pharm Assoc* 2001; 41:529.
22. Grover F, Wu HD, Blanford C,et al. *J Fam Pract* 2002; 51:570.
23. Felkey BG, Fox BI. *Pharmacotherapy Self Assessment Program*, 4th ed. Kansas City: American College of Clinical Pharmacy, 2001, Chap 7.
24. Field MJ, Grigsby J. *JAMA* 2002; 288:423.
25. Silverman M. *Allergy* 1999; 54(49):35.
26. Gostin LO. *JAMA* 2001; 285:3015.
27. Schaefer M. *Pharmacy World & Science* 2002; 24:120.
28. Tessier C. *Healthcare Informatics* 2003; 20:87.
29. Landis NT. *Am J Health-Syst Pharm* 1995; 52:584.
30. Levy S. *Drug Topics* 2001; (May 21):46.
31. Page D. *Drug Topics* 2000; (Mar 6):120.
32. Rupp MT. *America's Pharmacist* 2002; (Jan):11–13.
33. Ringold DB, Santell JP, Schneider PJ. *Am J Health-Syst Pharm* 2000; 57:1759.
34. Proceedings from the Sesquicentennial Stepping Stone Summit One: *J Am Pharm Assoc* 2003; 43:140.
35. Tucker SA. *Proceedings Bar Code Administration Conference*, April 25, 2003, 12–14.
36. Knapp DA. Professionally Determined Need for Pharmacy Services in 2020: Report of a Conference Sponsored by the Pharmacy Manpower Project, Inc. March 25, 2003, 1–22.
37. Kohn LT, Corrigan JM, Donaldson MS. *To Err Is Human*. Washington DC: National Academy Press, 1999.
38. Barker KN, Flynn EA, Pepper GA, et al. *Arch Intern Med* 2002; 162:1897.
39. Flynn EA, Barker KN, Carnahan BJ. *J Am Pharm Assoc* 2002; 43:191.
40. Barker KN. *Am J Hosp Pharm* 1969; 26:324.
41. Means BJ, Derewicz HJ, Lamy PP. *Am J Hosp Pharm* 1975; 32:186.
42. Barker KN, Pearson RE, Hepler CD, et al. *Am J Hosp Pharm* 1984; 41:1352.
43. Barker KN, Allan EL. *Am J Health-Syst Pharm* 1995; 52:400.
44. Borel JM, Rascati KL. *Am J Health-Syst Pharm* 1995; 52:1875.
45. Maliekal JJ. *J Pharm Technol* 1993; 9:47.
46. Flynn EA, unpublished, 2003.
47. Barker KN. *Am J Health-Syst Pharm* 1995; 52:2445.
48. Barker KN, Felkey BG, Flynn EA, et al. *Consult Pharm* 1998; 13:256.
49. ASHP. *Am J Health-Syst Pharm* 1998; 55:1403.
50. Technological Solutions to Standard Compliance: Automated Dispensing, Joint Commission on Accreditation of Healthcare Organization; Oakbrook Terrace, IL; 2000. Audiotape.
51. Hepler CD, Strand LM. *Am J Health-Syst Pharm* 1990; 47:544.
52. Hersh, WR. *JAMA* 2002; 288:1955.
53. Schacht HM, Dorup J. *J Med Internet Res* 2001; 3:4.

CHAPTER 96

The Patient: Behavioral Determinants

Bonnie L Svarstad, PhD

Dara Bultman Sitter, PhD, RPh

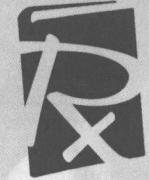

Health professionals often assume that the process of health care simply involves a patient to seek care for his/her symptoms, a physician to prescribe appropriately, a pharmacist to dispense appropriately, and a patient to follow directions and take the medication properly. Similarly, it is tempting to believe that patients, upon following physician and pharmacist suggestions, readily experience symptom improvement and better health. The reality is that many individuals needing health care do not receive it, receive it late, or do not follow through with directions. For example, a National Health Survey shows that at least 30% of those considering help for emotional problems do not actually seek care.[1] In other cases, there may be a considerable delay in seeking care. While most breast cancer symptoms are discovered by women, at least one third of breast cancer patients will be aware of their symptoms for 3 months or more before seeking an initial provider evaluation.[2] In addition, 30% to 60% of all individuals who obtain medical care do not follow through with prescribed treatment[3] and almost half of those taking medications do not ask any questions when visiting the physician.[4]

Why do some people seek medical advice while others with similar symptoms do not? Why do some individuals who obtain medical care follow recommendations and take an active role in their care, while others with similar diagnoses and treatments not follow through with recommendations and not ask any questions about their treatment. To answer these questions, we need to understand the determinants of patient behavior. This chapter begins with a section on theories related to patient behavior in health. Four sections describe how patient behavior is influenced by characteristics of the patient, drug regimen, environmental factors, and interaction with providers. Finally, a health collaboration model is presented as a tool to help pharmacists understand how they can positively affect patient behavior and health outcomes.

TYPES OF PATIENT BEHAVIOR IN HEALTH

The three main areas in the study of patient behavior are: (1) preventing illness or detecting it in an asymptomatic stage, (2) obtaining a diagnosis and discovering suitable treatment, and (3) undertaking or maintaining treatment aimed at restoring health or halting disease progression. Kasl and Cobb[5] defined these health-related behaviors and labeled them health behavior, illness behavior, and sick-role behavior, respectively. The definitions are still useful today, although some terminology has changed to reflect contemporary theory and research on health behavior.

Health behavior that is preventive in nature generally is referred to as *preventive health behavior*. Expanding on the original definition, preventive health behavior is defined as actions taken to prevent illness and maintain physical, emotional, intellectual, spiritual, and social well-being. Examples of preven-

tive health behaviors include participation in health screening programs, following healthy diet recommendations, participation in relaxation and cardiovascular exercises, and creating and maintaining close personal relationships.

Illness behavior is any activity undertaken by individuals who perceive themselves to be ill that defines the state of their health and aids in discovering a suitable remedy.[6] Illness behavior is the way persons respond to bodily indications that they experience as abnormal; thus it involves the manner in which persons monitor their bodies, define and interpret their symptoms, and seek health care.[7] Individuals attempt to ascribe cause and meaning to their illness symptoms and may self-diagnose and treat. Alternatively, individuals may visit a doctor or another prescriber and a pharmacist in order to obtain a prescription drug.

Actions taken to restore health or halt disease progression traditionally have been referred to as sick-role behaviors and now are referred to as *treatment behaviors*. Originally, the conceptualization of sick-role behavior[8] offered a systematic approach for analyzing the behavior of sick individuals in the US and other modern Western societies. This functionalist perspective regarded illness as dysfunctional to society and considered sick-role behavior as seeing the physician, passively following his or her prescription, and regaining health. This traditional view of the patient as a passive individual has been criticized extensively in recent years.[9]

Patients today are considered to be thinking, able decision makers who can play an important role in the treatment process.[10] Because patients are now recognized as active individuals, more attention is being paid to ways of restoring health or slowing illness progression through improved provider-patient communication and patients' involvement in their own treatment. Emphasis therefore is placed on a range of patient treatment behaviors including sharing beliefs and expectations, asking questions, adhering to regimens, using home monitoring devices, keeping appointments, identifying and reporting side effects and drug-taking problems, and other valuable forms of communication that are necessary in contemporary health care.

MODELS OF PREVENTIVE BEHAVIOR AND HEALTH UTILIZATION

People experience illness and treatment at many levels. Physiological, intellectual, social, and emotional processes are all a part of an individual's illness experience. A patient's understanding of illness or symptoms, the information provided by health-care providers, how the illness and treatment affect usual daily activities as well as the individual's previous experiences and beliefs with illness all influence behavior. Behavioral scientists have attempted to understand human responses to illness by using a number of different theoretical perspectives and models of health behavior.[11–16] The two models commonly referred to in the study of patient behavior are the Health Belief Model developed by Rosenstock[14] and Andersen's Model of Health Service Utilization.[11]

The Health Belief Model was developed when studying preventive health behaviors. The model suggests that individuals seek preventive care if they possess some relevant health motivation and view themselves as vulnerable, if they view the condition as threatening, and if they believe action will be beneficial. In other words, these individuals believe themselves to be susceptible, the condition to be serious, and the benefits of action to outweigh the potential barriers. In addition, some cue to action must occur, either as a symptom or as an outside motivational message, thus inspiring the individual to take action. This model focuses on individuals, placing decision-making in their hands, and suggests that individuals determine how to balance the intricacies of their own lives.

The study of illness behavior often is examined using Andersen's Model of Health Services Utilization. Andersen suggested that three main factors affect an individual's use of health services:

1. Predisposing factors
2. Enabling factors
3. Need factors

Predisposing factors are those factors that vary an individual's inclination to use services. Andersen suggested that prior to illness, individuals have a measure of propensity toward use of medical services. These predisposing factors include demographic variables such as age and gender; social structure variables such as education, occupation, and ethnicity; and health beliefs about medical care, physicians, disease, and medication use. Enabling factors are those factors influencing the individual's ability to use services, thus they reflect the fact that an individual's ability to use services depends on individual family and community resources. Finally, need factors are those factors related to the individual's belief in the seriousness of illness symptoms and the necessity of intervention. Need factors are separated into two categories, perceived need and evaluated need.

Both the Rosenstock and Andersen models of health utilization include the patient perspective, patient demographics, patient resources, and provider variables. As previously stated, these models are very useful when focusing on preventive health behavior and initial use of health services. In cases of chronic illness requiring ongoing treatment, the models could be improved. At the very least, additional influencing factors such as drug characteristics and the treatment environment must be incorporated into a model of health behavior. Ongoing treatment also requires continual interaction between the patient and the provider, and that aspect must be incorporated into a health behavior model, as discussed later. Because patient behavior and outcomes are influenced by the patients themselves, provider characteristics, drug factors, and the treatment environment, the discussion begins here.

PATIENT FACTORS INFLUENCING BEHAVIOR

Many patient factors have been examined in relation to behavior and health. Although study findings vary, the two demographic factors continually observed are patient age and sex. The relationship between age, sex, and health is in part physiological and in part a social construct. Age and gender influence health experiences through life. Survey information related to age, sex, illness, and drug use gives evidence to this point.

Older people tend to use health services more than younger people. While the elderly represent 12% of the population, they account for 34% of total pharmaceutical expenditures.[17] The relationship between age and drug use is in part related to more chronic illnesses in old age. Approximately 36% of the elderly have three or more chronic conditions, while about one third of the nonelderly have at least one chronic condition.[17] Biological age is not the only reason for increased use of health services among the elderly. Gerontologists argue that age often brings loss of customary resources and thus changes the way individuals are attended to and the way they cope with stress.[18]

Women tend to use health services more than men. In a survey of 1360 elderly rural individuals, women reported taking twice as much medication as men.[19] The self-reported use of OTC medications in the rural older population also shows that women take more OTC medications than men.[20] A longitudinal study of 488 healthy, community-dwelling, elderly volunteers show that female subjects, those older than 80 years or those who reported themselves to be in fair or poor health on initial health self-report have a significantly increased use of prescription medications. Moreover, increased medication use did not predict mortality over the next 10 years in this population.[21]

Sex also makes a difference in psychotropic medication use. In the case of children, the gender effect on psychotropic drug use varies across child age.[22] At younger ages, male children are more likely to use psychotropic drugs. However, at older ages, female children were more likely to use psychotropic drugs. Use of psychotropic drugs varies by gender in adults.[23] After controlling for statistically significant factors such as demographic and health services, presenting complaints, and psychiatric diagnoses, women were still 37% more likely than men to receive a prescription for an anxiolytic and 82% more likely than men to receive an antidepressant prescription. Conversely, Sleath et al[24] found that men were more likely to receive psychotropic medications than women, in a poorer, older, and more nonwhite sample of patients.

Age and gender make a difference in the number of visits made to the doctor's office per year. Across age groups males visit the doctor less often than females do.[9] The greatest difference occurs in the reproductive years, when women make about twice the number of office visits of men (3.1 versus 1.7). Men and women 65 years or older make the most office visits, followed by middle-aged persons and children under 15 years.[9]

Age and gender make a difference in experiences at the community pharmacy. Schommer and Wiederholt[25] report that male patients and older patients are more likely to be solicited for feedback and have drug use monitored by pharmacists. A separate survey from 2135 randomly selected respondents also suggests that men receive more consultation from pharmacists; however, individuals younger than 40 years reported receiving more consultation from pharmacists than older respondents.[26] In another study, younger patients were more likely than older patients to know how their prescribed antidepressant worked, when it started working, common side effects, how to manage side effects, and how long their physician wanted them to take the medication.[27]

The influence of social factors may explain the consistent finding that males report fewer physical symptoms than females and typically have a lower level of drug use. Physical differences only partially explain gender differences in symptom reporting and medication use.[28] Studies of children's illness behavior suggest that boys and girls acquire different beliefs and ways of coping with pain through the process of socialization into traditional male and female roles: girls are encouraged to express their pain, whereas boys are encouraged to deny their pain and avoid feminine or sissy-like behaviors.[29] Consequently, men may be less likely to complain about, and seek relief from, pain unless they are encouraged to do so by their caregivers.

Other important patient factors examined in relation to behavior and health include socioeconomic level, race, and ethnicity. Socioeconomic level is a measure used to reflect income, education, and occupation; it describes social class within a community. Differences between socioeconomic groups in accessibility, use, and quality of care are contributing factors to the widening gap in rates of morbidity and mortality. Recent evidence of the inequality that persists comes from the National Longitudinal Mortality Study; higher levels of both income and education are associated with lower rates of mortality.[30] Race and ethnicity are associated with differences in health-related problems, including access to health-care services. Socioeconomic resources also influence children's health behavior, with uninsured children being more likely than insured children to have gone without needed medical, dental, and other health care (22% versus 6%).[31] Health-care providers may find it useful to be aware of and explore potential differences in health beliefs, diet, and other health behaviors.

In a classic sociological study, Zborowski[32] demonstrated that patients from different ethnic backgrounds had very different reactions to pain, even though they were suffering from similar physical problems (ie, herniated disks and spinal lesions). For example, Jewish and Italian patients tended to have a more emotional response to pain; they felt freer to discuss their pain, complain about it, groan and cry, and ask for relief. In contrast, patients from other backgrounds tried to deny their pain and appear more stoic. Based on observational and interview data, Zborowski concluded that the patients had learned different ways of reacting to pain and that they simply were behaving in a manner that was expected, accepted, and approved by their families and others in their community.

The primary chronic health problem among Mexican Americans in the US is non-insulin-dependent diabetes mellitus. In fact, diabetes is the fifth leading cause of death among Latino women and seventh among men.[33] The US Hispanic populations experience diabetes complications such as nephropathy leading to end-stage renal disease, retinopathy and blindness, neuropathy, and nontraumatic lower extremity amputations.[34] While access to medical care or extent of medical care may not be the reason for the differences in complications in Hispanics and African Americans, the researchers suggest that the quality of medical care is a likely determinant of morbidity.

Health-care providers interviewed about perceived barriers to treating Latino patients have mentioned a number of problems, including communication barriers, financial problems, and cultural barriers.[35] Specifically, Latino patients are often very polite to doctors, so polite that rather than discuss their diabetes care, the patients nod their heads and agree with the doctor. Patients often do not believe that the medication supplies are free and therefore do not take the necessary diabetic supplies as often as needed. Other patients believe that receiving government assistance in medical supplies will decrease chances of US citizenship. For the families that do pay for medical supplies, a different problem arises. Expenses for a woman's needs often are considered secondary to the good of her family, and therefore expenditures for diabetes medications and supplies are considered less important than other family necessities. Finally, traditional folk remedies, such as aloe, cactus, and garlic, compete with the use of prescribed diet and medications, because patients (and possibly providers) are not aware that treatments can be combined.

Understanding patient behavior requires an attention to possible and common emotional experiences. Emotional factors of concern to patients include uncertainty of what to expect with this new illness or symptom; dependency on providers to give the best treatment and on family to help with daily life; fear of change and death; pain and discomfort; lack of privacy in physical examinations; loss of identity as a healthy person; isolation from usual support systems such as coworkers, teammates, and friends; and a search for meaning on how to put all of these experiences into perspective. Emotional factors are of particular concern when the patient has been diagnosed with a terminal illness, an illness with a social stigma, or an illness that requires change in daily behavior.

A look at some empirical work emphasizes the importance of health beliefs, perceptions, and expectations. In a study focused on medication adherence, using patient interview and record reviews, researchers found that the best predictor of treatment

adherence was previous patient experience with the medication.[36] In addition, patients were more likely to adhere to the medication treatment when they had been told more about taking the medication, were asked about prior experience with antidepressants, and discussed other things they could do to make their life more pleasant. It is not understood if these messages influenced patient beliefs or if these messages allowed enough communication between the patient and provider to influence patient beliefs. In another study of patients receiving treatment for depression, positive patient beliefs at the beginning of treatment were the best predictor of continued antidepressant use and a positive evaluation of the medication at followup.[27]

The meaning of insulin treatments differs for patients and providers. For example, surveys suggest that most Hispanic patients recognize positive aspects of insulin treatment, but virtually all report negative effects, and nearly one third believe that receiving a prescription for insulin indicates that the disease has advanced into a very serious stage.[37] Forty-three percent of patients were concerned that insulin causes serious health problems. In fact, 25% of Hispanic patients report fear that insulin causes blindness. Patients need information that may not appear obvious to providers.

Patient expectations of pharmacist care affects patient behavior.[38] Pharmacy clients may not ask pharmacists questions because of client embarrassment or because they are not aware that it is appropriate to seek information from pharmacists. Clients may not realize that pharmacists check for drug interaction and that patient consultation is required by law in some states, while an offer to counsel is required in others.

In general, patient age, sex, ethnicity, socioeconomic level, and health beliefs affect patient behavior in health. Older individuals and women tend to use more health resources. Ethnicity affects health beliefs, diagnosis, and treatment. Socioeconomic level affects health service use, morbidity, and mortality. Social distance may exist between patients and providers with different ages, gender, ethnicity, and socioeconomic level and is a potential barrier to effective treatment. Barriers to more appropriate patient health behaviors can be reduced by providers.

DRUG FACTORS INFLUENCING PATIENT BEHAVIOR

Drug regimens can be complex. The complexity of a drug regimen often is measured in the total number of medications taken daily, number of daily doses, duration of treatment, the extent to which the regimen is tailored to daily routines, and the side-effect profile. Medications may require special behaviors, for example having to take a dose 1 hr before or 2 hr after a meal, avoiding foods that are common in the diet, taking doses three or more times in a day, refrigerator storage, or skill in administration. In addition, just learning the name of the drug prescribed, purpose of the drug, proper dose, when to begin taking it, frequency of dosing, and when to stop treatment is complex.

The complexity of a therapeutic regimen may prevent patients from adhering completely. Complex regimens may produce information overload. Alternatively, medications requiring behaviors that are difficult to fit into regular daily activities are less likely to be taken as prescribed by a patient. A drug adherence study using an electronic monitoring device to measure dose compliance shows that patients adhere better to once-daily dosing than twice-daily dosing.[39]

Medication treatment often is accompanied by adverse drug effects. Antidepressant and antipsychotic medication nonadherence has been related to adverse drug experiences.[40,41] Blackwell[42] suggests that it is mainly unexpected or alarming side effects of treatment that patients offer as the reason for stopping treatment and that a discussion of side effects along with an explanation of the therapeutic benefits of the medication would be helpful to patients. Myers and Calvert[43] found that patients given information on antidepressant benefits and adverse effects were less likely to report side effects than patients given only adverse effect information or almost no information. In another study of treatment with antidepressants, 27% the patients were bothered by the medication and their dissatisfaction with the medication significantly increased the number of medication omissions.[27]

ENVIRONMENTAL FACTORS INFLUENCING PATIENT BEHAVIOR

CHOICE AND CONTROL—Patients given more autonomy and opportunities for self-determination tend to show greater health and morale improvements. Rodin and Janis[44] suggest that asking patients for their opinions during the medical encounter increases their feelings of involvement and self-efficacy. The researchers believe that internalization of treatment plans and feelings of greater control result in better adherence to recommendations and improved health status. Social and environmental restrictions in choice and control over daily activities can have negative effects on physical health and well-being of nursing-home residents.[45]

Allowing patients a choice in their medication regimen also can affect patient adherence positively.[46] Patients were randomly allocated to one of three treatment groups: group A received one dose of medication (75 mg) at night; group B received three doses of medication (25 mg each) during the day; group C were allowed to choose either A or B above. Researchers report the greatest rate of adherence occurred in the group who chose to take 1 tablet three times a day.

PHARMACY ENVIRONMENT—The structural layout of many community pharmacies does not include an area for private consultation and dialog between the patient and the pharmacist. In addition to this lack of privacy, pharmacists often experience other environmental barriers to meaningful interaction with their patients, including insufficient supportive personnel, a heavy workload and backlog, people waiting to present prescriptions or receive pharmacist assistance, incoming phone calls and requests for information or help from co-workers, interns, and other staff, and inadequate computer technology, software, and preparation for new consultation roles. The impact of these environmental factors are not well studied, but they are believed to be major barriers to pharmacist and patient interaction.[47] For example, a recent observational study in 306 pharmacies found that pharmacists working in busy versus non-busy environments are less likely to talk with patients, to give oral information to patients, and to ask questions assessing patients' understanding.[48] Patients also have reported that pharmacy site barriers (including pharmacist time limitations and lack of privacy) are among the most common reasons why they do not ask the pharmacist their questions.[38] Research examining the effects of these environmental factors on patient behavior is rich in potential for improving patient care.

EFFECTS OF PROVIDER-PATIENT INTERACTION ON PATIENT BEHAVIOR

The relationship between patient and health-care provider has been studied much more extensively between patient and doctor than between patient and pharmacist. Research using observation, audio-transcriptions, and interventions suggests that both physician-patient interactions and pharmacist-patient interactions are related to patient behaviors and outcomes.[49,50] Patients use three main sources of information when making decisions about their illness and treatment: their personal experience with the illness and various treatments; information obtained from family, friends, and the larger culture; and their interaction with health professionals.[12] In recent years, there have been increased efforts to understand and improve the ways in which providers and patients interact with

each other, because of changing societal views about the patient's role in health care and growing evidence that provider-patient interaction plays a central role in the safe and effective use of medications and health behavior change.[51–53] For example, many consumer and professional groups have criticized the lack of drug information provided by physicians and pharmacists and advocated a new *health culture* in which patients take a more active collaborative role in their health care.[52] Scientific studies also have found that the quality of provider-patient communication about drugs varies greatly and that efforts to improve communication can affect the patient's health behavior and quality of life in multiple ways, suggesting new goals and models of communication.[10,16,52]

In the sections below, scientific research is briefly reviewed, examining the different ways in which provider-patient interaction can affect the patient's health behavior. A new model of interaction called the Health Collaboration Model (HCM) then is presented. This new model incorporates current research and philosophies of care and can be used to guide pharmacists' efforts to understand and improve collaboration processes and outcomes in their practice. In contrast to traditional models of medical care, the HCM emphasizes the importance of patient feedback and participation in treatment decisions. It also clarifies the different ways in which providers can enhance patient comprehension and recall of regimens, patient motivation and satisfaction with care, patient feedback, and collaborative problem-solving and resolution of conflicts.

EFFECTS OF PROVIDER INSTRUCTION ON PATIENT COMPREHENSION AND RECALL—Physicians and pharmacists continue to be the main sources of drug information and advice given to patients. However, observational studies of provider-patient interaction point to a number of problems. Patients often receive information about the drug name and recommended dose and dosage frequency, but the majority of patients still receive no specific oral counseling about the purpose of therapy, how long to take their medication, side effects, other precautions, and when the medication will begin to work.[26,48] Studies also have demonstrated a direct link between the *provision of explicit or specific instructions* and patient comprehension of the regimen and its components; patients whose providers do give them more explicit or specific instructions clearly have a better understanding of how they are supposed to take their medication.[16,27] In fact, the quality of medication instruction by a provider is a better predictor of patient comprehension and recall than the patient's age and education.[27]

Research in psychology suggests that people are more likely to comprehend and recall those items that are considered important or relevant to them. Studies of health communication support this notion; patients whose providers communicate the *purpose or importance* of drug therapy are more likely to have an accurate interpretation and recall of the regimen than patients whose providers do not discuss these points.[49] Emphasizing the importance of certain recommendations also enhances patient recall of these particular recommendations, according to experimental studies conducted by Ley.[54] Another proven method of improving patient recall of advice is *repetition* of those items that are likely to be misinterpreted or forgotten. While repetition does not always have the predicted effect, it generally produces a 20% to 30% improvement in patient recall of advice.[55]

Research also has shown that there are substantial gains in patient comprehension and recall when providers use *written reinforcement* and *visual aids,* including printed leaflets or information sheets, expanded prescription labels and stickers, calibrated liquid measuring devices, and special containers or calendars that indicate exactly when each dose is to be taken.[56]

Several qualifications must be noted, however. First, none of these techniques is effective by itself. In fact, provision of written information without oral review and discussion by a pharmacist or physician usually fails to achieve desired outcomes.[56] Written information and memory aids cannot eliminate side effects and other problems that undermine patients' motivation

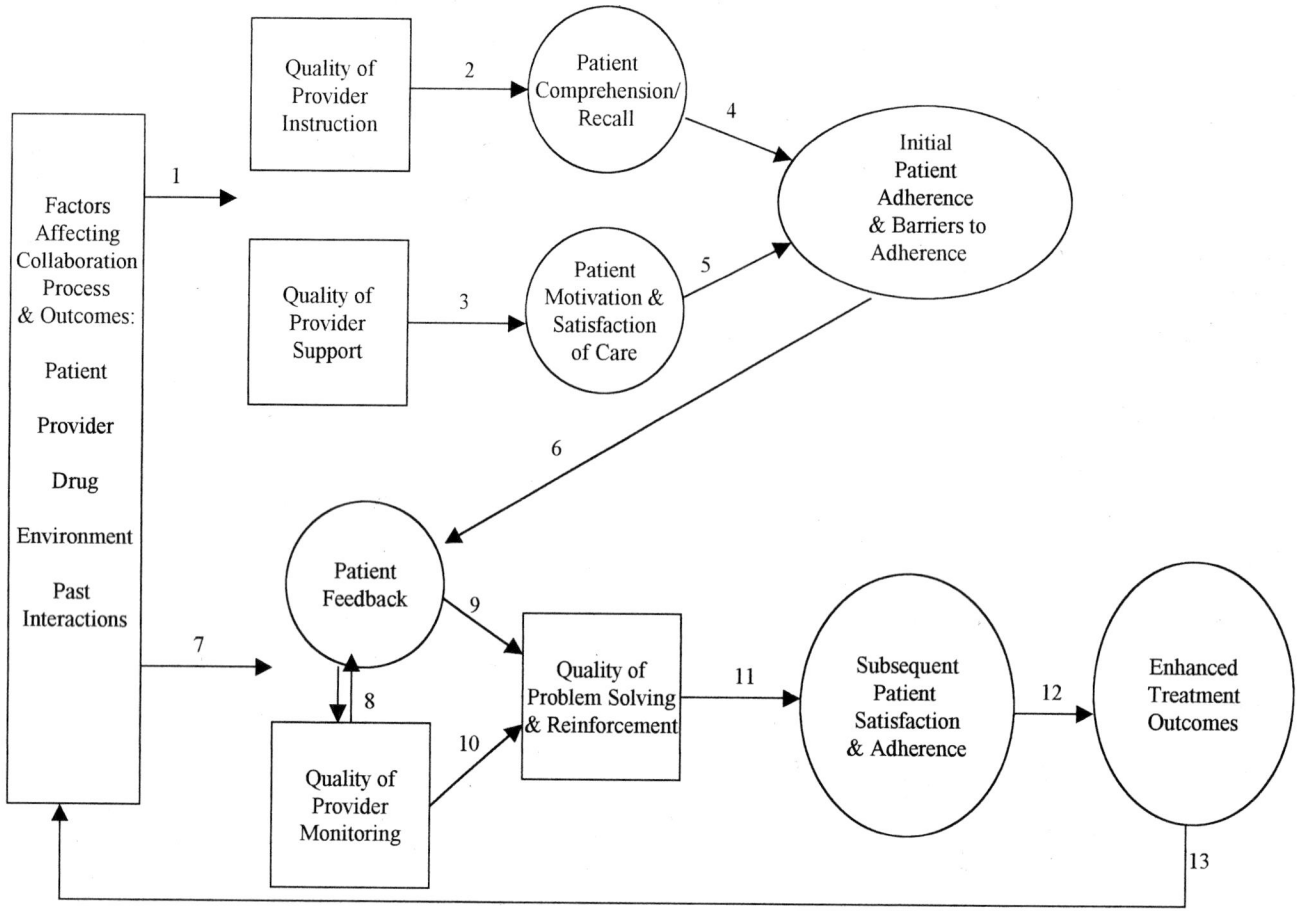

Figure 96-1. Health collaboration model.

and concerns. The provider who is able to solicit accurate patient feedback is then able to resolve patient-specific problems and provide appropriate reinforcement as necessary (arrows 9–10). This type of two-way communication and collaborative problem-solving leads to greater patient satisfaction and adherence (arrow 11) and enhanced treatment outcomes (arrow 12). The final arrow (14) illustrates the importance of past interactions and treatment experiences in establishing and maintaining a trusting relationship that is the cornerstone of effective health and pharmaceutical care.

Like other conceptual tools, the Health Collaboration Model can play an important role in pharmacy practice and research. First, it enables pharmacy practitioners and researchers to organize large amounts of information that would otherwise be confusing or difficult to interpret and use. Second, it enables pharmacists to identify potential connections and implications that are not obvious when examining results from a single study or set of observations. Finally, it can be used as a stimulus and guide for further discussion, evaluation, and practice development. It helps us see that the patient's behavior depends more upon the patient's beliefs, feelings, and interactions than on the patient's medical diagnosis or severity of illness. It also helps us see pharmacists who have a good understanding of patient behavior can have a positive impact on treatment outcomes by providing quality instruction, support, monitoring, and collaborative problem-solving and reinforcement.

REFERENCES

1. Silverman MM, Eichler A, Williams GD. *Public Health Rep* 1987; 102(Jan-Feb):47.
2. Facione NC, et al. *Cancer Pract* 1997; 5(4):220.
3. Meichenbaum D, Turk DC. Facilitating Treatment Adherence: A Practitioner's Guidebook. New York: Plenum Press, 1987.
4. Sleath BL, et al. *Med Care* 1999; 37:1169.
5. Kasl SV, Cobb S. *Arch Environ Health* 1966; 12:246, 531.
6. Green LW, Krueter MW. *Health Education Planning: An Educational Environmental Approach.* Mountain View, CA: Mayfield, 1991.
7. Mechanic D. In *Handbook of Health, Health Care, and the Health Professions.* Mechanic D, ed. New York: Free Press, 1983, p 591.
8. Parsons T. *The Social System.* New York: Free Press, 1951.
9. Wolinsky FD. *Principles, Practitioners, and Issues,* 2nd ed. Belmont, CA: Wadsworth, 1988.
10. Chewning B, Sleath B. *Soc Sci Med* 1996; 42(3):389.
11. Andersen R. *A Behavioral Model of Families' Use of Health Services.* University of Chicago: Center for Health Admin Studies, 1968.
12. Leventhal H, Zimmerman R, Guttman M. In Gentry WD, ed. *Handbook of Behavioral Medicine.* New York: Guilford Press, 1984.
13. Mechanic D. *Medical Sociology: A Selective View.* New York: Free Press, 1968.
14. Rosenstock IM. *Milbank Mem Fund Q* 1966; 44:94.
15. Suchman E. *J Health Hum Behav* 1965; 6:114.
16. Svarstad BL. In Aiken LH, Mechanic D, eds. *Applications of Social Science to Clinical Medicine and Health Policy.* New Brunswick, NJ: Rutgers University Press, 1986, p 438.
17. Mueller C, Schur C, O'Connell J. *Am J Public Health* 1997; 87(10):1626.
18. Markides KS. *Aging and Health Perspectives on Gender, Race, Ethnicity, and Class.* Newbury Park, CA: Sage, 1989, p 12.
19. Lassila HC, et al. *Ann Pharmacother* 1996; 30:589.
20. Stoehr GP, et al. *J Am Geriatr Soc* 1997; 45(2):158.
21. Hershman DL, et al. *J Am Geriatr Soc* 1995; 43(4) 356.
22. Hong SH, Shepherd MD. *Am J Health-Syst Pharm* 1996; 53(16):1934.
23. Hohmann AA. *Med Care* 1989; 27(5):478.
24. Sleath B, Svarstad B, Roter D. *Patient Educ Couns* 1998; 34:227.
25. Schommer JC, Wiederholt JB. *Pharm Res* 1997; 14:145.

26. Wiederholt JB, Clarridge BR, Svarstad BL. *Med Care* 1992; 30(2):159.
27. Bultman DC. Svarstad BL. *Patient Educ Couns* 2000; 40:173.
28. Svarstad BL, et al. *Med Care* 1987; 25(11):1088.
29. Lewis CE, Lewis MA. *N Engl J Med* 1977; 297:863.
30. Rogot E. A mortality study of 1.3 million persons by demographic, social and economic factors (1979–1985 followup, US Natl Longitudinal Mortality Study). Bethesda, MD: NIH, Natl Heart, Lung, and Blood Inst, 1992.
31. Newacheck PW, et al. *N Engl J Med* 1998; 338:513.
32. Zborowski M. *J Soc Issues* 1952; 8:16.
33. *Building Understanding to Prevent and Control Diabetes Among Hispanics/Latinos* (selected annotations). Atlanta, GA: CDCP, 1996.
34. Cowie CC, Harris MI. *Diabetes Care* 1997; 20(2): 142.
35. Lipton RB, et al. *Diabetes Educ* 1998; 24(1):67.
36. Lin EHB, et al. *Med Care* 1995; 33(1):67.
37. Hunt LM, Valenzuela MA, Pugh JA. *Diabetes Care* 1997; 20(3):292.
38. Chewning B, Schommer JC. *Pharm Res* 1996; 13(9):1299.
39. Kruse W, et al. *Int J Pharm Pharmacother Ther* 1994; 32(Sep):452.
40. Montgomery SA, et al. *Int Clin Psychopharmacol* 1994; 9:47.
41. Windgassen K. *Acta Psychiatr Scand* 1992; 86:405.
42. Blackwell B. *N Engl J Med* 1973; 289:245.
43. Myers ED, Calvert EJ. *Br J Clin Pharmacol* 1984; 17:21.
44. Rodin J, Janis IL. In Interpersonal Issues on Health Care. Friedman HS, DiMatteo MR, eds. Orlando, FL: Academic Press, 1982, p 33.
45. Ryden M. Nurs Res 1984; 33:130.
46. Myers ED. Branthwaite A. *Br J Psychiatry* 1992; 160:83.
47. Kimberlin CL, et al. *Med Care* 1993; 31:451.
48. Svarstad BL, Bultman DC, Mount JK. *J Am Pharm Assoc* 2004; 44:22.
49. Svarstad BL. In Mechanic D, ed. *The Growth of Bureaucratic Medicine: An Inquiry into the Dynamics of Patient Behavior and the Organization of Medical Care.* New York: Wiley, 1976.
50. Hall JA, Roter DL, Katz NR. *Med Care* 1988; 26:657.
51. DiMatteo MR, DiNicola DD. *Achieving Patient Compliance.* New York: Pergamon, 1982.
52. Lilja J, Larsson S, Hamilton D. *Drug Communication. How Cognitive Science Can Help the Health Professionals* Kuopio Univ Publ A. Pharm Sci 24 Sweden, 1996.
53. Roter DL, et al. *Med Care* 1998; 36:1138.
54. Ley P. *J Health Hum Behav* 1972; 13:311.
55. Ley P. *J Soc Clin Psychol* 1979; 18:245.
56. Morris LA, Halperin JA. *Am J Public Health* 1979; 69: 47.
57. Ley P. In *Contributions to Medical Psychology.* Rachman S, ed. Oxford: Pergamon, 1977, p 9.
58. Ley P, et al. *Psychol Med* 1976; 6:599.
59. Cohen F, Lazarus RS. In Mechanic D, ed. *Handbook of Health, Health Care, and the Health Professions.* New York: Free Press, 1983, p 608.
60. Joos SK, Hickam DH. In Glanz K, Lewis FM, Rimer BK, eds. *Health Behavior and Health Education: Theory, Research, and Practice.* San Francisco: Jossey-Bass, 1990, p 216.
61. Inui TS, Carter WB. *Med Care* 1985; 23:521.
62. McKenney JM, et al. *Circulation* 1973; 48:1104.
63. Haynes RB, et al. *Lancet* 1976: 1265.
64. Nessman DG, Carnahan JE, Nugent CA. *Arch Intern Med* 1980; 140:1427.
65. Levine D, et al. *JAMA* 1979; 241:1700.
66. Bond CA, Salinger R. *J Clin Psychiatry* 1979; 40:501.
67. Kelly GR, Scott JE. *Med Care* 1990; 28:1181.
68. Johnson Al, et al. *Can Med Assoc J* 1978; 119:1034.
69. Svarstad BL, et al. *Patient Educ Couns* 1999; 37:113.
70. Morris L. *Med Care* 1982; 20:596.
71. Bultman DC, Svarstad BL. Patient Educ Couns 2000; 40:173.
72. Rickles NM. A randomized, controlled study evaluating the impact of an antidepressant monitoring program on consumer outcomes. Unpublished PhD dissertation, University of Wisconsin–Madison, School of Pharmacy, 2003.
73. Greenfield S, Kaplan S, Ware JE. *Ann Intern Med* 1985; 102:520.
74. Greenfield S, et al. *J Gen Intern Med* 1988; 3:448.
75. Freidson E. *Profession of Medicine: A Study in the Sociology of Applied Knowledge.* New York: Harper & Row, 1970.
76. Swain MA, Steckel SB. *Res Nurs Health* 1981; 4:213.

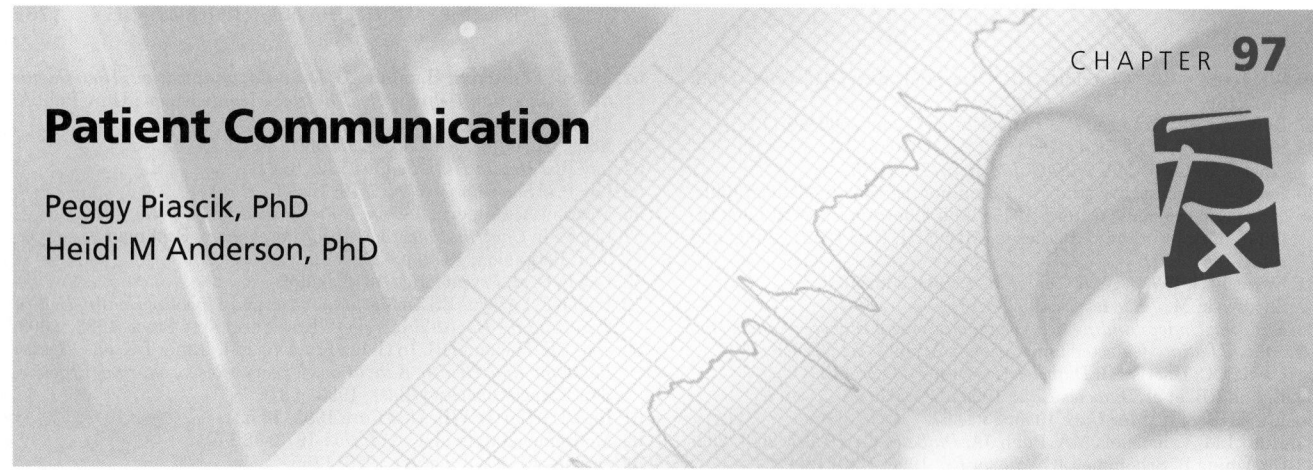

CHAPTER 97

Patient Communication

Peggy Piascik, PhD
Heidi M Anderson, PhD

A constructive pharmacist-patient relationship is essential to sound health care practice and the optimal well-being of the patient. These pharmacist-patient relationships begin and develop with effective communication, both verbal and nonverbal. Mutual trust and respect are basic characteristics of this relationship. Ineffective communication may reduce the accuracy of the medical diagnosis.

Mock asserts that "the concept of effective clinician-patient communication is a necessity, not an option. Because communication is both a science and an art that can be learned and mastered, there are many resulting benefits for those who work diligently to improve their technique, not the least of which is increased clinician satisfaction."[1] Therefore, health care professions education, and specifically pharmacy education, should include specific training in patient communication skills and an understanding of the psychological reactions to illness and treatment.

To provide quality patient care, pharmacists must have the desire and ability to communicate effectively with patients, other health care professionals, and the public. This chapter will describe the factors a pharmacist must consider and techniques that are useful in effective patient communication.

THE COMMUNICATION PROCESS

Communication is the sharing of information, ideas, thoughts, and feelings. It involves not just the spoken word, but also what is conveyed through inflection, vocal quality, facial expression, body posture, and other behavioral responses. As a first step toward communicating more effectively, pharmacists must understand the communication process.

The goal of all communication is understanding. For one person to understand a message composed by another, the receiver must do more than recognize the words used in the message by the sender. Effective communication occurs only when the meaning of a message is held in common by the participants. Human nature makes it difficult to attain this point of understanding between two or more people because each person's view of reality is influenced by past life experiences, the current situation, and perceptions of each other. This individualistic perception influences both the way in which a message is sent and the way in which it is received.

When a person wishes to share information with another, the sender must choose how to transmit that message. The medium of the message can be written, oral, nonverbal, or electronic. If the sender decides to transmit the message through words, the sender must encode the message by choosing words that best convey the intended meaning to the receiver.

Once the information is encoded, the sender loses control of the message because its meaning comes from the receiver's de-

coding of it. If the receiver responds to the message, that response acts as feedback to the sender. This gives the sender an opportunity to clarify and correct any misunderstanding. This sequence of encoding, transmitting, and decoding messages continues so long as sender and receiver continue to communicate.

Communication usually takes place through multiple nonverbal channels as well. For example, as the words of a message are transmitted, facial expressions, gestures, vocal quality, and other nonverbal cues also are sent. These nonverbal signs may modify the intended meaning of a message. A mixed message may result when the intended verbal and nonverbal messages are not understood as meaning similar things.

INFORMATION GATHERING AND PATIENT EMPOWERMENT

The interactions of a pharmacist and a patient usually can be categorized as either an information-gathering or information-giving session.[2] Information gathering usually is done during a medication-history interview, which is a conversation with a multifaceted purpose. Pharmacists initiate the interaction to investigate and acquire data about a patient's medication-taking experiences, assess a patient's understanding of past and current medication-taking experiences, assess a patient's motivation for complying with the medication regimen, and possibly suggest to the prescriber a change in regimen if the information gathered warrants such an action. The direct patient-pharmacist interaction during a medication-history interview frequently provides the pharmacist with an opportunity to begin a professional relationship with the patient.

Research has revealed that a patient who is involved in deciding on his or her treatment is more likely to comply with the treatment.[3,4] Patient empowerment is a concept that refers to patients having the right to make their own choices about their health care.[5] Feste argues that "the empowerment model has evolved out of the realization that patients cannot be forced to follow a lifestyle dictated by health-care professionals."[5] The patient empowerment model is based on the assumption that to be healthy, people must be able to bring about changes not only in their personal behavior but also in their social situations and the institutions that influence their lives.

Effective communication should involve patient empowerment in the health care-patient relationship. Patient empowerment posits that since patients are the ones who experience the consequences of both having and treating their illness, they have the right to be the primary decision makers regarding their medical condition. This philosophy further asserts that although the health care provider should be involved in the decision, the final determination of what is best for the pa-

Table 97-1. Outline of a Patient Empowerment Program

1. Health care professional assess current status (physical, emotional, cognitive, etc.)
   - Review patient's actual self-care practices
   - Reviews patient's recommended self-care practices
2. Health care professional provides relevant medical information
   - Describes various treatment options
   - Reviews costs and benefits for each option
3. Health care professional acknowledges patient's responsibility for self-care
   - Helps patient clarify personal values specific to their illness
   - Helps patient assess level of personal responsibility for their care
   - Helps patient select treatment goals
4. Patient identifies barriers and strengths related to achieving self-care
   - Assesses medical barriers and sources of support
   - Assesses life/social barriers and sources of support
5. Patient assumes problem-solving responsibility
   - Develops skills to optimize support (eg, communication and assertiveness skills to enhance support from family and friends; increases support networks)
   - Identifies potential barriers
   - Learns strategies/skills to overcome barriers (eg, negotiation, self-care agreements and plans, conflict resolution)
6. Patient establishes plan with assistance from provider
7. Patient carriers out plan
8. Patient and provider evaluate and review plan using problem-solving model

Adapted from Funnell MM, et al. *The Diabetes Educator* 1991; 17(1):37.

tient is both the right and responsibility of the individual patient.[5]

Feste further states that "the empowerment model speaks of self-awareness, personal responsibility, informed choices and quality of life. Therefore, in the empowerment view, the primary purpose of the health care professional is to prepare patients to make informed decisions about their own [medical] care."[5]

Funnell and associates also explain the process and outcome of patient empowerment.[6] They suggest that "people are empowered when they have sufficient knowledge to make rational decisions, sufficient control and resources to implement their decisions, and sufficient experience to evaluate the effectiveness of their decisions. Empowerment is more than an intervention or strategy to help people make behavior changes to adhere to a treatment plan. Fundamentally, patient empowerment is an outcome. Patients are empowered when they have knowledge, skills, attitudes, and self-awareness necessary to influence their own behavior and that of others in order to improve the quality of their lives."[6] Table 97-1 provides an outline of patient empowerment as adapted from Funnell's model.

WHY PHARMACISTS COUNSEL PATIENTS

Communicating with patients about their medications provides significant benefits to both the patient and the pharmacist. The patient will have a better understanding of the purpose for the prescribed therapy and the appropriate use of the medication. This leads to several potential benefits:

- Improved therapeutic outcomes and decreased adverse effects
- Improved patient adherence to the treatment plan
- Decreased medication errors and misuse
- Enhanced patient self-management by involving the patient in designing the therapeutic plan
- Potential for decreased health care costs due to appropriate use of medications and prevention of adverse events

The pharmacist also benefits in this process. Potential benefits to the pharmacist in this process include:

- Enhanced professional status in the view of patients and other health care providers
- Establishment of an essential component of patient care that cannot be replaced by technicians or automation
- Enhanced job satisfaction through improving patient outcomes
- A value-added service to offer patients
- Revenue generation through payment for counseling services–limited at present but growing
- Fulfillment of legal responsibility to counsel patients according to the OBRA 90 guidelines

The Ad Hoc Panel on Medication Counseling Behavior Guidelines of the USP has identified six desired outcomes of patient counseling.[7] It is expected that, as a result of a properly conducted counseling interaction, the patient will:

- Recognize why a prescribed medication is helpful for maintaining or promoting well-being
- Accept the support from the health care professional in establishing a working relationship and foundation for continual interaction and consultation
- Develop the ability to make more appropriate medication-related decisions concerning compliance or adherence
- Improve coping strategies to deal with medication side effects and drug interactions
- Become a more informed, efficient, active participant in disease treatment and self-care management
- Show motivation toward taking medications to improve his or her health status

OPTIMIZING THE ENVIRONMENT FOR PATIENT COMMUNICATION

The optimal setting for communicating with patients is a private consultation room adjacent to the dispensing area. A private setting has been shown to enhance patient retention of the counseling information, increase patient adherence to the drug regimen, and increase patient satisfaction with the counseling experience[8]; however, many pharmacy settings lack sufficient space to create this type of environment. The pharmacist must be aware of the physical barriers that exist in the pharmacy and work to minimize them.

The physical layout of the pharmacy may include a prescription counter that separates the pharmacist from the patient, a partition made of glass or other materials, a raised floor that puts the pharmacist on a higher level than the patient, floor or counter displays that add to congestion and separate the patient from the pharmacist, or inadequate lighting. Use of the following techniques may overcome these physical barriers:

- Come out from behind the counter to greet the patient
- Face the patient and maintain eye contact
- Position yourself a comfortable distance from the patient, usually 1 1/2 to 4 feet from the patient

The noise and distractions in a busy pharmacy can be handled using the following techniques:

- Move away from the pharmacy counter when possible to a more private area of the pharmacy
- Ask other employees in the pharmacy not to interrupt during a patient session
- Face the patient and speak clearly and distinctly in a tone loud enough to be heard but not so loud as to be heard by others in the pharmacy

PHARMACIST BARRIERS TO COMMUNICATION

Pharmacists who are uncomfortable interacting with patients or who have had little training in patient interaction may engage in inappropriate nonverbal behaviors that interfere with good pharmacist-patient communication. Examples of such behaviors include nervous movements or "fidgeting," crossed arms or legs, turning or leaning away from the patient, failure to maintain eye contact, and obvious distractedness. Techniques that improve patient interaction have been described by Muldary[9] using the acronym CLOSER. The suggested techniques include:

- Control distractions, such as nervous habits
- Lean toward patient
- Open body posture, uncross arms and legs
- Squarely face patient
- Eye contact 50–75% of the time
- Relax

Other barriers to effective communication cited by pharmacists include lack of time, economic considerations, poor communication skills or lack of confidence in those skills, lack of knowledge about current drugs or patient history, and the patient's failure to value the counseling session or pharmacist expertise.[10,11] Lack of time and economic considerations in patient counseling can be overcome by increasing the use of technical personnel to relieve pharmacists from dispensing functions and allowing the pharmacist to spend time with patients. Poor communication skills or lack of expertise about recent drug advances can be overcome by appropriate choice of continuing professional education opportunities to improve knowledge and skills in areas of identified weakness. The patient's failure to appreciate the value of consultation with the pharmacist can be overcome by advertising the service provided and personally offering the consultation to each patient with a brief description of the importance of this process in improving patient medication therapy outcomes. Another barrier to effective communication is taking into account the patient's cultural perspective.

CULTURE AS A BARRIER TO COMMUNICATION

Galanti states that a problem that is beginning to receive attention in the United States is the cultural gap between the medical system and the huge number of ethnic minorities served by the health care system.[12] Galanti asserts that "the goal of the medical system is to provide optimal care for all patients."[12] In a multiethnic society, this can be accomplished only if the health care providers understand cultural differences " . . . that create conflicts and misunderstandings and that may result in inferior medical care".[12]

All health care professionals are finding themselves faced with an increased number of patients from various cultures. Cultural diversity challenges health care providers to facilitate bridging cross-cultural gaps with patients. The patient-health care provider relationship may be seriously disrupted by misunderstandings due to different beliefs, values, or language. It is through providing culturally relevant care that health care professionals truly serve the needs of all patients in our diverse society.

Health care providers must find effective ways to communicate with patients from diverse backgrounds. In an effective patient communication session, the pharmacist gathers not only objective information about the patient's health condition, but also an understanding of the patient's own perspective regarding his or her health. This perspective may include the patient's viewpoint from his or her own cultural perspective. Discovering the patient's perspective can help diagnosis and make for a more effective and efficient health care process.

Galanti identifies several cultural areas in which communication may be misunderstood.[12] A few of these areas are identified in Table 97-2 and briefly discussed below. The reader is encouraged to read Galanti's book to learn more about other cultural aspects and practices that may affect a patient's health care.

Table 97-2. Cultural Factors that May Affect Health Care

- Verbal and Nonverbal Communication
  Idioms
  Same Word, Different Meaning
  Format for Names
  Eye Contact
  Touching
- Time Orientation
  Patients may operate with a present orientation, past orientation, or future orientation
- Religion & Spirituality
  Blood Beliefs
    Transfusions
    Drawing Blood
  Prayer
  Holy Days
  Sacred Symbols
  Lucky and Unlucky numbers
- Dietary practices
  Specific diets
  Special holiday preparations
  Taboos for certain foods
  Nutritional deficiencies
- Folk Medicine
  Fevers
  Coin Rubbing
  Medications

Verbal and Nonverbal Communication

Verbal and nonverbal communication may lead to misunderstandings. Miscommunication may occur when individuals use idioms (eg, patient has 'cold feet'). Avoid using idioms. Different words have different meanings in the same language (eg, 'horita' means right now in Mexico; it means an hour in Puerto Rico). Using a first name of anyone other than a friend is considered inappropriate or discourteous in most cultures. Still other cultures consider it disrespectful to look someone directly in the eye especially if that person is in a superior position, and some cultures may not be comfortable with casual touching and hugging that many Americans do without even thinking.

Time Orientation

Time orientation varies among cultures. When scheduling an appointment with a patient who has a different time orientation, be sure to specify clock time instead of scheduling in relation to an activity. For example, for some patients, lunchtime means between 1:00 and 2:00 PM rather than 12:00, and some European countries eat dinner at 10:00 in the evening. Be aware that not every culture eats meals at the same time.

Religion and Spirituality

Religion and spirituality are common sources of miscommunication. Some religions do not accept blood transfusions; others may refuse to have blood drawn because of beliefs about getting bad fortune or death if blood is drawn. Some cultures have certain times of day that prayer is mandated and holy days may dictate that certain behaviors are restricted, such as driving on the Sabbath. Various cultures have symbols that are sacred. These may be worn (eg, rosary) or be placed in the patient's room. If the patient is hospitalized, health care professionals need to respect the item and explain the reason the item may need to be removed from the individual. Finally, certain cultures believe that there are lucky and unlucky numbers (eg, Chinese regard 8 and 9 as lucky; the number 4 is seen as unlucky by some Japanese). Therefore, health professionals need to respect patients' religious beliefs and try to accommodate their practices as much as possible.

Dietary Practices

Dietary practices may include such activities as Ramadan by Muslim patients. Some ethnic groups cannot tolerate certain foods or are forbidden to eat certain foods (eg, Hindu are forbidden to eat beef). Health care providers need to be aware of the patient's diet, both in terms of content and preparation.

Folk Medicine

Many cultures have developed local methods for treating illnesses and diseases. Galanti reminds us that "some techniques, such as coin rubbing may produce marks that appear to be signs of child abuse or are unrelated to symptoms. It is important to recognize these before jumping to unwarranted conclusions."[12]

In summary, health professionals must consider the patient's cultural perspective to provide effective communication and thus effective health care. Some final suggestions are:

- Be aware of the customs and beliefs of religious, ethnic, and recent immigrant groups in your area
- Try to work within the health belief system of the patient and family
- Respect patients' viewpoints; listen to them
- Learn about the customs of the patient, alternate health care methods and medications
- Explain risks of not taking medication

A MODEL PATIENT COUNSELING SESSION FOR A NEW PRESCRIPTION

A correct diagnosis and appropriately prescribed drug therapy will be ineffective unless the patient understands the reasons for the therapy, how it is to be used, and the outcomes of the therapy. In addition, it is critical that the patient is motivated to adhere to the prescribed regimen so that he or she will experience optimal effectiveness of the drug therapy.

The pharmacist should view the patient counseling interaction as a two way sharing of knowledge. The pharmacist is the expert in drug therapy. The patient is the expert with regard to the personal medical history, past medication use, life-style issues, and patient attitudes toward medication use. The pharmacist must first assess the patient's knowledge and attitudes about the prescribed medication and adjust the counseling session to assist the patient in achieving the best possible outcome.

Each pharmacist should develop a personal patient counseling routine to ensure that all important issues are discussed with each patient. It is useful to work from a checklist, at least until the process becomes second nature to the pharmacist. The essential elements described below should be considered for each counseling session. The pharmacist must then tailor the steps to the particular patient and the situation. For example, a patient interaction with a new patient who is receiving a medication for the first time will be significantly different than a session with a well-known patient who has been taking the same medications for a period of time.

PREPARING FOR THE SESSION

Pharmacists should spend a few moments mentally preparing for the interchange about to occur. Preparation greatly enhances the experience for both parties and, ultimately, the quality of the interaction. The pharmacist should know as much as possible about the patient before approaching the patient or caregiver. This is easier in a hospital setting where the patient's medical record and other health care providers can provide valuable background information about the patient. In the community setting, the pharmacist can review the prescription as well as the patient's medication record if the patient has been to the pharmacy before. It rarely is possible to know much about a patient before a first pharmacy visit, but

the patient can be asked to fill out a medication history form if there is not time to complete a medication history interview at the time the prescription is dispensed. Review of the prescription tells the pharmacist the patient name, when the prescriber was seen, whether it is a new medication or a refill, and the name of the medication. This may provide clues to the patient's medical condition if that information is not available from the patient's profile information.

Another important issue to consider before a session actually begins is the physical state of the patient. Observation of the patient prior to the counseling session can reveal many clues about the patient's physical and mental state.

STEPS TO A SUCCESSFUL PATIENT COUNSELING SESSION

The following steps represent a logical outline for counseling a patient on a new prescription (Fig 97-1).

1. **Introduce yourself and identify the patient.** Greet the patient. Smile and offer your hand in greeting if appropriate. Provide your name as well as your position in the pharmacy and identify the person with whom you are speaking. If the person is not the patient, determine the relationship between the patient and person picking up the prescription. A counseling session may

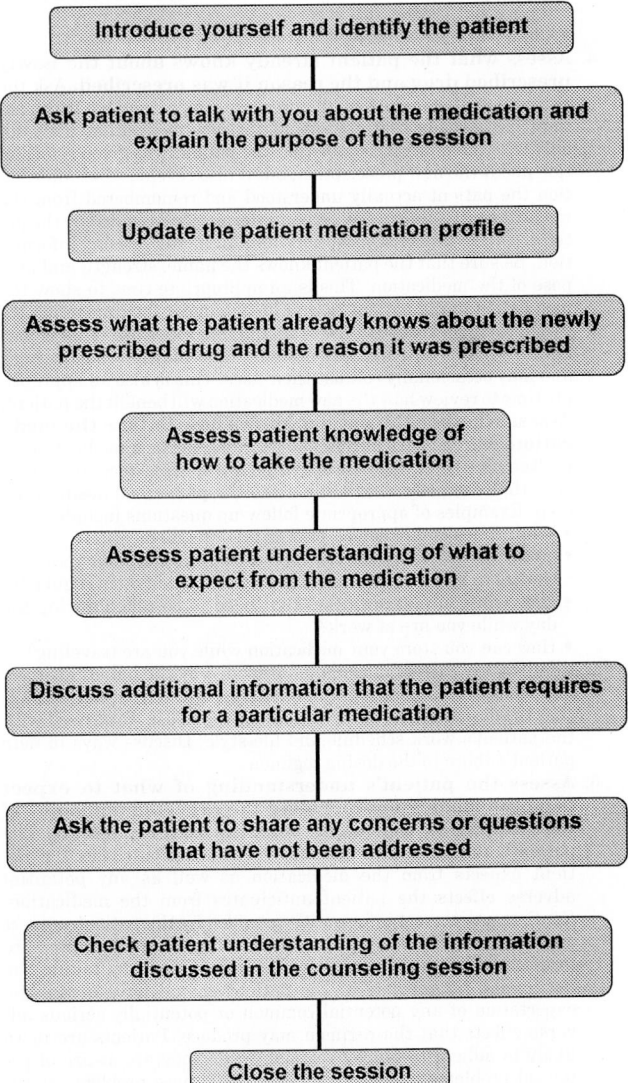

Figure 97-1. Steps in a patient counseling session.

not be appropriate if the person picking up the prescription is merely a friend or neighbor rather than a caregiver. In this case, arrangements should be made for phone consultation or provision of written counseling materials.

2. **Ask patient to talk with you about the medication. Explain the purpose and the importance of the counseling session.** Determine that the patient has sufficient time for a conversation. A distracted patient will not listen to any information provided in the session. Explaining the purpose and importance of the counseling session in terms of the benefits to the patient will increase the effectiveness of the session. Many patients do not receive patient counseling regularly and are not aware of the benefits to be gained. It is helpful to ask the patient if he or she has any concerns about the new medication before you start through the counseling process. This allows you to deal with any issues that are bothering the patient first so that the patient is not distracted by other concerns while you are providing drug information to her. For example, the patient may be wondering if the drug will be covered by her health plan or whether she will have to pay the full cost of the medicine. Answering that question first will relieve the patient's mind and allow her to concentrate on what you are saying to her.

3. **Update the patient medication profile.** Review with the patient any profile information relevant to the new prescription. This ensures that the pharmacist knows about any recent changes that would affect the patient's current therapy. This may include the following:
   - Allergy and disease state status
   - New or discontinued prescription drugs that may not be included in the patient record
   - New or discontinued non-prescription drugs including dietary supplements and herbal products that may not be included in the patient record
   - Changes to social/lifestyle history

4. **Assess what the patient already knows about the newly prescribed drug and the reason it was prescribed.** Ask the patient why he or she saw the prescriber today and what the patient has already been told about the new medication. This not only tells the pharmacist whether the patient was given information about the new prescription, but it also reveals what information the patient actually understood and remembered from the medical visit. Confirm any correct information provided by the patient, correct any misconceptions and fill in any missing information. Be sure that the patient knows the name, strength and purpose of the medication. This is an appropriate time to show the medication to the patient so that he will make the connection between the appearance of the drug and its proper use. This is particularly important for patients who take multiple medications and may occasionally confuse their uses. This is also an appropriate time to review how the new medication will benefit the patient.

5. **Assess whether the patient knows how to take the medication.** Ask the patient how she will take the new medication. It is often necessary to follow up with a few specific questions to ensure that the patient will adhere to the prescribed dosing regimen. Examples of appropriate follow-up questions include:
   - What times of day do you plan to take the medication?
   - How can you schedule the medication around your daily activities to help you remember to take the medication regularly?
   - How will you plan for doses that need to be taken during the day while you are at work?
   - How can you store your medication while you are traveling?

   Confirm any correct information provided by the patient, correct any misconceptions and fill in any missing information. Be sure that the dosing regimen the patient agrees to use works well with the patient's work schedule and life-style. Discuss ways to help patient adhere to the dosing regimen.

6. **Assess the patient's understanding of what to expect from the medication including the expected outcomes of the therapy as well as its potential adverse effects.** The patient's response tells the pharmacist what outcomes the patient expects from the medication as well as any potential adverse effects the patient anticipates from the medication. Confirm any correct information provided by the patient, correct any misconceptions and fill in any missing information. Be sure to discuss the therapeutic benefits to be gained by taking the medication appropriately. The patient should have a realistic expectation of any potential common or potentially serious adverse effects that the regimen may produce. Patients are more likely to adhere to a drug regimen when they are aware of potential problems and know what to do if those problems occur. The patient should know if the adverse effect will resolve by itself and how long that may take, whether there are any steps a

patient should take to relieve or resolve adverse effects, or if an adverse effect should be reported to the prescriber or pharmacist. Offering solutions to resolve drug-related problems relieves patient anxiety and empowers the patient to deal with the problem directly. Patients who are not prepared to deal with adverse effects often quit taking medication and do not report it to a health care provider.

7. **Discuss any additional information that the patient requires for a particular medication.** Examples of additional information that the pharmacist may provide to the patient includes:
   - Potential interactions with other drugs, foods or diseases
   - Missed doses
   - Monitoring information–how will the patient know the medication is working, any testing that should be done to assess the therapy, follow-up appointments with health care providers
   - Refill information
   - Storage information
   - Life-style changes to implement–changes in diet, exercise, avoid sun, etc.

   The pharmacist must use professional judgment in determining what information is essential to provide to a particular patient in a given situation and when to stop talking so that "information overload" does not become a problem.

8. **Ask the patient if he or she has any concerns or questions that have not been addressed in the previous discussion.** Patients usually do not bring up these concerns unless they are asked directly by the pharmacist. The patient may be distracted by these concerns while the pharmacist is providing information. It is best to address concerns as soon as they are identified. A follow-up question about unresolved issues and problems ensures that the patient has had an opportunity to voice any concerns that may be a barrier to medication use.

9. **Check patient understanding of the information discussed in the counseling session.** Perhaps the most critical step in the process is to check patient understanding of the newly prescribed medication and its use. This can be accomplished by putting the question in the context of checking the pharmacist's success in communicating the information clearly to the patient. This avoids putting the patient "on the spot" or making him feel that he is being quizzed. An example question might be the following:

   "Mrs. Jones, we've discussed a lot of information about your new prescription today. To be sure that I did a good job explaining everything, would you recap for me what you learned today about your new medication?"

   As the patient recaps her understanding of the information, the pharmacist can assess the patient's knowledge and retention of the information. This provides the opportunity to reinforce any critical information, correct any misinformation, and fill in any information that the pharmacist may have omitted during the counseling session. This also gives the pharmacist the opportunity to praise and encourage the patient.

10. **Closing the session.** To close the counseling session:
    - Provide written counseling information you have used during the session.
    - Tell the patient how to reach you if other questions or concerns arise.
    - Confirm when you expect the patient to return for a refill or follow-up with health care provider.
    - Reinforce the value to the patient of appropriate medication use and the positive outcomes possible for the patient.
    - Thank the patient for spending the time to discuss the new medication with you.

COUNSELING PATIENTS ON THE USE OF REFILL PRESCRIPTIONS

The basic principles of a patient counseling session do not change whether the patient is starting a new medication or refilling an ongoing prescription. However, the focus of the discussion is somewhat different during a counseling session for a refill. A refill counseling session should concentrate on the following three areas:

- Confirm that the patient has been taking the correct medication and knows the indication for its use. Show the medication to the patient to determine that there is no confusion with a different prescription.
- Ask how the patient has been taking the medication. This tells the pharmacist whether the patient has adhered to the regimen. Ad-

ditional evidence of the patient's compliance comes from the medication profile information. Has the patient returned at the appropriate time for a refill? When the patient describes how he or she has been taking the medication, does he appear sure of the information? Praise appropriate medication use and assist the patient in resolving any issues that have interfered with adherence to the regimen.

- Ask how the medication is working for the patient. What benefits has the patient gained from taking the medication? What problems have arisen while taking the medication? How has the patient handled these problems? Provide potential solutions to any unresolved problems. Encourage the patient by reiterating the benefits of continued medication use. Confirm the appropriate follow-up steps for monitoring the patient.

For sample dialogues between pharmacists and patients that illustrate the process described above, the reader is referred to the Bibliography at the end of the chapter.

APPROPRIATE TECHNIQUES TO USE DURING A COUNSELING SESSION

Throughout the patient counseling session, the following techniques for good communication should be utilized.

1. **Nonverbal cues.** Pharmacists and patients alike communicate emotions and other information in nonverbal ways. Blank stares, inattentiveness, nervous speech patterns, and interruptions are distracting and detrimental to effective communication. The verbal and nonverbal aspects of an interaction cannot be separated if one wishes to appreciate fully the nature of the interaction.

   Eye Contact—Facial features, as well as facial expressions, are assumed to reveal personality traits. A great deal of information is communicated through head and facial movements, but perhaps the movement of another person's eyes provides more clues than any other facial structure. Therefore, a gaze is a major nonverbal signal to others.

   Patients vary in the amount of eye contact that makes them comfortable, so interviewers should take cues from them. The best a pharmacist can offer is frequent and attentive eye contact, avoiding blank stares. Eye contact helps assess the meaning that is behind the patient's words and conveys the message "I'm listening." Thus, eye contact represents an important building block toward establishing patient trust and rapport.

   Mannerisms—The study of nonverbal facilitation has led to the marketing of provocative bestsellers that promise readers "You'll be able to read people like a book." Gestures, vocal qualities, body movement, clothing, and hygiene can provide information about interviewers and patients, but ferreting out clues to hidden meanings can be more damaging than helpful to professional relationships.

   The pharmacist needs to make the patient feel comfortable by enhancing physical and psychological privacy. The pharmacist communicates a posture of involvement by facing the patient directly and leaning forward at a slight angle, which is a sign of attentiveness to the patient's needs. If the patient is seated or lying down, the interviewer should sit, if possible. Some other examples of nonverbal facilitation are an inclined head, a head nod, and hand gestures that suggest understanding or the desire for more information.

   Taking notes is appropriate so long as it is not the major focus of attention for either the pharmacist or patient. Excessive writing of notes has disadvantages. It is distracting to patients, impairs interpersonal dynamics, and provides a convenient and absorbing escape for pharmacists. Novice interviewers should take whatever notes are needed to achieve accuracy, but they should strive to improve their listening skills by recording only selected information at the moment and then completing the notes immediately after the interview.

   Vocal Qualities—Pitch, range, tone, clarity, and tempo are vocal qualities. Pitch refers to the frequency level of the voice. Pitch level influences patient attitudes toward pharmacists and the content of the message. While a monotone is generally disliked by most individuals, exaggerated pitch changes are disliked even more. Speakers with naturally spontaneous voices using neither a wide nor narrow range of pitch tend to be perceived more favorably.

   Voice clarity is an important attribute for effective communication. To ensure that the patient can hear and comprehend, the

pharmacist should assess the patient's language and hearing abilities and then change speech patterns, if necessary.

Tempo is the speed of vocal production. Inappropriate delays may irritate patients, while interruptions may rush patients and interfere with the smooth flow of conversation. Fast tempo and frequent pauses often are associated with emotions such as fear or anger. Slow tempo also often is associated with anger, as well as sadness and depression. A slow tempo with frequent pauses and utterances such as "uh," "er," and "um" can indicate uncertainty; perhaps the pharmacist is stalling while waiting for the patient's response or while formulating the next question to ask.

People often express their emotions by talking too fast. Pharmacists should keep their rate of speech conversational.

Touch—Touch can enhance verbal communications and facilitate social interactions with patients. For example, a greeting handshake by a pharmacist may be part of the introduction to the patient session. Touch can also be used to attend to the patient's comfort, and the appropriate touch can display sympathy, empathy, concern, and even be used to get a patient's attention.

The patient's cultural background should be used as a guide to help any health care professional know when to use touch. It is important to keep in mind that not everyone is comfortable being touched. Some cultures consider it inappropriate for men and women to touch, even in a professional setting. Patients from these cultures would not even shake the hand of someone from the opposite sex. In the patient-pharmacist relationship, observe the patient's behavior, and if possible the behavior of the family, to see what they are comfortable with.

2. **Listening.** Listening appropriately to the patient is hard work, but it is extremely important to effective communication. The pharmacist must allow the patient to speak without interruption and concentrate on the words and meaning of the patient's message. The pharmacist should rid himself or herself of distractions, ask clarifying questions where appropriate, and avoid jumping to conclusions or judging the patient's words.

3. **Open-ended questions.** Ask the patient open-ended questions when gathering information. An open-ended question is one that cannot be answered with a yes or no. It requires that the patient provide information to you rather than merely telling you they know the answer to the question. A yes or no answer tells you whether the patient thinks she knows the information but does not allow you to assess the accuracy of the information. Open-ended questions start with who, what, where, when, why, or how. Avoid leading or restrictive questions. Leading or restrictive questions cue the patient to respond with answers predetermined by the questioner rather than allowing the patient to determine the answer to the question. A leading question usually supplies a hint to the patient about the answer the pharmacist is expecting. Like closed-ended questions, leading or restrictive questions do not provide complete information about what the patient knows or thinks. To illustrate the difference between these types of questions, look at the following example:

   Mrs. Woods comes into the pharmacy with a new prescription for metoprolol. The pharmacist wishes to determine Mrs. Woods' understanding of the use of this drug. She asks the question in one of the following ways:

   Closed question: Did Dr. Hart tell you what this medication is to be used for?

   Leading question: Did you see Dr. Hart for your high blood pressure today?

   Open question: Why did you see Dr. Hart today?

   The answer to the closed question will tell whether the prescriber talked to Mrs. Woods about the purpose of the new medication. But it will not reveal anything about her understanding and recollection of the information. The leading question tells Mrs. Woods that the expected answer is to say that she saw the doctor about her high blood pressure and she is likely to answer yes regardless of her true reason for seeing the doctor. The open question allows the patient the freedom to tell, in her own words, exactly why she visited the doctor today.

4. **Use paraphrasing to clarify what the patient says.** Paraphrasing is a technique in which the pharmacist reframes what the patient has said in his own words. This tells the patient that the pharmacist has listened to the information provided and is confirming that the message was received accurately. Use of paraphrasing is sometimes also called active listening. An example of paraphrasing is provided below.

   Patient comment: "I have so many medicines. It is hard to keep them all straight. Sometimes I get confused and I might take them wrong."

Pharmacist paraphrasing: "It sounds like you have a hard time managing all of your medications and that you worry you sometimes might confuse them and take them incorrectly."

Use of paraphrasing allows the patient to check the pharmacist's understanding of the information provided and correct any misinformation.

5. **Avoid technical jargon.** Jargon is the language of specialized terms used by a group or profession. The unnecessary use of technical terms may increase patient anxiety. If use of technical terms is necessary, they should be explained after assessing the patient's understanding of the terms.

The language of pharmacy is filled with medical terminology, drug names, and abbreviations. Words with Latin or Greek prefixes that are commonly used in health communication are particularly confusing. Examples might include prenatal, postprandial, antimicrobial, and dysmenorrhea. The partnership for Clear Health Communication has published a fact sheet called *Words to Watch.*[13] This fact sheet identifies four kinds of words that cause the majority of misunderstanding in health literacy. The types of words that have been identified as easily misunderstood are:

• Medical words—frequently used by health care professionals and in health care instructions
• Concept words—used to describe an idea, metaphor, or notion
• Category words—describe a group or subset, and may be unfamiliar
• Value judgment words—may need an example or visual to convey their meaning with clarity

Table 97-3 provides examples of words in each category that are easily misunderstood by patients and suggests alternative wording to increase patient comprehension.

6. **Organize the session in a logical manner.** The session should be organized so that the information flows logically from one issue to the next. Information should be structured to begin with simple concepts and progress to more complex issues. The most important information should be presented first and then reiterated at the end of the session. Patients will retain information longer when it is presented this way.

Using a standard format to the session helps the pharmacist develop techniques to address each essential element in the process. A disorganized approach increases the likelihood that important questions or information are omitted. In addition, the patient is more likely to become confused if the pharmacist jumps around from one topic to another.

7. **Maintain control of the session.** Time is usually a critical factor in a counseling session. The pharmacist must be sure to permit sufficient time to gather all necessary information and discuss pertinent drug-related issues. The pharmacist must direct the session efficiently and assertively to bring the conversation back to the topic when the patient strays too far from the purpose of the session or dwells on particular concerns too long.

8. **Use written information to supplement verbal counseling.** Research shows that using multiple methods of communication is most effective in delivering the message and having that message understood and retained by the patient. The pharmacist can use the prescription vial as a source of written communication. After showing the medication to the patient, the pharmacist can refer to the directions on the label as well as any ancillary information contained in auxiliary labels. Plain language written counseling materials can be used during the discussion to highlight important information. The pharmacist may use a highlighter to accent the most critical pieces of information and provide the highlighted copy to the patient for later reference. The materials should also contain contact information for the patient to call the pharmacist with any questions that arise later.

TECHNIQUES FOR COUNSELING PATIENTS WHO PRESENT BARRIERS

Patient counseling is a difficult process when performed in ideal circumstances. The process becomes even more challenging when the patient presents barriers that must be overcome to achieve effective communication. Patient barriers generally fall into two categories—functional or emotional.[14]

Functional barriers occur because the patient has difficulty receiving and understanding the communication provided by the pharmacist. Examples of this type of barrier include low illiteracy, hearing or visual impairment, and non-English speaking patients.

Emotional barriers occur when the patient is experiencing strong emotions that may interfere with the patient's thought processes and prevent her from listening to communications or responding appropriately. Examples of emotional barriers would be anger, frustration, sadness, worry, or embarrassment.

The pharmacist must be able to recognize the presence of these barriers and should be prepared to use appropriate strategies to overcome the barrier presented by the patient. Observation of the patient prior to beginning the counseling session, review of the patient medication profile for notes about the patient, and the patient's behavior during the counseling session will usually reveal the presence of a barrier to a watchful pharmacist. Each type of barrier will be addressed individually to provide clues to identifying the patient barrier that may exist and provide potential strategies to assisting the patient to overcome the barrier.

Table 97-3. Words Easily Misunderstood by Patients

	PROBLEM WORD	REPLACE WITH:
Medical Word Examples	Benign	Won't cause harm; is not cancer
	Condition	How you feel; health problem
	Lesion	Wound; sore
	Oral	By mouth
Concept Word Examples	Avoid	Stay away from; do not use or eat
	Intake	What you eat or drink; what goes into your body
	Option	Choice
	Referral	Ask you to see another doctor; get a second opinion
Category Word Examples	Adverse (reaction)	Bad
	Hazardous	Not safe; dangerous
	Generic	Product sold without a brand name, like ibuprofen (Advil is brand name)
	Noncancerous	Not cancer
Value Judgment Word Examples	Adequate	Enough *Example (adequate water): 6–8 glasses a day*
	Excessive	Too much *Example (bleeding): if blood soaks through the bandage*
	Increase gradually	Add to *Example (exercise): add 5 minutes a week*
	Moderately	Not too much *Example (exercise): so you don't get out of breath*

Adapted from *Words to Watch Fact Sheet.* Partnership for Clear Health Communication, available at http://www.askme3.org, accessed 6/10/03.

Functional Barriers

Functional barriers can be grouped into four subcategories:[14]

1. Sensory abnormalities–visual and hearing impairment
2. Language differences–low literacy, non-English speaking
3. Comprehension difficulties–psychiatric conditions, mental retardation, dementia.
4. Alternative health beliefs were discussed earlier in the chapter under *Culture as a Barrier to Communication.*

The pharmacist must remember to treat patients who have functional impairments with respect and avoid patronizing, talking down to the patient, or directing comments to a third party as if the patient is not present. The pharmacist must exercise patience in identifying and solving the patient barrier to communication.

1. **Sensory abnormalities**

   The Visually-Impaired Patient. Clues to visual impairment such as a seeing-eye dog, dark glasses, or a cane may be obvious if the patient is blind. Other patients may have unusually thick glasses or may hold written materials very close to their eyes. For patients who cannot use written materials, verbal communication with a follow-up to recap the session is critical.

   Suggested techniques to improve counseling include:
   - Large type labels and written materials, use of bold print and pastel-colored background on paper to improve contrast
   - Braille label or instructions
   - Well-lighted counseling area
   - Shape, size, and smell of medication and container to distinguish medicines from each other; mark containers with something to set them apart
   - Devices such as a magnifier for a syringe
   - The local Society for the Prevention of Blindness for more tips or suggestions

   The Hearing-Impaired Patient. Clues to hearing impairment may be age, presence of a hearing aid, use of sign language, loud speech, asking for frequent repetition, ignoring questions, or failing to respond to sounds in the pharmacy.

   Suggested techniques to improve counseling include:
   - Face the patient and speak slowly and distinctly; use low pitch, higher volume voice, but do not yell
   - Quiet area for counseling; this is especially helpful for patients with hearing aids
   - Sign language (flash cards for basic words are available) or gestures to explain
   - Facial expressions to communicate
   - Notes to patient or written counseling materials
   - Pictograms or auxiliary labels to convey ideas
   - TDD technology to communicate by phone when appropriate

2. **Language barriers**

   The Low Literacy Patient. Patients who have difficulty reading or writing are often embarrassed and attempt to hide the problem. Pharmacists may not be able to detect this problem quickly or easily. Some clues that may indicate poor literacy in a patient include making excuses for not reading or writing due to a headache or having forgotten reading glasses. The patient may ask the pharmacist to fill out a check or write down information to take with him. The patient usually appears eager to follow the verbal instructions given and asks few questions. He or she may also ignore written information during the counseling session.

   If the pharmacist suspects that a patient has low literacy skills, he or she might say to the patient, "A lot of people have trouble reading and remembering these instructions. Does this ever happen to you?" Another strategy is to ask the patient, "Does anyone help you at home to take your medicine correctly?" That person usually reads for the patient also. In that case, the surrogate reader, who is usually another family member, should be present at the counseling session to understand the instructions so that he or she can reinforce the counseling information for the patient at home. Finally, the pharmacist may suggest peer-group literacy or health education classes where the patient can interact with other patients who have the same literacy issues.

   Suggested techniques to improve counseling include:
   - Careful verbal instructions; slow down if necessary; ask for recap of information
   - Pictograms or auxiliary labels that provide pictorial reminders to patient
   - Rewritten materials prepared for the appropriate reading level

- Video instructions
- Use of numbers, colors and shapes to distinguish meds
- Pill containers to keep medicines organized by day and time of dose
- Phone number for follow-up if patient forgets any verbal information provided

Preparing written materials for the low literacy patient. Most patients need help understanding the written counseling information that pharmacies provide from their computer systems or through other sources. Research has shown that health care materials are written at or above the 10th grade level.[15] However, the average American reads at the 8th or 9th grade level, and one in five patients read at or below the 5th grade level. According to the Center for Health Care Strategies, minorities, immigrants, and the elderly have a greater problem with literacy than the general population. More than 66% of Americans over the age of 60 have either marginal or inadequate literacy skills.[15]

Patients with low literacy skills have health care costs four times higher than patients with adequate literacy skills.[16] This is likely due to an increased rate of hospitalization because these patients make more medication errors, are less compliant with prescribed drug regimens, and have great difficulty working through the cumbersome health care system.[17]

Simple words, short sentences, large type, and use of "white" or unprinted space are useful techniques when preparing written materials for low literacy patients. Complicated medical or technical words should be replaced with simpler choices as previously described. Comic-strip formats may be useful for presenting drug information or demonstrating techniques to patients with low health literacy skills.[18]

However, it is important when using comic-strips or other types of illustrations that the materials do not appear to be condescending. The objective for a picture is the same as for written materials, to communicate an important concept. Therefore, pictures should focus on desired behaviors rather than on drug facts, and the information should be both culturally sensitive and relevant to the patient situation.[19,20]

The Foreign-Speaking Patient. The patient who does not speak English or understands very little English somewhat resembles both the hearing-impaired and the low literacy patient. This patient will have difficulty understanding both the verbal and the written communication provided by the pharmacist. The patient's name and dress may indicate that they are originally from another country and are not native English-speaking patients. The patient may respond in a foreign language or with a heavy accent to her English. The patient may seem confused or may respond inappropriately, either verbally or with inappropriate body language.

Suggested techniques to improve counseling include:
- Nonverbal cues and body language to communicate ideas to the patient
- Speak slowly; use simple, basic terminology
- Substitute numbers and calendars for written instructions
- Pictograms and auxiliary labels containing pictures or draw pictures for the patient
- Ask open-ended questions to see if the patient has understood your communication
- Reinforce information with accompanying family member whose English is more proficient

If a large percentage of the pharmacy's patient population speaks the same language, the following steps would be worth investigating:
- Learn the language or, at least, learn some key words
- Employ a translator, live or computerized; use printed instructions in other languages or manufacturers' videos in other languages

Comprehension Difficulties. Patients who have poor comprehension, whether it is caused by a psychiatric illness or mental retardation, are unable to process the information communicated and respond appropriately. Clues to the nature of the barrier may include psychiatric medications in the patient profile, patient address that indicates the patient lives in an institutional setting, inappropriate behavior, dress, or responses. While the patient barrier may be readily apparent, some patient behaviors may be easily confused with other types of barriers and will be evident only with time and repeated interactions with the patient.

Suggested techniques to improve counseling include:
- Patience, kindness, and extra attention to the nonverbal message since patients usually interpret nonverbal messages well
- Rephrase or carefully repeat when necessary; speak slowly and face patient

- Reassure patient as needed
- Ask for feedback from patient to assess level of understanding
- Keep it simple; use no jargon
- Prioritize the information to be given, stress the most important points, break into small segments of information
- Use association to daily activities
- Use calendar or containers to help organize and remember when to take medications
- Use demonstrations when appropriate
- Include caregiver or family member in conversation when possible

Counseling Children and Adolescents

The USP Pediatrics Advisory Panel and its *Ad Hoc* Advisory Panel on Children and Medicines have developed a position paper entitled *Ten Guiding Principles for Teaching Children and Adolescents About Medicines*.[21] These principles encourage activities that help children and adolescents to become active participants in their own health behavior, particularly with regard to medication use. The basic principles are provided in Table 97-4.

Suggestions for talking to children about their medications include:

- Talk to parents and children about how to protect young children from accidental poisoning and what to do if it occurs.
- When children are old enough to understand, speak directly with them about their medicines. Tell children what you expect them to do and why.
- Encourage children to ask you questions about their illness and treatment.

Health care professionals are often unsure of what information is appropriate to share with pediatric patients. Table 97-5 provides examples of questions children have about their medications classified by age. This provides some guidance about the type of information that is appropriate at different ages.

Table 97-4. Ten Guiding Principles for Teaching Children and Adolescents About Medicines

1. Children, as users of medicines, have a right to appropriate information about their medicines that reflects the child's health status, capabilities, and culture.
2. Children want to know. Health care providers and health educators should communicate directly with children about their medicines.
3. Children's interest in medicines should be encouraged, and they should be taught how to ask questions of health care providers, parents, and other caregivers about medicines and other therapies.
4. Children learn by example. The actions of parents and other caregivers should show children appropriate use of medicines.
5. Children, their parents, and their health care providers should negotiate the gradual transfer of responsibility for medicine use in ways that respect parental responsibilities and the health status and capabilities of the child.
6. Children's medicine education should take into account what children want to know about medicines, as well as what health professionals think children should know.
7. Children should receive basic information about medicines and their proper use as a part of school health education.
8. Children's medicine education should include information about the general use and misuse of medicines, as well as about the specific medicines the child is using.
9. Children have a right to information that will enable them to avoid poisoning through the misuse of medicines.
10. Children asked to participate in clinical trials (after parents' consent) have a right to receive appropriate information to promote their understanding before assent and participation.

From Doak CC, Doak, LG, Root JH. *Teaching Patients with Low Literacy Skills.* Philadelphia: JB Lippincott, 1996.

Table 97-5. What Children Want to Know about Medicines at Different Ages

Grades K-1
1. Why some medicines are only for children
2. How they can tell the difference between medicines for children and medicines for adults
3. The therapeutic purposes of medicines
4. Dose forms and ways of taking medicines
5. Importance of complying with the treatment regimen
6. The side effects of some medicines
7. That whether a medicine helps is not related to its color, size, or taste

Children Grades 2–5
1. What the ingredients (active and inactive) are in medicines
2. How medicines work and where medicines go in the body
3. How doctors know that a medicine works
4. Why there are different medicines for different illnesses
5. Why the same medicine can be for different illnesses
6. Why there are different medicines for a single illness
7. Why you should not take other people's medicines
8. How to ask questions of health care professionals about medicines
9. How to read labels
10. Difference between licit and illicit ("good" and "bad") drugs

Children Grades 6–8
1. Difference between prescription and OTC medicines
2. Meaning of dependency and addiction
3. How medicines are made
4. Why medicines come in different forms
5. Reasons for a special diet and time schedule when taking a medicine
6. Potential for drug interactions with other medicines and foods
7. Lack of a relationship between the efficacy of a medicine and its source or price
8. Difference between brand and generic medicines
9. Difference between medicines, botanicals/herbals, and homeopathics
10. How to select an appropriate over-the-counter medicine
11. *For children born outside of the US or whose parents are recent immigrants,* differences between medicines produced in their country of origin and medicines produced elsewhere

Concepts are based on information obtained in 1996 in focus groups of schoolchildren grades K-8 in Baltimore, MD, New York City, and Worcester, MA.
Adapted from Doak CC, Doak, LG, Root JH. *Teaching Patients with Low Literacy Skills.* Philadelphia: JB Lippincott, 1996.

Counseling the Elderly Patient

The most rapidly growing segment of the population, the elderly, present a great number of challenges to the communication skills of a pharmacist. The elderly patient may have several functional barriers. Vision and hearing are often impaired, and the patient may have difficulty removing child-proof tops, self-injecting insulin, or applying creams and ointments. Many elderly have low literacy skills as previously discussed. Additionally, cognitive impairments become more common with increasing age. As patients age, chronic conditions and the number of medications prescribed increase. Many of the techniques previously discussed with other barriers are useful when counseling elderly patients. In addition, pharmacists should consider the following:

- Additional time may be required to address the needs of the patient.
- Written information and compliance reminder aids are particularly helpful with large numbers of prescription products.

Studies indicate that an effective way to provide counseling to elderly patients is to provide small pieces of specific information coupled with a reminder aid and verbal reinforcement of the information.[23] It is also important for pharmacists to consider their own feelings about aging. One recommendation to increase empathy for elderly patients is to consider what the patient and the world were like when he or she was younger and to remember that the patient was not always old.[24]

Emotional Barriers

Regardless of the type of emotion the patient exhibits, dealing with a highly emotional patient is challenging for the pharmacist. Often the pharmacist is uncomfortable with the emotions expressed by the patient and responds inappropriately by ignoring the issue at hand or by focusing on trying to solve the patient's problem. When the pharmacist recognizes that a patient is in an emotional state, it is important to deal with the emotional barrier first. Discussing the patient's current medication needs will be ineffective while the patient is distracted by other issues. It is important, at the very least, to acknowledge the patient's concerns.

The most effective way to address patients' emotional concerns is to use empathic responses, also called reflective responding. Use of this technique requires that the pharmacist truly listens to what the patient is saying, both in words and nonverbal communication. Additionally, to be successful using this technique, the pharmacist must have a desire to understand and help the patient.

It is important to understand the meaning of empathy, a concept that is often confused with sympathy. When expressing sympathy, the pharmacist feels sorry for the patient. Empathy is a neutral process in which the pharmacist identifies with the feelings of the patient. This is sometimes described as putting yourself into the other person's shoes. It is not necessary to actually have experienced the same situation or emotion, but rather to try to understand how the patient feels. Using empathy tells the patient that the pharmacist is interested in him, and it is a positive step in building the pharmacist-patient relationship. Over time, the patient is more willing to voice questions and concerns to the pharmacist thereby improving the quality of care the pharmacist can provide.

Expressing empathy to the patient is accomplished through the use of a reflective response. A reflective response is the pharmacist's way of communicating to the patient his or her understanding of the patient's feelings. It acknowledges the patient's feelings and usually has a calming effect on the patient that may allow the pharmacist to proceed with the counseling session.

How to Formulate a Reflective Response

The starting point for formulating a reflective response is to mentally paraphrase what the patient has expressed and to state that for the patient. Examples of phrases that often begin a reflective response include the following:

- "It sounds like . . . "
- "I gather that . . . "
- "What I hear you saying is . . . "
- "It seems that . . . "
- "In other words . . . "
- "If I understand you correctly . . . "
- It appears that you are saying . . . "

Use of this type of response tells the patient that the pharmacist is listening and is trying to understand the patient's concerns. It also tells the patient what the pharmacist thinks he or she is feeling. This allows the patient the opportunity to reply affirmatively or gesture that the pharmacist has correctly understood the situation. If the pharmacist has misinterpreted the patient's feeling, he or she will usually correct the pharmacist's misimpression.

What Reflective Responses Are Not

It is often easier to understand a good reflective response by looking at statements that are not truly empathic. The most common errors in attempting to express empathy are to offer advice or judge the patient. Some examples will illustrate the most common errors pharmacists make in attempting empathic responding.

Mr. Roberts, a regular patient in the pharmacy (looking worried and upset): *"My doctor says I might need to have surgery if this drug doesn't work."*

Pharmacist 1: *"Oh, there is no need to worry. I'm sure this medication will work and everything will be fine."*

Pharmacist 1 makes a judgment about the patient's concerns and tells the patient that he is wrong to be concerned. This response may actually make the patient feel worse and lets him know that the pharmacist does not understand his concerns.

Pharmacist 2: *"You should get a second opinion from another doctor before you think about having surgery. Maybe it won't really be necessary."*

Pharmacist 3: *"You shouldn't think that far ahead. Maybe the medication will work and you would have worried for nothing."*

Pharmacist 2 and 3 provide advice to the patient about what he should do but do not acknowledge his current feelings and concerns. Advice, even when it is appropriate, should be deferred to a later time in the conversation if at all.

Pharmacist 4: *"I know how you feel. My mother just went through the same experience. But it all ended up okay."*

Pharmacist 4 is engaging in deflecting behavior. This pharmacist takes the focus from the patient to himself. While it may seem appropriate to give an example of a similar experience that tells the patient you have experienced the same feelings, this type of response brings the pharmacist's feelings into the conversation rather than focusing on the patient concerns.

Pharmacist 5: *"Have you asked your doctor about one of the new medications for this condition?"*

When pharmacists feel uncomfortable dealing with the patient's emotions and concerns, they frequently concentrate on facts and question asking. While information gathering is important in a patient counseling session, it is not appropriate at this point in the conversation when calming the patient is the primary goal.

While each of these responses seems like a sincere attempt to be helpful to the patient, none of them is a reflecting response. Remember that the primary purpose of empathic responding is understanding and acknowledging the patient's feelings not solving the patient's problem. Examples of appropriate reflecting responses for Mr. Roberts include:

Pharmacist: It sounds like you are worried about the possibility of having surgery.

Pharmacist: I can see that you are concerned about whether the new medicine will work so you won't need surgery. Let's take a few minutes to talk about how to use the new medicine so that you can get the best possible effect from it.

These responses acknowledge the patient's worry and the pharmacist's understanding of why he is worried. The second response continues after addressing the patient's concern to offering patient counseling and the benefit to the patient in participating in that process. Ultimately, the purpose of empathic responding is to move the patient to a mental and emotional state that will allow the pharmacist to continue with the patient counseling session.

It takes time and practice to become proficient in using reflective responses. Pharmacists may choose to practice these techniques on family, friends, and patients with whom they already have good relationships prior to attempting these techniques on difficult patients.

When Reflective Responses Don't Work

Obviously, reflective responses will be unsuccessful if the pharmacist is not skillful at this process. As stated previously, this skill can be improved through practice. Sometimes, the process will not work regardless of the skill of the pharmacist. The patient's emotional state may be too highly charged to respond to a brief interaction with a pharmacist. The patient may be irrational due to psychiatric illness or the influence of drugs. The pharmacist must maintain a cool demeanor and utilize assertiveness techniques when required. When it is obvious that these techniques will be unsuccessful, the pharmacist may terminate the interaction.

THE ANGRY PATIENT—Perhaps the most common and difficult emotional situation a pharmacist faces on a daily basis is the angry patient. Patients may be angry when they arrive at the pharmacy for a variety of reasons—time spent at the doctor's office, concerns over health or health care costs, or frustration over dealing with the complexities of the health care system, just to name a few. It may be helpful to recognize that anger is a secondary emotion.[16] The patient may begin by feeling fear, hurt, anxiety, or frustration over events not under the person's control. The most effective techniques to deal with patient anger are assertive.

Assertiveness is a neutral expression of one's personal rights, feelings, and beliefs that does not violate the rights of others. It sets boundaries for what behavior is acceptable. Assertiveness techniques that may be useful in dealing with patients who are angry or aggressive include the following:

- Language ownership–This is the demonstration of owning your feelings and emotions. Rather than using nonspecific terms, speak in the first person. For example, when speaking to a verbally abusive patient, don't respond with:
  "Everyone one in the pharmacy hates it when you talk to them in that tone."
  To use ownership language, say *"I feel angry and uncomfortable when you speak to me in a condescending tone and use inappropriate words."*
- Specificity–Clearly state what your needs and expectations of the other person are. For example, when speaking to a patient who has made several unreasonable demands, don't respond with:
  "You are being totally unreasonable."
  To use language specificity, say *"It is not appropriate to ask me to refill a prescription that is not authorized for refills without an approval from your doctor. That would be a violation of pharmacy laws."*

WHEN PATIENTS REFUSE PATIENT COUNSELING

Patients may decline the offer of patient counseling because they don't value taking the time to participate in the counseling process. Other patients may be rushed for time or distracted by other concerns that prevent them from listening to information about their prescription medications. When this happens, the pharmacist should be sure to give the patient written counseling materials along with the phone number of the pharmacy. The patient should be encouraged to call the pharmacy to discuss any concerns that she has at a more appropriate time. The pharmacist may offer to make an appointment with the patient for counseling over the telephone at a later date.

CONDUCTING A PATIENT MEDICATION INTERVIEW

In order to provide the best possible patient care, a pharmacist must collect information from the patient about current and past medication use as well as medical conditions and life-style information (Fig 97-2). This information serves as a database for the pharmacist to help patients achieve the best possible

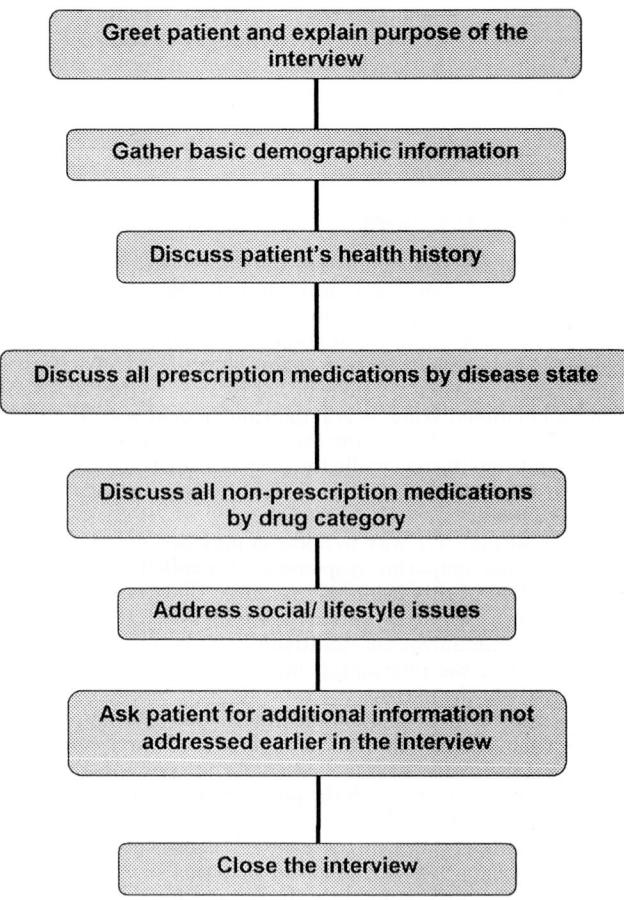

Figure 97-2. Steps in a patient medication history interview.

outcomes of drug therapy. This process has several purposes for the pharmacist and patient:

- Helps to establish the pharmacist-patient relationship
- Provides a basis for assessing the appropriateness and effectiveness of past and present medications
- Assists the pharmacist in solving current drug-related problems and preventing future problems

It is preferable to conduct medication interviews by appointment since this process will take a minimum of 20–30 minutes and possibly longer for patients who have extensive medication histories. The interview should take place in a private setting due to the confidential nature of information to be discussed. Some pharmacists prefer to give the patient a blank medication profile and ask the patient to fill out the form and bring it to the interview. If this technique is used, the pharmacist should work through the form with the patient to confirm and complete the information provided by the patient.

Utilizing a standard format when conducting medication interviews ensures that important information is not overlooked in the process. A logical structure for the patient interview is suggested below.

Steps in the Patient Medication Interview

1. *Greeting and purpose of the interview*
   The patient should be greeted and the pharmacist should make introductions if the patient is not already known to the pharmacist. The patient should be put at ease with some small talk. The

purpose of the session and the benefits to the patient should be outlined. The patient should be assured that the information gathered will be held in confidence.

2. *Gathering of basic information*
Basic information such as complete name, address, phone number, birth date, all regular health care providers, insurance information, and occupation should be gathered.

3. *Patient's health history*
The patient should be asked about all current and past medical conditions including the symptoms experienced and the duration of the illness. Female patients of child-bearing age should be asked if they are pregnant or breastfeeding. Allergies and the type of reaction the patient experienced upon exposure to the substance should be determined.

4. *Prescription medication use*
Each medical condition identified above should be addressed in turn. The patient should be asked to describe all medications in current use including the name, strength of the drug, prescriber, dosage form and route of administration, dosing schedule including how the patient adheres to the prescribed regimen, the patient's perception of how well the medication works, adverse effects that the patient has experienced and the steps taken to relieve those effects. The patient should also describe all past medications used for a particular condition and the reasons why the medication was discontinued. The medications used for each condition should be discussed in turn.

5. *Nonprescription medication use*
The patient should be asked to describe the use of all products purchased without a prescription. This includes all typical over-the-counter products as well as dietary supplements and herbal products. Patients often have difficulty remembering these products and their use. Prompters that the pharmacist might use include asking in turn about the major categories of products. For example, "Mrs. Jennings, do you take any products to treat symptoms of cough, cold, or allergies?" The pharmacist should ask the same follow-up questions about how the products are used that are asked for the prescription products.

6. *Life-style issues*
Asking patients about life-style issues as well as the use of recreational drugs is best left until the end of the interview when the patient has become comfortable with the pharmacist and the process. The pharmacist should explain that use of these products may affect drug therapy and a clear understanding of the extent of use of these products is necessary for the best patient care. Remind the patient that this information is strictly confidential. The patient should be given the option of refusing to provide this type of information. The patient should be asked about use of tobacco products and alcohol as well as recreational drugs.

7. *Closing the interview*
After completing the systematic collection of information, the pharmacist should offer the patient the opportunity to add any additional information he or she wishes to share or to ask any questions. The pharmacist should reiterate that all information collected will be held in confidence unless there is a need to discuss some of the information with another health care provider in the course of providing care for the patient. The pharmacist will need time to review the information and formulate any recommendations that should be made to the patient. A follow-up appointment should be scheduled with the patient for this purpose. The patient should be thanked for taking the time to complete the interview.

SUMMARY

In summary, the pharmacist-patient relationship is an important one in health care. The relationship that is built on effective communication and trust and established over time may be related to better patient health outcomes. This chapter explained the communication process, introduced the concept of patient empowerment, described pharmacist counseling and communication skills, reviewed a model patient counseling session, a model medication history process and presented steps and techniques for counseling patients who present to the pharmacy with barriers. It is imperative that future health care professionals and pharmacists understand the need for effective communication and the link with patient health behavior.

REFERENCES

1. Mock KD. *Physician's News Digest* February 2001. http://www.physiciansnews.com/law/201.html. accessed February 7, 2003.
2. Ranelli PL, Svarstad BL, Boh L. *Am J Hosp Pharm* 1989; 46:267.
3. Meichenbaum D., Turk DC. *Facilitating Treatment Adherence: Practitioner's Guidebook.* New York: Plenum Press; 1987.
4. Britten N, Stevenson, FA, Barry, CA, et al. *BMJ* 2000; 320 (8233):484.
5. Feste C. *Diabetes Care* 1992; 15(7):922.
6. Funnell MM, et al. *The Diabetes Educator* 1991; 17(1):37.
7. *USP Medication Counseling Behavior Guidelines.* Rockville, MD: USP Convention, Inc., Feb 1997.
8. Beardsley RS, Johnson CA, Wise G. *J Am Pharm Assoc* 1977; NS17:366.
9. Muldary TW. *Interpersonal Relations for Health Professionals—A Social Skills Approach.* New York: MacMillan, 1983.
10. Knapp DA. *Am J Pharm Educ* 1979; 43(4):357.
11. Rantucci MJ. *Pharmacists Talking with Patients: A Guide to Patient Counseling.* Philadelphia: Williams and Wilkins, 1997.
12. Galanti G. *Caring for Patients from Different Cultures.* Philadelphia: University of Pennsylvania Press, 1997.
13. *Words to Watch Fact Sheet.* Partnership for Clear Health Communication, available at http://www.askme3.org, accessed 6/10/03.
14. *The Pharmacist-Patient Consultation Program PPCP-Unit 2, How to Counsel Patients in Challenging Situations:* New York: Pfizer, 1993.
15. Doak CC, Doak, LG, Root JH. *Teaching Patients with Low Literacy Skills.* Philadelphia: JB Lippincott, 1996.
16. Weiss BD. *20 Common Problems in Primary Care.* New York: McGraw-Hill. 1999.
17. Baker DW, Parker RM, Williams MV, et al. *J Gen Intern Med* 1998; 13:791.
18. Hohn MD. *Empowerment Health Education in Adult Literacy: A Guide for Public Health and Adult Literacy Practitioners, Policy Makers and Funders.* System for Adult Basic Education Support at Northern Essex Community College. Lawrence, MA, 1998.
19. Ad Hoc Committee on Health Literacy for the Council on Scientific Affairs, American Medical Association. *JAMA* 1999; 281: 552–57.
20. Center for Health Care Strategies, Inc. "Provider Strategies to Help Low-Literate Patients," 1998. Available at: http://www.chcs org/resource/hl.html
21. *Ten Guiding Principles for Teaching Children and Adolescents About Medicines, A Position Statement of the United States Pharmacopeia.* Rockville, MD: Division of Information Development, United States Pharmacopeia, Feb 1997.
22. Berger BA. Communication Skills for Pharmacist. Washington DC: Jobson Publishing, 2002.
23. Ascione F, Shimp L. *Drug Intell Clin Pharm* 1984; 18(11):926.
24. Currie CT. *Talking with Patients: A Basic Clinical Skill.* Oxford: Oxford University Press, 1992.

BIBLIOGRAPHY

Tindall W, Beardsley RS, Kimberlin, CL, et al. *Communication Skills in Pharmacy Practice: A Practical Guide for Students and Practitioners.* Baltimore: Lippincott Williams & Wilkins, 2002.
Rantucci MJ. *Pharmacists Talking with Patients: A Guide to Patient Counseling.* Baltimore: Lippincott Williams & Wilkins, 1997.
Berger BA. *Communication Skills for Pharmacists: Building Relationships, Improving Patient Care.* Washington DC: Jobson Publishing, 2002.
Meldrum H. *Interpersonal Communication in Pharmaceutical Care.* New York: Pharmaceutical Products Press, 1994.
The Pharmacist-Patient Consultation Program PPCP-Unit 1, An Interactive Approach to Verify Patient Understanding; New York: Pfizer, 1993.
The Pharmacist-Patient Consultation Program PPCP-Unit 2, How to Counsel Patients in Challenging Situations: New York: Pfizer, 1993.
The Pharmacist-Patient Consultation Program PPCP-Unit 3,Counseling to Enhance Compliance: New York: Pfizer, 1995.

WEBSITES

http://www.usp.org
http://www.askme3.org/
http://www.plainlanguage.gov/

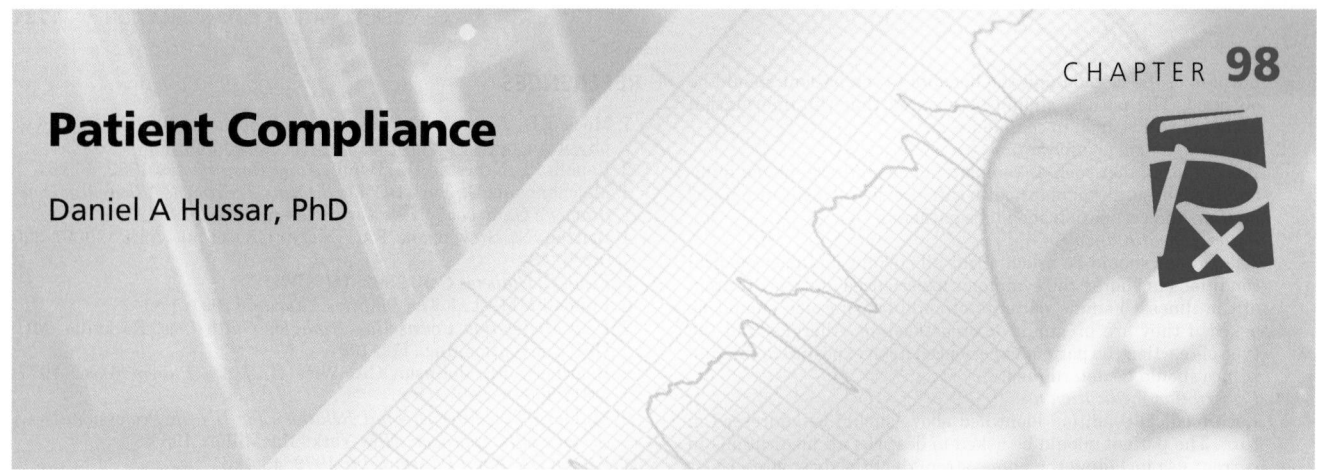

CHAPTER 98

Patient Compliance

Daniel A Hussar, PhD

The important advances that have been made in the understanding of the etiology of many disease states, and the development of many new therapeutic agents, have made it possible to cure or provide symptomatic control of many clinical disorders. However, accompanying the increasing sophistication relative to diagnostic and therapeutic knowledge and skills has been the recognition that in many circumstances, drugs are not being used in a manner conducive to optimal benefit and safety. In many situations, efforts to maintain or improve health fall short of the goals that are considered attainable, and frequently, the failure to achieve the desired outcomes has been attributable to patient noncompliance or partial compliance.

With regard to the provision of health care, the concept of compliance can be viewed broadly, as it relates to instructions concerning diet, exercise, rest, return appointments, etc, in addition to the use of drugs. However, it is in discussions concerning drug therapy that the designation *patient compliance* is employed most frequently. It is in this context that it will be used in this discussion, and compliance can be defined as the extent to which an individual's behavior coincides with medical or health instructions/advice.

Compliance with therapy implies an understanding of how the medication is to be used, as well as a positive behavior in which the patient is motivated sufficiently to use the prescribed treatment in the manner intended, because of a perceived self-benefit and a positive outcome (eg, enhanced daily functioning and well-being). Some have recommended the use of the terms *adherence* or *concordance* rather than the designation *compliance;* however, the latter term continues to be the most widely accepted and used.

The term *persistence* is also used to identify the duration of time over which a patient continues to take prescribed medication.

Problems concerning patient compliance with instructions have been recognized for years and, indeed, Hippocrates once cautioned, "Keep watch also on the fault of patients which often makes them lie about the taking of things prescribed." Twenty-three centuries later, attaining patient compliance in the use of their medications continues to represent a formidable challenge for health care providers.

When the complexity of the patient's illnesses and the actions of potent therapeutic agents are taken into account, the physician, pharmacist, and other health professionals easily can become preoccupied with the diagnosis of the disease state as well as the selection and implications of drug therapy and assume that the patient will follow the instructions provided. After all, since the medication is being provided to improve and/or maintain the patient's health, why would the patient not follow instructions? Yet, studies continue to show that a large percentage of patients, for a variety of reasons, do not take their medication in the manner intended.

Although some patients make a conscious decision to deviate from the prescribed regimen (ie, *intentional* noncompliance), many intend to take their medication according to instructions and, in some cases, even may be unaware that their use of medication differs from what the prescriber intended.

The term *patient noncompliance* suggests that the patient is at fault for the inappropriate use of medication. Although this is often the case, in a number of situations, the physician and pharmacist have not provided the patient with adequate instructions or have not presented the instructions in such a manner that the patient understands them. The most basic questions regarding drug usage must be addressed—Has the patient been provided with adequate instructions? Does the patient understand how the medication is to be taken? Nothing should be taken for granted regarding the patient's understanding of how to use medication, and appropriate steps must be taken to provide patients with the information and counseling necessary to use their medications as effectively and as safely as possible.

NONCOMPLIANCE

Types

The situations most commonly associated with noncompliance with drug therapy include failure to have the prescription dispensed or renewed, omission of doses, errors of dosage, incorrect administration, errors in the time of administration, and premature discontinuation.

Some patients for whom medication has been prescribed do not even take their prescriptions to a pharmacy, and some others who do take their prescriptions to a pharmacy fail to pick them up when they are completed. In a survey[1] of consumers, 2% responded that they had brought prescriptions to the pharmacy but failed to pick them up. The most common explanations for not taking the prescriptions to a pharmacy or not picking them up are that patients feel that they have recovered from the condition or otherwise don't need the medication, they think they have a similar medicine at home, they don't like to take medicine, the cost is too high, or they forget to pick up the prescription from the pharmacy. In the many situations in which infection is associated with fever and local discomfort, patients already may be taking nonprescription medications, such as acetaminophen. The ability of these agents to provide some, if not complete, relief of the symptoms of early infection may lead some patients to conclude that the condition is improving, or better, and that it is not necessary to have a prescription dispensed.

The omission of doses is one of the most common types of noncompliance and is more likely to occur when a medication is to be administered at frequent intervals and/or for an extended period of time. Errors of dosage include situations in which the amount of an individual dose or frequency of administration is incorrect.

Examples of the incorrect administration of medication include not using the proper technique in using metered-dose inhalers and, in some cases, giving medication by the wrong route of administration. Errors in the time of administration of the drug may include situations in which medication is administered in an inappropriate relationship to meals. Certain drugs—eg, tetracycline, alendronate (Fosamax)—should be administered apart from meals to achieve optimal absorption. The time of day at which a drug is administered also may be important in the use of some medications; eg, diuretics are best administered in the morning.

The premature discontinuation of treatment occurs commonly with the use of antibiotics as well as medications used in the treatment of chronic disorders such as hypertension. Patients must be apprised of the importance of taking the medication in the manner instructed, even though their condition may be asymptomatic or, as in the case of infections, the symptoms may have subsided soon after the initiation of therapy.

Studies reflect a wide variation in the degree of noncompliance. Many reports indicate that at least one-third of patients failed to comply with instructions, and for patients with chronic illnesses on long-term treatment regimens the results suggest a rate of noncompliance of approximately 50%.

Consequences

The importance and scope of the difficulties that result from the failure to use medications in the manner intended have resulted in the National Council on Patient Information and Education designating noncompliance as *America's other drug problem,* and others have described it as an "invisible epidemic."[2] Others have noted that noncompliance may be the most significant problem that faces medicine today[3] and that "knowledge of patient compliance is of critical importance in interpreting drug response, whether it be in the individual patient or in a clinical trial."[4] In response to concerns regarding mismedication among elderly patients, including observations that 55% of this patient population is noncompliant, the Office of the Inspector General conducted a study to determine why elderly people fail to follow prescription medication regimens.[5]

"Drugs don't work if people don't take them." This observation made by former Surgeon General C Everett Koop in his keynote address at a symposium on *Improving Medication Compliance,*[6] provides a clear statement of one of the consequences of noncompliance. In many cases noncompliance results in *underuse* of a drug, thereby depriving the patient of the anticipated therapeutic benefits and possibly resulting in a progressive worsening or other complications of the condition being treated.

Noncompliance also may result in the *overuse* of a drug. When excessive doses are employed or when the medication is given more frequently than intended, there is an increased risk of adverse reactions. These problems may develop rather innocently, as when a patient recognizes that he has forgotten a dose of medication and doubles the next dose to make up for it. Some other patients appear to believe that if the one-tablet dose that has been prescribed provides some relief of symptoms, two or three tablets will be even more effective.

Numerous hospital admissions and nursing-home admissions are related to noncompliance. In a study of 315 consecutive medical admissions of elderly patients to a community hospital, 28% were medication-related—17% because of adverse reactions and 11% because of noncompliance.[7] A review of published studies of drug-related hospital admissions noted that 11 reports indicated that 22.7% of adverse drug reaction hospitalizations were induced by noncompliance.[8]

Hypertension is the most frequently studied disease with regard to compliance. Although educational and screening programs have significantly reduced the number of individuals who are unaware that they have hypertension, it is thought that most of the more than 50 million Americans with high blood pressure do not have their condition under good control. For those hypertensive patients for whom treatment has been prescribed, many do not have their blood pressure under effective control, and a major reason for the failure to control hypertension is noncompliance with regimens that would work if administered as intended. Noncompliance is one of the most commonly missed diagnoses, and the manner in which patients use their medication should be evaluated before the therapeutic regimen is changed. In one study it is reported that the underuse of antihypertensive medications may be associated with hospitalization that could have been prevented if patients had complied with their treatment regimens.[9]

The statins (eg, atorvastatin [Lipitor], simvastatin [Zocor]) have been shown to significantly reduce morbidity and mortality in patients with coronary heart disease and in patients with hyperlipidemia, when they are used on a continuing basis. However, in two recent studies, compliance with statin therapy declined more than 25% in the first 6 months after the original prescription, with further declines in compliance occurring the longer the patients were followed.[10,11]

Noncompliance has major implications for those with HIV infection/AIDS. The complexity of the treatment regimens used in the treatment of HIV infection/AIDS and its complications results in a "pill burden" that is often associated with noncompliance. Surveys have demonstrated that approximately one-third of the patients missed doses during the 3-day period prior to the surveys. The Guidelines for the Use of Antiretroviral Agents in HIV-1-Infected Adults and Adolescents include the following observations:

"Adherence is a key determinant in the degree and duration of virologic suppression. Among studies reporting on the association between suboptimal adherence and virologic failure, nonadherence among patients on HAART (highly active antiretroviral therapy) was the strongest predictor for the failure to achieve viral suppression below the level of detection."[12]

An additional concern is that the irregular treatment that results from noncompliance appears to accelerate the emergence of resistant strains of HIV.

It has been observed that about one-half of patients with schizophrenia are noncompliant in using their medications and experience a relapse of symptoms within a year of initiation of antipsychotic treatment. The inadequate control of schizophrenia has, in some situations, been associated with violent actions.

One report[13] has called attention to the hazards of noncompliance with antiepileptic drug regimens. In examining autopsy records pertaining to 11 cases of unattended, unexpected deaths of epileptic patients, no antiepileptic drugs were found in 4 patients and subtherapeutic concentrations were noted in 6 others. It is suggested that a number of these deaths may have been preventable had there been better compliance with the instructions for using the medication(s).

Similarly, a leading cause of death in transplant patients, some of whom had waited for years for a donor organ, is the rejection that results from noncompliance in using immunosuppressant medication.[14]

The economic consequences of noncompliance also are alarming, and some have estimated that the costs associated with noncompliance in the US exceed $100 billion a year. The cost of noncompliance and the capacity of improved compliance to reduce health-care expenditures are the subject of a review of a number of studies in which it is observed that the benefits realized from improved compliance outweigh, in some cases far outweigh, the costs of programs designed to improve compliance."[15]

Noncompliance also may take other forms. The problems associated with drug misuse and abuse, whether unintentional or deliberate, are well recognized. Although usually not thought of in terms of noncompliance, drug-abuse problems sometimes result from excessive use of medications that have been prescribed for existing clinical disorders.

Another implication relates to the storage of drugs that are not used completely during the intended period of treatment. Keeping these drugs may result in their inappropriate use at some later time. Accidental poisonings have resulted, and stockpiled medications have been used to commit suicide.

The recognition that noncompliance is so prevalent has raised questions regarding the attention this variable has received in clinical studies of therapeutic agents. For example, an analysis of the sources and the amount of overt and hidden bias in reports of double-blind studies of nonsteroidal anti-inflammatory drugs published between 1966 and 1985 revealed that only 13% of the studies measured compliance.[16] The potential changes in therapeutic response resulting from noncompliance dictate that close attention be given to this aspect of the study of the action of therapeutic agents.

Although the consideration of the consequences of noncompliance should focus primarily on the problems that may develop, there also should be an awareness of situations in which some patients may benefit from being noncompliant. Designated by one investigator[17] as *intelligent noncompliance,* it is noted that certain individuals have a rational basis (eg, avoiding adverse effects) for altering the dosage of their medication, and that good treatment outcomes are still attained. However, the fact that certain patients may benefit from not complying with a treatment regimen must not be considered a reason for health professionals to be less diligent in detecting noncompliance and initiating the appropriate corrective measures, as any situation in which noncompliance occurs requires careful evaluation.

Detection

Like the diagnosis of medical disorders, detection of noncompliance is a necessary prerequisite for adequate treatment. In addition, like many diseases, compliant or noncompliant behavior is not stable and may change over time, necessitating the regular use of detection methods to measure this behavior as part of the assessment of treatment efficacy.

The ideal detection method would measure compliance at the time and place of the medication-taking (or other treatment) event. Direct observation of the patient would come closest to providing this ideal measure of compliance. However, this method usually is not practical.

Current detection methods include indirect measures, such as self-report, interview, therapeutic outcome, pill count, change in the weight of metered-dose inhaler canisters, medication-refill rate, insurance prescription claims databases, and computerized compliance monitors, and direct measures, such as biological markers, tracer compounds, and assay of body fluids. In general, the direct methods of detection have a higher sensitivity and specificity than the indirect methods. However, all of these methods have their limitations. To help overcome limitations of the assessment methods and to provide corroborative information, it is recommended that at least two different detection methods be used to measure compliance.

INDIRECT METHODS—Self-reports and interviews with patients are the most common and simplest methods of attempting to determine compliance with therapy. However, many studies have demonstrated that even the most skilled and highly refined interviewing techniques substantially overestimate medication compliance. In spite of the limitations of interviews, asking carefully constructed questions (eg, "Most people have trouble remembering to take their medicine. Do you have trouble remembering to take yours?")[18] in a nonthreatening manner will help to identify some noncompliant patients.

Pill counts are another detection method used to measure compliance and frequently are used in clinical drug studies. A patient's compliance with a medication regimen can be assessed by the difference between the number of dosage units initially dispensed and the number remaining in the container on a return visit or during an unscheduled home visit. However, *pill dumping* (ie, attempts by patients to misrepresent their compliance by discarding medication) is common, and several studies have shown that return counts grossly overestimate actual compliance rates.[19,20]

The achievement of treatment goals sometimes has been used as a measure of a patient's compliance. When a particular treatment is associated with a successful outcome (eg, normal blood pressure, glucose concentration, or intraocular pressure), satisfactory compliance with the regimen may be inferred. However, patients may *load-up* on medication or comply with other treatment regimens (eg, diet) just before their return visit. Such behavior has been called the *toothbrush effect,* after the way people brush their teeth just before seeing a dentist. The toothbrush effect can invalidate almost completely the health-outcome strategy, as well as certain other detection methods (eg, determination of drug concentrations in a body fluid).

Computerized compliance monitors are the most recent and reliable of the indirect-detection methods, but their cost may preclude their use in most practice settings. The Medication Event Monitoring System (MEMS) is a microprocessor housed in the cap of the medication container. Each time the patient removes the cap, the time and date are recorded. Data are retrieved by connecting the microprocessor unit to a computer. The data not only provide an indication of individual dosing patterns, but also allow correlations with clinical events. Such data might be useful to the clinician in understanding why treatment has not been fully successful. Although the computerized monitors provide no direct information on whether or how much medication was actually taken, their use helps to supplement other methods. For example, in one study[21] in which pill counts indicated near-perfect compliance, the monitor in the cap showed that fewer than half of all cap openings occurred at the prescribed interval of 12 ± 2 hr.

In a study designed to compare multiple measures of compliance with the use of HIV protease inhibitors, it is noted that compliance may be underestimated by MEMS and overestimated by pill count and interview.[23] These investigators also combined these three measures to determine a composite adherence score (CAS) that was more clearly related to clinical outcome than any of the three measures used individually.

DIRECT METHODS—Biological markers and tracer compounds indicate patient compliance over an extended period. For example, measurement of glycosylated hemoglobin in patients with diabetes mellitus gives an objective assessment of metabolic control during the preceding 3-month period. Tracer compounds—small amounts of agents with long half-lives such as phenobarbital—have been added to drugs in some studies and measured in biological fluids as pharmacological indicators of compliance.

Finally, compliance also has been measured through determination of drug concentrations in patients' biological fluids. However, the usefulness of data on drug concentrations in biological fluids is limited because (1) concentrations of drugs are affected by individual differences in absorption, distribution, metabolism, and excretion, and low or erratic drug concentrations are not necessarily an indication of noncompliance[22]; (2) drug concentrations do not provide data regarding the timing of doses consumed; and (3) brief intake of rapidly cleared drugs before testing can produce results that show adequate drug concentrations, erroneously suggesting regular medication use.

The Noncompliant Patient

Efforts have been made to demonstrate the relationship of noncompliance to a number of variables such as age, education, occupation, socioeconomic status, personality factors, physiological variables, and the number, types, and severity of illnesses. Although certain patterns have been noted in some studies, the results, in general, have been inconsistent, and it continues to be difficult to identify which patients are most likely to be noncompliant.

A distinction has been made between attitudinal and behavioral compliance, since often the attitude and behavior of a patient may be incongruent. For example, patients fully may intend to take the medication according to instructions but actually not do so because they are forgetful or really do not understand the instructions. On the other hand, some patients may have no intention of complying but nevertheless do so.

Some individuals are intentionally noncompliant, and this further underscores the complexity of the challenge to develop strategies to improve compliance. Although considerable progress has been made in recognizing and addressing the problems associated with noncompliance, an observation made in an early discussion of this subject continues to be valid today—"It has not proved possible to identify an uncooperative type. Every patient is a potential defaulter; compliance can never be assumed."[24] In a recent commentary on the challenge of attaining compliance, the authors observe: "Bluntly, we are very human physicians in corruptible institutions treating fallible patients. Everyone takes shortcuts. This is the ragged edge of medicine in the 21st century."[25]

Considerable attention has been directed toward the sociobehavioral determinants of compliance, and a number of models based on behavioral principles have been described.[26] A *health-belief model*, which initially was developed[27] to explain preventive health behaviors such as obtaining immunizations and prophylactic dental care, was revised subsequently[28] to apply to compliance with prescribed medical regimens. A *third-generation* model was then proposed[3] that focuses more specifically on health decisions. This *health-decision* model combines decision analysis, behavioral decision theory, and health beliefs to yield a model of health decisions and resultant behavior. The components of this model and the manner in which they are interrelated are outlined in Figure 98-1.

With respect to the relationship between health beliefs and compliance, if compliance is to be achieved, patients must believe that

They actually have the illness that has been diagnosed.
The illness could cause severe consequences with regard to their health and daily functioning.
The treatment prescribed will reduce the present or future severity of the condition.
The benefits of the regimen prescribed outweigh the perceived disadvantages and costs of following the recommended action.

In addition, there must be a stimulus to trigger the advocated health behavior, which can be either internal (eg, concern about the disease) or external (eg, interaction with the physician or pharmacist).

Patient education and counseling initiatives should be designed to encourage the beliefs noted above, particularly since many patients believe that "you only need to take medication when you are ill and experience symptoms" and/or "you need to stop taking medication once in awhile or else your body becomes dependent on it or the medication will become less effective."

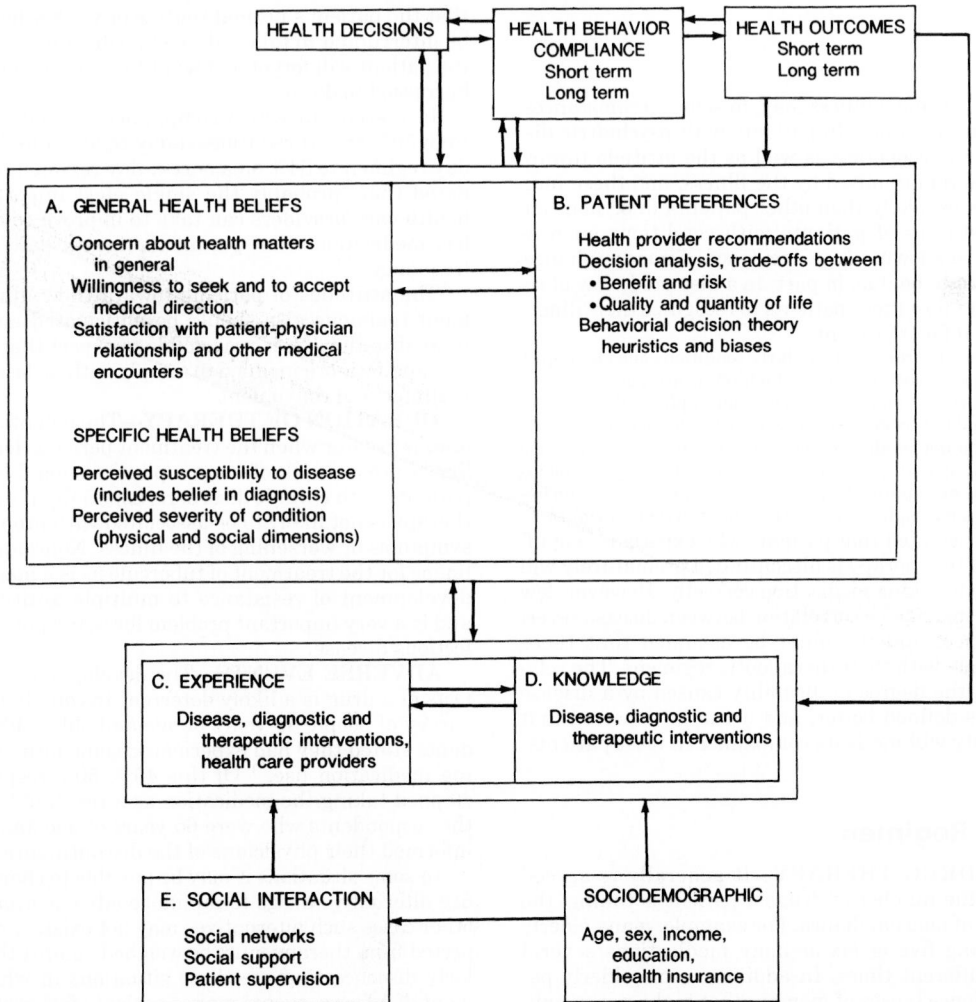

Figure 98-1. The health-decision model, combining the health-belief model and patient preferences, including decision analysis and behavioral decision theory. (From Eraker SA, et al. *Ann Intern Med* 1984; 100:258.)

There are also other *patient factors* that may contribute to noncompliance. Patients who live alone are less likely to comply than those who live with another family member who can take an interest in and/or supervise their therapy. The increasing problems of drug abuse and addiction have increased the awareness and concern about becoming dependent on agents that are prescribed for legitimate medical reasons. Although drugs that carry a potential for abuse and development of dependence often are prescribed and used too casually, some patients develop a fear of dependence regarding use of any drug that is to be employed for a prolonged period. To avoid such a possibility or to prove to themselves that they are not dependent, they may interrupt or stop therapy or use the medication in smaller amounts.

Numerous other factors have been suggested to contribute to patient noncompliance, and the most important of these are considered in the following discussion.

FACTORS ASSOCIATED WITH NONCOMPLIANCE

In addition to the patient factors previously considered, a number of other determinants of patient compliance have been cited. Some of the more important and/or commonly considered factors are discussed below. Although the relationship of some of these factors to the occurrence of noncompliance has not been proven, there should be an awareness of the potential implications in selected patients.

Disease

The nature of the patient's illness may, in some circumstances, contribute to noncompliance. In patients with psychiatric disorders, the ability to cooperate as well as the attitude toward treatment may be compromised by the illness, and these individuals may be more likely than other patients to be noncompliant. Several studies of patients with conditions such as schizophrenia have shown a high incidence of noncompliance, and this is thought to be due, in part, to a distorted view of reality that does not allow these patients to recognize their illness as well as the need for treatment.

Patients with chronic disorders, particularly conditions such as hypertension and hypercholesterolemia, which often are not associated with symptoms are also more likely to be noncompliers. Patients understandably tend to become discouraged with extended therapeutic programs that do not produce cures of the conditions. Even when cures can be anticipated as a result of long-term therapy, problems still can occur, as exemplified by patients with tuberculosis who frequently become noncompliant as the treatment period continues.

It might be anticipated that patients who experience significant symptoms if the therapy is discontinued prematurely will be more attentive to taking medication correctly. However, few studies have demonstrated a correlation between disease severity and compliance, and it cannot be assumed that these patients will comply with their therapeutic regimens. The relationship between the degree of disability caused by a disease and compliance is defined better, and it can be expected that increased disability will motivate compliance in most patients.

Therapeutic Regimen

MULTIPLE DRUG THERAPY—It generally is agreed that the greater the number of drugs a patient is taking, the higher is the risk of noncompliance. For example, many elderly patients are taking five or six or more medications several times a day at different times. In addition, some elderly patients may experience lapses of memory that make noncompliance even more likely. Even when specific dosage instructions for the medications are provided, problems still can occur.

The similarity of appearance (eg, size, color, or shape) of certain drugs may contribute to the confusion that can exist in the use of multiple drugs. It is desirable that there be an awareness of the physical characteristics of the drugs used, so that the patient will not be taking, for example, only small white tablets.

The observations in an editorial[29] provide a perspective that is helpful in understanding the challenge for the patient who is to take a number of medications.

"A common consequence of too many pills is organizational breakdown. Given a regimen of four pills once a day, one pill twice a day, three pills three times daily, and two pills four times daily, compliance suffers. Even the best intentions struggle under such complexity. Day-to-day pill-taking becomes a little like a church dinner, at which no one takes exactly the same foods or the same portions. An assortment of dishes bewilders the senses. Except for the most compulsive patient, a regimen of many pills many times a day breeds more variety than regularity. Reducing pills and reducing intervals helps minimize the randomness of taking drugs. Potluck becomes a balanced diet."

Although combination drug products have certain disadvantages, their use may help improve compliance with therapy, since only one product need be administered rather than several. Therapy usually should not be initiated with a combination product but rather with the individual agents. Once the optimal dosages of the individual drugs have been determined, if they correspond to the amounts included in the combination, these products can be used to advantage.

FREQUENCY OF ADMINISTRATION—The administration of medication at frequent intervals makes it more likely that the patient's normal routine or work schedule will have to be interrupted to take a dose of medication, and in many cases the patient will forget, not want to be inconvenienced, or be embarrassed to do so.

In a study in which compliance was observed to improve from 59% on a three-times-a-day regimen to 75% on a twice-a-day regimen to 84% on a once-a-day regimen, the investigators noted that "probably the single most important action that health-care providers can take to improve compliance is to select medications that permit the lowest daily prescribed dose frequency."[30]

The attitudes of patients toward their illnesses and treatment regimens also should be anticipated and addressed. In most situations, it is reasonable to expect that patients will favor, and be more inclined to comply with, a dosage regimen that is simple and convenient.

DURATION OF THERAPY—The potential for noncompliance is greater when the treatment period is long. As noted earlier, a greater risk of noncompliance should be anticipated in patients with chronic disorders, especially if discontinuation of therapy is not likely to be associated with prompt recurrence of symptoms or worsening of the illness. Noncompliance with regimens for the treatment of tuberculosis is a major reason for the development of resistance to multiple antitubercular agents and is a very important problem for many patients with this infectious disease.

ADVERSE EVENTS—The development of unpleasant effects of a drug is a likely deterrent to compliance. In an AARP survey of people 45 years of age and older, 40% of the respondents stated they had experienced some form of side effect during medication use.[31] Of this 40%, 50% responded that they stopped taking the medication as a result of the side effect. Of the respondents who were 65 years of age and older, only 47% informed their physicians of the discontinuation.

In some situations it may be possible to change the dosage or use alternative drugs to minimize adverse events. However, in other cases such alternatives may not exist, and the benefits expected from therapy must be weighed against the risks. Particularly disconcerting are those situations in which the development of adverse events makes patients feel worse than they did before therapy was initiated, as often occurs in hypertensive patients.

The adverse events (eg, nausea, vomiting, hair loss) associated with the use of many antineoplastic drugs are sufficiently distressing to a number of patients with cancer that they do not take their medication in the manner intended. The reduction in the quality of life resulting from effects such as severe nausea and vomiting may be of such importance to some individuals that they do not comply with a regimen that in some cases may even offer the hope of being curative.

The ability of certain drugs to cause sexual dysfunction is a reason for noncompliance by some patients, with the antipsychotic agents, antidepressants, and antihypertensive agents being implicated most frequently.

Even a *warning* about possible adverse events may result in some individuals not complying with instructions. It is inadvisable for patients being treated with sedatives or other agents with a central nervous system depressant effect to consume alcoholic beverages, because of the possibility of an excessive depressant response. However, there should be a realistic recognition that some patients, if faced with a mandate not to drink while on drug therapy, will choose not to take their prescribed medication. Although problems of combined alcohol-drug usage are well known, this situation continues to present a challenge of effectively communicating with the patient so that optimal benefit can be achieved at minimal risk.

PATIENTS MAY BE ASYMPTOMATIC OR SYMPTOMS SUBSIDE—It is understandably difficult to convince a patient of the value of drug therapy when the patient has not experienced symptoms prior to initiation of therapy. Such is often the case in the treatment of hypertension, and the lack of previous symptoms coupled with the probable lack of appearance of symptoms if therapy is discontinued contributes to the high rate of noncompliance in these patients.

In other circumstances patients may feel better after taking the drug and feel that they no longer need to take it once the symptoms subside. Situations frequently occur in which patients do not complete a full course of antibiotic therapy once they feel that the infection has been controlled. This practice increases the likelihood of a recurrence of the infection and increased resistance of the microorganisms causing the infection, and patients must be advised to take the full course of antibiotic therapy.

COST OF MEDICATION—Noncompliance may occur with the use of drugs that have a relatively low cost; however, it might be anticipated that patients may be even more reluctant to use the entire prescribed quantity of more-expensive agents. The expense involved has been cited by some patients as the reason for not having prescriptions dispensed at all, whereas in other cases the medication is taken less frequently than intended or prematurely discontinued because of the cost.

Concerns regarding the consequences of noncompliance or partial compliance that result because patients are not able to afford their prescribed medications are an important reason for the high level of attention that has been devoted to the development of Medicare coverage of prescription drugs for outpatients, as well as initiatives to import medications from Canada and other countries in which they are available at lower costs.

ADMINISTRATION OF MEDICATION—Although patients may fully intend to comply with instructions, they may inadvertently receive the wrong quantity of medication because of incorrect measurement of medication, use of inappropriate measuring devices, or incorrect use of medication-administration devices. The inaccuracy of using teaspoons to administer liquid medications is well known and is compounded by the possibility of spillage and asking the patient to measure a fraction of a teaspoonful. This problem has been long recognized, but problems still occur. The importance of providing the patient with measuring cups, or calibrated droppers for the use of oral liquids is evident.

Some patients do not use metered-dose aerosol inhalation devices correctly, and this could result in inadequate control of the conditions (eg, asthma) for which their use are intended. The provision of oral instruction by the pharmacist has resulted in better patient understanding and performance of the correct steps for inhaler use.

TASTE OF MEDICATION—Medication taste problems are encountered most commonly with the use of oral liquids by children. Getting a child to take a dose of medication may be such a difficult task for a parent that doses may be missed or administration of the drug discontinued as soon as the parent sees any sign of improvement. Experiences such as these have resulted in initiatives to flavor liquid medications so that they are acceptable to children. FLAVO Ŗ has used more than three dozen flavors in the development of a medication-flavoring formulary system that has been used successfully in pharmacies around the country. This system also has been extended for use in medications prescribed for pets.

Compliance problems relating to the taste of medication are not limited to children. Objections to the taste of liquid potassium chloride preparations often are raised; a number of patients discontinue taking the medication for this reason.

Patient/Health Professional Interaction

The circumstances surrounding the visit of a patient with a physician and pharmacist and the quality and effectiveness of the interaction of these health professionals with the patient are major determinants of the patient's understanding of, and attitude toward, the illness and therapeutic regimen. One of the patient's greatest needs is psychological support provided in a compassionate manner, and it has been observed that patients are more inclined to comply with the instructions of a physician they know well and respect and from whom they receive information and assurance about their illnesses and medications.

The patient-physician interaction has been described as a negotiation between two active and equal participants with a strategy that includes the elements of "putting the ill at ease," respect, positive attitude, information, translation, feedback, patient response, and negotiation. Respect for the patient and a realistic appraisal of the circumstances of the individual patient are essential if therapeutic goals are to be achieved.

In a discussion of the influence of the patient-physician relationship on compliance, the following observation was made:

"Our only true influence on the patient is based on the strength of our professional relationship with that patient. And it is this relationship that is central to improving patient compliance with both medication and treatment regimens."[32]

These observations are equally important with respect to the interaction between the pharmacist and the patient. The following factors are among those that could influence compliance adversely if inadequate attention is given to the scope and quality of the interaction with the patient.

FAILURE TO COMPREHEND THE IMPORTANCE OF THERAPY—A major reason for noncompliance is that the importance of the drug therapy and the potential consequences if the medication is not used according to instructions have not been impressed upon the patient. Patients usually know relatively little about their illnesses, let alone the therapeutic benefits and problems that could result from drug therapy. Therefore, they establish their own beliefs and expectations with respect to their drug therapy. If the therapy does not meet these expectations they are more likely to become noncompliant. Greater attention to educating patients about their conditions as well as the benefits and limitations of drug therapy will contribute to better compliance with therapeutic regimens.

POOR UNDERSTANDING OF THE INSTRUCTIONS—Prescriptions that state that medication should be taken *as directed* can be the source of misunderstanding as well as serious consequences. Even when instructions are more specific, confusion still may occur, and there have been many errors of interpretation of instructions that the prescriber considered to be clear. For example, many prescriptions are written and labeled to indicate how many doses are to be taken each day with no additional clarification as to how the doses are to be scheduled. How should instructions to take one tablet three times a day be interpreted? Does this mean every 8 hr, or with meals, or possibly some other schedule? If the drug is to be given with meals or at a specified time before or after meals, it usually is assumed that the patient eats three meals a day. Yet this is not always the case. In one study,[33] patients being treated with medications with instructions to take them three times a day were interviewed with respect to the times at which they administered the individual doses of medication. Of 137 patients, only 1 was administering the medication at regular 8-hr intervals between doses, and 79% of the patients reported taking all three doses within 12 hr, leaving a dosage interval of 12 hr or more.

A patient may be knowledgeable about the dosage and the specific times at which the medication is to be administered but not understand the meaning of *auxiliary* instructions. Some patients have received prescriptions for a tetracycline derivative in a container to which is affixed an auxiliary label with a precaution about exposure to sunlight. However, in the absence of additional explanation, some have concluded that it is the medication that needs to be protected from sunlight (and have placed the container in the refrigerator) and have not recognized that the information applies to an adverse event for which *they* are at risk.

Pharmacists should be certain that patients are familiar with special considerations pertaining to the particular dosage form dispensed, such as the importance of not chewing or crushing controlled-release capsules or tablets. In one report the death of a patient is suspected to be due to chewing diltiazem extended-release capsules (Cardizem CD) because she thought the capsules were too big to swallow whole.[34]

In some cases the uncertainty or confusion on the part of the patient is such that medications are given by the wrong route of administration (eg, instilling oral pediatric antibiotic drops into the ear for an ear infection or administering suppositories by the oral route).

A patient being prepared for an electrocardiogram was observed to have 20 transdermal nitroglycerin patches at various locations on his body. Although he had understood the instructions to apply one patch a day, no instruction had been provided regarding their removal.

Although not a complete listing of all factors that result in noncompliance, those discussed give an indication of the difficult challenge of assuring optimal drug therapy.

IMPROVING COMPLIANCE

It often is assumed that health professionals recognize the importance of noncompliance and will take the steps necessary to achieve the compliance of their patients with the instructions provided. However, this assumption may not always be valid. In one study, physician compliance with public health recommendations for tuberculosis control was evaluated.[35] The study revealed poor compliance by physicians with recommended policies for the prevention of tuberculosis in health-care workers, thereby raising concerns about the personal risk of tuberculosis for these physicians, as well as questions about how effectively such physicians will promote preventive actions among their patients. An accompanying editorial[36] noted that "one might wonder how much patient noncompliance is fostered by a less than enthusiastic endorsement by the health-care provider." For strategies to improve compliance to be effective, health professionals must not only believe that noncompliance is an important problem, but also be willing to make a greater commitment to the steps that will help their patients be compliant.

A number of strategies to enhance compliance have been proposed. Inherent in many of the factors considered is the matter of communication of the physician and pharmacist with the patient. This communication is, in many cases, not only incomplete and ineffective, but often there is also the impression that

physicians and pharmacists are too busy or not interested in talking with the patient. Improving communications must be considered the key to increasing compliance and some of the approaches and recommendations directed toward this goal are reviewed in the following discussion. Pharmacists have a particularly valuable opportunity to encourage compliance since their advice accompanies the actual dispensing of the medication, and they usually are the last health professional to see the patient prior to the time the medication is to be used.

Identification of Risk Factors

All patients should be viewed as potential noncompliers. A first step in efforts to improve compliance should be to recognize individuals who are most likely to be noncompliant, as judged by a consideration of the risk factors noted earlier. These factors should be taken into account in planning the patient's therapy so that the simplest regimen that is, to the extent possible, compatible with the patient's normal activities can be developed.

Development of Treatment Plan

The more complex the treatment regimen, the greater is the risk of noncompliance, and this must be recognized in the development of the treatment plan. The use of longer-acting drugs in a therapeutic class, or dosage forms that are administered less frequently, also may simplify the regimen.

The treatment plan should be individualized on the basis of the patient's needs, and when possible, the patient should be a participant in decisions regarding the therapeutic regimen. Compliant patients see themselves as active members of the team involved in their care, not as passive victims of a disease and the health-care system. Involving patients in the development of a treatment plan will help them view the regimen as something that increases their control and options, rather than something that is done to them.

To help reduce inconvenience and forgetfulness, the regimen should be *tailored* so that the doses of medication are administered at times that correspond to regular activities in the patient's daily schedule. When prescriptions are written, the instructions should be as specific as possible.

Instructions such as *"as directed"* or other directions that are subject to misinterpretation should be avoided. Even such seemingly specific instructions as *one tablet three times a day* often are misinterpreted, as discussed previously. Where possible and with a recognition of the patient's normal routine, the specific times of day at which the patient is to take the medication should be indicated.

The APhA and the American Society of Internal Medicine have developed a statement on prescription writing and prescription labeling (Appendix A). Not only do the guidelines provide important information and suggestions, but the statement reflects the type of interdisciplinary cooperation that also must be achieved in practice if patient needs are to be served best.

The prescription can be used as the organizing instrument of instruction. However, "most often the prescription slip simply is handed over as the closing act of the encounter, while the patient or parent is outward bound."[37] The prescription should signal the start of an alliance, and it behooves the physician to emphasize its importance.

Many prescriptions that patients receive from their physicians are never dispensed. Little progress has been made in detecting and correcting these occurrences, further emphasizing the need for more-effective communication and a closer working relationship between physicians and pharmacists.

Patient Education

One of the findings of the report of the Office of the Inspector General is "education is the best way to improve compliance."

However, former FDA Commissioner David Kessler has expressed concern that "the nation also is facing a communications gap that has serious implications for the public health. This gap extends from what patients want to know about their medicines to what they actually learn from their physicians and pharmacists."[38] He further observes that "physicians . . . need to re-examine the amount of information they give their patients and the way they deliver it. In addition, they need to acknowledge that pharmacists should have a larger role in patient education and advise their patients to expect counseling when they fill their prescriptions."[38]

Many factors influence the effectiveness of educational efforts and a patient's development of compliant behavior. Decisions must be made as to what information should be provided to patients about their illnesses and drug therapy. It must be recognized that when the information is too comprehensive or detailed or is presented inappropriately (eg, a discussion of adverse events that alarms the patient), the patient actually may be discouraged from taking the medications. Thus, compliance may be compromised rather than enhanced.

In discussing an illness or drug therapy with a patient, a distinction should be made between *information* and *education*. Patients may receive information but not understand it and use it correctly, whereas education implies understanding and behavioral change. Patients should be encouraged to participate in the discussion, and when possible, they should be brought in on the decision-making process.

The goal of patient education is to provide information that the patient is able to understand and use. The anticipated benefits of the therapy should be explained, as should the importance of complying with the provided instructions. Complex terms and unnecessary jargon that can interfere with patient understanding should be avoided. Patients should be asked to repeat the instructions for administering their medications to show that they understand them, and they also should be encouraged to ask questions. At the least, the questions noted in Table 98-1 should be addressed. It is recommended by the National Council on Patient Information and Education (NCPIE) that these questions be discussed each time a patient obtains prescription medication.

ORAL COMMUNICATION/COUNSELING—Communication between the pharmacist and patient regarding the use of medication can be both oral and written. Although it may be supplemented and reinforced by written instructions, oral communication is the most important component of patient education because it directly involves both the patient and the pharmacist in a two-way exchange and provides the opportunity for the patient to raise questions. For such communication to be most effective it should be conducted in a setting that provides privacy and is free of distractions.

Although many pharmacies do not presently have a separate patient consultation area, this is a desirable goal. Not only will this emphasize to the patient the importance the pharmacist attaches to the information being discussed, but it also will strengthen further the recognition of the pharmacist as one who is contributing to the patient's health care.

Medication often is obtained in a manner that does not lend itself to oral communication. For example, the pharmacist may

receive a telephoned prescription from a physician that is to be delivered to the patient's home or picked up at the pharmacy by a relative or friend. In these circumstances, when appropriate, the pharmacist might call the patient to discuss the use of the medication.

The effect of pharmacist counseling on patient compliance has been evaluated in a number of studies. Studies assessing pharmacist counseling of patients with hypertension have demonstrated a significant increase in the patients' knowledge of hypertension and its treatment, their compliance with prescribed therapy, and the number of patients whose blood pressures were maintained in the normal range.

A *compliance clinic* has been described[39] in which pharmacists endeavored to improve the compliance of patients referred to the clinic by physicians. Six of the 14 patients seen on a regular basis demonstrated a significant reduction in emergency room visits, and 8 patients exhibited reduced hospitalizations, as determined by a comparison of pre- and postclinic records. In addition to the therapeutic benefits most patients will experience as a result of improved compliance, there is a considerable cost savings to be achieved as a result of the reduced hospitalization.

WRITTEN COMMUNICATION—The emphasis on oral communication should not be interpreted to indicate that written communication is not important. Although at the time of the visit to the physician or pharmacist patients may understand how the medication is to be used, later they may not remember the details relating to administration of the drug. Therefore, specific instructions for use should be placed on the prescription label.

It is also desirable and sometimes required to provide supplementary written instructions or other information pertaining to the patient's illness or drug therapy, and many pharmacists provide patients with medication instruction cards or inserts. Information that pertains to the specific medication/formulation being dispensed is preferred to information that applies to a therapeutic class of agents or a general statement that applies to all dosage forms of a particular medication. The provision of supplementary written information appears to be most effective in improving compliance with short-term therapeutic regimens (eg, antibiotic therapy). For drugs used on a long-term basis, written information as a sole intervention has not been shown to be sufficient for improving patient compliance.

Although the supplemental instructions and information may be thorough and well written, it must be recognized that many patients cannot read. Millions of adults in the US are functionally illiterate (ie, they cannot perform the basic reading tasks required to function in society) and millions more are only marginally literate. In one study[49] of more than 2600 predominantly indigent and minority patients, 42% were unable to comprehend directions for taking medication on an empty stomach. Written instructions and information also must be viewed as one-way communication unless patients are permitted to discuss and ask questions about their therapy. Therefore, oral and written communication should be used to complement each other, and both should be viewed as important components of the effort to educate patients regarding their drug therapy.

AUDIOVISUAL MATERIALS—The use of audiovisual aids may be particularly valuable in certain situations because patients may be better able to visualize the nature of the illness or how their medication acts or is to be administered (eg, the administration of insulin, the use of a metered-dose inhaler). An increasing number of health-care professionals have used such aids effectively by making them available for viewing in a patient waiting area or consultation room and then answering questions the patient may have.

CONTROLLED THERAPY—It has been proposed that hospitalized patients be given the responsibility for self-medication prior to discharge. Usually, patients go from a complete dependence on others for the administration of their medication while hospitalized to a situation in which they are given the full responsibility when discharged, often with the assump-

Table 98-1. Patient Questions Regarding Medication[a]

1. What is the name of the medicine, and what is it supposed to do?
2. How much of the medicine should I take, when should I take it and for how long?
3. What foods, beverages, and other medicines should I avoid while taking it?
4. What are the possible side effects, and what should I do if they occur?
5. What written material is available about the medicine?

[a] Questions that patients should ask, as recommended by the NCPIE.

tion that they know about their drugs because they were taking them in the hospital. Similarly, many ambulatory patients who are expected to be responsible for their own treatment have not been provided with adequate information.

The suggested arrangement would permit patients to start using the medications on their own before discharge, so that health-care professionals can more directly identify problems or situations that might undermine compliance, and answer patient questions.

Special programs for providing information about medication are needed for some individuals including sight-impaired and hearing-impaired patients. Some pharmacists prepare prescription labels in Braille for the blind and use a telecommunication device for the deaf (TDD) to communicate with hearing-impaired patients over telephone lines. The Medifier is a molded plastic device (in four sizes) into which a prescription vial is placed. A clear lens magnifies the print on the label so that patients with vision problems can read the instructions.

Patient Motivation

Many health care professionals assume that patients who are knowledgeable about their illness and therapeutic regimen are likely to be compliant. Although this premise is valid for many patients, increased patient knowledge does not necessarily alter patient behavior and compliance. Therefore, there must be an awareness of the need to motivate patients to use the knowledge they have acquired to achieve optimum benefit from their therapy.

Information must be provided to patients in a manner that is not coercive, threatening, or demeaning. The best intentioned, most comprehensive educational efforts will not be effective if the patient cannot be motivated to comply with the instructions for taking the medication. In addition to counseling the patient and providing specific written instructions, supplying cues for appropriate behavior (prompting) may be of value in motivating the patient to be compliant. Cues may be verbal or nonverbal, with examples of the latter including the use of special packaging or reminder systems.

The physician-patient interaction has been characterized as a *negotiation*. This concept may be extended further by the development of *contracts* between patients and health-care providers in which the agreed-upon treatment goals and responsibilities are outlined. As summarized in a review,[3] contracts offer "a written outline of expected behavior, the involvement of the patient in the decision-making process concerning the regimen and the opportunity to discuss potential problems and solutions with the physician, a formal commitment to the program from the patient, and rewards . . . which create incentives for achieving compliance goals." Although such a structured approach will not be needed with most individuals, it may be effective for patients who have not responded to other initiatives to ensure compliance.

Noncompliance is the greatest challenge in the control of tuberculosis, and the difficulties currently encountered in the management of this infection have prompted one clinician to make the following observations: "Sometimes it takes a little imagination. Give them a cup of coffee. Talk to them. Pay them an honorarium to come in and take the medicine. If the public doesn't want drug-resistant TB, and if bribing people is the way to get them to take their medicine, then I say bribe them."[41]

Compliance Aids

LABELING—The importance of the accuracy and specificity of the information on the label of the prescription container has been noted. Auxiliary labels that provide additional information regarding the use, precautions, and/or storage of the medication also will contribute to the attainment of compliance. The inclusion of pictograms in labeling and patient information

leaflets has been demonstrated to have a positive effect in the acquisition and understanding of information regarding medications prescribed for patients with limited literacy skills.[43]

MEDICATION CALENDARS AND DRUG REMINDER CHARTS—Various forms, such as medication calendars, have been developed and are designed to assist patients in self-administering drugs. In addition to their use in helping patients understand which medication to take and when to take it, the forms on which patients are to check the appropriate area for each dose of medication they take, can be evaluated by the pharmacist or physician when the patients return for more medication or have their next appointment.

SPECIAL MEDICATION CONTAINERS, CAPS, AND SYSTEMS—Several types of medication containers have been developed to help patients organize their medications and to monitor self-administration of the drugs. An example is the 28-compartment MEDISET container that contains four compartments for different time periods (ie, morning, midday, evening, bedtime) for each day of the week. The Med Light Tablet Organizer also has 28 compartments as well as an alarm and flashing light.

Specially designed caps for prescription containers also have been developed to facilitate compliance, and include features such as a digital timepiece that displays the time and day on which the last dose of medication was taken, and an alarm and flashing light when it is time to take the next dose. Containers/caps that contain all or some of these features include The Prescript Time Cap, The Pill Timer, and Remind Cap Closures. The use of microelectronic medication monitors (Medication Event Monitoring System) in the caps of prescription containers has been described earlier.

For patients with vision impairment or who otherwise have difficulty reading information on prescription labels, products such as Talking Rx, ScripTalk, and Aloud Talking Prescription Labels have been developed to play a prerecorded message when activated. Instructions for using the medication are recorded in a small electronic unit or microchip that is attached to the bottom of the container or embedded in a label.

Although these special prescription containers, caps, and systems are not needed by most patients, they may be effective in achieving compliance by patients who forget doses or who are confused by the complexity of the regimen.

COMPLIANCE PACKAGING—The manner in which medication is packaged also has an influence on patient compliance. A *compliance package* has been defined as a prepackaged unit that provides one treatment cycle of the medication to the patient in a ready-to-use package, and a comprehensive review of the use of such packaging as a patient education tool has been published.[43] This type of packaging usually is based on blister packaging using unit-of-use dosing and is designed to serve as a patient-education tool for health professionals and to make it easier for patients to understand and remember to take their medications correctly at home. Specially designed packaging for oral contraceptives was one of the first initiatives of this type and has been valuable in increasing patient understanding of how these agents are to be taken.

Special packages of certain corticosteroids (eg, *Medrol Dosepak*) also have been designed to facilitate the use of steroids in dosage regimens that may be difficult to understand or remember.

The Medicine-On-Time system is an example of a packaging system that provides unit-of-use dosing with specific labeling in a plastic card that is set up like a calendar. In addition to simplifying the use of medications for patients who self-administer their medications, these systems also have been very useful in the distribution and administration of medications in assisted-living and other patient-care facilities.

A possible negative effect of drug packaging on patient compliance is seen with the use of the child-resistant containers. Some patients, particularly the elderly and those with conditions like arthritis and parkinsonism, have difficulty opening some of these containers and may not persist in their efforts to do so. There also may be difficulty opening some foil-packed drugs. Pharmacists should be alert to problems of this type and, when appropriate, suggest use of standard containers or caps.

DOSAGE FORMS—New dosage forms of certain drugs also have been developed, in large part in recognition of problems of noncompliance. For example, the development of longer- acting, controlled-release dosage forms of numerous medications (eg, calcium channel blocking agents) has permitted less frequent administration of these agents, which facilitates compliance. The use of transdermal delivery systems permits less-frequent administration of the drugs (eg, nitroglycerin, fentanyl) given by this route.

Monitoring Therapy

SELF-MONITORING—Patients should be apprised of the importance of monitoring their own treatment regimen and, in some situations, the response parameters. The attention to the responsibility that patients must personally assume also has been considered in consumer publications, as illustrated by an article in *Good Housekeeping* titled "If your medicine isn't working.... It may not be the medicine at all. It could be *you!*"[44]

PHARMACIST MONITORING—The pharmacist's role in minimizing noncompliance does not end when the prescription is dispensed. The pharmacist is in an excellent position to detect noncompliance pertaining to drugs used in the management of chronic conditions, such as hypertension and diabetes, by being alert to situations in which the frequency of requested refills is not consistent with the directions for use. Pharmacist follow-up with telephoned or mailed refill reminders has been found to increase compliance.

One approach in which both health professionals and patients have collaborated effectively in reviewing/monitoring the use of medication has been the *brown bag* program. The Administration on Aging and National Council on Patient Information and Education (NCPIE) have encouraged older consumers to put all their medicines in a bag and take them to their health professional for a personalized medicine review.

DIRECTLY OBSERVED TREATMENT (DOT)—Even when many of the steps described earlier have been taken, noncompliance may still result. For example, there is great concern about the high rates of treatment failure in patients with tuberculosis and the increasing prevalence of drug-resistant tuberculosis. In one study that used self-administered treatment, 39% of patients were lost from the study with a 6-month antitubercular regimen and 49% with a 9-month regimen.[45] In contrast, in a study that used a 6-month regimen of directly observed treatment (ie, giving patients their medications and seeing that they are swallowed), fewer than 10% of the patients were lost to further treatment.[46] A commentary advocating the use of directly observed treatment regimens for patients with tuberculosis observed that "we can't afford not to try it."[47]

Many of the recommendations for improving patient compliance are included in a comprehensive set, *Recommendations for Action to Advance Prescription Medicine Compliance* that has been developed by NCPIE (Appendix B). A meta-analysis of 153 studies published between 1977 and 1994 that evaluated the effectiveness of interventions to improve patient compliance with medical regimens has been published.[48] The authors conclude that "no single strategy or programmatic focus showed any clear advantage compared with another. Comprehensive interventions combining cognitive, behavioral, and affective components were more effective than single-focus interventions."

CONCLUSION

Considerable time, effort, and expense often have gone into the diagnosis of a patient's illness and the development of a treatment program. Yet the goals of therapy will not be reached unless the patient understands and follows the instructions for use of the drugs prescribed. One also cannot help but wonder how often patients have been categorized as treatment failures and have had their therapy changed, possibly to more potent and toxic agents, when the reason for the lack of response or an unanticipated altered response was noncompliance.

Despite the increasing attention directed to the issue of noncompliance, the problem continues to be prevalent. Although not uniformly successful, the approaches taken and suggestions advanced in an effort to improve compliance have contributed substantially to recognition of the problem and provided a valuable base on which to develop modified or new approaches to the problem. Certain approaches that involve a significantly increased commitment of time on the part of health-care professionals may be viewed by some as impractical. Yet can this increased commitment of time compare with the time and money that are currently being wasted as a result of noncompliance?

The improvement of compliance will result in a situation in which all parties benefit. Most importantly patients benefit from the enhancement of the efficacy and safety of their drug therapy. Pharmacists benefit because there is an increased recognition and respect for the value of the advice and service that they provide. Pharmaceutical manufacturers benefit from the favorable recognition that accompanies the effective and safe use of their drugs as well as from the increased sales resulting from the larger number of prescriptions being dispensed. Finally, society and the health care system benefit as a result of fewer problems associated with noncompliance. Although an increase in compliance will result in more prescriptions being dispensed and a higher level of expenditures for prescription medications, this increase in costs will be more than offset by a reduction in costs (eg, physician visits, hospitalizations) attributable to problems due to noncompliance.

For too long patients have been deprived of close attention to, and monitoring of, their drug therapy. An excuse that health-care professionals are too busy to advise patients regarding their drug therapy cannot be accepted; the highest priority must be assigned to taking the steps to ensure that patients will use their medications in the appropriate manner.

REFERENCES

1. *Schering Report XVIII.* 1996.
2. Smith MC. In Smith MC, Wertheimer AI, eds. Social and Behavioral Aspects of Pharmaceutical Care. New York: Pharmaceutical Products Press, 1996.
3. Eraker SA, et al. *Ann Intern Med* 1984; 100:258.
4. Peck C. *Medic Event Monit Overview* 1991; 3:1.
5. Kusserow RP. Office of the Inspector General, OEI-04-89-89121, Mar 1990.
6. Koop CE. *Proc Symp Natl Pharm Council* 1984; 1.
7. Col N, et al. *Arch Intern Med* 1990; 150:841.
8. Einarson TR. *Ann Pharmacother* 1993; 27:832.
9. Maronde RF, et al. *Med Care* 1989; 27:1159.
10. Benner JS, et al. *JAMA* 2002; 288:455.
11. Jackevicius CA, et al. *JAMA* 2002; 288:462.
12. Guidelines for the Use of Antiretroviral Agents in HIV-1-Infected Adults and Adolescents. Department of Health and Human Services, July14, 2003:9.
13. Bowerman DL, et al. *J Forensic Sci* 1978; 23:522.
14. Rovelli M, et al. *Transplant Proc* 1989; 21:833.
15. Smith M. *Proc Symp Natl Pharm Council* 1984; 35.
16. Gotzsche PC. *Controlled Clin Trials* 1989; 10:31.
17. Weintraub M. *Contemp Pharm Pract* 1981; 4:8.
18. Sackett DL. In *Compliance in Health Care.* Haynes RB, Taylor DW, Sackett DL, eds. Baltimore: Johns Hopkins University Press, 1979, p 286.
19. Rudd P, et al. *Clin Pharmacol Ther* 1989; 46:169.
20. Pullar T, et al. *Clin Pharmacol Ther* 1989; 46:163.
21. Rudd P, et al. *Clin Pharmacol Ther* 1990; 48:676.
22. Kossoy AF, et al. *J Allergy Clin Immunol* 1989; 84:60.
23. Liu H, et al. *Ann Intern Med* 2001; 134:968.
24. Porter AMW. *Br Med J* 1969; 1:218.
25. Powsner S, Spitzer R. *Lancet* 2003; 361:2003.

26. Svarstad BL. *NARD J* 1986; Feb: 75.
27. Rosenstock IM. *Milbank Mem Fund Q* 1966; 55(Jul): 94.
28. Becker MH, et al. *Med Care* 1977; 15(Suppl 5):27.
29. Kroenke K. *Am J Med* 1985; 79:149.
30. Eisen SA, et al. *Arch Intern Med* 1990; 150:1881.
31. Prescription drugs: A survey of consumer use, attitudes and behavior. Washington DC: AARP, 1984.
32. Sbarbaro JA. *Ann Allergy* 1990; 64:325.
33. Norell SE, et al. *Am J Hosp Pharm* 1984; 41:1183.
34. Ballard DB. *Am J Health-Syst Pharm* 1996; 53:1962,
35. Geiseler PJ, Nelson KE, Cripsen RG. *Am Rev Respir Dis* 1987; 135:3.
36. Miller B, Snider DE. *Am Rev Respir Dis* 1987; 135:1.
37. Yaffe SJ, et al. *Drug Ther* 1977; 7(11):64.
38. Kessler DA. *N Engl J Med* 1991; 325:1650.
39. Cable GL, et al. *Contemp Pharm Pract* 1982; 5:38.
40. Williams MV, et al. *JAMA* 1995; 274:1677.
41. Reichman L. *Newsweek* 1992; (Mar 16):57.
42. Mansoor LE, Dowse R. *Ann Pharmacother* 2003; 37:1003.
43. Smith DL. *Am Pharm* 1989; NS29(2):42.
44. Dawson ML. *Good Housekeeping* 1991; Apr:235.
45. Combs DL, et al. *Ann Intern Med* 1990; 112:397.
46. Cohn, DL, et al. *Ann Intern Med* 1990; 112:407.
47. Iseman MD, et al. *N Engl J Med* 328: 576, 1993.
48. Roter DL. *Med Care* 1998; 36:1138.

Statement on Prescription Writing and Prescription Labeling[a]

INTRODUCTION

Historically, the pharmaceutical and medical professions have devoted considerable time and effort to the development and rational utilization of safe and effective drugs for the treatment and prevention of illness. Today, that successful effort continues, helping to achieve the highest standards of health in the world for the American people. But in order to gain maximum benefit from the use of drugs while minimizing their adverse side effects, prescribers and pharmacists must maintain effective communications not only among themselves, but with their patients as well. The directions for drug use and other information which prescribers indicate on prescription orders and which pharmacists transfer to prescription labels are critical to safe and effective drug therapy. In order to assure that this information is conveyed clearly and effectively to patients, the following guidelines have been developed by the American Pharmaceutical Association and the American Society of Internal Medicine.

GUIDELINES FOR PRESCRIBERS

The following guidelines are recommended for prescribers when writing directions for drug use on their prescription orders:

1. The name and strength of the drug dispensed will be recorded on the prescription label by the pharmacist unless otherwise directed by the prescriber.
2. Whenever possible, specific times of the day for drug administration should be indicated. (For example, *Take one capsule at 8:00 am, 12:00 noon, and 8:00 pm* is preferable to *Take one capsule three times daily.* Likewise, *Take one tablet two hours after meals* is preferable to *Take one tablet after meals.*)
3. The use of potentially confusing abbreviations, ie, *qid, qod, qd,* etc, is discouraged.
4. Vague instructions such as *Take as necessary* or *Take as directed* which are confusing to the patient are to be avoided.
5. If dosing at specific intervals around-the-clock is therapeutically important, this should specifically be stated on the prescription by indicating appropriate times for drug administration.
6. The symptom, indication, or the intended effect for which the drug is being used should be included in the instructions whenever possible. (For example, *Take one tablet at 8:00 am and 8:00 pm for high blood pressure,* or *Take one teaspoonful at 8:00 am, 11:00 am, 3:00 pm, and 6:00 pm for cough.*)
7. The Metric System of weights and measures should be used.
8. The prescription order should indicate whether or not the prescription should be renewed and, if so, the number of times and the period of time such renewal is authorized. Statements such as *Refill prn* or *Refill ad lib* are discouraged.
9. Either single or multi-drug prescription forms may be used when appropriately designed, and pursuant to the desires of local medical and pharmaceutical societies.
10. When institutional prescription blanks are used, the prescriber should print his/her name, telephone number and registration number on the prescription blank.

GUIDELINES FOR PHARMACISTS

1. Pharmacists should include the following information on the prescription label: name, address and telephone number of pharmacy; name of prescriber; name, strength and quantity of drug dispensed (unless otherwise directed by the prescriber); directions for use; prescription number; date on which prescription is dispensed; full name of patient and any other information required by law.
2. Instructions to the patient regarding directions for use of medication should be concise and precise, but readily understandable to the patient. Where the pharmacist feels that the prescription order does not meet these criteria, he should attempt to clarify the order with the prescriber in order to prevent confusion. Verbal reinforcement and/or clarification of instructions should be given to the patient by the pharmacist when appropriate.
3. For those dosage forms where confusion may develop as to how the medication is to be administered (for example, oral drops which may be mistakenly instilled in the ear or suppositories which may be mistakenly administered orally), the pharmacist should clearly indicate the intended route of administration on the prescription label.
4. The pharmacist should include an expiration date on the prescription label when appropriate.
5. Where special storage conditions are required, the pharmacist should indicate appropriate instructions for storage on the prescription label.

CONCLUSION

Communicating effective dosage instructions to patients clearly and succinctly is a responsibility of both the medical and pharmaceutical professions. Recent studies documenting the low order of compliance with prescription instructions indicate that poor communication between the medical and pharmaceutical professions and poor comprehension by the public may be causative factors.

The American Pharmaceutical Association and the American Society of Internal Medicine believe that the guidelines as stated above will serve as an initial step toward patients achieving a better understanding of their medication and dosing instructions. The two associations urge state and local societies representing pharmacists and prescribers to appoint joint committees for the purpose of refining these guidelines further as local desires and conditions warrant. The associations believe that such cooperative efforts between the professions are essential to good patient care and that significant progress can be made in other areas by initiating discussions between the two professions concerning common interests and goals.

---

[a] By American Pharmaceutical Association/American Society of Internal Medicine (revised March 1976).

NCPIE Recommendations for Action to Advance Prescription Medicine Compliance

ADVANCING COMPLIANCE: NCPIE PANELS MAKE RECOMMENDATIONS

In December 1994, the National Council on Patient Information and Education (NCPIE) sponsored a conference, "Advancing Prescription Medicine Compliance: New Paradigms, New Practices." The most important objective of this conference was to produce realistic recommendations for advancing compliance across health care professions and practice settings.

To develop recommendations, commissioned speakers addressed prescription medicine compliance issues relating to: physicians, pharmacists, nurses, manufacturers, patients, managed care organizations, NCPIE and other groups. Each speaker suggested what could be done to improve compliance. Six complementary working groups then used the speakers' ideas as a springboard in developing recommendations for each group and for groups in collaboration. These were then presented to the full conference for participants' response and consideration.

The following recommendations are directed to the varied organizations and individuals who can advance compliance; however, many recommendations apply to more than one category under which they are listed:

1. Physicians and Medical Schools

   - Involve the patient in treatment decisions.
   - Monitor compliance with prescribed treatment at every patient visit; follow up outside of scheduled visits as appropriate. Give the patient an alternate contact person at your office if you might be unavailable when he/she calls between visits.
   - Document patient compliance using a compliance-monitoring form that can be incorporated into the patient's record.
   - Coordinate patients' medication regimens with health professionals providing remote site care, including visiting nurses, physician assistants and nurses in satellite clinics or offices, and pharmacists working with patients in care facilities or in the pharmacy.
   - Include patient communication skills in medical training and continuing education curricula.
   - Train physicians to communicate with other members of the health care team to ensure continuity of care.

2. Pharmacists, Pharmacy-Providers and Educators

   - Become proactive about gathering and providing medicine information. Ask questions that stimulate dialogue, discuss care plans with patients, and use information about patients to make better decisions.
   - Provide compliance monitoring and documentation for at least one at-risk patient per month. Share your findings with the patient and with his/her other health care providers.
   - Work with management to redesign facilities to increase pharmacist/patient contact, and to provide a private counseling area.
   - Incorporate patient communication skills and new teaching methods into undergraduate courses and continuing education programs.
   - Work with other health professional schools/organizations to develop interdisciplinary compliance education programs.
   - Integrate behavioral and clinical sciences in educating pharmacists about compliance.

3. Individual Nurses and Educators

   - Integrate into each patient encounter an educational assessment of patient medicine knowledge.
   - Collaborate with other health care providers, including prescribers and pharmacists, about patient compliance issues.
   - Develop programs to increase nurses' knowledge and skills for compliance-enhancement.
   - Include compliance questions in examinations for professional degrees, licensing, and continuing education.

4. All Health Professionals

   - Individualize patient care, including medication management, considering factors such as age, culture, gender, attitudes, and personal situation.
   - Specifically ask patients about use of over-the-counter drugs, including vitamins and dietary supplements.
   - Engage in a dialogue with patients and involve them as partners in the treatment process. Explain why you think a treatment plan is most appropriate for your patient.
   - Use written materials to reinforce oral counseling, not as a substitute for it.
   - Respect a patient's right to confidentiality when sharing medication compliance experience with the patient's other health care providers, including nurses, pharmacists, physicians, and physician assistants.

5. Pharmaceutical Manufacturers

   - Individually and as an industry, develop a public service advertising campaign promoting patient medication compliance with therapy.
   - Support health professionals' education to develop effective communicators in a patient-centered health care system.
   - Recognize and promote role models who can demonstrate improved compliance from a patient-centered approach.
   - Provide NCPIE's "Get the Answers" brochure with all responses to consumer information requests or "800" program responses.
   - Support interdisciplinary teams that provide patient education and programs for compliance and health promotion.

6. Patients

   - Become an active participant in making treatment decisions and solving problems that could inhibit proper medicine use.
   - Talk to your health professionals about why and how to use your prescription medicines. Give them information about your medicine use (prescription and over-the-counter medicines, vitamins and dietary supplements) and health. If you stop or change a prescribed treatment, tell them and explain why you did this. Get the answers to any questions you have.
   - Recognize, accept, and carry out your responsibilities in the treatment regimen.

7. Managed Care Organizations and Hospitals

- Use existing databases to profile the extent of medicine noncompliance among your health plan members.
- Develop and implement programs for patient compliance support (e.g., group support programs, educational interventions, monitoring clinics, compliance packaging aids, and brown bag reviews). Keep health care providers informed about these programs so they can refer appropriate patients as part of an individualized compliance regimen.
- Develop and implement innovative programs that teach patient's responsibility for and involvement in his/her health care.
- Identify, implement, and evaluate compliance-promoting organizational practices and policies.
- Review drug use policies, such as formulary policy guidelines, from a patient compliance perspective. Revise policies accordingly to facilitate compliance.
- Develop and implement computerized systems that allow departments to share clinical patient information electronically.

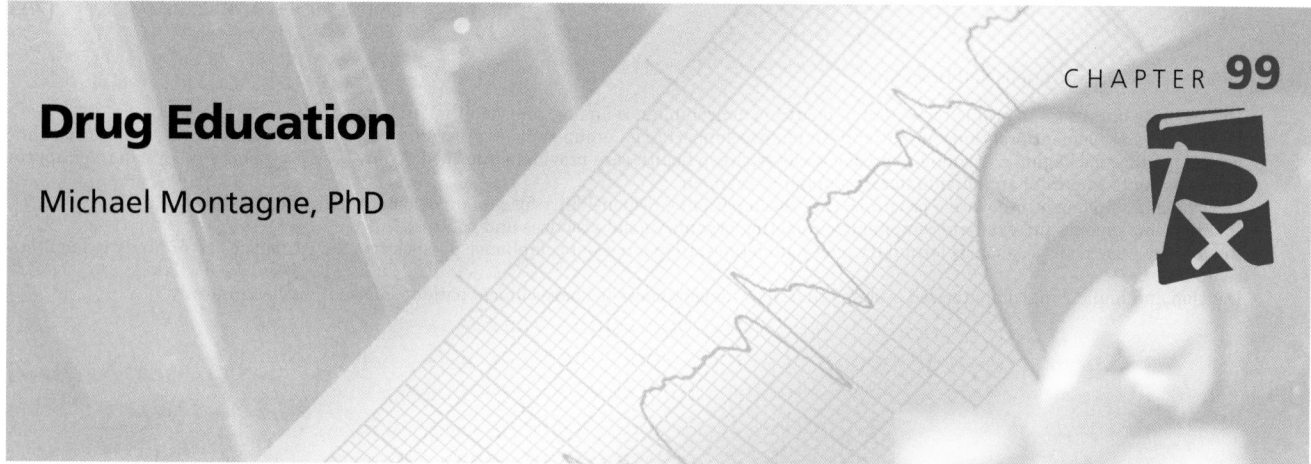

CHAPTER **99**

Drug Education

Michael Montagne, PhD

Drug use occurs in virtually every society and culture. Whether the use of a particular drug is for a medical or a nonmedical reason, problems resulting from use often arise. Preventing drug use problems is a major concern of most societies, and it usually is highlighted when specific outbreaks of problems or inappropriate use occur. As pharmacy is the profession to which the control of drugs is attributed, it should be involved intimately with those activities aimed at preventing or reducing drug use problems. In fact, the pharmaceutical profession should be providing the leadership and directing the research in this area. It is unfortunate that, on the whole, pharmacy has been lacking in its social responsibility for the chemical substances it develops, promotes, and dispenses.

Most pharmacists are aware of the important problems that potentially can occur with the appropriate use of prescription medications, such as adverse reactions and drug interactions. Many pharmacists also are knowledgeable about potential problems inherent in self-medication with a nonprescription drug, though they probably are less familiar with the use of herbal remedies and homeopathic medications in the same context. Few pharmacists, however, are aware of potential problems that can arise with social-recreational drug use. Regardless of the situation, the problem of poisoning or overdose by a drug should be delegated to poison-control centers and hospital emergency rooms. The individual pharmacist, particularly one working in a community setting, may not feel capable of consulting or educating a particular drug consumer in these problem areas.

Most societies are in great need of learning more rational and appropriate uses of all types of drugs and of gaining control over the products (drugs) of their own technology. Humans have learned how to create (extract and/or synthesize) drug products, yet humans have not learned fully how to use these products in an optimal manner. The primary importance of drug education is its benefit to the drug user (patient or consumer); such education can improve the appropriateness of drug taking behaviors to achieve optimal health and well-being. At the center of any educational effort is the provision of drug information, the strategy with which pharmacists and pharmacy students are most familiar. In today's highly complex, technological world, the availability of current and precise information allows one to understand, to make better choices, and to prevent or solve problems.

The individual best suited to assist people in preventing drug use problems and in achieving optimal, desired experiences from their drug taking is the pharmacist. The pharmacist is an accessible source of high-quality information and educational programs and should be concerned with a person's drug-taking behavior. Whether it be the use of a prescription medicine or an herbal remedy to achieve or maintain a state of health, the use of a drug for its socially oriented effects in a recreational setting, or the ingestion of a chemical substance to enhance a religious or aesthetic experience, the perspective presented herein considers the pharmacist to be the leader in efforts to prevent or limit drug use problems.

In this chapter, the basic principles of drug education are presented with the underlying premise that these principles and strategies are applicable to any type of drug use. Although information about, and inherent problems resulting from, specific types of drug taking might vary from drug to drug or among reasons for use, the fundamental approach to educating people and fostering changes in drug use is the same. The word *drug* refers to any substance, other than food, which by its chemical or physical nature, alters structure or function in a human being, resulting in physiological, behavioral, or social changes. This includes all medicinal agents (whether defined legally as prescription or nonprescription), herbal and home remedies, alcohol and caffeine (and other substances that are often considered *food* by consumers, but are used for their pharmacological activity), substances used primarily in a nonmedical context, and even poisons.

Many approaches have been developed for designing drug information and drug education programs in medical settings, and many of these are described in other chapters of this book. The majority of the examples in this chapter, therefore, come from the realm of *drug abuse* prevention. These techniques and strategies, and their basic principles, are also applicable to educating patients about medicines or providing drug education programs in any context. It is important to realize that, conversely, ideas, strategies, and programs from the field of patient drug education can be relevant to the development of programs on the nonmedical use of drugs, and some examples of this broader view of drug education are provided.

DRUG USE AND DRUG EDUCATION

Human beings engage in a great variety of drug taking behaviors, but one of the most important and rudimentary considerations involves the definition of what constitutes a drug and which situations characterize drug taking. In a 1972 nationwide survey of drug use, adults and youths were asked to indicate which substances they regarded as drugs.[1] More than 80% of the respondents regarded substances such as heroin, cocaine, marijuana, and psychotherapeutic agents to be drugs. One should realize, however, that a small proportion of the general public (5–20%, depending on the specific drug) did not regard these substances to be drugs. Alcohol and tobacco were regarded as drugs by less than one-third of the respondents. Most of the adolescent respondents (84%) did not consider tobacco to be a drug, although we might expect that if the survey were repeated today, the results would be different.

The key point is that individuals can hold different beliefs or perceptions about which chemical substances they regard as being drugs. In fact, this type of survey can be a useful and interesting exercise in a drug education program. The audience is shown a list of chemical substances and asked to indicate which ones are drugs and which ones are not. Not only can this exercise, and its results, provide the educator with a better idea of the opinions and level of drug knowledge of an individual or group, but it also can be used as a focal point for discussion at that time or subsequent sessions. The belief that certain substances may be drugs is important in understanding why and how people use such substances, and it should be a primary consideration in the development of any drug education program.

The nature and extent of certain types of drug taking vary by drug, availability (or accessibility), and the reason for use. In the medical realm, drug taking may be initiated by the patient, as in self-medication, or it may be directed by another person, usually a physician, who writes a prescription for it. Studies of self-medication are limited. The research done in this area indicates that self-diagnosis, rather than making contact with the health-care delivery system, occurs in the majority of illness episodes and that self-medication occurs from 60% to 90% of the time in these situations.[2] Studies of nonprescription-drug consumption indicate that, in general, approximately one-third of a population could be defined as current users of such substances and that from 25% to 60% of a population may be users of such drugs during any specific period.[2] The prevalence of nonprescription drug use is even higher in the older adult population (ranging from 50% to 90%), in addition to their extensive use of prescription drugs.[2]

The recent Slone Survey studied medication use of all types at the population level.[3] This study determined that during 1998–99, 81% of adults had used at least one medication in the week prior to the study interview; 50% used at least one prescription medication; and 7% used five or more. The highest prevalence of medication use was among older women; 57% used at least five medications and 12% used at least ten. Herbal products were used by 14% of the population, and 16% of prescription users also used an herbal concurrently. Vitamin and mineral supplements were used by 40% of the population.

When a drug is prescribed for a patient, health professionals expect that the drug will be taken precisely as directed. Compliance with medication regimens is another type of drug taking considered of major importance in a successful treatment plan. There have been many studies in this area (see *Compliance* chapter for a thorough review); their results have shown that anywhere from 5% to 90% of patients may be noncompliant in some manner. Although there is a wide variation in noncompliance, caused by various factors as well as the research design of particular studies, the rate of noncompliance, in general, probably ranges from 33% to 50% in any given population. This situation represents a different behavior; many patients are not taking drugs when they should be.

Drug taking also occurs in a nonmedical context. Although cigarette smoking has declined steadily among adults, tobacco use has increased in young people during the past few years.[4] The prevalence of alcohol use has remained stable for many years, but there is an increase in binge drinking among young adults, especially college students.[4] Nationwide surveys of drug use, conducted by the National Institute on Drug Abuse in 2001, found that 18% of youths (less than 18 years), 35% of young adults (18–25 years), and 25% of adults (26 years or older) were current users of tobacco, whereas 20% of youths, 58% of young adults, and 56% of adults were current users of alcohol.[4]

The nonmedical use of most other types of psychoactive drugs has declined during the past decade, but there have been increases in the use of some substances over the past couple of years.[4] The nonmedical use of marijuana, cocaine, and some psychedelic drugs (eg, LSD) has increased in the past 2 years in all age groups, but especially in the 12–17 age group. The greatest increase in the use of a specific nonmedical drug has occurred with marijuana. The nonmedical use of prescription psychotherapeutic drugs also has increased in the past year.

The misuse of drugs, including the development of an addiction, also has increased in the past couple of years.[4] Among 12–17 year olds, the misuse of or dependence on any drug (including alcohol) has increased from 7.7% to 7.8%; among 18–25 year olds, from 15.4% to 18.4%; and for people 26 years of age and older, from 4.8% to 5.4%. Alcohol is the biggest problem, by far, followed by marijuana and then the nonmedical use of a prescription psychotherapeutic agent (primarily pain relievers). Drugs are also the cause of almost one-half of all poisoning episodes (see *Poisons* chapter), a type of drug taking behavior that is usually unintentional, except in cases of suicide.

Drugs clearly are used appropriately in certain situations for beneficial reasons, are not used in some instances when they should be, and are used inappropriately on many occasions. In all three circumstances, though most often in the last two examples, problems can result from drug use. The prevention or recognition and management of problems resulting from drug use are the main reasons for developing and providing drug education programs.

Two additional aspects of drug use important in assisting drug users are their type of drug use behavior and their reasons or motivations for use. The focus of many drug education programs is on the drug itself and not the behavior (drug use). This has led to programs that focus on illegal drugs, but not legal drugs; on "hard" drugs, but not "soft" drugs; and on the pharmacology of the drug, but not on how that drug is used. Instead of focusing on these ill-defined or irrelevant terms, the focus of drug education should be on behavior, how and why the drug is being used. A typology of drug taking behaviors was developed by the National Commission of Marijuana and Drug Abuse,[1] and it can be very useful in orienting both the educator's and audience's focus on drug use, rather than on a drug (Table 99-1). Reasons or motivations for using drugs are the key to understanding why individuals use drugs. These reasons also should be addressed in developing and offering drug education programs (Table 99-2).

Drug education in a medical context has occurred for some time. The earliest health promotion movement occurred in the 19th century, and educational activities were an important part of the effort. Patient counseling always has been a part of the health professional's role, though the assumption of this role has varied from time to time, especially within pharmacy. The principle strategies have been to provide either drug information or drug education to patients through verbal interaction. Structured educational programs have been developed throughout the 20th century, but it was only after World War II that concerted efforts to develop and implement health education programs began to occur in public health. In the 1950s and 1960s, several attitudinal and behavioral approaches were studied to expand the traditional information-based approach and improve on the effectiveness of information only programs. At the beginning of the 21st century, the behavioral approach has become popular in health education programs, and the use of the mass media has increased dramatically.

Early efforts in education about nonmedical drug use consisted of negative portrayals of drugs and moralizing about drug use in the classroom and through the mass media, with little objective information being presented. Such an approach unfortunately still can be found in many contemporary drug education programs. These early efforts evolved into the drug education programs of the late 1960s and early 1970s, which claimed to provide relatively objective information, mostly pharmacological in nature, to children in the health, social science, or some other part of a school's curriculum. In most of these cases, the information was provided, but ways of using and incorporating it into one's life-style were not presented and discussed. Several studies in the 1970s found that informational programs in this area aroused the student's curiosity about drugs and increased the likelihood of experimentation with drugs.[5,6]

Table 99-1. Typology of Drug Taking Behaviors

TYPOLOGY OF DRUG TAKING BEHAVIORS

Intensity - how much (single dose)
Frequency- how often (dosing schedule)
Duration - how long (length of use)

Experimental
   Short-term, non-patterned trial
   Variable intensity but minimal frequency
   Reason: curiosity about effects
   May be a shared social activity or individual
   Low risk to individual and society
   Limited long-term problems

Social-Recreational
   Patterned use
   Variable intensity, frequency, and duration
   Social setting of use
   Reason: for effects or group acceptance
   Voluntary act
   May not escalate, but can lead to habit formation
   Low-high individual risk (differs by drug and dose)
   Low-moderate societal risk

Circumstantial-Situational
   Patterned use
   Variable intensity and frequency, limited duration
   Reason: task-specific and usually self-limiting
   Achievement of effect to cope with symptom,
     condition, situation, or need
   Personal (individual) use (setting)
   Moderate risk to individual (dose-dependent)
   Moderate societal risk
   Can lead to escalation in drug taking behaviors
   (Self-medication hypothesis)

Intensified
   Long-term patterned use (duration)
   At least daily use (freq.) with moderate-high intensity
   Reason: Achievement of relief from symptoms, situation,
     personal problems, possibly to prevent withdrawal
   All settings
   Drug is a part of everyday life
   Moderate-high risk for individual (dependence)
   Moderate-high risk for society

Compulsive
   Long-term patterned use (duration)
   High intensity and frequency
   Reason: Dependence and loss-of-functioning, lifestyle
   Drug and Its Use Become Central Focus of Life
   High individual and societal risk

From National Committee on Marijuana and Drug Abuse, 1972.

There came, consequently, a shift in educational programming toward the goal of enhancing social competencies (ie, a person's communication and interpersonal skills and ability to make decisions and to solve problems). The reasoning was that a stable, well-adjusted, socially competent individual surely would have little need for drugs, and in those cases when drugs were used, it would be only socially approved substances in socially accepted and appropriate ways. Such programs usually were effective in enhancing these competencies, but the subsequent influence on drug taking was usually negligible. It was soon realized, however, that the effectiveness of these programs indicated a general lack of social competency training in the family, schools, religious settings, and other places. These programs have value in an educational plan, but mostly when incorporated with drug information, alternatives to drugs, recognition of drug use problems, and other related activities.

In the mid-1970s, in the US, several *responsible drug use* programs were created, mainly in response to the dominant approach, which implied that a successful drug education program would result in abstinence from socially disapproved drugs, and of course, a reduction in drug use problems. The *responsible drug use* movement accepted the notion that people will always want to take chemical substances, and so programs were designed to foster appropriate drug taking behaviors, rational decision-making in the use of drugs, and skills for preventing or recognizing drug use problems.

Programs employing the responsible drug-use approach ranged from responsible drinking-awareness activities, to drug-overdose first-aid training, to the suggestion that some individuals who had alcohol-use problems could reintegrate social drinking into their lives after chemical dependency treatment and counseling. Such programs, however, were not of value to all individuals and groups who engaged in drug taking, and the relative utility and effectiveness of these programs still are not well known.

A few researchers and educators more recently have suggested a rather different drug education and drug prevention approach in which drug taking is considered a *natural behavior*.[7] In this context, educational programs focus on the need to alter one's state of consciousness in an acceptable way and to use drugs in a responsible manner consistent with one's lifestyle. The drug taker is alerted additionally to the importance of values and the influence of societal attitudes on drug taking. These two notions are extremely important in presenting programs or for counseling patients with regard to drug use.

Differences in opinion about and the actual use of many drugs may vary considerably between different individuals and groups. Tobacco (nicotine) and coffee (caffeine) were considered dangerously toxic and addictive substances in earlier times, whereas few people today call either a drug, although renewed interest in combating cigarette smoking has led to the labeling of nicotine as being as addictive as heroin.

In some societies, alcohol is the social drug of choice by adults, whereas marijuana is the social drug of the young people despite its being socially unaccepted or illegal. In other societies, alcohol use is forbidden, whereas marijuana use is socially accepted. As a result of these differences, specific needs for information, education, or consultation to resolve problems in drug taking may not be met; it might be that what we are now doing in the name of stopping the drug problem *is* the drug problem.

Table 99-2. Reasons/Motivations for Drug Use

For drug's effects (therapeutic or otherwise)
Accessibility and availability of drugs
Peer pressure/ modeling/social acceptance
Genetic predisposition
Suggestibility
Curiosity
User set (personality, past experiences, attitudes and perceptions, expectations, motivations for use)
Information, instructions, and accounts of drug effects and experiences (including other users, mass media and advertising)
Meanings of drug effects
Labels for describing drug effects (symbols, metaphors)
Inherent behavior in humans
Rituals of preparation, administration, use
Religious reasons
Social and communication networks
Group/social interaction dynamics
Prior mood and body state
Symptom sensitivity
Coping response
Physical and social setting
Social-cultural background of user
Political and social control
Body image/ideology
Escape
"I don't know" & "As an excuse" (for other behavior)

In the 1980s, there was a backlash against the *responsible drug use* approach and a reorientation of prevention efforts from a supply-reduction strategy (ie, preventing or limiting the supply and flow of drugs at the source) to a demand-reduction strategy (ie, preventing or limiting the need, and thus actual use, of drugs in an indigenous population). Popular contemporary trends are the *Just Say No* campaign and the use of the mass media to inform and educate. The refusal skill technique (eg, *Just Say No* campaign) is an abstinence-based approach, which was developed in the area of smoking prevention research. The use of peers in educational programs also increased in the 1990s. Much of the effort started in the field of alcohol education as attempts were made to move away from authoritarian, moralistic programs with abstinence as a goal to peer-facilitated strategies based on the concept of self-discovery and the fact that alcohol use is socially approved and engendered in most societies, even if it is an illegal activity for certain segments (eg, by age) of the population. Regardless of these trends, *fads*, or new approaches in drug-education programming, there are a few basic principles that always should be considered.

BASIC PRINCIPLES OF DRUG EDUCATION

Various strategies and techniques exist for use in counseling and educating patients, but before these are considered, the process through which learning takes place is reviewed. The process of learning occurs in three domains or in three different ways[8] (Fig 99-1). The basic domain is cognitive, where facts and information are assimilated. A person's knowledge is built through a process of acquiring, understanding, retaining (memory), and reinforcing specific bits of information. The next domain (affective) involves the formation of attitudes such as feelings, beliefs, perceptions, emotions, and appreciations. These are constructed through an interactive process, combining knowledge (from the cognitive domain) and real-life experiences during which the person's knowledge is applied and evaluated to see if it fits that of reality. The behavioral domain (eg, actions, decision-making, physical abilities) is developed from what the person knows and feels, in conjunction with the nature and requirements of their social environment.

Values may affect all domains of learning. One's viewpoint, ethical orientation, or way of life influences drug taking,[9] and it also influences educators as they develop and provide programs. The classic philosophical approach is to consider beliefs and decision-making in one of two ways. The deontological approach focuses more on the action or motive behind the decision, whereas the teleological approach focuses more on the results or consequences of the action or decision.

Decisions to give or take drugs can follow the same philosophical lines of thought. In health care, for instance, the outcome or result of therapy usually is more important than the nature of the therapy itself. In many cases, a vast array of drugs is used to continue the patient's life (the primary *result* of therapy) even when the drugs themselves lead to various negative effects and problems, sometimes worse than the disease itself. Medical and drug research in the past also followed the teleological approach. The emphasis was on the results of research (ie, finding a drug that would cure a disease) and less on what happened to the patients in the experiment. Contempo-

rary clinical drug trials are much more ethical, but the emphasis on results or the outcome of therapy still remains.

The influence of values also can be seen in the development and provision of drug education programs. As described by Dembo,[10] the two current views or frames of reference in drug prevention and treatment differ in their emphasis on drug use. The positivist view focuses on drug use problems and drug education attempts to alter the user's attitudes and behaviors in the direction of total abstinence. The interactionist view stresses the importance of sociocultural and environmental factors leading to drug taking as a valued activity, and drug education focuses on the development of social sanctions and rituals to prevent or limit dysfunctional drug taking. Each viewpoint would result in the development of perhaps different types of drug education programs.

The importance of values in drug taking and drug education even has been considered a primary facet in the development of programs. One approach is known as values clarification, which was developed as a strategy to improve an adolescent's general social skills and which has been adapted to drug education and drug prevention programs.[11] The idea behind values clarification is that an individual's beliefs and ability to make decisions are influenced greatly by values. The clearer these values and the process of valuing are, the more self-directed and consistent the individual is in making optimal decisions and choices in life. The values-clarification strategy has become an important part of some drug education efforts.

The main problem that educational theorists and researchers have had is in determining what and how much of what is learned in one domain influences the learning process in another domain. There is a dominant notion, based in part on common sense, that the provision of drug information will improve appropriate drug-taking behaviors in most situations (eg, increased compliance, responsible self-medication, or decreased social-recreational use). Various research in different areas of drug education suggests that this relation *does not necessarily* hold true.

Many studies on patient package inserts (PPIs), for instance, have found that this form of printed information can lead to reliable gains in drug knowledge, but they seem to have little effect on how patients use a drug.[12] Although the patients' knowledge and understanding (cognitive domain) of the drug and drug regimen were improved, their initial decisions regarding drug therapy, their intention of using the drug (attitudinal domain), and their actual compliance with the regimen were not changed greatly. The same also holds in educating people about nonmedical drug use. The relation between what a person knows about the nonmedical use of drugs and whether a person actually uses drugs in such a way is not very strong, according to most of the research in this area.[13] This body of research also suggests that the relation between knowledge, attitudes, and behavior is unclear and may be weak or inconsistent for some individuals or in some drug taking situations.

On the other hand, some studies of drug knowledge, attitudes, and behavior in the area of social-recreational drug use have shown a relationship between these three domains in some educational situations. The strongest relationship seems to exist between attitudes and behaviors with regard to smoking behavior (and to a limited extent, alcohol use), but even this appears to be a complex and difficult connection to describe and predict in educational efforts. Interactions with individual patients in practice settings also might show that improving patients' knowledge about their drug therapy, in fact, directly influences their compliance behavior. It is obvious that some things we know do influence our attitudes about them, and what we feel about them will influence how we act toward them.

The relationships illustrated in Figure 99-1 are assumed to exist, but not necessarily for everyone in all possible situations, and the relations are shown to occur in either direction. The most important point to realize is that for achieving a particular type of effect, the best approach is to focus on the domain of learning where the desired effect or change should occur. If the

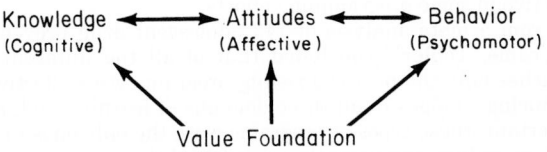

Figure 99-1. Domains of learning.

goal of the educator's efforts is a negative attitude toward the use of certain drugs, then the educational program should focus its activities more on attitudes and less on increasing drug knowledge or on discouraging drug taking. If the goal of the program is to prevent or limit certain types of drug use, the focus should be on building skills and directing behavior away from use and not so much on increasing drug knowledge or on developing attitudes against drugs and their use.

Truly effective drug education occurs by individualizing the learning process to the particular needs of the patient or consumer. The pharmacist should become aware of a particular person's situation and be ready to help as needed. Not only is this a part of effective counseling and drug education, but most people indicate that this approach (ie, being considered as a unique human being) is what they desire and expect in interactions with health professionals.

Individualized attention, not surprisingly, is also one of the major factors in a consumer's selection and patronage of a particular pharmacy. In terms of drug education, then, the best way to approach the learning process is to:

Assess the person's level of knowledge and provide relevant information in those areas where there is a deficiency.
Counsel the person and encourage positive attitudes toward the appropriate and controlled use of drugs.
Evaluate the person's drug taking and general health over time to verify appropriate patterns of use and optimal outcomes from use and to reinforce positive attitudes and behaviors.

This individualized approach also raises an extremely important concept that has attracted much attention recently: the importance of literacy in reading and understanding health and drug information. About 18% of the US adult population reads at the 5th grade level or lower, and almost half of the population reads at less than the 10th grade level, with the average reading level at the 8th to 9th grade.[14] It is imperative that health and drug counselors and educators become more aware and educate themselves about this major problem.

The concepts and principles presented in this chapter apply to people who use a chemical substance for a medical or nonmedical reason in any setting. The delineation of educational effects or outcomes is most productive when it is based on the idea that people learn and act on what they know in different ways.

EFFECTS AND OUTCOMES OF DRUG-EDUCATION PROGRAMS

The most important concept, which surprisingly often is not stated explicitly in educational programs, is the behavior or problem that is the target of the educational or prevention effort. This is unfortunately the case with most drug education programs. There is sometimes a general sense of what should be achieved, but the specific results or outcomes are not clearly delineated. Several different, though not necessarily mutually exclusive, goals for drug education programs are:

An increase in drug knowledge
A change in attitudes about drugs and their use
An improvement in social functioning (eg, social competency), which might lead to better decision making in drug taking situations
A change in drug use in general
A change in the use of specific types of drugs
A reduction in the occurrence of specific drug-use problems

Once the overall goals of the program are determined, more specific results and outcomes may be identified and characterized.

This degree of generality appears to occur most often in educational programs on the nonmedical use of drugs. Most programs list a primary goal of prevention of drug abuse, but the question of what constitutes *abuse* of a chemical substance usually is not well defined. This results in the adoption of complete abstinence from drug use as the goal of the educational or prevention program.

What, then, are the effects and outcomes of drug education programs? The most effective type, in relation to one specific level of learning, addresses drug knowledge. The provision of drug information, and the receipt and understanding of that information, leads to increases at the cognitive level most of the time; patients or consumers show an improvement in their knowledge about drugs, as measured by some cognitive test. This increase in knowledge, however, may not lead to a change in attitudes or behaviors. For instance, the effectiveness of PPIs and other programmed medication instruction sheets are variable. Studies of PPIs by the Rand Corporation provided a better idea of the use and effectiveness of patient drug information.[12] The principle findings of those studies were that:

PPIs are likely to be read widely.
PPIs are used as reference documents by many patients.
PPIs lead to reliable gains in drug knowledge.
PPIs seem to have little effect on how patients use a drug.
PPIs do not, in general, lead patients to report more side effects.
PPIs are unlikely to change the frequency with which patients contact their physicians.
Patients find written drug information helpful.
The amount of explanation provided in a PPI makes little difference in how much information patients understand or remember.
The simplicity with which a PPI is written has little effect on understanding.

Other studies, as well as comprehensive reviews of the literature in this area, have arrived at similar conclusions.[15,16] In a medical context, the provision of drug information often leads to measurable gains in knowledge about drugs, but corresponding changes in drug taking (eg, improved compliance or more appropriate self-medication) may not occur, especially if learning also does not take place in the attitudinal or behavioral domain.

Drug education programs directed at these other domains of learning most often have their effect in those specific domains. The general lack of effectiveness of drug information programs in improving compliance motivated educators to develop other techniques. In the area of compliance, several attitudinal and behavioral strategies have been developed (see *Compliance* chapter). For example, health beliefs have been found to influence an individual's decision making about seeking health care and complying with prescribed therapy. In educational efforts, the Health Belief Model[17] has been used to design specific techniques and strategies, which have been found to be effective in increasing compliance in some patients. Behavior modification techniques also have been effective in helping patients to adhere to dieting plans, to comply with complex or difficult therapeutic regimens, and even to stop smoking.

In the area of nonmedical drug education, the informational approach also has been found to have a short-term effect on drug knowledge and little effect on nonmedical drug use. The interesting and somewhat unfortunate exception is that the provision of information or lecturing solely on the pharmacology of the *drugs of abuse* was found in some studies actually to increase students' curiosity and their desire to experiment with these substances.[5,18] In these studies, drug use increased slightly for a short time after the educational program, and then it fell back to the level measured before the educational activity. Early efforts using fear-arousal messages and scare tactics were found to have an immediate effect, when compared with the provision of factual information or discussions of attitudes, but the effect usually only lasted for a short period. The consensus of researchers is that fear as a part of punishment is not an effective approach, but positive reinforcement might be effective in some programming efforts.

From a meta-analysis of 143 adolescent drug prevention programs, Tobler[19] concluded that of all the different approaches only the peer counseling programs were effective in producing changes in all three domains of learning and, most important, these types of programs were the only ones to prevent or reduce significantly nonmedical drug use in adolescents. Programs using alternatives to drugs were found to be effective in reducing drug use for *high-risk'* adolescents. In general, this large-scale analytical review found that multimodality programs were much more effective than programs that used only a single approach or strategy. A review and analysis of 35 drug-education programs, which employed specific outcome measures, found that the *new generation* of prevention strategies may produce more positive and fewer negative results than did the older drug-information approaches.[20] Even when positive changes were noted in a particular program, those changes were usually small and short term. Other studies and reviews have arrived at similar conclusions; most educational programs, regardless of the approach or strategy, seem to produce changes in drug knowledge, but few are capable of leading to significant changes in drug taking behaviors.[21]

Some educators, however, have argued and shown through research that the relation among knowledge, attitudes, and behavior might be a complex one, and although changes in the cognitive domain can occur quickly, changes in attitudes and behaviors take longer to be internalized by the learner and put into everyday, real-life practice.[22]

Strategies and approaches that have been developed more recently have not been shown to be more effective. The refusal-skills approach (eg, *Just Say No*) appears to be most effective in smoking prevention, but even then, the effect is short term. Mass-media approaches to drug education and prevention also have been shown to have a noticeable, short-term effect on drug use, especially in terms of smoking prevention. The use of written drug information, as a supplement to the media content, seems to improve slightly the effectiveness of the mass media.

DRUG EDUCATION IN A MEDICAL CONTEXT

The range of audiences for medical drug education programs can vary from the one-to-one interaction with an individual patient to comprehensive programming for groups of people or whole communities. Drug information and consultation are educational activities that pharmacists have been using for some time. Providing information, presenting drug education programs and consulting with patients and health professionals represent the major prevention efforts requiring pharmacy involvement (see Appendix A).

Drug taking in a medical context often is influenced or directed by a health professional. The drug educator should not forget this audience in planning and developing drug education programs. The primary group is the drug prescriber, mostly physicians. Research has shown that prescribing behaviors are influenced by numerous factors, including: prescriber education and training; drug advertising and promotion; interactions with colleagues; control and regulatory mechanisms in health care; and the demands of patients and society.

These factors should be considered in developing programs to educate physicians and others about drugs and to improve the appropriateness of their prescribing behaviors.[23] Drug information newsletters and other services, counter detailing and screening pharmaceutical representatives, in-service seminars and presentations and drug utilization review with feedback and consultation are the most commonly used approaches to improve drug knowledge and change prescribing practices.

The actual education of patients about their prescribed medications covers a wide range of complex and involved strategies (see Appendix A). At one end of the spectrum, a drug information sheet (also called a study instruction sheet), education card, or PPI is given to the patient along with the medication. Information sheets in languages other than English, and in a pictorial format for those who cannot read, also have been designed. Programmed instruction sheets, which provide both information and auto-tutorial learning with reinforcement, also have been developed and used in pharmacy. The value and effectiveness of sheets is variable, with the greatest degree of learning occurring in the cognitive domain.

Written drug information obviously is important, and used by many patients. The best manner to provide such information, however, may not be through mandatory distribution of standardized information, but by individualization of the information to the patient's needs. Supplementing written information with verbal counseling usually increases its effectiveness and utility. The *Omnibus Budget Reconciliation Act of 1990* (OBRA 90) mandates patient counseling. The pharmacist also may help patients' informational needs by being aware of and providing some of the many consumer-oriented drug books now on the market.

Experience suggests that the vast majority of patients' questions and needs can be answered fairly immediately from one's knowledge and experience. The optimal distribution of drug information should be based on the old adage: the right information, in the right form and amount, to the right person or place at the right time.

One concept that has emerged recently as an effective learning strategy is social support. Some programs have been designed to include social support in the educational process, and this concept even can be applied to individual counseling situations in health-care settings. The pharmacist and a significant other, such as a spouse, family member, or friend, help in motivating the patient toward a positive health behavior by monitoring drug use, noting problems, and reinforcing appropriate drug taking behaviors. In the context of motivation, another technique, called motivational interviewing, has been developed in patient education. Motivational interviewing is a patient-centered counseling approach for initiating behavior change by helping patients resolve ambivalence or confusion in understanding their treatment regimens. It is an approach that helps patients to increase their motivation to change.

Another strategy involves the use of behavior modification to assure appropriate drug use. This problem solving process employs the observation of behavior, cueing (some type of motivator or reminder to initiate behavior), and rewards to define and modify behavior in a specific way. The patient learns about the medical condition and drug regimen, and then implements a self-management program related to his particular therapy. The patient becomes a partner in the planning of therapy, and consequently feels responsible for following the agreed-upon regimen. These two techniques, social support and behavior modification programs, have been found to be effective in improving patient compliance with medication regimens.

There is one type of drug taking behavior for which few educational programs have been developed. Self-medication and related practices involving home remedies have not been well studied in the past, and consequently, ideas and theories for how to change and improve self-medicating behavior are limited. Some investigators are working on the application of the *Health Belief Model*[17] to situations involving self-diagnosis and self-medication. For the most part, educational activities in self-medication have consisted of drug information, usually in the form of consumer-oriented books on drugs. A perusal of the health and medical sections of local bookstores should give the reader an idea of the range and quality of this information.

Basic principles in the provision of drug information apply to the evaluation and use of these materials as well, before they are suggested or distributed to consumers. In addition to consumer-oriented books and materials, the only other strategies developed in this area are simple, structured educational presentations on self-medication trends, fads, and problems, and the use of algorithms or flow charts to assist consumers in their decision making.[24]

DRUG EDUCATION IN A NONMEDICAL CONTEXT

Various programs have been designed to provide information and education on drug taking in a nonmedical context (see Appendix A). The classic approach is to provide drug-specific (eg, pharmacology) and drug-related (eg, drug laws or alternatives) information to individuals or groups. The affective or attitudinal approach consists of training in communication skills, values clarification, self-esteem and coping with stress. Informational and affective strategies often are combined in a single program or a series of workshops.

The behavioral approach focuses on the building of skills, such as refusal skills to counter peer pressure, assertiveness, decision making and problem solving, or employs behavioral modification techniques to help identify and change inappropriate behaviors. Comprehensive programming involves complex, multisession educational experiences that are designed to have an effect on all domains of learning. Examples of these types of programs include peer-counselor and teacher training, curricular design in school settings, and community-based approaches such as parenting and parent–child interaction workshops and the use of the local mass media.

Research has shown that the best point in a curriculum to begin or to expand *drug abuse* education programming is approximately at the fifth- or sixth-grade level.[5] Student populations may differ greatly from one school setting to another, thus necessitating the use of a needs assessment survey to determine their level of experience and understanding. Drug-related information (eg, drug laws, alternatives to drugs) also should be presented and discussed as part of any drug education program, particularly if the program goal is abstinence from drug use.

Social competencies are those skills and abilities that promote healthy personal and social functioning. It has been suggested that people who are not socially competent (ie, those with low levels of trust, confidence, self-esteem, identity, directionality, and interpersonal skills) are more likely to engage in inappropriate drug use. On the other hand, the socially competent person is more likely to make better decisions about drug use, prevent problems from drug use, or recognize such problems and solve them. In fact, the strategy of enhancing social competencies is a major part of Alcoholics or Narcotics Anonymous.

The training of gatekeepers and other key people to assist in recognizing drug use problems and in referring people to appropriate health and social agencies has been the focus of some educational programs. Gatekeepers are those individuals to whom a person might turn for help in dealing with drug use problems. Such individuals can be family members, school personnel, religious leaders, local officials, criminal-justice workers, bartenders (with regard to alcohol use problems), civic organizations, and health professionals. Pharmacists perhaps are qualified best to be gatekeepers for individuals who have drug-use problems.

Being a gatekeeper essentially means being able to recognize potential or actual drug-use problems, being empathic in understanding the different attitudes or motivations that might have led to the problem, and being able to assist the person in solving the problem or making a referral. Such skills are not difficult to learn and actually enhance one's ability to help family, friends, patients, and even one's self with all kinds of problems.

DEVELOPING DRUG-EDUCATION PROGRAMS

The provision of drug education programs occurs to varying degrees, according to the motivations of the pharmacist and the nature of the pharmacy-practice setting. Many factors should be considered in developing a drug education service:

What types of educational programs can be provided?
How involved the pharmacist is willing to become, given the constraints of personal knowledge and skills, space, time, manpower, availability of resources, and financial considerations?

It is good practice to define the exact role one plans to assume as a drug educator, including the specific programs and services to be provided. This provides a framework upon which

skills and abilities may be built and acts as a point of reference from which to work. It also delineates how and what to promote, and makes it clear to patients and consumers what is being offered.

It is important to recognize that each pharmacist becomes a drug educator to a different degree of involvement. One pharmacist may wish to provide only verbal and written information at his pharmacy, whereas another may be willing to give structured drug education presentations before groups of people. Neither should be forced to do more or less. In essence, the type of education required by the patients and consumers must be determined, and a personal educational style best suited to meet those needs must be developed.

In using any particular educational strategy or program, the pharmacist should be familiar with its goals and content, the target audience for whom it is intended, its biases and flaws, the results of any evaluation studies performed on it, its known effect on actual use and practical considerations such as costs, time and manpower requirements, materials and equipment, and extra training.

Whether an individual or group effort, drug education activities require an interactive and structured approach, such as described by the framework illustrated in Figure 99-2. This general approach is useful during education of individual patients in practice settings or during presentation of formal programs before groups of people. The approach basically delineates the important steps one should consider in the conceptualization, development, and implementation of any activity intended to educate patients and consumers about drugs.

The first step is the identification or presentation of a specific question, problem, or need. This might consist of anything from a patient's noncompliance with prescribed drug therapy to a community's need for comprehensive programming in the area of alcohol use and alcoholism. The problem is identified and defined through interaction with the pharmacist. Once the need has been stated and defined, appropriate strategies can be selected and combined into a specific educational or prevention program. The activity may be as simple as the provision of written and verbal drug information to the patient, or it might be as complex as a multisession drug education program involving various strategies. The effect of the activity that has been implemented always should be monitored and evaluated to assure relevance and usefulness in fulfilling the need. In the instance of an ineffective strategy or program, then, the pharmacist can add or drop specific strategies to improve the overall program.

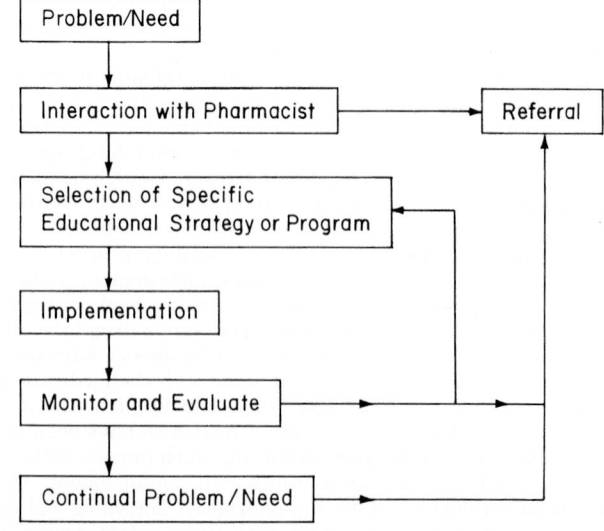

Figure 99-2. Pharmacist-oriented approach to drug education.

Table 99-3. Guidelines for Developing a Drug Education Program

I. Identify Audience and Educational Need or Problem
  1. Receive request for program
  2. Determine need or problem and individual or group at risk
II. Set Goals and Objectives for the Program
  1. Clarify needs, interests, and expectations
  2. Determine outcomes
  3. Define specific goals and objectives
  4. Identify specific topics and content areas based on needs and objectives
  5. Determine focus and philosophical approach
III. Develop Resources and Materials
  1. Identify sources of information and gather and evaluate these materials
  2. Identify key people with expertise
  3. Prepare new materials
IV. Select Appropriate Educational Techniques
  1. Choose teaching approach and strategies
  2. Identify educational setting, time-frame, equipment, and other technical needs
V. Design, Implement, and Evaluate the Program
  1. Structure the program format
  2. Make a complete outline
  3. Pretest components, content, and educational approach
  4. Implement the program
  5. Evaluate and refine

If there is a continual need or problem or if the pharmacist feels that the nature of the stated problem is outside of his or her area of expertise or comfort, a referral should be made.

A stepwise approach also should be used in developing drug education programs, but the educator must realize that a list of guidelines (Table 99-3) represents only those decisions and activities that should be considered in the planning and developmental stages. These guidelines, and program outlines and curricula from other sources, must never be used in a cookbook fashion, with little or no critical thought about what is being done.

Flexibility in program design and tailoring the program to the individual needs of the audience are most essential for a successful educational endeavor. One procedure for improving the match between the audience's needs and expectations and the educational program's content and approach is to perform a needs assessment. A short questionnaire is prepared to elicit the needs, suggestions, and expectations of the target audience, as well as the demographic information on the group's charac-

teristics. The results from such a survey then are used to design the content and format of the educational program.

In addition to the program's content and educational materials, there are a few technical matters that need to be considered (Table 99-4). The provision of drug information and drug education programs always entails the use of time, money, and equipment. More complex and involved programs often are more effective in changing drug taking behaviors, but they also can be more costly and time consuming. The provider of a drug education program also must make certain that specific types of equipment (eg, audiovisuals or computers) are available and in good working order for the program. Finally, in most situations, the consent or permission of the audience or their representative, such as in school settings, is necessary prior to the actual implementation of any educational activity.

Developing and providing educational services involves four steps: design, implementation, evaluation, and promotion. Each step should be directed by the specific situation. The design of educational services consists of assessing patients' needs, collecting and developing resources and program materials, being trained in their appropriate use, and planning their distribution to the target person or audience.

Patient or consumer needs may be determined by recalling past experiences with specific problems, being aware of the mass media and the concerns of consumer-advocacy groups, and surveying the local population for current and future needs. Many pharmacists periodically have used patient-need surveys (which simply can consist of a single page of general, open-ended questions soliciting a written response from the person or a listing of services and programs that the person can check off) to assist them in the design process. They have found that besides being useful for that purpose, it also builds greater trust and loyalty among their patients and gives the pharmacist an idea of what the patients think about the pharmacy and pharmacist in general.

Once the educational services are defined and developed, they can be implemented whenever a need or problem arises. On many occasions, the pharmacist might have to take the initiative, particularly if it is perceived there are potential drug-use problems occurring in a person or in the community. Most of what is involved in implementation has already been described. Local and regional resources (eg, drug information and poison-control centers, mental health and chemical-dependency facilities, hospitals, libraries, bookstores, and media centers) should be identified beforehand to determine what services or information they can provide, and to know when they are available and how to reach them if necessary. One should consider evaluating the educational services used to make sure that they are both ef-

Table 99-4. Technical Aspects of Drug Education Programs

APPROACH	GROUP SIZE	AUDIENCE	TIME	COSTS	OUTCOMES
Cognitive only	any number	nonspecific heterogeneous unless content specific	short	low except material costs	short-term gains in knowledge
Affective (Social Competencies)	small groups (<20)	nonspecific or target groups	short	low	short-term changes in attitudes
Cognitive and Affective	small to medium size (depends on activities)	nonspecific or target groups	short to medium (depends on content)	low	short-term changes in knowledge and attitudes
Skills Building	small groups (<15)	focused on specific skill or activity homogeneous	time consuming multi-session	high*	significant changes in attitudes and reductions in drug use (medium to long-term impact)
Comprehensive Programming	small groups directly large groups indirectly for certain activities (mass media)	very focused on specific goals or tasks homogeneous for direct programs heterogeneous for indirect programs	very time consuming multi-session	high*	significant changes in attitudes and reductions in drug use, esp alcohol, tobacco, and marijuana

*High cost involves personnel, materials, and multi-media, all over multiple sessions, so dependent on number of sessions in the specific program.

fective and efficient and that the information and services provided are understandable and of use in meeting the problem or need. Evaluations can be performed in the same manner as the aforementioned patient-need surveys.

The pharmacist also should consider the promotion of educational programs and services, so that the patients and consumers become aware of and use them. The promotion of such services is similar, in concept, to the promotion of any product or service. Detailed descriptions may be found in any reference book on marketing, advertising, or business practices. There are many specific techniques that can be used in promotion. Some are free of cost and involve only a small amount of time, whereas the willingness to spend more time and money leads to more intricate and diverse promotional schemes. One comprehensive way is through the local mass media. It is not difficult to contact the local town or neighborhood newspaper, local TV or radio station, and local cable networks and ask for a news story or even request an interview that would describe the new educational services that will be provided to the community.

If the services are significantly new in nature or potentially beneficial to the community, such as presenting structured drug education programs, free news stories and public service announcements about these services and their provider could result. Word-of-mouth communication from current users of the services also is important. It is good to end an episode involving counseling and education with the statement, "If you, or anyone else you know, needs further help or information, please don't hesitate to contact me." Advertising in the phonebook and through the media, and placing signs in the pharmacy's window and at key spots around the community also may be effective.

Single-page consumer-oriented drug information sheets may be produced for distribution. Assistance for the printing of such materials may be obtained from local agencies and businesses as a show of community support. There is also the accepted practice of promoting a new service by informing lay people or community groups about them. Through a process of diffusion, this information is shared with a larger number of people who come in contact with those who have been informed. In most communities, key people or groups include teachers and counselors at local schools, the Jaycees and Chamber of Commerce, the PTA, women's clubs, consumer groups, governmental agencies, social and welfare organizations, chemical-dependency agencies, and other health professionals in the area.

FUTURE EFFORTS

The nature and focus of most drug education and drug prevention programs will not change greatly in the near future. Numerous different strategies and techniques have been developed, but what is really needed are more concerted efforts to design and evaluate programs in a rational manner. In a philosophical way, our ability to prevent drug use problems can be improved in several ways. Drugs should not be categorized as being "hard" or "soft," licit or illicit, or addictive or nonaddictive, but instead it should be stressed that the use of any chemical substance carries with it a certain potential for the development of problems, depending on the pattern and setting of use, the reason for use, past experiences with the drug, and various additional social and pharmacological factors. Future efforts should focus more on preventing or limiting drug use problems.

Some educators[25] have even argued that a health promotion, rather than the more traditional disease prevention, approach should be used. Also, a need exists to become more cognizant of attitudes, values, and motivations—especially those that differ from our own—in people's drug taking, because these factors are most important in recognizing and char-

acterizing the nature and the extent of drug-use problems. For instance, some educators have argued that it is time to view drug use as a motivated, adaptive behavior that is pursued in the consummation of valued experience, and then to develop strategies and programs based on this notion.[7,10]

In practical terms, the success of future programs and activities depends on a clearer and more coordinated effort in using the strategies and techniques that have been developed and tested. Health professionals, the family, schools, and communities should combine their efforts and integrate drug- education strategies into ongoing activities, instead of just adding them onto irrelevant courses and programs. Attitudinal strategies and basic drug information should be combined in educational programs. The various structured and prepackaged materials and techniques should be selected and synthesized into programmatic formats that best meet the needs of the target audience.

It is important to identify individuals or groups at high risk for developing drug-use problems and to focus educational and prevention efforts on their needs. Finally, a humanistic approach, in which drug taking is considered a natural kind of behavior and in which an awareness of different values is stressed, should be brought into educational programming. Regardless of the degree of involvement, it is time for pharmacists and the pharmaceutical profession to provide more drug education programs for their patients and all of society.

Acknowledgment—The author acknowledges the pharmacists and pharmacy students of Kentucky, Massachusetts, Minnesota, New Hampshire, and Pennsylvania who have been involved in the development and use of many ideas, materials, and programs described herein.

REFERENCES

1. National Commission on Marijuana and Drug Abuse. *Drug Use in America: Problem in Perspective.* Washington, DC: USGPO, 1973.
2. Montagne M, Basara L. In: Smith MC, Wertheimer AI. *Social and Behavioral Aspects of Pharmaceutical Care.* New York: Pharmaceutical Products Press, 1996.
3. Kaufman DW, Kelly JP, Rosenberg L, et al. *JAMA* 2002; 287:337.
4. National Institute on Drug Abuse. *National Household Survey on Drug Abuse.* Washington, DC: USGPO, 2002.
5. Tennant FS, et al. *Pediatrics* 1973; 52:246.
6. Blum RH. *Drug Education: Results and Recommendations.* Lexington, MA: Heath, 1976.
7. Einstein S, ed. *Drugs in Relation to the Drug User.* New York: Pergamon, 1980.
8. Bettinghaus EP. *Prev Med* 1986; 15:475.
9. Veatch RM. *J Drug Issues* 1977; 7:253.
10. Dembo R. *Int J Addict* 1981; 16:1399.
11. Simon SB. *Beginning Values Clarification: A Guidebook for the Use of Values Clarification in the Classroom.* San Diego: Pennant Press, 1975.
12. Kanouse DE, et al. *Informing Patients about Drugs.* Santa Monica: Rand Corporation, 1981.
13. Montagne M, Scott DM. *Int J Addictions* 1993; 28:1177.
14. Doak CC, Doak LG, Root JH. *Teaching Patients with Low Literacy Skills,* 2nd ed. Philadelphia: JB Lippincott, 1996.
15. Mullen PD, Green LW. *Measuring Patient Drug Information Transfer: An Assessment of the Literature.* Washington DC: PMA, 1984.
16. Glanz K, et al. *Med Care* 1981; 19:141.
17. Becker MH, ed. *The Health Belief Model and Personal Health Behavior.* Thorofare, NJ: Slack, 1974.
18. Goodstadt M, ed. *Research on Methods and Programs of Drug Education.* Toronto: Addict Res Found, 1974.
19. Tobler NS. *J Drug Issues* 1986; 16:537.
20. Schaps E, et al. *Int J Addict* 1980; 15:657.
21. Anon. *Promising Community Drug Abuse Prevention Programs.* Rockville, MD: USGAO, 1991.
22. Gonzalez GM. *J Alcohol Drug Educ* 1982; 27:2.
23. Segal R, Wang F. *PPMQ* 1999; 19:30.
24. Vickery DM, Fries JF. *Take Care of Yourself: A Consumer's Guide to Medical Care.* Reading, MA: Addison-Wesley, 1976.
25. Room R. *Public Health Rep* 1981; 96:26.

Specific Strategies and Programs in Drug Education[a]

COGNITIVE (INFORMATION) PROGRAMS

Drug Information

Corry JM, Cimbolic P. *Drugs: Facts, Alternatives, Decisions*. Belmont, CA: Wadsworth, Belmont CA, 1985.
Julien RM. *Primer on Drug Action*, 8th ed. New York: WH Freeman, 1995.
Weil A, Rosen W. *From Chocolate to Morphine: Everything You Need to Know About Mind-Altering Drugs*. Rev. ed. Boston MA: Houghton-Mifflin, 1998.
Goldberg R. *Taking Sides: Clashing Views on Controversial Issues in Drugs and Society*. 3rd ed. Guilford CT: Dushkin/McGraw-Hill, 1998.
Hartzema AG. *Optimizing Patient Comprehension through Medicine Information Leaflets*. Rockville MD: U.S. Pharmacopeia, 1999.
Morris LA. *Communicating Therapeutic Risks*. New York: Springer-Verlag, 1990.

Computer-Assisted Instruction

Gustafson DH et al. *Ann Rev Publ Health* 1987; 8: 387.
Anon. *Healthcare CAI Directory*. Alexandria VA: Stewart Publ., 1991–2002.

Drug Information Services

Montagne M et al. *Am J Hosp Pharm* 1980; 37: 1211.
Rolett V, Kinney, J. *How to Start and Run an Alcohol and Other Drug Information Centre: A Guide*. Rockville, MD: Office of Substance Abuse Prevention, 1990.
Snow B. *Drug Information: A Guide to Current Resources*. Lanham MD: Scarecrow Press, 1999.

Health Literacy

Doak CC, Doak LG, Root JH. *Teaching Patients with Low Literacy Skill*. 2nd ed. Philadelphia PA: JB Lippincott, 1996.
Dowse R, Ehlers MS. *Int J Pharm Pract* 1998; 6: 109.
Zimmerman M, Newton N, Frumin L, Wittet S. *Developing Health & Family Planning Print Materials for Low-Literate Audiences: A Guide*. Seattle WA: Program for Appropriate Technology in Health (PATH), 1989.

AFFECTIVE (ATTITUDINAL) PROGRAMS

Interpersonal Skills

Begin S et al. *Traditional Ties: Cultural Awareness and Listening Skills*. White Plains, NY: Longman, 1992.
Tindall WN, Beadsley RS, Kimberlin CL, Speziale HS. *Communication Skills in Pharmacy Practice*. 4th ed. Philadelphia PA: Lippincott Williams & Wilkins, 2002.

Values Clarification

Dembo R. *Int J Addict* 1981; 16: 1399.
Simon SB, Howe LW, Kirschenbaum H. *Values Clarification: A Handbook of Practical Strategies for Teachers and Students*. New York: Dodd, Mead, 1978.

Social Competencies

Bell C, Battjes R, eds. *Research: Deterring Drug Abuse among Children and Adolescents*. Rockville, MD: National Institute on Drug Abuse, 1985.
Masters R, Houston J. *Mind Games*. New York: Viking, 1972.

Parenting

Ezetoye S et al. *Childhood and Chemical Abuse: Prevention and Intervention*. New York: Haworth,1986.
Manatt M. *Parents, Peers and Pot II*. Rockville, MD: National Institute on Drug Abuse, 1983.

---

[a] These citations contain specific program descriptions.

Coping with Stress

Kleinke CL. *Coping with Life's Challenges*. Cambridge, MA: Course Tech, 1997.
Shiffman S, Wills TA, eds. *Coping and Substance Use*. Orlando, FL: Academic, 1985.

BEHAVIORAL (SKILLS-BUILDING) PROGRAMS

Refusal Skills and Peer Pressure

Adolescent Peer Pressure: Theory, Correlates, and Program Implications for Drug Abuse Prevention. Rockville, MD: National Institute on Drug Abuse, 1986.
Goldstein AP, Reagles KW, Amann LL. *Refusal Skills: Preventing Drug Use in Adolescents*. Champaign IL: Research Press, 1990.

Fear-Arousal Messages

Leathar DS et al, eds. *Health Education and the Media II*. New York: Pergamon, 1986.

Alternatives to Drugs

Cohen S. *JAMA* 1977; 238:1561.
NIDA. *A Review of Alternative Activities and Alternative Programs in Youth Oriented Prevention*. Rockville, MD: NIDA, 1996.

Social-Control Mechanisms

Einstein S, ed. *Drugs in Relation to the Drug User*. New York: Pergamon, 1980.
Zinberg NE, Harding WM, eds. *Control Over Intoxicant Use: Pharmacological, Psychological, & Social Considerations*. New York: Human Sciences Press, 1981.

Social Support/Group Activities

Glynn TJ et al, eds. *Preventing Adolescent Drug Abuse: Intervention Strategies*. Rockville, MD: National Institute on Drug Abuse, 1983.
Gottlieb BH. *Social Support Strategies: Guidelines for Mental Health Practice*. Thousand Oaks, CA: Sage, 1983.

Behavior Modification

Kaplan JS, Drainville B. *Beyond Behavior Modification: A Cognitive-Behavioral Approach to Behavior Management in the School*. Austin TX: Pro-Ed, 1990.
Stuart RB, ed. *Adherence, Compliance, and Generalization in Behavioral Medicine*. New York: Brunner/Mazel, 1982.
Sundel SS, Sundel M. *Behavior Modification in the Human Services*. Thousand Oaks, CA: Sage, 1993.

Motivational Interviewing

Emmons KM, Rollnick S. *Amer J Prev Med* 2001; 20: 68.
Miller WR, Rollnick S. *Motivational Interviewing: Preparing People for Change*. New York: Guilford Press, 2002.

Decision Making and Problem Solving

Botvin GJ. *Life Skills Training*. Princeton NJ: Princeton Technical, 1996.
Goodstadt MS, Sheppard MA. *J Studies Alcohol* 1983; 44: 362.
Koberg D, Bagnall J. *The Universal Traveler: A Soft-Systems Guide to Creativity, Problem-Solving, and the Process of Reaching Goals*. Los Altos, CA: William Kaufmann, 1972.

PROGRAM PLANNING

Program Development

Edwards G, Arif A. *Drug Problems in the Sociocultural Context: A Basis for Policies and Programme Planning*. Geneva: WHO, 1980.
Moskowitz JM. *J Stud Alcohol* 1989; 50: 54.

Needs Assessment

Claydon PD, Johnson ME. *J Alcohol Drug Educ* 1985; 31: 51.
World Health Association. *Assessment of Public Health and Social Problems with the Use of Psychotropic Drugs*. Geneva: WHO, 1981.

Program Outcomes

Schaps E et al. *J Drug Issues* 1981; 11: 17.
National Institute on Drug Abuse. *Meta-Analysis of Drug Abuse Prevention Programs*. Rockville, MD: NIDA, 1997.

Program Evaluation

Hawkins JD, Nederhood B. *Handbook for Evaluating Drug and Alcohol Prevention Programs*. Rockville, MD: Substance Abuse Prev, 1987.
Montagne M. *Eval Health Prof* 1982; 5: 477.

Role of the Educator

Dembo R. *Int J Addict* 1981; 16: 1399.
Oshodin OG. *J Alcohol Drug Educ* 1984; 29: 1.

COMPREHENSIVE PROGRAMMING

Mass Media

Flay BR. *J School Health* 1986; 56: 401.
Resnick H. *Youth and Drugs: Society's Mixed Messages*. Rockville, MD: NIDA, 1990.

Holistic/Integrated Approaches

Embry D, McDaniel R. *Reclaiming Wyoming: A Comprehensive Blueprint for Prevention, Early Intervention and Treatment of Substance Abuse*. Cheyenne, WY: Wyoming Department of Health, 2002 (access at http://wdhfs.state.wy.us/WDH or through Wyoming House Bill 83).
Nebelkopf E. *Psychoactive Drugs* 1981; 13: 345.
Winkelman DL, Harbet SC. *J Alcohol Drug Educ* 1985; 31: 17.

School-Based Program

Anon. *Drug Abuse Resistance Education (D.A.R.E.)*. Revised program, 2002, access at http://www.dare.com.
Bangert-Drowns RL. *J Drug Educ* 1988; 18: 243.
Pentz MA et al. *JAMA* 1989; 261:3259.

Community-Based Programs

Giesbrecht N, et al, eds. *Research, Action, and the Community: Experiences in the Prevention of Alcohol and Other Drug Problems*. Rockville, MD: Office of Substance Abuse Prevention, 1989.
NIDA. *The Future by Design. A Community Framework for Preventing Alcohol and Other Drug Problems*. Rockville, MD: USGPO, 1991.
Project Alert (middle grades): www.projectalert.best.org.
Project Success (high school): www.modelprograms.samhsa.gov.

Peer Counseling

Arkin EB, Funkhouser JE. *Communicating about Alcohol and Other Drugs: Strategies for Reaching Populations at Risk*. Rockville, MD: Office of Substance Abuse Prevention, 1990.
Office of Substance Abuse Prevention. *Preventing Adolescent Drug Use: From Theory to Practice*. Rockville, MD: OSAP, 1991.

Health-Professional Training

Ewan CE, Waite A. *Int J Addict* 1982; 17: 1211.
Lewis DC et al. *JAMA* 1987; 257: 2945.

Gatekeeper Training

Jensen K. *Int J Health Educ* 1981; 24 (suppl): 1.
Schaps E et al. *J Alcohol Drug Educ* 1984; 29: 35.

Curricular Guides and Bibliographies

Cornacchia HJ et al. *Drugs in the Classroom: A Conceptual Model for School Programs,* 2nd ed. St. Louis: Mosby, 1978.
Anon. *Learning to Live Drug Free: A Curriculum Model for Prevention*. Rockville, MD: NIDA, 1990.
Anon. *Prevention Plus II*. Rockville, MD: Office of Substance Abuse Prevention, 1989.

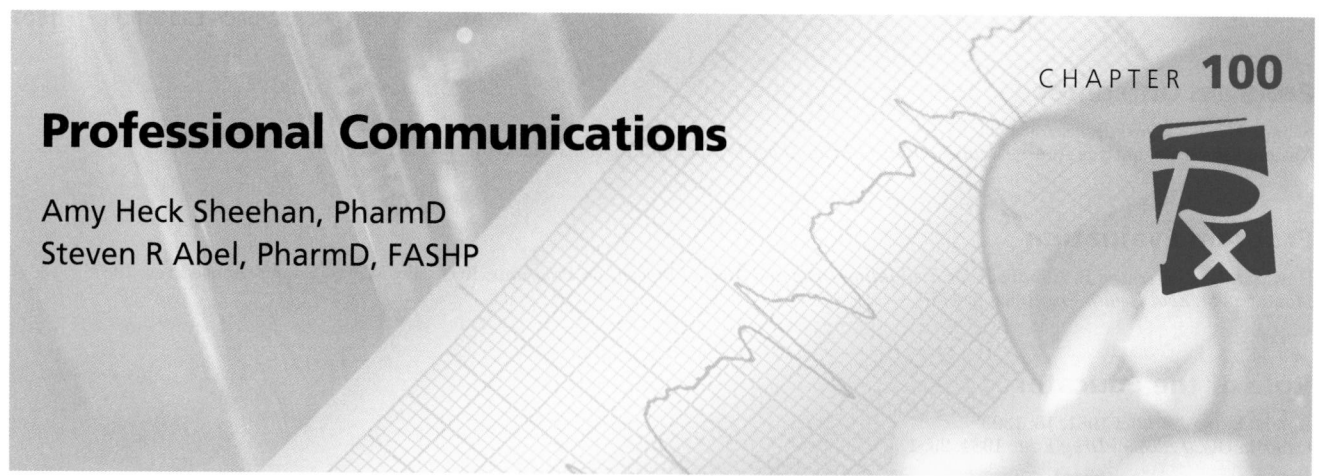

CHAPTER 100

Professional Communications

Amy Heck Sheehan, PharmD
Steven R Abel, PharmD, FASHP

Communication is a vital skill, necessary for success in personal and professional settings. Pharmacists often serve as the guardians of appropriate drug therapy. Therefore, communicating effectively is key to reinforcing the value of the pharmacist within the health care system. Pharmacists communicate with patients and a wide variety of health care professionals on a daily basis. The type of information that is communicated may be the same. However, the knowledge level and expectation of the audience dictate the delivery of the message. Regardless of knowledge or expertise, pharmacists cannot actively participate in patient care unless they can communicate effectively.

Pharmacy career options have expanded into multiple, different settings including hospital, community, managed care, academia, and industry. In all of these settings, communication is critical. Whether verbally responding to a physician's question during patient care rounds, providing an educational program to nursing staff, or publishing results of a research project in a biomedical journal, communication skills are paramount to effective pharmacy practice. This chapter will discuss appropriate professional communication skills related to verbal and written drug therapy recommendations, oral presentations, formulary communications, published manuscripts, poster presentations, professional and personnel issues, and communicating with the media.

COMMUNICATING WITH HEALTH CARE PROFESSIONALS

Verbal Communications

Regardless of the practice setting, verbal communication is the most common type of communication that pharmacists utilize. It is common for a pharmacist to be approached by several different individuals (with varying backgrounds), regarding a multitude of situations, in a single day. As practitioners, pharmacists should be encouraged to remember that any type of question or interaction, regardless of how informal it may seem, is an important method of professional communication. Whether responding to a question concerning compatibility of intravenous medications from a nurse, a drug dosing question from a physician, or a request about the adverse effects of a medication from a patient; all of these interactions require excellent verbal communication skills. The most common verbal communications that pharmacists engage in involve responding to drug therapy questions and receiving verbal drug orders.

RECEIVING DRUG THERAPY QUESTIONS

A major challenge in responding to requests for drug therapy recommendations is determining the unique situation that prompted the request. Often, the original request posed by a requestor does not represent the actual information needed.[1,2] Requestors of information are sometimes unclear when asking questions pertaining to specific-patient needs. This most likely occurs because they are not aware of the specific information that pharmacists need to provide a comprehensive response. Therefore, pharmacists should recognize this potential challenge and use appropriate listening and questioning skills to collect pertinent background information to determine the exact context of the question. Questions that often appear simplistic in nature at first glance may actually be more complex when all appropriate background is considered. If pertinent background is not determined and the pharmacist does not have a clear understanding of why the question is being asked, patient care could be jeopardized. For example, if a physician asks a pharmacist a question regarding the dose of a medication, inaccurate and potentially harmful information may be provided if patient-specific factors such as age, weight, and renal or hepatic function, are not considered.[1]

Consider the example of a middle-aged man who approaches a community pharmacist and asks the question "Is Advil good for muscle pain?"[2] At first glance this appears to be a relatively simple question. Advil contains ibuprofen, which is a common over-the-counter (OTC) analgesic. Therefore, it would appear that a reasonable answer to the man's request would be "yes". However, what if the pharmacist further questions the man about his medical history to determine why he was asking this question? After further questioning, the pharmacist realizes that the man had recently started lovastatin therapy. This additional background information suggests that the patient may be experiencing symptoms of lovastatin-induced myopathy. Instead of answering the question at face value, the pharmacist in this situation is able to identify a potential drug-related adverse event by collecting important background information to determine "why" the man was asking the question.

The previous example illustrates the importance of questioning strategies to collect pertinent background information and determine the true information need. Pharmacists should apply the appropriate skills to ask logical background questions in a reasonable sequence to clarify each question. This is especially important when confronted with an impatient requestor who may not realize the value of gathering background information.

When receiving drug-related information requests from health care professionals, it is particularly useful to ask the information requestor if his or her question is about a specific patient.[1,2] This allows the pharmacist to ascertain key patient data immediately and usually prompts the requestor to describe more information about the patient. Another helpful questioning strategy is to use open-ended questions.[2] Open-ended questions cannot be answered by one-word, short answers; but require responses with detailed descriptions, and enhance information exchange about the context of the question. In the previous example about Advil and muscle aches, an appropriate open-ended question could be, "Can you describe your muscle pain to me?" This question allows the patient to provide more details about the circumstances surrounding his question. There are situations however, when the pharmacist will need to ask direct questions to obtain certain types of factual information like patient age, weight, or current medications. For pharmacists to gain a clear understanding of the actual question, a mixture of different types of questioning strategies should be used.

In addition to asking appropriate questions, it is important to have strong listening skills. Pharmacists should avoid all possible distractions when gathering background information. If the interaction is in person, the pharmacist may use non-verbal cues such as facial expressions, eye contact, and other forms of body language to interpret the requestor's response to his or her background questions. Communicating over the telephone is inherently more difficult, and in these situations, pharmacists must be especially skilled in gathering background information. It is very important to ask for clarifications when necessary to ensure a complete understanding of the situation. Finally, an important last step to collecting appropriate background information is to repeat the question or request to verify the inquiry. This will help clarify any discrepancies between the requestor and pharmacist. Pharmacists should remember that it is their professional responsibility to collect pertinent background information to fully understand the true information request. Providing drug therapy recommendations without a complete understanding of the pertinent background is simply negligent. Table 100-1 is a list of important background questions to consider when receiving a drug-related request. These questions allow the pharmacist to formulate the most appropriate response. Care also should be taken to identify when a response is needed. Providing timely and accurate responses establishes the value of pharmacists as drug therapy experts.

RESPONDING TO DRUG THERAPY QUESTIONS

After a complete and accurate response to the request is developed, communicating the information clearly and concisely is critical. Utilization of appropriate information resources, data analysis, and formulation of responses is beyond the scope of this chapter. However, the reader is referred to *Drug Information: A Guide for Pharmacists* for more information on this topic.[1]

In the clinical pharmacy practice setting, verbal communications may be more common than written communications. Therefore, it is very important for pharmacists to have the necessary skills to communicate information verbally in an effective manner. Oral responses are generally preferred because they are more personal than written responses, and they allow for prompt clarification of information that may be unclear. Verbal responses may also be favored in situations that are of high priority (emergency situations when a prompt response is needed) or when a sensitive issue is being discussed. It is important to note that when pharmacists effectively communicate drug information in a face-to-face manner, they promote the profession of pharmacy by being recognized as valuable members of the health care team. However, when information is communicated orally, the risk for misinterpretation exists.[3]

When communicating important drug therapy information, one should always make sure to identify him- or herself professionally as pharmacist. This provides the requester with confidence that a professional with appropriate educational background is responding to their request. If responding to a question that was posed during a previous interaction, it is recommended to review briefly what the initial drug therapy question was for the purpose of refreshing the memory of the requester. For questions that are specific to a certain patient, the patient should be identified to avoid any potential confusion.[3]

When verbally communicating the specifics of the response, the pertinent facts should be stated, limitations to the literature should be acknowledged, and a final conclusion and recommendation should be provided.[1,3] Pharmacists should make sure to focus on the key points in a clear and concise manner and reinforce the major point again at the end of the conversation. All relevant information should be presented. However, describing large amounts of minor details should be avoided. It may be helpful to write a brief outline using bullet points with the major issues to be communicated. This helps to ensure that pertinent information is not forgotten and that the information is communicated in a clear and concise manner. Once the response has been communicated verbally, verification should be made to make sure that the information provided to the requestor was sufficient to meet his or her needs. An offer to provide written documentation of the response should also be made.[3] Proper methods for documenting drug therapy recommendations will be reviewed later in this chapter.

Displaying confidence is obviously very important during the delivery of the response. If the pharmacist does not appear confident in his or her response, the requester may certainly have reservations about the information provided. Additionally, the vocabulary and terminology that is used should be appropriate for the given audience. For example, when communicating with a physician, professional terminology should be used and all medical terms should be pronounced correctly. However, when communicating with a patient, terminology that a layperson can easily understand should be used. Finally, follow-up questions should be expected and addressed in advance to save valuable time.

USING THE TELEPHONE FOR COMMUNICATION

Pharmacists are often asked to respond to questions and provide drug therapy recommendations using the telephone. Therefore, all pharmacists should be familiar with professional phone etiquette. Face-to-face interactions are preferred, as they are more personal; however, in many situations telephone interactions are necessary.

Regardless of the professional setting, the telephone should always be answered by providing a greeting that identifies the pharmacist's name and affiliation (eg, "Pharmacy Department, this is John, a pharmacist, speaking"). It is also helpful for pharmacists to have a pen and paper readily available before answering the telephone to document any notes that are necessary during the conversation. Many pharmacists find it helpful to write down the exact date and time that a call is received. The hold option should always be used when asking someone to wait

Table 100-1. Questions to Consider When Collecting Pertinent Background Information

What is the requestor's name, profession, and affiliation?
Does the question pertain to a specific patient?
Do I have a clear understanding of the question or problem?
Do I know if the correct question is being asked?
Do I know why the question is being asked?
Do I understand the requestor's expectations?
Do I know pertinent patient history and background information?
Do I know what unique circumstances generated the question?
Do I have insight about how the information I provide will actually be used?

Adapted from Calis KA, Heck AM. In: Malone PM, Mosdell KW, Kier KL, eds. *Drug Information- A Guide for Pharmacists*, 2nd ed. Stamford, CT: Appleton and Lange, 2001.

on the telephone line. This maintains a professional setting and avoids the potential for the caller to overhear background conversations while waiting for the pharmacist to return to the telephone line. Repeating information to clarify any discrepancies is also especially important to avoid any confusion.

FOLLOW-UP AND DOCUMENTATION

Follow-up is extremely important to maintaining professional practice. This allows pharmacists to verify if their recommendations were taken and to investigate patient outcomes while demonstrating dedication to patient care. Additionally, pharmacists can learn from their experiences and develop more confidence when they conduct regular follow-up to drug therapy recommendations.[1]

Although verbal recommendations do not always include a formal written response, it is important to document oral drug therapy recommendations for several reasons including in the event that legal questions arise. Documentation also reinforces the usefulness of pharmacists to other health care professionals and contributes to pharmacist workload assessment. Proper methods for documenting drug therapy recommendations in patient medical charts are reviewed in the next section of this chapter.

RECEIVING VERBAL DRUG ORDERS

Pharmacists may be asked to receive medication orders over the telephone. A licensed prescriber, or an agent of the prescriber, can communicate a patient-specific order directly to the pharmacist. This process challenges the pharmacist to dictate the information necessary to accurately fill the prescriber's order, as well as quickly ascertain if the prescription will be an appropriate medication for the patient.

The pharmacist should ask the prescribing party to identify him or herself and to provide the appropriate contact information to verify authenticity and to ensure a method of contact in case follow-up questions are necessary. Asking questions and directing the conversation can assist the pharmacist in controlling the rate and extent of information exchange. Patient-specific information must be obtained along with a complete and accurate description of the medication regimen. The patient's medication order should always be verbally repeated back to the prescriber to verify accuracy. Repeating information to clarify any discrepancies is especially important when taking verbal medication orders from a prescriber over the telephone. The Institute for Safe Medication Practices (ISMP) recommends that all verbal orders and telephone prescriptions be repeated back to the prescriber to reduce the likelihood of medication errors.[4] It should also be documented that the verbal order was repeated back to the prescriber. Verbal drug orders may not be the ideal means of communicating drug therapy orders, but this method is sometimes employed for urgent institutional orders or as a means of convenience in community settings. Verbal drug orders emphasize the importance of excellent communication skills to allow accurate and rapid decision-making processes.

Written Communications

DOCUMENTATION OF PATIENT CARE IN THE PERMANENT MEDICAL RECORD

OBRA-90 legislation set forth the requirements for patient education and maintenance of records, which reflect the thought process of the pharmacist as it relates to patient care. For practitioners who previously did not formally document their therapeutic recommendations, OBRA-90 formalized the requirement for completion of that task. The OBRA-90 legislation requires that pharmacists maintain a database inclusive of patient diagnosis, pertinent demographics, and perhaps most im-

portantly that documentation regarding input into patient care may be located such that review by an impartial, external reviewer will clearly identify the intent of the pharmacist's actions in terms of patient care.

The American Society of Health-System Pharmacists (ASHP) has recently published guidelines on documenting pharmaceutical care in patient medical records.[4] In developing these guidelines, it was emphasized that recommendations made by pharmacists on behalf of their patients should be documented in a permanent manner, such that information is accessible to all health care professionals caring for the patient.[4] These recommendations may include the patient's medication history, allergies, consultations to other health care professionals regarding drug therapy management, verbal orders, order clarification, drug-related problems, drug-therapy monitoring findings, and patient education. It is stressed that documentation by pharmacists should incorporate a standard format and be written in a legible, clear, and complete manner.[4]

The Weed method of documentation has been most utilized and accepted by health care professionals including pharmacists.[5,6] The Weed method consists of the development of a patient problem list and SOAP note, which organizes written patient care communications into subsections related to Subjective, Objective, Assessment, and Plan components for the identified problem(s). In addition to the components, each chart note should be appropriately titled (eg, Pharmacy Note), dated, timed, and signed with the appropriate professional designation of the pharmacist (eg, RPh) along with the method for follow-up contact from the recipient (eg, pager or telephone number). The components of each of the sections of a soap note are included in Table 100-2.

The authors have expanded this methodology to include two additional components, Education and Outcomes. These were incorporated into the authors' formalized documentation program because of the belief that most patients require some type of educational support to optimize therapy and because pharmacists often provide recommendations without identifying the desired specific endpoint in terms of outcomes. Addition of the latter component serves as a mechanism for follow-up to determine whether or not therapeutic goals have been met. It also provides a basis for understanding when care is passed from one pharmacist to another. Figure 100-1 contains an example SOAPEO note.

An alternative method to SOAP charting is Focused Documentation. Focused Documentation is a simplified method of charting, which reduces repetition, uses components reflective of Focus, Data, and Action. In the authors' practice, Focused Documentation is the preferred method for charting except in situations where the physician requests or the pharmacist initiates a comprehensive review of a patient's medication regimen. This may be the case if polypharmacy is an issue, or if a patient demonstrates symptoms consistent with sub- or supratherapeutic response(s) to medications and/or an adverse drug event. An example of Focused Documentation for the above scenario is included in Figure 100-2.

Table 100-2. Components of the SOAP Note[5,6]

S – Subjective: Patient's complaints or symptoms; data provided by family members should be characterized as such.

O – Objective: Patient data including age, sex, race, height, weight, vital signs, results of laboratory and diagnostic tests, and physical exam findings.

A – Assessment: The pharmacist's evaluation of therapeutic alternatives or resolution of drug-therapy problems which may define the necessity for all drugs in the patient's regimen, evaluate the potential for drug interactions, document the appropriateness of the drug regimen and/or evaluate the patient's previous response to pharmacotherapy.

P – Plan: The plan should include specific drug therapy recommendations (drug, dose, route, frequency, duration), monitoring parameters and the necessity for further studies or tests.

Scenario:

AW is a 38YOWM with duodenal ulcer diagnosed this admission following extensive work-up. PMH is significant for epilepsy, controlled since childhood with phenytoin. AW weighs 68 kg and is 5'10" tall. He is employed as a financial analyst in a high-stress, demanding firm. AW reports NKDA. The physician has ordered ranitidine 150 mg PO BID. Ranitidine is a nonformulary drug.

Pharmacist Documentation:

3/9/03 Pharmacy Note
1100
S: AW is a 38YOWM with duodenal ulcer. Dr. Jones has ordered ranitidine, a nonformulary drug.
O: AW receives daily maintenance therapy with phenytoin, to control a seizure disorder.
A: Ranitidine is a nonformulary item. In light of concurrent phenytoin therapy, cimetidine is not considered a viable alternative. Suggest initiating therapy with famotidine.
P: Begin famotidine 20 mg PO BID
E: Educate patient that ranitidine is not available and famotidine has been prescribed as an alternative. Therapy should be administered BID, with a 12-hour dosing interval being most desirable.
O: Control and resolution of patient's duodenal ulcer while avoiding drug-drug interactions.

Figure 100-1. Example of a SOAPEO note.

Formal Presentations

Pharmacists are routinely involved in the delivery of formal presentations, including continuing education and inservice programs. The pharmacist should evaluate the specific needs of the audience and target the level of the educational program accordingly. Pharmacists who know their audience can then prepare specific objectives that include content consistent with the expectations of the recipients. Presentations should be organized based upon the objectives and should not include excessive information that detracts from the key points. Because pharmacists frequently present to other health care professionals, provision of examples, stories, or analogies that include application of the information shared may facilitate the learning process for the participants. Although there is not one approved method for formal presentations, it is clear that "practice makes perfect." The presenter should be certain to prepare his/her talk well in advance of the presentation date, to allow ample time for practice.

In most settings, it is recommended that the presenter use some type of visual aid, which would include slides, overheads or transparencies, or flip charts. Given current technology, the development of a Microsoft PowerPoint presentation is common, as slides can quickly be converted to handouts for program participants. Whether using slides or transparencies, several formatting recommendations exist that have been summarized in Table 100-3.[7]

When properly developed, visual aids should serve as a prompt for the speaker, which should minimize the need for note cards or a complete presentation text. Presenters should be cautioned to speak from their slides or visual aids, but not to read. Other keys to effective presentation include the use of voice inflection to maintain listener interest, incorporating gestures, which accentuate voice inflection, and allowing a pause when emphasizing key points. It is important to dress consistently with the audience. Thus, a formal presentation requires formal (eg, business suit) attire. Nonverbal communication enhances the relationship with the audience. If possible, the speaker should try to move away from the lectern or walk about the front of the room, to make a connection with a greater portion of the audience. Eye contact brings the audience into the presentation. If uncomfortable looking directly at individuals, the speaker should try looking at the top of heads. In a large room, participants will still feel the presenter is making contact with them. In a smaller setting, speakers can try to identify three or four "friendly" faces throughout the audience and use them as a gauge to the presentation as well as a link to the audience.[7]

Most presentations will include time for questions and answers. If time allows, in some settings, it is more effective to allow the audience to interrupt the formal presentation and ask questions instead of waiting until the end. This can enhance the presentation, but the speaker must be careful not to allow excessive time for discussion. Effective presenters should repeat

---

3/9/03 Pharmacy Note
1100

Focus: Ranitidine, a nonformulary drug, has been prescribed for AW.

Data: AW receives daily maintenance therapy with phenytoin, to control a seizure disorder. Therefore, cimetidine is not a viable alternative.

Action: Begin famotidine 20mg BID. Educate patient regarding alternative therapy and monitor response.

Figure 100-2. Example of Focused Documentation.

Table 100-3. Characteristics of the Ideal Slide/Transparency Text

Horizontal with 2:3 ratio
Content limited to main point
Black or dark blue background
Title in all capitals
Outline format in lowercase
Maximum of seven lines of text
No more than seven words per line
Readable font such as Helvetica or Arial
Limited use of capitals and italics
Graphic slide will have no more than 5–7 bars, columns, or pieces of a pie chart; clear labels or legends in corresponding colors

Adapted from Casella PJ. In: *Writing, Speaking, and Communication Skills for Health Professionals*. The Health Care Communication Group. London: Yale University Press, 2001.

questions to assure that everyone in the audience has heard and understands the inquiry. As in all aspects of health care, if one does not know the response to a question, it is best to admit this freely and offer to follow-up or defer to an expert colleague in the audience who may know the answer. If questions do not relate to the presentation topic, the speaker should respond to the best of his or her ability and redirect the conversation to a point that does relate. The authors recommend the text *Writing, Speaking, and Communication Skills for Health Professionals* to any pharmacist who wishes to strengthen his or her presentation skills.[7]

Formulary Communications

Written communication skills are extremely important for pharmacists who participate in formulary management. A drug formulary can be defined as a continually revised compilation of medications that indicate the current clinical judgment of the medical staff and are readily available for use within an institution.[8] Drug formularies serve the purpose of providing decreased inventory and allow practitioners to gain familiarity with certain drug products. Formularies also promote a decreased risk for medication errors and help the institution provide cost-effective therapy. Ideally, a drug formulary should contain the most cost-effective medications to treat all disease states likely to be encountered within a given institution. A comprehensive review of the issues related to formulary management is beyond the scope of this chapter. However, the most common ways that pharmacists use professional communication skills to contribute to formulary management are through the preparation of drug evaluation monographs (or drug class reviews), medication-use evaluations, clinical pathways, drug alerts, and newsletters. Basic guidelines for the preparation of these documents are listed below.

DRUG EVALUATION MONOGPAPHS

A drug evaluation monograph is an objective, written appraisal of a medication (or class of medications in the case of drug class reviews) under consideration for formulary addition.[9] Drug evaluation monographs are almost always prepared by pharmacists. The following sections are commonly used as a general template in preparing a drug evaluation monograph.[8,9] However, the specific template used by an institution may be modified to meet the institution's needs.

Title: This section includes basic information such as generic and trade names, manufacturer, available dosage forms, and the corresponding national drug code (NDC) numbers, the American Hospital Formulary Service (AHFS) Pharmacologic-Therapeutic Classification, and any important storage instructions. The AHFS Pharmacologic-Therapeutic Classification number is found in the classification index of the *AHFS Drug Information* reference book. *AHFS Drug Information* is published by the American Society of Health-System Pharmacists and is commonly used as an important reference book for practicing pharmacists. The AHFS Pharmacologic-Therapeutic Classification method indexes medications by pharmacologic and therapeutic effects by assigning numerical values to each drug class. Many institutions use the AHFS Pharmacologic-Therapeutic Classification system to index the medications available on the drug formulary. Use of a classification system helps organize an institution's formulary list.

Description and Pharmacology: This section includes a description of the compound including the therapeutic mechanism of action. Important differences in the pharmacological effects of the monograph drug as compared to current formulary agents of the same class should be discussed as well.

Pharmacokinetics: This section includes a brief review of the available pharmacokinetic data (ie, absorption, distribution, metabolism, excretion), including information about potential pharmacokinetic changes in pediatric and geriatric patients or patients with renal or hepatic dysfunction or other disease states. For this data, a chart format is commonly preferable. This is especially helpful for drug class reviews when several agents within a given drug class are being compared.

FDA-Approved Indications: A list of all the FDA-approved indications and any significant differences between the monograph drug and similar products within the same drug class should be provided. Because many medications are used for indications that are not officially approved by the FDA, it is also important to list pertinent off-label uses of the medication as well.

Clinical Efficacy: A thorough review of available literature pertinent to the efficacy and safety of the requested drug as it relates to the FDA-approved and off-label indications should be presented. Studies that are reviewed should include placebo-controlled and comparative trials, with emphasis on comparative trials when available. It is important to note that clinical trials, which do not assess the safety and efficacy of the drug product, should not be included. For example, pharmacokinetic evaluations in healthy subjects or animal toxicology studies are not appropriate for inclusion in the clinical efficacy section of a drug evaluation monograph. These types of studies may be referenced in other sections of the monograph (such as the pharmacokinetic section or the safety section), but they do not provide clinical efficacy information.

Typically, it is best to follow a general template when abstracting clinical trial data within a drug monograph evaluation. This improves readability, ensures consistency, and allows comparisons to be made between different clinical trials in a relatively simple format. The citation, objective, and study design should always be stated in a clear and concise manner. Detailed information describing the inclusion/exclusion criteria, randomization process, study treatments, and the efficacy and safety assessments should be included in the description of the methods. Within the results section, the writer should report specific numbers to describe the efficacy and safety of the drug. For example, instead of simply reporting a "statistically significant difference between groups," the writer should report the quantitative difference in the outcome measure between study groups (eg, 160 mg/dL versus 110 mg/dL). This allows the reader to interpret the potential clinical significance of the results. In addition to a short conclusion, the writer should provide a brief commentary regarding the potential strengths and limitations that should be considered when interpreting the results of the study. An example of a clinical trial summary that would be appropriate for inclusion in a drug evaluation monograph is shown in Figure 100-3.

Safety and Tolerability: This section should include information regarding manufacturer-labeled contraindications, warnings, and precautions (including pregnancy and lactation information). Adverse event data should be presented in a manner that emphasizes the most common and most serious adverse events, with suggested strategies to prevent or manage these events if they occur. Potential drug-drug, drug-food, drug-laboratory, and drug-herb interactions should also be presented with suggested management approaches. As with all sections of the drug monograph, comparative data should be presented when available.

Medication Error Possibility: Information should be included about potential medication errors that could occur in dosing, medication preparation, medication administration, or concerns with look-alike/sound-alike names. If potential risks exist, methods for preventing medication errors should be introduced.

Dosing and Administration: The recommended doses for specific indications and patient populations (eg, geriatric, pediatric, obese, renal failure) should be clearly listed. If applicable, a description of dosage titration should be included. For parenteral medications, it is important

Citation: Kane JM, Carson WH, Saha AR, et al. Efficacy and safety of aripiprazole and haloperidol versus placebo in patients with schizophrenia and schizoaffective disorder. *J Clin Psychiatry* 2002; 63:763-771.

Objective: To determine the efficacy and safety of aripiprazole and haloperidol compared to placebo.

Design: Multicenter, randomized, double-blind, placebo-controlled, parallel clinical trial

Methods: Subjects included men and women aged 18 to 65 years with a primary diagnosis of schizophrenia or schizoaffective disorder who were hospitalized for an acute relapse. A Positive and Negative Syndrome Scale (PANSS) total score of at least 60, with scores of at least 4 on any two items of the psychotic subscale, was required. Additionally, all subjects were required to have documented prior responsiveness to antipsychotic medication. Exclusion criteria included pregnancy, breastfeeding, psychiatric disorders other than schizophrenia or schizoaffective disorder, or a history of violence, suicidal attempts or serious suicidal ideation. Patients were also excluded if they had a clinically significant neurologic abnormality, drug or alcohol abuse, or any acute or unstable medical condition. All subjects underwent a 5-day placebo washout period, and were randomly assigned to treatment if they continued to meet inclusion criteria after the washout. Patients were randomly assigned to one of four treatment groups for four weeks: 15 mg aripiprazole, 30 mg aripiprazole, 10 mg haloperidol, or placebo given once daily after breakfast. Doses were fixed without titration, and patients were hospitalized throughout the trial. PANSS and the Clinical Global Impressions scale were used to measure efficacy. Adverse events were monitored and graded on intensity each week. Extrapyramidal symptoms (EPS) were evaluated using the Simpson-Angus Scale, Barnes Akathesia Scale, and the Abnormal Involuntary Movement Scale (AIMS) on a weekly basis.

Results: A total of 414 patients were randomized for treatment; 102 patients in the placebo group, 102 patients in the aripiprazole 15 mg group, 102 patients in the aripiprazole 30 mg group, and 104 patients in the haloperidol 10 mg group. The 15-mg and 30-mg doses of aripiprazole and haloperidol 10-mg dose showed significant improvements compared to placebo in the PANSS total score (aripiprazole 15 mg –15.5 vs. placebo –2.9, $P < 0.001$; aripiprazole 30 mg –11.4 vs. placebo –2.9, $P = 0.009$; and haloperidol –13.8 vs. placebo –2.9, $P = 0.001$), the PANSS positive subscale (aripiprazole 15 mg –4.2 vs. placebo –0.6, $P < 0.001$; aripiprazole 30 mg –3.8 vs. placebo –0.6, $P = 0.001$; and haloperidol –4.4 vs. placebo –0.6; $P < 0.001$), the CGI-S score (aripiprazole 15 mg -0.6 vs. placebo –0.1, $P < 0.001$; aripiprazole 30 mg –0.4 vs. placebo –0.1, $P = 0.019$; and haloperidol –0.05 vs. placebo –0.1, $P = 0.002$), and the PANSS-derived BPRS core score (aripiprazole 15 mg –3.1 vs. placebo –1.1, $P < 0.001$; aripiprazole 30 mg –3.0 vs. placebo –1.1, $P = 0.001$; and haloperidol –3.5 vs. placebo –1.1; $P < 0.001$). Statistically significant improvements were also reported for the PANSS negative subscale score in the 15-mg aripiprazole group, but not for the 30-mg dose of aripiprazole. Study drop out rates were similar between treatment groups (11% in the haloperidol group, 9% in the aripiprazole 15 mg group, and 8% in the aripiprazole 30 mg group). The most common adverse events associated with aripiprazole were headache, anxiety, insomnia, nausea, dizziness, and vomiting. Fifteen percent of patients in the aripiprazole 15 mg group and 14% of patients in the aripiprazole 30 mg group reported nausea, compared to only 7% and 6% of patients in the placebo and haloperidol 10-mg groups, respectively. Vomiting was reported by 8% and 17% of patients receiving 15 mg and 30 mg of aripiparazole, respectively compared to 10% in both the placebo and haloperidol groups. Aripiprazole was not associated with significant changes in EPS, body weight, serum prolactin levels or ECG readings.

Conclusions: Aripiprazole, at doses of 15 and 30 mg daily, was found to be more effective than placebo and similarly effective to haloperidol 10 mg in patients with schizophrenia and schizoaffective disorder following four weeks of treatment. Both doses of aripiprazole were generally well tolerated.

Comment: Although aripiprazole demonstrated efficacy and safety in the treatment of schizophrenia over placebo in the four-week study, the role of aripiprazole therapy cannot be established at this time due to a lack adequate long-term comparative data. Additionally, the haloperidol-dosing schedule in this study does not reflect current clinical practice (ie, once daily compared to divided into 2 to 3 doses.)

Figure 100-3. Example of a clinical trial summary for a drug evaluation monograph.

to list information about reconstitution techniques, appropriate diluents, long-term stability, and compatibility with other medications. Special administration issues such as infusion rate or the need for in-line filters should also be addressed in this section.

Patient Monitoring Parameters and Patient Information: Information regarding recommended patient monitoring parameters with suggested time intervals for assessments should be presented. Additionally, patient information written in lay terms for the monograph drug should be provided.

Budget Impact: This section should provide a quantitative description of the health system's cost for the new product based on the typical dosage regimen (eg, Q8h × 10 days). The cost per bottle (or package) is not always helpful, because it does not take into account the typical dosage regimen. It is best to provide this data in a tabular format that compares the new product to currently available agents. Additionally, it is helpful to include projected use and how the item will affect the health system's total drug budget.

Summary and Recommendations: The summary should briefly review the pertinent data presented throughout the document including a concise discussion of the drug class and information regarding the efficacy, safety, and cost of the new drug product in comparison to currently available formulary agents. Any important advantages of the new drug should also be highlighted in this section. Finally, the recommendation should be stated with appropriate rationale. Recommendations for the deletion of alternative agents from the drug formulary should also be included in this section. In some institutions, the summary and recommendation are listed on the front page of the drug evaluation monograph to make it easier for reference and discussion during the Pharmacy and Therapeutics (P&T) Committee meeting.[9]

Authorship: The pharmacist who prepared the monograph should be listed along with the date that the final document was completed. Additionally, pharmacists who served as document reviewers should be listed.

References: All references should be footnoted and listed at the end of the document in the order that they appear within the text. References should be cited using the Uniform Requirements of Manuscripts Submitted to Biomedical Journals.[10]

Some P&T Committees use a one-page summary in lieu of the entire drug evaluation monograph. Pharmacists typically present the summary of the drug evaluation monograph or drug class review verbally during the P&T Committee meeting.[9]

MEDICATION-USE EVALUATION

Medication-use evaluation (MUE) is a continuous improvement method used to evaluate the use of medications within a health system to identify areas for improvement in medication-related outcomes.[8] Medication-use evaluation is frequently completed based upon evidence-based clinical practice guidelines and clinical pathways. In addition, MUE may be based upon approved criteria for use of an individual drug or drugs within a therapeutic class. While MUE is no longer required by regulatory agencies such as the Joint Commission on Accreditation of Healthcare Organizations, it is completed as an ongoing indicator of continuing quality improvement.

There are several key communication issues related to MUE. First, it is imperative that the criteria for MUE are approved by the medical staff and/or any other group of health care providers who are expected to apply the criteria in the care of their patients. Following completion of an MUE, results should be shared through appropriate channels. Within health care organizations, MUE is often a function of the Pharmacy and Therapeutics Committee. The most common communication-related problems in the MUE process generally occur after results have been discussed by the committee. Discussion frequently culminates in recommendations for the improvement of care. These recommendations are often not shared with practitioners, nor is there subsequent assessment to determine the results of the recommended improvements. Thus, the 360-degree cycle associated with study completion and process improvement is not completed, and recommendations for improved care are not implemented. It is essential that the pharmacist assume accountability for completion of this process, in its entirety.

The following sections provide a general template to follow when reporting results of an MUE.

Background: This section should provide background information about why the MUE was conducted. For example, the reason may be that the medication being evaluated has been associated with medication errors, or because the medication may be associated with a serious adverse event. Pertinent literature or national guidelines that support the need for an MUE should also be reviewed. This section should end with a statement describing the primary objective of the MUE.

Methods: A detailed description of exactly how the MUE was conducted should be included. The methods for patient selection, identification, and data collection should be listed; as well as the study time period and sample size. Justification for the selected sample size should be provided. It may be helpful to list the types of data that were collected. For example, if the MUE assessed appropriate use of a particular medication with regards to renal function, serum creatinine would be recorded for all patients.

Results: Detailed results for each type of data that was collected should be presented in a tabular format. The presentation of results should include patient demographics and numerical values for all data.

Summary: The results of the MUE should be briefly summarized, highlighting the most important findings.

Recommendations: Finally, the recommendations to improve medication use should be presented. These should be specific to the health system.

CLINICAL PRACTICE GUIDELINES AND PATHWAYS

Evidence-based clinical practice guidelines have been defined as, "systematically developed statements to assist practitioner and patient decisions about health care for specific circumstances."[11] Guidelines should include specifications for care, which may be disease-based (eg, hypertension, asthma, diabetes) or process-focused (eg, guidelines for the use of serum levels in monitoring aminoglycoside therapy). Clinical pathways reflect the details that support practice guidelines. For example, guidelines which focus on the use of serum levels in monitoring gentamicin therapy might state that patients with an elevated serum creatinine of greater than 2 mg/dL or those receiving daily dosages in excess of 6mg/kg be candidates for serum level monitoring. The corresponding clinical pathway would state the exact manner in which the serum levels should be monitored, such as obtaining the trough level within 30 minutes prior to the infusion of a gentamicin dose, and the peak 30 minutes after the end of a one-half hour infusion.

Clinical practice guidelines and pathways should be specifically and succinctly written, such that there is no confusion regarding the intent of the guideline or the exact process for application of the guideline. Health care organizations with sophisticated information systems (including computer-generated physician order entry) frequently incorporate guidelines and pathways into their software to provide guidance to practitioners in the care of their patients.

DRUG ALERT NOTIFICATIONS

In many cases, there may be situations that require the pharmacy department to alert the medical and nursing staff of an important medication-related issue. Examples requiring drug alert notifications include critical drug product shortages, change in pharmacy procedures, or withdrawal of a drug from the market. Typically, pharmacists are responsible for developing these types of communications. The most effective method is generally the preparation of a one-page communication that clearly states the problem or issue and provides a recommendation for managing the problem. The notification should provide contact information for potential questions or concerns. An example of a drug alert notification is shown in Figure 100-4.

NEWSLETTERS

Most health systems have a pharmacy newsletter that is published on a regular basis to communicate important formulary decisions that have been made by the P&T Committee. As drug therapy specialists, the main writers and editors of pharmacy newsletters are pharmacists. When preparing a pharmacy newsletter the primary factors to consider are the target audience, the primary goal of publication, and professional appearance.[12] The specific format used varies greatly depending on these primary factors. Professional writing strategies will be discussed in detail later in this chapter. Pharmacy newsletters serve a valuable purpose for communicating important information to the medical staff and provide visibility for the pharmacy department.

Writing Manuscripts For Publication

Pharmacists may be involved in writing a wide variety of manuscripts for publication. These include book chapters, editorials, case reports, review articles, and clinical research studies. Publishing these types of manuscripts is essential to enhance communication among peers and advance/promote the

DRUG ALERT
PHARMACY AND THERAPEUTICS COMMITTEE
CLARIAN HEALTH HOSPITALS

-MORPHINE PCA –
Concentration Change

Effective Tuesday, September 3rd, 2002, the concentration of Morphine PCA
stocked at all Clarian hospitals will be standardized to

30mg/30ml (1mg/ml)

This change is being implemented due to medication safety concerns of carrying two
different concentrations and due to availability problems with the 2mg/ml Morphine PCA
concentration.

For more information, contact a pharmacist or the
Drug Information Service at 962-1750

Figure 100-4. Example drug alert notification.

profession. Generally, pharmacists are not trained to be writers; for this reason, preparing a manuscript for publication can sometimes appear to be an overwhelming, daunting task. However, publishing is a very fulfilling accomplishment that can lead to professional advancement and recognition.

PREPARATION

Preparation is the first step to any project. Because writing an article for publication is typically a long process, the first hurdle for pharmacists to overcome is the anxiety associated with the project. Because anxiety can sometimes lead to procrastination, it is very important to overcome any apprehensions as soon as possible. A good way to deal with this is to begin the initial preparation process by conducting background research, gathering all necessary resources, and developing an outline for the manuscript.[12] It is also helpful to develop a working plan for completion of the project.[13,14] The writing project should be divided into small sections and attainable deadlines for the completion of each section should be made. Time for working on each section should be planned, similarly to other scheduled daily activities. This strategy can help avoid postponing the writing process due to an already busy schedule.

After all necessary resources have been collected, the items should be organized in a systematic fashion. This will enable the writer to locate references quickly when they are needed during the writing process. This can eliminate frustration and save valuable time later. An outline should also be developed to define the project clearly. When developing an outline, it is best to consider the primary objective of the manuscript and the target audience. Knowing this information will help determine which topics or sections should be included in the manuscript. An effective outline should help make the writing process easier because it determines focus areas. With computer word-processing packages, the outline can be used as a working template for the final manuscript. If the manuscript is intended for a specific medical journal or book, the publishers will customarily have requirements for the various sections that must be included. This will allow organization and provide a framework to follow during the writing process. Many biomedical journals follow *The Uniform Requirements for Manuscripts Submitted to Biomedical Journals*.[10] This is a document prepared by a group of editors to provide guidelines for manuscripts that are submitted to medical journals for publication. Table 100-4 lists the general sections that should be included in the publication of a research project.[13]

WRITING THE FIRST DRAFT

Once the outline has been prepared and all information resources have been gathered, the next step is to begin writing. Professional writing is a skill that requires continued practice. Because most pharmacists are not trained writers, this step is often quite difficult. One potential difficulty is finding the time necessary to devote to writing. As stated above, a helpful strategy to manage this problem is to reserve short blocks of time each day that are devoted to writing the manuscript. This approach may be easier for a busy practitioner than to reserve an entire day for completing the project. Progress can be made using short blocks of time, even if the daily goal is to write only one or two paragraphs. During this time, it is helpful to use a technique known as freewriting.[13,14] Freewriting involves taking about 20 to 30 minutes to write your ideas continuously without stopping to check grammar, spelling, or references.[13] Once a few paragraphs have been written in this manner, then content revisions and clarifications can made. In general, is it best to complete a first draft in its entirety before beginning the editing process.[12] However, it is sometimes difficult to avoid becoming engaged in the minor details of correcting grammatical and typographical errors in paragraphs that have already been written. This habit can lead to frustration and slow down the entire writing process. Strategies such as disabling the spelling and grammar check programs of the word-processing program and turning the computer screen off have been recommended to avoid the temptation of making corrections instead of writing new paragraphs.[13,14] Professional writing also follows a certain set of rules that are different from other types of writing.

Table 100-4. Basic Sections of a Research Project Publication[10,13]

Introduction:	Background information to support "why" the project was conducted (written in present tense)
Methods:	Detailed description of all study procedures (written in past tense)
Results:	Detailed description of study findings (written in past tense)
Discussion:	Description of the clinical implications and limitations of the study findings (written present tense)
Conclusions:	A statement of the final conclusions (written in present tense)

General rules for professional writing are listed in Table 100-5.[12] An excellent reference for general stylistic considerations including the rules of proper punctuation and grammar, and avoiding commonly misused words is *The Elements of Style*, written by William Strunk and EB White.[15]

EDITING

After the first draft has been completed, editing is the final critical step. When a manuscript is submitted for publication, or any type of written communication for that matter, it represents an image of the writer. If a written manuscript is full of typographical and grammatical errors, this reflects poorly upon on the author. Because is it sometimes difficult for the author to identify noticeable errors, it is especially useful to ask colleagues to help proofread one's manuscript. Other strategies that have been suggested to aid the editing process include reading sentences out loud slowly, reading sentences in reverse chronological order, and enlarging the font on the computer screen.[13] It is also useful for the author to put the manuscript away from view for several days, and then come back to it at a later date.

REFERENCING

It is very important for authors to be familiar with proper referencing techniques to give credit when appropriate and avoid committing plagiarism. Plagiarism is defined as using the ideas or words of another, in a way that represents them as one's own. Authors should always be vigilant of the potential for plagiarism when writing manuscripts for publication. If copying words verbatim from another authors' work, quotation marks should be used around the material and the appropriate authors should be cited. A good general rule to follow is to use quotation marks around three or more words in a row that are taken directly from a source without modification. If paraphrasing another author, the original publication should always be cited. Specific instructions for citing various types of publications can be found in the *Uniform Requirements for Manuscripts Submitted to Biomedical Journals*.[10]

Preparing Poster Presentations

Poster presentations are a common method for sharing information at national meetings. At most national pharmacy meetings, there is an opportunity to present research ideas in a poster format. The basic components of a scientific poster are similar to the basic sections of a written research project. These sections include background, methods, results, limitations, and conclusions (see Table 100-4). Posters differ from written manuscripts in the amount of detail presented. With the exception of the background and conclusion sections, posters should not contain full sentences.[16] Information should be presented in at least 18-point font and bullet points and boxes should be used to emphasize the main points. This makes it easier for passersby to read and interpret. There are two different methods to make

a poster. The first is to use separate slides (or panels) for each section. This can be done using Microsoft® PowerPoint slides. Alternatively, some word-processing programs allow presenters to make single page posters. These posters still contain different slides for each section, but can be printed as a one-page sheet. This can make the poster easier to transport and arrange at the meeting. The general rules of professional writing discussed above and the importance of proofreading also apply to the preparation of poster presentations. A suggested format for a poster presentation is shown in Figure 100-5.

Written Professional Communication

Given the diverse responsibilities and practice locations of pharmacists, effective written communication is essential. This type of communication encompasses interpersonal interactions among peers and other health care professionals, as well as administrative functions.

ELECTRONIC MAIL

While the introduction of e-mail has greatly facilitated contact and reduced telephone messages for many, this type of communication must be appropriately utilized in the professional environment. Within this environment, e-mail should be for professional use only. Attention should be given to one's chosen e-mail sign-on. If a pharmacist's given name is not utilized for e-mail communication, care should be taken to choose a name that reflects positively on the character of the pharmacist as a professional. Professional e-communication should be utilized in situations where the messenger has concluded that a face-to-face meeting or telephone (ie, direct) communication would not communicate the message more effectively. When communicating by e-mail, it is important to remember that any message may be either saved or forwarded for viewing by others. Accordingly, close attention should be paid to content and format. For example, use of capital letters could be interpreted as "yelling."

The subject line should clarify the intent of the message. The content of messages should be concise but thorough enough to be understood. Given that messages may be printed or shared, one should refrain from including confidential or controversial information. E-mail users are advised to compose professional communications with a word processing program initially, to facilitate spelling and grammar checks. When e-communication is utilized, it is most appropriate to respond within the same business day, but a goal would be to respond in no longer than 24 hours. It is recognized that this may be a challenge, depending on the setting.

MEMORANDA (MEMOS)

Most pharmacists will find a need to communicate with other health care providers via memos, whether or not they have administrative positions. Written memos are frequently used to

---

Table 100-5. General Rules for Professional Writing

Use proper grammar and spelling
Keep sentences simple and direct
Avoid writing in the first person (eg, I, we, us)
Avoid using the passive voice
Avoid using contractions
Avoid using abbreviations or acronyms
Proofread

Adapted from Malone P. In: Malone PM, Mosdell KW, Kier KL, eds. *Drug Information: A Guide for Pharmacists,* 2nd ed. Stamford, CT: Appleton and Lange, 2001.

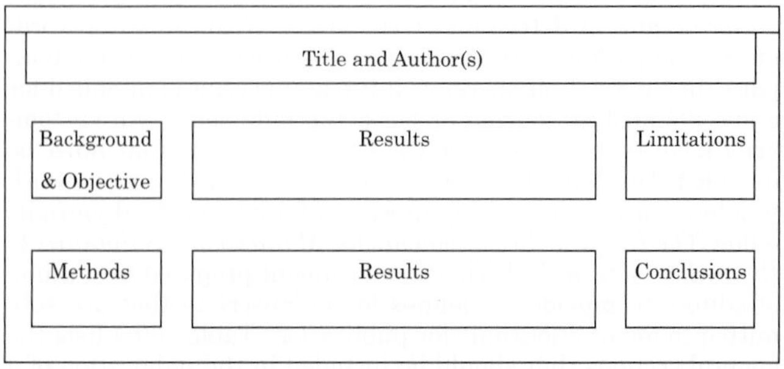

Figure 100-5. Suggested format for poster presentation.

communicate drug information, policy changes, or in the evaluation/discipline of employees. Memos should be formal in format and should be addressed to a specific individual or group of individuals, whenever possible. The format for a professional memorandum is included in Figure 100-6.

COVER LETTERS

Cover letters should accompany applications for employment. As such they offer a written "first impression" to the recipient. Much like e-mail and memos, cover letters should be addressed to a specific individual whenever possible. The cover letter should be written in standard business format, as referenced in any primary or secondary school English text. The first paragraph of the cover letter should include the purpose for writing the letter. For example, the letter may be written to introduce a pharmacist as a candidate for employment. The content would then reflect the pharmacist's background and training and his or her current position. The middle paragraph should contain a brief summary of the key strengths, which make the pharmacist a strong and/or unique candidate for a particular employment opportunity. The last paragraph should close with identification of the mechanism for follow-up. For example, the author may wish to indicate that if the letter recipient does not provide follow-up contact within a two-week time frame, the author will initiate such contact. The letter should also specify the preferred mechanism for contact (eg, e-mail, telephone with specific number).

RESUME

The resume should serve as a one-page summary or snapshot of an individual's education and work experience. Frequently, the resume contains a professional objective, as it is often used to facilitate an employment opportunity. Resumes are designed to highlight professional accomplishments and hopefully entice the recipient to make an offer for an interview. Within today's professional environment, resumes are frequently requested of individuals seeking positions in community pharmacy. Individuals seeking employment within academia, the pharmaceutical industry or hospitals are most frequently requested to submit a curriculum vitae as part of their application package. Figure 100-7 contains an example of potential resume content.

CURRICULUM VITAE

The curriculum vitae is intended to be a comprehensive chronology of the education, training, and work experience which also reflects professional presentations and publications. The health care professional should maintain a curriculum vitae that is inclusive of all types of professional activities. Potential categories for a curriculum vitae are included in Figure 100-8. Some accomplished professionals maintain an abbreviated curriculum vitae that represents the most recent 5 to 10 years of accomplishments.

```
Date:  March 10, 2003

To:    Jane A. Doe, PharmD, RPh
       Director of Pharmacy

From:  Samuel T. Smith, PharmD, RPh
       Associate Director of Pharmacy

Re:    Staffing Patterns for Outpatient Pharmacy
```

Figure 100-6. Example of memo header.

```
               Name (centered, top)

Business address              Permanent address (if desired)
Employment objective
Education
Skills
Professional experience (perhaps selected, most relevant)
Other work experience (as applicable)
Activities and honors (most relevant)
```

Figure 100-7. Content of the resume.

Personnel Communication

Position Description

Pharmacists, particularly those in management positions, are frequently required to write position descriptions for other pharmacists, technicians, and/or other supportive personnel. The position description should delineate the required qualifications, experience, and an overview of job responsibilities. Most position descriptions also include an overview of the required competencies for successful job performance.

The types of positions for which pharmacists might prepare position descriptions include:

Clerical: Individuals who complete tasks including word processing, filing, bookkeeping, and serving as a receptionist.

Service: Individuals involved with equipment and/or building maintenance.

Administrative: Individuals who may complete some clerical functions, with the addition of budgeting/financial management or supervision of clerical staff.

Technical: Individuals involved with product procurement and preparation, along with certain levels of customer interaction

Professional: Including pharmacists, nurses, etc.

Educational requirements may include the ability to read/write English or another language, high school diploma, vocational training, certification, college course work, associate degree, BS degree, advanced degree, or postgraduate training. Required experience should include the number of years and type of experience (ie, directly related to the position). Other related skills might include word processing, accounting, supervision, prescription processing, and perhaps work with automated dispensing systems, to name a few. The position description should include essential duties and the percent of effort that is designated to each duty. Figure 100-9 contains an example position description for a pharmacist.

```
               Name (centered, top)

Business address              Permanent address (if desired)
Education (post high-school, chronological order)
Licensure/certification
Professional experience (list most current first)
Other work experience (as applicable)
Organizational and committee appointments (where applicable)
Affiliations (eg, professional organizations, includes offices held)
Awards/honors
Service (eg, professional, community)
Grants (where applicable)
Presentations
Publications (by category, eg, refereed articles, book chapters)
Date of most recent revision
```

Figure 100-8. Content of the curriculum vitae.

POSITION DESCRIPTION

AMBULATORY CARE PHARMACIST

PROFESSIONAL PHARMACY SYSTEMS
300 NORTH CARLETON BLVD.
INDIANAPOLIS, IN 44444-4444

Qualifications:

1. Doctor of Pharmacy (PharmD) degree and/or a BS in Pharmacy

2. Minimum of 3 years experience in progressive pharmacy practice

3. Eligibility for and attainment of pharmacy licensure in the State of Indiana

4. Involvement with disease state management programs (eg, diabetes, asthma, hyperlipidemia, anticoagulation) preferred

5. Strong organizational and interpersonal skills

6. Ability to communicate effectively with patients of varying educational backgrounds

Position Responsibilities:

1. Assist with prescription processing and patient education

2. Provide direct disease management services for patients with diabetes, asthma, hyperlipidemia, coagulation disorders

3. Assist in the development and marketing of additional disease management programs to support community-based physician practices

4. Serve as a preceptor for PharmD students completing experiential learning rotations within the practice site

Required Core Competencies:

Knowledge

1. Knowledge of procedures and laws pertaining to the processing and dispensing of prescriptions

2. Knowledge of disease state management including diabetes, asthma, hyperlipidemia, coagulation disorders

Skills

1. Ability to modify disease state recommendations based upon patient lifestyle

2. Ability to individualize education for each patient

Behaviors

1. Monitors indicators of response including disease-based parameters and understanding

Figure 100-9. Example of position description.

2.   Provides individualized follow-up for patients to optimize outcomes

It is anticipated that the ambulatory care pharmacist will have responsibilities that mirror the following:

Prescription Processing (50%)

The ambulatory care pharmacist will assist with prescription processing for clinic patients. This activity includes provision of education relative to prescribed therapies and advising patients regarding the appropriate use of over-the-counter and alternative therapies.

Disease State Management (30%)

The ambulatory care pharmacist will provide direct disease state management for patients with asthma, diabetes, hyperlipidemia, and coagulation disorders through established protocols.

Program Development/Marketing (10%)

In conjunction with practice management, the ambulatory care pharmacist will assist with the identification, program development, and marketing of additional disease state management programs.

Experiential Learning (10%)

The ambulatory care pharmacist will assist with supervision of advanced clerkship students from state colleges of pharmacy.

Figure 100-9. *(continued)*

Ambulatory Care Pharmacist Position
Professional Pharmacy Systems
Ambulatory Clinic

Professional Pharmacy Systems invites applications for a full-time pharmacist position in its Indianapolis, Indiana ambulatory clinic site. Applicants should possess a PharmD or BS in pharmacy. Candidates should have a minimum of three years experience in progressive pharmacy practice. Involvement with disease state management programs (eg, diabetes, asthma, hyperlipidemia, anticoagulation) is preferred. The candidate should be able to demonstrate strengths in organization and communication with both patients and other health care professionals. The ability to speak a second language (preferably Spanish) is highly desirable. Salary will be commensurate with qualifications and experience. Review of applications will begin upon receipt and continue until the position is filled. Applicants should send a letter of intent with curriculum vitae and the names and addresses of three references to:

Steven R. Abel, PharmD, FASHP
Pharmacy Director
Professional Pharmacy Systems
300 North Carleton Blvd.
Indianapolis, IN 44444-4444
sabel@professionalpharmacysx.org

Figure 100-10. Example job posting.

JOB POSTINGS

Once a position description has been developed, job postings reflecting abbreviated qualifications and responsibilities for the successful applicant are prepared. Job postings are commonly used to advertise for candidates in local newspapers, professional journals, and/or via the Internet. Position descriptions should include contact information for the individual responsible for recruitment and should also reflect the status of an equal opportunity employer, where applicable. An example position description is included in Figure 100-10.

INTERVIEWING

Interviewing is an essential skill for pharmacists, whether they serve in administrative positions and are responsible for hiring staff that will enhance their services or apply their skills in obtaining a fulfilling professional position. It is important for pharmacists to be aware of the different types of interviews in which they might participate. These include the following:

Structured Interview: An interview that utilizes a predetermined list of questions that are designed to facilitate comparison among the candidates. This format is good for a naive interviewer, because it provides a "script" for the interview process, but it may not offer enough flexibility to allow complete assessment of a candidate's strengths and liabilities.

Unstructured Interview: An interview that is unorganized, spontaneous, and flexible. This format tests the listening skills of the interviewee while challenging the interviewer to remain on task and ascertain pertinent information from the candidate.

Stress Interview: An interview designed to determine the emotional stability of the interviewee. Questions are asked in a direct, sometimes offensive manner in an effort to strike an emotional chord and evaluate the candidate's response.

Behavioral Interview: An interview that is focused on identifying how the interviewee reacted in certain situations. Questions may focus on stressful, frustrating, or positive scenarios. The interviewer asks how the candidate reacted to the scenario, and what they learned or might do differently as a result. The interviewee's past experiences are the focus for specific examples, which offer the interviewer a chance to determine strengths and weaknesses based upon "lessons learned."

Regardless of the interview technique, interviewers and interviewees alike should be prepared to discuss topics including personal interests, education, experience, and career goals. Skills related to interpersonal interactions, communication, and technical/practical competence will also be evaluated. Topics that may not be discussed in an interview are included in Table 100-6.

PERFORMANCE APPRAISAL

Pharmacists will have the responsibility to provide input into or prepare performance appraisals. The primary purpose of the performance appraisal is to enhance employee development. Performance appraisals are also frequently utilized to distribute rewards (eg, salary increases). When communicating with the employee regarding performance, the discussion should focus on four characteristics of good performance criteria. Performance criteria should be achievable, measurable, unbiased, and significant to the work of the individual. It is suggested that performance criteria be developed jointly by the supervisor and employee, including the method for assessment.

Table 100-6. Inappropriate Interview Topics

Age
Arrest or conviction record
Credit rating
Disabilities
Marital/family status
Military record
Name, national origin, or religion
Request for a photograph

This approach should make the review process most valuable for the involved parties.

Several general guidelines exist for conducting the appraisal interview. Appraisals should be conducted in a quiet setting that is removed from the general workplace and other employees. The frequency and timing of performance evaluations should be known to the employee. In most settings, evaluations occur on an annual basis (eg, at the end of each year) or on the anniversary of employment. Presentation of the appraisal is critical to its success. Managers should begin their assessment by citing specific examples or instances in which the employee made positive contributions to the site. Criticism is acceptable, but should be offered as opportunities for employee development and should always be presented after at least some positive statements are made. The evaluation should be offered as the manager's interpretation of the available facts. If opportunities for improvement are recommended, these should be delivered in a tactful, but direct manner.

Verbal evaluations should always be supported by paper documentation of performance. The employee and manager should sign the written document. This does not imply that the employee agrees with the assessment, simply that they have read and understand its content. Evaluations should not be changed, but the employee should be offered the opportunity to prepare a written addendum or response that can be appended to the written document and retained in the employee record.

PROGRESSIVE DISCIPLINE

Unfortunately, the process of progressive discipline is a necessary component of most professional work environments. Progressive discipline occurs when there are identified problems with an individual's work habits or performance. There are five steps in the progressive discipline process. The first involves verbal counseling of the employee by the supervisor, with written documentation that the verbal counseling occurred. The written documentation simply serves as a record for the employee's file. The second step in progressive discipline is provision of a written warning. Should performance not improve, there is a follow-up to the written warning issued, which may subsequently lead to suspension and finally discharge. Supervisors should be aware of the process for progressive discipline and should carefully document all events. Without documentation, the poor performer may not be able to be terminated.

When communicating with an employee throughout the progressive discipline process, the supervisor should describe the problem(s) specifically, including the implications of why the problem(s) are of concern to the supervisor and/or within the workplace. The employee should be given a chance to provide his or her explanation, and the supervisor should actively listen during this process. The employee should be asked for input on problem resolution. When completed effectively, the act of progressive discipline should put the onus for improvement on the individual employee. At each step within the progressive discipline process, specific action should be agreed upon, and a date identified for follow-up to review progress. In general, no more than two weeks should pass between discussions. Supervisors should express confidence that the employee can improve, except at discharge. Again, the importance of documentation throughout this process cannot be overemphasized.

POLICIES AND PROCEDURES

Policies and procedures are required in virtually all practice settings. When written properly, policies and procedures should serve as the basis for completion of each function or activity within the workplace. Policies and procedures should be written such that a naive employee should be able to read the policy and procedure and successfully complete a given task. It is virtually impossible for policies and procedures to be too detailed. For example, if a particular task requires use of a computer, the procedure should begin by instructing the participants to turn on the computer using the green switch on the side of the processor. The participant might next be instructed that, once the screen is visible, the cursor should be used to select the appropriate icon for execution of the task, etc. It is common for policies and procedures to be prepared by managers or individuals most familiar with the individual activity. New employees or individuals from other areas within the work environment are frequently utilized to test the depth and detail of written policies and procedures.

COMMUNICATING WITH ADMINISTRATORS

Effective communication with administrators is critical to the success of pharmacists and managers, regardless of the practice setting. It is important to remember that administrators are inundated with information from various sources. Accordingly, communication should be concise and appropriately detailed such that the administrator can effectively understand the situation without being forced to wade through unnecessary paperwork.

Project Proposals

Project proposals require careful thought to detail and are frequently lengthy documents including flow diagrams, policies/procedures, treatment algorithms, etc. Although administrative support is essential to the advancement of any project proposal, it is unrealistic to expect that an administrator will wade through the levels of detail common to most project proposals. Therefore, such proposals should be accompanied by an executive summary that is a maximum of 2 pages in length. The executive summary should enable the administrator to see the "big picture" of the proposal and to refer to the detailed attachments for clarification of key points, without complete review of the proposal. The executive summary should consist of the following subsections (where applicable): goal, target market, required equipment, market research information, action plan, and conclusion.

Presentation of Data

The most common method of sharing data is through presentation of information in tabular format. Unfortunately, this method does not allow the recipient to compare and contrast data for trends, key points, etc. quickly. Alternative methods of data presentation are often overlooked, although they have the potential to augment significantly the display and communicate the intended message more effectively.

For example, line charts, including run and control charts, display discreet data points over time. Bar charts are utilized to compare items. Column charts assist with display of data over time (eg, annual pharmacy expenses 1998–2003). Pie charts, which are commonly utilized display a comparison, but really show the components of a whole at some point of time (eg, static data). Dot charts facilitate evaluation of a relationship between two variables, such as the correlation of years of pharmacy practice experience with a lower incidence of medication errors. An example of the use of a bar chart *versus* a table to display data is included in Figure 100-11.[17]

COMMUNICATING WITH THE MEDIA

In the current information age, public demand for health-related news is greater than ever before. As a result, there is also an increased need for the expertise of health care professionals to help communicate this information accurately. Pharmacists, as drug therapy specialists, are often asked to provide information to the media about drug-related safety and efficacy. Media interviews may be conducted in a face-to-face manner, as the case with television interviews, or via the telephone or e-mail, as in cases of written publications such as newspapers or magazines. Although communication with the media can be very challenging, it is important for pharmacists to communicate accurate information using an effective style and to represent the profession of pharmacy in a positive manner.

Collecting Background Information

When contacted for a potential media interview, the first step is to collect background information before agreeing to an interview. If contacted directly by a journalist, it is best to avoid the urge to respond to his or her questions immediately. General information should be gathered about the nature of the interview such as the name and affiliation of the reporter, the type of interview (eg, television, radio, telephone), when and where the interview will take place, the types of questions that will be asked, and the target audience.[18] This will help the pharmacist determine if he or she is the most qualified person to respond to the reporter's inquiries. For example, if the reporter is asking a policy question, it may be best to defer the questions to an appropriate administrator. Most institutions have a pubic relations department that is responsible for screening requests for media interviews and contacting the most qualified individual to respond. This department should be contacted prior to any media interaction.

Preparation

Once the context of the interview is understood, the next step is to prepare. Although time may be limited, effective preparation is one of the most critical steps to successful communication with the media.[18] As a general rule, it is best to avoid answering impromptu questions without first doing some homework. This is especially the case when pharmacists are responding to the mass media. It is often necessary to gather or confirm the facts and to consult with colleagues before formulating a response to media questions. This helps to ensure that accurate and up-to-date information is communicated.

After sufficient research has been conducted, the pharmacist should determine the major message that they wish to convey.[18] Depending on the situation, there may be more than one message a pharmacist wishes to communicate. During preparation, it is helpful to write down the major message and

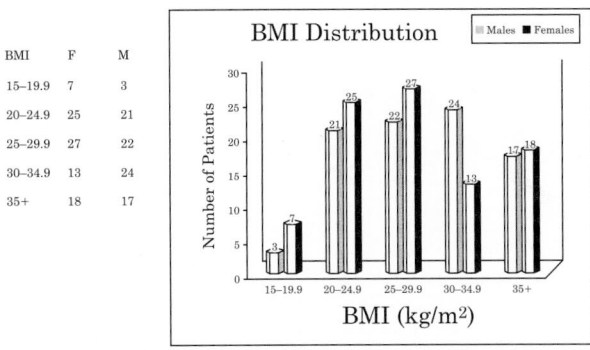

Data Presentation

BMI	F	M
15–19.9	7	3
20–24.9	25	21
25–29.9	27	22
30–34.9	13	24
35+	18	17

Figure 100-11. Use of a bar chart versus a table to display data.

list key talking points under each message. Key talking points should include the relevant facts, statistics, or supporting details.[18] This will help refine the major message to only the most important pieces of information. Preparing in this manner is particularly important, because most media interviews are conducted during a very short period of time. There simply may not be enough time for the pharmacist to communicate all of the pertinent details. Therefore, preparing a major message with supporting talking points can make a huge difference in delivery during the interview. If the pharmacist is not appropriately prepared, he or she may run out of time and not be able to communicate the most important facts. In addition, pharmacists should consider the characteristics of the target audience when developing the major message and key talking points; this will help to make sure they are providing relevant information at an appropriate level of understanding.[18] Being organized and prepared is the key to successfully communicating an important message in a clear and concise manner.

Delivery of the Message

Delivery is critical during a media interview. The same concepts that apply when delivering formal presentations should be considered when communicating during a media interview. These include using an open body position, maintaining eye contact with the reporter, using vocal inflections and pauses to emphasize key talking points, exhibiting confidence, and using a relaxed and steady pace.[18] If being interviewed over the telephone, many of these same principles apply. Pharmacists should be aware that interviewers most likely will quote statements that are made. Therefore, it is important to speak is a manner that is both professional and quotable. Pharmacists should never make statements that they do not want to read in print because reporters are not required to respect the statement "this is off the record."[18] If interviewing for information that will be presented in a printed article, it is good practice to request permission to review the article to make any necessary corrections prior to publication.

SUMMARY AND CONCLUSION

Communication is a vital skill for pharmacists, which is utilized multiple times each day, regardless of practice setting.

This chapter provides a broad overview of the most common types of written and verbal communication skills that are necessary for successful pharmacists.

REFERENCES

1. Calis KA, Heck AM. In: Malone PM, Mosdell KW, Kier KL eds. *Drug Information- A Guide for Pharmacists*, 2nd ed. Stamford, CT: Appleton and Lange, 2001.
2. Galt KA. In: *Clinical Skills Program: Module 1 Drug Information*. Bethesda, MD: American Society of Health-System Pharmacists, 1995.
3. Galt KA, Calis KA, Turcasso NM. In: *Clinical Skills Program: Module 3 Drug Information*. Bethesda, MD: American Society of Health-System Pharmacists, 1995.
4. ASHP Council on Professional Affairs. *Am J Health-Syst Pharm* 2003; 60:705.
5. Weed LL. *N Engl J Med* 1968; 278:593.
6. Weed LL. *N Engl J Med* 1968; 278:652.
7. Casella PJ. In: *Writing, Speaking, and Communication Skills for Health Professionals*. The Health Care Communication Group. London: Yale University Press, 2001.
8. Formulary Management. In: *Best Practices for Health-System Pharmacy. Positions and Guidance Documents of ASHP 2002–2003 Edition*. Bethesda, MD: American Society of Health-System Pharmacists, 2003.
9. Malone P. In: Drug Information- A guide for pharmacists, 2nd Edition. Malone PM, Mosdell KW, Kier KL eds. Stamford, CT: Appleton and Lange, 2001.
10. International Committee of Medical Journal Editors. Uniform requirements for manuscript submitted to biomedical journals. *JAMA* 1997; 277:927.
11. Field JM, Lohr KN, eds. *Guidelines for Clinical Practice: From Development to Use*. Washington, DC: National Academy Press, 1992.
12. Malone P. In: Malone PM, Mosdell KW, Kier KL, eds. *Drug Information: A Guide for Pharmacists,* 2nd ed. Stamford, CT: Appleton and Lange, 2001.
13. Coffin C. In: *Writing, Speaking, and Communication Skills for Health Professionals*. The Health Care Communication Group. London: Yale University Press, 2001.
14. Browner WS. In: Hiscock T, ed. *Publishing and Presenting Clinical Research*. Baltimore, MD: Williams and Wilkins, 1999.
15. Strunk W Jr, White EB. *The Elements of Style*, 4th ed. Boston, MA: Allyn & Bacon; 2000.
16. Browner WS. In: Hiscock T, ed. *Publishing and Presenting Clinical Research*. Baltimore: Williams & Wilkins, 1999.
17. Murry S, Murry O. *Total Quality Tools for Health Care*. PQSystems Inc, 1997.
18. Tolbert N, Sims S. *Media Matters*. Washington, DC: The Communications Center. Susan Peterson Productions, 2001.

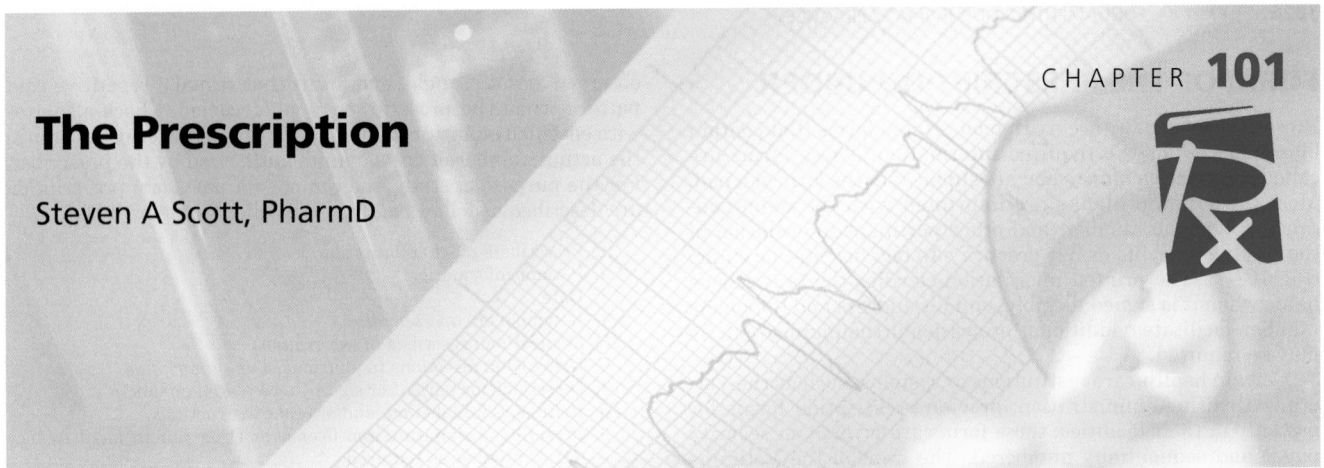

CHAPTER 101

The Prescription

Steven A Scott, PharmD

A *prescription* is an order for medication issued by a physician, dentist, or other properly licensed medical practitioner. Various states also have licensed other prescribers who have limited scopes of practice. For example, a veterinarian may prescribe only for animals; a podiatrist can prescribe only for conditions of the human foot; and optometrists have been given authority, in some states, to use drugs for diagnostic purposes, whereas in others they have received authority to use and prescribe drugs for disorders of the eye. In certain states, nurse practitioners, optometrists, psychologists, and even pharmacists, can issue prescriptions under protocol or with certain restrictions. Prescriptions designate a specific medication and dosage to be administered to a particular patient at a specified time. Commonly, the prescribed medication also is referred to as the *prescription* by the patient.

The prescription order is a part of the professional relationship among the prescriber, the pharmacist, and the patient. It is the pharmacist's responsibility in this relationship to provide quality pharmaceutical care that meets the medication needs of the patient. The pharmacist must be precise in the manual aspects of filling the prescription order and must provide the patient with the necessary information and guidance to assure the patient's compliance in taking the medication properly. It is also the pharmacist's responsibility to advise the prescriber of drug sensitivities the patient may have, previous adverse drug reactions (ADRs), and/or other medications that the patient may be taking that may alter the effectiveness or safety of the newly or previously prescribed medications. Pharmacists now find themselves frequently contacting physicians to suggest alternative drug products for individual patients as dictated by the formularies used by third-part prescription insurance plans. To meet these responsibilities, it is essential that the pharmacist maintains a high level of practice competence, keeps appropriate records on the health status and medication history of his/her patients and develops professional working relationships with other health professionals.

Pharmacists must establish and maintain the trust of the prescriber and the patient. Pharmaceutical care cannot optimally occur until the pharmacist has established a relationship with the patient. An important part of this relationship includes maintaining confidentiality. The medication being taken by a patient and the nature of his illness is a private matter that must be respected. The Health Insurance Portability and Accountability Act of 1996 (HIPAA) mandated the development of standards and requirements to control the flow of health information throughout the healthcare system. The act, which went into effect in April 2003, places additional restrictions and safeguards on how medical information can be utilized and disclosed. Pharmacists must now take special care to avoid discussing patient information where others not directly involved in the care of the patient can overhear the conversation and must obtain written permission from the patient to disclose certain types of medical information.

There are two broad legal classifications of medications: those that can be obtained only by prescription and those that may be purchased without a prescription. The latter are termed *nonprescription* drugs or *over-the-counter* (OTC) drugs. Medications that may be dispensed legally only on prescription are referred to as *prescription* drugs or *legend* drugs. The latter term refers to the *legend* that must appear on the label of the product as it is provided to the pharmacist by the manufacturer—*Caution: Federal Law Prohibits Dispensing Without Prescription*. Occasionally, physicians may issue prescriptions for nonlegend drugs that they desire the patient to receive.

Prescriptions may be written by the prescriber and given to the patient for presentation at the pharmacy, may be telephoned or communicated directly to the pharmacist by means of a fax machine, or may be electronically sent from a physician's computer to a pharmacist's computer. Prescription orders received verbally should be reduced to proper written form immediately or entered directly into a prescription computer by the pharmacist.

In the future, electronic prescribing may become the dominate means by which pharmacists receive prescriptions. In an attempt to minimize medication errors and enforce the use of the institution's drug formulary, numerous large hospitals now require physicians to enter orders directly into at a computer terminal or through a PDA. These orders are screened for potential errors and sent directly to the pharmacy for processing. This practice has been implemented on a much smaller scale in retail pharmacies in some geographic areas. As systems that interface between physician offices and pharmacies are further developed and refined, the practice of electronic prescribing will likely to become widespread.

Potential advantages associated with electronic prescribing include: (1) reducing or eliminating the errors associated with illegible handwriting; (2) prescribers can receive on-screen prompts for drug-specific dosing information; (3) information from the patient's medical record can be linked with information from the patient's prescription records; (4) prescribers would be notified if a drug product is covered by the patient's insurance plan when the order is being generated rather than when it is presented at the pharmacy; (5) refill requests can be expedited; and (6) computers can facilitate data exchange between the physician and pharmacist allowing individuals to better manage their time and facilitate interactions with their patients.[1]

FORM OF THE PRESCRIPTION ORDER

Prescriptions usually are written on printed forms that contain blank spaces for the required information. These forms are called *prescription blanks* and are supplied in the form of a pad. Most prescription blanks are imprinted with the name, address, telephone number, and other pertinent information of the physician or his or her practice site (eg, hospital or clinic) (Fig 101-1). The printed information clarifies the prescriber's name when it is signed illegibly, and his address and telephone number facilitates additional professional communication, as may be required.

Certain health-care institutions or systems, such as the Veterans Health Administration, provide prescription forms for use only in their facilities; these forms are printed on security paper and sequentially numbered. The front of the Veterans Administration (VA) form, printed in gray tone, has checkoff blocks to indicate patient status (eg, inpatient) as well as check-off blocks to override the general authority to allow drug substitution and require the product name, strength, and quantity to be placed on the label. The back of the form, in white, which must be completed before dispensing an original or refill prescription, provides space to enter the manufacturer and control number of the product, the date dispensed or mailed, the signature or initials of the dispensing pharmacist, and any calculations or written notations.

Prescription blanks that are used by the pharmacist in his/her transposition of verbally received prescriptions commonly are imprinted with the name, address, and telephone number of the pharmacy. These blanks also may be used by physicians to write prescriptions when visiting the pharmacy. Specially imprinted prescription blanks are not required legally for prescriptions; any paper or other writing material may be used. Most states allow prescription orders to be faxed to a pharmacy *directly from* the prescriber, and even allow direct computer transmission of a prescription order from the prescriber to the pharmacy's computer.

Some states require prescription blanks for controlled substances (especially *Schedule II*) to include certain security features. These include triplicate prescription forms, sequentially numbered forms, forms with special watermarks that can only be observed at a 45° angle, and forms that reveal a repetitive *void* pattern when the prescription is photocopied. Check-off boxes with specified quantities also may appear on the forms to confirm the actual number of dosage units authorized by the prescriber. For the purpose of study, the component parts of a prescription are described as follows and are identified in Figure 101-1.

1. Prescribers office information
2. Patient information
3. Date
4. ℞ symbol or *superscription*
5. Medication prescribed or *inscription*
6. Dispensing directions to pharmacist or *subscription*
7. Directions for patient or *signa* (to be placed on label)
8. Refill, special labeling, and/or other instructions
9. Prescriber's signature and license or Drug Enforcement Agency (DEA) number as required

In practice, some of the above information (such as the patient's address) may be absent when the prescription is received by the pharmacist. In these instances the pharmacist obtains the necessary information from the patient or physician, as is required.

PATIENT INFORMATION—The full name and address of the patient are necessary on the prescription for identification purposes. Names and addresses written illegibly should be clarified on acceptance of the prescription. Incorrect spelling of a patient's name on a prescription label might cause concern in the patient's mind as to the correctness of the medication and possibly would hamper the desired professional relationship between the pharmacist and patient.

Federal law requires that the full names and addresses of the prescriber and the patient be included on prescriptions for certain controlled substances. The physician's DEA registration number also is required on the prescription. Controlled substances are drugs that, because of their potential for abuse, are controlled under special regulations by the federal government. The address of the patient is useful for identification purposes as well as for delivery of medication to the patient's home.

Some prescription blanks used by medical specialists, particularly pediatricians, include a space for insertion of the patient's age, weight, or body surface area. This information is placed on the prescription by the physician when medication dosage is an important function of age or weight. This information assists the pharmacist in interpreting the prescription, checking the dose prescribed for the child and is particularly useful when a child has the same name as one of his/her parents.

DATE—Prescriptions are dated at the time they are written and also when they are received and filled in the pharmacy. The date is important in establishing the medication record of the patient. An unusual lapse of time between the date a prescription was written and the date it is brought to the pharmacy may be questioned by a pharmacist to determine if the intent of the physician and the needs of the patient can still be met. The date prescribed is also important to a pharmacist in filling prescriptions for controlled substances. The *Drug Abuse Control Amendments* specify that no prescription order for controlled substances may be dispensed or renewed more than 6 months after the date prescribed.

℞ SYMBOL OR SUPERSCRIPTION—The ℞ symbol generally is understood to be a contraction of the Latin verb *recipe*, meaning *take thou* or *you take*. Some historians believe this symbol originated from the sign of Jupiter, ♃, employed by the ancients in requesting aid in healing. Gradual distortion through the years has led to the symbol currently used. Today, the symbol is representative of both the prescription and the pharmacy itself.

MEDICATION PRESCRIBED OR INSCRIPTION—This is the body or principal part of the prescription order. It contains the names, dosages, and quantities of the prescribed ingredients.

Today, the majority of prescriptions are written for medications already prepared or prefabricated into dosage forms by industrial manufacturers. The medications may be prescribed

(1) **CLARKE COUNTY HEALTH DEPARTMENT**
345 NORTH HARRIS STREET
ATHENS, GA 30610
PHONE 542-8600

(2)(3) Patient's Name *Samantha Ericson*   Date 4/18/94

Address *27 Fifth St.*

(4)(5) ℞   *Ampicillin*   *250 mg.*

(6)   *Disp: #40*

(7)   *Sig: One q.i.d.*

(8)   Label ☑
Do Not Label ☐
Refill 1 2 3 4
PRN

(9)   *Walter J. Brown Jr. M.D.* M.D.

Dea. # _____

Figure 101-1. Example of a physician's prescription showing typical form and content.

under their trademarked or manufacturer's proprietary name or by their nonproprietary or *generic* names.

Pharmacists are required to dispense the trademarked product when prescribed, unless substitution of an equivalent product is permitted by the prescribing physician or by state law. Most states have generic substitution laws that mandate the use of a generically equivalent product for certain patients. In some instances, the patient also must consent to the drug substitution. Some states require the prescriber to write specific instructions or sign a specific line on the prescription to allow or disallow product substitution. Many health maintenance organizations and prescription benefit plans have strict formularies for which only certain drug products within a therapeutic class may be dispensed. Thus, the pharmacists may be directed by the prescription plan to dispense a similar but different drug product than was prescribed for the patient.

Prescription orders requiring the pharmacist to mix ingredients are termed *compounded* prescriptions. Prescriptions requiring compounding contain the names and quantities of each ingredient required. The names of the ingredients generally are written using the nonproprietary names of the materials, although occasionally proprietary names may be employed. Quantities of ingredients to be used may be indicated in the metric or apothecary system of weights and measures; however, the use of the apothecary system is dramatically diminishing to becoming nonexistent. These systems are described in Chapter 11.

In the use of the metric system, the decimal is often replaced by a vertical line that may be imprinted on the prescription blank or drawn by the prescriber. The symbols *g* or *mL* often are eliminated, as it is understood that solids are dispensed by weight (in grams) and liquids by volume (in milliliters).

DISPENSING DIRECTIONS TO PHARMACIST OR SUBSCRIPTION—This part of the prescription consists of directions to the pharmacist for the preparation of the prescription. With diminished frequency of compounded prescriptions, such directions are likewise less frequent. In a majority of prescriptions, the subscription serves merely to designate the dosage form (eg, tablets, capsules, inhaler, transdermal patch) and the number of dosage units to be supplied. Examples of prescription directions to the pharmacist include the following among others:

M ft caps dtd no xxiv (Mix and make capsules. Dispense 24 such doses).
Ft supp No xii (Make 12 suppositories).
M ft ung (Mix and make an ointment).
Disp tabs No c (Dispense 100 tablets).

DIRECTIONS FOR PATIENT OR SIGNATURA—The prescriber indicates the directions for the patient's use of the medication in the portion of the prescription termed the *Signatura*. The word, usually abbreviated *Signa* or *Sig* means *mark thou*. The directions in the signa commonly are written using abbreviated forms of English or Latin terms or a combination of each. Examples include:

Tabs ii q4h (Take two tablets every 4 hours).
Caps i 4xd pc & hs (Take one capsule four times a day after meals and at bedtime).
Instill gtts ii od (Instill two drops into the right eye).

The directions are transcribed by the pharmacist onto the prescription label of the container of dispensed medication. A list of some prescription abbreviations is presented in Table 101-1.

It is advisable and required by law in most states for the pharmacist to reinforce the directions to the patient when dispensing the medication because the patient may be uncertain or confused as to the proper method of use. Some pharmacists and physicians provide their patients with written directions outlining the proper use of the medication prescribed. Frequently, these directions include the best time to take the medication, the importance of adhering to the prescribed dosage schedule, what to do if a dose is missed, the permitted use of the medication with respect to food, drink, and/or other medications the patient may

be taking, as well as information about the drug itself. As a requirement of law, certain manufacturers have prepared patient package inserts (PPIs) for specific products for issuance to patients (Fig 101-2). These present to the patient information regarding the usefulness of the medication as well as its side effects and potential hazards. Other PPIs are available to pharmacists for use in their practices from professional and commercial sources. For example, The United States Pharmacopeial Convention provides patient education leaflets containing supplementary printed instructions on many drugs and drug categories to physicians, pharmacists, and other health professionals for distribution to patients (Fig 101-3). The information is also available on computer software, allowing leaflets to be printed in the pharmacy as needed and with a compatible computer and standard line printer. Similar computer software programs are available from various other sources, designed to generate personalized patient-counseling information for use by the pharmacist in patient education.[2] Numerous sources of information for consumers are now available via the Internet. Pharmacists can refer patients to these web sites but may want to caution patients that all of the information on these sites may not apply to their individual situation.

In addition to instructions to the patient, most prescribers desire and laws dictate that the name and strength of the prescribed drug be included on the label of the dispensed medication. Prescribers indicate this to the pharmacist by including the name and strength of the drug in the signa or by simply writing in the word *label* in the signa. Some prescription blanks have the word *label* printed for circling or checking by the prescribing physician (see Fig 101-1). The advantages to having the name and strength of the drug identified on the prescription label include the facilitation of communication among the patient and the pharmacist and the physician and the rapid identification of the medication in times of accidental or purposeful overdose. When a generic drug product is dispensed, it is customary to include the manufacture of the product on the label as well.

The date after which the medication will be subpotent (expiration date) may be placed on the label based on information included on the original manufacturer's package. This precaution is important for certain drugs that rapidly deteriorate and lose their potency. For example, many oral liquid formulations of antibiotics remain stable for only a period of 14 days under refrigeration, and one-half that time when nonrefrigerated after their preparation by the pharmacist. Certain ophthalmologic preparations and most parenteral dosage forms have relatively short shelf lives once removed from refrigeration and thus containers must include the expiration date.

Physicians generally do not specify that expiration dates be noted on the label because they recognize that the pharmacist provides this information when dispensing such preparations. Statements on auxiliary labels such as *do not use after __ days* or *discard after __ days* serve this purpose. Some state laws require that pharmacists place the expiration date on the label of all medications dispensed, even those with no special stability problems.

SPECIAL LABELING AND OTHER INSTRUCTIONS—The number of authorized refills should be indicated on each prescription by the prescriber. In the event that no refill information is provided, it is understood that no refills have been authorized; however, it is advised that the label state such to avoid confusion. Most prescription blanks include a section where this information may be indicated (see Fig 101-1). Most states limit refills on a prescription to one year after the prescription was written originally. When a prescriber indicates that a prescription can be refilled *prn* "as needed," the pharmacist should refill it only with a frequency consistent with the directions. No refills are permitted for *Schedule II* controlled substances.

HOSPITAL MEDICATION ORDERS

Medication orders for inpatients in hospitals and other institutions are written by the physician on forms called the *Physi-*

Table 101-1. Commonly Used Abbreviations in Prescriptions and Medication Orders

ABBREVIATION	MEANING	ABBREVIATION	MEANING
aa	of each	MS	morphine sulfate
abd	abdomen	MTX	methotrexate
ac	before meals	MVI	multivitamin
ad	To, up to	m	Mix
a.d.	Right ear	N&V	Nausea and vomiting
ad lib	At pleasure, freely	non rep/NR	Do not repeat
AM	morning	noct	At night
amp	Ampul of medication	NS	normal saline
aq	Water	NTG	nitroglycerin
a.s.	left ear	OA	osteoarthritis
ASA	aspirin	OCD	obsessive compulsive disorder
ATC	Around the clock	OJ	orange juice
au	each ear	O2	oxygen
BCP	birth control pill	ou	Each eye
bid	Twice a day	od	Right eye
BM	Bowel movement	os	Left eye
BP	Blood pressure	P	pulse
BPH	benign prostatic hypertrophy	pc	After eating
BS	Blood sugar	PEFR	peak expiratory flow rate
BSA	Body surface area	pm	evening
c	with	po	by mouth
Ca	calcium	postop	after surgery
CAD	coronary artery disease	pr	rectally
caps	Capsule	prn	when necessary
cc	cubic centimeter [milliliter]	pulv	A powder
CHF	congestive heart failure	PVCs	premature ventricular contractions
COPD	chronic obstructive pulmonary disease	PVD	peripheral vascular disease
CP	chest pain	q	every
CRNP	Certified Registered Nurse Practitioner	qd	every day
dil	dilute	qid	four times daily
dtd	Let such doses be given	qod	every other day
DC	discontinue medication	qs	as much as is sufficient
DDS	Doctor of Dental Surgery	qs ad	a sufficient quantity to (prepare)
DMD	Doctor of Medical Dentistry	qh	every hour
disp	dispense	RA	rheumatoid arthritis
div	divide	RN	Registered Nurse
DJD	degenerative joint disease	Rect	Use rectally
DM	diabetes mellitus	s	without
DO	Doctor of Osteopathy	ss	One-half
DW	distilled water	SC	subcutaneous injection
Dx	diagnosis	Sig	write on label
elix	elixir	SL	sublingual
EtOH	ethanol	SLE	systemic lupus erythematosus
Ft	Make, let it be made	SOB	shortness of breath
g or gm	gram	sol	Solution
GERD	gastroesophageal reflux disease	SQ or SubQ	subcutaneous injection
GI	Gastrointestinal	sq m, m^2	square meter
GU	Genitourinary	stat	immediately
gr	Grain	supp	Suppository
gtt	A drop	Susp	Suspension
HA	headache	Sx	symptom
HBP	High blood pressure	syr	Syrup
HCTZ	hydrochlorothiazide	T	temperature
HR	heart rate	tab	tablet
HRT	hormone replacement therapy	TB	tuberculosis
hs	at bedtime	TCN	tetracycline
HTN	Hypertension	TED	thromboembolic disease
inj	An injection	TIA	transient ischemic attack
IV	Intravenous injection	tid	three times a day
IM	Intramuscular injection	tiw	three times a week
ID	Intradermal injection	tbsp	tablespoon
IU	international units	TMP-SMX	trimethoprim-sulfamethoxazole
JRA	juvenile rheumatoid arthritis	tsp	teaspoon
KCL	potassium chloride	top	(Use) topically
kg	kilogram	Tx	treatment
L	liter	U	unit
mcg	microgram	UA	uric acid, urinalysis
MD	Doctor of Medicine	UC	ulcerative colitis
mEq	milliequivalent	ud	as directed
mg	milligram	ung	ointment
mg/kg	milligrams/kilogram	URI	upper respiratory infection
mg/m²	milligrams/square meter	ut dict	as directed
mL	milliliter	UTI	urinary tract infection
mOsmol	milliosmole	WA	while awake
m or min	Minimum	wk	week
MOM	Milk of Magnesia		

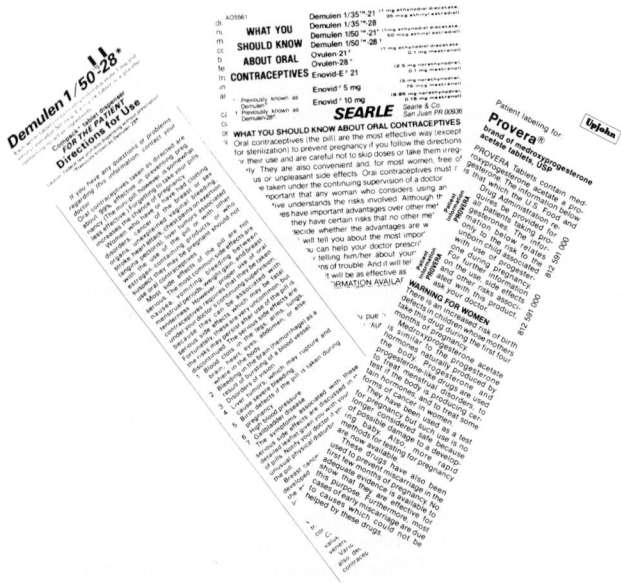

Figure 101-2. Example of manufacturers' patient package inserts intended to enhance patient understanding of the medication prescribed.

cian's Order Sheet. The type of form used varies between institutions and even within the institution, depending on the unit rendering the care. Because these orders are written in a controlled environment, many of the requirements and restrictions placed on prescription orders for outpatients do not apply in the institutional setting. Institutional pharmacy practice is discussed in Chapter 127.

PROCESSING THE PRESCRIPTION ORDER

The manner in which a pharmacist processes a prescription order is important in fulfilling his/her professional responsibilities and can enhance his/her image with the physician and the patient. Proper procedures are given below for receiving, read-

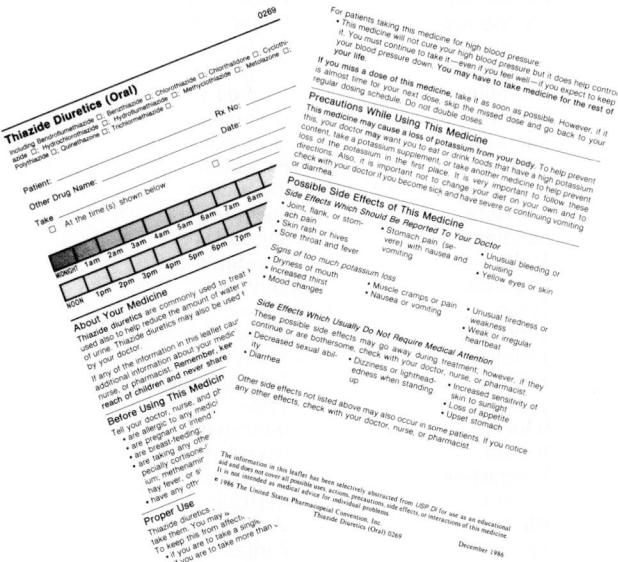

Figure 101-3. Examples of USP Patient Education Leaflets. The information also is available on computer disk for use in the pharmacy (courtesy, The USPC).

ing and checking, numbering and dating, labeling, preparing, packaging, rechecking, delivering and counseling, recording and filing, and pricing the prescriptions.

RECEIVING THE PRESCRIPTION—It is desirable that the patient present the prescription order directly to the pharmacist because this enhances the pharmacist–patient relationship and facilitates the gathering of essential disease and drug information from the patient. This is critical for the provision of quality pharmaceutical care. In situations in which this is not practical, the individual receiving the prescription should be trained to accept it in a professional manner and obtain the correct name, address, and other pertinent patient information. Patients having a prescription filled for the first time at a pharmacy may be asked to complete a brief health and medication history to establish a database in the pharmacy's computer for the patient. It is important to determine if the patient's medications are provided through insurance coverage and whether the patient wishes to wait, call back, or have the medication delivered. If the pharmacist is unable to receive the prescription order personally, he/she should be available to provide an estimate of the length of time required for filling the prescription and to price it if requested by the patient. Many pharmacists make it a practice to price prescriptions before dispensing, especially in the case of unusually expensive medication, to avoid subsequent questions concerning the charge.

READING AND CHECKING THE PRESCRIPTION—The prescription order first should be read completely and carefully. There should be no doubt as to the ingredients or quantities prescribed. From the pharmacy's prescription computer (or other record of the patient's medication history), the pharmacist should determine the compatibility of the newly prescribed medication with other drugs being taken by the patient and also consider if any drug–food or drug-disease interactions may exist. Most prescription computer software programs identify possible drug–drug interactions. However, these software programs do not always identify the potential significance of the drug–drug interaction. This is the point at which the pharmacist must use information specific to this patient to determine the significance of the interaction and to determine if the prescriber should be contacted. In addition, references may be used for this purpose, such as *USP Dispensing Information (USP DI)* or *Drug Interaction Facts.* Should the probability or likelihood of a drug interaction exist, the pharmacist should first consider alternative drug products that might be used and then consult with the prescriber to determine best therapeutic alternative for the patient and be prepared to make recommendations. The same would apply when a medication is prescribed for a patient who has a known drug allergy or sensitivity to the prescribed drug or to other drugs of the same chemical class. If something is illegible or if it appears that an error has been made, the pharmacist should consult another pharmacist or the prescriber. *A pharmacist should never guess at the meaning of an indistinct word or unrecognized abbreviation.* Unfamiliar or unclear abbreviations represent a source of error in interpreting and dispensing prescriptions.[3] No *official* or standard list of prescription abbreviations exists. Many of those in use are derived from the Latin and generally are recognized (see Table 101-1). However, many others may be simply shorthand creations of the individual prescriber.

Common prescriber abbreviations for drug names include *Pb* for phenobarbital, *HCTZ* for hydrochlorothiazide, *MTX* for methotrexate, and *ASA* for aspirin. Diseases and conditions also are commonly abbreviated (eg, *CHF* for congestive heart failure, *BPH* for benign prostatic hypertrophy, *URI* for upper respiratory tract infection, *HBP* for high blood pressure). Other abbreviations, such as *ATC* for around-the-clock, *WA* for while awake, and *BM* for bowel movement, also are used in prescription writing.

The use of Latin words, phrases, and abbreviations in prescriptions is a carryover from the time that Latin was considered the international language of medicine. Latin was used extensively in writing prescription orders until the early part of the 20th century. Although its use gradually has diminished, it is still used widely, in the form of abbreviations, in the subscription and signa portions of prescriptions.

Pharmacists are frequently confronted in their interpretation of the prescription order with the names of drugs that look alike or sound alike. These similar names are a potential source for errors. Knowledge of the patient's medical problems and diagnoses can often provide the pharmacist with insight into which of the look-alike or sound-alike drugs is intended for the patient. There have been numerous cases in which the brand name of a drug product has been changed after several months on the market subsequent to confusion with other marketed drugs with similar brand names. Examples of drugs with similar names are listed in Table 101-2.

The pharmacist must take great care and use his/her broad knowledge of drug products to prevent dispensing errors. A telephone call to the physician, made so as not to alarm the patient, serves to verify the meaning of a prescription that is unclear and at the same time bolster the professional reputation of the pharmacist as a careful practitioner and valuable member of the health team.

Omissions, such as the failure to specify the desired strength of a medication or its dosage form, must be corrected. In such a case, the pharmacist should never elect to dispense the usual dose or dosage form but instead should consult the prescriber. To detect such omissions and provide the physician with the necessary information, the pharmacist must be familiar with available strengths and dosage forms of prefabricated drug products. Knowledge of available dosage forms also enables the pharmacist to suggest a more appropriate or easy-to-use method of drug delivery for a particular patient.

The amount and frequency of a dose must be noted carefully and checked. In determining the safety of the dose of a medicinal agent, the age, weight, and condition of the patient (eg, liver function, kidney function), dosage form prescribed, possible influence of other concomitant drugs being taken, and the frequency of administration all must be considered. Several guides are available to the pharmacist in evaluating the safety of a prescribed dose. The *USP DI* provides usual doses and dosage ranges for many drugs in use. Manufacturers' catalogs, file cards, and package inserts provide dosage information on their products. References such as *Physicians' Desk Reference, AMA Drug Evaluations, American Hospital Formulary Service Drug Information, Drug Facts and Comparisons, Handbook of Clinical Drug Data, Pharmacist's Drug Handbook,* and *Pediatric Dosage Handbook* are useful general sources of such information. Some computer software programs now can check doses for pediatric patients when the child's weight is entered. In the case of a suspected error in dose, appropriate references should be checked prior to consulting the physician.

Measurement of liquid medication may lead to dosage variation caused by differences in the capacity of household spoons and interpretation of which measuring device to use by the patient. The problems associated with teaspoonful dosage have long been recognized. A standard teaspoon has been established by the American National Standards Institute as containing 4.93 ± 0.24 mL. For practical purposes, the standard teaspoonful is considered to be equivalent to 5 mL, although different household teaspoons vary widely in capacity. Thus, 1 fl oz (29.57 mL) of a medicated liquid is considered to provide approximately six standard teaspoonful doses.

Table 101-2. Examples of Look-Alike and/or Sound-Alike Drug Names

Adriamycin	Achromycin	Methotrexate	Metolazone
Albuterol	Atenolol	Myleran	Mylicon
Alupent	Atrovent	Nicardipine	Nifedipine
Amikin	Amicar	Orinase	Ornade
Apresoline	Priscoline	Pediapred	PediaProfen
Brevital	Bretylol	Penicillin	Penicillamine
Carafate	Cafergot	Percodan	Percocet
Cefoxitin	Cefotaxime	Phenobarbital	Pentobarbital
Chlorpromazine	Chlorpropamide	Physostigmine	Pyridostigmin
Clonidine	Klonopin	Pitressin	Pitocin
Cyclosporine	Cycloserine	Prazepam	Prazosin
Digitoxin	Digoxin	Prednisolone	Prednisone
Dilantin	Dilaudid	Prednisone	Primidone
Diphenhydramine	Diphenhydrinate	Prilosec	Prozac
Dopamine	Dobutamine	Quinamm	Quinidine
Doriden	Doxidan	Quinidine	Clonidine
Doxirubicin	Daunorubicin	Quinine	Quinidine
Dyazide	Diazoxide	Ramapril	Enalapril
Enalapril	Anafranil	Regroton	Hygroton
Enduronyl	Inderal	Ritodrine	Ranitidine
Esimil	Estinyl	Salsalate	Sucralfate
Florinal	Florinef	Sandimmune	Sandostatin
Florinal	Fioricet	Stelazine	Selegiline
Fluocinolone	Fluocinonide	Tegretol	Tegopen
Folic Acid	Folinic Acid	Tenex	Xanax
Glipizide	Glyburide	Timolol	Atenolol
Haldol	Halcion	Timolol	Tylenol
Hydralazine	Hydroxyzine	Tolazamide	Tolbutamide
Hydroxyzine	Hydroxyurea	Tylenol	Tylox
Imferon	Interferon	Vanceril	Vancenase
Inderal	Isordil	Vicodin	Hycodan
Indocin	Lincocin	Vinblastine	Vincristine
Isomil	Isordil	Vistaril	Restoril
Lanoxin	Xanax	Wellbutrin	Wellcovorin
Lithobid	Lithotabs	Xanax	Zantac
Lorazepam	Alprazolam	Zarontin	Zaroxolyn
Mesantoin	Mestinon	Zofran	Zantac
Metaproterenol	Metoprolol	Zovirax	Zostrix
		Zyloprim	ZORprin

To avoid errors in liquid dosing, pharmacists often dispense calibrated measuring devices with liquid medication. Some of these devices are shown in Figures 101-4 and 101-5.

NUMBERING AND DATING—It is a legal requirement to number the prescription order and to place the same number on the label. This serves to identify the bottle or package and to connect it with the original order for reference or to renew the prescription. Consecutive numbers are assigned by prescription computers or manually by use of numbering machines.

Dating of the prescription on the date filled is also a legal requirement. This information is important in determining the appropriate refill frequency, patient compliance, and as an alternate means of locating the prescription order should the prescription number be lost by the patient. The prescription computer may be employed for these purposes.

LABELING—The prescription label may be typewritten or prepared by computer, using the information entered by the pharmacist or pharmacy assistant. Figure 101-6 demonstrates a computer-prepared prescription, including the label, patient-counseling information, and receipt. The type and quality of computer printer used by a pharmacy can have a major effect on the readability of a prescription label. Newer laser printers produce a label with a type font and boldness that is much easier for most patients to read.

A prescription should have an aesthetic and professional-appearing label. If the label and the container are not neat and professional in appearance, the patient may conclude that the prescription medication itself was also prepared in a careless manner. This may result in a loss of confidence in the pharmacist or pharmacy.

The name and address of the pharmacy are legally required to appear on the label; the telephone number is also commonly included. The prescription number, prescriber's name, patient's name, directions for use (in easy to understand language for the patient), and the date of dispensing also are legally required; and the name and strength of the medication are also frequently included.

Some state laws require that the name or initials of the pharmacist dispensing the medication appear on the label. Some pharmacists indicate the refill or renewal status of the prescription on the primary label or use an auxiliary label to indicate this information. Occasionally, the manufacturer's lot number for the medication dispensed is entered on the label to aid in rapid identification of medication that might be recalled.

Labeling requirements for controlled substances are presented in Chapter 111. Auxiliary labels are used to emphasize important aspects of the dispensed medication, including its proper use, handling, storage, refill status, and necessary warnings or precautions. A *shake-well* label is indicated for a prescription containing ingredients that may physically sepa-

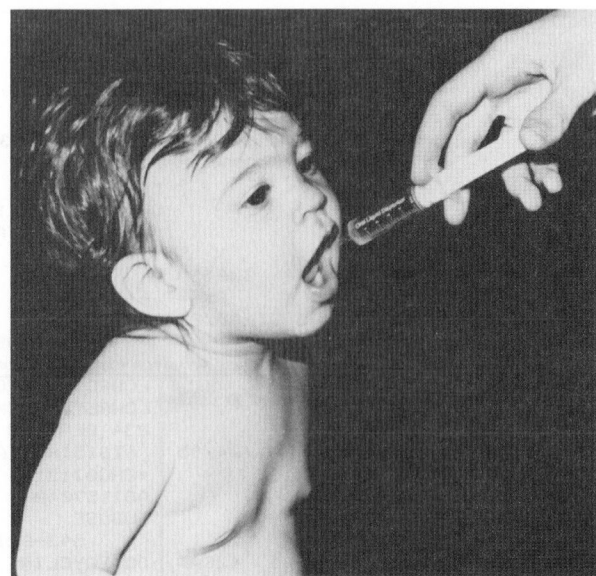

Figure 101-5. An oral liquid dispenser for the accurate delivery of small doses of liquid medication to infants (courtesy, Baxa).

rate on standing (eg, suspensions, lotions, and emulsions). The use of labels such as *For the Ear, For the Eye*, and *External Use* is recommended because of the added safety these offer, even when the primary directions indicate their proper use. Other precautionary labels may be used to warn that the medication should not be swallowed, used internally or should be kept out of reach of children and others for whom it is not intended.

Auxiliary labels are available in various colors to give them special prominence. They should be placed in a conspicuous spot on the prescription container. Examples of some auxiliary labels in English and Spanish are shown in Figure 101-7.

In certain circumstances it may be desirable for the pharmacist to supplement the instructions or directions of the prescriber. Some states have passed regulations that recognize that a need may exist for the pharmacist to add to the directions of the prescriber to either clarify or expand the prescriber's instructions. Such regulations indicate that when, in the judgment of the pharmacist, directions to the patient are necessary, either for clarification or for insurance of proper administration of the medication, the pharmacist may add such directions or cautionary messages to those indicated by the prescriber on the original prescription. For example, a pharmacist might advise that a medication be taken with a large volume of water or that certain foods or activities are to be avoided when taking the medication.

The federal government has required that patient product information be provided with the dispensing of certain drugs to ensure that the patient is apprised of proper use of the medication, its benefits and risks, and the signs of adverse reaction. Examples of these are shown in Figure 101-2. Other types of patient information sheets have been noted in this chapter and may be used by pharmacists in their practice. Virtual all prescription computer systems are programmed to provide supplemental instructions to patients (see Fig 101-6). These printed instructions may be used by the pharmacist to reinforce his or her personal efforts in patient counseling. Pharmacists may need to assist some patients interpret the information contained in these product information sheets. This is especially the case when dealing with poorly educated patients, patients who have impaired cognitive function, or when dispensing a drug product that has many potential indications.

PREPARING THE PRESCRIPTION—After reading and checking the prescription order, the pharmacist should decide on the exact procedure to be followed in dispensing or com-

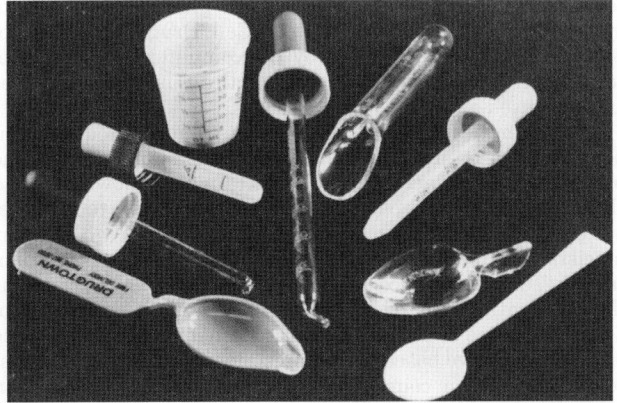

Figure 101-4. Examples of medicinal spoons of various capacities, calibrated medicine droppers, an oral medication tube, and a disposable medication cup.[4]

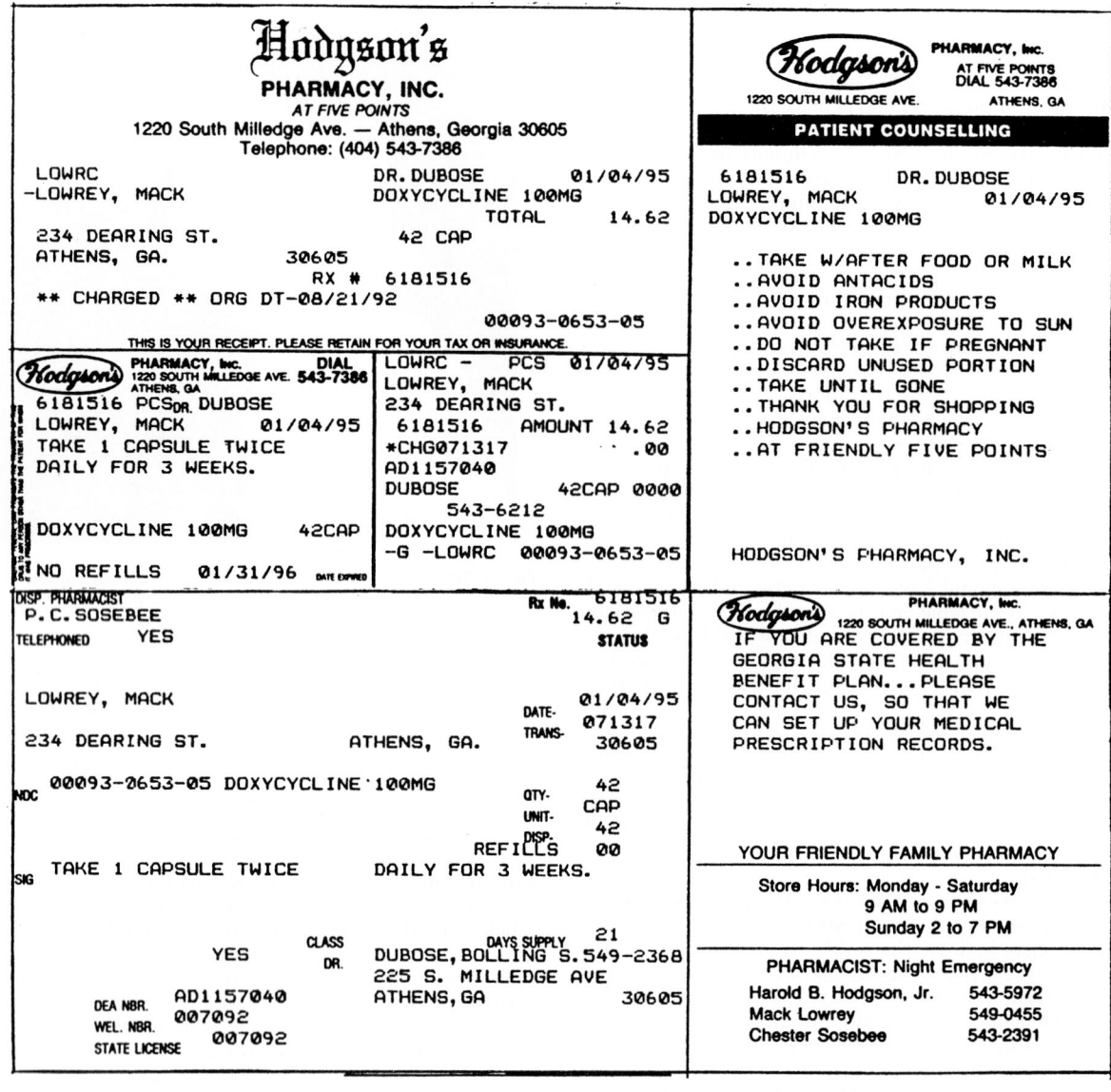

Figure 101-6. Example of a computer-prepared prescription record, label, patient receipt, and patient-counseling information.

pounding the ingredients. Most prescriptions call for dispensing medications already prefabricated into dosage forms by pharmaceutical manufacturers. Care must be exercised by the pharmacist in making certain that the product dispensed is of the prescribed dosage, form, strength, and number of dosage units. As noted above, when substitution is permitted, the pharmacist is responsible for the selection of the manufacturer's product to use in filling the prescription. He/she performs this responsibility on the basis of his knowledge of the quality, effectiveness, and cost to the patient of the selected product.

In preparing prescriptions with prefabricated products, the pharmacist should check the manufacturer's label, comparing it with the prescription order, before and after filling the order, to make certain of its correctness. Products that show signs of poor manufacture, which look deteriorated or are past the stated expiration date on the label should never be dispensed.

Solid, prefabricated dosage forms generally are counted in the pharmacy using a device such as that shown in Figure 101-8. Such a device facilitates the rapid and sanitary counting and transferring of medication from the stock packages to the prescription container. To prevent contamination of tablets and

capsules, the counting tray should be wiped clean after each counting, as powder, especially from uncoated tablets, tends to remain on the tray. Many high volume pharmacies use automated counting machines (eg, Baker Cell, Drug-O-Matic, AutoScript III) that are activated by the computer when the prescription order is entered. In some practices, unit dose packages are dispensed as shown in Figure 101-9.

Although the number of prescriptions that now require compounding represents only a small percentage of the total, the pharmacist must acquire and maintain the knowledge and skills necessary to prepare them accurately. The extemporaneous compounding of prescriptions is an activity for which pharmacists are qualified uniquely by virtue of their education, training, and experience. *Pharmacy compounding* is defined as the preparation, mixing, assembling, packaging, or labeling of a drug or device as a result of a practitioner's prescription-drug order or initiative based on the prescriber–patient–pharmacist relationship in the course of professional practice.[5] In addition to the compounding of individual prescriptions when received, guidelines of the FDA permit the preparation of small quantities of compounded products in anticipation of prescriptions for individual patients based on regularly observed prescribing

ENGLISH

SHAKE WELL

FOR EXTERNAL USE ONLY

THIS PRESCRIPTION CAN ONLY BE REFILLED BY AUTHORITY OF YOUR PHYSICIAN

NOT TO BE TAKEN BY MOUTH

KEEP IN REFRIGERATOR DO NOT FREEZE

POISON

FOR THE eye

KEEP OUT OF REACH OF CHILDREN

SPANISH

AGITESE

USO EXTERNO

SOLO SE PUEDE REPITIR CON AUTORIZACIÓN DE SU MÉDICO.

NO SE TOME

Mantengalo en la nevera. NO CONGELARO.

VENENO

PARA LOS OJOS

MANTENGASE FUERA DEL ALCANCE DE LOS NIÑOS

Figure 101-7. Examples of pharmacy auxiliary labels in English and Spanish. Actual labels available in color (courtesy, PHARMEX).

patterns. However, unless licensed as a manufacturer, pharmacies may not engage in the large-scale preparation of drugs for other pharmacies or entities for resale.[6]

Extemporaneous compounding is essential in the course of professional practice to prepare drug formulations in dosage forms or strengths that are not otherwise commercially available. The process may include the use of readily available bulk pharmaceutical chemicals, or it may require the use and conversion of a commercially available dosage form into another form. For example, it is not uncommon to fortify or reduce the strength of an active ingredient in a dermatological preparation, to reformulate adult dosage forms, such as tablets or capsules, into an oral suspension for use by pediatric patients, or to prepare intravenous admixtures in the hospital, nursing home, or home-care setting.[7] In each instance of compounding, the pharmacist must apply his/her technical and scientific knowledge and use available informational sources to assure product efficacy and stability. Information about the preparation and stability of drugs into suspension formulations can often be obtained from pharmacists' colleagues at pediatric hospitals where the preparation of such formulations may be commonplace.

When a prescription requiring compounding is received, the pharmacist should take into consideration the chemical and physical compatibility of the ingredients, the proper order of mixing, the need for special adjuvants or techniques, and the mathematical calculations required.

Once deciding on the procedure, the pharmacist assembles the necessary materials in a single location on the prescription counter. As each ingredient is used, it is transferred to another

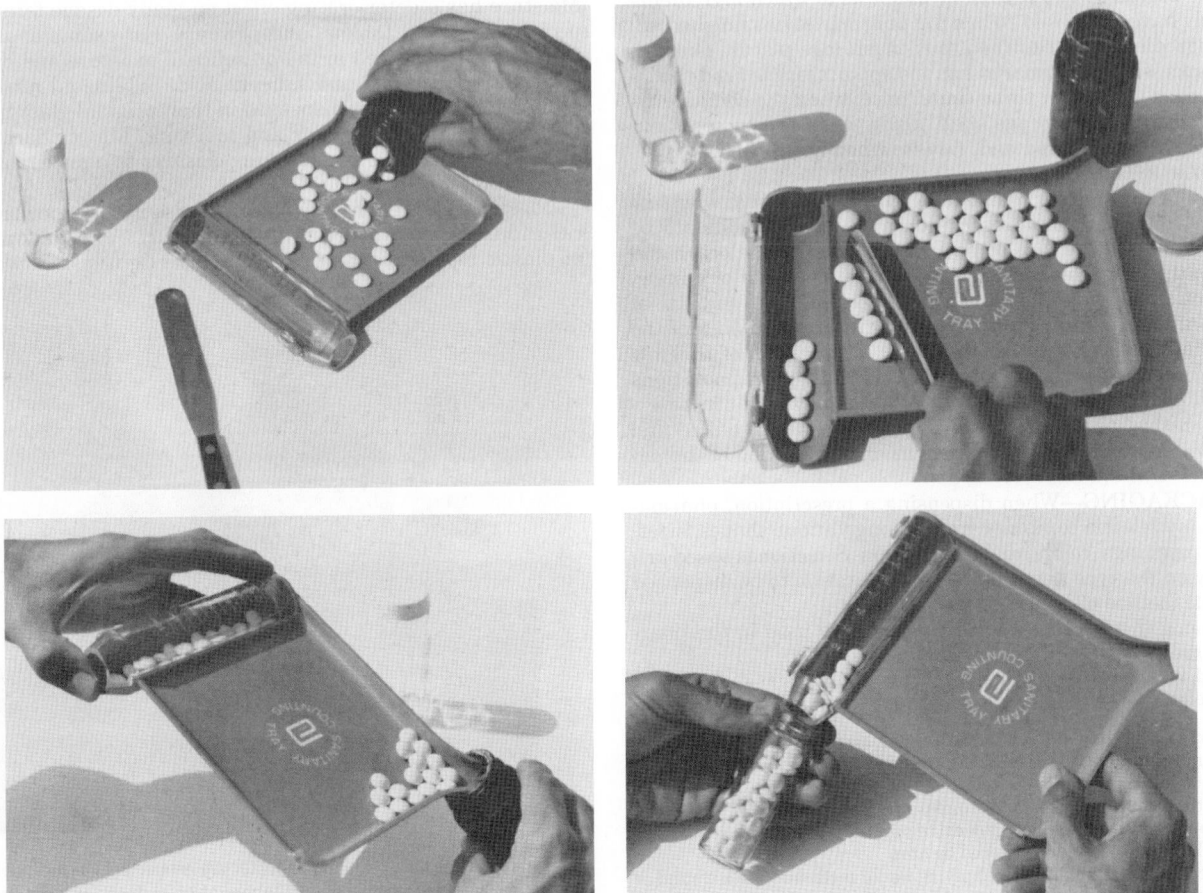

Figure 101-8. Steps in the hygienic counting of solid dosage units with the Abbott Sanitary Counting Tray: (1) placing units from the stock package onto the tray, (2) counting and transferring the units to the trough, (3) returning the excess units to the stock container, and (4) transferring the counted units into the prescription container.

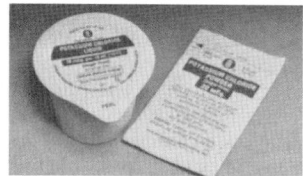 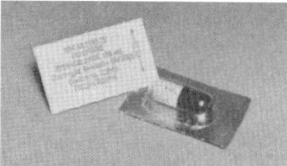

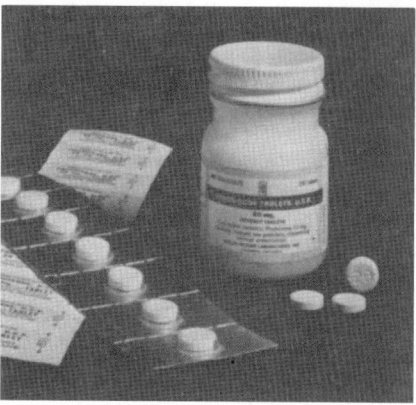

Figure 101-9. Examples of multiple-unit and single-unit packaging, including patient cup, unit dose of powder, blister packaging of single capsule, and strip packaging of tablets (courtesy, Roxane).

location away from the workstation. The use of this technique provides the pharmacist with a mechanical check on the introduction of each ingredient. If the pharmacist is interrupted during the process, there is then no doubt as to which ingredients already have been used. When the pharmacist has finished, all the ingredients are returned to their storage places. Through this process, the pharmacist has the opportunity to read the label of each ingredient three times: once, when the container is removed from the storage shelf, again when the contents are weighed and measured and, finally, when the container is returned to the shelf.

Any calculations or compounding information that would be useful in refilling the prescription at a later date should be noted either on the face or back of the prescription order and also in the computer system. Adjuvants used, order of mixing, amount of each ingredient, capsule size used, type and size of the container, name and product identification number of the manufacturer, auxiliary labels used, clarification of illegible words or numbers, price charged, and any special notations should be recorded. The failure to do this may result in differences in the appearance of the prescription when refilled and possibly create doubt and apprehension in the mind of the patient.

PACKAGING—When dispensing a prescription, pharmacists may select a container from among various shapes, sizes, mouth openings, colors, and composition. Selection is based primarily on the type and quantity of medication to be dispensed and the method of its use.

Among the types of containers generally used in the pharmacy are

Round vials: Used primarily for solid dosage forms as capsules and tablets

Prescription bottles: Used for dispensing liquids of low viscosity

Wide-mouth bottles: Used for bulk powders, large quantities of tablets or capsules, and viscous liquids that cannot be poured readily from the narrow-necked standard prescription bottles

Dropper bottles: Used for dispensing ophthalmic, nasal, otic (ear), or oral liquids to be administered by drop

Applicator bottles: Used for applying liquid medication to a wound or skin surface

Ointment jars and collapsible tubes: Used to dispense semisolid dosage forms, such as ointments and creams

Sifter-top containers: Used for topical powders to be applied by sprinkling

Hinged-lid or slide boxes: Used for dispensing suppositories and powders prepared in packets

Aerosol containers: Used for pharmaceutical aerosol products (These are pressurized systems dispensed by the pharmacist in the original container.)

Most of the prescription containers usually are available in colorless or amber-colored glass or plastic. Amber-colored containers are most widely used because these provide maximum protection of their contents against photochemical deterioration. Plastic amber containers are generally used except in situations where moisture sensitive drug products dictate the use of glass bottles of vials. The containers shown in Figure 101-10 are examples of such containers. The use of outer wrappings or cartons also may be used to protect light-sensitive pharmaceuticals. Pharmaceutical manufacturers select and use containers that do not affect the composition or stability of their products adversely. Similar types of containers should be used by the pharmacist in dispensing the medication to the patient. FDA regulations require pharmaceutical manufacturers to include in their prescription-product labeling the type of container to be used by the pharmacist when dispensing the prescription drug to preserve its *identity, strength, quality, and purity.* The regulation does not apply to products intended to be dispensed in the manufacturer's original container. Many manufacturers now package their products in quantities which correspond to 30 or 90 day supplies which allows the pharmacist to affix a label directly on the container thus streamlining the drug packaging and dispensing process.

The closure on a prescription container is as important as the container itself. By law, prescription containers must be moisture-proof and thus the ability of the closure to restrict entrance of moisture into the container is of prime importance. Moisture has a deteriorating effect on many dosage forms, especially capsules, tablets, and powders. For example, aspirin tablets are hydrolyzed in the presence of moisture and broken down into acetic acid and salicylic acid. Sublingual nitroglycerin tablets are always dispensed in their original glass bottles to minimize exposure to air and moisture. Many pharmacies use screw-cap glass or tight-fitting closures to reduce moisture penetration (Fig 101-11).

Plastic containers have widespread use in the pharmaceutical industry and in prescription practice. The advantages of plastic over glass containers include lightness of weight,

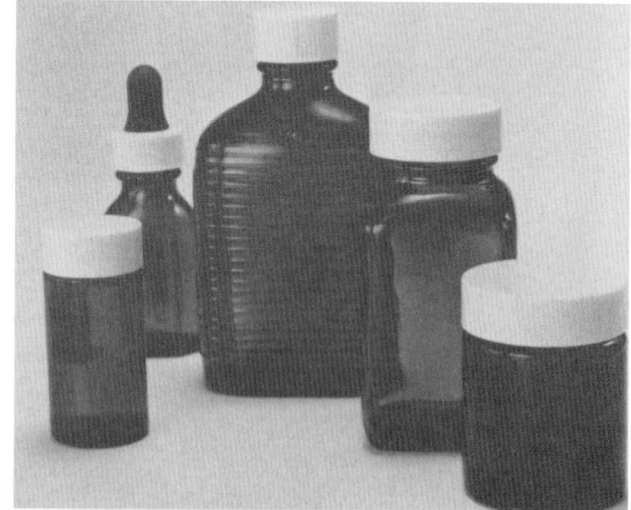

Figure 101-10. Examples of light-protective amber prescription containers for, from left to right: small numbers of solid dosage forms, such as tablets and capsules; liquid preparations administered by drops; liquid preparations; powders or large numbers of solid dosage forms; and semisolid preparations, such as ointments and creams (courtesy, Armstrong Cork).

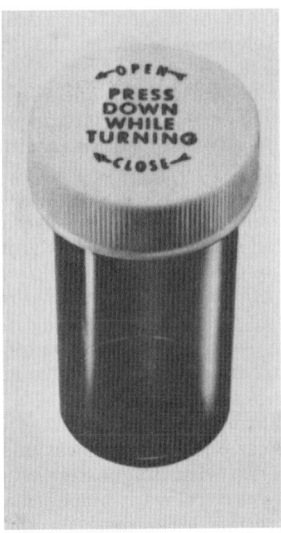 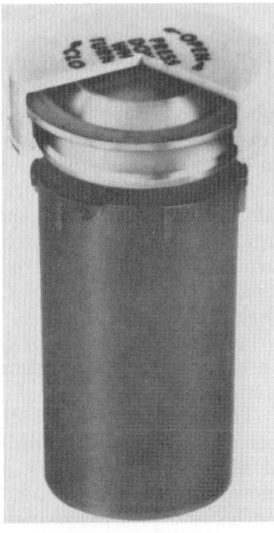

Figure 101-11. Gross and cutaway views of moisture-tight prescription container (courtesy, Kerr Glass).

resistance to breakage on impact and greater versatility in container design. Flexible polyethylene is used widely in the packaging of squeeze bottles for medication to be administered as drops or as a spray. Nose drops, eye drops, and throat sprays, as well as oral medication to be administered in a dropwise manner, frequently are packaged and dispensed in these containers. Lotions, medicated shampoos, and creams also are packaged conveniently in flexible polyethylene containers. Pliable ointment tubes and flexible plastic containers for intravenous fluids also are used widely.

Rigid polystyrene vials are employed commonly by pharmacists to dispense capsules and tablets. This type of plastic also is used widely in ointment jars and box packages for suppositories. The modern compact-type container used for oral contraceptives, which contain sufficient tablets for a monthly cycle of administration and permit scheduled removal of one tablet at a time, is a prime example of the imaginative packaging possible with plastic. Examples of these containers are shown in Figure 101-12. These prepackaged containers, as obtained from the manufacturer, are labeled properly by the pharmacist and dispensed in the original container to the patient. Several manufacturers now market antibiotics and other medications used for a limited number of days packaged as individual dosage units on cards with the instructions for administration indicated next to each dose. This approach to drug packaging is designed to help assure compliance to the prescribed regimen.

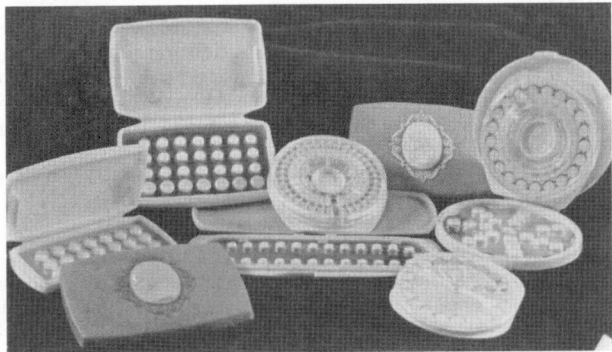

Figure 101-12. Examples of plastic packaging used for oral contraceptive products. (From Ansel HC. *Introduction to Pharmaceutical Dosage Forms,* 4th ed. Philadelphia: Lea & Febiger, 1985.)

The increased responsibilities of pharmacists in drug distribution and inventory control in hospitals, nursing homes, and other patient-care facilities have had an effect on the development of the single-unit drug package, such as the strip package, the blister package, and the plastic disposable syringe. These single-unit packages are termed unit-dose packages at the time of administration to a specific patient. Examples are shown in Figure 101-9.

CHILD-RESISTANT CONTAINERS—The high number of accidental poisonings after ingestion of medication and other household chemicals by children led to the passage of the *Poison Prevention Packaging Act in 11010.* The initial regulation called for use of *childproof* closures for aspirin products and certain household chemical products shown to have significant potential for causing accidental poisoning in youngsters. As the technical capability in producing effective closures was developed, the regulations were extended to include the use of such safety closures in the packaging of both legend and OTC medications.

The Consumer Product Safety Commission has ruled that manufacturers must place prescription drugs in child-resistant packages if the original package is intended to go directly from the pharmacist to the patient. However, manufacturers need not place drugs in safety packaging if the drugs are intended to be repackaged by pharmacists.

All legend drugs intended for oral use must be dispensed by the pharmacist to the patient in containers having safety closures unless the prescribing physician or the patient specifically requests otherwise. A request for a non-child-resistant container may be applied to a single prescription or to all of a patient's dispensed medications. The pharmacist should clarify the patient's desires, obtain and file a signed waiver request, and maintain the information in the prescription computer for future reference.[9] There are some exceptions to the overall requirements, such as oral contraceptive packages because of their unique and useful design, and certain cardiac drugs (eg, nitroglycerin) because of the importance to the patient for direct and immediate access to the medication.

Exemptions also are permitted in the case of OTC medication for one-package size or specially marked packages to be available to consumers for whom safety closures might be unnecessary or too difficult to manipulate. These consumers include childless persons, arthritic patients, and the debilitated.

Further, drugs that are used or dispensed in inpatient institutions, such as hospitals, nursing homes, and extended-care facilities, need not be dispensed with safety closures unless they are intended for patients who are leaving the confines of the institution. Examples of child-resistant containers are shown in Figures 101-11 and 101-13.

RECHECKING—The importance of this step cannot be overemphasized. Every prescription should be rechecked and the ingredients and amounts used verified by the pharmacist. All details of the label should be rechecked against the prescription order to verify directions, patient's name, prescription number, date, and prescriber's name. Rechecking is especially important for those drug products available in multiple strengths.

DELIVERING AND PATIENT COUNSELING—The pharmacist personally should present the prescription medication to the patient (or family member, caregiver) unless it is to be delivered to the patient's home or workplace. Suggested questions to ask the patient when dispensing a new prescription include:

1. What did the doctor tell you the medication is for?
2. How did the doctor tell you to take the medication?
3. What did the doctor tell you to expect from the medication?

Appropriate responses to these questions by the patient gives the pharmacist assurance that the patient knows how to use the medication properly. When presenting the medication to the patient, the pharmacist should reinforce the information the patient already is aware of, call attention to any auxiliary

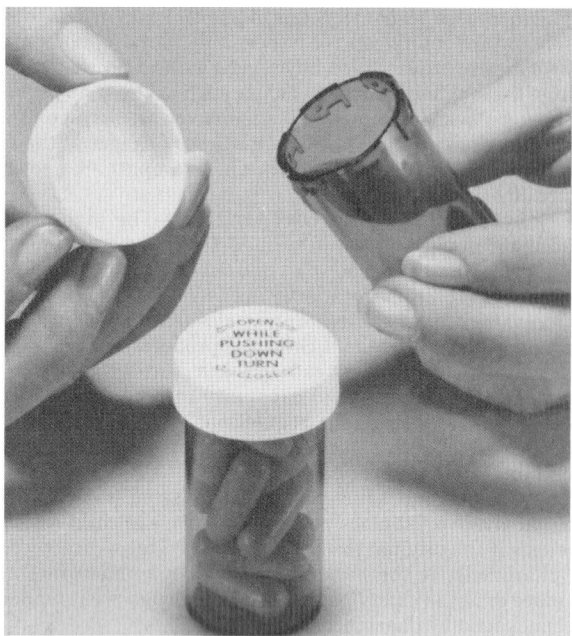

Figure 101-13. Example of child-resistant safety closure on a prescription container (courtesy, Owens-Brockway).

labeling instructions, and provide further information regarding the medication as may be desirable. When personal delivery of the prescription is not possible, the pharmacist should make certain that the appropriate instructions are provided to the patient and that the patient is encouraged to telephone the pharmacy should there be any questions. The pharmacist should take the initiative to telephone the patient when a product is dispensed with unusual or complicated dosing instructions and when specific precautions need to be reviewed.

There is an increased awareness that labeling instructions frequently are inadequate to ensure patient understanding of his/her medication and his/her adherence or compliance with recommended instructions. The responsibility that the patient receive specific instructions, precautions, and warnings for safe and effective use of prescribed drugs is the shared responsibility of the prescriber and the pharmacist. Reinforcement of the labeled instructions is through verbal communication among the prescriber, pharmacist, and patient, or as supplemental printed instructions, as noted previously (see Fig 101-3).

The *Omnibus Budget Reconciliation Act of 1990* (OBRA 90) amended the 1965 Medicaid law and, among other things, required the development of state drug-use review (DUR) programs and patient counseling activities by pharmacists. Although the law applies specifically to pharmaceutical care rendered to persons receiving Medicaid benefits, the individual states have developed and adopted similar pharmacy practice standards to apply uniformly to all patients.

The specific requirements of the Act are presented in Chapter 111; however, in brief, pharmacists must offer to discuss with each eligible patient—or caregiver of such individual—who presents a prescription, information on the drug, dosage form, route of administration, any special directions for use, common side effects or interactions and therapeutic contraindications that may apply, techniques for self-monitoring drug therapy, proper storage, prescription refill information, and action to be taken in the event of a missed dose. Written information may be used to supplement but not replace the oral counseling requirement.

Under the Act, the pharmacist also must make a reasonable effort to obtain, record, and maintain patient profiles of the patient's disease states, known allergies, and drug sensitivities; a comprehensive list of medications taken and medical devices used; pharmacists' comments relevant to the patient's drug therapy; and the name, address, telephone number, date of birth or age, and gender of the patient.

The state DUR programs must be prospective and retrospective to ensure that the medications are appropriate, medically necessary, unlikely to result in adverse medical results, and based on predetermined standards.

To assist the pharmacist in having up-to-date and pertinent information available for the counseling of his patients, several organized and conveniently arranged sources of dispensing information for patients are available. For example, *USP Dispensing Information, Vol I, Drug Information for the Health Care Professional*, and Vol II, *Advice for the Patient* (drug information in lay language), provide useful information on officially recognized medications for use by pharmacists in counseling their patients.

These references provide the pharmacist with resource information, including clinical indications and applications, ADRs, drug interactions, interference with diagnostic tests, known effects on the fetus and newborn, relevant biopharmaceutics and pharmacokinetics, excretion of the drug through breast milk, sugar and/or alcohol content of the medication, and other information deemed important.

RECORDING AND FILING—A record of the prescriptions dispensed is maintained in the pharmacy through the use of computer and hard copy prescription files. Newer centralized computer systems used by many chain drug stores allow pharmacists from anyplace in the system to access a patient's records and refill a prescription previously dispensed at another store.

Various prescription file types are available to maintain original prescription orders. Metal or cardboard units, which conveniently store approximately 1000 prescriptions are common. When these files are used, holes are punched in the prescription orders; the files are then slipped onto two metal rods firmly attached to the file and placed in a designated compartment in numerical order for safe storage and rapid retrieval.

Suitably partitioned drawers sometimes are used for filing. The partitions may be placed between every 100 or 1000 prescriptions, plainly marked with the numbers of the prescriptions filed in that section. This method permits the removal of a single prescription without preventing ready access to others, as normally occurs when metal rod files are used.

PRICING THE PRESCRIPTION—For a prescription practice to be successful, the pharmacist must be an effective manager of the financial aspects of his practice. To maintain the types of pharmaceutical services desired by his patients, the pharmacist must make a fair and equitable profit.

Each pharmacy should have a method for pricing prescriptions that is applied consistently by each pharmacist practicing in that pharmacy. The pricing method should be established to ensure the profitable operation of the prescription department. A uniform and consistently applied system is beneficial to the pharmacist and helps to avoid misunderstandings from patrons.

The charge applied to a prescription should cover the costs of the ingredients, including the container and label, the time of the involved pharmacist and auxiliary personnel, the cost of inventory maintenance and other operational costs of the department, as well as providing a reasonable margin of profit on investment.

Although many methods of pricing prescriptions have been used through the years, the most common are as follows:

1. *% Markup:.* Cost of ingredients + (cost of ingredients × % markup) = dispensing price
2. *% Markup + Minimum Fee:* Cost of ingredients + (cost of ingredients × % markup) + minimum fee (the minimum fee usually is established to recover the combined cost of the container, label, overhead, and professional services) = dispensing price
3. *Professional Fee:* Cost of ingredients + professional fee = dispensing price. The professional fee includes all the dispensing costs and professional remuneration. A true professional fee is in-

dependent of the cost of the ingredients and thus does not vary from one prescription to another. Some pharmacists use a variable or sliding professional-fee method, whereby the magnitude of the fee is varied somewhat on the cost of the ingredients.

In practice, the professional fee may vary widely between pharmacies, depending on the cost and types of pharmaceutical services rendered (eg, family record systems, delivery service, home health-care needs, cognitive services) and the professional desires of the pharmacist. Pharmacies using the professional fee commonly make adjustments for prescriptions requiring compounding to compensate for the extra time, materials, and equipment. Some pharmacies may charge their patients an annual fee for professional services. This fee then might entitle the patient to the following: routine professional service each time a prescription is filled, a yearly record of prescriptions, regular blood pressure checks, plus a yearly one-on-one consultation.

Governmental units, such as state human services agencies and most insurance companies and prescription card services, have adopted the professional-fee method for the reimbursement of pharmacists in filling prescriptions covered under their programs. Such third-party payers negotiate the professional fee to be used with pharmacists interested in participating in the programs. This practice has resulted in lower fees being paid to many pharmacists as large-volume pharmacies attempt to maintain profits by increasing prescription volume. Most of these programs have a *copayment* provision that requires the patient to pay a portion of the charge for each prescription he/she has filled. As the cost of prescription drugs has increased, most prescription drug plans have implemented a tiered *copayment* system where the percentage the patient must pay is reduced if generic drug or preferred formulary products are prescribed and dispensed.

PRESCRIPTION REFILLING—Instructions for refilling a prescription are provided by the prescriber, on the original prescription or by verbal communication. Although prescriptions for noncontrolled substances have no limitation according to federal law as to the number of refills permitted or the date of expiration, state laws may impose such limits. Many states limit refills to 1 year after the prescription was written. Refilling prescriptions for controlled substances is limited as described in Chapter 111.

Physicians and pharmacists should work together so that prescriptions are renewed only with the frequency consistent with directions for use, and the pharmacist should check with the prescriber after a reasonable time to assure himself/herself that his/her intent is being met. No prescription should be renewed indefinitely without the patient being reevaluated by the prescriber to assure that the medication as originally prescribed remains the medication of choice.

Renewals should be noted on the reverse side of the prescription order or in the prescription computer with the date, the quantity dispensed if different from the original, and the name or initials of the pharmacist dispensing the medication. If verbal authorization has been obtained from the prescriber, this should be recorded.

The maintenance of accurate records of renewals is important for following federal and state laws and for providing information on the patient's medication history.

COPIES AND TRANSFERS OF PRESCRIPTION ORDERS—Occasionally, these are requested by the patient or a pharmacist on behalf of the patient. In some instances, the intention is to provide information, and in other instances, the patient is desirous of having the copy refilled at another pharmacy. Patients who change residences either temporarily or permanently may request their prescriptions be transferred to another pharmacy. Chain pharmacies that have centralized computer systems can access a patient's prescription records from any of their pharmacies throughout the US and can easily transfer any remaining refills on the original prescription order.

Although the FDA maintains that a copy of a prescription order has no legal status and should not be honored, the agency has opened the door for honoring copies under certain circumstances. The FDA does not object to the exchange of prescription copies between pharmacies for the purpose of renewal, provided that certain safeguards are taken: (1) the original order is voided and marked to indicate that a copy has been issued, the individual to whom it has been issued, and the date of issuance; (2) the copy should be so marked and the location and number of original noted; (3) the copy shows the date of original dispensing, the date of the last renewal, and the number of renewals remaining.[8]

This procedure does not apply to *Schedule II* controlled drugs or if individual states prohibit such a procedure. In instances in which copies of prescriptions are provided by the pharmacist and in which the copy may not be refilled legally, the pharmacist supplying the copy should write *Copy—Not to be Dispensed* or a similar designation across the top. A copy should be made exactly like the original, including all pertinent information that a pharmacist might require in dispensing the medication as originally provided. The copy preferably should be written or typed on a preprinted form identifying the pharmacy.

The DEA amended the *Code of Federal Regulations* (CFR) in 1981 to permit the transfer of prescription orders between two pharmacies for controlled-substance prescriptions that may be renewed lawfully. The amendment allows for the transfer of an original prescription order for controlled substances listed in *Schedules III, IV,* or *V* between pharmacies on a one-time basis only.

To comply with these regulations, pharmacists first must ascertain if the transfer of a prescription order for renewal dispensing purposes is permissible under state or other applicable law. When a prescription order is transferred, it must be communicated directly between two licensed pharmacists, and the transferring pharmacist must record the following information:

Write *VOID* on the face of the invalidated prescription order.
On the back of the invalidated prescription order, the name, the address, and the DEA registration number of the pharmacy it was transferred to and the name of the pharmacist who received the information.
The date of transfer and the transferring pharmacist's name.

The pharmacist receiving the transferred prescription order must reduce to writing the following:

The word *transfer* on the face of the transferred prescription order.
All information required on a controlled-substance prescription order as it appears on the original prescription order.
The date of issuance of original prescription order.
The original number of renewals authorized on the original prescription order.
The date of the original prescription order.
The number of valid renewals remaining and the date of the last renewal.
The pharmacy's name, address, DEA registration number and the original prescription number for which the prescription order was transferred.
The name of the transferring pharmacist.

The DEA requires that the original and the transferred prescription orders must be maintained for 2 years from the date of the last renewal. Most states now allow the transfer of prescriptions via computers within their states, whereas some allow computer transfers from other states. Pharmacies electronically accessing the same prescription record must satisfy all information requirements of a manual mode for prescription transferral.

PATIENT COMPLIANCE WITH PRESCRIBED MEDICATION

When a prescriber writes a prescription, it is with the intent that the patient fills the prescription promptly and begins using the medication according to directions. Patient adher-

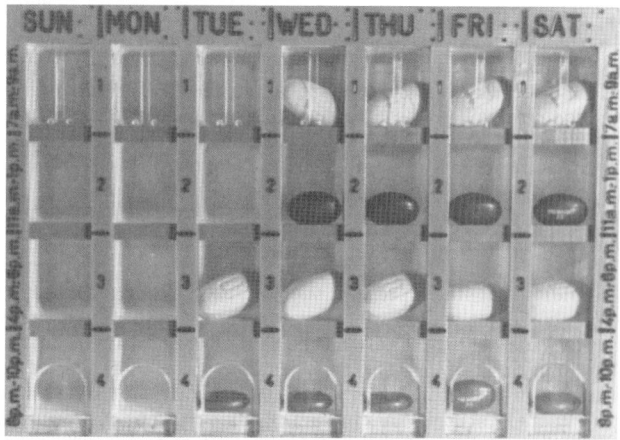

Figure 101-14. Example of the MEDISET medication container designed to assist patient compliance with prescribed medication schedule (courtesy, Drug Intelligence).

ence or compliance with the prescribed medication schedule has been a source of concern to the physician and the pharmacist.

Patients may unnecessarily delay the initiation of drug therapy or may wait to see if they *feel better* before having the prescription filled. Some patients discontinue their medication prematurely because they are feeling better and see no particular need to continue taking the medication. Other patients may take excessive doses of the medication believing that they will get better faster, whereas others take their medication at incorrect intervals or whenever they remember.

On refilling a prescription, a pharmacist generally can determine the compliance of the patient in taking his/her medication by comparing the dosage units dispensed *versus* the dosage units apparently taken over the treatment period. Pharmacists can often gain a great deal of useful information about compliance by simply having the patient describe how he/she takes the medication on a daily basis. Pharmacy computer systems are useful in determining patient compliance and can be used to generate refill reminder cards or telephone lists for courtesy calls to remind patients about the need to comply with their medication.

Specially designed medication containers are useful in assisting patients to adhere to their medication schedule. These containers have individual compartments for daily medication and generally hold a week's supply (Fig 101-14). Containers for oral contraceptive medication, previously discussed and shown in Figure 101-12, have proved effective in patient compliance during the monthly medication cycle. See also Chapter 98.

USE OF COMPUTER SYSTEMS TO PROCESS PRESCRIPTIONS

The use of computer systems in pharmacy practice is now standard because of the expanded informational needs of the pharmacist, the need for on-line prescription plan approval, the increased amount of paper work required in the practice, the need for efficiency, and the availability of computer technology and expanded databases to provide the necessary support. Most chain pharmacies are linked together by dedicated telephone lines or satellites, thus facilitating the sharing of information between pharmacies (Fig 101-15).

In general, computerized systems in pharmacy are used in three areas: prescription dispensing and associated record maintenance, clinical support and accounting, and business management. Most insurance and prescription plans now require on-line verification and authorization prior to the dispensing of any medication. Pharmacists can now use the Inter-

net to obtain and download information about disease states and drug therapy for their patients.

Prescription Dispensing and Associated Record Maintenance

LABEL PREPARATION—Once basic prescription information is entered, the computer produces an error-free label or multiple labels if required.

PRESCRIPTION NUMBER ASSIGNMENT—Consecutive numbers are assigned to prescriptions by the computer, and the problem of lost and duplicate numbers virtually is eliminated.

RECEIPT PREPARATION—Prescription computers calculate the price of the prescription and store information. Thus, it is simple for the computer to prepare a receipt automatically for the patient that may include the amount paid for an individual prescription or for the total prescriptions filled over a given period. This information may be important to the patient for insurance or tax purposes.

PRESCRIPTION NOTATION—As a prescription order is processed, the pharmacist typically makes several notations, including the initials of the dispensing pharmacist, the drug cost and product dispensed, and special entries such as *dispensed only one-half at patient request*. This information may be retained by the computer and used in renewal processing.

RENEWAL PROCESSING—The computer-assisted renewal processing of prescriptions is almost automatic. If the computerized records indicate that the prescription renewal is allowable, the computer automatically prepares the new label and receipt, updates the renewal status of the prescription, recalculates the price on the basis of current cost information, and adds the entire transaction to the patient's medication profile. See also Chapter 117.

Clinical Support

PATIENT MEDICATION PROFILES—On command, the computer presents on its monitor the most recent medications that have been dispensed to the individual patient. This information is used by the pharmacist in ascertaining potential drug–drug interactions. Information pertaining to the patient's drug allergies and primary illnesses also permits the pharmacist to assess the drug therapy and dispense only rational and effective medications.

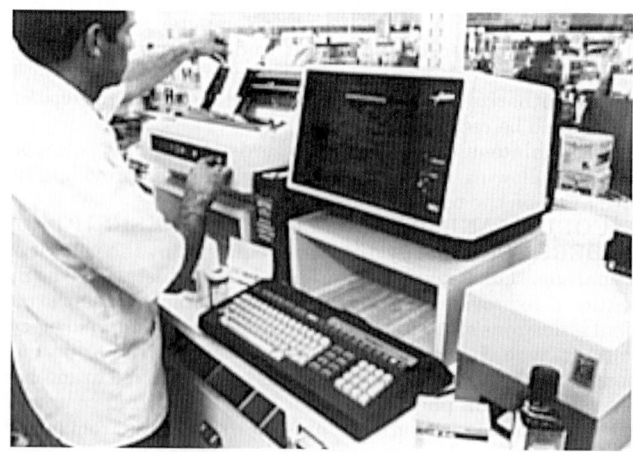

Figure 101-15. Pharmacist using a prescription computer system in his professional practice (courtesy, General Computer).

PATIENT EDUCATION INFORMATION—Computer-printed information is provided to the patient on the medication dispensed. The information generally includes the proper use and administration of the medication, precautions, possible side effects, a brief description of the purpose of the medication, and how to proceed if a dose is missed. Some computer programs also may generate a picture of the dosage form.

DRUG UTILIZATION MONITORING—By tracking the dispensing dates and quantities dispensed, a pharmacist can determine a patient's compliance in taking the prescribed medication properly.

Accounting and Business Management

BUSINESS RECORDKEEPING—The computer may be programmed to provide accounts receivable, payroll, general ledger, accounts payable, third-party claims processing and records, inventory control and ordering, sales analysis functions, and daily summary of business.

PRESCRIPTION ANALYSIS—The computer provides retrievable information on daily, monthly, or yearly prescription totals; new *versus* refilled prescriptions; medication costs per prescription filled; and profit per prescription filled.

DRUG-PRODUCT DEFECT AND ADVERSE-REACTION REPORTING PROGRAMS

Monitoring Drug-Product Quality

Monitoring drug-product quality is an important function of the practicing pharmacist. The medications dispensed on prescription and those sold OTC should meet high standards of manufacturing quality to assure safety and efficacy when used properly.

As contained in the *Code of Federal Regulations* (21 CFR 211), manufacturers of pharmaceutical products must comply with FDA standards for *Current Good Manufacturing Practice (CGMP) for Finished Pharmaceuticals* to ensure product quality. A section of these regulations includes provisions for the reporting and handling of drug-product complaints. A complaint or concern regarding product quality may arise from a patient or from a health professional and may be communicated directly to the manufacturer or brought to the attention of the FDA. In either case, the information is shared between the agency and the manufacturer, and each complaint is evaluated to determine whether corrective action is required. Complaints or concerns may relate to any factor of product quality or effectiveness, including dosage form integrity, stability, appearance, odor, taste, color, packaging, and labeling.

Pharmacists play an important role in the detection and reporting of product defects through participation in the FDA's *Medical Products Reporting Program* (MedWatch), a voluntary program for the reporting of concerns regarding the quality of distributed prescription and nonprescription drug products. Since the program's initiation in 1993, both the number of serious events reported has increased and the quality of adverse-event reporting to the FDA has improved, primarily owing to the efforts of pharmacists.[10] Information provided through this program becomes useful to the manufacturer and the FDA in maintaining quality standards.[11] Pharmacists may report drug-product quality concerns by telephone (1-800-FDA-1088), on the FDA's web site [www.fda.gov], or by mail using the MedWatch form provided for this purpose (Fig 101-16).

Specific information requested on the FDA MedWatch form includes product name, dosage form, strength, and size; National Drug Code Number, if available; lot number and expiration date; name and address of manufacturer, distributor, or labeler; name, address, and profession of person reporting the suspected product defect; a description of the problem noted or suspected and the date and the signature of the person filing the report. The option is given to the person filing the report to remain anonymous in the subsequent FDA communication to the affected manufacturer or distributor.

Monitoring Adverse Drug Reactions

The FDA has specific requirements for drug manufacturers of investigational and marketed pharmaceutical products to report adverse drug reactions (ADRs) or adverse drug experiences (ADEs).[12] Pharmacists have the opportunity to participate in reporting such incidents through practices in the institutional and community pharmacy settings. Observations of reactions to investigational drugs generally are observed in the clinical (usually institutional) setting during controlled clinical studies as investigational drugs are evaluated prior to FDA approval for marketing. Reactions to marketed drugs may be observed during any postmarketing clinical studies and through surveillance by health professionals during the course of their practice.

The postmarketing surveillance of pharmaceuticals for adverse reactions is essential in establishing a complete safety profile for marketed drugs. Once marketed, the number and diversity of patients receiving a new drug is far greater than during the controlled clinical trials. Thus, some ADRs and drug interactions that escape detection during the clinical trials are seen initially after the drug product is marketed. During the past decade, there are several examples of newly marketed drug products that subsequently have been removed from the market after postmarketing surveillance by the FDA and the manufacturer has detected the occurrence of rare but potentially lethal adverse reactions or drug interactions.

Pharmacists and other health-care providers who observe suspect reactions to drugs are encouraged to report these to the FDA. Serious reactions, observations of events not described in the package insert, and reactions to newly marketed products are of particular importance. The FDA provides the MedWatch form for filing a voluntary—or in the case of user facilities, distributors, or manufacturers, a mandatory—report. The form includes space for entering patient information; adverse reaction information, including a description of the reaction experience and relevant laboratory tests or data; suspect drug information, such as the drug name, manufacturer, lot number, daily dose, route of administration, dates of administration and duration of administration; concomitant drugs taken and record of administration; and name and contact information for the person or manufacturer filing the report. In some institutions in which clinical studies are conducted, computer programs are used to record, monitor, and report suspected ADEs.[13] ADR reports may result in changes in product labeling, warning letters to health-care professionals regarding safe conditions of use, requirements for further clinical or safety studies or, in some instances, withdrawal of the product from the market.[14]

LEGAL CONSIDERATIONS

All aspects of manufacture, distribution, and possession of drugs are controlled by both state and federal laws and regulations. State laws and regulations governing the practice of pharmacy generally are administered by state boards of pharmacy composed of varying numbers of pharmacy practitioners and in some instances by consumer representation. These boards generally regulate the licensing of pharmacy interns, pharmacists, and pharmacies, and enforce rules and regulations pertaining to the legal and ethical practice of pharmacy within the state. State regulations regarding drugs frequently include and extend the federal law. Federal laws are administered by various federal agencies and pertain primarily to products considered interstate commerce.

MEDWATCH

THE FDA MEDICAL PRODUCTS REPORTING PROGRAM

For VOLUNTARY reporting by health professionals of adverse events and product problems

Form Approved: OMB No. 0910-0291 Expires:12/31/94
See OMB statement on reverse

FDA Use Only

Triage unit sequence #

Page ___ of ___

A. Patient information

1. **Patient identifier** In confidence
2. **Age at time of event:** or **Date of birth:**
3. **Sex** ☐ female ☐ male
4. **Weight** ___ lbs or ___ kgs

B. Adverse event or product problem

1. ☐ **Adverse event** and/or ☐ **Product problem** (e.g., defects/malfunctions)
2. **Outcomes attributed to adverse event** (check all that apply)
   - ☐ death ___ (mo/day/yr)
   - ☐ life-threatening
   - ☐ hospitalization – initial or prolonged
   - ☐ disability
   - ☐ congenital anomaly
   - ☐ required intervention to prevent permanent impairment/damage
   - ☐ other: ___
3. **Date of event** (mo/day/yr)
4. **Date of this report** (mo/day/yr)
5. **Describe event or problem**
6. **Relevant tests/laboratory data,** including dates
7. **Other relevant history, including preexisting medical conditions** (e.g., allergies, race, pregnancy, smoking and alcohol use, hepatic/renal dysfunction, etc.)

PLEASE TYPE OR USE BLACK INK

C. Suspect medication(s)

1. **Name** (give labeled strength & mfr/labeler, if known) #1 #2
2. **Dose, frequency & route used** #1 #2
3. **Therapy dates** (if unknown, give duration) from/to (or best estimate) #1 #2
4. **Diagnosis for use** (indication) #1 #2
5. **Event abated after use stopped or dose reduced**
   #1 ☐ yes ☐ no ☐ doesn't apply
   #2 ☐ yes ☐ no ☐ doesn't apply
6. **Lot #** (if known) #1 #2
7. **Exp. date** (if known) #1 #2
8. **Event reappeared after reintroduction**
   #1 ☐ yes ☐ no ☐ doesn't apply
   #2 ☐ yes ☐ no ☐ doesn't apply
9. **NDC #** (for product problems only) – –
10. **Concomitant medical products** and therapy dates (exclude treatment of event)

D. Suspect medical device

1. **Brand name**
2. **Type of device**
3. **Manufacturer name & address**
4. **Operator of device** ☐ health professional ☐ lay user/patient ☐ other: ___
5. **Expiration date** (mo/day/yr)
6. **model #** ___ **catalog #** ___ **serial #** ___ **lot #** ___ **other #**
7. **If implanted, give date** (mo/day/yr)
8. **If explanted, give date** (mo/day/yr)
9. **Device available for evaluation?** (Do not send to FDA) ☐ yes ☐ no ☐ returned to manufacturer on ___ (mo/day/yr)
10. **Concomitant medical products** and therapy dates (exclude treatment of event)

E. Reporter (see confidentiality section on back)

1. **Name, address & phone #**
2. **Health professional?** ☐ yes ☐ no
3. **Occupation**
4. **Also reported to** ☐ manufacturer ☐ user facility ☐ distributor
5. **If you do NOT want your identity disclosed to the manufacturer, place an " X " in this box.** ☐

FDA

Mail to: MEDWATCH **5600 Fishers Lane Rockville, MD 20852-9787** *or* **FAX to: 1-800-FDA-0178**

FDA Form 3500 (6/93) **Submission of a report does not constitute an admission that medical personnel or the product caused or contributed to the event.**

Figure 101-16. FDA MedWatch Reporting Form.

The laws governing the practice of pharmacy are presented in Chapter 111.

REFERENCES

1. Ukens C, *Drug* Topics 2000; 34–39.
2. Poirier TI, Giudici RA. *Hosp Pharm* 1992; 27:408.
3. Cohen MR, Davis NM. *Am Pharm* 1992; NS32:112, 1992.
4. Ansel HC. *Introduction to Pharmaceutical Dosage Forms*, 4th ed. Philadelphia: Lea & Febiger, 1985.
5. Resolution 88-4-92, NABP.
6. *Compliance Guidelines, Manufacturer, Distribution, and Promotion of Adulterated, Misbranded, or Unapproved New Drugs for Human Use by State-Licensed Pharmacies,* FDA, 1992.
7. Crawford SY, Dombrowski SR. *AJHP* 1991; 48:1205.
8. *Pharm Pract* 11018; 13(3):18.
9. *Pharm Today* 1992; Dec 21:3.
10. Bolger G, Goetsch R. *Am Pharm* 1992; NS32:139.
11. Piazza-Hepp TD, Kennedy DL. *AJHP* 1995; 52:1436.
12. 21 CFR §312.32; 21 CFR §314.80.
13. *Profiles Hosp Pharm* 1991; 5(3):12.
14. Sills JM, Tanner LA, Milstien JB. *AJHP* 1986; 43:2764.

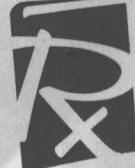

CHAPTER 102

Providing a Framework for Ensuring Medication Use Safety

Karen E Smith, MS, RPh, CPHQ

Sharon Murphy Enright, MBA, RPh

The US health care system is paradoxical, offering at once the promise of death-defying state of the art care, and also the threat of injury, and even death, resulting from flawed and sometimes dysfunctional performance. In 1998, the Institute of Medicine sponsored National Roundtable on Health Care quality, published a report that called attention to an alarming problem[1]:

"Serious and widespread quality problems exist throughout American medicine. These problems . . . occur in small and large communities alike, in all parts of the country, and with approximately equal frequency in managed care and fee-for-service systems of care. Very large numbers of Americans are harmed as a result."

This realization was brought sharply to public and professional attention with the publication in November 1999, of *To Err is Human: Building a Safer Health System*, the first report of the Institute of Medicine (IOM) Committee on Quality. This benchmark report reframed medical error as a chronic threat to public health, and galvanized media attention to the issue. Some startling findings included[2]:

- 98,000 Americans die annually as a result of preventable medical errors.
- National costs (including lost income, lost household production, disability and health care costs) of preventable adverse events–medical errors resulting in injury–are estimated between $17 and $29 billion, of which health care cost represents over half.
- More Americans die of medication errors annually than from workplace injuries.
- Even medication errors that do not result in actual harm have a cost, calculated at as much as $2 billion annually.

Because these hospital-based studies do not even account for errors in other settings where they occur with at least equal frequency, the figures offer only a modest estimate of the real target of actual errors. *Err* recommended a comprehensive approach to improving patient safety, which would demand a broad-based response. There was no magic bullet, no single solution, no single recommendation as *the answer*. Preventing errors means designing the health care system to build in safety at all levels.

Eighteen months later, IOM followed with a second–even more comprehensive–report, *Crossing the Quality Chasm: A New Health System for the 21st Century,* that calls for nothing less than redesign of the US health care system.[3] *Chasm* paints a graphic and detailed picture of how and where the health care system fails to meet the needs and expectations of the patients it serves. The report addressed three problem categories introduced in *To Err is Human*: overuse, underuse, and misuse that contributed to problems with patient care. Misuse–failures to execute clinical care plans and procedures properly. Overuse–use of health care resources and procedures in the ab-

sence of evidence. Underuse–failure to employ health practices of proven benefit. Among the observations[3]:

- Health care today harms too frequently and routinely fails to deliver its potential benefits.
- Tens of thousands of Americans die each year from errors in their care, and hundreds of thousands suffer or barely escape from nonfatal injuries that a truly high quality care system would largely prevent.
- During the last decade, more than 70 publications in leading peer-reviewed clinical journals have documented serious quality shortcomings.
- Waste, medical error, lack of access to clinical information, unnecessary duplication of services, long waiting times and delays, and overuse of services where the harm outweighs the benefit, contribute to a system that, as a whole does not make the best use of its resources. The current system cannot do the job. Trying harder will not work. Changing systems of care will.

With a current annual investment of over $1 trillion in the health care sector expected to grow to $2 trillion or 16% of Gross Domestic Product by 2007, *Chasm* reports that a sizable commitment on the order of $1 billion over 3 to 5 years, will be required for the rapid and significant change that is needed.[4]

Err offered a similar conclusion relative to safety: flaws are unacceptable and common. The effective remedy is not to browbeat the health care workforce by asking them to try harder to give safe care, when in fact, the courage, hard work, and commitment of health care workers are the only real means to stem the tide of errors latent in the health care system.[5] Unfortunately, workers must rely on outmoded systems and poor workflow design that sets them up to fail, despite efforts to the contrary.

Growth in knowledge and technologies has never been so profound and prolific. However, research on the quality of care demonstrates that the health care system falls short in its ability to translate knowledge to practice and to apply new technologies safely and appropriately. One realizes that knowledge of best practice is not applied systematically or rapidly, in fact the diffusion of innovation of best practice is frustratingly slow. An average of 17 years is required for new evidence-based knowledge to be incorporated into common practice.[6] System redesign, more rigorous information technology to support clinical and administrative processes and improved knowledge management capabilities will be required.

The IOM committee sets forth six Aims for Improvement, establishing what should be attainable common goals: care should be safe, effective, timely, patient-centered, and efficient. Yet, *Chasm* reports that as it exists, the American health care system is incapable of providing the public with the quality it expects and deserves and offers few of these basic aims consistently. Quality problems occur typically not because of failure of goodwill, knowledge, effort, or resources, but rather because of fundamental shortcomings in the way care is organized.[7] If, as *Err* suggests, exhortation, blaming, and trying harder cannot get the necessary job done, what system redesign considerations must be considered?

Chasm calls for change at four levels (Fig 102-1):

Experience of patients and communities. The focus for improvement must shift from the health care system itself to being patient-centric, tying quality issues more closely to patient's values and expectations, actual experiences, cost and social justice.

Microsystems of care. The small work units that actually give care to patients represent the microsystem level. This team of people, with their information system, client population of patients, and a defined set of work processes represents where *work* or *care* happens, where quality occurs or does not. Care at the microsystem level must be knowledge-based, patient-centered, and systems-minded. The quality of a microsystem is its sustained ability to provide ever-improving levels of care: safe, effective, patient-centered, timely, efficient, and equitable.

Health care organizations (or macrosystems). The quality of an organization lies in its ability to support microsystem's ability to sustain ever-improving care levels. Through their culture, policies, and the tools provided for work, health care organizations frame the capacity for microsystems to achieve care improvements. Organizations need to develop more robust and persistent systems for identifying, diffusing, and adopting best practice. Access to information and decision support systems must be available to create a supporting network of knowledge at the microsystem level. Because human assets are a fundamental differentiating factor, organizations need to invest in recognition and development in the persistent improvement of knowledge, skills, and competency within the workforce. Beyond individual knowledge, skills, and competency, effective and collaborative teams and teamwork will be essential to achieving improvement goals, as will coordination of care among services, departments and across the continuum of care, particularly with respect to patients with chronic illnesses. Finally, organizations need to commit philosophically and in practice to a data-driven measurement and assessment of performance and outcomes.

Health care environment. Sweeping and difficult changes will be necessary in the external environment, including capital and operating financing, regulation, accreditation, litigation and tort reform, professional education, and social policy. Needed change at microsystem and organizational levels reflect *toxicities* resulting from the external environment. Who would pay for telephone-based or e-mail care? What will be the source of capital for much needed information technologies? A safety culture functions on the basis of openness, transparency, and trust but without tort reform to ease pressures of litigation and in an environment of *blame and shame* can that be a reality? The quality of the health care environment may determine how well organizations and microsystems can achieve their quality goals.

Err and, to an even greater extent *Chasm*, reflect a solid base in systems thinking. Solidly tying experiences of patients to the fundamental definitions of quality, judgments of performance, delivery systems, organizations, and policies and procedures can only be made in the context of health status, satisfaction, and reduction of morbidity and mortality. Improving patient safety relies on an understanding of systems thinking, complex adaptive systems, and learning in complex systems.

While *Chasm*, has provided the framework for improvement, additional work by the IOM, through the *Quality Chasm Series* continues to build the body of evidence, understanding, and necessary action steps to keep patients safe. In January 2003, the IOM released the report entitled *Priority Areas for National Action Transforming Health Care Quality* that clearly identified 20 priority areas that collectively address preventive measures, care coordination, patient self-management, and health literacy issues that cross acute, chronic, and palliative care domains.[8] A subsequent report, *Fostering Rapid Advances in Health Care: Learning from System Demonstrations* identified the need for primary care redesign, improved information and technology infrastructures, insurance coverage changes, and malpractice reform strategies necessary to make care patient-centered and safety focused.[9]

In *Leadership by Example: Coordinating Government Roles in Improving Health Care Quality,* the IOM goes further to recommend a multi-pronged approach to care improvement by suggesting the federal government take advantage of the influence it has to set the standards for national health care quality.[10] Specifically, the report indicates that clinical data reporting requirements, purchasing strategies, standardized performance measures, and quality reports should be developed to accelerate the development of knowledge and tools that have been demonstrated to improve quality. An additional report, *Patient Safety: Achieving a New Standard For Care* outlines the IOM recommendations for enhancing knowledge, developing tools, disseminating results in order to build the necessary health data interchange and work plan to develop data standards applicable to the collection, coding, and classification of patient safety information.[11]

The IOM also identified that to provide safe and effective care, health professional education requires a major overhaul to address changing health system expectations, evolving practice requirements, new information and technologies and staffing arrangements. The first report released by the IOM, *Health Professions Education: A Bridge to Quality* provides a mix of approaches necessary to improve training environments, research, public reporting and leadership.[12] The focus of this report identifies the need to integrate a core set of competencies—patient-centered care, interdisciplinary teams, evidence-based practice, quality improvement and informatics—into health professions education. A second report, addressed nursing workforce issues, *Keeping Patients Safe: Transforming the Work Environment of Nurses*, identifies necessary safeguards for safe and effective care.[13] While specifically focused on an evaluation of nursing practices, resources, and environment, the report highlights changes that could impact all care professionals and patient safety efforts: effective leadership, adequate staffing, organizational support for ongoing learning, interdisciplinary collaboration, appropriate work design, and organizational support through governance and culture that supports safety as a priority.

The IOM and other groups continue to build the body of evidence necessary to identify strategies for sustainable and effective care improvement. What has been identified to date? There are clear conditions and priorities for care improvement action that requires attention. A need exists for leadership to be passionate and engaged for safety improvement to occur. Comprehensive strategies must be implemented to develop the workforce to provide the sustainable, change needed to improve care delivery. The findings in the Quality Chasm Series to date highlight the breath and diversity of issues that must be addressed to improve local as well as natural health care quality.

DEFINING THE SCOPE OF THE SAFETY PROBLEM

Safety is an implied minimum standard in providing health care. Yet many Americans are harmed as a result of medical error. While the horrific cases such as Betsy Lehman, a health reporter for the Boston *Globe* who died as a result of a chemother-

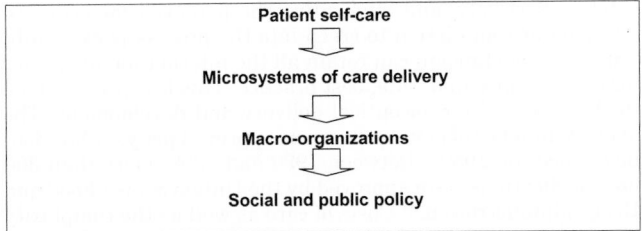

Figure 102-1. Levels of quality-focus in health care. Data from Berwick DM. A user's manual for the IOM's "quality chasm" report. *Health Aff (Millwood)* 2002; 21(3):80.

apy overdose or Ben Kolb, an 8-year-old boy who died during *minor surgery* due to a medication mix up make headlines, these events provide only the tip of an iceberg describing concerns regarding the safety of medication use.[14]

Research in the area of medication safety and error prevention has identified some serious concerns for patients and care providers. As health care delivery systems become more complex, it is evident that the opportunities for error abounds. A national, concerted effort by health professionals, organizations, purchasers, and regulators will be required to deal with this complex issue.

Reports published indicate that errors involving medications are responsible for an immense burden of patient injury, suffering, and death. Those involved in caring for patients and those who receive care agree that the errors observed should not happen. Current research has identified some issues, previously only discussed behind closed doors, regarding the scope and seriousness of the problem of medication errors:

- The costs of medication-related morbidity and mortality are high.
- Many medication errors are preventable, and physicians, nurses, and pharmacists can play a vital role in diminishing medication errors.
- The medication use process is highly complex, problem-prone, and requires a systematic approach for improvement.

Reports indicate that adverse drug events (ADEs)–injuries caused by the use (or nonuse) of a medication–affects as many as 1.3 million hospitalized patients annually.[15]

Several large studies have identified that medication-related errors occur frequently in hospitals. In 1993, medication errors were estimated to account for 7,000 deaths annually in the US.[16] In a second study conducted in New York, adverse events due to medications accounted for 19.4% of all injuries.[17] A third study evaluated 39 prospective studies utilizing a data set obtained from the literature between 1966 and 1996. The overall incidence of serious adverse drug reactions in hospitalized patients was 6.7% and of fatal ADRs was 0.32%. In 1994, it was estimated 2,216,000 hospitalized patients experienced serious ADRs and 106,000 had fatal ADRs making these reactions the fourth and sixth leading causes of death in the US.[18] A final study that requires discussion is a matched case-control study of patients admitted to a tertiary care institution in Salt Lake City. Classen et al identified that adverse drug events represented 2.43 of 100 admissions to their facility. The occurrence of an adverse drug event was associated with an increased length of stay of 1.91 days and an increased cost of $2,262. The increased risk of death among patients experiencing and ADE was 1.88.[19]

Not all medication errors that occur result in actual harm to patients, but evidence suggests that those that do cause harm are also costly. One study conducted found that nearly 2% of admissions experienced a potentially preventable ADE resulting in an increased hospital cost of nearly $4,700 per admission.[20] When that cost is annualized for the 700-bed teaching facility, this results in an overall cost of $2.8 million. If the findings are placed in the context of national admission rates, ADEs in inpatients could result in costs of $2 billion for the nation as a whole.[20]

Hospitals only represent a fraction of the total population at risk for an adverse drug event. Injuries from medication use have been documented during the vulnerable peri-discharge period. An evaluation by Forster et al evaluated 400 consecutive patients discharged home from a general internal medical service.[21] The patient's post hospital course was determined by conducting a medical record review and a structured telephone interview approximately 3 weeks after the discharge. A total of 76 (19%) were found to have some type of adverse events after discharge. Of interest is that adverse drug events were the most common type of adverse event reported at a frequency of 66%.[21]

Additional studies frame the issue of medication-related errors in other settings by identifying errors in prescribing and dispensing of prescriptions in an outpatient environment. There is evidence that ADEs account for a sizable number of admissions to inpatient facilities; however, it is unknown how many of these ADEs are directly associated with error. One study found that between 3% and 11% of hospital admissions were attributable to ADEs.[22] ADEs are often identified as a reason to seek care at a physician office or emergency room. In a study evaluating 1,000 patients in a community, office-based medical practice, patients were observed for adverse drug events. It was determined that 42 patients presented with an ADE of which 23 were found to be potentially avoidable.[23] In another evaluation, 1.7% of 62,216 patients seen in an emergency department visits were identified as associated with medication noncompliance or inappropriate prescribing.[24]

Adverse drug events can also occur in nursing homes. A study by Bootman et al in 1997 demonstrated that for every dollar spent on medications in nursing facilitites, $1.33 is consumed in the treatment of medication-related morbidity and mortality.[25] Total costs for the nation were estimated to be $7.6 billion, with a significant portion of the costs, $3.6 billion estimated to be avoidable.

Patient nonadherence with medication regimens also appear to be a significant quality issue. However, the extent to which nonadherence contributes to error is not known. With a greater emphasis on community-based, long-term care, increased ambulatory surgery, shorter hospital stays and greater complexity in therapy, patients themselves play an increasingly more important role in the administration of medications. Greenberg et al identified that 4.3% of the elderly enrolled in Medicare social HMOs in 1988 required assistance in administering medications.[26] In a meta-analysis conducted by Sullivan et al in 1986, it was estimated that 5.5% of admissions can be attributed to medication therapy noncompliance, resulting in 1.94 million admissions and potentially $8.5 billion in hospital costs.[27]

It has been estimated that for every dollar spent on ambulatory medications, another dollar is spent to treat new health problems caused by the medication.[28] This has resulted in projections that the health care cost of treating medication-related morbidity and mortality in the ambulatory setting to be as high as $76.6 billion in 1994.[29] Not all of this medication-related morbidity and mortality has been identified as preventable. However, numerous evaluations in population-based studies of patients in the community, health plans, hospitals, and nursing homes suggest that prescribing, dispensing by pharmacists, and unintentional nonadherence on the part of patients contribute significantly to this problem.[30–33]

Appropriate medication use is a complex process involving multiple organizations and professions from various disciplines combined with a working knowledge of medications, access to accurate and complete patient information and integration of interrelated decisions over a period of time. The growing complexity of science and technology requires health care providers to know more, manage more, monitor more, and involve more care providers than every before. Current methods of organizing and delivering care are not able to meet the new expectations of patients and families because the knowledge, skills, care options, devices, and medications have advanced more rapidly than the health care system's ability to deliver them safety, effectively, and efficiently. The potential for errors of omission or commission to creep into the process is extraordinary. No one clinician can retain all the information necessary for overseeing sound, safe, best practice. This is especially true in the case of pharmaceutical delivery and development. The average number of new medications approved per year has doubled since the 1980s. Between 1990 and 1999, more than 300 new medications were approved by the United States Food and Drug Administration.[34] Costs of care as well as the complexity of managing the use of existing and new pharmaceuticals are only expected to intensify as a result.

One of the consequences of these advances in medicine and technology is that people are now living longer. Changing mortality patterns, increasing numbers of individuals 65 years of age and older, and increases in incidence in prevalence of chronic conditions have important implications for the health care delivery system. Unlike the episodic care that occurs in acute care, effective care of the chronically ill requires a high degree of collaboration. Delivery of care must include joint development of care plans, goals, targets, implementation strategies, patient self-management training, sustained follow up and monitoring, and decision support systems. This collaboration requirement adds another layer of complexity to the delivery of care. The potential for the development of medication errors, adverse events, and mismanagement issues within and along the care system is enormous.

Access to treatments and use of best practice guidelines have lead to national quality improvement initiatives and priority action items to assure that change and improvements are made. As medical science and technology has advanced at a rapid pace, the system used to support and distribute care has not been able to keep up with the pace. Research indicates that the health care system currently falls short of being able to translate knowledge into practice. Variation of health system performance varies greatly. Many patients remain without health care insurance and have little to no access to basic health care services. For those without insurance, care is unobtainable except in emergency situations. A highly fragmented system lacks information capabilities, frequently provides duplication of services, long waiting times and delays.

Despite the vast range of available guidelines, best practices, standards, and evidence-based practice recommendations, a gap exists between the care people should receive and care they do receive. This is the case for acute, chronic, and preventive care and whether overuse, underuse, or misuse of resources are evaluated. Medication use examples can emphasize this point. Influenza vaccine is recommended as a preventive measure in adults over the age of 65, yet vaccination rates seldom occur over 60% of those at risk.[35] Antibiotic overuse continues to be a concern, which has lead to increase bacteriologic resistance. Antibiotics are not considered appropriate care for patients exhibiting symptoms of the common cold. Several studies in the 1990s identified that for 44–60% of patient visits diagnosed with a common cold were treated with antibiotics.[36] In other studies, such as those conducted by the Center for Medicare and Medicaid Services (CMS, formally known as the Health Care Financing Administration or HCFA), these identify that for patients suffering from myocardial infarction, use of aspirin, beta blockers, and other agents used to preserve or improve cardiovascular performance are not used as frequently as they should be and vary based on regional factors.[37]

National estimates indicate that as many as 70% of adverse drug events are due to errors and may be preventable.[38] Yet, since the reports of these findings it appears that little progress has actually been made. Clearly, a new approach is needed within health care organizations to improve the safety of medication use. Building the required safer medication system will mean redesigning processes of care to ensure patients are safe from accidental injury. A number of practices have been shown to reduce error in the medication process and are recommended to be in place in health care settings. Recommendations for building a safer medication use system include redesigning processes that govern medication use, involving all members of the medication use team and creating a new culture that identifies medication safety as a priority for the organization. Despite the availability of tested methods in health care and other industries, regulatory mandates, and published resources, gaps continue to exist between current recommendations and actual practice in organizations due to a variety of attitudinal, educational, and system barriers.

What issues are preventing organizations from improving the safety of medication use? Inconsistent reporting and fear of sanction for identifying errors can make it difficult to identify what is contributing to an adverse event. As a result, organizations are not able to track and trend information that could yield effective strategies for adverse event prevention within a care setting.

If errors occur, but are not reported, investigation and prevention strategies cannot be developed. Because some published studies indicate that as many as 95% of medication errors go unreported, this could be a significant issue for any organization.[39] Having a clear understanding of error, error theory, risks, and capabilities influencing safe and effective medication use is essential to impact and transform the current systems in place for providing care. Understanding human system interactions and elements that have been identified in other industries may hold the cues and clues needed for the system overhaul required by health care.

UNDERSTANDING ERROR

Health care systems have traditionally operated under the assumption that if care providers are well educated and follow well-developed policies, procedures, or guidelines, errors will not happen. That is in fact, not the case. Errors reoccur despite the best educational and planning efforts.

To understand what is or is not known about medication-related adverse events, common definitions must be established and understood. Organizations must come to a common understanding regarding medication errors, reporting requirements, and risks to capture and act upon error potential within their own medication use systems. While the literature has provided practitioners with a series of operational definitions, the following, developed by the Institute of Healthcare Improvement, reviews some commonly accepted definitions associated with medication use safety.[40]

Adverse Event: An injury caused by medical treatment, not necessarily due to an error.

Adverse Drug Event (ADE): An injury, large or small, caused by the use (including nonuse) of a drug. It can be as harmless as a rash or as serious as death from an overdose. There are two types of ADEs: (1) those caused by errors and (2) those that occur despite proper usage of a medication. If an ADE is caused by an error, it is by definition, preventable. Nonpreventable ADEs (injury, but no error) are called adverse drug reactions.

Preventable Adverse Drug Event: An injury due to an error in the use of a drug (including failure to use).

Potential Adverse Drug Event (PADE): A potential ADE is a serious medication error—one that has the potential to cause an ADE, but did not, either by luck (eg, the patient was not allergic to the drug despite a note in the record stating so) or because it was intercepted (eg, the nurse recognized an order for a medication to which the patient was allergic and called the physician to get it changed). Examining potential ADEs helps to identify both where the system is failing (the error) and where it is working (interception).

Adverse Drug Reaction (ADR): Further defined by the World Health Organization, to characterize injuries caused when drugs are used in the usual accepted fashion. By definition then an ADR does not result from an error. Unfortunately many have used this term as synonymous with ADE, which blurs an important distinction.

These definitions provide the following insights regarding adverse events and medication use:

- Medication errors are considered preventable while adverse drug reactions are generally are not.
- If an error occurs, but is intercepted by someone in the process, it might not result in an adverse event. These potential adverse events are often referred to as *near misses*.
- Capturing information regarding *near misses* could yield vital information regarding system performance.

IDENTIFYING RISK

Research indicates that perhaps one of the best ways to address the problem of adverse drug events and medication errors is to recognize that inherent risk exists with use of medications in patient care. This view is based on two concepts:

- Medications are inherently toxic, and there is a risk to taking them and, perhaps, not taking them. Each time a practitioner prescribes a product, a treatment risk *versus* benefit must be assessed. If a patient takes prescribed medications in a different manner than prescribed or if over-the-counter products and alternative agents are added, there are additional risks. Side effects and tragic rare reactions are also difficult to anticipate.
- Health care professionals are human and can make mistakes. Yet, during training and practice, they are immersed in an environment where there is no room for error. Reporting an error is often viewed as professional failure or negligence and is followed by sanction or punishment of the individuals involved. A zero error standard is demanded in health care. However, it is sobering to consider that each time care is provided many potential serious adverse events are possible. Increased patient complexity and decreased numbers of health care staff contribute to potential error. This results in health care workers worrying constantly about the ever-present reality of error.

Because errors are thought to be preventable, examining what happened when an error occurs is the natural response, a means to develop future prevention strategies. Unfortunately, in many organizations, the response to error targets the people rather than the system involved in the production of an error.

What is an Acceptable Error Rate?

Finding an *acceptable* rate of error consumes many organizations. What is an acceptable rate of error might just be the wrong question entirely. Is any error really acceptable? Is there really a target? What individual would truly desire to be involved in any significant error?

Everyone seems to be looking (unsuccessfully) for benchmarks for error rates related to medication use. Unfortunately, there are none! The Center for Medicare and Medicaid Services suggested several years ago that a 2% error rate was an acceptable target for health care systems for which to strive.[41]

- Is a 2% error rate acceptable to care providers?
- How would patients feel about an error rate of 2%?
- Would health systems reward staff for seriously injuring only 30 people a year?

Perhaps the best answer to these questions comes from a Deming example of the impact of errors.[42] Deming suggests that if the following systems were 99.9% safe, the United States would encounter:

- 84 unsafe plane landings daily
- 16,000 lost pieces of mail per hour
- 32,000 bank check errors per day

Literature reports have attempted to apply this concept of 0.1% error as a 'safe enough' system. Leape et al suggest that even a health care error rate of 0.1%, a 99.9% safe system, is simply not good enough.[43] Leape's work describes how an error rate of 0.1% effects the medication use process. He has noted that at a minimum, 10 to 14 steps commonly exist between a physician prescribing a medication and a patient receiving a medication.[44] Assuming each person involved in every step of a 10-step medication use process was operating at a peak efficiency of 99.9%, 10% of patients receiving medications within that system would be involved in some type of medication-related error.

Clearly, trying to predict an *acceptable* rate of error is not a reasonable approach. Goals should center on elimination of all error: a focus of zero error is the target, even while recognizing the impossibility of that goal. This creates an interesting paradox for care providers. Health systems often act like ostriches with heads buried in the sand, denying the likelihood of error that exists in the increasingly complex health care delivery system, expecting zero defect performance and yet continue to allow members of health care teams (physi-

cians, nurses, and pharmacists) to operate as *captains of their own professional ships* in the care delivery process. No one individual alone has the scope of control or information to absolutely prevent error, yet each individual acts as if they can, with a growing fear that in fact control of the next accident waiting to happen is an individual's responsibility. When an error does occur, organizations have a fairly typical response: shame and blame, retrain and/or reorganize, then return to business as usual.

For the sake of argument and improved patient care, it is important to maintain a zero error standard. The focus, however, must shift from blaming individuals to prevention of future errors by designing safety as a component of the system to accomplish this. If blame and sanction continues in health care, reporting will not occur. Inconsistent reporting makes identifying patterns of occurrence difficult or impossible. This eliminates hope for creating effective prevention strategies. This does not imply that individuals can be careless. If in fact, to err is human and caregivers are expected to be vigilant and responsible, creating systems that minimize risk and error are paramount for advancing an agenda of safety.

Organizational Vs. Individual Error

When reviewing error types and error theory in the literature, one finds descriptions of individual and organizational errors. Individual errors in health care are far more common. Organizational errors are rare, but can occur in complex technologies such as health care. Complete system failures, such infectious or hazard exposures that affect large populations of patients and health care workers may occur in health care systems. Most examples of organizational errors include accidents in the aviation industry, nuclear power plants, banks, stadiums, etc, where the result of a system failure impacts a significant portion of the population or community.

Part of the challenge with preventing or resolving error is having a true understanding the development of errors within the organizational construct, the logic or chain of events, and methods to evaluate beyond the surface detail to identify potential solutions or mitigation strategies.

In most industries, including health care, built in protections and defenses are put into place to assure that safe, effective care of people and assets occur. Reason has identified that there are a variety of defenses put into systems to provide the following functions[45]:

- Create understanding or awareness of hazards
- Give guidance on how to operate safely
- Provide alarms and warnings when risk or danger is evident
- Place barriers between hazards and individuals or other systems
- Restore system to a safe state when conditions are not normal
- Contain or eliminated hazards if the barrier is not adequate
- Establish methods of escape and rescue should hazard containment fail

As Reason defines these, there is some implied depth to the layers of protection so that it makes in nearly impossible for something to go awry. In the case of medication use, these points of defense are often in place, although the depth and scope of their implementation may vary. Medication information, policies and procedures, guidelines, and restrictions are often in place to assure that medication use hazards are evaluated or mitigated. Dosing adjustments, review of orders by multiple, skilled practitioners, use of dosing thresholds, alarms on medication administration devices all present opportunities to alert the need for change or modification of a medication use process. When those barriers fail, often antidotes or rescue protocols are available to contain potential adverse events. The rigor with which these principles are applied can mean the difference between a fatal error or successful treatment process.

In an ideal world, all the defensive layers would be intact and no penetration of a possible failure could occur. Unfortunately, in the real world, each defense layer can have weaknesses and gaps. Holes in defenses can occur. To identify how these failures can occur, the concepts of latent conditions and active failures must be described. These models hold the key to understanding methods to redesign the medication use process to control, contain, or mitigate errors within health care.

Latent Conditions and Active Failures

Complex systems such as those involved in health care are inherently hazardous by their very nature. It is not unexpected that all complex systems may have minor faults. When failures do occur, they are often the result of multiple apparently innocuous faults (referred to in the literature as latent error) that occur simultaneously or in clusters. Yet, the concept of latent error is not routinely evaluated in health care. This is error that has been defined as beyond the individual. It implies faulty design, poor maintenance, or error in overall management. Interaction between this system-related problem and individual may not be discernable and effect not immediate.

The Swiss Cheese metaphor has been utilized by Reason and others to represent a dynamic, moving picture of defensive layers (Fig 102-2).[46]

These defenses within an organization or process often move around based on local conditions. Consider how routine defenses in the medication use process could be removed deliberately (violation of procedure) or inadvertently (error) during calibration, maintenance, or testing of a medication delivery device. Each of these *holes* could be coming and going, shifting, shrinking, and expanding in response to the environmental condition or operator activity. Consider an example of an intravenous infusion device not adequately calibrated, not maintained, or with no maintenance plan in place. Continued use of the inadequately calibrated equipment could be producing small, relatively indistinguishable readings that could lead to decisions for care that could be problematic. Some operators of the equipment may recognize the variation and modify the device to override a problem; others may be unaware that any problem exists. Reporting of the concern may not occur or go unnoticed if no underlying plan for maintenance evaluation is in place. Other examples of latent conditions in the health care system might include:

- Lack of adequate patient information (eg, no information about prior treatments or allergies)
- Lack of appropriate communication (eg, failure to fully communicate order changes and ambiguous or misleading medication orders)
- Lack of medication information (eg, no maximum dose warnings)
- Lack of adequate medication labeling (eg, a syringe with no description of route of administration, IM or IV)
- Lack of adequate training or resources on a topic area

How are these types of latent failures identified by members of the health care team? How would a pharmacist or other care provider know if these failures are possible? What has been de-

signed as a system safety net to capture possible accidents before they happen? The design of many care systems for patient have *built-in* features that pose latent error potential:

- Interruptions
- Workload and/or poor delineation of responsibilities
- Work schedules that are inappropriate and stress-producing
- Lack of standards leading to workarounds
- Lack of information
- Lack of training leading to variation in work habits and abilities

Health care is a complex system involving the interaction of large numbers of highly trained personnel in many diverse, interrelated, and interdependent activities. Redefining and redesigning what each team member does is necessary to reduce or prevent errors from occurring.

It is important to note that these types of latent failures can be present at any level of the organization. Latent conditions are present in all systems. They are a part of organizational life. This is not to say that latent conditions are always a result of bad decisions. The original design and allocation of resources to support the medication use process may have been based on sound information. System inequities can be unforeseen and create quality, reliability problems at some point within the process. No one individual or leader can possibly foresee all the future ramifications of current system design. Latent conditions, by definition, are seeded within the infrastructure of the organization and are often related to production or service design, contracting, regulatory, or governmental mandates. They can remain dormant. Development of these failures and exposure of latent conditions only become visible when they are instigated by humans at the front line or sharp end of the process; when the decisions are tested and applied. The concept of latent error demonstrates a new way of thinking for health care systems. Rather than being derived from a single massive failure, single component or person, system failures truly do arise from an insidious accumulation of individual faults. A series of defenses can fail *together* even in an extraordinarily safe system.

Because people design, operate, maintain, and manage complex systems such as medication use, it is hardly surprising that often people are implicated first in errors. Humans contribute to the breakdown of systems. Making decisions, juggling time, and weighing the evidence are common and necessary day-to-day, minute-to-minute health care worker activities. Practitioners and others are provided resources, data, and tools to care for patients. They apply knowledge and make judgments about care activities. Health care providers operate at the sharp end of the care process—the hazardous end that interacts directly with the patient. Care providers must interact with equipment, environments, other people and change each day.

In reality, the limiting steps to moving to a redesigned health care system that would minimize latent failures has less to do with technology than with the human aspect. When things go wrong, the technology is "blamed", but the social, behavioral, psychological, and cultural factors associated with the technology are the more likely culprits. Both simple fixes and more complex technology innovations have unintended consequences. In short, it is not possible to introduce a new technology into a system without changing behavior and altering outcomes, often in unanticipated ways, intentionally or not.

Sharp End, Blunt End Interactions

Reason provides another model for consideration regarding the role of systems and supports for human interactions with those systems (Fig 102-3).[47]

Practitioners are directly influenced and affected by the *blunt end of the system*—the institutional structure, policy, other resources, regulations, and technology—but are truly working at the *sharp end* where care situations often vary. Work by Cook and Woods identifies that human functioning at

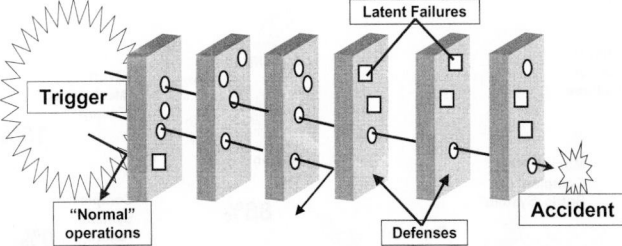

Figure 102-2. Latent failure: The Swiss Cheese diagram. Adapted from Reason J. *Human Error.* Cambridge, UK: Cambridge University Press, 1990:208.

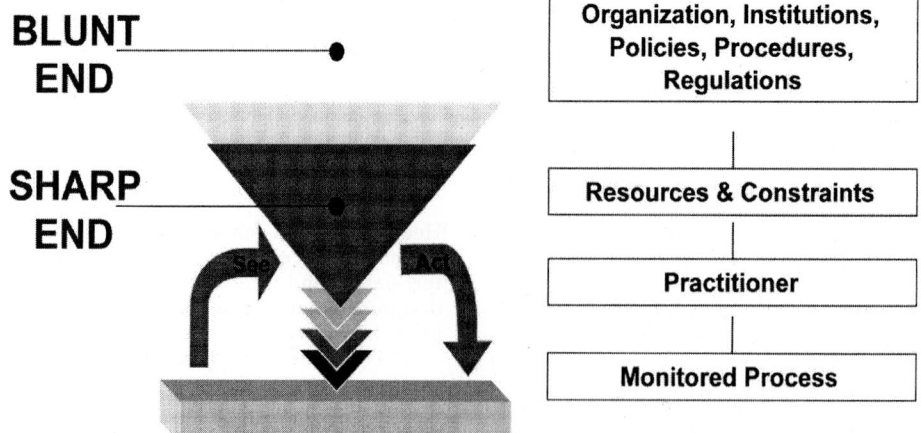

Figure 102-3. Sharp end / blunt end interaction. Adapted from Bogner MS, ed. *Human Error in Medicine.* Hillsdale, NJ: Lawrence Erlbaum Associates, 1994:295.

the sharp end in systems and health care in particular is extremely complex. Success or failure of a process, such as medication use, is dependent on:[48]

- The context in which the process occurs and how the practitioner is expected to perform in an environment that can vary
- The technology impact on the practitioner performance, because it has the potential to create new forms of error and failure
- Practitioner action usually involves a set of people affecting the medication use process
- Individuals who have shaped the *blunt end supports* for practitioners can create dilemmas or tradeoffs among goals that can compete at the sharp end of the process
- Attribution of the error at the sharp end is often a process of social judgment rather than a scientific conclusion

Consider what happens if blunt end components are absent or not well defined for medication use? A patient presents for treatment with co-morbidities that have the potential to affect medication use selection, dosing, and monitoring, but consequences and information are not clearly known by the care providers. What about a new scenario where policy has not yet been defined or distributed? A patient with a functional or cognitive impairment is potentially unable to self-administer his/her own medication with the administration equipment provided. What if the sharp end need does not match the blunt end support? The policy doesn't match the patient or the situation, as in the case of the prescribing of a medication for an unapproved use.

Practitioners of course must act and react at the sharp end. Resources and constraints at this sharp end can impact how the process actually plays out. As a result, resources are applied and outcomes occur based on what is available and what the sharp end user knows about.

When evaluating the medication use process or investigating an error, simply focusing on the sharp end interaction may lead to inappropriate and inaccurate conclusions. Investigations must consider how the blunt end of the process contributes to what was executed at the sharp end by the practitioner. Issues that contribute to errors and adverse events are often difficult to see because current tools use to evaluate health care systems are inadequate. Measurement and evaluation of all aspects of the medication use system does not routinely occur. Organizations may only collect and report selected information and reflect observations solely at the sharp end of the process. An understanding of optimal system performance and system vulnerabilities are part of the new-look understanding needed to identify safety hazards within the medication use process.

The Cycle of Error

A noted expert in the area of systems analysis, anesthesiology, and error theory, Dr. Richard Cook has visually described a cycle of error and what the investigation process looks like in a health care organization (Fig 102-4).[49]

Typically, reactions to a health care error involve associating a person with blame. It is easy to identify and blame a person present at the time the error occurred. In general, people involved in complex health care processes really do a great job managing at the point of their interaction with the process. Members of the health care team troubleshoot and react or modify when needed to reacting to changing patient conditions. In most cases, these skills of adaptation are rewarded and encouraged in health care.

Despite this balancing act by health care team members, actions after an adverse event usually focus on training or retraining those involved or accused. New rules, regulations or sanctions are implemented. Although these steps may result in heightened awareness of possible error prone processes, research suggests that these changes alone do not provide long lasting improvements.

Consider the following common response to an error associated with the overdose of chemotherapy. Typically, the action steps include:

- Development of new order forms
- Retraining of staff

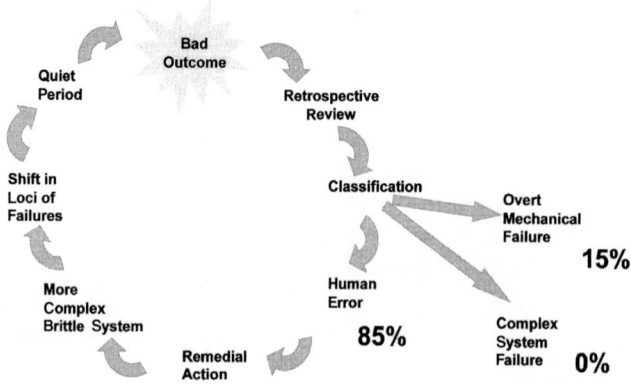

Figure 102-4. Error cycle. Bogner MS, ed. *Human Error in Medicine.* Hillsdale, NJ: Lawrence Erlbaum Associates, 1994:29.

- Development of new policy, including restricting the use of the medications involved to specific physician groups
- Purchase or standardization of infusion devices and/or new calculation checking process is mandated

Oftentimes, these interventions alone may only increase complexity and introduce new opportunities for failure. As the previous diagram suggests, the error cycle tends to repeat itself when the usual quick fixes or incremental modifications are made in isolation within the system.

Cook suggests that in health care it is also highly unlikely that after an event occurs the correction of one set of specific flaws will be of value in preventing future errors. In fact, Cook describes that it is more likely that a combination of flaws actually contribute to the development of the problem within the system. If only one or two isolated steps are modified, the system may in fact become more vulnerable by shifting the locus of where the error may occur the next time.[49]

This new way of thinking about error analysis and system repair highlights the fact that the health care system is highly complex and interactive. This necessitates a true system view of the medication use process before rushing to an isolated solution or fix.

Factors that Contribute to Error in Health Care

Several specific factors have been identified that contribute to health care system error and provide some additional challenges for resolving the issues.[43] The culture of medical practice itself: complex, heroic, and focused on an expectation of perfection. Physicians and others fear implications of negligence and reporting may not occur as a result. In this environment, the physician is seen as the controller or gatekeeper of all aspects of care. Blaming activity is thus promoted when things don't go as planned.

Additionally, because of the complex nature of health care, adjustments and changes, of any type, often occur seemingly in a vacuum. Miscommunication or no communication can result.

When it comes to error investigation in health care, postaccident reviews often identify human error as the cause due to hindsight bias. This knowledge of the outcome makes the path to failure appear obvious to the investigator. It implies that individuals involved in the process could have foreseen what was about to happen even if they could not. In fact, the conclusion that practitioners should have known that the factors involved would inevitably lead to an accident actually poses some real obstacles to a thorough, unbiased investigation. Human performance analysis at this point may be far from fair or accurate as a result, yet this is the common method for accident investigation.

Error and Human Capacity

Human error can occur as a result of human capacity itself. Errors can be made by teams or by individuals. Some errors occur as a result of misinterpreting speech or written communication. The probability of an error increases with increased workloads and long or rotating shifts. Stress and fatigue also affect performance. Human capacity elements that affect decision-making and have error potential include memory, skill, rule, and knowledge.[50]

Human Error Types

Action errors attributed to an error of subconscious or automatic behavior are called "slips."[51] These have been referred to as errors that occur when individuals are in the automatic mode. "Slips" occur as a result of distraction. An example might be getting into a hospital service elevator and intending to go to the laboratory for medication blood level results, but walking off the elevator on the floor where the cafeteria is instead.

Errors associated with conscious thought are termed "mistakes."[51] These types of errors are often identified as individuals *not thinking straight*. Mistakes are rule-based and knowledge-based cognition errors. Essentially, a wrong rule is chosen and applied. This may reflect a lack of information, a misinterpretation of the situation, or an inability to apply information to a new scenario. As an example, consider how a health care provider addresses look-alike labels or sound-alike medication names. These examples are accidents waiting to happen.

Errors that people make are often traceable to extrinsic factors that affect capacity and set the individual up to fail, rather than intrinsic factors such as forgetting or inattention.

Preventing Error

Error prevention in health care has not focused on addressing these types of human factors. Instead it has relied almost exclusively on the training of personnel to perform perfectly. Conventional wisdom suggests that if something goes wrong, someone *goofed*. The presumption is that people are unreliable. As a result finding the culprit and assigning blame is the solution to combating future error.

The assumption has been that if clinicians are well educated and follow policies, procedures, or other guidelines, errors will not happen. It is believed that highly trained people will not make errors. In fact, this is not true. Highly trained people make mistakes. If the organization has the belief that people are intrinsically unreliable, it would follow that elimination of error could only be resolved by replacing humans with automation. Some organizations are moving in this direction; however, automation is not able to cope with infrequent situations and variable environments. Consideration of human factors and the humanness of care must still be evaluated and planned for even in highly automated environments.

Error Investigation in Other Industry

Other industries have identified these issues and have modified their approach to error analysis and prevention. Improving safety in these environments has been focused on understanding how the details of economic, organizational and technological factors create vulnerabilities and paths to failure. Because health care is also dynamic, improving safety may also require this new look perspective.

Safety can only be achieved by learning how system components interact. Organizations that have shown progress on safety have an understanding about how technical and organizational factors play out in real work and how people act and react in the face of these changes. Error theories in other industries focus on the following concepts:

- Errors are common
- Errors are a result of complex cognitive mechanisms
- Psychologists, human factors specialists, and engineers are critical to the investigation of error and development of error prevention strategies
- Man-machine interfaces need investigation for error potential
- Defining complex systems and their component interactions are crucial
- Work environment redesign, including ergonomic factors, must be included

Decision-making regarding medication use is complex and minor variations from patient case to case do not always allow for simple rules or routines to be followed. Safety engineers view workflow, interactions, distractions, coupling activities, handoffs, and timing as a part of an error generating system that must be evaluated and designed for safety. Members of other industries define systems clearly and focus on the whole rather on an isolated segment of the system.

Aviation Safety System Design

The aviation industry has made great advances in the area of error prevention and human factors research based on these key elements for change. The recognition of the role that human factors play in error development has produced a system that is focused on identification and prevention. The Federal Aviation Administration (FAA) and National Aeronautics and Space Administration (NASA) established the Aviation Safety and Reporting System (ASRS) in 1975. This program collects and responds to voluntary submitted aviation safety reports.[52] Data from these reports are used to:

- Alert authorities regarding deficiencies and discrepancies
- Support policy development and improvement planning
- Strengthen foundation of human factors safety research. This last component is probably the most important since it is generally realized that two-thirds of aviation accidents root causes are human performance error

Safety Advances in Anesthesia Practice

The medical specialty of anesthesia has embraced some of these ASRS techniques and incorporated a systems-approach regarding error analysis and prevention. As early as 1968, some fundamental changes in anesthesia practice were instituted to reduce the morbidity and mortality associated with anesthesia. A fundamental change was needed for this high-risk, problem-prone activity. Anesthesia supported investigation of workload, effects of stress and fatigue, incorporating a team approach, and a focus on error prevention.

The result of initiating change in these areas significantly reduced mortality. Groups such as the American Society for Anesthesia (ASA) have continued this effort by developing and establishing practice/treatment guidelines, as well as supporting continued research in the areas of workload analysis/fatigue. Additionally, ASA efforts focus on a team approach to care as well as providing for checks and balances in anesthesia activities. Advancement of credentialing activities/standards for the practice, development of position papers regarding safety, and educational programming are also provided by ASA.[53]

These ASA efforts have had a significant impact on mortality. Ten years ago, death rates associated with anesthesia were 1 in 10,000 to 20,000; now these rates have dropped to 1 in 200,000.[54–56] Anesthesia has led the medical profession in recognizing that system factors cause errors. Advances have been made because there has been a focus on designing fail-safe systems and in training to avoid errors.

This view also seems relevant to other health care environments. Consider a nursing unit at shift change or a pharmacy located in a high traffic area with multiple distraction points. There are many risks for misinterpretation or poor communication in this environment. Clearly, the nursing unit or a pharmacy in a bustling chain practice environment is a difficult place for high-level complex care to occur. Simply redesigning a component of the work (eg, a reporting form or format) will not be sufficient to address the complexity of the systems that influence how nurses conduct shift reports. Potential for error is great. With caseloads increasing and staffing shortages looming, the potential for error can escalate.

Factors Associated with Human Error Development

Three general factors have been identified that contribute to the development of human errors. Each item contributes to the development of human stress and fatigue. Organizations should incorporate strategies to address these factors to identify potential adverse drug event prevention strategies. These aspects are summarized in below[57]:

Psychological Precursors: These are associated with issues such as excessive care assignments, excessive work schedules, long shifts, inad-

equate physical working conditions, and strained work relationships. Development of physical stress and fatigue in these scenarios can lead to the individual being vulnerable to error.

Team Function: A lack of supportive leadership encouragement and group cohesion can lead to dysfunctional performance. Individuals will be unable to communicate effectively and function effectively. If power relationships exist, decision-making and communication may also be impaired. It is unlikely that suggestions for improvement will be made. Errors, if identified, may go unchecked or unreported in this environment.

Training: A lack of adequate training can predispose individuals to errors. Simply providing educational materials, however, is not enough. A method for assessing individual competency and capacity to apply new knowledge is also essential. Individuals must also be trained for teamwork and be willing to learn and teach each member on the team. If individuals do not understand their responsibility or have the necessary skills, errors are more likely to occur.

Organizational and Environmental Factors Contributing to Human Error

Additionally, many organizational and environmental factors contribute to the development of human error and must be identified and addressed within the organization. These factors include:

- Lack of a supportive environment
- A culture based on fear and retribution for mistakes
- Lack of teamwork
- Inadequate or limited training

To assess system performance, it is also necessary to understand the complex cognitive processes that health care providers use to perform their individual jobs. Plans for care are created and followed by individuals and as a team of care providers. Problem-solving activities can occur by individuals or as a team. Gaba provides a process model of anesthetist's real time decision-making and actions while providing care (Fig 102-5).[58]

Although focused on anesthesia care specifically, the model identifies critical action loop of care that can be applied to any health care provider activity[58]:

- Observation
- Decision
- Action
- Re-evaluation

In addition, this loop of activity must operate under several controls:

Resource allocation: including delegation of tasks and responsibilities during the procedure, monitoring and cross-checking activities, and attention to process.

Supervisory control: reviewing data, prioritizing activities, reacting to change/ interruptions and actions if necessary.

Sensory and motor control: routine observations, problem recognition, prediction of needs and outcomes, action planning regarding both abstract and procedural issues.

The anesthetist must have overall vigilance and sustained attention to detail. Ongoing observation and problem recognition is vital. Having a plan and a response for acute and unexpected situations is also necessary. Making sure that the plan is reviewed, data is evaluated and re-evaluated and that others are informed of the steps necessary for an optimal outcome are also essential components. All of these activities within the process model can be subject to human error and failures of the human capacity itself. The following items must be considered as medication use plans are developed:

- Infrequent or inadequate medication use data observation
- Responses to false medication use data
- Inadequate planning or forecasting responses to medication use problems
- Inadequate workload management for medication use process
- Inadequate crosschecking of activities
- Poor communication
- Poor leadership
- Increased fatigue and reduced vigilance

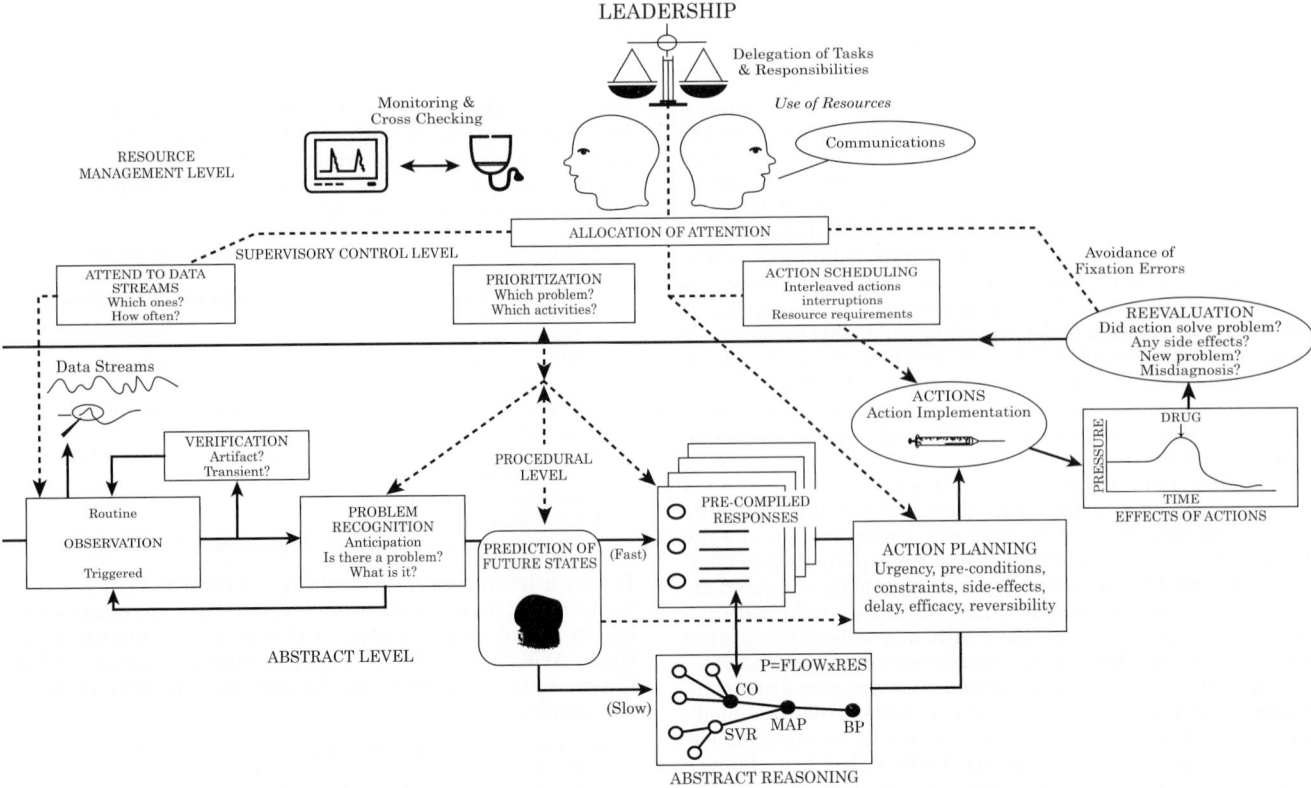

Figure 102-5. Anesthesia decision model. From Bogner MS, ed. *Human Error in Medicine.* Hillsdale, NJ: Lawrence Erlbaum Associates, 1994:209.

Certainly, lack of knowledge and skill can contribute to error in this environment, but suboptimal performance of these processes resides in how decisions and actions of humans are linked together in this complex care area. Many tradeoffs and decisions must be continuously balanced and refined. Although these activities might be slightly different for other areas of medicine, the concepts for improvement and attention for development of safer performance are similar:

- Training and competency assessment of practitioners is vital, but a new focus on problem-solving, supervisory control, and resource management is needed for assuring safety
- Ergonomics of the work environment must be evaluated to reduce the possibility of "slips"
- Communication and vigilance by the use of effective teamwork and crew coordination are essential for reducing risk
- Workload management, distribution of workload, and standards are necessary for safe performance
- Optimum planning of action and monitoring activities are needed

THE ROLE OF THE PATIENT IN MEDICATION USE

The Institute of Medicine identified 10 new rules to transition the general health care system to better meet patient care needs.[59] These rules and recommendations require partnerships between patients and care providers to improve health care processes, including medication use. These care rules have been adapted below to identify opportunities in medication improvement and include:

- Care based on continuing relationships that measure and monitor effects of medications
- Customization of medication treatments based on patient needs and values
- Patients as the source of control for medication use decisions
- Shared knowledge and free flow of information regarding risks and benefits of medication use

- Decision-making based on evidence of medication use findings
- Safety as a medication use system property
- Need for transparency so that all care providers and those involved in care have adequate and appropriate medication use information while respecting patient confidentiality
- Anticipation of medication use and monitoring needs associated with treatment and conditions
- Continuous decrease in waste of services, time, and expenses
- Cooperation among clinicians to focus toward a common goal for treatment based on patient's wishes

These rules are consistent with other quality initiatives and medication use improvement strategies that have as its focus providing safe, effective, timely, efficient, and equitable care that is designed and focused on meeting individual patient medication use needs.

The patient-clinician encounter is also a potential source for error, adverse events, or misaligned therapeutic goals. The unfamiliar environment of diagnosis, treatment, and information regarding use of medications is often intimidating and unsettling for patients. Pharmacies, hospitals, or outpatient examination rooms are often locations where pieces of health information and assessment are exchanged. Use or evaluation of prescription efficacy or toxicity may also occur over a telephone call. Information is not always conveyed by words alone during an exchange. Miscommunication, verbal and nonverbal, can occur in a conscious or unconscious fashion.

The two participants, the patient and the clinician, often have asymmetrical discussions. The provider often contributes to the discussion as an authority figure; the patient as a subordinate. Both participants often come from different socioeconomic backgrounds and educational experiences. Each participant may use different terms and vocabulary to describe symptoms, outcomes, and concerns. Additionally, cultural, ethnic, racial, gender, age, and religious differences contribute to differing sets of beliefs and values.

The environment along with social, educational, and personal factors can all contribute to miscommunication or misinterpretation of clinical findings and plans. While a common goal might be agreed upon, improving patient's quality of life through the use of medications, this goal could be perceived differently by each partner in the exchange and not fully realized by either party. Misunderstandings could lead to serious errors. Practitioners need to have an understanding of the patient's cognitive capability and competence, environmental and social situation as well as values and beliefs in order to effectively communicate and design safe and effective medication use plans. Patients should also be encouraged to be better health care consumers and become better informed. Patients should be encouraged to express their needs and concerns and receive as much information on medications and options as desired. Above all, there needs to be a dialog regarding their need for solutions to their perceived problems that respect their own wishes while respecting their independence whenever possible. For the practitioner, this means combining some common sense as well as innovative strategies to assess, adapt, and improve communication strategies for patients.

Patients, families, and health care providers often must make difficult and complex care decisions including those involving use or nonuse of medications. Unfortunately, despite regulations, guidelines, and research, many patients and families do not get the information they need to make informed decisions and practitioners often fear discussing risks with patients. Practitioners often have difficulty determining what risks to share and finding the words to convey the potential for risk with treatments. This communication can pose great challenges for physicians, nurses, or pharmacists involved in medication use. Some or all of the risks may not be known or understood. Perceptions of risk also vary. Is the risk of liver damage or headache from the use of a medication for diabetes more significant than the development of renal disease associated with diabetes disease progression?

Patients have a right to information regarding any proposed treatment as well as risks involved. This includes informing the patient regarding their condition, treatment plan, prognosis, complications, risks, benefits, alternative treatments, and other vital pieces of information regarding possible treatment in order to give consent to a specific care plan. Health systems and individual practitioners need to identify and implement a strategy for risk discussions with patients. Pichert and Hickson suggest the following framework for communications with patients[60]:

- Identify patient preferences for information (amount and format)
- Evaluate patient and family's desired decision-making role
- Provide assessment and response to patient ideas, concerns, and expectation
- Discuss clinical issue
- Review and define decision needed
- Identify all alternatives (include patient's ideas as well)
- Present and evaluate evidence available
- Discuss pros and cons (benefits and risks) and work with patient to explore impacts on values, life-style
- Ask patient to identify a preference
- Identify with patient any conflicts or concerns
- Determine methods to resolve conflicts and make or negotiate a final decision
- Agree on an action plan and a follow up plan
- Document the discussion and plan

In addition to discussing risks and benefits in advance, health care providers need to identify methods to disclose errors or adverse events to patients when they occur. Telling patients and families about unwanted outcomes and errors is not easy. Dealing with their response and reactions can be challenging as well. Accepting responsibility, investigating the event and possibly changing practice as a result of the investigation and findings requires a plan. When dealing with errors or adverse events, practitioners and health care organizations need to provide the necessary care, compassion and concern to create a climate that will help patients. Failing to communicate a concern or an adverse outcome can routinely lead to pursuit of legal counsel and malpractice litigation. Organizations must be will-

ing to share and act upon findings of error investigations and make patients and families aware of actions that will be taken to mitigate or resolve the adverse outcome for their loved one. Patients are also often interested in knowing that strategies are put into place to assure that the same event will not recur for another patient. Health care organizations should have a plan to provide this information by taking the initiative in explaining adverse event. Recommendations for initiating these difficult conversations include[61]:

- If possible, seek counsel from the health care organization's risk manager
- Select a setting that will preserve dignity and confidentiality
- Deliver a clear message
- Discuss support options
- Wait silently for a reaction from patient and/or family
- Deal with the reaction
- Express empathy, but be careful that it is not interpreted as negligence
- Conclude interaction by reviewing discussion and asking if patient has understanding
- Document the discussion
- Consider a follow-up meeting
- Share findings with necessary organizational personnel

For each interaction or consultation with a patient receiving medications, there are some methods that practitioners can utilize to provide ongoing support of safe medication use by patients. Wiegman and Cohen suggest that patients must have the answers to the following 12 questions in order to ensure safe medication use[62]:

- What are the brand and generic names of the medication?
- What is the purpose of the medication?
- What is the strength and dosage?
- What are the possible side effects and what should be done if they occur?
- Are there medications that should be avoided while using this product?
- How long should this medication be used? What outcomes are expected?
- When is the best time to take this medication?
- How should this medication be stored?
- What should be done if a dose is missed?
- What foods should be avoided while taking this medication?
- Does this medication replace another medication currently prescribed?
- What written information is available to explain this medication?

Patients can and should play an important role in their medication therapy. Patients have a right to know about their medication therapies and practitioners have to assess that the information they are providing reflects not only the best scientific evidence available regarding risks and benefits but also considers alternatives, values, and concerns presented by patients. To assure that all options are discussed, practitioners should assure that medication information for patients are current and reflect clear goals and monitoring plans. Additionally, efforts should be undertaken to assure that communication is two-way and conducted so that messages sent are understood by all parties.

HEALTH CARE AS A SYSTEM

"The problems we have created will not be solved by the level of thinking that created them." **Albert Einstein**

Improving patient care safety requires a systems view of the care delivery process, a unique perspective on reality that sharpens awareness of the system as a whole, including how its parts interrelate. Systems thinking teaches us that interactions between parts are often more important than actions of individual parts because interactions often produce valuable new and unpredictable capabilities that are beyond the capabilities of any single component.

One thinks and speaks of health care as a system. Yet, while the term *health care system* is in common use, there is no specific vocabulary that is commonly used to express the dynamic complexity of what the term means, either discretely in discussing an organizational entity (tightly or loosely coupled sites of care across the continuum) or globally to refer to the care delivery process available in America. In fact generically, *system* can typically have at least three meanings:

- *THE* system, the way things get done, how it works, the powers that be
- Groupings of elements for classification or analysis
- A functionally related group of interacting, interrelated, or interdependent elements forming a complex whole with a common aim

By definition, systems of things are complex. How the elements function together defines *systemness*. For purposes of this discussion, interdependence is a key feature. Deming defines a system as a group of interdependent people, items, processes, products, and services with a common aim.[63] Complex adaptive systems–slime mold, termite mounds, ant colonies, bee hives, flocks of birds, pods of whales, or health care organizations–must adjust to fluctuating environmental conditions to survive. Individual agents within the system are free to act in ways not always predictable and the actions of those agents change the context of the other agents in the system. No amount of data-driven forecasting, top-down strategic planning, management controls or policies and procedures can account for all the possible variables of fluctuation and change. As a result, complex adaptive systems must be continually emergent and self-organizing in response to the internal and external stimuli. Health care leaders have begun to recognize the wisdom of the basis of systems thinking: *The whole is greater than the sum of its parts.*

Complex adaptive systems have been described in a growing body of research, literature, and theory known as complexity science. Despite complexity, and apparent randomness, these intricate and leaderless operations and maneuvers–like flocks of geese flying south to the same destination at precisely the right time in response to changing conditions–don't descend into chaos and in fact demonstrate a stunning nimbleness, precision and efficacy.[64] As with ants in search of food for the nest, or birds migrating, humans have the capacity to self-organize to apply knowledge, experience, organizational support, and resources in delivering care.

Complex systems have *fuzzy* boundaries. Membership can change and agents can simultaneously be members of several systems, which can create unexpected actions. Internalized rules sets drive actions. Schooling fish, migrating birds, stampeding herds of animals need to follow only three instinctive rules: match your speed to your neighbor's, avoid collisions, and always move toward the center of the mass. Similar rules exist on a human level within health care, reflecting instincts, constructs, and mental models based on knowledge and experience. However, there is no need for them to be shared, explicit, or logical when viewed by another agent.[65] In everyday life, many complex behaviors emerge from relatively simple rules.[66] While no one directs our actions, one knows how to behave adaptively in commuting to work, to get where one wants to go.

Because the *rules* are not fixed, elements are changeable and may be simultaneously part of multiple systems, relationships are nonlinear, behavior is emergent and sensitive to small changes in conditions, complex systems are inherently unpredictable over time.[67] Paradox, tension, and anxiety are natural products of complex systems. Plsek identifies questions that aid in exploring the paradox[68]:

- How can we provide direction without issuing directives?
- How can we lead by serving?
- How can we maintain authority without control?
- How can we set direction when we don't know the future?
- How can we oppose change by accepting it? How can we accept change by opposing it?
- How can we be both a system and independent parts?

Systems naturally seem to resist imposed change, yet system behavior follows natural attractor patterns. Resistance is really poorly understood attractor patterns; dialog, listening, appre-

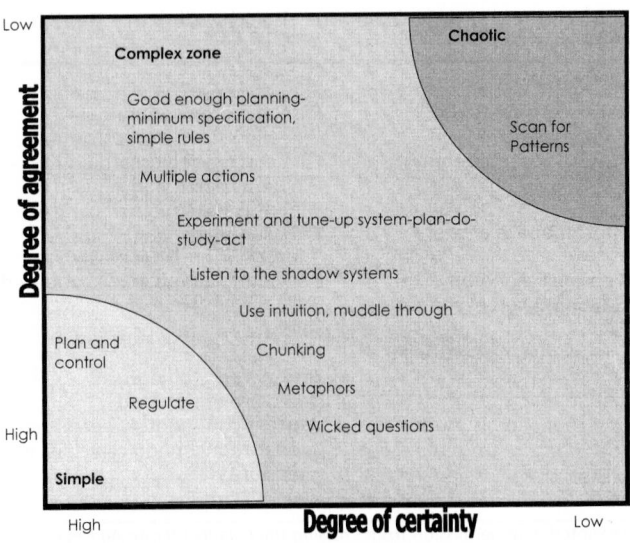

Figure 102-6. Certainty agreement. Adapted from Wilson T, Holt T. Complexity and clinical care. *BMJ* 2001; 323:687.

ciative inquiry and a trust environment build understanding, shift attractor patterns, increasing the tension for change and the likelihood of success for complex change initiatives.

Too often in complex adaptive systems, individuals are expected to produce definitive answers to questions or issues in conditions of high uncertainty and low agreement. Figure 102-6 displays certainty-agreement diagram, reflecting the edge of chaos notion of complexity.

The middle zone reflects the lack of certainty and agreement so evident in clinical practice decision-making and in many of the decisions facing health care organizations, including patient safety improvement. View the system through a lens of complexity, learning flexibility, and adaptability as a leadership strategy. This zone of complexity is managed with a few simple rules, minimum specifications to provide direction and sense making opportunity, experimentation, including the Plan–Do–Study–Act (PDSA) cycle for testing improvement. In this zone, a *good enough* vision and the *next best step* in the right direction is more likely than perfection. In uncertainty, one balances data and intuition, safety and risk, control and acceptance of the unknowable. Techniques such as *chunking* (ie, creating categories of events to understand the underlying patterns of behavior) or analogy and metaphor are useful to understand behaviors. The result is the adaptive behavior of system elements reacting to the change around them.

One of the most compelling calls for the application of the principles of complexity science to health care appears in *Chasm*, which offers 10 simple rules for the 21st Century of Health Care (Table 102-1).

Systems thinking methods define a process for analysis, reflecting seven basic skills. Each skill plays a role in supporting one or more of the steps. The skills are not difficult, but are often counterintuitive to traditional thinking and organizational behavior. Figure 102-7 displays seven systems thinking skills and illustrates the process and the individual skills that must be mastered.

Systems thinking begins with the definition of a problem or issue of concern. Once that is defined, it is necessary to construct a model or hypothesis, which represents one's assumptions about how a particular part of the system works. The hypothesis is then tested by simulating the model. If the model can generate the problem, it is a valid hypothesis; if not, it needs to be modified and retested. Once a valid model exists, it can be communicated to others to begin the change process. It is important to realize that all models are always wrong to some degree, hence the value is not in how *right* the model is, but how

Table 102-1. Simple Rules for the 21st Century Health Care System

CURRENT APPROACH	NEW RULES
Care based primarily on visits	Care based on continuous healing relationships
Professional autonomy drives variability	Care customized according to patient needs and values
Professionals control care	Patient is the source of control
Information is a record	Knowledge is shared and information flows freely
Decisionmaking based on training and experience	Decisionmaking is evidence-based
"Do no harm" is an individual responsibility	Safety is a system property
Secrecy is necessary	Transparency is necessary
System reacts to needs	Needs are anticipated
Cost reduction is sought	Waste is continuously decreased
Preference is given to professional roles over the system	Cooperation among clinicians is a priority

Reprinted with permission from *Crossing the Quality Chasm: An New Health System for the 21st Century.* © 2001 by the National Academy of Sciences, Courtesy of the National Academies Press, Washington, DC.

useful it is helping to clarify and understand the reality of the system. Every model is only as good as the thinking that goes into creating it and the seven basic thinking skills play significant roles in improving the quality of the thinking that leads to the hypothesis and model.

The seven skills are typically applied sequentially, to address three separate aspects of problem/issue identification and resolution[69]:

1. *Specifying the problem or issue and setting boundaries for the model*
   - Dynamic thinking
   - System as cause thinking
   - Forest thinking
2. *Constructing the model*
   - Operational thinking
   - Closed-loop thinking
   - Quantitative thinking

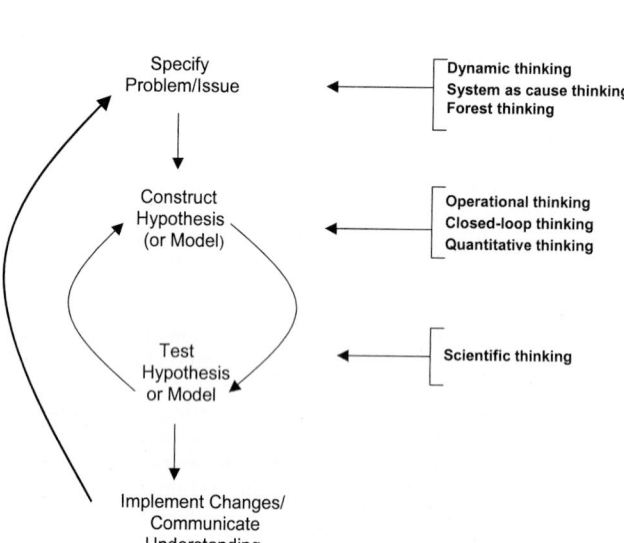

Figure 102-7. Seven system thinking skills. Adapted from Richmond B. *The "Thinking" in Systems Thinking.* Waltham, MA: Pegasus Communications, 2000.

3. *Testing the mode.*
   - Scientific thinking

Each skill brings a unique perspective to the analysis. Systems thinking and complexity theory reframe one's view of systems that are only partially understood by traditional methods.[70] These concepts allow for insights into organizational behavior and evolution, demonstrating sustainability, viability, health, and the capacity to innovate. They offer an alternative view and options for new approaches to complex issues like patient safety. Applying systems thinking and skills at the microsystems level offers the potential for new perspectives to target safety improvement where it matters most–at the point of care (Table 102-2).

TARGETING MEDICATION SAFETY AT THE MICROSYSTEM LEVEL

What to do about safety and performance is the key question for many professionals and health care organizations. How can individuals make a difference? What is the best first step? Will someone come up with a grand master plan that provides a roadmap? IOM's *Chasm* offers four recommendations for a tiered strategy[71]:

- Establish a national focus on patient safety by creating a center for patient safety within the Agency for Healthcare Research and Quality (AHRQ)
- Identify and learn from errors by establishing nationwide mandatory and voluntary reporting systems
- Raise standards and expectations for improvement in safety through the actions of oversight organizations, group purchasers, and professional groups
- Create safety systems inside health care organizations through the implementation of safe practices at the delivery level

For the most part, medical safety research, including research on medication safety, has focused on identification, quantification, and exploration of causal pathways of error, as well as well as the concept of safety culture and the structure that supports a safety culture. Organizations and individuals have been the focus of growing scrutiny, yet until recently, little attention has been addressed at the microsystem level of care delivery, where the vast majority of care is delivered to patients. In relative isolation, researchers have studied medical and surgical staff, interdisciplinary teams and specialty practice to discern what characteristics enhance safety. How structures and strategies of care delivery at the microsystem level affect performance and outcomes holds a promise for vast improvement opportunity. Additional research will be needed to develop and test better ways to prevent errors and improve safety at the microsystem level–the sharp end–of health care organizations.

The microsystems concept is based on systems theory and the work of Deming, Senge, Wheatley, and others who applied systems thinking to concepts of organizational development, improvement, and leadership discussed elsewhere in this chapter.[72–74]

The notion of a microsystem in health care springs from Quinn's theory of the smallest replicable unit, stemming from research of highly successful organizations that continually engineered the frontline interface relationship that connected the organization's core competency with customer need.[75]

Microsystems are defined as small, organized groups of providers and staff caring for defined populations of patients. Nelson et al define clinical microsystems in health care as[76]:

"A small group of people who work together on a regular basis to provide care to discrete subpopulations of patients. It has clinical and business aims, linked processes, and a shared information environment, and it produces performance outcomes. Microsystems evolve over time and are often embedded in larger organizations. They are complex adaptive systems, and as such they must do the primary work associated with core aims, meet the needs of internal staff and maintain themselves over time as clinical units."

Table 102-2. Traditional Thinking VS. System Thinking Skills

TRADITIONAL SKILLS	SYSTEMS THINKING SKILLS
Static thinking Focusing on particular events	**Dynamic Thinking** Framing a problem in terms of a pattern of behavior over time
System as effect thinking Viewing behavior generated by a system as driven by external forces	**System as cause thinking** Placing responsibility for behavior on internal actors who manage the policies and plumbing of the system
Tree by tree thinking Believing that really knowing something means focusing on the details	**Forest thinking** Believing that to know something, you must understand the context of relationships
Factors thinking Listing factors that influence or are correlated with some result	**Operational thinking** Concentrating on getting at causality and understanding how a behavior is actually generated
Straight line thinking Viewing causality as running one way, with each cause independent from all other causes	**Closed loop thinking** Viewing causality as an ongoing process, not a one time event, with the "effect" feeding back to influence the causes, and the causes affecting each other
Measurement thinking Searching for perfectly measured data	**Quantitative thinking** Accepting that you can always quantify, though you can't always measure
Proving truth thinking Seeking to prove models to be true by validating them with historical data	**Scientific thinking** Recognizing that all models are working hypotheses that always have limited applicability

Adapted from Richmond B. *The "Thinking" in Systems Thinking*. Waltham, MA: Pegasus Communications, 2000.

Focus on the microsystem offers the potential for greater standardization of common activities, while still offering needed customization of care for individual patients. An increased use and analysis of information and medical evidence to support daily work is a key component of improvement efforts at the microsystem level. Constant measurement and feedback of data to providers and patients offers the infrastructure and information flow that supports shared learning, understanding, and improvement of process, performance, and outcome. Open dialog, collaborative teamwork and multifunctional/multidisciplinary cooperation, respect, and caring are the hallmark of a highly reliable microsystem of care. Learning within and among microsystems offers an unsurpassed opportunity to identify and spread best practices. The results of interactions between patients, staff, and support processes produce results–clinical, economic, health status, and satisfaction outcomes—that combine to represent a relative value. There is also a gestalt, *what it feels like*, that includes relationships, culture, and climate. The structure, process, and patterns of behavior, sentiment, and results contribute to capability and reliability.

Weick and Sutcliffe have written extensively about highly reliable systems that function in highly complex environments, engage highly sensitive technologies, and have high demand for failure free results.[77] Air traffic control, nuclear reactor sites, and naval carrier commands are among the examples offered for organizations that operate with very low error rates and virtually no failures over many years. Among the behavioral characteristics noted in these highly functioning microsystems are awareness of the unit as a microsystem with its inherent responsibility of purpose and mindfulness of the need for reliability.

Mindfulness is demonstrated by a virtual preoccupation with failure and its consequences as a potential event. Operating in such an environment typically means that simple answers and solutions aren't readily accepted; the team takes deliberate steps to create a rich and detailed view of issues and problems, with full recognition of the complexity, unpredictability, and unknowability of the environment. Highly reliable microsystems fully understand and accept Reason's concept of *latent failures*, loopholes in the system's defenses,

barriers, and safeguards and are attentive to these imperfections that can combine for calamitous results. These microsystems are resilient and have developed capacity to detect, contain, and bounce back from those inevitable errors. They are not error-free, but errors don't disable them. Through a combination of keeping errors small and improvising workarounds, they keep the system functioning. Finally, such systems defer to the expertise demanded by the situation and transfer leadership to the most appropriate team member for the situation. The more richly these practices are adopted and shared within the microsystem, the more mindful it becomes. The result is a radical *presentness*, a connection to the actual demands of the moment and current situation, coupled with a chronic unease that catastrophe might actually occur at any time.

Mohr and Donaldson studied clinical microsystems with the objective of identifying the characteristics that support these organizational units to achieve the success they do.[78] Their findings were reported in an IOM publication and outlined eight attributes associated with high quality, including:

- Constancy of purpose.
- Investment in improvement.
- Alignment of role and training for efficiency and staff satisfaction.
- Integration of information technology into workflow.
- Ongoing measurement of outcomes.
- Supportiveness of the larger organization.
- Connection to the community to enhance care delivery and extend influence.

Nelson et al studied 20 high performing clinical systems characterized by superior performance and initially identified nine, but updated their work to reflect 10 characteristics shared by the systems.[76,79] These characteristics interact and interrelate to support the delivery of outstanding performance, and no single feature can stand alone to produce high quality, high value results (Fig 102-8 and Table 102-3).

Leadership of the microsystem must maintain constancy of purpose, establish clear goals and expectations, foster positive culture, and advocate for the microsystem in the larger organization. Formal leaders, informal leaders, and on the spot leaders are all part of a shared web of leadership that is based on empowering individual autonomy and accountability. Leaders must balance selling and reaching collective goals

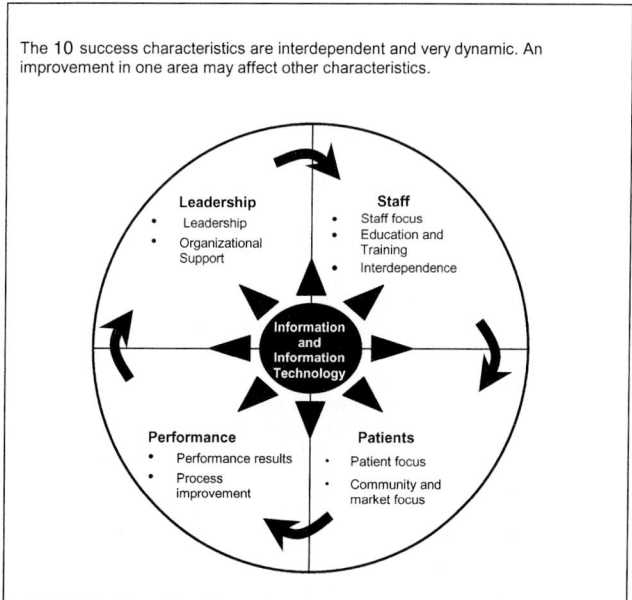

The 10 success characteristics are interdependent and very dynamic. An improvement in one area may affect other characteristics.

Figure 102-8. Clinical microsystems' 10 success characteristics. Adapted from Nelson EC, et al. Microsystems in health care: Learning from high-performing front line clinical units. *Joint Commission Journal on Quality and Safety* 2002; 28(9). Reprinted with permission.

with this autonomy through building knowledge, respectful action, thoughtful review, and reflection.

Organizational support is provided by the larger organization through recognition, information, and resources to legitimize the work of the microsystem. Coordination between microsystems is facilitated, and opportunities to connect and facilitate the work of the microsystem to the larger organization are fostered. Supports are in place to coordinate hand-offs between microsystems.

Staff focus includes attention to hiring the right people for the job, actively integrating new staff into work roles as well as the culture, and aligning competencies with the work. Expectations of staff are high: performance, continuing education, professional growth, and networking are part of the concept of human value chain, linking the microsystem's vision with people. Hiring, orienting, education and (re)training, incentives, and retention are priorities.

Education and training is the ongoing responsibility of the microsystem. There is a team-based approach to training and recognition that continuing education and development of competencies aligning with work roles is recognized as vital for success.

Interdependence is established and maintained through the development of trusting and collaborative relationships of staff based on willingness to help others on the team, understand and appreciate complementary roles and a belief that all contribute individually to a shared purpose. The team is multidisciplinary, and there is respect for each role on the team.

Patient focus is a primary concern, meeting all patient needs through caring, listening, educating, and in response to special requests. Patient focus is exhibited through innovation in response to patient need, provision of a smooth and timely service flow, and the ongoing nurturing of a relationship with the community and other health care resources. The patient is our reason for existence.

Community and market focus should be understood and served by microsystem. The relationship, how the microsystem serves the community, and how the community is a resource to the microsystem must actively connect patients to all available resources to meet their needs. A focus on excellence, partnerships, and innovative collaboration should be part of the individual microsystem and organizational outreach plan.

Performance results should focus on achieving high quality outcomes, reducing costs, streamlining care delivery processes, using feedback effectively, promoting positive competition, and establishing useful dialog about current practice performance and future goals for improvement.

Process improvement must be supported by resources. Within the microsystem and organization, an atmosphere for learning and redesign is supported by a plan for continuous system and practice monitoring, use of benchmarking, change assessment, and an empowered staff focusing on innovation and improvement.

Information and information technology IS THE CONNECTOR of staff to patients, staff to staff, needs with actions to meet needs. Technology can facilitate effective communication and both formal and informal channels must be used to keep everyone informed all the time to assure that learning and knowledge is linked to patient care. Communication, with reliance on technology and redundancy of communication channels keep everyone on the team informed, facilitate open dialog and keeps all team members in the loop on important topics and issues, with information access at the point of need.

Awareness of the need for change is a first step. Nelson et al have developed a short self-assessment instrument for use within clinical microsystems to evaluate development against the characteristics identified for microsystem success (See Appendix 1). Self-assessment should begin with introduction of the concept of clinical microsystems and completion of the evaluation by all staff members. Informational findings should be collated and distributed to the team. Then discussion of the results should occur using the findings as an opportunity to identify the strengths and development opportunities for the microsystem. Develop a plan for change based on the results. Focus on improving the level of microsystem performance: establish a few simple rules or minimal specifications, select a small number of measures, and provide regular, performance-focused data as feedback to gauge the level of performance. Develop a clear and compelling sense of organizational purpose. Find ways to recognize, promote, and reward performance, innovation, and improvement that supports the mission. Establish shared leadership, decentralized decision-making, and autonomy. Exercise *tight-loose-tight* controls; tight alignment of the mission, vision, and strategies, flexibility at the microsystem level to allow individuals and teams to achieve the mission as they see fit, tight control over accountability to deliver safety and performance results.[80,81]

Nelson and colleagues suggest that understanding and nurturing clinical microsystems may create an opportunity for leverage toward the goal of a safety and more effective health care system.[76] But, there is reason for caution. Galvin noted[82]:

"New ideas in health care have a tendency to oversimplify and overpromise. Whether it be managed care, continuous quality improvement, or defined contribution, proponents seem to subscribe to the domino theory of health policy: if only this one idea could be applied appropriately, the great stack of complicated issues in health care would fall into place one by one."

The domino effect only works when all the dominoes are aligned. As described previously, attention to microsystem level activity and alignment has been a critical gap, but it is no silver bullet. Mastery at the clinical microsystem level can make a significant contribution to performance improvement for safety and outcomes, but it cannot effect the totality of change without equally effective attention at the self care (patient), relationship (patient-caregiver), macrosystem (organizational), and social (community and public policy) levels described in *Chasm*. There is no simple, quick fix to a complex, immense, and dysfunctional health care system dilemma like medication safety.

At the sharp end—microsystem level—one needs to understand the medication use process and the performance results it produces.

UNDERSTANDING THE MEDICATION USE PROCESS

While not all medication use systems are exactly the same, there are some constant and essential components of the medication use process that appear across the continuum of patient

Table 102-3. Scope of Ten Success Characteristics, Underlying Principles, and Safety Impact

SCOPE OF SUCCESS CHARACTERISTIC	UNDERLYING PRINCIPLE	SAFETY IMPACT
Leadership - Maintain constancy of purpose - Establish clear goals/expectations - Foster positive culture - Advocacy with in macro organization - Formal, informal, on-the-spot	Leader balances setting and reaching collective goals with empowering individual autonomy and accountability	- Define safety vision - Identify constraints for safety improvement - Allocate resources for plan development, implementation, monitoring and evaluation - Build input of microsystem to plan development - Align quality and safety goals - Provide update to Board of Trustees
Organizational support - Recognition, resources, information - Enhance and legitimize work of microsystem	Larger organization finds ways to connect and facilitate work of microsystem, including coordination and handoffs between Microsystems	- Work with clinical Microsystems to identify patient safety issues and make relevant local changes - Put the necessary resources and tools into the hands of individuals without making it superficial
Staff focus - Selective hiring - Integration into culture and roles - Aligning work with training competencies - High expectations for performance, continuing education, professional growth, networking	Human resource value chain that links microsystem's vision with real people for hiring, orienting, continuously educating, retraining and providing incentives	- Assess current safety culture - Identify gap between current culture and safety vision - Plan cultural interventions - Conduct periodic assessments of culture
Education and training - Ongoing education - Organizational learning - Work roles and competencies aligned - Best use of people and resources	Team approaches to training create learning that is collaborative and focused on quality, safety and integrated into work flow	- Develop patient safety curriculum - Provide training and education of key clinical and management leadership - Develop a core of people with patient safety skills who can work across microsystems as a resource
Interdependence of care team - Trust - Collaboration - Willingness to help others - Appreciation of complimentary roles - Recognition of inputs to shared purpose	Multidisciplinary team provides care and every person is respected for individual vital role	- Build PDSA into debriefings - Use daily huddles for AARs (after action reviews) and celebrate identifying errors
Patient focus - Caring - Listening - Educating - Response to special requests - Innovating - Providing smooth service flow - Relationship with community resources	The patient is the common focal point, it's why we're all here	- Establish patient and family partnerships - Support disclosure and truth about medical error
Community and market focus - Partnership with community for resource exchange - Outreach - Innovation and excellence	Resource exchange and information sharing to assure that patient needs are met	- Analyze safety issues in community and partner with external groups to reduce risk to population
Performance patterns - Patient outcomes - Cost avoidance - Streamlined delivery - Data feedback - Positive competition - Open dialog about performance	Outcomes are routinely measured, with feedback to Microsystems leading to change based on data	- Develop key safety measures - Create the "business case" for safety
Process improvement - Learning and redesign focus - Continuous care monitoring - Benchmarking - Tests of change - Staff empowered to innovate	Studying, measuring and improving care are essential elements of daily work	- Identify patient safety priorities based on assessment of key safety measures - Address the work that will be required at the microsystem level - Establish patient safety "demonstration sites" - Transfer the learning
Information and IT - Information is key - Technology links information and care - Communication and channels	Information is a connector designed to support work of the unit for the right information at the right time	- Enhance error reporting system - Build safety concepts into information flow (e.g. checklists, reminder systems, etc)

Adapted from Nelson EC, et al. Microsystems in health care: learning from high-performing front-line clinical units. *Joint Commission Journal on Quality and Safety 2002;* 28(9). Reprinted with permission.

care. These same steps occur in the inpatient, outpatient, acute care, long-term care, and home care settings. Medication use complication and errors can occur in all patient care settings; no patient care arena is immune.

Describing Medication Use

Medication use is a complex process involving, at times, multiple organizations and professionals from various disciplines. Risk factors can be identified along the medication use continuum. Knowledge of medications and timely access to accurate and complete information contribute to a series of interrelated decisions executed at various times throughout the patient care process. Error can creep in at any point. Safe medication use is dependent on a number of well-executed, sequential steps. Some errors are errors of commission (eg, administration of an improper medication); other errors are of omission (eg, failure to administer a medication that was prescribed). The diagram below depicts the steps involved in the medication use process. Consider how error may interfere with the appropriate and safe execution of the steps shown in Figure 102-9.

These steps involve participation of a variety of individuals and can range from expertly trained health professionals to the layperson in the ambulatory setting. At each step of the process, multiple factors can determine whether or not the step will be performed without error. An error-free final result depends upon error-free performance throughout the entire process. Thus, focusing on system change, rather than the individual practitioner, can yield more long-standing, predictable, and effective development of safety improvements.

Collaboration Across the Medication Use Process

Collaboration is essential to minimize patient risk in the medication use process. Health care providers within the organization need to understand and identify how these components function and who is involved in making these steps safe. Clear understanding of the critical safety issues at each one of these steps is of particular importance because the primary goal of adverse event identification is adverse event prevention. Each step can be considered a risk point and provides opportunities for internal checks and balances.

At each step in the medication use process, it is often assumed physicians, nurses, pharmacists, and other health care providers in the organization play a role in patient evaluation. This evaluation would include assessing patient characteris-

tics, medication selection, concurrent medications, medication dosage selection, and medication administration methods appropriate for the condition to be treated. Additionally, it is also believed that by having this collaboration, each set of practitioner eyes can protect patients by catching a mistake made earlier in the process or by correcting for another individual's lack of understanding or poor judgment.

Despite this practitioner-centered safety system, errors can—and do—occur.

This is not to suggest that the vital role of health care professionals should be ignored. Physicians, nurses, pharmacists, and others will continue to play an important role in ensuring the safe and appropriate use of medications. The current system of prescribing, dispensing, administering, and monitoring, however, often places the responsibility on the individual to avoid making the mistake. Because this expectation seems unreasonable, organizations should focus efforts to improve medication use safety by using a systems-based approach that identifies:

- Errors that occur most frequently
- Possible root causes of errors
- Error prevention strategies to make it harder for the same or similar errors to occur
- If the organization has a system that makes it harder to commit an error, it will be more difficult for mistakes to go on undetected and for harm to come to patients

System Failures Identified in the Medication Use Process

Varieties of systems failures have been identified in hospitals that have studied factors associated with adverse events.[83] These system failures are listed below:

- Deficiencies in medication knowledge, including prescribing of incorrect medications, doses, forms, frequency, or routes of administration
- Failure to verify the identity or dose of medication administered, often due to look-alike packaging or similarities between medication names
- Inaccessibility of patient information including laboratory test results, current medications, and information on the patient's current condition
- Incorrect transcription of orders, often due to illegibility of the physician's handwriting
- Failure to note known medication allergies
- Inefficient order tracking, making it difficult to determine when a medication has been given, missed/discontinued or changed
- Poor communication between services, including between nurses and pharmacists
- Improper use of administration devices
- Lack of standardized dosing schedules or disregard of existing standards
- Lack of standardized system for medication distribution
- Lack of standardized procedure across units
- Errors in preparation of intravenous medications (when performed in the patient care area)
- Poor information transfer when patients are moved from one patient care area to another
- Inadequate or nonexistent system for resolving conflicts related to medication orders
- Deficiencies in staffing or work assignments leading to excessive workloads, inconsistent availability of staff or inadequate management
- Lack of feedback and follow-up information on observed adverse drug events

As a result of this identification, a variety of improvement recommendations have been made for health care systems to consider as they identify methods to reduce adverse drug events.[84] Strategies include:

- Elimination of handwritten medical records and physician orders
- Institute fail-safe tracking of medications and laboratory tests to ensure that patients receive correct medications and tests on time

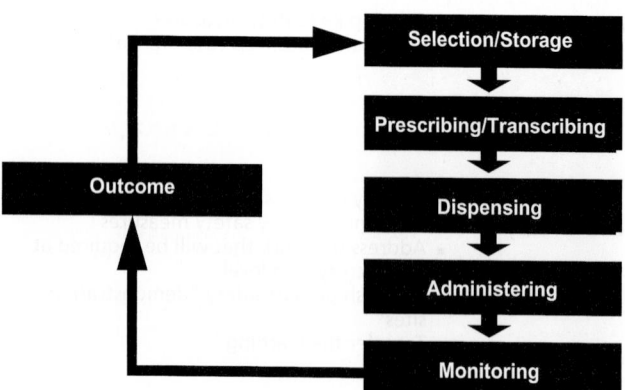

Figure 102-9. Medication use process. Adapted from JCAHO. JCAHO 2003 Hospital Accreditation Standards. Oakbrook, IL: Joint Commission Resources, 2004:175. Reprinted with permission.

- Establish protocols and guidelines that outline standardized practices
- Provide all medications in unit dose packaging, ready for patient administration
- Standardize medication procedures such as protocols for the use of hazardous medications, medication terminology, and medication names
- Make it difficult for someone to do something wrong by error proofing
- Implement bar-coding
- Make relevant patient information available at the point of patient care
- Improve the patient's knowledge about treatment

Although, most of the suggestions provided could be implemented promptly and have been demonstrated to greatly reduce certain types of errors, these are not routinely incorporated into practice within organizations. Organizations must develop a systematic approach to evaluate their own medication use processes and establish a plan for improvement at each step: storage and selection, prescribing, dispensing, administering, and monitoring. Many recommendations have been provided in the literature for consideration to improve medication use safety.

Recommendations for Storage and Selection

Organizations of all types should develop a list of medications (a formulary) that is maintained and based on patient need and safety as well as economics. As this list is developed, proper storage and control of medications must be established. How medications are selected for routine use should consider parameters of need, given the type of diseases and conditions treated; effectiveness in terms of toxicities, pharmacokinetic properties; therapeutic or pharmaceutical equivalence; risk potential such as known incidence of adverse drug events or potential for error in the medication use process (prescribing, preparation, dispensing, and administering), and acquisition cost or patient cost impact.

Practitioners should also identify methods to reduce the chance of medication error causes by medications with similar names or similar packaging. It is not enough to *tell* practitioners to *be careful* as they select or store medications for use. Reading the label and product name selected out loud may help serve as a double check. For each product, repeating name of the medication, dose, and route may help identify if the wrong product is selected. Human nature leads practitioners to identify items by color, shape, font type on packaging, symbology as well as other visual characteristics. As practitioners select medications for use within their health care organization, an evaluation of reported safety alerts due to labeling and packaging should be considered. Known look-like or sound-alike products should be avoided. At a minimum, placing these look-alikes, sound-alikes in different locations and apart from each other in the storage area with additional labeling or signage warning of similarities may also assist in promoting correct product selection.

Manufacturers have also been called upon to improve the readability of medication labeling and packaging. Reducing label clutter on packaging, use of color coding along with distinctive background patterns or borders, providing two-sided labeling and assuring contrast of important medication name, dose and route information on packaging have all been suggested as methods to improve the medication labeling process.[85] Additional suggestions for standardizing display of medication concentration, strength, or terminology such as single dose and multi-dose packaging has also been advocated.[85] Often a display of additional advertising information and a display of company name and logo can interfere with product identification. Just as the medication ordering process can be improved by including standardizing terminology and warning information, use of

standards could also improve safety. Some manufacturers have begun using distinctive typeface, serif or sans serif and upper- or lower-case letters to convey distinctive portions of look-alike or sound-alike names.

Recommendations for Prescribing Improvements

Many opportunities exist to improve the safety of the medication use process. The prescribing phase of the medication use process, however, encompasses the majority of medication errors that result in preventable ADEs. The knowledge that ADEs can be prevented compels organizations to identify the factors or system failures that contribute to the errors in the prescribing phase. Such factors identified in the prescribing phase include[86,87]:

- Availability of medication information at time of prescribing
- Access to patient information at time of prescribing
- Availability of dosing information at time of prescribing
- Availability of allergy information at time of prescribing
- Accuracy or completeness of order by prescriber
- Legibility of handwriting
- Use of abbreviations
- Use of decimals in expressions of weight and measure
- Use of varied units of measure
- Medication name look-alikes or sound-alikes

Error Potential in the Prescribing Phase

The three most common forms of prescribing errors include dosing errors, prescribing medications to which the patient had an allergic history, and errors involving the prescribing of inappropriate dosage forms.[87] In the examples listed, timely access and use of information is essential to avoid adverse drug events. Although not a panacea, use of a computerized medication order entry system can significantly contribute to the prevention of medication errors. The type of health care information that is best suited for computerization includes[88]:

- General information storage (eg, patient or medication information, retrieval)
- Repetitive functions (eg, dosage guidelines, medication names, allergy information)
- Complex processes that depend on reproducible results
- Items where legibility is essential
- Items that require timely attention
- Items where accuracy is vital

In the prescribing stage, lack of medication knowledge and lack of patient information account for the majority of errors. Many physicians find it a challenge to keep up with this data flood and often prescribe on the basis of incomplete or obsolete information, greatly increasing the risk of error. In addition, an enormous volume of new medical information is generated each year, including information on powerful medications available for acute and chronic disease. Dosing calculations are a well-recognized cause of medication errors. Performing routine, independent cross-checking of dosing calculations are useful when verifying dosages for pediatric, geriatric, oncology, transplant, or other populations with special medication requirements. For verifying dosages, use of both mg/kg and mg/m^2 (or other expressions as unit per weight or body surface area) in addition to actual dose calculated is recommended. Another potential safety improvement includes standardizing dosages whenever possible as well as the use of commercially available dosage forms. This will require prescriber approval and cooperation. However, avoiding complex calculations is one way to avoid calculation errors. If transcription of medication orders is part of the health care organization's practice to transfer prescribing information to a medication administration record, similar guidelines and standards for evaluating standards, completeness, and accuracy should be put into place with a routine evaluation of practice compliance.

Other practices (eg, the use of verbal orders, electronic order transmission via facsimile machine, use of global prescription orders such as *resume all previous orders*) provide many opportunities for miscommunication. Whenever possible, verbal orders should be avoided. Only specific personnel (eg, physicians, pharmacists, nurses) should be allowed to dictate and receive verbal medication orders and only in approved circumstances. When used, verbal orders should be enunciated slowly and distinctly. Difficult medication names and instructions should be spelled out. Ambiguity should be clarified. The individual receiving the order should transcribe the order and then immediately read the information back to the prescriber. In the inpatient or long-term care setting, the prescriber should countersign and verify the verbal order as soon as possible.

Many health care organizations now use facsimile transmissions for prescription order transmission. Streaked, blackened, or faded areas and phone line *noise* appearing as random markings are often present on facsimile transmissions. Careful inspection of the copy is necessary to evaluate if extraneous markings interfere with the actual order. Transmission of prescription orders in this manner still can contain illegible, ambiguous, or improper abbreviations.

Failure to write a prescription order can also provide many opportunities for error. When medications are held or resumed or patient care is transferred to another location or provider, it is imperative that a complete review of medications is occurs. Simply stating *resume all, hold all,* or *continue all previous medications* is not acceptable practice. Reviewing all medications for appropriateness is good practice and also a systematic method to review the indication for use and monitoring plan in place for the patient.

Another technique used to assure safe and effective prescribing practice is the use of a medication formulary. While physicians often consider a medication formulary as simply a method to control expenditures, formularies can be used as instructional and quality tools to assure that only agents that are safe, effective, and necessary for use are provided for patients under care. An organized formulary process comprises of a systematic peer review of medications for use and monitoring within a health system. Medications are typically evaluated for safety, effectiveness, policy implication, and practice requirements. Use of a formulary can assure that information is provided in a timely fashion, because the product has been thoroughly evaluated for use.

Executing a safe and effective prescription order requires communication of complete information to all intended readers. A complete order should contain, at a minimum:

- Patient name
- Patient specific data
- Generic and brand name (ideally, both names should be provided; if only one name used, generic is preferred)
- Medication strength, in metric units by weight
- Dosage form
- Amount to be dispensed, in metric units (terms such as bottle, tube or ampule should be avoided)
- Complete directions for use including route of administration, duration, dosing frequency, medication purpose, and number of authorized refills

While abbreviations might appear to be a time saver, their use can lead to confusion, misinterpretation, and increase the potential for error. Misplaced or missing decimal points also pose concerns. Recommendations for improving orders requiring fractions or decimal indications include adding a zero before a decimal point and eliminating trailing decimal points and zeros. Various organizations, including the Institute for Safe Medication Practices, have published lists of abbreviations and decimal point miscommunications that have been associated with medication errors and should not be used.[89] To reduce error potential, preprinted order forms have been suggested to reduce error potential. It is important to note that if preprinted orders are not carefully developed, they may actually induce errors. As standard orders, algorithms or preprinted guidelines are developed, all disciplines involved in the ordering process, should be involved in the development, review, and approval of these documents.

Prescribing improvement efforts should include development of policies and procedures that support safe medication use and ordering. Practitioners should routinely be required to assess and document the need for and selecting the correct medication. Regimen selection should assure that specific, individual treatment goals are identified. Improvement efforts should also include attention to avoiding delay in treatment or in responding to a medication use concern, including inappropriate indication (or no clear treatment indication) and failure to provide preventive care or prophylactic treatment. Prescribing plans should include monitoring or follow up treatment.

Prescribing can be improved if prescribers have the necessary data to assure that decisions can be made (ie, indications for use, potential for interactions, risks and benefits, monitoring concerns). The process of medication prescribing via computer order entry would greatly affect the rate of errors associated with ADEs. A computerized medication ordering system could provide alerts regarding specific prescribing concerns in the medication ordering process (eg, identifying dose, allergy, drug-drug interactions). Having a routine approach to detect, intercept, and prevent these problems will reduce the potential for an adverse event to occur.

Clinical information systems can also assist in reducing adverse drug events and medication errors by:

- Increasing patient profile access and systematic screening of medication orders
- Alerting medical staff of abnormal doses, medication interactions, or allergies (based on patient profile)
- Generating 24-hour patient medication updates
- Recording medication administration

Computer support in the prescribing process is beneficial due to the fact that this process demands attention to detail related to the medication product, patient, and population characteristics, clinical information, and administrative issues.

It is important to remember that practitioners receiving the information within the organization are still required to use the appropriate skills to determine the relevance of this information for the patient. Simply automating the prescriptive process does not in and of itself make it safer.

Lessons have been learned in other domains regarding the impact and implications of technology.[90] If one thinks technology can solve security problems, then the person doesn't understand the problems and the technology. New technologies have enormous capacity, but what is seldom thought about is not how well it works, but how well it fails.

The most important element of any safety measure is people, not technology. The trick is to remember that technology can't save the day. The system has to be built around the people. Highly trained and motivated people bring to a task a quality not found in and technology: human judgment. Human beings do make mistakes of course, but they can recover from failure in ways that machines and software cannot. The well-trained mind is ductile. It can understand surprises and overcomes them. It fails well. *Key Learning*: Automating the process may, in fact, introduce new errors into the process. There is no substitute for human judgment within the medication use process.

Recommendations for Dispensing

In general, pharmacies and pharmacists are responsible for assuring that medications are dispensed correctly. Most dispensing errors involve providing an incorrect medication, dosage strength, or dosage form to a patient.[91,92] Other common dispensing errors are dosing calculation errors or lack of interaction or contraindication with other prescribed medications. Typically, these errors are due to commission or omission and as a result of a "slip" or a "mistake" as identified by Reason.[51]

Error Potential in the Dispensing Phase

Dispensing is a complex process requiring a series of sequential tasks including preparation and processing of the prescription, locating and preparing the product, delivering the product to the end user and potentially providing counseling, screening and assessment activities at the time the medication is provided to the end user. The dispensing process has both mechanical and judgmental components. As a result, prevention of dispensing errors will require a comprehensive approach including evaluation of:

- Work environment: workload, distractions, physical location of service, hours of operation
- Inventory management: outdated or unused products, look-alikes, sound-alikes, clutter, labeling, purchasing of unit of use products
- Information resources: available references, updates, consultants, computer or decision support technology
- Performance evaluation: evaluation of staff competency and practice skill, knowledge and behaviors, cross-checking redundancies
- Patient involvement: patient education and review with *show and tell* techniques

This includes developing policies and procedures that support safe dispensing and distribution of medications. Methods to assure complete review and processing of the order should be defined. Other recommendations include controlling the distribution of medications through the use of a patient medication dose system. In cases where dosing can be standardized, every attempt should be made to provide the medication in the most ready to use format to decrease the potential for error. If necessary, specific guidelines for compounding or preparing medications should be clearly outlined and evaluated for compliance. Medications should be provided for patients in a timely manner while including safeguards such as the review of all prescription orders by a pharmacist. Products should be safely labeled, adhering to appropriate law and regulation as well and using a standardized method.

Several critical steps have been advocated for improving dispensing accuracy[93,94]:

- Secure or sequester high-risk medications
- Develop and implement standardized storage procedures
- Reduce distraction potential and improve workflow in dispensing environment
- Use reminders (labels, computer alerts) to prevent look-alike, sound-alike mix-ups
- Keep prescription order, label, medication and the medication container together throughout dispensing process
- Perform a final check on prescription content including verification with original prescription order and label
- Enter a manufacturer identification code into the computer profile and on prescription label
- Perform a final check on the prescription label, if possible, using automation such as bar-coding
- Provide patient counseling

Use of automation to improve the safety of dispensing in the inpatient and outpatient settings has been on the increase. In the 1980s, automated dispensing devices became available with hopes to reduce medication error rates, increase pharmacy and nursing department efficiency, improve availability of medication access on inpatient units, and enhance pharmacy inventory and billing capability. These systems are essentially medication storage devices that electronically control and dispense medications as well as track medication use. Many commercial systems are available. These devices require user identifiers, passwords, and track access by health care provider and use of medications by patient. Some systems include medication information support and integrate with internal and external systems such as medication profiling systems, clinical information databases, and the Internet.

The goal for utilizing such devices is to provide a *closed loop system*. It is a system that allows integration of prescribing information, medication information, real time clinical screening, intervention, and medication administration activities.

Recently, the Food and Drug Administration proposed rules that would require the use of bar codes on medication labels. This regulatory action would require manufacturers to provide linear bar code labels for prescription and over the counter products. While the rule will require approximately 3 years to be implemented after the final rules are published at the end of 2003, it is anticipated that this action will result in 413,000 fewer adverse events over 20 years as well as a significant reduction in costs associated with injury, litigation, and malpractice insurance.[95]

While automation has the potential for controlling, standardizing, and distributing medications in a timely and monitored fashion, human intervention can prevent systems from functioning as designed. Practitioners can override some patient safety features. When automated systems are replenished with stock or when returns are made, refilling mix-ups can occur. If verification of the prescription order, access to only the medication required or real time patient verification cannot be performed at the same time as medication dispensed (ie, not a closed loop system for medication use), error can still occur within the medication use process. While this type of automation has great potential for decreasing medication errors, it also has the potential to increase the opportunity for error if not applied or maintained appropriately. Certainly, judgment in the dispensing process cannot be adequately automated or replaced by use of such as device.

Recommendations for Administration

Responsibility for safe medication administration is often inappropriately placed on one individual, the person performing the actual administration activity. In fact, safe medication administration is a team effort, relying on all of the individuals involved in the medication use process to detect and evaluate clinical practice as the decision is made to provide a medication for a patient.

Error Potential in the Administration Phase

The administration phase, serves as a last final check on processing the entire medication order itself and includes:

- Evaluating the written order for appropriateness and completeness
- Assuring appropriate indication for use
- Evaluating and interpreting use of terminology and order method (abbreviation, units of measure, use of verbal orders)
- Dosing calculation or verification
- Identification of the patient
- Timing of treatment in context of other therapies
- Preparation and possibly dispensing of medication
- Proper use of medication devices
- Patient education
- Documentation of treatment

Efforts to improve medication administration safety should include addressing all these aspects of administration through appropriate policies and procedures. This would include methods to assure that the right medication is administered to the right patient at the right dose, right time, right route, and for an indicated reason. Informing the patient about the medication and whenever possible including the patient in the medication administration. Prescription orders should be verified and patients identified prior to administration. Processes to assure that medications are retrieved from the patient supply when they are discontinued from the regimen or recalled by the manufacturer should also be in place. Staff must also be evaluated regarding their skills, knowledge, and behaviors expected for safe medication use. This includes their capabilities in the use of medication devices, ability to complete or verify dosage calculations and prepare medications. An assessment of documentation, communication, and clinical problem-solving capabilities as well as other medication use competencies are necessary to assure application of knowledge at this final point of care to assure safe medication use.

Recommendations for Monitoring and Outcomes

Ongoing measurement and monitoring of medication use is essential to assure safe and effective medication use. As part of any safety improvement initiative, this would include developing policies and procedures that support monitoring of medication effects. Use of guidelines and clinical pathways are common methods to assure a systematic approach to monitoring therapy. Documentation and exchange of these medication use outcomes findings should be shared with patients and other care providers as required. Systems should be in place to assure that patient responses are monitored and that both benefits of therapy and unexpected outcomes are documented. This necessitates identification and reporting of adverse drug events as well as methods of re-evaluating medication selection, regimen, frequency, and duration. Efforts to collaborate and communicate between care providers and for including patients in the process should be established to allow for complete review and management of patients medication regimens. Including patient perceptions along with information from the medical record and medication profile or list is essential. The primary concerns that exist with current monitoring systems include lack of:

- Guideline use
- Therapeutic monitoring plans
- Collaboration on common goal or of therapy
- Patient involvement

Gaps in the monitoring process, design, or follow-through have the potential to cause medication use errors.

CHANGING SYSTEMS WITHIN ORGANIZATIONS

Improving organizational and environmental factors in health care, as demonstrated in the aviation industry, enables system change to occur. If teams in an organization can work effectively, communication improves, resulting in the motivation to understand error. Unless an organization has a culture that supports understanding and reducing errors, system changes may only be minimally effective. Ideally, a strategy to improve error prevention should be coupled with organizational transformation and structured process changes. Optimizing a work environment for safety, increasing mechanisms for communication, having a leadership agenda, and commitment for medication safety improvement are essential components for an organization.

The Institute for Healthcare Improvement has identified that prevention must be the organizational focus and has provided strategies that should be included in the plan for medication use safety. The following items have routinely been identified as a top 10 list for improvement in the literature[96]:

- Improving knowledge about medications (availability, access and timeliness)
- Dose/identity tracking of medications (process understanding of distribution)
- Available patient information (availability, access, accuracy and timeliness)

- Order transcription (elimination of process)
- Allergy defense (hard stop capabilities, access to patient information)
- Medication order tracking (streamlining and effective communication of patient needs)
- Communication (patient information, system performance, medication use)
- Device use (standardization and competency regarding use)
- Standardization of medication dose
- Standardization of medication distribution

The challenge of a list like this is simple: it does not represent a one-time fix. Rather, it is a life-long agenda that requires ongoing and persistent attention. Reducing errors within an organization requires mindfulness (ie, diligence, attention to detail, and ongoing re-evaluation of this very dynamic medication use process).

However, strategies that have been put into place to reduce error potential have traditionally focused solely on the following items:

- Unit dose or unit of use medications
- Protocol and checklist development
- Computerization of patient information
- Standards including dosing times, specific medications for specific procedures or guidelines
- Training and education programs
- Decentralized or increased availability of pharmacists

These system redesign efforts have been recommended in the literature for years and appear insufficient to address the latent error potential within the health care system. Although this list identifies an array of systems improvements, an organization must understand that people make safety possible within the system. Organizations must routinely investigate and identify their own risk potentials. Having discussions regarding *near misses* may help identify where potential risks exist. Ongoing staff dialog, creating a sense of mindfulness, or even a preoccupation with safety is necessary to assure that organizational membership will take the lead in identifying next steps for improving medication use . . . and where the true risks lie.

The ongoing challenge for leadership is that there is a need for operational diligence. Identifying the careful balance between describing and supporting system change and integrating a human factors approach regarding how to implement and use these system improvements. In a sense, this is about understanding and designing a practitioner-medication use system interface at an organizational level and measuring and monitoring its performance.

How are adverse events identified and discussed within organizations? What prevents learning from occurring? How are prevention strategies developed? Literature suggests that members of a health care organization are more likely to discuss their errors when provided protection from disciplinary action. This is important in light of the fact that 95% of all medication errors go unreported because staff fears punishment.[97]

By establishing a method for all health care professionals to contribute information on medication use safety and errors in a nonthreatening fashion, an environment can be created to focus on improving patient care. If teams are allowed to work in an effective and efficient environment, communication can be improved and personnel can become motivated to understand the cause of errors along with methods to report and prevent them. Process redesign is essential, but unless the organization has a culture that supports understanding and reducing error, the effects of process change will be minimal. The team is the critical component for implementing a successful safety strategy. Leadership must focus on creating vision and collaboration that will allow the team to be successful.

Leadership for Safety

Medical and health care professions have experienced a sharp shift of attention in recent years, and patient safety is the new focus for what ails the system. Leadership is a critical and recurring theme for the improvement of patient and medication use safety. In *Chasm,* the IOM calls for strong and clear leadership for patient safety throughout the system. Baldridge award criteria charge an organization's senior leadership to set directions and create a patient focus, clearly visible values, and high expectations. Leaders seeking Baldridge recognition must ensure the creation of strategies, systems, and methods for achieving excellence in health care, stimulating innovation, and building knowledge and capabilities.[98]

Leadership is an attribute that allows some people to attract the loyalty and trust of followers by the simple fact of existing. Their resonant message, created infrastructure, amassed commitment, evidence, and rightness of vision captures follower's minds. While it is not the only, or even the most important factor, charismatic ability to communicate a heart-felt belief in a goal, the passion of commitment and the certainty of success serves to capture the hearts of followers. Capturing their souls with a belief system cements the bond of a shared goal and begins the distribution of leadership more widely.

Leadership is a term that has traditionally been used to identify formal leaders who are designated by position, and whose responsibilities include setting directional vision, mission, and achievement targets for the organization. They are also responsible for the setting and maintaining the culture, climate, and values that define how the organization behaves, grows, and interacts, internally and externally.

It is misleading to think that leadership is only provided by a few highly positioned people in the organization. This is particularly true for achievement of complex objectives like improving patient and medication use safety. Increasingly, the concept of leadership is becoming *democratized,* to recognize situational, informal, and *on-the-spot* leadership, and the growing notion that leadership must exist in everyone, to varying degrees, as health care organizations (*Read:* complex adaptive systems) learn to learn in a complex and evolving environment.

Leadership inspired by complexity theory acknowledges that change occurs naturally and continually within systems and that individuals engage in that change for a variety of reasons and to varying degrees. In the systems view, the leader's primary responsibility is to create systems that widely disseminate rich and credible information about better practices in ways that are meaningful to the various target audiences– those individuals who can influence performance and outcomes at the sharp end of the system, where care is delivered to the patient.

Fundamentally, health care organizations must, therefore, evolve to be learning organizations and to implement a strategy to eliminate *blaming* behavior, transitioning to the ubiquitous *safety culture.* Senge defines leadership as being about creating a domain in which human beings continually deepen their understanding of reality and become more capable of participating in unfolding the world.[99] Ultimately, leadership is about creating new realities.

There is no question that leadership for safety needs to start at the top. The real value is to commit to investment in the organization–from the board of trustees to the caregiver to the security guard (whether physical or information) to the support staff–and to build a belief that with a concerted and best effort on the part of every individual, that the organization can survive and triumph, and that patients will be the real winners in the process. To accomplish this, leaders need to allow themselves to be vulnerable, to admit they don't possess all the answers, acknowledging that patient safety is a mutual and joint quest for innovation and solutions that reside in the collective minds of everyone (all the stakeholders.) This need starts with trustee leaders, who must ask:

- What initiatives are in place to assess quality?
- How is medication use safety addressed in the organization's mission statement?
- Is there an overall approach or plan for medication use safety?
- Does the plan include senior level leadership, provide defined objectives, commitment to the necessary personnel, and budget sufficient for goals?

- Is there a need for a chief medication use safety officer? Is the role focused on the importance of the medication use process? How closely is that role tied to the medication use process and delivery system?
- What commitments have been made to developing a safety of culture? What is the current state of the culture relative to safety?
- What measures are in place to ensure accurate, timely and relevant reporting for safety, with measures against progress?

This *starting at the top* will require change in attitudes and beliefs. Trust evolves from vulnerability (ie, the admission that no one has all the answers). Collaboration means letting go of insecure competition that assumes that one's gain is another's loss; being right destroys value. Communication must be ramped up and skills honed; this is the key to solving problems. Communication is also key to relationship building, which translates to understanding and openness; it is a lot harder to oppose what one understands. While there is some measure of risk associated with taking an untested course, there are no tested courses of action to improve safety, no guarantees. Leaders who will contribute to improvement and learning will be forced to take risks, to become the change they envision, reflecting a Gandhian philosophy. Finally, leaders need to personalize the need to change. If there are insurmountable problems, imposed external issues, the leader must assume the need to change the way the problem is framed, to change context, to assume that as some level, the organization, the leader, individuals are contributing to the problem or could behave differently to avoid it, minimize impact, or eliminate it.

Creating a learning organization requires a shared vision, inspiring individual workers–at every level, in every discipline–to embrace the effort and commit their best individual effort. This vision must be patient-focused, expectations set high but not impossible, sufficiently tangible, so that individual workers can identify with the vision and translate it to the context of their own day-to-day activities. Leaders, formal and dispersed, must take responsibility for fostering learning, through the use of champions, traditional education and training infrastructure and a culture-building that values, and rewards, innovative new applications of knowledge for performance and safety improvement. Learning opportunities should be designed to transcend passive assimilation of information, focusing on double-loop learning that is applied and reinforced by feedback of information that is close to the work and performance outcomes in both time and proximity.

It is a popular but confounding truism that every system is perfectly designed to get the results it gets. How then does one learn to redesign systems, to learn to change, to take action by deploying a plan to improve patient safety, particularly as it relates to medication use? To create change, leaders at every level of the organization will need to build knowledge, take action, and assess information to determine an enduring course of action.

Leaders–and every individual committed to improving the safety of the health care system–will need to commit to gaining new knowledge and skills that are not taught in the average health care–or pharmacy–curriculum. Needed knowledge and skills will include:

- Health care as a process, systems thinking, and a holistic view of managing and coordinating care
- Science of variation, measurement, assessment, data collection, analysis and reporting, including the concept of the balanced scorecard, statistical process control (eg, flow charting, graphing, pareto charts, run or control charts, RCA/FMEA, etc.)
- Customer and beneficiary knowledge and insight including what are the expectations and preferences of customers vs. what is possible given system constraints to influence the scope and boundaries of care decisions and to plan for the future
- Leading, following, and making changes, including change management, knowledge of assessment and influence of climate and culture, and the fine art of managing knowledge workers in an environment of scarce human resources
- Collaboration and reinforcement of individual capability for maximal impact, working effectively in teams to optimize the culture, climate and knowledge management of the organization, to create

the best work place environment, attract and retain the best employees and to become a world class example of quality and results
- Social context, reflecting community and organizational values, and fiscal and ethical accountability for responsible action
- Learning to develop new, useful knowledge based on empiric testing and application of evidence-based information for improvement
- Support and enhancement of individual professional discipline's subject matter with specific attention to evolving core competencies

Geller suggests that leaders need to focus transactionally on another, parallel agenda[100]:

- Focus on process
- Educate, train, and retrain
- Use conditional statements, not absolutes, and always leave the door open
- Listen, first, last, always
- Promote personal and individual ownership
- Create and encourage choice
- Set and enforce expectations
- Maintain a paradoxical balance between confidence and uncertainty
- Create more distinctions (not fewer) to generate a continuum of performance and value that will spread performance improvement opportunities and targets
- LOOK BEYOND THE NUMBERS; not everything can be measured

The IOM report, *Health Professions Education: A Bridge to Quality*, issued in 2003, recommended an overarching vision for the education and competency base needed for health professionals to be successful in a commitment to redesigning the health care system[12]:

"All health professionals should be educated to deliver patient-centered care as members of an interdisciplinary team, emphasizing evidence-based practice, quality improvement approaches and informatics."

Figure 102-10 depicts the overlap and relationship of these core competencies.

Leadership begins with vision, a full and in-depth understanding of the organization, its challenges in clinical quality and satisfaction, and the ability to create a culture that sustains quality and excellence in delivering health care to patients.

Culture begins with a commitment to lifelong learning, process redesign, and a belief that no one can ever know it all. In the safety culture, leaders support and sustain the belief that performance and outcomes must be continually measured and evaluated, that collaboration and teamwork must be the norm and are valued, and that organizational expectations demand care coordination and anticipated patient need to provide consistent and predictably high levels of care. Education must be transformed so that it is not solely focused on competence, but for ca-

pability (the ability to adapt to change, generate new knowledge, and continuously improving performance).[101] Successful, safe health systems will depend on organizations that focus on providing care that keeps up with the ever-changing context and landscape of health care delivery. Education for capability must focus on supporting learners who can identify and construct their own learning goals, receive feedback, reflect and move forward with new ideas to support best practices. Learning capability must be nurtured and supported. Reflective learners can transform as the environment around them changes; poor, ill equipped learners simply complain about the change, the demands and their involvement in the complexity of the care process.

Leaders, *even capital L* traditional ones, are not out there, alone. They rely on a powerful coalition of people who believe in the same vision, value, culture, and who share a time frame for achievement. This larger view of collective leadership in each individual delivers strength, rebound, and sustainability. Positional leaders need to act to:

- Remove obstacles
- Learn from mistakes
- Ask questions, listen and learn

Every system is perfectly designed to get the results it gets. Leaders must continually redesign the system for an emerging set of expectations, influenced substantially by existing culture and recognition of the value cultural change can bring.

Over the next 20 years, the health care system will have to treat proportionately more people, with more illnesses, using fewer dollars and health care workers. In the face of declining resources and growing demand, the health care system will have to be explicitly designed to implement new systems of care that are fundamentally sustainable. This reinvention will require a groundswell of leadership support to engage the consumer to maintain good health and actively manage illness, to employ technology where appropriate for improvement, and to assure systems that are intended to meet explicit needs, in contrast to the incremental and band-aid patched system in place today. Above all, as has occurred in other industries, these designed processes will need to be certifiably safe and efficient. By 2020, the current situation in which health care delivery actually contributes to morbidity and mortality through unavailable error, should be seen as a wretched historical anomaly.[102]

To redesign the system this dramatically, one will need to understand the behavior of complex systems and the science of system design, including informatics. Recognizing the complex interrelationships of technical and social systems, is the first step.[102] Whether enraptured by the promise of technology, or fear it, technology itself will not drive direction as much as the will and commitment of people. Cultural beliefs and values will shape the future of safety successes.

SAFETY CULTURE

"It must be considered that there is nothing more difficult to carry out, nor more doubtful of success, nor more dangerous to handle than to initiate a new order of things."—**Machiavelli**

Systemic change doesn't occur on command, nor is it a quick fix. It requires a long-term commitment. Typically, systemic change transitions require a period of 3 to 5 years, with the major factors of complexity, ambiguity, and the power of organizational culture contributing to the lengthening of the transition period. All too often the culture of an organization dictates success or failure of a change initiative.

Culture is a somewhat fuzzy concept. Schein defines it as the combined rituals, climate, values, and behaviors that shape what life is like within an organization. He further characterizes culture as define by six properties (1) shared basic assumptions, (2) that are invented, discovered, or developed by a group as it (3) learns to cope with its problem of external adaptation and internal integration in ways that (4) have work well enough to be considered valid, and therefore (5) can be taught to new group members as the (6) correct way to perceive, think, and feel

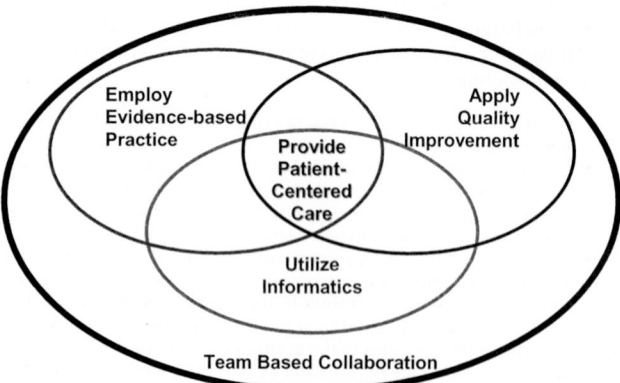

Figure 102-10. Overlap of core competencies for health professionals. Reprinted with permission from *Health Professions Education: A Bridge to Quality*. © 2003 by the National Academy of Sciences, courtesy of the National Academies Press, Washington, DC.

in relation to the problems.[103] Culture provides basic assumptions, shared values, and artifacts–visible markers and activities–that guide the way organizational members behave toward each other and approach their work. On one level, culture is a very simple concept, nothing elusive or magical: simply decide what the desired attitudes and behaviors are, identify the expectations and how people will be measured against norms. But as with many things in life, it really isn't that simple.

Culture is based on values. It reflects the vision and mission of the organization, as well as the goals that are set and the strategies that it employs to reach its goals. Leaders and top management must set the tone and expectation for the culture in the beliefs, values and actions that define expectations.

Communication from the top down must be credible, consistent, and relevant to be received and acted upon by workers, without any perception of hypocrisy. The perceived messages must resonate with workers, build in intensity toward a consensus and belief system. Reward systems must be aligned to support and reinforce the culture concept. Promotions, salary adjustment, approval, and reinforcement mechanisms should all flow in the direction of individuals acting on and supporting the culture, values, and beliefs, to avoid saying one thing, only to do another.

Individual roles and decision-making processes influence culture. Organizational systems–how training occurs, appraisal and reinforcement mechanisms, how goals are set–contribute to defining a culture. Job design, the complexity of technologies an organization adopts, and the interdependence of people in the culture play a significant role. Culture shapes what one expects from individual behaviors. Leadership, communication, and power distribution signal when and how cultures change.

Culture gives us a set of *felt* meanings in an orderly pattern, creating significance that provides individuals in the organization with a sense of belonging, order, and predictability. Culture is not what people do; it is what they feel. If people allow themselves to believe that culture is what people do, it becomes too easy to assume that parts, procedures, or goals can be changed without people being affected. Nothing could be further from the truth. Cultural symbols, rituals, and myths are not easily replaced.

Culture is a holistic concept. It is not one facet of work life, rather it is a complete set of feelings, affecting all individuals and groups, their attitudinal and structural behavior patterns. Cultures emerge to help cope with life's challenges and to teach the correct, accepted way to think, act, and behave in the larger organization. Every organization and group has a culture, no matter how dysfunctional it may be.

The prevailing culture in most health care organizations is an impediment to acknowledging error. Improving medication use safety will require cultural change.

Culture change is hard, slow, and subject to relapse. Schein suggests:

> Never start with the idea of changing culture. Start with the issue the organization faces in this case medication use safety; only when those business issues are clear should one ask the role of the culture in resolving the problem. . . .

If changes need to be made, try to build on cultural strengths rather than attempting to change those elements that may be weaknesses.[104] Creation or enhancement of a safety culture is dependent on deliberate manipulation of organizational characteristics believed to impact safety management.

Much attention has been devoted to the notion of a *safety culture*. A safety culture creates a perspective focused on minimizing exposure to danger or injury. Safety cultures are characterized by communications that are founded on mutual trust, shared perceptions of safety's importance, and confidence in efforts to ensure it is a high priority. The term *safety culture* first entered public awareness in the aftermath of the Chernobyl nuclear power disaster and quickly spread to the aviation and chemical processing industries. *Err*, which focused to closely on medication errors, reported[105]:

Health care organizations must develop a culture of safety such that an organization's care processes and workforce are focused on improving the reliability and safety of care for patients.

Reason suggests that a safety culture is an informed culture, one where those who manage and operate the system have current knowledge about the human, technical, organizational, and environmental factors that determine the safety of the system as a whole.[106] Reason identified four subcultures that underpin a safety culture:

A *reporting culture* focuses on what gets reported when errors or near misses occur since safety cultures depend heavily on what can be learned from mistakes and near misses. Reporting cultures protect the safety and confidentiality of those who report, and they steadfastly trust the reports of those closest to the knowledge of the event. A safety culture must be informed and cannot exist with a flawed reporting relationship, where reports either do not exist or cannot be trusted.

How an organization apportions blame determines if it is a *just culture*, characterized a trusting environment that encourages, and even rewards, reporting of safety information. A just culture also has a clear line of demarcation between acceptable behavior that offers learning opportunity and does not deserve disciplinary action, and unacceptable behavior. In an environment where it is unclear what falls into the unacceptable range–about 10% of all events according to Reason–people are afraid and ashamed of error, only compounded in organizations that deal with errors inconsistently or routinely assigning blame. Trust is a pivotal factor in the just safety culture, with the solid knowledge that only clearly identified unsafe behavior is punished.

A *flexible culture* adapts to changing demands. In flexible cultures, information and decision-making tend to flow to technical expertise, hence they are less hierarchical. Mindfulness and its preoccupation with the potential for failure, creates an environment where any small symptom of concern is clue that safety may be at issue. When data are inconclusive, the default is to assume a safety risk, and to seek more data.

Knowledge changes culture, therefore, the concept of a *learning culture* is an important concept for safety. Learning cultures evolve when information is generated by knowledgeable people, and that information is widely shared. This access to information, coupled with a just and flexible environment, allows workers to become aware of best practices and to take action to adopt them. Dialog and open discussion about issues of controversy, where answers are not absolute and where variability is high, is characteristic of a learning culture. Learning can easily be stifled when management dismisses or *reasons away* issues that are raised, where promises are made and commitments are not kept or when individuals have a growing sense of the issues being far outside their control.

There is no absolute *cookbook* for building a safety culture. Several steps are important and support the development[107]:

Notice everything. Try to concentrate on mindful attention to patterns of the expected and unexpected events of routine operations. One might miss the unexpected unless you are looking for it.

Track down bad news. Try to understand the issues and causal factors, and just as importantly, notice what happens to bad news and the people who report it.

Clarify the onus of proof. Is the system assumed to be safe until disaster strikes? Or, dangerous until proven safe? Who decides? How many indicators would have to line up before there is a perceived problem?

Watch for unusual events and patterns. Encourage others to discuss and report unusual events. What are individuals not seeing? Try not to deny or rationalize the unusual event.

Define the near miss. Consider whether a near miss is a signal that safeguards are working, or that the system is vulnerable. Raise the comfort level to increase discussion of near miss events in the workplace.

Keep a holistic view and consolidate *explanations* for individual small deviations to avoid *de minimus* errors that cause us to explain away individual symptoms, and miss the diagnosis. Keep track of symptoms, diagnoses and alternative explanations.

Culture eats strategy for lunch. Don't overlook the power of social influence and the dominance of cultural systems, where strength is gained from mutual reinforcement.

Learning occurs and behavior changes when feedback is available, particularly when that feedback is proximate to the event. How does feedback occur? Is it passive or active? Is there an expectation that action will occur? Are feedback mechanisms and results a focus on ongoing attention and discussion?

Put individuals out there to actively stand for a safety culture. Public, irrevocable and actively chosen behavior with good purpose and aim, substantiated with values and reason, attract attention and often shape future behaviors.

Feelings are the engine of culture. Culture is about approval and disapproval, pride, despair, happiness, hypocrisy, shame and failure. It pumps intensity into what could be cool and impersonal ideas, and it makes one wince when something goes terribly wrong, fully knowing that it should not have occurred. Understand the feelings of your culture. Try to articulate what the culture means in terms of feelings and encourage others to express their perceptions. It will help to understand culture, to identify areas for improvement and to act to strengthen the influence culture has on behaviors and results.

Keep values simple. It may be as simple as do the right thing, do the right thing well, and continually improve. Keep it simple to ensure diligent attention, and to minimize confusion, dilution and a breakdown of consensus around the values.

Think safety first. Dwell on the mindfulness of failure, discover limits, uncover shortcomings and system flaws. Focus on the fear of failure, blaming behavior, the anxiety about errors that exists in the workplace. Provide supportive resources, training, positive role models, mentors, coaches, and a positive vision for what can be better in the future if some change occurs. Ask for and give help to move toward realization of the vision.

Realize that building a safety culture is an iterative process that will be reinforced as a result of ongoing continuous attention and activity focused on safety. Risk and hazards will not magically disappear one day when the goal is reached. This is a continual, endless quest toward a definitive victory that will require every part, every player's mindful attention, and the effective management of the team process.

TRAINING FOR TEAMWORK

Improving medication use safety will require substantial change in most health care organizations including change in culture, systems, and processes. Individuals and systems change because they learn. Adult learners choose to learn because they want to change, and in that learning process, they use existing competencies as a base for building new capabilities. Behavior change among adults derives from a complex mix of goal setting, deliberate action, feedback, and reinforcement, which is facilitated by appropriate education and training.[108] Culture changes over time, based on shared knowledge.

Learning, and therefore change, occur in a zone of complexity, where individuals engage items of knowledge in an unfamiliar and uncertain context and create a meaningful mental framework to make a transition from unfamiliar to familiar. This learning process is not passive, nor is it taught. Existing competencies are transformed and retuned for new circumstances within each individual.

As previously discussed, health care organizations are complex adaptive system. This perspective provides a point of reference to consider the learning process, where the behavior of individuals and the system itself evolves based on feedback regarding the actual and immediate impact of actions. Existing competencies become the base for transformational learning, and new capability evolves when new information is provided to learners about the impact of their own actions and those of others. The most successful educational processes offer feedback as it takes place. Not all learners transform feedback to capability at the same rate, in the same way. Reflective learners are open to this feedback and adapt their behaviors, transforming themselves and their impact as the world changes. Less adept learners are either not receptive to the feedback, or adapt inappropriately and complain.

In the past, knowledge was a scarce commodity, accessed by scholars and experts, held tightly in memory and brain capac-

ity. Today everyone drowns in information. Knowing and acknowledging that one cannot commit all of the information to which one has access to memory–can't know it all–offers some relief from the burden of guilt that makes one feel that he/she should. Knowing what we don't know is an important step to understanding complex system events and finding a path to change. Beyond what we don't know, there is a frontier of unknowable and emerging information that represents uncertainty. This is information that is not yet integrated into a useful context to build knowledge and capability. In today's incessant flow of information, an expert's value lies in the ability to access *known* knowledge efficiently and with speed, to explore *new* knowledge to create new and relevant context, learning to create mental links between seemingly disparate ideas.

Because learning often occurs in the cracks between systems and system elements, understanding the interrelationships and connections between the elements can be more valuable than knowing the details of the individual parts. Yet health care organizations tend to *teach* in a more traditional, curricular, disciplinary, and fact-driven manner, the tendency is to provide factual content without context. It is no surprise that many learners don't understand the relevance, can't associate the new knowledge to other related information or their work, and as a result, fail to apply the learning to build competency and capacity for change.

Most education and training is planned to be formal and relies on narrowly defined learning objectives. Knowledge is presented as static, finite, and linear. The objective is to provide factual information that should be of interest to build knowledge, but traditional approaches seldom *connect the dots* to demonstrate how information can and should be applied, what the impact can be and how the information can create positive change for performance improvement. Alternatively, knowledge transfer can be dynamic, based on analysis, synthesis, and problem solving.

Learning tools–*cookbooks*, checklists, and reminder systems–are becoming more prevalent, and they are–no question–useful adjuncts, but they are only useful after learning has occurred, not as a substitute for it. In contrast to what is typically offered, what is needed in adult learning is context. Learning occurs when the information is immediately relevant and applicable and where social interaction is a component of the format and reinforces the learning. Rich use of examples, stories, and metaphors fire one's intuition and imagination to build relational connectivity between what is known and learning, fostering a sort of *sensemaking* that stimulates the mental leap to assimilate and apply new knowledge. Shared experience and dialog reinforce the applicability and capacity to use the new information. Small group problem-based learning involving a facilitator provides the opportunity for positive and negative feedback, allows ownership of the idea to evolve, and creates confidence and the motivation to act to use the new knowledge. Consider a range of methods including informal and unplanned learning, self-directed learning, and nonlinear approaches focused on process (Table 102-4).

Given the complexity of driving and restraining forces for medication use safety change, it is essential to consider and design related education and training with a system focus rather than targeting individual deficiencies or failures. The organization must honor learning above blame, and this must be clearly reflected in education and training. Interventions should reflect a range of methods to change behavior of physicians, nurses, pharmacists, and other health workers because multiple approaches are more likely to succeed than a single intervention or approach.[109]

Education and training are likely to be needed and are not interchangeable. Core knowledge of systems thinking, complexity concepts and principles of complex adaptive systems, aspects of teamwork, safety culture, conflict resolution, human factors must be provided. Training using experiential learning, practice with feedback, simulations, and reinforcement are just as necessary.

Table 102-4. Process-Oriented Learning Methods

Informal and Unplanned Learning
- *Experiential learning*–Shadowing, apprenticeship, rotational attachments
- *Networking opportunities*–Conferences and workshops, poster sessions, extended breaks
- *Learning activities*–reflection exercises, suggestions for group discussions
- *Buzz groups* submerged in lectures–turn to neighbor dialog opportunities
- *Facilitated email list servers* for professional interest groups
- *Teachback opportunities*–newly skilled workers training others in new techniques to share understanding
- *Feedback*–response to provide the learner with information on the real or projected outcome of their actions

Self-directed Learning
- *Mentoring*–named individuals provide support and guidance to self-directed learners
- *Peer supported learning groups*–small group process used for mutual support and problem solving
- *Personal learning log*–structured form for identifying and meeting new learning needs as they arise
- *Appraisal*–regular, structured review of progress and goals
- *Modular courses*–offer high degree of variety and choice

Non-linear Learning
- *Case-based discussions*–grand rounds, clinical case presentations, significant event audit
- *Simulations*–opportunities to practice unfamiliar tasks in unfamiliar contexts by modeling complex situations
- *Role play*
- *Small group problem-based learning*
- *Team building exercises*

Adapted from Fraser SW, Greenhalgh T. Coping with complexity: educating for capability. *BMJ* 2001; 323: 802.

It is important to find opportunities for small wins and build on them. Use problems as treasured opportunities to test ideas for improvement, learn and share learning more widely. Small wins become long-term gains as they aggregate and rebound in the organization. Focus on the microsystem level of the organization with teams as the essential unit. Teams offer flexibility, redundancy and consistently outperform individuals, but they must function effectively to do so. Team training is an essential investment to establish an important building block for safety improvement.

Team cohesiveness, effective collaboration, and team processes are essential to having an effective, collaborative safety plan. The team must see itself as part of the bigger organization. They must be aware of the need for their independence as well as interdependence within the organization.

Team training must have an emphasis on safety. The focus of all team initiatives should be from the perspective of hazard avoidance. If well integrated into all aspects, the team can assist as the transformational leaders for an idea, relying on upstream supportive sponsorship for the vision and goals that drive the organizational initiative.

Creating team stability is also important, especially in those areas that are high-risk. Teams in emergency departments (eg, Code Blue situations, disaster response) allow for well-established relationships that produce smooth communication and decision-making in stressful circumstances.

Increasing Feedback

The team should be encouraged to monitor effectiveness of activities and report findings. Within the organization, the staff needs a mechanism to showcase their activities and actions for patient care safety improvement. The team should also be encouraged to identify problems and potential areas for improvement. These activities should be incorporated into standard communication systems (eg, common reporting processes, quality improvement, staff meetings, shift reports).

Improving Communication

Communication is the glue that holds the medication use process together. Therefore, organizations should focus on training all staff to avoid indirect communication involved in patient care activities. This can include activities to deal with difficult situations such as the emotions that occur during stressful, emergent events. Additionally, a focus on reduction of verbal orders or encouragement of *hear back* or *repeat back* processes with verbal orders to reduce the potential for error should be included in the communication training plan.

Development of Competencies Focused on Safety

Providing training opportunities for staff on safety is simply not enough. The IOM report, *Health Professions Education: A Bridge to Quality* clearly identified that clinical education practices have not kept pace or been responsive to the demands of shifting patient demographics and desires, changing health system expectations, evolving practice requirements, new staffing arrangements, new information, new technology, and the needed focus on quality improvement. In fact, the report identified the need to integrate a core set of competencies—ones shared across all professions—to provide the necessary leverage for safety and care improvement.[12] The committee proposed five core competencies that all clinicians should possess, regardless of discipline, to meet the needs of the 21st-century health system[12]:

- Provide patient-centered care—identify, respect, and care about patients' differences, values, and preferences are expressed needs.
- Work in interdisciplinary teams—cooperate collaborate, communicate, and integrate care in teams to assure that care is continuous and reliable
- Employ evidence-based practice—integrate best research with clinical expertise and patient values.
- Apply quality improvement—identify errors, risks, and hazards in care to continuously understand and measure the quality of care provided and use that information to understand and implement basic safety design principles.
- Utilize informatics—communicate, manage knowledge, mitigate error and support decision-making information technology.

Organizations must include methods for staff to demonstrate their knowledge and skills regarding safety, including these core competencies, as part of their routine competency evaluation. Additionally, staff should be able to demonstrate their ability to communicate, identify, and report adverse events. As part of the organization's routine staff competency evaluation process, organizations should identify method of evaluating the staff's ability to:

- Focus on risk reduction activities within the work environment
- Assess patient risk and selection for treatments
- Monitor effects of care
- Identify ADEs
- Respond to ADEs when identified

Collaboration for Change

Change efforts are often designed and implemented by individual departments, frequently with little or no integration with other departmental efforts. Change can be difficult for many reasons:

- The wide variety of styles, needs, and change preparedness within departments and individuals require collaboration on a regular basis
- Collaboration, communication, and working together as a team will help to achieve harmonious results with change efforts

Once an organization has accepted the idea that errors do happen, a focus on prevention, systems improvement and human factors is needed. But, what needs to happen within the organization?

For a new focus for change within health care to be sustainable, positive changes regarding safety improvement are necessary. These changes include:

- An ongoing focus and learning from safety and human factors research and its application to health care
- Specific leadership and organizational culture initiatives
- Ongoing scientific measurement of safety and safety practice conformance

ORGANIZATIONAL ISSUES

Health care professionals often wait for accidents to occur before taking appropriate preventive action. Too often, the focus is on the person involved in the error. Reactions include methods to hold the individual up as an example and to invoke discipline and educate others regarding what went wrong. Other high-risk industries (eg, aviation, nuclear energy) scrutinize their systems for error potential in an ongoing, proactive fashion while focusing on the relationship between man and system.

Experts indicate that errors are, in fact, rarely due to faulty people. Individuals rarely err on purpose. In fact, the systems in which people work have a marked effect on the incidence of human error.

A number of industries outside the health care system have developed and implemented strategies to prevent errors by correcting and avoiding system failures. The aviation industry, as an example, also strives for zero defects. To ensure safety, the airline industry has developed a wide array of systematic and organizational safeguards for safety improvement.

As a result of these strategies, the risk for passengers is greatly diminished. Health care, like aviation, involves a highly complex interaction of highly skilled personnel who provide diverse yet interrelated and interdependent functions.

Applications of aviation principles to health care practice may provide a fresh look at safety and vulnerabilities within the medication use process. In fact, many of the ideas embraced by pilots (eg, the use of checklists and standards) have been utilized within health care as a means to reduce variation and risk in the treatment of patients.

Health care organizations tend to make the same medication mistakes over and over because members tend to accuse individual employees rather than consider the real root cause of the error, a faulty system.

Implementing new strategies will require a profound change in the way health care does business. A new framework for guiding organizations will be needed to transition health systems to better meet patient needs. *Chasm*, highlights methods to guide these transitions and help organizations remain focused on the true agenda: safer care for patients.[110]

- Redesign care practices based on best practice
- Use information technologies to improve access to clinical information and support decision-making
- Develop effective teams
- Incorporate new knowledge and skills management
- Coordinate care across patient conditions, services and settings over time
- Incorporate performance and outcomes measures for improvement and accountability

Some distinct observations and conclusions have been made as a result of these adverse event studies:

- ADEs are common, more common than previously recognized
- ADEs resulting from error are preventable
- For each preventable error, three more near misses occur
- Ordering and administration of medications are most likely to be identified as error prone
- Costs of ADEs are significant and include injury, malpractice, additional care and work and overall damage to organization.

- Organizational redesign is needed
- There are costs for implementing safe systems; but the costs of inaction are much higher
- Error reduction strategies will require a systems oriented approach
- Many errors that are preventable are also often not reported; organizations must identify methods for health care providers to report and engage in prevention activities

A variety of factors can influence individual and team performance. Of growing concern are the effects of burnout, stress, and fatigue.

Burnout, Stress, and Fatigue

Providing health care is a highly complex and demanding process that is affected by a variety of psychological and workplace factors that can combine to create an environment conducive to errors.

Burnout—emotional exhaustion, depersonalization, and reduced personal capacity to accomplish—can be a contributing factor to medical errors. Research conducted to measure burnout and its effects, define the condition as[111]:

"A state of emotional exhaustion in which service providers view recipients impersonally and their own performance disparagingly."

Workload demands, erosion in professional respect, limited resources, manpower shortages, heavier practice demands, industry consolidation, and many other stressors all contribute to the growing sense of frustration, discouragement, and disenchantment, and eventually to cynicism and despair. All of this contributes to a lack of effectiveness in the job, a declining focus, and gives rise to absenteeism, turnover, physical illness, and in some cases substance abuse. There is also significant deterioration in relationships with coworkers and patients, both of which further contribute to the conduciveness to error and sometimes, disastrous results for patients. Some more subtle stress factors must also be considered.

Health care is uncertain by its very nature, characterized by ambiguous data, an incomplete understanding of some biologic functions, variability in response to treatment, and the frequent need to act on incomplete information. And, the stakes are high. Clinical uncertainty can have a long-term negative effect on clinical caregivers and their performance.[112]

In today's health care environment, virtually all providers feel a sense of diminished control as a result of consolidation and reorganization, changing incentives, managed care and growing insurance restrictions. In conditions of perceived lack of control, individuals are more subject to the pressures of stress and distraction.

Research also demonstrates that crowding and the social density of the environment affects performance. Workers in a crowded space are less tolerant of frustration and less able to perform routine tasks reliably.[113]

Most organizations are facing the reality of doing more with less—people, budget dollars, and time—and this growing task load also has a negative effect on performance.

Stress impacts job performance and social interactions, and predisposes health professionals to medical errors. The cause of this is unclear, but three theories offer insight. The cognitive fatigue hypothesis suggests that prolonged stress reduces attention capacity because disproportionate resources are devoted to the stressor, reducing the capacity left for performance. Alternatively, learned helplessness teaches the individual over time that a response does not influence the stressor, and over time motivation to perform is eroded. Finally, the frustration mood theory suggests that building frustration resulting from stress establishes irritation and anger that diminishes ability to perform and effects interpersonal relationships.[114] Regardless of the theory, the resulting impact is that highly trained, well-meaning, dedicated health professionals can have performance impacted to the extent of being involved with a medical error. Perhaps most disturbing is the effect of stress and burnout on social interaction and communication within the team or work group given the importance of the effectiveness of the team at the microsystem level.

Fatigue and sleep deprivation has been a long-standing concern in health care. The provision of health care has a 24/7 demand with round the clock staffing for continuous care, which naturally necessitates standard shift work as well as *ad hoc* nonroutine scheduling in response to demand.

Significant research efforts have demonstrated beyond a doubt that fatigue impairs performance.[115,116] An Office of Technology Assessment report documents that nonstandard work schedules and night shift work disrupt circadian rhythms and that frequently extended hours beyond a normal 8-hour shift has a negative impact on the worker's health, safety, and performance.[117] Night shifts lead to loss of sleep, difficulty performing specific tasks in the middle of the night, disrupted social and family life, and loss of concentration.

Beyond the difficulties associated with night shift work, a number of other factors contribute to fatigue. Whether due to manpower shortages, scheduling convenience preferences or the goal of amassing overtime benefits, long shifts, back-to-back and successive shifts, and extra shifts/moonlighting are common practice for health care workers. Inadequate rest, sleep loss, displaced or disrupted feelings of tiredness and continuous mental of physical activity all contribute to feelings of fatigue. But there are predictable consequences associated with fatigue, including slowed reaction time, lapses of attention to critical detail, compromised problem solving skills, decreased motivation, and overall lower level of vigor for completing important tasks. Overall, there is a diminished ability to do work and a subjective sense of tiredness.

Everyone is familiar with physical fatigue that produces a temporary loss of power to respond to demands. Often a result of continued physical stimulation over an extended work period, physical fatigue is characterized by muscle tiredness, diminished physical performance, back discomfort, and cognitive impairment. But there is also general or mental fatigue that produces subjective feelings of weariness after hours of repeated performance of nonphysical tasks. This type of fatigue triggers a decrease in afferent nerve impulses or decreased feedback from the cortex to the reticular activating system, which results in a lack of novel stimuli producing monotony or boredom. Combined with sleep deprivation, drowsiness contributes to the overall sense of fatigue. Reaction time and performance decline, mood and motivation drop precipitously, as do initiative and enthusiasm.

Fatigue can also be classified as acute or chronic. Fatigue from intense and excessive cognitive work is short-lived and can be reversed with sleep and rest. Chronic mental fatigue is the result of excessive cognitive work over weeks or months, coupled with cumulative stress, and is not relieved by rest. Time away from the work is needed, either in the form of a vacation or change of job responsibilities. This type of chronic sleep debt builds gradually and may be imperceptible. However, the individual is seldom maximally alert. While physical activity is not impaired to a great extent, mental acuity and performance degrade quickly. Initially speed of performance and response slows perceptibly. Continue sleep loss leads to the occurrence of brief mental lapses–or microsleeps of 1-10 second duration that contribute substantially to slowed response and errors of omission.[118] Mood, motivation, morale, and initiative erode dramatically. In combination, less work gets done, and attention to detail is lacking, potentially leading to mistakes, accidents, and errors.

Sleep loss has immediate negative effects. Loss of one night's sleep, followed by 18 hours of work can result in a 25% decrease in cognitive ability. At 24 hours, it can drop to 70% of baseline, remain stable for 18 hours, then fall dramatically to again about 40% of baseline.[119] The real problem is that the individual is seldom aware of the diminished capacity. Because both sustained workloads (8–12 hours or longer on the job) and shift work changes lead to loss of sleep and disrupted circadian rhythms,

this is prevalent problem in society, and in particular among health care workers, who may be chronically sleep deprived.

With increasing sleep loss, there is growing difficulty actively monitoring static or slowly changing stimuli (eg, vital signs displays), as our ability to be vigilant decreases. Typically, decreases in reaction time and lower likelihood of identifying visual or auditory alarms occur as quickly as 20 to 30 minutes into the task. Sustained vigilance and mindfulness can fall victim to microsleeps, described earlier, resulting in slower response time, errors of omission and very long reaction times. As time on task increases, lapses increase in frequency and duration, and performance between lapses erodes as well. Vigilance decrements prompt job designers to build rest pauses, breaks, and rotational job assignment into such work as naval carrier command, air traffic control, and nuclear control centers. For health care workers, a failure of vigilance can lead to slowed recognition of changes in patient status, missing important signs and information or failure to deliver a treatment sequence in a timely fashion. While the effects of shift duration and recommended limits have not been clearly established, consideration must be given to the potential impact of back-to-back shifts, routine staffing with 7 days on 7 days off with 12-hour shifts, and other *creative* solutions to manpower issues within health care professions.

Clearly, the human side of performance and performance capacity must be evaluated in addition to system and process capability. Safe medication use requires a delicate balance of factors to achieve best care. How do organizations construct the framework to evaluate how man, machine and system interact? Planning, executing, evaluating, and assuring safe medication use requires a systematic approach. Incorporating medication use improvement activities into the health care organization's performance improvement and strategic planning process is one way to assure ongoing attention to this critical health care issue.

LINKING SAFETY AND PERFORMANCE IMPROVEMENT

Medical error prevention approaches have focused primarily on protocol development, training of care providers, and punishment when things go wrong. Although these approaches have an effect, they are not *the answer*. These efforts alone cannot be relied upon to create perfect performance in health care.

Clearly, implementation of these strategies alone are not greatly reducing error rates. Simply creating plans and policies has not proven to completely resolve the problem. A fine balance of integrating a wide range of strategies, identifying how staff implement and use these strategies and measuring their effects are necessary.

The quality of health care in the United States falls short of what it could be. Literature documents some serious quality problems. There is a gap, for some a *chasm*, between services that should be provided based on current professional knowledge, technology, and services that patients actually receive. This wake-up call for health care has inspired many organizations to rededicate their focus on identifying, measuring, and implementing performance improvement strategies to strive for better care services.

THE PERFORMANCE IMPROVEMENT PROCESS

All safety improvement efforts require making a change. Not all changes, however, result in an improvement. Therefore, it is essential that health systems identify the changes most likely to result in a sustainable improvement. One particular model for improvement, the Plan-Do-Study-Act learning cycle, has been advocated for use by health care systems to improve processes affecting patient care. The model was initially developed by Thomas Nolan and his colleagues at Associates in Process Improvement.[120] This model has a demonstrated framework for a variety of system contexts including health care and can be used alone or in conjunction with other change models that are utilized within a health care system to accelerate improvement efforts. The Plan-Do-Study-Act (PDSA) process is dependent upon the work of a team that has an interest in evaluating a change and has knowledge of what the current process is and is capable of being (Fig 102-11).

The model has two parts. First a series of three questions must be answered.

1. What is the aim of the change initiative? A system cannot be improved without a clear and firm intention. The health system should clearly identify, in numerical or specific terms, what is to be accomplished by the change effort. Agreement on this aim by the organization or health system is crucial. The answer to this question can help determine the people, time, money, and other resources necessary to accomplish the desired goal. An example might be a goal of reducing adverse drug events that lead to injury by 50% on a hospital nursing unit.

2. How will the health system know if the change has resulted in the desired improvement? Knowing and articulating the current process serves as the foundation for the measurement process. Identifying clear, objective measurements are crucial to the improvement process. Health systems should identify quantitative measures to determine if the change resulted in an actual improvement. Another example might be to measure how many incomplete prescription orders were received in the pharmacy after an initiative to preprint routine prescription orders in an outpatient chemotherapy clinic.

3. What changes should be made to result in the improvement? Ideas for changing the medication use process can come from a variety of sources: results of root cause analysis or failure mode and effects investigations, scientific literature, a hunch, among others. The goal is to identify a change or series of changes to be tested in a real world setting to find out if the change improves care as the aim has described.

Second, use of a learning cycle, referred to as the PDSA cycle is used to test and implement the identified change. This cycle is really based on a systematic, trial and learning approach. The PDSA is a shorthand way of describing how a change is tried, observed, and then evaluated for future modification. The completion of a PDSA cycle leads directly to a next cycle. The team learns from the test, identifies what works or doesn't, and then determines what should be kept, changed, or abandoned for improvement. The challenges of each step of the PDSA process are as highlighted below:

Step 1 PLAN: The team should state the objective of the PDSA cycle. How will the change be tested? Who will be involved? What will be measured? Where will these observations be made? What data will be collected? How will training occur? This is the greatest challenge of the change initiative and the most time consuming, but it clearly sets the context and framework for the team to evaluate the change.

Step 2 DO: This is the phase where the test or change is actually carried out. Documentation of the observations and findings begin at this stage. Data collection is occurring

Step 3 STUDY: At this point, evaluation of the data occurs. The team needs to compare the findings of the change initiative to the predictions made. A summary of learnings and findings must be provided.

Step 4 ACT: At this point, analysis of findings is complete and the team needs to determine what modifications are necessary, what gains should be held and what new knowledge has been identified. The team then must plan for the next change cycle. The team continues to link PDSA cycles to continue refinement of the change until it is ready for broader implementation. Linking small cycles of change and improvement can help overcome the natural resistance to change often felt by health systems. People are far more willing to test change if they know that modifications will be made as needed based on findings.

From the perspective of safe medication use, the improvement process must include a strategy to prevent ADEs at every step in the medication use process and methods to identify the prevalence of system failures versus individual negligence within the organization.

Several recommendations have been identified to minimize the risks in the medication use process. Reviewing recommendations in and of themselves are not the answer. If an organization is investing time, energy, and resources into implementing change, the expectation is to observe the result of measurable improvements. Organizations expecting to reach their objectives must implement performance improvement strategies.

Improving patient safety is a complex undertaking. Organizing a team of individuals with diverse skills, characteristics, and knowledge is an essential first step. Deciding who should be on the team begins with a focus on the strategic initiative.

The overall plan for the organizational safety initiative includes three steps that allow the organization to determine the aim or goal of whatever it is trying to accomplish. These steps include:

- Developing a strategy
- Analyzing organizational capabilities
- Developing an action plan

The first step in developing a strategy means asking the questions that uncover where the organization is currently when it comes to medication errors. Each organization must:

- State the aim of the project targeting medication use improvement
- Identify measures that will identify safety improvement
- Describe current practice, compare to the desired state or condition and predict changes likely to occur (gap analysis)
- Plan for the implementation of the improvement strategy
- Pilot the desired changes
- Check and restudy the results
- Act to improve
- Reflect on learning

This model is consistent with the Joint Commission as well as other national mandates on continuous improvement regarding medication use:[121]

- A system of continuous medication monitoring
- Medication use documentation system
- Plan for data aggregation and analysis
- Focus on high volume, problem prone medication use
- Assessment of all significant ADEs

TOOLS TO IDENTIFY, CONTROL, CONTAIN OR MITIGATE RISK

Failure detection, reduction, and prevention strategies are receiving new attention as the health care industry moves to respond to the challenges established in the IOM reports and in the literature. Since instances of medical errors have been reported with increasing regularity in the media, the public trust of health care systems appears to be eroding. Often health systems skip vital problem solving steps and *jump to*

AIM

CURRENT KNOWLEDGE

CYCLE FOR LEARNING AND IMPROVEMENT

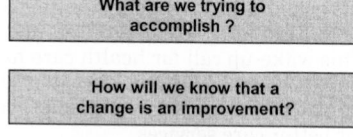

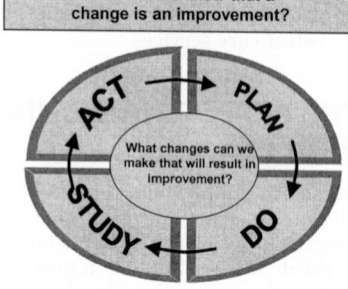

Figure 102-11. The Plan-Do-Study-Act learning cycle. Adapted from Nelson EC, Batalden PB, Mohr J, Plume SK, et al. *Joint Commission Journal on Quality and Safety.* 1996;22(4):243. Reprinted with permission.

solutions when a critical incident or error occurs. When adverse events occur, health systems must identify the causes of the event, the interrelationship of these causes, and implement improvement or redesign efforts to eliminate causes of error. Since errors are thought to be preventable, organizations must also identify methods to design or redesign systems *proactively*. These proactive efforts are aimed to prevent, or at least minimize, the likelihood that failures occur and also protect patients from the effects of failures when they do occur.

Regulatory and accreditation agencies have galvanized around the issue of responding to events and providing strategies to implement prevention initiatives. Two strategies, root cause analysis and failure mode and effects analysis have been identified as systematic methods for error investigation, reduction and prevention.

Identifying Errors and Cause

Variation in performance can produce unexpected and adverse outcomes. Sentinel events, as defined by the Joint Commission on Accreditation of Health Care Organizations (JCAHO), are unexpected occurrences involving death or serious physical or psychological injury or the risk thereof.[122] Error investigation requires a rigorous, systematic approach to evaluate basic or causal factors for variation in system performance. Root cause analysis, a technique utilized to identify the fundamental reason for system failure, focuses on systems and processes rather than on individuals involved in the system.

Root cause analysis (RCA) is not a single tool or strategy, but an investigative approach that utilizes many tools in combination to solve a problem.[123] The use of RCA helps identify clear factors or causes that result in, at best, performance variation, and at worst, adverse events or errors within a system. A root cause, by definition, is a single element that is directly attributed to starting a cause and effect chain that creates the problem observed. A root cause is the most fundamental reason a failure or situation where performance does not meet expectations, has occurred. The word *cause* does not imply or assign blame as part of the definition. Instead, *cause* refers to a relationship or potential relationship between factors that enable a failure or error to occur.

Now while it is possible that one single cause exists, it is often found that there are many causes of variation when failures occur and no one root cause can be identified as solely responsible for an error or bad outcome. Several causes might be identified. It is important that identification of all possible causes occur so that effective strategies to reduce these variations and their impact can be considered.

When an error occurs, health systems are charged with identifying:

- Why the event occurred
- How to prevent the event from occurring in the future

To do this, identification of proximate causes (obvious or immediate cause) and underlying causes (cause that lead to proximate cause) and their relationships *must be identified*. Root cause analysis helps to identify the apparent proximate causes to get at that root cause of interest.

Conducting a root cause analysis requires a team effort. Assembling a multidisciplinary team that understands the process under investigation is essential. The team assigned to conducting a root cause analysis works to understand the process(es) under investigation, the causes or potential causes of variation, and the process changes that would make variation less likely to occur. As part of the investigation, a root cause analysis examines common causes and special causes within clinical and organizational processes to identify potential system improvements.

Common cause variation is inherent within a system and a consequence of process design.[124] This type of variation is systemic and endogenous within the system. As an example, a health system might be investigating the length of time required to dispense a prescription to an outpatient in an ambulatory clinic. The time required might vary depending on how busy the pharmacy is, whether the prescription is a refill or new order, if the patient is new to the clinic, if the product requires compounding, or even the time of day the prescription is presented to the pharmacy staff. Variation in the process of providing a prescription is inherent, resulting from common causes such as staffing levels, availability of patient information, or access to medication supply. A process that varies only because of common causes is said to be stable. The level of performance of a stable process, or the range of the common cause variation, can only be changed by redesigning the process. If an organization desires to improve prescription wait time, what is expectation for improvement? If data collected suggests that wait times can be as short as 5 minutes or as long as 50 minutes, is that acceptable? Would further investigation of the 50-minute wait time yield valuable insight for process change? To reduce any variation, it is necessary to determine cause. If the variation is unexpected or unacceptable, redesign of the system may be necessary.

A special cause is variation which occurs from unusual circumstances or events that are difficult to predict.[124] Special cause is not inherent as part of the system; it is usually as a result of external influence and not part of the system as designed. The results of special cause variation often leads to process instability which is best described as intermittent and unpredictable. Examples of special cause variation in the medication use process might include manufacturer recalls, compounding equipment or automation failure, widespread professional staff sick calls, environmental/natural disaster or other *acts of God* that lead to failure. These special causes should be identified and eliminated. However, this will only affect the abnormal performance in that process. It cannot prevent the special cause from recurring.

Health care, however, is part of a larger system. In health care, special cause variation in performance may be a signal that common cause variation is occurring within the larger system context. In the example of manufacturer recall of a medication, is there a failure in the system that provides communication, support, or alternatives when a recall occurs? When automation fails, could that signal an outmoded or nonfunctional equipment maintenance program? In the case of a tornado, does the response plan provide adequate pharmaceutical care support for victims? By conducting a thorough root cause analysis and identifying common and special cause variation within the process, an opportunity exists to reduce special cause variation in one process by redesigning the larger system of which it is a part.

Root cause analysis is used reactively—to investigate the reason for a bad or unexpected outcome. That means that a failure has already occurred. Root cause analysis techniques, however, can also be used to probe near miss events or as a part of other performance improvement initiatives that focus on system redesign. A near miss is defined as an event that *almost occurred*. An example might be an overdose of a medication that was dispensed by a pharmacy. The patient did not receive the medication because a nurse or family member identified the dosing error and did not receive the product. Adverse consequences to the patient were avoided. A root cause analysis in this case could yield useful information about process failure. The best root cause analyses look at entire processes and support systems involved in an event to minimize risk as well as the potential for recurrence of the failure being investigated. All root cause analysis efforts should produce clear action plans for implementation to reduce the risk of similar events occurring in the future.

Steps for Conducting a Root Cause Analysis

There are several key features for health care organizations to consider as the conduct a root cause analysis[125]:

- Identify a multidisciplinary team to assess the error, failure, or adverse event of interest
- Establish a way to communicate findings and data elements required to conduct the analysis
- Create a plan with target dates, responsibilities, and measurement/data collection strategies required for the investigation
- Define all elements of the process and issues clearly
- Brainstorm all possible causes or potential causes
- Identify interrelationships of causes or potential causes
- Sort, analyze and prioritize cause list
- Determine which processes and systems are part of the investigation
- Determine special and common causes
- Begin the design and implementation of the change while engaging in the root cause analysis
- Repeat each of the steps listed previously as appropriate
- Focus on being thorough (Ask *why*) and credible (Be consistent, dig deep, and leave no stone unturned!)
- Target system improvement . . . particularly the larger systems
- Redesign to eliminate root cause(s)
- Measure and assess new design

Benefits of Conducting a Root Cause Analysis

Root cause analysis can help organizations identify risk or weak points in processes, underlying or systemic causes, and corrective actions. Information from root causes can be shared with practitioners to help prevent future failures. This knowledge can be shared in within health care systems to contribute to proactive improvement activities. The systematic approach outlined by root cause analysis techniques allows organizations to[126]:

- Focus on systems and processes, not individuals
- Use multidisciplinary participation to include views and values of process participants, customers and leaders
- Make links between special and common cause variation findings
- Allow root cause team to dig deep by asking *why* repeatedly
- Evaluate chain of causation, identifying both proximate and direct cause
- Determine risk points and their contribution to failure
- Identify change potential to reduce risk
- Create an action plan with assignments, timelines, and responsibilities
- Implement action or redesign consistent with other performance improvement efforts to test impact of change effort

Although a useful and essential tool to assist health care providers, root cause analysis is only part of the problem solving process. Analyzing processes only after bad outcomes occur must be joined with a prospective look at what could go wrong before failures occur. The use of failure mode and effects analysis (FMEA) is a proactive, prospective technique used to prevent process, system or product problems before they occur. This activity can provide a safety next to identify problems that could occur, provide prediction of failure severity and the health care system's ability to detect potential failures before they occur. Clearly the goal of utilizing FMEA in combination with RCA is to assure that harm to patients could be avoided, managed, or eliminated.

Preventing Errors and Cause

The concept of failure mode and effects analysis comes from the engineering industry. The technique has been around for over 40 years.[127] Industries such as aerospace, nuclear power, electronics, and food processing have utilized FMEA strategies to reduce or eliminate after-the-event correction strategies when failures occur.

FMEA is also a team based and systematic approach like RCA, but instead of used to investigate an error after it occurs, it is a proactive approach used to identify why a process or design can fail, why it might fail and how it can be made safer. If a particular failure is identified by a FMEA cannot be pre-

vented, the technique then focuses on protections that can be put into place to prevent the failure from reaching the patient or mitigating the effects of the failure if it reaches the patient. FMEA requires a clear understanding of its component word parts.[128]

Failure: When a system, process or service performs in a way that is not intended or desirable. The failure could be evident as a lack of success, nonperformance, nonoccurrence, or complete breakdown or cessation of function.

Mode: The manner or method in which something, like a failure can occur. The term *failure mode*, is then the manner in which something can fail. A single failure may have many failure modes.

Effects: The results or consequences of a failure mode.

Analysis: An examination of the elements or structure of a process or service.

Conducting a failure mode and effects analysis also requires a team effort. Assembling a multidisciplinary team that understands the process undergoing redesign or newly implemented is essential. The team assigned to conducting a failure mode and effects analysis must work to understand the process(es) under analysis, the causes or potential causes of failures, and the necessary steps to assure that failures are less likely to occur. As part of analysis the team will identify many potentials for failure. Some may be very real others only hypothetical. The team will need to determine what failures to address and assign priority to these action steps. This activity, or prioritization, requires what is called a criticality analysis.

A criticality analysis is a method used to identify relative measures of importance for a failure mode.[129] For each failure mode identified, a rank is determined for its importance based on a combined evaluation of three factors:

- Severity: this rating estimates how serious the effect would be if in fact the failure occurred
- Probability of occurrence: this rating estimates the likelihood that the failure would happen
- Detectability: this rating estimates the degree to which the failure could be detected.

The team needs to agree on a scoring method to assist with this process. A numerical scale, such as 1 to 10 or qualitative scale, such as high, medium, or low, could also be utilized. In any case, the team must agree on definitions of the scales and how the scoring will occur. As part of this scoring discussion, it is a good idea to identify how disagreement on scoring or rating will be handled and how this will be resolved and consensus reached.

Because teams must focus their energies on addressing failures most likely to cause harm, the ranking process allows for evaluation of these three factors simultaneously. If a qualitative scale is used to determine priority, the group must agree which ratings or combination of ratings will require attention. If a numerical scale is used, a risk priority number (RPN) can be calculated. In some texts, an RPN is also referred to as a criticality index (CI).[129] An RPN is calculated as follows:

$$RPN = severity \times occurrence \times detectability$$

Failure modes with high RPNs require immediate attention. It might be helpful for organizations to identify a score that serves as a cutoff point for action.

This concept of FMEA is a relatively new one for health care organizations, but is growing in acceptance. In 1994, the Institute for Safe Medication Practices (ISMP) began recommending use of FMEA medication use process improvement and redesign.[130] As an example, the Department of Veteran's Affairs National Center for Patient Safety (NCPS) has introduced a prospective analysis model called Health care Failure Modes and Effects Analysis (HFMEA) which combines FMEA characteristics with the Hazard Analysis and Critical Control Point (HACCP) model developed to ensure food safety.[131] All VA facilities received training and moved forward with utilization of this tool in 2001. These efforts are contributing to a shift toward a new way of thinking, describing, and evaluating errors within health care systems.

The term *error* is being utilized less because of the implication of human involvement and perception of blame or fault. Failure has been the preferred term because it can be utilized to describe latent or hazardous conditions that could result in harm to an individual without assigning blame. FMEA is a technique that assumes that no matter how knowledgeable or careful people are, failures will occur in some situations. The focus is on *WHAT* could allow the failure to occur, not *WHO*.

Conducting a Failure Mode and Effects Analysis

There are several key features for health care organizations to consider as the conduct a failure mode and effects analysis[132]:

- Select a high-risk process to evaluate and assemble a team. Consider a process that is likely to impact the safety of patients within the health care organization.
- Diagram the new or existing process of interest. Include the all the steps and identify the actual v expected performance.
- Brainstorm all potential failure modes within the process and determine their effects.
- Prioritize the list of failure modes identified. The basis for identifying priority actions should be based on the severity, occurrence, and detectability capability within the health care organization.
- Identify the root causes of failure modes.
- Redesign the current or create the new process.
- Analyze or test the changes or new process identified.
- Implement and monitor the redesigned or new process.

Benefits of Conducting a Failure Mode and Effects Analysis

The primary benefit of conducting an FMEA is that this technique has been used successfully to reduce the risk of errors and failures and increase the successful performance of a process. For medication use, this means a decrease in the likelihood of untoward or sentinel medication events. A true advantage is that this process can also provide protection for patients and evaluate systems for potential risk reduction strategies. FMEA can serve as an effective quality improvement tool in any health care organization with out the use of complicated tools or statistical analysis. Data can be evaluated for real or perceived failure potential and identify clear opportunities for improvement through a group process. FMEA explores how processes, design, or service can be improved or redesigned to reduce the likelihood of failure.

Data Collection and Reporting

Reporting and data capturing processes must be well defined and understood within the organization. Having a systems approach to reporting is another necessary component for improving safety. Consider the following tips for improving the reporting process:

- Define medication errors within the organization
- Provide automatic report distribution to key leadership within the organization
- Make reporting voluntary to encourage near miss reporting
- Consider use of an outside group to review reports and identify trends and trouble-spots
- Create a paperless system for ease of reporting
- Allow free-form reporting to capture all information
- Ensure that system for reporting is nonpunitive
- Involve the patient
- Evaluate ways to improve informed consent process and disclosing risks to patients
- Use benchmarking data
- Provide timely feedback regarding information collected from reports

- Identify actionable strategies for follow-up . . . and then *FOLLOW-UP*

Methods must be in place to measure, monitor, evaluate, and improve performance even in the face of an adverse event. Further, organizations should not wait until a problem arises in the organization to respond to this safety agenda. Organizations need to identify safety activities that are proactive and ensure that information regarding patient and staff incidents, measurement and monitoring activities, and communication plans are in place. The following items should be identified in a safety plan for medication use improvement:

- Incorporate measurement into performance improvement activities
- Trend data and create a dashboard of indicators of interest
- Focus on safety as a priority in job descriptions and performance appraisals
- Incorporate team safety training into orientation programs and ongoing competency assessments
- Create a plan to communicate information learned from reporting an error throughout the entire organization

IMPLEMENTING ACTION STEPS FOR CHANGE

Creating steps for successful implementation of medication safety improvements could be the most important part of an effective safety initiative. First and foremost, it is important for an organization to define the aim of a safety initiative. It is critical that all team members understand and can explain what the aim is of the improvement, and also the reason for implementing the change. Organizations must identify and involve key players who will assist in the implementation of the change. Teamwork and collaboration are essential at all organizational levels.

Define and Provide Resources

Organizations must find and allocate the resources that will be needed. Think of time as a resource, including time for team members to participate on the team, completing team assignments and communicating with other team members and target audiences. Identifying and securing resources for safety initiatives must be a part of the leadership and organization's priority.

Define the Change Needed

The desired changes for safety improvement should be well outlined in clear, measurable terms. Organizations must determine initial measures that will help assess if the change is an improvement. The team should identify how data will be collected, analyzed, displayed, and reported. Organizations should also identify resources to assist in the process. Many national support groups and resources exist. The Institute for Safe Medication Practices (ISMP-www.ismp.org), American Society of Health-System Pharmacists (ASHP-www.ashp.org), Institute for Healthcare Improvement (IHI-www.ihi.org), Joint Commission on Accreditation of Healthcare Organizations (JCAHO-www.jcaho.org) and others offer opportunities for dialog and exchange and have tools, tips, and networks to share the success strategies as well as examples of common problems encountered with medication use.

Communicate Findings

Utilize existing systems to communicate the change as well as reporting the results of safety performance improvement initiatives. Organizations must dedicate resources to create the message that will be delivered when introducing and implementing the change, including who will deliver the message, the content, timing, and the audience that will be targeted. All too often, data points, such as error rates, percentages or other factoids are shared, but little context provided. As a result, people who receive this information and are charged to act upon the data, are often unable to *connect the dots* and identify how to use the data for improvement to achieve sustainable performance results. If the organization fails to utilize the data collected in a way to demonstrate a commitment to medication use, individuals may lose their enthusiasm for reporting important findings and progress toward improving medication safety within the organization impaired or impossible.

As part of this communication planning process, it is important to identify barriers and potential solutions. These issues must be discussed openly and honestly. Every opportunity *must be used* to encourage reporting, promote safety, and reward prevention strategies. Additionally, identify opportunities to review improvement activities, results, and key learnings in leadership meetings, staff meetings etc.

Adopting Change

Assess mechanisms available to educate target audiences and to promote adoption of the change. It is important to remember that diffusion, dissemination, and adoption of any new innovation or change is dependent on each individual's capability and ability to make change happen—implementation of change occurs at different rates in different people. Everett Rogers described this phenomenon of how people accept adopt and influence change in his text *Diffusion of Innovations* in 1962.[133] His research sought to identify how and why innovations in agriculture, family planning, public health, and nutrition became adopted in developing countries of Latin America, Africa, and Asia. The goal was to identify how to speed up rates of infusion of new ideas since it was found that it often years passed before progress had been made. What Rogers found was that efforts for change should be directed toward those people who are most likely to accept new ideas and trial innovations. Efforts and energy should not be wasted on individuals who resist or fight against change. Within health care systems, it is important to identify who needs to be part of the safety improvement effort. Identifying those who are willing to lead the safety charge, be a willing team participant, and help with creative design are likely to help fuel process improvement success. It is important not to waste time on those who will never be convinced of the need for the change.

Determine what exists and what else may need to be developed. This plan should include all care providers including medical staff. In order to adopt change, find opportunities for medical staff to be involved in the peer review of adverse events, the credentialing process as well as involvement in safety initiatives. Methods to assess competency of staff providing care should also be included. Identify methods to integrate safety skill and action assessment into day-to-day activities of staff. This may include creating mentors in the area of best practices that support safe medication use.

Achieving Optimal Outcomes

Change may not always be desirable. To manage the health care environment to provide for optimal outcomes (ie, clinical, economic, health status, patient satisfaction) the organization must maintain an action plan that supports a continuous, prospective or concurrent, data-driven and measurable improvement process.[134] Organizations must understand that error can and will occur. The environment that the medication use process operates in is influenced and modified continually by external and internal forces. These forces must be evaluated and managed. Asking the question, "How will we know if we have implemented a medication use safety strategy that has re-

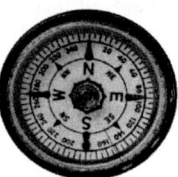

Clinical Outcomes

Satisfaction Outcomes

Economic Outcomes

Health Status Outcomes

Figure 102-12. Outcomes Compass. Adapted from Nelson EC, Batalden PB, Mohr J, Plume SK, et al. *Joint Commission Journal on Quality Improvement* 1996; 22(4):243. Reprinted with permission.

sulted in an improvement?" is a critical one. It is important to note that this is an iterative process . . . and that additional questioning to determine if the change is STILL an improvement over time, is necessary (Fig 102-12).

This outcomes compass depicts the breadth of outcomes associated with medication use. Adverse events can also be described as negative impacts in any of these outcome areas:

- Clinical: an undesired physical response, drop in blood pressure, altered lab test
- Health status: patient unable to return to previous or improved level of functioning
- Economic: delayed discharge, use of other agents to resolve symptoms
- Satisfaction: lack of meeting patient or other medication use process customer expectations

The impact of medication safety initiatives should include evaluations of these global aspects as part of your design.

BARRIERS ASSOCIATED WITH SAFETY IMPROVEMENT

There are many reasons why organizations struggle with improving safety within their organization. Often, traditional methods such as medication error or adverse drug event reporting are cumbersome. Organizations have not adequately defined the process, the scope of collection, and members of the health care team do not understand why there is a need to collect and discuss the data. Many involved in the reporting end of the process never hear about the information gleaned from the analysis.

Additionally, data collection and discussion about medication errors or adverse events are often fragmented. Pharmacy might collect and discuss some of the data, while nursing may be responsible for other parts and risk management or QA may get involved for other issues. As a result, frustration occurs due to a lack of communication, integration, and input. Documentation systems are also cumbersome and often do not fit in well with other day-to-day care responsibilities. What happens with all these events reported? Fear that individuals will be blamed for the error and that punitive action will be taken also limits individual participation in the process.

Having a plan and an organizational understanding of the aim regarding safety improvement is essential. Many parts of the health care team contribute to the use of medications within the organization. All members within the organization must be aware of the importance of medication use safety, mindful of the potential for error and their role in averting it and what the organization has in place to assure that safety is a priority.

Integration of all data and associated knowledge regarding medication use is needed. The integration of existing data, including ADR, medication error, pharmacy/nursing interventions, and medication interaction data, into one organization-wide database is the key to an effective ADE quality management program.

The overall impact of the database could be measured by examining the impact that the reduced incidence of ADEs has on health outcomes: clinical, economic, patient satisfaction, and health status outcomes. Specific goals for adverse event improvement activities generally include:

- Increase documentation
- Aggregate data effectively
- Organizational education and training regarding prevention and detection
- Use data to improve the medication use system
- Minimize patient risk
- Maximize health outcomes
- Create an open and honest environment where there is a focus on system improvement and reporting
- Remove focus on individual and punitive process
- Meet regulatory standards

Many groups have identified methods to improve the safety of the medication use process. National and local groups have strategies to share and stories to tell. It is important to learn and replicate best practice and build on the success of others.

SOURCES OF LEARNING ABOUT PATIENT SAFETY

The following descriptions of organizations and initiatives for patient safety improvement are provided as background for this critical and dynamic field of endeavor. Many of these organizations are headed or staffed by physicians and other health care professionals, giving them a unique prospective on ways to improve on patient safety. All are accompanied by the website address for that organization's home page. This is not intended to be an exhaustive list, there are many pharmacy, nursing and other discipline-focused initiatives contributing to national safety improvement initiatives, but this provides a sample of what is available.

The Agency for Healthcare Research and Quality (AHRQ)

The AHRQ, a division of the Department of Health and Human Services, is the lead federal agency on quality of care research. Its mission is to support, conduct, and disseminate research that improves access to care and the outcomes, quality, cost, and utilization of health care services. The AHRQ has been fulfilling this mission since 1998 through its leadership role in the Federal Quality Interagency Coordination Task Force (http://www.quic.gov). This task force is spearheading the initiation of a number of federally funded research projects on patient safety. The AHRQ spends approximately 80% of its budget ($270 million in FY2001) funding research grants. It allocated $50 million for patient safety research grants in FY2001. Web site: http://www.ahcpr.gov/qual/errorsix.htm

The American Hospital Association (AHA)

The AHA makes available a wide variety of tools and resources to assist in improving care (http://www.aha.org/Patient Safety/Safe home.asp). One tool, *Strategies for Leadership: Hospital Executives and Their Role in Patient Safety*, was developed by James B. Conway, chief operations officer at Dana-Farber Caner Institute in Boston, specifically for executives' personal use and reflection on their efforts to develop a culture of safety. Web site: http://www.aha.org/PatientSafety/Culture Safety.asp

Anesthesia Patient Safety Foundation (APSF)

The APSF was established in 1984 "to assure that no patient shall be harmed by the effects of anesthesia," as set forth in its mission statement. The APSF is noteworthy because it has been instrumental in the dramatic improvements in anesthesia safety. As such, it represents a good source of insight and precedence for activities-such as clinical investigations and communications programs-that can be undertaken to improve patient safety. Web site: http://www.gasnet.org/societies/apsf/index.html

Annenberg Patient Safety Conferences

The *Examining Error in Health Care Conferences* were held in October 1996, November 1998, and May 2001. The meetings were sponsored by a myriad of organizations, including the American Association for the Advancement of Science, American Society of Health-System Pharmacists, American Medical Association, and Annenberg Health Sciences Center at Rancho Mirage, CA. Ongoing, annual conferences provide updates and rigorous reviews of the collaborative system improvements necessary to improve health care safety. The Web site contains listings and descriptions of the disparate organizations involved in this interdisciplinary topic, names and titles of presentations, and order forms for proceedings and audiotapes of the sessions: http://www.mederrors.org

Institute for Healthcare Improvement (IHI)

The IHI is a Boston-based, independent, nonprofit organization founded in 1991 to foster systematic improvements in health care in the United States, Canada, and Europe. The IHI is a leading force in promoting and facilitating teamwork and collaborative care in a variety of health care reform initiatives. Its mantra is that people and organizations who share a common goal (eg, patient safety improvement) can achieve more by working together than by working separately. The activities of the IHI embody a systems thinking approach toward the goal of creating health care systems that are accessible, safe, easy to use, and satisfying for patients and communities. Web site: http://www.ihi.org/

Institute for Safe Medication Practices (ISMP)

The ISMP is a nonprofit organization that works with the major stakeholders in health care to provide information education about adverse drug events and their prevention. The ISMP works closely with the U.S. Pharmacopoeia (USP) to analyze data gathered through the Medication Error Reduction Program (MERP), which was launched by the USP in 1991. (The USP shares MERP data with the U.S. Food and Drug Administration, which operates its own adverse drug event reporting system, called MedWatch.) Web site: http://www.ismp.org/

Joint Commission on Accreditation of Healthcare Organizations (Joint Commission, JCAHO)

The patient safety standards that the Joint Commission has put into place address a number of significant patient safety issues including the implementation of patient safety programs, the responsibility of organization leadership to create a culture of safety, the prevention of medical errors through the prospective analysis and redesign of vulnerable patient systems (eg, the ordering, preparation, and dispensing of medications), and the hospital's responsibility to tell a patient if he or she has been harmed by the care provided. The Joint Commission is in the process of standardizing and implementing similar patient safety standards throughout its accreditation programs across the care continuum. In addition to standards changes highlighting safety improvement, the JCAHO has established a list National Patient Safety Goals (NPSGs) for organizations to implement to assure that best practices are implemented to drive safety improvement. The JCAHO is also collaborating with the National Quality Forum (NQF) and others to establish national best practices and expectations. It is anticipated that one of the best practices, the use of barcoding for medication administration, will be required for all hospitals by 2007 as part of an NPSG. Web site: http://www.jcaho.org

Leapfrog Group

Established in 1990, the Leapfrog Group is a coalition of large, self-insured employers seeking to leverage their purchasing power to drive improvements in health care quality. Their strategy is to monitor the quality of health care services in communities in which their employees work and live, focusing initially on hospitals, and channel their employees to those facilities that achieve those objective measures of high-quality care. The group currently is focusing on three initiatives for quality improvement in hospital-based care: (1) evidence-based hospital referral, (2) use of intensivists, and (3) computerized physician order entry (CPOE). The CPOE initiative is of particular interest of this curriculum because research to date indicates that general use of CPOE can significantly reduce medical errors and their attendant costs. Web site: http://www.leapfroggroup.org

Malcolm Baldrige National Quality Program

The MBNQ Program has developed a questionnaire to assess how an organization is performing and learn what can be improved. The questionnaire is based on the Baldrige Criteria for Performance Excellence and is available at their Web site: http://www.quality.nist.gov/Progress.htm

Massachusetts Coalition for the Prevention of Medical Errors

The coalition participants include senior leadership and expert staff from organizations with a longstanding commitment to quality and public accountability. This includes professional associations representing hospitals, physicians, nurses, nurse executives, and long-term care institutions; state and federal agencies with responsibility for licensure and oversight; accrediting bodies; and clinical researchers. The coalition's goals are to identify and implement best practices to reduce medical errors in Massachusetts and to facilitate professional and public education regarding patient safety. Web site: http://www.macoalition.org/

Minnesota Hospital and Healthcare Partnership (MHHP)

The MHHP leads a coalition on patient safety within Minnesota's health care community to improve and enhance patient safety in all aspects of care delivery and strengthen public trust. The Patient Safety Committee address public policy, leadership, and best practices to position MHHP and its mem-

ber facilities ad demonstrated leaders in patient safety. Web site: http://www.mhhp.com/psafety/leaderkit.htm

National Academy for State Health Policy (NASHP)

NASHP is at the forefront of examining how states monitor and respond to quality and patient safety issues. Areas of focus have included the state government's role in patient safety, actions the states have taken to improve patient safety, and other steps states are taking to improve quality of care. Web site: http://www.nashp.org

National Coalition on Health Care (NCHC)

The NCHC is the nation's largest and most broadly representative alliance working to improve health care in America. The coalition-which is nonprofit and nonpartisan-was founded in 1990 and comprises more than 90 groups employing or representing approximately 100 million Americans. Members are united in the belief that we need and can achieve better more affordable health care for all Americans. Web site: http://www.americanshealth.org/

National Committee for Quality Assurance (NCQA)

The NCQA is a private, nonprofit organization dedicated to improvement of health care quality, with its primary focus being on managed care organizations. Activities performed by the NCQA include oversight of health care quality, conducting quality improvement initiatives, and recognition of providers that demonstrate excellence in health care. The most widely known program run by the NCQA is its Health Plan Employer and Data Information Set (HEDIS), a body of standardized performance measures designed to insure that purchasers and consumers have the information they need to reliably compare the performance of managed care plans. HEDIS report cards are now made available online at MedScape and CBS Health Watch. In addition to HEDIS, the NCQA administers a physician organization certification program, launched in 1997; to help managed care organizations and purchasers assess physician organizations. Web site: http://www.ncqa.org/

National Patient Safety Foundation (NPSF)

The NPSF was established in 1997 by the American Medical Association with the mission to help health care systems achieve measurable improvements in patient safety. It seeks to identify, create, and facilitate the application of a core body of knowledge about patient safety; to foster a culture of receptivity to patient safety initiatives; and to raise public awareness about patient safety. Among the activities sponsored by the NPSF are the national and regional educational conferences and dissemination of publications. Their online bibliography (http://www.npsf.org/clearinghouse2001.htm) contains a wealth of citations in the patient safety literature dating back to 1939, from peer-reviewed publications and authoritative textbooks. Web site: http://www.npsf.org

National Quality Forum (NQF)

The National Quality Forum is a private, not-for-profit membership organization created to develop and implement a national strategy for healthcare quality measurement and reporting. The mission of the NQF is to improve American healthcare through endorsement of consensus-based national standards for measurement and public reporting of healthcare performance data that provide meaningful information about whether care is safe, timely, beneficial, patient-centered, equitable and efficient. The NQF, in collaboration with several other organizations and stakeholders, has identified 30 healthcare safe practices that should be universally utilized in applicable clinical care settings to reduce the risk of harm to patients. This list is provided in Appendix 2, with the full report available at the NQF website. Web site: http://www.qualityforum.org.

United States Pharmacopeial Convention (USP)

The United States Pharmacopeial Convention (USP) was established to promote public health and benefit practitioners and patients by disseminating authoritative standards and information developed by its volunteers for medicines, other healthcare technologies, and related practices used to maintain and improve health and promote optimal healthcare delivery. The USP establishes enforceable standards and provides recommended guideline on the production, purity, content and quality of medications, diagnostic agents and nutritionals. While many of the individual standards established by the USP affect safety and quality of medications, the USP has three major areas that contribute to the general body of safety evidence for medication use:

Safe Medication Use Expert Committee: The USP Safe Medication Use Expert Committee (SMU EC) was established as a member of the Council of Experts at USP's meeting in April 2000, and is thus, a formal constituent of the standards-setting process. This Expert Committee represents medicine, nursing, and pharmacy and includes representation from academia, research, government, and consumer interest. The SMU EC functions to promulgate patient safety and safe medication use by proposing standards for incorporation in the United States Pharmacopeia-National Formulary (USP-NF), identifying "better practices", reviewing the MEDMARX[SM] Annual Reports and analyzing medication error data to determine priority areas such as CPOE, imprint and bar-codes, errors in non-hospital settings, good products and labeling practices, consumer and clinical education, best practices, recommendations for pediatric medications, neuromuscular blocking agents and others, and high alert drugs such as insulin and potassium chloride concentrate. As an example of their ongoing work to improve medication safety, standards for safe pharmaceutical compounding for sterile preparations (USP NF 797) were established for implementation in 2004.

The National Coordinating Council for Medication Error Reporting and Prevention (NCC MERP): This is an independent body comprised of 25 national and international organizations. In 1995, USP spearheaded the formation of the National Coordinating Council for Medication Error Reporting and Prevention. This nationwide program allows for health professionals who encounter actual or potential medication errors to report confidentially and anonymously, if preferred, to USP. USP reviews each report for health hazards and forwards all information to the Food and Drug Administration and the product manufacturer. The MER Program is presented in cooperation with the Institute for Safe Medication Practices

MEDMARX Program[SM]: A national database, MEDMARX allows subscribing facilities to access and share information. This landmark program has nearly 500,000 medication error records submitted by more than 700 participants. The MEDMARX[SM] program is a comprehensive, Internet-accessible, anonymous medication error reporting program and quality improvement tool. The program facilitates efficient documentation, tracking, and trending of data to identify medication error prevention strategies. Web site: http://www.usp.org.

SUMMARY AND CONCLUSIONS

The IOM reports–*To Err is Human* and *Crossing the Quality Chasm* paint a vivid landscape of the crisis in the American health care system and offer recommendations to point to a path for change. Mindful that the Chinese word for crisis contains two elements, danger and opportunity, we are reminded that that the edge of chaos is where change occurs, where systems unfreeze and reform with renewed capacity to respond to environmental forces, and to adapt.

The path to safer medication use and improvements in patient safety is not about a destination. This is a journey that must involve iterative learning. There are no absolute solutions, no mystical pronouncements that will tell the profession of pharmacy what to do to fix the system. The problems it faces will not be solved by the level of thinking that created them. The profession is forced to consider new approaches, new knowledge and to consider ways of thinking, acting and being that are outside our traditional approaches.

Some hard lessons learned from other transformational change initiatives, health care, and other industries provide insight and wisdom for the journey:

- Gather and use evidence to define the path and to persuade others to follow it.
- Realize that if you build it, they may not come. People always do want what makes sense to them in their own context, in their own time. The context cannot be overlooked because it is believed that content is impressive and persuasive. Allow some time for sense-making and learning to occur, but remember to front-end-load the learning with vision, direction and feedback.
- Wanting to do the right thing is not the problem. The aggregated consequences of how things are done creates the outcomes, morbidity, mortality, and cost experienced. Redesign will be essential. Make it easy to do the right thing, not harder. Simplification is a key.
- Engage the culture. Do not wait for it to change. Miracles happen when knowledge and context are shared through feedback. Build on best knowledge to engage the culture, with the realization that culture changes when knowledge shifts occur.
- Knowledge is sticky. Without a systematic process, enablers, and system supports, it doesn't move easily. Posters, senior leader's speeches, newsletters, and slogans typically do not cause knowledge *to blow*. Use data, make personal connections, use champions to move knowledge to influence culture to create change.
- Think about absorptive capacity. What issues might compete or conflict with the priority of the safety issue. Consider timing, how full individual plates are and craft a compelling message to engage people in the process.
- Consider ways to increase the dialog about safety. Communities of practice and successful microsystems are powerful tribes. When they work, knowledge flows and best practices can be replicated. Dialog is the key to effective information flow and to uncovering tacit knowledge that holds keys to success strategies.

Ultimately, the judge of the quality of work, the services delivered and the outcomes of care is an increasingly well-informed patient, as well as their payors and regulators from the public and private sectors. Focus on patient needs and wants, less on how we do it around here.

Enjoy the journey.

REFERENCES

1. Chassin MR, Galvin RW. *JAMA* 1995; 280(10):29.
2. Institute of Medicine. *To Err Is Human: Building a Safer Health System.* Kohn LT, Corrigan JM, Donaldson MS, eds. Washington, DC: National Academy Press, 2000.
3. Committee on Quality Health Care in America. *Crossing the Quality Chasm: A New Health System for the 21st Century.* Institute of Medicine, ed. Washington, DC: National Academy Press, 2001.
4. HCFA1999. 1998 National Health Expenditures, Department of Health and Human Services, Washington, DC. Available at: http://www.hcfa.gov/stats/nhe-oact/hilites.htm. Accessed January 10, 2000.
5. Institute of Medicine. *To Err Is Human: Building a Safer Health System.* Kohn LT, Corrigan JM, Donaldson MS, eds. Washington, DC: National Academy Press, 2000.
6. Committee on Quality Health Care in America. *Crossing the Quality Chasm: A New Health System for the 21st Century.* Institute of Medicine, ed. Washington, DC: National Academy Press, 2001.

7. Committee on Quality Health Care in America. *Crossing the Quality Chasm: A New Health System for the 21st Century.* Institute of Medicine, ed. Washington, DC: National Academy Press, 2001.
8. Committee on Identifying Priority Areas for Quality Improvement. *Priority Areas for National Action: Transforming Health Care Quality.* Institute of Medicine, ed. Washington, DC: National Academy Press, 2003.
9. Committee on Rapid Advance Demonstration Projects: Health Care Finance and Delivery Systems. *Fostering Rapid Advances in Health Care: Learning From System Demonstrations.* Institute of Medicine, ed. Washington, DC: National Academy Press, 2003.
10. Committee on Enhancing Federal Healthcare Quality Programs. *Leadership by Example: Coordinating Government Roles in Improving Health Care Quality.* Institute of Medicine, ed. Washington, DC: National Academy Press, 2003.
11. Committee on Data Standards for Patient Safety: Board on Health Care Services. *Patient Safety: Achieving a New Standard for Care.* Institute of Medicine, ed. Washington, DC: National Academy Press, 2004.
12. Committee on the Health Professions Education Summit: Board on Health Care Services. *Health Professions Education: A Bridge to Quality.* Institute of Medicine, ed. Washington, DC: National Academy Press, 2003: 45–69.
13. Committee on the Work Environment for Nurses and Patient Safety. Board on Health Care Services. *Keeping Patients Safe: Transforming the Work Environment of Nurses.* Institute of Medicine, ed. Washington, DC: National Academy Press, 2004.
14. Cook R, Woods D, Miller C. *A Tale of Two Stories: Contrasting Views of Patient Safety.* Chicago, IL: National Patient Safety Foundation, 1998. Available at: http://www.npsf.org/exec/npsf rpt.pdf. Accessed April 30, 2003.
15. Leape LL, Kabcenell A, Berwick DM, et al. *Reducing Adverse Drug Events.* Boston MA: Institute for Healthcare Improvement; 1998.
16. Phillips DP, Christenfeld N, Glynn LM. *Lancet* 1998; 351:643.
17. Leape LL, Brennan TA, Laird N, et al. *N Engl J Med* 1991; 324:337.
18. Lazarou JL, Pomeranz BH, Corey PN. *JAMA* 1998; 279:1200.
19. Classen DC, Pestotnik SL, Evans RS, et al. *JAMA* 1997; 277:301.
20. Bates DW, Spell N, Cullen DJ, et al. *JAMA* 1997; 277:307.
21. Forster AJ, Murff HJ, Peterson JF, et al. *Ann Intern Med* 2003; 138:161.
22. Beard K. *Drug Aging* 1992; 2:356.
23. Burnum JF. *Ann Intern Med* 1976; 85:80.
24. Schneitman-McIntire O, Farnent TA, Gordon N, et al. *Am J Health Syst Pharm* 1996; 3:1416.
25. Bootman JL, Harrison DL, Cox E. *Arch Intern Med* 1997; 157:2089.
26. Greenberg J, Leutz W, Greenlick M, et al. *Health Aff (Millwood)* 1998; 7:66.
27. Sullivan SD, Kreling DH, Hazlet TK, et al. *J Res Pharm Econ* 1990; 2:19.
28. Alliance for Aging Research. *When Medicine Hurts Instead of Helps.* Washington, DC: Alliance for Aging Research; 1998. Available at: http://www.agingresearch.org/brochures/medicinehurts/when-medicinehurts.html. Accessed April 30, 2003.
29. Johnson JA, Bootman JL. *Arch Intern Med* 1995; 155:1949.
30. Halas J, Haghfelt T, Gram LF, et al. *J Intern Med* 1990; 228:379.
31. Wilcox SM, Himmelstein DU, Woodhandler S. *JAMA* 1994; 272:292.
32. Knox R. Prescription errors tied to lack of advice: pharmacists skirting law, Massachusetts study finds. Boston Globe. February 10, 1999: (Metro); BI. Available at: http://www.bostonglobe.com. Accessed November 26, 2002.
33. Einarson TR. *Ann Pharmacother* 1993; 27:832.
34. United States Food and Drug Administration. CDER New and Generic Drug Approvals. Available at: http://www.accessdata.fda.gov/scripts/cder/drugcat. Accessed April 30, 2003.
35. Centers for Disease Control and Prevention. *Morbidity and Mortality Weekly Report* 1995; 44:506.
36. Gonzales R, Steiner JF, Sande MA. *JAMA* 1997; 278:901.
37. Ellerbeck EF, Jencks SF, Radford MJ, et al. *JAMA* 1995; 273:1509.
38. Leape LL, Lauthers AG, Brennan TA, et al. *QRB* 1993; 8:144.
39. Hume M. *The Quality Letter* 1999; 11(3):2.
40. Leape LL, Kabcenell A, Berwick DM et al. *Reducing Adverse Drug Events.* Boston MA: Institute for Healthcare Improvement; 1998: 175.
41. Institute for Safe Medication Practices. Proposed HCFA rule may cause increase in medication errors. ISMP Medication Safety Alert, January 28, 1998. Available at: http://www.ismp.org/MSAarticles/HCFA.html. Accessed on April 23, 2003.
42. Deming WE. *Out of the Crisis.* Cambridge, MA: Massachusetts Institute of Technology, 1986.
43. Leape LL. Error in medicine. *JAMA* 1994; 272(23):1851.

44. Leape LL, Kabcenell A, Berwick DM, et al. *Reducing Adverse Drug Events.* Boston, MA: Institute for Healthcare Improvement, 1998:84–91.
45. Reason J. *Managing the Risks of Organizational Accidents.* Aldershot, UK: Ashgate, 1997:7.
46. Reason J. *Human Error.* Cambridge, UK: Cambridge University Press, 1990:208.
47. Reason J. *Managing the Risks of Organizational Accidents.* Aldershot, UK: Ashgate, 1997.
48. Cook R, Woods D. In: Bogner MS, ed. *Human Error in Medicine.* Hillsdale, NJ: Lawrence Erlbaum Associates, 1994:257.
49. Cook R, Woods D. In: Bogner MS, ed. *Human Error in Medicine.* Hillsdale, NJ: Lawrence Erlbaum Associates, 1994:287.
50. Reason J. *Human Error.* Cambridge, UK: Cambridge University Press, 1990:42.
51. Reason J. *Human Error.* Cambridge, UK: Cambridge University Press, 1990:8.
52. Beardsley D, Woods K, eds. *First Do No Harm: A Practical Guide to Medication Safety and JCAHO Compliance.* Marblehead, MA: Opus Communications, 1990:12.
53. American Society of Anesthesiologists. Position paper. Available at: www.asahq.org. Accessed on April 30, 2003.
54. Gaba DM. Human error in anesthetic mishaps. *Int Anesthesiol Clin* 1989; 27(3):137.
55. JCAHO. *Jt Comm J Qual Improv* 1998; 24(4):175.
56. Chassin MR. *Millbank Q* 1998; 764:565.
57. Leape LL, Kabcenell A, Berwick DM, et al. *Reducing Adverse Drug Events.* Boston, MA: Institute for Healthcare Improvement, 1998:52.
58. Gaba DM. In Bogner MS, ed. *Human Error in Medicine.* Hillsdale, NJ: Lawrence Erlbaum Associates, 1994:208.
59. Committee on Quality Health Care in America. *Crossing the Quality Chasm: A New Health System for the 21st Century.* Institute of Medicine, ed. Washington, DC: National Academy Press, 2001:66.
60. Pichert JW, Hickson GB. In: Vincent C, ed. *Clinical Risk Management: Enhancing Patient Safety,* 2nd ed. London: BMH Books, 2001:274.
61. Pichert JW, Hickson GB. In: Vincent C, ed. *Clinical Risk Management: Enhancing Patient Safety,* 2nd ed. London: BMH Books, 2001:277.
62. Wiegman S, Cohen M. In: Cohen M, ed. *Medication Errors.* Washington, DC: American Pharmaceutical Association, 1999:14.2.
63. Batalden PB, Mohr JJ. *Qual Manag Health Care* 1997;5(3):3.
64. Weber DO. *Health Forum J* 2002; Mar/Apr:10.
65. Stich SP. Rationality. In: Osherson DN, Smith EE, eds. *An Invitation to Cognitive Science: Thinking.* Vol 3. Cambridge, MA: MIT Press, 1990.
66. Plsek PE, Greenhalgh T. *BMJ* 2001; 323:625.
67. Lorenz E. *The Essence of Chaos.* Seattle: University of Washington Press, 1993.
68. Zimmerman B, Lindberg C, Plsek P. *Edgeware: Insights From Complexity Science for Healthcare Leaders.* Irving, TX: VHA Publishing, 1998:34.
69. Richmond B. *The "Thinking" in Systems Thinking: Seven Essential Skills. Toolbox Reprint Series.* Waltham, MA: Pegasus Communications Inc, 2000.
70. Zimmerman B, Lindberg C, Plsek P. *Edgeware: Insights From Complexity Science for Healthcare Leaders.* Irving, TX: VHA Publishing, 1998:33.
71. Committee on Quality Health Care in America. *Crossing the Quality Chasm: A New Health System for the 21st Century.* Institute of Medicine, ed. Washington, DC: National Academy Press, 2001:5.
72. Deming WE. *Out of the Crisis.* Cambridge, MA: Massachusetts Institute for Technology, 1986.
73. Senge PM. *The Fifth Discipline: The Art and Practice of the Learning Organization.* New York: Doubleday, 1990.
74. Wheatley MJ. *Leadership and the New Science: Learning About Organization From an Orderly Universe.* San Francisco: Berrett-Koehler, 1992.
75. Quinn JB. *Intelligent Enterprise: A Knowledge and Service Based Paradigm for Industry.* New York: The Free Press, 1992.
76. Nelson EC, Batalden PM, Huber TP, et al. *Jt Comm J Qual Improv* 2002; 28:472.
77. Weick KE, Sutcliffe KM. *Managing the Unexpected: Assuring High Performance in an Age of Complexity.* San Francisco: Jossey-Bass, 2001.
78. Donaldson MS, Mohr JJ. *Exploring Innovation and Quality Improvement in Health Care Microsystems: A Cross-Case Analysis. A Technical Report on the Quality of Health Care in America.* Washington, DC: Institute of Medicine, 2000.
79. Godfrey MM, ed. *Clinical Microsystem Action Guide: Improving Healthcare by Improving Your Microsystem Version 2.1.* Lebanon,

NH: Trustees of Dartmouth College; 2004. Available at: www.clinicalmicrosystem.org/actionGuide.htm. Accessed July 1, 2004.

80. Health Care Advisory Board. *Run to Rigor.* Washington, DC: Health Care Advisory Board, 1997.

81. Caldwell C. *Frontiers Health Serv Manag* 1998; 15:35.

82. Galvin RS. *Health Aff (Millwood)* 2001; 20:57.

83. Leape LL, Bates DW, Cullen DJ, et al. *JAMA* 1995; 274:35.

84. Fairclough J, ed. *Briefings on JCAHO* 1996; (Dec):9.

85. Cohen M. *Medication Errors.* Washington, DC: American Pharmaceutical Association, 1999:13.1–13.21.

86. Leape LL, Bates DW, Cullen DJ, et al. *JAMA* 1995; 274:38.

87. Bates DW, Cullen DJ, Laird N, et al. *JAMA* 1995; 274:29.

88. Cohen M. A Call to Action to Eliminate Handwritten Prescriptions Within 3 Years. Available at: http:// www.ismp.org. Accessed April 30, 2003.

89. Institute for Safe Medication Practices. Do not use these dangerous abbreviations or dose designations. Available at http:// www.ismp.org/msarticles/specialissuetable.html. Accessed April 30, 2003.

90. Mann CC. *Atlantic Monthly* 2001; 290(2):81.

91. Cohen M. *Medication Errors.* Washington, DC: American Pharmaceutical Association, 1999: 9.1.

92. Leape LL, Brennan TA, Laird N, et al. *N Engl J Med* 1991; 324:337.

93. Ukens C. *Drug Topics* 1997; (Mar):100.

94. Cohen M. *Medication Errors.* Washington, DC: American Pharmaceutical Association, 1999: 9.1–9.19.

95. US Food and Drug Administration. Questions and answers regarding the bar code proposal. Washington, DC: US Food and Drug Administration, March 13,2003. Available at: www.fda.gov. Accessed March 13, 2003.

96. Institute for Healthcare Improvement. *Medical Practice Communicator* 1998; 5(2):6.

97. Hume M. *The Quality Letter* 1999; 11(3):4.

98. Baldrige National Quality Program. Healthcare criteria for performance excellence. Gaithersburg, MD: National Institute of Standards and Technology. Available at http://www.quality.nist.gov/healthcare_criteria.htm. Accessed April 30, 2003.

99. Jaworsky J. *Synchronicity.* San Francisco: Barrett-Koehler; 1996:5.

100. Geller ES. *Professional Safety* 2000; 45(5):38.

101. Fraiser SW, Greehalgh T. *BMJ* 2001;323:799.

102. Coiera E. *BMJ* 2004;328:1197.

103. Schein E. *Organizational Culture and Leadership,* 2nd ed. San Francisco: Jossey-Bass, 1992.

104. Schein E. *The Corporate Culture Survival Guide.* San Francisco: Jossey-Bass, 1999:189.

105. Kohn LT, Corrigan JM, Donaldson MS, eds. *To Err Is Human: Building a Safer Health System.* Institute of Medicine, ed. Washington, DC: National Academy Press; 2000:14.

106. Reason J. *Managing the Risks of Organizational Accidents.* Aldershot, UK: Ashgate, 1998:194.

107. Weick KE, Sutcliffe KM. *Managing the Unexpected: Assuring High Performance in an Age of Complexity.* San Francisco: Jossey-Bass, 2001:138.

108. Errickson KA, Krampe RT, Tesch-Romer C. *Psych Rev* 1993; 100:363.

109. Greco PJ, Eisensberg J. *N Engl J Med* 1993; 329:1271.

110. Committee on Quality Health Care in America. *Crossing the Quality Chasm: A New Health System for the 21st Century.* Institute of Medicine, ed. Washington, DC: National Academy Press; 2001:117.

111. Leiter M. *Canadian Psychology* 32:547.

112. Anderson JD, Jay SJ, Weng HC, et al. Studying the effect of clinical uncertainty on physician's decision-making using ILIAD. *MEDINFO 8,* Part 2: 869.

113. Cohen S. *Psych Bulletin* 88:82–108.

114. Campbell DA, Cornett PL. How stress and burnout produce medical mistakes. In: Rosenthal MM, Sutcliffe KM, eds. *Medical Error: What Do We Know? What Do We Do?* San Francisco: Jossey-Bass; 2002:46.

115. VanDongen HPA, Dinges DF. Circadian rhythm in fatigue, alertness and performance. In: Kryger MH, Toth T, Dement WC, eds. *Principles and Practice of Sleep Medicine,* 3rd ed. Philadelphia: WB Saunders, 2000:391.

116. Dinges DF, Pack F, Williams K, et al. *Sleep* 1997; 20:267.

117. Liskowsky DR, ed. Biological rhythms: Implications for the worker. US Office of Technology Assessment, Rep. NO. OTA-BA-463. Washington, DC: US Govt. Printing Office, 1991.

118. Kreuger GP. Fatigue, performance and medication error. In: Bogner MS Ed. *Human Error in Medicine.* Hillsdale, NJ: Lawrence Erlbaum Associates, 1994:316.

119. Angus RG, Heslegrave RJ, Myles WS. *Psychophysiology* 1985; 22(3):276.

120. Langley G, Nolan K, Nolan T, et al. *The Improvement Guide: A Practical Approach to Enhancing Organizational Performance.* San Francisco: Jossey-Bass, 1996.

121. The Joint Commission on Accreditation of Healthcare Organizations. *JCAHO 2004 Hospital Accreditation Standards.* Oakbrook IL: Joint Commission Resources, 2004:175.

122. The Joint Commission on Accreditation of Healthcare Organizations. *JCAHO 2004 Hospital Accreditation Standards.* Oakbrook IL: Joint Commission Resources, 2004:73.

123. Anderson B, Fagerhaug T. *Root Cause Analysis: Simplified Tools and Techniques.* Milwaukee: ASQ Press, 2000: 2.

124. Murray SK, Murray OB. *Total Quality Tools for Healthcare.* Dayton, OH: PQ Systems Inc, 1997:230.

125. Joint Commission on Accreditation of Healthcare Organizations. *Root Cause Analysis in Healthcare: Tools and Techniques,* 2nd ed. Oakbrook Terrace, IL: Joint Commission Resources, 2003:17.

126. Joint Commission on Accreditation of Healthcare Organizations. *Root Cause Analysis in Healthcare: Tools and Techniques,* 2nd ed. Oakbrook Terrace, IL: Joint Commission Resources, 2003: 8.

127. Joint Commission on Accreditation of Healthcare Organizations. *Failure Mode and Effects Analysis in Health Care: Proactive Risk Reduction.* Oakbrook Terrace, IL: Joint Commission Resources, 2002:1.

128. Joint Commission on Accreditation of Healthcare Organizations. *Failure Mode and Effects Analysis in Health Care: Proactive Risk Reduction.* Oakbrook Terrace, IL: Joint Commission Resources, 2002:7.

129. Stamatis DH. *Failure Mode and Effect Analysis: FMEA from Theory to Execution.* Milwaukee, WI: ASQ Quality Press, 1995:33.

130. Cohen MR, Davis NM, Senders J. *Hosp Pharm* 1994; 29:319.

131. DeRosier J, Stalhandske E, Bagian JP, et al. *Jt Comm J Qual Imp* 2002; 28(5):248.

132. Joint Commission on Accreditation of Healthcare Organizations. *Failure Mode and Effects Analysis in Health Care: Proactive Risk Reduction.* Oakbrook Terrace, IL: Joint Commission Resources, 2002:9.

133. Rogers EM. *Diffusion of Innovations,* 4th ed. New York: The Free Press, 1995.

134. Nelson EC, Mohr JJ, Batalden PB, et al. *Jt Comm J Qual Safety* 1996; 22(4):243.

Appendix 102-1. Clinical Microsystem Assessment Tool

Instructions: Each of the following characteristics (eg, leadership) is followed by a series of descriptors. For each characteristic, please check the description that best describes your current microsystem and delivery of care OR a microsystem YOU are most familiar with.

	Characteristic	Descriptions			
Leadership	***Leadership:*** The role of leaders is to balance selling and reaching collective goals, and to empower individual autonomy and accountability, through building knowledge, respectful action, reviewing and reflecting.	☐ Leaders often tell me how to do my job and leave little room for innovation and autonomy. Overall, they don't foster a positive culture.	☐ Leaders struggle to find the right balance between reaching performance goals and empowering the staff.	☐ Leaders maintain constancy of purpose, establish clear goals and expectations, and foster a respectful positive culture. Leaders take time to build knowledge, review and reflect, and take action about Microsystems and the larger organization	☐ Can't Rate
	Organizational Support: The larger organization looks for ways to support the work of the microsystem and coordinate the hand-offs between microsystems.	☐ The larger organization isn't supportive in a way that provides recognition, information and resources to enhance my work.	☐ The larger organization is inconsistent and unpredictable in providing the recognition, information and resources needed to enhance my work.	☐ The larger organization provides recognition, information, and resources that enhance my work and makes it easier for me to meet the needs of patients.	☐ Can't Rate
Staff	***Staff Focus:*** There is selective hiring of the right kind of people. The orientation process is designed to fully integrate new staff into culture and work roles. Expectations of staff are high regarding performance, continuing education, professional growth, and networking.	☐ I am not made to feel like a valued member of the microsystem. My orientation was incomplete. My continuing education and professional growth needs are not being met.	☐ I feel like I am a valued member of the microsystem, but I don't think the microsystem is doing all that it could to support education and training of staff, workload and professional growth.	☐ I am a valued member of the microsystem and what I say matters. This is evident through staffing, education and training, workload, and professional growth.	☐ Can't Rate
	Education and Training: All clinical Microsystems have responsibility for the ongoing education and training of staff and for aligning daily work roles with training competencies.	☐ Training is accomplished in disciplinary silos, eg, nurses train nurses, physicians train residents, etc. The educational efforts are not aligned with the flow of patient care, so that education becomes an "add on" to what we do.	☐ We recognize that our training could be different to reflect the needs of our microsystem, but we haven't made many changes yet. Some continuing education is available to everyone.	☐ There is a team approach to training, whether we are training staff, nurses or students. Education and patient care are integrated into the flow of work ina way that benefits both from the available resources. Continuing education for all staff is recognized as vital to our continued success.	☐ Can't Rate
	Interdependence: The interaction of staff is characterized by trust, collaboration, willingness to help each other, appreciation of complementary roles, respect and recognition that all contribute individually to a shared purpose.	☐ I work independently and I am responsible for my own part of the work. There is a lack of collaboration and a lack of appreciation for the importance of complementary roles.	☐ The care approach is interdisciplinary but we are not always available to work together as an effective team.	☐ Care provided by a interdisciplinary team characterized by trust, collaboration, appreciation of complementary roles, and a recognition that all contribute individually to a shared purpose.	☐ Can't Rate

	Characteristic	Descriptions			
Patient	***Patient Focus:*** The primary concern is to meet all patient needs—caring, listening, educating, and responding to special requests, innovating to meet patient needs and smooth service flow.	☐ Most of us, including our patients, would agree that we do not always provide patient centered care. We are not always clear about what patients want and need.	☐ We are actively working to provide patient centered care and we are making progress toward more effectively and consistently learning about and meeting patient needs.	☐ We are effective in learning about and meeting patient needs—caring, listening, educating, and responding to special requests and smooth service flow.	☐ Can't Rate
Patient	***Community and Market Focus:*** The microsystem is a resource for the community; the community is a resource to the microsystem; the microsystem establishes excellent and innovative relationships with the community.	☐ We focus on the patients who come to our unit. We haven't implemented any outreach programs in our community. Patients and their families often make their own connections to the community resources they need.	☐ We have tried a few outreach programs and have had some success, but it is not the norm for us to go out into the community or actively connect patients to the community resources that are available to them.	☐ We are doing everything we can to understand our community. We actively employ resources to help us with the community. We add to the community and we draw on resource from the community to meet patient needs	☐ Can't Rate
Performance	***Performance Results:*** Performance focuses on patient outcomes, avoidable costs, streamlining delivery, using data feedback, promoting positive competition, and frank discussions about performance.	☐ We don't routinely collect data on the process or outcomes of the care we provide.	☐ We often collect data on the outcomes of the care we provide and on some processes of care.	☐ Outcomes (clinical, satisfaction, financial, technical and safety) are routinely measured, we feed data back to staff and we make changes based on data.	☐ Can't Rate
Performance	***Process Improvement:*** An atmosphere for learning and redesign is supported by the continuous monitoring of care, use of benchmarking, frequent tests of change and a staff that has been empowered to innovate.	☐ The resource required (in the form of training, financial, support, and time) are rarely available to support improvement work. Any improvement activities we do are in addition to our daily work.	☐ Some resources are available to support improvement work, but we don't use them as often as we could. Change ideas are implemented without much discipline.	☐ There are ample resources to support continual improvement work. Studying, measuring, and improving care in a scientific way are essential parts of our daily work.	☐ Can't Rate
Information/Info Technology	***Information and Information Technology:*** Information is THE connector—Staff to patients, staff to staff, needs with actions to meet needs. Technology facilitates effective communication and multiple formal and informal channels are used to keep everyone informed all the time, list to everyone's ideas and ensure that everyone is connected on important topics.	A ☐ Patients have access to some standard information that is available to all patients.	☐ Patients have access to standard information that is available to all patients. We've started to think about how to improve the information they are given to better meet their needs.	☐ Patients have a variety of ways to get the information they need and it can be customized to meet their individual learning styles. We routinely ask patients for feedback about how to improve the information we give them.	☐ Can't Rate
Information/Info Technology	Given the complexity of information and the use of technology in the microsystem, assess your microsystem on the following three characteristics:	B ☐ I am always tracking down the information I need to do my work.	☐ Most of the time, I have the information I need, but sometimes essential information is missing and I have to track it down.	☐ The information I need to do my work is available when I need it.	☐ Can't Rate
Information/Info Technology	A. Integration of information with patients B. Integration of information with providers and staff C. Integration of information with technology	C ☐ The technology I need to facilitate and enhance my work is either not available to me or it is available but not effective. The technology we currently have does not make my job easier.	☐ I have access to technology that will enhance my work, but it is not easy to use and seems to be cumbersome and time consuming.	Technology facilitates a smooth linkage between information and patient care by providing timely, effective access to a rich information environment. The information environment has been designed to support the work of the clinical unit.	☐ Can't Rate

From Nelson EC, et al. Microsystems in health care: learning from high-performing front-line clinical units. *Joint Commission Journal on Quality and Safety* 2002;28(9). Reprinted with permission.

Available at: http://www.clinicalmicrosystem.org/actionGuide.htm.

Appendix 102-2. NQF-Endorsed Set of Safe Practices

1. Create a healthcare culture of safety.
2. For designated high-risk, elective surgical procedures or other specified care, patients should be clearly informed of the likely reduced risk of an adverse outcome at treatment facilities that have demonstrated superior outcomes and should be referred to such facilities in accordance with the patient's stated preference.
3. Specify an explicit protocol to be used to ensure an adequate level of nursing based on the institution's usual patient mix and the experience and training of its nursing staff.
4. All patients in general intensive care units (both adult and pediatric) should be managed by physicians having specific training and certification in critical care medicine ("critical care certified").
5. Pharmacists should actively participate in the medication-use process, including, at a minimum, being available for consultation with prescribers on medication ordering, interpretation and review of medication orders, preparation of medications, dispensing of medications, and administration and monitoring of medications.
6. Verbal orders should be recorded whenever possible and immediately read back to the prescriber—i.e., a healthcare provider receiving a verbal order should read or repeat back the information that the prescriber conveys in order to verify the accuracy of what was heard.
7. Use only standardized abbreviations and dose designations.
8. Patient care summaries or other similar records should not be prepared from memory.
9. Ensure that care information, especially changes in orders and new diagnostic information, is transmitted in a timely and clearly understandable form to all of the patient's current healthcare providers who need that information to provide care.
10. Ask each patient or legal surrogate to recount what he or she has been told during the informed consent discussion.
11. Ensure that written documentation of the patient's preference for life-sustaining treatments is prominently displayed in his or her chart.
12. Implement a computerized prescriber order entry system.
13. Implement a standardized protocol to prevent the mislabeling of radiographs.
14. Implement standardized protocols to prevent the occurrence of wrong-site procedures or wrong-patient procedures.
15. Evaluate each patient undergoing elective surgery for risk of an acute ischemic cardiac event during surgery, and provide prophylactic treatment of high-risk patients with beta blockers.
16. Evaluate each patient upon admission, and regularly thereafter, for the risk of developing pressure ulcers. This evaluation should be repeated at regular intervals during care. Clinically appropriate preventive methods should be implemented consequent to the evaluation.
17. Evaluate each patient upon admission, and regularly thereafter, for the risk of developing deep vein thrombosis (DVT)/venous thromboembolism (VTE). Utilize clinically appropriate methods to prevent DVT/VTE.
18. Utilize dedicated anti-thrombotic (anti-coagulation) services that facilitate coordinated care management.
19. Upon admission, and regularly thereafter, evaluate each patient for the risk of aspiration.
20. Adhere to effective methods of preventing central venous catheter-associated blood stream infections.
21. Evaluate each pre-operative patient in light of his or her planned surgical procedure for the risk of surgical site infection and implement appropriate antibiotic prophylaxis and other preventive measures based on that evaluation.
22. Utilize validated protocols to evaluate patients who are at risk for contrast media-induced renal failure and utilize a clinically appropriate method for reducing risk of renal injury based on the patient's kidney function evaluation.
23. Evaluate each patient upon admission, and regularly thereafter, for risk of malnutrition. Employ clinically appropriate strategies to prevent malnutrition.
24. Whenever a pneumatic tourniquet is used, evaluate the patient for the risk of an ischemic and/or thrombotic complication and utilize the appropriate prophylactic measures.
25. Decontaminate hands with either a hygienic hand rub or by washing with a disinfectant soap prior to and after direct contact with the patient or objects immediately around the patient.
26. Vaccinate healthcare workers against influenza to protect both them and patients from influenza.
27. Keep workspaces where medications are prepared clean, orderly, well lit, and free of clutter distraction and noise.
28. Standardize the methods for labeling, packaging and storing medications.
29. Identify all "high alert" drugs (eg, intravenous adrenergic agonists and antagonists, chemotherapy agents, anticoagulants and antithrombotics, concentrated parenteral electrolytes, general anesthetics, neuromuscular blockers, insulin and oral hypoglycemics, narcotics and opiates).
30. Dispense medications in unit-dose or, when appropriate, unit-of-use form, whenever possible.

From: National Quality Forum. *Safe Practices for Better Healthcare: A Consensus Report.* Washington, DC: National Quality Forum, 2003.

Available at:
http://www.qualityforum.org/txsafeexecsumm+order6-8-03PUBLIC.pdf

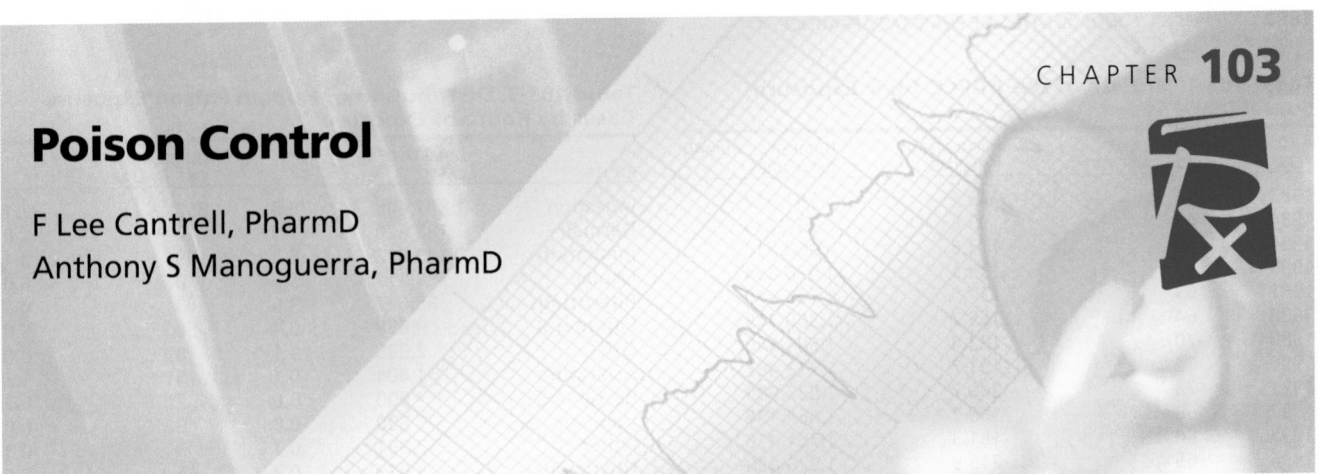

Poison Control

F Lee Cantrell, PharmD

Anthony S Manoguerra, PharmD

Annually, it is estimated that there are between 5 and 10 million toxic exposures in the United States. Among children older than one year, accidents cause more deaths than do the five leading fatal diseases combined. Also, among the most common causes of death of preadolescents, adolescents, and adults is suicide. Frequently, accidents and suicides involve poisons. Another important cause of morbidity and mortality, especially among the young, is the deliberate abuse of drugs and chemicals for their effects on the central nervous system. Even though the reporting undoubtedly is incomplete, especially of suicides and abuses, there are known to be more than 10,000 deaths annually in the US attributable to poisoning.

In addition to the fatalities caused by poisoning, there are staggering numbers of nonfatal cases requiring treatment. The toll in terms of manpower, expense, and occupation of medical facilities cannot be estimated but must be tremendous.

In most instances, accidental poisonings should be preventable. This is especially true of accidental poisonings of young children by drugs and chemicals found in the home. This is a problem of great public-health significance, the solution of which requires efforts of individuals in many disciplines. Among these are pharmacists, who can play a key role in preventing or mitigating the consequences of accidental poisonings, especially those caused by drugs.

EPIDEMIOLOGY

Effective preventive measures require a knowledge of who and what are involved, how it happened, and any predisposing or contributory factors. For delineating some of these factors, a description of the experiences of those poison-control centers who report to the Toxic Exposure and Surveillance System (TESS) of the American Association of Poison Control Centers (AAPCC) may be instructive. The TESS of the AAPCC was established in 1983. The data collected by this system constitutes the largest body of data about poisoning exposures in the world. Table 103-1 summarizes the growth of this system. Since its inception in 1983, when it represented approximately 11% of the US population with slightly more than 250,000 reported human exposure cases from 16 reporting centers, the system has grown continually. In 2001, 2,267,979 human exposure cases were reported from 64 centers representing approximately 99% of the US population.

Poisoning exposure calls (Table 103-2) make up approximately 80% of all calls reported to the system. Poison centers also receive calls that are informational in nature in which no poisoning victim is involved. The majority of information calls are toxicology or drug-information requests, but they also include requests for medical and veterinary information. Of the

human poisoning exposure cases reported in 2001, 85% were unintentional in nature. Suicidal or intentional poisonings made up 10%, whereas poisonings involving drug abuse amounted to 1%. Environmental or industrial exposures accounted for 4% of the human poisoning exposure cases.

Of the 2,267,979 exposure cases reported in 2001, 75.8% involved ingestions as the route of exposure. The remainder of exposures were:

Dermal, 7.9%
Ophthalmic, 5.3%
Inhalation, 6.3%
Bites and stings, 3.6%
Parenteral, 0.4%
Miscellaneous or unknown, 0.7%

Children 5 years of age and younger were involved in 51.6% of the cases. Ages 6 through 19 were involved in 14.2%, whereas 33.5% involved adults aged 19 and older. In terms of gender, males and females were represented equally.

In terms of the severity of exposures handled by poison-control centers, 20% had no effect, and 15.5% had only a minor effect. Major toxicity was observed in only 0.6%.

In cases of a poisoning exposure, approximately 75% of poisonings were managed at home or in some other non-health-care facility. Generally, treatment consisted of dilution, irrigation, or rarely emesis. Of the remaining exposure cases, 22% were managed in a health-care facility, and 3.5% either refused referral to a health care facility or the situation was unknown (Tables 103-3 to 103-6).

In the AAPCC database, the substances most frequently involved in human poisoning exposures were over-the-counter and prescription analgesics, cleaning substances, cosmetics and personal care products, foreign bodies, plants, sedatives-hypnotics, antipsychotics, over-the-counter and prescription cough and cold preparations, topical preparations, bites or envenomations, antidepressants, pesticides, foods, antihistamines, alcohols, oral antimicrobials, hydrocarbons, and chemicals (Table 103-7). A wide variety of agents made up the remaining cases. In contrast, the most frequent category of toxic substances involved in reported fatalities was over-the-counter and prescription analgesics, followed by sedatives-hypnotics-antipsychotics, antidepressants, stimulants and street drugs, cardiovascular drugs, alcohols, chemicals, anticonvulsants, gases and fumes, antihistamines, muscle relaxants, hormone and hormone antagonists, cleaning substances, automotive products, asthma therapies, and pesticides. Among those categories causing the most fatalities, there is a wide variation in the percentage of fatalities with respect to all exposures in that category.

Table 103-1. Growth of the AAPCC Toxic Exposure Surveillance System

YEAR	NUMBER OF POISON CENTERS	POPULATION (MILLIONS)	NUMBER OF HUMAN EXPOSURES
1983	16	43.1	251,012
1984	47	99.8	730,224
1985	56	113.6	900,513
1986	57	132.1	1,098,894
1987	63	137.5	1,166,940
1988	64	155.7	1,368,748
1989	70	182.4	1,581,540
1990	72	191.7	1,713,462
1991	73	200.7	1,837,939
1992	68	196.7	1,864,188
1993	64	181.3	1,751,476
1994	65	215.9	1,926,438
1995	67	218.5	2,023,089
1996	67	232.3	2,155,952
1997	66	250.1	2,192,088
1998	65	257.5	2,241,082
1999	64	260.9	2,201,156
2000	63	270.6	2,168,248
2001	64	281.3	2,267,979

Adapted from Litovitz TL et al. 2001 Annual Report of the American Association of Poison Control Centers Toxic Exposure Surveillance System. *Am J Emerg Med* 2002; 20:391.

Therapeutic overdosage has important preventive implications for the pharmacist. It is not uncommon for a parent who has never been told of the toxic potential of such a common drug as acetaminophen to administer several times the safe dose to a small infant over a period of several days. In fact, such unintentional overdoses are responsible for many of the most serious cases of poisoning.

Particularly tragic are accidental poisonings caused by materials that are either outmoded, excessively toxic for their intended use, or for which there is only questionable rationale. Also, household chemicals, solvents, cleaners, and some pesticides, although valuable to the professional user, are excessively toxic for routine household use. There is little reason for employing highly dangerous materials such as arsenic, phosphorus, or strychnine as rodenticides when warfarin-type com-

Table 103-2. Typical Pattern of Human Poison Exposure Cases Reported to AAPCC

TYPE OF POISONING	NUMBER OF CASES	TOTAL %
Unintentional	1,931,841	85.2
General	1,455,602	64.2
Therapeutic error	167,014	7.4
Bite/sting	85,713	3.8
Misuse	82,867	3.7
Environmental	57,209	2.5
Food poisoning	41,319	1.8
Occupational	35,472	1.6
Unknown	6,645	0.3
Intentional	262,703	11.6
Suicidal	176,221	7.8
Abuse	38,640	1.7
Misuse	37,078	1.6
Unknown	10,764	0.5
Adverse Reaction	49,198	2.2
Drug	35,646	1.6
Other	9,519	0.4
Food	4,033	0.2
Unknown	7,986	0.4
Total	2,267,979	100

Adapted from Litovitz TL et al. 2001 Annual Report of the American Association of Poison Control Centers Toxic Exposure Surveillance System. *Am J Emerg Med* 2002; 20:391.

Table 103-3. Distribution of Human Poison Exposure Cases by Route of Exposure

ROUTE	NUMBER OF CASES	%	NUMBER OF FATALITIES	%
Ingestion	1,807,448	75.8	893	77.1
Dermal	188,620	7.9	12	1.0
Inhalation	149,812	6.3	109	9.4
Ocular	126,117	5.3	0	0.0
Bites/stings	85,627	3.6	3	0.3
Parenteral	9,658	0.4	58	5.0
Otic	2,336	0.1	0	0.0
Aspiration	1,404	0.1	15	1.3
Rectal	900	0.0	2	0.2
Vaginal	800	0.0	0	0.0
Other	2,851	0.1	3	0.3
Unknown	8,025	0.3	63	5.4

Multiple routes of exposure were observed in many poison-exposure victims. Percentage is based on the total number of exposure routes (1,932,106) for all patients, 822 for fatal cases, rather than the total number of human exposures (1,837,939) or fatalities (764).
Adapted from Litovitz TL et al. 2001 Annual Report of the American Association of Poison Control Centers Toxic Exposure Surveillance System. *Am J Emerg Med* 2002; 20:391.

pounds, which possess very low acute human toxicity, work equally well.

Influential Factors

Several factors are important in the consideration of poisoning risk and in poison prevention.

AGE—Approximately two-thirds of poisonings occur in children and are accidental, whereas a large portion of the poisonings in adolescents and adults represent suicide attempts. Poisonings do occur in adults from the inadvertent ingestion of some material other than the intended medication or accidental overdosage of proper medication. Although these accidents are rare, people should be cautioned to carefully read labels before taking medications, not to take medications in the dark, not to transfer medications from their original containers, to protect medication labels against destruction, and to follow the recommended dosage schedules carefully.

Accidental poisoning is less common in children older than 5 years of age. The most critical age period is between 1 and 3 years, where nearly one-half of poisonings occur. Poisoning is among the most common reasons to bring a child to the hospital for emergency treatment. The reasons for the high incidence in that age range relate to certain characteristics of child development. During these early years the youngster is inquisi-

Table 103-4. Distribution of Human Poison Exposure Cases by Age of Victim

AGE (YR)	% OF CASES	AGE (YR)	% OF CASES
<1	6.1	30–39	7.9
1	16.7	40–49	6.0
2	16.2	50–59	3.5
3	7.1	60–69	1.9
4	3.3	70–79	1.4
5	1.9	80–89	0.8
6–12	6.9	90–99	0.1
13–19	7.3	Unknown	3.9
Child, unknown age	0.4	adult Unknown age	0.5
20–29	7.9	Total	100.0

Adapted from Litovitz TL et al. 2001 Annual Report of the American Association of Poison Control Centers Toxic Exposure Surveillance System. *Am J Emerg Med* 2002; 20:391.

Table 103-5. Medical Outcome of Human Exposure Cases

OUTCOME	NUMBER	%
No effect	453,975	20.0
Minor effect	351,191	15.5
Moderate effect	102,540	4.5
Major effect	13,918	0.6
Death	1,074	0.0
No follow-up, nontoxic	405,568	17.9
No follow-up, minimally toxic	776,728	34.2
No follow-up, potentially toxic[a]	99,294	4.4
Unrelated effect	63,691	2.8
Total	2,267,979	100.0

[a] Patient lost to follow-up. Exposure was assessed as potentially toxic.
Adapted from Litovitz TL et al. 2001 Annual Report of the American Association of Poison Control Centers Toxic Exposure Surveillance System. *Am J Emerg Med* 2002; 20:391.

Table 103-7. Substances Most Frequently Involved in Human Poison Exposures

SUBSTANCE	NUMBER	%[A]
Analgesics	240,757	10.6
Cleaning substances	216,102	9.5
Cosmetics/personal care products	208,171	9.2
Foreign bodies	115,320	5.1
Plants	105,560	4.7
Sedatives/hypnotics/antipsychotics	100,141	4.4
Cough and cold preparations	97,710	4.3
Topicals	95,854	4.2
Bites/envenomations	93,821	4.1
Antidepressants	92,675	4.1
Pesticides (includes rodenticides)	90,010	4.0
Food products, food poisoning	67,149	3.0
Antihistamines	67,053	3.0
Alcohols	64,462	2.8
Antimicrobials	61,357	2.7
Hydrocarbons	59,738	2.6
Chemicals	56,381	2.5

[A] Percentages are based on total number of known ingested substances rather than the total number of human exposures cases.
Note: Despite a high frequency of involvement, these substances are not necessarily the most toxic, but rather reflect only ready availability.
Adapted from Litovitz TL et al. 2001 Annual Report of the American Association of Poison Control Centers Toxic Exposure Surveillance System. *Am J Emerg Med* 2002; 20:391.

tive. By one year of age, the child also usually can either crawl or walk, yet is too young to recognize danger. It is to be expected that attempts will be made to mouth or ingest any substance left within reach.

No matter how distasteful a product may be, a child still will make an initial attempt to eat or taste it. Although pleasant flavoring may be influential in a child's ingesting a larger dose, it has little bearing on whether or not an initial attempt to ingest the material will be made. During the first 2 to 3 years of life, texture is at least as important as flavor in determining acceptability of something to be ingested. The young child may ingest materials that would readily gag or dissuade an older individual. At this age, children ingest even highly caustic substances such as acids and alkalis without hesitation.

Children younger than one year old may be given a toxic material by an older sibling. Thus, it is important to keep potentially toxic materials inaccessible to young children and also to their older brothers and sisters. In addition, children should be educated not to give things to the baby without parental permission. Preschool education programs teach children these principles to reinforce parents' instructions.

Among children older than 3 years of age, ingestions may occur as group activities. Occasionally, two or more children share the material in some form of play, where they might otherwise be unlikely to ingest it by themselves. Again, at this age, children are more educable than earlier, so instruction to avoid potentially toxic nonfood substances (eg, cleaning products, personal care products, plants) should be given in the home and in the educational environment.

Some of the supposedly accidental poisonings in teenage and younger children are actually suicide attempts or gestures, or attempts at drug abuse. It is important to realize that serious suicide attempts may occur as young as 9 or 10 years of age. Among the adolescent population, suicidal attempts or gestures are not uncommon and also occur several years immediately before and after this important transitional stage of life.

Table 103-6. Management Site of Human Poisoning Exposure Cases[a]

MANAGEMENT SITE	NUMBER	%
Non-health facility	1,689,907	74.5
Health-care facility	498,524	22.0
Refused referral	46,103	2.0
Other	21,017	0.9
Unknown	12,428	0.5
Total	1,837,939	100

Adapted from Litovitz TL et al. 2001 Annual Report of the American Association of Poison Control Centers Toxic Exposure Surveillance System. *Am J Emerg Med* 2002; 20:391.

ACCIDENT PRONENESS—Only a small number of patients treated for poisoning have had a history of having been involved in similar accidents. Thus, although some children may be involved in repetitive episodes, they account for a small percentage of these cases. Nonetheless, a child who has ingested something once, especially if some effort was required in the act, may be at greater future risk and should be treated accordingly. The idea that there are accident-prone children probably is less valid than the fact that there are accident-prone situations and surroundings. Parental education about poison-prevention techniques and what to do in case of a poisoning should be considered part of the routine follow-up in all childhood poisoning episodes.

LOCATION—The majority of childhood accidental poisonings occur in the home. At the time they were ingested, materials that become involved in accidental childhood poisoning usually have been left out after being used rather than being returned to their usual place of storage. The most common areas for poisoning within the home are the kitchen, bathroom, and bedroom.

The highest incidence of accidental childhood poisoning is in the late afternoon and around the dinner hour or in the early-morning hours. However, poisonings occur with regular consistency during a child's waking hours. Poisonings in the late-morning hours often occur in the kitchen, and the substances most frequently involved are common household products (eg, cleaning agents, polishes, and other materials commonly kept in the kitchen). Poisonings that occur in the bedroom may involve cosmetics and, to a lesser extent, medications. Bathroom incidents usually involve either medications or topical antiseptics. The more often a consumer product is used and stored in the home, the more likely it is to be involved in an accidental poisoning exposure.

Among cases that occur outside the home, the garage and automobile are common sites of accidental poisoning in young children. Medications found either in the glove compartment or in mother's purse are most frequently involved in the automobile. Pesticides, petroleum products, cleaning agents, and paint products are often stored in the garage and thus involved in poisoning. An increasing percentage of cases occurring inside or outside the home involve plants kept for decorative purposes or those growing in the yard or wild in the fields. Parents should be reminded that children may be poisoned when they visit the homes of others (especially grandparents) who leave medications and household items within reach because they are not accustomed to having children about.

ACCESSIBILITY—Poison-prevention campaigns often focus on the provision of a locked medicine cabinet. The availability of a safe storage place for medicines is desirable, but this probably would prevent less than one-half the cases of accidental childhood poisoning.

In up to 75% of accidental childhood poisoning cases, the materials involved has been left within reach of a child. In many instances, ingestion occurs when the individual responsible for the care of a child is interrupted during his or her use of the material in question.

People must be instructed to provide a secure storage place for potentially toxic materials and to return these materials immediately after use.

THE CONTAINER—Removal of potentially toxic materials from their original containers is a significant factor in increasing risk of accidental poisoning, especially with certain compounds. The common practice, for example, of storing a small quantity of gasoline or solvents in a soft-drink bottle is especially hazardous. Other hazardous materials where this approach is employed are automobile products, paint products, cleaning solutions, and pesticides. Sometimes the container used to transfer the offending substance is a drinking glass or dish. In all such instances, toxic substances are easily confused as food or other edible items. In addition, transfer of materials from their original containers creates problems of accurate identification when a poisoning does occur. A similar problem exists when materials, particularly medications, are not identified properly in their original containers. All prescription containers should identify the contents on the label accurately.

SUPERVISION—Many children are under the supervision of one or both parents at the time an accidental poisoning occurs. However, usual adult supervision is not adequate to prevent poisoning accidents in young children. This may, in part, be because parents underestimate the child's ability to move quickly and ingest a potentially toxic material. A common error is to leave medications on a bedside stand after administering them. The child for whom it was intended or a sibling may ingest a portion or the entire contents.

A significant number of childhood poisonings occur when there is a disruption in the normal household routine. Times of moving, painting, holidays, visits by friends or relatives, or death or illness in the family are occasions when increased caution should be exercised. Other circumstances that invite unsupervised access of children to potentially toxic materials are when items are sent through the mail or have been discarded into a waste container.

When deteriorated or unwanted materials are to be discarded, the safest procedure for potentially toxic liquids or powders is either to pour them down a drain or flush them down a toilet. With some highly concentrated, toxic materials, such as pesticide concentrates, even the amount remaining in an *empty* bottle may be sufficient to cause serious poisoning. Those containers should be rinsed thoroughly before being discarded and placed carefully in closed waste containers as far from normal access of children as possible.

Optimal supervision also involves attention to detail in the legitimate use of potentially hazardous materials. As previously noted, drug labels should always be examined carefully to ensure accurate identification before a medication is administered or taken. Self-medication, use of another individual's medications for the "same problem," and unsupervised self-diagnosis and prescription of a child's treatment by the parents should only be encouraged with appropriate education and potential for consumer understanding.

There is a tendency for many to believe that if a material were significantly hazardous it would not be available for over-the-counter (OTC) sales, but this is untrue. Frequently, parents may overmedicate a child, either because they underestimate the potential hazard or are given inadequate instructions. It is important that physicians who order and pharmacists who dispense or recommend over-the-counter medications provide and emphasize specific instructions concerning proper use. The pharmacist plays a key role in patient education, even if the intervention is only a minute or two.

Although seemingly unlikely, it is not uncommon for a patient who has been advised to take or administer "some aspirin every once in a while" to use two or three times the safe dose every few hours for several days or to take concurrent medications containing salicylates until serious intoxication occurs. Instructions on the label are meaningful to the cautious and the concerned, but they are rarely the people who become poisoned. Person-to-person discussion is far more effective and can easily take place at the time a material is prescribed or dispensed.

TREATMENT

The most important treatment measure for poisoning is prevention. Once a poisoning occurs, it is important to be able to provide highly skilled supportive medical care. It is insufficient to focus only on simple first-aid measures, antidotal therapy, or home remedies.

Actually, there are few poisons for which there are effective antidotes. Even in the instances in which antidotes are available, supportive care is equally as important; indeed, the best antidote in the world is of little value without good supportive care. Most of the home remedies that have been recommended from time to time are actually of little value or are even potentially dangerous. Most tend to waste valuable time that could better be devoted to proper treatment under adequate medical supervision.

Unfortunately, many lay publications, including first-aid texts, are outmoded in this respect and continue to recommend all sorts of elaborate but ineffective procedures to be carried out in the home. The same criticism can be leveled at the instructions provided on the many rather complicated antidote lists and first-aid treatment charts that are disseminated for use by the public, often by well-meaning professional organizations.

FIRST-AID PRINCIPLES

The cardinal rule for first-aid treatment of poisoning is to remove the poison from contact with the patient (unless such removal is contraindicated) and to obtain further definitive medical care at the earliest possible moment if warranted.

The more simplified instructions for home treatment are, the more likely they will be followed and the less likely they are to either delay or be substituted for proper care by a physician. Thus, general procedures that are simple and applicable regardless of the nature of the poison are to be recommended until medical help can be obtained.

Recommended procedures for lay use in the first-aid treatment of poisoning are outlined in Table 103-8. The principal elements are knowing what to do before you call someone, obtaining medical advice immediately to determine what to do next, and terminating contact of the victim with the poison by dilution, washing or, in increasingly rare instances, through induction of vomiting. In regard to the latter point, note that induction of vomiting with ipecac syrup is the only method of vomiting in use today. Many measures recommended in the past for the induction of vomiting, such as mechanical stimulation of the posterior pharynx or giving mustard water or salt water, appear to be less effective and may be dangerous. The most widely used emetic for first-aid use is ipecac syrup. However, a lack of scientific data demonstrating a positive impact on patient outcome has led to a substantial decline in the use of ipecac syrup.

Activated charcoal is a highly effective adsorbent of many poisons and appears to be more effective than ipecac-induced vomiting at decreasing the absorption of materials from the gastrointestinal tract. This material adsorbs most organic and inorganic materials. Thus, its routine use in cases of poisoning by ingestion is worthwhile. Remember, however, that if activated charcoal is given before ipecac syrup, it will inactivate the latter. Consequently, if one is going to both induce vomiting and administer activated charcoal, it is advisable to induce vomiting first and then, after the vomiting has subsided, administer the charcoal. As the use of ipecac-induced emesis has declined in popularity, the use of activated charcoal as the sole method of gastrointestinal decontamination has increased substantially. Activated charcoal is worthwhile as a nonspecific antidote for home use and for use in hospitals and in poison treatment centers. It is best given as a slurry in water.

In recent years parents have been encouraged to keep ipecac syrup and activated charcoal in homes where there are children of poisoning-prone age. If such items are to be used, it is important that a prominent part of the label instructions is to call the local poison-control center, an emergency department, or a physician before administering either.

ANTIDOTES—Note that although activated charcoal is an effective, nonspecific adsorbent of many materials, there is no true *universal antidote*. The classic universal antidote, which was in use for a long period, consisted of activated charcoal, tannic acid, or magnesium oxide (or, in the home: burnt toast, strong tea, or milk of magnesia). It now has been established that the last two constituents have no significant efficacy and may actually impede the one active ingredient, activated charcoal. The long-advocated preparation of burnt toast and strong tea in the home has no merit.

Because they are not used often, it is important for information concerning antidotes to be readily available so that they can be used properly and at the earliest possible moment. It is important not to waste time searching for nonexistent antidotes. For a few poisons, there are chemical antidotes that react with the poison in the stomach either to inactivate it or to retard its absorption. Such local antidotes are sufficiently innocuous that they can be administered safely.

The most useful antidotes are those available for systemic administration to counteract the effects of poisons that have been absorbed. Table 103-9 summarizes the use and administration of antidotes that currently are recommended.

OTHER MEASURES—Aside from removal or inactivation of the poison and use of antidotes when available, the treatment of poisoning is supportive. The symptomatic or supportive approach to treatment does not differ significantly from that encountered in other medical problems. Common problems requiring supportive care include coma, respiratory insufficiency, convulsions, shock, vomiting, diarrhea, fluid and electrolyte disturbances, cerebral edema, kidney failure, and damage to other organs.

Additionally, several procedures exist that may be used to hasten elimination of a poison. In some instances, drugs can be eliminated more rapidly with diuresis induced by use of pharmacological or osmotic diuretics along with alkalinization of the urine. With poisons that are dialyzable, extracorporeal hemodialysis (use of artificial kidney) is preferred. Also, charcoal hemoperfusion is effective with many agents. These procedures are indicated when normal excretory processes fail or

---

Table 103-8. First-Aid Treatment for Poisoning

I. DO THESE THINGS BEFORE YOU CALL SOMEONE
  A. Remove poisons from contact with eyes, skin, or mouth.
    1. Eyes: Gently wash eyes with plenty of water (or milk) for 10 to 15 minutes with the eyelids held open. Remove contact lenses and again wash the eyes. Do not allow victims to rub their eyes.
    2. Skin: Wash poisons off the skin with large amounts of plain water. Then wash the skin with a detergent if it is possible. Remove and discard all contaminated clothing.
    3. Mouth: Look into victim's mouth and remove all tablets, powder, plants, or any other material that is found. Also examine for cuts, burns, or any unusual coloring. Wipe out mouth with a cloth and wash thoroughly with water.
  B. Remove victim from contact with poisonous fumes or gases.
    Get the victim into fresh air.
    Loosen all tight-fitting clothing.
    If the victim is not breathing, one should start artificial respiration immediately. Do not stop until the victim is either breathing well or emergency assistance arrives. Use oxygen if available. Send someone else to call for help.

II. CALL FOR INFORMATION ABOUT WHAT TO DO NEXT:
  A. Call the poison control center or your physician.
    1. Identify yourself and your relationship to the victim.
    2. Describe the victim by name, age, and sex.
    3. Have the package or poison in your hand and identify as best as you can what and how much the victim ingested.
  B. Call for information even if you are unsure. Keep calm. You have enough time to act, but don't delay unnecessarily.

III. IF YOU ARE INSTRUCTED TO INDUCE VOMITING
    Never induce vomiting until you are instructed to do so.
  A. If you live more than one hour from the closest medical facility, have syrup of ipecac available to induce vomiting. The use of this drug has declined substantially in recent years, but there still may be instances where the use of ipecac syrup may be suggested. The poison center or your doctor will instruct you in how to administer the ipecac syrup.
  B. Don't waste time trying other ways to make the victim vomit.
    Tickling the back of the throat with your fingers, a spoon, or some other object is not effective. Do not use salt water. It is potentially dangerous.
  C. Never induce vomiting if the patient:
    Is unconscious
    Is having convulsions (seizures)
    Has swallowed strong caustics or corrosives
    Has swallowed petroleum products, cleaning fluids, gasoline, lighter fluid, etc, unless specifically instructed to do so

IV. IF YOU GO TO THE HOSPITAL:
  A. Take with you or send the poison container, poisonous plant, etc
  B. Take any vomitus you collect
  C. Do not administer substances such as coffee, alcohol, stimulants, or drugs to the victim

Table 103-9. Summary of Antidotes and Stocking Levels[a]

GENERIC/BRAND NAME	USE	NOTES	SUGGESTED STOCKING LEVEL
Atropine	Organophosphate/Carbamate insecticide poisoning, bradycardia induced by a variety of toxins	Requires very large amounts in severe organophosphate/ carbamate insecticide poisoning	1,000 mg total Preservative free
Antivenin Crotalidae Polyvalent (equine) Wyeth-Ayerst	Rattlesnake envenomation	Different dosing from Cro-Fab™	20 vials
Antivenin Crotalidae Polyvalent Immune FAB-Ovine/Cro-Fab	Rattlesnake envenomation	Different dosing from Wyeth-Ayerst polyvalent antivenin	18 vials
Antivenin, Black Widow Spider/Antivenin (Latrodectus Mactans)	Black Widow spider envenomation		1 × 6000u vial
BAL (Dimercaprol)/BAL in oil 10%	Heavy metal poisoning		4 × 3ml 10% in oil amps
Calcium chloride injection	Calcium channel blocker poisoning		20 × 10ml 10% vials
Calcium gluconate powder	Hydrofluoric acid skin exposures	For compounding topical gel	1 × 100gm powder bottle
Calcium gluconate injection	Calcium channel blocker poisoning, hydrofluoric acid poisoning or skin exposure, toxin-induced hypocalcemia		20 × 10ml 10% vials
Cyanide Antidote Kit/Taylor Cyanide Antidote Kit	Cyanide poisoning		2 kits
Deferoxamine/Desferal	Iron poisoning		12 × 500mg vials (6 grams total)
Digoxin Immune FAB (ovine)/ Digibind, DigiFab	Digitalis glycoside poisoning		20 vials
DMSA (Succimer)/Chemet	Heavy metal poisoning		1 × 100 capsule bottle
EDTA, Calcium/Versenate	Heavy metal poisoning		18 × 1000mg/5ml amps
Ethanol IV 10%	Ethylene glycol, methanol poisoning		3 × 1000ml (10%) bottles in 5% dextrose
Flumazenil/ Romazicon	Benzodiazepine poisoning		5 × 0.5mg/ml vial
Fomepizole (4-MP)/Antizol	Ethylene glycol, methanol poisoning		4 × 1.5ml (1gm/ml) vials
Glucagon	Beta blocker, calcium channel blocker poisoning		100 × 1mg vials
Methylene Blue	Methemoglobinemia		5 × 10ml 1% amps
N-Acetylcysteine (NAC)/ Mucomyst	Acetaminophen poisoning	Use orally. Dilute (at least by a 3:1 ratio) in juice or soda to increase palatability	7 × 30ml 20% vials
Naloxone/ Narcan	Narcotic overdose		20 × 0.4mg/2ml amps
Octreotide acetate/ Sandostatin	Sulfonylurea poisoning		2 × 1ml (0.1mg/ml) amp or 1 × 5ml (.2mg/ml) MDV
Physostigmine/Antilerium	Anticholinergic poisoning		10 × 2ml 1mg/ml vials
Pralidoxine (2-PAM)/ Protopam	Organophosphate pesticide poisoning		12 × 1gm 20ml vials
Pyridoxine (Vitamin B$_6$)/ Beesix	Isoniazid (INH) poisoning	Very large amounts needed (20 grams total)	20 × 10ml (100mg/ml) vials
Vitamin K$_1$ (Phytonadione)/ Mephyton, AquaMephyton	Warfarin and super-warfarin (rodenticide) anticoagulant poisoning		100 × 5mg tabs 10 × 10mg/ml amps

[a] Based on dose to treat a 70-kg patient for 24 hours.
Adapted from California Poison Control System Antidote Chart, California Poison Control System, University of California San Francisco, School of Pharmacy, 2002.

prove to be inadequate or when the degree of poisoning portends a fatal outcome unless the level of poison in the body is rapidly reduced.

Centers that are likely to be called on to treat cases of poisoning generally have the necessary supplies and equipment for performance of peritoneal dialysis, hemodialysis, and hemoperfusion. If such is not available in a given hospital, the poison center should have information concerning the nearest location of such equipment.

PREVENTION

Many preventive measures have been suggested or alluded to previously. Total prevention through education is an ideal worth striving to accomplish. To date, educational programs have eliminated only a portion of the problem. One concern is that educational efforts may be too general, so the public does not know precisely what it should do and has no specific actions to implement. Instruction is most effective when it includes specific directions that can and should be followed. For instance, announcing to parents that they should "keep things out of the reach of small children" helps little until they are told what to keep out of reach.

It is not uncommon in cases of childhood poisoning that parents are unaware that the material was potentially poisonous, that they took no special precautions because their child had been no problem previously, or that they thought the material was inaccessible to the child. Aiming educational efforts at specific actions (see below) has far more chance of being effective. General admonitions about preventing poisoning are much less likely to be effective.

Consonant with the theory of specific instruction is the need to provide specific directions with individual products. This is an important role for the pharmacist. There is a tendency for precautionary labeling to be ignored until after an accident. Labels may be effective in directing individuals to proper treatment, but their preventive value depends on the consumer's interest and concern in reading the label in the first place. Person-to-person instruction by the physician or the dispensing pharmacist is much more effective.

Limiting the availability of highly toxic materials or directing the consumer to the least toxic material that will serve the intended purpose are of potential value. Outmoded materials that have higher degrees of toxicity should be eliminated as safer substitutes become available. Pharmacists should be in a position to advise about comparative safety as well as efficacy of the products that they dispense or sell.

THE *POISON PREVENTION PACKAGING ACT*— Enacted in 1970, this legislation (PL 91-601; 16CFR 1700) calls for the packaging of specified potentially hazardous household chemicals and drugs in *safety* containers. The latter include safety-capped vials or bottles or *strip, blister,* or other unit packaging. Child-resistant packaging must be demonstrated through the use of standardized tests in target-age populations to resist opening by children but not by adults. Such testing demonstrates the particularly effective barrier these packages provide to the poison-prone-age child. Drugs designated thus far as requiring such packaging include, with certain specific exemptions, aspirin-containing preparations, those containing high concentrations of methyl salicylate, prescription drugs, caustics, petroleum distillates, glycols, alcohols, acetaminophen, and iron. Additional drugs may be regulated similarly by the time of this publication. For the benefit of the elderly and infirm, the law provides that a single size of regulated products may, at the request of the consumer or prescribing physician, be packaged in conventional containers that are labeled as being intended for households without young children.

Although the manufacturer provides the safety packaging for over-the-counter drugs, the pharmacist is responsible for complying with the regulations for prescription products that are repackaged and plays a key role in implementation of this important poisoning-prevention measure. The pharmacist is the person to select and employ appropriate packaging for prescription items and is in an excellent position to promote the effectiveness of the Act. The Act can succeed only to the extent that purchasing adults accept and use the special packaging. The pharmacist should assure that people are aware of the availability of such packaging for regulated products, that they are instructed as to its importance and proper use, and that substitutions of conventional packaging are restricted to legitimate and informed requests. This is particularly important as long as reversible or dual function closures are used because their comparative safety has yet to be demonstrated.

POISON-CONTROL CENTERS

The poison-control concept was initiated in Chicago in 1953. After the impetus of local health officials, pediatricians, and other interested physicians, a single center for collecting product data was established. The idea soon caught on and numerous other centers were established. To provide a coordinating agency for these centers, the then Bureau of Product Safety in the Food and Drug Administration (FDA) established the National Clearinghouse for Poison Control Centers. This clearinghouse served as a center for collecting and standardizing product toxicology data and for distributing this data in the form of 5- by 8-inch index cards to recognized poison-control centers. State health departments were given the responsibility for identifying poison centers within their states. The great interest in poison control eventually resulted in more than 580 officially recognized poison-control centers and numerous additional unofficial centers, including drug-information services, bringing the total to well over 600. Unfortunately, many poison centers have had little if any capability for providing sophisticated information or treatment for poisoning, because they handle as few as one call per week.

From the beginning, studies of poison-control center operations demonstrated a wide variability in the manner by which services were provided. Some centers provided information solely to physicians or health-care facilities, whereas others provided information to the public or both. Staffing of poison-control centers likewise was variable. The staff of a poison center may have consisted only of full- or part-time clerks, nurses, or pharmacists without any direct medical supervision, or they have consisted of a full-time clinical toxicologist-medical director and specially trained, full-time professional staff, such as clinical pharmacists or nurses. Other centers have included pharmacologists, emergency room physicians, ambulatory pediatricians, or other scientifically trained personnel as staff or consultants.

The questions facing the poison-control center movement, now in the sixth decade after its inception, are to whom to provide services, how best to provide services, how to improve services, how to standardize or monitor services, and how to organize such services on a regional or a national basis. The question of how to organize these services has been resolved to a great degree over these past several years. Consolidation of manpower and resources into centralized or regional services is crucial. In centralized or regional poison-control centers, sophisticated information can be provided to health professionals and the public. Treatment facilities are generally an integral part of the regional poison-control center, and the staff, particularly the medical staff, can provide the treatment for poisoning victims. In addition, active supervision and even bedside consultation of poisoning cases admitted to other health-care facilities ought to be provided.

Optimally, there should be 50 to 60 regional programs in the US. A regional poison-control center should be one that, in less densely populated areas, serves a single or multistate region or that, in heavily populated areas, serves a portion of a state. Generally, a regional center serves no fewer than one million people, but could serve as many as 5 to 10 million people in areas of high-population density. A regional center would provide:

Comprehensive poison information, both to health professionals and consumers
Comprehensive poisoning treatment services
A toll-free communication system
Access to a full range of analytical toxicological services
Access to transportation facilities for critically ill patients
Professional and public education programs
Collection and dissemination of poisoning experience data

In essence, these regional centers are capable of assuming ultimate responsibility, which includes the functions mentioned above, for the provision of poisoning consultations and patient care for all poisonings brought to its attention within its region. The AAPCC has developed standards for regional poison-control centers and provides a process to evaluate a poison center's capabilities and to designate centers as *regional poison centers*. The types of services and equipment recommended for various types of centers are described in more detail in references noted in the *Bibliography*.

NATIONAL POISON PREVENTION WEEK

Since 1962 the third week of March has been designated National Poison Prevention Week. In addition to giving annual emphasis to the problem of poison control, this week provides an opportunity for concentrated educational efforts directed to the public. Pharmacists should play an active role in the activities of this period. Special displays in pharmacies have been one type of effective strategy. Other worthwhile activities have included television or radio messages, special meetings, and newspaper articles, all of which can be made more effective by involved pharmacists. By joining forces with the regional or local poison-control centers, this week can be used to highlight the year-round educational activities of the center and the community.

ROLE OF THE PHARMACIST

There is much that a pharmacist can do to help prevent poisoning and to improve the treatment thereof. Pharmacists direct and staff many regional poison centers. They actively provide consultation to physicians treating poisoned patients to assure quality care.

Undoubtedly, the most important role played by a pharmacist is in the area of prevention. This role, relative to poison-prevention packaging of prescription drugs, was mentioned previously. However, the role of the pharmacist is particularly critical with regard to nonprescription or OTC items. With prescription medications, there is involvement of a physician who may provide instructions and precautionary advice. However, with over-the-counter products, the pharmacist is often the only person who is in a position to serve these functions.

The pharmacist can and should provide, explain, and amplify directions for proper use of potentially toxic materials, bearing in mind that the concern is for the safety of the patient and for other household individuals. Thus, the dispensing of a toxic medication provides an opportunity to warn the buyer about the hazards of leaving the material within reach of unsuspecting children.

In some instances, it is desirable to affix warning labels on the products that a pharmacist dispenses or to hand out patient information materials. The dispensing of a drug also provides an opportunity to inquire and give advice about facilities for safe storage. Because of this contact, the pharmacist can play a personalized role in cautioning about prescription and commercial products.

The pharmacist can do much to reduce the aforementioned limitations of labeling. Although the public often may not read or appreciate precautions on labels, the effectiveness of the latter are increased significantly if a pharmacist takes time to explain them. The pharmacist also has a unique role to play in detecting product or labeling defects and an obligation to call to the attention of appropriate manufacturers or regulatory agencies potential labeling or product defects.

There has been a tendency in the past for the development of too many small and ineffectual poison centers, the activities of which could be carried out more effectively and efficiently if they were amalgamated with others in the same area. Local pharmacy associations should support the trend toward centralization and regionalization of poison information and treatment facilities.

Finally, pharmacists can assist greatly in the educational efforts of a community by distributing literature and by providing space for displays related to poisoning prevention.

REFERENCES

1. Litovitz TL, et al. 2001 Annual Report of the American Association of Poison Control Centers Toxic Exposure Surveillance System. *Am J Emerg Med* 2002; 20:391.
2. California Poison Control System Antidote Chart, California Poison Control System, University of California San Francisco, School of Pharmacy, 2002.

BIBLIOGRAPHY

Ellenhorn MJ, et al, eds. *Medical Toxicology: Diagnosis and Treatment of Human Poisoning.* Baltimore: Williams & Wilkins, 1997.

Goldfrank LR, et al, eds. *Goldfrank's Toxicologic Emergencies,* 3rd ed. New York: McGraw-Hill Professional, 2002.

Haddad LM, Winchester JF, eds. *Clinical Management of Poisoning and Drug Overdose,* 2nd ed. Philadelphia: WB Saunders, 1990.

Henretig FM, Cupit GC, Temple AR, et al. In: Fleisher G, Ludwig S, eds. *Textbook of Pediatric Emergency Medicine.* Baltimore: Williams & Wilkins, 1988.

Litovitz TL, Manoguerra AS. *Pediatrics* 1992; 89:999.

Manoguerra AS. In: Haddad LM, Winchester JF, eds. *Clinical Management of Poisoning and Drug Overdose,* 2nd ed. Philadelphia: WB Saunders, 1990.

Manoguerra AS. *Vet Human Toxicol* 1991; 33:131.

Manoguerra AS, Temple AR. *Emerg Med Clin North Am* 1984; 2:185.

Rumack BH, et al, eds. *Poisindex.* Denver: Micromedex, 1989.

Temple AR. *Ann Rev Pharmacol Toxicol* 1977; 17:215, 1977.

Temple AR. *Pediatrics* 1984; 5:964.

Temple AR. *Vet Human Toxicol* 1982; 24 (suppl):2,1982.

Temple AR, Mancini RE. In: Yaffe SJ, ed. *Pediatric Pharmacology.* New York: Grune & Stratton, 1980.

Temple AR, Veltri JC. One year's experience in a regional poison control center. *Clin Toxicol* 1978;12:277.

Veltri JC, Temple AR. *Clin Toxicol* 1976; 9:407.

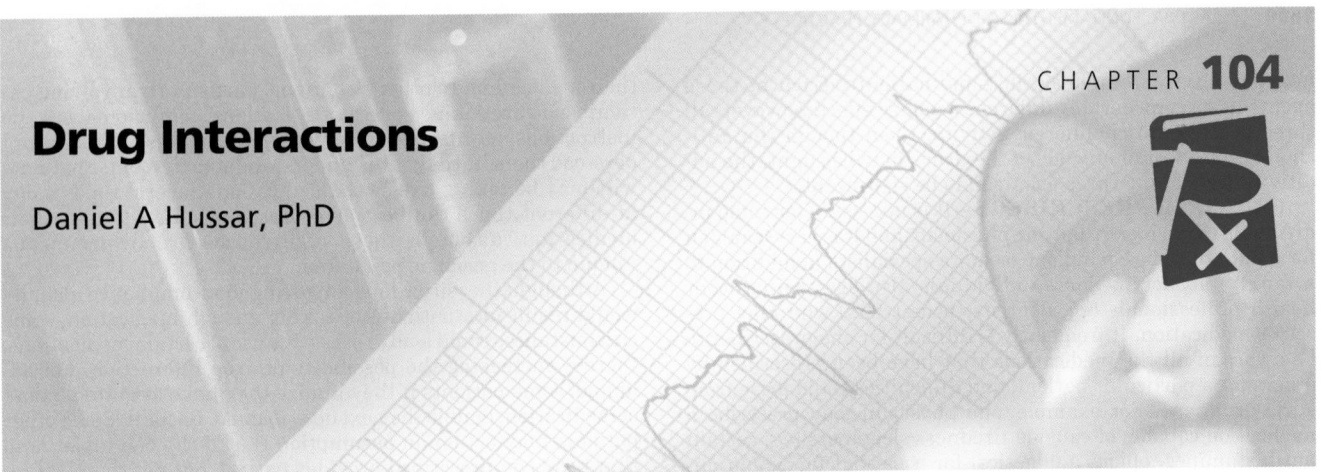

Drug Interactions

Daniel A Hussar, PhD

Although some drug-related problems develop unexpectedly and cannot be predicted, many are related to known properties and actions of the drugs and reasonably can be anticipated. However, as drug therapy becomes more complex and because many patients are being treated with two or more drugs, the ability to predict the magnitude of a specific action of any given drug diminishes. These circumstances point to a need not only for maintenance of complete and current medication records for patients but also for closer monitoring and supervision of drug therapy so that problems can be prevented or detected at an early stage in their development. The pharmacist is in a unique position to meet these needs, and opportunities exist for greater involvement in, and contribution to, provision of drug therapy that is both efficacious and safe.

Many drug-related problems are caused by drug interactions. As a basis for this discussion a drug interaction may be considered a situation in which the effects of one drug are altered by prior or concurrent administration of another drug (ie, drug-drug interactions). The concept of drug interaction often is extended to include situations in which

1. Food or certain dietary items influence the activity of a drug (ie, drug-food interactions) or
2. Herbs or other natural products influence the activity of a drug or
3. Environmental chemicals or smoking influences the activity of a drug or
4. A drug causes alterations of laboratory test results (ie, drug-laboratory test interactions) or
5. A drug causes undesired effects in patients with certain disease states (ie, drug-disease interactions).

Considerable attention has been focused on the subject of drug interaction, and information pertaining to these occurrences has been widely publicized. Several comprehensive references, such as *Drug Interaction Facts* (Tatro DS, ed. St Louis: Facts and Comparisons, 2005) and *Drug Interactions Analysis and Management* (Hansten PD, Horn JR, eds. St Louis: Facts and Comparisons, 2005) deal exclusively with this subject, while other references give extensive attention to it. Computerized databases that provide drug interaction information are also widely used.

Problems that may result from drug interactions also have been publicized to the public. In addition to cautions given to patients by physicians and pharmacists, articles on the subject have appeared in many publications widely read by the public. Many have observed that drug interactions are an important cause of concern for consumers as reflected, in part, by the number of inquiries regarding these drug-related problems initiated to Internet and other drug information sources.

One of the most important consequences of a drug interaction is an excessive response to one or more of the agents being used. For example, a significantly enhanced effect of agents like digoxin and warfarin can result in serious adverse events. Not as well recognized, but also very important, are those interactions in which drug activity is decreased, resulting in a loss of efficacy. These interactions are especially difficult to detect, since they may be mistaken for therapeutic failure or progression of the disease.

Some drug interactions continue to occur even though they are well documented and recognized. Digoxin and a diuretic often are given concurrently, and rationally so, in treating patients with congestive heart failure. It is well known that most diuretics can cause potassium depletion that if uncorrected could become excessive and lead to an increased action of digoxin and adverse events. Yet problems continue to occur as a result of this interaction.

Even with the extensive publicity that drug interactions have received, it is still often difficult to determine their incidence or clinical significance. However, numerous studies have demonstrated that many patients receive multiple drug therapy with agents of recognized potential for interaction. As the number of drugs in a patient's therapeutic regimen increases, the greater is the risk of occurrence of a drug interaction. Although there are only limited data regarding many of the potential drug interactions that have been suggested, considerable progress has been made in defining the level of risk attending the use of a number of combinations of drugs. Indeed, the risk of serious interactions involving the use of terfenadine, astemizole, cisapride, and mibefradil was sufficiently important for these drugs to be withdrawn from the market in the US.

FACTORS CONTRIBUTING TO THE OCCURRENCE OF DRUG INTERACTIONS

A number of factors contribute to the occurrence of drug interactions.

MULTIPLE PHARMACOLOGICAL EFFECTS—Most drugs used in current therapy have the capacity to influence many physiological systems. Therefore, two drugs concomitantly administered will often affect some of the same systems.

When considering the potential for interactions between drugs there often is a tendency only to be concerned with the primary effects of the drugs involved and to overlook the secondary activities they possess. Combined therapy with a phenothiazine antipsychotic (eg, chlorpromazine), a tricyclic antidepressant (eg, amitriptyline), and an antiparkinson agent (eg, trihexyphenidyl) is employed in some patients. Each of these agents has a considerably different primary effect; however, all three possess anticholinergic activity. Even though the anticholinergic effect of any one of the drugs may be slight, the additive effects of the three agents may be significant.

MULTIPLE PRESCRIBERS—It is necessary for some individuals to see more than one physician, and it is very common for a patient to be seeing one or more specialists in addition to a family physician. Some individuals also are seeing other health professionals (eg, dentists, podiatrists) who may prescribe medication. It frequently is difficult for one prescriber to be aware of all the medications that have been prescribed by others for a particular patient, and difficulties could arise from such situations. For example, one physician may prescribe a medication capable of causing tiredness/sleepiness (eg, certain antihistamines, opioid analgesics) for a patient for whom another physician has prescribed an antianxiety agent, with the possible consequence of an excessive depressant effect.

Even though the patient is seeing different physicians, he or she often will have the prescriptions dispensed by the same pharmacy. Therefore, the pharmacist has an important role in the detection and prevention of drug-related problems.

USE OF NONPRESCRIPTION PRODUCTS—Many reports of drug interactions have involved the concurrent use of a prescription drug with a nonprescription drug (eg, aspirin, antacids, decongestants) or herbal (St John's wort) or other natural product. When a physician questions patients about medications that they are taking, the patients often will neglect to mention the nonprescription products that they have purchased. Many patients have been taking preparations such as antacids, analgesics, laxatives, dietary supplements, and herbal products for such long periods and in such a routine manner that they do not consider them to be drugs or to be important with respect to the effectiveness and safety of medications. This information often may be missed in questioning a patient, and some physicians and pharmacists prefer to use a list of symptoms that might ordinarily be treated with nonprescription products in trying to obtain this information from the patient.

Interactions also may result from the concurrent use of two or more products available without a prescription. In some situations two nonprescription products promoted for different purposes contain the same active ingredient(s), increasing the risk of an excessive response to these agents. Diphenhydramine is included in many products for its antihistaminic action but also is included for its sedative effect in many nonprescription sleep-aid formulations. Patients often are unaware that products they purchase for different conditions may contain the same active ingredients and that they, therefore, are at increased risk of problems with the use of products they might assume to be safe because they do not require a prescription.

Although many individuals will have their prescriptions dispensed in their local pharmacy, they often purchase nonprescription drugs elsewhere, thus making identification of potential problems extremely difficult for the pharmacist as well as the physician. For this reason, patients should be encouraged to obtain both their prescription and nonprescription medications at a pharmacy. Such advice is justified, however, only when the pharmacist personally supervises the sale of nonprescription medications with which problems may develop.

The precautions observed with respect to potential interactions involving products that are typically designated as nonprescription drugs also apply to the use of herbal products, dietary supplements, and other related products that are available without a prescription. Although much is still to be learned about the properties of these products, many appear to have a potential to interact with prescription medications, and patients should be asked whether they are using such products.

PATIENT NONCOMPLIANCE—For a variety of reasons many patients do not take medication in the manner intended by the prescriber. Some have not received adequate instruction from the prescriber and pharmacist as to how and when to take

their medication. In other situations, particularly involving patients who are taking several medications, confusion about the instructions may develop even though the patient may have understood them initially. It is understandable that older patients who may be taking five or six medications several times a day at different times can become confused or forget to take their medication, although these occurrences are by no means unique to the geriatric population.

Although the situations involving noncompliance usually would result in a patient not taking enough medication, some circumstances could lead to excessive use of certain medications, thereby increasing the possibility of drug interaction. For example, some patients if they realize they have forgotten a dose of medication, double the next dose to make up for it. Some other patients may act on an assumption that if the one tablet-dose that has been prescribed provides partial, but not complete relief of symptoms, a two-tablet dose will be even more effective.

DRUG ABUSE—The tendencies of some individuals to abuse or deliberately misuse drugs also may lead to an increased incidence of drug interactions. The antianxiety agents, opioid analgesics, and amphetamines are among the agents most often abused, and the inappropriate use of these drugs can result in a number of problems, including an increased potential for drug interaction.

Many interactions that occur are undetected or unreported. Koch-Weser (*Drug Inform J* 1972; 6: 42) observed that detection of drug interactions by clinicians is inefficient and cited six reasons for existence of this situation. Although initially noted in 1972, many of these observations are just as valid today.

1. In most cases the clinical situation is too complex to allow recognition of an unexpected event in a patient's course as related to his or her drug therapy.
2. With few exceptions, the intensity of action of drugs in the therapeutic setting cannot be quantitated accurately.

One reason for the many reports of interactions involving anticoagulants, antidiabetic agents, and antihypertensive agents is that there are specific parameters such as prothrombin time, blood glucose concentrations, and blood pressure that can be measured and provide a quantitative indication of drug activity. Therefore, any change in these values that may be caused by introducing another drug into therapy can be measured with relative ease. In contrast, when one considers drugs like the antipsychotic agents and analgesics with which it is far more difficult to measure degree of activity, it becomes increasingly difficult to observe and measure the effect of other drugs on their activity.

3. Even when a deficient, excessive, or abnormal response to one or both drugs is recognized clearly during concomitant administration, it is attributed usually to factors other than drug interaction.

When an unexpected response to a drug develops, it often is attributed to something other than a drug interaction, such as patient idiosyncrasy in the case of an excessive response, or tolerance in the case of a deficient response.

4. The index of suspicion of most clinicians concerning drug interactions is quite low, and many practicing physicians are hardly aware of the phenomenon.
5. Practicing physicians tend to doubt their observations concerning drug interactions unless the same interaction has been reported previously.

Although physicians are now well aware of the occurrence of drug interactions, there are situations in which a drug interaction may be occurring but there are other factors that also could contribute to the altered response noted. Therefore, physicians often accept a reasonable explanation, albeit incomplete, based on information with which they are familiar, rather than suspect a possibility that has not been reported previously. Although many interactions that have been reported via case reports have not been confirmed by other observations or additional study, many single-case reports have served as the stimulus for additional study that has resulted in warnings about potentially dangerous interactions.

6. Physicians frequently fail to report drug interactions even when they have unequivocally recognized them.

Several factors, no doubt, contribute to this situation. The time it would take to write up a case report to submit to a journal is a deterrent to many physicians and pharmacists. Also, since drug interactions often represent an undesirable experience for the patient, health professionals often are reluctant to expose themselves to possible criticism, or even liability, regarding the therapy. However, it is important that health professionals communicate information that will be useful to others or will help others to avoid the same problems.

USING DRUG-INTERACTION INFORMATION

Although there has been considerable progress in identifying drug interactions, a careful analysis of the literature reveals that some of the information is conflicting, incomplete, and misleading. Too frequently, the suggested clinical importance of an alleged drug interaction is greatly overstated and publicized.

The use of some of this information unfortunately has led, in some situations, to an undue degree of alarm characterized by some observers as *drug-interaction hysteria* or a *drug-interaction anxiety syndrome*. Caution is needed, therefore, in evaluating and using the information available, because by overreacting to a possible problem, a more difficult situation may result than might have occurred if nothing were done. In some situations patients have been deprived unnecessarily of therapy from which they could benefit as a result of concern about a potential interaction with other medication they are taking. Conversely, some health-care practitioners have found so many of the reports and commentaries regarding drug interactions to be lacking in clinical relevance that their skepticism has precluded adequate attention to those interactions that are clinically relevant. Recognition of the importance of exercising the appropriate clinical perspective is essential if optimal therapy is to be achieved.

In using the literature on drug interactions and deciding what action is appropriate, a number of factors should be kept in mind.

INTERACTING DRUGS USUALLY CAN BE USED TOGETHER—In most cases, two drugs that are known to interact can be administered concurrently so long as adequate precautions are taken (eg, closer monitoring of therapy, dosage adjustments to compensate for the altered response). Although there are some situations in which the use of one drug usually is contraindicated while another is being given, such combinations are not likely to be employed frequently, and there may even be exceptions to the contraindication under certain circumstances. In those situations, though, where another agent with similar therapeutic properties and a lesser risk of interacting could be used, such a course of action would be preferable.

Serious reactions have been reported to occur following the concurrent use of a monoamine oxidase inhibitor (MAOI) (eg, tranylcypromine) with a tricyclic antidepressant (eg, amitriptyline), and the literature for most of these products warns that use of such combinations is contraindicated. However, it has been indicated by some that such reactions do not occur commonly and that these combinations, when used under close supervision, may be of benefit in some patients when conventional drug therapy has failed. The fact that these combinations may be used beneficially in some patients does not excuse the pharmacist from responsibility in checking the therapy with the physician. However, the pharmacist should be aware that certain circumstances may justify the concomitant use of even *contraindicated* drugs.

BENEFICIAL INTERACTIONS—It should be recognized that sometimes a second drug is prescribed intentionally to modify the effects of another. Such an approach might be used in an effort to enhance the effectiveness or to reduce the adverse effects of the primary agent. In these situations the efficacy and/or safety of a drug is increased, indicating that interactions are not always harmful as frequently thought, but also can be beneficial.

The ability of probenecid to increase the serum concentrations and prolong the activity of penicillin derivatives has been known for many years, and this interaction has been used to therapeutic advantage in certain infections. Probenecid also is used to reduce the risk of toxicity to certain agents such as cidofovir. By inhibiting the renal tubular secretion of cidofovir, probenecid reduces its renal clearance as well as the risk of nephrotoxicity. For this reason orally administered probenecid must accompany each IV infusion of cidofovir.

Another example of a situation in which one drug is given to minimize the undesirable effects of another is seen with the use of an antiparkinson drug with an antipsychotic agent in an effort to reduce the extrapyramidal effects of the latter.

By inhibiting the metabolism of levodopa in the peripheral tissues, carbidopa and entacapone have been used to both increase the effectiveness and reduce the occurrence of adverse events of levodopa.

NATURE OF REPORTS—Reports and reviews of interactions sometimes attach importance to isolated observations of problems in one patient or a limited number of patients. On several occasions a suspected interaction that was observed in a single patient has been reported in a number of reviews, tables, and computer databases without qualification as to the nature of the report or the possible significance of the interaction. The fact that such an interaction now is included in a number of references can result in an impression that the problem is well documented and clinically significant.

DEPTH OF INFORMATION—Many of the charts, tables, and computer databases of drug interactions do not provide detailed information about specific situations. The mere mention of an increased or decreased effect of one drug in the presence of another is not enough to form a judgment as to the clinical importance and potential severity of the situation. Because of this, most references of this type should be used only to screen initially for possible interactions, and more comprehensive reference sources should be consulted for further information.

CURRENT LITERATURE—It is important to review the current literature constantly, since new information may change the significance of earlier reports. The existence of conflicting reports regarding some interactions also will become evident as the literature is carefully searched. Although there is no assurance that more-recent information is more accurate or pertinent, the date of publication of a particular reference should be noted, and, when appropriate, more current references consulted. The importance of having access to the current literature is reflected in the decisions of the publishers of the most widely used comprehensive drug-interaction references to issue updates at frequent intervals (eg, four times a year).

It is also important to be aware of warnings about medications that are issued by the FDA and pharmaceutical manufacturers as well as pertinent revisions in product labeling. Several warnings regarding drug interactions involving terfenadine and mibefradil preceded the withdrawal of these drugs from the market.

RECOMMENDATIONS AND THERAPEUTIC ALTERNATIVES—There is not enough information available on many reported interactions to permit the development of specific guidelines to govern such combination therapy. When such guidelines are presented they can be extremely helpful, and there is an increasing number of such statements in the package inserts for various products. Where possible, the pharmacist should not only identify a potential problem but also be prepared to make a recommendation to the physician and/or patient as to how problems best can be avoided or minimized.

For example, it is known that aspirin may enhance the anti-coagulant activity of warfarin. Although many patients taking the two drugs concurrently will not experience a problem, ac-etaminophen usually would be preferred to aspirin for use as an analgesic in patients on anticoagulant therapy because it is not likely to alter the activity of agents such as warfarin. However, before making a recommendation that a patient on anticoagu-lant therapy use acetaminophen instead of aspirin, there should be an awareness of the purpose for which the aspirin is to be used. Although acetaminophen is comparable to aspirin with regard to analgesic and antipyretic activity, it possesses little anti-inflammatory activity and, unlike aspirin, has not been shown to reduce the risk of problems such as transient is-chemic attacks and myocardial infarction. Therefore, it should not be used as an alternative to aspirin in the conditions in which one of these actions is needed.

The use of tetracycline by a patient also taking antacids pro-vides an example of a situation in which a specific recommen-dation can be made to avoid a problem. If taken at the same time, the antacid can decrease the absorption and effectiveness of the tetracycline. However, if the two agents are given at least 1 hr apart, the problem should be avoided.

VIEWING INTERACTIONS IN PERSPECTIVE—Even after the previously discussed factors have been considered and the data have been analyzed critically, the possibility of inter-actions developing must be viewed in perspective. Although an altered response appears likely, it might not be clinically sig-nificant in many patients. In these situations a patient should not be deprived of needed therapy because of the possibility of an interaction, but such therapy should be monitored closely.

Most health-care practitioners do not have rapid access to a large number of primary literature sources. Therefore, the use of an authoritative and comprehensive reference source such as *Drug Interaction Facts* or *Drug Interactions Analysis and Man-agement* is recommended, and these references can be very helpful in identifying potential problems and in making judg-ments as to their clinical importance and therapeutic alterna-tives. However, even though certain interactions are well docu-mented, it often is difficult, if not impossible, to predict the severity of an interaction, if indeed it does develop. The many variables that may influence the activity of a drug and its abil-ity to interact with other agents contribute to the existing un-certainty. Many of these variables pertain to the drugs being used and include dosage, route of administration, time of ad-ministration, sequence of administration, and duration of ther-apy, whereas other variables, which are considered in the fol-lowing discussion, pertain to the patient.

PATIENT VARIABLES

There are many factors that influence the response to a drug in man. A number of reports have indicated how these factors may predispose a patient to the development of adverse events to a drug, and it can be anticipated that many of these considera-tions also apply to the development of drug interactions.

AGE—When considering the risk of drug-related problems, age is an important factor. Studies indicate that there is an in-creased incidence of adverse drug events in both young and geriatric patients, and it is reasonable to expect that the occur-rence of drug interactions also is highest in these patient groups.

Drug-related problems in young patients are encountered most frequently in newborn infants. Newborn infants do not have fully developed enzyme systems that are involved in the metabolism of certain drugs, and they also have immature re-nal function.

Several factors point to an increased risk of interactions in the elderly. Most elderly patients have at least one chronic ill-ness (eg, hypertension, diabetes), and this is reflected in the prescribing of a larger number of medications for this patient group. The types of diseases more frequently experienced by el-derly patients (eg, renal disorders) may contribute to an altered drug response, and there appears to be an increased sensitivity to the action of certain drugs with advancing age. In addition, there may be aging-related changes in the absorption, distribu-tion, metabolism, and excretion of certain drugs, which in-crease the possibility of adverse events and drug interactions. Accordingly, drug therapy in elderly patients must be moni-tored especially closely.

GENETIC FACTORS—These may be responsible for the de-velopment of an unexpected drug response in a particular patient. Isoniazid is metabolized by an acetylation process, the rate of which appears to be under genetic control. Some individuals me-tabolize isoniazid rapidly, whereas others metabolize it slowly, thus necessitating careful dosage adjustment, as the dose that provides satisfactory concentrations in rapid acetylators may cause toxicity in slow acetylators. For example, isoniazid causes peripheral neuritis in a number of patients, and this effect has been noted most frequently in slow acetylators.

It has been observed that isoniazid may inhibit the metabolism of phenytoin, possibly resulting in the development of adverse events (nystagmus, ataxia, lethargy) of the latter. However, studies have indicated that those patients who devel-oped phenytoin toxicity when also receiving isoniazid were slow acetylators of isoniazid. It is likely that this interaction will be of significance only in patients who metabolize isoniazid at a very slow rate.

DISEASE STATES—A number of disease states, other than the one for which a particular drug is being used, may in-fluence patient response to a drug. Impaired renal and hepatic function are the most important conditions that may alter drug activity. However, other disorders also may bring about a change in the activity of a drug. Since many drugs are bound ex-tensively to plasma proteins and only the unbound fraction of the drug is active, a decreased concentration or amount of pro-tein conceivably could change the availability of drugs and, thus, their activity. This possibility must be recognized in pa-tients with conditions that may be associated with hypoalbu-minemia.

RENAL FUNCTION—Renal function is one of the most important determinants of drug activity. The patient's renal status should be known, particularly when drugs that are ex-creted primarily in an active form by the kidney are to be used for long periods of time. If there is renal impairment and the usual dose of a drug that is excreted by the kidney is given, there can be an increased and prolonged effect, since it is not being excreted at the normal rate. As additional doses are given, serum concentrations will increase, possibly resulting in toxicity. Therefore, a need exists for careful dosage adjustment and particular caution when other potentially interacting drugs are added to the therapeutic regimen.

The alteration of renal excretion as a mechanism by which a number of drug interactions develop is considered later, and the status of the patient's renal function is an important deter-minant of the rate of excretion of the drugs involved and the oc-currence of interactions.

HEPATIC FUNCTION—Many drugs are metabolized in the liver by a number of mechanisms. Therefore, when there is hepatic damage, these drugs may be metabolized at a slower rate and exhibit a prolonged effect. Although each situation should be evaluated to determine whether a reduction in dosage is necessary, it should be recognized that some drugs will be metabolized at the normal rate even though hepatic function is impaired. A number of studies of drug metabolism in patients with liver disease have been conducted. However, the results vary considerably, and it is difficult to predict with certainty whether the rate of metabolism will be altered in a given patient.

Many therapeutic agents are metabolized by hepatic enzymes. If other drugs alter the amount and/or activity of these enzymes, a modified response to the drugs that depend on these enzymes for their metabolism might occur. For example, many agents (eg, barbiturates, rifampin) are known to stimulate the activity of hepatic enzymes (enzyme induction). The result would be a more rapid metabolism and excretion of concurrently administered agents that are metabolized by these enzymes. This mechanism of drug interaction is discussed in greater detail later as are the situations in which the action of hepatic enzymes is inhibited.

ALCOHOL CONSUMPTION—Several studies have shown that chronic use of alcoholic beverages may increase the rate of metabolism of drugs such as warfarin and phenytoin, probably by increasing the activity of hepatic enzymes. However, in contrast, acute use of alcohol by nonalcoholic individuals may cause an inhibition of hepatic enzymes.

Concurrent use of alcoholic beverages with sedatives and other depressant drugs could result in an excessive depressant response. The fact that the use of such combinations is commonplace cannot be cause for failing to exercise the caution that must be observed if problems are to be averted.

SMOKING—A number of investigations have suggested that smoking increases the activity of drug-metabolizing enzymes in the liver, with the result that certain therapeutic agents (eg, diazepam, propoxyphene, theophylline, olanzapine) are metabolized more rapidly, and their effect is decreased.

DIET—Food often may affect the rate and extent of absorption of drugs from the gastrointestinal (GI) tract. For example, many antibiotics should be given at least 1 hr before or 2 hr after meals to achieve optimal absorption.

The type of food may be important with regard to the absorption of concurrently administered drugs. For example, dietary items such as milk and other dairy products that contain calcium may decrease the absorption of tetracycline and fluoroquinolone derivatives by forming a complex with them in the GI tract that is absorbed poorly.

Some dietary items, such as certain cheeses and alcoholic beverages, have a relatively high content of the pressor amine tyramine. Tyramine is metabolized by MAO, and normally these enzymes in the intestinal wall and liver protect against the pressor actions of amines in foods. However, if these enzymes were to be inhibited by an MAOI, large quantities of unmetabolized tyramine could accumulate, which could lead to the development of a severe hypertensive reaction.

Certain dietary items contain an appreciable amount of vitamin K. A change in dietary habits that would significantly alter the intake of these foods could cause problems in patients on warfarin therapy.

Diet also may influence urinary pH values. One study has compared the excretion of amphetamine in two groups of patients maintained on different diets. One group was placed on a balanced protein diet that provided an acidic urine (average pH of 5.9), whereas the other group was put on a low-protein diet that provided an alkaline urine (average pH of 7.5). Each group was given a dose of amphetamine, and those with the acidic urine excreted 23 to 56% of unchanged amphetamine in the first 8 hr and 5 to 13% in the next 8 hr. In comparison, in those with an alkalinized urine, there was a 2 to 6% excretion in the first 8 hr, followed by a 0.5 to 3% excretion in the next 8 hr.

INDIVIDUAL VARIATION—Even after the preceding factors have been considered, wide variations in the response of patients to drugs will be seen that are often difficult to explain. Plasma concentrations of certain drugs may vary widely among individuals using the same dosage regimen over the same time period. When recognition is taken of the difficulty in predicting the response to many therapeutic agents when they are given alone, the challenge and limitations in endeavoring to anticipate the response with a multiple-drug regimen clearly become apparent.

MECHANISMS OF DRUG INTERACTION

An understanding of the mechanisms by which drug interactions develop will be valuable in anticipating such situations and dealing with problems that do develop. Although the circumstances surrounding the development of some drug interactions are complex and poorly understood, the mechanisms by which most interactions develop are well documented and relate to the basic processes by which a drug acts and is acted upon in the body.

These mechanisms often are categorized generally as being pharmacokinetic or pharmacodynamic types. *Pharmacokinetic interactions* are those in which one agent (designated by some as the *precipitant drug*) alters the absorption, distribution, metabolism, or excretion (ADME) of a second agent (the *object drug*), with a resultant change in the plasma concentration of the latter agent. Included among the *pharmacodynamic interactions* are those in which drugs having similar (or opposing) pharmacological effects are administered concurrently and situations in which the sensitivity or responsiveness of the tissues to one drug is altered by another. Pharmacodynamic interactions also have been viewed as situations in which there is a change in drug effect without a change in drug plasma concentration.

Although the pharmacokinetic interactions often present challenging clinical problems that have been publicized widely, the pharmacodynamic interactions are encountered more frequently. It also should be recognized that several mechanisms may be involved in the development of certain interactions.

Pharmacokinetic Interactions

ALTERATION OF GI ABSORPTION

Interactions that involve a change in the absorption of a drug from the GI tract may develop through different mechanisms and be of varying clinical importance. In some situations the absorption of the drug may be reduced, and its therapeutic activity compromised. In others, absorption may be delayed, but the same amount of drug is absorbed eventually. A delay in drug absorption can be undesirable when a rapid effect is needed to relieve acute symptoms, such as pain. The slower absorption rate also may prolong the effects of a drug and may present difficulty. For example, if the effects of a hypnotic agent are prolonged, the patient may experience excessive residual sedation or *hangover* in the morning. A slower rate of absorption may preclude achievement of effective plasma and tissue concentrations of drugs that are metabolized rapidly and excreted.

Conversely, a delay in drug absorption may not be clinically significant; this is usually the case when a drug is being used on a chronic basis and therapeutic concentrations in the body have already been achieved.

As a general guideline, it is the drugs that are not absorbed completely under *optimum* circumstances that are most susceptible to alterations of GI absorption.

ALTERATION OF PH

Since many drugs are weak acids or weak bases, the pH of the GI contents may influence the extent of absorption. It is recognized that the nonionized form of a drug (the more lipid-soluble form) will be absorbed more readily than the ionized form. Acidic drugs exist primarily in the nonionized form in the upper region of the GI tract (having a lower pH). If a drug such as an antacid is ingested, which will raise the pH of the GI contents, it is possible that the absorption of such acidic drugs can be delayed and/or inhibited partially.

Although changes in absorption might be predicted for many acidic and basic drugs on a theoretical basis, it would appear that clinically important interactions are likely to occur in only a few situations, and factors other than pH seem to be more important determinants of GI absorption.

KETOCONAZOLE–ANTACIDS—An acidic medium is required to achieve dissolution of ketoconazole following oral administration. Therefore, an antacid, a histamine H_2-receptor antagonist (eg, cimetidine, ranitidine), or a proton pump inhibitor (eg, lansoprazole, omeprazole) is likely to reduce the dissolution, absorption, and effectiveness of the antifungal agent. An antacid should be administered at least 2 hr after ketoconazole; the concurrent use of ketoconazole and a histamine H_2-receptor antagonist or proton pump inhibitor is best avoided, and alternative agents having a lesser potential for interaction should be considered.

BISACODYL–ANTACIDS—A change in the pH of the GI contents also may cause another type of problem. For example, oral dosage forms of the laxative bisacodyl are enteric-coated because the drug can be extremely irritating. It has been suggested that this agent should not be given orally within an hour of antacid therapy or ingestion of milk because an increase in the pH of the GI contents may cause disintegration of the enteric coating in the stomach, resulting in release of the drug in this area, which could cause irritation and vomiting.

Antacids also may alter the GI absorption of drugs through other mechanisms, and additional examples are considered in the following discussion.

Complexation and Adsorption

TETRACYCLINES–METALS—The interaction between tetracycline derivatives and certain metal ions is well known. Tetracycline can combine with metal ions such as calcium, magnesium, aluminum, iron, bismuth, and zinc in the GI tract to form complexes that are absorbed poorly. Thus, the simultaneous administration of certain dietary items (eg, milk, other products containing calcium) or drugs (eg, antacids, iron preparations, products containing calcium salts) with tetracycline could result in a significant decrease in the amount of antibiotic absorbed.

The absorption of doxycycline and minocycline is influenced to a lesser extent by simultaneous ingestion of food or milk. However, the concurrent administration of aluminum hydroxide gel will decrease absorption of these analogs, as is seen with other tetracyclines.

When two drugs are recognized as having a potential to interact there is often a tendency to believe that one of them should be discontinued. In the case of the antacid-tetracycline interaction, problems can be avoided by allowing an appropriate interval of time to separate administration of the two agents. This interval should be as long as possible, but a minimum period of 1 hr should elapse between administration of the drugs.

The interaction between doxycycline and iron salts calls attention to another factor that must be considered, as the results of one study suggest that the interaction cannot be avoided completely by allowing an interval of 3 hr (or even a longer period) to separate administration of the two drugs. It is noted that a significant amount of doxycycline is transported back to the GI tract via the enterohepatic circulation, and the unabsorbed iron still present in the GI tract prevents reabsorption of the antibiotic.

FLUOROQUINOLONES–METALS—Aluminum- and magnesium-containing antacids, as well as certain dietary items (eg, milk, yogurt), have been reported to reduce markedly the absorption and serum concentrations of fluoroquinolones, probably as a result of the metal ions complexing with the anti-infective agent. Even allowing a long interval to separate the administration of the two drugs may not be sufficient to avoid the interaction, and as long an interval as possible should separate the administration of the fluoroquinolone and metal-containing product. For example, in the product labeling for moxifloxacin, it is recommended that this antibacterial agent be taken at least 4 hours before or 8 hours after antacids containing magnesium or aluminum, as well as sucralfate, metal cations such as iron, and multivitamin preparations with zinc.

CHOLESTYRAMINE AND COLESTIPOL—Other interactions involving complexation might be anticipated when the drugs cholestyramine and colestipol are used. These resinous materials, which are not absorbed from the GI tract, bind with bile acids and prevent their reabsorption. In addition to binding with bile acids, cholestyramine and colestipol can bind with drugs that are present in the GI tract, and these agents may reduce the absorption of drugs such as thyroid hormone, warfarin, digoxin, and thiazide diuretics. To reduce the possibility of an interaction, the interval between the administration of cholestyramine or colestipol and another drug should be as long as possible.

The naturally occurring human bile acid, ursodiol, is used in the dissolution of gallstones composed primarily of cholesterol. Because of the affinity of cholestyramine and colestipol for bile acids, the administration of these agents should be separated by as long an interval as possible.

It also should be recognized that prolonged administration of cholestyramine and colestipol can decrease the absorption of fat-soluble vitamins such as vitamin K. This could lead to increased bleeding tendencies in some patients if the vitamin K intake is not increased. When cholestyramine or colestipol is administered to a patient on warfarin therapy, it is understandably difficult to predict the eventual response, since conceivably the absorption of both the anticoagulant and its antagonist, vitamin K, could be reduced.

A newer bile acid-binding agent, colesevelam, appears less likely than cholestyramine and colestipol to interact with other medications or fat-soluble vitamins. Accordingly, colesevelam would be preferred to the other agents in situations in which the potential exists for these interactions.

An interesting application of this interaction is seen with the use of leflunomide in the treatment of rheumatoid arthritis. Leflunomide can cause fetal harm if administered during pregnancy, and it has an active metabolite that can persist in the system for up to 2 years. If a woman of childbearing potential discontinues use of leflunomide, it is recommended that cholestyramine (8 g, three times a day, for 11 days) be used to accelerate the elimination of the drug and its active metabolite.

PENICILLAMINE–METALS—Aluminum and iron salts have been reported to reduce the absorption of penicillamine significantly, probably through chelation and/or adsorption mechanisms. An interval of at least 2 hr should separate the administration of an antacid or iron salt and penicillamine. Food also will decrease the absorption of penicillamine, and the drug should be administered apart from meals.

Alteration of Motility/Rate of Gastric Emptying

CATHARTICS—A cathartic, by increasing GI motility, may increase the rate at which another drug passes through the GI tract. This could result in a decreased absorption of certain drugs, particularly those that normally are absorbed slowly and require prolonged contact with the absorbing surface or those that are absorbed only at a particular site along the GI tract. Similar problems might be noted with enteric-coated and controlled-release formulations.

ANTICHOLINERGICS—Anticholinergics, by decreasing GI motility, also may influence drug absorption. The effect may be one of *decreased* absorption, since the reduced peristalsis may retard dissolution and the slowing of gastric emptying may delay absorption from the small intestine, or *increased* absorption if a drug is retained for a longer period of time in the area from which it is optimally absorbed.

METOCLOPRAMIDE—Because metoclopramide increases motility of the upper GI tract, it should be anticipated that it may influence the absorption of other drugs administered concurrently.

The Effect of Food

It is known that food can influence the absorption of a number of drugs. In some situations, absorption may be delayed but not reduced, whereas in other circumstances the total amount of drug absorbed may be reduced. The effect of food in influencing drug absorption sometimes is due to its action in slowing gastric emptying. However, food also may affect absorption by binding with drugs, decreasing the access of drugs to sites of absorption, altering the dissolution rate of drugs, or altering the pH of the GI contents. The drug-administration time schedules used in many hospitals and long-term care facilities may correspond closely to the times at which meals are served. It is important that a specific dosage schedule be established for those drugs that should be administered apart from meals or with food.

ANTI-INFECTIVE AGENTS–FOOD—The presence of food in the GI tract will reduce the absorption of many anti-infective agents. Although there are some exceptions (eg, penicillin V, amoxicillin, doxycycline, minocycline), it generally is recommended that the penicillin and tetracycline derivatives as well as certain other anti-infective agents be given at least 1 hr before meals or 2 hr after meals, to achieve optimum absorption.

Erythromycin stearate formulations should be administered at least 1 hr before meals or 2 hr after a meal, whereas formulations of erythromycin ethylsuccinate may be given without regard to meals.

The formulations of erythromycin base should be considered on an individual basis because the information for some products indicates they may be given without regard to meals, whereas for other products it is noted that optimum absorption is achieved when given apart from meals.

THEOPHYLLINE–FOOD—It generally has been felt that food does not alter the activity of theophylline significantly when the drug is administered in an immediate-release formulation (ie, those formulations that are not controlled-release).

However, considerable variation is seen among the controlled-release formulations of theophylline with respect to their potential to interact with food. If data are insufficient to assess the potential for a particular theophylline formulation to interact with food, the medication preferably should be administered apart from meals.

CAPTOPRIL–FOOD—The presence of food in the GI tract has been reported to reduce the absorption of captopril by 30 to 40%. Although more-recent investigations suggest that food is unlikely to alter significantly the effects of captopril, it is advisable to administer the drug 1 hr before meals. Food does not appear to alter the absorption of most of the other angiotensin-converting enzyme inhibitors (eg, enalapril, lisinopril).

ALENDRONATE AND RISEDRONATE–FOOD—Food and even orange juice, coffee, and mineral water may markedly reduce the bioavailability of alendronate and risedronate, and it is recommended that these drugs be administered soon after arising at least 1/2 hr before any food, beverage, or medication, with plain water only.

ACARBOSE AND MIGLITOL–FOOD—In some situations it is important that a medication be administered with food to obtain optimum benefit. Acarbose and miglitol are effective in the treatment of diabetes mellitus because they delay the digestion of ingested carbohydrates and reduce the elevation of blood glucose concentrations following meals. Maximum effectiveness is attained when doses are administered at the start (with the first bite) of each main meal.

Alteration of Metabolism in the GI Tract

The absorption of certain agents is influenced by the extent to which they are metabolized in the GI tract.

MAOIs–TYRAMINE—There have been reports of serious reactions (hypertensive crisis) occurring in people being treated with an MAOI (eg, isocarboxazid, phenelzine, tranylcypromine) following ingestion of certain foods with a high content of pressor substances, such as tyramine.

Tyramine is metabolized by MAO, and normally these enzymes in the intestinal wall and in the liver protect against the pressor actions of amines in foods. However, when these enzymes are inhibited, large quantities of unmetabolized tyramine can accumulate and act to release norepinephrine from adrenergic neurons where greater-than-usual stores of this catecholamine are concentrated as a result of MAO inhibition. Among the foods having the highest tyramine content are aged cheeses (eg, cheddar; in contrast, cottage and cream cheeses contain little or no tyramine and need not be restricted), certain alcoholic beverages (eg, Chianti wine), pickled fish (eg, herring), concentrated yeast extracts, and broad-bean pods (also known as fava beans or Italian green beans).

The pharmaceutical companies that market the MAOIs have developed lists of dietary items that patients taking one of these agents should avoid. This information should be provided to, and discussed with, each patient for whom an MAOI is prescribed.

GRAPEFRUIT JUICE—The consumption of grapefruit juice has been reported to increase the serum concentration and activity of a number of medications such as certain calcium channel blockers (eg, amlodipine, felodipine, nisoldipine), certain HMG-CoA reductase inhibitors (eg, lovastatin), and cyclosporine. The bioavailability of most of these agents is generally low, primarily as a result of extensive first-pass metabolism. It has been suggested that components of grapefruit juice reduce the activity of the cytochrome P-450 enzymes (primarily CYP3A4) in the gut wall that are involved in the metabolism of these agents. As a result, larger amounts of unmetabolized drug is absorbed, and serum concentrations are increased.

Alteration of GI Flora

Changes in the microbial flora of the GI tract caused by antibiotics may alter the production or metabolism of certain agents, with a resultant change in the amount of agent being absorbed and available to produce a clinical response.

ANTICOAGULANTS–ANTIBIOTICS—A number of anti-infective agents have been reported to enhance the effect of concurrently administered anticoagulants. It has been suggested that this effect develops, in part, as a result of interference by the anti-infective agent with production of vitamin K by microorganisms in the GI tract. Broad-spectrum antibiotics such as the tetracyclines are most likely to cause problems of this type, although similar effects also may be seen with other antibiotics. The clinical importance of this mechanism has been questioned, and if it is a factor, it is likely that problems will occur only in patients who have a low dietary intake of vitamin K.

It is also probable that other mechanisms may be involved in some of these interactions. For example, the increased anticoagulant effect noted when sulfonamides and anticoagulants are given concurrently may be due, in part, to displacement of the anticoagulant from protein-binding sites and/or inhibition of its hepatic metabolism.

DIGOXIN–ANTIBIOTICS—It is estimated that approximately 10% of patients being treated with digoxin convert a significant portion of the parent compound to inactive reduction metabolites in the GI tract. The bacterial flora of the intestine contributes to this metabolic process. Elevated serum digoxin concentrations have been observed in patients receiving erythromycin or tetracycline concurrently, and it is suggested that these antibiotics, by reducing the bacterial flora, decrease the extent to which digoxin is metabolized in the GI tract, resulting in the higher serum concentrations of the cardiac glycoside.

ORAL CONTRACEPTIVES–ANTIBIOTICS—Several antibiotics (eg, ampicillin) have been suggested to decrease the effectiveness of oral contraceptives. The estrogen component of the contraceptive formulation is conjugated to a large extent in the liver and excreted in the bile. Bacteria in the intestine hydrolyze the conjugated form of the estrogen, permitting the free drug to be reabsorbed, and contribute to the serum concentration of the estrogen. Antibiotics, by reducing the bacterial flora, may interrupt the enterohepatic circulation, with a resultant reduction in serum estrogen concentrations.

Although questions have been raised regarding the significance of this interaction, it would be desirable for patients to use supplementary contraceptive measures in addition to the oral contraceptive, during cycles in which antibiotics are used.

Malabsorption States

Certain drugs, such as laxatives, colchicine, cholestyramine, and colestipol, have been reported to cause malabsorption problems that result in decreased absorption of vitamins and nutrients from the GI tract. It should be recognized that these agents may alter absorption of other drugs that are administered simultaneously, and several examples with cholestyramine already have been considered.

ALTERATION OF DISTRIBUTION

Displacement from Protein-Binding Sites

An interaction of this type may occur when two drugs that are capable of binding to proteins are administered concurrently. Although they may bind at different sites on the protein, the binding characteristics of one of the drugs may be altered (noncompetitive displacement). Probably more significant are situations in which two drugs are capable of binding to the same sites on the protein (competitive displacement). Since there are only a limited number of protein-binding sites, competition will exist, and the drug with the greater affinity for the binding sites will displace the other from plasma or tissue proteins. It is recognized that the protein-bound fraction of a drug in the body is not pharmacologically active. However, an equilibrium exists between bound and unbound fractions, and as the unbound or *free* form of the drug is metabolized and excreted, bound drug is released gradually to maintain the equilibrium and pharmacological response.

The binding of acidic drugs to serum albumin represents the type of drug-protein binding that has been studied most extensively. The binding to albumin is readily reversible, and the albumin-drug complex essentially serves as a reservoir that releases more drug as the free drug is metabolized and/or excreted. The importance of the binding of basic drugs (eg, propranolol, lidocaine) to α_1-acid glycoprotein (AAG) also has been recognized. Even small increases in the reactant protein concentration, such as might be associated with infection and inflammation, can result in significant changes in the concentration of free drug.

The risk of an interaction occurring is greatest with drugs that are highly protein-bound (more than 90%) and also have a small apparent volume of distribution. Since only a small fraction of the drug ordinarily would be available in the *free* form, the displacement of even a small percentage of the amount that is bound to proteins could produce a considerable increase in activity.

The risk of interactions resulting from protein displacement appears to be greatest during the first several days of concurrent therapy. It has been suggested that drugs having the greatest capability of displacing a highly bound drug such as warfarin can increase the anticoagulant response within 24 hr

and exhibit maximum potentiation in 3 to 5 days. After this period the effect levels off, since the drug, as a result of greater amounts being available in the unbound form, also is being metabolized more rapidly and excreted. Therefore, the anticoagulant usually has a shorter half-life when a displacing agent is given concurrently.

METHOTREXATE—Methotrexate is highly bound to plasma proteins, and it has been suggested that agents such as the salicylates may be capable of displacing it from binding sites. Studies also indicate that salicylates may increase the action of methotrexate by inhibiting its renal excretion. Although data pertaining to this interaction are limited, the potential for toxicity with methotrexate dictates extreme caution in any situation in which it is used.

PHENYTOIN–VALPROIC ACID—Valproic acid has been reported to displace phenytoin from plasma protein–binding sites, and some studies suggest it also may inhibit the metabolism of phenytoin. In some patients the result may be significantly increased free phenytoin concentrations and the occurrence of adverse events, even when the total phenytoin serum concentrations are within what would ordinarily be considered the desired therapeutic range. The evaluation of the potential for these agents to interact is made even more complex by reports that phenytoin may decrease valproic acid plasma concentrations. Combination therapy with these agents should be monitored closely, with dosage adjustments made as needed, in an effort to achieve effective control of the disorders for which they have been prescribed with as low a risk of adverse events as possible.

REDUCED ALBUMIN CONCENTRATIONS—Because many drugs are bound extensively to plasma proteins, a decreased concentration or amount of protein could change the availability of drugs and thus their activity. Although the type and incidence of clinical problems have not been determined conclusively, several reports suggest that the incidence of adverse events with certain drugs may be higher in patients with conditions associated with hypoalbuminemia (eg, renal, hepatic, and GI diseases).

A relationship between prednisone dosage, frequency of adverse events, and serum albumin concentrations has been shown in one study. When the serum albumin concentration is less than 2.5 g/100 mL, the frequency of prednisone adverse events is almost doubled, and this is attributed to an increased concentration of prednisolone, an active metabolite of prednisone.

In another study it was noted that the incidence of adverse events to phenytoin was greater in patients with low serum albumin concentrations. It is suggested that the higher incidence of adverse events in the hypoalbuminemic patients is probably due to increased circulating concentrations of unbound phenytoin.

STIMULATION OF METABOLISM

Drug metabolism occurs primarily in the liver and most commonly involves oxidation, reduction, hydrolysis, and conjugation (eg, with glucuronic acid) reactions. Quantitatively, the most important hepatic enzymes are the cytochrome P-450 enzymes, which have been divided into families and subfamilies (eg, CYP3A4) on the basis of the similarity of their amino acid sequences. These enzymes are responsible for the oxidation—often, hydroxylation—of a large number of drugs (Table 104-1). Several comprehensive reviews of the clinically significant cytochrome P-450 drug interactions have been developed (Michalets EL. *Pharmacotherapy* 1998; 18:84; Flockhart DA. www.drug-interactions.com).

Many drug interactions have resulted from the ability of one drug to stimulate the metabolism of another, most often by increasing the activity of hepatic enzymes that are involved in the metabolism of numerous therapeutic agents. The increased activity probably is due to enhanced enzyme synthesis, resulting in increased amounts of drug-metabolizing enzymes, an effect fre-

Table 104-1. Examples of Substrates, Inhibitors, and Inducers of Certain Cytochrome P450 Enzymes

CYP ENZYME	SUBSTRATES	INHIBITORS	INDUCERS
CYP1A2	caffeine clozapine olanzapine theophylline	cimetidine ciprofloxacin	cigarette smoke
CYP2C9	celecoxib ibuprofen losartan phenytoin warfarin	fluconazole fluoxetine	rifampin
CYP2C19	diazepam	cimetidine fluoxetine omeprazole	rifampin
CYP2D6	amitriptyline codeine imipramine metoprolol mexiletine propafenone propranolol risperidone tramadol	cimetidine fluoxetine paroxetine quinidine	

CYP3A4	atorvastatin
	carbamazepine
	cyclosporine
	dexamethasone
	diltiazem
	felodipine
	HIV protease
	  inhibitors
	
	lovastatin
	midazolam
	nifedipine
	quinidine
	sildenafil
	simvastatin
	tacrolimus
	tadalafil
	triazolam
	vardenafil
		amiodarone
		clarithromycin
		erythromycin
		fluconazole
		grapefruit juice
		HIV protease
		  inhibitors
		  (eg, indinavir,
		  ritonavir)
		itraconazole
		ketoconazole
			carbamazepine
			efavirenz
			phenobarbital
			phenytoin
			rifampin
			St John's wort

quently referred to as *enzyme induction*. These situations have been documented well, with barbiturates, phenytoin, carbamazepine, and rifampin being among the agents best recognized as causing enzyme induction. The ability of the herbal product St John's wort to cause enzyme induction is also well documented.

In most situations, drugs are converted to less active, water-soluble metabolites, and enzyme induction usually will result in an increased metabolism and excretion and a reduced pharmacological action of the agent being metabolized by hepatic enzymes. Less frequently, a drug may be converted to a metabolite that is more active than the parent compound, and there may be an enhanced response. However, the initially increased effect may subsequently diminish, since the drug will be excreted more rapidly and have a shorter duration of action.

The stimulation of hepatic enzyme activity is not only a factor in the development of drug interactions, but also may be responsible for a drug (eg, carbamazepine) stimulating its own metabolism. With continued use, the half-life of the drug will decrease, possibly resulting in a need to increase the dosage.

WARFARIN–PHENOBARBITAL—By causing enzyme induction, phenobarbital can increase the rate of metabolism of warfarin. The result of this interaction is a decreased response to the anticoagulant since it is being more rapidly metabolized and excreted, possibly leading to an increased risk of thrombus formation if the interaction is not recognized. To compensate for this loss of effect, the dose of warfarin would have to be in-

creased until the desired activity was obtained. If the dose of warfarin has been increased to compensate for loss of activity, it will have to be reduced when phenobarbital is discontinued. Otherwise, the readjusted higher dosage that was necessary when phenobarbital was given concurrently may be excessive when it is withdrawn and possibly result in hemorrhaging.

It is probable that all barbiturates have the ability to cause enzyme induction, although phenobarbital may be a more potent inducing agent than analogs having a shorter duration of action. Several studies indicate that the effect of barbiturates in decreasing anticoagulant activity is evident within 2 to 5 days, and it is suggested that the administration of a barbiturate for a week or longer is likely to produce this effect in most patients. There have been varying reports as to how rapidly enzyme activity returns to pretreatment levels when the barbiturate is discontinued. However, it is probable that in most situations normal enzyme activity will be restored in 2 to 3 weeks.

Although close monitoring of combined barbiturate-anticoagulant therapy usually will prevent problems from developing, it would seem unwise to expose the patient unnecessarily to the risk of an interaction when therapeutic alternatives are available. The benzodiazepines (eg, diazepam, temazepam) are not likely to interact with warfarin and one of these agents might be useful as an alternative to a barbiturate. These alternatives apply to the use of a barbiturate as a sedative-hypnotic. Although some benzodiazepines have been used in certain types of seizure disorders, they would not be adequate alternatives to phenobarbital when the latter is used in the treatment of these conditions.

ORAL CONTRACEPTIVES—Phenobarbital, rifampin, and other drugs are known to increase the metabolism of steroid hormones, including estrogens and progestins that are used in oral contraceptive formulations. The high rate of effectiveness of oral contraceptives may suggest that other agents are not likely to reduce their effect significantly. However, there is concern that agents capable of causing enzyme induction indeed may reduce the effectiveness of oral contraceptives, possibly resulting in an unplanned pregnancy. This possibility takes on increased significance in view of the fact that the dosages of the hormones included in these products have been decreased in the interest of minimizing the risk of adverse events. It is possible that the lower dosages of the hormones used in certain products could be approaching the minimum effective concentration and that addition of another agent that can reduce their action is sufficient to compromise their effectiveness. Although the potential for such an interaction is low, the importance of the possible consequences warrants extra caution, and additional contraceptive measures should be used during the period of time that the enzyme- inducing drug is used.

HIV PROTEASE INHIBITORS—All of the HIV protease inhibitors (eg, amprenavir, atazanavir, lopinavir, nelfinavir) are extensively metabolized via CYP3A/3A4 pathways, and the concurrent use of an enzyme inducer could reduce their action and compromise the effectiveness of the antiretroviral regimen for HIV infection/AIDS of which they are a component. Rifampin is such a strong enzyme inducer that its concurrent use with most of the HIV protease inhibitors is contraindicated.

SMOKING—A number of studies have indicated that the effects of certain drugs may be decreased in individuals who are heavy smokers, presumably because of increased hepatic enzyme activity resulting from the action of polycyclic hydrocarbons that are present in cigarette smoke. Among the drugs whose metabolism is increased and therapeutic activity likely to be reduced are diazepam, propoxyphene, theophylline, pentazocine, and olanzapine. In addition to careful monitoring of therapy with drugs that are metabolized by hepatic enzyme systems in patients who are moderate or heavy smokers, caution also must be exercised if a patient treated with such a medication discontinues smoking. For example, if therapy with olanzapine is initiated in a patient who is a heavy smoker, the maintenance dosage will be determined during the time period in which the enzyme-inducing action of smoking is decreasing the effect of the medication. If the patient stops smoking and is still taking the medication, the dosage that had been appropriate is now likely to be excessive and will have to be reduced.

In the examples noted, the effect of smoking is to increase the rate of metabolism of other agents being used, and a decreased response to these agents can be anticipated. In contrast, a significant risk of toxicity exists when oral contraceptives are used by women who smoke, as it has been noted that smoking markedly increases the risk of serious cardiovascular effects (eg, myocardial infarction), especially in women over 35 years of age.

ALCOHOL—Alcohol may either stimulate or inhibit the activity of hepatic enzymes, depending on the circumstances of use. An increased rate of metabolism of warfarin and phenytoin has been reported in alcoholic patients. This was attributed to increased liver enzyme activity caused by chronic administration of alcohol.

In contrast, acute use of alcohol by nonalcoholic individuals may cause inhibition of hepatic enzymes. This may decrease the rate of metabolism, thereby increasing the effect of other agents administered concurrently, and may be responsible, at least in part, for the enhanced sedation experienced when alcoholic beverages and sedative drugs are taken together by individuals who are not alcoholics. The extent to which the mechanisms of enzyme inhibition and central nervous system (CNS) summation or synergism are involved in this interaction remains to be clarified.

LEVODOPA–PYRIDOXINE—Pyridoxine has been shown to reduce the action of levodopa by accelerating its decarboxylation to dopamine in the peripheral tissues. Consequently, less levodopa reaches and crosses the blood-brain barrier, with the result that less dopamine is formed in the brain and the therapeutic effect is diminished. Doses of pyridoxine of 10 to 25 mg have been reported to rapidly reverse the effect of the antiparkinson drug.

The combination product *Sinemet* contains both levodopa and carbidopa, the latter agent acting as an inhibitor of decarboxylase enzymes. When administered with levodopa, carbidopa permits the use of significantly lower doses of the former, since it now is metabolized to a lesser extent in the peripheral tissues. The decrease in dosage often is accompanied by a decreased incidence of adverse effects. Since carbidopa does not cross the blood-brain barrier, it will not hinder the conversion of levodopa to dopamine in the brain.

Levodopa is metabolized also in the peripheral tissues in a pathway that is catalyzed by catechol-*O*-methyltransferase (COMT). When the decarboxylation pathway is inhibited by carbidopa, the *O*-methylation pathway becomes the primary pathway through which levodopa is metabolized in the peripheral tissues. The COMT inhibitor entacapone was developed to inhibit this metabolic pathway and has been used in conjunction with levodopa and carbidopa. A combination product (Stalevo) that includes these three agents has been recently marketed.

INHIBITION OF METABOLISM

A number of situations have been reported in which one drug has inhibited the metabolism of another, usually resulting in a prolonged and intensified activity of the latter (Table 104-1).

ALCOHOL–DISULFIRAM—A well-known example of inhibition of metabolism that has been used to advantage is the use of disulfiram in the treatment of alcoholism. Disulfiram inhibits the activity of aldehyde dehydrogenase, thus inhibiting oxidation of acetaldehyde, an oxidation product of alcohol. This results in accumulation of excessive quantities of acetaldehyde and development of the unpleasant effects characteristic of the disulfiram reaction. A similar noteworthy reaction occurs between metronidazole and alcohol.

Disulfiram is not a selective inhibitor of aldehyde dehydrogenase but exhibits several inhibitory actions that can result in the development of drug interactions. It has been reported that it can enhance the activity of warfarin and phenytoin, presumably by inhibiting their metabolism.

MERCAPTOPURINE OR AZATHIOPRINE–ALLOPURINOL—Allopurinol, by inhibiting the enzyme xanthine oxidase, reduces production of uric acid, which is the basis for its use in the treatment of gout. Xanthine oxidase also has an important role in the metabolism of such potentially toxic drugs as mercaptopurine and azathioprine, and when this enzyme is inhibited by allopurinol, the effect of the latter agents can be increased markedly. When allopurinol is given in doses of 300 to 600 mg/day concurrently with either of these drugs, it is advised that the dose of mercaptopurine or azathioprine be reduced to about 1/3 to 1/4 the usual dose.

CIMETIDINE—Because cimetidine is known to inhibit hepatic oxidative enzyme systems, it should be anticipated that the action of other agents that are metabolized extensively via these pathways will be increased. There are reports of such interactions with carbamazepine, diazepam, phenytoin, theophylline, warfarin, and other agents, and it may be necessary to reduce the dosage of these agents when cimetidine is included in the therapeutic regimen. Although ranitidine also binds to a limited extent to the cytochrome P-450 enzymes involved in the metabolism of these agents, it appears to have a lesser affinity for the enzymes than does cimetidine. Consequently, clinically significant interactions are less likely to occur with ranitidine. Studies of the other histamine H$_2$-receptor antagonists (famotidine and nizatidine) suggest that they are not likely to inhibit oxidative metabolic pathways and to interact with other drugs via this mechanism.

THEOPHYLLINE–MACROLIDE ANTIBIOTICS—Erythromycin has been reported to increase significantly serum theophylline concentrations by inhibiting its hepatic metabolism. Patients receiving high doses of theophylline or who are otherwise predisposed to theophylline toxicity should be monitored closely if erythromycin is administered concurrently. It also should be anticipated that clarithromycin and telithromycin will inhibit the metabolism of theophylline, whereas azithromycin is unlikely to interact.

THEOPHYLLINE–FLUOROQUINOLONES—Ciprofloxacin has been reported to increase the plasma concentrations and activity of theophylline markedly, presumably by inhibiting its hepatic metabolism, and concurrent use is best avoided. Certain other fluoroquinolones, such as levofloxacin, are not likely to inhibit hepatic enzyme systems and interact with theophylline.

MAOIs—There have been many reports of drug interactions involving use of an MAOI with another drug or with certain dietary items. It is likely that MAOIs enhance the effect of drugs such as the barbiturates and opioid analgesics by inhibiting hepatic enzyme systems involved in their metabolism. However, other mechanisms are involved in some of the more publicized problems with these compounds and are considered elsewhere in this chapter.

CALCIUM CHANNEL BLOCKING AGENTS—The calcium channel blocking agents (eg, diltiazem, nifedipine, verapamil) have been reported to interact with a number of drugs, although the mechanisms through which these interactions occur are not completely defined. It has been suggested that verapamil and diltiazem may inhibit the hepatic metabolism of carbamazepine, thereby increasing the activity of the latter agent. Because the calcium channel blocking agents are metabolized themselves in the liver, they may interact with certain drugs because they are competing for the same metabolic pathways.

ALTERATION OF EXCRETION

Although some therapeutic agents are eliminated via other mechanisms, most drugs and their metabolites are excreted, at least in part, via the kidneys. The most important clinical implications of altering renal excretion involve the use of drugs that are excreted in their unchanged form or in the form of an active metabolite. Thus, substances with pharmacological activity are being reabsorbed or excreted to a greater extent when renal excretion is altered. In contrast, when only inactive metabolites are being excreted, changes in therapeutic activity are less likely to be associated with the use of other drugs that can influence renal excretory pathways.

Alteration of Urinary pH

SALICYLATES–ACIDIFYING AND ALKALINIZING AGENTS—A change in urinary pH will influence the ionization of weak acids and weak bases and thus affect the extent to which these agents are reabsorbed and excreted. When a drug is in its nonionized form it will diffuse more readily from urine back into blood. Therefore, for an acidic drug, there will be a larger proportion of drug in the nonionized form in an acid urine than in an alkaline urine—where it will exist primarily as an ionized salt. The result is that from an acid urine more of an acidic drug will diffuse back into the blood and produce a prolonged, and perhaps intensified, activity. In one study it was noted that a salicylate dosage regimen that provided a serum concentration of 20 to 30 μg/mL in a patient when the urinary pH was approximately 6.5 produced serum concentrations that were approximately twice as high when the urinary pH was decreased to 5.5. The risk of a significant interaction is greatest in patients who are taking large doses of salicylates (eg, for arthritis).

AMPHETAMINES–ALKALINIZING AGENTS—Converse effects will be seen for a basic drug like dextroamphetamine. In one investigation the excretion of a dose of dextroamphetamine at urinary pH values of approximately 5 and 8 was studied. When the urinary pH was maintained at approximately 5, 54.5% of the dose of dextroamphetamine was excreted within 16 hr, compared with a 2.9% excretion in the same period when the urinary pH was maintained at approximately 8.

Similar observations have been made with other basic drugs. One report calls attention to the possible development of quinidine toxicity when urine becomes alkaline, since excretion of quinidine was shown to decrease considerably as urinary pH was raised. In another investigation, when the urinary pH was increased to about 8 with sodium bicarbonate, the plasma half-life of pseudoephedrine was approximately double that in normal subjects. When urinary pH in the same subjects was decreased to 5.2, using ammonium chloride, the plasma half-life decreased markedly from control values.

Alteration of Active Transport

PENICILLINS–PROBENECID—A number of organic acids undergo active transport from the blood into the tubular urine and *vice versa*. In some situations these agents interfere with the excretion of each other. It is well-recognized that probenecid can increase serum concentrations and prolong activity of penicillin derivatives by blocking their tubular secretion. Often there will be a 2-fold to 4-fold elevation of serum penicillin concentrations, although the degree to which these concentrations are increased and the duration of activity prolonged depend on a number of factors.

Probenecid also has been reported to decrease renal excretion of other agents, including methotrexate.

METHOTREXATE–NONSTEROIDAL ANTI-INFLAMMATORY DRUGS—A number of nonsteroidal anti-inflammatory drugs (NSAIDs) have been reported to increase the activity and toxicity of methotrexate. There have been several reports of fatal methotrexate toxicity in patients also receiving ketoprofen, and it has been suggested that ketoprofen inhibited the active renal tubular secretion of methotrexate. However, other mechanisms probably also contribute to an increase in serum methotrexate concentrations. Most of the patients in whom these interactions have been reported were receiving high-dose methotrexate therapy for neoplastic disorders. However, caution also should be exercised in patients receiving lower doses, particularly since low-dose methotrexate regimens are used in patients with rheumatoid arthritis who also are taking an NSAID.

LITHIUM–NONSTEROIDAL ANTI-INFLAMMATORY DRUGS—The serum concentrations and incidence of adverse effects of lithium salts have been reported to be increased by the concurrent administration of anti-inflammatory agents such as ibuprofen, indomethacin, and piroxicam. It is suggested that the renal clearance of lithium is reduced as a result of the action of these anti-inflammatory agents to inhibit renal prostaglandin synthesis. This interaction should be anticipated when any NSAID is administered concurrently with a lithium salt.

ALTERATION OF DRUG TRANSPORT

There has been increased recognition of the importance of P-glycoprotein in the absorption, distribution, metabolism, and excretion of certain drugs. P-glycoprotein functions as a transport system that may act as a barrier for certain agents and as a pump that facilitates the transport of certain agents across membranes. For example, it limits cellular uptake of certain drugs from the blood into the brain and from the intestinal lumen into epithelial cells. The role of P-glycoprotein in the overall absorption of a drug that is administered orally in high milligram doses is not likely to be clinically important because this transport system is quickly saturated by the high concentrations of drug in the intestinal lumen. However, its role may be important in the absorption of drugs that are administered orally in very small doses (eg, digoxin). Numerous medications have been shown to be substrates for P-glycoprotein including agents such as cyclosporine, digoxin, diltiazem, verapamil, atorvastatin, lovastatin, simvastatin, doxorubicin, paclitaxel, HIV protease inhibitors, and loperamide.

There is overlapping substrate specificity between P-glycoprotein and CYP3A4, and many of the drugs that inhibit or induce CYP3A4 also inhibit or induce P-glycoprotein. Therefore, drug interactions that result from inhibition or induction of CYP3A4 often also involve inhibition or induction of P-glycoprotein. Inhibitors of P-glycoprotein include agents such as clarithromycin, erythromycin, itraconazole, ketoconazole, quinidine, and verapamil. Inducers include such agents as rifampin and St John's wort.

DIGOXIN–QUINIDINE OR VERAPAMIL—The concurrent use of quinidine or verapamil with digoxin has resulted in significantly greater serum digoxin concentrations. Both quinidine and verapamil are inhibitors of P-glycoprotein and it is thought that this action results in increased absorption, decreased elimination, and higher concentrations of digoxin. Conversely, inducers of P-glycoprotein such as rifampin and St John's wort would be expected to decrease serum concentrations of digoxin.

LOPERAMIDE–P-GLYCOPROTEIN—The antidiarrheal agent loperamide is very unlikely to cause central nervous system adverse events, in part because P-glycoprotein prevents it from crossing the blood-brain barrier and gaining access to the central nervous system. However, if a patient using loperamide is also treated with a P-glycoprotein inhibitor, CNS effects that are characteristic of the opioids may be experienced.

Pharmacodynamic Interactions

Although pharmacokinetic interactions often present challenging clinical problems and are publicized widely, pharmacodynamic interactions are the type that occur most frequently.

DRUGS HAVING OPPOSING PHARMACOLOGICAL EFFECTS

Interactions resulting from the use of two drugs with opposing effects should be among the easiest to detect. However, these sometimes are due to the secondary effects of certain drugs and this and other factors may preclude early identification of such situations.

DIURETICS—The ability of the thiazides and certain other diuretics to elevate blood glucose concentrations is well known. When the diuretic is prescribed for a diabetic patient being treated with insulin or one of the oral antidiabetic agents, this action may partially counteract the glucose-lowering action of the antidiabetic drug, necessitating an adjustment in dosage. Similarly, many diuretics may produce a hyperuricemic effect. Therapy in patients with gout should be monitored closely, as the hyperuricemic action of a diuretic may necessitate an adjustment in dosage of the agent being used in the treatment of gout.

DRUGS HAVING SIMILAR PHARMACOLOGICAL EFFECTS

An excessive response attributable to the concurrent use of drugs having similar actions is the type of interaction that occurs most often, and these potential problems warrant particular attention.

CNS DEPRESSANTS—An excessive CNS depressant effect resulting from the concurrent use of two or more drugs exhibiting a depressant action represents one of the most dangerous drug-related problems. Older patients should be viewed as being especially susceptible to this type of response, and patients experiencing effects such as sedation and dizziness are at increased risk of falls and injuries, such as hip fractures. Patients also must be advised of the risks of operating motor vehicles or machinery. In considering multiple drug regimens, recognition must be taken of the large number of agents (eg, sedative-hypnotics, antipsychotics, tricyclic antidepressants, opioid analgesics, and most antihistamines) that can exhibit a depressant effect that will be at least additive to the effect contributed by other drugs. If it is considered necessary to use agents with a CNS depressant action concurrently, it should be anticipated that a lower dosage of at least one of the agents should be used.

ALCOHOL–OTHER CNS DEPRESSANTS—The increased CNS depressant effect that is experienced by individuals being treated with depressant drugs when they consume alcoholic beverages is among the best-known interactions. However, this interaction also illustrates the difficulties in trying to predict the magnitude of the response that will be experienced by a particular patient, as the response will depend on many variables, including the patient's tolerance to alcohol. How then should the patient be instructed when he or she is to take a depressant medication? Certainly it would be most desirable not to consume alcoholic beverages during the period the medication is being taken. However, there should be a realistic recognition that many patients if faced with a mandate not to drink while on drug therapy will decide not to take the drug. Every patient should be alerted to the fact that the depressant effect of the drug prescribed may be increased by alcohol. If it is anticipated that a patient would not completely avoid alcoholic beverages, that patient should be urged to use them in moderation, particularly when therapy is initiated or the dosage is increased, and cautioned to observe his or her own tolerance when such combinations are employed. The fact that many individuals can take depressant drugs and consume relatively large amounts of alcoholic beverages with no apparent difficulty should not be cause to forget that such combinations have been lethal in some individuals and the cause of injury in others. Thus, there is an important need to caution all patients for whom such drugs are prescribed.

DRUGS HAVING ANTICHOLINERGIC ACTIVITY—Drugs that differ considerably in their primary pharmacological actions may exhibit the same secondary effects. Some patients being treated with antipsychotic agents such as chlorpromazine also are given an antiparkinson agent such as trihexyphenidyl to control the extrapyramidal effects of the former. In addition, a number of these patients experience symptoms of depression, and a tricyclic antidepressant such as amitriptyline might be added to the therapy. Each of these three agents possesses anticholinergic activity, and the additive effect could result in side effects such as dryness of the mouth, blurred vision, urinary retention, constipation, and elevation of intraocular pressure.

Even an effect such as dryness of the mouth, which most health professionals would consider as a minor problem, could be troublesome in certain patients. For example, persistent dryness of the mouth could make the use of dentures more difficult and also cause other dental complications. In addition, there may be increased difficulty in chewing and swallowing, an important factor with respect to the problem of malnutrition in many elderly individuals. Dryness of the mouth also may result in other problems as illustrated by a case report of a patient treated with imipramine. The patient experienced persistent dryness of the mouth and when nitroglycerin tablets were administered sublingually for the management of exertional angina, the relief of the symptoms was delayed because of the slower dissolution of the sublingual tablets.

It has been observed that an excessive anticholinergic effect can cause an atropine-like delirium, particularly in geriatric patients. This effect could be misinterpreted as an increase in psychiatric symptoms, which might be treated by increasing the dosage of the therapeutic agents that are actually responsible for causing the problem. This example points out the difficulty that often can exist in distinguishing between the symptoms of the condition(s) being treated and the effects of the drug(s) being employed as therapy.

Several studies call attention to other potential problems associated with the use of drugs having anticholinergic activity. In one investigation using volunteers aged 60 to 72, trihexyphenidyl was found to cause substantial memory impairment. In another study of 22 demented nursing-home patients, it was noted that those with high serum anticholinergic concentrations had greater impairment in self-care capacity than patients with low concentrations.

The blurring of vision, which also may be associated with the use of drugs having anticholinergic activity, may be especially distressing for older patients, particularly those whose physical activities may be limited and for whom reading is a favorite activity.

Several reports have described the development of severe hyperpyrexia in patients taking phenothiazine–antiparkinson combinations who were exposed to high environmental temperature and humidity. These investigators call attention to the ability of these combinations to interfere with the thermoregulatory system of the body and recommend that physicians treating patients in hot and humid climates should minimize outdoor exposure of patients receiving high doses of these agents.

DRUGS EXHIBITING HYPOTENSIVE EFFECTS—Certain antihypertensive drugs as well as some other classes of medications (eg, tricyclic antidepressants) can cause orthostatic hypotension, resulting in symptoms such as dizziness, lightheadedness, and, in more severe cases, syncope. Older patients are more susceptible to this type of response and the associated risks such as falls and injuries, and appropriate precautions should be exercised whether these agents are given alone or in combination.

The use of sildenafil, tadalafil, and vardenafil in the treatment of erectile dysfunction is contraindicated in patients treated with nitrates because these agents may potentiate the hypotensive effect of the nitrates.

NSAIDs—Several situations exist in which a patient unknowingly may be taking several different products that contain the same NSAID. An arthritic patient whose condition has been managed with ibuprofen obtained via prescription (often at dosage levels at or near the recommended maximum) may purchase an ibuprofen product available without a prescription for pain/discomfort not associated with the arthritis, without recognizing that the two products contain the same drug and that there is an increased risk of adverse effects.

ALTERATION OF ELECTROLYTE CONCENTRATIONS

Several important drug interactions occur as a result of the ability of certain therapeutic agents to alter the concentration of electrolytes such as potassium and sodium. When these drugs are included in a therapeutic regimen, it is important that electrolyte concentrations be monitored periodically.

DIGOXIN–DIURETICS—One of the problems associated with the use of most of the commonly employed diuretics (eg, the thiazide derivatives) is that they can cause an excessive loss of potassium. Particular caution is necessary in patients also being treated with digoxin, many of whom would be candidates for diuretic therapy. If potassium depletion remains uncorrected, the heart may become more sensitive to the effects of the cardiac glycoside and arrhythmia may result.

Although potassium supplementation will be necessary in many individuals being treated with a potassium-depleting diuretic, the initiation of therapy with such a diuretic must not be viewed as a mandate also to provide potassium supplementation. This decision should be based on a consideration of the individual patient situation, and the appropriate parameters should be monitored periodically. It must be recognized that dangers also exist if hyperkalemia occurs as a result of excessive supplementation. This risk of such complications is greatest in patients with diminished renal function.

In addition to the diuretics, other agents also can cause potassium depletion. Prolonged therapy with cathartics and corticosteroids may cause potassium depletion, although this is not likely to occur as quickly or to the same extent as with diuretics.

Interest has developed also in the clinical implications of magnesium depletion. Concern has been expressed that this condition occurs much more commonly than is recognized and that some clinical problems may continue or worsen despite seemingly adequate electrolyte therapy because magnesium deficiency has not been identified and corrected.

Diuretic therapy may lead to development of magnesium depletion, and as observed when potassium is depleted, the activity of digoxin may be increased and possibly result in toxicity. In some patients with digoxin toxicity, low serum-magnesium concentrations may coexist with normal potassium values.

ANGIOTENSIN-CONVERTING ENZYME IN-HIBITORS–POTASSIUM-SPARING DIURETICS—The angiotensin-converting enzyme (ACE) inhibitors (eg, enalapril, lisinopril, ramipril) may cause an elevation of serum potassium concentrations. Potassium-sparing diuretics (amiloride, spironolactone, and triamterene) or potassium supplements should be used concurrently with caution, because of the risk of hyperkalemia and associated complications. Salt substitutes containing potassium also should be used with caution.

LITHIUM–DIURETICS—Sodium depletion is known to increase lithium toxicity, for which reason it generally has been recommended that lithium salts should not be used in patients on diuretic therapy or on a sodium-restricted diet. Even protracted sweating or diarrhea can cause sufficient depletion of sodium to result in decreased tolerance to lithium.

The sodium depletion caused by diuretics reduces the renal clearance and increases the activity of lithium. However, if preferable therapeutic alternatives are not available, concurrent therapy need not be contraindicated so long as the interaction is recognized and steps are taken to monitor therapy and adjust dosage.

INTERACTIONS AT RECEPTOR SITES

MAOIs–SYMPATHOMIMETIC AGENTS—MAO functions to break down catecholamines such as norepinephrine. When the enzyme is inhibited, the concentrations of norepinephrine within adrenergic neurons increase, and a drug that can stimulate its release can bring about an exaggerated re-sponse. It is by this mechanism that interactions between MAOIs and indirectly acting sympathomimetic amines (eg, amphetamine) develop. Thus, if amphetamine is administered to patients whose stores of norepinephrine have been increased by MAO inhibition, they may experience severe headache, hypertension (possibly a hypertensive crisis), and cardiac arrhythmias. The serious consequences associated with these interactions contraindicate use of these agents in combination.

Although most sympathomimetic amines, such as amphetamine, are available only by prescription, others such as phenylephrine, which also has been reported to interact similarly with MAOIs, are found in many nonprescription cold and allergy preparations. It is important that patients being treated with MAOIs avoid using products containing these agents.

MAOIs–TRICYCLIC ANTIDEPRESSANTS—Cautions in the product literature, as well as case reports, warn against concurrent use of an MAOI with a tricyclic antidepressant (eg, amitriptyline, imipramine) because severe atropine-like reactions, tremors, convulsions, hyperthermia, and vascular collapse have been reported to result from such use. It is recommended in the labeling for most of these products that therapy with an MAOI or a tricyclic antidepressant should not be initiated until at least 7 to 14 days after therapy with the other has been discontinued.

Although the labeling for most MAOIs and tricyclic antidepressants notes that concurrent use is contraindicated, there is debate as to the degree of risk involved. Several studies of the combined use of these agents have revealed little evidence of interaction, and the growing impression that serious interactions are uncommon, coupled with the reports of favorable results with such combinations in selected patients who did not respond to either agent given alone, have led some to conclude that these combinations can be employed cautiously. In patients who are refractory to single antidepressants and who are not candidates for alternative therapeutic approaches, the potential benefits of combination therapy may outweigh the risks. However, such therapy should be undertaken only by those who are thoroughly familiar with the risks involved and under circumstances in which therapy can be monitored closely.

MAOIs–SELECTIVE SEROTONIN REUPTAKE INHIBITORS—Serious consequences may result from the combined use of an MAOI and a selective serotonin reuptake inhibitor (SSRI, citalopram, escitalopram, fluoxetine, fluvoxamine, paroxetine, sertaline), and concurrent use or use within 14 days before or after most of these agents is contraindicated.

There have been several reports of deaths of patients in whom therapy with an MAOI was initiated shortly after discontinuation of fluoxetine. Because of the long half-lives of fluoxetine and its active metabolite, it is recommended that at least 5 weeks should elapse between discontinuation of fluoxetine and initiation of therapy with an MAOI.

It should be noted that the antineoplastic procarbazine and the anti-infectives furazolidone and linezolid, also can inhibit MAO enzymes, and warnings applying to the use of other MAOIs should be heeded for these drugs also.

GUANETHIDINE–TRICYCLIC ANTIDEPRESSANTS—Guanethidine is transported to its site of action within adrenergic neurons by a transport system that also is responsible for uptake of norepinephrine, as well as several indirectly acting sympathomimetic amines such as ephedrine and the amphetamines. Concentration of guanethidine in these neurons is necessary for its antihypertensive action. Tricyclic antidepressants can inhibit uptake of guanethidine into the neuron terminal, thereby preventing its concentration at these sites and reducing its activity. Other studies suggest that antipsychotic agents such as chlorpromazine and haloperidol can act similarly to the tricyclic antidepressants in reducing the antihypertensive effect of this agent.

Although other mechanisms may be involved in the development of drug interactions, the ones cited are the most important. As often stated, more than one mechanism may be responsible for certain interactions; these mechanisms may work in concert or in opposition as determinants of the resulting effect. Still other drug interactions develop by mechanisms yet to be identified.

However, an awareness of the factors predisposing to the development of drug interactions, as well as the mechanisms by which many of them occur, will be of value in the identification and prevention of potential problems.

It is evident that significant limitations still exist in trying to predict the results of combination therapy. In the following section, guidelines are provided to reduce the risk of the occurrence of drug interactions.

REDUCING THE RISK OF DRUG INTERACTION

The reduction of the risk of drug interactions is a challenge that embraces a number of considerations. Although they could be applied to drug therapy in general, the following guidelines to reduce and manage drug interactions are offered to assist health professionals who have the responsibility of selecting and monitoring therapeutic regimens.

Identify the Patient Risk Factors Factors such as age, the nature of the patient's medical problems (eg, impaired renal function), dietary habits, smoking, and problems like alcoholism will influence the effect of certain drugs and should be considered during the initial patient interview.

Take a Thorough Drug History An accurate and complete record of the prescription and nonprescription medications a patient is taking as well as products such as herbal products and dietary supplements must be obtained. Numerous interactions have resulted from a lack of awareness of prescription products prescribed by another physician or nonprescription medications the patient did not consider important enough to mention.

Be Knowledgeable about the Actions of the Drugs Being Used The knowledge of the properties and the primary and secondary pharmacological actions of each of the agents used or being considered for use is essential if the interaction potential is to be assessed accurately.

Consider Therapeutic Alternatives In most cases, two drugs that are known to interact can be administered concurrently as long as adequate precautions are taken (eg, closer monitoring of therapy or dosage adjustments to compensate for the altered response). However, in those situations in which another agent with similar therapeutic properties and a lesser risk of interacting is available, it should be used.

Avoid Complex Therapeutic Regimens When Possible The number of medications used should be kept to a minimum. In addition, the use of medications or dosage regimens that permit less-frequent administration may help avoid interactions that result from an alteration of absorption (eg, when a drug is administered in close proximity to meals).

Educate the Patient Patients often know little about their illnesses, let alone the benefits and problems that could result from drug therapy. Individuals who are aware of, and understand, this information can be expected to be in greater compliance with the instructions for administering medications and more attentive to the development of symptoms that could be early indicators of drug-related problems. Patients should be encouraged to ask questions about their therapy and to report any excessive or unexpected responses. There should be no uncertainty on the part of patients as to how to use their medications in the most effective and safest way.

Monitor Therapy The risk of drug-related problems warrants close monitoring, not only for the possible occurrence of drug interactions but also for adverse events occurring with individual agents and noncompliance. Any change in patient behavior should be suspected as being drug-related until that possibility is excluded.

Individualize Therapy Although the development of a therapeutic regimen that meets the specific needs of individual patients is inherent in many of the above guidelines, the importance of individualization of therapy cannot be emphasized too strongly. Wide variations in the response of patients to the same dose of certain individual drugs is well-recognized. It is difficult to predict the response of many therapeutic agents when they are given alone; the challenge and limitations in anticipating the response with a multiple-drug regimen are even greater. Therefore, priority should be assigned to the needs and clinical response of the individual patient, rather than to the usual dosage recommendations and standard treatment and monitoring guidelines.

The pharmacist will be involved actively in the observance of the guidelines described above. In addition, the need to not only maintain complete and current patient medication records, but also to supervise and monitor drug therapy more closely, places the pharmacist in a strategic position to detect and prevent drug interactions. By observing the preceding guidelines and recommendations and by strengthening communication with patients and other health professionals, the pharmacist has a valuable opportunity to make a significant contribution toward the further enhancement of the efficacy and safety of drug therapy.

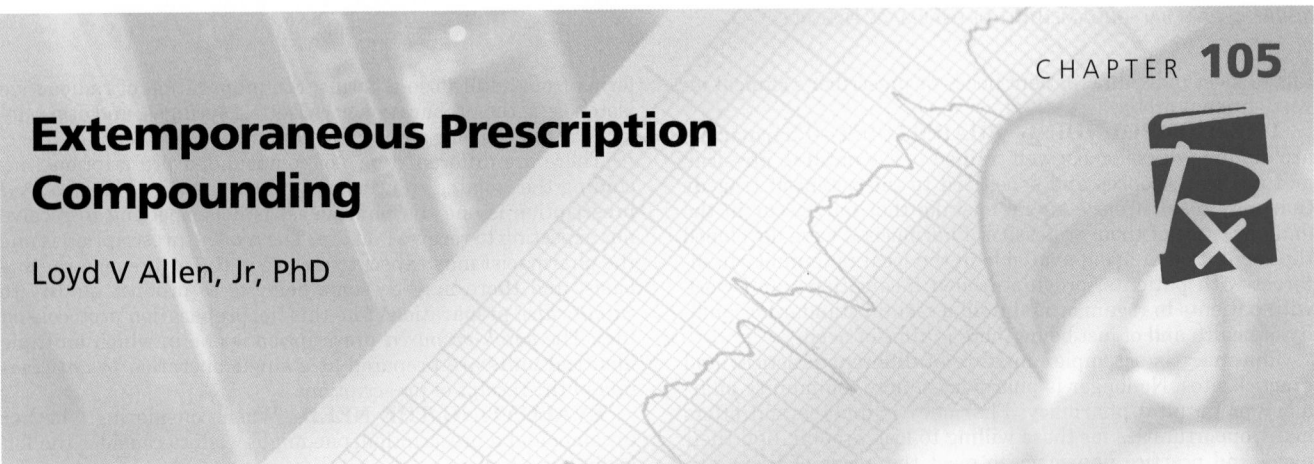

CHAPTER 105

Extemporaneous Prescription Compounding

Loyd V Allen, Jr, PhD

Historically, *pharmaceutical compounding* has been an integral part of pharmacy practice as shown by some definitions and references to pharmacy, such as

Pharmacy is the art or practice of preparing and preserving drugs and of compounding and dispensing medicines according to the prescriptions of physicians.[1]

Pharmacy is (1) the art or practice of preparing, preserving, *compounding,* and dispensing drugs or (2) a place where medicines are *compounded* or dispensed.[2]

Pharmacy is the science, art, and practice of preparing, preserving, *compounding*, and dispensing medicinal drugs and giving instructions for their use.[3]

And thou shalt make it an oil of holy ointment, an ointment *compounded* after the art of the apothecary; it shall be an anointing oil.[4]

Compounding is a professional prerogative that pharmacists have performed since the beginning of the profession. Even today, the definitions of pharmacy include the *preparation of drugs*.[5,6]

The heritage of pharmacy, spanning some 5000 years, has centered around the provision of pharmaceutical products for patients. Pharmacists are the only health care professionals that possess the knowledge and skill required for compounding and preparing medications to meet the unique needs of patients. The responsibility of extemporaneously compounding safe, effective prescription products for patients who require special care is fundamental to the pharmacy profession.

The 19th century did not see an end to the art of compounding, but the art did give way, however grudgingly, to new technology. In the 20th century, it has been estimated that a *broad knowledge of compounding* was still essential for 80% of the prescriptions dispensed in the 1920s. Although pharmacists increasingly relied on chemicals purchased from the manufacturer to make up prescriptions, there still remained much to be done *secundum artem*.[1]

Pharmaceutical industry began to take over the production of most medications used by the medical profession. In many ways this has provided superior service, new methods, and a vast array of innovative products that could not have been provided in a one-on-one basis. Research and development have been the hallmarks of the pharmaceutical manufacturers. However, the very nature of providing millions of doses of a product requires that the dosage forms (eg, capsules, tablets, suppositories) and doses (individual strengths of each dose) be limited and results in a one-sided approach to therapy. In the 21st century, it is simply not economical for a pharmaceutical company to produce a product in 10 different conceivable doses or in 5 different dosage forms to meet the needs of the entire range of individuals receiving therapy. Windows of activity are determined that meet the majority of patient needs, but the very nature of the process cannot meet all patient needs.

We also must recognize that some individuals and their health care needs do not fall in the windows of theoretical dosage strength and dosage forms and that large-scale manufacturers cannot tailor-make a medication for a handful of patients and do so cost effectively and meet the ever-changing needs of a given patient or institution. The skills of pharmacists in practicing their art of compounding fills in this gap to meet individualized needs. By this assessment the pharmacist may, through understanding of the principals of compounding and recognition of their skill level in working secundum artem, recommend that therapy be provided that is not provided by pharmaceutical industry but that is individualized for a specific patients' needs at a specific time.

Compounding has always been a basic part of pharmacy practice; the drugs, dosage forms, and equipment or techniques used are the variables. Pharmacists possess knowledge and skills that are unique and are not duplicated by any other profession. Pharmacy activities to individualize patient therapy include compounding and clinical functions. Either function in the absence of the other results in placing pharmacy in a disadvantaged position. It is important to use a pharmacist's expertise to adjust dosage quantities, frequencies, and even dosage forms for enhanced compliance. All pharmacists should understand the options presented by compounding.

Pharmaceutical compounding is increasing for a number of reasons, including the availability of a limited number of dosage forms for most drugs, a limited number of strengths of most drugs, home health care, hospice, the non-availability of drug products/combinations, discontinued drugs, drug shortages, orphan drugs, new therapeutic approaches and special patient populations (pediatrics, geriatrics, bioidentical hormone replacement therapy for postmenopausal women, pain management, dental patients, environmentally and cosmetic sensitive patients, sports injuries and veterinary compounding, including small, large, herd, exotic, and companion animals).

Newly evolving dosage forms and therapeutic approaches suggest that compounding of pharmaceuticals and related products specifically for individual patients will become more common in pharmacy practice. Compounding pharmacy is unique as it allows one to use much of their scientific, math, and technology background to a fuller extent than some of the other types of practices. Compounding pharmacists develop a special and unique relationship with the patients they serve. They work hand in hand with physicians to solve problems not addressed by commercially available dosage forms.

In the hospital and home health-care environments, there has been a noticeable increase in the *batch production* of sterile products. Reasons for this increase may include the changing patterns of drug therapy, such as home parenteral therapy and patient-controlled parenteral administration and the use of noncommercially available injectable drug products in hospitals to meet individual patient needs or prescriber's clinical investigational protocols.

THE COMPOUNDING PHARMACIST—Pharmacists are unique professionals: well trained in the natural, physical, and medical sciences and sensitized to the potential tragedy that may result from a single mistake that may occur in the daily practice of their profession. Pharmacists have developed the reputation of being available in the local community to interact with patients, provide needed medications, and work with patients to regain or maintain a certain standard or quality of health and of just being there in time of need.

Pharmacy is a complex mixture of different practices and practice sites. No longer is pharmacy simply community pharmacy or hospital pharmacy. Pharmacy is diverse and offers many opportunities for those willing to look around, find their niche and practice pharmacy to meet the needs of their own community of patients. Most compounding pharmacists appear to be interested and excited about their practices. In fact, many pharmacists intimately involved in pharmaceutical care have now realized the importance of providing *individualized patient care* through the preparation of *patient-specific products*. Compounding pharmacy is not for everyone, but as it grows, it will provide an increasingly significant number of pharmacists the excitement and fulfillment of using their innovative and creative skills to solve patient problems. This is compounding pharmacy.

As mentioned, pharmaceutical compounding requires the use of one's training in mathematics, science, and technology more than some of the other practices of pharmacy. It has been stated:

"The sciences are what support pharmacy's expertise in drug distribution and drug use. Recent history leads one to question whether we in the profession, and some in pharmaceutical education, recognize and appreciate the contribution that the pharmaceutical sciences have made and continue to make to the pharmacy profession and health care. The pharmaceutical sciences are what make us unique. They provide us the special value that we bring to the bedside. No other health professional is capable of bringing to the pharmacotherapeutic decision-making table such concepts as pH, particle size, partition coefficient, protein binding, structure-activity relationships, economics, and epidemiology. The pharmaceutical sciences, combined with pharmacy's infrastructure, including pharmaceutical education, are what make the pharmacist an indispensable participant on the health care team."[7]

And what area of pharmacy practice has the opportunity of using the scientific education and training as much as pharmacists involved in individualizing patient care through extemporaneous compounding? The pharmaceutical sciences, especially chemistry and pharmaceutics, serve as the foundation for pharmacists' ability to formulate specific dosage forms to meet patients' needs.

DEFINITIONS—Pharmacy is united in the sense that pharmacists have a responsibility to serve their patients and compound an appropriately prescribed product in the course of their professional practice. It is the right and responsibility of pharmacists to compound medications to meet the specific needs of patients. Pharmacists are ultimately responsible for the integrity of the finished product prepared under their immediate supervision.

Compounding has been defined by the National Association of Boards of Pharmacy:

"Compounding means the preparation, mixing, assembling, packaging, or labeling of a drug or device (i) as the result of a practitioner's Prescription Drug Order or initiative based on the pharmacist/patient/prescriber relationship in the course of professional practice, or (ii) for the purpose of, as an incident to research, teaching, or chemical analysis and not for sale or dispensing. Compounding also includes the preparation of drugs and devices in anticipation of Prescription Drug Orders based on routine, regularly observed patterns."[8]

Compounding may hold different meanings to different pharmacists. It may mean the preparation of oral liquids, topical creams/ointments, suppositories; the conversion of one dose or dosage form into another; the preparation of select dosage forms from bulk chemicals; the preparation of intravenous admixtures, parenteral nutrition solutions, pediatric dosage forms from adult dosage forms; the preparation of radioactive isotopes; or the preparation of cassettes, syringes, and other devices with drugs for administration in the home setting.

There are different types of compounded prescriptions, including the isolated, routine and batch prepared. The *isolated* prescription is one the pharmacist is not expecting to receive nor expecting to receive it again. The *routine* prescription is one the pharmacist may expect to receive in the future on a routine basis, and there may be some benefits to product quality to *standardize* preparations like this (ie, preparation protocols on file). The *batch-prepared* prescription is one in which multiple identical units are prepared as a single operation *in anticipation* of the receipt of prescriptions.

EVALUATING THE NEED—When considering whether to compound a prescription, one might wish to consider the following questions:

1. Is the product commercially available in the exact dosage form, strength, and packaging?
2. Is the prescription rational concerning the ingredients, intended use, dosage, and method of administration?
3. Am I qualified to prepare this prescription by education, skill development, and expertise?
4. Do I have the proper equipment, supplies, and chemicals or drugs?
5. Is there documentation for assigning a *beyond-use* date for the prescription, or do I use the guidelines delineated in US Pharmacopeia (USP) Chapters <795> and <797>, *Pharmacy Compounding-Nonsterile Preparations* and *Pharmacy Compounding-Sterile Preparations,* respectively?
6. Is there an alternative by which the patient will receive a benefit?
7. Will this compounded product satisfy the intent of the prescribing physician and meet the needs of the patient?
8. Is there a bona fide prescriber–pharmacist–patient relationship?
9. Does the patient have the necessary storage facility, if required, to assure potency of the product until its beyond-use date?
10. Can I perform the necessary calculations to prepare the product?
11. Am I willing to complete the necessary documentation to prepare the product?
12. Is there a literature reference that might provide information on use, preparation, stability, administration, etc?
13. How long will the patient be using the product and is the expected duration of therapy consistent with an appropriate beyond-use date? Alternatively, should the product be prepared in small quantities and dispensed to the patient in short intervals?
14. Can I do some basic quality control to check the product prior to dispensing (eg, capsule weight variation, pH, visual observations)?
15. Am I assured of ingredient identity, quality, and purity?
16. What procedures do I have for investigating and correcting failures?
17. Are the physical, chemical and therapeutic properties of the individual ingredients consistent with the expected properties of the ordered drug product?[9]

Evaluating the Feasibility of Batch Compounding

The following questions may be considered prior to batch compounding activities:

1. Will the processes, procedures, compounding environment, and equipment used to prepare this batch produce the expected qualities in the finished product?
2. Will all the critical processes and procedures be carried out exactly as intended for every batch of the prepared product to produce the same high-quality product in every batch?
3. Will the finished product have all the qualities as specified, on completion of the preparation and packaging of each batch?
4. Will each batch retain all the qualities within the specified limits until the end of the labeled beyond-use date?
5. Can I monitor and trace the history of each batch, identify potential sources of problems and institute appropriate corrective measures to minimize the likelihood of their occurrence?[9]

Pharmacists who perform batch compounding should be capable and willing to do it properly, particularly when sterile drug products are involved. Trends indicate that more batch compounding may be occurring in more pharmacies in the future.

ECONOMIC CONSIDERATIONS—There are at least two different economic considerations in making the decision to compound prescriptions; these include (1) pharmacist compensation and (2) health-care costs.

Pharmaceutical compounding is a cognitive service, hence cognitive services reimbursement is justified. As a surgeon uses both cognitive and technical, manipulative skills, so does the pharmacist use cognitive, technical, and manipulative skills in extemporaneous compounding to meet individualized patient needs. The pricing of a compounded prescription should include consideration for pharmacodynamic and pharmacotherapeutic decision making, formulation expertise, time, and reimbursement of materials. Compounding prescriptions can be attractive professionally and financially. Historically, it has been said that compounding is an act whereby the professional and scientific knowledge of a pharmacist can find its expression. For those pharmacists dedicated to doing a quality job in compounding, the professional, psychological, and financial rewards can be substantial.

Compounding prescriptions can be a way of lowering the cost of drug therapy. In some cases, it is less expensive for the pharmacist to prepare a specific prescription for the patient, which may mean the difference between the patient actually obtaining the drug or doing without it. If compounding a prescription results in a patient being able to afford the drug therapy, it must be considered.

Another example concerns the economic use of expensive drug products. Some drug products are expensive and may have short shelf lives. If a patient does not need the entire contents of a vial or dosage unit, in many cases, the remaining drug product is discarded and wasted. However, there are numerous instances in which the pharmacist can divide the commercial product into smaller, usable units, store it properly and dispense the required quantity on individual prescriptions.

Another obliquely related economic question can also be addressed about the commercialization of compounded products. Over the years it has been interesting to note that many compounded products eventually become commercially available products. Examples include:

Fentanyl Lozenges
Minoxidil Topical Solution
Nystatin Lozenges
Clindamycin Topical Solution
Tetracaine-Adrenalin-Cocaine (TAC) Solution
Dihydroergotamine Mesylate Nasal Spray
Buprenorphine Nasal Spray
Buffered Hypertonic Saline Solution
Erythromycin Topical Solution

as well as numerous other dermatological and pediatric oral liquids and some premixed intravenous solutions. It is inevitable that a product will be manufactured when a product becomes economically profitable for a pharmaceutical manufacturer to produce it.

COMPOUNDING FACTORS

STABILITY—One key factor in compounding prescriptions is stability. The more common types of stability of which compounding pharmacists should be aware include chemical, physical, and microbiological. Whereas commercially manufactured products are required to possess an *expiration date*, compounded products are assigned a *beyond-use date*. There are numerous sources of information that can be used for determining an appropriate beyond-use date, such as chemical companies, manufacturers literature, laboratory data, journals, and published books on the subject. Generally, most pharmacists prepare or dispense small quantities of compounded products; recommend storage at room, cool, or cold temperatures; and use a conservative beyond-use date.

The guidelines published in the USP 26/NF 21 Section <795>, *Pharmacy Compounding*, state that

"In the absence of stability information that is applicable to a specific drug and preparation, the following maximum beyond-use dates are recommended for non-sterile compounded drug precautions that are packaged in tight, light-resistant containers and stored at controlled room temperature unless otherwise indicated."

For nonaqueous liquids and solid formulations (for which the manufactured drug product is the source of active ingredient)—The beyond-use date is not later than 25% of the time remaining until the product's expiration date or 6 months, whichever is earlier.

A USP or NF substance is the source of active ingredient—The beyond-use date is not later than 6 months.

For water-containing formulations (prepared from ingredients in solid form)—The beyond-use date is not later than 14 days when stored at cold temperatures.

For all other formulations—The beyond-use date is not later than the intended duration of therapy or 30 days, whichever is earlier.

These beyond-use date limits may be exceeded when there is supporting valid scientific stability information that is directly applicable to the specific preparation (ie, the *same* drug concentration range, pH, excipients, vehicle, water content).[10]

QUALITY CONTROL—One of the fastest growing and most important areas of pharmaceutical compounding is that of quality control. Quality must be built-in to the preparation from the beginning steps to evaluating the final preparation. There are several quality control tests that can be done within the pharmacy and others can be sent to a contract laboratory. The following quality control tests can be considered for the respective dosage forms.

1. Oral and topical liquids (solutions, suspensions, emulsions): Weight/volume, pH, specific gravity, active drug assay, globule size range, rheological properties/pourability, physical observation (color, clarity), physical stability (discoloration, foreign materials, gas formation, mold growth).
2. Hard Gelatin Capsules: Weight-overall average weight, weight-individual weight variation, dissolution of capsule shell, disintegration and/or dissolution of capsule contents, active-drug assay, physical appearance (color, uniformity, extent of fill, locked), physical stability (discoloration, changes in appearance).
3. Ointments, Creams and Gels: Theoretical weight compared to actual weight, pH, specific gravity, active drug assay, physical observations (color, clarity, texture-surface, texture-spatula spread, appearance, feel) and rheological properties.
4. Suppositories, Troches, Lollipops and Sticks: Weight, specific gravity, active drug assay, physical observation (color, clarity, texture of surface, appearance, feel), melting test, dissolution test, physical stability.
5. Parenteral preparations: Weight/volume, physical observation, pH, specific gravity, osmolality, assay, color, clarity, particulate matter, sterility, pyrogenicity.

COMPOUNDING SUPPORT—Numerous agencies, companies, organizations, etc, are available to assist pharmacists in compounding. Information, chemicals, supplies, and equipment are readily available. Chemical and supply companies have increased in size and number in recent years and many provide information on compounding, incompatibilities, and stability. Specialty compounding organizations have developed over recent years and generally provide full-line services and products to the compounding pharmacist. Many national organizations provide continuing professional education programs in both non-sterile and sterile compounding.

These entities provide services to compounding pharmacists ranging from selling only compounding aids to providing only chemicals. Others offer additional services to include formulas as well as consulting expertise by telephone or via the internet. This service can assist in the process of compounding a particular product that may be difficult.

TRAINING AND EXPERIENCE—Pharmacists involved in upgrading and increasing the traditional aspects of extemporaneous compounding need to keep current with all the new tools of their trade, retrieve the old from storage, and put in a bit of practice using their scientific background and their art before they will be comfortable in exhibiting their skills. When considering providing additional services of compounding in an institution, pharmacists should not expect that this will change a great deal of their practice in time consumed for compounding. The majority of the time, pharmaceutical manufacturers do provide what patients need. They do an excellent job, as they have invested money and effort into research and development, and are entitled to the sales of products that they are approved to produce. The extemporaneous compounding by pharmacists meets the additional needs of patients that traditionally manufactured products do not meet.

Because there is an expectation that pharmacists can compound, there is a need that pharmacists be able to compound. Because of the decrease in instruction in compounding pharmacy in colleges of pharmacy, graduating pharmacists may not feel comfortable in their ability to compound. They can be advised to seek training if their practice may encompass compounding activities. The need for compounding training and experience is addressed by short courses, continuing education, increased curricular requirements, and apprenticeships. Additional training areas for compounding are needed to provide the experience needed to compound prescriptions accurately and safely. Many pharmacists who compound become actively involved in the practicums and rotations of the colleges of pharmacy in their respective states.

Only properly educated pharmacists should be involved in pharmaceutical compounding. If pharmacists wish to compound, but do not possess the required techniques or skills, they should participate in continuing professional education programs that have been designed to train them properly, including the scientific basis and practical skills necessary for sound, contemporary compounding.

EQUIPMENT—The equipment needed will be determined by the type and extent of the services one chooses to provide. Many pharmacies already have clean air environments (eg, laminar air flow hoods, isolation barrier systems) where aseptic compounding of sterile solutions is performed. These same units can be used to compound other sterile preparations such as eye drops. A balance, preferably electronic, is essential. Ointment slabs (ie, pill tiles), along with spatulas of different types and materials, should be purchased. A few mortars and pestles (ie, glass, ceramic, plastic) and some glassware should be secured. It may not be necessary to buy a roomful of equipment, but one should purchase what is needed to start the service and should build on it as the service grows and expands to different arenas.

Much of the equipment used today in compounding has changed. Today, electronic balances are used more often than torsion balances; micropipets are commonplace; and ultrafreezers are sometimes required in addition to standard refrigerator freezers. This area is constantly changing and the compounding pharmacist should be aware of the available technology to prepare accurate and effective prescriptions. Becoming acquainted with the local representative for a laboratory supply company is helpful.

ENVIRONMENT—A separate area for traditional compounding is recommended, rather than simply cleaning off a small area of the dispensing counter. The compounding pharmacist needs a clean, neat, well-lit and quiet working area. If aseptic compounding is considered, a clean air environment (e.g., laminar air flow hood, isolation barrier system) should be used. The actual facility to be used depends on the level and volume of compounding to be done.

FORMULAS—Consistency of the compounded product is important. Formulas should be developed or obtained and tried to assure that each time an extemporaneous product is prepared, the methods used, ingredients added, and the order of steps is documented. This accomplishes three things. First, it provides the methodology for each person involved or requested to provide such service the information necessary to

do so properly. Second, it provides consistency from batch to batch. Third, if the product does not turn out the way expected, a stepwise methodology exists for reviewing and determining what happened and if revisions and improvements are needed.

CHEMICALS AND SUPPLIES—If one is going to prepare a topical product, a vehicle (eg, cream, ointment, gel) and the active ingredients (eg, either finely ground product from an available tablet or injection or pharmaceutical-grade chemicals) would be required. One needs proper dispensing containers for the medication. In short, a relationship with providers that carry chemicals and supplies is important.

Pharmacists have been using chemicals and other materials for prescription compounding throughout history. In the past, these chemicals and materials have been obtained from natural products, raw materials, and household ingredients. Today, compounding pharmacists use chemicals from various reliable commercial sources, depending on their availability.

Some chemical companies place a disclaimer on their chemicals for various reasons, including, but not necessarily limited to

1. The companies do not want to be required to provide complete labeling of the materials as required by the *Food Drug and Cosmetic (FD&C) Act*; consequently, they state they are not to be used as drugs. This exempts the companies from having to comply with the FD&C regulations.
2. The source of the chemicals may not be companies meeting current Good Manufacturing Practices; consequently, when the drugs are repackaged, only selected information concerning the level of potency, impurities, and other miscellaneous characterization data is provided.
3. The disclaimer is to protect the companies from the use of their products without the full safety and effectiveness testing as required by the Food and Drug Administration (FDA) for drug products for manufacturing.

Historically, the *FD&C Act* has not applied to chemicals used for pharmaceutical compounding, but it does apply to chemicals used for manufacturing. The selection of the chemical source for compounding is a judgment call on the part of pharmacists. When selecting a supplier of compounding chemicals, certificates of analysis should be obtained and reviewed for purity, impurities, etc, as part of the decision-making process.

Chapter <795>, *Pharmacy Compounding*, in the USP 26/NF 21 is reprinted here as follows[10]:

"A USP or NF grade drug substance is the preferred source of ingredients for compounding all drug preparations. If that is not available, the use of another high-quality source, such as analytical reagent (AR) or certified American Chemical Society (ACS) grade, is an option for professional judgment. If the substance is not an official preparation or substance, additional information, such as a certificate of analysis, needs to be obtained by the pharmacist to ensure its suitability."

A manufactured drug product may be a source of active ingredient. Only manufactured drugs from containers labeled with a batch control number and a future expiration date are acceptable as a potential source of active ingredients. When compounding with manufactured drug products, the pharmacist must consider all ingredients present in the drug product relative to the intended use of the compounded preparation.

In summary, it is the responsibility of the pharmacist to select the *most-appropriate* quality of chemical for compounding, beginning with the USP/NF as the first choice and, if this is not available, then descending the list of purity grades (Table 105-1) using professional judgment and discretion. A certificate of analysis for the chemicals should be obtained and kept on file in the pharmacy for these selected chemicals.[10,11]

COMPOUNDING INFORMATION SOURCES

Numerous sources are now available for compounding information, including books, journals, pamphlets, brochures and elec-

Table 105-1. Description of Chemical Grades

GRADE	DESCRIPTION
Technical or commercial	Indeterminate quality
CP (chemically pure)	More refined, but still of unknown quality
USP/NF	Meets minimum purity standards; conforms to tolerances set by the SP/NF for contaminants dangerous to health
ACS reagent	High purity; conforms to minimum specifications set by the Reagent Chemicals Committee of the American Chemical Society
Analytical reagent	Very high purity
HPLC	Solvents purified for use in high-performance liquid chromatography (HPLC); very high purity
Spectroscopic grade	Very high purity
Primary standard	Highest purity; required for accurate volumetric analysis) (for standard solutions)

tronic media. Some of these reference sources should be accessible by compounding pharmacies, including the following:

1. **Pharmacy and medical libraries**
2. **References**
   Allen Jr LV. The Art, Science and Technology of Pharmaceutical Compounding, 2nd ed. Washington DC: American Pharmaceutical Association; 2002.
   Allen Jr LV, Popovich NG, Ansel HC. Pharmaceutical Dosage Forms and Drug Delivery Systems. Media, PA: Lippincott Williams & Wilkins, 2004.
   Merck Index. 13th ed. Whitehouse Station, NJ: Merck & Co, 2001.
   Remington: The Science and Practice of Pharmacy. 21st ed. Lippincott Williams and Wilkins, 2004.
   Trissel LA. Trissel's Stability of Compounded Formulations, 2nd ed. Washington DC: American Pharmaceutical Association; 2000.
   Trissel LA. Handbook on Injectable Drugs. Bethesda, MD: American Society of Health-Systems Pharmacists.
   United States Pharmacopeia 26/National Formulary 21. United States Pharmacopeial Convention, Rockville, MD, 2003.
3. **Journals**
   International Journal of Pharmaceutical Compounding
   Journal of the American Society of Health-System Pharmacists
   Lippincott's Hospital Pharmacy
   Pharmacy Times
   US Pharmacist
4. **Package insert information from pharmaceutical manufacturers**

COMPOUNDING TYPES

AMBULATORY-CARE COMPOUNDING—If individuals can walk, they are considered mobile or ambulatory (ie, they are not bedridden). Consequently, most pharmacists are involved in ambulatory care, and most ambulatory patients are *outpatients*. Actually, the term can also be applied to home-care patients and even institutionalized patients who are mobile. One general characteristic of ambulatory patients is that they are generally responsible for obtaining their own medication, storing it, preparing it (if necessary), and taking it.[12] It seems almost incongruous that in health care today as we become more aware that patients are *individuals*, respond as *individuals,* and must be treated as *individuals* that some health-care providers appear to be grouping patients into *categories*. They are grouped in categories for treatment, for reimbursement from a third party, or for determining levels of care in managed-care organizations and using *fixed-dose products* provided by pharmaceutical manufacturers that are available because the marketing demand is sufficiently high to justify their manufac-

ture and production. Why should the availability or the lack of availability of a specific economically profitable commercially available product dictate the therapy of a patient?

Pharmacists have an opportunity to extend their activities in patient care as the emphasis continues to shift from inpatient care to ambulatory care. Ambulatory care, however, is so diverse and involves so many disciplines that sometimes it is difficult to understand it; and, it changes rapidly. Also, ambulatory care could generally encourage a team approach to health improvement, prevention, health maintenance, risk assessment, early detection, management, curative therapy, and rehabilitation.[13] Ambulatory care offers various opportunities for individualizing patient care through pharmaceutical compounding. In fact, it is the area where most compounding pharmacists practice.

Pharmacists' roles in ambulatory care patients can include, among others

1. Dispensing
2. Compounding
3. Counseling
4. Minimizing medication errors
5. Compliance enhancement
6. Therapeutic drug monitoring
7. Minimizing expenditures[12–14]

Most reimbursement for ambulatory patients comes from the dispensing or the compounding process. Little financial consideration is given to counseling, minimizing medication errors, compliance enhancement and therapeutic monitoring. However, these activities are important and should be performed. Because of the unique nature of compounded medications, counseling is an absolute must for these patients.

From the above discussion of the activities of ambulatory care pharmacists, it should be evident that extemporaneous compounding can be vitally important in ambulatory patient care.

HOSPITAL PHARMACY COMPOUNDING—The ever-present responsibility of the health-care industry is to provide the best available care for the patient, using the best means to do so, and providing that care in a conducive environment. This must be sufficiently economical to not put the institution in jeopardy of being unable to continue to provide the services to the community they serve. This requires cooperation on the part of the hospital administration, the medical staff, and the employees (nurses and pharmacists in particular as regards to medication usage) and must involve the patient. One of the effective means by which hospitals, and therefore hospital pharmacies, can meet these challenges is to consider expanding extemporaneous compounding services within the hospital pharmacy. Pharmaceutical care and pharmaceutical compounding can provide cost savings to the hospital while providing needed options to the physician through problem-solving approaches and stimulating the hospital pharmacist through new challenges that allow the expression of both their skills and their art.

Hospital pharmacists have always been actively involved in compounding, or producing medications for the patient. Daily intravenous (IV) therapy is provided through compounding of medications. Antibiotic piggybacks, total parenteral nutrition (TPN) solutions, IV additives, and many others are daily calculated, compounded, dispensed, and then generally administered by the nursing staff. The preparation of pediatric dosage forms has also been an area of extensive activity in some hospitals.

To assist hospital administrators in supporting the provision of extemporaneous compounding services, they should be aware that[15]

1. The patients' needs are better served
2. The economic implication is favorable to the institution, or at least no less favorable than other alternatives
3. The provision of such alternative care improves and does not detract from the image of the institution for the purpose of public relations

4. Making such services available enhances the abilities of the physician to meet the patients' specific needs
5. The services fall within regulatory guidelines
6. The pharmacy staff is capable of performing such services

Members of the hospital staff are constantly reading journal articles and are generally aware of innovative thought and practice by their peers. When physicians become aware of the skill, availability, and awareness of pharmaceutical compounding and that they can literally have almost any medication they need, in the form and strength they need for a specific situation, they generally request it more often. As the hospital pharmacy staff demonstrates their expertise and problem-solving skills, the medical staff consistently depends upon them.

Guidelines are essential in determining any changes that go on within a hospital pharmacy. Policies and procedures must be written to indicate the types of services that are made available. The two most important aspects to consider when making both the decision and the guidelines are[15]:

1. Keep intact the triad relationship. The medical staff (physician), the hospital staff (pharmacist and nurse), and the patient should all be informed of the decision to approach patient care by the use of institutionally compounded products. The patient is already aware that much of this occurs in the preparation of their TPN solutions or their IV antibiotic piggybacks. Patient awareness that the institution has recognized a special need they might have and that the institution is going the extra mile to meet those needs enhances public relations. The patient, recognizing that they are being treated as an individual, is receiving treatment benefit that may have a placebo effect in enhancing their improvement, especially when handled in a caring manner.
2. Do not overstep one's bounds. When products are commercially available to meet the needs of the institution, the patient, and the physician use them. When the physician desires a product that is different for any number of reasons than anything commercially available, then one should consider extemporaneous compounding.

In consideration of meeting patient specific needs, the hospital pharmacist must look at various modalities as potential solutions. When traditional hospital processes and procedures are not meeting the patient's need, extemporaneous compounding should be a consideration. Improving outcomes, getting patients well and out of the hospital as quickly as possible, should be the end goal. Individualized dosage forms, dosage strengths, and alternative routes of administration can often help attain these goals. There are many easily accessible organizations specializing in helping meet these needs. The public relations aspect of meeting these needs may enhance community support. Improving outcomes assists the medical staff by allowing them to spend their time dealing with new problems as hospital pharmacy meets the challenge of past problems. Nursing and pharmacy have the enhanced opportunity to use the skills they have developed and to provide opportunities for pharmacy to have more patient involvement and job satisfaction.

VETERINARY COMPOUNDING—The first symposium on veterinary compounding was a significant forum for discussion by experts and was a pivotal point in the history of veterinary compounding, occurring in September 1993.[16] The meeting was important because it assembled an impressive group of experts on veterinary compounding, who then set about explaining and defining the roles of the veterinarian and the pharmacist.

The FDA's interest in compounding by veterinarians dates back to the beginning of the1990s. The avowed purpose of the symposium was to provide a forum for a comprehensive, public debate in response to the American Veterinary Medical Association (AVMA) position on compounding prior to the issuance of the FDA *Compliance Policy Guide* on veterinary compounding. Numerous speakers presented views on (1) compounding by veterinarians, and (2) compounding for veterinarians by pharmacists. Topics such as conflicts of interest, lack of compounding training by veterinarians, the *new-drug* issue, and bioequivalency standards were discussed in detail.[16]

Veterinary compounding is necessary for many reasons. For example, with multiple species ranging from small to large it would be impossible to practice effective medicine without compounded products! Do we simply refuse to treat exotic species or small animals? Do we abandon oncology in veterinary medicine?

Also commented on was a more specific area of need: the lack of an ideal anesthetic drug, which has led veterinarians to devise anesthetic combinations inducing good-quality anesthesia, with minimal risk to the animal. Compounding is essential for safe and effective veterinary anesthetic practice. Veterinarians need to administer anesthetic drugs to a wide variety of animals with a wide variety of temperaments in settings that are less than ideal. They are called on to anesthetize elephants, gorillas, tigers, ostriches, sharks, horses, cows, and poisonous snakes, among others.

Other reasons why veterinary compounding is necessary included:

The necessity for multiple injections in the absence of a compounded multi-ingredient product

Rapid changes in management and disease problems in veterinary medicine

Problems associated with the treatment of large numbers of animals with several drugs within a short period

Cost-prohibitive factors associated with the large volume of some large-volume parenterals required for animals

The need for previously prepared antidotes for use in cases of animal poisoning

There are unique considerations involved with veterinary compounding compared with compounding for human patients. A few examples follow:

1. If compounding for food-producing animals, what is the potential effect on human health? Are appropriate "washout" times established to minimize exposure of the public to any drug residues in the animal?
2. There is a large variability in response to drugs by different animal species. It is sometimes difficult to find dosing information on a mg/kg basis.
3. Some animals cannot metabolize certain chemicals (cats cannot metabolize "benzoates").
4. There is a large difference in animal sizes from small birds to large elephants.
5. Flavoring is a unique problem with some finicky animals (eg, cats).
6. Selection of a dosage form for different animals can sometimes be challenging.
7. A "batch" of a compounded preparation may be 1000 pounds for a herd of animals.

The summarized ideas expressed at the aforementioned veterinary meeting were

- Veterinarians have a definite need for drug compounding
- Drug compounding was reported to be necessary in all areas of veterinary medicine
- The necessity of compounding poisoning antidotes (eg, sodium nitrite, sodium thiosulfate, methylene blue, or CaEDTA) was expressed

Compounding will continue to exist in the future for the same reason as it does now, to fulfill therapeutic needs in veterinary medicine, as well as in medicine for human patients. Difficulties and costs associated with the veterinary drug-approval process make compounding necessary to fulfill therapeutic needs not being met by the introduction of therapeutic agents.

An increasing interdependence between the veterinarian and the pharmacist is developing, resulting in higher standards of veterinary care. As to the future of compounding for veterinary patients, it was reported that

1. It is virtually inconceivable that there will ever be FDA-approved drugs labeled for every therapeutic need in every species of animal.
2. It appears that compounding for veterinary medicine will become more prevalent, as it has in human medicine, especially with the future introduction of biotechnology-derived products with limited stability.[16]

NUCLEAR PHARMACY COMPOUNDING—Nuclear pharmacy is a specialty practice of pharmacy that has been defined as a patient-oriented service that embodies the scientific knowledge and professional judgment required for improving and promoting health through assurance of the safe and efficacious use of radioactive drugs for diagnosis and therapy. Radioactive drugs, commonly referred to as radiopharmaceuticals, are a special class of drugs that are regulated by the FDA. They are unique in that they contain an unstable nuclide (radioactive nuclide) as a part of the compound designed to localize in an organ or tissue. Since radiopharmaceuticals are radioactive, the Nuclear Regulatory Commission or a similar state agency is involved in regulatory matters relevant to radiopharmaceuticals.

A nuclear pharmacist is expert at preparing (compounding) radiopharmaceuticals with Tc-99m sodium pertechnetate and reagent kits. The kits are multidose vials containing the compound to be *labeled* with the radioactive nuclide Tc-99m to create the radiopharmaceutical. The contents within the vial are sterile and pyrogen free as is the Tc-99m sodium pertechnetate. Most radiopharmaceuticals are administered intravenously so a nuclear pharmacist must be proficient at maintaining aseptic conditions during compounding.

The most common setting for the provision of radiopharmaceuticals by nuclear pharmacists is a commercially centralized nuclear pharmacy. Radiopharmaceuticals are generally prepared early in the morning and unit doses delivered to hospitals in the region surrounding the nuclear pharmacy. The nuclear pharmacy provides economic benefit to the hospital by use of all the doses of a radiopharmaceutical produced in a multidose vial plus reduction in space required for radiopharmaceutical preparation and radioactive waste containment. Other benefits include the availability of infrequently used radiopharmaceuticals, specialized products requiring extensive compounding, and the resources of pharmaceutical care available through professionals in nuclear pharmacy. Today there are several hundred commercial centralized nuclear pharmacies providing a significant fraction of radiopharmaceuticals used in nuclear medicine procedures. What started as limited service in large medical centers and universities by a few pharmacists with education beyond the entry-level pharmacy degree has grown to extensive services provided by several hundred first-professional-degree pharmacists. Truly a remarkable change in a time period of 20 to 25 years, resulting from dedicated entrepreneurs working to make a difference in patient care through quality products and pharmaceutical care.[17]

JOB SATISFACTION

Job satisfaction among independent community pharmacists who were classified as compounders and noncompounders has been measured.[18] Two previously validated survey instruments that measured job satisfaction were used with additional questions to determine the volume of compounded prescriptions the respondent dispensed. Questionnaires were mailed to randomly selected independent community pharmacists in the US and Canada with a response rate of 53.4% ($n = 391$).

The results indicate that pharmacists' job satisfaction levels may be improved if intrinsic factors are satisfied in their job role. Because prescription compounding provides satisfaction with several intrinsic factors such as variety, challenge, and use of skills, independent community pharmacists may improve their job satisfaction levels by providing prescription compounding services.

In the past 25 years, studies on pharmacist job satisfaction have provided descriptive information on job satisfaction or have attempted to assess the relationship between factors and job satisfaction. One factor that studies have shown positively influences pharmacist job satisfaction is the provision of clinical services by the pharmacist. From these clinical services, the following intrinsic job characteristics were identified:

1. Opportunities for self-expression and self-actualization
2. Autonomy
3. Variety
4. Skill
5. Responsibility
6. Feelings of confidence, pride and accomplishment

All of these characteristics can enhance an individual's satisfaction with job situations. Several of these intrinsic job characteristics describe the activities of those pharmacists who do compounding in their daily work tasks, and thus a study into the relation between job satisfaction and prescription compounding seemed warranted.

One of the responsibilities of a compounder requires that the pharmacist become actively engaged in the clinical assessment of a patient to assist the prescriber in determining the customized patient specific formula to be extemporaneously compounded. In addition, this responsibility requires the pharmacist to interact with prescribers and the patient as the customized formulation and dosage form are determined. The use of clinical skills and physician–patient interaction have been identified in previous studies as intrinsic factors that enhance a pharmacist's job satisfaction. Therefore, a compounder using clinical skills and interacting with prescribers and patients may be predisposed to a higher job satisfaction than would be noncompounders whose responsibilities may not require such activities. The objective of the study was to determine and compare the job satisfaction of pharmacists who are classified as compounders and noncompounders.

This study supports findings of earlier studies that show that job satisfaction is influenced by pharmacist activities that include intrinsic job characteristics. Because a compounder is typically required to use his or her professional skills to meet the challenges of preparing a variety of formulations, such intrinsic job characteristics may have a positive influence on job satisfaction of compounders.

The two statistically and probably practical significant differences between compounders and noncompounders was in career satisfaction and overall job satisfaction. The professional challenges of the practice activities of a compounder (ie, prescriber–patient interaction to determine customized dosage form, art, and skill in compounding an elegant dosage form and patient monitoring) are intrinsic factors that may have influenced respondents' opinions.

REGULATIONS AND GUIDELINES[8]

Two documents are of special importance in providing guidelines and standards for pharmaceutical compounding; these include the:

1. *National Association of Boards of Pharmacy Good Compounding Practices Applicable to State Licensed Pharmacies, and*
2. USP 26/NF 21 Chapter <795>, *Pharmacy Compounding-Nonsterile Preparations* and Chapter <797>, *Pharmacy Compounding-Sterile Preparations,*

as well as numerous other portions of the USP/NF. Of these, the National Association of Boards of Pharmacy *Good Compounding Practices Applicable to State Licensed Pharmacies* and a summary of the USP/NF Chapters <795> and <797> will be discussed.

GOOD COMPOUNDING PRACTICES APPLICABLE TO STATE-LICENSED PHARMACIES—The following Good Compounding Practices (GCPs) are meant to apply only to the compounding of drugs by state-licensed pharmacies.

SUBPART A—GENERAL PROVISIONS The recommendations contained herein are considered the minimum current good compounding practices for the preparation of drug products by state-licensed pharmacies for dispensing or administration to humans or animals.

The following definitions from the *NABP Model State Pharmacy Act* apply to these GCPs. States may wish to insert their own definitions to comply with *State Pharmacy Practice Acts*.

Compounding—The preparation, mixing, assembling, packaging, or Labeling of a Drug or Device (i) as the result of a Practitioner's Prescription Drug Order or initiative based on the Practitioner/patient/Pharmacist relationship in the course of professional practice, or (ii) for the purpose of, or as an incident to, research, teaching or chemical analysis and not for sale or Dispensing. Compounding also includes the preparation of Drugs or Devices in anticipation of Prescription Drug Orders based on routine, regularly observed prescribing patterns.

Manufacturing—The production, preparation, propagation, conversion or processing of a Drug or Device, either directly or indirectly, by extraction from substances of natural origin or independently by means of chemical or biological synthesis, and includes any packaging or repackaging of the substance(s) or Labeling or relabeling of its container, and the promotion and marketing of such Drugs or Devices. Manufacturing also includes the preparation and promotion of commercially available products from bulk compounds for resale by pharmacies, Practitioners, or other Persons.

Component—Any ingredient intended for use in the compounding of a drug product, including those that may not appear in such product. Based on the existence of a Pharmacist/patient/Prescriber relationship and the presentation of a valid Prescription, Pharmacists may Compound, in reasonable quantities, Drug products that are commercially available in the marketplace.

Pharmacists shall receive, store, or use drug substances for compounding that have been made in an FDA-approved facility. Pharmacists shall also receive, store, or use drug components in compounding prescriptions that meet official compendia requirements. If neither of these requirements can be met, pharmacists shall use their professional judgment to procure alternatives.

Pharmacists may compound drugs in very limited quantities prior to receiving a valid prescription based on a history of receiving valid prescriptions that have been generated solely within an established pharmacist/patient/prescriber relationship, and provided that they maintain the prescriptions on file for all such products compounded at the pharmacy (as required by State law). The compounding of inordinate amounts of drugs in anticipation of receiving prescriptions without any historical basis is considered manufacturing.

Pharmacists shall not offer compounded drug products to other State-licensed persons or commercial entities for subsequent resale, except in the course of professional practice for a prescriber to administer to an individual patient. Compounding pharmacies/pharmacists may advertise or otherwise promote the fact that they provide prescription compounding services; however, they shall not solicit business (eg, promote, advertise, or use salespersons) to compound specific drug products.

The distribution of inordinate amounts of compounded products pursuant to a legitimate prescription out of state without a prescriber/patient/pharmacist relationship is considered manufacturing. Pharmacists engaged in the compounding of drugs shall operate in conformance with applicable State law regulating the practice of pharmacy.

SUBPART B—ORGANIZATION AND PERSONNEL As in the dispensing of all prescriptions, the pharmacist has the responsibility and authority to inspect and approve or reject all components, drug product containers, closures, in-process materials, labeling and the authority to prepare and review all compounding records to assure that no errors have occurred in the compounding process. The pharmacist is also responsible for the proper maintenance, cleanliness and use of all equipment used in prescription compounding practice.

All pharmacists who engage in compounding of drugs, shall be proficient in the art of compounding and shall maintain that proficiency through current awareness and training. Also, every pharmacist who engages in drug compounding must be aware of and familiar with all details of the Good Compounding Practices.

Personnel engaged in the compounding of drugs shall wear clean clothing appropriate to the operation being performed. Protective apparel, such as a coat/jacket, apron or hand or arm coverings, shall be worn as necessary to protect drug products from contamination.

Only personnel authorized by the responsible pharmacist shall be in the immediate vicinity of the drug compounding operation. Any person shown at any time (either by medical examination or pharmacist determination) to have an apparent illness or open lesion(s) that may adversely affect the safety or quality of a drug product being compounded shall be excluded from direct contact with components, drug product containers, closures, in-process materials and drug products until the condition is corrected or determined by competent medical personnel not to jeopardize the safety or quality of the products(s) being compounded. All personnel who normally assist the pharmacist in compounding procedures shall be instructed to report to the pharmacist any health conditions that may have an adverse effect on drug products.

SUBPART C—DRUG COMPOUNDING FACILITIES Pharmacies engaging in compounding shall have a specifically designated and adequate area (space) for the orderly placement of equipment and materials to be used to compound medications. The drug compounding area for sterile products shall be separate and distinct from the area used for the compounding or dispensing of non-sterile drug products. The area(s) used for the compounding of drugs shall be maintained in a good state of repair.

Bulk drugs and other materials used in the compounding of drugs must be stored in adequately labeled containers in a clean, dry area or, if required, under proper refrigeration.

Adequate lighting and ventilation shall be provided in all drug compounding areas. Potable water shall be supplied under continuous positive pressure in a plumbing system free of defects that could contribute contamination to any compounded drug product. Adequate washing facilities, easily accessible to the compounding area(s) of the pharmacy, shall be provided. These facilities shall include, but not be limited to, hot and cold water, soap or detergent, and air-driers or single-use towels.

The area(s) used for the compounding of drugs shall be maintained in a clean and sanitary condition. It shall be free of infestation by insects, rodents and other vermin. Trash shall be held and disposed of in a timely and sanitary manner. Sewage, trash and other refuse in and from the pharmacy and immediate drug compounding area(s) shall be disposed of in a safe and sanitary manner.

Sterile Products/Radiopharmaceuticals—If sterile (aseptic) products are being compounded, conditions set forth in the *NABP Model Rules for Sterile Pharmaceuticals* must be followed.

If radiopharmaceuticals are being compounded, conditions set forth in the *NABP Model Rules for Nuclear/Radiologic Pharmacy* must be followed.

Special Precaution Products—If drug products with special precautions for contamination, such as penicillin, are involved in a compounding operation, appropriate measures, including either the dedication of equipment for such operations or the meticulous cleaning of contaminated equipment prior to its return to inventory, must be used in order to prevent cross-contamination.

SUBPART D—EQUIPMENT Equipment used in the compounding of drug products shall be of appropriate design, adequate size, and suitably located to facilitate operations for its intended use and for its cleaning and maintenance. Equipment used in the compounding of drug products shall be of suitable composition so that surfaces that contact components, in-process materials, or drug products shall not be reactive, additive or absorptive so as to alter the safety, identity, strength, quality or purity of the drug product beyond that desired.

Equipment and utensils used for compounding shall be cleaned and sanitized immediately prior to use to prevent contamination that would alter the safety, identity, strength, quality or purity of the drug product beyond that desired. In the case of equipment, utensils and containers/closures used in the compounding of sterile drug products, cleaning, sterilization and maintenance procedures as set forth in the *NABP Model Rules for Sterile Pharmaceuticals* must be followed.

Previously cleaned equipment and utensils used for compounding drugs must be protected from contamination prior to use. Immediately prior to the initiation of compounding operations, they must be inspected by the pharmacist and determined to be suitable for use.

Automatic, mechanical or electronic equipment, or other types of equipment or related systems that will perform a function satisfactorily may be used in the compounding of drug products. If such equipment is used, it shall be routinely inspected, calibrated (if necessary) or checked to assure proper performance.

SUBPART E—CONTROL OF COMPONENTS AND DRUG PRODUCT CONTAINERS AND CLOSURES Components, drug product containers and closures, used in the compounding of drugs shall be handled and stored in a manner to prevent contamination. Bagged or boxed components of drug product containers and closures used in the compounding of drugs shall be stored off the floor in such a manner as to permit cleaning and inspection.

Drug product containers and closures shall not be reactive, additive or absorptive so as to alter the safety, identity, strength, quality or purity of the compounded drug beyond the desired result. Components, drug product containers and closures for use in the compounding of drug products shall be rotated so that the oldest stock is used first. Container closure systems shall provide adequate protection against foreseeable external factors in storage and use that can cause deterioration or contamination of the compounded drug product. Drug product containers and closures shall be clean and, where indicated by the intended use of the drug, sterilized and processed to remove pyrogenic properties to assure that they are suitable for their intended use.

Drug product containers and closures intended for the compounding of sterile products must be handled, sterilized, stored, etc in keeping with the *NABP Model Rules for Sterile Pharmaceuticals*. Methods of cleaning, sterilizing and processing to remove pyrogenic properties shall be written and followed for drug product containers and closures used in the preparation of sterile pharmaceuticals, if these processes are performed by the pharmacist, or under the pharmacist's supervision following *the NABP Model Rules for Sterile Pharmaceuticals.*

SUBPART F—DRUG COMPOUNDING CONTROLS There shall be written procedures for the compounding of drug products to assure that the finished products have the identity, strength, quality and purity they purport or are represented to possess. Such procedures shall include a listing of the components (ingredients), their amounts (in weight or volume), the order of component addition and a description of the compounding process. All equipment and utensils and the container/closure system, relevant to the sterility and stability of the intended use of the drug, shall be listed. These written procedures shall be followed in the execution of the drug compounding procedure.

Components for drug product compounding shall be accurately weighed, measured or subdivided as appropriate. These operations should be checked and rechecked by the compounding pharmacist at each stage of the process to ensure that each weight or measure is correct as stated in the written compounding procedures. If a component is removed from the original container to another (eg, a powder is taken from the original container, weighed, placed in a container and stored in another container) the new container shall be identified with the:

(a) component name, and
(b) weight or measure.

To assure the reasonable uniformity and integrity of compounded drug products, written procedures shall be established and followed that describe the tests or examinations to be conducted on the product being compounded (e.g., compounding of capsules). Such control procedures shall be established to monitor the output and to validate the performance of those compounding processes that may be responsible for causing variability in the final drug product. Such control procedures shall include, but are not limited to, the following (where appropriate):

(a) capsule weight variation;
(b) adequacy of mixing to assure uniformity and homogeneity;
(c) clarity, completeness or pH of solutions.

Appropriate written procedures designed to prevent microbiological contamination of compounded drug products purporting to be sterile shall be established and followed. Such procedures shall include validation of any sterilization process.

SUBPART G—LABELING CONTROL OF EXCESS PRODUCTS In the case where a quantity of a compounded drug product in excess of that to be initially dispensed in accordance with Subpart A is prepared, the excess product shall be labeled or documentation referenced with the complete list of ingredients (components), the preparation date, and the assigned expiration date based upon professional judgment, appropriate testing, or published data. It shall also be stored and accounted for under conditions dictated by its composition and stability characteristics (eg, in a clean, dry place on a shelf or in the refrigerator) to ensure its strength, quality and purity.

At the completion of the drug finishing operation, the product shall be examined for correct labeling.

SUBPART H—RECORDS AND REPORTS Any procedures or other records required to be maintained in compliance with these Good Compounding Practices shall be retained for the same period of time as each State requires for the retention of prescription files.

All records required to be retained under these Good Compounding Practices, or copies of such records, shall be readily available for authorized inspection during the retention period at the establishment where the activities described in such records occurred. These records or copies thereof shall be subject to photocopying or other means of reproduction as part of such inspection.

Records required under these Good Compounding Practices may be retained either as the original records or as true copies, such as photocopies, microfilm, microfiche or other accurate reproductions of the original records.

USP 26/NF 21—The following are summaries of Chapters <795>, *Pharmacy Compounding-Nonsterile Preparations*[10], and <797>, *Pharmacy Compounding-Sterile Preparations*[11], in the USP/NF.

Chapter <795>—This material is divided into (1) Compounding Environment, (2) Stability of Compounded Preparations, (3) Definitions, (4) Ingredient Selection and Calculations, (5) Checklist for Acceptable Strength, Quality and Purity, (6) Compounded Preparations, (7) Compounding Process, (8) Compounding Records and documents, (9) Quality Control and (10) Patient Counseling.

The Compounding Environment section discusses the standards for the facility and the equipment that is used. Both should be adequate and appropriate for the compounding activities that will be performed.

The area should be separate from other functions that occur in the pharmacy and should be maintained in a clean and sanitary condition.

The Stability of Compounded Preparations section has been previously discussed in this chapter. Special attention is given to the "Beyond-Use Labeling that is required for compounded preparations.

The Definitions include terms such as preparation(s), official substance(s), active ingredient(s) and added substances.

Ingredient Selection and Calculations discuss the sources of the ingredients, a topic that has also been covered in this chapter along with the compounding of non-drug preparations. The calculations area is a brief summary of what is involved to obtain, theoretically, 100% of the amount of each ingredient in compounded preparations.

The Checklist for Acceptable Strength, Quality and Purity emphasizes the USP/NF hallmarks of standards of acceptable Strength, Quality, and Purity and is presented in a series of questions to be answered.

Compounded Preparations discusses examples of compounded dosage forms along with some precautionary statements as appropriate. Some of the dosage forms discussed include tips on compounding procedures.

The Compounding Process section is a step-by-step presentation on the compounding process to ensure uniformity of activities in preparing each formulation.

Compounding Records and Documents describes the *Formulation Record*, the *Compounding Record*, and the *Material Safety Data Sheets* (MSDS) files that should be maintained. The rationale and purpose of the documents is explained.

Quality Control is included to ensure the accuracy and completeness of the compounding process. Compounded preparations must meet the USP/NF standards and the pharmacist should review each procedure in the compounding process as a final check.

The section ends with various aspects for Patient Counseling involving the proper use, storage, and evidence of instability of the compounded preparation(s).

Chapter <797>—involves procedures and requirements for compounding sterile preparations (CSPs). This chapter has been completely revised, formerly known as Chapter <1206> Sterile Drug Products for Home Use. It is divided into the following sections: (1) Introduction, (2) Responsibility of Compounding Personnel, (3) CSP Microbial Contamination Risk Levels, (4) Compounding Accuracy and Sterilization, (5) Personnel Training and Evaluation in Aseptic Manipulation Skills, (6) Environmental Quality and Control, (7) Processing, (8) Verification of Automated Compounding Devices for Parenteral Nutrition Compounding, (9) Finished Preparation Release Checks and Tests, (10) Storage and Beyond-Use Dating, (11) Maintaining Product Quality and Control After the CSP Leaves the Pharmacy, (12) Patient or Caregiver Training, (13) Patient Monitoring and Adverse Events Reporting, and (14) The Quality Assurance Program.

The Introduction discusses the intent and organization of the chapter and emphasizes that it is the ultimate responsibility of all personnel who prepare CSPs to understand these fundamental practices and precautions and to develop and implement appropriate procedures.

The section on the Responsibility of Compounding Personnel discusses the various procedures, requirements, and performance responsibilities of those involved in compounding sterile preparations.

CSP microbial Contamination Risk Levels includes a discussion on the various risk levels determined by the corresponding probability of contaminating a CSP with (1) microbial contamination, and (2) chemical and physical contamination. Three risk levels are identified; Low, Medium and High. The characteristics described for each level are intended as a guide to the breadth and depth of care necessary in compounding. The section discusses the conditions, examples and quality assurance associated with each risk level.

Verification of Compounding Accuracy and Sterilization includes a discussion of the methods of sterilization (filtration, steam) and their characteristics and requirements.

Personnel Training and Evaluation in Aseptic Manipulation Skills describes the requirements for training of the personnel involved as well as how these individuals are validated in aseptic manipulations.

Environmental Quality and Control involves critical site exposure, clean rooms and barrier isolators, environmental controls, the CSP environment, cleaning and sanitizing the workspaces, personnel cleansing and gowning, suggested standard operating procedures and environmental monitoring.

Processing includes a discussion on aseptic technique, components, sterile ingredients and components, nonsterile ingredients and components, and equipment standards.

The compounding of parenteral nutrition preparations often involves automated devices, which are discussed in the Verification of Automated Compounding Devices for Parenteral Nutrition Compounding and includes sections on accuracy and precision.

Finished Preparation Release Checks and Tests describes physical inspection, compounding accuracy checks, sterility testing, bacterial endotoxin (pyrogen) testing and identity and strength verification of ingredients.

Storage and beyond use dating provides information on the determination of beyond-use dates for CSPs. The beyond-use dates for CSPs is associated with the end-product testing for these preparations as well as the monitoring of controlled storage areas.

The section on Maintaining Product Quality and Control After the CSP Leaves the Pharmacy discusses both sterile preparations for institutional use and packing and transporting CSPs. Topics included in these sections include packaging, handling and transportation, administration, education and training and storage in locations outside CSP facilities (in patients homes).

Patient or Caregiver Training provides detailed topics that should be a part of a training program to ensure the patient or caregiver understands and complies with the many special and complex responsibilities involving the storage, handling and administrations of CSPs.

Patient Monitoring and Adverse Events Reporting explains standards for monitoring patients and any adverse events that might occur, including the establishment of standard operating procedures for reporting these events.

The Quality Assurance section describes the standard of a formal program that is intended to provide a mechanism for monitoring, evaluating, correcting and improving the activities and processes involved with CSPs.

There are two additional General Chapters in the USP/NF prepared specifically for pharmacy compounding; <1160> Pharmaceutical Calculations in Prescription Compounding, and <1075> Good Compounding Practices.

USP General Chapter <1160> Pharmaceutical Calculations in Prescription Compounding is provided as a reference and review of pharmaceutical calculations that may be used in compounding pharmacies.[19] It discusses topics such as weighing, buffer solutions, dosage calculations, percentage concentrations, specific gravity, dilution and concentration, potency units, reconstitution, alligation, molar, molal and normal concentrations, milliequivalents and millimoles, isoosmotic solutions, flow rates in intravenous sets, temperature, and others related to pharmaceutical compounding.

USP General Chapter, <1075> Good Compounding Practices is designed to provide compounders with guidance on applying good compounding practices for the preparation of compounded formulations for dispensing and/or administration to humans or animals.[20] It covers definitions, responsibilities, training, procedures and documentation, drug compounding facilities, equipment, packaging and product containers, controls, labeling, records and reports, office-use compounding and the compounding of veterinarian products and pharmacy-generated products.

Numerous other General Chapters in the USP/NF are related to compounding and directly impact it, such as Chapters <1151> Pharmaceutical Dosage Forms, <1176> Prescription Balances and Volumetric Apparatus, <12191> Stability Considerations in Dispensing Practice, and <1231> Water for Pharmaceutical Purposes.

SUMMARY

Pharmacy compounding is providing pharmacists with a unique opportunity to practice their time-honored profession. It will become an even more important part of pharmacy practice in the future, including those involved in community, hospital, nursing home, home health care, veterinary, and other specialty practices. Pharmaceutical compounding is a practice in which the clinical expertise of pharmacists can be merged with the scientific expertise of pharmacists to make pharmaceutical care a reality.

Pharmacists should not hesitate to become involved in pharmacy compounding but should be aware of the requirements and uniqueness of formulating a specific drug product for a specific patient. This is an important component in providing pharmaceutical care. After all, without the pharmaceutical product, there is no pharmaceutical care.

REFERENCES

1. *Webster's Revised Unabridged Dictionary of the English Language.* Springfield, MA: Merriam, 1913, 1075.
2. *Webster's Seventh New Collegiate Dictionary.* Springfield, MA: Merriam, 1963, 633.
3. *International Dictionary of Medicine and Biology.* Vol. III. New York: John Wiley, 1986.
4. Exodus 30:25. *Holy Bible.* King James Version.
5. *The Compact Oxford English Dictionary,* 2nd ed. New York: Oxford University Press, 1991.
6. *American Heritage Dictionary of the English Language,* 3rd ed. Microsoft Corp, 1992 [in electronic form in Microsoft Bookshelf '95, 1995].
7. Penna R. *Am J Pharm Educ* 1997; 61(Spring):103.
8. *Good Compounding Practices Applicable to State Licensed Pharmacies.* Park Ridge, IL: NABP, 1993.
9. Allen LV Jr. *Int J Pharm Compound* 1997; 2:71.
10. United States Pharmacopeia 26/ National Formulary 21. Rockville, MD: USP Convention, Inc., 2002, pp 2197–2201.
11. Allen LV Jr. *Int J Pharm Compound.* 1997;1:46.
12. Popovich NG. In: Gennaro AR, ed. *Remington: The Science and Practice of Pharmacy,* 19th ed. Easton, PA: Mack Publishing Co, 1995.
13. Raehl CL, Bond CA, Pitterle ME. *Pharmacotherapy* 1993; 13(6):618.
14. Goode MA, Gums JG. *Ann Pharmacother* 1993; 27:502.
15. Sundberg JA. *Int J Pharm Compound* 1997; 1(5):314.
16. Anonymous. *J Am Vet Med Assoc* 1994; 204(2):189.
17. Shaw SM. *Int J Pharm Compound* 1998; 2(6):424.
18. Letendre WR, Shepherd MD, Brown CM. *Int J Pharm Compound* 1998; 2(6):455.
19. *Pharmacopeial Forum* 2003; 29(3):750.
20. *Pharmacopeial Forum* 2003; 28(2):476, 640.

CHAPTER 106

Nuclear Pharmacy Practice

Stanley M Shaw, PhD

James A Ponto, MS, BCNP

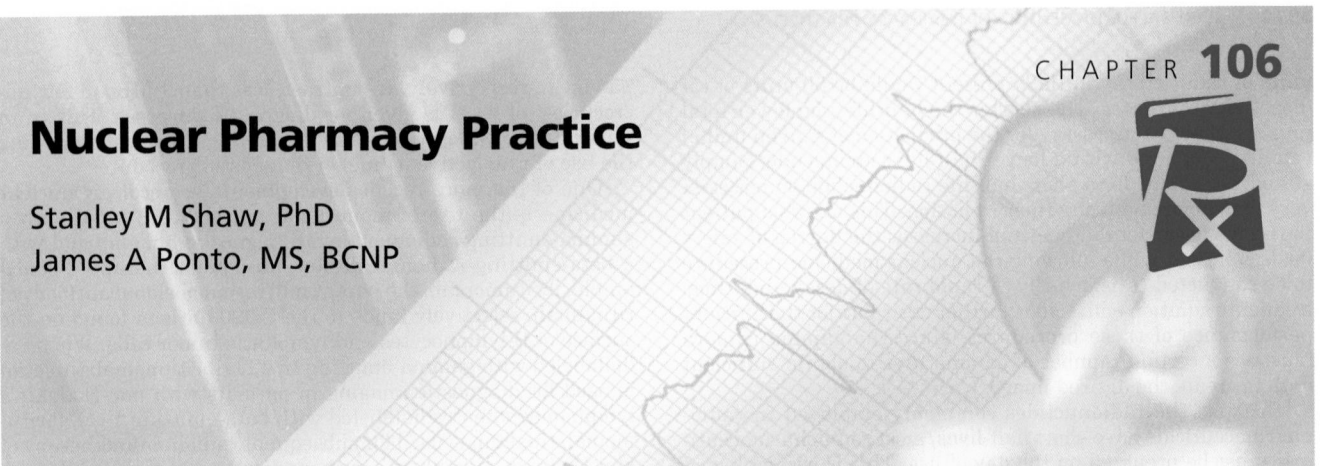

Nuclear pharmacy (also referred to as radiopharmacy) is the specialty practice of pharmacy that focuses on the safe and efficacious use of radioactive drugs. Radioactive drugs, usually referred to as radiopharmaceuticals, constitute a special class of drugs according to the Food, Drug, and Cosmetic Act (FD&C Act). The Food and Drug Administration (FDA), in Title 21 of the Code of Federal Regulations (CFR), defines a radioactive drug as a drug that exhibits spontaneous disintegration of unstable nuclei with the emission of nuclear particles or photons and includes any nonradioactive reagent kit or nuclide generator that is intended to be used in the preparation of any such substance. From this definition, it is apparent that a radiopharmaceutical consists of both a drug component and a radioactive component. The drug component is responsible for localization in specific organs or tissues. The radioactive component is responsible for the emission of gamma rays for external detection in diagnostic imaging and/or particulate radiation for radionuclide therapy. Radioactive *in vitro* diagnostic kits for radioimmunoassays and brachytherapy sources for radiotherapy implants are classified by the FDA as devices, in contradistinction to radiopharmaceuticals which are classified as drugs.

A distinctive feature of radiopharmaceuticals, in contrast to traditional drugs, is their lack of pharmacological effects. Radiopharmaceuticals typically are employed as tracers of physiological functions. Their small amounts of mass produce negligible effects on biological processes, while their radioactivity allows noninvasive external monitoring or targeted therapeutic irradiation.

Some radiopharmaceuticals are simply salts of radioisotopes of elements (eg, I-131 sodium iodide, Tl-201 thallous chloride, Sr-89 strontium chloride[1]), but most radiopharmaceuticals consist of radioactive atoms attached to, or incorporated into, other chemical compounds that serve to carry the radioactive atoms to the intended tissues or organs. Some radiopharmaceuticals are manufactured and commercially marketed by pharmaceutical companies in their final, ready-to-use dosage forms. Because of their short half-lives, however, most radiopharmaceuticals require preparation of the final product either on-site, such as in a hospital, or in a local commercial nuclear pharmacy that then delivers the finished products to surrounding hospitals and clinics.

Radiopharmaceuticals can be categorized as either diagnostic or therapeutic. Diagnostic radiopharmaceuticals are intended for use in the diagnosis and/or monitoring of various disease states. Relatively small radiation doses are delivered, similar in magnitude to radiation doses from diagnostic X-ray procedures. Examples of diagnostic radiopharmaceuticals include Tc-99m diphosphonates for bone imaging procedures, Tc-99m macroaggregated albumin for lung imaging procedures, and Tl-201 thallous chloride for myocardial perfusion imaging procedures. Therapeutic radiopharmaceuticals, on the other hand, are intended for use in the treatment of various disease states. Relatively large radiation doses purposefully are delivered to cause localized radiation damage, similar in magnitude to radiation doses from teletherapy irradiation. A common example of a therapeutic radiopharmaceutical is I-131 sodium iodide for treatment of hyperthyroidism or thyroid cancer.

Radiopharmaceuticals are employed in the discipline termed "nuclear medicine." Nuclear medicine may be a separate unit or found as a part of radiology. In some situations, limited groups of radiopharmaceuticals may also be employed in specialty practices such as radiation oncology, cardiology, or endocrinology. In a diagnostic nuclear medicine procedure, the radiopharmaceutical is administered to the patient most often by IV injection, although sometimes by oral, inhalation, or other routes. The localization, disposition, and/or clearance of the radiopharmaceutical is then determined by detection of the radiation emitted from the radionuclide with a sophisticated instrument termed a "gamma camera." Obviously, the type of radiation detected is gamma, and the data exhibited by the detector will be an image or picture. Quantitative information can be obtained by using computers associated with the radiation detector. Normal versus abnormal images will vary depending upon the procedure. For example, a normal image with a radiopharmaceutical designed to be phagocytized by the liver will appear as a rather uniform uptake and distribution of the radiopharmaceutical throughout the liver. A space-occupying lesion such as a tumor lacks phagocytic cells so does not concentrate the radiopharmaceutical. Thus, the image of the liver will show a *cold* area (ie, an area with less radioactivity than the surrounding liver). The opposite effect will be noted in the case of a radiopharmaceutical designed to localize metastatic lesions in the bone. Excessive amounts of the radioactivity will occur in the area of the metastatic lesion, in comparison to the surrounding normal bone. This is termed a *hot* spot on the image.

The radionuclides typically used for radiopharmaceuticals employed in diagnostic nuclear medicine studies have short physical half-lives. Half-life is defined as the time that it takes for one-half of the radioactive atoms to undergo radioactive decay with emission of their characteristic radiation. For example, technetium Tc-99m has a physical half-life of 6.0 hr, so 100

---

[1] In practice, most radiopharmaceuticals usually are referred to by common names, such as abbreviated chemical names, rather than by nonproprietary drug names established by the United States Adopted Names Council (USAN).

units of radioactivity initially present would be 50 units of radioactivity 6 hr later. The shorter the half-life, the fewer total number of atoms necessary for the production of a given unit of activity, compared with a longer half-life radionuclide. Simply stated, the atoms for a short-half-life radionuclide do not exist very long before emitting their radiation. This allows a patient to receive fewer total atoms and increases the degree of safety for the patient while allowing the nuclear medicine procedure to be conducted satisfactorily. A rapid rate of decay and, thus, frequent radiation emission is further desirable for the efficient performance of these procedures, since the gamma camera must *see* a certain number of gamma rays to obtain sufficient data to create the desired image.

Because the radionuclides commonly employed in radiopharmaceuticals have short half-lives, most radiopharmaceuticals must be prepared on the day of use. This is accomplished most frequently with the aid of a nonradioactive reagent kit and radioactivity obtained from a radionuclide generator. The reagent kit is usually a multidose vial that contains the compound (ligand) to be labeled (ie, attachment of the radionuclide to the compound) and other components necessary to accomplish the labeling process and allow administration of the final product. The radionuclide generator most often employed is the technetium generator. The radionuclide technetium Tc-99m is produced by the decay of molybdenum Mo-99. Molybdenum-99 has a half-life of 67 hr and allows the generation of Tc-99m over a period of 1 to 2 weeks. The Tc-99m is separated from the Mo-99 by passing a sterile saline solution through a column containing the Mo-99 and the Tc-99m that has been generated. The Tc-99m eluate, in the chemical form of sodium pertechnetate, is collected in a sterile vial. Aliquots of this eluate are then used to prepare radiopharmaceuticals with the reagent kits.

Quality-control issues are important in this process. The possibility of the presence of Mo-99 in the eluate must be determined, because this radionuclide has a longer half-life, emits a more damaging form of radiation (beta), and is in the wrong chemical form. The half-life of Tc-99m is 6.0 hr, and only gamma radiation is emitted from these radioactive atoms. Gamma radiation is less likely to produce damage to cells than is beta or alpha radiation. The purity of the desired compound must be determined following preparation of the radiopharmaceutical with the sodium pertechnetate and a reagent kit. This generally is accomplished using paper or thin-layer chromatography procedures. A specified percentage of the radioactivity must be incorporated in the specified compound (ie, the radiopharmaceutical). If a significant fraction of the radioactivity remains as sodium pertechnetate, the radiopharmaceutical product will not distribute in the body as expected and might cause confusion or even an improper diagnosis.

A few radiopharmaceuticals are employed in the treatment of disease. Like diagnostic radiopharmaceuticals, these compounds are designed to localize in the diseased tissue. Instead of employing the emitted radiation to trace the distribution of the radiopharmaceutical as is done for diagnosis, however, the radiation is intended to destroy cells in the diseased area. The radiation deposits its energy in a very localized area and in a manner that leads to the enhanced probability of causing some deleterious effect to a key component of the cell such as DNA. Beta radiation is the most common type of radiation employed to treat diseases.

Perhaps the best known approach to therapy with a radiopharmaceutical involves the use of radioactive iodine, I-131, administered as sodium iodide to the patient. The I-131 is taken up by the thyroid gland and incorporated into thyroid hormones. Whereas small, diagnostic dosages of I-131 produce negligible biological damage, the beta radiation emitted by large, therapeutic dosages of I-131 destroys thyroid tissue. Depending upon the disease state, hyperthyroidism or cancer, the amount of radioactive iodide given to the patient varies considerably. The usual dosage ranges for treatment of hyperthyroidism (partial destruction) and thyroid carcinoma (total destruction) are 140 to 370 MBq (4–10 mCi) and 3700 to 5550 MBq (100 to 150 mCi), respectively. In contrast, less than 1 MBq (a few microcuries) of I-131 is given for diagnostic purposes. This is an important consideration when counseling a patient regarding the use of radioactive iodine for diagnostic procedures.

One of the more recent developments in oncologic nuclear medicine is the use of monoclonal antibodies labeled with a gamma-emitting radionuclide for diagnostic imaging and with a beta-emitting radionuclide for subsequent therapy. For example, ibritumomab, the parent murine monoclonal antibody of rituximab, selectively binds to the CD20 antigen found on the surface of B-lymphocytes and lymphatic tumor cells. When radiolabeled with gamma-emitting In-111, ibritumomab tiuxetan is used for diagnostic imaging in patients with non-Hodgkin's lymphoma; when radiolabeled with beta-emitting Y-90, ibritumomab tiuxetan is used for subsequent radioimmunotherapy of non-Hodgkin's lymphoma in these same patients.

To practice nuclear pharmacy, pharmacists must have specialized training in several areas such as nuclear physics, radiation detection instrumentation, radiochemistry, and radiation protection. An experiential component of this training in a practice setting is essential as well. The level of knowledge and experience necessary, as well as services provided, vary with the practice site. The majority of nuclear pharmacists practice in a commercial nuclear pharmacy. Most practitioners in this setting have a first professional degree, while nuclear pharmacists in an institutional site commonly have received an advanced degree (eg, an MS). The basic functions are similar; however, the pharmacist in the larger hospital may be more involved with clinical service, investigational products, and teaching. The pharmacist in a commercial nuclear pharmacy inherently spends considerable time preparing and dispensing radiopharmaceuticals, because one pharmacy generally services 10 to 15 different hospitals and clinics.

The main objectives of this chapter are to review the development of nuclear pharmacy and describe functions of a nuclear pharmacist regardless of the practice site. Regulatory restrictions and the specialized training required to practice nuclear pharmacy are addressed. The relevance of pharmaceutical care to nuclear pharmacy is considered as well as the importance of various diagnostic imaging modalities to the management of patients and to the assessment of therapeutic outcomes.

DEVELOPMENT OF NUCLEAR PHARMACY

Natural radioactivity was first observed in 1867 by Niepce de Saint-Victor, who noticed *fogging* in a silver chloride emulsion while working with uranium salts. He attributed this effect, however, to luminescence phenomena. While performing similar phosphorescence experiments in 1896, Antoine Henri Becquerel, now credited as the discoverer of radioactivity, noted that uranium emitted penetrating rays that were similar to the x-rays identified a year earlier by Wilhelm Roentgen. However, it was not until 1898, after Marie and Pierre Curie had determined that these emissions were originating from the unstable elements radium and polonium, that the phenomenon of radioactivity truly was recognized. By 1899, Ernest Rutherford had determined the existence of two distinct types of radiation, which he called alpha and beta. A year later, Paul Villard identified a third type of radiation, which was called gamma. The theory of radioactive disintegration was advanced in 1902 by Ernest Rutherford and Frederick Soddy. The discovery of artificially produced radioactive nuclides occurred on New Year's Eve, 1933, in an experiment conducted by Frederic Joliet and Irene Curie. They noticed that positrons continued to be emitted, but at an inverse exponential rate, following irradiation of aluminum foil with a polonium preparation. By the end of July 1934, Enrico Fermi had produced radioisotopes of 40 elements by neutron bombardment. Also in 1934, Ernest O Lawrence invented the cyclotron and produced numerous radionuclides by bombarding stable atoms with artificially accelerated particles. In 1946, radionuclides produced in the Oak Ridge National Laboratory reactor were made widely available for biological and medical purposes.

Shortly after the discovery of radium, Henri Becquerel reported a skin burn received from a vial of radium that he carried in his pocket. Following additional experiments on his own skin, Pierre Curie suggested that the destructive biological effects from radium might have a possible medical use. Consequently, Paul Oudin first used an external source of radium in the treatment of uterine cervical cancer in 1904. By 1911, clinical trials using *Curie therapy* with parenteral injections of radium also were carried out in attempts to cure arthritis, lupus erythematosus, various cancers, and several other poorly defined diseases. Unfortunately, these initial attempts at internal therapeutic use of a radionuclide proved to be valueless and may have actually contributed to the induction of leukemia in some patients given very high doses. In 1938, following his brother's invention of the cyclotron, John Lawrence made the first clinical therapeutic application of an artificial radionuclide when he used P-32 to treat leukemia. By 1942, several investigators were using I-131 to treat hyperthyroidism, and successful treatment of thyroid cancer with I-131 was first reported in 1946.

The diagnostic use of radionuclides had its beginning in the development of the tracer concept, pioneered by Georg de Hevesy. In 1923, Professor de Hevesy used tracer principles for the first time by employing Pb-212 to study the absorption of lead nitrate in bean plants. In what was probably the first human application of a radionuclide in a diagnostic study, Herman Blumgart and associates, in 1927, determined the arm-to-arm circulation time in patients following an antecubital injection of Rn-222 in one arm and detecting its presence some time later in the other arm. The introduction of an improved radiation detector by H Geiger and W Müller in 1929 stimulated further *in vivo* applications using radioisotopes. Development of imaging devices during the 1950s and 1960s, including the rectilinear scanner, the scintillation camera, and the coincidence positron emission tomographic (PET) scanner, together with an explosive growth in radioisotope production and radiopharmaceutical development, propelled the clinical applications of radionuclides into the modern era of nuclear medicine.

The rapid increase in the medical use of radionuclides during these early years corresponded to the increased production and availability of radionuclides produced by cyclotrons and by nuclear reactors. Abbott Laboratories began marketing a line of radioactive pharmaceuticals in 1948. Two years later, the vice-chairman of the Joint Committee on Atomic Energy suggested that atomic energy should be a matter of concern to practicing pharmacists. In that same year, John E Christian, a professor of pharmacy at Purdue University, stated unequivocally that hospital pharmacists should be prepared to provide information and assistance in the establishment of radioisotope facilities and programs. In 1954, GB Hutchinson indicated that preparations containing radioactivity that are intended for human use are indeed pharmaceuticals and should fall under the purview of pharmacists. A report of the first Committee on Isotopes of the American Society of Hospital Pharmacists (ASHP), appointed in 1954, presented pictorially the first functional nuclear pharmacy in this country, established at the University of Chicago Clinics. In 1957, Captain William H Briner, a pharmacist at the National Institutes of Health (NIH), recognized the expanding applications of radiopharmaceuticals for the diagnosis of disease and the necessary involvement of pharmacists to ensure the formulation of radioactive chemicals into radioactive pharmaceuticals. After obtaining intensive training at the Oak Ridge National Laboratory, Captain Briner established a small unit in the NIH Pharmacy Department for the receipt, preparation, and control of radiopharmaceuticals. This was the second nuclear

pharmacy established in the country and the longest still in existence (the first was closed after 1 year). For his many pioneering contributions to the field, Captain Briner often is referred to as the father of nuclear pharmacy practice.

With the advent of the Tc-99m generator in the late 1960s, a source of a versatile radionuclide became readily available to thousands of hospitals. As technetium was found to be complexed and chelated by numerous organ-specific compounds, pharmaceutical manufacturers began supplying reagent kits designed for the simplified preparation of Tc-99m-labeled radiopharmaceuticals. Technetium-99m radiopharmaceutical use spread rapidly, and pharmacists increasingly became involved in the preparation and dispensing of short-lived radiopharmaceuticals for human use. In 1969, the first postgraduate program in nuclear pharmacy was established by Walter Wolf at the University of Southern California. Other early university educational programs for nuclear pharmacy included Purdue, Michigan, Tennessee, and New Mexico. Although Purdue University did not initiate a formally designated program in nuclear pharmacy until 1972, John E Christian created the Department of Bionucleonics in the School of Pharmacy at Purdue in 1959. The focus of the department was education and research in radiotracer methodology. Several early leaders in nuclear pharmacy used their training in bionucleonics to develop radiopharmaceutical services.

The decade of the 1970s witnessed tremendous growth in nuclear medicine, new radiopharmaceuticals, and nuclear pharmacy. Institutional nuclear pharmacies were established at many academic/tertiary medical centers. In 1972, the first commercial nuclear pharmacy was created in Albuquerque, NM, by Richard Keesee, an assistant professor in the University of New Mexico College of Pharmacy. The facility was affiliated with the College of Pharmacy and located in the Bernalillo County Medical Center. Sixteen hospitals in the city of Albuquerque and surrounding cities in New Mexico were serviced by the nuclear pharmacy. The nuclear pharmacy also served as a teaching facility for the College's pharmacy students. Within a short time graduates from the program established commercial nuclear pharmacies in many major cities. Today, there are several hundred commercial nuclear pharmacies providing the major fraction of radiopharmaceuticals used in nuclear medicine procedures.

During this same decade, nuclear pharmacy matured and emerged as a true specialty in pharmacy practice. Nuclear pharmacists first met as a clearly recognized group on August 6, 1974, in Chicago at the *Nuclear Pharmacy '74* Symposium conducted under the auspices of the APhA's Academy of General Practice of Pharmacy. The Section on Nuclear Pharmacy in the APhA's Academy of General Practice of Pharmacy was established in 1975. In that same year, a Special Interest Group on Nuclear Pharmacy Practice was formed within the ASHP. Nuclear Pharmacy was recognized officially as a specialty in pharmacy practice, the first specialty so recognized, by the Board of Pharmaceutical Specialties in 1978. The first examination for board certification in nuclear pharmacy was administered on April 24, 1982, to 72 practitioners. More than 500 nuclear pharmacists have since become Board Certified Nuclear Pharmacists (BCNPs).

In the decades of the 1980s and 1990s, nuclear pharmacy saw fluctuating periods of maintenance and growth, as major changes in health care took place. Primarily related to cost considerations, there was a steady shift by hospitals from preparing radiopharmaceuticals in-house to purchasing radiopharmaceuticals as unit doses from commercial nuclear pharmacies. It is estimated that today 70–80% of all radiopharmaceutical doses are dispensed through commercial nuclear pharmacy channels. In a fashion similar to conventional retail pharmacy, commercial nuclear pharmacy has evolved from predominately independent pharmacies to major chains. Currently, there are approximately 350 commercial nuclear pharmacies in the US. Of these, approximately, 70% are members of one of several chains, and the other 30% are independents.

Nuclear pharmacy remains a dynamic and vital field, which requires communication and networking. Dissemination of information is achieved through publication in professional newsletters, journals, and books and presentations at professional meetings. Nearly ubiquitous internet access allows rapid communication via e-mail and interactive group sites and provides unlimited opportunities for searching and retrieving specific information. "The Nuclear Pharmacy" web site, established in 1997 and continuously updated, serves as the unofficial site for the nuclear pharmacy profession.

PRACTICE OF NUCLEAR PHARMACY

The practice of nuclear pharmacy is composed of several domains related to the provision of nuclear pharmacy services. These domains, determined by formal task analyses, serve as the basic structure for the APhA's Nuclear Pharmacy Practice Guidelines (nee Standards). The Guidelines include lists of tasks and their related knowledge statements for each domain to aid in the further description and interpretation of nuclear pharmacy practice. Because of differences in practice setting, job responsibilities, and other factors, all of the Guidelines are not applicable to all nuclear pharmacists. Moreover, the Guidelines are not all-inclusive of this dynamic field. Hence, the pharmacist's professional judgment should be used when interpreting or applying the Guidelines.

The nine general domains involved in nuclear pharmacy practice are

1. Procurement
2. Compounding
3. Quality assurance
4. Dispensing
5. Distribution
6. Health and safety
7. Provision of information and consultation
8. Monitoring patient outcome
9. Research and development

Procurement of radiopharmaceuticals and other drugs, supplies, and materials necessary for nuclear pharmacy practice involves determining product specifications, initiating purchase orders, receiving shipments, maintaining inventory, and storing materials under proper conditions. Although these tasks appear similar to those involved in community and hospital pharmacy practice, special characteristics and requirements associated with radiopharmaceuticals present some unique demands. For example, radiopharmaceuticals or radioactive components, because of their short half-lives, are not available through conventional wholesalers; rather, they typically are ordered directly from the manufacturers.

Ordering of radiopharmaceuticals or radioactive components requires knowledge of calibration time, shipping/delivery schedule, and radioactive decay before receipt and use. Because of the necessity for overnight delivery, shipping charges are frequently a substantial portion of the acquisition cost for many radioactive items. Receipt of radioactive materials involves following regulatory procedures for opening packages, including performing surveys for radioactive contamination. Inventory control of radioactive materials is complicated by their distinctive, continuous radioactive decay; fortunately, repetitive manual calculations have been replaced by computer software programs developed for this purpose. Storage of radioactive materials must incorporate appropriate radiation shielding in addition to traditional requirements for light, temperature, and humidity.

Compounding of radiopharmaceuticals involves a wide variety of activities ranging from relatively simple tasks such as reconstituting reagent kits with Tc-99m sodium pertechnetate to complex tasks such as operating a cyclotron and synthesizing new radiochemical entities from raw materials. As with compounding activities performed by community and hospital pharmacists, compounding of radiopharmaceuticals requires receipt (or anticipation) of a valid prescription/drug order; appropriate components, supplies, and equipment; a suitable environment, especially for sterile dosage forms; appropriate recordkeeping, including written procedures and lot-specific information to ensure traceability; and validation or verification of the compounding procedure, storage conditions, and expiration.

Compounding of radiopharmaceuticals is complicated by the issues of radioactivity and of chemical reactions. Radioactivity during preparation and delay prior to patient administration must be addressed both in terms of radioactive decay (ie, exponential loss of radioactivity over time) and in terms of radiation protection (eg, shielding). Unlike the vast majority of traditional compounding, which involves mixing of ingredients, compounding of radiopharmaceuticals typically involves chemical reactions to *label* a molecule with a radionuclide. For most Tc-99m-labeled compounds, stannous reduction of Tc(VII) pertechnetate to a lower oxidation state is followed by chelation of technetium atoms by multidentate ligands. Chemical reactions involved for other radiopharmaceuticals include covalent bonding, transchelation, and coordination complexation.

The radionuclides used in compounding radiopharmaceuticals typically are obtained from three sources. Some radionuclides (eg, In-111, I-123) are purchased directly from the manufacturer; unfortunately, these tend to be expensive and have somewhat limited availability and shipment schedules. Some radionuclides (eg, F-18, C-11) are created on-site using a cyclotron; unfortunately, these tend to be expensive and on-site cyclotrons are available in only a limited number of facilities. Most radiopharmaceuticals use Tc-99m that is produced in, and eluted from, an on-site Mo-99/Tc-99m generator. Advantages of generator-produced Tc-99m are its relatively low cost, ready availability, and simplicity of use. However, because not all radiopharmaceuticals can be labeled with Tc-99m, other radionuclides obtained from the former two sources continue to be important.

The vast majority of radiopharmaceuticals are intended for parenteral administration; thus, aseptic technique is an important skill observed in nuclear pharmacy compounding and dispensing. Nuclear pharmacists also compound radiolabeled biologicals such as autologous blood cells, monoclonal antibodies, and peptides. Strict adherence to *universal precautions* (also referred to as standard precautions) and proper infection control handling is essential when radiolabeling patient blood cells, especially those obtained from patients harboring blood-borne pathogens (eg, hepatitis, human immunodeficiency virus, communicable microorganisms).

The term "compounding," as originally used in the Nuclear Pharmacy Practice Guidelines, referred to both preparation of radiopharmaceuticals according to manufacturer instructions and to extemporaneous compounding of products not commercially available. Section 127 of the Food and Drug Administration Modernization Act (FDAMA) of 1997[2] defined compounding in such a way that excluded mixing, reconstituting, or other such acts performed in accordance with directions contained in the approved product labeling. However, this section on pharmacy compounding expressly did not apply to radiopharmaceuticals. To proactively address issues related to radiopharmaceutical compounding, the APhA Section on Nuclear Pharmacy Practice established a Nuclear Pharmacy Compounding Practice Committee to develop a set of professional guidelines for the compounding of radiopharmaceuticals. These *Nuclear Pharmacy Compounding Guidelines* were approved and published in 2001. As described in these Guidelines, radiopharmaceutical compounding does not include mixing, recon-

---

[2] Section 127 of FDAMA 1997, which addressed application of federal law to the practice of pharmacy compounding, was nullified in 2002 by a US Supreme Court ruling in the case of Thompson, Secretary of Health and Human Services, et al. *v.* Western States Medical Center et al.

stitution, or other such acts performed in accordance with directions contained in the approved product labeling. Furthermore, these Guidelines advocate that radiopharmaceutical compounding does not include any deviation(s) from directions contained in approved product labeling which result in a final radiopharmaceutical product that is of the same quality and purity as that produced with adherence to the product labeling.

Compounding of PET radiopharmaceuticals requires more extensive controls and validation procedures than those for most other radiopharmaceuticals; hence, a supplemental document entitled *Nuclear Pharmacy Guidelines for the Compounding of Radiopharmaceuticals for Positron Emission Tomography* has been developed and published by the APhA. Similarly, a general chapter on *Radiopharmaceuticals for Positron Emission Tomography—Compounding* was published in the Eighth Supplement to USP 23 and has been included in subsequent revisions of the USP.

Quality assurance of radiopharmaceuticals involves performing the appropriate chemical, physical, and biological tests on radiopharmaceuticals to ensure the suitability of the products for use in humans. These activities include not only the completion of the test, but also interpretation of the results, evaluation of analytical test methods, calibration or functional checks of equipment and instruments used, and appropriate recordkeeping. Radiopharmaceuticals must meet all specifications described in their respective USP monographs, including such parameters as radionuclidic purity, radiochemical purity, chemical purity, pH, particle size, sterility, bacterial endotoxin, and specific activity. Often these standards are guaranteed by the manufacturer, but especially for compounded products and products for which preparation involves deviations from directions contained in their approved labeling, verification of purity specifications is the responsibility of the nuclear pharmacist.

Radionuclidic purity (ie, the fraction of radioactivity as the specified radionuclide) typically is determined by gamma spectroscopy or differential photon attenuation. A common example of a radionuclidic impurity is the presence of Mo-99 in a Tc-99m generator eluate. Radiochemical purity (ie, the fraction of the radionuclide in the specified chemical form) generally is determined by paper, thin layer, or column chromatography. A common example of a radiochemical impurity is Tc-99m pertechnetate in a Tc-99m-labeled product. Chemical purity (ie, specified amounts of nonradioactive chemicals) typically is determined by various chemical detection techniques such as color change when mixed with certain reagents. One example of a chemical impurity is aluminum (leached from the generator column) in a Tc-99m generator eluate. Hydrogen-ion concentration typically is determined with a pH meter or pH paper. Particle size of macroaggregated albumin products typically is determined by microscopic inspection of a sample placed on a hemocytometer slide. Sterility and bacterial endotoxin testing typically are performed using microbial growth media and Limulus Amebocyte Lysate methods, respectively. Specific activity (ie, ratio of radioactivity per mass) is calculated on the basis of radioactivity measurements and masses of components/products.

Dispensing radiopharmaceuticals occurs upon the receipt of a valid prescription or drug order from an authorized physician. In contrast to traditional pharmacy practice, radiopharmaceuticals are rarely dispensed directly to patients; rather, they are dispensed to hospitals or clinics for administration to patients by trained health professionals. Although multidose vials may be dispensed as a sort of *ward stock* system, radiopharmaceuticals generally are dispensed in *unit doses* ready for administration to the patient. In addition to radiopharmaceuticals, certain other drugs, such as those used in pharmacological intervention studies, frequently are dispensed by nuclear pharmacists.

The nuclear pharmacist is responsible for ensuring that the radiopharmaceutical dosage is not only consistent with the prescription order, but is also appropriate based on patient history and other factors such as age, weight, sex, surface area, and gamma camera sensitivity. Radioactive decay between prepara-

tion and dispensing times and between dispensing and administration times must be taken into account. Most of these calculations, historically done manually, routinely are incorporated in specialized computer software programs. Because most radiopharmaceuticals are parenteral products, the nuclear pharmacist must adhere to aseptic technique. With some radiopharmaceuticals, it is necessary for the nuclear pharmacist also to consider the total mass, the number of particles, or the amount of nonradioactive chemical that is present in the dispensed product. Radiopharmaceuticals also are subject to special labeling requirements such as inclusion of the standard radiation symbol and the words *Caution—Radioactive Material.*

Distribution of radiopharmaceuticals within an institution is subject to institutional policies and procedures, generally involving lead-lined boxes or other shielded containers labeled with identifying information. Distribution of radiopharmaceuticals from a commercial nuclear pharmacy to other institutions is subject to local, state, and federal regulations, including those promulgated by state boards of pharmacy, the Department of Transportation (DOT), and the Nuclear Regulatory Commission (NRC). These requirements generally relate to packaging, labeling, shipping papers, and other recordkeeping, as well as general issues related to shipper and carrier licensing and personnel training.

Health and safety are crucial elements of nuclear pharmacy practice. Radiation safety standards, including limits for radiation doses, levels of radiation in an area, concentrations of radioactivity in air and waste water, waste disposal, and precautionary procedures have been established and are enforced by the NRC. Although radiation protection may be the most visible and most regulated, other aspects of health and safety are also important. Hazardous chemicals, such as chromatography solvents, must be stored, handled, and disposed of using proper techniques, personal protective devices, containers, and environment. Biological specimens, such as blood samples obtained for preparation of labeled red cells or leukocytes, must be handled as potentially infectious, using *universal precautions.* Lastly, physical exertion, such as lifting heavy lead shields, must be done with appropriate care.

Provision of information and consultation is a highly important function of nuclear pharmacists. Employing oral and written communication skills, nuclear pharmacists convey their expert knowledge to physicians, technologists, other pharmacists, patients, and others. In addition to just reciting facts, the nuclear pharmacist should provide appropriate context and perspective so that the information is useful. Basic science information provided by nuclear pharmacists includes the biological effects of radiation, radiation physics, radiation protection, and radiopharmaceutical chemistry. Radiopharmaceutical product information provided by nuclear pharmacists includes radiopharmaceutical compounding and quality assurance, availability of radiopharmaceutical products, and radiopharmaceutical product defects. Radiopharmaceutical use information provided by nuclear pharmacists includes clinical applications of radiopharmaceuticals, radiopharmaceutical selection and dosing, pharmacological interventions and drug interactions associated with radiopharmaceuticals, adverse reactions to radiopharmaceuticals, and regulatory requirements. Such information may be of general applicability (eg, teaching), of organizational value (eg, policies and procedures), or of pertinence to the care of specific patients (eg, pharmaceutical care).

Monitoring patient outcome is an important component in the concept of pharmaceutical care. In a broad sense, this encompasses many different activities that, taken together, ensure optimal outcomes for individual patients. Within the scope of his or her practice, a nuclear pharmacist can assist in:

1. Ensuring that patients are appropriately referred to nuclear medicine.
2. Developing institutional standards for the rational use of radiopharmaceuticals and ancillary medications and conducting drug use evaluations for these drugs.

3. Prospectively screening patients regarding appropriate use of radiopharmaceuticals and ancillary medications.
4. Evaluating the safety and efficacy of radiopharmaceutical and ancillary medications.
5. Ensuring that patients receive proper preparation prior to receiving radiopharmaceuticals and ancillary medications.
6. Ensuring that appropriate interventions are used to enhance nuclear medicine procedures.
7. Ensuring that clinical problems associated with the use of radiopharmaceuticals or ancillary medications are prevented or recognized, investigated, and rectified.
8. Monitoring the safety and efficacy or outcomes of individual patients' drug regimens, surgical interventions, and other therapeutic measures using imaging modalities and radiometric technology.
9. Administering therapeutic or diagnostic radiopharmaceuticals and ancillary medications and performing nuclear medicine procedures.
10. Ensuring that information gained through the use of diagnostic radiopharmaceuticals is included as an integral component of a patient's therapeutic care plan.

While some of these activities (eg, conducting drug use evaluations) have an indirect impact on patient care, most have a direct impact on the care of the individual patients and, hence, their healthcare outcomes.

Research and development of new radiopharmaceuticals and clinical applications are vital for the viability and future growth of nuclear medicine and the nuclear pharmacy profession, let alone improvements in patient care. Nuclear pharmacist involvement may include participation in the development of new radiopharmaceuticals, including product design and laboratory testing. Similarly, nuclear pharmacists may participate in developing new compounding procedures or quality-control testing methods for existing radiopharmaceuticals. A frequent area of nuclear pharmacy involvement is participation in clinical trials of investigational radiopharmaceuticals and in the evaluation of new uses for existing radiopharmaceuticals. In addition, nuclear pharmacists often serve as members on institutional radiation safety and radioactive drug research committees.

REGULATIONS

Regulation of nuclear pharmacy practice has a fairly complex history due largely to the dichotomous nature of radiopharmaceuticals, which are viewed as both radioactive materials and as drug products. During the formative years of nuclear medicine, radiopharmaceuticals were controlled chiefly by the Atomic Energy Commission (AEC), because they typically contained *by-product* (ie, produced in a nuclear reactor) radionuclides. The 1954 Atomic Energy Act authorized the AEC to license the possession, use, and transfer of by-product materials, including radiopharmaceuticals. The AEC was replaced, in part, in 1975 by the NRC, which continues to have responsibility for licensing and other regulatory functions pertaining to by-product radioactive materials. Accelerator (eg, cyclotron) produced radionuclides have increasingly been used in radiopharmaceuticals. Because the NRC has authority to regulate by-product materials only, individual states are responsible for regulating accelerator-produced materials in a manner similar to their regulation of X-ray-producing machines. In addition, the NRC has entered into agreements with 34 states, referred to as *Agreement States,* whereby authority to control by-product materials has been transferred to the analogous state agencies. Hence, under the current regulatory scheme, the NRC regulates by-product materials only in non–agreement states, the non–agreement states regulate X-ray-producing machines and accelerator-produced materials only, and agreement states regulate all radioactive materials and X-ray-producing machines.

The primary responsibility of the NRC (and analogous state agencies) is to provide for the radiation safety of workers and the general public, to protect their health and minimize danger to life and property. In a series of chapters in Title 10 of the CFR, the NRC promulgates standards for radiation protection, licensing of facilities handling radioactive materials, the medical use of radioactive materials, and the packaging and transportation of radioactive materials. Each of these chapters has an impact on the practice of nuclear pharmacy. For example, 10 CFR Part 19 delineates requirements for providing instructions to workers regarding radiation safety practices, for reporting to workers their radiation exposures, and for notifying workers of their rights regarding inspections. 10 CFR 20 specifies radiation protection standards including maximum radiation dose limits to workers, the general public, and pregnant women; radiation monitoring of physical facilities and of personnel; proper use of radiation symbols, signs, and labels; receiving and opening packaging containing radioactive materials; and storage, control, and waste disposal of radioactive materials. 10 CFR 30 and 32 describe, respectively, rules involved with licensing for the handling and use of radioactive materials and for the manufacture and/or distribution of radioactive materials. Nuclear pharmacies, as commercial distributors of radioactive materials, are generally licensed pursuant to Part 32 regulations. 10 CFR 35 details requirements for the medical use of radioactive materials, including general administrative requirements for the radiation safety program; general technical requirements for maintenance and use of radiation instruments, for handling radiopharmaceutical dosages, for radiation surveys, for release of patients containing radioactive materials, and for storage and disposal of radioactive waste. 10 CFR 35 also details specific procedural requirements involved in the use of radiopharmaceuticals for uptake, dilution and excretion studies, for imaging and localization studies, and for therapy; training and experience requirements for radiation safety officer, authorized user physician, authorized medical physicist, and authorized nuclear pharmacist; and specific records and reports. 10 CFR 71 specifies standards for packaging of radioactive materials for transport.

An important philosophy mandated in these regulations is ALARA, an acronym for maintaining radiation exposures *As Low As Reasonably Achievable*. In practice, this means that management and workers must strive to keep radiation exposures well below maximum permissible limits. Typical ALARA goals are radiation exposures that are no more than 10% or 30% of the applicable limit, depending on type of worker activity. ALARA is achieved by judicious application of radiation protection principles (*viz*, time, distance, and shielding) and contamination control.

The regulation of radiopharmaceuticals as drug products has an interesting history. The enactment in 1962 of the Kefauver-Harris Amendments to the FD&C Act significantly increased federal control of the development, production, and premarket testing of drugs. These new requirements severely threatened the availability of radiopharmaceuticals, which many considered to be not *real drugs* because of their lack of pharmacological effects. This potential problem was averted, however, when the FDA promptly issued a temporary exemption for radioactive new drugs from these regulations, provided they were distributed in complete compliance with existing AEC regulations. The temporary exemption was rescinded, in part, in 1971 and subsequently totally revoked in 1975. Thereafter, radiopharmaceuticals have been regulated by the FDA in the same manner as all other drugs. This includes testing for safety and efficacy under Investigational New Drug (IND) provisions, approval for marketing drugs or biologicals through the New Drug Application (NDA) process, production under Current Good Manufacturing Practices (cGMPs), and information contained in labeling and promotional materials.

Although the legislative intent of the FD&C Act was that it would not interfere with the practices of medicine and pharmacy, the highly specialized practice of nuclear pharmacy led to confusion and uncertainty as to which compounding activities constituted manufacturing and which were included in the traditional practice of pharmacy. Hence, in 1984, the FDA published its *Nuclear Pharmacy Guideline: Criteria for Determin-*

ing When to Register as a Drug Establishment. In addition to common nuclear pharmacy preparation activities, such as those involving generator-produced Tc-99m and reagent kits, this FDA document specifically stated that a nuclear pharmacy that "operates an accelerator or nuclear reactor to provide radionuclides and radiochemicals to manufacture radioactive drugs to be dispensed under a prescription" does not have to register as a drug establishment. This statement has been especially important for the compounding of PET radiopharmaceuticals, whose short half-lives (eg, 2, 10, 20, and 110 minutes for O-15, N-13, C-11, and F-18, respectively) effectively preclude traditional bulk manufacturing and wide distribution and thus require preparation in close proximity to the location of use.

During the 1990s, as PET evolved from predominantly research applications to routine clinical use in patient care, the FDA began viewing the preparation of PET radiopharmaceuticals as being more complex, requiring special facilities and controls, compared to other radiopharmaceuticals. Hence, the FDA announced in 1995 that it intended to regulate PET radiopharmaceuticals as manufactured new drugs rather than as compounded products. The FDAMA of 1997 specifically addressed preparation of PET radiopharmaceuticals in its Section 121, authorizing FDA to develop procedures and requirements for cGMPs and for submission of new drug applications and abbreviated new drug applications specific for PET radiopharmaceuticals. At the time of this writing, FDA has developed draft proposed rules and guidance documents for PET radiopharmaceuticals, but finalization and implementation remain in process. Nonetheless, over the next few years, the preparation of PET radiopharmaceuticals is expected to transition from state-regulated professional compounding to FDA-regulated manufacturing.

With regard to non-PET radiopharmaceuticals, the FDAMA of 1997 expressly excluded radiopharmaceuticals from its Section 127 which dealt with pharmacy compounding.[2] The associated Conference Report stated that "nothing in [the radiopharmaceutical exclusion clause] is intended to change or otherwise affect the current law with respect to radiopharmaceuticals." Thus, it appears that the FDA's 1984 Nuclear Pharmacy Guideline continues to apply for the compounding of non-PET radiopharmaceuticals.

Radiopharmaceuticals, because of their radioactivity, also are classified as hazardous materials. Consequently, they are subject to regulation by a variety of other federal and state agencies. For example, the DOT regulates the transport of hazardous [radioactive] materials, the Occupational Safety and Health Administration (OSHA) regulates the handling of hazardous [radioactive] materials in the workplace, and the Environmental Protection Agency (EPA) regulates the disposal of hazardous [radioactive] waste.

Regulation of nuclear pharmacists also reflects the dichotomous nature of their practice involving radiopharmaceuticals as both radioactive materials and drug products. Nuclear pharmacy practice, being highly technical and specialized, has presented a rather unique challenge to the state boards of pharmacy. The National Association of Boards of Pharmacy (NABP) has assumed a leadership role in assisting individual state boards with guidance in this area. Since 1977, the NABP has published *Model Regulations for Nuclear Pharmacy,* a document that was developed and is maintained through timely revisions in consultation with the FDA, NRC, pharmacy professional organizations, and individual practicing nuclear pharmacists. Although variable, most state boards of pharmacy tend to follow, in large part, these NABP Model Regulations. One important part of these regulations is the recognition of a *Qualified Nuclear Pharmacist.* A recent version of the NABP Model Regulations contains the following definition:

"Qualified Nuclear Pharmacist" means a currently licensed Pharmacist in the State of practice, who is certified as a Nuclear Pharmacist by the State Board of Pharmacy or by a certification Board recognized by the State Board of Pharmacy, or who meets the following standards:

1. Minimum standards of training for "authorized user status" of radioactive material [cite State Radiation Control Agency or NRC licensure guide.].
2. Completed a minimum of 200 contact hours of instruction in nuclear pharmacy and the safe handling and the use of radioactive materials from a program approved by the State Board of Pharmacy, with emphasis in the following areas:
   a. radiation physics and instrumentation;
   b. radiation protection;
   c. mathematics of radioactivity;
   d. radiation biology; and
   e. radiopharmaceutical chemistry.
3. Attained a minimum of 500 hours of clinical nuclear pharmacy training under the supervision of a qualified nuclear pharmacist.

Nuclear pharmacists also are regulated with regard to handling of radioactive materials by the NRC and/or analogous state agencies. Initially, training and experience requirements to be named as an authorized user on a commercial nuclear pharmacy license were based on the criteria used for physicians or radiation safety officers. In 1994, the NRC revised its regulations to add a definition for *Authorized Nuclear Pharmacist* along with specific criteria for individuals to be recognized as such. The training requirements for an Authorized Nuclear Pharmacist established in 1994 were revised slightly by NRC in its 2002 revision of 10 CFR 35, and currently require an Authorized Nuclear Pharmacist to be a pharmacist who:

a. Is certified as a nuclear pharmacist by a specialty board whose certification process includes all of the requirements in paragraph b of this section and whose certification has been recognized by the Commission or an Agreement State; or

b.1. Has completed 700 hours in a structured educational program consisting of both:
Didactic training in the following areas–
   • radiation physics and instrumentation;
   • radiation protection;
   • mathematics pertaining to the use and measurement of radioactivity;
   • chemistry of byproduct material for medical use; and
   • radiation biology; and
Supervised practical experience in a nuclear pharmacy involving–
   • shipping, receiving, and performing related radiation surveys;
   • using and performing checks for proper operation of instruments used to determine the activity of dosages, survey meters, and, if appropriate, instruments used to measure alpha- or beta-emitting radionuclides;
   • calculating, assaying, and safely preparing dosages for patients or human research subjects;
   • using administrative controls to avoid medical events in the administration of byproduct material;
   • using procedures to prevent or minimize radioactive contamination and using proper decontamination procedures; and

b.2. Has obtained written certification, signed by a preceptor authorized nuclear pharmacist, that the individual has satisfactorily completed the requirements in paragraph b.1. of this section and has achieved a level of competency sufficient to function independently as an authorized nuclear pharmacist.

Prior to 1994, associated NRC regulations restricted radiopharmaceutical preparation and dispensing to FDA-approved products. However, along with the recognition of authorized nuclear pharmacists in its 1994 rule revisions, the NRC rescinded these restrictions to thereafter permit authorized nuclear pharmacists to prepare and dispense extemporaneously compounded radiopharmaceuticals in addition to commercially manufactured products.

Nuclear pharmacists who are involved in performing nuclear laboratory tests (eg, plasma and/or red cell volume determinations, Schilling tests for vitamin B-12 absorption) are subject to certain laboratory regulations. The Clinical Laboratory Improvement Amendments (CLIA) were passed by Congress in 1988 to establish quality standards for all laboratory testing to ensure the accuracy, reliability, and timeliness of patient test results regardless of where the testing is performed. A laboratory is defined as any facility that performs laboratory testing on specimens derived from humans for the purpose of providing information for the diagnosis, prevention, treatment of disease, or impairment of, or assessment of health. Implementation of the CLIA program, including inspection and certification of laboratories, is the responsibility of the Division of Laboratory Services of the Centers for Medicare and Medicaid Services (CMS).

EDUCATION AND CERTIFICATION

Nuclear pharmacists are specialists who must gain certain knowledge and skills beyond those of generalist practitioners. To aid educators and to ensure compliance with regulations regarding the training of nuclear pharmacists, documents have been prepared that describe the didactic knowledge base and the practice experience components that should be included in a nuclear pharmacy training program. The ASHP has developed standards for residency training in nuclear pharmacy. These standards include the qualifications of the training site, the nuclear pharmacy service, and the program director and preceptors, as well as the qualifications of the applicant. Standards for the residency program itself also are presented, including detailed goal statements and associated educational objectives in areas such as practice foundation skills, direct patient care, drug information and drug policy development, and practice management. The Section on Nuclear Pharmacy, APhA has prepared guidelines for the training of nuclear pharmacists. The guidelines encompass a detailed syllabus for didactic instruction in:

1. Radiation physics and instrumentation;
2. Mathematics of radioactivity use and measurement;
3. Radiation protection and regulations;
4. Radiation biology;
5. Radiopharmaceutical chemistry;
6. The clinical use of radiopharmaceuticals.

A detailed listing of experiential components also is described within the document, along with the suggested number of contact hours for each major area.

Pharmacists may receive the training necessary to enter the practice of nuclear pharmacy by several approaches. A few schools of pharmacy offer a series of undergraduate elective courses to fulfill the didactic requirement. Practice experience is attained either through a nuclear pharmacy within the school or through a summer internship program. Postgraduate education through an MS degree program or a residency in nuclear pharmacy provides another route by which a pharmacist can enter nuclear pharmacy practice. Many of the nuclear pharmacists in hospital practice have this type of educational background. A certificate program is another option by which a pharmacist can obtain the didactic training required by the NRC or State Board of Pharmacy. These are available through some schools of pharmacy and can vary in length from five consecutive weeks on site followed by experiential training to several months in which didactic and experiential training are intermixed. In some programs, the didactic coursework is available via videotapes or the internet, thus allowing the trainee the flexibility of learning at home or work and customizing his/her own schedule.

Regardless of the educational approach to training, nuclear pharmacists can demonstrate their competency by gaining certification in nuclear pharmacy. The Board of Pharmaceutical Specialties (BPS), established in 1976 by APhA, recognized nuclear pharmacy as the first specialty in pharmacy practice in 1978. Since 1982, the BPS has offered certification examinations in nuclear pharmacy, with successful applicants earning the status of Board Certified Nuclear Pharmacist (BCNP). Prerequisites for the certification examination include graduation from an accredited school of pharmacy, valid license to practice pharmacy, and at least 4000 hours of experience in nuclear pharmacy practice, of which:

- Up to 2000 hours may be obtained from nuclear pharmacy course work completed in academic settings;
- Up to 2000 hours may be obtained from nuclear pharmacy residency programs;
- Up to 2000 hours may be obtained from internships in licensed nuclear pharmacies or health-care facilities;
- Up to 4000 hours may be obtained from nuclear pharmacy practice in a licensed nuclear pharmacy or health-care facility.

Certification in nuclear pharmacy is issued for a period of 7 years. Recertification for an additional 7 years can be gained by successful completion of one of two processes, either by re-examination or by participation in a BPS-approved professional development (continuing education) program.

PHARMACEUTICAL CARE

Pharmaceutical care has been described as foundational to *generalist* practice. Moreover, pharmaceutical care typically has been defined as a practice in which the practitioner takes responsibility for a patient's *drug therapy* needs for the purpose of positive patient outcomes. Hence, on the surface, the *specialty* of nuclear pharmacy, which deals primarily with *diagnostic* radiopharmaceuticals, may appear to fall outside the precepts of pharmaceutical care. However, when viewed more broadly, many activities routinely performed by nuclear pharmacists directly or indirectly contribute to positive patient outcomes.

As noted in the introduction, nuclear medicine procedures are commonly employed to aid in the diagnosis of disease as well as to monitor therapeutic outcome. Both endeavors may be considered relevant to the concept of pharmaceutical care. Nuclear pharmacists and pharmacists in general provide pharmaceutical care through their knowledge of applications of radiopharmaceuticals in nuclear medicine. Bone imaging to stage cancer followed by monitoring of the course of therapy is an example of the importance of a nuclear medicine procedure to pharmaceutical care. Determination of the ejection fraction of the heart prior to and during the course of therapy with doxorubicin, to monitor the cardiotoxicity of the cancer chemotherapy agent, is another important application of nuclear medicine relevant to the role of a pharmacist in the care of a patient. Nuclear medicine procedures also are applied to patients with various types of cancer prior to and following surgical, radiation, and/or chemotherapy to monitor therapeutic response, detect residual or recurrent malignant disease, and to differentiate viable tumor from necrosis and scar.

The pharmacologic actions of therapeutic drugs frequently are used to increase the specificity or the sensitivity of nuclear medicine procedures as well as to reduce the time necessary to conduct certain procedures. These procedures are termed "drug intervention" or "pharmacological nuclear medicine" procedures. A few examples of therapeutic drugs used as interventions include sincalide and morphine sulfate in hepatobiliary imaging procedures, acetazolamide in cerebral blood flow imaging procedures, dipyridamole, adenosine, and dobutamine in myocardial perfusion imaging procedures, and furosemide and captopril in renal imaging procedures. Furosemide, for instance, is used to aid in the identification of a problem in the urinary tract. Following administration of a renally excreted radiopharmaceutical to the patient, a gamma camera monitors its accumulation in the renal collecting system. Once the collecting system is filled, furosemide is injected intravenously. If the problem in the collecting system is caused by a ureteral obstruction, most of the radioactive urine will remain in the collecting system. Conversely, if there is a nonobstructive condition, such as dilation of the renal pelvis due to prior urinary tract surgery or a previous obstruction, radioactive urine will flow out of the collecting system down the ureter to the bladder as a result of the diuretic action of the furosemide.

These interventional procedures, employing pharmacological drugs with radiopharmaceuticals, are useful in assessing the need for surgery or other aggressive therapy versus a less drastic, more conservative medical treatment. The outcome of the procedures, as well as any subsequent follow-up procedures, will be very important in the management of the patient. The nuclear pharmacist can help develop protocols for drug intervention procedures. Dosing, storage, drug interactions, treatments for adverse reactions, and information on contraindications for interventional drugs are other traditional services that the nuclear pharmacist can provide. When several therapeutic drugs are available for the same interventional procedure, the nuclear pharmacist may become a member of the medical team responsible for selection of the optimal agent for the patient population or the individual patient.

While some therapeutic drugs are useful in nuclear medicine, others may adversely affect the localization and/or kinetics of the radiopharmaceutical. For example, drugs listed in Table 106-1 may decrease the thyroidal uptake of radioiodide given to a patient to determine thyroid function. If the drug reduces the amount of radioactivity taken up by the thyroid, a patient with hyperthyroidism might be underdiagnosed as having less severe disease or misdiagnosed as normal. This could lead to inadequate treatment of the patient's condition or, if the interference was recognized, delay appropriate treatment until valid testing could be repeated. The need to monitor for medications and other therapies prior to a bone imaging procedure is important also. As is noted in Table 106-2, unexpected organ uptake or a decrease in skeletal uptake of the bone-imaging radiopharmaceutical may occur from several different types of drugs or therapies administered to the patient before the nuclear medicine procedure.

The nuclear pharmacist provides pharmaceutical care by monitoring for interfering drugs and other factors prior to a nuclear medicine procedure or following the procedure if questions arise concerning unusual or unanticipated outcomes. Although nuclear pharmacists are not always present within the hospital or clinic, they may provide care by developing and sharing information with nuclear medicine personnel or hospital pharmacists involved in drug monitoring. Prescreening for potential problems can be helpful in preventing additional costs incurred by repeat procedures as well as limiting the radiation dose to the patient. Pharmaceutical care also is practiced by nuclear pharmacists when they utilize their knowledge of poten-

tial problems in the formulation, preparation, and dispensing of radiopharmaceutical products to prevent suboptimal results of nuclear medicine procedures due to product-related problems.

The basic clinical activities of a nuclear pharmacist are similar to those conducted by pharmacists in other areas of practice. The nuclear pharmacist is the product information specialist for nuclear medicine personnel and patients. In-service presentations on new products, drug information, and drugs or therapies that may compromise a nuclear medicine procedure are the responsibility of the nuclear pharmacist. Information on trade name versus generic products, chemical names, dosage forms, common dosages, and sources of products are provided by the nuclear pharmacist. Cost and availability are important considerations in nuclear medicine. This is especially true because of the short half-lives of radionuclides used in radiopharmaceuticals. Scheduling of patients and the timely availability of the radiopharmaceutical needed for the procedure are critical to conducting nuclear medicine services at an economically acceptable level. Counseling patients, ensuring discontinuation of medications or other therapies that may interfere with the biodistribution of a radiopharmaceutical, and individualized dosage calculations are examples of pharmaceutical care supplied by nuclear pharmacists.

The nuclear pharmacist must be aware of the route of elimination of a radiopharmaceutical and conditions that may adversely affect elimination. The status of kidney function (or dialysis therapy) can be of significance for radiopharmaceuticals eliminated by the kidneys. The bilirubin level may affect the elimination of radiopharmaceuticals employed in hepatobiliary procedures, such as those conducted in infants to distinguish biliary atresia from neonatal hepatitis. Radiopharmaceutical dosage calculations are important in such situations and, thus, constitute an important role for nuclear pharmacists. The potential absorbed radiation dose to the patient may be affected by the status of the route of elimination and, of course, pediatric versus adult population. Also, radiation dosimetry is of significance in radiation exposure to the fetus in the pregnant woman. A routine question for women of childbearing age is, "Are you pregnant or is there a possibility that you might be pregnant?" If the woman later found that she was pregnant or if the nuclear medicine procedure on a known pregnant woman is considered beneficial relative to the risk, the nuclear pharmacist can calcu-

Table 106-1. Drugs That May Decrease the Thyroidal Uptake of Radioiodide

Adrenocorticosteroids	Lugol's solution
Aminosalicylic acid	Meglumine diatrizoate
Androgens	Meprobamate
Anticoagulants (heparin, warfarin)	Methimazole
Antihistamines	Morphine
Antithyroid drugs	Para-aminosalicylic acid
Antitussives	Perchlorates
Benzodiazepines	Phenylbutazone
Cholecystographic agents (oral)	Phenytoin
Cimetidine	Propylthiouracil
Clioquinol	Resorcinol
Competing anions (Br$^-$, ClO$_4^-$, BF$_4^-$, SCN$^-$)	Salicylates
Corticotropin	Sodium diatrizoate
Epinephrine	Sodium nitroprusside
Estrogens	Sulfonamides
Expectorants (iodine-containing)	Sulfonylureas
Fluorides (inorganic)	Thiocyanates
Iodides (inorganic & topical)	Thiopental
Iodinated radiopaque contrast media	Thyroglobulin
Iodine tincture	Thyroid extracts
Iodine-containing collyria	Thyroxine
Iodoquinol	Tolbutamide
Liothyronine sodium	Sulfobromophthalein
Liotrix	Vitamin/mineral supplements
Lithium	

Table 106-2. Drugs and Therapies That May Affect the Disposition of Technetium-99m Phosphate and Diphosphonate Bone Agents

Unexpected organ uptake of the radiopharmaceutical due to the presence of

Allopurinol	Methotrexate
Aluminum-containing antacids	Penicillamine
Amphotericin B	Pentamidine
Bleomycin	Radiation therapy
Calcium gluconate	Red blood cell transfusions
Cisplatin	Sodium diatrizoate
Cocaine	Sodium iothalamate
Cyclophosphamide	Stannous ions
Dextrose (intravenous)	Verapamil
Doxorubicin	Vincristine
Iron therapy	

Decreased bone uptake of the radiopharmaceutical due to the presence of

Calcitonin	Indomethacin
Calcium	Iodinated contrast media
Corticosteroids	Parathyroid hormone
Dichloromethane	Iron therapy
Estrogens	Inorganic phosphates (enema)
Etidrenate disodium	
Ferrous salts	Steroid therapy
Glucocorticoids	Vitamin D_3

late the potential radiation dose to the fetus, knowing the specific organ distribution for the radiopharmaceutical, the dosage of radioactivity given, and the type of radiation emitted by the radionuclide, as well as other factors.

Nuclear pharmacists provide pharmaceutical care to breast-feeding women. There is concern for radiation exposure to the nursing child and increased exposure to the woman's breast from the radiopharmaceutical. Knowledge of the true risk is critical because the benefit of the procedure would be lost if the procedure was not conducted when the risk was minimal and, conversely, if the procedure was conducted when the risk was excessive in comparison to the benefit. The radiation risk to the child from ingestion of the radioactivity is influenced by many factors, such as the radiopharmaceutical, the characteristics of the radionuclide, the amount of radioactivity given to the mother, and the frequency and volume of feeding. Several guidelines, including NRC's Regulatory Guide 8.39, have been published that address the course of action to be taken, which may be interruption for a given time interval or total cessation of breastfeeding. Using patient-specific data and certain assumptions, the nuclear pharmacist can determine the appropriateness and applicability of these guidelines and formulate specific recommendations for individual patients.

Although documented adverse reactions to radiopharmaceuticals are comparatively rare, the nuclear pharmacist provides pharmaceutical care by monitoring for adverse reactions. Adverse reactions to radiopharmaceuticals, if they do occur, are usually mild and transient and require little medical treatment. The most common of these is a skin rash associated with Tc-99m diphosphonate bone agents. However, a few life-threatening reactions (eg, anaphylaxis) have been reported for some radiopharmaceuticals such as Tc-99m sulfur colloid. The nuclear pharmacist should ensure that epinephrine, pressor amines, corticosteroids, antihistamines, and advanced cardiopulmonary life-support systems are readily available in the unlikely event that a severe reaction was to occur. Also, the nuclear pharmacist can dispel unrealistic fears of allergic reactions to radiopharmaceuticals, such as a patient scheduled for a diagnostic thyroid procedure using radioactive iodine who has a history of reactions to iodinated X-ray contrast media or to seafood. In this instance, the nuclear pharmacist can reassure the patient that the radiopharmaceutical and iodinated X-ray contrast media are distinctly different in chemical structure and that the amount (mass) of radioactive iodine to be admin-

istered is only one millionth of the average daily ingestion of iodine from dietary sources.

Drug Utilization Evaluation (DUE) and Drug Utilization Review (DUR) are important functions for nuclear pharmacists, especially in a larger institutional setting. A prime example is associated with the nuclear medicine procedure employed to differentiate between an infarcted and ischemic condition in the heart. A radiopharmaceutical that localizes in myocardial muscle in proportion to coronary perfusion is injected during *stress,* commonly induced by graded exercise on a treadmill. Imaging is performed after this stress and also, separately, while the patient is in a resting state. Differentiation between an infarcted and an ischemic area can be obtained by comparison of images at rest and images at stress. If the patient has experienced a myocardial infarct, the damaged tissue will contain less radioactivity than the healthy tissue both when the heart is at rest and when it is stressed. If, however, the patient has ischemic heart disease, the affected area will appear normal at rest but will show significantly less than normal radioactivity at stress, because of stress-induced ischemia. The pharmacologically induced coronary vasodilatory effect of dipyridamole or adenosine can substitute for exercise stress in patients who are unable to exercise adequately. Patients who are elderly or obese, who have peripheral vascular disease or orthopedic problems, or who are on beta-blocker therapy are examples of candidates for pharmacological stress. In some of these patients, however, use of dipyridamole or adenosine is contraindicated due to severe bronchopulmonary disease, certain cardiac conduction disorders, or the presence of methylxanthines (eg, theophylline, caffeine). In such patients, cardiac stress can generally be achieved using dobutamine, whose pharmacologic effects include positive inotropic and chronotropic cardiac responses. The nuclear pharmacist can be extensively involved in DUE or DUR activities associated with these pharmacologic stress procedures.

With an increasing number of therapeutic radiopharmaceuticals being developed, marketed, and used, new opportunities are becoming available for nuclear pharmacists to provide pharmaceutical care to patients receiving radiopharmaceutical therapy. Expanded roles for nuclear pharmacists in these situations include activities such as calculating individual patient dosages, counseling patients regarding their therapy, and monitoring patients for adverse or toxic effects. Nuclear pharmacists can also determine patient eligibility for early release from the treatment facility, in compliance with NRC requirements, based on patient specific measurements and calculations. Counseling of such patients regarding radiation safety precautions to be followed after release can also be provided by nuclear pharmacists.

Patient-specific pharmaceutical care presents a major challenge for nuclear pharmacists practicing in a commercial nuclear pharmacy. These pharmacists typically dispense unit dose radiopharmaceuticals to physicians in hospitals or clinics; they have little if any direct patient interaction and have only limited, if any, access to patient medical records. In most states, these nuclear pharmacists are exempted from mandatory requirements for patient counseling. Hence nearly all pharmaceutical care activities, either general or patient-specific, are undertaken indirectly through physicians and other healthcare providers. This situation could be improved by establishing convenient mechanisms for nuclear pharmacists to access patient information (eg, by electronic networking) and to communicate directly with patients (eg, video teleconferencing). Another viable approach could be to establish a close working relationship with one or more on-site hospital or clinic pharmacists. This partnering between an on-site pharmacist and a nuclear pharmacist specialist, somewhat analogous to a physician generalist consulting with a physician specialist, could be an efficient way for nuclear pharmacist specialists to provide enhanced pharmaceutical care to many more patients.

EXPANDED SERVICES

Nuclear pharmacists traditionally provide radiopharmaceuticals and professional services to nuclear medicine. However, some nuclear pharmacists have encouraged the expansion of services into other areas of medical imaging. Imaging modalities such as computerized tomography (CT), magnetic resonance imaging (MRI), ultrasound, and other radiographic procedures as well as nuclear medicine are used commonly to aid in the determination of a disease state and to monitor therapeutic outcomes. Each of these diagnostic imaging modalities often employs some form of *contrast agent* to enhance the utility of the imaging procedure. All of these contrast agents are classified as drugs. They have specified indications, contraindications, warnings, precautions, and dosages. They may cause adverse reactions ranging from minor to life-threatening effects, and may be involved in various drug interactions or otherwise interfere with subsequent procedures. Specific preparation for a patient, including pretreatment with certain drugs, prior to an imaging procedure may be necessary. Pharmacologic drug interventions may also be important in performing some of these imaging procedures. Patient counseling is another concern for those who conduct imaging procedures. Based on these drug-related issues, it is obvious that the services of a pharmacist should be provided to patients and personnel in diagnostic imaging areas. While the nuclear pharmacist may be the logical person to provide this service, the physical location and time constraints of many nuclear pharmacists do not allow the full extent of pharmaceutical care that should be provided. Nonetheless, even the nuclear pharmacist in a commercial nuclear pharmacy can serve as a valuable source of information and can partner with institutional pharmacists. Pharmacists in community and hospital settings can establish working relationships with nuclear pharmacists who can provide consultation in these areas.

Some nuclear pharmacists have also encouraged the expansion of services into therapeutic radiology or radiation oncology. For example, brachytherapy uses radioactive devices (also called sources) that are inserted into cancerous tissues to deliver localized radiation therapy. These radioactive devices are generally solids (eg, seeds or wires) but in some cases may be a liquid contained in a balloon. Nuclear pharmacists can be involved in providing device product services including ordering, storage, inventory, dosage assay, and dispensing. As applicable, nuclear

pharmacists can determine patient eligibility for early release from the treatment facility, in compliance with NRC requirements, based on patient specific measurements and calculations and can provide counseling of such patients regarding radiation safety precautions to be followed after release.

SUMMARY

Nuclear pharmacy is a specialized practice of pharmacy focusing on radiopharmaceuticals. Nonetheless, the basic functions and responsibilities of the nuclear pharmacist are the same as those for others who practice pharmacy. The nuclear pharmacist is an expert in a specific class of drugs but also must remain current on all medications employed in the treatment of disease, especially those used for interventional studies, those that potentially interfere with nuclear medicine procedures, and those whose effectiveness or toxicity may be monitored by nuclear medicine studies. The knowledge and capabilities of a nuclear pharmacist build upon the basic skills and knowledge imparted to all pharmacists through the education required to enter the practice of pharmacy. The additional training needed to become a nuclear pharmacist can be attained by several routes. Although some nuclear pharmacists practice in a hospital setting, most nuclear pharmacists practice in commercial nuclear pharmacies that provide services to numerous nearby hospitals and clinics.

Pharmaceutical care activities are an important aspect of nuclear pharmacy practice. The majority of these activities are indirect, often performed in consultation with nuclear medicine staff. Direct, patient-specific pharmaceutical care is difficult for nuclear pharmacists practicing in commercial settings; in these situations, partnering between a nuclear pharmacist and an on-site pharmacist may be a viable option. Some nuclear pharmacists have also expanded their roles to provide services in other diagnostic imaging areas and in radiation oncology regarding contrast media drugs and radioactive devices for brachytherapy, respectively.

The specialty practice of nuclear pharmacy has been instrumental in leading pharmacy into the development and the recognition of specialties in pharmacy. The dedication of early pioneers and the support of professional pharmacy organizations have been of great significance in the development of nuclear pharmacy to the degree of excellence experienced today. Practitioners, educators, and other professionals are challenged by the past to build on and surpass the success of those that have gone before. As is true for all of pharmacy, the future of the profession cannot stand upon the past, but only on innovative care and services provided by those with a vision for the future.

BIBLIOGRAPHY

ASHP Supplemental Standard and Learning Objectives for Residency Training in Nuclear Pharmacy Practice. Bethesda, MD: ASHP, 1997.
Augustine SC, Norenberg JP, et al. *J Am Pharm Assoc* 2002; 42:93.
Brucer M. *A Chronology of Nuclear Medicine 1600–1989.* St Louis: Heritage, 1990.
Callahan RJ. *Hosp Pharm* 1990; 25:697.
Callahan RJ. *Semin Nucl Med* 1996; 26:85.
Callahan RJ, Dragotakes SC. *Clin Pos Imag* 1999; 2:211.
Chilton HM. *J Pharm Pract* 1989; 2:302.
Clanton JA. *J Pharm Pract* 1989; 2:191.
Glatcz G, Ponto JA, Hladik WB III. *Am J Health-Syst Pharm* 1990; 47:1628.
Gobuty AH. *Am J Health-Syst Pharm* 1989; 2:171.
Gregorio N, Hladik WB III, Kavula MP. *J Pharm Pract* 1989; 2:284.
Hammes RJ, Laven DL, Catizon C. *J Pharm Pract* 1989; 2:314.
Hilliard N. *The Nuclear Pharmacy.* Little Rock, AR: University of Arkansas for Medical Sciences; 2003. (Available at: http://nucle-arpharmacy.uams.edu/)
Hinkle GH, Beightol RW, et al. *J Pharm Pract* 1989; 2:177.

Hung JC, Augustine SC, et al. *J Am Pharm Assoc* 2002; 42:789.
Hung JC, Ponto JA, Hammes RJ. *Semin Nucl Med* 1996:208.
Kowalsky RJ, Ponto JA. *J Pharm Pract* 1989; 2:139.
Laven DL, Shaw SM. *J Pharm Pract* 1989; 2: 287.
Manning RG, Wolfangel RG. *J Pharm Pract* 1989; 2:185.
Nuclear Pharmacy Practice Guidelines. Washington DC: Section on Nuclear Pharmacy, APhA, 1994.
Petry NA. *J Pharm Pract* 1989; 2:306.
Ponto JA. *J Pharm Pract* 1989; 2:299.
Ponto JA. *Hosp Pharm* 1996; 31:190.
Ponto JA. *Radiographics* 1998; 18:1395.

Ponto JA, Hung JC. *J Nucl Med Technol* 2000; 28:76.
Rhodes BA, Hladik WB III, Norenberg JP. *Semin Nucl Med* 1996; 26:77.
Rotman M, Laven DL, Levine G. *Semin Nucl Med* 1996; 26:96.
Schmelter RF, Godat JF, Cole CN. *J Pharm Pract* 1989; 2:280.
Shaw SM. *Am J Pharm Ed* 1994; 58:190.
Shaw SM. *J APhA* 1997; NS37:99.
Shaw SM, Ice RD. *J Nucl Med Technol* 2000; 28:8.
Silberstein EB, Ryan J, et al. *J Nucl Med* 1996; 37:185.
Swanson DP, Jurgens RW. *J Pharm Pract* 1989; 2:162.
Syllabus for Nuclear Pharmacy Training, developed by the Section on Nuclear Pharmacy, APhA, Washington, DC, 1994.

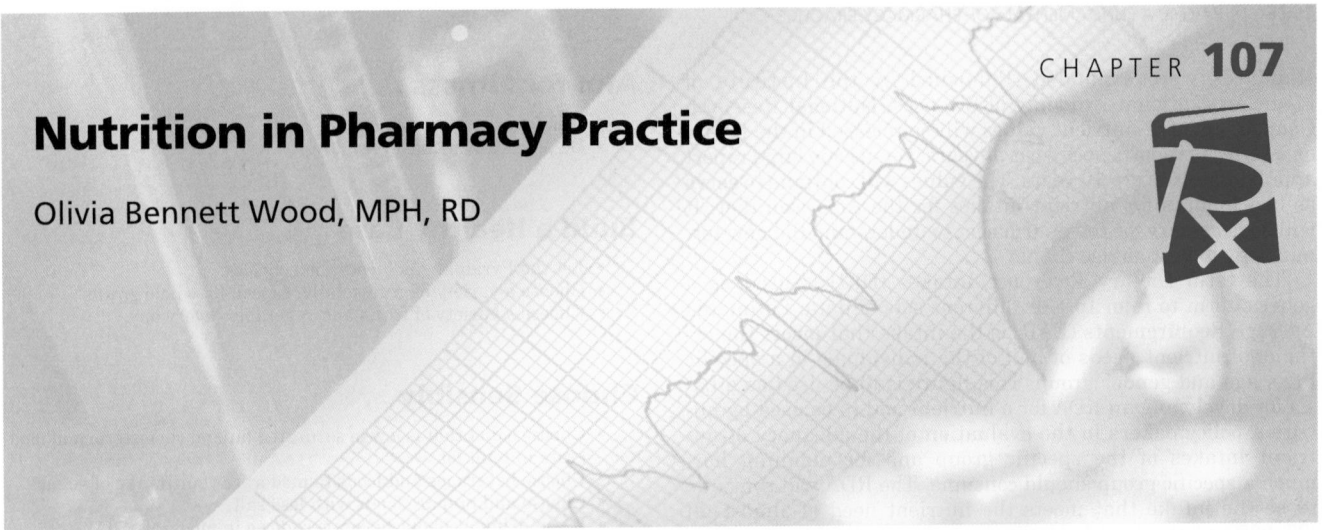

CHAPTER 107

Nutrition in Pharmacy Practice

Olivia Bennett Wood, MPH, RD

Practicing pharmacists are asked many questions about foods and nutrition, including specific questions about which products or supplements a client may be considering for purchase and what amount of a product to ingest. A review of basic nutrition and knowledge of dietary standards and guidance helps provide the pharmacist with sound information to supply the client.

NUTRITION 101

Nutrients are chemical substances found in food that are needed for life. The realization that nutrients are chemicals helps the pharmacist understand why there are interactions with drugs, which also are composed of chemicals. Putting together the chemicals from food and drugs is more potentially reactive because of the introduction into the complex system of the body.

There are over 40 different nutrients needed by the body for growth, reproduction, and maintenance of tissue and body regulations. For classification purposes nutrients are divided into six basic categories: proteins, carbohydrates, lipids, vitamins, minerals, and water. The only additional substance needed for life is oxygen. Nutrient groups providing kilocalories (kcal) and thus supplying a source of energy for the body are carbohydrates, proteins, and fat. The Dietary Reference Intakes lists a wide range of acceptable percent of total kilocalories for carbohydrate, 45–65%, for protein, 20–35%, and for fat, 10–35%. Currently in the average US diet, the percent of total kilocalories provided by carbohydrate, protein, and fat is approximately 50, 16, and 34, respectively with much individual variation due to personal diet patterns and behaviors. Another additional source of energy in the US diet is alcohol.

Each category of nutrients performs different, but interrelated, functions in the body. Carbohydrates provide kilocalories for energy and dietary fiber for bulk. Often divided into complex and simple, carbohydrates are found in many food groups, including grains, milk, fruits, and vegetables. Complex carbohydrates include starchy vegetables such as corn and potatoes, many foods prepared from grains such as breads, cereals and pastas and legumes, dried beans, and peas. Simple carbohydrates are the main sugars found in fruit, fructose, and in milk, lactose, and in foods made from sugar such as jellies and syrups. Proteins play the major role in growth, maintenance, and repair of body tissue. Protein can be used by the body to supply kilocalories when carbohydrates and fats are not supplied in adequate amounts, but this is not a desirable function of proteins. Proteins are supplied by both animal and vegetable sources. Animal sources include meats, poultry, fish, eggs, milk, and milk products such as cheese and yogurt. Vegetable sources include nuts, seeds, legumes and smaller amounts in grains and some vegetables. Lipids provide the primary source of kilocalories in the US diet. The term *lipid* is used to encompass both fats and oils, terms that simply indicate the nature of the lipid at room temperature. Fats are solids and oils are liquid at room temperature. Lipids provide essential fatty acids, are components of cell membranes, are involved in synthesis of some hormones, and surround and cushion internal organs as adipose tissue. Vitamins are organic compounds needed in small amounts to help the body function in normal growth, reproduction, and maintenance. They do not supply kilocalories but do facilitate chemical reactions that extract energy from the metabolism of carbohydrate, fat, and protein. Minerals function in a wide array of metabolic roles in the body ranging from enzyme components to electrolyte balance to providing structure for hard tissues. Vitamins and minerals are more fully discussed in Chapter 92. Water is also a nutrient and, next to oxygen, the most important substance needed for life. Approximately two-thirds of the weight of the body is water. Water is important in the proper removal of waste products from the body, is a component of body secretions, helps to regulate body temperature, and provides for lubrication of the body.

Nutrient needs are estimated by balance studies on both animals and humans that compare nutrient intake and excretion, by biochemical markers of a nutrient in the body components and excreta, and by clinical and physical evaluation of humans in both health and disease. Not all types of study are possible on humans; thus a variety of studies is used to estimate a single requirement or a range in the requirement for the nutrient. Nutrients can be consumed in quantities that are too little for good health, a range that is generally thought to be conducive to good health, and an amount, for some nutrients, that cannot only be detrimental to good health, but could be toxic to life. Current research is focused on identifying which nutrients and in what amount have a protective effect in preventing or reducing the risk of chronic diseases.

FOODS AND NUTRITION STANDARDS AND DIETARY GUIDANCE

DIETARY REFERENCE INTAKES—The Recommended Dietary Allowances (RDA) have been recognized universally as the standard for levels of nutrients recommended in the American diet. In 1997, new terminology was introduced and the standards were expanded. Published by the Institute of Medicine, National Academy of Sciences, National Research Council, updated nutrient values will be released in the future as a series of reports over several years, versus one large report approximately every 10 years. The values will continue to serve as benchmarks for nutrient intakes for the American diet. It will be necessary for the pharmacist to understand the new terminology to best advise clients.

The term Dietary Reference Intakes (DRI) is used as a generic term to refer to four different sets of data. Estimated Average Requirements (EAR) is the intake that meets the estimated nutrient needs of half of the individuals in a specific life stage and gender group. This figure is to be used as a basis for developing an RDA for a nutrient and to be used by nutrition policymakers in the evaluation of the adequacy of nutrient intakes of the specific group and for planning how much a specific group should consume. The RDA will continue to be the intake that meets the nutrient need of almost all (97–98%) of the healthy individuals in a specific age and/or gender group. The RDA should be used in guiding individuals to achieve adequate nutrient intake aimed at decreasing the risk of chronic disease. It is based on estimating an average requirement plus an increase to account for the variation within a particular group.

Adequate Intake (AI) is used when sufficient scientific evidence is unavailable to estimate an average requirement. AIs can be used by individuals and professionals as a goal for intake when a RDA cannot be determined for the nutrient. The AI is derived through experimental or observational data that show a mean intake that appears to sustain a desired indicator of health. Tolerable Upper Intake Level (UL) is used to indicate the maximum intake by an individual that is unlikely to pose risks of adverse health effects in almost all healthy individuals in a specified group. The UL is not intended to be a recommended level of intake, and there is no established benefit for individuals to consume nutrients at levels greater than those given by the RDA or the AI.

The DRIs have been under continual revision since 1997, with electrolytes and water recommendations to be released in September 2003. Table 107-1 includes the most recent values for elements, Table 107-2 for vitamins, Table 107-3 for the macronutrients, and Table 107-4 for electrolytes and water. **DIETARY GUIDANCE**—Numbers associated with the DRI standards, reported as grams, milligrams, and micrograms, are not easily interpreted to consumers unless they are related to food and a diet pattern. The practicing pharmacist needs to know acceptable guidelines that are consumer friendly to assist the client. Dietary guidance is meant to be individualized to the client, and it is the individualization that can take a simplistic educational tool and make it fit within an individual's complex need. Dietary guidance fosters time-honored concepts of good nutrition: variety, balance, and moderation. Variety refers to choosing different foods each day from within different food groups; balance refers to including foods from all food groups daily; and moderation refers to controlling serving size to allow for variety and balance within a kilocalorie allowance.

THE DIETARY GUIDELINES FOR AMERICANS AND THE FOOD GUIDE PYRAMID—The Dietary Guidelines for Americans[1] provide advice about nutrition and food choices related to disease prevention for healthy Americans age 2 years and older. The guidelines have been published every 5 years since 1980 by the US Department of Agriculture (USDA) and the US Department of Health and Human Services (DHHS). This standard is also helpful in advising clients with modified diets, as all diets, normal and modified, are based on the same general principles. The current edition of the Dietary Guidelines, released in 2000, is in Figure 107-1. There are 10 Dietary Guidelines, listed under three overall themes. It is intended that all 10 be used together to plan appropriate nutritional care for individuals and groups. The 2000 Dietary Guidelines for Americans include

Aim for Fitness . . .

- Aim for a healthy weight.
- Be physically active every day.

Build a Healthy Base . . .

- Let the Pyramid guide your food choices.
- Choose a variety of grains daily, especially whole grains.
- Choose a variety of fruits and vegetables every day.

Choose Sensibly . . .

- Choose a diet that is low in saturated fat and cholesterol and moderate in total fat.
- Choose beverages and foods to moderate your intake of sugars.
- Choose and prepare foods with less salt.
- If you drink alcoholic beverages, do so in moderation.

Words such as *variety, low*, and *moderate* have different meanings to different people. A review of each of the guidelines assists the practitioner in helping clients interpret this standard guidance. Specific issues of current debate are integrated within this review of the guidelines.

Aim for Fitness

AIM FOR A HEALTH WEIGHT—The 2000 edition of the Dietary Guidelines placed greater emphasis on the importance of maintenance of a healthy weight. The practicing pharmacist is asked multiple questions about weight gain and loss by consumers. These questions range from asking for interpretation of standards associated with weight to selection of products or programs to assist in weight gain or loss. Clients may be most comfortable with standard weight and height charts (Table 107-5), but a National Institutes of Health (NIH) panel suggests health care providers use the Body Mass Index (BMI) as a standard. The BMI is calculated by weight in kilograms divided by height in meters, squared. This measure minimizes the effect of height and correlates with other more precise measures of body fatness. The BMI standard is increasingly used in the professional and lay literature (Table 107-6).

Excess weight can be detrimental to good health, and the desire for weight loss is a major concern of many Americans. The current increase in the prevalence of overweight in the US is a major public health concern, particularly in children. Co-morbidities associated with excess weight include commonly known ones such as coronary heart disease (CHD), stroke, hypertension, diabetes mellitus, gout, dyslipidemias, cholecystitis, and gallstones. Less commonly known co-morbidities include obstructive sleep apnea, osteoarthritis of weight-bearing joints, reduced fertility, increased risk of accidents caused by less physical agility, and impaired obstetrical performance.

Pharmacists often are asked to help the consumer select specific food products or supplements advertised to assist with weight loss or gain, as these products are frequently available in the pharmacy setting. A well-balanced diet for weight loss should not require the purchase of any special product. In general, clients wishing to lose weight need professional advice if they wish to select any weight loss product or regimen. Table 107-7 lists NIH guidelines for choosing a weight-loss program, and Table 100-8 lists a means to analyze weight-loss approaches. The minimum number of servings of the Food Guide Pyramid provides approximately 1200 to 1400 kcal. This amount of kilocalories would be an acceptable weight-loss regimen for most adults. **BE PHYSICALLY ACTIVE EACH DAY**—In the fall of 2002, the DRI report addressed activity for the first time. No doubt this was in response to the increasing public health concern regarding overweight and obesity. The recommendation is for one hour per day of total activity time, which correlates with

Table 107-1. Food and Nutrition Board, Institute of Medicine-National Academy of Sciences Dietary Reference Intakes: Elements

DIETARY REFERENCE INTAKES: ELEMENTS

NUTRIENT	FUNCTION	LIFE STAGE GROUP	RDA/AI*	UL[a]	SELECTED FOOD SOURCES	ADVERSE EFFECTS OF EXCESSIVE CONSUMPTION	SPECIAL CONSIDERATIONS
Arsenic	No biological function in humans although animal data indicate a requirement	Infants	ND[b]	ND	Dairy products meat, poultry, fish, grains and cereal	No data on the possible adverse effects of organic arsenic compounds in food were found. Inorganic arsenic is a known toxic substance.	None
		0–6 mo	ND	ND			
		7–12 mo					
		Children					
		1–3 y	ND	ND		Although the UL was not determined for arsenic, there is no justification for adding arsenic to food or supplements.	
		4–8 y	ND	ND			
		Males					
		9–13 y	ND	ND			
		14–18 y	ND	ND			
		19–30 y	ND	ND			
		31–50 y	ND	ND			
		50–70 y	ND	ND			
		>70 y	ND	ND			
		Females					
		9–13 y	ND	ND			
		14–18 y	ND	ND			
		19–30 y	ND	ND			
		31–50 y	ND	ND			
		50–70 y	ND	ND			
		>70 y	ND	ND			
		Pregnancy					
		≤18 y	ND	ND			
		19–30 y	ND	ND			
		31–50 y	ND	ND			
		Lactation					
		≤18 y	ND	ND			
		19–30 y	ND	ND			
		31–50 y	ND	ND			
Boron	No clear biological function in humans although animal data indicate a functional role	Infants		(mg/d)	Fruit-based beverages and products, potatoes, legumes, milk, avocado, peanut butter, peanuts	Reproductive and developmental effects as observed in animal studies.	None
		0–6 mo	ND	ND			
		7–12 mo	ND	ND			
		Children					
		1–3 y	ND	3			
		4–8 y	ND	6			
		Males					
		9–13 y	ND	11			
		14–18 y	ND	17			
		19–30 y	ND	20			
		31–50 y	ND	20			
		50–70 y	ND	20			
		>70 y	ND	20			
		Females					
		9–13 y	ND	11			
		14–18 y	ND	17			
		19–30 y	ND	20			
		31–50 y	ND	20			
		50–70 y	ND	20			
		>70 y	ND	20			
		Pregnancy					
		≤18 y	ND	17			
		19–30 y	ND	20			
		31–50 y	ND	20			
		Lactation					
		≤18 y	ND	17			
		19–30 y	ND	20			
		31–50 y	ND	20			

NOTE: The table is adapted from the DRI reports, see www.nap.edu. It represents Recommended Dietary Allowances (RDAs) in **bold type**. Adequate intakes (AIs) in ordinary type followed by an asterisk (*), and Tolerable Upper Intake Levels (ULs)[a]. RDAs and AIs may both be used as goals for individual intake. RDAs are set to meet the needs of almost all (97 to 98 percent) individuals in a group. For healthy breastfed infants, the AI is the mean intake. The AI for other life stage and gender groups is believed to cover the needs of all individuals in the group, but lack of data prevent being able to specify with confidence the percentage of individuals covered by this intake.

[a]UL = The maximum level of daily nutrient intake that is likely to pose no risk of adverse effects. Unless otherwise specified, the UL represents total intake from food, water, and supplements. Due to lack of suitable data, ULs could not be established for vitamin K, thiamin, riboflavin, vitamin B12, pantothenic acid, biotin, or carotenoids. In the absence of ULs, extra caution may be warranted in consuming levels above recommended intakes.

[b]ND = Not determinable due to lack of data of adverse effects in this age group and concern with regard to lack of ability to handle excess amounts. Source of intake should be from food only to prevent high levels of intake.

SOURCES: *Dietary Reference intakes for Calcium, Phosphorous, Magnesium. Vitamin D, and Fluoride* (1997); *Dietary Reference Intakes for Thiamin, Riboflavin, Niacin, Vitamin B6, Folate, Vitamin B12, Paniothenic Acid, Biotin, and Choline* (1998); *Dietary Reference Intakes for Vitamin C, Vitamin E, Selenium, and Carotenoids (2000);* and *Dietary Reference Intakes for Vitamin A, Vitamin K, Arsenic, Boron, Chromium, Copper, Iodine, Iron, Manganese, Molybdenum, Nickel, Silicon, Vanadium, and Zinc* (2001). These reports may be accessed via www.nap.edu.

Table 107-1. *(continued).*

DIETARY REFERENCE INTAKES: ELEMENTS

NUTRIENT	FUNCTION	LIFE STAGE GROUP	RDA/AI*	UL[a]	SELECTED FOOD SOURCES	ADVERSE EFFECTS OF EXCESSIVE CONSUMPTION	SPECIAL CONSIDERATIONS
Calcium	Essential role in blood clotting, muscle contraction, nerve transmission, and bone and tooth formation	Infants	(mg/d)	(mg/d)	Milk, cheese, yogurt, corn tortillas, calcium-set tofu, Chinese cabbage, kale, broccoli	Kidney stones, hypercalcemia, milk alkali syndrome, and renal insufficiency	Amenorrheic women (exercise- or anorexia nervosa-induced) have reduced net calcium absorption
		0–6 mo	210*	ND[b]			
		7–12 mo	270*	ND			
		Children					There is no consistent data to support that a high protein intake increase calcium requirement.
		1–3 y	500*	2,500			
		4–8 y	800*	2,500			
		Males					
		9–13 y	1,300*	2,500			
		14–18 y	1,300*	2,500			
		19–30 y	1,000*	2,500			
		31–50 y	1,000*	2,500			
		50–70 y	1,200*	2,500			
		<70 y	1,200*	2,500			
		Females					
		9–13 y	1,300*	2,500			
		14–18 y	1,300*	2,500			
		19–30 y	1,000*	2,500			
		31–50 y	1,000*	2,500			
		50–70 y	1,200*	2,500			
		<70 y	1,200*	2,500			
		Pregnancy					
		≤18 y	1,300*	2,500			
		19–30 y	1,000*	2,500			
		31–50 y	1,000*	2,500			
		Lactation					
		≤18 y	1,300*	2,500			
		19–30 y	1,000*	2,500			
		31–50 y	1,000*	2,500			
Chromium	Helps to maintain normal blood glucose levels	Infants	(μg/d)		Some cereals, meats, poultry, fish, beer	Chronic renal failure	Individuals with Wilson's disease, Indian childhood cirrhosis and idiopathic copper toxicosis may be at increased risk of adverse effects from excess copper intake.
		0–6 mo	0.2*	ND			
		7–12 mo	5.5*	ND			
		Children					
		1–3 y	11*	ND			
		4–8 y	15*	ND			
		Males					
		9–13 y	25*	ND			
		14–18 y	35*	ND			
		19–30 y	35*	ND			
		31–50 y	35*	ND			
		50–70 y	30*	ND			
		>70 y	30*	ND			
		Females					
		9–13 y	21*	ND			
		14–18 y	24*	ND			
		19–30 y	25*	ND			
		31–50 y	25*	ND			
		50–70 y	20*	ND			
		>70 y	20*	ND			
		Pregnancy					
		≤18 y	29*	ND			
		19–30 y	30*	ND			
		31–50 y	30*	ND			
		Lactation					
		≤18 y	44*	ND			
		19–30 y	45*	ND			
		31–50 y	45*	ND			

NOTE: The table is adapted from the DRI reports, see www.nap.edu. It represents Recommended Dietary Allowances (RDAs) in **bold type**. Adequate intakes (AIs) in ordinary type followed by an asterisk (*), and Tolerable Upper Intake Levels (ULs)[a]. RDAs and AIs may both be used as goals for individual intake. RDAs are set to meet the needs of almost all (97 to 98 percent) individuals in a group. For healthy breastfed infants, the AI is the mean intake. The AI for other life stage and gender groups is believed to cover the needs of all individuals in the group, but lack of data prevent being able to specify with confidence the percentage of individuals covered by this intake.

[a]UL = The maximum level of daily nutrient intake that is likely to pose no risk of adverse effects. Unless otherwise specified, the UL represents total intake from food, water, and supplements. Due to lack of suitable data, ULs could not be established for vitamin K, thiamin, riboflavin, vitamin B₁₂, pantothenic acid, biotin, or carotenoids. In the absence of ULs, extra caution may be warranted in consuming levels above recommended intakes.

[b]ND = Not determinable due to lack of data of adverse effects in this age group and concern with regard to lack of ability to handle excess amounts. Source of intake should be from food only to prevent high levels of intake.

SOURCES: *Dietary Reference intakes for Calcium, Phosphorous, Magnesium. Vitamin D, and Fluoride* (1997); *Dietary Reference Intakes for Thiamin, Riboflavin, Niacin, Vitamin B₆, Folate, Vitamin B₁₂, Paniothenic Acid, Biotin, and Choline* (1998); *Dietary Reference Intakes for Vitamin C, Vitamin E, Selenium, and Carotenoids (2000);* and *Dietary Reference Intakes for Vitamin A, Vitamin K, Arsenic, Boron, Chromium, Copper, Iodine, Iron, Manganese, Molybdenum, Nickel, Silicon, Vanadium, and Zinc* (2001). These reports may be accessed via www.nap.edu.

Table 107-1. *(continued).*

DIETARY REFERENCE INTAKES: ELEMENTS

NUTRIENT	FUNCTION	LIFE STAGE GROUP	RDA/AI*	UL[a]	SELECTED FOOD SOURCES	ADVERSE EFFECTS OF EXCESSIVE CONSUMPTION	SPECIAL CONSIDERATIONS
Copper	Components of enzymes in iron metabolism	Infants	(μg/d)	(μg/d)	Organ meats, seafood, nuts seeds, wheat bran cereals, whole grain products, cocoa products	Gastrointestinal distress, liver damage	None
		0–6 mo	200*	ND[b]			
		7–12 mo	220*	ND			
		Children					
		1–3 y	**340**	1,000			
		4–8 y	**440**	3,000			
		Males					
		9–13 y	**700**	5,000			
		14–18 y	**890**	8,000			
		19–30 y	**900**	10,000			
		31–50 y	**900**	10,000			
		50–70 y	**900**	10,000			
		>70 y	**900**	10,000			
		Females					
		9–13 y	**700**	5,000			
		14–18 y	**890**	8,000			
		19–30 y	**900**	10,000			
		31–50 y	**900**	10,000			
		50–70 y	**900**	10,000			
		>70 y	**900**	10,000			
		Pregnancy					
		≤18 y	**1000**	8,000			
		19–30 y	**1000**	10,000			
		31–50 y	**1000**	10,000			
		Lactation					
		≤18 y	**1300**	8,000			
		19–30 y	**1300**	10,000			
		31–50 y	**1300**	10,000			
Fluoride	Inhibits the initiation and progression of dental caries and stimulates new bone formation	Infants	(mg/d)	(mg/d)	Fluoridated water, teas, marine fish, fluoridated dental products	Enamel and skeletal fluorosis	None
		0–6 mo	0.01*	0.7			
		7–12 mo	0.5*	0.9			
		Children					
		1–3 y	0.7*	1.3			
		4–8 y	1*	2.2			
		Males	2*	10			
		9–13 y					
		14–18 y	3*	10			
		19–30 y	4*	10			
		31–50 y	4*	10			
		50–70 y	4*	10			
		>70 y	4*	10			
		Females					
		9–13 y	2*	10			
		14–18 y	3*	10			
		19–30 y	3*	10			
		31–50 y	3*	10			
		50–70 y	3*	10			
		>70 y	3*	10			
		Pregnancy					
		≤18 y	3*	10			
		19–30 y	3*	10			
		31–50 y	3*	10			
		Lactation					
		≤18 y	3*	10			
		19–30 y	3*	10			
		31–50 y	3*	10			

NOTE: The table is adapted from the DRI reports, see www.nap.edu. It represents Recommended Dietary Allowances (RDAs) in **bold type.** Adequate intakes (AIs) in ordinary type followed by an asterisk (*), and Tolerable Upper Intake Levels (ULs)[a]. RDAs and AIs may both be used as goals for individual intake. RDAs are set to meet the needs of almost all (97 to 98 percent) individuals in a group. For healthy breastfed infants, the AI is the mean intake. The AI for other life stage and gender groups is believed to cover the needs of all individuals in the group, but lack of data prevent being able to specify with confidence the percentage of individuals covered by this intake.

[a]UL = The maximum level of daily nutrient intake that is likely to pose no risk of adverse effects. Unless otherwise specified, the UL represents total intake from food, water, and supplements. Due to lack of suitable data, ULs could not be established for vitamin K, thiamin, riboflavin, vitamin B12, pantothenic acid, biotin, or carotenoids. In the absence of ULs, extra caution may be warranted in consuming levels above recommended intakes.

[b]ND = Not determinable due to lack of data of adverse effects in this age group and concern with regard to lack of ability to handle excess amounts. Source of intake should be from food only to prevent high levels of intake.

SOURCES: *Dietary Reference intakes for Calcium, Phosphorous, Magnesium. Vitamin D, and Fluoride* (1997); *Dietary Reference Intakes for Thiamin, Riboflavin, Niacin, Vitamin B6, Folate, Vitamin B12, Paniothenic Acid, Biotin, and Choline* (1998); *Dietary Reference Intakes for Vitamin C, Vitamin E, Selenium, and Carotenoids (2000);* and *Dietary Reference Intakes for Vitamin A, Vitamin K, Arsenic, Boron, Chromium, Copper, Iodine, Iron, Manganese, Molybdenum, Nickel, Silicon, Vanadium, and Zinc* (2001). These reports may be accessed via www.nap.edu.

Table 107-1. *(continued).*

DIETARY REFERENCE INTAKES: ELEMENTS

NUTRIENT	FUNCTION	LIFE STAGE GROUP	RDA/AI*	UL[a]	SELECTED FOOD SOURCES	ADVERSE EFFECTS OF EXCESSIVE CONSUMPTION	SPECIAL CONSIDERATIONS
Iodine	Component of the thyroid hormones; and prevents goiter and cretinism	Infants	(μg/d)	(μg/d)	Marine origin, processed foods, iodized salt	Elevated thyroid stimulating hormone (TSH) concentration	Individuals with autoimmune thyroid disease, previous iodine deficiency, or nodular goiter and distinctly susceptible to the adverse effect of excess iodine intake. Therefore, individuals with these conditions may not be protected by the UL for iodine intake for the general population.
		0–6 mo	110*	ND[b]			
		7–12 mo	130*	ND			
		Children					
		1–3 y	90	200			
		1–4 y	90	300			
		Males					
		9–13 y	**120**	600			
		14–18 y	**150**	900			
		19–30 y	**150**	1,100			
		31–50 y	**150**	1,100			
		50–70 y	**150**	1,100			
		>70 y	**150**	1,100			
		Females					
		9–13 y	**120**	600			
		14–18 y	**150**	900			
		19–30 y	**150**	1,100			
		31–50 y	**150**	1,100			
		50–70 y	**150**	1,100			
		>70 y	**150**	1,100			
		Pregnancy					
		≤18 y	**220**	900			
		19–30 y	**220**	1,100			
		31–50 y	**220**	1,100			
		Lactation					
		≤18 y	**290**	900			
		19–30 y	**290**	1,100			
		31–50 y	**290**	1,100			
Iron (mg/d)	Component of hemoglobin and numerous enzymes; prevents microcytic hypochromic anemia	Infants	(mg/d)	(mg/d)	Fruits, vegetables and fortified bread and grain products such as cereal (nonheme iron sources), meat and poultry (heme iron sources)	Gastrointestinal distress	Non-heme iron absorption is lower for those consuming vegetarian diets than for those eating nonvegetarian diets. Therefore, it has been suggested that the iron requirement for those consuming a vegetarian diet is approximately 2-fold greater than for those consuming a nonvegetarian diet. Recommended intake assumes 75% of iron is from heme iron sources.
		0–6 mo	0.27*	40			
		7–12 mo	11	40			
		Children					
		1–3 y	7	40			
		4–8 y	10	40			
		Males					
		9–13 y	**8**	40			
		14–18 y	**11**	45			
		19–30 y	**8**	45			
		31–50 y	**8**	45			
		50–70 y	**8**	45			
		>70 y	**8**	45			
		Females					
		9–13 y	**8**	40			
		14–18 y	**15**	45			
		19–30 y	**18**	45			
		31–50 y	**18**	45			
		50–70 y	**8**	45			
		>70 y	**8**	45			
		Pregnancy					
		≤18 y	27	45			
		19–30 y	27	45			
		31–50 y	27	45			
		Lactation					
		≤18 y	10	45			
		19–30 y	9	45			
		31–50 y	9	45			

NOTE: The table is adapted from the DRI reports, see www.nap.edu. It represents Recommended Dietary Allowances (RDAs) in **bold type**. Adequate intakes (AIs) in ordinary type followed by an asterisk (*), and Tolerable Upper Intake Levels (ULs)[a]. RDAs and AIs may both be used as goals for individual intake. RDAs are set to meet the needs of almost all (97 to 98 percent) individuals in a group. For healthy breastfed infants, the AI is the mean intake. The AI for other life stage and gender groups is believed to cover the needs of all individuals in the group, but lack of data prevent being able to specify with confidence the percentage of individuals covered by this intake.

[a]UL = The maximum level of daily nutrient intake that is likely to pose no risk of adverse effects. Unless otherwise specified, the UL represents total intake from food, water, and supplements. Due to lack of suitable data, ULs could not be established for vitamin K, thiamin, riboflavin, vitamin B₁₂, pantothenic acid, biotin, or carotenoids. In the absence of ULs, extra caution may be warranted in consuming levels above recommended intakes.

[b]ND = Not determinable due to lack of data of adverse effects in this age group and concern with regard to lack of ability to handle excess amounts. Source of intake should be from food only to prevent high levels of intake.

SOURCES: *Dietary Reference intakes for Calcium, Phosphorous, Magnesium. Vitamin D, and Fluoride* (1997); *Dietary Reference Intakes for Thiamin, Riboflavin, Niacin, Vitamin B₆, Folate, Vitamin B₁₂, Paniothenic Acid, Biotin, and Choline* (1998); *Dietary Reference Intakes for Vitamin C, Vitamin E, Selenium, and Carotenoids (2000);* and *Dietary Reference Intakes for Vitamin A, Vitamin K, Arsenic, Boron, Chromium, Copper, Iodine, Iron, Manganese, Molybdenum, Nickel, Silicon, Vanadium, and Zinc* (2001). These reports may be accessed via www.nap.edu.

Table 107-1. (continued).

NUTRIENT	FUNCTION	LIFE STAGE GROUP	RDA/AI*	UL[a]	SELECTED FOOD SOURCES	ADVERSE EFFECTS OF EXCESSIVE CONSUMPTION	SPECIAL CONSIDERATIONS
Magnesium	Cofactor for enzyme systems	Infants	(mg/d)	(mg/d)	Green leafy vegetables, unpolished grains, nuts, meat, starches, milk	There is no evidence of adverse effects from the consumption of naturally occurring magnesium in foods	None
		0–6 mo	30*	ND[b]			
		7–12 mo	75*	ND		Adverse effects from magnesium containing supplements may include osmotic diarrhea.	
		Children					
		1–3 y	**80**	85			
		4–8 y	**130**	110		The UL for magnesium represents intake from a pharmacological agent only and does not include intake from food and water.	
		Males					
		9–13 y	**240**	350			
		14–18 y	**410**	350			
		19–30 y	**499**	350			
		31–50 y	**420**	350			
		50–70 y	**420**	350			
		>70 y	**420**	350			
		Females					
		9–13 y	**240**	350			
		14–18 y	**380**	350			
		19–30 y	**310**	350			
		31–50 y	**320**	350			
		50–70 y	**320**	350			
		>70 y					
		Pregnancy					
		≤18 y	**400**	350			
		19–30 y	**350**	350			
		31–50 y	**360**	350			
		Lactation					
		≤18 y	**360**	350			
		19–30 y	**310**	350			
		31–50 y	**320**	350			
Manganese	Involved in the formation of bone, as well as in enzymes involved in amino acid, cholesterol, and carbohydrate metabolism	Infants	(mg/d)	(mg/d)	Nuts, legumes, tea, and whole grains	Elevated blood concentration and neurotoxocity	Because manganese in drinking water and supplements may be more bioavailable than manganese from food, caution should be taken when using manganese supplements especially among those persons already consuming large amounts of manganese from diets high in plant products.
		0–6 mo	0.003*	ND			
		7–12 mo	0.6*	ND			
		Children					
		1–3 y	1.2*	2			
		4–8 y	1.5*	3			
		Males					
		9–13 y	1.9*	6			
		14–18 y	2.2*	9			
		19–30 y	2.3*	11			In addition, individuals with liver disease may be distinctly susceptible to the adverse effects of excess manganese intake.
		31–50 y	2.3*	11			
		50–70 y	2.3*	11			
		>70 y	2.3*	11			
		Females					
		9–13 y	1.6*	6			
		14–18 y	1.6*	9			
		19–30 y	1.8*	11			
		31–50 y	1.8*	11			
		50–70 y	1.8*	11			
		>70 y	1.8*	11			
		Pregnancy					
		≤18 y	2.0*	9			
		19–30 y	2.0*	11			
		31–50 y	2.0*	11			
		Lactation					
		≤18 y	2.6*	9			
		19–30 y	2.6*	11			
		31–50 y	2.6*	11			

NOTE: The table is adapted from the DRI reports, see www.nap.edu. It represents Recommended Dietary Allowances (RDAs) in **bold type**. Adequate intakes (AIs) in ordinary type followed by an asterisk (*), and Tolerable Upper Intake Levels (ULs)[a]. RDAs and AIs may both be used as goals for individual intake. RDAs are set to meet the needs of almost all (97 to 98 percent) individuals in a group. For healthy breastfed infants, the AI is the mean intake. The AI for other life stage and gender groups is believed to cover the needs of all individuals in the group, but lack of data prevent being able to specify with confidence the percentage of individuals covered by this intake.

[a]UL = The maximum level of daily nutrient intake that is likely to pose no risk of adverse effects. Unless otherwise specified, the UL represents total intake from food, water, and supplements. Due to lack of suitable data, ULs could not be established for vitamin K, thiamin, riboflavin, vitamin B_{12}, pantothenic acid, biotin, or carotenoids. In the absence of ULs, extra caution may be warranted in consuming levels above recommended intakes.

[b]ND = Not determinable due to lack of data of adverse effects in this age group and concern with regard to lack of ability to handle excess amounts. Source of intake should be from food only to prevent high levels of intake.

SOURCES: *Dietary Reference intakes for Calcium, Phosphorous, Magnesium. Vitamin D, and Fluoride* (1997); *Dietary Reference Intakes for Thiamin, Riboflavin, Niacin, Vitamin B_6, Folate, Vitamin B_{12}, Paniothenic Acid, Biotin, and Choline* (1998); *Dietary Reference Intakes for Vitamin C, Vitamin E, Selenium, and Carotenoids (2000);* and *Dietary Reference Intakes for Vitamin A, Vitamin K, Arsenic, Boron, Chromium, Copper, Iodine, Iron, Manganese, Molybdenum, Nickel, Silicon, Vanadium, and Zinc* (2001). These reports may be accessed via www.nap.edu.

Table 107-1. *(continued).*

DIETARY REFERENCE INTAKES: ELEMENTS

NUTRIENT	FUNCTION	LIFE STAGE GROUP	RDA/AI*	UL[a]	SELECTED FOOD SOURCES	ADVERSE EFFECTS OF EXCESSIVE CONSUMPTION	SPECIAL CONSIDERATIONS
Molybdenum	Cofactor for enzymes involved in catabolism of sulfur amino acids, purines and pyridines.	Infants	(μg/d)	(μg/d)	Legumes, grain products and nuts	Reproductive effects as observed in animal studies.	Individuals who are deficient in dietary copper intake or have some dysfunction in copper metabolism that makes them copper-deficient could be at increased risk of molybdenum toxicity.
		0–6 mo	2*	ND[b]			
		7–12 mo	3*	ND			
		Children					
		1–3 y	**17**	300			
		4–8 y	**22**	600			
		Males					
		9–13 y	**34**	1,100			
		14–18 y	**43**	1,700			
		19–30 y	**45**	2,000			
		31–50 y	**45**	2,000			
		50–70 y	**45**	2,000			
		>70 y	**45**	2,000			
		Females					
		9–13 y	**34**	1,100			
		14–18 y	**43**	1,700			
		19–30 y	**45**	2,000			
		31–50 y	**45**	2,000			
		50–70 y	**45**	2,000			
		>70 y					
		Pregnancy					
		≤ 18 y	**50**	1,700			
		19–30 y	**50**	2,000			
		31–50 y	**50**	2,000			
		Lactation					
		≤ 18 y	**50**	1,700			
		19–30 y	**50**	2,000			
		31–50 y	**50**	2,000			
Nickel	No clear biological function in humans has been identified. May serve as a cofactor of metalloenzymes in microorganisms.	Infants	(mg/d)	(mg/d)	Nuts, legumes, cereals, sweeteners, chocolate milk powder, chocolate candy	Decreased body weight gain Note: As observed in animal studies	Individual with preexisting nickel hypersensitivity (from previous dermal exposure) and kidney dysfunction are distinctly susceptible to the adverse effects of excess nickel intake
		0–6 mo	ND	ND			
		7–12 mo	ND	ND			
		Children					
		1–3 y	ND	0.2			
		4–8 y	ND	0.3			
		Males					
		9–13 y	ND	0.6			
		14–18 y	ND	1.0			
		19–30 y	ND	1.0			
		31–50 y	ND	1.0			
		50–70 y	ND	1.0			
		>70 y	ND	1.0			
		Females					
		9–13 y	ND	0.6			
		14–18 y	ND	1.0			
		19–30 y	ND	1.0			
		31–50 y	ND	1.0			
		50–70 y	ND	1.0			
		>70 y	ND	1.0			
		Pregnancy					
		≤ 18 y	ND	1.0			
		19–30 y	ND	1.0			
		31–50 y	ND	1.0			
		Lactation					
		≤ 18 y	ND	1.0			
		19–30 y	ND	1.0			
		31–50 y	ND	1.0			

NOTE: The table is adapted from the DRI reports, see www.nap.edu. It represents Recommended Dietary Allowances (RDAs) in **bold type.** Adequate intakes (AIs) in ordinary type followed by an asterisk (*), and Tolerable Upper Intake Levels (ULs)[a]. RDAs and AIs may both be used as goals for individual intake. RDAs are set to meet the needs of almost all (97 to 98 percent) individuals in a group. For healthy breastfed infants, the AI is the mean intake. The AI for other life stage and gender groups is believed to cover the needs of all individuals in the group, but lack of data prevent being able to specify with confidence the percentage of individuals covered by this intake.

[a]UL = The maximum level of daily nutrient intake that is likely to pose no risk of adverse effects. Unless otherwise specified, the UL represents total intake from food, water, and supplements. Due to lack of suitable data, ULs could not be established for vitamin K, thiamin, riboflavin, vitamin B12, pantothenic acid, biotin, or carotenoids. In the absence of ULs, extra caution may be warranted in consuming levels above recommended intakes.

[b]ND = Not determinable due to lack of data of adverse effects in this age group and concern with regard to lack of ability to handle excess amounts. Source of intake should be from food only to prevent high levels of intake.

SOURCES: *Dietary Reference intakes for Calcium, Phosphorous, Magnesium. Vitamin D, and Fluoride* (1997); *Dietary Reference Intakes for Thiamin, Riboflavin, Niacin, Vitamin B6, Folate, Vitamin B12, Paniothenic Acid, Biotin, and Choline* (1998); *Dietary Reference Intakes for Vitamin C, Vitamin E, Selenium, and Carotenoids (2000);* and *Dietary Reference Intakes for Vitamin A, Vitamin K, Arsenic, Boron, Chromium, Copper, Iodine, Iron, Manganese, Molybdenum, Nickel, Silicon, Vanadium, and Zinc* (2001). These reports may be accessed via www.nap.edu.

Table 107-1. *(continued).*

		LIFE STAGE			SELECTED FOOD	ADVERSE EFFECTS OF	
NUTRIENT	FUNCTION	GROUP	RDA/AI*	UL[a]	SOURCES	EXCESSIVE CONSUMPTION	SPECIAL CONSIDERATIONS
Phosphorus	Maintenance of pH, storage and transfer of energy and nucleotide synthesis	Infants	(mg/d)	(mg/d)	Milk, yogurt, ice cream, cheese, peas, meat, eggs, some cereals and breads	Metastalic calcification, skeletal porosity, interference with calcium absorption	Athletes and others with high energy expenditure frequently consume amounts from food greater than the UL without apparent effect.
		0–6 mo	100*	ND[b]			
		7–12 mo	275*	ND			
		Children					
		1–3 y	**460**	3,000			
		4–8 y	**500**	3,000			
		Males					
		9–13 y	**1,250**	4,000			
		14–18 y	**1,250**	4,000			
		19–30 y	**700**	4,000			
		31–50 y	**700**	4,000			
		50–70 y	**700**	4,000			
		>70 y	**700**	3,000			
		Females					
		9–13 y	**1,250**	4,000			
		14–18 y	**1,250**	4,000			
		19–30 y	**700**	4,000			
		31–50 y	**700**	4,000			
		50–70 y	**700**	3,000			
		>70 y	**700**				
		Pregnancy					
		≤18 y	**1,250**	3,500			
		19–30 y	**700**	3,500			
		31–50 y	**700**	3,500			
		Lactation					
		≤18 y	**1,250**	4,000			
		19–30 y	**700**	4,000			
		31–50 y	**700**	4,000			
Selenium	Defense against oxidative stress and regulation of action, and the oxidation status of vitamin C and other molecules	Infants	(μg/d)	(μg/d)	Organ meats, seafood, plants (depending on content)	Hair and nail brittleness and loss	None
		0–6 mo	15*	45			
		7–12 mo	20*	60			
		Children					
		1–3 y	20	90			
		4–8 y	30	150			
		Males					
		9–13 y	40	280			
		14–18 y	55	400			
		19–30 y	55	400			
		31–50 y	55	400			
		50–70 y	55	400			
		>70 y	55	400			
		Females					
		9–13 y	40	280			
		14–18 y	55	400			
		19–30 y	55	400			
		31–50 y	55	400			
		50–70 y	55	400			
		>70 y	55	400			
		Pregnancy					
		≤18 y	60	400			
		19–30 y	60	400			
		31–50 y	60	400			
		Lactation					
		≤18 y	70	400			
		19–30 y	70	400			
		31–50 y	70	400			

NOTE: The table is adapted from the DRI reports, see www.nap.edu. It represents Recommended Dietary Allowances (RDAs) in **bold type.** Adequate intakes (AIs) in ordinary type followed by an asterisk (*), and Tolerable Upper Intake Levels (ULs)[a]. RDAs and AIs may both be used as goals for individual intake. RDAs are set to meet the needs of almost all (97 to 98 percent) individuals in a group. For healthy breastfed infants, the AI is the mean intake. The AI for other life stage and gender groups is believed to cover the needs of all individuals in the group, but lack of data prevent being able to specify with confidence the percentage of individuals covered by this intake.

[a]UL = The maximum level of daily nutrient intake that is likely to pose no risk of adverse effects. Unless otherwise specified, the UL represents total intake from food, water, and supplements. Due to lack of suitable data, ULs could not be established for vitamin K, thiamin, riboflavin, vitamin B[12], pantothenic acid, biotin, or carotenoids. In the absence of ULs, extra caution may be warranted in consuming levels above recommended intakes.

[b]ND = Not determinable due to lack of data of adverse effects in this age group and concern with regard to lack of ability to handle excess amounts. Source of intake should be from food only to prevent high levels of intake.

SOURCES: *Dietary Reference intakes for Calcium, Phosphorous, Magnesium. Vitamin D, and Fluoride* (1997); *Dietary Reference Intakes for Thiamin, Riboflavin, Niacin, Vitamin B6, Folate, Vitamin B12, Paniothenic Acid, Biotin, and Choline* (1998); *Dietary Reference Intakes for Vitamin C, Vitamin E, Selenium, and Carotenoids* (2000); and *Dietary Reference Intakes for Vitamin A, Vitamin K, Arsenic, Boron, Chromium, Copper, Iodine, Iron, Manganese, Molybdenum, Nickel, Silicon, Vanadium, and Zinc* (2001). These reports may be accessed via www.nap.edu.

Table 107-1. *(continued).*

		DIETARY REFERENCE INTAKES: ELEMENTS					
NUTRIENT	FUNCTION	LIFE STAGE GROUP	RDA/AI*	UL[a]	SELECTED FOOD SOURCES	ADVERSE EFFECTS OF EXCESSIVE CONSUMPTION	SPECIAL CONSIDERATIONS
Zinc	Component of multiple enzymes and proteins; involved in the regulation of gene expression.	Infants	(mg/d)	(mg/d)	Fortified cereals, red meats, certain seafood	Reduced copper status	Zinc absorption is lower for those consuming vegetarian diets than for those eating nonvegetarian diets. Therefore, it has been suggested that the zinc requirement for those consuming a vegetarian diet is approximately 2-fold greater than for consuming a nonvegetarian diet.
		0–6 mo	2*	4			
		7–12 mo	3	5			
		Children					
		1–3 y	**3**	7			
		4–8 y	**5**	12			
		Males					
		9–13 y	**8**	23			
		14–18 y	**11**	34			
		19–30 y	**11**	40			
		31–50 y	**11**	40			
		50–70 y	**11**	40			
		>70 y	**11**	40			
		Females					
		9–13 y	**8**	23			
		14–18 y	**9**	34			
		19–30 y	**8**	40			
		31–50 y	**8**	40			
		50–70 y	**8**	40			
		>70 y	**8**	40			
		Pregnancy					
		≤18 y	**12**	34			
		19–30 y	**11**	40			
		31–50 y	**11**	40			
		Lactation					
		≤18 y	**13**	34			
		19–30 y	**12**	40			
		31–50 y	**12**	40			

NOTE: The table is adapted from the DRI reports, see www.nap.edu. It represents Recommended Dietary Allowances (RDAs) in **bold type.** Adequate intakes (AIs) in ordinary type followed by an asterisk (*), and Tolerable Upper Intake Levels (ULs)[a]. RDAs and AIs may both be used as goals for individual intake. RDAs are set to meet the needs of almost all (97 to 98 percent) individuals in a group. For healthy breastfed infants, the AI is the mean intake. The AI for other life stage and gender groups is believed to cover the needs of all individuals in the group, but lack of data prevent being able to specify with confidence the percentage of individuals covered by this intake.
[a]UL = The maximum level of daily nutrient intake that is likely to pose no risk of adverse effects. Unless otherwise specified, the UL represents total intake from food, water, and supplements. Due to lack of suitable data, ULs could not be established for vitamin K, thiamin, riboflavin, vitamin B$_{12}$, pantothenic acid, biotin, or carotenoids. In the absence of ULs, extra caution may be warranted in consuming levels above recommended intakes.
[b]ND = Not determinable due to lack of data of adverse effects in this age group and concern with regard to lack of ability to handle excess amounts. Source of intake should be from food only to prevent high levels of intake.
SOURCES: *Dietary Reference intakes for Calcium, Phosphorous, Magnesium. Vitamin D, and Fluoride* (1997); *Dietary Reference Intakes for Thiamin, Riboflavin, Niacin, Vitamin B$_6$, Folate, Vitamin B$_{12}$, Paniothenic Acid, Biotin, and Choline* (1998); *Dietary Reference Intakes for Vitamin C, Vitamin E, Selenium, and Carotenoids (2000);* and *Dietary Reference Intakes for Vitamin A, Vitamin K, Arsenic, Boron, Chromium, Copper, Iodine, Iron, Manganese, Molybdenum, Nickel, Silicon, Vanadium, and Zinc* (2001). These reports may be accessed via www.nap.edu.

maintenance of a healthy weight. Total activity time includes cumulative activities such as an exercise plan as well activities associated with daily life such as climbing stairs. The report suggests a moderate to higher intensity exercise plan for those in a sedentary occupation.

Build a Healthy Base

LET THE PYRAMID GUIDE YOUR FOOD CHOICES— No single food supplies all the nutrients needed by the body. Therefore, it is important to eat a variety of foods, on a daily basis, to meet all the nutrient needs of the body. The Food Guide Pyramid[2], Figure 107-2, was developed by the USDA to help interpret the Dietary Guidelines. It is anticipated the Food Guide Pyramid will be revised in the near future. Multiple versions of the Food Guide Pyramid are available for many different cuisines and ethnic food patterns. Both the Dietary Guidelines for Americans and the Food Guide Pyramid support the concept that all foods can fit in a well-balanced diet and help to eliminate the negative and untrue perception that there are good foods and bad foods. There are no good foods and bad foods, but there are good diets and bad diets. The pyramid shape emphasizes

that the foundation of a sound diet should be foods from the bread, cereal, rice, and pasta group. Build on this foundation by adding foods from the vegetable and fruit groups, and then from the milk and meat groups. Each group suggests a range of servings to consume each day. Fats, oils, and sweets are to be used sparingly and are represented in the top section of the pyramid. The top section is not considered a group of foods, and there are no suggested serving ranges for the fats, oils, and sweets. It should be remembered that fats and sweets can often be "hidden" in some baked foods such as muffins, etc. The complete name of the milk and meat groups identifies food alternatives within each group that provide many of the same basic nutrients as milk or meat. For example, calcium, an important nutrient supplied by the milk group can be obtained through other foods (eg, yogurt, hard cheeses such as cheddar, cottage cheese, or even cheese foods). Not all alternatives supply the same amount of calcium. It takes 2 cups of cottage cheese and 2 oz of a processed cheese food to equal the amount of calcium in only 1 cup of milk or yogurt. Calcium alternatives also are found in the vegetable group and in legumes. Basic nutrition texts and educational information about the Dietary Guidelines and the Food Guide Pyramid from the USDA and the HHS are helpful in interpreting specifics about these educational tools.

Table 107-2. Food and Nutrition Board, Institute of Medicine-National Academy of Sciences Dietary Reference Intakes: Vitamins

DIETARY REFERENCE INTAKES: VITAMINS

NUTRIENT	FUNCTION	LIFE STAGE GROUP	RDA/AI*	UL[a]	SELECTED FOOD SOURCES	ADVERSE EFFECTS OF EXCESSIVE CONSUMPTION	SPECIAL CONSIDERATIONS
Biotin	Coenzyme in synthesis of fat, glycogen, and amino acids	Infants	(µg/d)		Liver and smaller amounts in fruits and meals	No adverse effects of biotin in humans or animals were found. This does not mean that there is no potential for adverse effects resulting from high intakes. Because data on the adverse effects of biotin are limited, caution may be warranted.	None
		0–6 mo	5*	ND[b]			
		7–12 mo	6*	ND			
		Children					
		1–3 y	8*	ND			
		4–8 y	12*	ND			
		Males					
		9–13 y	20*	ND			
		14–18 y	25*	ND			
		19–30 y	30*	ND			
		31–50 y	30*	ND			
		50–70 y	30*	ND			
		>70 y	30*	ND			
		Females					
		9–13 y	20*	ND			
		14–18 y	25*	ND			
		19–30 y	30*	ND			
		31–50 y	30*	ND			
		50–70 y	30*	ND			
		>70 y	30*	ND			
		Pregnancy					
		≤18 y	30*	ND			
		19–30 y	30*	ND			
		31–50 y	30*	ND			
		Lactation					
		≤18 y	35*	ND			
		19–30 y	35*	ND			
		31–50 y	35*	ND			
Choline	Precursor for acetylcholine, phospholipids and betaine	Infants	(mg/d)	(mg/d)	Milk, liver, eggs, peanuts	Fishy body odor, sweating, salivation, hypotension, hepatotoxicity	Individuals with trimethylaminuria, renal disease, liver disease, depression and Parkinson's disease, may be at risk of adverse effects with choline intakes at the UL.
		0–6 mo	**125***	ND			
		7–12 mo	**150***	ND			Although AIs have been set for choline, there are few data to assess whether a dietary supply of choline is needed at all stages of the life cycle, and it may be that the choline requirement can be met by endogenous synthesis at some of these stages.
		Children					
		1–3 y	200*	1000			
		4–8 y	250*	1000			
		Males					
		9–13 y	375*	2000			
		14–18 y	550*	3000			
		19–30 y	550*	3500			
		31–50 y	550*	3500			
		50–70 y	550*	3500			
		>70 y	550*	3500			
		Females					
		9–13 y	375*	2000			
		14–18 y	400*	3000			
		19–30 y	425*	3500			
		31–50 y	425*	3500			
		50–70 y	425*	3500			
		>70 y	425*	3500			
		Pregnancy					
		≤18 y	450*	3000			
		19–30 y	450*	3500			
		31–50 y	450*	3500			
		Lactation					
		≤18 y	550*	3000			
		19–30 y	550*	3500			
		31–50 y	550*	3500			

NOTE: The table is adapted from the DRI reports, see www.nap.edu. It represents Recommended Dietary Allowances (RDAs) in **bold type**, Adequate intakes (AIs) in ordinary type followed by an asterisk (*), and Tolerable Upper Intake Levels (ULs)[a]. RDAs and AIs may both be used as goals for individual intake. RDAs are set to meet the needs of almost all (97 to 98 percent) individuals in a group. For healthy breastfed infants, the AI is the mean intake. The AI for other life stage and gender groups is believed to cover the needs of all individuals in the group, but lack of data prevent being able to specify with confidence the percentage of individuals covered by this intake.

[a]UL = The maximum level of daily nutrient intake that is likely to pose no risk of adverse effects. Unless otherwise specified, the UL represents total intake from food, water, and supplements. Due to lack of suitable data, ULs could not be established for vitamin K, thiamin, riboflavin, vitamin B$_{12}$, pantolhenic acid, biolin, or carotenoids. In the absence of ULs, extra caution may be warranted in consuming levels above recommended intakes.

[b]ND = Not determinable due to lack of data of adverse effects in this age group and concern with regard to lack of ability to handle excess amounts. Source of intake should be from food only to prevent high levels of intake.

SOURCES: *Dietary Reference Intakes for Calcium, Phosphorous, Magnesium, Vitamin D, and Fluoride* (1997); *Dietary Reference Intakes for Thiamin, Riboflavin, Niacin, Vitamin B$_6$, Folate, Vitamin B$_{12}$, Pantolhenic Acid, Biotin, and Choline* (1998); *Dietary Reference Intakes for Vitamin C, Vitamin E, Selenium, and Carotenoids* (2000); and *Dietary Reference Intakes for Vitamin A, Vitamin K, Arsenic, Boron, Chromium, Copper, Iodine, Iron, Manganese, Molybdenum, Nickel, Silicon, Vanadium, and Zinc* (2001). These reports may be accessed via www.nap.edu.

Table 107-2. (continued).

DIETARY REFERENCE INTAKES: VITAMINS

NUTRIENT	FUNCTION	LIFE STAGE GROUP	RDA/AI*	UL[a]	SELECTED FOOD SOURCES	ADVERSE EFFECTS OF EXCESSIVE CONSUMPTION	SPECIAL CONSIDERATIONS

Folate
 	
Also known as:
Folic acid
Folacin
Pteroylpoly-
glutamates
 	
Note: Given as dietary folate equivalents (DFE). 1 DFE = 1 μg food folate = 0.6 μg of folate from fortified food or as a supplement consumed with food = 0.5 μg of a supplement taken on an empty stomach.
	Coenzyme in the metabolism of nucleic and amino acids; prevents megaloblastic anemia	Infants
		  0–6 mo
		  7–12 mo
		Children
		  1–3 y
		  4–8 y
		Males
		  9–13 y
		  14–18 y
		  19–30 y
		  31–50 y
		  50–70 y
		  >70 y
		Females
		  9–13 y
		  14–18 y
		  19–30 y
		  31–50 y
		  50–70 y
		  >70 y
		Pregnancy
		  ≤18 y
		  19–30 y
		  31–50 y
		Lactation
		  ≤18 y
		  19–30 y
		  31–50 y
			(μg/d)
			65*
			80*
			
			150
			200
			
			300
			400
			400
			400
			400
			400
			
			300
			400
			400
			400
			400
			400
			
			600
			600
			600
			
			500
			500
			500
				(μg/d)
				ND[b]
				ND
				
				300
				400
				
				600
				800
				1,000
				1,000
				1,000
				1,000
				
				600
				800
				1,000
				1,000
				1,000
				1,000
				
				800
				1,000
				1,000
				
				800
				1,000
				1,000
					Enriched cereal grains, dark leafy vegetables, enriched and whole-grain breads and bread products, fortified ready-to-eat cereals	Masks neurological complication in people with vitamin B_{12} deficiency.
						
						No adverse effects associated with folate from food or supplements have been reported. This does not mean that there is no potential for adverse effects resulting from high intakes. Because data on the adverse effects of folate are limited, caution may be warranted.
						
						The UL for folate applies to synthetic forms obtained from supplements and/or fortified foods.
							In view of evidence linking folate intake with neural tube defects in the fetus, it is recommended that all women capable of becoming pregnant consume 400 μg from supplements or fortified foods in addition to intake of food folate from a varied diet.
							
							It is assumed that women will continue consuming. or fortified food until their 400 μg from supplements pregnancy is confirmed and they enter prenatal care, which ordinarily occurs after the end of the periconceptional period—the critical time for formation of the neural tube.

Niacin
 	
Includes nicotinic acid amide, nicotinic acid (pyridine-3-carboxylic acid), and derivatives that exhibit the biological activity of nicotinamide.
 	
Note: Given as niacin equivalents (NE). 1 mg of niacin = 60 mg of tryptophan; 0–6 months = preformed niacin (not NE).
	Coenzyme or cosubstrate in many biological reduction and oxidation reactions—thus required for energy metabolism	Infants
		  0–6 mo
		  7–12 mo
		Children
		  1–3 y
		  4–8 y
		Males
		  9–13 y
		  14–18 y
		  19–30 y
		  31–50 y
		  50–70 y
		  >70 y
		Females
		  9–13 y
		  14–18 y
		  19–30 y
		  31–50 y
		  50–70 y
		  >70 y
		Pregnancy
		  ≤18 y
		  19–30 y
		  31–50 y
		Lactation
		  ≤18 y
		  19–30 y
		  31–50 y
			(mg/d)
			2*
			4*
			
			6
			8
			
			12
			16
			16
			16
			16
			16
			
			12
			14
			14
			14
			14
			14
			
			18
			18
			18
			
			17
			17
			17
				(mg/d)
				ND
				ND
				
				10
				15
				
				20
				30
				35
				35
				35
				35
				
				20
				30
				35
				35
				35
				35
				
				30
				35
				35
				
				30
				35
				35
					Meat, fish, poultry, enriched and whole-grain breads and bread products, fortified ready-to-eat cereals	There is no evidence of the adverse effects from consumption of naturally occuring niacin in foods.
						
						Adverse effects from niacin containing supplements may include flushing and gastrointestinal distress.
						
						The UL for niacin applies to synthetic forms obtained from supplements, fortified foods, or a combination of the two.
							Extra niacin may be required by persons treated with hemodialysis or peritoneal dialysis, or those with malabsorption syndrome.

NOTE: The table is adapted from the DRI reports, see www.nap.edu. It represents Recommended Dietary Allowances (RDAs) in **bold type**, Adequate intakes (AIs) in ordinary type followed by an asterisk (*), and Tolerable Upper Intake Levels (ULs)[a]. RDAs and AIs may both be used as goals for individual intake. RDAs are set to meet the needs of almost all (97 to 98 percent) individuals in a group. For healthy breastfed infants, the AI is the mean intake. The AI for other life stage and gender groups is believed to cover the needs of all individuals in the group, but lack of data prevent being able to specify with confidence the percentage of individuals covered by this intake.

[a]UL = The maximum level of daily nutrient intake that is likely to pose no risk of adverse effects. Unless otherwise specified, the UL represents total intake from food, water, and supplements. Due to lack of suitable data, ULs could not be established for vitamin K, thiamin, riboflavin, vitamin B_{12}, pantolhenic acid, biolin, or carotenoids. In the absence of ULs, extra caution may be warranted in consuming levels above recommended intakes.

[b]ND = Not determinable due to lack of data of adverse effects in this age group and concern with regard to lack of ability to handle excess amounts. Source of intake should be from food only to prevent high levels of intake.

SOURCES: *Dietary Reference Intakes for Calcium, Phosphorous, Magnesium, Vitamin D, and Fluoride* (1997); *Dietary Reference Intakes for Thiamin, Riboflavin, Niacin, Vitamin B₆, Folate, Vitamin B₁₂, Pantolhenic Acid, Biotin, and Choline* (1998); *Dietary Reference Intakes for Vitamin C, Vitamin E, Selenium, and Carotenoids* (2000); and *Dietary Reference Intakes for Vitamin A, Vitamin K, Arsenic, Boron, Chromium, Copper, Iodine, Iron, Manganese, Molybdenum, Nickel, Silicon, Vanadium, and Zinc* (2001). These reports may be accessed via www.nap.edu.

Table 107-2. (continued).

DIETARY REFERENCE INTAKES: VITAMINS

NUTRIENT	FUNCTION	LIFE STAGE GROUP	RDA/AI*	UL[a]	SELECTED FOOD SOURCES	ADVERSE EFFECTS OF EXCESSIVE CONSUMPTION	SPECIAL CONSIDERATIONS
Pantothenic Acid	Coenzyme in fatty acid metabolism	Infants	(mg/d)	(mg/d)	Chicken, beef potatoes, oats cereals, tomato products, liver, kidney, yeast, egg yolk, broccoli, whole grains	No adverse effects associated with panthothenic acid from food or supplements have been reported. This does not mean that there is no potential for adverse effects resulting from high intakes. Because data on the adverse effects of panthothenic acid are limited, caution may be warranted.	None
		0–6 mo	1.7*	ND[b]			
		7–12, mo	1.8*	ND			
		Children					
		1–3 y	2*	ND			
		4–8 y	3*	ND			
		Males					
		9–13 y	4*	ND			
		14–18 y	5*	ND			
		19–30 y	5*	ND			
		31–50 y	5*	ND			
		50–70 y	5*	ND			
		>70 y	5*	ND			
		Females					
		9–13 y	4*	ND			
		14–18 y	5*	ND			
		19–30 y	5*	ND			
		31–50 y	5*	ND			
		50–70 y	5*	ND			
		>70 y	5*	ND			
		Pregnancy					
		≤18 y	6*	ND			
		19–30 y	6*	ND			
		31–50 y	6*	ND			
		Lactation					
		≤18 y	7*	ND			
		19–30 y	7*	ND			
		31–50 y	7*	ND			
Riboflavin Also known as: Vitamin B$_2$	Coenzyme in numerous redox reactions	Infants	(mg/d)	(mg/d)	Organ meats, milk, bread products and fortified cereals	No adverse effects associated with riboflavin consumption from food or supplements have been reported. This does not mean that there is no potential for adverse effects resulting from high intakes. Because data on the adverse effects of riboflavin are limited, caution may be warranted.	None
		0–6 mo	0.3*	ND			
		7–12 mo	0.4*	ND			
		Children					
		1–3 y	**0.5**	ND			
		4–8 y	**0.6**	ND			
		Males					
		9–13 y	**0.9**	ND			
		14–18 y	**1.3**	ND			
		19–30 y	**1.3**	ND			
		31–50 y	**1.3**	ND			
		50–70 y	**1.3**	ND			
		>70 y	**1.3**	ND			
		Females					
		9–13 y	**0.9**	ND			
		14–18 y	**1.0**	ND			
		19–30 y	**1.1**	ND			
		31–50 y	**1.1**	ND			
		50–70 y	**1.1**	ND			
		>70 y	**1.1**	ND			
		Pregnancy					
		≤18 y	**1.4**	ND			
		19–30 y	**1.4**	ND			
		31–50 y	**1.4**	ND			
		Lactation					
		≤18 y	**1.6**	ND			
		19–30 y	**1.6**	ND			
		31–50 y	**1.6**	ND			

NOTE: The table is adapted from the DRI reports, see www.nap.edu. It represents Recommended Dietary Allowances (RDAs) in **bold type**, Adequate intakes (AIs) in ordinary type followed by an asterisk (*), and Tolerable Upper Intake Levels (ULs)[a]. RDAs and AIs may both be used as goals for individual intake. RDAs are set to meet the needs of almost all (97 to 98 percent) individuals in a group. For healthy breastfed infants, the AI is the mean intake. The AI for other life stage and gender groups is believed to cover the needs of all individuals in the group, but lack of data prevent being able to specify with confidence the percentage of individuals covered by this intake.

[a]UL = The maximum level of daily nutrient intake that is likely to pose no risk of adverse effects. Unless otherwise specified, the UL represents total intake from food, water, and supplements. Due to lack of suitable data, ULs could not be established for vitamin K, thiamin, riboflavin, vitamin B$_{12}$, pantolhenic acid, biolin, or carotenoids. In the absence of ULs, extra caution may be warranted in consuming levels above recommended intakes.

[b]ND = Not determinable due to lack of data of adverse effects in this age group and concern with regard to lack of ability to handle excess amounts. Source of intake should be from food only to prevent high levels of intake.

SOURCES: *Dietary Reference Intakes for Calcium, Phosphorous, Magnesium, Vitamin D, and Fluoride* (1997); *Dietary Reference Intakes for Thiamin, Riboflavin, Niacin, Vitamin B$_6$, Folate, Vitamin B$_{12}$, Pantolhenic Acid, Biotin, and Choline* (1998); *Dietary Reference Intakes for Vitamin C, Vitamin E, Selenium, and Carotenoids* (2000); and *Dietary Reference Intakes for Vitamin A, Vitamin K, Arsenic, Boron, Chromium, Copper, Iodine, Iron, Manganese, Molybdenum, Nickel, Silicon, Vanadium, and Zinc* (2001). These reports may be accessed via www.nap.edu.

Table 107-2. (continued).

					SELECTED	ADVERSE EFFECTS OF	
NUTRIENT	**FUNCTION**	**LIFE STAGE GROUP**	**RDA/AI***	**UL[a]**	**FOOD SOURCES**	**EXCESSIVE CONSUMPTION**	**SPECIAL CONSIDERATIONS**
Thiamin Also known as: Vitamin B$_1$ Aneurin	Coenzyme in the metabolism of carbohydrates and branched-chain amino acids	Infants 0–6 mo 7–12 mo Children 1–3 y 4–8 y Males 9–13 y 14–18 y 19–30 y 31–50 y 50–70 y >70 y Females 9–13 y 14–18 y 19–30 y 31–50 y 50–70 y >70 y Pregnancy ≤18 y 19–30 y 31–50 y Lactation ≤18 y 19–30 y 31–50 y	(mg/d) 0.2* 0.3* **0.5** **0.6** **0.9** **1.2** **1.2** **1.2** **1.2** **1.2** 0.9 1.0 **1.1** **1.1** **1.1** **1.1** **1.4** **1.4** **1.4** **1.4** **1.4** **1.4**	ND[b] ND ND ND ND ND ND ND ND ND ND ND ND ND ND ND ND ND ND ND ND ND	Enriched, fortified, or whole-grain products; bread and bread products, mixed foods whose main ingredient is grain, and ready-to-eat cereals.	No adverse effects associated with thiamin from food or supplements have been reported. This does not mean that there is no potential for adverse effects resulting from high intakes. Because data on the adverse effects of thiamin are limited, caution may be warranted.	Persons who may have increased needs for thiamin include those being treated with hemodialysis or paritoneal dialysis, or individuals with malabsorption syndrome.
Vitamin A Includes provitamin A carotenoids that are dietary precursors of retinol. Note: Given as retinol activity equivalents (RAEs), 1 RAE = 1 μg retinol, 12 μg β-carotene, 24 μg α-carotene, or 24 μg β-cryptoxanthin. To calculate RAEs from REs of provitamin A carotenoids in foods, divide the REs by 2. For pre-formed vitamin A in foods or supplements and for provitamin A carotenoids in supplements, 1 RE = RAE.	Required for normal vision, gene expression, reproduction, embryonic development and immune function	Infants 0–6 mo 7–12 mo Children 1–3 y 4–8 y Males 9–13 y 14–18 y 19–30 y 31–50 y 50–70 y >70 y Females 9–13 y 14–18 y 19–30 y 31–50 y 50–70 y >70 y Pregnancy ≤18 y 19–30 y 31–50 y Lactation ≤18 y 19–30 y 31–50 y	(μg/d) 400* 500* **300** **400** **600** **900** **900** **900** **900** **900** **600** **700** **700** **700** **700** **700** 750 **770** **770** **1,200** **1,300** **1,300**	(μg/d) 600 600 600 900 1,700 2,800 3,000 3,000 3,000 3,000 1,700 2,800 3,000 3,000 3,000 3,000 2,800 3,000 3,000 2,800 3,000 3,000	Liver, dairy products, fish	Teratological effects, liver toxicity Note: From preformed Vitamin A only.	Individuals with high alcohol intake, pre-existing liver disease, hyperlipidemia or severe protein malnutrition may be distinctly susceptible to the adverse effects of source excess preformed vitamin A intake. β-carotene supplements are advised only to serve as a provitamin A for individuals at risk of vitamin A deficiency.

NOTE: The table is adapted from the DRI reports, see www.nap.edu. It represents Recommended Dietary Allowances (RDAs) in **bold type**, Adequate intakes (AIs) in ordinary type followed by an asterisk (*), and Tolerable Upper Intake Levels (ULs)[a]. RDAs and AIs may both be used as goals for individual intake. RDAs are set to meet the needs of almost all (97 to 98 percent) individuals in a group. For healthy breastfed infants, the AI is the mean intake. The AI for other life stage and gender groups is believed to cover the needs of all individuals in the group, but lack of data prevent being able to specify with confidence the percentage of individuals covered by this intake.

[a]UL = The maximum level of daily nutrient intake that is likely to pose no risk of adverse effects. Unless otherwise specified, the UL represents total intake from food, water, and supplements. Due to lack of suitable data, ULs could not be established for vitamin K, thiamin, riboflavin, vitamin B$_{12}$, pantolhenic acid, biolin, or carotenoids. In the absence of ULs, extra caution may be warranted in consuming levels above recommended intakes.

[b]ND = Not determinable due to lack of data of adverse effects in this age group and concern with regard to lack of ability to handle excess amounts. Source of intake should be from food only to prevent high levels of intake.

SOURCES: *Dietary Reference Intakes for Calcium, Phosphorous, Magnesium, Vitamin D, and Fluoride* (1997); *Dietary Reference Intakes for Thiamin, Riboflavin, Niacin, Vitamin B$_6$, Folate, Vitamin B$_{12}$, Pantolhenic Acid, Biotin, and Choline* (1998); *Dietary Reference Intakes for Vitamin C, Vitamin E, Selenium, and Carotenoids* (2000); and *Dietary Reference Intakes for Vitamin A, Vitamin K, Arsenic, Boron, Chromium, Copper, Iodine, Iron, Manganese, Molybdenum, Nickel, Silicon, Vanadium, and Zinc* (2001). These reports may be accessed via www.nap.edu.

Table 107-2. (continued).

NUTRIENT	FUNCTION	LIFE STAGE GROUP	RDA/AI*	UL[a]	SELECTED FOOD SOURCES	ADVERSE EFFECTS OF EXCESSIVE CONSUMPTION	SPECIAL CONSIDERATIONS
Vitamin B_6	Coenzyme in the metabolism of amino acids, glycogen and sphingold bases	Infants	(mg/d)	(mg/d)	Fortified cereals, organ meats, fortified soy-based meat substitutes	No adverse effects associated with Vitamin B_6 from food have been reported. This does not mean that there is no potential for adverse effects resulting from high intakes. Because data on the adverse effects of Vitamin B_6 are limited, caution may be warranted. Sensory neuropathy has occurred from high intakes of supplemental forms.	None
Vitamin B_6 comprises a group of six related compounds: pyridoxal, pyridoxine, pyridoxamine, and 5'-phosphates (PLP, PNP, PMP)		0–6 mo	0.1*	ND[b]			
		7–12 mo	0.3*	ND			
		Children					
		1–3 y	**0.5**	30			
		4–8 y	**0.6**	40			
		Males					
		9–13 y	**1.0**	60			
		14–18 y	**1.3**	80			
		19–30 y	**1.3**	100			
		31–50 y	**1.3**	100			
		50–70 y	**1.7**	100			
		>70 y	**1.7**	100			
		Females					
		9–13 y	**1.0**	60			
		14–18 y	**1.2**	80			
		19–30 y	**1.3**	100			
		31–50 y	**1.3**	100			
		50–70 y	**1.5**	100			
		>70 y	**1.5**	100			
		Pregnancy					
		≤18 y	**1.9**	80			
		19–30 y	**1.9**	100			
		31–50 y	**1.9**	100			
		Lactation					
		≤18 y	**2.0**	80			
		19–30 y	**2.0**	100			
		31–50 y	**2.0**	100			
Vitamin B_{12} Also known as: Cobalamin	Coenzyme in nucleic acid metabolism; prevents megaloblastic anemia	Infants	(mg/d)	(mg/d)	Fortified cereals, meat, fish, poultry	No adverse effects have been associated with the consumption of the amounts of vitamin B_{12} normally found in foods or supplements. This does not mean that there is no potential for adverse effects resulting from high intakes. Because data on the adverse effects of vitamin B_{12} are limited, caution may be warranted.	Because 10 to 30 percent of older people may malabsorb food-bound vitamin B_{12}, it is advisable for those older than 50 year to meet their RDA mainly by consuming foods fortified with vitamin B_{12} or a supplement containing vitamin B_{12}.
		0–6 mo	0.4*	ND			
		7–12 mo	0.5*	ND			
		Children					
		1–3 y	**0.9**	ND			
		4–8 y	**1.2**	ND			
		Males					
		9–13 y	**1.8**	ND			
		14–18 y	**2.4**	ND			
		19–30 y	**2.4**	ND			
		31–50 y	**2.4**	ND			
		50–70 y	**2.4**	ND			
		>70 y	**2.4**	ND			
		Females					
		9–13 y	**1.8**	ND			
		14–18 y	**2.4**	ND			
		19–30 y	**2.4**	ND			
		50–70 y	**2.4**	ND			
		>70 y	**2.4**	ND			
		Pregnancy					
		≤18 y	**2.6**	ND			
		19–30 y	**2.6**	ND			
		31–50 y	**2.6**	ND			
		Lactation					
		≤18 y	**2.8**	ND			
		19–30 y	**2.8**	ND			
		31–50 y	**2.8**	ND			

NOTE: The table is adapted from the DRI reports, see www.nap.edu. It represents Recommended Dietary Allowances (RDAs) in **bold type**, Adequate intakes (AIs) in ordinary type followed by an asterisk (*), and Tolerable Upper Intake Levels (ULs)[a]. RDAs and AIs may both be used as goals for individual intake. RDAs are set to meet the needs of almost all (97 to 98 percent) individuals in a group. For healthy breastfed infants, the AI is the mean intake. The AI for other life stage and gender groups is believed to cover the needs of all individuals in the group, but lack of data prevent being able to specify with confidence the percentage of individuals covered by this intake.

[a]UL = The maximum level of daily nutrient intake that is likely to pose no risk of adverse effects. Unless otherwise specified, the UL represents total intake from food, water, and supplements. Due to lack of suitable data, ULs could not be established for vitamin K, thiamin, riboflavin, vitamin B_{12}, pantolhenic acid, biolin, or carotenoids. In the absence of ULs, extra caution may be warranted in consuming levels above recommended intakes.

[b]ND = Not determinable due to lack of data of adverse effects in this age group and concern with regard to lack of ability to handle excess amounts. Source of intake should be from food only to prevent high levels of intake.

SOURCES: *Dietary Reference Intakes for Calcium, Phosphorous, Magnesium, Vitamin D, and Fluoride* (1997); *Dietary Reference Intakes for Thiamin, Riboflavin, Niacin, Vitamin B_6, Folate, Vitamin B_{12}, Pantolhenic Acid, Biotin, and Choline* (1998); *Dietary Reference Intakes for Vitamin C, Vitamin E, Selenium, and Carotenoids* (2000); and *Dietary Reference Intakes for Vitamin A, Vitamin K, Arsenic, Boron, Chromium, Copper, Iodine, Iron, Manganese, Molybdenum, Nickel, Silicon, Vanadium, and Zinc* (2001). These reports may be accessed via www.nap.edu.

Table 107-2. (continued).

DIETARY REFERENCE INTAKES: VITAMINS

NUTRIENT	FUNCTION	LIFE STAGE GROUP	RDA/AI*	UL[a]	SELECTED FOOD SOURCES	ADVERSE EFFECTS OF EXCESSIVE CONSUMPTION	SPECIAL CONSIDERATIONS
Vitamin C Also known as: Ascorbic acid Dehydro-ascorbic acid (DHA)	Cofactor for reactions requiring reduced copper or iron metallo-enzyme and as a protec-tive antioxi-dant	Infants 0–6 mo 7–12 mo Children 1–3 y 4–8 y Males 9–13 y 14–18 y 19–30 y 31–50 y 50–70 y >70 y Females 9–13 y 14–18 y 19–30 y 31–50 y 50–70 y >70 y Pregnancy ≤18 y 19–30 y 31–50 y Lactation ≤18 y 19–30 y 31–50 y	(mg/d) 40* 50* **15** **25** **45** **75** **90** **1.3** **1.7** **1.7** **45** **65** **75** **7.5** **75** **75** **80** **85** **85** **115** **120** **120**	(mg/d) ND[b] ND 400 850 1,200 1,800 2,000 2,000 2,000 2,000 1,200 1,800 2,000 2,000 2,000 2,000 1,800 2,000 2,000 1,800 2,000 2,000	Citrus fruits, tomatoes, tomato juice, potatoes, brussel sprouts, cauliflower, broccoli, strawberies, cabbage, and spinach	Gastrointestinal disturbances, kidney stones, excess iron absorption	Individuals who smoke require an additional 35 mg/d of vitamin C over that needed by nonsmokers. Nonsmokers regularly exposed to tobacco smoke are encouraged to ensure they meet the RDA for vitamin C.
Vitamin D Also known as: Calciferol Note: 1 µg calciferol = 40 IU vitamin D The DRI values are based on the absence of adequate exposure to sunlight	Maintain serum calcium and phosphorus concentra-tions.	Infants 0–6 mo 7–12 mo Children 1–3 y 4–8 y Males 9–13 y 14–18 y 19–30 y 31–50 y 50–70 y >70 y Females 9–13 y 14–18 y 19–30 y 31–50 y 50–70 y >70 y Pregnancy ≤18 y 19–30 y 31–50 y Lactation ≤18 y 19–30 y 31–50 y	(µg/d) 5* 5* 5* 5* 5* 5* 5* 5* 10* 15* 5* 5* 5* 5* 10* 15* 5* 5* 5* 5* 5* 5*	(µg/d) 25 25 50 50 50 50 50 50 50 50 50 50 50 50 50 50 50 50 50 50 50 50	Fish liver oils, flesh of fatty fish, liver and fat from seals and polar bears, eggs from hens that have been fed vitamin D, fortified milk products and fortified cereals	Elevated plasma 25 (OH) D concentration causing hypercalcemia	Patients on glucocorticoid therapy may require additional vitamin D.

NOTE: The table is adapted from the DRI reports, see www.nap.edu. It represents Recommended Dietary Allowances (RDAs) in **bold type**, Adequate intakes (AIs) in ordinary type followed by an asterisk (*), and Tolerable Upper Intake Levels (ULs)[a]. RDAs and AIs may both be used as goals for individual intake. RDAs are set to meet the needs of almost all (97 to 98 percent) individuals in a group. For healthy breastfed infants, the AI is the mean intake. The AI for other life stage and gender groups is believed to cover the needs of all individuals in the group, but lack of data prevent being able to specify with confidence the percentage of individuals covered by this intake.

[a]UL = The maximum level of daily nutrient intake that is likely to pose no risk of adverse effects. Unless otherwise specified, the UL represents total intake from food, water, and supplements. Due to lack of suitable data, ULs could not be established for vitamin K, thiamin, riboflavin, vitamin B$_{12}$, pantolhenic acid, biolin, or carotenoids. In the absence of ULs, extra caution may be warranted in consuming levels above recommended intakes.

[b]ND = Not determinable due to lack of data of adverse effects in this age group and concern with regard to lack of ability to handle excess amounts. Source of intake should be from food only to prevent high levels of intake.

SOURCES: *Dietary Reference Intakes for Calcium, Phosphorous, Magnesium, Vitamin D, and Fluoride* (1997); *Dietary Reference Intakes for Thiamin, Riboflavin, Niacin, Vitamin B$_6$, Folate, Vitamin B$_{12}$, Pantolhenic Acid, Biotin, and Choline* (1998); *Dietary Reference Intakes for Vitamin C, Vitamin E, Selenium, and Carotenoids* (2000); and *Dietary Reference Intakes for Vitamin A, Vitamin K, Arsenic, Boron, Chromium, Copper, Iodine, Iron, Manganese, Molybdenum, Nickel, Silicon, Vanadium, and Zinc* (2001). These reports may be accessed via www.nap.edu.

Table 107-2. (continued).

NUTRIENT	FUNCTION	LIFE STAGE GROUP	RDA/AI*	UL[a]	SELECTED FOOD SOURCES	ADVERSE EFFECTS OF EXCESSIVE CONSUMPTION	SPECIAL CONSIDERATIONS
Vitamin E Also known as: α-tocopherol Note: As α-tocopherol α-Tocopherol includes *RRR*-α-tocopherol, the only form of α-tocopherol that occurs naturally in foods, and the 2R-stereoisomeric forms of α-tocopherol (*RRR*-, *RSR*-, *RRS*-, and *RSS*-α-tocopherol) that occur in fortified foods and supplements. It does not include the 2S-stereoisomeric forms of α-tocopherol (*SRR*-, *SSR*-, *SRS*-, and *SSS*-α-tocopherol), also found in fortified foods and supplements.	A metabolic function has not yet been identified. Vitamin E's major function appears to be as a non-specific chain-breaking antioxidant.	Infants 0–6 mo 7–12 mo Children 1–3 y 4–8 y Males 9–13 y 14–18 y 19–30 y 31–50 y 50–70 y >70 y Females 9–13 y 14–18 y 19–30 y 31–50 y 50–70 y >70 y Pregnancy ≤18 y 19–30 y 31–50 y Lactation ≤18 y 19–30 y 31–50 y	(mg/d) 4* 5* **6** **7** **11** **15** **15** **15** **15** **15** **11** **15** **15** **15** **15** **15** **15** **15** **15** **19** **19** **19**	(mg/d) ND[b] ND 200 300 600 800 1,000 1,000 1,000 1,000 600 800 1,000 1,000 1,000 1,000 800 1,000 1,000 800 1,000 1,000	Vegetable oils, unprocessed cereal grains, nuts, fruits, vegetables, meats	There is no evidence of adverse effects from the consumption of vitamin E naturally occuring in foods. Adverse effects from vitamin E containing supplements may include hemorrhagic toxicity. The UL for vitamin E applies to any form of α-tocopherol obtained from supplements, fortified foods, or a combination of the two.	Patients on anticoagulant therapy should be monitored when taking vitamin E supplements.
Vitamin K	Coenzyme during the synthesis of many proteins involved in blood clotting and bone metabolism	Infants 0–6 mo 7–12 mo Children 1–3 y 4–8 y Males 9–13 y 14–18 y 19–30 y 31–50 y 50–70 y >70 y Females 9–13 y 14–18 y 19–30 y 31–50 y 50–70 y >70 y Pregnancy ≤18 y 19–30 y 31–50 y Lactation ≤18 y 19–30 y 31–50 y	(μg/d) 2.0* 2.5* 30* 55* 60* 75* 120* 120* 120* 120* 60* 75 90* 90* 90* 90* 75* 90* 90* 75* 90* 90*	ND ND ND ND ND ND ND ND ND ND ND ND ND ND ND ND ND ND ND ND ND ND	Green vegetables (collards, spinach, salad greens, broccoli), brussel sprouts, cabbage, plant oils and margarine	No adverse effects associated with vitamin K consumption from food or supplements have been reported in humans or animals. This does not mean that there is no potential for adverse effects resulting from high intakes. Because data on the adverse effects of vitamin K are limited, caution may be warranted.	Patients on anticoagulant therapy should monitor vitamin K intake.

NOTE: The table is adapted from the DRI reports, see www.nap.edu. It represents Recommended Dietary Allowances (RDAs) in **bold type**, Adequate intakes (AIs) in ordinary type followed by an asterisk (*), and Tolerable Upper Intake Levels (ULs)[a]. RDAs and AIs may both be used as goals for individual intake. RDAs are set to meet the needs of almost all (97 to 98 percent) individuals in a group. For healthy breastfed infants, the AI is the mean intake. The AI for other life stage and gender groups is believed to cover the needs of all individuals in the group, but lack of data prevent being able to specify with confidence the percentage of individuals covered by this intake.

[a]UL = The maximum level of daily nutrient intake that is likely to pose no risk of adverse effects. Unless otherwise specified, the UL represents total intake from food, water, and supplements. Due to lack of suitable data, ULs could not be established for vitamin K, thiamin, riboflavin, vitamin B12, pantolhenic acid, biolin, or carotenoids. In the absence of ULs, extra caution may be warranted in consuming levels above recommended intakes.

[b]ND = Not determinable due to lack of data of adverse effects in this age group and concern with regard to lack of ability to handle excess amounts. Source of intake should be from food only to prevent high levels of intake.

SOURCES: *Dietary Reference Intakes for Calcium, Phosphorous, Magnesium, Vitamin D, and Fluoride* (1997); *Dietary Reference Intakes for Thiamin, Riboflavin, Niacin, Vitamin B6, Folate, Vitamin B12, Pantolhenic Acid, Biotin, and Choline* (1998); *Dietary Reference Intakes for Vitamin C, Vitamin E, Selenium, and Carotenoids* (2000); and *Dietary Reference Intakes for Vitamin A, Vitamin K, Arsenic, Boron, Chromium, Copper, Iodine, Iron, Manganese, Molybdenum, Nickel, Silicon, Vanadium, and Zinc* (2001). These reports may be accessed via www.nap.edu.

Table 107-3. Food and Nutrition Board, Institute of Medicine-National Academy of Sciences Dietary Reference Intakes: Macronutrients

NUTRIENT	FUNCTION	LIFE STAGE GROUP	RDA/AI* G/D	AMDR	SELECTED FOOD SOURCES	ADVERSE EFFECT OF EXCESSIVE CONSUMPTION
Carbohydrate— Total digestible	RDA based on its role as the primary energy source for the brain; AMDR based on its role as a source of kilocalories to maintain body weight	Infants			Starch and sugar are the major types of carbohydrates. Grains and vegetables (corn, pasta, rice, potatoes, breads) are sources of starch. Natural sugars are found in fruits and juices. Sources of added sugars are soft drinks, candy, fruit drinks, and desserts.	While no defined intake level at which potential adverse effects of total digestible carbohydrate was identified, the upper end of the adequate macronutrient distribution range (AMDR) was based on decreasing risk of chronic disease and providing adequate intake of other nutrients. It is suggested that the maximal intake of added sugars be limited to providing no more than 25 percent of energy.
		0–6 mo	60*	ND[b]		
		7–12 mo	95*	ND		
		Children				
		1–3 y	**130**	45–65		
		4–8 y	**130**	45–65		
		Males				
		9–13 y	**130**	45–65		
		14–18 y	**130**	45–65		
		19–30 y	**130**	45–65		
		31–50 y	**130**	45–65		
		50–70 y	**130**	45–65		
		>70 y				
		Females				
		9–13 y	**130**	45–65		
		14–18 y	**130**	45–65		
		19–30 y	**130**	45–65		
		31–50 y	**130**	45–65		
		50–70 y	**130**	45–65		
		>70 y	**130**	45–65		
		Pregnancy				
		≤18 y	**175**	45–65		
		19–30 y	**175**	45–65		
		31–50 y	**175**	45–65		
		Lactation				
		≤18 y	**210**	45–65		
		19–30 y	**210**	45–65		
		31–50 y	**210**	45–65		
Total Fiber	Improves laxation, reduces risk of coronary heart disease, assists in maintaining normal blooed glucose levels.	Infants			Includes dietary fiber naturally present in grains (such as found in oats, wheat, or unmilled rice) and functional fiber synthesized or isolated from plants or animals and shown to be of benefit to health	Dietary fiber can have variable compositions and therefore it is difficult to link a specific source of fiber with a particular adverse effect, especially when phylate is also present in the natural fiber source. It is concluded that as part of an overall healthy diet, a high intake of dietary fiber will not produce deleterious effects in healthy individuals. While occasional adverse gastrointestinal symptoms are observed when consuming some isolated or synthetic fibers, serious chronic adverse effects have not been observed. Due to the bulky nature of fibers, excess consumption is likely to be self-limiting. Therefore, a UL was not set for individual functional fibers.
		0–8 mo	ND			
		7–12 mo	ND			
		Children				
		1–3 y	19*			
		4–8 y	25*			
		Males				
		9–13 y	31*			
		14–18 y	38*			
		19–30 y	38*			
		31–50 y	38*			
		50–70 y	30*			
		>70 y	30*			
		Females				
		9–13 y	26*			
		14–18 y	26*			
		19–30 y	25*			
		31–50 y	25*			
		50–70 y	21*			
		>70 y	21*			
		Pregnancy				
		≤18 y	28*			
		19–30 y	28*			
		31–50 y	28*			
		Lactation				
		≤18 y	29*			
		19–30 y	29*			
		31–50 y	29*			

NOTE: The table is adapted from the DRI reports, see www.nap.edu. It represents Recommended Dietary Allowances (RDAs) in the **bold type,** Adequate Intakes (AIs) in ordinary type followed by an asterisk (*). RDAs and AIs may both be used as goals for individual intake. RDAs are set to meet the needs of almost all (97 to 98 percent) individuals in a group. For healthy breastfed infants, the AI is the mean intake. The AI for other life stage and gender groups is believed to cover the needs of all individuals in the group, but lack of data prevent being able to specify with confidence the percentage of individuals covered by this intake.

[a]Acceptance Macronutrient Distribution Range (AMDR)[a] is the range of intake for a particular energy source that is associated with reduced risk of chronic disease while providing intakes of essential nutrients. If an individual consumes in excess of the AMDR, there is a potential of increasing the risk of chronic diseases and/or insufficient intakes of essential nutrients.

[b]ND = Not determinable due to lack of data of adverse effects in this age group and concern with regard to lack of ability to handle excess amounts. Source of intake should be from food only to prevent high levels of intake.

SOURCES: *Dietary Reference Intakes for Energy, Carbohydrate, Fiber, Fat, Fatty Acids, Cholesterol, Protein, and Amino acids (2002).* This report may be accessed via www.nap.edu.

Table 107-3. *(continued).*

					DIETARY REFERENCE INTAKES: MACRONUTRIENTS	
NUTRIENT	FUNCTION	LIFE STAGE GROUP	RDA/AI* G/D	AMDR[b]	SELECTED FOOD SOURCES	ADVERSE EFFECT OF EXCESSIVE CONSUMPTION
Total fat	Energy source and when found in foods, is a source of *n-6* and *n-3* polysaturated fatty acids. Its presence in the diet increases absorption of fat soluble vitamins and precursors such as vitamin A and pro-vitamin A carotenoids.	Infants 0–6 mo 7–12 mo	31* 30*		Butter, margarine, vegetable oils, whole milk, visible fat on meat and poultry products, invisible fat in fish, shellfish, some plant products such as seeds and nuts, and bakery products.	While no defined intake level at which potential adverse effects of total fat was identified, the upper end of AMDR is based on decreasing risk of chronic disease and providing adequate intake of other nutrients. The lower end of the AMDR is based on concerns related to the increase in plasma triacylglycerol concentrations and decreased HDL cheolesterol concentrations seen with very low fat (and thus high carbohydrate) diets.
		Children 1–3 y 4–8 y		30–40 25–35		
		Males 9–13 y 14–18 y 19–30 y 31–50 y 50–70 y >70 y		25–35 25–35 20–35 20–35 20–35 20–35		
		Females 9–13 y 14–18 y 19–30 y 31–50 y 50–70 y >70 y		25–35 25–35 20–35 20–35 20–35 20–35		
		Pregnancy ≤18 y 19–30 y 31–50 y		20–35 20–35 20–35		
		Lactation ≤18 y 19–30 y 31–50 y		20–35 20–35 20–35		
n-6 polyunsaturated fatty acids (linoleic acid)	Essential component of structural membrane lipids, involved with cell signaling, and precursor of eicosanoids. Required for normal skin function.	Infants 0–6 mo 7–12 mo	4.4* 4.6*	ND[b] ND	Nuts, seeds, and vegetable oils such as soybean, safflower, and corn oil.	While no defined intake level at which potential adverse effects of *n-6* polyunsaturated fatty acids was identified, the upper end of the AMDR is based the lack of evidence that demonstrates long-term safety and human in vitro studies which show increased free-radical formation and lipid peroxidation with higher amounts of n-6 fatty acids. Lipid peroxidation is thought to be a component of in the development of atherosclerotic plaques.
		Children 1–3 y 4–8 y	7* 10*	5–10 5–10		
		Males 9–13 y 14–18 y 19–30 y 31–50 y 50–70 y >70 y	12* 16* 17* 17* 14* 14*	5–10 5–10 5–10 5–10 5–10 5–10		
		Females 9–13 y 14–18 y 19–30 y 31–50 y 50–70 y >70 y	10* 11* 17* 17* 14* **14***	5–10 5–10 5–10 5–10 5–10 5–10		
		Pregnancy ≤18 y 19–30 y 31–50 y	13* 13* 13*	5–10 5–10 5–10		
		Lactation ≤18 y 19–30 y 31–50 y	13* 13* 13*	5–10 5–10 5–10		

NOTE: The table is adapted from the DRI reports, see www.nap.edu. It represents Recommended Dietary Allowances (RDAs) in the **bold type,** Adequate Intakes (AIs) in ordinary type followed by an asterisk (*). RDAs and AIs may both be used as goals for individual intake. RDAs are set to meet the needs of almost all (97 to 98 percent) individuals in a group. For healthy breastfed infants, the AI is the mean intake. The AI for other life stage and gender groups is believed to cover the needs of all individuals in the group, but lack of data prevent being able to specify with confidence the percentage of individuals covered by this intake.

[a]Acceptance Macronutrient Distribution Range (AMDR)[a] is the range of intake for a particular energy source that is associated with reduced risk of chronic disease while providing intakes of essential nutrients. If an individual consumes in excess of the AMDR, there is a potential of increasing the risk of chronic diseases and/or insufficient intakes of essential nutrients.

[b]ND = Not determinable due to lack of data of adverse effects in this age group and concern with regard to lack of ability to handle excess amounts. Source of intake should be from food only to prevent high levels of intake.

SOURCES: *Dietary Reference Intakes for Energy, Carbohydrate, Fiber, Fat, Fatty Acids, Cholesterol, Protein, and Amino acids (2002).* This report may be accessed via www.nap.edu.

Table 107-3. *(continued).*

DIETARY REFERENCE INTAKES: MACRONUTRIENTS

NUTRIENT	FUNCTION	LIFE STAGE GROUP	RDA/AI* G/D	AMDR[a]	SELECTED FOOD SOURCES	ADVERSE EFFECT OF EXCESSIVE CONSUMPTION
n-3 polyunsaturated fatty acids (α-linoleic acid)	Involved with neurological development and growth. Precursor of elcosanoids.	Infants			Vegetable oils such as soybean, canola, and flax seed oil, fish oils, fatty fish, with smaller amounts in meats and eggs.	While no defined intake level at which potential adverse effects of n-3 polyunsaturated fatty acids was identified, the upper end of AMDR is based on maintaining the appropriate balance with n-6 fatty acids and on the lack of evidence that demonstrates long-term safety, along with human in vitro studies which show increased free-radical formation and lipid peroxidation with higher amounts of polyunsaturated fatty acids. Lipid peroxidation is thought to be a component of in the development of atherosclerotic plaques.
		0–6 mo	0.5*	ND[b]		
		7–12 mo	0.5*	ND		
		Children				
		1–3 y	0.7*	0.6–1.2		
		4–8 y	0.9*	0.6–1.2		
		Males				
		9–13 y	1.2*	0.6–1.2		
		14–18 y	1.6*	0.6–1.2		
		19–30 y	1.6*	0.6–1.2		
		31–50 y	1.6*	0.6–1.2		
		50–70 y	1.6*	0.6–1.2		
		>70 y	1.6*	0.6–1.2		
		Females				
		9–13 y	1.0*	0.6–1.2		
		14–18 y	1.1*	0.6–1.2		
		19–30 y	1.1*	0.6–1.2		
		31–50 y	1.1*	0.6–1.2		
		50–70 y	1.1*	0.6–1.2		
		>70 y	1.1*	0.6–1.2		
		Pregnancy				
		≤18 y	**1.4***	0.6–1.2		
		19–30 y	**1.4***	0.6–1.2		
		31–50 y	**1.4***	0.6–1.2		
		Lactation				
		≤18 y	1.3*	0.6–1.2		
		19–30 y	1.3*	0.6–1.2		
		31–50 y	1.3*	0.6–1.2		
Saturated and *trans* fatty acids, and cholesterol	No required role for these nutrients other than as energy sources was identified; the body can synthesize its needs for saturated fatty acids and cholesterol from other sources.	Infants			Saturated fatty acids are present in animal fats (meat fats and butter fat), and coconut and palm kernel oils. Sources of cholesterol include liver, eggs, and foods that contain eggs such as cheesecake and custard pies. Sources of *trans* fatty acids include stick margarines and foods containing hydrogenated or partially-hydrogenated vegetable shortenings.	There is an incremental increase in plasma total and low-density lipoprotein cholesterol concentrations with increased intake of saturated or *trans* fatty acids or with cholesterol at even very low levels in the diet. Therefore, the intakes of each should be minimized while consuming a nutritionally adequate diet.
		0–6 mo	ND			
		7–12 mo	ND			
		Children				
		1–3 y				
		4–8 y				
		Males				
		9–13 y				
		14–18 y				
		19–30 y				
		31–50 y				
		50–70 y				
		>70 y				
		Females				
		9–13 y				
		14–18 y				
		19–30 y				
		31–50 y				
		50-70 y				
		>70 y				
		Pregnancy				
		≤18 y				
		19–30 y				
		31–50 y				
		Lactation				
		≤18 y				
		19–30 y				
		31–50 y				

NOTE: The table is adapted from the DRI reports, see www.nap.edu. It represents Recommended Dietary Allowances (RDAs) in the **bold type**, Adequate Intakes (AIs) in ordinary type followed by an asterisk (*). RDAs and AIs may both be used as goals for individual intake. RDAs are set to meet the needs of almost all (97 to 98 percent) individuals in a group. For healthy breastfed infants, the AI is the mean intake. The AI for other life stage and gender groups is believed to cover the needs of all individuals in the group, but lack of data prevent being able to specify with confidence the percentage of individuals covered by this intake.

[a]Acceptance Macronutrient Distribution Range (AMDR)[a] is the range of intake for a particular energy source that is associated with reduced risk of chronic disease while providing intakes of essential nutrients. If an individual consumes in excess of the AMDR, there is a potential of increasing the risk of chronic diseases and/or insufficient intakes of essential nutrients.

[b]ND = Not determinable due to lack of data of adverse effects in this age group and concern with regard to lack of ability to handle excess amounts. Source of intake should be from food only to prevent high levels of intake.

SOURCES: *Dietary Reference Intakes for Energy, Carbohydrate, Fiber, Fat, Fatty Acids, Cholesterol, Protein, and Amino acids (2002).* This report may be accessed via www.nap.edu.

Table 107-3. *(continued).*

			DIETARY REFERENCE INTAKES: MACRONUTRIENTS			
NUTRIENT	FUNCTION	LIFE STAGE GROUP	RDA/AI* G/D*	AMDR[a]	SELECTED FOOD SOURCES	ADVERSE EFFECT OF EXCESSIVE CONSUMPTION
Protein and amino acids	Serves as the major structural component of all cells in the body, and functions as enzymes, in membranes, as transport carriers, and as some hormones. During digestion and absorption dietary proteins are broken down to amino acids, which become the building blocks of these structural and functional compounds. Nine of the amino acids must be provided in the diet; these are termed indispensable amino acids. The body can make the other amino acids needed to synthesize specific structures from other amino acids.	Infants			Proteins from animal sources, such as meat, poultry, fish, eggs, milk, cheese, and yogurt, provide all nine indispensable amino acids in adequate amounts, and for this reason are considered "complete proteins". Proteins from plants, legumes, grains nuts, seeds, and vegetables tend to be deficient in one or more of the indispensable amino acids and are called 'incomplete proteins'. Vegan diets adequate in total protein content can be "complete" by combining sources of incomplete proteins which lack different indispensable amino acids.	While no defined intake level at which potential adverse effects of protein was identified, the upper end of AMDR based on complementing the AMDR for carbohydrate and fat for the various age groups. The lower end of the AMDR is set at approximately the RDA.
		0–6 mo	9.1*	ND[c]		
		7–12 mo	13.5	ND		
		Children				
		1–3 y	13	5–20		
		4–8 y	19	10–30		
		Males				
		9–13 y	**34**	10–30		
		14–18 y	**52**	10–30		
		19–30 y	**56**	10–35		
		31–50 y	**56**	10–35		
		50–70 y	**56**	10–35		
		>70 y	**56**	10–35		
		Females				
		9–13 y	**34**	10–30		
		14–18 y	**46**	10–30		
		19–30 y	**46**	10–35		
		31–50 y	**46**	10–35		
		50–70 y	**46**	10–35		
		> 70 y	**46**	10–35		
		Pregnancy				
		≤18 y	**71**	10.35		
		19–30 y	**71**	10.35		
		31–50 y	**71**	10.35		
		Lactation				
		≤18 y	**71**	10.35		
		19–30 y	**71**	10.35		
		31–50 y	**71**	10.35		

NOTE: The table is adapted from the DRI reports, see www.nap.edu. It represents Recommended Dietary Allowances (RDAs) in the **bold type,** Adequate Intakes (AIs) in ordinary type followed by an asterisk (*). RDAs and AIs may both be used as goals for individual intake. RDAs are set to meet the needs of almost all (97 to 98 percent) individuals in a group. For healthy breastfed infants, the AI is the mean intake. The AI for other life stage and gender groups is believed to cover the needs of all individuals in the group, but lack of data prevent being able to specify with confidence the percentage of individuals covered by this intake.
[a]Based on 1.5 g/kg/day for infants, 1.1 g/kg/day for 1–3, 0.95 g/kg/day for 4–13 y, 0.85 g/kg/day for 14–18 y, 0.8 g/kg/day for adults, and 1.1 g/kg/day for pregnant (using pre-pregnancy weight) and lactating women.
[b]Acceptable Macronutrient Distribution Range (AMDR)[a] is the range of intake for a particular energy source that is associated with reduced risk of chronic disease while providing intakes of essential nutrients. If an individuals consumed in excess of the AMDR, there is a potential of increasing the risk of chronic diseases and insufficient intakes of essential nutrients.
[c]ND = Not determinable due to lack of data of adverse effects in this age group and concern with regard to lack of ability to handle excess amounts. Source of intake should be from food only to prevent high levels of intake.
SOURCES: *Dietary Reference Intakes for Energy, Carbohydrate, Fiber, Fat, Fatty Acids, Cholesterol, Protein, and Amino acids (2002).* This report may be accessed via www.nap.edu.

Meat alternatives that supply the same amount of protein as a 2-oz, cooked serving of meat include 2 eggs, 1 cup dried beans or peas (cooked), 4 tablespoons peanut butter, 2 oz hard cheese, or 1/2 cup cottage cheese. Although these foods substitute for the protein in a 2-oz serving of meat, poultry, or fish, they do not substitute for all the other nutrients found in meat such as iron, zinc, and B vitamins.

Appropriate use of the Food Guide Pyramid requires knowledge of what constitutes a serving. Evidence indicates consumers are more confused about serving sizes and how they relate to the amount of food eaten. This likely is contributing to the overconsumption of food and the increased prevalence of obesity in our society. The Food Guide Pyramid gives suggested servings and defines the serving size. A "serving" is very different from a portion as a portion is an amount of food eaten in one setting, is often more than a serving, and may contribute unwanted calories. Consider today's 20 to 46 oz beverage versus a traditional serving size of 8 oz. Table 107-9 reviews what is considered a serving.

Two specific guidelines further emphasize the foods at the first and second level of the pyramid base.

CHOOSE A VARIETY OF GRAINS DAILY, ESPECIALLY WHOLE GRAINS—Foods from grains form the base of the Food Guide Pyramid, thus illustrating that this should be the foundation of a healthy diet. These three food groups provide fewer kilocalories than many foods in the top two pyramid groups, are important sources of vitamins and minerals, and are the only food sources of dietary fiber. Grains include foods such as pasta, breads, cereals, and rice. When selecting a diet high in grains, especially bread and baked products, look for those labeled *whole grain* or that list *whole-grain* flours as one of the first ingredients on the label. Also be aware that many baked items can also be high in fat and sugar.

CHOOSE A VARIETY OF FRUITS AND VEGETABLES DAILY—The Five-A-Day campaign was initiated by the National Cancer Institute in the early 1990s to call attention to ingesting a minimum of five fruits and vegetables a day.

Evidence suggests this simple recommendation could help to reduce the risk for some cancers because of the vitamin, mineral, and fiber content of fruits and vegetables. Evidence is mounting to indicate a protective role for nutrients especially associated with fruits and vegetables. This includes the antioxidant nutrients (vitamin C, vitamin E, beta carotene, and the mineral selenium) and the B vitamin folic acid. Fruits and vegetables are the primary sources of beta-carotene, as well as vitamins A and C, whereas selenium is found in meat, fish, and eggs but also in the grains of whole-wheat bread and oatmeal. Vitamin E is found in oils used in salad dressings and margarines. Antioxidants help to prevent the oxidation of

Table 107-3. *(continued).*

		DIETARY REFERENCE INTAKES: MACRONUTRIENTS		
NUTRIENT	FUNCTION	IOM/FNB 2002 SCORING PATTERN[a]	MG/G PROTEIN	ADVERSE EFFECTS OF EXCESSIVE CONSUMPTION
Indispensable amino acids:				
Histidine	The building blocks of all proteins in the body and some hormones. These nine amino acids must be provided in the diet and thus are termed indispensable amino acids. The body can make the other amino acids needed to synthesize specific structures from other amino acids and carbohydrate precursors.	Histidine	18	Since there is no evidence that amino acids found in usual or even high intakes of protein from food present any risk, attention was focused on intakes of the L-form of these and other amino acid found in dietary protein and amino acid supplements. Even from well-studied amino acids, adequate dose-response data from human or animal studies on which to base a UL were not available. While no defined intake level at which potential adverse effects of protein was identified for any amino acid, this does not mean that there is no potential for adverse effects resulting from high intakes of amino acids from dietary supplements. Since data on the adverse effects of high levels of amino acid intakes from dietary supplements are limited, caution may be warranted.
Isoleucine		Isoleucine	25	
Lysine		Lysine	55	
Leucine		Leucine	51	
Methlonine & Cysteine		Methionine & Cysteine	25	
Phenylalanine & Tyrosine		Phenylalanine & Tyrosine	47	
Threonine		Threonine	27	
Tryptophan		Tryptophan	7	
Valine		Valine	32	

NOTE: The table is adapted from the DRI reports, see www.nap.edu.
[a] Based on the amino acid requirements derived for Preschool Children (1–3 y): (EAR for amino acid + EAR for protein); for 1–3 y group where EAR for protein = 0.88 g/kg/d.
SOURCES: *Dietary Reference Intakes for Energy, Carbohydrate. Fiber, Fat, Fatty Acids, Cholesterol, Protein, and Amino Acids* (2002). This report may be accessed via www.nap.edu.

substances in the body, including free radicals. Free radicals are compounds with an unpaired electron that can be especially destructive to electron-dense areas of the cell such as the DNA and the cell membrane. Lipids are components of cell membranes. Oxidation of lipids occurs freely in the body and in foods. The antioxidant nutrients help to decrease the amount and rate of oxidation. The oxidation of lipids is implicated in the development of arterial plaque in CHD and in the DNA changes in the cell during the initiation of a cancer. Oxidation of lipids in foods causes rancidity and spoilage. Folic acid, a member of the B vitamin family, is found in some fruits and vegetables as folate. Adequate amounts of folic acid have been proved to reduce the risk of neural-tube defects, such as spina bifida, in the developing fetus. This role of folic acid is so strong that in 1992, the US Public Health Service (USPHS) issued a recommendation for all women of childbearing age to take the vitamin as a supplement. It is important to take folic acid before conception because neural-tube development occurs in the first trimester of pregnancy. This is a time when many women would not yet know they were pregnant. To further foster the consumption of folic acid in the diet, the nutrient was added to enriched bread products starting in January 1998 and is believed responsible for the reduction of related neural tube defects. Folic acid also may be related to reduction of risk of cardiovascular disease through a role in reducing homocysteine levels.

Fiber is an important component of plant carbohydrates in our diet, and the best sources are the whole grains, fruits and vegetables, and legumes. Dietary fiber is defined as plant parts that are not digested by the human digestive tract. Animal foods such as dairy foods and meats do not contain any dietary fiber. For the first time, the DRI report in September 2002 recommended to eat 14 g of dietary fiber for every 1000 calories. This represents approximately double what most Americans currently consume. Increasing dietary fiber would decrease the incidence of diverticulosis and potentially problems associated with constipation. Table 107-10 includes a representative fiber content of selected types of foods.

Not all food fiber acts the same in the body. Contributing a smaller part of the total fiber content of foods are soluble fibers that act in the small intestine. Soluble fiber is related to less absorption of dietary cholesterol and also plays a role in the control of blood glucose. Insoluble fibers act in the large intestine where they add bulk and foster regular elimination of wastes. Food sources have a mixture of soluble and insoluble. When asked about fiber supplements, the clinician should first stress food sources such as grains, fruits, vegetables, and legumes because food sources offer the added benefit of the vitamins and minerals associated with these foods. Additionally plant foods carry a variety of phytochemicals, substances in plants that increasingly are being found to offer benefits related to good health.

KEEP FOOD SAFE TO EAT—The addition of this dietary guideline in the 2000 edition illustrates the increasing concern over food borne illness and the importance of handling food safely in the home. Basic hygiene practices such as washing hands before handling food and washing surfaces in contact with food, such as cutting boards and counters, seem common sense, but lack of these practices contributes to food-borne illness. Although these practices are recommended for everyone, they are especially important for the vulnerable population groups such as pregnant women and those with a compromised immune system.

Choose Sensibly

CHOOSE A DIET THAT IS LOW IN SATURATED FAT AND CHOLESTEROL AND MODERATE IN TOTAL FAT—With all the increased emphasis on fats in the diet, it is important for the professional to understand that some dietary fat is needed for good health. Fats provide essential substances such as essential fatty acids and are sources of the fat-soluble vitamins A, E, D, and K. The Dietary Guidelines counsel Americans to choose a diet low in total fat, and particularly low in saturated fat and cholesterol. Many pharmacy clients are on medications to reduce their cholesterol or triglyceride levels. Although blood lipids and dietary lipids are not always directly associated, in general, medications intended to alter blood lipids work best if the client also is following a diet modified in fat. Dietary fat often is referred to as saturated, polyunsaturated, or monounsaturated, which refers to the degree of saturation of the fatty acid, the basic chemical unit in fat. Although the DRIs recommended a wide range for the percent of kcal from fat, the current version of the Dietary Guidelines suggests less than 30% of total kilocalories

Table 107-4. Food and Nutrition Board, Institute of Medicine-National Academy of Sciences Dietary Reference Intakes: Electrolytes and Water

DIETARY REFERENCE INTAKES: ELECTROLYTES AND WATER

NUTRIENT	FUNCTION	LIFE STAGE GROUP	AI	UL[a]	SELECTED FOOD SOURCES	ADVERSE EFFECTS OF EXCESSIVE CONSUMPTION	SPECIAL CONSIDERATIONS
Sodium	Maintains fluid volume outside of cells and thus normal cell function.		(g/d)	(g/d)	Processed foods to which sodium chloride (salt) /benzoate/phosphate have been added; salted meats, nuts, cold cuts; margarine; butter; salt added to foods in cooking or at the table. Salt is ~ 40% sodium by weight.	Hypertension; increased risk of cardiovascular disease and stroke.	The AI is set based on being able to obtain a nutritionally adequate diet for other nutrients and to meet the needs for sweat losses for individuals engaged in recommended levels of physical activity. Individuals engaged in activity at higher levels or in humid climates resulting in excessive sweat may need more than the AI. The UL applies to apparently healthy individuals without hypertension; it thus may be too high for individuals who already have hypertension or who are under the care of a health care professional.
		Infants					
		0–6 mo	0.12	ND[b]			
		7–12 mo	0.37	ND[b]			
		Children					
		1–3 y	1.0	1.5			
		4–8 y	1.2	1.9			
		Males					
		9–13 y	1.5	2.2			
		14–18 y	1.5	2.3			
		19–30 y	1.5	2.3			
		31–50 y	1.5	2.3			
		50–70 y	1.3	2.3			
		>70 y	1.2	2.3			
		Females					
		9–13 y	1.5	2.2			
		14–18 y	1.5	2.3			
		19–30 y	1.5	2.3			
		31–50 y	1.5	2.3			
		50–70 y	1.3	2.3			
		>70 y	1.2	2.3			
		Pregnancy					
		14–18 y	1.5	2.3			
		19–50 y	1.5	2.3			
		Lactation					
		14–18 y	1.5	2.3			
		19–50 y	1.5	2.3			
Chloride	With sodium, maintains fluid volume outside of cells and thus normal cell function.		(g/d)	(g/d)	See above; about 60% by weight of salt.	In concert with sodium, results in hypertension.	Chloride is lost usually with sodium in sweat, as well as in vomiting and diarrhea. The AI and UL are equal-molar in amount to sodium since most of sodium in diet comes as sodium chloride (salt).
		Infants					
		0–6 mo	0.18	ND[b]			
		7–12 mo	0.57	ND[b]			
		Children					
		1–3 y	1.5	2.3			
		4–8 y	1.9	2.9			
		Males					
		9–13 y	2.3	3.4			
		14–18 y	2.3	3.6			
		19–30 y	2.3	3.6			
		31–50 y	2.3	3.6			
		50–70 y	2.0	3.6			
		>70 y	1.8	3.6			
		Females					
		9–13 y	2.3	3.4			
		14–18 y	2.3	3.6			
		19–30 y	2.3	3.6			
		31–50 y	2.3	3.6			
		50–70 y	2.0	3.6			
		>70 y	1.8	3.6			
		Pregnancy					
		14–18 y	2.3	3.6			
		19–50 y	2.3	3.6			
		Lactation					
		14–18 y	2.3	3.6			
		19–50 y	2.3	3.6			

NOTE: The table is adapted from the DRI reports. See www.nap.edu. Adequate Intakes (AIs) may be used as a goal for individual intake. For healthy breastfed infants, the AI is the mean intake. The AI for other life stage and gender groups is believed to cover the needs of all individuals in the group, but lack of data prevent being able to specify with confidence the percentage of individuals covered by this intake; therefore, no Recommended Dietary Allowance (RDA) was set.

[a]UL = The maximum level of daily nutrient intake that is likely to pose no risk of adverse effects. Unless otherwise specified, the UL represents total intake from food, water, and supplements. Due to lack of suitable data, ULs could not be established for potassium, water, and inorganic sulfate. In the absence of ULs, extra caution may be warranted in consuming levels above recommended intakes.

[b]ND = Not determinable due to lack of data of adverse effects in this age group and concern with regard to lack of ability to handle excess amounts. Source of intake should be from food only to prevent high levels of intake.

SOURCE: *Dietary Reference Intakes for Water, Potassium, Sodium, Chloride, and Sulfate.* This reports may be accessed via www.nap.edu.

Table 107-4. *(continued)*.

NUTRIENT	FUNCTION	LIFE STAGE GROUP	AI	UL[a]	SELECTED FOOD SOURCES	ADVERSE EFFECTS OF EXCESSIVE CONSUMPTION	SPECIAL CONSIDERATIONS
Potassium	Maintains fluid volume inside/ outside of cells and thus normal cell function; acts to blunt the rise of blood pressure in response to excess sodium intake, and decrease markers of bone turnover and recurrence of kidney stones.		(g/d)	No UL.	Fruits and vegetables; dried peas; dairy products; meats, and nuts.	None documented from food alone; however, potassium from supplements or salt substitute can result in hyperkalemia and possibly sudden death if excess is consumed by individuals with chronic renal insufficiency (kidney disease) or diabetes.	Individuals taking drugs for cardiovascular disease such as ACE inhibitors, ARBs (Angiontensin Receptor Blockers), or potassium sparing diuretics should be careful to not consume supplements containing potassium and may need to consume less than the AI for potassium.
		Infants					
		0–6 mo	0.4				
		7–12 mo	0.7				
		Children					
		1–3 y	3.0				
		4–8 y	3.8				
		Males					
		9–13 y	4.5				
		14–18 y	4.7				
		19–30 y	4.7				
		31–50 y	4.7				
		50–70 y	4.7				
		>70 y	4.7				
		Females					
		9–13 y	4.5				
		14–18 y	4.7				
		19–30 y	4.7				
		31–50 y	4.7				
		50–70 y	4.7				
		>70 y	4.7				
		Pregnancy					
		14–18 y	4.7				
		19–50 y	4.7				
		Lactation					
		14–18 y	5.1				
		19–50 y	5.1				
Water	Maintains homeostasis in the body and allows for transport of nutrients to cells and removal and excretion of waste products of metabolism.		(L/d)	No UL.	All beverages, including water, as well as moisture in foods (high moisture foods include watermelon, meats, soups, etc.).	No UL because normally functioning kidneys can handle more than 0.7 L (24 oz) of fluid per hour; symptoms of water intoxication include hyponatremia which can result in heart failure and rhabdomyolysis (skeletal muscle tissue injury) which can lead to kidney failure.	Recommended intakes for water are based on median intakes of generally healthy individuals who are adequately hydrated; individuals can be adequately hydrated at levels below as well as above the AIs provided. The AIs provided are for total water in temperate climates. All sources can contribute to total water needs; beverages (including tea, coffee, juices, sodas, and drinking water) and moisture found in foods. Moisture in food accounts for about 20% of total water intake. Thirst and consumption of beverages at meals are adequate to maintain hydration.
		Infants					
		0–6 mo	0.7				
		7–12 mo	0.8				
		Children					
		1–3 y	1.3				
		4–8 y	1.7				
		Males					
		9–13 y	2.4				
		14–18 y	3.3				
		19–30 y	3.7				
		31–50 y	3.7				
		50–70 y	3.7				
		>70 y	3.7				
		Females					
		9–13 y	2.1				
		14–18 y	2.3				
		19–30 y	2.7				
		31–50 y	2.7				
		50–70 y	2.7				
		>70 y	2.7				
		Pregnancy					
		14–18 y	3.0				
		19–50 y	3.0				
		Lactation					
		14–18 y	3.8				
		19–50 y	3.8				

NOTE: The table is adapted from the DRI reports. See www.nap.edu. Adequate Intakes (AIs) may be used as a goal for individual intake. For healthy breastfed infants, the AI is the mean intake. The AI for other life stage and gender groups is believed to cover the needs of all individuals in the group, but lack of data prevent being able to specify with confidence the percentage of individuals covered by this intake; therefore, no Recommended Dietary Allowance (RDA) was set.

[a]UL = The maximum level of daily nutrient intake that is likely to pose no risk of adverse effects. Unless otherwise specified, the UL represents total intake from food, water, and supplements. Due to lack of suitable data, ULs could not be established for potassium, water, and inorganic sulfate. In the absence of ULs, extra caution may be warranted in consuming levels above recommended intakes.

[b]ND = Not determinable due to lack of data of adverse effects in this age group and concern with regard to lack of ability to handle excess amounts. Source of intake should be from food only to prevent high levels of intake.

SOURCE: *Dietary Reference Intakes for Water, Potassium, Sodium, Chloride, and Sulfate.* This reports may be accessed via www.nap.edu.

Table 107-4. *(continued).*

						ADVERSE EFFECTS OF	
		LIFE STAGE			SELECTED FOOD	EXCESSIVE	
NUTRIENT	FUNCTION	GROUP	AI	UL[a]	SOURCES	CONSUMPTION	SPECIAL CONSIDERATIONS
Inorganic Sulfate	Required for biosynthesis of 3'-phosphoadenosine-5'-phosphate (PAPS), which provides sulfate when sulfur-containing compounds are needed such as chondroitin sulfate and cerebroside sulfate.	Infants 0–6 mo 7–12 mo Children 1–3 y 4–8 y Males 9–13 y 14–18 y 19–30 y 31–50 y 50–70 y >70 y Females 9–13 y 14–18 y 19–30 y 31–50 y 50–70 y >70 y Pregnancy 14–18 y 19–50 y Lactation 14–18 y 19–50 y	No recommended intake was set as adequate sulfate is available from dietary inorganic sulfate from water and foods, and from sources of organic sulfate, such as glutathlone and the sulfur amino acids methionine and cysteine. Metabolic breakdown of the recommended intake for protein and sulfur amino acids should provide adequate inorganic sulfate for synthesis of required sulfur-containing compounds.	No UL	Dried fruit (dates, raisins, dried apples), soy flour, fruit juices, coconut milk, red and white wine, bread, as well as meats that are high in sulfur amino acids.	Osmotic diarrhea was observed in areas where water supply had high levels; odor and off taste usually limit intake, and thus no UL was set.	

NOTE: The table is adapted from the DRI reports. See www.nap.edu. Adequate Intakes (AIs) may be used as a goal for individual intake. For healthy breastfed infants, the AI is the mean intake. The AI for other life stage and gender groups is believed to cover the needs of all individuals in the group, but lack of data prevent being able to specify with confidence the percentage of individuals covered by this intake; therefore, no Recommended Dietary Allowance (RDA) was set.
[a]UL = The maximum level of daily nutrient intake that is likely to pose no risk of adverse effects. Unless otherwise specified, the UL represents total intake from food, water, and supplements. Due to lack of suitable data, ULs could not be established for potassium, water, and inorganic sulfate. In the absence of ULs, extra caution may be warranted in consuming levels above recommended intakes.
[b]ND = Not determinable due to lack of data of adverse effects in this age group and concern with regard to lack of ability to handle excess amounts. Source of intake should be from food only to prevent high levels of intake.
SOURCE: *Dietary Reference Intakes for Water, Potassium, Sodium, Chloride, and Sulfate.* This reports may be accessed via www.nap.edu.

and a saturated fat content of less than 10% of total kilocalories. Saturated fats are found primarily in animal sources such as butter, lard and the fat associated with red meats, and in milk (other than skim) and milk products such as cheese. Poultry and fish also have some saturated fat, but, in general, less than red meats. Polyunsaturated fats primarily come from plant sources of which sunflower, corn, soybean, cottonseed, and safflower oils are primary sources; products, such as some margarines, are made from these plants oils. Monounsaturated fatty acids are of both plant and animal origin with olive oil and peanut oil the most common examples. Cholesterol is a type of fat found only in animal foods, such as butter, lard, eggs, whole and 2% milk, and milk products from these sources. Cholesterol also is produced by the body and is not a dietary essential. Lowering dietary cholesterol does not necessarily mean that the cholesterol level in the blood will correspond. Generally, approximately one third of American's blood cholesterol levels respond to a diet lower in cholesterol. Generally, less total fat, less saturated fat, and less cholesterol are associated with a reduction in the risk of cardiovascular diseases, including stroke. Following the Food Guide Pyramid is the starting place for a diet plan lower in fat. Be-

cause most saturated fat is found in animal sources and cholesterol is only found in foods of animal origin, if the diet foundation is based on grains, fruits, and vegetables, with only the suggested serving sizes from the meat and milk groups, the resulting diet is naturally low in total fat, saturated fat, and cholesterol. As apparent in Figure 107-2, the Food Guide Pyramid also helps consumers identify where fats are located in the food groupings through the use of icons to represent fats that are both naturally occurring and are added to foods.

There will always be issues regarding lipids! Current ones include *trans* fatty acids and the role of several specific fatty acids. *Trans* fatty acids refer to the orientation of the molecule when fats are hydrogenated for the purpose of providing the food industry and the consumer with fats of differing consistencies. For example, hydrogenation is used to change the physical state of oil, which is a liquid, to the physical state of a solid, as in making a solid margarine from a liquid vegetable oil. The addition of hydrogen to the molecule increases the saturation of the molecule, but also alters the structural orientation of the organic molecule from the more naturally occurring *cis* form to a *trans* form, thus a *trans* fatty acid. Estimated ranges of the

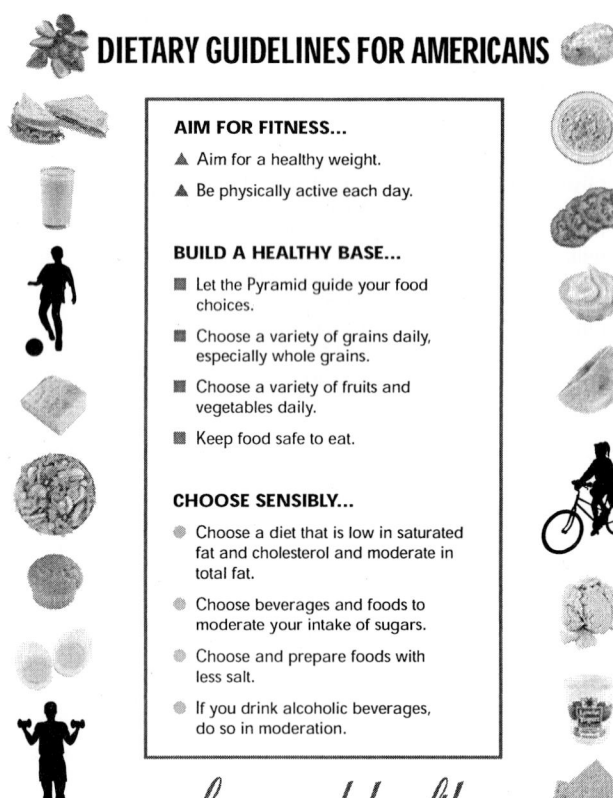

Figure 107-1. Dietary guidelines for Americans.

Table 107-5. Suggested Weight for Adults

| HEIGHT[b] | WEIGHT (LBS)[a] | |
	19–34 YEARS OLD	35 YEARS OLD AND OLDER
5′0	97–128	108–139
5′1	101–132	111–143
5′2	104–137	115–148
5′3	107–141	119–152
5′4	111–146	122–157
5′5	114–150	126–162
5′6	118–155	130–167
5′7	121–160	134–172
5′8	125–164	138–178
5′9	129–169	142–183
5′10	132–174	146–188
5′11	136–179	151–194
6′0	140–184	155–199
6′1	144–189	149–205
6′2	148–195	164–210
6′3	152–200	168–216
6′4	156–205	173–222
6′5	160–211	177–228
6′6	164–216	182–234

The higher weights in the ranges generally aplpy to men, who tend to have more muscle and bone; the lower weights more often apply to women, who have less muscle and bone.
[a] Without shoes.
[b] Without clothes.

amount of *trans* fatty acids in the diet of Americans range from 3% to 8% of total kilocalories. There is not general agreement among scientists and health professionals on. a specific amount of *trans* fatty acids thought to be harmful, and no DRI. For 2003, the FDA is considering requiring *trans* fatty acids to be listed on food labels. The DRIs recommend intakes for 2 specific types of fatty acids, an omega-3 fatty acid, alpha-linolenic acid, and an omega-6 fatty acid, linoleic acid, both polyunsaturated fatty acids essential in the diet. Omega-3 fatty acids are commonly found in fatty fish such as salmon and tuna and in some oils such as canola or soybean oil. Through a role in reducing the tendency of blood to clot, omega-3 fatty acids may reduce the risk of CVD. These essential fatty acids also have functions related to vision, the immune system, and the hormone-like compounds they produce called eicosanoids. A general recommendation is to consume fish several times a week. Omega-6 fatty acids are found in milk and some oils such as soybean and flaxseed oils.

CHOOSE BEVERAGES AND FOODS TO MODERATE YOUR INTAKE OF SUGAR—Of all the scientific evidence associating various components of the diet with disease, there is little, if any, to support a direct role of sugar. Sugar in the diet does not cause diabetes or hyperactivity and is only indirectly associated with the promotion of dental decay. Sugars are added to the diet in popular ingredients added to food and occur naturally in some foods such as milk and fruit. The 2002 DRI report suggested added sugars not be more than 25% of total calories consumed. Consumers who eat higher amounts of

Table 107-6. Body Weight According to Height and Body Mass Index

| HEIGHT (INCHES) BODY WEIGHT (LBS) | BODY MASS INDEX | | | | | | | | | | | | | | | |
	19	21	23	25	27	29	31	33	35	37	39	41	43	45	47	49
58	91	100	110	119	129	138	148	157	167	176	186	195	205	214	224	233
59	94	104	114	124	134	144	154	164	174	184	193	203	213	223	233	243
60	97	107	117	127	138	148	158	168	178	188	199	209	219	229	239	250
61	101	111	122	132	143	154	164	175	185	196	207	217	228	238	249	260
62	103	114	125	136	147	158	168	179	190	201	212	223	234	245	255	266
63	107	119	130	141	152	164	175	186	198	209	220	231	243	254	265	277
64	111	123	135	146	158	170	182	193	205	217	228	240	252	264	275	287
65	114	126	138	150	162	174	186	198	210	222	234	246	258	270	282	294
66	118	131	143	156	168	180	193	205	218	230	243	255	268	280	292	305
67	121	134	147	159	172	185	198	210	223	236	248	261	274	287	299	312
68	125	139	152	165	178	191	205	218	231	244	257	271	284	297	310	323
69	128	142	155	169	182	196	209	223	236	250	263	277	290	304	317	331
70	133	147	161	175	189	203	217	231	244	258	272	286	300	314	328	342
71	136	150	164	179	193	207	221	236	250	264	279	293	307	321	336	350
72	140	155	170	185	199	214	229	244	258	273	288	303	317	332	347	362
73	143	158	174	189	204	219	234	249	264	279	294	309	324	340	355	370
74	148	164	179	195	210	226	242	257	273	288	304	319	334	351	366	382
75	151	167	183	199	215	231	247	263	279	294	310	326	342	358	374	390
76	156	172	189	205	222	238	255	271	287	304	320	337	353	370	386	402

Table 107-7. NIH Guidelines for Choosing a Weight Loss Program

The diet should be safe and include all of the Recommended Dietary Allowances for vitamins, minerals, and protein.

The program should be directed toward a slow, steady weight loss unless a more rapid weight loss is medically indicated.

A doctor should evaluate health status if the client's weight loss goal is greater than 15 to 20 pounds, if the client has any health problems, or if the client takes medication on a regular basis.

The program should include plans for weight maintenance.

The program should give the prospective client a detailed list of fees and costs of additional items.

NIH = National Institutes of Health.

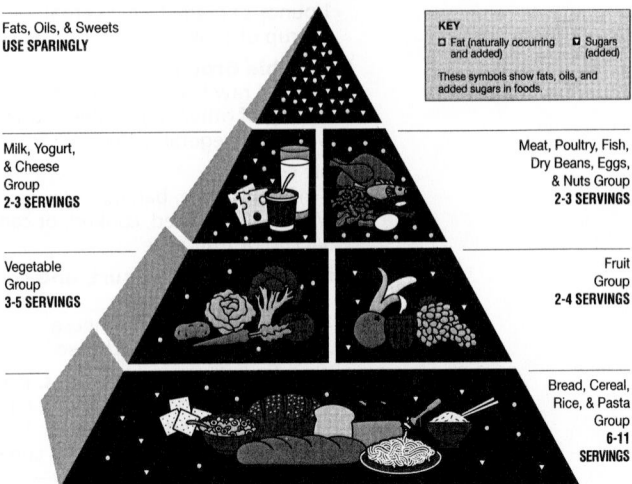

Figure 107-2. Food guide pyramid. A guide to daily food choices.

sugar in their diet may be lacking a good balance of vitamins and minerals but are not necessarily more likely to be overweight. The Food Guide Pyramid uses icons to represent added sugars to foods. Unlike the icons representing fats, the sugar icons only include added sugars because this is where additional kilocalories would occur in the diet, versus the naturally occurring sugars found in fruit or milk (see Fig 107-2).

CHOOSE AND PREPARE FOODS WITH LESS SALT— Sodium in the American diet comes primarily from salt or sodium chloride. Most of the salt and sodium comes from the addition of salt, or other ingredients containing salt, at the table, in cooking, and from the salt added to foods during processing. Examples of foods that receive salt during processing are salad dressings, soups, most snack foods such as chips and dips, cured meats, and most packaged foods. Sodium plays an important role in the body to help regulate body fluids and blood pressure. Most Americans consume more salt and sodium than is needed for daily balance, but most individuals simply excrete it. For this reason there is some controversy on having a general guideline for all Americans to limit the consumption of sodium.

For some Americans excess consumption of salt and sodium contributes to hypertension, kidney disease, heart disease, and a host of other problems. The taste for salt is acquired, and the general advice is to be more moderate in our consumption.

Salt-sensitive people will see a reduction in blood pressure with a reduction in sodium in the diet, but not all people are salt sensitive. A means to identify salt sensitivity is a current area of nutrition research. Many clients maintained on diuretics also follow a diet lower in sodium. The most common lower sodium diet plans are for a 2- to 3-g sodium restriction. A diet without added salt generally provides approximately 3 g of sodium, whereas a diet without added salt and the reduction of foods especially high in sodium generally provides approximately 2 g of sodium. A new DRI for sodium was released in 2004 (see Table 107-4).

IF YOU DRINK ALCOHOLIC BEVERAGES, DO SO IN MODERATION—Alcohol supplies kilocalories but no nutrients. Although some nutrients may be present in a beverage mixed with the alcohol, this is a dietary guideline because many

Table 107-8. Analysis of Weight Loss/Management Approaches

DOES THE WEIGHT LOSS MAINTENANCE APPROACH	YES	NO
1. Promise weight loss greater than 1/2 to 1 lb per week?	☐	☐
2. Claim a single or few foods are crucial to the diet?	☐	☐
3. Advocate a single source of foods, eg, a fortified beverage?	☐	☐
4. Eliminate any one or more of the food groups associated with the Food Guide Pyramid?		
Bread, cereal, rice, and pasta	☐	☐
Fruit	☐	☐
Vegetables	☐	☐
Milk, yogurt, cheese	☐	☐
Meat, poultry, fish, dry beans, eggs, and nuts	☐	☐
5. Advise less than he minimum number of servings for		
Bread, cereal, rice, and pasta (6–11)	☐	☐
Fruit (2–4)	☐	☐
Vegetables (3–5)	☐	☐
Milk, yogurt, cheese (2–3)	☐	☐
Meat and its alternatives	☐	☐
6. Suggest fewer than three meals per day?	☐	☐
7. Suggest a requirement for fewer specific foods in combination with other specific foods?	☐	☐
8. Sell a product?	☐	☐
9. Suggest the diet is all you need without reference to behavior modification?	☐	☐
10. Suggest a program without exercise?	☐	☐

If the answer to any one of these questions is "YES," you should be aware the approach does NOT conform to generally accepted standards for appropriate weight loss or weight maintenance.

Table 107-9. What Counts as a Serving?[a]

Grain Products Group (bread, cereal, rice, and pasta)
1 slice of bread
1 ounce of ready-to-eat cereal
1/2 cup of cooked cereal, rice, or pasta

Vegetable Group
1 cup of raw leafy vegetables
1/2 cup of other vegetables—cooked or chopped raw
3/4 cup of vegetable juice

Fruit Group
1 medium apple, banana, orange
1/2 cup of chopped, cooked, or canned fruit
3/4 cup of fruit juice

Milk Group (milk, yogurt, and cheese)
1 cup of milk or yogurt
11/2 ounces of natural cheese
2 ounces of processed cheese

Meat and Beans Group (meat, poultry, fish, dry beans, eggs, and nuts)
2–3 ounces of cooked lean meat, poultry, or fish
1/2 cup of cooked dry beans or 1 egg counts as 1 ounce of lean meat.
2 tbsp of peanut butter or 1/3 cup of nuts count as ounce of meat.

[a] Some foods fit into more than one group. Dry beans, peas, and lentils can be counted as servings in either the meat and beans group or vegetable group. These "crossover" foods can be counted as servings form either one or the other group, but not both. Serving sizes indicated here are those used in the Food guide Pyramid and based on both suggested and usually consumed portions necessary to achieve adequate nutrient intake. They differ from serving sizes on the Nutrition Facts Label, which reflect portions usually consumed.

Americans need guidance regarding alcoholic beverages. Moderation is defined as no more than one drink per day for women and no more than two drinks per day for men. Many clients on medications may be advised not to consume alcohol and pregnant and lactating women are advised to avoid all alcohol.

Other Dietary Guidance

Many other appropriate dietary guidance standards exist. The US Dietary Guidelines is a generic set of guidelines, whereas many standards are for specific purposes. For example, an appropriate set of guidelines is published by The American Heart Association with more focus on prevention of CVD. The American Institute for Cancer Research has a global report with a focus on a plant-based diet for prevention of cancer, and The American Cancer Society also has a set of guidelines aimed at cancer reduction risk. The American Diabetes Association releases recommendations specific to persons who have diabetes. All these guides have many components in common, namely, to follow a food pattern consistent with a variety of foods from different food groups, to maintain weight within an acceptable range, and to alter any over consumption of food components determined to be detrimental to an individual's health such as kilocalories, fat, saturated fat, cholesterol, sugar, sodium, and alcohol.

Table 107-10. Average Fiber (g) in Food Types

Legumes (1/2 cup)	8
Cereals, bran (1/2 cup)	8
Cereals, whole grain (1/2 cup)	3
Nuts and seeds (1 oz)	3
Starchy vegetables (1/2 cup)	3
Vegetables (1/2 cup)	2
Breads and crackers, whole grain (1 slice, 5 crackers)	2
Fruit (1 piece or 1/2 cup)	2
Meats, poultry, fish	0
Dairy products	0

FOOD AND SUPPLEMENT LABELING

LABELS—Food items and supplements are often sold in the pharmacy, making it important for the pharmacist to understand nutrition labeling regulations. A current labeling focus is to have more accurate and less misleading labeling on diet supplements. The *Nutrition Labeling and Education Act* of 1990 requires most packaged foods to list a specified set of nutrition facts on the label. Standard setting and enforcement for nutrition labeling is a responsibility of the Food and Drug Administration (FDA). Nutrition labels are helpful in complying with the Dietary Guidelines. Figure 107-3 is an example of a current food label with the minimum required facts. All the nutrition information on the label is based on the stated serving size. Larger packages, such as cereal boxes, often include additional information not required by law. At the bottom of the panel is located percent daily values based on a standard diet of 2000 kcal. Daily Values (DV) represent another standard used primarily only on nutrition labels. The DV is based on either a DRI or, in the case of dietary components without a current DRI such as fiber and cholesterol, the DV follows a generally acceptable standard such as the Dietary Guidelines. DVs give a quick analysis for those diet components of current concern. Because it takes years for labels to catch-up when standards change, the 2003 label information is not yet based on the most current DRIs.

Nutrition labeling for raw fruits, vegetables, and fish is voluntary, but the standards are consistent with those required on packaged foods in terms of the required set of information and the format in which it is presented. The FDA provides the retailer with the factual data for the voluntary listing of the 20 most commonly consumed raw fruits, vegetables, and fish, and they are posted in the store at the point of purchase. At the current time, the FDA does not plan to require labeling for fresh foods unless less than 60% of retailers do not adhere to the voluntary listing.

DESCRIPTIVE TERMINOLOGY ON LABEL—Some of the terms on labels are approved by the FDA, in conjunction with the Food Safety and Inspection Service (FSIS), to describe a food product. Other terms, such as *dietetic*, are not regulated, are discouraged by the FDA, and are not needed

Nutrition Facts

Serving Size

Servings Per Container

Amount Per Serving

Calories   Calories from Fat

% Daily Value*

Total Fat g	%
Saturated Fat g	%
Cholesterol mg	%
Sodium mg	%
Total Carbohydrate g	%
Dietary Fiber g	%
Sugars g	
Protein g	

Vitamin A	%	•	Vitamin C	%
Calcium	%	•	Iron	%

* Percent Daily Values are based on a 2,000 calorie diet. Your daily values may be higher or lower depending on your calorie needs:

	Calories	2,000	2,500
Total Fat	Less than	65g	80g
Sat Fat	Less than	20g	25g
Cholesterol	Less than	300mg	300mg
Sodium	Less than	2,400mg	2,400mg
Total Carbohydrate		300g	375g
Fiber		25g	30g

Calories per gram:

Fat 9   •   Carbohydrate 4   •   Protein 4

Figure 107-3. The representative content of a current food label with minimum required facts.

when regulated terms are used on labels. Eleven core terms form the basis of the descriptions. The eleven are *free, low, lean, extra lean, high, good source, reduced, less, light, fewer,* and *more.* Additionally synonyms are approved for the terms. Approved synonyms for *free* include *without, trivial source of, negligible source of, insignificant source of, no,* and *zero.* A food meets the definition for *low* if a large amount of the food could be eaten without exceeding the DV for the nutrient. Synonyms allowed for *low* are *contains a small amount of, low source of, little,* and *few.* A product can claim a specific food is a *good* source of a nutrient only if the food contains 10-19% of the DV for the nutrient or *high* only if the product contains

20% or more of the DV for the nutrient. Some terms cannot be used unless additional characteristics of the product also support the claim. For example products that bear claims related to *percent fat free* also must meet the definition for *low fat* and must accurately reflect the amount of fat in 100 g of the food. Table 107-11 includes the terms commonly used on products as related to specific nutrients.

ADDITIONAL LISTINGS ON LABELS—The section on a food label that lists the ingredients is not considered part of the nutrition labeling regulations, but it does conform to other regulations. Generally, ingredients are listed by their chemical to allow consumers to identify a substance they may need to avoid because of a food sensitivity or allergy. Ingredients also are listed in descending order of their amount. When looking for a whole-grain product, the words *whole grain*, should be among the first in the ingredient list.

All food labels must bear the name and address of the manufacturer and the weight. Universal bar codes allow the product to be traced to the exact place, date, and time it was manufactured. Consumers are encouraged to contact the manufacturer with any specific questions about the product. Many products also have dates on them, but, at the present time, dating is neither required or regulated.

HEALTH CLAIMS ON FOODS—Health claims are only allowed if there is sufficient scientific basis for a relation between nutrient and health or disease. All health claim wording must be pre-approved by the FDA and must state the relationship of the claim to the total daily diet. As of February 2003, health claims were allowed for the following diet and health relationships:

- Calcium and osteoporosis
- Dietary lipids (fat) and cancer
- Dietary saturated fat and cholesterol and risk of coronary heard disease
- Dietary sugar alcohol and dental caries
- Fiber-containing grain products, fruits, and vegetables and cancer
- Folic acid and neural tube defects
- Fruits and vegetables and cancer
- Fruits, vegetables, and grain products that contain fiber, particularly soluble fiber, and risk of coronary heart disease
- Sodium and hypertension
- Soluble fiber from certain foods and risk of coronary heart disease
- Soy protein and risk of coronary heart disease
- Stanols/sterols and risk of coronary heart disease

The regulation of organic foods, and rules for labeling, became effective in October 2002. Foods may now be labeled *organic* if no chemical fertilizers, sewage sludge, or synthetic pesticides are used, and if the food has not been genetically modified or irradiated.

LABELS ON DIETARY SUPPLEMENTS—The *Dietary Supplement Health and Education Act of 1994* required the FDA to develop labeling requirements specifically designed for products containing ingredients such as vitamins, minerals, herbs, or amino acids intended to supplement the diet. Information similar to the Nutrition Facts panel on foods is now required. Health claims on supplements must follow the same regulations as health claims on foods and may not claim to diagnose, mitigate, treat, cure, or prevent a specific disease or class of diseases. However, unlike drugs, and even foods, dietary supplements are not currently required to follow quality control measures. Therefore, the supplement may or may not have the amount of ingredients as stated on the label, and may even contain ingredients, including contaminants, that are not listed on the label. Unlike foods, dietary supplements are also allowed to make structure and/or function claims. These claims are not pre-approved by the FDA and can be immensely confusing to the consumer.

Labeling regulations for supplements were first on a voluntary basis, with requirements becoming effective in March 1999 for all products labeled after that date. Products on the market before March 1999 that carried the voluntary labeling as suggested by the FDA can remain on the market shelf. Those prod-

Table 107-11. Meanings of Descriptive Words for Specific Nutrients

Sugar
Sugar free: less than 0.5 grams (g) per serving
No added sugar, Without added sugar, No sugar added:
- No sugars added during processing or packing, including ingredients that contain sugars (for example, fruit juices, applesauce, or dried fruit).
- Processing does not increase the sugar content above the amount naturally present in the ingredients. (A functionally insignificant increase in sugars is acceptable from processes used for purposes other than increasing sugar content.)
- The food that it resembles and for which it substitutes normally contains added sugars.
- If the food doesn't meet the requirements for a low- or reduced-calorie food, the product bears a statement that the food is not low-calorie or calorie-reduced and directs consumers' attention to the nutrition panel for further information on sugars and calorie content.
Reduced sugar: at least 25 percent less sugar per serving than reference food

Calories
Calorie free: fewer than 5 calories per serving
Low calorie: 40 calories or less per serving and if the serving is 30 g or less or 2 tablespoons or less, per 50 g of the food
Reduced or Fewer calories: at least 25 percent fewer calories per serving than reference food

Fat
Fat free: less than 0.5 g of fat per serving
Saturated fat free: less than 0.5 g per serving and the level of trans fatty acids does not exceed 1 percent of total fat
Low fat: 3 g or less per serving, and if the serving is 30 g or less or 2 tablespoons or less, per 50 g of the food
Low saturated fat: 1 g or less per serving and not more than 15 percent of calories from saturated fatty acids
Reduced or Less fat: at least 25 percent less per serving than reference food
Reduced or Less saturated fat: at least 25 percent less per serving than reference food

Cholesterol
Cholesterol free: less than 2 milligrams (mg) of cholesterol and 2 g or less of saturated fat per serving
Low cholesterol: 20 mg or less and 2 g or less of saturated fat per serving and, if the serving is 30 g or less or 2 tablespoons or less, per 50 g of the food
Reduced or Less cholesterol: at least 25 percent less and 2 g or less of saturated fat per serving than reference food

Sodium
Sodium free: less than 5 mg per serving
Low sodium: 140 mg or less per serving and, if the serving is 30 g or less or 2 tablespoons or less, per 50 g of the food
Very low sodium: 35 mg or less per serving and, if the serving is 30 g or less or 2 tablespoons or less, per 50 g of the food
Reduced or Less sodium: at least 25 percent less per serving than reference food

Fiber
High fiber: 5 or more per serving. (Foods making high-fiber claims must meet the definition for low fat, or the level of total fat must appear next to the high-fiber claim.)
Good source of fiber: 2.5 g to 4.9 per serving
More or Added fiber: at least 2.5 g more per serving than reference food

ucts with no voluntary labeling will be subject to the new rules. Words such as *high potency* will be required for the product to meet the standard of 100% or more of the DRI or the DV established for that nutrient. *High potency* also can be used with multi-ingredient products if two thirds of the nutrients that are in the product are present at levels that are more than 100% of the DRI or the DV. The term "antioxidant" may be used in conjunction with previously defined terms of *good*, *high*, or *good and high* for products for which scientific evidence shows that after absorption of a sufficient quantity, the antioxidant nutrient or nutrients inactivate free radicals or prevent radical-initiated chemical reactions in the body.

ISSUES RELATED TO SUPPLEMENTS—General agreement on taking nutritional supplements is lacking among medical and nutrition professionals. In general a wise nutritional strategy is to obtain nutrients from foods as part of a well-balanced diet, and supplements should not be taken as an excuse for not obtaining sufficient nutrients from the daily diet. However, supplementation, including the amount to be taken, is appropriate when the supplement has been shown to be safe through sound scientific discovery. Supplementation is needed when food intake may be variable, such as in childhood; when needs may be temporarily increased, such as in pregnancy and lactation; when a specific recommendation from an appropriate source has been made, such as the USPHS recommending folic acid for all women of childbearing age; or when the client has a medical condition that is altering digestion, absorption, metabolism, or excretion of nutrients, such as malabsorption

syndromes, renal disease, etc. Surveys have associated supplement users with higher intake of nutrients from foods, with whites, women, older persons, those who have higher education and incomes, and more common among persons who believe diet affects disease. In general, large epidemiological studies have demonstrated supplement use has not lowered overall mortality but has sometimes been associated with a reduced risk of a specific disease.

Over-the-counter (OTC) supplements continue to offer the client a wide variety of substances, including nutrients, packaged in many different combinations. Labeling regulations on supplements help to interpret the information, but the pharmacist should not rely solely on the label in giving advice. The pharmacist can best answer specific questions about supplements and their claims if the scientific literature is thoroughly understood, including all possible advantages and disadvantages of the supplement. An important concept to remember is that nutrients do not function individually, but rather in complex interrelations. Single doses of nutrients can upset natural balances and interrelations. Because of nutrient interrelations, the best advice when a supplement is warranted or desired, is to take one that supplies an acceptable amount of all the nutrients and does not exceed the DRI standard for any one nutrient. This suggestion is consistent with recommendations of the American Medical Association, the Food and Nutrition Board of the National Academy of Sciences, the American Dietetic Association (ADA), the American Society for Clinical Nutrition, and the National Council Against Health Fraud.

FUNCTIONAL FOODS, PHARMACOTHERAPY, AND NUTRACEUTICALS—As scientific evidence has advanced the knowledge of beneficial relations among food, nutrition, health, and disease, a new arena for foods, and food technology, has emerged. Terms such as functional foods, pharmafoods, pharmaceuticals, pharmacotherapy, and nutraceuticals now exist with little current agreement on standardized definitions and many different definitions published in the literature. The terms have in common that nutrients may have a beneficial effect in the prevention and treatment of disease. The public is aware of some of the terms owing to use in the popular press. Literally hundreds of food components exist, and through bioengineering, those components proved of benefit could be increased in the food supply. For example, the antioxidant beta-carotene could be increased in a food or even added to foods that normally would not have this precursor to vitamin A. Strong research is needed to help answer which nutrients need to be increased in the diet whether in the form of foods or as a supplement and what level is needed to gain a benefit and cause no harm. As the media reports suspected benefits, pharmacists are increasingly asked for recommendations about supplements and foods. Until solid evidence is generated, including amounts to recommend, the best advice remains to eat a wide variety of foods with an emphasis on plant foods to form the foundation of the diet.

ADDITIVES IN FOOD AND SUPPLEMENTS—A food additive is any substance that becomes part of a food product. Technically speaking, supplements could be considered additives because they become part of the diet even when they are not in a food product.

Food additives can be intentionally added, such as salt or cinnamon, or unintentionally added, such as when a pesticide used to treat crops unintentionally is incorporated into the plant or when a drug given to an animal unintentionally ends up in the food product supplied by that animal. Even chemical substances that migrate from package materials can become unintentional additives. Generally, additives intentionally added to foods impart properties that yield an improved food supply.

Broad purposes of food additives include maintaining or improving nutritional value such as the addition of vitamins and minerals to a food product. The surge in the addition of calcium to juices and other foods is a good example of this function. A second broad purpose of additives is to maintain freshness in the food. The addition of antioxidants to foods processed with fat, such as potato chips, helps to prevent the fat from becoming rancid, and preservatives help to prevent spoilage as well as changes in color, texture, and flavor of food. A third broad purpose of additives is to help in the processing and preparation of foods such as when emulsifiers are added to peanut butter and mayonnaise to keep the product smooth or to salad dressings and chocolate milk to keep the product in a homogenous solution rather than allowing it to separate. A fourth broad purpose of additives is to make food more appealing. This represents the most widely used additive examples and includes coloring agents, natural and synthetic flavors, flavor enhancers, and sweeteners. The flavor of strawberries in ice cream can come from a strawberry or a chemical flavoring, and the pink color is added because consumers expect strawberry ice cream to be pink. Consumers use additives in the home preparation of food through the use of salt, pepper, sugar, and other ingredients. The most widely used food additives by the food industry are sugar, salt, and corn syrup. These three plus citric acid, baking soda, vegetable colors, mustard, and pepper account for more than 98%, by weight, of all food additives used in the US.

Food additives are regulated under the same basic law as are drugs; the *Food, Drug & Cosmetics (FD&C) Act*. Food and color additive amendments occurred in 1958 and 1960. Only two groups of additives were exempt at that time from a strict testing and approval process. Additives already in use and found to cause no harm when the amendments were added, in 1958 and 1960, were placed on a *generally recognized as safe* (GRAS) list, and a second list of prior sanctioned additives were exempt be-

cause of previously meeting the regulatory requirements. However, if questions should arise about the GRAS substances, the testing required would meet all current regulations. Colors used in drugs are the same colors approved for use in foods. All new additives must undergo years of testing, similar to the testing required for new drugs, before being approved by the FDA.

Unintentional additives are monitored through collection and analysis of foods at their point of production and through the FDA Total Diet Study. The Total Diet Study purchases all types of regular foods from the grocery four times a year and in four regions of the US. These foods are then prepared in their usual manner and tested for all substances present in the final product, including nutrients as well as additives. The incidence of unintentional additives, such as pesticides, must be less than amounts established by the FDA, FSIS, and the Environmental Protection Agency (EPA). One approved food process, the irradiation of foods, is regulated as an additive. This is to assure consumers that any changes in the food from irradiation are monitored by the same strict regulations as all other substances added to foods.

FOODS AND NUTRITION MISINFORMATION—In this chapter, several recommendations from reputable sources about eating healthfully have been discussed, but all the recommendations from reputable sources do not begin to compare in number to the abundance of misinformation that exists about foods and nutrition. Notwithstanding the immense cost of purchasing foods and supplements for which no added benefit is known, foods and nutrition misinformation may be harmful when it contributes to false hope and delay of appropriate treatment for an ailment. Misinformation may occur because of a cultural influence, misinterpretation of scientific studies, or as a result of fraudulent business practice. The dietary supplements labeling regulations should help control the latter. Pharmacists should know general ways to spot misinformation and the most common myths related to foods and nutrition. Of the top health frauds listed by the FDA, many are related to nutrition. These included instant weight-loss schemes; supplements to boost sexual ability; fraudulent arthritis products; megavitamin and mineral therapies for cancer, AIDS, and other ailments; false nutritional schemes such as bee pollen, OTC herbal remedies, wheat germ capsules, and protein supplements; chelation therapy; and specific diets and vitamin and mineral supplements to treat candidiasis. In general, suspect misinformation when the following has occurred

- *Recommendations promise a quick fix, such as loss of 5 lb a week.* Use Table 107-7 as a way to determine the merit of a diet program.
- *Dire warnings of danger are listed for a single food or product or regimen.* Hundreds of foods and approximately 90,000 meals are eaten over a normal lifetime. It would take a lot of any one food for it to severely affect health. Avoiding specific foods does not guarantee a healthy diet. A healthy diet is about what is eaten, not what is avoided.
- *A single food is recommended as superior to all other foods.* No one food, or even several foods, has all the nutrients needed for life.
- *The nation's food supply is reported as being unable to provide adequate nutrients through overprocessing, requiring the purchase of special products or supplements to overcome the deficit.* The US has the best, safest, and most regulated food supply in the world.
- *Claims that sound too good to be true such as an increase in metabolism simply by taking a supplement.* Activity is needed to get any significant increase in metabolism to burn kilocalories.
- *Recommendations based on a single study, a study with few subjects, a study that was not conducted as a double blind, a study that was not confirmed by other studies, a study that was not peer reviewed, or a study that was complex but is listing simplistic recommendations.* Professionals must learn how to interpret scientific studies.
- *A list of good or bad foods.* There are no good or bad foods, but there are good and bad diets.
- *Recommendations made to help sell a product.* A well-balanced diet does not require the purchase of a specific product.
- *Recommendations from studies that ignore differences among individuals, treating all people the same.* People come in all sizes and shapes and are individual in their diet patterns and behaviors.

Table 107-12. Usual Medical Nutrition Therapy in Selected Health Conditions

HEALTH CONDITION	USUAL NUTRITION THERAPY
Coronary Heart Disease	Achievement and maintenance of appropriate weight range.
	Optimization of serum lipid levels by alteration of dietary total fat, saturated fat, polyunsaturated fat, monounsaturated fat, cholesterol, and carbohydrate content of diet. May include sodium modification.
Diabetes Mellitus	Achievement and maintenance of appropriate weight range.
	Food intake to achieve normalized blood glucose values in conjunction with, or without, insulin therapy.
	Optimization of serum lipid levels via dietary lipid alterations listed under Coronary Heart Disease.
HIV/AIDS	Maintenance of appropriate weight range, including use of meals replacement supplements as necessary. May require parenteral nutrition and repletion of specific nutrients as assessed. Management of nutrition-related issues, ie, food safety, drug/nutrient/food interactions, and food regimens and general guidance to help offset related problems ie, nausea, vomiting, satiety, dysphagia. Attention to the social aspects of food as well as restorative and maintenance aspects. Clients need assistance in evaluating supplement information and nutrition products.
Hypertension	Achievement and maintenance of appropriate weight range.
	Attention to adequate amounts of fruits and vegetables, calcium, magnesium customary limitation of salt, sodium, and alcohol. and potassium with
Neoplastic Disease	Same as HIV/AIDS listed above.
Obesity	Achievement and maintenance of appropriate weight range. Alteration of serum parameters often associated with Obesity, ie, blood lipids.
Chronic Renal Disease	General nutrition therapies include varying levels of protein, depending on the disease stage; decreasing dietary phosphorus, potassium, sodium, and fluids and increasing calcium via the diet and/or supplements. Weight maintenance within a normal range and vitamin and mineral supplements are also concerns when individually warranted.

MEDICAL NUTRITION THERAPY—The assessment and development of nutrition care plans, along with monitoring and evaluation, for clients who have diseases that could benefit from nutrition intervention is termed Medical Nutrition Therapy (MNT). The MNT process is effective in treating disease and preventing disease complications, resulting in health benefits and cost savings for the public. Many health-care advocacy and government groups have published recommendations that include MNT. These include, but are not limited to, the National Cholesterol Education Program, the National High Blood Pressure Education Program, the American Diabetes Association, the American Cancer Society, the National Academy of Sciences Committee on Nutritional Status During Pregnancy and Lactation, and the Nutrition Screening Initiative. Many health problems that warrant MNT also include medication(s).

Foremost in any MNT is the individualization of a nutrition care plan to the client. The client should be assessed as to their nutritional status and how it may be compromised by the specific disease process. Assessment includes attention to anthropometric measures (ie, height, weight, and adipose deposits), biochemical measures (ie, all pertinent laboratory values), clinical evaluations (ie, a physical assessment of the body), and a diet evaluation to assess the usual diet and factors that affect eating behavior. After a thorough assessment, the nutrition professional can determine the best nutrition care plan for the individual, taking into account the medical and drug therapy the client will be receiving during their illness. All diet plans for MNT use the Dietary Guidelines for Americans and the DRIs as basic guidelines. An appropriate nutrition care plan first attempts to feed the client in as normal a fashion as possible, using enteral nutrition or the gut for entry of nutrients. In some cases the client may require the administration of nutrition outside the gut, parenteral nutrition, to achieve the nutrition goal. When the client is in a stage of growth, (ie, childhood), a major goal of MNT is to foster a normal growth pattern. Many chronic diseases result in anorexia, presenting feeding challenges to the client and nutrition professional.

The individualization of the nutrition care plan is important, but general aspects can be listed as customary with specific conditions (Table 107-12). When a client has multiple conditions (ie, both hypertension and diabetes mellitus), the MNT must include aspects related to the control of both disease entities.

RESOURCES—The practicing pharmacist can benefit immensely from making contact with nutritional professionals. Ultimately, it is the client who benefits from the teamwork of all health professionals. The Registered Dietitian (RD) is the nutrition counterpart to the Registered Pharmacist. The RD provides general nutrition guidance as well as MNT individualized to the client's specific needs. Through its National Center for Nutrition and Dietetics, the ADA maintains a Nutrition Hot Line for professionals and consumers at 1-800-366-1655. Callers can listen to prerecorded food and nutrition messages, locate RDs in their area for nutrition counseling, and seek answers to questions from RDs. The information is available in both English and Spanish and also via telecommunications device for the deaf. The ADA also publishes refereed position papers on issues of importance about foods and nutrition. Many of the position papers related to information in this chapter are included in the chapter bibliography. Increasingly, the worldwide web (www) is being used by consumers and professionals for information. The professional must be able to evaluate all resource information, including the www, as to its validity and usefulness. In the bibliography are several resources to provide information on evaluation of nutrition information.

REFERENCES

1. *Nutrition and Your Health: Dietary Guidelines for Americans* (HGB #232), 5th ed. Washington DC: USDA, DHHS, 2000.
2. *The Food Guide Pyramid* (HGB #252), Washington DC: USDA, 1996.

GOVERNMENT PUBLICATIONS

CDC. Folic acid and prevention of spina bifida and anencephaly: 10 years after the US Public Health Service Recommendation. *MMWR* 2002; 51 (No. RR-13).

CDC. Spina bifida and anencephaly prevalence–United States, 1001–2001. *MMWR* 2002; 51 (No. RR-13).

Kurtzweil P. Food label close-up. *FDA Consumer* 1994; (Apr):15.

Kurtzweil P. 'Daily values' encourage healthy diet. *FDA Consumer* 1993; (May):29.

Kurtzweil P. Answers to consumer questions about the food label. *FDA Consumer 1995;* (Jul): 6.

Thomas PR, ed. *Weighing the Options: Criteria for Evaluating Weight-Management Programs.* Committee to Develop Criteria for Evaluating the Outcome of Approaches to Prevent and Treat Obesity. Washington DC: National Academy Press, 1995.

JOURNAL ARTICLES

Committee Report: Summary of Revisions for the 2002 Clinical Practice Recommendations for Diabetes. *Diabetes Care* 2002;25:3.

Coulston AM, Johnson RK. Sugar and sugars: Myths and realities. *J Am Diet Assoc* 2002; 102:351.

Davis CA, Britten P, Myers E. Past, present, and future of the Food Guide Pyramid. *J Am Diet Assoc* 2001;101:881.

Lewis C. Nutrient intakes and body weights of persons consuming high and moderate levels of added sugars. *J Am Diet Assoc* 1992; 92:708.

Pennington JAT, Wilkening VL. Final regulations for the nutrition labeling of raw fruits, vegetables, and fish. *J Am Diet Assoc* 1997; 97:1299.

Radimer K, Subar A, Thompson F. Nonvitamin, nonmineral dietary supplements: Issues and findings from NHANES III. *J Am Diet Assoc* 2001; 100:447.

Voelker R. Getting the story straight on nutrition. *JAMA* 1998; 279:417.

Wood OB. Popovich NG. Non-drug treatment of obesity. *JAPhA* 1996; NS36:636.

POSITION PAPERS OF THE AMERICAN DIETETIC ASSOCIATION

Cost-effectiveness of medical nutrition therapy. *J Am Diet Assoc* 1995; 95:88.

Food and nutrition misinformation. *J Am Diet Assoc* 2002; 102:260.

Food fortification and dietary supplements. *J Am Diet Assoc* 2001; 101: 115.

Food and water safety. *J Am Diet Assoc* 1997; 97:184.

Health implications of dietary fiber. *J Am Diet Assoc* 2002; 102:993.

Medical nutrition therapy and pharmacotherapy. *J Am Diet Assoc* 1999; 99:227.

The role of nutrition in health promotion and disease prevention. *J Am Diet Assoc* 2002; 102:1680.

The total diet approach to communicating food and nutrition information. *J Am Diet Assoc* 2002; 102:100.

Weight management. *J Am Diet Assoc* 2002; 102:1145.

Food and Nutrition Science Alliance (FANSA) Statements

Note—FANSA is made up of The American Dietetic Association, The American Society for Clinical Nutrition, Inc., American Society for Nutrition Sciences, and Institute of Food Technologists. For information contact National Center for Nutrition and Dietetics, American Dietetic Association, 120 South Riverside Plaza, Suite 2000, Chicago, IL 60606.

Making sense of risks associated with diet.

Making sense of scientific research about diet and health.

What does the public need to know about dietary supplements?

BOOKS

Coulston A, Rock CL, Monsen ER. *Nutrition in the Prevention and Treatment of Disease.* San Diego: Academic Press, 2001.

Insel P, Turner RD, Ross D. *Nutrition.* Boston: Jones and Bartlett, 2001.

Institute of Medicine. *Dietary Reference Intakes for Calcium, Phosphorus, Magnesium, Vitamin D and Flouride.* Food and Nutrition Board. Washington DC: National Academy Press, 1997.

Institute of Medicine. *Dietary Reference Intakes for Energy, Carbohydrate, Fiber, Fat, Fatty Acids, Cholesterol, Protein, and Amino Acids.* Food and Nutrition Board. Washington DC: National Academy Press, 2002.

Institute of Medicine. *Dietary Reference Intakes for Thiamin, Riboflavin, Niacin, Vitamin B6, Folate, Vitamin B12, Pantothenic Acid, Biotin, and Choline.* Food and Nutrition Board. Washington DC: National Academy Press, 1998.

Institute of Medicine. *Dietary Reference Intakes for Vitamin A, Vitamin K, Arsenic, Boron, Chromium, Copper, Iodine, Iron, Molybdenum, Nickel, Silicon, Vanadium and Zinc.* Food and Nutrition Board. Washington DC: National Academy Press, 2001.

Institute of Medicine. *Dietary Reference Intakes for Vitamin C, Vitamin E, Selenium, and Carotenoids.* Food and Nutrition Board. Washington DC: National Academy Press, 2000.

Institute of Medicine. *Dietary Reference Intakes: Use in Dietary Assessment.* Food and Nutrition Board. Washington DC: National Academy Press, 2000.

Bowman B, Russell R, eds. *Present Knowledge in Nutrition.* Washington DC: ILSI Press, 2001.

Institute of Medicine. *Recommended Dietary Allowances.* Foods and Nutrition Board. Washington DC: National Academy Press, 1989.

Shils ME, Olson JA, Shike M, Ross, AC. *Modern Nutrition in Health and Disease,* 9th ed. Baltimore: Williams and Wilkins, 1999.

WEB SITES

American Dietetic Association (position papers) http://www.eatright.org/

American Society for Nutritional Sciences: http://www.asns.org

Center for Nutrition Policy and Promotion http://www.usda.gov/cnpp

Dietary Reference Intakes http://www.nas.edu

Food and Drug Administration (FDA) http://www.fda.gov

Food and Nutrition Information Center (FNIC) http://www.nalusda.gov/fnic/

Food Safety and Inspection Service (FSIS) http://www.fsis.usda.gov

Healthfinder—US Government (A gateway consumer health information web site from the US Government. Find selected online publications, clearinghouses, databases, web sites, and support and self-help groups, as well as the government agencies and not-for-profit organizations that produce reliable information for the public) http://www.healthfinder.gov/

National Council Against Health Fraud http://www.ncahf.org/

National Organic Program. http://www.ams.usda.gov/nop

Tufts University Navigator (Reviews websites using set criteria and a panel of nutrition professionals) http://navigator.tufts.edu/

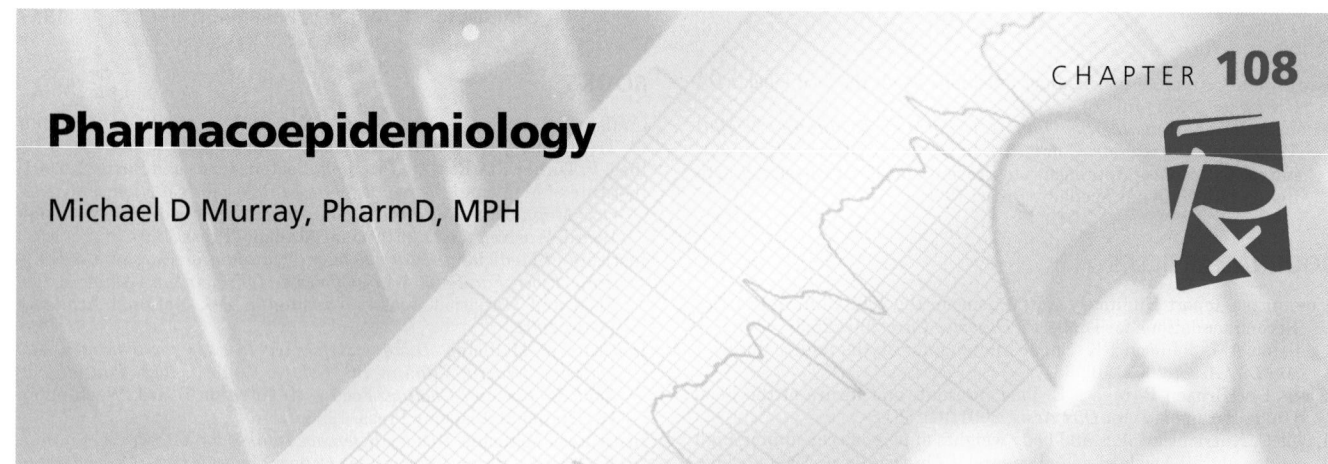

CHAPTER 108

Pharmacoepidemiology

Michael D Murray, PharmD, MPH

Pharmacoepidemiology, or drug epidemiology, is the study of the effects of drugs in populations of people. The discipline is an amalgam of clinical pharmacology, clinical epidemiology, medical informatics, and biostatistics. There are a number of reasons why pharmacoepidemiology has recently emerged as a discipline. Traditional clinical pharmacology directs much of its attention to the pharmacokinetics and pharmacodynamics of drugs. These studies usually involve small numbers of subjects (6–25) who are studied intensively to obtain an understanding of drug absorption, distribution, metabolism, or excretion. Studies of these parameters determine the dose and frequency of administration of new drugs in the treatment of patients and are required before drugs are marketed. However, such studies tell us little about certain experiences of drugs after they are marketed. It is in this postmarketing phase that the tools of clinical epidemiology come into play, especially in determining the frequency of adverse drug effects.

Though new drug products undergo the careful scrutiny of Phase I through III testing, some drug products are recalled soon after they are marketed. There are a litany of such experiences including phocomelia from thalidomide, Guillain-Barré syndrome from influenza vaccine, endometrial cancer from diethylstilbestrol, cardiac valve disorders from the combination use of fenfluramine and phentermine (Fen-Fen), anaphylaxis from zomepirac, hepatic failure from bromfenac, and cardiac arrest from interactions from drugs like mibefradil or terfenadine when administered with drugs that inhibit P-450 CYP 3A4 such as ketoconazole and erythromycin. A major reason for these drug product recalls is that premarketing studies treat too few patients (typically 3000–4000) to detect uncommon drug effects. An adverse effect that occurs in only 1 in 25,000 persons would go unnoticed in only 4000 treated patients in the premarketing phase. Yet once the drugs are marketed, they often reach millions of patients and rare events can become manifest. Hence, premarketing studies have insufficient statistical power to detect rare adverse effects.

The effect of sample size on the statistical power of a study is shown in Figure 108-1. In general terms, the *power* of a test is the ability of a statistical test used in a study to detect a relationship between an exposure (drug) and an event or outcome. The highest value the power can have is one, and the lowest is zero. The figure shows the power curve for a clinical trial in which the outcome of interest occurs in 4 of every 1000 patients in one treatment group and in 1 in every 1000 patients in another treatment group. For clinical trials, it is generally desirable to keep the power of a study above 0.80. From the figure it can be seen that fewer than 4000 patients in each group would yield insufficient power to detect a difference between groups when alpha is 0.05 and a two-tailed test is performed. Another way to interpret the curve is to consider that an adverse effect occurred in 0.4% of patients receiving a drug, and the same adverse effect occurred in 0.1% of patients receiving placebo; more than 8000 patients would need to be recruited into the study to detect such an effect. The cost of such a study would be prohibitive.

Another important reason that important adverse events are not identified in the premarketing drug experience is that although subjects in premarketing studies have the disease that the drug is targeted to treat, they are otherwise healthy people. Typically, premarketing studies exclude patients who have complicating factors such as renal or hepatic insufficiency, diabetes mellitus, or heart failure. But once the drugs are marketed, they often reach patients with a multitude of comorbidities and complicating conditions. In this real world setting of care, treated patients are sicker, and adverse drug reactions are more common.

Because adverse effects of drug products are more commonly observed after marketing, the Food and Drug Administration (FDA) created the MedWatch Medical Products Reporting Program, which is the largest drug and device surveillance program in the US (see below). A similar program is operated by the World Health Organization (WHO). Such drug surveillance programs are important ways for drug regulatory agencies to keep their fingers on the pulse of the adverse drug experiences of countries.

Now that the interface between pharmacoepidemiology and clinical pharmacology and clinical epidemiology is clearer, the question remains as to how medical informatics and biostatistics enter into the mix. Health systems such as managed-care organizations, hospitals, clinics, and medical centers generate a large volume of data on patients. Increasingly, such data are being captured and stored in huge databases. Data found in these warehouses often come from many sources including the pharmacy, laboratory, radiology, and patient-care clinics and wards. To conduct studies of outcomes of patients who have been prescribed drugs requires merging these large files from disparate sources. Such integrated databases are becoming larger and richer. When such data are available through time and are linked using a unique patient identifier, a variety of studies of the effects of drugs in large populations of patients (ie, pharmacoepidemiologic studies) are possible.[1] The analysis of such large data sets requires the tools of biostatistics. The types of statistical procedures used in the analysis of data for pharmacoepidemiologic studies can range from simple counts of events to sophisticated mathematical models. Some of the procedures that apply to pharmacoepidemiology are described in this chapter.

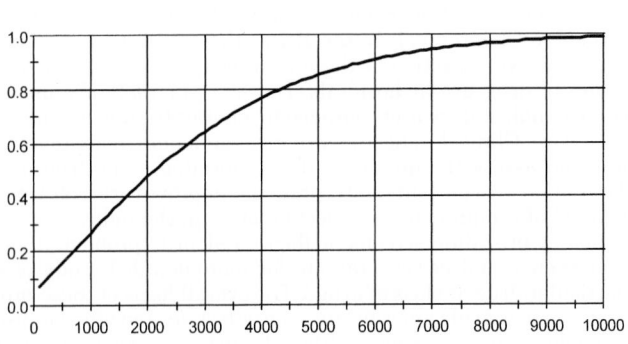

Power as a Function of Sample Size

Figure 108-1. Power as a function of sample size in two treatment groups. The study was designed to detect an event that occurs in 4 out of 1000 patients in one group and 1 patient in 1000 in the other group.

TYPES OF STUDIES

Table 108-1 lists the various types of studies that are used in pharmacoepidemiology. There are two fundamental types of pharmacoepidemiologic studies—experimental and nonexperimental. These are distinguished by the method in which subjects are assigned to treatments. Nonexperimental studies can be further categorized as descriptive and analytic studies.

In experimental studies, the investigator assigns treatments to subjects, or patients may be randomly assigned to treatment in some forms of experimental or analytic studies.

Patients enrolled in *randomized clinical trials* have their treatment assigned at random. It is the most common experimental method for testing drug effects and is considered the best available evidence in clinical research. Important characteristics of the randomized clinical trial are described below.

Field trials are another form of experimental study, used to study dietary factors and vaccines. In field trials the investigator makes the treatment available and then determines how well it works with careful follow up. Examples of field trials include studies of ascorbic acid in preventing the common cold, studies of poliomyelitis vaccines, and the Multiple Risk Factor Intervention Trial (MRFIT). MRFIT studied the effect of preventives such as diet and drugs on the incidence of myocardial infarction in 12,866 high-risk persons. It has been estimated that the MRFIT study would cost more than $500 million to conduct in 1997 dollars. Community intervention trials are similar to field trials, but the treatment intervention is directed at a town or community such as fluoridation of drinking water to prevent dental caries.

In nonexperimental studies, patients are not assigned to treatments by the investigator. Most of these studies enroll patients who are receiving care, including medications, from conventional settings of care such as clinics and hospitals. Nonexperimental studies are usually descriptive. Descriptive studies are conducted to describe or summarize data. For example, an investigator may wish to know the types of drugs prescribed at an outpatient pharmacy by drug class. These data would help the investigator determine what types of drugs could be studied more rigorously using the prescription data from this setting. Clearly, if there were only five prescriptions for a particular drug, then the investigator might only be able to conclude that the drug is not used very often. Descriptive data are helpful in *hypothesis-generation* and determining whether there are

Table 108-1. Types, Characteristics, and Examples of Pharmacoepidemiology Studies

STUDY TYPE	DESCRIPTION	NUMBER OF PATIENTS (PER TREATMENT GROUP)	RELATIVE COST	EXAMPLE
Experimental studies				
Randomized clinical trials	Study patients with specific disease	50 to 5000	$$ to $$$$	Efficacy of alteplase and reteplase in preventing death after a myocardial infarction
Field trials	Study subjects to prevent disease	>5000	$$$$	Vaccination to prevent polio
Community intervention trials	Study communities to prevent disease	>5000	$$$	Fluoridation of water to prevent dental cavities
Nonexperimental studies				
Prospective cohort	Observe groups of patients treated with the same drug	>5000	$$$$	Nurses Health Study Cohort
Retrospective cohort	Extract data from an existing repository to look at outcomes of exposed groups	>5000	$	Risk of renal insufficiency from NSAIDs
Case-control	Determine the association between a drug and rare event	20 to 1000	$$ to $$$	Risk of Alzheimer's disease and vitamin use
Cross-sectional	Determine the prevalence of drug use in a patient population at a given time	50 to 1 million	$	Profile of calcium-channel antagonists in a managed-care organization
Ecological	Determine the association between drug use of a population or group and an event	5 to 100 groups	$	Deaths from asthma and the quantities of metered-dose inhalers dispensed
Case series	Reveal the common experiences of a number of patients following drug exposure	3 to 30	$	Valvular heart disease associated with fenfluramine-phentermine (Fen-Phen)
Case report	Reveal the experience of a single patient following drug exposure	1	$	Toxic epidermal necrolysis from phenytoin

sufficient numbers of patients, prescriptions, events, etc, to conduct a more rigorous study. Such studies might include profiles of drug use, drug surveillance, patient types, or disease types.

Analytical nonexperimental studies are often used to *test hypotheses*. For example, one might find from a descriptive study that patients prescribed one type of nonsteroidal anti-inflammatory drug (NSAID) have a greater prevalence of gastropathy than those receiving other NSAIDs. One might then ask whether this is because this NSAID is truly more gastrotoxic or whether sicker patients who are prone to develop gastropathy are also more likely to be prescribed this drug. To tease-out the answer to this question would require a study that gives rates of gastropathy that control for illnesses that increase the likelihood of gastropathy and use of other drugs and foods that might also increase the risk of gastropathy among these patients.

DRUG SURVEILLANCE—The FDA's MedWatch is a drug surveillance program that looks for signals of adverse drug effects among all marketed drugs and then provides careful follow up when necessary. A benefit of surveillance programs is that there is early recognition of important problems. For example, who would have anticipated the recent problem involving the anorectic drugs Fen-Phen that resulted in heart valve abnormalities in those who took this weight-reducing combination? Other events that were identified by such post-marketing surveillance (PMS) programs that led to drug withdrawals include the sometimes fatal arrhythmias from CYP 3A4 drug interactions involving mibefradil (Posicor), terfenadine (Seldane), astemizole (Hismanal), and cisapride (Propulsid). Hence, the benefit of PMS is in monitoring for signals in the population of patients being treated day-to-day with drugs.

MedWatch and similar sentinel programs are important tools for the detection of rare effects, but they have several important limitations. Foremost among the limitations is that these programs depend on voluntary reporting. Because the signal comes from submissions to the FDA, predominantly by pharmacists, it is important for pharmacists to complete MedWatch forms when major new and unusual problems are identified in the care of patients. Reports of known adverse effects of marketed drugs are not required. A MedWatch form can be found in Figure 108-2. Reports may also be submitted online at https://www.accessdata.fda.gov/scripts/medwatch/. The big problem is that such forms are often not completed for heretofore unknown drug misadventures, and thus the signal is not generated or is generated later, only after many patients may have suffered. Pharmacist participation in drug surveillance programs is a central way to contribute to pharmacoepidemiology. See also Chapter 115.

DRUG USE—In pharmacoepidemiology, one needs to know two numbers to calculate the rates of events of interest. First, one needs to know the numerator (eg, numbers of adverse events). When reporting of such events is consistent and complete, one can then estimate this numerator using drug surveillance programs such as MedWatch. Again, it is important to realize that the estimate of events is only as good as the reporting of events. However, surveillance programs cannot provide an accurate estimate of the denominator, namely, the number of patients exposed to the drug product. These denominator data can be accessed by drug use.

Drug use data are improving, largely because of increasing use of computer information systems in health care. Computerization of pharmacy is ubiquitous owing largely to the need to process and store prescriptions. The increase in pharmacy benefit management companies has further consolidated prescription data. Moreover, there are corporations that can provide national estimates of drug use. One such corporation, IMS America, has prescription data for the US and many of the Western European countries. These data can be used to provide estimates of drug use and as such provide an estimate of the denominator when calculating the rates of events.

On a smaller scale, pharmacists employed by hospitals and managed-care organizations are familiar with the drug use review programs that have roots in pharmacoepidemiologic

method and are required by the Joint Commission on the Accreditation of Healthcare Organizations. Such programs are described in Chapter 127. In the 1970s, these programs involved the intensive collection of the indications, processes, and outcomes of drug use at hospitals. However, in 1989, the use of clinical indicators was encouraged to monitor the delivery of patient care. Clinical indicators are measurements made to monitor and assess the quality and appropriateness of drug use. The notion is to measure, interpret, and improve care over time. Instead of comprehensive collection of data, the indicators are aimed at providing screens or flags to identify problem areas that then would become targets for more-detailed study of a particular drug or class of drugs. The overall focus of these programs is to provide appropriate, safe, effective, and efficient use of medications.[2] However, although such programs aimed at measuring clinical indicators are too small in scope to measure rare events, they are very effective in studying indications for drug use and monitoring processes.

There are several key points to address concerning institutional programs to improve drug use. First, these are very important studies to improve the use of drugs at a particular institution. When such programs are formally conducted within the framework of continuous quality improvement, the benefits to the institution and its patients are endless. However, these programs involving drug use measurement and quality indicators are not usually conducted as formal research studies that address explicit study questions or test hypotheses. It would be a mistake to assume otherwise. This is a common error made when collecting data for such programs. The biggest problem is that such programs monitor too few patients to conclude that a particular outcome of interest does or does not occur. For example, suppose that an investigator is interested in the incidence of vomiting in patients prescribed a new antibiotic. If 10 consecutive patients are monitored and no vomiting occurs, perhaps there were too few patients monitored to observe this adverse effect, the dose administered was too low to elicit the effect, or vomiting was not among the parameters being monitored during the period of patient observation. Thus, surveillance, drug use, and continuous quality improvement programs may not be designed appropriately or have sufficient numbers of patients to address a specific research question. Instead, other epidemiologic approaches must be employed.

THE RANDOMIZED CONTROLLED TRIAL—The gold standard in determining the beneficial and adverse effects of drugs is the prospective, blinded, randomized clinical trial. It is helpful to understand the merits and drawbacks of the randomized clinical trial for better understanding of the advantages and disadvantages of the various types of epidemiologic studies. When patients are randomly assigned to treatments, many biases are controlled that would otherwise preclude valid results. Ideally, neither the patient nor the physician is able to distinguish between the drug products being tested because they are "blinded." Persons performing assessments or measurements of interest should also be blinded to treatment. Typically, randomized clinical trials are conducted when comparing the efficacy of two drugs or of one drug against a placebo. Rarely, is a randomized clinical trial conducted to determine whether drugs differ in their propensity to cause adverse drug reactions.

One may wonder, why not just use randomized clinical trials for all studies of drugs? There are four primary reasons.

Randomized clinical trials often are prohibitively expensive (ie, costing millions of dollars). Unless the issue is of the utmost importance, federal monies are not made available to conduct the study. If it is a new drug product, the innovator drug company must be certain that after doing the study, it can recoup its investment.

Randomized clinical trials are often unethical for studies of the adverse effects of drugs. How many patients would enroll for a study with the sole purpose of determining the incidence of gastrointestinal (GI) perforation from a new drug?

Large numbers of patients are needed to conduct studies of rare events. Even after the moral and ethical issues for a study

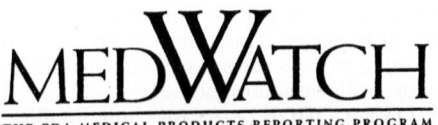

For **VOLUNTARY** reporting
by health professionals of adverse
events and product problems

THE FDA MEDICAL PRODUCTS REPORTING PROGRAM

Page ____ of ____

Form Approved: OMB No. 0910-0291 Expires: 8/31/00
See OMB statement on reverse

FDA Use Only

Triage unit
sequence #

A. Patient information

1. Patient identifier	2. Age at time of event: or Date of birth:	3. Sex	4. Weight
In confidence		☐ female ☐ male	____ lbs or ____ kgs

B. Adverse event or product problem

1. ☐ **Adverse event** and/or ☐ **Product problem** (e.g., defects/malfunctions)

2. **Outcomes attributed to adverse event**
(check all that apply)

☐ death _____ (mo/day/yr)
☐ life-threatening
☐ hospitalization – initial or prolonged

☐ disability
☐ congenital anomaly
☐ required intervention to prevent permanent impairment/damage
☐ other: _____

3. Date of event (mo/day/yr)	4. Date of this report (mo/day/yr)

5. **Describe event or problem**

6. **Relevant tests/laboratory data,** including dates

7. **Other relevant history, including preexisting medical conditions** (e.g., allergies, race, pregnancy, smoking and alcohol use, hepatic/renal dysfunction, etc.)

PLEASE TYPE OR USE BLACK INK

C. Suspect medication(s)

1. **Name** (give labeled strength & mfr/labeler, if known)
#1

#2

2. **Dose, frequency & route used** #1 #2	3. **Therapy dates** (if unknown, give duration) from/to (or best estimate) #1 #2

4. **Diagnosis for use** (indication) #1 #2	5. **Event abated after use stopped or dose reduced** #1 ☐ yes ☐ no ☐ doesn't apply #2 ☐ yes ☐ no ☐ doesn't apply

6. **Lot #** (if known) #1 #2	7. **Exp. date** (if known) #1 #2	8. **Event reappeared after reintroduction** #1 ☐ yes ☐ no ☐ doesn't apply #2 ☐ yes ☐ no ☐ doesn't apply

9. **NDC #** (for product problems only)
____ – ____

10. **Concomitant medical products** and therapy dates (exclude treatment of event)

D. Suspect medical device

1. **Brand name**

2. **Type of device**

3. **Manufacturer name & address**	4. **Operator of device** ☐ health professional ☐ lay user/patient ☐ other: _____
6. model # _____ catalog # _____ serial # _____ lot # _____ other # _____	5. **Expiration date** (mo/day/yr) 7. **If implanted, give date** (mo/day/yr) 8. **If explanted, give date** (mo/day/yr)

9. **Device available for evaluation?** (Do not send to FDA)
☐ yes ☐ no ☐ returned to manufacturer on _____ (mo/day/yr)

10. **Concomitant medical products** and therapy dates (exclude treatment of event)

E. Reporter (see confidentiality section on back)

1. **Name & address**	phone #

2. **Health professional?** ☐ yes ☐ no	3. **Occupation**	4. **Also reported to** ☐ manufacturer ☐ user facility ☐ distributor

5. **If you do NOT want your identity disclosed to the manufacturer, place an "X" in this box.** ☐

Mail to: MEDWATCH
5600 Fishers Lane
Rockville, MD 20852-9787

***or* FAX to:**
1-800-FDA-0178

FDA Form 3500

Submission of a report does not constitute an admission that medical personnel or the product caused or contributed to the event.

Figure 108-2. MedWatch program report form (FDA Form 3500, Expires 3/31/2005).

are resolved, if it is a rare event, then the numbers of patients needed to determine the true incidence of the effect or address a specific study question would be enormous.

Randomized clinical trials take a long time to conduct. If a question must be addressed in a timely fashion, such as for regulatory action, clearly a randomized clinical trial conducted over 3 years could not provide an answer to a question soon enough.

Primarily, for these reasons, pharmacoepidemiologic methods have been the preferred method of inquiry, especially for determining the adverse effects of drugs.

Because many relevant and important drug-related questions cannot be addressed with randomized clinical trials, the nonexperimental methods of pharmacoepidemiology are especially important. For such clinically important and relevant questions, nonexperimental methods of pharmacoepidemiology must be used. Among such methods are the cohort and case-control studies as shown in Figure 108-3. These and other common pharmacoepidemiologic methods are described below.

THE COHORT STUDY—Cohorts are groups. Cohort studies are, therefore, studies of groups of patients having some common drug exposure of interest. For example, one may wish to learn about the benefits and risks of the NSAIDs on the population of patients likely to be prescribed them. The cohort or group would be defined on the basis of patients' exposure to NSAIDs. There are two types of cohort studies: prospective and retrospective.

PROSPECTIVE COHORT—In terms of scientific evidence and control over the factors of interest, the prospective cohort study is often the preferred type of cohort study. As implied in its name, the prospective study looks forward in time (Fig 108-3). Doing so allows the investigator maximum control over the study definition and its conduct.

The event of interest or dependent variable (eg, development of aplastic anemia) can be specifically defined, and its occurrence carefully monitored.

The potential confounding factors and variables that must be controlled in the analysis can also be defined and measured.

Despite these advantages, prospective cohort studies can be very expensive to conduct and in similar fashion to the randomized clinical trial can cost millions of dollars to assemble and follow the cohort over time. An example of a prospective cohort study is the Nurse's Health Study, which began in 1976.

The cohort comprises 121,700 female nurses who completed life-style and medical histories. This cohort study has proved valuable in determining various aspects of female health, especially as it relates to cardiovascular disease.[3,4]

RETROSPECTIVE COHORT—As its name implies, the retrospective cohort study looks back on existing data. These data usually come from large, computer databases. However, data can also come from paper charts or medical records. In these studies, cohorts are assembled in the same way as in prospective cohort studies, namely, on the basis of exposure to certain drugs of interest. The major advantage of retrospective cohort studies is lower costs. These are much less expensive to conduct than either clinical trials or prospective studies. The major disadvantage is that there are many forms of bias (see below) that are found in retrospective studies.

Conceptually, retrospective cohort studies are conducted the same way as prospective cohort studies.

The cohort is defined by determining the index date when the drug of interest was first prescribed. Although the index date will differ for each patient, it acts as the anchor for two key viewpoints: (1) for looking forward in time for the occurrence of the outcomes of interest (eg, myocardial infarction or renal insufficiency) and (2) for looking backward in time for the baseline factors that must be controlled in the analysis.

Data on the outcomes and baseline factors are extracted from the database or charts for all patients in the cohort. Fundamentally, the extraction process is similar whether performed by computer or by hand.

Regardless of whether cohort studies are prospective or retrospective, there are a number of critical characteristics to such studies. Drug exposure should be verified to prevent misclassification of cohort membership. A common problem in pharmacoepidemiologic studies is that patients could get a medication from a pharmacy that is not among those from which data are derived, physicians may provide the drug as a sample from their office, or the drug may be available as an OTC drug and as such can be directly available to the patient. If a drug is available from multiple sources, then the investigator should demonstrate that all sources were included in the cohort formed for study.

THE CASE-CONTROL STUDY—Methodologically, case-control studies are the diametric opposite of cohort studies (Fig 108-3). Generally, case-control studies are conducted when the outcome of interest is rare. Instead of beginning with a group of patients using the same drug (with a common exposure) and following them until they have a specific event, as with the cohort study, in the case-control study one first identifies a group of patients with a common event or disease. These are the *cases*. For example, if an investigatory wished to determine whether a certain drug caused aplastic anemia (a rare event), first, patients with aplastic anemia would be identified. The *controls* would be people who are representative of the underlying population from which the cases came but who did not have the outcome of interest. In the aplastic anemia example, the investigator would search for patients who came from the same setting of care as the cases or from the same community. Sometimes controls are matched to cases on certain background factors that predict or confound the outcome, such as age, gender, or smoking status.

The idea of the case-control study is to compare the prevalence of exposure between the cases and controls. This is the difficult aspect of such studies and is often a contentious issue that results in plenty of debate. A single report of a case-control study in a journal can result in using twice as much journal space publishing the letters to the editor than used for the original report. The main reason for this is that there are many ways in which bias can enter into the design, conduct, and interpretation of these studies. When obtaining data directly from patients pertaining to the exposure, there may be a major difference between patients' memories of their drug use in the case and those of control groups. This recall bias is described below.

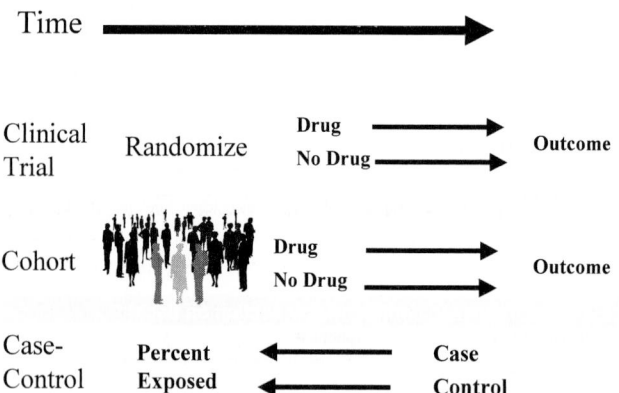

Figure 108-3. Orientation of studies relative to time. In the clinical trial, patients are randomly assigned to treatment groups and monitored prospectively for the outcome of interest. In the cohort study, treatment groups are assembled on the basis of their treatments or other distinguishing characteristics and followed until the occurrences of the outcome. With the prospective cohort study the outcome of interest occurs after the study onset and with the retrospective study the outcome has already occurred when the study starts. In the case-control study, the prevalence of past treatments is compared in a group of patients with the outcome of interest (cases) and a control group of patients who did not experience the outcome at the time data were collected.

THE CASE REPORT—The case report is the presentation of the experience of a single patient. It is usually presented in a way that supports a hypothesis or an answer to a question of interest. Case reports are often referred to as *hypothesis-generating* because these bring forth evidence that supports a hypothesis or conclusion. For example, the presentation of the medications for a patient that were administered until the development of aplastic anemia might suggest that one or more of these drugs could have caused the aplastic anemia. However, it could not be concluded that another patient who took one or more of the same drugs would be at equal risk, because of the many other factors that also cause aplastic anemia, such as viral infections or exposure to insecticides, which may not be part of a patient's medical record or their recollection and would, therefore, not be reported.

When the common experiences of more than one patient are presented, this is referred to as a *case series*. Obviously, the greater the number of common experiences, the stronger the evidence to support a conclusion. For example, if five patients developed aplastic anemia after exposure to the same medication, this would raise suspicion beyond that for only one such patient. A good example of the impact of the case series is the 24 patient reports describing valvular heart abnormalities from concurrent fenfluramine and phentermine use.[5] These data were compelling enough for the withdrawal of fenfluramine from the market.

THE CROSS-SECTIONAL STUDY—This is a study conducted to obtain the prevalence of an outcome in a given set of patients such as those being treated with a drug at a single time point. Cross-sectional studies are often referred to as *snapshot* studies. Because data are collected all at once, the temporal relationship between the use of the drug and the outcome of interest cannot be determined in cross-sectional studies. This is a problem if the investigator is trying to make cause-and-effect inferences.

THE ECOLOGICAL STUDY—There are times when data are not available at the patient level, but there is interest in getting a preliminary understanding of the relationship between the use of a drug and an outcome. This may entice an investigator to use aggregate data to compare the gross amount of drug used and the rate of occurrence of an event for a community, state, or country. In other words, the unit of analysis in ecological studies is a population instead of a patient. An example of such an approach is the comparison of the numbers of prescriptions of β-adrenergic agonist inhalers dispensed in a country and the numbers of deaths from asthma. Such a relationship would be confounded by the increasing use of medications with increasing severity of illness (ie, sicker patients use more β-adrenergic agonist inhalers and are more likely to die of their disease, regardless). Another problem is that the investi-

gator might not even know whether the patients who died were even prescribed the medication, a dilemma known as the *ecological fallacy*. Hence, it can be observed that although ecological studies are easy to conduct, there may be major problems when using the data to make cause-and-effect inferences.

MEASUREMENTS

As with any scientific discipline, valid measurements are critical for accurate interpretation of the results of pharmacoepidemiologic studies. There are several fundamental metrics helpful to understand. For descriptive studies these include frequencies, distributions, prevalence, and incidence rates. For analytical studies these include the rate difference, rate ratio, relative risk, and odds ratio. A description of these measurements and how they are calculated are found in Table 108-2.

FREQUENCIES—In epidemiology, the prevalence and incidence of events are the most commonly used metrics; they are also the most commonly confused. The primary issue that distinguishes *prevalence* from *incidence* is the types of patients counted per unit time. As can be seen in Figure 108-4, the prevalence of an event is equal to the number of patients with the outcome of interest at a single point (cross-section) in time. Prevalence is often reported as a proportion or percentage (eg, the prevalence of asthma was 12%). If the measurement is made on all patients at a single moment in time (a snapshot), then it is referred to as a *point prevalence*. For example, consider the vertical dashed line in Figure 108-4. At that point in time, the prevalence of drug use is 4/1000 patients or 0.4%. If the measurement is made on all patients during a specific time interval, for example one year, then this is called a *period prevalence*. As shown in Figure 108-4, the period prevalence is 0.7%, 0.7%, 0.7%, and 0.8% for 1996, 1997, 1998, and 1999, respectively.

However, if an investigator begins with a group of patients naïve to an outcome and go forward in time and count all patients who contracted the disease or had the event, this is called the *incidence*. Incidence is measured as counts of patients with the outcome per unit time (12 per 100,000 person-years). The incidence of drug use in Figure 108-4 is 8/996 persons over the 4 years or 2/1000 person-years. The reason that 996 persons is used instead of 1000 persons is that one must remove from the denominator the patients who already have had the event of interest.

Accurate numerators and denominators are needed to calculate accurate prevalence and incidence rates. Though simple to say, depending on the data available for analysis, they may be impossible to compute accurately. Sometimes both the numerator and denominator are poorly ascertained. This is often

Table 108-2. Types of Measurements in Pharmacoepidemiology Studies

MEASURE	DEFINITION	COMMENTS
Prevalence	Frequency of cases at a given time or period	Often confused with incidence; reported as a percentage
Point prevalence	Frequency of cases at an instant	Used in cross-sectional studies
Period prevalence	Frequency of cases within a period such as 1 yr	Often confused with point prevalence
Incidence	Frequency of new cases in a population over a period	Mostly reported as a rate, such as 10/100,000 person-years
Relative risk or risk ratio	Incidence in the exposed group divided by the incidence in the unexposed	Addresses the number of times greater risk in exposed than in the unexposed; a relative risk of 1 means that the risk is equal with and without exposure
Odds ratio	An odds is the probability of an outcome happening divided by the probability of the event not happening; an odds ratio is the odds of the event in those exposed divided by the odds in the unexposed	Provides an estimate of the relative risk for rare outcomes; an odds ratio of 1 means that there is no association between exposure and outcome
Attributable risk or risk difference	Incidence in the exposed group minus incidence in the unexposed	Addresses the incidence of a disease attributed to an exposure

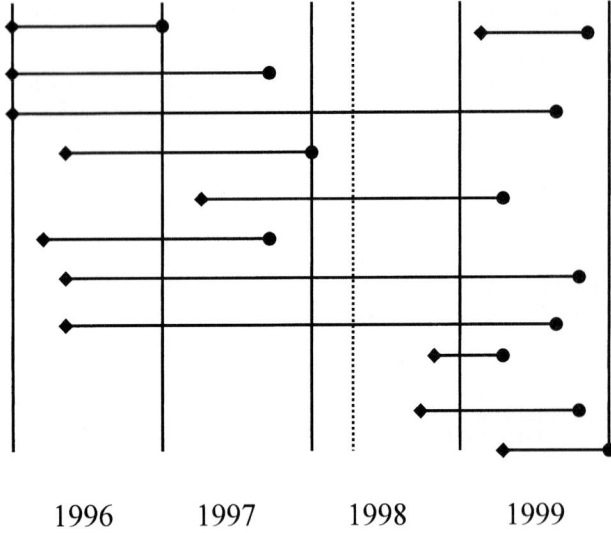

Figure 108-4. Distribution of the experiences of 12 patients prescribed a medication over a 4-year period, to illustrate the difference between prevalence and incidence. *Diamonds* indicate the date of the first prescription; *circles* indicate the stop date.

observed in sentinel surveillance programs such as MedWatch in which the numerator contains only those patients who had the outcome of interest *and* were reported. The denominator can only be estimated on the basis of national drug-use data, which must often be found in the literature or purchased from a vendor. Often the numerator is carefully calculated, but the denominator is unknown. For example, one may know when a certain event such as hospitalization for a specific reason occurs in patients prescribed a specific drug or drug class, but the investigator may not be able to estimate accurately the number of patients in the underlying population. This occurs in open health-care systems in which patients are free to switch healthcare plans. Lack of an accurate denominator can limit the usefulness of large databases such as those found in managed-care organizations. Investigators have often resorted to using the client enrollment file for denominator data. However, fluctuations in the numbers of clients can make enrollment data misleading, even over short intervals such as one year.

PREDICTION—Occasionally, an investigator wants to know whether a certain drug predicts a future benefit or adverse effect. For such studies, one needs to know whether the benefit or risk occurred for all patients and also the status of factors of interest before the patients were first prescribed the drug. An example of such a study would be determining the risk of renal impairment from a drug. It would be important to know patients' renal function before the drug of interest was administered. These data would allow one to adjust the predictive model on the basis of baseline renal function for these patients. If the investigatory was comparing two drugs, it would be important to have such data to know that renal function was similar in the two groups at baseline or whether this was taken into account.

BIAS

Bias is deviation from the truth. It affects all forms of experimentation and is described in Chapter 12. However, a number of biases that are unique to pharmacoepidemiology differ conceptually from those in laboratory studies and merit special attention. Generally, these can be classified as selection bias, measurement bias, and confounding bias. Because clinical studies cannot be controlled as carefully as laboratory studies, many forms of bias must be considered as possible explanations

for the results of pharmacoepidemiologic studies. Indeed, Sackett has catalogued 35 biases that can occur in analytic studies.[6]

SELECTION BIAS—Selection bias is a major problem of all nonrandomized clinical studies. It becomes manifest when groups for comparison are not balanced in terms of important background characteristics. When lopsided groups are compared, the investigator has difficulty interpreting the result because it is not known whether results are because of a drug exposure or because imbalances in one or more background characteristics have affected the results.

Pharmacoepidemiologists who conduct research using existing medical records need to realize that physicians' prescribing habits create biased groups. A common example of selection bias involves the prescribing patterns of physicians after the marketing of new drug products. As one might imagine, there is avid interest in learning as much as possible about the "realworld" experiences of recently marketed drugs. Soon after marketing, new drugs become the focus of inquiry. However, a big problem immediately becomes apparent when investigators compare the background characteristics of patients prescribed the newer and older drugs. What usually occurs is that patients prescribed the new drug are those who were not responding to the older therapies, and they are often sicker patients. This makes any comparison of recent and existing drugs inherently difficult.

Another example from the Regenstrief research center further illustrates selection bias. It is known that NSAIDs worsen renal function of patients with renal insufficiency. There were several reports that the NSAID sulindac was a renal-sparing NSAID, meaning that it did not worsen renal insufficiency in patients at risk of this effect as the other NSAIDs did. After reading these reports, some physicians began prescribing sulindac to their patients with preexisting renal insufficiency. When patients' baseline renal function was compared before they were prescribed NSAIDs, it was found that the patients who were prescribed sulindac had worse baseline renal function (ie, higher serum creatinine values) than patients prescribed other NSAIDs. Hence, physicians' preference for prescribing sulindac for patients with renal insufficiency created a bias in interpreting the true effect of the various NSAIDs. The end result was a bias that may have made sulindac look worse than the other NSAIDs.

There are ways to deal with selection bias for studies of existing data. Most notable among them are matching, mathematical modeling, and use of propensity scores. In matching, a control subject is matched with each case subject on important background characteristics. Using the previous example, an investigator could match patients with preexisting renal insufficiency who were prescribed sulindac with patients with preexisting renal insufficiency who were prescribed ibuprofen and look at the changes in serum creatinine afterward. Likewise, one would match those with normal prior renal function prescribed sulindac with those with normal prior renal function before they were prescribed ibuprofen.

With analysis of covariance, an investigator would put into a mathematical model a parameter that controls for differences in important background characteristics. Again, from the previous example, one would put patients' baseline serum creatinine or creatinine clearance into the model to adjust for baseline differences among the various NSAIDs being compared. Doing so would provide the estimated effect of the NSAID controlling for patients' prior renal function. The general idea is to balance comparison groups so a fair comparison is made.

Finally, propensity scores adjust for the probability that a patient will be prescribed one drug over another. To do so, a single score is calculated using logistic regression that includes all of the background characteristics that are important to a physician who was trying to decide between drugs. This score could then be used as a covariate in a mathematical model that looked at the outcome of interest. In calculating the propensity score in the example above, an investigator would want to include not only patients' baseline renal function, but perhaps age, gender, race, indication for the NSAID (eg, rheumatoid arthritis, osteoarthritis), and other factors that would predict which NSAID physicians prescribe. Hence, though selection bias is a problem in such studies, there are ways to deal with this form of bias.

An example of how propensity score methods are used to adjust for important background characteristics is demonstrated in Figure 108-5, Panels a and b. This study used propensity scores to adjust for age and other relevant variables to determine the effects of various NSAIDs on renal function.[7] It is clear from Figure panel a, that there is an important imbalance of the mean age of patients prescribed ibuprofen and sulindac. Because renal function declines with increasing age and sulindac is more commonly prescribed for older adults than ibuprofen, such a comparison is confounded. A more appropriate comparison is shown in Figure panel b, where age subgroups of patients prescribed ibuprofen and sulindac have been matched using propensity scores. Doing so permits comparison of ibuprofen and sulindac by age-matched subgroups, which is a much more intuitive and fair comparison.

Selection bias creeps into other areas of measurement in epidemiology. It has recently become popular to use *benchmarking* to compare the experiences of one hospital with those of another. If various aspects of the underlying characteristics of hospitals being compared are not controlled, then such a comparison will be faulty. A wild extrapolation of this would be to compare the rates of death in a hospice where terminally ill patients are cared for in their final days with those of patients from an acute-care hospital. Obviously, such a comparison is

fraught with error. It can also enter into the process of selecting the papers for inclusion in meta-analysis (see Chapter 12).

MEASUREMENT BIAS—Measurement bias results when comparison groups are measured differently. Misclassification of the event of interest can obviously be a problem. This requires careful definition of the characteristics of a case. If the case definition is based on a diagnosis or diagnostic code (ICD-9 code), some cases may be missed or be inappropriately included. For example, using only the diagnosis of *congestive heart failure* may be too broad if the disease of interest is left ventricular systolic dysfunction. Using *congestive heart failure* only would also include patients with diastolic dysfunction, which is treated entirely differently from systolic dysfunction. A related issue is the date of onset of a disease or disorder. Which is the date of onset of diabetes for a patient—the data of the diagnosis or the date of the first fasting or random blood glucose that was over the upper critical value of normal? These issues require careful consideration in the planning stages of the study.

A common problem is that patient follow up may be inadequate and incomplete. When patients are lost to follow up, it may appear in the analysis as though they did not have the interest. This commonly occurs when patients have access to multiple-care settings. An admission to a hospital that does not contribute data to the analytic database would go unnoticed. This could be a major problem if hospital admission is the primary dependent variable for the study. Patients unable to obtain a needed (perceived or real) drug will seek care elsewhere. If this drug is a study drug of interest, then patients may be differentially lost, which can result in an important bias.

Unmeasured or missing data on key confounders and effect modifiers can destroy the validity of cohort studies. It is not feasible for large population cohort studies such as the Framingham Study or Nurses Health Study to measure everything. The data collected depend upon the types of studies anticipated. If data are not collected pertaining to a key confounder, then the results of a study in which that variable is important may not be valid.

Finally, a pharmacoepidemiologic study that has excellent *internal* validity may have limited *external* validity. Internal validity deals with how well the results of the study represent the truth for the patients who were studied. External validity addresses the question of whether the results of the study extrapolate to other settings. Persons willing to participate in clinical studies may differ from other persons in meaningful ways. A study of drug-related hospital admission in one setting of care may differ from the findings in another because of the system for remuneration at each setting instead of drug factors *per se*.

There are methods for reducing measurement biases. Most important is making certain that groups being compared derive from the same underlying population and that the instruments of measurement are the same. As mentioned previously, a major problem with the use of observational data to make inferences about drugs is that physicians may preferentially prescribe some drugs more than others for sicker patients and, subsequently, conduct laboratory tests more frequently on the sicker patients. When cohorts are assembled on the basis of use of a certain drug and the outcome of interest is a laboratory measurement, patients prescribed the drug for sicker patients will likely appear to be doing worse. This is because the drug was prescribed for the sicker patients, and those patients were more likely to have received the laboratory test. The healthier patients could have been prescribed another drug, but never been tested.

RECALL BIAS—Recall bias occurs in case-control studies and can profoundly distort the results. It occurs because of differential recall of medications between cases and controls. Recall bias occurs because cases have better recollection of the drugs that they have been prescribed than the controls, and as such the prevalence of exposure to drugs of interest will be inflated excessively in the cases compared with the controls. This

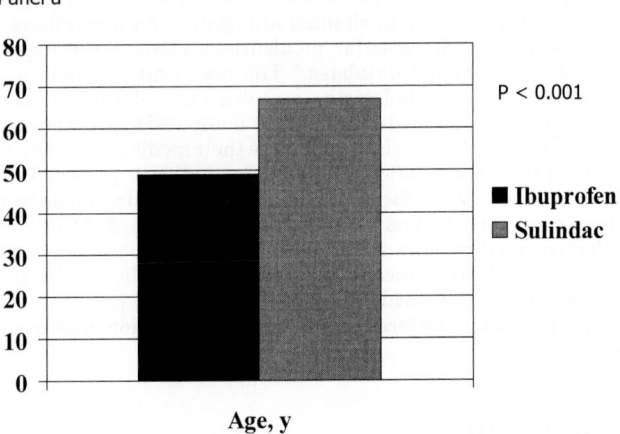

Panel a

P < 0.001

■ **Ibuprofen**
■ **Sulindac**

Age, y

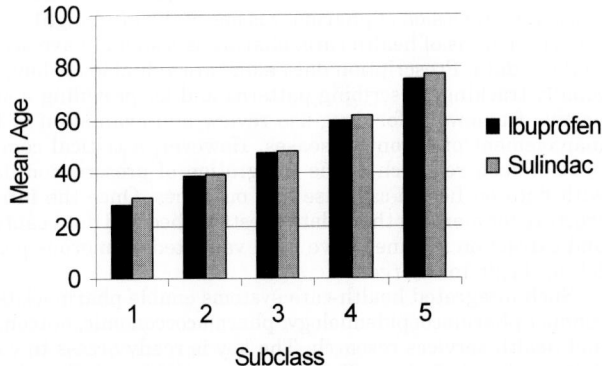

Panel b

■ Ibuprofen
■ Sulindac

Subclass

Figure 108-5A. An example of how propensity score methods are used to adjust for important background characteristics. **B.** Age subgroups of patients prescribed ibuprofen and sulindac have been matched using propensity scores.

falsely increases the association between the drug and the outcome of interest. For example, if an investigator was interested in knowing the drugs associated with developing cancer, the recall of drug histories might be more complete in the patients with cancer (cases) than in the controls. If one used the medical records instead of patient recall, it might be found that physicians of patients with cancer kept more-complete drug histories than the physicians caring for control patients. Because case-control studies depend on past exposures and the recording of exposures can be lopsided between cases and controls, an investigator might find that many drugs are associated with cancer owing to these measurement errors.

Another example that makes it easy to understand this bias is to think about the last time you were nauseated and then vomited (the outcome). In this circumstance, you might be inclined to think carefully about all of the foods and drinks consumed over the last day or so, in an attempt to pinpoint the causative food and avoid it in the future. However, few people reflect on the food eaten from day to day, and often fail to remember a diet as readily when we are not ill. This is recall bias. It occurs when women who have malformed infants are compared with those with normal births; the mothers of malformed infants reflect carefully on all of the medications that were taken during pregnancy, and the mothers of normal infants pay less attention to medications used.

CONFOUNDING—Confounding is a form of bias that confuses the results of pharmacoepidemiologic studies. A confounder is a factor that is associated with the outcome of interest and that if not considered will change the results so dramatically that it could result in erroneous study conclusions. A commonly used example is that of the investigation of the relationship between alcohol use and cancer. The data support such a relationship. However, it must be realized that smoking is known to cause cancer and people who drink alcohol also are more likely to smoke. Therefore, the relationship between alcohol consumption and cancer is confounded by smoking.

There are three requisites of confounding:

- The confounder is a risk factor for the outcome of interest.
- The confounder is associated with the drug being studied.
- The confounder is not a temporary step between the drug exposure and the outcome of interest.

In the preceding example, it can be observed that

1. Smoking is a risk factor for cancer.
2. Smoking and alcohol consumption are correlated.
3. Smoking is not an intermediate step in the causal pathway between alcohol use and cancer.

Taken together, the confounder is a factor that creates a bias or lopsided study result because it is not accounted for or ascertained in the investigation. The degree of confounding is important; the confounding bias could be so small that it does not affect the study conclusions, or it could be so large that results are entirely wrong and misleading.

There are three ways to control confounding:

1. Before the study is conducted, certain types of patients could be excluded from participation. In the example above, smokers could be *excluded* to estimate the effect of alcohol on the development of cancer.
2. If the study is executed and the data on the appropriate factors were obtained, patients could be *stratified* or *grouped* according to the factor of interest. For example, the effects of alcohol on cancer could be determined in both smokers and nonsmokers.
3. If there are multiple confounders this can be accomplished by mathematical modeling. Here, the investigator would estimate the risk of cancer by retaining extra variables in the mathematical model to distinguish smokers and nonsmokers as well as other potential confounders.

The best way to deal with confounding is to avoid it, and the only way to avoid it is with randomization. Patients randomly assigned to treatments are usually balanced on factors that result in bias, including confounders. This is the key reason why randomized clinical trials are preferable for determining differences between treatments. However, randomization to exposure or treatment is not performed in nonexperimental studies.

NEWS BREAKS AND FANATICISM

Besides participating in the conduct of research, another way pharmacists participate in pharmacoepidemiology is in patient education when news (good or bad) about a drug is released by the media about pharmacoepidemiologic studies. Keeping pace with the latest news stories requires some vigilance. Almost weekly, the public hears a news report about a drug product that leads to a barrage of telephone calls to pharmacists and physicians. Often these are pharmacoepidemiologic studies. From these news reports, patients hear that the drug they are taking is associated with an adverse outcome. This strikes fear into the hearts of these patients, who promptly call their pharmacists and physicians. Alert pharmacists will be able to anticipate the rash of calls and prepare themselves to spend time alleviating patients' fears until they can arrange to visit their physicians. Unless the risk is severe (eg, arrhythmia or death) or the patient has not tolerated the drug, then the patient should continue to take the medication. An exception would be in those instances in which the drug's benefits are not well documented and there are no withdrawal symptoms, in which case the drug could be discontinued. Patients could put themselves at great risk when breaking news results in their prompt discontinuation of medications that are life-sustaining (eg, antiarrhythmics) or produce adverse withdrawal phenomena (eg, β-adrenergic antagonists or clonidine).

The author and his colleagues have examined the effects of a prepublication presentation about the hazards of *immediate-release* forms of calcium channel antagonists on prescribing of a variety of cardiovascular medications using prescriptions stored in a national database.[8] The presentation—held at a large meeting of cardiologists—received a considerable amount of coverage in the media prompting many calls by patients to pharmacies and physicians to change their medications. The results of this study indicated that many patients' prescriptions for *sustained-release* forms of calcium channel antagonists were discontinued as well as immediate-release forms. Further, less effective medications such as alpha-adrenergic antagonists were instead prescribed. This experience highlights the profound and sometimes aberrant effect of media to presentations at professional conferences before a publication undergoes peer-review.

THE FUTURE

As health care becomes more automated with computer systems, the availability of large volumes of data will increase. Because the profession of pharmacy is one of the most highly computerized areas of health care, pharmacists should have access to these data. Prescription data alone are valuable for longitudinally tracking prescribing patterns and for providing a supportive framework for drug-use review and evaluation of the management of chronic diseases. However, a critical component of such research is the integration of prescription data with data on health-care use and outcomes. Once the infrastructure for merging these data is established and data capture and extraction routines have been validated, numerous possibilities begin to emerge.

Such integrated health-care systems enable pharmacists to conduct pharmacoepidemiology, pharmacoeconomic, outcomes, and health services research. The key is ready access to valid data in a timely fashion. This requires a solid foundation of support constituted by automated information experts, programmers, administrators, clinicians, and researchers. Many health-care systems have all of these individuals in place, but they have not yet directed their attention to the value of conducting pharmacoepidemiologic research. The primary reason for that is that most information systems have been created for billing purposes, with little attention to the use of their data for research. However, this position is slowly changing.

Pharmacists frequently are called upon to help health-care administrators understand the use of drugs in their care setting. Increasingly, administrators are requesting information on the value of pharmaceuticals being prescribed that in turn is requiring pharmacists and researchers to request prescription data that are integrated with resource-utilization data and cost or charge data. As ordinarily occurs with any new process, the first attempts to extract integrated data from huge databases are slow. However, with repeated applications of integrated data, new efficiencies occur, which make future data extractions and studies easier to conduct.

SUMMARY

Pharmacoepidemiology is a valuable contribution to the pharmaceutical sciences. It runs a spectrum from case reports that are sentinels of problems to labor-intensive and expensive randomized clinical trials considered the gold-standard of therapy. Pharmacists use the methods of pharmacoepidemiology when conducting drug-use reviews and evaluations. Pharmacoepidemiologic studies reveal little more than fodder for debate when studies are done without considering the numbers of biases that can occur. More frequently, however, pharmacoepidemiology provides the best available evidence supporting or refuting a hypothesis otherwise lacking data so that health policy can be written. The increasing use of automated databases provides pharmacists with access to large volumes of data that can be used to address many important issues. Access to these data coupled with an understanding of the principles of pharmacoepidemiologic research will permit pharmacists to contribute to society's growing need for timely answers to important questions in drug therapy.

REFERENCES

1. Murray MD, Smith FE, Fox J, et al. Structure, functions, and activities of a research support informatics section. *JAMA* 2003; 10:389.
2. *Qual Rev Bull* 1989; 15(9):330.
3. Stampfer MJ, et al. *N Engl J Med* 1991; 325:756.
4. Stampfer MJ, et al. *N Engl J Med* 1993; 328:1444.
5. Connolly HM, et al. *N Engl J Med* 1997; 337:581.
6. Sackett DL. *J Chronic Dis* 1979; 32:51.
7. Perkins, SM, Tu W, Underhill MG, et al. *Pharmacoepi Drug Safety* 2000; 9:931.
8. Brunt ME, Murray MD, Hui SL, et al. *J Gen Intern Med* 2003;18: 84.

BIBLIOGRAPHY

Textbooks

Bernier RH, Mason VM, eds. *Episource: A Guide to Resources in Epidemiology.* Roswell, GA: The Epidemiology Monitor, 1998.
Fletcher RH, Fletcher SW, Wagner EH. *Clinical Epidemiology: The Essentials,* ed 3. Baltimore: Williams & Wilkins, 1996.
Hartzema AG, Porta MS, Tilson HH, eds. *Pharmaco Epidemiology: An Introduction,* 3rd ed. Cincinnati: Harvey Whitney Books, 1997.
Kleinbaum DG, Kupper LL, Morgenstern H. *Epidemiologic Research: Principles and Quantitative Methods.* New York: Van Nostrand Reinhold, 1982.
Omenn GS, Fielding JE, Lave LB, eds. *Annual Review of Public Health,* vol 15. Palo Alto, CA: Annual Reviews, 1994.
Rothman KJ, Greenland S, eds. *Modern Epidemiology,* 2nd ed. Philadelphia: Lippincott-Raven, 1998.
Sackett DL, et al. *Clinical Epidemiology: A Basic Science for Clinical Medicine,* 2nd ed. Boston: Little, Brown, 1991.
Schlesselman JJ, ed. Case-Control Studies: Design, conduct, and analysis. New York: Oxford University Press, 1982.
Strom BL. *Pharmacoepidemiology,* 3rd ed. New York: John Wiley, 2000.

Software

Kleinbaum DG, Sullivan KM, Barker ND. ActivEpi Introductory Epidemiology Course. Data Description, Inc. Springer.
Borenstein M, Rothstein H, Cohen J, et al. Power and Precision, Biostat, Teaneck, NJ or www.PowerAnalysis.com.
SAS Institute Inc, Cary, NC or www.sas.com.
SPSS, Chicago, IL or www.spss.com.
S-Plus, Mathsoft, Data Anal Prod Div, Seattle, WA or www.mathsoft.com.

Associations

American Society of Clinical Pharmacology and Therapeutics (ASCPT), Section on Pharmacoepidemiology, Drug Safety, and Outcomes Research, Sharon J. Swan, CAE, Executive Director, 528 North Washington Street, Alexandria, VA 22314, Phone: (703) 836-6981, Fax (703) 836-5223 or www.ascpt.org.
International Society for Pharmacoepidemiology (ISPE), Mark Epstein, ScD, Executive Secretary, 4340 East West Highway, Suite 401, Bethesda, MD 20814-4411, Phone: (301) 718-6500, Fax: (301) 656-0989 or www.pharmacoepi.org.

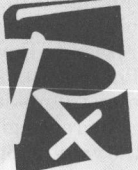

CHAPTER 109

Surgical Supplies

Thomas A Barbolt, PhD, DABT
Sylvia H Liu, BVM, DACVP

A professional service rendered by many pharmacists consists of supplying surgical instruments, sutures, surgical dressings, and other equipment employed by the surgical personnel during and after a surgical operation. Some pharmacists who have obtained the necessary background of information carry a complete line of such supplies and even are able to provide operating tables and other heavy equipment.

There are comparatively few such completely equipped pharmacies; the major outlet is through surgical supply houses.

Every pharmacist, however, should be familiar with two of the products mentioned above, namely, *Surgical Dressings* and *Sutures,* which are discussed in detail below. The selection of the correct type of surgical dressing or suture is a critical factor in safeguarding the welfare of the patient undergoing surgery. Many items in these categories are handled routinely by pharmacists, and all of these items come within the purview of their professional responsibility.

SURGICAL DRESSINGS

DEFINITION—*Surgical dressing* is a term applied to a wide range of materials used for dressing wounds or injured or diseased tissues. Dressings may serve to

Provide an environment for moist wound healing. Desiccation of a wound is a major factor in retarding wound healing and increasing scarring. Dressings that prevent desiccation provide an optimal environment for autolysis cell migration, granulation, and reepithelialization.

Prevent maceration by permitting evaporation or absorption. In highly exudative wounds, excessive moisture and autolytic enzymes will damage repairing tissue and will provide a perfect culture medium for microbes.

Promote hemostasis.

Protect the wound from further damage (mechanical damage, microbial invasion, dehydration, maceration, chemical damage, alteration in pH).

Reduce heat loss.

Control microbial growth (by incorporation of antimicrobial drugs).

Promote autolysis.

Promote healing.

Provide compression, promoting hemostasis, and reducing edema.

Provide support.

Reduce pain, increase patient comfort, and improve functional use of wound site.

Reduce odor.

Improve the appearance of the wound site.

Reduce overall costs associated with wound treatment.

SELECTION OF A WOUND DRESSING—Dressing selection should be made on the basis of the degree of exudation, presence or likelihood of infection, presence of necrotic tissue, and anatomical site. The correct selection of a wound dressing depends not only on the type of wound but also on the stage of repair. The use of a wound dressing cannot be considered in isolation, but rather in the context of an integrated wound-care program.

CLASSIFICATION—Functionally, the simplest method of classification uses the terms *primary* and *secondary* dressing. A primary dressing directly contacts the wound. It may provide absorptive capacity and may prevent desiccation, infection, and

adhesion of the secondary dressing to the wound. A secondary dressing is placed over a primary dressing, providing further protection, absorptive capacity, compression, or occlusion. Although some dressings are solely primary or secondary in nature, others have the characteristics of both. The following classification is used here:

TYPES OF WOUND DRESSINGS

Primary/secondary wound dressings
Secondary dressings
   Absorbents
   Bandages
   Adhesive tapes
Protectives

Within this classification, dressings are considered on the basis of composition.

SPECIFICATIONS—Surgical dressings and sutures are required to meet specific requirements of the USP for many characteristics. For these specific requirements and the performance of several of the official tests, eg, *Absorbency test* and *Fiber length* of cotton, *Diameter* of sutures, and *Tensile strength* of sutures, textile fabrics, and films refer to the detailed instructions provided in the USP.

PRIMARY WOUND DRESSINGS

Plain Gauze has been used as a primary dressing but will stick to all but clean, incised wounds. Although this property has been used to debride exudative, infected, and necrotic wounds, this practice may be painful and is often counterproductive, causing the removal of granhhulation tissue and new epithelium.

Impregnated Gauze is used to reduce its adherence to wounds. Cotton, rayon, or cellulose acetate gauze has been impregnated with a variety of substances such as petroleum or paraffin (Aquaphor, *Beiersdorf,* Vaseline (*Sherwood*), KY jelly (*Johnson & Johnson*), petrolatum emulsion (Adaptic, *Johnson & Johnson*), zinc saline (NutraDress, *Derma Sciences*), or sodium chloride (mesalt, *SCA Molnlycke*). Coatings may wear off, allowing epithelial ingrowth and necessitating a dressing change. A secondary dressing should be used with these dressings to prevent desiccation, provide absorbency, and prevent the entrance of pathogens. When used with an appropriate secondary dressing, these dressings may be used in heavily exuding wounds.

Film Dressings (transparent film, occlusive or semiocclusive) are films of polyurethane with acrylic or polyether adhesives that provide a semipermeable membrane to water vapor and oxygen yet are waterproof. In lightly exuding wounds they permit enough evaporation to promote moist wound healing and prevent maceration. Film dressings exclude bacteria from wounds and permit bathing and observation of the wound. Film dressings will adhere well to intact skin and have a low adherence for wound tissue. They should not be used in infected or heavily exuding wounds.

Film dressings may wrinkle, forming channels for microbial entrance. Difficulty in handling film dressings has been overcome by special design of various application systems. In addition to their use as wound dressings, adhesive films have been used to protect areas vulnerable to pressure, friction, or shear ulceration or for infusion or cannulation sites. Examples of transparent film dressings are Bioclusive (R) Transparent Dressing *(Johnson & Johnson)*, Opsite *(Smith & Nephew)*, Tegaderm *(3M)*, and Dermasite *(Derma Sciences)*.

PRIMARY/SECONDARY WOUND DRESSINGS

Composite Dressings have primary and secondary components that prevent adherence to the wound, with some degree of absorbency. The degree of occlusion provided by these dressings varies. Release *(Johnson & Johnson)*, Telfa *(Kendall)*, and Melolin *(Smith and Nephew)* consist of lightly absorbent rayon or cotton pads sandwiched between porous polyethylene films. Nu-Derm *(Johnson & Johnson)* and Lyofoam A *(Seton Healthcare Group)* consist of polyurethane foams with a film backing.

Hydrogels are complex lattices in which the dispersion medium is trapped rather like water in a molecular sponge. The *hydrogel* is typically a cross-linked polymer such as polyvinylpyrrolidone, cross-linked polyethylene oxide gel, or polyacrylamide. Hydrogels are nonadherent dressings that through semipermeable film allow a high rate of evaporation (and cooling) without compromising wound hydration. This makes them useful in burn treatment. Hydrogels are also very useful in hairy areas where entrapment of hair into the dressing would not be traumatic. Examples of hydrogels are Geliperm *(Geistlich)*, Vigilon *(Bard)*, Flexderm *(Dow Hickam)*, and Nu-Gel *(Johnson & Johnson)*. The latter is held together with a fusible fiber scrim.

Hydrocolloid Dressings combine the benefits of occlusion and absorbency. Hydrocolloids are dispersions of particles around which water molecules and solvated ions form a shell-like structure. Fluid absorption occurs principally by particle swelling and enlargement of this structure. The *hydrocolloid* mass of these dressings consists of gum-like materials, such as guar or karaya, sodium carboxymethylcellulose, and pectin, bound by an adhesive such as polyisobutylene.

Hydrocolloid dressings display wet tack (adhesion to a wet surface) because of particle swelling. This property facilitates atraumatic removal. The dry tack of hydrocolloid dressings is due to an adhesive such as polyisobutylene, which is inactivated by moisture. The dry tack retained by the dressing around the wound preserves the edge seal. Exudate absorption by most hydrocolloid dressings results in the formation of a yellow/brown gelatinous mass that remains on the wound after dressing removal. This may be irrigated from the wound and should not be confused with pus.

Because hydrocolloids absorb water slowly, they are of little use on acutely exuding wounds. They are, however, very useful for moderately to highly exudative chronic wounds. Examples of hydrocolloid dressings include Duoderm *(ConvaTec)*, Comfeel Plus *(Coloplast)*, and RepliCare *(Smith & Nephew)*.

CALCIUM ALGINATE DRESSINGS—Alginic acid is a naturally occurring polysaccharide derived from brown seaweeds. As the calcium salt, these fibrous nonwoven dressings are highly absorbent and are used on moderately to highly exuding wounds. They may be held in place with gauze tape or a film dressing. They also may be used to pack wounds. Examples of calcium alginate dressings are Sorbsan *(Dow Hickam)*, Algosteril *(Johnson & Johnson)*, and Kaltostat *(Calgon Vestal)*.

SECONDARY WOUND DRESSINGS

Absorbents

SURGICAL COTTON—Cotton is the basic surgical absorbent. It is official Purified Cotton USP.

Domestic cotton grown in the Southern US is suitable for surgical purposes. The domestic cotton plant reaches a height of 2 to 4 ft. Growing from the seeds is a pod or boll that bursts open upon ripening, exposing a mass of white cotton fibers. Each of these fibers is a minute, hair-like tube, the outer wall being pure cellulose, the opening filled with plant fluids. When the boll bursts open, the fiber collapses into a flat ribbon-like form, twisted and doubled upon itself more than 100 times from end to end.

The raw cotton fiber, mechanically cleaned of dirt and carded into layers but not otherwise treated, has a limited use for paddings and coverings of unbroken surfaces. This form is supplied under the name *nonabsorbent cotton*. It also is used frequently as cotton plugs in the bacteriological laboratory because of its nonabsorbency.

Absorbent Cotton is prepared from the raw fiber by a series of processes that remove the natural waxes and all impurities and foreign substances and render the fibers absorbent. It is a practically pure, white cellulose fiber.

Besides the familiar roll form, Purified Cotton may be obtained in various prepared forms such as cotton balls or cotton-tipped applicators.

Absorbent balls made of a uniform surgical viscose-rayon fiber also are available. These absorb fluids faster and retain their shape better than cotton balls.

Nonabsorbent Bleached Cotton, prepared by a modified bleaching process that retains the water-repellent natural oils and waxes, also is available. This cotton is identified easily by its silky feel. Because it is repellent to water, it does not become matted or inelastic. Consequently, it is well-adapted to packing, padding, and cushioning of dressings over traumatized areas and as nonabsorbent backing on sanitary napkins, combines, and drainage dressings.

Rayon, or regenerated cellulose, is made from wood or cotton linters. After dissolving it in a mixture of alkali and carbon disulfide, cellulose thread is reprecipitated in an acid-coagulating bath by passage through fine holes in a metal plate. Because plant lignins have been removed, as well as the more circular cross section, rayon fibers are softer and more lustrous than cotton.

SURGICAL GAUZES—The function of surgical gauze is to provide an absorbent material of sufficient tensile strength for surgical dressings. It is known as *Absorbent Gauze USP*.

In the process of making surgical gauze, the raw cotton fiber is cleaned mechanically and then spun or twisted into a thread, and the thread in turn is woven into an open-mesh cloth that is gray and nonabsorbent. It is bleached white and rendered absorbent by much the same processes as those used in the preparation of surgical cotton.

The gauze thus treated is dried by passing a continuous length through a tentering machine. Tenterhooks straighten, stretch, and hold it taut as it is dried. When it leaves this apparatus, the dried gauze is cut into lengths, folded, rolled, and packaged.

Gauze is classified according to its mesh, or number of threads per inch. Some types of surgical dressing require a close-meshed gauze for extra strength and greater protection, while other uses such as primary wound dressings, absorbent secondary dressings, and larger dressings to absorb purulent matter or other drainage require softer, more absorbent gauzes with a more open structure.

Various forms of pads, compresses, and dressings are made from surgical gauze, alone or in conjunction with absorbent cotton, tissue paper, and other materials.

Filmated Gauze is a folded absorbent gauze with a thin, even film of cotton or rayon distributed over each layer. This filmation fluffs up and gives ample dressing volume, yet costs less than gauze alone of equivalent volume. It possesses quick absorption and unusual softness.

Nonwoven Surgical Sponges—Nonwoven fabrics have been developed that are suitable alternatives to woven cotton gauze for use in wound cleaning, wound dressing, and tissue-handling. These nonwoven fabrics depend on dense entanglement of their synthetic fibers (Dacron, rayon, etc) to provide the fabric with an acceptable tensile strength approaching that of woven cotton gauze. They typically offer greater absorbent capacity than cotton gauze sponges of comparable bulk, while generating less lint. Specialty versions of the nonwoven sponges are available prefenestrated for IV tubing or drain-dressing procedures. One manufacturer *(Johnson & Johnson)* provides both a nonwoven sponge for wound dressing (Sof-Wick: very soft texture, very absorbent or Topper: highly absorbent, fewer dressing changes) and a nonwoven general-purpose cleansing/prep sponge (NuGauze: gauze-like texture, more absorbent than gauze). Additionally, a new universal sponge which combines the best attributes of woven and nonwoven gauze, has been created from a new fabric technology. Mirasorb *(Johnson & Johnson)* is made from a cotton blend, is more absorbent and resilient than woven gauze, provides less adherence to healthy tissue, and reduces wound damage and tissue trauma upon removal.

Selvage-Edge Gauze Strips in widths of 1/4 to 2 inches are designed specially and woven for use both as packing strips in surgery of the nose and sinuses, nasal hemostasis, etc, and as drainage wicks in the treatment of boils, abscesses, fistulas, and other draining wounds. The ravelproof, selvage edges on both sides eliminate all loose threads. These gauzes are available unmedicated or medicated with 5% iodoform. These strips are obtainable in sterile form packed in sealed glass jars. Nu Gauze Packing Strips are packaged in polystyrene containers.

Gauze Pads or Sponges are folded squares of surgical gauze. These are so folded that no cut gauze edges or loose threads are exposed. This prevents loose fibers from entering the wound. The pads are folded such that each size may be unfolded to larger sizes without exposing cut edges or loose threads. Sterilized packages of these frequently used all-gauze sponges are available in tamper-proof packages. Such sterile units particularly are well-suited to the numerous tray sets prepared in hospitals.

X-ray Detectable Gauze Pads are similar to all-gauze pads but contain inserts treated with barium sulfate. They are nontoxic, soft, and nonabrasive. They remain permanently detectable because they neither deteriorate in the body nor are affected by either sterilization or time. Examples of X-ray detectable sponges include Vistec and Kerlix (unique, crinkle-weave, soft, and absorbent), both manufactured by Kendall. Ray-Tec X-Ray Detectable Sponges *(Johnson & Johnson)* contain a nonabrasive vinyl plastic monofilament that gives a characteristic pattern in the X-ray.

Composite absorbent dressings have been developed for specific purposes. They usually consist of layers of absorbent gauze or nonwoven fabric with fillers of cotton, rayon, nonwoven fabric, or tissue paper in suitable arrangements. Composite sponges have gauze or nonwoven fabric surfaces with fillers of cotton, rayon, nonwoven fabric, or absorbent tissue.

Dressing Combines are designed to provide warmth and protection and to absorb large quantities of fluid that may drain from an incision or wound. Each combine consists of a nonwoven fabric cover enclosing fiber with or without absorbent tissue. They also may incorporate a nonabsorbent layer of cotton, tissue, or plastic film to prevent fluid from coming through to soil liners and bedding, though some combined dressings are entirely absorbent.

Laparotomy Sponges, also known as *Abdominal Packs, Tape Pads* or *Packs, Walling-Off Mops, Stitched Pads, Quilted Pads, Gauze Mops,* etc, are used to form a nonabrasive wall that will prevent abdominal or other organs from entering into the field of operation and to help maintain body temperature during exposure. They are made of four layers of 28-×-24 mesh gauze. The edges are folded in and hemmed. The entire pack is cross-stitched, and a looped tape 1/2-inch wide and 20-inches long is attached to one corner. A desirable feature of one type is an X-ray-detectable insert so firmly incorporated into the gauze that it cannot become detached. Treated with barium sulfate, the monofilament is nontoxic, and, were it to be left inadvertently *in situ*, would cause no more foreign-body reaction than an ordinary dressing.

Sanitary Napkins intended for special hospital use, otherwise known as *V-Pads, Obstetrical (OB) Pads, Perineal Pads, Maternity Pads,* etc, are used in obstetrical, gynecological, or maternity cases. Napkins that have repellent tissue on the side and back surfaces of the napkin usually are preferred because of their greater fluid-holding capacity. Sanitary napkins generally come with two sizes of filler, 3 × 9-inch or 3 × 11-inch. The napkin cover generally is made from a nonwoven fabric or a nonwoven fabric supported with an open-mesh scrim. Packaged, sterilized napkins are available and used generally to reduce cross-contamination possibilities.

Disposable Cleaners made from various types of nonwoven fabrics are available. They generally offer advantages over paper in wet strength and abrasion resistance, plus having better cleaning ability. Their advantages over cloth are reduced laundry expense and cross-contamination possibilities.

Eye Pads are scientifically shaped to fit comfortably and cover the eye completely, thus protecting the eyebrow when taped. These pads are made using nonwoven fabric. Two sides are enclosed to prevent the cotton from escaping and the pad from distorting. When desired, the pad may be folded and used as a pressure dressing. Eye pads especially are useful in the outpatient clinic of the hospital, the industrial medical department, and the physician's office. They are sealed in individual sterile envelopes.

Nursing Pads are designed in a contour shape to fit comfortably under the nursing brassiere or breast binder.

Disposable Underpads are used for incontinent, maternity, and other patients with severe drainage. Such pads cost less than the average hospital-made product and provide a neat, clean, easy-to-handle pad that is changed quickly and easily disposed. Disposable briefs are available (*Johnson & Johnson, Kendall*).

Cotton-Tipped Applicators are used to apply medications or cleanse an area. Machine-made cotton-tipped applicators are uniform in size, resulting in no waste of cotton or medications. The cotton is attached firmly to the stick and may be sterilized readily without affecting the anchorage of the cotton. They are available in 3- or 6-inch lengths.

Bandages

The function of bandages is to hold dressings in place by providing pressure or support. They may be inelastic, be elastic, or become rigid after shaping for immobilization.

Common Gauze Roller Bandage is listed in the USP as a form in which *Absorbent Gauze* may be provided. It is prepared from *Type I Absorbent Gauze* in various widths and lengths. Each bandage is in one continuous piece, tightly rolled and substantially free from loose threads and ravelings.

Muslin Bandage Rolls are made of heavier unbleached material (56×60 mesh). They are supplied in the same widths as the regular gauze bandage. Muslin bandages are very strong and are used wherever gauze bandages do not provide sufficient strength or support. They frequently are used to hold splints or bulky compression dressings in place.

Elastic Bandages are made in several types:

1. **Woven Elastic Bandage** is made of heavy elastic webbing containing rubber threads. Good support and pressure are provided by this type of rubber elastic bandage.
2. **Crepe Bandage** is elastic but contains no rubber. Its elasticity is due to a special weave that allows it to stretch to practically twice its length, even after repeated launderings. This elasticity makes it especially serviceable in bandaging varicose veins, sprains, etc, because it conforms closely to the skin or joint surfaces, lies flat and secure, yet allows limited motion and stretches in case of swelling so that circulation is not impaired.
3. **Conforming Bandage** is made from two plies of specially processed, high-quality, 14×8-inch cotton gauze folded to the center. This type is much easier to use and apply than ordinary roller bandage, since it tends to cling to itself during application, thus preventing slipping. It readily conforms to all body contours without the necessity of *reversing* or twisting. A further advantage is the fact that there can be no rough or frayed edge. Kling Conforming Gauze Bandage and Sof-King Conforming Bandage *(Johnson & Johnson)* are available in a variety of sizes up to 6 inches wide. This gauze is used widely to hold dressings or splints firmly in place and occasionally as a primary dressing when sticking to the wound is not a problem. A mercerized cotton Conforming Gauze Bandage clings to itself and thus remains in place better than gauze made of other materials. Sof-King is a one-ply rayon and polyester blend bandage that provides greater bulk for cushioning and greater absorbency.
4. **High-Bulk Bandage** is made of multiple layers (typically six) of crimped cotton gauze. The high bulk of this bandage type is designed to provide padding protection in wound dressing applications. It also provides the absorbent capacity of a cotton dressing component. One version (Sof-Band High Bulk, *Johnson & Johnson*) is made of mercerized cotton to help the bandage cling to itself, which facilitates application and improves dressing stability.
5. **Compression Bandage** is composed of cotton knitted or woven with either viscose, polyurethane, nylon, or elastane threads. The bandage is comfortable and easy to apply. Its use is primarily to maintain controlled levels of pressure when compression therapy is required. As with all compression bandages, these products should be utilized with caution on patients with marked peripheral ischemia or impaired arterial blood supply. Examples of compression bandge include Tensopress *(Smith and Nephew)*, Yeinopress *(Moliner)*, and Setopress *(Seton Healthcare)*.

Triangular Bandages usually are made by cutting a square of bleached muslin diagonally from corner to corner, forming two right triangles of equal size and shape. The length of the base is approximately 54 inches. These bandages were brought into prominence by Esmarch and still bear his name. They are used in first-aid work for head dressings, binders, and arm slings and as temporary splints for broken bones.

Orthopedic Bandages are used to provide immobilization and support in the treatment of broken bones and in certain conditions of bones and joints. Plaster of Paris–impregnated gauze has been the standard material for this purpose. More recently introduced are synthetic cast materials made of polyester cotton or fiberglass. Various types of plastic sheets also are offered that can be shaped easily and hardened to a rigid form by cooling or chemical reaction. These are useful chiefly for splints and corrective braces.

Individually packaged plaster of Paris bandages and splints are available in a wide variety of sizes. The Specialist brand *(Johnson & Johnson)* is made from specially treated plaster, uniformly spread and firmly bonded to the fabric. This results in a high strength-to-weight ratio in casts made from such bandages. Synthetic casts are applied like plaster of Paris. The Delta-Lite Synthetic Casting System *(Johnson & Johnson)* offers both polyester, cotton fabric impregnated with a polyurethane resin, and fiberglass casting materials. Scotchcast Softcast *(3M)* consists of a knitted fiberglass substrate impregnated with a polyurethane resin containing a surface-modifying agent (reduce tack, facilitate application). The casts are water-resistant, light weight, and durable.

Orthoflex Elastic Plaster Bandages *(Johnson & Johnson)* are plaster of Paris bandages containing elastic threads in the fabric and are intended for specialized prosthetic uses.

Stockinette Bandages are made of stockinette material knitted or woven in tubular form without seams. Surgical stockinette is unbleached. Because it is soft and will stretch readily to conform comfortably to the arm, leg, or body, it is used to cover the skin prior to the application of a plaster of Paris or synthetic cast.

Cast Paddings are soft, absorbent, protective paddings, applied like a bandage to the areas affected, before application of a cast. They are composed of various fiber constructions that conform and cling, absorb moisture, and allow the skin to breathe.

Adhesive Tapes

Surgical adhesive tapes are made in many different forms, varying both in the type of backing and in the formulation of the adhesive mass according to specific needs and requirements. The tapes available today may be divided into two broad categories: those with a rubber-based adhesive and those with an acrylate adhesive. Both types have a variety of uses. When strength of backing, superior adhesion, and economy are required (eg, athletic strapping), rubber adhesives commonly are used. Acrylate adhesives on a variety of backing materials are used widely in surgical dressing applications, when reduced skin trauma is required, as in operative and postoperative procedures; they are supplied in various strength and adhesion levels.

ACRYLATE ADHESIVES—Acrylate adhesives on a nonwoven or fabric backing have been accepted widely for use as surgical tapes, owing largely to what may be termed their hypoallergenic nature. Because acrylate adhesives are basically a unipolymeric system, they eliminate the use of a large number of components in rubber-based adhesives. In poly(alkyl-acrylate) adhesives, the desired balance between adhesion, cohesion, and flow properties is determined by the choice of monomers and the control of the polymerization reactions. Once the polymer is made, no other formulating or compounding is needed. In addition, the acrylics have an excellent shelf-life because they are not affected readily by heat, light, or air, factors that tend to degrade rubber-based adhesives.

Acrylate adhesives combine the proper balance of tack and long-term adhesion. Their molecular structure permits the passage of water vapor so they are nonocclusive and thus when coated on a porous backing material do not cause overhydration in the stratum corneum. Traumatic response to surgical tapes is minimized substantially when tapes are constructed to allow normal skin moisture to pass through adhesive and backing material. With this construction, the moisture content and strength of the horny cell layers remain relatively normal. When a porous tape is removed, the planes of separation develop near the surface of the stratum corneum, in the region of the naturally desquamating cells. This allows repeated use of tape over the same site with minimal damage to the skin.

Hypoallergenic Surgical Tapes with acrylate adhesive are available with a variety of porous backing materials. Rayon taffeta cloth backing provides a high-strength tape well-suited for affixing heavy dressings. Lighter dressing applications can be accomplished with lower-strength, economical, paper-backed surgical tapes. A knitted backing tape (Dermiform, *Johnson & Johnson*) provides some of the economies of paper surgical tape with the strength and conformability of a cloth backing. Other tapes feature elastic cloth or foam backing materials for special taping needs.

RUBBER-BASED ADHESIVES—A second group of surgical adhesive tapes is the cloth-backed and plastic-backed rubber adhesives. These are used principally where heavy support and a high level of adhesion are required. Modern rubber-based adhesive tape masses consist of varying mixtures of several classes of substances and are composed of an elastomer (para or pale crepe rubber in the case of natural rubber tapes, and synthetic elastomers made from polymers of isobutylene, alkylacrylate, or similar materials), one of several types of rosin or modified rosin, antioxidants, plasticizers and fillers, and coloring agents to give the tape the desired tint or whiteness.

ADHESIVE TAPE REACTIONS—While skin reactions formerly were accepted by the medical profession as almost predictable sequelae to the use of adhesive tape, with better understanding of the mechanisms of such reactions and progress in research and technology, the long-sought-for objective of hyporeactivity has, in large degree, been attained.

Because adhesive tape masses historically have consisted of heterogeneous and complex mixtures of organic compounds, it is not surprising that many workers have ascribed adhesive tape reaction to allergy. More-recent work, however, has shown that a true allergic response to the modern adhesive tape mass or its components is a factor in only a small proportion of clinical reactions and that most observed reactions are ascribed properly to other factors, mainly mechanical irritation and, to a lesser degree, chemical irritation. There apparently is no significant difference in reaction between patients with or without a history of allergy, but true specific dermatitis may occur more readily in persons who have manifested some other form of contact dermatitis.

Adverse manifestations produced by adhesive tape are characterized by erythema, edema, papules, vesicles, and in severe cases, desquamation. Itching may be intense, or it may be absent. The reaction may be demonstrated readily by patch-testing, and usually manifests itself early—within 24 to 48 hr. Characteristically, the reaction becomes more severe the longer the tape is left in place and continues to increase in intensity for some time after the tape is removed. This type of reaction is long-lasting and requires days for its complete subsidence.

Two distinct types of irritation can result from the mechanical dynamics of removing tape from the skin. One response—induced vasodilation—is a relatively nontraumatic, transitory effect in which no actual damage to the skin occurs. A second type—skin stripping—is a traumatic response in which skin is removed with the tape and actual damage to the epidermal layers results. Such mechanical skin removal is possibly the dominant cause of clinical reactions seen with the use of adhesive tape.

Chemical irritation from adhesive tape results when irritating components in the mass or backing of the tape permeate the underlying tissues of the skin. The tape construction can influence the reactivity of such ingredients substantially. For example, many compounds that normally do not penetrate intact stratum corneum can penetrate overhydrated corneum.

When portions of the stratum corneum are removed, the barrier capacity of the skin is damaged substantially. In this situation, any irritating components of the tape have ready access to underlying tissues. These substances then can cause a degree of irritation that is far greater than would be observed on intact skin.

PROTECTIVES

Until recently, protectives included only the various impermeable materials intended to be used adjunctively with other dressing components to prevent the loss of moisture or heat from a wound site or to protect clothing or bed liners from wound exudate. Film dressings are excellent devices to protect against infection and dislodgement of vascular cannulae and drainage sites. In addition, they may be used to protect vulnerable areas against pressure sores.

Protectives also are employed to cover wet dressings and hot or cold compresses. In common use as protectives are plastic sheeting and waxed or plastic-coated paper. These prevent the escape of moisture or heat from the dressing or the compress and protect clothing or bed linens. Rubber sheeting is a rubber-coated cloth, waterproof and flexible, in various lengths and widths for use as a covering for bedding. A so-called *nursery sheeting* is supplied, coated only on one side.

PRODUCTS FOR ADHESION PREVENTION—Adhesions are abnormal connections between organs or tissues that form after trauma, including surgery. They consist of organized fibrin and fibrovascular scar tissue and complicate all areas of surgery. In gynecological surgery, adhesions may result in infertility and pelvic pain; in intestinal surgery they may result in intestinal obstruction; in cardiac surgery they may render a second sternotomy hazardous, and in tendon surgery they will prevent mobility.

Although careful tissue handling and good hemostasis may reduce adhesion formation, there are few proven entities designed for the prevention of adhesions. Gynecare Interceed Absorbable Adhesion Barrier *(Ethicon)* is a knitted fabric of oxidized regenerated cellulose that is placed at a site where adhesions are suspected to occur. It swells and gels to form a barrier between two adjacent surfaces, allowing remesothelialization to take place. The fabric then degrades grossly by about 14 days and microscopically by about 28 days. Interceed Barrier is indicated for reducing the incidence of adhesions in pelvic gynecological surgery. Other mechanical barriers used for the prevention of adhesions include Seprafilm *(Genzyme)* and Gore-Tex Surgical Membrane *(Gore)*. Newer products available for the prevention of postoperative adhesions that are not site-specific for application include Gynecare Intergel Adhesion Prevention Solution, a ferric hyaluronate gel *(Lifecore Biomedical)* and Sepracoat, a dilute hyaluronic acid solution *(Genzyme)*.

OPERATING ROOM SUPPLIES

Hemostatic Products accelerate hemostasis by providing a thrombogenic surface that promotes platelet aggregation and fibrin polymerization. These topical hemostatic agents include collagen, gelatin, cellulose, and thrombin. These include collagen sponges and powders (Instat, *Johnson & Johnson;* Helistat, *Integra Life Sciences;* Actifoam, *Bard;* Avitene, *Davol;* Helitene, *Integra Life Sciences*), gelatin sponges (Surgifoam, *Johnson & Johnson;* Gelfoam, *Upjohn*), and Oxidized Regenerated Cellulose USP (Surgicel, *Johnson & Johnson*). Both oxidized cellulose and oxidized regenerated cellulose are agents whose actions depend on the formation of a coagulum consisting of salts of polyanhydroglucuronic acid and hemoglobin. When applied to a bleeding surface, they swell to form a brown gelatinous mass that is absorbed gradually by the tissues, usually within 7 to 14 days. They are employed in surgery for the control of moderate bleeding when suturing or ligation is impractical or ineffective.

Thrombin (USP) solutions of bovine origin (Thrombinar, *Jones Medical*) promote hemostasis by catalyzing the conversion of fibrinogen to fibrin. They may be used in conjunction with fibrinogen concentrates prepared from autologous cryoprecipitate or from pooled donor blood.

Tissue sealants are absorbable and are used for a variety of indications including sealing of arterial punctures, sealing of air leaks during pulmonary surgery, and supporting wound healing. The area of tissue sealants is expanding rapidly, with new products reaching the market for numerous indications. Angio-seal *(Kendall),* an absorbable material, is used as a sealant for arterial punctures. AdvaSeal *(Focal),* a synthetic absorbable sealant, is used to seal air leaks during pulmonary surgery. Tissell *(Immuno AE),* a two-component fibrin sealant, is used to promote wound healing as well as achieve hemostasis and tissue adhesion. BioGlue, *(Cryolife)* is a bovine albumin-based glue used to seal aortic aneurysms and anastomotic sites.

Tissue glues are used for topical skin adhesives and replace the need for sutures, staples, or adhesive strips for certain types of lacerations requiring closely approximated wound edges. Dermabond *(Closure Medical),* an octyl cyanoacrylate, is used as a topical skin adhesive that sloughs from the wound as reepithelialization of the skin occurs, providing sufficient time for wound healing. Indermil (Tyco Healthcare), a butyl cyanoacrylate, is another topical skin adhesive.

Disposable Sterile OR and OB Packs are prepared, packaged, and sterilized assemblies of diapering and gown units, designed to fulfill the operating and delivery room needs. They eliminate the problems of laundering, storage, assembly, and sterilization of muslin drapes and gowns. They introduce many special materials with particular properties of porosity; repellency to water, alcohol, blood and other fluids; abrasion resistance; and other desirable attributes.

Double packages of contamination-resistant paper have been developed to permit opening and use without compromising sterility. Retention of sterile characteristics until used, eliminates the need for resterilization.

Face masks for use in the operating room and where contamination must be controlled generally are made of plied, fine-mesh gauze, shaped to cover the nose, mouth, and chin. They are laundered and autoclaved. Disposable face masks with special filtration material giving high retention of particulate matter and designed for more effective fitting are available from several manufacturers. Surgine Face Mask *(Johnson & Johnson)* claims a 94% filtration efficiency with high user comfort.

SURGICAL DRESSINGS

ADHESIVE BANDAGE

Adhesive Absorbent Compress; Adhesive Absorbent Gauze

A compress of four layers of Type I absorbent gauze, or other suitable material, affixed to a film or fabric coated with a pressure-sensitive adhesive substance. It is sterile. The compress may contain a suitable antimicrobial agent and may contain one or more suitable colors. The adhesive surface is protected by a suitable removable covering.

Description—The compress is substantially free from loose threads or ravelings; the adhesive strip may be perforated, and the back may be coated with a water-repellent film.

GAUZE BANDAGE

Type I absorbent gauze; contains no dye or other additives.

Description—One continuous piece, tightly rolled, in various widths and lengths and substantially free from loose threads and ravelings.

OXIDIZED CELLULOSE

Absorbable Cellulose; Absorbable Cotton; Cellulosic Acid; Hemo-Pak *(Johnson & Johnson);* Oxycel *(Deseret Medical)*

Sterile gauze or cotton that has been oxidized chemically to make it both hemostatic and absorbable; contains 16% to 24% carboxyl (COOH) groups.

Description—In the form of gauze or lint. Is slightly off-white in color, is acid to the taste, and has a slight charred odor.

Solubility—Insoluble in water or acids; soluble in dilute alkalies.

Comments—The value of oxidized cellulose in various surgical procedures is based upon its properties of absorbability when buried in tissues and its remarkable hemostatic effect. Absorption occurs between the second and seventh day following implantation of the dry material, depending on the adequacy of the blood supplied to the area and the degree of chemical degradation of the implanted material. Complete absorption of large amounts of blood-soaked gauze may take 6 weeks or longer, and serious surgical complications and cyst formation have been reported as the result of failure to absorb. Hemostasis depends upon the marked affinity of *cellulosic acid* for hemoglobin. When exposed to blood, either *in vitro* or in surgical conditions, the oxidized gauze or cotton turns very dark brown or black and forms a soft gelatinous mass that readily molds itself to the contours of irregular surfaces and controls surgical hemorrhage by providing an artificially induced clot. Pressure should be exerted on the gauze or cotton for about 2 min to facilitate the sealing off of small, bleeding vessels.

Two factors require emphasis: (1) cellulosic acid does not enter the physiological clotting mechanism *per se* but forms what might be termed an *artificial clot* as described and, therefore, is effective in controlling the bleeding hemophiliac and (2) the hemostatic action of cellulosic acid is not enhanced by the addition of other hemostatic agents, such as thrombin (which in any case would be destroyed by the pH of the gauze unless some means of neutralization were practicable). The hemostatic effect of either one alone is greater than the combination.

It is useful as a temporary packing for the control of capillary, venous, or small arterial hemorrhage, but since it inhibits epithelialization, it should be used only for the immediate control of *hemorrhage* and not as a surface dressing. A purer and more uniform product prepared from oxidized regenerated cellulose has been developed and is available as Surgicel Absorbable Hemostat. This offers many advantages over the older, less-uniform oxidized cellulose derived from cotton and, because of its chemical uniformity, ensures dependable performance and overcomes many of the difficulties encountered with the older type of cotton product. The knitted fabric strips do not fragment, may be sutured in place easily if necessary, and provide prompt and complete absorption with minimum tissue reaction.

OXIDIZED REGENERATED CELLULOSE

Surgicel; Surgicel Nu-Knit; Surgicel Fibrillar *(Johnson & Johnson)*

Contains 18–24% carboxyl groups (COOH), calculated on the dried basis. It is sterile.

Preparation—Cellulose is dissolved and regenerated by a process similar to the manufacture of rayon, which is then oxidized.

Description—Creamy white gauze, lint, or woven material.

Solubility—Insoluble in water; soluble in alkali hydroxides.

Comments—Absorbable hemostatic.

PURIFIED COTTON

Gossypium Purificatum; Absorbent Cotton

The hair of the seed of cultivated varieties of *Gossypium hirsutum* Linné or other species of *Gossypium* (Fam *Malvaceae*), freed from adhering impurities, deprived of fatty matter, bleached, and sterilized in its final container.

Description—White, soft, fine, filament-like hairs appearing under the microscope as hollow, flattened and twisted bands, striate and slightly thickened at the edges; practically odorless and practically tasteless.

Solubility—Insoluble in ordinary solvents; soluble in ammoniated cupric oxide TS.

DEXTRANOMER

Debrisan (Johnson & Johnson)

Dextranomer is a three-dimensional cross-linked dextran polymer prepared by interaction of dextran with epichlorohydrin.

Description—White, spherical beads, 0.1 to 0.3 mm in diameter; hydrophilic. Also available dispersed in polyethylene glycol, as a paste.

Solubility—Insoluble in water or alcohol. Each gram absorbs about 4 mL of aqueous fluid, the beads swelling and forming a gel.

Comments—Topically to cleanse secreting lesions such as venous stasis ulcers, decubitus ulcers, infected traumatic and surgical wounds, and infected burns. It absorbs the exudates, including the components that tend to impede tissue repair, and thereby retards eschar formation and keeps lesions soft and pliable.

ABSORBABLE DUSTING POWDER

Starch-derivative Dusting Powder

An absorbable powder prepared by processing cornstarch and intended for use as a lubricant for surgical gloves; contains not more than 2% magnesium oxide.

Description—White, odorless powder; pH (1 in 10 suspension) between 10 and 10.8.

ABSORBENT GAUZE

Carbasus Absorbens; Gauze

Cotton, or a mixture of cotton and not more than 53.0%, by weight, of purified rayon, in the form of a plain woven cloth. If rendered sterile, it is packaged to protect it from contamination.

Description—White cotton cloth of various thread counts and weights; may be supplied in various lengths and widths and in the form of rolls or folds.

PURIFIED RAYON

A fibrous form of bleached, regenerated cellulose. It may contain not more than 1.25% titanium dioxide.

Preparation—By the viscose rayon process.

Description—White, lustrous or dull, fine, soft, filamentous fibers, appearing under the microscope as round, oval, or slightly flattened translucent rods, straight or crimped, striate and with serrate cross-sectional edges; practically odorless and practically tasteless.

Solubility—Very soluble in ammoniated cupric oxide TS or dilute H_2SO_4 (3 in 5); insoluble in ordinary solvents.

Comments—Hemostatic.

ADHESIVE TAPE

Sterile Adhesive Tape

Fabric and/or film evenly coated on one side with a pressure-sensitive, adhesive mixture. If rendered sterile, it is protected from contamination by appropriate packaging.

SUTURES AND SUTURE MATERIALS

A surgical suture is a strand or fiber used to hold wound edges in apposition during healing, and the process of applying such a strand is called *suturing*. When such material, without a needle, is used to stop bleeding by tying off severed blood vessels, the strand is called a *ligature,* and the process is known as *ligating*. Suture materials, however, have uses beyond those involved in the repair of wounds in that they often are used in reconstructive procedures.

Surgical sutures were first listed in the second supplement of USP XI in a monograph on catgut sutures, which then were designated officially as *Surgical Gut*. USP XII carried a similar monograph on surgical silk. USP XVI contained, in addition to surgical gut, a generalized monograph designed to cover all sutures in addition to catgut, and this is also true of USP XX. USP 23 additionally describes synthetic absorbable sutures.

At one time or another, nearly every form of fibrous material or wire that offered any promise at all has been used as a suture, and indeed many materials that by present standards offer no promise at all have been evaluated.

Cotton and linen were among the earliest suture materials, but the use of animal intestines and sinews also claims great antiquity. As in many other fields of science, there have been fads, and numerous materials have enjoyed varying favor through the centuries. Frequently, the acceptance of a given suture material depended on its successful use by an eminent surgeon whose authority encouraged emulation, and in many cases, there appeared to be legitimate scientific justification for such use.

Possibly the most important factor in the acceptance of suture materials has been their characteristics in the presence of infection. As knowledge of bacteriology increased and methods of sterilization improved, the earlier disadvantages of certain sutures have been overcome, so that currently a wide variety of surgical suture materials may be sterilized conveniently and effectively.

Among the widely accepted methods for the sterilization of sutures are autoclave sterilization with free access of water vapor, applicable only for those sutures that are not harmed by this process; dry heat at 310°F; ethylene oxide; and irradiation sterilization using either beta or gamma rays.

Irradiation sterilization has many advantages over the older methods insofar as commercial production is concerned. The sutures are sterilized in their final sealed packages, eliminating any danger of recontamination. The radiation dose is greater than necessary to kill even the most resistant spore-forming organisms. One great advantage of this method lies in the relative lack of deteriorating effect upon many sutures. Irradiation-sterilized surgical gut is stronger, more pliable, and easier to handle than dry-heat-sterilized surgical gut sutures.

Suture materials may be divided into two principal classes: absorbable and nonabsorbable. In the first class are found those materials that are capable of being broken down or digested by the body. Catgut, the classic absorbable suture derived from collagen-rich animal tissue, is proteinaceous in nature, and it appears that certain proteolytic enzymes in tissues are responsible for the digestion of catgut and its disappearance from the wound area. New forms of absorbable sutures based upon synthetic polyesters such as polyglycolic acid, copolymers of lactide and glycolide, polydioxanone, copolymers of glycolide and caprolactone, and a blend of glycolide, trimethylene carbonate, and dioxanone have been introduced as alternative absorbable materials.

Nonabsorbable sutures are manufactured from various materials such as polyester, nylon, or polypropylene. These materials incite a minimal foreign-body reaction at the site of placement, which resolves over time. Nonabsorbable sutures are used frequently for cardiovascular, ophthalmic, and neurological procedures.

ABSORBABLE SUTURES

SURGICAL GUT—Catgut is still used in surgical procedures, but its use, especially in the US, has declined because of the availability of new, synthetic, absorbable suture materials. Its basic constituent is collagen derived from the serosal or submucosal layer of the small intestine of healthy ruminants (cows, sheep, goats). The intestines from the freshly killed animals are cleaned of their contents and split longitudinally into ribbons. Mechanical processes remove the innermost mucosa and the outer muscularis layers, essentially leaving only the submucosal or serosal collagenous layers. This appears as a thin, strong network consisting chiefly of collagen, whose orientation and strength are increased markedly by subsequent processing. From one to five or six such ribbons are stretched, spun, or twisted under tension and dried under tension to form a uniform strand. These strands are polished to a uniform diameter and cut into appropriate lengths for packaging and sterilization.

In another method, collagen sutures are produced from collagen derived from beef tendon. The tendons are suitably treated and dispersed. The dispersed collagen is extruded, precipitated, and reconstituted as fine strands that are then twisted, stretched, tanned, and otherwise treated to give absorbable sutures with the desired characteristics.

Diameter and strength requirements for absorbable surgical suture (surgical gut) are specified in the USP, in which will be found descriptions of the suture as well as the apparatus and methods for measuring diameter, tensile strength, and sterility and other tests.

Plain and Chromicized Surgical Gut—Two varieties of catgut, distinguished by their resistance to absorptive action by tissue enzymes, are described in the USP as *Type A,* plain or untreated, and *Type C,* medium treatment. The availability of both types reflects the surgeon's requirements for catgut that will retain its tensile strength for varying periods of time or that will show an increased resistance to the proteolytic substances found in certain body tissues. This is accomplished by the incorporation of chromium salts or other chemicals to prolong its survival in tissues. Such products formerly were designated as 10-, 20-, or 40-day catgut, on the assumption that these sutures would remain for such periods in normal tissue. The variations in catgut as a natural product, as well as the variations in patients and in sites of implantations, make such designations qualitative, so they were replaced by the more general statement of type. While many tests for the expected duration of resistance have been proposed, none is accepted fully as comparable to digestion in animal tissues, and none has been included in the USP.

Approximately half the surgical gut used in the US has been either chromicized or otherwise treated. Raw catgut is analogous to rawhide, while chromicized catgut is comparable to chrome-tanned leather. The tanning process is applied either to the ribbons before they have been twisted into the strand form or to the finished twisted strand. Treatment in the ribbon form is reported to result in a more uniform deposition of chromium salts throughout the entire cross-section of the suture, while string chromicization sometimes causes the deposition of relatively heavier concentrations of the tanning agent near the periphery of the strand, with less penetration to its center. Deficient tanning of catgut may result in its premature absorption with possible wound disruption, although such incidents now are recognized often as the effects of nutritional or other inadequacies, with resultant weakness of the tissues themselves. Excessive chrome concentration in surgical gut may produce sutures that digest slowly. Since they survive in normal tissues for a long time, they occasionally may extrude through the skin some months following surgery. The mechanism of such extrusion by highly tanned catgut or by nonabsorbable sutures is not clear, although it probably reflects the natural tendency of the body to eliminate or reject foreign material.

Tissue Reaction—Following any surgical incision, there is an outpouring of blood and lymph into and through the wound. These fluids coagulate or clot, forming a network upon which new cells may build. The capillaries in the area dilate, and the blood supply in the vicinity of the wound is increased. Leukocytes in the area also increase in number.

The absorption of surgical gut takes place along with the tissue repair processes. The leukocytes, which appear early in any wound, produce proteolytic enzymes that, among other functions, carry out the digestion of absorbable catgut sutures. After this process is well along, fibroblasts appear and begin to lay down the collagen fibers essential for the increasing strength and healing of the wound. In the first phase of wound healing, the number and character of the debriding cells, together with such secondary effects as swelling, pain, and redness, constitute *tissue reaction*. Chromic catgut elicits a less intense tissue reaction of a leukocytic or exudative type than does the plain variety.

Plain gut is digested by enzymes at a faster rate than chromic gut. The surgeon chooses either plain or chromic gut, depending on the type of tissue involved, the condition of the patient, and the estimated healing time of the wound. Small sizes of surgical gut cause less tissue reaction and irritation than large sizes. There is less digestive work for the enzymes to do. For this reason surgeons try never to use a suture that is stronger than the tissue in which it is to be used. The larger sutures merely add to tissue irritation without supplying any needed strength to the wound.

Sterilization and Packaging—Disappointing experiences with many attempts to sterilize gut by chemical means have created widespread distrust of the effectiveness of most chemicals. The exception has been the use of ethylene oxide, which has provided an effective means for sterilizing sutures. The more common methods are dry-heat sterilization (after first dehydrating the catgut) and irradiation sterilization in the final sealed packet.

At one time most surgical gut was produced and labeled as *boilable*. It was packaged in glass tubes with the strands immersed in a water-free, high-boiling tubing fluid—usually xylene. The exteriors of the tubes could be sterilized at the hospital by autoclaving—hence, the term *boilable*.

The disadvantage of boilable catgut has been that the drying necessary to permit high-temperature sterilization produces a stiff strand, which is still stiff as removed from the tube, and which requires soaking for several minutes in sterile water before surgeons find it pliable enough to use. This process no longer is used (with isolated exceptions).

The present method of packaging provides sutures ready for use as removed from the packet. The catgut, designated *nonboilable,* is contained in either a foil or plastic packet, immersed in a pliabilizing fluid that generally consists of an alcohol or mixtures of an alcohol with a small percentage of water. The water has a pliabilizing effect but would ruin the gut if the latter was subjected to high temperatures—therefore, the designation *nonboilable*.

Irradiation and ethylene oxide sterilization techniques, as described in the USP, largely have replaced the older accepted method of dry-heat sterilization. These methods have permitted the development of more-convenient packaging innovations that were not practical with the older methods.

For even greater convenience, all foil or plastic packets are now overwrapped in a secondary package. Both the contents and the outside of the inner packet are rendered sterile. By peeling open the overwrap package, the inner packet can be delivered ready for use in a sterile condition on the operating table.

Sterility Testing—Freedom from contamination is the most important property of any suture. Every lot of sutures furnished by reputable manufacturers is subjected to a series of physical and chemical tests, in accordance with prescribed USP sterility test procedures as well as validated sterilization processes. No lot of sutures is released until all of these tests have been passed successfully; hence, the surgeon has developed a justified confidence in the adequacy and sterility of these products. Because of the extraordinary reliability of radiation sterilization, acceptance of product sterility based on validated measurement and control of the radiation process is becoming more widespread.

Operating Room Procedures—Before a scheduled operation, the nurse usually selects the necessary types of sutures designated by the operating surgeon. The required number of overwrapped packages is opened by peeling apart the outer package and flipping or otherwise removing in an aseptic manner the inner sterile packets and placing them on the Mayo stand. The packets are opened by tearing, if foil, and by cutting with sterile scissors, if plastic. Straightening the nonboilable suture is accomplished by a gentle pull. They commonly are used as removed from the packet. Abuse of catgut sutures may lead to their failure in tissues, with possible serious consequences to the patient.

SYNTHETIC ABSORBABLE SUTURES—The combination of high tensile strength and absorbability that makes catgut so useful as a suture has been incorporated into synthetic fibers. Polymers derived from condensing the cyclic derivative of glycolic acid (glycolide), mixtures of glycolide and lactide (derived by cyclicizing lactic acid), dioxanone, glycolide with trimethylene carbonate, mixtures of glycolide and caprolactone and blends of glycolide, trimethylene carbonate, and dioxanone have been shown to possess properties that make them suitable for many surgical procedures. Dexon II (*Davis & Geck*), a polyglycolic acid homopolymer, and Vicryl (*Ethicon*) and Polysorb (*US Surgical*), glycolide and lactide copolymers, are melt-extruded into multifilament yarns that then are braided into various sizes of sutures. Such braids have high tensile strength and, unlike catgut, must be packaged without fluid and sterilized with ethylene oxide to avoid degradation. PANACRYL suture (*Ethicon*) is another glycolide and lactide copolymer that has long-term strength retention found useful for various orthopedic procedures. Polymers such as dioxanone (*PDS II, Ethicon*), glycolide and caprolactone (*Monocryl, Ethicon*), glycolide with trimethylene carbonate (*Maxon, Davis & Geck*), and blends of glycolide, trimethylene carbonate, and dioxanone (*Biosyn, US Surgical*) are provided as pliable monofilaments. Synthetic absorbable sutures do not undergo the enzymically mediated absorption process that is well-known for catgut. Rather, the suture is broken down completely by simple bulk hydrolysis as it resides in the tissue, and the tissue reaction is minimal. A new device that represents the first generation of "active" sutures is VICRYL Plus Antibacterial suture (*Ethicon*). This suture has an antibacterial coating containing triclosan that inhibits the colonization of the suture by bacteria known to be associated with surgical site infections.

CARGILE MEMBRANE—This is a thin sheet of pliable tissue obtained from the appendix *(blind gut)* of the steer or ox. It is designed primarily to cover surfaces from which the peritoneum has been removed, especially where a sterile membrane would lessen the formation of adhesions. The membrane is available in sterile sheets of approximately 4 × 6 inches and sometimes is used as a packing or protective sheath. At present, the use of such material is limited.

FASCIA LATA—This is obtained from ox fascia and is designed for use as a heavy suture or repair in hernia or similar cases. It usually is attached firmly to a strong structure by means of a nonabsorbable suture. It is supplied in the form of sterile strips approximately 1/2 inches wide and 8 inches long and also in sheets about 3 × 5 inches.

It should be emphasized, in connection with the above, that catgut strands and ribbons are the only ones that are completely and readily absorbable. The other materials may be absorbed very slowly or may be incorporated in the tissues by invasion of fibroblasts.

NONABSORBABLE SUTURES

The second principal class of suture consists of natural and synthetic nonabsorbable suture materials that are relatively resistant to attack by normal tissue fluids. Several of these materials remain, apparently unchanged, for many years in tissue and usually will be found encapsulated in a thin sheath of fibrous connective tissue. When nonabsorbable sutures are used for skin closure, they usually are removed after the incision or wound has healed to the point where suture support is no longer necessary.

Silk is an important nonabsorbable surgical suture. Selected grades of degummed commercial silk fibers are used and consist chiefly of the protein fibroin as extruded by the silkworm. Many such fibers are twisted into a single strand of various diameters, as specified in the USP, and sold in the natural color or after dyeing. By far the most popular construction is braided silk, in which several twisted yarns are braided into a compact structure favored for its firmness and strength. Most braided silk is dyed and also given a treatment to render it noncapillary. In use as a skin suture this minimizes the rise of tissue fluids to the surface and thus the counterpassage inward of organisms from the surface. Further objectives of such treatments are to impart a degree of stiffness to improve the handling and tying properties, to minimize attachment of tissue cells that would cause pain on removal of the suture and to lubricate the implantation and removal of the silk. When silk or any other suture is dyed, the USP requires that it be done with a color additive approved by the FDA.

Specifications—The USP describes in the monograph for Nonabsorbable Surgical Suture (which now includes cotton, linen, metallic wire, nylon, rayon, Dacron, and silk) the respective sizes, diameters, and tensile strengths.

Uses—Silk sutures are handled easily and tolerated well by body tissue, although they may cause significant tissue reaction. In the presence of infection, however, the interstices of silk strands protect organisms from antimicrobial agents and from the body's defense mechanisms, so that chronic sinuses may form that do not heal until the silk is removed or is sloughed by the tissues. Silk, as well as any other nonabsorbable suture, occasionally migrates from the site of implantation and comes to the surface to be extruded months after the operation. In certain sites, the suture knots or ends may serve as centers for the formation of concretions or for other irritating action. Silk usu-

ally becomes encapsulated and remains in the tissues for extended periods of time as the protein slowly degrades.

DERMAL SILK—These sutures consist of natural twisted silk encased in an insoluble coating of tanned gelatin or other protein. This coating must withstand autoclaving without stripping, and its purpose is to prevent the ingrowth of tissue cells, which would interfere with its removal after use as a skin or dermal suture.

COTTON AND LINEN—Sutures derived from cellulose are among the oldest known but currently are used to a limited extent. These are twisted from fiber staple, have moderately high tensile strength, and are stable to heat sterilization. Cotton sutures prepared by suture manufacturers are uniform and have reproducible strength and largely have replaced the household sewing cotton used by many surgeons years ago. These are desirable because of their handling properties but are not used widely in critical areas where strength must be maintained for long periods of time because they slowly degrade.

Synthetic Nonabsorbable Sutures

Nylon, the first modern synthetic fiber, came into use as a suture partly as a result of World War II shortages of high-grade silk and partly because of its own merits. It is a synthetic polyamide obtained from the condensation of adipic acid and hexamethylenediamine or from the condensation-polymerization of caprolactam. It is available in the form of monofilaments (Ethilon, *Ethicon;* Dermalon, *Davis & Geck*) in the useful range of sizes, as well as in the form of multifilament fibers (Nurolon, *Ethicon;* Surgilon, *Davis & Geck;* Nylon, *Deknatel;* Bralon, *US Surgical*) braided into strands of comparable diameter. It is strong and water-resistant and has come into use for all suturing or ligating. Monofilament nylon is used as a skin or stay suture or for plastic surgery. Braided nylon more often is buried in tissues and is subject to the same limitations as braided silk in the presence of infection.

POLYESTER FIBER—Of the numerous multifilament synthetic fibers introduced after the success of nylon, only polyester has been accepted as a suitable braided nonabsorbable suture, while polypropylene has enjoyed increasing popularity as a nonabsorbable monofilament suture. Polyester suture is prepared by melt-extruding polyethylene terephthalate into fine filaments that then are braided into various sizes. In general, the tensile strength of polyester braided sutures is superior to that of braided silk and nylon and twisted cotton. Examples of braided polyester sutures include Ethibond Excel *(Ethicon),* Surgidac *(US Surgical),* TiCron *(Davis & Geck),* Tevedek II, and Polydek, both manufactured by *Deknatel.* Novafil *(Davis & Geck),* a copolymer of polybutylene terephthalate and polytetramethylene ether glycol, is available as a monofilament polyester suture.

The polyester sutures, in contrast with most other materials except polypropylene and stainless steel, do not lose strength significantly when in contact with water or body fluids. For this reason, they have become a suture of choice when there is a critical need for permanent reinforcement as, for example, in the installation of artificial heart valves. They have the advantage of excellent knot-holding characteristics and are available in the natural color or dyed to enhance visibility in the surgical field.

Recent developments have seen the commercialization of braided polyester fiber sutures coated or impregnated with nontoxic lubricants such as polytetrafluoroethylene or silicone resins. Polybutilate, a lubricant especially designed for polyester suture use, has been derived from a condensation polymer of butanediol and adipic acid. These sutures exhibit the advantage of a smoother surface, which gives the suture improved handling properties and permits an easier and more gentle passage through tissue.

POLYOLEFIN FIBERS—Of increasing interest in the nonabsorbable suture field is the development of fibers based on polyolefins. Although polyethylene sutures have been available, the use of polypropylene monofilament (Prolene, *Ethicon;* Surgipro, *US Surgical;* Surgilene, *Davis & Geck;* Deklene II, Deknatel) has increased greatly during recent years. Polypropylene sutures, compared to monofilament nylon, tie more secure knots and have a very low order of tissue reactivity. Because of the smoothness of polypropylene sutures, they slip through tissue easily and, because there is no tissue ingrowth, they may be removed easily when necessary. They have found wide application in cardiovascular and other surgical specialties. Another member of this family of sutures is Pronova suture (*Ethicon*) which is based on a blend of polyvinylidene fluoride and a copolymer of polyvinylidene fluoride and hexafluoropropylene. This monofilament suture is noted for its resistance to damage in the surgical field and may be useful in robotic surgery.

Polytetrafluoroethylene (PTFE) suture (Gore-Tex, *Gore*) has been recommended for use with vascular grafts derived from the same material, as well as in other surgical procedures.

Metallic Sutures

For some years increased attention has been paid to the use of various metal wire sutures and other metallic devices to assist surgical repair.

SILVER—Among the older materials that still are used to some extent are silver wire, foil, and other forms. Relatively little work has been reported recently on these items. Silver is available readily and is alleged to have some antiseptic action but in some tissues is definitely irritating. Irritation has been shown by a great many metals and alloys and now is regarded as a controlling consideration in the choice of substances for implantation in tissues.

STAINLESS STEEL—This ferrous alloy, which so long has been employed usefully in industrial and other applications in which resistance to chemical attack is essential, has been used widely in the form of wire sutures, fixation plates, screws, and other items. Stainless steel is a rather general term covering a wide variety of materials, and many of the early alloys were attacked by body fluids. The proper selection of stainless-steel compositions seems to provide a material essentially inert in tissues and free from the earlier disadvantages. Stainless-steel sutures are available as both twisted and monofilament strands and represent the strongest available material. However, they are relatively difficult to use and are employed most commonly in areas where great strength is required, such as in the repair of the sternum after chest surgery.

Surgical Meshes

Surgical meshes are used as reinforcement material to aid in tissue repair and encourage ingrowth of fibrous connective tissue. Meshes are used for umbilical, abdominal, and inguinal hernia repair procedures. Meshes can be knitted or woven of absorbable or nonabsorbable suture materials. Some examples of the variety of meshes available for surgical use include absorbable woven or knitted Vicryl flat mesh (*Ethicon)* and knitted Dexon flat mesh *(Davis & Geck);* nonabsorbable knitted polypropylene flat mesh (Prolene, and Prolene Soft Mesh, lighter-weight and more flexible, *Ethicon;* Marlex, *Bard;* Trelex, *Meadox;* Surgipro, *US Surgical;* Artrium, *Artrium*), nonabsorbable PTFE mesh manufactured by *Gore* (Mycromesh, Dual Mesh, Soft Tissue Patch), and nonabsorbable knitted polyester mesh (Mersilene, *Ethicon).* Many of these mesh products are available in preshaped forms designed for ease of use for the specific surgical repair procedure (Prolene Hernia System, and Prolene 3D Patch, *Ethicon;* Prefix Plug, *Bard).* Other mesh devices are composites of absorbable and non-absorbable components that have the advantage of good intra-operative

handling with a light-weight and flexible substrate that provides permanent wound support (Vypro I and Vypro II, *Ethicon).*

Surgical Needles

Suture materials may be threaded on eyed needles for suturing. While formerly only eyed needles were available, there is an overwhelming trend to the use of eyeless needles, one or two being attached to each individual strand. One such needle is manufactured with an open channel into which the suture can be placed, and the channel is then swaged around the strand. Another type, known as *seamless,* has a very delicate hole drilled in the shank. To prevent pullout, the shank is pressed firmly about the suture. These sutures offer great advantage in minimizing trauma. With an eyed needle an opening in tissue must be made large enough to accommodate the needle and two thicknesses of suture, but with the eyeless needle, the opening need only accommodate the needle, slightly larger than the single suture that follows. This is greatly esteemed in fine surgery such as plastic and ophthalmic work. A wide variety of eyeless needles on different sutures are now available to meet most of the demands of the surgeon. By a recent innovation, it has been possible to control the release of a suture from an eyeless needle by a gentle tug so that the surgeon need not take the time to cut the needle from the suture when it is no longer required.

VITALLIUM—This metal, which is an alloy of cobalt, chromium, and molybdenum, has been applied to many surgical problems in various forms since 1937, although not in the form of sutures or ligatures. The alloy has shown some variability in strength and stiffness and is incapable of much modification at the time of operation, but generally shows negligible tissue reactions. In addition to some use for dentures, surgical forms of vitallium include fracture plates, screws, bolts, nails and appliances, orbital implants, nasal skeletal supports, tendon rods, tubes for blood vessel anastomosis or bile duct repair, and skull plates.

Other Suturing Techniques

Although sutures and ligatures have remained the most effective and popular devices for closing wounds and hemostasis, other techniques are being used with increasing frequency. Surgical stapling devices are available that automatically approximate tissue with rows of steel staples. Such devices exist for closing skin and anastomosing blood vessels as well as for reconstructing other organs such as stomach and intestines. Some surgical staplers are designed to cut tissue before or after the staples are applied.

During the last several years, V-shaped steel, tantalum, or titanium clips have been used to clamp small blood vessels, and this alternative to ligation is becoming increasingly popular as the application instruments become more convenient and easier to use. Stainless-steel clips or staples have been used frequently to coapt skin incisions. More recently, strips of fabric or plastic material coated with a suitable adhesive have been used for the same application.

New approaches to ligating clips are represented by absorbable materials, polydioxanone and lactomer. Ligating clips made from these substances absorb after their function is completed and do not remain in the patient permanently as do metallic clips. Thus, interference with diagnostic imaging techniques such as X-ray and CAT scans is avoided.

With the advent of minimally invasive surgical procedures, the industry faces significant challenges. Several new needles and other devices have been introduced to the market, facilitating the ease with which the surgeon can approximate and suture tissue through a trocar port.

SUTURE MONOGRAPH

ABSORBABLE SURGICAL SUTURE

Surgical Catgut; Catgut Suture; Surgical Gut; Sterilized Surgical Catgut BP; Sterilized Surgical Ligature

A sterile strand prepared from collagen derived from healthy mammals or from a synthetic polymer. Its length is not less than 95.0% of that stated on the label. Its diameter and tensile strength correspond to the size designation indicated on the label, within the limits prescribed herein. It is capable of being absorbed by living mammalian tissue but may be treated to modify its resistance to absorption. It may be modified with respect to body or texture. It may be impregnated or coated with a suitable antimicrobial agent. It may be colored by a color additive approved by the FDA.

Description—Flexible strand varying in treatment, color, size, packaging, and resistance to absorption, according to the intended purpose. The collagen suture is either *Type A* Suture or *Type C* Suture. Both types consist of processed strands of collagen, but *Type C* Suture is processed by physical or chemical means to provide greater resistance to absorption in living mammalian tissue.

NONABSORBABLE SURGICAL SUTURE

Surgical Sutures; Surgical Silk; Sterile Surgical Silk

A strand of material that is suitably resistant to the action of living mammalian tissue. Its length is not less than 95.0% of that stated on the label. Its diameter and tensile strength correspond to the size designation indicated on the label, within the limits prescribed herein. It may be nonsterile or sterile. It may be impregnated or coated with a suitable antimicrobial agent.

It may be modified with respect to body or texture, or to reduce capillarity, and may be suitably bleached. It may be colored by a color additive approved by the FDA.

Description—Flexible, monofilament or multifilament, continuous strand, placed in an envelope, tube, or other suitable container or wound on a reel or spool. If it is a multifilament strand, the individual filaments may be combined by spinning, twisting, braiding, or any combination thereof. Nonabsorbable Surgical Suture is classed and typed as follows: *Class I* Suture is composed of silk or synthetic fibers of monofilament, twisted or braided construction. *Class II* Suture is composed of cotton or linen fibers or coated natural or synthetic fibers in which the coating forms a casing of significant thickness but does not contribute appreciably to strength. *Class III* Suture is composed of monofilament or multifilament metal wire.

CHAPTER 110

Health Accessories

Donald O Fedder, DrPH, FAPhA, BOCO

Mary Lynn McPherson, PharmD, BCPS, CDE

Thomas G Pettinger, BSP, BOCO

For too long, many pharmacists treated Home Medical Equipment (HME) as merely a convenience for their prescription patients. Physicians and other health professionals may have been convinced that the pharmacist had neither the necessary expertise nor equipment and sent their patients elsewhere for such services. In recent years, however, few aspects of professional practice have changed as much or grown as rapidly as the pharmacy's HME departments. The specially trained pharmacist is becoming recognized more widely as an expert in this area by other health professionals and can provide a professional and profitable adjunct to the pharmacy's other services.

A comprehensive HME department may include a wide variety of surgical dressings and supplies; and convalescent aids including wheelchairs, walkers, hospital beds, hydraulic patient lifters, urology and incontinence supplies, ostomy appliances, elastic supports, mastectomy breast forms, and orthopedic braces. In addition, many pharmacies specialize in home health-care equipment such as traction devices, blood-glucose monitors, blood-pressure-monitoring devices, suction machines, oxygen and respiratory-therapy equipment, nerve and muscle stimulators, phototherapy lights, apnea monitors, and rehabilitation equipment. Some pharmacies may even specialize in providing intravenous medications and supplies for enteral or parenteral nutrition.

Even more important than merely providing large varieties of health accessories is the pharmacist's growing involvement in selecting and fitting them and in instructing the patient in their proper use and maintenance. It is essential that pharmacists are not only knowledgeable and skilled, but recognize their own limitations. Professionals must prepare themselves for services that are not usually subsumed under the "practice pharmacy" definitions. HME products and services, in many cases, require specialized training if the patient is to be properly served. It is not a weakness to admit to patients, physician or others of one's need to refer to a more qualified source.

To provide these services the pharmacist must acquire new skills and expertise that can be obtained through a large variety of sources, such as special courses given by health-accessory distributors and manufacturers, professional associations, and some college or university-based programs.

The initial step in selecting the appropriate health product is a thorough evaluation of the patient's needs and then matching these needs to the available options. Note that the option may very well be referral to another source for care.

Age	Disability-related factors
Life-style	Patient and equipment measurements
Diagnosis	Patient ability for self-care
Prognosis	Reimbursement sources

Each of these factors should be considered when selecting the most appropriate health accessory for the patient. It is often necessary to verify insurance coverage, including whether particular equipment is mandated by an HMO and which equipment will be considered for reimbursement by Medicare, Medicaid, or insurance companies. Although a standard "prescription" may not be required, most third parties will expect some indication that the product/service is a medical necessity to be reimbursed.

Other steps may include consulting with the patient, physician, and family; selecting the accessory from stock or ordering it from the manufacturer or distributor; and checking the accessory to ensure that it meets the appropriate specifications. Usually, follow-up adjustments or modifications are necessary.

Useful forms (eg, certificates of medical necessity CMN), disability analysis, measurement, prescription and ordering forms—are usually available from health-accessory manufacturers, insurance companies, and government agencies. In fact, some insurance companies and government agencies may mandate the use of their special forms. Documentation of patient analysis, measurements, and what was sold/dispensed is an essential part of record keeping, especially in this litigious society.

WHEELCHAIRS

Wheelchairs range from the most simple self-propelled devices used to provide independence of movement for a person temporarily inhibited in walking,to specially built models. The battery-powered "scooter" has become quite popular, especially because the development of longer lasting battery chargers. There are literally hundreds of different wheelchairs to serve the patient's different needs. Figure 110-1 shows one example. The importance of an individualized prescription cannot be overemphasized. A carefully prescribed chair has a prolonged and useful life and promotes the patient's maximal physical independence.

The general loss of body functions in aged or infirmed patients serves as a guide to providing the best chair for their needs. They may have less strength and endurance than a younger or healthier person and, therefore, may require safety and convenience features. This point reemphasizes the general rule when fitting any wheelchair: the primary considerations in fitting are the user's physical limitations and lifestyle.

MEASUREMENTS—Following the disability analysis, the measurements of the patient and the chair should be considered when preparing a prescription for the proper chair.

The Patient—Ideally, the patient should be sitting when measured, preferably in a chair that allows good body alignment.

Side-to-Side (widest area of hips while sitting)—It is important to determine the chair seat width. To avoid pressure on the hips or thighs, yet help maintain good seating posture and stability, the chair-seat width should be 2 inches more than the width straight across the hips.

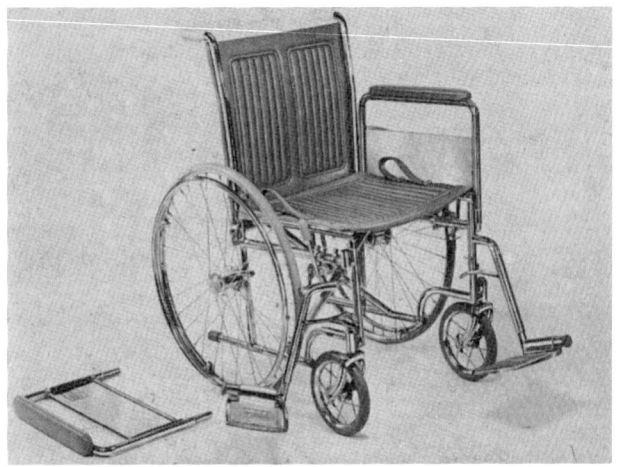

Figure 110-1. Adult wheelchair with full-length, removable arms and swing-away, detachable footrests (courtesy, Everest & Jennings).

Knee-to-Hip—This measurement is critical to determine the actual chair-seat depth. Normally, the seat depth will be approximately 2 to 3 inches less than this measurement to provide adequate support, yet avoid pressure behind the knee. If a back panel or back cushion is to be inserted, its thickness must be considered.

Seat-to-Elbow—This measurement serves as an indicator for armrest height. Depending on seating posture, armrest height should provide proper body support. (*Danger signals:* drooping or hunched up shoulders when the patient's elbows are resting on the armrests.) It should be noted that an armrest height 1 inch more than the patient's seat-to-elbow measurement will force the patient's elbows slightly forward, providing a natural brace against forward body slumping, especially when descending ramps.

Floor-to-Knee—This measurement is used to determine footrest adjustments from seat level and/or special seat height. The minimum footrest adjustment should be at least 2 inches less than this measurement to avoid pressure against the underside of the legs. A good visual guide for proper footrest adjustment (especially when using a standard chair) is to make sure that the tops of the patient's thighs are horizontal and parallel to the floor. To obtain greater-than-standard maximum footrest adjustment, a special seat height must be considered. Sometimes the use of a solid insert seat and/or seat cushion will solve this problem, although it should be remembered that optimum seat height allows patients to place their feet on the floor without excessive pressure behind the knees.

Seat-to-Armpit—Used to determine back-upholstery height on standard-back chairs. This is important because many patients must be able to put their arms over the back upholstery and hook their elbows under the push handles to achieve leverage when reaching for things.

Other Measurements—May be required for more-involved or custom wheelchairs. Consult manufacturer product literature.

The Chair—Certain wheelchair dimensions (Fig 110-2) are important in preparing an individualized prescription. The following are some of the components and measurements that should be considered.

Arms—Full-length, nondetachable arms are available. Desk- or full-length detachable styles are needed if the user must do a lateral transfer. Because detachable arms are offset from the main frame of the wheelchair, they also provide 1 1/2 to 2 inches of additional seat width. Thus, a wheelchair with 18 inches of upholstery and detachable arms actually yields 19 1/2 to 20 inches of seat width. Just as this feature widens the seat, it also widens the overall width of the wheelchair. If this additional overall width results in an architectural restriction, *wraparound* or *space-saver* arm styles must be considered. They are mounted behind the back uprights instead of between the uprights and the rear wheel. This design allows the additional seat width and removable convenience but keeps the overall width to that of a standard-frame wheelchair.

Another consideration of the arm is its height in relation to the seat. Standard arm height is approximately 10 inches. The arm can be manufactured to any specified height; however, a more convenient option is the adjustable-height arm, which is available in the detachable styles.

Seat and Back Width—A determination of seat and back width is the most important and fundamental part in selecting the proper wheelchair. A standard adult wheelchair has an 18-inch seat and back upholstery. Wheelchairs are typically available in 2-inch increments from 12 to 24 inches. When considering seat width, remember the effect of detachable arms. A wheelchair that is too wide will promote leaning to one side or limit the ability of the user to propel the chair. Too narrow a wheelchair can result in pressure sores.

Foot Supports—There are two basic types of foot supports: the footrest and the elevating legrest. Both are adjustable in length. To determine which type would be more beneficial to the user, consider the condition of the legs. If there is swelling or infirmity involving the leg or reduced flexion in the knee, elevating legrests might be indicated. A new concept, the articulating elevating leg rest, extends automatically as the leg rest is raised, to fit the outstretched leg correctly (Fig 110-3). In most other cases the simple footrest will suffice. At this point, also consider options such as removable versus fixed assemblies, quad-release levers, heel-and-toe loops, and oversized or nonskid footplates.

Seat Height—The standard seat height is approximately 19 to 20 inches from the floor. Hemi- or low-seat wheelchairs run about 2 inches lower. Seat height is important to those users who propel the wheelchair with one or both feet. A higher seat may be required for users with long legs so the footrest-to-ground clearance will not be less than 1 1/2 to 2 inches.

Seat Depth—The standard seat depth is 16 inches. The seat should be deep enough to support the thighs properly without putting pressure on the back of the calf.

Back Height—The standard back height is 16.5 inches. A higher back height provides more support for a weak upper body. A lower back height provides less support but allows greater freedom of movement. To determine which is best, consider overall physical strength and lifestyle. Try to keep the height of the back to a minimum, i.e., high enough to provide adequate support, yet still allow upper-body mobility.

Wheels—Standard wheelchairs use a 24-inch rear wheel with an 8-inch front caster. Hemi wheelchairs have a 22-inch rear wheel. The rear wheel generally is aligned with the back upright. In the case of a reclining or amputee chair the wheels are set back to provide a larger base of support, which is needed to prevent tipping backward.

Note: Additional Precautions during measurement

1. When taking measurements and adjusting the wheelchair always consider the effects of cushions and body positioners if they are to be used.

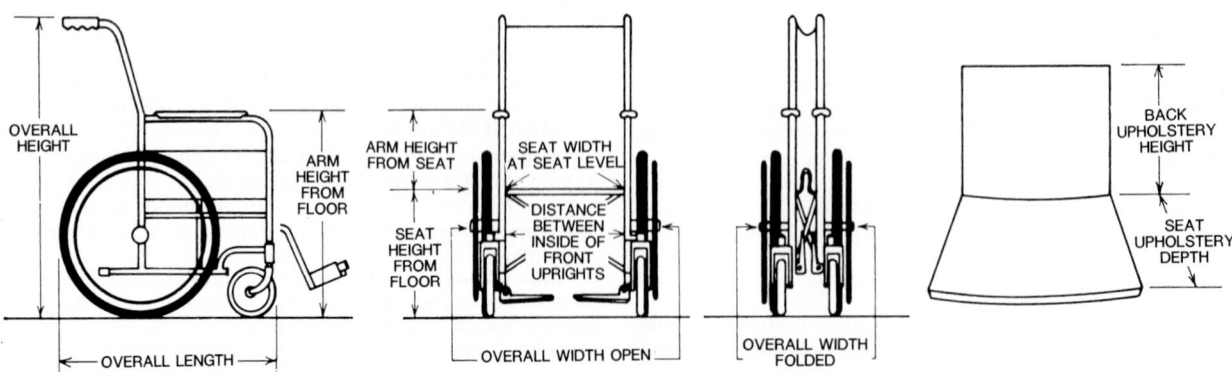

Figure 110-2. Key to wheelchair dimensions (courtesy, Everest & Jennings).

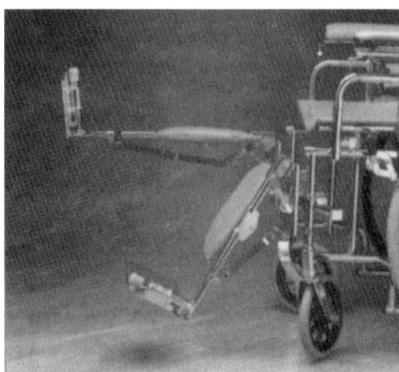

Figure 110-3. Articulating, elevating leg rest (courtesy, Invacare).

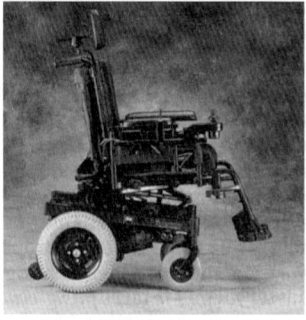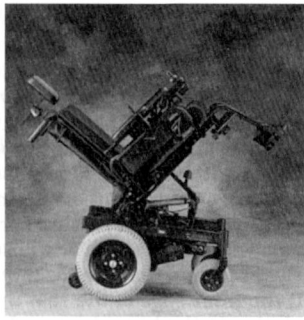

45° of tilt

Figure 110-4. Action Jarsys weight-shifting tilt system moves the seat to optimize the client's center of gravity during the tilt cycle (courtesy, Invacare).

2. Always fit the wheelchair for the user's present condition. Make some allowances for progressive diseases but never overfit a wheelchair. Extra, added features add weight and can make the wheelchair cumbersome to its user.

When the pharmacist has completed the measurements and evaluations and actually has the patient sitting in the chair, there are three quick *hand checks* the pharmacist can make.

1. An extended hand should fit between the hip and the skirt guard of the chair.
2. Three or four fingers should fit between the seat upholstery and the back of the calf.
3. Three or four fingers should fit between the top of the back upholstery and the underarm.

This kind of a quick double-check is the type of professional activity that will differentiate a pharmacist as an authority on health accessories.

While most patients will be able to use the manually operated wheelchairs described previously, a growing number will need a battery-powered wheelchair. This will include some quadriplegics and any patients who lack the ability to propel a chair manually. In some cases when the patient has no hand or arm movement a chair can be operated by chin control or a sip-and-puff control, in which the controls may be operated by the patient inhaling or exhaling into a straw-like device. Recently, even dental controls have become available, and wheelchairs controlled by vocal commands are under development and may soon be on the market. For wheelchair-bound patients who do not have the ability to reposition themselves in the chair, tilt-in-space wheelchairs (Fig 110-4) are available. Shifting the weight-bearing areas of the body can provide relief from or prevent formation of decubitus ulcers.

Because patients using an electric wheelchair usually spend the major part of their waking hours in their chair, it is especially important that the chair and its accessories be fitted properly to them. Manufacturers can provide specialized measuring and fitting guides for power wheelchairs.

One other health-accessory product that may be included in the wheelchair category is the three- or four-wheeled, battery-operated scooter. These are often useful for people with limited mobility. Persons who can walk a short distance in the home environment may be unable to spend several hours on their feet in a shopping center or on a trip to a museum or zoo. A battery-operated scooter may be the perfect answer to such a situation, and many health-accessory dealers include three- or four-wheeled scooters in their product mix (Fig 110-5).

CUSHIONS AND SUPPLIES FOR PRESSURE SORES

Many types of cushions are available for a variety of purposes. Some are used to simulate a hospital bed's gatch spring. These enable the patient to eat and work in bed in relative comfort, while others are used to bolster the patient's legs to achieve flexion of the lumbar spine during traction. The most important use is to protect the patient from bruises and prevent the occurrence of pressure sores (ie, decubitus ulcers, bed sores).

Pressure sores result from pressure at the thinly covered bony prominences of the body such as the sacrum, tuberosities of the ischium (below the buttocks), heels, elbows, shoulder blades, and ears and back of the head in children. When pressure interferes with the normal circulation of capillary blood in the tissues, it can cause localized ulceration and gangrene.

A pressure sore begins as a reddened area that, if left untreated, will develop into an open sore; if not corrected early, surgery may be the only feasible remedy. The best cure is prevention. According to Richard M Meer, Founder and Executive Director of the Center for Tissue Trauma Research and Education (Jensen Beach, FL), "all pressure sores are preventable," a notion that unfortunately still is denied by some health professionals in institutions where pressure sores continue to occur. As health-care consultants to their customers, community pharmacists are in a unique position to facilitate an understanding of pressure sore–prevention techniques that can be used in the home-care environment.

Pressure sores most commonly occur after long-term confinement in either a bed or a wheelchair. In institutions where nursing services are provided or at home where family members are available, the following measures will prevent their occurrence:

1. Keep the bed dry and clean.
2. Thoroughly pat the skin dry.
3. To increase circulation, regularly and gently massage the skin.
4. Change the position of the patient in bed as frequently as possible, at least a minimum of every 2 hours.
5. Relieve pressure as soon as the first signs of redness appear.

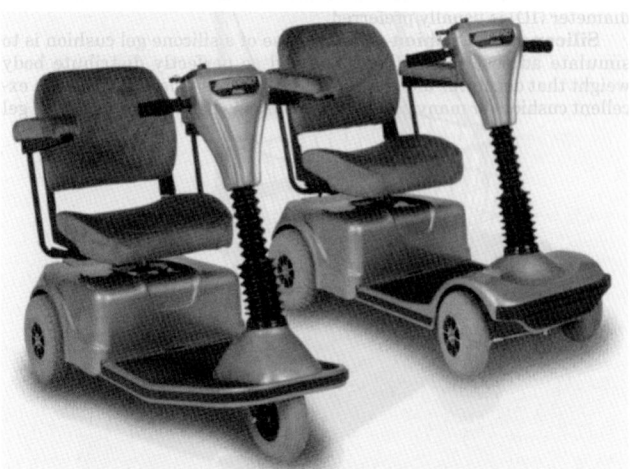

Figure 110-5. Three- and four-wheeled scooters (courtesy Pride Health Care).

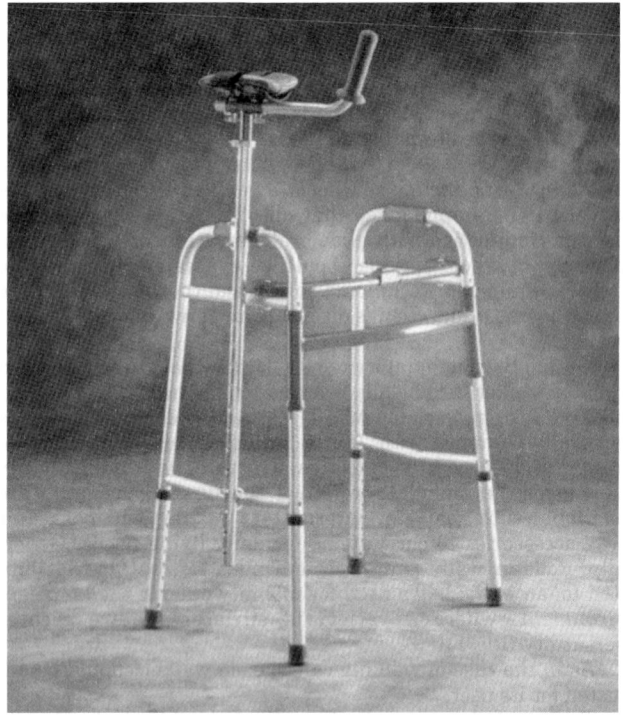

Figure 110-10. Walker with platform attachment (courtesy, Invacare).

tachment that allows the forearm to bear the weight instead of the hand or wrist (Fig 110-10).

Crutches

FOREARM CRUTCHES—Neither walking canes nor walkers provide support to the patient's wrists and elbows. The forearm crutch, however, is designed specifically to provide such support in that it has a vertical member that extends above the wrist and is secured reasonably well to the fleshy part of the forearm by a collar or cuff.

The term forearm crutch is generic. They commonly are referred to as Canadian crutches or Lofstrand crutches. All can be recognized by the collar or cuff that encircles the patient's forearm. The cuff usually is open, and the opening may face either the side or front. It is important that the cuff be open so the crutches may be thrown out of the way if the patient falls. The handgrip projects from the main shaft, and unless specifically instructed by the physician or physical therapist to the contrary, the patient should be instructed to hold the handgrip so that it points forward.

If only one crutch is used, it should be used on the side opposite the weak leg. When two crutches are used, the patient should be instructed to step forward with the right leg and the left crutch, followed by the left leg and right crutch, and so on. Commonly known as the two-point gait, it is recommended for persons using forearm crutches unless, of course, the physician or physical therapist suggests a different gait.

In fitting the forearm crutch, the patient should stand normally erect, with arms at the sides. The forearm cuff is flipped back out of the way, and the handgrip is brought to the crease in the wrists by adjusting or cutting the main shaft. The length of the vertical member between the handgrip and the forearm cuff also should be adjusted so that the cuff comes to the middle of the patient's forearm, usually over the fleshiest part. Care should be taken to make sure that the cuff does not interfere with the elbow when it is fully bent. The cuff can be opened or closed by bending and shaping by hand, with very little effort. Patients should be shown how to do this as they

may want the cuff larger or tighter, depending on their clothing.

AXILLARY CRUTCHES—More common than the forearm crutch is the ordinary wooden or aluminum underarm crutch—the axillary crutch. It provides more support than the forearm crutch because it braces both wrist and elbow.

Adjustable crutches are preferred, as they offer better and easier fitting. First, the patient should stand normally erect with arms at the sides. The crutch is placed under the arms, with the crutch tip on the floor at a point approximately 6 to 8 inches ahead of the patient's toes and 6 to 8 inches to the side. The main shaft is lengthened or shortened so that the top of the crutch is about 1.5 inch (two finger-widths) from the armpit. This fitting should be done with crutch tips and axillary cushions in place on the crutch.

The second step is to adjust the position of the handgrip on the crutch so that it comes to the crease in the wrist. The crutch should be in the same position for this handgrip adjustment as it was during the fitting of its entire length. The arm then is brought out alongside the crutch for the handgrip adjustment.

A flexed elbow is important when using an axillary crutch. If the handgrip is not positioned at the wrist so that the elbow bends when the patient takes hold of the handgrip, the tops of the crutches would push up into the armpits with each swing. But with the elbows bent initially, the crutch tops are safely below the armpits, since the patient must straighten his or her arms on the swing through. When underarm crutches are fitted properly, there is little or no danger of injury to the lymph glands, blood vessels, or radial nerves in the armpits, which can lead to *crutch paralysis*. The primary danger signal is an elevation in the patient's shoulders with each swing through the crutches. When that happens, it is clear that the patient's weight is bearing on the crutch tops and not on the handgrips as it should be.

There are several axillary crutch gaits. The safest, most stable, and most common is the four-point gait. The patient begins by moving the left crutch forward. Next, the patient moves the right leg forward. The right crutch then is brought up to the right foot, and finally, the left leg is brought up to the left crutch.

The two-point gait, the principal gait used when two canes are employed, is also used commonly with forearm and axillary crutches. Simply, both the left crutch and right leg are brought forward; then the right crutch and left leg are brought forward.

The three-point gait has two variations: the swing-to gait and the swing-through gait. In either form, the patient begins by moving both crutches forward simultaneously. In the swing-to gait, both feet (or one foot for an amputee or when one leg is in a non-weight-bearing cast) are swung to a point between the two crutches. In the swing-through gait, the feet (or foot) are swung through the crutches to a point ahead of the two crutches—it helps to visualize a triangle made by the two crutchtips and foot, and flipping that triangle end-over-end.

Another common crutch gait is the hemiplegic gait. It is nothing more than the use of a single axillary crutch in exactly the same manner as one would use a single cane. The crutch is carried on the strong side and is moved forward together with the weak limb, alternating with the good leg.

Accessories

TIPS—The most important accessory is the tip, which makes contact with the floor. No cane or crutch should ever be sold or rented without a good tip. Safety requires that cane and crutch tips have the following minimum characteristics: they must fit the cane or crutch shaft snugly, have a suction-grip bottom, and have a flexible neck so the bottom of the tip will stay in complete contact with the floor when the cane or crutch rocks through a gait. The suction-grip bottom of a crutch or cane tip should be as large as possible—the more rubber in contact with the floor, the less chance of slippage.

AXILLARY CUSHIONS—These are designed to protect the underarm from bruises and inhibit slippage of the crutch top from under the arm. They should not be weight-bearing, as the top of the crutch should be fitted to be 1 1/2 inches from the armpit.

HANDGRIPS—These are more varied in type and style because they are designed for various purposes. The most common kinds of handgrips are dense foam-rubber sleeves that fit over the standard crutch grip. The split handgrips should be used for nonadjustable crutches only, as they tend to slip around the handgrip. Taping them tightly will secure them somewhat. The nonsplit, often called closed, handgrip is better for the patient, but it requires removal of the crutch's handgrip to put it on.

Other contoured handgrips and *palmgrips* are available. Because the natural palm line is not horizontal, they are designed to alleviate problems such as hand discomfort and wrist soreness associated with the traditional horizontal crutch handgrip.

SEAT-LIFT CHAIRS—Another aid to mobility being used in homes today is chairs with electrically powered seat-lift mechanisms. Designed for the patient who can ambulate (often only with the assistance of a cane or walker) but is unable to get out of a chair unassisted, the seat-lift chair can add greatly to the independence and mobility of a patient at home. This may simplify the job of a primary caregiver, who may be a frail spouse who has great difficulty assisting the patient out of a chair (Fig 110-11).

STAIRWAY SYSTEMS—A home stairway system can aid a patient living in a two-story home who has difficulty using the stairs. Models are available for straight, angled, or curved stairways. Some models, such as the Electra-Ride II (Fig 110-12) are battery-operated and will continue to work even during a power outage.

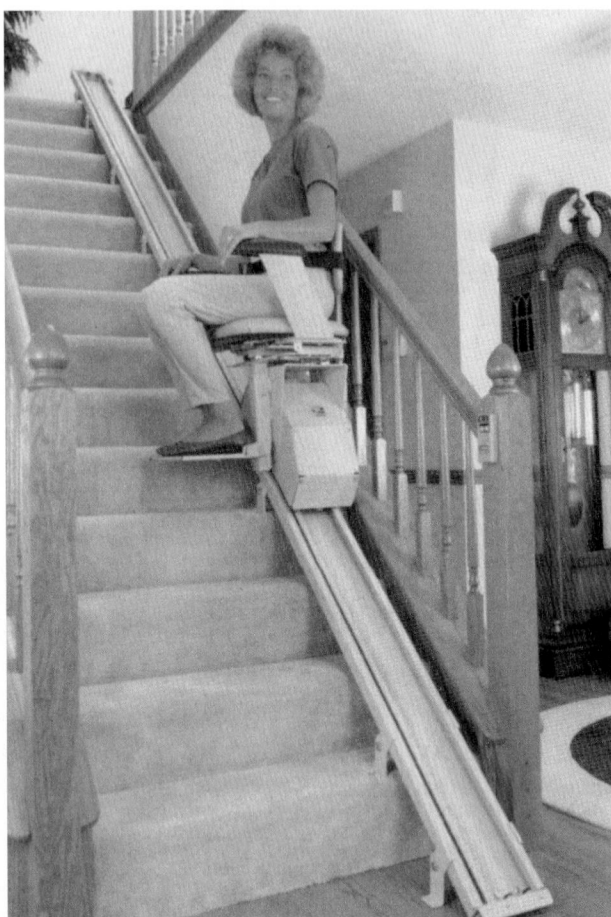

Figure 110-12. Electra-Ride II stairlift (courtesy, Bruno Independent Living Aids).

COMMODES

A commode is little more than a portable toilet, and yet there are a variety of different types. More than a convenience, a commode can mean the difference between coming home or staying in the hospital. Whenever the patient is unable to ambulate from the bed to the bathroom or to be transported via wheelchair, there is a need for a commode.

Perhaps the most common type is the steel- or aluminum-frame commode with a toilet seat and cover plus a removable plastic pail and cover. Adjustable legs are desirable, since some patients need a rather tall one to aid them both in sitting and in getting up more easily. The *Drop-arm* commode enables easier lateral transfer to and from the commode seat. Some patients also find this innovation helpful when there is a need to insert suppositories. Depending upon the attitude of the patient and, more often, that of the family, an aluminum folding commode can be removed from view when it is not in use.

The common aluminum- or steel-frame commode uses its uplifted toilet seat cover as a backrest. Commodes are available with padded and nonpadded backs, an upholstered seat and armrests, and casters for moving about easily (Fig 110-13); others are made of wood and resemble furniture—eg, the disguised, Danish Modern commode. Some commodes are designed to be used both in the bedroom and in the bathroom. These are either backless or have a removable back, so as not to interfere with the toilet tank.

Although commodes may be rented in most states, it is unwise to reuse the commode pail; it should be sold to the customer during the first month's rental. It also is helpful to advise the patient's family that a pail filled to one-third with water

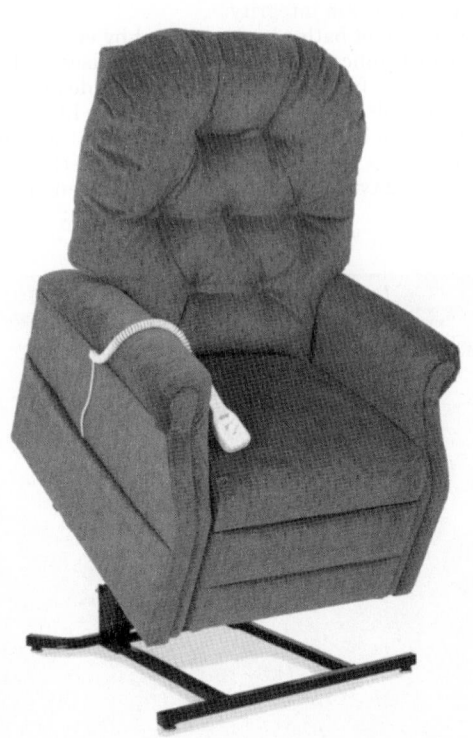

Figure 110-11. Seat-lift chair (courtesy, Pride Health Care).

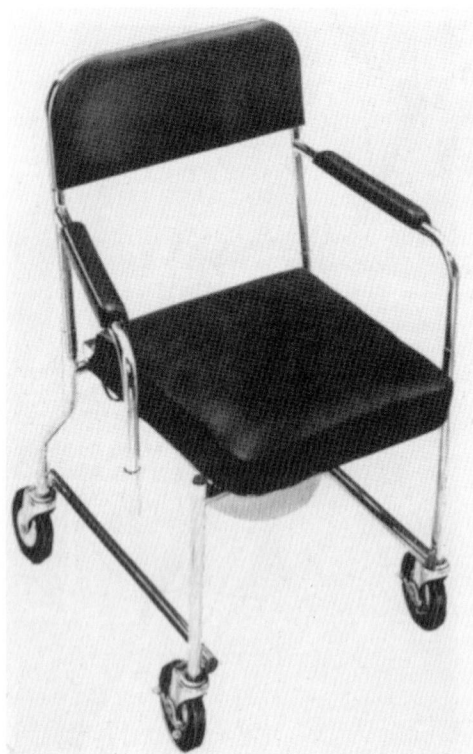

Figure 110-13. Padded commode on casters with pivot arms (courtesy, Lumex).

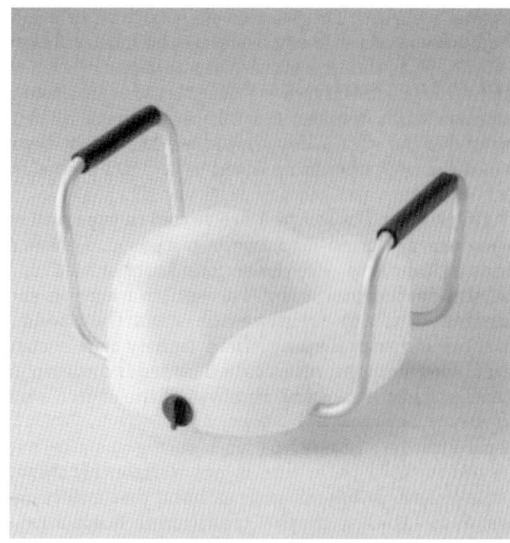

Figure 110-14. Elevated toilet seat with arm rails (courtesy, Invacare).

will be easier to keep clean. Deodorant tablets and drops are also appropriate as an accessory to any commode rental or sale.

A commode with wheels should be used with caution.

BATHROOM SAFETY AIDS

Before dispensing any bathroom safety aid that is weight-bearing (or for that matter, any medical equipment that is designed to support the partner's full weight), it is advisable to ask the patient's height and weight and document that information on the receipt, invoice, or intake sheet that is kept in the patient's file. Most bathroom safety aids list the weight capacity of that product on the package, on a tag, or in a catalog.

Safety in the bathroom primarily means safety in the tub or at the toilet. An elevated toilet seat makes it easier for patients to sit or stand and suggests the need for some kind of toilet guard rail. Attaching-type toilet rails can connect to the bowl with the regular toilet seat bolts. Some attaching types are designed with detachable sides, permitting the use of one side only, as well as easier cleaning of the rail in general.

Elevated toilet seats vary considerably with respect to the materials from which they are fabricated, whether or not they have full or partial splash guards, to what extent they are adjustable in height, and whether or not they are padded for softness or, like any normal toilet seat, quite hard. The full splash guard may be preferred by many people, but the pharmacist should keep in mind that persons without good legs and body control (paraplegics and quadriplegics, particularly) need the open sides that only the elevated toilet seat with the partial splash guard has, to administer to their personal cleanliness independently and to insert suppositories without assistance. The least expensive, and by far the most popular, elevated toilet seats are one-piece molded plastic. Combination elevated toilet seats with attached hand rails are available, but may *tip* if equal pressure is not applied to both sides when rising (Fig 110-14).

Safety aids for the bathtub include adhesive strips and spots for the tub bottom, mats for preventing slips, and a variety of tub seats and safety grab bars. Tub seats are either bench types with legs or seats that straddle the tub sides.

One type of bench has either fixed (standard)- or adjustable-height legs and is available with or without a back. A transfer bench (Fig 110-15) is used with two legs in the tub and two legs on the floor outside the tub. The patient can sit down on the portion of the seat that is outside the tub, swing his or her legs over the edge of the tub, and slide across the bench until the entire body is *inside* the tub. Transfer benches are available with solid seats or with a commode opening to facilitate perineal cleansing. Some models of transfer benches have suction-cup footpieces or clamp onto the side of the tube for security and stability and are available with a plastic or a padded seat for comfort and protection of skin integrity.

Another type of bath seat is powered by either water pressure or a hydraulic pump that actually raises or lowers the height of the seat from the height of the tub side to near the bottom. This seat also can be classified as a bath lift.

Bathtub grab bars range from those that attach to the side of the bathtub to wall-mounted grab bars. Perhaps the most frequently used type is one that extends high enough to give a

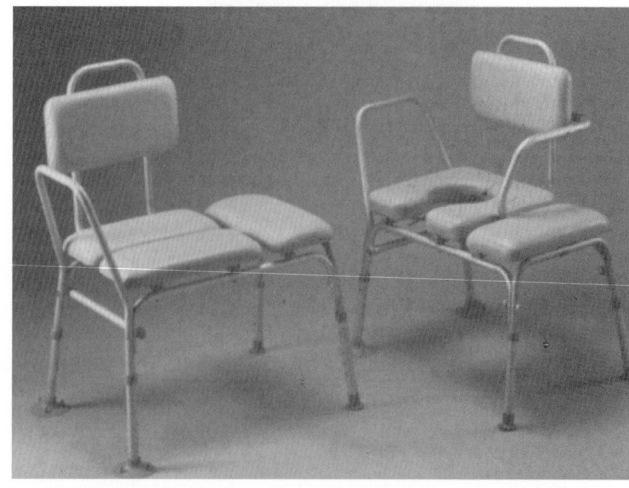

Figure 110-15. Transfer bath benches (courtesy, Lumex).

person standing outside the tub a firm support before stepping into the tub. Wall grab bars take a variety of shapes, angles, and lengths. Finishes of vinyl coating, smooth chrome, and a knurled texture for grip security are all available. True grab bars extend from the wall at least 4 to 5 inches, enabling a falling person to slip the forearm behind the bar and hook the elbow over it. Patient and/or family members should be cautioned to have the grab bars mounted to wood or metal studs within the walls. Using toggle bolts drilled in tile or plaster walls, but not securely anchored must be avoided at all costs!

Pharmacists should know how the bars they stock are mounted best for safety and either be able to instruct the customer in the mounting procedure, provide such service, or have someone who will provide installation services on call. Caution: be aware of liability when doing so.

HOSPITAL BEDS

The health-accessories department of a pharmacy also may have hospital beds for sale or rental, including manual or electrically operated beds. The bed can be either fixed or variable height, and its spring should have an adjustable head and foot section that raises the patient's knees as well as permits the feet to be elevated.

The electrically operated bed may be either the full-electric or semielectric type. The height of the full-electric bed is adjustable from the floor and permits positioning of both the head and foot sections. The semielectric bed may have a manual crank to adjust the height. Caution the patient or family member that electric hospital beds may not be reimbursable unless a clear indication of medical necessity can be determined.

MATTRESSES—Polyfoam mattresses with waterproof ticking are excellent for rental purposes, especially with split-spring hospital beds, as one person can handle them easily. An innerspring mattress should be used with an electrically operated bed or when the heavier mattress is preferred; however, not every innerspring mattress will work well on a hospital bed, since the springs must be hinged to have the mattress flex properly when the spring is adjusted. Sometimes the selection of the type of mattress is influenced by the diagnosis or the insurance coverage

Any mattress used for rental purposes should be constructed with a waterproof covering, and it is advised also to provide plastic mattress covers. The pharmacist should be aware of local or state regulations regarding the sanitizing of rental mattresses, as well as Occupational Safety and Health Administration (OSHA) regulations that might apply for infection control.

BEDSIDE SAFETY RAILS—It is recommended to stock three types of bedside safety rails, full-length and half-length rails for use on a hospital bed and the other for use on any kind of bed normally used in the home. Rails for use with a hospital bed have clamps that attach to the steel parts of the spring. Rails used on home-type beds are attached by connecting rods placed between the regular mattress and box spring. This *any-bed* type of safety rail usually is made of aluminum, with cross-members of steel. Hospital bed rails may be constructed of aluminum or steel. Bed rails used on home beds are to provide safety and should not be used as repositioning aids or transfer-assist devices.

BED HANDLES—A newer product to assist patients in getting into or out of their own beds is the Bedside Assistant *(Bed Handles, Inc)*. Installed by just sliding them between the mattress and box spring, they provide extra stability for anyone who feels dizzy or unsteady as they get into or out of bed (Fig 110-16).

ALTERNATING PRESSURE PADS—The alternating pressure pad (APP) is a thin air-mattress pad arranged in longitudinal tubes and connected to an air pump that alternately inflates and deflates alternate rows of tubes. To eliminate

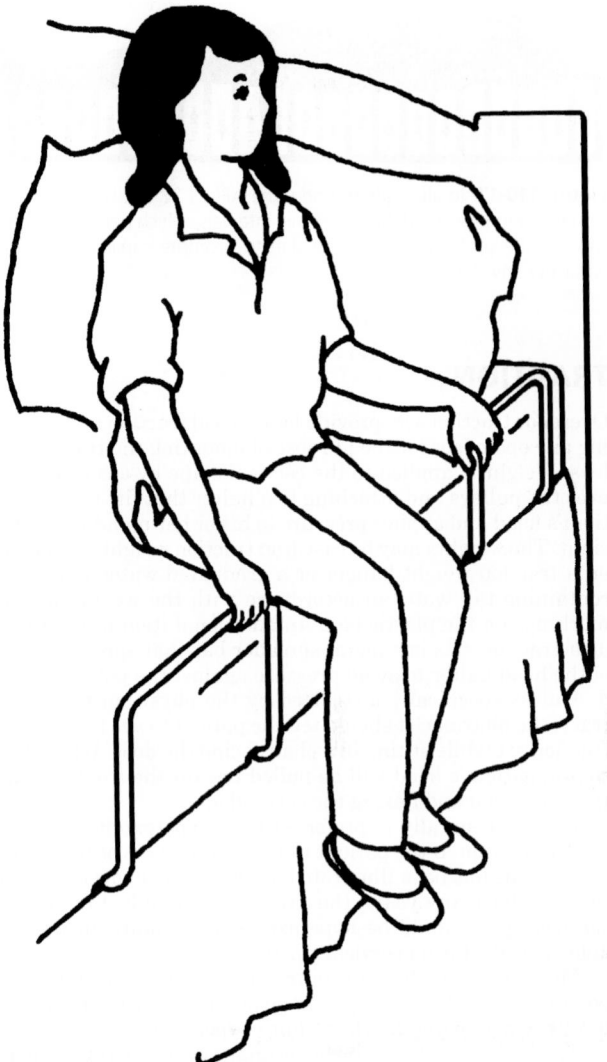

Figure 110-16. Patient using the Bedside Assistant (courtesy, Bed Handles).

counterpressure, sometimes created by the smooth long tubes in earlier APP pads, newer configurations may include small pillows arranged longitudinally in lieu of straight tubes. It works on the principle that circulation in the tissue occurs in the absence of pressure.

A newer product, the alternating pressure mattress (APM) by Invacare, features a full 7-inch-deep system with a variety of settings that can reduce interface pressure for treatment of Stage I through Stage IV pressure sores (Fig 110-17). A moisture-permeable covering also can help prevent skin breakdown by removing moisture from the skin.

TRAPEZE BARS—The typical overbed trapeze bar is used by the patient as an assist in sitting up and getting into and out of bed. It usually is made of steel and, by means of clamps, is attached to the headboard of a hospital bed. A trapeze-bar floor-stand, which enables the trapeze to be used over any bed, is also available.

Trapeze bars are adjustable in height, and some models also provide adjustability in the position of the bar over the bed. A special clamp permits the bar to be swung to various positions and locked for security. A pivoting trapeze bar should never be used with the floor stand, as accidents may occur unless the bar is suspended properly.

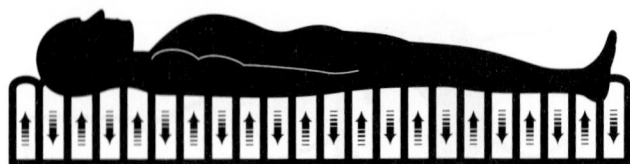

Figure 110-17. In alternating mode, the APM's 22 adjacent air cells alternatively inflate and deflate at 5-min intervals, which periodically redistributes the pressure against the skin to promote capillary circulation (courtesy, Invacare).

TRACTION

Overdoor traction sets provide for cervical traction at home, using any open door for the purpose of mounting the traction pulleys. Weight is applied to the cervical spine by a cord running over the pulleys and attaching to a halter that fits over the patient's head and applies pressure to his or her mandible and occiput. The weights may be cast-iron traction weights suspended on a traction-weight hanger or a graduated water-weight bag containing tap water in accordance with the weight-of-water markings on the plastic bag. An additional item in most overdoor traction sets is a metal spreader bar that spreads the top of the head halter to avoid pressure against the patient's ears.

Unless specifically instructed by the physician to the contrary, the pharmacist should tell the patient to use the overdoor traction set while sitting in a chair facing the door. When doing so, the patient's head will be pulled toward the front, bending the chin down and flexing the cervical spine.

Flexion generally is preferred over hyperextension in any type of traction. If the patient were to sit with his or her back to the door, as has been illustrated on the covers of overdoor traction sets for many years, the chin would be pulled up and the cervical spine would be hyperextended—usually an undesirable attitude during cervical traction.

Most patients who require traction will need it in a flexion posture; the rest need hyperextension. It may be dangerous to use flexion on patients who require hyperextension.

Any traction set—even the ordinary overdoor type—should be sold or rented only on the written prescription of a physician who specifies the frequency of treatment, the length of each treatment, the weight to be applied, whether the traction is to be static or intermittent, and special instructions as to positioning of the patient with respect to flexion and hyperextension. It is often necessary for the pharmacist or the patient to call either the physician or the physical therapist to clarify the amount of weight to be used or the length of time of each treatment.

TRACTION IN BED—While cervical traction may be given while the patient is either sitting in a chair or reclining in bed, pelvic traction is administered at home only when the patient is in prone position. There are two basic types of applied-in-bed traction sets: one is for use with a hospital bed and the other for use with any bed. The any-bed traction device has the typical vertical adjustments and pulleys and is mounted on a floor stand. Buck's extension traction or a mattress clamp set may require a sturdy headboard or footboard, as it has no floor stand. Either type is used for both pelvic and cervical traction.

When applying cervical traction to a patient lying in bed, unless specifically instructed by the physician to the contrary, traction pulleys usually are mounted quite high so as to develop flexion of the cervical spine and mildly depress the patient's chin.

When pelvic traction is applied, flexion is also important, and the pulleys should be mounted quite high to produce flexion of the lumbar spine. It also may be helpful to raise the head section of the hospital bed or bolster the ordinary bed with a wedge cushion or mattress elevator. Additionally, the patient's knees should be elevated either with the knee adjustments of the hospital bed spring or ordinary pillows placed under the knees. These recommendations must have the approval of the physician.

A complete traction department also will have pelvic traction belts in a variety of sizes, without which pelvic traction cannot be applied. A universal (one size fits all) belt with Velcro fasteners is also available.

PATIENT LIFTERS

Among a wide range of hydraulic and screw-type patient lifters, the floor-model hydraulic patient lifter is used most commonly (Fig 110-18). All lifters have an adjustable boom to which a patient-carrying sling or seat is attached. Lifter bases differ, though they are typically U-shaped and may be either adjustable or nonadjustable in width. The adjustable base may be spread wide and moved around almost any chair or commode so that the patient sling is suspended directly over the seat to which the patient will transfer.

Sling design is an important consideration when choosing a patient lifter. Slings in all fabrics come as one- or two-piece units, with and without head supports; they also may be had with a commode opening.

Positioning the sling under the patient who is in bed is accomplished in much the same way that bed linens are changed under a patient. The patient is rolled on one side while half the sling is folded accordion fashion and tucked up against him or her. The sling should be so positioned that on rolling back, the spine will rest on the middle of the sling. The patient is rolled back over the folded portion of the sling and to his or her other side while the folded part of the sling is unfolded; then the patient is returned to his or her back. Attention should be paid to the vertical positioning of the sling also—the bottom edge of the sling should not extend to the middle of the patient's knee, but rather should come just to the knee.

When the sling is placed properly under the patient, the lifter is brought to the bed, the chains or straps are hooked up, and the boom is raised slowly and gently until the patient is

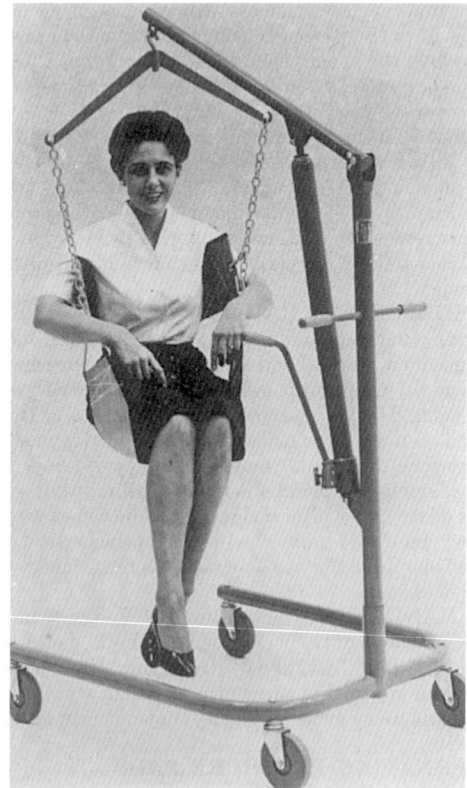

Figure 110-18. Painted hydraulic patient lifter with nonadjustable base and two-piece canvas patient sling (courtesy, Ted Hoyer & Co).

lifted off the mattress. Patients should never take hold of the lifter chains; their arms should be safely inside the sling. To avoid swinging of the sling when moving the lifter, the attendant should cross the patient's ankles and hold the bottom heel with one hand while pulling the lifter with the other. Patients should always be facing the lifter when they are suspended by the lifter sling.

When a patient is ready to be lowered into a chair, commode, or bed, the attendant should release the hydraulic valve carefully and slowly, guiding the patient into position by the heel. A common mistake is to remove the sling from beneath the patient after transferring him or her to a chair or commode. It is considerably easier, and safer too, to let patients sit on the sling, and remove only the chains and lifter from their view.

When it's time to pick the patient up again, the lifter only need be brought into position, the chains hooked up, and the patient lifted slowly out of the chair.

A patient lifter with a special type of base must be used for bathtub transfers.

BEDPANS

Bedpans, used for the collection of feces, may be round but are predominantly oval and are constructed of plastic, stainless steel, enamelware, or porcelain. Single-patient-use plastic bedpans (nonautoclavable) are considerably less expensive than their metal and porcelain counterparts. Plastic, like rubber, also tends to be warmer to the touch and therefore much more comfortable than steel, porcelain, or enamelware. There is also available a smaller, sloping, flatter bedpan, called a fracture bedpan, for use, primarily for urine, with immobilized or overweight patients.

It is helpful to the patient for the pharmacist to suggest that when a hospital bed is available, the back rest and knee section of the gatch spring should be elevated when using the bedpan. The backrest should be elevated substantially while the knee section should be elevated only slightly. When a hospital bed is not available in the patient's home, four or five pillows behind the back will make using a bedpan much easier.

ACCESSORIES FOR THE BEDFAST PATIENT

Special tables and trays for spill-preventing, safety, and patient comfort are near-essentials in any sickroom (Fig 110-19). The common overbed table is an ideal accessory whether or not the patient has a hospital bed. Some overbed tables have a center section that can be raised to a slanted position for the support of a book or magazine; others have a vanity tray and mirror that slide out from beneath the tabletop for use by the bedfast patient. Sturdy breakfast trays that straddle the patient's hips while he or she is in bed, special folding tables, and trays with contoured fronts that enable the wheelchair user to get comfortably close contribute to the nonambulatory patient's comfort and convenience in the sickroom at home.

Easy-reachers are devices that enable the bedfast patient to reach out and pick up things normally beyond his reach.

A solid or inflatable plastic shampoo tray facilitates shampooing for patients who cannot leave their beds. The tray fits across the mattress where a pillow normally goes and is designed to carry shampoo water to a drain at the side of the bed, where it may be collected in a plastic bucket. The patient's head rests in the shampoo tray, which, though it has quite high sides, has a depression for the back of the neck.

Folding backrests with or without arms, wedge-shaped foam cushions, bedboards, and footboards with adjustable cushions for the prevention of foot rotation are additional articles for the comfort and convenience of the bedfast patient. When it is necessary to keep bed linens and blankets off the patient's feet and legs, a blanket support, sometimes referred to as a leg or body

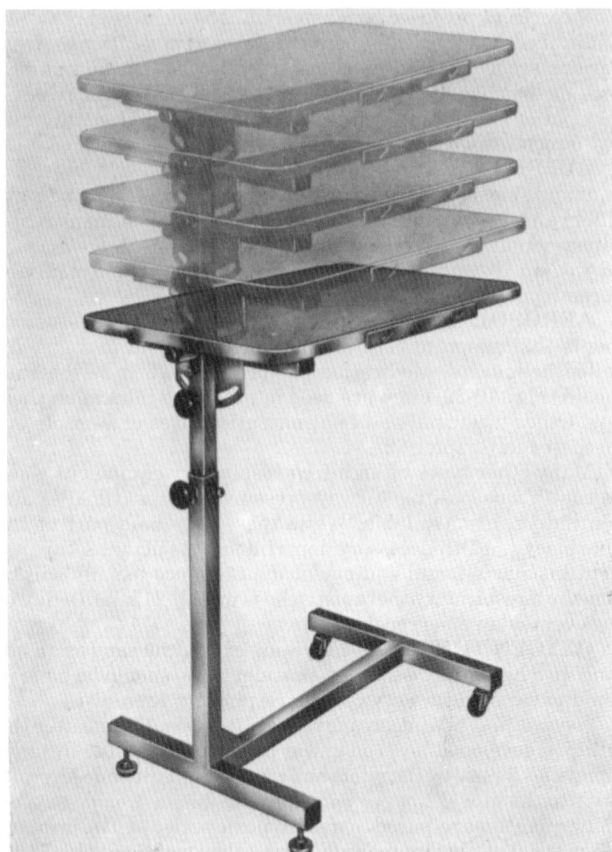

Figure 110-19. Adjustable overbed table with tilt-top for books or magazines (courtesy, Lumex).

cradle, is desirable. Holding mitts, built-up forks and swivel spoons, food guards, feeding cups, pencil and cigarette holders, and simple drinking straws with accordion hinges that bend without collapsing are some of the devices that make patient home-care effective.

Folding patient-privacy screens are a frequently requested sickroom accessory, especially when the patient will be using a bedside commode.

Finally, a health-accessories department also may stock a modest assortment of safety vests and belts, crib nets, and restraints for use by nursing homes and extended-care facilities, as well as by the patient at home.

RESPIRATORY THERAPY

STEAM VAPORIZERS—The modern steam inhaler is essentially the same as the now nearly forgotten croup kettle, except that it uses electricity to generate heat and steam. The advantage of this more modern adaptation lies in the attainment of a constant temperature. Also, most forms of this apparatus are equipped with a regulator so that when they run dry, the heating unit shuts off simultaneously. These are easier to handle in the home, especially at night.

The familiar vaporizer provides the conventional hot-steam therapy for the relief of upper respiratory illnesses. Physicians recommend it for colds, sinusitis, and similar ailments.

The portable room humidifier, on the other hand, provides a cool mist to compensate for the lack of sufficient moisture in the air and occasionally is used for its expectorant effect in liquefying tenacious mucus in the airway. An additional advantage is that since no heater is used, it is entirely safe for small children.

Vaporizers are used extensively in the home today to humidify bedrooms or chambers where patients suffering from various bronchial conditions may rest. Cool-vapor humidifiers provide effective high-humidity inhalation therapy for respiratory patients and can be used as well to restore proper humidity to rooms dried out by winter heating.

AIR PURIFIERS—The removal of dust, pollen, spores, secondhand smoke, and other irritants from room air by an air purifier can be a valuable adjunct to the treatment of many respiratory conditions. Models using a true HEPA (*high efficiency particulate arresting*) filter can remove up to 99.97% of all airborne room particles.

AEROSOL THERAPY AND NEBULIZERS—Instruments that generate very fine particles of liquid in a gas are called nebulizers. Medication compressors, such as the Pulmoaid (Fig 110-20) often are used in providing inhalation therapy. Other medicinal and pharmaceutical uses of aerosols are discussed in Chapter 69.

Many other types of high-tech respiratory equipment, such as continuous positive airway pressure devices (CPAPs) and ventilators, are available. While these may be a part of the pharmacy's health-accessory department, the actual setup, patient instruction, and equipment maintenance usually will be done by a respiratory therapist, who is on call 24 hours a day in the event of an emergency.

OXYGEN THERAPY—Providing oxygen therapy as an adjunct to a health-accessories department also should be done in conjunction with the services of a respiratory therapist.

Oxygen first became available as a therapeutic gas after the military developed an economical process to distill it in large quantities for use by the pilots and crew of high-altitude aircraft. Prior to this it was not economically feasible to provide oxygen in the quantities required to treat hypoxic patients. The primary commercial method of manufacturing therapeutic oxygen is by the liquification of air followed by fractional distillation.

Supplemental oxygen is used to treat various clinical disorders, both respiratory and nonrespiratory in nature.

Oxygen often is prescribed at a rate of 2 L/min for the relief of arterial hypoxemia and any of its secondary complications. Oxygen also has proved to be therapeutic in treating pulmonary hypertension, polycythemia secondary to hypoxemia, chronic disease states which may be complicated by anemia, cancer, migraine headaches, coronary artery disease, seizure disorders, sickle-cell crisis, and sleep apnea.

Some adverse effects and hazards of oxygen therapy include oxygen-induced hypoventilation, absorption atelectasis, and oxygen toxicity. Oxygen-induced hypoventilation is probably the greatest potential hazard of oxygen therapy.

In certain clinical situations the respiratory therapy drive that results from carbon dioxide stimulation of the respiratory center is blunted. This phenomenon may be the consequence of

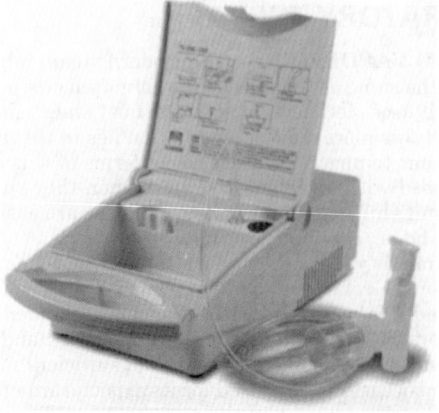

Figure 110-20. DeVilbiss Pulmo-Aide LT compressor (courtesy, Sunrise Medical).

a drug overdose such as with a barbiturate or heroin or, more commonly, chronic hypercarbia. Hypoventilation is of particular importance in patients with severe chronic obstructive pulmonary disease (COPD) in which carbon dioxide retention and hypoxemia have developed over a long period of time. The respiratory drive of most of these patients results from hypoxic stimulation of the carotid chemoreceptors. Thus, the main stimulus for respiration is hypoxemia. If this hypoxic drive is relieved through the advent of excessive oxygen therapy, hypoventilation may occur, and further carbon dioxide retention with possible cessation of ventilation could result.

Absorption atelectasis is the result of collapsed alveoli from a high concentration of oxygen in the inhaled air. Nitrogen, an inert gas that makes up 79% of our atmosphere, maintains the residual volume of space in the alveoli as the oxygen component of inhaled air is diffused through the pulmonary membrane and absorbed into the bloodstream. When a high concentration of oxygen is inhaled into the alveoli, the oxygen is absorbed rapidly into the blood, potentially leaving the alveoli empty and collapsed. This is particularly significant in patients with pulmonary disease that involves narrowing or obstructing the airways and a low ventilation-perfusion ratio.

Oxygen toxicity is not a significant hazard until oxygen concentrations are greater than 50% for prolonged periods of time. Oxygen toxicity can affect the pulmonary system, central nervous system, retina, and endocrine organs adversely. Pulmonary changes are usually the first to manifest, with increased permeability of capillary endothelial cells resulting in alveolar congestion, intraalveolar hemorrhage, and fibrinous exudation of the hyaline membrane. Normally, the first symptoms include substernal burning discomfort, cough, paresthesia, nausea, and vomiting.

A prescription of 2 L/min is generally considered sufficiently therapeutic without a great increase in risk of the previous hazards.

For the home-care patient on oxygen therapy, there are basically three different types of delivery systems available: the liquid system, compressed gas system, and oxygen concentrator. Each has its own distinct advantages and disadvantages. Choosing a system that is most applicable is based on the patient's needs, lifestyle, mobility, convenience, frequency of use, and volume of oxygen consumed. Reimbursement criteria set up by Medicare or an HMO also may dictate which type of system is used.

The oxygen in a liquid system has been compressed and cooled at −184.4° (−300°F). The resulting volume is less than 0.2% of an equivalent amount of oxygen at atmospheric pressure and temperature. The system consists of a large reservoir vessel and a lightweight portable unit. Both are designed to protect the extremely cold contents from heat and to regulate a consistent rate of evaporation from a liquid to a gas for subsequent use by the patient. Most large reservoirs will hold 75 to 100 lb of liquid oxygen and require filling once every week or so. Although considered stationary units, some patients have secured them in vehicles for travel. The portable unit is light enough, at approximately 8 lb when filled, to be transported over the shoulder by its carrying strap.

Compressed-gas oxygen systems consist of a basic high-pressure tank and a pressure regulator with an attached flow meter graduated in liters per minute. The most stable and reliable form of oxygen delivery and storage systems, it is most applicable for patients who predominantly are confined to their home with an occasional need for mobility or patients who require oxygen on an *as needed* basis. Compressed oxygen is available in a variety of tank sizes (Fig 110-21).

The largest, the H tank, holds 244 ft^3 or 6900 L of oxygen and is the standard stationary unit of the system. Smaller tanks, some of lightweight aluminum construction, are available for use as portable systems. The most common tanks are the E with 22 ft^3 or 622 L of oxygen, often used with a small pull cart, and the D with 12.6 ft^3 or 356 L of oxygen, easily carried in a shoulder bag.

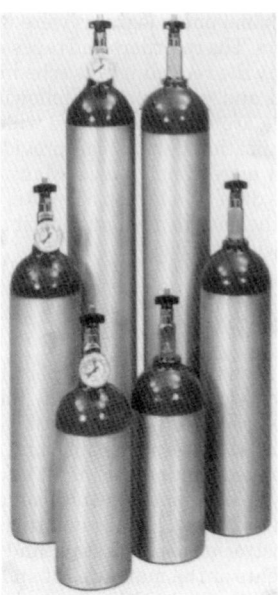

Figure 110-21. Portable oxygen tanks (courtesy, DeVilbiss).

OXYGEN CONCENTRATOR AND ENRICHER— Electrically powered by standard 110-V household current, these devices pump in ambient room air and then preferentially separate oxygen from nitrogen and deliver approximately 95% oxygen at maximum flows of 3 to 6 L/min. Much improved in efficiency and reliability over the last few years, all concentrators still require inspection by a trained technician, preferably quarterly but at least annually, to verify the percentage of oxygen delivered and perform a scheduled, routine maintenance program. This type of system never needs refilling and is extremely convenient for the homebound patient. The disadvantage of older systems is that the system cannot store any oxygen for portable or emergency use during an electrical outage. Patients should be advised to have a separate source of oxygen, such as a compressed tank, available. Newer units actually are capable of filling portable tanks. One brand of concentrator (Fig 110-22) can produce a liter flow of 0 to 6 L/min and also can fill any backup tank at 3 L/min while still providing oxygen for the patient. The most commonly used backup tank, the E tank, takes about 2 hr to fill. The use of this type of unit, where practical, and the use of oxygen-conservation devices can reduce the number of service and delivery calls normally associated with providing oxygen therapy.

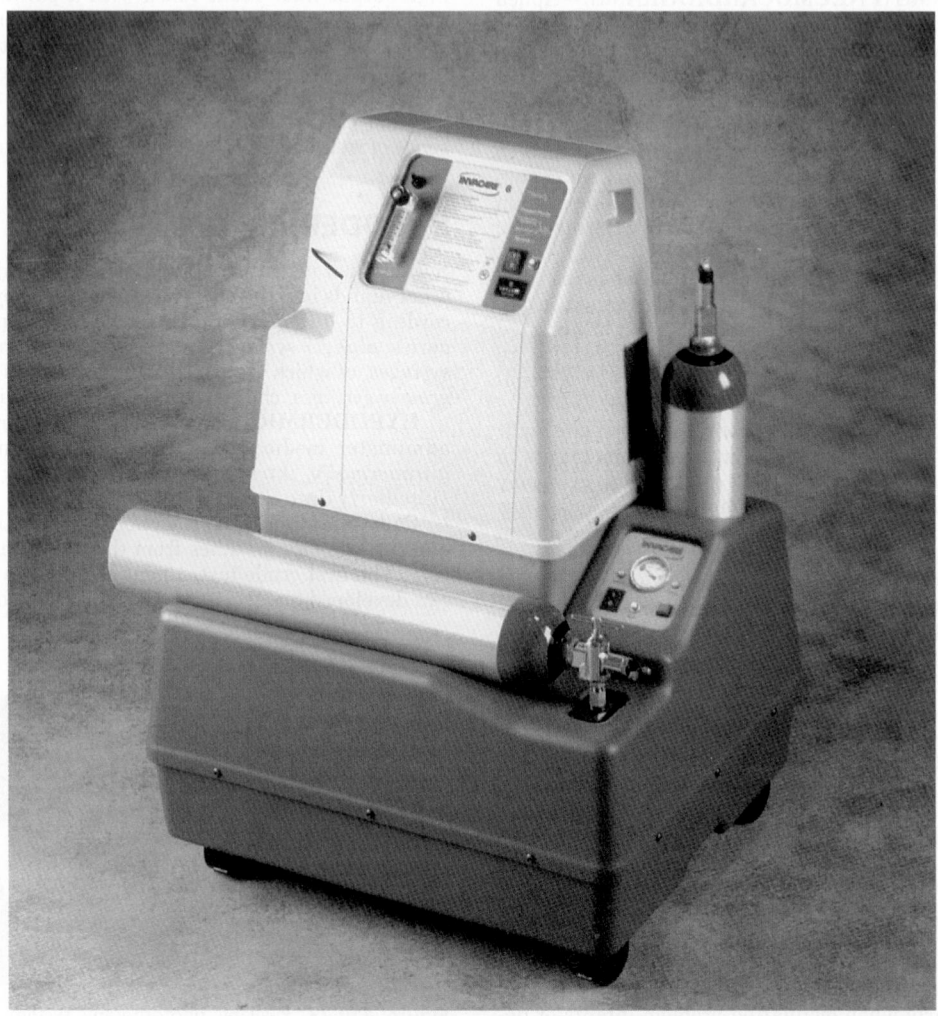

Figure 110-22. Venture HomeFill complete home oxygen system (courtesy, Invacare).

APNEA PROGRAMS

Sudden infant death syndrome (SIDS) is the number one cause of death in the US for infants under the age of 1 year. The relationship between SIDS and apnea (a pause in respiration of 15 to 20 sec or longer) is not exactly clear and is still somewhat controversial. However, a large portion of the pediatric medical community has begun home-monitoring in infants who have experienced episodes of prolonged apnea.

In the last few years a great deal of medical research has been devoted to improving understanding of the relationship between SIDS and apnea. This has resulted in the publication of a large number of journal articles about apnea and SIDS, the establishment of an annual medical conference on the subject, the startup of numerous hospital-based apnea programs, and a general increased awareness in the medical community about the problem.

As the interest in the medical community has increased, so has the number of physicians prescribing home monitors. Apnea programs were once the domain of a select few physicians and hospitals nationwide. Now, most hospitals with a Level II or III nursery have developed their own apnea-monitoring programs, staffed with a team of medical professionals. These programs evaluate infants at risk for apnea and prescribe the use of a home monitor. Typically, a neonatologist heads up the team and is assisted by nurses and respiratory therapists specializing in the treatment of infants.

The increased interest in SIDS and apnea by the medical community has stimulated tremendous growth in the number of home-health-care dealers offering apnea-monitoring programs.

PNEUMOGRAMS (PNEUMOCARDIOGRAMS)—Apnea monitoring has become much more sophisticated in the last few years. Very specific and detailed evaluation and screening programs have been established by hospitals to determine which infants will need to go home with an apnea monitor. Once in the home, more followup work now is being done. Historically, 12 hour recordings known as pneumograms were performed to evaluate an infant's progress in the home environment. Long-term event recordings are now commonplace for documentation of the types of alarms an infant is having and to determine the proper time for monitor discontinuance.

Pneumograms are two-channel recordings of heart rate (ECG) and respiration. Typically, these are performed in the home for a 12 hour period. These recordings then are printed out and analyzed by a physician or technician. The results are used to determine if the infant needs further study at a hospital apnea center or no longer needs to be monitored.

A 12-hour pneumogram is a *snapshot* recording of one night in an infant's life. The recording may include apnea events in combination with normal activity *(well information)* or it may include only *well information*. If an infant who previously has had a number of serious problems while being monitored has an unusual evening during a 12-hour pneumogram, with no events occurring, the physician has a recording that is not an accurate reflection of the infant's true condition.

An event recorder provides the caregiver with long-term information about the events that are causing the monitor to alarm. This provides the physician important documentation about the number and type of events an infant is having over a long period of time. An event recording provides a physician with a more realistic record of an infant's condition. The physician can alter the infant's monitoring program or discontinue monitoring altogether based on the results of the recording.

Event recordings, normally taken for a period of 72 hr or longer, are similar to two-channel pneumograms. They record heart rate and respiration data, but rather than continuously recording this information over a 12-hr period, they only record information when the monitor sounds an alarm. An event recording provides the caregiver with information about alarm events occurring in the home. This information is extremely valuable, particularly when evaluating problem infants or determining when to discontinue monitoring.

Traditionally, home pneumograms were made on small cassette-tape recorders. The recorders and tapes would be delivered to the home the day the recording was scheduled, and the readings were printed and analyzed the following day. Multiple-channel recordings are being used more widely, and improved electronic communication devices can provide physicians with results on a much more timely basis. Many units can be connected to store the data on a laptop computer or, through a modem, to transmit the data to a neonatologist at a hospital or directly to the physician's office.

PHOTOTHERAPY

The treatment of neonatal jaundice (hyperbilirubinemia) often involves the use of a phototherapy light. Phototherapy treatment also may be provided by a fiberoptic system, which consists of an illuminator, a fiberoptic cable, and a fiberoptic panel, which can be wrapped around an infant's torso (Fig 110-23). Phototherapy may be done in the hospital or, at the doctor's and parent's option, in the home. Home phototherapy costs can be a fraction of the cost of a hospital stay, and the financial resources of the parents or the mandates of an HMO may require home treatment. While the health-accessories pharmacist may stock and set up these units, a nursing service usually will provide the everyday blood-testing required.

LIGHT THERAPY—Studies have shown that during the winter months, especially in the northern climates, up to 20% of the population may suffer from sunlight affective disorder (SAD). Three-fourths of these will be women. By combining high-output fluorescent tubes with a parabolic reflector, one company has designed a light unit that can produce up to 10,000 lux (a unit of measure of light intensity) of light, similar to that of a very bright and sunny spring day (Fig 110-24). By contrast, normal indoor lighting levels may range from 200 to 700 lux. Usage for only 15 to 30 min a day may increase the sense of well-being for those affected by this disorder.

HYPODERMIC EQUIPMENT

Syringes are instruments intended for the injection of water or other liquids into the body or its cavities. They are classified according to differences in principle of action into three categories: *plunger syringes,* such as the hypodermic syringes; *bulb syringes,* of which the ear and ulcer syringes are one type, and *gravity syringes,* characterized by the fountain syringes.

HYPODERMIC SYRINGES—These syringes are used to administer medication *subcutaneously* (under the skin) or *intradermally, intravenously* (into a vein or artery), or *intramuscularly* (into the muscle).

Parenteral therapy or injection of medication under the skin and through tissues dates from the beginning of the 19th century. The first crude instrument of this type was a needle trocar, developed to deposit morphine in paste form. The principle

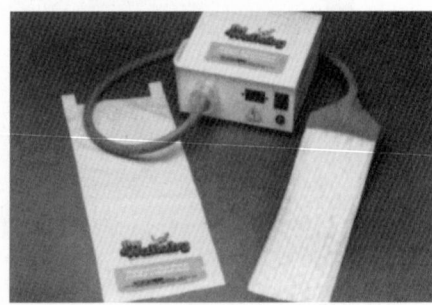

Figure 110-23. Wallaby phototherapy system (courtesy, Medical Products).

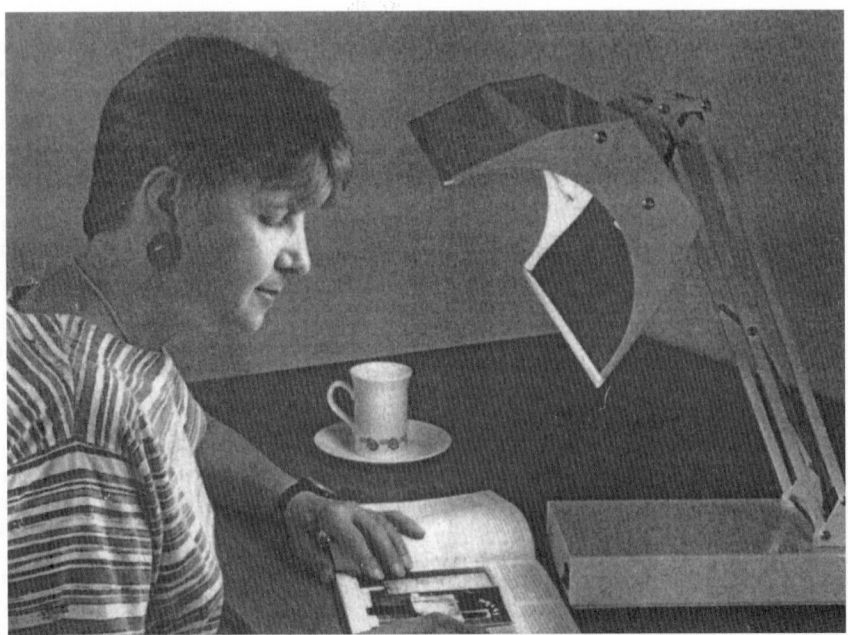

Figure 110-24. Satellite light system (courtesy, Northern Light Techologies).

of introducing medication under the skin, however, became popular in the first half of the 20th century.

Luer Syringes—The inventor of this type of apparatus, Dr Luer, patented his syringe; the letters patent have long since expired but today most hypodermic syringes of this style bear his name. The outstanding feature of the Luer syringe was its ground-glass surfaces. In many instances, the inside of the glass barrel and the outside of the glass plunger were ground individually. Later, they were ground together so that they would provide a perfect fit and prevent back leakage.

Hypodermic syringes are always of the plunger type, characterized by the type of piston and difference of size or capacity. The *tuberculin syringe* is a small syringe not exceeding 1 mL in capacity and graduated in 0.1- or 0.01-mL divisions. The *hypodermic syringe* is usually of 2- to 50-mL capacity. There are larger piston syringes, ranging up to 200 mL, for various purposes such as transfusions and in veterinary medicine. Graduations may be in fractions of a mL or in *minims*. Syringes also may be prepared with special graduations, such as *units* of insulin.

DISPOSABLE HYPODERMIC SYRINGES—Most hypodermic syringes used outside of a hospital setting are of the disposable variety. Various types of disposable hypodermic syringes, each carrying a single dose of sterile medication, now are supplied as a standard dosage container by many pharmaceutical manufacturers.

HYPODERMIC NEEDLES—Hypodermic needles used with Luer syringes are of metal and consist of a hub, which locks to the ground-glass tip by friction, and a needle point that varies in diameter and length. Needles also are called *cannulas*. Hypodermic needles have been made of stainless steel, hyperchrome steel, carbon steel, chromium, nickeloid, platinum, platinum-iridium, silver, or gold.

Hypodermic needles are characterized by their different points, which have a long, tapering reinforced point and beveled cutting edges of varying degree. A *long-bevel* or *long-taper* needle is used for local anesthesia, aspirating, hypodermoclysis, and subcutaneous administration. A *short-bevel* needle is used for intravenous administration, infusions, and transfusions. A *special short-bevel* needle is employed for intradermal and spinal administration (Fig 110-25).

Size—Selection of a size is governed by four factors—safety, rate of flow, comfort of patient, and depth of penetration. There are three standard dimensions—length, outside diameter of the

cannula, and wall thickness. Regular needles are measured for length from where the cannula joins the hub to the tip of the point (hub not included).

The gauge of a needle is measured by the outside diameter of the cannula or needle shaft. The usual range of diameter for needles is from 13-gauge (largest diameter) to 27-gauge. Needles seldom are less than $\frac{1}{4}$-inch long or longer than $3\frac{1}{2}$ inches.

There are many special needles, designed for a variety of purposes. Various *biopsy* and *bone-marrow transfusion* needles range from 16- to 19-gauge and $\frac{1}{2}$ to $3\frac{1}{2}$ inches long. They are characterized by their heavy-shaped hubs.

Needles for *local anesthesia* range from 26-gauge, $\frac{1}{2}$ inch to 20-gauge, 6 inch. *Intravenous, blood transfusion* needles, some with fitted cannulas, range from 19-gauge, $1\frac{1}{4}$ inch to 15-gauge, $2\frac{1}{2}$ inch.

There are also special needles and cannulas for *abscess, eye, hemorrhoidal, tonsil, laryngeal,* and *pneumothorax* use.

These many types of special-purpose hypodermic needles are of varying diameters and varying lengths. Examples of some of these are shown in Figure 110-26.

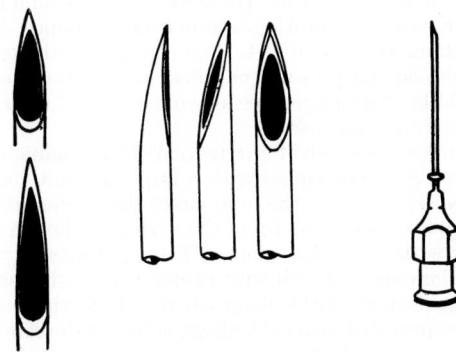

Figure 110-25. Hypodermic needles. *Left,* short-bevel and long-bevel needle points; *left center,* the Huber point with closed bevel and side opening to avoid producing tissue plugs; *right center,* regular point showing features that ensure less cutting, more distention of tissue, and reduced trauma, seepage, and after-pain; *right,* needle with security button that prevents a broken cannula from becoming lost in the tissues.

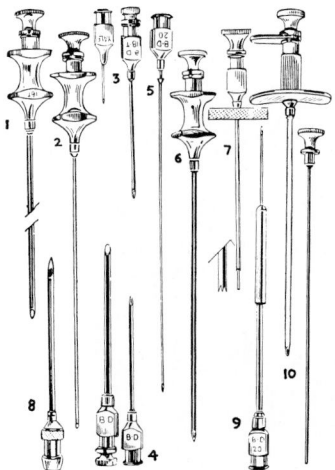

Figure 110-26. Special hypodermic needles. 1, caudal needle; 2, epidural needle for single-shot anesthesia; 3, intravenous anesthesia short-bevel and long needles (with vinyl tubing); 4, blood transfusion needles (with vinyl tubing); 5, short-bevel beaded local anesthesia needles; 6, spinal needle with large spool hub; 7, biopsy needle for bone-marrow aspirations; 8, infusion needle, with female Luer slip; 9, hemorrhoidal needle with threaded adjustable gauge to adjust depth of puncture; 10, cerebral angiography needle with thin-walled outer cannula, corrugated shield, and inner cannula (courtesy, Becton-Dickinson).

BULB SYRINGES

Bulb syringes frequently are preferred for use where sterility is not necessary or where plunger-type syringes, because of their force, would be dangerous to use. Bulb syringes are of particular value in the nose and ear and for wound and urinary irrigation.

These syringes customarily are known by the name of the part of the body for which they are intended.

Nasal syringes or *nasal aspirators* are soft rubber bulbs of about 1-oz capacity, with an acorn-shaped nasal tip to fit the nostril. The tip may be either glass, plastic, or hard rubber. A glass tip allows visual examination of the mucus removed from the nostril.

Ear syringes and *ulcer syringes* are one-piece molded bulbs of soft, flexible rubber, with long, narrow nozzles and are employed in treating the eye, ear, and nose and for irrigation of any open cavity or ulcer.

If necessary, bulb syringes should be sterilized with germicidal solutions. Prolonged boiling will injure the rubber.

Rectal syringes are customarily of the bulb type, with a long narrow nozzle. They frequently are employed in the administration of enemas to infants. These are the safest and least expensive of syringes requiring minimal maintenance. Such syringes customarily are of 1- to 4-oz capacity. Although many syringes provide hard-rubber or vulcanite tips, the use of hard tips should be discouraged because of occasional injury to the soft tissues from their use.

Vaginal syringes, used for irrigation of the vagina, are 8- to 10-oz capacity bulb syringes with a large vulcanite or rubber spray tube. Pressure on the bulb forces the medicated or irrigating liquid through the tip of the syringe either in a direct stream or with a *whirling* motion. These syringes in white or various colors are provided with rubber, sleeve-shaped, round or oval shields to prevent leakage when in use. Caps sealing the nozzles are provided to avoid leakage or loss of the contents before use. One model has a convenient plastic stopper at the bottom of the bulb opening, with a removable strainer, which permits mixing of medications.

ENEMA SYRINGES—Fountain syringes consist of a reservoir with a capacity of 1 to 3 qt, a 5-ft rubber tube, and a vaginal or rectal nozzle. These are used for irrigation with water, salt solution, soap suds, or special medications.

Pharmacists should caution users of enema syringes as follows: the *drop* must not exceed 4 ft to prevent excessive gravity pressure, the fluid should be maintained at body temperature to avoid chills or burns, and the tube customarily is closed with a mechanical pinchcock. Before using the syringe, the cutoff should be released for a moment until some liquid issues from the nozzle. The user must be certain that no air remains that might be forced from the tube into the body cavity. Hard-rubber nozzles are supplied frequently with enema syringes, but as they may cause damage to the rectum, they preferably are replaced by catheters or tubes of soft rubber, about 3/16 inches in diameter and 15 inches in length.

Enemas—In simple constipation, whenever evacuation of the lower bowel is indicated, and when proctological examination or surgery is indicated, an enema customarily is given because of its local, comfortable, and safe action in a relatively short period of time.

Enemas should not be used when nausea, vomiting, or abdominal pain is present nor more often than necessary, to avoid dependence. Prepared enemas are available for use in simple constipation or whenever evacuation of the lower bowel is indicated, such as in proctological or sigmoidoscopic examinations; small, disposable units consisting of flexible plastic bottles of 6- to 50-mL aqueous or oil solutions, with self-fitted comfortable plastic or rubber tip are available.

DRESSINGS AND FIRST-AID SUPPLIES

Pharmacists are the proper distributors of sterile materials for treating wounds. Their training enables them to appreciate the care necessary in their handling and storage, and they often are called upon for advice or instruction on their use. The following items fall in this class: absorbent cotton, cotton balls and buds, sterile rolls and pads of gauze, elastic bandages, disposable fabric tissues and underpads, eye pads, sponges, tissues and towels, adhesive elastic bandages, aerosol adherent, spray dressings, first-aid kits, scissors, tweezers, and applicators. Various types of oxygen and moisture-permeable transparent dressings such as *Tegaderm* or hydroactive dressings such as *Duoderm* serve specialized needs.

The pharmacy with a comprehensive health-accessories department will stock bulk packages of these items for use by nursing homes, visiting nurses services, and patients who consume quantities sufficient to warrant their making larger purchases, in addition to the smaller packages for the pharmacy's usual customers.

THE FAMILY MEDICINE CABINET—There is a place in every home where medicines are kept. The medicine cabinet should be either locked or completely out of the reach of children. Every bottle or box within should be labeled clearly. Unused prescription medications, outdated over-the-counter drugs, and empty bottles do not belong in the medicine cabinet and should be removed. Some community pharmacists provide folders containing information on first-aid, poison antidotes, and simple home medication for use by their patients so that the pharmacy's name is always in view in the medicine cabinet. This also is accomplished by providing a gummed *family prescription record* for the inside of the cabinet door or an *emergency label* bearing space for entering telephone numbers for the doctor, pharmacy, hospital, and fire and police departments, to be attached to the telephone or telephone book.

In addition, the pharmacist should urge that every family car, camper, and boat be equipped with an adequate first-aid kit in addition to a flashlight, flares, and a hand-held fire extinguisher.

SNAKE-BITE KITS—Anyone in snake, bee, or wasp country should carry a snake-bite kit. Usually, these are available in a compact plastic or metal case containing a tourniquet rubber or other lymph constrictor, antiseptic, razor blade or knife, and one or more suction cups or syringes. These are available from Cutter or Becton-Dickinson. Many lives are saved each year by prompt action at the spot where the snake attacks, and relief from the pain and swelling of severe insect stings is also important. Snake bites are medical emergencies that require immediate treatment.

Every hospital pharmacist should have a chart of disaster-unit equipment required for a hospital, and all pharmacists should be familiar with the requirements and needs of disaster units.

HOT-WATER BOTTLES—The best instruments for applying dry heat are the hot-water bottle and the electric heating pad. Hot-water bottles may be of the usual 2-qt size or of the 1-pt capacity in the form of a *face bottle* for neuralgia of the head and for infant conditions. Each hot-water bottle has an opening through which warm water is added and a stopper securely sealed with a washer. It is more convenient to attach the stopper permanently to the bottle to prevent its loss. Some have screw-stopper attachments that permit conversion of the bottle into a fountain syringe.

When filling a hot-water bottle, it should be held against the back of the hand or forearm to ensure that the temperature is not too high. The hot-water bottle should never be allowed to come in contact with the skin, or burns may result. Flannelette bags or even a towel wrapped around the hot-water bottle will give adequate passage of heat and comfort and convenience.

After use, the empty hot-water bottle should be hung by the tap at its bottom for thorough draining. Water of boiling temperature, oil, grease, alcohol, or turpentine should not be permitted to come in contact with the material of the hot-water bottle.

MOIST-HEAT PACKS—Various commercial moist-heat packs are in common use in hospitals and nursing homes and are also available for use at home. These steam packs appear as compartmented, cloth bean bags when new and are filled with tiny beads. When boiled in water or heated in a microwave oven, however, the beads become hydrated and combine into a gelatinous substance that has the unique property of holding its temperature far longer than any other pack—about 30 to 40 min.

Moist-heat packs such as these must be wrapped in layers of Turkish towel to prevent burns and should never be used in direct contact with the skin. They are available in a variety of sizes, including a contoured pack designed specifically for the neck and shoulders. The neck-contour steam pack, as well as others, also has optional terry-cloth covers, lined with foam rubber, which takes the place of layers of toweling. Heating units are also available, but the patient at home can prepare a steam pack in an ordinary pot of boiling water. They can be used over and over again without loss of effectiveness if care is taken to avoid dehydration—easily accomplished by wrapping the steam pack in a plastic bag and storing it in the refrigerator. For long-term storage, these packs can be kept in the freezer (ie, again, sealed in a plastic bag) to prevent drying out.

ELECTRIC HEATING PADS—The advantage of the electric heating pad over the hot-water bottle is that there is no possibility of leaking or spilling, and the temperature is controlled constantly and indefinitely. Most are wet proof for wet or dry application and have soft-foam padding and washable flannel covers. Most have adjustable heating elements that permit the temperature to be set at the desired level and an illuminated temperature-control panel. One of the more popular electric moist-heating pads is manufactured by Battle Creek under the trade name *Thermophore*. These are controlled by means of a handheld switch that automatically turns the unit off when released, eliminating the possibility of burns caused by a patient's falling asleep. The Thermophore heating pad creates moist heat without preboiling or using large amounts of water, hence, its desirability in the home environment. The unit's flannel cover is dipped into water and then wrung dry. Intermittent applications of heat create *fomentation,* or intense moist heat. The manufacturer recommends that treatments not exceed 30 minutes in length. Customarily, all such electrical devices are inspected to ensure safe operation. However, short circuits and breakage of the heating element may result from constant use.

Automatic heat bonnets for scalp treatments; heat bandages for sprains, bursitis, or arthritis; neck and throat heating pads for stiff neck or whiplash cases; sinus masks for heat therapy of sinus areas; and even thermal massagers are available. The pharmacist always should caution the patient *not* to sleep while using an electric heating pad.

Still another modality for providing heat therapy are systems that pump temperature-controlled heated water through a special pad or pads. The pads can be applied to the areas of the body that require heat therapy. A key-operated temperature set point maintains the circulating water at a constant, preset temperature (Fig 110-27).

PERSONAL HEAT WRAPS OR PATCHES–Personal heat therapy products are useful in the management of mild to moderately self-limiting sprains, strains, and chronic conditions. These products contain iron and other natural materials that undergo an exothermic oxidative reaction when exposed to air. These products have been shown to be useful in treating low back pain, neck and shoulder pain, wrist pain, and abdominal menstrual cramps.

PARAFFIN BATHS—Heat also can be applied uniformly to feet, hands, or elbows by using a paraffin bath. By dipping the foot, hand, or elbow into the warm paraffin a number of times, a soft *glove* is formed that will release its heat slowly and uniformly. After the treatment the *glove* is just peeled off (Fig 110-28).

COLD APPLICATION—In deep inflammation the effects of external application of either heat or cold are essentially similar, owing to reflexes arising from the stimulation of the nerves conducting temperature sensation. Experience has shown that there are some conditions (eg, appendicitis) in which the application of cold is more desirable.

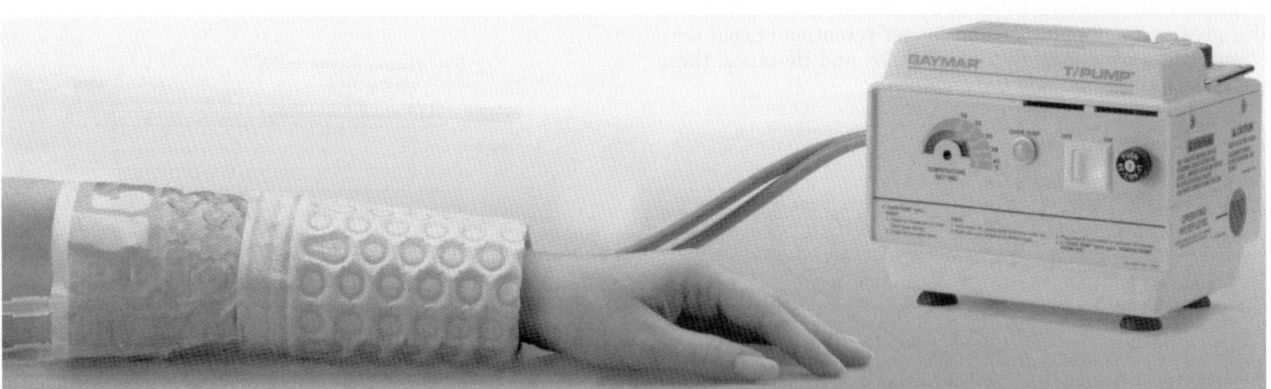

Figure 110-27. Gaymar T/Pump heat therapy system (courtesy, Gaymar Industries).

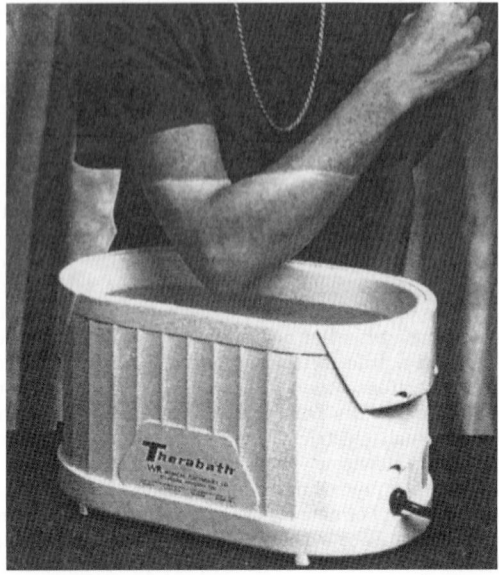

Figure 110-28. Paraffin heat therapy system (courtesy, Therabath).

Appliances for local application of cold are reusable cold packs and the familiar ice bag or ice cap (Fig 110-29). The latter is usually a circular rubber or rubberized cloth bag, circular in shape, with a large opening to admit cracked ice. Occasionally thick rubber, similar to that used in hot-water bottles, is employed. Usually, ice caps require a cover of some type to protect the skin. The contents of an ice cap are less flaccid than the liquid in hot-water bottles. Therefore, thin-rubber or cloth construction is preferable, to ensure better conformation with the body. The pleated shape common to many ice caps avoids bulginess and allows the introduction of large amounts of ice. The English Ice Cap is an example of an ice bag with an cloth, ornamental covering.

An adaptation of the ice cap is used for throat inflammation. It is the collar-shaped rubber bag known as a tonsillectomy bag. It fits snugly around the neck. Ice bags also are made in a long, narrow shape for use around the throat and along the spine.

COLD PACKS—Instead of using ice, some hospitals keep *redi-freeze ice packs* that are stored in refrigerators until needed and are exchanged for bags that have become warm in use. Thus, cold packs are immediately available at all times, and the liquid contents conform more readily to the contours of the body.

Ice packs of soft rubber or plastic, filled with a nontoxic solution of 10% propylene glycol and water, are available in the usual designs. When stored in the freezing compartment of the refrigerator, the contents freeze to a semisolid or slush that provides greater comfort in use and longer retention of cold temperature than ice cubes. Fitted with tabs and tie-tapes, these are available in throat and body shapes.

In addition, instant hot and cold packs are available that provide a portable modality for heat and cold therapy, ideal in situations when refrigeration or heating units are not accessible. To activate the packs, they are struck firmly, which breaks an inner packet containing an activating fluid. This fluid comes into contact with the base chemical, and the resulting chemical reaction is either endothermic, producing cold, or exothermic, producing heat. They maintain heat or cold for about 30 minutes and then must be discarded.

Another type of cold therapy circulates iced water through a special pad next to the part of the body being treated. Temperature control can be adjusted from 45° to 55°F for continuous use or below 45°F for sessions of 20 minutes or less.

THERMOMETERS

Hippocrates in 460 BC recognized that abnormal human temperature was a disease symptom. In 1610 AD Sanctorius developed the first clumsy oral thermometer. The thermometer was unreliable until 1714, when Fahrenheit developed the first dependable scale and instrument. It had standard gradations, and mercury was used as the heat-measuring liquid. In 1835, two Frenchmen, Becquerel and Breschet, established the mean, or average, temperature of a healthy man as 98.6° on the scale devised by Fahrenheit. A Hollander, Antoon Van Haen, in 1754 developed the first practical clinical thermometer. Thermometers were seldom depended on in medical practice until about 1865, when a Scottish physician named Aitken invented a self-registering thermometer.

THERMOMETERS FOR HOME USE—The types of thermometers usually employed in the home are the *household thermometer,* or common type for reading interior or outside air temperature, and *clinical* or *fever* thermometers (Fig 110-30). The temperature of the atmosphere at the surface of the earth varies more than 200°F, but man's body temperature rarely varies beyond 97° to 104°F, with the portent of danger at either extreme.

The change in temperature of the patient is one of the important symptoms upon which physicians base their diagnoses and treatments. The instrument employed for body-temperature determination is the *clinical,* or more popularly called *fever,* thermometer.

An abnormal temperature is nature's warning sign that something is wrong or amiss. A rapid rise or fall and substantial deviations from normal are danger signals. Every home should have a fever thermometer available at all times.

The essential difference between an ordinary thermometer and one designed for determining body temperature is the self-registering feature of the fever thermometer. When the mercury column has risen to the maximum temperature, it remains until shaken back into the reservoir at the bottom of the instrument. This is due to a constriction that acts as a tiny check-valve in the thermometer bore, just above the bulb, and permits

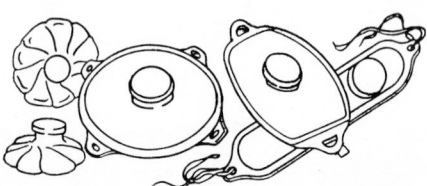

Figure 110-29. Ice caps and bags. *Left,* mackintosh cloth and rubber collapsible ice cap; *center,* ice bags; *right,* spinal and throat ice bags.

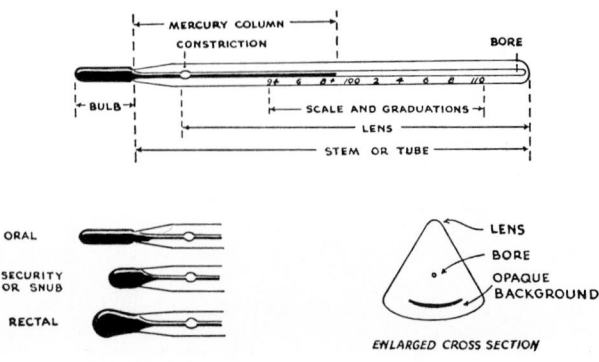

Figure 110-30. Diagram of thermometer construction.

passage of the mercury on expansion but does not permit its return on contraction.

CLINICAL OR FEVER THERMOMETERS—Three bulb types of fever thermometers are available:

The *oral type,* characterized by the slender mercury reservoir, is the most sensitive for mouth use.

The *rectal type* has a blunt, strong, pear-shaped bulb for safety and to ensure retention in the rectum.

A small, sturdy *universal, security, snub,* or *stubb* type with a short, stubby bulb, for oral or rectal use and safer for babies or irrational patients (Fig 110-30).

All fever thermometers have a magnifying-lens front that renders the mercury column visible against an opaque background. Some have a colored line that by reflection helps detect the mercury column, or guidelines that center the eye on the image of the column. Others are flat so that the markings are on the same plane as the mercury when the thermometer is held in normal reading position.

TAKING BODY TEMPERATURE—Fever thermometers should always be sterilized and shaken down below 97°F before taking a reading. For *oral* temperatures, the thermometer should be placed in the mouth, with the bulb under the rear edge of the tongue, and rotated once or twice to ensure complete contact. The transfer of body heat to the thermometer is speeded by then shifting the bulb to the opposite rear edge of the tongue. The lips should be kept closed, and the thermometer left in the mouth for at least 3 min. Regardless of length of initial oral exposure, it is always well after the initial reading to return the thermometer to the patient's mouth for another minute, to provide a check or verification of the original reading. Oral temperatures should not be taken for 30 minutes after exercising, smoking, eating, or taking hot or cold drinks.

Rectal temperature should be taken only with a rectal or stubby bulb thermometer. The bulb should be lubricated with a water-soluble jelly and gently inserted deeply enough to pass the constricting muscle, leaving about half the thermometer exposed. Babies should be held firmly face down, their buttocks separated with one hand, and the thermometer held in place with the other. The thermometer should be left in place at least 4 minutes.

A longer time may be necessary for temperature readings if the thermometer is cold or if the patient is anemic or aged, with poor blood circulation. Axillary (underarm) temperature measurement is not recommended except when all other methods are impossible.

NORMAL TEMPERATURES—The average normal oral temperature is 98.6°F, but some variations are natural. Healthy persons may have temperatures as much as 1°F above or below the average normal temperature. One's temperature may range from about 97.3°F at 2 to 5 am to about 98°F in the morning and to about 99°F in the late afternoon. One should determine his or her normal temperature by a series of readings while in good health, for comparison as a personal standard when one is ill.

Normal rectal temperatures are usually 1°F higher, or 99.6°F, though the *normal* mark on all types of fever thermometers, including the rectal type, is at 98.6°F.

BASAL TEMPERATURE GRAPH—A woman who wishes to become pregnant may increase her chances of conception greatly by having intercourse at the time of ovulation, or she may decrease the chance of contraception by avoiding intercourse then. She may use her knowledge of the fertile interval for avoidance of conception for some time by natural means, then use it for a planned pregnancy (*natural child spacing*).

Basal temperature graphs are helpful in determining whether and when ovulation occurs. Ovulation is the release of an egg (ovum) from the ovary; ordinarily it occurs only once in each menstrual cycle. Conception can take place only if intercourse takes place at or near this time, during the interval of transition between low- and high-temperature levels.

The basal temperature graph reflects slight body changes taking place during the menstrual cycle; charts for plotting the daily temperatures are available from Schering, Becton-Dickinson, and elsewhere. The *basal resting* temperature in the first part of the cycle is usually well below normal; in the last 2 weeks or so of the cycle the basal temperature is closer to 98.6°F. Most important, *the shift from the lower to the higher temperature occurs about the time of ovulation* (Fig 110-31).

The variations in the temperature before and after ovulation are slight, often only a few tenths to a half degree, so it is important that the temperature be taken carefully and recorded accurately. Special thermometers are available for this purpose. They record temperatures within the usual range of cyclic variations (from 96° to 100°F only) and are graduated in tenths of a degree and are easier to read than the ordinary fever thermometers, although the latter may be used.

TEMPERATURE COMPARISONS—Throughout the US the Fahrenheit scale still is employed, although the use of the Celsius scale is increasing rapidly in medical circles. Some hospitals and physicians prefer the latter scale, and clinical thermometers graduated in Celsius degrees are available. Normal body temperature on the Celsius scale is 37°. A comparison of temperature equivalents of the two scales, in the range of body temperatures below and above normal, is given in Table 110-1.

ACCURACY—The critical factors in obtaining maximum accuracy are that the thermometer must be designed properly, it must be sufficiently accurate to meet each specific requirement, and it must be used properly.

In general, the accuracy of fever thermometers is established either by federal standards, or by states, local authorities, and sometimes private institutions, usually operating for hospital groups.

Thermometers offered for sale that exceed the standards usually bear specific information on the certificate indicating special accuracy or selection for other factors beyond the minimum requirements. They are valuable for critical temperature use, such as in diagnosis of certain pulmonary diseases and infectious diseases, both surgical and medical, and for basal-temperature studies, now being used widely in the study of human fertility.

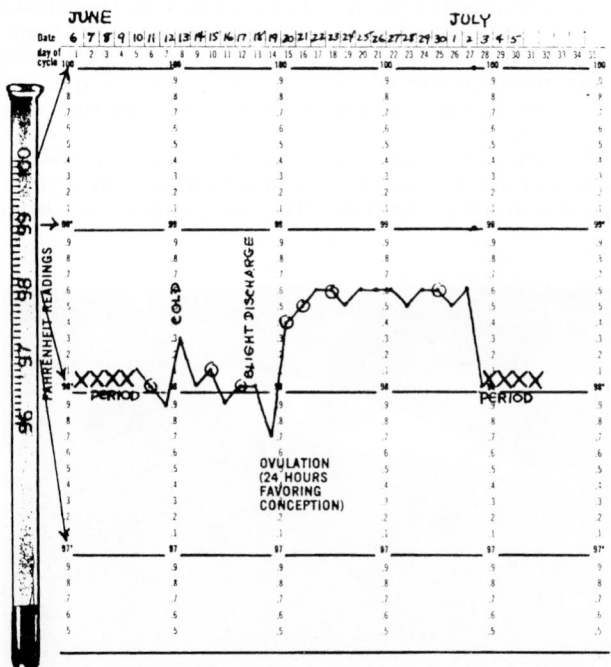

Figure 110-31. Basal temperature graph for determination of ovulation period in the female.

Table 110-1. Temperature Comparison

FAHRENHEIT	CELSIUS
96.0	35.55
97.0	36.11
97.6	36.36
98.0	36.65
98.6	37.0
99.0	37.22
99.5	37.50
100.0	37.77
101.0	38.33
102.0	38.88
103.0	39.44
104.0	40.0

READING THE THERMOMETER—Next to accuracy, the most important feature of a fever thermometer is its ease of reading. This is especially true for the inexperienced home user, who will appreciate being shown thermometers with easy-reading features, as offered by many manufacturers. Always demonstrate how to hold the thermometer for reading, which should be done with the back to good light and the instrument held horizontally in the right hand, about 12 inches from the eyes. The bulb should never be held while reading, but the thermometer may be steadied by the left-hand index finger placed behind it. With the markings to the front, the thermometer should be rotated slowly until the mercury is visible.

CARE OF THE THERMOMETER—After the thermometer has been read and the temperature recorded, it always should be shaken down so that it is ready for use the next time it is needed. In shaking down the mercury column, the thermometer should be grasped firmly between the thumb and the forefinger at the scale end and shaken vigorously by several snaps of the wrist until the reading is below 97°F. This is effective, and a good way to describe this method is to liken it to shaking water off the bulb, which the customer can visualize. The thermometer should *never* be held in the fingers while the hand is struck upon a solid surface to jar down the mercury column. Such rough handling is almost certain to cause a breakage or rupture of the constriction, even though it may appear unbroken. If dropped, even though apparently unbroken, the thermometer should be tested before using. Fever thermometers should never be exposed to heat, the sun's rays, or a heat unit or be displayed in a pharmacy display window.

Currently, there are also available a variety of low-cost, battery-operated electronic fever thermometers, with a visible gauge, that sell for under $10. The most popular is the digital type (Fig 110-32); however, models with analog indicators are available. This type of thermometer gives precise temperature readings within a minute and is safe to use. Most have a *peak hold* feature, so that the maximum temperature attained can be read, and use disposable probe covers for sanitation.

A thermometer designed to make quantitative temperature measurements directly from the surface of the skin has been developed at the University of Colorado, Craig Rehabilitation Hospital. Known as a temporal scanner, this instrument is accurate to within one-tenth of a degree when measuring the difference in heat generated by an arthritic joint and that generated by a healthy tissue. Its probe is about 6 inches long and has about a 5/8 inch diameter. Its hollow aluminum barrel holds a spring mechanism—like a ballpoint pen—that permits the user to exert uniform pressure when measuring skin temperatures.

The new tympanic thermometer (Fig 110-33) can be used on virtually every patient, newborn to elderly. The contoured safety probe of the thermometer is placed snugly into the patient's ear. A sensor on the tip of the probe measures the infrared emissions from the tympanic membrane. The thermometer converts this information into an accurate temperature reading and displays it on a clear liquid-crystal display (LCD) panel in approximately 3 sec.

Color-change thermometers are easy to use, but frequently inaccurate and unreliable. The thermometer is an adhesive strip placed on the skin, usually the forehead, and a heat-sensitive material in the strip changes color in response to the temperature gradient. Skin temperature does not always reflect core temperature, however, and may be influenced by a variety of factors such as the environmental temperature and skin perfusion.

BLOOD-PRESSURE MONITORS

While pharmacies near hospitals and in clinics or large professional buildings have long sold stethoscopes to doctors and nurses and sometimes to patients, increased public interest in health and fitness in general and hypertension in particular has created an ever-growing interest in blood-pressure monitoring devices. Once plain, nurses' stethoscopes now come in many colors and styles, and the sale of stethoscopes and replacement chestpieces, tubing, diaphragms, and eartips to nurses not only brings in additional revenue but also introduces them to all the other health-related accessories offered by the pharmacy.

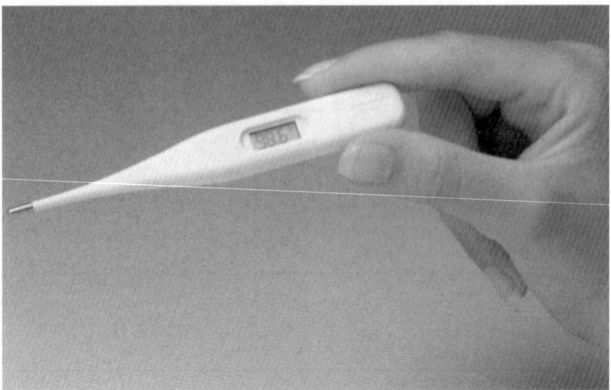

Figure 110-32. Digital electronic thermometer (courtesy, Omron Healthcare).

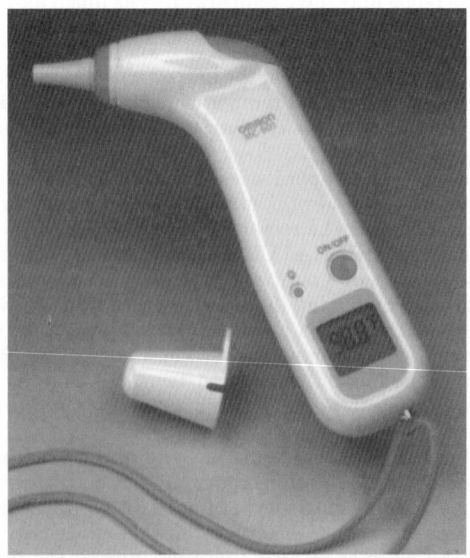

Figure 110-33. Tympanic thermometer (courtesy, Omron Healthcare).

Desk-type mercury sphygmomanometers are still used in professionals' offices, but aneroid models are much more popular. Inexpensive self-taking aneroid models can be purchased for home use. More expensive digital models are available and easy to use, and some even come with printers. Other digital models take systolic and diastolic measurements from the index finger or from compact wristband monitors (Fig 110-34).

A pharmacist can highlight the blood-pressure monitor department by offering free blood-pressure screenings, either on an as-needed basis or specifying a certain morning or afternoon each week. Training in proper techniques for measuring blood pressure may be offered by a local chapter of the American Heart Association.

After taking a subject's blood pressure, the pharmacist or a properly trained associate may choose to record the measurement on a folding wallet card (Fig 110-35). The patient can be advised to return at regular intervals for further readings or encouraged to consult a physician if appropriate. By having the pharmacy name and logo on the opposite side of the folding card, patients are carrying a reminder of the pharmacy in their wallets. Also, if patients show the readings to their physicians, physicians may become more aware of the professional level of services provided by the pharmacy.

BLOOD-GLUCOSE MONITORS

A pharmacy can expand its services to diabetic patients by offering blood-glucose monitoring devices and providing training in proper usage. Models are available that are inexpensive and easy to use at home. Ongoing purchases of the test strips and other supplies used with these monitors can provide opportunities for patients to return to the pharmacy on a regular basis. For more detailed coverage of these devices, their usee and maintenance, the reader is referred to Chapter 125.

TENS

Transcutaneous electrical nerve stimulation (TENS) is an electrical method of controlling pain. It is a safe, nonaddictive, and noninvasive alternative to drug therapy. A TENS unit delivers

Name _____

DATE	TIME	BLOOD PRESSURE	INITIALS
		/	
		/	
		/	
		/	
		/	
		/	
		/	
		/	
		/	
		/	
		/	
		/	
		/	
		/	
		/	

Figure 110-35. Wallet blood-pressure record card.

mild electrical signals through the skin to the underlying nerves to relieve pain by blocking the pain message before it reaches the brain or by causing the body to release pain-relieving endorphins.

A small battery-powered stimulator generates low-intensity electrical impulses to electrodes adhering to the skin. A physician or therapist will determine the stimulation parameters. The pharmacist (who has been trained in TENS usage) will instruct the patient in placement of electrodes and use of lead wires to connect the electrodes to the unit, give instructions on adjusting the level of intensity and the treatment schedule, and advise the client on proper skin care.

Also available are muscle stimulators, which use an electric current to stimulate an atrophied or weakened muscle. This should be done in conjunction with a physical therapist, under the direction of a physician.

BREAST PUMPS

Every year more working mothers who want to continue breast-feeding their babies when they return to work after maternity leave are learning of the availability and advantages of breast pumps. The emergence of women's health issues in the public consciousness has led many employers to accommodate the needs of new mothers who need to breast pump during the workday.

Breast pumps may be used occasionally, as in a day or evening away from the baby, or more regularly, as by a mother who pumps once or twice a day while at work. Babies who are unavailable for any feedings for a period of time (such as premature babies kept in the hospital after the mother is released) may necessitate the mother breast pumping until the baby comes home.

Simple manual pumps are available for occasional use. Electric pumps, including models with convenient compact carrying cases, are recommended for regular pumping. The electric models also can be used with time-saving double-pumping kits that pump both breasts at the same time (Fig 110-36).

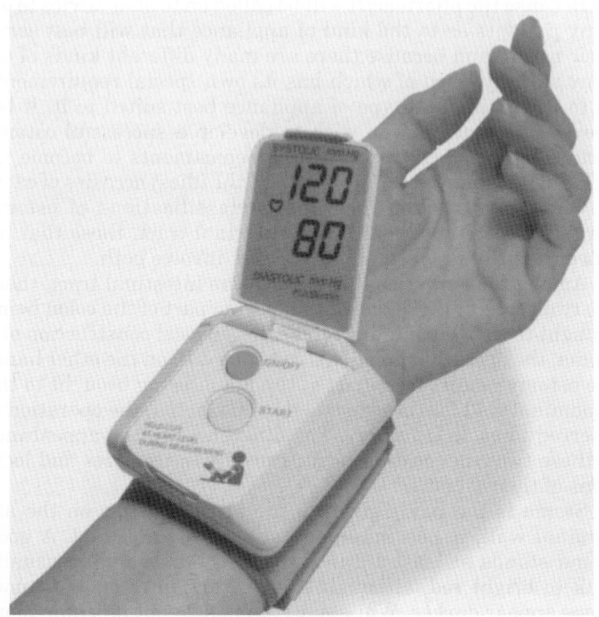

Figure 110-34. Wrist blood-pressure monitor (courtesy, Omron Healthcare).

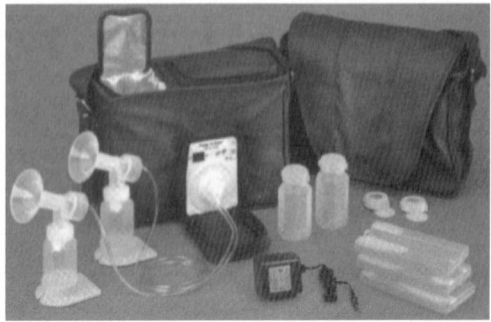

Figure 110-36. Breast pump (courtesy, Medela).

VACUUM CONSTRICTION DEVICES

A nonsurgical solution to impotence is vacuum constriction therapy. Many men are silent, embarrassed, or uneasy about discussing their impotence. Pharmacists can provide the confidential and professional advice essential for the successful use of these devices.

Impotence may result from inadequate blood flow into the penis and/or the inability of blood vessels to retain the blood flowing into the penis. *Osbon Medical Systems* defines therapy as follows: Vacuum constriction involves placing the penis in a patented vacuum cylinder. An erection is achieved by creating a vacuum that generates blood flow into the penis, causing engorgement and rigidity. Similar to the natural erection process, blood flow from the penis then is reduced, using a simple retention device. In this manner an erection can be maintained safely and easily for up to 30 min (Fig 110-37).

IV PHARMACY

Historically, parenteral preparations (see Chapter 41) and IV admixtures (see Chapter 42) were not a normal component of community pharmacy practice. With the rapid increases both in technology and in the demand for care in the home, many pharmacies now prepare and dispense enteral nutrient solutions

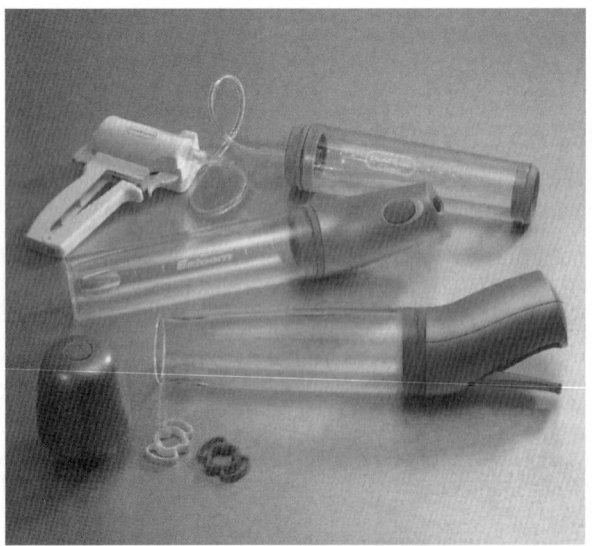

Figure 110-37. ErecAid System Classic, ErecAid System Esteem battery and manual models, and Easy Action ring applicator (courtesy, TIMM Medical Technologies).

and IV solutions such as antibiotics, TPN (total parenteral nutrition), biological modifiers, and other IV solutions.

Because of technological advances, many of the functions of providing IV therapy that traditionally have been provided in a hospital setting can now be replicated in the home, up to and including the complex therapy required by a patient who has been discharged from a hospital after a bone marrow transplant.

Different types of infusion pumps also may be supplied by the pharmacist. Newer models are able to provide for continuous flow (hydration), intermittent flow, or PCA (patient- controlled analgesia). With an intermittent flow, the home-care nurse, on a once-a-day visit, could set the pump to provide a 1-hr medication flow every 4 or 6 hr, or however the physician directs, often with a *keep open* between treatments. Thus, exact treatment schedules set by the physician can be maintained. A pump with a PCA function also should have a lockout device so that patients cannot give themselves more than a specified number of doses within a predetermined time-frame. Some pumps can be connected to a modem so that a pharmacist or nurse off-site can change the dosage. Pumps may have video screens (which can be connected to a laptop computer or a printer) that can monitor how often PCA patients give or attempt to give themselves more medication.

Pharmaceuticals given IV always should be provided with the assistance of a home-care nurse (either on staff or from a home-nursing agency). It is essential that there are always open lines of communication between the physician, the pharmacist, and the home-care nurse.

OSTOMY APPLIANCES AND SUPPLIES

UNDERSTANDING THE OSTOMY—An ostomy is a surgical procedure whereby parts of the intestinal and/or urinary tract are removed from the patient, the remaining end(s) then are brought to the abdominal wall and a stoma (Gk, mouth) or artificial opening, is constructed surgically through which urine or feces will pass from then on.

It is estimated that more than 80,000 such operations are performed annually in the US, most resulting in the saving of lives. There are approximately a million Americans now living who have had such surgery, and each one of them is buying appliances and supplies on a regular basis.

Because the pharmacist will be called on to offer advice to ostomy patients as to the kind of appliance that will best serve their needs, and because there are many different kinds of ostomy surgery, each of which has its own special requirements as to the fitting and type of appliance best suited to it, it behooves pharmacists who wish to develop a successful ostomy section in their health-accessories departments to become familiar with every type of surgery and the idiosyncrasies of each.

One could develop three basic classifications of ostomy surgery: those that involve the intestinal tract, those that involve the urinary tract, and those that involve both.

Among the surgeries that involve the intestinal tract, there are two types. If the ostomy results from part of the colon being brought to the abdominal wall for the surgical construction of a stoma, the operation is called a *colostomy*. If, on the other hand, the ostomy results from part of the ileum being brought to the abdominal wall for the construction of a stoma, the operation is referred to as an *ileostomy*. The differences in the appearance of these two categories consist primarily in the sizes and locations of their stomas.

Stoma is the name given to the artificial anus on the abdominal wall; it has the appearance of a small bud. A good stoma stands at least 1/2 inch above the skin and is usually pink to bright red, although stomas vary in color and sometimes appear darker. While most stomas do not protrude more than about 1/2 inch, there are some that may have been constructed so that they protrude an inch or more. But a pharmacist who observes a stoma that protrudes more than 1 1/2 inch should question the patient as to whether it was that long shortly following the surgery. In cases in which the length of the stoma has changed drastically since the surgery, the chances are that it has become prolapsed, and the patient should be advised to consult his/her physician for possible corrective surgery to avoid the potentiality of strangulation of the intestine. It also is possible for a stoma to *shrink* back into the body. When it becomes inverted, management can become very difficult, and corrective surgery may be indicated. Also, corrective surgery may be necessary if intestinal stomas become too small. An indication that this is happening might be a patient needing appliances with smaller and smaller openings.

Stomas appear red because surgeons invert the end of the intestine slightly when they bring it to the outside of the abdominal wall. After suturing the intestine to the abdominal skin, it becomes an integral part of the body wall, and all tissues live normally. Actually, the red surface of an ostomy stoma is the intestinal capillary bed; it stays red because blood continues to flow through it. As it is also a mucous membrane, it will continue to stay wet.

As most ileostomies result in the entire colon being separated from the small intestine at a point just behind the ileocecal valve (where the ileum joins the cecum), that is usually where the incision is made in the abdominal wall and where the ileum is brought to the outside of the body. The location of the ileocecal valve is near the appendix, in the abdomen's lower-right quadrant, and where an ileostomy stoma typically is located. Because the stoma in an ileostomy is constructed from the small intestine, it will be smaller than the colostomy stoma, which is made from the colon. However, it is important to note that the location of stomas on the outside of the body cannot be standardized as colostomy on the left side and ileostomy on the right side.

Placement of the stoma is determined by body folds, the waistline, bony prominences, old scar tissue, and the person's occupation. The fecal matter or output indicates what type of surgery was performed.

In a colostomy, only part of the colon is removed from the body. The types of colostomies depend upon where the diseased part of the colon is separated from the healthy part of the colon. When only the juncture of the sigmoid colon with the rectum and anus is involved, the surgeon brings the sigmoid colon to the surface of the abdomen and the surgery is termed a *sigmoid colostomy*. When the separation occurs along the length of the descending colon, anywhere between the splenic flexure (the bend where the transverse colon meets the descending colon) and the sigmoid flexure, the operation is called a *descending colostomy*. Accordingly, when the surgeon makes the separation along the length of the transverse colon anywhere between the splenic flexure and the hepatic flexure (where the transverse and ascending colon meet), the surgery is termed a *transverse colostomy;* an *ascending colostomy* occurs between the hepatic flexure and the cecum. Finally, when the stoma is constructed with that part of the colon called the cecum, the surgery is simply called a *cecostomy*.

These five surgeries, while they are all colostomies, are distinctly different from each other in that different lengths of colon remain in patients having different types of colostomies. Because a primary function of the colon is the removal of water from the feces as it passes through it, it is understandable that the feces produced at a cecostomy stoma will be quite loose and watery, while the feces produced at a sigmoid colostomy stoma are generally quite solid. Likewise, the ascending, transverse, and descending colostomies produce feces, within the extremes just described, of varying degrees of consistency. The additional fact that all colostomies, because of the reservoir effect of the colon still remaining, can be managed better than ileostomies in which there is no reservoir remaining has implications for the pharmacist with regard to the types of appliances that are best suited for each type of ostomy.

The implications are that different colostomies in particular, and intestinal ostomies in general, because of differences in fe-

cal products, create nonidentical problems for the patient, i.e., not all colostomies can be irrigated successfully, they require different types of appliances, and they use different kinds of accessories. There is very little difference in the size of the stomas of each of the five colostomies, but they may be located on the abdominal wall differently. Colostomy stomas, which usually are located in the lower-left quadrant of the patient's abdomen tend toward more-solid feces, while those usually located in the lower-right quadrant tend toward feces that contain more water and are, therefore, of looser consistency. The most common reasons for performing a colostomy are cancer of the lower bowel, trauma, and ruptured diverticula.

When the entire colon must be removed, the surgeon performs an *ileostomy* by separating the colon from the small intestine behind the ileocecal valve. The result is a stoma much smaller than any colostomy stoma, located in the lower-right quadrant and producing fecal material that is always loose and watery. Most ileostomies are performed on people between the ages of 18 and 40 and are usually the result of an ulceration of the inner lining of the colon that is called ulcerative colitis.

There are several types of urinary diversions, the most common being those in which the patient's bladder must be removed. The preferred surgical procedure brings the two ureters together, implants them in an artificial bladder, and enables the patient to have but one stoma to manage and one appliance to wear instead of the usual two.

This operation is frequently referred to as an *ileal bladder, ileal conduit,* or *urinary diversion*. All three names indicate the same operation, however.

During this operation, the surgeon removes a piece of the healthy small intestine at the ileum and then performs a resection of the two ends of the ileum, joining them together again. The missing piece is usually between 6 and 8 inches and is a relatively insignificant loss to the small intestine, which measures nearly 24 ft in the average adult. One end of the piece of ileum is closed, and the other is brought to the outside of the body to become the single stoma. Once the two ureters are implanted in the closed end of the piece of ileum, that piece becomes a conduit for the urine—actually a substitute bladder. Because this conduit or bladder is made from a piece of the ileum, it has earned the names ileal conduit and ileal bladder.

The stoma has the appearance of an ileostomy stoma and, usually, is located within the same quadrant, the lower right, but its product is only urine. While most ileostomy stomas are located in the lower half of the lower-right quadrant of the abdomen, most ileal conduit stomas are located in the upper half of the lower-right quadrant. The only way to be sure which ostomy is which is to determine the nature of the waste product.

When the two ureters are severed or cannot be brought forward to the abdominal wall for any reason, the surgeon is forced to bring the ureters to the nearest outside surface—the patient's back. Stomas appearing on the dorsal side or openings through which renal catheters lead directly to the kidneys, indicate an operation called a *nephrostomy*. Persons with bilateral nephrostomies wear two appliances.

In a cystostomy, the bladder wall is brought to the skin, and a stoma is formed. This often is done for paraplegics and quadriplegics. The stoma is just above the symphysis pubis. The stoma for a vesicotomy, in which the urethra is brought directly to the surface of the skin, would be very similar in appearance to that of a cystostomy. Vesicotomies are often temporary operations and are rarely of concern to the pharmacist. There are two other ostomies that are temporary and with which the pharmacist should be familiar. One is a modified kind of descending colostomy in which the lower portion of the descending colon, sigmoid colon, and rectum are not removed from the patient. After the surgical separation is made, both ends of the colon are brought to the outside and two stomas are constructed, one active and the other inactive.

This operation, the *double-barrel colostomy,* results in two stomas, side-by-side, normally located in the lower-left quadrant and producing solid fecal material exactly like the ordinary descending colostomy. This condition may last from 1 month to a year or longer, depending entirely on when the surgeon is satisfied that a resection can be performed without further complication. Sometimes the double-barrel colostomy is performed in the hope that the lower bowel can be brought back to normal with treatment and rest. On occasion, a patient with a double-barrel colostomy must return to the hospital for a permanent colostomy.

The second kind of temporary colostomy is called a *loop colostomy*. Normally, patients who have a loop colostomy performed will have the colon repaired and back to normal within a few weeks and before they leave the hospital. Loop-colostomy appliances are applied during surgery by the physician and are the only ostomy appliances that are packaged sterile, besides the common postoperative drain. This ostomy gets its name from the fact that, unlike the double-barrel colostomy, the loop colostomy doesn't result in the complete separation of the intestine but, rather, a loop of intestine is brought through an incision and temporarily is secured to the abdominal wall by means of a plastic or silicone rod that is slipped under the loop and across the incision; the loop then is perforated surgically to relieve the impaction. The wound stays open, and the loop remains visible until the perforation in the intestine is closed and the loop is returned to its normal position within the visceral cavity. It is highly unlikely that a pharmacist will ever be called upon to fit a loop-colostomy appliance although he or she may still want to stock the appliances for use by the hospital.

CHOOSING THE RIGHT APPLIANCE—The various ostomies described above can be grouped into three major categories for the purpose of understanding which kinds of appliances are most appropriate for each.

1. Those ostomies that only produce solid waste at their stomas. They include the sigmoid colostomy, descending colostomy, transverse colostomy, double-barrel colostomy, and often the loop colostomy.
2. Those ostomies that only produce urine at their stomas. They include the cutaneous ureterostomy, nephrostomy, cystostomy, vesicotomy, and urostomy.
3. Those ostomies that, for one reason or another, produce liquid or semisolid fecal matter at their stomas. They include the ileostomy, cecostomy, ascending colostomy and sometimes the loop colostomy.

In real life, neat and perfectly reliable categories such as the ones just described do not exist. People differ, their digestive processes are different, and their diets are different. The consistency of the waste matter in any one individual also varies from day to day. Yet these categories are useful generally, and in addition, they point up the fact that an appliance should be chosen primarily for the nature of the waste matter it will have to collect.

Further, the groupings do indicate that among a host of ostomy appliances presently on the market from numerous manufacturers, there are just three basic types, categorized primarily by the nature of the waste material for which they are intended: those designed for pure urine, for semisolids, and for solid waste matter. Other considerations in choosing the right appliance for each patient include the size of gasket openings that fit around the stoma, method of attaching the appliance around the stoma, patient's financial resources (including what reimbursement limits may be placed either on types, quantities, or cost of appliances by government agencies such as Medicare and medical-assistance programs or by HMOs or insurance companies), and activities in which the patient engages at work or at play (Fig 110-38).

OSTOMY APPLIANCES FOR SOLID WASTES—The colostomy appliance, so-called because most colostomies are solid-waste-producing, is the appliance used for most colostomies. There are many types of colostomy appliances on the market, recognizable by larger-size gasket openings to accommodate the larger stomas characteristic of all colostomies and by detachable, throwaway pouches made of thin polyethylene plastic; some are sealed at their bottoms. However, some

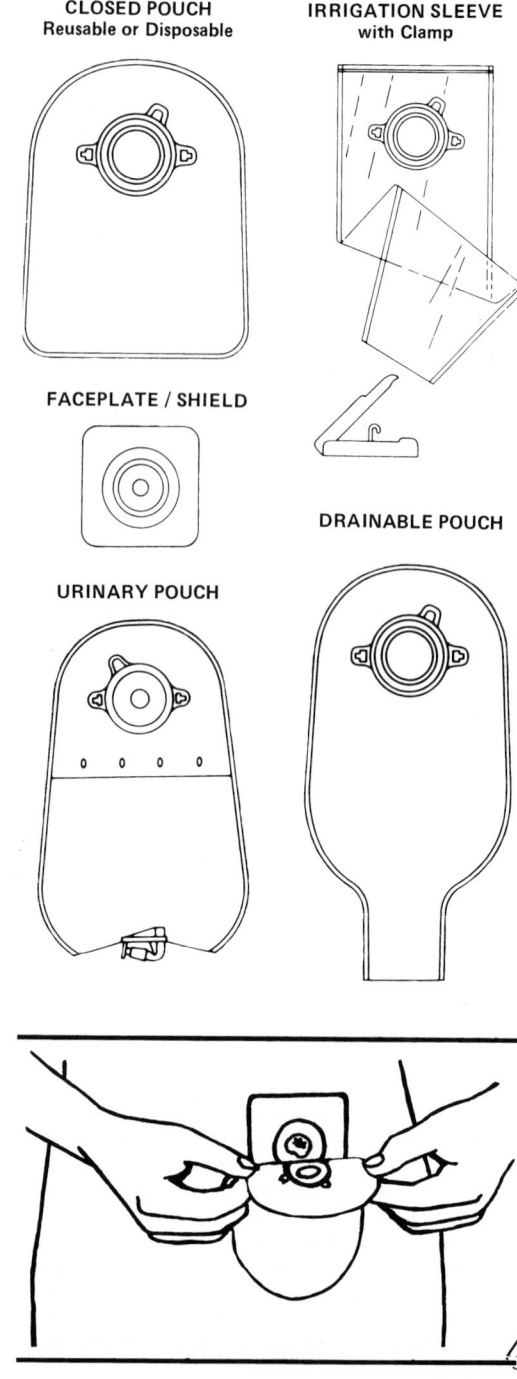

Figure 110-38. Ostomy appliances (courtesy, Convatec).

colostomates do use open-ended pouches. The fact that these pouches are sealed at the bottom and are disposable indicates the impracticability of bottom drains for solid wastes generally. By and large, colostomy appliances are not the permanent type, since the ostomies that produce solid wastes do not cause the problems with skin excoriation typical of the wetter ostomies.

The self-adhesive colostomy appliance is more of a collection bag with adhesive around the stoma opening than it is an appliance. The openings may be cut with scissors to fit the stoma precisely, though most manufacturers provide several sizes. The advantages with this type of appliance are that it is lightweight and quite flat against the body so it is less likely to show through clothing. Those colostomates who irrigate regularly find this type of appliance perfect for safety's sake.

Some colostomates are urged by their physicians to irrigate on a regular basis. Irrigation is the process of administering an enema to the colon via the stoma for the purpose of establishing regular, conveniently timed, evacuation of the bowel—in other words, to become relatively stool-free. It is necessary just once a day at the most and may be scheduled in the morning before dressing or in the evening before retiring. It is a highly individual thing, and some persons need to irrigate only every other day or two to three times a week. Some persons have quite irritable bowels and cannot remain stool-free.

After irrigation, the colostomate can expect to have no bowel activity until the next irrigation, except perhaps for slight dripping now and then. Many ostomates, after irrigation, wear only a gauze pad over the stoma for safety and psychological confidence. The pad can be taped over the stoma or secured with a two-way stretch wraparound.

The irrigation process is quite simple and takes up to an hour for completion. The important steps include:

The stoma should be dilated with a gloved finger (finger cot) and a bit of lubricating jelly prior to insertion of the irrigator cone.

About 1 quart of tepid water (some patients add a couple of tablespoons of salt) is placed in the irrigating bag—never hung more than head high. About 15 min should be allowed before permitting evacuation; after the initial gush it normally takes another 20 to 25 min before the colon is really empty.

Most people close the end of the irrigating sleeve with a clamp and then shower or shave during this period.

Sometimes drinking a cup of strong black coffee or a glass of ice-cold water will start the intestinal peristalsis necessary for complete evacuation.

Irrigation is a technique for accomplishing regularity and security throughout the day but is only useful in those ostomies that produce solid wastes. Many physicians and enterostomal therapists now are recognizing the importance of diet in gaining control and regularity of bowel movements and irrigation. The question of whether or not a particular colostomy patient should irrigate should be answered only by the physician or enterostomal therapist (ET) nurse. Irrigation usually is not advised when the possibility of reconnecting the intestine at a later date exists.

APPLIANCES FOR URINE AND SEMISOLIDS—The appliances used for urinary diversions and ileostomies are both similar to the appliances used for colostomies (Fig 110-38). A notable difference is in the size of the stoma openings (because urostomy and ileostomy stomas are usually much smaller than colostomy stomas). Also, since the discharge from either a urinary diversion or an ileostomy is more liquid than that from most colostomies, there is more often a need for skin barriers and protectants such as karaya, Stomahesive, and similar products to maintain a waterproof seal.

The real difference between a urinary appliance and an appliance for semisolids is in their bottoms, however. Where the urinary appliance has a nylon twist-drain plug in the bottom, the *ileostomy* appliance merely narrows down to between 1½ to 2½ inches and is just open. The bottom is closed with a clip. To drain, the clip is removed, and the bottom of the appliance unfolded.

Different manufacturers make appliances that, although basically similar in design or function, differ with respect to method of securing to the skin. In the past, urinary and ileostomy appliances often were made of rubber and secured to the skin with adhesives. Periodically, these appliances had to be removed, often with the help of an adhesive remover. The appliances then had to be cleaned, dried out, and reapplied. Some ostomates still use permanent appliances of this type, but most new ostomates choose the disposable type.

OSTOMY APPLIANCE ACCESSORIES—Most popular among a host of accessories for ostomy appliances of all kinds are pectin-based or karaya gum washers, Stomahesive powder,

and Stomahesive and similar barrier pastes. These pastes can be used to fill in irregularities in skin surfaces to protect against leakage.

Varieties of deodorant drops, tablets, and sprays are available; some are applied to the outside of the appliance, while others are dropped into the bag prior to applying it. Most ostomy appliances now have odorproof barriers. Silicone and benzoin tincture sprays also may be used to prepare the skin around the stoma. In addition, racks for drying an appliance after washing, abdominal dressings and cover sponges, gloves and wipes, and even zippered, purse-size pouches for supplies are available to make things easier for the ostomate. Some manufacturers now offer new easy-to-apply appliances featuring synthetic materials to reduce skin irritation and prevent leakage.

But perhaps the most helpful things that pharmacists can provide their patients who have ostomies are suggestions and ideas on how to manage themselves with a minimum of difficulty. Knowledge of these things will come from the ostomates themselves, and it is therefore wise to spend some time asking them questions. It is also important for a pharmacist featuring ostomy-care products to develop a good working relationship with an ET, a nurse specially trained in ostomy care. The ET can advise the pharmacist or the patient when unexpected problems occur. Membership in a local ostomy club or the United Ostomy Association is another way to increase your knowledge of the problems ostomates often encounter.

UROLOGY AND INCONTINENCE SUPPLIES

URINALS—These containers are employed to collect urine. They differ in shape according to male or female use. They ordinarily are made of white enamelware or plastic, which is by far the most common, especially for use at home. Plastic urinals come in two basic types: single-patient use or autoclavable.

CATHETERS—To collect urine from the patient unable to void naturally or when incontinence pants and external catheters are inadequate, indwelling catheters are employed.

The insertion of catheters is a dangerous procedure, customarily handled by physicians or trained nurses and orderlies. Serious infections of the bladder and damage to the urethral and bladder tissues may result from improper insertion.

Flexible soft-rubber catheters consist of small rubber tubes with a closed solid tip. At one end is a flaring funnel-shaped opening to facilitate attachment of the catheter to a plastic junction or another tube leading to a collection unit. At the inserted end is a wide opening that leads to the channel through which urine flows to the collection unit. This is referred to as a straight catheter, in contrast to the indwelling catheter, which is designed to remain in the urethra for long periods of time.

The indwelling retention catheter, or Foley catheter as it is commonly known, is characterized by a balloon at its insertion end (Fig 110-39). The balloon is designed to secure the catheter tip within the patient's bladder to keep it from slipping or being pulled out. There are two channels that run from the insertion tip to the end of the Foley catheter—one for the passing of urine and the other for the injection of sterile water that inflates the balloon.

Foley catheters are available with either 5- or 30-mL balloons. The 30-mL balloon catheter, which also is known as a hemostatic catheter, is used commonly in nursing homes for patients whose urethras have become dilated or for those patients who have pulled the 5-mL balloon catheter out. A common

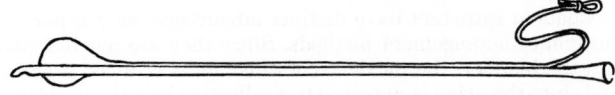

Figure 110-39. Balloon catheter, for prolonged insertion through the urethra into the bladder.

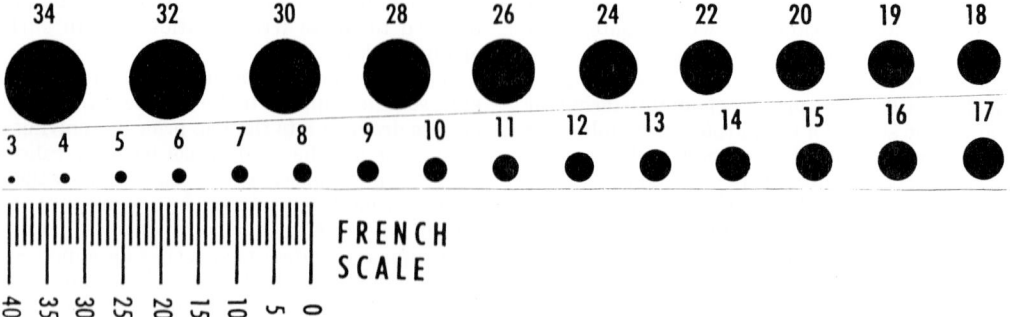

Figure 110-40. Standard French scale for hospital tubing and catheters as well as rectal and colon, stomach-feeding, suction, urinary drainage, and oxygen tubes (courtesy, Becton-Dickinson). To determine the French size if instruments are oval or other shape, use a strip of paper to measure the periphery—then lay on the scale at the left.

mistake in filling a balloon catheter is to use too little water. It takes about 10 mL to inflate a 5-mL Foley balloon because nearly 5 mL is held in the filling lumen that runs the length of the catheter. The diameters of the catheter also vary in size. Though their use is limited somewhat, 75-mL balloon retention catheters are also available. The French scale is employed most commonly (Fig 110-40).

Other innovations in the urinary catheter include a Foley catheter with its own supply of sterile water for balloon inflation. With these catheters, a valve is released following insertion of the catheter, and the sterile water, which is under pressure, runs up its channel and inflates the balloon. They are especially convenient, as there is no need to prepare a syringe for balloon inflation, but they are considerably more expensive than the typical Foley catheter. Another improvement is the silicone and Teflon coatings on the outside and inside of Foley catheters. Such coatings not only cut down friction during insertion and removal of the catheter, but also inhibit buildup of deposits on catheter walls, thus extending the time between catheter changes and reducing irritating infection and leakage problems. The newest improvement is the all-silicone catheter, now manufactured by Kendall, Bard, and others.

The pharmacy also may stock a variety of urine-collection units and catheter administration trays. The bladder-care tray, sometimes called a *cathtray*, is a sterile package containing the items required during the administration of a Foley catheter, packed sequentially with those things needed first on top.

Male condom catheters and female external catheters are designed to be worn by the patient. They allow mobility and discrete urinary collection without the use of pads or an indwelling catheter. These external types of collection systems are becoming more widely used and are available in a number of different styles. The style selected is usually a matter of personal preference, activity level, and size and capacity requirements.

The male condom catheter system consists of two parts: the penile sheath, which resembles a condom with a drainage opening, and a collection bag. The single-use condom catheter may be self-adhesive or attach with an adhesive foam strap. The reuseable style is secured with an adjustable rubber or foam strap worn over the catheter. These are not as secure, but are considerably more cost-effective.

External female catheters are not reliably successful in containing urine. The device consists of a pouch with a sticky wafer that is attached to the vulva; the end of the pouch is connected to a larger drainage bag.

Condom catheters have distinct advantages over other incontinence management methods. Since they are not inserted into the bladder, the incidence of infection is reduced greatly. And since the urine is conveyed to a collection bag, the problems of odor and skin breakdown associated with diapers and absorbent pads are minimized.

It is advisable for the pharmacist to inquire as to whether the patient has an allergy to latex. Finding the right urological products is a big problem for patients with latex allergies.

URINARY BAGS—There are two basic types of urinary bags: leg bags and night urinary collection bags. Both can be used with external or indwelling catheter systems.

Leg bags vary in size and capacity and are used by a patient who is ambulatory. The bag is connected to the catheter by a length of plastic or rubber tubing (usually sold separately). The bag itself is worn on the inside of the thigh or lower leg, whichever is most comfortable and least conspicuous. It is secured in place by use of adjustable elastic straps. A common error is to fasten the leg straps so they encircle the bag, thus restricting its volume.

Night urinary collection bags vary in style. The standard is a bag that hangs from the side of the bed or the back of the wheelchair. The standard capacity is 2000 mL. Night bags are also available in a cube or a bottle form.

INCONTINENCE PANTS—A variety of body-contoured incontinence pants are available for both men and women. Disposables are the most popular, with a variety of absorbancies being available.

Other products helpful for the incontinent patient include disposable underpads, adult diapers, rubber sheeting, silicone skin sprays, and body lotions and deodorants. Perineal washing solutions are available for cleaning skin. Their advantages are deodorizing, disinfecting, and maintaining the skin's normal acidity and moisture content and ease of use. The skin may be protected with skin barriers.

TRUSSES

Hernias and trusses are as old as mankind. A truss is defined as a supportive device, usually consisting of a pad with a belt, worn to prevent enlargement of a hernia or the return of a reduced hernia. A hernia is defined as the protrusion of an organ or bodily structure through the wall that normally contains it.

The first trusses were nothing more than a rope or strap and a rock. Celsus developed the use of a plate, and in medieval times a form of plaster and plate were used. The spring-and-belt-type truss, practically as it is today in principle, was developed by the Netherlands physician Camper in 1785.

There are several types of hernias. One is the protrusion of the intestine and its surrounding membrane, the peritoneum, through a natural opening in the abdominal wall and may be inguinal, scrotal or femoral, depending upon the site of the protrusion. Other hernias, incisional hernias, are the result of a protrusion through the muscles of the abdomen usually occurring at a point previously weakened. An incisional hernia occurs at the site of a previous surgical incision. The natural openings in the abdominal musculature through which a true

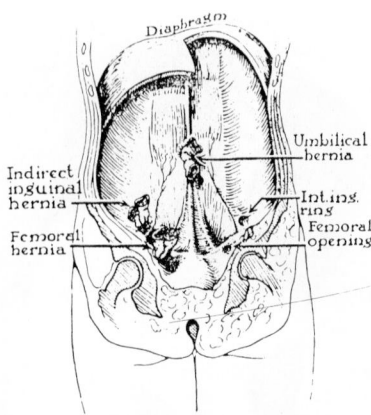

Figure 110-41. Looking toward the front of the abdominal wall, from within the cavity, showing the five congenitally weak points.

hernia may occur include the umbilical opening; the inguinal openings, through which, in the male, the spermatic cord passes, and in the female, the round ligament passes; and the openings for the femoral arteries (Fig 110-41).

Abdominal or umbilical hernias are common. Infants in the first year of life show an incidence of 19.6/1000. Between ages 20 and 24, the incidence is lowest, rising to 24.2/1000 in the 70- to 74-year age group.

Of all males afflicted with hernias, 96% suffer from the inguinal type. The corresponding incidence of inguinal hernias among females is just 44.3%. While surgery is the preferred treatment for all hernias, it is not always the best solution for all patients. Some will require trusses in lieu of surgery.

Hernia trusses of all kinds vary from soft-fabric supports (not actually capable of holding a true hernia!) to models containing a metal or steel band and requiring experienced judgment on the part of the fitter. The type and location of truss pads and the weight and build of the patient are important considerations in truss fitting. All trusses should be fitted while the patient is lying down and the hernia is reduced (the protruding intestine has been returned to the abdominal cavity) or the truss itself may cause strangulation.

A well-fitted truss, appropriate to the specific patient and the specific type of hernia, may be tested by having the patient bend, stoop, and cough. If the patient can do those things without having a protrusion of the intestine past the truss pad, it is likely that it is fitted properly. Finally, it is important for pharmacists to teach patients how to properly put on the truss and test its security while they are in the fitting room, so they can remove it with confidence when they are on their own.

FITTING SCHOOLS—The pharmacist who will be in charge of the truss and orthopedic department should attend a fitting school. This may require time and travel, but it basically trains the pharmacist in the anatomy involved, and appliance selection and fitting skills, which are absolutely necessary. Several good schools are conducted by surgical-appliance manufacturers and typically run 3 to 5 days. Such programs are presented by the Camp Institute of Applied Technology, Surgical Appliance Industry, Freeman, and others. Professional organizations such as the National Community Pharmacists Association (an ACPE provider) also conduct continuing education programs.

No pharmacist or pharmacy employee should attempt any truss or orthopedic fitting involving shaping metal without proper training.

Attendance at one of these schools provides background on the definition, location, varieties, frequency, symptoms, causes, complications, and treatment of conditions that could result in the use of these types of surgical appliances:

Orthopedic corsets
Spinal braces
Cervical collars and braces
Knee, ankle, and foot orthoses
Traction equipment
Compression hosiery
Trusses
Mastectomy prostheses
The interested pharmacist should refer to literature available from appliance manufacturers.

ORTHOPEDIC SUPPORTS AND BRACES

The spinal column can be divided into five major sections:

The cervical spine, consisting of 7 vertebrae, supports the head and is characterized by an anterior curve.
The thoracic spine, consisting of 12 vertebrae with a pair of ribs attached to each, is characterized by a posterior curve.
The lumbar spine, consisting of 5 vertebrae, is characterized by an anterior curve.
The sacrum, consisting of 5 vertebrae that are joined so tightly as to appear as one bone, is situated beneath the fifth lumbar vertebra and between the two innominate bones of the pelvis forming the sacroiliac joints and is characterized by a posterior curve.
The coccyx, consisting of 3 to 5 vertebrae is immediately beneath the sacrum and continues its posterior curve (Fig 110-42A).

Apart from the cervical spine, anomalies of the spinal column include lordosis, a hyperextension of the lumbar spine recognizable as swayback; kyphosis, a flexion of the lumbar spine and/or hyperextension of the thoracic spine, often appearing as hunchback; and scoliosis, an S-shaped lateral curve of the spine (Fig 110-42B). Each of these conditions, in varying degree, often requires use of supportive garments or braces. Sometimes ruptures of the intervertebral discs, the cartilaginous shock-absorbing cushions between separate vertebrae, interfere with the spinal cord or the nerves leading from it. An example is sciatica, in which a ruptured intervertebral disc causes compression or trauma at the base of the sciatic nerve resulting in extreme pain at the back of the thigh and running down the inside of the leg along the course of the sciatic nerve. This condition also may require the use of a spinal garment or brace and, occasionally, the occurrence of spondylolisthesis (the slippage of lower vertebrae usually against the sacrum) will bring the patient to the pharmacy with a prescription for a garment or brace-fitting.

These and other conditions create a need for spinal braces and orthopedic garments to limit motion in the spine and permit healing. While pharmacists should be knowledgeable about them, they should never diagnose such conditions or prescribe

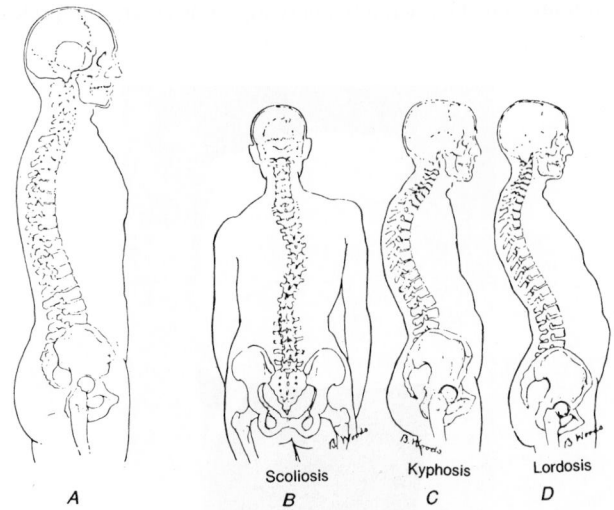

Figure 110-42. *A,* Curves of the normal spine; *B–D,* abnormal curves of the spine.

the wearing of an orthopedic appliance. That should be left entirely to the physician. Unhappy consequences can be avoided and the surgical-appliance business strengthened if the pharmacist will adhere to the simple rule of never fitting any brace or support except on the prescription of a physician.

The most commonly prescribed back supports fitted in a pharmacy setting are the industrial back supports made of neoprene or heavy elastic (sometimes with shoulder straps). They provide support to, and somewhat limit mobility of, the lower spine. Orthopedic back corsets have a back length of 12 to 15 inches and are made of heavy, cloth material or elastic (Fig 110-43). They often feature two or four rigid metal stays that the fitter will shape to the physician's order, usually to the contour of the patient's back. Readymade spinal braces often are similar in principle to corsets but are generally of heavier construction. Braces limit mobility to a greater degree than orthopedic corsets. A custom-made or fitted body jacket would limit mobility even more than a spinal brace. The proper fitting of spinal braces and body jackets would probably require the expertise of a skilled orthotist.

The procedures for fitting different orthopedic supports and braces are quite involved and are better covered in the week-long schools presented by manufacturers than in a few paragraphs in this text.

Conditions affecting the cervical spine often result in a prescription for a cervical collar or brace. The most popular type is a soft-foam collar with a *Velcro* closure. Unless the prescriber specifies flexion or extension, the fitter usually would select a collar that provided support to hold the head in a neutral position. A more rigid plastic collar (Philadelphia type) can be adjusted to the contours of the patient's neck, chin, and shoulders. This type will provide a greater degree of immobilization than a soft collar. Still more immobilization can be obtained by the application of a properly fitted metal cervical brace.

The use of cervical-traction devices also is specified often in the treatment of conditions affecting the cervical spine.

Supports for the knee can vary from a simple pull-on elastic type as found in many pharmacies, to 10- or 11-inch-long braces with shaped metal hinges and leather straps, to complex braces such as an ACL knee orthosis (Fig 110-44).

COMPRESSION THERAPY—Many types of compression hosiery are available in pharmacy health-accessory departments. Lightweight, fashion-sheer elastic hosiery is very popular but does not give as much support as heavier, surgical-weight hosiery. For severe or unusual conditions, custom-made elastic supports for arm or leg (such as Jobst, Fig 110-45) can be ordered. Antiembolism hosiery is intended primarily for bedfast patients.

Taking the patient into a private fitting room, measuring the limb, and then actually applying the hose are the profes-

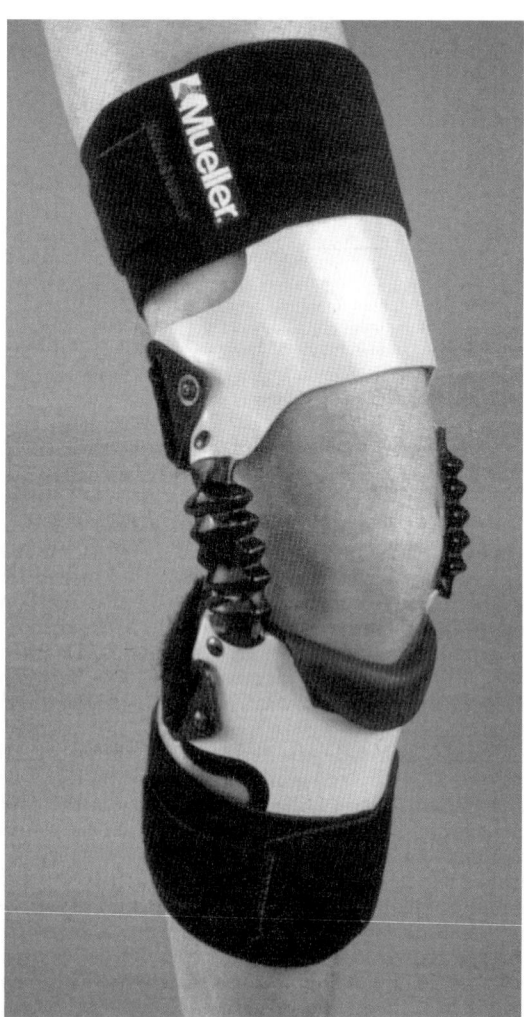

Figure 110-44. Magnum competition ACL knee brace (courtesy, Mueller Sports Medicine).

sional activities that will differentiate qualified health-care-accessories pharmacists from their peers. It should be noted that the best time to measure and fit elastic compression hosiery is early in the morning when the affected limb is likely to be the least distended.

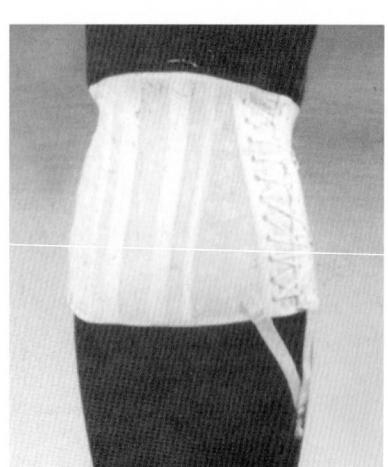

Figure 110-43. Lumbosacral support (courtesy, Camp).

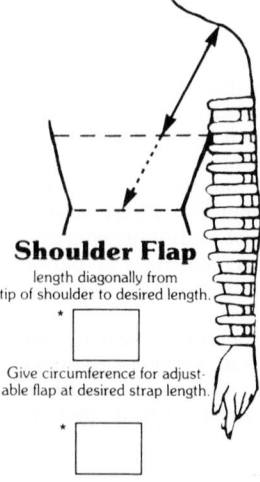

Figure 110-45. Custom-made elastic support (courtesy, Jobst).

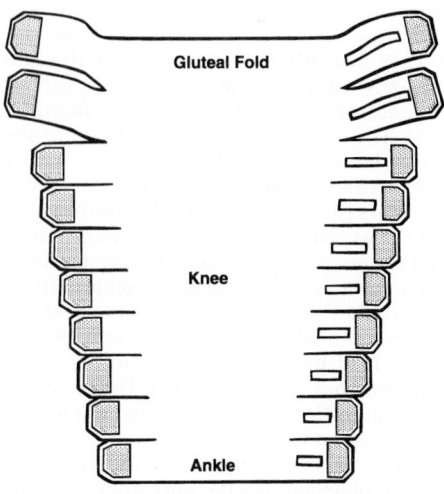

**Inside view
Quick-Fit Thigh-High Legging**

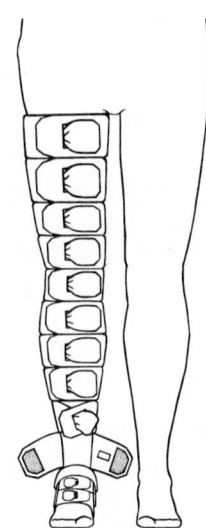

**Quick-Fit Thigh-High Legging
with Ankle-Foot Wrap**

Figure 110-46. Circ Aid Quick-Fit thigh-high legging (courtesy, Circ Aid Medical Products).

A nonelastic form of compression therapy is the CircAid system of nonelastic, adjustable, interlocking bands that give patients the ability to maintain compression levels regardless of changes in limb size or physical ability (Fig 110-46).

Recent advances in the treatment and management of primary and secondary lymphedema with the use of multicompartmental pneumatic compressors has done much to improve the quality of life for people suffering from lymphedema. Pneumatic compression devices are designed to reduce lymphedema in the extremity by applying pressure sequentially through a multicell pneumatic arm or leg sleeve. The pneumatic sleeve inflates in a distal to proximal direction, promoting the flow of lymph fluid through existing lymphatics by exerting pressure on the interstitial tissue. Because the sequential milking pattern is soothing and comfortable, it results in excellent patient compliance.

To maintain the results obtained by home treatments with a multicell compression device, graduated compression hosiery is recommended. The lymphedema garments should be worn during periods of activity to prevent the rapid reaccumulation of lymphatic fluid. Patients should be measured after they have begun their treatments and have achieved some reduction in swelling. Periodic remeasuring is necessary to monitor further reduction.

In some cases, such as severe edema, the physician also may prescribe a lymphedema pump and sleeve to reduce the edema prior to applying compression hosiery. Usually, pumps are rented, although sales are not uncommon. Lymphedema pumps, particularly the sequential types, should be rented or sold only by qualified professionals who are very familiar with their uses and contraindications.

The Reid Sleeve is an alternative method of providing compression therapy. The Reid Sleeve applies a gentle gradient pressure with a unique, soft-foam insert. Compression is tailored to the patient's needs by a series of adjustable straps. The sleeve easily slides over the affected limb, and then the compression bands are adjusted. A specially designed gage is as easy to use as a blood-pressure cuff. This simple procedure ensures that compression applied to the patient's limb is applied consistently and in the proper range to provide optimal results. Patients can fit the sleeve in minutes without assistance and have the confidence of knowing they are applying the pressure prescribed by their doctor. As the patient improves, the Reid

Sleeve can be adjusted to the new arm size, thereby maintaining the proper pressure range (Fig 110-47).

MASTECTOMY PROSTHESES—The fitting of mastectomy prostheses and bras is often a logical adjunct to an orthopedic corset and compression hosiery section in a pharmacy's health-accessories department. It is essential to have a female fitter for this department.

In most cases, breast surgery is the result of breast cancer. Some surgeries, such as a lumpectomy, remove only a portion of the breast. A *simple* mastectomy results in the removal of breast tissue. More-involved surgery results in removal of breast tissue and additional underlying tissue.

A variety of breast forms are available to fit a woman after each type of surgery, although it is often difficult to fit a woman after a lumpectomy. (Note: Male breast cancer, while rare, does occur.) The breast form is designed not only to help restore a woman's shape, but also to replace the weight lost and restore proper balance.

Although more women are selecting reconstruction each year, external breast forms remain a safe alternative. There have been many advances in the technology of manufacturing the forms, resulting in more-comfortable, natural-feeling breast prostheses. Although some forms are made with polyester fiberfill or foam, most are made with silicone. Conventional silicone forms generally are designed to be worn in conjunction with a specially designed pocketed bra that holds the breast form securely in place.

A new development in silicone breast prostheses allows the form to attach safely and securely directly to the chest wall by means of an adhesive skin support. This new option gives a woman greater freedom for an active lifestyle as well as fashion flexibility (Fig 110-48).

THE FITTING ROOM—For such a department, an adequate, private fitting room and stock space nearby are an absolute necessity. The fitting room need be no more than 8 × 8 ft but should be clean, be free of any stock or display, and have an inward-swinging door to shield the fitting table from view. The fitting room also should be soundproofed to provide privacy and enable a patient to feel comfortable discussing his or her condition. As many fittings are done with the patient in a horizontal position, a table 72 by 26 and 30 inches high, padded with moisture-proof vinyl and a pillow is needed, as well as a chair, coat hooks and clothes hangers, four-legged stool, small dressing

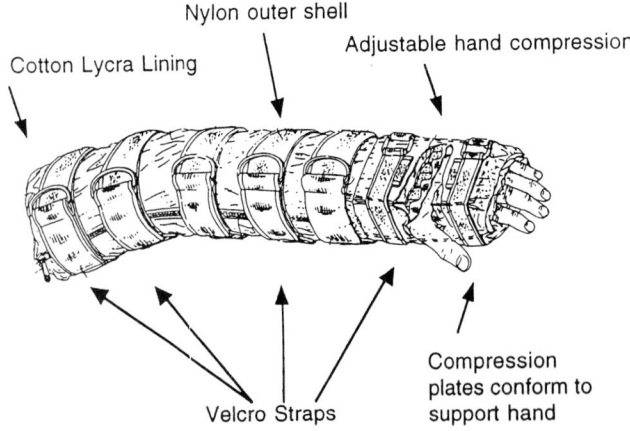

Cotton Lycra Lining

Nylon outer shell

Adjustable hand compression

Velcro Straps

Compression plates conform to support hand

Figure 110-47. The Reid Sleeve (courtesy, Peninsula Medical).

table, and a full-length mirror. Professional simplicity and cleanliness are exceedingly important. The use of rolled paper on the table is practical and economical. If the pharmacy also has a comprehensive ostomy center, a second chair, so both the patient and the pharmacist can sit, is recommended. As a health-accessories department grows and prospers, more than one fitting room may be needed. Additional fitting rooms may not all need fitting tables, especially if a large portion of the expected clientele will be there for mastectomy or elastic hosiery fittings.

Conveniently near the fitting room should be the orthopedic inventory. It depends on the volume of sales, types and number of physicians prescribing appliances, and extent of the pharmacy's promotion. An estimate of the required initial stock space is about 30 to 40 ft^2. Also near the fitting room should be a sink with antiseptic soap and disposable paper toweling for use by the pharmacist before and after each fitting. Where ostomy fittings are concerned, it is advisable to have such a sink inside the fitting room.

Each pharmacy should keep a service record for each patient, with data on physician's instructions, appliances fitted, and any reorders.

WHAT TO STOCK

There are perhaps as many opinions as to which items should be represented within the pharmacy's surgical supplies and convalescent aids department as there are pharmacies, manu-

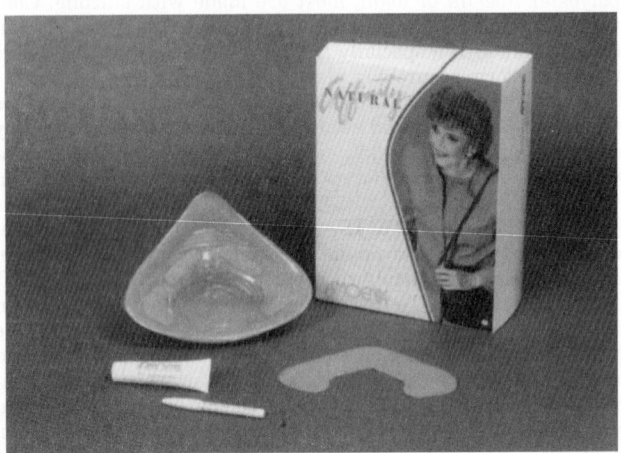

Figure 110-48. Breast form (courtesy, Amoena).

facturers, and wholesale distributors with experience in this field. Pharmacies differ, one from the other, in a multitude of ways. They face different limitations with regard to the available space within their pharmacies for the establishment of health-accessories departments. Their financial resources are different. The markets they purport to serve are different, with respect to both size and demographics. With regard to their drawing areas, differences exist due to various, specific economic factors reflecting distinctively different kinds of demand.

In an area with a heavy coal-mining industry, the market demand for respiratory therapy equipment might be very high relative to that in a rural farming community.

The extent to which hospital outpatient departments and home-care-oriented health agencies provide the thrust for a viable home health-care market within the community is vastly different from one town to another. Different pharmacies in different communities face widely divergent forms of competition, in both degree and kind.

All these considerations affect different pharmacies differently. Each pharmacist who contemplates the development of a surgical supplies and convalescent aids department must take these considerations into account when making decisions about what to stock. These are the issues that ultimately determine the optimum variety and depth of in-stock inventory for any given pharmacy.

Pharmacists must first decide which type or types of health accessories they want to specialize in handling. If they want to start with durable medical equipment such as canes, crutches, walkers, wheelchairs, commodes, and hospital beds, they should contact manufacturers of that type of equipment for advice on which products to stock. The same would be true for ostomy, urological, and incontinence supplies. Before opening a department for either orthopedic or mastectomy fitting, it would be necessary to attend a manufacturer's or wholesaler's school to obtain proper instruction. The manufacturer or wholesaler again would be a valuable source of information to assist in selecting those products best suited to an individual pharmacy. Before establishing a comprehensive respiratory-services department, it would be advisable to affiliate with a respiratory therapist who could assist in dealing with manufacturers in selecting the products most suited to a particular market area.

In many pharmacies, it is the actual experience of having capital tied up in slow moving inventory that has led many owners to the unfortunate practice of choosing a stocking inventory policy for health-accessories departments solely on the basis of the kind and number of requests received for various types of medical equipment in the past.

Thus, a vicious cycle ensues. For example, a pharmacist has no calls for specialized kinds of wheelchairs, and therefore, stocks only four or five basic wheelchair types. Then, when someone comes into the pharmacy for a wheelchair, because of a lack of wheelchair expertise and because more-specialized types of wheelchairs are not immediately available, he or she buys one of the wheelchairs that is in stock. Sometime then in the future, when visiting his or her physician or physical therapist, that person reports, often without realizing it, that the pharmacy was unable to meet his or her specific wheelchair needs. The result is that the physician or therapist will not send patients to the pharmacy for further wheelchair fittings.

From then on, the only persons who come to the pharmacy for wheelchairs are those who are either that pharmacy's regular patients or those who are largely uncounseled and self-initiate their visits to the pharmacy. And so, based on the past experience of not having had calls for specialized types of wheelchairs, the pharmacist concludes there is not much demand for them.

Without question, pharmacists who are interested in developing a successful surgical supplies and convalescent aids department within their pharmacies face a very serious dilemma. Either they play it safe and continue to stock those supplies for which they know they will have calls or they decide to expand their inventory and expertise in an effort to become relatively sophisticated. By doing the latter, pharmacists run the risk of raising their operating costs in an industry about which, at the very least, they are uncertain.

Many pharmacists who are involved successfully in providing a comprehensive health-accessories service are discovering that when they give better service with the more specialized kinds of equipment, they also do better with ordinary kinds of equipment. That is because their pharmacies become recognized as *the* places where patients should be sent for a wheelchair, a walker, and other kinds of durable medical equipment and surgical supplies. It is also true that an improvement in health-accessories service tends to boost a pharmacy's prescription volume as well.

In preparation for the development of a list of inventory items for a health-accessories department, pharmacists should formulate guidelines for themselves that incorporate those variables discussed previously regarding space available within the pharmacy for such a department, financial resources, etc. It is also helpful to categorize the kinds of equipment and merchandise pharmacists might want to stock and then rank the various articles within each category as to the relative importance of each in meeting the health needs of their community.

One of the very first things pharmacists must do is to familiarize themselves with the industry's manufacturers and become knowledgeable about the products manufactured. While their local wholesaler may have many of the items they will need in their health-accessories department, pharmacists will have to establish direct-buying relationships to be able to obtain the scores of things their wholesaler does not stock. They should begin an alphabetical file of manufacturers' catalogs and price lists and develop an index that cross-references products with their manufacturers. An index of this type will save hours of time and possible embarrassment before their customers as well by enabling them to go quickly to appropriate information when faced with questions for which they don't have ready answers. Questions of this type will come frequently, and pharmacists will realize it as they become aware of how broad this field really is. Simply, too, pharmacists should admit an ignorance about certain products and be able to suggest to the patient where to go to have their questions answered and their needs addressed.

REIMBURSEMENT

A pharmacist would not accept a prescription for medication from a new customer without first asking if the patient is covered by an insurance plan. It is even more important to do this when dealing with health-care accessories.

Every year, more and more health-care accessories are being billed to third-party payers, and pharmacists providing these services must be sure to follow all the rules of the various government and insurance plans if they expect to be reimbursed for their services. The pharmacist must first determine whether the pharmacy can be a provider for the requested services under a particular plan. Then it must be determined if the patient is indeed a covered beneficiary under that plan. It is also often necessary to determine if the physician is an authorized prescriber for that plan. Finally, the pharmacist must verify that the prescribed item or service is indeed a covered benefit and at what level benefits will be paid.

Since Medicare and many insurances pay only 80% (or some other portion) of the allowed claim, it is often necessary to determine if there is a second or even third insurance and verify these benefits. It may even be necessary to check to be sure which insurance is primary and which is secondary. A retired patient on Medicare whose spouse is still working may have Medicare coverage that is secondary to the spouse's insurance coverage at work. The primary insurance coverage on a minor child is determined by which parent's birthday comes earlier in the year.

It is also necessary to have a qualifying prescription and/or Certificate of Medical Necessity (CMN) before submitting a claim. Medicare has developed CMNs which are required to be used for many products, a few of which are wheelchairs, hospital beds, seat lift chairs, and even oxygen. HCFA (the Health Care Finance Administration) has set up a system of HCPCS codes (the HCFA Common Procedure Coding System) for every item that may be considered for reimbursement by Medicare. These codes are matched with the diagnosis code (ICD-9), which must be included on the claim, and Medicare and many insurance companies will match the item being dispensed with the diagnosis code to help determine if coverage will be approved.

Sometimes Medicare or an insurance company will contact the doctor for further information before paying a claim. (This is called *developing the claim*.) Sometimes a claim will be down-coded to a code that results in lower payment. For example, a physician may prescribe a semielectric hospital bed but with documentation that only qualifies the patient for a manually adjustable bed. If the pharmacist dispenses the semielectric bed as ordered and submits a claim to Medicare for it, the claim may be down-coded to a manual bed and paid accordingly.

While some insurance companies still pay claims in full (or a fixed percentage of the claim) as billed, more and more insurance companies, HMOs, and PPOs as well as Medicare and Medicaid base their payments on fee schedules and/or maximum allowable payment levels. Routinely, many insurance companies will not pay full price for a brand-name drug when a lower cost generic equivalent is available. So too, they will not pay a higher price for items they consider "deluxe" or not medically necessary. An example is the hospital bed in the preceding paragraph. While the doctor, patient, and pharmacist may all agree that a particular product or feature is really medically necessary, the insurance company or Medicare may not agree.

It is very important that the pharmacist providing health-care accessories take the time to learn the intricacies of billing for these items and keep up with the constant changes occurring. As the pharmacy's business in health accessories grows, it is often advisable to have at least one person dedicated to obtaining proper prescriptions, billing, posting payments, billing secondary insurances, reviewing denied or reduced payments, and in general keeping up-to-date on reimbursement issues.

PROMOTION

The first form of promotion the pharmacist can use is a well-stocked and attractive floor display (Fig 110-49).

Prior to deciding on other kinds of promotion to undertake, pharmacists must determine from where most of their health-accessories volume is likely to come. Pharmacists who are involved successfully in comprehensive surgical supplies and convalescent aids departments are finding is that the greatest share of their surgical business is not done with their regular patients, but with new ones coming to their pharmacies specifically for medical supplies. There is little doubt that the reason most of these new patrons find their way to these pharmacies is that they were sent there by medical and allied health professionals in their own communities.

Referrals for wheelchairs, walkers, ostomy supplies, breathing equipment, and other health accessories come from physicians, hospitals, nursing homes, and a wide variety of community health professionals, among whom are therapists (physical, occupational, enterostomal, respiratory), nurses, medical social workers, social service directors, home-care coordinators, visiting nurses, and trainers in organized athletics. Physicians in most major specialties will make referrals. It is important that each health professional be approached about products or services relevant to his or her specific discipline. Organizations in which these and other health professionals can be found include hospitals and nursing homes, visiting nurse associations, private physical therapy associations, state departments of vocational rehabilitation, insur-

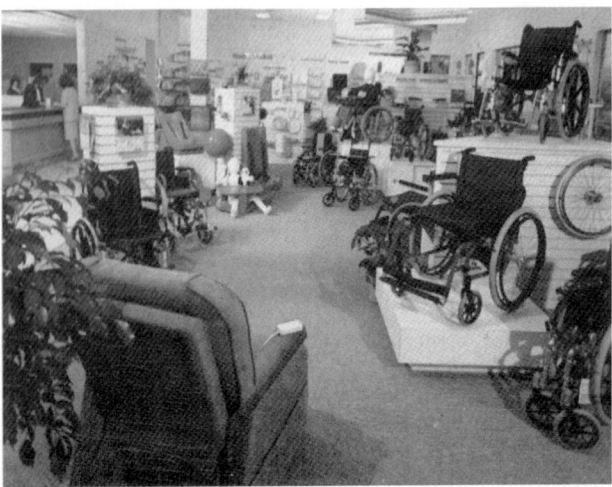

Figure 110-49. Floor display and wall space. This very common arrangement can be most productive. With the advantage of being able to display all the wheelchairs and walkers open, it gives the consumer a total and comprehensive picture of your home-care department at once.

ance companies, athletic departments in schools, commercial and manufacturing plants, rehabilitation centers, home-health agencies, clinics and agencies such as the Easter Seal Society, American Cancer Society, Multiple Sclerosis Association, Muscular Dystrophy Foundation, National Paraplegia Foundation, United Cerebral Palsy, United Ostomy Association, and many others. These, then, are the people and the organizations at which the pharmacy's principal promotional programs must be aimed. And while promotion to the general public is still very important, it is crucial that the pharmacist develop effective promotional programs aimed at the professional community.

Because it is quite common for many of these *new* patrons to begin to patronize their *new* pharmacy for other health needs, it is not surprising that the very existence of a comprehensive health-accessories department is regarded by the pharmacies who operate them as an excellent means for promoting the pharmacy as a whole.

Since the largest part of surgical supplies and health accessories volume originates with medical and allied health professionals within the community, the question must be asked: What prompts these professionals to recommend one dealer over another?

Aspects about the retail distribution of medical equipment and supplies that most concern a community's medical and allied health professionals are

1. That the supplier have the academic background and practical know-how to recommend the right equipment for each patient need and be able to show the patient how the equipment should be used.correctly.
2. That the supplier not practice medicine, physical therapy, etc, but call on practitioners of these professions for consultation and guidance when appropriate.
3. That the supplier have in stock an adequate inventory, in kind and quantity, to meet the immediate needs of his or her patients.
4. That the supplier, in addition to having ample stock, have access to wide varieties of medical equipment and supplies from numerous manufacturers, to service the special and unique needs of patients.
5. That the supplier distribute only merchandise of good quality and stand behind what he or she rents and sells. Many medical professionals are name-brand conscious also.
6. That the supplier have the capability of providing basic maintenance and repair services for what he or she sells and rents.
7. That the suppliers' equipment be priced competitively in rentals and sales.

8. That the supplier operate the business in an immaculate, well-organized, efficient, and thoroughly professional manner.

Advertising in professional journals, direct-mail campaigns, newspapers, and television commercials are all effective and commonly used methods of proclaiming that a pharmacy has the attributes that the professional community expects.

Attending and sponsoring meetings of groups, such as the local ostomy or diabetes associations, or working with public service groups, such as *Reach to Recovery,* allows the pharmacist to interact with health-care professionals and volunteers who are influential in these areas.

Sending a doctor or other referral source a written *Thank You* for each new referral also helps to remind the doctor of the professional services provided by the pharmacist. Even a simple note stating that a patient was fitted with a particular type of orthopedic support on a certain date as prescribed by the physician may end up in the patient's file where the doctor may see it several times.

One of the most effective ways of promoting a health accessories department, especially one that features the fitting of orthopedic and mastectomy appliances, is direct physician detailing. Calling on them in their offices is one sure way of promoting one's health accessories department. Even if it is not possible to visit the physician each time, contacts with his/her office personnel, especially a nurse, often can be very effective. Many times patients will ask the receptionist, while making the next appointment, where they can purchase or rent the item that has just been prescribed.

Another effective method to communicate that the pharmacy has the expertise and inventory to meet the community's health-care needs is by a developing a program of regular hospital displays. Further, in-service training classes for the staffs in hospitals and nursing homes as well as presentations at universities, social-service organizations, and special-interest groups are effective.

How better to demonstrate one's expertise in selecting, and when necessary measuring and fitting, health accessories than by providing instruction to groups of health professionals in a hospital or nursing home in the basic principles and proper use of the accessories, particularly those that serve as aids in convalescence or home care of the patient. Thus, for example, the important subject of walking aids—canes, forearm crutches, axillary crutches, and walkers—should include a discussion of the physiological factors of ambulation; the selection, measurement, and fitting of the devices to provide maximum leverage and comfort; and the manner of their use in walking on level areas as well as ascending or descending stairs. Many other subjects can be presented similarly by pharmacists knowledgeable in the use of convalescent aids and other health accessories.

Various equipment manufacturers offer in-service training programs that may be used as a guide to developing training programs for hospitals, nursing homes, visiting nurse associations, and schools.

With the advent of various managed-care programs, including plans for Medicare beneficiaries, another type of promotion has become necessary. Pharmacists may have taken many or all of the previous steps to promote their health-accessory department and still see meager results because most of the physicians who might recommend the pharmacy's services are required to refer to other providers who are in a particular health-care network, while the pharmacy is not. Pharmacists must actively pursue those health-care organizations for whom they want to provide services.

While some organizations deal only with capitated providers or may have an exclusive provider, many will work with several preferred providers. Often it is difficult to find the actual decision maker who may allow the pharmacy to become a preferred provider, but as the pharmacy becomes a provider for a few organizations, gradually other doors may be opened because of the excellent service provided. Often being exceptionally good in a small niche market may *open the door* to becoming a provider of other services as well.

All of the above-listed methods of promotion have one thing in common, relationship-building, a key element in forming a strong health-accessory department in the pharmacy.

PROFESSIONAL APPROACH

Pharmacists should not conclude hastily that they will be successful in this field, regardless of their estimate of the local market, their inventory, and their display facilities. Unless the pharmacist is willing to devote time and intelligent effort to the venture, he or she will fail. Pharmacists should be interested in helping the aged, the infirm, and the sick. Their attitude must be professional, and their approach to prospective referring physicians and the public must be made on that basis, not on mere availability or price. They must become knowledgeable in the areas of reimbursement and accreditation. Most important, they must have developed the expertise to recommend the right equipment and supplies and instruct their patrons in their proper use.

Pharmacists who seriously are considering developing this specialty will need to expand their reading list of relevant professional journals and periodicals. In addition to the major pharmacy journals, the following publications will broaden their knowledge and perspective concerning convalescent aids and surgical supplies: *HomeCare, HME News, Home Health Care Dealer, Medical Product Sales, Today's Home Healthcare Provider, Home Health Products, Ostomy Quarterly, The Journal of Care Management,* and journals in specialty fields such as physical therapy, occupational therapy, or respiratory therapy.

The National Community Pharmacists Association (NCPA) created a special division of Home Health Care Pharmacy Services. This division can provide additional information to pharmacists on changes in government programs that affect pharmacists providing home-health-care accessories. The NCPA publishes a newsletter, the *Alternative Pharmacist Monthly.* The NCPA, an accredited APCE provider, also provides educational programs concerning ostomy, incontinence, wound management, orthotics, and prosthetics. An advanced certificate program in orthotics and prosthetics is offered by the NCPA, and a number of other certification programs are available.

The surgical-supply department of the modern community pharmacy is recognized by physician and layman alike as a proper extension of the pharmacist's professional service. Physicians and allied health professionals quickly assess this new service as an important contribution to the health-team concept.

CERTIFICATION

Pharmacists who provide orthotic services should consider qualifying for credential, the Certified Orthotic Fitter, issued by the Board for Orthotists/Prosthetist Certification (BOC). Information regarding BOC certification may be attained from their website, www.bocusa.org. BOC Facility Accreditation is also available for pharmacies providing a wide array of Home Medical Equipment and services.

ACCREDITATION

The final step that pharmacists can—and should—take to demonstrate their competence as providers of health-care accessories is to become accredited. There are a number of accrediting bodies. The best known is the JCAHO (Joint Commission on Accreditation of Healthcare Organizations).

To become accredited, the pharmacy must, among other things, pass an on-site inspection in which the surveyor determines the firm's competency in such areas as:

1. Patient rights and responsibilities
2. Care, treatments, and service
3. Education
4. Environmental safety
5. Equipment management
6. Management of human resources
7. Management of information
8. Infection control
9. Quality assurance

The survey will include interviews with staff and clients, *riding along* on equipment deliveries, and spot checks of patient files. Accreditation extends for a period of 3 years, at which time the firm must be resurveyed.

The Accreditation Commission for Home Care, Inc, also can provide accreditation for firms that qualify. It has a specialty section dealing with the fitting of mastectomy prostheses. After successfully passing an on-site survey, a firm may be accredited for 3 years.

Other organizations that provide accreditation are CHAP (the Commission on Health Accreditation Programs), CARF (the Commission on Accreditation of Rehab Facilities), and NCQA (the National Committee for Quality Assurance).

THE FUTURE

Increased life expectancy has produced an increase in the number of aged persons and a corresponding increase in the number of ill and infirm persons in this segment of our population. The growing number of aged persons, the trend toward their greater subsidization, and the rapid increase in services from home-health-care agencies and hospital outpatient departments portends an ever-increasing number of potential candidates for surgical supplies and convalescent aids in the future. This is also true of many persons who are not aged but still are ill or infirm.

Though nursing homes do care for a substantial number of such patients, more of them want to remain at home and avoid the upward, spiraling costs of institutional care. Hospitals are reluctant to provide services to persons not in need of acute-care facilities, except on an outpatient basis, as it is too costly for both the patient and the hospital. As a result, the trend is to transfer the patient to home care as soon as possible. Encouraged to do so by the principal health-insurance companies such as Blue Cross and by developing home-health-care agencies, the demand for surgical appliances and medical equipment for use in the patient's home is growing daily.

This chapter was prepared as an overview of many, but not all, of the avenues pharmacists might take to expand their professional horizons. To be really successful in any, let alone all, of the areas, a sincere commitment of time, energy, and other resources may be required, but the professional rewards can make it all worthwhile.

ACKNOWLEDGMENT—The authors acknowledge the contributions of Barry N Eigen, MBA; Cindy Ciardo, Certified Fitter and BOC Orthotist; and Janet Lutze, RN, BSN, CETN to the development and enhancement of this chapter.

Social, Behavioral, Economic, and Administrative Sciences

Nicholas G Popovich, PhD

Professor and Head

Department of Pharmacy Administration

University of Illinois at Chicago

College of Pharmacy

Chicago, IL

Social, Behavioral, Economic, and Administrative Sciences

CHAPTER 111

Laws Governing Pharmacy

Jesse C Vivian, BS Pharm, JD
Joseph L Fink III, BS Pharm, JD

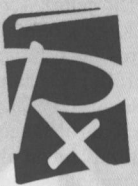

Pharmacists—whether community practitioners, employed by an institution or working for a pharmaceutical manufacturer—must be aware of the legal requirements that apply to their daily professional activities. The laws pertaining to the practice of pharmacy arise from a variety of different sources, including statutory laws such as the Food Drug and Cosmetic Act (FD&CA), the Controlled Substances Act (CSA), the Poison Prevention Packaging Act (PPPA), at the federal level and Pharmacy Practice Acts or Codes at the state level. In addition, several regulatory agencies in the federal government including the Food and Drug Administration (FDA), the Consumer Product Safety Commission (CPSC) and the Drug Enforcement Administration (DEA) have the authority to promulgate regulations that have the force of law. State agencies such as a Board of Pharmacy

also adopt rules or regulations that have the force of law. Another source of law comes from court decisions the either interpret statutory and regulatory laws or make new laws based on judicial decisions; the later type of rulings are often called "judge made" or "common" laws derived for the English court system.

Beside the various *sources* of laws, there are a multitude of *types* of law. Civil law governs the relationship between individuals within society, whereas criminal law governs the relationship of the individual to society as a whole. Two important subdivisions of civil law are the law of contracts and tort law. The former concerns relationships that the individuals enter into voluntarily, while the latter embodies relationships that exist automatically by virtue of law. Each *type* and *source* of law is applicable to pharmacists and pharmacy practice.

LAWS GOVERNING THE PRACTICE OF PHARMACY

Relationship between State and Federal Laws

Differentiating between state and federal laws governing the practice of pharmacy can be a daunting task because some areas of the law are reserved exclusively to state governments while other topics are governed exclusively by federal authorities. Complicating the subject even more, there are numerous issues that both the state and federal laws address. In the later case, when both federal and state laws speak to the same issue, the governing bodies are said to have "concurrent jurisdiction." Determining which of the two sets of laws to apply to any given situation is sometimes difficult, especially in cases where the two laws differ in their obligations or prohibitions. As a general rule, when there is a "conflict of laws" it is usually safer to apply and follow the stricter law. An example will help illustrate the point. DEA regulations require pharmacies to keep controlled substances records, including prescriptions for at least two years. Several states have laws that all prescriptions be stored in a pharmacy for a longer period. In Michigan, for example, pharmacies must retain prescriptions a minimum of five years from the date of last refill. Because record retention is a subject of "concurrent jurisdiction" between state and federal governments, a pharmacist would follow the "stricter" law and, at least in Michigan, keep all prescriptions, including those for controlled substances, for a minimum of five years from the date of the last refill. Another area of "concurrent jurisdiction" that has sparked over a decade of controversy involves the compounding of drugs by pharmacists. Historically, compounding was thought to be exclusively in the realm of state jurisdiction. In the early 1990s, the FDA began an aggressive approach to regulate

pharmacies that were engaging in large scale compounding more akin to manufacturing. Viewed another way, the FDA was attempting to regulate pharmacies that were manufacturing, and therefore subject to federal laws, under the guise of state regulated compounding practices. The furor over the subject led to an amendment to the FD&CA that gave the FDA some regulatory authority over compounding while leaving other aspects of compounding subject to state law. This in turn led the National Associations of Boards of Pharmacy (NAPB) to adopt model guidelines for states to enact. Animosities between the FDA and compounding pharmacies finally cumulated in a Unites States Supreme Court decision in April, 2002 that should have settled the issue in favor of state authority to regulate compounding. Undaunted by the Supreme Court decision, within days, the FDA reissued guidelines to its field officers to distinguish between acceptable compounding activities and unlawful manufacturing by pharmacies without a federally issued manufacturing license. The topic is addressed in more detail under the *Compounding* subsection below.

The authority for states to regulate pharmacy originates in the Tenth Amendment to the United States Constitution, which reserves most "police powers" to the states. The terminology could be misleading if "police power" were thought to refer to law enforcement officers only. In fact, as the term is used in the law, the "police power" reserved exclusively to the states means that the states have the authority to pass laws designed to protect the health, safety and welfare of its citizens. Note that the Constitution reserves *most* "police powers" to the states. As might be expected, there are exceptions that permit the federal government to "preempt" inconsistent state laws if the federal government determines it will "occupy the field" of a particular subject matter. Another example is offered to clarify the point. Every state has laws regarding the labeling and packaging of drugs dispensed pursuant to a prescription. Some states even have laws regarding the type of container used to contain prescription drugs. The Consumer Product Safety Commission (CPSC), a federal agency, acting under the auspices of the federal Poison Prevention Packaging Act (PPPA) has "preempted" inconsistent state laws dealing with the packaging of "household substances," which include prescription drugs. Under the applicable regulations, every drug dispensed by prescription must be in a child resistant container unless the patient or prescriber requests otherwise. Because of the preemption, any state law not consistent with the demands of the CPSC regulations would have no force of law and pharmacists are required to follow the federal mandates.

Perhaps it is too simplistic to put it this way, but another general rule to use in determining which jurisdictional body controls a subject matter is to think of state laws as regulating the *practice of pharmacy* and the federal government as regulating *pharmaceuticals* including their marketing, production and distribution. As with all laws, there are exceptions to this general rule. Nonetheless, it should help readers better comprehend the scope of the jurisdictional authority of the different governmental bodies.

STATE LAWS

As mentioned, the regulation of the *practice of pharmacy* is primarily a function of the states and not of the federal government. Accordingly, states are relatively free to enact laws and Board of Pharmacy rules independent of the federal government (so long as the regulations are not in conflict or inconsistent with federal law). While pharmacy laws of the different states do vary among themselves, they are in agreement with respect to the fundamental principles, purposes, aims and objectives of pharmacy practice. In a Chapter of this magnitude, it is impossible to consider the vast array and nuances of every state pharmacy practice law. Therefore, the focus will be on the commonalities among state laws.

Like every profession, the practice of pharmacy is a privilege bestowed by the state. However, this is a privilege available only to a class of persons who satisfy stated minimal qualifications. No one may practice pharmacy without a license, except for those who are licensed according to state law. However, anyone may achieve such licensure by successfully completing the statutory pattern of qualification that the state has established and as administered by an agency given the regulatory authority. Not every state has a Board of Pharmacy as the regulatory agency with this authority; however because that is the term used by the majority of states, hereafter the governing administrative agency will be referred to as the Board of Pharmacy. In some instances the Board of Pharmacy is a sub-agency that exists as part of a larger state agency, such as a department of health or licensing.

Once licensure is gained it may not be easily revoked. The state may suspend, revoke or terminate it but only after due process and for just cause as set out in the appropriate legislation. At the same time, the state undertakes to protect the public and the licensed pharmacists from practice by unlicensed (hence, unqualified) parties in its jurisdiction. As to licensed pharmacists, they have gained what constitutes a "monopoly" to practice pharmacy safeguarded by the Federal and state constitutions as a property right. While they must abide by the legislation to preserve it, pharmacists must pay fees required to accomplish initial and continuing licensure, and must satisfy the legal, moral and ethical standards of their peers, as set out in law and regulations. They do have the right to legal redress against any who would seek unjustifiably to deprive them of the benefits and prerogatives of licensure. Pharmacy practice acts specifically must identify the conduct for which sanctions can be imposed.

State pharmacy laws generally provide for:

1. The educational and experiential qualifications that pharmacists must meet at the time of an examination for licensure (or "registration"). The vast majority of states require that applicant for licensure to have graduated from an "accredited" school or collage of Pharmacy or take a "foreign licensure" exam to show that the applicants knowledge and credentials match graduates of an accredited institution.
2. Establishment of an administrative agency (Board of Pharmacy) charged with enforcement and administration of the pharmacy practice laws. This agency will have powers delegated by the legislature in pharmacy practice statutes to promulgate rules or regulations to implement the statutes. A certain amount of enforcement discretion will be vested in a Boards of Pharmacy. While the board is authorized to make rules and regulations for the enforcement and administration of the pharmacy law, such rules and regulations must be strictly in accord with the expressed or implied purposes of the law. The board is an administrative, not a legislative, agency. It may not exercise any power or authority not clearly delegated to it. The Board of Pharmacy will grant licenses to qualified pharmacists and pharmacies, and also have the power to impose sanctions against those who do not follow the applicable laws. The conditions under which licensure or registration may be canceled, revoked, suspended, or put on probation must be specified in a statute or regulation. Many Boards of Pharmacy have other disciplinary sanctions available including civil fines and the imposition of a community service requirement. Some state laws specify that violations of the pharmacy act are punishable as a criminal misdemeanor.
3. The granting of licenses for the conduct of a community and institutional pharmacy. In most states permits are issued for one or two years and application must be made for renewal at a specified time.
4. Periodic re-licensure of pharmacists. In most states, certificates of licensure or registration are granted for the period of one or two years.
5. The prominent display of the certificate of licensure or registration in the pharmacy in which the holder is employed.
6. Reciprocal registration whereby a pharmacist licensed by examination in one state may, by conforming to more or less nominal rules, becomes registered in another state without full licensure examination. In almost all states and jurisdictions within the United States, reciprocating pharmacists must take the pharmacy law exam in the state they wish to become licensed in.

Every state has a pharmacy practice act that regulates the profession, but there is significant variation in the detail of these acts from state to state. Many of the states statutes are antiquated, with amendments being added in a haphazard manner. Many of these early acts regulated an older and traditional profession that was primarily product-oriented and involved in the preparation and delivery of drugs.

Nuclear pharmacy, clinical pharmacy, pharmaceutical care, mandated counseling and drug-product selection are just some of the developments impacting upon regulation of pharmacy since most of the laws were originally developed. These changes, along with the need to provide more uniformity among the states, caused the National Associations of Boards of Pharmacy (NABP) to develop a *Model State Pharmacy Practice Act* (MSPPA). The Model Act is intended to provide both uniformity and flexibility to the states that adopt it. Many states have adopted some of the Model Act's provisions while formulating unique regulations to address issues of particular concern in individual states.

The NABP's MSPPA is online at http://nabp.net and is available for downloading without fee. Readers who are interested in seeing how a model act is organized and the suggested topics that should be covered in a state act are advised to visit the NABP site or contact the NABP (700 Busse Hwy., Oak Ridge, IL 60068; Phone: 847-698-6227). Because there are so many variations in the pharmacy laws between states, readers should consult the laws of the particular state in interest.

One of the more common sections contained in nearly every state pharmacy act is a definition of the "practice of pharmacy." The MSPPA includes a broad interpretation of the term:

The Practice of Pharmacy means the interpretation, evaluation, and implementation of Medical Orders; the Dispensing of Prescription Drug

Orders; participation in Drug and Device selection, Drug Administration, Drug Regimen Reviews, and drug or drug-related research; provision of Patient Counseling and the provision of those acts or services necessary to provide Pharmaceutical Care in all areas of patient care including Primary Care; and the responsibility for Compounding and Labeling of Drugs and Devices (except Labeling by a Manufacturer, repackager, or distributor of Non-Prescription Drugs and commercially packaged Legend Drugs and Devices), proper and safe storage of Drugs and Devices, and maintenance of proper records for them.

In contrast, many state statutes are so out of date in that they limit the practice of pharmacy to the preparation and distribution of a dosage form. The MSPPA adopts very broad language to allow boards of pharmacy to promulgate rules and regulations with considerable flexibility as the profession changes to meet future needs.

Definitions

No matter which state laws are being considered, the best place to start is with definitions contained within the statutes or acts. Many words in laws are used in ways that differ from common everyday usage. Basic definitions are essential to the clarity, administration and enforcement of any law. For example, comments to the MSPPA indicate that the *practice of pharmacy* includes the selection of therapeutic agents in accord with institutional protocols or some other legal authority. The definition also encompasses the concept of consulting with, or providing information to, both the prescriber and the patient regarding drug therapy. Patient counseling and pharmaceutical care are further defined in the model rules.

The following definitions from the MSPPA are provided as examples of important terms often included in pharmacy acts:

(a) *Administer* means the direct application of a Drug to the body of a patient or research subject by injection, inhalation, ingestion, or any other means.

(b) *Automated Pharmacy Systems* include, but are not limited to, mechanical systems that perform operations or activities, other than compounding or administration, relative to the storage, packaging, dispensing, or distribution of medications, and that collect, control, and maintain all transaction information.

(c) *Beyond-Use Date* means a date determined by a Pharmacist and placed on a prescription label at the time of Dispensing that is intended to indicate to the patient or caregiver a time beyond which the contents of the prescription are not recommended to be used.

(d) *Compounding* means the preparation, mixing, assembling, packaging, or Labeling of a Drug or Device (i) as the result of a Practitioner's Prescription Drug Order or initiative based on the Practitioner/patient/Pharmacist relationship in the course of professional practice, or (ii) for the purpose of, or as an incident to, research, teaching, or chemical analysis and not for sale or Dispensing. Compounding also includes the preparation of Drugs or Devices in anticipation of Prescription Drug Orders based on routine, regularly observed prescribing patterns.

(e) *Confidential Information* means information accessed, maintained by, or transmitted to the Pharmacist in the patient's records or that is communicated to the patient as part of patient counseling, which is privileged and may be released only to the patient or, as the patient directs, to those Practitioners, other authorized health care professionals, and other Pharmacists where, in the Pharmacist's professional judgment, such release is necessary to protect the patient's health and well being; and to such other Persons or governmental agencies authorized by law to receive such Confidential Information, regardless of whether such information is in the form of paper, preserved on microfilm, or is stored on electronic media.

(f) *Dispense* or *Dispensing* means the interpretation, evaluation, and implementation of a Prescription Drug Order, including the preparation and Delivery of a Drug or Device to a patient or patient's agent in a suitable container appropriately labeled for subsequent Administration to, or use by, a patient.

(g) *Distribute* means the Delivery of a Drug or Device other than by Administering or Dispensing.

(h) *Drug* means:
(1) Articles recognized as Drugs in any official compendium, or supplement thereto, designated from time to time by the Board for use in the diagnosis, cure, mitigation, treatment, or prevention of disease in humans or other animals;
(2) Articles intended for use in the diagnosis, cure, mitigation, treatment, or prevention of disease in humans or other animals;
(3) Articles (other than food) intended to affect the structure or any function of the body of humans or other animals; and
(4) Articles intended for use as a component of any articles specified in clause (1), (2), or (3) of this subsection.

(i) *Emergency Situations*, for the purposes of authorizing an oral Prescription Drug Order of a Schedule II controlled substance, means those situations in which the prescribing Practitioner determines (1) that immediate Administration of the controlled substance is necessary for proper treatment of the patient, (2) that no appropriate alternative treatment is available, including Administration of a drug that is not a Schedule II controlled substance, and (3) that it is not reasonably possible for the prescribing Practitioner to provide a written Prescription Drug Order to be presented to the person Dispensing the substance, prior to the Dispensing.

(j) *Equivalent Drug Product* means a Drug product that has the same established name, active ingredient(s), strength or concentration, dosage form, and route of Administration and that is formulated to contain the same amount of active ingredient(s) in the same dosage form and to meet the same compendial or other applicable standards (ie, strength, quality, purity, and identity), but that may differ in characteristics such as shape, scoring, configuration, packaging, excipients (including colors, flavors, preservatives), and expiration time.

(k) *Intern* means an individual who is:
(1) currently licensed by this State to engage in the Practice of Pharmacy while under the personal supervision of a Pharmacist and is satisfactorily progressing toward meeting the requirements for licensure as a Pharmacist; or
(2) a graduate of an approved college of pharmacy or a graduate who has established educational equivalency by obtaining a Foreign Pharmacy Graduate Examination Committee (FPGEC) Certificate, who is currently licensed by the Board of Pharmacy for the purpose of obtaining practical experience as a requirement for licensure as a Pharmacist; or
(3) a qualified applicant awaiting examination for licensure; or
(4) an individual participating in a residency or fellowship program.

(l) *Labeling* means the process of preparing and affixing a label to any Drug container exclusive, however, of the labeling by a Manufacturer, packer, or distributor of a Non Prescription Drug or commercially packaged Legend Drug or Device. Any such label shall include all information required by federal and state law or rule.

(m) *Non Prescription Drug* means a drug that may be sold without a prescription and that is labeled for use by the consumer in accordance with the requirements of the laws and rules of this State and the Federal Government.

(n) *Patient Counseling* means the oral communication by the Pharmacist of information, as defined in the rules of the Board, to the patient or caregiver, to ensure the proper use of Drugs and Devices.

(o) *Person* means an individual, corporation, partnership, association, or any other legal entity including government.

(p) *Pharmaceutical Care* is the provision of drug therapy and other patient care services intended to achieve outcomes related to the cure or prevention of a disease, elimination or reduction of a patient's symptoms, or arresting or slowing of a disease process as defined in the Rules of the Board.

(q) *Pharmacist* means an individual currently licensed by this State to engage in the Practice of Pharmacy.

(r) *Pharmacist-in-Charge* means a Pharmacist currently licensed in this state who accepts responsibility for the operation of a Pharmacy in conformance with all laws and rules pertinent to the Practice of Pharmacy and the distribution of Drugs, and who is personally in full and actual charge of such pharmacy and personnel.

(s) *Pharmacy* means any place within this State where Drugs are Dispensed and Pharmaceutical Care is provided and any place outside of this State where Drugs are Dispensed and Pharmaceutical Care is provided to residents of this State.

(t) *Practice of Telepharmacy Across State Lines* means the provision of Pharmaceutical Care through the use of telecommunications and information technologies that occurs when the patient is physically located within the jurisdiction and the Pharmacist is located outside the jurisdiction.

(u) *Practitioner* means an individual currently licensed, registered, or otherwise authorized by the appropriate jurisdiction to prescribe and Administer Drugs in the course of professional practice.

(v) *Preceptor* means an individual who is currently licensed as a Pharmacist by the Board of Pharmacy, meets the qualifications as a Preceptor under the Rules of the Board, and participates in the instructional training of pharmacy Interns.

(w) *Prescription Drug* or *Legend Drug* means a Drug that is required under Federal law to be labeled with either of the following statements prior to being Dispensed or Delivered: (i) *Caution: Federal law prohibits dispensing without prescription or Rx Only*; or (ii) *Caution: Federal law restricts this drug to use by, or on the order of, a licensed veterinarian*; or (iii) a Drug that is required by any applicable Federal or State law or rule to be Dispensed pursuant only to a Prescription Drug Order or is restricted to use by Practitioners only.

The definitions of a device or a drug in state law are often similar to those included in the FD&CA, but their application will be different under state law as the Board of Pharmacy is interested primarily in the dispensing aspects of such drugs or devices as opposed to the Federal orientation to the purity, strength and appropriate labeling of drugs.

The various states will also include a variety of individuals within the definition of a "practitioner" who is permitted to prescribe prescription only drugs. Such provisions anticipate that those persons other than pharmacists who are permitted to prescribe and administer drugs will be specifically authorized in other legislation.

Each state pharmacy practice act, as well as state controlled substances legislation, must be examined carefully to determine the legality of pharmacists filling prescription orders written by practitioners or prescribers in other states. The majority of the states do not prohibit the dispensing of prescription orders that originate out-of-state, but some states prohibit the dispensing of prescriptions from all out-of-state prescribers except those living in *border states*. Pharmacists should consult state statutes carefully and with the board of pharmacy to determine the legal status of prescription orders originating in another state.

Rules and Regulations

There are vast differences in the rules (or "regulations" as they are called in some states) between the states. Fortunately, the NABP, through its MSPPA, has provided some basic rules that every state should follow. The following is a restatement from Article II of the MSPPA:

"The Board of Pharmacy shall make, adopt, amend, and repeal such rules as may be deemed necessary by the Board from time to time for the proper administration and enforcement of this Act. Such rules shall be promulgated in accordance with the procedures specified in the Administrative Procedures Act of this State.

(a) The Board of Pharmacy shall be responsible for the control and regulation of the Practice of Pharmacy in this State including, but not limited to, the following:

(1) The licensing by examination or by license transfer of applicants who are qualified to engage in the Practice of Pharmacy under the provisions of this Act;

(2) The renewal of licenses to engage in the Practice of Pharmacy;

(3) The establishment and enforcement of compliance with professional standards and rules of conduct of Pharmacists engaged in the Practice of Pharmacy;

(4) The determination and issuance of standards for recognition and approval of degree programs of schools and colleges of pharmacy whose graduates shall be eligible for licensure in this State, and the specification and enforcement of requirements for practical training, including internship;

(5) The enforcement of those provisions of this Act relating to the conduct or competence of Pharmacists practicing in this State, and the suspension, revocation, or restriction of licenses to engage in the Practice of Pharmacy;

(6) The licensure and regulation of the training, qualifications, and employment of Pharmacy Interns and Pharmacy Technicians;

(7) The collection of professional demographic data;

(8) The right to seize any such Drugs and Devices found by the Board to constitute an imminent danger to the public health and welfare;

(9) Establishing minimum specifications for the physical facilities, technical equipment, environment, supplies, personnel, and procedures for the storage, Compounding and/or Dispensing of such Drugs or Devices, and for the monitoring of drug therapy;

(10) Establishing minimum standards for the purity and quality of such Drugs, Devices, and other materials within the Practice of Pharmacy;

(11) The issuance and renewal of licenses of all Persons engaged in the manufacture and distribution of Drugs and Devices;

(12) Inspection of any licensed Person at all reasonable hours for the purpose of determining if any provisions of the laws governing the legal distribution of Drugs or Devices or the Practice of Pharmacy are being violated. The Board of Pharmacy, its officers, inspectors, and representatives shall cooperate with all agencies charged with the enforcement of the laws of the US, of this State, and of all other states relating to Drugs, Devices, and the Practice of Pharmacy; and

(13) Establishing minimum standards for maintaining the integrity and confidentiality of prescription information and other patient health-care information.

(b) The Board of Pharmacy shall have such other duties, powers, and authority as may be necessary to the enforcement of this Act and to the enforcement of Board rules made pursuant thereto, which shall include, but are not limited to, the following:

(1) The Board may join such professional organizations and associations organized exclusively to promote the improvement of the standards of the Practice of Pharmacy for the protection of the health and welfare of the public and/or whose activities assist and facilitate the work of the Board.

(2) The Board may receive and expend funds, in addition to its [annual/biennial] appropriation, from parties other than the State, provided:

(i) Such funds are awarded for the pursuit of a specific objective that the Board is authorized to accomplish by this Act, or that the Board is qualified to accomplish by reason of its jurisdiction or professional expertise;

(ii) Such funds are expended for the pursuit of the objective for which they are awarded;

(iii) Activities connected with or occasioned by the expenditures of such funds do not interfere with the performance of the Board's duties and responsibilities, and do not conflict with the exercise of the Board's powers as specified by this Act;

(iv) Such funds are kept in a separate, special account; and

(v) Periodic reports are made concerning the Board's receipt and expenditure of such funds.

(3) The Board may establish a Bill of Rights for patients concerning the health-care services a patient may expect in regard to Pharmaceutical Care.

(4) Any investigation, inquiry, or hearing that the State Board of Pharmacy is empowered to hold or undertake may be held or undertaken by or before any member or members of the Board and the finding or order of such member or members shall be deemed to be the order of said Board when approved and confirmed as noted in Section 210(d).

(5) Embargo

(i) Notwithstanding anything in this Act to the contrary, whenever a duly authorized representative of the Board finds, or has probable cause to believe, that any Drug or Device is adulterated or misbranded within the meaning of the (State) Food and Drug Act, he shall affix to such Drug or Device a tag or other appropriate marking giving notice that such article is or is suspected of being adulterated or misbranded, has been detained or embargoed, and warning all Persons not to remove or dispose of such article by sale or otherwise until provision for removal or disposal is given by the Board, its agent, or the Court. No Person shall remove or dispose of such embargoed Drug or Device by sale or otherwise without the permission of the Board or its agent or, after summary proceedings have been instituted, without permission from the Court.

(ii) When a Drug or Device detained or embargoed under Paragraph (i) of this subsection (5) has been declared by such representative to be adulterated or misbranded, the Board shall, as soon as practical thereafter, petition the Judge of the Court in which jurisdiction the article is detained or embargoed for an order for condemnation of such article. If the judge determines that the Drug or Device so detained or embargoed is not adulterated or misbranded, the Board shall direct the immediate removal of the tag or other marking.

(iii) If the court finds the detained or embargoed Drug or Device is adulterated or misbranded, such Drug or Device, after entry of the decree, shall be destroyed at the expense of the owner under the supervision of a Board representative and all court costs and fees, storage, and other proper expense shall be borne by the owner of such Drug or Device. When the adulteration or misbranding can be corrected by proper Labeling or processing of the Drug or Device, the Court, after entry of the decree and after such costs, fees, and expenses have been paid and a good and sufficient bond has been posted, may direct that such Drug or Device be Delivered to the owner thereof for such Labeling or processing under the supervision of a Board representative. Expense of such supervision shall be paid by the owner. Such bond shall be returned to the owner of the Drug or Device on representation to the Court by the Board that the Drug or Device is no longer in violation of the embargo and the expense of supervision has been paid.

(iv) It is the duty of the Attorney General [State's Attorney] to whom the Board reports any violation of Section 213(b)(5) to cause appropriate proceedings to be instituted in the proper court without delay and to be prosecuted in the manner required by law. Nothing in this subparagraph (iv) shall be construed to require the Board to report violations whenever the Board believes the public's interest will be adequately served in the circumstances by a suitable written notice or warning.

(6) The Board may place under seal all Drugs or Devices that are owned by or in the possession, custody, or control of a licensee at the time his license is suspended or revoked or at the time the Board refuses to renew his license. Except as otherwise provided in this section, Drugs or Devices so sealed shall not be disposed of until appeal rights under the Administrative Procedures Act have expired, or an appeal filed pursuant to that Act has been determined. The court involved in an appeal filed pursuant to the Administrative Procedures Act may order the Board, during the pendency of the appeal, to sell sealed Drugs that are perishable. The proceeds of such a sale shall be deposited with that court.

(7) Except as otherwise provided to the contrary, the Board shall exercise all of its duties, powers, and authority in accordance with the State Administrative Procedures Act.

(8) In addition to the fees specifically provided for herein, the Board may assess additional reasonable fees for services rendered to carry out its duties and responsibilities as required or authorized by this Act or Rules adopted hereunder. Such services rendered shall include, but not be limited to, the following:

(i) Issuance of duplicate certificates or identification cards;

(ii) Mailing lists, or reports of data maintained by the Board;

(iii) Copies of any documents;

(iv) Certification of documents;

(v) Notices of meetings;

(vi) Licensure transfer;

(vii) Examination administration to a licensure applicant; and

(viii) Examination materials.

(9) Cost Recovery

(i) If any order issues in resolution of a disciplinary proceeding before the Board of Pharmacy, the Board may request the to direct any licensee found guilty of a charge involving a violation of any drug laws or rules, to pay to the Board a sum not to exceed the reasonable costs of the investigation and prosecution of the case and, in any case, not to exceed twenty-five thousand dollars ($25,000).

(ii) In the case of a Pharmacy or Wholesale Distributor, the order may be made as to the corporate owner, if any, and as to any Pharmacist, officer, owner, or partner of the Pharmacy or Wholesale Distributor who is found to have had knowledge of or have knowingly participated in one or more of the violations set forth in this section.

(iii) The costs to be assessed shall be fixed by the and shall not be increased by the Board; where the Board does not adopt a proposed decision and remands the case to a(n) _____, the _____, shall not increase any assessed costs.

(iv) Where an order for recovery of costs is made and timely payment is not made as directed in the Board's decision, the Board may enforce the order for payment in the Court in the county where the administrative hearing was held. This right of enforcement shall be in addition to any other rights the Board may have as to any Person directed to pay costs.

(v) In any action for recovery of costs, proof of the Board's decision shall be conclusive proof of the validity of the order of payment and the terms for payment."

Licensure Exams

Passing an examination is a necessary prerequisite prior to licensure. Each state administers two exams, one dealing with the clinical and practice knowledge of the licensure applicant and the other dealing with state and federal law. The later test is often referred to as the "pharmacy jurisprudence" exam. All but a few states (at the time of publication, the two exceptions are California and Hawaii) administer the NAPLEX that was developed by the NABP to test clinical and practice-based knowledge skills. The NAPLEX consists of a combined format that determines a candidate's competency to practice through an integrated test, rather than dividing the material into separate subject areas. Most states now administer the NABP's Multistate Pharmacy Jurisprudence Exam (MPJE) to test the applicant's knowledge of individual state and federal laws. The MPJE provides flexibility to permit each state to test on its unique state laws while incorporating the federal laws common across the country. Detailed information about the MPJE is available in the NABP Registration Bulletin and at the NABP website: www.nabp.net. The MPJE has several questions involving federal laws pertinent to the practice of pharmacy. For this reason, applicants must know both federal and state laws. Applicants should take special care to learn both federal and state controlled substances laws because these are usually emphasized in the examinations. It is important to understand that there is no distinction between federal and state laws in the questions. Applicants are advised to answer all questions according to prevailing state law unless there is a stricter or preemptive federal law on point.

The MPJE is administered over a two-hour period in the computer-adaptive format similar to the NAPLEX. Each examination is unique to the individual applicant. One of the most important things to realize when sitting for this exam is that answers cannot be changed once they are entered. Unlike the traditional pencil and ink exam, the applicant cannot review questions and change answers later. Likewise, it is important to understand that a question cannot be skipped and referred to at later time. These factors make taking this test very different from the experiences of most pharmacy students.

While the test consists of 90 questions, only 60 are graded. A score of 75% or higher on the graded questions is needed to earn a passing mark. There is no distinction in the exam between graded and ungraded questions so the applicant has no way of knowing which of the 90 questions actually counts towards the final score.

Applicants should also be aware that the state MPJE scores may only be used for obtaining a pharmacist license in the state where the applicant is applying for a pharmacist license. Each state that uses the MPJE has its own separate version of the exam. However, applicants for a license in another state may actually take the exam for that state in another sate and have the results reported to the state where licensure is sought. Applicants are not allowed to take the examination before graduation.

Reciprocity

As an alternative to licensure by examination, some applicants also may seek licensure by the reciprocal or license transfer process. Such an applicant must:

(1) Have submitted a written application in the form prescribed by the Board of Pharmacy;

(2) Have attained the age of majority;

(3) Have good moral character;

(4) Have possessed at the time of initial licensure as a Pharmacist all qualifications necessary to have been eligible for licensure at that time in this State;

(5) Have engaged in the Practice of Pharmacy for a period of at least one (1) year or have met the internship requirements of this State within the one (1) year period immediately previous to the date of such application;

(6) Have presented to the Board proof of initial licensure by examination and proof that such license is in good standing;

(7) Have presented to the Board proof that any other license granted to the applicant by any other state has not been suspended, revoked, or otherwise restricted for any reason except non-renewal or for the failure to obtain the required continuing education credits in any state where the applicant is currently licensed but not engaged in the Practice of Pharmacy; and

(8) Have paid the fees specified by the Board.

(9) No applicant is be eligible for license transfer unless the state in which the applicant was initially licensed as a Pharmacist also grants licensure transfer to Pharmacists duly licensed by examination in this State, under like circumstances and conditions.

At the time of publication only California and Hawaii do not reciprocate with any of the other 48 states. In the past Florida was also a non-reciprocating state but it was removing some of the reciprocity restrictions at press time and is expected to participate in the reciprocity process in the near future.

The NABP acts as a clearinghouse for the reciprocation process. The applicant provides information to the NABP that in turn verifies these facts relating to licensure and provides that information to the reciprocating state. The reciprocating state reviews the application, and it is highly likely that before it will issue a license it will require the applicant to pass a jurisprudence examination (either the MPJE or its own jurisprudence exam) on the state laws where licensure is sought.

Interstate Practice

One of the more recent developments in pharmacy regulation involves practices that cross state borders such as in mail-order and internet dispensing where a pharmacist in one state may be dispensing prescriptions and counseling patients in another state. This presents a challenge to Boards of Pharmacy that do not have any legal authority or jurisdiction over the pharmacist located out of state. The MSPPA has a provision to address this situation:

(a) An applicant applying for registration to engage in the Practice of Telepharmacy Across State Lines shall:
    (1) present to the Board proof of licensure in another jurisdiction and proof that such license is in good standing;
    (2) submit a written application in the form prescribed by the Board of Pharmacy;
    (3) pay the fee(s) specified by the Board of Pharmacy for the issuance of the license; and

(4) comply with all other requirements of the Board of Pharmacy.

(b) Application
    (1) The written application required under Section 304(a)(1) of the Act shall request of the applicant, at a minimum, the following information:
        (i) Name, address, and current pharmacist licensure information in all other jurisdictions, including jurisdiction(s) of licensure and license number(s);
        (ii) Name, address, phone number, and (if applicable) jurisdiction of licensure and license number of the site where the Practice of Telepharmacy will originate;
        (iii) A statement of the scope of patient services that will be provided;
        (iv) A description of the protocol or framework by which patient care will be provided, including any collaborative practice arrangements with other health-care practitioners; and
        (v) A statement attesting that the applicant will abide by the pharmacy laws and regulations of the jurisdiction in which the patient is located.

A few states have adopted the model act language and others have taken a different approach. One example involves the "long arm jurisdiction" approach in which a state requires any out of state pharmacy that sends prescription drug into the state be licensed and comply with that state's laws. In either event, states still have jurisdictional and practical limits on seeking to discipline pharmacists and pharmacies located out of the state. This could be an area where the federal government may have to intervene to set up some uniform enforcement laws.

Institutional Pharmacy

The NABP also has developed model rules for institutional pharmacy. These regulations may be applied to facilities such as a hospital, nursing home, psychiatric center, health maintenance organization and others. These regulations include special provisions for the distribution of drugs when the institutional pharmacy is unattended by a licensed pharmacist. The model rules include provisions for night cabinets, emergency kits, investigational drugs, quality assurance and other items that particularly are applicable to the institutional practice of pharmacy.

Central to the issue of regulating institutional pharmacy practice is the definition of *institution*. The Model Rules for Institutional Pharmacy (MRIP) veloped by NAPB provides:

(a) *Institutional Facility* means any organization whose primary purpose is to provide a physical environment for patients to obtain health-care services, including but not limited to a(n):
    (1) Hospital;
    (2) Convalescent Home;
    (3) Nursing Home;
    (4) Extended Care Facility;
    (5) Mental Health Facility;
    (6) Rehabilitation Center;
    (7) Psychiatric Center;
    (8) Developmental Disability Center;
    (9) Drug Abuse Treatment Center;
    (10) Family Planning Clinic;
    (11) Penal Institution;
    (12) Hospice;
    (13) Public Health Facility;
    (14) Athletic Facility.

(b) *Institutional Pharmacy* means that physical portion of an Institutional Facility where Drugs, Devices, and other materials used in the diagnosis and treatment of injury, illness, and disease (hereinafter referred to as Drugs) are Dispensed, Compounded, and distributed and Pharmaceutical Care is provided; and that is registered with the State Board of Pharmacy pursuant to Article V of the Pharmacy Practice Act.

The MRIP contemplates that a *Pharmacist-in-Charge* will direct pharmacy practice in the institution. Absences are addressed in another provision:

(a) During such times as an Institutional Pharmacy may be unattended by a Pharmacist, arrangements shall be made in advance by the Pharmacist-in-Charge for provision of Drugs to the medical staff and other authorized personnel of the Institutional Facility by use of night cabinets and, in emergency circumstances, by access to the Pharmacy. A Pharmacist must be *on call* during all absences.

(b) In the absence of a Pharmacist, Drugs shall be stored in a locked cabinet or other enclosure constructed and located outside of the pharmacy area, to which only specifically authorized personnel may obtain access by key or combination, and that is sufficiently secure to deny access to unauthorized persons. The Pharmacist-in-Charge shall, in conjunction with the appropriate committee of the Institutional Facility, develop inventory listings of those Drugs to be included in such cabinet(s) and determine who may have access, and shall ensure that:

(1) Drugs are properly Labeled;

(2) Only prepackaged Drugs are available, in amounts sufficient for immediate therapeutic requirements;

(3) Whenever access to the cabinet occurs, written Practitioner's orders and proofs-of-use are provided;

(4) All Drugs therein are inventoried no less than once per week;

(5) A complete audit of all activity concerning such cabinet is conducted no less than once per month; and

(6) Written policies and procedures are established to implement the requirements of this Section 4.

(c) Whenever any Drug is not available from floor supplies or night cabinets, and such Drug is required to treat the immediate needs of a patient whose health would otherwise be jeopardized, such Drug may be obtained from the Pharmacy in accordance with the requirements of this Section 4. One supervisory nurse in any given 8-hr shift is responsible for obtaining Drugs from the Pharmacy. The responsible nurse shall be designated in writing by the appropriate committee of the Institutional Facility. Removal of any Drug from the Pharmacy by an authorized nurse must be recorded on a suitable form showing patient name, room number, name of Drug, strength, amount, date, time, and signature of nurse. The form shall be left with the container from which the Drug was removed.

(d) For an Institutional Facility that does not have an Institutional Pharmacy, Drugs may be provided for use by authorized personnel by emergency kits located at such Facility, provided, however, such kits meet the following requirements:

(1) Emergency kit drugs are those Drugs that may be required to meet the immediate therapeutic needs of patients and that are not available from any other authorized source in sufficient time to prevent risk of harm to patients by delay resulting from obtaining such Drugs from such other sources;

(2) All emergency kit drugs shall be provided and sealed by a Pharmacist;

(3) The supplying Pharmacist and the medical staff of the Institutional Facility shall jointly determine the Drugs, by identity and quantity, to be included in emergency kits;

(4) Emergency kits shall be stored in secured areas to prevent unauthorized access, and to ensure a proper environment for preservation of the Drugs within them;

(5) The exterior of each emergency kit shall be labeled so as to clearly indicate that it is an emergency drug kit and that it is for use in emergencies only. The label shall contain a listing of the Drugs contained in the kit, including name, strength, quantity, and expiration date of the contents, and the name, address(es), and telephone number(s) of the supplying Pharmacist;

(6) Drugs shall be removed from emergency kits only pursuant to a valid Prescription Drug Order;

(7) Whenever an emergency kit is opened, the supplying Pharmacist shall be notified and the Pharmacist shall restock and reseal the kit within a reasonable time so as to prevent risk of harm to patients; and

(8) The expiration date of an emergency kit shall be the earliest date of expiration of any Drug supplied in the kit. Upon the occurrence of the expiration date, the supplying Pharmacist shall replace the expired Drug. (MSPPA)

Drug distribution and control are also to be assigned responsibility of the Pharmacist-in-Charge:

(a) The Pharmacist-in-Charge shall establish written procedures for the safe and efficient distribution of Drugs and for the provision of Pharmaceutical Care. An annual updated copy of such procedures shall be on hand for inspection by the Board of Pharmacy.

(b) Drugs brought into an Institutional Facility by a patient shall not be Administered unless they can be identified and the quality of the Drug assured. If such Drugs are not to be Administered, then the Pharmacist-in-Charge shall, according to procedures specified in writing, have them turned into the Pharmacy, which shall package and seal them and return them to an adult member of the patient's immediate family, or store and return them to the patient upon discharge.

(c) Investigational Drugs shall be stored in and Dispensed from the Pharmacy only. All information with respect to investigational Drugs shall be maintained in the Pharmacy.

Licensing of Facilities

In most states community, as well as institutional, pharmacies may be operated only under permits issued by the board of pharmacy. State law normally will require an annual fee, provisions for inspection of the premises, proper prescription records and the maintenance of certain minimums of equipment or stock. The licensure of facilities provides a Board of Pharmacy with knowledge of all premises involved in the storage, distribution and sale of drugs and devices within the state and those located outside the state that are shipping drugs into the state. These requirements permit a Board of Pharmacy to better to insure against drug diversion from legitimate channels of commerce.

Nuclear Pharmacy

Nuclear pharmacy, recognized as the first specialty area in the profession, also may have special regulations at the state level. Most regulations make it unlawful for any person to provide nuclear pharmaceutical services unless under the supervision of a qualified nuclear pharmacist. The MSPPA defines *a Qualified Nuclear Pharmacist* as a currently licensed pharmacist in the State of practice, who is certified as a Nuclear Pharmacist by the State Board of Pharmacy or by a certification board recognized by the State Board of Pharmacy, or who meets the following standards:

(1) Minimum standards of training for *authorized user status* of radioactive material.

(2) Completed a minimum of 200 contact hours of instruction in nuclear pharmacy and the safe handling and the use of radioactive materials from a program approved by the State Board of Pharmacy, with emphasis in the following areas:

(i) Radiation physics and instrumentation;

(ii) Radiation protection;

(iii) Mathematics of radioactivity;

(iv) Radiation biology; and

(v) Radiopharmaceutical chemistry.

(3) Attain a minimum of 500 hr of clinical nuclear pharmacy training under the supervision of a qualified nuclear pharmacist.

Pharmaceutical Care

The NABP has developed comprehensive model rules to implement the patient-care concepts embodied in the definition of the practice of pharmacy. The rules provide for the age-old requirements of a prescription- drug order with provisions for the electronic transmittal of the prescription to the pharmacist. The transfer of prescriptions between unrelated pharmacies also is addressed in these rules.

The model rules include provisions for drug-product selection, prescription labeling and patient records. These sections provide an important background for the central focus of the pharmaceutical care rules—the requirement for patient counseling and prospective drug review by the pharmacist. Following a review of the patient's records for therapeutic duplication, drug interactions, over- or under-use and a number of other considerations, the pharmacist personally must initiate discussion with the patient or the patient's caregiver regarding the prescription.

Minimum Requirements for a Pharmacy

The physical facilities housing a pharmacy are addressed in the Model Rules for Pharmaceutical Care:

(1) Each Pharmacy shall be of sufficient size to allow for the safe and proper storage of Prescription Drugs and for the safe and proper Compounding and/or preparation of Prescription Drug Orders.

(2) Each Pharmacy shall maintain an area designated for the provision of Patient Counseling services. This area shall be designed to provide a reasonable expectation of privacy.

(3) Each Pharmacy shall maintain on file at least one current reference in each of the following categories:
 (a) State and Federal drug laws relating to the Practice of Pharmacy and the legal distribution of Drugs and any rules or regulations adopted pursuant thereto;
 (b) pharmacology;
 (c) dosage and toxicology;
 (d) general.

(4) Each Pharmacy shall maintain patient-oriented reference material for guidance in proper drug usage.

(5) All areas where Drugs and Devices are stored shall be dry, well-lighted, well-ventilated, and maintained in a clean and orderly condition. Storage areas shall be maintained at temperatures that will ensure the integrity of the Drugs prior to their Dispensing as stipulated by the USP/NF and/or the Manufacturer's or distributor's Labeling unless otherwise indicated by the Board.

(6) Each Pharmacy shall have access to a sink with hot and cold running water that is convenient to the Compounding area for the purpose of hand scrubs prior to Compounding.

(7) Security
 (a) Each Pharmacist, while on duty, shall be responsible for the security of the Pharmacy, including provisions for effective control against theft or diversion of Drugs and/or Devices.
 (b) The Pharmacy shall be secured by either a physical barrier with suitable locks and/or an electronic barrier to detect entry at a time when the Pharmacist is not present. Such barrier shall be approved by the Board of Pharmacy before being put into use.
 (c) Prescription and other patient health-care information shall be maintained in a manner that protects the integrity and confidentiality of such information as provided by the rules of the Board.

(8) Equipment/Supplies
 (a) The Pharmacy shall carry and use the equipment and supplies necessary to conduct a Pharmacy in a manner that is in the best interest of the patients served and to comply with all State and Federal laws.

(9) The Pharmacy shall provide a means for patients to prevent disclosure of Confidential Information or personally identifiable information that was obtained or collected by the Pharmacist or Pharmacy incidental to the delivery of Pharmaceutical Care other than as authorized by law or rules of the Board. (MSPPA)

Duties of the pharmacist and pharmacy personnel are also delineated:

Duties and Responsibilities of the Pharmacist-in-Charge

(1) No Person shall operate a Pharmacy without a Pharmacist-in-Charge. The Pharmacist-in-Charge of a Pharmacy shall be designated in the application of the Pharmacy for license, and in each renewal thereof. A Pharmacist may not serve as Pharmacist-in-Charge unless he is physically present in the Pharmacy a sufficient amount of time to provide supervision and control. A Pharmacist may not serve as Pharmacist-in-Charge for more than one Pharmacy at any one time except upon obtaining written permission from the Board.

(2) The Pharmacist-in-Charge has the following responsibilities:
 (a) Developing quality assurance programs for pharmacy services designed to objectively and systematically monitor and evaluate the quality and appropriateness of patient care, pursue opportunities to improve patient care, and resolve identified problems. Quality assurance programs shall be designed to prevent and detect drug diversion.
 (b) The Pharmacist-in-Charge shall develop or adopt, implement, and maintain a Pharmacy Technician Training Manual for the specific practice setting of which he is in charge. He shall supervise a training program conducted pursuant to the Pharmacy Technician Training Manual for all indi-

viduals employed by the Pharmacy who will assist in the Practice of Pharmacy. The Pharmacist-in-Charge shall be responsible for maintaining a record of all technicians successfully completing the Pharmacy's Technician training program and shall attest to the Board of Pharmacy, in a timely manner, those persons who, from time to time, have met the training requirements necessary for registration with the Board.
 (c) Establishing policies and procedures for the procurement, storage, security, and disposition of Drugs and Devices.
 (d) Establishing policies and procedures for the provision of pharmacy services.
 (e) Assuring that the Automated Pharmacy System is in good working order and accurately dispenses the correct strength, dosage form, and quantity of the drug prescribed while maintaining appropriate record keeping and security safeguards.
 (f) Implementing an ongoing quality assurance program that monitors performance of the Automated Pharmacy System, which is evidenced by written policies and procedures developed by the pharmacy.
 (g) Assuring that all Pharmacists and Interns employed at the Pharmacy are currently licensed and that all Pharmacy Technicians employed at the Pharmacy are currently registered with the Board of Pharmacy.
 (h) Notifying the Board of Pharmacy immediately of any of the following changes:
  (i) Change of employment or responsibility as the Pharmacist-in-Charge;
  (ii) Change of ownership of the Pharmacy;
  (iii) Change of address of the Pharmacy; or
  (iv) Permanent closing of the Pharmacy.
 (i) Making or filing any reports required by State or Federal laws and rules.
 (j) Responding to the Board of Pharmacy regarding any minor violations brought to his/her attention.
 (k) Establishing policies and procedures for maintaining the integrity and confidentiality of prescription information and patient health-care information, or verifying the existence thereof and ensuring that all employees of the Pharmacy read, sign, and comply with the established policies and procedures.
 (l) Assuring that the means provided for as stipulated in Section 1.A.(9) have been established and implemented.
 (m) Providing the Board with prior written notice of the installation or removal of Automated Pharmacy Systems. Such notice must include, but is not limited to:
  (i) The name and address of the pharmacy;
  (ii) The location of the automated equipment; and
  (iii) The identification of the responsible pharmacist.

(3) The Pharmacist-in-Charge shall be assisted by a sufficient number of Pharmacists and Pharmacy Technicians as may be required to competently and safely provide pharmacy services.
 (a) The Pharmacist-in-Charge shall maintain and file with the Board of Pharmacy, on a form provided by the Board, a current list of all Pharmacy Technicians assisting in the provision of pharmacy services.
 (b) The Pharmacist-in-Charge shall develop and implement written policies and procedures to specify the duties to be performed by Pharmacy Technicians. The duties and responsibilities of these personnel shall be consistent with their training and experience. These policies and procedures shall, at a minimum, specify that Pharmacy Technicians are to be personally and directly supervised by a Pharmacist stationed within the same work area who has the ability to control and who is responsible for the activities of Pharmacy Technicians, and that Pharmacy Technicians are not assigned duties that may be performed only by a Pharmacist.

(4) The Pharmacist-in-Charge shall develop and implement a procedure for proper management of Drug recalls that may include, where appropriate, contacting patients to whom the recalled Drug product(s) have been Dispensed. (MSPPA)

Processing of prescription orders are described in detail:

A. *Prescription Drug Order.* A Prescription Drug Order shall contain the following information at a minimum:
 (1) Full name and street address of the patient;
 (2) Name, address, and, if required by law or rules of the Board, DEA registration number of the prescribing Practitioner;

(3) Date of issuance;

(4) Name, strength, dosage form, and quantity of Drug prescribed;

(5) Directions for use;

(6) Refills authorized, if any; and

(7) If a written Prescription Drug Order, prescribing Practitioner's signature.

B. *Manner of Issuance of a Prescription Drug Order.* A Prescription Drug Order, to be effective, must be issued for a legitimate medical purpose by a Practitioner acting within the course of legitimate professional practice.

(1) A Prescription Drug Order must be communicated directly to a Pharmacist in a licensed Pharmacy. This may be accomplished in one of the following ways. A Prescription Drug Order, including that for a controlled substance listed in Schedules II through V, may be communicated in written form. A Prescription Drug Order, including that for a controlled substance listed in Schedules III through V, and, in certain situations, that for a controlled substance listed in Schedule II, may be communicated orally (including telephone voice communication) or by way of Electronic Transmission.

(2) If communicated orally or by way of Electronic Transmission, the Prescription Drug Order shall be immediately reduced to a form by the Pharmacist that may be maintained for the time required by laws or rules. . . .

C. *Transfer of a Prescription Drug Order.* Pharmacies using automated data processing systems shall satisfy all information requirements of a manual mode for Prescription Drug Order transferal, except as noted in subsection (4) below. The transfer of original Prescription Drug Order information for the purpose of refill dispensing is permissible between Pharmacies subject to the following requirements:

(1) The information is communicated directly between two Pharmacists and the transferring Pharmacist records the following information:

(a) Write the word *VOID* on the face of the invalidated Prescription Drug Order;

(b) Record on the reverse side of the invalidated Prescription Drug Order the name and address of the Pharmacy to which it was transferred and the name of the Pharmacist receiving the Prescription Drug Order;

(c) Record the date of the transfer and the name of the Pharmacist transferring the information; and

(d) The computer record shall reflect the fact that the original Prescription Drug Order has been voided and shall contain all the other information required above.

(2) The Pharmacist receiving the transferred Prescription Drug Order information shall reduce to writing the following:

(a) Write the word *TRANSFER* on the face of the transferred Prescription Drug Order;

(b) Provide all information required to be on a Prescription Drug Order pursuant to State and Federal laws and rules, and include:

(i) Date of issuance of original Prescription Drug Order;

(ii) Original number of refills authorized on original Prescription Drug Order;

(iii) Date of original Dispensing;

(iv) Number of valid refills remaining and date of last refill;

(v) Pharmacy's name, address, and original prescription number from which the Prescription Drug Order information was transferred; and

(vi) Name of transferring Pharmacist.

(c) Systems providing for the electronic transfer of information shall not infringe on a patient's freedom of choice as to the provider of Pharmaceutical Care.

(3) Both the original and transferred Prescription Drug Order shall be maintained for a period of 5 yr from the date of last refill.

(4) Pharmacies accessing a common electronic file or database used to maintain required Dispensing information are not required to transfer Prescription Drug Orders or information for Dispensing purposes between or among Pharmacies participating in the same common prescription file, provided, however, that any such common file shall contain complete records of each Prescription Drug Order and refill Dispensed, and, further, that a hard copy record of each Prescription Drug Order transferred or accessed for purposes of refilling shall be generated and maintained at the Pharmacy refilling

the Prescription Drug Order or to which the Prescription Drug Order is transferred.

D. *Drug Product Selection by the Pharmacist.*

(1) A Pharmacist Dispensing a Prescription Drug Order for a Drug product prescribed by its brand name may select any Equivalent Drug Product provided that the Manufacturer or distributor holds, if applicable, either an approved New Drug Application (NDA) or an approved Abbreviated New Drug Application (ANDA), unless other approval by law or from the FDA is required.

(2) The Pharmacist shall not select an Equivalent Drug Product if the Practitioner instructs otherwise, either orally or in writing, on the Prescription Drug Order.

(3) The Pharmacist shall notify the patient or patient's agent if a Drug other than the brand name Drug prescribed is Dispensed.

(4) Whenever Drug Product Selection is performed by a Pharmacist, the Pharmacist shall Dispense the Equivalent Drug Product in a container Labeled in accordance with Section 3.E (Labeling).

E. *Labeling.*

(1) All Drugs Dispensed for use by inpatients of a hospital or other health-care facility, whereby the Drug is not in the possession of the ultimate user prior to Administration, shall meet the following requirements:

(a) The label of a single-unit package of an individual-dose or unit-dose system of packaging of Drugs shall include:

(i) The nonproprietary or proprietary name of the Drug;

(ii) The route of Administration, if other than oral;

(iii) The strength and volume, where appropriate, expressed in the metric system whenever possible;

(iv) The control number and expiration date;

(v) Identification of the re-packager by name or by license number shall be clearly distinguishable from the rest of the label; and

(vi) Special storage conditions, if required.

(b) When a multiple-dose Drug distribution system is used, including Dispensing of single unit packages, the Drugs shall be Dispensed in a container to which is affixed a label containing the following information:

(i) Identification of the Dispensing Pharmacy;

(ii) The patient's name;

(iii) The date of Dispensing;

(iv) The nonproprietary and/or proprietary name of the Drug Dispensed; and

(v) The strength, expressed in the metric system whenever possible.

(2) All Drugs Dispensed to ambulatory or outpatients shall contain a label affixed to the container in which such Drug is dispensed including:

(a) The name and address of the Pharmacy Dispensing the Drug;

(b) The name of the patient for whom the Drug is prescribed; or, if the patient is an animal, the name of the owner and the species of the animal;

(c) The name of the prescribing Practitioner;

(d) Such directions as may be stated on the Prescription Drug Order;

(e) The date of Dispensing;

(f) Any cautions that may be required by Federal or State law;

(g) The serial number of the Prescription Drug Order;

(h) The name or initials of the Dispensing Pharmacist;

(i) The proprietary or generic name of the Drug Dispensed and its strength, if more than one strength of the Drug is marketed;

(i) When Dispensing an Equivalent Drug Product, the word *INTERCHANGE* or letters *IC* must appear on the label affixed to the container in which such Drug is Dispensed, followed by the generic name and Manufacturer, or reasonable abbreviation, and/or distributor of the chosen product.

(ii) The requirements of (i) only apply to single-entity, multiple-source Drugs.

(iii) When Dispensing a single-entity, single-source Drug, the trade name of the prescribed Drug may also appear on the label, and the generic name of the prescribed Drug may also appear on the label.

(iv) When Dispensing a fixed combination product, the USP's publication of Pharmacy Equivalent Names

(PEN) for fixed combination products is the official list of abbreviations for such Labeling, and will be the approved abbreviation for identifying the combination product Dispensed. If no PEN has been officially issued by the USP, the Practitioner or Pharmacist will label the medication secundum artem.

    (v) Subsection (i) - (iv) apply in all cases of Dispensing by Practitioners or Pharmacists.

  (j) The name of the Manufacturer or distributor of the Drug;

  (k) The Beyond-Use Date. . . .

F. *Patient Records.*

(1) A patient record system shall be maintained by all Pharmacies for patients for whom Prescription Drug Orders are Dispensed. The patient record system shall provide for the immediate retrieval of information necessary for the Dispensing Pharmacist to identify previously Dispensed Drugs at the time a Prescription Drug Order is presented for Dispensing. The Pharmacist shall make a reasonable effort to obtain, record, and maintain the following information:

  (a) Full name of the patient for whom the Drug is intended;

  (b) Street address and telephone number of the patient;

  (c) Patient's age or date of birth;

  (d) Patient's gender;

  (e) A list of all Prescription Drug Orders obtained by the patient at the Pharmacy maintaining the patient record during the (number) years immediately preceding the most recent entry showing the name of the Drug, prescription number, name and strength of the Drug, the quantity and date received, and the name of the Practitioner; and

  (f) Pharmacist comments relevant to the individual's drug therapy, including any other information peculiar to the specific patient or Drug.

(2) The Pharmacist shall make a reasonable effort to obtain from the patient or the patient's agent and shall record any known allergies, drug reactions, idiosyncrasies, and chronic conditions or disease states of the patient and the identity of any other Drugs, including over-the-counter Drugs or Devices currently being used by the patient that may relate to Prospective Drug Review.

(3) A patient record shall be maintained for a period of not less than 5 years from the date of the last entry in the profile record. This record may be a hard copy or a computerized form.

(4) Confidential Information or personally identifiable information may be released to the patient or the patient's authorized representative, the prescriber or other licensed Practitioner then caring for the patient, another licensed Pharmacist, the Board or its representative, or any other person duly authorized by law to receive such information. Confidential Information or personally identifiable information in the patient medication record may be released to others only on written release of the patient.

G. *Prospective Drug Review.* A Pharmacist shall review the patient record and each Prescription Drug Order presented for Dispensing for purposes of promoting therapeutic appropriateness by identifying:

(1) Over-utilization or under-utilization;

(2) Therapeutic duplication;

(3) Drug-disease contraindications;

(4) Drug-Drug interactions;

(5) Incorrect Drug dosage or duration of Drug treatment;

(6) Drug-allergy interactions;

(7) Clinical abuse/misuse.

Upon recognizing any of the above, the Pharmacist must take appropriate steps to avoid or resolve the problem and if necessary, include consultation with the Prescriber.

H. *Patient Counseling.*

(1) Upon receipt of a Prescription Drug Order and following a review of the patient's record, a Pharmacist shall personally initiate discussion of matters that will enhance or optimize drug therapy with each patient or caregiver of such patient. Such discussion shall be in person, whenever practicable, or by telephone and shall include appropriate elements of patient counseling. Such elements may include the following:

  (a) The name and description of the Drug;

  (b) The dosage form, dose, route of Administration, and duration of Drug therapy;

  (c) Intended use of the Drug and expected action;

  (d) Special directions and precautions for preparation, Administration, and use by the patient;

  (e) Common severe side or adverse effects or interactions and therapeutic contraindications that may be encountered, including their avoidance, and the action required if they occur;

  (f) Techniques for self-monitoring Drug therapy;

  (g) Proper storage;

  (h) Prescription refill information;

  (i) Action to be taken in the event of a missed dose; and

  (j) Pharmacist comments relevant to the individual's Drug therapy, including any other information peculiar to the specific patient or Drug.

    Alternative forms of patient information shall be used to supplement Patient Counseling when appropriate. Examples include written information leaflets, pictogram labels, video programs, etc.

(2) A Pharmacist providing Telepharmacy services across state lines shall:

  (a) Identify himself or herself to patients as a *licensed pharmacist*;

  (b) Notify patients of the jurisdiction in which he or she is currently licensed to Practice Pharmacy and registered to Practice Telepharmacy Across State Lines; and

  (c) Provide patients with that jurisdiction's board of pharmacy address and/or phone number.

(4) Patient Counseling, as described above and defined in this Act, shall not be required for inpatients of a hospital or institution where other licensed health-care professionals are authorized to Administer the Drug(s).

(5) A Pharmacist shall not be required to counsel a patient or caregiver when the patient or caregiver refuses such consultation.

The Model Rules for Pharmaceutical Care also address unprofessional conduct.

Unprofessional conduct shall include, but is not limited to, the following acts of a Pharmacist or Pharmacy:

(1) The publication or circulation of false, misleading, or otherwise deceptive statements concerning the Practice of Pharmacy.

(2) Unreasonably refusing to Compound or Dispense Prescription Drug Orders that may be expected to be Compounded or Dispensed in Pharmacies by Pharmacists.

(3) Attempting to circumvent the Patient Counseling requirements, or discouraging the patient from receiving Patient Counseling concerning their Prescription Drug Orders.

(4) Divulging or revealing to unauthorized Persons patient or Practitioner information or the nature of professional Pharmacy services rendered without the patient's express consent, or without order or direction of a court. The following are considered authorized Persons:

  (a) Patient or patient's agent, or another Pharmacist acting on behalf of a patient;

  (b) Practitioner who issued the Prescription Drug Order;

  (c) Certified/licensed health-care personnel who are responsible for the care of the patient;

  (d) A member, inspector, agent, or investigator of the Board of Pharmacy or any Federal, State, county, or municipal officer whose duty is to enforce the laws of this State or the US relating to Drugs and/or Devices and who is engaged in a specific investigation involving a designated Person or Drug; and

  (e) An agency of government charged with the responsibility of providing medical care for the patient, upon a written request by an authorized representative of the agency requesting such information.

(5) Selling, giving away, or otherwise disposing of accessories, chemicals, or Drugs or Devices found in illegal Drug traffic when the Pharmacist knows or should have known of their intended use in illegal activities.

(6) Engaging in conduct likely to deceive, defraud, or harm the public, or demonstrating a willful or careless disregard for the health, welfare, or safety of a patient, or engaging in conduct that substantially departs from the standards of care ordinarily exercised by a Pharmacist, with proof of actual injury not having to be established.

(7) Selling a Drug for which a Prescription Drug Order from a Practitioner is required, without having received a Prescription Drug Order for the Drug.

(8) Willfully and knowingly failing to maintain complete and accurate records of all Drugs received, Dispensed, or disposed of in compliance with the Federal laws and regulations and State laws and rules.

(9) Obtaining any remuneration by fraud, misrepresentation, or deception, including, but not limited to, receiving remuneration for amending or modifying, or attempting to amend or modify, a patient's Pharmaceutical Care, absent a clear benefit to the patient, solely in response to promotion or marketing activities.

All states that intend to remain in compliance with Federal Medicaid requirements need to adopt some form of patient counseling. The Omnibus Budget Reconciliation Act (OBRA) of 1990 provides that pharmacists must offer to counsel, in person or by telephone, all Medicaid recipients who receive prescription drugs. The model rules provide a framework for the states to adopt so that the concepts of pharmaceutical care might be extended to all patients, not just those on Medicaid.

Computer Regulations

Computerization has become an important component of the profession as more and more pharmacies keep a wide variety of records on computers. Model rules have been developed by the NABP for states who wish to use them to facilitate the inspection of pharmacies employing computers. These computer systems must have adequate security and systems safeguards to maintain the confidentiality of patients and to prevent unauthorized access or manipulation of patient-profile data.

The computer system must provide for on-line retrieval of original information for those prescription orders that are currently authorized for refilling. The MSPPA states:

The computerized system shall have the capability of producing a printout of any prescription-drug order information. The systems should provide a refill-by-refill audit trail for any specified strength and dosage form of any drug. Such an audit trail must be by printout, and include name of the prescribing practitioner, name and location of the patient, quantity dispensed on each refill, date of dispensing of each refill, name or identification code of the dispensing pharmacist and unique identifier of the prescription.

The model rules also provide for special backup procedures when the automated system becomes temporarily inoperative. This auxiliary system must insure that all refills are authorized and that the maximum number of refills is not exceeded, and it must! be maintained until the automated system becomes operational. The proposed model rules provide that nothing shall preclude the pharmacist from using professional judgment for the benefit of the patient's health and safety when the computerized system is not working. When the computer returns to operation, all information regarding prescriptions filled and refilled during the inoperative period must be entered into the computer within 96 hours.

Pharmacy Ownership

Few states have ownership restrictions on pharmacies. Some states have attempted to legislate against physician-owned pharmacies or any other type of non-pharmacist owned pharmacies. The US Supreme Court in 1928 held that laws restricting pharmacy ownership only to pharmacists violated the Fourteenth Amendment of the US Constitution. Forty-four years later, the same issue again was raised in the North Dakota courts. The North Dakota Pharmacy Act required that the majority of stock of a pharmacy corporation be owned by registered pharmacists in good standing in North Dakota. The statute was challenged by an out-of-state chain operation, and the case

eventually was appealed to the US Supreme Court. The nation's highest court reversed its earlier decision and held that pharmacy-ownership laws were constitutionally sound if such a requirement could be related reasonably to the public's health and welfare. The case was returned to the North Dakota Supreme Court and that court identified seven possible reasons for ownership restrictions:

1. The professional and ethical standards of pharmacy demand the pharmacist's concern for the quantity and quality of stock and equipment. A drug that has deteriorated because of improper storage can be a detriment to public health. A drug not in stock poses a threat to the individual who needs it now. Decisions made in conjunction with the quantity and quality of stock and equipment by non-registered pharmacist-owners could be detrimental to the public health and welfare.
2. Supervision of hired pharmacists by registered-pharmacist-owners would be in the best interests of public health and safety.
3. Responsibility for improper action could be pinpointed more readily when supervision is in registered pharmacist-owners.
4. The dignity of a profession, and the morale and proficiency of those licensed to engage therein, is enhanced by prohibiting the practitioner from subordinating himself to the direction of untrained supervisors.
5. If control and management is vested in laymen unacquainted with pharmaceutical service, who are untrained and unlicensed, the risk is that social accountability will be subordinated to the profit motive.
6. The term pharmacy was intended to identify a particular type of establishment within which a health profession is practiced, and thus was intended to be more than a mere means of making a profit. He who holds the purse strings controls the policy.
7. Doctor-owned pharmacies with built-in conflict-of-interest problems could be restricted.

Although this case cleared the way for state legislatures to develop restrictions on the ownership of pharmacies, there has not been a great deal of momentum in this area. Consumer groups and large national pharmacy corporations have lobbied successfully against such proposals.

Hypodermic Needles and Syringes

Some states restrict the sale of hypodermic needles and syringes to a pharmacist on an over-the-counter (OTC) basis. The pharmacist of course must use good professional discretion to ensure that the devices are not to be used illegally. Other states will require that these devices be sold only upon a physicians order. Other states restrict the sale of these devises to prescription only status but make exception to permit their sale without a prescription order when they are to be used by diabetics, for the administration of adrenaline or for veterinary use. In these latter cases a registry is often required as evidence of the OTC sale.

Compounding

As mentioned in the *Relationship Between State and Federal Laws* section in the introductory remarks to this chapter, the issue of states rights versus federal rights on the issue of which government controls the practice of pharmacy compounding has been controversial since the early 1990s. Before that period of time, compounding was considered to be part of the practice of pharmacy and therefore regulated exclusively bt the states. Policy makers at the FDA began rethinking the issue when some of the large, brand name drug manufacturers that belong to the Pharmaceutical Research and Manufacturers of America (PhRMA) group decided that community pharmacists should not be permitted to compound drugs that are available in commercial preparations. In public, the FDA claimed that many retail pharmacies were purchasing large quantities of bulk drug substances and combining those substances into specific drug products before ever receiving any valid prescriptions. The FDA speculated that these pharmacies engaged in this large-scale compounding to circumvent the drug, adulteration, and misbranding provisions of the Food, Drug, and Cosmetic Act (FD&CA), discussed further below, that regulate the manufacture of drugs.

The mechanism chosen for this newly developed attempt to regulate pharmacy practice was to declare compounded preparations to be unapproved new drugs even when all of the ingredients in the compounded product had pre-approval from the FDA. There was no consideration given to the fact that first half century after enactment of the FDCA, the FDA left regulation of compounding to state governments. During those approximately 50 years, pharmacists regularly compounded products without applying to the FDA for an NDA (new drug approval). The FDA justified its authority by claiming unapproved compounds could be a dangerous threat to public health. It also reasoned that the availability of commercial products that had been through a rigorous NDA process could satisfy the needs of the vast majority of patients, and pharmacist compounding was no longer necessary.

To give field agents some standards for searching out pharmacists engaged in this illegal public endangerment, the FDA developed Compliance Policy Guide (CPG) 7132.16 in 1992. The guideline contained nine "factors" that agents were to take into account before deciding if a pharmacist was engaged in illegal manufacturing under the pretext of normal compounding. One of the factors was whether the pharmacy advertises compounding services or solicits prescriptions requiring compounding from physicians for commercially available products. It may only be a historical quirk, but 1992 was also the year that Congress passed the Prescription Drug User Fee Act (PDUFA). This law changed the FDA from being a exclusive taxpayer supported agency to one that is funded, at least in part, by the commercial manufacturers who are subject to its regulations. The FDA did not take into consideration that some patients might have unique needs that commercial preparations could not address. Several enforcement actions were taken against small pharmacies taking care of one patient at a time. The FDA also took enforcement actions against some of the larger operations that solicited prescriptions from across state lines and compounded large batches of medications in anticipation of receiving prescriptions.

Soon after the guideline went into effect, a group representing pharmacies that engaged in widespread compounding activities known as Professionals and Patients for Customized Care (P2C2) sought to prevent its enforcement. They claimed that the FDA violated federal rulemaking procedures because the Compliance Policy was really a new rule that affected substantive rights and therefore should have been subject to formal procedures and public comment under the federal Administrative Procedures Act. They claimed that this was a new attempt by the federal government to regulate the practice of pharmacy. In 1995, a federal court of appeals affirmed a lower court finding that the FDA was well within its authority to use the guidelines in the manner it choose. In doing so, the court noted that the FDA had some limitations imposed on it by Congress. The law has been that pharmacists who dispense drugs upon prescriptions of practitioners for their patients, and do not manufacture or compound drugs for sale other than in the regular course of their business of dispensing or selling drugs, are exempt from FDA registration requirements for manufacturing and the misbranding provisions of the FD&CA. The court also noted that although the FD&CA does not expressly exempt "pharmacies" or "compounded drugs" from the new drug, adulteration, or misbranding provisions, the FDA as a matter of policy had not historically brought enforcement actions against pharmacies engaged in traditional compounding. In the court's view the Compliance Policy does not change that law; it simply announces factors for deciding when pharmacies have overstepped the authority to compound.

Despite that governmental victory, the acrimony between compounding pharmacies and the FDA continued. At the time, Congress was engaged in hearings to reform other FDA practices. This effort culminated in the Food and Drug Administration Modernization Act of 1997 (FDAMA), which, among other things, added a new section to the FD&CA. This new part, §503a, attempted to accommodate the FDA's need to prevent unsafe products from being marketed and at the same time prevent the agency from overreaching into the normal practice of pharmacy. A majority of the factors contained in the Compliance Policy were incorporated into FDAMA. The statute stated, in essence, that pharmacist-compounded drugs are exempt from the FD&CA's standard drug-approval requirements as long as the pharmacies refrain from advertising or promoting particular compounded drugs.

Before the law was scheduled to take effect, another group of pharmacies specializing in compounding services sought an injunction to prevent its enforcement. They claimed that the advertising ban violates the Constitution's free speech guarantee in the First Amendment. Both the district court and the court of appeals found the statute unconstitutional.

Supreme Court Decision

The US Supreme Court agreed to hear the FDA's appeal. The high court rendered its decision in *Thompson v. Western States Medical Center*, 70 USLW 4275 on April 30, 2002. With a narrow majority of five justices agreeing over the vigorous opposition of the four justices in the minority, the Supreme Court agreed that the entire statute (§503a) is unconstitutional and must be stricken because it infringes on commercial speech rights. The decision rebuked the unsound position of the FDA that average pharmacists working in the community cannot be trusted to safely compound drug products. It also questioned the integrity of the FDA when it claimed the ban on the advertising of these products is necessary to prevent the public from demanding drugs they do not otherwise need and pressuring doctors who cannot resist prescribing them.

While there are a number of salient points in the majority opinion, one of the more striking is the court's focus on the fact that the attempted restrictions on pharmacy compounding only applies to products that are otherwise commercially available. The FDA attempted to justify this application by claiming the new drug approval process that manufacturers are subject to results in scientifically sound conclusions about the safety and efficacy of commercial products. The FDA also complained that the impressions of the individual doctors who think a patient might benefit from a compounded alternative to a commercial product cannot be relied upon because these physicians are incapable of compiling sufficient safety data. Ignoring the irony of the situation, the FDA claimed in the same breath that it did not want to end all compounding for individual patients by pharmacists because compounding is "sometimes critical to the care of patients with drug allergies, patients who cannot tolerate particular drug delivery systems, and patients requiring special drug dosages." Apparently those doctors who cannot be trusted to make adequate safety assessments if a product is commercially available can be trusted when a commercial product is not as desirable. What is so striking about the attempted distinction is that it is exactly when a physician thinks there is an alternative to the commercially available product that a compounded product is called for. A majority of the justices concluded that this argument puts the FDA into an untenable position. Preserving the integrity of the new drug approval process is an important governmental interest, but no more important than its interest in encouraging a system that permits patients access to the particular drugs needed to treat individual conditions.

The majority of the justices also rejected the FDA's argument that advertising, or the lack thereof, is somehow tied to the quality of the product produced by compounding pharmacies. Justice O'Connor seemed especially perplexed by the FDA's position that it is perfectly fine for compounded drugs that have not undergone safety and efficacy testing to be sold by compounding pharmacies that do not advertise, but not all right if the products or services are advertised. The government justified its position by claiming that advertising is not necessary for traditional small scale compounding legally performed by pharmacists for individual patients where commercial products are not available. It claimed that pharmacies that do advertise are the ones engaged in the large-scale operations that look more like manufacturing than compounding. In other words, the FDA used advertising as proxy for the large-scale production of compounded drugs to meet marketplace needs as opposed to individual needs determined on a case-by-case basis. According to the FDA, the ban on advertising closes a loophole that would allow unlicensed manufacturing under the notion that the pharmacy was merely compounding. Justice O'Connor did not buy into the claim that without advertising it would not be possible to market a drug on a large scale to make safety and efficacy testing economically feasible. Nor did she accept the idea that conditioning an exemption from the FDA approval process on refraining from advertising is an acceptable way to permit compounding and yet also guarantee that compounding is not conducted on such a scale as to undermine the FDA approval process.

She went on to complain that the amount of beneficial speech prohibited by the FDAMA is forbidding enough to hold it unconstitutional. Her concern centered around the intimidation effect the ban would have on pharmacists wanting to advertise legitimate compounding services. She noted that forbidding the advertisement of compounded drugs altogether would prevent pharmacists with no interest in mass-producing medications, but who serve clienteles with special medical needs, from telling the doctors treating those clients about the alternative drugs available through compounding. She set forth an example involving a pharmacist serving a children's hospital, where many patients are unable to swallow pills, would be prevented from telling the children's doctors about a new development in compounding that allowed the drug to be administered another way. In her opinion, the ban would also prohibit a pharmacist from posting a notice informing customers that if their children refuse to take medications because of the taste, the pharmacist could change the flavor. The net result of the *Thompson* decision is to render §503a unconstitutional and unenforceable.

Despite that holding, within days of the *Thompson* decision by the Supreme Court, the FDA "re-issued" its 1992 Compliance Policy Guidance (Guidance) (CPG Ch. 4 § 460.200 (May, 2002) with minor alterations to give the FDA and pharmacists notice of what factors will be taken into account to determine whether the pharmacy is engaged in legal compounding as opposed to unlawful manufacturing of drugs under the guise of compounding. It is noteworthy that the Guidance was published as FDA policy without any advance public notice or comment period. The irony of that action is that it was the original 1992 Guidance on compounding issued by the FDA (CPG Ch. 4 § 7132.16 (March, 1992) renumbered to § 460.200) that underlies the Thompson decision. Taking these developments into account, it should be clear the pharmacies may advertise compounding services but still not "manufacture" large quantities of drugs under the guise of compounding.

Both the current 2002 and original 1992 versions of the Guidance are presented below in the hope that comparing the "current thinking" of the FDA with its thought process over a decade ago may be instructive in determining the agency's priorities. Although there are places that the two versions do not line up exactly, the 1992 version has been reordered with its original factor number to match the 2002 version as close as possible. In both versions, the preamble states that in deciding whether the FDA will initiate an enforcement action, it will consider whether the pharmacy engages in *any* of the following acts (emphasis added):

2002 COMPLIANCE POLICY GUIDE	1992 COMPLIANCE POLICY GUIDE (REORDERED)
1. Compounding of drugs in anticipation of receiving prescriptions, except in very limited quantities in relation to the amounts of drugs compounded after receiving valid prescriptions.	6. Compounding inordinate amounts of drugs in anticipation of receiving prescriptions in relation to the amounts of drugs compounded after receiving valid prescriptions.
2. Compounding drugs that were withdrawn or removed from the market for safety reasons.	
3. Compounding finished drugs from bulk active ingredients that are not components of FDA approved drugs without an FDA sanctioned investigational new drug application (IND).	
4. Receiving, storing, or using drug substances without first obtaining written assurance from the supplier that each lot of the drug substance has been made in an FDA-registered facility.	3. Receiving, storing, or using drug substances without first obtaining written assurance from the supplier that each lot of the drug substance has been made in an FDA-approved facility.
5. Receiving, storing, or using drug components not guaranteed or otherwise determined to meet official compendia requirements.	4. Receiving, storing, or using drug components not guaranteed or otherwise determined to meet official compendia requirements.
6. Using commercial scale manufacturing or testing equipment for compounding drug products.	5. Using commercial scale manufacturing or testing equipment for compounding drug products.
7. Compounding drugs for third parties who resell to individual patients or offering compounded drug products at wholesale to other state licensed persons or commercial entities for resale.	7. Offering compounded drug products at wholesale to other state licensed persons or commercial entities for resale.
8. Compounding drug products that are commercially available in the marketplace or that are essentially copies of commercially available FDA-approved drug products. In certain circumstances, it may be appropriate for a pharmacist to compound a small quantity of a drug that is only slightly different than an FDA-approved drug that is commercially available. In these circumstances, FDA will consider whether there is documentation of the medical need for the particular variation of the compound for the particular patient.	2. Compounding, regularly, or in inordinate amounts, drug products that are commercially available in the marketplace and that are essentially generic copies of commercially available, FDA-approved drug products.

At approximately the same time that the federal Congress was considering the FDAMA amendment to the FDCA that added the compounding statute, the NAPB was adopting language for its MSPPA that could serve as the basis for states to adopt regulations that would compliment the federal provisions. In that spirit, the NAPB developed *Good Compounding Practices* guidelines to assist pharmacists who engage in the practice of compounding drugs. Given the legal developments surrounding the issue, it is difficult to predict how much applicability it will have in influencing FDA inspectors equipped with the 2002 FDA Guidance on compounding. A few of the relevant portions of the NABP's are reproduced here so that readers can view a slightly different approach than used by the FDA. The following definitions are excerpted from the NABP *Good Compounding Practices* section of the MSPPA:

Compounding—the preparation, mixing, assembling, packaging, or Labeling of a Drug or Device (i) as the result of a Practitioner's Prescription Drug Order or initiative based on the Practitioner/patient/Pharmacist relationship in the course of professional practice, or (ii) for the purpose of, or as an incident to, research, teaching, or chemical analysis and not for sale or Dispensing. Compounding also includes the preparation of Drugs or Devices in anticipation of Prescription Drug Orders based on routine, regularly observed prescribing patterns.

Manufacturing—the production, preparation, propagation, conversion, or processing of a Drug or Device, either directly or indirectly, by extraction from substances of natural origin or independently by means of chemical or biological synthesis, and includes any packaging or repackaging of the substance(s) or Labeling or re-labeling of its container, and the promotion and marketing of such Drugs or Devices. Manufacturing also includes the preparation and promotion of commercially available products from bulk compounds for resale by pharmacies, Practitioners, or other Persons.

Component—any ingredient intended for use in the compounding of a drug product, including those that may not appear in such product.

THE FEDERAL FOOD, DRUG AND COSMETIC ACT

Regulation of Pharmaceuticals

Congress has the authority to regulate drugs pursuant to its powers under the "commerce clause" (Article 1, Section 8) of the US Constitution, which grants Congress authority to regulate commerce among the states. This type of transaction is known as "interstate commerce." Transactions occurring within only one state are called "intrastate commerce." The federal government's control over interstate commerce extends to control over intrastate commerce in many instances. For example, the FD&CA regulates the distribution of drugs between states, but it also regulates the distribution of drugs within a state (eg, the selling and dispensing of drugs by a neighborhood pharmacist whose transactions are entirely intrastate). The federal intrastate regulation is constitutional because the courts have decided that intrastate transactions may have a significant effect on interstate commerce.

In the introductory remarks, it was mentioned that the basic focus of federal regulations affecting pharmacy practice are laws that deal with the safety and efficacy of drugs, their production, labeling and distribution. The history of federal regulation of pharmaceuticals makes the understanding of current laws significantly easier to understand.

Summary of Important Points About the FD&CA

The FD&CA is designed to protect the public health by requiring that:

Only safe, effective, and properly labeled drugs may be introduced into interstate commerce.

The food and cosmetic preparations subject to the Act be safe and properly labeled.

The manufacturing, processing, packaging, and holding of drugs comply with the Current Good Manufacturing Practices (CGMP) set by the FDA.

The FD&CA be enforced by the FDA.

OTC (nonprescription) drugs be labeled for safe use by consumers in self-medication.

Prescription drugs be dispensed to an individual only pursuant to a prescription or administered directly by the physician or other authorized prescriber.

Drug prescriptions be refilled only as authorized by a physician or other authorized prescriber.

Specific labeling be used for both prescription and nonprescription drugs.

Dispensing a drug for distribution in violation of the Act's labeling requirements is "misbranding" the drug.

Drugs containing filthy, putrid, and decomposed substances and drugs packed and held under unsanitary conditions be deemed "adulterated."

Seizures of misbranded or adulterated drugs can be made by the FDA.

Interpretations of the Act show that lack of knowledge or lack of criminal intent will not excuse a violation.

An employer or other responsible person may be prosecuted for violations of the Act committed by an employee.

FDA has broad inspection powers over factories, warehouses, and establishments where drugs, food, medical devices, and cosmetics are made or processed.

The FDA is authorized to perform limited inspection of pharmacies in certain circumstances.

Manufacturers or re-packagers of drugs must register with the FDA.

Historical Background of the Act

The first federal statute designed to protect US citizens from harmful drugs was the Import Drug Act of 1848 (9 Stat. 237), which prohibited the importation of adulterated drugs. It was passed because anti-malarial medication for US troops in Mexico was found to be grossly adulterated and lacking in potency.

The next federal legislation concerning adulterated articles was enacted on August 30, 1890, when Congress adopted a law to prevent importation of dangerously adulterated articles for food and drink. The law worked by permitting the President of the United States to issue a proclamation prohibiting importing of adulterated articles. In 1902, Congress passed a law (32 Stat. 632) prohibiting the introduction of falsely labeled dairy products into interstate commerce (21 U.S.C §16).

The primary forerunner of today's FD&CA was enacted on June 30, 1906, with the passing of the Wiley-Heyburn Act, or the Federal Pure Food and Drug Act of 1906, which took effect in 1907. The Act was prompted, in part, by public concern over unsanitary practices in the drug and food industries, resulting in lack of purity. The 1906 Act was a major advancement in prohibiting adulteration and misbranding of food and drugs in interstate commerce. Drug adulteration was defined in the 1906 Act to prohibit the marketing of drugs of substandard strength or purity (below United States Pharmacopoeia (USP) or National Formulary (NF) standards unless the drugs were labeled to show how their strength, quality, and purity differed from those of the formulary standard). This concept of adulteration is carried through to present law (see §501(b) of the Act). The 1906 Act, with several minor amendments, lasted until 1938 (shortly after what has become known as the sulfanilamide tragedy, described below) when Congress adopted new legislation.

The Sulfanilamide Tragedy

In 1937, the S.E. Massengill Company marketed Sulfanilamide Elixir, which contained 40 grains of sulfanilamide per fluid ounce in a solution with diethylene glycol. The diethylene glycol solvent was suggested by the firm's chief chemist in response to its marketing department's demand for a liquid preparation of sulfanilamide, a "sulfa" drug used to treat hemolytic streptococcal infections. Toxicity tests of the product were not conducted and very little was known about the inherent toxicity of diethylene glycol (a deadly poison now used as a type of permanent automotive antifreeze). More than 100 individuals reportedly died from ingesting Sulfanilamide Elixir before the FDA removed it from the market under a technical labeling violation under the 1906 Act. This incident propelled the passage of the 1938 FD&CA.

The FD&CA (21 U.S.C. §301 et seq.) is divided into 9 chapters, many of which are not discussed here because they deal exclusively with food and cosmetics. Only specific provisions of the Act concerning pharmacists and pharmacy practice are provided here. Further, only a few select portions of the Act are reproduced. For those interested, the entire Act may be found online at http://www.gpo.gov.

The 1938 Federal FC&C Act remains as the basis of today's law. It requires anyone who wishes to market a drug product to prove its safety to the FDA before it could be marketed. This was the beginning of the "pre-market approval process" for drugs in the United States—requiring the submission of a New Drug Application (NDA). Any compound that falls within the definition of a "new drug" under the act requires an NDA to be submitted to the FDA. The Act, as it was originally passed, did not require a manufacturer to prove the efficacy of the drug product. That requirement came about in a later amendment to the Act.

Definition of Drug

The definition of a "drug" as set forth in Section 201 (g)(1) of the FD&CA (21 U.S.C. §321(g)(1)) does not differentiate between prescription and nonprescription drugs, nor does it distinguish legal or lawful drugs from illicit ones:

The term "drug" means (A) articles recognized in the official United States Pharmacopeia, official Homeopathic Pharmacopeia of the United States, or official National Formulary, or any supplement to any of them; and (B) articles intended for use in the diagnosis, cure, mitigation, treatment, or prevention of disease in man or other animals; and (C) articles (other than food) intended to affect the structure or any function of the body of man or other animals; and (D) articles intended for use as a component of any articles specified in clause (A), (B), or (C). A food or dietary supplement for which a claim, subject to Sections 403(r)(1)(B) and 403(r)(3) or Sections 403(r)(1)(B) and 403(r)(5)(D), is made in accordance with the requirements of Section 403(r) is not a drug solely because the label or the labeling contains such a claim. A food, dietary ingredient, or dietary supplement for which a truthful and not misleading statement is made in accordance with Section 403(r)(6) is not a drug under clause (C) solely because the label or the labeling contains such a statement.

Intended Use

Often, a key element in determining whether a particular item is a drug is the "intended use" of the manufacturer or distributor of the article. The classifications under the FD&CA are not mutually exclusive. For example, an item may meet the criteria to be classified as both a drug and a cosmetic under the legal framework of this statute.

The Grandfather Clause

The 1938 Act contains a loophole known as the "grandfather clause." This provision exempts certain drugs that were on the market the day prior to the effective date of the Act (in 1938) from having to meet the FDA's pre-approval marketing requirements. Although few of those drugs are still marketed, today, many of them have now obtained "approval" via an NDA or an Abbreviated New Drug Application (ANDA).

Before the 1938 FD&CA, there was very limited federal or state control over the retail sale of non-narcotic and non-poisonous drugs. The 1914 Harrison Narcotic Act regulated the distribution of narcotics, and there were various state laws restricting the retail sale of poisons. However, there was no federal comprehensive law that regulated the dispensing of controlled substances or other drugs. Community pharmacists were at liberty to dispense all manner of non-narcotic and non-poisonous drugs without a prescription.

In the 1930s, sensational drug abuse cases contributed to the enactment of the FD&CA. The Act restricted certain drugs to be dispensed only by the pharmacist, and dispensed pursuant to a prescription only. The prescriptions were non-refillable. However, some pharmacists did not take the Act seriously, especially in light of their history of relatively free dispensing powers. Furthermore, it was believed that the Act's labeling requirements only applied to *interstate* drug distribution as opposed to *intrastate* distribution.

The 1948 US Supreme Court case of *United States v. Sullivan*, 332 U.S. 689 (1948), helped to clarify the real effect of the Act. That case involved a community pharmacist who sold sulfathiazole tablets over-the-counter, labeled with only the drug name and dispensed in the pharmacist's own container. The Court held that his action, which in effect constituted dispensing a drug without a prescription, violated a misbranding (§301(k)) of the FD&CA. More importantly, the Act was applied judicially to an intrastate transaction, which extended the powers of the Federal Act over intrastate as well as interstate commerce.

The Durham-Humphrey Amendment Provision

After the *Sullivan* case, pharmaceutical organizations worked for an amendment to the Act to clarify the dispensing obligations of pharmacists. The new provision, enacted in 1951, as the Durham-Humphrey Amendment was named for Carl Durham, a pharmacist representing North Carolina in the US House of Representatives, and Hubert Humphrey, a pharmacist representing Minnesota in the US Senate. The Durham-Humphrey Amendment (FD&CA §503(b)(1); 21 U.S.C. §353(b)(1)) took effect in 1952. The amendment distinguished drugs requiring a prescription from Over the Counter (OTC) drugs. The amendment accomplished this goal by defining the kinds of drugs that cannot be used safely without medical supervision. The amendment restricted the sale of such drugs by requiring a prescription from a practitioner licensed by state law to prescribe drugs and dispensing pursuant to only a prescription. In addition to requiring a prescription for specific drugs, the Durham Humphrey Amendment also provided statutory provisions for the receipt of oral prescriptions as well as provisions allowing for the refilling of prescriptions. Refilling the prescription is allowed only if it specifically is authorized in the prescription or if authorization is obtained subsequently from the prescribing practitioner or from another licensed practitioner. If the original prescription does not contain an indication of refills, it is by law deemed to be a "no refill."

The terms "physician," "prescriber," and "practitioner," when used in this discussion, refer to the individual who is permitted by the jurisdiction or state in which he or she practices to prescribe or administer drugs in the course of professional practice. The determination of who may prescribe/administer is made by the state, not by the federal government.

The Thalidomide Tragedy

In late 1961, the "thalidomide disaster" began to unfold. Thalidomide was marketed in 1958 and was sold without prescription as a tranquilizer in the West German Federal Republic until April 1961, when the drug was recognized as causing polyneuritis in adults. In November 1961, the drug first was believed to cause the severe birth defect phocomelia, or "seal limbs." By that time thousands of infants had been born in West Germany without one or both arms or legs or with only partially formed extremities. The manufacturer withdrew the drug from the West German market on November 26, 1961.

A number of drug firms had obtained licenses to market thalidomide worldwide. In the United States, the William S. Merrell Company had distributed the drug experimentally in 1960 under the trade name Kevadon, but the FDA never gave final approval to the NDA the company had submitted.

The FDA's timely action in withholding Kevadon approval was because an FDA medical officer refused approval while seeking data on further proof of safety. Even so, 29,413 patients in the United States had been involved in the human clinical trial testing of Kevadon. When the evidence that thalidomide was teratogenic (causing harm to the human fetus) was established, the FDA agents seized almost all of the Kevadon on the market. Consequently, only a very small number of phocomelia cases were reported in the United States. Thalidomide had been widely tested around the world as a sedative and tranquilizer. It was later found to act as an anti-nauseant in pregnancy, and its widespread use for that indication brought the horrible side effect to the surface. The lesson of the thalidomide tragedy is that serious side effects caused by certain new drugs, or caused by new uses for old drugs, may not be discovered until the drug has had very wide clinical use—after some damage already has occurred.

Kefauver-Harris Amendment

The thalidomide tragedy was the impetus for the Kefauver-Harris Amendment, otherwise known as the 1962 Drug Amendments, to the FD&CA. In the late 1950s and early 1960s, Senator Estes Kefauver of Tennessee led Congressional hearings concerning antitrust legislation and drug pricing. The Kefauver-Harris Amendment, which became effective in 1963, required substantiation to the FDA of both the *safety and efficacy* of all drugs introduced after 1962 and of drugs for which NDAs had been approved between 1938 and 1962. Any compound falling under the revised definition of a "new drug" as defined in §201(p) of the Act required this substantiation. The amendments required a positive act of approval by the FDA (as opposed to automatic approval if not disapproved by the FDA under the previous version of the Act). The amendments also contained a typical grandfather clause exempting from both safety and efficacy requirements the drugs on the market from 1906 to the day prior to the effective date of the 1938 Act, as those drugs were never subject to NDAs.

Drug Approval Process

NEW DRUGS—New drugs simply refer to those that have not yet received general recognition by medical experts as being both safe and effective for the intended use. A new drug may not be commercially marketed in the United States unless it has been approved as safe and effective. Such approval is based upon an NDA, which must contain acceptable scientific data, including the results of tests, to evaluate its safety. There must be substantial evidence of effectiveness for the conditions for which the drug is to be sold. Often, the question of whether a drug is recognized as "safe and effective" is a question of fact that must be decided in a legal action.

Newly discovered chemicals are not the only subjects of NDAs. A drug may be legally regarded as a "new drug" if it is an old, established drug (pre-1938 FD&C) which is offered in a new dosage form, with new medical claims, in new dosage levels, or if the drug is to be used on a different patient population. An NDA may also be required if a new combination of old drugs is used.

SYNOPSIS OF NEW DRUG APPLICATION PROCEDURES—Before a new drug can be marketed, federal law requires the submission and approval of form FDA-356h. Before

the NDA is filed, an Investigational New Drug (IND) form (form FDA-1571) for the drug must be filed. The specific FDA regulations regarding INDs and NDAs are contained in 21 CFR §§312 and 314. The FDA also has provided for the electronic submission of NDAs. A Guidance Document entitled Guidance for Industry Providing Regulatory Submissions in Electronic Format-NDAs may be found on the Internet at: http://www.fda. gov/cder/guidance/index.htm. In addition, copies of forms required for such submissions may also be found on the Internet at http://aosweb.psc.dhhs.gov/forms/fdaforms.htm. If the FDA does not reject the IND request within 30 days of submission, clinical testing of the investigational drug on humans may begin by the IND sponsor. The IND application must include proof of preclinical testing of the new drug on animals to substantiate the safety of clinical testing in humans.

The sponsor of the IND can be a drug manufacturer, hospital, pharmacy, physician, pharmacist, or anyone who submits the application. However, the individuals (investigators) who conduct the clinical trials must be trained and experienced, and a statement of their respective qualifications must be attached to the IND. The investigators submit to the IND sponsor a completed and signed "Statement of Investigator" Form FDA-1572.

Phase 1 of clinical investigation involves a small number of patients in carefully controlled studies of the drug toxicity, metabolism, absorption, and elimination, to determine the preferred route of administration and safe dosage.

Phase 2 involves use of the investigational drug on a limited number of patients for specific disease treatment or prevention, along with additional pharmacology studies on animals to further determine the drug's safety.

Phase 3 trials evaluate whether information obtained from phase 1 and 2 studies can reasonably ensure the safety and efficacy of the drug or if the drug has a potential value outweighing its possible hazards.

"Phase 4," as it is unofficially termed, involves post-marketing surveillance of approved drugs to detect adverse effects or other problems not encountered in the 3 prior phases of drug testing due to the limited number of patients using the medication (see 21 CFR §314.80).

Before a human being may be involved as a subject in research, the investigator must obtain legally effective "informed consent" of the patient or his or her representative (21 CFR Part 50).

In April 1996, the FDA released a Guidance Document entitled Guidance for Industry Good Clinical Practice: Consolidated Guidance that may be obtained on the Internet at http:// www.fda.gov/cder/guidance/index.htm or from the Drug Information Branch CDER, 5600 Fishers Lane, Rockville, MD 20857, telephone 301-827-4573. This guidance discusses the informed consent process of "trial subjects" in depth.

If, during the clinical testing of a new drug, the data furnished to the FDA indicate that the drug is too toxic under the criteria of the FDA's risk/benefit ratio, the FDA will terminate the IND approval. In this instance, the FDA's action is not subject to court review or appeal and, as such, it is one of the rare examples in the law in which administrative action is not judicially reviewable. If all goes well with the clinical testing, the sponsor of the drug (usually the manufacturer or supplier at this point) submits a voluminous NDA (form FD-356H) to the FDA wherein the proposed labeling (package insert) is contained. If approved by the FDA, the package insert will accompany the marketed drug product in its package.

After the NDA is approved by the FDA, the drug is marketed, but the drug manufacturer's reporting does not end there. The 1962 amendment to the Act requires that the manufacturer submit periodic reports to the FDA, containing samples of current labeling and advertisements, summaries of medical journal articles on the drug, and information on adverse reactions.

EFFICACY AND THE DEFINITION OF A "NEW DRUG"—Disputes arose between pharmaceutical firms and the FDA as to how the 1962 Drug Amendments affected the efficacy requirement for new drugs approved by the FDA between 1938 and 1962. The issue was determined somewhat in three separate United States Supreme Court cases all decided on the same day—June 18, 1973. In the first case, the Court ruled that the 1962 efficacy proof requirement (well-controlled and adequate clinical studies) retrospectively applied to all NDAs approved from 1938 to 1962. The Court also held that the FDA had the power to decide whether a drug is a new drug as defined in §201(p) of the FD&CA. Thus, the Court held that the FDA had the authority to withdraw the NDA of any drug on the market. In the second case, the court held that generic drugs are subject to the FDA's requirements for proof of safety and efficacy. In the third case, the Court concluded that the FDA has authority to determine what comprises a "new drug" under the Act.

GENERIC DRUG APPROVALS—In the late 1970s and early 1980s, a series of cases arose that challenged the FDA's authority to determine the "new drug" status of generic versions of brand name drugs. FDA policy at the time allowed the marketing of generic products as long as an Abbreviated New Drug Application (ANDA) had been filed. Although it had not been "officially" approved the "paper NDA," as it was called at the time, required only data on labeling and manufacturing, but not data relating to safety and efficacy. This policy was based on the theory that the active ingredients in such products had become generally recognized as safe and effective and therefore, the FDA need only require assurance of proper labeling and manufacturing. However, there was concern by some about bioavailability and bioequivalence of these generic drugs. In 1975, a district court judge ruled that the FDA could not permit drugs to be marketed unless an NDA or ANDA had been approved. Two Court of Appeals cases split on the issue of whether a generic version of an approved pioneer drug is considered a "new drug" under the Act and therefore subject to the NDA or ANDA approval process. Because of this split among the circuits, the issue ended up in the United States Supreme Court. The landmark Supreme Court case of *United States v. Generix Drug* (1983) resolved the issue. The Court held that the definition of "drug" under the Act included inactive as well as active ingredients, and, therefore, a generic version of a pioneer drug would require its own NDA or ANDA if it differed in any significant respect from the pioneer drug.

Drug Efficacy Study

As mentioned above, the 1962 Kefauver-Harris Amendment to the Act required proof of efficacy in addition to proof of safety before a drug product could be introduced into interstate commerce. The issue of how these provisions should be applied to drugs approved between 1938 and 1962 was controversial.

In 1966, the FDA commissioned the National Academy of Sciences/National Research Council to evaluate drug products introduced between 1938 and 1962. Some 16,000 claims for 4000 drug products were reviewed. Approximately 15% were reported to be ineffective (ie, lack of substantial evidence of effectiveness), 34.9% were reported to be possibly effective, 7.3% were reported to be probably effective, 19.1% were reported to be effective, and 24% were reported to be "effective but....". The FDA initiated an action to remove from the market those drug products that lacked proof of efficacy. This process was known as the Drug Efficacy Study Implementation (DESI) project. The process of removing ineffective drugs from the market took several years. The DESI project in now concluded.

Current Good Manufacturing Practices (CGMP)

The FDA's CGMP regulations apply to a pharmacy only if it is engaged in repackaging and re-labeling drugs beyond the usual conduct of dispensing and selling them at retail. Such activities, outside the usual scope of pharmacy practice, would sub-

ject the pharmacy to FDA registration (FDCA §510) and to FDA inspection at regular intervals.

The FDA, in its introductory comments to the CGMP regulations, gave 3 situations in pharmacy practice that require the pharmacy to comply with FDA registration, inspections, and CGMPs:

If the pharmacy in hospital repackages drug products for its own use as well as for that in other hospitals;

if a pharmacy chain repackages and re-labels quantities of drug products from the manufacturer's original commercial containers for shipment to an individual chain location; and

if similar repackaging and re-labeling are conducted by individual pharmacists as members of an informal buying group (43 Fed. Reg. 45028).

If a hospital pharmacy confines repackaging of drug products to those used solely within the hospital, the hospital would not be subject to the FDA registration, regular inspections or the CGMP compliance requirements. Similarly, the usual type of repackaging and re-labeling of drug products done for on-premises dispensing or retail sale would not subject a pharmacy to FDA registration, regular inspections, and CGMP compliance requirements.

The FDA has also stated that CGMP requirements apply to shared service operations servicing HMOs and hospital groups. FDA Guideline 7356.002B states:

For the purposes of differentiating whether an establishment is acting as a pharmacy or as a re-packager/re-labeler, the repackaging of drug products by licensed pharmacists, (ie, filling prescriptions for identified patients), is within the regular practice of pharmacy. The repackaging of drug products by pharmacists, or any other entity, for resale or distribution to hospitals, other pharmacies, nursing homes, health care facilities, etc., are beyond the practice of pharmacy, and these re-packaging/re-labeling facilities are thus required to register and list all such products with the FDA. Thus, hospitals packaging drugs provided to other hospitals, nursing homes, or other entities are subject to the FDA's CGMP requirements.

The FDA's authority for its position on manufacturing practices can be found in the FD&CA. §501(a)(2)(B) of the Act (21 U.S.C. §351(a)(2)(B) which provides that a drug will be deemed adulterated if the methods used in or the facilities or controls used for its manufacture, processing, packing, or holding do not conform to CGMP regulations. This section of the law is applicable to wholesalers, retailers, pharmacies, and hospitals as well as to drug manufacturers. However, the FDA states the CGMP regulations only apply to organizations engaged in the preparation of a drug product and, therefore, do not apply to wholesalers, retailers, pharmacies, and hospitals engaged in activities that are traditional to them. Pharmacies are exempt from FDA manufacturer registration only if they do not manufacture, prepare, propagate, compound, or process drugs for sale other than in the regular course of dispensing and selling drugs at retail (21 U.S.C. §510(g)(1). The exemption from regular FDA factory inspection is given to pharmacies by 21 U.S.C. §704(a)(2)(A); again, the pharmacy may engage only in the regular business of dispensing and selling drugs at retail. Consequently, repackaging and re-labeling of drugs for off-premises sale can be interpreted as out of the regular course of the pharmacy's business and, hence, nullify the exemptions in §§510(g) and 704(a) and the FDA exemption of the pharmacy from CGMP compliance.

The Drug Price Competition and Patent Term Restoration Act of 1984

The legislation known as the Hatch-Waxman Act (Pub. L. No. 98-417, and 98-427, 98 Stat 1585 (1984) (21 U.S.C. §355 (j), FD&CA §505 (j) was a congressional effort to strike a balance between the competing forces of generic firms and innovator (pioneer or brand name) drug firms. Title I of the Act extended the ANDA process to generic versions of drugs first approved and marketed after 1962. It required the FDA to approve generic drugs shown to be "bioequivalent" to a previously approved drug. This eliminated the requirement for generic manufacturers to duplicate expensive clinical and animal research to demonstrate the safety and efficacy of the products. In essence, this act codified the "paper NDA" process that the FDA had been using for several prior years. Title II of the Act compensated pioneer companies for losses caused by competition from the generic companies by extending the patent terms of some pioneer drugs.

The Prescription Drug User Fee Act of 1992

The Prescription Drug User Fee Act of 1992 (PDUFA), (Pub. L. 102-571; 106 Stat. 4491) authorized the FDA to charge fees to cover the costs incurred for review of human drug applications and supplements, inspection of prescription drug establishments, and other activities. The intent of this legislation was to make additional funds available to the FDA to expedite the review of human drug applications. The PDUFA authorized three different types of user fees: drug application fees, annual establishment fees, and annual product fees. Fees are assessed at different rates depending on whether an application requires a review of clinical data on safety and efficacy as opposed to review of only bioavailability or bioequivalence studies. All or part of the fees may be waived at the FDA's discretion. While this Act has been vital to the economic survival of the FDA and has been renewed several times, it has not been without controversy. Consumer advocate groups have noted that the Act turned the FDA into a manufacturer-funded group as opposed to a taxpayer supported agency. This has led to complaints that the FDA is now more oriented to manufacturer's interests instead of an agency designed to protect the public health and safety.

The Food and Drug Administration Modernization Act of 1997 (FDAMA)

The first major overhaul of the Food, Drug, and Cosmetic Act in over 30 years occurred with the passage of the Food and Drug Administration Modernization Act of 1997 (FDAMA) (Pub. L. No. 105-115, 111 Stat. 2296). FDAMA made major changes in the regulation of foods, drugs, and devices. Documents related to FDAMA implementation can be found on the Internet as part of FDA's Web site, http://www.fda.gov or http://www.fda.gov/cder/fdama. Some of the major changes of FDAMA that impact pharmacy include:

PEDIATRIC STUDIES OF DRUGS—§111 of FDAMA (§505A FD&CA) authorized the FDA to determine that a particular drug may produce health benefits in a pediatric population. The first step in this process required that the FDA, after consultation with experts in pediatric research, develop, prioritize, and publish a list of approved drugs for which additional pediatric information may produce health benefits in the pediatric population. If such a determination was made, the FDA could then request pediatric studies of the drug from the manufacturer. Once the manufacturer completed these studies and they were accepted by the FDA, the FDA had the ability to grant an additional 6 months of marketing exclusivity for the drug. The additional 6 months of marketing exclusivity did not apply to drugs for which an NDA was submitted after January 1, 2002.

The FDA began to implement these provisions on May 20, 1998 ((63 Fed. Reg. 27733) when it announced the availability of a "List of Drugs for Which Additional Pediatric Information May Produce Health Benefits in the Pediatric Population." On June 1998, the FDA made available a "Guidance for Industry Qualifying for Pediatric Exclusivity" However, at the time that this publication was going to press, the federal government ordered a halt to the Pediatric testing program. Readers are urged to consult the web sites listed above to determine the current status to this program.

PHARMACY COMPOUNDING—As detailed in the **Compounding** subsection above, FDAMA also contained §127 (21 U.S.C. §503a) that attempted to clarify that compounding of pharmaceutical products was appropriately regulated by the states and exempted pharmacies from requirements for compliance with NDAs and current good manufacturing requirements when compounding drugs for an identified individual patient. As noted, the United States Supreme Court held that provision unconstitutional because there is no rational relationship between the ban on advertising compounding services as a condition for exemption from the NDA mandates.

ELIMINATION OF CERTAIN LABELING REQUIREMENTS—Section 126 of FDAMA changed the requirement for the "prescription legend" that commercial containers had to bear on the label for prescription drugs packaging. A drug is now required to bear, at a minimum, the symbol "Rx only." In addition, this provision repealed Section 502(d) of the FDC Act, which required the labels of certain habit-forming drugs to bear the statement, "Warning—May Be Habit Forming."

DISSEMINATION OF OFF-LABEL TREATMENT INFORMATION—Section 551 of FDAMA provides incentives for manufacturers to conduct research on new uses of drugs and to file supplemental NDAs (SNDAs) for these uses by allowing manufacturers to disseminate limited information on unapproved uses of drugs. It required that information on an unapproved use must be in the form of a peer-reviewed article, and the information must include a statement disclosing, among other things, that the information concerns a use that has not been approved or cleared by the FDA. In addition, it required that notice was to be provided to the FDA 60 days before any information was disseminated under these provisions. A manufacturer could not disseminate information under this section unless the it had submitted a supplemental NDA for the new use or certified that studies to support the new use had been done or were going to be done, and an application submitted. The application was to be filed no later than 6 months after the date of the initial dissemination of the information if the studies had already been completed and no later than 36 months if studies had yet to be completed. These provisions have been found to be unconstitutional by the courts under the First Amendment right to commercial speech.

Liability Under The FD&CA

The FD&CA imposes a form of strict liability (liability without fault) on all who are affected by its provisions. (The specific prohibited acts involving misbranding and adulteration of drugs are discussed in the next section.) This concept is illustrated in the case of *United States v. Vitamin Industries*, 130 F.Supp. 755 (D Neb 1955), which indicated that criminal intention is not essential for one to violate the Act. In other words, it is not a defense for the accused to claim lack of knowledge or lack of intent to violate the law. Although this may seem rather harsh, if lack of knowledge or specific intent were an acceptable defense, every violator would avail himself or herself of this claim and the Act would become unenforceable *United States v. Dotterweich*, 320 U.S. 277 (1943) and *United States v. Park*, 421 U.S. 658 (1975).

Doctrine of Respondeat Superior

Under the FD&CA, an employer can be convicted for a violation committed by an employee. The legal term for this doctrine is *Respondeat Superior*. There are several situations where this doctrine applies:

(1) The employer know or should know of the employee's illegal action;
(2) the employer participated in or willfully authorized or consented to the employee's illegal act; or
(3) the employer has a responsible share in the employee's illegal act.

Any one of these situations will impute liability to the employer; all three need not be present.

Strict liability of a proprietor under the FD&CA exists if it is proven in court the defendant is the sole proprietor of a business, and the offense committed was committed by an employee of that business during the course of business duties. Although the proprietor may not have violated the law personally, he or she may still be found guilty. Responsibility for the acts of the employee rests with the proprietor. Strict liability of the member of a partnership under the FD&CA exists if it can be proven in court the defendant is a member of a partnership and is responsible, in part, for the conduct of its activities. If it can be proven that an employee of the partnership, during the course of business duties, violated the law, the defendant will be found guilty, although he or she did not personally commit the offense.

Recordkeeping under the FD&CA

Recordkeeping for the pharmacist under the FD&CA is similar to the recordkeeping required under the Controlled Substances Act (CSA) (discussed in detail below) but is not so precisely defined or detailed. Probably the most important distinction between the recordkeeping under the CSA as opposed to that under the FD&CA is, for the pharmacist, the required documents for the CSA are more quantitative while those for the FD&C Act are more qualitative. The recordkeeping under the CSA is concerned with accountability for the receipt and disposition of drugs, whereas recordkeeping under the FD&CA is concerned with the ability to trace a specific drug product, usually in response to drug recall.

Nonetheless, the basic type of records is the same under the two Acts. For example, purchase invoices are considered records of drug receipt, prescriptions are records of drug disposition, and inventories furnish a record of drugs on hand. Sales or other disposals of drugs to physicians or pharmacists, returns to wholesalers or manufacturers, drug destruction, and thefts should be documented by some type of written or other reliable memorandum.

Drug records should be kept at least for the running of state or federal statute of limitations on crimes. In most cases, this is a period of 5 or 6 years from the date of the alleged felony offense. Although federal or state drug control laws often provide for a lesser period of time (usually 3 years) for retention of drug records, the reason for preserving the records for the length of the statute of limitations is that they furnish proof of the transactions involved in a lawsuit, some of which may provide a valid defense to a prosecution arising out of an alleged drug law violation.

Prescription Drug Labeling

LABELS ON COMMERCIAL CONTAINERS—FDA regulations require that the following information appear on the manufacturer's or distributor's container of prescription drugs (21 CFR §§201.1 to 201.55):

The name and address of the manufacturer, packager, or distributor;
ingredient information;
a statement of identity (ie, the generic and the proprietary names);
quantity in terms of weight or measure applicable to drug (eg, 0.5 g);
the net quantity of the package contents (eg, 100 tablets);
a statement of dosage or a reference to the package insert for dosage information;
the expiration date of the drug;
the lot number; and
the National Drug Code (NDC) number (requested, not required, by FDA regulations).

PACKAGE INSERTS/PROFESSIONAL PRODUCT LABELING—The package insert is the part of a prescription drug product's approved labeling directed to health care professionals. It is the primary mechanism by which the FDA and drug manufacturers communicate essential, science-based prescribing information to health care practitioners.

Historically, the contents and format of package insert labeling are imposed by FDA regulations (21 CFR §201.56). FDA regulations §§201.56 and 201.57, as they affect the prescription drug labeling described in FDA regulation 201.100 (d) (21 CFR §201.100 (d), were revised in June 1979. Under the regulations, the package insert labeling must contain a summary of essential scientific information that is needed for the safe and effective use of the drug. The labeling must be informative, accurate, and neither promotional in tone nor false or misleading. The labeling must be based, whenever possible, on data derived from human experiments. Implied claims and suggestions for drug use may not be made if there is inadequate evidence of safety or lack of substantial evidence of effectiveness. Conclusions that are based on animal data are permitted if they are necessary for safe and effective use of the drug in humans; however, they must be identified as animal data. There is no law or regulation that prohibits the pharmacist from giving a package insert to a patient.

21 CFR §201.56 requires that the package insert for a prescription drug product contain the following specific information under the following section headings and in the following order:

Description (proprietary and generic names);
Clinical pharmacology;
Indications and usage (the use of the drug in the treatment, prevention, or diagnosis of a recognized disease or condition);
Contraindications;
Warnings;
Precautions;
Adverse reactions;
Drug abuse and dependence;
Overdosage;
Dosage and administration; and
How supplied.

Other FDA Regulations

On December 22, 2000, the FDA proposed new regulations that would significantly change the "labeling" (ie, the package insert) of prescription drugs. The proposal may be found at 65 FR 81082 and at http://www.fda.gov/OHRMS/DOCKETS/98fr/122200a.pdf.

The FDA's intent in making this proposal is to "make it easier for health care practitioners to access, read, and use" the package insert information, and to "enhance the safe and effective use of prescription drug products." By making the information easier to find, read, and use, the FDA hopes to reduce medical errors caused by inadequate communication. The labeling change would require the addition (at the beginning of the insert) of a "Highlights of Prescribing Information" section. This section is intended to be a concise extract of the most important information that is contained in the Comprehensive Information" section that would follow. The Highlights section would contain the following categories:

boxed warnings;
recent substantive labeling changes;
indications and usage;
dosage and administration;
how supplied;
contraindications;
warnings/precautions, including a subsection for the most common adverse reactions;
drug interactions; and
use in specific populations.

In addition, "R_x" should be present to indicate the product is sold only by prescription. A triangular icon appears for drugs that have been approved for marketing within the past 3 years. In addition to proposing changes to the package insert, the rule also provides for some changes to the label of the prescription drug itself. The agency hopes that by reducing the amount of required information on product labels and simplifying them, the number of medications errors will be reduced.

Patient Package Inserts

HISTORICAL BACKGROUND OF PATIENT PACKAGE INSERTS—The first patient warning of a prescription drug was in 1968 when the FDA required that the following statement appear on the dispensing package of an isoproterenol inhalation drug product (21 CFR §201.306): "Warning: Do not exceed the dose prescribed by your physician. If difficulty in breathing persists, contact your physician immediately." Isoproterenol aerosols and nebulizer solutions (eg, Aerolone Solution, Isuprel HCl Solution, Medihaler-Iso) are prescription-only drugs. The package warnings were required because repeated use of isoproterenol inhalation preparations occasionally causes airway resistance or a refractory state (commonly known as "concrete of the nasal passages"). Cardiac arrest and death also were noted in several instances of excessive use of the drug therapy.

In 1970, the FDA issued a regulation (21 CFR §310.501) requiring that certain information about oral contraceptive drugs be included in each package of the prescription drug dispensed to the patient. Again, the patient labeling informed the patient of the possible adverse effects (eg, thrombophlebitis, pulmonary embolism, retinal artery thrombosis, MI, benign hepatic adenomas, induction of fetal abnormalities, gallbladder disease). In 1977, a regulation (21 CFR §310.515) was issued requiring that information regarding the newly discovered hazards of estrogen be provided for estrogenic drug products (eg, diethylstilbestrol, Premarin, Tace, and Estinyl tablets) and for combination preparations containing estrogens. Essentially, the PPI listed the risk of estrogens leading to endometrial carcinoma and risks encountered when estrogens are taken during pregnancy. Similar labeling requirements were promulgated for contraceptive intrauterine devices (IUDs), which were regulated as prescription drugs or medical devices, and for progestational drug products (see 21 CFR §310.516). (When diethylstilbestrol or progestational drug products are intended for contraceptive use, labeling requirements under 21 CFR §310.501 apply.)

It is required that the manufacturer of a drug requiring a PPI provide the pharmacist with a sufficient amount of PPIs to provide one to each patient to whom the drug is dispensed. Sample forms of PPIs are provided by the FDA, and the manufacturer is, additionally, obligated to provide a PPI in Spanish upon the request of the distributor or dispenser.

The FDA requires the pharmacist to provide the PPI to the patient upon dispensing of the drug that is subject to the PPI requirements. PPIs for products dispensed in acute care hospitals or long-term care facilities are considered to have been provided if given to the patient before the first administration of the drug and every 30 days thereafter. Outpatient prescriptions are subject to the same requirements as are applicable to those dispensed by the community pharmacist.

UNIT-DOSE LABELING—Unit-dose (or individual-dose) packaging of drug products is done routinely, especially in the institutional setting. Individually wrapped and labeled single doses of drug products in tablet or capsule form have resulted in an efficient institutional drug distribution system. The main advantages of the unit-dose system are: it reduces errors because each dose is labeled with the drug identity and strength, and it permits the return and recycling of unused doses provided the sealed package has not been opened. However, the unit-dose system is more expensive than multi-dose drug distribution systems.

The FDA, in Compliance Policy Guide 7132b.10, specifies its requirements for unit dose labeling for solid and liquid oral dosage forms of both prescription and nonprescription drugs. For prescription drugs, the label of the actual unit-dose container must contain:

The established name of the drug and the quantity of active ingredient per dosage unit;
The expiration date (21 CFR §§201.17, 211.137)
The lot or control number (see 21 CFR §§201.100(b), 211.130);

The name and place of business of the manufacturer, packer, or distributor as provided for in 21 CFR §201.1;
For official drugs, any statement required by the compendia; for unofficial drugs, any pertinent statement bearing on special characteristics of the dosage form.

The Compliance Policy Guide (CPG) does not require, but strongly recommends, that the label contain:

Any pertinent statement bearing on the need for special storage conditions;
Information to alert a health professional that a procedure(s) is necessary prior to patient administration;
If more than one dosage unit is contained, the number of dosage units per container and the strength per dosage unit.

Because most commonly prescribed drugs are available in commercially marketed unit-dose packaging, it is prudent the pharmacist use the commercial unit-dose drug product, rather than repackaging the drug.

LABELING OF CUSTOMIZED MEDICATION PACKAGES—In lieu of dispensing 2 or more drug products in separate containers, a pharmacist may, with the consent of the patient, his or her caregiver, or prescriber, provide a customized medication package (Patient Med Pak).

Regulation of Dietary Supplements

Traditionally, the FDA considered dietary supplements to be foods and regulated them accordingly. The focus of the agency was on ensuring safety and wholesomeness as well as ensuring the labeling was truthful and not misleading.

DIETARY SUPPLEMENT HEALTH AND EDUCATION ACT OF 1994—In 1994 Congress enacted the Dietary Supplement Health and Education Act (DSHEA), amending several portions of the FD&CA pertaining to dietary supplements and ingredients of dietary supplements. The most important point for pharmacists to understand about dietary supplements is that they are not regulated as "drugs" by the FDA and are exempt from the safety and efficacy requirements for drugs as well as the Current Good Manufacturing Practices (CGMPs) applicable to drugs. The CGMP exemption may be coming to an abrupt halt for dietary supplements. On March 7, 2003 the FDA issued a 527 page proposed rule that would bring dietary supplements under most, but not all, of the CGMP regulations. The proposed regulations contained a 90 day comment period. As such, at the time that this publication was going to press, the future of the proposed regulation was not finalized. Readers who are interested in the final regulation are urged to consult to FDA's web site at http://www.fda.gov for updated information.

DSHEA defines "dietary supplements" and treats them as a special class that falls somewhere in between foods and drugs. The legislation prohibits Congress from regulating "dietary supplements" as food additives or as drugs. It places the burden on the FDA to prove a dietary supplement is unsafe before it can be removed from the market. The intent of Congress in passing this legislation was to protect "the right of access of consumers to safe dietary supplements" and to remove "unreasonable regulatory barriers limiting or slowing the flow of safe products and accurate information to consumers." The passage of this legislation has had a significant impact on the marketing of dietary supplements in this country. Under DSHEA (§201(ff)), a "dietary supplement" is defined as:

A product (other than tobacco) intended to supplement the diet that bears or contains one or more of the following dietary ingredients:

A vitamin;
A mineral; an herb or other botanical; an amino acid; a dietary substance for use by man to supplement the diet by increasing the total dietary intake;
A concentrate, metabolite, constituent, extract, or combination of any ingredient above;
A product intended for ingestion in tablet, capsule, powder, softgel, gel cap, or liquid form; or if not intended for ingestion in such a form, is

not represented as conventional food and is not represented for use as a sole item of a meal or of the diet; and

Labeled as a dietary supplement.

Probably the most significant result of DSHEA is that it allows dietary supplement manufacturers to make certain claims on their products' labels. These claims cannot constitute a "disease claim" (ie, the type of claim made for a drug that claims it is effective to treat a disease). However, certain "structure/function" claims are allowed under the law. This type of claim describes, for example, the role the nutrient or dietary supplement plays in affecting the normal structure or function of the human body (as opposed to affecting the structure or function of the human body in a disease state). When such a claim is made on the label, the following "disclaimer" must also appear: "This statement has not been evaluated by the Food and Drug Administration. This product is not intended to diagnose, treat, cure, or prevent any disease." The manufacturer must have substantiation that such a statement is truthful and not misleading, and must notify the FDA within 30 days of the marketing of the dietary supplement with such a statement.

DSHEA also modified the law with regard to what constitutes "labeling" of a dietary supplement. Scientific publications and other types of information marketed along with dietary supplements are not defined as "labeling" as long as certain conditions are met.

Under DSHEA, a dietary supplement manufacturer may place a claim that the product affects the "structure/function" of the body on its product without pre-approval of the FDA. On January 6, 2000, the FDA issued final regulations regarding types of "structure/function" claims allowed to be made under DSHEA (65 FFR 1000). In general, claims that a product affects the normal structure or function of the human body are allowed. Any claim that explicitly or implicitly says the product can be used to "prevent, treat, cure, mitigate, or diagnose disease" are considered "disease claims" and would subject the product to the drug requirements under the Act. The rule clarifies that such prohibited express or implied claims are made through the name of a product, through a statement about the formulation of a product (contains aspirin) or through the use of pictures, vignettes, or symbols (EKG tracings). The rule allows for claims that do not relate to disease, including health maintenance claims ("maintains a healthy circulatory system"), other non-disease claims ("for muscle enhancement," "helps you relax"), and claims for common, minor symptoms often associated with life stages ("for common symptoms of PMS," "for hot flashes"). A detailed Continuing Education article on the subject may be accessed at: http://www.uspharmacist.com/ce/healthclaims/default.cfm.

Drug Recalls

There are essentially 3 classifications of FDA drug recall:

Class I exists where there is a reasonable possibility that the use of or exposure to a product will cause either serious adverse effects on health or death.

Class II exists where the use of or exposure to a product may cause temporary or medically reversible adverse effects on health or where the probability of serious adverse effects on health is remote.

Class III exists where the use of or exposure to a product is not likely to cause adverse health consequences.

Note that no statutory provision expressly authorizes the FDA to order a drug product recall. Manufacturers do know, however, that if the FDA requests or suggests a drug product recall, and the manufacturer does not comply, the product is subject to the ultimate FDA sanction: withdrawal of the product's NDA and seizure of all products on the market.

LABELING OF OTC AND DISPENSED DRUGS—The regulations for drug labeling are contained in §§502 and 503 of the FD&C (21 U.S.C. §§352 and 353). Labeling of controlled substances is discussed in detail in the Controlled Substances

section. The emphasis in this section is on the basic labeling required for both prescription and OTC drugs.

The FDA regulations differentiate between the terms "label" and "labeling." Label means the printed, written, or graphic material that is literally affixed to the container of the drug (21 CFR §1.3(b)). Labeling means the printed, written, or graphic material that is enclosed with or accompanies the drug once it enters interstate commerce and is put up for sale after shipment (21 CFR §1.3(a)).

Much of the authority of the FD&C over the manufacture and distribution of food, drugs, medical devices, and cosmetics is through the labeling requirements of the FDA regulations implementing the statute.

The FDA promulgates regulations dealing with specific labeling requirements authorized by the FD&CA. In addition, the FDA issues labeling requirements pursuant to the authority of the Fair Packaging and Labeling Act (15 U.S.C. §1047 et seq.), which concern truthfulness in labeling as applicable to consumer packaging (eg, defining "economy size," "king size," etc.).

Of importance to the pharmacist are those FDA regulations relating to the general labeling of drugs and to specific labeling of prescription and nonprescription drugs. The FDA also has specific labeling requirements applicable to veterinary drugs. Applicable FDA regulations on labeling can be found at 21 CFR §201.

"Adequate *directions* for use" refers to the labeling of nonprescription drugs. The directions must be written clearly so the layperson can use a drug safely for the purposes for which it is intended (see 21 CFR §201.5). "Adequate *information* for its use" differs from the term previously discussed. It is defined in 21 CFR §201.100(c)(1) in reference to prescription drugs and applies to the promotional labeling and the package inserts accompanying the drugs in commercial containers. The labeling must include the medical indication, effects, and dosage; the route, method, frequency, and duration of administration; and any relevant hazards, contraindications, side effects, and precautions.

SPECIAL LABELING—Special labeling for certain drugs is contained in 21 CFR Part 201 Subpart G. These include specific requirements for certain prescription and certain OTC drugs. One example is the statement required by 21 CFR §201.314 for salicylate preparations that says: "Warning: Keep out of reach of children."

LABELING OF NONPRESCRIPTION DRUGS—On March 17, 1999, the FDA issued final regulations regarding the labeling of OTC drug products. The latest regulation is based on the FDA's success with standardizing food labeling. The General Requirements for the OTC label are contained in 21 CFR Part 210 Subparts A and C. Generally, the label of an OTC drug must contain:

a principal display panel, including a statement of identity of the product (21 CFR §201.60 and 201.61);

the name and address of the manufacturer, packager, or distributor (21 CFR §201.1);

the net quantity of contents (21 CFR §201.62);

the National Drug Code number is requested, but not required, to be on the label (21 CFR §201.2);

cautions and warnings that are needed for the protection of the user (this requirement varies by the type of product);

adequate directions for safe and effective use (21 CFR §201.5);

content and format of OTC product labeling in "Drug Facts" panel format (21 CFR §201.66).

The regulations are designed to simplify OTC drug product labeling to enable consumers to make informed decisions about the medications they use and give their families. The regulations require the labeling to be in a standardized format that clearly shows the drug's active ingredients, uses, warnings, directions, and inactive ingredients. The FDA also recommends that manufacturers include a phone number for consumers to call for more information. The regulations set requirements for minimum type sizes and other graphic features for the standardized format, including options for modifying the format for various package sizes and shapes.

The Drug Facts panel must contain the following information in the following order:

Drug Facts—title
Active ingredient(s)—including amount in each dosage unit
Purpose—pharmacologic class
Use(s)—indications
Warnings
> Do not use—absolute contraindications, when the product should not be used under any circumstances
> Ask a doctor before use if you have—warnings for persons with certain pre-existing conditions and for persons experiencing certain symptoms
> Ask a doctor or pharmacist before use if you are—drug-drug and food-drug interactions
> When using this product—side effects that could occur and substances or activities to avoid
> Stop use and ask a doctor if—signs of toxicity and other serious reactions that would require consumers to stop using the product immediately
> Pregnancy/breast-feeding warning
> Keep out of reach of children/Accidental overdose warnings
> Direction—dosage when, how, or how often to take
Other information
Inactive ingredients
Questions? (Optional)—followed by telephone number

On December 1, 1999, the FDA announced the availability of a Guidance Document entitled "Draft Guidance for Industry on Labeling of Over-the-Counter Human Drug Products Using a Column Format" (21 CFR §201.5). It can be found on the Internet at http://www.fda.gov/cder/guidance/index.htm. By way of a "negative prohibition," it requires OTC drug labeling to contain the following information:

statements of all cases, conditions, and purposes for which the drug is intended, except those restricted under medical supervision;
the normal dose for each intended use of the drug and the doses for individuals of different ages and different physical conditions;
both the frequency and duration of administration or application;
the administration or application in relation to meals, onset of symptoms, or other time factors;
the route or method of administration or application; and
the preparation for use (ie, shaking, dilution, etc.).

When adequate directions for common use of an OTC drug are known to the ordinary individual (which would be unlikely) there is an exemption under 21 CFR §201.116 from both the adequate directions for use requirement of labeling and from the prescription-only requirement, although not from the other labeling requirements of law, such as ingredient information and the manufacturer's name.

The individual who repackages or re-labels an OTC drug from bulk supply must comply with all of the FDA labeling regulations that are applicable to labeling OTC drugs. Failure to do so will render the product misbranded. 21 CFR §201.66(e) provides a mechanism to request an exemption or deferral from the standardized format. It requires documentation of why a particular requirement is inapplicable or contrary to public health and requires a copy of the proposed labeling also be submitted.

Because a pharmacist is licensed, he or she is considered an expert on drugs and, as such, must be able to professionally answer all queries that his or her patients may have concerning the active ingredients and the labeling of the OTC drugs sold in the pharmacy. The patient is ultimately responsible for reading and following the drug labeling; however, the pharmacist should draw attention to the directions for and warnings on use of the drugs.

While the pharmacist may not legally diagnose or prescribe in most states, he or she may recommend a nonprescription drug product in response to the patient's request for a remedy. When recommending a drug product, the pharmacist must be careful not to give an express warranty or guarantee for the preparation so as not to be involved in a civil liability suit should the "guaranteed remedy" prove ineffective.

When nonprescription drugs are dispensed pursuant to a prescription, the prescription label satisfies the FDA labeling requirements applicable to consumer self-medication labeling.

Prescription Drug Marketing Act

The Prescription Drug Marketing Act of 1987 (PDMA), which became law in 1988 (P.L. 100-293), amended the FD&CA to reduce the potential public health risks that may result from diversion of prescription drugs from legitimate commercial channels (see 21 U.S.C. §353[c]-[e]). Congress found the reintroduction of these drugs into commercial channels could lead to the distribution of mislabeled, adulterated, and subpotent or counterfeit drugs to the American public. The PDMA requires that states license wholesale distributors of prescription human drugs in conformance with federal guidelines that provide minimum standards for prescription drug storage, handling, and recordkeeping. It also requires wholesale distributors who are not authorized manufacturers' distributors to provide a written statement to the purchaser identifying each prior sale.

The PDMA, sometimes known as the Drug Diversion Act, amended several sections of the FD&CA to:

Ban the reimportation of federal legend human drugs manufactured in the United States, except when reimported by the manufacturer or for emergency medical care with permission of the Secretary;
prohibit, with certain exceptions, the sale, purchase, or trade (including the offer to sell, purchase, or trade) federal legend human drugs by hospitals or health care entities;
prohibit, with certain exceptions, the sale, trade, or purchase (including the offer to sell, purchase, or trade) federal legend human drugs donated or sold at reduced cost to charitable institutions;
ban the sale, purchase, or trade, and the counterfeiting of drug coupons;
ban the sale, purchase, or trade (including the offer to sell, purchase, or trade) of drug samples;
require practitioners to request samples in writing;
mandate storage, handling, and recordkeeping requirements for drug samples;
require state licensing of wholesale distributors of federal legend human drugs under federal guidelines that include minimum standards for storage, handling, and recordkeeping;
require unauthorized drug distributors to provide a statement of origin ("pedigree") as part of certain sales of drugs; and
set forth criminal and civil penalties for violations of these provisions.

The re-importation of prescription human drugs produced in the United States is banned, except when re-imported by the manufacturer or, after FDA approval, for emergency use. The PDMA also bans sale, trade, or purchase of drug samples and the trafficking in and counterfeiting of drug coupons (forms that may be redeemed for a prescription drug at no cost or reduced cost). For purposes of this legislation, a drug sample is defined as "a unit of drug, which is not intended to be sold, that is intended to promote the sale of the drug." The PDMA requires all requests for drug samples be made in writing by licensed practitioners. It also requires drug samples be properly stored and handled, and certain recordkeeping be followed. With certain specific exceptions, the resale of prescription drugs purchased by hospitals or health care facilities or donated or supplied to charitable institutions is prohibited.

On December 3, 1999, the FDA issued its final regulations implementing this legislation (see 64 Fed. Reg. 67720-67731). The final rule set forth requirements for re-importation and wholesale distribution of prescription drugs, the offer of, or the sale, purchase, or trade of prescription drugs purchased by hospitals or health care entities, or donated to charitable organizations, and the distribution of prescription drug samples. In this rulemaking, the FDA also amended certain sections of the regulations entitled "Guidelines for State Licensing of Wholesale Prescription Drug Distributors." However, on May 3, 2000, at 65 FR 25639, the FDA announced it was delaying the effective date for certain requirements related to wholesale distribution of prescription drugs by distributors who were not authorized distributors of record. Another portion of the final regulation being stayed was one prohibiting blood centers functioning as "health care entities" to act as wholesale distributors of blood derivatives. The PDMA provision prohibits wholesale distribution of drugs in interstate commerce unless the wholesaler is licensed by a state in accordance with the guidelines.

Key points with regard to the PDMA and its final implementing regulations with regard to samples and pharmacies are:

A "drug sample" is defined as "a unit of a prescription drug that is not intended to be sold and is intended to promote the sale of the drug."

The FDA's position is that starter packs, which are distributed free to pharmacies, are not samples because they are intended to be sold by the pharmacy. Also, vouchers or other similar systems for indigent patients filled out of pharmacy's stock at the manufacturer's expense are not considered samples.

Samples only may be distributed by a practitioner licensed to prescribe, or to the pharmacy of a hospitals or health care entity (at the written request of a prescriber).

The proposed rule stated that drug samples found in a retail pharmacy would be considered evidence that the sample was obtained by the pharmacy in violation of the Act. The final rule excludes this provision, but if the pharmacy is not part of a health care entity, the presumption probably can still be made.

Drug Price Competition and Patent Term Restoration Act of 1984

When President Ronald Reagan signed the Drug Price Competition and Patent Term Restoration Act (DPCPTRA) into law on September 24, 1984, he stated "this legislation will speed up the process of federal approval of inexpensive generic versions of many brand-name drugs, make the generic versions more widely available to consumers, and grant pharmaceutical firms added incentives to develop new drugs." The law converts the drug approval process that had been used for pre-1962 generic drugs and makes that process a formal requirement for moving post-1962 drugs to ANDA status. All generic drugs approved under this process must be bioequivalent to the brand name reference drug. The DPCPTRA provides pioneer drug firms 5 years of patent restoration or at least 5 years of exclusive marketing once their drug is approved. Generic companies may not submit an application until 5 years after the approval of the brand-name product.

Some pharmacists and consumers have raised concerns about the equivalence of generic copies marketed under the new law. Particular concerns have been raised regarding substituting generic drug products for brand name products that still have exclusivity over certain indications. Another concern is that the FDAs criteria for bioequivalence may not be sufficient to guarantee safety and efficacy for a class of drugs commonly called Narrow Therapeutic Index (NTI) drugs.

Misbranding and Adulteration

§§501 and 502 of the Act prohibit the introduction into interstate commerce of any article that is "misbranded" or "adulterated," as those terms are defined under the FD&CA. The misbranding and adulteration provisions apply to action taken after shipment in interstate commerce.

The United States Pharmacopoeia and National Formulary

The majority of drugs marketed in the United States have monographs in The United States Pharmacopoeia/National Formulary (USP/NF). The FD&CA recognizes the USP/NF as an "official compendia." If a drug product that appears in a monograph in the USP/NF fails to meet the standards for strength, quality, purity, packaging, or labeling contained in the monograph, the drug may be deemed "misbranded" or "adulterated"

under the Act. For example, USP's monograph for nitroglycerin tablets requires that prescriptions be labeled for sublingual use and that they be dispensed in the original unopened container. In addition, the USP/NF's standards for packaging and storage of prescription drugs are widely recognized by individual state Food, Drug, and Cosmetic acts as well as by state pharmacy practice acts and regulations.

Adulterated Drugs

In most instances, adulteration violations would be committed by the pharmaceutical manufacturer. For example, if a drug is manufactured under conditions that do not conform to Current Good Manufacturing Practices, the drug is deemed adulterated under the Act. Section 502(a)-(d) states that:

A drug or device shall be deemed to be adulterated:

(a)(1) If it consists in whole or in part of any filthy, putrid, or decomposed substance; or (2)(A) if it has been prepared, packed, or held under insanitary conditions whereby it may have been contaminated with filth, or whereby it may have been rendered injurious to health; or (B) if it is a drug and the methods used in, or the facilities or controls used for, its manufacture, processing, packing, or holding do not conform to or are not opeerated or administered in conformity with current good manufacturing practice to assure that such drug meets the requirements of this Act as to safety and has the identity and strength, and meets the quality and purity characteristics, which it purports or is represented to possess; or (C) if it is a compounded positron emission tomography drug, and the methods used in, or the facilities and controls used for, its compounding, processing, packing, or holding do not conform to or are not operated or administered in conformity with the positron emission tomography compounding standards and the official monographs of the United States Pharmacopeia to assure that such drug meets the requirements of this Act as to safety and has the identity and strength, and meets the quality and purity characteristics, that it purports or is represented to possess; or (3) if its container is composed, in whole or in part, of any poisonous or deleterious substance which may render the contents injurious to health; or (4) if (A) it bears or contains, for purposes of coloring only, a color additive which is unsafe within the meaning of Section 721(a), or (B) it is a color additive the intended use of which in or on drugs or devices is for purposes of coloring only and is unsafe within the meaning of Section 721(a); or (5) if it is a new animal drug which is unsafe within the meaning of Section 512; or (6) if it is an animal feed bearing or containing a new animal drug, and such animal feed is unsafe within the meaning of Section 512.

(b) If it purports to be or is represented as a drug the name of which is recognized in an official compendium, and its strength differs from, or its quality or purity falls below, the standards set forth in such compendium. Such determination as to strength, quality, or purity shall be made in accordance with the tests or methods of assay set forth in such compendium, except that whenever tests or methods of assay have not been prescribed in such compendium, or such tests or methods of assay as are prescribed are, in the judgment of the Secretary, insufficient for the making of such determination, the Secretary shall bring such fact to the attention of the appropriate body charged with the revision of such compendium, and if such body fails within a reasonable time to prescribe tests or methods of assay which, in the judgment of the Secretary, are sufficient for purposes of this paragraph, then the Secretary shall promulgate regulations prescribing appropriate tests or methods of assay in accordance with which such determination as to strength, quality, or purity shall be made. No drug defined in an official compendium shall be deemed to be adulterated under this paragraph because it differs from the standard of strength, quality, or purity therefore set forth in such compendium, if its difference in strength, quality, or purity from such standards is plainly stated on its label. Whenever a drug is recognized in both the United States Pharmacopeia and the Homeopathic Pharmacopeia of the United States it shall be subject to the requirements of the United States Pharmacopeia unless it is labeled and offered for sale as a homeopathic drug, in which case it shall be subject to the provisions of the Homeopathic Pharmacopeia of the United States and not to those of the United States Pharmacopeia.

(c) If it is not subject to the provisions of paragraph (b) of this section and its strength differs from, or its purity or quality falls below, that which it purports or is represented to possess.

(d) If it is a drug and any substance has been (1) mixed or packed therewith so as to reduce its quality or strength or (2) substituted wholly or in part therfore.

Misbranded Drugs

Misbranded or mislabeled drugs are those that are sold, dispensed, or distributed in violation of the labeling requirements of the FD&CA. The courts have held that when a pharmacist sells a prescription drug at retail without a prescription or refills a prescription without the prescriber's authorization, he or she has in effect "misbranded" the drug. *United States v. Carlisle*, 234 F.2d 196 (5th Cir. 1956).

Section 502 (a)-(p) of the Act provides that:

A drug or device shall be deemed misbranded—

(a) If its labeling is false or misleading in any particular. Health care economic information provided to a formulary committee, or other similar entity, in the course of the committee or the entity carrying out its responsibilities for the selection of drugs for managed care or other similar organizations, shall not be considered to be false or misleading under this paragraph if the health care economic information directly relates to an indication approved under Section 505 or under Section 351(a) of the Public Health Service Act for such drug and is based on competent and reliable scientific evidence. The requirements set forth in Section 505(a) or in Section 351(a) of the Public Health Service Act shall not apply to health care economic information provided to such a committee or entity in accordance with this paragraph. Information that is relevant to the substantiation of the health care economic information presented pursuant to this paragraph shall be made available to the Secretary upon request. In this paragraph, the term "health care economic information" means any analysis that identifies, measures, or compares the economic consequences, including the costs of the represented health outcomes, of the use of a drug to the use of another drug, to another health care intervention, or to no intervention.(b) If in a package form unless it bears a label containing (1) the name and place of business of the manufacturer, packer, or distributor; and (2) an accurate statement of the quantity of the contents in terms of weight, measure, or numerical count: Provided, That under clause (2) of this paragraph reasonable variations shall be permitted, and exemptions as to small packages shall be established, by regulations prescribed by the Secretary.

(c) If any word, statement, or other information required by or under authority of this Act to appear on the label or labeling is not prominently placed theron with such conspicuousness (as compared with other words, statements, designs, or devices, in the labeling) and in such terms as to render it likely to be read and understood by the ordinary individual under customary conditions of purchase and use.

(d) (Repealed by Pub. L. 105-115, November 21, 1997.)

(e)(1)(A) If it is a drug, unless its label bears, to the exclusion of any other nonproprietary name (except the applicable systematic chemical name or the chemical formula)—(i) the established name (as defined in subparagraph (3)) of the drug, if there is such a name; (ii) the established name and quantity, or, if determined to be appropriate by the Secretary, the proportion of each active ingredient, including the quantity, kind, and proportion of any alcohol, and also including whether active or not the established name and quantity or if determined to be appropriate by the Secretary, the proportion of any bromides, ether, chloroform, acetanilide, acetophenetidin, amidopyrine, antipyrine, atropine, hyoscine, hyoscyamine, arsenic, digitalis, digitalis glucosides, mercury, ouabain, strophanthin, strychnine, thyroid, or any derivative or preparation of any such substances, contained therein, except that the requirement for stating the quantity of the active ingredients, other than the quantity of those specifically named in this subclause, shall not apply to nonprescription drugs not intended for human use; and (iii) the established name of each inactive ingredient listed in alphabetical order on the outside container of the retail package and, if determined to be appropriate by the Secretary, on the immediate container, as prescribed in regulation promulgated by the Secretary, except that nothing in this subclause shall be deemed to require that any trade secret be divulged, and except that the requirements of this subclause with respect to alphabetical order shall apply only to nonprescription drugs that are not also cosmetics and that this subclause shall not apply to nonprescription drugs not intended for human use.

(B) For any prescription drug the established name of such drug or ingredient, as the case may be, on such label (and on any labeling on which a name for such drug or ingredient is used) shall be printed prominently and in type at least half as large as that used thereon for any proprietary name or designation for such drug or ingredient, except that to the extent that compliance with the requirements of subclause (ii) or (iii) of clause (A) or this clause is impracticable, exemptions shall be established by regulations promulgated by the Secretary.

(2) If it is a device and it has an established name, unless its label bears, to the exclusion of any other nonproprietary name, its established name (as defined in subparagraph (4)) prominently printed in type at least half as large as that used thereon for any proprietary name or designation for such device, except that to the extent compliance with the requirements of this subparagraph is impracticable, exemptions shall be established by regulations promulgated by the Secretary.

(3) As used in subparagraph (1), the term "established name" with respect to a drug or ingredient thereof, means (A) the applicable official name designated pursuant to Section 508, or (B) if there is no such name and such drug, or such ingredient, is an article recognized in an official compendium, then the official title thereof in such compendium, or (C) if neither clause (A) nor clause (B) of this subparagraph applies, then the common or usual name, if any, of such drug or of such ingredient, except that where clause (B) of this subparagraph applies to an article recognized in the United States Pharmacopeia and in the Homeopathic Pharamcopeia under different official titles, the official title used in the United States Pharmacopeia shall apply unless it is labeled and offered for sale as a homeopathic drug, in which case the official title used in the Homeopathic Pharmacopeia shall apply.

(4) As used in subparagraph (2), the term "established name" with respect to a device means (A) the applicable official name of the device designated pursuant to Section 508, (B) if there is no such name and such device is an article recognized in an official compendium, then the official title thereof in such compendium, or (C) if neither clause (A) nor clause (B) of this subparagraph applies, then any common or usual name of such device.

(f) Unless its labeling bears (1) adequate directions for use; and (2) such adequate warnings against use in those pathological conditions or by children where its use may be dangerous to health, or against unsafe dosage or methods or duration of administration or application, in such manner and form, as are necessary for the protection of users, except that where any requirement of clause (1) of this paragraph, as applied to any drug or device, is not necessary for the protection of the public health, the Secretary shall promulgate regulations exempting such drug or device from such requirement.

(g) If it purports to be a drug the name of which is recognized in an official compendium, unless it is packaged and labeled as prescribed therein. The method of packing may be modified with the consent of the Secretary. Whenever a drug is recognized in both the United States Pharmacopeia and the Homeopathic Pharmacopeia of the United States, it shall be subject to the requirements of the United States Pharmacopeia with respect to packaging and labeling unless it is labeled and offered for sale as a homeopathic drug, in which case it shall be subject to the provisions of the Homeopathic Pharmacopeia of the United States, and not to those of the United States Pharmacopeia, except that in the event of inconsistency between the requirements of this paragraph and those of paragraph (e) as to the name by which the drug or its ingredients shall be designated, the requirements of paragraph (e) shall prevail.

(h) If it has been found by the Secretary to be a drug liable to deterioration, unless it is packaged in such form and manner, and its label bears a statement of such precautions, as the Secretary shall by regulations require as necessary for the protection of the public health. No such regulation shall be established for any drug recognized in an official compendium until the Secretary shall have informed the appropriate body charged with the revision of such compendium of the need for such packaging or labeling requirements and such body shall have failed within a reasonable time to prescribe such requirements.

(i)(1) If it is a drug and its container is so made, formed, or filled as to be misleading; or (2) if it is an imitation of another drug; or (3) if it is offered for sale under the name of another drug.

(j) If it is dangerous to health when used in the dosage or manner; or with the frequency or duration prescribed, recommended, or suggested in the labeling thereof.

(k) (Repealed by Pub. L. 105-115, November 21, 1997.)

(l) (Repealed by Pub. L. 105-115, November 21, 1997.)

(m) If it is a color additive the intended use of which is for the purpose of coloring only, unless its packaging and labeling are in conformity with such packaging and labeling requirements applicable to such color additive, as may be contained in regulations issued under Section 721.

(n) In the case of any prescription drug distributed or offered for sale in any State, unless the manufacturer, packer, or distributor thereof includes in all advertisements and other descriptive printed matter issued or caused to be issued by the manufacturer, packer, or distributor with respect to that drug a true statement of (1) the established name as defined in Section 502(e), printed prominently and in type at least half as large as that used for any trade or brand name thereof, (2) the formula showing quantitatively each ingredient of such drug to the extent required for labels under Section 502(e), and (3) such other information in brief summary relating to side effects, contraindications, and effectiveness as shall be required in regulations which shall be issued by the Secretary in accordance with the procedure specified in Section 701(e) of this Act, except (A) in extraordinary circumstances, no regulation issued under this paragraph shall require prior approval by the Secretary of the content of any advertisement, and (B) no advertisement of a prescription drug, published after the effective date of regulations issued under this paragraph applicable to advertisements of prescription drugs, shall, with respect to the matters specified in this paragraph or covered by such regulations, be subject to the provisions of Sections 12 through 17 of the Federal Trade Commission Act, as amended (15 U.S.C. 52-57). This paragraph (n) shall not be applicable to any printed matter which the Secretary determines to be labeling as defined in Section 201(m) of this Act. Nothing in the Convention on Psychotropic Substances, signed at Vienna, Austria, on February 21, 1971, shall be construed to prevent drug price communications to consumers.

If it was manufactured, prepared, propagated, compounded, or processed in an establishment in any State not duly registered under Section 510, if it was not included in a list required by Section 510(j), if a notice or other information respecting it was not provided as required by such section or Section 510(k), or if it does not bear such symbols from the uniform system for identification of devices prescribed under Section 510(e) as the Secretary by regulation requires.

(p) If it is a drug and its packaging or labeling is in violation of an applicable regulation issued pursuant to Section 3 and 4 of the Poison Prevention Packaging Act of 1970.

To understand the meaning of the term "misbranded," the term must be read in light of the requirement of §502(f)(1) of the FD&CA (21 U.S.C. §352(f)(1) stating that the labeling of a drug contain "adequate directions for use." That is to say, prescription drugs are such because medical experts agree adequate directions for consumer self-medication cannot be provided for these drugs. Regardless of what directions a pharmacist or other dispenser might give when a legend drug is dispensed in absence of a prescription, the directions are, by law, not adequate for consumer use. Only the practitioner licensed to prescribe drugs is allowed to give directions adequate for the patient's safe and effective use of the federal legend drug product.

The Prescription Label

The directions and supervision of the prescribing or administering prescriber suffice in lieu of the adequate directions for use requirements of §502(f)(1) of the FD&CA. However, this does not mean a drug may be dispensed without labeling by the pharmacist. Section 503(b)(2) of the Act (21 U.S.C. §353[b][2]) requires the prescription label have the following information:

The name and address of the dispenser (pharmacy);
the serial number of the prescription;
the date of the prescription or the date of its filling (or refilling)—state law often determines which date is to be used;
the name of the prescriber;
the name of the patient, if stated in the prescription; and
directions for use, including precautions, if any, as indicated on the prescription.

State law may require the following further information including:

The name and address of the patient;
the initials or name of the dispensing pharmacist;
the telephone number of the pharmacy;
the drug name, strength, and manufacturer's lot or control number;
the beyond-use date, if any; and
the name of the manufacturer or distributor.

Receipt of Misbranded or Adulterated Drugs

If a pharmacy receives a misbranded or adulterated drug from a manufacturer or drug wholesaler, there is protection from federal penalty if the drug is then sold to a consumer. The FD&CA provides a number of exemptions from prosecution for the sale of misbranded or adulterated products that are received from outside sources, although civil liability may not be avoided because of implied warranty under state laws.

Section 303(c) of the Act states that a retail dealer can escape criminal penalty for receipt and subsequent delivery (sale) of misbranded or adulterated drugs if the delivery is in good faith and if, on request, he or she furnishes the FDA with records of the source of the interstate shipment. When the pharmacist purchases drugs from a wholesaler or manufacturer, he or she should look for a guaranty that the drugs are not adulterated or misbranded on the invoice. Consequently, a pharmacy may obtain protection from its drug suppliers by obtaining a "continuing guaranty" (as part of its original purchase contracts). Again, if the guaranty is not obtained, the retailer has some protection under §303(c)(1). The drug wholesaler generally is limited to obtaining a guaranty from its suppliers since the §303(c)(1) exemption usually does not apply because the wholesaler puts drugs into interstate commerce.

Prescription Drugs

FDA regulations define "prescription drugs" as drugs subject to the requirement of §503(b)(1) of the FD&CA, which states:

A drug intended for use by man which (A) because of its toxicity or other potentiality for harmful effect, or the method of its use, or the collateral measures necessary to its use, is not safe for use except under the supervision of a practitioner licensed by law to administer such drug; or (B) is limited by an approved application under Section 505 to use under the professional supervision of a practitioner licensed by law to administer such drug; shall be dispensed only (i) upon a written prescription of a practitioner licensed by law to administer such drug, or (ii) upon an oral prescription of such practitioner, which is reduced promptly to writing and filed by the pharmacist, or (iii) by refilling any such written or oral prescription if such refilling is authorized by the prescriber either in the original prescription or by oral order which is reduced promptly to writing and filed by the pharmacist. The act of dispensing a drug contrary to the provisions of this paragraph shall be deemed to be an act which results in the drug being misbranded while held for sale.

and as those exempt from the requirement of §502(f)(1), which states that drugs must bear adequate directions for use or be considered misbranded and subject to seizure under certain conditions. A drug is limited by the Act to dispensing by or upon a prescription because it is habit-forming, toxic, or has a potential for harm, or the NDA limits it to use under a physician's supervision. 21 CFR Part 201 Subpart D.)

Previously, one of the conditions of the FDA regulations for exempting a prescription-only drug from the §502(f)(1) requirement of adequate directions for safe use was that the label of the prescription drug, prior to dispensing, required the statement: "Caution: Federal law prohibits dispensing without a prescription." (This phrase is known as the "federal legend," and, hence, prescription drugs have historically been known as "legend" drugs.) Section 126 of the FDAMA amended Section 503(b)(4) of the FD&CA to require, at a minimum, that prior to dispensing, the label of prescription products contain the phrase "Rx only." The intent of this change was to simplify the labeling of prescription drug products in an effort to help reduce the incidence of medication errors in which product labeling and package design had been identified as a contributing factor. While the new requirement does not prohibit manufacturers from including other language on the label (ie, the "old" federal legend), the FDA believes that in the interest of simplification, it is preferable to have only the "Rx only" statement. The FDA has published a Guidance for Industry addressing the implementation of Section 126 of FDAMA. The Guidance Document, which may be accessed at http://www.fda.gov/cder/guidance/index.htm states the FDA intends to exercise its enforcement discretion and not object if a manufacturer does not comply with the labeling provisions until the next revision of its labels, or by February 19, 2003, whichever comes first.

Nonprescription (Over-the-Counter) Drugs

Nonprescription drugs (OTCs)are defined as drugs recognized among experts to be safe and effective for use (21 CFR §330.10). These drugs must be manufactured in accordance with the FDA's current good manufacturing standards and be labeled with directions for the layperson that indicate their safe and effective use.

POISONS

A poison has been defined as any drug known to the pharmaceutical or medical profession that is liable to be destructive to adult human life if taken in quantities of 60 grains or less. This general definition is helpful in indicating the substances customarily regarded as poisonous, but it is not followed in many of the state poison laws. Regulation of the sale of poisons usually falls within the jurisdiction of the state governments and governmental limits in this area may vary widely from state to state.

State statutes regulating the sale of poisons usually require that the purchaser be of a certain minimum age and that he know, or be informed, that the substance being purchased is a poison. Moreover, the pharmacist frequently has a responsibility to determine that the substance will be used for a lawful purpose. Recordkeeping requirements usually are specified in state statutes. For example, the pharmacist may be required to record the date of sale, name and address of the purchaser, name or initials of the seller, name and quantity of the poison and purpose for which it is intended. Some states require that the purchaser sign the record book to form a receipt and impress upon the purchaser the dangerous nature of the substance. The book in which this information is recorded frequently is referred to as the Poison Register and there may be a requirement that the book be used exclusively for recording sales of poisons. Most states specify a time period during which the sales records must be preserved and made available for inspection by appropriate state authorities.

Special labeling requirements for poisons frequently are encountered. The usual minimum requirement is that the container bear the name of the substance, the word poison, and the name and place of business of the seller. Such state requirements may be supplemented by federal requirements concerning labeling with information about toxicity, cautionary statements and information about treatment. Poisons are not permitted to be mailed without specific authorization from the US Postal Service.

Poison Prevention Packaging Act

The Poison Prevention Packaging Act was enacted by Congress during 1970 and authorizes the Consumer Product Safety Commission (CPSC) to establish standards for child-resistant packaging. The agency also enforces the statute at the pharmacy level.

Under this statute, prescription drugs, and some nonprescription medications, are considered to be hazardous household substances and, consequently, must be dispensed with a child-resistant closure. However, there are some exceptions to this requirement under the Act.

Most nonprescription medications are not required to be packaged in a child-resistant fashion. However, the CPSC has ordered, for example, that aspirin and products containing more than 500 mg of iron per package must be in safety packages. Yet manufacturers of aspirin products may produce one size of a package containing the drug that has a standard closure. Such non-safety packages are required to bear the warning statement, *This package for households without young children.* Other nonprescription products may be added to the list of drugs requiring safety packaging and pharmacists should watch for such developments.

Some prescription drugs are not required to be dispensed in child-resistant packages either. For example, the CPSC has stated that safety packaging is not required for sublingual dosage forms of nitroglycerin as well as sublingual and chewable dosage forms of isosorbide dinitrate in strengths of 5 mg or less. Other prescription drugs may be considered for exemption from the requirements of the Act and, while under consideration, child-resistant packaging is not required.

The prescriber may request that a drug, which otherwise would be required to be in a child-resistant package, be dispensed with a standard closure. The patient also has this option under the Act. The legislation does not require any specific fashion for communicating this waiver, ie, it is not required to be in writing. For example, a prescriber transmitting a prescription by telephone could indicate orally that standard packaging is requested. Nonetheless, the pharmacist may desire to have requests by prescribers or patients for noncomplying packaging in writing to document the transaction; this could prove to be invaluable in case of an adverse occurrence.

At the outset of the enforcement of this statute, the CPSC took the position that the pharmacist could not advise the patient of the option of standard packaging. This position was taken in furtherance of the agency's view that non-safety packaging should be the rare exception, not the rule, and a feeling that if pharmacists were to advise patients of their options widely, the Act would be undermined. The APhA challenged this position of the agency and the CPSC now adopts the position that pharmacists may advise patients of their right to request non-safety packaging.

Drugs dispensed for use by inpatients, be they in a hospital or a nursing home, are not required to be in child-resistant containers because the patients usually do not have access to them.

Manufacturers are not required to use child-resistant closures on stock bottles of medication that are not intended to reach the patient. However, if the packaging provided by the manufacturer is that which will be dispensed to the patient, eg, packages bearing antibiotic powders for reconstitution, safety tops must be used.

Federal Hazardous Substances Act

The Federal Hazardous Substances Act is the standard for the cautionary labeling of hazardous substances, including poisons. That Act provides that no state or political subdivision (municipality) may establish or continue to effect a cautionary labeling requirement that is applicable to hazardous substances or their packaging unless the cautionary labeling requirement is identical to that of the federal act, or unless the state labeling requirements provide a higher degree of protection than the federal requirements [15 U.S.C. §§1261(p) and §1262(b)]. However, not all state poison sale laws are pre-empted by federal law; only the labeling requirements are affected by the federal pre-emption. A number of state poison control laws contained provisions for the recording of the sale and inquiry into the purchaser's intended use and knowledge of the substance. These provisions may still be the legal standard, although the author does not know of a current court case illustrating the point. The practicing pharmacist should be aware of the general nature of the recording and warning proviso and should be knowledgeable of the exact requirement in the state in which he or she practices.

Federal Anti-Tampering Act

The Federal Anti-Tampering Act, passed by Congress as a result of a deliberate contamination of Tylenol capsules in 1982, makes it a federal offense to tamper with consumer products and gives regulatory authority to the Federal Bureau of Investigation, US Department of Agriculture, and FDA. The term tamper, when used in a criminal statute, has the limited meaning of improper interference "as for the purpose of alteration and to make objectionable or unauthorized changes." Tampering involves changing a product from what it was intended to be by the manufacturer. There are 5 sections of the Act:

Tampering with a consumer product that affects interstate or foreign commerce with reckless disregard for the risk of death or bodily injury to another person;

Tainting a consumer product with the intent of injuring a business;

Communicating false information that a consumer product has been tainted;

Threatening to tamper with a consumer product; and

Conspiring to tamper.

By regulation, tamper-resistant packaging is required for certain OTC drug products, cosmetics, and medical devices (contact lens solutions and lubricants). Dentifrices, dermatologics, lozenges, and insulin are excluded. A tamper-resistant package is defined as "one having an indicator or barrier to entry which, if breached or missing, can reasonably be expected to provide visible evidence to consumers that tampering has occurred." The regulations do not require the use of specific packaging technologies; any technology that achieves the required effect is acceptable. For tamper-resistant packaging to be fully effective, consumers need to examine the packaging carefully before consuming the contents, and they must be aware of the specific tamper-resistant features that have been used. FDA regulations require that the labeling of products with tamper-resistant packaging bear a statement alerting the consumer to the tamper-resistant feature. This labeling statement must be placed so it remains intact even if the tamper-resistant feature is breached or missing. If tampering is suspected, the closest FDA district office should be immediately notified.

The tamper-resistant packaging regulations for OTC drug products (21 CFR §211.132) are part of the CGMP's for finished drug products. For devices, the tamper-resistant packaging regulations are in 21 CFR §800.12, and those for cosmetics are in 21 CFR §700.25. A Compliance Policy Guide (7132a.17) that describes specific tamper-resistant packaging technologies is available from the National Technical Information Service, 5285 Port Royal Road, Springfield, VA 22161.

Electronic Signatures in Global and National Commerce Act (E-Sign)

In June 2000, President Bill Clinton signed the "E-Sign" Law (Public Law 106-229). Most of its provisions went into effect on October 1, 2000. While this law is not pharmacy specific, it may have great impact on the way pharmacy is practiced. The essence of the law is to spur the growth of electronic commerce by ensuring electronic contracts, signatures, and records will have the same legal status and effect as their ink and paper counterparts. Because E-Sign applies to all "transactions" (with few exceptions) in interstate commerce, it clearly encompasses the filling of prescriptions. This legislation has the potential to propel the electronic transmission of prescriptions. It is also important to note that the legislation is "technology neutral." It does not predetermine what technology to use or standards for such technology.

The legislation has 2 parts—one addressing primarily electronic signatures, and the other addressing electronic records. E-Sign states that electronic contracts, signatures, and records cannot be denied legal effect because the signature or record is in electronic form. E-Sign also declares that all other statutes, regulations, or rules of law requiring written signatures or written records are invalid or "pre-empted" in most circumstances. However, E-Sign does not require anyone (except governmental agencies) to accept an electronic signature or record. So, individuals still have a choice in determining whether to conduct business electronically.

ELECTRONIC SIGNATURES—By declaring that an electronic signature "may not be denied legal effect, validity, or enforceability solely because it is in electronic form," E-Sign effectively voids requirements that prescriptions be on paper or printed as a hard copy. In addition, E-Sign eliminates requirements that prescriptions be "hand-signed" or signed by the practitioner "in writing" or in the practitioner's "own handwriting." These types of handwriting requirements often are contained in state pharmacy practice acts and regulations but also appear in federal law through DEA requirements.

ELECTRONIC RECORDKEEPING—The recordkeeping portion of E-Sign states that any recordkeeping requirement related to transactions involving interstate commerce may be met by keeping electronic records—as long as the record accurately reflects the information to be retained and that it remains accessible to all who have a right to see the information. This portion of E-Sign is in direct conflict with many or most state pharmacy regulations. To avoid the provisions of E-Sign, a federal agency that attempts to require written signatures or records must show there is a "substantial justification" for making an exception.

THE COMPREHENSIVE DRUG ABUSE PREVENTION AND CONTROL ACT OF 1970

Current laws and regulations pertaining to controlled substances are online at www.deadiversion.usdoj.gov. The Federal *Comprehensive Drug Abuse Prevention and Control Act* became effective on May 1, 1971. Title II of that Act is known as the *Controlled Substances Act* (CSA) and it regulates the manufacture, distribution and dispensing of controlled substances. This law supersedes most previous narcotic and drug-abuse control laws, and places the enforcement of this Act with the Drug Enforcement Administration (DEA), which is part of the US Department of Justice. The DEA has promulgated extensive regulations to implement the Act, and these regulations appear in 21 CFR §§1300–end.

The statute provides a *closed* system for virtually every person who legitimately handles controlled substances other than the ultimate user. Over 500,000 individuals and institutions, such as hospitals, pharmacies, researchers, drug manufacturers and physicians are included in the class of persons subject to direct regulation through registration with the DEA. In addition to replacing or amending the numerous Federal laws relating to the control of drugs, the CSA is intended to aid in reducing the widespread diversion of these substances from legitimate channels.

When enacting the CSA Congress no longer relied upon the tax clause of the US Constitution, as had been done in the past. The authority for Congress to enact this legislation was derived from the interstate commerce clause of the Constitution. The power to regulate the health, safety and welfare of the American people has been left primarily within the jurisdiction of the individual states through the *police powers* that were reserved to the states via the Tenth Amendment of the US Constitution. However, Congress determined that the Federal control of intrastate incidents of the traffic in controlled substances is essential to the effective control of the interstate incidents of such traffic, and it thereby felt compelled to enter into the regulation of subject matter that previously had been left to the states. It must be remembered that if a provision of state or local law is inconsistent or conflicts with a provision of the CSA, the state or local law must yield to the Federal provision. However, if the state or local law augments or strengthens the Federal act, the more stringent state provision must be followed. To provide uniformity with the Federal Government, the majority of the states have adopted a *Uniform Controlled Substances Act*.

IMPORTANT DEFINITIONS

The following selected definitions are derived from the CSA or from the DEA regulations. These definitions must be read carefully for their language will affect greatly the use of the words within the Act. The following definitions are those that bear most heavily upon pharmacy practice:

Administer refers to the direct application of a controlled substance to the body of a patient or research subject.

Dispenser means an individual practitioner, an institutional practitioner, pharmacy or pharmacist who dispenses a controlled substance.

Individual practitioner means a physician, dentist, veterinarian or other individual licensed, registered or otherwise permitted, by the US or the jurisdiction in which he or she practices, to dispense a controlled substance in the course of professional practice, but does not include a pharmacist, a pharmacy or an institutional practitioner.

Institutional practitioner means a hospital or other person (other than an individual) licensed, registered or otherwise permitted, by the US or the jurisdiction in which it practices, to dispense a controlled substance in the course of professional practice, but does not include a pharmacy.

Narcotic drug means any of the following, whether produced directly or indirectly by extraction from substances of vegetable origin, or independently by means of chemical synthesis: (a) opium, coca leaves and opiates; (b) a compound, manufacture, salt, derivative or preparation of opium, coca leaves or opiates; (c) a substance that is chemically identical with any of the substances referred to in a or b.

Person includes any individual, corporation, government or governmental subdivision or agency, business trust, partnership, association or other legal entity.

Pharmacist means any pharmacist licensed by a State to dispense controlled substances, and shall include any other person (eg, pharmacist-intern) authorized by a State to dispense controlled substances under the supervision of a pharmacist licensed by such State.

Prescription means an order for medication that is dispensed to or for an ultimate user but does not include an order for medication that is dispensed for immediate administration to the ultimate user (eg, an order to dispense a drug to a bed patient for immediate administration in a hospital is not a prescription).

Readily retrievable means that certain records are kept by automatic data processing systems or other electronic or mechanized recording systems in such a manner that they can be separated from all other records in a reasonable time and/or records are kept on which certain items are asterisked, redlined or in some other manner visually identifiable apart from other items appearing on the records.

SCHEDULES

The drugs that come under the jurisdiction of the CSA have been categorized according to their potential for abuse and are divided into five schedules. Procedures for controlling a substance under the CSA are set forth in Section 201 of the Act. Scheduling requests may be initiated by the DHHS, by the DEA or by petition of a manufacturer, medical society, pharmaceutical association, public interest group or an individual citizen.

Once the DEA receives a request to control a drug or remove a substance entirely from the schedules, the agency must request that the DHHS conduct a scientific and medical evaluation. The Secretary of the DHHS then consults with the FDA and the other affected agencies regarding recommendations whether the drug or other substance should be controlled or removed from control. The medical and scientific evaluations are binding on the DEA with respect to scientific and medical matters and, if the DHHS recommends that a drug not be controlled, the DEA may not control the substance.

After the DEA receives the DHHS report, it then will proceed to make a final decision. If it has determined to control the drug, a proposal will be published in the *Federal Register* setting forth the proposed schedule and inviting all interested parties to file comments. At this point the affected parties may request a hearing before an administrative law judge. If no hearing is requested, the DEA will evaluate all the comments received and publish a final order in the *Federal Register*.

In reaching a final decision, the DEA is required by the Act to consider a number of factors with respect to each drug proposed to be controlled or removed from the schedules. These include potential for abuse; pharmacological effects; risk to public health; the history, scope, duration and significance of the abuse and the potential for psychic or physiological dependence.

The drugs that come under the jurisdiction of the CSA are divided into five schedules based upon their potential for abuse as follows:

SCHEDULE I—These drugs have a high potential for abuse and no accepted medical use in the US. The three broad categories of substances found in this schedule are the opiates, opium derivatives and hallucinogens. Some examples are heroin, marihuana, LSD, peyote, mescaline, psilocybin, tetrahydrocannabinols (THC) and dihydromorphine and others.

Properly registered persons may use Schedule I substances for research purposes. The FDA has approved the marketing of the THC product, dronabinol (Marinol), and the synthetic cannabinoid, nabilone (Cesamet), for the treatment of the nausea and vomiting associated with cancer chemotherapy. Both agents have been placed in Schedule II. All other tetrahydrocannabinols and marihuana remain in Schedule I.

SCHEDULE II—These drugs also have a high potential for abuse, but do have a currently accepted medical use in treatment in the US. It has been determined that the abuse of a drug, or other substances included in this schedule, may lead to severe psychological or physical dependence. The broad categories of Schedule II drugs include opiates and opium derivatives, derivatives of coca leaves and certain CNS stimulants and depressants. Some examples of Schedule II controlled narcotic substances are opium, morphine, codeine, hydromorphone (Dilaudid), methadone (Dolophine), pantopon, meperidine (Demerol), cocaine, oxycodone (Percodan—in combination with aspirin), anileridine (Leritine) and oxymorphone (Numorphan). Also in Schedule II are amphetamine (Benzedrine, Dexedrine) and methamphetamine (Desoxyn), phenmetrazine (Preludin), methylphenidate (Ritalin), amobarbital, pentobarbital, secobarbital, etorphine hydrochloride, diphenoxylate and phencyclidine.

The quantity of the substance in a drug product often determines under which schedule it will be controlled. For example, amphetamines and codeine generally are included in Schedule II. However, certain products containing smaller quantities, most often in combination with a noncontrolled substance, are controlled in Schedules III and V.

SCHEDULE III—These drugs have accepted medical use in the US, but they have a lower potential for abuse than Schedule I and II drugs. Schedule III drugs include compounds containing limited quantities of certain narcotic drugs, and non-narcotic drugs such as derivatives of barbituric acid except those that are listed in another schedule, glutethimide, methyprylon (Noludar), nalorphine, benzphetamine, chlorphentermine, clortermine, phendimetrazine and paregoric. Any suppository dosage form containing amobarbital, secobarbital or pentobarbital is in this schedule.

SCHEDULE IV—These drugs have a low potential for abuse relative to those in Schedule III. Abuse of Schedule IV drugs or substances may lead to limited physical dependence or psychological dependence as compared to those included in Schedule III. Schedule IV drugs are generally the long-acting barbiturates, certain hypnotics and the minor tranquilizers. For all practical purposes there are no regulatory differences between Schedule III and IV. Some of the more common drugs found in Schedule IV are barbital, phenobarbital, methylphenobarbital, chloral betaine, chloral hydrate, ethchlorvynol (Placidyl), ethinamate (Valmid), meprobamate (Equanil, Miltown), paraldehyde, methohexital, fenfluramine, diethylpropion, phentermine, chlordiazepoxide (Librium), diazepam (Valium), oxazepam (Serax), clorazepate (Tranxene), flurazepam (Dalmane), clonazepam (Clonopin), prazepam (Verstran), lorazepam (Ativan), mebutamate, propoxyphene (Darvon) and pentazocine (Talwin-NX).

SCHEDULE V—These drugs have the lowest abuse potential of the controlled substances and consist of preparations containing limited quantities of certain narcotic drugs generally for antitussive and antidiarrheal purposes. As a general rule, Schedule V items are OTC preparations that might be sold without a prescription. There are notable exceptions, and the pharmacist should always check the label to see if the FDA has determined the item to be a prescription-only item. For example, Lomotil is a Schedule V item, but it is prescription-only.

Manufacturers of nonnarcotic substances that may be sold OTC under the terms of the FD&C Act may apply to the DEA to have their product excluded from any schedule. Phenobarbital is the most common substance found in those products that are excluded from the scheduling process. One of the prime factors considered in determining whether to exclude a product would be the amount of the controlled substance involved. Once a product is excluded under Section 201 (g)(1) of the CSA it is no longer subject to DEA control. However, the pharmacist always should consult state and local laws to determine if any of the federally excluded products have been given more restrictive controls.

Schedule V Retail Distribution Restrictions

Controlled substances listed in Schedule V, which are not prescription only drugs, may be dispensed without a prescription by a pharmacist to a purchaser at retail, provided the following conditions are met:

1. Such dispensing is made only by a pharmacist (which, by definition, also includes a pharmacy intern unless prohibited by state law). However, after the pharmacist has fulfilled his professional and legal responsibilities, the actual cash, credit transaction or delivery may be completed by a nonpharmacist.
2. Not more than 240 mL (8 oz) or 48 solid dosage units of any substance containing opium, or more than 120 mL (4 oz) or 24 solid dosage units of any other controlled substance may be dispensed at retail to the same purchaser in any given 48-hr period without a prescription.
3. The purchaser at retail is at least 18 years of age.
4. The pharmacist requires every retail purchaser of a controlled substance, who is not known to him, to furnish suitable identification (including proof of age where appropriate).
5. A bound record book is maintained that contains the name and address of the purchaser, name and quantity of controlled substance purchased, date of each sale and initials of the selling pharmacist. This record book shall be maintained for a period of 2 years from the date of the last transaction entered in the record book, and it must be made available for inspection and copying by officers of the US, authorized by the Attorney General.
6. Other federal, state or local law does not require a prescription.

The pharmacist must be cautioned that in some states certain, or all, Schedule V substances have been placed on prescription-only status. In these states the more restrictive state law would apply and prohibit the OTC sale of Schedule V items.

Symbols and Labeling

Each commercial container of controlled substances will have on its label a symbol designating to which schedule it belongs. The symbol for Schedule I through V controlled substances will be as follows:

I or C-I
II or C-II
III or C-III
IV or C-IV
V or C-V.

The symbols will be at least twice as large as the largest letter printed on the label. There are exceptions to these labeling requirements. In those cases where the commercial container is too small to accommodate the label, only the box and the package insert must contain the *C* symbol.

As a general rule, these symbols are not required on prescription containers dispensed by a pharmacist to a patient in the course of his professional practice, although laws of some states may require such symbols on prescriptions dispensed to extended-care facilities.

Registration

Every "person" who manufactures, distributes, or dispenses any controlled substance or who proposes to engage in the manufacture, distribution or dispensing of any controlled substance must obtain a registration unless exempted. Registrations vary in length from 1 to 3 years. Most pharmacy registrations will be issued for a three year period. A unique DEA number is assigned to those who must register under the law including manufacturers, distributors, wholesalers and practitioners such as physicians, dentists, veterinarians, scientists, pharmacies, podiatrists and hospitals. There are, however, seven general categories of persons who are exempt from registration under the statute or the regulations, including civil defense officials, law enforcement officials, certain government employees, practitioners affiliated with registered institutions and agents or employees of registrants. It is this latter exemption that permits individual pharmacists not to register with the DEA since such pharmacists serve as agents of the registered pharmacies.

In other words, pharmacies must register with the DEA to dispense controlled substances but pharmacists do not. The one exception is for a pharmacist who owns a pharmacy as a sole proprietor; in such a case, the pharmacist would be required to register. The certificate of registration must be maintained at the registered location and kept available for official inspections. If an individual owns and operates more than one pharmacy, each place of business must be registered separately.

Applications for reregistration will be mailed by the DEA to each registered person approximately 60 days before the expiration date of the registration. If a registered pharmacy does not receive such forms within 45 days prior to the expiration date of the registration, it must give notice of such fact and request the reregistration forms.

New Registrations

Pharmacies that seek to become registered for the first time must request a registration application from the DEA. No pharmacy may engage in any activity for which registration is required until its application for registration has been granted and a certificate issued to it by the DEA. However, a pharmacy may not dispense controlled substances if it has not been issued a valid state license, even though the DEA already may have registered the pharmacy and authorized it to obtain controlled substances. See *Wedgewood Village Pharmacy v. Ashcroft*, 2003 US Dist Lexis 22401 (Dec 15, 2003).

Modifications such as change of address, location or name by existing registrants may be made without going through the new registration process. To make such a modification, the registrant should submit a letter to the DEA requesting it. No fee is required. A registrant also may apply to modify his registration to authorize the handling of additional schedules of controlled substances, but may not modify his registration to transfer it to another party.

Termination

The DEA has the authority under the CSA to suspend or revoke a registration where the registrant has falsified his application, or has been convicted of a felony under the federal or state CSA or has had his state license or registration suspended and no longer is authorized by state law to dispense controlled substances. Except in emergency situations, registrants are assured of a hearing and due process of law prior to suspension or revocation of registration. In addition, the registration of any person terminates if and when such a person dies, ceases legal existence or discontinues business or professional practice.

Distribution

As a general rule a separate DEA registration is required for each activity a registrant wishes to engage in such as manufacturing, distributing, dispensing or conducting research. However, a pharmacy registered to dispense a controlled substance may distribute (without being registered as a distributor) a quantity of controlled substances to a physician, another pharmacy, hospital or nursing home for the purpose of general dispensing by that practitioner provided the following conditions are met:

1. The pharmacy or practitioner to which the controlled substance is being distributed is registered under the Act to dispense that controlled substance.
2. The distribution is recorded as being distributed by the pharmacy and the pharmacist, or practitioner, records the substance being received. The pharmacy distributing a controlled substance must record the name of the substance, the dosage form, the quantity and the name, address and DEA registration number of the pharmacy or practitioner to whom it is distributed as well as the date of distribution.
3. If the substance is listed in Schedule I or II, the transfer must be made on official DEA order form 222.
4. The total number of dosage units of controlled substances distributed by a pharmacy may not exceed 5% of all controlled substances dispensed by the pharmacy during the 12-month period in which the pharmacy is registered. If at any time it does exceed 5% the pharmacy is required to register as a distributor as well as being registered as a pharmacy.

As an incident to this distribution, a pharmacist may manufacture (without being registered to manufacture) an aqueous or oleaginous solution or solid dosage form containing a narcotic controlled substance in a proportion not exceeding 20% of the complete solution, compound or mixture.

The regulations also permit a person lawfully in possession of controlled substances to return them to the supplier without registering as a distributor. Registrants would have to use official DEA order forms for the return of Schedule I and II substances to a supplier.

Records and Reports

Every pharmacy handling controlled substances must keep complete and accurate records of all receiving and dispensing transactions that must be maintained for a period of at least 2 years. Many states require that the records be kept for as long as 5 years from the date of the last dispensation.

All inventories and records of controlled substances in Schedule II must be maintained separately from all other records of the registrant. All inventories and records of controlled substances in Schedules III, IV, and V must be maintained separately or must be in such form that they are readily retrievable from the ordinary professional and business records of the pharmacy.

All records pertaining to controlled substances must be made available for inspection and copying by duly authorized DEA officials and state authorized agents.

When a registrant first engages in business, and every 2 years thereafter, a complete and accurate inventory of all stocks of controlled substances on hand must be completed and kept by the registrant for a period of 2 years. Pharmacies are not required to submit a copy of the inventory to the DEA; however, many states require a copy of the inventory be sent to the regulatory agency.

Continuing Records

Every pharmacy must maintain, on a current basis, a complete and accurate record of each controlled substance received. Copy 3 of executed DEA order form 222 retained by the pharmacy, which have been completed as described under the section entitled *Order Forms*, will constitute a pharmacy's receiving records for Schedule II controlled substances. Invoices for Schedule III, IV, and V controlled substances will be considered as complete receiving records if the actual date of receipt is recorded clearly on the invoices by the pharmacist or other responsible individual.

Filing Prescriptions

Under federal law, prescription orders for controlled substances must be filed in one of the following three ways:

1. A pharmacy can maintain three separate files—a file for Schedule II drugs dispensed, a file for Schedules III, IV, and V drugs dispensed and a file for prescription orders for all other drugs dispensed.
2. A pharmacy can maintain two files—a file for all Schedule II drugs dispensed, and another file for all other drugs dispensed, including those in Schedules III, IV, and V. If this method is used, the prescription orders in the file for Schedules III, IV, and V must be stamped with the letter *C* in red ink, not less than 1-inch high, in the lower-right corner. This distinctive marking makes the records *readily retrievable* for inspection.
3. A pharmacy can maintain two files—one file for all controlled drugs in all schedules and a second file for all prescription orders for noncontrolled drugs dispensed. If this method is used, the prescription orders for drugs in Schedules III, IV, and V in the controlled drug prescription file must be stamped with the red letter *C* not less than 1-inch high in the lower-right corner, as previously mentioned. This latter requirement is waived for pharmacies using electronic record keeping methods. State requirements vary widely but usually do not permit as many options for maintaining prescription records as permitted under federal law. State laws may impose additional considerations.

Inventory

The CSA requires each registrant to make a complete and accurate record of all stocks of controlled substances on hand every 2 years. The DEA no longer specifies a date on which the inventory must be performed. Many states do, however, specify a date or provide for a window of time when the inventory must occur. The actual taking of the inventory should not vary more than 4 days from the biennial inventory date. The inventory record must:

1. List the name, address, and DEA registration number of the registrant.
2. Indicate the date and time the inventory is taken, ie, opening or closing of business.
3. Be signed by the person or persons responsible for taking the inventory.
4. Be maintained at the location appearing on the registration certificate for at least 2 years.
5. Keep records of Schedule II drugs separate from all other controlled substances.

When taking the inventory of Schedule II controlled substances, an exact count or measure must be made. When taking the inventory of Schedules III, IV, and V controlled substances, an estimated count may be made unless the container holds more than 1000 dosage units, in which case an exact count must be made if the container has been opened.

NEWLY CONTROLLED SUBSTANCES—Occasionally a drug that has not been controlled previously will be placed in one of the drug schedules or a controlled substance will be moved into a higher or lower schedule. In either case the drug must be inventoried as of the effective date of transfer, and this inventory should be added to the biennial inventory. Note that many states require pharmacies to perform an audit of CS drugs annually.

Order Forms

The order form system developed by the DEA is a completely closed system of drug distribution. The DEA permits only authorized persons to obtain or distribute *Schedule I* or *II* controlled substances and only pursuant to official DEA order form 222. The regulations set forth those instances where official order forms are not required to transfer *Schedule I* or *II* controlled substances, eg, transfer to a patient pursuant to a written prescription, administration to a patient by a registered practitioner, procurement by civil defense officials or delivery by a common carrier to a warehouse.

A pharmacy desiring official order forms may requisition the appropriate ones from the DEA. Such forms are numbered serially and issued with the name, address and registration number of the pharmacy, the authorized activity and authorized schedules with respect to that pharmacy. Each triplicate form is contained in a book of seven. Up to six books may be ordered at one time unless the pharmacy can show that it needs to exceed this limit. There is no charge for these forms.

The pharmacist must prepare and execute the order form in triplicate using a typewriter, pen or indelible pencil. One must enter the name and address of the supplier from whom the controlled substances are being ordered. Only one supplier may be listed on any one form. There are ten lines in the *item* section of each form. Each of the ten lines must contain a different drug or *item*. The number of lines completed must be totaled at the bottom. This is the total number of lines or items and not the total number of commercial containers ordered. The order form must be completed properly and have no material alterations or erasures or a distributor will be obligated to refuse the form, and may elect to do so in other cases as well, if the order form is not completed correctly.

The purchaser must sign his name and date the order form on the day he places the order. If his name is different from the authorized registrant, ie, if the pharmacist has been given a power of attorney to complete order forms, he also must include the name of the authorized registrant in the signature space. When the form is completed, the purchaser separates the three copies in the following manner: Copies 1 and 2 must be kept intact with the carbon in between them. These are sent in with the registrant's order to his supplier. Copy 3 is retained by the purchaser separately from other records. When the registrant receives the items he must record, on the retained Copy 3, the number of packages and the date such packages were received. A space is provided for this.

Power of Attorney

Any registered pharmacy may authorize one or more individuals, whether or not they are at the registered location of the pharmacy, to obtain and execute order forms on its behalf by executing a power of attorney for each such individual. This must be signed by the same person who signed the most recent application for registration or reregistration and must contain the signature of the individual being authorized to obtain and execute order forms. The power of attorney is not submitted to the DEA but must be retained by the pharmacy with the executed forms. It must be available for inspection together with the order form records. A power of attorney may be revoked at any time by filing a notice of revocation, signed by the individual who signed the most recent application for registration or reregistration and by filing it with the power of attorney being revoked. Many states have restrictions on who may sign order forms under a power of attorney. For example only a licensed health-care worker such as a pharmacist may be permitted to sign the forms under such restrictions.

Lost or Theft

When unfilled order forms are lost, the pharmacy must execute a new form 222 in triplicate. The pharmacy also must execute form 106 containing the serial number and date of the lost form, stating that the drugs in it were never received, and attach a copy of that statement to Copy 3 of the lost form. A copy of that statement also should be attached to Copies 1 and 2 of the newly executed order form.

Whenever any used or unused order forms are stolen or lost, upon discovery, the pharmacy must report this immediately to the Drug Enforcement Administration on form 106, stating the serial numbers of each form lost or stolen. If an entire book or books of order forms are lost or stolen, and the pharmacist is unable to state the serial numbers, he shall report, in lieu of the serial numbers, the date or approximate date of issuance. Lost or stolen order forms also should be reported to the state board of pharmacy or other state controlled substance agency.

Prescriptions

WHO MAY ISSUE—To issue a prescription an individual practitioner must be both (1) authorized to prescribe controlled substances by the jurisdiction, usually a state, where licensed to practice and (2) either registered or exempted from registration by the DEA.

PURPOSE OF ISSUE—A prescription for a controlled substance to be effective must be issued for a legitimate medical purpose by a practitioner acting in the usual course of professional practice. The responsibility for the proper prescribing and dispensing of controlled substances is upon the prescribing practitioner, but a corresponding liability rests with the pharmacist who dispenses the prescription. An order purporting to be a prescription issued not in the usual course of professional treatment, or in legitimate and authorized research, is not a prescription within the meaning and intent of Section 309 of the CSA. The person knowingly dispensing such a purported prescription, as well as the person issuing it, will be subject to the penalties provided for violations of the provisions of law relating to controlled substances.

A prescription by which a practitioner attempts to resupply an office stock or maintain drug-dependent individuals is not a valid prescription and, therefore, is void.

EXECUTION OF PRESCRIPTIONS—All prescriptions for controlled substances must be dated as of, and signed on, the day when issued and bear the full name and address of the patient and the name, address and registration number of the practitioner. A practitioner may sign a prescription in the same manner as a check or legal document, eg, J. H. Smith or John H Smith. Where an oral order is not permitted, prescriptions must be executed using a typewriter, ink or an indelible pencil and must be signed manually by the practitioner. The prescription may be prepared by a secretary or agent for the signature of a practitioner, but the prescriber is responsible in case the prescription does not conform, in all essential respects, to the law and regulations.

Prescription orders that are written for controlled substances in Schedule II must be executed using a typewriter, ink or indelible pencil and must be signed by the practitioner issuing such prescription orders. In an emergency, Schedule II drugs may be dispensed upon an oral or facsimile (fax) authorization (see below). Prescription orders for controlled substances in Schedules III, IV, or V may be issued either orally or in writing by a practitioner or his authorized agent. Federal law also permits facsimile transmission of Schedule III, IV, and V prescriptions.

EMERGENCY DISPENSING-SCHEDULE II—In the case of a bona fide emergency, as defined by the Secretary of Health and Human Services, a pharmacist may dispense a Schedule II controlled substance upon receiving oral or facsimile authorization of a prescriber provided that:

1. The quantity prescribed and dispensed is limited to the amount adequate to treat the patient during the emergency period. Prescribing or dispensing beyond the emergency period must be pursuant to a written prescription order.
2. The oral prescription order is reduced immediately to writing by the pharmacist and contain all information, except for the prescriber's signature.
3. If the prescriber is not known to the pharmacist, he must make a reasonable effort to determine that the oral authorization came from a prescriber, by verifying his telephone number against that listed in the directory and other good-faith efforts to insure his identity.
4. Within 7 days after authorizing an emergency oral prescription order, the prescriber must cause a written prescription order for the emergency quantity prescribed to be delivered to the dispensing pharmacist. The prescription order shall have written on its face *Authorization for Emergency Dispensing*. The written prescription order may be delivered in person or by mail, but if delivered by mail it must be postmarked within the 7 day period. Upon receipt, the dispensing pharmacist must attach this prescription order to the oral emergency prescription order that had been reduced to writing earlier. The pharmacist shall notify the nearest office of the DEA, if the prescriber fails to deliver a written prescription order to him. Failure of the pharmacist to do so shall void the authority conferred by the subsection to dispense without a written prescription order of a prescriber.

Definition of Emergency—For the purpose of authorizing an oral prescription order of a controlled substance listed in Schedule II of the *Controlled Substances Act,* the term *emergency situation* means those situations in which the prescriber determines that:

1. Immediate administration of the controlled substance is necessary for the proper treatment of the intended user.
2. No appropriate alternative treatment is available, including administration of a drug that is not a controlled substance under Schedule II of the Act.
3. It is not reasonably possible for the prescriber to provide a written prescription order to be presented to the person dispensing the substance, prior to the dispensing.

TRANSMISSION OF PRESCRIPTION FACSIMILE- DEA regulations do permit facsimile transmission of prescriptions for medications in Schedules II-V directly from the prescriber to the pharmacy. However, this authorization is contingent upon such activity also be authorized under relevant state law.

Schedule II medications may be dispensed pursuant to faxed authorization only if the patient is [a] receiving home infusion treatment, [b] in a long-term care facility, or [c] a hospice patient. Detailed regulations regarding this are located at 21 CFR §1306.

With Schedule III and IV medications the transmitted facsimile may serve as authority for dispensing the controlled substance.

REFILLS AND RENEWALS—No prescription for a Schedule II controlled substance may be refilled; however, in certain limited circumstances, federal law allows the partial filling of Schedule II prescriptions. (See below) Prescriptions for Schedule III or IV controlled substances may be refilled if so authorized. These prescriptions may not be filled or refilled more than 6 months after the date issued or be refilled more than five times after the date issued. After five refills or after 6 months, the practitioner may renew the prescription. A renewal of any such prescription must be recorded on a new prescription blank and a new prescription number assigned. Oral prescriptions must be committed to writing by the pharmacist who receives the oral order.

Prescriptions for a Schedule V controlled substance may be refilled only as authorized by the prescribing practitioner on the prescription. If no such authorization is given, the prescription may not be refilled. However, if the item may be sold over the counter legally, the burden of determining the propriety of the sale will be upon the pharmacist.

Recording Refills—A pharmacist, after refilling a prescription for any controlled substance in Schedules III, IV, or V, must enter on the back of that prescription his initials, the date the prescription was refilled and the amount of drug dispensed. If the pharmacist merely initials and dates the back of the prescription, he shall be deemed to have dispensed a refill for the full face amount of the prescription.

Computerization—A pharmacy is permitted to use a data processing system as an alternative method for the storage and retrieval of prescription refill information for controlled substances in Schedules III and IV.

The computerized system must provide immediate retrieval, (via CRT display or hard-copy printout) of original prescription information for those prescriptions that currently are authorized for refilling. The information that readily must be retrievable must include, but is not limited to, data such as the original prescription number, date of issuance of the prescription by the practitioner, full name and address of the patient, practitioner's name and DEA registration number, name, strength, dosage form, quantity of the controlled substance prescribed, quantity dispensed if different from the quantity prescribed and the total number of refills authorized by the prescriber.

In addition, the system must provide immediate retrieval of the current refill history for Schedule III or IV controlled substance prescriptions that have been authorized for refills during the past 6 months and backup documentation to show that the refill information is correct. The backup documentation must be stored in a separate file at the pharmacy and maintained for a 2-year period from the dispensing date.

TRANSMITTAL OF ORAL AUTHORIZATION—A practitioner's nurse, or other member of the staff, cannot authorize the renewal of a prescription for a controlled substance that has been refilled five times or is 6-months old. The authority for prescribing controlled substances is vested only with the practitioner, and cannot be delegated to anyone else. However, nurses or staff members receiving calls from pharmacies regarding renewals may act as the practitioners agent and transmit the practitioners order. In other words, once the practitioner authorizes the order, an agent may communicate that order to the pharmacy.

PRACTITIONERS OFFICE STOCK—A pharmacist may not dispense a controlled substance on the order of a prescription that is issued by a practitioner and is intended for the office use of the practitioner. Distribution must be made on invoice and/or order form, if required.

LABEL REQUIREMENTS—The pharmacist filling a prescription for controlled substances listed in Schedules II, III, IV or V must affix to the package a label showing the pharmacy name and address, serial number and date of initial filling, name of the patient, name of the practitioner issuing the prescription, directions for use and cautionary statements, if any. This labeling requirement does not apply to institutionalized patients.

The label of any drug listed as a controlled substance in Schedules II, III, or IV of the CSA must, when dispensed to a patient, contain the following warning:

CAUTION: Federal law prohibits the transfer of this drug to any person other than the patient for whom it was prescribed.

PARTIAL FILLING-*SCHEDULE II*—The partial filling of a *Schedule II* controlled substance prescription is permissible if the pharmacist is unable to supply the full quantity called for in a written or emergency oral prescription. The pharmacist may supply a portion of the quantity called for provided a notation of the quantity supplied is made on the face of the written prescription (or written record of the emergency oral prescription). The remaining portion may be filled within 72 hr of the first dispensing; however, if the remaining portion is not, or cannot be filled within the 72-hour period, the pharmacist must notify the prescriber. No further quantity may be supplied beyond the 72 hours except on a new prescription. However, the partial dispensing of a prescription for Schedule II controlled substances beyond the 72-hour limitation is permissible for patients in long-term care facilities.

A prescription for a Schedule II controlled substance written for a patient in a Long Term Care Facility (LTCF) or for a patient with a medical diagnosis documenting a terminal illness may be filled in partial quantities to include individual dosage units. If there is any question whether a patient may be classified as having a terminal illness, the pharmacist must contact the practitioner prior to partially filling the prescription. Both the pharmacist and the prescribing practitioner have a corresponding responsibility to assure that the controlled substance is for a terminally ill patient. The pharmacist must record on the prescription whether the patient is *terminally ill* or an *LTCF patient*. A prescription that is partially filled and does not contain the notation *terminally ill* or *LTCF patient* shall be deemed to have been filled in violation of the Act. For each partial filling, the dispensing pharmacist shall record on the back of the prescription (or on another appropriate record, uniformly maintained, and readily retrievable) the date of the partial filling, quantity dispensed, remaining quantity authorized to be dispensed, and the identification of the dispensing pharmacist. The total quantity of Schedule II controlled substances dispensed in all partial fillings must not exceed the total quantity prescribed. Schedule II prescriptions for patients in a LTCF or patients with a medical diagnosis documenting a terminal illness shall be valid for a period not to exceed 60 days from the issue date unless sooner terminated by the discontinuance of medication.

PARTIAL FILLING-*SCHEDULE III* AND *IV*—Partial filling of prescriptions for controlled substances in Schedules III and IV is permitted if the pharmacist filling or refilling the prescription sets forth the quantity dispensed and his initials on the back of the prescription. In addition, the partial fillings may not exceed the total amount authorized in the prescription and the dispensing of all refills must be within the 6-month limit.

TRANSFERS—Prescriptions for Schedules III, IV, and V drugs may be transferred between pharmacies for refill purposes. The transfer of original prescription information for a controlled substance listed in Schedules III, IV, or V for the purpose of refill dispensing is permissible between differently owned pharmacies on a one time basis only. However, pharmacies electronically sharing a real-time, on-line database may transfer up to the maximum refills permitted by law and the prescriber's authorization. Transfers are subject to the following requirements:

The transfer is communicated directly between two licensed pharmacists and the transferring pharmacist records the following information:

Write the word *VOID* on the face of the invalidated prescription.

Record on the reverse of the invalidated prescription the name, address and DEA registration number of the pharmacy to which it was transferred and the name of the pharmacist receiving the prescription information.

Record the date of the transfer and the name of the pharmacist transferring the information.

The pharmacist receiving the transferred prescription information is required to reduce to writing the following:

Write the word *transfer* on the face of the transferred prescription.

Provide all information required to be on a prescription pursuant to 21 CFR §1306.05 and include:

- Date of issuance of original prescription;
- Original number of refills authorized on original prescription;
- Date of original dispensing;

- Number of valid refills remaining and date(s) and locations of previous refill(s)
- Pharmacy's name, address, DEA registration number and prescription number from which the prescription information was transferred;
- Name of pharmacist who transferred the prescription;
- Pharmacy's name, address, DEA registration number and prescription number from which the prescription was originally filled.

The original and transferred prescription(s) must be maintained for a period of 2 years from the date of last refill.

Distribution on Discontinuance or Transfer

Any registrant desiring to discontinue business activities altogether, or with respect to controlled substances (without transferring such business activities to another person), must return, for cancellation, the registrant's certificate of registration and any unexecuted order forms in his possession to the location as instructed by the DEA Field Office.

Any controlled substances in possession of the registrant may be disposed of in accordance with instructions under the section on drug Disposal (below).

Any registrant desiring to discontinue business activities altogether, or with respect to controlled substances (by transferring such business activities to another person), must submit in person or by registered or certified mail, return receipt requested, to the nearest DEA office at least 14 days in advance of the date of the proposed transfer:

1. The name, address and registration number of the pharmacy discontinuing business.
2. The name, address and registration number of the person acquiring the pharmacy.
3. Whether the business activities will be continued at the location registered by the person discontinuing business or moved to another location (if the latter, the address of the new location should be listed).
4. The date on which the transfer of controlled substances will occur.

On the day of transfer a complete inventory of all controlled substances being transferred must be taken in accordance with 21 CFR §§1304.11–1304.19. This inventory serves as the final inventory of the registrant transferor and the initial inventory for the registrant transferee. A copy of the inventory must be included in the records of each person. It is not necessary to file a copy with the DEA unless requested by the Regional Director. Transfers of any Schedule II substances require the use of order form 222.

On the day of transfer all records required to be kept by the registrant transferor, with reference to the controlled substances being transferred, are to be transferred to the registrant transferee. Responsibility for the accuracy of records prior to the date of transfer remains with the transferor, but responsibility for custody and maintenance shall be upon the transferee.

Miscellaneous Requirements

SECURITY—Pharmacies must keep Schedules II, III, IV, and V controlled substances in a locked cabinet or dispersed throughout the noncontrolled stock in such a manner as to deter theft. A combination of these two methods is permissible. For example, many pharmacies lock Schedule II drugs in a drawer or cabinet while dispersing Schedule III, IV, and V drugs alphabetically throughout the nonscheduled drug inventory.

DISPOSAL—A pharmacy wishing to dispose of any excess or undesired stock of controlled substances must contact its nearest DEA Office and request the necessary form (DEA-41). A cover letter from the pharmacy must be attached to the report stating that the controlled substances are not desired and the pharmacy wishes to dispose of them.

Upon the receipt of the letter from the pharmacy, one of four courses of action will be chosen by the DEA; this will be stated in letter form, attached to the original copy of the DEA-41 form and returned to the pharmacy.

The four courses of action are:

1. The drugs may be destroyed by two responsible parties employed or acting on behalf of the registrant. This course of action will be used when there are factors that preclude an on-the-site destruction witnessed by DEA personnel, such as the firms history of compliance and the abuse potential of the drugs involved.
2. The excess or undesired stocks of controlled substances should be forwarded to the appropriate state agency for destruction. In lieu of actual surrender to the state agency, destructions witnessed by state personnel are acceptable.
3. The substances should be held until DEA personnel arrive at a mutually convenient time to witness their destruction. DEA personnel will date and sign the reports or forms after witnessing the destruction.
4. The substances should be forwarded to the DEA Field Office that serves the area in which the registrant is located. Upon receipt of the substances, the DEA Field Office will verify the actual substance submitted. If errors are found, a corrected form must be prepared and the registrant duly notified. The original form will be returned to the registrant.

DRUG THEFT—Any pharmacy involved in loss of controlled substances must notify the nearest DEA office of the theft or significant loss upon discovery. The pharmacy must make a report regarding the loss or theft by completing DEA-106 form. Such reports shall contain the following information: name and address of firm, DEA registration number, date of theft, local police department notified, type of theft, listing of symbols or cost code used by the pharmacy in marking containers and listing of the controlled substances missing. Four copies of this report should be made. The pharmacy should keep the original copy for its records and forward two copies to the nearest DEA office. Most states require a copy be sent to the Board of Pharmacy as well. Local ordinances may require notification be provided to the appropriate police authority.

Mailing

Title 39 of the Code of Federal Regulations contains the US Postal Service Regulations regarding nonmailable matter and special mailing rules for various articles and substances. Controlled substances may be mailed to a patient's home if they are sent in a reasonable quantity intended for personal use. Controlled substances may also be transmitted in the mail between persons registered with the DEA or between persons who are exempted from registration such as military, law enforcement or civil defense personnel in the performance of their official duties.

Parcels containing controlled substances must be prepared and packaged for mailing in accordance with the regulations set forth in 39 CFR §124. Regular mail may be used for these parcels.

DEA Inspections

The CSA specifically requires an administrative search warrant for most nonconsensual DEA inspections. Therefore, for an agent of the DEA to enter any DEA-registered premise, the agent must state the purpose for the inspection and present appropriate identification. In addition, the agent must either obtain an informed consent from the registrant, secure an administrative inspection warrant or fit into one of the special exceptions set forth in the statute. The Act recognizes certain exigent circumstances in which an inspection warrant is not required such as the initial registration inspection, inspection of mobile vehicles, emergency situations or dangerous health situations.

TORT LAW

Tort law is that subdivision of the civil law that deals with relationships between individuals created by law rather than by the parties themselves. A tort is a private injury or wrong arising from a breach of a duty created by law. It may involve harm to a person, as well as damage to property, caused negligently or intentionally.

Negligent torts are those that arise because the tort-feasor (the person doing the act) breached a duty or level of care expected of him. Intentional torts are those that the actor does purposefully or with an intention of achieving the desired result.

NEGLIGENCE

Negligence has been defined as the omission to do something that a reasonable person, guided by those ordinary considerations that ordinarily regulate human affairs, would do, or the doing of something that a reasonable and prudent individual would not do. As is obvious from this statement, one can be negligent either by doing or failing to do something. A more direct description is that negligence occurs when a person under a duty to another to use due care breaches that duty, resulting in the other party suffering damages as a direct result of that breach. Using this statement as a point of departure, each element of negligence shall be considered in order.

In the normal situation, the existence of a legal duty will be created by the activities of other persons. The jury will be charged with determining what the fictional reasonable and prudent person mentioned above would have done under the circumstances. To do this, the jurors receive testimony from a number of people to determine what they would have done. The jury then decides what the reasonable and prudent person would have done, and that creates the existence of a legal duty. In the ordinary circumstance, the duty will be created by the actions of laymen. Yet, when pharmacists are acting within the scope of their professional calling, their performance will be evaluated in light of what professional peers would have done. Generally, pharmacists will be held liable for negligence only if they departed from the practice of other reputable practitioners of pharmacy. For the general practitioner of pharmacy, the reference standard to be used is other general practitioners of pharmacy. While there may be individuals within the profession with greater knowledge or skill in a particular area, eg, the detection of drug interactions, the general practitioner of pharmacy will be required to discharge only that amount of skill exhibited by peers, not the experts.

Nonetheless, this does not mean that the members of a profession can lag unduly in adopting new methods or procedures. A number of courts have ruled that while in the usual case the law will recognize the standard of care established by the members of the trade, industry or profession, the entire group may have lagged in adopting an innovation. In such cases the courts will not be bound by the standards used by the profession, but rather the court will establish the standard of care to be exercised under the circumstance.

The concept of duty is not fixed but constantly evolving and changing. An example of this is the doctrine of the pharmacists duty to consult with patients about proper drug use. Through a number of cases decided during the past 40 years, various courts have ruled that the pharmacist does have the legal duty to instruct the patient about safe and proper use of medication. This duty is owed to the patient, and should a pharmacist fail to fulfill this responsibility, he may be held answerable in court.

A second requirement for the existence of negligence is damage. The party who is alleging negligence must prove that he suffered legally sufficient damages. Generally, these damages must be substantial, not slight, eg, a temporary skin rash would be insufficient.

The party bringing the suit next must prove that the damages were the direct result of the pharmacist's breach of a legal duty. This may be quite difficult. In some cases it is known that the patient suffered legally cognizable damages, but it cannot be established by a preponderance of the evidence that damages flowed directly from a breach of duty.

The plaintiff has the burden of establishing those first three elements. Once they have been shown in a legally sufficient manner, the pharmacist has a number of defenses that may be available to result in a verdict of not liable. One such defense may be contributory negligence. That is the rule that a person who has in some way contributed to his own injury will not be entitled to recover. In a majority of states the rule is one of comparative negligence. While contributory negligence is a total bar to recovery by the plaintiff, in states that follow the comparative negligence rule the jury engages in an allocation of responsibility and bases the amount of damages awarded on the parties' relative contributions to the injury.

Another defense that the pharmacist has is known as voluntary assumption of the risk. This is the doctrine that states that a patient who understands the risk inherent in a transaction or procedure, and who voluntarily gives his informed consent to assume the risk, cannot sue to recover for damages that occur from the defined risk. An unresolved issue is whether presenting a patient with a patient package insert or leaflet that outlines the potential hazards of a certain medication results in informed consent and, consequently, voluntary assumption of the risk. Generally the procedure required for informed consent is a lengthy discussion covering the alternatives and the relative incidence of the various risks. This point probably will be litigated in the future.

Another defense that may be available to the pharmacist is the statute of limitations. The legislature imposes a time limit on filing suits for negligence. Generally, the statute of limitations in this area is 2 years, meaning that the suit must be filed within 2 years of the time of reasonable discovery of the damage. Note, however, that a person may suffer some damage and not be able to discover it until some time long after the incident, as in the diethylstilbestrol cases that were litigated. In those cases, the injured parties, daughters of women who took the drug during pregnancy, developed precancerous lesions 15 to 20 years after the drug was consumed. The statute of limitations would begin to run at the time of reasonable discovery, not the time when the drug was dispensed.

The issue of liability of the pharmacist for negligence has been raised in conjunction with a number of developments and innovations in pharmacy practice in recent years. A consideration of the application of the above discussion to these developments is in order. Of necessity, a detailed discussion of these areas is impossible in this chapter. The professional literature contains a number of articles that address these issues in detail, and the interested reader may wish to refer to those.

Patient medication records (PMRs) have been adopted widely in community pharmacy practice. This is largely attributable to the requirements of federal legislation adopted during 1990 known as OBRA '90. This mandated that pharmacists maintain records of medication dispensed to Medicaid patients and offer to consult with those patients at the time of dispensing. Most states expanded this dictate to include all patients.

Some states have mandated by statute that PMR's be maintained. In such a case a special rule of negligence may apply. The doctrine of negligence *per se* is that where a statute mandates that a certain activity be performed to protect an identifiable group of people from an identifiable type of harm and one does not do it, that fact and the statute may be introduced into evidence at trial to establish the duty and breach of it. This facilitates the case of the plaintiff. Note that this rule of negligence per se is applicable only in the case where the activity is required by a statute. A regulation of a board of pharmacy, for example, would not suffice to establish the duty in and of itself. Nonetheless, such a regulation could be introduced into evidence to buttress the testimony of pharmacists on this point.

All states have now enacted drug product selection legislation that frees the pharmacist from the restrictions of the anti-substitution laws, enabling him to use his professional judgment in selecting products to be dispensed on certain prescriptions. Naturally, because these statutes give pharmacists greater responsibility, they increase their potential liability. However, so long as they discharge this responsibility in a prudent fashion, the potential for legal entanglements will be minimal. In some states the government has provided guidance for the pharmacist in the form of a positive formulary, designating those drugs for which interchange is permissible. The FDA also has published such a list. In the case of pharmacists who selects a product from the formulary for brand interchange, they then should have a fairly good defense based on a reliance on such governmental lists.

There has not been a successful law suit based on negligence in drug product selection. This even more is significant in light of the fact that pharmacists have been selecting extensively the brand of product to be dispensed for years pursuant to prescriptions written using generic terminology.

Pharmacists should not be concerned unduly with their potential liability exposure as they move into new areas of practice. So long as they are competent to assume the new responsibility and perform the task in a diligent fashion, their liability problems should continue to be minimal.

INTENTIONAL TORTS

The law distinguishes intentional acts from those that are negligent or careless in nature. Intentional wrongs to persons or property involve such torts as assault, battery, and false imprisonment. At the onset, it is important to distinguish between a tort and a crime. The same act may give rise, but not necessarily, to both a tort and a crime. The criminal violation will be prosecuted in the name of the state, but the same act also may result in a separate civil lawsuit between the individuals involved. Quite naturally, intentional torts require a showing of the element of intent, but it is not necessary to demonstrate harmful or hostile design.

ASSAULT—An intentional act, other than the mere speaking of words, which places another individual in apprehension of harmful or offensive contact is an assault. The danger must be of an immediate nature and the individual must be aware of the defendant's apparent intent. Bodily contact is not necessary to establish a claim for relief and, thus, damages for an assault alone are likely to be nominal.

BATTERY—A battery is defined as an intentional act that, directly or indirectly, is the cause of harmful or offensive contact with another person. Assault and battery are separate torts but very often will appear together. A person may be liable for battery even though he intended only to play a practical joke or intended to confer a benefit on the other party. In patient-care settings it is possible for a cause of action based upon battery to arise during unauthorized surgical operations.

A number of defenses exist for the torts of assault and battery. An individual who consents to physical contact may not claim a battery successfully. Consent to physical contact may be expressed or implied in nature. Consent to surgical procedures also will negate an action based upon assault and battery, but the consent obtained from the patient should be an informed consent, ie, the patient must have a sufficient understanding of that to which he is consenting. The use of investigational drugs also will require informed consent.

DEFAMATION—Defamation is a false communication that injures the good name or reputation of another. Defamatory statements that are communicated in a permanent form such as the written word, pictures, statues, etc, are called libel. Communications that are more transient in nature such as the spoken word or a gesture are termed slander.

A defamatory statement, either libel or slander, must be communicated to a third person, ie, one other than the person defamed. The statement will be deemed defamatory if it harms the reputation of another or exposes an individual to scorn, ridicule or contempt.

Because of its historical background, special rules have been developed regarding the showing of actual damages in a case of defamation. Almost any action based upon libel will be able to proceed regardless of whether actual monetary damages have been suffered by the plaintiff. Most courts have held that special harm or actual dollar loss must be shown in cases of slander unless the slander fits into established exceptions.

As is true with the other tort situations, several defenses exist to actions for libel and slander. Truth is always a defense to actions based upon defamation of character. The burden is on the defendant, in a defamation action, to prove that the statement was true.

Certain individuals are said to be privileged to defame, or free from liability for slander or libel. An absolute privilege exists for defamatory remarks made during the course of judicial, legislative or executive proceedings. Many states have enacted statutes that provide immunity from civil lawsuits for pharmacists and other health-care professionals who file charges or present evidence against another member of their profession regarding alleged incompetence or gross misconduct. The immunity often is extended to claims filed with a board of pharmacy or with the regularly constituted review committee of a pharmaceutical society or hospital. In addition, most states also will provide immunity for those individuals, including pharmacists, who are required to report suspected cases of child abuse.

Pharmacists may subject themselves to litigation for careless remarks made about patients or other health-care professionals in the community. Oral statements that accuse another of improper conduct of a business or unprofessionalism are slanderous per se, and subject the maker to liability without the necessity of showing actual damages. A pharmacist's untrue imputation of certain loathsome diseases also could result in litigation based upon slander *per se*.

RIGHT TO PRIVACY—A relatively new tort is invasion of another's privacy. The oral or written dissemination of private information about an individual, even if true, may give rise to an action based on invasion of privacy. Information contained in patient medication records or prescriptions is confidential in nature and should be released only with the consent of the patient or pursuant to a warrant, subpoena or other statutory authority. The invasion must be objectionable and not too trifling. Truth is not a defense to this type of action nor is the absence of malice.

The right to privacy often conflicts with the state's authority to exercise its power to protect the public health, safety and welfare, known as the "police power." An example of this right was the subject of a lawsuit. Certain individuals in the state of New York filed a lawsuit against that state for the inclusion of prescription information in a computerized data bank. The plaintiffs alleged that the inclusion of the names of patients, who receive Schedule II prescription drugs, in a centralized computer file violated their rights to privacy. The case eventually was decided by the US Supreme Court, which ruled that the New York statute did not impair any privacy interest. The court found that the requirement was a reasonable exercise of the state's police powers. This decision led to the implementation of triplicate prescription requirements for Schedule II prescriptions now in place in a number of states.

Liability based upon the tortious invasion of privacy should not be confused with the constitutional right of privacy that protects an individual from unconstitutional intrusions by government. The constitutional right of privacy increasingly is being used by courts as the basis for allowing health-care decisions to be made by patients.

Recent statutory law adopted by the federal congress and implemented through regulations promulgated by various federal agencies codifies the common law rights of privacy and confidentiality with regards to medical records. The Health Insurance Portability and Accountability Act (HIPAA) was signed into law on August 21, 1996. It took the federal agencies charged with enforcement of the statutes several years to adopt regulations that explain the rights and duties of those affected by the law. The final rule can be found at www.hhs.gov/ocr/hipaa/finalreg.html. Questions and answers from OCR can be found at www.hhs.gov/ocr/hipaa/privacy.html.

Most of the regulations took effect in April 2003. The regulations and statutes include significant new protections for individuals who have preexisting medical conditions or might suffer discrimination in health coverage based on a factor that relates to the individual's health. This part of HIPAA, Title I (Health Care Access, Portability, and Renewability) amends the Employee Retirement Income Security Act of 1974 (ERISA). Portions of the Internal Revenue Code and the Public Health Service Act are also affected. The new rules place requirements on employer-sponsored group health plans, insurance companies, and health maintenance organizations (HMOs). In addition, these HIPAA provisions require that certain employers and individuals must guarantee the renewability and availability of health coverage and protect many workers who lose health coverage by providing better access to individual health insurance coverage.

Title II (Preventing Health Care Fraud and Abuse; Administrative Simplification; Medical Liability Reform) is intended to reduce the costs and administrative burdens of health care by replacing the many non-standard formats currently used nationally, with a single set of electronic standards that would be used throughout the health care industry.

Title II, Subtitle F (Administrative Simplification) presents implications for all health providers. The goals of these HIPAA regulations are to improve the efficiency and effectiveness of health care, to improve the Medicaid and Medicare programs, to control fraud and abuse with regard to health plans, and to simplify administrative aspects of health care. According to the federal Department of Health and Human Services that oversees this part of the regulations, the rules set forth standards for each of the following areas:

- Electronic Data Interchange (EDI) for Claims/Transaction Administration. The standards relate to claims data forms and attachments; plan enrollment and disenrollment; premium payments; claims status; referral certification and authorization. The law mandates the use of national standards for electronic exchange of health care data—to help reduce the volume of paperwork and facilitate efficient processing of health care claims.
- National Unique Identifiers. The standards will facilitate the creation and adoption of the use of a national identification system for health care providers, payers (or plans), and employers. Each provider will be assigned its own unique identifier to be used for all transactions.
- Standardized Code Sets. These standards specify the medical and administrative code sets for diagnoses, procedures, pharmaceuticals and other health care data Standardized codes will streamline the processing of health care claims/transactions.

- Security. These standards establish measures that ensure the security of health care information maintained by health care providers, health plans, hospitals, health insurers, and health care clearinghouses.
- Electronic Signatures. The standards specify procedures for electronic transmission and authentication of signatures.
- Transfer of Information among Health Plans. Set standards for transferring across health plans the data elements needed for coordination of benefits and processing of claims.
- Privacy. The law stipulates the standards for privacy of individually identifiable medical and health information.

It is the privacy rights that will likely have the most impact on the practice of pharmacy. While pharmacists have always respected the confidentiality duties imbedded in the profession's Code of Ethics, HIPAA sets forth specific regulatory mandates about what kind of information may or must be disclosed and the entities to whom the information may or must be disclosed. In most instances pharmacies will have to obtain prior consent, or at least make a good faith effort, from patients before releasing any "protected health information" (PHI) for "treatment, payment and health care operations" (TPO). Providers are also required to give notice to patients about their privacy rights within the institution or location where the information is stored.

The HIPAA law is complicated and extensive. Pharmacists and pharmacy interns as well as all technicians and others who may have access to PHI data should be well versed in the mandates of the law. Breaches of duties mandated by these regulations carry significant and severe sanctions that could result in heavy fines and, in some circumstances, prison time. Prevention of even innocent or accidental disclosures requires all providers to invest time in learning about HIPAA rules and regulations.

COMMERCIAL LAW

The pharmacist should understand the general principles of the law of contracts to realize the responsibility he undertakes when entering a business obligation or an employment relationship. The law of advertising has a direct bearing on the day-to-day activities of pharmacists, both as professionals and as consumers. Questions concerning ownership of prescriptions and application of the federal antitrust laws to the pharmacist's relationships with third-party prescription program administrators may be encountered frequently by pharmacists.

It is impossible in a general treatise of this kind to describe in detail the legal subjects on which the pharmacist should keep posted. All that can be attempted is a general outline.

Because the US is composed of 50 individual jurisdictions, the law may vary from state to state. Nonetheless, it is possible to provide an overview of the law applicable to pharmacists in the operation of their practices. To a certain extent the laws applicable to commercial activities have been rendered uniform in most of the states through enactment of the Uniform Commercial Code (UCC); it was drafted in the early part of the last century by a group of noted legal scholars to bring some order out of the patchwork quilt of states laws applicable to business affairs. Enacted nearly intact in almost all states, the UCC has done a great deal to facilitate the flow of commerce among the states.

CONTRACT LAW

A contract may be defined as a promise or set of promises for the breach of which the law provides a remedy, or the performance of which the law, in some way, recognizes as a duty. Yet, the law requires much more for a contract to result than a mere exchange of promises. Perhaps a more complete definition of a contract is an agreement between legally competent individuals based on genuine assent of the parties and supported by consideration, made for a lawful purpose and in the form required by law, if any. This definition provides a framework for discussion of these elements of a contract.

The agreement between the parties, which forms a basis for the contract, is composed of both an offer and an acceptance. For an offer to be legally sufficient the party making it must have the intention of entering into an agreement with the other party. For example, an offer made in jest would not indicate the required contractual intent. Moreover, an invitation to make an offer or an offer to negotiate is not a legally cognizable offer for it, too, lacks contractual intent. Advertisements are not an offer of sale but, rather, an indication of willingness to consider an offer made by the potential purchaser. The offer must be communicated to the other party prior to acceptance for an agreement to result.

An additional requirement for an offer is that it be definite. This means that the offer must be detailed sufficiently to provide a basis for the agreement. Courts will not add an essential element to an offer, agreement or contract. At the time of acceptance the offer must still be viable. An offer may be withdrawn prior to acceptance, in the absence of an option having been granted. An option is a binding promise to keep an offer open for a stated period of time. If an option exists, the person making the offer may not withdraw it until the option period has expired. An offer also may be terminated by rejection or by lapse of a period of time stated in the offer.

Acceptance is assent by the recipient of the offer to the terms of the offer. No particular form of acceptance is required, eg, in writing, unless specified in the offer. However, the acceptance must be absolute and unconditional. Any variation of the terms or conditions in the acceptance will result in rejection of the offer.

The parties entering into a contract must be competent legally to do so. This means that each party must have contractual capacity. Minors generally lack contractual capacity and contracts they enter into are subject to their avoidance. The other party may not be able to enforce the contract against a minor because the contract can be voided by the minor due to his lack of contractual capacity. However, parents may be liable under contract theory for necessaries provided to their minor dependents. Necessaries are those things relating to the health, education or comfort of the minor. Prescription drugs probably would fall within this category and a pharmacist providing them to a minor would, in all likelihood, be able to collect the reasonable value of the medication from the parents.

Insane persons also may be under a contractual incapacity. If a person is so mentally deranged as not to know that a contract is being made or does not understand the consequences of what he is doing, the contract may be voided on recovering sanity. The same is true of a person who is so intoxicated as to be unaware that he is making a contract.

The requirement of genuineness of assent relates to mistake, misrepresentation, concealment, fraud or exercise of undue influence or duress over one of the parties. Each of these activities has a different effect on the enforceability of the contract, and a full discussion of each is beyond the scope of this discussion. Nonetheless, the pharmacist should be aware that each bears a possibility for interference with the enforceability of the contract.

Consideration is essential for a contract to be enforceable. It may be defined as an act or forbearance, or the promise of either, which is offered by one party to an agreement and accepted by the other as an inducement to the others' act or promise. When you have given consideration you have agreed to do something that you were not bound to do or you have agreed to refrain from doing that which you have the right to do.

Consideration must be provided by both parties to the contract. If only one is providing consideration, no contract results. It is a mere gift and not legally enforceable.

Ordinarily, courts will not inquire into the adequacy of the consideration exchanged by the parties. The fact that the amount of consideration may appear to be small in the eyes of one person does not necessarily mean that the amount is inadequate or inappropriate. Hence, if some consideration is provided, the contract will be enforceable. One sometimes hears of employment contracts for a dollar-a-year person, as in the case of a wealthy individual working for the government or a charity. Such an employment contract will be enforceable even though the value of a person's services will be much greater than the amount of compensation provided.

For a contract to be enforceable it must be made for a lawful purpose, and this must be achieved in a lawful manner. If this were not so, the courts might be placed in the uncomfortable situation of compelling one party to a contract to commit a crime to have the contract performed. An example of this doctrine is the rule that contracts of an unlicensed operator cannot be enforced. Hence, one who practices pharmacy without being licensed to do so, is likely to be charged with the crime of violating the state pharmacy practice act, and also will be unable to enforce the contracts he made while practicing pharmacy, ie, he will be unable to sue to collect for his services.

Contracts for the sale of prohibited articles also are unenforceable. The sale of a prescription drug without valid authorization would fall in this category. Contracts that unreasonably restrain trade also are unlawful and, consequently, unenforceable. When a pharmacist sells a pharmacy it is customary for the purchaser to request that the contract contain a noncompetition clause that bans the seller from owning a pharmacy within certain geographic and time limits. The purpose is to prevent the seller from selling and immediately opening up a pharmacy, attracting all his prior patients. If such a clause is drafted to include too large a geographic area, or for too long a time, it will be unenforceable due to its restraint on trade. However, note that only contracts that unreasonably restrain trade are unlawful. Consequently, if the noncompetition clause is drafted carefully it will be enforceable. Such provisions increasingly are being seen in employment contracts for pharmacists as well.

Most contracts are not required to be in writing to be enforceable. Obviously, though, it is much easier to prove the existence of and enforce one that is written. Each state has a Statute of Frauds that dictates which types of contracts must be in writing to be enforceable. Generally, contracts for creation of an interest in land, which run for more than 1 year, must be in writing. Those that involve employment for more than 1 year and those that are for sale of goods of a value of $500 or more also must be in writing. Each state may have additional categories, and the minimum limits just mentioned may vary from state to state.

When a contract is breached, the nonbreaching party has the right to bring legal action against the breaching party to recover that sum of money that will place him in the same position as he would have been had the contract been performed. There are a number of types of damages that may be assessed against the breaching party. Nominal damages are awarded when the injured party did not suffer an actual loss. They usually are of minimal magnitude. Compensatory damages are those that are designed to compensate the injured party for his loss. Liquidated damages also may be encountered; these are those for which provision was made in the contract itself by the contracting parties when they entered into the agreement. Liquidated-damage clauses generally will be enforced if the amount specified is not excessive and if the contract is of such a nature that it would be difficult to determine the actual amount of damages.

The UCC addresses a special category of contracts known as sales. A sale may be defined as a transaction wherein a seller transfers title for personal property to a buyer for a price (consideration).

Of particular interest to pharmacists is the law applicable to warranties in sales transactions. A warranty is an assurance or guarantee, by a seller, that the goods sold are, or will be, as represented. Warranties may be divided into two general categories: express and implied.

Express warranties are those based on an affirmation of fact or promise relating to the goods, whereas an implied warranty is one that exists by virtue of law, not because of an express statement by the seller. Express warranties may be made about almost any attribute of the goods, but the warranties implied by law are more limited in scope. One such implied warranty is the implied warranty of merchantability. It is seen only with sellers who usually deal in goods of that type and means that the goods provided must be fit for the ordinary purposes for which such goods are used.

The implied warranty of fitness for a particular purpose is present when the seller knows the use to which the goods will be put and has reason to know that the buyer is relying on the sellers' skill and judgment to select suitable goods for the purpose. These implied warranties automatically are present in a transaction without any action on the part of the seller to place them there. They can be removed from the sale but require a specific type of action.

Goods sold *as is* are sold with no implied warranties. To remove the implied warranty of merchantability those specific words must be used, but the disclaimer can be made orally. Removal of the implied warranty of fitness for a particular purpose can be done only by written words, but no special language is required. However, the statement that the warranty is absent must be conspicuous. Naturally, express warranties can be kept out of a transaction merely by not making an express statement about the goods.

PRESCRIPTION OWNERSHIP

A question arises from time to time regarding ownership of the prescription. When it is issued by the prescriber, the patient gains ownership of the document. When it is transferred to the pharmacist for purposes of dispensing the medication, ownership then passes to the pharmacist, pursuant to the contract between the pharmacist and the patient. However, the patient retains certain rights with regard to the document.

While the document itself is the property of the pharmacist and must be retained by law for recordkeeping purposes, the patient has the legal right to refills that the law and the prescriber have authorized. Moreover, the patient may have a right to obtain a copy of the prescription, except in those cases where the giving of a copy is prohibited or limited. For example, in some states copies provided to patients must be marked with a statement indicating that the prescription copy is provided for informational use only and cannot serve as the basis for dispensing medication.

In some situations, such as with prescriptions that are suspected to be forgeries or those that bear the potential for a harmful drug interaction, the pharmacist may wish to deface or retain the document even though the medication will not be dispensed. Such action does, however, present the risk that the prescription might be legitimate or that the drug interaction would not result. In such a case a suit for damages that resulted from his action may result because he does not own the document. Should the pharmacist receive a prescription that he does not intend to follow, the problem should be handled through communication with either the patient or the prescriber, not by defacing the document that he does not own.

Because the pharmacist owns the prescription records reflecting medication that he has dispensed, they are assets of the pharmacy that may be transferred on the cessation of the practice. Prescription records should be maintained for a minimum of 5 years, the statute of limitations of the FD&C Act.

ANTITRUST AND PRESCRIPTION INSURANCE PLANS

Third-party prescription drug insurance programs have burgeoned in the US in recent years, and a substantial portion of Americans now have insurance coverage for their medication expenditures. This brief discussion shall center on the legal problems associated with private third-party prescription plans, not those administered by governmental agencies.

In the typical third-party plan, the pharmacy owner receives an offer to participate in the insurance plan and a contract to be signed. This usually provides for reimbursement of the pharmacist's cost in acquiring the drug product dispensed and the addition of a dispensing fee of fixed magnitude. Other provisions may relate to what products are compensable, eg, many plans will not pay for nonprescription medication, or limit quantities that may be dispensed. Provisions also are seen dealing with claims submission, services the pharmacist is required to provide and access to the pharmacists financial records for purposes of program accountability. Often, the offer to participate in such plans is distributed to many pharmacies in an area for the insurer to offer the subscriber maximum flexibility in selecting a pharmacist with whom to deal or to offer enrollees a variety of options for service.

When such offers to participate are disseminated widely, the possibility of the offers being discussed collectively arises. This may run afoul of the Sherman Antitrust Act of 1890, which provides that

> Every contract, combination . . . or conspiracy, in restraint of trade or commerce among the several States . . . is declared to be illegal.

Thus, collective action by pharmacists to withhold entering into contracts with the insurer because the professional fee is too low or because other provisions of the contract are objectionable may violate this federal statute. Individual penalties may be assessed under this statute. Applicability of this statute to pharmacy was affirmed in the 1962 case of *US v. Northern California Pharmaceutical Association*. In that case the activity that brought federal sanctions was publication of a recommended fee schedule in an attempt to encourage the adoption of uniform pricing.

With prescription drug insurance plans, the activity that may violate the statute is collective action by pharmacists (combination . . . or conspiracy) to withhold their participation (restrain trade) in the insurance plan until the contract is worded in terms acceptable to them as a group. While such action is legally permissible if done by an individual acting alone, collective action toward the same end would be unlawful.

In addition to the criminal penalties mentioned above, the patients who are injured by such unlawful activity may bring a civil suit to recover damages. Of importance is the fact that in an antitrust claim, the award is for treble damages, ie, the amount of damages is calculated and then multiplied by three to yield the amount the party engaging in the unlawful activity must pay.

ADVERTISING

The regulation of the advertising and promotion of drugs on an interstate commerce basis is a shared commitment of numerous federal agencies, including the Postal Service, FCC, FTC and FDA. The latter two bear the brunt of the responsibility. The FTC is involved actively in the regulation of OTC drug advertising while the FDA exercises its jurisdiction primarily over matters involving the labeling and advertising of prescription drugs. There is, however, considerable overlap between the two agencies because of statutory definitions and by mutual agreement.

States can also regulate drug advertising. However, state limitations imposed primarily by budget give these controls much less effect in comparison to federal activities. The pharmacist, therefore, will be bound primarily by federal restrictions in the area of advertising.

FEDERAL TRADE COMMISSION—The FTC derives its authority over advertising in general and drug advertising in particular from the Federal Trade Commission Act. Section 5 of that statute provides

> "Unfair methods of competition in commerce and unfair or deceptive acts or practices in commerce are hereby declared unlawful."

In addition, Section 12 makes it unlawful to disseminate a false advertisement for the purpose of inducing, or that is likely to induce, the purchase of food, drugs, devices or cosmetics. The Wheeler-Lea Amendment to the Act defines *false advertising* as follows:

> "The term 'false advertisement' means an advertisement, other than labeling, which is misleading in a material respect; and in determining whether any advertisement is misleading, there shall be taken into account (among other things) representations made or suggested by statement, word, design, device, sound or any combination thereof, and also the extent to which the advertisement fails to reveal facts, material in the light of such representations or material with respect to consequences, which may result from the use of the commodity to which the advertisement relates under the conditions prescribed in said advertisement, or under such conditions as are customary or usual."

Based on the above provision, the FTC has authority to move against false advertisements for OTC drug products and also advertisements that operate in an unfair or deceptive way. The Commission can use its powers by either promulgating a Trade Regulation Rule or by issuing a complaint against an advertiser when there is reason to believe that the law has been violated.

In most cases in which a complaint is issued by the FTC, the advertiser is willing to enter into an agreement to cease and desist from the use of the acts and practices being investigated. Such an agreement is for settlement purposes only, and it does not constitute an admission by the advertiser that the law has been violated. The FTC has been successful in obtaining consent agreements from a number of corporations, including those practicing pharmacy, which require all items advertised to be available for sale readily at or below the advertised price. Displays of advertised items must be marked conspicuously by a sign or other means disclosing that the item is *as advertised* or *on sale*. In addition, many of the consent orders provide that if the advertised item is unavailable, the consumer may either be given a rain-check or be allowed to purchase a similar product of equal or better quality at or below the advertised price. Phrases such as *regular price* or *manufacturers suggested list price* and words of similar import should not be used unless they can be documented. Whenever a *free, 2-for-1, half price sale, 1¢ sale* or similar type of offer is made, all of its terms and conditions to the consumer should be made clear at the outset.

If the parties are unable to agree to a consent order, an FTC complaint will result in a trial before an administrative law judge who will determine if a violation has occurred and, if so, the appropriate remedies. This decision may be appealed by either party to the full Commission sitting as an appellate body. Thereafter, review can be pursued to a US Court of Appeals and possibly to the US Supreme Court. A case involving a well-known mouthwash followed just such a procedure. An administrative law judge ruled that the advertisements for the mouthwash had made claims that were false, misleading and deceptive. Under the administrative ruling, the manufacturer was ordered to stop making such claims and also to institute corrective advertising to inform consumers that the product would not help prevent colds or sore throats or lessen their severity. This ruling was upheld by the full Commission and by a federal appeals court, and the US Supreme Court rejected the manufacturer's petition for further review.

In another action, a 1975 FTC complaint alleging false and misleading advertising included a pharmacy as a defendant even though the ads were prepared by the manufacturer's advertising agency. The administrative law judge held that although the retailer did not know whether the ad claims were true or false, it was not relieved of responsibility simply because the ad copy and content were prepared by others. The full FTC bench ruled that the Act does not exempt the seller of a product from investigating the truthfulness of claims set forth over the retailers own name. The lack of knowledge of the falsity of the ad was found not to be a defense.

FOOD AND DRUG ADMINISTRATION—Prior to 1962 the FTC was vested with sole authority for regulating the advertising of drugs. The Kefauver-Harris Amendments of 1962 to the FD&C Act gave the FDA control over prescription drug advertising. Thus, the FDA regulates the labeling of prescription drugs and their advertising as well. All advertisements and other descriptive printed matter issued by the manufacturer must include a statement of the established name, quantitative formula and other information such as side effects, contraindications and effectiveness.

The FDA's authority over the regulation of prescription drug advertising extends to advertising directed to professionals and also to that presented to the lay public. Up until 1997, the FDA required manufacturers to include a *brief summary* of important information health-care professionals and patients need about use of prescription drugs in any advertising. This rule effectively banned any television or radio advertising. In late 1997 the FDA changed its policy and began permitting direct to consumer advertising of prescription drugs on broadcast media as long as the manufacturer includes a *major statement* that discloses significant risks associated with the drugs use. The new approach presumes the advertising is truthful and not misleading. Under the proposed guidelines broadcast advertising will have to include:

Providing a toll-free telephone number for consumers to access detailed product information in a timely fashion—either by mail, fax or phone.

Referring to direct-to-consumer print ads that contain a brief summary of the product labeling. Reference to brochures containing similar information would also be acceptable if the brochures were distributed in a variety of publicly available sites such as doctors' offices, libraries and stores.

Providing an Internet web page (URL) address with full access to the approved product labeling.

Containing a statement that pharmacists, and/or physicians and/or veterinarians (in the case of animal drugs) may provide additional information about the product.

At the time of this revision, the proposed guidelines were not adopted. By internal policy decision, the FDA permits broadcast advertising of prescription drugs as long as the content conforms to the proposed guidelines. Print advertising still must comply with the *brief summary* requirement.

STATE REGULATION—For some time, many states had pharmacy act provisions or pharmacy board regulations that prohibited or severely restricted prescription drug advertising. Numerous state court decisions had been handed down regarding the permissibility of such prohibitions, but their dictate was anything but clear. To obtain an ultimate decision on this controversy, a group of consumers filed suit against the Virginia State Board of Pharmacy alleging a First Amendment right to receive prescription price information. The case of Virginia State Board of Pharmacy v Virginia Citizens Consumer Council, Inc. eventually reached the US Supreme Court. The court, basing its decision on the First Amendment, held that even speech that primarily is commercial in nature is protected. The consumer should have the freedom to obtain the price information necessary to make a choice regarding prescription drugs. The FTC previously had proposed a Trade Regulation Rule that would preempt and override all state statutes and regulations that prohibited prescription drug advertising, but with the advent of the Virginia case the FTC did not feel it was necessary to move further in this area.

BIBLIOGRAPHY

Abood RR, Brushwood DB. *Pharmacy Practice and the Law*, 3rd ed. Gaithersburg, MD: Aspen Publishers, 2000.

Brushwood DB. *Pharmacy Malpractice: Law and Regulations*, 3rd ed. Gaithersburg, MD: Aspen Publishers, 2000.

Fink III JL, Vivian JC, Bernstein IG. *Pharmacy Law Digest*. St Louis: Facts & Comparisons, (latest annual revision).

Merrill RA, Hutt PB. *Food and Drug Law: Cases and Materials*, 2nd ed. Mineola, NY: Foundation Press, 1991.

Vivian, JC. *Michigan Pharmacy Law: A Guide to the Statutes and Regulations*, 2nd ed. Lansing, MI: Michigan Pharmacists Association, 2003.

CHAPTER 112

Re-Engineering Pharmacy Practice

Robert W Bennett, MS, RPh

Sara J Beis, MS, RPh

Caring practitioners are of crucial importance to all health professions. Most individuals attracted to a career as a health professional desire and expect to provide patient care. These attitudes remain despite the tremendous changes that are occurring in health care. In fact, the one constant in health care in the last century has been change. This change has led to a re-engineering of the health care system, fueled by the explosion of technological advances and the movement toward patient-focused health care. The nature of pharmacy practice also must change to a focus on pharmaceutical care in response to the advancements in the health care environment. For the pharmacist to be recognized as a health professional, pharmaceutical care and the direct patient contact it requires must be fully implemented. There must be a focus of the caring pharmacist's abilities and responsibilities on achieving optimal therapeutic outcomes to improve a patient's quality of life.[1,2]

Re-engineering pharmacy practice to provide pharmaceutical care assumes that a pharmacy core value is caring for the patient; advancing the good of every patient in a caring, compassionate, and confidential manner.[3] Caring assumes that the pharmacist has an emotional commitment to the well-being of the patient who needs and deserves the pharmacist's compassion and attention.[3]

This adaptation to pharmaceutical care requires a major shift in the essential skills, education, and mindset of pharmacists. The pharmacy professionals who have been successful in this endeavor have successfully changed the way they work and think about the use of drugs in the patients they serve. They have developed interpersonal skills, collaborated with other health professionals, and implemented programs that provide care to individual patients. However, while the provision of pharmaceutical care is the goal, it has not yet been achieved in the majority of practices. Thus, practice re-engineering for pharmaceutical care is necessary. To make suggestions for where re-engineering should take pharmacy practice in the future, it is important to look back at where pharmacy has been and how it has evolved to its present position.

THE EVOLUTION OF PHARMACY PRACTICE

Over the last 150 years, the profession of pharmacy has advanced from a practice focused on manufacturing and compounding, to distribution of drug product, to clinical practice with an eventual role as providers of pharmaceutical care.[4] In considering these changes, it appears that the profession has truly changed completely from one focused on a drug product to one focused on the patient. The only common thread that ties today's pharmacists with those who practiced at the turn of the last century seems to be drug therapy itself. Each of these steps in the evolution of pharmacy practice requires different skill sets of the practitioner and even a different type of personality for the individual to find a personal fit with the tasks involved. The various levels of pharmacy services provided have also held a different perceived value to the patient and other decision-makers involved in the provision of health care.

STAGES OF EVOLUTION OF PHARMACY PRACTICE (1860 TO 2000s)

In the late 1800s, the pharmacist was serving the social role of apothecary by manufacturing drug products; preparing elixirs and powders for individual patients. Pharmacists learned these skills through apprenticeships. Patients came to see the pharmacist whose primary role was to provide pure, unadulterated medication while meeting a secondary role of providing advice as to how the specific remedy was to be used. Society valued the pharmacist's ability to prepare the drug and advise those in need of their product as well as the care provided by the pharmacist.

As the industrial age took hold in the United States, companies whose sole purpose was bulk and mass production of drug productions grew and propagated. The development of these commercial products left community pharmacy practice to focus on compounding preparations that were not commercially available. By providing these compounding services to patients along with advice on how to use the compounds to care for illness, the pharmacist working in the apothecary continued to provide a valued service to society.

Though World War I took place thousands of miles away in Europe, this conflict played an important role in shaping the course of pharmaceutical education in the United States. The War Department refused to commission pharmacists as officers. This decision pushed the profession to formalize their education process by requiring a four-year bachelor's degree for entry to the profession. When World War II began, pharmacists felt they were in a better position to achieve commission as officers in the new conflict. However, the War Emergency Department Advisory Committee decided pharmacists entering military service would not be commissioned while nurses would be granted rank as officers.[5] Unfortunately, this decision along with opinion surveys indicated that society considered the pharmacy profession of little value.

During the post-war period, a review of the profession by the American Council on Education's Pharmaceutical Survey indicated that pharmaceutical education was quite conservative and obsolescent, providing knowledge in current skills rather than future needs or professional skills. Tension developed in the various practice areas of pharmacy when the survey encouraged the profession to adopt a 6-year doctor of pharmacy degree as a standard across the country. Only California colleges/schools followed the recommendation, while the rest of the nation settled for a 5-year degree that fell short of the suggested requirements for teaching skills needed for future professional expansion. Thus, compromise set the stage for future debates over the educational requirements needed for pharmacists.

At the same time of change, the discipline of hospital pharmacy developed as a service to manage the drug product inventory for use in the inpatient setting. Hospital growth was spurred by the passage of the Hill-Burton Act, and the result was increased expansion and new construction of hospitals in underserved areas. This growth and expansion attitude in the hospital industry was reflected in pharmacy practice as the pharmacist's role expanded beyond the distribution of medication. Hospital pharmacists became involved in a variety of tasks including nursing education regarding the administration of drugs, and participation in Pharmacy and Therapeutics Committees that selected drug products for use in the institution. Through these activities, hospital pharmacists preserved some of their educational focus in the scientific use of medications acquired in pharmacy school. However, consistent with their community practice colleagues, the emphasis of practice remained on a drug product.

In 1951, the Durham-Humphrey Amendment to the 1938 Food, Drug and Cosmetic Act required that drugs which cannot be safely used without medical supervision be dispensed only by prescription of a licensed practitioner. Until this amendment, there was no requirement that any drug be labeled for sale by prescription only. The amendment defined prescription drugs as those unsafe for self-medication and should, therefore, be used only under a doctor's supervision. With this legislation, the pharmacist's role in the provision of care was dramatically limited by removing any latitude the pharmacist may have had in selecting (a) drug(s) for the individual patient. The pharmacist became only the dispenser of the drugs ordered by the physician. Even the 1952 American Pharmaceutical Association's (APhA) Code of Ethics prohibited the pharmacist from discussing in detail the nature of the drug dispensed and its therapeutic effect. With this changing attitude and legislation, the pharmacists in the community setting lost their social purpose and became merely suppliers of drug orders and not the providers of the service of care. Without the ability to help the patient select drug therapy and discuss medication use, those successful in the profession called upon skills of managing a business and shifted away from a focus on scientific skills previously mentored in their pharmacy school training or apprenticeship.

In the 1960s, as laws changed, community pharmacists again began counseling their patients on the use of drug products. In 1969, APhA revised its Code of Ethics, eliminating the old restrictions on patient counseling. Pharmacists were encouraged to provide the necessary information to assure the patient's health and safety. Some pharmacies branched into other areas of practice such as durable medical equipment that required the pharmacist to educate patients in the use of these items for self-care. During this time, drugs available for over-the-counter or nonprescription use expanded, and community pharmacists found a niche educating patients on the proper use of nonprescription drugs. However, as pharmacists focused their skills on the business of running the pharmacy, the education needed for scientific assessment of new medication and counseling skills was limited in most pharmacy school curricula. For pharmacists who had been in practice for some time, the therapeutic skills that were present upon graduation had declined over time due to lack of use. Thus, the move to counseling in the community setting was limited by the pharma-

cist's skill set and also by the work environment which varied from employment as an owner or employee of an independent or a chain community pharmacy. Due to the limited move to providing education on medication use to the patients, pharmacists at this time continued to have a weak social value in the provision of health care.

Unfortunately, this lack of perceived social value of pharmacy services occurred at a critical time in the development of health care benefits in the United States. In 1965, amendments to the Social Security Act created Medicare and Medicaid to provide health benefits to Americans 65 years of age or older, low-income children lacking parental support, their caretaker relatives, the blind, and individuals with disabilities. Hospital pharmacists benefited from the enactment of the legislation that required the pharmacy department to be directed by a pharmacist to receive reimbursement. However, Part B of Medicare, the elective portion of this federal insurance that covers outpatient treatment such as physician office visits, did not include coverage for outpatient prescription medications. Besides leaving prescription coverage out of this Federal insurance program, pharmacists were not included as providers of health care services while nurses, physical therapists, occupational therapists, and allied health care professionals were considered providers eligible to be reimbursed for services rendered. This exclusion of the pharmacist was simply a mirror of the societal value placed on pharmacy services in the early 1960s. It was not until the late 1980s and early 1990s that procedures were developed for documentation and billing of outpatient counseling and patient monitoring by pharmacists. Using these procedures, some community pharmacists were paid for services by private insurance companies when the pharmacy could justify the value of its services to company officials. However, due to lack of support within the Medicare program for coverage, general support of payment for these services has been severely limited. Outside of the hospital setting, expansion of counseling and medication monitoring and management services has occurred very slowly in the last quarter of the 20th century.

During this same period, pharmacists practicing in hospitals were expanding the application of their scientific knowledge of drug therapy by providing clinical services. These clinical services provided physicians with information about pharmacokinetics and the nature of drug action to improve the prescriber's ability to effectively select and utilize appropriate drug therapy. Thus, pharmacists in hospitals were better able to use and expand their knowledge of drug therapy gained during their education. However, while these new services moved the pharmacist to the bedside, their focus continued to be on the drug therapy rather than on the patient being treated. In providing these new services, these pharmacists began to have a social value to other the health care providers in the institutional setting. This value allowed hospital pharmacy managers to find support in their organization to develop or adopt training programs to aid staff pharmacists in the understanding, adoption, and provision of these new clinical services. The addition of Medicare and Medicaid coverage for hospital care in the 1960s caused hospitals to experience immense growth that fueled expansion and the emergence of technology. During this period, the development of hospital-based clinical pharmacy services was encouraged and well received. Fortunately, clinical pharmacy practice became established and proved its value to hospital administration before the controls on health care spending were implemented with prospective payment system in the mid 1980s. Pharmacists had shown that they could decrease the length of stay for the hospitalized patient through clinical services, a critical factor in controlling costs. However, with continuing trends at the end of the century to cut hospital costs, clinical pharmacy services are often considered as areas for potential cuts in funding, especially where the value of the service is not truly embraced by the administration.

Pharmacy at the beginning of the 21st century continues to finds itself in transition as the profession moves from a focus on the drug product to the actual use of the agents by patients to control and eliminate disease. Discussions in the 1980s looking at the future of pharmacy in the next century called for the shift in the profession's focus and thus curricular change in the education of pharmacy practitioners. Hepler and Strand presented these concerns in the early 1990s and called for a movement to the pharmaceutical care model as a commitment to true growth and change in the pharmacy profession.[6] They defined pharmaceutical care as "the responsible provision of drug therapy for the purpose of achieving definite outcomes that improve the patient's quality of life." These outcomes include the cure of disease, reduction or elimination of symptoms, arresting or slowing a disease process, and preventing a disease or symptom. The major functions the pharmacist performs in this care model include identifying any drug-related problems, and resolving or preventing these problems. As previously stated, Hepler and Strand called for pharmacists to accept responsibility for care, not merely perform functions that provide care. Thus, a serious change in mindset is required for pharmacists to work within this new professional model. They are no longer just providing a service; they are responsible for the outcome of the medication use process. Hepler and Strand go so far as to indicate that a pharmacist who does not accept this responsibility is not performing a professional role, and thus has not achieved professional maturation. For the pharmacists already involved the clinical practice, acceptance of pharmaceutical care primarily requires a shift in attitude. For those still practicing in the dispensing mode, a significant change in knowledge and skills will be necessary to move to pharmaceutical care.

Higby and Hepler describe an evolutionary process that has occurred in pharmacy where the adoption of the pharmaceutical care model takes place as opportunities arise.[5,7] Because these isolated opportunities happen sporadically, there is no true expansion to the new practice model. Before the opportunity to provide such care arises, the pharmacist must become skilled in the techniques to provide such care. Depending on the nature of their original educational experience, the mid-career pharmacist may need additional education or additional practice using skills that were acquired in school, but have become weak due to lack of exercise. Further, the individual pharmacists may embrace the notion of pharmaceutical care, but their work environment and assignment may not support or nurture the pharmaceutical care model. These pharmacists need the support of their employers, be that a hospital or a retail pharmacy organization, to "re-engineer" their practice. It is important that these employers come to understand the value in the provision of pharmaceutical care as this practice provides a safer medication use system that optimizes the investment in drug therapy.

Re-engineering practice requires a problem-solving approach to identify and define the barriers that are impeding incorporation of pharmaceutical care into practice. Once the barriers are identified, strategies can be developed to overcome them. In some instances, careful identification of problems raises the level of awareness and sets in motion the processes needed for resolution. In other cases, the problems are so deeply rooted that resolution is very difficult.

CURRENT BARRIERS TO THE PROVISION OF PHARMACEUTICAL CARE

Numerous barriers frustrate the provision of pharmaceutical care to patients by pharmacists. Practice-related issues such as lack of time, insufficient knowledge and confidence, conflicting job functions, poorly designed workflow, physical layout problems, and lack of institutional or corporate support are commonly stated as important barriers to the provision of pharmaceutical care. However, education-related issues in pharmacist training and development also contribute to the lack of incorporation of pharmaceutical care into the practice setting. These education-related issues are at the root of this problem.

Education-Related Barriers

The professional socialization of pharmacy students and pharmacists is influenced by two conflicting roles.[2] One role is that of pharmacy operations/business person while the other is health care professional. In its attempts to re-engineer pharmacy practice to the provision of pharmaceutical care, pharmaceutical education has often come into direct conflict with the operations side of pharmacy practice. This conflict has led to what Manasse et al termed "inconsistent socialization" to describe the incompatibility between the operations/business and professional forces of socialization.[8]

While professional socialization involves learning the knowledge and skills needed to practice as a pharmacist, it also involves the important acquisition of appropriate behaviors, attitudes, and values. Socialization of a future pharmacist begins when the individual selects pharmacy as a career. However, the extent of professional socialization develops rapidly once the individual is accepted to pharmacy school. During their years in school, pharmacy students are exposed to numerous influences on the role of the pharmacist through interactions with other influential people including basic and applied science faculty, practice and clinical faculty, pharmacists, patients, family members and friends, fellow students, and allied health care professionals. The absence of uniformity or agreement among these influences causes the student to develop conflicting behaviors, beliefs, and values regarding their practice role.

Longitudinal studies on the socialization of pharmacy students have identified this inconsistent socialization.[9–13] The clashes of socialization forces lead to differences between student's and recent graduate's expectations about their role in providing pharmaceutical care and others' expectations of their role.[9] This incomplete socialization of the neophyte pharmacist is thought to carry over and the majority of pharmacists in active practice have not been adequately prepared to take on the pharmaceutical care role.[14,15] While efforts to improve the development of caring attributes in pharmacy students have been incorporated into the accreditation standards for pharmacy schools and of active pharmacists through certificate and non-traditional doctor of pharmacy programs, pharmaceutical education has a long way to go to socialize professionally students and pharmacists as providers of pharmaceutical care. The longitudinal studies also found that pharmacy students have a reduced sense of calling to the profession in their last year of pharmacy school compared to prior years. The students develop "disillusionment" or "realistic disenchantment" with their professional role *versus* their operations/business role as they progress through the curriculum.[10,16,17] Students enter school with a level of idealism or are given this idealism early in their training, only to have it diminish over time. It has been argued that students are presented the patient-focused pharmaceutical care perspective of professional practice by pharmacy educators, only to have this perspective largely unsupported as they gain experience in the real world and enter a practice where pharmacy operations and the business role are the main emphasis. When students and pharmacists are unclear about what is expected of them, their perceived role can be easily swayed by the opinions of powerful others (eg, employers, patients, physicians). This role conflict results in dissatisfaction with practice for pharmacists whose expectations of practice were to serve as health professionals and provide pharmaceutical care. Over time, these pharmacy practitioners become socialized into the pharmacy operations role. Many are unable to assume the professional role of pharmaceutical care provider even though they participate in pharmaceutical care credentialing programs and are provided opportunities by their employer to implement patient-focused programs at their practice. Therefore, if pharmaceutical care is going to be fully implemented in practice, it is important for pharmaceutical education, pharmacy associations, and corporate and institutional pharmacy to work together and develop a common vision for the professional role of the pharmacist; a role that is complimentary to, not in conflict with, the business/operations side of the pharmacy.

Physicians are professionally socialized to provide medical care to individual patients and view it as their primary role even though they also manage their office operations and are under increasing stress to treat more and more patients. Nurses often have a heavy load of patients plus documentation and other operations-related functions but still view provision of nursing care for the individual patient as their primary role.[18–20] Medical and nursing students are attracted to their chosen profession because there is an expectation that the practitioners will have an emotional caring for the individual patient.[21–23] Because this role is supported consistently by their power figures throughout training and entry into practice, a physician or nurse that is socialized to provide patient care is usually produced. If the profession of pharmacy is able to come together and create a climate where its practitioners are viewed by the public and allied health care professionals as a providers of care to individual patients, schools will attract individuals with that expectation and their training and entry into practice will better prepare them for this role.[24,25]

Practice-Related Barriers

Before discussing barriers in practice that prevent the pharmacist from providing care to individual patients, the process of pharmaceutical care must be reviewed in more detail. The process to provide pharmaceutical care to the patient requires several steps. The first step is to identify and define the patient's disease- and drug-related problems. For instance, a problem might be identified that a child with asthma is overusing his albuterol inhaler. Defining the problem would require investigation of the factors leading to the overuse. Perhaps the presence of three asthma triggers were defined: the child received a cat for Christmas, his parents started smoking in the house again, and the family is short of money so his Serevent prescription was not refilled.

The next step in the pharmaceutical care process would be to review the patient's medication regimen and available information on medical treatment, peak flow meter results, laboratory values, etc. The information gathered from all of these activities would then be used by the pharmacist as a basis for an assessment of the patient's pharmaceutical care needs. For the child with asthma, the assessment would include the increased number of daily asthma problems, noncompliance with his/her Serevent® inhaler, and lack of parent understanding of asthma triggers and medication use. Based on the assessment, the pharmacist would develop and implement a care plan to help the patient and his caregivers (parents). The plan should be recorded and include desired outcomes of the care to be provided including education for the child and parents concerning all asthma medications and their role in preventing/controlling exacerbations, help with prioritizing medication purchase and possibly, information on programs that could assist with lowering medication cost. The plan also would include education on asthma triggers, especially cat dander and second hand smoke. In implementing this plan, the pharmacist is establishing a covenant to provide care to the child and his parents. This is the emotional caring referred to above. The pharmacist should document the care provided and provide a report to the primary care provider of patient needs identified and pharmacist actions taken to help the patient. Using this approach will allow the pharmacist to be viewed by allied health care professionals as a care provider. In addition, the pharmacist will be viewed as a caring individual by the patient and caregiver that will hopefully motivate and empower him/her to take an active role in asthma self-management. The last step in the process is to monitor the patient to determine if the desired outcomes are being met. The first important monitoring function is to determine if the patient is receiving therapeutic benefit. Because the pharmacist is justifiably concerned with untoward effects (eg,

adverse drug effects, drug interactions) and other drug-related problems (eg, over/under use, noncompliance), (s)he may not gather sufficient information to determine the degree of therapeutic benefit the patient is receiving from his drug therapy. This can lead to conflict because the primary care provider is usually most concerned with therapeutic benefit. The pharmacist must take this issue into careful consideration in recommendations for changes in care. For example, if in the eyes of the physician, the child with asthma has benefited from Serevent, the physician would likely not be inclined to accept any recommendation to replace it in the regimen. If the pharmacist felt a change in therapy was needed, recommending Advair, a combination product containing Serevent and an inhaled steroid, might be the best way to impact the patient's care. Thus, monitoring requires the pharmacist to view the total patient.

It is also essential that the pharmacist be conscientious in following up on all matters concerning the patient. If the patient has questions or concerns that the pharmacist is unable to satisfy when meeting with the patient, the pharmacist should get back to the patient with the answers or educational information as soon as feasible. Whenever possible, it also is important that the pharmacist personally follow up with the primary care provider on concerns or recommendations rather than just suggesting to the patient to talk to the provider. One reason is because if the patient is not complying with the provider's previous advice, (s)he may be reluctant to admit it to the provider. A second reason is that it is difficult to predict how the patient will convey the pharmacist's concern or recommendation to the provider. Some patients may even tell the provider, "The pharmacist said your treatment is wrong." Another reason is that the patient may simply not understand the information in a way to communicate it properly to the physician. It is difficult to reach many providers and compliance with HIPAA privacy regulations may complicate the process further. However, if the information is imperative to the patient's treatment plan, the pharmacist should gain the patient's permission by explaining the importance of informing the provider.

The pharmaceutical care process outlined above requires a great time commitment by the pharmacist and considerable interpersonal and communication skills are required. Diplomacy is a must, and significant skills as an educator are required. Thus, pharmaceutical care provision requires a knowledgeable, highly skilled practitioner who has a passion for taking care of patients.

Numerous practice-related barriers stand in the way of the pharmacist's ability to provide individualized patient care to optimize the patient's therapeutic outcomes to the prescribed drug therapy. Table 112-1 shows the barriers to providing pharmaceutical care among a group of Indiana community pharmacists participating in a one-year pharmaceutical care certificate program.[26] The pharmacists' perceptions at the beginning of the program (baseline) are typical of most pharmacists. Their perceptions after one year of training will be discussed later. Time to provide care is the major barrier for pharmacists. Lack of time is based on the pharmacist's involvement in processing a high volume of prescriptions/drug orders. Poor workflow design and staffing shortages often contribute to this problem. Studies have shown that pharmacists spend the majority of their time processing and dispensing prescriptions.[27–29] A Midwestern study found that staff pharmacists in high-volume community pharmacies interacted with patients at a rate of once every 3 to 4 minutes.[30]

Most pharmacists are busy and pharmacies are staffed based on drug order/prescription processing needs. No standardized staffing formula has been developed for pharmacy workload allocation. The State of North Carolina has set limits of 150 prescriptions and 12 work hours per pharmacist, but each pharmacy will have unique staffing needs and this formula may or may not be applicable to specific pharmacies depending on other activities required of the pharmacist and staffing of technicians and other personnel.[31] In many settings,

Table 112-1. Perceived Barriers to Providing Pharmaceutical Care—Pharmacists' Responses at Baseline and 1-year Follow-up

BARRIER	BASELINE (%)	1 YEAR (%)
High-volume store	83	32
Poor workflow	23	23
Patients do not want pharmaceutical care	23	27
Lack of data/documentation systems	20	50
Pharmacist has too many interruptions	17	41
Pharmacist needs more education on pharmaceutical care	14	14
Lack of support from management	11	9
Physical layout of the pharmacy	11	32
Lack of sufficient clinical reference resources	9	9
Lack of patient continuity	6	6
Third party will not reimburse for care services	3	5
Management responsibilities take too much time	3	9
Pharmacist colleagues do not believe in care services	3	9

improved workflow, increased use of automated dispensing systems and technicians have allowed the same number of pharmacists to dispense more prescriptions. This improved prescription processing has not contributed to increased opportunities for pharmacists to provide pharmaceutical care because that is not their purpose. The measures have not even freed up time for most pharmacists to counsel patients on new and/or refill prescriptions despite OBRA '90. In the Midwestern study, low rates of personal interaction with patients also occurred with hospital pharmacists. These practitioners tended to focus on medication dispensing, telephone interactions with providers, and population-based drug use management.[30] If pharmaceutical care is going to become a priority, system development for pharmaceutical care services and outcomes must be given the same attention that prescription-processing operations currently receive.

The pharmaceutical care process described above dictates that pharmacists work with other health professionals, identify and solve problems, and communicate orally and in writing. Many neophyte and experienced pharmacists are not adequately prepared to perform these new roles. For some, it is lack of knowledge and skills. For others, it is lack of confidence in their ability. Others prefer to be involved in more passive activities. A study of Ohio pharmacists divided pharmaceutical care practice into four dimensions: Drug Information Source, Information Gathering, Patient Counseling, and Drug Monitoring.[15] The first two dimensions were operationalized by the researchers as "passive" activities of pharmaceutical care meaning they can be completed without much direct patient contact, follow-up activities or anticipation of problems that might be encountered. Pharmacists wait for questions to arise then answer the question or process the prescription drug order. The last two dimensions were operationalized by the Ohio investigators as "active" functions because they dictate proactive involvement by the pharmacist with the patient and other health care providers. They also require the pharmacist to anticipate potential problems that might be encountered. Both of the active functions demand relationship building, problem solving and implementing strategies for optimizing drug outcomes.

The results of the study found that pharmacists were engaged in mostly passive activities suggesting that current pharmaceutical care activities involve being an information resource and maintaining medication records. Even hospital clinical pharmacists tend to be more involved with drug infor-

mation centers, pharmacokinetic monitoring programs, drug management programs, and adverse drug and medication error analysis reporting where direct patient contact is limited. Even many of the pharmacists who participate on rounding teams serve as information resources rather than providers of direct patient care. Further, in some schools of pharmacy, clinical faculty that have been professionally socialized to serve as passive resource models create clerkship rotations for students who also function as information sources to their rounding teams. These information resource pharmacists work very hard and perform valuable services; they just are not involved in providing individualized pharmaceutical care to patients. Only a small percentage of students have the vision and confidence to seek opportunities to be involved in direct patient care. A desperate need exists for preceptors to serve as direct patient care pharmacist role models. The best examples of pharmacists who have transitioned to the active dimensions of care are the disease management pharmacists involved in collaborative care such as diabetes self-management programs, anticoagulation clinics, and asthma, hypertension or dyslipidemia management programs. These pharmacists also serve as excellent role model preceptors for advanced clerkship students. Fortunately, this practitioner group is a growing percentage of practicing pharmacists.

Lack of demand by patients for these services is also cited as a significant barrier. The image portrayed by pharmacy is one of prescription processing and patients do not know to expect pharmaceutical care. In addition, patients often view their prescriptions as expensive and do not want to pay for additional care services. Another factor is that pharmacists are reluctant and shy away from asking patients to pay for care services and typically fail to train pharmacy staff to fulfill these functions. Also, marketing efforts have not been directed educating the public on the value of individualized pharmacist care. Finally, there is debate on the best approach for pharmacy to gain compensation.[32] Some feel that free services have value to the pharmacy and market them as free to gain a competitive edge. They contend that high patient loyalty and improved store traffic pays for the expenses through increased store revenue. For example, a patient with type-1 diabetes will purchase a large number of diabetes supplies each year in addition to their other store purchases. Another important consideration is that pharmacist participation in patient care programs increases job satisfaction and retention. Pharmacist job retention is important due to the high cost of training new employees.

Other pharmacists favor developing programs and marketing them to patients who are willing to pay for them as an out-of-pocket expense. There are groups of patients who value the pharmacist and are willing to pay, if asked. Making these patients aware that the service exists is of primary importance. However, many patients only want pharmacist care services when most of the cost is covered by insurance. While pharmacy organizations and pharmacists are working to obtain insurance coverage for its services, broad acceptance by the insurance companies may result in the same problems currently faced by pharmacy with prescription reimbursement; insurers who drastically discount the fees for pharmacist services.[32] The most effective approach is that the pharmacists develop relationships with insurers to provide specific services to their patients. The pharmacist provides specific documentation for the services provided and the insurer can track the patients' total medical costs to determine if the pharmacist services are cost effective. A major barrier to this approach is the tremendous effort required of the pharmacist to develop the relationship, service structure and payment mechanism. An alternative approach is for the pharmacist to develop a relationship with an employer to provide services to their employees. This can be a win-win for both the pharmacy and the employer. The pharmacist receives payment for services provided while the employer is viewed by the employee as interested in his health. The success of the service will be improved employee health, productivity and work attendance.

The barriers to this approach are the effort and patience required to put a disease management program into place and the complex issue of demonstrating improved patient outcomes. Development of outcome measures can be completed by partnering with a faculty member skilled in pharmacoeconomics research at a school/college of pharmacy.

Community and outpatient clinic pharmacists struggle with three additional barriers (ie, lack of an adequate patient database, lack of disease management resources, lack of a private patient consultation area). Most of these settings do not have a system that allows them access to patient medical records, treatment protocols, lab values, and diagnostic test results. Health Care Smart Cards containing pertinent patient medical information have been proposed for many years but the concept has never been operationalized for a variety of reasons. While the lack of medical information does put the pharmacist at a disadvantage, pharmacists also contribute to the problem. Even when pharmacists interact with patients and their providers to solve drug- and disease-related problems, these interactions are seldom documented. Documentation is limited to interactions involving the processing of the prescription. Building a patient pharmacy chart by keeping a record of patient and provider interactions, problem assessments and plans developed to solve problems, monitoring results and follow-up interactions with the patient would form a valuable patient database. Again, the emphasis is placed on pharmacy operations instead of pharmaceutical care provision.

Most pharmacists are at a distinct disadvantage with respect to having sufficient resources available for pharmaceutical care provisions. Most in-pharmacy references are limited to drug compendia such as the *Red Book, Physician's Desk Reference*, or *Facts and Comparison's*, and possibly a drug interactions text. Medical and therapeutics texts are seldom available. The Internet is a rich source of information that can satisfy nearly all informational needs, but the majority of pharmacies do not have a personal computer and/or an Internet connection dedicated to this use.

A huge problem for many community pharmacies and outpatient clinics is lack of a private patient consultation area. Newer pharmacy layouts provide plenty of semiprivate space for consultation with patients but the high ceilings, open counters and patients waiting all along the counter do not allow for complete privacy. Thus, patients are not inclined to discuss the private issues of their medical conditions when others can easily overhear. The new HIPAA privacy guidelines implemented on April 14, 2003, call for the pharmacist to make every attempt in this semiprivate environment to protect each patient's privacy. However, the semiprivate nature of the environment may discourage an open-relationship between many pharmacists and patients. In the past, private consultation rooms were included in some pharmacy designs, but these were largely abandoned. The rooms were not utilized because emphasis was on prescription processing, not on providing individualized care to patients. Perhaps it is time to revisit this design concept in the pharmaceutical care model.

The final barrier pertains to a variety of cultural, language, financial, and attitudinal factors that affect the ability of the pharmacist to interact with the patient. For certain ethnic groups, it is important to include the father in educational programs pertaining to treatment of a child's disease because the father has the final say on meal plans or even the acceptability of drug treatment. Populations of non-English speaking patients (eg, Hispanic, Vietnamese, Russian) may have difficulty accessing pharmaceutical care in many areas of the country. Many patients have difficulty identifying the resources needed to purchase medications, let alone paying for care, education, and monitoring. A variety of attitudinal problems result in patients not receiving pharmaceutical care. Many people do not like to take medication and will only do so when convinced it is absolutely necessary. Others simply do not understand the importance of taking medication or just take it while they feel ill, stopping as soon as they feel better.

Noncompliance is a vast problem that has been well described.[33,34] Pharmacy has contributed to the problem through insufficient patient counseling and the failure to implement in-pharmacy programs to identify and correct patient noncompliance with medications.

If pharmacies and pharmacists want to commit to pharmaceutical care provision, systems must be designed to provide pharmacists the opportunity to provide care. In a study in which Indiana community pharmacists participated in a 12-month pharmaceutical care certificate program, pharmacist's perception of the importance of time due to excessive prescription volume as a barrier changed (Table 112-1).[26] At the beginning of the training, a vast majority of the pharmacists (83%) felt prescription volume was the major barrier to pharmaceutical care provision. After completing the year-long certificate program, major perceived barriers were lack of data and documentation systems, poor physical layout of the pharmacy, and excessive interruptions. The perception of prescription volume as a barrier fell to 32% of the participants. For pharmacy to be in a position to provide pharmaceutical care, all barriers must be addressed and strategies developed to overcome them.

STRATEGIES TO OVERCOME IDENTIFIED BARRIERS

It has been well documented that pharmaceutical care improves therapeutic benefit and patient outcomes, decreases negative untoward effects, and avoids the financial costs of negative therapeutic outcomes.[33–36] However, as previously discussed, the main pharmacist job function revolves around routine prescription processing *in lieu* of pharmaceutical care functions.

In describing pharmaceutical care, Strand asserted that essentials for its success included pharmacists with a passion for providing care, technicians and other pharmacy support staff trained to perform the tasks associated with prescription processing, and a change in mindset in which the pharmacist's role is perceived as providing care to patients.[37,38] A 2003 White Paper endorsed by 12 prominent national pharmacy organizations states that "implementation of pharmaceutical care requires a fundamental change in the way pharmacies operate. Pharmacists must relinquish routine product-handling functions to competent technicians and technology."[39] This paradigm shift will not be completed easily. Even pharmacists who want to be pharmaceutical care providers may have difficulty turning over prescription processing to others because pharmacists have been taught that this function is critical to safe medication use. Most caring pharmacists are "recovering dispensers" because dispensing is an integral part of their professional socialization process and training. To make the transition to being a pharmaceutical care practitioner, many pharmacists will need substantial training in a wide range of subject areas. Examples of the range of areas would include: working effectively with technicians and partner pharmacists, adult education techniques, disease state management, pharmacist-patient communication techniques, documentation of care, and marketing techniques for pharmaceutical care. Gaining these skills will require a multifaceted approach to educational opportunities. The pharmacists will need support, reassurance, mentors, role models, and networks of pharmacists who are working toward a common goal of pharmaceutical care. Thus, strategies must be devised to overcome the myriad of barriers needed to implement and evaluate the effectiveness of pharmaceutical care practice models. This approach is to get the pharmacists in practice "up to speed." The Schools/Colleges of Pharmacy must also continue to improve curricula to professionally socialize students to have an expectation and commitment to pharmaceutical care provision. Strategies to overcome practice barriers will be presented first followed by approaches to overcome pharmaceutical education barriers.

Strategies to Overcome Practice Barriers

The pharmacy must create, implement, and evaluate a plan for pharmaceutical care service provision. Planning is multifaceted and getting started with plan development is often the hardest part. Most pharmacies provide many services to patients but the services are random, provided only when a patient presents or when the pharmacist has time. To develop an organized program of care, the pharmacy must first organize its services by developing a plan. Key questions to answer during plan development include: what service is to be offered, what policies and procedures will be followed, who is going to staff it, how will other pharmacy operations be staffed, how will potential patients be identified, what computer hardware and software is needed, what information will need to be documented, what forms will be used, what other records will be needed, how will the program be evaluated, what will the program cost to operate, how will the program be financed, will there be a charge to the patient? Coming up with the answers to these questions and many others may appear to be a daunting task, but a team of enthusiastic pharmacists, pharmacy managers, and business people can accomplish the task. Patience and persistence will be required.

For all of the above reasons, it is often best to start with a pilot program on a small, controllable project to gain experience without making a huge time or financial commitment. If the pilot program proves successful, it can be expanded and refined. An example program on compliance improvement for new antihypertensive patients is described below.

Example Compliance Improvement/ Antihypertensive Callback Program

An extremely important service that could start out on a small scale and expand as experience in gained is a Compliance Improvement Program. Noncompliance with prescribed medications and the resulting hospitalizations and physician office visits were estimated in a 1995 study to cost between $75 and $150 million dollars per year in unnecessary expenditures.[33] These costs do not include lost work time and decreased productivity as a result of illness. Noncompliance continues to be a huge problem, and most pharmacies have no programs to identify and manage noncompliance in their patient population. Implementing a service that encourages a patient to take medications as prescribed is good for patient care and it is good for business. A pilot could be initiated in one particular area. For example, it is not uncommon for patients receiving a new antihypertensive agent to not have the prescription refilled because they do not understand the need or may experience a problem that causes them to discontinue the agent. A pharmacy-based pilot Antihypertensive Callback Program to contact the patient 3 weeks after the fill date for the new blood pressure lowering agent may help to identify and correct these problems and improve compliance. The purpose of this telephone call would be to ascertain if the patient is still taking the drug, find out if he has been checking his blood pressure regularly using the proper techniques, and to point out the importance of regular refills, monitoring, and physician visits. The first step in establishing the service would be to develop a list of antihypertensive agents and a procedure to identify patients with a diagnosis of hypertension, because many of these agents may be used to manage other conditions. The next step is to establish a protocol for informing patients about the purpose of the program and that the pharmacist will be in contact in three weeks. Forms would need to be developed to record the patient's contact information (phone and fax numbers, email address) and to document the pharmacist-patient interaction. It also must be decided which pharmacist(s) will do the calling and what times will be allocated to make the calls and complete the documentation. Some practice calls might be even necessary to help the pharmacist feel comfortable and to establish the information to be covered at each call. At this point, the program can be implemented. Because a patient record has been generated, the pharmacy can continue to follow these patients on a regular basis to provide support and solve problems. This service would be invaluable to helping antihypertensive patients comply with their medication and over the long term prevent complications of untreated hypertension. In addition, it would support the pharmacy's refill business and open the door for sales of blood pressure measurement kits or bring the patient into the pharmacy to use the BP kiosk, which may lead to additional purchases. It also would improve patient loyalty for the pharmacy. Surveys can be used to collect information on patient satisfaction. The compliance rates of patients that receive the service should be measured and recorded. It also would be important to collect data on the patients' blood pressure readings. Many blood pressure kiosks will maintain a record of a patient's blood pressure readings or the pharmacy may want to invest in a Dynapulse blood pressure kit, a BP cuff and software that allows measurements to be banked in a computer so that graphs can be generated for use by health care providers. Summation of the data collected can be used in marketing efforts to patients and health care providers and to support requests for payment from insurers or employees. Summation of data collected and debriefing of pharmacists and other care service staff is also important to program evaluation. The evaluation results are used to improve the service and make continuous changes.

Strategies to Overcome Practice Barriers (Continued)

The next step in the planning process is to determine what opportunities exist to provide care to patients in the pharmacy's service area. For example, if the pharmacy is considering the development of services to patients with diabetes, it would be important to determine the number of patients with diabetes presently served by the pharmacy, the estimated diabetes population in the pharmacy's service area, and other diabetes education programs offered to this population. It would also be important to generate a report from the pharmacy's prescription database to identify current patients with prescriptions for euglycemic agents and/or other diabetes-related products. Other necessary data would be important to collect. Many states have disease-related statistics on web sites that can be accessed to determine the estimated number of persons with diabetes in each county. For example, the Access Indiana government web site is a valuable resource.[40] The existence of other diabetes education programs would require evaluating programs offered through hospitals, regional diabetes centers, doctor's offices, and other pharmacies. Even though other programs are offered, it should be ascertained if there are unmet needs that a new diabetes care service can satisfy. For instance, many hospital-based programs have diabetes classes for newly diagnosed patients. However, once the patient is discharged, little follow-up care may be available. A diabetes self-management education program that offers the patient an opportunity for regular interaction with a caring pharmacist may satisfy this unmet need. It will be essential for the pharmacy to document the services provided. Data to be collected would include: blood glucose monitoring and glycosylated hemoglobin results, patient quality of life, patient satisfaction with the service, amount of time spent with the patient, and problems identified and solved. This data would be important in demonstrating the value of the service and marketing the service to key employers and insurance providers in an effort to gain payment and show cost-benefit. It is advisable for the pharmacy to partner with other pharmacies and faculty members with expertise in pharmacoeconomics from a nearby pharmacy school to design the study, collect data, and analyze it for positive outcomes of the pharmacists' contribution to patient care. The Asheville Project, a community pharmacy diabetes care program in Asheville, NC, is a partnership of pharmacists and faculty members. One of the benefits of this partnership is a group of publications in the *Journal of the American Pharmaceutical Association* that demonstrate the value of the community pharmacist in the provision of diabetes care.[41–44]

At the same time, the plan for a care service is being developed and refined, it is important to prepare a vision and mission statement for the pharmacy and the service. The pharmacy's vision is a guiding image of success, formed in terms of a contribution to society. It answers the question, "What will success look like?" For example, the vision for a pharmacy's diabetes self-management education program might be: "To partner with diabetes patients to show improved therapeutic outcomes and reduce long-term disease complications." The entire pharmacy staff must reach a consensus on this vision and work as a team to achieve it. It also is important to note that the vision has measurable components that can be used to demonstrate success.

The mission statement answers the question, "Why does our service exist?" All members of the pharmacy staff also must be in agreement on the mission. For example, the mission of a pharmacy's Diabetes Self-Management Training (DSMT) that has been implemented is: "To provide quality educational services to persons with diabetes in order to assist in improving their quality of life."[45] This mission should be prominently posted in the pharmacy for all to read. In addition, all patients who enroll in the service should be provided a copy of the mission and how the mission will be accomplished by the pharmacy. For example, to accomplish the DSMT mission stated above, the pharmacy informs its patients that it help them understand: (1) diabetes and its acute and long-term complications; (2) monitoring techniques and goal levels for blood glucose and hemoglobin A1c; (3) one's diabetes medications; (4) healthy eating concepts and your meal plan; (5) one's exercise plan and how it fits with daily activities.[45]

Another important part of the plan involves staffing and workflow. Retention of staff is a constant problem that causes considerable stress in most pharmacies. Just as it is important to develop a plan to staff the prescription processing activities and devise a workflow that uses the pharmacist's knowledge and skills effectively, pharmaceutical care activities must be properly staffed with an efficient flow of work. Many pharmacies try to fit the care service into the prescription processing workflow. In a low volume operation that may work, but medium and high-volume pharmacies put so many demands on the pharmacist to oversee the dispensing aspects, it is difficult for the pharmacist to comply with OBRA '90 patient counseling activities, let alone implement a care service. Therefore, a good staffing plan must be developed and managers and staff pharmacists on both the dispensing and service side must reach a consensus on the roles of all members of the pharmacy staff in this plan. The first step in the process is to determine the staff members who will be involved and estimate the amount of their time that will be spent on the project. As with any new project, much of the developmental work may require some of the pharmacist's personal time to create the service. This is not too much to ask of a career-oriented professional and would be expected of any salaried employee. However, once the service has been approved and implemented, the pharmacist must be freed from other work activities to staff the service. In the beginning, it will likely be possible to schedule overlap with partners to free the care pharmacist to provide the service. However, as the service grows, specific pharmacist care hours must be scheduled. All members of the pharmacy staff must buy into this concept and understand that each staff member has an important role in keeping both distributive and care areas of the pharmacy functioning smoothly. In addition, everyone who works in the pharmacy, store, clinic, or hospital (checkout clerks, receptionists, anyone who will come into contact with patients seeking service or health professionals seeking consultation) must be aware of the care service and be able to refer inquiries correctly. In case the pharmacist is not on duty at the time, a calendar should be in the pharmacy showing the pharmacist's schedule and available appointment times.

Another important part of the planning process is to calculate the cost of the service. The pharmacist's time will be a large part of the cost, thus calculating the time involved will be important. There are many ways to calculate this cost based on the method used to pay the pharmacist (eg, hourly or salaried). As an example, assume the pharmacist spends 5.0 hours per week on a new care service and the pharmacist's salary/fringe is $100,000 based on 2080 work-hours per year. Thus, the rate for the pharmacist (100,000/2080) is $48 per hour and the pharmacist cost is $240 for 5.0 hours. In the same fashion, the cost of other staff involved in the service also must be calculated. Other expenses must be estimated such as computer hardware/software, Internet service providers, office and copying charges, costs for designing brochures and/or program materials, equipment and supplies, demonstration devices (many of these can be donated by the manufacturer), and telephone tolls. It is important to estimate as many of the expenses as possible. This gives the pharmacy a handle on how many dollars the service must earn to break-even. Once the break-even point is determined, the desired profit can be added to determine the total revenue projection for the service. This projection can be divided by the number of patients expected to utilize the service allowing one to calculate a per visit patient fee. If the patient were self-pay, this amount would be the fee charged. It also is the usual and customary charge that would be submitted to an insurance carrier. Finally, if the pharmacy is expecting to pay for all or part of the service by increased volume, the pharmacy must have a special key function or store card that allows a patient's spending to be tracked.

The fee setting approach described above is preferable to the one used by many pharmacies to determine care service fees. Many pharmacies charge a fee based on $1.50 to $2.50 per minute. Unless, the pharmacy has calculated its expenses and desired profit, how is it to know if $1.50 to $2.50 per minute is appropriate?

The planning process should determine if special permits (eg, a CLIA waiver) are required? The CLIA waiver applies to laboratory tests excluded from regulatory oversight by the FDA. It must be obtained if these tests will be performed in the pharmacy. Common CLIA waived tests include including blood glucose, hemoglobin A1c, and cholesterol tests measured by approved monitors. The purpose of obtaining the waiver is to assure that the pharmacy's policies and procedures include safe handling and disposal of biohazardous testing materials.

The planning process should also include evaluation of pharmacy staff abilities and identification of the training required to provide the planned service. Training should include all preparation required to perform the service. If the pharmacy were implementing a lipid monitoring and consultation service, training would certainly include use of the cholesterol monitor, knowledge and skills on dyslipidema, and its management. However, training might also correct other weaknesses such as interpersonal skills, marketing, and documentation techniques. Technicians and other pharmacy personnel must understand and be trained in job functions that will allow the pharmacist the freedom to provide care. In some situations, the pharmacy may hire another health professional (eg, a nurse or dietician) to provide monitoring functions thus freeing the pharmacist time to provide drug therapy management services. A pharmacist and nurse can, for example, form an effective team in providing care to patients.

Proper training for pharmacists is a must to improve knowledge, skills, and confidence. As mentioned above, pharmacists should take a careful inventory of their strengths and weaknesses then search for (a) training program(s) that will bring them up to the necessary level. Training is available through academic course work, continuing education programs, and certificate programs. Academic course work is directed at a specific topic area. For example, a class in Spanish for Health Professionals, Professional Leadership and Supervision, Marketing of Professional Services, or Outcomes Assessment may satisfy a specific pharmacist need for a developing a care service. A course in pathophysiology, pharmacology, or therapeutics would be useful to update the knowledge of a pharmacist who has been out of school for a while.

Continuing education programs are usually limited in scope. The purpose of most CE programs is to update knowledge in a particular area via lectures at live seminars or teleconferences or readings for online or home study programs. To implement a care service, development of skills in addition to knowledge is also required. For skill development to occur, the CE program must be interactive (usually in a workshop format) and provide an opportunity for the participant to practice and problem-solve.

Many certificate programs are marketed to help practitioners develop the knowledge and skills needed to provide a care service. In deciding on which certificate program to select, the pharmacist must look at the topics covered and at the method of delivery. Most certificate programs are designed to be interactive combining lectures and home study to improve knowledge and skills. However, many certificate programs fail to provide a mechanism that allows the pharmacist to apply the knowledge and skills to his/her practice setting. This application of the knowledge and skills to the actual practice setting is crucial to implementing a care service. Thus, certificate programs that include assignments to be completed on actual patients or within the practice setting enable the pharmacist to adapt the information presented to a real situation.

Once sufficient planning has occurred, the next step is to implement the program and continuously evaluate it. Program planning is actually a circular process that consists of identifying a need → creating a mission → designing a program to carry out the mission → implementing the program → and evaluating the results. The experience gained in program delivery and evaluation is used to refine/expand the need → adjust the mission → redesign the program → implement the revised program→ and evaluate the new offering. This circular process is repeated each time the program is offered. It is important to understand that evaluation of a service is not the end of the program. The results of the evaluation process are used for continuous quality improvement and program expansion.

It is important to note that the program does not have to be planned to perfection or have every detail complete before it is implemented. Many programs have never been implemented because the pharmacist felt the need to complete one more task, certificate program, or pharmacy staff hire before beginning the program. Planning is crucial, but it is also important to start, gaining experience along the way, then make refinements based on that experience. Setting a start date and sticking to it may avoid this pitfall.

Strategies to Overcome Educational Barriers

The American Association of Colleges of Pharmacy (AACP) and American Council on Pharmaceutical Education (ACPE) have worked closely with member Schools/Colleges of Pharmacy over the past several years to focus curricula on the pharmaceutical care provision. Accreditation standards require each school to be able to document its progress in implementing a curriculum that addresses the professional socialization of the students and allows them to integrate the knowledge, skills, and attitudes from all of the disciplines that contribute to preparation of a pharmaceutical care practitioner.[46,47] While there is still much work to do in this regard, much progress has been made. The conversion to the Doctor of

Pharmacy as the first professional degree was a major step in the process. In addition, schools have incorporated a patient-centered, ability-based outcome approach that provides consistent assessment and feedback for each student in his/her learning and application of basic and applied sciences, pharmacy practice principles, pharmaceutical care provision, and professional development. A program of continuous quality assessment and improvement must be in place and demonstrated to ACPE as each school's accreditation is reviewed every six years.[46] Advanced clerkship rotations must be rigorous, and core objectives for inpatient and ambulatory care rotations must be met.[46] Introductory practice experiences (IPEs) are now a curricular requirement by ACPE.[46] IPEs are experiential coursework that fall early in the professional curriculum (ie, the 1st and 2nd professional year).[9] A major purpose of the IPE is for the school/college to develop educational outcomes that establish what the students can perform, not just what they know.[9] The educational experiences needed to achieve these outcomes can be designed to socialize the student with a caring attitude, internalize the components of pharmaceutical care, and develop a passion for lifelong learning. As new practitioners are trained in these programs, enter practice, and become preceptors, the expectation is that they will have the leadership and interpersonal skills to re-engineer practice to pharmaceutical care provision and be able to instill this process in the students they precept.

TOTAL PHARMACY CARE: A MODEL FOR THE FUTURE

The strategies discussed previously have proved useful to many pharmacies as they move from traditional distribution to pharmaceutical care provision. It is a difficult and time-consuming undertaking. For complete practice re-engineering to occur, a model is needed that can focus a pharmacy and its staff on all aspects of the job at hand. In the late 1990s, Holland and Nimmo studied the nature and extent of the shift in pharmacy practice to the pharmaceutical care model.[4] They discovered continuing reports of widespread failure to persuade pharmacists to become involved in clinical pharmacy and pharmaceutical care roles despite efforts by management to motivate this change through application of traditional managerial theory regarding motivation in the workplace. Holland and Nimmo found that while many managers urged the move to the new model of care, individual pharmacists did not have an understanding of how the pharmaceutical care work in their own practice environment. Thus, in an attempt to communicate effectively the needed transition to pharmaceutical care to those working at the forefront of patient care, Holland and Nimmo proposed a descriptive model of practice they referred to as Total Pharmacy Care (TPC).[4] This model was intended to help pharmacists understand how they fit into the larger scheme while accommodating individual differences in health care delivery systems and individual practice sites, and account for ongoing need for change as we move to the pharmaceutical care model.

TPC describes the state of pharmacy practice in the late 1990s as a combination of five distinct practice models: drug information, self-care, clinical pharmacy, pharmaceutical care, and distribution. All components of TPC operate concurrently to provide a comprehensive range of services to maximize the outcome of drug therapy defined as the provision of pharmaceutical care.

In the Drug Information practice model, the pharmacist provides general advice to health care consumers by, for example, participating in the design and provision of wellness campaigns. These pharmacists participate in the formulary decision-making process and evaluate and monitor the use of medication once it is accepted to the formulary. In the Drug Information model, the pharmacist is involved in educating physicians and allied health care professionals, as well as the patient, regarding selection and safe use of medication.

In the Self-Care practice model, the pharmacist provides general advice to the consumer on health care matters. These pharmacists assess individual patient needs, recommend effective and safe drug therapies, and provide the patients with referrals when the treatment is outside the pharmacist's scope of practice.

Pharmacists working in the clinical practice model contribute to the physician's therapeutic management of the patient by providing the physician with drug information, pharmacokinetic calculations and interpretations, taking patient drug histories, or by designing, monitoring, and evaluating the patient's specific drug treatment.

The Pharmaceutical Care practice model allows the pharmacist to take the responsibility as part of the patient care team for modifying, designing, recommending, monitoring, or evaluating pharmacotherapy, and most importantly, to ensure the desired outcomes of the selected drug therapy.

The Distributive practice model includes the roles traditionally assigned to the pharmacist to ensure the integrity of the prescription through proper handling of records and dispensing of the drug product. While one would expect that this role would have lessened with the move to pharmaceutical care and the introduction of automated dispensing systems at the end of the 20th century, distribution and its associated technical tasks are still a major role of the most pharmacists in practice today.

The TPC model acknowledges the numerous ways that pharmacists provide the various components of practice needed to assure safe medication use. It also allows for the varying amount of time individual pharmacists spend in different practice models and how that will change as the need and opportunity arises. The model assumes that, if the concept of pharmaceutical care is widely adopted by the profession, individual pharmacists will influence their environment to allow the provision of this type of care. Thus, the proportion of pharmacists who practice pharmaceutical care will ultimately increase.

TPC does not suggest that pharmaceutical care will be the only accepted practice model; it requires all five models to meet a population's need. Even Hepler in discussing issues raised by the pharmaceutical care model acknowledged the need for a pharmacy services that fall outside the definition of pharmaceutical care.[48] TPC says it is the sum of all models that will maximize pharmacy's contribution to the nation's health and well-being. However, the hope is that all pharmacists will adopt the idea that pharmacists are at least partially responsible for the outcome of drug therapy regardless of the five models in which the pharmacist is practicing.

Pharmacists can use the TPC model to identify current practice characteristics. Once these characteristics are identified, they can use it to plan what they need to accomplish in their environment to provide TPC. They also can use it to determine how the proportions of pharmacists working in the various practice models would change if pharmacy were contributing maximally to positive patient care outcomes. Thus, TPC can be used as a long-range planning tool for individual pharmacists and pharmacy managers.

TPC indicates that the number of pharmacists engaged in the distributive model will decrease, although the nature of the pharmacists' involvement is likely to change dramatically as automation takes over the process. As health care moves to more managed care, the drug information practice model will likely increase, especially as the focus of care moves to drug selection for the population, instead of the individual. As the patient mix shifts to ambulatory care and as patients view themselves as the primary managers of care, especially with the shift of drugs in major therapeutic care areas switching to over-the-counter status, the portion of pharmacists involved in the self-care practice model will increase. As patients begin to value pharmaceutical care, demand for the assistance of pharmacist will increase.

TOTAL PHARMACY CARE: VARYING KNOWLEDGE, SKILLS, AND ATTITUDES

The tasks required in each of the five practice models each require a different set of skills and abilities to function successfully. Thus, each has differing needs of professional competency. Professional competence is defined as the degree to which the individual can use the knowledge, skills, and judgment associated with the profession to perform effectively in the domain of possible encounters defining the scope of professional practice.[49] Nimmo and Holland furthered their discussion of the TPC model with a description of the pharmacist's professional competency equation that was intended to provide a framework for the review of the prerequisites for success in each of the five practice models.[50] Their professional competence equation has three components: skills, professional socialization, and judgment.

Skills include consideration of psychomotor skills and the intellectual problem-solving skills. This would include conducting an effective literature search and drawing the appropriate conclusions for pharmacists practicing in the drug information model. For those working in self-care, the ability to determine the diagnosis for a stage of a common cold and recommending the correct OTC medications is a required competence. Problem-solving skills depend on the possession of content-matter knowledge, a procedural knowledge, and appropriate thinking strategy for working toward a solution.[51] Different methods of communication are required when talking with patients, discussing care with teams, or influencing prescriber drug choice because these involve intellectual problem-solving skills.

Professional socialization is defined as the attitudes and values associated with pharmacists' expectation of themselves as a professional. The attitudes and values instilled in pharmacists during early education and skill development in the classroom and through experiential training form a mindset as to whom they are as professionals. This mindset establishes what the person considers as appropriate job responsibilities for a pharmacist, to whom they considers themselves responsible, their social purpose, their relationship with other health care providers, their responsibility to the profession, and the nature of their relationship with patients. Professional socialization differs in each of the five components in the Total Pharmacy Care Model.

The remaining component of professional competency is judgment. A professional does not just perform routine tasks, but applies a critical decision-making process to his/her work. Judgment results from continuous practice of the required psychomotor and problem solving skills that reflect the nature of one's attitudes and values (ie, professional socialization). Over time, the pharmacist develops a wealth of experience that allows him/her to deal with situations by going beyond just applying rules or protocols, but to exercise creativity and intellectual problem solving to the situation. Judgment has also been referred to as tacit knowledge. Judgment is developed in a specific practice model by giving the pharmacist an opportunity to perform activities required while at the same time providing constructive feedback. Pharmacists with high standards of professional socialization will reflect on their daily practice and constantly judge the quality of their work while continuing to seek additional knowledge and skills to improve their performance.

DIFFERENTIATING THE PRACTICE MODELS

As we review the tasks performed in each of the five practice models considered in the TPC model, it becomes clear the variation in professional competence required for those successful in each model. There is one skill that is consistent in all five models, that being communication. However, the type and intensity of communication vary. As pharmacists move from the distributive model to the pharmaceutical care model, the communication skills become more important and more extensively involved in the success of the pharmacists.

The Drug Information model requires pharmacists to be skilled in literature evaluation and able to apply analytical skills to influence medication policy decisions. These pharmacists must be effective presenting information to groups and should function well in committees. Pharmacists working in this model enjoy searching the compendia of drug and disease knowledge for answers and do not require a high degree of social interaction. Their primary role is on the analysis and provision of drug information to groups, be that for patients as health promotion information or as drug monographs for health care professionals.

The pharmacist practicing in the Self-Care model must possess skills required to perform health screening and make basic diagnosis to aid in the selection of nonprescription drug use or for referral for more complete care. Besides disease and care knowledge, these pharmacists must have well-developed communication skills to allow them to communicate effectively with patients about their condition. These pharmacists enjoy solving technical problems and enjoy a high level of social interaction.

The Clinical Pharmacy model requires the pharmacist to have highly developed technical problem-solving skills as they assess chronic and acute diseases and monitor drug therapy. Communication in this model is concentrated between the pharmacists and the physician as well as other members of the health care team. While some of these pharmacists may be involved in taking medication histories, communication skills required for these pharmacist-patient interactions are minimal. These pharmacists enjoy technical problem-solving, but generally do not require a high level of social interaction.

The Pharmaceutical Care model is similar to the Clinical Pharmacy practice model in that it requires the technical skills to design, implement and monitor drug therapy. However, it differs in required communication skills because the Pharmaceutical Care model now adds the requirement high level of communication with the patient in addition to the health care team. The pharmacist becomes the patient advocate in this model, communicating the patient's concerns, condition, and problems to allied health care professionals. This model requires the highest level of commitment to the patient as the pharmacist takes on an ethical responsibility to the patient for the outcome of drug therapy.

The Distributive model focuses on the technical knowledge of drugs and their storage, preparation, and delivery. Pharmacists successful in this model enjoy the daily routine, solving technical problems, and working alone. Requirements for communication skills focus on conveying their knowledge of drug therapy to patients and providing information on the administration of medication to other health care providers.

FACILITATING PRACTICE CHANGE, THE HOLLAND-NIMMO PRACTICE CHANGE MODEL

To assure the pharmacy profession's shift to the more patient care focused models of Pharmaceutical Care and Self-Care, individual pharmacists must be encouraged to embrace the concept of changing their practice and make the commitment to acquire the professional competency (ie, the knowledge, skills, and professional judgment) to function effectively in their new chosen model. The direct facilitator of the change is most frequently the employer, whether an institutional or community pharmacy manager, acting in the leadership role to ensure that the vision for change is realized.

In the late 1990s, Holland and Nimmo found that although well-developed educational programming exists to allow phar-

macists to acquire the skills needed to make changes in their daily practice, few actually implemented these changes.[52] An intensive examination of the process needed for changes resulted in the Holland-Nimmo practice change model. The model is an analytic tool that can be used regardless of the practice change desired. The model proposes that there are three components that must be satisfied simultaneously before the change is likely to be implemented, regardless of the nature of a change in practice desired. If any of the components is missing or not provided simultaneously, the likelihood of successful change is limited. The three required components are a favorable practice environment, appropriate learning resources, and viable motivational strategies.

Pharmacists are unlikely to follow through on a personal commitment to change their practice unless they work in an environment where they can use the new practice model. While they may wish to practice pharmaceutical care and find personal time to acquire the new skills they may need, they are unlikely to make the effort if they will not be able to apply their new skills and commitment to care in their daily practice. If the desire to change and the work environment are conducive, the pharmacist must have access to resources that will allow him/her to acquire any new knowledge and skills required to function in the new practice model. If the environment is conducive and the learning resources are available, the pharmacist must be motivated to take the necessary steps to make the changes needed to implement the new practice model.

The first element required for practice change is a practice environment that allows the pharmacist to function in the new practice model as a routine part of his/her work. Creating a new environment may require an acceptance of the new role for pharmacists at the higher administrative levels in the organization in which the pharmacist is employed. It may require pharmacy management to demonstrate cost-savings or at least show that the new practice model will be cost neutral to win corporate administrations support for the change. With this support, necessary financial resources will be available to provide the workspace redesign, personnel, and equipment required to redesign the work environment to facilitate the new practice model. Additionally, there must be support for the new services among the other health care providers in the patient care area. As previously stated, in the Clinical Pharmacy and the Pharmaceutical Care models, the pharmacist becomes a member of the health care team. Acceptance of the pharmacist's new or expanding role by the other members of the patient care team, including the patient, is prerequisite to success of the new model.

Once these are in place, pharmacy management can set out to make the specific changes within their own departments to facilitate change. These will include a re-working of the specific jobs in the department to allow the pharmacists time to undertake their new professional responsibilities. This may include training technicians to take on additional responsibilities to free pharmacist time. It may also require additional technology such as automated dispensing machines or computer support to streamline traditional dispensing processes to free the pharmacists for time with patient care. These changes should culminate with a new position description written to reflect the new duties and responsibilities for the pharmacist taking on patient care roles.

Learning resources will be necessary to allow the pharmacists to acquire the new knowledge and skills required with the new practice model. The quest for knowledge should begin by systematically comparing the skills required in the new job description with the pharmacist's current set of skills, knowledge, and attitudes. Once the determination of the needed skills is complete, educational programs to fill these gaps must be accessible and affordable for the pharmacist. Employers can help facilitate this process by providing educational programs at the workplace or providing financial support to allow the pharmacist to attend programs on their own time. In addition, employers may consider allowing pharmacists to undertake the educational programs during work hours to further encourage the acquisition of these new skills. Finally, employers can encourage or sponsor membership and active involvement in state and national pharmacy associations.

The motivation to make the change must be present in the individual pharmacist. Pharmacists will vary in their motivation to change in that some will embrace the new practice model and actively seek any necessary means to facilitate change. Others will sit back and watch the situation and contemplate the effects of the change before deciding to make the change themselves. Still other pharmacists will never adopt the new practice model. These differences point to the important concept that motivation is very complex and involve one's personality, values, and attitudes. Managers wishing to influence their staff must account for the mindset of each practitioner and apply a systematic motivational process that will maximize the possibility of a decision to change.

The two major factors influencing a pharmacist's receptiveness to change are personality and professional socialization.[53] Personality is defined long before the pharmacist enters the profession. It may be difficult for pharmacists whose personalities do not match the practice models make the changes needed to be successful. However, professional socialization while it begins to take shape during pharmacy school continues to be shaped and molded throughout the professional's career.

Personality is the characteristic ways in which an individual thinks, feels, and behaves while reacting to the environment. Its makeup includes a person's major traits, motivations, self-concept, and emotional behaviors. The sources of these components are multifaceted and include hereditary and constitutional tendencies, training, and identification with parents and cultural environment, along with person's experiences and major relationships in early life. Personality in an adult is usually considered to be stable, and change only occurs if there is some alteration in fundamental perceptual, ideational, or responsive tendencies. People tend to choose a vocation they consider to be consistent with their personality traits. Gross dissatisfaction in the workplace, ineffective coping behavior on the job, and job changing is common when the personality and the work situation do not match with personality type. It is important to consider the personality of an individual pharmacist when changing practice models.

The studies suggest personality types among pharmacists characterized by a strong sense of responsibility, conscientiousness, practicality, logic, and, in about one in five, fear of personal communication. This personality profile represents a match between type and the profession of pharmacy when it was an occupation that mostly required technical problem solving with limited interaction with patients and allied health care professionals. Thus, it was considered that these practitioners chose pharmacy because they preferred well-planned, routine work found commonly in the traditional dispensing model of practice. Communication apprehension, described as avoidance of verbal interaction with others due to anxiety, occurs in 20% of pharmacists. This is consistent with the general population.[54]

When these prevalent personality types found in current practitioners are compared to the types required in the newer practice models, one finds potential for major mismatch of personality when a move to a new practice model is attempted. Pharmacists with personalities lacking the traits of independent decision-making, original thinking, patience and understanding, and sociability will have difficulty functioning in the pharmaceutical care model where these characteristics are required. The one in five with communication apprehension is unlikely to find comfort in a practice role requiring additional communication with physicians or patients. However, the common traits of logic and practicality can serve pharmacists well in all practice models when they take on complex problem-solving and analysis. Their conscientiousness can help to assure that all-important information, be it drug information

for professionals or patient information, is considered in complex decision making processes. Those who find comfort in communicating with others may be able to make the transition to practices in the Drug Information model or the Clinical Pharmacy model as their communication requirements focus on interaction with like individuals (ie, allied health care providers). Those communicators who do have an extroverted nature will find comfort working in the Self-Care and Pharmaceutical Care models once they acquire the skills and knowledge to handle the complex problem-solving required. Thus, it is important for the pharmacist to understand his/her role personality type. Completion of the Myers-Briggs Personality Test may be worthwhile exercise to help these pharmacists gain a better understanding of their personality. It is not uncommon for personality testing to be sponsored by employers at retreats and other job-related functions to help employees determine their personality types and work within some team-building exercises to learn how individuals of different types can work together to accomplish the company's objectives. For an individual who has never had personality testing available, the test can be taken online (a fee is involved) at www.cpp.com.

With this understanding, the individual can best determine the areas of practice where he/she will best function and, thus, find satisfaction and comfort. If the individual wishes to function in a practice model unsuited for his/her personality type, corrective measures do exist to the individual overcome certain personality deficiencies. For instance, assume that an introverted practitioner is interested in becoming a Drug Information specialist, but has a fear of speaking to groups. Participating in Toastmasters or another public speaking organization may be sufficient to help overcome this fear.

For practicing pharmacists to make a change in their practice model they must re-formulate their practice values and attitudes - or be "resocialized." While personality characteristics are relatively set in early life, professional socialization continues to develop throughout the course of one's career. Traditional management methods to facilitate work changes have failed because their focus is on the performance of a "job" rather than an actual change in the way a professional accepts the values and attitudes required by the new practice model. Thus, there is an opportunity here to employ new methods to facilitate the changes needed in attitudes and values—or in professional socialization—to be successful in the new practice model.

Nimmo and Holland proposed a systematic process to assist managers to motivate their staffs to be "resocialized" into the new pharmacy practice models.[53] The process adapted accepted educational and psychological theories including Krathwohl's taxonomy of learning,[55] Roger's diffusion of innovation,[56] and instructional psychology.[57] The use of the learning theory encourages the managers to facilitate actively the change in values and attitudes and does not use passive or nonassertive methods to accomplish the change which needs to progress rapidly throughout the profession.

Krathwohl's taxonomy suggests that affective learning has a five-level hierarchy of stages that include Receiving, Responding, Valuing, Organization, and ultimately Characterization by a value or value complex. To relate this model to the changes in pharmacy practice, the pharmacist working in the distributive model begins to change by *receiving* information about the practice of pharmaceutical care. If the change progresses, these practitioners will actively *respond* to the information they received about the new model and then will *value* pharmaceutical care as an appropriate model for their practice. As they value the new model they will *reorganize* their practice to incorporate these new values. Ultimately, the new values will be so strongly embraced that they will *characterize* the pharmacist's overall approach to the profession.

As a prerequisite to engaging in the motivational strategy, managers should consider the existing characteristics of their staff. The development of new attitudes and values is most effective in the presence of an understanding of each practitioner's personality and previous professional socialization. In some cases, personality and the strength of previous professional socialization may not allow the pharmacist to make the change to a new practice model despite use of the very best motivational strategy.

To begin the change process, the manager should determine the current professional orientation of staff members to understand which attitudes and values require nurturing and any variance between the current and desired situations. With this background, an effective motivational strategy can be customized for individual staff members by apply the following process to "resocialize" the pharmacists to provide care under the new model.

LEVEL 1.0: RECEIVING

To begin the process of professional resocialization, the pharmacist must "receive" the information about the new practice model. The three stages in this step are awareness, willingness to receive, and controlled or selected attention. Here the practitioner moves from an awareness of the new practice model, to becoming interested in learning the new model, and finally to actually actively seeking or paying attention to information the new model.

FACILITATING LEVEL 1.0 RECEIVING

Before change can be considered, knowledge of the new practice model must be available to understand what change might be considered. Due to variations in the original professional socialization of pharmacists, some practitioners look routinely for information about new practice opportunities. Others who consider pharmacy a job, not a profession, tend not to seek additional knowledge. Thus, at this step of the change process the manager should focus on providing information about the new practice model to those who would not be looking for it.

Practitioners bring their personalities and professional socialization that form their mindset with which the new practice model will be considered. The mindset may facilitate or hinder willingness to recognize AND consider the implications of the new model. Those trained in school when the focus was on technical problem-solving and limited patient interaction may find the new Pharmaceutical Care practice model incongruous with in their mindset. To deal with this situation, the educational technique using an interactive lecture to provide information including a clear concept of the new model and allow discussion of critical information guided with carefully framed questions can help provide understanding. Guided discussions can also help to reach this desired effect. The facilitator of the discussion or lecture should be an opinion leader among the pharmacists, and not necessarily the supervisor. Included in the presentations should be demonstrations of the bridge between the current practice model and the proposed one, as well as examples of success with the transformation. The discussion should be conducted to include all participants because only through dialogue can the discussion leader be sure that the participants have secured an understanding of the information. These lectures or discussion should occur in an environment conducive to learning because the acceptance of this information is critical to begin the change process needed for the profession. An off-site meeting (eg, retreat, away from distractions is a good way to generate enthusiasm for a new model.

Once the pharmacists have shown awareness and willingness to receive the information, management should be sure to provide opportunities for them to do so. Providing printed material, access, and time to connect to the Internet for information searches facilitates learning for those who have now moved to the controlled or selected attention stage. The phar-

macists should be encouraged to observe and encouraged to converse with pharmacists who are already practicing in the new model, whether it is locally or through visits to other institutions or educational meetings. In addition, membership in and attending meetings of professional associations is an excellent method to network with practitioners involved in changing practice. Understanding of the new model is improved through these opportunities to network and learn. Management should encourage and provide the opportunity for these discussions to take place. By participating in the discussions, management can determine if the pharmacists are ready for the next step. However, management must walk a fine line between dominating the discussions in an attempt to force the pharmacists to accept its point of view, and leading the discussions to help the pharmacists arrive and the desired point of view.

LEVEL 2.0: RESPONDING

As pharmacists pass through the responding phase, they advance from complying with a request that they learn more about the new model of practice to deriving personal pleasure and psychic reward from the learning. In this step the pharmacist has a limited commitment to the new practice model because it is value is not yet realized. However, interest in the possibility of expanding practice is enough to stimulate learning. When the pharmacist becomes willing to consider the new model as a possible method of accepted practice the development of motivation to change has begun.

FACILITATING LEVEL 2.0 RESPONDING

In this step, the practitioner determines if he/she can fit into the new practice model and most importantly does he/she consider this an option for his/her practice. The pharmacist will consider what (s)he has to gain by adopting the new model and if (s)he will fit in the new type of practice. Nimmo and Holland suggest that a trial of the new practice behavior at this stage can speed up the formation of attitudes and values needed to facilitate the new practice model. Witnessing the new practice model in action provides the pharmacist with a personal sense of the new practice model and is critical to a change in attitudes and values. However, pharmacists are socialized to require accuracy in their work. If introduced to a practice situation in which (s)he feels incompetent, the pharmacist will likely reject rather than accept the new practice model. Coaching to recognize personal competence is a must.

LEVEL 3.0: VALUING

The practitioner comes into this level with a belief in the values of the new practice model that becomes a mindset. Over time a mindset develops that reflects a complete transformation to the required new values and attitudes. The pharmacist now has a preference for the new model and wishes to become more involved in the new practice. Once a preference is established, there is a true commitment to the new concept where formation of the new attitudes and values associated with the new practice model is complete and the pharmacist is truly ready to make the change in practice.

FACILITATING LEVEL 3.0 VALUING

At this level, pharmacists are engaged in an internal process of evaluation. They enter this level with a full understanding of the proposed form of practice and have tested it against their capacity to perform it and their interest in doing it. Now they begin an internal analysis comparing their old paradigm against the new one and resolve any remaining uncertainty of the value and fit of the new model. Because personal evaluation and decision is the activity here, it is difficult for the pharmacy manager to be involved in this step–except to provide support and encouragement to the pharmacist undertaking this evaluation.

LEVEL 4.0: ORGANIZATION

Once there is a commitment to the change, the pharmacist must reorganize professional and personal priorities to allow a change in practice to occur. First, the pharmacists must grasp the value by understanding how the new practice model relates to all other methods of practice and why it is the preferred model for practice. Once the understanding takes place, the pharmacist commits to organizing priorities–whether there be educational or work process needs–to allow for the change to a new practice model to truly occur.

FACILITATING LEVEL 4.0: ORGANIZATION

While the manager's role in facilitating the reorganization of the practitioner's value system remains limited as the pharmacist determines his/her own priorities, it can be useful to facilitate conversations with peers who are involved actively in the new practice. This can help the pharmacist understand the fit of his/her own values and attitudes into the new model and begin to understand the organization needed to allow his/her practice to convert to the new model. This interaction can be helpful for those who are having difficulty determining how to handle the change when conflicts exist with personal priorities.

It is while organizing these priorities that pharmacists will determine what new skills or knowledge they will need to acquire to become competent providers in the new model. The manager can be most helpful by providing the learning resources needed and providing financial assistance and work time or release from work to allow for training and studying. By providing these educational opportunities, management can remove an important barrier that many times has prevented pharmacists from moving forward to the advanced practice models of clinical pharmacy and pharmaceutical care.

LEVEL 5.0: CHARACTERIZATION BY A VALUE OR VALUE COMPLEX

At this level resocialization is complete. Here the positive values and attitudes about the new practice model go beyond being just being adopted, they become the definition of the person as a professional. This occurs as the pharmacist internalizes the new practice to the point that the attitudes and values are considered part of the mindset without thinking. Beyond becoming part of the mindset, the new practice model characterizes the personal values of the individual where the new practice behavior has come to characterize the individual.

FACILITATING LEVEL 5.0

As a person internalizes values and moves to characterization, management has little role in this step. The best way to facilitate the progression to this highest level of learning is to facilitate the steps along the way, allowing the individual to progress to this point of characterization.

FACILITATING MOTIVATION

Reflecting on Krathwohl's Taxonomy of Affected Learning can help managers find areas where they can encourage the changes in attitudes and values pharmacists must make to become effective practitioners in the new practice models. Success in motivating pharmacists to develop new values as a part of their professional socialization will help advance the profession as providers of pharmaceutical care to all patients in the 21st century.

REFERENCES

1. Hepler CD, Strand LM. *Am J Pharm Ed* 1989; 53: 7S.
2. Chalmers RK, Adler DS, Haddad AM *et al. Am J Pharm Ed* 1995; 59: 85.
3. Fjortoft NF, Zgarrick DP. *Am J Pharm Ed* 2001; 65: 335.
4. Holland RW, Nimmo CM. *Am J Health-Syst Pharm* 1999; 546: 1758.
5. Higby GJ. *Am J Health-Syst Pharm* 1997; 544: 1805.
6. Hepler CD, Strand LM. *Am J Hosp Pharm* 1990; 47:533.
7. Hepler CD. *Am J Pharm Educ* 1987;51:369.
8. Manasse HR, Stewart JE, Hall RH. In: Wertheimer AI, Smith MC, eds, *Pharmacy Practice: Social and Behavioral Aspects*, 2nd ed. Baltimore, University Park Press, Baltimore, 1981, Chap 2.
9. Beck DE, Selby SG, Janer AL. *Am J Pharm Ed* 1996; 60: 122.
10. Schwirian PM, Facchinetti NJ. *Am J Pharm Ed* 1974; 38: 18.
11. Speranza KA, McCook WM. *Am J Pharm Ed* 1978; 42: 11.
12. Smith M, Messer S. *Am J Pharm Ed* 1991; 55: 30.
13. Hatoum HT, Smith MC. *Am J Pharm Ed* 1987; 51: 7.
14. Hatwig CA, Crane VS, Hayman JN. Topics Hosp Pharm Mgmnt 1993; 13(3): 1.
15. Schommer JC, Cable GL. *Am J Pharm Ed* 1996; 60: 36.
16. Knapp DE, Knapp DA. *Soc Sci Med* 1968; 1: 455.
17. Buerki RA. *Am J Pharm Ed* 1977; 41: 28.
18. Von Essen L. *Int J Nurs Stud* 1991; 28: 267.
19. Kelly B. *J Nurs Educ* 1992; 31: 121.
20. Rognstad MK. *J Nurs Educ* 2002; 41: 321.
21. Armstrong D. *Soc Sci Med* 1983; 17: 457.
22. Rawnsley M. *Adv Nurs Sci* 1990; 13, 41.
23. Pellegrino ED. *JAMA* 1974; 227: 1288.
24. Murawski MM, Miederhoff PA. *Am J Pharm Ed* 1994; 58: 310.
25. Hepler CD. *Am Pharm* 1990; NS30 (10): 28.
26. Barner JC, Bennett RW. *J Am Pharm Assoc* 1999; 39: 362.
27. Arthur Andersen. Pharmacy activity cost and productivity study. November 1999. Accessed February 21, 2003 at www.nascd.org/user-assets/PDF_files/arthur_andersen.pdf.
28. Ringold DJ, Santell JP, Schneider PJ. *Am J Health-Syst Pharm* 2000; 57: 1759.
29. Dupclay L, Rupp MT, Bennett RW. *J Am Pharm Assoc* 1999; 39: 74.
30. Schommer JC, Pedersen CA. *J Am Pharm Assoc* 2001; 41: 760.
31. Wick JY, Zanni GR. *Consultant Pharmacist* 2003; 18: 105.
32. Ganther JM. *J Am Pharm Assoc* 2002; 42: 875.
33. Johnson JA, Bootman JL. *Arch Int Med* 1995; 155: 1949.
34. Johnson JA, Bootman JL. *Am J Health-Syst Pharm* 1997; 54: 554.
35. American Pharmaceutical Association. Project ImPACT. Accessed February 23, 2003 at www.aphafoundation.org/Project_Impact/Impact.htm.
36. Bootman JL, Harrison DL, Cox E. *Arch Int Med* 1997; 157: 2089.
37. Strand LM. *Pharm J* 1998; 260: 874.
38. Johnson JA, Bootman JL. *Am J Health-Syst Pharm.* 1997; 54: 554.
39. American Pharmaceutical Association. Project ImPACT. Accessed February 23, 2003 at www.aphafoundation.org/Project_Impact/Impact.htm
40. Access Indiana. Analysis of Diabetes Morbidity and Mortality in the State of Indiana, 1989–1993. Accessed March 24, 2003 at http://www.in.gov/isdh/programs/diabetes/summery.htm.
41. Cranor CW, Christensen DB. *J Am Pharm Assoc* 2003; 43: 149.
42. Cranor CW, Christensen DB. *J Am Pharm Assoc* 2003; 43: 160.
43. Cranor CW, Bunting BA, Christensen DB. *J Am Pharm Assoc* 2003; 43: 173.
44. Garrett DG, Martin LA. *J Am Pharm Assoc* 2003; 43: 185.
45. Personal communication. Diabetes self-management training program. Kroger Pharmacy, Central Marketing Area, Indianapolis, IN, February 25, 2003.
46. American Council on Pharmaceutical Education. Standards for Curriculum, Accreditation Standards for the Professional Program in Pharmacy Leading to the Doctor of Pharmacy Degree. Adopted June

14, 1997. Accessed March 20, 2003 at www.acpe-accredit.org/frameset_ProfProg.htm.
47. Hammer DP, Paulsen SM. *Am J Pharm Ed* 2001; 65: 77.
48. Hepler CD. *J Pharm Teach* 1996;5(1–2): 19.
49. Kane MT. *Eval Health Prof* 1992; 15(2):163.
50. Nimmo CM, Holland RW. *Am J Health-Syst Pharm* 1999; 56: 1981.
51. Anderson JR. *The Architecture of Cognition.* Cambridge, MA: Harvard Univ. Press; 1983.
52. Holland RW, Nimmo CM. *Am J Health-Syst Pharm* 1999; 56:2235.
53. Nimmo CM, Holland RW. *Am J Health-Syst Pharm* 1999; 56:2458.
54. Anderson-Harper HM, Berger BA, Noel R. *Am J Pharm Educ* 1992; 56:252–8.
55. Krathwohl DR, Bloom BS, Masia BB. *Taxonomy of Educational Objectives; the Classification of Educational Goals, Handbook II: Affective Domain.* White Plains, NY: Longman; 1964.
56. Rogers EM. *Diffusion of Innovations.* 4th ed. New York: Free Press; 1995.
57. Prochaska JO, DiClemente CC. *The Transtheoretical Approach: Crossing Traditional Boundaries of Therapy.* Homewood, IL: Dow Jones-Irwin; 1984.

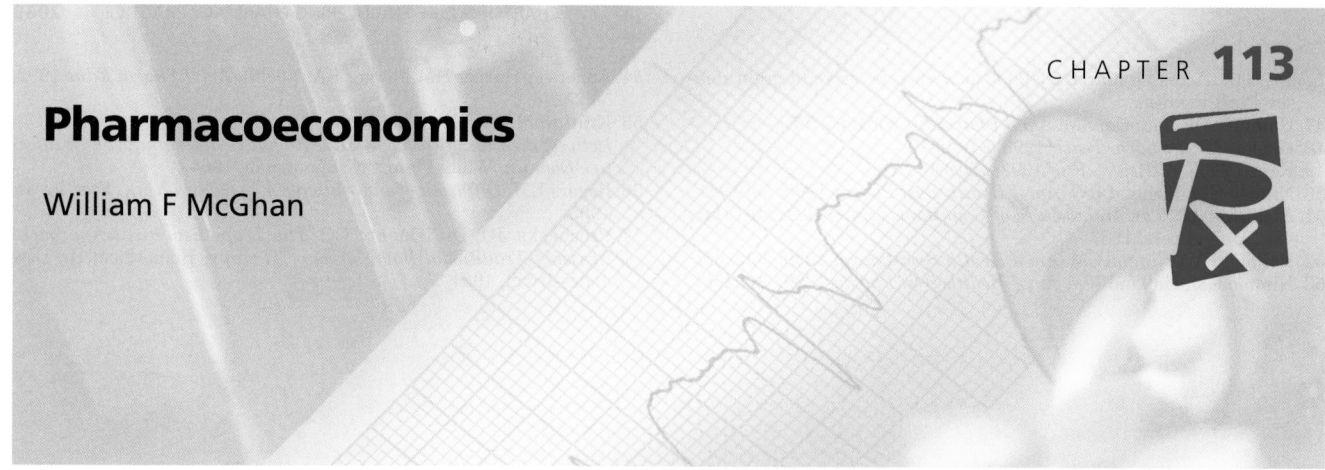

CHAPTER 113

Pharmacoeconomics

William F McGhan

Practitioners and managers face a multitude of economic challenges as the ability to discover new therapies seems boundless while patients' resources to purchase these cures remains limited. How does one decide which are the best medicines to use within restricted budgets? The continuing impact of cost-containment is causing administrators and policymakers in all health fields to examine closely the costs and benefits of both proposed and existing programs. It is increasingly evident that private employers and public agencies are demanding that health programs be evaluated in terms of clinical and social outcomes related to costs incurred.

Cost-benefit analysis and other pharmacoeconomic tools are ways to analyze the value of the service to the public. These methods supplement the traditional marketplace value as measured by the prices that the patient or patron is willing to pay. As third parties continue to pay for a higher percentage of prescriptions dispensed, pharmacy managers are very cognizant that pharmacy services require continual cost-justification to survive and thrive in the future.[1-3]

Pharmacy entrepreneurs have established numerous innovative roles for pharmacists, such as home intravenous therapy, drug-level monitoring, parenteral nutrition management, hospice care, and self-care counseling, among others. The use of valid economic evaluation methods (eg, cost-benefit and cost-effectiveness analysis) to measure the value and impact of new services can increase acceptance of such programs by the medical profession, third-party payers, and consumers.[4-6]

There is increasing competition among health professionals for the limited dollars and resources available. Within institutions and communities, pharmacists will have to compete increasingly with nursing, medical, and other groups for adequate reimbursement and payment.[7,8] Therefore, pharmacy must document the cost-benefits of distinct pharmacy services and develop priorities for those services to compete successfully in the ever-changing health care landscapes.

The purpose of this chapter is to present the fundamental concepts of pharmacoeconomics and to suggest how these concepts can be applied in justifying, evaluating, and improving pharmacy programs and services.

As a general background, it is important to appreciate the types of evaluations that are involved when examining costs and consequences in health interventions. To facilitate an understanding of terminology used in this chapter, the reader is referred to the glossary of terms in Table 113-1. In addition, Table 113-2 provides a framework from Drummond et al[9] emphasizing that full economic evaluations involve the comparison of at least two interventions and an examination of all costs and consequences.

ANALYTICAL PERSPECTIVES

Point of view is a vital consideration in pharmacoeconomics. If a pharmacy service is providing a positive benefit to cost in terms of value to society as a whole, the service may not be valued in the same way by separate segments of society. For example, a drug therapy that reduces the number of admissions or patient-days in an acute care institution is positive from society's point of view but not necessarily from that of the institution's administrator who depends upon a high number of patient admissions to meet expenses. One must determine whose interests are being served when identifying outcome criteria for evaluation. When considering pharmacoeconomic perspectives, one must always consider who pays the costs and who receives the benefits. For example, a proposal to start a new pharmacy service that is funded by a hospital administrator would usually want to demonstrate that based on the projected number of inpatients, the revenues to the hospital would outweigh the pharmacy service costs. However, a pharmacy proposal to be funded by an outside employer group, such as an automobile manufacturer, would probably want to attempt to decrease hospital admissions and that could decrease the normal revenue for the hospital. A favorable economic analysis that showed savings in hospital expenditure from the employer perspective would probably not be viewed positively from the hospital perspective. More broadly, what is viewed as saving money for society may be viewed differently by third-party payers, administrators, health providers, governmental agencies, or even the individual patient. It is generally agreed among health economists that the societal perspective should always be discussed in an evaluative report, even though the focus of the report might deal with other segments such as hospitals or insurance agencies.

OVERVIEW OF ECONOMIC METHODS

This section will acquaint the reader with some of the methodological issues regarding two common pharmacoeconomic analyses including cost-benefit analysis (CBA) and cost-effectiveness analysis (CEA). Table 113-3 provides a basic comparison of these methods along with cost of illness, cost-minimization, and cost-utility analysis. One can differentiate between the various approaches according to the units used to measure the inputs and outcomes, as shown in the table. In classic operations research (inputs versus outputs), the inputs would be measured in "pharmacy hours" and the output "production" units would be "number of prescriptions dispensed" or "number of patients monitored." In general, the outputs in CEA are related to vari-

Table 113-1. Glossary

Contingent valuation: a method for evaluation of benefit or value to individuals of therapy that uses survey methods to establish willingness-to-pay.

Cost-benefit analysis (CBA): a type of analysis that measures costs and benefits in pecuniary units and computes a net monetary gain/loss or a cost-benefit ratio.

Cost-effectiveness analysis (CEA): a type of analysis that compares interventions or programs having a common health outcome (eg, reduction of blood pressure; life-years saved) in a situation where, for a given level of resources, the decision maker wishes to maximize the health benefits conferred to the population of concern. This type of analysis can be used to assess cost-effectiveness efficiency.

Cost-utility analysis (CUA): a type of analysis that measures benefits in utility-weighted life-years (QALYs) and which computes a cost per utility-measure ratio for comparison between programs.

Decision analysis: an explicit quantitative approach for prescribing decisions under conditions of uncertainty.

Decision tree: a framework for representing alternatives for use in decision analysis.

Direct costs: those that are wholly attributable to the service in question, for example, the services of professional and paraprofessional personnel, equipment, and materials.

Discount rate: rate of discount used to convert future costs and benefits into equivalent present values; typically 2% to 6% per annum.

Equity: fairness in the allocation of resources or treatments among different individuals or groups.

Indirect costs: (1) indirect costs are societal, economic, and productivity losses due to morbidity and early mortality; also (2) indirect cost is sometimes used to refer to overhead costs that are based on costs that are shared by many services concurrently, for example maintenance, electricity, and administration.

Net benefit: total benefit (in monetary units) minus total cost (in monetary units); a basic decision criterion in cost-benefit analysis.

Opportunity cost: the opportunity cost of a commodity is the value of the best alternative use to which those resources could have been put; the value of the productive opportunities foregone by the decision to use them in producing that commodity.

Pharmacoeconomics: the study of how individuals and societies choose to allocate scarce pharmaceutical and health resources among competing alternative uses and to distribute the products and services among members of the society.

Quality of life (QOL): physical, social, and emotional aspects of a patient's well being that are relevant and important to the individual.

Quality-adjusted life year (QALY): a common measure of health improvement used in cost-utility analysis; combines mortality and quality of life gains (outcome of a treatment measured as the number of years of life saved, adjusted for quality).

Sensitivity analysis: a process through which the robustness of an economic model is assessed by examining the changes in results of the analysis when key variables are varied over a specified range.

Utility: a measure of value of an outcome that reflects attitudes toward risk.

Willingness-to-pay: the maximum amount of money that an individual is prepared to give up to ensure that a proposed health care measure is undertaken.

---

ous outcome measures, such as lives saved, life-years added, disability-days prevented, and so on. CBA is differentiated from CEA because CBA uses monetary values, dollars to measure the output of the respective program. Further discussion and examples of these techniques have been presented elsewhere.[1-3,10-18] It is hoped that the evaluation mechanisms delineated here may be helpful in managing pharmaceutical services toward improved societal value and generate greater acceptance by health care providers, administrators, and the public.

COST-BENEFIT ANALYSIS

The use of CBA is not a new concept in evaluating health programs. CBA is a basic tool that can be utilized to improve the decision-making process in the allocation of funds to health and other programs.[10,19-28] While the overall concept of CBA is simple, many of the methodological considerations require a certain degree of technical expertise, that will be introduced below, to apply CBA appropriately.

CBA evolved from the need to ascertain estimates of the costs and benefits of public investment projects. Expenditures

for health care should produce net social benefits for the public. CBA techniques can be applied to make such resource allocation decisions in the health care field. Economists have indicated that medical care is an investment good and consumption good. When considered as an investment good, medical care is an investment in human capital.[29] As Pigou has pointed out, "the most important investment of all is the investment in health, intelligence, and character of the people."[30] In economic terms, the present value of a person's lifetime productivity is generally considered the appropriate measure of the benefit from investment in human capital.[31,32]

A major function in any pharmacy planning process is the formulation of alternative ways to achieve desired objectives and then choosing between those alternatives. Many times, decisions are made on the basis of intuition and personal judgment. By requiring one to state precise definitions and objectives (eg, to identify criteria for judging results, to quantify the results of each alternative, to provide formal exposition of alternatives and examination of the effects of assumptions and uncertainties), cost-benefit analysis provides a more solid basis for decision-making.

Table 113-2. Types of Pharmacoeconomics Evaluations

		ARE BOTH COSTS AND CONSEQUENCES OF THE ALTERNATIVES EXAMINED?		
		NO		YES
		Examines only Consequences	Examines only Costs	Examines both
IS THERE A COMPARISON OF TWO OR MORE ALTERNATIVES	N O	Outcome Description	Cost Description	Cost-Outcome Description
	Y E S	Efficacy Description	Cost Analysis	Full Economic Evaluation CBA, CEA, CUA, (etc.)

Adapted from Drummond MF, O'Bien BJ, Stoddart GL, et al. Methods for the Economic Evaluation of Health Care Programs. Oxford: Oxford University Press, 1997.

Table 113-3. Comparison of Pharmacoeconomic Methods and Calculations

METHOD	ABBR	BASIC FORMULA	DISCOUNTING MATH	INPUT	OUTPUT	RESULTS EXPRESSED	GOAL Determine:	Advantage / Disadvantage	EXAMPLE
COST OF ILLNESS	COI	$(DC+IC)$	$\sum_{t=1}^{n}[C_t/(1+r)^t]$	$	$	Total cost of illness.	Total cost of illness.	Does not look at TXs separately.	Cost of migraine in U.S.
COST MINIMIZATION ANALYSIS	CMA	C_1-C_2 Or [Preferred Formula] $(DC_1+IC_1)-(DC_2+IC_2)$	$\sum_{t=1}^{n}[C_t/(1+r)^t]$	$	Assumed Equal	Net cost savings.	Lowest cost TX.	Assume both TXs have same effectiveness.	Assume two antibiotics have same effects for killing bugs but differ on RN & IV cost.
COST EFFECT-IVENESS ANALYSIS	CEA	$(C_1-C_2)/(E_1-E_2)$ or [Preferred Formula] $(DC_1+IC_1)-(DC_2+IC_2)/(E_1-E_2)$	$\sum_{t=1}^{n}[C_t/(1+r)^t]/$ $\sum_{t=1}^{n}[E_t/(1+r)^t]$	$	Health Effect	Incremental cost against change in unit of outcome.	TX attaining effect for lower cost.	Compare TXs that have same type of effect units.	Compare two HTN Rxs for life yrs.
COST BENEFIT ANALYSIS or NET BENEFIT	CBA	$(B_1-B_2)/$ $(DC_1+IC_1)-(DC_2-IC_2)$ or [Preferred Formula] NET BENEFIT = (B_1-B_2)	$\sum_{t=1}^{n}[B_t/(1+r)^t]/$ $\sum_{t=1}^{n}[C_t/(1+r)^t]$ or $\sum_{t=1}^{n}[(B_t-C_t)/(1+r)^t]$	$	Dollars	Net benefit or ratio of incremental benefits to incremental costs.	TX giving best net benefit or higher B/C ratio (or Return on Investment).	TXs can have diff effects, but must put into dollars.	Compare two cholesterol Rxs and convert life yrs to wages.
COST UTILITY ANALYSIS	CUA	$(DC_1+IC_1)-(DC_2+IC_2)$ $(C_1-C_2)/(U_1-U_2)$ or [Preferred Formula] $(DC_1+IC_1)-(DC_2+IC_2)/(U_1-U_2)$	$\sum_{t=1}^{n}[C_t/(1+r)^t]/$ $\sum_{t=1}^{n}[U_t/(1+r)^t]$	$	Patient Preference	Incremental cost against change in unit of outcome adjusted by patient preference.	TX attaining effect (adjusted for patient preference) for lower cost.	Preferences are difficult to measure.	Compare two cancer Rxs & use QOL adjusted life years gained.

Although it may not be easy to conduct a full economic evaluation, an important advantage of cost-benefit analysis is that it forces those responsible to quantify input (costs) and outputs (benefits) as thoroughly as possible rather than rest content with vague qualitative judgments or personal hunches.[30,31]

Cost-benefit analysis consists of identifying all the societal benefits that will accrue from a health program of interest and converting them into equivalent dollars in the year in which they will occur. This stream of benefit dollars is then discounted to its equivalent present value at the selected interest rate. On the other side of the equation, all costs of the program are identified and allocated to a specific year in the future and, again, the costs are discounted to their present value at usually the same interest rate. Then, other things being equal, the program with the largest present value of benefits minus costs is the "best" in terms of its economic value.

Ideally, all benefits and costs caused by the program should be included. This presents considerable difficulty, especially on the benefits side of the equation because many of the benefits are either difficult to measure, difficult to convert to dollars, or both. For example, benefits such as improved patient comfort, improved patient satisfaction with the health care system, improved working conditions for the physician, among others are difficult to measure and extremely difficult to convert into dollars.[33–38]

Another problem in cost-benefit analysis is how one determines the proper interest rate for discounting future benefits and costs. Prest and Turvey recommend that the selection of an interest rate be based on similar projects, followed by sensitivity analysis of the problem to determine the effect of a range of discount rates as the final solution. The problem of selecting an appropriate discount rate and other methodological considerations will be discussed in further detail later in the chapter.

MEASURING BENEFITS AND COSTS

The economic benefits of a health program are defined as the reduction in costs realized because of the implementation of that program. The conventional classification of these benefits and costs are threefold: direct, indirect, and intangible. There is sometimes disagreement on where to include a cost or benefit value in various economic equations, especially those dealing with CBA ratios where all benefits are on top of the equation as the numerator and all input costs are on the bottom as the denominator. For example, if a new drug allows you to use that one drug instead of two different drugs for patients, should the savings of not having to use the second drug be considered a minus value in the input costs of the numerator or should it be a positive figure on the benefit side of the ratio equation in the denominator? To resolve this ratio dilemma, it has become more popular to calculate net benefits (B−C) in place of the traditional CBA ratio (B/C).

DIRECT COSTS

Direct costs include those costs incurred prior to diagnosis and hospitalization, during hospitalization, during convalescent care, and during continued medical surveillance. Rice suggested that these costs include "expenditures for prevention, detection, treatment, rehabilitation, research, training, and capital investments in medical facilities as well as professional services, drugs, medical supplies, and nonpersonal health services." Direct benefits are defined as "that portion of averted costs currently borne that are associated with spending for health services; they represent potential savings in the use of health resources."[39,40] In other words, direct benefits are estimations of savings on direct costs. These terms are often subdivided into direct medical costs as described above and then direct nonmedical costs that include patient telephone expenses, taxi and parking fares, etc.

INDIRECT COSTS

Rice[39,40] provided a systematic method of measuring indirect costs. Her estimates include wage and productivity losses resulting from illness, disability, and death based on age and sex for major causal categories of morbidity and mortality. Indirect benefits represent the potential savings on indirect costs. Despite extensive treatment in the literature, indirect benefits can be difficult to quantify. They are the result of the avoidance of earnings and productivity losses that would have been borne without the health program in question.

INTANGIBLE COSTS

Intangible costs of ill health are difficult, if not impossible, to measure. These costs may be described as the "psychic" costs of disease such as those incurred from pain, suffering, and grief.[41,42] The measurement of such intangible benefits poses a most challenging task. Mishan[43] emphasizes that attempts should be made to account for these valuable "spillover" effects, if at all possible.

DISCOUNT RATES

All benefits and costs that occur at different times must be adjusted to reflect comparable values. This is accomplished by converting dollar amounts into present values through the use of an interest rate referred to as the discount rate. Although most economists agree that discounting is essential, there is much discussion as to the appropriate rate for any given situation. The consequences of choosing a high or a low discount rate are clear: a low discount rate favors projects with benefits accruing in the distant future, while a high rate favors projects with costs in the distant future.[44–47] One commonly used rate is the current yield rate on long-term government bonds. This seems practical because it represents a riskless long-term alternative use of funds by a tax-free institution and, therefore, appears valid for use by hospitals in evaluating long-term investment proposals. Theoretical support can be found in the literature for practically any figure between the pure time-reference (riskless) rate, as low as 4%, and the corporate return on capital, approximately 20%.[48–50]

Cost-benefit methodology is based upon certain assumptions. It is important to have these assumptions clearly in mind before proceeding. The basic assumptions of CBA are as follows:

1. It is possible to separate one service from another service in a sensible way.
2. There is a possibility of choice between the interventions.
3. It is possible to estimate the outcomes associated with each service.
4. It is possible to value these outcomes.
5. It is possible to estimate the cost of providing each service.
6. These costs and benefits can be weighed against each other.
7. The goal should be to provide only those services/treatments in which the benefits outweigh the costs.

Using these assumptions, there are several mathematical methods for developing the classic benefit to cost ratio. All have the same objective, but they differ in the way in which they handle the data mathematically.[51,52] The most common method is the following calculation:

$$\text{Cost Benefit Ratio} = \frac{\sum_{t=1}^{n}[B_t/(1+r)^t]}{\sum_{t=1}^{n}[C_t/(1+r)^t]}$$

where B_t = total benefits for time period t, C_t = total costs for time period t, r = discount rate, and n = number of time periods. The decision criterion is as follows:

If B/C > 1, then benefits exceed costs and program is socially valuable.

If B/C = 1, then benefits equal costs.

If B/C < 1, then benefits are less than costs; therefore, program is not socially beneficial.

Table 113-4. Sample Comparison Using Three Different Cost-Benefit Equations

	COSTS STARTUP $t(0)$	BENEFITS END OF FIRST YEAR $t(1)$	1 COST BENEFIT RATIO (B/C)	2 NET PRESENT VALUE (B−C)	3 INTERNAL RATE OF RETURN (B−C)/C
Program A	$10,000	$15,000	1.5:1	$5,000	50%
Program B	$100,000	$180,000	1.8:1	$80,000	80%

A major problem with any economic analysis is in choosing "r," the discount rate that was discussed earlier.

The more popular equation used in cost-benefit analysis relates to the logical concept of net benefit and net present value (NPV) represented in the equation below.

$$\text{Benefit-Costs} = \text{NPV} = \sum_{t=1}^{n}[(B_t - C_t)/(1+r)^t]$$

The results of these equations can be misleading, depending on the potential differences in the magnitude of dollars and time involved when comparing the costs and benefits of competing programs. In Table 113-3, there is comparative information about the formulae and factors for pharmacoeconomic calculations. In Table 113-4 simplified versions of three different cost-benefit approaches have been presented to illustrate how the decision factors may vary. The third approach presented in the table includes calculation of a "rate of return" on the investment, which is a rearrangement of the above equations to allow calculation of the "rate of return" from an initial program investment over a potential stream of benefits over time. From these various calculation options, one must select which formula is most appropriate in their institution or setting and perhaps the calculated answers from all three CBA equations should be presented in the report. Many economists recommend the net present value (NPV) approach because of the problems with comparing ratios.

In the example provided in Table 113-4, Program A might represent a proposal for a medium-size computer in the pharmacy while Program B might represent a large computer system with multiple decentralized terminals. Although Program B has a higher cost-benefit ratio and rate of return, it is an expensive system and the pharmacy may not be able to commit such a substantial amount of funds. Numerous other examples could be considered here which change the results from the various formulas and make it more difficult to select between programs.

It should be emphasized that, for the numbers presented in this example, the calculations have been greatly simplified. The calculations and comparisons become more complex as benefits are accrued at different increments of time and as costs and benefits are properly discounted with the more complete formulas presented earlier.

If a new project involves start-up costs, such as a laminar flow hood for a home IV service, calculations from the above formulas can be considered. If there are extra benefits accrued by an efficient distribution system, the amount of money that must be saved as benefits each year becomes similar to paying off a start-up loan (SL) over time (t) with interest rate (r) and with extra yearly benefits (Bx). Therefore:

$$Bx = SL[r/1 - (1+r)^{-t}]$$

COST-EFFECTIVENESS ANALYSIS (CEA)

Requirements for Cost-Effectiveness Analysis[53–55] are that:

1. The optimal alternative (not necessarily the least costly) for accomplishing an objective should be possible;
2. At least two alternative interventions should be possible;
3. It need not be cost-reduction analysis but rather an optimizing process; and

4. The outcomes of the alternatives can be quantified using a common unit of measurement.

In CEA, costs are calculated in dollars but alternative ways are then compared for achieving a specific set of results such as blood pressure or life expectancy changes. The objective is not just how to use funds most wisely; CEA also includes the constraint that similar output measurements must be obtained in order to properly compare interventions. Thus, CEA is applied to health matters in situations where the program's inputs can be readily measured in dollars, but the program's outputs are more appropriately stated in terms of the health improvement created (eg, life-years extended). Weinstein and Stason provided an explanation of the use of CEA for the practicing physician as well as for the physician-administrator.[10]

Basic mathematical examples of various economic analyses are presented for cost benefit (Table 113-5), cost-effectiveness (Table 113-6), cost-utility (Table 113-7), and cost-minimization (Table 113-8).[59]

QUALITY OF LIFE OUTCOMES AND PATIENT PREFERENCES

Equally significant and equally misunderstood in pharmacoeconomics and patient outcomes management is the issue of quality of life.[56,57] Although it is recognized that there are physical, mental, and social impairments associated with disease, there is not strong consensus on how to accurately measure these factors. Consequently, the concept of satisfaction with care is often overlooked in cost-effectiveness studies and even the approval process of the Food and Drug Administration (FDA). However, pharmacoeconomics and outcomes research considers quality of life an important predictor in creating a full model of survival and improvement. Quality of life (QOL) is related to clinical outcomes as much as drugs, practitioners, settings, and types of disease. The question is how to select and utilize the most appropriate instruments (sample titles listed in Table 113-9) for measuring quality of life and satisfaction with care in a meaningful way.

Another important aspect of quality of life research is the number of healthy years within life extension. In an average life span of 73 or 74 years, people may have about 11 or 12 dysfunctional years. Therefore, whenever one examines the pharmacoeconomic impact of pharmaceuticals, one should adjust for the

Table 113-5. Cost-Benefit Analysis Example

	COST OF THERAPIES	
	DRUG A	DRUG B
Costs		
Acquisition Cost	300	400
Administration	50	0
Monitoring	50	0
Adverse Effects	100	0
Subtotal	500	400
Benefits		
Days at Work ($)	1000	1000
Extra Mos of Life ($)	2000	3000
Subtotal ($)	3000	4000
Benefit to Cost Ratio:	3000/500	4000/400
	= 6:1	=10:1

Table 113-6. Cost-Effectiveness Analysis Example

	COST OF THERAPIES ($)	
	DRUG A	DRUG B
Costs		
Acquisition Cost	300	400
Administration	50	0
Monitoring	50	0
Adverse Effects	100	0
Subtotal	500	400
Outputs		
Extra Years of Life	1.5	1.6
Cost-Effectiveness		
Ratio:	500/1.5	400/1.6
	=$333[a]	=$250[a]

[a] Per extra year of life.

Table 113-8. Cost Minimization Analysis Example

	COST OF THERAPIES ($)	
	DRUG A	DRUG B
Costs		
Acquisition Cost	250	350
Administration	75	0
Monitoring	75	25
Adverse Effects	100	25
Subtotal	500	400
Outcomes		
Antibiotic Effectiveness	90%	90%
Result = Cost of Drug A > Cost of Drug B		

Note: In cost minimization, both interventions (drugs) are considered to be equally effective; and in this example, the cost minimization question is answered by stating that Drug B is $100 less than Drug A.

quality of life of any extra years to reflect whether this increase leads to full, healthy years or includes some dysfunctional adjustments as well. Likewise, if adjustments are not made for comorbidities, the resulting health profile may be skewed. For example, untreated hypertension may escape a quality-of-life measurement because it does not overtly affect daily life. But a myocardial infarction, for example, would definitely lessen quality of life. The FDA has been leery of drugs that make patients feel better while life expectancy is reduced. Nevertheless, one must be able to present to patients the different probabilities between perfect health and death, the compromises associated with different treatments, and then administer care accordingly. To present these probabilities, though, one must monitor what happens to patients during clinical treatments over time and collect data on their utilities. This means that one should ask patients how they feel about their therapy options, which therapies they prefer, and how their quantity and quality of life are affected. Pharmaceutical companies have sponsored work that examines probabilities, utilities, and cost-effectiveness and then charts the results over time.

QALY (quality adjusted life year) has become a major term in pharmacoeconomics. It is a measure of health improvement used in cost utility analysis (CUA). It combines mortality and QOL gains and considers the outcome of a treatment measured as the number of years of life saved, adjusted for quality. See Table 113-7 for a cost-utility example that illustrates the basic calculations on how the number of life years is adjusted for quality.

DECISION ANALYSIS

Weinstein and Fineberg define decision analysis as ". . . a systematic approach to decision making under conditions of uncertainty." Decision analysis is an approach that is: explicit, quantitative, and prescriptive.[5]

It is explicit in that it forces the decision maker to separate the logical structure into its component parts so they can be analyzed individually then recombined systematically to suggest a decision. It is quantitative in that the decision maker is compelled to be precise about values placed on outcomes. Finally, it is prescriptive in that it aids in deciding what a person should do under a given set of circumstances. The basic steps in decision analysis include identifying and bounding the decision problem; structuring the decision problem over time; characterizing the information needed to fill in the structure; and then choosing the preferred course of action.

Table 113-7. Cost-Utility Analysis Example

	COST OF THERAPIES ($)	
	DRUG A	DRUG B
Costs		
Acquisition Cost	300	400
Administration'	50	0
Monitoring	50	0
Adverse Effects	100	0
Subtotal	500	400
Utilities		
Extra Years of Life	1.5	1.6
Quality of Life	.33	.25
QALYs[a]	0.50	0.40
Cost to Utility Ratio:	500/0.5	400/0.4
	= $1000[b]	= $1000[b]

[a] QALYs = Quality Adjusted Life Years.
[b] Per extra quality adjusted life year.

Table113-9. Outcomes and Quality of Life Measurement Approaches

I. Basic Outcomes List
   A. Death
   B. Disease
   C. Disability
   D. Discomfort
   E. Dissatisfaction
II. Major Quality of Life Domains
   A. Physical status and functional abilities
   B. Psychological status and well-being
   C. Social interactions
   D. Economic status and factors
III. Expanded Outcomes List
   A. Clinical End Points
      1. Symptoms & Signs
      2. Laboratory Values
      3. Death
   B. Functional Parameters
      1. Physical (activities)
      2. Mental (depression)
      3. Social (fiends)
      4. Role (work)
   C. General Well Being
      1. Pain
      2. Energy/Fatigue
      3. Health perceptions
      4. Opportunity (future)
      5. Life satisfaction
   D. Satisfaction with Care
      1. Access
      2. Convenience
      3. Financial Coverage
      4. Quality
      5. General
III. Sample of Instruments for Outcomes Measurement
   A. Generic Instruments—SIP, Nottingham, QWB, SF-36, EQ-5D
   B. Specific Instruments—Pain, Arthritis, Epilepsy, Cancer, COPD, GI

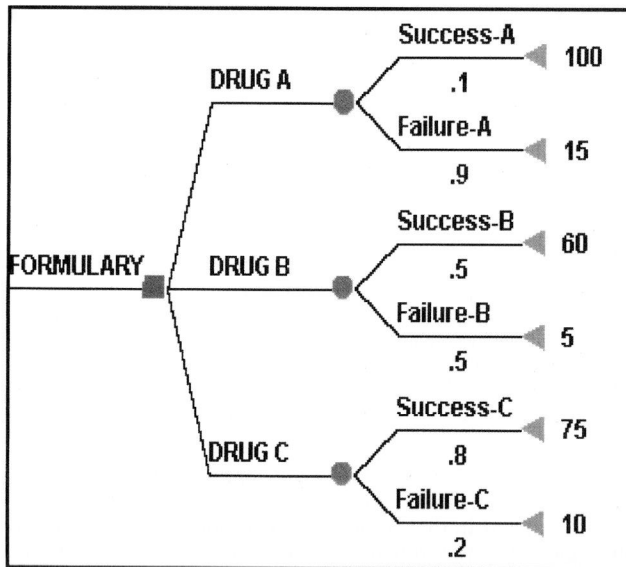

Figure 113-1. Decision tree. Note: this decision tree is constructed from the same numbers in Table 113-10. For example, the numbers listed on the far right of this tree are utility values which could represent quality of life scores or cost. The calculations in basic trees are performed the same

Decision trees, as illustrated in Figure 113-1 may be considered by the reader to be the most familiar image for decision analyses. It is important to remind ourselves that the mathematics along a horizontal "branch" in decision trees can be converted to rows in a spreadsheet (Table 113-10).[61] Even more importantly we must realize that there are other, theory related, alternative mechanism (in addition to the traditional decision trees) that are being utilized and published in the health care evaluations.[58,59]

In this example, quality of life and cost data may be incorporated into the utility score (U). Utility scores can be ascertained from previous research, expert panels, practitioners, and/or from patients themselves. If desirable and possible, the utility score could in fact be replaced with "net benefits" in dollars (benefits minus costs) of one therapy over another. As the table shows, one is seeking the therapy that generates the highest expected utility. If the outcome of the study is focused on cost, then one is usually seeking the intervention with the lowest expected value. Using decision-analysis concepts, researchers can construct decision tree models of what actually happens to the patient from diagnosis to cure. As a result of utilizing such analytical approaches, one can more clearly see not only costs, but also the probability of entering one health state over another. For example, with the visual decision tree in Figure 113-1, one should be able to more clearly understand the pharmacoeconomic implications of the health states related to success or failure with different therapies.

Another alternative decision-making approach is Multi-attribute Utility Theory (MAUT). MAUT is a procedure for identifying, characterizing, and comparing the variables that may affect a decision. Each criteria in a MAUT decision is usually given a different weight, often provided from an expert panel, and the total scores for each intervention option are mathematically calculated. MAUT has been used to analyze managerial and policy decisions and it is used in health care publications for providers and patients.[60] MAUT methods are useful when conducting cost-consequence analysis where multiple outcomes are included in the analysis.

From computer modeling, one can develop treatment protocols. Each branch of a decision tree designates specific treatments for patients at specific health states. In a simplified form, a decision tree can double as an educational tool for presenting available therapy options and probable consequences to the patient.[61,62]

Wennberg has been exploring ways to involve patients in a shared decision-making process.[62] One of his projects involved a computer interactive program on prostrate surgery education. The program explains to patients the probability of success, what degree of pain that might be encountered at each step, and what the procedure actually entails. After viewing this program with visual graphic depictions of the surgery, many of the patients changed their decisions about wanting surgery over watchful waiting. This reduction in a major procedure resulted from a greater focus on quality of life and patient satisfaction. With further evaluation and perhaps modification of the computer program, it should also produce more cost-effective care. Wennberg's work is an application of outcomes research which helped to weigh costs, utilities, and quality of life for the patient.

DEVELOPING A FORMULARY LIST–RANKING PRIORITIES

Table 113-11 illustrates how cost ratios can be used to rank alternative therapies as one might do for a drug formulary. The numbers in the second column of the table lists the total quality-adjusted life years (QALYs) for all of one's patient population benefiting from the treatment options in each row. The numbers in the third column lists the total cost of treatment for all of one's targeted patient population for each treatment option in each row. For the next step in the selection process, rank the therapy options by their cost-effectiveness ratios. Options have already been ranked appropriately in this table. For the final selection step, add each therapy option into one's formulary, moving down each row until your allocated budget is exhausted. In other words, if you have only $420,000, you would be able to fund therapies A, B, and C. These options have the best cost-utility for one's population given one's available budget. Cost effectiveness and cost utility ratios are sometimes presented in similar fashion and are called League Tables. Tengs et al[63] have published an extensive list of interventions (Table 113-12) and Neumann and

Table 113-10. Example of Expected Utility Calculations Often Seen in Decision Tree Analysis

	OUTCOME	UTILITY (U)	PROBABILITY (P)	EXPECTED UTILITY (U × P)	TOTAL EXPECTED UTILITY	RANK
DRUG A	Success	100	0.1	10		—
	Fail	15	0.9	13.5	23.5	Third
DRUG B	Success	60	0.5	30		
	Fail	5	0.5	2.5	32.5	Second
DRUG C	Success	75	0.8	60		
	Fail	10	0.2	2	62	First

Note: The drug with the highest expected utility is the preferred therapy (ie, Drug C).

Table 113-11. Health Economic Selections With Fixed Budget

THERAPY OR PROGRAM	QALYS[a]	COST[b] ($THOUSAND)	C/U RATIO ($THOUSAND)
A	50	100	2
B	50	200	4
C	20	120	6
D	25	200	8
E	10	120	12
F	5	80	16
G	10	180	18
H	10	220	22
I	15	450	30

[a] Total Quality Adjusted Life Years (QALYs) for all of patient population benefitting.
[b] Total cost of treatment for all of targeted patient population.
Selection procedure: first, rank therapies by cost-effectiveness ratios, then add therapy options until budget is exhausted.

colleagues[64] maintain a website with a substantial list of cost utility ratios based on health economic studies.

These listings must be used with caution, because there are a number of criticisms of rankings with cost outcome ratios, often called league tables, including[9]:

- Different reports use different methods
- What were the comparators (eg, which drugs, which surgeries)?
- Difficult to be flexible about future comparators
- Orphan and rare disease consideration
- Randomized trials versus epidemiology
- Regional and international differences in resource use
- Regional and international differences in cost
- Confidence intervals of findings
- Difficult to test statistical significance between treatments but can consider financial impact

INCREMENTAL ANALYSIS

Whether one is dealing with cost analyses or decision analysis, it is important to properly compare one treatment to another, and one should understand the concepts in incremental analysis. Incremental analysis does not mean that one is adding a second therapy to the patient's regimen, but it is a technique for

Table 113-12. Comparison of Interventions—Cost per Life Year Gained

INTERVENTION CATEGORY	NUMBER OF STUDIES	MEDIAN COST PER LIFE-YEAR ($)
Child Immunization	6	<0
Drug & EtOH Tx	4	<0
Beta-Blocker post MI	4	2,000
Tuberculosis Tx	2	9,000
Smoking Advice	15	6,000
Hypertension Tx	6	15,000
HIV/AIDS Tx	6	23,000
Hormone Replacement	13	42,000
Renal Dia. &/or Transplant	22	44,500
Heart Transplant	2	54,000
Radon Control	7	141,000
Cholesterol Tx	19	154,000
Vinyl Chloride Control	2	1,614,000
School Bus Safety	8	1,757,000
Asbestos Control	41	1,865,000
Benzene Control	27	14,153,000
Radiation Control	28	27,386,000

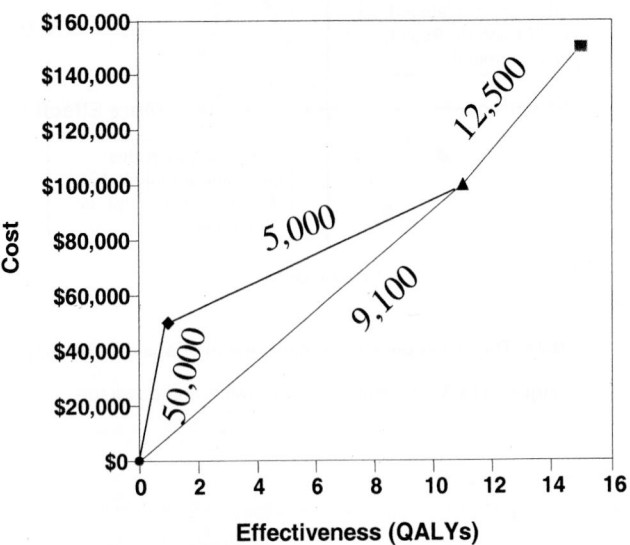

Incremental Cost-Effectiveness Analysis At Various Treament Options

- • Control ($0, 0 QALYs)
- ◆ A1 ($50000, 1 QALYs)
- ▲ A2 ($100000, 11 QALYs)
- ■ A3 ($150000, 15 QALYs)

- ◆ Dominated treatment

Figure 113-2. Incremental analysis and slopes.

comparing one therapy to another. The basic incremental formulas are as follows:

$$\text{CEA: } (\text{Cost}_1 - \text{Cost}_2) / (\text{Effectiveness}_1 - \text{Effectiveness}_2) \text{ or}$$

$$\text{CUA: } (\text{Cost}_1 - \text{Cost}_2) / (\text{Utility}_1 - \text{Utility}_2) \text{ or}$$

As illustrated in Figure 113-2 and explained by Drummond et al, suppose one is interested in program treatment A2 which could be a new vaccination program or a new drug proposed for formulary adoption and reimbursement. Compared to placebo or doing nothing, A2 costs an additional $100,000 and provides 11 extra QALYs in the population, with an incremental cost-effectiveness ratio of $9,100 per QALY. This might be the figure included in a league table for comparison to other interventions or formulary drugs. The cost per QALY ratio between two points is given by the slope of the line. But suppose current practice is to have program A1. This costs $50,000 but generated only 1 QALY. If one compares A2 with A1, a more acceptable incremental cost-effectiveness ratio of $5000 per QALY is obtained. But A1 is a "dominated" program and should not be considered in the relevant set of alternative therapies. This illustrates that the incremental analysis of A2 over A1 could be misleading.

An interesting way of presenting this information is illustrated in Figure 113-3. By thinking of this information in quadrants, one can more easily visualize the relationship between therapies. Drugs that are cheaper and more effective would fall in the "accept" or "dominant" sector, while drugs that are more expensive and less effective would be "dominated" (ie, overshadowed, discouraged from use) by better treatments that are more cost-effective. The slopes of the lines represent the incremental cost ratios and, in general, therapies between $20,000

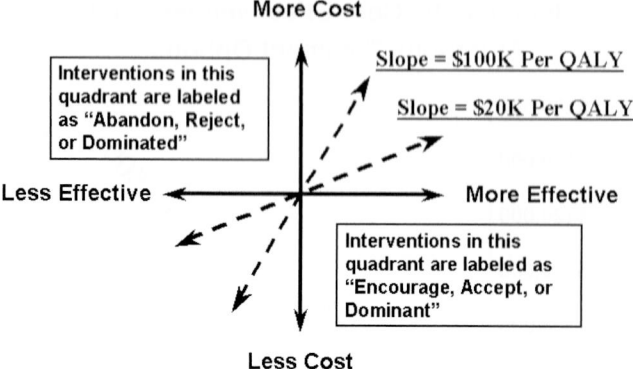

Note: The center point is the comparison or standard therapy

Figure 113-3. Pharmacoeconomic ratios and quadrants.

to $100,000 per life year saved (or per QALY) are often considered acceptable in public policy reports.

A classic manuscript involving incremental analysis deals with the comparison of tissue plasminogen activator (TPA) to streptokinase.[65] In this study, the important question did not involve looking at the CEA ratio of each drug individually; but instead, it analyzed the incremental differences of the new drug TPA over the standard therapy at the time. The analysis demonstrated that TPA, when compared to streptokinase, had an incremental cost per life year saved of about $40,000 which was considered a socially acceptable value.[65]

PHARMACOECONOMIC CONSULT FORM

Figure 113-4 provides a basic consult form that suggests a framework for pharmacoeconomic assessments. If a decision needs to be made between alternative treatments, this form could help structure the calculations and considerations related to pharmacoeconomics. This consult worksheet is a template for evaluating therapy options for a drug formulary, framing a formal pharmacoeconomic study, or the worksheet could be used for a basic pharmacoeconomic calculation sheet to be discussed with a physician or patient and then placed in a patient's record. At an individual patient level, it might be difficult to have the time with each patient to consider complicated discounting calculations.

CHECKLIST AND SCORING FORM FOR A PHARMACOECONOMIC STUDY

In Table 113-13 the reader is provided with an evaluation checklist that includes a weighting system for evaluating an article or a research proposal. This form could be utilized for an external review or self-assessment of a research proposal. It could also be utilized to compare several articles to determine which articles are more rigorous than others. This comparison might be useful in formulary decisions when comparing several articles on alternative treatments.

DISCUSSION

A key impact that the profession of pharmacy needs to give more attention to is the idea that the greatest benefit we can generate for society as a whole is to target and take more responsibility toward decreasing mortality, not just decreasing morbidity. Giving extra years of life to a patient population can be converted to dollars for society, which greatly enhances the benefit-to-cost ratio of a program. Substantially more research remains to be performed on the potential impact of pharmacists and their services on mortality rate. Computer technology and the Internet are tremendous resources for learning and applying these evaluation techniques, and then continually documenting outcomes for practitioners and patients.[66] It is expected that reimbursement plans will include more incentives for documented decreases in patient morbidity and mortality.

Pharmacy practitioners and managers must consider cost-benefit and cost-effectiveness based on the outcomes of the services that pharmacy delivers and the impact that pharmacy services can provide. There are a number of ways that the profession of pharmacy can produce positive outcomes on hospital services. For example, pharmaceutical services can:

- Decrease morbidity in patient populations
- Increase the percentage of patients in therapeutic control
- Reduce the overall costs of the treatment by utilizing more efficient modes of therapy
- Reduce the number of physician visits
- Reduce the rate of hospitalization attributable to or affected by the improper use of drugs
- Contribute to better use of health manpower by utilizing computers and technicians
- Decrease the incidence and intensity of iatrogenic disease, such as adverse drug reactions

Other examples of the types of pharmacy services and their potential benefits and effects include patient consultation, which improves patient compliance, reduces medication errors, reduces misuse of medication, and provides efficient use of all personnel. A unit dose distribution program can improve patient therapy while reducing drug waste and, perhaps, nursing personnel costs.

By monitoring drug therapy in acute care situations, pharmacy can provide early detection of therapy failure or adverse reaction. Admixture programs provide better intravenous therapy and possibly more efficient use of personnel. Under patient and therapy responsibilities, drug prescribing by pharmacists might be added, which can be highly cost-effective. What is being performed in defined patient care situations is substituting a pharmacist's salary for that of a physician, which may be two or even three times greater. Pharmacists can be very beneficial in the areas of patient discharge interviews and in recording patient histories. Under personnel substitutions, one can look at ways that pharmacists can increase physician productivity and, by using computers and technicians, how the pharmacy salary budget can be best allocated.

In this chapter, a general explanation of pharmacoeconomics has been provided with the intent of helping the reader in cost-justification efforts and providing cost-effective outcomes. There are encouraging reports in the literature that demonstrate that pharmacists can have cost-beneficial effects in a numerous areas. Still, it must be realized that even though this research is positive, there is a need to continue to develop programs that maximize the benefit-to-cost ratio to society and to institutions. Even though a pharmacy endeavor can demonstrate a positive ratio of benefit to cost, society or the institutions will ultimately invest their resources in programs that have the higher benefit-to-cost or the best cost-utility ratio. Similarly, the health system must be convinced that these beneficial pharmacy services are worth utilizing with modification or even deletion of other less effective programs if necessary. Pharmacy managers must fully understand these evaluation tools if their programs are to thrive in the future.[67]

PHARMACOECONOMICS CONSULT:
BASIC CALCULATION SHEET

I. ID NUMBER:

II. TREATMENT OBJECTIVES:

III. PERSPECTIVE:	☐ Society	☐ Patient	☐ Payer	☐ Provider	☐ Hospital	☐ Other
IV. TYPE OF ANALYSIS:[a]	☐ COI	☐ CMA	☐ CBA	☐ CEA	☐ CUA	☐ Other

V. TREATMENT OPTIONS:

	Treatment A	Treatment B
Names of Treatment:		
Disease/Symptom:		
Major Outcome Measure:		

VI. COST FACTORS

	Treatment A	Treatment B	Incremental
A. DIRECT COSTS: (HEALTH CARE RESOURCES)			
Practitioner			
Clinic/Hospital			
Acquisition			
Administration			
Monitoring			
Managing			
ADRs			
_____			
_____			
B. DIRECT COSTS: (NON-HEALTH CARE RESOURCES)			
Transport			
Telephone			
_____			

	Treatment A	Treatment B	Incremental
C. INDIRECT COSTS			
Morbidity Costs (time lost from work in dollars)			
Mortality Costs (time lost from work in dollars)			
D. INTANGIBLE COSTS (difficult to put in dollars)			
Discomfort/Pain			
Emotional			
QOL Quality of Life Index (as percentage of full health)			
TOTAL COST			

VII. MEASUREMENT CONSIDERATIONS
of effectiveness, benefit, or utility.

Unit of measurement
COI	(direct and indirect costs of illness)
CMA	(input costs only, outcomes assumed equivalent)
CBA & NB	(input = $, outcomes all in dollars)
CEA	(input = $, outcomes in natural units, mmHg, etc.)
CUA	(input = $, outcomes in utiles, QALYs)
Other	

VIII. CALCULATED RESULTS:
(Ratios are results of Outcomes divided by Inputs.)

		Treatment A	Treatment B	Incremental
COI	(direct & indirect costs of illness)			
CMA:	(total direct & indirect costs)			
CBA:	(benefit over cost ratio)			
[NB:	(benefit minus cost)]			
CEA:	(cost over effectiveness over ratio)			
CUA:	(cost over utility ratio)			
Other:				

[a] See calculation formula table for definitions.
From McGhan WF, Smith MD. *Pharmacy Business* 1993; (Spring):6.

Figure 113-4. Pharmacoeconomic consult template.

Table 113-13. Evaluation Criteria for Assessing a Pharmacoeconomic Study

EVALUATION CRITERIA	RELATIVE CRITERIA WEIGHT/IMPORTANCE (SCALE 0 'NOT APPLICABLE' TO 10 'VERY IMPORTANT')	ITEM QUALITY SCORE (SCALE 1 'NOT AT ALL SATISFACTORY' TO 10 'TOTALLY SATISFACTORY')
1. APPROPRIATE QUESTION? Was a well-defined question posed in answerable form? Did the study examine both costs and effects of the service(s) or program(s)? Did the study involve a comparison of alternatives? Was a viewpoint for the analysis stated and was the study placed in any particular decision-making content?	_____	_____
2. PROPER ALTERNATIVES? Was a comprehensive description of the competing alternatives given? Were any important alternatives omitted? Was (Should) a do-nothing alternative (be) considered?	_____	_____
3. EFFECTIVENESS DETERMINED? Was there evidence that the program's effectiveness had been established? Has this been done through a randomized, controlled clinical trial? If not, how strong was the evidence of effectiveness?	_____	_____
4. ALL COSTS AND CONSEQUENCES? Were all the important and relevant costs and consequences for each alternative identified? Was the range wide enough for the research question at hand? Did it cover all relevant viewpoints? (Possible viewpoints include the community or social viewpoint, and those of patients and third-party payers. Other viewpoints may also be relevant depending upon the particular analysis.) Were capital costs, as well as operating costs, included?	_____	_____
5. ACCURATE MEASUREMENT? Were costs and consequences measured accurately in appropriate physical units? (eg, hours of nursing time, number of physician visits, lost workdays, gained life-years) Were any of the identified terms omitted from measurement? If so, does this mean that they carried no weight in the subsequent analysis? Were there any special circumstances (eg, joint use of resources) that made measurement difficult?	_____	_____
6. PROPER VALUES ASSIGNED? Were costs and consequences valued credibly? Were the sources of all values clearly identified? Were market values employed for changes involving resources gained or depleted? Where market values were absent (eg, volunteer labor) or market values did not reflect actual values (such as clinic space donated at a reduced rate), were adjustments made to approximate market values? Was the valuation of consequences appropriate for the question posed? (ie, has the appropriate type or types of analysis—cost-effectiveness, cost-benefit, cost-utility–been selected?)	_____	_____
7. DISCOUNTING & TIME ADJUSTMENTS? Were costs and consequences adjusted for differential timing? Were costs and consequences that occur in the future "discounted" to their present value? Was any justification given for the discount rate used?	_____	_____
8. INCREMENTAL ANALYSIS? Was an incremental analysis of costs and consequences of alternatives performed? Were the additional (incremental) costs generated by one alternative over another compared to the additional effects, benefits, or utilities generated?	_____	_____
9. SENSITIVITY ANALYSIS? Was a sensitivity analysis performed? Was justification provided for the ranges of values (for key study parameters) employed in the sensitivity analysis? Were study results sensitive to changes in the values (within the assumed range)?	_____	_____
10. ALL ISSUES DISCUSSED? Did the presentation and discussion of study results include all issues of concern to users? Were the conclusions of the analysis based on some overall index or ratio of costs to consequences (eg, cost-effectiveness ratio)? If so, was the index interpreted intelligently or in a mechanistic fashion? Were the results compared with those of others who have investigated the same question?	_____	_____
Did the study discuss the generalizability of the results to other settings and patient/client groups?	_____	_____
Did the study allude to, or take account of, other important factors in the choice or decision under consideration (eg, distribution of costs and consequences or relevant ethical issues)	_____	_____
TOTAL WEIGHTED SCORE FOR A STUDY IS CALCULATED BY MULTIPLYING EACH OF THE TEN IMPORTANCE WEIGHTS BY ITS CORRESPONDING QUALITY SCORE	_____	_____

REFERENCES

1. McGhan WF. *Hospital Formulary* 1993; 28:365.
2. McGhan W, Rowland C, Bootman JL. *Am J Hosp Pharm* 1978; 35:133.
3. Gold MR, et al. *Cost-Effectiveness in Health and Medicine.* Oxford: Oxford University Press, 1996.
4. Ray M. Am J Hosp Pharm 1979; 36:308.
5. Bootman JL, McGhan WF, Schondelmeyer SW. *Drug Intelligence and Clinical Pharmacy* 1982; 16:235.
6. McGhan WF, Lewis NJ. *Clinical Therapeutics* 1992; 3:486.
7. Enright SM. *Am J Hosp Pharm* 1983; 40:835.
8. Curtiss FR. *Am J Hosp Pharm* 1983; 40:586.
9. Drummond MF, O'Brien BJ, Stoddart GL, et al. *Methods for the Economic Evaluation of Health Care Programs.* Oxford: Oxford University Press, 1997.
10. Weinstein MC, Stason B. *N Engl J Med* 1977; 296:716.
11. Shepard DS, Thompson MS. *Publ Health Rep* 1979; 94:535.
12. Crystal R, Brewster A. *Inquiry* 1966; 3:3.
13. Acton J. *Law Contemporary Problems* 1976; 40:46.
14. Emlet HE Jr. *Analysis in Solutions to National Health Problems.* Presented at the 1968 Joint National Meeting of the Operations Research Society of America, San Francisco, May 1–3, 1968.
15. Gellman DD. *Cancer Med Assoc J* 1974; 4:998.
16. Goldschmidt PG. *Inquiry* 1976; 13:29.
17. Bootman JL, et al. *J Pharm Sci* 1979; 68:267.
18. Bootman JL, et al. *Am J Hosp Pharm* 1979; 36:368.
19. Strange PV, Sumner AT. *N Engl J Med* 1978; 298:372.
20. Cretin S. *Health Serv Res* 1977; 12:174.
21. Mattsson W, et al. *Acta Radiology and Oncology* 1979; 18:509.
22. Stason W, Weinstein M. *N Engl J Med* 1977; 296:732.
23. Estershan RJ Jr, et al. *Cancer* 1976; 37:646.
24. Bryers F, Hawthorne VM. *J Epidemiol Comm Health* 1978; 32:171.
25. Kissick WL. *Health Econ* 1969; 39:44.
26. Klarman H. *Int J Health Serv Res* 1974; 4:325.
27. Klarman H. *Am J Public Health* 1967; 57:1948.
28. Smith W. *Public Health Rep* 1979; 68:267.
29. Mushkin S, d'Accolings F. *Public Health Rep* 1959; 74:338.
30. Pigou AC. *Socialism Versus Capitalism.* London: Macmillan Press, 1947.
31. Prest AR, Turvey R. *Economist Journal* 1965; 75:683.
32. Peters GH. *Cost / Benefit Analysis and Public Expenditures, Paper 8.* London: Institute of Economic Affairs, 1968.
33. Osteryoung J. *Capital Budgeting: Long-Term Asset Selection.* Columbus, OH: Grid Inc., 1974.
34. Silvers JB, Praholed CK. *Financial Management of Health Institutions.* New York: Spectrum Publications, 1974.
35. Van Horne JC. *Financial Management and Policy.* Englewood Cliffs, NJ: Prentice-Hall, 1974.
36. Torrance G. *A Generalized Cost-Effectiveness Model for Evaluation of Health Programs.* Ph.D. Dissertation, State University of New York at Buffalo, 1971.
37. Klarman H. *J Occup Med* 1974 (March):172.
38. Schulbert HC, Sheldon CA, Baker F. *Program Evaluation in the Health Field.* New York: Behavioral Publications, 1969.
39. Rice DP. *Public Health Rep* 1969; 84:91.
40. Rice DP. *Estimating the Cost of Illness.* Health Economics Series No. 6. Washington DC: US Government Printing Office, 1966.
41. Rinehard K, Felsman F, Moody L. *Public Health Rep* 1970; 85:402.
42. Ridker RG. *Economic Cost of Air Pollution.* New York: Praeger, 1967.
43. Mishan EJ. Evaluation of life and limb: A theoretical approach. In Harberger A, et al. *Benefit / Cost Analysis.* Chicago: Aldine-Atherton, 1971.
44. Packer AH. *Operations Research* 1968; 16:227.
45. Klarman H. *Economics of Health.* New York: Columbia University Press, 1965.
46. Marglin SA. *J Econ* 1963; 77:95.
47. Baumol WJ. On the discount rate for public projects. In Haveman R, Margolia J, eds. *Public Expenditures and Policy Analysis.* Chicago: Markham, 1970.
48. Amadio J, Mueller J, Grey R. *Benefit / Cost Ratio.* In Public Health Report, Illinois Department of Public Health, Southern Illinois University: Carbondale and Jackson County Health Department, 1976.
49. Joehnk M, McGrail GR, Degal NJ. *Application of a Benefit / Cost Model to Family Practice.* Prepared by the Department of Health, Education and Welfare. National Technical Information Service No. HRP-0007312, 1975.
50. Cohn E. *Public Expenditures Analysis.* Lexington, MA: DC Heath, 1972.
51. Ruchlin HS, et al. *Economics and Health Care.* Springfield, IL: Charles C Thomas, 1973.
52. Mishan EJ. *Cost-Benefit Analysis.* New York: Holt, Rinehart and Winston, 1976.
53. Goldman TA. *Cost-Effectiveness Analysis.* New York: Praeger, 1967.
54. Goldman TA. *Cost-Effectiveness Analysis.* New York: Praeger, 1967.
55. Bootman JL, Townsend RB, McGhan WF. *Principles of Pharmacoeconomics*, 3rd ed. Cincinnati, OH: Harvey Whitney Books 2004.
56. Ellwood PM. *N Engl J Med* 1988; 318:1549.
57. MacKeigan LD, Pathak DS. *Am J Health Syst Pharm* 1992; 49: 2236.
58. www.treeage.com
59. www.healthstrategy.com
60. Schumacher GE. *Am J Hosp Pharm* 1991; 48:301.
61. Einarson TR, McGhan WF, Bootman JL. *Am J Health Syst Pharm* 1985; 42:364.
62. Wennberg JE. *JAMA* 1987; 258:2568.
63. Tengs TO, Adams ME, Pliskin JS, et al. *Risk Analysis* 15(3):369.
64. www.hsph.harvard.edu/organizations/hcra/cuadatabase/intro.html
65. Mark DB, et al. *N Engl J Med* 1995;332:1418.
66. McGhan W. *Expert Reviews in Pharmacoeconomics and Outcomes Research* 2002; 2(4):89.
67. McGhan WF, Smith MD. *Pharmacy Business* 1993; (Spring):6.

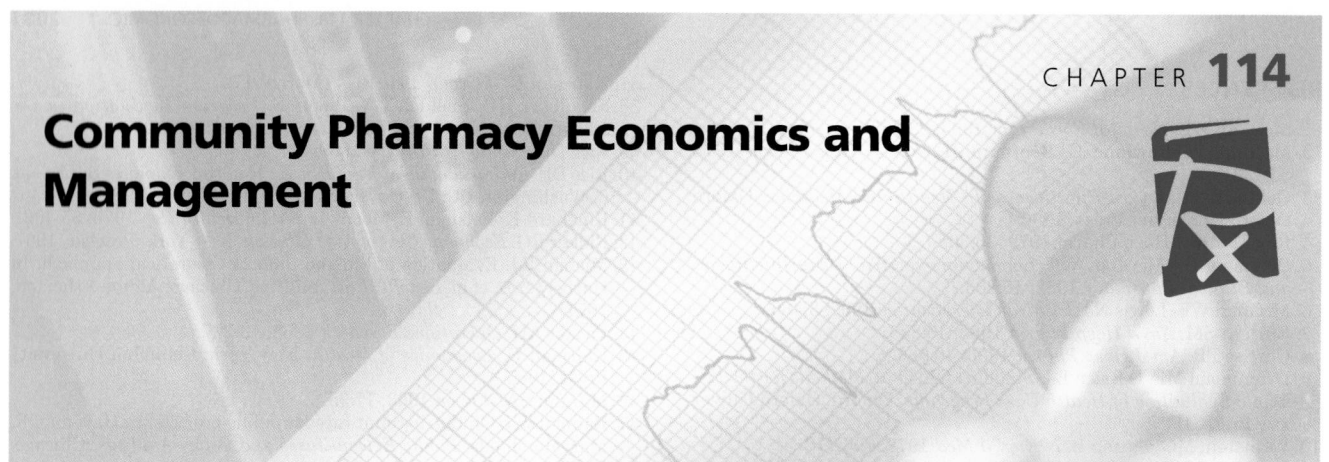

CHAPTER 114

Community Pharmacy Economics and Management

The economic effect of the health-care industry on our society is difficult to evaluate. However, recognizing that health care currently represents over 13% of National Gross Domestic Product (GDP) should give some indication of its effect. It is accepted that advances made by the industry during the past few decades have reduced morbidity and mortality rates that, in turn, have increased productivity and added to the gross domestic product. At the same time, the cost of health care is rising at a faster rate than is the consumer price index (CPI) for all items, and this cost continues to represent an increasingly larger share of the GDP.

ECONOMICS OF HEALTH CARE

According to the US Health Care Financing Administration, Americans spent $969 billion on personal health care in 1997. Projections based on historical trends indicate that personal health-care expenditures may exceed $1.8 trillion by the year 2007. However, the actual level of future expenditures will be determined by the outcome of current efforts to reform the US health-care system. The increase in expenditures for personal health care is the result of a number of factors, including

Population increases and aging of the population.
Inflation (general and medical).
Increased use of facilities and services.
Increased governmental involvement in health care.
Increased quality of care from new technologies, equipment, and drugs.

Further analysis of national health expenditures reveals that a significant portion of personal health costs are paid with public funds. In 1997, governmental outlays represented more than 46% of all health-care expenditures. Medicare payments accounted for a major portion of governmental health-care expenditures. However, state Medicaid programs and other social welfare programs also contributed to the public expenditures for health care.

The magnitude of health-care expenditures in the US and the growing governmental involvement as a third-party payer of health-care costs are evidence of society's commitment to providing the best care possible for all citizens. Those involved in the delivery of health care share society's commitment and, therefore, must be concerned with the economics of the delivery system.

The pharmaceutical segment of the health-care industry entails a significant expenditure. In 1997 more than $108 billion was spent at the retail level for drugs and other medical nondurables in the United States. The 1997 expenditure for prescription drugs represented 7.2% of the nation's personal health bill.

In view of the level of expenditures for drugs and pharmaceutical services and given the trend of health-care costs, it is apparent that those involved in the delivery of pharmaceutical services must be aware of their responsibility to provide high-quality services in the most economical way. Although some look on third-party payment as a mechanism for solving the high cost of health care, including the drug-cost segment, it should be understood that third-party payment does not reduce the cost. It simply spreads it over a larger population.

Actually, third-party payment may increase the total cost of health care as additional administrative costs and increased use of services are inherent in these programs. It follows that third-party payers, whether governmental or private, have an obligation to their constituents to ensure the delivery of quality services at reasonable prices. In this regard, health professionals find their services under scrutiny by a sophisticated group of agencies representing a large portion of the general public.

In recent years, concern over increasing personal health-care expenditures has led to the development of various alternative delivery systems for prepaid health care. These systems, sometimes referred to as managed-care programs, include Health Maintenance Organizations (HMOs), Preferred Provider Organizations (PPOs) and Administrative Service Organizations (ASOs) sponsored by providers of health care.

The objectives of all of the managed-care programs are to provide quality health services while attempting to reduce the rate of increase of health-care expenditures. The cost-containment objective of managed-care programs has generated increased competition among providers, as only the most cost-effective providers are eligible to participate in some programs.

With the development of managed-care programs, those who provide pharmacy services must consider economic and professional factors as they make decisions about participation in the programs. Pharmacy owners and managers face the challenge of maintaining the economic practicality of their pharmacies as participants in managed-care programs.

Participation in such programs often increases administrative expenses for the pharmacy while providing reimbursement that may not be adequate to cover the costs of providing quality pharmacy services. In response to the move to managed-care programs, several pharmacy organizations have formed Pharmacy Services Administrative Organizations (PSAOs) that are attempting to provide an alternative system that balances the public need for cost-effective services with the professional and economic needs of those who provide pharmacy services.

In the past, the cost of health care was given little attention by the providers of health services. It was assumed that the primary obligation of the provider was to ensure the physical well-being of the patient, without regard to cost. It is now apparent that it does little good to develop a level of health care that is unsurpassed in the world if a sizable segment of the population cannot afford to pay for it.

The obligation of health professionals to consider the economic dimensions of health care is now recognized. For example, pharmacy practice laws in all states have been amended to allow pharmacists to practice drug-product selection. These amendments allow the pharmacist, under specified conditions, to choose drug products with due regard for both the physical and the economic well-being of the patient. The drug-product selection amendments are tangible evidence of societal concern with the cost of health care. The concern of health professionals with the cost of health care now reinforces the efforts of consumer groups, government, and others involved in financing health care, to the end of providing the best care for all, regardless of economic status.

According to the Health Insurance Council, comprehensive health-service planning and delivery should be based on the following guidelines.

Health services cost money, and good health service costs a good deal of money. Agencies that spend money on behalf of others have a responsibility to get their money's worth for their beneficiaries.
Financing methods for health service should encourage efficient organization and management of the professional personnel and institutions.
Financing methods should distribute the burden of medical care costs in the way that best assures proper care of the entire population.
Health personnel and institutions must be reimbursed in amounts and by methods that permit them to maintain standards and achieve efficiency.

Although these guidelines are intended for the total health-care system, they may be applied to any segment of the system. The guidelines include concepts that are applicable to pharmacy practice. The guidelines suggest that health insurers promote efficient organization and management of personnel and facilities. It follows that pharmacists should promote efficient organization and management. Using carefully developed organizational plans and modern management techniques, pharmacists in community practice can contribute to the efforts being made to contain health-care costs.

THE COMMUNITY PHARMACY

The majority of consumer expenditures for prescription drugs, proprietary medicines and health appliances are channeled through the over 51,000 community pharmacies in the United States. Although heterogeneous in some respects, as in type of ownership and type of goods and services offered, community pharmacies generally are recognized by the public as the most accessible source of drugs and of information about drugs.

Community pharmacy, as used here, is defined broadly to include all of those establishments that are privately owned and whose function, in varying degrees, is to serve society's need for both drug products and pharmaceutical services. It is difficult to characterize or describe the typical pharmacy because of the great variance among them. They range from the corporately owned chain pharmacy, to the pharmacy department in a supermarket, to the independently owned pharmaceutical center that provides prescription service plus a relatively few lines of health-related products.

According to the operating data submitted to the National Community Pharmacist Association Searle Digest (NCPA; Alexandria, VA) by community pharmacy owners, the average independent community pharmacy generated sales of $1,649,052 in 1997. These data represent a summary of individual pharmacy operating figures that were supplied voluntarily by pharmacy managers and owners.

Note that the editors of the NCPA-Searle Digest make no attempt to structure the sample that comprises the data input and, therefore, their citations are subject to the statistical limitations inherent in the collection of unstructured voluntary

data. It appears, however, that the figures serve to describe fairly accurately the financial profile of the independent community pharmacy.

The data from the 1996 NCPA-Searle Digest indicate that approximately 75% of the revenues of the pharmacies reporting are derived from prescription medications and services. The average prescription charge in 1991, as reported in the NCPA-Searle Digest, was $30.53, compared with an average charge reported 6 years earlier of $22.44. Note that the average prescription charge is not an accurate measure of the price changes for prescription medications. Over a period of years, the types of drugs dispensed have changed with the introduction of new products that usually provide improved drug therapy at a higher cost. In addition, there has been an increase in the number of maintenance drugs prescribed with a corresponding increase in the average number of dosage units per prescription order. Therefore, the average prescription charge in 1997 was for a different mix of prescription products, in larger quantities, than was represented by the average charge in 1991.

CHAIN PHARMACIES—The foregoing discussion dealt mainly with the independent pharmacies that represent approximately 43% of the community pharmacies in the United States. Chain pharmacies also are an important factor in the delivery of pharmaceutical services and products to the public.

There is no consensus on the definition for a chain pharmacy, as there appears to be a question as to what criteria are appropriate for classifying a group of centrally owned pharmacies as chain pharmacies. To some, the matter of central ownership, alone, is sufficient to classify the individual units as chain pharmacies. Another approach is to classify individual units that are owned centrally as chain pharmacies only when there also is centralized organization and management.

The number of centrally owned units also has been used as a method of defining chain pharmacies. However, this criterion does not provide a satisfactory answer to the question, as many multiple-unit pharmacies are owned centrally and yet each unit functions independently from the central ownership. In mode of operation these pharmacies are more similar to individually owned community pharmacies. On the other hand, as the number of units under a central ownership increases, at some point there must be some coordination of policies and activities that results in more central management.

Although it is not possible to establish an exact number of units as the point at which all units assume the characteristics of a true chain pharmacy operation, it appears that there is some relation between the number of units owned and the definition of a pharmacy chain. The US Department of Commerce defines a pharmacy chain as those units with prescription departments that are centrally owned by individuals or organizations who own 11 or more units.

The typical chain pharmacy operates from a broader base in the variety of goods offered for sale than does the independent pharmacy. The kinds of goods offered for sale in chain pharmacies are almost limitless and include durable consumer goods in addition to health-related products.

In this regard it may be somewhat misleading to compare sales in the chain pharmacy with sales in the independent community pharmacy. However, when trends over the past few years are studied, it is apparent that the chain pharmacies have improved their relative position in such areas as revenues from prescription medications and over-the-counter (OTC) drugs.

Establishment of a Community Pharmacy

The pharmacist considering the establishment of a new pharmacy should subject the basic decision to an objective analysis that should include a consideration of community needs—does the community really need another facility for pharmaceutical services? This question may have both a quantitative and a qualitative dimension. Perhaps a given community has a sufficient number of pharmacies and yet none of them is providing the full scope of needed services. If a community need is identified, the analysis should continue in terms of evaluating the various alternatives that are available for satisfying it. Perhaps an existing pharmacy could be purchased and made to provide more-extensive pharmaceutical services or there may be an opportunity to join with another pharmacist in the ownership of an existing pharmacy and establish a group practice. Such alternatives provide the opportunity for improving services to the community while promoting the most efficient use of professional personnel and facilities.

If the analysis indicates that a new pharmacy should be established, the pharmacist must consider a number of questions, some of them simultaneously, eg

What is the appropriate legal organization for the enterprise?
What specific location should be chosen?
How may the necessary capital be obtained?

Although each of the foregoing questions is related to the others and cannot be isolated in a practical situation, each will be treated by itself for purposes of this discussion.

ORGANIZATION

The pharmacist may choose from three widely recognized forms of legal organization for the community pharmacy enterprise. Traditionally, the majority of these have been organized as individual or sole proprietorships, with little governmental control applied to the organizational structure.

In recent years, because of the increase in the joint ownership of pharmacies by two or more individuals, the partnership and corporate forms of organization have become more significant. The partnership, as a form of business organization, enjoys relative independence from governmental control. The corporation, as a creation of the state government, is subject to rather strict governmental regulation. Each form presents advantages that must be weighed against the disadvantages and limitations that become apparent when compared with the alternative forms of organization.

UNINCORPORATED SOLE PROPRIETORSHIPS— The business enterprise owned and managed by an unincorporated sole proprietor is not considered in law a separate legal entity; rather, the owner and the enterprise are considered one. It follows that the risk inherent in establishing a business enterprise in this way has implications for the nonbusiness assets of the proprietor.

The unincorporated sole proprietor has unlimited personal liability. Personal assets are available to satisfy business obligations, and business assets may be used to satisfy personal debts. In return for assuming unlimited liability, the sole proprietor enjoys the freedom to conduct the enterprise in any lawful manner he or she deems appropriate.

Except for the required licenses, the sole proprietor may begin or quit operations without legal formality or governmental permission. Some states do require that a statement of ownership be filed with a designated office when the owner's name is not indicated in the name of the enterprise. The sole proprietor receives all profits from the enterprise.

The size or scope of the operation is not necessarily a determining factor in the decision to organize as a sole proprietorship, as opposed to one of the other forms of organization. However, because of the risks involved and the fact that few persons possess all of the abilities and capacities necessary for carrying on a large complex enterprise, the sole proprietorship most often is associated with smaller, less complex operations.

Historically, the majority of community pharmacists are independent by nature and have chosen this rather informal form of organization. The typical community pharmacy being geographically local and only moderately complex in scope of operation generally succeeds under the unincorporated sole-ownership system.

PARTNERSHIPS—When the resources of one individual are not sufficient to provide a proper base for establishing a pharmacy or when the individual does not wish to assume the entire risk associated with the entrepreneurial function, joint ownership may be considered. Partnership arrangements and incorporation are mechanisms that may be used to broaden the financial or talent base for an enterprise and also may serve to spread the risk. The partnership may be described as an association of two or more individuals based on an expressed or implied contract. They combine their resources as co-owners of an enterprise for their mutual profit. This provides a way for the individuals to do jointly what they could not do separately.

As to liability, a partnership may be described as an association of sole proprietors, because at law the partnership is not considered separate from those who compose it. As with the sole proprietorship, each partner is liable for all debts of the partnership, even to the extent of personal assets. Within the scope of partnership activities, each general partner is considered an agent of the other general partners and, as such, each has the right to bind or commit the partnership in business affairs. Because of the mutual-agency concept and the unlimited liability inherent in partnership associations, it is especially important that the full implications of such an arrangement be understood before adopting this form.

Although it is a contractual arrangement, there are few legal restrictions or regulations applied to the partnership association. No expressed governmental consent is required for establishing or dissolving a partnership, and the contract may be written or simply based on a handshake, as long as the elements of a valid contract are present. This is not to imply that the partnership should be consummated on the basis of an informal verbal agreement. The contractual relation between partners should be verified by a written agreement drafted with the assistance of a lawyer.

The close personal relationship among partners tends to foster a disregard for formalized written documents relating to the operation of the partnership. In the interest of producing a smoothly functioning organization and helping to prevent disagreements among the partners, it is most important that a written partnership agreement be prepared at the outset.

Such matters as the investment, duties, responsibilities, and division of profits and losses of each partner should be considered and incorporated into the partnership agreement. The agreement not only provides a reference for solving future misunderstanding but also serves to compel the partners, at the inception of the agreement, to consider matters that might otherwise remain hidden until a specific problem arises.

The partnership as a form of business organization provides a mechanism for joint ownership of an enterprise that is relatively free of governmental regulation and that embodies the same flexibility of operation enjoyed by the sole proprietorship. As the partnership is not considered a legal entity, it is not required to pay income taxes on profits; rather, the individual partners are assigned their share of profits and pay income taxes on them as individuals.

When compared with the corporate form of joint ownership, the partnership usually presents an advantage to the co-owners with regard to income tax liability. The partnership has been a popular form of organization for the co-ownership of community pharmacies.

CORPORATIONS—Co-ownership also may be effected through a more formal organization known as the corporation, which is a separate legal entity, created by the expressed authority of the state. A properly constituted corporation offers the stockholders the advantage of limited liability for business debts.

In contrast to the sole proprietorship and the partnership, the incorporated business enterprise is considered a separate entity from the persons who own it. Consequently, in the absence of a statute to the contrary, corporate stockholders are liable only to the extent of their contributions to the capital of the enterprise. As a general rule, creditors of the corporation cannot proceed against the individual stock holders for debts of the corporation.

As a legal entity created by the state, the corporation enjoys continuity of life subject only to the limitation(s) included in its charter. The death or incapacity of a stockholder or the transfer of ownership in no way affects the corporate existence.

The corporation provides a way for individuals to invest in a business venture without placing their personal assets in jeopardy. It also provides a convenient, highly organized mechanism for accumulating a large amount of capital from several individuals to establish a business enterprise.

In terms of initial organization, the formation of a corporation is more complex and formal than other types of ownership. Each state has a required procedure to be followed in the creation of a corporation, and once franchised, it is subject to regulation and control by the state.

By definition, the corporation only has those powers and can do those things that are authorized by the state, in contrast to the partnership, which may do any lawful thing agreed to by the partners. The corporation may be dissolved only by or with the expressed consent of the state.

The status of the corporate enterprise as a legal entity makes it subject to local, state, and federal income taxes on its earnings. When the earnings after corporate income taxes are distributed as dividends, the individual stockholders are required to pay personal income taxes on them. As a result, the owners of corporations are said to be subject to double taxation, a factor that in many cases has deterred sole proprietorships and partnerships from adopting the corporate form of organization. However, under special conditions the owners of a corporation may avoid double taxation of profits by requesting designation as a Subchapter S corporation under provisions of the US Internal Revenue Code. If Subchapter S status is granted, profits are not subject to corporate income taxes but are passed through to stockholders and taxed as part of their personal income.

In the field of community pharmacy, the majority of chain organizations are corporations. The corporate form provides the protection of limited liability, which is especially important for larger multiunit operations. In addition, a fair number of the larger nonchain pharmacies are also incorporated, although it should be noted that neither size nor scope of operation is necessarily the only determinant in the decision to incorporate.

In establishing a new pharmacy, the prospective owner(s) must decide at the outset which form of organization to follow. The factors of liability, flexibility of operations, governmental regulation, continuity of life, and income taxes should be considered in relation to the scope of the operation and the personal circumstances of the organizers. It is especially important to seek legal counsel in arriving at a decision.

SITE SELECTION

Much has been written on the criteria that should be employed in choosing a specific community as the site for a new pharmacy. Such factors as population in the trading area, distribution of income among the population, type of industry, and the competitive climate have been cited as being important.

Sometimes a pharmacy is established in a community because the pharmacist-owner is determined to own a pharmacy in a specific community because of personal factors such as family ties, climate, or other appeals of the community. In such cases the decision often is made without regard to the key issue of whether the community needs another facility for pharmaceutical services.

If a need is identified in a given town or city, the selection of a specific site requires careful consideration. The degree of success of a community pharmacy may depend on the choice of the location most suitable among those available. In some cases, the choice of a specific site is extremely limited; the pharmacist must choose from what is available rather than that which is most desirable.

The majority of consumers choose the pharmacy they will patronize on the basis of convenience and accessibility, so long as the pharmacy offers adequate service and fair prices. Therefore, the primary emphasis in site selection should be on obtaining a location that is central to the population to be served. The modern pharmacy must provide easy access and adequate parking. The growth of shopping centers may be cited as evidence of the importance of these factors.

As a general rule, shopping centers are located centrally in relation to the neighborhood, community or region they serve. They provide easy access and adequate free parking.

Interestingly, as a general rule, community pharmacies are more successful in neighborhood and community shopping centers than in the larger regional centers. This tends to substantiate the impression that consumers wish to obtain pharmacy services near home.

Although a site in a neighborhood or community shopping center may be considered a choice location for a new pharmacy, as a practical matter, few independent community pharmacists are able to obtain such locations. Because of the nature of the system used to finance new shopping centers, preference is given by the developers of the centers to large well-established chain pharmacies. However, it appears that there are other suitable locations for a traditional pharmacy that emphasized professional services rather than the sale of non-health-related merchandise.

The island type of location, where the pharmacy sits by itself on a main traffic artery into a suburb and surrounded by adequate parking facilities, has proved to be attractive to consumers. A location within a large medical clinic also may prove to be valuable, although, because of the tendency of patients to obtain prescription service near home, the clinic location may not be so important as some believe.

The selection of a site solely because it is available readily or inexpensively, should be avoided. Usually, a bargain location in terms of rent proves to be a liability rather than an asset in the long run.

The selection of the proper site for a new pharmacy is important especially as it is a decision that the pharmacist may have to live with for 5, 10, or more years, depending on the terms of the lease, if the pharmacy is operated in a rented facility. Whenever possible, advice should be obtained from others regarding site selection. Some wholesale drug firms provide counsel in this regard, or a business consulting firm may be engaged to assist in making an objective evaluation of alternatives.

CAPITAL

Planning and assembling the capital requirements for a new pharmacy are predicated on careful evaluation of projected sales volume, breadth and depth of inventory requirements, and estimated operating expenses. The amount of capital required for the operation of a successful pharmacy is a function of its productivity.

Although certain of the assets required represent a fixed core necessary for any pharmacy, regardless of sales volume, beyond these, the amount of assets required largely depends on the scope of operation and the volume anticipated. As illustrated in Table 114-1, as sales volume increases, investment in inventory, fixtures, and other assets also increases.

Other factors also have an effect on capital requirements. For example, the policy of the owner toward offering credit may require more or less working capital. The mix of sales volume also may affect capital requirements.

The problem of determining capital requirements for a new pharmacy is difficult. Most of the underlying factors are based on conjecture and forecasts regarding the future, for which there is no reliable basis at the outset. However, some

Table 114-1. Balance Sheets for NCPA-Searle Digest Pharmacies under 5 Years Old: 1996 (Averages per Pharmacy)[a]

	SALES UNDER $750,000	SALES $750,000 TO $1,500,000
Assets		
Current assets		
Cash	$ 14,473	$ 35,379
Accounts receivable	15,353	40,097
Inventory	68,113	132,223
Total current assets	$ 97,939	$ 207,699
Fixed assets		
Fixtures and equipment and leasehold improvements (net after reserve for depreciation)	11,019	18,438
Other assets		
Prepaid expenses, deposits, etc.	4,823	8,210
Total assets[b]	$114,781	$ 234,347
Liabilities		
Current and accrued liabilities		
Accounts payable	$ 19,344	$ 47,063
Notes payable (within 1 yr)	9,830	20,573
Accrued expenses and other liabilities	7,173	8,343
Total current and accrued liabilities	$ 36,347	$ 75,979
Long-term liabilities		
Notes payable (later than 1 yr)	40,513	77,181
Total liabilities	$ 76,860	$ 153,160
Net Worth	37,921	81,187
Total liabilities and net worth[b]	$114,781	$ 234,347
Net working capital	$ 61,592	$ 131,720
Sales	$500,014	$1,113,921
Purchases	$363,613	$ 816,748
New profit (before taxes)	$ 10,308	$ 47,101

[a] Source: The NCPA-Searle Digest for 1997.
[b] Excludes land, building, investments and goodwill plus corresponding liabilities.

judgment must be made as to what assets are required for a specific venture, so that the pharmacist may explore the feasibility of assembling a definite amount of capital.

When making the forecasts and estimates needed to establish the basis from which to estimate capital requirements, a sense of conservatism should prevail. The projected sales volume should be estimated at minimum level and operating expenses, at maximum level. It is usually easier to add new capital if sales exceed expectation than it is to recall committed capital if sales are less than anticipated. When operating expenses are estimated on the high side and planned for accordingly with adequate capital, a margin of safety is provided. If expenses are estimated at a level lower than is actually realized, financial difficulty may be encountered.

The method of estimating the capital requirements for a new pharmacy can be described by example. Assume that a conservative estimate indicates that a new pharmacy can produce $750,000 in sales volume during the first year of operation. The question becomes, What kinds of capital will be necessary to support the estimated volume and in what amounts? The answer is as follows: cash, inventory, fixtures, and equipment. The assumption made here is that the owner will not own the building or land used for the pharmacy. The

amount of capital required in each category is related, in varying degrees, to the anticipated sales volume and may be estimated as follows.

CASH—Sufficient cash is needed to pay preopening expenses, operating expenses for a stated period, and some excess for emergency use. Preopening expenses include license fees, legal fees, utility deposits, and advertising. These expenses, with the possible exception of advertising, are fixed relatively for any new pharmacy and are not related to sales volume. They are determined easily and usually total $2000 to $3000. The higher figure will be assumed here.

It is considered good practice to start a new business venture with sufficient cash to pay the first 2 to 3 months of operating expenses, on the theory that the first months of operation may be extremely slow. For a new pharmacy, the amount required may be determined by relating estimated monthly sales volume to operating expense statistics, available from such sources as the NCPA-Searle Digest. Only cash expense items are used in the calculation. Such noncash expenses as depreciation and bad debt losses are not considered.

For a pharmacy in the volume category of this example, the NCPA-Searle Digest indicates that approximately 25% of sales go to cover cash operating expenses, including a salary for the pharmacy owner. Applying this percentage to 3-month sales of a pharmacy with annual sales of $750,000 gives a figure of $46,875 needed to pay operating expenses for a 3-month period. The total amount of cash required for preopening expenses and early operating expenses equals $49,875. In addition, cash is needed to provide the other kinds of capital described below.

INVENTORY—The amount of inventory necessary to support a $750,000 sales volume may be determined by referring to data that give averages for cost of goods sold and annual stock-turnover rates. Again referring to the NCPA-Searle Digest, the cost of goods sold for a pharmacy with sales of $750,000 is approximately 73%, or $547,000. The average annual stock-turnover rate is given as 4.7 for a pharmacy with this sales volume and is determined by division of the cost of goods sold by the average inventory at cost. Knowing the cost of goods sold and the stock-turnover rate, it is possible to estimate the average inventory; in this case it is approximately $116,400.

FIXTURES AND EQUIPMENT—The fixtures and equipment necessary for a new pharmacy also are related to estimated volume. Larger volume means more inventory, which, in turn, requires more fixtures and equipment to facilitate storage and display. The size of the building to be furnished and the quality of fixtures chosen also affects the total expended. On occasion, savings may be realized by purchasing good, used fixtures and equipment, usually available at a fraction of the cost of new ones. A reasonable expenditure for these items for a pharmacy properly equipped to generate annual sales of $750,000 would be approximately $30,000.

TOTAL INVESTMENT AND SOURCES OF CAPITAL—The total investment required for a new pharmacy with estimated sales per year of $750,000 would be approximately $196,275, broken down as

Cash (for preopening and operating expenses)	$ 49,875
Inventory	116,400
Fixtures and equipment	30,000
Total investment	$ 196,275

The total represents the cash value of the assets required to establish the new pharmacy in this example. However, the amount of actual cash needed will be somewhat less than the total amount stated. In most cases, the owner can assemble the required assets by using a combination of equity capital, borrowed capital, and credit.

Equity capital consists of the investment of the owner or owners, and it comes from personal savings or from other sources that require no security and no commitment as to date of repayment. Relatives may be a source of equity capital, either on a co-ownership basis or simply by providing unsecured, undated loans. It is thought that at least one-half to two-thirds of the total requirement should be equity capital, although many successful pharmacies have been established with lower amounts. The amount of equity capital provided influences the availability of borrowed capital and the level of credit that may be obtained by the owner.

Commercial lending institutions, such as banks and savings and loan associations, usually require a substantial equity interest in a new business venture before they consider lending the funds necessary to supplement the owner's contribution. Generally, commercial lending institutions should not be depended on for a significant portion of initial capital needs. Such institutions are limited in the amount of risk they are willing to assume, especially for new ventures.

Trade sources, such as suppliers of fixtures and wholesale drug firms, present the best opportunity for obtaining nonequity capital for the new pharmacy. It is common for wholesalers to supply the opening inventory requirements for a new pharmacy on the basis of approximately 50% of the total cost as a down payment, with the balance to be paid over an extended period that varies with the individual circumstances. Usually, if the time exceeds 90 to 180 days, the supplier attaches an interest charge to the unpaid balance.

The amount of cash required for inventory may be further reduced by cutting back the level of inventory at the outset and then building it up to the required level as operations continue and sales volume increase. Two cautions should be considered in obtaining any significant amount of capital through the use of trade credit:

The interest factor should be studied; depending on the rate and the method of calculation, interest charges can be surprisingly high.
The use of credit simply postpones the underlying obligation to some future date or dates. Repayment of credit obligations should be considered in terms of the practical feasibility of meeting the obligations when they are due.

Fixtures and equipment may be obtained by relatively long-term financing through suppliers, or in some cases through finance companies by a mechanism similar to the one used to finance a personal automobile. Underlying this form of financing is a chattel mortgage that places title to the fixtures and equipment in the hands of the lender as security.

The interest charges from this type of financing may be especially significant, often reaching an effective rate of 15% or more annually. Usually a down payment of one-quarter to one-third of the value of the fixtures is required, with the balance to be paid in installments over as many as 5 years. The scheduled installment payments should be included in long-range financial budgeting and planning.

After the potential sources of capital have been evaluated carefully, it may be necessary to make compromises or adjustments regarding the amounts estimated originally. In some cases the owner will reduce his withdrawals or salary during early operations to reduce the amount of cash needed for operating expenses. Inventories also may be reduced at the outset. In fact, it is considered good practice to hold approximately 20% of the amount budgeted for inventory in abeyance until the needs of the particular community are identified.

The amount required for fixtures and equipment may be reduced by purchasing some used fixtures and equipment. It also is possible to lease fixtures and equipment, although this may increase the cost of fixtures and equipment over the long term. However, such arrangements also reduce initial capital requirements. By these means and through the judicious use of borrowed funds and credit, a new pharmacy may be established with less cash than is indicated by the figure for the total investment.

MANAGEMENT

In general terms, the management function may be described as all those activities involved in the organization and direction of the elements of an economically productive enterprise.

Money, material, equipment, and people must be brought together in the proper relations to one another to achieve the objectives and goals that management has identified. Management practices predicated on predetermined goals and objectives provide for more efficient operation and provide a basis for measuring the effectiveness of management activities.

The management activities of the pharmacist too often consist of handling day-to-day problems and crises. Much of the activity labeled management in the typical community pharmacy is actually routine administrative work that can and should be delegated to nonmanagement personnel. Perhaps this point is best illustrated by the axiom "management's job is not to do, but to get others to do."

The traditional approach to community pharmacy management consisting of the ad hoc handling of problems as they arise is inconsistent with the nature or responsibilities of modern practice. The total of all activities in a pharmacy is becoming increasingly complex, because of increased volume of operations and outside pressures for more efficient delivery of pharmaceutical services and products.

All health workers are being called on to develop a social conscience and assume more responsibility for the economic effect of their activities. Although technological changes may relieve some of the pressure on health-care costs, better management and administrative techniques also can contribute significantly to solving the problem.

The effect of more effective management also may be reflected in improved professional services to the public. For example, a management decision to assign certain record-keeping functions in the prescription department to nonprofessional personnel allows a more economical use of professional staff. At the same time, it provides the pharmacist with more time for consultation with the patient.

The Role of Management

OBJECTIVES AND GOALS—The first role of management for any business enterprise should be to establish the objectives and goals for the organization. Concurrently, management must provide the policies that serve as the framework for accomplishing the stated objectives. For example, one objective might be an atmosphere of patient orientation, the elements of which would need to be identified. Proper record-keeping procedures, facilities for consultations, and patient-oriented personnel would be prerequisite for carrying out this objective.

Working with predetermined objectives provides the manager with a basis for establishing policy and assists in decision making. As in the example cited, the objective has implications in the area of personnel policies and practices. Recruitment and selection techniques geared toward obtaining professional and supporting staff who can function effectively in a patient-oriented environment would have to be developed by the manager.

The kinds of objectives to be established by management might be divided into two categories:

1. A set of rather basic, almost philosophical objectives need to be developed; for example, will the pharmacy stress low prices rather than full service?
2. Objectives concerned with more specific operational matters are needed, as meeting a projected sales volume level during a given year.

In either case, it is management's responsibility to provide a sense of direction by setting forth both basic and specific objectives as guidelines for current and future activities.

Objectives lie in the future and, therefore, are subject to adjustments dictated by forces outside the control of management. Management personnel should keep abreast of those technological, economic, and social changes that relate to stated organizational objectives. In this regard the role of management in establishing objectives and goals must include a mechanism for continuing re-evaluation and updating of objectives.

MATERIAL AND HUMAN RESOURCES—The organization of these resources to pursue the objectives of the enterprise represents the second management function. The kinds and amounts of resources required are largely dictated by the nature of the objectives. The ability to obtain capital, generally considered an entrepreneurial rather than a managerial function, also may influence this management responsibility.

For the typical independent community pharmacy, it is neither possible nor practical to divorce acquisition of capital from its application and management. In most cases, the same person is charged with both functions. Assuming that the required inventories, equipment, and people can be assembled, it remains for management to provide the organizational structure and the coordination necessary to mold these resources into an efficiently functioning community pharmacy.

PLANNING AND CONTROLLING OPERATIONS—Although a major share of the manager's time must be devoted to controlling day-to-day operations, it is important to maintain a balance between the present and the future. Control of current operations far too often becomes the sole function of many managers, who devote little or no time to planning for future operations.

The lack of planning often compounds the problems associated with day-to-day operations, resulting in a situation in which the controlling function requires all of the management effort. For example, many managers spend a disproportionate amount of time ordering merchandise and maintaining inventory when, through a properly planned inventory-control program, this routine activity could be delegated to others.

The brief and simplistic description of management functions given here tends to understate their complexity and significance. Management may be considered an art rather than a science. There are few established laws or formulas for solving the problems inherent in conducting an economically productive enterprise. It especially is difficult to make the numerous and varied decisions required in exercising the management functions. Although there have been attempts to quantify these decisions through the use of mathematics and mathematical models, in the last analysis the human element still dominates the decision-making process.

As management decisions are made and implemented by human beings to affect human beings, it is apparent that those who manage need to consider and study the behavioral and social sciences so they may function effectively. For the community pharmacist who performs the dual role of health professional and manager, such a background especially is appropriate.

Essentially, management is an exercise in group dynamics. The manager must be able to organize, direct, and control a group of individuals toward the stated objectives of the organization. The manager who is unable to obtain the cooperation of his subordinates or who fails to delegate the responsibility for routine operational matters to others is not functioning effectively.

In the community pharmacy the human dimension of management especially is crucial. The nature of the typical community pharmacy is such that the manager constantly is in close personal contact with his employees, suppliers, and patrons.

In such an environment it is difficult to make consistently objective decisions. Further, the dual role of the pharmacist-manager tends to create situations involving conflicts between sound management decisions and professional responsibilities. For example, as a manager, the pharmacist establishes policies regarding the extension of credit to patrons. Yet when a patron with a poor credit rating has an immediate need for prescription medication, the established policies may be waived or adjusted to satisfy the professional obligation of the pharmacist to the patron.

These rather unique characteristics and the need for the pharmacist-manager to be more flexible than those performing the management function in other types of organizations should not be construed to minimize the importance of effective management in the community pharmacy. In the current socioeconomic climate, with increasing costs of operation and pressures to reduce the costs of health care, the management function takes on greater, rather than lesser, significance.

The functions of management provide a somewhat theoretical basis for understanding the overall role of management in the continuing operation of an economically viable enterprise. For practical purposes, however, it may be more valuable to examine the role of management as it relates to the various resources and activities that go to compose the business entity.

In the community pharmacy the following items require effective management: money, inventory, facilities, personnel, credit, and risk. Establishing objectives, organization, planning, and control apply to each of these items, as well as to the pharmacy as a unit. At this level the objectives are more specific, and the organization, planning, and control more definitive.

Consideration of the management of the specific elements that in total represent the community pharmacy does not imply that each element is managed in isolation. There are many interrelations among the various elements, and a decision regarding one element often has an effect on one or more of the others. For example, the decision to expand the inventory may have implications to the management of money, facilities, personnel, and risk.

Money

To a large extent, the success of a community pharmacy depends on the ability to obtain money from various sources in sufficient quantity to acquire and support the resources necessary for operation. Once the money is obtained it becomes management's function to employ it in the most appropriate way to achieve the objectives of the pharmacy.

In its simplest and most pragmatic form, the objective of money management is to maximize the rate of return on investment. Such an objective may appear inconsistent with the responsibilities of professionals engaged in providing health services, yet in the long run the economical use of money is beneficial to society.

In theory, money is in limited supply and demand usually exceeds supply. In the competition for the limited supply, only the most efficient users of money can obtain it. Applying this concept to community pharmacy practice would suggest that only those owners who can manage money effectively, in all its forms, succeed. In a sense, the foregoing concept simply is a statement of the basis of our economic system in which efficiency is rewarded and inefficiency is not.

In the broad sense, money management applies not only to cash but to all those materials and services that are used in the operation of a pharmacy and are purchased with money. Given a limited amount, the manager must make judgments and decisions about the use of the money in terms of the stated objectives.

In this regard conflicts may develop between basic objectives. For example, the objective of maximizing return on investment may conflict with the objective of offering full services, as in the case in which a decision must be made regarding the purchase of a delivery vehicle. The money invested for this purpose represents an inefficient use of money for many pharmacies and thus is contrary to the objective of maximizing return on investment. Yet, for the goal of providing full services to the patrons of the pharmacy to be met, such an investment may be necessary.

The effectiveness of money management may be measured to some extent by the progress made toward meeting noneconomic objectives. For the most part, however, the most meaningful measure of effectiveness is in economic terms, specifically, by the return on investment, which for a pharmacy may be expressed in two ways:

Return on Total Assets—The rate of return on total assets is determined by dividing the total of all assets employed in the pharmacy into the net profit. No distinction is made between owner's equity and borrowed capital in this calculation. This ratio describes the productivity of the total asset investment.

Return on Owner's Equity—The rate of return realized on the owner's investment in the pharmacy is determined by division of the difference between total assets and total liabilities (owner's equity) into the net profit. This ratio describes how well the funds provided by the owners are being used.

The manager may calculate these rates and compare them with national data to obtain some idea of the effectiveness of the money management policies. Rates below the national averages, such as those reported in the NCPA-Searle Digest, may indicate too much investment for the level of operation or the inefficient management of the pharmacy.

In either event, by using the return on investment concept and analyzing the operation of the pharmacy, the manager can identify a problem requiring attention and can take appropriate steps to correct it.

The management of money in terms of both the total commitment of capital and the application of the owner's equity represents only one dimension of the management function in this area. In a narrower sense, money management also is concerned with day-to-day inflow and outflow of cash from operations. The maintenance of balanced cash flow requires the application of the management functions of planning and control.

Budgeting is necessary to assure that sufficient cash is available to meet such obligations as accounts payable, wages, and taxes. To a large extent, cash needs can be anticipated by an analysis of past experiences combined with projections of future operations.

The inflow of cash may be estimated in the same way. Matching cash revenues with cash expenditures is of more than academic significance: both excessive and deficient cash balances may prove to be uneconomical. When more cash is maintained than is necessary for normal operations, the excess represents earning power that is not being used.

For the pharmacy that consistently maintains a balance of several thousand dollars in its checking account, it may be possible to transfer some of the cash to a savings account or to convert the cash into high-quality marketable securities. In this way, the excess cash earns interest or otherwise appreciates and yet still is available easily for emergency use. A deficient cash position presents some obvious problems, including the possible impairment of the firm's credit rating that may have long-term implications.

One problem associated with an unfavorable cash position is inability to pay bills on time. In many cases this results in a loss of cash discounts. It is a common practice for suppliers to allow a 1% or 2% discount for the payment of invoices within a given time. The usual terms allow the discount to be taken if the amount is paid within 10 days of a specified date; otherwise, the full amount is due in 30 days. The buyer is offered what appears to be a small discount for paying the bill 20 days early. In terms of interest rates, however, the 2% cash discount for paying 20 days early represents an annual interest rate of approximately 36%.

For the typical pharmacy, cash discounts can amount to thousands of dollars each year. Too often, managers do not recognize the significance of taking advantage of all cash discounts, and consequently they do not devote sufficient thought to alternative courses of action when faced with an unfavorable cash position. It may be possible to borrow money on a short-term basis at a low annual interest to take advantage of a 2% cash discount representing an effective annual interest rate of approximately 36%.

To some extent, the manager can control the cash flow in the pharmacy. Although certain obligations such as payrolls and taxes are fixed as to time of payment, the manager may be able to influence other aspects of cash flow. Good management of credit and collection procedures, for example, can increase inflow. Proper scheduling of purchases of inventory can effect a degree of control over the timing of the outflow for such purposes.

The manager makes the decisions regarding acquisition of new fixtures and equipment that requires outflows of cash either in a lump sum or in installments. Depending on future prospects for cash inflow, the manager can decide whether to proceed with such acquisitions.

In actual practice, inflow for a given period should be estimated, and known fixed obligations for the same period should be deducted. If a balance remains, this represents discretionary cash available for expenditure. If a negative figure results, it is management's responsibility to attempt to increase inflow or decrease outflow to achieve a balance.

During periods of temporary cash deficiencies, management may be required to obtain additional funds through borrowing. Knowledge of the sources of funds and the cost of such funds is a prerequisite for effective money management.

Inventory

The merchandise inventory represents the largest single asset on the balance sheet for the typical community pharmacy. More than 50% of all assets, excluding real estate holdings, were reported as merchandise inventory for NCPA-Searle Digest pharmacies in 1996. The extent of this investment plus the fact that the inventory requirements for a given pharmacy are in a constant state of flux forces a need for continuing management attention to this area of operation.

It has been stated that the community pharmacist is the buying agent in the community for health-related products. He or she must provide the right products, in the right quantities, at the right time, and at the right prices to serve the needs of patrons.

Because of varying consumer preferences and geographical differences in prescribing habits of physicians, the management of inventory becomes a highly individualized function in each community pharmacy. Given a limited amount of capital and the responsibility to use the capital economically, the manager must develop systems and policies that ensure a continuous flow of needed goods while avoiding the problems of excessive inventory levels.

Although the objective of effective inventory management is stated simply here, in practice it represents one of the most challenging responsibilities of management. In the community pharmacy the management of inventory is complicated by a major portion of the inventory consisting of prescription (legend) drugs. This makes the problem of inventory control in the pharmacy unique in comparison with control in other enterprises that distribute products at the retail level.

The demand for prescription drugs is generated by physicians and other health practitioners rather than by the ultimate consumer. When dealing directly with the consumer, it is easier to manage inventory. Excessive inventory levels can be reduced by special sales and markdowns. These techniques cannot be used to effect reduction in overstock of prescription drugs.

On the other hand, the successful pharmacy depends on maintaining a breadth and depth of prescription drug inventory that is adequate to handle all prescription orders received. Usually, the need for a prescription drug is immediate. The patient cannot wait until it is ordered or is delivered in a few days. The dilemma of the manager in this situation is apparent—that of providing a continuous supply of products that are characterized by an unpredictable and uncontrollable demand.

The management of other segments of the inventory such as OTC drugs, cosmetics, and sundry items, although not subject to the limitations inherent in the prescription drug segment, presents no less a problem to the manager. Changing consumer preferences and pressures by suppliers to buy greater quantities and assortments of OTC drugs and nondrug items increase the need for careful attention to this area of management.

Three basic decisions are required for the effective management of inventory. They are as follows: the specific items to be included in the inventory, the quantity of each item required, and the best source of supply.

The specific items included in the inventory should be chosen according to the needs of the community. Although there is a core of items common to every pharmacy, a significant portion of the inventory is dictated by local demand. In this regard the manager must be objective in the selection of goods and ignore those personal preferences that might influence purchasing decisions. For the newly established pharmacy it is important that a portion of the capital budgeted for the initial inventory is held in reserve until the preferences of the local community are identified. As operations continue, the manager is constantly faced with decisions on additions to the original selection.

Some managers adopt the policy of stocking all new items immediately, as long as the items are related to current merchandise assortments. Other managers adopt the wait-and-see policy, stocking new items only when a local demand is established. Both approaches have advantages and drawbacks.

The wait-and-see manager runs the risk of losing considerable sales volume and, perhaps more importantly, develops a reputation for not having in stock what the patrons desire. On the other hand, the manager who indiscriminately adds all new items to the inventory runs the risk of an overcommitment of capital to inventory, with its serious economic implications. Striking a balance between these two extremes presents a challenge to the manager.

Perhaps as important as the specific items to be included in the inventory is the quantity of each item carried in stock. Assuming that a given item should be stocked, the manager must decide what quantity is necessary. At this point, several decisions must be made, based on a consideration of sources of supply, extent of demand, and such financial factors as quantity discounts and buying terms.

In most instances the manager may choose from alternative sources of supply. Some manufacturers of prescription drugs and many producers of the other goods distributed through pharmacies sell directly to the pharmacy. The pharmacist also may obtain inventory needs from indirect sources, such as wholesale drug companies.

Direct sources offer the advantage of lower prices, whereas indirect sources offer the advantage of faster delivery. Generally, direct purchasing requires a larger commitment to inventory investment because of minimum order requirements established by the manufacturer and increased delivery time.

Indirect sellers, such as wholesale drug firms, usually do not establish a minimum order level and emphasize rapid and frequent delivery service. The quantity of a given item carried in the pharmacy's stock, therefore, is influenced, to some degree, by the source of supply.

Quantity-purchase discounts play an important role in decisions regarding inventory levels. Generally, the purchase of larger numbers or sizes of the items stocked in the pharmacy effects a lower cost per item or unit. Such cost savings can be beneficial to both the owner of the pharmacy and to the public being served. However, note that cost savings on the purchase of goods in larger quantities can be offset by additional expenses that accrue from excessive inventory levels.

The costs associated with maintaining a merchandise inventory include implicit and explicit interest, obsolescence, deterioration, storage, property taxes, and insurance. Generally, these costs increase in direct proportion to the level of inventory.

The capital invested in inventory represents money that could be used in other ways to earn a return. To the extent that such an investment is necessary to generate sales and to earn a profit, it may be said that the investment is economically

sound. However, when the investment in inventory exceeds what is actually required for the level of operation realized, the excess represents an uneconomical use of capital.

For example, assume that a pharmacy has $90,000 invested in inventory. The safest alternative use of this capital might be to buy time-savings certificates at an effective annual rate of 5%. At this rate, the $90,000 would earn $4,500 per year and it can be said that this inventory investment has an implicit interest cost of $4,500. To the extent that the inventory produces net profit in excess of $4,500 the capital represented is being used economically.

Assume further that it can be shown that the $90,000 inventory could be reduced to $80,000 without adversely affecting sales or net profit. In terms of the safest alternative use of funds, the excess inventory of $10,000 is costing $500 per year in interest that could be earned and added to net profit.

An explicit interest cost also may result from excess inventory levels if the capital tied up in inventory is needed to pay other operational expenses. To support current activities, the pharmacy owner may be forced to borrow money at current interest rates. To the extent that the need to borrow is caused by excessive inventory investment, the cost of borrowing should be considered a cost of the excess inventory.

The possibility of obsolescence and deterioration are risks associated with the maintenance of an inventory, and although such risks may result in some unavoidable losses, they are minimized at optimum inventory levels. When the costs of storage, insurance, and taxes are added to the interest factors and to the risk of obsolescence and deterioration, the cost of each dollar invested in inventory can be significant. An awareness of the costs associated with inventory investment proves useful to the manager as he or she makes decisions regarding the types and quantities of goods to be included in the merchandise inventory.

The effectiveness of inventory management traditionally has been measured by the stock-turnover rate (the annual rate of turnover for the inventory). The rate is calculated with the following formula:

cost of goods sold for the year/average inventory at cost
= stock-turnover rate

This rate denotes the number of times, on the average, that the inventory has been sold and replaced during a given year. It represents the turnover of dollars invested in inventory but tells nothing of the turnover of specific items or units that go to make up the inventory. As presented here, the rate relates to the entire inventory of the pharmacy. However, the same concept may be applied to departments if appropriate data are available.

The stock-turnover rate may be calculated for a specific pharmacy and then compared with national averages such as those reported in the NCPA-Searle Digest. The average rate reported by the NCPA-Searle Digest pharmacies for 1996 was 6.6. It generally is assumed that a rate of approximately 5 to 6 times per year is indicative of adequate management of inventory. Rates considerably below this level may indicate an overinvestment in inventory.

Note that pharmacies with rather low sales volumes typically have stock-turnover rates much lower than the average. For these pharmacies, increased sales represent the only real opportunity for improving their position in this area.

The typical community pharmacy with a sales volume near the national average should show an annual stock-turnover rate of at least 5 times/year. If it falls significantly below the average, the management of inventory should be reexamined.

The rate may be improved in two ways. Attempts can be made to increase sales while keeping the inventory level constant. Generating more sales with the same inventory increases the rate. In the event it is not possible to increase sales, the alternative is to reduce the inventory level. With constant sales, this produces a faster rate of turnover.

A combination of the two alternatives, increasing sales while reducing inventory, can have a profound effect on the stock-turnover rate. As a practical matter, the manager may best be able to work toward a reduction of the inventory level as an immediate means of improving the rate. Certain items in the inventory may be returned to suppliers for refunds or credit. Items that cannot be returned may be sold at reduced prices. Most important, buying practices should be reviewed with the objective of reducing purchases until a more favorable rate is achieved.

If a stock-turnover rate of 5 is adequate, a rate of 7 or 8 might appear to be excellent. In some cases this is a valid assumption. However, unless the inventory is managed carefully, high rates may cause problems that are as serious as those resulting from low rates. An extremely high rate may be achieved by ultraconservative buying policies.

Conservative buying betters the rate for capital invested in inventory, but the improvement may prove to be uneconomical in the long run. When undue emphasis is placed on maintaining a high stock-turnover rate, quantity discounts may be lost, resulting in an increase in cost of goods sold. Usually, a pharmacy can afford to do at least some quantity buying, thus realizing the benefits accruing from quantity discounts.

Frequently, buying in small quantities increases the time and effort involved in the buying process. More orders must be submitted and checked in, and more accounting time is required for processing several small orders as compared with a few large ones.

Finally, and perhaps most important, the manager who attempts to control the inventory level too closely runs the risk of frequently being out of items. The disadvantages of this include a reduced sales volume and accompanying gross margin. Further, a reputation for being out of stock may result in a loss of patrons to other pharmacies where their needs are met more consistently.

Through good management, however, it is possible to realize an annual stock-turnover rate higher than the accepted norm without creating the problems described here, and many successful pharmacies do this. However, unusually high rates reduce the likelihood of meeting the objective of having on hand the right goods at the right time, in the right quantity, and at the right price.

In the final analysis, the key to effective management of merchandise is stock control on a day-to-day basis. The manager is responsible for designing policies, procedures, and systems for controlling and maintaining the proper selection and level of goods carried in stock. Proper training of employees in the importance of stock control and proper use of established control systems are the responsibilities of management.

There are several formal systems that may be employed to assist in inventory control. Many pharmacies, for example, maintain and control stock by using computer-based reorder systems. Other firms use the perpetual inventory method of stock control.

The pharmacy manager also can effect reasonable control over inventory by implementing a well-organized visual stock-control system. By predetermining the number of units of each item to be carried in stock, based on estimated sales and adequate turnover, the manager can establish minimum and maximum stock levels for each item. The indicated levels for each item are recorded in an inventory-control book or on the shelf where the item is stored. It becomes a simple task for an employee to check the stock on a regularly scheduled basis and to note those items that should be reordered.

There is nothing profound about such a system, but it does formalize an important function and provides a mechanism for the maintenance of inventory levels. Such a system also forces the manager to think in terms of the minimum and maximum stock levels for each item. This in itself effects a degree of control over the total inventory.

Often, overcommitment of capital to inventory is not apparent until the end of an accounting period, when a physical inventory is made. In many cases the inventory level creeps upward without a corresponding increase in sales.

When little attention is given to a comparison of the inflow of goods against the outflow, it is easy to accumulate excessive inventory. One mechanism that may be used to combat this problem is the buying budget. In its simplest form the buying budget provides a means of dollar control of inventory on the basis of matching purchases with sales. In a pharmacy, each dollar of sales generally represents approximately $0.70 in inventory at cost prices. Assuming a balanced inventory level at the outset, approximately $700 would be needed to restore the inventory level after $1000 worth of goods had been sold at retail.

The buying budget concept is most effective when used to plan purchases in the near future. The manager determines a budget by estimating sales for a future period, as for the next month, then calculating the amount of new inventory that is necessary to support the anticipated sales. The resulting figure becomes the buying budget for the period involved.

As purchases of inventory items are made during the period, they are subtracted from the budgeted amount. The balance is termed the open-to-buy allowance for the remainder of the period. Although the budgeted figure represents neither an absolute minimum nor maximum, it does provide a guide for management control of the dollars invested in inventory.

The real advantage of the buying budget lies in the fact that continuing management attention is directed toward an important operating problem.

Facilities

On the average, approximately 15% of the capital required for a typical community pharmacy is invested in fixtures, equipment, and leasehold improvements. Charges for housing the pharmacy are second only to wages among the costs of operation. Expressed as a percentage of annual net sales, rent represents approximately 2.0%.

Overall, the cost of facilities necessary to operate a pharmacy represents a significant portion of total costs. Management of these costs is difficult, especially because they are based on long-term commitments from which there is little opportunity for retreat. Rent, for example, most often is agreed on in advance for a 5- to 10-year period. The lease that establishes the level of rent to be paid is a legal contract that, once agreed to, is enforceable for its term. Fixtures and equipment, once purchased, represent costs that only can be recovered by longtime use.

Management's main role in the effective and economical use of facilities lies in a careful consideration of the original commitment to these assets. In a sense, facilities must be managed in advance.

RENTAL AGREEMENTS—As is the case in most areas of management, decisions regarding the types and amounts of facilities depend in large measure on projections and forecasts of future operations. Basic decisions on the size of the building and quantities of fixtures and equipment are related intimately to anticipated sales volume. The nature of the pharmacy also plays a role in these decisions. An exclusively prescription pharmacy usually requires less space than does a pharmacy that emphasizes general merchandise.

In negotiating the rental agreement the manager must have some notion of anticipated sales and the relation of rent to sales. Although such information may be useful as a guideline for negotiating with potential landlords, generally, landlords refuse to be bound by statistics.

In many cases rental figures for two or more pharmacies are difficult to compare because the services provided by landlords may vary. A pharmacy located in a medical clinic may pay rent considerably in excess of the average figure for a pharmacy doing a similar volume in another location. However, it may be that the rent includes janitorial services, centralized heating, air conditioning, or other services normally not provided.

When negotiating a rental agreement or renewing a lease, the manager may be able to get a stabilization of the rental charge as a percentage of sales by obtaining a percentage lease arrangement. This provides that the landlord receives rent based on a percentage of net sales. Such an arrangement is attractive, especially for a new pharmacy for which there is doubt about the level of sales volume that may be realized.

Landlords increasingly are receptive to percentage lease arrangements. In most cases, however, they insist on a guaranteed minimum rent, with a percentage to be added after a specified sales volume has been realized. If the guaranteed minimum rent is set at a modest figure, this may prove to be advantageous for the pharmacy.

It would be inaccurate to infer that the manager has significant command of the alternatives and terms of the rental agreement. Most often, the landlord dictates the terms of the lease. Management's main role is to avoid gross errors in judgment, resulting in long-term overcommitments for space and rent.

FIXTURES AND EQUIPMENT—The original commitment for fixtures and equipment should be made only after careful analysis of requirements and after searching the market for the most economical and suitable fixtures and equipment. The manager has options regarding quantity, quality, and sources of supply for these facilities. It is good practice to secure bids from several sources before making the final decision on the purchase of fixtures and equipment. Further, many suppliers provide counsel and advice.

Once acquired, the problem of proper arrangement of fixtures and equipment requires additional management decisions. For example, should the prescription laboratory be located in the front or the rear of the pharmacy? When located in the front, it is visible from the street and tends to emphasize prescription service to passersby; when located in the rear, it provides a private atmosphere, free from congestion and activity.

Numerous other decisions regarding layout must be made. Thus, the manager is well-advised to make use of the services of experts in store design before making these decisions.

Studies have demonstrated that the arrangement of fixtures and proper departmentalization of goods can help increase sales volume, promote employee efficiency, and make the pharmacy more pleasant and convenient for patrons. With modern fixtures designed for flexibility, the manager can experiment with various arrangements and layouts until the most efficient combination is achieved. Proper management of facilities can play a significant role in efficient and profitable operation.

Personnel

One of the most important aspects of developing an efficiently operating community pharmacy is a well-conceived program of personnel management. The uniquely personal nature of the atmosphere in the typical community pharmacy dictates that the proper selection, training, and maintenance of employees be given top priority as management functions.

Each employee represents the pharmacy in daily interaction with patrons, physicians, and suppliers. Their ability to reflect and to carry out the objectives of the pharmacy may mean the difference between financial success and failure.

In view of the obvious benefits of sound personnel management, it is surprising to observe that many managers look on good personnel administration as an area for which they have neither the inclination nor the time. Deficiencies in this area arise in part from the numerous and diverse responsibilities assumed by most pharmacy managers. Yet, time and attention devoted to personnel management would, in the long run, free more time for other management functions. The properly selected and well-trained employee can assume many duties that otherwise may be the responsibility of the manager.

The nature of retail employment also contributes to the complexity of personnel management in the pharmacy. In general, retail concerns experience significant variations in the demand for employees. Seasonal variations in sales require adjustments in staff needs. Further, retail activity often is concentrated during certain days of the week and certain hours of the day. Under such conditions, it is difficult to manage payroll costs without the extensive use of part-time help.

Because of the extensive use of part-time employees, many of the people employed by retail firms are young people without previous work experience. Often they have little understanding of the economic value of the services they are expected to render. Personnel of this type present special problems in training and orientation, not only to a specific job but also to the general obligation of an employee to an employer.

Attracting competent employees is made more difficult by the need to cater to the desires of the public regarding store hours. Modern consumers expect to shop 7 days a week and into the late evening hours. The retail employee, therefore, is expected to work during hours and on days when others in society are free to shop and play.

Other problems associated with obtaining good employees are inherent in the nature of retailing. Retail employees are meeting the public continually, so they must be of at least average intelligence, present a good appearance, and have an acceptable personality. Also, wages paid to retail employees ordinarily are well below those paid in other industries.

SELECTION—Although the nature of retail employment is unique in many respects, the basic principles of personnel management may be applied in the development of a program for selecting, training, and maintaining employees for the retail field and specifically for the community pharmacy. Proper selection techniques must be developed to ensure that employees are compatible with the job to be done and with the objectives of the pharmacy.

A high turnover rate in a pharmacy often makes the attitude of management toward selecting employees rather casual. Managers rationalize that the employee will not be staying long, therefore, why worry about selectivity?

Further, the manager frequently is faced with the problem of replacing employees on relatively short notice. In such emergencies selectivity often is ignored.

Improper selection of employees has the effect of perpetuating and intensifying the turnover problem, and the employee who is not suited to his job can be detrimental to the operation of the pharmacy. Two general rules should be incorporated into the personnel policies regarding selection.

1. Minimum standards for qualifications of employees should not be allowed to fall below the minimum standards for service established for the pharmacy. To "underhire" for a given position can serve only to undermine the reputation of the pharmacy.
2. "Overhiring" should be avoided; obviously superior people should not be hired for inferior jobs. Such personnel rapidly become discontented and may have an adverse effect on staff morale and efficiency.

Proper selection of personnel for a specific job is predicated on an understanding of the duties and responsibilities involved and on knowledge of the individual characteristics required for efficient performance. The manager should develop a job description and a job specification for each position in the pharmacy.

The job description is a brief summary of the scope of the job, its relation to other jobs, and such details as working hours and pay scales. It also serves to prevent misunderstandings about the nature or duties of a particular job. The job specification sets forth the characteristics and competencies necessary in the individual who fills the position.

With these materials, the manager is in a position to evaluate objectively the candidates who apply for the position. Selection also requires a knowledge of the sources of potential employees. For some jobs, promotion from within the pharmacy staff may be appropriate. In most cases external sources must be used, such as employment agencies, placement offices of schools, and universities or classified newspaper advertising.

A growing source of part-time employees are the co-op work-study programs of many high schools. An availability file should be established in the pharmacy—a record of qualified people who applied for jobs when no openings existed.

The manager should develop an application form to assist in the selection process. Although the application form serves basically to provide information about the applicant, it can serve other purposes as well; for example,

It provides a means for observing the applicant's ability to follow simple written instructions.

It serves as a guide in the employment interview. If no openings currently are available, it can go into the availability file.

It serves a practical purpose as a part of the employee's permanent record and as a source of information for social security and withholding tax reports.

A properly designed application form can serve as an effective screening device for prospective employees. The information supplied on the application form often indicates that the applicant does not meet the job specifications and, thus, should not be considered further. If the information suggests that the applicant is a good prospect, the selection procedure should continue with an interview.

Often the employment interview is the sole selection procedure used by pharmacy managers, and this is not advisable. At the least, the references provided by the applicant should be checked thoroughly to substantiate the impressions generated by the interview. The interview, however, is a key step in most selections. It should be conducted in an unhurried manner, in privacy and in a relatively informal atmosphere. Much can be learned about the prospective employee through a properly conducted interview.

The manager also might consider developing some simple tests to be used in the selection process. Testing is used as a selection technique by many larger firms and can be most useful. In the pharmacy, simple arithmetic tests can be used in selecting personnel for sales or clerking positions that may require that the person be able to handle the simple problems involved in making change and computing sales taxes.

Note that all employment policies and procedures must be consistent with applicable federal and state laws governing equal employment opportunity. In general such laws prohibit discrimination in selection and hiring practices.

ORIENTATION AND TRAINING—Proper selection needs to be followed by adequate orientation and training of the employee. These can serve to increase productivity and to reduce employee turnover. The orientation process should include a give-and-take discussion with the employee on the following questions:

What are the basic philosophies of the pharmacy (toward patrons, other health professionals, and employees)?

What are the hours the employee is expected to work (evenings, weekends, and holidays)?

How long is the lunch hour?

How is overtime handled?

What is the policy regarding coffee breaks?

What are the regulations about smoking?

What are the rules regarding punctuality?

Are uniforms required? If so, who buys them and who pays for laundering?

What are the safety and security regulations?

May this employee answer the telephone? If so what information is he or she authorized to give?

Can the telephone be used for personal calls?

What is the vacation policy?

What is the policy regarding leave (sick or personal business)?

What are the opportunities and procedures for advancement?

What are the policies on employee purchases and discounts?

These questions are by no means all-inclusive on those matters that might be of concern to both the employer and the employee, but the use of such a list provides a basis for posing additional specific questions. Although some of the questions may appear to be trivial, these are the kinds of matters that often cause problems between employers and employees.

In an extreme case disagreements over such matters may lead to termination of employment. In other cases, employee resentment may be reflected in attitudes toward and dealings with patrons of the pharmacy, and this could be the most serious consequence of such disagreement. If these matters are discussed in advance, misunderstandings may be minimized, to the mutual benefit of both parties.

After a general orientation to the pharmacy the employee needs specific training in the duties and responsibilities of the job. Too often the new pharmacy employee is trained by the sink-or-swim method. The employee is simply put to work and is expected to pick up knowledge on the job. Obviously, such a method of training is inefficient and in the long run costly, although it does offer the advantage of requiring little or no management time or effort.

Although the typical community pharmacy has neither the staff nor the facilities for sophisticated training programs, there are effective, simple, training methods that can be used. The sponsor system of training is the most appropriate for a pharmacy. A new employee is assigned to a capable experienced employee who explains and demonstrates the job in question. The conference method also may be used, by itself or to supplement the sponsor system. Here, the new employee meets privately with the pharmacy manager or a designated employee to discuss the techniques of the job. In either case the management responsibility lies in organizing and structuring the training so that all aspects of the employee's duties are considered.

COMPENSATION—Retaining good employees is one of the most difficult problems faced by the community pharmacy manager. There are many elements in the employment environment that may help in keeping employees, but most important is the compensation plan. Adequate compensation is necessary, not only to retain employees but also to encourage them to work toward the overall goals and objectives of the pharmacy. The basic elements of a sound plan are

Adequacy—The amount of compensation should be commensurate with the responsibilities of the job. Adequacy also may be viewed in a legal sense in terms of state and federal minimum wage laws.

Simplicity—Plans that are uncomplicated are understood easily by the employee and have the further advantage of being easy to administer.

Progressiveness—A plan should recognize and reward initiative, productivity, and increasing value of the employee to the pharmacy. It should provide incentive for doing a better job. Periodic review of performance and salary should be provided for in the plan.

Patron Protection—The plan should not encourage acts that are detrimental to the best interests of the patrons of the pharmacy. For example, it is inappropriate to offer extra commissions for promoting the sale of OTC drugs. If commissions are paid on these drugs, the employee may be tempted to place personal economic gain ahead of the real needs of the patron.

Traditionally, the compensation plan for pharmacy employees has consisted of an hourly or weekly salary plus the legally required social security contribution by the employer for each employee. Modern personnel management calls for a broader compensation plan to compete effectively for the limited number of good employees.

Increasingly, even small pharmacies are offering plans that include not only salary but such fringe benefits as health insurance, life insurance, paid vacation, and sick days plus supplemental retirement benefits. When such benefits are provided, the employer should calculate their value in terms of preincome tax dollars, thus demonstrating to the employee their real economic value.

Credit

The need for credit is apparent especially when health products and services are involved. The need for drugs and pharmaceutical services often is immediate and independent of the cash position of the patient. Further, a charge account statement provides the patient with a mechanism for keeping track of expenditures for drugs for insurance and income tax purposes.

Credit management in the community pharmacy, on occasion, presents a conflict between sound business practice and professional responsibility. Sound business practice may indicate that credit should not be given to a particular patron, whereas professional responsibility may dictate that credit must be given. It is not possible to develop inflexible credit policies that solves such problems. However, it is possible to develop policies and procedures that are effective in a majority of such situations. There are two general areas that require attention in credit management.

POLICIES AND PROCEDURES—Included here are the matters of eligibility, limits on credit, credit terms, maintaining accurate records and identification of credit patrons. Deciding which patrons are eligible for credit is the most troublesome problem for the pharmacy manager.

It is difficult to make a decision without knowing the credit history of the patron. Data on past credit experiences must be obtained and should be checked. The patron can be asked to supply the necessary information and usually will do so.

However, verification presents a serious practical problem. Some managers attempt to verify the information personally by contacting each credit reference. Such a procedure is time consuming, and the information received is often incomplete.

A better approach appears to lie in the use of professional credit bureaus. Most localities are now served by such bureaus that, for a fee, investigates prospective credit customers and supplies a report on their ratings. With this information the manager can make better decisions and minimize the problems associated with granting credit.

COLLECTION—The best policies can be thwarted by careless collection procedures. The terms of credit granted should be made clear to the grantee at the outset. If the terms are not met, appropriate and prompt action should be taken.

The manager is responsible for establishing the guidelines and procedures necessary to ensure prompt payment of credit accounts. Collection policies that result in prompt payment offer a number of advantages.

Prompt payment means rapid turnover of capital invested in accounts receivable, and this permits a given level of operations to be supported with less capital. Operating expenses are lower when accounts are paid on time as delinquent accounts cost money in terms of employee time and supplies required for follow-ups.

Finally, there is a definite relation between the length of time accounts are outstanding and bad debt losses; usually, the longer an account is outstanding, the less likely it is to be collected.

Although guidelines and procedures should be established for collecting past-due accounts, rarely is the same procedure appropriate for all such accounts. New accounts, for example, should be handled firmly to impress the patron with the importance of prompt payment. Casual handling or lack of follow-up of delinquent new accounts sets a precedent that may be hard to overcome.

For established accounts, more individualized treatment is indicated. Some patrons fail to pay promptly simply out of negligence. Usually a simple reminder stimulates payment. Others may be willing to pay their debts but for reasons beyond their control are unable to do so. The manager may be able to work out a budget plan for those to help solve their problems.

A small group of patrons may fall into the category of those who simply do not wish to pay. Outside collection agencies or legal action may be the only alternative for this group. In any event, policies and procedures for collection should be included as part of the credit management function.

Credit also may be provided to patrons by means of various credit card systems operated by banks. The credit card system involves the establishment of a line of credit for an individual with a participating bank or group of banks. The individual is issued a credit card that is honored by participating businesses for goods or services. The participating business then forwards the receipts for sales of goods or services to the bank and receives immediate payment, less a service charge based on the amount of the sale.

The advantages of this system lie in the fact that bad-debt losses are reduced almost to zero, and the cost of billing is assumed by the bank. Even though the amount realized from the sales transaction is reduced by the amount of the service charge, some pharmacy owners view the bank credit card system as the answer to problems associated with credit transactions. In fact, many pharmacies use such systems as their only credit program.

As a practical matter, however, many people who require drugs and pharmaceutical services cannot qualify, and some people refuse to participate in the credit card system. As a result, some pharmacies use such systems simply as a supplement to their own charge-account system. In addition, increasing numbers of pharmacies are accepting nationally recognized credit cards.

Most, if not all, community pharmacies today also extend credit for prescription drugs and pharmacy services to private and government third-party programs. In 1997 it was estimated that 71% of all outpatient prescriptions were paid for, either in full or in part, by third-party programs. As a result, a significant portion of the accounts receivable for the typical community pharmacy represents payments due from third-party payers. Generally, credit extended to third-party payers involves minimal risk of bad-debt losses if services are provided to patients who are eligible for benefits, program requirements are met, and accurate claims are submitted. However, the payment cycle from the submission of a claim to receipt of reimbursement varies greatly among third-party payers. Some process claims within 15 to 20 days, whereas others may take a month or more. To minimize delays in reimbursement, the pharmacy manager must implement systems that assure the prompt submission of accurately prepared claims to all third parties.

Fortunately, increasing numbers of third-party payers are using electronic systems that provide for on-line processing and adjudication of claims for pharmacy services. The electronic transmission of claims directly from the pharmacy to the third-party payer provides for instant verification of patient eligibility, confirms whether the service provided is a payable benefit and confirms the amount to be paid to the pharmacy provider. Electronic submission of claims also may shorten the payment cycle and reduce the average collection period for accounts receivable from third-party payers.

To measure the effectiveness of management control over credit sales, it is useful to calculate the average collection period of customers' accounts receivable. Average daily credit sales are divided into the total of accounts receivable at the end of a period, giving the average collection period for accounts receivable. In theory, this figure should be approximately 40 days if all accounts are paid on time. Figures in excess of 60 days indicate deficiencies in credit policies and credit management, and call for prompt action.

Risk

As a commercial enterprise, a community pharmacy presents numerous risks in terms of economic gain or loss. Some risks inherent in the operation are speculative in nature. For example, will operations produce a profit or a loss? With this type of risk there is an uncertainty that may work either to the detriment or to the benefit of the pharmacy owner. Such risks can be managed only indirectly by careful attention to the management of all of the elements comprising the pharmacy. Even then there is no guarantee of success.

Other risks associated with the operation of a pharmacy may be termed pure risks. These involve uncertainty and chance of loss but do not provide a gain directly if the loss is not realized. Tangible destructible property is subject to pure risk; its destruction always is possible but not certain.

For example, there is a risk that the merchandise inventory owned by the pharmacy may be destroyed by fire. If a fire occurs a loss surely will be suffered, but if it does not occur no direct increase in value or profit is realized. Pure risk may be controlled or protected against by appropriate direct management action.

TYPES—The first function of management related to controlling pure risk is to identify and analyze the several perils to which business assets are subject. Some perils are common to all pharmacies; others are unique to specific situations. It is important, therefore, that the analysis of risk be individualized. There are four common categories of perils to be considered.

Actual Loss of Property—All tangible property is subject to being lost. For the pharmacy, most such losses are due to dishonesty such as shoplifting, burglary, robbery, or embezzlement.

Damage or Destruction of Property—Most tangible property is exposed to possible destruction or damage by fire, the elements, civil commotion, and various other causes.

Civil Liability—Every pharmacy is subject to various risks associated with dealing with the public and with employing people. Negligence or breach of responsibility, alleged or proven, can cause financial losses. Injuries to individuals in the pharmacy, malpractice by pharmacists, and product liability are examples of these perils.

Contractual Liability—Legal liability beyond that imposed by the law may be assumed in a contractual relationship between a pharmacist and other persons. The lease signed by the pharmacist to obtain the building for the pharmacy is an example of contractual liability.

RISK MANAGEMENT—Each peril identified by the pharmacy manager must be further analyzed to determine the probability of occurrence of an actual loss as follows: the loss must be quantified in terms of its effect on the total assets of the pharmacy and the ability to handle the loss; the manager must decide which of the alternative methods or combination of methods should be utilized to protect against each peril or loss. The three commonly recognized ways to handle risks are

Self-Insurance—This may be used to protect against small losses with a low probability of occurrence. A reserve is established and, in the event such losses occur, they are paid for out of the reserve that is created by systematically setting aside money for this purpose. A major danger is that a large loss may occur before a sufficient reserve has been established. Except for large, multiunit pharmacies, self-insurance is not practical for community pharmacies.

Assumption of Risk—When the probability of loss is low and the loss is of small magnitude, it may be economically advantageous for the owner to assume the risk. For example, when the cost of insuring plate glass against perils other than fire and the elements is compared with the probability of loss from these perils, most owners decide to assume the risk. Assumption of risk differs from self-insurance in that no reserve is established. Obviously, this method of risk management must be used carefully.

Insurance through Others—The majority of pure risks associated with community pharmacy practice are of sufficient magnitude to dictate the placement of risks with other parties such as insurance companies. They offer service to the insured and provide indemnity in the event a loss is suffered. Such firms provide the technical knowledge and the legal experience required for settling losses quickly and efficiently. Often the services of insurance companies are as important as the indemnification they provide, as is the case in liability suits.

Too often the management of risk is considered adequate when proper provision has been made to insure indemnification in the event of a loss. A complete risk-management program should include a consideration of loss prevention as well as protection. An attempt to prevent losses can be beneficial in many ways.

Insurance companies are beginning to recognize clients with good records and to reward them by reductions in premiums. A direct cash savings thus is effected by reduction of prevention of losses. More important, most tangible losses result in other losses that cannot be handled by insurance. For example, when an error is made in dispensing prescription medication and a malpractice suit is brought, the tangible dollar cost of such a suit may be paid by the insurance company.

The intangible loss caused by damage to the reputation of the pharmacy cannot be alleviated by cash payment. Prevention of such occurrences is the best way to avoid all of the losses

involved. Loss prevention, both philosophically and practically, should be an integral part of risk-management programs.

The services of an insurance counselor may prove valuable to the manager of a pharmacy in developing a risk-management program. The complexities involved in evaluating risks and in understanding the various types of insurance policies and terminology call for expert advice. The insurance counselor generally is the best source of unbiased information.

The insurance counselor usually does not order policies. The counselor's function is to evaluate the risks of a specific individual or firm and to make recommendations regarding the best way to deal with them. The fee for these services is paid by the insured rather than the insurer. Expenditures of money for this service may prove to be extremely economical in the long run.

INSURANCE—Among the types of coverage required for the community pharmacy are

Fire insurance
Malpractice insurance
General public liability insurance
Products liability insurance
Employer's liability or worker's compensation
Crime insurance
Business interruption insurance

These specific coverages may be acquired separately or several of them may be included in a package policy, similar to the well-known homeowner's policy. Package policies have the advantage of offering broader coverage at the same or even at a lower cost than do the individual policies purchased separately. Such policies should be evaluated carefully; the multiple coverage involved may leave gaps in protection that are not apparent until a loss occurs. It often is difficult to know exactly what is covered, and to what extent, under package, all-risks policies.

Perhaps the most important coverage for the tangible assets of the pharmacy is fire insurance. Although most pharmacies are protected to some degree, often the amount of the fire insurance falls below the actual value of the property.

This is particularly important because most fire insurance policies contain a co-insurance clause. This clause requires that insurance equal to a specified percentage of the value of the property be carried at all times. A common requirement is 80% of the value.

Under co-insurance if, at the time of a loss, the amount of insurance carried is below the required amount, the insured must bear part of the loss. For example, if the insurable value of the property owned by a pharmacist is $50,000 and the fire insurance policy has an 80% co-insurance clause, the pharmacist must carry $40,000 worth of insurance on the property. If only $30,000 is carried and a $10,000 loss is suffered, the insurer is required to pay only $7,500. The pharmacist must assume the balance of the loss because only 75% of the required amount of insurance was maintained.

The standard fire insurance policy should be supplemented by an extended coverage endorsement. For a small additional fee this endorsement has the effect of extending protection to cover damage by windstorm, hail, explosion, riot, smoke, and from land vehicles and aircraft. Note that usually neither the standard fire insurance policy nor the extended coverage endorsement covers losses of documents, accounts receivable, prescription files, or currency.

Several types of liability insurance are becoming increasingly important in modern practice. Pharmacy owners may be required to answer a suit arising out of the negligence or alleged negligence of them or of their employees. In addition, the pharmacy is a public facility where there are innumerable opportunities for injury to patrons.

Product liability may arise out of claims of patrons that have suffered injuries from products purchased in the pharmacy. Although the pharmacist may be able to fall back on the manufacturer under the concept of implied warranty, such claims must be answered by the pharmacist. Insurance can provide the financial and legal resources necessary to answer suits of this type.

The owner must obtain coverage of sufficient scope and amounts adequate to protect against liability claims. Without insurance coverage, an unfavorable judgment from one such claim may be sufficient to bankrupt the owner.

Insurance coverage against criminal acts also should be obtained. In addition, the manager is in an excellent position to use loss prevention as a means of minimizing these risks. Minimizing the amount of cash carried on the premises, installation of burglar alarm systems, and carefully observed security measures can greatly reduce losses in this area.

The dishonesty of employees can be controlled best by adequate systems and policies regarding handling of cash and other assets. Shoplifting losses can be reduced by proper surveillance and proper training of employees. As a rule, insurance is not available to cover these losses.

When a pharmacy suffers losses because of fire or other causes that interrupt operations, the actual loss goes beyond the property that is damaged or destroyed. Profits are lost while the pharmacy is closed. Certain business expenses continue, even during interrupted operations. Key employees may be forced to seek other employment. Such losses may be covered by business interruption insurance. This is designed to indemnify the owner for lost profits, continuing expenses, and salaries of key employees during a reasonable period of interrupted operations.

Life insurance also may have a role in a comprehensive risk-management program for a community pharmacy. If a pharmacist is the sole owner of a pharmacy, insurance on his life can provide funds to take care of the debts of the pharmacy in the event of the owner's death. If the pharmacist is the co-owner of the pharmacy as a partner, arrangements should be made for life insurance on each partner with the other partner(s) named as beneficiaries. The amount of such insurance should be sufficient to pay for each partner's equity in the enterprise.

In the event of the death of a partner, the surviving partner(s) can use the proceeds from the insurance to buy a deceased partner's interest in the pharmacy from the heirs. Such an arrangement reduces the possibility that the enterprise would be dissolved to settle the estate of a deceased partner. The premium payments made for partnership life insurance policies are regarded as a business expense.

There are various other risks that may be covered effectively by insurance. Some of these are peculiar to individual circumstances and must be analyzed and managed in terms of the specific pharmacy. Effective management of all the insurable risks associated with modern community pharmacy practice must be combined with effective management of the uninsurable speculative risks inherent in entrepreneurial activity.

Records

For various reasons—some legal, some financial, and some professional—the maintenance of records in the pharmacy is becoming increasingly important. The types of records required may be classified as

Records required by law regarding the acquisition and disposition of drugs.
Records regarding patient utilization of drugs.
Records regarding the past and the present financial status of the pharmacy.

Management's role in this function is to identify the specific records required, develop systems for keeping them, and delegate the responsibility for day-to-day record keeping to capable personnel.

LEGAL RECORDS—According to federal and state law, the pharmacy owner or manager is charged with maintaining accurate up-to-date records on specific classes of drugs and poisons. Under the provisions of the *Federal Controlled Substances Act of 1970*, the pharmacist is charged with maintain-

ing accurate records related to the acquisition and disposition of certain drugs that are deemed to be subject to possible misuse or abuse. Several states have enacted legislation that requires accurate records on the distribution of poisons and other hazardous substances.

The legal implications of record keeping, as it relates to these drugs, are serious. Improperly maintained or incomplete records can bring legal action and penalties.

PATIENT RECORDS—In recent years many pharmacists have broadened their record-keeping activities to include patient drug histories. Although the form of patient record varies, the basic idea is to establish a record (usually on a family-unit basis) that allows the pharmacist to monitor the drug usage of each member of the family. It increasingly is apparent that, because of the kinds and amounts of drugs being taken by the average patient, there is need for a drug history for each individual.

To reduce the problems associated with drug interactions and individual idiosyncrasies to drugs, the pharmacist has a professional obligation to maintain records of this type. In addition, these records also may serve economic purposes, as sources of information for insurance claims and for income tax deductions of the patient.

FINANCIAL RECORDS—Properly collected and organized accounting data serve various important uses and are of value to the pharmacy owner in the following ways:

Providing the basic tools for efficient management and measuring its effect.
Making sound decisions regarding future cash needs, inventory requirements, personnel matters, and expansion of facilities.
Evaluating past operations, controlling current operations, and providing information for planning and forecasting.
Analyzing revenues and expenses.
Measuring return on investment.
Providing the required information to potential grantors of credit and loans as well as to federal, state, and local governmental agencies regarding income and business taxes.
Helping to ensure a profitable operation.

Generally, the manager no longer acts as bookkeeper in the community pharmacy. Considering the complexities of contemporary business and the importance of good financial records, the pharmacist is well advised to employ experts to assist in the development and the maintenance of his or her accounting system. The experts can help to develop an individualized system that meets the accepted criteria for good financial records: objectivity, conservatism, consistency, and comparability.

Financial records should reflect, insofar as is possible, an objective evaluation of the transactions and data on which they are based. Personal opinion and judgment should not be allowed to prevail over an objective analysis of financial data. For example, the cost of fixtures in the pharmacy should be reported in the financial statement on the basis of acquisition cost as evidenced by a bill of sale or an invoice.

The value of these fixtures should not be increased on the statements simply because management feels they are worth more than the original cost because of increasing price levels. Convincing objective evidence of the dollar amounts reported on the financial statement is a prerequisite to maintaining the integrity of such statements.

The general optimism of many owners and managers may be in conflict with the principle of conservatism as it relates to financial records. A moderately conservative approach should be employed in reporting financial data; otherwise, the data may tend to overstate earnings and assets and to understate liabilities. The consequences of overstated earnings include the possibility of excess income tax liability in a given year.

If a choice must be made between understatement or overstatement of income or assets, the principle of conservatism would dictate understatement. This does not imply that earnings or assets should be understated deliberately. However, when estimates or opinions must be used in making decisions regarding financial records, a conservative attitude should prevail. For example, many managers are reluctant to admit that a certain percentage of accounts receivable will prove to be uncollectable.

They are inclined to report accounts receivable in the financial records without a realistic reduction for bad debts. To do this without adjustment based on recognition of the likelihood of some not being collected is to violate the principle of conservatism.

Although there is no hard and fast rule for accounting for financial transactions, it is important that a given enterprise be consistent in its accounting system. This also is linked closely to the final criterion for good financial records: comparability.

There are various methods of recording and reporting financial transactions, and decisions must be made regarding the best method. Once chosen, it should be applied consistently throughout the life of the enterprise so that financial records will be comparable from period to period. For example, there are several ways to allocate depreciation charges to expense. If the policy on depreciation is changed from one period to the next, the net income may be altered significantly. Such a change would have an effect on the comparability of the financial statements for the two periods.

Attention to consistency and comparability should not necessarily rule out all changes in accounting methods. When valid reasons dictate a change in method, it should be made. However, the nature of the change should be indicated clearly on future financial statements.

Comparability of financial records also is important in the broader sense to compare records between firms in the same field. It is advantageous to be able to compare the financial statements for the pharmacy with similar statements such as those reported in the NCPA-Searle Digest and other references. Such comparisons are facilitated if relatively standard accounting systems are used. The manager could instruct his or her accountant to classify expenses according to the NCPA-Searle Digest system. He or she then would be able to analyze the expenses of their pharmacies in relation to national trends and averages.

The day-by-day financial transactions are summarized in the statements prepared at the end of the accounting period. Among the statements most important to those concerned with the financial progress of the pharmacy are the balance sheet and the income statement. Assuming that the underlying data have been treated objectively and conservatively, the balance sheet should represent fairly accurately the financial position of the pharmacy at the end of a given period. It reflects the basic accounting equation:

$$\text{assets} = \text{liabilities} + \text{owner's equity}$$

Assets are the items of value owned by the enterprise, listed at cost prices less any allowances for depreciation or doubtful accounts. The liabilities and owner's equity represent the claims against the assets.

The balance sheet is of interest to the owners in terms of the total value of their investment and the value of specific assets that make up the total investment. Managers especially are interested in such items as total merchandise inventory and accounts receivable.

Future management decisions regarding inventory control and credit policies may be influenced by the information included on the balance sheet. Those who are asked to grant credit to the pharmacy will be interested in the current liabilities and the owner's equity, as reported on the balance sheet. A formal detailed balance sheet should be prepared at least once a year. One commonly used format for reporting balance-sheet information for community pharmacies is illustrated in Table 94-1.

The income statement details the effects of revenue and expense transactions during a given accounting period. Unlike the balance sheet, which describes the financial position of an enterprise on a given date, the income statement summarizes only those transactions directly related to income production for a specific period, usually a year. For most purposes the income statement is used in concert with the balance sheet, each supplementing the other.

The owners of the pharmacy are interested not only in total investment but also in the net profit, which represents return on investment. The manager cannot accurately judge the appropriateness of the level of merchandise inventory reported in the balance sheet without knowing the sales revenue generated by the inventory as reported in the income statement.

The information included in the income statement can be used by the manager to plan for future operations and as a means for controlling current operations. When the information is compared against past years and national averages, trends are observed and problem areas may be identified. The manager then can make decisions and take actions intended to improve the profit-making potential of the pharmacy.

BIBLIOGRAPHY

Marino FA, Zabloski EJ, Herman CM. *Principles of Pharmaceutical Accounting*. Philadelphia: Lea & Febiger, 1980.

Smith HA. *Principles and Methods of Pharmacy Management*, 3rd ed. Philadelphia: Lea & Febiger, 1986.

Tharp CP, Lecca PJ. *Pharmacy Management for Students and Practitioners*, 2nd ed. St. Louis: Mosby, 1979.

Hoffman DC. *Effective Pharmacy Management*, 6th ed. Kansas City, MO: Marion Merrell Dow, 1990.

The NCPA-Searle Digest (1998 and 1997 eds). Alexandria, VA: National Community Pharmacists Association.

IMS Class-of-Trade Analysis 1997. Plymouth Meeting, PA: IMS America, Ltd, 1998.

Carrol NV. *Financial Management for Pharmacists: A Decision Making Approach*. Lippincott Williams & Wilkins, Baltimore, 1998.

DiLima SN, Eutsey DE. *Pharmacy Practice Management Forms, Guidelines and Checklists*. Aspen, 1998.

ACKNOWLEDGMENT—Joseph Thomas III, PhD is acknowledged for his contributions in previous editions of this work.

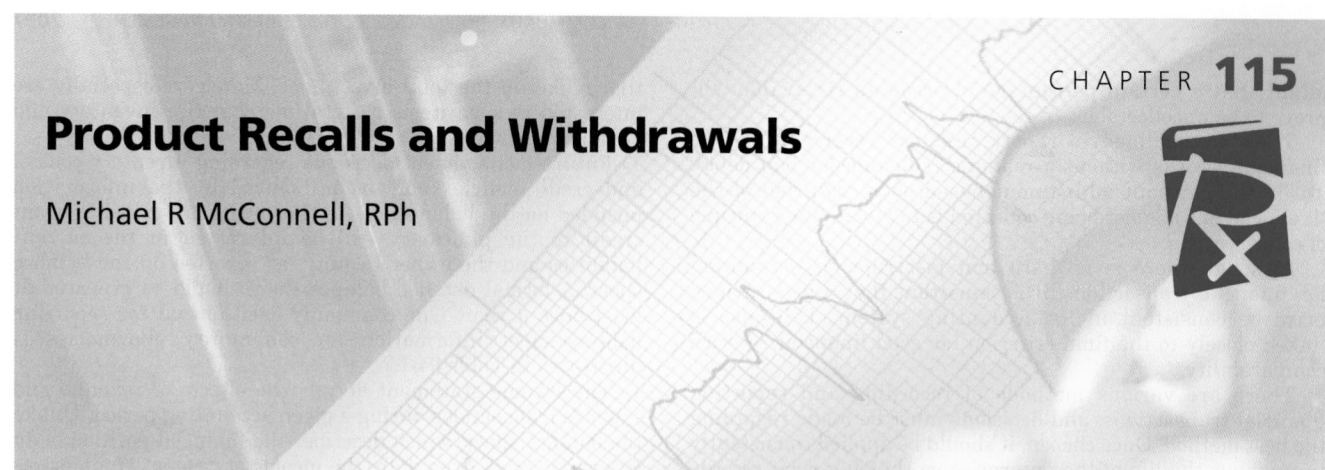

CHAPTER 115

Product Recalls and Withdrawals

Michael R McConnell, RPh

Occasionally, pharmaceutical manufacturers must recall or withdraw products from wholesalers, pharmacies, and/or patients. There are approximately 200 pharmaceutical recalls every year. The reasons for recalls and withdrawals range from life-threatening situations (eg, a product that is supposed to be sterile but is instead contaminated with bacteria) to situations where there is no health hazard or risk, but simply, the product does not measure up to the quality control standards that the pharmaceutical community wishes to present to the public (eg, a label that appears upside-down on its container).

The purpose of this chapter is to offer guidelines and background information for practicing pharmacists to handle efficiently and in a professional manner recalls and withdrawals. It is impossible to anticipate every possible situation, and it is unwise to have a "cookie cutter" solution for every recall or withdrawal.[1] It is hoped that pharmacists will take these guidelines and then enhance or modify them to fit their particular practice. This chapter is divided into several sections: (1) Recall Procedures; (2) Action When a Recall Happens; and (3) Background Information, Future Directions, and Implications of Recalls.

RECALL PROCEDURES

Documenting Recall Procedures

The lack of documentation for quality systems seems to be a typical condition for many American companies. In the 20th century, America seems to have been successful without having to write everything down, without keeping extensive records, without issuing many standard operating procedures. Now, everyone is faced with the challenge of documenting what it is that we do. The watchwords for the future seem to be: *"If you do it, write it. If you write it, do it!"*[2]

The purpose of any written procedure is to provide a documented plan for what to do in a certain situation. Pharmacists may well find that it is better to create procedures (eg, Policies and Procedures) prior to a crisis situation, when a "cooler" head and more time allows for better quality consideration. The middle of a life-threatening recall is not the time to try and think of everything to do. Established written procedures better ensure that policies are carried out consistently and with the same level of quality from event to event. In large institutions, there may be dozens of pharmacy personnel, and written procedures are essential if the pharmacy department is to function as a cohesive unit. Written procedures are also valuable in a one-pharmacist facility. Even in the case of a sole-practitioner community pharmacist working most of the hours the pharmacy is open, recalls may not happen with enough regularity for the pharmacist to remember exactly what to do from one recall to another. Never mind that Murphy's Law says that the "worst

recalls will happen when the sole-practitioner pharmacist is on a rare vacation and a relief pharmacist is on duty." In a situation such as this, written procedures can help to ensure the smooth delivery of high quality patient services, and lessen the risk of legal liability.

In developing the procedures' documentation, the pharmacist may want to *create forms* or templates to guide pharmacy personnel through the recall procedures. A form is simply a printed or typed document with blank spaces for insertion of required information. Creating a form does not have to involve deluxe design skills. In the interest of getting a procedure form created in a timely manner, a simple handwritten layout may be the most efficient way to get it accomplished in today's environment.

Elements Of A Recall Procedure

There may be many elements of a recall procedure. A simple list includes the following three major elements:

1. Communication
2. Product handling
3. Recordkeeping

A pharmacist may discover that for a particular pharmacy institution, facility, or type of pharmacy practice, there needs to be additional elements. There is probably no one right answer.

COMMUNICATION

After becoming aware of a product recall or withdrawal, one of the first things a pharmacist will probably need to do is to communicate the recall to someone else. It may be helpful to think in terms of:

who to contact (who needs to know about this recall event? ie, other pharmacists, physicians, patients, etc.);
what to communicate (what facts, options, advice, etc., need to be communicated?);
when to send out communication (how quickly does the communication need to take place?);
how to communicate (what are the appropriate methods to send communication quickly, accurately, etc.?).

Regarding to **whom** a communication should be forwarded, the pharmacist may wish to make a list of those who could be affected by a recall. Here, the idea is not that all those who might possibly be affected by any recall need to be notified about every aspect of every recall. As will be discussed later (ie, in the background discussion on recalls), recalls vary in importance, and there may be situations where it is perfectly reasonable **not** to communicate a recall to a wide audience. A sample checklist of *Who to Contact* is shown in Figure 115-1. In preparing the *Who to Contact* list, the pharmacist may want to list actual specific facilities in the area for which he/she feels a responsibility to notify about recalls. For example, even if a recall is being carried out only to the pharmacy level (more about *levels* later), the pharmacist may want to notify some physicians's offices, nursing homes, and other similarly interested parties.

Regarding **what** should be communicated, the pharmacist may wish to think in terms of the following:

1. Identifying the **product**
2. Stating the **reason** for recall
3. The **action** to be taken by the person being contacted

Also, when considering what should be communicated, one should think about the audience. For example, to communicate the product identity *within a pharmacy* the pharmacist should include the product name, strength, manufacturer, package size, NDC, and lot number. To communicate product identity *to a patient*, things such as package size, NDC, and lot number may have little meaning and may be confusing. Likewise, when communicating the reason for a recall to a patient, it may be factual to say that a product "contains *Pseudomonas aeruginosa*," but it may have more meaning for the patient if the pharmacist said that the product is "contaminated with bacteria." Care must be taken when communicating the original reason for the product recall, especially when communicating to patients.

Although it can be said that everyone (eg, other pharmacists, physicians, patients) has a right to know the reason for the recall, pharmacists should keep in mind the ramifications that a recall communication may have for patients. For example, will the wording used when stating the reason for a recall possibly cause a patient to stop taking a life-saving medication and, thus, be subject to a possibly greater harm than if the recalled product was continued? A patient who discontinues an anticonvulsant or an antiarrhythmic drug may place himself/herself in a greater danger than by continuing to take a recalled medication that may only be slightly subpotent at the end of its expiration date. This leads to the next consideration.

What course of *action* should be communicated? In general, if a recall is being communicated officially to the patient level, then it is usually, but not always, serious enough that the patient will probably be instructed to stop taking the product. Sometimes a patient will be instructed to continue his/her medication but to see his/her physician as soon as possible. The original recall communication from the pharmaceutical manufacturer or the Food and Drug Administration (FDA) will probably have presented actions to communicate to patients. In any case, the impact of a recalled product on any individual patient's health and exactly what action an individual patient should take is a matter best addressed by the patient's physician.

Pharmacists play a very important role in one aspect of what action to take after a recall, and that regards the availability of alternative therapy. In preparing for consultations with physicians and patients regarding possible alternative therapy, the pharmacist may want to consider such questions as follows:

- Is the same product available in a different strength? For example, taking two 5 mg tablets instead of the recalled 10 mg tablet?
- Is the same product available in an alternative dosage form (eg, oral liquid, subcutaneous injection)?
- Is the same chemical entity available from a different manufacturer? If so, are there any important differences in the formulation (eg, different color dyes, different preservatives)?
- If no alternative identical chemical entity is available, then what products are in the same therapeutic class as the recalled product and, therefore, might be viable options for alternative patient therapy?

The pharmacist who is prepared with answers to these questions can be instrumental in helping a physician work through the implications of whether or not a patient should discontinue a recalled product.

More mundane, but still important, considerations involve product disposition and reimbursement. Regarding disposition, should the product be returned to the pharmacy, sent directly to the manufacturer, disposed of down the drain, or handled with some other action? If it should be returned to the manufacturer, should it be sent by secured carrier (which may be important for legal liability reasons)? If product tampering is suspected, then the patient may be asked to hold the product pending imminent retrieval by an agent of the FDA or the Federal Bureau of Investigation (FBI). A patient may be tempted to just dispose of a product "down the drain" and forego reimbursement. But, if the product is potentially hazardous, then disposing down the drain may have environmental ramifications. This is usually a consideration only when large quantities of product are involved (eg, in a pharmacy or wholesaler), but environmental regulations may state that *any* quantities of certain substances (eg, chemotoxic agents or heavy metals) are forbidden to be dumped into a sanitary sewer.

Regarding reimbursement, questions may include the following:

- How much will the patient be reimbursed for the actual product (eg, full price paid vs full price minus any amount used, or minus any co-pay or deductible)?.
- Will reimbursement be given for follow-up physician visits, and if so, what kind of receipts or documentation will the patient need to secure?

The matter of *when* to communicate a recall can be naively answered with "as soon as possible." But, one must recognize the effect that the decision of *when* to communicate has on *how* a communication is then made. For example, if the recall communication should be made as soon as possible, does that imply that sending a letter by first class mail is unacceptable and that everyone should be contacted by telephone or by facsimile (fax)? And, what is a practical time frame for a pharmacy to contact hundreds of patients, even if it is an urgent matter? Within hours? The same day? Within a few days?

The target date or time for completing recall communications to patients, physicians, or other pharmacists should be commensurate with the degree of health hazard of the recall. For example, in the case of a minor product mislabeling that does not pose a serious health risk and the recall is to be carried out only to other pharmacies that may have purchased the product from the pharmacy, then it may be perfectly reasonable to set a notification goal of a few days. In the case of a sterile product that is contaminated with bacteria where the recall is being carried out to the patient level, it may be more prudent to set a goal of notifying all patients within a 24-hour time period.

The methods that a pharmacist chooses for *how* to communicate recalls should follow directly from the above considerations of the *whos*, *whats*, and *whens* of communication. Again, using the present examples, if communication of a recall with no health hazard needs to be completed within a few days, then sending a first class mail letter may be the most appropriate method. If a recall communication involves potential health risks, using the telephone or faxing to communicate more quickly and have some degree of confirmation that the recall notice was received, may be the more appropriate method. The pharmacy's written procedures for how to communicate may include considerable details, such as whether or not the pharmacist should leave a message on a patient's answering machine, and if a message is to be left on an answering machine, whether or not the message mentions details about a recalled product, or just a message for a particular person to call the pharmacy. HIPAA regulations regarding patient confidentiality would be a consideration in these instances.

PRODUCT HANDLING

Establishing written procedures for how product is to be handled should address such items as:

1. Identifying the recalled product
2. Locating the product in the pharmacy
3. Quarantining and returning the product

Identifying the recalled product is accomplished most reliably if its NDC number is used. Reliance on identifying factors such as name, manufacturer, etc. can be confusing in the modern pharmaceutical marketplace considering repackaging, contract manufacturing, and group purchasing and labeling. The other identifier necessary in most pharmaceutical recalls is the product lot number. The lot number identifies which manufactured batch of the product is affected by any particular recall. Some recalls affect all lots manufactured, but most are limited to certain lots.

In locating the recalled product within the pharmacy or facility, it is vital that pharmacists establish a checklist of all locations where a recalled product might possibly reside (Fig. 115-3). In addition to the obvious answer of looking for a recalled product on the main shelves, the pharmacist should consider other locations, such as, the fast mover section, refrigerator, special section categories (eg, otics, ophthalmics, dermatologicals), returns box, and prescriptions in will-call, just to identify a few. In the case of hospital or institutional pharmacies, it is important that written procedures clearly delineate the locations where the pharmacy is responsible for managing the inventory. These will vary from institution to institution, but may include such locations as satellite pharmacies, clinic pharmacies, nursing stations, automated dispensing units (eg, Pyxis machines), emergency rooms, and operating rooms. It may be that the pharmacy department is *not* responsible for all pharmaceuticals in all locations throughout the facility, and that is all the more reason why the locations for which the pharmacy department *is* responsible should be clearly identified in the written procedures.

Once all of the affected recalled product has been identified and located, it must be collected and labeled as *recalled*. While immediate removal of the recalled product from the facility may be desirable, as a practical matter it is often the case that the return instructions from the manufacturer have not been finalized. It may take several days before return shipping instructions and the attendant materials such as inventory forms and shipping labels, arrive in the pharmacy. In the meantime, it is vital that all the recalled product be clearly labeled in some manner as not for use and quarantined. A procedure for this may include such means as using bright orange tape to secure the recalled bottles (boxes, etc.) and then marking the tape with words such as "*RECALLED - DO NOT USE*" or "*QUARANTINE*." This procedure is very important. It cannot be assumed that just because the recalled product has been removed from shelves, there is no danger of dispensing it to patients. Unfortunately, the FDA has many anecdotal reports of recalled merchandise that was removed from pharmacy shelves and placed in a "safe" location only to have another pharmacist pick up the recalled product and dispense it later.[3]

A pharmacy's written procedure for product return should include where the product is to be forwarded and how it should be packaged and shipped. For most pharmacies, it will probably be that the product will be returned to a location as described in the pharmaceutical manufacturer's recall letter. This may be a manufacturer's warehouse, distribution center, or an approved third-party reverse distribution handler. Or, the manufacturer may instruct that the product be returned through the wholesaler where the product was initially purchased. The importance of established written procedures comes into play when the case arises that a pharmacy will choose *not* to return product according to the manufacturers instructions. An example of this situation occurs with many community chain pharmacies who are required by their corporate headquarters to return recalled product to, perhaps, a chain warehouse where all recalled product will be consolidated and handled as one big return. Deviating from the manufacturer's recommendation can be reasonable and acceptable, however, it is important for the pharmacist to be able to reference the pharmacy's own standard operating procedures as justification.

When packaging the product for return shipping, good packaging practices should be followed, such as allowing for sufficient cushion packing so that liquids do not break in shipment. The choice of a return shipping method should be carefully considered. The manufacturer may provide pre-paid shipping labels that dictate that a certain carrier be used. If no carrier is chosen by the manufacturer, pharmacists may wish to choose a carrier that can provide proof of pickup and proof of delivery. This can be very important in situations where the product may be hazardous or where product has a high monetary value.

Special Note—There may be some instances where the product should not be sent by common carrier or the US Postal Service at all. One example occurs when product tampering is suspected. If it is possible that a prosecution could result, then the government may want to establish an *unbroken chain* of custody of the product. Another example occurs in those situations of major adverse health consequences whereby the causative agent (eg, bacterial contamination, wrong product in bottle) has not been definitively established and immediate investigation is warranted. If the product has been returned through a ground or air carrier, it may be days before it is received by the FDA or the manufacturer. Instead, the pharmacist should hold the product for pickup. The FDA will gladly send its own agents, or local law enforcement agents, to the pharmacy to pick up the product when the situation is warranted.[4]

RECORDKEEPING

The reasons that a pharmacist would want to document the actions in a recall range from the simple determination of fact (eg, which product was affected, whether patients were notified) to lessening of legal liability (ie, good records may show a pattern of a pharmacist's diligent concern for patient health). Documenting a pharmacist's actions during a recall can be greatly facilitated by forms and checklists. Examples of forms that may be appropriate are demonstrated in Figures 115-1, 115-2, and 115-3. In addition to using forms to establish documentation of a pharmacist's own actions, copies of documents created by others should also be kept (eg, the original recall letter from the manufacturer, a copy of the pre-paid shipping label,). A simple pocket file folder can be labeled with the name of the particular recall and then all documents, forms, letters, responses, etc., can be kept in one place.

Action When a Recall Happens

Once a recall event has begun, the pharmacist should proceed in a step-by-step manner. A good outline that the pharmacist may wish to customize might include:

1. Receiving the initial notification
2. Listing further action steps
3. Carrying out further notification
4. Responding to the initial notification
5. Product handling
6. Reimbursement

INITIAL NOTIFICATION

By definition, the first thing that will occur in any particular recall is that the pharmacist will learn about that recall for the first time. This may be by one of several methods. Most common is a notice from a pharmaceutical manufacturer, a wholesaler, or a community chain headquarters. This can be by letter, facsimile, or automated telephone voice message. However, other methods include reading a report in pharmacy journals, on an Internet webpage, learning about it from a pharmacist at another pharmacy, a mass media news report, or (frustratingly) hearing about it from a patient. In any case, the pharmacist should make a note of the date and time that the notice was received. If the notice was not received in writing, then the pharmacist should consolidate in writing the pertinent facts known at that time and date that piece of paper (it has now become the first document of that recall).

Recalled Product Name _____Today's Date _____

Manufacturer _____

NDC #   __ __ __ __ __ - __ __ __ __ - __ __

Contacted for this Recall ?

Yes (date & initial)	No	INTERNAL PHARMACY PERSONNEL	NOTES
☐ _____	☐	Director of Pharmacy	
☐ _____	☐	Staff Pharmacists	
☐ _____	☐	Pharmacy Interns / Technicians	
☐ _____	☐	Front-end Clerks / Window Clerks / Receptionist	
☐ _____	☐	Materials Management / Inventory Clerks	
☐ _____	☐	Other _____	

Yes (date & initial)	No	EXTERNAL PHARMACY PERSONNEL
☐ _____	☐	Other Pharmacy of Same Ownership
☐ _____	☐	Other Pharmacist to whom product sold or loaned
☐ _____	☐	Other _____

Yes (date & initial)	No	HEALTHCARE PROFESSIONALS
☐ _____	☐	Local Physicians
☐ _____	☐	Nurses / Physician's Assistants
☐ _____	☐	Other _____

Yes (date & initial)	No	PATIENTS
☐ _____	☐	Patients Identified having Rx filled within _____ months
☐ _____	☐	All Patients / Customers
☐ _____	☐	Other _____

Yes (date & initial)	No	
		_____
☐ _____	☐	_____
☐ _____	☐	_____

Personnel Name _____ Title _____ Date _____

Personnel Name _____ Title _____ Date _____

Figure 115-1. Recall or Withdrawal WHO to CONTACT LIST.

	Date	Product	In Stock ?	Notify Patients?	Date Returned	RPh/Tech notes
1.	1/11/2005	amoxicillin 250mg caps 100s Acme Pharma NDC 99999-888-77 4 lots (see folder)	Yes 2 btls of lot# THX1188	No	1/13/2005	MJ Smith, RPh
2.	1/26/2005	meperidine inj 50mG/mL 20mL Wonderful Labs NDC 11111-2222-33 lot# BR549	No	N/A	N/A	MJ Smith, RPh
3.	2/6/2005	furosemide tabs 20mg 1000s November Pharmaceuticals NDC 98765-4321-00 4 lots (see folder)	Yes 1 full btl + 1/4 btl	Yes see folder for list	2/10/2005	K Ashby, Tech
4.	3/7/2005	infant glycerine suppos 24s August Products Co. NDC 12345-6789-10 6 lots (see folder)	No	N/A	N/A	MJ Smith, RPh
5.						
6.						
7.						
8.						
9.						

Figure 115-2. An example of a pharmacy recall log for calendar year 2005.

Recalled Product Name _____ Today's Date _____

Manufacturer_____

NDC #   __ __ __ __ __ - __ __ __ __ - __ __

Check & Initial	**Location**	**Number of units found**
_____	Main Shelves (Alphabetical)	_____
_____	Fast Mover Section	_____
_____	Refrigerator	_____
_____	Specialty Section (Otics, topicals)	_____
_____	Returns Box	_____
_____	Will Call Prescriptions	_____
_____	Satellite Stations	_____
_____	_____	_____
_____	_____	_____
_____	_____	_____
_____	_____	_____

Personnel Name _____ Title _____ Date _____

Personnel Name _____ Title _____ Date _____

Figure 115-3. Recall or withdrawal PRODUCT LOCATOR CHECKLIST.

ACTION STEPS

The next step the pharmacist should perform is to make a list of action steps dictated by that particular recall. If there are no written recall procedures for the pharmacist's particular facility, it is recommended that the pharmacist should first simply write down all the action steps that he/she can think of. The list may include items discussed in the paragraphs above, as well as instructions from the recall notice received from the manufacturer, wholesaler, or headquarters.

Then, the pharmacist should prioritize the actions' steps according to their urgency. For example, carrying out further notification to other pharmacists (and possibly patients) is more urgent than packaging the recalled product for return shipment.

FURTHER NOTIFICATION

Carrying out further notification, sometimes called a sub-recall, may be an important part of a particular recall. In the case

where patient notification is required, the pharmacist will have to identify any patients who may have received the recalled product and then communicate the recall instructions to them. The timeliness of communicating to the patient could be a matter of life and death in the worst case, or could simply spare confusion and anxiety in the least case.

RESPONSE TO NOTIFICATION

An important aspect of the recall process is responding back to the manufacturer, wholesaler, or whomever initiated the recall notification. The pharmacist should promptly respond that the notice was received and that the pharmacist is carrying out the actions instructed in the recall communication. This response can be fulfilled by different methods. In the case of a letter sent by US mail, usually there is a postage-paid business reply card. Some manufacturers have a toll-free fax number, and the recall response can be transmitted by fax. If the notification was forwarded by automated telephone voice messaging, then the pharmacist should listen to the entire message and press the appropriate button on the telephone keypad to respond.

Pharmacists must respond to the recall notification to indicate how many packages of the recalled product they have in stock. Also, pharmacists must respond **even if they do not have any of the recalled product, and even if they do not carry the recalled product in stock**. This is a requirement of the Code of Federal Regulations.[5]

PRODUCT HANDLING

As described in the procedures section on product handling, the recalled product must be identified, located, quarantined, and returned.

REIMBURSEMENT

The pharmacist will want to monitor when reimbursement is received from the manufacturer. Although product reimbursement is not an urgent health-related issue, many patients may be understandably anxious about how much and when they will be reimbursed. Pharmacists should attempt to ascertain what the manufacturer's reimbursement policy will be, and, failing that, at least, reassure the patient that some form of reasonable compensation could be expected from most major manufacturers.

Long-Term Record Keeping

As stated in previous sections, the importance of long-term record keeping cannot be overemphasized. If, unfortunately, litigation ensues because of a recall, it probably will not happen in the weeks or months immediately following the recall. It will probably happen a year or more later. The pharmacist will be well served to have copies of all internal recall documents (eg, lists of contacts, when contacts were made), as well as copies of all documents created by others (eg, original recall letter from manufacturer, copy of business reply card returned to manufacturer).

BACKGROUND INFORMATION, FUTURE DIRECTION, AND IMPLICATIONS OF RECALLS

Importance of Lot Numbers

The overwhelming majority of pharmaceutical products are not manufactured in a continuous manner like automobiles rolling off an assembly line. Rather, pharmaceuticals are manufactured in batches (ie, synonymously "lots") like how one's mother might make chocolate chip cookies. Each lot manufactured is coded with a specific Lot Number so that if there is any need (eg, as in a product recall), then that particular lot can be traced back to discover such things as which raw materials were used, what equipment was used, and which personnel were on duty during the manufacture of that lot. The configuration of the lot number (eg, combination of letters and/or numbers) is at the discretion of each individual manufacturer. However, regulations require that the lot number be printed on each package. Recalls can affect one lot, multiple lots, or all lots that have ever been manufactured. The pharmacist can help the recall process by paying close attention to which lots are affected by a particular recall. Occasionally, to spare time and resources, some pharmacists have simply returned all product in stock even though only certain lots were affected in that recall. Besides being generally wasteful, this can create an unnecessary product shortage.

Classes of Recalls and Withdrawals

The difference between a recall and a withdrawal is that the word *recall* applies if the product in question could potentially violate the FD&C (Food, Drug and Cosmetic) Act. A recall is defined as "a firm's removal or correction of a marketed product that the FDA considers to be in violation of the laws it administers and against which the agency would initiate legal action (eg, seizure)."[6] A withdrawal is defined as "a firm's removal or correction of a distributed product which involves a minor violation that would not be subject to legal action by the Food and Drug Administration or which involves no violation, eg, normal stock rotation practices, routine equipment adjustments, and repairs, etc."[6] It is not clear what is meant by "a minor violation that would not be subject to legal action" because the term "minor violation" is not defined in the Food, Drug and Cosmetic Act.[7]

One example of a withdrawal that would not violate the Act would be in that instance when a manufacturer changed the formulation from, for example, a green tablet to a blue tablet and desired to pull all of the old green tablets to avoid confusion in the marketplace. Another example would occur after the introduction of an approved new drug. A manufacturer may experience an unacceptable number of adverse drug reactions and decide to withdraw the product from the market.

Another recent (and unfortunate) example is the situation involving product tampering (including product counterfeiting). For reasons that may seem counterintuitive, situations involving product tampering or counterfeiting are usually classified as *withdrawals*, not recalls. This involves legal definitions regarding whether the manufacturer may be responsible for violations of the FD&C Act. If no manufacturing responsibility exists, then the definition of recall does not apply and the action is termed a withdrawal (Note: the legal intricacies associated with this example are beyond the scope of this chapter).

For legal liability reasons, a manufacturer may prefer to characterize a particular event as a *withdrawal* rather than a *recall*. This has occurred a few times in recent years when manufacturers have quickly taken the initiative to send out notifications (without conferring with the FDA) and describe the event as a withdrawal, when it really should have been termed a recall. This prompted the FDA to issue statements warning manufacturers to confer with the FDA on whether an event should be a recall or a withdrawal, or risk having to send out a corrective notice.[8,9] In any case, the following statement may be one of the most important of this chapter:

> **Whether a removal event is termed a *recall* or a *withdrawal*, the pharmacist should follow basically the same procedures.**

Officially, recalls are listed by the FDA in the FDA Enforcement Report. It is published weekly and can be viewed free on the Internet at http://www.fda.gov or a written version can be subscribed to at a cost of approximately $100 per year. The Enforcement Report is the official listing of FDA actions. However, it only includes *violative* actions, that is, it only lists recalls (seizures, etc.), not withdrawals. Also, any particular recall may not appear in the Enforcement Report for many weeks or even months after a recall was issued. The FDA is moving toward an Internet-based posting system for recall notices. It is anticipated that with this new system, recall notices might be posted within 1 to 2 days from the time a manufacturer first notifies the FDA of a problem.[13]

Strictly speaking, all recalls of drug products are *voluntary*. Through what might be described as a "loophole" in the law, the FDA has no authority under the Federal Food, Drug, and Cosmetic Act to order a recall without the aid of a court.[10] The FDA (more specifically, the Secretary of Health and Human Services) does have the authority to order a recall of medical devices, infant milk formulas, and some biologicals, but pharmaceutical product recalls are voluntary.

If a pharmaceutical manufacturer refuses to recall a product, then the only immediate enforcement tool the FDA has is to initiate a *seizure*. Seizures are slow, costly, and generally inefficient. However, there are some pharmaceutical seizures every year. Outside of the legal realm, the FDA has one very potent tool for inducing the manufacturer to conduct the recall, and that is the power of the press release. If the manufacturer is "dragging its heels" about doing a recall, essentially, the FDA will inform the manufacturer that the FDA has no choice but to issue a general press release naming the company, the product, and describing the potential for health hazard, etc. As a practical matter, the threat (whether explicit or implicit) of a press release usually prompts the manufacturer to initiate a *voluntary* recall.

> **Recall communications from manufacturers to pharmacists very often state that the recall is *voluntary* for the manufacturer, but pharmacists should NOT make the mistake of concluding that the recall is in any way voluntary for the pharmacist. Pharmacists should carry out all recall procedures with all due diligence.**

The overwhelming number of things that can go wrong during the manufacture of a product, regardless how unintentional or minor, will usually result in the product being "misbranded" or "adulterated" under the Food Drug and Cosmetic Act, and thus subject to a "recall." Recalls are classified as follows:

Class I is a situation in which there is a reasonable probability that the use of, or exposure to, a violative product will cause serious adverse health consequences or death.

Class II is a situation in which the use of or exposure to a violative product may cause temporary or medically reversible adverse health consequences or where the probability of serious adverse health consequences is remote.

Class III is a situation in which the use of, or exposure to, a violative product is not likely to cause adverse health consequences.[11]

Of the approximately 200 drug recalls per year, about 45% are Class III; about 50% are Class II, and less than 5% are Class I.[12]

Usually, a health hazard evaluation committee within the FDA determines the Class of a recall. The committee is composed of physicians and other appropriate scientific personnel who may consult with private practice physicians, the Centers for Disease Control and Prevention, and the manufacturer's medical department. The Committee then makes a recommendation for that particular recall. Although the FDA will try to expedite this process, it can still take several days. This is the reason why some recall notifications have been sent to pharmacists directly without a Class of recall listed.

In an effort to streamline the process, the FDA has taken an initiative to have recall officers in local FDA offices make classification decisions. Whether this initiative will result in all future recall communications containing a classification remains to be seen. In any case, the lack of an official recall classification should in no way inhibit the pharmacist from implementing the recall process. The pharmacist's individual recall policies and procedures should be carried out forthwith. The possibility of a lack of official classification does, however, imply that *pharmacists should NOT write recall procedures that are dependent on knowing the Class of recall*. For example, having a procedure that instructs to notify patients in the case of a Class I recall but not in the case of a Class II recall, would be an inappropriate recall procedure because the class of recall may not be known for days or weeks after an initial recall announcement is made. Whether or not to notify patients about a recall should be based on the degree of health hazard, not on the official classification. The initial recall announcement from the manufacturer almost always has instructions for "if-and-when" to notify patients. However, if those instructions are absent or unclear, then the pharmacist should take whatever appropriate action that good judgment dictates (ie, as he/she performs many times a day).

Level of Recall and Distribution Channels

When a recall is announced by a manufacturer, there should be a statement about at what *level* the recall is being carried out. In its simplest form, the levels of pharmaceutical distribution system in the US can be charted thus:

Pharmaceutical Manufacturer > Drug Wholesaler > Pharmacy > Patient.

Additional distributors of pharmaceutical products, such as repackagers and nursing homes, complicate the distribution channel and do not always fit neatly into the definition of what is a wholesaler or pharmacy, but the above is a reasonable model. The initial recall notice issued by the manufacturer should state the level of the recall, but unfortunately, this is not always the case.

Some pharmacists make the erroneous assumption that the Class of recall correlates perfectly with the level of distribution (ie, that Class I = patient level, Class II = pharmacy level, and Class III = wholesaler level). This is NOT true. Many Class III recalls are carried out to the pharmacy level, some Class II recalls have been carried out to the patient level, and a few Class I recalls did not involve notifying patients because the product was caught before it was fully distributed.

Sometimes, wholesalers contribute to the confusion about recall level by sending pharmacies copies of recall letters that were sent to the wholesaler and were meant by the manufacturer to be a "wholesaler-only" recall. It might be said that the wholesaler is simply erring "on the side of caution" by sending the recall notice to the pharmacy. But if that is taken to its logical conclusion by all wholesalers then there would be a *de facto* elimination of the wholesaler-only recall and there would be two levels of recall: wholesaler/pharmacy and patient. There is some sentiment within the FDA that this should actually be the case (ie, if a product is worth recalling from the wholesaler, then it is worth recalling from the pharmacy). At this time there is no final word on the situation and pharmacists will just have to use their best judgment. Pharmacists must determine the *level* of the recall independently of the *class* of the recall and then take appropriate action.

Reasons for Recalls

The approximately 200 pharmaceutical recalls issued every year happen for a variety of reasons. Table 115-1 shows some major reasons and a rough approximation of what percentage of all pharmaceutical recalls these represent.[12]

Table 115-1. Reasons for, Descriptions of, and Approximate Incidence of Pharmaceutical Recalls

REASON	DESCRIPTION	% ALL DRUG RECALLS[a]
Potency	Failure to maintain potency at certain time points during the "in date" period.	20 %
Labeling/ packaging mixups	Incorrect strength on label; wrong product in bottle; etc.	25 %
Misc. product problems	Discoloration; leaking bottles; particulate matter; etc.	5 %
Dissolution	Failure to dissolve at certain time points during the "in-date" period.	5 %
Manufacturing discrepancies	Deviations from official manufacturing procedures	5 %
Contamination	Contamination with bacteria or general lack of sterility	45 %

[a] Approximate percentages based on data from 2002.

Future Directions and Implications

Some potential legal developments may affect pharmacists directly in coming years. Legislation (ie, state, federal) changes constantly, and pharmacists must keep abreast of new regulations. One possible legislative initiative may require pharmacists to notify patients in the case of certain recalls. While this chapter has stated that proper patient notification should be good normal practice for the pharmacist, currently there is no specific law or regulation that states that pharmacists must notify patients of a drug recall. Pending federal legislation may codify that item. This situation may be analogous to the patient counseling situation. Conscientious pharmacists tried to do patient counseling in a conscientious manner as part of overall professional responsibility, but legislation then required counseling, and rules and regulations spelled out specifics of how it should be performed (eg, some pharmacists would claim there are too many specifics while others would claim there are not enough specifics). If new legislation passes requiring that pharmacists notify patients of a recall, it is unclear whether that legislation will really make any difference in the conscientious pharmacist's day-to-day practice.

One outgrowth of recalls that may affect pharmacists' future practice is the topic of tracking dispensed drugs by lot number. For each manufactured lot of a pharmaceutical product, the manufacturer is required to track exactly where each bottle of that lot has been shipped. The overwhelming majority of wholesalers and pharmacies do not track by lot number where product has gone. Tracking by lot number is an enormous data management burden for manufacturers. However, it does have the benefit that when a product needs to be recalled and the product defect can be traced to specific lots only, then the manufacturer has to recall only those lots and not all of the product in the marketplace. With modern computerized shipping and billing records, wholesalers can determine if a particular product has been sold to a particular pharmacy. Because a wholesaler does not track by lot number, for each recall it must notify every pharmacy that purchased the product even though the pharmacy may have only purchased unaffected product. But, at least the pharmacy can check inventory, return only the affected product, and keep any unaffected product in stock to serve patients.

In the case where the pharmacist has dispensed the product, unless it was dispensed in the original container, currently, there is no way to determine whether the patient is holding product from a recalled lot or from an unaffected lot. Thus, patient level recalls involve removing *all* product from *all* patients. Theoretically, if pharmacists tracked dispensed product by lot number, then they could notify and recall product only from those patients with affected product, and patients with unaffected product would not necessarily even have to know that a recall took place. There are other problems with whether or not this scenario would work. Some overall *pros* and *cons* are apparent. A significant *con* is the detailed record keeping that

would be required. Improved computer software might make it possible. The *pros* are that with detailed lot number records, a pharmacist might receive a recall notice and quickly be able to determine that he/she never stocked the product nor dispensed the recalled lot. Their recall obligations would be quickly concluded.

SUMMARY

Important steps for a pharmacist to take to handle recalls effectively are as follows:

1. Establish **procedures.** This should be performed before a recall occurs. If one is not sure how to start, one should just think of whatever one can, and write it down. Keep it simple and brief. As experience is gained and better methods are found, these can be incorporated into the procedure. Whatever can be performed before an actual recall hits, the "smoother" the recall will go.
2. **Document** what is performed. This may save a life. Legally, it may demonstrate and prove that the pharmacist acted with due diligence.
3. Use good **judgment.** Laws are not always clear; Definitions are not always exact. Instructions can be confusing. In the end, do what is best for the patient.

Thankfully, most recalls do not involve life-threatening situations. Occasionally, they will. The pharmacist is on the front line and plays a most important, crucial role in protecting the patient from potentially unsafe products.

REFERENCES

1. Pendergast MK, Deputy Commissioner, FDA. Seminar on Strategic Planning for Crisis Management, The Food and Drug Law Institute, Washington DC, Jun 7, 1995.
2. MacLean GE. Documenting Quality for ISO 9000 and Other Industry Standards. Milwaukee: ASQC Quality Press, 1993.
3. Bryant WR, Recall Officer, Office of Regulatory Affairs, FDA [personal communication]. Mar 1998.
4. Morrison EF, Deputy Director, Div of Emergency and Investigations Operations, FDA, at Crisis Management, Drug Information Assoc, Philadelphia, Oct 6, 1997.
5. 21 CFR 7.49(d) (Apr 1997).
6. Regulatory Procedures Manual, Pt 5 (Recall Procedures), FDA, 1988.
7. Parket BR, Valentino G. *Drug Info J* 1994; 28:899.
8. Pendergast MK, Deputy Commissioner, FDA, at A Meeting on Notification of Product Withdrawals and Recalls, NIH, Bethesda MD, Nov 19, 1996.
9. Simmons JC, Director Office of Compliance, CBER, FDA [Ltr], May 29, 1997.
10. Fed Reg 43(117): 26202, Jun 16, 1978.
11. Background and Definitions: http://www.fda.gov/oc/po/firmrecalls/recall_defin.html Apr 2003.
12. FDA Enforcement Reports for 2002.
13. Williams S, District Compliance Officer, FDA, at Drug and Device Recalls Conference, CBI, Nov 2002.

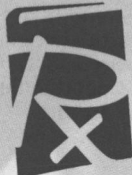

CHAPTER **116**

Marketing Pharmaceutical Care Services

Randal P McDonough, PharmD, MS
William R Doucette, PhD

"Marketing is the business function that identifies customer needs and wants, determines which target markets the organization can serve best, and designs appropriate products, services, and programs to serve these markets. However, marketing is much more than just an isolated business function—it is a philosophy that guides the entire organization."[1]

Marketing is a proven approach for stimulating consumers to purchase new services. As pharmacists work to expand their role by providing new services, marketing can be used to create demand for these services. In recent years, practitioners have worked hard to re-engineer their practices to incorporate a philosophy of pharmaceutical care into their practices. This re-engineering has resulted in pharmacies presenting a *new look* to their patients by incorporating patient consultation areas, workflow improvements, and the increased use of pharmacy technicians within the practice. In addition, pharmacists are performing new activities in their practices as new services are offered to their patients. To reach their full potential, pharmacists can market their services.

An understanding of patient needs and wants is essential for developing and implementing a successful plan for marketing pharmacy services. The need for most of our patients is to have good health. If their health deteriorates, a need exists to return to a healthy state. Patients have many options for products, services, and providers to help them achieve this healthy state, including pharmacists and pharmacy-care services. Patients choose the resources that they believe best fit their needs. To be successful, a pharmacy can incorporate a marketing management process as a basic component of their operation.

MARKETING MANAGEMENT PROCESS

A marketing management process should include three primary steps: (1) evaluating a market, (2) planning marketing strategies and tactics, and (3) implementing and controlling marketing effort. A market can be viewed as containing buyers and sellers that react to each other and to other influences acting in the market. In this case, the actors in a market for pharmacy services usually include service providers, patients, payers, and employers. They interact in a local setting under the influence of a mix of external factors such as the socioeconomic conditions and the level of medical technology present in the community.

Evaluating a market entails consideration of both a macroenvironment and a microenvironment. A macroenvironment refers to forces that affect the parties in a market, and encompasses five sectors: economic, competitive, technological, social, and regulatory. Economic considerations can affect the likelihood that patients will be able to pay for a pharmacy ser-

vice. For example, the closing of a large local employer can greatly limit the demand for services, perhaps by eliminating health insurance coverage.

Competitive factors such as consolidation of ownership can be important. For instance, the presence of a large chain usually affects pricing levels and could affect supply of pharmacists. Technology can support new services. For example, some pharmacists are incorporating personal digital assistants (PDAs) into their service provision. Social factors should be considered, such as the percentage of elderly without family support in the community. Regulatory issues can include state or federal regulations. For example, many states allow collaborative practice agreements between pharmacists and physicians.

In addition to identifying important influences in the macroenvironment, the microenvironment should be evaluated. This means that important stakeholders should be identified and appraised. Such an assessment can result in identification of parties that will facilitate, hinder, or not affect the pharmacy's marketing efforts. Types of parties to evaluate include patient groups, competitors, suppliers, and payers. One way to assess a pharmacy's microenvironment is to perform a SWOT analysis (Table 116-1) that can be used to assess the internal strengths and weaknesses of the pharmacy in context with the opportunities and threats that may exist in its external environment.[2,3]

Strengths can include the clinical expertise of pharmacists in certain disease-state management programs, the positive image of the pharmacy in the community, and the diversity of services offered by the practice. Weaknesses can include workflow issues, shortage of technician help, and lack of time to provide pharmaceutical care services. The opportunities of a practice may be with physician groups, collaborative practice strategies with certain physicians, and the needs of the community for innovative health-care services. When one identifies the threats to the practice, competitive programs should be distinguished, turf issues with other health-care providers need to be recognized, and lack of reimbursement for clinical services should be considered.

Through this analysis, pharmacists can determine what services or programs they offer or can offer in the future to gain a competitive or differential advantage in the marketplace. In addition, pharmacists within the practice need to identify their weaknesses and develop strategies that either minimize these factors or convert them into strengths.

After completing the SWOT Analysis, pharmacists can match the strengths of their pharmacy with the opportunities in the marketplace and minimize the threats (or competition) to a profitable practice. Examples of threats to the pharmacy can include a competitor with superior services, the lack of reimbursement for cognitive services, and increased costs to implementing and sustaining a clinical service.

Table 116-1. SWOT Analysis

S = Strengths of the practice (Internal environment)	W = Weaknesses of the practice (Internal environment)
O = Opportunities for the practice (External environment)	T = Threats to the practice (External environment)

A stakeholder analysis can be part of the SWOT analysis. A *stakeholder* is anyone who can affect the success of the practice. They include other health-care providers, community resources such as hospitals and clinics, community leaders, public agencies, employers, and third-party payers. Other potential stakeholders to the practice may include other pharmacists not employed by the pharmacy but who have created some type of alliance with the pharmacy. Stakeholders influence the practice by providing a support structure for new ideas, identifying key targets for marketing efforts, and providing a process that helps to improve the quality of the services provided by the pharmacy.

To better understand the external environment of their pharmacy, pharmacists may use marketing research techniques. This provides them with additional information about their marketplace and assists them in the development of strategies to increase sales, improve the practice, assess the competition, and determine the needs of patients. Market research can encompass several techniques that may include questionnaires, telephone surveys, focus groups, casual conversation, observation, and published data. This information should be collected and updated annually and the necessary adjustments made to the marketing plan.

The information gathered from this market research can be continually incorporated into the practice's SWOT analysis. The research provides new information regarding external opportunities and threats to the practice. Using this information, along with an internal inventory of the strengths and weaknesses of their pharmacy, provides an excellent starting point to develop a comprehensive marketing plan.

PLANNING OF MARKETING

The second phase of the marketing management process is to plan marketing strategies and tactics. A marketing plan should contain key elements that are essential for successful implementation. The marketing plan should be consistent with the mission of the practice and should incorporate analyses performed during the evaluation phase, especially the SWOT analysis. From the analyses, target markets may be identified, the marketing mix determined, and the marketing strategies developed. Included in the marketing plan should be a process to monitor the results of the plan. The key elements of a marketing plan include[4]

SWOT analysis (see Table 92-1)
Goals and objectives
Target markets
Marketing mix
Control processes

Goals and Objectives

After the SWOT analysis is written, a set of goal statements can be prepared. These statements lead to objectives that a pharmacy wants to accomplish. They should reflect the mission statement for the practice, which is the underlying philosophy of the pharmacy. Goal statements are general and provide direction for the practice to meet the mission of the pharmacy. Each goal statement has its own specific *objectives* that are the outcomes needed to meet the goals. The objectives that are developed for the practice should be clearly stated, realistic, and

measurable. It is through the objectives that pharmacists can determine the success or failure of their marketing plan. Some common objectives that have been used by pharmacists include improved profitability, sales growth of a particular service or product, market share improvement, risk diversification, and practice innovation. A well-written marketing plan with clear, quantifiable goals and objectives can provide the pharmacist with the feedback mechanism to change and refine specific components of the plan. To achieve the goals and objectives, one must accomplish *specific tasks* in accordance with a *timeline* that provides a reasonable period for completion of each task. Table 116-2 provides examples of a mission statement, a goal statement, and objectives.

Once the goals and objectives are developed, time should be spent thinking about the persons (target markets) who can benefit from the services offered by the practice. The goal of a pharmacy's marketing activities is to stimulate exchanges with patients who are likely to benefit from services provided. A marketing approach focuses the marketing efforts on those groups in the market, known as target markets.

Target Markets

Target markets are those customers who behave in similar patterns and can benefit from the pharmacy care services offered by the practice.[5] It is important to identify key targets for the marketing efforts because it is neither efficient nor cost effective to market to the general public. Customers who are the targets of the marketing process should have needs and wants that the pharmacy services can meet. When initiating the market plan, it is beneficial to consider how customers behave. Research in this area shows that subgroups of consumers can be identified based on their adoption (ie, use of) new services.[6,7]

ADOPTION GROUPS—Five groups can be considered, based on their likelihood of trying new services. A list of these is as follows:

1. Innovators—less than 5% of customers.
2. Early adopters—10–15% of customers.
3. Early majority—30–35% of customers.
4. Late majority—30–35% of customers.
5. Late adopters—15–20% of customers.

Table 116-2. Mission, Goals Statements, and Objectives

Mission Statement of the practice	To enhance health status and provide innovative and high-quality pharmacy services by being sincere, compassionate, and focused on the individual needs of each patient.
Goal Statement	To market and promote the pharmacy services effectively to physicians and other health-care providers to increase the referrals to the practice.
Objectives	Within 3 months, identify key decision makers in each medical group.
	In the next 3 months, identify the key 100 primary-care physicians and develop a newsletter that provides information about the programs and pharmacy-care services offered by the practice.
	Identify 100% of the physicians (specialists and primary care) who care for a large percentage of diabetes and asthma patients.
	In the next 3 months, identify competing programs/services within the community.
	Within 1 month, develop promotional tools to use when marketing to physicians and other health-care providers.

Innovators represent the smallest percentage of customers, but they are the first to try a new service, if they believe it meets their needs. They are considered risk takers and venturesome. Early adopters, who often are opinion leaders in the community, need to hear the marketing message several times because they carefully evaluate new ideas and services. This group accepts a new service early in the marketing efforts.

The early majority, though not leaders, do adopt a new service earlier than the average consumer. Repeat marketing efforts need to stay focused on this group because they need to hear the marketing message several times before purchasing a new service. In addition, this group represents a large proportion of a market.

The late majority are consumers who question new products and services. However, they adopt a new service once the majority of consumers buy. This group is not likely to respond to early marketing efforts.

The last group is the late adopters who not only question a new innovation, but remain suspicious. This group buys only after the service has a well-proven record. Again, this group is not likely to be responsive to early marketing activities.

By understanding the characteristics of each of these groups, marketing plans can be created to focus on the appropriate group. For new pharmacy services, innovators and early adopters would be of most interest. Typically, consumers in these two groups are younger, have more education, and have higher income than other consumers.[6,7] Because they trust their own judgment, they are more willing to try new services and to respond to promotional strategies that attract them to such services.

Relationship Marketing

Relationship marketing is a strategy that pharmacists can use to improve their marketing efforts. The focus of this strategy is developing long-term and lasting relationships with like-minded customers who share a common desire or concern. In other words, pharmacists should focus their marketing efforts on those customers who are most likely to benefit from their services. Pharmacists who embrace the philosophy of relationship marketing realize that each patient encounter builds on the previous one. In this approach, pharmacists are more likely to identify the explicit health needs of their patients and provide a service that helps them achieve their therapeutic goals.

Marketing Mix

The term for the variables that are under the pharmacists' control is marketing mix. The variables are selected strategically to increase the likelihood of successful marketing. The elements of the marketing mix, also called the 4 P's of marketing include:[4,8–10]

1. Product
2. Price
3. Promotion.
4. Place

A fifth P, positioning, often is included as well.

The **product** refers to what is being marketed. With pharmaceutical care services, it is not a physical product that needs promoting but rather intangible services. Services have certain characteristics that differentiate them from products. These differences are referred to as the 4 I's in service marketing.[4,11]

1. Intangible
2. Inconsistent
3. Inseparable
4. Non-Inventoried

Because patients cannot physically see or touch a service (*intangible*), they must experience the services to receive the benefits. This experience and the quality of the interaction with the pharmacist provide the basis for patient satisfaction with the services. It may be useful to try to raise the tangibility of a service by adding a tangible component such as a paper report or some other materials.

Pharmacy services typically are delivered by individual pharmacists. This results in variability in delivery among different practitioners (*inconsistency*). The clinical competencies, knowledge base, communication skills, and personalities of the pharmacists are all key factors for provider performance in service delivery. Proper training of pharmacy personnel and use of a consistent service process can constrain problems with inconsistent service delivery.

Because pharmacy care services cannot be separated from the pharmacists who perform them (*inseparability*), quality programs need to be delivered by quality providers. Kotler[12] discussed the need for service providers to focus on the technical quality of the service (was the service successful?) and its functional quality (did the pharmacist demonstrate concern, empathy, and competence in providing the care?). In other words, providers that deliver *high-touch* as well as *high-tech* services are more likely to have satisfied customers. In addition, the development of protocols, policies and procedures, and standard educational materials helps to enhance pharmacists' performance with service delivery. Last, continuous quality-improvement activities should be implemented to keep the quality of the service at a high level.

The fourth characteristic of services is the concept of *inventory*. Unlike goods, services do not have a physical presence in the practice, and thus cannot be stored. Rather, to provide pharmacy-care services, a practitioner needs to be prepared to deliver services when purchased by the patient. There is a cost of inventory associated with the pharmacist who is working but who may not always be delivering pharmacy-care services. The challenge in this situation is to provide sufficient pharmacist coverage to provide services when needed but, at the same time, to minimize pharmacist overlap and costs. By understanding the patient flow in the pharmacy throughout the day, strategies can be developed to improve the efficiencies of the practice. The use of appointments for pharmacy services has become more common in pharmacies that have attained sufficient service volume.

Often, marketing a program or service involves making a major change in the perceptions of a patient of a pharmacy and the pharmacists who are employed there. For example, if patients view pharmacists as doing little more than dispensing, it is unlikely that they will want to participate in pharmacy-care activities. Increasing the expectations of patients can be accomplished by making changes, ranging from simply improving the workflow to becoming certified in a particular area of expertise. If a pharmacist wants to create the image of being knowledgeable about diabetes education, for example, he or she may want to become a Certified Diabetes Educator (CDE) or to enroll in a certificate program that focuses on that disease. Patients who perceive a service as new and different are more likely to see the benefit of those services. Another strategy to increase patient awareness of a service is to stock a variety of products related to the service (ie, a diabetes supply display). Helping patients select appropriate products can offer a unique opportunity to market the service of the pharmacy on a personal level. Pharmacists can also indirectly change patients' perceptions by partnering with physicians and other health-care providers who may serve as a referral source for the practice. This helps to give the practice credibility and an improved public image.

FEATURES VERSUS BENEFITS OF A PHARMACY SERVICE

Changing perceptions and expectations of the practice are important, but not the sole activity that guarantees success for marketing a service. It is equally important to examine the

Table 116-3. Features and Benefits

FEATURES	BENEFITS
One-on-one patient education	Providing you with the information necessary to help you make better decisions about your own health care.
	Helping you take charge of your own health.
Medication review and assessment	Making sure your medications are working appropriately to improve your health.
	Reducing problems associated with medications, such as side effects and interactions with other medications.
Communication with other health-care providers	Keeping your physician informed about the education provided so he/she can better care for your health-care needs.
	Providing feedback about your medications to make sure you are receiving the benefits needed to keep you healthy.

needs of the persons identified as targets of the marketing efforts. Once these needs are recognized, the marketing message can focus on the features and benefits (Table 116-3) of the services that are specific for that group (target market or stakeholder).

The *features* of the service are the elements that describe what the service offers the patient. In contrast, the *benefits* of the service to the individual patient or the stakeholder help describe why that person should be interested in the service. Understanding these key principles in service marketing helps to develop effective marketing strategies and promotional materials. More important, it provides the pharmacist with a focus to discuss services to patients during one-on-one consultations.

Using features and benefits to market services may be helpful for patients, health-care providers, and third-party payers. However, the features and benefits for these other groups and payers may be different depending on their needs. For example, a medication review service feature may be used for discussing a disease management service with physicians as well as third-party payers, but the benefits are different. The benefit to physicians may be to relieve the time constraints they experience in their own practices. For example, it would be useful to discuss how the services can reduce the number of unnecessary calls from patients regarding their medications. Also, by providing this service, patient compliance and other issues related to the medications can be assessed by the pharmacist, with progress reports forwarded to the physician on a regular basis. This can complement the physician's educational efforts with the patient regarding proper medication use. In contrast, the benefit to the payer would focus on cost issues and how this service could potentially save them money by reducing the additional use of health-care resources (eg, hospitalizations and increased physician visits) due to inappropriate medication use.

Price considerations are difficult for most pharmacists because they have limited experience pricing pharmacy services. Nonetheless, setting an appropriate price that remains competitive yet profitable is important. Being aware of the pricing strategies of competing programs such as a diabetes center can provide information that helps to guide fees. If a competitive program does not exist or if an innovative program is developed, setting a fee structure then becomes more difficult. It is important to think about the resources and time (ie, costs) consumed by offering the service and set prices accordingly. By concentrating on the value of the service and creating the per-

ception of expertise to the customer, fees can be set higher and adjusted only after the market has had time to respond. It is important to assess the prices for services continually to make sure the practice remains profitable and competitive.

Promotion, the third marketing principle is more than just advertising. Promotional strategies include publicity, public relations, direct mail, sales promotions, advertising, and personal selling (Table 116-4). To be cost effective, the strategies used should focus on customers who can benefit from the services offered. Using the features and benefits to describe the services to these customers helps in developing effective promotional material. The effectiveness of each strategy should be determined by measuring the outcomes associated with the promotional effort. This evaluation helps to determine which methods are worthwhile or ineffective and also provides the information needed to make adjustments in the overall plan.

The development of effective promotional materials requires much time and thought. When using *direct mail* as a strategy, developing a mailing list should be the first step in the process. Mailing lists can be created from the pharmacy computer record, a membership list from service groups and support groups, as well as from lists developed from special promotions when information is collected. There are certain guidelines that can be followed to create direct-mail pieces.[5] Keeping focused on the features and benefits for that particular target market helps organize the message.

Publicity is another form of promotion that should be considered in the marketing plan. Some of the strategies that are effective and inexpensive include newsletter articles, opinion editorials, and news and press releases. The same principles are important for these promotional materials: emphasize features and benefits, keep focused on the reader, and avoid complex medical terminology that may confuse the reader.

Providing presentations to support groups can be part of the promotional mix. The presentations should be well planned in advance. The pharmacist should know what points he/she wants to discuss with the group and how one will promote the services of the pharmacy. Avoid lecturing, and keep the presentation as much of a discussion as possible. By listening to the participants, information can be gathered about their needs and wants. The pharmacist should make sure to bring brochures, business cards, and other promotional materials that can be handed out to the group during the presentation. Attendees should be invited to visit the practice or call if they have any questions about the services or programs that the pharmacy offers.

Participating in special events or community-wide events can augment the overall marketing strategy. A goal when participating in events such as health fairs is to increase the good will of the pharmacy, to generate interest in the clinical programs developed, and to demonstrate the competence and skills of the pharmacists to potential patients. Creating special events such as health promotions and screenings, *brown bag* days, and open houses allow potential patients and local healthcare providers to learn about and experience the new services offered at the practice.

Other promotional strategies such as sales promotions and personal selling should be considered in the marketing plan. Sales promotions include any materials or efforts developed to assist the pharmacist in selling his/her clinical services, such as

Table 116-4. Promotional Strategies

PROMOTIONAL STRATEGY	TARGETS/STAKEHOLDERS	FREQUENCY
List the promotional strategies that will be used by the practice.	Identify the Target Markets and Stakeholders the promotional strategies are targeting.	How frequent will this promotional strategy be used, ie, quarterly, monthly, weekly, etc.

coupons or discounted service trials. Another promotional technique is personal selling, which occurs when someone describes the pharmacy service to a patient or stakeholder. During such a selling process, a pharmacist can use a series of questions to identify explicit needs of the patient. The explicit needs relate to the benefits that a patient might be able to achieve, in part, through receiving a pharmacy service. For example, a patient with asthma might be able to spend more time jogging or hiking after participating in an asthma management service at the pharmacy. Personal selling can help a patient recognize such an opportunity.

A skill that may help pharmacists in their personal selling efforts is learning to identify the needs of their patients. By identifying the needs, pharmacists can apply the personal selling process during their consultations with patients. This personal selling process is need(s) identification, a brief description of the clinical service or program that can satisfy the need(s), an explanation of its benefits and the cost to the patient. Because many pharmacists do not think of themselves as salespeople, training programs in personal selling techniques may provide additional skills to help them excel in this effort. One strategy that can be used by pharmacists to improve their abilities to uncover their patients' explicit needs is the SPIN model.[13] In this model pharmacists use four different types of probes to identify their patients' needs and wants: situating, problem, implication, and need-payoff questions.

Situation questions are used during the initial encounter with the patient. These types of probes are used to gather background information about the patient. The next types of probes in the SPIN model are the problem questions. These questions probe the patient for any dissatisfactions or concerns that they have with their health or medications. Problem questions help to uncover the patients' implicit needs, but at this point, the patient may not fully realize the impact their concerns have on their health or quality of life. Implication questions are used to help the patient become more aware of the true impact their health or medications concerns have on their daily lives. In answering these questions, patients may realize that their problem or dissatisfaction has significant implications and may require some action (eg, a pharmacy service) to resolve. Lastly, need-payoff questions help patients articulate their explicit needs about their health concerns or dissatisfactions. By answering these questions, patients begin to focus on possible solutions to their problems. Pharmacists can now discuss how a particular service they have can address the patients' problems. Table 116-5 provides examples of the four types of probes used for the SPIN model.

Table 116-5. Probing Questions Using the SPIN Model

SITUATION QUESTIONS:
What are your current complaints related to your health?
What medications are you taking?
What current medical conditions to you have?
How are you feeling?
PROBLEM QUESTIONS:
Have you experienced any drowsiness or other side effects with this medication that you are taking?
How have your blood pressures been since starting on your new blood pressure medication?
IMPLICATION QUESTIONS:
Has the drowsiness that you experienced with your new medication affect your daily activities?
What are your concerns about controlling your blood pressures?
NEED-PAYOFF QUESTIONS:
Would it be beneficial for you if a medication review service can identify alternative medications that may have less side effects such as drowsiness?
Did you know that keeping your blood pressures within goal range will substantially reduce your risk of developing long term complications?

Advertising, another promotional technique, includes the paid efforts of the practice to deliver the marketing message to a broader audience. Radio, television, and newspapers are effective media to market programs and services. The media selected depends on the message that the pharmacist wants to promote, the audience he/she wants to reach, and his/her budget. It is important to find out about the readership or viewership of the media and the costs of advertising because this information helps in deciding which promotional strategies fit within one's marketing plan and budget. It is possible that a local cable TV sponsorship can be cost-effective in reaching a particular target market.

The best promotion is providing quality care to the patient. Patients can be the greatest advocates of a pharmacy by sharing their experiences with their friends and other healthcare providers. If they discuss the services with their physicians and their satisfaction with those services, this could enhance the physician's image of the practice. Such an enhanced image could translate to an increased likelihood that the physician will refer patients to the pharmacy. It is important to assess the quality of the practice continually by receiving feedback from patients. This can be in the form of patient satisfaction surveys; the information collected from these surveys may be incorporated into new promotional materials. Table 116-4 can be used to generate a list of promotional strategies employed by a pharmacy.

Place refers to where and how the services are delivered. When providing services, it is important to make it available at the right place and at the right time. Convenience to the patient or customer needs to be assessed to assure success of the service. Within the pharmacy, an area that is considered private and professional helps in improving the perception of the patient. If possible, it may be necessary to deliver the service outside the pharmacy such as at a physician clinic or at the work site of the employer who contracts out for the services. The use of the telephone as an element of service delivery should be considered, especially with follow-up monitoring that may be associated with a service. If the practice has a delivery service, this service may be used to provide patient care and should be included in the marketing plan.

Positioning is the final element of marketing that needs to be considered. Positioning refers to creating a favorable image of the pharmacy in the minds of potential targets and stakeholders so they want and demand your services.[4] In a competitive environment, positioning helps to create a niche for the practice that addresses unmet needs of a group of patients. For example, some patients who have been newly diagnosed with diabetes prefer a one-on-one educational session with a health care provider instead of group sessions commonly seen in diabetes centers. A pharmacist can position his/her practice as one that provides individualized sessions to attract those patients to his/her practice. The messages contained in promotional materials are vital to establishing a favorable position in a market. Once a marketing plan is prepared, attention can be turned to implementing it and controlling the marketing activities.

IMPLEMENTING AND CONTROLLING MARKETING ACTIVITIES

Two components of implementing and controlling of marketing activities can be considered: rollout of the service and monitoring of activities. Pharmacy service rollout should be guided with an action plan that identifies the activities that need to be performed, when each activity will occur, and who will be responsible for getting it done. A starting place is to generate a task list for the service rollout. Tasks can address a variety of areas that are likely to require some change to accommodate a new pharmacy service. Such areas include: workflow and staffing, staff training, materials and systems for service

Table 116-6. Tasks and Timeline

TASK	PERSON RESPONSBILE	OBJECTIVES MET	DEADLINE TO COMPLETE TASK
List the tasks that need to be completed.	Identify who the person is responsible for specific tasks; this can be a pharmacist, technician, or clerk.	From the goal and objective statements listed, identify which one corresponds to each task.	Have a deadline for each task to be completed. Once completed have the person responsible for the task initial and date this form.

provision and documentation, pharmacy layout, and marketing materials (Table 116-6).

The workflow of a pharmacy service can be mapped out using a service blueprint.[14] A service blueprint is a map of service processes that depicts the steps that will occur during the service and details the roles of patients, service providers, and supporting services. By mapping the entire service process, a comprehensive view of the workflow can be assessed. Perhaps a new layout needs to be developed or new equipment needs to be purchased and then incorporated into the practice.

Another common need for service rollout is staff training. Some training may be needed to sharpen the clinical knowledge of the pharmacists. In addition, the actual service process should be learned by the pharmacists and other staff. Even if technicians do not provide a service, they will need to know its process to be able to coordinate activities with pharmacists who are providing services. Staff should be trained to fully utilize any documentation system that is used for new services.

Initially, not all marketing strategies, nor all promotional materials, provide the results anticipated. It is important to test, monitor, and refine strategies and tools continually and to minimize costly approaches to the marketing plan that are marginally effective. During evaluation of the effectiveness of new materials, it is also important to allow adequate time for testing. The marketing plan, timeline, and budget help to provide the boundaries or limits to the marketing process. Predefined outcome measures of the marketing plan provide the goals or the results of the marketing process. By referring to the written marketing plan, one can make an accurate assessment of marketing materials.

As the action plan is executed, the first day of service will draw nearer. A specific day should be set, on which the pharmacy is able to provide the new service. Some promotional efforts can create awareness for the service. The staff and facility should be ready to go, once the service goes live. A good approach is to spend special attention on the first few service patients to get an initial assessment of the service process. This will allow early identification of problems, which can be addressed before large problems develop.

To monitor the marketing activities, an information system should be utilized. Commonly, such a system needs to be developed as new pharmacy services are offered. The system should allow the evaluation of performance at achieving marketing objectives. Performance indicators should be identified, and processes for collecting and reporting this information can be established. Then, regular reports can be used to assess service quality and other marketing performance objectives.

A number of performance indicators can be monitored. These indicators should be established before implementation and processes are in place to collect the data. The outcomes may include:

Number of services or programs sold
Increase in pharmacy service revenue
Increase in referrals
Number of contracts with employers
Improved patient satisfaction surveys
Quality of the services

By assessing these outcome data from the marketing efforts, one can make decisions about future marketing efforts and the cost-effectiveness of certain strategies. For example, low pa-

tient satisfaction with a service can be used to guide improvements in the service delivery. Any performance shortfalls should lead to identification for the cause of the shortfall. All of the marketing mix should be considered. Once a potential cause is found, adjustments can be made in the marketing effort to address it.

Budgeting for the marketing plan will need to be addressed at this time as well. Several strategies can be used to determine the appropriate amount that should be spent for marketing and advertising.[15,16]

One common approach is to determine a fixed percentage of sales to set aside for advertising (*percentage of sales*). Although this method is easily applied, it has some inherent problems. Its major shortcoming is the implication that sales cause advertising. Instead, marketing and advertising should be seen as increasing sales.

A second method is to establish a marketing budget based on the competition or industry norms (*competitive parity*). This is not an optimal approach because the competition may be reaching a different target market or may not have appropriated sufficient funds for marketing. In addition, these figures may not be readily available.

The next approach is the *affordable method*. This strategy takes the marketing budget into consideration only after funds have been allocated to other important operations or projects to the pharmacy. The remaining funds then are applied to the marketing budget. This approach does not take into account the goals and objectives of the marketing plan and how to complete the tasks of the marketing plan effectively.

The last strategy, *objective and task approach*, is the most cost-effective method for determining a budget. This *bottom-up* method determines the goals and objectives of the marketing plan, the tasks that need to be completed, and the costs associated with each task. The marketing budget is created by determining what investment is needed to implement the marketing strategies developed during the planning process. Assessments of the effectiveness of each strategy allow adjustments to be made in the plan and budget.

Decisions about the amount spent on marketing should be evaluated routinely by looking at the return on investment. One should contact various sources to determine the most cost-effective methods of advertising. Certain promotional strategies may prove to be more effective than others, causing the need to reassess the investment in these strategies. Some pharmacies may invest a larger amount in the marketing budget earlier in the planning stages and hire a consultant. Once the plan is put into place and the consultant is no longer needed, the practice can decrease the budget to usual levels. Regardless of which strategies are used, developing and refining a budget is a dynamic process and helps guide decisions for the marketing plan.

Another key part of monitoring marketing effort is to seek feedback from patients. Receiving feedback from patients and stakeholders regarding promotional materials before market testing helps in the development of these marketing tools. One approach is to recruit a small group of patients and stakeholders to preview materials regularly. During the market testing, carefully evaluate patient and stakeholder response to the marketing strategies. It is during this time that feedback about the effectiveness of certain marketing materials and tools can be collected to help revise and refine these materials. For example, asking all new service customers how they found out about the services can help identify effective promotions. Once this step is accomplished, implementation of the marketing plan follows.

Once decisions are finalized regarding each aspect of the marketing process, implementation of the plan is next. The goal is to follow the written action plan and timeline created during the planning process. Expect minor problems as new activities are undertaken. For example, territory battles may arise with other health-care providers and within one's own pharmacy. Delegating tasks and responsibilities to individuals within the practice distributes the workload associated with each task and can include all the staff. It is important that pharmacists remain supportive and realistic when assigning tasks to other employees in the practice, because each employee must feel that his or her contributions are equally important. Use of a monthly planner or calendar to assign responsibility to individuals to complete certain tasks can assist the pharmacist in the implementation process. Employees should date and initial each task as it is completed. Providing incentives for employees encourages their participation and creates a sense of ownership in the marketing process.

The different promotional strategies should be implemented at this time as well. Promotion and advertising dollars should be kept within the established budget. Because an increase in sales may not be immediate, cash-flow considerations should be part of the implementation plan. The practice may need to stagger activities to assure sufficient funds when needed. When the pharmacist is determining costs associated with certain tasks, economic considerations are important, as well as time constraints on the staff. Both are equally significant. The time and cost of the implementation phase can be substantial; pharmacists and staff need to remain committed to the marketing plan to help ensure its success. In addition, pharmacists should remain flexible and make adjustments to the plan if expected results are not realized.

CONCLUSIONS

To successfully implement pharmacy-care services, pharmacists can market their services. The three steps of the marketing process outlined in this chapter provide a basic framework that can be applied to any practice. Each step of the marketing process may be individualized to a particular practice site, demographic area, patient base, competitive environment, and financial constraint. Regardless of the pharmacy involved, however, the importance of adequate market research and planning should not be underestimated. A thorough analysis of one's environment is essential to identify key targets and stakeholders, recognize opportunities and threats to the practice's success, and ensure that marketing resources are used in the most cost-effective manner.

When implementing the marketing plan in an individual pharmacy, pharmacists should use goals, objectives, and individual tasks to give direction to the marketing process. Including all employees in this process, from clerks to pharmacist, helps to ensure consistency and commitment from all involved. During the implementation phase of the marketing plan, regularly scheduled meetings should be held to keep employees updated and informed on the marketing efforts. By careful consideration of the concepts described in this chapter and by involving all employees of the pharmacy in the process, pharmacists can achieve the optimal results from their marketing plan.

REFERENCES

1. Kotler P, Armstrong G. *Principles of Marketing*. Upper Saddle River, NJ: Prentice Hall, 1996.
2. Kotler P. *Marketing Management*. Upper Saddle River, NJ: Prentice Hall, 1997; 84.
3. Berkowitz EN. *Essentials of Health Care Marketing*. Gaithersburg, MD: Aspen 1996; 44.
4. Schwartz A, Sogol E. *Drug Topics* 1987; 6:69.
5. Rovers JP et al. *A Practical Guide to Pharmaceutical Care*. Washington, DC: APhA, 1998, chap 9.
6. Kotler P. *Marketing Management*. Upper Saddle River, NJ: Prentice Hall. 1997; 336.
7. Kotler P, Armstrong G. *Principles of Marketing*. Upper Saddle River, NJ: Prentice Hall, 1996; 167.
8. Berkowitz EN. *Essentials of Health Care Marketing*. Gaithersburg, MD: Aspen, 1996; 6.
9. Kotler P. *Marketing Management*. Upper Saddle River, NJ: Prentice Hall, 1997; 92.
10. Kotler P, Armstrong G. *Principles of Marketing*. Upper Saddle River, NJ: Prentice Hall, 1996; 48.
11. Berkowitz EN. *Essentials of Health Care Marketing*. Gaithersburg, MD: Aspen 1996; 202.
12. Kotler P. *Marketing Management*. Upper Saddle River, NJ: Prentice Hall, 1997; 473.
13. Rackham N. SPIN Selling. New York: McGraw-Hill, 1988.
14. Holdford DA, Kennedy DT. *JAPhA* 1999; 39:545.
15. Berkowitz EN. *Essentials of Health Care Marketing*, Gaithersburg, MD: Aspen 1996; 314.
16. Kotler P. *Marketing Management*. Upper Saddle River, NJ: Prentice Hall, 1997; 620.

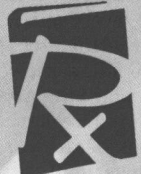

CHAPTER 117

Documenting, Billing, and Reimbursement for Pharmaceutical Care Services

Michael T Rupp

THE ROLE OF DOCUMENTATION IN PHARMACEUTICAL CARE

The role of clinical documentation in pharmaceutical care is often underappreciated or misunderstood entirely. Documentation is viewed by some pharmacists as an activity that detracts from care by consuming time that could otherwise be spent with the patient. In fact, accurate and consistent documentation of clinical observations, decisions, and actions improves the quality of care delivered to patients in several important ways:

1. It imposes a logical structure on the clinician's thinking. Essentially, documentation requires the pharmacist to ask and answer the questions, "What did I do, and why did I do it?" Over the course of time, the same critical reasoning is incorporated into the process of planning and delivering care. This continuous critical self-assessment translates into a more logical, deliberate, and consistent approach to providing care.
2. It enhances the quality of care through improving the continuity of care. This effect is particularly pronounced in the community practice setting, where systems to ensure continuity of patient care are often not as fully developed as institutional practice settings. Properly integrated into a practice, written documentation provides a mechanism for assuring the consistent flow of patient information from encounter-to-encounter and from provider-to-provider. Like other health care providers, pharmacists often develop close relationships with their patients. As a result, some may erroneously conclude that documenting the services they perform is unnecessary because "they will remember." However, such a casual approach increases the risk that important patient information will be overlooked. When this happens, the quality of care inevitably suffers.
3. In addition to supporting patient care, clinical documentation also creates a permanent written record of observations made and actions taken for legal purposes. As Cohen has noted, "if it isn't documented, it wasn't done."[1] Perhaps more to the point is the admonition found on a nurses' station in a large hospital: "In God We Trust, All Others Must Document!"
4. Documentation of activities is useful in workload management to maximize the use of existing personnel and justify the need for additional positions.[2] Additionally, documentation of key professional activities, such as pharmacists' interventions to correct prescribing errors, can serve to establish the need for, and value of, the pharmacist in the channel of distribution for prescription medications.[3–6] Indeed, the importance of documenting pharmacist interventions has been recognized by the Joint Commission on Accreditation of Healthcare Organizations (JCAHO) who have included it as a key clinical quality indicator in a medication-use monitoring system.[7]

Portions of this chapter were excerpted with permission from: Rupp MT. *Pharmacist Care Claim Form User's Manual: A Guide to Pharmacist Care Compensation,* 3rd ed. Alexandria, VA: National Community Pharmacists Association, 2000.

5. It may be performed for purposes of billing and getting paid for care provided to patients.[8] In November 1990, the Office of HHS Inspector General, Richard P Kusserow, released a report titled *The Clinical Role of the Community Pharmacist.*[9] The report concluded, "there is strong evidence that clinical pharmacy services add value to patient care," but that "in the community pharmacy setting, significant barriers exist that limit the range of clinical services generally provided." Among the most formidable of these barriers, the report concluded, is "a transaction-based reimbursement structure [which] links pharmacists' reimbursement to the sale of a product rather than provision of services."

Thus, the development of compensation strategies that recognize the value of professional services and equitably reward pharmacists who competently and consistently provide them, represents a clear and urgent priority for the profession. As a result, developing accurate and efficient documentation and billing systems represent a clinical, legal, and economic mandate for the pharmacy profession.

NARRATIVE DOCUMENTATION: THE SOAP SYSTEM

Many of the seminal advances in clinical documentation can be traced to the work of Dr Lawrence Weed, a physician and pioneer in creating systematic approaches to organizing the collection, storage, and use of clinical information.[10] Weed's intuitive problem-oriented medical record (POMR) represented a significant advance from the fragmented source-oriented record that had preceded it, in which notes were filed according to the source from which they had come, such as physician orders, nursing notes, laboratory reports, and so on.

As described by Weed, the POMR consisted of four essential components:

1. The defined data base
2. The complete problem list
3. The initial plan
4. The progress notes

Weed recommended that progress notes be further organized to reflect the four types of information that are commonly found in clinical documentation. This has come to be known as the SOAP approach to clinical documentation, SOAP representing an acronym for Subjective, Objective, Assessment, and Plan.

Subjective information includes a description of the problem and the associated symptoms in the patient's own words. These notes often contain verbatim quotes from the patient, *"I feel hot and achy, and I have a splitting headache,"* and/or those close to the patient such as a relative or friend, *"She has been complaining of fever and headache for a couple of days."*

Objective information includes observations made and data collected and/or considered by the caregiver that is relevant to the problem including physical exam or assessment, laboratory data, and so on (eg, *Patient presents to the pharmacy in acute distress complaining of flu-like symptoms for the past 2 days. Complexion is pale, skin is warm and dry to the touch, temperature is 101° F orally*).

The assessment component of the note allows the caregiver to express his/her net conclusion or opinion about the problem based on the subjective and objective information that is available (eg, *Patient's symptoms are consistent with flu*). The assessment note may be seen as a diagnosis, clinical impression, or a change in the condition of the patient for better or worse.

The plan component of the progress note describes the recommended course of action based on the new information being considered by the caregiver. This may include revising a previous plan or establishing a new one and may contain recommended treatment, patient education/instruction, and/or the need for additional information (eg, *Recommended acetaminophen 650 mg every 4–6 hours, push fluids, and bed rest. If symptoms worsen, or if not improved in 48 hours, patient instructed to see physician*).

Although the SOAP approach provides a simple, logical structure for documenting clinical encounters with patients, there are some elements that are not applicable to every care-related service performed by the pharmacist. For example, subjective patient information is usually only relevant to situations involving direct patient care. In other situations, such as an intervention to correct a prescription-related problem that is identified during prescription screening and dispensing, subjective patient information would often be unnecessary or irrelevant.[12]

Many permutations of the SOAP approach to clinical documentation have appeared over the years. However, even under different acronyms, most are essentially minor derivations of Weed's simple, yet effective approach. By organizing clinical documentation in a logical and consistent format, SOAP maintains significant advantages over unstructured approaches for ensuring greater accuracy and completeness of a care encounter. Additionally, since the SOAP approach is widely used in the clinical training of many health professionals, it is likely to be more familiar, and therefore more acceptable, to health professionals and claims administrators working for third party payers.

USING ABBREVIATIONS AND SYMBOLS—It is not uncommon for pharmacists and other health professionals to use symbols and abbreviations in their clinical documentation. Used appropriately, symbols and abbreviations can improve the accuracy of documentation while conserving provider time and documentation space. However, used inappropriately, these shortcuts can increase the likelihood of medication errors and other adverse patient outcomes.

Consider the following note: *Pt c/o PND × 5d*. In this note, *PND* could refer to either *paroxysmal nocturnal dyspnea*, or *post nasal drip*. Without additional information, it is impossible to say which with any certainty. Documentation should clarify, not obscure. Ambiguous or equivocal clinical documentation is simply unacceptable. Many commonly used acronyms, symbols, and medical abbreviations have multiple uses and interpretations. For this reason, it is prudent to avoid using them whenever possible. If they are to be used, however, it is important that their meaning is clear and unambiguous. Pharmacists who wish to use symbols and abbreviations in their documentation should adopt and strictly adhere to a standard set of approved symbols and abbreviations in their practices. Excellent references are available to assist in establishing an approved list of symbols and abbreviations for a pharmaceutical care practice.[13]

STANDARDIZED CODING SYSTEMS

The advantage of narrative documentation is that it allows the caregiver to provide detail and nuance to the documentation of clinical observations, impressions, and activities. However, a significant limitation of narrative documentation is the difficulty in transforming it into quantifiable data that are consistent with contemporary computer-based information management and claims administration systems. To do this, it is necessary to create ways to codify key data related to the care provided to the patient. This, in turn, has given rise to standardized coding systems that allow for more efficient documentation and billing of health services.

CODING SYSTEMS TO DOCUMENT PHARMACEUTICAL CARE—The National Council for Prescription Drug Programs (NCPDP) is a standards development organization (SDO) whose membership includes representation from virtually every relevant segment in the US prescription drug delivery system. Since its inception in 1976, the mission of NCPDP has been to create and promote voluntary standards for information transfer in prescription drug benefit program administration. In this capacity, the Council has historically concerned itself primarily with the creation and maintenance of standards for the exchange of information related to the delivery of prescription drug products. NCPDP's Universal Claims Form that was released in 1977 and its more recent electronic counterparts are familiar to most community pharmacists.

In November 1993, NCPDP recognized the need to add the ability to document and bill for pharmaceutical care services to its electronic telecommunication standard. It responded to this emerging need by creating WG-10, the Professional Pharmacy Services (PPS) Work Group. The mission of WG-10 was to:

"create a standardized, practical framework that will allow the electronic documentation, storage and transmission of clinical and billing data that describe the delivery of professional pharmacy services."

Essentially, the mission of the work group was to define and operationalize the pharmacist's prescription-related professional services in a uniform coding system and integrate this system into the electronic claims administration process through the creation of an electronic data interchange (EDI) standard. This standard could then serve as the basis for the efficient communication of information related to the delivery of pharmacists' care-related services to patients. This, in turn, would provide an essential prerequisite for the creation of efficient mechanisms by which pharmacists could routinely document their professional services and, where covered by a patient's health insurance or pharmacy services benefit plan, bill and receive compensation for these services.

In 1995, the NCPDP approved the addition of the new PPS code set, and billing for professional services became part of NCPDP's electronic telecommunication standard.[14,15] Following NCPDP's approval, the National Community Pharmacists Association (NCPA) modified their popular Pharmacist Care Claim Form (PCCF) to support the NCPDP coding standard, thereby taking an important step toward creating uniformity in how pharmacists document and bill for their professional services. Since this alignment occurred, all subsequent versions of the PCCF have continued to support the PPS coding system. The most recent version of this claim form appears in Figure 117-1. In addition, NCPA publishes a manual on the use of the PCCF.[16]

The core of the PCCF consists of six fields of information:

1. Reason for Service
2. Professional Service
3. Result of Service
4. Level of Service
5. Drugs Involved
6. Billing Codes/Professional Fees

As illustrated on the PCCF in Figure 1, the *Reason for Service* codes are further classified into one of five code groups to better reflect their shared content:

1. Administrative
2. Dosing/Limits
3. Drug Conflict
4. Disease Management
5. Precautionary

PHARMACIST CARE CLAIM FORM

Subscriber Information

Name | Phone

Address

City | State | Zip

Birthdate | Sex M / F | Social Security/Subscriber I. D. No. | Date of Service

Employer | Employer I. D.

Group No. | Plan No.

Patient

Name | Birthdate | Sex M / F

Relationship of Patient to Subscriber □ Self □ Spouse □ Child □ Other

SUBMIT TO ▶

REFERENCE #

HCFA-1500 attached □

PATIENT AUTHORIZATION
I hereby authorize release of information to health care providers, institutions, and/or payers that may pertain to my illness and/or treatment received. I certify that the information I have reported with regard to my insurance coverage is correct, and I have received the pharmacist care/service rendered.

Patient Signature | Date

FAX (937) 438-8361
Reorder From: **MED-PASS** 800-438-8884
Version 5 (Rev. 4/00)
Med-Pass Form # **ND1203**
© 1993-2000 National Community Pharmacists Association (NCPA)
XFM 011497

Pharmacist Care Information

I. REASON FOR SERVICE

ADMINISTRATIVE

Call Help Desk	CH
Drug Not Available	NA
Lock-In Recipient	LK
Missing Information/Clarification	MS
New Patient Processing	NP
Non-Covered Drug Purchase	NC
Non-Formulary Drug	NF
Payer/Processor Question	TP
Prescription Authentication	AN
Product Selection Opportunity	PS

DOSING/LIMITS

Excessive Duration	MX
Excessive Quantity	EX
High Dose	HD
Insufficient Duration	MN
Insufficient Quantity	NS
Low Dose	LD
Overuse	ER
Suboptimal Compliance	SC
Suboptimal Dosage Form	SF
Suboptimal Regimen	SR
Underuse	LR

DRUG CONFLICT

Additive Toxicity	AT
Drug-Age Precaution	PA
Drug-Allergy	DA
Drug-Disease (Reported)	MC
Drug-Disease (Inferred)	DC
Drug-Drug Interactions	DD
Drug-Gender	SX
Drug Incompatibility	DI

Drug-Pregnancy	PG
Iatrogenic Condition	IC
Ingredient Duplication	ID
Lactation/Nursing Interaction	NR
Prior Adverse Drug Reaction	PR
Therapeutic Duplication	TD

DISEASE MANAGEMENT

Additional Drug Needed	AD
Adverse Drug Reaction	AR
Apparent Drug Misuse	DM
Chronic Disease Management	CD
Health Provider Referral	RF
Laboratory Test Needed	TN
New Disease/Diagnosis	ND
Patient Complaint /Symptom	CS
Patient Education/Instruction	ED
Patient Question/Concern	PC
Plan Protocol	PP
Preventive Health Care	PH
Prescriber Consultation	PN
Suboptimal Drug/Indication	SD
Suspected Environmental Risk	RE
Unnecessary Drug	NN

PRECAUTIONARY

Alcohol Precaution	OH
Drug-Food Interaction	DF
Drug-Lab Conflict	DL
Side Effect	SE
Tobacco Use Precaution	DS
Other (specify below)	97

II. PROFESSIONAL SERVICE

ADMINISTRATIVE

Formulary Enforcement	FE
Generic Product Selection	GP
Literature Search/Review	SW
Patient Medication History	PH
Payer/Processor Consulted	TC
Therapeutic Product Interchange	TH

PATIENT CARE

Coordination Of Care	CC
Dosing Evaluation/Determination	DE
Medication Administration	MA
Medication Review	MR
Patient Assessment	AS
Patient Consulted	PØ
Patient Education/Instruction	PE
Patient Monitoring	PM
Perform Laboratory Test	PT
Pharmacist Consulted Other Source	RØ
Prescriber Consulted	MØ
Recommended Laboratory Test	RT
Self-Care Consultation	SC
Other (specify below)	98

III. RESULT OF SERVICE

DISPENSED

Brand-to-Generic Change	1H
Filled As Is, False Positive	1A
Filled Prescription As Is	1B
Filled, With Different Directions	1D
Filled, With Different Dosage Form	1K
Filled, With Different Dose	1C
Filled, With Different Drug	1E
Filled, With Different Quantity	1F
Filled, With Prescriber Approval	1G
Rx-to-OTC Change	1J

NOT DISPENSED

Not Filled, Directions Clarified	2B
Prescription Not Filled	2A

PATIENT CARE

Compliance Aid Provided	3M
Discontinued Drug	3C
Drug Therapy Unchanged	3G
Follow-Up Report	3H
Instructions Understood	3K
Medication Administered	3N
Patient Referral	3J
Recommendation Accepted	3A
Recommendation Not Accepted	3B
Regimen Changed	3D
Therapy Changed	3E
Therapy Changed - Cost Increase Acknowledged	3F
Other (specify below)	99

IV. LEVEL OF SERVICE

Level 1 (Lowest) = 11   Level 4 = 14
Level 2 = 12   Level 5 (Highest) = 15
Level 3 = 13

V. DRUGS INVOLVED (IF APPLICABLE)

NDC: | NDC:

VI. BILLING CODE/PROFESSIONAL FEE

FEE

DISCUSSION

I am certified to provide pharmacist care for:

□ Anticoagulation
□ Arthritis
□ Asthma/Resp. Condition
□ Diabetes
□ Immunizations
□ Infectious diseases
□ Hormone Replacement Therapy
□ Hypertension
□ Lipid Disorders
□ Mental Health
□ Nutrition/wellness
□ Orthotics/prosthetics
□ Osteoporosis
□ Ostomy/incontinence/wounds
□ Pain Management
□ Reproductive Health
□ Other

Pharmacy Imprint

NAME | TELEPHONE

ADDRESS

NCPDP/NABP NO. | SSN/TIN

I hereby certify that the pharmacist care rendered as indicated has been completed and the fee submitted is the actual fee I have charged and intend to collect for this service.

Signature of Pharmacist ▶

Date | Pharmacist I.D.

WHITE - PAYER   YELLOW - PATIENT   PINK - PHARMACY/OTHER

Figure 117-1. Pharmacist care claim form (version 5).

Codes in this field are used to indicate the problem or need that stimulated the pharmacist's professional service.

Adjacent to this field on the PCCF are the *Professional Service* codes that describe the professional service(s) that were performed in response to the problem or need that was identified. These services are divided into two groups: administrative and patient care.

The *Result of Service* codes are used to describe the immediate outcomes of the service that was performed. Clearly, many things can and do result from professional services that pharmacists perform during their delivery of care. However, some of these results, such as improved patient health outcomes, can only be determined at some point well after the performance of the service. For this reason, the measurement and recording of true patient health outcomes—while an important part of clinical documentation—is inconsistent with most billing and claims administration systems in which documentation and billing is performed contemporaneously with the delivery of care. As a result, the codes in the *Result of Service* field primarily reflect process or procedural outcomes of the service that was performed, rather than true patient health outcomes.

Values in the *Level of Service* field may be used to describe the intensity of the service that was performed. For any pharmacist service (ie, Reason-Service-Result combination), a number of different levels of service are possible. In contrast to the other fields of information, the definition and rules of assignment for codes in this field are left to the decision of users and their trading partners. In some cases, the level of service may be best represented by the amount of time the pharmacist required to perform the service. Alternatively, it may be based on the complexity of the problem, the level of professional judgment that was required, or the risk that the identified problem represented to the patient. Most pharmacists use the Level of Service field to record the amount of time that was required to perform the service in question. If so, it is important to note that in some cases a pharmacist's service to a patient may be interrupted. This may occur, for example, when a physician is not immediately available and the pharmacist must wait for a return telephone call. When such an interruption occurs, the delay that results should not be considered when assigning level of service unless the pharmacist was actively engaged in the performance of the service during the elapsed time period. For additional guidance on this and other issues, the reader is directed to the *Pharmacist Care Claim Form User's Manual*.[16]

Although not always the case, one or more drug products may be involved in the delivery of a pharmacist service to a patient. If so, the *Drugs Involved* field allows for the identification of up to two specific drug products using the standard 11-character NDC (National Drug Code) as the product identifier. Although many pharmacist services/interventions involve only a single drug product, circumstances may arise in which the pharmacist wishes to identify two drug products with a particular service. Such situations may include the following medication conflicts (ie, Reason for Service):

Additive Toxicity (AT)
Drug-Drug Interactions (DD)
Drug Incompatibility (DI)
Ingredient Duplication (ID)
Prior Adverse Drug Reaction (PR)
Therapeutic Duplication (TD)

In cases of formulary enforcement (NF) or discretionary product selection (PS), this field allows for the identification of both the originally prescribed product and the product that was eventually dispensed.

The *Billing Code* for a pharmacist service on the PCCF is created by transferring the two-character codes from columns I through IV to the appropriately numbered boxes in this field. The resulting 8-character code represents a complete professional pharmacist service. Also included on the PCCF is a section called *Discussion* within which the pharmacist could include a brief narrative summary of the service and/or provide additional information not captured in the codes selected.

THE PHARMACY PRACTICE ACTIVITY CLASSIFICATION—Although NCPDP's PPS code set captures many services pharmacists may perform, it cannot be considered exhaustive in terms of its representation of the pharmacist as a healthcare professional. The single greatest challenge that has historically faced those who would create standard coding systems to document and bill for pharmaceutical care services has been the absence of a comprehensive and widely embraced list of specific activities that pharmacists may perform in the course of fulfilling their professional responsibilities. An important step toward overcoming this barrier was taken in 1998, when ten national professional associations jointly issued the Pharmacy Practice Activity Classification (PPAC).[17]

The PPAC is intended to be an exhaustive classification of activities performed by practicing pharmacists across the continuum of health care settings. Much like a biological taxonomy, the PPAC is organized as a hierarchy. In descending order, they are: domain, class, activity, task and step.

At the highest level in the PPAC are four broad domains of pharmacist activity:

1. Ensuring Appropriate Therapy and Outcomes
2. Dispensing Medications and Devices
3. Health Promotion and Disease Prevention
4. Health Systems Management

Within each domain are more specific classes of activity. Within each class are individual activities, and so on, down to the most specific level in the system which are discrete steps involved in performing a particular activity-related task. An example of the increasingly specific hierarchical nature of the PPAC is

Domain A Ensuring Appropriate Therapy and Outcomes
Class A.2 Ensuring Patient's Understanding And Adherence to His or Her Treatment Plan
Activity A.2.1 Interview patient
Task A.2.1.4 Verify patient understanding and knowledge of treatment plan
Step A.2.1.4.1 Verify that patient can describe the use of new and/or existing medication

Note that the presence of an activity on the PPAC does not necessarily mean it is performed exclusively by pharmacists. Indeed, some activities listed in the system are routinely performed by automated systems or delegated to supportive personnel in many pharmacy practices. These activities were included in the PPAC because it was thought that they remain the professional responsibility of the pharmacist to ensure they are performed correctly, whether the pharmacist is personally performing them, or merely supervising others in their performance.

It is too early to determine what affect, if any, the PPAC will have on future documentation and billing systems for pharmaceutical care. However, its potential to serve as the foundation for a common language with which pharmacists and the pharmacy profession may articulate the professional roles and responsibilities of the pharmacist is significant. It is not unlikely that the PPAC, or some derivative thereof, may eventually serve as the basis for future standardized documentation and billing systems in pharmacy.

FEE SETTING AND THE RESOURCE-BASED RELATIVE VALUE SCALE—To the right of the billing code on the PCCF, an area is provided for the pharmacist to assign a professional fee for the service that was performed. At present, there exists no widely accepted standard for assigning professional fees to pharmacist services. For private pay patients, professional service fees will be set by pharmacists in much the same way that other products and services are priced. Where these services are covered by insurance or third party benefit plans, the pharmacist's professional fees will be determined in negotiation with payers.

Many pharmacists who routinely bill major medical carriers for their services know that under the Medicare program, physicians' fees are set by a Resource-Based Relative Value Scale (RBRVS). Because some have suggested that a similar approach may be used in future payment systems that are created for pharmaceutical care, it is useful to describe the RBRVS system briefly within the context of this discussion.

By the early 1980s, government third party payers had concluded that the UCR (usual, customary and reasonable) method of compensating physicians and other medical care providers was financially unsound and encouraged abuse. This opinion was particularly prevalent in the Medicare program, where it was decided that a standard fee schedule was needed for physician services. The result was the creation of an ongoing research project at Harvard University known as the Resource-Based Relative Value Scale project.[18]

Essentially, the RBRVS project was an attempt to create a method of reimbursing physician services that is based on the estimated resource input costs required to perform the services. The RBRVS that is used by Medicare to determine physicians' fees defines the resource input costs as consisting of four components:

1. The time required by the physician before, during, and after the service
2. The intensity with which the time was spent
3. The practice costs necessary to supply the service
4. The opportunity costs of additional training or specialization the physician may have been required to complete in order to provide the service.[19]

The RBRVS combines these resource inputs into a model that is intended to reflect the relative costs that efficient physicians would incur in providing a given service if a perfectly competitive market existed. Since it was not considered feasible to gather data on all 7,000 Medicare procedure codes, the researchers surveyed 3,000 physicians in 18 specialties to determine the work necessary to perform over 400 medical services. They then grouped the procedures into broad classes of services that were assumed to be relatively similar in terms of resource inputs and extrapolated the results to procedures that were not surveyed.

The general approach used in the RBRVS has received widespread support from policymakers, and even some physician organizations. As a result, it has been suggested that a similar approach may eventually be applied to determine the professional fees of other providers, including pharmacists.

PHARMACIST CREDENTIALING—It now appears likely that programs to certify pharmacist competency in the performance of certain specialized patient care services will increase in the future. Already, some third party payers require certified evidence of advanced proficiency as a condition of compensation for certain services.

In 1998, two groups were formed to develop consensus and create standards for credentialing pharmacists.[20] The National Institute for Standards in Pharmacist Credentialing (NISPC) was formed through a consortium agreement between the National Association of Chain Drug Stores (NACDS), the National Community Pharmacists Association (NCPA), and the National Association of Boards of Pharmacy (NABP) to create standards for a series of examinations to credential pharmacists in various specific disease states. A separate group, the Council on Credentialing in Pharmacy (CCP), includes representation from the Academy of Managed Care Pharmacists (AMCP), the American Association of Colleges of Pharmacy (AACP), the American College of Apothecaries (ACA), the American College of Clinical Pharamcy (ACCP), the American Pharmaceutical Association (APhA), the American Society of Consultant Pharmacists (ASCP), and the American Society of Health-System Pharmacists (ASHP). The focus of this group appears to be the certification of generalist practitioners who are capable of providing pharmaceutical care.

Thus, although some disagreement still exists with respect to whether pharmacy should credential practitioners in focused areas of specialty expertise or general pharmaceutical care, there seems to be growing agreement about the need for, and value of, credentialing as a way to ensure a certain minimally acceptable level of proficiency.

The PCCF anticipated this trend and includes a field on the form that allows pharmacists to indicate their certification status in the management of specific disease states. Also included on the PCCF are fields to document the identity of both the pharmacy organization at which the service was provided, and the individual pharmacist who performed the service. Currently, SDOs are working with governmental agencies to create a system of unique provider identification numbers (UPIN) that will allow for the tracking of virtually any billed health care service to the individual who provided the service. This is in keeping with a growing interest among payers for more individual accountability from providers of all health care services.

LIMITATIONS OF THE PPS STANDARD

It is important for potential users to recognize the limitations of the PPS coding standard as it is currently configured. It is not the intent of the standard to represent the entirety of pharmaceutical care and the professional roles and responsibilities of pharmacists in all practice settings. The PPS standard was created to support those professional activities and responsibilities that are now, or may be anticipated to soon be included in third party pharmacy service benefit plans in the ambulatory practice setting, especially those services that are traceable to a particular prescription drug claim. It is recognized that pharmacists in certain specialized settings (eg, long-term care, consulting, radiopharmacy) have additional roles and responsibilities that may not be adequately captured in this first version of the PPS standard. Moreover, many professional services of community pharmacists are not performed in relation to a particular prescription drug claim. As discussed below, these limitations of NCPDP's PPS codes has led to the recent adoption of an alternative system that pharmacists may use to bill their professional services that are not traceable to a particular prescription drug claim, the CMS-1500 form and its electronic equivalent, the X12N 837 Health Care Claim.

While not strictly a limitation, an important caveat of the PPS coding standard is that it is not intended to replace more comprehensive narrative documentation by pharmacists of care delivered to their patients. Rather, like all coding systems, the standard is intended to provide an efficient and uniform mechanism for electronically communicating key aspects of this care, primarily for billing purposes. A complete clinical picture should always be recorded by the pharmacist in the patient's pharmacy-based medical record *before* any claims coding mechanism is consulted or applied.

USING THE CMS-1500 TO FILE PHARMACIST CARE CLAIMS—First issued in the early 1980s, the Centers for Medicare and Medicaid Services' (formerly the Health Care Financing Administration) CMS-1500 (ie, *universal*) claim form is the most widely recognized and accepted format for billing third party payers for health care services. It is required by Medicare and many other third party payers for payment of health care services. Still commonly referred to as the "HCFA-1500" (pronounced hick-fa), the most recent version was released in December, 1990 and is illustrated in Figure 117-2.

In deciding whether to use the CMS-1500 to bill for pharmacist care services, the pharmacist should consider the nature of the service provided, as well as the payer to whom the claim will be submitted. Many pharmacist care services are discrete events that occur during the routine process of providing care, particularly prescription care, to patients. For some of these services, the value that is created is confined primarily to the prescription benefit plan. For example, when a pharmacist recommends a therapeutically equivalent but less expensive product to a prescriber, the value created by the pharmacist is restricted to the differential in the ingredient costs of the two drug products.

In other cases, the value of the pharmacist's professional service goes beyond, or is less likely to be recognized as directly relevant to, the prescription drug benefit. An example would be the pharmacist's involvement in patient education, instruction, or disease state management activities. Since there are often no

PLEASE
DO NOT
STAPLE
IN THIS
AREA

CARRIER

HEALTH INSURANCE CLAIM FORM

PICA | | PICA

1. MEDICARE   MEDICAID   CHAMPUS   CHAMPVA   GROUP HEALTH PLAN   FECA BLK LUNG   OTHER | 1a. INSURED'S I.D. NUMBER (FOR PROGRAM IN ITEM 1)

(Medicare #)   (Medicaid #)   (Sponsor's SSN)   (VA File #)   (SSN or ID)   (SSN)   (ID)

2. PATIENT'S NAME (Last Name, First Name, Middle Initial) | 3. PATIENT'S BIRTH DATE MM DD YY   SEX M ☐ F ☐ | 4. INSURED'S NAME (Last Name, First Name, Middle Initial)

5. PATIENT'S ADDRESS (No., Street) | 6. PATIENT RELATIONSHIP TO INSURED   Self ☐ Spouse ☐ Child ☐ Other ☐ | 7. INSURED'S ADDRESS (No., Street)

CITY | STATE | 8. PATIENT STATUS   Single ☐ Married ☐ Other ☐ | CITY | STATE

ZIP CODE | TELEPHONE (Include Area Code) ( ) | Employed ☐ Full-Time Student ☐ Part-Time Student ☐ | ZIP CODE | TELEPHONE (INCLUDE AREA CODE) ( )

9. OTHER INSURED'S NAME (Last Name, First Name, Middle Initial) | 10. IS PATIENT'S CONDITION RELATED TO: | 11. INSURED'S POLICY GROUP OR FECA NUMBER

a. OTHER INSURED'S POLICY OR GROUP NUMBER | a. EMPLOYMENT? (CURRENT OR PREVIOUS)   YES ☐ NO ☐ | a. INSURED'S DATE OF BIRTH MM DD YY   SEX M ☐ F ☐

b. OTHER INSURED'S DATE OF BIRTH MM DD YY   SEX M ☐ F ☐ | b. AUTO ACCIDENT?   PLACE (State)   YES ☐ NO ☐ | b. EMPLOYER'S NAME OR SCHOOL NAME

c. EMPLOYER'S NAME OR SCHOOL NAME | c. OTHER ACCIDENT?   YES ☐ NO ☐ | c. INSURANCE PLAN NAME OR PROGRAM NAME

d. INSURANCE PLAN NAME OR PROGRAM NAME | 10d. RESERVED FOR LOCAL USE | d. IS THERE ANOTHER HEALTH BENEFIT PLAN?   YES ☐ NO ☐   If yes, return to and complete item 9 a-d.

READ BACK OF FORM BEFORE COMPLETING & SIGNING THIS FORM.
12. PATIENT'S OR AUTHORIZED PERSON'S SIGNATURE I authorize the release of any medical or other information necessary to process this claim. I also request payment of government benefits either to myself or to the party who accepts assignment below.

SIGNED _____ DATE _____

13. INSURED'S OR AUTHORIZED PERSON'S SIGNATURE I authorize payment of medical benefits to the undersigned physician or supplier for services described below.

SIGNED _____

14. DATE OF CURRENT: MM DD YY   ILLNESS (First symptom) OR INJURY (Accident) OR PREGNANCY(LMP) | 15. IF PATIENT HAS HAD SAME OR SIMILAR ILLNESS. GIVE FIRST DATE MM DD YY | 16. DATES PATIENT UNABLE TO WORK IN CURRENT OCCUPATION MM DD YY   FROM   TO MM DD YY

17. NAME OF REFERRING PHYSICIAN OR OTHER SOURCE | 17a. I.D. NUMBER OF REFERRING PHYSICIAN | 18. HOSPITALIZATION DATES RELATED TO CURRENT SERVICES MM DD YY   FROM   TO MM DD YY

19. RESERVED FOR LOCAL USE | 20. OUTSIDE LAB? $ CHARGES   YES ☐ NO ☐

21. DIAGNOSIS OR NATURE OF ILLNESS OR INJURY. (RELATE ITEMS 1,2,3 OR 4 TO ITEM 24E BY LINE)
1. _____ . ___   3. _____ . ___
2. _____ . ___   4. _____ . ___ | 22. MEDICAID RESUBMISSION CODE   ORIGINAL REF. NO.
23. PRIOR AUTHORIZATION NUMBER

24. A DATE(S) OF SERVICE						B Place of Service	C Type of Service	D PROCEDURES, SERVICES, OR SUPPLIES (Explain Unusual Circumstances)		E DIAGNOSIS CODE	F $ CHARGES	G DAYS OR UNITS	H EPSDT Family Plan	I EMG	J COB	K RESERVED FOR LOCAL USE
From MM	DD	YY	To MM	DD	YY			CPT/HCPCS	MODIFIER							
1																
2																
3																
4																
5																
6																

25. FEDERAL TAX I.D. NUMBER   SSN ☐ EIN ☐ | 26. PATIENT'S ACCOUNT NO. | 27. ACCEPT ASSIGNMENT? (For govt. claims, see back)   YES ☐ NO ☐ | 28. TOTAL CHARGE $ | 29. AMOUNT PAID $ | 30. BALANCE DUE $

31. SIGNATURE OF PHYSICIAN OR SUPPLIER INCLUDING DEGREES OR CREDENTIALS (I certify that the statements on the reverse apply to this bill and are made a part thereof.)

SIGNED _____ DATE _____ | 32. NAME AND ADDRESS OF FACILITY WHERE SERVICES WERE RENDERED (If other than home or office) | 33. PHYSICIAN'S, SUPPLIER'S BILLING NAME, ADDRESS, ZIP CODE & PHONE #

PIN#   GRP#

(APPROVED BY AMA COUNCIL ON MEDICAL SERVICE 8/88)   *PLEASE PRINT OR TYPE*   APPROVED OMB-0938-0008 FORM HCFA-1500 (12-90),   FORM RRB-1500, APPROVED OMB-1215-0055 FORM OWCP-1500,   APPROVED OMB-0720-0001 (CHAMPUS)

Med-Pass Form # ND1001

PATIENT AND INSURED INFORMATION

PHYSICIAN OR SUPPLIER INFORMATION

Figure 117-2. CMS-1500 claim form.

"hard dollar" savings to the prescription benefit plan from such services, the value created by the pharmacist is likely to be better recognized and appreciated by that component of the patient's medical insurance plan that is concerned with the total care of the patient, and the total cost of that care. This is usually what is commonly referred to as the *major medical* component of the patient's health insurance plan.

Pharmacists should consider filing their claim with the patient's major medical insurance carrier whenever they provide a service whose primary value is likely to be realized through positive patient health outcomes, or the prevention of negative health outcomes and their related economic sequelae. While each carrier will have its own policies and procedures for filing major medical claims, many require a CMS-1500 to be submitted in the claims packet.

Billing Using the CMS-1500

The CMS-1500 claim form is the most widely recognized and accepted format for billing third party payers for health care services. It is required by Medicare and many other third party payers for payment of health care services. The form consists of 33 boxes or fields of required information. Fields 1–13 contain information about the patient and the insured beneficiary. The remaining 20 fields 14–33 contain information about the provider or supplier of the service. Two fields on the form are particularly important for ensuring prompt and correct payment, field 21 and field 24D.

The first rule of third party payment for health care services is there must have existed a demonstrated medical need for the service that was performed. On the PCCF, need is established by the Reason for Service code that the pharmacist selects. On the CMS-1500, need is established by the patient's diagnosis and related background facts about the condition being treated.

INTERNATIONAL CLASSIFICATION OF DISEASES CODING—Field 21 on the CMS-1500 form is labeled 'Diagnosis or Nature of Illness or Injury.' This field contains four slots, numbered 1–4, for entering patient diagnostic information using the ICD-9-CM (*International Classification of Diseases, 9th Revision, Clinical Modification*) coding system, commonly referred to simply as "ICD-9." This reference is available through a variety of medical publishers.

At least one diagnosis code must be reported on each claim. Up to four codes may be reported if needed to accurately represent the reason for the service that was provided. When more than one is reported, the code which represents the disease, condition or problem that was primarily responsible for the service provided should be listed first, with any additional or supplementary codes listed afterward in order of their proximal relationship to the primary code.

The ICD-9 coding system contains nineteen categories of codes. Categories 1–15 (codes 001–779) identify diseases and related medical conditions. Category 16 (codes 780–799) designates symptoms, signs, and ill-defined conditions. Category 19 (codes 800–999) relates to injury and poisoning. Each of these categories contain numerical codes of 3 to 5 digits, depending upon the level of specificity and precision. For example, undifferentiated asthma is coded as 493 in the ICD-9 system. For asthma with an allergic cause, 493.9 would be the appropriate selection. An additional fifth digit is also available if the patient does or does not have a history of status asthmaticus (ie, 493.91 or 493.90, respectively).

Thus, with each successive digit, the level of diagnostic precision increases. With few exceptions, payers generally require the submission of diagnoses that are coded to at least the fourth digit. Failure to do so will often result in payment delay or rejection. In addition, other common coding problems are:

- The patient's chronic diagnosis which is not the reason for the encounter is incorrectly billed as the primary diagnosis;
- The ICD-9 code that is selected is inaccurate or insufficiently precise (ie, not coded to the fourth or fifth digit when appropriate); and

- A supplementary code is used inappropriately as the primary reason for the encounter.

In addition to the above 17 categories of numerical codes, the ICD-9 system provides two categories of supplementary codes. The first of these is the Supplementary Classification of Factors Influencing Health Status and Contact with Health Services (V01–V82), more commonly known as the "V codes." Of particular interest to pharmacists within the V codes are a series (V73–V82) that are used to classify routine screening examinations, such as those that might be part of a preventive care assessment. For example, there is a special code that is used when screening for diabetes mellitus (V77.1).

The final category of ICD-9 codes is the Supplementary Classification of External Causes of Injury and Poisoning (E800–E999) commonly known as the "E codes." This category allows the classification of environmental events, circumstances, and conditions as the cause of the patient's illness and is generally not used by pharmacists to code for their services.

Because there is no place for narrative description of the patient's condition on the CMS-1500, it is particularly important that code selection is as accurate and specific as possible. It is also for this reason that many pharmacists who bill major medical carriers for their services routinely append additional clinical documentation when they submit a CMS-1500.

CPT CODING—Field 24D on the CMS-1500 form is labeled "Procedures, Services or Supplies." Payers who require the CMS-1500 will usually require the use of Physician's Current Procedural Terms (CPT) codes or CMS's Common Procedure Coding System. Although CMS recently changed its name from the former HCFA, these codes are still commonly referred to as HCPCS (pronounced "hick-picks") codes. As with diagnosis, it is essential that pharmacists thoroughly understand the codes that are used in this field to describe the service that was performed.

The relationship between HCPCS and CPT is illustrated in Figure 117-3. The CPT codes were created by the American Medical Association in 1966 to be a listing of descriptive terms and identifying codes for reporting medical services and procedures performed by physicians. In 1983, HCFA developed HCPCS as a uniform method for health care providers and medical suppliers to code professional services, procedures, and supplies to meet the operational needs of the Medicare and Medicaid programs.

The HCPCS classification is organized into three numbered levels of codes, each of which represents a unique coding system.

Level I of HCPCS is the CPT codes, the maintenance of which continues to be performed by the AMA.

Level II codes were created by HCFA to cover medical services and supplies that are not covered in the CPT codes. Although these codes were primarily intended for use with government payers, they are also recognized by many private insurers.

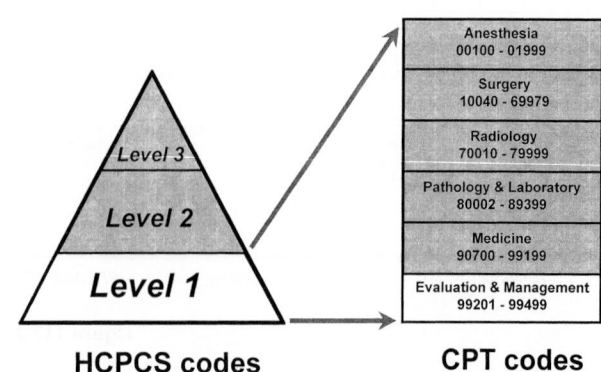

Figure 117-3. Medical care coding systems.

Level III codes were historically assigned by Medicare carriers in individual states and are therefore not common across all insurance carriers. Level III codes are being discontinued under the provisions of the recently enacted HIPAA legislation (see below).

Most pharmacists who wish to bill for their patient care activities will find the CPT codes to be the most useful, especially that section known as the *Evaluation and Management*, or *E&M* codes. As illustrated in Figure 117-3, the E&M codes occupy one of six sections within the CPT coding structure. Each five-digit numerical E&M code begins with a *99* prefix (ie, 99201–99499). The codes are divided into several categories including office visits, hospital visits, and consultations. These categories are further subdivided into two or more subcategories. For example, separate codes are available for an outpatient office visit with a provider depending on whether the patient is established or new to the practice.

E&M code selection is usually based on three key components, with additional considerations becoming relevant only under special circumstances. Once the appropriate category is selected (eg, outpatient office visit with an established patient), the proper code is determined on the basis of:

1. The level of **History** that is taken on the patient (the four levels of History include: Problem Focused, Expanded Problem Focused, Detailed, and Comprehensive.
2. The extent of the **Examination** that was performed (the four Levels of Examination include: Problem Focused, Expanded Problem Focused, Detailed, and Comprehensive).
3. The level of **Medical Decision Making** that was required to perform the service (the four levels of Medical Decision Making include: Straightforward, Low Complexity, Moderate Complexity, and High Complexity.

Selection of the level of medical decision making that was required is itself determined on the basis of three additional considerations:

1. The number of diagnosis or management options
2. The amount and/or complexity of data reviewed
3. The risk of complications and/or morbidity or mortality

Five different codes are available to describe an office visit with a new patient (99201–99205). Likewise, five codes are available to describe an office visit with an established patient (99211–99215). Many pharmacists in the community practice setting will find that these 10 codes most of their needs related to completing a CMS-1500 claim form.

Table 117-1 illustrates how a provider would use the three key components of history, examination, and medical decision making to select the code that best represents the nature of a patient care encounter. For example, 99213 would be the most appropriate code to describe an office visit with an established patient that required expanded problem-focused history and examination and a relatively low level of medical decision making.

Under special circumstances, other considerations become operative in code selection. For example, when counseling or coordination of care activities account for more than 50% of a patient encounter, selection of the proper E&M code from among a sequence involving different levels of care is based exclusively on the amount of time the provider spent with the patient. For example, 99204 would be the most appropriate code to describe an office visit with an established patient that was dominated by counseling and required about 45 minutes to complete.

Also illustrated in Table 117-1 are the *Relative Value Unit* scores (RVUs) that CMS has assigned to each of the codes using the RBRVS discussed above. The resulting RVU score is then regionally adjusted and multiplied by a monetary conversion factor to determine the dollar amount that a provider will be paid for a particular service or procedure under Medicare.

In addition to the 99201–05 and 99211–15 series, there are several sets of CPT codes that are commonly used to report preventive medicine or health services that some pharmacists find useful. Two series of codes, 99381–99387 (new patient) and 99391–99397 (established patient), are used for preventive medicine evaluation and management that includes a comprehensive history and examination, as well as counseling and/or risk factor reduction interventions. However, most pharmacists will find two other series of codes to be more applicable for their preventive health services. The series 99401–99404 are for preventive medicine counseling and/or risk factor reduction intervention(s) provided to an individual patient, with separate codes reflecting increasing amounts of time required for the service (eg, 99402 for approximately 30 minutes). Two additional codes are available when similar services are provided to more than one person in a group setting, such as a class. In this case, the code 99411 is used if the service required approximately 30 minutes, while 99412 is available if the service required approximately 60 minutes.

Additional information about CPT/HCPCS coding is available through The American Medical Association, CMS, and various commercial publishers of medical coding materials.

GENERAL PAYMENT PRINCIPLES

As discussed previously, some pharmacist care services are isolated activities that pharmacists perform to correct problems or fulfill needs that have arisen unexpectedly during the course of the practice day. In these cases, it is often unrealistic for the pharmacist to have prenegotiated payment coverage for the service with the payer. As a result, the pharmacist must submit a "cold" claim to the payer in hopes that the information contained on the claim will make a persuasive case for payment. Unfortunately, while proper completion of the required claims forms and aggressive follow-up with the payer can significantly improve the likelihood of receiving at least partial payment, the submission of cold claims to third party payers for pharmacist care activities is still a risky venture under the best of circumstances.

Table 117-1. Selected E&M Codes Used to Bill Pharmaceutical Care

E & M CODES	HISTORY	EXAMINATION	MEDICAL DECISION MAKING	TIME	RVUS
CODES FOR A NEW PATIENT OFFICE VISIT					
99201	Problem Focused	Problem Focused	Straightforward	10 min	.82
99202	Exp. Problem Focused	Exp. Problem Focused	Straightforward	20 min	1.32
99203	Detailed	Detailed	Low Complexity	30 min	1.80
99204	Comprehensive	Comprehensive	Mod. Complexity	45 min	2.66
99205	Comprehensive	Comprehensive	High Complexity	60 min	3.33
CODES FOR AN ESTABLISHED PATIENT OFFICE VISIT					
E & M CODES	HISTORY	EXAMINATION	MEDICAL DECISION MAKING	TIME	RVUS
99211	Minimal problems			5 min	.40
99212	Problem Focused	Problem Focused	Low Complexity	10 min	.71
99213	Exp. Problem Focused	Exp. Problem Focused	Low Complexity	15 min	1.00
99214	Detailed	Detailed	Mod. Complexity	25 min	1.55
99215	Comprehensive	Comprehensive	High Complexity	40 min	2.53

Recognizing this reality, some pharmacists have developed and implemented cohesive pharmacist care *products* in their practices. These products often take the form of specific disease state management or patient education/instruction programs.[21] For these types of services, it is both possible and desirable for the pharmacist to have prenegotiated authorization for payment with selected insurers or managed care organizations whose patients are potential candidates for the service or program in question. These agreements will dramatically improve the efficiency and effectiveness of the claims process.

When it is not possible to prenegotiate payment, the pharmacist has two options. First, the pharmacist can deliver the service and explain to the patient that payment will be sought from their insurer. In this case it is important the patient understands that the ultimate responsibility for payment rests with the patient. Alternatively, it is sometimes possible to delay provision of the service until the payer can be contacted to confirm or deny coverage for the service in question.

HIPAA AND RELATED RECENT EVENTS

In 1996, the 104th Congress passed Public Law 104-191 entitled the "Health Insurance Portability and Accountability Act of 1996." Known informally as HIPAA ("hip-ah"), this law directed the Secretary of HHS to adopt national standards to enable health information, including claims transactions, to be exchanged electronically. The law also requires the creation of regulations to ensure the privacy and security of patients' health information. The final rule for HIPAA was published in August 2000 and was originally set for implementation in October 2002. However, due to the complexity of standardizing the electronic exchange of health information, Congress passed legislation in late 2001 to extend the deadline for compliance of transactions and code sets until October 2003.

While it is still too early to know what the full impact of HIPAA will be, there is little question that it will have a profound affect on how the business of health care is transacted in the electronic environment. Within the context of professional pharmacy services, a particularly interesting development has occurred. As noted above, NCPDP is the standards development organization (SDO) that has historically maintained electronic data interchange standards in pharmacy. In recognition of this status, the HIPAA Final Rule on Standards For Electronic Transactions adopted the NCPDP Telecommunication Standard Format, Version 5.1 as the standard for pharmacy claims. However, another electronic standard, the ASC X12N 837 Health Care Claim, was adopted for professional health care claims that are billed to major medical carriers, including those of pharmacists. X12N is the insurance subcommittee of X12, a standards development organization that is involved in the development of electronic data interchange standards in a variety of industries.

As discussed earlier in this chapter, most pharmacists who are successfully billing third party payers for their professional services are doing so through the major medical carrier using the CMS-1500 universal claim form. Routine payment for professional pharmacy services has simply not made its way into prescription benefit plans in any meaningful way, since most PBMs continue to consider these services beyond the scope of the prescription benefit plans they manage. Since, the X12N 837 claim represents the electronic equivalent of the CMS-1500 form, the HIPAA ruling effectively eliminates NCPDP and its code sets from relevance in the future electronic billing for professional pharmacy services, except where the service is traceable to a particular prescription drug claim, and is billed to a prescription benefit manager (PBM).

As this chapter was being completed, HHS had rejected a petition by NCPDP to add their standard to that of ASC X12N 837 as a HIPAA-compliant standard for professional pharmacy services billing. Although it is possible that this decision may eventually be reconsidered, it now appears that the future of billing for pharmacy-related services will be clearly split between prescription-related services (NCPDP) and the myriad other professional cognitive services that pharmacists perform in their care of patients (X12N).

In preparing for the implementation of HIPAA in early 2002, the NCPA sought collaboration from other national pharmacy associations to join the X12 Pharmacy Advisory Panel it had established. As this chapter was nearing completion, the Panel had been joined by APhA, ASCP, ACCP, and ASHP, with NACDS also considering membership. The Panel was created to advance professional pharmacy services billing via the X12N 837 standard, and to provide oversight and maintenance of the HIPAA-compliant *X12N 837 Health Care Claim: Pharmacy Professional Services Companion Guide* that had been released by NCPA several months earlier. The *Guide* contains the EDI transaction segments and data elements that are germane to pharmacy professional services as billed using the X12N 837 claim, the electronic version of the CMS-1500 claim.

In May 2003, the American Medical Association signaled its acceptance of the X12 Pharmacy Advisory Panel as representing the coding interests of pharmacists by its vote to include the Panel on its Health Care Professionals Advisory Committee (HCPAC). The HCPAC was formed to allow participation by nonphysician health professionals in the AMA's CPT Editorial Panel process which is responsible for maintaining the CPT code set. The addition of pharmacy to the HCPAC represents an important step in the recognition of pharmacists as providers of patient health care services beyond the scope of prescription drug delivery. Membership on the HCPAC also gives pharmacy a vote in the future direction of the CPT codes that most pharmacists use to bill their professional services.

Another event of potentially profound significance to the future of compensation for pharmacist care services occurred on May 25, 2001, when Senator Tim Johnson (D-SD) introduced S. 974 entitled the "Medicare Pharmacist Services Coverage Act" to the 107th Congress. If passed, this legislation would amend Title XVIII of the Social Security Act to provide beneficiaries with coverage for pharmacists' drug therapy management services under Part B of the Medicare program. By recognizing pharmacists as eligible health care providers, an oversight in the original 1965 legislation, this bill would allow pharmacists to obtain provider numbers to bill Medicare directly for their professional services. The bill received two readings before being referred to the Finance Committee where it remained as this chapter neared completion.

CONCLUSIONS

Like pharmacy practice itself, documentation is a learned skill. Increasingly, technology is assisting the pharmacist to accurately and consistently document the care they provide. However, good documenters are not born, they are made. Until recently, pharmacy curricula provided relatively little opportunity for students to develop their written communication skills. The same can be said for the professional careers of most pharmacists. Due to the pharmaceutical care movement and the economic imperatives now facing the profession, these conditions are rapidly changing. Pharmacists who wish to participate fully in the movement toward patient-centered care, and who expect to be paid for their activities, must master the art of clinical documentation and billing.

Pharmacists who wish to pursue compensation for their professional services must recognize that they are still entering largely uncharted waters. Most government and private third party payers still do not have well-defined policies for paying pharmacists for their professional services. This is not to say that payers have no interest in pharmaceutical care. Rather, for the most part they simply do not understand what it is, or how it will benefit them and their beneficiaries.

In his economic treatise, *Wealth of Nations*, Adam Smith commented on pharmacists and the value of their professional services:

> Apothecaries' profit is become a bye-word, denoting something uncommonly extravagant. This great apparent profit, however, is frequently no more than the reasonable wages of labour. The skill of an apothecary is much nicer and more delicate matter than that of any artificer whatever; and trust which is reposed in him is of much greater importance. He is the physician of the poor in all cases, and of the rich when the distress or danger is not very great. His reward, therefore, ought to be suitable to his skill and his trust, and it arises generally from the price at which he sells his drugs. But the whole drugs which the best employed apothecary, in a large market town, will sell in a year, may not perhaps cost him above thirty or forty pounds. Though he should sell them, therefore, for three or four hundred, or at a thousand percent profit, this may frequently be no more than the reasonable wages of his labour charged, in the only way in which he can charge them, upon the price of his drugs. The greater part of the apparent profit is real wages disguised in the garb of profit.[22]

Although the practice of pharmacy has changed dramatically in the two centuries since those words were written, the basis for compensating pharmacists has not. In general, the value of pharmacists' professional services is still interwoven with, and obscured by, the price of the products they sell. The future of compensation for professional cognitive services must break from this tradition.

The creation of pharmacy services terminology and related electronic claims transmissions standards will help speed the evolution of new payment systems. Likewise, the growing body of research in outcomes assessment and pharmacoeconomics will allow the pharmacy profession to better understand the economic value of pharmaceutical care and better communicate this value to payers. Indeed, demonstrating to payers the value of pharmacists' services represents a priority—perhaps *the* priority—for pharmacy practice-related research in the years ahead.

REFERENCES

1. Cohen MR. *Hosp Pharm* 1989; 24:180.
2. Pugh CB. *Top Hosp Pharm Manage* 1992; 11(4):30.
3. Rupp MT, Schondelmeyer SW, Wilson GT, et al. *Am Pharm* 1988; NS28:30.
4. Rupp MT. *Am Pharm* 1988; NS28:22.
5. Rupp MT, DeYoung M, Schondelmeyer SW. *Medical Care* 1992; 30:926.
6. Rupp MT. *Annals of Pharmacotherapy* 1992; 26:1580.
7. Schaff RL, Schumock GT, Nadzam DM. *Hosp Pharm* 1991; 26:326.
8. Rupp MT. *Am Pharm* 1992; NS32:79.
9. US Department of Health and Human Services Office of the Inspector General. *The Clinical Role of the Community Pharmacist,* 1990.
10. Weed LL. *Medical Records, Medical Education and Patient Care.* Case Western Reserve University Press, 1971.
11. Berni R, Readey H. Problem-Oriented Medical Record Implementation. St Louis: CV Mosby, 1974.
12. Rupp MT. Screening for prescribing errors. *Am Pharm* 1991; NS31:71.
13. Hensyl WR, ed. *Stedman's Abbreviations, Acronyms & Symbols.* Baltimore: Williams & Wilkins, 1992.
14. Rupp MT. Standardizing documentation for filing pharmaceutical care claims. *Am Pharm* 1995; NS35:26.
15. Rupp MT. *Council Connection: Journal of the NCPDP* 1995; (Jan/Feb):16.
16. Rupp MT. *Pharmacist Care Claim Form User's Manual: A Guide to Pharmacist Care Compensation,* 2nd ed. National Community Pharmacists Association, 1997.
17. The American Pharmaceutical Association. *Pharmacy Practice Activity Classification.* 1998.
18. Hsiao WC, et al. A National Study of Resource-Based Relative Value Scales for Physician Services: Final Report. September 27, 1988. Boston: Harvard University Press.
19. Becker ER, et al. *Am J Pub Health* 1990; 80:799.
20. English T. Groups team up to coordinate credentialing. *Pharmacy Today* 1998; 4:6.
21. Rupp MT, McCallian DJ, Sheth KK. Developing and marketing a community pharmacy-based asthma management program. *JAPhA* 1997; NS36:694.
22. Smith A. 1776. In: Campbell RH, Skinner AS, eds. *Adam Smith: Inquiry into the Nature and Causes of the Wealth of Nations.* Indianapolis: Liberty Classic Press, 1981.

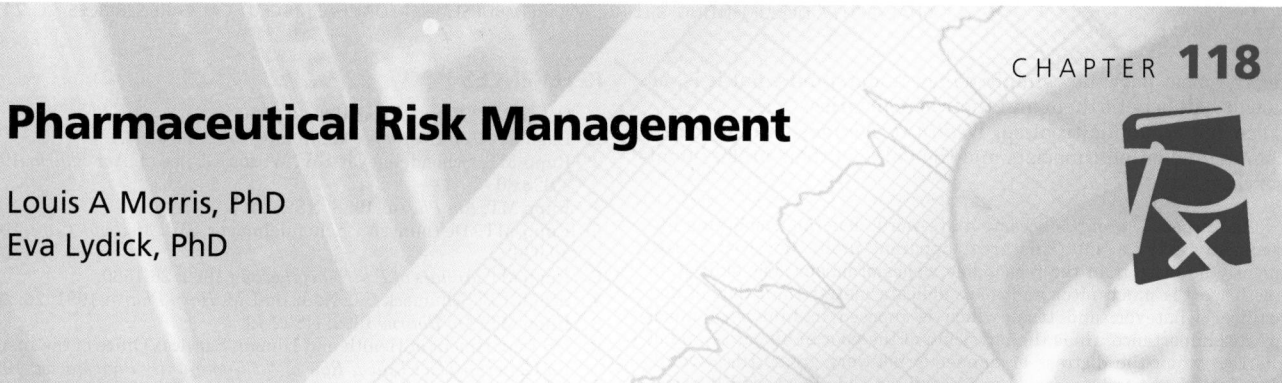

CHAPTER 118

Pharmaceutical Risk Management

Louis A Morris, PhD

Eva Lydick, PhD

THE NEW ERA OF RISK MANAGEMENT

In the United States, drugs are approved only if they are determined to be safe to use for the conditions described in their label. This basic tenet of the Food, Drug and Cosmetic Act has not changed. What has changed though in recent years is the interpretation of the term "safe." Modern concepts of pharmaceutical risk management are based on the premise that drug manufacturers, health care professionals, and patients have a responsibility to minimize the risks of using pharmaceutical products. It is not enough to make drugs minimally safe, they must be as safe as possible over the lifecycle of the product's use.[1–3]

Historically, the Food and Drug Administration (FDA) has interpreted the requirement that a drug must be "safe" to mean that the benefits of a drug outweigh its risks. The determination was made on a "categorical" basis, where the totality of risks was weighted against the totality of benefits when considered for the purposes outlined in the drug product's labeling. If a drug did not meet this criterion, it was not approved or its label was rewritten to narrow the conditions for use. This logic was endemic in the FDA for most of the 20th century. On average, two to four drugs over each 5-year period were withdrawn from the marketplace after post-marketing surveillance data uncovered new risks.[4] Similarly, on occasion, the FDA would require some special "tool" or intervention to improve a product's safety profile. For example, patient package inserts were used to warn women about the risk of birth control pills and a special distribution system was used to limit the dispensing of Clozaril (clozapine) to patients who underwent blood testing that demonstrated that they were not having a serious adverse reaction. However, starting in the early 1990s, this philosophy started to change, as the FDA began to take a more active role in post-marketing surveillance and began instituting a more aggressive "management" process to assure greater safety in the use of marketed drugs. No longer do the manufacturer and FDA provide passive oversight and labeling changes to control risks, now the manufacturer must actively monitor for suspected, but unquantified risks and actively manage and minimize known risks.

PRECURSOR HISTORY

FDA's new concepts for risk management amount to a "cultural shift" in the logic of drug approval and the FDA's role. The key events that led to this change can be traced to a series of reports that highlighted the need for improved medical safety. In 1999, the Institute of Medicine (IOM) released a report entitled, "To Err is Human."[5] This report reviewed the nature and cause of medication errors, estimating that up to 98,000 people died each year due to these errors. In their assessment the IOM included both adverse drug reactions and human errors in drug administration. The report captured the attention of news reporters and the government. Headlines proclaimed alarm at the larger number of fatalities caused by medical errors. Consequently, there was a government-wide initiative started to develop methods and institute procedures to reduce medical errors.

For its part, the FDA was already concerned about medical safety and sought to increase its oversight and control of the safe use of marketed drugs. The IOM report provided impetus and support for an already developing policy of increasingly active intervention. During the 4-year period from 1998 to 2001, at least 10 drugs were withdrawn from the market (Table 118-1). For each preceding 5-year period from 1979 to 1998, on the average only two to four drugs were withdrawn.

Statements made by FDA officials regarding some of these withdrawals suggested that the FDA no longer believed that passive oversight and re-labeling drugs with new warnings was sufficient. Furthermore, the FDA no longer believed that it was sufficient to identify safe conditions of use in the label and that healthcare professionals and patients had to comply with advocated directions of use for the drug to remain on the market.

As a summary of this new philosophy of risk management, the FDA staff issued a report to the Commissioner that highlighted processes for developing risk management systems and signaled new ideas for measuring and intervening to manage risks.[6] (US FDA, 1999). Entitled, "Managing the Risks of Medical Products," the FDA report borrowed heavily from risk management philosophies in other fields, such as environmental risk management and airline safety. It emphasized the process of developing risk management plans to control and manage drug safety.

The risk management "revolution" at the FDA continues today. Under FDA regulations and the Food and Drug Administration's Modernization Act, the FDA may approve new drugs with new restrictions that are intended to assure safe use (Subpart H). These restrictions include limiting distribution to certain facilities or physicians with special training or experience or limiting distribution based on the condition of the performance of specified medical procedures. The regulations specify that the limitations must be commensurate with the specific safety concerns presented by the product. In addition, drugs continue to be approved with restrictions imposed by manufacturers seeking FDA approval.

As discussed below, in March 2003, the FDA released a series of "draft concept papers" focusing on premarketing risk assessment, risk management and pharmacovigilance. After reviewing comments on the concept papers, in May 2004, FDA released a series of Guidances for industry. The risk management guidance contained several revisions that addressed concerns from industry. The draft guidance stated that for certain drugs that pose risk management concerns, there must be a

Table 118-1. Drugs Withdrawn from 1998 to 2001

DRUG	DATE WITHDRAWN
Seldane (terfenadine)	2/98
Posicor (mibefradil)	6/98
Duract (bromphenac)	6/98
Hismanal (astemizole)	6/99
Roxar (grepafloxacin)	11/99
Propulsid (cisapride)	3/00
Rezulin (troglitazone)	3/00
Lotronex (alosetron HCl)	8/00
Raplon (rapacuronium)	3/01
Baycol (cerivaxtatin)	8/01

Risk Minimization Action Plan (Risk MAP) that describes what risks are faces and how they will be handled. The plan must identify a series of "tools" or interventions used to control risk. These tools include a series of informational interventions (to health care providers, patients, or the public) and distribution controls that specific conditions or populations of patient or providers that limit the prescribing or dispensing of the medication. The tools must be pretested, and the plan must be evaluated periodically.

THE FOUR PILLARS OF RISK MANAGEMENT

With the release of the risk management draft guidance the FDA has come to the conclusion that it is necessary to fully consider the risk management process for certain products considered for approval and for continuous marketing. The authors will categorize this process into four key elements: (1) Risk Assessment, (2) Risk Quantification, (3) Development and Implementation of Risk Management Tools (eg, Risk Communication and Distribution and Behavioral Control Systems), and (4) Evaluation of the Effectiveness of these tools and the implementation of design modifications, if necessary. In the section following, the authors review each of these elements in depth.

Risk Assessment

Before even beginning development on a risk management program, it is necessary to understand the nature and magnitude of risks associated with a therapy. Thus, the first part of any risk management program is good risk assessment. The initial step is often referred to as *signal detection*. This means that an analyst must sift through the vast number of real or potential adverse events that can occur to individuals receiving a drug to identify those likely to be a true consequence of taking the drug. This requires careful review of all the available data from multiple sources, good understanding of the underlying disease processes and consequences, non-clinical (animal studies or *in vitro*) experiments, information from similar products, clinical studies including clinical pharmacology trials, and any post-marketing experience, if available.

Risk assessment should be a continuous, on-going effort throughout drug development and needs to involve individuals from multiple disciplines, eg, clinical research, clinical pharmacology, toxicology, and epidemiology). Non-clinical studies provide information on the pharmacological effects of drug (eg, potential molecular targets other than the one desired, cytochrome P450 metabolism). Animal models are often, but not always, consistent with effects in humans and may demonstrate injury in specific organ systems that will heighten concern over a similar effect in humans. However, there is a need to validate all animal models and evaluate results carefully from these models as they may yield both false negatives and false positives.

Clinical trials constitute the bulk of the information available on the safety and efficacy of a new product prior to launch. Usually, these studies are designed to provide the maximum amount of information in a limited time frame while exposing a limited number of individuals to an investigational product. Because of their short time frame and small sample size, these studies are limited in the amount of information they provide about the safety of a new medicine. Current International Conference on Harmonization (ICH), an international regulatory body, requirements for trials of long-term medications to mandate that studies supporting a new drug application include at least 1500 patients on the new drug with 300–600 exposed for at least 6 months and 100 exposed for 12 months or more. With 1500 patients, it is possible to rule an event rate of 1/500, but many of the more serious adverse events that have been highlighted in recent news reports and product withdrawals occurred at less 1/1000 and some even at less than 1/ 10,000.

Phase I studies provide a metabolic profile of the product as well as adverse event potential in special populations (eg, the elderly, those with renal or hepatic impairment). Phase II / III studies can provide information on moderately common adverse events and perhaps provide a signal for the possibility of some less common, but serious, adverse events. In addition to reported adverse events, their number, frequency, and nature, important information can be obtained from inspection of discontinuations due to adverse events, changes in laboratory results, vital signs or symptoms. Careful analyses of phase IIb/III trials can help identify those at highest risks for harm as well as those patients that will receive the most benefit. This information should be included into the package insert to inform the prescriber of the appropriate use of products. Because of their large size, phase IIIb/IV have the potential to identify less common, but not rare, serious adverse events.

Evaluation of a drug's safety is quite a different process than evaluating its efficacy. As opposed to efficacy endpoints, which are well defined and defined with great care to preserve the level of significance, safety endpoints can take many forms, including some previously unrecognized. Instead of one or a very few number of endpoints, safety considerations, including combinations and varying levels of sensitivity, are infinite. If the nominal significance of efficacy of 0.05 is used as a standard, safety comparisons in clinical trials will always yield a number of significant differences. Determining which associations are causal and which are spurious is not a simple process.

Following drug launch, individual occurrences of adverse events in connection with drug use are reported to either the FDA or the drug manufacturer. This voluntary reporting is an excellent signal generating system and has been responsible for the majority of safety alerts that occur in marketed products.[7] However, there is no denominator associated with these events, as the likelihood of a particular drug-event combination being reported has been shown to vary by the nature of the event, length of time the drug is on the market, the drug's market share, the quality of the surveillance system instituted by of the manufacturer, publicity, new knowledge, secular trends, as well as reporting regulations. Another source of difficulty in detecting a possible source of concern is that what is defined as an "event" can be ambiguous. By combining related adverse reaction reporting terms, it is possible to amplify weak safety signals or by separating out individual, but related, reported terms, it is possible to obscure important toxicities. Dividing adverse event terms into sub-terms can divide the same event into many terms, decreasing the magnitude of the signal.

To deal with these confounding effects, spontaneous reports are reviewed on an individual basis for biological/medical plausibility, timing of event in relationship to exposure, possibility of other explanations, and re-challenge and de-challenge effects. Systematic review of large numbers of reports often includes comparing the proportional reporting rates for one drug against the proportional reporting rates of all products.[8] This convention requires generating a proportion or percentage for each named event or effect compared to total reports for that product and comparing this proportion to a similar proportion developed for all drugs, or specified subset of all drugs.

The FDA maintains an Adverse Event Report System (AERS) of voluntary reports submitted by health care professionals. In addition, all manufacturers are required to submit all domestic adverse drug experiences, whether or not considered drug-related, all serious and unlabeled events from foreign reports and the scientific literature, and all serious, unlabeled events observed in post-marketing studies deemed to be possibly related to the drug under study. The term for this practice of continual monitoring for unwanted, untoward effects of drugs already on the market is pharmacovigilance. Thus, pharmacovigilance refers almost exclusively to analyses of data in spontaneous reporting systems.

Consequently, whether before or after launch of a drug, signal detection rests on careful review, judgment, and experience. Hallmarks of a causal relationship are appropriate time order, consistency, specificity, strength of the association, as well as coherence or medical plausibility.[9]

Risk Quantification

Risk assessment also implies that there is a need to confirm the association between the event and drug exposure and to estimate the magnitude of the risk. These next steps involve an entirely different set of activities and processes. This quantitative exercise can only occur after a signal has been identified, and there is a clear definition of the suspected event. Like measures of efficacy, quantitative estimates of association between a drug and an event requires formal study and analyses. Pharmacoepidemiology is defined as the study of the utilization and effects of drugs in the population at large and usually provides the scientific processes necessary to accurately estimate the probability of these adverse effects (as well as beneficial effects) in the population.

For relatively common events, clinical trials provide a rich source of data with the advantage of an obvious and comparable control group, known exposure, and consistent information on disease severity and co-morbid conditions. Phase IIIb or IV studies, which often are much larger than phase IIb and III studies, can be designed to capture specific information on the event in question. In addition, large, simple studies can be fielded to evaluate the occurrence of a single or very small number of events in a very large number of patients (ie, tens of thousands). However, it is necessary to adequately and accurately "frame the question" (ie, design the study to meet specific objectives) for these or any study looking at a specific association. In randomized studies conducted after the product is on the market, decisions on control or comparison group may be difficult due to ethical or logistical considerations.

One of the most useful developments over the past 20 years has been the advent of computerized billing and payment. These administrative records leave a paper trail of the occurrence of specific events that can be analyzed to provide insights into specific exposure–event relationships. Whether in private insurance, Medicaid or Medicare plans, records of specific prescriptions and specific events can be linked for the same individual. Comparing event rates in those exposed to specific drugs with a similar group not exposed provides evidence for a causal link between drug and adverse event. Because of their vast size, accessibility, and collection of information unbiased by the relationship in question, administrative databases provide the source for the majority of pharmacoepidemiology studies on the risks and benefits of drugs. However, there are other forms of studies, such as a prospective documentation of drug exposure and follow-up for adverse events (ie, often seen in registries) and a case-control methodology that selects patients on the occurrence or non-occurrence of an event and then either searches a database for record of specific drug exposure or queries the individual or surrogate for exposure.

Patient registries are one of the most confusing topics in the realm of risk management as the term is used in many different ways. A registry is merely a group of individuals assembled (and, generally, followed over time) with some common attribute. Common registries are for individuals with specific diseases or specific "exposures," for example, taking a drug. What makes analysis of registries complicated is that often there is no obvious control or comparison group. If the registry is formed because of exposure to a particular drug, there is usually no corresponding cohort of similar individuals unexposed, first, because of the expense in forming and following a cohort may make it extremely costly to create a comparison group (such as a no treatment control group) and, second, even if such a group were formed, it may not provide unbiased data because registries differ from trials in that there is no randomization. People who refuse to take a medicine may be quite different in many ways to people who do. Comparing these two groups may produce "non-equivalent" comparisons where differences among the groups are due to a variety of factors unrelated to the drug in question. For example, patients or their physicians can choose to continue with a drug or switch to another. Likewise those who do not take the drug at the time of initiation of a registry may do so at a later date. On the other hand, a registry offers the advantage of providing prospective and established data for a specific purpose. The desired and necessary information is collected from all members of the cohort with a specific purpose rather than relying on the medical system to collect appropriate information in a consistent manner.

Registries can provide information on the occurrence of specific events, but often lack the ability of generalizing this information to a broader group of patients or groups. Further, many patients may differ in a significant fashion from those that participate in a registry. Information on the absolute risk can be estimated, but the risk differences or risks relative to an unexposed group are difficult to estimate.

Because of the relatively few ways the biologic organism can respond to insults, most drug adverse events fall into a relatively small number of categories.[10] Thus, when patients are taking a number of different medications, it may be very difficult to assign suspicion to one particular product. Also, these events do occur in the absence of exposure to any drug.[11,12] Understanding the background rate of specific events, especially the background rate in patients with specific disease states, is essential for assessing the contribution of drugs to these events. Thus, most analyses provide information on the statistical patient. For example, patients taking statins are more likely to experience liver test elevations than those not on these drugs. But, it is actually difficult to attribute an abnormal test result in an identified patient to their specific use of a statin.

Rigorous risk management plans and post-marketing surveillance can help products in a number of ways. They can dispel suspicion of an association. For example, at the time of the launch of lovastatin, there was concern that it may be associated with lens opacities. This concern arose from a study in dogs. A number of other products had produced a spurious signal in dogs, but this particular result was accompanied by an increased reporting of opacities in a human study population. The results of the latter were confounded by the fact that the report from the dog study occurred between baseline and follow-up lens examinations. The concern raised by the animal study resulted in more intense examination at follow-up and greater reporting of opacities. However, large, carefully designed follow-up studies revealed no increase in opacities with lovastatin.[13,14] Consequently, this resulted in the removal from the package insert of the need to perform slit lamp examination on individuals prescribed lovastatin.

At times, medical and biologic understanding will lag behind application and adverse events will not be reported because they are not believed to have any association with the product. For example, there were little or no reports of renal adverse events for indomethacin during the first 10 years it was on the market. Only with the increased understanding of a relationship between non-steroidal anti-inflammatory drugs (NSAIDs) and prostaglandin synthesis and prostaglandin and renal function was there recognition that NSAIDs may indeed have an adverse effect on the renal system.[15] Today, there is a clear acceptance that NSAIDs can produce renal failure in a small minority of patients.[16,17]

Because of the need for benefits to exceed the risks with specific products, those products that may most require a comprehensive risk management program are those for treating individuals with non-life-threatening conditions. Of the 16 drugs withdrawn from the market between 1975 and 2000,[18] 10 were for symptomatic or preventive therapies (one for psoriasis, two anti-hypertensive, four NSAID, two antihistamine, one acid/peptic disorders). The remaining six were antibiotics (two) and one each for treatments for congestive heart failure, arrhythmia, depression and type 2 diabetes. In 1997, dexfenfluramine (Redux) made the headlines and caused a major pharmaceutical company to suffer huge losses. This product was indicated for obesity, but a sizeable number of those prescribed the drug were less than 20% overweight and at a much lower risk for major health problems associated with obesity. The fact that the majority of those taking dexfenfluramine were not expected to have a major health impact as a result of their condition meant that the belatedly discovered effect of the drug on heart valves was unacceptable.[19]

No drug is absolutely safe. Relative safety means benefits exceed risks for a defined population and use. Relative benefits and risks differ depending on patient characteristics. Thus, positive benefits *versus* risks may not apply to off-label use. Risks are often classified as pharmacological, that is, those that are the result of the pharmacologic properties of the drug, or idiosyncratic, ie, the mechanism of event is not understood or may result because of some characteristic of the individual.

Risk Communication

It is not enough to learn about risks and quantify their occurrence. One must communicate that information to health care professionals and patients. If the communication is successful, people will become aware of the risk and modify their behavior to avoid safety hazards. Without such communication, there is no hope that patients will change their behavior. The challenge of risk communication is to make people aware of risk issues and to develop messages and select communication channels that will lead to behavior change or adaptation, and the maintenance of those protective behaviors that will avoid adverse safety outcomes continuously.

Risk communication may be conceptualized at a *macro* and a *micro* level. On the macro level, companies must develop a risk communications plan targeted to induce and maintain safe use behaviors. For example, if a drug can be abused/misused, the risk communication plan must convince the individual not to abuse the medication or if the drug may dangerously interact with another medication, the company must develop a communication plan to assure that the patient knows which drugs to avoid. These communications must make people aware of risks. These must also help people understand and identify the conditions that must be avoided. They must persuade people that they are personally susceptible to these dangers. They must convince people of the importance of adopting risk avoidance behaviors. Often, multiple communications (or multiple exposures to the same communication) are necessary to "break through the clutter" of other communications and provide a memorable and convincing message.

The physician and pharmacist have a critical role in this process. They provide the first line of communication for the safe use of drugs. Oral communication is credible, memorable,

and may be phrased in an understandable and convincing manner tailored to each individual patient. Written communication is also necessary. Written communication is needed to educate and to remind health professionals of the importance of counseling. Written communication is also important to reinforce the counseling messages of physicians and pharmacists.

In recent years there are several forms of communications developed for patients (often referred to as patient information tools). Many of these tools have slightly different roles in the communications process. Table 118-2 describes some of these tools as well as their distribution method and their purpose. Often, various combinations of these tools are used to reinforce and stimulate conditions necessary for behavioral compliance. For example, some drugs that require medication guides also require the use of wallet cards, patient agreements, informed consent, brochures and/or videos.

The design of a risk communications plan should be based on accomplishing a specific set of goals and objectives. The number, type, and timing of risk communications interventions should be based on a theoretical model of successful communications as well as practical advice gained from understanding the audience for the communications (eg, current beliefs, barriers and facilitators of communications, the skills needed to undertake and maintain behavioral compliance, sub-cultural variations in perceiving and understanding risks, situational constraints in displaying desired behaviors). When developing a risk minimization plan, the FDA requests that companies specify the goals and objectives of the plan and to select and justify the choice of tools. The justification may be based on research supporting the effectiveness of the tool or it may be based on some logic or external (audience) statement of support for the tool.

On a micro level, the individual tools must be designed to accomplish the desired communication goals. To develop risk communication tools, it is essential that there is a clear set of communication objectives (COs). These communication objectives must be enumerated explicitly to assure that the tool is focused on achieving the most important goals. The COs also serve as the basis for evaluation of the tool's impact.

Once the COs are set, the document (or script) is written. There are important document design principles to be followed. Clearly, the documents must be presented in a simple and understandable format. Clear writing principles must be followed such as use of short sentences, avoidance of complex terminol-

Table 118-2. Patient Communications Forms Designed for Risk Communication

FORM (TOOLS)	DISTRIBUTION	PURPOSE
Brochure	Physician	General education (knowledge)
Patient package insert	Package or pharmacist	Risk communication
Medication guide	Package	Risk communication and methods of avoidance
Informed consent	Physician	Acknowledgement of risks
Warning stickers	Package	Risk "signal"
Wallet card	Starter kit	Reminder
Stickers for medication vial	Pharmacist on medication vial	Reminder
Patient agreement or contract	Physician	Behavioral commitment
Decision aid	Physician	Choice of therapy
Video tape or CD	Physician or starter kit	Persuasion or choice of therapy
Recurring interventions (telephone calls)	Telephone	Behavioral maintenance

ogy and emphasizing the most important messages with formatting and graphics. However, the presentation must not be so simplified that the important messages are lost. Further, the information presented must be sufficient to provide the reader with an understanding of what are the meaningful risks, why such risks are significant and how they may be avoided. Human factors psychologists advocate that a complete warning message must contain a clear "signal word" (eg, "warning" or "attention"), it must explicitly cite the risk involved (eg, the drug may cause birth defects), how to avoid the risk (eg, to avoid use if pregnant) and a rationale for the risk to convince readers of the significance of the problem (eg, informing readers that the drug crosses the placental barrier).[20]

To assure that the designed communication delivers the intended messages as defined by the COs, it is important to pretest communications. Qualitative tests (ie, one-on-one interviews) are often used to help formulate question wording and pretest initial questionnaire designs. More formal quantitative comprehension tests use individuals in the target population (ie, consumers in the target market or actual patients). Respondents are asked to read the test materials and answer questions (ie, based on the COs) to test their understanding, interpretation, decision-making, and beliefs about the medication and the material tested. Questions that demonstrate a lack of understanding may lead to design changes in the test materials. However, other considerations, such as the amount and complexity of the materials presented and the nature of the questions themselves must be taken into consideration to determine the meaning of various test scores. Once designed, justified, and tested, the risk communication tools can be produced and distributed in various forms. Eventually, they must be delivered to and read by the intended audience for them to have any impact. According to the FDA's concept paper, the nature of the impact of these tools in the "real world" must be tested (note *Evaluation* below).

DISTRIBUTION AND BEHAVIORAL CONTROL SYSTEMS

Whereas much of what one hopes to accomplish in managing pharmaceutical risks may be realized through carefully designed communications, information dissemination may not be sufficient to lead to behavior change. Often, information is viewed as a "weak intervention." For information to have an impact it must be received, read, understood, motivational, persuasive, remembered and implemented for behavior change to be effective. Furthermore, longer term behavior maintenance means that information must be effective over the long term, often for many years. While voluntary adaptations are viewed as the most positive method of influencing health behavior, it may also be necessary to institute distribution or behavioral control systems that influence risk avoidance behavior.

A distribution system is necessary for a drug to be delivered to the patient. For all prescription drugs, it is necessary for the physician to order a prescription (eg, in writing or verbally) and a pharmacist to dispense the drug. Certain drugs, such as scheduled medicines, also require limits on refills and additional record keeping. For certain risk minimization programs, there have been additional controls developed to minimize "risky" behaviors. For example, for Clozeril (clozapine),where certain blood disorders may resulted from taking the drug, patients are required to submit to monthly blood tests that demonstrate the drug is not having an undesirable effect. This "no blood, no drug" policy has minimized the impact of these problems and permitted a helpful drug to remain on the market. Another example of a distribution control system is the use of a verification sticker program. These are used for certain acne drugs, most notably, Accutane (ie, isotretinoin). In this instance, the drug may have important adverse consequences (eg, causing birth defects if taken during pregnancy). A woman taking Accutane must, therefore, have a monthly pregnancy test to demonstrate that she is not pregnant, and the physician must date and affix a sticker to the prescription (no refills are permitted) that communicates to the pharmacist that the woman is not pregnant. The pharmacist may only dispense the medication if the sticker is attached to the prescription and appropriately dated within 7 days of dispensing.

Other distribution control systems, such as obtaining a prescription for the medication only from a physician who has been certified to prescribe the medicine or providing medication only to a patient who has been certified to receive the prescription have been suggested or implemented by various companies. The logic underpinning such designs is derived from "systems theory," which has been used by various industries (eg, the aircraft industry) to design "safety" into the "systems" used.

Systems theory relies on a number of "design" elements to force an individual to behave in a prescribed fashion. According to systems theory, any activity may be conceived as a "system" that requires actions to occur for the activity to be accomplished. For example, the issuance of a prescription requires the doctor to diagnose an illness (or prescribe a drug to prevent an illness), to choose the medication (along with dosage and directions), to provide the prescription to a patient (or surrogate). Upon delivery to the pharmacy the review and checking of the prescription by pharmacy staff must take place, the retrieval of the medication from storage occurs, the counting of tablets, the labeling of the vial, the temporary storage of the prescription and the dispensing of the prescription to the patient (or surrogate) must take place. There may (and should) be additional stages in this model, such as counseling of patients by physicians and pharmacists, information collection and retrieval, administrative activities for reimbursement and compliance with various laws and regulations and additional risk management activities). However, even this simplified "system" requires many different activities, and mistakes may occur at several different points. To prevent such errors, various procedures may be instituted and controls or design changes implemented. For example, to prevent taking the wrong bottle off the shelve, color-coded bottles may be used or bar codes utilized that necessitate being checked or the institute may implement a mandatory check list of actions to prevent dispensing the wrong medication.

There are a number of "forcing functions" (ie, design features that build in safety) such as having drug names be of a certain font size or that constitute a certain percentage of the front display panel and multiple redundancies (eg, having the drug name on multiple places on the bottle of medicine) that help design safety. At the heart of systems theory is the logic that such procedures must be followed every time an activity is undertaken, or the resulting action cannot take place.

FDA AND THE RISK MANAGEMENT PROGRAM (RMP)

As discussed previously, once the FDA guidance is finalized, certain new drug applications will require a Risk MAP. The purpose of this program will be to propose, design, implement and evaluate a number of interventions intended to minimize the risks of using the drug. In similar fashion to a clinical development program, the Risk MAP will have a defined set of goals and objectives, developed specifically for the drug in question. It is anticipated that this will occur by the end of 2004.

Each Risk MAP must specify the overall goals of the program, (eg, specifying that no pregnant woman be prescribed a specific drug). For each goal, one or more objectives should be specified. These are intermediate steps necessary for achieving the overall goal, for example, specifying that all physicians must fully inform women patients about the risks of taking a drug if pregnant. Finally, a number of tools or interventions must be specified that will aid in obtaining the specified goals and objectives, for example, specifying that there will be a brochure and a video drafted for physicians to distribute to patients. Each of these tools should be justified and pretested to help assure that they will achieve their intended purpose(s).

Evaluation of the Effectiveness of These Tools

One of the important contributions of the FDA draft guidance on risk management was the proposal to evaluate fully the impact of the entire risk minimization program and the impact of the individual tools intended to control risks.

Three types of evaluations are possible. First, individual tools may be pretested as part of the development process. For example, comprehension tests, as discussed previously, may be used to help design impactful communications. Second, a series of interventions may be instituted in a field test (ie, likely, a phase IIIB study). This study may be in the form of a clinical trial where various distribution sites are randomized to deliver various combinations of interventions. By comparing outcomes among sites, the impact of various interventions may be judged. However, care must be taken to assure sufficient power to determine differences among sites and avoiding confounding sites with intervention biases.

Third, the FDA proposed that all Risk MAPs be evaluated fully once implemented. The FDA suggested the use of two different measures of Risk MAP impact and the use of well-defined and validated measures. Based on the evaluation of the Risk MAP, there is a consequent obligation to modify or increase interventions, if not successful. However, few of the interventions implemented in the past to reduce the risks of a drug have been rigorously evaluated. Too often, those that have been evaluated have demonstrated that for all their good intentions, the effect was less than desired. For example, package insert requirements for liver enzyme monitoring are not well followed, even in the face of major media coverage of the risks of hepatic failure.[21] Risk minimization programs must eventually be able to show that they decrease or mitigate the likelihood of adverse events.

Ideally, intervention effectiveness should be evaluated based on ability to decrease actual health outcomes (eg, cases of jaundice, liver disease, and / or liver failures). Often, however, this is impractical, and it may be necessary to monitor surrogates (eg, increases in ALT/AST levels) or process measures (eg, frequency of testing for liver enzyme elevations) or even the comprehension, knowledge, and attitude among patients, prescribers, and pharmacists about the risks and consequences. For outcomes and process measures, the same tools that allow the estimation of risk can be used to estimate the change in risk under a given set of risk management interventions.

The term *registry* often throws terror into the heart of a pharmaceutical marketing director. A very strict risk management program can require all individuals receiving the drug to be followed for appropriateness of treatment and monitoring and/or specific outcomes under conditions of a registry. However, more broadly, the use of a registry provides information on a sample of individuals receiving the medication in question. This sample of individuals can be followed for specific monitoring and/or outcomes such as compliance with laboratory monitoring and/or the effectiveness of that monitoring in preventing one or more clinical adverse events.

In this instance, the criteria for entering the registry is exposure to a particular drug. Although one may wish to recruit all such individuals exposed into the registry, while in all likelihood, one will only be able to recruit a percentage of those individuals. Thus, more commonly, a registry is composed of a sample of willing individuals who have received the drug or have the underlying disease for which the drug may be prescribed.

The same type of observational studies used in assessment of the magnitude of risks, can (and should) be used to monitor the effectiveness of specific interventions. Administrative databases can be used to answer routine queries on the occurrence of contraindicated co-prescribing or overdosing, appropriate monitoring, and associations between prescribing of selected drugs and specific events. Note that such associations do not imply causality. Identical to the analyses for estimating magnitude of risk, analyses should be conducted to estimate the risk under the management program(s). When it is not clear which invention(s) would be most effective, it may be worthwhile to use an experimental design comparing different interventions.

Regardless of evaluation study, interventions need to be assessed on their effectiveness of preventing serious adverse events and on the basis of their cost and burden on the health care system. Too rigorous an intervention may result in many additional visits, tests, and other forms of monitoring. This, in turn, may result is increased mistakes due to increased tasks. Increased costs may make the new therapy of less value than other, less effective therapies and/or raise patient privacy concerns. Other possible decreased benefits that follow from risk management interventions that are too stringent may be decreased patient compliance and decreased drug access to patients that would benefit.

CONCLUSION AND SUMMARY

Risk management is a new and evolving discipline. It is difficult to argue that drugs should be provided to patients in a manner that minimizes potential hazards. The FDA has advanced the public health by fostering greater attention over the discovery, quantification, and management of risks. However, any policy that results in new activities to control one set of hazards may result in creating new, unexpected, hazards. Thus, continuing to evaluate the hazards of drugs and the interventions intended to control these hazards, is essential to assure that the benefits of a Risk Minimization Program will, itself, outweigh its risks.

REFERENCES

1. US Food and Drug Administration. Concept paper: Premarketing risk assessment. www.fda.gov/cder/meeting/riskmanagment.hrm, March 2003a.
2. US Food and Drug Administration. Concept paper: Risk management programs. www.fda.gov/cder/meeting/riskmanagment.hrm, March 2003b.
3. US Food and Drug Administration. Concept paper: Risk assessment of observational data: good pharmacovigilance practices and pharmacoepidemiologic assessment. www.fda.gov/cder/meeting/riskmanagment.hrm, March 2003c.
4. US Food and Drug Administration. Report to the Nation: Improving the public health through human drugs. *CDER*, 2002.
5. Institute of Medicine. *To Err is Human: Building a Safer Healthcare System.* Kohn L, Corrigan JM, Molla S (eds). Washington DC: National Academy Press, 2000.
6. US Food and Drug Administration, Report to the FDA Commissioner from the Task Force on Risk Management. *Managing the Risks from Medical Product Use: Creating a Risk Management Framework,* May 1999.
7. Venning GR. *BMJ* 1983; 286:458–460.
8. Bruinsma W. *Dermatologica* 1972; 145:377–388.
9. Hill AB. *Proc Roy Soc Med* 1965; 58:295–300.
10. Benichou C. *A Practical Guide to Diagnosis and Management.* Chichester, England: John Wiley & Sons, 1995.
11. Clark JM, Brancati FL, Diehl AM. *Am J Gastroenterol* 2003; 98:955–956.
12. Erbey JR, Silberman C, Lydick E. *Am J Med* 2000; 109:588–590.
13. Laties AM, Shear CL, Lippa EA, et al. *Am J Cardiol* 1991; 67: 447–453.
14. Chylack LT Jr, Mantell G, Wolfe JK, et al. *Optometry and Visual Science* 1993; 70:937–943.
15. Lydick E, Blumenthal SJ, Guess HA. *J Clin Res Pharmacoepidemiol* 1990; 4:183–189.
16. Ahmad SR, Korepeter C, Brinker A, et al. *Drug Safety* 2002; 25: 537–544.
17. Pirson Y, van Ypersele de Strihou C. *Am J Kidney Dis* 1986; 8:338–344.
18. Lasser KE, Allen PD, Woohandler SJ, et al. *JAMA* 2002; 287:2215–2220.
19. Connolly HM, Crary JL, McGoon MD, et al. *N Engl J Med* 1997; 337: 581–588.
20. Morris LA, Aikin KJ. The "pharmacokinetics" of patient communications. *Drug Information Journal* 2001; 36:509–527.
21. Graham DJ, Drinkard CR, Shatin D, et al. *JAMA* 2001; 286:831–833.

CHAPTER 119

Integrated Health Care Delivery Systems

Mark A Touchette, PharmD, BCPS

Barbara J Zarowitz, PharmD, FCCP, BCPS

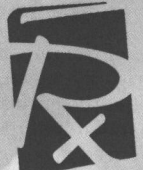

BACKGROUND

The changing forces responsible for driving the integration of health care systems has led to considerable confusion about integrated health systems (also known as organized health systems), their functions, structure, and processes. In 1996, Shortell et al defined an integrated health system as "a network of organizations that provides or arranges to provide a coordinated continuum of services to a defined population and is willing to be held clinically and fiscally accountable for the outcomes and health status of the population serviced."[1] This definition was stimulated by the belief that the movement toward global capitation and provider-owned health plans would continue to grow. Because, in some cases, there has been movement away from global capitation and provider-owned health plans, Coddington et al defined integrated health systems as those which "provide a comprehensive spectrum of high quality, well-coordinated health care services on a cost-effective basis to residents of its service area.[2] To accomplish this, physicians and hospitals and other health care providers work together for the benefit of the customers. The medical care provided will be enhanced by a commitment to education and research." Although integrated systems in existence today vary widely in their composition, many are comprised of a parent corporation that manages several dissimilar subsidiaries such as hospitals, medical groups, specialty clinics, health plans, home health services, and ambulatory pharmacies as well as components dedicated to improving care through research and education. Systems such as these types are referred to as "vertically integrated" and were formed with the goals of providing high quality, low cost care to populations of patients in broad geographic areas, eliminating duplication of services, and providing care across the continuum (referred to as "seamless" health care).

The impetus for the formation of today's integrated health systems can be traced back to the 1970s when Certificate of Need laws and inpatient care cost ceilings were introduced with the intent of restraining uncontrolled growth in the number of inpatient hospitals beds and resultant increases in health care spending. This led to more care being provided in the outpatient environment as hospitals partnered with private practice physicians in areas such as ambulatory surgery and other outpatient treatment centers to maintain financial viability. In 1982, Diagnosis Related Groups were introduced which resulted in further decreases in hospital census by limiting reimbursement to standard lengths of stay for each condition. To maintain profitability, hospitals sought to capitalize on economies of scale, to increase their patient base, and to leverage purchasing opportunities. Also, in response to inflation in health care spending, the mid-1980s witnessed an increase in the number of patients covered under managed care contracts.

Through the mid-1990s further movement toward integration was driven by several factors.[2] These included a perceived shortage of primary care physicians, the potential for health care reform under the Clinton administration, the perceived need to provide broad geographic coverage, and the desire to offer "single signature contracting" that allows alignment of financial incentives among physicians and hospitals. In addition, it was believed that health plans would not contract with individual physicians or small groups. Larger organized groups capable of capitalizing on the economies of scale and of accepting financial risks for the population developed as "global capitation" was believed to be the future trend. It therefore made sense for physicians and hospitals to work together to compete for dollars awarded on a "per member per month" basis.

Beginning about 1995, forces driving integration of health systems began to change.[2] It became clear that many medical groups and hospitals were not capable of assuming financial risk as evidenced by many large integrated systems experiencing significant financial short falls. Also, declining provider and consumer sentiments regarding managed care and the consumer's desire for increased freedom of choice began to favor larger numbers of specialists or specialty groups, putting organized systems with an emphasis on primary care at a disadvantage. Large integrated systems began to struggle with the complexity of the infrastructure required to manage systems that include such dissimilar entities such as medical groups, hospitals and health plans. Competing interests coupled with the significant challenge and time required to develop successful corporate culture made it difficult for these systems to survive. It is increasingly recognized that discretionary consumer spending on "quality of life" services such as cosmetic surgery, laser eye surgery, complimentary and alternative medicine, infertility treatment, and hearing aids is increasing; integrated systems with a primary care focus may have not have been positioned to meet this demand.

The changing environment of health care has led many integrated systems to re-evaluate their priorities.[2] Current drivers favoring the continued integration of health care systems have been identified. The concept of seamless care continues to be important as consumers appreciate "one stop shopping" where health care is coordinated. Economies of scale, where clinical and administrative services are combined continue to drive integration as well as the ability of integrated systems to provide care to broad geographic areas. This is especially true when integrated systems offer outreach programs to patients in rural areas where such services would not be available otherwise. Improved access to service for patients needs to be addressed, with the goal being to shorten the time required to get an appointment. A strong regional or national brand name is important in attracting patients and providers alike, and the ability to be recognized for continuous quality improvement has received attention as much focus has been trained on the ability of organizations to provide safe, error-free care. Another factor favoring large integrated systems is that these systems are large enough to have the financial capability to develop information technologies that allow information sharing and automation across the organization. One recent major shift in priority of many integrated health systems is the divestiture of their health plan and a shift toward payer neutral strategies, as it is believed that consumers will play a larger role in selecting their health plans and providers in the future. Although the drivers favoring the integration have changed in recent years, there is still strong rationale favoring an integrated approach to delivering health care.

PHARMACY SERVICES—In a fully integrated system, the pharmacists all work for the same corporation, with the same mission to provide quality, cost-efficient care across the continuum. Ideally, the patient's medical record is available to all caregivers within an integrated system. Pharmacists are then able to assure that the patient's pharmacotherapy plan follows them from the inpatient to the outpatient arena and vice-versa. This gives the integrated health system pharmacist the ability to play a role in the development of care plans in the hospital that will be carried out in the ambulatory arena by another pharmacist who will continue to provide care for the patient. Likewise, information on the patient's pharmacotherapy plan and educational needs that have been assessed and documented by pharmacists working in specialty clinic settings, such as anticoagulation clinics, can be provided by inpatient pharmacists when necessary. This working arrangement allows pharmacists to shift their attention to assuring appropriate pharmacotherapy outcomes from the use of medications as opposed to the traditional focus on drug dispensing and drug price control.

Pharmacists are important leaders in formulary development in integrated systems, as their knowledge and experience in therapeutics and pharmacoeconomics add value to formulary decision-making, development of disease management guidelines, and evaluation of pharmacotherapy outcomes for the system. Formularies and disease management guidelines are not limited to drugs needed for inpatient care, but expand to include agents needed in the outpatient and home-care setting.

An integrated health care system uses the economies of scale to secure contract pricing on pharmaceutical purchases. Because of the structure of an integrated system, just-in-time delivery can be used to provide drugs to the numerous locations where care is provided. This decreases inventory and stocking costs to the system. In this situation, it is essential for the pharmacists to review medication orders and manage the drug use process. The focus of the pharmacist in the integrated system moves from the traditional dispensing activities to the provision of pharmaceutical care.

The pharmacy services in an integrated system may be organized into an assortment of reporting structures. The structure of the Group Health Cooperative of Puget Sound has been described as a matrix. In this integrated system, the pharmacists in the clinics and hospitals report directly to the managers of the facility. There is a matrix relationship between these manager pharmacists and the director of pharmacy administration. In this arrangement the pharmacy administration provides support services, including purchasing and contracting, information system support, development of policies and procedures, support for Pharmacy & Therapeutics Committee activities, long-range planning, and overall support of operations.[3] In the Henry Ford Health System, the pharmacy director of each hospital reports to hospital administration. All ambulatory services are brought together as a product line under the Community Care Services business unit of the system. While the pharmacists in the system are all supportive of the continuum of care, there is no corporate organizational structure supporting the various pharmacy services. The pharmacy directors and managers from the system hospitals, Ambulatory Pharmacy Product Line, and health maintenance organization (HMO) have taken it upon themselves to meet monthly to discuss clinical and operational issues that concern pharmacy services for all patients of the system. It is their goal to support pharmacists as providers of cost-efficient pharmaceutical care and to ensure that optimal patient outcomes are achieved in the integrated system if pharmacists are to continue to play a role in the delivery of health care.

PATIENT-SPECIFIC CARE

Primary Care

Primary care is the provision of integrated, accessible health care services by clinicians who are accountable for addressing a large majority of personal health care needs, developing a sustained partnership with the patient, and practicing in the context of family and community.[4] Primary care is the point-of-entry of patient into the health system, where continuity of care is provided over a period of time, and care is comprehensive (medical specialties, nutrition, social) and highly personalized. As such, primary-care practice generally is devoted to internal medicine, family practice, and pediatrics.

Ambulatory care refers more broadly to care that can be delivered in very specific or more general clinic environments and includes emergency rooms and specialty and subspecialty clinics. Primary care serves an important *gatekeeper* role for the health system. The Primary Care team, composed of doctors, nurses, pharmacists, and other health professionals, identifies and manages the patients' health and wellness, intervening to remedy acute illnesses as they occur and referring the patient to more-specialized practitioners or services when needed. As such, the Primary Care team regulates and controls access of the patient to more-specialized health services within the system.

The role of pharmacists has evolved in outpatient environments within integrated health systems. Initially, pharmacists had selective roles within specific clinics, such as anticoagulation or hypertension, which generally developed because of a close working relationship between the physician leadership and the pharmacist. Pharmacists' activities were limited to the therapeutic area of interest of the physician mentor for the clinic. Often, pharmacists started seeing patients with the physician and gradually became recognized by the physician as a capable provider of care. These positions usually were funded through colleges of pharmacy and were limited to pharmacy faculty. The clinics operated as separate functional units, not integrated into the rest of the care of the patient or into the rest of the system of care, for example, the hospital. When outpatient clinics became part of integrated health systems, some traditional models of pharmacist-managed clinics survived. However, the role of pharmacists in primary care clinics in integrated health systems has been expanded to include other activities of focus that meet newly defined patient care or health system needs.

Today, primary-care roles have been chosen deliberately to complement patient-care needs in large, integrated systems. There are several reasons why pharmacist's roles have changed. Health care is now being driven by continuous improvement. Primary-care clinics are chosen carefully, based on quality-driven analyses to improve the quality of patient care. In 1999, the American Society of Health-System Pharmacists defined minimum practice standards for pharmaceutical services in ambulatory care environments.[5]

HEDIS (Health Plan Employer Data and Information Set) was developed by the National Committee for Quality Assurance (NCQA), an independent, not-for-profit organization dedicated to assessing and reporting on the quality of managed-care plans. The NCQA surveys and accredits managed-care plans much as the Joint Commission on Accreditation of Healthcare Organizations (JCAHO) accredits hospitals and home-care agencies. HEDIS incorporates measures related to outcomes or results, as well as the process measures, utilization, and financial data. There are indicators in several domains. Overall outpatient drug use, β-blocker treatment after acute myocardial infarction, appropriate medications for patients with asthma, and antibiotic treatment for children with otitis media are four drug-related indicators. Pharmacists are involved in assimilating overall drug use data and delivering and assessing quality of care delivered to post myocardial infarction, asthma, diabetes, depression, and otitis media patients.

Pharmacists have been identified as one of the important members of the health care team who affect the quality and cost of care.[6] Systems of care, individual patient care, and management of large populations have been improved through pharmacists' involvement. Integrated systems are responsible for the totality of care from birth to death, during wellness and disease, with an emphasis on health wellness and disease prevention. Because of this, pharmacists find themselves in new roles, serving as partners with the patient to encourage the promotion of health and wellness. Table 119-1 compares pharmacist roles in traditional ambulatory-care clinics with those commonly found in integrated health systems.

Quality monitors in place in health systems are designed for continuous assessment of opportunities to improve care of patients across the system. For example, when the Food and Drug Administration (FDA) approved several drug-therapy regimens for the eradication of *Helicobacter pylori* as a cause of peptic ulcer disease, it became clear that health systems, particularly those with managed-care populations, could both improve the quality of care provided and lower the total costs of care by treating patients with antibiotics to eradicate *H. pylori* rather than treating each new ulcer that developed. An appropriate mechanism to identify and treat these patients did not exist. Patients continued to present to their doctors when symptoms of peptic ulcer disease caused them to go to their doctor or emergency room.

Many integrated systems offer *H. pylori* services consisting of teams of nurses and pharmacists, trained to identify patients eligible for treatment from the overall population of patients served by the health system. Identification occurs through the use of large databases on patient characteristics and computerized searches of patient records to identify patients who have had a history of peptic ulcer disease and who may be a candidate to test for the presence of the bacteria. These patients are then called, proactively, into the clinic to be tested for the presence of *H. pylori*. If they are positive, patients are treated with a course of antibiotics and a proton pump inhibitor to eradicate the organism and prevent further recurrence of disease, decline in health, and greater costs associated with acute disease intervention.

The pharmacist-nurse team selects the therapy, usually from a previously developed care plan, algorithm, or care map, and then monitors the patients, interacting with them several times during the course of therapy to ensure compliance and answer any drug- or disease-related questions the patient poses. Patients are followed until their course of therapy is complete, symptoms are resolved, and chronic proton pump inhibitor or histamine-2 antagonist therapy is no longer required. When necessary, reevaluation for the presence of *H. pylori* can occur to determine the possibility of therapeutic failure due to antimicrobial resistance or previously undetected nonadherence to the first eradication regimen.

Pharmacists are participating in smoking cessation programs. Smoking is associated with over $110 billion in annual medical costs in the US. Managed-care systems implement programs to help participating members quit smoking, thereby enhancing their health, decreasing illness risk, and improving quality of life. Pharmacists' roles include identifying patients who may be candidates for nicotine replacement therapy, referring patients with chemical addiction for treatment, teaching patients how to use nicotine patches, lozenges, or gum, and providing realistic expectations about the need for behavioral modification with nicotine replacement products or bupropion (Zyban). Patients are taught to watch for adverse effects in one-on-one contact when the product is dispensed and in-group sessions. As members of the smoking cessation teams, pharmacists work closely with nurses, psychologists, and physicians to monitor patient progress throughout their treatment and for a year following their smoking cessation.

Recently, the role of pharmacists in lipid clinics has been described. Deaths from cardiovascular consequences of hyperlipidemia account for over $100 million annually. While lipid-lowering drugs are being prescribed with increasing frequency, it has been shown that fewer than 50% of treated patients reach and sustain the National Cholesterol Education Program (NCEP) target cholesterol values. There are numerous reports of pharmacist-managed lipid clinics where pharmacists are asked to manage patients on lipid-lowering therapy, educate the patients, adjust doses according to repeat laboratory evaluation, and assess compliance to diet and drug-therapy regimens. While long-term outcome data, such as morbidity and mortality reduction, are not known, improved attainment of cholesterol and triglyceride values has been shown in these disease-specific clinics.

CARE MAPS AND CLINICAL PATHWAYS—Most primary or ambulatory care clinics do not have a specific disease focus. In primary care settings, health care personnel provide more comprehensive care across the complete spectrum of health and disease from birth to death. However, to provide care of this comprehensive magnitude, most integrated health systems have attempted to reduce practice variance by guiding routine diagnosis, intervention, and drug treatment through the use of practice guidelines, clinical pathways, or care maps, coupled with the measurement of achieved outcomes. Reduction in process variance helps to improve the quality of care while decreasing the cost.

In a sense, algorithms, guidelines, and care maps define *best practice* within a range of acceptable choices and allow clinicians to select the patient intervention and monitor the patient's progress through the disease process as guided by the care map's guidelines. Clinical pathways have been referred to in the medical literature by more than 30 different names. Clinical pathways or care maps incorporate goals of treatment based on standards of care, current practice guidelines, scientific evidence, and benchmarking against systems of management used in other health systems.[7]

Table 119-1. Primary Care Roles of Pharmacists

TRADITIONAL PRIMARY CARE ROLES	PRIMARY CARE ROLES IN INTEGRATED HEALTH SYSTEMS
Specific, limited in scope	Broad, integrated into a system of care
Based in a traditional medical specialty	Part of an overall disease management strategy
Chosen by practice interest	Chosen by patient/health system need
Usually single providers of care	Teams of providers delivering care
Monitoring of patients by provider	Measurement of quality and success of service by health system
Unaffected by cost	Driven by value to the patient and health system; quality at lowest cost
Examples: anticoagulation, hypertension,	Examples: smoking cessation, travel, diabetes clinics lipid, *Helicobacter pylori* clinics

**Table 119-2. Protocol-Driven Care:
Situations Using Care Maps, Algorithms,
Guidelines**

	REDUCES VARIANCE IN	OUTCOME MEASURES
Primary Care		
Anticoagulation	INR targets	Days therapeutic
	Time to therapeutic	INRs in Range
Asthma	Drug choices	FEV1
	Emergency Room visits	Readmission rate
	Monitoring therapy	
	Patient education	
Acid peptic disease	Drug choices	*H Pylori* Eradication
	Diagnosis	Days to pain relief
	Cost of therapy	
	Side effects	
	Retreatment	
Acute Care		
Pneumonia	Drug and treatment choices	Time to defervescence
Deep vein thrombosis	Monitoring, dosing	Time to therapeutic APTT/INR, time to ambulation
Myocardial infarction	Thrombolytic protocol	Time to treatment
	Testing	Length of stay
	Rehabilitation	
Tricyclic Overdose	Interventions	Time to recovery

Table 119-2 summarizes examples of situations in which care maps are used as a tool to direct care. Care maps describe pharmacological as well as nonpharmacological therapies, interventions, activities, and outcomes, often throughout the entire course of care (from diagnosis, through admission, and after discharge). They usually are developed for high-cost, high-volume, and/or high-risk diagnoses or procedures. The goals of care maps are to decrease practice variance and, thus, enhance the quality of care, provide continuity of care, decrease care fragmentation (particularly when patient care is handed-off from one service to another), guide the family and patient through expected treatment and progress, optimize cost-effectiveness of health care delivery, and increase satisfaction of patients, families, staff, and physicians.

Importantly, care maps create common expectations and goals previously agreed-upon by the patient and his/her care team. They increase the likelihood that all members of the health care team share responsibility for the care and final outcome of the patient, enhance communication, and promote early problem detection and resolution. Care maps serve as a useful educational tool for new staff and patients.

Care maps generally include specific goals, desired outcomes, and interventions for several domains of care that may include patient education, activity level, discharge planning, medications, nutrition, elimination, diagnostic tests and procedures, and treatments. Table 119-3 depicts standard care map components with example goals, interventions, and documentation strategies shown for deep vein thrombosis (DVT). The goal of the care map is to diagnose, treat and monitor low-risk patients with deep vein thrombosis without hospitalization and to have a rapid, accurate process in place to identify and hospitalize patients with more complex or serious complications of deep vein thrombosis. In both treatment settings, achievement of the desired therapeutic outcome is paramount and assured through a clear delineation of responsibilities and interventions that lead to the desired outcome.

Care maps are developed by a team of individuals who will be involved in the various stages of care of the patient during his or her flow through the process. For the care map depicted in Table 119-3, team members may involve a nurse, pharmacist, physician, social worker, dietitian, and diagnostic radiologist. Each of the team members has responsibility for a component of the care delivered, yet all have shared responsibility for the daily outcomes of interest and the overall treatment outcome. In paperless systems with electronic medical records, team members chart progress electronically; documentation can be performed manually on wall charts.

The care map serves to decrease redundant charting and recording activities and is an easily accessible monitoring and communication tool. At the end of the episode of care, the care map is stored as a permanent part of the medical record.

The role of pharmacists on clinical pathway teams may be as simple as providing consultative advice regarding the drug, intravenous fluids, nutritional products, or their sequencing or as complicated as a day-by-day defined caretaker role of educating the patient and remaining team members about the drug-therapy component of the care map, administering medications, adjusting medication doses, identifying drug-therapy endpoints and monitoring parameters, and performing drug-related monitoring (eg, blood pressure or blood sugar checks). Certain care maps are more conducive to active pharmacist's roles, while others, such as an appendectomy pathway, may leave little need for pharmacist involvement other than the selection and monitoring of analgesic therapy.

DISEASE MANAGEMENT—Disease management deserves mention in primary-care environments, as it is becoming a focal point around which care delivery models of care are developing. To many, disease management is a natural extension of care maps, clinical pathways, and guidelines. Disease management is an evaluative approach to health care delivery that attempts to improve outcomes for patients with a specific disease while optimizing the overall use of health care resources. Outcomes research is a rapidly evolving field that incorporates epidemiology, health services research, health economics, and psychometrics. Measurement of clinical and other outcomes has become important to patients, insurance companies, pharmaceutical companies, and purchasers of health care.

Disease management uses an explicit, systematic, population-based approach to proactively identify patients at risk, intervene with specific programs of care, and measure clinical and other outcomes. The most frequently instituted disease management programs within health systems are for diabetes (83%), asthma (71%), immunization (68%), drug therapy monitoring (58%), hypertension (44%), depression (50%), wellness (36%), anticoagulation management (30%), migraine management (23%), HIV/AIDS (19%), refill clinic (12%), and alternative care (8%). The driving impetus behind disease management programs is reduction of costs, improvement of patient outcomes, improvement of the process of care, and attainment and retention of members.

Candidate diseases for disease management programs are those that consume 80% of the resources and drive up the overall health-system costs. It is estimated that 20% of a selected diseased population is responsible for 80% of the total cost of care for that disease. This concept of 20% of the patients driving 80% of the cost is referred to as the 80-20 rule. The high-use group is the focus of disease management programs that look for opportunities to improve the process of care, education of the patient, drug therapy, and use of expensive resources. The 20% of patients who are high users are often further subdivided to identify the top 5% of patients responsible for 60% of the cost or claims submitted. The top 5% of patients are directed into case management, described in the following section. The remaining high-user patients are managed to obtain the most positive effects on outcomes and cost through innovative monitoring and follow-up.

Disease management tools include guidelines, algorithms, care maps, and a wide variety of patient tools to enhance treatment and drug-therapy adherence. Patients are provided with tools that change behavior, such as participation in support groups, discounts on health club memberships, access to weight-control programs, and episodic telephone reminder calls to take their medicine and measure the parameter of interest (eg, peak flow for asthma, blood sugar for diabetes).

Selected conditions for disease management programs usually meet several criteria. The total cost of the disease is high; it is prevalent in the population and definable by specific criteria; variation in practice and patient management exists; treatment methods are known, and it is possible to intervene to improve care; and opportunities exist within the system to improve the management of the condition or disease. Once the disease or condition has been selected, preparatory work involves understanding the natural course and cost drivers for the disease, developing guidelines for diagnosis and treatment, modifying patient and physician behavior, and identifying cost-effective care strategies. A measurement system must be in place to determine the effectiveness of implemented strategies and modify approaches for continuous improvement of the management of the condition in question. Figure 119-1 depicts the components of disease management.

In outpatient settings, pharmacists participate in disease management programs through their involvement in patient education, monitoring, and follow-up, as well as by performing tests (eg, blood-pressure monitoring, INR, blood-sugar or cholesterol monitoring). These activities may occur in multidisciplinary clinics or through pharmacies. Even in network pharmacies, technicians are doing more of the dispensing process while the pharmacist's roles are expanding to include reviewing prescriptions, educating patients and other health care workers about drug therapy, and monitoring or enhancing drug-therapy adherence.

Certificate programs are available for pharmacists to provide them with the tools, education, and training necessary to participate effectively in disease management programs. Even without advanced training, pharmacists can participate in disease awareness days and help teach patients about their medications. The National Institutes of Health has defined the pharmacist's role in the management of patients with asthma, in six steps as outlined in Table 119-4.

CASE MANAGEMENT—Case management is a process by which an experienced professional (nurse, doctor, social worker, pharmacist) works with patients, providers, and insurers to coordinate all services deemed necessary to provide the patient with medically appropriate health care. The goals of case management are to provide quality health care while decreasing the cost of providing such care. There are two types of case management: primary-care case management and catastrophic, or high-cost, case management.

In primary-care case management, a physician–care manager, acting as an informed purchaser, coordinates all patient care, referring the patient to specialists or alternative-care providers as needed. This is what has been described previously as primary care. Catastrophic case management usually is conducted by a registered nurse on behalf of the payer. The nurse typically works with the patient, providers, and pharmacists to ensure that care is rendered in a coordinated fashion, according to an established and agreed-upon treatment plan. Candidates for case management are identified through disease management programs or by their primary-care provider and may be patients who fail routine follow-up, who continue to consume an exceptionally high proportion of medical and financial resources, or those for whom the quality of care has been adversely affected by circumstances beyond the management of the routine delivery system.

Case managers often follow patients over the full course of their treatment, which may improve the continuity of care and increase patient compliance with care methods while reducing costs. The financial goals of most case management programs are to keep patients out of the hospital and emergency department by appropriately increasing the ambulatory care support and drug therapy. Thus, outpatient drug costs may increase to decrease other healthcare costs. Case managers in-

volve pharmacists in redesigning drug-therapy regimens to offer equally effective, lower-cost alternatives for patients who consume high resources, for example, generic equivalents rather than branded drugs and first-generation products rather than high-cost new-release and potentially unproven therapeutic alternatives.

Case management, disease management, guidelines, care maps, and other tools of organizing the provision of care have arisen as a result of managed care. Managed care attempts to offer a coordinated approach to the delivery and financing of health care services that balance price restraint and resource management with access to quality health care. Aspects of managed care are prevalent in primary-care settings of large integrated health systems. Even those without his/her own HMO is focused on providing best value to their patients; best value is highest quality at the lowest cost.

DATA REPORTING AND MEASUREMENT—Pharmacists and other health care providers need access to data and information to have an effective impact on care in a population of patients served by a large integrated health system. On a micro-level, individual practitioners can improve the quality of care of their own patients. To evaluate and improve individual patient care, pharmacists need access to the medical record, drug-dispensing records, laboratory results, and diagnostic reports. These are readily available in most systems. On a macro-level, an individual can improve the quality of care in a population of patients. When health systems are responsible for the lives and outcomes of their patients and they assume the financial risk for providing the care to these patients, health care is managed. Managed care requires access to databases that reveal information about the patients, the way that treatments and drugs are used, and their outcomes, so that global decisions about care delivery can be made. Databases generally fall into four major areas: medical claims data, pharmacy claims data, member eligibility data, and provider data.[8] Protection of patient privacy, as required by the Health Insurance Portability and Accountability Act (HIPAA), must be assured whenever health care workers access or utilize patient data. Health systems are required to notify patients of their rights to privacy and document that patients have received notification. HIPAA requirements are discussed more fully in Chapter 111: *Laws Governing Pharmacy.*

A claim is information submitted by a provider (doctor) or a covered person to establish that medical services were provided, from which processing for payment to the provider or covered person is made. Claims databases allow health systems, including managed-care organizations, to generate descriptive statistics on patients, providers, and diseases; to conduct comprehensive cost and resource-use analyses; and to build economic models of diseases.

Health care databases allow pharmacists to examine the effectiveness of a treatment to be assessed and the effects of drug-switching patterns within disease categories to be measured. These data are used to determine the cost and outcome implications of new treatments and formulary changes, as well as for monitoring disease management programs. Data are formatted in rows of transactions each time a service is provided to a patient. The medical claims data may outline claims related to hospitalization, procedures, diagnostic tests, use of medical facilities, and visits to clinics or emergency rooms. The pharmacy claims data outline each prescription date written, date filled, drug, dose, patient information, prescribing physician, ingredient cost, amount paid, and copayment for plans in which the patient pays a portion of the total prescription fee.

Member eligibility data pertain to the patient's enrollment history, benefit plan and code, employer, primary-care provider, and personal data such as address, telephone number, gender, dependents in the household, and social security number.

The provider information includes multiple physician identifiers such as state license numbers, drug enforcement administration (DEA) numbers, and federal tax identification numbers as well as physician demographic information.

Table 119-3. Care Map Template: Deep Vein Thrombosis

			Patient Presents with Signs and Determine risk of complications and	
	LOW RISK: OUTPATIENT DIAGNOSIS, MANAGEMENT AND TREATMENT			
DOMAIN OF CARE	PRE-ADMISSION	DAY 1	DAY 5 TO GOAL INR	GOAL INR TO END OF TREATMENT
Outcomes	Prepare to send the patient home and arrange follow-up	Confirm diagnosis	Attain therapeutic INR. Swelling and discomfort alleviated.	INRs Q2 week, then monthly
Level of Care	Moderate	Minimal	None	None
Patient Education	Discuss possible diagnosis and OPD management.	Discuss doppler results and duration of LMWH. Dietary and warfarin drug interaction counseling. Training for LMWH self-injection.	Duration of oral anticoagulation.	Reinforce dietary and drug interactions
Activity Level Discharge Planning	As tolerated Identify insurance coverage for LMWH and Home Health Care	As tolerated Confirm that patient has necessary resources for OPD management. Triage to anticoagulation clinic.	As tolerated None	As tolerated None
Medications	LMWH admin: _____	Continue LMWH for 5 days or until INR at goal. Administer first dose of warfarin. Time warf: _____	Adjust warfarin dose daily in response to INR. Continue LMWH.	Warfarin to Goal INR
Nutrition	Regular oral diet	Regular oral diet. Counsel food interactions	Regular oral diet. Reinforce food interactions.	Regular oral diet. Reinforce food interactions.
Elimination	Stool softeners ordered as needed.	Normal elimination	Normal elimination	Normal elimination
Diagnostics/ Procedures	Schedule venous doppler for next day (Day 1). Appoint time: _____	Perform doppler. Baseline LFTs, CBC, INR.	INR	INR
Treatments	Recommend leg elevation for next 12–24 hours.	None	None	None

There are many limitations to health care databases. Services not covered by the health plan may be omitted, coding errors can and do occur, and specific information about disease severity is not available, thus requiring chart review or other patient-specific inquiries to evaluate true efficacy. Because of these limitations, many health systems have developed additional, more specific and probing reporting systems to key into areas of focus. A summary of sample pharmacy-related reports for a large integrated health system is outlined in Table 119-5.

The reports in Table 119-5 are reviewed by pharmacists and used to educate prescribers about their drug use. Opportunities are identified to reduce drug costs and increase formulary compliance and quality, using methods referred to as counter detailing. Large databases are useful for describing patient, provider, and disease characteristics and estimating the implications of a change in the formulary; measuring the effects of treatment guidelines; and monitoring disease management programs.

Data and measurement are an important part of the role that pharmacists play in integrated health systems, not only because of access to necessary data, but also because of understanding of the relationships between the data and patient, provider, or health system. Colleagues ask pharmacists to evaluate how drugs are being used and to assist them in interpreting data to identify opportunities to change prescribing guidelines, modify a care map or disease management program, and assess overall compliance with system guidelines.

DOCUMENTATION—"If it isn't documented, it didn't happen." In every role within health systems including primary care, acute care, long-term care, and home care, pharmacists need to document their activities, findings, interventions, and outcomes of interventions. There are regulatory, ethical, and communication-mandated reasons for documentation. Documentation may be as simple as jotting a note to a physician to remind him or her to change the dose of a drug at the patient's next visit or be a formal summary of a drug-therapy plan in a patient's chart. Much documentation is now electronic.

Pharmacy order entry systems allow for free text entry to note specific information regarding a patient or prescription, such as allergy, brand preference, characteristics, or name clarifications. However, most pharmacy order entry systems fall short of facilitating complete documentation of the provision of care or advice to a patient, patient's family, provider, or other health professional. Pharmacy departments often design their own systems to capture the activities and ensure that employee productivity can be measured and strategic decisions about deployment of personnel and development of new services can occur. In fee-for-service environments, documentation systems are used to generate bills for reimbursement of services. Docu-

Symptoms Consistent with DVT

underlying conditions

| | HIGH RISK: ADMIT FOR DIAGNOSIS, INITIAL MANAGEMENT AND TREATMENT | | | |
PRE-ADMISSION	DAY 1	DAY 2-GOAL INR	DISCHARGE	DISCHARGE TO END OF TREATMENT
Admission, diagnostics, drugs within 1 hr; Time to ER: _____ Time of Admiss: _____	Ambulation; Maintain therapeutic APTT; Initiate warfarin; APTT: ___; Time war:___	Maintain therapeutic APTT until INR therapeutic.	Educated patient at INR goal without DVT symptoms.	Maintain goal INR
High	Moderate	Moderate	None	None
Orientation to the unit and disease process and diagnostics	Drugs and monitoring tests. Teaching done: _____	Reinforce risk of bleeding, frequency of monitoring on warfarin. Post-test score:_____	Reinforce risk of bleeding and anticoagulation clinic process.	Reinforce dietary and drug interactions
Restricted	As tolerated once APTT at goal.	As tolerated	As tolerated	As tolerated
Identify insurance and living environment	Provision for home care as needed. Disposition:_____	Triage to anticoagulation clinic for OPD follow-up.	Plan for discharge medications and family pick-up.	None
I.V. heparin protocol. Target APTT 1.5 – 2.5 x control within 16 hr; Time Heparin: _____	I.V. heparin per protocol. P.O. warfarin per protocol. Goal INR: 2–3	I.V. heparin per protocol. P.O. warfarin per protocol. Goal INR: 2–3	Warfarin Rx written and filled.	Warfarin to goal INR
Regular diet ordered & initiated	Regular oral diet. Counsel food interactions	Regular oral diet. Reinforce food interactions.	Regular oral diet. Reinforce food interactions.	Reinforce dietary and drug interactions
Evaluated and stool softeners ordered as needed	Normal elimination	Normal elimination	Normal elimination	Normal elimination
Venous doppler within 6 hours. Doppler: ___	Monitor for signs of PE; VQ scan or angiogram if indicated	INR	INR	INR
Leg elevated until heparin APTT therapeutic	Upper body exercises	None	None	None

mentation is an important part of every practicing pharmacist's activities. Each of the following aspects should be documented for every intervention:

1. The nature of the pharmacist intervention (eg, prescribing error, prescribing omission, drug-therapy monitoring, or drug interaction);
2. What service the pharmacist performed;
3. The outcome of the intervention; and
4. What drugs were involved in the intervention.

Most pharmacists in primary-care settings are actively identifying, preventing, resolving, and documenting adverse drug reactions. Documentation involves system-specific reporting mechanisms, such as to a quality committee, and then the use of the FDA's MedWatch form for serious adverse drug or device reactions. In particular, the FDA is interested in drugs and devices that have been released within the last 24 months and those associated with therapeutic interchange programs.

Table 119-6 summarizes activities performed by primary-care pharmacists in the US and their frequency, based on type of integrated health system practice. Most of the activities listed in Table 119-6 have been discussed or are covered under

System Supportive Roles for Patient Care. Academic detailing, or counter detailing, is a common function in managed-care settings of integrated health systems as a means to educate prescribers about system-wide formulary drugs and approved guidelines.

Pharmacists are trained to make appointments with physicians to review new drug guidelines and formulary additions. They emphasize the proper use, dosing, and supportive data, much as a pharmaceutical company representative would for a new drug. More importantly, health system pharmacists discuss drugs that are not on formulary and patterns of drug use that are inconsistent with system guidelines, to seek conformance of practice. Counter detailing, used in conjunction with prescribers' profiles or report cards, are effective methods to drive drug use toward system-chosen options.

Acute Care

The term *acute care* embraces the hospitalization phase of health and disease. It represents a very short time and small

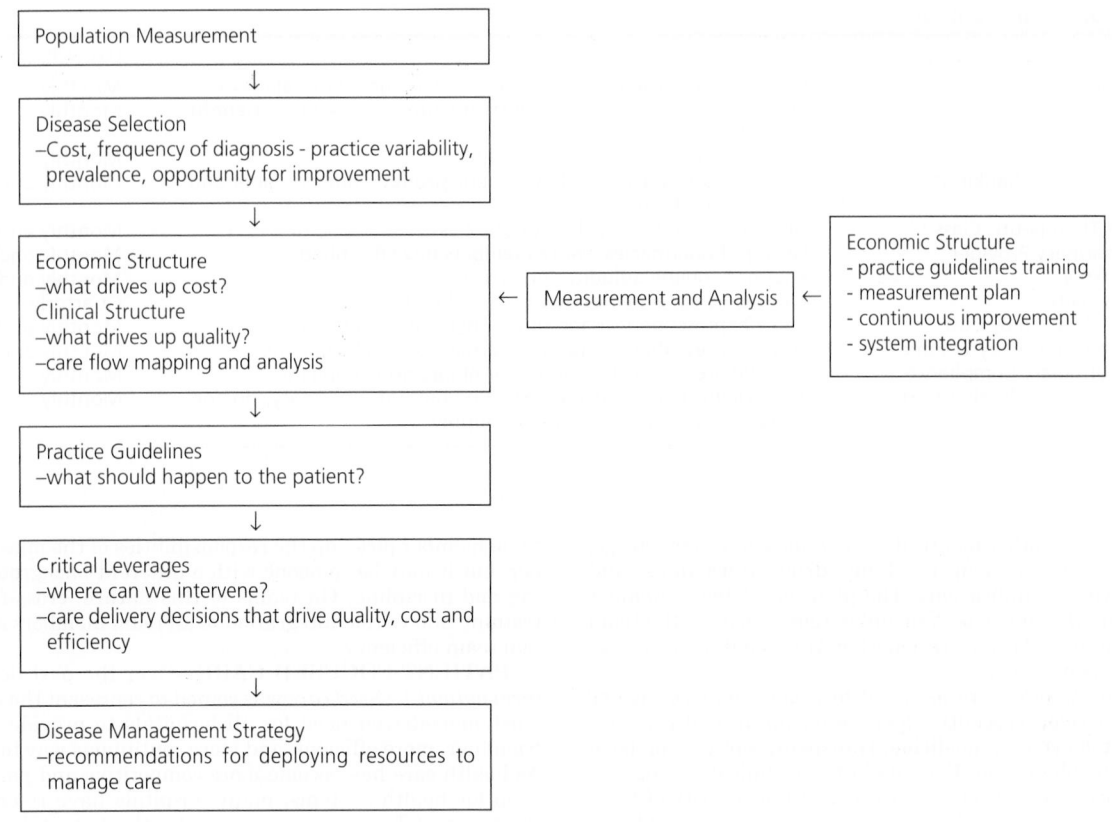

Figure 119-1. Disease management.

component of the total spectrum of health care management for most people. The goals of integrated health systems and managed-care organizations are to optimize health and wellness programs to minimize the number of occasions people need acute care. Acute-care needs may arise at any time from birth to death, but generally are concentrated toward the end of life. High costs result from hospitalizations and use of specialized services and technology. Therefore, the impetus is on disease prevention and health promotion to keep people out of the hospital. In integrated health systems, costs are shifted from inpatient (acute care) to outpatient (primary care) to manage patients in their homes and community settings.

Although the acute-care, or hospital, component of most integrated systems is being decreased to control costs, it remains

Table 119-4. Asthma Management

Educate the Patient
- Proper use of inhalers, and peak flow meters
- Drug information

Assess and Monitor Disease Severity
- Discuss symptoms and monitoring of symptoms

Avoid or Control Precipitating Factors
- Advocacy to limit allergen exposure

Establish Medication Plans for Chronic Management
- Review medication plan with team to optimize drug therapy

Establish plans for Monitoring Exacerbations
- Outline steps for caregiver and patient to take when exacerbations occur

Provide Regular Follow-up Care
- Participate in follow-up visits to reinforce drug therapy principles

the most sophisticated clinical segment of any health care system and cares for patients during the most acutely ill phases of their lives. Likewise, the sophistication of acute-care pharmacy services is high, with significant areas of expertise and specialization in both the distributive and the clinical roles assumed by pharmacists.

MULTIDISCIPLINARY TEAMS—As in primary care, the process of care delivery in acute-care settings is often organized around teams of providers, which may consist of nurses, physicians, respiratory therapists, and pharmacists. Whereas centralized pharmacy or decentralized pharmacy satellites provide unit-dose intravenous and oral medications to patients, clinical pharmacists are redeployed from these operational areas to serve as members of multidisciplinary-care teams. Pharmacists may be assigned to teams based on therapeutic focus, geographical proximity, or service-alignment and serve important roles to ensure that quality pharmaceutical care is achieved. While they may enter or verify the entry of drug orders into the computer, they typically do not distribute, admix, or dispense drugs. The distributive functions are generally performed centrally and supported by automated devices and technical support staff.

Clinical acute-care pharmacists have evolved into roles that have been shown to contribute significantly to the overall quality of the care delivered to hospitalized patients. The major focus of care, independent of the therapeutic focus area, is to ensure that optimal pharmaceutical care is delivered. Pharmacists are held accountable by their team and pharmacy administration to ensure that the drugs are given responsibly for the purpose of achieving a definite outcome that will improve the patient's quality of life, cure disease, eliminate symptoms, slow disease progress, or prevent disease.[9]

Pharmacists work proactively with their health care team to identify, solve, prevent, and document drug-related problems. Drug-related problems include untreated indications, improper

Table 119-5. Database Reports

REPORT NAME	REPORT DESCRIPTION	FREQUENCY OF REPORTING
MAC Savings	Maximum allowable cost vs. HCFA vs. average wholesale price	Monthly
Member Utilization	Top 100 members with highest utilization ranked by benefit value	Monthly
Brand Generic	Generic utilization summary by clinic	Monthly
Drug Usage Product Ranking*	Top 2000 drugs dispensed by generic product index number and total ingredient cost	Monthly and quarterly
Drug Usage Therapeutic Class	Drug usage ranked by therapeutic class	Monthly and quarterly
Financial Pharmacy Provider	Listing of pharmacies where members have Rxs filled	Monthly and quarterly
Pharmacy Errors	Pharmacy online adjudication errors	Monthly and quarterly
Prescriber Activity	Prescribers' Rx activities by DEA # and # of members	Quarterly
Prescriber Utilization by Cost	Top 200 prescribers' usage of pharmaceuticals by cost	Monthly and quarterly
Prescriber Utilization* by Volume	Top 200 prescribers' usage of pharmaceuticals by volume	Monthly and quarterly
Prescriber Formulary Compliance	Top 200 prescribers ranked by formulary noncompliance	Monthly
Prescriber Detail by Member Cost of Claims*	Total claims paid exceeding $500 by patient, pharmacy, doctor, drug name, quantity and days supply	Monthly

drug selection, subtherapeutic dosage, failure to receive drugs, overdosage, adverse drug reactions, drug interactions, and drug use without indications. The pharmacist team member has the drug-therapy expertise and is relied upon by the team for information and collaboration when treatment plans are being made and modified.

Pharmacists often are assigned to a particular service or team and develop specialty expertise for an area of practice, such as intensive-care medicine, transplant surgery, or bone marrow transplantation. Patients in these clinical settings require intense, specialized care because of the severity of their illness. Pharmacists on these teams are often responsible for writing drug and nutrition orders and monitoring the patients continuously during their acute phase. In this team structure, pharmacists may cover for each other when one is scheduled off, but the service coverage is continuous.

Other predominant roles for hospital pharmacists have included alignment with a service that cares for only one aspect of the patients' needs during their hospitalization. Teams such as the nutrition or pain team focus on a narrow aspect of the patient needs, while the primary team provides the overall patient care. On these teams, nurses, pharmacists, dietitians, or physician's assistants may have interchangeable roles that complement each other. When one is scheduled off, another team member picks up the responsibilities of the missing member, but it may be someone with a different background training and discipline. On teams of this nature, cross-functional training allows role integration of all team members and maximal team efficiency.

PATIENT-FOCUSED CARE—Over the past decade, the term *patient-focused care* was coined to represent the consumer (customer)-driven need for all hospitals to provide care in a friendlier, more efficient, and more continuous way to patients. As health care has become more competitive and patients can shop for health systems, many hospitals have re-engineered their care-delivery process to make the hospital stay more pleasant for the patients and easier for the staff. The goal of patient-focused care is to provide high-quality, compassionate, and cost-effective care to patients and improve customer satisfaction. The goal is accomplished through bringing the services to the bedside of the patient rather than taking the patient off the unit to other services.

A common theme of the patient-focused care model involves the use of small interdisciplinary teams responsible for continuity of care of the patient from admission to discharge. A key component of patient-focused care is the creation of multi-skilled teams of individuals who share responsibility and expertise in providing care and making care decisions at the bed-

Table 119-6. Percentage of Ambulatory Pharmacists Performing Function by Health-System Type

FUNCTION	STAFF OR GROUP HMO	IPA	HOSPITAL-BASED	PHYSICIAN-BASED
Make pharmaceutical decisions for large populations	55	67	37	46
Monitor patient outcomes	80	74	68	62
Monitor medication compliance	93	77	75	76
Conduct wellness and prevention programs	63	61	57	56
Conduct specialized clinics	46	28	36	29
Track adverse drug reactions	98	66	89	82
Prepare home infusion medications	43	26	50	41
Use pharmacoeconomic data for formulary decision-making	73	86	70	79
Provide written information with each new Rx	87	53	83	82
Provide oral counseling with each new Rx	88	54	84	79
Collect HEDIS* Data	69	71	24	18
Provide physician profiles or report cards	71	76	38	47
Design pharmacy benefits	61	71	26	41
Negotiate pharmaceutical contracts	61	57	44	50
Write medication orders	22	15	50	41
Conduct medication management programs (DUE)	90	74	76	71
Have prescribing authority	20	6	20	12
Conduct academic detailing	65	69	44	56

* HEDIS = Health Plan Employer Data and Information Set.

side. The patient's exposure is maximized to a smaller number of caretakers, and the number of care steps is minimized to reduce fragmentation of services. Care partners are cross-trained to draw blood, perform x-rays, change and bathe patients, and assist the nurse in other patient-related activities. The pharmacist, nurse, and physician collaborate to formulate drug-therapy plans, diagnostic testing, follow-up, and endpoints. Much of the care is directed by care maps and monitored by flow charts in each patient's room. Patient-focused care is an operational restructuring that centers on the patient as opposed to the current emphasis on departments and caregivers.

A 2000 survey, published by Raehl and Bond, revealed that 26% of US hospital pharmacy departments were operating in a predominant patient-focused system, with traditional departments remaining as core (ie, smaller, flatter) structures.[10] The survey demonstrated that pharmacists were involved in providing direct patient care in 85% of the hospitals operating in a patient-focused model, and pharmacy personnel almost always reported through traditional pharmacy department channels.

In some patient-focused care implementation projects, pharmacy roles and responsibilities were significantly expanded to include obtaining a complete medication history, assisting in the development of drug treatment plans, implementing drug-therapy plans, assisting in evaluating and modifying drug therapy, educating patients throughout their hospital stay about their drug therapy, preparing patients for discharge, and follow-up by telephone after discharge. A small decentralized pharmacy was located on each patient care unit. First doses and urgently needed medications were prepared by a technician and checked by the patient-focused care pharmacist before they are given to the patient with the remaining doses are prepared centrally and redistributed to the patient-focused care unit on a 24-hour schedule. Expanded responsibilities led to increased numbers of pharmacists and pharmacy technicians required to perform the defined work.

Although data have shown that patients on patient-focused care units have shorter average hospital stays, have fewer follow-up emergency room visits and are readmitted less often than control patients, severe economic pressures and workforce shortages have forced the dissolution of patient-focused care models in some cases. This has been due primarily to the unfavorable reimbursement environment in health care, the labor intense nature of the patient-focused care model as well inefficiencies and the inability to realize anticipated savings resulting from decentralization of care processes.

PROTOCOL-DRIVEN CARE—The opportunity for variance in practice exists in the hospital as it does in the primary-care setting. Guidelines, protocols, and decision algorithms have been in use in hospitals for many years to attempt to improve the consistency of care, reduce the likelihood of errors, and reduce costs. Care maps that outline care steps from admission to discharge are in place for all facets of care in most hospitals. Care maps can be a helpful bridge between the acute-care and primary-care settings.

The pharmacist's role in acute-care protocols can be quite extensive. In the inpatient treatment arm of the deep vein thrombosis care map shown in Table 119-3, the pharmacist takes a complete medication history, works collaboratively with the team to initiate and optimize heparin therapy, educates the patient daily about various aspects of heparin and warfarin therapy, ensures early initiation of warfarin therapy with a sufficient heparin overlap period, and performs discharge medication counseling and follow-up with the patient's local pharmacy. In each step, the pharmacist, just like other team members, documents the outcomes she/he is responsible for achieving, on the care map.

Protocol-driven care facilitates drug-therapy decisions within a range of acceptable choices predicted to include 90% of patient situations. For example, the deep vein thrombosis protocol denotes starting and maintenance dosing of heparin, the frequency of APTT monitoring, and suggested dosing adjustments in response to resultant APTT values. With this infor-

mation and their professional training and background, pharmacists can make dosing and monitoring adjustments without necessarily consulting with the rest of the team. Protocol-driven prescribing is effective because the protocols are developed in advance for noncontroversial treatments, within which clear-cut decisions can be made.

When patients deviate from the range of choices outlined in the protocol, the team reassembles to discuss alternative treatment choices and designs a new plan to get the patient back on course. Protocols do not cover all possible clinical situations, but are designed to provide a framework of care for most situations that arise. Protocol-driven prescribing allows autonomy of choice within a range of acceptable choices outlined in the protocol but prevents aberrant decisions that may jeopardize patient care.[7]

In large integrated health systems, the opportunity exists to make the transition from inpatient (acute care) to outpatient (primary care) as seamless as possible. The patient should not experience an interruption in the way care is delivered or the level of knowledge and sophistication of the team members at each phase of care. To provide seamless care, sophisticated technology and information systems are needed to share medical and drug information through the transition. Corporate alignment of the financial and reporting structures of individuals in acute-care and primary-care environments is necessary to facilitate smooth patient transition. Successful integration is difficult to achieve, even in the most highly developed health systems, because of the magnitude and complexity of the components.

COST-JUSTIFICATION Documentation is an essential component of the pharmacist's responsibilities in the acute phase of care. Through years of careful documentation of the impact of pharmacy services on overall care of patients, it has been shown that care is improved and costs are reduced. For every dollar spent on pharmacists, anywhere from 1.7 to 17 times that much money is saved in drug-therapy-related expenses.[6] Documentation allows effective communication between services, teams, and health care providers. Documentation provides a mechanism to create optimal staffing patterns for patients of different acuity of illness and therapeutic focus. Through documentation, pharmacists can verify the impact they have for promotion, annual performance review, and internal recognition.

Many approaches have been taken to document acute-care pharmacy services. Both manual and automated systems exist that summarize problems identified, interventions taken, and outcomes associated with the interventions. In most cases, the problems and interventions relate to the drug-related problems described by pharmaceutical care. However, in certain areas of practice, pharmacists have developed extended patient-care roles and may be administering medications or performing procedures. Pharmacists may have a role in research protocols that must be documented in the patient's medical record and the research records. Pharmacists routinely leave notes in patients' charts and care maps and consult notes, and many are involved in writing drug orders. Each of these mechanisms is important documentation of care rendered. Documentation is critical in all facets of pharmacy practice.

Long-Term, Hospice, and Home Care

Home care is the provision of resources for medical care in the patient's home. Services include skilled nursing care, intravenous medications and nutrition, physical and occupational therapy, rehabilitation care, and respiratory care. Pharmacists work with home care nurses to streamline drug therapy and minimize the risk of drug-related problems. Hospice care is any comprehensive program that provides specialized care to terminally ill patients. Hospice programs offer medical, sociological, and psychological services to patients in the institutional and home setting. Long-term care's goal is to help people with disabilities be as independent as possible; thus it is focused more on caring than on curing. Long-term care provides assistance and care for persons with chronic disabilities and is needed by persons who require help with the activities of daily living or who suffer from cognitive impairment. Long-term care is not limited to the elderly, but the need for long-term care is more prevalent in the elderly. Pharmacists provide dispensing and clinical services to hospice and long-term care facilities. Given that medication safety is of great concern in elderly and compromised patients, drug therapy should be evaluated carefully to assure that the fewest possible drugs at the lowest effective doses are used.

Integrated health systems usually offer these areas of care to patients, as well as primary and acute care. Home care is becoming increasingly important to facilitate the transfer from acute care back to the home and primary-care setting. Pharmacists have important roles in all three care phases, as drug therapy is usually involved. Table 119-7 summarizes predominant pharmacy roles in home care, hospice, and long-term care settings.

Education

The role that pharmacists have in educating patients, physicians, and other health care workers in health systems is so important that it warrants separate mention. The educational role spans all facets of practice in integrated systems.

PATIENTS—Many physicians leave patient's drug education to the pharmacist, as their direct contact time with patients is limited increasingly by the need to enhance productivity. The pharmacist is the patients' last professional contact before they take a medication and has the opportunity and responsibility to safeguard the patients' health and to help ensure the success of the drug therapy. In the past, pressure to educate patients came from the federal government via the Omnibus Budget Reconciliation Act of 1990 (OBRA 90) and FDA Guidelines. Now, patients demand information about the safe and effective use of their medications. It is desirable for pharmacists to provide credible, accurate information rather than allowing the patient to default to easily available and potentially suspect drug information available through the Internet.

The simplest form of patient education is counseling at the time of dispensing the prescription. At minimum patients should know how to take their medicine, how often, how much, what to do if a dose is missed, what side effects to watch for, food and drug interactions of significance, and how to store the medication. Consumers are being told that the pharmacist should answer questions about prescription and over-the-counter products, that they will discuss drug-therapy concerns privately with the patient that pharmacy systems screen for potentially serious drug interactions and that pharmacy prices should be reasonably competitive. While written materials can supplement the oral personal communication between the pharmacist and patient, they should not substitute for one-on-one interaction. Only through probing and the use of open-ended questions can pharmacists determine true patient understanding about their medications and reinforce important concepts.

Nonadherence to prescription medications has been estimated to cost $50 billion in the US annually, with another $50 billion in indirect costs, such as lost productivity and time lost from work or school. Pharmacist counseling has been shown to improve adherence to medications. Six important factors in ensuring patient compliance to drug therapy are stage of therapy, literacy level, age, cultural and language issues, gender, and readiness to comply. When filling first prescriptions or for newly diagnosed patients is the best time to ask the three "prime", important questions:

What did your doctor tell you this medicine is for?
How did he or she tell you to take the medication?
What did the doctor tell you to expect the medication?

For patients who have been taking the same medication for years, it is simple to reinforce compliance and elicit any problems the patient may have been having with their drug therapy.

A second important factor is the literacy level of the patient. As many as 40 million American adults are functionally illiterate, and 50 million more are marginally literate. There are several age-related factors that affect medication compliance. Children need to be supervised by their parents when taking medications, teenagers need to understand the importance of proper use, middle- and older-age patients may have special communications needs and consume a higher proportion of medications in society. Increased age is associated with memory problems, hearing and physical impairments, and comprehension issues, all of which can interfere with medication compliance.

Patients from different cultural backgrounds may have different perceptions about health care, and language barriers further compound the conveyance of clear concise directions about medications. Lastly, gender and readiness to comply are inherent characteristics that pharmacists must assess before developing an approach to communicating with patients.

Once information about these six important factors affecting medication compliance is known, pharmacists are prepared to counsel patients effectively about their medication. These six factors pertain to all pharmacy practice settings within integrated systems. Whether in a clinic pharmacy, inpatient, or home setting, the pharmacist should seek a quiet, private area where the patient can be seated comfortably (or lie down if still infirm). Patients must be comfortable to be prepared to receive information and ask questions or they will not listen, go elsewhere for information, or fail to comply.

Pharmacists participate in a wide variety of patient educational experiences other than counseling at the time of dispensing. Brown bag lunches are used when the patients bring in their medication and pharmacists discuss what the drugs are and how they are used and answer questions patients may have about their drug therapy. Therapeutically focused workshops

Table 119-7. Home Care, Hospice Care, and Long-Term Care

FUNCTIONS	HOME CARE	HOSPICE CARE	LONG-TERM CARE
Intravenous admixture	X	X	X
Medication preparation and dispensing	X	X	X
Therapeutic drug monitoring	X		X
Drug therapy review	X	X	X
Dosing, monitoring and follow-up of medications and nutrition therapy	X		X
Tracking adverse drug reactions	X	X	X
Development of drug therapy protocols	X	X	X
Develop of team-based treatment plans	X	X	X
Drug use evaluation	X	X	X
Patient/family education	X	X	X
Protocol-driven prescribing	X	X	X
Communication liaison between acute care and primary care	X		

or lectures are offered to patients recovering from stroke, myocardial infarction, and other disabilities to offer information about drug therapy for these disorders. Large group sessions for recovering alcoholics, smokers, diabetics, asthmatics, and patients with other conditions are used to bring several health care professionals together and offer information to patients. Dietitians, pharmacists, nurses, and others lead discussions with patients and answer questions they have about their disease process, diet, and drugs. All of these formats in which pharmacists share information with patients help to establish the pharmacist as a trusted professional and reputable source of information.

Other important educational topics for patients who receive care in integrated health systems are to improve overall understanding about medication programs, benefits, formularies, and cost considerations. Physicians often are asked to prescribe drugs listed on a formulary of choices, to use generic alternatives whenever possible, and less expensive branded drugs when the health system is at risk for the cost of care delivered. Managed-care organizations employ therapeutic substitutions or switch programs to increase the use of *best-value* medications for their patients. Most patients have insufficient understanding about these processes and decisions and frequently label them managed-care *rip-offs* that cheapen health care. Proactive educational mailings, brochures, and discussions with patients often allay their concern that less-expensive drug choices are inferior. Seminars, use of the Internet, and video summaries of this information can be helpful adjunctive ways of conveying information to patients in this high-technology era of medicine.

Particularly useful tools for patient education are the telephone, fax machines, and electronic mail (e-mail). Patients really appreciate personal follow-up and inquiry regarding their medications. In many integrated systems in which pharmacists are truly and responsibly providing pharmaceutical care, follow-up telephone calls asking how the patient is doing, if he or she is having any problems with the medication or has any other questions are a service that greatly enhances customer satisfaction, loyalty, and compliance. A surprisingly large number of patients have access to fax machines and e-mail, which provides another electronic avenue for communication and follow-up without interfering with their day or inconveniencing the pharmacist.

PHYSICIANS AND OTHER HEALTH CARE WORKERS—Ongoing education to physicians and other health care workers allows a bond of learning, growth, and service to develop that is valued and deeply respected by other health-system colleagues. Physicians rely on pharmacists, other colleagues, and pharmaceutical representatives for most of their updates on new drugs and therapeutics. They attend professional meetings infrequently enough that this form of continuing education is of limited use. Unfortunately, the pharmaceutical industry has been very effective in scheduling visits and employing strategies to educate physicians about new drugs and motivate their use, even in instances where the new drug adds little value to available treatments. Pharmacists can be effective in conveying a balance between the drug company's marketing information and the medical literature and help to ensure that the information prescribers receive is consistent with health-system guidelines on drug use.

As a part of the health care team, pharmacists may be asked to convey information more formally, in lectures or journal clubs, to the prescribers and the rest of the team. Pharmacists benefit from honing their presentation skills (the ability to design and convey information effectively with limited time), in oral and written formats. Interpretation of the medical literature, biostatistical design, and trial methodologies are important features of providing drug information accurately and effectively.

Information to prescribers can take the form of newsletters, written guidelines, monographs, or electronic transmissions. All communication media should be explored to ensure maximal exposure for transmission of educational materials to prescribers and other health care professionals. As health professionals who subscribe to lifelong learning, pharmacists can contribute meaningfully to the education of other professionals and patients in their system.

SYSTEM SUPPORT FOR PATIENT CARE

Information Systems

One important asset in an integrated system is the information about patient health care usage and the cost of health care. Today this information is best stored, sorted, and analyzed through the use of computers. Medical informatics is an information science specialty that is defined as the use of a computer-assisted systems approach to obtain, process, store, retrieve, manipulate, analyze, and distribute data.[11] In an integrated system, the availability of data allows the information to be placed on a network that can be accessed by all providers in the system and further facilitate care across the continuum.

With system computer access a pharmacist in a satellite ambulatory site can access the patient's hospital records, get information regarding the nature of a drug reaction, and thus take action to avoid an allergic reaction. Computerization and information systems can be used to streamline medication dispensing, freeing the pharmacist for more involvement in providing patient care. Additionally, computers and information systems can assist pharmacists in the provision of cognitive services, as the rapid availability of current, accurate medical information is the basis for these services.

Network computers can facilitate communication with system employees. Workers can send e-mail to each other detailing specific encounters with patients. Frequently in integrated systems, employees are distributed over a large geographic area that limits communication between these providers of care over the continuum. Network e-mail provides an open line of communication between these workers and can lead to better working relationships. Managers can use mail lists to inform all employees quickly of procedural changes or other necessary information that can aid in the efficient provision of patient care. This electronic exchange of information allows faster and less cumbersome exchange of information.

In some cases the Internet may be used to provide access to system information. There is great concern regarding the use of the Internet as a conduit to supply patient and medical information because of the ability of unauthorized persons to access the information. Thus, information provided on the Internet by integrated systems is presented in three levels of complexity.

Some systems only maintain a Web page that provides general information about the system and the services provided. At the next level of complexity the system provides guidelines and policies in a password-protected area to limit access to authorized users. It is on this level that systems are most likely to provide information. The highest level of complexity also requires the highest level of security, as here access to patient medical information is available to authorized employees with passwords. It is becoming common for patients to have access to their own health page through secure sites that integrate appropriate medical, drug, and financial information. Given the raised conscientiousness regarding protected health information, health systems have improved confidentiality to assure compliance with HIPAA.

There are three types of databases that are used by pharmacists in an integrated system: administrative, bibliographic, and point-of-care.[12]

ADMINISTRATIVE DATABASES—Hospital and ambulatory pharmacies have used computers regularly for prescription order entry since the 1970s. These information systems were first developed to perform the administrative task of providing accurate billing for medication. The costs for these computer systems were offset by the capture of lost charges. In addition, the computers provided accurate labels and work lists for medication cart filling and IV admixture preparation. Reports that assess drug quantity use for inventory control can be generated with this information. From a clinical standpoint, early programs began providing patient profiles for pharmacists to review for drug interactions and allergies.

In the hospital setting, computer administrative databases can provide information about which agents are carried on the formulary. Similarly, in the ambulatory setting computer links can verify the insurance eligibility of the patient as well as identify formulary agents that are covered by the patient's insurance plan. In both settings, computer programs can be used in billing the insurance company for the drug costs. While pharmacy administrative databases developed separately in inpatient and ambulatory settings, the information available and the use of the computer hardware are similar.

While these computers are expensive, the economy of scale provided by the integrated system allows the large amount of capital needed to purchase this equipment. The volume of units dispensed in an integrated system also justifies the expenditure on the computerized equipment that can dispense medications for cost-efficiency while allowing the implementation of just-in-time inventory to control drug costs further. Besides controlling drug costs, these computerized systems can add efficiency and accuracy to work performed by caregivers, further improving the quality of the health care services provided by the integrated system.

Administrative databases also can be used by pharmacists for medication use review. Through the use of prescription data, reports can be run that identify prescribing patterns of physicians. This information can be used to determine if the physician is adhering to formulary or to practice prescribing recommendations, and proper follow-up education can take place. In some integrated health systems, an individual physician's compensation may be tied to the adherence to formulary or guidelines.

Administrative databases can be used to identify patients needing specific interventions. For example, pharmacists may feel there is a need for additional counseling of patients with hyperlipidemia. To locate these patients, the pharmacy database can be queried to identify all patients taking an anti-hyperlipidemic agent. This query may identify more patients than one pharmacist can counsel in a reasonable amount of time. The pharmacist may further choose to work with only the patients taking these agents who have coronary heart disease. These patients can be identified by crossing the prescription database information with a diagnostic code. As the pharmacist only wishes to work with the patients who have not reached goal values, the identified lipid test results can be extracted from the system's laboratory database. The pharmacist has identified the system's patients who will be best served by the pharmaceutical intervention through the use of database queries.

BIBLIOGRAPHIC DATABASES—Bibliographic databases provide pharmacists with easy access to medical information that previously required a trip to a medical library and hours of exhausting searching. By placing these databases on the system's network, pharmacists and other caregivers can access this information at their particular site. MEDLINE and International Pharmaceutical Abstracts are examples of databases that track the biomedical literature. There is an assortment of similar databases available to search specific areas of interest, which include allied health care journals.

The literature citations found through the database searches can serve to support clinical decision-making for individual patients as well as the development of treatment guidelines for the integrated delivery system.

POINT-OF-CARE DATABASES—Point-of-care databases provide clinical decision support at the patient's bedside or in the clinic setting and can be useful tools for pharmacists providing pharmaceutical care. These databases use information derived from administrative databases, bibliographic databases, and official FDA labeling. Clinical screening databases and references databases are the two types of point-of-care databases that pharmacists find useful.

The clinical screening databases are used to screen for drug-related problems such as drug interactions and allergy contraindications. For example, the patient's administrative data may contain information indicating the presence of a penicillin allergy. With the link to the clinical screening database, when an order for penicillin is entered on this patient, a flag will appear alerting the pharmacist to the problem and will not permit dispensing of the penicillin without further action by the pharmacist. At this point, the cognitive function of the pharmacist is activated, as the problem must be investigated and needs decisions by the pharmacist to verify the allergy and discuss an alternate drug choice with the physician. The same scenario would take place if the clinical screening database identified a drug interaction. Clinical screening databases can aid in the direction of pharmacist interventions.

The earliest reference database was Micromedex, which provides an assortment of drug and poison control information in database form. Other reference databases are electronic versions of commonly used pharmacy reference books, such as the *American Hospital Formulary Service, Facts and Comparisons,* and *USP Drug Information.*

There are several advantages to common databases. All system caregivers have access to the same information, which can be updated at one central location in a timely manner with placement of the database on the network. With published information, updates are usually only available once a year, and the work required to distribute a large number of books through a system can be cumbersome. Thus, the process of disseminating information is improved through computerization. Databases allow quick retrieval of the needed information through the use of search engines, thus allowing a decision to be made quickly at the point-of-care. It is important to note that patient information is also available in several of these databases. Network availability of patient instruction sheets allows all caregivers access to the same teaching tools, so the information given to patients will be common wherever they are seen in the system.

THE MEDICAL RECORD—As the integrated health care system is the keeper of all data associated with the care of the patient, the use of computerized patient medical records on the system's network makes this information readily accessible to caregivers across the system. Previously, patient's paper charts were delivered from site to site as the patient was seen as an inpatient and in the outpatient clinic. The paper method requires time and resources to transport patient information, and often the chart and the patient are not in the same place at the same time. Without valuable historic care information, the clinician is forced to provide care based on limited information, thus sometimes providing fragmented care. With the use of computerized, networked medical records, an integrated system can deliver seamless, efficient care.

Further efficiencies can be realized in an integrated system, as all data developed using different information systems can be organized in one location. For example, the laboratory and pharmacy databases can be programmed to dump their data directly into the medical record's database, eliminating the need to access a different computer system or different software to gain access to test results and prescription information. Pharmacists can enter notes in the medical record about pharmaceutical care provided to the patient, so that physicians and other caregivers can review these valuable activities.

COMPUTERIZATION—As an integrated system is the provider of *seamless* health care, information systems provide the backbone to this provision of care. By the virtue that information of all types is available on patients for caregivers to use, the expense of network computerization is required to use this data efficiently in providing patient care. It is important for pharmacists to be involved with the development and use of information systems in the integrated system. Computerization and automated dispensing systems can be used for accurate dispensing of medication. With dispensing tasks provided by technology, the pharmacist can use information in the decision-making functions required to provide pharmaceutical care.

INTEGRATION OF TECHNOLOGY AND AUTOMATION INTO PRACTICE

As technology and automation continue to be increasingly used in health care and other industries, so has the responsibility of pharmacists to understand and integrate these systems into their practice. When used appropriately, automation and information technology can be powerful tools in integrating and managing data, increasing quality and efficiency and assuring safety while helping contain costs. In addition to incorporating automation and information technology into individual practice areas such as inpatient and ambulatory pharmacy practices, integrated health systems face the additional challenge of assuring that these technologies complement practice in all areas and assist in the provision of seamless care throughout the continuum.

In the inpatient acute care environment, several types of automation are employed for medication dispensing and compounding. Automated medication dispensing cabinets (eg, SurMed, others) are frequently employed to make many medications available on the patient care unit while offering a degree of medication control. Some institutions use these devices for dispensing controlled substances or floor stock medications only, while others use them for up to 90% of all first doses dispensed. Ideally, these devices communicate with the pharmacy information management system via an interface so that all orders may be reviewed and approved by a pharmacist prior to being removed by a nurse for administration to a patient. The main advantage of these cabinets is that medications are immediately available on the patient care unit and medication charge capture and inventory record keeping is enhanced. They also improve the accountability of controlled substances. These advantages must be balanced against the increased potential for medication errors to occur, the need to maintain several locations for medication inventories, the workload associated with maintaining and stocking the cabinets as well as the impact on nursing workload. Although these devices allow access to the medication more quickly, they may actually require the nurse to do more work as he or she must spend time accessing the machine for each dose. This can be especially problematic if insufficient numbers of cabinets are available in each area, requiring the nurse to travel significant distances to retrieve medications.

Some pharmacists believe that automated medication dispensing devices should be used only in conjunction with Point-of-Care medication administration error prevention (eg, Bridge Drug Management System, Acu-Scan Rx) systems. Point-of-Care systems employ palm-size devices that provide the nurse with real-time access to the patient's medication profile and/or medication administration record. Through the use of barcode technology, the system assists the caregiver in verifying that the right drug is given in the right dose to the right patient at the right time. With this system, the nurse scans the barcode on the medication as well as the barcode on the patient's wristband. Using a radio frequency telecommunications network, the hand held device communicates with the pharmacy computer system to verify the dose to be administered against the patient's medication profile and allergies. Once verification takes place, the nurse administers the medication and uses the hand held device to record that the dose has been administered. One of the major hurdles to implementation of Point-of-Care technology is that not all medications are bar coded and no standard symbology for bar coding of drugs has been adopted. In addition, radio frequency

networks are not yet installed in many hospitals. Once these problems have been sufficiently addressed, the use of Point of Care error prevention systems are likely to gain more widespread use and allow the increased use of automated dispensing cabinets.

Another widely used automated methodology in the inpatient environment is the use of robotics for packaging and dispensing of unit-dose medications and total parenteral nutrition (TPN) solutions. Robot Rx and the ATC Profile are examples of machines employed in central pharmacy environments. The Robot Rx has the capability of packaging and bar coding of medications, dispensing first doses, filling unit dose medication carts as well as handling medication returns and removing outdated inventory. It also is capable of preparing supplies of medications for restocking of automated dispensing cabinets. Disadvantages of this system include large space requirements and the "double-packaging" medications to assure that a bar code is affixed. The ATC profile is capable of packaging and bar coding of medications in patient-specific single or multiple dose strips, which are easy for the nurse to find and identify. This machine is used primarily to increase the efficiency of unit dose cart filling, although the potential for first dose dispensing exists. The main disadvantage of the ATC profile is the large number of medication returns that must be put away manually.

Many inpatient pharmacy areas employ automation for preparation or IV solutions or TPN solutions. These systems allow mass production of TPN base solutions and are also capable or adding electrolytes and other additives. These systems reduce the amount of technician time required to prepare solutions and reduce the amount of pharmacist time required for checking of final products. The cost-effectiveness of such devices depends on the number of TPN solutions prepared by any given institution.

One of the most exciting forms of technology now beginning to be employed by inpatient clinical pharmacists is the use of clinical decision support algorithms for drug therapy monitoring. Through the integration of databases such as the patient's medication profile, lab information, and demographic data, users are able to create "rules" which identify drug therapy-related problems. An example would include identification of a patient on a drug such as cefotetan (which interferes with production of carboxylated clotting factor) whose INR becomes elevated. Violation of this "rule" results in a clinical alert, which appears on the pharmacy computer system, notifying the clinical pharmacist that intervention may be warranted. This system has the potential to reduce dramatically the amount of time a clinical pharmacist spends manually reviewing databases and patient profiles to identify actual or potential problems, and allows pharmacists to spend more time making actual interventions. Ideally, the same system utilized to identify drug-related problems is also used to document and tabulate pharmacist interventions, resulting in further efficiency gains.

Automation and other technologies are also employed in the ambulatory setting of integrated health systems. Automation in ambulatory pharmacies range from systems designed to count tablets and capsules to nearly full automation of the dispensing process. Some systems offer visual imaging to assist the pharmacist in verifying the accuracy of the filling process while other systems employ bar code technology to verify the NDC barcode on the labeled package matches the NDC on the manufacturer's package. These features reduce the possibility of a product picking error from reaching the patient.

Technology is available that allows dispensing of prescriptions within medical clinics or physician offices. Some systems allow physicians to transmit medication orders electronically to a pharmacy, where the pharmacist enters the information into the patients medication profile, then electronically activates an automated dispensing machine located in the medical clinic or physician's office, which results in the dispensing of prepackaged and labeled prescriptions which are then provided to the patient by the physician or his representative. The person dispensing the prescription scans a barcode on the dispensed product, which allows verification that the correct drug has been dispensed. Other systems bypass the pharmacist altogether and allow the physician to dispense pre-packaged, prelabeled, bar-coded medications directly to the patient. These systems also allow the physician to adjudicate claims with the patient's third party payer. A drawback to the above systems includes the requirement to fill relatively large numbers of prescriptions to cost-justify the technology. Also, because not all drugs are stocked in these machines, and because some medications must still be provided by traditional pharmacies, patient profiles maintained by stand alone systems in physician offices will not allow drug interaction checking against a complete patient profile in many instances.

Computerized Prescriber Order Entry (CPOE) is a technology whereby a prescriber directly enters orders into a computerized database. These orders are then sent to a pharmacy computer system via an interface. The pharmacist then reviews the order, and if appropriate, approves the order and dispenses the medication or allows the medication to be dispensed or retrieved from an automated dispensing device. Some CPOE systems allow for screening of drug interactions and identify and correct potential errors such as incorrect doses, routes, or frequencies before they occur. The time taken for the order to be received in the pharmacy is reduced, and legibility problems are avoided. In the inpatient environment, CPOE offers the advantage of selection of predefined treatment order sets, increasing compliance with disease management guidelines. In both the inpatient and ambulatory settings, CPOE can enhance prescriber compliance with system and payer formularies. The ideal CPOE system integrates the patient's medication profile, laboratory and other pertinent patient information into one database to allow the clinician access to all pertinent information at the time the prescription is written.

Implementation of automation impacts the manner in which pharmacy is practiced, in both the inpatient and outpatient settings. Most enhanced automated technologies, if implemented appropriately, will reduce the number of pharmacists and technicians required to perform basic functions associated with medication dispensing and distribution. This is thought by many as an opportunity to spend more time providing direct patient care activities such as patient counseling, performing pharmacotherapy histories, participating in patient care rounds, or participating in disease management activities. The extent to which pharmacists are successful in these endeavors is dependent on their willingness and ability to market the value of providing such services to institutional administrators and payers. Also, it is important that pharmacists assure that automation is implemented and utilized appropriately and that policies and procedures designed to assure safe and appropriate use of these systems.

Outcomes Management

Pharmacoeconomics can be thought of as the description and analysis of the cost of drug therapy to health care systems and society.[13] Further, pharmacoeconomics identifies, measures, and compares the costs, benefits, and risks of drugs and pharmacy services. These techniques are used in an integrated health care system to ensure selection of quality, cost-efficient treatment.

Traditionally, medical decision-making was focused on the clinical indicators of disease and the outcomes of treatment. In other words, this information answered the question, *Did the patient get better with the treatment?* If the answer was *yes,* the treatment was considered acceptable and useful. The issues of quality and cost-efficiency were not addressed with this type of analysis. Indeed, information currently presented to the FDA for drug product approval does no more than illustrate that the drug made the patient *better* or at least caused no harm.

In an integrated health care system interested in providing the best quality and cost-efficient care, decision-making based solely on clinical outcomes is limited in its usefulness and may in fact be detrimental to the overall health of the system. Thus, the framework for decision-making is broadened to include measures of economic and humanistic outcomes to deal with the limitations of the traditional approach. Here the drug or pharmacy intervention is analyzed not just to determine if the patients got better but how much better they got in terms of health care resource use (economic outcomes) and patient satisfaction (humanistic outcomes). This broadening of approach is synonymous with the broadening of approach to health care taken by an integrated system. In a fragmented health care delivery system decisions are made only on the basis of their effect on the care given. It is only appropriate that integrated systems adopt the new, broader decision-making framework, as it is concerned about delivery of quality, cost-efficient across the continuum.

THE OUTCOMES MANAGEMENT MODEL—The outcomes management model combines the techniques of outcomes research with the Plan-Do-Check-Act (PDCA) process model for quality improvement. Outcome management allows the important issues of efficiency, capability, efficacy, and productivity to be addressed.[14] Outcomes research is aimed at building theories and models for evaluating effective drug treatment protocols, successful treatment interventions, and optimal therapeutic outcomes. Outcomes researchers translate these theories into models for measuring the effectiveness of drugs and procedures as summarized by Vermeulen et al, in 2000.[15]

Outcomes management is the daily application of these models in the integrated health care delivery system. Outcomes management can be used to identify areas of patient care in which a treatment guideline, a clinical pharmacy service, or an operational improvement is needed to ensure the delivery of quality, cost-efficient patient care. It can identify best-practice options that can be implemented throughout the system.

Once a guideline, service, or operational improvement is designed, a parallel research design should be developed to collect and analyze the outcomes of the intervention. Both the process improvement and its evaluation should be launched simultaneously. This allows outcomes data to be collected to determine the effect of the intervention from the beginning of the process. Analysis of the data is conducted using accepted statistical techniques. Feedback is provided to the decision-makers as well as those involved in the planning and implementation of the process-improvement plan so that modification can be made to further this process. When changes are made, the outcomes management model begins again and continuously cycles, providing continuous improvement to the process.

APPLICATIONS—*Guidelines, Critical Pathways, and Treatment Protocols*—Outcomes data such as treatment failures, overuse of laboratory tests, or prolonged lengths of stay in the hospital are measures of treatment outcomes that can signal a need for a guideline, pathway, or protocol. These outliers in care can indicate the need for structured use of medication to optimize effectiveness. For example, one institution noted increasing costs for low-osmolality contrast media. Evaluation of use indicated that the use of this agent over the conventional high-osmolality contrast media had not affected the rate of adverse drug reactions reported to be a benefit of the low-osmolality agent. A guideline was implemented regarding the targeted use of these agents to ensure that those who would benefit most from the more-costly agents would receive them. At the time the guidelines were implemented, an outcomes study also was begun. The outcomes study indicated that drug costs were decreased by limiting the use of the agent, without negative effect on patient outcomes.[16]

Medication Safety—Although the benefits of clinical pharmacy services may be obvious to pharmacists, the use of the outcomes management model allows demonstration of the beneficial impact of these services on clinical, economic, and humanistic outcomes. In an integrated system the impact of these services over the continuum of care can be measured, and cost savings can be captured. For example, a high number of inpatient admissions (economic outcome) for bleeding among patients on warfarin therapy (clinical outcome) can signal the need for better patient education on the monitoring and use of the drug. With this information, a pharmacy manager can identify and assemble a multidisciplinary team to improve the process of outpatient warfarin. When the intervention is implemented, the clinic pharmacist can collect outcomes data on the patients participating in the modified clinic process. A decrease in bleeding episodes after implementation can be attributed to the process improvement.

OPERATIONAL IMPROVEMENTS—The need to change the organization of pharmacy tasks can be identified through economic outcomes such as increased overtime payroll. The pharmacy manager also may determine the need for a reorganization of work assignments when work is not being accomplished and the departmental goals are not being met. For example, the manager may be interested in the purchase of a robotic dispensing machine to free up pharmacists for clinical functions. To develop the plan for the purchase of the robot, an economic model can be developed to determine if the traditional methods of dispensing or the robotic dispensing machine is the most efficient use of capital. Once the decision is made, continuous collection of outcomes data relating to dispensing as well as clinical services can be gathered. Outcomes assessment can be used to support the continuation of the program or signal other changes that need to be made in the process.

BENEFIT MANAGEMENT—The activities involved in pharmacy benefit management began when insurance companies decided to pay for prescription medication as part of the covered benefits. Early management included activities involved with prescription dispensing and the payment to the retail drug stores for prescription costs covered under the plan. The management of this benefit became more important as insurance providers found that the costs of the pharmacy benefit continued to climb. Today, pharmacy benefit management entails a host of activities that now span the scope from dispensing drugs to the management of outcomes.

As controlling drug costs is important to insurance carriers, it likewise has become important to integrated health care systems that wish to provide cost-efficient care. Also, as most integrated systems are involved with managed-care plans that capitate the pharmacy benefit, the importance of maximizing the investment in prescription drugs for the provision of optimal health care outcomes becomes critical.

The degree of system integration and resources available will determine whether the integrated system entirely manages the benefit itself or contracts with a company that offers various services for pharmacy benefit management. These companies are called pharmacy benefit managers (PBMs). A survey conducted in 2001 revealed that PBMs are primarily involved in claims adjudication, while some are involved in providing disease management programs for their managed care organization or integrated system.[17] The activities involved in pharmacy benefit management have been described in four levels of sophistication.[18] There are varying degrees of each level of activity used in the management in an integrated system. Systems may pick and choose which services will be provided internally and externally through contracts with PBMs.

Level 1 (Managed Costs)—At this basic level of service, the focus is on managing costs of prescription drugs and handling the technical aspects of paying pharmacy claims, including reporting usage information. While an integrated system usually provides ambulatory prescription services through system-owned pharmacies, in most systems there are some patients who receive medication through retail pharmacies. In either case, the pharmacists filling the prescription need access to information about the insurance coverage—whether the patient and the particular medication are covered—before the service is rendered. Further, the pharmacist also needs a mechanism to process the claim for payment of the service.

All of these activities are best carried out through the use of a computerized system. As this is a highly technical function, it is less expensive for a system to contract with a PBM or other company with these skills and equipment for claims processing. For the integrated system to try to set up its own claims-processing activities would require huge capital costs for a hardware system that by the nature of the advances in computer systems would become obsolete quickly. Additionally, PBMs have provider customer-support personnel to handle problems arising from equipment problems and verification of coverage.

Another activity involved in managing the cost of prescriptions at Level 1 of benefit management involves controlling the costs of the drugs themselves. An integrated health system usually represents a large patient population and thus a significant amount of prescription usage. This fact can be used as leverage with pharmaceutical companies to secure product discounts. Additionally, the use of formularies can ensure that the patients only receive coverage for prescriptions for agents with low contract prices. Encouragement to use generic products is another way to hold down prescription drug prices. Limiting the quantities of drugs available for a given period of time, controls individual prescription costs. For example, new prescriptions may be limited to a 30-day supply.

A copayment often is used to interest patients in holding down the price of prescriptions. In some cases tiering of copayments is used to encourage patients to accept a less expensive alternative. For example, a drug may be available as a branded drug and a generic. The copayment is higher if the patient insists on receiving the branded product and reduced if the generic is accepted.

Level 2 (Managed Utilization)—At this point of managing the pharmacy benefit, the emphasis shifts to utilization review, optimal use, and standards of care. Here information about the types and volume of drugs prescribed and the prescribing patterns of individual physicians is shared with the payers and the physicians. The use of this information is intended to educate the physician about the use of cost-effective therapy. In some integrated systems, physician compensation is tied to compliance with prescription formularies and the use of lower-cost medications.

Therapeutic interchange of medication is implemented at this level to ensure that products chosen as the most cost-effective in their class are used. In some cases, the dispensing pharmacist is required to call prescribing physicians to inform them of the change in medication. In some integrated systems, with the appropriate legal arrangements with medical staff, therapeutic interchange can be automatically implemented much like is performed currently in hospitals under the authority of the Pharmacy and Therapeutics Committee and the hospital's Medical Executive Board.

While activities in Level 2 do not require the equipment of Level 1, they do require expertise in drug use evaluation and physician education. Integrated-system pharmacists with a background in hospital pharmacy may be likely candidates to provide these services to the system. These pharmacists understand the work required in performing utilization review and the techniques for presenting this information to physicians, which easily can be expanded to take on the additional aspect of ambulatory care. However, if personnel with this expertise are not available in the system, these functions can be contracted to a PBM.

Level 3 (Managed Therapy)—Level 3 focuses on disease management and how drug therapy is integrated into overall management. This approach is more comprehensive than the drug-focused approach of Level 2. In disease management, the front-line health care provider and the patients become involved in the care program. With disease management, providers develop guidelines or treatment pathways to reflect best practice in the treatment of a specific disease. It is important that pharmacists, as the integrated delivery system's drug experts, become involved in these activities. Patients also are given the responsibility of carrying out their treatment at home and learning how to manage their disease.

Integrated systems with pharmacists who have expertise in the development of guidelines and experience in working with patient-care teams can provide these services internally. It is important for the pharmacy manager to claim these activities for the pharmacy, as this is the future of pharmacy practice. As the patient is involved in the disease management process, the pharmacist has long been established as the patient's ongoing contact within health care. This relationship should be nurtured and used as a mechanism to establish system pharmacists as important participants in disease management.

Level 4 (Managed Outcomes)—The managed outcomes phase occurs when the integrated health system is able to apply treatment guidelines for multiple disease states across the patient base and use outcomes analysis to demonstrate the value of the care. This level of activity requires that the first three levels of pharmacy benefit management be firmly in place. This requires integrated data links of prescription and medical information that is often only available in an integrated system. Success at this level is not merely defined as the ability to manipulate data for outcomes analysis, but the ability to use this information to ensure the provision of quality care. As this level provides assurance of the provision of quality, cost-efficient care, integrated systems are striving to reach this level of function in the management of the pharmacy benefit.

FORMULARIES—Formularies represent a tool for pharmacy benefit management at its basic level and have been used since the 1950s to control drug costs and reduce performance variance in hospitals. Formularies in hospitals have developed from a list of drugs stocked in the institutions to an entire system to optimize patient care through effective, safe, and cost-effective use of drugs.[19] As the integrated system is interested in providing quality, cost-efficient drug therapy, the use of pharmacoeconomic techniques in the formulary decision-making process is necessary. Pharmacoeconomics goes beyond the traditional analysis of efficacy and safety to include costs of treatment and thus provide a global assessment of the medication. This type of analysis assigns a value to drug treatment so that the agent can be compared more equitably with other therapies.

These techniques for drug evaluation and formulary decision-making have been adopted in the integrated health care systems and managed-care organizations and outlined in detail in a 2000 publication of the Academy of Managed Care Pharmacy.[20] The changes in the drug evaluation process include the concerns of providing care across the continuum. The structure of the Pharmacy and Therapeutics Committee is changed for the integrated system to include an appropriate balance of primary-care physicians and specialists. Often the pharmacy representation will be expanded to include institutional and ambulatory pharmacists. Administrators involved with the managed-care plans for the system are often included. In some cases a PBM is contracted to provide formulary management. In this case, the PBM has its own Pharmacy and Therapeutics Committee and formulary of approved agents.

Formularies are described according to access the prescribers have to various drug entities. The control over access originally was intended merely to control drug costs; today the control is maintained to ensure the use of the most cost-effective agents and reduce process variation through statistical process control.

Open Formulary—This formulary is usually a comprehensive list of prescription products available, without restrictions on the choice of agent. Often within the open formulary, certain products are considered preferred as more cost-effective agents. These products are promoted for use to prescribers through newsletters and preferred products lists. Dispensing pharmacists may receive computerized messages encouraging them to contact the prescriber to switch to these agents when a nonpreferred agent is prescribed. Because there are no restrictions enforced, this type of formulary has limited impact on prescribing and thus little effect in managing the pharmacy benefit.

Closed Formulary—This formulary is a limited list of drugs chosen for inclusion by the Pharmacy and Therapeutics Committee. Typically, these formularies limit selection to between 300 and 1000 dosage forms. Usually, these formularies offer several choices of agents in each therapeutic category. In a health plan using the closed formulary, only drugs on the formulary drug list will be covered.

A mechanism must be in place to provide authorization when a patient requires a nonformulary agent. A letter of medical necessity from the prescribing physician or documentation of treatment failure on the covered agents may be needed to gain authorization for use.

Closed systems require more efforts to administer than the open system. The physician must be educated as to which medications are acceptable. The dispensing pharmacists become involved in contacting the physician if a nonformulary agent is prescribed. While this physician contact may take time, this provides the pharmacist an opportunity to work with the physician to improve care. Thus, these additional activities at the prescribing and dispensing phases contribute to more-effective drug choices and the control of costs, thus better control of the benefit.

For many years employers were required to provide open formularies as part of their employee benefit packages, because of union demands. However, as the pressure to control drug costs is increasing, more plans and in turn integrated systems are closing their formularies.

Restrictions—Within either formulary structure, other mechanisms of restriction may be used to direct therapeutic use and control costs. Restrictions often are placed on specific agents that are not considered to be used for problems covered by the health care insurance. For example, retinoic acid is used for both acne and age-related skin wrinkling. This drug treatment may not be covered for patients over 35 who would be suspected of using the product for wrinkles. As many plans do not cover plastic surgery for the same problem, it may be determined that use of this agent also is not covered. Some medications may have a lifetime cap, such as nicotine patches. In this way, the attempt is made to cover patches only for patients who are truly making an effort to stop smoking and not for those who are using the patches in situations in which smoking is not allowed.

A common restriction is the requirement for generic dispensing when the agents are available. Generic drug usage can provide the same therapeutic outcome at as much as a 60% saving in drug costs. In some cases, the branded drug may be available to patients if they are willing to pay the difference in price.

Prior authorization is used to direct proper care and control costs of drugs. In this case the prescriber must contact the insurer with specific information about the patient's condition. If previously set requirements are met, the prescription is authorized for coverage.

Drugs are sometimes restricted to specific physicians for use. These are usually very expensive medications that require a high level of expertise to prescribe and monitor the treatment. In many cases these restrictions require the primary-care physician to attempt treatment with a commonly used drug before referral to the specialist who has access to the restricted agent. While this may have limited effect on drug costs, it helps ensure safe and effective use of these specialized agents for the appropriate patients.

Incentives—The use of economic incentives to the integrated system or patient to promote use of preferred agents is one way to manage the pharmacy benefit. For the integrated system, the incentive is some form of risk-sharing agreement with the managed-care organization. In this case, part of the capitation for the patient is withheld to cover prescription costs. If the actual prescription costs are less than the withheld amount, the remainder is returned to the system.

The incentive for pharmacists may be an increase in the dispensing fee when generic drugs are used. A newer trend is to provide pharmacists incentives for cognitive services employed when changing an agent to a formulary or preferred product.

Patients may receive an incentive though a graduated system of copayments. Use of generic drugs may come with a lower copayment than use of branded agents. Preferred agents have a lower copayment than nonpreferred agents. Nonformulary agents may not be covered at all, thus encouraging the patient to have the prescriber select a covered medication.

The impact of these various incentives will influence drug costs to varying degrees. For physicians who are employees of integrated system and not direct recipients of the capitation fees, the shared risk incentive may have little effect unless the system explains the impact on the revenues and financial health of the system. The incentive will only influence pharmacists if the money offered is seen as a sufficient amount to cover the time involved in contacting the physician to switch a prescription. Patients who have no direct control on what is prescribed may in fact be irritated when they present a prescription for a nonformulary agent and are asked to pay for their medication.

BENEFIT MANAGEMENT COMPANIES—While PBMs can provide the total scope of services to the integrated health care system, there are many things to be considered when contracting for business services. Although there is little question that PBMs can provide claims processing with their computer systems, the practicality of using their services for some of the higher levels of pharmacy benefit management is less certain.

Much of the expertise needed to develop treatment protocols and disease-management plans often lies in the integrated health care system itself. The practitioners know their own unique patient population and, through personal interaction, understand local needs. This understanding can be valuable in developing the correct treatment plans to optimize outcomes in the specific patient population. While there is always a cost involved in developing these programs, the system has to determine whether internal development or external development (PBM) will provide the best product for the investment.

It is important to consider that whoever develops the treatment plan it will be the system's caregivers who will implement it. They must understand the plan and take ownership of it to implement the plan for optimal patient outcomes.

When pharmacy benefit management moves to Levels 3 and 4, there is a great deal of internal system information that must be used in decision-making and analysis. When this is done internally the issues of confidentiality remain in the system. When a PBM is involved in these activities, the system's confidential information must be provided to the PBM. While these confidentiality issues can be dealt with in contracts, the sharing of proprietary information in the competitive field of health care becomes a significant concern to the administrators of an integrated health care system.

HEALTH PROFESSIONAL EDUCATION—This chapter has discussed numerous mechanisms that are developed in integrated health care systems to ensure the provision of quality, cost-efficient care. These mechanisms are only helpful to this end if they are understood and adopted by practitioners at the point of care. To make these tools useful, the integrated system must develop an educational program for physicians, pharmacists, other health care providers, and patients. Pharmacists have an assortment of skills that can be used for these tasks. Pharmacy managers in integrated systems should work with administration to establish pharmacists as leaders in these educational roles.

Group Meetings—An efficient way to reach a large number of people is through group meetings. These educational meetings should be conducted throughout the integrated system for physicians, allied health care professionals, pharmacists, and patients. If geographically, it is not practical to have all department personnel in one place, the use of multimedia in the form of teleconferencing or videotape presentations can provide an education forum.

Medical staffs in integrated health care systems meet on a regular basis to discuss clinic procedures and day-to-day operational activities. This forum provides an opportune time for pharmacists to present information regarding formulary procedure, formulary agents, treatment guidelines, and disease management. As the practitioners are discussing the operation of their clinic, it is an easy transition to provide clinical information for incorporation into their daily treatment practices.

In the integrated health care system, patients are important players in their own care, and education of patients also must be considered. Often support groups meet, providing a forum to provide new information about services and treatment to a significant number of patients.

One-on-One Meetings—The pharmaceutical industry has long used this method to educate physicians about the use of their products. When pharmacists use this forum, it has been referred to as academic, or counter, detailing. The use of the term *counter* is meant to indicate the pharmacist is speaking against the information provided by the manufacturer. This is not always the case. The difference between detailing by the pharmaceutical sales force and that by the integrated-system pharmacist usually involves the purpose of the detailing activity. The salesperson is encouraging the use of the product for company profit, whereas the pharmacist is encouraging the use of the product that will provide quality, cost-efficient care for the patient. Sometimes the same product meets these two objectives, and then the two detailing activities do not run *counter* to each other. When this situation occurs it may be helpful for the system to use pharmaceutical sales representatives to educate the physicians on the use of agents. However, caution is advised, as their ultimate goal is maximal usage of their product, and the system's goal is optimal use of the proper treatment.

Pharmacists can use the same techniques used by the sales representatives in detailing activity. However, the discussion between the pharmacist and the physician can be more open, as topics for discussion are not governed by federal law as they are with the pharmaceutical representative. Pharmacists can provide the physician with system documents describing treatment as well as journal articles. Pharmacists can discuss actual system costs and use patterns to illustrate which drugs can provide care at lower costs. These educational sessions can serve to bolster the physician-pharmacist relationship and demonstrate the pharmacists' expertise in drug therapy.

Patient counseling frequently takes place in a one-on-one manner at the time of prescription dispensing. While this is an excellent time to educate the patient, it may not be optimal, as the pharmacy is often the last stop in the patient visit. Pharmacists in integrated health care systems are frequently in the clinic areas. Patient educational sessions can take place during the course of the office visit. This situation may prove optimal, as the physician, pharmacist, and patient are in the same locale to address treatment goals and changes in therapy.

Materials—In the hospital setting, the term *the formulary* has not only referred to the list of approved drug products, but also to a published document. Most formulary books not only contained the list of approved drugs, but also policies and procedures regarding pharmacy services and prescription writing along with guidelines and protocols. Encouraging the use of this book as a source of prescribing information can be helpful in educating physicians and other health care practitioners about the use of drugs in the system.

As integrated health systems computerize information systems, formularies can be placed in this environment for easier access by practitioners around the system. Besides the benefit of access, this electronic information can be more easily updated than the traditional printed format, which was updated usually once a year. Besides access to the formulary, other information regarding disease management and patient care can be provided in this format.

In systems where computer access is not readily available to all system care providers, a newsletter can be helpful in providing practical information in the patient-care areas. This document provides information in a short, easy-to-read format that can be posted in the patient-care work areas for easy access.

Many prescribers have integrated electronic drug information and hand-held prescribing technology in personal device assistants (PDAs). Comprehensive drug information databases that provide drug doses, side effects, indications, cost, contraindications and formulary alternatives are available for a wide range of national and statewide insurance plans. For example, in Michigan the formularies of all of the large HMOs are available at no cost to the users through ePocrates as a simple download from http://www.ePocrates.com. Other programs have established direct links to CPOE applications such that the physician can step out to dictate his/her patient note and send the prescription to the patient's pharmacy through infrared wireless technology (Fig 119-2).

Patient education materials should not be limited to those handed out at the time the drug is dispensed, nor limited to information on drugs alone. Information should be provided to patients on their disease and how their treatment plan works to control or eliminate their health problem. Much of this information is available from the various disease research and ad-

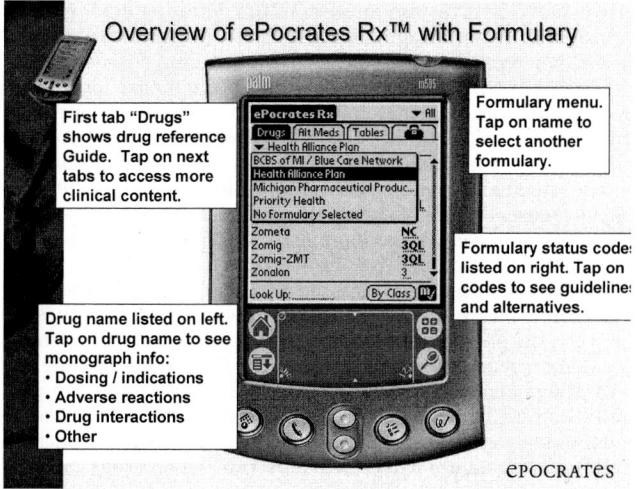

Figure 119-2. Personal device assistant with formularies (courtesy, ePocrates, Inc.).

vocacy groups such as the American Heart Association and American Diabetes Association and through government agencies. This information can be provided to patients in the clinics or mailed to the patient's home as a method of follow-up to one-on-one counseling. Physicians can download and print relevant materials from the Internet to support the patient's educational needs or refer them to high-quality web sites where credible information about their disease process or drug therapy is available.

ACHIEVING BUSINESS RESULTS

Pharmacy as a Business

HEALTH CARE BUSINESS—Business is a system of inputs and outputs in which monetary, human, and material resources are converted into the output or product. To continue to do business those outputs must be of value to the market in which they are sold, so that more resources can be purchased and more products can be produced. In other words, you have to make money to stay in business. While relating this to health care at one time seemed less than ethical, in today's health care environment this statement rings true. It is to this end that integrated health care systems have developed for the purpose of providing a quality product (health care) for a price that is considered competitive in the marketplace.

Pharmacists in integrated health care systems have the same mission to provide quality, cost-efficient care to the patients of the system. In pharmacy, the inputs include the skills of the pharmacists, medications, equipment, and supplies. The outputs include the products used, the goods (prescription and other medications) and services (drug-therapy monitoring) needed to provide patients with pharmaceutical care. In an integrated system the pharmacists must work to ensure seamless delivery of this care across the continuum. The coordination of these functions is the responsibility of the pharmacy management. If management is successful, it will have used the resources available, provided the proper patient care, and generated a profit to the system to save on overall costs. By understanding this concept it is easy to deduce that the concept of providing pharmaceutical care goes hand-in-hand with the business concept of serving the patient's needs with the resources available.

TOTAL QUALITY MANAGEMENT—While business is still defined as a system of inputs and outputs, the way business is conducted in the US has changed over the past several decades as foreign competition has entered and taken a front seat in world markets. The industry hit hardest by these chang-

ing concepts was the automobile manufacturers. The once world leaders in the industry, General Motors, Ford, and Chrysler, found that the Japanese were beginning to steal market share from them easily, in the late 1970s. As the problem grew, the industry giants realized that the competition was producing a better-quality, more cost-efficient product that the customers wanted. The carmakers realized that the way the Japanese handled the process of inputs and outputs was different. The Japanese after World War II sought the help of an American, Edward Demming, who helped them reconstruct the way business was run with a system called Total Quality Management (TQM). With this concept, business runs in a streamline manner. Employees who work daily with the product are asked for input about how to make the product better. Customers are asked how they feel about the product or service. The information from both these parties is taken into consideration and implemented to improve the product continuously. Efficiency in production is stressed. Just-in-time inventory concept is embraced. *Benchmarking* is used. This practice identifies the best practices of business and uses them as a standard for comparison with how a specific company is performing. As the auto industry adopted these concepts, it began to regain lost business in world markets. These concepts of running a quality, cost-efficient business are shared by integrated health care delivery systems, thus the adoption of TQM and the associated techniques was natural for the modern health care business. The Malcolm Baldridge Awards are now given to businesses for their achievement in the implementation and adoption of the TQM concepts. The health care industry participates in this awards process, and thus health care systems that achieve these highly prized honors are considered leaders in the field.

As health care delivery embraces the concept of customer satisfaction, it is important to consider who customers of an integrated system are. Health care is a unique industry in that the consumers of the service often do not pay for the service—someone else does. Although the patients are the customers of the service, their satisfaction with the service is still important, as there are competitors for their business. These customers have personal concerns for quality.

The other very important customer is the payer, who may be an employer group or health plan. This customer's focal concern is the cost of health care. If the payer is not satisfied with the cost of health care products and services provided by the system, it will take its business elsewhere. In this case, the payer looks at health care as a business commodity and expects the health care system to operate under the same business constraints as the payer does. That is, to provide a quality product in a cost-efficient manner. Thus, again this concept of using the structure of an integrated health care system as a quality, cost-efficient method to provide health care is in concert with the concerns of the potential customers, which is good business.

Many large employer groups have embraced exceptionally high standards of quality in their manufacturing and engineering areas. Health care, unlike manufacturing, is struggling to achieve "zero defect" outcomes. Corporations like General Electric, Ford Motor Corporation, and Motorola have adopted a quality philosophy and methodology called *Six-Sigma*. In *Six-Sigma,* systematic and statistically-based processes are applied to relevant defects in performance, driven by customer expectations. *Six-Sigma* methodologies aim to reduce the variation in clinical and business process which give rise to long cycle times, high cost and poor outcomes.[21] A process that operates at true *Six-Sigma* levels is producing acceptable quality levels over 99.99% of the time or producing no more than 3.4 defects per million events. In health care, 19% of medications dispensed in hospitals result in an error equating to a Sigma level of 2.4. Integrated delivery systems have far to go to achieve the level of quality performance expected by purchasers of health care. Pharmacists can have a pivotal role in achieving *Six-Sigma* quality due to the ease of access to data, knowledge of statistics and high ethical standards.

FUNCTIONAL AREAS—Pharmacy managers in an integrated system are faced with balancing the various inputs and demand for the different outputs to provide a quality, cost-efficient pharmacy service. There must be a business focus that ensures that monetary, human, and material resources (inputs) are allocated to the areas where they are most needed. Sound business practices of budgeting and quality control, among others, can be used to identify, monitor, and suggest change in pharmacy operations. Use of business plans, including long-range planning, is important for pharmacy managers to keep pharmacy practice on course with its goals and the goals of the integrated system. When pharmacy services are running smoothly, the system has another service that it can point to in its constant effort to stay competitive in the marketplace.

For the pharmacy manager, there is much to juggle to allow pharmaceutical care to establish and maintain its place in an integrated system. The plan may be for pharmacists to become involved in an academic detailing program with the system's physicians. In an effort to run a streamlined operation, no additional personnel will be made available for this task. The pharmacy manager then must use business skills to analyze the current work patterns, locate inefficiencies, and improve the process so that the existing pharmacists have time to take on these new tasks.

Accounting and Finance—Just as pharmacy departments in integrated systems take a different form, accounting in these systems takes a different approach to what is considered fiscally sound operations. In an integrated system, the money spent on expensive medications in the inpatient setting can save money in the consumption of the outpatient dollar. As the integrated system handles care through the continuum, the value of these expensive medications can be realized. Expensive drugs, which are given to inpatients, may save money for the system's ambulatory business units or *vice versa*.

Because of the ability of an integrated system to spread costs as well as savings across these systems, pharmacists working in these systems must broaden their fiscal management. In a system, pharmacy managers must have an understanding of purchasing, billing, and accounting as it applies to pharmacy throughout the system. Justification of fiscal losses in one site must be balanced in pharmacy savings at another point of care, and as saving health care use dollars in other facets of care, for example, office visits or decreased readmission rates.

Managed care has been an important driving force in the establishment of integrated systems for the provision of quality because of payment methods offered by the plans to health care providers who wish to contract with the plan. In this contractual agreement, the health care provider agrees to provide health care services in return for payment from the managed-care plan. This differs from the traditional relationship between providers and traditional insurance in that payment is not made on an occurrence basis, but on a monthly basis. Managed-care payment is made on a monthly basis for an agreed-upon fee that is called a per member per month (PMPM) fee. Under this structure the variation in the plan's costs only depend on the number of members enrolled, not on the number of services or complexity of services provided. Thus, if the patients use fewer services or the integrated system can run more efficiently, the system makes money. On the other hand, care is based on a PMPM for all care, it is common to if the patients require more services, the managed-care plan pays out no more money.

While the overall coverage in managed care is based on a PMPM for all care, it is common to have the pharmacy fees carved out from the total health-care benefit payment. The principles of services utilization under managed care apply to the pharmacy benefit as they did to the total health care benefit. If pharmacy services can provide prescription and pharmaceutical care at costs less than the amount paid by the managed-care plan, the pharmacy makes money. Thus, it is important for the pharmacy manager to understand this concept and understand why it is important to select the most cost-efficient agents for use in the managed-care population.

Human Resources—Efficiencies across the system are important to reach the goal of quality, cost-efficient care. This principle holds true when it comes to handling human resource issues in the pharmacy. To provide cost-efficient care, the system cannot afford to employ personnel who are not equipped to perform the tasks required. As integrated systems have changed the way health care is delivered, it is important for pharmacy managers to understand that these changes may be difficult for employees to understand and, thus, are not working to their optimal efficiencies. The pharmacy manager must find new ways to find qualified people, develop and motivate staff, and retain qualified people. These requirements do not differ from the human resource function of any business; however, as health care is rapidly changing, it becomes critical for the integrated system pharmacy management to be quicker and more innovative in these human resource functions.

Operations—Operations management is the organizing of the process that turns the inputs into the outputs. In the case of pharmacy services in the integrated system, pharmacy management is required so that the process takes the skills of the pharmacist and the medications and turns them into a quality, cost-efficient product of pharmaceutical care.

To provide these services the managers must look at pharmacy activities across the system and determine if all operations are running efficiently. In those areas where weaknesses are found, the operation is evaluated, and changes are made to improve services. The benefit from an integrated system is that pharmacists with various types of expertise can be called upon for assistance.

An integrated system is usually in a better position to adopt the use of computers and automation for dispensing medication and information to help the pharmacist. With computer links and automated dispensing units, pharmacist time can be freed up for patient counseling and physician education. In this way, the pharmacists can assist physicians in the choice of the most cost-efficient medication and help the patient use the drug for the best health care outcome. Thus, better operational management can play an important role in ensuring that quality, cost-efficient pharmaceutical care is delivered by the system.

Marketing—Marketing usually is associated with advertising or personnel selling a product or services. Marketing of pharmacy services in an integrated health care system is of critical importance for the survival of pharmacists as health care providers. A key factor in a successful business is to provide goods or services that have value to the customer. As integrated health care systems are run in a cost-efficient manner, any service or product that is not viewed as adding value to health care will be eliminated. In discussing marketing of pharmacy services it is important to consider the customers of pharmacy services in the integrated system.

Marketing plays an important role in developing the trust of health care providers. If the health care team sees the pharmacist as someone providing a valued service by working as a member of the team, the value of pharmacy involvement in patient care is accepted. In an integrated health care system, this involvement may be as simple as providing information regarding drug interactions to avoid negative outcomes or as complex as a pharmacist overseeing the complete care of a patient in a warfarin clinic. Through pharmacy marketing these services are accepted by the decision-makers of the system as quality, cost-efficient efforts needed to maintain the level of care demanded by the integrated system.

To ensure that pharmacy services are being provided to meet patient needs, marketing activities include identifying target markets for services, developing a product mix to satisfy these target markets, ensuring convenience and competitive pricing of products and services, and promoting pharmacy services. This reflects mostly on the quality initiative of an integrated health care system.

THE MANAGEMENT PROCESS—Bringing these functions together to run a quality, cost-efficient pharmacy service in one setting is a challenge. When the various types of pharmacy services provided in an integrated health care system are considered, the task appears overwhelming. Thus, the management process requires a directed, organized effort that can be sustained over the continuum of care for a long period of time. A good pharmacy manager prepares plans and organizes resources, especially the staff, in a way to bring together the talents to achieve the goal of providing quality, cost-efficient pharmaceutical care by directing their activities and controlling their activities. In an integrated system the use of TQM concepts indicates that the manager solicits input from the employees and customers of the service to ensure the best process.

PLANNING—Planning is the most critical element to ensure a successful operation. It requires that internal strengths and weaknesses of pharmacy services in the system be evaluated. In an integrated system, this review is expanded beyond the pharmacy alone and must include evaluation of pharmacy's interactions with the overall provision of health care. The operation and plans for expansion for the health care system as a whole must be understood for the pharmacy manager to plan for the pharmacy operations required over the continuum of care. Once the pharmacy's place in the overall business plan for the integrated system is understood, the manager can set goals for the department and develop policies, procedures, and business strategies to carry out the plan.

Organizing—Once the plan for action is determined, the pharmacy manager must organize pharmacy resources to accomplish the stated objectives. This involves identifying the tasks to complete, assigning tasks to individuals, and defining methods of accountability. Cooperation of pharmacists around the system is often required to complete a single process, thus organizations take on a broader scope than in the traditional health care delivery.

Staffing—Staffing involves identifying and providing the human resource needs for the system's pharmacy services. While the hiring and training of pharmacists in an integrated system is parallel to the process in any business, it is important to employ personnel who grasp the concepts of providing care across the continuum. In this situation, the qualified employees possess good communication skills and interest in working with the entire health care team to provide quality, cost-efficient care.

Directing—Directing involves keeping personnel focused on attaining system goals. This can be difficult in an integrated system, as sometimes it is difficult for employees to understand that the small part of the overall care process to which they contribute plays an important function in ensuring that quality, cost-efficient service is provided. While planning and organizing are management functions that usually take place before a process is implemented, directing the process is a continuing function of the pharmacy manager. Further, it is important to direct employee focus to the accomplishments required to reach the long-term plan. Integrated systems experience constant change as they grow through mergers and acquisitions. It is during these times of change that the manager must be especially diligent in directing the focus of integrated health care system pharmacy personnel.

Control—The controlling process involves periodic assessment of the work process. While directing activities is a day-to-day activity of business management, control through the use of reports and reviews ensures that the pharmacy's activities are on the correct course to achieve goals. This periodic assessment also is important because change in integrated health systems is continual. These periodic assessments can allow for review of the pharmacy process goals alongside the system's changing goals. This management function can signal the need to return to planning or organization to meet the new situation.

DEVELOPING A BUSINESS PLAN—If an integrated system is to use its resources for the best achievable outcomes, clear goals and a clear plan to achieve these goals are critical.

A universal goal of integrated health care delivery systems is to provide quality, cost-efficient health care services to all patients. With this clearly understood system goal in mind, pharmacy management can develop a strategic plan that allows the manager to focus on the pharmacy's strengths, reduce weaknesses, bring together resources, and direct pharmacy to initiate a process that will ensure the delivery of quality, cost-efficient pharmaceutical care. Business goals generally are categorized as outcomes management, expense management, and profit. As managed care and its concern with quality play a major role in the provision of care in the integrated system, outcomes management that uses traditional measures of economic and clinical outcomes along with humanistic outcomes is becoming the benchmark method for determining if an integrated system is meeting its goals.

Outcomes—By using the outcomes management model, the pharmacy manager can determine the need for a pharmacy intervention to improve patient care. By assessing clinical, economic, and humanistic outcomes, the pharmacists can determine if treatment is being maximized throughout the integrated system. Once the diagnosis is completed, a plan of action can be implemented. An important component of the plan is a method of collecting specific outcome information that will allow measurement of the effect of the intervention on outcomes. With this outcome data in hand, the manager can perform an analysis to determine the success or failure of the process. This analysis can reveal where improvement is needed. After improvements are made, the cycle of analysis continues to repeat itself. This technique allows managers to identify what works and what does not and to improve the planning and the process over time. As the outcomes management model involves continuous process improvement, it is recognized as an important tool to ensure quality, cost-efficient service in integrated health care delivery systems.

Expenses—In traditional pharmacy practice, expense management was tied solely to meeting an assigned budget for pharmacy purchases and personnel costs. In an integrated health care system, these remain important, but the costs and savings in other health care costs, such as additional office visits or decrease in length of hospitalization, can be factored into the pharmacy budget. As the integrated system recognizes savings across the system, pharmacy managers must be in tune with system accounting to identify savings in other costs that can be attributed to the use of expensive drugs or pharmacy services.

Profit—Profit is a simple concept of business, in which the cost to produce the product is less than the value the product is sold for in the marketplace. In the traditional pharmacy setting, pharmacists worked hard to procure drugs for the least possible cost while ensuring that the payers paid more for drugs than the purchase price and the cost to run the pharmacy. While this concept of pharmacy profit is still important today, it is measured differently because of the influence of managed care. While some customers of an integrated system may still pay for individual services, more and more patients have managed pharmacy coverage by which the pharmacist is paid a set PMPM. The key to profits here is to ensure that drug and business expenses are less than the PMPM payment. As always, the pharmacy manager who can best control the costs of doing business has the best chance of maintaining the profit needed to stay in business.

SECURING THE FUTURE—While the basic principles of business apply to the operation of any pharmacy service, diligence in applying these principles to pharmacy services in an integrated health care system is critical. While drugs are an acceptable product used to treat disease and illness, the services of a pharmacist may not be understood as clearly and thus valued by either those who are running the health care system or those paying for the pharmacy benefit. If pharmacy is viewed only as a service that delivers drugs, integrated-systems managers will see the economy of replacing pharmacists with technicians who can operate automated dispensing machines.

In an integrated system, an effective pharmacy manager uses sound business principles to show the systems administrator that pharmacists are the most appropriate managers of the pharmacy business within the organization. To do this, the manager must begin by using sound business principles to procure drug stock efficiently at the best price. While a pharmacy focus on drug-inventory management may seem misdirected, one must understand that those running integrated systems are often businessmen first. It is efficient spending of health care dollars on drugs, which is the quickest, easiest, and most traditional measure of an efficient business operation. A pharmacy manager who can use business principles to establish sound drug-inventory management will establish credibility with the system administrators.

This credibility establishes a foundation from which the pharmacist can work to establish or expand pharmacy services in the direct patient-care arena. This is where the use of sound business techniques becomes particularly important to pharmacists. For example, if it were proposed that a pharmacist be placed in a clinic to monitor patients on warfarin therapy, this would make good business sense, as it would be less expensive to have a pharmacist monitor these patients than the physician. Further, twice as many patients could be cared for, as both physicians and pharmacists see patients; that would increase patient satisfaction with access to health care providers. However, a nurse could be seen as able to provide the same care as the pharmacist at a lower cost. This is where the pharmacy manager can use techniques of outcomes research and pharmacoeconomics to give support to the sound business decision that a pharmacist can provide quality, cost-efficient care in this role. The outcomes management model further provides the tools to reaffirm the soundness of this decision, as the actual intervention is continually monitored and improved to ensure continuing quality, cost-efficient patient care. It is only through the use of sound business techniques that the pharmacist will win and keep a place within the integrated health system's provider team.

Pharmacy managers in integrated health care systems are running a pharmacy business as part of a very large business that delivers health care across the continuum. As part of this integrated business, the pharmacy manager is required to interact with many business managers who handle other facets of health care delivery. It is important for the pharmacy manager to understand what these other managers value in the operation of the delivery system, to function as a team player to ensure the provision of quality, cost-efficient health care, the product of the integrated health care delivery system. It is through the marriage of leadership skills with data and measurements, continuous quality improvement, employee-mindedness, and strategic thinking that business results are achieved and customer satisfaction is optimized.

CHALLENGES

Integrated health delivery systems face enormous future challenges. Many of these are in various stages of integration. During the process of integration through mergers, acquisitions, and joint ventures, vision and strategy must be communicated clearly to employees, the community, and health system stakeholders. Change is occurring rapidly in health care. Communication plans are essential to allay the anxiety of pharmacists and other health care workers. Organizational structures must be designed to achieve both vision and strategy. Relationships between system components must be well defined and understood. In professions such as pharmacy, corporate committees can be developed to help develop a strategy and vision for pharmacy throughout the health system. Physician involvement is needed to align pharmacy services with medical need and to ensure medical staff support of system wide formulary and drug use policies and guidelines. Information systems must be integrated, and common databases are needed for shared informa-

tion across facilities. Physician order entry systems with links to physician offices, clinics, and the hospitals in the system are needed to reduce practice variance and enhance quality. Cross-functional training of pharmacists to bridge clinical roles in acute and primary-care settings with common goals defined and clear time lines are needed. Staff development, education, and retooling are needed to ensure shared expectations, skills, and competence. A process for evaluation and continuous process improvement will help to ensure continued alignment of processes with visions and goals. Pharmacists in health systems are part of the continuing vortex of change and as such must be prepared for dynamic, responsive role shifts as system goals are defined and redefined, and functions merged.

Another future challenge for pharmacists in health systems is the change in the delivery of services and care. The term *era of telemedicine or cybermedicine* has been coined to represent the way that patients seek and receive information about their health and medications. Electronic and Internet capabilities have put vast information in the hands of the consumer. This represents both an advantage and a challenge. As discussed, the electronic and cyber educational opportunities are enormous. Patients can be directed to databases and Web pages of the health system where guidelines, helpful hints, and online chat rooms with pharmacists and other professionals facilitate the exchange of information and knowledge. The opportunity may represent a threat to health systems that have not prepared for this wave of communication, as patients may find erroneous sources of information. The public wants to be educated about drugs and will find a means of gaining necessary information. The challenge to pharmacists in health systems is to ensure that patients are provided with accurate information consistent with safe, effective drug use.

The pharmaceutical industry is positioned to continue advertising directly to consumers. Television, magazines, direct-to-home mailings, help-lines, and other strategies are used to gain access to consumers. While physicians previously were seen as the customers of the pharmaceutical industry, patients are now the target. Lay people, with no medical training, are being barraged with information about drugs and messages to ask their physician to prescribe new drug therapies. Direct-to-consumer advertising presents a large challenge to health-system pharmacists. It forces pharmacists to stay up-to-date on all newly released drugs and devices, because often patients will question pharmacists about new entrants to the market. Pharmacists may have to counter consumer requests with alternative formulary choices and provide sufficient explanation to satisfy patients about the choices made by health-system formulary committees. Pharmacists are asked about new drugs about which little or no information is known, and they are expected to have answers.

In a more global sense, drug-purchasing agreements and formularies will continue to merge to gain increasingly larger market shares. As a result of increasing costs of providing medical and pharmacy services to patients, employers may begin contracting directly with health systems for health services rather than going through an insurance plan. For systems that own their own HMOs, this may be happening already, but future alliances will occur to cut out the middle provider. Contracts may be negotiated this way to reduce the cost of providing care and improve access of the purchaser's employees to the medical care by ensuring exclusivity with the health system. Pharmacists will be asked to provide pharmacy services directly to large companies (eg, General Motors, IBM, General Electric) rather than to individual patients. As a part of this service, the pharmacy benefits, drugs provided, educational offerings, and clinical services will all have to be tailored to meet the needs of the new purchasers of health care.

Pharmacists continue to play a pivotal role in the evolution of care delivered by health systems. To prepare for future challenges, pharmacists will need enhanced development of analytical, business, and financial skills. Knowledge of marketing strategies may be important, as direct-to-consumer advertising from pharmacies to patients may play a role in maintaining and growing business. Customer satisfaction will be improved through extended clinical and educational services offered to patients. System-wide integration will require that pharmacists serve on committees and teams ensure alignment of financial, informational, and technological systems; clinical services; job descriptions; and care delivery. Pharmacists with leadership skills will help shape the vision for corporate pharmacy integration and are needed to plan for pharmacy in the 21st century.

REFERENCES

1. Shortell SM et al. *Remaking Health Care in America: Building Organized Delivery Systems.* San Francisco: Jossey-Bass, 1996.
2. Coddington DC et al. *The Changing Dynamics of Integrated Health Care.* Colorado: Medical Group Management Association, 2000.
3. Penna PM. *Am J Health-Syst Pharm* 1996; 53(suppl 1):S7.
4. *Defining Primary Care. An Interim Report.* Washington, DC: NAS Inst of Med, 1994.
5. ASHP Reports. *Am J Health-Syst Pharm* 1999; 56:1744.
6. Schumock G, et al. *Pharmacother* 2003; 23:113.
7. ACCP. *Pharmacother* 1996; 16;723.
8. Armstrong EP, Manuchehri F. *Am J Health-Syst Pharm* 1997; 54:1973.
9. Hepler CD, Strand LM. *Am J Health-Syst Pharm* 1990; 47:533.
10. Raehl CL, Bond CA. *Pharmacother* 2000; 20:436
11. Barker KN, Allan EL, Swenson ES. *Am J Pharm Educ* 1989; 53:27.
12. Felky BG, Barker KN. *Am J Health-Syst Pharm* 1995; 52:537.
13. Sanchez LA. *Am J Health-Syst Pharm* 1999; 56:1630.
14. McGhan WF, Briesacher BA. *Pharmacoeconomics* 1994; 6:412.
15. Vermeulen LC, Beis SJ, Cano SB. *Am J Health-Syst Pharm* 2000; 57:2277.
16. Grant KL, Canamo JM. *Am J Health-Syst Pharm* 1997; 54:1395.
17. Knapp KK, Blalock SJ, Black BL. *Am J Health-Syst Pharm* 2001; 58:2151.
18. Flagstad MS. *Am J Health-Syst Pharm* 1996; 53(suppl 1):S10.
19. Goldberg RB. *J Manage Care Pharm* 1997; 3:565.
20. Gricar JA et al. http://www.amcp.org/publications/index_publications.asp. Accessed on January 26, 2003.
21. International Organization for Standardization, at http://www.iso.ch/iso/en/iso9000–14000/tour/9000pub.html. Accessed on February 23, 2002.

Patient Care

Nicholas G Popovich, PhD

Professor and Head
Department of Pharmacy Administration
University of Illinois at Chicago
College of Pharmacy
Chicago, IL

CHAPTER 120

Specialization in Pharmacy Practice

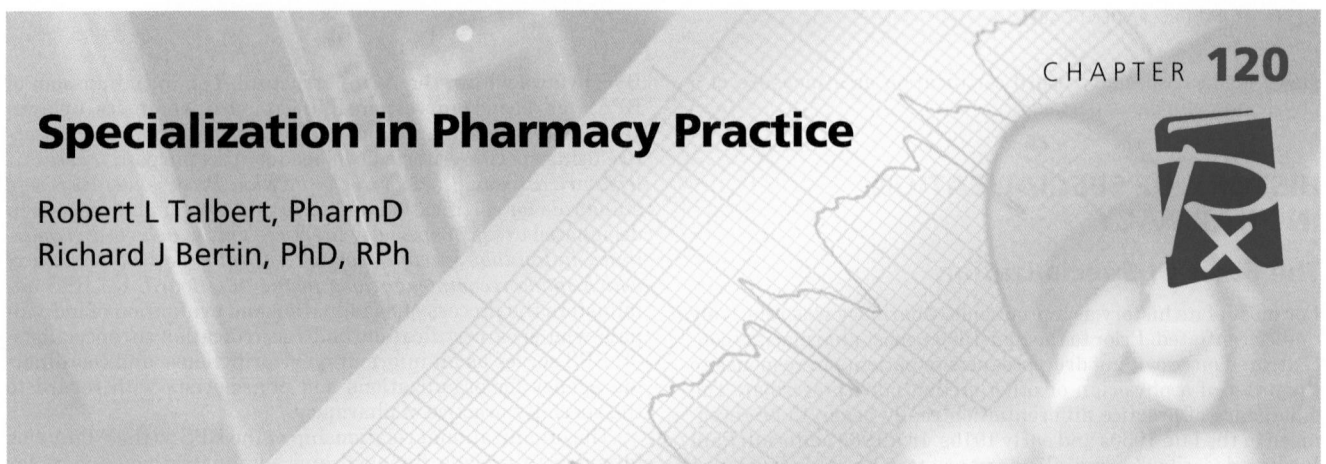

Robert L Talbert, PharmD

Richard J Bertin, PhD, RPh

Compared with many other professions, only recently has the profession of pharmacy entered the arena of advanced level credentialing. Formally, the medical profession has been recognizing specialty practice for nearly 100 years. Several other health professions (eg, nursing, optometry, dentistry) also demonstrate a long history of advanced level credentialing of qualified members. In fact, specialization in the healing arts is probably as old as the first declaration by a priest or shaman that he possessed special knowledge, insight, and power to heal. Therefore, he differed from other members of the tribe and was so recognized.[1]

HISTORY OF SPECIALIZATION IN MEDICINE

Specialization in medicine enjoys a long history. Medicine's evolution to its currently high credentialed state provides an interesting study in the professional, economic, and political forces that influence such a transformation. While there are major differences between medicine and many other health professions, medicine can serve as a model for other professions seeking to have credentialed specialists.

In medicine, the growth of specialization began in the 1920s and 1930s and is directly connected to the development of medical science and the resulting improvements made in medical care delivery. In the US, the growth of medical specialization is largely due to the physician's need to master the special tools and skills needed to deliver quality health care and the intricacies of social, political, and economic forces.

Most specialty areas developed around organ systems (eg, ophthalmology, otolaryngology, urology, neurosurgery, gastroenterology, cardiology); however, physicians were the only assessors of their own qualifications to practice a given specialty. There was no formal system to assure the public that the heart specialist was different from the general practitioner or that a physician claiming to be a specialist was indeed qualified. Consequently, specialty societies and medical education institutions collaborated on developing boards to define specialty qualifications and to issue credentials that would assure the public of the specialist's qualifications. The American Board of Ophthalmology established in 1917 was the first specialty board in the US.[2] It established the guidelines for the education, training, and evaluation of candidates desiring certification to practice ophthalmology. The second specialty board, the American Board of Otolaryngology was established in 1924. The third and fourth boards, the American Board of Obstetrics and Gynecology and the American Board of Dermatology and Syphilology, were established in 1930 and 1932, respectively. These were followed by several other specialties, such as, the American Board of Internal Medicine in 1936 and the American Board of Surgery in 1937.

The objectives of each specialty board were to elevate the standards of a specialty area, to familiarize the public with its aims and ideals, to protect the public against irresponsible and unqualified practitioners, to receive applications for examinations in a specialty area, to conduct examinations of such applicants, and to issue certificates of qualification in a specialty area. Since 1934, official recognition of specialty boards in medicine has been achieved by the collaborative efforts of the American Board of Medical Specialties and the American Medical Association (AMA) Council on Medical Education. The American Board of Medical Specialties (ABMS) approves 24 medical specialties. This organization has become the standard by which the profession and the public recognize physician specialists in the US.[3] In addition to the 24 ABMS member boards, approximately 180 non-ABMS boards issue specialty certification.

The establishment of board certification for physician specialists was based on the concept that a physician, who successfully met certain predetermined qualifications and attained the requisite level of knowledge, skill, and experience in a well-defined specialized area of medicine, would be a better practitioner than one who did not meet these qualifications. The implication was that a specialist would produce better health care outcomes, less morbidity, and/or greater efficiency in providing health care. However, while intuitively logical, this concept has not been validated by any studies.[4] One may argue that physicians with specialties provide state-of-the-art knowledge and that the patients ultimately benefit from specialist-dominated care. On the other hand, there may be instances where the sophisticated, expensive, specialist-dominated care may not produce any better health outcomes than did other, simpler, less-expensive health care delivery systems.

VALUE OF SPECIALIZATION IN MEDICINE

Although board certification is not required for an individual physician to practice medicine, the value of specialty certification in medicine, at least in medically sophisticated societies, is quite clear. Most hospitals and managed care organizations require that at least a certain percentage of their staff be board certified. Specialty board certification status for a physician is often used as a standard of excellence. Most hospitals, managed care organizations and health insurance plans require board certification for physicians for them to obtain clinical privileges and hospital appointments. Furthermore, the Joint Commission on Accreditation of Healthcare Organizations (JCAHO) and the National Committee for Quality Assurance embrace medical specialty board certification by incorporating it into their accreditation standards.[5] Commonly, the public also views medical specialty board certification as a measure of a physician's clinical expertise.

HISTORY OF SPECIALIZATION IN PHARMACY

The Basis of Specialization

For most of its history as a profession, pharmacy was relatively undifferentiated. Prior to the mid-1900s, most pharmacists concentrated on providing drug products to patients in response to the order of a physician or other credentialed prescriber. The emergence of practice differentiation really began to be recognized in the late 1960s and early 1970s. In a 1968 editorial, Paul Parker described hospital pharmacists who had developed unique roles that were distinctive from the traditional dispensing roles of the pharmacist.[6] These pioneering "clinical pharmacists" participated with physicians in therapeutic decision-making, and Parker suggested that their level of knowledge and practice skills required special educational and experiential preparation. Further, he encouraged hospital pharmacists to organize their departments to recognize and utilize these emerging "specialists" and proposed that the medical model of service organization might be applicable to pharmacy.[6] Shortly thereafter, the Study Commission on Pharmacy, known synonymously as the Millis commission, was commissioned by the American Association of Colleges of Pharmacy (AACP). Its report, published in 1975, acknowledged that differentiation in pharmacy practice was occurring and that this differentiation was, in general, expected and desirable. While not specifying specialty practice areas, the commission suggested that a structure be established to oversee all pharmacist credentialing.

In a series of editorials between 1974 and 1976, Donald Francke outlined his concept of a structure for the practice of pharmacy.[7] Specialization was addressed as part of the continuum of education, and he identified the pharmacotherapeutic specialist, the clinical radiopharmacist specialist, the drug information specialist, the pediatric clinical pharmacy specialist, and the pharmacy practice specialist, among others.[7]

Task Force on Specialization in Pharmacy–Role of APhA

Perceiving the evolving interest in differentiated practice within the pharmacy profession, the Board of Trustees of the American Pharmaceutical Association (APhA; now the American Pharmacists Association) appointed a Task Force on Specialties in Pharmacy in early 1973. This group was charged to (1) identify existing or potential areas of specialization (or, alternatively, to determine that there were no specialties and that the practice of pharmacy was not likely to become specialized); (2) propose a means by which specialties could be identified; and (3) develop the means by which individuals could become recognized as specialists, as well as recommendations for recertification.

The Task Force published its report in 1974.[8] While not concluding whether specialties existed at that time, it did determine that one or more specialties would develop in the near future and that there was need for an independent agency to recognize these specialists. It made several recommendations concerning the recognition process and proposed the establishment of a Board of Pharmaceutical Specialties (BPS) to develop the mechanism to identify specialty practice areas and recognize individual specialists.

Development of the Board of Pharmaceutical Specialties

The Board of Pharmaceutical Specialties was officially established on January 5, 1976, when APhA members approved the

BPS bylaws within the APhA structure. The initial mission of BPS was based on responsibilities outlined in its bylaws. (1) BPS recognizes appropriate specialties in pharmacy practice using specific criteria developed for this purpose. *These criteria are discussed below in the Petition Process.* (2) BPS sets standards for certification and recertification of pharmacists in designated areas of specialty practice. *This is achieved primarily by individual specialty councils, within the BPS structure, which make recommendations to the full Board.* (3) BPS administers the process of examination and evaluation of individuals who seek certification and recertification as specialists. (4) BPS serves as an information clearinghouse and coordinating agency for organizations and pharmacists with regard to the specialty practice of pharmacy.

The organizational relationship of the BPS to the APhA was intended to provide financial and administrative support for the young organization, while ensuring that decisions regarding recognition of specialties and specialists would be independent. To this end, BPS bylaws provide for a nine-member Board, comprised of six pharmacists and three non-pharmacists (ie, two other health professions members and one public/consumer member). The Board is appointed by the APhA Board of Trustees, but is independently responsible for administering the specialty certification process. This Board is advised by Specialty Councils, representing each recognized specialty. The Specialty Councils are comprised of six pharmacists from the specialty practice area itself, and three pharmacists representing the profession in general. The Specialty Council Chairs (ie, currently numbering five and representing the specialties of Nuclear Pharmacy, Nutrition Support Pharmacy, Oncology Pharmacy, Pharmacotherapy, and Psychiatric Pharmacy) as well as the Executive Director/Secretary of BPS (an administrative staff position) serve as *ex-officio* members of the Board of Pharmaceutical Specialties.

The initial membership of the Board of Pharmaceutical Specialties included:

R. Paul Baumgartner, Jr., PharmD
Carl G Britto, BS
Maureen M Fink, BS (Vice Chair)
Thomas D Foster, PharmD
John D James, BS
Warren E Weaver, PhD (Chair)
Erma Angevine, BA
Charlotte Cumbie-Doster, RN, EdD
Rosemary A Gellene, MD

BPS New Specialty Petition Process

A key role of the Board of Pharmaceutical Specialties is the recognition of new specialties within the profession. To its credit, the founders of BPS sought to make this a very formal and participative process for the pharmacy profession. Seven criteria for recognition of a new specialty were established, which remain in effect today.[9] These criteria must be addressed in detail in a petition that is submitted to BPS by an organization or group seeking recognition of a new specialty in pharmacy. A more detailed description of the petition process is available from BPS and on its web site, which provides additional guidelines for needed supporting information under each criterion. The BPS criteria that must be met for a new specialty are as follows:

1. The profession of pharmacy **needs** specifically trained practitioners in the specialty practice area to fulfill the responsibilities of the profession in improving the health and welfare of the public. Licensed pharmacists or other health care professionals cannot provide the level of services that pharmacist specialists can, and pharmacy's responsibilities may not be fulfilled effectively without their contributions.
2. A **clear, significant demand** for the specialty is made by the public and health care systems.
3. A **reasonable number** of pharmacist specialists practice in and **devote significant time** to provision of services in the specialty area.

4. Practice in the specialty area requires **specialized knowledge** of pharmaceutical sciences based upon the biological, physical, and behavioral sciences. The specialty may not be based solely on the practice environment or managerial, procedural, or technical services.
5. Pharmacists in the specialty practice area perform **specialized functions**, acquired through education and training beyond the basic level attained by licensed pharmacists.
6. Pharmacy schools and other organizations offer **education and training** in the specialty practice area.
7. **Transmission of knowledge** in the specialty practice area occurs through books, journals, symposia, professional meetings, and other formal media or mechanisms.

Petition Review and Approval

When the BPS receives a petition proposing a new specialty, a formal review process begins. If an initial staff and Board review indicate that the petition is complete and reasonably addresses the criteria, the petition is released for review and comment by the profession and the public. At least two open hearings, usually at major pharmacy meetings, are held to solicit input from the pharmacy profession, other health professions, third-party payers, and the public. Finally, the Board will consider the detailed information in the petition and any comments provided during the review period to determine whether the criteria for establishment of a new specialty have been met. The Board's decision is appealable in accordance with established BPS appeals policy. Once a new specialty has been approved, the initial Specialty Council is appointed. The organization or group that submitted the petition appoints the six specialist members to the Council, and BPS appoints the three non-specialist pharmacist members. After the first certification examination is administered and the first group of specialists is certified, all new specialist members of a Specialty Council are required to hold the certification. One of the initial charges to this Council is to work with the BPS, the sponsoring organization and others within and outside the profession to develop initial funding to establish the specialty. The other major charge is to work with the BPS testing consultant to develop the process itself.

Establishment of a Specialty Certification Process

Across all professional fields, there are relatively consistent procedures that need to be followed in the development and implementation of an advanced practice certification process. To be respected and successful, a certification examination must be psychometrically sound and legally defensible. This process begins when the BPS, and the profession determines that the legitimate criteria for the establishment of the specialty have been met. An early responsibility of the Specialty Council is to work with the testing consultant to conduct a role delineation study, also known as a job analysis. Usually, this is a very comprehensive survey designed to identify what specific knowledge, skills, and tasks characterize the specialty and can be used to differentiate between practitioners who are and are not at the specialist level. This is administered to a large group of pharmacists, some of whom are generally believed to be practicing at the specialist level, and some who are thought not to be practicing at that level.

When appropriately analyzed, the results of this study form the Content Outline or Examination Specifications for the specialty's certification examination, which determines what types of questions should comprise the examination. Next, the Council convenes groups of knowledgeable individuals to draft questions (also known as test items) that meet established test specifications. When appropriate, test items are based on evidence-based clinical practice guidelines and randomized clinical trial data, and each item is referenced for validation purposes. Following an extensive review, these questions are used to create the specialty examination itself. All BPS specialty certification examinations consist of 200 multiple-choice questions. Each has four possible answers, only one of which is correct. After the first examination has been drafted, the Council and other experts conduct a passing point study, which results in a psychometrically valid passing score. A passing point study involves determining what fraction of minimally competent practitioners would likely select the correct answer for each item. BPS and most similar advanced practice certifications utilize a Criterion referenced scoring system, rather than the more familiar Norm referenced system more common in academic institutions. Detailed discussion of these systems in included on the BPS website (http://www.bpsweb.org) and educational testing references. Recertification in all five BPS specialties is required every 7 years. Recertification examinations consist of 100 multiple choice questions in the same format as the original certification examination. When available, a BPS-approved professional development program may be substituted for the written recertification examination.

Evolution of Specialties

In the pre-BPS discussions across the pharmacy profession, several potential specialties were identified. It was not surprising that Nuclear Pharmacy emerged as the first petition to be submitted to the BPS. A section on Nuclear Pharmacy had been established within the APhA structure in 1975, and there was little debate that specialized knowledge and skill was required to practice nuclear pharmacy safely and competently. The community of nuclear pharmacy practitioners was relatively small and close-knit, and the APhA was in an excellent position to assist BPS to develop the specialty.[10] It was nearly 12 years, however, before any other specialties were proposed. Since that time, however, four additional specialties have been recognized. Those petitions were submitted by three other major professional organizations, marking the profession's recognition that the BPS could ideally serve the entire pharmacy profession as its specialty certification body. Although other certifications have emerged in recent years under other auspices, BPS remains the only organization in pharmacy offering specialty level certification.

The bar graph (Fig 120-1) illustrates the development and growth of specialties in pharmacy since 1995. Note that numbers represent individuals currently certified by BPS as of the year indicated. Individuals who failed to recertify when required are removed from these totals.

CURRENT SPECIALTIES IN PHARMACY

Nuclear Pharmacy

1. Supporting Organization(s)
   American Pharmaceutical Association
2. Year of Specialty Recognition: 1978
3. Description of the Specialty:
   Nuclear Pharmacy seeks to improve and promote the public health through the safe and effective use of radioactive drugs for diagnosis and therapy. A nuclear pharmacist, as a member of the nuclear medicine team, specializes in the procurement, compounding, quality control testing, dispensing, distribution, and monitoring of radiopharmaceuticals. In addition, the nuclear pharmacist provides consultation regarding health and safety issues, as well as the use of non-radioactive drugs and patient care. Those who are granted certification in this specialty may use the designation Board Certified Nuclear Pharmacist and the initials BCNP, as long as certification is valid.
4. Eligibility Requirements:
   The minimum requirements for certification in nuclear pharmacy are:
   - Graduation from a pharmacy program accredited by the American Council on Pharmaceutical Education (ACPE) or an alternative educational program accepted by BPS (eg, pharmacy school outside of USA)

Pharmacists Certified by the Board of Pharmaceutical Specialties

The table below illustrates the numbers of pharmacist specialists holding BPS certification in each of the years noted. This graph demonstrates the growth in specialization in the five recognized areas for which testing programs have been implemented.

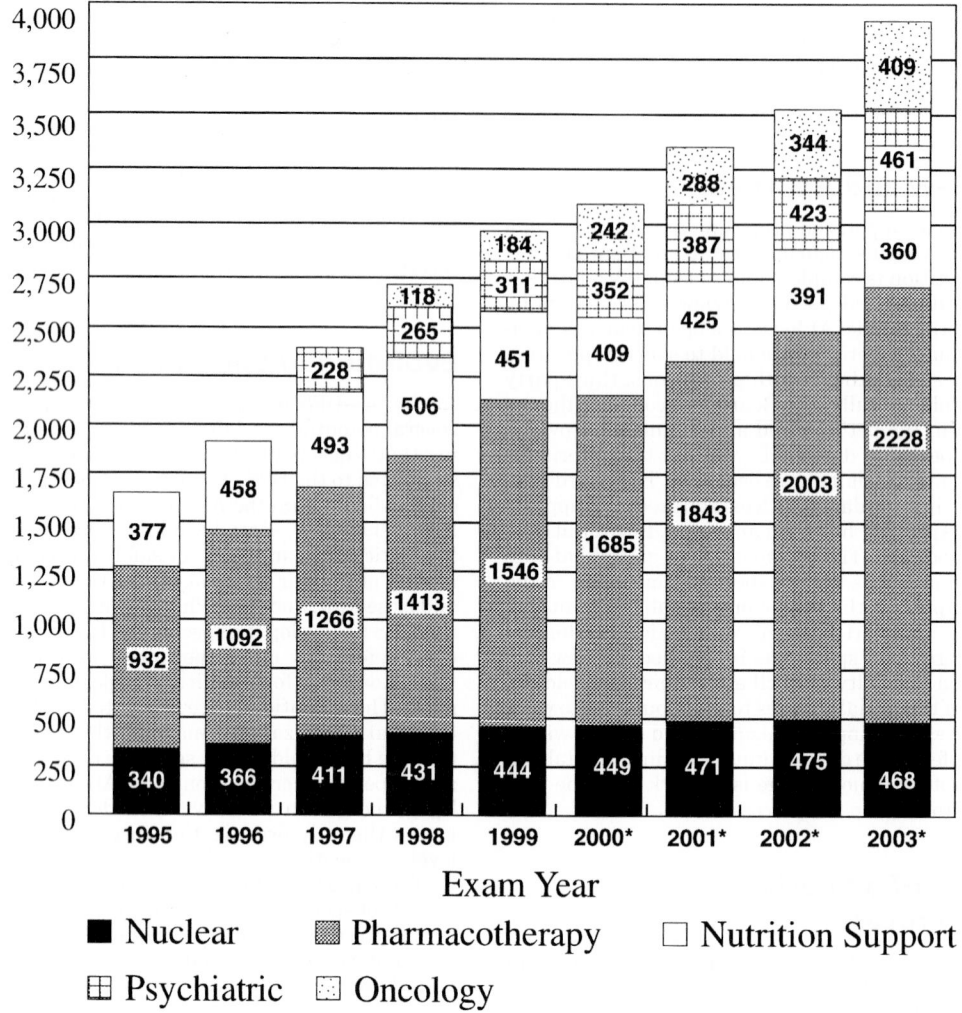

*individuals who failed to recertify have been excluded from these figures.

Figure 120-1. Pharmacists certified by the Board of Pharmaceutical Specialties.

- Current, active license to practice pharmacy
- 4,000 hours of training/experience in nuclear pharmacy practice
- Achieving a passing score on the Nuclear Pharmacy Specialty Certification Examination.

The required 4,000 hours of experience may be earned in a variety of settings.

Academic-up to 2,000 hours:
- Undergraduate courses in nuclear pharmacy: up to 100 hours experience for every quarter credit hour or 150 hours experience for every semester credit hour, to a maximum of 1,500 hours
- Postgraduate courses in nuclear pharmacy: up to 100 hours experience for every quarter credit hour or 150 hours experience for every semester credit hour, to a maximum of 1,500 hours
- MS or PhD degree in nuclear pharmacy: 2,000 hours
- Successful completion of the Nuclear Pharmacy Certificate Program offered by Purdue University (217 hours) or The Ohio State University (214 hours). Credit for other courses will be assessed on a case-by-case basis.

Training/Practice-up to 4,000 hours:
- Residency in nuclear pharmacy: hour-for-hour credit to a maximum of 2,000 hours
- Internship to satisfy requirements of state boards of pharmacy: hour-for-hour credit in a licensed nuclear pharmacy or facility authorized to handle radioactive materials, to a maximum of 2,000 hours
- Nuclear pharmacy practice: hour-for-hour credit in a licensed nuclear pharmacy or health care facility approved by state or federal agencies to handle radioactive materials, to a maximum of 4,000 hours.

5. Examination Content
- Procurement of radiopharmaceuticals (6% of the examination)
- Compounding of radiopharmaceuticals (20% of the examination)
- Quality Assurance of radiopharmaceuticals (15% of the examination)
- Dispensing of radiopharmaceuticals (20% of the examination)
- Distribution of radiopharmaceuticals (5% of the examination)

- Health and Safety associated with radiopharmaceuticals (15% of the examination)
- Provision of Information and Consultation (15% of the examination)
- Monitoring Patient Outcomes (2% of the examination)
- Research and Development (2% of the examination)

6. Recertification
Recertification for Board Certified Nuclear Pharmacists (BCNP) is a three-step process:
- Self-evaluation: Review of the nuclear pharmacy practice activities/functions that have changed since initial certification or last recertification.
- Peer review: Documentation of nuclear pharmacy practice over the seven year certification period.
- Formal Assessment: This assessment of a practitioner's knowledge and skills will be accomplished through one of two methods: 1) achieving a passing score on the 100-item, multiple-choice objective recertification examination, based on the content outline of the certification examination; OR 2) earning 70 hours of continuing education credit provided by a professional development program approved by BPS.
- A current, active license to practice pharmacy is required for recertification.
- As part of the recertification process, every BCNP is asked to complete an annual practice report form provided by BPS. At time of recertification, the BCNP must also certify that the candidate is not under suspension by the Nuclear Regulatory Commission or their state radiation control organization.

7. Members of the first Specialty Council
All appointed in 1978: (* = non-specialist member)
David R. Allen, PhD
*Horace Aslin, BS
Ronald J. Callahan, MS
James R. Cooper, PharmD
Thomas Deutsch, BS
Rodney D. Ice, PhD
*John Romankiewicz, PharmD
Stanley M. Shaw, PhD
*Margaret C. Yarborough, BS

Nutrition Support Pharmacy

1. Supporting Organization(s)
American Society of Health-System Pharmacists and American Society for Parenteral and Enteral Nutrition
2. Year of Recognition: 1988
3. Description of the Specialty:
Nutrition support pharmacy addresses the care of patients who receive specialized nutrition support, including parenteral and enteral nutrition. The nutrition support pharmacist has responsibility for promoting maintenance and/or restoration of optimal nutritional status, designing and modifying treatment according to the needs of the patient. The nutrition support pharmacist has responsibility for direct patient care and often functions as a member of a multidisciplinary nutrition support team. Those who are granted certification in this specialty may use the designation Board Certified Nutrition Support Pharmacist and the initials BCNSP, as long as certification is valid.
4. Eligibility Requirements
The minimum requirements for this specialty certification are:
- Graduation from a pharmacy program accredited by the American Council on Pharmaceutical Education (ACPE) or an alternative educational program accepted by BPS (eg, pharmacy school outside of USA).
- Current, active license to practice pharmacy.
- Completion of three (3) years practice experience with substantial time spent in nutrition support pharmacy activities
OR
Completion of a specialty residency in nutrition support pharmacy practice plus one (1) additional year of practice with substantial time spent in nutrition support pharmacy activities
OR
Completion of a nutrition support fellowship plus one (1) additional year of practice experience with substantial time spent in nutrition support pharmacy activities
OR

Completion of BOTH a specialty residency in nutrition support pharmacy practice AND a nutrition support fellowship (no additional year of experience required).
- Achieving a passing score on the Nutrition Support Pharmacy Specialty Certification Examination

5. Examination Content
Domain 1: Provision of individualized nutrition support care to patients
- Subdomain A: Assessment of the patient (17% of the examination)
- Subdomain B: Development and Implementation of a therapeutic plan (22% of the examination)
- Subdomain C: Monitoring and Management of the patient (39% of the examination)
Domain 2: Management of nutrition support services (13% of the examination)
Domain 3: Advancement of nutrition support pharmacy practice (9% of the examination)

6. Recertification
Recertification for Board Certified Nutrition Support Pharmacists (BCNSP) is based on the following activities:
- Earning a minimum of 3.0 continuing education units (CEU) in nutrition support with no less than 1.0 CEU earned every two years. These CEUs must be from providers approved by the American Council on Pharmaceutical Education (ACPE). NOTE: 1.0 CEU equals 10 hours of approved continuing education.
- Achieving a passing score on the 100-item, multiple-choice recertification examination, which is based on the content outline of the certification examination
- A current, active license to practice pharmacy is required for recertification.

7. Members of the first Specialty Council
All appointed in 1989: (* = non-specialist member)
Joseph S. Bertino, PharmD
Lawrence A. Robinson, PharmD
*Stephen M. Caiola, MS
Michael D. Reed, PharmD
Deborah B. Thorn, MBA
*Ellen A. Leitinger, PharmD
Beverly J. Holcombe, PharmD
Kathleen M. Strausburg, MS
*James A. Ponto, MS

Pharmacotherapy

1. Supporting Organization(s)
American College of Clinical Pharmacy
2. Year of Recognition: 1988
3. Description of the Specialty:
Pharmacotherapy is that area of pharmacy practice that is responsible for ensuring the safe, appropriate, and economical use of drugs in patient care. The pharmacotherapy specialist has responsibility for direct patient care, often functions as a member of a multidisciplinary team and is frequently the primary source of drug information for other healthcare professionals. Those who are granted certification in this specialty may use the designation Board Certified Pharmacotherapy Specialist and the initials BCPS, as long as certification is valid.
4. Eligibility Requirements
The minimum requirements for this specialty certification are:
- Graduation from a pharmacy program accredited by the American Council on Pharmaceutical Education (ACPE) or an alternative educational program accepted by BPS (eg, pharmacy school outside the USA)
- Current, active license to practice pharmacy
- *Bachelor of Science in Pharmacy degree (or equivalent) plus a, b, or c below.
  a. Five (5) years of practice with substantial component (>50%) of patient care activities in pharmacotherapy
OR
  b. Completion of a Pharmacy Practice or Specialty Residency and three additional years of practice with a substantial component (>50%) of patient care activities in pharmacotherapy
OR
  c. Completion of BOTH a Pharmacy Practice Residency and a Specialty Residency with a substantial component (>50%) of patient care activities in pharmacotherapy
*Doctor of Pharmacy degree plus a or b below.

a. Three (3) years of practice experience with a substantial component (>50%) of patient care activities in pharmacotherapy

OR

b. Completion of a Pharmacy Practice or Specialty Residency with a substantial component (>50%) of patient care activities in pharmacotherapy

- Achieving a passing score on the Pharmacotherapy Specialty Certification

    Examination

    *One of these two requirements must be met in order to be certified.

5. Examination Content

    Domain 1: Collect and interpret data to design, recommend, implement, monitor, and modify patient-specific pharmacotherapy in collaboration with other health care professionals to optimize drug therapy (55% of the examination)

    Domain 2: Retrieve, generate, interpret, and disseminate knowledge in pharmacotherapy (30% of the examination)

    Domain 3: Design, recommend, implement, monitor and modify system specific policies and procedures in collaboration with other professionals/administrators to optimize health care (15% of the examination)

6. Recertification

    Recertification for Board Certified Pharmacotherapy Specialists (BCPS) is an assessment of a practitioner's knowledge and skills through one of two methods:

    - Achieving a passing score on the 100-item, multiple-choice objective recertification examination, based on the content outline of the certification examination;

        OR

    - Earning 120 hours of continuing education credit provided by a professional development program approved by BPS.

    - A current, active license to practice pharmacy is required for recertification.

7. Members of the first Specialty Council

    All appointed in 1989: (* = non-specialist member)

    David R. Rush, PharmD

    Robert L. Talbert, PharmD

    *William C. Porter, PharmD

    Peter Gal, PharmD

    Peter H. Vlasses, PharmD

    *William A. Smith, PharmD

    George E. Dukes, PharmD

    Barbara J. Zarowitz, PharmD

    *William A. Miller, PharmD

Psychiatric Pharmacy

1. Supporting Organization(s)

    American Society of Health-System Pharmacists

2. Year of Recognition: 1994

3. Description of the Specialty:

    Psychiatric pharmacy addresses the pharmaceutical care of patients with psychiatric-related illnesses. As a member of a multidisciplinary treatment team, the psychiatric pharmacy specialist is often responsible for optimizing drug treatment and patient care by conducting such activities as monitoring patient response, patient assessment, recognizing drug-induced problems, and recommending appropriate treatment plans. Those who are granted certification in this specialty may use the designation Board Certified Psychiatric Pharmacist and the initials BCPP, as long as certification is valid.

4. Eligibility Requirements

    The minimum requirements for this specialty certification are:

    - Graduation from a pharmacy program accredited by the American Council on Pharmaceutical Education (ACPE) or an alternative educational program accepted by BPS (eg, pharmacy school outside the USA)

    - Current, active license to practice pharmacy

    - Completion of four (4) years of practice with substantial time spent in psychiatric pharmacy practice

        OR

    - Completion of a specialty residency in psychiatric pharmacy plus one (1) additional year of practice with substantial time spent in psychiatric pharmacy

    - Achieving a passing score on the Psychiatric Pharmacy Specialty Certification Examination

5. Examination Content

    Domain 1: Collaborate with other health professionals in pursuing optimal drug therapy for neuropsychiatric patients; this requires that the psychiatric pharmacist collect and interpret pertinent clinical data, and assume personal responsibility for successful drug therapy outcomes (ie, through the recommendation, design, implementation, monitoring, and modification of pharmacotherapeutic plans for the patient) (75% of the examination)

    Domain 2: Interpret, generate and/or disseminate knowledge in neuropsychiatric pharmacy (20% of the examination)

    Domain 3: In collaboration with other professionals/administrators, recommend, design, implement, monitor, and modify systems and policies to optimize the use of drugs in the treatment of neuropsychiatric patients (5% of the examination)

6. Recertification

    Recertification of Board Certified Psychiatric Pharmacists (BCPP) requires an assessment of a practitioner's knowledge and skills through one of two methods:

    - Achieving a passing score on the 100-item multiple choice recertification examination, based on the content outline of the certification examination;

        OR

    - Earning 120 hours of continuing education credit provided by a professional development program approved by BPS.

    - A current, active license to practice pharmacy is required for recertification.

7. Members of the first Specialty Council

    Appointed in 1994: (* = non-specialist member)

    M. Lynn Crismon, PharmD

    Martha P. Fankhauser, MS

    *George H. Hinkle, MS

    Michael W. Jann, PharmD

    *Howard A. Juni, PharmD

    Raymond C. Love, PharmD

    *Max D. Ray, PharmD

    Glen L. Stimmel, PharmD

    Barbara G. Wells, PharmD

Oncology Pharmacy

1. Supporting Organization(s)

    American Society of Health-System Pharmacists

2. Year of Recognition: 1996

3. Description of the Specialty:

    Oncology pharmacy specialists recommend, design, implement, monitor and modify pharmacotherapeutic plans to optimize outcomes in patients with malignant diseases. Those who are granted certification in this specialty may use the designation Board Certified Oncology Pharmacist and the initials BCOP, as long as certification is valid.

4. Eligibility Requirements

    The minimum requirements for this specialty certification are:

    - Graduation from a pharmacy program accredited by the American Council on Pharmaceutical Education (ACPE) or an alternative educational program accepted by BPS (eg, pharmacy school outside the USA)

    - Current, active license to practice pharmacy

    - Completion of three (3) years of practice with substantial time spent in oncology pharmacy

        OR

    - Completion of a specialty residency in oncology pharmacy plus one (1) additional year of practice with substantial time spent in oncology pharmacy

    - Achieving a passing score on the Oncology Pharmacy Specialty Certification Examination

5. Examination Content

    Domain 1: Collaborate with other health professionals in pursuing optimal drug therapy for patients with cancer. This requires that the oncology pharmacist collects and interprets pertinent clinical data, and assumes personal responsibility for successful drug therapy outcomes. (60% of the examination)

    Domain 2: Interpret, generate and/or disseminate knowledge in oncology as it applies to oncology pharmacy practice. (20% of the examination)

    Domain 3: In collaboration with other professionals, patients, and the public, recommend, design, implement, monitor, and modify systems and policies to optimize the use of drugs in patients with cancer. (15% of the examination)

Domain 4: Collaborate with other professionals and the public in addressing public health issues (eg, risk factors, prevention, screening, cancer survivorship) as they relate to oncology pharmacy practice. (5% of the examination)

6. Recertification

Recertification for Board Certified Oncology Pharmacists (BCOP) requires achieving a passing score on the 100-item, multiple-choice recertification examination, which is based on the content outline of the certification examination. As of the summer, 2003, a professional development option for recertification of BCOP is under development.

A current, active license to practice pharmacy is required for recertification.

7. Members of the first Specialty Council

Appointed in 1997: (* = non-specialist member)

*Samuel C. Augustine, PharmD
Carol M. Balmer, PharmD
*Toby Clark, MS
Rebecca S. Finley, PharmD
Barry R. Goldspiel, PharmD
Robert J. Ignoffo, PharmD
Jim M. Koeller, PharmD
Celeste M. Lindley, PharmD
*Kathleen M. Strausburg, MS

ADDED QUALIFICATIONS PROCESS AND CURRENTLY RECOGNIZED AREAS

In 1997, BPS approved a process for the recognition of Added Qualifications in an existing specialty. Added Qualifications provides a method to document further differentiation of practitioners within BPS-recognized specialties.[11] BPS issued its *Petitioner Information for Added Qualifications in Infectious Diseases* document in August 1997. This was followed by the publishing of several articles, meetings with interested organizations, and other informational activities. Conferral of added qualifications requires submission of a $100 fee and a structured portfolio, which is reviewed by the pertinent BPS Specialty Council and scored in accordance with published criteria. Added Qualifications must be reaffirmed every 7 years, just as BPS certification in a primary specialty.

In May 1998, the Society of Infectious Diseases Pharmacists submitted a petition for Added Qualifications in Infectious Diseases Pharmacotherapy. The petition, including the portfolio review process, was approved by BPS in March 1999. In March 2000, the American College of Clinical Pharmacy (ACCP) submitted a petition to BPS, requesting designation of cardiology as a second area of Added Qualifications within Pharmacotherapy. The petition, including the portfolio review process, was approved by BPS in October 2000.

As of spring 2003, 40 Board Certified Pharmacotherapy Specialists held Added Qualifications in Infectious Diseases, and 21 held Added Qualifications in Cardiology. To date, no other petitions for Added Qualifications have been presented to BPS, although pharmacist groups have expressed interest in establishment of a program for Pediatrics (within pharmacotherapy), Positron Emitting Tomography (within Nuclear Pharmacy), bone marrow transplant (within Oncology), and some others.

THE BPS SPECIALTY CERTIFICATION PROCESS

Currently, BPS specialty certification and recertification examinations are administered once annually, on the first Saturday in October. The application deadline is the preceding August 1. Examination sites are established in approximately 18 cities in the continental United States. Additional, "alternate sites" may be established in other US cities, at the request of 10 or more candidates, and in foreign countries. In recent years, BPS has had a total of approximately 28 sites each year worldwide.

Complete examination information, including a Candidate's Guide, Specialty Content Outlines, current fees, and application materials are available upon request from BPS or at the website, www.bpsweb.org. First-time applicants are encouraged to apply on-line.

As previously described, each BPS specialty certification examination consists of 200 multiple choice questions, each having only one correct answer. Written recertification examinations consist of 100 questions. Short practice tests for each specialty are posted on the BPS website to illustrate the construction of the questions and their content.

Candidates are informed in writing of their performance on each domain of the examination, and successful candidates are awarded a BPS certificate. A BPS certification or recertification examination may be retaken if necessary at reduced fee.

THE VALUE OF SPECIALTY CERTIFICATION IN PHARMACY

As in other professions where specialty certification has become established, this rigorous process provides value and benefit to society, to the pharmacy profession, and to the certified individuals.

Society

The existence of pharmacists who have demonstrated an advanced level of practice knowledge and skill has clearly resulted in improved pharmaceutical care for patients. Numerous studies have investigated the positive impact of clinically trained pharmacists in inpatient and ambulatory care settings.[12] Pharmacists who are able to interact with other health professionals in planning and implementing therapy contribute special expertise in areas that complement the skills of their colleagues. As the recognized "drug experts," they can also help to ensure that patients maximize the potential benefits of therapy. While there have been few direct studies of the impact of specialty certification in pharmacy (or in medicine, for that matter) on patient outcomes, available evidence suggests that training and experience are important determinants of quality care. Specialty certification provides an objective, independent measure of knowledge and experience against an established standard. High quality certification programs in all fields maintain that their first obligation is to society, and ensure that their programs meet that goal.

The Pharmacy Profession

As the numbers of BPS-certified pharmacists have grown within the pharmacy profession, the value of this credential has been increasingly recognized. Just as in other health professions, increasingly, specialty board certification is viewed as an important qualification for clinical faculty in pharmacy schools.[13] BPS certification has also been accepted by several schools as a measure of the clinical expertise of applicants to non-traditional PharmD programs, often exempting them from certain didactic requirements. Specialty board certification is a respected model of clinical expertise in institutional settings where clinical privileges are required to perform some patient-care services. When other health professionals understand that pharmacists can also meet this rigorous standard, the status of the profession and pharmacists' ability to participate fully in patient care increases.

The Individual

Specialty certification confers many potential benefits for the pharmacist. Positive recognition by patients, colleagues, and employers often brings psychological "enrichment" and reward to pharmacists who have worked hard to develop and document their expertise. There are also increasing instances of monetary reward for specialty certification. Some examples include: Bonus pay for members of the uniformed services and pharmacists in many institutional systems; hiring or promotion preference, particularly for professionally challenging clinical specialist positions; reimbursement of costs for certification and/or recertification; eligibility for participation in collaborative practice or other arrangements where payment for pharmaceutical services is possible. As specialty certification becomes more common in pharmacy, recognition of its value to the individual pharmacist will also increase, just as it has for medicine and other health professions.

OTHER CREDENTIALS IN PHARMACY

Specialty certification is but one of several options open to pharmacists seeking to advance professionally after their initial entry into practice. Other credentials available include:

- Formal post-graduate degree programs
- Residency or fellowship training
- Certificate training programs
- Multi-disciplinary certification programs (eg, Certified Diabetes Educator)
- Non-specialty certification programs (eg, Certified Disease Manager; Certified Geriatric Pharmacist)

Detailed discussion of these opportunities is beyond the scope of this chapter. Attainment of some of these credentials may help prepare or qualify a pharmacist for BPS Specialty Certification.

COUNCIL ON CREDENTIALING IN PHARMACY

Because of the multiplicity of credentials available to pharmacists, several of the major membership organizations in pharmacy joined to establish the Council on Credentialing in Pharmacy in 1997. This organization provides a forum for discussion, planning, and dissemination of information within and outside the pharmacy profession on the topic of credentialing for pharmacists and pharmacy technicians. The Council's Reference paper on Pharmacy Credentialing has become an important resource on the topic.[14]

FUTURE OF SPECIALIZATION

Pharmaceutical care and the services offered by pharmacists will continue to evolve and increase in complexity and sophistication. For example, between 1993 and 2003, the Food and Drug Administration approved more than 300 new drugs, biologicals, and vaccines that prevent and treat over 150 conditions.[15] Many of these are new molecular entities and not oral dosing forms, and require greater expertise in their preparation and administration than older products. Furthermore, as pharmacy and the rest of medicine move into the era of pharmacogenomics and gene therapy, new and expanded skills and knowledge will be required to utilize new tools in the therapeutic armamentarium safely and effectively. As has occurred with other health professions, pharmacy will most likely respond to

these challenges by increasing specialization. Further, health care systems, payers, and patients will continue to demand greater knowledge and skill *and documentation of that knowledge and skill* from those professionals responsible for drug therapy management.

In less than a decade (1995–2003) the number of board certified specialists in pharmacy has grown by nearly 240% (ie, from 1649 to 3926); however, many pharmacists have not sought specialty credentialing. As of the year 2004, fewer than 5% of practicing pharmacists have sought any type of advanced practice certification, and optimal recognition and acceptance of specialization has clearly not yet arrived. The future of specialty certification will ultimately be defined by many factors, including attainment of provider status for pharmacists to be recognized by Combined Medicare-Medicaid Services, continued development of collaborative prescriptive practices (ie, currently, more than 40 states have such legislation), further expansion of postgraduate training programs including new degrees and specialty practice residencies, employer practices, and society's acceptance of new roles and practices for pharmacists. Over the past two decades, the growth in pharmacy residents has been impressive, from 356 to 1080 or approximately 300%.[16] As more and more students continue to seek postgraduate training to differentiate themselves from the typical graduate, the number of pharmacy practice residencies and specialty practice residencies will expand. A new cadre of specialty-trained practitioners will help drive the process of specialty recognition.

While it is uncertain which areas of pharmacy practice will be recognized as specialties for the future, discussion has centered around compounding, pain management or palliative care, and perhaps, ambulatory or primary care. Each new specialty must satisfy all seven criteria for recognition by BPS and ultimately the pharmacy profession, and this process will maintain the high standards set forth by the visionaries who began this process nearly three decades ago.

REFERENCES

1. Fenninger LD. *JASHP* 1991; 43:746.
2. Stevens R. *American Medicine and the Public Interest: A History of Specialization.* Berkeley: University of California Press, 1998, p 113.
3. American Board of Medical Specialties. www.abms.org/about.asp. Accessed October 10, 2003.
4. Sologoff S, et al. *Acad Med* 1994; 69:740.
5. Sharp LK, et al. *Acad Med* 2000; 77:534.
6. Maddox RR. *AJHP* 1991; 48:480.
7. Francke DE. *Drug Intel Clin Pharm* 1976; 10:593.
8. Cohelan, J, et al. *JAPhA* 1974; NS14:618.
9. Board of Pharmaceutical Specialties. www.bpsweb.org/New. Specialty.Recognition/shtml. Accessed 2003 October 10, 2003.
10. Grussing P, et al. *Am J Pharm Ed* 1983; 47:11.
11. Bertin RJ. *Ann Pharmacotherapy* 1997; 31:1532.
12. Pradel FG, Palumbo FB, Flowers L, et al. *JAPhA* 2004; 44 (in press).
13. Wells B. *Am J Pharm Ed* 1999; 63:106.
14. Council on Credentialing in Pharmacy. White Paper on Pharmacy Credentialing, www.pharmacycredentialing.org/ccp/CCPWhitePaper2003.pdf. Accessed December 10, 2003.
15. Pharmaceutical Research and Manufacturers of America. New Drug Approvals series, Washington, DC: PhRMA 1994–2003 www.phrma.org/newmedicines. Accessed December 29, 2003.
16. American Society of Health-System Pharmacists, Accreditation Services Division, Personal Communication (Bruce Nelson), December 29, 2003.

CHAPTER 121

Pharmacists and Disease State Management

Matthew K Ito, PharmD, FCCP, BCPS

James Palmieri, PharmD

Doug Geraets, PharmD, FCCP, BCPS

Disease state management (DSM) is a systematic population-based approach to medical care that is being used with increased frequency in a variety of health care systems in an effort to standardize and improve provider adherence to treatment guidelines. The goal of DSM is to improve treatment outcomes while controlling health care costs. The historical patient care model in medicine has been an individualized physician-patient approach that can result in fragmented and suboptimal care. Although individual clinicians incorporate information gained from their training, personal experience, and the medical literature into their daily patient care activities, this does not always translate into optimal care. As an example, in a multicenter survey from five regions of the United States, only 18% of adult patients with coronary artery disease (CAD) receiving cholesterol-lowering medication for at least 3 months achieved their National Cholesterol Education Program (NCEP)[1] low-density lipoprotein (LDL) cholesterol target of $\leq$ 100 mg/dL.[2] This suboptimal treatment does result in higher vascular events, death, and health care costs.[3] Patients with hypertension face a similar problem. Based on the Third National Health and Nutrition Examination Survey (NHANES III), only 34% of all patients with hypertension were at or below a systolic blood pressure of 140 mmHg.[4]

DSM has been defined by Zitter as "a comprehensive integrated approach to care and reimbursement based fundamentally on the natural course of a disease with treatment designed to address the illness with maximum effectiveness and efficiency."[5] Therefore, in this management system, each patient may be proactively triaged at different stages in his/her disease process using a defined care plan established from evidence-based protocols or guidelines, rather than a series of fragmented encounters with various parts of the health care system. This integrated approach is developed with a quantifiable economic structure and a defined quality improvement process.

The Disease Management Association of America (DMAA) is a nonprofit membership organization founded in 1999 to represent the disease management community. The DMAA has defined those components needed for a full-service disease management program as shown in Table 121-1.[6] Programs consisting of fewer components are considered disease management support services.

As part of a prescription drug management program, DSM can be used as one of the methods to control medication utilization and pharmacy expenditures. Other methods include utilization management (eg, quantity limitations, prior authorizations), formulary management (open or closed), delivery systems, (eg, retail, mail order), and benefit design and consumer cost sharing (eg, copayments, coinsurance). This chapter will focus on DSM and steps involved in developing an effective program.

HISTORICAL BACKGROUND

Until the 1970s, the primary mode of health care reimbursement was through fee-for-service. In this model, health care costs skyrocketed, physicians relied largely on accumulated individual practice experience for disease treatment, and patient care interventions, rational or not, were reimbursed. New technologies added to the cost of health care, and in a fee-for-service environment their values were rarely assessed. Managed care was 'born' as the diagnosis-related groups (DRG) system was instituted in the early 1980s by the federal government as a means to reign in health care costs, with beneficial results observed by the early 1990s (Fig. 121-1).[7] Private payers, while watching their bottom line, also demanded that costs be curtailed. Neither the public nor private sectors, however, were willing to forego quality. Therefore, managed care is ever evolving to adapt to the seemingly diametric opposition of cost and quality. DSM is both an example of and a microcosm for this evolution. Managed care first targeted hospital and physician costs, as these were and are the most costly components of health care. After hospital and physician cost containment, managed care organizations (MCOs) addressed prescription drug costs (ie, the third most costly budget item) and by the mid-1980s most large MCOs had prescription drug management programs, either internally developed or contracted, with cost containment as their primary focus.[8] The skyrocketing cost of pharmaceuticals continues to be a driving force behind cost containment measures employed by MCOs.

Although quality and cost containment have always been mutual goals of managed care, skyrocketing costs, coupled with a 'silo' approach to hospital, physician, and pharmaceutical cost containment had a neutral—and sometimes negative effect on quality care delivery. Consumers of health care began to perceive a sacrifice in the quality of care to maintain the bottom line. The health care industry responded with the development of DSM programs that would, if effective, integrate health care services across the patient care continuum, positively influence quality care, and maximize efficiencies that would lead to cost containment. Initially, DSM programs were offered as outsourced products developed by stand-alone vendors or, more often, by pharmaceutical manufacturers. Justly or unjustly, however, the DSM programs developed by pharmaceuticals manufacturers were hurt by the perception that they were offered as a means through which pharmaceutical manufacturers could market their drugs and gain an increase in market shares. Many of these programs have since been abandoned, merged with other programs, or sold outright. Increasingly, DSM programs are developed and or operated through health care systems that work to identify proven processes and apply these to the care of patients enrolled in their system.

Table 121-1. Disease Management Association of America (DMAA) Definition of What Components Need to be Included for Full Service Disease Management Programs

COMPONENTS OF A DISEASE MANAGEMENT PROGRAM

- Population Identification processes
- Evidence-based practice guidelines
- Collaborative practice models to include physician and support-service providers
- Patient self-management education (may include primary prevention, behavior modification programs, and compliance/surveillance)
- Process and outcomes measurement, evaluation, and management
- Routine reporting/feedback loop (may include communication with patient, physician, health plan and ancillary providers, and practice profiling)

Full Service Disease Management Programs must include all six components. Programs consisting of fewer components are **Disease Management Support Services.**

Pharmacy benefit management (PBM), itself an industry with the main function of effectively managing the drug benefit program of MCOs through unit cost containment and utilization management, may also offer DSM as a means of increasing the quality and value of their services. PBM companies maintain a complete database of medications dispensed for enrolled patients. This information is very useful to anyone attempting to maximize drug efficacy and minimize cost. As an example, adherence to a medication regimen can be inferred through a patient's refill history, which is maintained in the PBM database; for another, a member-patient's medication list used to treat a particular disease state is available through this same mechanism.

Finally, another way in which DSM is evolving is through consolidation of programs and services. Although DSM pro-

Table 121-2. Appropriate Medical Conditions or Characteristics to be Targeted for a Disease State Management Program

CHARACTERISTICS

- Well-defined disease course
- High cost
- Chronic diseases or conditions
- High frequency
- Available outcomes benchmarks
- Measurable outcomes
- Treatment methods variable
- High incidence of non-adherence
- Preventable therapeutic misadventure is common or catastrophic
- Rare occurrence

grams focused on one disease has demonstrated cost and quality improvements, further efficiencies can be obtained if patient care is less piecemeal. It is believed that this "patient-centered" approach may allow synergistic benefits if the co-morbidities being treated are related.[9]

DSM QUALIFIERS

Certain diseases or treatments lend themselves to DSM (Table 121-2). They include those in which the disease course is well-defined, and/or propel health care costs. Chronicity, prevalence, those with available benchmarks or definable, measurable outcomes, variability in treatment methodology, expensive therapies, and high incidence of nonadherence or preventable therapeutic misadventure are common characteristics. "Rare" diseases may qualify, because DSM programs can take advantage of economies of scale if cases from a broad geographic area are managed from a central location. Table 121-3 is an adaptation of the list of most costly medical conditions treated in the United States in 1997 to show DSM-appropriate conditions. Table 121-4 lists diseases or conditions successfully managed through a DSM program.[10] Many require drug therapy, providing the opportunity for pharmacists to play a key role in DSM.

PHARMACISTS AND DISEASE STATE MANAGEMENT

It is fairly well documented that pharmacotherapy-related outcomes can be improved by implementation of protocol-driven disease specific management programs by pharmacists collaborating with other health care providers. Noteworthy examples include an increased percentage of patients achieving NCEP LDL cholesterol targets following lipid-optimization,[11] a reduction in the length of hospitalization in patients taking warfarin guided by a pharmacist,[12] and a reduction in all-cause mortality in patients with heart failure receiving medication evalua-

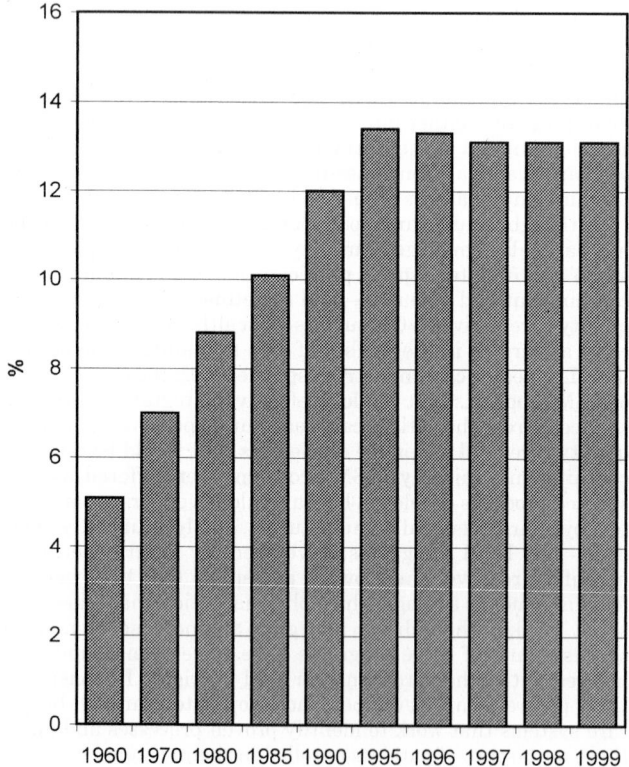

Figure 121-1. Total Health Expenditures as a Percentage of Gross Domestic Product, 1960–1999

Table 121-3. Selected Medical Conditions Among the Most Costly in 1997–Focus on Chronic Conditions Appropriate for Disease Management[7]

CONDITION	RANKING ($ MILLIONS)	TOTAL EXPENDITURE (THOUSANDS)	NO. OF PEOPLE AFFECTED
Heart disease	1	57,506	17,019
Mental disorder	4	29,731	20,152
Pulmonary disease	5	28,974	41,475
Diabetes	6	19,660	9,938
Hypertension	7	18,241	27,430
Cerebrovascular	8	16,333	2,252

Adapted from Cohen JW, Krauss NA. *Health Affairs* 2003; 22:129.

Table 121-4. Published Reports of Pharmacist Involved in Disease State Management (DSM) Programs

DISEASE STATES	FINDINGS	REFERENCE
Asthma	Significant reduction in ER visits and hospital admissions	Wantanabe et al.
Anticoagulation	Significant reduction in length of hospitalization	Dager et al.
	Significant reduction in total hospital costs	Mamdani et al.
Heart Failure	Significantly lower all-cause mortality	Gattis et al.
	Significant decrease in hospital readmissions	Riegel et al.
ICU Patients	Increase in cost savings related to pharmaceuticals	Baldinger et al.
	Significant reduction in preventable ADEs	Leape et al.
H. pylori	Cost-avoidance of $95 per patient	Segarra-Newnham et al.
Hyperlipidemia	Significant increase in patients meeting LDL-c goals	Ito et al.
Diabetes Mellitus	Reduction in mean HbA$_{1c}$ by 0.7% vs 0.1% in controls	Grace et al.
	Decrease in total health care costs	Gerber et al.
Hypertension	Significant improvement in BP, QOL, and patient satisfaction	Carter et al.
General DSM	Decrease total monthly medical costs	Munroe et al.

H = *Helicobacter*; ICU = intensive care unit; ER = emergency room; ADEs = adverse drug effects; LDL-c = Low density lipoprotein cholesterol; QOL = quality of life; BP = blood pressure.

tion by pharmacy.[13] These examples employ outcome-related pharmacist cognitive services that were made possible from the fairly recent evolution of the profession over the past 35 years or so.

In 1976, the American Pharmaceutical Association (APhA, recently renamed the American Pharmacists Association) established the Board of Pharmaceutical Specialties given the charge of developing and administering board certification examinations to pharmacists with specialized training or experience. To be visionary for the future needs such as these, schools and colleges of pharmacy voted in 1992 to adopt the six-year Doctor of Pharmacy degree as the only professional degree in pharmacy.

Around the same time, the profession of pharmacy was moving toward the pharmaceutical care model of patient-centered, outcome-oriented practice (as first outlined by Hepler and Strand) and away from product-oriented procurement as its primary focus.[14] This patient-centered practice resulted from advances in information technology, the increased role of pharmacy technicians, and the evolution of pharmacy automation. These changes place pharmacists in a unique position to broaden their scope of practice and increase services where appropriate as collaborative care providers aimed at maximizing health-related outcome and minimizing drug-related misadventures—all the while assuring cost-effective use of pharmaceuticals. Health care administrators, physicians, ancillary care providers, and the public are increasingly recognizing the unique training and knowledge that pharmacists have in support of these activities.

Requirements for pharmacists who are involved in DSM vary from state to state and among health care organizations. Typically, pharmacists who are involved in DSM have advanced skill development either through a residency or fellowship program or have acquired skills from years of experience. Other methods of development are available through various certification programs that will provide some of the foundations needed to participate effectively in DSM. The National Institute for Standards in Pharmacist Credentialing (NISPC) offer programs in Certified Disease Management (CDM) for anticoagulation, asthma, diabetes, and dyslipidemia. The NISPC is a credentialing organization composed of the APhA, the National Association of Boards of Pharmacy (NABP), the National Association of Chain Drug Stores (NACDS), and the National Community Pharmacists Association (NCPA). Each set of DSM standards is created by a panel of experts composed of practitioners, academicians, PBM managers, and board of pharmacy members. The development of additional DSM standards will be based upon the needs and recommendations of practitioners, schools of pharmacy, payers, and the general health care community. The goals of the CDM credential program are to assist in validating the pharmacists specialized knowledge and skills.

Credentialing earns pharmacists national recognition in specific disease states, increases revenue potential, and acknowledges their achievement and commitment to the profession and patient care. Further information is available at www.nispc-net.org.[15]

A Pharmacist's Role

Three strategies have been described[16] that, if followed, should help pharmacists develop practices that embody pharmaceutical care and DSM. First, careful planning of provided services should be carried out with buy-in from third party payers, physicians, and plan members. Second, close communication with the primary care physician regarding each patient's care should be maintained. And last, clear documentation of processes and outcomes should be maintained and measured against a reasonable benchmark.

The activities performed by pharmacists in managed care are not unique to this methodology and are discussed in more detail elsewhere in this book; however, it is interesting to note the ways in which these activities may benefit a DSM program. Pharmacists may provide primary care to patients in DSM programs through providing vaccinations, glucose and cholesterol screening and blood pressure monitoring in either the ambulatory care setting or in community pharmacy. In this role, pharmacists apply "pharmaceutical care" principles to manage patients with chronic medical problems, either making recommendations to a primary care or specialty physician, or prescribing under protocol. State law authorizes the latter, and rules may vary between states. In California, upon a physician's patient-specific authorization, pharmacists are authorized to initiate or adjust a drug regimen, order or perform routine drug therapy-related patient assessments such as vital signs, order drug therapy-related laboratory tests, and administer drugs and biologicals by injection, including immunizations.[17] In certain circumstances, pharmacists may be required to achieve advanced certification to perform these functions. For example, performing a fingerstick to assess blood sugar or cholesterol is beyond the scope of practice of pharmacists without first being certified to do so.

Pharmacists receive extensive training in pharmacology, pharmacokinetics, pharmacodynamics, and pharmacotherapeutics that makes them uniquely qualified to evaluate drug literature. Drug information activities performed by managed care pharmacists are used to support drug utilization review or medication use evaluation, as well as formulary management. All are important components for devising cost containment and utilization management strategies. These activities are also used to support an evidenced-based approach to DSM for developing population-based treatment plans and protocols. Further, physician and allied health professional education by pharmacists is conducted to provide a balanced assessment of supporting literature and facilitate acceptance of the treatment plans.

The public also values educational functions the pharmacists provide. Patient counseling to educate patients on the proper use of medications as well as their risks and benefits, is a necessary function both ancillary to, and within a DSM program to maximize pharmacotherapeutic regimens. Pharmacists' patient counseling activities have been demonstrated to improve adherence to the therapeutic regimen, increase therapeutic efficacy and outcomes attainment, and potentially harmful medication errors.[15]

Pharmacists may serve as case managers in a DSM program. This is particularly advantageous when the drug therapy regimen used to treat the disease is susceptible to drug-drug, drug-food, or drug-disease complications. DSM programs incorporating pharmacists as case managers have been successfully deployed to care for patients with among others, diabetes mellitus, depression, smoking cessation, cardiovascular risk reduction, anticoagulation, and hypertension.

Careers in pharmacoeconomics and outcomes research are being pursued by pharmacists in academic and industrial settings. These activities are undertaken to determine the value of medications for the treatment and prevention of disease, and the research may involve either a drug-specific focus or population-based health care delivery. Most pharmacy schools provide a solid background in science, therapeutics, and economics required to produce pharmacist graduates equipped with the skills necessary to make a valuable contribution in this developing field. Postgraduate training (eg, graduate study, fellowships) enhances these skills and prepares pharmacists for independent research.

COMPONENTS OF A SUCCESSFUL DISEASE MANAGEMENT PROGRAM

DSM programs tailor population-based outcomes to individualized patient care. The challenge for successful management of patients using the DSM format is to demonstrate that the benefits derived from this form of patient care (in the form of cost and quality improvements) outweigh the resources used. There are certain characteristics that successful DSM programs share. A reliable and extensive medical informatics infrastructure allows for easy access to patients and their medical records. This includes telecommunications, computer networking, and data storage. Case managers working within a DSM program may monitor patients' progress using telephone surveillance and/or web-based telephone data collection devices. Integrated data collection and storage across the continuum of care, though not required, best serves the practitioners of DSM for patient follow-up and for reporting cost and quality outcomes. Complete data that is accurate and timely is essential to the success of a DSM program. Data collected should be analyzed and compared to benchmarked data points when available [as, for example, from the National Committee for Quality Assurance's (NCQA) Health Plan Employer Data and Information Set HEDIS)] to demonstrate quality outcomes. Medical claims, clinical and humanistic (satisfaction) data are all useful data points to benchmark.

As mentioned previously, one of the basic principles of DSM is identifying and offering a patient the best care for their disease. Successful DSM programs base goals on evidence-based outcomes. They incorporate treatment guidelines (eg, national guidelines if available or those developed by the health system after critical assessment of the literature) to reduce the amount of variability in practice that can lead to cost and quality inefficiencies. Development of treatment guidelines should be a cooperative consensus of all disciplines involved, as well as expert opinion and evidence from the scientific literature (eg, using published evidence grading).

Care in a DSM program should be physician-directed, yet take advantage of the expertise of a multi-disciplinary ancillary health care team (mid-level providers and pharmacists) to improve care and cost efficiency. Proper use of ancillary care for patient monitoring and management not requiring diagnostic skills of a physician can improve quality, reduce care costs, and have a positive effect on physicians workload, making room for patient visits requiring diagnosis-related activities.

Acceptance of the program by the primary care physician and/or health plan is of paramount importance to the success of a DSM program. Authorization from one or both entities is required for patients to have access to the DSM program. A key to acceptance may include shared risk, which also includes shared cost savings. Changing prescribing patterns and adherence to treatment guidelines might be enhanced by reasonable financial incentive. In addition, the practitioners affected by DSM programs need to be included early in development of the program to gain their support.

DSM programs should be financially viable. As such, demonstrable outcomes are only part of the story. They must be couched within a reimbursement system that acknowledges benefit of integrated care delivery. For example, payers should recognize that the costs for pharmaceuticals (eg, beta-blockers, angiotensin converting enzyme inhibitors) may increase in a DSM program targeting congestive heart failure, but that other, offsetting costs (eg, hospitalizations, surgical procedures, lost productive time, patient discomfort) should be reduced. In contrast, a DSM program that increases total health care costs with improvement in outcomes may be at odds with the goal of the heath care system.

Patient and physician education helps ensure that a DSM program is successful. Patients are empowered through learning about their disease. Signs of proper therapeutic management as well as therapeutic misadventure enable the patient to stay out of trouble, if they are taught how to identify these. Likewise, physicians are more apt to incorporate proven therapeutic modalities into patient care if they are informed of evidenced-based best practices as eluded to earlier.

Finally, continuous quality improvement (CQI) processes should be incorporated into the practice model to monitor and enhance care practices. Compliance with guidelines and assessment outcomes (humanistic, clinical, and economic) should be evaluated periodically and new evidenced-based information needs to be incorporated into the treatment guidelines as well.

DEVELOPMENT OF A DISEASE STATE MANAGEMENT PROTOCOL

The Protocol

One of the first tasks for the pharmacist planning to provide DSM is a detailed and specific protocol. Generally, this would be specific to a particular disease condition or area. The protocol should spell out in detail the responsibility of the pharmacist and specific endpoints for drug therapy.

The pharmacist wishing to develop such a protocol need not start from "ground zero." Numerous examples of DSM services and protocols have been published or are readily available from national organizations (see examples Table 121-2).[11–13, 18–27] In addition, extensive reviews on establishing and evaluating clinical pharmacy services providing DSM have recently been published.[28–31]

The protocol should clearly define pharmacist responsibility, including prescriptive privileges, authority to order and monitor selected laboratory indices, and consultation privileges. In addition, patient follow-up intervals and outcomes expected of pharmaceutical care should be included. Quality improvement measures may also be included as part of the protocol and are highly recommended as discussed above.

Documentation of the DSM activities is also a key element. Without proper documentation, the pharmacist will be unable to manage accurately and safely the patient's disease condition. In addition, without adequate documentation, the pharmacist will be unable to obtain compensation for services as well as determine the economics of the program. Finally, programs with poor or absent documentation of patient care activities may run afoul of various regulatory bodies such as the Centers for Medicare and Medicaid Services (CMS; formerly the Healthcare Financing Administration, or HCFA), the Department of Health and Human Services (DHHS) and the Joint Commission on Accreditation of Healthcare Organizations (JCAHO). Documentation of the complexity of the interventions (eg, such as amount of time spent with a patient, extent of an examination, the medical decision making involved) should be included.

Most of all, objectives within DSM protocols should be realistic. Unrealistic objectives that have a low likelihood of being attained will serve to frustrate the pharmacist and disappoint the patient. Of equal importance, failure to meet one's objectives while increasing the utilization of resources will be a conflict for one's health care system.

As mentioned in the previous section, when developing DSM protocols and determining objectives for such services, pharmacists should consult clinical practice guidelines established by government agencies, professional organizations, or international bodies. Historically, such guidelines are evidence-based and compose a consensus of experts in a disease area or diagnosis group. A comprehensive database of evidence-based clinical practice guidelines and related documents is available online through the National Guideline Clearinghouse at: www.guidelines.gov supported by the Agency for Healthcare Research and Quality (formerly Agency for Health Care Policy and Research, AHCPR).

The protocol should make some effort to define the organizational structure of the DSM program or clinic. The schedule of the clinic (days meeting, hours of clinic), how patients are checked in/out and screened, and the time periods allotted for appointments should be included. Consideration must be given for the amount of time necessary to consult new patients versus returning patients. Policies for patients who do not keep appointments, rescheduling patients, and how many times a patient can be rescheduled prior to being dropped from the service need to be established.

The ultimate goal is a DSM protocol that is dynamic and designed to minimize difficulty for the pharmacist and other practitioners. Efforts should be made, most commonly on a yearly basis, to review the protocol, update those areas based on management guidelines, and to reassess overall structure, function, and objectives.

Collaborative Agreement with Health Providers

Pharmacists who desire to establish DSM programs must be willing to invest time and energy to establish strong professional working relationships with other providers (eg, physicians, nurses, nurse practitioners, physician assistants) and staff members. Several keys to building working relationships is being responsive, doing more than what is expected of the pharmacist, and being willing to spend time with patients. Most often, examples of pharmacists providing DSM involve the pharmacist having identified a physician "champion" or advocate for their activity. Often this individual is a general practitioner in primary practice or a specialist in a particular disease area (eg, cardiologist, endocrinologist). In addition, support from physicians higher up the administrative hierarchy (Chief of Staff, Associate Chief of Ambulatory Care) can be invaluable in allowing the pharmacist to establish and manage disease-specific clinic activities and/or clinics.

Collaborative practice agreements with a provider should be established as part of the DSM protocol. When establishing collaborative practice agreements, pharmacists and physicians must evaluate their needs to determine the types of services the pharmacist will provide. The majority of states have passed legislation that allow pharmacists to practice collaborative drug therapy management with physicians. However, even without legislation, most medicine and pharmacy practice acts are broadly worded to allow collaborative practice arrangements (including drug therapy management) to exist between pharmacists and physicians. Some states may require pharmacists credentialing (as discussed above) in DSM to practice under a collaborative agreement with a physician. The pharmacist will need to evaluate his/her own individual state requirements.

Promoting/Influencing Stakeholders

Once the DSM protocol has been developed, the pharmacist must consider promoting their services and influencing stakeholders (eg, patients, physicians, and the MCO). This will require in some cases tremendous educational efforts. As mentioned in the previous section, a physician "champion" will be essential in most cases to develop a favorable partnership with the stakeholders. The pharmacist must be prepared and flexible enough to meet the concerns of all stakeholders. The collection of member and provider satisfaction data will help to ensure the longevity of the program.

Requisite Equipment and Set-Up

The minimum equipment and space required to practice DSM is a private area to interview and examine the patient. An examination room in a clinic or physicians office will usually be available for this purpose. In the case of a clinic that is telephone surveillance-based, a private desk area that includes a telephone and personal computer is necessary. If not already available in the examination area, a small desk, several chairs, and electrical power access will be required. This additional space would be required for equipment, such as computers, and to allow for processing of paperwork. In addition, a combination television/VCR is a very helpful option in case instructional videos need to be viewed by the patient. The ideal situation would be a separate interview/counseling room that would also double as the pharmacist's office.

Documentation and Forms

As previously emphasized, documentation is a key element of DSM. Before initiating the service, forms that document accurately and adequately all activities of the pharmacist should be available. There is little reason, in this era, to utilize paper forms for processing this information. Every effort should be made to computerize all documentation and interventions of the pharmacist. Many institutions and physician clinics are progressing rapidly to a paperless "electronic" medical record, and the pharmacist should embrace this in his/her DSM practice. The Veterans Affairs Medical Centers, for example, have been utilizing electronic medical notes and medical record for several years. There are numerous examples of commercial systems available for documentation and maintaining a medical record. The pharmacist is encouraged to research these and consider their use. If paper documentation is utilized in patient care, the pharmacist should make sure to develop forms which adequately document the complexity of the interventions (eg, amount of time spent with a patient, extent of an examination, the medical decision making involved) to allow good patient management and appropriate billing to occur.

Billing and Reimbursement

Billing and reimbursement issues have been the pharmacist's curse when attempting to make DSM pay for itself. Pharmacists are restricted in their ability to bill for services and there are discrepancies in compensation for their services.[32] The pharmacist is at a disadvantage in that the Social Security Act does not recognize the pharmacist as a provider of health care management services. Efforts are underway to change this. However, legislation will be required at a federal level, and this will likely take years to accomplish. At the current time, there are essentially three mechanisms to obtain reimbursement through the federal government and that is through the CMS that oversees Medicare and Medicaid financing. These include "incident to" billing, under an outpatient technical component using ambulatory patient classification (APC) codes, or for outpatient diabetes self-management training as part of a multidisciplinary team.

In institutions and physicians offices, the pharmacist can use the physician provider number ("incident to" billing) to seek payment for professional services. In most cases the pharmacist would bill under CPT code 99211 (this reflects a 5 to 15 minute consultation). However, this reimbursement rate is low and likely inadequate to support a pharmacists position in most cases. Also there are specific requirements (eg, the encounter must occur in a physicians office or clinic, physician must be present) that must be met to allow the pharmacists to use this type of billing. This may vary from state to state and by regional Medicare payers.

Billing at a higher CPT code for services such as 99212–99215 is controversial and may be determined by regional payers. For example, pharmacists in some states providing pharmacy DSM services are billing at the higher CPT codes and getting reimbursement from payers (eg, Medicare).

Medicare initiated a prospective payment system for reimbursement of outpatient visits in July 2000. The outpatient reimbursement is procedure-based (versus inpatient which is diagnosis-related reimbursement). Medicare-approved providers continue to bill professional services, but the outpatient technical component (ie, facility fee) is replaced by the new reimbursement system. This new system sets consistent reimbursement rates for outpatient services and charts nonprofessional procedures performed to known patient-care level APC codes known. As pharmacists cannot bill as a provider, their services become part of the overall facility reimbursement. The pharmacist's time to provide care increases the technical level allowing reimbursement which is often several times higher than the lowest "incident to" physician fee.

Finally, in January 2001 CMS (then HCFA) finalized rules on Medicare coverage of outpatient diabetes self-management training that allows payment of the pharmacist for diabetes training as part of a multidisciplinary team.

Unfortunately, payment for professional services for community pharmacists is more challenging and serves as a disincentive for the pharmacist to engage in DSM activities. Some possibilities are summarized below. Pharmacists approved by CMS as immunization providers may bill for immunizations. The first step in billing for services is to obtain a Medicare provider number to allow for billing. This can be accomplished by securing the necessary forms or submitting electronically at www.cms.hhs.gov. At the current time, the pharmacist is limited to billing insurance and third party carriers for in-person management only. No reimbursement is allowed for any form of telephone management. For in-person DSM, the pharmacist will be able to bill for laboratory services and for the non-MD health care provider visit. For example, if billing for anticoagulation management services, the pharmacist can bill a fee for obtaining the blood sample using a CPT code. For venipuncture-only the Medicare CPT code is G0001 and for venipuncture or finger stick it is 36415. The prothrombin time/International Normalized Ratio can be billed using CPT code 85610QW.

Other options are to charge a professional fee. Some pharmacists, particularly in community pharmacy, have found some success directly billing the patient a professional fee. Generally, attempts at billing private insurance carriers have been disappointing with many declining to reimburse the pharmacist based on lack of provider status at the federal level.

Potential Barriers

Potential barriers to DSM practices have been alluded to or discussed in some detail in previous sections of this chapter. The main barriers are acceptance by other providers of the services of the pharmacist and the reimbursement issues covered above. Each discipline that participates in the DSM program will have different interests, goals, and views. It is not paramount that there is total agreement on every issue. However, trust is one of the most important elements that needs to be established and confirmed.

Acceptance of other providers must be earned by investing the time and energy to create strong professional relationships with other providers and staff members. The pharmacist must be friendly, do beyond that what is expected, and be agreeable to spend time with patients.

As for reimbursement, success is a moving target, however documentation is a key element along with billing appropriately and adhering to legal requirements.

BUSINESS PLANS

It is common for pharmacists in managed care and at private health care facilities to create a business plan. Business plans are often very detailed and is beyond the scope of this chapter. The business plan may contain some background and description of the service, market analysis and strategy, operational structure and process, financial projections, milestones, schedule, action plan, risks, opportunities, conclusions, and any supportive documents. The business plan should be written in a manner to deemphasize or shift away from a "drug silo" cost assessment to an emphasis of the total direct health care costs. Some DSM programs may increase drug utilization, but lower total health care costs by reducing hospitalizations and emergency room visits.

QUALITY ASSURANCE

Evaluation of Outcomes

Evaluation of health outcomes is the ultimate measure of success of DSM. Measures of health outcomes should be an essential part of the management protocol. Usually, the initial step is a baseline evaluation of current indicators of performance for disease control and outcome. Measured outcomes of the DSM program may include well-known indicators of disease control such as glycosylated hemoglobin, blood pressure, or lipid concentrations, as well as secondary complications, hospitalizations, QOL, patient and physician satisfaction, mortality, or health care costs. As mentioned previously, these outcomes should be benchmarked to measures such as those from NCQA HEDIS or JCAHO.

In addition, measuring process-oriented outcomes, such as percentage of patients treated to established guidelines which are a component of the DSM protocol may be another useful measure of service quality. After implementation of the program, outcomes assessment leads to continuous modification of the program from feedback and constantly updated practice standards.

Ironically, one of the dichotomies of pharmacist's activities in DSM is that increasing the overall quality of care may require the need for increased prescription costs (ie, through maximization of existing prescriptions and new prescription orders) to improve overall patient health and outcomes. Fortunately, studies have shown that pharmacists are able to ensure overall appropriate use of medications resulting in improved disease control, reduced health care use, and overall decreased health care costs.[11,8–21,25]

More difficult measures of quality of care associated with DSM include reduction of disease events and affects on survival (reduced mortality). Because long-term outcomes require longer-term data collection and a concurrent control group (using historical controls have their own inherent problems), which are not always practical, intermediate outcomes (ie, LDL cholesterol) may be more practical.

Final measures of quality of DSM services are humanistic (patient-specific) outcome measures such as patient satisfaction, quality of life (QOL) measures, and functional status. Recent study findings[33,34] have suggested more data or more specific questionnaires are required to document possible benefit of pharmacy care on humanistic outcomes. Patient satisfaction may assess numerous aspects of a DSM services including satisfaction with clinic process and waiting times, pharmaceutical care, disease control and endpoint attainment, and provider communication.

SUMMARY

Many diseases go untreated or are not managed optimally in the United States and other countries. DSM programs can be used as an effective strategy for enhancing patient outcomes and reducing management cost of diseases by ensuring consistent care using evidence-based treatment algorithms or protocols. In addition, education of patients and physicians is one key element in the success of a DSM program. The type and depth of training pharmacists receive during their formal pharmacy education and postgraduate training programs as well as enhanced recognition through board certification has opened up opportunities for collaborative care and other cognitive services within DSM programs. DSM programs are becoming more popular with health care systems and MCO and exemplify the unique expertise of the pharmacist toward making them effective. Thus the opportunity for pharmacists to enhance their role in disease-oriented approaches is here.

REFERENCES

1. Pearson TA, Laurora I, Chu H, et al. *Arch Intern Med* 2000; 160:459.
2. Executive summary of the third report of the National Cholesterol Education Program (NCEP) expert panel on detection, evaluation, and treatment of high blood cholesterol in adults (Adult Treatment Panel III). *JAMA* 2001; 285:2486.
3. Ito MK, DeLucca GM, Aldridge MA. *J Cardiovasc Pharmacol Therapeut* 2001; 6:129.
4. DiTusa L, Luzier AB, Jarosz DE, et al. *Am J Manage Care* 2001; 7:520.
5. Zitter M. *Med Interface* 1995; 7:70.
6. http://www.dmaa.org/definition.htlm
7. Data from the Centers for Medicare and Medicaid Services, National Health Statistics Group, Office of the Actuary, National Health Expenditures, 2000.
8. Navarro RP. In: Navarro RP, ed. *Managed Care Pharmacy Practice.* Maryland: Aspen, 1999.
9. Carroll J. *Managed Care.* www.managedcaremag.com/archives/0009/0009.dm_consolidate.html. September, 2000.
10. Cohen JW, Krauss NA. *Health Affairs* 2003; 22:129.
11. Ito MK, Lin JC, Morreale AP, et al. *Am J Health-Syst Pharm* 2001; 58:1734.
12. Dager WE, Branch JM, King JH, et al. *Ann Pharmacother* 2000; 34:567.
13. Gattis WA, Hasselbad V, Whellan DJ, et al. *Arch Intern Med* 1999; 159:1939.
14. Hepler CD, Strand LM. *Am J Hosp Pharm* 1990; 47:533.
15. http://www.nispcnet.org
16. Navarro RP, Chrstensen D, Leider H. In: Navarro RP, ed. *Managed Care Pharmacy Practice.* Maryland: Aspen, 1999.
17. California Business and Professions Code, Chapter 9, article 3, section 4052
18. Wantanabe T, Ohta M, Murata M, et al. *J Clin Pharm Ther* 1998; 23:303.
19. Mamdani MM, Racine E, McCreadie S, et al. *Pharmacotherapy* 1999; 19:1064.
20. Riegel B, Thomason T, Carlson B, et al. *Congest Heart Fail* 1999; 5:164.
21. Baldinger SL, Chow MS, Gannon RH, et al. *Am J Health-System Pharm* 1997; 54:2811.
22. Leape LL, Cullen DJ, Clapp MD, et al. *JAMA* 1999; 282:267.
23. Segarra-Newnham M, Siebert WF. *Hosp Pharm* 1998; 33:205.
24. Grace KA, McPherson MI, Burstein AH. *Am J Health-System Pharm* 1998; 55:S27.
25. Gerber RA, Liu G, McCombs JS. *Am J Managed Care* 1998; 4:991.
26. Carter BL, Barnette DJ, Chrischilles E, et al. *Pharmacotherapy* 1997; 17:1274.
27. Munroe WP, Kunz K, Dalmady-Israel C, et al. *Clin Ther* 1997; 19:113.
28. The ACCP task force on ambulatory care clinical pharmacy practice. *Pharmacotherapy* 1994; 14:743.
29. Kassam R, et al. *J Am Pharm Assoc (Wash)* 1999; 39:843.
30. Lepinski PW, Woller TW, Abramowitz PW. *Top Hosp Pharm Manage* 1992; 11:86.
31. Skledar SJ, Hess MM. *Am J Health-Syst Pharm* 2000; 57:S23.
32. Speer A, Bess DT. *Am J Health-Syst Pharm* 2003; 60:78.
33. Malone DC, Carter BL, Billups SJ, et al. *Med Care* 39:113.
34. Funderburk FR, Pathak DS, Pleil DS. *Pharm Pract Manag Q* 1998;17(4):54.

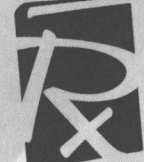

CHAPTER 122

Development of a Pharmacy Care Plan and Patient Problem Solving

Deepika Vadher, PharmD, BCPS

Bradley C Cannon, PharmD

INTRODUCTION

The practice of pharmacy has undergone several evolutionary leaps in the last four decades. Emphasis on the creation, preparation and dispensing of pharmaceuticals has given way to pharmacotherapeutic decision making and measurable patient outcomes, with increasing focus on patient safety. As this emphasis has shifted, academic pharmacy has adopted new paradigms and approaches in its preparation of future practitioners. Examples include introductory clinical pharmacy experiences, problem-based learning, and service learning opportunities. Students must understand their current and future roles in the ever-changing health care system, Further, students' didactic experience should include elements that develop and nurture their knowledge, skills, attitudes, and values. One central concept that often forms the framework for this approach to learning is that of pharmaceutical care.

Pharmaceutical care is a straightforward concept. It involves the pharmacist working in concert with his/her patients and other healthcare providers to identify, monitor, and achieve desirable health-related outcomes through the appropriate use of medications. While many consider the first reference to modern-day pharmaceutical care to be in 1989,[1] the theoretical construct was described several years before.[2] This expanded approach to care has been the subject of much discussion ever since, as well as recognized and supported in recent years by other healthcare providers.[3] And, while this advance appears to be logical and sensible, pharmaceutical care remains very difficult to define. At times, pharmaceutical care is perceived to include only a specific set of practitioners or practice settings. Further, in spite of a variety of excellent models for the provision of this care (ie, inpatient and outpatient), the delivery of pharmaceutical care is far from uniform within the profession.

In spite of our advancing knowledge and technology, drug-related problems and adverse drug events are a major source of morbidity and mortality in the United States. In a recent study, 4.4 adverse drug events were found to have occurred per 100 patient days in an inpatient setting, with 58% deemed to be preventable.[4] These results appear to be consistent with other studies.[5,6] Further, medication-related errors have been identified as a significant cause of emergency room visits and subsequent hospitalizations.[7-10] Thus, new approaches to the safe and effective use of medicinal products should be considered. One way this may be accomplished is through the enhanced utilization of the pharmacist in the drug delivery and utilization process.

Comparison to Clinical Pharmacy

Recently, the American College of Clinical Pharmacy (ACCP) has proposed the definition of clinical pharmacy to be "A health science discipline that embodies the application and develop-

ment, by pharmacists, of scientific principles of pharmacology, toxicology, therapeutics, clinical pharmacokinetics, pharmacoeconomics, pharmacogenomics, and other life sciences for the care of patients."[11] The origin of the phrase appears to be related closely to the development of cognitive services in the inpatient setting[12] as well as concentrating on patients and their needs. As these services are intended to optimize the care provided to patients by pharmacists, there appears to be a significant amount of overlap with the provision of pharmaceutical care. In fact, all providers of pharmaceutical care may be considered to be practicing as clinical pharmacists. However, the explicit definition of pharmaceutical care requires the provider to assume a shared responsibility for therapeutic outcomes, as well as the communication of their efforts with other healthcare professionals. This requires an expanded view of pharmaceutical care as a strategy rather than a discipline. Further, while clinical pharmacy is, by definition, provided by pharmacists, it has been proposed that pharmaceutical care may be provided by a variety of healthcare professionals.[1]

This chapter is intended to contribute toward the pharmacy student and the practitioner's ability to provide pharmaceutical care. The care provided must be based upon a logical, effective, and patient-specific pharmaceutical care plan. This chapter is written to demonstrate what constitutes a pharmaceutical care plan and how it is created by the pharmacist.

Who Provides It?

Pharmaceutical care is an equally appropriate practice model for independent community practice, chain community practice, institutional practice, among other settings. While the specific services provided may differ among these practice environments, the underpinning philosophy of pharmaceutical care remains the same: achieving definitive outcomes for patients. Some examples of the various care settings include: outpatient clinics, emergency patient care centers, and specific inpatient units such as medical/surgical intensive care, infectious disease, transplant, pediatrics, trauma, internal medicine, and cardiac, among others. Indeed, several of these are featured in other chapters of *Remington*.

A central feature of pharmaceutical care is to identify, prevent and resolve drug-related problems (DRPs). Pharmaceutical care and pharmacist-managed drug-related problems may differ among practice settings and from patient to patient. Examples of pharmaceutical care services offered include: generic and therapeutic interchange, pharmacokinetic and therapeutic consultation, patient interviewing, patient counseling, team rounding, drug information, laboratory monitoring, and monitoring drugs with either high costs, narrow therapeutic windows, or potential adverse effects, to list just a few.

ROLE OF A PHARMACIST

The profession and roles of pharmacists are continuously evolving. There is a consensus among all major pharmacy organizations that pharmaceutical care is a viable and justifiable option and goal for the profession of pharmacy. Pharmaceutical care is defined by Hepler and Strand[1] as the responsible provision for providing drug therapy for the purposes of achieving definite outcomes. Pharmaceutical care focuses on activities that lead to positive patient outcomes, and accepting end results of medication therapy remains important in providing such services. According to Penna and colleagues,[13] to practice pharmaceutical care, a pharmacist must be a scientific problem solver, a good communicator, educator and learner. Primary activities involved in pharmaceutical care include: obtaining a medication history, identifying real and potential drug-related problems, developing a pharmacy care plan to include implementing and monitoring parameters to resolve and prevent drug-related problems, and evaluating the plan to determine if clinical outcomes have been achieved through documentation, patient consultation follow-up to determine if the desired clinical outcomes have been achieved. All this is achievable through competent skills and knowledge gained to provide reliable cognitive services. Cognitive services or value-added services (eg, patient drug or disease counseling) allow pharmacists to attain positive outcomes.[14]

Cognitive services are closely linked with the concepts of clinical pharmacy and pharmaceutical care. Key components of both include application of one's judgment, knowledge, and ability to solve DRPs. To practice effectively, pharmaceutical care focus must be placed on patient satisfaction. It is important to conduct a one-on-one patient session to review past disease and medical histories, current drug, herbal, dietary supplement, and non-drug therapies; related signs and symptoms; and desired outcomes. Collection of this information allows the pharmacist to identify patient drug-related problems and develop a pharmacy care plan to help resolve these problems.[15,16] Table 122-1 demonstrates the proposed nine steps to Pharmaceutical Care for Pharmacists.

In carrying out daily responsibilities, identifying DRPs or developing a pharmacy care plan, pharmacists must also address societal needs. Societal needs may be identified by providing value-added services for patients and performing these activities with ethical and professional prerogatives in mind. On a daily basis, pharmacists may be confronted with professional dilemmas that are legally, ethically and/or morally challenging (eg, patient confidentiality issues, pro-life issues). One must learn to balance these challenges while maintaining a level of personal comfort to practice successfully and deliver optimal care on behalf of the patient.[17]

Table 122-1. Nine Steps to Pharmaceutical Care

1. Develop a covenantal relationship between the pharmacist and the patient
2. Collect relevant drug, disease, and patient information
3. Interpret this information to identify all the patient's drug-related problems
4. Prioritize the patient's drug-related problems
5. Identify those drug-related problems for which the pharmacist will assume responsibility
6. Identify patient-specific outcomes for each drug-related problem for which the pharmacist has assumed responsibility.
7. Develop a therapeutic plan to attain the desired patient-specific outcomes for each drug-related problem
8. Develop a monitoring plan to assess whether predetermined outcomes have been attained
9. Implement and follow the pharmacy care plan, which consists of desired outcomes, therapeutic plan, and monitoring plan.

Adapted from Winslade NE, Bajcar JM, Bombassao A: Pharmacist's Management of Drug-related Problems: A Tool for Teaching and Providing Pharmaceutical Care. Pharmacotherapy 1997; 17(4):805; with permission.

STUDENT RESPONSIBILITIES

Education

According to the AACP Commission, the goal of pharmaceutical education is to "inculcate students with values necessary to serve society as caring, ethical, learning professional and enlightened citizens."[17] This is accomplished by providing a curriculum which enables students to learn, develop skills, and nurture values necessary to meet the needs of patients and society. Pharmacy education lays the foundation for students to acquire the knowledge and abilities required to be successful pharmacists in the future. Students are responsible for becoming active participants in this process, incorporating knowledge and developing skills in their career while embracing life-long learning.[17]

IMPORTANCE OF SKILLS

Skills necessary for the delivery of pharmaceutical care include patient care skills, clinical skills, application of drug knowledge and drug information skills, and professional skills (eg, interpersonal skills, service orientation). Collecting, collating, and organizing patient information from medical charts and computer databases is necessary. Equally important is the personal time a pharmacist invests in obtaining the information directly from the patient. The concept of patient-centered practice or patient care skills becomes evident when the pharmacist attempts to build a relationship of trust with the patient. This interaction will help identify and determine patients' preferences for their health-care outcomes. Patient encounters for students are planned to occur during internship and/or the experiential component (eg, fourth professional year clerkship rotations) of their curriculum. Routinely, students on rotation provide clinical pharmacy services under the direct supervision of a clinical pharmacy preceptor. The goal of the preceptor is to bridge classroom learning to real-life clinical experiences, enhance students' drug knowledge, and help develop the students' professional judgment and values. Clinical skills (eg, being capable to interpret blood levels and lab data, assess the patient's needs, apply therapeutic data to drug-related problems) are key factors for an optimal drug regimen. Furthermore, drug knowledge and information skills, as well as the ability to rationalize therapeutic decisions are equally important in achieving optimal patient care. Finally, professional skills remain essential for a successful, future practicing pharmacist. Professional responsibilities, whether learned through school during courses or heightened during clerkship rotations, distinguishes all health care professionals.[17] Examples of professional responsibilities for pharmacists may include holding high professional aspirations for the practice of pharmacy, a commitment to serve the community and humanity, serving as mentors for future pharmacists, and maintaining personal standards of integrity, competency, reasoning, and life-long learning.

For one to be proficient with skills gained or acquired, one must demonstrate competency or mastery of the skills learned. In pharmacy school, competency may be ascertained through successful outcomes on examinations, quizzes, and simulated patient exercises, among others. To test student competency and skill sets in a clinical setting, the use of algorithms and flow charts may be used on clerkship rotations. Flow charts (Fig. 122-1) encourage a uniform approach to problem solving and assist students in identifying DRPs, learning to ask appropriate questions, and becoming capable of formulating recommendations for monitoring and follow-up planning.[18]

Experiential practice and the work environment also help students gain experience toward identifying and resolving DRPs, not all of which will be clear-cut textbook scenarios. Awareness of such ambiguities exists throughout pharmacy practice and in other healthcare arenas. Professional prerogatives, ethical dilemmas, and the balance of both may be quite challenging. The American Pharmacists Association (APhA)

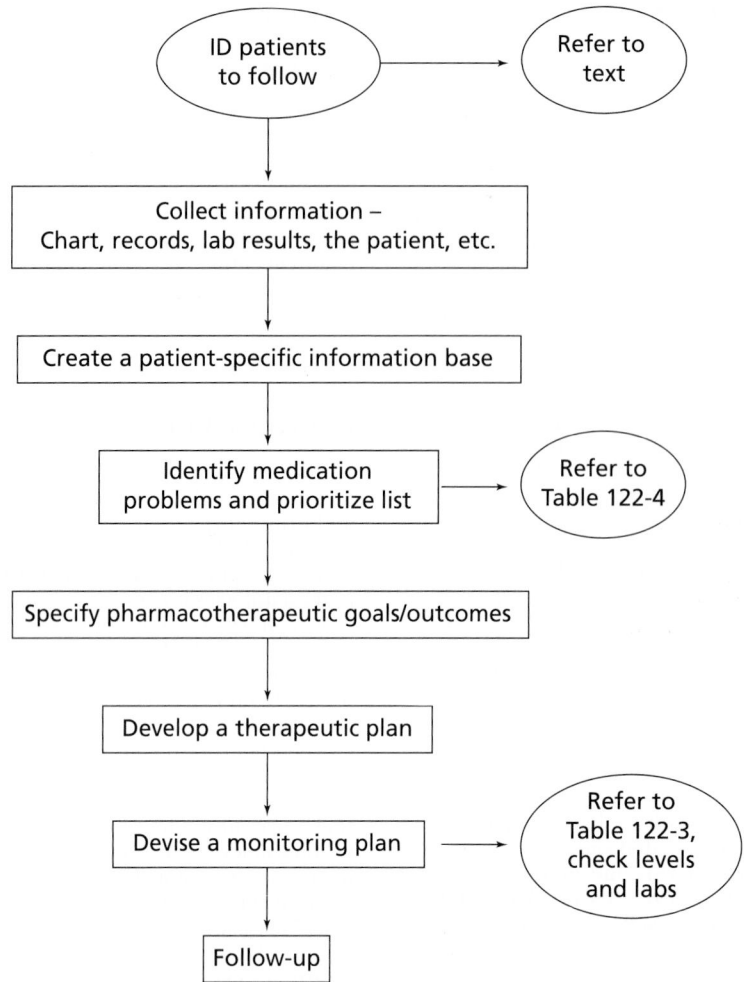

Figure 122-1. Example of a Flow Chart

Code of Ethics, states "a pharmacist should hold the health and safety of patients to be of first consideration and should render to each patient the full measure of professional ability as an essential health practitioner."[17] In some instances, a pharmacist's moral and ethical beliefs may conflict with his/her professional duty. For this reason, as a future pharmacist, it is important to be comfortable making decisions in the face of these uncertainties.[19]

Identifying Patients to Follow

To develop a pharmacy care plan and problem solve, the student will need to identify patients with DRPs to follow. Numerous studies have indicated that elderly patients (eg, older than 65 years of age) are at an increased risk for DRPs because, typically, they have multiple medical problems, have multiple drug therapies, and the physiological effects of aging on the disposition of drugs warrants close monitoring. Greater than three concomitant diseases, five or more medication regimens, twelve or more doses of drugs a day, and frequent medication regimen changes in the past year can lead to nonadherence and demand further investigation. Students may also learn by monitoring patients with compromised renal or hepatic function, those that demonstrate abnormal clinical laboratory values, and those who present with potential drug-drug interactions or duplicate therapies. Sometimes regulatory or

reimbursement issues dictate or necessitate tracking the care of certain patients (eg, high cost drugs and therapies). By this selective process, one can effectively concentrate his/her activity on those patients who have the greatest potential for benefit from clinical services.[20]

DEVELOPING A PHARMACY CARE PLAN

Pharmacy care plan notes help to formalize and document a specific course of treatment for the patient. For example, when a patient is admitted to the hospital, the physician formulates a medical care plan for that patient. In parallel, the clinical pharmacist develops a pharmacy care plan for the patient. It is important that the plan be evaluated and revised according to the changing needs of the patient on a continuing daily basis.[21] Strand and colleagues developed a framework for the provision of a pharmaceutical care plan in their practice site, termed the pharmacist's workup of drug therapy (PWDT). Care plans will vary somewhat depending upon specific pharmacy settings. The PWDT allows the pharmacist to gather data, prevent or identify and resolve DRPs, and monitor the selected therapy (see Fig. 122-2A,B).[22]

The first step in formulating a care plan is to build a caring relationship with the patient, collect and organize information relevant to the patient, and create a patient-specific database. This relationship should be predicated on an honest and open

Example A: Documentation Form Used by PharmD Students for Interventions

COMMUNITY PHARMACY CLINICAL CONSULTATION

Patient's initials ________________ Approximate age ________________

Physician's initials ________________ Date ________________

Illness/conditions from profile or history (check):

___ Arthritis	___ Hyperlipidemia	___ Diabetes
___ Hypertension	___ Angina	___ Pregnancy
___ Asthma/COPD	___ CHF	Other ________________

Current Rx/OT medicatons and dose (from patient and profile):

________________ ________________

________________ ________________

Medications with which patient has had past problems (allergies, reactions):

____

Drug-related problem(s): ________________

____

Subjective: ________________

____

Objective: ________________

____

Assessment: ________________

____

Plan: ________________

____

Follow-up with physician and/or patient: ________________

____

Consultation peformed at:

________________ ________________

PharmD Student Pharmacist

Adapted from Anderson RJ, et al. Documentation of pharmaceutical care activities in community pharmacies by doctor of pharmacy students. *Journal of Pharmacy Practice* 1995;8:83–88.

Example B: **Patient initials**

Student name:

Allergies/Reactions:

Write up date:

Deepika Vadher, PharmD, BCPS

CC:

HPI:

Emergency Room

Admit vitals: T   BP   HR   RR

Ht: Wt: IBW: CrCl (est):

Admit Labs: Other labs:

Treatment in ER:

PMH:

Family Hx:

Social Hx:

Studies/Labs Pending:

Consults:

Home medications/ OTCs/ Herbals: (List drug, dose, frequency and indication)

Differential Diagnosis:

ROS: Findings

GEN:

HEENT:

NECK:

CV:

PULM:

ABD:

GI:

GU:

EXT:

NEURO:

Prioritized Problem List:

Hospital Course (Day ___)

♦ *Include problem, all supporting data/labs, pharmaceutical care plan, vitals, recent labs, recommendations, medications added or deleted, monitoring plans for efficacy and toxicities, consults, pending labs and discharge plans, etc*

Problems:	**Progress, supporting studies, labs, treatment regimens** (started, continued, discontinued, etc.)**and plans**	**Monitoring/ pending labs**	**Your Interventions**

Discharge Plans (Focus on new medications started, old medications deleted, disease state education, etc.)

Mercy Fitzgerald General Medicine Form – D. Vadher (rev.9/04)

Figure 122-2. *Continued.*

exchange of information to aid in solving patient problems and making recommendations to the attending physician or interventions on behalf of the patient. Both parties (pharmacist and patient) must mutually respect the pharmacist-patient relationship to address and provide optimal care. To provide such service, the pharmacist must communicate with the patient to ascertain his/her needs, wants, desires and goals, and evaluate if his/her wishes will be met with the prescribed or recommended treatment regimens.[23] Addressing patient-specific problems requires asking appropriate questions to help gain insight about the patient's understanding of his/her disease states, drugs and his/her attitude toward drugs, drug therapy, and drug usage patterns. Asking appropriate open-ended questions to gain comprehensive information is useful to help create a patient-specific database. Also, interviewing the patient helps build a rapport with the patient. However, before interviewing the patient, the pharmacist should review the patient's chart, medical card-ex, or prescription databases to determine the diagnosis, past medical history, medication history, and any other pertinent data (eg, recent labs, family and social history).[21] In an institutional setting, the pharmacist may examine the medical record and collaborate with the medical staff and patient to collect needed information. In a community setting, data collection may be limited to observations, conducting an interview with the patient, and in some circumstances, communicating with the physician or healthcare professional.

The next step in the development of a pharmacy care plan includes identifying DRPs and their subsequent prioritization. Collecting and processing relevant data should result in a list of patient-specific DRPs. This is accomplished by listing the patient's potential and actual medication-related problems and then ranking them by severity. The classic priority of problems, from most to least severe, first includes acute and then chronic problems. Finally, historical problems and other health-related risk factors are listed from most to least immediate. The medication history interview provides information regarding patient medication prior to admission and often will identify drug problems that will necessitate a change in drug therapy. Throughout this process, modifications must be made daily to address patient-specific problems.[23]

After collecting the information, the pharmacist should address the patient's needs, identify any potential problems and establish desired therapeutic goals and outcomes. The pharmacist's main responsibility is to maximize positive outcomes of drug therapy and minimize drug misadventures. Patient therapy should result in the achievement of definite outcomes that improve the patient's quality of life. Definite and desired outcomes that improve a patient's quality of life are (1) cure of a disease; (2) elimination, amelioration, or reduction of the patient's symptoms; (3) arresting or slowing the disease process; (4) preventing further disease or symptoms; and (5) returning the patient's physiological status to a normal healthy state. Pharmaceutical care is patient-oriented, and it involves developing, implementing, and monitoring a therapeutic plan that is designed to achieve these outcomes.[21,24]

The next step in the development of a pharmacy care plan involves therapeutic planning to achieve patient-specific outcomes or endpoints. The pharmacist's recommendation should incorporate therapeutic efficacy, safety, comfort and convenience, adherence, and cost considerations to the regimen. The best pharmacotherapy regimen for the patient should involve patient-specific, individualized drug dosing, frequency of drug administration, and duration of treatment. Most therapeutic problems will demonstrate more than one empirically acceptable solution. Thus, alternatives should always be considered and included in the plan. Viable alternatives require comparative analysis and critical review of the medical literature to reveal which agent(s) is(are) best suited for the patient based on clinical efficacy, safety, patient satisfaction, and cost.

The processes of problem-solving and the development of a care plan are incomplete until monitoring produces data that serves to empirically support the recommended solutions. One

Table 122-2. Example of Drugs with Narrow Therapeutic Indices Requiring Pharmacist Monitoring [14]

EXAMPLES OF DRUGS WITH NARROW THERAPEUTIC INDICES	RECOMMENDED THERAPEUTIC SERUM LEVELS
Warfarin	INR 2-3 or 2.5-3.5 (dependent on indication)
Heparin	aPTT = 1.5-2.5 × the normal (ie, baseline 30 s → 45-75 s)
Aminoglycoside	Gent/tobra: <2-5-6 (8-10) Amikacin: {9-}15-24
Vancomycin	5-10 (trough)–20-50 (peak)
Digoxin	0.8-2 OR 1.5-2.5 (arrhythmia) mcg/ml
Theophylline	10–20 mcg/ml
Phenytoin	10–20 mcg/ml
Others:	
Valproic Acid	50–100 mcg/ml
Procainamide	3–10 mcg/ml

must assess specific, desired endpoints to document the attainment of outcomes and resolution/prevention of DRPs through a monitoring plan. The next step focuses on the monitoring parameters of serum drug levels or surrogate markers for the drug. Monitoring for efficacy and toxicity reflects the active involvement by the pharmacist. Monitoring for efficacy assesses whether a given drug regimen is working to achieve the therapeutic goals previously identified, and monitoring for toxicity determines if the patient is experiencing any unwanted adverse effects from the regimen (see Table 122-2 for a listing of representative drugs to monitor with therapeutic levels for each).[25]

The final step in the development of a pharmacy care plan involves following up on one's recommendations and re-evaluating the patient's problem list. It is imperative to continue to monitor the patient after discharge or counseling session as this act provides continuity of patient care. Times, dates, and mechanisms of follow up (ie, consultation in person or via a telephone call) should be documented in the care plan note. This allows the pharmacist-patient relationship to flourish and continue building toward a trusting, meaningful relationship.[14]

PREVENTION

A central feature of pharmaceutical care is to identify, resolve and prevent DRPs. Throughout the process of problem solving and identifying DRPs, importance should also be placed on the prevention of future, potential problems. Preventing future DRPs involves identifying: drug allergies, inappropriate dosages, drugs with narrow therapeutic indices that require frequent monitoring, exacerbation of disease due to suboptimal doses, patient nonadherence, herbal/dietary supplement product use, suspected drug abuse, and potential for drug-drug interactions. The presence of these DRPs leads to less-than-optimal therapeutic patient outcomes and could result in future hospitalizations. The cost to society of drug-induced hospitalization can be immense in morbidity, mortality, and treatment, and therefore, is a topic of great importance to clinicians, health care administrators, and society in general.

Drug-related hospital admissions may be precipitated by a host of factors including adverse drug reactions, drug-drug interactions, drug misuse, inadequate or improper therapy, and nonadherence leading to disease exacerbation or complications. To date, numerous studies have found an increased rate of hospital admission rates secondary to medication noncompliance and/or adverse drug reactions. The actual number of DRPs necessitating hospital admission may be higher than reported because of lack of documentation, further underestimating the problem.[24] Table 122-3 demonstrates examples of Pharmacy Care Plan notes.[26]

Table 122-3. Example of a Documentation Form for Drug Related Problems Used by PharmD Students on Rotation with Deepika Vadher Pharmacy Care Plan/Clerkship Rotation Worksheet

Patient initials _____ Student Name: _____ Date Written: _____

DRUG-RELATED PROBLEM	OUTCOMES	ASSESSMENT	THERAPEUTIC PLAN	THERAPEUTIC PLAN END POINTS	MONITORING PLAN	PLAN END POINT MET?
List problem and all supporting data (labs, review of symptoms, vitals, etc.)	Address the following: • Clinical or outcome • Pharmacother-peutic	List and assess all drug and non-drug treatment related to problem.	Which drug or non-drug treatment should be instituted or changes made to existing drug therapy? (drug, dose, frequency, route, etc.)	List parameters for each outcome: (Goal BP, SCr, etc.)	For each desirable endpoint— what should be monitored and frequency of monitoring	Any interventions?
1)						
2)						
3)						
4)						

PROBLEM SOLVING

Initially, collecting and interpreting relevant patient information, identifying patient health-care needs, and formulating a DRP list may be challenging for the pharmacy student. These steps require that the student learn to recognize, obtain, and process relevant drug, disease, and patient information in a problem solving format. Problem solving involves identifying drug-related problems, suggesting interventions, and documenting patient outcomes. Each patient is unique, and how one approaches each particular problem is specific for that individual patient. Problem solving is a learned and developed skill which frequently requires fine tuning over time. As the saying goes, "the road to success is always under construction" and with due time one will sense a level of comfort in approaching and solving problems.[27]

Identifying Drug-Related Problems

As discussed earlier, the primary focus of pharmaceutical care is placed on the patient. Properly-educated, skilled and developed pharmacists have familiarity and knowledge of prescription medications, over-the-counter medications, and herbal/dietary supplements. This knowledge base serves as a very thorough and reliable method of obtaining the patient's mediation history. Once one has identified which patients to monitor, the next step involves identifying medication-related problems for the specific patient. After obtaining a thorough patient history, review the current medication regimen for allergies; drug-drug and drug-food interactions; nonprescription and herbal/dietary supplement medication use; adverse reactions; therapeutic duplication; and appropriate drug selection, dose, duration, and dose frequency to aid in processing a medication-related problem list.

The type of pharmaceutical problem identified in the community pharmacy setting may differ from that reported in the hospital practice environment. Therefore, it is important to be cognizant about one's practice site setting before identifying and focusing on related problems. In a study evaluating drug-related problems in the hospital and community settings, it was found that underdosing comprised 31.5% of student interventions in hospital settings versus 3% in the community setting. The incidence of potential drug interactions and adverse drug reactions was found to be four-fold greater in the community setting when compared to the hospital setting.[28] Table 122-4 demonstrates a listing of drug-related problems.[22,29]

Making Recommendations

Assessing the DRP list and making therapeutic recommendations or interventions requires clinical knowledge and a strong pharmaceutical foundation. Staying abreast of clinical knowledge and continually striving for improvement will aid in the transition from student learning to application of knowledge gained during clerkship rotations and the work environment. Access to information and becoming familiar and knowledgeable of where to obtain information may help address and resolve DRPs. Reliable and validated internet resources, drug information resources, the primary medical/science literature, and national guidelines may help guide the management of one's patient. In 1989, the federal government was charged with the development of guidelines (which were later endorsed by specialty groups and other organizations) to aid clinicians in the proper management and treatment of specific, clinical problems. Guidelines are educational tools that serve as a source of guidance to aid clinicians in their decision-making.

Table 122-4. Drug-Related Problems Encountered by Pharmacist Monitoring[16]

• Untreated condition
• Improper drug selection
• Underdose
• Failure of patient to receive drug
• Overdose
• Adverse drug reaction
• Drug-drug interaction
• Drug-food interaction
• Drug without indication
• Nonadherence
• Duplicate therapy
• Allergies
• Requiring renal or hepatic adjustments
• Miscellaneous-
• Poly-pharmacy

Another approach to aid in clinical decision making is to use the results of patient care research or literature, or, in other words, practice evidence-based medicine. Evidence-based medicine includes decision making regarding pharmacotherapy that has been found to be beneficial for the group of patients being studied. Making recommendations in conjunction with guidelines and practicing evidence-based medicine helps provide optimal patient care.

Documenting Recommendations

After identifying the DRPs and making clear, concise recommendations, the next step is to document the intervention. As a profession, pharmacists must share responsibility for patient outcomes and record their recommendations, defend/support their reasons, and demonstrate expected outcomes. Medical and nursing documentation is widely accepted. Routinely, physicians and nurses document clinical patient care activities. To justify continued clinical services in the past, pharmacists have documented administrative projects and protocols. However, these have not been necessarily related to direct patient care. The trend towards pharmaceutical care focuses on patient care and documentation, which will help develop and improve services rendered by pharmacists. Such services should include written or verbal documentation of recommendations.[29] Either form of documentation is appropriate, however, it is important to be clear and succinct. During one's initial experience with documentation, the student's preceptor will have to proofread and approve all documentation of recommendations prior to its transmission to allied healthcare practitioners. As students become more comfortable and proficient with documenting actions and plans, they may be able to act more independently—depending on the preceptor and practice setting.

SOAP NOTES

The suggested format for organizing patient notes in medical charts is to use the SOAP note. Written SOAP notes include **S**ubjective and **O**bjective data, **A**ssessment of the problems, and appropriate **P**lans. A strong database that includes information about the patient, the disease, and any drugs is necessary for effective clinical decision making and documentation.

Subjective data is elicited by interviewing the patient. General subjective patient data includes, among others, the patient's chief complaint, history of present illness, previous medical problems, current medications, allergies, social (eg, smoking, alcohol, illicit drug use) and family history, and history of adherence to medications. Objective data includes all pertinent patient vital signs, physical examination notes, and pharmacological review of systems and clinical laboratory values. The assessment portion includes primary and secondary diagnoses, which encompasses a comprehensive and relevant explanation of the DRPs, therapeutic alternatives, and the rationale for the recommended therapeutic plan. Finally, the plan should contain a description of the desired clinical and pharmacotherapeutic outcomes. The plan is developed based on the subjective and objective information and the final assessment of each problem. The therapeutic plan should include a detailed monitoring plan for each DRP and future patient education initiatives. Written recommendations are then incorporated into the patient's chart, which is a legal document.[27, 29]

Verbal documentation may entail direct communication with the healthcare provider about one's concerns and recommendations for a patient. Problems involving drug therapy should be discussed in a clear and concise manner with the proper healthcare team member. At times, the physician may be too distracted focusing on acute patient issues and may not have an opportunity to read a written recommendation, but may be available for verbal consultation. Verbal communication followed by chart documentation of the care plan helps to emphasize your concerns

for the patient's wellbeing. Whether a recommendation is written or verbal, the pharmacist is an integral part of a healthcare team, whose focus is achieving positive optimal patient outcomes. Numerous studies indicate that physicians accept 80% to 90% of pharmacist-generated recommendations. This strongly supports the pharmacist's role in a patient care team.[30]

IMPORTANCE OF DOCUMENTATION

"If it is not documented, it has not been done." For the profession of pharmacy to evolve toward cognitive services and away from distributive functions, and to secure reimbursement for all new services, pharmacists must document value-added pharmacy services. Reimbursement from the provision of pharmaceutical care that is beyond customary dispensing and counseling should be an incentive for all practicing pharmacists. In the future, a successful pharmacist will be recognized by their impact on cost savings and the number of pharmaceutical interventions, rather than the number of prescriptions filled per day.[28]

IMPORTANCE OF PHARMACEUTICAL CARE

Throughout this chapter, much emphasis has been placed on the importance of pharmaceutical care. However, as with any change to a profession and how it is practiced, one encounters many barriers for implementation. Such barriers include: inadequate education and less-than-optimal skill development of pharmacists, pharmacist reluctance "to become involved and patient oriented," unnecessary and overly restrictive legal requirements, limited access to and communication of patient-specific information among practitioners, lack of time to implement new practice designs, limited market-driven demand, current lack of compensation for professional services, facility design and space utilization, and restriction issues. Legal and risk management issues with documentation may deter future pharmacists from providing and charting pharmaceutical care. However, with appropriate education and practical experience, these barriers will be overcome and pharmacists will learn to become comfortable with documentation and accept responsibility for patient care outcomes. Success requires dedication, personal effort, motivation, and energy to provide competent pharmaceutical care.

PATIENT EDUCATION

To provide adequate patient education, it is important that the patient knows the drug name, indication, dosage or strength, and frequency of his/her medication(s). Focus may be placed on patients with a history of nonadherence, new prescriptions, new diagnosis, chronic diseases, potential drug-drug interactions, or multiple daily medications. In some hospitals, the nursing staff is mainly responsible for medication counseling. However, pharmacists are better qualified to offer such services. Some hospitals have pharmacists conducting discharge counseling. Restructuring pharmacist responsibilities to provide pharmaceutical care will make the opportunity to provide discharge counseling for the profession attainable in healthcare settings. Through discharge counseling, the pharmacist, along with allied healthcare team members, may help the patient make the difficult transition from the controlled hospital environment to his/her home. Most states mandate outpatient counseling and this is a wonderful encouragement, inducement, and opportunity for the pharmacy student to develop this skill during the experiential component of the curriculum.

PATIENT ADHERENCE

Adherence to one's medication regimen is essential to optimize therapeutic outcomes and achieve maximum benefit to the patient. The pivotal role of the pharmacist toward optimizing adherence encompasses many actions: assessing adherence problems, identifying predisposing factors contributing to non-adherence, providing comprehensive counseling, and recommending specific adherence strategies targeted to individual patient needs. Nonadherence can be a result of many factors including, but not limited to, medication regimen complexity (eg, how a dosage is administered, timing, form of medication), other existing conditions or diseases, and personal values and healthcare beliefs. Pharmacists remain uniquely positioned to assess and treat adherence-related problems that may adversely affect patients' health outcomes.

Adherence Assessment

Patients may be selective in the information they wish to receive. Nonadherence is a multivariant, complex problem, which may be influenced by patient's health beliefs, the extent to which they feel in control of their own health, their cultural norms, and strategies they have developed to cope with their illnesses. There are two methods to assess adherence: direct and indirect methods. The direct method employs blood-level monitoring and urine assay for the measurement of the drug and/or its metabolites/markers. Indirect methods of assessing adherence utilize, among others, patient interviews, tablet/capsule counts, refill records, and drug reminder sheets or tables, list a few.[31]

SUMMARY AND CONCLUSION

Pharmaceutical care may be provided by a wide range of practitioners and all pharmacists involved in the provision of patient care. Many of the principles of pharmaceutical care are also embraced in the practice of clinical pharmacy, making the two difficult to distinguish. Both approaches require the use of knowledge and skills gained in formal academic training and with experience, as well as a determined approach to life-long learning. Essential skills include oral/written communication and problem solving, and should be an integral part of the student's professional, on-campus education, and reinforced in the Advanced Practice Experience portion of the curriculum.

Often the end product of this care is the creation of a pharmaceutical care plan. Examples include a pharmacist's work-up of drug therapy (PWDT) or SOAP note, and should include a prioritized list of issues, monitoring parameters, and specific outcomes to be achieved. This plan is built on trust and understanding between patient and provider, and focuses on mutually developed goals. The documentation of all provided services is critical, and serves to demonstrate the professional responsibility pharmacists assume in the provision of pharmaceutical care. This also serves to justify the need for, and reimbursement of, cognitive services.

As the role of a pharmacist continues to evolve, so too will the reality of pharmaceutical care. To date, the consuming public largely considers pharmacists to be knowledgeable and trusted, and often turns to them for advice and information. However, there are still many more of the public who are unaware of the skills of the pharmacist beyond those of dispensing. As pharmacist cognitive services are developed, implemented, and expanded to impact more of the general public, it is possible that the monitoring of many chronic diseases will be accomplished in the community or ambulatory setting. The continued, active participation in the identification, resolution, and prevention of drug-related problems will continue to impact patients positively and serve to define further the role of the pharmacist in the healthcare system.

REFERENCES

1. Hepler CD, Strand LM. Opportunities and responsibilities in pharmaceutical care *Am J Pharm Ed* 1989;53(suppl):S7–15.
2. Brodie DC, Parish PA, Poston JW. Societal needs for drugs and drug related services. *Am J Pharm Ed* 1980;44:276–8.
3. Pharmacist scope of practice. American College of Physicians–American Society of Internal Medicine [position paper]. *Ann Intern Med* 2002;136:79–85.
4. Forster AJ, Halil RB, Tierney MG. Pharmacist surveillance of adverse drug events. *Am J Health-Syst Pharm* 2004;61:1466–72.
5. Classen DC, Pestotnik SL, Evans RS, Lloyd JF, Burke JP. Adverse drug events in hospitalized patients. Excess length of stay, extra costs, and attributable mortality. *JAMA* 1997;277(4):301–6.
6. Bates DW, Spell N, Cullen DJ, Burdick E, Laird N, Petersen LA et al. The costs of adverse drug events in hospitalized patients. Adverse Drug Events Prevention Study Group. *JAMA* 1997;277(4):307–11.
7. Winterstein AG, Sauer BC, Hepler CD, Poole C. Preventable drug-related hospital admissions. *Ann Pharmacother* 2002;36(7–8):1238–48.
8. Hafner JW, Belknap SM, Squillante MD, Bucheit KA. Adverse drug events in emergency department patients. *Ann Emerg Med* 2002;39(3):258–67.
9. Schneitman-McIntire O, Farnen TA, Gordon N, Chan J, Toy WA. Medication misadventures resulting in emergency department visits at an HMO medical center. *Am J Health Syst Pharm* 1996;53(12):1416–22.
10. Dennehy CE, Kishi DT, Louie C. Drug-related illness in emergency department patients. *Am J Health Syst Pharm* 1996;53(12):1422–6.
11. http://www.accp.com/report/rpt0204/art01.php Defining Clinical Pharmacy. Accessed 11/12/04.
12. Lipman AG. Integrating clinical and distributive pharmaceutical services: implications for clinical pharmacy education. *Am J Pharm Educ* 1986;50(1):63–6.
13. Penna RP. Pharmaceutical care: Pharmacy's mission for the 1990s. *AJHP* 1990; 47:543–9.
14. Kassam R, Farris KB, Burback L. Pharmaceutical care research and education project: Pharmacists' interventions. *J Am Pharm Assoc* 2001; 41:410–10.
15. Barnett CW, Nykamp D, Hopkins W. Provision and documentation of cognitive services by pharmacy students and their preceptors in the community setting. *J Pharm Teaching* 1994; 43:63–75.
16. Winslade NE, Bajcar JM, Bombassaro A. Pharmacist's management of drug-related problems: A tool for teaching and providing pharmaceutical care. *Pharmacotherapy* 1997; 17(4):801–809.
17. Buerki RA, Vottero LD. The changing face of pharmaceutical education: Ethics and professional prerogatives. *Am J of Pharm Educ* 1991; 55:71–74.
18. Robertson KE. Process for preventing or identifying and resolving problems in drug therapy. *AJHP* 1996; 53:639–50.
19. Briceland LL, Hamilton RA, Kane MP. Pharmacy students' experience with identifying and solving drug-related problems during clinical clerkship. *AJHP* 1993; 50:294–6.
20. Koecheler JA, Abramowitz PW, Swim SE. Indications for the selection of ambulatory patients who warrant pharmacist monitoring. *AJHP* 1989; 46:729–32.
21. Bennett RW, Bryant BG, Kelly AL. Development of a pharmacy care plan. *AJHP* 1973; 30:698–701.
22. Strand LM, Cipolle RJ, Morley PC. Documenting the clinical pharmacist's activities: back to basics. *Drug Intell Clin Pharm* 1988;22(1):63–7.
23. Binyon D. Pharmaceutical care: its impact on patient care and the hospital community interface. *The Pharmaceutical Journal* 1994; 253:344–49.
24. Johnson JA, Bootman JL. Drug-related morbidity and mortality. *Arch Intern Med* 1995; 155:1949–56.
25. Drug Information Handbook. Individual Drug Monographs. Lexi-Comp. 2004
26. Bajcar JM, Wichman K. Implementing the practice functions of pharmaceutical care–a pilot study in critical care. *CJHP* 1999; 52:234–239.
27. Briceland LL, Kane MP, Hamilton RA. Evaluation of patient-care interventions by Pharm.D. Clerkship students. *AJHP* 1992; 49:1130–32.
28. Anderson RJ, Nykamp D, Miyahara RK. Documentation of pharmaceutical care activities in community pharmacies by doctor of pharmacy students. *J of Pharm Prac* 1995; 8:83–88.
29. Strand LM, Cipolle RJ, Morley PC. Documenting the clinical pharmacist's activities: Back to basics. *Drug Intell Clin Pharm* 1988; 22:63–7.
30. Klopfer JD, Einarson TR. Acceptance of pharmacists' suggestions by prescribers: a literature review. *Hosp Pharm* 1990; 25:830–2.
31. Nichols-English G, Poirier S. Optimizing adherence to pharmaceutical care plans. *J Am Pharm Assoc* 2000; 40:475–85.

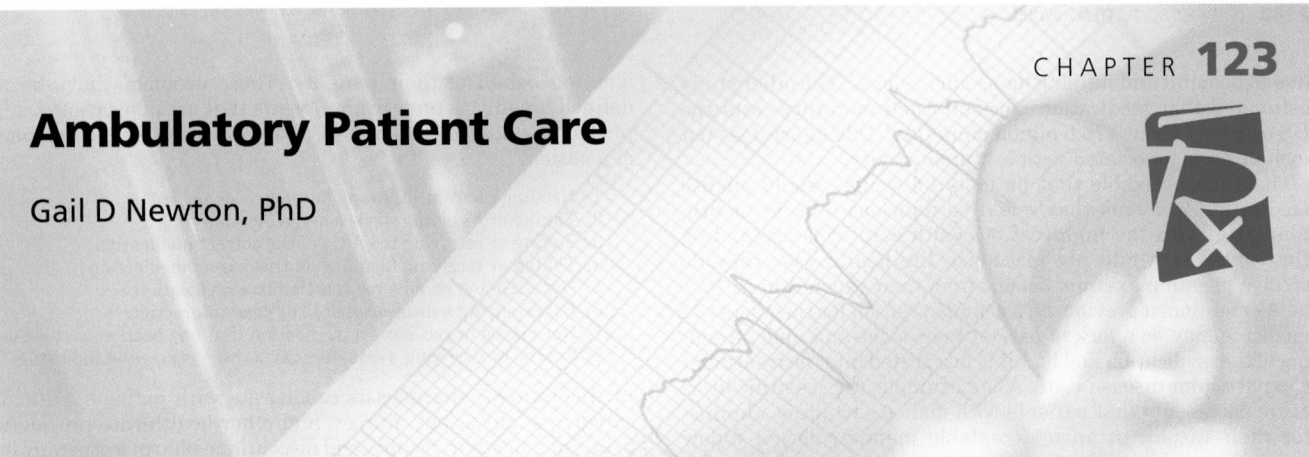

CHAPTER 123

Ambulatory Patient Care

Gail D Newton, PhD

Various designations are used to categorize patients: institutionalized, noninstitutionalized, inpatient, outpatient, bedridden, and ambulatory. Strictly speaking, ambulatory patients are those who are able to walk (ie, those who are not bedridden). Therefore, ambulatory patients may be inpatients of an institution, such as a hospital or extended-care facility, if they are not confined to bed. However, the term ambulatory patient has become more restrictive in its modern usage simply to mean a noninstitutionalized patient.

Ambulatory patients referred to here are noninstitutionalized patients who have the responsibility for obtaining their medication, storing it, and taking it. They may or may not be outpatients, depending upon where they receive their treatment. They may even be in a wheelchair and, strictly speaking, not ambulatory, but if they are not institutionalized they will have the same basic responsibility for their medication as *walking patients*.

Whether patients consult a physician who may prescribe medication or whether they decide to treat themselves, the community pharmacist more than likely will come into contact with them. It is important, therefore, for the pharmacist to have an understanding of these patients so that as a pharmacist and member of the health-care team, the best possible health care for ambulatory patients may be provided through proper use of knowledge and judgment.

MEDICATION-RELATED NEEDS OF AMBULATORY PATIENTS

It is known that the ambulatory patient does not adhere always to the directions for taking medicine. There are a number of reasons for this, and the reader is advised to consult Chapter 115 for a thorough and enlightening discussion of patient compliance. Through the decade of the 1970s, numerous studies demonstrated that patients widely misuse medications, with frequency ranges between 20% and 82%.[1] This wide variation reflects study differences, medication class differences, and investigator interpretation of patient misuse of medication.

In one of the earliest studies, Latiolais and Berry[2] compiled a number of ways in which patients may misuse medications. Many of these same problems exist today and are

1. Overdosage
   a. Taking more than the prescribed dose at any one administration
   b. Taking more than the prescribed number of doses in any one day
   c. Taking a dose, prescribed as needed, at a time other than when needed
   d. Taking the same medication from two or more different bottles simultaneously

2. Underdosage
   a. Taking less than the prescribed dose at any one administration
   b. Omitting one or more doses
   c. Discontinuing the drug before the prescribed duration of time
   d. Omitting the dose of a medication, prescribed as needed, when it is needed
3. Taking a dose at a different time if a time has been specified in the directions
4. Taking a dose in a form other than that specified in the directions
5. Using the wrong route of administration
6. Taking medication that has been discontinued
7. Taking outdated medications
8. Taking someone else's medications
9. Taking two or more medications that are contraindicated therapeutically
10. Failing to get the prescription filled
11. Failing to understand how to use the administration unit properly (eg, inhaler)
12. Failing to understand how to use or administer the dosage form properly

Using the above criteria, the authors found that 42.8% of the patients sampled were misusing their medications and that 4.4% misused their medicine in such a manner as to pose a serious threat to their health. The types of misuse committed most frequently were overdosage and omission of doses. Overdosage represented 41.3% of the total misused prescriptions. Omitting one or more doses occurred in 23.6% of the misused prescriptions. Another result of this study showed that of the prescriptions being misused, patients actually were aware they were misusing about one-half of them.

This apparently deliberate misuse perhaps is more understandable when viewed with respect to the single most often mentioned reason, occurring fully one-third of the time, that the patient did not understand the instructions. The second most frequent reason given by the patients for not following directions was that they thought they needed another dose. Another frequent reason was that the patient thought he or she was cured and stopped taking the drug before the prescribed time.

In 1992, a study by Clepper estimated that one-half of the 1.8 billion prescriptions dispensed on an annual basis are taken incorrectly.[1] It also estimated that 90% of all outpatients make mistakes taking their medications. Further, these mistakes account for 10% of all hospital admissions in the general population and 25% of all hospital admissions in the elderly. As a result, health-care costs increase and work productivity decreases. However, the most alarming finding of this study was that patient noncompliance may be linked to more than 125,000 deaths annually.

Two of the most recent studies have provided estimates of the actual cost of medication misuse in the US. One study estimated these costs to be approximately $100 billion, with more than one-half due to loss of productivity and nearly one-third due to hospital and nursing home admissions.[3] The other study estimated that medication morbidity and mortality costs the US economy about $76.6 billion annually.[4] This figure does not include costs associated with lost productivity.

It is inconceivable that patients knowingly would misuse medication in a way that would be injurious to their health. Similarly, with the high cost of health care, it is astounding that patients would not maximize the health care they do receive to gain maximum benefit from their expenditures.

As mentioned previously, a common reason for the misuse of medicine may be a lack of patient knowledge and understanding of the medication and how it is integrated into the treatment of a particular disease state. As an example, the scientific literature documents that patients with diabetes mellitus administer their insulin in an unacceptable manner, do not follow their diets, exhibit poor foot care, and do not test their urine and/or blood correctly.[5] Although bad habits and/or a lack of responsibility on the part of patients may account for some of these behaviors, lack of patient understanding of the importance of each treatment component for the prevention of disease complications is also a factor in many instances.

Other patient misconceptions also contribute to medication misuse. For example, *If one tablet is good, two will be even better,* is a common patient belief that is fraught with danger. Patients also frequently discontinue medicines inappropriately for a variety of reasons. In this context, a recent study identified the most common reasons for patients not having prescriptions refilled.[6] These reasons, in decreasing order of importance were that the

1. Medication was not working.
2. Medication was causing side effects.
3. Condition improved.
4. Patient received negative information about the medication.
5. Cost of the medication was too high.
6. Patient was confused about how to take the medication.

The noted philosopher and educator in medicine, Sir William Osler, in 1891, captured the essence of man and medicine when he stated that, "the desire to take medicines is perhaps the greatest feature that distinguishes man from animals." Unfortunately, his statement did not capture the mode in which man takes medicine, as demonstrated by the findings of the investigations described previously. These results clearly demonstrate the need for skilled professionals to assist patients to gain optimal benefit from their drug therapy. As medication experts who are often the most accessible health-care providers, community pharmacists are uniquely positioned and professionally obligated to fulfill this need for ambulatory patients.

THE PHARMACIST'S RESPONSIBILITY

In years past, the responsibility of the pharmacist was to dispense prescriptions accurately, provide medication counseling, and answer questions of concern to the patient. Recently, however, the profession of pharmacy has adopted pharmaceutical care as its mission and thereby extended the responsibility of the pharmacist.[7] Pharmaceutical care focuses pharmacists' attitudes, behavior, commitment, concern, ethics, functions, knowledge, responsibilities, and skills on the provision of drug therapy to individual patients. The goal is to achieve optimal outcomes that improve the patient's quality of life. These outcomes may include

1. Cure of the disease
2. Elimination or reduction of symptoms
3. Arresting or slowing the disease process
4. Prevention of disease
5. Diagnosis of disease
6. Desired alterations in the physiological processes

Pharmacist providers of pharmaceutical care assume responsibility to identify, prevent, and resolve medication-related prob-

lems on behalf of their patients. These problems have been defined broadly as undesirable events that are of psychological, physiological, social, or economic origin and may be the function of a patient:

1. Needing pharmacotherapy but not receiving it
2. Taking or receiving the wrong medication
3. Taking or receiving too little of the correct medication
4. Taking or receiving too much of the correct medication
5. Experiencing an adverse reaction to a medication
6. Experiencing a drug-drug or drug-food interaction
7. Not taking or receiving a medication that has been prescribed or
8. Taking or receiving a drug for which there is no valid indication.[8]

In this context, pharmacists collaborate with patients, patient caregivers, physicians, nurses, and other health-care providers to initiate, monitor, modify, and discontinue pharmacotherapy to avoid or resolve these medication-related problems. To that end, pharmacist providers of pharmaceutical care engage in a series of sequential steps to ensure that individual patients receive cost-effective pharmacotherapy that results in optimal therapeutic outcomes. These steps include having the pharmacist

a. Establish a committed relationship with individual patients
b. Collect, synthesize and interpret relevant patient information
c. Define and prioritize the potential and actual medication-related problems of the patient
d. Establish a desired pharmacotherapeutic outcome for each medication-related problem
e. Determine feasible pharmacotherapeutic alternatives to achieve each desired outcome
f. Select the best pharmacotherapeutic solution based upon individual patient circumstances
g. Design a monitoring plan to determine if the desired pharmacotherapeutic outcome has been achieved and
h. Implement the individualized pharmacotherapeutic and monitoring plans and evaluate and document the results of pharmacotherapeutic and monitoring plans.[8]

An advantage of pharmaceutical care over previous definitions of pharmacy practice is its applicability to all practice settings and to prescription *and* nonprescription therapies (see Chapter 114). Further, research demonstrates that pharmaceutical care services provided by pharmacists add value to the care of both institutionalized and ambulatory patients. This added value includes improvements in patient outcomes, enhanced patient compliance, and reduced health-care costs associated with medication misadventuring/misuse.[9]

In spite of these findings, realization of pharmaceutical care roles has been slow, particularly in ambulatory practice settings. To encourage further evolution of pharmaceutical care in ambulatory settings, the US Department of Health and Human Services' (DHHS's) Office of the Inspector General in 1990 summarized the current status of clinical services available in community settings, described barriers that limit the availability of these services, provided recommendations to reduce these barriers, and strongly recommended the establishment of strategies to deliver pharmaceutical care comprehensively in the ambulatory setting.[10]

Subsequently, the Omnibus Budget Reconciliation Act of 1990 (OBRA 90) was enacted and required each state Medicaid Agency to institute a Drug Use Review (DUR) program for covered outpatient drugs by no later than January 1, 1993. This act also required pharmacists to provide prospective utilization (ie, patient profile) review and counseling for Medicaid patients. It is hoped that societal and professional pressure will be such to ensure that all patients and not just Medicaid patients will receive these services. In fact, a number of states have legislated that these services will be provided to all patients.[11]

These legislative developments indicate a need for pharmaceutical care services in ambulatory practice settings. It is the intent of this chapter to operationalize further the concept of pharmaceutical care in this context so that community pharmacists may continue to evolve toward the realization of pharmaceutical care roles in their practices.

Establishment of a Committed Relationship with Individual Patients

The first step in the provision of pharmaceutical care is the establishment of a committed relationship with the patient. To that end, pharmacists must seek and be granted authority by their patients to intervene on their behalf. Pharmacists also may need to secure permission from other health-care providers and patient caregivers (eg, in cases in which the patient is a child or unable to visit the pharmacy in person) to provide pharmaceutical-care services. The key to doing so in all instances is effective communication.

Building a committed relationship cannot occur at a distance. The pharmacist must interact directly with the patient to earn his or her trust and to obtain permission to take responsibility for the outcomes of drug therapy. Thus, pharmacists in an ambulatory setting must take the initiative to introduce themselves and their services at the time the patient first presents a prescription.

Ideally, the pharmacist should invite the new patient into a private or semiprivate area of the pharmacy to explain the proposed relationship, it's benefits, and his or her commitment to the patient's well-being. Realistically, it may be impossible for the pharmacist to interview the patient at the time the prescription is originally dispensed, because of time constraints imposed by other professional responsibilities. In this case, the pharmacist should arrange to meet with the patient at another, mutually convenient time.

Committed relationships are rarely the result of a single interaction. In addition, by its very nature, pharmaceutical care is an iterative and ongoing process, as long as the patient has unresolved medication-related problems. Therefore, once a rapport has been established, the pharmacist must interact regularly with the patient to strengthen the relationship and to collect additional data necessary to ensure that the patient's pharmaceutical-care needs continue to be met.

COLLECTION, SYNTHESIS, AND INTERPRETATION OF RELEVANT PATIENT INFORMATION

As mentioned previously, the pharmacist's primary responsibility in the delivery of pharmaceutical care is to identify, prevent, and resolve medication problems. A key factor in the fulfillment of this obligation is the availability of essential patient data. These data have been categorized in various ways by dif-

ferent authors. The specific framework used to categorize patient data is less important than the consistent use of a single method to do so. This ensures that all potentially useful information is considered for each patient.

For the purposes of the present discussion, patient information is organized into three categories. Specific data items are grouped within each category as illustrated in Table 123-1. To make appropriate decisions about patient therapy, pharmacists must understand the utility of different types of information in the decision-making process. Further, they must realize that different decisions require different types of patient information. Thus, an appropriate and comprehensive database for a specific patient may or may not include all of the information included in Table 123-1.

In the context of ambulatory patients, useful demographic information includes the patient's name, age, gender, and race. Age, gender, and race are often important factors in the selection of medications and dose determinations. For example, medication doses are often lower in elderly patients because of diminished renal or hepatic function. Gender is important in the case of a female of childbearing age if medications that are being considered for treatment are potentially harmful to unborn children. Finally, race is an important factor in the treatment of hypertension in African-American patients because a number of antihypertensive medications are ineffective in this population.

Core medical information includes past medical problems and all current acute and chronic diseases, including assessments of their severity, prognoses, and associated patient complaints. In some instances, it also may be appropriate to collect information about a patient's physical impairments or disabilities. For example, a patient with limited manual dexterity secondary to an arthritic condition may have difficulty using a medication administration device such as a metered-dose inhaler.

It also may be appropriate in some cases for the pharmacist to collect additional medical information for a specific patient. For example, information relative to a patient's immune status would be important when the selected drug therapy can cause further immunosuppression. Similarly, home blood-glucose and blood-pressure measurements would be useful to assess the effectiveness of therapy for patients who suffer from diabetes mellitus and hypertension, respectively.

Essential therapeutic information includes the names of all prescription and nonprescription drugs used by the patient and their frequency of use and therapeutic indications. Drug allergies, previous adverse drug reactions, and intolerances also should be noted for each patient. In addition, because of the rising popularity of alternative therapies, pharmacists should inquire about the use of home remedies, vitamin/mineral sup-

Table 123-1. Patient Information for the Provision of Pharmaceutical Care

LIFESTYLE	DEMOGRAPHIC/MEDICAL	THERAPEUTIC
Ethnic background	Age	Past therapies[b]
Sexual history	Gender	Prescription drugs
Living arrangement	Race	Nonprescription drugs
Social support	Health status[a]	Alternative therapies
Health beliefs	Impairments/disabilities	Present therapies[b]
Expectations of care	Past medical problems	Prescription drugs
Financial/insurance status	Current medical problems	Nonprescription drugs
Daily activities	Severity	Alternative therapies
Tobacco, alcohol, caffeine use	Prognoses	Allergies
Dietary/exercise practices	Chief complaints	Adverse drug reactions
Perceptions of current diseases	Physical assessment data	Physicians
Perceptions of current therapy	Laboratory data	Other care providers
Compliance with current therapy		
Concerns about current therapy		

[a] Includes cardiac, hepatic, immune, nutritional, and renal status.
[b] Includes therapeutic regimens.

plements, herbal preparations, and other nontraditional therapeutic modalities (eg, acupuncture, aroma therapy).

Perhaps the most often overlooked category of information includes details related to the patient's life-style. Information in this category can be crucial under a variety of circumstances. Patient health beliefs and perceptions of illness and prescribed therapy are known to influence patient compliance strongly.[12] As a result, pharmacists should attempt to collect information about these perceptions and beliefs in all patient care situations.

In some situations, additional life-style information becomes important. As an example, the abuse of alcohol by a female patient who needs treatment for trichomoniasis would be important because the drug of choice for this disease (ie, metronidazole) causes a disulfiram-like reaction when alcohol is consumed. The sexual history of the patient in this situation also would be pertinent because treatment of male partners is necessary to prevent recurrence of the disease in the female. Because each patient presents with a unique set of circumstances, pharmacists must use professional judgment to determine which types of lifestyle information are essential for optimal patient care.

The pharmacist also must determine an appropriate source of each type of information. Common sources include the patient, the patient's caregiver or family, the pharmacy patient profile, medical records, laboratories, physicians, nurses, and other health-care providers. Appropriate sources vary from situation to situation. In each case, the pharmacist must consider a source's ability to provide accurate, reliable information and the ease with which the source may be accessed.[13]

As an example, consider the case of a retired, 67-year-old man who has suffered from diabetes mellitus for 30 years. When the patient and his wife visited the pharmacy for the first time to pick up prescriptions for insulin and syringes and to purchase test strips for his blood-glucose meter, the pharmacist on duty asked the patient to complete a new patient information form. Upon inspection of the completed form, the pharmacist concluded that blood-glucose measurements also would be important to obtain in this case to determine how well the patient's blood sugar is currently controlled. Alternative information sources in this instance would include the patient, the patient's wife, the patient's medical record, and the patient's blood-glucose meter, assuming it has dedicated memory to store test results, and the patient tests his blood regularly using correct technique.

The pharmacist may be able to obtain blood-glucose and glycosylated hemoglobin results for the patient by calling the patient's physician and asking for this information from the patient's medical record. However, these results may not be up-to-date unless the patient had recently visited the physician. Further, locating the physician for a consult may be difficult. The pharmacist could ask the patient directly or he could ask the patient's wife. In these instances, however, it is unlikely that either individual could remember more than one or two measurements. Moreover, the reliability of the reported results could be influenced by the memory or veracity of the person who reports them. Thus, the pharmacist in this instance concluded that if available, the most reliable and - accessible source of blood-glucose measurements would be those stored in the memory of the patient's home bloodglucose meter.

In many instances, the most appropriate information sources are the patient or other individuals involved in the patient's care (eg, physicians). Thus, pharmacists must develop exemplary communication skills and prepare for interactions with these individuals in advance to obtain accurate and complete information in an efficient manner. Specifically, the pharmacist must be a skilled listener, speaker, and observer who formulates questions in advance to elicit the desired information about the patient.

Because pharmacists in ambulatory practice settings rarely have access to patient medical records, it is often necessary to conduct an interview with the patient to obtain critical background information. To save time, some pharmacists ask patients to complete an intake questionnaire prior to being interviewed. This instrument asks the patient for basic background health and demographic information that is elaborated further as appropriate during the interview process.

A successful interview begins with an organized approach that is driven by the nature and amount of information that is needed from the patient. For example, the approach taken during an initial patient visit to the pharmacy would be much different from subsequent visits when baseline information is typically updated.

Ideally, patient interviews should be conducted face-to-face in a quiet, relatively private area of the pharmacy. In addition, patients feel more comfortable when the pharmacist is seated at the same level near them, rather than behind a desk or high prescription counter. The pharmacist should begin the interview by greeting the patient, introducing himself or herself, and briefly explaining the purpose of the interview and the expected amount of time required for its completion.

Following this introduction the pharmacist should proceed with the interview, using an appropriate mix of question types to obtain the desired information. Generally, open-ended questions followed by appropriate probes are effective in this regard. Pharmacists also should attend to information communicated nonverbally by themselves and by the patients. In this context, note taking should occur only after the patient is finished speaking. This is because breaking eye contact while the patient is talking may be interpreted by the patient as disinterest on the part of the pharmacist and may limit patient responses. Further, pharmacists may miss important nonverbal cues if they are looking at their notes while a patient is speaking.

Pharmacists also must be aware of, and sensitive to, the influence of age, gender, and cultural, educational, family, and socioeconomic variables on patient responses during the interview. For example, a patient who is illiterate would be unable to complete a written patient information form. Rather the instrument would need to be administered verbally to the patient. As a further example, studies have demonstrated that patients in lower socioeconomic classes tend to seek medical attention and report bothersome symptoms less frequently than wealthier patients.[14] In this context, pharmacists may need to use more probing questions to obtain information from patients of lower socioeconomic status.

Occasionally, the most appropriate source of patient information is the patient's physician. Although the interaction between the pharmacist and physician is not considered to be an interview, many of the interview techniques outlined previously can facilitate the collection of patient information. Specifically, similar to the patient interview, the pharmacist should have a clear idea of the desired information and a logically sequenced set of questions to obtain this data prior to contacting the physician. In addition, pharmacists should begin the conversation by greeting the physician; introducing themselves and briefly explaining the nature of the desired information before asking specific questions is also appropriate.

Regardless of the source or type, patient information must be recorded in an organized and systematic manner. Recording systems vary widely. However, the system that is used should ensure that patient information is readily retrievable, provide for efficient evaluation of medication-related problems, and permit recording of pharmacist evaluations, recommendations, and patient-monitoring information.

Most community pharmacies employ computer-based medication profiles to record and maintain patient information. While the specific format of these records varies from program to program, an example of a typical patient medication profile is illustrated in Figure 123-1. These records typically include basic patient demographic and medical information and a list of all prescriptions filled at a particular pharmacy. However, because they typically do not provide for documentation of other therapies, monitoring information, and pharmacist recommendations, their utility for the provision of comprehensive pharmaceutical care is limited.

PATIENT'S NAME: Stacy Smith		KNOWN DISEASES	ALLERGIES/ SENSITIVITIES	ADDITIONAL INFORMATION
ADDRESS: 313 Hummingbird Lane		Asthma Sinusitis	Aspirin	multiple vitamin daily
PHONE NO.: 694-8374				
DATE OF BIRTH: 3/17/69				

Date	Rx#	Medication	Strength	Quantity	Dosage Regimen	R.Ph. Init.	Physician	Refills
9/21/97	12543	Ventolin	90mcg/act.	17g	ii puffs q6h prn	AR	Jones	6
9/21/97	20199	Serevent	25mcg/act.	13g	ii puffs bid	TS	Jones	1
10/19/97	20199	Serevent	25mcg/act.	13g	ii puffs bid	RS	Jones	0
10/19/97	12543	Ventolin	90mcg/act.	17g	i-ii q4h prn	RS	Jones	5
10/19/97	34578	Azmacort	60mg/act.	20g	ii puffs tid	AR	Jones	1
10/30/97	12543	Ventolin	90mcg/act.	17g	ii puffs q6h prn	AR	Jones	4
11/11/97	12543	Ventolin	90mcg/act.	17g	ii puffs q6h prn	AR	Jones	3
11/20/97	12543	Ventolin	90mcg/act.	17g	ii puffs q6h prn	AR	Jones	2

Figure 123-1. A typical patient profile.

A more useful alternative to the traditional patient profile is illustrated in Figure 123-2*A* and *B* and was developed for use in an ambulatory wellness clinic by the author. This pharmacist's patient data record provides fields to record all of the data contained on a patient profile. In addition, this record includes fields for the documentation of the patient's past medical and social histories and space for the pharmacist to record additional, patient-specific data, including monitoring information, interventions made on behalf of the patient, and the associated outcomes.

A variety of manual and computer-based tools are commercially available to overcome the limitations of patient medication profiles. For example, Problem-Oriented Medical Record (ie, POMR) cards were recently marketed by Global Publishing Network, Inc, as a manual system for monitoring and documenting patient care. An example is included as Figure 123-3. These cards include sections for patient background characteristics, medical history, medication profile, lab data, medication-related problems, progress notes, and pharmacist's recommendations. Although marketed primarily as a tool for institutional pharmacists, POMR cards also may be a cost-effective alternative for community practitioners.

Comprehensive, computer-based pharmaceutical-care systems also have become available recently from a number of vendors. CarePoint has developed a Windows-based system (ie, Guardian™) that enables pharmacists to collect detailed patient medical and medication histories and to document individual patient needs, interventions, outcomes, and impressions, using the SOAP format, eg, *S*ubjective patient data, *O*bjective patient data, data *A*ssessment and therapeutic *P*lan. The software also includes features to facilitate patient counseling, outcome monitoring, and third-party billing for pharmacists' cognitive services. A representative screen from the software is included as Figure 123-4.

HealthCare Computer Corporation's AlphaPC is a similar system that also has the capability to interface with a large number of other computer-based resources. For example, the system supports a variety of intake questionnaires, enabling pharmacists to choose the format that best suits their patients' needs. In addition, the system creates a series of patient education materials and pharmacist directions for their use when the patient suffers from a common, chronic condition (eg, asthma, diabetes). Finally, the system also can be connected to medical devices to record blood pressure, peak flow, and blood-glucose and blood-cholesterol measurements.

The recent development of innovative systems to collect, maintain, and analyze patient information clearly illustrates the profession's movement toward the realization of new, patient-centered practice roles. Further, as technology evolves, sophisticated tools to support additional pharmacist functions during the provision of pharmaceutical care likely will become available.

Definition and Prioritization of the Patient's Potential and Actual Medication-Related Problems

Evident in the previous section are the benefits of systematic collection and organization of patient databases (ie, efficient recording, retrieval, and evaluation of information). Similarly, the definition and prioritization of patients' medication-related problems requires a systematic approach to prevent problems from being overlooked. A variety of approaches have been developed and are described in the following paragraphs. More important than the specific approach chosen by the pharmacist, however, is the consistent application of a single approach to the evaluation of patient information. This also helps to avoid omissions in the patient's medication-related problem list and in the subsequent formulation of therapeutic goals.

Demographic Information

Name: Tina Smith	Primary Care Physician: Bert Walker
Address: 2090 Mosside Drive	Occupation: Retail Sales Associate
Telephone #: 693-3148	Height: 5'8"; Weight 156lbs (actual 10/97)
Date of Birth: 8/11/65	Rx Insurance: $200.00 deductible then 80% covered

Date	Rx #	Medication	Regimen	R.Ph.	Physician	Refills
5/23	974	Hismanal 10mg #30	i po daily during allergy season	RW	Walker	2
4/10	328	Sporanox 100mg #30	ii daily	HS	Pitman	0
3/25	110	Imitrex 25mg #20	i po at onset of HA then i in 2 hours if needed	GR	Walker	0
3/10	328	Sporanox 100mg #30	ii daily	HS	Pitman	1
2/10	328	Sporanox 100mg #30	ii daily	HS	Pitman	2
12/2	110	Imitrex 25mg #20	i po at onset of HA then i in 2 hours if needed	GR	Walker	1

Acute/Chronic Medical Problems

migraines, hayfever, onychomycosis

Allergies/Intolerances (Reaction)

penicillin (rash)

Past Medical History

GERD 1995
shingles 1991

Social History

married 1990
divorced 1995

Lab/Monitoring Data

migraine diary suggests chocolate is a trigger

Pharmacist Notes/Interventions

5/23 - The patient brought in a new prescription for Hismanal which can interact with Sporanox to produce cardiac arrhythmias....questioned patient if she still is using the Sporanox....she said she sucessfully completed her treatment earlier this month. The diary is unremarkable for additional migraine triggers.

R.W.

3/10 - The patient brought in the migraine trigger diary that she has been keeping since 12/3. It appears that chocolate may be a migraine trigger. Evaluate diary again at the time of next visit.

B.T.

12/2 - The patient was given a migraine trigger diary and instructed on how to use it. She was also encouraged to bring it with her at the time of each visit to the pharmacy.

B.T.

Figure 123-2. *A*, A pharmacist's patient data record.

Demographic Information

Name: Barry Sommers	Primary Care Physician: Steven Marshall
Address: 1341 Sinclair Drive	Occupation: Retired Prison Guard
Telephone #: 593-3078	Height: 6'1"; Weight 230lbs
Date of Birth: 7/21/35	Rx Insurance: $8.00 copay

Date	Rx #	Medication	Regimen	R.Ph.	Physician	Refills
7/15	890	HCTZ 25mg #30	i daily	MH	Spandel	2
7/15	110	Glipizide 10mg #30	i po qd	MH	Spandel	5
6/24	890	HCTZ 25mg	i daily	RT	Spandel	3
6/4	110	Glipizide 10mg #30	i po qd	JL	Spandel	6
6/4	328	Sular 20mg #60	ii daily	JL	Spandel	6
5/10	328	Sular 20mg #60	ii daily	MH	Spandel	7
5/10	110	Glipizide 10mg #30	i po qd	MH	Spandel	7

Acute/Chronic Medical Problems

NIDDM, hypertension, CHF (new 6/24)

Allergies/Intolerances (Reaction)

Past Medical History

left knee replaced 1998
right knee replaced 1995

Social History

married 1958, lives with wife, smokes 1 ppd x 40yrs

Lab/Monitoring Data

BP 135/85, Blood Glucose 180mg/dL on 7/15
BP 127/80, Blood Glucose 111mg/dL on 6/4

Pharmacist Notes/Interventions

7/15 - The patient returned to the pharmacy today for refills and brought his meter and log book. The test performed here was unusually high for him. The logbook revealed a trend toward higher readings over the last 10 days. The meter appears to be operating appropriately. I will investigate further and follow-up with the patient/physician as needed. *M.S.*

6/4 - The patient brought in his meter today and performed a test while I observed - fasting measurement was 111mg/dL. Patient reported that readings have generally been in the 100-135mg/dL range since last visit but forgot to bring his log. His technique is fine. *J.L*

5/10 - The patient purchased and was trained to use an Accu-Check Easy blood glucose meter and agreed to bring the meter with him on refill visits so pharmacist can reassess technique/obtain a measurement for the patient record. *M.S.*

Figure 123-2. *(Continued) B,* A pharmacist's patient data record.

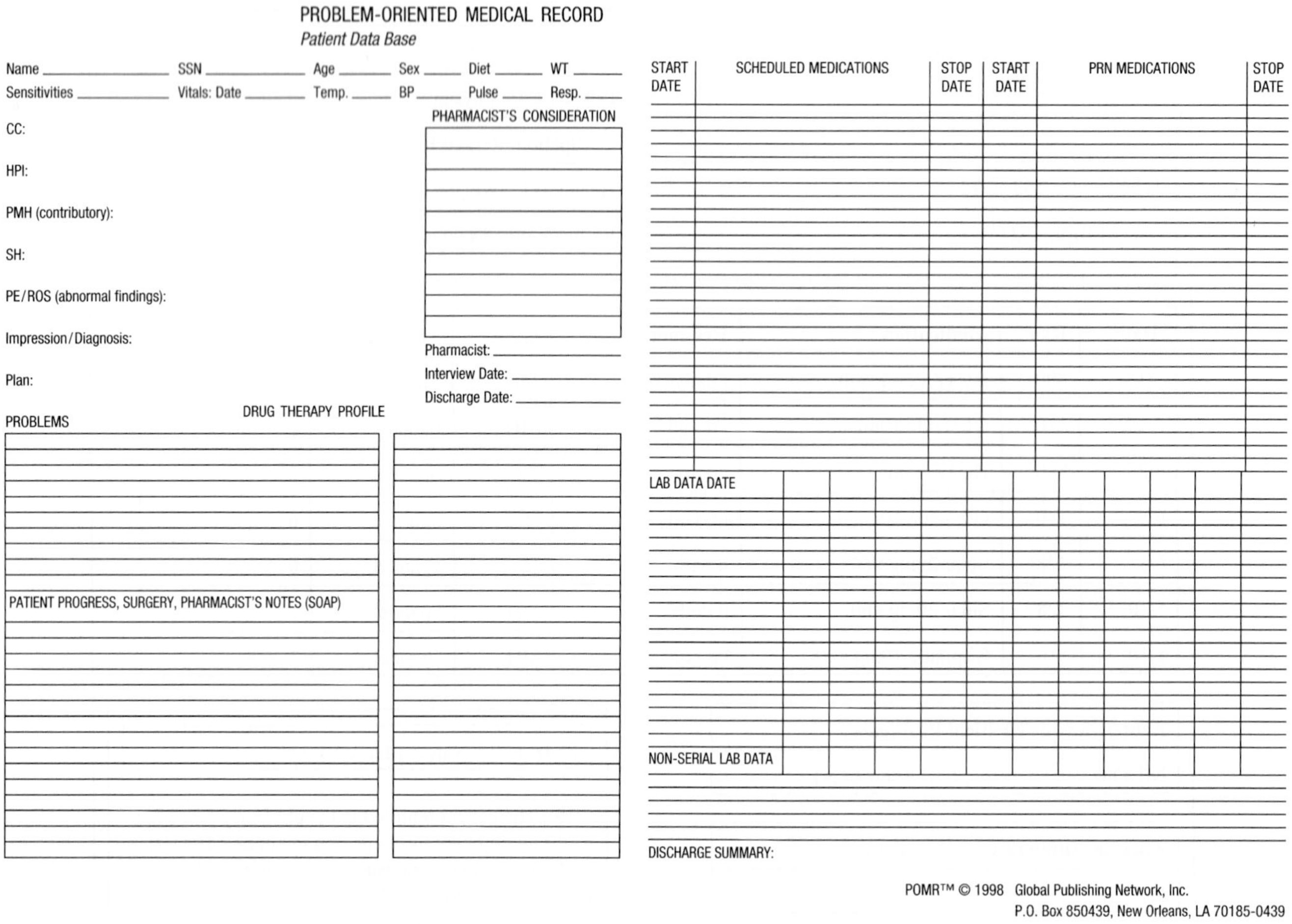

PROBLEM-ORIENTED MEDICAL RECORD
Patient Data Base

Name _____ SSN _____ Age _____ Sex ____ Diet _____ WT _____
Sensitivities _____ Vitals: Date _____ Temp. _____ BP _____ Pulse _____ Resp. _____

CC:

HPI:

PMH (contributory):

SH:

PE / ROS (abnormal findings):

Impression / Diagnosis:

Plan:

PROBLEMS

DRUG THERAPY PROFILE

PATIENT PROGRESS, SURGERY, PHARMACIST'S NOTES (SOAP)

PHARMACIST'S CONSIDERATION

Pharmacist: _____
Interview Date: _____
Discharge Date: _____

START DATE	SCHEDULED MEDICATIONS	STOP DATE	START DATE	PRN MEDICATIONS	STOP DATE

LAB DATA DATE

NON-SERIAL LAB DATA

DISCHARGE SUMMARY:

POMR™ © 1998 Global Publishing Network, Inc.
P.O. Box 850439, New Orleans, LA 70185-0439

Figure 123-3. The Problem-Oriented Medical Record (POMR).

One of the earliest approaches for the identification of medication problems is the 10-step method adapted from the work of Srnka and Self.[15] Using this method, pharmacists examine individual patient databases for actual and potential problems in the following 10 categories.

History of adverse effects
Potentially unwarranted/unintended changes in therapeutic regimen
Potential quantitative misuse (noncompliance, misuse, overuse)
Duplication of medications
Additive effects from similar medication use
Inappropriate dosage, route of administration, dosing schedule, or dosage form
Potential current adverse effects
Drug-drug interactions
Drug-disease interactions
Irrational therapeutic regimen

For example, the patient whose profile is illustrated in Figure 123-1 began receiving refills of her Ventolin more frequently than usual, beginning in October. In addition, she stopped having her other two asthma medications (ie, Serevent and Azmacort) refilled at the same time. Both of these potential problems would fall into the category of quantitative misuse. It would be important for the pharmacist to ask the patient tactfully about the reasons for these changes. Increased use of Ventolin may indicate that her condition is worsening. Further, the patient may be receiving sample units of Serevent and Azmacort from her physician or may be using another pharmacy to have prescriptions for these medications filled. Both scenarios could account for the apparent underuse of Serevent and Azmacort. In any case, the potential problem would be recorded by the pharmacist for further investigation.

The authors of the 10-step method suggest that pharmacists have a pocket card with the 10 categories available to aid the review of the patient profile each time they dispense a prescription. This pocket card provides them with a framework in which to review the profile and, with time, ultimately is committed to memory.

Strand et al advocate use of the eight medication-related problem categories outlined previously in the definition of pharmaceutical care.[8] These authors also stress the importance of clear and explicit problem statements. This is because problems stated in specific terms provide more guidance for the selection of an optimal problem solution. In this context, the authors recommend statements that describe each of two problem components:

1. The illness, symptoms, or risk factors
2. The actual or potential relationships to drug therapy.

To clarify the rationale behind this recommendation, consider the pharmacist's patient data record for Tina Smith, which is illustrated in Figure 123-2A. On 5/23 the pharmacist on duty noted a problem with the patient's new prescription. If this problem was defined simply as a drug interaction, the pharmacist would not know whether the solution is to

1. Discontinue a drug and recommend a new one
2. Increase the dose
3. Decrease the dose
4. Add a new drug
5. Discontinue all therapy
6. Implement some other appropriate action (eg, stagger medication doses)

In contrast, if the problem is stated as significant risk of serious cardiac arrhythmia due to an interaction between two med-

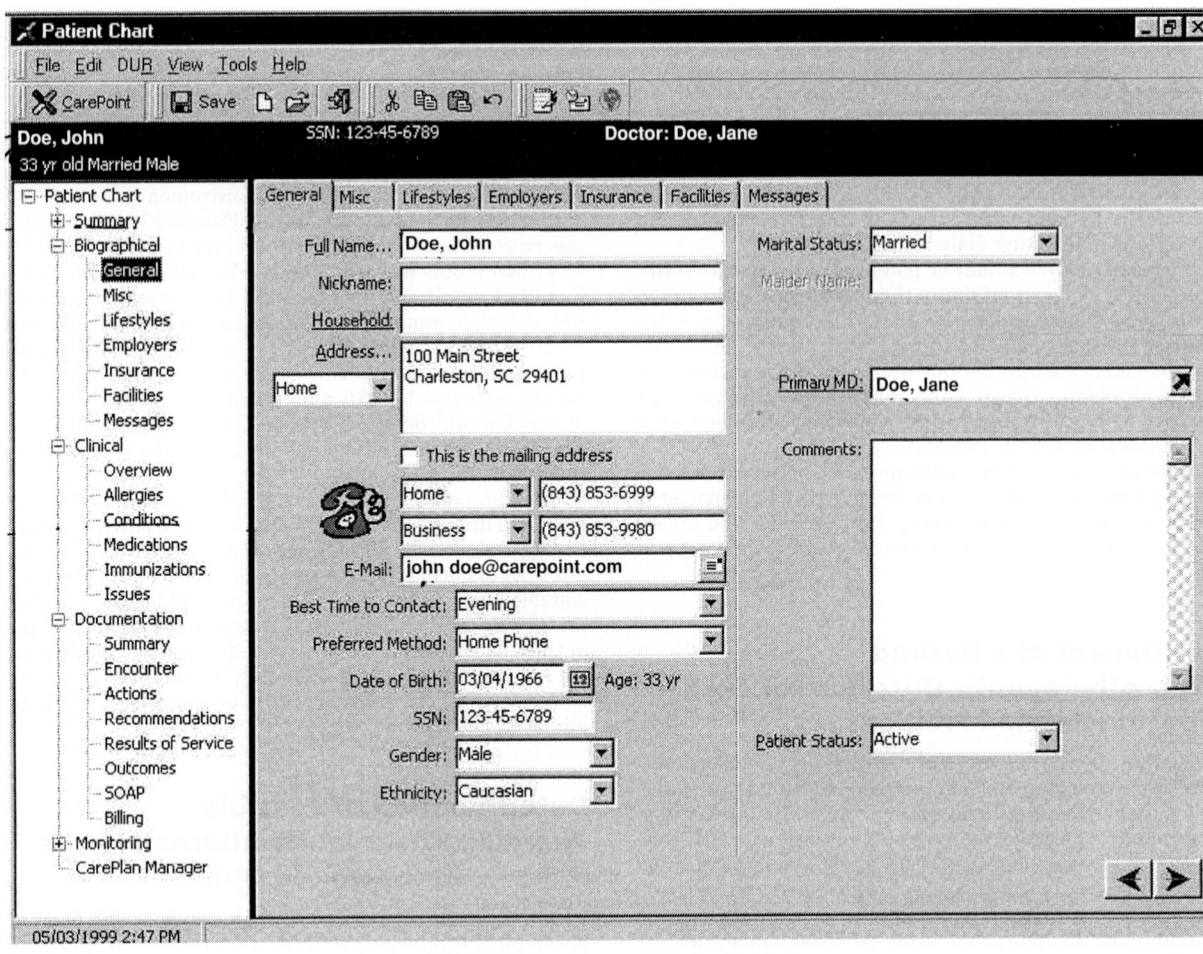

Figure 123-4. A Guardian patient chart.

ically necessary therapies (ie, Sporanox and Hismanal), the solution is much clearer. That is, under no circumstances should the two medications be used together by the patient. If the patient was still taking Sporanox, either the Hismanal or the Sporanox therapy must be discontinued and an alternative medication recommended as a replacement.

One of the most comprehensive systems for the assessment of medication problems was developed by Shimp and Mason as part of the American Society of Health System Pharmacists' Clinical Skills Program.[16] The system consists of two instruments. The Drug Therapy Assessment Worksheet (DTAW) prompts the pharmacist with a series of *guiding* questions to determine if problems exist in any of the following 11 drug-therapy problem categories:

Correlation between drug therapy and medical problems
Appropriate drug selection
Drug regimen
Therapeutic duplication
Drug allergy or intolerance
Adverse drug events
Interactions: drug-drug, drug-disease, drug-nutrient, and drug-laboratory test
Social or recreational drug use
Failure to receive therapy
Financial impact
Patient knowledge of drug therapy

Problems identified during completion of the DTAW then are transferred to a Drug Therapy Problem List (DTPL). This in-strument consists of three columns that provide space for pharmacists to record the

1. Date on which the problem was identified
2. Drug-therapy problem
3. Actions or interventions employed to solve the problem

To illustrate how a pharmacist might use this system, consider the pharmacist's patient data record for Mr Sommers, illustrated in Figure 123-2B. For the drug-therapy category interactions: drug-drug, drug-disease, drug-nutrient, and drug–laboratory test, the DTAW prompts the pharmacist to answer the following questions.

a. Are there any drug-drug interactions?
b. Are they clinically significant?
c. Are any medications contraindicated (relatively or absolutely) given patient characteristics and current/past disease states?
d. Are there drug-nutrient interactions?
e. Are they clinically significant?
f. Are there drug-laboratory interactions?
g. Are they clinically significant?

The pharmacist who assesses the profile in Figure 123-2B using the DTAW would notice that the patient began receiving hydrochlorthiazide (HCTZ) following the diagnosis of congestive heart failure (CHF). Although HCTZ is commonly used to treat CHF, it is not usually a drug-of-choice in patients with concomitant diabetes mellitus because it can increase blood-glucose levels. In fact, inspection of the patient's blood-glucose measurements in the Lab/Monitoring section of his record suggests that this drug-disease interaction may be occurring. Thus, the pharmacist would indicate on the DTAW that a problem exists and record his rationale for this belief in the column reserved for comments and notes. A specific statement of the problem would then be transferred to the DTPL. In this context, the pharmacist may formulate the problem as a clinically significant glucose intolerance possibly due to an interaction between the patient's therapy for CHF and hypertension (ie, HCTZ) and his preexisting diabetes mellitus.

After identifying all actual or potential medication-related problems in the patient database, the pharmacist must determine which problems to address first. For this purpose, the pharmacist must consider the probability that a particular problem will occur and the seriousness of the consequences if it does ensue. Problems that have the highest likelihood of causing the patient significant harm (eg, a patient with a history of anaphylaxis secondary to penicillin who has been prescibed amoxicillin) are generally ranked highest. The prioritized list of problem statements would then be used by the pharmacist to develop a specific goal for resolving each problem and subsequently to design pharmacotherapeutic regimens to achieve each goal.

Establishment of a Desired Pharmacotherapeutic Outcome for Each Medication-Related Problem

Pharmacotherapeutic outcomes are predefined medication-related goals for the resolution of problems identified in the previous step of the pharmaceutical-care process. Similar to problem statements, these outcomes should be clearly articulated to help the pharmacist identify feasible problem solutions and to evaluate results of the alternative that is ultimately chosen. Typically, these statements are simply the mirror image of the problem and fall into one of the three following categories:[8]

The patient is receiving appropriate pharmacotherapy for each definitively diagnosed disease.
The patient is receiving the appropriate dose of each medication at appropriate time intervals.
The patient is free from adverse drug reactions, side effects, and drug interactions.

In this context, a pharmacist would initially conclude from Tina Smith's pharmacist patient data record in Figure 123-2A (ie, prior to determining that the patient no longer takes Sporanox) that one of the patient's potential problems was a significant risk of serious cardiac arrhythmia due to an interaction between two medically necessary therapies (ie, Sporanox and Hismanal). Thus, the corresponding goal would be to provide the necessary pharmacotherapy for hay fever symptoms and onychomycosis without the risk of a serious drug interaction. Similarly, a pharmacist would determine from Mr Sommers' patient record in Figure 123-2B that the patient was experiencing clinically significant glucose intolerance due to an interaction between his therapy for CHF and hypertension (ie, HCTZ) and his preexisting diabetes mellitus. The corresponding goal in this instance would be to provide the necessary pharmacotherapy for CHF and hypertension without impairing glucose tolerance.

Once the pharmacist has articulated the desired pharmacotherapeutic outcome for each medication-related problem, he or she must define appropriate indicators for each goal. Indicators are measurable variables that can be used to monitor the effectiveness of the pharmacotherapeutic solutions to medication-related problems. To be optimally useful in this regard, indicators must be designed to include:

1. A patient factor
2. A progress factor
3. A time factor[8]

Patient factors are variables that can be measured to determine the impact of therapy and include reports of symptoms, laboratory values, and the results of quality-of-life assessments. Progress factors explicitly describe the degree of improvement in patient variables that can reasonably be expected to result from the pharmacotherapy. Finally, time factors characterize the time frame in which the pharmacotherapy should have achieved the desired degree of improvement.

For the patient illustrated in Figure 123-2A, an appropriate patient factor would be the severity of the patient's hay fever symptoms as measured by the patient on a scale of 1 to 5, with 1 signifying no relief and 5 representing complete relief of each symptom. An appropriate progress factor might be a value greater than 3 for each symptom, because complete relief of allergy symptoms secondary to antihistamine therapy occurs infrequently. An appropriate time factor for this level of relief would be 4 to 8 weeks. This is based on the time to reach steady state, which is indicated in the product's package insert.[17]

For the patient in Figure 123-2B, who has CHF, hypertension, and diabetes mellitus, an appropriate patient factor would be blood-glucose levels. The associated progress factor would be a return to normal fasting levels, ie <140 mg/dL. Finally, a reasonable time period for return to normal fasting blood-glucose levels would be approximately 2 days following discontinuation of therapy with HCTZ. This was determined by multiplying the average elimination half-life for HCTZ (ie, 10 hr) by five; ie, an estimate of the number of half-lives required for a drug to be eliminated from the body.[18]

Determination of Feasible Pharmacotherapeutic Alternatives to Achieve Each Desired Outcome

Following articulation of a goal for each medication-related problem, the pharmacist must generate a list of all feasible problem solutions. The reason for this brainstorming step is to ensure that all possible solutions have been considered before any one is chosen. It is also a useful backup tool when the first alternative selected is ineffective for a particular patient.

Generally, pharmacotherapeutic goals may be achieved by correction of a system problem, adjustment of current pharmacotherapy, or development of an entirely new pharmacotherapeutic plan. Thus, the pharmacist should begin the development of a list of feasible solutions by considering alternative solutions within each of these categories.

An example of a system problem would be a patient who has difficulty having prescriptions refilled regularly because of lack of transportation to and from the pharmacy. In this case, the pharmacist would work with the patient and other individuals (eg, caregivers, transportation services) to ensure that the patient receives medication refills in a timely fashion. An example of a minor therapeutic adjustment could be the downward adjustment of the theophylline dose for a patient who suffers from chronic bronchitis and is prescribed another medication known to impede theophylline metabolism, eg, an oral contraceptive. Finally, an example of a situation in which a new therapeutic plan would be appropriate involves a patient who has been prescribed erythromycin for a minor infection and who has previously suffered from intolerable nausea and vomiting when this medication was prescribed.

To facilitate the subsequent determination of an optimal solution in the next step, the pharmacist should take care to list alternatives in a consistent format. Strand et al recommend listing alternatives according to distinguishing characteristics.[8] This makes the advantages and disadvantages of each alternative more visible and therefore easy to compare with one another. In the context system problem described previously, a list could be developed to distinguish alternative

Table 123-2. Therapeutic Alternatives for the Treatment of CHF and Hypertension in a Diabetic Patient

CATEGORY	GLUCOSE	INSULIN SENSITIVITY	LD CHOLESTEROL	HDL CHOLESTEROL	TRIGLYCERIDES
ACE inhibitors	↓^{a}	↑	(↓)	↔	↔
α-Blockers	↔	↑	(↓)	(↑)	↔
β-Blockers	↑	↓	↔	↓	↑
Calcium channel blockers	↔	(↑)	(↓)	↔	↔
Direct vasodilators	?	↔	↔	↔	↔
Thiazide diuretics	↑	↓	↑	(↓)	(↑)

^{a} ↑, increase; ↓, decrease; (↑), possible increase; (↓), possible decrease; ↔, no effect; ?, unknown.

sources of patient assistance. For alternatives in the therapeutic adjustment example, the list might be created to distinguish alternative theophylline products according to available product strengths or dosage forms to accomplish the adjustment. In the final example, in which a new therapeutic plan was indicated, alternative medications could be listed according to available dosage forms, mechanisms of action, clinical efficacy, incidence of adverse reactions (eg, nausea and vomiting), or even cost.

To illustrate the generation of a comprehensive list of feasible alternatives for a specific example, consider the Mr Sommers' pharmacist's patient data record in Figure 123-2B. Using the recommendations of Strand et al and appropriate references,[19] the pharmacist could begin by listing alternatives to HCTZ for the treatment of hypertension and CHF according to mechanism of action, as illustrated in the first column of Table 123-2. Next, the pharmacist could further distinguish these six categories by listing the general effect each has on blood glucose and insulin sensitivity, as shown in the second and third columns of Table 123-2. Finally, because patients who suffer from diabetes mellitus are at increased risk for the development of atherosclerotic heart and brain disease, the pharmacist could determine and list the effects of each category on serum lipids.

In many instances it is also appropriate to list the approximate cost of individual medications in each category. However, in this instance, the patient has prescription coverage with a small copay. Thus, this information is not as useful as it might be in the case of an uninsured or underinsured patient.

Selection of the Best Pharmacotherapeutic Solution Based upon Individual Patient Circumstances

During this step, the pharmacist must determine which therapeutic alternative is best for the patient. In this context the pharmacist's recommendation for the solution of each medication-related problem should include the chosen medication, dosage form, dose frequency and duration, and any special instructions (eg, uncommon administration procedures) for the patient. At this point it is especially important to involve the patient in the selection of appropriate therapy. This helps to ensure that the patient is able and willing to comply with all associated therapeutic and monitoring instructions.

In the case of Mr Sommers, the pharmacist concluded from his research that an ACE inhibitor would be most appropriate. Upon questioning by the pharmacist, Mr Sommers expressed his desire to continue to be able to take all of his medications once daily in the morning. Upon further investigation, however, the pharmacist learned that it would be more appropriate to initiate therapy with a shorter-acting ACE inhibitor such as captopril, initally with 6.25 mg 3 times a day. Once the effective dose of captopril is achieved, the patient can then be switched to a once-daily ACE inhibitor such as lisinopril.[20] After the pharmacist explained this, the patient agreed that he would be able to manage multiple daily doses of captopril if they were only necessary for a short period of time.

Design of a Monitoring Plan to Determine If the Desired Pharmacotherapeutic Outcome Has Been Achieved

Prior to implementing any therapeutic recommendation, the pharmacist must develop a plan to monitor the patient's progress toward each goal established in a previous step. This plan should include appropriate pharmacotherapeutic monitoring parameters, realistic endpoints for each parameter, and the frequency with which each parameter will be assessed. The number and nature of each plan component depends on the

1. Properties of the recommended medications
2. Patient's background characteristics
3. Availability of practical, cost-effective monitoring methods.

Pharmacotherapeutic monitoring parameters are either quantitative or qualitative assessments of patient progress toward specific therapeutic goals. Quantitative assessments are objective measures of a particular variable and include blood pressure, pulse, temperature, serum drug levels, and blood-glucose determinations. Qualitative assessments are subjective determinations of change in a particular variable. Examples include patient self-reported changes in symptoms such as nausea, pain, and sedation.

It is important to note that some pharmacotherapeutic goals may necessitate the identification of multiple monitoring parameters while others will require only one. For example, a number of parameters could be used to monitor the resolution of a bacterial infection of the upper respiratory tract. These might include temperature, sputum color, cough, and/or white blood cell counts, depending on the patient's situation. In contrast, achievement of serum theophylline levels in the therapeutic range could only be determined by performing serum theophylline assays.

It is also important to mention that pharmacists must take care to ensure that the desired endpoint specified for each pharmacotherapeutic goal is realistic and achievable, based upon individual patient characteristics. For example, a score of 0 on a pain scale (ie, indicating no pain) may be achievable for a patient who has just undergone a tooth extraction, but would likely be unreasonable for a patient suffering from metastatic bone cancer. Similarly, an appropriate endpoint for chemotherapy in a patient in the earliest stage of breast cancer may be remission of the disease. However, a more appropriate endpoint for a similar patient in the terminal stage of the disease would be to reduce pain scale scores through the use of analgesics.

When choosing appropriate monitoring parameters for a given patient, the pharmacist must take into account the therapeutic efficacy of the selected medication and the potential for the medication to cause new problems (ie, side effects and adverse reactions). In the context of the pharmacist's recommendation of captopril to treat Mr Sommers' CHF and hypertension, blood pressure would be an example of a quantitative measure of therapeutic efficacy, and the severity of dyspnea on exertion would be a qualitative measure. Desired endpoints might be blood pressure measurements in the normal range for Mr Sommers' age and, at the very least, no change in the level of dyspnea on exertion.

Monitoring parameters to identify new problems as a result of captopril therapy might include the development of a maculopapular rash on the trunk or extremities (the most common side effect of captopril), alteration of taste perception, and the onset of a dry, hacking cough in the absence of other respiratory pathology. Realistic endpoints might be that symptoms, if they occur at all, do not interfere with Mr Sommers' daily activities. Monitoring data for all of the aforementioned parameters could be collected by the pharmacist each time Mr Sommers returns to the pharmacy for prescription refills.

Patient-specific characteristics also should be taken into consideration by the pharmacist when selecting appropriate monitoring parameters. Of particular importance are patient characteristics that may influence the pharmacokinetic disposition of the recommended medication. For example, captopril has been associated with the development of proteinuria and decreased renal function in some patients. Twenty percent of patients treated with captopril develop stable elevations in BUN and serum creatinine levels that may reach as high as 20% over baseline measurements. Others experience a more accelerated deterioration in renal function that necessitates discontinuation of captopril. However, most of these patients had evidence of preexisting renal disease.[21]

Although Mr Sommers does not apparently suffer from renal dysfunction at the present time, he is at risk for its development secondary to his diabetes mellitus. In addition, he suffers from CHF. Thus, the pharmacist in this situation also may recommend monitoring Mr Sommers' BUN and serum creatinine levels in addition to the parameters described previously. The pharmacist may recommend baseline measurement of BUN and serum creatinine and regular measurments (eg, every 3 months) for the first year of therapy.

Implementation of Individualized Pharmacotherapeutic and Monitoring Plans

The next step in the pharmaceutical-care process is to implement the pharmacotherapeutic and monitoring plans developed by the pharmacist. This involves securing physician approval for any changes in the originally prescribed therapy, counseling the patient about the proper use of the recommended therapy, and collecting monitoring data to evaluate the efficacy of the pharmacotherapeutic plan.

In some instances, it is necessary for pharmacists to secure authorization from a physician to initiate or modify a patient's pharmacotherapy. In the case of Mr Sommers, the pharmacist would need to contact Dr Spandel to seek approval to discontinue HCTZ and initiate therapy with captopril. The pharmacist in this case also would recommend monitoring Mr Sommers' BUN and serum creatinine and would request regular access to these laboratory results. In any situation in which the physician must be contacted, pharmacists can maximize the likelihood that their requests will be approved by following a few simple guidelines.

First, and most important, the pharmacist must prepare thoroughly prior to consulting with the physician. All necessary references must be checked, and relevant information, including citations, should be recorded in advance for rapid retrieval as needed during the consultation. Upon contacting the physician, the pharmacist should present a detailed but concise description of the problem. This should be followed by a specific solution for the problem, the pharmacist's rationale for the recommended solution, and supporting references. At the conclusion of the consultation, all information, including the outcome of the consult, should be documented in the patient's record.

The next implementation step is to educate the patient relative to the proper use of the chosen therapy. Effective counseling helps to ensure that patients adhere to prescribed therapies

and enables pharmacists to identify and resolve medication-related problems as expediently as possible.[22–26]

OBRA 90 establishes minimum requirements for counseling individuals receiving benefits, consistent with applicable state laws and the pharmacist's professional judgment. At a minimum, the pharmacist should ensure that the patient knows

The name and description of the medication.
The dosage form, dosage, route of administration, and duration of drug therapy
Special directions and precautions for preparation, administration, and use by the patient
Common severe side or adverse effects or interactions and therapeutic contraindications that may be encountered—including their avoidance—and the action required if they occur
Techniques for self-monitoring drug therapy
Proper medication storage
Prescription refill information
Action to be taken in the event of a missed dose

In this context, the pharmacist who counsels Mr Sommers about his captopril therapy should tell the patient the following:

The name of the medication is captopril.
The strength of each tablet is 12.5 mg.
The doctor wants you to take one-half tablet by mouth 3 times a day.
This medication is being used to treat high blood pressure and congestive heart failure. It should be continued until the doctor decides otherwise.
The tablets should be broken or cut in half at the score mark in the center of each tablet. This medicine works best when it is taken on an empty stomach 1 hr before a meal. Ideally, this medication should be taken at the same time each day.
If you miss a dose, take it as soon as you remember unless it is close to the time of your next dose. In this instance, simply skip that dose and resume therapy with the next scheduled tablet.
Do not double doses.
This medication may cause dizziness or lightheadedness, especially after the first dose. Make sure you know how you will react to the medication before driving or operating dangerous machinery.
Minor side effects include coughing, changes in taste perception, and mild diarrhea and stomach upset.
Contact your physician if any of these symptoms become severe enough to interfere with daily activities.
Call your physician immediately if you experience fever, swelling of the face or extremities, trouble breathing, irregular heartbeat, nervousness, or tingling/heaviness in your legs.
Keep regularly scheduled appointments for laboratory tests and physician appointments. Consider use of a home blood-pressure-monitoring device for blood-pressure monitoring between physician visits.
Store this medication in a cool, dry place that is out of the reach of children.
Your doctor probably will adjust your dose before you run out of this medication; therefore, there are no refills on your current prescription.[27]

When taken at face value, the minimum counseling requirements set forth by OBRA 90 may be misleading because they may be interpreted as a one-time, one-way communication of information from the pharmacist to the patient. Indeed, while this type of interaction may fulfill the legal requirements of OBRA 90, it will not always, if ever, be sufficient to provide the level of professional service intended in the definition of pharmaceutical care.[28]

In fact, if the intent of pharmaceutical care is to optimize therapeutic outcomes, a one-way communication of drug information to the patient at the time of purchase rarely makes sense. This is apparent when one considers the frame of mind of patients at the time they pick up a prescription. In the worst case, the patient is feeling sick and is concentrating on little more than returning home to rest and recuperate. In less extreme circumstances, patients may be annoyed after having to take time off from work to perhaps spend hours in a physician's office followed by another period of waiting in the pharmacy. As a result, they are probably not overly enthusiastic about learning all there is to know about the prescribed medication in a few minutes of verbal counseling from the pharmacist.

In this context, some may argue that printed information to be read at a more convenient time would suffice as adequate counseling for the patient. In fact, this approach has been used by some pharmacists as a means of dealing with the relative lack of time for verbal counseling at the time of dispensing. In addition, in an effort to increase the availability of prescription drug information to the public, the FDA proposed a rule commonly known as MedGuide in 1995. This rule set forth goals for the distribution of printed prescription drug information to consumers and would have required pharmaceutical manufacturers to include drug information for products that posed a serious health risk.

Although Congress passed legislation in 1996 that put the MedGuide proposal on hold, health professionals are being asked to voluntarily provide prescription drug information in the form of leaflets written in simple language. Consistent with DHHS's goal under its Healthy People 2000 program, this information must reach 75% of patients by the year 2000 and 95% of patients by 2006.[29] However, pharmacists should be cautioned not to rely entirely on printed drug information to educate their patients.

When used alone, written information may actually be less effective than a one-time, one-way communication of information from the pharmacist.[12] This is because there is no way to ensure that the patient will actually read the information prior to initiating the prescribed therapy. Further, there is no guarantee that the patient will contact the pharmacist with any questions that may arise after reading it. Even worse, the patient may be illiterate and unable to read the information at all. This is a real concern in the US, where over 20% of adults read at or below the fifth-grade level.[30]

A more effective approach to patient counseling would include two-way communication between the pharmacist and patient and would be augmented by printed information as needed, depending upon the specific situation. In addition, the approach must make efficient use of the pharmacist's and the patient's valuable time. Pharmacists employed by the Indian Health Service (IHS) have used one such approach for many years.

While traditional approaches to patient counseling focus on providing information, the goal of the IHS method is to verify that patients have acquired requisite drug information, using an interactive approach. For counseling on new prescriptions, the pharmacist asks the patient to answer the following questions.

What did the doctor tell you the medication is for?
How did the doctor tell you to take the medication?
What did the doctor tell you to expect?

Answers to these questions are then used by the pharmacist to determine the patient's specific information needs. The approach saves time, because the pharmacist must only supply the information that the patient does not already have. In fact, IHS studies have found the time required to counsel a patient about a new prescription takes a little under 2 minutes using this approach.[31]

To promote patient adherence and to monitor patient progress toward medication-related goals, IHS pharmacists use a second technique for refill prescriptions that takes only about 30 seconds. Using this approach, the pharmacist removes the cap from the prescription, shows the medication to the patient and asks, "What do you use this medication for? How do you take it? What kinds of problems are you having? Is there anything else I can do for you today?" Both techniques encourage pharmacist-patient interaction. Again, the pharmacist's questions are used to verify patient understanding and fill in any information gaps.[31]

Follow-up Evaluation and Documentation of the Results of Pharmacotherapeutic and Monitoring Plans

At predetermined intervals, the pharmacist must review collected monitoring data to determine if satisfactory progress is being made toward the desired medication-related goals. At the same time, the pharmacist must ascertain if any new problems have developed since the last review. If the desired outcomes have not been met or if new problems have occurred, the pharmacist, physician, and patient may need to make changes in the original pharmacotherapeutic and monitoring plans.

Changes are made following reconsideration of relevant information from earlier steps in the pharmaceutical-care process or from the collection of new information as needed. Suppose, for example, that Mr Sommers returned to the pharmacy 1 week after initiation of captopril and complained of intolerable coughing. In this case, the pharmacist would review the alternative therapies originally considered and select another medication to treat Mr Sommers without causing a cough. If the pharmacist, physician, or patient was not satisfied with any of the alternatives considered previously, the pharmacist would consult the literature to identify a more suitable therapy.

In any event, the final step in the pharmaceutical-care process requires that the pharmacist document all interventions and outcomes in the patient's record. This information then becomes baseline information upon which subsequent adjustments and/or new therapeutic decisions are made. This information also may be required if the pharmacist attempts to obtain reimbursement for pharmaceutical-care services from a third party.

BARRIERS TO PHARMACEUTICAL CARE

Although the profession of pharmacy has embraced pharmaceutical care as its new mission, the implementation of pharmaceutical care, particularly in ambulatory practice settings, has been slow. A variety of factors have impeded pharmacists' ability to implement pharmaceutical care and can be grouped into four general categories.

Individual pharmacist characteristics
Practice-setting constraints
Intraprofessional barriers
System impediments

An awareness of the potential barriers to pharmaceutical care and a working understanding of alternatives for surmounting these constraints may assist pharmacists during the transition to pharmaceutical-care practice.

Individual Pharmacist Characteristics

Individual pharmacist attitudes and background knowledge and/or skill deficiencies may hamper the implementation of pharmaceutical care in any practice setting. For example, some pharmacists have grown quite comfortable with traditional practice functions and may be fearful about changing to assume new, unfamiliar roles. In addition, they may be concerned that expanding professional practice roles will place them in conflict with patients who do not feel the need for pharmaceutical care and/or with other health-care professionals who believe they are more qualified to provide these services. Finally, some pharmacists might lack confidence in their educational preparation to provide an advanced level of care to their patients.

Indeed, the provision of pharmaceutical care will require many pharmacists to update their professional knowledge and skill base. First and foremost, pharmacists must develop a thorough understanding of what it means to provide pharmaceutical care. Many pharmacists mistakenly believe that they always have provided the level of professional service embodied in the definition of the concept. In reality, however, many fail to realize that pharmaceutical care is more than occasional interventions on behalf of the patient. Thus, pharmacists must take it upon themselves to develop an accurate understanding of the pharmaceutical-care process. Only then, will they be able to shift the focus of their practices from dispensing medications to the provision of patient-oriented, professional services.[32]

Pharmacists who commit to managing the pharmacotherapy of their patients must be familiar with current advances in the treatment of common diseases and with literature resources/databases that are available to assist them to make sound therapeutic decisions. Thus, some pharmacists may find it necessary to update their knowledge of therapeutics and drug information resources/capabilities.

Similarly, the provision of pharmaceutical care requires that pharmacists develop strong, effective problem-solving skills.[33] Most pharmacists have already developed basic problem-solving abilities. However, they may not have regularly applied these skills to the resolution of their patients' medication-related problems. As a result, some pharmacists may benefit from additional instruction on clinical problem solving.

Finally, oral and written communication skills are central to the provision of pharmaceutical care.[33] Among other things, strong communication skills are crucial for eliciting important information from patients, documenting pharmacists' therapeutic decisions, and counseling patients about the proper use of medications. Strong communication skills are also essential to convey information about patients' pharmacotherapy to physicians and other health-care providers. Because the levels of communication proficiency and frequency entailed for the provision of pharmaceutical care are generally higher than the requirements for traditional roles, some pharmacists may benefit from additional instruction prior to fully implementing pharmaceutical-care services.

One strategy for coping with the aforementioned barriers is for pharmacists to transition gradually to the provision of patient-oriented professional services. Adapting to change and the development of advanced practice abilities must develop over time. Thus, pharmacists should initially focus on the provision of limited pharmaceutical-care services to a specific group of patients. The group should be chosen to reflect an area of disease/therapeutics (eg, asthma care, diabetes care) in which pharmacists feel comfortable with their current level of expertise. Then, as pharmacists gain confidence and develop additional expertise, they can extend pharmaceutical-care services to additional patients.

An especially useful resource for pharmacists who want to develop new skills for the provision of pharmaceutical care is *The Pharmacists' Learning Assistance Network (PLAN)*. The *PLAN* is a continuing pharmaceutical education information service that is provided to pharmacists through the American Council on Pharmaceutical Education (ACPE). It was developed to enable pharmacists to pursue a curricular approach to professional development through organization and planning of their continuing pharmaceutical education needs. A computerized compilation of all continuing pharmaceutical education programs offered by ACPE-approved providers serves as the database for the service. The *PLAN* service may be contacted by telephone between 9:00 a.m. and 4:00 p.m. (Central Time) Monday through Friday by dialing (800) 533-3606. During this time professional staff members are available to discuss pharmacists' personal educational needs and available continuing education programs that may be useful to meet those needs.[34]

Practice-Setting Constraints

Resource constraints and other factors associated with a particular practice setting also are mentioned frequently as barriers to the provision of pharmaceutical care. For example, pharmacists often complain that they do not have time to provide pharmaceutical care in addition to their normal responsibilities.[32] When taken at face value, the assessment of these pharmacists relative to time available to provide pharmaceutical care is accurate. Upon closer scrutiny, however, other variables may be contributing to the perceived lack of time.

It is possible that pharmacists who perceive a lack of time for pharmaceutical-care services have not delegated enough nontechnical pharmacy functions to available support personnel or may not have taken full advantage of available technology (eg, fax machines, documentation software, automated dispensing equipment) in the dispensing process. In this context, pharmacists should scrutinize the tasks routinely performed to determine if any functions can be accomplished more efficiently through the use of technology or support personnel. Tasks that are reassigned to support personnel should then be added to the appropriate job descriptions. Training also must be instituted to enable support personnel to perform these new responsibilities. In this way, although time will be required to complete the aforementioned measures, pharmacists may be able to free additional time to provide patient care services in the long run.

Similarly, pharmacists should examine the workflow pattern in the pharmacy to make sure that departmental personnel can complete their assigned duties as efficiently as possible. Each dispensing station should provide easy access to prescription containers, labels, prescription files, patient records, telephones, and fast-moving prescription products. Space for direct, confidential pharmacist-patient interaction also should be located as close to the dispensing area as possible. These measures also may help to free pharmacist time for the provision of pharmaceutical care.[35]

A lack of financial resources also is mentioned often as a barrier to the provision of pharmaceutical care.[32] Purchasing additional equipment, hiring and training additional personnel, and redesigning the pharmacy can be quite expensive. A further complication exists when the management of the pharmacy organization is not committed to the provision of pharmaceutical care. In that situation, support for even minor modifications of the practice environment may be completely absent.

A gradual transition to the provision of pharmaceutical care also may be an effective means for pharmacists to contend with barriers in the practice setting. Most pharmacists should be able to offer pharmaceutical care to a limited number of patients without incurring large expenses. Then, as the number of patients receiving care is expanded, pharmacists can gradually modify the environment to be more conducive to patient-oriented services. The documented impact of these early efforts to provide pharmaceutical care also may be useful to persuade pharmacy management to provide resources for the transition.

Intraprofessional Barriers

Professional organizations, regulatory bodies, and schools/colleges of pharmacy also may be perceived as barriers to the implementation of pharmaceutical care insofar as their efforts fail to support practitioners adequately in their transition efforts. For example, until very recently professional pharmacy organizations have become increasingly fragmented into groups with widely different interests and competing agendas.[36] The resultant lack of consensus has weakened the profession politically. This is important because many debates relative to the profession are settled in the political arena (eg, OBRA 90). Thus, pharmacists from all practice settings and the organizations that represent them must work cooperatively to develop a common agenda for the implementation of pharmaceutical care if this new mission is ever to be fully realized by the profession.

As the practice of pharmacy transitions to pharmaceutical care, legislation governing the practice of the profession also must evolve to permit pharmacist provision of expanded patient care services. Outdated board of pharmacy regulations such as limitations on the nontechnical functions that can be performed by technicians or the restrictions on modes of prescription transmission can actually impede pharmacists in their efforts to implement pharmaceutical care. To prevent such obstacles, state boards and associations must work cooperatively with local colleges/schools of pharmacy and practitioners to identify and correct problematic rules and regulations.[32]

Schools/colleges of pharmacy must assume a variety of roles to support the transition to pharmaceutical care. They must continually evaluate and modify their professional curricula to ensure that pharmacy graduates are prepared to assume contemporary patient care roles.[9,33] Similarly, they must assess the continuing education needs of their alumni and provide instructional opportunities for practicing pharmacists to develop further the professional knowledge and skills required to render pharmaceutical care.[9,33] Educational programs also should be developed to prepare practitioners to precept pharmacy students during the experiential component of professional curricula. Finally, colleges/schools of pharmacy must conduct research to demonstrate the value of pharmaceutical care to society.[32]

System Impediments

Several characteristics of the health-care system in the US also impede the provision of pharmaceutical care. Among these are the general lack of pharmacist reimbursement for pharmaceutical-care services, a lack of patient demand, and a lack of acceptance of pharmaceutical-care roles by other health professionals.

At present, pharmacists are not often reimbursed for pharmaceutical-care services. Rather, they receive remuneration for the drug products dispensed. However, as outlined previously, the body of evidence supports the feeling that pharmaceutical-care services add value to patient care by enhancing patient compliance, improving patient outcomes, and reducing health-care costs.

Consumers are beginning to recognize the value of pharmaceutical-care services. In addition, there is evidence to support the notion that patients are willing to pay for consultation if they know it is available, is of potential benefit, and what it costs. For example, one enterprising pharmacist in Indiana successfully offers families who purchase prescriptions at his pharmacy professional consultation services for a flat annual fee. The cost of the prescription then is based upon the cost to the pharmacy plus a handling charge. This pharmacist also, with some success, has billed insurance companies for pharmaceutical-care services that were provided to his patients.[37]

Third-party purchasers of health care also are beginning to recognize the value of pharmaceutical care and to compensate pharmacists who provide these services. As an example, a recent amendment to the Mississippi Medicaid plan permits reimbursement for disease-state management services provided by appropriately credentialed or certified pharmacists. Eligible pharmacists receive $20.00 for each 15- to 30-min patient consultation for the management of diabetes mellitus, asthma, hyperlipidemia, or coagulation disorders in that state.[38,39]

Although compensation for pharmaceutical-care services is still the exception rather than the rule, pharmacists should consistently bill patients and third-party payers for these services. Some pharmacists may be reluctant to ask patients for direct payment for pharmaceutical care. However, if they do not, patients will not demand coverage for these services from third-party payers for health care. In this context, third-party coverage of pharmaceutical coverage will not change.

Pharmacy organizations also must work with third-party payers to develop standardized pharmacy service terminology and universal systems for billing and claims transmission (see Chapter 93). This is because standardized third-party compensation policies are necessary for widespread pharmacist reimbursement for pharmaceutical-care services.[32,37]

Initially, patient demand for pharmaceutical-care services may be low. Patients may resist the adoption of pharmaceutical care for a variety of reasons. Some may be reluctant to spend additional time consulting with a pharmacist. Others may be concerned about cost. Some patients may feel that the pharmacist is trying to take over a portion of the physician's role and want to avoid angering their own doctor. Regardless of the specific explanation given by a patient for refusing pharmacist services, the underlying issue is that patients generally are unaccustomed to this level of service and do not fully understand the concept of pharmaceutical care.[32]

In this context, pharmacists should take the time to explain their services thoroughly to each patient. They should emphasize that pharmaceutical care complements rather than duplicates services provided by other health professionals. In addition, pharmacists should describe how patients benefit from pharmaceutical-care services. Pharmacists also may generate demand for pharmaceutical care through effective marketing of their services to their communities and through participation in national public relations and educational campaigns such as the annual *National Pharmacy Week* sponsored every fall by the APhA.

Finally, it is likely that some health-care professionals will resist pharmacists' assumption of patient care roles. For example, nurses and physicians may view pharmacist management of pharmacotherapy as an encroachment on their professional territory. Pharmacists should not be intimidated and/or discouraged by this lack of acceptance. Rather, they should forge relationships with health professionals one at a time, beginning with those individuals who are open to collaboration. Realistically, not all health professionals will completely accept pharmacists' expanded role. However, over time and with perseverance, most pharmacists will be able to establish themselves as integral members of the health-care team.

A Systematic Approach For Overcoming Barriers To Pharmaceutical Care

In a recent book, Hagel and Rovers et al advocate the use of a strategic planning process to assist pharmacists in the transition from a product-oriented business to a patient-centered practice. The authors assert that the primary reason that many pharmacists are still struggling to implement patient-centered care is because the system they work in is not conducive to the changes they desire to bring about. Thus, the authors' approach targets the practice rather than individual pharmacists and assists service implementers to answer the following fundamental planning questions.

- Where am I now?
- Where do I want to be?
- How do I get there?
- How will I know when I have arrived?

To that end, the book includes detailed chapters to assist implementers with everything from patient care planning to adjusting infrastructure, staff development and outcome evaluation.[40]

HEALTH EDUCATION

A primary concern of the pharmacist should be the welfare of humanity and the relief of human suffering. In fact, one oath contains the passage, "I will use my knowledge and skills to the best of my ability in serving the public and other health professionals." Today, there is little doubt that the continuing *buzzword* in contemporary pharmacy practice is *information*—specifically, consumer health information.

By virtue of the pharmacists' accessibility and familiarity with the community, it is obvious that they can exercise a dynamic impact, which can be translated into not only the triage function but also the dissemination of effective and useful health education. One study revealed that over 90% of those interviewed visited a pharmacy at least once a month, and 60%, at least once a week. The hours a pharmacy is open per week greatly exceed those of all other health facilities with the possible exception of the hospital emergency room. Although many consumers continue to view the pharmacist as *an invisible man behind a secret counter who delegates responsibility to technicians and clerks to deal directly with the public,* this attitude is being changed positively to reflect the pharmacist as a source of health information along with the physician. A vast majority of the public does not hesitate to ask the pharmacist about a health matter and usually he or she is the first person, other than family or friends, who is consulted.

Frequently, the pharmacist is confronted with a variety of inquiries:

- A telephone call from a frantic mother whose child has just swallowed a number of chewable vitamin-iron tablets and wants to know what to do.
- A nervous teenage girl who wants to know how to use a home pregnancy kit.
- A habitual smoker who is interested in the success rate of the nicotine transdermal patches.
- An expectant mother who is afraid for her baby because she may have been exposed to a neighborhood child with German measles.

The situations are endless but typify the need for the pharmacist to be approachable and willing to help.

To answer these people or synthesize a plan of action, pharmacists must maintain professional competence and keep abreast of developments of drugs and disease states. At the same time they should serve as expeditors to solve patient problems. The familiarity of the pharmacist with the community lends itself to proper referral of patients to other health-care professionals, including providing addresses and telephone numbers. Indeed, the pharmacist is in a position to assess physicians on the basis of personal experience, the types of prescriptions they write or telephone, patient comments about the care they receive, and inquiries about physician follow-up. Beyond health-care assistance, the pharmacist also should be able to recommend nonmedical facilities that provide effective care (eg, a shoe store that exercises judgment and care in fitting jogging shoes). Further, pharmacists should know that pharmaceutical companies do offer physicians free drugs for needy patients. While individual manufacturer requirements for assistance may differ, the following are some common requirements:

- Eligible patients cannot be covered by Medicaid or a private insurance plan that has prescription-drug coverage.
- Physicians must initiate the request on behalf of the patient and, in some instances, provide a statement of the patient's financial hardship.
- No more than a 3-months' supply is available at one time, although requests may be renewed.

Pharmacists can advise interested patients to seek an alphabetical listing of drugs covered by specific pharmaceutical companies, including information on assistance for acquired immunodeficiency syndrome (AIDS) drugs, by contacting The Senate Special Committee on Aging, Dirksen Senate Office Building, Room G-31, Washington, DC 20510 (1-202-224-5364). Similarly, physicians can be advised to contact the Pharmaceutical Manufacturers' Association, 1100 15th St, NW, Washington, DC 20005 for a directory of manufacturers' assistance programs.

In 1993 there were 100 regional poison control centers in the US (of which 38 were certified through the American Association of Poison Control Centers), and every pharmacy should have the telephone numbers and addresses of those in the local area for quick patient referral. Although unintentional poisonings and deaths have dropped dramatically since child-resistant packaging was introduced, tragedies continue to occur among young children. The pharmacist must be able to deal effectively with these emergencies, exercise judgment, and be decisive with such inquiries.

Another alarming problem that has surfaced within recent years is child and spousal abuse. This is of concern to all communities, and pharmacists, by their involvement, can serve in several ways to help alleviate the problem. For example, be aware of the warning signs of abuse and neglect from the perspective of the child (eg, seems unduly afraid of parents, shows evidence of repeated skin or other injuries, shows signs of poor overall care) and the parent (eg, makes no attempt to explain the child's most obvious injuries or offers absurd, contradictory explanations; shows a lack of control or fear of losing control). Given the warning signs of child abuse and neglect, the pharmacist can coax information from the parent gently when either

taking the initiative to do so or provided the opportunity. A simple conversation may be sufficient encouragement for an abusive parent to admit the need for assistance and guidance. At this point the pharmacist must have the name of an individual at the community abuse center with whom the parent can talk both before and during a crisis. Given uncooperative parents the pharmacist must exercise professional judgment and report the matter to local authorities. The pharmacist, like all citizens, is immune from civil and/or criminal liability when reporting any knowledge or suspicion of child abuse.

By participation with local authorities and professionals in information forums conducted by social workers, the pharmacist can provide information to the abusive parent on how drugs, including alcohol, can affect one's behavior, change one's mood, effect depression with long-term use, and induce psychotic reactions. When this information is blended with the physician-nurse discussion of physical injury incurred from abuse and with teacher awareness of reporting suspicions, it adds immeasurably to the dimension of such a symposium.

The pharmacist also should recognize the need for health education on a broader scale. Many of the health problems encountered by communities can be prevented or alleviated with proper education. But it must be the pharmacist who is willing to share the wealth of knowledge and information he or she has accrued. All persons are not knowledgeable about the extent of pharmacists' education and thus automatically do not think of them as a source of information. Thus, pharmacists must provide the impetus to focus attention toward the capability they have relative to health education. There are several ways they can achieve this.

One method is to make the pharmacy the health center of the community. The willingness to participate in *Poison Prevention Week* or *National Diabetes Month* focuses consumer education toward the pharmacy. Coupled with this is the distribution of pamphlets of public interest on health information for the community. A display of free health literature in the pharmacy demonstrates a commitment to effective health care. There are myriads of pamphlets available on a variety of topics (eg, *Diabetes, Dry Skin and You,* or *The Professional Treatment of Constipation*) from pharmaceutical manufacturers that can be used effectively to promote health care. This encourages inquiries from consumers and, if displayed neatly in the prescription waiting area of the pharmacy, may afford the opportunity to the patient to read health-related information while waiting for a prescription. The pharmacist should make an effort to question pharmaceutical manufacturers' representatives about the availability of such pamphlets for the community. Many times pamphlets are available, but unless requested, they remain confined to the box in which they are contained.

In the event there is an outbreak of a communicable disease (eg, pediculosis capitis at a local elementary school), the pharmacist should obtain and disseminate useful patient-related information. If this type of information is provided directly to the patient/caregiver at the time of medication puzrchase or in conjunction with the local school nurse, needless parental worry and confusion is avoided.

The AIDS crisis continues and ranks as the most significant global health concern of the 1990s. The impact of AIDS on society and on the health-care system is significant, and it is incumbent upon pharmacists to become knowledgeable about this disease process and to identify their role in efforts to stop its spread. Pharmacists can play two major roles in the community human immunodeficiency virus (HIV) disease effort:

1. They can actively participate in the provision of care, treatment, and information to people afflicted with HIV/AIDS.
2. By virtue of their accessibility, they are in an excellent position to provide HIV prevention information to consumers and the general public.

The provision of care for HIV and AIDS patients is similar to the treatment of other patients. However, the treatment of these patients is more complex, the disease can be debilitating, and the emotional impact upon the patient, family, and health-care providers can be substantial. Aside from normal distributive functions, it is important that the pharmacist provide patient counseling and educational services (eg, treatment options, side effects, transmission information, risk reduction guidelines for sexual activity), emphasize patient compliance (including keeping scheduled medical appointments), provide emotional support, and provide referrals to appropriate resources (eg, financial, housing, health-care providers, or therapists).

The AIDS patient provides a unique opportunity for pharmacists, and they should interact with these patients in a way that encourages communication and confidence. It is very important that the patient feel *safe* with the pharmacist. Patients must feel that they are not being judged or scorned because of their disease or sexual orientation. Confidentiality is important to the AIDS patient; protecting it is a particularly important role for the pharmacist. Many patients have legitimate concerns that they may lose their jobs and/or be alienated from family and friends if their HIV status becomes known.

Pharmacists should be prepared to listen to a patient's desire to participate in nontraditional therapies. They should be open to discussing with patients the pros and cons of traditional and nontraditional options. It is estimated that health fraud in the US approaches $40 billion on an annual basis. Health fraud knows no bounds and frequently targets certain groups of people, including those with serious illnesses. Products and therapies of quackery waste people's limited financial resources, may offer ineffective or harmful therapy, predispose a patient to harmful adverse effects, and even persuade a patient to forgo traditional therapy that might be more beneficial. To help patients identify credible clinical trials, pharmacists can encourage them to call the AIDS Clinical Trials Information Service hotline (1-800-874-2572).

A key attribute to being a professional is being accessible to those one serves. In this context, the role of the pharmacist is illustrated aptly in the area of family planning. By sharing knowledge and information about oral contraceptive therapy, nonprescription modes of contraception control, prevention of venereal disease, and pregnancy testing and by assisting couples dealing with fertility impairment, the pharmacist demonstrates accessibility and increases the awareness of the public that the pharmacy is the place where knowledge and informed advice are available.

Pharmacy school curricula recognize the need for effective oral communication both on an individual patient basis and to larger numbers of assembled people (eg, civic and church groups, clubs) by implementing effective course work in the undergraduate curriculum. However, if the pharmacist does not accept the challenge and communicate information, then other, less-qualified persons may be asked by the consuming public to fill this informational void. Sometimes pharmacists are fearful of presenting talks or having discussions with interested groups because of a lack of self-confidence. At the same time they may feel that they do not have the capability to discuss a topic because of a lack of information.

Recognizing these shortcomings in its past graduates, schools/colleges now have electronic literature-searching programs in their libraries to educate and heighten students' awareness of literature resources. Schools/colleges are committing toward outcome-based curricula that are anchored toward the development of student oral communication skills, decision-making skills, and problem-solving abilities, among others. It is hoped that this will encourage greater involvement of the pharmacist in community discussion on health issues. However, one must still deal with the current situation, and pharmacists in practice should look to their local public libraries for information support or consider contacting either their alma mater or state/local pharmaceutical associations for meaningful information.

It is essential that pharmacists contribute to public informational forums and make the community aware of public-health problems. Information and guidance should not be confined solely to drugs and their use, but also should include health-related issues (eg, sexually transmitted diseases, hazards of smokeless tobacco). A true concern must center around the casual attitude of the public toward drugs, a concept that unfortunately is reinforced through commercial advertising and communication media.

Whenever possible, pharmacists must help restore consumer confidence when it has been put in a position of doubt. The classic examples occurred in 1982 and in 1986 with Tylenol-tampering incidents and in 1991 with a Sudafed-tampering incident. Several persons were killed because of the deliberate introduction of cyanide into capsules on the shelf. Pharmacists responded by displaying posters and informational bulletins that instructed consumers to complete the following:

- Read the label. The labels on OTC medicines with tamper-evident packages tell what seals and other features a person should look for.
- Inspect the outer packaging. Check for loose, torn, sliced, or missing wrappings as well as discolored products and unusual odors.
- Inspect the medication once it is opened. Look at it again before taking it. If it looks suspicious, be suspicious.
- Never take medications in the dark.
- The label should be read and medication inspected at every dose.

Unfortunately, there are innovative and creative individuals in the community who may create new problems. Thus, the pharmacist must maintain constant surveillance and be willing to allay fears.

In response to the initial event, the federal government passed amendments to its laws (18 USC 65) to provide for tamper-evident and tamper-resistant packaging of OTC products. This amendment (PL 989-127, Oct 1983) calls for several measures. While the act is complicated, it leaves the impression that there is not a thing that can be done to a commercial package that is not prohibited, and that is as it should be. The pharmacist must be careful not to destroy the tamper-evident or tamper-resistant component of the packaging inadvertently. To do so may bring the pharmacist under the Act as a violator. Products that have been opened by consumers (often for the purpose of noting how big the tablets are, or for comparing the product with one that is already being used by that individual) are rendered unsalable, and they must be removed promptly from the shelf and returned to the supplier.

Most OTC products are covered by the Act. Specifically excluded are insulin, dermatologicals, dentifrices, and lozenges. While nothing prevents manufacturers from placing those products into tamper-resistant or tamper-evident packaging, it is not required at this time.

Pharmacists always should remain above reproach in the eye of the public. They should avoid even the appearance of professional impropriety and thereby not create questions of ethics within the mind of the patient. The most important means pharmacists have in educating society on health matters is the personal contact they have with the public. Whenever possible, they should volunteer health information and encourage people to exercise proper judgment to maintain good health. Some have been very creative and have developed and written patient-oriented newsletters on timely subjects that reinforce the attitude that the pharmacist is both a drug information specialist and health-care educator and provider. Others have achieved this same end by writing health information columns for local newspapers or participating in local media programs to provide health-care information. Professional organizations (eg, NCPA) have been helpful, too, through the provision of print-based health information (eg, Pharm/alert) that the pharmacist can use and disseminate for public education.

Finally, by showing a professional interest in, and attitude toward, the clientele that frequents the pharmacy, the pharmacist makes people feel they are important and that they have someone upon whom they can depend for help. A notable example of this is in ostomy care. There are over 1.1 million ostomates in the US, with new ones increasing by about 90,000 each year. In the end, though, it is the pharmacist who really benefits by the intangible return of fulfillment and enrichment from using skills and information learned through formal and continuing education and practical experience.

CONCLUSION

Pharmacy is evolving from a product-oriented to a patient-oriented profession. This role modification is extremely healthy for the patient, the pharmacist, and other members of the health-care team. However, the evolution will present pharmacists with a number of new challenges. Now, more than in the past, pharmacists must make the acquisition of contemporary practice knowledge and skills a high priority, to render the level of service embodied in the concept of pharmaceutical care. Pharmacy educators organizations and regulatory bodies must all work together to support pharmacists as they assume expanded health-care roles. Pharmacy and the health-care industry must work to ensure that the pharmacist is compensated justly for all services. But before this can happen it will be necessary for pharmacy to demonstrate *value-added* to the cost of the prescription. Marketing of the purpose of pharmacy in the health-care morass and of the services provided by the pharmacist is needed to generate an appropriate perceived value among purchasers and users of health-care services. Pharmacists should view themselves as dispensers of therapy and drug-effect interpretations as well as of drugs themselves. Service components of pharmacy should be identified clearly to third-party payers and be visible to consumers, so that they know what is available at what cost and how it may be accessed. In the future, pharmacy services must be evaluated on patient outcome (ie, pharmaceutical care) rather than the number of prescriptions dispensed, and pharmacy must evolve toward interpretation and patient consultation, related to the use of medication technologies.

REFERENCES

1. Clepper I. *Drug Topics* 1992; 136(16):44.
2. Latiolais CJ, Berry CC. *Drug Intell Clin Pharm* 1969; 3:270.
3. Berg JS, et al. *Ann Pharmacother* 1993; 27:S3.
4. Johnson JA, Bootman JL. *Arch Intern Med* 1995; 155:1949.
5. Rosenstock IM. *Diabetes Care* 1985; 8(6):610.
6. Cardinale V. *Drug Topics* 1995; 139(10):35.
7. *The Role of the Pharmacist in Comprehensive Medication Use Management. The Delivery of Pharmaceutical Care* (white paper). Washington, DC: APhA, Mar 1992.
8. Strand SM, Cipple RJ, Morley PC. *Pharmaceutical Care: An Introduction.* Kalamazoo, MI: Upjohn Co, 1992.
9. Cipolle RJ, Strand LM, Morley PC. *Pharmaceutical Care Practice.* New York: McGraw-Hill, 1998.
10. *The Clinical Role of the Community Pharmacist.* Washington, DC: OIG, DHHS, Nov 1990.
11. *1997–1998 Survey of Pharmacy Law.* Park Ridge, IL: NABP 1997.
12. Haggard A. *Handbook of Patient Education.* Rockville, MD: Aspen, 1989.
13. Mason NA, Shimp LA. *Building a Pharmacist's Patient Data Base. Module 2: Clinical Skills Program.* Bethesda, MD: ASHP, 1993.
14. Jones NJ, Campbell S. *Designing and Recommending a Pharmacist's Care Plan. Module 4: Clinical Skills Program.* Bethesda, MD: ASHP, 1994.
15. Srnka QM, Self TH. *Systematic Medication Profile Review,* ed 3. Alexandria, VA: American College of Apothecaries, 1991.
16. Mason NA, Shimp LA. *Constructing a Patient's Drug Therapy Problem List. Module 3: Clinical Skills Program.* Bethesda, MD: ASHP, 1993.
17. *Hismanal* [pkg insert]. Titusville, NJ: Janssen Pharmaceutica, 1996.
18. Ritschel WA. *Handbook of Basic Pharmacokinetics,* ed 4. Hamilton, IL: Drug Intell Publ, 1992.
19. *Med Lett Drugs Ther* 1996; 38(985):92.
20. DiGregorio RV. *US Pharmacist* 1998; 23(6):101.
21. *American Hospital Formulary Service: Drug Information.* Bethesda, MD: ASHP, 1998.
22. Hussar DA. *Am J Pharm Sci Supp Public Health* 1994; 166(1):1.
23. Baskin L. *Hosp Formul* 1998; 33(1):S64.
24. Todd WE, Ladon EH. *Dis Manage Health Outcomes* 1998; 3(1):1.
25. Kehoe WA, Katz RC. *Ann Pharmacother* 1998; 32(12):1076.
26. Murphy J, Coster G. *Drugs* 1997; 54(12):797.
27. *USP DI Vol II. Advice for the Patient,* ed 18. Rockville, MD: USPC, 1998.
28. Beardsly RS. *J Pharmacoepidemiol* 1995; 3(2):49.
29. Nordenberg T. *FDA Consum* 1997; (Jul-Aug):1.
30. *National Adult Literacy Survey,* US Dept of Educ, Natl Cntr for Educ Stats, Sep 1993.
31. Conlan MF. *Drug Topics* 1991; 135(8):66.
32. Rovers, JP et al. *A Practical Guide to Pharmaceutical Care.* Washington, DC: APhA, 1998.
33. Meyer SM, Trinca CE. In Knowlton CE, Penna RP, eds. *Pharmaceutical Care.* New York: Chapman & Hall, 1996, p 283.
34. *Approved Providers of Continuing Pharmaceutical Education.* Chicago: ACPE, 1998.
35. Portner TS. *Effective Pharmacy Managment,* ed 7. Alexandria, VA: NARD Manage Inst, 1994.
36. Hatoum HT, Valuck RJ. In *Pharmaceutical Care.* In Knowlton CE, Penna RP, eds. New York: Chapman & Hall, 1996, p 68.
37. Rupp MT. In *Pharmaceutical Care.* In Knowlton CE, Penna RP, eds. New York: Chapman & Hall, 1996, p 257.
38. Anon. *AJHP* 1998; 55(12):1238.
39. Landis NT. *AJHP* 1998; 55(23): 2452.
40. Hagel HP, Rovers, JP, eds. *Managing the Patient-Centered Pharmacy.* Washington, DC: American Pharmaceutical Association.

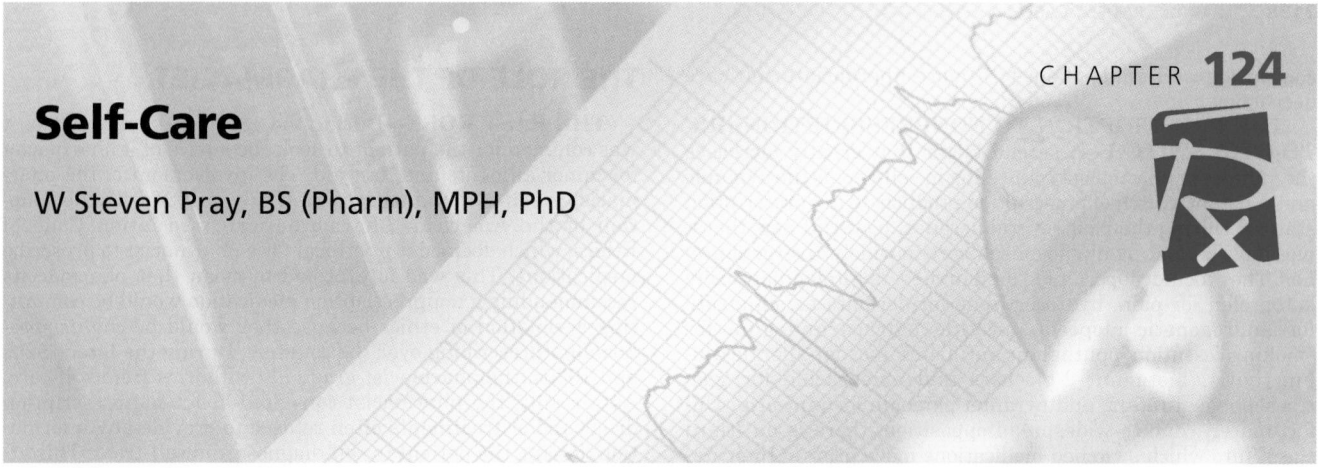

Self-Care

W Steven Pray, BS (Pharm), MPH, PhD

CHAPTER **124**

PHARMACISTS AND SELF-CARE WITH NONPRE-SCRIPTION PRODUCTS—Pharmacists are in a unique position because of their education, training, and ready accessibility to the public when it comes to self-medication by the public with nonprescription (over-the-counter or OTC) drugs. Experts estimate that the number of nonprescription products is in excess of 100,000, but the accuracy of this estimate is unknown. In the United States, nonprescription product sales exceeded $14 billion in 2001.[1]

Like other businesses, pharmacies are in a fight for survival. Recent years have seen closings of many small independent stores. Third-party plans have reduced prescription profits so dramatically that some retailers have turned to high volume strategies in an attempt to survive. One unfortunate result of high volume is decreased patient interaction time. Pharmacists are forced to spend long hours behind the prescription counter with no scheduled lunch hour and little patient contact. Even though counseling is required, it is often cursory and hurried. Management demands more work with less help, because hiring additional pharmacists and pharmacy technicians further reduces shrinking profits. This dismal picture is more prevalent in high volume chain stores.

Fortunately, some pharmacies realize that pushing for high volume is self-defeating in the long run, because it appeals to the patient who wants cheap products at the expense of quality. Some of these more enlightened locations have realized that another route key to survival is to cultivate a specialty or "niche."

There are several viable and profitable specialties, such as compounding. Unfortunately, articles in pharmacy journals and textbooks (eg, *Handbook of Nonprescription Drugs*) often advise embracing ethically and scientifically indefensible areas such as herbal supplements and homeopathic products. This is especially regrettable when the pharmacist has a wide range of nonprescription products that are ethical, safe, and effective.

Marketing one's practice location as a center for self-care through intense counseling on nonprescription products and devices is a logical and profitable specialty. Self-care is especially appealing because of several factors:

- Minor medical conditions can be advised competently by the pharmacist who has expertise and education in these areas.
- Most pharmacists have had a nonprescription products/self-care course as part of the professional pharmacy curriculum.
- The typical pharmacy already stocks a wide range of nonprescription products and devices, so that there is no need to purchase a special group of products.
- The nonprescription market contains many ingredients lacking proof of efficacy and/or safety. Pharmacist counseling helps patients choose products whose safety and efficacy is demonstrated.
- Effective counseling in the nonprescription area allows the pharmacist to extend the concept of pharmaceutical care.

- Although nonprescription products are available in non-pharmacy outlets, the patient will not be able to obtain legitimate self-care advice at these locations.
- Many pharmacies locate nonprescription products away from the immediate location of the pharmacy. The pharmacist cannot advise patients who need help with these items, which seriously compromises their ability to offer self-care counseling. Those who choose to place nonprescription products in close proximity to the pharmacy enhance their credibility as experts in self-care.
- In other stores, nonprescription products are positioned close to the pharmacy, but shelving is parallel to the pharmacy, rather than perpendicular, which also makes it impossible to see patients who need help. Choosing a store layout that allows the pharmacist to visualize the patients in the self-care aisles allows the pharmacist to render assistance when necessary.

The pharmacist who wishes to develop this niche should obtain current information on the various self-treatable conditions, as well as all of the nonprescription ingredients and the many precautions associated with their use.

THE MOVEMENT TOWARD SELF-CARE—During the 1960s, this country experienced a growing distrust of established entities, such as the government, organized religion, and legitimate medicine. One of the consequences was a compelling consumer desire to rebel against the traditional provider/patient relationship, in which the consumer meekly and unquestioningly followed the directions of the provider. Patients began to demand a greater personal involvement and responsibility for health-care maintenance and treatment, a trend that continues today.[2] Direct-to-consumer advertising of prescription products enhanced this by indirectly communicating to consumers an innovative medical paradigm in which patients should demand a particular prescription product from the physician based on the advertisements they had seen. Consumers also feel competent to guide their own medical therapy based on past personal experience or anecdotal information from friends and relatives in regard to a particular prescription or nonprescription product. This is partly due to the common myth that any nonprescription product or device advertised in the media is safe and effective for self-use without any medical supervision. Further, some patients feel that the nonprescription product label contains all information of importance and deny the possibility that a pharmacist consultation can add any value to the purchase. Partially as a result of these various market forces and misconceptions, nonprescription products cause many episodes of morbidity and mortality that might have been prevented with judicious pharmacist counseling.[3] It is an uncomfortable truth that the patient who enters a pharmacy with a preconceived self-care opinion about a particular product or course of action is often manifestly and profoundly incorrect, and it is in the highest tradition of pharmaceutical care that the concerned pharmacist correct the patient's mis-

2197

conception and guide them to a more appropriate self-care decision.

THE PRESCRIPTION TO NONPRESCRIPTION (RX-TO-OTC) SWITCH—A second factor that greatly increases the validity of pharmacist counseling in self-care is the dynamic and constant switch of prescription products to nonprescription status.[4] During the past several decades, powerful new therapies have become available for self-care in widely divergent arenas. They include loperamide for diarrhea, ibuprofen/naproxen/ketoprofen for pain, hydrocortisone for dermatoses, minoxidil for androgenetic alopecia, nicotine patches and gum for smoking cessation, ophthalmic antihistamines for allergic conjunctivitis, histamine-2-blockers and omeprazole for gastroesophageal reflux, and pyrantel pamoate for pinworm. Unfortunately, due to widespread opposition, there is no "third class" into which switched medications move prior to their unsupervised release to the American public. This leads to the uncomfortable realization that a particular medication awaiting a switch is only available under a physician's prescription, requiring pharmacist counseling and refill authorization until midnight the day before the switch occurs. At 12:01 am on the day of the switch, the ingredient is suddenly deemed safe enough to be sold to any consumer in any location at any time, with no professional monitoring or advice being necessary. It can be purchased in any gas station, beauty shop, airport lobby, or hotel vending machine. Since there is no requirement for professional counseling prior to purchase of nonprescription products, the manufacturer assumes the full burden of communicating all of the risks and other information that was formerly provided by the pharmacist. Thus, the manufacturer of nonprescription products has a higher duty to directly warn the patient of risks associated with their use than the does manufacturer of prescription products. Pharmacists must embrace these products, stressing the value to the consumer of purchasing them in a pharmacy in order to obtain the counseling that enhances appropriate use.

CAN PATIENTS READ NONPRESCRIPTION PRODUCT LABELS?—Another major rationale for pharmacist involvement in self-care is the issue of patients and their ability to read and/or comprehend nonprescription product labels. The FDA mandated a new label that is intended to more clearly communicate issues in use of products to patients. However, the pharmacist can still add value to the purchase of nonprescription products by acting as a "learned intermediary." In this role, the pharmacist can point out specific contraindications to use of certain products, answering questions about dosing, adverse effects, and appropriate use.

There are still some patients who will be unable to properly read and/or interpret the label. Some suffer impaired vision (eg, glaucoma damage, detached retina, macular degeneration) that does not allow them to read the small print. Others suffer from tremor or other conditions that make it difficult to hold the container still for reading prior to purchase. Others cannot understand the terminology used on labels, perhaps because English is not their primary language. Still other patients have limited reading comprehension or may be completely illiterate. In all of these cases, pharmacist counseling can be of immense value.

HOW PATIENTS CHOOSE NONPRESCRIPTION PRODUCTS AND DEVICES—Persons do not always seek the advice of a physician with every illness. Symptoms of the ailment may be deemed minor enough to treat with a nonprescription product. The decision of the patient concerning which product to purchase often is based on prior experience with the product; advice received from a neighbor or relatives; and commercial advertisements by manufacturers. However, the pharmacist is the only expert in self-care with nonprescription products and devices. Pharmacists can develop an enduring self-care specialty by making defensible patient triage decisions that are based on scientific principles. Through this practice, it is often necessary to guide incorrect patient purchase decisions into a more suitable and appropriate path.

THE ROLE OF THE PHARMACIST

THE PAST ROLE—During the 1800s and early 1900s, it was common for the patient to seek the advice of a pharmacist for minor ailments and first aid. The involvement of the pharmacist in self-care changed dramatically in 1921 with the adoption of the American Pharmaceutical Association Code of Ethics, which deemed it unethical for a pharmacist to prescribe medications. This was interpreted to mean that pharmacists recommending a nonprescription medication would be committing a violation of ethics because they would be *counter-prescribing* (prescribing over the counter). During the later 1920s and 1930s, the pharmacist gradually withdrew from self-care. As a result, the pharmacist consulted about nonprescription drugs and/or treatments often refused to provide any information, forcing the patient to self-diagnose and self-treat. This attitude continued into the early 1970s, when pharmacists were taught not to tell patients the intended use or potential adverse effects of their prescription medications. Prescriptions were not labeled routinely with the contents so that the patient would be forced to ask the physician for additional information.

During this time, many pharmacists also felt uncomfortable counseling patients about minor ailments. Patients were often referred to the physician for all problems. Few colleges of pharmacy included any coursework involving nonprescription products. Pharmacists were not required to communicate to patients with any degree of skill, and could actually pass an entire work day without being asked to move to the front of the pharmacy to talk to the patient. The profession attracted a certain number of communication-apprehensive individuals, and the pharmacy curricula of the day did not include any training in communication. Thus, their communication skills were rudimentary and untested.

PHARMACY CHANGES IN THE 1970s—During the mid-1970s pharmacy was rejuvenated with the promotion and gradual introduction of clinical and *patient-oriented* concepts into the practice of pharmacy. Advising the patient on health matters not only became fashionable but was recognized as a responsibility of the pharmacist, ethically and legally. The pharmacist was encouraged to question the patient who had decided to self-medicate and triage the patient (ie, recommend a nonprescription medication or recommend that the patient seek medical attention). By 1969 the membership of the APhA voted to adopt a new Code of Ethics that held the health and welfare of the patient to be of first consideration for the pharmacist.

This brief historical perspective explains why the older, more mature pharmacist in practice today may feel somewhat uncomfortable in providing advice to persons who decide to treat themselves and why pharmacists may simply decline to offer this professional service. A number of pharmacists may have to be educated, or re-educated, on how to counsel the patient who elects to pursue self-care. Continuing-education providers should strive to educate pharmacists who did not have the benefit of a formal course in nonprescription drug therapy through intensive lectures replete with case studies and treatment algorithms.

THE PHARMACIST'S POTENTIAL ROLE TODAY—The move to self-care, the ongoing switch of potent medications to nonprescription status, and the inability to read and understand nonprescription labels effectively, all point to the potential importance of the pharmacist as a nonprescription product information source. It is clear that the pharmacist is in an ideal position to help consumers with their self-care needs, but the pharmacist *must* take a proactive role. Consumer trends indicate that the pharmacist slowly is gaining recognition as a legitimate source of information about nonprescription drugs/products. Consumers seek pharmacists who provide service, and media advertisements tout the pharmacist as a source to consult.[5] The factors (in descending order of importance) germane to the patient/consumer selection of a pharmacist were:

1. Actively discussing instructions for the use of the pharmaceutical product, including effectiveness, anticipated side effects, and duration of treatment.
2. Being available for consultation.
3. Providing willingness to offer advice on general health problems.
4. Being friendly and approachable.

THE NONPRESCRIPTION PRODUCT LABEL—The FDA supports the concept of self-medication but, unfortunately, has not embraced the concept of the pharmacist as the first professional that the patient should consult before using the product. As pharmacists struggled to be included on the label of nonprescription products, they faced opposition from the nonprescription industry (who wished their marketing messages to reach the public undiluted by any "learned intermediary") and physicians (who balked at pharmacists being given co-equal status on the labels). Only in addressing drug interactions is the pharmacist's advice specifically mentioned on nonprescription product labels.

RESPONSIBILITIES OF THE PHARMACIST IN SELF-CARE

Self-care counseling is a primary-care activity that carries with it a great amount of professional responsibility. Communicating information about OTC products requires the same basic skills used for prescription medications and does not mandate additional specialized education/training or vast financial expenditures to be well done.

Many commercial enterprises use the old business maxim, "The customer is always right." However, in pharmacy, the customer is often not right in the potential choice of a self-care product or device. They may be mistaken in the need for a product, the choice of a product, and often the need to consult a physician or other primary care practitioner. It is the pharmacist's responsibility to correct the patient's misconceptions tactfully as a component of pharmaceutical care. To provide proper advice, the pharmacist must gather relevant information needed to decide whether the patient should not select a specific product, should choose a nonprescription product or device, or should be referred to the physician. This process is referred to as *pharmacist triage*.

THE TRIAGE FUNCTION OF THE PHARMACIST

Patients who wish to treat themselves may not seek the services of a pharmacist. Nonprescription products and devices are freely available in food stores, variety stores, vending machines in hotel lobbies, airports, and gasoline stations. The drawback to these purchases is that these venues lack a pharmacist to provide medically sound recommendations to the patient. Thus, the consumer then may choose a product or advice on the basis of recommendations from friends or family, the attractiveness of the packaging, or perhaps the memory of an entertaining media advertisement. While the vast majority of advertisements sponsored by nonprescription drug and device manufacturers are factual and accurate, patients are bombarded with hundreds of ads from less reputable manufacturers urging consumers to purchase products or devices that lack proof of safety and/or efficacy. Thus, without a pharmacist, patient safety may be seriously compromised. The presence of an educated/trained pharmacist is the value-added benefit of purchasing nonprescription drug products and devices at a pharmacy. Of course, this argument assumes that the pharmacist has embraced the concept of triage, moving from a protected area behind the prescription counter to engage patients actively. The pharmacist who talks to patients about nonprescription medications re-

ceives many questions daily.[6] The simplest of these questions is "Where can I find (name of product)?" However, the prudent pharmacist must learn to get *behind* this type of question, asking what type of problem has prompted this particular visit to the pharmacy. Failure to discover the nature of the medical condition can lead the patient to inappropriate use of a product. However, the pharmacist must understand that some patients are hesitant to provide any details and must be prepared for a cool rebuff from some patients. Other patients refuse to consider any advice from the pharmacist. This may be due to the greater relative influence of their friends, the advertising, or their own perception of the quality of the pharmacist interaction. However, the pharmacist should still make an attempt to educate the patient regarding a safer course of action.

In certain circumstances, the patient may ask about a specific medical condition where more complicated questions will be asked and triage decisions become critical. Patients can be placed into one of the following three categories.

No Need for a Product—The patient may have no perceptible need for a nonprescription product or device (eg, the healthy patient who has become convinced that unproven dietary supplements such as gingko and noni juice are necessary for everyday use). At times, another intervention will fit the concept of pharmaceutical care more closely than selling a product (eg, educating a patient about sleep-hygiene methods to treat insomnia rather than purchasing a nonprescription sleep-aid).

A Minor Medical Condition That Will Benefit From a Nonprescription Product or Device—There are numerous medical conditions that may be improved with self-care products and devices (eg, the common cold or athletes' foot).

A Medical Condition That Places the Patient Beyond the Realm of Self-Care—When the medical condition cannot be classified as minor or is clearly beyond the capacity of nonprescription products or devices, the patient must be referred for care from another practitioner (eg, MD, DO, podiatrist, optometrist, or dentist) who is able to properly diagnose and treat the condition through ordering lab tests and diagnostic examinations, and providing prescription medications when necessary. In the most severe cases, the patient should be instructed to go to the nearest emergency room and given directions if they are unfamiliar with its location.

Thus, many times in the average work day, the pharmacist who is willing to assist patients in self-care must implement pharmaceutical care through recognizing medical conditions, deciding whether they are self-treatable, knowing which products are appropriate for those conditions, and being able to persuade the patients which courses of action are most suitable. To carry out these sophisticated decisions, the pharmacist must possess a vast body of knowledge. The information needed to properly triage a patient can be divided into two categories: those related to the product and those related to the patient.

PRODUCT-RELATED DECISION FACTORS

The foremost factors to consider in nonprescription products and devices are safety and efficacy, both of which must be present. Safety without proven efficacy is a waste of money. Conversely, efficacy without proven safety presents an unacceptable risk to the patient.

Prior to the 1970s, objective data regarding safety and efficacy of nonprescription products and devices were difficult to find in professional medical literature. In the early 1970s, the U.S. Congress remedied that unfortunate situation by mandating a sweeping review of all nonprescription drug products and devices. This review dramatically improved the information available, but the downside has been the slow pace at which the review has been conducted. It is still proceeding one-quarter of a century later. Nevertheless, the Nonprescription Drug Review process of the FDA has been highly beneficial to pharmacists. It has provided a knowledge base that facilitates sound decisions regarding comparative product effectiveness and safety. The review process has generated substantial scientific research, producing impressive amounts of new information on nonprescription medications. At the same time it has placed a burden upon the pharmacist to keep current about new information in this important subject area. A real handicap for the diligent pharmacist is obtaining factual, current information. Current pharmacy literature often provides synopses of the latest FDA rulings.

The major strength of the FDA review of nonprescription drug products and devices has been its objectivity. Full approval for any ingredient requires overwhelming evidence of safety and efficacy. Proof of efficacy must be demonstrated in placebo-controlled, double-blind studies with sample sizes sufficient to ensure statistical significance when the correct statistical tests are used. FDA personnel carefully examine each study submitted to uncover such shortcomings as bias in patient recruitment, poor questionnaire construction, insufficient blinding, and use of parametric statistics on nominal or ordinal data. The study must have been replicated in a nonrelated research center. Thus, strict adherence to the scientific method ensures that medications are proved efficacious. Proof of safety is determined through a comprehensive literature search to uncover studies that list adverse reactions and through examinations of all other extant literature on the specific ingredient. While no medication is free of adverse reactions, the risk must be small in relation to the proven benefit the consumer can expect from the product when used as directed.

If a nonprescription medication is proven safe and efficacious, it is given a designation known as Category I. These ingredients can be recommended by the pharmacist with confidence as long as all label warnings and dosing directions are carefully read and adhered to, and as long as all patient-related decision factors are taken into consideration.

Ingredients that lack proof of safety and/or efficacy are referred to as Category III ingredients. The pharmacist should take great caution in recommending these ingredients. If their efficacy remains unproven, any possible risks to which the patient would be exposed are unacceptable. If, on the other hand, their safety is unproved, any possible benefit is not worth the risk to patient safety.

Category II ingredients were determined to be unsafe and/or to lack efficacy. The FDA is usually able to force their removal eventually, but an article in the lay press exposed situations in which pharmacies continued to sell these banned products freely.[7] Selling products containing these ingredients exposes patients to chemicals already proven to be unsafe, or ineffective, or both, an indefensible business decision.

There are several reasons why pharmacists might recommend products that lack proof of safety and/or efficacy. For instance, companies have sponsored promotions in which an unidentified *mystery shopper* enters pharmacies and asks for help with a certain medical condition. These shoppers are actually acting for a certain company, and the pharmacist who recommends that company's product may win a cash prize, a free trip, or a new vehicle. Advertising campaigns encourage the pharmacist to suggest that company's product to all who ask, just in case the person might be the mystery shopper. Thus, the pharmacist might suggest a specific product out of selfish self-interest. Pharmacists are also approached by *rack jobbers,* who often ask to place a rack of merchandise in the pharmacy on consignment. The pharmacist does not purchase the items on the rack and has no cash outlay. When products sell, the pharmacist receives a set fee. The rack jobbers promise to restock the rack as needed. These products should be inspected carefully to ensure that their ingredients are actually safe and effective. This seductive approach may have been used by the manufacturers of Cal-Ban 3000, a diet aid that was marketed nationally. The ingredient in Cal-Ban 3000 had not been approved by the FDA.[8] Its labeling was confusing in listing its ingredient as *Cyamopsis tetragonolobus,* which was the scientific name of guar gum, a complex sugar that swells when wetted. The FDA was advised by health professionals of adverse reactions and discovered that ten hospitalizations from intestinal or esophageal obstruction had occurred. One death occurred from a blood clot that reached the lungs following surgical removal of a guar gum throat obstruction. The FDA forced the company to recall the product, levying a heavy fine. Had pharmacists been more wary about selling a product of unknown efficacy/safety, perhaps the medical problems could have been prevented. Some pharmacists sell unproven products out of a desire to please the customer. It is uncomfortable to have a confrontation with a patient who is convinced that an unproven product is the best choice for them. For example, a patient may be convinced that ginseng has helped him feel younger or that ginkgo has helped improve his memory. After many months of use, patients may become extremely upset with the pharmacist who then counsels them to discontinue these unproved products and seek legitimate medical care if their symptoms return.

Pharmacists also fear that they will lose business if they refuse to sell unproven products. They may not want to be viewed as an impediment to the patient. They also realize that patients may listen to the pharmacist, then purchase the products they wanted in the first place at a store down the street. Of course, pandering to the patient's every whim is ultimately self-defeating. The pharmacist must instead strive to build a reputation for professional integrity by refusing to sell questionable products and by offering logical reasons for such refusals. Such a refusal is in the highest traditions of pharmaceutical care and professional ethics.

Pharmacists may sell unproven products out of a belief that the product may actually work, even though data are lacking, or from the mistaken belief that "It can't hurt, can it?" These pharmacists will evidently continue to sell unproven products until they cause overt patient harm or until there is overwhelming evidence of a lack of efficacy. Unfortunately, congressional legislation has burdened the overworked FDA so that unscrupulous companies can continue to market their unproven products for a long period without making the barest pretense of carrying out legitimate scientific studies. The patient often has no idea that the products lack proof of safety and/or efficacy despite the fact that they are sold freely on the shelf of the pharmacy.

An example of the extreme care pharmacists should take in recommending nonprescription products is provided by phenylpropanolamine (PPA). PPA was first developed to maintain blood pressure, but was included in nonprescription products meant for oral nasal decongestion and weight control by the 1970s. PPA was first reviewed in 1976 by the FDA review panel for oral nasal decongestants, which recommended Category I status.[9] However, in 1985 the FDA published its tentative final monograph on OTC nasal decongestants.[10] In this publication, the agency placed PPA in regulatory limbo, declining to assign it any status because of concerns over blood pressure elevation. Out of concern for the safety of consumers, a prudent manufacturer should have withdrawn products containing PPA at that point or reformulated to a safer alternative (eg, pseudoephedrine), since the FDA was not convinced the ingredient was safe; but they continued to market PPA; they could have warned of the risk of PPA-associated hypertension and stroke, but did not do so. In 1990, Congress held hearings on PPA, causing the FDA to reopen the administrative record on PPA in 1991.[11] During the 1990s, debate raged over the safety of PPA, but patients continued to use PPA and pharmacists continued to recommend it. Many billions of doses were sold. Finally, a report (the Yale Hemorrhagic Stroke Project) demonstrated to the satisfaction of the Nonprescription Drugs Advisory Committee of the FDA that PPA caused hemorrhagic strokes in users, and the FDA in 2000 asked the pharmaceutical industry to discontinue marketing it.[12,13] Industry should have placed a voluntary warning about stroke on the label to fully warn consumers of its occurrence; in failing to do so they never clearly explained the potential risk of stroke to patients on the product labels to allow them to weigh the benefits of use against the risk of stroke before use (most packages had no mention of stroke on the label at all). Further, once the FDA requested a voluntary cessation on manufacturing of PPA-containing products, industry never issued an immediate active recall of all PPA-containing products (sold and unsold) with a widely publicized public health alert targeted to all potential consumers warning of the risk of hemorrhagic stroke. As a result, many millions of doses remained in medicine cabinets. Also, products containing PPA were found in secondary markets (eg, flea markets, deep discounters) several years later, often having passed their expiration dates. The FDA estimated PPA might have caused as many as 500 strokes yearly, so manufacturer refusal to withdraw products containing it in 1985 might have caused as many as 7500 stokes from 1985 to 2000.[14,15] According to a 2001 report from FDA personnel, the actual number of strokes yearly could have been far higher due to underreporting.[16] If pharmacists had recommended against the product starting in 1985 and refused to stock it, many of these strokes would have been prevented. The pharmacist must take a strong stand for patient advocacy in situations such as this where ingredients lack evidence of proven safety and/or efficacy and manufacturers refuse to withdraw the products or add voluntary warnings to fully apprise patients of the potential risks to the products they sell.

PATIENT-RELATED DECISION FACTORS

The pharmacist who sells only safe and effective ingredients may feel there is no need to counsel patients seeking self-care. This is a mistaken assumption, as the safe and effective ingredients have many restrictions on their use that must be observed to ensure that patient health is not compromised.

AGE OF THE PATIENT—The FDA and its panels have established the minimum ages above which nonprescription ingredients may be administered safely. Certain guidelines are still preliminary, but major changes in the lower age cutoffs are unlikely.

As a general rule, nonprescription products are not to be recommended to patients below the age of two years. (Teething products are an exception, being approved down to four months of age; there is also a pediatric ibuprofen product approved down to the age of six months.) Some products are not safe for dosing under the age of 6, 12, or 16, or 18 years (Table 124-1). These age cutoffs are not arbitrary. With each age cutoff, there is overwhelming evidence that providing the ingredient to those younger than indicated on the label without the supervision of a prescribing professional can be extremely dangerous. For instance, pharmacists are routinely asked about dosing of antihistamine-containing cold and allergy products for patients as young as one month of age. However, administration of antihistamines to those below the age of six years can result in paradoxical excitation (with the exception of loratadine). Similarly, use of antidiarrheals in those under the age of three years can result in life-threatening fluid and electrolyte abnormalities. Despite these warnings, various companies have distributed pediatric dosing charts that purport to provide safe doses for acetaminophen, loperamide, pseudoephedrine, and antihistamines down to ages as young as newborns.

DURATION/SEVERITY OF THE CONDITION—The range of conditions for which patients seek self-care is nothing short of amazing. The author has been asked to recommend nonprescription products for heavy-metal toxicity from inhalation of fumes from welding nickel pipe, brown recluse spider bites, nail and scalp fungi, loose teeth, boils, and eyeballs bruised so completely that the whites were totally blackened. Fortunately, these incidents are the exception, and most minor medical conditions for which self-care is sought will resolve regardless of whether a nonprescription product is used or not.

The pharmacist must remember that even a seemingly minor condition or symptom may reflect an underlying cause that is beyond self-treatment. For instance, while simple headache

Table 124-1. Selected Nonprescription Products and the Ages Below That These Should NOT be Recommended for Self-Care (According to FDA-Approved Labeling)[3]

AGE	PRODUCT(S)
None	Diaper rash products, topical protectant products
4 months	Gingival analgesic products for teething
6 months	Ibuprofen drops, sunscreen products
2 years	Glycerin suppositories, hydrocortisone, antacid products, dimenhydrinate (motion sickness), fluoride toothpastes, pyrantel pamoate, oral nasal decongestant products, sore throat products, antitussive products (except codeine), expectorant products, acetaminophen, children's loratadine syrup
3 years	Antidiarrheal products (except for loperamide)
5 years	Oral sodium phosphate/biphosphate products
6 years	Loperamide, anticavity rinse products, cyclizine (for motion sickness), psyllium (for constipation), methylcellulose, bisacodyl, antihistamine products (except loratadine, meclizine, and dimenhydrinate), cromolyn sodium nasal, codeine, ophthalmic vasoconstrictor/antihistamine combination products
12 years	Hypersensitive tooth products, meclizine, H2-blockers, hemorrhoid products, naproxen, caffeine, insomnia products, cerumen impaction products, skin hyperpigmentation products, topical terbinafine and butenafine, ketoconazole shampoo, vaginal antifungal products, ibuprofen 200 mg tablets
16 years	Ketoprofen
18 years	Minoxidil, nicotine cessation therapies

is usually benign, a headache that lasts for a certain period may indicate serious underlying pathology (eg, bacterial meningitis). Additionally, constipation of sufficient duration may indicate fecal impaction and/or megacolon/megarectum. For these reasons, many nonprescription products and devices carry a labeled safe maximal time cutoff for unsupervised use in self-care (Table 124-2). For instance, nonprescription diarrhea products carry the warning "Do not use for more than 2 days unless directed by a physician." The FDA seldom clarifies the exact meaning. For instance, how should the pharmacist handle the patient who already has had diarrhea for 3 days when seeking self-care products? Should the pharmacist advise an additional 2 days of therapy prior to seeking medical care? How about the patient who has a chronic diarrhea for 2 months? Obviously, both patients are in greater need of rehydration and electrolyte replacement than the patient with only a single diarrheal episode and both should be referred for physician care.

When examining the FDA-labeled maximal durations for self-use, the pharmacist should err on the side of patient safety. First, it is vital to ask "How long have you had this condition?"

Table 124-2. Selected Medical Conditions and the Duration of Time Beyond Which the Patient Should be Referred for Professional Care (eg, Physician, Dentist, Podiatrist) (According to FDA-Approved Labeling)[3]

DURATION	MEDICAL CONDITION
2 days	Diarrhea, migraine
3 days	Fever, dry eye, red eye
4 days	Excessive earwax
7 days	Oral mucosal injury, canker sores, constipation, hemorrhoids, muscular injury, burns, vaginal irritation
10 days	Pain in an adult
14 days	Stomach upset, insomnia

or "When did the symptoms begin?" A judicious judgment allows appropriate triage decisions to be made. Diarrhea products only allow two days of self-care, so a strict interpretation of this timeline is preferable because of the potentially serious nature of diarrhea. In other words, the patient who has already had diarrhea for two days or more is beyond the realm of safe self-care and should be referred immediately to a physician (an emergency room visit may be required if a primary care physician is unavailable). Intraoral topical analgesics (eg, benzocaine) are only to be used for one week to ensure that the patient seeks professional care for a more serious cause of oral sores, such as an oral tumor. Again, a strict interpretation is needed, and the patient with an oral lesion of one week or more in duration should be referred immediately for an oral evaluation without being sold a product. On the other hand, corn and callus products caution against use for more than 14 days. Obviously, typical patients have had the corn or callus for many months to years and may be allowed to use the product for 2 weeks from the point they begin self-care.

CONTRAINDICATIONS—Just as is the case with prescription products, certain nonprescription products are unsafe for unsupervised self-use when the patient also has other medical conditions (Table 124-3). For instance, antihistamines are contraindicated in the patient with glaucoma, because they can cause a rise in intraocular pressure in a patient with narrow (acute or angle-closure) glaucoma, causing irreversible visual loss. Laxatives are contraindicated with rectal bleeding, since this is a cardinal sign of colorectal carcinoma. Oral nasal decongestants are contraindicated in the patient with hypertension. The typical patient seldom reads these warnings, and those that do may not understand them. The pharmacist can perform a particular service in explaining the warnings and offering alternative FDA-approved products that would be safer, when they exist. If there is no ingredient that is safe and effective, patients should be urged to seek the advice of the physician or other prescriber monitoring their condition.

CURRENT USE OF MEDICATIONS, FOODS, AND DRUGS—Some nonprescription ingredients have FDA-labeled precautions regarding drug interactions or warnings against concomitant ingestion with other medications, foods, or drugs of abuse (eg, alcohol, nicotine) (Table 124-4). The pharmacist might inspect a patient's profile or ask about routine medications to discover whether or not these precautions pertain to a

Table 124-3. Selected Nonprescription Products and Medical Conditions That Contraindicate Their Use (According to FDA-Approved Labeling)[3]

NONPRESCRIPTION	PATIENT CONDITION(S) OR SYMPTOM(S) THAT CONTRAINDICATE PRODUCT/CLASS SELF-CARE WITH THE SPECIFIC PRODUCT/CLASS
Teething Products	Fever, nasal congestion
H2-Blocker Products	Persistent abdominal pain
Aspirin	Flu, chickenpox, in children and teenagers
Antihistamine Products (except Loratadine)	Emphysema, chronic bronchitis, glaucoma, difficulty in urination due to an enlarged prostate
Loratadine	Liver or kidney problems
Loperamide	Fever over 101°F, blood or mucus in the stool, liver disease
Pyrantel Pamoate	Pregnancy, liver disease
Hemorrhoid Products	Bleeding from the rectum
Nasal Decongestant Products	Heart disease, high blood pressure, thyroid disease, diabetes mellitus, difficulty in urination due to an enlarged prostate
Sore Throat Products	Fever, headache, rash, swelling, nausea and/or vomiting
Cerumen Impaction Products	Ear drainage or discharge, ear pain or irritation, rash in the ear dizziness; perforation of the eardrum, recent ear surgery

Table 124-4. Selected Nonprescription Products and Medications/Foods/Drugs With Which They Are Contraindicated or With Which Concurrent Use Should be Avoided (According to FDA-Approved Labeling)[3]

NONPRESCRIPTION	MEDICATIONS/FOODS/DRUGS WITH WHICH THEY ARE CONTRAINDICATED
Cimetidine	Theophylline, warfarin, phenytoin
Cyclizine, Meclizine	Alcohol, sedatives, tranquilizers
Mineral Oil	Meals, stool softeners
Oral Bisacodyl	Antacid or milk (within 1 hour)
Bismuth Subsalicylate	Medications for anticoagulation, diabetes, gout or arthritis
Diphenhydramine	Any other product containing diphenhydramine
Oral Nasal Decongestant Products, Dextromethorphan	Monoamine oxidase inhibitors (current use or within two weeks of stopping the MAOI)
Internal Analgesic Products	Three or more alcoholic beverages a day
Nicotine Cessation Products	Any other form of nicotine

specific patient. For instance, nonprescription cimetidine carries a label warning against concomitant use with theophylline, warfarin, and phenytoin. For patients taking these medications, the pharmacist could point out the other three alternative H₂ blockers, which do not carry this warning. Another example is nonprescription salicylates, which carry a warning against concomitant use of anticoagulants, as well as medications for gout, arthritis, and diabetes. At times, the pharmacist may choose to provide drug interaction warnings that exceed those the manufacturer includes. For instance, the risks of phenylpropanolamine-associated hypertension and hemorrhagic stroke were heightened if the patient also ingested caffeine; the manufacturers should have warned patients of this simple additive effect but failed to do so. Only those patients purchasing their products in a pharmacy might have been warned of this interaction.

DEMOGRAPHIC VARIABLES—Occasionally, a patient's demographic variables (other than age) may contraindicate a certain nonprescription product. For instance, nonprescription diuretics (eg, pamabrom, ammonium chloride) carry FDA approval only for menstrual-related water retention.[3] They are never to be recommended for any other cause of fluid retention (eg, possible congestive heart failure or renal dysfunction). Thus, gender disqualifies any male from the safe purchase and use of nonprescription diuretics. As another example, nonprescription hypopigmenting products containing hydroquinone are used legitimately for lightening skin that has darkened in response to sun exposure (eg, solar lentigines or sun-induced freckles), usage of oral contraceptives or estrogens, or during pregnancy. African-Americans and Hispanic Americans have used these products incorrectly in misguided attempts to lighten overall skin color. This may result in exogenous ochronosis, a paradoxical darkening of the skin. Thus, the pharmacist should counsel these patients against use of skin-hypopigmenting agents for overall skin lightening. Miscellaneous demographic patient factors should also be elicited, such as allergies to the specific ingredients present in the medication, and whether the patient is pregnant or breast-feeding.

PAST MEDICATION USE—As the pharmacist questions the patient, it is also important to ask about the products or devices already used to alleviate the condition. This also provides a clue regarding the duration of the condition. Instances of the improper use of unproven products (eg, homeopathic) or of application of home remedies can be uncovered and discouraged. The pharmacist also can discourage the use of unapproved and unsafe products such as those sold in health-food stores. Assuming the patient still has a few days of self-care remaining, the pharmacist can then recommend an appropriate product.

EXACT NATURE OF THE CONDITION—It is vital for the pharmacist to elicit a detailed history of the condition, even if the patient has formulated a self-diagnosis. This ability requires a thorough understanding of the minor medical conditions that are self-treatable and also of the various *red flags* that indicate a serious condition that requires referral to another health care professional. The pharmacist is hampered in discovering the exact nature of the condition for several reasons:

- The pharmacist typically has not undergone formal training in physical assessment, so that judgments must be rendered without a full spectrum of medical information being available. At times the disorder can be confirmed visually (eg, warts or athlete's foot), but in other situations (eg, vaginal candidiasis or hemorrhoids), the pharmacist depends wholly on the verbal information imparted by lay persons who may be fundamentally mistaken regarding certain aspects of their condition (eg, its appearance).
- The legality of pharmacist assessment is questionable, and the boundaries are vague and ill-defined. While the pharmacist can easily recognize poison ivy dermatitis, should the pharmacist examine throats to differentiate viral from bacterial pharyngitis? While the pharmacist can easily check a patient's head for head lice, should the pharmacist also check pubic areas for pubic lice? It has been suggested that retail pharmacists should conduct ear inspections for perforated eardrum, peer into the nostrils to recognize sinus congestion, and look into the fundus of the eye to recognize arteriovenous nicking.[17] But where does this stop? Would a pharmacist be justified in peering down the esophagus to recognize gastroesophageal reflux–induced esophagitis or conducting a digital rectal exam to differentiate hemorrhoidal bleeding from colorectal carcinoma? On what basis can the individual pharmacist decide what distinguishes acceptable assessment from the unacceptable? One must examine state pharmacy practice acts to remove these decisions from their seemingly arbitrary designations. The pharmacist is cautioned to ensure that the pharmacy practice act for that state allows pharmacist assessment prior to beginning to assess patients. In Oklahoma, a pharmacist's license was suspended because he did not "refrain from attempts at diagnosis and treatment that infringe upon the legally constituted rights and obligations of practitioners of the healing arts."[18,19] Resistance from the local medical society should be anticipated. Finally, the pharmacist should check malpractice insurance to ensure that these nontraditional but emerging pharmacist roles are covered in the case of legal complications.
- The typical pharmacy lacks otoscopes and equipment for appropriate assessments. Also, while many pharmacies have added areas for OBRA-mandated patient counseling, few pharmacies have examining rooms with a door for patient privacy. Male pharmacists may not fully understand the legal necessity of having a female employee present when examining a female patient.

The difficulties involved in pharmacists' assessment demonstrate that the pharmacist should not hesitate to triage the patient to a medical practitioner if there is any doubt about the condition being appropriate for self-care or if the validity of the patient's self-diagnosis is questionable.

There are many conditions that require referral, including nail and scalp fungi, boils or any other bacterial skin infection, sinus infection, ear pain, dental pain, swimmer's ear, eye infections, thumbsucking, nailbiting, nocturnal leg cramps, urinary tract pain/infection, and vomiting caused by anything other than motion sickness.

PAST EXPERIENCE WITH THE CONDITION—The pharmacist should discover whether the patient has experienced the condition previously. If so, was a physician or other legitimate practitioner consulted, and was a diagnosis made? For instance, consider the patient who enters the pharmacy with conjunctival redness and tearing. If the patient has been diagnosed with perennial allergic rhinitis, these symptoms constitute part of the syndrome and nonprescription products are appropriate. On the other hand, if the patient has not been diagnosed with allergic rhinitis, viral conjunctivitis is possible, necessitating referral.

As another example, corneal edema causes the patient to experience halos around lights and blurred vision. If previously diagnosed by a physician as due to some benign cause (eg, prolonged wearing of contact lenses), it is easily self-treat-

able with nonprescription 2–5% sodium chloride products. However, if the patient has not sought medical advice, the condition may be due to glaucoma, which requires immediate referral.

The female with a vaginal fungal infection is yet another example. If she has never had a physician-diagnosed vaginal fungal infection, she must obtain a physician diagnosis prior to using a nonprescription product. However, once she has received such a diagnosis, she can self-differentiate fungal vaginitis from other causes (eg, trichomonal) and can begin self-treatment. Thus the pharmacist must discover whether she is competent to self-treat, with judicious questioning prior to the sale of vaginal antifungals.

THE REASON FOR A SPECIFIC MEDICATION REQUEST—When patients have a product in mind, the pharmacist should discover why that specific medication is requested. Was the decision due to a previous successful experience with that product? Did they observe or read an advertisement? Did they hear a testimonial from a relative or friend?

The patient's motivation to purchase a specific product can have a profound impact on the pharmacist's actions, because previous use with positive results is one of the most potent arguments. Unless the product is not safe and effective, it is in the patient's best interest to switch to an alternate product, because of loss of confidence in a potential cure (eg, switching from a systemic analgesic to a topical analgesic for sore throat). On the other hand, if the motivation is simply an advertisement or advice from a well-meaning friend or relative, the pharmacist may be better able to offer an alternative product that may be a better choice.

COUNSELING TIPS

In the perfect pharmacist-patient self-care situation, the pharmacist always approaches the patient with a friendly "May I help you find something?" This lets the patient know that the pharmacist is available to provide the needed advice, facilitating communications. However, in busy retail establishments, pharmacists often cannot cruise the nonprescription aisles to converse with patients at their leisure. More often, it is the patient who seeks assistance and initiates the dialog when considering purchase of an OTC remedy. In these cases, pharmacists may give the unfortunate impression that they have been interrupted while carrying out a more important duty.

The patient may initiate the self-care conversation with several general types of questions that call for different types of pharmacist aid. For example:

What do you have for diarrhea? (provide relief for a patient's symptom)
What is the best antacid? (choose a specific product from a category of nonprescription products and/or devices)
Do you carry Lotrimin AF Cream? (locate a product for the patient)

As the pharmacist assesses the question and brings the various product- and patient-related decision-making factors to that specific situation, several important tips can be used.

EXERCISE ACTIVE LISTENING—The patient should be allowed to state the problem completely, and the pharmacist should provide the undivided attention that is necessary to minimize misperception and misunderstanding. The pharmacist should mentally summarize what the patient has said and provide positive feedback that conveys an understanding of the problem, with empathy and concern. Using the patient's own words or paraphrasing them demonstrates a full understanding of his problem(s). Rewording and paraphrasing also force the pharmacist to focus on the situation and understand its various aspects. This process also facilitates and enhances personal relations between the pharmacist and patient by exhibiting the concern expected of a caring professional.

QUESTION THE PATIENT THOROUGHLY—Quite often, the patient provides incomplete or contradictory information, much of which is necessarily subjective. To make the appropriate triage decision, the pharmacist must thoroughly cover the patient-related decision-making factors listed previously (eg, age, duration of the condition, or exact nature of the condition). Other helpful information includes:

Does the condition come and go at certain times during the day?
How severe is the problem? If it is recurrent, is it worsening?
Do you have any other symptoms?
Have you noticed a specific trigger that worsens your symptoms or causes them to recur?

Questioning should be direct and to the point. With experience, the pharmacist should be able to gather needed information in a period of minutes. If the situation is more complex and time-consuming, the pharmacist can ask patients to return at a mutually agreeable time, contact them by telephone, or refer them directly to a physician.

INTERPRET VERBAL AND NONVERBAL COMMUNICATION—Every question asked of the patient should be phrased carefully to facilitate interpretation. The patient should be able to understand that the questions asked come from a genuine interest and desire to help. The pharmacist may ask two types of questions:

1. Open-ended questions, which draw forth information regarding the medical problem. For instance, " Can you tell me about your symptoms?" This question type provides flexibility for patient response and encourages more than a simple yes-or-no answer.
2. A direct question, which is useful when the information is a specific inquiry, eg, "How long have you noticed the burning sensation in your stomach?"

Nonverbal communication skills also serve a vital role in this situation. Body posture, facial expression, and distance maintained by the patient all provide perception of the patient as a whole. At the same time it is important to be aware of the patient's nonverbal behavior. Physical barriers to communication should be eliminated whenever possible. The pharmacist should make every effort not to talk down to the patient, neither verbally (ie, use the vernacular) nor physically (ie, the pharmacist and patient should be at the same eye level). These exchanges should be as private and uninterrupted as possible. Many pharmacies lack a private consultation area, but privacy can be achieved readily without expense by simply forming a triangle using the patient, the pharmacist, and the wall shelf or gondola as partitions. This automatically signals others that the consultation is private and should not be interrupted.

Whenever possible, the pharmacist should assess the patient physically, through observation or inspection. For example, the skin is assessed easily by inspection and palpation. However, the lung requires percussion and auscultation, not a realistic practice for the practicing retail pharmacist. The clear majority of pharmacists obtain physical data (eg, number of comedones per side of the face) exclusively through the use of observation. Further, there are clues to the overall state of health of the patient, and these provide insight into the seriousness of the problem. Facial expressions mirror pain and discomfort, pallor and lethargy may indicate an infectious process, and persistent coughing may be a sign of some systemic illness.

SPEAK TO A RESPONSIBLE CAREGIVER—When counseling the patient, the pharmacist may hear phrases such as:

"I can't do that without talking to my parents."
"My husband won't let me go to the doctor; we don't have insurance."
"I'm not sure what it looks like; it's for my grandmother."

In these situations, it may be prudent to call the individual from whom more information is necessary or who needs to be convinced of the serious nature of the problem.

GAINING THE PATIENT'S COOPERATION

After the pharmacist has questioned the patient thoroughly and considered various courses of action, the time comes when

a recommendation must be made. The triage decision and its ramifications fall into several categories.

THE PHARMACIST CHOOSES NOT TO RECOMMEND ANY PRODUCT OR DEVICE—Many patients are simply worried that a product might be necessary. The pharmacist may inform them of the fact that their condition is likely to recede without any intervention and that no product will relieve their symptoms. An example would be to discourage smoking cessation to help coughing symptoms rather than purchasing a cough product. Some patients will be dissatisfied with this type of advice and remain convinced that a product will help them. They may simply purchase the product in another establishment in an effort to ignore the helpful advice of the pharmacist.

RECOMMENDING A SPECIFIC NONPRESCRIPTION PRODUCT OR DEVICE—When the pharmacist recommends a specific nonprescription product or device, most patients take the advice and purchase that product. However, a small group of patients insist on their first product choice, even though it clearly may be inappropriate. The pharmacist may urge them to reconsider, with the precaution that it is not the best product. When pharmacists recommend a drug treatment for a condition amenable to self-therapy, they should tell the patient of the condition itself, the monitoring guideposts to remember, and the duration of time before the patient should notice the benefit of treatment.

With acne vulgaris, for example, the objectives of topical treatment are to control an existing condition, impede acne in the developmental stages, and relieve the discomfort (ie, physical or psychological). The patient should be advised that continual, daily application of the medication to the entire face will gradually reduce the number of lesions, but that 2 to 3 weeks may elapse before any noticeable improvement. Indices that demonstrate acne may be worsening and require medical attention should be incorporated into the discussion. Adverse effects and potential toxicities should be noted. Using benzoyl peroxide as an example, the acne patient should understand that some skin redness and irritation may develop.

RECOMMENDING REFERRAL—This is one of the most difficult groups for which to provide advice. They enter the pharmacy asking for relief from what they perceive as a *minor* complaint, but are confronted with unwelcome advice to consult another health care professional. The pharmacist may even insist that they make an immediate visit to an emergency room. These medical alternatives involve an expenditure of money and time. All of the persuasive powers of the pharmacist must be brought to bear in this situation. Phrases such as the following may be used:

"If he were my child, I would take him to the emergency room immediately."
"The consequences of this could be as severe as loss of sight."
"I have heard of this type of problem resulting in a ruptured appendix if it is not diagnosed by a physician."

The goal of these and similar phrases is to impress upon the patient the potential gravity of the problem.

Patient harm may ensue when a pharmacist recommends a product until a patient can be checked by another health care professional. Some patients simply will not follow through and make the appointment, particularly if the product seems to work initially for his/her condition. An example is the patient who requests a nonprescription analgesic for tooth pain, promising to "visit the dentist tomorrow."

FOLLOW-UP—Whenever possible, the pharmacist should follow up with the patient, consistent with the concept of pharmaceutical care. To facilitate follow-up, pharmacists might note the patient's name and telephone number, after requesting permission to make a follow-up call. Patients might also be asked to share the results of the suggested triage decision back to the pharmacist. If the patient does not respond to the treatment plan, additional information and data assessment (eg, did the patient follow instructions correctly, taking the correct dose for the recommended duration?) may help determine a new course of action. Frequently, this reevaluation culminates with the referral of the patient to the physician for further treatment. If at all possible the pharmacist should share information attained from the initial and the follow-up evaluation with the physician.

PRECAUTIONS

The pharmacist providing advice in self-care must take great caution in recommending products that lack proof of safety and/or efficacy. Examples include the numerous herbs and "dietary supplements," ear candles, athletic aids, obesity treatments, and other quack products and devices.

Another example of products that should not be recommended is homeopathic products. Homeopathy is an outdated branch of medicine that was developed in the early 1800s.[20] Among its theories are:

A. One treats a condition by administration of a product that causes the same symptoms. Thus, cockroach extract is used for asthma, candidal suppositories for vaginal *Candida,* caffeine for insomnia, ipecac for vomiting, and bronchial cancer extract for bronchial cancer.
B. If one drop of active ingredient is diluted with 99 drops of water and the flask is struck against a firm surface repeatedly in a process known as *succussion,* the water molecules will allegedly use the medication as a template and align themselves so that the diluted medication supposedly becomes stronger.
C. Each 1/10 dilution is known as 1X. Supposedly, the more diluted the medication is, the stronger it becomes, according to homeopathic practitioners. Some homeopathic remedies are as "strong" as 60X, by which time Avogadro's number has been surpassed, and there is no active ingredient in the final preparation.

All of these homeopathic theories directly contradict basic principles of pharmacology and the dose-response curve.[21] Further, there is no conclusive evidence that they work when subjected to the exhaustive and rigorous scrutiny required in double-blinded, placebo-controlled trials with sample sizes sufficient to ensure statistical and clinical significance.

Through a loophole intentionally placed in the 1938 federal law, homeopathic products are not required to prove efficacy as legitimate medication must. This double-standard should cause the pharmacist to pause when considering sales of these products. Several lawsuits against chain stores that sell these products have been settled out of court.

SUMMARY

Self-care is one of the most daunting challenges retail pharmacists face. This is partly because patients can purchase nonprescription products and devices for self-care in virtually any location. The problem is worsened because the patient is bombarded by advertisements from nonprescription product/device, herbal, and homeopathic manufacturers that promote one product to the exclusion of all others. When patients choose to purchase these items in a pharmacy, the pharmacist is challenged to discover product-related and patient-related factors that facilitate appropriate triage. In doing so, the pharmacist must use the highest principles of pharmaceutical care, employing a balanced and rational approach that rests on the precepts of legitimate scientific evidence rather than the seductive lure of expensive advertisements.

REFERENCES

1. OTC facts and figures. www.chpa-info.org. Accessed 3/26/2002.
2. *Self-care in the new millennium.* Washington, DC: Consumer Healthcare Products Association, 2001.
3. Pray WS. *Nonprescription Product Therapeutics.* Baltimore: Williams & Wilkins, 1999.
4. Newton G, Popovich NG, Pray WS. *JAPhA* 1996; NS36(8):489.
5. Epstein D. *Drug Topics* 1997; 141(12):45.
6. Pray WS. *JAPhA* 1996; NS36(5):329.
7. *The Clinical Role of the Community Pharmacist.* Washington, DC: OIG, DHHS, Nov 1990.
8. Clepper I. *Drug Topics* 1992; 136(16):44.
9. *Federal Register* 1976; 41(176):38311.
10. *Federal Register* 1985; 50(10):2220.
11. *Federal Register* 1991; 56(156):38391.
12. Kernan WN, Viscoli CM, Brass LM, et al. *New Engl J Med* 2000; 343(25):1826.
13. http://www.fda.gov/cder/drug/infopage/ppa/qa.htm
14. Noonan D. *Newsweek* 2000;(October 30):59.
15. Smith IK. *Time* 2000;(October 30):101.
16. LaGrenade L, Graham DJ, Nourjah P. *JAMA* 2001; 286:3081.
17. Pauley T, Marcrom R, Randolph R. *Am Pharm* 1995; NS35:40.
18. *1992–1993 Survey of Pharmacy Law.* Park Ridge, IL: NABP, 1992:48.
19. Brown GH, Kirking DM, Ascione FJ. *Am Pharm* 1983; NS23: 25.
20. Pray WS. *Am J Pharm Educ* 1996; 60(Summer): 198.
21. Pray WS. *Am J Pain Manage* 1992; 2(2):63.

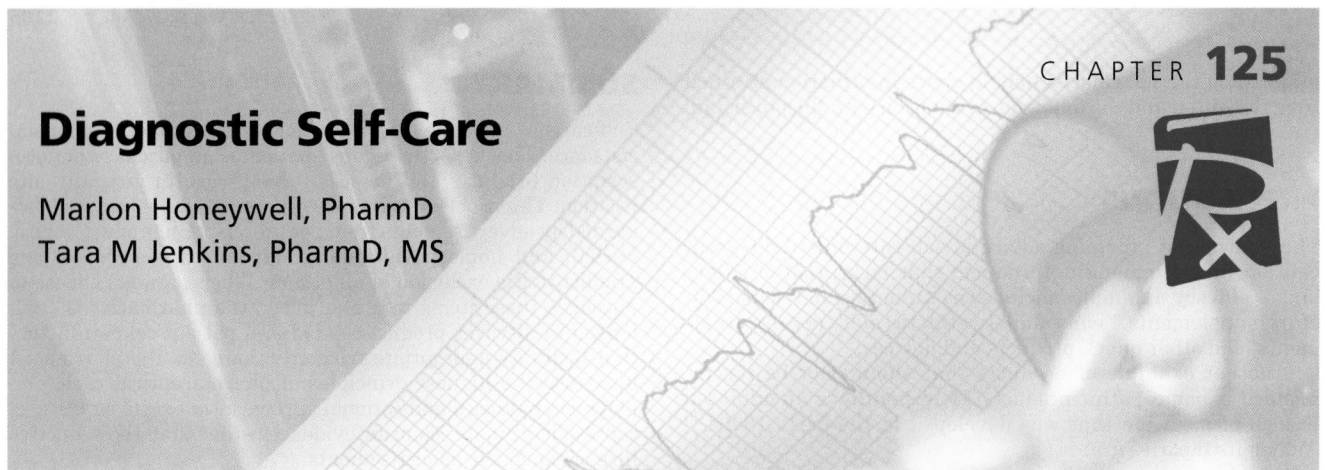

CHAPTER 125

Diagnostic Self-Care

Marlon Honeywell, PharmD

Tara M Jenkins, PharmD, MS

Since the introduction of the first home pregnancy test in 1977, diagnostic aids and devices have expanded self-care into an information-based and profitable market. In one year, patients spend approximately $650 million on home tests and monitors.[1] In addition to nonprescription products, the pharmacist must also have a working knowledge of diagnostic aids and devices currently available to consumers. The market for these products has an average growth rate of 17% attributable to the relatively low cost, reliability, and user-friendliness of the exams.

Diagnostic devices have revolutionized the self-care industry. Consumers benefit from their easy accessibility. These devices include blood pressure monitors, home blood glucose monitors, HIV exams, cholesterol exams, and home tests for colorectal cancer. They help monitor chronic diseases, diminish doctor visits and associated costs, decrease hospitalizations, and allow consumers to become an active part of their own health care. With the trend toward pharmaceutical care and preventive medicine, the pharmacist can perform a vital public health role by counseling the consumer on newer diagnostic devices, thereby contributing to a reduction in deaths from colon cancer, helping patients monitor blood glucose, and aiding in the detection of drug abuse, among others.

Even though they have become more user-friendly, patients may still encounter problems with even the simplest devices. Consequently, pharmacists are often summoned to educate patients on proper use, and the validity and application of the results. It is essential that pharmacists ask questions about the disease or exam and make any appropriate recommendations based upon the available information. The pharmacist should remind the patient that any information attained as a result of counseling shall remain strictly confidential. The pharmacist should also mention that these test kits/devices must be used in collaboration with health-care professionals who can interpret and discuss the test results and their implications.

Diagnostic aids and tests are complex to use; patient understanding is maximized when a pharmacist is involved in the purchase and use of these products. If these products are purchased in a non-pharmacy outlet, the consumer does not have the opportunity to ask questions or receive reliable recommendations from an educated professional, thereby increasing the chances for product misuse.[1] Pharmacist counseling has direct benefits to the patient. The pharmacist is a highly educated drug-information specialist in over-the-counter (OTC) products. This, in conjunction with practical experience, makes the pharmacist the only health professional who understands the limitations of self-treatment with OTC products and who is also uniquely positioned to encourage the patient to seek the professional advice of a physician when necessary.

OBJECTIVES

Recently, the pharmacy profession enhanced the emphasis of pharmaceutical care, which encompasses proper self-care, preventive medicine, and follow-ups. Because of the increasing utilization of diagnostic test kits, it becomes necessary to discuss the issues surrounding these devices. The objectives of this chapter shall be to promote reader awareness of the following: the function of diagnostic test kits; pharmacist and consumer responsibility as it relates to counseling and utilization, respectively; the professional responsibility of pharmacists to contribute not only to consumer comprehension, but to other patient issues; the Food and Drug Administration's (FDA) concerns about these devices and any related recommendations; the scope of the marketplace for these items; and the various categories of in-home test kits and pertinent information regarding these devices. Pharmacists can enhance consumer understanding of the devices by gaining a thorough understanding of their use and counseling patients at every opportunity. The pharmacist has the ability to answer any consumer-related questions and recommend solutions to any problems, which will increase the effectiveness of the test kits and the impact of pharmaceutical care in the eye of the consumer.

FUNCTION

The function of testing devices is to provide accurate and reliable information to the patient in a short period of time. The exam must be easy to read and use, thus allowing the patient to make an informed decision based on exam results. The device should also carry label instructions that are understandable to a variety of patients regardless of their level of education or literacy. Instructions should be provided in a step-by-step approach, which may encourage confidence in self-administration and interpretation. The device should also instruct the patient on the next appropriate step to take after obtaining exam results. For example, if a blood glucose meter determined a blood glucose level that required the expertise of a clinician, this must be clearly explained to the patient. In some instances, a phone number may be included for professional consultation about any consumer-related questions or misconceptions. Manufacturer support may ensure that the device is utilized properly and that results are not tainted by misuse.

THE PHARMACIST

Clinicians must take the lead role in protecting patients, their peers, and themselves from the unfortunate consequences of medication errors and device mishandling. Errors occur for a variety of reasons in every aspect of the health profession, including inaccurate communication between the clinician, the patient, or deficits in the knowledge and performance of the health care professional. Hence, the pharmacist's role in aiding with selection of the appropriate device, counseling about proper use, and interpretation of results is indispensable. The pharmacist is constantly accessible to the public, providing the opportunity to make a profound impact in the effectiveness of this growing market. It is the responsibility of the pharmacist to be familiar with these devices and to examine constantly any new literature related to the disease state or apparatus so that appropriate advice may be provided to the consumer. For example, product manufacturers should be periodically contacted to inquire about any recent developments and offer demonstrations to the pharmacy staff to guarantee proper training and application. Although most devices will include information booklets from the manufacturer, the pharmacist should take an active role in explaining the information to the patient. Proactively approaching the consumer may save money by detecting potential problems early, thus decreasing the likelihood of the patient purchasing a second exam because of mishandling. This "show and tell" theory will promote effectiveness and help perfect the patient's use of the product.

THE CONSUMER'S RESPONSIBILITY

Studies demonstrate that self-care is compromised by therapeutic failure of medication regimens, testing devices, and compliance tactics.[2] Strategies involving careful labeling, simplification of regimens, device instructions, and enhanced patient-pharmacist interaction may remedy this problem. Therefore, the consumer also has a shared responsibility in the correct use of these devices. First of all, any pertinent information related to the patient's physical examination or the disease state itself should be conveyed to the pharmacist. The pharmacist should be made aware of any allergies or potential adverse reactions. If the consumer has difficulty in reading materials or does not understand the instructions, that information should be relayed to the pharmacist, affording the opportunity for personal assistance. The consumer should ensure that all questions are documented, which will consequently promote constructive use of time and permit the pharmacist to respond to all concerns appropriately. It is important for the consumer to be patient and understanding because the pharmacist might be busy upon his/her arrival, necessitating a wait before counseling may occur. Towards the end of the consultation, the consumer should repeat the directions to the pharmacist to ensure understanding, and demonstrate proper use of the product.

PROFESSIONAL OPPORTUNITY

Martin and Pigarelli suggest that some diagnostic devices may produce 99% accuracy when administered properly.[3] This presents the pharmacist with an opportunity to make a difference in enhancing the device productivity. Pharmacists fit into a model in which the cost and benefits of medication and device usage are carefully managed to increase the quality of care. The precision of these devices will rely on the communication between the health care professional and the consumer. Unfortunately, the major productivity gap lies in the adherence of the patient to counseling and device instructions. Greater patient interaction with pharmacists has been recognized as a key component in solutions to medication errors and device misuse. A second study estimated that nearly 25% of hospital and long-term care admissions were attributable to non-adherence of advice or directions.[4] Therefore, reinforcement of instructions by the pharmacist during the interaction may be crucial for patient compliance with directions or counseling (eg, package insert or counseling), and may have a profound impact on the potential effectiveness of the device.

The pharmacist should seize the opportunity to converse with the patient about other ailments unrelated to the diagnostic exam. In some cases, patients may be reluctant to speak to a doctor or pharmacist in regards to clinically insignificant medical disorders. This unwillingness usually leads to self-diagnosis and treatment. Ferris et al conducted a study involving 95 women who were purchasing over-the-counter products used to self-treat vulvovaginal candidiasis.[5] The time period was September 1997 through December 1999, and the patients were required to answer an in-depth survey and complete a clinical examination. Laboratory tests were performed. Only 32% of patients made the correct self-diagnosis and an additional 19% had mixed vaginosis involving candidiasis and bacteria. One patient actually required hospitalization for her condition. Misdiagnosis in most cases, leads to inappropriate treatment. In turn, misdiagnosis and treatment has the potential to increase the severity of the patient's condition due to the delay in treatment with suitable medication. Although self-treatment may prove to be a less expensive option for the patient, it may also be detrimental to the patient's health. By asking open-ended questions, the pharmacist may be able to discover problems and aid the patient in selecting a suitable option for treatment or refer the patient to a physician.

FDA REGULATORY CENTERS

In 1982, an agreement prepared by the FDA detailed the working relationships between the organizations previously identified as the Bureau of Medical Devices (BMD), the Bureau of Radiologic Health (BRH), and the Bureau of Biologics (BOB). The purpose of this agreement was to identify the responsibilities of each entity for medical device activities.[6] Since then, there have been several major organizational modifications within the FDA. In 1982, BMD and BRH were joined to form the Center for Devices and Radiologic Health (CDRH). Also in 1982, BOB and the Bureau of Drugs were merged to form the Center for Drugs and Biologics (CDB), with biological products regulated by the Office of Biologics Research and Review (OBRR). However, in 1987, the CDB was divided into two major centers, with biological products regulated by the Center for Biologics Evaluation and Research (CBER).

Because both centers were responsible for similar regulations regarding diagnostic devices, the Intercenter Agreement between the CDRH and CBER was developed and became effective October 31, 1991. CDRH was designated as the lead Center in the FDA for regulating medical devices to ensure their safety and effectiveness. CDRH will use the device authorities of the federal Food, Drug and Cosmetic Act (FDC Act) as well as other authorities delegated to it for the devices regulated in that Center. For example, home diagnostic exams that do not require blood banking are controlled by the CDRH (eg, blood glucose monitors, pregnancy tests, or infertility exams).

The CBER was delegated the lead center for regulating certain medical devices utilized in or indicated for the collection, processing, or administration of biological products that utilize blood banking or blood extraction as a primary means of sample collection. This Center also uses the FDC Act and the Public Health Service Act (PHSA), as well as any other authorities delegated to it. *In vitro* tests, which are required for blood donor screenings and related to blood banking practices, (such as donor re-entry) are licensed under the PHSA. The CBER is also responsible for regulating all *in vitro* tests (including diagnostic tests which are not performed in association with blood bank practices, and any other medical devices intended for use with human immunodeficiency virus, type 1 (HIV-1) and type 2 (HIV-2), and any other retroviruses). Examples of *in vitro* reagents may include Hepatitis B Surface antigen, Hepatitis C Viral Encoded antigen, HIV-1, HIV-2, and Human T-Lymphotropic virus. These devices may include but are not limited to the following: collection devices, specimen containers, hospital or home test kits, and support kits intended for the inactivation of these viruses. For a product that is a combination of a device and a biological product, the determination of the regulating Center is made based upon the primary mode of action.

FDA CONCERNS

Self-testing diagnostic and monitoring devices are often seen as a less expensive and more convenient alternative compared to a trip to the doctor's office. These devices are sold in increasingly high numbers. Self-monitoring for conditions such as diabetes mellitus and hypertension are made easier using these devices. However, this technology is not without its limits and could result in life-threatening problems for those who rely solely on the test without the expertise of a health-care provider.

Home test kits are inexpensive compared to a co-payment to the doctor and a great deal less time-consuming. An advantage is that they provide quick results. Women often use home pregnancy test kits for these reasons, as well as for the convenience of testing at home. Some women prefer a definite diagnosis prior to visiting their physician and home pregnancy tests may aid in confirmation. Early verification may enable clinicians to counsel women about their options and discourage any harmful behaviors such as smoking or alcohol consumption.

Because these exams offer early confirmation of problems, disease, or pregnancy, they have become increasingly popular among consumers. One sign of their popularity is the fact that many pharmacists are moving the home diagnostic exams from behind the counter onto freestanding displays. The Internet also makes these devices more accessible by offering direct home delivery.

Steve Gutman, MD, director of the FDA's clinical laboratory devices division, stated that consumers need to be wary about buying and using the kits on their own. "People need to carefully read the test-kit labeling and instructions, where important information and warnings about the product are listed," he says. Labeling demonstrates how the test works and steps to take in case of product failure. Home diagnostic exams are meant to be adjunctive to physician visits, not a replacement for them. "Although the menu of home testing products has expanded," Gutman says, "the advice is still the same."[7]

Although home test kits provide convenience, confidentiality, and cost-savings, physicians seem concerned about the availability of medical tests that may encourage self-diagnosis because of the possibility of result misinterpretation. For example, Sandy Stewart, PhD, a research engineer in the FDA's CDRH says that blood pressure monitors should be employed to track blood pressure readings between physician visits. "Users should never change their medications or spontaneously stop use based upon home blood pressure readings." If there are significant variations in the readings, the user should contact their physician immediately. "The blood pressure reading taken at the doctor's office must be the final word."[7]

The benefit of having a clinician involved is that the results may be evaluated within the context of the whole health picture and the decision for treatment options will not rely on one test result. Furthermore, receiving news of pregnancy, illness, or infection over the phone, or from the color of a test strip, may be overwhelming. "The first 72 hours following a positive HIV diagnosis is when people are most likely to hurt themselves," says Edward Geraty, a licensed clinical social worker with Behavioral Science Associates in Baltimore. It is imperative to have face-to-face contact when delivering a HIV diagnosis. "Without it," he says, "there is a psychological component of the person's illness that is completely negated from the process."

Accuracy is a critical consideration when it comes to home testing. False-positive results indicate that a condition is present when, in fact, it is not. Likewise, false-negative results may give the consumer a sense of security and lengthen the time until a patient obtains a valid diagnosis and treatment, if needed.

The Federal Trade Commission has the distinct responsibility of enforcing consumer protection laws. Recently, they have evaluated the results of several unapproved HIV home exams advertised and sold on the Internet for self-diagnosis. In each incident, the kits displayed a negative result when a known positive sample was applied. Similarly, the FDA recently examined a number of unapproved home HIV tests sold on the Internet that were confiscated during a criminal investigation.[8] None of the HIV tests produced accurate results. The FDA concluded that the outcome could have serious consequences for a user resulting in mental and emotional stress, lack of access to proper medical treatment, and possible transmission of disease to unaffected individuals. The CBER continues to investigate people and firms involved in the illegal sale of unapproved HIV home test kits in the United States.

FDA RECOMMENDATIONS

Follow Directions

In most cases, home diagnostic exams involve relatively simple procedures with straightforward instructions. The FDA requires that all test kits be simple enough for the average consumer to utilize the exam at home without direct supervision. For example, some pregnancy exams only require a stream of urine to produce colored indicator lines, whereas glucose monitors usually require placing a small blood sample onto a reagent strip. The consumer should carefully follow the directions as recommended by the manufacturer. If any questions exist, a health care professional should be contacted for clarification. Modification of directions or test kit samples is not recommended.

Storage

Home test kits should not be stored in places where they might be exposed to extreme temperatures. This may result in deterioration of the product over time. By storing the kits properly as recommended by the manufacturer, the consumer will lessen the probability of false results.

Expiration Date

Patients should check the expiration date before purchasing a diagnostic exam. Expired test kits may produce inaccurate results.

Nonadherence to Directions

Failure to follow directions with home test kits can compromise the integrity of the results. Non-compliance with device instructions, improper storage, shipment, or collection of specimens may diminish effectiveness. Inaccurate readings may be produced if urine samples are not collected at the appropriate time of day or if foods ingested mimic metabolites being measured. Extracted samples (eg, blood or urine) not applied within the recommended manufacturer time frame or exposed to severe temperature changes could generate false positive or false negative results.

FDA-Approved Devices

FDA-approved tests have undergone extensive analysis and review by the manufacturer of the product. For an in-home exam, the manufacturer must demonstrate to the FDA that the result of the test will benefit consumers and the kit is simple enough for consumers to decide whether the test is appropriate for their condition.[8] On the other hand, unapproved devices lack the guarantee of accuracy or sensitivity and they have no documented history of dependability. Proper training to interpret results is not provided with the kits and they do not have a validated record of precision. Because of the aforementioned problems, the FDA has determined that unapproved tests may be inconsistent and inaccurate.

Internet Purchasing

The consequences of consumer health fraud range from significant financial loss to consumer avoidance of legitimate treatment.[7] The FDA wants consumers to be aware of a number of unapproved test kits available on the Internet, in magazines, or newspapers, for home use. Internet sites advertise test kits that falsely claim everything from FDA approval to detecting illness within 15 minutes or less. Consumers who purchase via the Internet may receive contaminated or counterfeit products, an improper test kit, or no product at all. The FDA confidently endorses home test kits available in reputable pharmacies or drugstores. Many of these products have undergone extensive review and testing by the CDRH or CBER divisions. Consumers may browse the FDA's web site at www.fda.gov/oc/buyonline/ for tips and warnings concerning Internet purchasing. Furthermore, www.fda.gov/cdrh/ode/otclist.html is an FDA site that contains a regularly updated list of approved home diagnostic exams sold over-the-counter.

GROWING MARKET

The marketplace for *in-vitro* diagnostic (IVD) products is among the most complex of all medical device sectors, involving public and private payers, prescribers and laboratory specialists, and an increasing variety of clinical and home use settings.[9] Making headway in this market requires manufacturers to undertake an intense period of research to understand their target market.

Currently in the realm of OTC diagnostic devices, the most active segments of the industry in terms of sales are clinical laboratory instruments and the emerging point-of-care (POC) testing systems (Table 125-1).[10] POC systems include automated testing devices, bedside diagnostic testing devices, and in-home diagnostic exams. The major clinical diagnostic laboratory instrument sectors include clinical chemistry, immunoassay, hematology, blood banking, urinalysis, microbiology, and emerging DNA and molecular testing. The average annual growth (AAGR) for the POC is expected to be 8.1% through 2007, while the laboratory instrument segment will grow at an estimated 6.4%.

Table 125-1. Point-of-Care System Sales

TESTING SEGMENT	2000		2005	
	SALES US ($ MIL)	MARKET SHARE	SALES US ($ MIL)	MARKET SHARE
Glucose	625	26	800	22
Pregnancy	500	20	700	19
Infectious disease	335	14	425	12
Critical care	275	11	375	10
Cholesterol	250	10	400	11
Coagulation	150	6	275	7
Cardiac markers	50	2	100	3
Drugs of abuse	50	2	55	1
Bilirubin	30	1	50	1
Other[a]	15	1	20	1
Total ($)	2280		3200	

[a]Other = fecal occult blood, *C. difficile*, prostate-specific antigen (PSA).
Adapted from Recognition and Initial Assessment of Alzheimer's disease and related dementia's. Clinical Practice Guideline 19. Rockville, MD: Department of Human Services, Public Health Service, Agency for Healthcare Policy and Research, 1996. AHCPR publication 97-0702.

United States

The United States is the largest IVD market in the world, with market shares and revenue totaling 9.7 billion dollars in 2000. In addition to being the largest market, the US is the largest IVD manufacturer, accounting for nearly 85% of all IVD products worldwide. Although the market share is enormous, there are two factors that may hamper continued economic growth. Consumer pressure to reduce prices has squeezed profits in the past. Undoubtedly, this trend will continue in the future. Another factor is the constantly challenging reimbursement issues for these devices. The US government is pursuing the establishment of reimbursement for various routine or esoteric exams.[11] Even with the projected 39% decline in market share in the US, IVD's largest companies are still expected to maintain healthy growth from international sales.

Point-of-Care Systems

Over the past couple of years, the market for POC diagnostics has experienced double-digit growth.[10] Researchers agree that future growth in this field will continue to be strong; however, not everyone agrees that double-digit growth can be sustained because of the Clinical Laboratory Improvement Amendment (CLIA). Approximately 95% of in-home diagnostic kits were CLIA-waived by the FDA. Some individuals believe that the market setting for POC diagnostics is severely constrained by the demand of physicians to designate that some new diagnostic exams be delegated as CLIA-waived, even if the device has not been designated for in-home use or to revisit to the requirements for CLIA-waiving.

In 1988, the CLIA law specified that laboratory requirements be based on the complexity of the test performed and established provisions for categorizing a test as waived.[12] On February 28, 1992, regulations were published to implement CLIA. In the regulations, waived tests were defined as simple laboratory examinations and procedures that were cleared by the FDA for home use. It had been determined that these test kits employ methodologies so simple and accurate so as to render the likelihood of erroneous results negligible and these exams would pose no reasonable harm to the patient if the test was performed incorrectly. Examples of CLIA-waived exams include but are not limited to: glucose monitors, ovulation tests, urine pregnancy exams, and urine ketone exams. Because more of these test kits are being marketed for in-home use, experts believe that the global IVD market will change and more dollars will be spent on these items.

ALZHEIMER'S DISEASE

Alzheimer's disease (AD) is a progressive debilitating disease that has a devastating effect on the lives of affected individuals and their families. Approximately 4 million Americans over the age of 65 suffer from AD.[13] AD can be divided into four stages of dementia, known as the forgetful stage, confused stage, demented stage, and end-stage dementia. The classic triad of clinical changes includes memory impairment, visuospatial defects and language changes. These may occur in the absence of confusion (unlike delirium), mental retardation, or other neurological disorders. They cause a considerable decline in the patient's ability to function.

Patients with AD have an inability to perform basic activities of daily living. Early forgetfulness and problems performing basic tasks (eg, balancing check book, making complex decisions) occur, while social functioning often remains intact. The ability to accomplish familiar tasks (eg, driving, using a telephone) is usually preserved in AD. However, patients with AD have been noted to lose olfactory function (anosmia). Their sense of smell becomes distorted and familiar fragrances, in a variety of cases, cannot be distinguished. Eventually, they develop behavioral changes, such as wandering, getting lost, and repeating the same questions. Visuospatial disturbances may manifest as a propensity to get lost and copy instructions.[14] In latter stages, patients may be unable to recall familiar objects or newly learned information. As the disease advances, they may develop irritability, psychosis, or disorientation and eventually, patients become completely dependent.

Diagnosis

Early diagnosis is the key to initiation of effective treatment options. Interviewing the patient and conducting a comprehensive clinical assessment usually reveals the most important diagnostic information. The clinician must extensively interview the patient to distinguish AD from other forms of dementia using the Diagnostic and Statistical Manual on Mental Disorders (DSM-4).

Screening

In an effort to provide an earlier diagnosis for AD patients, the development of a screening technique was devised. Knowing that anosmia and AD are linked, researchers began to conduct clinical studies on their relationship. In 1994, Soloman concluded that 90% of patients with AD showed varying degrees of anosmia.[15] In another experiment, the smell sensitivity of 80 normal elderly patients was compared with 80 AD elderly patients and the AD patients were found to have significantly poorer sense of smell. It was reported that 74% of the AD elderly claimed to have normal sensitivity after smelling the sample, yet, to recognize an aroma, they required a sample with an average concentration of *nine* times more than that needed by a normal elderly patient. It is noteworthy that the AD victims were not aware of the onset of anosmia, and, therefore, did not recognize their loss of olfactory sensitivity.

Home Diagnostic Exam

Subsequent to the development of the Pocket Smell Test (PST) and the Pennsylvania Smell Identification Test (PSIT), FMG Innovatives developed the Early Alert Alzheimer's Home Screening Test. This is the first home exam, based on the research involving the PSIT and PST, offered to patients as a non-invasive, self-administered test to screen for possible anosmia secondary to dementia. In 2003, the exam costs approximately $19.00 and affords patients the opportunity for early diagnosis.

Procedure

1. Open the screening booklet to the first page which is entitled ODOR #1.
2. Using the pencil provided, scratch the odor strip several times in a zigzag fashion to release the odor.
3. Place the odor strip directly under both nostrils and sniff.
4. Look for choices provided above odor strip. If patient is unsure or no smell is present, the closest answer choice should be selected.
5. Turn to the second page entitled ODOR #2. Repeat steps 2–4.
6. Continue this process until all 12 strips have been sniffed and an answer has been circled for each odor.

Scoring

After selecting the number of incorrect answers and placing them in the "TOTAL NUMBER INCORRECT" box, the patient or caregiver can read the results. Afterwards, if 4 or more incorrect answers exist, the patient should contact a physician. If there are less than 4 incorrect answers and symptoms of AD are present, a physician should still be contacted. This exam is

intended as a screening tool and further testing is recommended.

Storage

1. Store test kit in a dry place below 86° Fahrenheit or 30° Celsius.
2. Do not scratch the odor strips until ready to use.
3. Do not allow odor strips to come into contact with any liquids.
4. Discard after use. Do not reuse.

HEPATITIS C

Over the last decade, Hepatitis C Virus (HCV) has emerged from obscurity as a disease (originally known as non-A, non-B Hepatitis) familiar only to a few experts, to one recognized as a major public health problem in the US and worldwide.[16] Responsible for a number of hepatic manifestations, HCV emerged in 1989 and was isolated through modern techniques of molecular cloning. The virus belongs to the flavivirus family and contains a single-stranded RNA genome approximately 10,000 nucleotides in length. Unfortunately, in approximately 80% of patients, infection with the virus is asymptomatic, and a physician may not discover abnormal liver function enzyme values upon examination of a blood specimen. Therefore, screening high-risk individuals is imperative in controlling the spread of this disease.

During the latter half of the last decade, the Centers for Disease Control (CDC) recommended that certain individuals be screened for HCV infection based upon their risk for infection (Table 125-2).[17] Those who inject legal or illicit drugs, patients on long-term hemodialysis, and individuals who received blood or blood components should all be tested routinely for HCV infection. Health care workers and infants born to seropositive mothers should also be tested. Infants born to seropositive mothers should not be tested until they have reached 12 months of age.[16] Immediate testing is not recommended because the infant will passively acquire antibodies to the virus and test positive even if he or she is not infected.

One of the largest obstacles in screening and diagnosing is the need to ask sensitive questions. In most cases, patients are not likely to come forward to be screened, but it is vital to reduce the cost associated with attempting to diagnose every high-risk patient. One strategy is to ask these questions in a standardized exam, which may remove the patient's anxiety associated with answering these questions. There are a variety of diagnostic tests used for screening patients at a physician's office (Table 125-3).

Table 125-2. Persons Recommended for Routine HCV Testing

1. Persons with specific medical conditions, such as:
   - Those who received clotting factors concentrated before 1987
   - Those who were treated with long-term dialysis
   - Those with persistently high ALT levels
2. Persons who have injected illegal drugs, including those who only experimented once or a few times
3. Prior recipients of transfusions or organ transplants, including those:
   - Who were informed that they received blood from a donor who later tested positive
   - Who received blood transfusions or components before 1992
   - Who received an organ transplant before 1992
4. Healthcare, emergency medical, and public safety workers
5. Infants over 12 months of age born to a seropositive mother

Adapted from Honeywell M, Hollis A, Thornton A, et al. *US Pharmacist* 2002; 27(5):HS81.

Table 125-3. Diagnostic Tests for Hepatitis C

1. Anti-HCV
   - Best screening test for patients with abnormal ALT/and or identified risk factors for HCV infection
2. Recombinant immunoblot assay (RIBA)
   - Supplemental assay employed for low-risk populations with a seropositive anti-HCV
3. Qualitative PCR
   - Detects HCV
   - Results expressed as present or absent
4. Quantitative PCR
   - Detects HCV
   - Sensitivity 100 to 1,000 copies/ml

Adapted from Honeywell M, Hollis A, Thornton A, et al. *US Pharmacist* 2002; 27(5):HS81.

In-Office Exams

The anti-HCV exam is usually suggested as the initial exam for screening patients with abnormal liver enzymes (eg, ALT) or other HCV risk factors. This assay is inexpensive and reliable. Its sensitivity is >90%, but its specificity varies according to the population tested.[16] For example, if a patient from a high-risk group is tested, the predictive percentage is approximately 93%, but in a low-risk population it may be as low as 50%. Therefore, a second test may be required to support the diagnosis. The recombinant immunoblot assay (RIBA) may be applied in this instance. This test utilizes sections of the HCV genome embedded in a nitrocellulose strip. A positive reaction is recorded when black bands appear after the strip has been placed in the patient's serum. If two or more bands appear, the result is considered to be positive; two bands or less is considered to be indeterminate. In immunosuppressed patients or patients undergoing chemotherapy, an antibody presence may be absent. If the patient is strongly suspected to have HCV, the polymerase chain reaction (PCR) may be useful. One other virologic assay, the branched chain DNA (bDNA), is sometimes ordered to help quantify the number of HCV-RNA copies per milliliter of blood.

Home Diagnostic Exams

The Home Access Hepatitis C Test was developed as an in-home exam created by Home Access Health Company. It is used to screen whole blood for Hepatitis C. This exam has been proven clinically safe and effective and was approved by the FDA in 1999. Comparative studies demonstrate that this exam is 99% accurate when measured against in-office exams in seropositive individuals.

Prior to testing, the patient should call a toll free number to activate a 14-digit test code and to obtain anonymous counseling from professional clinicians to ensure understanding of instructions or to answer any questions. Using the lancet included in the test pack, the patient should deposit a sample of blood onto the test card. The sample test card is then sealed and mailed in a self-addressed postage-prepaid mailer. Four to 10 business days should be allotted to process the results. The access number should be called and using the 14-digit PIN, the patient is given the test results and, if necessary, offered professional counseling regarding the results.

The exam is offered in most pharmacies across the continental US, and in 2003, costs approximately $56 per test. The American Liver Foundation (ALF) has recognized Home Access as an important advancement in the fight against liver disorders. Individuals who may be exposed to HCV are encouraged by the ALF to obtain counseling, testing, and if appropriate, medical treatment.

INFERTILITY

Infertility affects more than 2 million couples in the US and may be attributed equally to both males and females. Many couples have problems conceiving due to a male's low sperm count, decreased sperm quality, or other medical conditions.[18] Unfortunately, there is no identifiable cause for this dilemma in approximately one-fifth of cases. Until recently, the OTC approach to infertility focused on the female chemistry. Lake Consumer Products created a new benchmark by developing FertilMARQ (BabyStart), a home infertility test kit specifically designed for males. Given FDA approval in 2001, it is sold in retail pharmacies for approximately $40.

Procedure

Each test kit contains materials for two separate exams. Prior to testing, consumers must purchase a spermicide-free condom. Once the semen sample is collected using the condom, the contents are emptied into the coated cup included in the kit. This cup contains a material which accelerates the process of converting the sperm from a viscous formulation into a liquid. After 15 minutes, the male places a drop of the liquefied semen into a well on the plastic test cassette, which resembles a home pregnancy test strip, adds two drops of the blue solution and then two drops of the clear solution and waits. If, after 5 minutes, the sample in the test well changes color to a darker blue than the reference blue shown on the test cassette, the result is positive. A positive result means that the sample contains greater than 20 million sperm per milliliter of ejaculate which the World Health Organization (WHO) has determined is required for fertility.[48] A blue lighter than the reference blue is a negative result indicating that the sperm count is below the mark.

The test usually requires about 30 minutes to complete. The patient should repeat the test within 7 days, but not within 3 days after ejaculation.[19] If the test is negative, the patient should be referred to a physician or fertility specialist to determine if other unknown factors are influencing the decline in sperm count. As a part of the FDA approval process, these examinations were offered to consumers and matched professional in-office exams 87% of the time.

Concerns

FertilMARQ does not inform consumers of any factors that may contribute to infertility such as alterations in urine pH levels, white blood cell count, speed, and mobility of sperm movement towards the egg. Nor does it provide any information about the sperms morphology (size and shape). Robert Stillman, a reproductive endocrinologist, states that the latter reason may be crucial in evaluating a male's capacity to conceive. Some physicians believe that FertilMARQ may be considered as a diagnostic tool by consumers and results may be used in lieu of consulting with a physician, thereby, circumventing the ability of a physician to find the actual cause of infertility.

This test should not be used as a diagnostic tool but as an initial screen in similar fashion to doctors who routinely administer in-office pregnancy exams to substantiate at-home testing. It is anticipated that women will be major supporters of the product. Many may purchase this product on behalf of their male counterparts to aid in determining the cause of a couple's inability to conceive.

ASTHMA

Asthma is the most common chronic illness in children, with a prevalence of 5.8% in the US. Hospitalization rates and morbidity continue to increase despite scientific advances that have improved our understanding of the pathophysiology of asthma, and the availability of new interventions. A recommended intervention to improve patient outcomes is the routine use of a peak flow meter (PFM). This device measures expiration from the lung and allows patients and caregivers to make informed therapeutic decisions. Although PFMs are not used in the initial diagnosis of asthma, these are commonly used at home to determine disease severity, thereby allowing the patient to decide whether treatment or hospitalization is required.

Introduced in the 1960s, PFM's have received increased attention in the recent past. In 1997, the National Asthma Education Program's Expert Panel recommended home monitoring of forced expiratory flow rate or Peak Flow Rate (PFR) for children with moderate to severe asthma to support clinicians in managing asthma more effectively.[20] The panel recommended PFM monitoring for the following: to detect asymptomatic deterioration in lung function, to monitor response to therapy, and to inform clinicians of needed changes in treatment, including emergency situations.

Peak Flow Rate

A normal PFR is based on the individual's age, height, sex, and race. A standardized "normal" may be obtained from a chart comparing the patient with a population without breathing problems. Interpretation of PFR is simplified for the patient by labeling three zones in the same manner akin to the colors of a traffic light. Be aware that the following zones are intended as a general guideline and a physician may alter these zones based upon the patient's specific condition.[21]

Green Zone. To be categorized in the green zone, the PFR should be between 80% and 100% of the baseline readings. In most cases, a measurement in this zone means that the patient's asthma is under reasonable control.

Yellow Zone. The yellow zone requires that the PFR be between 50% and 80% of the patient's baseline measurements. This may be indicative of airway narrowing and may require extra treatment. A therapeutic plan should be constructed, with the advice of a physician, allocating options for this zone. For example, if PFR is noted to be in the yellow zone, a physician may recommend that the patient inhale extra puffs of their prescribed Albuterol inhaler to help open the airways leading to the lungs.

Red Zone. Less than 50% of the baseline PFR signals a medical alert and immediate action should be taken. In some instances, a physician may decide that the red zone should be 80% or less of the baseline. In either case, severe airway narrowing may be occurring, and the patient should be instructed to take rescue medications immediately and possibly seek emergency care from a hospital emergency room. If the physician has developed a therapeutic emergency plan for the red zone, those instructions should be followed.

Peak Flow Meter Use

1. Before each use, make certain the sliding marker or arrow on the PFM is at the bottom of the numbered scale (zero or the lowest number on the scale).
2. Stand up straight. Any gum or food should be removed from the mouth. Take a deep breath (as deep as possible). The mouthpiece should be placed in the mouth, and the lips should be closed tightly around the mouthpiece. In one breath, the patient should blow out as hard and as quickly as possible.
3. The force of the air will cause the marker to move upward along a numbered scale. The number should be noted in a diary.
4. Repeat the entire routine three times. If the device has been used appropriately, the outcomes from all three trials should be similar.
5. The highest of three ratings should be recorded. The patient should not calculate an average of the ratings.
6. The PFR should be measured at the same time each day, and the clinician should help decide what time is appropriate (eg, between 7:00 and 9:00 AM and between 6:00 and 8:00 PM). Some individuals may need to measure PFR before and after the administration of medication. This may be an appropriate recommendation if daily testing times are inconsistent.

7. The patient should maintain a chart of PFR readings, and these should be discussed with clinicians during consultation.

Management Plan

It is important for the patient to measure the PFR consistently and to develop a therapeutic plan based on the readings. This may help to decrease the morbidity and mortality associated with asthma and also diminishes the number of hospitalizations and emergency care visits.

COLON CANCER

In 1998, an estimated 135,000 individuals were newly diagnosed with colon cancer, and of those people, 55,000 died from related complications. Colorectal cancer is the third most commonly diagnosed cancer and the second most deadly cancer in the US. The average American lifetime risk of developing colorectal cancer has been estimated to be about 5%.[22] Therefore, early detection has become vitally important and has been shown to reduce the mortality associated with this condition. The 5-year survival rate for patients with localized disease who are diagnosed early is estimated at 91%. This decreases to 60% in patients with regional spread and to 6% with distant metastases. These facts have encouraged pharmaceutical companies to develop self-care exams to facilitate earlier detection and treatment. Suggestions for colon cancer screening as recommended by the American Gastroenterological Association are found in Table 125-4.

Office Screening Techniques

Screening is most often applied to determine which individuals are more at risk for the development of colon cancer. Screening tools include the digital rectal examination (DRE), fecal occult blood test (FOBT), flexible sigmoidoscopy, colonoscopy, and double contrast barium exam (DCBE). The latter two generally have been recommended for individuals with a higher risk of colon cancer who have had abnormalities detected by other screening techniques.

The in-office examinations that test the stool for blood are Hemoccult, Hemoccult II, and Sensa. These tests consist of guaiac-impregnated cards that give a result regarding the

---

Table 125-4. Recommendations for Colorectal Cancer Screening

A. Screening is recommended if the following warning signs are noticed:
1. Bleeding from the rectum
2. Blood in the stool or in the toilet after a bowel movement
3. A change in the shape and/or color of the stool
4. Continuous cramping in the lower stomach
5. A feeling of discomfort or an urge to have a bowel movement when there is no need to have one

B. Screening at an earlier age should occur in the following conditions:
1. Past history of colorectal cancer or large polyps
2. A close relative (eg, parent, sister, child) has been diagnosed
3. A history of ulcerative colitis or Crohn's disease
4. A hereditary colon cancer syndrome

C. Screening programs (with a digital rectal exam at each screening) recommended beginning at age 50:
1. Fecal occult blood testing every year
2. Flexible sigmoidoscopy every 5 years
3. Double-contrast barium enema every 5–10 years
4. Colonoscopy every 10 years

Data from Mandel J, Bond J, Church T, et al. Reducing mortality from colorectal cancer by screening for fecal occult blood. *N Engl J Med* 1993; 328:1365.

presence or absence of blood when treated with a developer solution. In the US, the majority of FOBTs are performed using these methods. Because cancerous and precancerous polyps bleed intermittently, these tests need to be repeated so that multiple samples may be analyzed minimizing the possibility of missing blood in the specimen.

Home Diagnostic Exams

ColoCare

In 1980, Helena Laboratories developed the first OTC diagnostic exam used to detect colon cancer. Although it was widely marketed as a home diagnostic test, it is also available for in-office use. Originally marketed as ColoScreen Self Test (CST) in 1980, ColoCare is used to determine the presence of fecal occult blood in a stool sample without removing the specimen from the toilet. Eliminating the necessity of handling a stool specimen allays most of the patient's apprehension about self-administration. This leads to an increase in patient acceptance, earlier diagnosis, and greater success in treatment of this pathological condition.

ColoCare, a third generation test, incorporates tetramethylbenzidine and cumene hydroperoxide as reagents. These have been proven to be comparable to guaiac methodology with an increased sensitivity for hemoglobin. Varying levels of water in the toilet bowl do not affect this test. In addition, diarrhea does not affect the effectiveness of the exam because it has not been shown to interfere with surface hemoglobin.

This diagnostic test has been designed to serve as a preliminary screen. Therefore, results obtained from this exam should not be considered as conclusive evidence of the presence or absence of gastrointestinal abnormalities. It is not intended to replace a physician's examination or consultation in regard to this condition.

PRE-TEST DIRECTIONS—Remove all toilet cleaners, disinfectants, or deodorizers from the toilet bowl. Flush toilet bowl twice before the bowel movement to remove any chemicals. If a noticeable color remains, flush once again. For two days before and throughout the testing period, the patient should be instructed to eat a normal, well-balanced diet that may consist of cooked chicken, tuna, or fish (not rare or raw). No red meat is allowed. The following medications should be avoided: aspirin, corticosteroids, reserpine, indomethacin, and other gastrointestinal irritants as these may cause gastrointestinal bleeding in the tract. Eating red meats or taking one of the aforementioned medications may stimulate a change in color on the test pad. Ascorbic acid (in excess of 250mg/day) and laxatives (containing mineral oil) may prevent a color change in the test when blood is present, thereby producing a false negative outcome.[23]

PROCEDURE—Before beginning this exam, patients should have a bowel movement.

1. Open foil pouch by tearing along the dotted line.
2. Remove one ColoCare pad from the pouch. Hold the pad along the outer edges. Carefully fold the open end of the pouch and tape closed to protect the remaining pads from exposure to moisture.
3. Hold the ColoCare pad with the printed side up. Carefully release the pad, allowing it to float on the water in the center of the bowl.
4. Observe the ColoCare pad for 30 seconds and note any blue or green appearance on the pad.
5. The two smaller squares on the bottom of the ColoCare pad are control areas and help the patient determine if the ColoCare pad is working properly. In 30 seconds, the small box on the left should turn bluish/green in color to demonstrate what the test result should look like if it is positive. The control box on the right should not change color demonstrating what a negative test result will be. If these boxes do not work as described, the test pad needs to be discarded and the procedure should be repeated after the next bowel movement.
6. The test results are determined by examining the pad for the presence of a blue and/or green color in the ColoCare test area

(large square at the top of the pad). If color develops in this square, it may not be the same shade or intensity as the smaller square.

7. ANY BLUE OR GREEN DISCOLORATION IN THE LARGE SQUARE DENOTES THE POSSIBLE PRESENCE OF BLOOD, AND THE PATIENT SHOULD BE INSTRUCTED TO CONTACT A PHYSICIAN AS SOON AS POSSIBLE.
8. Using the first diagram on the reply card provided, the patient should be instructed to place an "X" in all areas (large and small) that changed color. The pad should be flushed along with the stool specimen and the examination should be repeated for the next two bowel movements.

ColoScreen/ColoScreen ES

Some individuals may still prefer the guaiac slide test as opposed to the ColoCare methodology. Therefore, Helena Laboratories also developed ColoScreen and ColoScreen ES to qualitatively detect fecal occult blood from a collected stool sample. Originally marketed in 1980, ColoScreen™ is a traditional guaiac test used to aid in the detection of a number of gastrointestinal disorders. It is composed of guaiac-impregnated paper enclosed in a cardboard frame, which permits sample application to one side, and development and interpretation on the other side. This process involves placing two fecal specimens, collected from each of three successive evacuations, onto the guaiac paper. This test is based on the oxidation of phenolic compounds, found in the guaiac, to quinines resulting in the production of a blue color. When a fecal specimen containing occult blood is applied to the test, hemoglobin will react with the guaiac. A psuedoperoxidase reaction will occur upon the addition of the developer solution, with a blue discoloration generated in direct proportion to the concentration of hemoglobin.

ColoScreen ES is an improvement over the original ColoScreen examination. It offers increased sensitivity and has been formulated to overcome the instability of guaiac solution and the hypersensitivity of benzidine and ortho-tolidine.

CHOLESTEROL

Cardiovascular disease is one of the leading causes of death in the US. In addition to hypertension, smoking, and diabetes mellitus, elevated serum cholesterol is considered an independent risk factor for the development of coronary heart disease (CHD) and cerebral vascular disease. Therapeutic life-style changes, early diagnosis, and improved management of dyslipidemia have the potential to reduce the impact cholesterol plays in the development of sequelae of cardiovascular disease. The Adult Treatment Panel III (ATP III) Guidelines[24] are found in Table 125-5.

When recommending patients for cholesterol screening, risk assessment becomes an important consideration. The major risk factors for CHD are age (>45 years for men and >55 years for women), smoking, hypertension, and a family history of premature heart disease. Recently, diabetes has been eliminated as a risk factor because it is now considered to be in the highest risk category for coronary events and has since been classified as a CHD risk equivalent. Other key changes in the new guidelines are located in Table 125-6[24]. Therefore, the pharmacist must continually be involved in monitoring for changes in patient medications, disease states, and dosages, which will allow patients at risk for CHD to be recognized and counseled regarding cholesterol screening and increase their familiarity with the devices used.

Home Diagnostic Exams

The BioScanner 2000 is the first home diagnostic exam that has the ability to perform multiple functions.[25] Currently, the

Table 125-5. Adult Treatment Panel III (ATP III) Guidelines for Life-Style Changes

1. Daily saturated fat intake below 7 percent of total calories and dietary cholesterol less than 200mg. The average American receives approximately 12 percent of total calories from saturated fat and has an average dietary cholesterol of 220–260mg in women and 360mg in men.
2. No more than 35 percent of daily calories from total fat, provided most are acquired from unsaturated fat, which does not raise cholesterol levels.
3. An increase intake of soluble fiber (grains, beans, peas, fruits, and vegetables) and plants stanols and sterols (found in certain margarines and salad dressings) that may lower low-density lipoprotein (LDL) levels.
4. Weight control and regular physical activity, which improves heart disease factors (eg, LDL).
5. All adults 20 years and older should test their cholesterol at least every 5 years, more often for individuals who are at a high risk for heart disease.

Adapted from Summary of the second report of the National Cholesterol Education (NCEP) Expert Panel on Detection, Evaluation, and Treatment of High Blood Cholesterol in Adults (Adult Treatment Panel III). 2001; http://www.nhlbi.nih.gov/guidelines/cholesterol/atp_iii.html. Accessed March 3, 2003.

BioScanner can screen for glucose, total cholesterol, HDL cholesterol, and ketones. Additional tests are being developed for this device including: triglycerides, LDL cholesterol, hemoglobinA_{1C}, hemoglobin, creatinine, and microalbumin. In 2003, the device retails for $172 and contains testing items as well as color-coded Memo chips, which contain the settings for each test. Memo chips are provided with each new pack of test strips and are responsible for the following:

a. Setting the device for the specific test to be performed (eg, glucose, ketones, and total cholesterol)
b. Identifying the lot number and expiration date of the strips
c. Setting the calibration curve for the specific lot

Table 125-6. Key Changes in NCEP Guidelines

Treat cholesterol more aggressively for those with diabetes.

Make a lipoprotein profile the first test for high cholesterol.

- Previous NCEP guidelines only recommended a screening test for total cholesterol and HDL or triglycerides. The newly suggested screenings will measure LDL, total cholesterol, HDL, and triglycerides.

Develop a new level at which low HDL becomes a major risk factor for disease.

- The new guidelines establish 40mg/dl as the benchmark for signaling possible heart disease, which was increased from 35 mg/dl. An HDL 60mg/dl or higher shall be considered cardioprotective against heart disease.

Identify a "metabolic syndrome" or risk factors for heart disease.

- Factors such as too much abdominal fat, elevated blood pressure, elevated triglycerides, and low HDL often occur simultaneously and dramatically increase the risk for coronary events.

Initiate more aggressive treatment for elevated triglycerides.

- Recent studies identified that triglycerides are linked to heart disease. The new guidelines recommend treating borderline-high levels (eg, life-style modifications, physical activity, and medications).

Advise against the use of hormone replacement therapy (HRT) as alternative to cholesterol-lowering medications.

- HRT reduces the risk for major coronary events or deaths among post-menopausal women with heart disease. Cholesterol-lowering agents have been found to reduce coronary events in women with or without heart disease.

d. Locking out all expired test strips
e. Establishing the accuracy range of the instrument

The cholesterol screening is fast, convenient, and requires no fasting. A sample of blood is placed on the test strip and results are available in one minute. BioScanner 2000 allows the storage of 250 glucose readings and 30 readings of any of the other exams. The device has a 2-minute automatic shut-off feature and is upgradeable for future exams.

Cardiocheck, also developed by Polymer Technology Systems, is another hand-held device that performs multiple functions. The health indicators available are total and HDL cholesterol, triglycerides, glucose, and ketones. The device costs $199 in 2003 and is also fully upgradeable. Cardiocheck is an updated version of the Bioscanner 2000 and is smaller, lighter, and consolidates lab testing affording multiple tests to be performed from a single needle stick.

Cholestrak, developed by Accutech, tests for cholesterol only. Results are available in approximately 15 minutes, and the exam costs approximately $20.00. It contains two foil-wrapped cholesterol tests, two lancets, and two result charts. The exam requires a finger prick with blood collection within 5 minutes of the finger prick. Results may be read within approximately 12–15 minutes.

Cholestrak Procedure

1. Thoroughly wash hands with soap and water.
2. Sit down and relax for 5 minutes (rub hands to warm them).
3. Prick the tip of middle or ring finger and withdraw a sample of blood.
4. Enough blood must be added to the well to cover the black "fill" circle within 5 minutes of pricking the finger.
5. Once the black fill circle is filled, wait for approximately 2–3 minutes.
6. Pull plastic tab on the right side of the testing device until the entire row is visualized.
7. The "OK" indicator will turn purple in 5 minutes, and the "END" indicator will turn green in approximately 10–12 minutes.
8. Using the Cholesterol Result Chart, match the number of the column labeled "test device reading" with the number to its right under the column labeled "Cholesterol mg/dl."
9. This is the measured cholesterol level. If the number is not on the card, call the CholesTrak Help Line.

Both Cardiocheck and Cholestrak must be sent to a laboratory to receive results. Although BioSafe developed Total Cholesterol and Cholesterol Panel, both measure total cholesterol. Cholesterol Panel Cholestrak also provides triglyceride, HDL and LDL cholesterol measurements. Results will be mailed to the patient within 1–2 weeks.

PREGNANCY TESTS

In the US, women are having more children than at any time in almost 30 years. In 1996, there were 6 million-plus pregnancies resulting in 3.9 million births.[26] It is believed that approximately one-third of all women, who believe they are pregnant, use a home pregnancy detection kit prior to seeking professional advice.

The FDA cleared the first home pregnancy detection kit in 1977. By July 1994, consumers spent $191 million on home pregnancy tests. Today, pregnancy detection tests are available for laboratory and in-home use.

Current pregnancy detection tests use monoclonal antibodies to detect human chorionic gonadotropin (hCG). The monoclonal antibodies are either antibodies or immunoglobulins that are capable of binding certain target chemicals, so that an extremely low amount of the target chemical can be detected. The "glycoprotein," hCG, can be detected once the fertilized ovum is implanted in the uterine wall.[27]

A sensitive blood or urine test may detect hCG as early as 8–9 days after ovulation. The plasma concentration of hCG doubles at least every 2 days, peaks between 60 and 70 days of pregnancy, and then declines. Urine hCG levels in pregnant women can reach 25 mIU/ml 7–10 days after conception and reach peak levels of up to 200,000 mlU/ml by the end of the first trimester.[28] Although concentrations of hCG vary in women, more sensitive tests measure lower levels of hCG.

Home Diagnostic Exams

Pregnancy tests use similar technology to detect hCG concentration in urine. Pregnancy tests, which are performed using a urine sample, often require the use of an absorbent wick stick. The stick may either be placed into the woman's urine stream for 2–10 seconds or placed into a collected cup of urine.

PROCEDURE FOR USING TEST STRIPS

1. Remove device from the package.
2. Immediately place a test strip into a collected sample of urine with the arrow end pointing towards the urine. Do not immerse past the MAX (Marker Line).
3. Remove the strip after 3 seconds and lay the strip flat on a clean, dry, non-absorbent surface.
4. Positive results may be observed in as little as 40 seconds.
5. In most cases, negative results are best confirmed after 5 minutes (the manufacturer's recommended reaction time).

PROCEDURE FOR USING A MIDSTREAM TEST

1. Remove device from the package.
2. Remove cap from device.
3. The consumer should turn the test stick so that the handle is facing her and the absorbent tip is located on the bottom. The consumer should not touch the reaction tip.
4. During a midstream of urine, hold the test stick for an average of 6 seconds so that a sufficient amount of urine contacts the absorbent tip.
5. Seal the absorbent window with the cap.
6. Lay the test flat while it is developing and read the result in 3 minutes.
7. In 2–5 minutes, a rose-colored control band will appear in the window to indicate the test is complete.
8. View the indicator window for the result.

The product produces a reading in approximately 2–5 minutes. Results are obtained by viewing the presence or absence of a line due to a second set of reactions, which produces a color change. Most products use a *Control* window or a *Not Pregnant* indicator to demonstrate a positive or negative test outcome.

Timing

Many home pregnancy detection tests market the use of their products as early as the first day of a missed period. Variability in the timing of ovulation among women exists, and it is important to note implantation does not always occur before the expected onset of next menses. According to Wilcox et al, pregnancy is not detectable before the blastocyst implants. This study used an extremely sensitive assay for hCG and concluded 10% of clinical pregnancies were undetectable on the first day of missed menses.[27] Most home pregnancy detection tests should be used any time of day as soon as a missed menses occurs and any day thereafter.

False Negatives

Home pregnancy tests average 97% accuracy.[29] Studies show a 25% rate of false negatives and a significant (though smaller) number of false positives. Women using these products should be aware of possible causes of false-positive or false-negative results and consider the possibility of poor technique, performing the test too close to conception, use of an outdated test, contaminated specimens, and concomitant drug therapy.

Availability

Home pregnancy detection tests are widely available in retail stores and via various online shopping venues. In 2003, the exams cost under $20.00. Prices vary depending on the product selected, the quantity of test products, and sensitivity specifications.

Storage

Home pregnancy detection tests should be stored at room temperature 15–30°C (59–86°F).

OVULATION PREDICTION TESTS

Ovulation prediction home test kits use monoclonal antibody technology to detect luteinizing hormone (LH). LH is a glycoprotein hormone that stimulates the final ripening of an ovarian follicle, its secretion of progesterone, its rupture to release the egg, and the conversion of the ruptured follicle into the corpus luteum.[30] Produced by the pituitary gland, LH is normally present in human urine. LH levels increase significantly prior to a women's most fertile day of the month.

Ovulation prediction test kits are intended to detect the LH surge, which usually occurs during the middle of a woman's menstrual cycle, approximately 1–1 1/2 days prior to ovulation. Ovulation typically occurs 10–12 hours after the peak of a LH surge.[31] The length of a LH surge varies among women.

Many studies have concluded that an egg can only be fertilized 6–24 hours after ovulation. Therefore, advanced detection of ovulation is very important to women seeking pregnancy. Proper timing is a key to ensuring sperm reaches a viable ovum.

Ovulation prediction tests may also measure estrone-3-glucuronide (E3G). Estrone is a metabolite of 17β-estradiol, commonly found in urine, ovaries, and placenta; it has less biological activity than the parent hormone.[30] Ovulation home detection kits are available in the following options: dipstick/test strip, midstream urine kit, and several saliva-based testing devices. Most kits contain materials to conduct several separate tests (as many as 9).

Midstream and Test Strip Ovulation Tests

Midstream and test strip ovulation detection kits are qualitative tests. They simply predict whether LH or E3G levels are elevated and do not confirm the ability of women to become pregnant. Midstream ovulation tests are calibrated to an analytical sensitivity of 25 mIU/ml and test strips are calibrated to 20 mIU/ml.[31]

All instructions should be read fully prior to starting each test. Instructions for ovulation prediction test strips vary slightly among available kits. Most package inserts warn against early morning urine testing and suggest the sample be obtained between 11:00 AM and 3:00 PM and 5:00 PM and 10:00 PM. Some suggest testing twice a day. Testing should begin before ovulation is predicted (day 12–14 in the average cycle). Various charts are included in the package insert to help determine the most favorable testing time frame based upon the patient's menstrual cycle. Tests should be carried out at the same time each day. Liquid intake should be reduced for 2 hours prior to testing to prevent urine dilution.

PROCEDURE USING AN OVULATION TEST STRIP

1. Remove product from packaging.
2. Collect urine in the included plastic cup.
3. Immerse test strip into urine with arrow pointing towards the urine.
4. Do not immerse past MAX (maximum) line.
5. Remove test strip after 5 seconds (no longer than 7 seconds).

6. Place on clean, dry, flat non-absorbent surface.
7. Wait for colored bands to appear. Positive results may be observed in as short as 40 seconds. Negative results may be confirmed after the full reaction time (5 minutes) has passed.
8. After interpretation, discard test strip

Some test strips have a control band, which is located in the upper section of the result window. In a positive result, the test band may be equal to or darker than the control band, and ovulation is predicted to occur in the next 24–48 hours. In a negative result, the test band may present lighter in color intensity than the control band. When testing, during the first few days the tests may be negative, and then a weak positive will result, followed by a strong positive.

Test devices are individually foil sealed to ensure test integrity and shelf half-life. The shelf life is approximately 1 year. Kits should not be used beyond expiration date. Foil packets should be opened immediately prior to the test.

Test Limitations

There are various limitations to using test strips for ovulation prediction. The test strips are for *in-vitro* diagnostic use only and are not reusable. Test results are truly valid only if instructions are followed precisely. Prescription medications such as menotropins may affect results. The onset of menopause and certain medical conditions can result in false-positive results due to elevated levels of LH.

Ovulation Microscope

An ovulation microscope observes visual changes evident in a woman's saliva. Prior to ovulation, a fern-like pattern is produced by the saliva due to an increase in the level of salt and estrogen. Most saliva-based ovulation predictors offer 40X to 60X magnification.[32] Studies imply that a higher the magnification may produce greater accuracy in predicting peak fertility.

Test Limitations

There are various limitations to using the microscope for ovulation prediction. Not all women produce a fern-like pattern in their saliva, and the pattern may not be easily visible to all women. Women, who produce the fern-like pattern during some days of their fertile period, generally do not fern all fertile days. Disruptions in the pattern may occur due to smoking, eating, drinking, toothbrushing, inappropriately placing saliva on slide, and conditions in the location where testing is performed.[33]

Ovulation prediction microscopes are convenient, discreet, compact, and easy-to-use. In 2003, the average cost for a microscopic ovulation detection device was approximately $28.00.

Storage

Ovulation tests are very sensitive to extreme temperatures. Most package inserts indicate the product should be stored at temperatures between 59° and 86° F. Users should be cautious when ordering these products via mail order. Many companies do not permit refunds and exchanges on products damaged due to improper temperature regulation. Any remaining tests in the kit are usable through the manufacturer's expiration date.

URINARY TRACT EXAMS

On an annual basis, in 2000, urinary tract infections (UTI) were reported to affect 11% of women.[34] In 1997, urinary tract infections resulted in 8.3 million doctor visits.[35] These statistics are astounding, but understandable considering the number of patients who request a recommendation for a product to assist

in the treatment of a UTI. Symptoms associated with UTI include pain on urination, urinary burning, urgency, or frequency.

Home Diagnostic Exams

The first urinary tract infection (UTI) detection product was marketed in 1997. The purpose of this test was to permit patients to detect a UTI or monitor the effectiveness of drug therapy after UTI diagnosis. Home UTI exams are qualitative tests. UTI detection home exams may detect either for the presence of nitrite (formed from bacteria), the enzyme catalase, or leukocyte esterase (formed from white blood cells) in the urine.[36] Nitrates taken in through dietary intake are normally excreted through the urine as nitrites. In patients with a Gram-negative UTI, the bacteria convert nitrate to nitrite. Positive results are identified as a dipstick color change or by the presence of foam in a sample test tube (Table 125-7).

Procedure for UTI Home Screening Test Kit

Prior to opening the test kit, patients should carefully read the directions and verify the product is not out of date. The testing environment is very important, and humid conditions should be avoided.

1. A test strip should be removed from the package quickly and the container top immediately replaced and closed tightly. The test strip should appear white, if not white it should be discarded.
2. Dip the test area of the strip into a freshly collected urine sample.
3. Tap the test strip against the edge of the cup to remove excess urine.
4. Wait 1 minute and then compare the test strip to the color strip located on the exterior of the vial of test strips.
5. A pink color indicates a positive result. Color changes that occur after 2 minutes should be ignored.

Concerns

Patients using home UTI diagnostic tests should be aware of the situations that can cause false-positive and false-negative test results. False positives may occur if patients have recently consumed phenazopyridine, rifampin, and other medications that discolor the urine and would interfere with test interpretation. If the patient ingests a medication that alkalinizes the urine, false-negative results are possible. Possible agents include ascorbic acid, fruit juices, and antibiotics. False negatives may also occur in patients who consume small amounts of nitrates (eg, vegetarians) and when urine has not had an adequate bladder retention time to form nitrites. There are a number of disease states that may increase the risk of UTI. These disease states include diabetes, neurological deficits, urinary calculi or obstruction, and a history of prior urinary tract infections.[37]

Table 125-7. Selected Home Diagnostic Urinary Tract Infection Exams

EXAM	REACTION TIME	POSITIVE RESULT INDICATOR
AZO	2 minutes	Dipstick color change
First Response Uriscreen	2 minutes	Foam present in sample tube
HealthCheck Uri-Test Urinary Tract Infection Screening Test	1 minute	Dipstick color change
UTI Home Screening Test Kit	<1 minutes	Dipstick color change (pink color)

Adapted from Boh LE. *Pharmacy Practice Manual: A Guide to the Clinical Experience*, 2nd ed. Baltimore: Lippincott, Williams & Wilkins, 2001.

HIV TESTS

Early detection of Human Immunodeficiency Virus (HIV) type-1 is important to reduce the spread of Acquired Immunodeficiency Syndrome (AIDS). Yet, a great deal of controversy exists on the appropriateness of home test kits for HIV detection. As a result, several detection kits have been introduced and withdrawn from the market in the US. Currently, Home Access HIV-1 Test System and Home Access HIV-1 Express Test System are the two tests available to patients today (Table 125-8). Test systems require patients to mail samples to the company for result processing.

The Home Access kits screen the blood specimen sample using an enzyme-linked immunoassay (ELISA) to test for antibodies to HIV-1. If a positive result is detected, an immunofluorescence assay (IFA) is used to confirm the result. Reliable results are only obtained if the patient follows the instructions carefully. Prior to performing the test, patients should locate the blood specimen collection card and remove the top page. The top page contains the confidential 11-digit Home Access Code Number. Users should read the informed consent section of the booklet and call the toll-free number included in the kit to register the confidential 11-digit number. This call indicates that the patient agrees to the informed-consent section of the booklet.

Procedure to Use the Home Access HIV-1 Detection Kit

1. Thoroughly wash hands with soap and water then dry hands completely.
2. Place the specimen collection kit on a clean, dry surface.
3. Unfold the blood specimen collection card to expose printed circle where blood should be placed.
4. Select a puncture site (preferred sites are middle and ring finger tips).
5. Patients should avoid the little finger and callused areas to ensure an adequate amount of blood may be collected.
6. Clean puncture site with alcohol pad and dry with gauze pad, which are included in the kit.
7. Hang hand by side of one's body for 30 seconds and shake it back and forth vigorously several times to stimulate blood flow to the fingers.
8. Place hand on table or countertop with palm up to avoid flinching or pulling away.
9. Hold lancet, included in kit, between first and second fingers of the other hand.
10. Press tip of lancet against target finger, use steady pressure to indent skin in selected location.
11. Use thumb to depress lancet trigger, using steady pressure.
12. Apply pressure to finger near puncture site. Allow large drops of blood to collect at site. Use thumb and first finger of other hand to increase blood flow.
13. Touch a large drop of blood to circle of blood specimen collection card. Additional drops may be placed around edges of primary drop to fill the circle completely.
14. Examine the back of card to ensure blood has completely soaked through. If it has not, place more blood on the front of the card.

To acquire more blood, use the second lancet in the kit to create another puncture site.

15. Place adhesive bandage provided in kit over the puncture site. Place used lancet(s) in the lancet disposal container included in the kit.
16. Write the Home Access Code Number on the blood specimen collection card.
17. Allow 30 minutes for blood to dry. Place blood specimen collection card inside the specimen return pouch included in the kit.
18. Tightly seal the specimen return pouch and place it in a cardboard U.S. Mail envelope included in the kit (Home Access); or seal in cardboard envelope and place it in a FedEx Overnight envelope (Home Access Express).
19. Call for results after seven business days (Home Access) or three business days (Home Access Express).

Concerns

As health care providers, pharmacists should be aware of the following precautions associated with HIV-1 home test kit use:

- False positives and false negatives are associated with the use of the kit.
- Patients taking anticoagulants and/or hemophiliacs should not use the kit.
- Blood samples not received within 10 days may not be tested due to perishability.
- The product is approved by FDA for individuals 18 years of age and older; studies do not support the use of the products in patients under 18 years of age.
- Only the individual being tested should use the lancets provided in the test kit. Lancets should not be reused nor given to another person using a testing kit. Used lancets should be disposed of properly in the container provided with the kit.

Home HIV-1 detection kits provide patients with an opportunity to test in the privacy of their own homes. Patients may use "Silent Purchase Slips," small slips of paper often located near the products to eliminate the embarrassment associated with purchasing a Home Access HIV-1 Test System. Testing is anonymous and confidential. Results may only be obtained by using a test kit code number. Test results, counseling, and referrals are available 24 hours a day. Patients who obtain positive results should schedule an appointment with a physician to confirm test results and seek medical attention.

DRUG ABUSE

The abuse of illicit drugs, a widespread problem in the US, is perhaps the most commonly missed diagnosis in adolescents. In 2001, 22.4% of high school seniors reported use of marijuana and 2.1% reported cocaine use. In 2000, 7% of youth ages 12–17 also reported use of marijuana.[38]

There are several nonprescription home test kits available to detect the usage of illicit substances, including hair and urine sample kits. Table 125-9 lists selected nonprescription drug abuse detection kits. Home drug abuse detection kits are qualitative tests that indicate the presence or absence of certain detectable agents.

Hair Sampling

Currently, urine sampling is the gold standard for drug testing; however, hair analysis is gaining popularity as an alternative to urine sampling due to the ability of hair to trap within its substances that were in the blood at the time the hair was formed in its follicle.[39] The chemical residues in hair cannot be removed by washing, bleaching, or carrying out any other hair-care routine. Because hair grows 0.5 inch per month, a 1.5-inch sample detects use of drugs within the last 90 days. This

Table 125-8. Available Home HIV-1 Detection Kits

KIT	NO. OF TESTS PER KIT	TIME PERIOD TO RESULT AVAILABILITY	APPROXIMATE COST
Home Access HIV-1 Test System	1	One week	$40
Home Access HIV-1 Express Test System	1	Three days (excluding Sunday or Holidays)	$50

Data from Pray WS, Popovich NG. In Gennaro AR, ed. *Remington: The Science and Practice of Pharmacy*, 20th ed. Baltimore: Lippincott Williams & Wilkins, 2000:1738–1745; and Home Access [package insert], 1996.

Table 125-9. Available Drug Abuse Detection Kits

DETECTION KITS	METHOD	DRUGS DETECTED	HOME/MAIL OPTION	TIME TO RESULT AVAILABILITY	DRUG DETECTION WINDOW	APPROX COST ($)
PDT-90 Personal Drug Testing Service	Hair	Amphetamines, barbiturates, benzodiazepines, cocaine, marijuana, methamphetamine, opiates, PCP	Mail	3–7 days	7–90 days	55.00
Rapid Drug Screen	Urine	Amphetamines, barbiturates, benzodiazepines, cocaine, marijuana, methamphetamine, methadone, opiates, PCP	Home	3 min	4 hours to 3 days	14.75
Parent's Alert	Urine	Amphetamines, cocaine/crack, barbiturates, benzodiazepines, marijuana, ecstasy, LSD, opiates/heroin, additives/diluents	Home	3–5 days		44.95

Data from Boh LE. *Pharmacy Practice Manual: A Guide to the Clinical Experience*, 2nd ed. Baltimore: Lippincott, Williams & Wilkins, 2001; Pray WS, Popovich NG. In Gennaro AR, ed. *Remington: The Science and Practice of Pharmacy,* 20th ed. Baltimore: Lippincott Williams & Wilkins, 2000:1738–1745; and PDT-90 Personal Drug Testing Service [package insert], 1997.

surveillance window yields valuable information regarding the long-term use of illicit substances.[40] Marketed in 1997, PDT-90 Personal Drug Testing Service was the first illicit drug detection product using hair analysis technology. This kit was developed for concerned parents interested in testing their children for illegal drug use.

Testing

Prior to sample collection, test kit directions should be read carefully. Obtaining a sample requires consent, both from an adult or the parental or legal guardian. Adult samples also require consent. The manufacturer does not recommend obtaining a sample without the consent of the individual. A hair sample should be collected from the crown of the head and mailed to the manufacturer of the product. Braided hair should be undone prior to collection. Toll-free telephone numbers are provided with kits to answer questions about sample collection, processing, or result notification.

Procedure for PDT-90 Personal Drug Testing Service

1. Remove all components from package.
2. Locate hair sample collection package, remove sample acquisition card, strip of foil, and integrity seal.
3. Remove strip of foil from sample collection package. Fold foil lengthwise to create a trough.
4. Using a sharp pair of scissors to take the sample, locate a small lock of hair that is 1/2 inch wide and one strand deep when held flat across the finger.
5. Cut the hair close to the scalp.
6. Place hair sample into foil trough, with the cut ends extending 1/4 inch beyond a slanted end of the foil. If the hair is short or curly, the hair should be wrapped before cutting it.
7. Press sides of foil together to trap hair sample inside. Remaining hair may be wrapped around foil.
8. Place the sample in the sample acquisition card. Remove the PDT-90 code card, containing a toll-free number and a confidential code number.
9. Place the integrity seal on the sample acquisition card, date it, and initial the card in the space provided.
10. Mail the sample acquisition card in the enclosed, first-class, postage-paid, return envelope.
11. Call the toll-free number after 5 business days to obtain the test result.

After 5 business days, the consumer calls a toll free number. During the telephone call, the consumer provides the code number that was located in the package. The company will then indicate which drugs, if any, were found in the hair sample.

Concerns

Drug testing should not be performed with hair samples obtained from a hairbrush to avoid sample contamination or the use of old dead hair samples.

Urine Sampling

Urine tests only detect usage within the last 2–3 days for most illicit drugs and do not provide an index of the degree of drug abuse over time.[39] Urine collection is objectionable due to its offensive nature and the ability for urine to be altered or substituted by devious subjects. Further, a urine test may not be feasible in patients unable to empty the bladder because of stress.[41]

Various agents may cause false-positive results including amphetamines, diphenoxylate, ephedrine, pseudoephedrine, methadone, chlorpromazine, dextromethorphan, promethazine, PCP, procainamide, doxylamine, thioridazine, and narcotics. False-negative results may occur due to ingestion of diuretics, excessive fluid intake, and urine contaminates such as bleach, lemon juice, salt, soap, or vinegar.[42]

DIABETES SELF-MONITORING TESTS

Diabetes is an extremely expensive disease for patients, their insurers, governments, and employers. Its direct and in-direct costs (eg, equipment, supplies, utilization of health facilities, and lost time from work) exceed $120 billion per year.[43] Home monitoring of blood glucose is critical to ensure proper management and treatment in insulin dependent diabetes mellitus (IDDM) and non-insulin dependent diabetes mellitus (NIDDM). Adequate treatment requires a continuous balance of insulin, oral medications, exercise, and diet. Successful modification of treatment requires patients to know and understand their blood glucose levels. Until the late 1970s, patients used urine glucose strips or glucose tablets to monitor the control of diabetes. Currently, self-monitoring blood glucose products (SMBGP) (Table 125-10) have replaced these items.

Blood Glucose Home Testing Devices

Technological advances in diabetes-testing have resulted in improved patient self-monitoring with the use of SMBGP. When performed correctly, self-monitoring is quick and accurate. Glucose testing requires a fingerstick using a lancet device to obtain a blood sample.

Table 125-10. Selected Home Blood Glucose Diagnostic Monitors

MONITOR	TIME TO RESULT (SECONDS)	NO. OF READINGS IN MEMORY	COMMENTS
Easy to use/Basic Monitors			
ExacTech RSG	30	~50	No calibration necessary
Glucometer Elite Basic	30	20	No buttons; no cleaning required
One Touch Basic	45	–	Large display; last result retrievable manually; possible to download previous 75 results; multilingual options
One Touch Fast Take	15	150	Large display; no cleaning required; possible to download previous results
Sophisticated Monitors			
Accu-Chek Advantage	40	100	No cleaning required; possible to download previous results; "Voicemate" option available
Glucometer Elite XL	30	120	Large display; possible to download previous results; multilingual options
Precision QID	20	10/~125	Large display; strips available for either whole blood or plasma; no cleaning required; Patient able to retrieve 10 readings; possible to download previous 125 results
One Touch Ultra	5	150	Large display; Product permits patient to obtain blood sample from the arm also
More Sophisticated Monitors			
Accu-Chek Complete	40	1000	No cleaning required; possible to download previous results; possible to display graphics and additional reports on meter screen
Glucometer DEX	30	100	Uses pre-filled cartridges with built-in strips; possible to download previous results
One Touch Profile	45	250	Permits user to record activities including meals, insulin dosing/timing; possible to download previous results; multilingual options

Data from Boh LE. *Pharmacy Practice Manual: A Guide to the Clinical Experience*, 2nd ed. Baltimore: Lippincott, Williams & Wilkins, 2001; Pray WS, Popovich NG. In Gennaro AR, ed. *Remington: The Science and Practice of Pharmacy*, 20th ed. Baltimore: Lippincott Williams & Wilkins, 2000:1738–1745; and PDT-90 Personal Drug Testing Service [package insert], 1997.

The process required to perform a blood glucose test using a SMBGP has been modified over time. Now, most SMBGPs are patient friendly, very easy to use, include large display screens, and provide multilingual options. Additional features may include audio readout, digital readout, memory, and printout capabilities.

Procedure for Applying Blood to Onetouch Ultra Test Strip

Prior to testing, the patient should read the directions carefully and code the meter to ensure the code number on the test strip bottle corresponds to the code number on the meter display. Control tests should be performed prior to using a new SMBGP and periodically thereafter as suggested in the product brochure. Patients using a SMBGP may obtain blood samples using one of several lancet devices (eg, Auto Lancet, Glucolet, Penlet, Penlet II, Softclix, and Soft Touch). Once the skin has been "pricked" with the lancet device, the following is a typical routine:

1. When the company symbol appears, touch and hold a drop of blood to the TOP EDGE of the test strip, where it meets the narrow channel.
2. The volume of the blood sample should correspond to the manufacturer's recommendation.
3. Hold the blood drop to the TOP EDGE until the confirmation window is completely filled. Then the meter will begin to count down.
4. Check the confirmation window.
5. If confirmation window does not fill completely before the meter begins to count down, do not add blood to test strip. Discard test strip and restart.
6. Read the results. Once the meter counts down from 5 to 1, the test result will display with date and time.

7. Used test strips, lancets, alcohol pads, and other supplies should be discarded properly.

Concerns

There are a number of concerns to keep in mind prior to suggesting an SMBG to a patient. Reliable results are best obtained by following the instructions carefully. Although patients may be required to draw blood samples as frequently as 5 times or more a day, the quality of information obtained out weighs this disadvantage. Patients should be advised to purchase and use the company recommended test strips for the equivalent meter. Patients should also be encouraged to wash and dry their hands thoroughly before and after testing.

Patients are often required to perform routine maintenance functions to ensure efficiency with their monitors. The routine functions may include: coding the meter, performing control tests, changing batteries, setting time and date, changing lancets, matching code numbers, and cleaning the meter. To aid with these tasks, patients should be referred to meter instructions and company toll free telephone numbers.

It is recommended that patients using SMBGP receive diabetes education prior to home testing and altering medication doses based on results. Typically, diabetes patients test 3–4 times a day.[44] In 2003, blood glucose test strips retail for approximately $60–$70 per box of 100.

Patients should be cautious of false-positive results due to anemia and false-negative results due to polycythemia.[45] Meters vary in blood drop sample size requirements. Glucose detection range varies among meters; the range is from 10 to 600 mg/dL. SMBGPs differ in price, and various insurance plans may not cover the cost of the meter and supplies. SMBGPs should be stored at room temperature.

Urine Glucose Tests

Urine glucose tests are noninvasive and provide a more economical option to patients unable to afford standard SMBGPs. Urine glucose strips use copper reduction or glucose oxidase for urine glucose detection. Urine glucose tests are problematic to use. They do not detect hypoglycemia, medication interferences, color vision abnormalities, and are unable to provide accurate specific values for results. For example, they only detect glucose in urine after the glucose threshold is exceeded in the kidneys. Further, they do not demonstrate what the current glucose level is but where it might have been several hours previously. Thus, diabetes patients should be discouraged from using urine glucose test strips as a primary marker. In 2003, prices varied from $7 to $10 per box of 50 strips.

Procedure for Using Urine Glucose Test Strips

1. Collect a fresh urine specimen in a clean, dry container.
2. Open diagnostic test bottle and remove one test strip. Hold the plastic end of test strip without touching the test area of the strip. Immediately replace cap on bottle.
3. Dip test area of strip into urine and remove it immediately (drawing edge of strip against the rim of the urine container to remove excess urine) or pass the test end of the strip through a stream of urine.
4. Begin timing.
5. Compare the glucose test area to the glucose color chart exactly 30 seconds after wetting.
6. Ignore any color changes that occur after 30 seconds.

Concerns

Urine glucose tests are affected by fluid intake. False-positive results may occur due to concomitant administration of ascorbic acid, cephalosporins, chloral hydrate, isoniazid, levodopa, methyldopa, high dose penicillins, probenecid, and salicylates. False negatives may occur due to ascorbic acid, aspirin, iron, levodopa, and methyldopa. Clinistix must be discarded 4 months after the bottle is first opened, and Diastix discarded after 6 months of opening. So, if patients use these, they should mark clearly on the label the date they open the product.

Urine Ketone Tests

Urine ketone testing is helpful when diabetes patients are ill or when blood glucose values exceed 250 mg/dL.[46] The presence of ketones (eg, acetone, acetoacetic acid, beta-hydroxybutyric acid) in the urine indicates that the body has attempted to break down stored body fat to use as a fuel source.[47] Diabetes patients are often advised to test periodically for ketones in the urine to assess the need for insulin dose adjustment.

Over the past decade, there has been an increased demand by patients on high protein diets for urine ketone test strips. Table 125-11 provides examples of urine ketone tests. Proper selection of urine ketone tests is based upon patients' needs. Urine ketone tests strips range between $7 and $32 per 50 test strips, in 2003.

Home HbA1C Tests

Measurement of glycosylated hemoglobin (HbA$_{1C}$) that has been altered by exposure to excess glucose allows physicians to obtain an estimate of patients' glucose control over the preceding 2–3 months.[48] HbA$_{1C}$ correlates with the likelihood of microvascular complications. Normal individuals should have a value of 4–6%; the goal for diabetics is less than 7%.[49]

Table 125-11. Selected Urine Ketone Detection Products

PRODUCT	DETECTABLE SUBSTANCES	COMMENTS
Ketostix	Ketones	Readily available in most retail settings
Keto-Diastix	Glucose, ketones	Readily available in most retail settings
Multistix	Bilirubin, glucose, ketones, occult blood, pH, protein, urobilinogen	Usually require retail setting to special order

Data from Boh LE. *Pharmacy Practice Manual: A Guide to the Clinical Experience*, 2nd ed. Baltimore: Lippincott, Williams & Wilkins, 2001; and Pray WS, Popovich NG. In Gennaro AR, ed. *Remington: The Science and Practice of Pharmacy*, 20th ed. Baltimore: Lippincott Williams & Wilkins, 2000:1738–1745.

Prior to purchasing a home HbA$_{1C}$ detection test, patients should ascertain their laboratory HbA$_{1C}$ value for comparison. Hemoglobin A$_{1c}$ test kits include the Accu-Chek Hemoglobin A$_{1c}$ Test Kit and the Biosafe™ Hemoglobin A$_{1c}$ Test Kit.[50] In 2003, the testing kits ranged between $35 and $40.

FUTURE INNOVATIONS IN DIAGNOSTIC PRODUCTS

Increased patient desire to be proactive through self-monitoring and self-management has sparked a consistent demand for new, advanced, and easy-to-use home diagnostic testing devices. Currently, there are many home diagnostic test kits in development. Kits originally created for commercial laboratories are now more patient-friendly and manufactured for home use.

Alzheimer's Disease

At the 8th Annual International Conference on Alzheimer's Disease and Related Disorders, world-renowned clinicians gathered to discuss the recent developments in the area of dementia. There were a variety of topics discussed. Dr. Relkin provided information regarding the advancements and future trends in the area of diagnosis. The topics presented were as follows: cerebrospinal fluid (CSF) markers, biological markers, imaging and the possibility of visualizing neurofibrillary tangles and plaques in living patients.

Studies have demonstrated that certain CSF markers are altered in AD, and their measurement may sometimes assist in diagnosis. Using proteomic techniques (eg, 2-dimensional gel electrophoresis coupled with mass spectroscopy), researchers have been able to identify sets of proteins in CSF associated with AD. Brain imaging has also been employed frequently for diagnostic purposes. Magnetic resonance imaging (MRI) and computed tomography (CT) have been used in addition to single photon emission studies such as the positron emission test (PET) and magnetic resonance spectroscopy (MRS). It is believed that serial imaging studies spaced 1–2 years apart may prove useful in the diagnosis of AD because of average brain shrinkage of 2.5% per year compared with 0.4% visualized in normal patients. Because there are so many new approaches to the diagnosis of AD, the next few years may show a considerable shift in the way clinicians diagnose AD.

Hepatitis C

Currently, the majority of research conducted on antibody-detecting assays is focused on HIV screening and diagnosis. In addition to the blood specimen examinations, there is a test that uses oral fluid collected from between the cheek and the gum of the mouth to screen for HIV infection. This exam has been extensively tested and reviewed, and there has been some inquiry about applying this technology to HCV exams. Unfortunately, this is not available for the detection of HCV, but it may be in the future.

Infertility

Current routine male semen analyses (eg, estimation of sperm concentration, motility, morphology) have limitations as fertility indicators. These analyses lack the potential to ascertain the functional capacity of spermatozoa, and they cannot predict the possible occurrence of *in-vivo* and *in-vitro* conception. In the last few years, efforts have been directed toward the development of the hypoosmotic swelling (HOS) and the acrosome reaction (AR) exam to assess the sperms functional capacity. Recently, progesterone receptor (PR) expression has also been discovered as a viable indicator of sperm function.

Asthma

Recently, investigators have studied the feasibility of using exhaled nitrous oxide to evaluate inflammation in mild to moderate asthma. Elevated nitrous oxide levels have been found in asthmatics because of their direct correlation to eosinophilic airway inflammation in both children and adults. Researchers suggested the possibility of applying this test as a marker for lung injury. Moreover, nitrous oxide has been successfully used as a marker for asthmatic response to treatment and is currently being investigated further for the possibility of other applications.

Recently, The FDA approved NIOX, a product developed by Aerocrine in Sweden, to be used in a physician's office to monitor asthma by recording changes in the levels of nitrous oxide obtained from a patient's breath. To use the device, a patient breathes into a mouthpiece that is connected by a tube to a special computer system that can give the physician an instant reading to facilitate making life-style recommendations or changing treatment parameters. Manufacturer-sponsored research demonstrated that most patients had a 30–70% decrease in nitrous oxide levels after 2 weeks of treatment with inhaled steroids. NIOX may prove to be of great benefit in adjusting treatment options in non- or mildly responsive asthmatics.

Colorectal Cancer

Early detection is the key to defeating colorectal cancer. If identified early, the 5-year survival rates improve 88%. For this reason, researchers are constantly developing new methods of detection. There are several new examinations being employed to screen patients for colorectal cancer and possibly afford patients effective treatment options early. The new examinations include: virtual colonoscopy, immunochemical fecal occult blood testing, and capsule video endoscopy.

Drug Abuse

Future home drug abuse detection kits are likely to be more consumer-friendly. There are consumer demands for more reliable saliva detection kits and home drug abuse detection kits that use blood samples. Forensic scientists are currently using a product, not for sale to consumers, which requires saliva samples to detect drug abuse. Company representatives indicated that they were performing clinical studies with the intent to seek FDA approval for sale of this product to consumers.

Diabetes

There are several companies experimenting with technologies to measure blood glucose levels with either minimal or no disruption to the skin. The following are diagnostic devices pend-

ing approval by the FDA: a device capable of using a low-level electrical current with a laser to produce virtually painless micropores through which glucose is extracted painlessly into a transdermal patch; a system that withdraws and tests interstitial fluid (ISF) on a disposable transdermal patch; an infrared glucose meter; a continuous glucose monitoring system using subcutaneous glucose sensors; a device using a transdermal patch and probe to measure ISF glucose; and a battery operated, hand-held meter that draws ISF from the body. These promising technologies offer the hope that improved monitoring devices could be developed to continuously provide blood glucose readings and even sound alarms warning of impending hypoglycemic reactions.

Additional Devices

Currently, additional diagnostic devices are in development for the following diseases: allergic disorders, cancer, glaucoma, infectious diseases, kidney disease, liver disease, and diabetes. Analyzers for home therapeutic drug monitoring by patients are also in development. Hand-held monitors, with changeable encoded computer chips, able to test blood chemistries including international normalized ratio (INR), lipids, glucose, HbA$_{1c}$, fructosamine, ketones, liver enzymes, and proteins, are all in the foreseeable future.

PHARMACISTS' RESPONSIBILITIES FOR DIAGNOSTIC SELF CARE

As the most accessible health care practitioner, the pharmacist plays a key role in recommending the most appropriate diagnostic device given the patient's circumstance. The development and FDA approval of new diagnostic devices requires pharmacists to remain abreast and understand the function and capabilities of these products.

A pharmacist must be patient and make certain the consumer understands how to use these products and know what to do when the test result is obtained. The patient-pharmacist relationship is important and a key element in ensuring the patient trusts that an appropriate recommendation will be provided and all information discussed shall remain confidential (Please refer to HIPAA regulations discussed in the *Laws Governing Pharmacy*, Chapter 111).

REFERENCES

1. Pray S, Popovich N. In Gennaro AR, ed. *Remington: The Science and Practice of Pharmacy,* 20th ed. Baltimore: Lippincott Williams & Wilkins, 2000:1738-1745.
2. McGraw C, Drennan V. *Nurs Stand* 2001; 15(18):33.
3. Martin B, Pigarelli D. Home test kits and monitoring devices. In Boh LE, ed. *Pharmacy Practice Manual*, 2nd ed. Baltimore: Lippincott Williams & Wilkins, 327–372.
4. American Society on Aging. *Pharmacy Management Can Reduce Medicare and Human Costs.* Forum. www.asaging.org/at/at-217/Forum.html. Accessed January 24, 2003.
5. Ferris D, Nyirjesy P, Sobel J, et al. *Obstet Gynecol* 2002; 99:419.
6. Food and Drug Administration. Intercenter Agreement between The Center for Biologics Evaluation and Research and The Center for Devices and Radiologic Health. Information Sheet. http://www.fda.gov/oc/ombudsman/bio-dev.htm. Accessed February 1, 2003.
7. Lewis C. Home Diagnostic Tests: The Ultimate House Call? FDA Consumer Magazine. 2001.Nov-Dec. http://www.fda.gov/fdac/features/2001/601_home.html. Accessed February 3, 2003.
8. Food and Drug Administration. FDA Warns About Two Unapproved Home-use Test Kits. Health and Human Services (HHS) News. http://www.fda.gov/bbs/topics/NEWS/NEW00592.html. Accessed February 7, 2003.
9. *The Worldwide Market for In Vitro Diagnostic Tests.* New York: Kalorama Information, 2002.
10. Business Communications Company, Inc. The U.S. Clinical Diagnostic Equipment Market. Press Release. http://www.bccreearch.com/editors/RB-168.html. Accessed February 8, 2003.

11. Halasey S, Park R. Making Sense of the Global IVD Market. Business and Marketing. Information Sheet. http://www.devicelink.com/ivdt/archive/02/09/001.html. Accessed February 9, 2003.

12. Food and Drug Administration. Information of CLIA Waivers. Center for Devices and Radiologic Health. Information Sheet. http://www.fda.gov/cdrh/clia/cliawaived.html. Accessed January 16, 2003.

13. Alzheimer's Association. About Alzheimer's. http://www.alz.org/aboutad/overview.html. Accessed February 6, 2003.

14. Recognition and Initial Assessment of Alzheimer's disease and related dementia's. Clinical Practice Guideline 19. Rockville, MD: Department of Human Services, Public Health Service, Agency for Healthcare Policy and Research, 1996. AHCPR publication 97–0702.

15. Soloman G. *Perceptual and Motor Skills.* 1994; 79(3 pt. 1):1249.

16. Honeywell M, Hollis A, Thornton A, et al. *US Pharmacist* 2002; 27(5):HS81.

17. Centers for Disease Control and Prevention. *Mortal Morbid Weekly Rep (MMWR)* 1998;47(RR=19):1.

18. Argo A, Nykamp D, Unterwagner W. Home diagnostics: on the shelf and in the future. *US Pharmacist* 2002; 27(4):36.

19. Baby Start [package insert]. Vernon Hills, IL. 2002.

20. McMullen A, Yoos L, Kitzman H. *J Pediatr Health Care* 2002; 16:67.

21. Medfacts. Educational Health Series. National Jewish Medical and Research Center. http://www.nationaljewish.org/medfacts/peak.html. Accessed March 1, 2003.

22. Mandel J, Bond J, Church T, et al. Reducing mortality from colorectal cancer by screening for fecal occult blood. *N Engl J Med* 1993; 328:1365.

23. Colocare Office Pack Insert. Helena Laboratories. Cat. No. 5651. 1993.

24. Summary of the second report of the National Cholesterol Education (NCEP) Expert Panel on Detection, Evaluation, and Treatment of High Blood Cholesterol in Adults (Adult Treatment Panel III). 2001; http://www.nhlbi.nih.gov/guidelines/cholesterol/atp_iii.htlm. Accessed March 3, 2003.

25. Bioscanner 2000 Home Blood Testing kit and Cholestrak Home Cholesterol Test. Information sheet. http://www.healthchecksystems.com/cholestrak.html. Accessed March 5, 2003.

26. Center for Disease Control and Prevention. Available at: http://www.cdc.gov/nchs/releases/00facts/trends.html. Accessed March 25, 2003.

27. Wilcox AJ, Baird DD, Dunson D, et al. *JAMA* 2001; 286:1759.

28. U.S. Food and Drug Administration Center for Devices and Radiological Health. Available at: http://www.fda.gov/cdrh/oivd/homeuse-pregnancy.html. Accessed March 18, 2003.

29. Clearblue Easy [package insert], 1996.

30. Dirckx JH, ed. Stedman's Concise Medical Dictionary for the Health Professions, Versailles: Lippincott Williams & Wilkins, 2001.

31. U.S. Food and Drug Administration Center for Devices and Radiological Health. Available at: http://www.fda.gov/cdrh/oivd/homeuse-ovulation-urine.html. Accessed March 20, 2003.

32. First Response Ovulation Predictor Test [package insert], 1991.

33. U.S. Food and Drug Administration Center for Devices and Radiological Health. Available at: http://www.fda.gov/cdrh/oivd/homeuse-ovulation-saliva.html. Accessed March 20, 2003.

34. Foxman B, Barlow R, D'Arcy H, Gillespie B, Sobel JD. *Annals of Epidemiology.* 2000; 10(8):509.

35. Ambulatory Care Visits to Physician Offices, Hospital Outpatient Departments, and Emergency Departments: United States, 1997. Atlanta, GA: NCHS, CDC, DHHS; November 1999. Vital and Health Statistics. Series 13, No. 143.

36. U.S. Food and Drug Administration Center for Devices and Radiological Health. Available at: http://www.fda.gov/cdrh/oivd/homeuse-urinary.html. Accessed March 23, 2003.

37. Munroe WP. *Am Pharm* 1994; NS34:50.

38. Center for Disease Control and Prevention. Available at: http://www.cdc.gov/nchs/fastats/druguse.htm. Accessed March 25, 2003.

39. Dupont RL, Baumgartner WA. *Forensic Sci Int* 1995; 70:63.

40. Moeller MR, Fey P, Sachs H. *Forensic Sci Int* 1993; 63:19.

41. Klonoff DC, Jurow AH. *JAMA* 1991; 265:84.

42. Boh LE. *Pharmacy Practice Manual: A Guide to the Clinical Experience,* 2nd ed. Baltimore: Lippincott, Williams & Wilkins, 2001.

43. Ziemer DC, et al. *Am J Med* 1996; 101:25.

44. Pray WS, Popovich NG. In Gennaro AR, ed. *Remington: The Science and Practice of Pharmacy,* 20th ed. Baltimore: Lippincott Williams & Wilkins, 2000:1738–1745.

45. Betschart J. *Nurs Clin North Am* 1993; 28:35.

46. Campbell RK. *Diabetes and the Pharmacist,* 2nd ed. Elkhart, IN: Ames Division, Miles Laboratories, 1986.

47. Lamb WH. *Br J Hosp Med* 1994; 51:471.

48. Anderson RM, et al. *Managing Your Diabetes.* Indianapolis: Eli Lilly, 1994.

49. PDT-90 Personal Drug Testing Service [package insert], 1997.

50. Home Access [package insert], 1996.

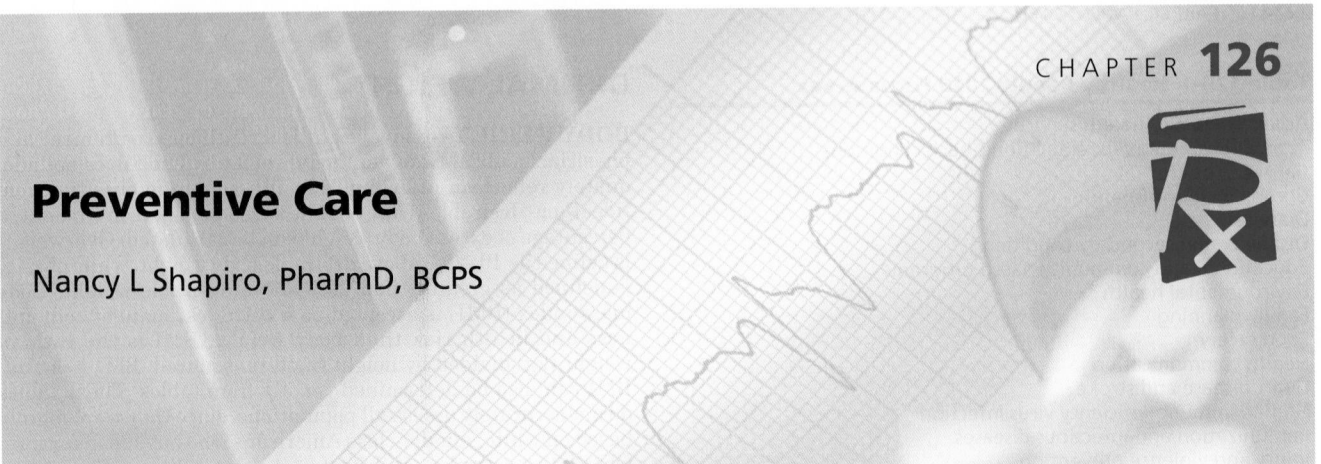

CHAPTER 126

Preventive Care

Nancy L Shapiro, PharmD, BCPS

There is an old saying, "an ounce of prevention is worth a pound of cure." This has never been more true than in health care. Routine follow-up with primary care physicians and other health care professionals can aid in the early detection of many medical conditions (eg, cancer, diabetes, hypertension) and can encourage healthy habits that prevent the development of other conditions (eg, lung cancer, obesity). This chapter seeks to point out areas of preventive care that are wide-reaching to the general population and are areas that pharmacists of all practices should be aware of when interacting with patients.

To begin with, it is appropriate to provide some definitions of prevention. Primary prevention refers to preventing a disease from occurring (eg, childhood vaccinations). Secondary prevention refers to trying to reduce morbidity in presymptomatic subjects with established disease by its early detection and treatment (eg, screening of asymptomatic women and early treatment of detected cervical cancer). Tertiary prevention is implemented on patients with a view of cure, palliation, rehabilitation, or prevention of recurrence or complications (eg, treatment of symptomatic cancer). There are numerous interpretations among individual practitioners about these three definitions, and their use is not recommended by all. Instead, it has been suggested clinical interventions be defined by their objective, target population, and type ("reduction of mortality by increased use of statins in patients with a history of myocardial infarction") instead of by level of prevention ("tertiary prevention of myocardial infarction").

Health promotion and disease prevention were not always priorities of health care. It was not until 1979 that the *Healthy People: The Surgeon General's Report on Health Promotion and Disease Prevention and Promoting Health/Preventing Disease: Objectives for the Nation* were published. In 1990, Healthy People 2000 recommendations were released, and in 2000, Healthy People 2010 objectives were released.[1] There are 28 focus areas of Healthy People 2010 (Table 126-1). The intent is to increase the quality and years of healthy life and to eliminate disparities among the overall health of various communities, ethnic groups, and classes. Ten leading health indicators were identified in Healthy People 2010 to address major public health concerns. These are the most important preventable threats to health and are the focus of national goals to minimize these threats. These indicators involve the following: physical activity, overweight and obesity, tobacco use, substance abuse, responsible sexual behavior, mental health, injury and violence, environmental quality, immunization, and access to care.

Providing cost-effective health care throughout the country is a huge challenge and is being undertaken by the US Preventive Service Task Force (USPSTF). This task force is an independent panel of experts in primary care and prevention that systematically reviews the evidence of effectiveness of, and develops recommendations for, clinical preventive services. The first task force started working in 1984 to 1989 to develop recommendations for primary care clinicians on the content of periodic health examinations. It published the *Guide to Clinical Preventive Services* based off of this work. In 1990, the second USPSTF updated these recommendations for preventive services and released the second edition of the guidelines in 1996. These recommendations were incorporated into Healthy People 2010. The Agency for Healthcare Research and Quality (AHRQ) convened the third task force (USPSTF III) in 1998. It continued its work that will create the *Guidelines to Clinical Preventive Services, 3rd edition*. New recommendations can be found on the web site www.ahcpr.gov/clinic/uspstfix.htm as these become available. These recommendations are modified by individual health plans for their use, endorsed by the American Association of Health Plans, incorporated into HEDIS (Health Plan Employer Data and Information Set) and may result in changes in laws regarding health coverage. Part of the challenge of the USPSTF is to make recommendations for care based on cost-effectiveness. Accordingly, they have developed ratings for their recommendations, based on the levels of evidence, which are listed in Table 126-2.

SCREENING FOR DISEASE PREVENTION—Disease screening is effective when the screening test can detect a disease or its precursor before it becomes symptomatic and when early treatment can improve the patient's outcome. Effective screening tests should be highly sensitive (ie, correctly identifying a high proportion of persons with the disease) and highly specific (ie, correctly identifying a high proportion of persons without the disease). Effective screening tests should not cause harm from the test itself. These should also be of an acceptable cost burden to society so as to be utilized by the patients that need it.

DISEASE PREVENTION INTERVENTIONS—The first method of prevention for a particular disease is to eliminate the risk factors that a patient possesses. When one considers risk factors to disease, these are often broken down into modifiable and nonmodifiable risk factors. Modifiable risk factors are actions that the individual can make to change his/her own behaviors, such as smoking cessation, weight loss, and dietary changes. Nonmodifiable risk factors often include the presence of genetic risk factors, concomitant disease states, and abnormal lab values, and cannot typically be changed by the actions of the patient. A key element to preventive care is to make patients aware of the risk factors that exist for various diseases and to minimize the presence of these risk factors.

CHEMOPREVENTION—Chemoprophylaxis is the use of natural or synthetic compounds to block, reverse, or prevent the development of a disease or undesirable outcome. Increasing evidence in the literature supports the role of chemoprevention to prevent the development of various diseases, such as the use of tamoxifen to prevent breast cancer development, as

Table 126-1. Healthy People 2010 Focus Areas

Access to quality health services
Arthritis, osteoporosis, and chronic back conditions
Cancer
Chronic kidney disease
Diabetes
Disability and secondary conditions
Educational and community-based programs
Environmental health
Family planning
Food safety
Health communication
Heart disease and stroke
Human immunodeficiency virus infection
Immunization and infectious diseases
Injury and violence prevention
Maternal, infant, and child health
Medical product safety
Mental health and mental disorders
Nutrition and obesity
Occupational safety and health
Oral health
Physical activity and fitness
Public health infrastructure
Respiratory diseases
Sexually transmitted diseases
Substance abuse
Tobacco use
Vision and hearing

From the Healthy People 2010 web site www.healthypeople.gov, accessed July 24, 2003.

will be discussed later. For patients that are at high risk for the development of a disease, because of underlying risk factors, consideration of drug therapy to help prevent the development of a disease may be necessary. Typically, clinicians think of antibiotics and antivirals because of their evidence against several infective illnesses (eg, isoniazid for tuberculosis, amoxicillin for dental prophylaxis against subacute bacterial endocarditis, and antiviral agents after needlestick injuries to prevent HIV transmission). The topics in this chapter will go beyond discussion of anti-infectives and will present agents with evidence to prevent noninfectious diseases.

CLINICAL GUIDELINES—Many organizations provide guidelines for screening of various diseases, actions to prevent disease, and effective chemoprevention methods. These recommendations can be found at the National Guideline Clearinghouse web site at www.guidelines.gov/index.asp, which is sponsored by the US Agency for Healthcare Research and Quality in partnership with the American Medical Association and the American Association of Health Plans. Interested readers can also search the internet home pages of major national organizations, such as the Centers for Disease Control and Prevention, American Diabetes Association, American Heart Association, and the American Cancer Society, or perform Medline searches for the individual recommendations. Readers are encouraged to search these guidelines routinely, because they are updated on a regular basis, as new research and evidence becomes available.

The focus of this chapter is on methods of disease prevention, including screening recommendations, identification and modification of known risk factors, chemoprotective measures, as well as interventions to help reduce the morbidity and mortality of the disease. The intent is not to provide a substitute for current therapeutic texts, but to supplement these resources by focusing on the preventive care aspects. Readers are referred to appropriate chapters within this text that will discuss in more detail the areas of smoking cessation and substance abuse, as well as the role of complementary and alternative medicine in disease treatment and prevention.

OPTIMAL WEIGHT

BODY WEIGHT—Body weight is a routine measurement at a physician's office. However, body weight by itself does not adequately reflect an individual's health risk from obesity. From "ideal" or "desirable" body weight based on a person's height, a percentage of excess body weight can be calculated. Overweight is defined as 10–20% above desirable body weight, while obesity is defined as greater than 20% above desirable weight. Body mass index (BMI) is accepted as a better estimate of body fatness and health risk than body weight. BMI is the ratio of weight (kg) divided by height (meters) squared: $BMI = kg/m^2$. BMI can also be determined readily from tables. These tables do not accurately assess all populations, since they were mainly based on white, middle-class Americans who buy life insurance. Obesity is a complex, multifactorial chronic disease. It involves interactions between genetics, metabolism, appetite regulation, food availability, behavior, physical activity, and cultural factors. The National Institutes of Health released guidelines on the evaluation and treatment of obesity in 1998. Their definitions for obesity and overweight are provided in Table 126-3.

Less than half of the US adult population maintains a healthy weight (BMI $\geq$19 but $\leq$25). Obesity has increased in every segment of the population, regardless of age, gender, income, ethnicity, or socioeconomic group. Being overweight or obese is a proven risk factor for diabetes, heart disease, stroke, hypertension, osteoarthritis, and some forms of cancer. Analy-

Table 126-2. USPSTF Recommendation Definitions

A	Strongly recommends that clinicians [the service] routinely provide to eligible patients. (The USPSTF found good that the service improves important evidence health outcomes and concludes that benefits substantially outweigh harms.)
B	Recommends that clinicians routinely provide [the service] to eligible patients. (The USPSTF found at least fair evidence that the service improves health outcomes and concludes that benefits outweigh harms.)
C	No recommendation for or against routine provision of [the service]. (The USPSTF found at least fair evidence that the service can improve health outcomes but concludes that the balance of benefits and harms it too close to justify a general recommendation.)
D	Recommends against routinely providing [the service] to asymptomatic patients.(The USPSTF found at least fair evidence that the service is ineffective or thatharms outweigh benefits.)
I	Evidence is insufficient to recommend for or against routinely providing [the service]. (Evidence that the service is effective is lacking, of poor quality,or conflicting and the balance of benefits and harms cannot be determined.)

The U.S. Preventive Services Task Force (USPSTF) grades the **quality of the overall evidence** for a service on a 3-point scale (good, fair, or poor).

Good	Evidence includes consistent results from well-designed, well-conducted studies in representative populations that directly assess effects on health outcomes.
Fair	Evidence is sufficient to determine effects on health outcomes, but the strength of the evidence is limited by the number, quality, or consistency of the individual studies; generalizability to routine practice; or indirect nature of evidence on health outcomes.
Poor	Evidence is insufficient to assess the effects on health outcomes because of limited number of power of studies, important flaws in their design or conduct, gaps in the chain of evidence, or lack of information on important health outcomes.

From www.ahcpr.gov/clinic/uspstfix.htm.

Table 126-3. Classification of Overweight and Obesity by BMI, Waist Circumference, and Associated Disease Risks

	BMI	OBESITY CLASS	MEN <40 INCHES WOMEN < 35 INCHES	>40 INCHES >35 INCHES
			DISEASE RISK[a] RELATIVE TO NORMAL WEIGHT AND WAIST CIRCUMFERENCE	
Underweight	<18.5		—	—
Normal[b]	18.5–24.9		—	—
Overweight	25.0–29.9		Increased	High
Obesity	30.0–34.9	I	High	Very High
	35.0–39.9	II	Very High	Very High
Extreme Obesity	>40	III	Extremely High	Extremely High

[a] Disease risk of type 2 diabetes, hypertension, and cardiovascular disease.
[b] Increased waist circumference can also be a marker for increased risk even in persons of normal weight.
From the National Heart, Lung, and Blood Institute, Obesity Guidelines, National Institutes of Health, 1998.

sis of data from NHANES III reveals that individuals with a body mass index ≥27 kg/m^2 have a greater than 70% chance of experiencing an obesity-related co-morbidity.[2] It has been estimated that 80–90% of people with type-2 diabetes are obese.[3] Increasing obesity in children has been linked to rising rates of childhood diabetes. More than one-third of all cases of hypertension in the US are related to obesity.[4]

OBESITY TREATMENT—Successful obesity treatment plans incorporate diet, exercise, behavior modification (with or without drug treatment), and/or surgical intervention. Prior to recommending any treatment, the clinician must evaluate the patient for the presence of secondary causes of obesity, such as thyroid dysfunction. If secondary causes are suspected, then a more complete diagnostic workup and appropriate therapy is important. The clinician should then evaluate the patient for the presence and severity of other obesity-related diseases, evaluating appropriate lab tests as indicated. Based on the outcome of this medical evaluation, the patient should be counseled on the risks and benefits of available treatment options. If obesity is present without other comorbid conditions, then the goal would be absolute weight loss. In the presence of comorbid conditions, relatively small reductions in total body weight can have significant effects on comorbidity. Weight loss of 5–10% of initial body weight has been shown in multiple studies to improve glucose intolerance and type-2 diabetes in obese individuals.[5–7] Weight loss has been shown to lower blood pressure, independent of sodium restriction in obese patients with hypertension.[8,9] The combination of diet and exercise-induced weight loss has shown favorable effects on lowering total cholesterol and increasing HDL cholesterol, and may eliminate the need for drug treatment.[10–12]

The average daily caloric intake for American men is 2800 kcal/day and 1800 kcal/day for women. Energy requirements are influenced by factors such as resting metabolic rate and activity level. The resting metabolic rate is higher at heavier weights, so larger people lose weight faster initially. As weight is lost, however, the resting metabolic rate decreases and intake must decline accordingly for weight loss to continue.

LONG-TERM BEHAVIORAL MODIFICATION—Long-term behavior modification is essential for successful weight loss. It may mean substituting undesirable habits with desirable ones (not using food as a reward, for example). To achieve weight loss, energy consumption must be less than energy expenditure. Because one pound of body fat contains about 3500 kcal, it is necessary to reduce the daily caloric intake by 500 kcal/day to achieve a weight loss of about 1 pound per week, or 1000 kcal/day to lose 2 pounds per week, both of which are considered reasonable goals. General recommendations for a balanced, low-calorie diet include limiting fat intake to 20–30% of total calories, and eating a minimum of five servings of fruits and vegetables daily. Choosing foods low in saturated fat and added sugars and high in nutritional value is important. Pharmacists should encourage patients to regularly eat an assortment of foods such as whole grains, low- or no-fat dairy products, and lean meat, fish, poultry, or beans. Appropriate portion-sizes for food is another behavior that needs to be re-

taught, as the "super-sizing" of American food portions is becoming more and more apparent.

For patients that have a BMI greater than 35 kg/m^2 and who are being followed by health care providers with specialized training, very-low calorie diets (VLCDs) may be useful. These VLCDs provide less than 800 kcal/day and produce a weight loss of 3.5–4 pounds per week. Surgical options such as gastric bypass or vertically banded laparoscopy are considered for patients with a BMI >40 kg/m^2. These procedures can cause weight loss of 1/3 of body weight, but are not without complications (eg, malabsorption, nausea/vomiting, gallstone formation). The long-term effects of these procedures on weight and overall health are still unknown.

There are three main mechanisms by which drugs can promote weight loss: (1) reduction of food intake, (2) blocking absorption of nutrients, and (3) increasing energy expenditure. Feeding behavior is influenced by the neurotransmitters serotonin, norepinephrine, and dopamine. These neurotransmitters inhibit feeding by suppressing appetite or producing feelings of satiety or fullness. Drugs such as amphetamines have been used for treatment of obesity since the 1930s, but because of their addictive component, became restricted as controlled substances in the 1970s. In the 1990s, the combination of fenfluramine and phentermine received much attention for its success in sustaining weight loss. Problems with cardiac valvular insufficiency and valvular structural abnormalities as a result of this combination, however, caused the FDA to withdraw fenfluramine, and a similar compound, dexfenfluramine, from the US market. Currently, there are two medications in the US approved for weight loss: sibutramine and orlistat. Sibutramine works by decreasing appetite and increasing metabolism through combined effects on serotonin and norepinephrine reuptake inhibition. Orlistat, on the other hand, works by selectively inhibiting gastrointestinal lipases, therefore, lowering dietary fat absorption. Several herbal products, such as chromium picolinate and ma huang, are also frequently used by patients for weight loss. However, evidence supporting these agents as safe and effective is sorely lacking.

EXERCISE—Increasing one's metabolism is a key component to weight loss. Unfortunately, in the US, citizens are increasingly becoming a nation of "couch potatoes." The increasing ease of food gathering and transportation has meant that there is a diminished opportunity to perform physical activity during our basic day-to-day living. In 1997, only 15% of adults performed the recommended amount of physical activity, and 40% of adults engaged in no leisure-time physical activity. One of the leading indicators of Healthy People 2010 is directed toward physical activity, and there are two objectives set forward.[1] The first objective is to increase the proportion of adolescents who engage in vigorous physical activity (defined as activity that promotes cardiovascular fitness on 3 or more days per week for 20 minutes or more per session) from the current 65% to 85%. The second is to increase the proportion of adults who engage in moderate physical activity (defined as activity for 30 minutes or more per day) from 15% to 30%.

Recommendations to increase physical activity in the community were released from the Task Force on Community Preventive Services in 2002.[13] Among the interventions that were strongly recommended based on the level of evidence were informational approaches such as community-wide campaigns that promote physical activity; behavioral and social approaches such as school-based physical education classes, social support interventions in community settings, and individually adapted health behavior change programs; and environmental and policy approaches such as creation of access to places to perform physical activity along with informational outreach activities.

CANCER

The most common causes of cancer and cancer death are shown in Figure 126-1. While it is beyond the scope of this chapter to discuss risk factors and preventive measures for all forms of cancer, the major ones, including colorectal, breast, skin, cervical, and prostate will be discussed.

Colorectal Cancer

INCIDENCE—For both men and women, colorectal cancer is the third leading cause of cancer-related deaths in the US.

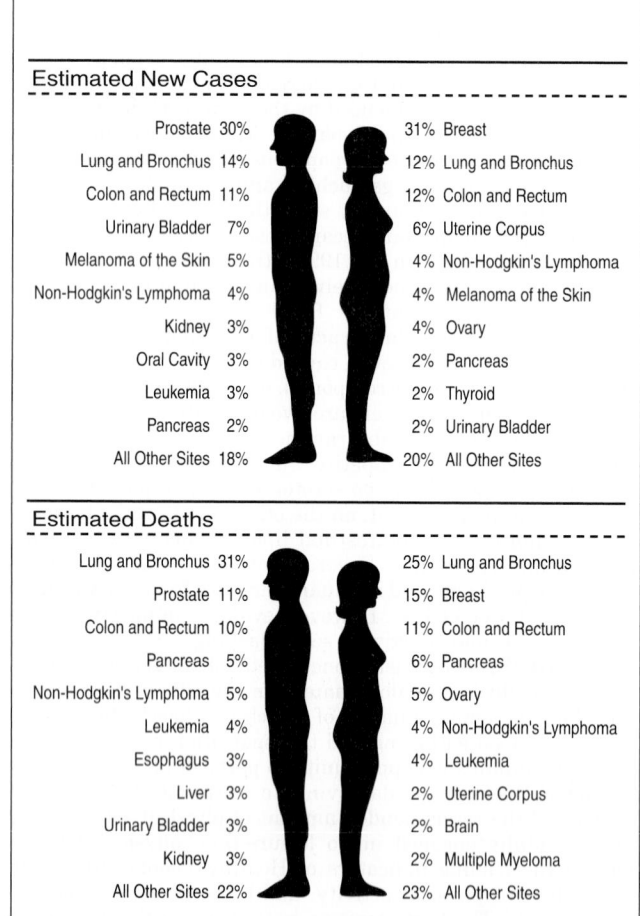

Figure 126-1. Ten leading cancer sites for the estimated new cancer cases and deaths by gender, US, 2002. (Excludes basal and squamous cell skin cancers and in situ carcinomas except urinary bladder. Percentages may not total 100% due to rounding.) (From Jemal A, Thomas A, Murray T, et al. Cancer statistics, 2002. *CA Cancer J Clin* 2002; 52:23. © 2002 Lippincott Williams & Wilkins.)

Table 126-4. American Cancer Society Dietary Recommendations

Have most of your foods come from plant sources
    Eat 5 or more servings of fruits and vegetables daily
    Eat other foods from plant sources, such as breads, cereals, grain products, rice, pasta, or beans several times each day
Limit intake of high fat foods, especially from animal sources
    Choose foods low in fat
    Limit consumption of meats, especially high-fat meats
Be physically active: achieve and maintain a healthy weight
    Be at least moderately active for 30 minutes or more most days of the week
    Stay within your healthy weight range
Limit consumption of alcoholic beverages, if you drink at all

Adapted from http://www.cancer.org/docroot/PED/content/ PED_3_2X_Diet_and_Activity_Factors_That_Affect_Risks.asp, accessed July 25, 2003.

The American Cancer Society estimates that 105,500 colon and 42,000 rectal cancers will be diagnosed in 2003, with about 57,100 deaths expected. Ninety-three percent of all colorectal cancers occur in patients older than 50 years of age. The median age at diagnosis is 72 years, and individual risk increases with increasing age. The American Cancer Society reports that the 1- and 5-year survival rates for patients with colon or rectal cancer are 83% and 62%, respectively. Even more importantly, when colorectal cancers are found early, in a localized state, the 5-year survival rate increases to 90%. However, only 37% of these cancers are detected at an early stage. Patients with colorectal cancer in the early stages may be asymptomatic or may have symptoms of rectal bleeding, persistent changes in bowel habits, with increased frequency or loose stools. Abdominal discomfort, pain, distention, constipation, and weight loss are all warning signs that deserve medical attention.

RISK FACTORS—Multiple risk factors are associated with the development of this malignancy, including genetic susceptibility, environmental, and life-style. It has been suggested that diets high in fiber are protective against the development of colorectal cancer. There has been conflicting data in support and against this recommendation. In addition, there is the suggestion, supported by numerous epidemiologic studies, that dietary fat increases one's risk of colorectal cancer. Most of the sources of fat in these studies were animal. But, it is unknown whether the source of fat is important, as is the question of saturated *versus* unsaturated fat. It is unclear whether the risk is associated with the fat source or the cooking or processing methods.[14] While current evidence indicates that animal meat and saturated fat intake appear to be associated with an increased risk of colorectal cancer, the magnitude of risk has not been determined. Dietary recommendations from the American Cancer Society are listed in Table 126-4.

Physical inactivity and elevated BMI are each independently associated with an increased risk of colon cancer.[15,16] Individuals with a total higher level of activity throughout life have the lowest risk. The risk of colon cancer may be increased as much as twofold in men who are in the highest quintile of body size. While the evidence is less consistent for women, the Iowa Women's Health Study showed that cancer risk for colorectal and breast cancer was 60% higher in women who were in the highest quartile of BMI compared to the cancer risk of women in the lowest quartile.[17] Potential mechanisms to this relationship include the observation that physical activity stimulates bowel peristalsis, resulting in decreased bowel transit time, and the possibility that exercise can alter levels of blood glucose, insulin, and other hormones, which may reduce tumor cell growth. Heavy alcohol consumption increases risk of rectal and colon cancer by as much as two to three times, although some studies have found no significant increase in risk.[14,16] The evidence is strongest for men, and no single source of alcohol is associated with a greater risk.

A prospective cohort of over 1 million Americans showed that long-term cigarette smoking is associated with an adjusted colorectal cancer mortality ratio of 1.32 (95% CI, 1.16–1.49) for men and 1.41 (95% CI, 1.26–1.58) for women smokers, compared to men and women who had never smoked.[18] Increased risk was evident after >20 years of smoking for men and women combined as compared with patients who never smoked. Risk among current and former smokers increased with duration of smoking and average number of cigarettes smoked per day; risk in former smokers decreased significantly with years since quitting. These authors suggested that as much as 12% of colorectal deaths were attributable to smoking.

SCREENING FOR COLORECTAL CANCER—Despite clear evidence to the benefit of screening for colorectal cancer, The Centers for Disease Control and Prevention estimated that in 1999 only 20.6% of US men and women over 50 had a fecal occult blood test in the year prior to the survey, and only 33.6% had a sigmoidoscopy or colonoscopy within the past 5 years.[19]

The US Multisociety Task Force on Colorectal Cancer released updated guidelines in 2003.[20] This panel recommends offering screening for colorectal cancer in average-risk men and women at age 50 (Fig 126-2). The strongest evidence-based recommendations include offering annual fecal occult blood testing (FOBT) or flexible sigmoidoscopy every 5 years. Each of these screening tests has been associated with reductions in mortality. FOBT uses a guaiac-based test of two samples from each of three consecutive stools. Patients with a positive specimen should be followed up with colonoscopy. Flexible sigmoidoscopy reduced mortality by two-thirds for lesions within reach of the sigmoidoscope. This panel found theoretical evidence supporting the combination of annual FOBT and flexible sigmoidoscopy every 5 years. No direct evidence of efficacy, but strong rationale, supports the recommendation of double-contrast barium enema every 5 to 10 years, or colonoscopy every 10 years. Both double-contrast barium enema and sigmoidoscopy are found to be less sensitive for detecting cancers than a colonoscopy and therefore are recommended at more frequent intervals. Colonoscopy is the most sensitive and specific of all of the available screening tests, but offers the disadvantage of greater cost, risk, and inconvenience to the patient. In 2001, Medicare rules allowed for a colonoscopy screening every 10 years to beneficiaries. While newer methods for screening for colorectal cancer are being developed, such as virtual colonoscopy and DNA analysis of stool samples, there is insufficient evidence to support these methods for screening tools.

Other recommendations have been made by the USPSTF, which in 2002 recommended screening all adults aged 50 and older. The panel found that benefits from screening substantially outweigh harms, but that the quality of evidence, magnitude of benefit, and potential harms vary with each method. Furthermore, it found that screening tests are cost-effective ($50,000 per year of life saved).[21] The American College of Gastroenterology recommends colonoscopy screening every 10 years as the preferred screening strategy, with an alternative being the flexible sigmoidoscopy every 5 years plus annual FOBT.[22] In contrast, the American Cancer Society recommends annual FOBT, flexible sigmoidoscopy every 5 years, annual FOBT plus flexible sigmoidoscopy every 5 years, double-contrast barium enema every 5 years, or colonoscopy every 10 years.[23] The American Cancer Society does not recommend digital rectal examination as a stand-alone screening test for colorectal cancer.

Pharmacists often have the opportunity to discuss colorectal screening when counseling patients on the use of polyethylene glycol purge products, such as Colyte and Nulytely. Careful attention should be paid to the timing of these products so that procedures can take place as scheduled. Pharmacists should be aware that there are differences in the guidelines with regards to method and frequency of colorectal cancer screening, but the

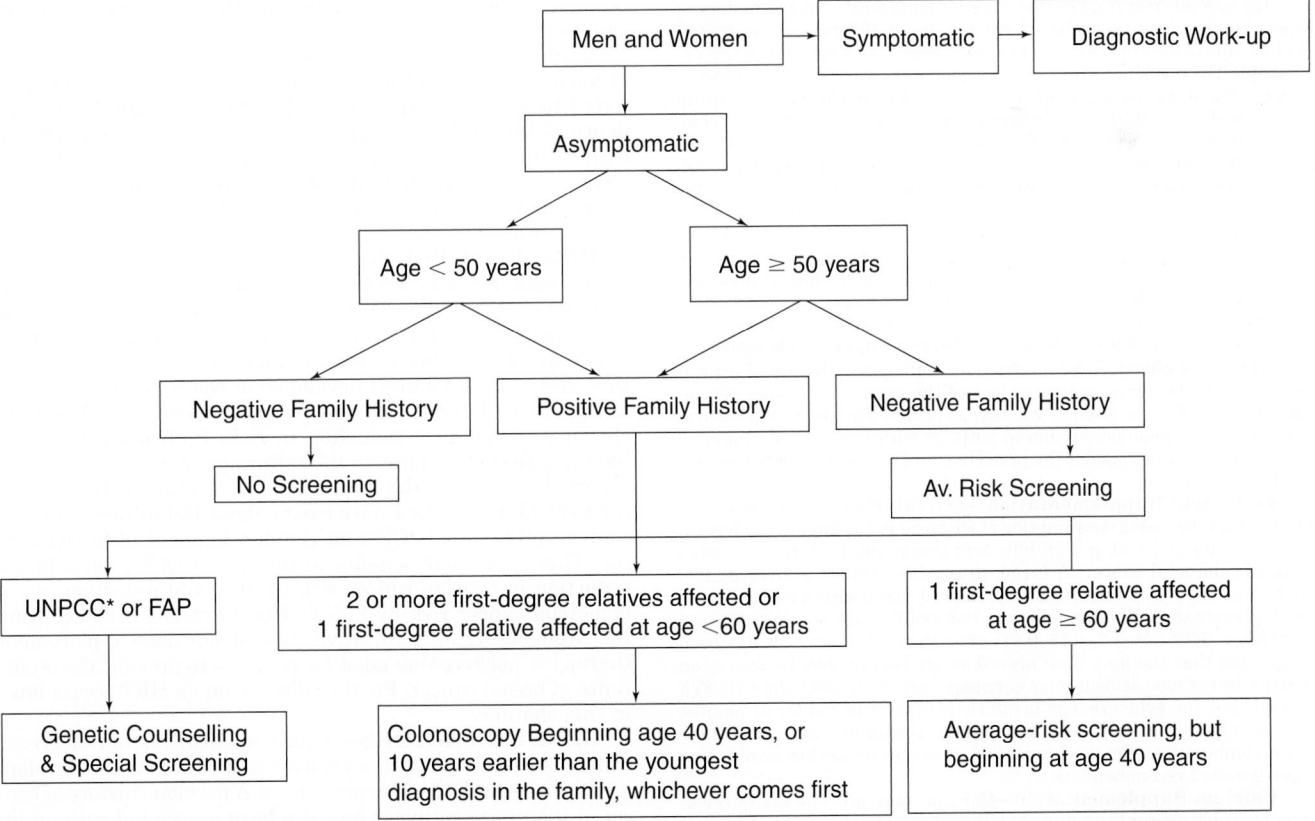

Figure 126-2. Algorithm for colorectal cancer screening. +, Either colorectal cancer or adenomatous polyp; *, HNPCC = hereditary nonpolyposis colorectal cancer and FAP = familial adenomatous polyposis. (Reprinted from Winawer S. Colorectal cancer screening and surveillance. *Gastroenterology* 2003; 124:544, with permission from the American Gastroenterological Association.)

accepted starting range for screening all adult patients at average risk is 50 years. Mass media campaigns have increased the awareness of the need for colon cancer screening, and counseling by pharmacists is a good way to help reinforce these recommendations. Additionally, pharmacists should be aware of patients displaying any of the colorectal cancer warning signs (eg, bleeding, changes in bowel habits, weight loss, abdominal pain) so that they can be referred to appropriate medical care and diagnostic work-up.

CHEMOPREVENTION OF COLORECTAL CANCER—

Aspirin—Regular use of non-steroidal anti-inflammatory drugs and aspirin use (at least two doses per week) is associated with a reduced risk of the development of colorectal cancer. In the Nurse's Health Study, colorectal cancer development was decreased in women who took aspirin regularly for 10 consecutive years, with the highest reduction occurring with an intake of four to six tablets per week.[24] A population-based study of non-aspirin NSAID users who had taken NSAIDs for at least 48 months in the previous 5 years revealed a relative risk of colorectal cancer of 0.49 (95% CI, 0.24–1.00) for users as compared to nonusers.[25] However, the Physician's Health Study, the first randomized trial of aspirin versus placebo, reported no decrease in colorectal cancer risk (RR = 1.03; 95% CI, 0.83–1.28) with aspirin 325 mg every other day for 12 years.[26] The potential mechanisms by which these agents exert their protective effects appear to be linked to their inhibition of cyclooxygenase-2 (COX-2) and free radical formation.

The question of whether aspirin should be recommended for patients with a prior history of colorectal cancer was recently addressed in two major trials. The first trial randomized 635 patients to 325-mg enteric-coated aspirin or placebo daily for a median duration of 31 months.[27] One or more adenomas were found in 17% of the aspirin patients and 27% of the placebo patients (p = 0.004). The mean (± SD) number of adenomas was lower in the aspirin group than the placebo group (0.3 ± 0.87 vs. 0.49 ± 0.99, p = 0.003). The adjusted relative risk of any recurrent adenoma in the aspirin group, compared to placebo was 0.64 (95% CI, 0.46–0.91). Time to the detection of a first adenoma was longer in the aspirin group than in the placebo group (hazard ratio for the detection of a new polyp 0.64; 95% CI, 0.43–0.94; p = 0.022). The authors concluded that aspirin use is associated with a significant reduction in the incidence of colorectal adenomas in patients with previous colorectal cancer.

The second trial randomized 1121 patients with a recent history of adenomas to receive placebo, 81 mg aspirin, or 325 mg aspirin daily.[28] Follow-up colonoscopy was performed 3 years after the qualifying endoscopy. The incidence of one or more adenomas was 47% in the placebo group, 38% in the 81 mg aspirin group, and 45% in the 325 mg aspirin group (global p = 0.04). Unadjusted relative risks of any adenoma compared to placebo were 0.81 for the 81 mg aspirin group (95% CI, 0.69–0.96) and 0.96 in the 325 mg aspirin group (95% CI, 0.81–1.13). Advanced neoplasms were found in 12.9% of placebo patients, 7.7% in the 81 mg aspirin group, and 10.7% in the 325 mg aspirin group. For advanced neoplasms, the relative risks were 0.59 (95% CI, 0.38–0.92) for the 81 mg group, and 0.83 (95% CI, 0.55–1.23) in the 325 mg aspirin group. The authors concluded that low-dose aspirin has a moderate chemoprotective effect on adenomas in the large bowel.

These trials suggest that aspirin reduces the risk of recurrent adenomas in patients with a history of colorectal cancer or adenomas. At this time, cost-effectiveness analyses do not support the use of aspirin for primary chemoprevention in lieu of the current screening recommendations. The question of whether aspirin should be recommended for secondary chemoprevention in patients with a history of colorectal neoplasm needs to consider the protective and harmful effects of aspirin with long-term use.

Folic Acid Supplementation—Several cohort trials have suggested that increased consumption of folic acid in the diet, in the form of supplements and eating high folic acid containing food, reduces one's risk of colorectal cancer. A large, prospective cohort of over 88,000 nurses in The Nurses Health Study, showed that taking a multivitamin with greater than 400 mcg folic acid reduced the risk of colorectal cancer (RR = 0.25, 95% CI, 0.13–0.51) after 15 years of use.[29] It has been suggested that the long time needed to see benefit may be due to an early effect of folic acid on colon carcinogenesis.[30] In 2003, the USPSTF stated that the evidence was insufficient to recommend for or against the use of vitamins A, C, or E, multivitamins with folic acid, or antioxidant combinations for the prevention of cancer or cardiovascular disease (Grade I recommendation).[31]

Calcium Supplementation—Calcium may prevent the development of colon cancer by binding to bile acids and fatty acids in the bowel lumen or by directly inhibiting the development of epithelial cells.[30] The exact benefit of calcium in the prevention of colon cancer has been questionable. One recent randomized trial in 930 patients with a history of colorectal adenomas demonstrated a significant reduction in the formation of new adenomas in patients receiving calcium supplements (3 gm calcium carbonate) compared to placebo (RR = 0.75 (95% CI, 0.60–0.96; p = 0.02).[32] Pooled results from the Nurses Health Study and the Health Professionals Follow-up Study, totaling 87,998 women and 47,344 men showed an inverse association between higher calcium intake of >1250 mg/day versus ≤500 mg/day and distal colon cancer (pooled RR = 0.65, 95% CI, 0.43–0.98), but incidence of proximal cancer was not significant.[33] There appeared to be minimal benefit in additional calcium carbonate intake beyond 700 mg/day, suggesting a possible threshold effect.

Although there is evidence supporting the use of hormone replacement therapy for the prevention of colorectal cancer, its use for this indication is no longer recommended (see HRT discussion later in this chapter). Results of a large American Cancer Society cohort do not support a substantial effect of vitamins C or E supplement use on overall colorectal cancer mortality.[34] Pharmacists should be aware of measures that patients can take to help prevent the development of colorectal cancer (eg, increasing physical activity, maintaining proper body weight, limiting fat intake, smoking cessation, minimizing alcohol intake, and using aspirin or an NSAID regularly). Further research is being conducted in this area to determine what other modifiable risk factors exist.

Breast Cancer

INCIDENCE—Breast cancer is the most common site of cancer and is second only to lung cancer as the leading cause of cancer death in American women. It is estimated that more than 192,000 new cases of breast cancer will be diagnosed and that more than 40,000 women will die of breast cancer each year. The incidence of breast cancer has been increasing over the last 4 decades. There are three main reasons for the increase in this incidence: an increase in the development of the disease itself due to changes in body hormones, body habitus, and dietary factors; increases in the detection because of mammography and regular clinical breast examinations; and because women are living longer and the mortality from other causes is decreasing.

While most people think of breast cancer as purely a disease of women, more than 1500 cases of male breast cancer were projected to be diagnosed in the United States in 2001. The incidence of breast cancer increases with increasing age. One in eight women will develop breast cancer during their lifetime. The cumulative probability of developing breast cancer increases with increasing age, but more than half of the risk occurs after age 60 years.[35]

RISK FACTORS—Risk factors for the development of breast cancer can be broken down into three categories: hormonal, genetic, and environmental. Hormonal factors such as early menarche, which is defined as menstruation beginning before age 12, has been shown to increase the cumulative lifetime risk of breast cancer development compared to menarche at age 16 or later.[36] Conversely, early menopause has been shown to result in a reduction in risk. Both nulliparity and having a first child later in life (after age 30 years) have been reported to increase the lifetime risk of developing breast cancer twofold. Conflicting data exists about the influence of oral contraceptive pills (OCPs) on the development of breast cancer. There are clear benefits to the use of OCPs, including a reduction in ovarian cancer risk by 40% and reduction in endometrial cancer risk by 60%.[37] Due to recent evidence from the Women's Health Initative, use of hormone replacement therapy is not recommended for patients to prevent the occurrence of breast cancer. Further discussion on HRT occurs later in this chapter.

GENETIC FACTORS—A past medical history of breast cancer is associated with a relative risk of 5.0 for the development of a contralateral breast cancer. A previous history of cancer of the uterus or ovary has also been associated with an increased risk. Family history of breast cancer has a strong association with a woman's own risk for developing the disease. The following statements about the estimates of the risks associated with family history include the following[38]:

1. Any first-degree relative with breast cancer increases a woman's risk of breast cancer 1.5–3-fold, depending on age;
2. Higher relative risk is associated with breast cancer with onset younger than age 45 years in one or more first-degree relatives;
3. Having multiple affected first-degree relatives has been inconsistently shown to elevate risks;
4. A second-degree affected relative increases a woman's risk of developing breast cancer by 50% (relative risk = 1.5); and
5. Affected family members on the maternal side and the paternal side contribute similarly to the risk.

Two breast cancer genes, BRCA1 and BRCA2, have been mapped to chromosome 17 and 13, respectively. Women with a strong family history of breast or ovarian cancer, or both, who are carriers of the BRCA1 have an estimated lifetime risk of 85% for breast cancer and 60% for ovarian cancer. Carriers of the BRCA2 mutation have similar risks for breast cancer, but much lower risks for ovarian cancer.[39] Current estimates of the risk of breast cancer in a woman who carries a BRCA1 or BRCA2 mutation and has a family history of multiple cases of breast or ovarian cancer, or both, range from 76% to 87%.[40–43] Estimates of the risk of ovarian cancer in a woman with such a history range from 32% to 84% for carriers of BRCA1 mutations, but are much lower for carriers of BRCA2 mutations.[41–43] These results were derived from studies of high-risk families and may not apply to all carriers of BRCA1 or BRCA2 mutations. There are no clear recommendations for prophylactic treatment for carriers of these mutations. Bilateral prophylactic mastectomy is one alternative, but this has failed to prevent cancer occurrence in some patients. Close follow-up (ie, mammography every 6 months) for carriers of the BRCA mutation is recommended by some.

ENVIRONMENTAL FACTORS—Case control and prospective studies in the US have generally failed to show an association between dietary fat and breast cancer risk. The relationship between vitamin A and breast cancer risk is unclear. In contrast, most studies suggest some benefit from β-carotene, vitamin C, and/or dietary fiber.[44] Other factors with conflicting evidence of their effects on breast cancer include obesity, alcohol intake, and radiation exposure.

PREVENTION AND EARLY DETECTION—Efforts at breast cancer prevention revolve around risk factor modification and identification. However, genetic risk factors including family history and previous history of other malignancies cannot be ignored. Isolation and screening for breast cancer genes in high-risk patients help identify candidates for prophylactic bilateral mastectomy. Chemoprevention includes interventions directed at inhibiting neoplastic development through pharmacologic measures. Retinoids and tamoxifen are two drugs being studied for their use in breast cancer chemoprevention.

MAMMOGRAPHY—Controversy exists in screening recommendations for annual mammography. It is generally accepted that annual mammograms should be performed in women ≥50 years of age, and reduction of mortality is associated with regular use of screening mammography. The controversy exists for women younger than 50 years of age. The American Cancer Society currently recommends a baseline mammogram for women between 35 and 40 years of age, and annual screening in women 40 years of age and older, while the NCI and USPSTF do not recommend routine screening in the 40–49 years age group, holding off on recommending annual mammography until age 50, due to finding no benefit to screening in the 40–49 year age group.[45–49] A summary of the differences in recommendations for the prevention of breast cancer can be found in Table 126-5. The results of the Canadian National Breast Screening Study-1, comparing (1) breast cancer mortality in 40–49-year-old women who received either screening annual mammography, breast physical examination, and instruction on breast self-examination on 4 or 5 occasions to (2) community care after a single breast physical examination and instruction on breast self-examination failed to show a reduction in breast cancer mortality in the annual mammography screening group (group 1) after 11 to 16 years of follow-up.[50]

BREAST SELF-EXAMINATIONS—Currently the American Cancer Society recommends that all women over the age of 20 years perform monthly breast self-examinations (BSEs). There is evidence to support this recommendation due to patients' ability to help diagnose the disease at an earlier stage and demonstrate a higher 5-year survival when compared to women who did not perform them.[51] However, reports from the published randomized clinical trial sponsored by the NCI in over 250,000 women in Shanghai, China, found that women who received intensive instruction in BSE did not reduce mortality from breast cancer and that programs to encourage BSE in the absence of mammography would be unlikely to reduce mortality from breast cancer. The BSE group was more likely to be diagnosed with benign breast lesions.[52] Although these results fail to show the benefit of BSE on mortality, it is still accepted as an effective screening tool for the discovery of breast cancers and is still generally recommended by most clinicians. Clinical breast examinations can occur during the course of a routine visit, but should occur no less often than every 2 years, beginning at age 35.

CHEMOPREVENTION—The Breast Cancer Prevention Trial P-1, part of the National Surgical Adjuvant Breast and Bowel Project (NSABP), was the main reason for the approval of tamoxifen for breast cancer risk reduction in high-risk women, defined as age >35 years with a 5-year predicted breast cancer risk of 1.67% as calculated by the Gail Model.[53,54] This trial showed that tamoxifen decreased the incidence of invasive and noninvasive breast cancer by about half when compared to placebo in high-risk patients treated for 5 years, and the authors felt that despite side effects, its use is appropriate in women at increased risk of the disease.[55] Previous trials for this indication had been less successful.[56,57] Initial results from the International Breast Cancer Intervention Study IBIS-1 have been released. These investigators compared tamoxifen 20 mg/day vs. placebo for 5 years in women at increased risk of breast cancer. They found a risk reduction of 32% for breast cancer, no increased risk for endometrial disease, and an increased risk of thromboembolic events in the tamoxifen group (OR 2.5, 95% CI, 1.5–4.4, p = 0.001). The authors concluded that overall risk *versus* benefit to prophylactic tamoxifen is still unclear, mortality from non-breast cancer causes is not increased from tamoxifen, and that temporary cessation of tamoxifen should be considered after major surgery or periods of immobility, in addition to appropriate antithrombotic measures. Patients at high risk of thromboembolic disease should not use prophylactic tamox-

Table 126-5. Guidelines for Early Detection of Breast Cancer

	AMERICAN CANCER SOCIETY	USPSTF	NATIONAL CANCER INSTITUTE
Breast self examination	Monthly (20+)	NR	NR
Clinical breast examination	Every 3 years (20–40)	Annual 50–69 with mammography	Every 3 years (20–40) annual (40+)
Mammogram	Annual (40+)	1–2 years (50–69)	NR (40–49)
			Annual (50+)

NR = not recommended.

ifen.[58] Data from the on-going STAR (Study of Tamoxifen and Raloxifene) trial is not yet available, but seeks to determine the incidence of breast cancer in high-risk patients receiving raloxifene 60 mg/day or tamoxifen 20 mg/day for 5 years. Clinicians will need to wait for these results before recommending raloxifene for this indication.[59] Readers interested in further information about the topic of tamoxifen for the prevention of breast cancer are referred to the following review.[60] For women at low or average risk of breast cancer, the USPSTF found fair evidence that tamoxifen and raloxifene may prevent some breast cancers. The panel concluded, however, that the potential harms of chemoprevention may outweigh the potential benefits in women who are not at high risk of breast cancer (Grade D recommendation). Clinicians should discuss chemoprevention with women at high risk for breast cancer and at low risk for adverse effects of chemoprevention, and inform patients of the potential benefits and harms of chemoprevention (B recommendation). For women at high risk of breast cancer, the USPSTF found fair evidence that treatment with tamoxifen can significantly reduce the risk of invasive estrogen-receptor-positive breast cancer and that the likelihood of benefit increases as the risk of breast cancer increases. Less evidence supports the benefit of raloxifene. The USPSTF found good evidence that tamoxifen and raloxifene increase the risk of thromboembolic events (eg, stroke, pulmonary embolism, and deep venous thrombosis) and symptomatic side effects (eg, hot flashes) and that tamoxifen, but not raloxifene, increases the risk of endometrial cancer. Their conclusion was that the balance of risks and benefits may be favorable in high-risk women, but will need to also consider individual patient preferences.

Prostate Cancer

INCIDENCE—Prostate cancer is the most common cancer in American men and is the second-leading cause of cancer-related deaths. Accepted risk factors for prostate cancer include age greater than 50 years, race, and family history. African Americans have a 5-year survival approximately 15% less than whites, perhaps due to the combination of higher levels of testosterone compared to white males and increased androgen receptor activation. Low-fat diets and other dietary considerations such as β-carotene, lycopene, and vitamin E may be protective, although these are still unproven. Smoking has not been associated with an increased risk of prostate cancer, but smokers with prostate cancer have an increase in mortality. Alcohol consumption does not appear to be associated with the development of prostate cancer. Many patients with localized prostate cancer are asymptomatic, while those with more invasive disease develop symptoms of alterations in urinary frequency, hesitancy, and flow, and new-onset impotence. Metastases from prostate cancer develop in the bone and lymph tissue. Some nonspecific signs of more advanced disease include anemia and weight loss. The prostate specific antigen (PSA) test involves taking a simple blood sample and detecting the enzyme levels. While it is simple and readily available, it does generate false-positives and false-negatives and cannot be recommended alone as a screening tool. Normal ranges for PSA differ by age and race (white vs. African American), and range from 0 to 6.5 ng/ml by some, while the American Cancer Society states that levels above 4 ng/ml are abnormal. Elevated PSAs occur commonly in patients with benign prostatic hypertrophy and prostatitis, making it difficult to distinguish the condition based on values alone. Diagnosis of prostate cancer is confirmed by transperianal or transrectal prostate biopsy.

SCREENING FOR PROSTATE CANCER—As with many other screening recommendations, controversy exists with regard to who should be screened for prostate cancer because clear-cut evidence on reductions in mortality are not yet available. The American Cancer Society recommends digital rectal examination (DRE) and prostate specific antigen (PSA)

be offered annually to men beginning at age 50 years with at least a 10-year life expectancy, and to younger men (45 years old) who are considered to be at high risk for prostate cancer development (eg, those with a strong family history, African Americans). If both tests are normal, no further diagnostic work-up is required. If either is abnormal, further work-up by transrectal ultrasound is indicated.[61] In contrast to this, the American College of Physicians recommends that instead of routinely screening all men, physicians should describe the potential benefits and harms of screening, diagnosis, and treatment, listen to the patient's concerns, and then decide on a course of therapy.[62]

The prognosis for prostate cancer depends on the extent of disease. A 5-year overall survival was estimated at 90% for whites and 75% for African Americans. Localized disease has survival rates as high as 100% in some studies, while more advanced disease has less favorable survival rates of around 30% for white males and slightly less for African American males. This is another example of a disease that is nearly always curable if detected early.

CHEMOPREVENTION—Evidence regarding chemoprevention against prostate cancer is currently limited. Selenium 200 mcg daily was associated with a significant (63%) reduction in the incidence of prostate cancer in 974 men with a history of either basal cell or squamous cell carcinoma. Thirteen prostate cancers occurred in the selenium-treated group and 35 cases in the placebo group. When results were restricted to patients with a PSA ≤4 ng/ml, a significant (74%) reduction was still found. There was no change in the incidence of the primary endpoint of basal and squamous cell carcinoma of the skin.[63] The benefit of finasteride in primary prevention of prostate cancer was shown in the Prostate Cancer Prevention Trial.[64] A total of 18,882 men ≥55 years of age with a normal digital rectal examination and a PSA ≤3ng/ml were randomized to treatment with finasteride 5 mg daily or placebo for 7 years. Prostate cancer was detected in 18.4% of men in the finasteride group, and in 24.4% in the placebo group, for a 24.8% reduction (95% CI, 18.6–30.6%, p <0.001). Of concern, however, was the fact that high-grade cancers were more common in the finasteride group, compared to placebo (37% vs. 22.2%; p < 0.001). Additionally, sexual side effects were more common in finasteride-treated men, while urinary symptoms were more common in placebo-treated men. While finasteride may prevent or delay the appearance of prostate cancer, the risk of side effects and increased risk of high-grade prostate cancer leaves the question regarding its place in therapy for routine primary prevention unanswered.

Cervical Cancer

INCIDENCE—The American Cancer Society estimates that in 2003 there will be 12,200 new cases of cervical cancer diagnosed, with 4,100 women dying from the disease. Risk factors for cervical cancer include having multiple sexual partners, age at first intercourse, exposure to human papilloma virus, and smoking. Cervical cytology, by way of Papanicolaou (Pap) smear screening can detect both precancerous lesions and presymptomatic invasive squamous cell cancer of the uterine cervix, both of which may be treated effectively. In the US between 1973 and 1998, age-adjusted incidence of invasive cervical cancer fell from 14.2 to 7.5 per 100,000 women, and mortality from 5.2 to 2.5 per 100,000 women.[65]

SCREENING—Although the efficacy of Pap smear screening has been well documented, the optimal interval at which repeat screening should be performed is not clear. Until recently, standard medical practice recommended annual screening of women who are sexually active, or age 21, whichever comes first, which some organizations still recommend.[66] Suggestions to increase the interval from 1 to 2 or even 3 years have been adopted by others.[67] Some guidelines recommend two or three annual smears to initiate screening, and if those are negative, intervals up to 3 years between smears may be appropriate.[68–70] The USPSTF recommends against routinely screening women over the age of 65 who are considered low risk as evidenced by previously negative Pap smears due to increased risks of potential harms and invasive testing compared to a low perceived benefit (Grade D recommendation), while the American Cancer Society recommends screening until age 70. Newer technologies, such as liquid-based cytology (eg, ThinPrep) and HPV DNA testing, may have improved sensitivity over conventional Pap smear screening, but are of a considerably higher cost and possibly lower specificity and there is insufficient evidence to support their use as the initial screening method (Grade I recommendation).

Skin Cancer

INCIDENCE—Non-melanoma skin cancer is the most common cancer in the United States, with an estimated annual incidence of more than 600,000 cases, and the majority of these cases occur as basal cell carcinoma. Squamous cell carcinomas represent 20% of non-melanoma skin cancers and are more significant because of their ability to metastasize. Non-melanoma skin cancers are very common, especially in the elderly. However, they cause limited morbidity and mortality. Melanoma is considered the deadliest of the skin cancers. The American Cancer Society estimates that in 2003 there will be 54,200 new cases of melanoma in this country, and about 7,600 people will die.[71]

Melanoma mortality ranks as the sixth leading cause of cancer deaths and is disproportionately higher in men and women over the age of 65 years. Roughly half of US deaths from melanoma occurred in men 50 years of age and older. While the incidence of melanoma is variable worldwide, it appears to be increasing universally. Once diagnosed, five-year survival rates are improving and are currently at 88%. The strongest predictor of prognosis is the thickness of the primary tumor. Melanomas less than 1 mm in depth have a small chance to metastasize.

RISK FACTORS—Patients with a strong genetic predisposition are at increased risk for the development of melanomas. Hereditary dysplastic nevus syndrome (HDNS) is characterized by a predisposition to develop dysplastic nevi and cutaneous melanoma. Heavy sun exposure increases one's chances of developing melanomas. It was previously thought that only exposure to UV-B rays increased one's risk of development, but now it is known that exposure to UV-A rays are also important. Melanoma incidence is related to the latitude and the intensity of the sun exposure. Patients at higher risk include those with fair hair color (red or blond) and light-colored eyes (blue, gray, or green), and who have a higher tendency to burn or hardly tan. Development of nonmelanoma skin cancers such as squamous cell and basal cell carcinomas is directly related to lifetime exposure to the sun. This association has not been found with melanomas, suggesting that the relationship to the development of melanoma is more complex than just related to total sun exposure. Patients with a history of severe sunburns appear to be at higher risk for development of melanoma than those with chronic sun exposure without sunburn. Intensive exposure to sunlight and subsequent sunburns is more hazardous during infancy and childhood than during adult life.

PRESENTATION—A normal mole is generally an evenly colored brown, tan, or black spot on the skin. It can be either flat or raised, and round or oval. Moles are generally less than 6 millimeters (1/4 inch) in diameter (about the width of a pencil eraser). A mole can be present at birth, or it can appear during childhood or young adulthood. Several moles can appear at the same time, especially on areas of the skin exposed to the sun. Once a mole has developed, it will usually stay the same size, shape, and color for many years. Moles may eventually fade away in older people. Most people have moles, and almost all moles are harmless. However, it is important to recognize changes in a mole that can suggest a melanoma may be developing.

The initial presentation of melanoma is often a lesion, which can be found anywhere on the body, but most commonly on the trunk of men and lower legs of women. Typically, melanomas are classified using the ABCD(E) system as follows: **A**symmetry; **B**order irregularity; **C**olor variability, **D**iameter greater than 6 mm, and **E**levation or enlargement. Once identified, suspicious lesions should be biopsied, and the diagnosis can be made.

SCREENING—There is some controversy as to the benefits of routine screening for melanoma. The USPSTF concludes that the evidence is insufficient to recommend for or against routinely screening for skin cancer using a total body skin examination for the early detection of cutaneous melanoma, basal cell cancer, or squamous cell skin cancer. Evidence is lacking that skin examination by clinicians is effective in reducing mortality or morbidity from skin cancer (Grade I recommendation). The American Cancer Society recommends skin examination as part of a cancer-related checkup every 3 years for people aged 20–40, and on a yearly basis for anyone over 40.[71] The American College of Preventive Medicine (ACPM) recommends that periodic total cutaneous examinations be performed, targeting populations at high risk for malignant melanoma, including individuals with family or personal history of skin cancer, predisposing phenotypic characteristics, and increased occupational or recreational exposure to sunlight, or clinical evidence of precursor lesions (eg, dysplastic or congenital nevi), but does not recommend routine screening.[72] However, the NIH Consensus Panel recommends screening for melanoma as part of routine primary care, while the American College of Obstetricians and Gynecologists recommends yearly, or as appropriate skin examination of women aged 13 and older based on risk factors.[73] There is agreement among the organizations of the need to educate the public to change behaviors that may decrease the risk of skin cancer, including sun avoidance, sun protection, and skin self-examination.

PREVENTIVE MEASURES—Sunscreens fall into two categories—thick paste-like ointments that block all solar rays, and light-absorbing sunscreens rated by "sun protective factor" (SPF). The SPF is a ratio of the number of minutes for treated *versus* untreated skin to redden with exposure to UV-B. An SPF of at least 15 is recommended and protects against 93% of UV-B. There is no scale for UV-A, which causes photoaging, or UV-C, the most carcinogenic ray that is blocked in the atmosphere by ozone. Sunscreens should be applied to all areas of skin exposed to the sun, particularly when the sunlight is strong. Advise patients to always follow directions when applying sunscreen, using a one-ounce, or palmful of sunscreen, 30 minutes before going outside, and to reapply it every 2 hours. Many sunscreens wear off with sweating and swimming and must be reapplied for maximum effectiveness. Patients should be advised to use sunscreen even on hazy days or days with light or broken cloud cover because the UV light still comes through.

The American College of Preventive Medicine finds insufficient evidence to recommend for or against sunscreen use. Nonmelanoma skin cancers may be reduced with regular, daily sunscreen use. There is insufficient evidence that chemical sunscreens protect against malignant melanoma, and they may, in fact, increase risk, due to increased sun exposure.[74]

Pharmacists can have a role in skin cancer prevention by encouraging patients to avoid sun exposure during peak times of the day (10 AM to 4 PM), wearing protective clothing, and wearing sunscreen with an SPF of at least 15 when outside. Special attention should be paid to those at highest risk, including children. Use of tanning beds, which contain mainly UV-A rays, should be discouraged, and patients should be educated about the risks of using them, including photoaging, ocular damage, and skin cancer. Pharmacists should be aware that fair-skinned men and women over age 65, patients with atypical moles, and those with more than 50 moles constitute known groups at substantially increased risk for melanoma. Clinicians should remain alert for suspicious skin lesions and help the patient seek appropriate medical care. A melanoma vaccine is currently in development.

DIABETES MELLITUS

INCIDENCE—Diabetes mellitus is a group of metabolic disorders characterized by hyperglycemia. It is associated with abnormalities in carbohydrate, fat, and protein metabolism, and long-term complications include microvascular complications such as retinopathy, nephropathy, and neuropathy, as well as macrovascular complications such as cardiovascular disease and stroke. Approximately 17 million people in the US, or 6.2% of the population, have diabetes. While an estimated 11.1 million have been diagnosed, unfortunately, 5.9 million people (or one-third) are unaware they have the disease.[75] Type-1 diabetes results from the body's failure to produce insulin, the hormone that "unlocks" the cells of the body, allowing glucose to enter and fuel them. It is estimated that 5–10% of Americans who are diagnosed with diabetes have Type-1 diabetes. Type-2 diabetes results from insulin resistance (a condition in which the body fails to properly use insulin), combined with relative insulin insufficiency. Approximately 90–95% (16 million) Americans have Type-2 diabetes. Gestational diabetes affects about 4% of all pregnant women, resulting in 135,000 cases in the United States each year.

DIABETES-RELATED COMPLICATIONS—Diabetes was the sixth leading cause of death listed on US death certificates in 1999, with heart disease as the leading cause of diabetes-related deaths. Adults with diabetes have heart disease death rates about 2 to 4 times higher than adults without diabetes. The risk for stroke is 2 to 4 times higher among people with diabetes. About 73% of adults with diabetes have blood pressure greater than or equal to 130/80 mmHg or use prescription medications for hypertension. Diabetes is the leading cause of new cases of blindness among adults 20–74 years old. Diabetes is the leading cause of treated end-stage renal disease, accounting for 43% of new cases. About 60–70% of people with diabetes have mild to severe forms of nervous system damage. More than 60% of non-traumatic lower-limb amputations in the United States occur among people with diabetes. Poorly controlled diabetes before conception and during the first trimester of pregnancy can cause major birth defects in 5–10% of pregnancies and spontaneous abortions in 15–20% of pregnancies. During the second and third trimesters, poorly controlled diabetes can result in excessively large babies, posing a risk to the mother and the child. People with diabetes are more susceptible to many other illnesses, and once they acquire these illnesses, often have a worse prognosis than people without diabetes. For example, they are more likely to die with pneumonia or influenza than people who do not have diabetes.

RISK FACTORS—Risk factors for Type-1 diabetes include autoimmune, genetic, and environmental factors. Risk factors for Type-2 diabetes are included in Table 126-6. Gestational diabetes occurs more frequently among African Americans, His-

Table 126-6. Risk Factors for Type 2 Diabetes

Age ≥45 years
Overweight (BMI >25 kg/m²)[a]
Family history of diabetes (parents or siblings with diabetes)
Physical inactivity
Race/ethnicity (African-Americans, Hispanic-Americans, Native Americans, Asian-Americans, and Pacific Islanders)
Previously identified IFG or IGT
History of GDM or delivery of a baby weighing >9 lbs
Hypertension (≥140/90 mmHg in adults)
HDL cholesterol ≤35 mg/dl and/or a triglyceride level ≥250 mg/dl
Polycystic ovary syndrome
History of vascular disease

[a] May not be correct for all ethnic groups.

Table 126-7. Categories of Glucose Tolerance

Fasting plasma glucose
  Normal: <110 mg/dl
  Impaired fasting glucose (IFG): ≥110 mg/dl and <126 mg/dl
  Diabetes mellitus: ≥126 mg/dl
Two-hour postload plasma glucose (oral glucose tolerance test)
  Normal: <140 mg/dl
  Impaired glucose tolerance (IGT): ≥140 mg/dl and <200 mg/dl
  Diabetes mellitus: ≥200 mg/dl

panic/Latino Americans, and Native Americans. It is also more common among obese women and women with a family history of diabetes.

DIAGNOSIS—The fasting plasma glucose test is the preferred way to diagnose diabetes. Normal fasting plasma glucose levels are less than 110 milligrams per deciliter (mg/dl). Fasting plasma glucose levels of more than 126 mg/dl on two or more tests on different days indicate diabetes. Sometimes, random blood samples may be used to test for diabetes when symptoms are present. A random blood glucose level of 200 mg/dl or higher indicates diabetes, but it must be reconfirmed on another day with a fasting plasma glucose or an oral glucose test. The oral glucose tolerance test begins with a fasting plasma glucose. After this test, 75 grams of glucose is ingested in a sweet-tasting liquid (100 grams for pregnant women). Blood samples are taken up to four times to measure blood glucose response. In a person without diabetes, the glucose levels rise and then fall quickly. In someone with diabetes, glucose levels rise higher than normal and fail to come back down as quickly.

People with glucose levels between normal and diabetic have impaired glucose tolerance (IGT). People with IGT do not have diabetes. Each year, only 1–5% of people whose test results show IGT actually develop diabetes. Upon retesting, as many as half of the people with IGT have normal oral glucose tolerance test results. Weight loss and exercise may help people with IGT return their glucose levels to normal. See Table 126-7 for Categories of Glucose Tolerance. A woman has gestational diabetes when she has any two of the following: a fasting plasma glucose of more than 95 mg/dl, a 1-hour glucose level of 180 mg/dl or higher, a 2-hour glucose level of 155 mg/dl or higher, or a 3-hour glucose level of 140 mg/dl or higher.

Once the diagnosis of diabetes is made, a glycosylated hemoglobin test (HbA1C) is used to monitor blood glucose control. Hemoglobin is the protein in red blood cells that carries oxygen. Glycosylated hemoglobin forms when glucose in the blood attaches to the hemoglobin. Because blood cells stay in circulation for 2–3 months, the glycosylated hemoglobin level is a good measure of a person's average blood glucose level over the previous 2–3 months. Although a high glycosylated hemoglobin level almost always means IGT or diabetes, people with IGT or diabetes can have normal levels. So this test is not used to diagnose diabetes. The goal for HbA1C is <7%.

COMMUNITY-BASED PROGRAMS—Although there is ample scientific evidence showing that certain risk factors predispose individuals to development of diabetes, there is insufficient evidence to conclude that community screening is a cost-effective approach to reduce the morbidity and mortality associated with diabetes in presumably healthy individuals. While community screening programs may provide a means to enhance public awareness of the seriousness of diabetes and its complications, other less costly approaches may be more appropriate, particularly because the potential risks are poorly defined. Thus, based on the lack of scientific evidence, community screening for diabetes, even in high-risk populations, is not recommended. The ADA Evidence Grading System for Clinical Practice Recommendations is listed in Table 126-8. Using this grading scale, and that of the USPSTF, The Recommendations for Screening for Diabetes for the two organizations are summarized in Table 126-9.

Table 126-8. ADA Evidence Grading System for Clinical Practice Recommendations

DESCRIPTION

A Clear evidence from well-conducted, generalizable, randomized controlled trials that are adequately powered, including:
Evidence from a well-conducted multicenter trial
Evidence from a meta-analysis that incorporated quality ratings in the analysis
Compelling nonexperimental evidence, ie, "all or none" rule developed by the Center for Evidence Based Medicine at Oxford*
Supportive evidence from well-conducted randomized controlled trials that are adequately powered, including:
Evidence from a well-conducted trial at one or more institutions
Evidence from a meta-analysis that incorporated quality ratings in the analysis

B Supportive evidence from well-conducted cohort studies, including:
Evidence from a well-conducted prospective cohort study or registry
Evidence from a well-conducted meta-analysis of cohort studies
Supportive evidence from a well-conducted case-control study

C Supportive evidence from poorly controlled or uncontrolled studies, including:
Evidence from randomized clinical trials with one or more major or three or more minor methodological flaws that could invalidate the results
Evidence from observational studies with high potential for bias (such as case series with comparison with historical controls)
Evidence from case series or case reports
Conflicting evidence with the weight of evidence supporting the recommendation

E Expert consensus or clinical experience

* Either all patients died before therapy and at least some survived with therapy or some patients died without therapy and none died with therapy.
Example: use of insulin in the treatment of diabetic ketoacidosis.
From *Diabetes Care* 26:S1–S2, 2003. Reprinted with permission from the American Diabetes Association.
Copyright © 2003 American Diabetes Association.

RECOMMENDATIONS FOR SCREENING OF COMPLICATIONS—Blood pressure should be measured at every routine diabetes visit. Patients found to have systolic blood pressure ≥130 mmHg or diastolic blood pressure ≥80 mmHg should have their blood pressures confirmed on a separate day. Orthostatic measurements of blood pressure should be performed to assess for the presence of autonomic neuropathy. Advise all patients not to smoke and include smoking cessation counseling and other forms of treatment as a routine component of diabetes care. In adult patients, test for lipid disorders at least annually and more often if needed to achieve goals. In adults with low-risk lipid values (LDL <100 mg/dl, HDL >60 mg/dl, triglycerides <150 mg/dl), repeat lipid assessments every 2 years. Perform an annual test for the presence of microalbuminuria in Type-1 diabetic patients with diabetes duration of ≥5 years and in all Type-2 diabetic patients, starting at diagnosis. Current recommendations for retinal screening include baseline screening in Type-1 diabetes when patients have had the disease for 5 years. Type-2 diabetics should have screening at the time of diagnosis. Subsequent examinations for Type-1 and Type-2 diabetic patients should be repeated annually by an ophthalmologist or optometrist who is knowledgeable and experienced in diagnosing the presence of diabetic retinopathy and is aware of its management. Examinations will be required more frequently if retinopathy is progressing. Annual foot ex-

aminations are recommended for all diabetics, and a visual inspection should be performed at each visit. Annual influenza vaccinations are recommended for all diabetics older than 6 months of age. They should also have one dose of pneumococcal vaccine, regardless of age. A one-time revaccination is recommended for individuals >64 years of age previously immunized when they were <65 years of age if the vaccine was administered >5 years ago. Other indications for repeat vaccination include nephritic syndrome, chronic renal disease, and other immunocompromised states, such as post-organ transplantation.

PREVENTION OF DIABETES—The hypothesis that Type-2 diabetes is preventable is supported by observational studies and two clinical trials on diet, exercise, or both in patients at high risk for the disease. In the Diabetes Prevention Program, a large prevention study of people at high-risk for Type-2 diabetes, 3,234 nondiabetic persons with elevated fasting and post-load plasma glucose were randomized to placebo, metformin 850 mg twice daily, or a life-style modification program with the goals of at least a 7-pound weight loss and at least 150 minutes of physical activity per week. The average follow-up period was 2.8 years. The incidence of diabetes was 11% for the placebo group, 7.8% for the metformin group, and 4.8% for the life-style group. The life-style intervention reduced the incidence by 58%, and metformin reduced the incidence by 31%, both of which were significant *versus* placebo. The life-style

Table 126-9. Recommendations for Screening for Diabetes

USPSTF:
The USPSTF concludes that the evidence is insufficient to recommend for or against routinely screening asymptomatic adults for Type 2 diabetes, impaired glucose tolerance, or impaired fasting glucose (Grade I).
The USPSTF recommends screening for Type 2 diabetes in adults with hypertension or hyperlipidemia (Grade B).

ADA:
Evaluation for type 2 diabetes should be performed within the health care setting. Patients, particularly those with a BMI ≥25 kg/m[2a], should be screened at 3-year intervals beginning at age 45; testing should be considered at an earlier age or be carried out more frequently in those who are overweight if additional diabetes risk factors are present. (Grade E)
The FPG is the recommended screening test. The OGTT may be necessary for the diagnosis of diabetes when the FPG is normal. The FPG is preferred for screenings because it is faster and easier to perform, more convenient, acceptable to patients, and less expensive. (Grade C)
Diagnostic testing should be performed in any clinical situation in which such testing is warranted; health care providers should not consider whether a person meets screening criteria in such cases. (Grade E)
Screening outside of health care settings, or community screening, has not been shown to be beneficial and may result in some harm; this type of screening is not recommended. (Grade E)

[a] May not be correct for all ethnic groups.
Data from US Preventive Services Task Force. Screening. Diabetes Mellitus, Adult Type II and American Diabetes Association. Screening for Type 2 Diabetes. *Diabetes Care* 2003; 26:S21.

group was significantly more effective than metformin in decreasing the incidence of diabetes. Treatment with metformin was most effective among younger, heavier people (those 25–40 years of age who were 50–80 pounds overweight) and less effective among older people and people who were not as overweight.[76]

The STOP-NIDDM Trial was a multi-centered, randomized, placebo-controlled trial comparing acarbose 100 mg three times daily to placebo in 1,429 patients with impaired glucose intolerance, with the primary endpoint being the development of diabetes using a yearly oral glucose tolerance test. A total of 221 of the 682 (32%) acarbose patients developed diabetes, whereas 285 of the 686 (42%) placebo patients developed diabetes after a mean follow-up period of 3.3 years, demonstrating a 25% risk reduction (p = 0.015). Weight loss contributed to the decreased risk of diabetes, but acarbose reduced the risk of diabetes even after adjustment for change in weight (p = 0.0063). The effects were consistent across age, sex, and body-mass index.[77] A follow-up of this study showed that treatment with acarbose in patients with impaired glucose tolerance decreased the risk of cardiovascular disease by 49% and hypertension by 34%.[78] There are no known methods to prevent Type-1 diabetes, although several clinical trials are currently in progress.

PREVENTION OF LONG-TERM COMPLICATIONS— Research studies in the United States and abroad have found that improved glycemic control benefits people with either Type-1 or Type-2 diabetes. In general, for every 1% reduction in HbA1C, the risk of developing microvascular diabetic complications (ie, eye, kidney, nerve disease) is reduced by 40%. Blood pressure control can reduce cardiovascular disease (ie, heart disease, stroke) by approximately 33% to 50% and can reduce microvascular disease (ie, eye, kidney, nerve disease) by approximately 33%. In general, for every 10 mmHg reduction in systolic blood pressure, the risk for any complication related to diabetes is reduced by 12%. Improved control of cholesterol and lipids (eg, HDL, LDL, and triglycerides) can reduce cardiovascular complications by 20–50%. Detection and treatment of diabetic eye disease with laser therapy can reduce the development of severe vision loss by an estimated 50–60%. Comprehensive foot care programs can reduce amputation rates by 45–85%. Detection and treatment of early diabetic kidney disease can reduce the development of kidney failure by 30–70%.

TREATMENT OF DIABETES—To survive, people with Type-1 diabetes must have insulin delivered by a pump or injections. Many people with Type-2 diabetes can control their blood glucose by following a careful diet and exercise program, losing excess weight, and taking oral medication. Many people with diabetes also need to take medications to control their cholesterol and blood pressure. Among adults with diagnosed diabetes, about 11% inject insulin and take oral medications, 22% inject insulin only, 49% take oral medications only, and 17% do not use either insulin or oral medications. As stated previously, the recommended goal for glycemic control is a HbA1C less than 7%. Once glycemic control has been reached, testing of HbA1C should continue every 3–4 months for those on insulin, and every 6–12 months for those not prescribed insulin. One quality assurance mechanism monitored through HEDIS is the percentage of patients with diabetes in a health plan who have HbA1C measured within the past year.

Blood pressure control is essential for prevention of complications of diabetes. Current goals of blood pressure are <130/80 mmHg for patients with diabetes. ACE inhibitors are the drugs of choice for hypertensive patients with microalbuminuria, proteinuria, or heart failure. Diabetics who smoke should be asked about their tobacco use at each visit, and should be strongly advised to quit. Diabetics who have known CHD should have annual lipid screening done, with treatment based on lipid profile. Aspirin is recommended for secondary prevention of CHD in patients with diabetes.

SELF-MANAGEMENT OF DIABETES—Diabetics should be encouraged to perform self-monitoring of blood glucose. It is useful to have values from all times of day, both fastings and nonfastings. Pharmacists in all settings can be involved in patient education of how to use blood glucose meters with the overall goal of preventing diabetes related complications.

ROLE OF THE PHARMACIST—Pharmacists can play an integral role in teaching patients about diabetes and its related complications. Reinforcement of the importance of management should be performed at every available opportunity, by educating patients on medications, proper control of blood sugars, control of hypo- and hyperglycemic symptoms, sick care management, vaccinations, and monitoring for signs of diabetes-related complications. Many pharmacists have gone on to become certified diabetes educators, and have practice sites in community pharmacies and ambulatory care clinics.

Pharmacists in ambulatory care are becoming more involved in the management of diabetes. Further discussion of this topic can be found in Chapter 121.

CARDIOVASCULAR DISEASE

INCIDENCE—Results from the AHA Heart and Stroke Statistical Update 2002 showed that 61.8 million Americans (1 in 5) have cardiovascular disease. Of these, 12.6 million have coronary artery disease, or CAD (angina, acute myocardial infarction). Each year, 1.1 million Americans will have a myocardial infarction and 600,000 will have a stroke. Death from cardiovascular diseases remains the number one killer of adult males and females.[79]

There are two screening strategies to reduce morbidity and mortality from CAD. The first involves screening for modifiable cardiac risk factors, such as hypertension, elevated serum cholesterol, cigarette smoking, physical inactivity, and diet. The second strategy is early detection of asymptomatic CAD. The principal tests for detecting asymptomatic CAD include resting and exercise ECGs, which can provide evidence of previous silent myocardial infarctions and silent or inducible myocardial ischemia. Thallium-201 scintigraphy, exercise echocardiography, and ambulatory ECG (Holter monitoring) are less commonly used for screening purposes.

Hypertension

INCIDENCE—It is estimated that more than 50 million Americans have hypertension. The etiology is usually unknown (primary or essential hypertension) and is rarely identified from a specific cause (secondary hypertension). Genetic factors have a role in the development of essential hypertension. Some secondary causes of hypertension include renal dysfunction, adrenal tumor, Cushing's syndrome, hyperthyroidism, pregnancy, and drug-induced causes. Drugs commonly associated with increased blood pressure include adrenocorticosteroids, amphetamines, oral decongestants, cyclosporine, non-steroidal anti-inflammatory drugs, and oral contraceptives. Herbal therapies such as ma huang, ginger, and licorice are associated with increases in blood pressure. If a secondary cause is found, treatment should target the underlying condition and any offending drugs should be discontinued.

RECOMMENDATIONS—Hypertension is a major risk factor for coronary heart disease, stroke, retinopathies, and renal dysfunction. The goals of treatment of hypertension are to limit target organ damage, thereby reducing the morbidity and mortality associated with the disease. Despite increases in awareness and treatment of hypertension, National Health and Nutrition Examination Survey III (NHANES III) results showed that only 29% of patients were controlled to below 140/90 mmHg. The Seventh Report of the Joint National Committee on Prevention, Detection, Evaluation, and Treatment of High Blood Pressure (JNC-7) was released in 2003.[80] These guidelines put a new emphasis on the importance of control of systolic blood pressure (BP) in persons older than 50 years, which has been recognized as a more important risk factor than diastolic BP. New to these guidelines is the classification of pre-hypertension, where systolic blood pressure is 120–139 mmHg, or diastolic blood pressure is 80–89 mmHg. Patients falling in this classification should have health-promoting life-style modifications to prevent CVD (discussed below). Target blood pressure for patients who do not have diabetes is <140/90 mmHg and is more aggressive at <130/80 mmHg in diabetics and patients with chronic kidney disease. Chronic kidney disease is defined by (1) reduced excretory function, with an estimated glomerular filtration rate of less than 60 ml/min per 1.73 m^2 (corresponding to a creatinine of >1.5 mg/dl in men or >1.3 mg/dl in women), or (2) the presence of albuminuria (>300 mg/day or 200 mg albumin per gram of creatinine). The classifications of Blood Pressure for Adults Aged 18 Years and Older is listed in Table 126-10.

LIFE-STYLE MODIFICATIONS—Non-drug therapies have been shown to lower BP, enhance antihypertensive drug efficacy, and decrease cardiovascular risk. Recommendations for non-drug therapy include weight reduction, with a goal of maintaining normal body weight; adopting a DASH eating plan (Dietary Approaches to Stop Hypertension), which includes having a diet rich in fruits, vegetables, and low-fat dairy products, with reduced saturated and total fat content; dietary sodium restriction to less than 100 mEq/L (2.4 g sodium or 6 g sodium chloride); physical activity, engaging in regular aerobic physical activity such as brisk walking at least 30 minutes per day on most days of the week; and moderation of alcohol consumption, limiting consumption to no more than 2 drinks per day in most men and no more than 1 drink per day in women and lighter-weight persons. All patients with hypertension and those in the prehypertensive category should be advised to make life-style modifications in addition to any pharmacologic treatment that they receive. Continued reinforcement and encouragement of these changes at health encounters may help patient adherence with these changes.

DRUG THERAPY CONSIDERATIONS—Some effective drug therapies for hypertension include β-blockers, diuretics, and ACE inhibitors. JNC-7 recommends thiazide-type diuretics as initial therapy for most patients with uncomplicated hypertension, either alone or in combination. There are certain high-risk conditions that are compelling indications for the initial use of other antihypertensive drug classes (ie, ACEI, ARBs, β-blockers, CCB). Many patients will require 2 or more antihypertensives to achieve their goal BP. If the BP is more than 20/10 mmHg above goal BP, consideration should be given to initiating two-drug therapy, one of which should be a thiazide. Support for the initiation of diuretics as first-line therapy for hypertension is based on the results of The Antihypertensive and Lipid-Lowering Treatment to Prevent Heart Attack Trial (ALLHAT), which showed that diuretics are as effective and safe as ACEI and calcium channel blockers.[81]

BLOOD PRESSURE MEASUREMENTS—Because hypertension is often termed a "silent killer," blood pressure measurements should be performed at each health care encounter. This includes visits to the doctor's office, but is increasingly becoming incorporated into regular pharmacy encounters as well, as pharmacists begin taking on an increasing role in disease state management. Further discussion of this topic can be found in the *Disease State Management* chapter of this text. Healthy People 2010 has a target to increase to 95% the percentage of Americans screened for hypertension within the past 2 years, and to increase to 50% the percentage of patients with controlled blood pressure, up from the 1990 rate of 27%.[1] Pharmacists in all settings should be aware of current recommendations for screening and management of hypertension so that they will be able to direct the care of patients appropriately. Additionally, pharmacists are involved in teaching patients how to check their blood pressures at home, as patients are taking on a larger role in their self-care.

Hyperlipidemia

RECOMMENDATIONS FOR TESTING AND MONITORING—Recommendations regarding the diagnosis and management of hyperlipidemia are provided by the National Cholesterol Education Program, which regularly updates these guidelines as new information becomes available. The current Adult Treatment Panel III recommendations state that all adults aged 20 years or older should obtain a fasting lipoprotein profile (total cholesterol, low density lipoprotein cholesterol (LDL-C), high density lipoprotein cholesterol (HDL-C), and triglycerides) once every 5 years.[82] If the testing opportunity is non-fasting, only the values for total cholesterol and HDL-C will be usable. In such a case, if total cholesterol is ≥200 mg/dl or high density lipoprotein is <40 mg/dl, a follow-up lipoprotein profile is needed for appropriate management based on LDL-C. The relationship between LDL-C levels and coronary heart disease risk is continuous over a broad range of LDL-C levels from

Table 126-10. Classification and Management of Blood Pressure for Adults Aged 18 Years or Older

| | | | | MANAGEMENT | | |
| | | | | | INITIAL DRUG THERAPY | |
BP CLASSIFICATION	SYSTOLIC BP, MMHG[a]		DIASTOLIC BP, MMHG[a]	LIFE-STYLE MODIFICATION	WITHOUT COMPELLING INDICATION	WITH COMPELLING INDICATION
Normal	<120	And	<80	Encourage		
Prehypertension	120–139	Or	80–89	Yes	No antihypertensive drug indicated	Drug(s) for the compelling indications[b]
Stage 1 Hypertension	140–159	Or	90–99	Yes	Thiazide-type diuretics for most; may consider ACEI, ARB, β-blocker, CCB, or combination	Drug(s) for the compeling indications Other antihypertensive drugs (diuretics, ACEI, ARB, β-blocker, CCB) as needed
Stage 2 Hypertension	≥160	Or	≥100	Yes	2-Drug combination for most (usually thiazide-type diuretic and ACEI or ARB or β-blocker or CCB)[c]	Drug(s) for the compelling indications Other antihypertensive drugs (diuretics, ACEI, ARB, β-blocker, CCB) as needed

[a] Treatment determined by highest BP category.
[b] Treat patients with chronic kidney disease or diabetes to BP goal of less than 130/80 mmHg.
[c] Initial combination therapy should be used cautiously in those at risk for orthostatic hypotension.
From Chobanian AV, Bakris GL, Black HR, et al. *JAMA* 2003; 289:2560.

Table 126-11. Adult Treatment Panel III Classification of Low-Density Lipoprotein (LDL-C), Total, and High Density Lipoprotein Cholesterol (HDL-C)

LDL-C (MG/DL)	
<100	Optimal
100–129	Near optimal/above optimal
130–159	Borderline high
160–189	High
≥190	Very High

TOTAL CHOLESTEROL (MG/DL)	
<200	Desirable
200–239	Borderline high
≥240	High

HDL-C (MG/DL)	
<40	Low
≥60	High

From NCEP III Guidelines, National Heart, Lung, and Blood Institute, National Institutes of Health.

low to high. Therefore, the Adult Treatment Panel III adopts the classification of LDL-C levels shown in Table 126-11; this also shows the classification of total and HDL-C levels.

The category of highest risk consists of coronary heart disease and coronary heart disease risk equivalents. The latter carry a risk for major coronary events equal to that of established coronary heart disease, ie, >20% per 10 years (more than 20 of 100 such individuals will develop coronary heart disease or have a recurrent coronary heart disease event within 10 years), based on large epidemiologic evidence from trials conducted in Framingham, Massachusetts. Coronary heart disease risk equivalents comprise: other clinical forms of atherosclerotic disease (peripheral arterial disease, abdominal aortic aneurysm, and symptomatic carotid artery disease), diabetes, and multiple risk factors that confer a 10-year risk for coronary heart disease >20%. Diabetes counts as a coronary heart disease risk equivalent because it confers a high risk of new coronary heart disease within 10 years, in part because of its frequent association with multiple risk factors. Furthermore, because persons with diabetes who experience an acute myocardial infarction (AMI) have an unusually high death rate either immediately or in the long term, a more intensive prevention strategy is warranted. Persons with coronary heart disease or coronary heart disease risk equivalents have the LDL-C goal (<100 mg/dl). The second category consists of persons with multiple (2+) risk factors in whom their 10-year risk score for coronary heart disease is ≤20%. Major Risk Factors that Modify LDL-C Goals are summarized in Table 126-12. Other life-habit risk factors for hyperlipidemia not included here are obesity, physical inactivity, and atherogenic diet; emerging risk factors consist of lipoprotein (a), homocysteine, prothrombotic, and proinflammatory factors, impaired fasting glucose, and evidence of subclinical atherosclerotic disease. These risk factors may be incorporated into future guidelines as more evidence develops.

The third category consists of persons having 0 to 1 risk factor; with few exceptions, persons in this category have a 10-year risk <10%. Their LDL-C goal is <160 mg/dl. See Table 126-13 for a summary of LDL goals.

EFFECTIVE TREATMENT—Effective drug treatment for hyperlipidemia consists of bile acid sequestrants, niacin, statins, fibric acid derivatives, and cholesterol uptake inhibitors. The largest amount of evidence on the benefits of lipid-lowering therapy is found with the statins. Results from large-scale trials of statin therapy have shown them to be effective for reducing total mortality, coronary mortality, revascularization rates, and stroke in patients with cardiovascular disease. For patients without underlying cardiovascular disease, statins are effective for reducing the incidence of first major coronary events, AMI, unstable angina, and revascularization proce-

dures. Despite adequate treatments available, results from NHANES III showed that only 28% of eligible patients are being treated with cholesterol-lowering therapy.[83] Recently, the results of the Heart Protection Study, a randomized trial of 20,536 adults with coronary disease, other occlusive arterial disease, or diabetes, to simvastatin 40 mg daily *versus* placebo, showed a significant reduction in all-cause mortality (12.9% vs. 14.7%; p = 0.0003).[84] Rates of AMI, stroke, and revascularization were all reduced by about one-third, when allowances were made for noncompliance. This is significant because it may demonstrate that statins produce a substantial reduction in major vascular events in patients without diagnosed coronary disease who have cerebrovascular disease, peripheral arterial disease, or diabetes, irrespective of the blood lipid concentrations when the treatment is initiated. These benefits were in addition to those of other treatments.

NON-DRUG TREATMENT—Therapeutic Life-Style Changes (TLC) are essential for reducing risk for CHD. Features recommended by the ATP III include reducing intake of saturated fat to <7% of total calories and reducing cholesterol to <200 mg/day; enhancing LDL lowering by addition of plant sterols/stanols (2 g/day) and soluble fiber (10–25 g/day); weight reduction; and increased physical activity. These life-style changes should be performed in addition to any pharmacologic treatment.

The National Committee for Quality Assurance (NCQA) has included cholesterol management after an acute event as one of its performance measures in the Health Plan Employer Data and Information Set (HEDIS). Managed care organizations will be scored on the percentage of their members screened for LDL-C and with LDL-C <130 mg/dl within 1 year after AMI, coronary artery bypass grafting (CABG), or percutaneous transluminal coronary angioplasty (PTCA).

Results from the Lipid Treatment Assessment Project (L-TAP) show that only 38% of patients are treated to their LDL-C target goals.[85] Reasons for this may include failure to initiate therapy, increase the dose, and monitor lipid levels; fear of combination of therapy; and non-adherence to drug therapy. Pharmacists in ambulatory clinics and community pharmacies have a role in helping to manage lipid-lowering therapy for their patients by providing interventions in treatment and monitoring and helping patients adhere to their medication regimens by educating them about their disease.

Aspirin and Anticoagulation

Decisions about aspirin therapy need to take into account the potential benefits compared to the risk for coronary heart disease, as well as the potential harms, such as gastrointestinal and intracranial bleeding. The optimum dose of aspirin for chemoprevention of heart disease is unknown. Primary and

Table 126-12. Major Risk Factors (Exclusive of LDL-C) that Modify LDL-C Goals[a]

Cigarette smoking
Hypertension (blood pressure >140/90 mmHg or on antihypertensive medication)
HDL-C <40 mg/dl[b]
Family history of premature CHD
    CHD in male first-degree relative < 55 years
    CHD in female first-degree relative <65 years
Age
    Men ≥ 45 years
    Women ≥ 55 years

[a] In Adult Treatment Panel III guidelines, diabetes is regarded as a coronary heart disease risk equivalent
[b] HDL-C ≥ 60 mg/dl counts as a "negative" risk factor; remove one risk factor from the total count
From ATP-III Guidelines, National Heart, Lung, and Blood Institute, National Institutes of Health.

Table 126-13. Risk Categories that Determine LDL-C Goals

RISK CATEGORY	LDL-C GOAL	LDL-C TO INITIATE TLC	LDL-C TO CONSIDER DRUG THERAPY
CHD or CHD risk equivalent 10-yr. risk >20%	<100 mg/dl	≥100 mg/dl	≥130 mg/dl 100–129 mg/dl: drug optional
2+ Risk Factors 10-yr. risk ≤20%	<130 mg/dl	≥130 mg/dl	10-yr. risk 10–20%: ≥130 mg/dl 10-yr. risk <10%: ≥160 mg/dl
0–1 Risk Factors	<160 mg/dl	≥160 mg/dl	≥190 mg/dl 160–189 mg/dl: drug optional

TLC = therapeutic life-style changes.
CHD = coronary heart disease.
From ATP-III Guidelines, National Heart, Lung, and Blood Institute, National Institutes of Health.

secondary prevention trials have demonstrated benefits with regimens ranging from 75 mg daily, 100 mg daily, to 325 mg every other day. Meta-analysis of 5 primary prevention trials showed that aspirin therapy reduced the risk for CHD by 28%. These trials also suggested that the rate of gastrointestinal bleeding is approximately 2–4 per 1,000 middle-aged individuals given aspirin for 5 years. Enteric-coated or buffered preparations do not clearly reduce the adverse gastrointestinal effects.

The USPSTF strongly recommends that clinicians discuss aspirin chemoprevention with adults who are at increased risk for coronary heart disease (Grade A recommendation). Men older than 40 years, postmenopausal women, and younger people with risk factors for coronary heart disease (hypertension, diabetes, or smoking) are at increased risk for heart disease and may wish to consider aspirin therapy. Currently, the American Diabetes Association recommends aspirin 75–325 mg daily in all adult patients with diabetes and macrovascular disease. The American College of Cardiology and the American Heart Association in 1997 recommended that daily aspirin therapy at 75–325 mg/day be considered for all patients at elevated risk of subsequent events due to a history of vascular disease. They stated that consideration should be given to a patient's particular cardiovascular risk profile, the demonstrated benefits of aspirin on reducing the risk of a first AMI, and aspirin side effects.[86] Aspirin is not generally recommended in patients less than 21 years of age due to the increased risk of Reye's syndrome.

ATRIAL FIBRILLATION AND STROKE—Atrial fibrillation (AF) is the most common sustained arrhythmia and is an important independent risk factor for stroke. It occurs in more than 2 million people in the United States. Prevalence increases after age 40 and rises rapidly after age 65. The median age of patients with AF is approximately 75 years. The rate of ischemic stroke in patients with AF and not treated with antithrombotic therapy averages about 5% per year. Management of AF is related to control of the arrhythmia itself, restoring and maintaining sinus rhythm, or ensuring that the ventricular rate is controlled, such as with the use of β-blockers, sotalol, or amiodarone, and prevention of thromboembolic complications. The risk for thromboembolism increases in patients with a prior stroke or TIA, history of hypertension, congestive heart failure, advanced age, diabetes mellitus, and coronary artery disease. Intensity of anticoagulation involves a balance between prevention of ischemic stroke and avoiding hemorrhagic complications. The American College of Chest Physicians recommendations for anticoagulation in patients with atrial fibrillation are found in Table 126-14. For patients that have suffered a recent stroke or TIA as a result of a cardioembolic event, oral anticoagulation (warfarin), with a target INR of 2.5 and range of 2–3 is recommended.[87] The Sixth ACCP Consensus Conference on Antithrombotic Therapy recommends that every patient who has experienced a noncardioembolic stroke or TIA and has no contraindications receive an antiplatelet agent regularly to reduce the risk of recurrent stroke or other vascular events. Aspirin, 50–325 mg daily, Aggrenox 200 mg twice daily,

or clopidogrel 75 mg daily are all acceptable options for initial therapy. Aggrenox is more effective than aspirin alone and may be more effective than clopidogrel, with a similarly favorable serious adverse effect profile.

CHRONIC STABLE ANGINA—For patients that have already suffered an AMI, therapy should be routinely prescribed in patients without contraindications. These agents should also be considered first-line therapy for patients with angina.

The ACC/AHA 2002 guidelines for the management of patients with chronic stable angina recommendations for drug therapy to prevent MI and death in asymptomatic patients are presented in Table 126-15. Recently, an important trial, called Heart Outcomes Prevention Evaluation (HOPE), showed that use of the ACE inhibitor ramipril (10 mg/d) reduced the incidence of cardiovascular death, AMI, and stroke in patients who were at high risk for, or had, vascular disease in the absence of heart failure.[88] The primary outcome in HOPE was a composite of cardiovascular death, MI, and stroke. However, the results of HOPE were so definitive that each of the components of the primary outcome by itself also showed statistical significance. Furthermore, only a small part of the benefit could be attributed to a reduction in blood pressure (22–23 mmHg). These results led to the addition of ACEI to these newest recommendations.

UNSTABLE ANGINA—The American College of Cardiology and the American Heart Association recommend that patients with unstable angina and non-ST-segment elevation MI be placed on aspirin as soon as possible after presentation of symptoms, and continued indefinitely. Recent changes to the guidelines were made to include the addition of clopidogrel, and the combination continued up to 9 months.[87a]

VITAMINS FOR CHD PREVENTION[87a]—Homocysteine is a sulfur-containing amino acid generated during the metabolism of methionine from dietary protein. Vitamins B6, vitamin B12, and folic acid are important cofactors in this metabolic process, and deficiencies of these vitamins may cause

Table 126.14. Recommendations for Patients with Atrial Fibrillation Considered for Chronic Oral Anticoagulation Therapy

AGE	MAJOR RISK FACTORS[a]	RECOMMENDATIONS FOR LONG-TERM THERAPY
<65	No major risk factors	Aspirin
<65	Major risk factors	Warfarin[b]
65 to 75	No major risk factors	Aspirin or Warfarin[b]
65 to 75	Major risk factors	Warfarin[b]
>75	All patients	Warfarin[b]

[a] Previous TIA, stroke, or systemic embolism; poor left ventricular function (moderate to severe left ventricular dysfunction on echocardiography, or recent CHF); hypertension
[b] Goal INR = 2.5; range = 2.0 − 3.0.
Data from Albers GW, Dalen JE, Laupacis A, et al Chest 2001;119:194S.

Table 126-15. Recommendations for Drug Therapy to Prevent MI and Death in Asymptomatic Patients

Class I
1. Aspirin in the absence of contraindication in patients with prior MI. *(Level of Evidence: A)*
2. Beta-blockers as initial therapy in the absence of contraindications in patients with prior MI. *(Level of Evidence: B)*
3. Lipid-lowering therapy in patients with documented CAD and LDL cholesterol greater than 130 mg/dL, with a target LDL of less than 100 mg/dL. *(Level of Evidence: A)*
4. ACE inhibitor in patients with CAD* who also have diabetes and/or left ventricular systolic dysfunction.*(Level of Evidence: A)*

Class IIa
1. Aspirin in the absence of contraindications in patients without prior MI. *(Level of Evidence: B)*
2. Beta-blockers as initial therapy in the absence of contraindications in patients without prior MI. *(Level of Evidence: C)*
3. Lipid-lowering therapy in patients with documented CAD and LDL cholesterol 100 to 129 mg/dL, with a target LDL of 100 mg/dL. *(Level of Evidence: C)*
4. ACE inhibitor in all patients with CAD[a] or other vascular disease. *(Level of Evidence: B)*

---

[a] Significant CAD by angiography or previous MI.
From Gibbons RJ, Abrams J, Chatterjee K, Daley J, Deedwania PC, et al. ACC/AHA 2002 guideline update for the management of patients with chronic stable angina—summary article: a report of the American College of Cardiology/American Heart Association Task Force on Practice Guidelines (Committee on the Management of Patients with Chronic Stable Angina). *Circulation* 2003;107:(1):149–58 © 2003 Lippincott Williams & Wilkins.

an elevated homocysteine level. Accumulation of homocysteine levels has been associated with increased risk of heart disease, and the American Heart Association has recognized homocysteine as a potential risk factor for vascular disease. Several studies have demonstrated an inverse relationship between folic acid consumption and homocysteine levels. In the Nurses Health Study, women who were in the lowest quintile of folic acid and vitamin B6 consumption had nearly a 2-fold increased risk of coronary heart disease.[89] For those patients that do not obtain adequate reduction of homocysteine through dietary measures, supplementation of folic acid, alone or with pyridoxine and cyanocobalamin, is useful. The optimal dose of folic acid is uncertain, but appears to be around 1 mg/day, causing a maximum reduction in homocysteine levels of about 25%. Currently there are no randomized controlled trials that demonstrate a benefit to homocysteine reduction on mortality, although trials are ongoing. As mentioned previously, in 2003, the USPSTF stated that the evidence was insufficient to recommend for or against the use of vitamins A, C, or E, multivitamins with folic acid, or antioxidant combinations for the prevention of cancer or cardiovascular disease (Grade I recommendation).[31] In 1999, A Statement from the American Heart Association was made stating that routine screening for hyperhomocysteinemia cannot be recommended at the present time due to lack of definitive evidence for clinical benefit. They stated that the clinician may consider determining levels in patients who are at "high risk" for hyperhomocysteinemia, including those with a strong family history of premature atherosclerosis, advanced age men and postmenopausal women, hypothyroidism, impaired kidney function, lupus, and those taking certain medications, such as niacin, theophylline, and methotrexate. A reasonable therapeutic goal for homocysteine levels in patients at risk for cardiovascular disease is <10 μmol/L.

The Heart Protection Study, a randomized trial of 20,536 patients with coronary disease, other occlusive arterial disease, or diabetes, compared placebo, vitamin E 600 mg, vitamin C 250 mg, and B-carotene 20 mg over a 5-year period. No significant differences were found in any of the outcome categories, including all-cause mortality, deaths from vascular or nonvascular causes, nonfatal myocardial infarction, or coronary death, nonfatal or fatal stroke, or coronary or noncoronary revascularization.[84] Results from the Physician's Health Study, a prospective cohort of 83,639 male physicians in the United States with no history of CVD or cancer, failed to show an association of self-selected supplement use (vitamin E, vitamin C, and multivitamins) on total CVD or CHD mortality after a mean follow-up period of 5.5 years.[90] These results suggest that while vitamin supplementation for patients at risk of coronary artery disease does not appear harmful, their use should not take the place of the proven therapies of aspirin, β-blockers, lipid-lowering therapy, and ACEI. There is currently no basis for recommending that patients take vitamin C or E supplements or other antioxidants for the express purpose of preventing or treating CAD.

HORMONE REPLACEMENT THERAPY

In 1993, the Postmenopausal Estrogen/Progestin Interventions (PEPI) Trial, which tested healthy postmenopausal women with no history of CHD with placebo, unopposed estrogen, or one of 3 combination estrogen/progestin combinations, had suggested that hormone replacement therapy may be beneficial for the prevention of coronary heart disease, due to benefits of increasing HDL-C, lowering LDL-C, and lowering fibrinogen levels.[91] Newer results from HERS suggested that patients with a history of CHD should not begin treatment with HRT for the prevention of AMI due to the increased incidence of CHD events during the first year of therapy, and a lack of overall benefit on the development of CHD and prevention of AMI.[92] In 2003, data was released from the Women's Health Initiative trial, comparing the safety and efficacy of estrogen plus progestin *versus* placebo for an average of 5.2 years in postmenopausal women without a history of CHD. Absolute excess risks per 10,000 person-years attributable to estrogen plus progestin were 7 more CHD events, 8 more strokes, 8 more PEs, and 8 more invasive breast cancers, while absolute risk reductions per 10,000 person-years were 6 fewer colorectal cancers and 5 fewer hip fractures. The absolute excess risk of events included in the global index was 19 per 10,000 person-years. Coronary heart disease mortality was not significantly increased. These results demonstrated that the risk-benefit profile of HRT is not a viable option for primary prevention of chronic diseases.[93] Also in 2002, the HERS II results (after an additional unblinded follow-up period of 2.7 years after the 4.1 year average duration of HERS) showed no significant decreases in rates of primary CHD events or secondary cardiovascular events among women treated with HRT compared with placebo.[94]

The results of the Women's Angiographic Vitamin and Estrogen (WAVE) trial found that postmenopausal women with heart disease who took hormone therapy either alone or in combination with high-dose antioxidant vitamins A and E did not have fewer heart attacks. Unlike the WHI study, WAVE participants did have prior evidence of heart disease, and although a much smaller study, adds to the evidence that HRT is not helpful in either preventing or treating heart disease.[95]

After evaluating evidence of both the benefits and harms of combined estrogen and progestin therapy, the U.S. Preventive Services Task concluded that HRT does not decrease and may increase the incidence of CHD. The effects of HRT on CHD mortality are less certain.[96] Further discussion of this topic will continue in the osteoporosis section.

OSTEOPOROSIS

DIAGNOSIS—Osteoporosis is a disease in which bones become fragile and more likely to break. In the absence of proper prevention or treatment, osteoporosis can progress painlessly until a bone breaks. Bone mineral density (BMD) reflects the balance between bone resorption and formation. Peak BMD is reached from age 20–35 for men and women. Osteoporosis occurs when resorption exceeds formation, with resultant bone loss. It is diagnosed based on T-scores, with the gold standard measurement being dual energy x-ray absorptimometry (DXA) of the hip and spine BMD. A T-score is the number of standard deviations away from the mean BMD for the young normal population. Patients with normal bone mass have T-scores greater than −1, osteopenia is a T-score of −1 to −2.5, and a T-score less than −2.5 is defined as osteoporosis by the World Health Organization. While skeletal x-rays demonstrate osteoporosis, they do not reliably do so until bone loss is greater than 20–30%. X-rays are of limited value in estimating bone mass.

SEQUELA—Annually, osteoporosis is responsible for 1.5 million fractures, typically in the hip, spine, and wrist. There are 10 million Americans (8 million women and 2 million men) with osteoporosis, and another 34 million Americans with low bone mass. Osteoporosis can be classified as postmenopausal (ie, due to estrogen deficiency), age-related, or secondary (ie, caused by certain medications such as steroids, or diseases such as malabsorption, cancer, or kidney or liver disease). Risk factors for osteoporotic fractures can be found in Table 126-16. Interested readers are referred to the National Osteoporosis Foundation website at www.nof.org.

Postmenopausal women who present with fractures should be evaluated by BMD testing to confirm the diagnosis and determine the disease severity. There is general consensus that measurement of BMD should be considered in patients receiving glucocorticoid therapy for 2 months or more and in patients with other conditions that place them at high risk for osteoporotic fractures. The USPSTF recommends that women age >65 years be screened routinely for osteoporosis and that patients with increased risk for osteoporotic fractures begin screening at age 60 (class B recommendation). No recommendation for or against routine screening is made for postmenopausal women younger than 60 or in women age 60–64 who are not at increased risk for osteoporotic fractures (class C recommendation).

Prevention of Osteoporosis

DIETARY APPROACHES—Adequate intake of calcium and vitamin D are important for the prevention of bone loss. It is recommended that adults age 19–50 years ingest 1000 mg of el-

Table 126-16. Risk Factors for Osteoporotic Fracture

Personal history of fracture after age 50
History of fracture in a first-degree relative
Current cigarette smoking
Low body weight (less than 127 pounds)
Estrogen deficiency (early menopause <45 years) or bilateral oviarectomy; prolonged premenopausal amenorrhea (>1 year)
Caucasian or Asian race
Advanced age
Female sex
Low calcium and vitamin D intake (lifelong)
Alcoholism
Impaired eyesight despite adequate correction
Recurrent falls
Inactive life-style
Poor health/frailty
Medications: glucocorticoids, excessive thyroid replacement, long-term heparin, lithium, chemotherapy

The four items in **bold** are key factors in determining risk of hip fracture independent of BMD.

emental calcium/day, while those older than 51 years should ingest 1,200 mg/day. Requirements of vitamin D increase as one gets older, going from 200 IU/day for those 19–50 years, to 400 IU/day for those 51–70 years, and 600 IU/day for those older than 71 years. Most Americans do not meet the requirements of calcium intake in their food, from sources such as milk, yogurt, cheese, ice cream, and fortified orange juice. Often these patients need to obtain calcium from one of the many available supplements. Between 5 and 15 minutes of casual daily exposure (without sunscreen) to sunlight is usually sufficient to produce one's vitamin D requirements. Patients who spend little time outdoors, or keep their bodies covered, with minimal sun exposure, need to find other sources. Dietary sources of vitamin D include fatty fish, dairy products, and liver. Milk is fortified with 400 IU/quart of vitamin D. Patients that have limited sun exposure and do not drink milk may need to use vitamin D supplements. Caffeine has been inconsistently associated with decreased bone mass. Teenage girls who drink a lot of carbonated beverages have an increased risk of fractures, in part due to decreased consumption of milk and therefore calcium, in favor of carbonated beverages.[97] Other possible dietary factors that influence risk for fractures include low vitamin K intake, low protein intake, and excessive vitamin A intake.

LIFE-STYLE MODIFICATIONS—Smoking increases one's risk of hip fracture and is associated with decreasing BMD. It is recommended to avoid tobacco use to help improve BMD. Alcohol use has been associated with a low BMD and an increased risk of fractures, but this has not been consistently demonstrated. Moderation of alcohol consumption is recommended despite this lack of evidence, especially when one considers the increased risk of falls associated with excessive alcohol intake. Physical activity for patients with osteoporosis should be encouraged. Regular exercise, especially resistance and high-impact activities, contributes to the development of high peak bone mass and may reduce the risk of falls in older individuals.

PHARMACOLOGIC INTERVENTIONS FOR PREVENTION AND TREATMENT—The National Osteoporosis Foundation suggests initiating therapy to reduce fracture risk in women with T-scores below −2 in the absence of risk factors and in women with T-scores below −1.5 if other risk factors are present. In patients over 70 with multiple risk factors, treatment may be warranted without BMD testing, due to the high risk of osteoporosis. The U.S. Food and Drug Administration has approved hormone replacement therapy, bisphosphonates, raloxifene, and calcitonin for osteoporosis prevention or treatment, or both. Bisphosphonates inhibit osteoclast-mediated bone resorption and have been shown to increase BMD at the spine and hip in a dose-dependent manner, as demonstrated from RCT. They consistently reduce the risk of vertebral fractures by 30–50%. Alendronate and risedronate reduce the risk of nonvertebral fractures in women with osteoporosis and adults with glucocorticoid-induced osteoporosis. Raloxifene, a selective estrogen-receptor modulator (SERM), has been shown to reduce the risk of vertebral fracture by 36% in large clinical trials. Salmon calcitonin has demonstrated increases in BMD at the lumbar spine, but exhibits less clear effects on the hip. RCT have demonstrated that estrogen therapy increases bone density and decreases bone resorption. The greatest benefit from HRT occurs during the first years following menopause. Unopposed estrogen should not be used in patients with an intact uterus due to the increased risk of endometrial cancer. Women with a history of unexplained vaginal bleeding, breast cancer, or thromboembolism should not take HRT. Results from the HERS II trial showed that treatment for 6.8 years with HRT in older women with coronary disease doubled the rate of venous thromboembolism and increased the risk of biliary tract surgery by 1.44 (95% CI, 1.10–1.90, p = 0.01).[98]

A meta-analysis of 22 trials of estrogen reported a 27% reduction in nonvertebral fractures (RR 0.73, 95% CI, 0.56–0.94).[99] The HERS trial found no reduction in hip, wrist, vertebral, or total fractures with hormone therapy (relative hazard for total fractures 1.04; 95% CI, 0.87–1.25).[92] The WHI trial found significant reductions in total fracture risk (RH 0.76; 95% CI, 0.63–0.92) in healthy women taking combined estrogen and progestin. The USPSTF concluded that there was good evidence that HRT increases bone mineral density and fair to good evidence that it reduces fractures.

In response to the release of the HERS and WHI trials, the North American Menopause Society (NAMS) updated its recommendations regarding the use of HRT. It recommends that alternatives should be considered to HRT due to the associated risks, weighing the risks and benefits of each, despite the fact that HRT is approved for treatment of postmenopausal osteoporosis. Additionally, the NAMS feels that lower than standard doses of HRT and estrogen therapy should be considered, based on the Women's Health, Osteoporosis, Progestin, Estrogen (HOPE) Trial.[100] This trial showed equivalent menopausal symptom relief and preservation of bone density without an increase in endometrial hyperplasia with lower doses of HRT.[101] Some authors feel that women using postmenopausal HRT for reasons other than control of menopausal symptoms should be advised to stop.[102] Other authors feel that long-term HRT should be offered to women at high risk of osteoporosis or with established osteoporosis.[103] Clinicians should carefully consider each individual patient's risks and benefits before deciding on the use of HRT for osteoporosis, as the debate will likely continue for some time. Pharmacists can help patients in their decision-making process by keeping informed about new research that is conducted and recommendations that are released.

ALZHEIMER'S DISEASE

INCIDENCE—Alzheimer's disease (AD) is the most common form of dementia among older people. It involves the parts of the brain that control thought, memory, and language.

AD usually presents in patients over age 65, but can occur as early as age 40. AD affects 3% of individuals aged 65–74 years, doubling every 5 years beyond age 65. Women are affected twice as often as men. Genetic factors for early onset cases (40–64 years) include chromosomal changes, including 1, 14, and 21. Late-onset AD (≥65 years) is primarily influenced by the apolipoprotein E (apo E) genotype, with the Apo E4 allele serving as a risk factor for development of AD. Environmental risk factors for AD include alcohol abuse, stroke, repeated or severe head trauma, lower levels of education, and small head circumference.

CHEMOPREVENTION—In a study looking at dietary intake of antioxidants in 5,395 people, higher intakes of vitamins C and E, flavinoids (found in cranberries, green and black tea, and peas and beans), and β-carotene were associated with reduced risk for Alzheimer's disease among smokers. In nonsmokers, vitamins C and E showed a potential protective effect, with risks reduced by 34% and 43%, respectively, among those with greatest intake of the vitamins, compared with those consuming the lowest amounts.[104]

In a second study, only dietary vitamin E was linked to reduced risk of Alzheimer's disease in a study of vitamin C, vitamin E, and β-carotene. Among 815 community-dwelling residents who were 65 years or older, increased intake of vitamin E from foods only was associated with a 70% lower risk of the disease. The protective effect was found only among people with a certain genotype, those without the apolipoprotein E4 gene.[105] It had been suggested from prospective and case-control trials that women taking estrogen lowered their risk of developing AD by 50%. However, results from the Women's Health Initiative Memory Study (WHIMS) contradict this. It randomly assigned 4,894 postmenopausal women aged 65 years or older and free of probable dementia at baseline to estrogen plus progestin or placebo. After an average of 4 years of follow up, 61 women were diagnosed as having dementia, 40/2229 women in the hormone group and 21/2303 in the placebo group.[106] In a re-

lated study, also from WHIMS, global cognitive function did not improve when compared with placebo. Most women on the hormone treatment did not experience clinically relevant adverse effects on cognitive function; however, a small increased risk of clinically meaningful cognitive decline occurred in the hormone group.[107] One possible explanation of this increased risk may be due to an increase in vascular-related dementia. This adds further fuel to the increased risks of HRT and that they should not be used for preventive measures.

THYROID DISEASE

DIAGNOSIS—Thyrotoxicosis, or hyperthyroidism, occurs when tissues are exposed to increased levels of thyroxine (T4), triiodothyronine (T3), or both. It occurs more commonly in women, with an annual incidence of 3 per 1,000. Hypothyroidism occurs in 1–2% of women, and 0.2% of men, with the incidence increasing with increasing age. Primary hypothyroidism (due to thyroid gland dysfunction) is the most common, with typical causes being Hashimoto's disease, or iatrogenic (due to exposure to radiation or thyroid surgery). Secondary hypothyroidism occurs as a result of diseases of the pituitary or hypothalamus. Common symptoms in hypothyroidism include fatigue, weight gain, cold intolerance, bradycardia, constipation, depression, and skin and hair dryness. Hyperthyroidism, on the other hand, presents with symptoms nearly opposite, including weight loss, heat intolerance, tachycardias or palpitations, hyperdefecation, nervousness, and hyperhydrosis.

SCREENING—The preferred method of screening for thyroid dysfunction is the thyroid stimulating hormone (TSH) test. A free thyroxine test should be done when the TSH level is undetectable or is ≥10 mU/L. Patients who have an undetectable TSH level and an elevated free thyroxine level have overt hyperthyroidism. Patients who have a TSH level >10 mU/L and a low free thyroxine level have overt hypothyroidism. Patients exhibiting either of these conditions are likely to benefit from appropriate treatment. In the case of hypothyroidism, treatment typically includes long-term thyroid replacement therapy. For thyrotoxicosis, treatment consists of propylthiouracil or methimazole, iodine-containing compounds, radioactive iodine, and surgery. Subclinical hypothyroidism occurs when patients exhibit slightly elevated TSH, but normal T4 and T3, and may or may not have symptoms. Currently there is insufficient evidence to recommend for or against treatment of subclinical hypothyroidism.

The exact age to begin screening for thyroid disease is debatable. The American College of Physicians and the American Society of Internal Medicine recommend screening women older than 50 years of age for unsuspected but symptomatic thyroid disease. However, the American Thyroid Association recommends that adults begin screening at the age of 35 years, and repeat screening every 5 years thereafter. The most compelling evidence is in women, but may be justified in men in the context of the periodic health exam.[108–111]

DEPRESSION

INCIDENCE—Approximately 20% of the US population is affected by mental illness during a given year. Of all mental illnesses, depression is the most common disorder, affecting more than 19 million adults in the United States. Major depression is the leading cause of disability and is the cause of more than two-thirds of suicides each year. Depression is associated with other medical conditions, such as heart disease, cancer, and diabetes as well as anxiety and eating disorders. Depression also has been associated with alcohol and illicit drug abuse. An estimated 8 million persons aged 15–54 years had coexisting mental and substance abuse disorders in 2002. The total estimated direct and indirect cost of mental illness in the United States in 1996 was $150 billion.

FACTORS CAUSING DEPRESSION—Certain drug therapy is associated with depression, eg, antihypertensive medications, (including reserpine, methyldopa, clonidine, hydralazine, and propranolol), and hormone therapy (oral contraceptives or corticosteroids). It has been suggested that isotretinoin may cause depression, although the mechanism is unknown. If a medication is suspected of causing psychiatric symptoms, patients should discuss their symptoms with their health provider so that the medication can be discontinued and an alternative therapy selected, if appropriate. Or the patient can begin treatment with a pharmacologic agent for depression.

Adults and older adults have the highest rates of depression. Major depression affects approximately twice as many women as men. Women who are poor, on welfare, less educated, and unemployed are more likely to experience depression. In addition, depression rates are higher among older adults with coexisting medical conditions. For example, 12% of older persons hospitalized for problems such as hip fracture or heart disease are diagnosed with depression. Rates of depression for older persons in nursing homes range from 15% to 25%. Seasonal affective disorder occurs commonly during winter months in patients who have reduced exposure to sunlight, possibly due to a disturbance in the natural circadian rhythm, which is sometimes treated with bright-light therapy.

DIAGNOSIS—The diagnosis of depression is made by qualified health professionals using the criteria in the Diagnostic and Statistical Manual of Mental Disorders, 4th edition (DSM-IV). Several screening tests are administered before a diagnosis is made, using various questionnaires such as the Beck Depression Inventory and the Zung Self-Rating Depression Scale (SDS). Questionnaires are also available for children.

TREATMENT—Depression is treatable. Available medications and psychological treatments, alone or in combination, can help 80% of those with depression. With adequate treatment, future episodes of depression can be prevented or reduced in severity. Treatment for depression can enable people to return to satisfactory, functioning lives. The Healthy People 2010 Leading Health Indicator is to increase the number of adults with recognized depression who receive treatment, from 23% in 1997, to 50% in 2010.[1] The USPSTF recommends screening adults for depression in clinical practices that have systems in place to assure accurate diagnosis, effective treatment, and followup (B recommendation). They found good evidence that screening improves the accurate identification of depressed patients in primary care settings and that treatment of depressed adults identified in primary care settings decreases clinical morbidity. However, the USPSTF concludes the evidence is insufficient to recommend for or against routine screening of children or adolescents for depression (I recommendation).[111a]

Pharmacists can be effective at identifying patients with risk factors for depression and observing patient behavior for signs of depression that may suggest the need for further evaluation and treatment. By identifying potential modifiable causes and encouraging patients to seek medical treatment, pharmacists can have an impact in reducing the morbidity and mortality of this disease.

RESPONSIBLE SEXUAL BEHAVIOR

Unintended pregnancies and sexually transmitted diseases (STDs), including infection with the human immunodeficiency virus that causes AIDS, can result from unprotected sexual behaviors. Abstinence is the only method of complete protection. If used correctly and consistently, condoms can help prevent both unintended pregnancy and STDs.

In 1999, 85% of adolescents abstained from sexual intercourse or used condoms if they were sexually active. In 1995, 23% of sexually active women reported that their partners used condoms. The Healthy People 2010 goal is to increase from 85% to 95% the number of adolescents in grades 9–12 who are not sexually active, or sexually active and use condoms, and to increase from 23% to 50% the number of sexually active unmarried women, age 18–44, who report condom use by their partners.[1]

Sexually transmitted diseases are common in the United States, with an estimated 15 million new cases of STDs reported each year. Almost 4 million of the new cases of STDs each year occur in adolescents. Women generally suffer more serious STD complications than men, including pelvic inflammatory disease, ectopic pregnancy, infertility, chronic pelvic pain, and cervical cancer from the human papilloma virus. African Americans and Hispanics have higher rates of STDs than whites. The total cost of the most common STDs and their complications is conservatively estimated at $17 billion annually in the US.

Human Immunodeficiency Virus (HIV)

INCIDENCE—Worldwide, 42 million people are estimated to be living with HIV/AIDS. Of these, 38.6 million are adults, 19.2 million are women, and 3.2 million are children under 15. Currently the Centers for Disease Control and Prevention (CDC) estimates that between 800,000 and 900,000 Americans are living with HIV. It is estimated that approximately 40,000 new HIV infections occur in the US each year. Also, the number of people living with AIDS is increasing, as effective new drug therapies are keeping HIV-infected persons healthy longer and dramatically reducing the death rate.

GUIDELINES FOR PREVENTION AND TREATMENT—The CDC regularly provides updates to their guidelines for the prevention and diagnosis of STDs, including HIV. These guidelines recommend testing for HIV in all patients who seek evaluation and treatment of STDs.[112] This should be performed in addition to counseling (both pretest and posttest counseling). HIV infection is diagnosed by tests for antibodies to HIV-1 and HIV-2. Antibody testing starts with a sensitive screening test such as enzyme-linked immunosorbent assay (ELISA). Reactive screening tests must be confirmed by a supplemental test, such as Western Blot, or by immunofluorescence assay. If confirmed by a supplemental test, a positive test indicates that a person is infected with HIV and is capable of transmitting the virus to others. HIV is detectable within 3 months after infection in at least 95% of patients. Although a negative antibody test result indicates that a patient is not infected, it cannot exclude the possibility of a recent infection. Patients with a new diagnosis should receive initial behavioral and psychosocial counseling on-site. Providers should be alert for medical or psychosocial conditions that might require immediate attention. Patients should be encouraged to notify their partners (including sex partners and needle sharing) and to refer them for counseling and testing.

Needlestick injuries are fairly common occurrences in the health care field. Guidelines are available from the US Public Health Service for the management of occupational exposure to HIV, HBV, and HCV and recommendations for postexposure prophylaxis. These guidelines are updated regularly, and include such topics as implementation of a bloodborne pathogen policy, treatment recommendations after needlestick injuries, monitoring for adverse effects, and laboratory testing to monitor for seroconversion.[113]

Health care providers should be knowledgeable about the symptoms and signs of acute retroviral syndrome, characterized by fever, malaise, lymphadenopathy, and skin rash, which occur within the first few weeks after HIV infection. This presentation occurs before the antibody test results become positive. Current guidelines suggest that patients with recently acquired HIV infection might benefit from antiretroviral drugs and may be candidates for clinical drug trials. Anyone with an acute HIV infection should be referred immediately to an appropriate HIV care provider. Once detection has been confirmed, this should prompt education efforts to reduce the spread of HIV to others. This includes counseling patients on high-risk behaviors (eg, sharing of intravenous needles, unprotected sexual behavior).

Chlamydia Infection

INCIDENCE—*Chlamydia trachomatis* is the most common sexually transmitted bacterial pathogen in the US, with an estimated 3 million new infections occurring each year. Chlamydia infections are a major cause of urethritis, cervicitis, and pelvic inflammatory disease (PID) in women and are an important cause of infertility, chronic pelvic pain, and ectopic pregnancy, as well as adverse pregnancy outcomes. Chlamydial infections are associated with a 3–5-fold increased risk for acquiring HIV. Perinatal transmission to infants can cause neonatal conjunctivitis and pneumonia. In men, chlamydia infections cause urethritis, epididymitis, and chronic complications including prostatitis and possibly infertility. Most women and men are asymptomatic, and chlamydia is readily transmitted between sexual partners, allowing for important reservoirs for new infections.

RISK FACTORS—Women and adolescents through age 20 years are at highest risk for chlamydia infection, but most reported data indicate that infection is prevalent among women aged 20–25. Age is the most important risk factor. Other patient characteristics associated with a higher prevalence of infection include being unmarried, African-American race, having a prior history of sexually transmitted disease, having new or multiple sex partners, having had cervical ectopy, and using barrier contraceptives inconsistently. Individual risk depends on the number of risk markers and local prevalence of the disease.

DIAGNOSIS—Clinicians should be observant for signs that suggest chlamydial infection during pelvic examinations of asymptomatic women (eg, discharge, cervical erythema, cervical friability). Positive results are found by cultures of endocervical or urethral samples, or by nucleic acid amplification tests. In patients where chlamydia is detected, assessment for the presence of other sexually transmitted diseases should occur.

TREATMENT—Effective and low-cost treatment of chlamydia is available, including a 7-day course of doxycycline or a single dose of azithromycin, with alternatives including erythromycin, ofloxacin, or levofloxacin. To minimize further transmission of infection, patients treated for chlamydia should be instructed to abstain from sexual intercourse for 7 days after single-dose therapy or until completion of a 7-day regimen. To minimize the risk for reinfection, patients should also be instructed to abstain from sexual intercourse until all of their sex partners are treated.

SCREENING—Repeat infection confers an elevated risk of pelvic inflammatory disease (PID) and other complications when compared with initial infection. Therefore, recently infected women are a high priority for repeat testing for chlamydia. For these reasons, clinicians and health care agencies should consider advising all women with chlamydial infection to be rescreened 3–4 months after treatment. Partners of infected individuals should be tested and treated if infected, or treated presumptively. Clinicians should be sensitive to the potential impact of diagnosing a sexually transmitted disease on a couple.

Screening for chlamydia is a HEDIS measure. The indicator is the proportion of sexually active women between the ages of 15 and 25 who were screened for chlamydia infection at least annually. The USPSTF strongly recommends that routine screening for chlamydial infection occur in all sexually active women aged ≤25 years, and other asymptomatic women at increased risk for infection (A Recommendation). The USPSTF found good evidence that screening for high risk women decreases the incidence of PID. For asymptomatic low-risk women in the general population, the USPSTF makes no recommendation for or against screening routinely for chlamy-

dial infection (C Recommendation), and concludes that the evidence is insufficient to recommend for or against routinely screening asymptomatic men for chlamydial infection (I Recommendation).[114]

Gonococcal Infections

INCIDENCE—In the United States, an estimated 600,000 new *Neisseria gonorrhoeae* infections occur each year. Most infections in men produce symptoms that cause them to seek treatment soon enough to prevent serious events, but this may not be soon enough to prevent spreading to others. Among women, many infections do not produce recognizable symptoms until complications (eg, PID) have occurred. Both symptomatic and asymptomatic cases of PID can result in tubal scarring that can lead to infertility or ectopic pregnancy. Because gonococcal infections among women often are asymptomatic, an important component of gonorrhea control in the US continues to be the screening of women at high risk for STDs. Recommended antibiotics for the treatment of gonococcal infections include single oral dose cefixime, ciprofloxacin, ofloxacin, or levofloxacin, or single dose intramuscular ceftriaxone.

DUAL THERAPY FOR GONOCOCCAL AND CHLAMYDIAL INFECTIONS—Patients infected with *N. gonorrhoeae* often are coinfected with *C. trachomatis*; leading to the recommendation that patients treated for gonococcal infection also be treated routinely with a regimen effective against uncomplicated genital chlamydia infection. Routine dual therapy without testing for chlamydia can be cost-effective for populations in which chlamydial infection accompanies 10–30% of gonococcal infections, because the cost of therapy for chlamydia (eg, $0.50–$1.50 for doxycycline) is less than the cost of testing. Some specialists believe that the routine use of dual therapy has resulted in substantial decreases in the prevalence of chlamydial infection.

PRENATAL CARE

STD SCREENING—Recommended screening tests for sexually transmitted diseases in all pregnant women include the following at the first prenatal visit: HIV, syphilis, and hepatitis B surface antigen. Screening for *Chlamydia trachomatis* is recommended in the first trimester and again in the third trimester in patients at increased risk for chlamydia, such as those with more than one sex partner. Screening for *Neisseria gonorrhoeae* and hepatitis C antibodies should be performed at the first prenatal visit in women at risk or those living in areas where the prevalence is high. Screening for bacterial vaginosis may be conducted at the first visit in asymptomatic patients at high risk for preterm labor, but routine testing in all patients is not currently supported.[115]

The USPSTF recommends that clinicians routinely screen all asymptomatic pregnant women aged 25 years and younger and others at increased risk for infection for chlamydial infection (B recommendation). The USPSTF makes no recommendation for or against routine screening of asymptomatic, low-risk pregnant women aged 26 years and older for chlamydial infection. (C recommendation).

FOLIC ACID DURING PREGNANCY—The American Academy of Pediatrics and the United States Public Health Service recommend that all women of childbearing age who are capable of becoming pregnant should consume 400 micrograms (0.4 milligrams) of folic acid daily to prevent neural tube defects. Because there is a high rate of unplanned pregnancies in the US, efforts at promoting food fortification to provide all women a daily intake of 400 mcg of folic acid is encouraged. In the absence of optimal fortification, women should consume 400 mcg of folic acid daily in addition to eating a healthy diet. Currently, the most convenient, inexpensive, and direct way to meet the recommended dosage is by taking a multivitamin containing 400 mcg of folic acid, but efforts to increase the availability of folic acid-only supplements should be encouraged for women who prefer not to take multivitamins. Because the risk for neural tube defects is not totally eliminated by folic acid use, routine prenatal screening for neural tube defects is still advisable.[116]

Women with a history of a previous pregnancy resulting in a fetus with a neural tube defect should be advised of the results of the British Medical Research Council (MRC) Vitamin Study.[117] This randomized trial compared one of four high-dose folic acid supplementation groups: 4 mg folic acid; multivitamin plus 4 mg folic acid; neither the multivitamin nor folic acid; or multivitamin without folic acid. Outcome information was available for 1,195 pregnancies. Folic acid supplementation was associated with a 71% reduction in the recurrence of neural tube defects. Multivitamins alone were not effective and did not contribute to additional benefit. During times in which a pregnancy is not planned, these high-risk women should consume 400 mcg of folic acid per day. However, they should be offered treatment with 4 mg of folic acid per day starting 1 month before the time they plan to become pregnant and throughout the first 3 months of pregnancy, unless contraindicated. Women should be advised not to attempt to achieve the 4 mg daily dosage of folic acid by taking multivitamins, which typically contain 400 mcg folic acid each, because of the possibility of ingesting harmful levels of other vitamins, such as vitamin A. It should be noted that 4 mg of folic acid did not prevent all neural tube defects in the Medical Research Council study. Therefore, high-risk patients should be cautioned that folic acid supplementation does not preclude the need for counseling or consideration of prenatal testing for neural tube defects.

No intervention or observational studies address prevention for other high-risk persons. Women with a close relative (eg, sibling, niece, or nephew) who had a neural tube defect (risk is approximately 0.3–1.0%), women with Type-1 diabetes mellitus (risk is approximately 1%), women with seizure disorders being treated with valproic acid or carbamazepine (risk is approximately 1%), and women or their partners who have a neural tube defect (risk may be 2–3%) and are planning a pregnancy should discuss with their physician the risk for an affected child and the advantages and disadvantages of increasing their daily periconceptional folic acid intake to 4 mg.

UNIVERSAL PRECAUTIONS

Universal precautions include the use of gloves, gowns, masks, and protective eyewear to prevent parenteral, mucous-membrane, and non-intact skin exposures to pathogens carried in the blood, such as HIV, hepatitis B, hepatitis C, and others. These pathogens may be carried in blood and body fluids such as semen, vaginal secretions, and cerebrospinal, pleural, synovial, peritoneal, pericardial, and amniotic fluids. When exposure to body fluids is expected, wearing proper protection is essential to infection control. Hand-washing is the single most important method to prevent transmission of infectious agents. Hands should be washed before and after each contact with patients, body fluids, and contaminated or soiled materials; between dirty and clean procedures on the same patient, after removing gloves; before and after performing invasive procedures; after using the rest room; and whenever hands are visibly soiled. The U.S. Occupational Safety and Health Administration (OSHA) and U.S. National Institute for Occupational Safety and Health (NIOSH) guidelines require use of special masks—National Institute for Occupational Safety and Health certified N-95 respirators—when caring for patients with contagious tuberculosis; use of these masks requires education to ensure proper fit.

HEPATITIS B—Immunization with hepatitis B vaccine is mandated by Occupational Safety and Health Administration for all persons whose job might involve exposure to blood or blood-containing body fluids. This consists of a series of three IM injections into the deltoid over a period of several months. Individual doses of the vaccine are dependent on the actual product used. If patients extend the interval beyond what is recommended, the series can simply be completed, with no need to start over. Response to the vaccine can be measured by anti-Hepatitis B levels (anti-HB) at 1–6 months after completion of the vaccine series. Vaccine nonresponders or inadequate responders may need subsequent booster vaccinations.

TUBERCULOSIS—In adults, screening for tuberculosis using the Mantoux skin test should be performed before health care employment to ensure active tuberculosis is detected early and treated. A test is considered positive in a healthy health care professional if an area of induration of at least 10 mm is detected. For persons with underlying conditions or known household exposure to tuberculosis, 5 mm of induration is considered positive. If the Mantoux test is positive, the employee is referred for evaluation and appropriate management. The frequency of repeat skin testing for purified protein derivative (PPD)-negative employees should be based on the risk of exposure to people with active tuberculosis. Risk factors will vary from employee to employee; yearly testing should be considered in practices where there has been a high rate of documented tuberculosis or skin test conversion among families and patients or among health care professionals. Consultation with local health departments is useful to determine the prevalence of tuberculosis in the local area.[118]

IMMUNIZATIONS

CHILDREN—Prior to the practice of routine immunizations, vaccine-preventable diseases were a major cause of morbidity and mortality in children. Recommendations for childhood vaccinations are approved by the Advisory Committee on Immunization Practices, the American Academy of Pediatrics, and the American Academy of Family Physicians.[119] Each year these guidelines are updated, and the recommendations from 2003 include vaccination against the following diseases: hepatitis B, diphtheria, tetanus, pertussis, Haemophilus influenzae Type b (Hib), polio, measles, mumps, rubella, varicella, and Streptococcus pneumoniae. For children in high-risk states and for certain high-risk groups, vaccination against hepatitis A is recommended. Annual vaccination against influenza is recommended for high-risk factors (eg, asthma, cardiac disease, sickle cell, HIV, diabetes) household members of persons in high-risk groups, anyone wishing to obtain immunity. The recommended vaccination schedule for adolescents and children can be found at www.cdc.gov.

The Healthy People 2010 Leading Health Indicator for vaccinations is to increase the proportion of young children who receive all vaccines that have been recommended for universal administration from 73% in 1998 to 80% by 2010: four or more doses of diphtheria/tetanus/acellular pertussis (DTaP) vaccine, three or more doses of polio vaccine, one or more dose of measles/mumps/rubella (MMR) vaccine, three or more doses of Hib vaccine, and three or more doses of hepatitis B (Hep B) vaccine.[1]

Barriers to childhood vaccinations include fear of adverse reactions, the unfounded fear that in fact vaccinations cause autism, concern over the long-term impact of the vaccine on the immune system, fear of multiple injections at one time, areas of poor access to vaccines, and lack of motivation by the parents. Strategies for high immunization levels include proper record keeping, recommendation to get the vaccine and reinforcement to return for follow up, reminder and recall messages to patients and providers, reduction of missed opportunities, and reduction in barriers to immunization within the practice.

ADOLESCENTS AND ADULTS—In 2002, the Advisory Committee on Immunization Practices approved for the first time a schedule for the routine vaccination of persons aged ≥19 years. It has been accepted by the American Academy of Family Physicians and the American College of Obstetrics and Gynecology, and will be updated annually.[120] This includes recommendations on tetanus, diphtheria, influenza, pneumococcus,

Table 126-17. Topics for Preventive Counseling in Adults and Adolescents

Tobacco use
Substance abuse, driving under impairment
Nutrition
Optimal body weight
Exercise
Injury prevention: seat belts, gun safety, household safety
Dental hygiene
Responsible sexual behavior
Stress management
Sleep hygiene

Hep B, Hep A, measles, mumps, rubella, varicella, and meningococcus. Included in these recommendations are recommendations for adults with certain medical conditions, such as pregnancy, diabetes, heart disease, renal failure, asplenia, and immunocompromised conditions such as HIV and malignancies. Both schedules can be found at www.cdc.gov.

Boosters against tetanus and diphtheria are recommended every 10 years by the CDC, while the American College of Physicians Task Force on Adult Immunizations supports giving a single Td booster at age 50 years for persons who have completed the full pediatric series.

Immunizations against influenza and pneumococcal disease can prevent serious illness and death. Pneumonia and influenza deaths together constitute the sixth leading cause of death in the United States. Influenza causes an average of 110,000 hospitalizations and 20,000 deaths annually; pneumococcal disease causes 10,000–14,000 deaths annually. For adults, the Leading Health Indicator is to increase the proportion of noninstitutionalized adults who are vaccinated annually against influenza (from 64% in 1998 to 90% by 2010) and ever vaccinated against pneumococcal disease (from 46% in 1998 to 90% by 2010). Coverage levels for immunizations in adults are not as high as those achieved in children, yet the health effects may be just as great. Low-income and minority children and adults are at greater risk for under-immunization. Barriers to adult immunization include not knowing immunizations are needed, misconceptions about vaccines, fear of injections, and lack of recommendations from healthcare providers.

TRAVEL IMMUNIZATIONS—With improvements in transportation, the ability to travel to far off lands is increasingly easy. With this comes the need for vaccination against infectious diseases found in these countries. Recommendations for travel vaccines are regularly updated by the CDC web site www.cdc.gov/travel. Pharmacists can assist patients planning to travel abroad to consult an international travel clinic weeks before their expected travel to identify the risks of the particular trip. Travel recommendations will be made based off of the length of the trip, previous travel to the area, the exact location of travel, the expected activities on the trip, the type of accommodations, the food supply that is available, and the health of the traveler. Additional information will be provided about food and water precautions to avoid diarrhea and insect-borne illnesses. Providing information such as boiling drinking water, avoiding uncooked foods or undercooked foods will help prevent the chances of diarrhea. Efforts to minimize getting bitten by mosquitoes, such as wearing light-colored clothing, minimizing perfume, avoiding outdoor activities at dusk or night time, and using insect repellants containing DEET, should be recommended. Vaccinations that may be recommended during international travel include malaria, typhoid fever, yellow fever, cholera, rabies, hepatitis A, hepatitis B, meningococcal, or Japanese encephalitis virus. Specific instructions for each vaccine with regard to timing and number of doses, and potential adverse effects should be reviewed with the patient.

OPPORTUNITIES FOR PHARMACISTS—Pharmacists in all settings are increasing their visibility as a provider of immunizations, as many states, ie, 30 in 2003, now allow pharmacists to administer vaccines within their practice. Training

programs such as those offered by the American Pharmacists Association have aided pharmacists in vaccination administration techniques, and have provided them with information to help develop this area of practice in their setting. Further, schools/colleges of pharmacy are now including immunization training in the curricula. The addition of pharmacists as vaccine providers can help achieve overall immunization goals, which are to reduce the morbidity and mortality associated with vaccine-preventable illnesses, and to improve overall vaccination rates.

SUMMARY AND CONCLUSIONS

Preventive care is a challenge that should be undertaken by health care providers in all practice settings. A summary of recommended preventive counseling topics can be found in Table 126-17. Pharmacists should "seize the moment" to educate and counsel patients regarding these various topics when the opportunities arise. Throughout this chapter, disease screening guidelines have been discussed. A current summary of recommendations can be found in Table 126-18. Several medications have evidence to their usefulness for chemoprevention of various diseases. A list of such medications and the diseases

Table 126-18. Preventive Services Screening Recommendations

MEN AND WOMEN

Colorectal cancer
Average risk: Age 50 and older
Higher risk: Age 40 and older
Depression
Screen adults in practices equipped to diagnose, treat, and follow up
Diabetes
Routine community screening is not recommended
Hyperlipidemia
Fasting lipid profile, starting at age 20 years, every 5 years
Hypertension
Screening at each health encounter
Influenza vaccine
Annually, beginning age 65, earlier in higher risk patients
Pneumococcal vaccine
At least one beginning at age 65
Skin Cancer
Variable; routine screening not recommended by some, while others recommend
Tetanus Booster
Every 10 years
Thyroid screening
Age 35 and every 5 years

MEN

Prostate cancer
PSA and DRE: Average risk: men age 50 and older; age 45 and older for higher risk

WOMEN

Breast cancer
Annual mammography: Age 50 and older; some recommend beginning at age 35
Breast self-examination: monthly, beginning at age 20
Clinical breast examination: At least every 2 years
Cervical cancer
Annual Pap smears: Begin when sexually active or age 21 (whichever comes first)
Chlamydia
Annually in sexually active women age 25 and older and others at increased risk
Pregnant women age 25 and younger and others at increased risk
Osteoporosis
Average risk: Age 65
Higher risk: Age 60

Table 126-19. Drugs with Evidence to Prevent Disease Development

DISEASE PREVENTED	DRUG OR DRUG CLASS
Alzheimer's	Vitamin E
Breast Cancer	Tamoxifen and Raloxifene
CAD	Aspirin, Statins
Colorectal cancer	Aspirin, COX-II Inhibitors
Prostate cancer	Finasteride, Selenium
Diabetes	Metformin and Acarbose
DVT	Heparin, LMWHs, Warfarin
Nephropathy	ACEI and ARBs
Osteoporosis	Bisphosphonates, Statins
Hip fracture	Calcium/Vitamin D, Bisphosphonates
NSAID-induced ulcer	Misoprostil and PPIs
Stress ulcer	H2 blockers, Sucralfate
CVD	ACEI
Exercise-induced asthma	Salmeterol, Formoterol
Pregnancy	OCPs
Emergency contraception	Mifepristone, Levonorgestrel
Neural tube defects	Folic acid
Vaccine-preventable illnesses	Vaccinations
Tobacco-related illnesses	Smoking cessation aids
Vitamin deficiencies	Various vitamins
Various infections (SBE, HIV, TB)	Various antibiotics, antivirals

they help prevent can be found in Table 126-19. Opportunities for pharmacists to help bring about awareness of recommendations and risk factors for the development of disease, and educate patients as to the benefits of prevention, occur daily. It is important for the pharmacists on the "front line" to have a general understanding of current recommendations for screening and disease prevention so that they can provide appropriate counseling and care for their patients.

REFERENCES

1. Healthy People 2010 Leading Health Indicators. www.healthypeople.gov/LHI. Accessed February 28, 2003.
2. Kuczmarski RJ, Carroll MD, Flegal KM, et al. *Obes Res* 1997; 5:542.
3. Kelley DE. *Nutr Clin Care* 1998; 1:38.
4. Rexrode KM, Manson JE, Hennkens CH. *Curr Opin Cardiol* 1996; 11:490.
5. Liu GC, Coulston AM, Lardinois CK, et al. *Arch Intern Med* 1985; 145:665.
6. Reaven GM, Staff of the Palo Alto GRECC Aging Study Unit. *J Am Geriatr Soc* 1985; 33:93.
7. Wing RR, Koeske R, Epstein LH, et al. *Arch Intern Med* 1987; 147:1749.
8. DeSimone G, Mancini G, Turco M, et al. *J Endocrinol Invest* 1992; 15:339.
9. Reisin E, Abel R, Modan M, et al. *N Engl J Med* 1978; 289:1.
10. Wood P, Stefanick M, Dreon D, et al. *N Engl J Med* 1988; 319:1173.
11. Svenson O, Hassager C, Christiansen C. *Am J Med* 1993; 95:131.
12. Wood P, Stefanick M, Williams P, et al. *N Engl J Med* 1991; 325:461.
13. Task Force on Community Preventive Services. *Am J Prev Med* 2002; 22(4 Suppl):67.
14. Potter JD. *J Natl Cancer Inst* 1999; 91:916.
15. Giovannucci E, Ascherio A, Rimm EB, et al. *Ann Intern Med* 1995; 12:327.
16. Kroser JA, Bachwich DR, Lichtenstein GR. *Hematol Oncol Clin North Am* 1997; 11:547.
17. Folsom AR, Kushi LH, Anderson KE, et al. *Arch Intern Med* 2000; 160:2117.\
18. Chao A, Thun MJ, Jacobs EJ, et al. *J Natl Cancer Inst* 2000; 92:1888.
19. Colorectal screening: www.cdc.gov/mmwr/preview/mmwrhtml/mm5009a2.htm.
20. Winawer S, Fletcher R, Rex D, et al. *Gastroenterology* 2003; 124:544.
21. U.S. Preventive Services Task Force. *Ann Intern Med* 2002; 137:129.
22. Rex DK, Johnson DA, Lieberman DA, et al. *Am J Gastroenterol* 2000; 95:868.
23. Smith RA, von Eschenbach AC, Wender R, et al. *CA Cancer J Clin* 2001; 51:38.
24. Giovannucci E, Egan KM, Hunter DJ, et al. *N Engl J Med* 1995; 333:609.
25. Smalley W, Ray WA, Daugherty, J, et al. *Arch Intern Med* 1999;159:161–66.
26. Sturmer T, Glynn RJ, Lee IM, et al. *Ann Intern Med* 1998; 128:713.
27. Sandler RS, Halabi S, Baron JA, et al. *N Engl J Med* 2003; 348:883.
28. Baron JA, Cole BF, Sandler RS, et al. *N Engl J Med* 2003; 348:891.
29. Giovannucci E, Stampfer MJ, Colditz GA, et al. *Ann Intern Med* 1998; 129:517.
30. Janne PA, Mayer RJ. *N Engl J Med* 2000; 342:1960.
31. U.S. Preventive Services Task Force. *Ann Intern Med* 2003; 139:51.
32. Baron JA, Beach M, Mandel JS, et al. *N Engl J Med* 1999; 340:101.
33. Wu K, Willett WC, Fuchs CS, et al. *J Natl Cancer Inst* 2002; 94:437.
34. Jacobs EJ, Connell CJ, Patel AV, et al. *Cancer Epidemiol Biomarkers Prev* 2001; 10:17.
35. Feuer EJ, Wun LM, Boring CC, et al. *J Natl Cancer Inst* 1993; 85:892.
36. Colditz GA, Stampfer MJ, Willett WC. *JAMA* 1990; 264:2648.
37. Abeloff MD, Lichter AS, Niederhuber JE, et al. In Clinical Oncology. New York: Churchill Livingstone, 1995; pp 1617–1714.
38. Weber BL, Abel JK, Brody LC, et al. *Cancer* 1994; 74:1013.
39. Struewing JP, Hartge P, Wacholder S, et al. *N Engl J Med* 1997; 336:1401.
40. Easton DF, Bishop DT, Ford D, Crockford GP, Breast Cancer Linkage Consortium. *Am J Hum Genet* 1993; 52:678.
41. Ford D, Easton DF, Bishop DT, Narod SA, Goldgar DE, Breast Cancer Linkage Consortium. *Lancet* 1994; 343:692.
42. Wooster R, Neuhausen SL, Mangion J, et al. *Science* 1994; 265:2088.
43. Easton DF, Ford D, Bishop DT. *Am J Hum Genet* 1995; 56:265.
44. Howe GR. *Cancer* 1994; 74:1078.
45. Leitch AM, Dodd GD, Costanza M, et al. *CA Cancer J Clin* 1997; 47:150.
46. Guide to Clinical Preventive Sciences, 2nd ed. Report of the US Preventive Services Task Force. Washington, DC, Department of Health and Human Services, 1995.
47. Fletcher SW, Black W, Harris R, et al. *J Natl Cancer Inst* 1993; 85:1644.
48. Kopans DB, Halpern E, Hulka CA. *Cancer* 1994; 74:1196.
49. National Institutes of Health Consensus Development Panel. *J Natl Cancer Inst* 1997; 89:1015.
50. Miller AB, To T, Baines CJ, et al. *Ann Intern Med* 2002; 137:305.
51. Huguley CM, Brown RL, Greenberg RS, et al. *Cancer* 1988; 62:1389.
52. Thomas DB, Gao DL, Ray RM, et al. *J Natl Cancer Inst* 2002; 94:1445.
53. Nolvadex (tamoxifen citrate) [package insert]. Wilmington, DE: AstraZeneca Pharmaceuticals, May 2002.
54. Gail MH, Brinton LA, Byar DP, et al. *J Natl Cancer Inst* 1989;81:1879.
55. Fisher B, Costantino JP, Wickerham DL, et al. *J Natl Cancer Inst* 1998; 90:1371.
56. Veronesi U, Maisonneuve P, Costa A, et al. *Lancet* 1998; 352:93.
57. Powles T, Eeles R, Ashley S, et al. *Lancet* 1998; 352:98.
58. IBIS investigators. *Lancet* 2002; 360(9336):817.
59. Jubelirer SJ, Crowell EB Jr. *W V Med J* 2000; 96(6):602.
60. Cersosimo RJ. *Ann Pharmacother* 2003; 37:268.
61. American Cancer Society. Prostate-Cancer Screening Guidelines, Cancer Facts and Figures 1997. Atlanta, GA: American Cancer Society, 1997.
62. American College of Physicians. *Ann Intern Med* 1997;126:480–484.
63. Clark LC, Dalkin B, Krongrad A, et al. *Br J Urol* 1998; 81:730.
64. Thompson IM, Goodman PJ, Tangen CM, et al. *N Engl J Med* 2003; 349:213.
65. Ries LAG, Eisner MP, Kosary CL, et al. SEER cancer statistics review, 1973–1998 http://seer.cancer.gov/csr/1973_1998/index.html, National Cancer Institute, Bethesda, Maryland (2001). Accessed July 25, 2003.
66. American Medical Association. *Arch Pediatr Adolesc Med* 1997; 151:123.
67. U.S. Preventive Services Task Force, Guide to clinical preventive services. Baltimore: Williams & Wilkins, 1996; 105–117.
68. American Academy of Family Physicians. *1997–1998 AAFP reference manual—clinical policies.* Kansas City, MO: American Academy of Family Physicians, 1997.
69. American College of Obstetricians and Gynecologists *Routine cancer screening. ACOG committee opinion number 185.* Washington, DC: American College of Obstetricians and Gynecologists, 1997.
70. Hawkes AP, Kronenberger CB, MacKenzie TD, et al. *Am J Prev Med* 1996; 12:342.
71. American Cancer Society. Melanoma: detection and symptoms. Available at http://www3.cancer.org/cancerinfo.
72. Ferrini RL, Perlman M, Hill L. *Am J Prev Med* 1998; 14:80.

73. NIH Consensus Development Panel on Early Melanoma. *JAMA* 1992; 268:1314.

74. Ferrini RL, American College of Preventive Medicine, Perlman M, Hill L. *Am J Prev Med* 1998;14:83.

75. American Diabetes Association. Diabetes Facts and Figures. Available at http://www.diabetes.org/main/info/facts/facts.jsp. Accessed July 25, 2003.

76. Diabetes Prevention Program Research Group. *N Engl J Med* 2002; 346:393.

77. Chiasson JL, Josse RG, Gomis R, et al. *Lancet* 2002; 359:2072.

78. Chiasson JL, Josse RG, Gomis R, et al. *JAMA* 2003; 290:486.

79. American Heart Association. *2002 Heart and Stroke Statistical Update*. Dallas: American Heart Association, 2001.

80. Chobanian AV, Bakris GL, Black HR, et al. *JAMA* 2003; 289:2560.

81. The ALLHAT Officers and Coordinators, for the ALLHAT Collaborative Research Group. *JAMA* 2002; 288:2981.

82. Expert Panel on Detection, Evaluation, and Treatment of High Blood Cholesterol in Adults. *JAMA* 2001; 285:2486.

83. Hoerger TJ, Bala MV, Bray JW, et al. *Am J Cardiol* 1998; 82:61.

84. Heart Protection Study Collaborative Group. *Lancet* 2002; 360:7.

85. Pearson TA, Laurora I, Chu H, et al. *Arch Intern Med* 2000; 160:459.

86. Hennekens CH, Dyken ML, Fuster V. *Circulation* 1997; 96:2751.

87. Albers GW, Dalen JE, Laupacis A, et al. *Chest* 2001; 119:1945.

87a. Braunwald E, et al. ACC/AHA 2002 guideline update for the management of patients with unstable angina and non-ST-segment elevation myocardial infarction: a report of the American College of Cardiology/American Heart Association Task Force on Practice Guidelines (Committee on the Management of Patients with Unstable Angina): 2002. www.acc.org/clinical/guidelines/unstable/unstable.pdf.

88. Yusuf S, Sleight P, Pogue J, et al. *N Engl J Med* 2000; 342:145.

89. Rimm EB, Willett WC, Hu FB, et al. *JAMA* 1998; 279:359.

90. Muntwyler J, Hennekens CH, Manson JE, et al. *Arch Intern Med* 2002; 162:1472.

91. Writing Group for the PEPI Trial. Effects of Estrogen or Estrogen/Progestin Regimens on Heart Disease Risk Factors in Postmenopausal Women. The Postmenopausal Estrogen/Progestin Interventions (PEPI) Trial. *JAMA* 1995; 273:199.

92. Hulley S, Grady D, Bush T, et al. *JAMA* 1998; 280:605.

93. Rossouw JE, Anderson GL, Prentice RL. Writing Group for the Women's Health Initiative Investigators, et al. *JAMA* 2002; 288:321.

94. Grady D, Herrington D, Bittner V, et al. *JAMA* 2002; 288:49.

95. Waters DD, Alderman EL, Hsia J, et al. *JAMA* 2002; 288:2432.

96. U.S. Preventive Services Task Force. *Hormone Replacement Therapy for Primary Prevention of Chronic Conditions: Recommendations and Rationale*. October 2002. Agency for Healthcare Research and Quality, Rockville, MD. http://www.ahrq.gov/clinic/3rduspstf/hrt/hrtrr.htm

97. Wyshak G. *Arch Pediatr Adolesc Med* 2000; 154:610.

98. Hulley S, Furburg C, Barrett-Connor E, et al. *JAMA* 2002; 288:58.

99. Torgerson D, Bell-Syer S. *JAMA* 2001; 285:2891.

100. Lindsay R, Gallagher JC, Kleerekoper M, et al. *JAMA* 2002; 287:2668.

101. NAMS Report. *Menopause* 2003; 10:6.

102. Solomon CG, Dluhy RG. *N Engl J Med* 2003; 348:579.

103. Rymer J, Wilson R, Ballard K. *BMJ* 2003; 326:322.

104. Engelhart MJ, Geerlings MI, Ruitenberg A, et al. *JAMA* 2002; 287:3223.

105. Morris MC, Evans DA, Bienias JL, et al. *JAMA* 2002; 287:3230.

106. Shumaker SA, Legault C, Rapp SR, et al. *JAMA* 2003; 289:2651.

107. Rapp SR, Espeland MA, Shumaker SA, et al. *JAMA* 2003; 289:2663.

108. American Thyroid Association. *Arch Intern Med* 2000; 160:1573.

109. American College of Physicians/American Society of Internal Medicine. *Ann Intern Med* 1998;129:141.

110. *Nelson HD, Helfand M, Woolf SH, et al. Ann Intern Med* 2002; 137:529.

111. American College of Physicians/American Society of Internal Medicine. *Ann Intern Med* 1998;129:144.

111a. U.S. Preventive Services Task Force. *Screening for Depression: Recommendations and Rationale*. May 2002. Agency for Healthcare Research and Quality, Rockville, MD. http://www.ahrq.gov/clinic/3rduspstf/depressrr.htm

112. Centers for Disease Control and Prevention. *MMWR Rec Rep* 2002; May 10;51(RR-6):2–5.

113. Updated US Public Health Service Guidelines for the Management of Occupational Exposures to HBV, HCV, and HIV and Recommendations for Postexposure Prophylaxis. *MMWR Rec Rep* 2001; 50(RR-11):1–52.

114. Berg AO. *Am J Prev Med* 2001; 20(3S):90–94.

115. Centers for Disease Control and Prevention. *MMWR Rec Rep* 2002; May 10;51(RR-6):5–7.

116. American Academy of Pediatrics. *Pediatrics* 1999; 104(2 Pt 1):325.

117. MRC Vitamin Study Research Group. *Lancet* 1991; 338:131.

118. American Academy of Pediatrics. The American Occupational Safety and Health Administration (OSHA). *Pediatrics* 2000; 105:1361.

119. The Centers of Disease Control and Prevention. *JAMA* 2002; 13:287(6):707.

120. Adult recommendations: Recommended adult immunization schedule—United States, 2002–2003. MMWR Morb Mortal Wkly Rep 2002; Oct 11;51(40):904.

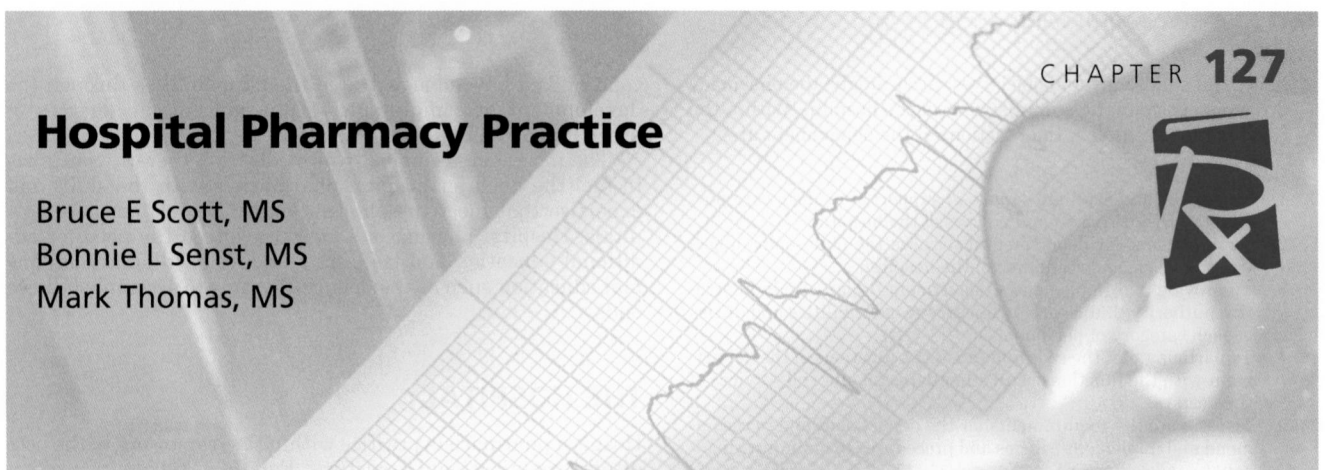

CHAPTER 127

Hospital Pharmacy Practice

Bruce E Scott, MS

Bonnie L Senst, MS

Mark Thomas, MS

The practice of hospital pharmacy has evolved in tandem with hospitals and the delivery of health care in the United States. A hospital is "an institution where the ill or injured may receive medical, surgical, or psychiatric treatment, nursing care, food and lodging, etc." as defined in Webster dictionary. While this definition continues to reflect accurately the purpose of today's hospitals, there has been an evolution in the scope of illness and injury care in hospitals, the services provided and the hospital organization itself. Major factors in this evolution have been the advances in medicine and technology and the changing medical needs and expectations of today's society.

The advancements in medicine and technology have allowed care that once required the intensive care of a hospital setting to be delivered in less intensive settings. As a result, we have witnessed the development of ambulatory surgery centers, skilled nursing facilities, home health services, outpatient treatment centers, and multiple chronic disease monitoring programs. Health care leaders continually search for the delivery model that meets the quality, safety, and access expectations of patients at an affordable cost. This quest led to a progression from individual stand-alone hospitals to health systems. These "health systems" include the acute care services that only hospitals are equipped to provide and a cadre of other services that may include primary care, specialty outpatient care, home care, nursing home facilities, hospice care, ambulatory surgery programs, and a network of physicians and other health care providers.

For this chapter, hospital pharmacy is defined as the practice of pharmacy in hospital settings and includes the organizationally related facilities or services. The pharmacy is defined as that department or division of the hospital wherein the procurement, storage, compounding, manufacturing, packaging, controlling, dispensing, and distribution of medications are performed by legally qualified, professionally competent pharmacists and their assistants. In addition to the traditional functions, the practice of pharmacy in a hospital also includes a broad responsibility for the safe and appropriate use of medications, which includes, among other things, the rational selection, dosing, and monitoring of the patients' overall medication-therapy. These professional responsibilities are fulfilled through collaboration with other health care professionals in the daily care of each patient. This collaboration often leads to the development of protocols, guidelines, formularies, policies, and safe medication practices in support of optimal medication use. The responsibilities of pharmacy services, role of hospital pharmacists, and the practice environment combine to make this a rewarding practice with unique characteristics.

UNIQUENESS OF HOSPITAL PHARMACY PRACTICE—A major factor making hospital pharmacy practice unique is the organizational structure of a hospital: a formalized pattern of authority, responsibility, and coordination that affects every department of the overall health care team. The administrator (highest hospital administrative position) implements the policies and philosophies of the governing board, delegates authority, and passes on responsibility to department leaders to carry out the patient care, teaching, research, and public-health objectives of the hospital. Department leaders, such as the director of pharmacy, are expected to coordinate their services and activities with other department leaders. The business and finance departments handle the financial affairs; the building services departments provide the essential maintenance and security functions; the human resources department implements personnel policies; the clinical laboratory department performs a multitude of patient laboratory tests and services; the nursing service provides continuous care; and dozens of other departments influence and affect the services of all hospital departments. Pharmacists work with various departments to assure the safe, efficient, and cost-appropriate distribution and use of medications, as well as practice as a team with physicians, nurses, and other health care professionals to care for patients of the hospital.

In addition to the internal forces operating within the hospital, the following is a listing of some external forces that affect the practice of pharmacy in the hospital setting:

- Accreditation agencies exert their influence on professional standards of practice as they affect patient care.
- Licensing agencies exert legal influences on hospital operations.
- The federal government imposes standards and regulations on hospitals, such as the *Conditions of Participation for Hospitals* under Medicare. Third-party payers exert their influence on the methods by which hospitals may bill and be reimbursed for services rendered to patients.
- The Office of Inspector General (OIG) establishes and enforces compliance standards for hospitals to detect and prevent fraud and abuse in the health care industry.
- Social agencies and governmental welfare agencies influence the services provided to medically indigent and totally indigent patients.
- The governing board and public opinion exert their influences over the policies, objectives, and philosophies of hospital operations and practices.

Because the hospital is an institution of and for the community, it is influenced heavily by the needs, expectations, and demands of the members of that community. These influences directly or indirectly impact the practice of pharmacy that must support the mission and goals of the hospital.

The hospital pharmacy has several basic general functions. These functions have been outlined in a document approved by the American Hospital Association (AHA), "Statement on Functions of a Hospital Department."[1] It reads as follows:

A department carries out its functions according to the philosophy and objectives of the hospital. The governing board establishes the philosophy and objectives. Accordingly, the pharmacy director reports to the administrator of the hospital. Within the organizational pattern, the functions of the department are:

1. To provide and evaluate service in support of medical care pursuant to the objectives and policies of the hospital.
2. To implement for departmental services the philosophy, objectives, policies, and standards of the hospital.
3. To provide and implement a departmental plan of administrative authority that clearly delineates responsibilities and duties of each category of personnel.
4. To participate in the coordination of the functions of the department with the functions of all other departments and services of the hospital.
5. To estimate the requirements for the department and to recommend and implement policies and procedures to maintain an adequate and competent staff.
6. To provide the means and methods by which personnel can work with other groups in interpreting the objectives of the hospital and the department to the patient and community.
7. To develop and maintain an effective system of clinical and/or administrative records and reports.
8. To estimate needs for facilities, supplies, and equipment and to implement a system for evaluation, control, and maintenance.
9. To participate in and adhere to the financial plan of operation for the hospital.
10. To initiate, utilize, and/or participate in studies or research projects designed for the improvement of patient care and the improvement of other administrative and hospital services.
11. To provide and implement a program of continuing education for all personnel.
12. To participate in and/or facilitate all educational programs that include student experiences in the department.
13. To participate in and adhere to the safety program of the hospital.

It is within this framework that the hospital pharmacist practices. The responsibility is to develop a high quality comprehensive pharmaceutical service, properly coordinate and meet the needs of the numerous diagnostic and therapeutic departments, the nursing service, the medical staff, and the hospital as a whole in the interest of continually improving patient care.

Hospital pharmacy has significantly grown in recent years that it has developed a body of specialized knowledge through its documented literature. It has created a workforce of well-qualified hospital practitioners who have adopted a sound philosophy of professional service and high standards of practice. There is special education and training at the graduate level; and there is a vigorous professional society—The American Society of Health-System Pharmacists (ASHP). This professional organization strives to meet the needs of pharmacists practicing in hospitals and other organized health care settings. The ASHP is actively involved in the provision of continuing education programs, publications, and other services designed to help the institutional practitioner in providing a high level of professional service. The ASHP Best Practices Standards provide documents that offer a point of reference for use by pharmacists in developing and evaluating their programs and services.

Curricula for the professional degree program, Doctor of Pharmacy (PharmD), include an experiential component in hospital practice. Most of the colleges/schools offer an undergraduate course in hospital pharmacy, while a few offer a graduate educational program leading to a Master of Science degree in hospital pharmacy. Concurrently, some of these graduate programs may be coordinated so students can complete a hospital pharmacy residency with their graduate work. The first programs of this type were at the Philadelphia College of Pharmacy and Science (1947), the Jefferson Medical College Hospital (1947), the University of Maryland (1947), the Johns Hopkins Hospital (1947), and the University of Michigan (1948). These combined educational and training programs have contributed much to develop and nurture career-minded, well-trained hospital pharmacists. Graduates of these programs have taken leadership positions in hospitals throughout the country and have demonstrated their capabilities through the development of comprehensive pharmaceutical services of broad scope and high quality.

The increasing complexity of medication therapy continues to fuel the need for hospital pharmacists with the skills and expertise that meet the pharmaceutical service needs of hospitals. Hospital pharmacists long recognized the need for additional education and training and developed additional formal education such as residency programs to accomplish these ends.

THE HOSPITAL

Hospital pharmacists practice within the framework of the hospital's organizational structure. For them to function effectively, it is essential that they understand what a hospital is, how it is organized, what its functions are, and how the pharmacy service fits into the overall patient care program.

DEFINITION—As stated by the AHA, the primary function of the institution is to provide patient services, diagnostic and therapeutic, for particular or general medical conditions.[2] Traditionally, a hospital has been defined in terms of its *form*, which includes its physical makeup and the quantitative nature of its services. This definition is exemplified best by the *Registration of Hospitals Program* of the AHA. To be registered under this program, an institution must meet certain requirements that constitute the definition of a hospital. Thus, the program differentiates between a hospital and other institutions such as extended-care facilities, convalescent homes, and homes for the aged.

REQUIREMENTS FOR REGISTRATION BY AHA AS A HOSPITAL[2]

1. The institution shall maintain at least six inpatient beds, which shall be continuously available for the care of patients who are nonrelated and who stay on the average in excess of 24 hours per admission.
2. The institution shall be constructed, equipped, and maintained to ensure the health and safety of patients and to provide uncrowded, sanitary facilities for the treatment of patients.
3. There shall be an identifiable governing authority legally and morally responsible for the conduct of the hospital.
4. There shall be a CEO to whom the governing authority delegates the continuous responsibility for the operation of the hospital in accordance with established policy.
5. There shall be an organized medical staff of fully licensed physicians that may include other licensed individuals permitted by law and by the hospital to provide independent patient care services in the hospital. The medical staff shall be accountable to the governing authority for maintaining proper standards of medical care, and it shall be governed by bylaws adopted by said staff and approved by the governing authority.
6. Each patient shall be admitted on the authority of a member of the medical staff who has been granted the privilege to admit patients to inpatient services in accordance with state law and criteria for standards of medical care established by the individual medical staff. Each patient's general medical condition is the responsibility of a qualified physician member of the medical staff. When nonphysician members of the medical staff are granted privileges to admit patients, a qualified physician makes provision for prompt medical evaluation of these patients. Any graduate of a foreign medical school who is permitted to assume responsibilities for patient care shall possess a valid license to practice medicine, or shall be certified by the Educational Commission for Foreign Medical Graduates, or shall have qualified for and have successfully completed an academic year of supervised clinical training under the direction of a medical school approved by the Liaison Committee on GAT Medical Education.
7. Registered nurse supervision and other nursing services are continuous.

8. A current and complete medical record shall be maintained by the institution for each patient and shall be available for reference.

9. Pharmacy service shall be maintained in the institution and shall be supervised by a registered pharmacist.

10. The institution shall provide patients with food service that meets the nutritional and therapeutic requirements; special diets shall also be available.

Hospitals are registered with the AHA as one of four types: general, special, rehabilitation and chronic disease, and psychiatric.

General: The primary function of the institution is to provide patient services, diagnostic and therapeutic, for a variety of medical conditions.

Special: The primary function of the institution is to provide diagnostic and therapeutic services for patients who have specified medical conditions, both surgical and nonsurgical.

Rehabilitation and Chronic Disease: The primary function of the institution is to provide diagnostic and therapeutic services to handicapped or disabled individuals requiring restorative and adjustive services.

Psychiatric: The primary function of the institution is to provide diagnostic and therapeutic services for patients who have psychiatric-related illnesses.

The broad purpose or mission to which that health system aspires also defines hospitals. Hospitals often serve as the focal point for the coordination and delivery of patient care to its community. Thus today, a hospital may be viewed as an organized structure that assembles the health professions, the diagnostic and therapeutic facilities, equipment and supplies, and the physical facilities into a coordinated system for delivering healthcare to the public.

Services provided by hospitals include those for patients in the institution itself (hospitalized patients) and also for patients in ambulatory-care clinics, emergency rooms, and emergency care centers, those in physicians' offices at hospitals, those in extended-care facilities and nursing homes either affiliated with or owned by the hospital, at home, through home health care services, those at wellness centers and those at community or neighborhood health clinics. In most communities, hospitals serve as the focal point of emergency care and treatment in the event of natural disasters, catastrophic accidents, and terrorist attacks.

Certain other definitions are required for proper understanding of the differences between hospitals and patient care institutions other than hospitals. In its accreditation program, the Joint Commission on Accreditation of Healthcare Organizations (JCAHO) defines long-term care facilities and divides them into two categories: a Long-Term Health Care Facility and a Resident-Care Facility.[3] These facilities are defined as follows:

Long-Term Health Care Facility—A facility for inpatient care other than a hospital, with an organized medical staff, medical staff equivalent, or medical director, and with continuous nursing service under professional nurse direction. It is designed to provide, in addition to the medical care dictated by diagnoses, comprehensive preventive, rehabilitative, social, spiritual, and emotional inpatient care to individuals requiring long-term health care and to convalescent patients who have a variety of medical conditions with varying needs.

Resident Treatment Facility—A facility providing safe, hygienic living arrangements for residents. Regular and emergency health services are available when needed, and appropriate supportive services, including preventive, rehabilitative, social, spiritual, and emotional, are provided on a regular basis.

These two broad categories cover the various types of long-term care designated by governmental agencies for licensure, certification, and/or reimbursement purposes, including skilled nursing care and intermediate care. Patient care is also delivered in other settings such as

Clinic: A facility or area where ambulatory patients are seen by appointment, treated by a group of physicians practicing together, and where the patient is not confined, as in a hospital. The term *clinic*

also is used to indicate the outpatient diagnostic facility operated by a hospital and also facilities operated by other agencies for the care of indigent and medically indigent patients. In the past, the term *clinic* usually has been reserved for facilities of a teaching nature where medical students and resident staff offered treatment to patients unable to afford private practitioners. While the concept of clinics caring for medically indigent patients continues today, networks of clinics are valuable components of today's health care delivery model in the United States.

Ambulatory Surgery Center: A facility where patients are admitted, surgical procedures are performed, and patients are discharged following assessment. Recovery from the procedure continues while the patient at home or in other settings.

DEVELOPMENT AND EXPANSION—Greek temples were forerunners of the modern hospital in the sense that they provided refuge and treatment for the sick and also provided for the teaching of young medical students. Temples as the Temple of Aesculapius (Greek god of Medicine) existed in 1134 BC, while the temple at Kos, Greece, was where Hippocrates (born about 460 BC) practiced. Hospitals had their origin in Indian and Egyptian culture during the 6th century BC. The evolution of the hospital is related to the sociological development of the individual's expansion of interest beyond himself and his family to the welfare of the community. Although early hospitals were instituted to remove certain people (eg, the insane, the incurable, the contagious) from society to protect it other hospitals were developed through religious and divine motives. The temples of the gods in early Greek and Roman civilization were used as hospitals where healing was associated with divine powers, while continued illness or death was associated with a lack of purity.

The first hospital on the American continent was built by the Spaniards (led by Cortez) in 1524—The Hospital of the Immaculate Conception in Mexico City. In 1663, the name was changed to The Hospital of Jesus of Nazareth. In the American colonies, a hospital was built in 1663 on Manhattan Island for sick soldiers. The first incorporated hospital in the United States was the Pennsylvania Hospital, established in 1751 through the efforts of Dr. Thomas Bond. It provided physicians in Philadelphia with a place to treat their private patients. Since 1873, the United States population has more than doubled, but the number of hospitals has increased from 149 to approximately 5,800.[4]

One of the major factors in the development and expansion of hospitals was the religious influence. Prior to the Christian era, hospitals were temples dedicated to the god of medicine in which the care of the sick was accompanied by magical, mystical, and religious ceremonies. The doctrines of Jesus Christ intensified the emotions and virtues of love, pity, and charity. These strong motivating forces toward one's fellow man gave impetus to the expansion of hospitals.

Another major factor in the development and expansion of hospitals was the military influence. Much of the stimulus toward medical and surgical progress over the centuries has come from the urgent need for care of the battlefield wounded. This was true during the Roman Empire; it was also true in the US before, during, and after the Civil War. The Civil War, however, focused attention on the inadequacy of hospital construction and also on the lack of nursing care. President Lincoln requested Catholic Sisters to care for wounded army personnel because hospital care was so poor. The Army's work set a pattern for improvement in patient care and combined the military and religious influences on hospital development.

Other factors that influenced the development and expansion of hospitals included:

- The Flexner report on medical education (1910), which caused revolutionary developments in medical education *per se* and in medical internship training, which helped the development of minimum standards for patient care in hospital surroundings.
- The activities of Florence Nightingale during and after the Crimean War, which served as the basis for revolutionizing the

quality of nursing care in hospitals and for the development of schools of nursing.

- The public interest in hospitals through greater dependence and improved confidence in hospital care.

With public dependence and confidence came public support, and this support provided the finances for further development, expansion, and improvement in hospital facilities. This public interest extended its influence into private hospitalization insurance and government participation in health care through Social Security and other health-related agencies. One of the most significant governmental programs that affected the development and expansion of hospital facilities in the United States was the adoption (in 1946) by the Congress of the Hospital Survey and Construction Act. Commonly known as the Hill-Burton program, this act provided federal funds for hospital construction on a matching basis with local communities. From 1946 to 1973, hundreds of new hospitals were built, while hundreds of other hospitals undertook major expansion programs of existing facilities through the availability of government finances through the Hill-Burton Act.

The Congress made funds available for construction and improvement of various health care facilities, including medical and nursing schools, outpatient and extended care facilities, and specialized diagnostic and therapeutic facilities in hospitals, and adopted a number of legislative amendments. In addition, the Social Security Amendments of 1965 (Medicare) had a long-range impact on the development and expansion of hospitals because funds are made available to pay for services of medically indigent patients.

In 1983, Congress enacted significant changes in the method by which hospitals are reimbursed for Medicare patients to hold down escalating hospital costs. A Prospective Payment System was developed to reimburse hospitals at a specific rate based upon the diagnosis of the patient, ie, the diagnosis-related group (DRG). This system of payment has influenced the mechanism by which private insurance companies reimburse the hospital for patient for care. This emphasis on cost containment has prompted a shift from care in hospital settings to care in less expensive ambulatory care settings for many medical services.

Beyond the three basic essentials of human existence (ie, food, clothing, shelter), the hospital has become a necessary instrument for providing a fourth basic element of survival—health. Health care in the United States has come to be defined as a right for all, rather than a luxury for a few. The hospital serves as a major instrument through which health professions are able to provide health care to the people of the community.

CLASSIFICATION—Hospitals may be classified in different ways, including

- type of service
- ownership
- length of stay
- bed capacity

Hospitals are classified by *type of service* such as general, special, rehabilitation and chronic disease, and psychiatric.

Hospitals are classified by *length of stay* as either short-term or long-term. A short-term hospital is one in which the average length of stay of the patient is less than 30 days. Patients with acute disease conditions and emergency needs are usually hospitalized for less than 30 days. General hospitals are short-term, because acutely ill patients usually recover in less than 30 days. Alternatively, a long-term hospital is one in which the average length of stay of the patient is 30 days or longer. Such patients have long-term illnesses, such as psychiatric conditions.

Hospitals are classified by *ownership* usually as governmental or nongovernmental. Hospitals falling into these categories of ownership are:

Governmental Hospitals
Federal
- Armed Forces,
- Veterans Administration
- US Public Health Service

Nongovernmental Hospitals
Nonprofit
- Church related or operated
- Other nonprofit

State
- County
- City (municipal)
- City-County

For profit
- Individual
- Partnership
- Corporation

Federal hospitals are owned and operated by various branches of the federal government. The United States Army, Air Force, and Navy hospitals are usually general medical and surgical hospitals, provided to care for military personnel, although there are specialized mental institutions within these groups. The Veterans Administration (VA) hospitals provide care for additional specialized groups of our population and operate general medical and surgical hospitals and also some mental hospitals.

State hospitals are owned by the state and controlled by a board of control or division of the state government or a similar organization responsible to state government. They are maintained by state appropriations and consist mainly of psychiatric hospitals. In some instances, state hospitals are general hospitals affiliated with a university involved in the training of physicians and other professional personnel, often referred to as teaching hospitals.

County hospitals are owned by the county and financed and controlled similarly to state hospitals, only on a county level. They are usually general hospitals caring for the indigent.

City hospitals are owned, financed, and controlled by the city government. They are usually general hospitals caring for the indigent.

In the nongovernmental hospital group, most institutions are general medical and surgical hospitals, varying only in their control and eligibility for receipt of state funds for charity or indigent patient care. The *proprietary* or *private hospital organized for profit* may be privately or publicly held. These hospitals often represent an investment interest of their owners, and profits are legally shared among the owners.

The *nonprofit,* nongovernmental hospitals are supported financially by fees from paying patients or by contributions from the several religious orders or churches. These hospitals are owned and controlled either by the religious order or diocese, as exemplified by the Catholic churches, by a separate governing board, as in churches of other denominations, or by a not-for-profit corporation in the community.

Community hospitals or private, nonprofit hospitals are owned and operated by members of the community, but with no relationship to the local government. Fees from patients from the community and surrounding area finance them. The cost of providing medical care for the indigent is a problem for the community hospital, and this cost is partially met through local, state, and federal assistance.

Hospitals generally are classified by *bed capacity* according to the following pattern:

Under 50 beds
50–99 beds
100–199 beds
200–299 beds
300–399 beds
400–499 beds
500 beds & over

Using these four general classifications, the approximately 5,800 hospitals in the United States are 85% nongovernmental, short-term, general or special hospitals. These 5,800 hospitals represent approximately 987,440 beds and admit about 35.6 million patients annually.[4]

FUNCTIONS—Traditionally, the hospital's basic purpose for existence has been the treatment and care of the sick and injured. In conjunction with this basic function, hospitals have been concerned with teaching, particularly of medical students, ever since the pre-Christian Era of Greek medicine. Research has been another function of the hospital. In modern times, a fourth function has been assumed by hospitals, namely, public health (ie, preventive medicine, wellness). Thus, the four fundamental functions of hospitals are patient care, education, research, and public health.

Patient Care—Patient care involves the diagnosis and treatment of illness or injury, preventive medicine, rehabilitation, convalescent care, and personalized services. The modern hospital is charged with maintaining and restoring health to the community that it serves through its patient care services. The other three functions are really the servants of patient care, because they contribute either directly or otherwise to the care of the sick and injured. Emergency care of the injured commands prime attention in any hospital—fully as important as the care of the inpatient. Outpatient care also has become an important part of the hospital's responsibility to the community.

Education—This is an important function of the modern hospital, whether it is or is not affiliated with a university. Education as a hospital function is of two major forms:

1. Education of the medical and allied health professions. This form includes physicians; nurses; medical social service workers; medical record librarians; dietitians; radiology and laboratory technicians; medical technologists; respiratory, physical, and occupational therapists; hospital administrators; pharmacists; and others. The hospital's educational program for these groups includes formal programs (such as medical, nursing, and pharmacy schools); in-service training programs for professional personnel, such as residencies; and on-the-job training programs for nonprofessional personnel. Such educational programs are essential; it is only in a hospital that such concentrated facilities are available to provide the necessary practical learning experience for dealing with saving human lives.
2. Education of the patient. This is an important hospital function, the scope of which is seldom realized by the public. It includes providing general education for children confined to long-term hospitalization; special education in the area of rehabilitation—mentally, socially, physically, and occupationally; and special education in health care, for example, teaching patients with diabetes or cardiac disorders to care for their ailment or teaching patients with colostomies to care for their personal needs.

Research—Hospitals conduct research as a vital function for two major purposes: the advancement of medical knowledge against disease and the improvement of hospital services. Both purposes are directed toward the basic aim of better health care for the patient. Examples of research activities in the hospital include devising new diagnostic procedures, conducting laboratory and clinical experiments, developing and perfecting new surgical procedures or techniques, and evaluating investigational medications. Other examples include research to improve administrative procedures for greater efficiency and lower cost to the patient; and designing, developing, and evaluating new equipment and facilities to improve patient care.

In the past, research in hospitals was performed primarily by medical staff. However, in recent years there has been a significant increase in research activities in the various hospital departments by other disciplines. Nursing, for example, is now engaged in significant research designed to improve patient care. Many medications are evaluated in hospitalized patients before they are marketed, and thus, the clinical evaluation of investigational medications presents many opportunities for the hospital pharmacist to participate in research. Pharmacists are involved in many other types of research, such as pharmacokinetic studies involving individualization of medication-dosing in patients, biopharmaceutical studies of medication products and radiopharmaceutical dosage formulations, and pharmacoeconomic studies, as well as administrative and professional studies on medication-distribution systems, the effectiveness of clinical roles of pharmacists, and medication utilization studies.

Public Health—The prime objective of this fourth and relatively new hospital function is to assist the community in reducing the incidence of illness and improving the general health of the population. Examples of public health activities are the close working relationships many hospitals have with public-health departments of communicable diseases; the participation in disease management or detection programs such as diabetes, hypertension, and cancer; the participation in mass public inoculation programs such as those against influenza and various childhood diseases; and the participation of hospital ambulatory care departments in teaching routine hygienic practices, wellness clinics, smoking cessation, and exercise and fitness programs, as well as ways in which patients should care for themselves when illness strikes. Hospital pharmacists have an opportunity to contribute to this function by providing health information brochures and services to outpatients and by instructing patients on the safe use of medications and poison prevention measures.

The terrorist attacks that took place in the United States on September 11, 2001, have redefined the hospital's relationship with public-health agencies. Historically, hospitals have taken part in responding to naturally occurring disasters or catastrophic accidents, such as tornadoes or train wrecks. Hospitals, in cooperation with local health authorities, had developed plans to handle a large number of casualties. However, communities now face a potential of orchestrated terrorism ranging from localized bombings to devastating scenarios such as the use of chemical or biological weapons or nuclear devices inflicting casualties on a massive scale. Hospitals in many communities are collaborating with local, state, and federal authorities to develop comprehensive emergency management plans that include response to large-scale chemical or bioterrorism attacks. The Department of Homeland Security and the Department of Health and Human Services work on a national level to respond to events such as public exposure to biological agents (eg, anthrax, botulism). Stockpiles of pharmaceuticals, including antibiotics and supportive care equipment such as ventilators and personal protective equipment, are warehoused and will be immediately delivered to an affected area. Locally, the disaster team must be prepared to respond to the immediate needs of the community until the supplies and therapeutic agents arrive and the contents are distributed. The pharmacy department should ensure needed supplies of pharmaceuticals are readily available. The pharmacist should work with their colleagues in other hospitals and drug wholesalers to establish a plan to treat their potential patients and the hospital's employees.

STANDARDS OF PRACTICE—In the United States, a level of protection for the public is provided through an accreditation process requiring that hospitals comply with certain standards of care. The accreditation program is conducted on a national basis, and its purpose is to determine the quality of care rendered to patients. This is achieved through the establishment of minimum standards of quality of patient care and the invitation to all hospitals to meet or surpass these standards by improving their services and facilities.

Accreditation of hospitals began in 1918 when The American College of Surgeons initiated its Hospital Standardization Programme. The purpose was to elevate the quality of surgical care provided in hospitals. The program involved setting up minimum standards of practice for the operating rooms, but it also identified the need for similar standards in all departments of the hospital. The first list of approved hospitals, published in 1919, contained 89 approved hospitals out of 692 surveyed. The American College of Surgeons standardization program was assumed by the Joint Commission on Accreditation of Hospitals (JCAH) in 1951.

The JCAH transitioned to a broader scope accreditation and in 1988 changed its name to the Joint Commission on Accreditation of Healthcare Organizations (JCAHO). The JCAHO establishes standards and provides accreditation services for other components of health care delivery including, home care, ambulatory care, behavioral health care organizations, as well as hospitals.

The JCAHO is an independent, voluntary agency, and its actions are not subject to ratification by the organizations represented by its component members. One of its objectives is to make known to the public the names of those hospitals that have invited its scrutiny and have been accredited by it through meeting the minimum standards established for good patient care. The net effect of the program is to enable the public to discriminate between hospitals that are accredited and those that are not.

During the years the American College of Surgeons administered the accreditation program, the pharmacy was not included among the essential divisions of the hospital but, rather, was listed as a complementary division. The JCAH continued this classification for several years. However, in 1956 the pharmacy department was included among the essential services of the hospital, and thus, official recognition was given to the importance of the pharmacy. In 1965, the JCAH amended its standards for medical staff functions by requiring a Pharmacy and Therapeutics Committee. Previously, the JCAH had only considered this committee to be a desirable one rather than an essential committee on the medical staff. This action placed a greater emphasis on medication use standards, was instrumental in expanding the role of pharmacists in the medication use process and medication safety.

Another major impetus to the development of standards of practice in hospitals came about with the enactment of the Social Security Amendments of 1965 (Medicare). This law set forth certain conditions that hospitals are required to meet for purposes of participating as providers of services to recipients of federally financed programs. These requirements are published as a manual entitled *Conditions of Participation—Hospitals* (available from the US Department of Health and Human Services, Social Security Administration, Washington, DC). Among the requirements for hospital participation is accreditation by an organization recognized by the Centers of Medicare and Medicaid Services including the JCAH and the American Osteopathic Association (AOA). This manual also includes the conditions of participation for the various departments of the hospital, including the pharmacy department. These conditions played a major role in challenging hospitals, particularly, small hospitals to consider appointing pharmacists to their staffs, providing comprehensive pharmacy services, and establishing pharmacy and therapeutics committees.

Standards of practice in hospitals are also influenced by other organizations. In 1999 and 2001, respectively, the Institute of Medicine, an advisory group to the National Academy of Sciences, issued reports titled "To Err is Human: Building a Safer Health System" and "Crossing the Quality Chasm: A New Health System for the 21st Century." These reports detailed the problem of medical errors in health systems and outlined improvement strategies. This resulted in a tidal wave of interest from the media, regulatory agencies, and the public in patient safety in hospitals. The outcome has been a renewed focus on patient safety in hospitals and organizations such as JCAHO as standards are continually revised.

ORGANIZATION AND ADMINISTRATION—The governing body has total accountability within the organization's structure in most hospitals. This board, commonly referred to as the board of trustees, board of directors, or board of regents, is accountable to provide direction for the organization and oversight of the operations. The board commonly hires a CEO to lead the organization and make recommendations to the board. This officer is commonly referred to as the CEO, President, or Superintendent. In the case of the federal hospitals, there is usually a federal structure through which local hospitals are organized and report. State, county, and city hospitals often have a governing board appointed by the designated political officer. In the nonprofit, nongovernmental hospital, there is usually a governing board, board of trustees, board of governors, or other titled group that assumes overall responsibility for the proper operation of the hospital so that adequate service can be rendered to the sick and injured at as low a cost as is compatible with efficiency.

The governing body has ultimate accountability for the operations, strategic direction, and appropriation of resources to fulfill the mission of the hospital. However, many duties to implement the policies and strategic plan of the Board are delegated to the responsibility of the CEO. These responsibilities include the selection of competent personnel including the medical staff, control of hospital funds, and supervision of the physical plant. By reason of certain court decisions, the responsibility for injury or other act by a member of the hospital staff on the hospital grounds reverts back to the governing board, although the individual hospital personnel is involved.

The governing board has its own internal organization, consisting of a president or chairman, vice-chairman, secretary, and treasurer. On many boards, the CEO of the hospital serves as the secretary. There are usually standing committees appointed, such as

- The executive committee
- The hospital committee dealing with personnel appointments, especially those of the medical staff, and with other activities of a departmental nature
- The finance committee, which is concerned with the hospital budget, room rates, and other financial matters
- A committee on public relations, which is concerned with educating the community on the value of the hospital and with maintaining a desirable relationship with the community

There may be other committees appointed as needs arise, such as an expansion and development committee when the hospital is concerned with the need for construction of additional hospital beds.

The CEO of the hospital must produce a two-way channel of communication between the board and the hospital staff and personnel. The CEO reports all essential facts concerning the operation of the hospital to the Board and receives from the Board all directives it issues.

For CEOs to carry out the overall responsibilities assigned by the governing board, they need assistance. Depending on the size of the hospital, there may be one or more administrators reporting to the CEO. The administrator responsible for that service also appoints a leader for each department. The department leaders have the responsibility of operating the departments effectively and properly, within the overall policies and philosophies established by the hospital's governing board.

Among the many departments that make up the modern hospital, there are some in which the services involve primarily the *professional care* of the patient, while the services of other departments involve mainly the *business management* of the hospital.

Some of the departments that deal with the professional care of the patient (diagnostic or therapeutic) include:

Ambulatory Care	Medical Records (HIMS)
Anesthesia	Medical Social Service
Blood Bank	Nuclear Medicine
Clinical Laboratories	Nursing Service
Dental Service	Occupational Therapy
Dietary and Nutrition Service	Pharmacy Service
Electrocardiograph Laboratory	Physical Medicine
Emergency Room	Radiology Therapy
Medical Library	Respiratory Therapy

Departments that deal with the business management or administrative side of the hospital include:

Accounting	Engineering & Maintenance
Admitting	Housekeeping
Biomedical Engineering	Information Systems
Business Office	Materials Management
Cafeteria	Patient and Employee Safety
Central Transportation	Patient Representatives
Credit & Collection	Personnel & Payroll
Public Relations	Risk Management
Marketing	Telecommunications
Care Improvement	Volunteer Service

THE MEDICAL STAFF—The medical staff of a hospital falls in a different category organizationally than the departments listed previously. In some cases, physicians are independent agents taking care of their patients, and they use the hospital, its departments, facilities, and services to care for these patients. The governing board of the hospital, and the community that it represents, exercises effective control over the medical staff. Although the governing board neither originates nor implements medical policy, it is responsible for the policy, and while the board members are not competent to pass judgment on the professional care of the patient, they are, as representatives of the ownership of the hospital, liable for dereliction of duties established by law. Thus, the board delegates a portion of its duties and responsibilities to its appointed medical staff to originate medical policy and carry out this policy in good faith. This requires that the medical staff be organized to govern itself and appraise its own work and yet be responsible to the governing board for the details of its work.

For a physician to be appointed to the medical staff of a hospital, an application for membership must be made. The credentials committee of the medical staff, which determines whether the physician is competent to practice in the claimed specialty, considers this application and appropriate credentials. The credentials committee also evaluates the qualifications of the physician to perform certain specialized procedures (eg, cardiac transplant, laser surgery, radiation oncology therapy). The credentials committee, if favorably impressed, makes its recommendation to the medical staff for appointment. Assuming this is approved, the recommendation goes to the governing board for final approval, upon which the physician is designated a member of the medical staff of the hospital for a specified period of time, usually one year, subject to renewal.

The organized medical staff of a hospital has certain duties:

- Providing professional care to patients of the hospital
- Maintaining its own efficiency
- Self-governance
- Participating in the educational program of the hospital
- Auditing its own professional work
- Advising and assisting the administrator and the governing board regarding medical policies

There are two main types of hospital staffs: *open* and *closed*.

An *open staff* is one in which certain physicians other than those on the attending or active medical staff are allowed to use the facilities, providing they comply with all rules and regulations of the institution. These physicians are termed members of the *courtesy* medical staff; the hospital is termed an *open-staff* hospital.

A *closed staff* is one in which all professional services, private and charity, are provided and controlled by the attending or active medical staff. A hospital with this type of staff is termed a *closed-staff* hospital. The closed staff, although it has minor drawbacks, is the more desirable for the average hospital and especially for the teaching hospital because it allows careful selection of a group of specialists with excellent reputations.

The medical staff may consist of any of the following groups: an honorary staff, a consulting staff, an active staff, an associate staff, a courtesy staff, and a resident staff. The *honorary medical staff* is composed of physicians who have been active in the hospital but who are retired and those whom it is desired to honor because of outstanding contributions. The *consulting medical staff* consists of specialists who are recognized as such by right of passing specialty boards or belonging to the national organization of their specialty and who serve as consultants to other members of the medical staff when called upon. The *active* or *attending medical staff* is the group primarily concerned with regular patient care. It is the group most actively involved in the hospital. In internal staff government, the medical staff is the authoritative body. The *associate medical staff* is composed of junior or less-experienced members of the staff. Appointment to this group is the first step toward active or attending staff membership. The *courtesy medical staff* consists of those physicians who desire the privilege of attending private patients, but who do not desire active staff membership. The *resident medical staff* is composed of residents, who are full-time employees of the hospital. These persons provide specific services in the care of the patient, for which they receive education and experience.

FINANCING HOSPITAL CARE—The technological developments of our industrialized society and the rapid advances of the medical sciences increase the financial burdens of hospitals annually. Hospitals, in their efforts to provide the best care available, must keep up with these advances by obtaining the newest diagnostic and therapeutic equipment, facilities, and products. In addition, the increasing cost of labor is reflected in the increased cost of the personalized services available in the modern hospital.

For centuries hospitals have struggled with the problem of finances adequate to cover operating expenses and fund capital purchases to improve services and care continually. At one time hospitals were a place where people went to die; the public cared little about their financial struggles. But, as the hospital developed into a place where people went to get well, the public took a more positive interest in the financial problems. In other words, the public has come to recognize that hospitals must have adequate funding to continue to provide patient care and protect the public health.

Sources of Income—There are several main sources of income for hospitals: patients, government, third-party hospitalization insurance, voluntary contributions, endowment funds, and investments.

Because most hospitals in the United States are private (nongovernmental operated), the bulk of income to these institutions is from the patient, either directly or indirectly. Funds may come from the patient directly, or they may come through hospitalization insurance (usually referred to as third-party payments). Most of the population is covered by hospitalization insurance commonly purchased by employers.

Another third-party principle involves the workmen's compensation regulations in the various states. These vary among the states, but essentially each involves the employer taking out an accident insurance policy that will pay for emergency treatment or hospitalization of the employee in case of accident or injury on the job.

Medically indigent patients are those who do not have sufficient income or insurance to pay for their own personal health needs. Although some private organizations provide assistance to this group of patients, the bulk of the financial assistance comes from tax funds through local, state, and federal agencies. The list of public, tax-supported programs for health-care assistance is formidable and becomes complex in determining what department, division, or agency of the federal, state, county, or city government is involved. In addition, dependents of members of the Armed Forces, members of the Public Health Service and their families, and the veterans of foreign wars receive health care through public tax funds.

The Social Security Amendments of 1965 and 1972 extended the benefits for hospitalization, physician's services, and outpatient services from the original Social Security Law. A substantial portion of hospital costs is provided under federal auspices.

Other sources of income for hospitals are the voluntary contributions of individuals, corporations, foundations, and community fund-raising campaigns. Some of these are direct contributions to the hospitals; others are made available in the form of grants for research; still others are given for major expansion or remodeling programs. Private health-assistance agencies assist individuals who need help by subsidizing the cost of their hospitalization and other health-care needs.

Many hospitals are fortunate in receiving substantial sums of money for the purpose of setting up endowment trust funds and for use by the hospitals in other ways. In addition, some hospitals receive some income through investments, such as in portfolios.

HEALTH MAINTENANCE ORGANIZATIONS—A health maintenance organization (HMO) is a public or private organization that provides and/or manages comprehensive health services to individuals enrolled win the HMO of the health plan. The purpose of such organizations is to provide high quality comprehensive or total health care services, emergency care, inpatient hospital and physician care, ambulatory physician care, prescription services, and preventive medical services while managing the cost of care. This type of comprehensive care while balancing the cost of care often is referred to as managed care.

In 1973, Congress passed the *Health Maintenance Organization Act of 1973* (Public Law 93-222), which provided new authority to the Department of Health, Education and Welfare (now Health and Human Services) to develop new HMOs. According to the Act, an HMO is an organizational entity that includes four essential attributes:

1. An organized system for providing health care in a geographic area that accepts the responsibility to provide or otherwise assure the delivery of health care;
2. An agreed-upon set of basic and supplemental health maintenance and treatment services to;
3. A voluntarily enrolled group of persons; and
4. For which services the HMO is reimbursed through a predetermined, fixed, periodic prepayment made by or on behalf of each person or family unit enrolled in the HMO without regard to the amount of actual services provided.

Among many other things, this legislation authorizes an HMO to "maintain, review and evaluate a drug use profile of its members receiving prescription drugs, evaluate patterns of drug utilization to assure optimum drug therapy and provide for instruction of its members and health professionals in the use of prescription and nonprescription drugs." Thus, opportunities for the development of challenging new roles for pharmacy have developed within HMOs in the broad areas of rational medication therapy including diagnostic and curative, as well as preventive therapy. Many would agree that pharmacy practice within these organized health-care facilities is characteristic of institutional pharmacy practice.

INTEGRATED HEALTH SYSTEMS—Recently, there has been a marked change in hospitals and their diversity of services. Many hospitals have merged with other hospitals and other patient care services such as home health care, ambulatory care clinics, long-term care, and wellness facilities. These systems often are known as *health systems,* because the overall governance of the system is unified. Directors of hospital departments are often administratively responsible for pharmaceutical services in multiple hospitals, ambulatory care pharmacies, long-term care pharmacy services, and home health care pharmacy services. As these *hospitals* evolve into health systems, various supportive systems such as computer systems, medication distribution systems, and clinical pharmacy services are provided and managed by one pharmacy administrative group for all units in the health system.

THE HOSPITAL PHARMACY

The separation of pharmacy from medicine took place in charitable institutions operated under governmental or ecclesiastic authority. The fact that business interests played no part in the delivery of care to patients in these institutions led to an eventual division of labor to improve the quality of care. This division of labor in the physician-apothecary function led to the recognition of pharmacy as a discipline separate from medicine. Because the division occurred in hospitals, the hospital pharmacist was the first recognized practitioner of the profession of pharmacy.

The development of hospital pharmacy in different countries was vitally affected by educational standards and the caliber of its practitioners. Thus, hospital pharmacy as an important professional specialty virtually was neglected in America for almost 168 years, from the time that Jonathan Roberts became the first hospital pharmacist at the Pennsylvania Hospital (Philadelphia) in 1752 to approximately 1920.

NATIONAL PROFESSIONAL SOCIETY—Although the existence of the American hospital covers a span of more than 200 years, only during the past four decades or so has there been a rapid expansion of pharmacy services leading to the present vast and complex hospital pharmacy system. As the movement toward the organization, expansion, and growth of the hospital pharmacy system in the US began to take shape, there also developed a movement toward the organization of hospital pharmacists. As Niemeyer et al[5] point out, the critical years for hospital pharmacy were the two decades from 1920 to 1940. The awakening in the 1920s came about as a result of a growing realization by hospital pharmacists of the problems, potentialities, and importance of their specialty. The advances in the 1930s resulted from their determination for organization, recognition, and establishment of higher standards of practice.[6]

The activities of hospital pharmacists during this critical period resulted in the formation of the American Society of Hospital Pharmacists in 1942, later renamed the American Society of Health-System Pharmacists (ASHP) in 1995. The development of the Society within the sphere of American pharmacy has been due in large part to the adoption of a philosophy of service by hospital pharmacists that places the patient as the focal point for the existence of pharmacy practice, as indicated in the ASHP Vision Statement for Pharmacy Practice in Hospitals and Health Systems (2001).[7] The unity that binds hospital pharmacists through their national professional society stems

from them being a goal-oriented group. The common bond among them is the development of higher standards of professional practice and service because *the patient needs them.* The membership, exceeding 30,000, represents a significant proportion of the pharmacists practicing in the institutional setting. Despite only being in existence since 1942, the ASHP has made significant contributions toward the improvement of hospital pharmacy through its leadership in the development of standards of practice, continuing education to maintain professional competency, various publications to support practice, standards for residency training, and residency accreditation services.

The Official Bulletin of the American Society of Hospital Pharmacists began in June 1943, which became the *American Journal of Hospital Pharmacy* in 1958. In addition, *Clinical Pharmacy* was published to provide in-depth articles dealing with clinical practice. In 1995, these two significant journals were combined to provide a journal on a semimonthly basis and were later merged into the *American Journal of Health-System Pharmacy.*

The *International Pharmaceutical Abstracts* (IPA) was introduced by the ASHP. This abstract service provides extensive coverage of the pharmaceutical literature and now is available for online computer searches.

AHFS Drug Information (American Hospital Formulary Service) is a comprehensive, unbiased source of current information on medications provided in print and electronic means. This is a comprehensive reference often used throughout the country and on an international basis. This reference supports pharmacists in their role as pharmaceutical consultants to the medical profession and other hospital staff.

The residency training programs in hospital pharmacy are accredited by the ASHP and serve as a basis for ensuring a high quality of training of future practitioners. In addition to a residency in pharmacy practice with emphasis on pharmaceutical care, specialized residencies in nuclear pharmacy, community pharmacy care, pediatric pharmacy, psychiatric pharmacy, geriatric pharmacy, drug information pharmacy practice, oncology pharmacy, primary care, internal medicine, clinical pharmacokinetics, critical care, nutrition support, pharmacotherapy practice, infective diseases practice, managed-care, home care, long-term care and management serve to provide a means to develop practitioners with specialized skills to meet future practice needs. Pharmacy technician training programs are also accredited by the ASHP, and these standards provide a basis for consistent technician training.

Other national organizations such as the American College of Clinical Pharmacists (ACCP), the American Association of Colleges of Pharmacy (AACP), and the American Pharmacists Association (APhA) have also supported the advancement of hospital pharmacy practice.

STANDARDS OF PRACTICE

The movement to develop standards of practice in the hospital was initiated by the American College of Surgeons during the early 1900s, when surgeons recognized the need to standardize and improve on surgical procedures, operating room techniques, and medical record keeping on surgical operations. The College found that to improve the overall care of surgical patients, standards needed to be developed in other departments of the hospital as well as in the operating room. As a result of their initiative, the first *Minimum Standard for Pharmacies in Hospitals* was presented to the 18th Hospital Standardization Conference of the American College of Surgeons in 1935. In 1942, when the ASHP was organized, a standing Committee on Minimum Standards was appointed for the purpose of maintaining and developing better minimum standards. The original standard of the American College of Surgeons was revised by the ASHP in 1950. This revised Standard was approved by the American Pharmaceutical Association, American Hospital Association, and Catholic Hospital Association and received editorial endorsement by the AMA. The *Minimum Standard for Pharmacies in Hospital,* evolved into a yearly publication called the *Best Practices for Health-System Pharmacy.* This publication provides a helpful set of principles on which to develop good professional practices within the hospital. *Best Practices for Health-System Pharmacy* is published annually, and the documents are available on the ASHP web site.

The JCAHO and the AOA continually revise their standards regarding the use of medications to assist hospital administrators and pharmacists review their pharmacy services. These standards, while not totally inclusive of a broad scope and high quality pharmacy service, do challenge the hospitals to meet optimum achievable standards of practice in providing high quality, safe, and effective medication use and services.

Another standard of practice relating to institutional pharmacy is the federal requirement imposed under the Social Security Amendments of 1965 (Medicare) and subsequent amendments. In addition, most state health departments have guidelines on hospital pharmacy and medication use systems.

ORGANIZATION—Within the organizational structure of the hospital, the director of pharmacy reports to an administrator of the hospital on the proper operation and management of the pharmacy. The director of pharmacy formulates and implements departmental administrative and professional policies of the pharmacy, subject to the approval of the administrator. The professional and clinical policies relating to hospital-pharmacy practice, which have a direct relationship to the medical staff, are formulated and developed through the pharmacy and therapeutics committee and are subject to administrative approval (see *Pharmacy and Therapeutics Committee*).

The organizational structure of the hospital pharmacy may be as illustrated in Figure 127-1. However, the structure differs significantly depending on the mission and services of the hospital. This chart attempts to illustrate the coordination and integration of all the technical elements of practice that must be implemented effectively into a total pharmaceutical service. For example, there are technical and professional elements of a clinical pharmacy service. On the other hand, there are clinical components of professional, technical, and support services. Likewise, there are educational, technical, and clinical implications to the research and supportive components to a pharmacy service. Therefore, the organizational structure of a modern hospital pharmacy in terms of the overall elements comprising its services and medication use leadership should be considered rather than viewing it from a clinical *versus* an operational standpoint. This philosophical approach to the organizational

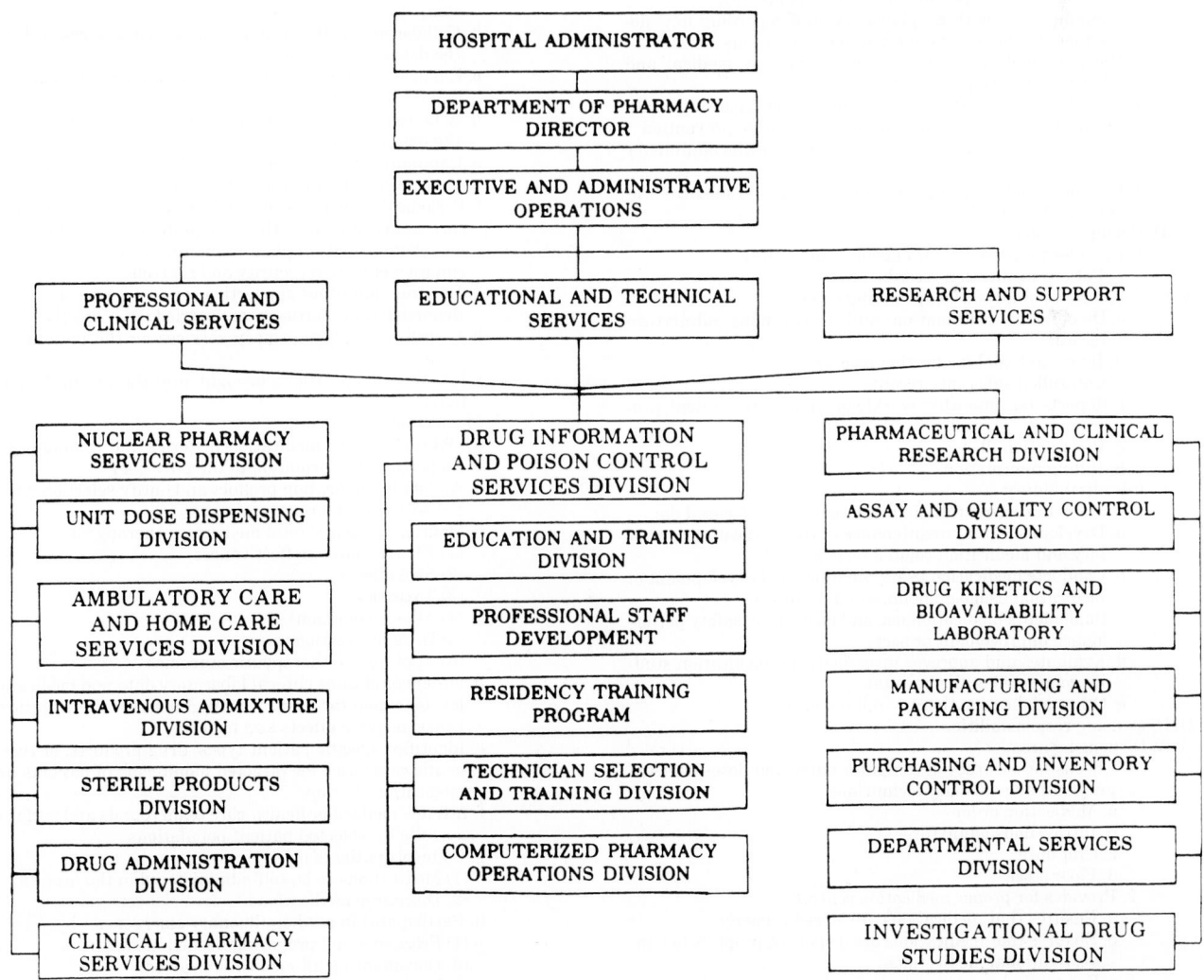

Figure 127-1. Typical organizational structure of a pharmacy department.

and operational aspects of hospital pharmacy is essential for effective use of all the pharmaceutical sciences that underlie the profession of pharmacy.

A close examination of this organizational chart shows the many ramifications of the practice of pharmacy in today's modern hospital. Hospital pharmacy staff primarily can be grouped into three categories: pharmacists, technicians, and clerical. The Pharmacist category includes those pharmacists who practice in medication distribution roles and those in clinical or direct patient care roles. Other pharmacists in the hospital include those who specialize in various areas of practice, such as leadership positions and pharmacy residents. The following is a comprehensive job description of the pharmacist's responsibilities in general hospital pharmacy activities and in clinical functions and responsibilities.

PHARMACIST RESPONSIBILITIES

I. General Responsibilities
   A. Policies and Procedures
      1. Ensures that policies and procedures are established and followed
      2. Ensures that all state and federal medication-related regulations and accreditation standards are followed
   B. Competence
      1. Maintains professional competence in areas of responsibility
   C. Training and Education
      1. Ensures that new personnel are trained properly
      2. Communicates with all pharmacy staff regarding new developments and assists in employee evaluations
      3. Provides medication information to pharmacy, medical, and other health-care personnel
      4. Provides patient education and counseling regarding medication therapy and medication-related disease prevention
      5. Assists in medication training of those staff who administer medications
      6. Provides education to pharmacy, nursing and medical students and residents
   D. Documentation
      1. Provides for proper record keeping and billing
         a. Patient medication records
         b. Extemporaneous compounding records
         c. Dispensing, automation and intravenous admixture records
         d. Investigational medication records
         e. Controlled substance records
         f. Reports (eg, monthly workload, financial, clinical programs)
         g. Prescription files
         h. Billing information
   E. Interdisciplinary
      1. Participates in multidisciplinary committees focused on:
         a. Development and maintenance of the medication formulary and medication-related policies
         b. Conducts medication use evaluations and development of medication usage guidelines and protocols
         c. Implements medication use and medication safety performance improvement projects
         d. Evaluates and approves investigational medication studies conducted in the hospital
         e. Other medication therapy-related issues
II. Dispensing responsibilities
   A. Dispensing area
      1. Checks for accuracy of computer entry and doses selected prepared by pharmacy technicians:
         a. Medication order
         b. Intravenous admixtures
         c. Unit dose
         d. Floor stock
      2. Provides for proper medication control:
         a. Ensures that medications are stored properly.
         b. Ensures that medications are dispensed properly (eg, investigational medications)
         c. Ensures adequate controlled substance procedures are in place

      3. Ensures that good techniques are used in compounding intravenous admixtures, chemotherapy, and extemporaneous preparations
      4. Coordinates the activities of the area with the available staff to make the best possible use of personnel and resources
      5. Keeps the dispensing area neat and orderly
      6. Coordinates the overall pharmaceutical needs of the patient-care areas with the dispensing area (eg, delivery schedules)
   B. Patient-care area
      1. Medication order review
         a. Reviews each medication and IV order for appropriate dosage, frequency, route, duration, monitoring parameters, and medication selection in combination with the patient's demographics, laboratory results, diagnosis, and other clinical parameters
         b. Reviews medication orders and the patient's current medication regimen to minimize adverse drug reactions, therapeutic duplication, drug interactions, and other contraindications
         c. Discusses medication order clarifications or recommendations with the prescriber and documents any changes
         d. Ensures that the medication orders are entered accurately into the appropriate pharmacy system
      2. Medication Administration
         a. Supervises medication administration and patient care area; Reviews each patient's medication administration form periodically to ensure that doses are being administered and charted correctly, that the transcription is accurate, and controlled substance documentation is complete
         b. Collaborates with nursing on missed doses, rescheduling the doses as necessary
         c. Ensures that proper medication administration techniques are used
         d. Acts as pharmacist liaison between the pharmacist and the patient care and medical staffs
         e. Communicates with nurses and physicians concerning medication administration problems
         f. Periodically, inspects the medication areas on the patient care areas to ensure that adequate levels of floor stock medications and supplies are maintained and ensures adequate medication security and controls
         g. Ensures that other supportive services performed by the department of pharmacy are carried out correctly
         h. Coordinates all pharmacy services on the patient care area
         i. Identifies medications brought into the hospital by patients
      3. Medication monitoring
         a. Obtains patient medication histories and communicates all pertinent information to the physician
         b. Assists in medication product and entity selection and in the selection of dosage regimens
         c. Monitors patients' total medication therapy for
            (1) Effectiveness/ineffectiveness
            (2) Side effects
            (3) Toxicities
            (4) Allergic reactions
            (5) Drug interactions
            (6) Appropriate therapeutic outcomes
         d. Orders or obtains clinical laboratory data and medication levels to monitor medication regimens for therapeutic efficacy, adverse effects and toxicity
         e. Identifies specific patient types, drug products, or therapeutic categories for targeted monitoring of patients and medication therapy
         f. Attends medical or health-care team rounds and performs consults for selected patient populations
         g. Counsels patients on
            (1) Medications to be self-administered in the hospital
            (2) Discharge medications
         h. Participates in cardiopulmonary emergencies by
            (1) Procuring and preparing needed medications.
            (2) Documenting all medications given
            (3) Performing cardiopulmonary resuscitation, if necessary

A growing number of hospital pharmacists specialize in specific patient populations (eg, geriatric, pediatric), patients with targeted therapeutic needs (eg, infectious disease, nutrition, pain management) or patients on a specific medical service (eg, oncology, cardiology). Pharmacists in hospitals are often given the authority by the hospital's Pharmacy and Therapeutics Committee and medical staff to write orders for alterations in medication therapy or associated laboratory orders according to established guidelines or protocols (eg, therapeutic substitutions, adjustment of selected medication doses or frequency based on patient conditions or laboratory values, ordering of laboratory tests to assist in monitoring medication therapy). In some hospitals, pharmacists and other allied health professionals must complete a hospital privileging process to provide selected patient services or perform medication prescribing. The privileging requirement occurs most frequently where there is a pharmacist-directed clinic in which the pharmacist provides direct patient care services in the ambulatory clinic areas (eg, pharmacist anticoagulation or hypertension clinic).

With continuing development of computer and pharmacy technology, automation and an automated medical record, the pharmacist's distributive and technical roles will be reduced continually, allowing more focus on patient care activities. The American Council on Pharmaceutical Education, the agency responsible for the accreditation of professional degree programs in pharmacy, has established the doctor of pharmacy (ie, PharmD) degree as the entry level degree for pharmacists. This degree program provides more clinical education and experiential preparation to fulfill these roles. Pharmacy residency programs provide additional training for pharmacists to practice in clinical roles or specialty areas of practice. For licensed pharmacists who wish to attain additional recognition for their knowledge in particular specialty areas, the Board of Pharmaceutical Specialties (BPS) has developed a certification process to recognize certain areas of specialty practice (eg, nuclear pharmacy, pharmacotherapy, nutritional support).

Pharmacy technicians provide the technical support for a hospital pharmacy. Technician roles are expanding to perform hospital pharmacy functions that do not require the skills and training of a pharmacist, allowing pharmacists to enhance their focus on assuring that the desired outcome of patients' medication regimen is achieved. Because individual state boards of pharmacy regulate and often specify the functions that technicians can perform under the supervision of a pharmacist, their roles vary among states. In addition, state boards may also specify the number of technicians relative to the number of pharmacists that can be utilized in the pharmacy.

The *White Paper on Pharmacy Technicians 2002: Needed changes can no longer wait*[8] discusses the functions, training, and regulation of technicians. Training of technicians is variable and certification is voluntary in most states. Less than half of technicians working in hospitals have received formal training, and the remainder have been trained primarily on the job. There are formal technician training programs nationwide, many of them at technical schools or community colleges, and there is a national accreditation service for pharmacy technician training programs. The Pharmacy Technician Certification Board (PTCB) started a voluntary national certification program for pharmacy technicians in 1995. In many states, technicians must be registered with the State Board of Pharmacy. Some states require certification for technicians, and many other hospitals are requiring technician certification as a condition for employment. With increased numbers of accredited training programs and expanding technician certification, technicians will be better prepared to move into roles of additional responsibility.

There follows a comprehensive job description of typical technician responsibilities.

TECHNICIAN RESPONSIBILITIES

I. General responsibilities
   a. Ensures that policies and procedures are followed
   b. Maintains competence in areas of responsibility
   c. Ensures new personnel are trained properly
II. Technical responsibilities
   a. Selects and prepares patient-specific unit dose and floor stock medications
   b. Utilizes aseptic technique to prepare and mix intravenous, parenteral nutrition and other admixtures
   c. Packages medications into unit dose and unit of use packaging
   d. Performs routine inspection of patient care and medication storage areas for medication control, security, and controlled substance accountability
   e. Orders, receives, and restocks medications and associated supplies into pharmacy and patient care inventory
   f. Collects patient demographic, laboratory, and other information to provide a complete medication profile and to provide data for pharmacist review
   g. Monitors the utilization of medications and IVs and reorders as necessary
   h. Returns outdated medications and tracks medication wastage
   i. Utilizes and manages computer software and medication related technology (eg, automated medication dispensing systems, parenteral nutrition admixture pumps, bar code technology)
III. Reporting and Documentation
   a. Documents medication preparation, packaging, and compounding
   b. Enters charges and credits to ensure billing accuracy
   c. Performs audits of medication processes and completes associated reports
   d. Completes controlled substance documentation

In smaller hospitals, sometimes staffed by only a single pharmacist, it is challenging for the pharmacists to maintain expertise in all areas of hospital pharmacy practice. In a large hospital, with a number of pharmacists who specialize in certain areas of practice, each may become expert in one or more disciplines. The staffing pattern in hospital pharmacy varies, with the scope and quality of pharmaceutical service being offered. Most hospitals with fewer than 50 beds employ at least one pharmacist and one technician. As the size of the hospital increases, so does the number of personnel in the pharmacy. For example, in a 300-bed progressive hospital, the pharmacy may be staffed with a director of pharmacy, an operations manager, a clinical specialist, from 10 to 20 staff pharmacists, 5 to 15 technicians, and a full-time department secretary. In the very large hospitals with several hundred beds, the staffing pattern in the hospital pharmacy may consist of a director of pharmacy, two or more associate or assistant directors, one or more managers, as many as 40 to 60 or more staff pharmacists (many of whom specialize in various clinical areas), 5 to 10 pharmacy residents, and about as many technical personnel as professional personnel. In addition, several clinical pharmacy faculty associated with a college of pharmacy also may be active within the department.

Pharmacy leadership provides management of pharmacy services and coordination of medication use throughout the hospital. This leadership role requires knowledge and the application of a variety of skills, including:

- Strategic planning
- Financial management
- Workload and productivity monitoring
- Budgeting and cost-containment
- Human resource management (eg, staffing, recruiting, performance evaluation, education, training)
- Quality assessment and performance improvement
- Policy, procedure, standard, and guideline development
- Customer satisfaction monitoring
- Medication safety monitoring and improvement
- Interdisciplinary and interprofessional partnership and collaboration

The director of pharmacy uses these skills and other management tools to ensure that all the services and functions are fulfilled adequately. Whereas, most hospital pharmacy managers have historically been pharmacists, non-pharmacist managers responsible for technicians, technology, and business managers are becoming more prevalent, especially in larger hospitals.

FACILITIES—There are great variations in the amount of floor space devoted to the pharmacy in hospitals of the same size and type. Such variations have a direct bearing on the scope of service that can be developed and conducted by the pharmacy. Helpful guides for planning hospital pharmacy facilities are available in the pharmacy literature.

In the small hospital with one pharmacist, only one room usually is required for the pharmacy (ie, a combination of dispensing, manufacturing, administrative, and all other features of a complete pharmaceutical service). When sterile products are to be prepared, there should be a separate room or area for such work. An area of this type is required for reconstituting lyophilized injections, ophthalmic preparations, packaging unit-dose injections into syringes, and preparing intravenous admixtures, all of which must remain sterile.

Hospitals of 200 beds and larger provide the opportunity for departmentalization of pharmacy activities. There should be a separate area for inpatient services and unit dose dispensing; outpatient service; an office for a manager; a compounding, repackaging, and labeling room; a storeroom; a sterile products and IV-admixture clean room; a room or area for a departmental computer; a separate area for drug information services; and space assigned on various patient care areas for unit dose medication storage, automated dispensing technology medication administration preparation, and clinical pharmacy services. As the hospital size advances to 500 to 1000 or more beds, the space requirements of pharmacy service will also increase.

MEDICATION SAFETY—Hospitals, independent of size and services offered, are highly complex organizations with multiple communication formats, interprofessional handoffs, and sophisticated yet complicated technology. Medication use within a hospital is subject to many opportunities for unintended results due to the combination of defects within this complex system and the reliance on human operators. The hospital pharmacist must assume a leadership role in developing a plan to eliminate or create awareness around system defects and to minimize the harm to the patient if an error occurs. Coordination with other hospital committees and departments such as the Pharmacy and Therapeutics Committee, Patient and/or Medication Safety Committees, Performance Improvement, and Risk Management departments is essential to preventing medication errors. The plan should incorporate key elements of:

1. Implementing best practices in medication use
2. Creating a medication use system that is fully understood by users and thus considered transparent
3. Maximizing safety with automation and technology
4. Conducting educational and training programs regarding medication safety
5. Reducing patient harm resulting from a medication accident

Establishing consensus around best practices in medication use at a hospital can be facilitated using a variety of resources such as ASHP's Best Practices in Hospital Pharmacy, and the Institute for Safe Medication Practices (ISMP) and National Patient Safety Foundation (NPSF) recommendations. Examples of actions to implement best practices include: eliminating the use of dangerous abbreviations, removing concentrated electrolytes from patient care areas, developing a mechanism to distinguish "look alike/sound alike" medications and creating a quality assurance program around high risk medications such as heparin or chemotherapy drugs.

Continually improving the safety of the hospital pharmacy systems requires that users have a complete understanding all system components and the system is considered "transparent." Transparency of the medication use system is important because it allows latent defects to become clear and easily un-

derstood by its human users. Transparency can be created proactively through the use of an open and blameless reporting system for errors. It can also be created by using a process known as a Failure Mode and Effects Analysis (FMEA). This tool is used to map out complex procedures carefully, breaking them down to each step, analyzing and prioritizing any identified risk or defect, and developing an action plan to address the defects. A simplified form of FMEA methodology can be used in evaluating new drugs for inclusion in the hospital's formulary. Automation and technology can be used to help eliminate or reduce medication errors by reducing reliance on human functions in the system. These technologies include bar code verification systems, robotics, smart IV pumps, clinical information support, and alerts and computerized physician order entry systems. The medication safety plan should incorporate a systematic program to evaluate new and existing technology, apply human factors design analysis or an FMEA, and create an implementation strategy that addresses the concerns of the end user prior to any installation so as to not inadvertently introduce risk into the system.

The plan should include the development of medication safety education programs for all relevant health care providers. Education should include recent developments in safety science as well as the lessons learned within the hospital's safety reporting system. Training programs should include orienting the new employee to identified areas of high risk within a given process, such as the compounding of medications for intravenous administration. Training should be conducted for any significant changes in processes or systems.

Finally, the hospital's medication safety plan should include a systematic and ongoing program to develop protocols to reduce variation and patient harm. These protocols may include communication and decision trees for patient transfers to the intensive care unit, the use of reversal agents, and the use of an extravasation kit.

The hospital's medication safety plan developed with pharmacy leadership and multidisciplinary professional participating can be an effective tool in reducing the likelihood of a medication error and improving the safety of patients.

PHARMACY AND THERAPEUTICS COMMITTEE— The American College of Surgeons recognized this need in 1935 when it adopted the first *Minimum Standard for Pharmacies in Hospitals*. The Pharmacy and Therapeutics (P&T) Committee also is recognized by the JCAHO as an essential committee of the hospital's medical staff. The P&T Committee is a committee of the medical staff and is chaired by a physician while the director of pharmacy commonly functions as secretary. Typically, it includes representation from medical staff specialties, pharmacy, nursing, administration, quality, laboratory, and other pertinent departments.

The ASHP has formulated and adopted a statement embodying the definition, purpose, organization, functions, and scope of a P&T Committee. This statement defines the primary purpose of the P&T Committee as policy development and education and is an effective guide to organizing such a committee.

Historically, some have thought that the sole purpose of a pharmacy and therapeutics committee was to develop a formulary and operate a formulary system. However, the function of this committee includes policy development and governance of the medication use process. Thus, the role is much broader than the formulary system. A hospital's medical staff could have an effective P&T Committee without having a formulary system. On the other hand, a hospital could not properly operate a formulary system without a P&T Committee unless the medical staff served as a *committee of the whole*.

During recent years, with the development of the clinical pharmacy movement, a number of clinical pharmacists on the staff of some departments have developed expertise in specific therapeutic specialty areas. Therefore, it was a logical development that a subcommittee structure could be developed under the pharmacy and therapeutics committee. For example, infectious disease physician specialists along with a clinical pharmacist who specialized in anti-infective pharmacology and therapeutics could provide the appropriate expertise to the pharmacy and therapeutics committee in this area of medication therapy. The organizational chart in Figure 127-2 illustrates an effective approach for the medical and pharmacy staffs to develop and implement a rational medication therapy program, a subcommittee structure of specialists in defined areas of therapeutics.

Another significant activity of the P&T Committee is performing Drug Usage Reviews (also known as Drug Usage Evaluations (DUEs) or Medication Use Evaluations (MUEs) studies). The committee, with active involvement by the pharmacy, determines the medications or therapeutic indication to be studied, determines the appropriate medication usage criteria, collects data, evaluates actual usage data against approval criteria, and makes recommendations for improvement in the appropriate use of the medication therapy studied. In addition, the Committee is charged by JCAHO to monitor Adverse Drug Reactions (ADRs) and medication errors, as a part of the quality assurance standards of the medical staff. The P&T Committee is involved in hospital medication safety prevention and management efforts and oversees medication use policies and systems.

FORMULARY SYSTEM—The formulary system and formularies have existed in the US since the days of the American Revolution and in European hospitals for centuries prior to this. The need for hospital formularies continues to increase due to:

- The increasing number and complexity of medications available
- Increased utilization due to direct-to-consumer and physician marketing strategies of the pharmaceutical industry
- The obligation of health care providers to exercise good stewardship in the appropriate use of medications

This is substantiated by the fact that the federal government requires the establishment of Professional Review Organizations (PROs), whose purpose it is to monitor and control the quality of services rendered to patients. The federal Maximum Allowable Cost (MAC) programs also are emphasizing cost control for patients on federally funded programs.

The formulary system—because it has attempted to outline the scientific data on a medication, including its toxicities, untoward side effects, safety profile, and beneficial effects—has been a controversial method of appraising medication therapy. While the pharmaceutical industry promotes the virtues of a brand name medication, the formulary system evaluates the virtues and defects of that medication in comparison with other brands with similar therapeutic uses. This often leads to therapeutic guidelines promoting the use of medications in various clinical situations.

The increasing use of alternative and complementary therapies by patients is creating challenges as hospitals make decisions on whether to include these agents on formulary. Often, adequate scientific data is not available, the products are not standardized, and since the products are not required to meet FDA medication formulation standards, the hospital cannot be assured of their content.

The ASHP has created several documents that can help physicians, pharmacists, and administrators with development of a formulary and with operating a hospital formulary system. Hospital pharmacists have viewed the hospital formulary system as a means to manage the medication inventory and provide high quality, safe, effective medications that meet the need of the patients. Essentially, the formulary system provided a mechanism to avoid brand duplication and therapeutic duplication, as well as promoting rational medication therapy. The success of this system is due to *peer review* in a hospital, whereby physicians agree to practice by the policies and procedures established by the committee process.

Many useful reference sources are available to assist the P&T Committee to develop an effective, ongoing rational medication therapy program and formulary system in the hospital. The knowledgeable drug-information specialist and the clinical pharmacist can use these reference sources effectively to encourage the medical staff of the individual hospital to select those medications its members consider most effective therapeutically, together with the preparations in which they may be administered most effectively. In addition, these committees have focused increasingly upon the pharmacoeconomics of medication therapy, prompting them to be more selective or restrictive in the medications available for patient care. According to the 2001 ASHP National Survey of Pharmacy Practice in Hospital Settings, more than 90% of hospitals use clinical, therapeutic, cost, and pharmacoeconomic information in the formulary management process, while nearly two thirds consider quality-of-life issues. Nearly 70% use clinical practice guidelines in the formulary management process, and 78% have a medication use evaluation program designed to improve prescribing.[9] The safety profile of the medication (eg, sound-alike medication, administration error potential) should be included in the formulary analysis.

An active P&T Committee with a well-developed formulary system provides assurance that the medical staff, the pharmacy staff, and the administration of the hospital have taken the necessary steps to assure the patient of an effective, safe, and cost-appropriate medication therapy program.

PURCHASING—The principal function in purchasing is to establish standards and specifications for all medications, chemicals, diagnostic agents, intravenous solutions, and pharmaceutical equipment. The pharmacist is responsible for the

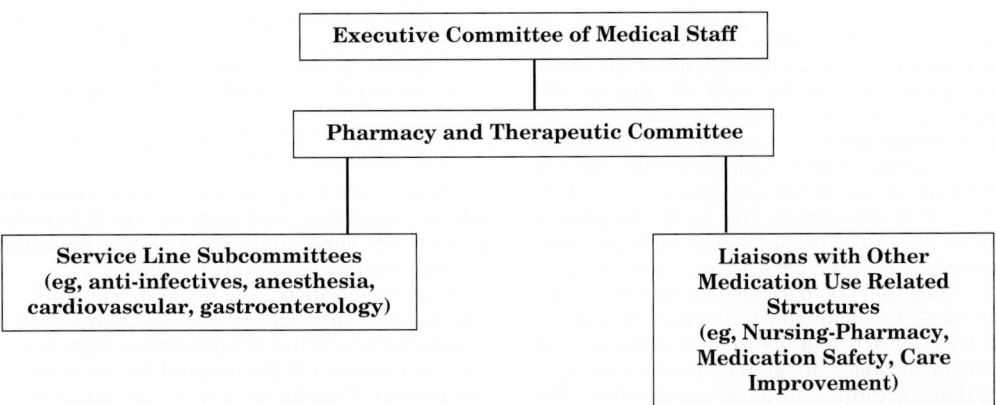

Figure 127-2. Organization of a Pharmacy and Therapeutics Committee.

quality of medications dispensed to patients. The P&T Committee serves as a potent force in helping the pharmacist establish adequate specifications for the purchase of quality pharmaceuticals.

Most hospitals have joined Group Purchasing Organizations (GPOs) or buying groups to pool their usage so that one uniform contract can be negotiated for all members of the group. Most hospital pharmacies now are obtaining all of their contract pharmaceuticals through one, single wholesaler, who provides the pharmaceuticals to the hospital for a small percentage fee. This system is known as the *prime-vendor* system and enables the hospital to order all pharmaceuticals from the prime vendor. Thus, multiple purchase orders are eliminated, and ordering is further facilitated through the use of a computer system. Most hospitals order electronically on a daily basis. This provides for a minimum inventory at the hospital and an optimum inventory rate of 10 to 20 times annually. In addition, the prime vendor can provide the hospital with coordinated purchase data and cost control reports. However, some pharmaceuticals must be obtained directly through the manufacturer.

Annual or semiannual inventories should be taken as a check on the theoretical inventory record maintained by either pharmacy or accounting. Various procedures are used to take a medication inventory. Many hospitals are using electronic data processing in inventory value determinations.

There has been an increasing frequency of drug product shortages in recent years, making it more difficult for pharmacies to maintain an adequate supply of select drug products. The Pharmacy Department and the P&T Committee have a role in determining and acquiring alternative pharmaceuticals to meet the needs of the hospital's patients and communicating this information to the medical and hospital staff.

MEDICATION-DISTRIBUTION SYSTEMS—The medication distribution system in hospitals is very complex and involves several health care professionals. The usual flow is physicians prescribe, pharmacists dispense, and nurses administer medications. However, to have this simple tripartite order executed, many steps must take place in between. The overall medication distribution and utilization process in the hospital involves an infinite number of procedures, personnel, departments, equipment, and storage. As an illustration, trace the path of a typical medication from procurement to administration to the patient.

Before a medication can be purchased, specifications must be prepared. This usually is performed through the medical staff and the pharmacist by means of a P&T Committee. Requisitions outlining the specifications for the medications selected are prepared and processed in the pharmacy. Medication shipments are accepted by the receiving department and distributed to the pharmacy, where they are checked and stored for future use. Inventory control procedures must be established. In the meantime, invoice for payment must be processed through the accounting department by a coordination of efforts among the pharmacy, purchasing, receiving, and accounts payable.

Physicians must prescribe medications before they can be administered. Upon receipt of the medication order (prescription), the pharmacist must review the order for appropriateness, given the patient's medication therapy regimen and clinical condition. Any recommendations due to patient condition, medication formulary status, or more appropriate therapy are communicated to the physician. In the pharmacy, the medications are transferred from the storage area to the dispensing area. There they may have to be prepackaged (for future use), compounded or manufactured, and have assay and control procedures performed. They must be packaged in correct quantities for use by the nurse to administer to the patient, labeled properly, checked for accuracy, and distributed to the patient care area. Here, the medications are stored again for continuous use by the patient, according to physicians' orders. The nurse obtains the necessary medication, prepares the medication for administration, brings it to the patient, ensures that the patient is the one who is to receive the medication, and records this information in the patient's record. Additionally, the nurse and pharmacist monitor the patient for therapeutic and adverse effects.

In the meantime, the pharmacy processes these medication orders for billing purposes and sends these charges electronically to the business office. There, they are posted to the patient's account. Then, through coordination between the pharmacy and the accounting department, data are accumulated and based on the cost of medications issued.

While the mechanics of this operation are taking place, other activities must be completed. Problems must be resolved in the procurement phase regarding medication shortages, overshipments, undershipments, or other shipping errors; errors in billing may have to be rectified. Outdated or deteriorated medications and/or drug product recalls may necessitate these having to be returned to the manufacturer. Recall procedures have to be established. Further information, such as dosage, toxicity, and side effects, may be required from the physician or nurse before the order or prescription can be filled.

The medication use cycle is complex and passes through many health care professionals to provide the appropriate medication to the patient. The average patient receives 20 doses of medication per day while in the hospital. At each step, there is an opportunity for a medication error that may or may not adversely affect the patient. Thus, the medication use system is subject to ongoing review by the P&T Committee and Safety Committee to optimize the safety of the system. Computers, automation, clinical pharmacist practitioners and bar-code technology can be incorporated into the medication system to optimize efficiency and safety.

Medication is administered to a hospital patient only upon the order of a physician (or designated allied health professional). Thus, a prescription order originates in the patient's medical record, where physicians write all the orders (prescriptions) for the patient. Because the patient's medical record remains at the patient care area, it is essential that some means be used to transmit the prescription order from the patient care area to the pharmacy. These orders are transmitted to the pharmacy usually in one of four ways:

- The medical record has a duplicate copy so that the pharmacy can obtain a carbon copy of the physician's original medication order.
- Patient care personnel transcribe the physician's order onto an inpatient prescription or requisition form; however, the transcription method is no longer recognized as acceptable practice.
- Physicians input the order into a computer terminal and the order is transmitted to the pharmacy.
- The physician writes the medication order on a separate blank, commonly for home use.

Most hospitals use procedures whereby the pharmacist obtains a direct copy of the physician's medication orders. The pharmacy department makes medications available at the patient care area for patient use usually in one of four ways:

1. A floor stock system
2. Individual labeled prescription for each patient
3. Patient-specific unit dose dispensing either filled in the central pharmacy or at the patient care area
4. Decentralized automation with a computerized link from the patient's profile to the automation to allow appropriate medication availability for the individual patient, or
5. A combination of the above.

Systems 1 and 2 are considered poor medication control methods in comparison with systems 3 or 4; however, until all hospitals adopt these unit-dose concepts, pharmacists often must operate with less desirable systems.

Medications dispensed under a *floor stock system* are of two classes: no charge and charge. No charge floor stock consists of a predetermined list of medications that are available on the patient care area of the hospital for use at no specific charge to the patient. Usually these items are inexpensive pharmaceuticals that have universal patient use (eg, alcohol, lotion, water for injection, normal saline injection). Usually, orders are received from each patient care area. In other hospitals, the pharmacy assumes the responsibility for restocking and maintaining the no charge floor stock medications. Under such a system, the nurse is relieved of having to maintain an inventory control, fill out a daily requisition order, and return the medication items to the shelves. Adequate controls can be set up on the basis of usage in relation to number of patient days per given interval of time. Some hospitals have adopted electronic data-processing procedures or bar code technology to handle the totaling and cost extension of medications issued and the preparation of monthly medication usage reports for each patient care area.

Charge floor stock is medication that is available at each patient care area of the hospital and for which a charge is made to the patient. Certain medications are required to be used almost immediately after the physician prescribes them, and it is not practical to obtain them from pharmacy in each instance, yet the cost and the volume of usage necessitate a charge to the patient. Such medications are usually injections or other single dose forms. A common method of handling charge floor stock medications is to attach a small removable label, bar code label, or pre-stamped pharmacy requisition form bearing the name of the medication to the charge floor-stock medication. When nurses access the medication, they merely remove the label and affix it to the usual inpatient prescription or requisition slip. This is then used for billing purposes and to replace the medication on the patient care area. The floor-stock system is also used in small hospitals where pharmacists are not available to dispense individual doses for patients. Most hospitals are switching to point-of-care automated dispensing technology for storage, charging, and inventory control of floor stock medications, particularly controlled substances. This eliminates the need for most of the manual inventory control, automates charging, and enhances controlled substance medication security and documentation.

Individual prescription patient medications are compounded and dispensed similarly to other prescriptions, except that the name and location of the patient is included on the label. The individual prescription method of distribution is used predominately in small hospitals where a pharmacist is not on the premises all the time.

In hospital pharmacy practice, medications are kept secure in a patient care area. The nurse or an assistant is responsible for administering the appropriate medication to each patient in the patient care area. Thus, it is important to know what medication is being administered. It is the nurse's professional responsibility to observe the patient for untoward adverse reactions and report this to the patient's physician. Individual prescriptions are commonly multiple doses of medications to be administered during the patient's hospital stay. A typical inpatient prescription label would contain the following information:

Mr. John Jones	Digoxin 0.25 mg	Room 608E
Number		#10
Lot #	Exp Date	
Doctor's name	Date	

To expedite the dispensing of inpatient prescription medications, hospital pharmacists have adopted the practice of prepackaging frequently used medications in standard administration quantities. It is not unusual for most of the inpatient prescription medications under this system to be prepackaged. Prepackaging medications requires accurate procedures, controls, and records to trace the identity of the medication at all time. Thus, a prepackaging control record form is used for documentation of manufacturer's control numbers, expiration date, pharmacy control number that appears on each prepackaged container label, and the pharmacist responsible for checking the prepackaging operation. In the case of a medication recalled by a manufacturer, the pharmacist easily can trace prepackaged quantities of the medication in question.

Hospitals pharmacies distributing medications use *the individual inpatient prescription system and the floor stock medication system* often use a combination of the two. Medications that are free floor stock are charged against the patient care service; however, in the final analysis, the patient does pay for the medications, because the cost is included as a part of the patient care service portion of the daily room rate.

Because of the large number and variety of medications stored on patient care areas—including individual patient prescriptions, free and charge floor stock, narcotics and other controlled medications, investigational medications, and emergency medication tray—it is an important responsibility of the pharmacist to inspect these medications routinely. Proper storage conditions must be adhered to, dated medications must be checked, narcotic medications must be safeguarded, and discontinued medications must be removed from the patient care area. To ensure proper control of medications in the patient care area, the pharmacist or the designated support person prepares a report to the nursing and pharmacy managers. The condition of a patient care area medication station may warrant attention by personnel from both departments. In some hospitals, pharmacists are assigned to specific patient care areas to coordinate the medications and address the medication therapy problems at the patient care area level. These pharmacists function as part of the patient care team.[10] Some hospitals also have technicians assigned to specific patient care areas to assist in the technical medication coordination activities.

The safest most accepted method of dispensing medications to hospitalized patients is called *unit dose dispensing* and has become the standard of practice in most hospitals today. In this system, the pharmacist prepares each dose of medication ready for administration, rather than issuing containers of medications to patient care areas where the nurse must prepare the medication for administration. For example, tablets and capsules are labeled and dispensed as a single dose for each patient, liquids are measured, lyophilized injections diluted and measured accurately into sterile syringes, parenteral medication admixtures added to intravenous solutions prior to use, and oral powders and other unusual dosage forms measured and mixed appropriately. Most of these procedures involve pharmaceutical techniques that are the pharmacist's responsibility. Hospital pharmacists use various models for the safe and efficient distribution of medications in their hospitals. Such distribution models may involve a centralized pharmacy and/or decentralized pharmacies in the patient care areas, centralized automation and/or decentralized automated dispensing technology, and information scheduling and retrieval.

The unit dose dispensing concept has changed many of the traditional functions of the hospital pharmacist. For example, the traditional prepackaging system of multiple doses of medications has evolved to the use of tablet and capsule strip packaging, labeling machines, and liquid unit dose packaging equipment. This is necessary since all medications are not available from the industry in unit dose packages. The traditional individual inpatient prescription also is eliminated and thereby eliminates prescription labeling. Free and charge floor-stock medication activities essentially are eliminated. A 2002 ASHP national survey of hospital-based pharmaceutical services in indicated that 89% of all hospitals employed the unit-dose-dispensing system; 81% dispensed more than three quarters of oral doses as unit doses and 63% of injectable doses to non-critical care patients.[11] This medication distribution system has become the standard of practice.

Unit dose dispensing lends itself to automation and the interface of that automation with various information systems supporting the medication use process. In practice there is a centralized philosophy and a decentralized philosophy to the use of automation. The centralized approach includes robotic technology operating from a central area. Medications are retrieved and placed in patient specific containers for transport to the patient care area and administration as directed by information received through an interface with the pharmacy information system. The decentralized approach involves the use of automated dispensing technology placed in the patient care areas. This technology is interfaced with the pharmacy information system and provides the caregiver access to medications prescribed for their patients. Both central and decentral technologies are capable of interfaces with information systems used in other components of the medication use process such as administration, documentation, and billing. This eliminates the traditional nurses' medication Kardex® (profile), medication ticket, and manual record of medication administered system of patients' medication therapy profiles. Additionally the creation of a single information source to support the medication use process eliminates the potential for conflicting information and provides a common record for all caregivers.

The General Accounting Office (GAO) studied several distribution systems in its *Study of Health-Care Facilities Construction Costs* (December 1972) and reported that in addition to safer and better patient care through minimization of medication errors, the unit-dose system was to be recommended because of its favorable life cycle cost-to-benefit ratio. The JCAHO also recommends the unit-dose distribution system. The ASHP *Statement on the Pharmacist's Responsibility for Distribution and Control of Drug Products* (1996) and the ASHP *Technical Assistance Bulletin on Hospital Drug Distribution and Control* (1981) provide the best demonstrated practices in hospitals for the medication use process.

PATIENT SELF-ADMINISTRATION OF MEDICATIONS IN HOSPITALS—Pharmacists have generally considered a unit-dose dispensing system as a panacea for hospital medication problems. However, unit-dose dispensing systems primarily have been *pharmacy-centered* rather than *patient-centered*. Many hospitals have developed patient self-administration programs as an alternative medication administration method for selected patients.

The self-administration of medications by patients in the hospital offers many advantages. It allows patients to assume more responsibility for their direct care, to learn how to use medications properly, and to be able to anticipate potential side effects and other medication-related problems. It provides a salient opportunity for the pharmacist to help educate patients on the safe and proper use of medications, and, thereby, alleviates much dedicated time spent by nurses and physicians performing this essential function. The objective is that patients should become more knowledgeable about their medication, thus enhancing proper and safe use of medications during hospitalization and after their discharge.

Self-administration of medications by patients can be implemented effectively on numerous hospital services, such as obstetrics, surgery, medicine, physical medicine and rehabilitation, and even in psychiatry.[12,13] Generally, patients with stable medication regimens, receiving chronic medications and in good physical and mental health are appropriate candidates for self-administration. Again, a procedural manual should be prepared that outlines the methods used to implement a patient self-administration program as part of a unit-dose distribution system. A self-administration medication program provides patients possession of their medication and makes them responsible for its administration. The nurse and pharmacist then make rounds to ensure that patients are using their medication properly.

A nurse-administered medication program is the appropriate system for most hospitalized patients. This program is used for patients who are not capable of self-administering their medications or for those medications that patients cannot administer by themselves.

INVESTIGATIONAL MEDICATIONS—These medications are often studied in the hospital setting where patients are supported by various diagnostic and treatment resources. The hospital pharmacist is in a strategic position to participate in the evaluation of investigational medications.

There are, however, many problems associated with the use of investigational medications in the hospital, some of which are as follows:

- Legal liabilities for the hospital if there is improper handling of investigational medications in the overall care of the patient.
- Nurses, as agents of the hospital, usually are responsible for administering investigational medications to patients. In performing this act, it is essential that sufficient information on the proper dosage, route of administration, possible adverse/toxic reactions and side effects, precautions, and proper labeling is available to them.
- Investigational medications, as they are made available from the manufacturer to the principal investigator, are not labeled sufficiently in many instances to prevent the possibility of error in their administration to patients.
- Because investigational medications fall in the area of research, in contrast to accepted methods of treatment, there are legal implications revolving around the need for written, informed consent by patients.
- In the case of double-blind studies, it is essential that the person holding the code be readily available 24 hours a day, 7 days a week, in the event a patient's condition warrants "breaking the code."

The FDA has delineated the legal requirements for proper records on the use of investigational medications. In case of a recall due to severe toxicity resulting from an investigational medication, it is essential that records of its use on specific patients in a hospital be readily available. In cases in which the lot number of the medication is a significant factor, such records also should be available.

In cases in which investigational medications are used for outpatients, it is essential that such medications be labeled and packaged to conform to legal requirements, such as child-proof packaging requirements and controlled substances requirements. Information must readily be available to assist physicians in other hospitals who may be required to treat patients suffering from over dosage, toxic symptoms, or illnesses or condition unrelated to the investigational medications.

It is essential that the supply of an investigational medication be available 24 hours per day if nurses are to maintain uninterrupted dosage schedules in the best interest of the patient. The hospital pharmacist needs to maintain adequate dispensing records (Fig 127-3) for all investigational medications dispensed.

Thus, the problems associated with the proper handling of investigational medications provide ample justification to warrant the establishment of sound policies and procedures governing their use in the hospital. This is a responsibility of the medical staff. The P&T Committee or Investigational Review Board (IRB) in collaboration with the P&T Committee should have the responsibility to formulate policies and procedures relative to the handling of investigational medications. To assist the committees, the ASHP developed a guideline on Pharmaceutical Research in Organized Heath-Care Setting and on Clinical Drug Research (1998) embodying basic principles applicable to the safe handling of investigational medications in the hospital. The International Conference on Harmonisation of Technical Requirements for Registration of Pharmaceuticals for Human Use (ICH) has developed a quality standard for designing, conducting, recording and reporting trials that involve the participation of human subjects.[14] The hospital pharmacist, as a key member of the P&T Committee, makes a real contribution to better patient care and safety by participating in formulating policies and procedures for handling investigational medications in the hospital. Often, pharmacists serve on the Institutional Review Board of a hospital and are involved with the review of all investigational studies involving humans. The pharmacist can provide valuable insight on the design, economics and ethics involved in medication studies in human patients.

Clinically, many hospital pharmacists are involved with the care of patients receiving investigational medications such as

THE UNIVERSITY OF KANSAS MEDICAL CENTER
PHARMACY DEPARTMENT

INVESTIGATIONAL DRUG DISPENSING RECORD

Name and Synonyms _____

Strength and Dosage Form _____

Manufacturer _____

Principal Investigator _____

Date	Patient Name	Case Number	Physician	Rx # or Location	Lot Number	Amount Dispensed	Amount on Hand

Figure 127-3. Investigational Drug Dispensing Record.

patients on an oncology medical service. These pharmacists often participate in patient monitoring, medication preparation and administration of investigational medications. Patient consent and patient information are essential in such activities. Pharmacists often provide specific written medication information to patients so that they may have a better understanding of their medication regimen and the various side effects or problems to expect.

A single prescription for a single patient does not raise the question of investigational medication use. Preparing large quantities of medications that have not been approved for human use by the FDA can violate the federal law. To avoid legal violation, a sponsor of a medication investigation must file a *Notice of Claimed Investigational Exemption for a New Drug* (IND) with the FDA. A pharmaceutical manufacturer usually files such a form; however, others may serve as the sponsor, such as a physician, pharmacist, an institution, such as a hospital, or the hospital pharmacy department.

An abbreviated form of IND is acceptable to the FDA when a physician wants to study a medication that is not sponsored by a manufacturer. The physician may serve both as sponsor and investigator, or the hospital pharmacy may serve as sponsor and the physician as investigator. Some hospital pharmacy departments serve as sponsors on many abbreviated INDs for special medication dosage forms that are not available commercially. The required forms for the sponsor and investigator plus the new-medication regulations are available from the FDA.

INTRAVENOUS ADMIXTURES—Hospital pharmacists are well trained to organize, develop, and operate a centralized pharmacy intravenous admixture service.[15] These services have been found to:

- Save nursing time for other professional nursing roles
- Provide a system for screening physical-chemical incompatibilities and dispensing stable preparations
- Minimize pharmaceutical calculation errors
- Reduce the risk of medication error by providing additional checks.[16]

- Centralize responsibility for preparation of parenteral admixtures.
- Label admixtures with rate of infusion as prescribed by the physician and provides a standardized label format
- Provide an aseptic environment for the preparation of admixtures
- Conform to the standards recommended by the JCAHO
- Conform to the guidelines established by the National Coordinating Committee on Large-Volume Parenterals
- Provide a mechanism for appropriately creating patient charges
- Provide for the preparation of solutions that are not commercially available

The JCAHO wisely promulgated the concept that the pharmacist should be involved in the preparation of medications preparing intravenous admixtures. In its 2004 *Standards for Accreditation,*[17] frequently, the JCAHO refers to the subject of the safe and accurate handling of all medications, including intravenous admixtures. One especially relevant statement is:

> When an on-site, licensed pharmacy is available, only the pharmacy compounds or admixes all sterile medications, intravenous admixtures, or other drugs except in emergencies or when not feasible (for example, the products stability is short).

In rising to the challenge posed by the JCAHO, it is essential that the pharmacist be involved in preparing intravenous admixtures. The responsibility for preparing intravenous admixtures is actually the same as that assumed for the unit-dose distribution system. It is important that specific guidelines for an effective intravenous admixture program are formulated.

The ASHP has furnished a document entitled *Quality Assurance for Pharmacy-Prepared Sterile Products* (1996).[18] These guidelines promote greater attention to clean-room technology, personnel training, validation, and quality assurance procedures. Specific guidelines for compounding cytotoxic and hazardous medications are also provided by the ASHP in a technical assistance bulletin. The intravenous admixture service can serve as a base for other pharmacy services such as chemotherapy compounding, allergy extract preparation, and parenteral home care programs.

AMBULATORY CARE SERVICES—As ambulatory care activities continue to increase within the institutional setting, the hospital pharmacist becomes more and more involved in providing services to these patients. These patients are often seen in clinic settings, by home care services, by hospice services, infusion centers, etc. Pharmacists practicing in ambulatory care settings have expanded many of the service concepts initiated in the hospital and the community pharmacy settings. They include special patient information brochures, patient dosing calendars, special packaging, patient education for home care, review of prescribing practices and recommendations for improvement, development of therapeutic protocols, etc. In addition, pharmacists in some clinics have collaborative practice agreements with physicians that allow the pharmacist to monitor selected patients and prescribe or adjust specific medication therapy in accordance with the agreement or protocol (eg, anticoagulation, hypertension, asthma, diabetes). These collaborative practice agreements can be established in most states. However, as of this publication, pharmacists are not currently recognized by the Center for Medicare and Medicaid as a provider, and therefore cannot bill independently for these services. The ASHP has promulgated a guideline to assist pharmacists entitled *Minimum Standard for Pharmaceutical Services in Ambulatory Care* (1999). These activities will continue to increase as more emphasis is placed on ambulatory care as part of the total patient care program by hospitals and, ultimately, when pharmacists achieve provider recognition.

TECHNOLOGY AND AUTOMATION IN PHARMACEUTICAL CARE—Significant progress has been made through the use of computers and hardware technology such as automation devices, robots, and point of care automated dispensing technology.[19,20] This development has been in concert with the pharmacist's responsibility for medication distribution and control. Intravenous solution compounders provide efficient methods of aseptically formulating various sterile solutions and additives into a final intravenous admixture product. Robotics connected to the pharmacy computer are able to package and select medications that are patient-specific for distribution by pharmacy. Other robots can select the appropriate medication, count a specified quantity, place the medications into a dispensing vial, and label the vial with patient-specific directions for ambulatory care pharmacy practice. Prescription dispensing machines can select the appropriate prescription medication vial, label the vial with the patient-specific information and instructions, and provide written patient teaching information upon receipt of electronic physician order. Decentralized point of care stations located on patient-care areas can provide the nurse access to medications for patient administration. These decentralized point-of-care systems are akin to bank automated teller machines (ATMs) in that they are controlled centrally and provide only restricted authorized access. They should be programmed only to allow access to medications for which that patient has an order on designated floor stock medications. As these new technology systems develop, the pharmacist must incorporate them safely into the hospital's medication distribution system to continue appropriate medication control throughout the hospital.

CLINICAL PHARMACY—The concept of *clinical* or *patient-oriented* pharmacy service has gained tremendous acceptance in hospital pharmacy. The hospital environment offers the hospital pharmacist a multitude of opportunities to develop meaningful clinical roles in the safe and rational use of medications in hospitalized, as well as ambulatory patients. This chapter does not include a detailed discussion of the hospital pharmacist's clinical roles and responsibilities because they are discussed elsewhere in this publication.

It is important to note that significant progress is being made in providing ongoing clinical pharmacy services in hospitals. Various service functions are described in the ASHP *Statement on the Role of the Pharmacist in Patient-Focused Care* (1995).

As increased emphasis is placed on cost containment in hospitals and improved medication-therapy utilization, the pharmacist has been valuable in monitoring patient medication utilization and promoting rational therapy. The pharmacist can best carry out the mandate of the P&T Committee relative to appropriate medication therapy. An evolution of clinical pharmacy practice is occurring in that pharmacists are embracing the concept of pharmaceutical care. In essence, the pharmacist is becoming a medication-therapy manager.

Pharmacists often document their clinical workload for various administrative purposes. This documentation often involves recording clinical interventions, financial impact of their interventions, and impact on patient care. Historically, pharmacists have used forms developed within hospital pharmacy departments, and, increasingly, are using computers or hand-held personal digital assistants (PDAs) to document workload numbers.

Documentation of clinical services, pharmaceutical care, and associated patient outcomes is important to illustrate the role and contribution of the pharmacist. The patient-specific information and the pharmacists' assessment, plan, recommendations and monitoring should be recorded in the patient's medical record so the information can be shared with other caregivers.

FUTURE PRACTICE—In reviewing the activities of hospital pharmacy practice, one must conclude that no two hospital practices are alike. Hospital pharmacy practice has made significant strides over the past three decades in changing the practice of pharmacists to provide a more patient-oriented pharmacy service. Medication distribution systems have been improved (unit dose and intravenous admixture services), and patient oriented clinical services have been implemented in large and small hospitals alike. Computerization and automation have increased efficiency and provide improved patient and management databases. Practice in hospitals has adjusted to the changing environment of health care. The challenge for the institutional pharmacist and the profession as a whole is to provide pharmaceutical care to all patients by shifting emphasis (not responsibility) from medication distribution to patient care. What the future holds for hospital pharmacy practice in the year 2010 is only speculation. However, it is very likely that dispensing automation, technology, automated medical records and prescriber order entry will free pharmacy staff time spent on technical activities. Technician roles and responsibilities will expand in overseeing medication automation and technical dispensing functions. Pharmacist roles will continue to focus on managing and optimizing medication therapy for inpatients and ambulatory patients, developing medication guidelines and protocols, and optimizing safe medication systems and services. With the significant progress in the last few years, one can be assured that the role of the hospital pharmacist on the health care team will be significant and will be directed at meeting the medication therapy needs of the patient. Thus, the hospital environment provides a rewarding career for the pharmacist.

REFERENCES

1. *Hospitals* 1964; 38(Jan 1): 109.
2. 2002 AHA Guide; Registration Requirements for Hospitals, A2-A3
3. 1992 AHA Guide tot he Healthcare Field, Chicago: Am Hosp assoc.
4. 2003 AHA Hospital Statistics
5. Niemeyer GF, et al. *Bull Am Soc Hosp Pharm* 1962; 9(4): 287.
6. Spease E, Porter RM. *JAPhA* 1936; 25: 65,
7. *AJHP* 2001; 58:1524
8. *AJHP* 2003; 60:37
9. *AJHP* 2001; 58:2251–66.
10. Hynniman C. AJHP 1991; 48:524.
11. AJHP 2003; 60:52–68
12. Roberts C, et al. *Drug Intel Clin Pharm* 1972; 6(12): 408.
13. Lucarotti RL, et al. *AJHP* 1973; 30(12): 1147.
14. International Conference on Harmonisation of Technical Requirements for Registration of Pharmaceuticals for Human Use (ICH) web site: (http://www.ich.org/pdfICH/e6.pdf)
15. Shoup LK, Godwin HN. *Implementation Guide for a Centralized Intravenous Admixture Program.* Travenol, 1977.
16. Thur MP, et al. *AJHP* 1972; 29(4): 298.
17. JCAHO 2004 Pre-publication Edition. www.jcaho.org/accredited+organizations/2004+standards.htm
18. *AJHP* 1993; 50:2386.
19. Felkey BG, et al. *JAPhA* 1996; NS36: 309.
20. Williams SJ, et al. *Hosp Pharm* 1996; 31: 1093.

BIBLIOGRAPHY

American Society of Health-System Pharmacists. Best Practices for Health-System Pharmacy: Positions and Guidance Documents of ASHP 2002–2003 Edition. ASHP Bethesda, MD. Also available on web site www.ashp.org.

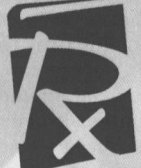

CHAPTER 128

Emergency Medicine Pharmacy Practice

Maria I Rudis, PharmD, DABAT, FCCM, BCPS
Payal Patel, BSc(Pharm), PharmD

OVERVIEW OF EMERGENCY MEDICINE AND EMERGENCY MEDICINE PHARMACY PRACTICE

Emergency medicine (EM) is an extremely exciting and rewarding area of pharmacy practice. The emergency department's (ED) unpredictability, potential chaotic activity, and patient complexity epitomize the specialty of EM.[1] Clinicians who work in the ED must be able to multi-task and identify the urgency of a task. Clinical services including nursing, pharmacy, social work, radiology, respiratory therapy, and home-care play a critical, central role in the optimal management of a patient presenting to the ED.

The ED serves as one of the first point of care destinations for any patient. A unique quality of EM is that no patient in extremis may be denied or refused care.[2] In this day of budget constraint and diminishing resources, the ED has become the safety net of last resort in a society with millions of underserved, uninsured patients.[1] There are various types of EDs ranging from relatively low-acuity to large trauma centers. Despite the differences in design, the one commonality is the wide spectrum of diseases that are encountered in the ED.

Pharmacists have played a key role in the ED since the 1970s.[3] Initial services focused on inventory control and cost-containment issues and the development of 24-hour pharmacy satellites to ensure accurate inventory of all medications and appropriate intravenous admixture preparation.[4] Clinical pharmacy services have evolved to include identification of drug-related problems, adverse drug reaction surveillance, pharmacokinetic and toxicology consultation, on-call pharmacy services, and provision of cardiopulmonary resuscitation.[3–8] However, a recent survey demonstrated an overall lack of pharmacy services in the ED. The authors surveyed hospital pharmacy departments with pharmacy practice residencies. They documented that only 3.4% of hospitals (n = 4/119)) reported having an ED satellite pharmacy. Further, only 13 (10.9%) of the remaining hospitals surveyed had a clinical pharmacist whose primary responsibility was to provide services to the ED.[4] These results illustrate that the majority of teaching hospitals in the US do not have pharmacy services in the ED. However, 30% (31/119) of the survey respondents stated that they planned to look for funding for ED pharmacy services in the future. This illustrates the potential growth and demand for pharmacists and pharmacy services in the ED.

DRUG-RELATED ISSUES IN THE EMERGENCY DEPARTMENT

Many ED visits and subsequent hospital admissions are in some part, if not entirely, related to a drug-related problem. Drug-related problems can be classified into eight categories: untreated indication, improper drug selection, subtherapeutic dosage, failure to receive drugs (includes patient noncompliance/nonadherence), overdosage, adverse drug reaction, drug interaction, and drugs used without an indication.[9] Although most drug-related problems can be resolved without a major impact on patient health, many are associated with significant morbidity and mortality.[10,11] A probability model estimated that morbidity and mortality associated with drug-related problems account for $76.6 billion in hospital costs, 17 million EM visits, and 8.7 million hospital admissions annually in the US.[12]

Several published reports have documented the problem of drug-related hospital admissions due to adverse drug reactions.[10,11,13] Hospital admissions secondary to all categories of drug-related problems as described above are likely much higher than those solely described for adverse effects.[9] A systematic search of reports published in the English language suggests drug-related problems account for as many as 28% of ED visits, of which as many as 24% result in hospital admissions. Approximately 70% of the drug-related visits to the ED were deemed preventable.[14] A clinical pharmacist in the ED may aid in identifying and resolving drug-related issues with subsequent reductions in recidivism, morbidity, mortality, and economic burden placed on the US health-care system.

SCOPE OF DISEASE

Some of the more common disease states presenting to a general adult ED include: acute stroke, sepsis, status epilepticus, acute respiratory exacerbations (eg, asthma, chronic obstructive pulmonary disease [COPD]), acute coronary syndromes (ie, both ST and non-ST-elevation myocardial infarction), congestive heart failure, cardiac arrhythmias, hypertensive urgencies/emergencies, thromboembolic disease (ie, deep vein and pulmonary thrombosis), acute peptic ulcer disease, acute pancreatitis, diabetic ketoacidosis, and various pain management issues. Depending on the location of the hospital (eg, proximity to an expressway, lower socioeconomic neighborhood), an ED pharmacist may also encounter patients presenting with trauma, various infectious diseases (eg, meningitis, malaria, tuberculosis, pneumonia, endocarditis, urosepsis, skin and soft-tissue infections) and drug overdoses.

PATIENT SELECTION

The ED clinician faces the challenge of addressing pharmacotherapeutic issues of diverse critically ill and non-critically ill as well as ambulatory patients simultaneously. One mechanism to help identify patients who would most benefit from a pharmacotherapeutic consultation is based on the general principle of triaging. In simplest terms, triage can be defined as the sorting or prioritizing of items (eg, patients, tasks).[15] Generally, patients with conditions requiring immediate stabilization involving drug therapy (eg, status epilepticus, diabetic ketoacidosis, acute coronary syndromes, cardiac arrhythmias, drug-overdose) should be assessed by the pharmacist first. Other situations, such as therapeutic drug monitoring, various infectious diseases, and patients on medications with a narrow therapeutic index, may be seen after the urgent patients are seen, with admitted or stable patients seen thereafter. Further triaging by the pharmacist may be quite different from that of a nurse or a physician. Another excellent triage mechanism is a direct referral by a fellow clinician (eg, physician, nurse, social work) for a pharmacotherapeutic consultation. In addition, the type of hospital and the individual priority programs identified at that particular institution might help guide the pharmacist in developing a triage system. Furthermore, a pharmacy clinician's skill set and training (eg, focus on trauma or critically ill patients, ambulatory care patients) may also influence the priority given to development of specific pharmacist-based programs in the ED (eg, toxicology consultation, pharmacist-driven medication refill program, asthma management).

EVALUATION OF THE ED PATIENT

Usually, time is a limiting factor in the ED. Thus, it is important to stress that the pharmacist's assessment or evaluation of the patient may occur concurrently with other clinicians. In general, when patients present to the ED, they have very limited formal medical information with them (ie, medical chart, consultation notes, laboratory data). However, if the patient is able to communicate effectively, his/her history is of great importance in patient assessment. Diagnosis of various conditions has been estimated to be based 76% on history, 12% on physical exam, with 12% attributed to ancillary studies (eg, laboratory, radiographic studies).[1] The initial patient examination should focus on the urgent, pharmacy-relevant concerns of the patient. Other medical problems not related to the patient's chief complaint should be addressed by a primary care provider, outside the scope of the ED visit.

Before the patient interview, the clinician should become familiar with the ambulance report, the triage nurse assessment, and the physician's evaluation to date and an old patient chart, if it is available. It is essential for the pharmacist to determine if the patient's chief complaint or reason for ED presentation may be related to particular medications/drug(s), and then develop a pharmaceutical care plan for management in the ED, and for continuation upon admission or discharge.

To this end, it is essential to perform a complete medication history focusing on prescription, over-the-counter medications, herbal and alternative therapies. The medication history should be performed in consultation with the patient or family members as many patients may take their medications differently than that indicated on the prescription vial. Another excellent resource is the patient's usual community pharmacy. For patients who tend to return to the same hospital, the ED pharmacy clinician should refer to medications prescribed/dispensed during previous visits to the ED or other clinics. Inpatient pharmacists on various clinical services may be able to provide a pharmacy-related history (eg, medication history, medication adherence, allergy status, medication-related issues, past medical history). By contacting the in-patient pharmacy clinician, the ED clinician can convey the patient's current medication-related concerns to the pharmacist that will be taking care of the patient if he/she is admitted.

In general, the medication assessment in conjunction with a head to toe evaluation of the patient will help ensure all the drug-related issues are identified/discovered. However, in the event the patient/family may be unable/unavailable to provide any medical or medication history, the physical examination and history from the scene (ie, obtained from the paramedics)

takes on even greater importance. In cases where no information is available, the pharmacy clinician, in similar fashion to the ED physician, must use 'detective' skills in combination with his/her knowledge of disease, pharmacology and toxicology to identify potential drug-related problems. In many cases, decisions regarding the ED management will need to be made without the benefit of an extensive work-up.

CONTINUITY OF CARE (SEAMLESS CARE) CONCEPT

Seamless care may be defined as the continuity of patient care between an institution and the community setting, with the goal of optimizing the patient's potential for wellness with as little disruption as possible to the patient's therapy.[16,17] Seamless care involves the transfer of relevant information between caregivers, with the overall intent to improve patient care and health outcomes.[18] Continuity of patient care can occur in a number of different ways (eg, ED to inpatient floor, ED to community partners, ED to patient). It is also important to remember that seamless care is a dynamic process, whereby information may also be transferred back to the ED to optimize patient care in the ED or during hospitalization.[17]

Seamless Care in the Hospital

Communication among health care providers within the hospital environment is a key component in striving to optimize patient care. The prompt initiation and continuation of optimal pharmacotherapy in the ED improves the likelihood of a faster resolution of disease and decrease the hospital length of stay.[19] It is routine for physicians and nurses to 'give report' from the point of origin of the patient (ie, ED) to the floor where the patient is to be admitted (ie, intensive care unit (ICU), in-patient, another institution to where the patient is transferred). A similar interaction should occur between the ED and in-patient pharmacists. Such communication should include details of the patient's presentation, ED course and treatment as well as the intended pharmacotherapeutic plan. The ED pharmacist may start a formal patient profile that is then transferred with the patient once he/she is admitted. This may occur electronically in a fully computerized medication administration record. This process reduces the likelihood of unnecessary medication changes upon admission and improves the continuity of care. In fact, increased communication among health professionals throughout the continuum of in-patient care has been shown to reduce the likelihood of errors.[20]

Seamless Care in the Community

Just as communication between the ED and other health care providers may improve care in the in-patient setting, the same can be accomplished in the outpatient setting upon ED discharge. Discharge from a hospital can be a very confusing and stressful experience for a patient, as he/she attempts to understand and recall elaborate medication changes and other directions despite feeling unwell.

Medication management is an especially important post-discharge issue. Many medications may have been added, deleted, or modified in some manner. This is confusing for the patient and for the health care providers in the community (ie, family physician, community pharmacist).[21] Furthermore, continuity of care (including monitoring of therapies started in the hospital) is more likely to occur if the community providers have a clear understanding of the reason for changes made in the patient's drug therapy.[22] For example, a pharmacy discharge letter is sent routinely to family physicians and community pharmacists for patients discharged from the geriatric unit at the Royal Victoria Hospital in Quebec, Canada. Specific information communicated in the discharge letter includes: medications upon admission, medications upon discharge, diagnosis (hospital admission), various laboratory values, reasons for treatment modification, and any required follow-up. Physicians, pharmacists, and nurses deemed the letter as being helpful in facilitating the transmission of pertinent information regarding the patient's drug regimen to the community health care providers.[22]

Telephone calls made to patients directly after an ED visit have been shown to increase patient satisfaction, increase patient adherence to follow-up appointments, and improved patient compliance to discharge instructions.[23-26] Dudas et al. demonstrated that follow-up telephone calls after discharge made specifically by pharmacists were associated with increased patient satisfaction, resolution of medication-related problems, and fewer return visits to the ED.[27] The authors also observed a trend toward fewer hospital readmissions within 30 days of discharge for patients receiving a telephone call. Approximately 15% of patients reported new symptoms or concerns during the follow-up telephone call, while 19% were unable to obtain all of their medications prescribed upon discharge. Therefore, the pharmacist who made the follow-up call may have been able to intervene and, subsequently, helped in preventing return ED visits.

PREVENTION OF HOSPITAL RE-ADMISSION

Effective means of sharing the pharmaceutical care plan with either in-patient clinicians or community health care providers is essential in helping to prevent re-admission or future ED visits.[14,17,18,22-27] Leaving a detailed note in the patient's medical record is an excellent means of sharing the care plan with multiple disciplines. For patients who are being discharged directly from the ED, a letter or note written in collaboration with the ED physician is also a great mechanism to provide useful information to the family physician and/or community pharmacist. Finally, the practitioner must remember to communicate the care plan to the patient. This care plan should include patient education and counseling regarding drug therapy and importance of compliance. Once patients understand why their medications are altered (and even understand why they take various medications), it is likely they will be adherent to the prescribed regimen. Ultimately, it is the patient who is responsible for the direction of their health care; hence, it is important to involve him/her in the decision-making process whenever possible.

PHARMACY SERVICES IN THE EMERGENCY DEPARTMENT

Scope and Standards of Practice

There are currently no standards of practice for ED pharmacy services. Pharmacists in the ED setting perform a broad range of distributive, clinical, teaching, and research activities. Some of these activities in teaching hospitals have recently been described by Thomasset et al. and are summarized in Table 128-1.[4] The nature and extent of pharmacy services and pharmacist activities vary from institution to institution.

Distributive Services

Traditionally, drug distribution services in the ED have involved ward stock supply of medications. Provision of unit dose packaging with a 24-hour supply of medication has been limited in the ED setting because a decision regarding patient disposition is usually made quickly. This has also meant that, traditionally, there has been inadequate accountability of medication use in the ED setting. In recent years, ED overcrowding has become a greater issue due to downsizing of hos-

TABLE 128-1. Clinical Pharmacy Services Provided to Emergency

SERVICE	NO. (%) HOSPITALS
Medication-error or adverse-drug-reaction reporting	71 (59.7)
Order clarification	64 (53.8)
Drug or toxicology information	60 (50.4)
Formulary adjustment	51 (42.9)
Cardiopulmonary resuscitation participation	42 (35.3)
Allergy screening	42 (35.3)
ED inservice meetings	44 (37.0)
Drug interaction screening	39 (32.8)
Antimicrobial dosing	36 (30.3)
Drug-use review	36 (30.3)
Renal dosing	33 (27.7)
Drug therapy recommendation	33 (27.7)
Pharmacokinetic dosing	29 (24.4)
Patient education and counseling	24 (20.2)
Research activities	23 (19.3)
Assessment of patient contraindications to therapy	22 (18.5)
Serving as preceptor for students and residents	22 (18.5)
Medication history review	11 (9.2)
Other	13 (10.9)

pital beds and a shortage of ICU beds (ie, due to nursing shortages). As a result, patients admitted to the hospital do tend to stay in the ED for prolonged periods of time waiting for a bed.[28-30] According to the Joint Commission on Accreditation of Healthcare Organizations (JCAHO) standards, a patient's medication profile should be reviewed once they are in the hospital for 24 hours.[31] This necessitates a pharmacist's review of medications in the ED, and also raises the issue of provision and accountability of medication use in this setting.

With the advent of technology, many institutions have elected to place automated drug dispensing machines (eg, Pyxis machines) in the ED setting as is common in the ICU or operating room (OR) settings. These are operational either 24 hours a day or only at night, when pharmacy services from either a central location or another satellite pharmacy are not available. These systems provide accountability for drug use and may be related to the individual obtaining the medication as well as the individual patient for whom the drug is intended. They may also facilitate evaluation of drug inventory levels as well as drug utilization reviews. However, pilfering and inappropriate drug selections are not prevented, nor is a patient's medication order reviewed prior to dispensing with this method.

An ED pharmacy satellite staffed with pharmacists and pharmacy technicians is likely the most optimal method of providing fast, accurate, and accountable drug distribution to ED patients. Pharmacy satellites in the ED have been described in the literature since 1985.[32] They have been shown to be cost-effective compared with traditional ward stock systems.[33] Having the pharmacy prepare IV admixtures in the ED pharmacy satellite removes this responsibility from the nurses whose time and effort should be directed to nursing patient care activities. Like the ICU and OR, the ED is a 24-hour operation and pharmacy services should be provided on a 24-hour, 7 days a week basis.[32] As such, most medications, particularly parenteral medications, are needed immediately for patient care and should be available within minutes in the ED setting. Pharmacists have the responsibility of ensuring appropriate stock of all medications used in the ED and, in particular, should be able to quickly provide adequate supplies of commonly used parenteral therapies and uncommonly used antidotes (for toxicological exposure and in instances of exposures to weapons of mass destruction), as well as other commonly used medications used in the ED.[34,35]

Clinical Services

Although there are published guidelines for the scope of practice for pharmacotherapy specialists,[36] clinical pharmacists in primary care,[37] and those practicing in the critical care setting,[38] there are no published guidelines regarding the optimal scope of pharmacy practice or pharmacy-related activities in the ED.[4] The applicability of the aforementioned guidelines to the ED setting may be limited for several reasons. First, the medication needs of patients in the ED may differ from those in the inpatient and primary care settings. Secondly, rapid patient turnover prevents pharmacists from providing standard clinical services and reduces their ability to perform activities that are routine in other settings.[4] Given these caveats, the American College of Clinical Pharmacy (ACCP) practice guidelines for pharmacotherapy specialists may nevertheless be applicable to EM pharmacy clinicians.[36] There are three areas of practice the Guidelines outlined: patient care, education, and research.

Direct Patient Care

The ACCP Guidelines outline the pharmacy clinician's patient care responsibilities in terms of designing, implementing, monitoring, evaluating, and modifying pharmacotherapy to ensure effective, safe, and economical care.[36] In the ED setting, this might involve obtaining a complete medication history including documenting non-prescription, vitamin, herbal, and alternative/complementary therapy use. The clinician should obtain a complete medication history making use of all available and appropriate resources including the patient, medical record, the hospital or community pharmacy, family members, family physician, or provincial/state prescription computer medication records (eg, PharmaNet system in Canada). Various physical assessment skills, interpretation of laboratory studies and diagnostic investigations are necessary to facilitate the implementation of the patient's pharmaceutical care plan. Patient education or counseling is another area of focus for the ED clinician. The pharmacist is a ready source of drug information for the other clinicians in the ED and should be able to retrieve information readily. All of these efforts may decrease the number or frequency of return visits to the ED.

Documentation of patient-specific issues or pharmacotherapeutic care plans in the medical record is also essential for medical-legal reasons and to help facilitate seamless care. Examples of ED pharmacist-driven activities include an ED-based medication refill clinic, toxicology consultation, participation in an acute stroke team, participation in the CPR team, outpatient deep vein thrombosis clinic, outpatient treatment protocol for skin and soft skin tissue infections, facilitation of procedural sedation, and acute pain management, as well as many others.

CHALLENGES TO PATIENT CARE

A variety of barriers may exist to the provision of patient care by the pharmacy clinician in the ED. Communication issues such as language barriers may initially present as a challenge to patient care depending on the ethnic diversity in the surrounding community. Although most hospitals provide interpretative services, these may not be available in a timely manner. In addition, patients who are unable to provide pertinent information, such as those who present with decreased level of consciousness may also pose a problem. These barriers are not unique to the pharmacist, and affect all ED clinicians, and thus, are usually surmountable. Using the patient's family or friends

is an excellent resource for obtaining a history or facilitating an assessment. Patients may also come in with prescription vials with their community pharmacy's name or phone number. The patient's community pharmacist is another resource as he/she can help inform the ED pharmacist of any on-going issues (eg, compliance). Accessing old medical charts (eg, paper charts or electronically through a computer system) may also prove to be a timely resource.

There may also be barriers to carrying out clinical pharmacy activities effectively. ED physicians and nurses may not be aware of the specialized knowledge base, training level and skills of an ED pharmacist. As with any new pharmacy service, the pharmacist may need to educate the other health care workers to overcome any resistance he/she may encounter. Full integration of the pharmacy clinician in the ED requires not only competence, skill, and confidence, but also administrative support from the ED and the pharmacy department or academic unit(s) involved. The pharmacist must also spend a considerable amount of time learning about the unique medications that are used in the ED and the unique 'culture' in the ED setting to be effective.

CRITICAL PATHWAYS

Critical pathways are comprehensive patient care plans incorporating all aspects of patient care relating to disease management based on standards of care, current literature, and benchmarking.[39] Critical pathways are also referred to as CarePath, CareMap, clinical pathway, clinical path of care, case management plan, multidisciplinary action plan, collaborative care tract, and Plan of Care in the literature.[40] Critical pathways describe the care of the patient in full including pharmacotherapy, non-pharmacological strategies, interventions, activities, and outcomes (ie, from diagnosis to post-discharge care).[39] Critical pathways standardize patient care and have been shown to reduce the length of hospital stay for coronary artery bypass patients[41,42] and community-acquired pneumonia.[19] They also improve quality of care for patients with acute stroke[43] and acute coronary syndromes.[44] Some of the general goals of the pathway are to aid in the continuity of care, to decrease fragmentation of services, to guide the patient and family through expected treatment and progress, to optimize cost-effectiveness of health care delivery, and to increase satisfaction of patients, families, staff, physicians, and third-party payers.[45]

The ED pharmacist should be involved in the development and implementation of pathways where drug therapy is extensive, expensive, or high risk (eg, ST-elevation myocardial infarction).[39] The pathway serves as an excellent tool not only for improving patient care but also for conducting pharmacy-driven research (eg, drug utilization reviews, pharmacoeconomic, outcomes research), which subsequently aids in establishing and justifying the pharmacy clinician's presence in the ED, and thus improving patient care.

EMERGENCY PREPAREDNESS

The ED pharmacist and pharmacy satellite have a unique responsibility to assist in the planning for, and to participate actively in, the coordinated response in the advent of an unintentional (eg, natural) or intentional (eg, bioterrorism) disaster. Because ED personnel are linked intricately with local and regional emergency medical services and local and regional disaster planning networks, the pharmacist in the ED has many key roles.

The American Society of Health-System Pharmacists (ASHP) Position Statement on this issue describes how a health-system pharmacist may help in this kind of event.[46] Briefly, the ED pharmacist should be involved in institutional and local disaster planning committees to assist in the selection of pharmaceuticals and related supplies for local and regional emergency inventories. The expertise of the pharmacist allows the planning committees to help develop and disseminate guidelines for the diagnosis and treatment of victims of terrorism attacks. For each biological agent, information should be readily available regarding symptom onset, treatment, post-exposure prophylaxis, patient isolation precautions, and the availability of antidotes at local hospitals. The pharmacist may help develop a procedure for obtaining and preparing antidotes that might not be available or stocked in sufficient quantities because national antidote stockpiles do not arrive quickly and are not designed to supplant local or regional resources.[47,48] The job of a pharmacist during a bioterrorism strike is to make and disseminate antidotes and information rapidly; provide dosage and vaccination schedules for both treatment and prophylaxis, and counsel patients.[34,49–51] During such an event pharmacists will need to find methods to meet the tremendous demand for various medications and to advise prescribers about treatment options. They will receive many telephone calls simultaneously asking for supplies and treatment alternatives.[52] To test the deployment of emergency preparedness plans, the ED pharmacist and pharmacy satellite should participate in organized, institutional disaster drills.

EDUCATION

The pharmacotherapy specialist is responsible for the education of other health care professionals and students, patients, and the public regarding rational use of medications in the ED.[36] The pharmacist is the expert in the field of pharmacotherapy. It is the pharmacy clinician's responsibility to keep current with cutting edge literature, including interpretation and its application to EM. Furthermore, it is also important to educate the rest of the pharmacy department staff regarding new practices in the field of EM to help keep them up-to-date. Most clinical pharmacy specialists will also have an affiliation or a cross-appointment with the faculty/college of pharmacy and/or the school of medicine, with ensuing formal teaching responsibilities. These formal teaching obligations may include coordination of a course or acting as a preceptor to pharmacy or medical students, residents and fellows.

Methods of Education

There are many different teaching opportunities in the ED. The choice of teaching method will depend on the audience and learning objectives. Pharmacist-directed educational activities may include regularly scheduled in-services, journal clubs, or pharmacology rounds. Pharmacists may also choose to participate in ED morbidity and mortality, toxicology, and follow-up rounds. The teaching session may be optimized when done in collaboration with other health care members (eg, nurse educator, physician).

In-services may be provided in traditional classroom style or in electronic format such as through e-mail distribution or web-based continuing education. E-mail is an excellent means of dissemination of information to an audience that is difficult to gather at a common meeting time (eg, due to shift work in the ED). Electronic in-services should be short, concise, and relevant. Avorn and Soumerai conducted a randomized controlled trial of "academic detailing," which involves non-biased information sent to a group of physicians combined with personal educational visits by clinical pharmacists.[53] The authors found academic detailing reduced the prescribing of target medications in addition to financial savings compared to the control group who only received written information. Furthermore, the effect persisted for at least nine months after the start of the intervention, with no significant increase in the use of expensive substitute medication. In a similar study conducted at an academic medical center, Solomon et al. found a reduction in the number of days of inappropriate levofloxacin and ceftazadime antibiotic administration from 8.8 to 5.5 days (p < 0.05).[54] The principles of academic detailing are easily applicable to the ED setting.

The pharmacy clinician is the ideal person to initiate and/or facilitate an ED journal club. The pharmacist has an excellent background in medical literature evaluation skills and, consequently, can teach others. The objective of a journal club is to impart basic literature evaluation skills and new clinically relevant knowledge to participants. The selected articles should be pertinent to the ED clinician. A fruitful benefit of a departmental journal club is to utilize evidence-based medicine to impact the choice of new therapies or optimize the use of existing drugs.

Morbidity and mortality rounds are an excellent teaching opportunity and an opportunity to showcase the pharmacy clinician's expertise. The pharmacist brings a unique perspective to patient care, which may enable him/her to identify and resolve drug-related issues that may not be obvious to the other health care team members.

The importance of patient education by pharmacists cannot be overstated. By educating patients in a variety of settings, pharmacists have been shown to improve patient compliance with pharmacotherapy and non-pharmacotherapeutic lifestyle changes in diseases such as asthma, diabetes, hypercholesteremia, heart failure as well as others. All of these diseases are associated with a high rate of recidivism and frequent ED visits. Patient education in the ED may decrease return ED visits and improve outcomes. This may be a very cost-effective investment to be undertaken by EDs and Departments of Pharmacy in the era of ED overcrowding.

Research and Publications

The third guideline the ACCP set forth for pharmacotherapy specialists is in the area of research.[36] The clinician is encouraged to participate in the generation of new knowledge, which pertains to pharmacotherapy affecting ED patients. The research may either be directed by the pharmacist or involve the pharmacist as a co-investigator. There are multiple examples of publications in the pharmacy and EM literature that documents pharmacists' involvement and leadership in conducting research in the ED setting.[52–55] As an example, Rudis et al. recently published several articles dealing with the optimal method of phenytoin loading in the EM.[55] Another example of pharmacist directed research affecting patient care was completed by Spina and Dillon focusing on the effect of dosing probenecid in combination with cefazolin in the ED.[56] Active pharmacist participation in research-related activities (eg, patient identification and recruitment, generation of research ideas and planned analysis for drug studies) in the ED is also very important.[57,58] Moreover, it is important to publish and present research, case reports, or topic summaries in journals and conferences that are read and attended by other clinicians who work in EM in an attempt to increase their exposure and experience with emergency room pharmacotherapy specialists.[55,57,59–63] The ED pharmacist may also be involved with providing input for clinical trials involving drug therapy in the ED, particularly as it relates to study design, data collection, and selection of appropriate outcome measures.

Preparation and Training

The practice of EM can be quite demanding and challenging, and, thus, requires a unique individual. Qualities of successful pharmacy clinicians in the ED include professional competence and confidence, 'tough skin,' compassion, and motivation. The individual should also possess excellent communication and presentation skills. The pharmacist must first have appropriate training regarding the clinical use of drugs ('at the bedside') in the ED. Electrocardiogram interpretation skills and advanced cardiac life support (ACLS) training as a provider and instructor is also an asset for clinicians working in the ED.

In Canada, in addition to completing an undergraduate baccalaureate degree in pharmacy, a post-baccalaureate professional degree (doctor of pharmacy) is strongly recommended. Further, prior to entering the doctor of pharmacy program in Canada, a hospital pharmacy residency program also aids in the preparation of the clinician. In the US, upon earning the entry-level doctor of pharmacy degree, the clinician may consider a one year's general residency and then complete a specialty residency program in his/her second year. For example, a one-year specialty residency program focusing in the area of EM, critical care, and toxicology is offered by Detroit Medical Center/Detroit Receiving Hospital, and accredited by the ASHP. There are other residency and fellowship programs that focus in critical care and toxicology, and place greater or lesser emphasis on EM. A list of specialty residencies that provide EM training can be found at www.accp.com.

The pharmacy student who wishes to explore a career as a pharmacist in the ED should choose experiential rotations that will allow for direct patient care in the acute care setting, such as in the ED, the ICU and in clinical toxicology. Coursework in acute care as well as courses in physical assessment will provide the student with much needed background for rotations in the ED and ICU. During their experiential training, students should develop clinical thinking and deductive reasoning skills in preparation for a clinical 'hands on' career in EM. The student should also seek out opportunities to shadow an ED clinician (ED physician, nurse, or pharmacist) or volunteer in an ED setting.

The EM pharmacist may also wish to seek certification (note Chapter 120) with the Board of Pharmaceutical Specialties in the area of pharmacotherapy (BCPS). Board certification implies that an individual possesses a high level of expertise in the area of pharmacotherapy. The American Board of Applied Toxicology (ABAT) was established to recognize exceptional knowledge, experience, and competence in the area of toxicology, which is of definite value for the EM clinician in dealing with toxicological exposures.

STRESS IN THE ED

One of the issues that any new health care provider in the ED will confront sooner or later—and may not be able to prepare for ahead of time—is the stress that is inherent in working in an ED. From one perspective, this 'stress' may be the price health care providers 'pay' for the privilege and gratification that comes from saving lives. All EM clinicians will face events which prove at one time or another to be stressful and/or traumatic.[64–67] Stress in the ED may result from a particularly severe patient presentation such as a death of a child, a case of domestic violence, or a mass casualty motor vehicle accident. Stress can also result from a chaotic or heavy workload, disruptive patients or inappropriate responses from health care providers. Several studies have found a neuroendocrine response (ie, cortisol secretion) to stressful situations and self-perceived work stress in the ED among physicians and nurses.[66,68]

Reaction to these stressful situations may vary from humor to frustration, anger, depression or dissociation. The response to stressors in the ED depends on the individual, their level of experience, training and exposure and the surrounding environment.[64–67,69,70] It is vital for all health professionals to be aware of stressors in the ED and to find positive and constructive outlets for feelings of frustration, stress or anxiety. Humor is often used in the ED setting to diffuse such events, to relieve tension, and to cope with often unspeakable trauma.[70] However, there must also be opportunities to either informally or formally discuss these events with other ED clinicians or psycho-behavioral professionals.[69,71–73] All of these resources may be helpful to promote a long career for health care providers in EM.

EVALUATION OF EM PHARMACY PRACTICE

The quality of patient care and pharmacy services provided to ED patients should be evaluated on a regular basis to ensure an optimal level of service is provided. According to the ACCP, there are different aspects of care that need to be evaluated including the process of delivering care and assessing health outcomes.[37] The rationale for establishing an acceptable or ideal process of delivering patient care is that the care should lead to better patient outcomes and quality of care. Furthermore, the information generated in the evaluation process will also likely serve as a source for potential publication or conference presentation.

LOGISTICS—HOW TO GET STARTED

Given that EM pharmacy practice may be intriguing and one may wish to become an EM practitioner, how does one proceed to secure such a position? The first step is to decide on the level of services and practice environment one wishes to work in. Is it at a trauma center or a teaching hospital, etc.? Then, one would have to gather information documenting the need for a pharmacist in the department. It is important to get the support of the pharmacy personnel, and also from clinicians in the ED and hospital administrators.

Writing a proposal is a crucial step, which should involve ideas of potential services or projects that will be implemented including time frame for completion and methods of assessment. Hospital administrators are usually interested in efforts that would optimize patient care and at the same time provide cost savings. Once the hospital or university is interested in having a pharmacy clinician in the ED, the question of funding will need to be addressed. Funding for most hospitals may be the limiting or complicating factor. However, proposing that the department of pharmacy and EM share the financial burden may be a reasonable option for both parties. Other potential sources of funding include grant money from various organizations. The proposal should include an adequate time frame for implementation and assessment of projects and establishing patient care. A 2-year "pilot" study is a reasonable time frame for implementation and evaluation of services.

Also, it is advantageous to review the medical and pharmaceutical literature to identify other practitioners who have been successful in developing and creating an EM service. Networking at conferences with these individuals is also an invaluable means to learn from others and gain their advice/guidance.

FUTURE

The demand and need for ED pharmacists is likely to grow in the near and distant future. The increasing focus on patient safety and optimization of pharmacotherapy; the recognition of the pharmacist as a key member of the healthcare team in the in-patient and outpatient settings; and the continual need to improve the cost-effectiveness of drug therapies in the acute care setting all will increase the demand for the services of an ED pharmacist to provide clinical, distributive, teaching and research services in the ED setting.

CONCLUSION

The ED is an exciting and ideal place for a pharmacist to practice pharmaceutical care, to conduct or participate in research, to educate allied health clinicians and students, and to be of service to patients. The ED is a nontraditional practice site and is emerging as a growing specialty area as the expertise of the pharmacist in this arena is becoming recognized. Further research is needed to determine the extent of existing pharmacy services and pharmacist activities in the ED so that outcomes of pharmacist interventions and activities may be quantified.

REFERENCES

1. Dailey RH. Approach to the patient in the Emergency Department. In: Rosen PBR, Danzl DF, Hockberger RS, et al eds. *Emergency Medicine: Concepts and Clinical Practice,* 4th ed. St Louis: Mosby-Year Book, 1998.
2. Consolidated Omnibus Budget Reconciliation Act of 1986, Pub L No 99-272, codified at 42 USC 1395dd (1988), as amended by the Omnibus Budget Reconciliation Act of 1989, Pub L No. 101-239, codified at 42 USC 1395 dd, as reprinted in 135 Cong Rec H9376 (Nov 21, 1989).
3. Czajka PA, Skoutakis VA, Wood GC, et al. *Am J Hosp Pharm* 1979; 36:1087.
4. Thomasset KB, Faris R. *Am J Health-Sys Pharm* 2003; 60:1561.
5. Schwerman E, Schwartau N, Thompson CO. *Drug Intell Clin Pharm* 1973; 7:299.
6. Elenbaas R. *N Engl J Med* 1972; 287:151.
7. Dennehy CE, Kishi DT, Louie C. *Am J Health-Sys Pharm* 1996; 53:1422.
8. Stoukides CA, D'Agostino PR, Kaufman MB. *Am J Hosp Pharm* 1993; 50:712.
9. Hepler CD, Strand LM. *Am J Hosp Pharm* 1990; 47:533.
10. Classen DC, Pestotnik SL, Evans RS, et al. *JAMA* 1997; 277:301.
11. Bates DW, Spell N, Cullen DJ, et al. *JAMA* 1997; 277:307.
12. Johnson JA, Bootman JL. *Arch Intern Med* 1995; 155:1949.
13. Lazarou J, Pomeranz BH, Corey PN. *JAMA* 1998; 279:1200.
14. Patel P, Zed PJ. *Pharmacotherapy* 2002;22(7):915–23.
15. Implementation guidelines for the Canadian emergency department triage & acuity scale (CTAS). Website found at http://www.caep.ca/002.policies/002-02.ctas.htm. Accessed February 20, 2003
16. Austin Z. *Hosp Pharm Pract* 1995; 3:17.
17. Cameron B. *Can J Hosp Pharm* 1994; 47:101.
18. Pegrum S. *The Pharmaceutical Journal* 1995; 254:445.
19. Cregin R, Segal-Maurer S, Weinbaum F, et al. *Am J Health-Sys Pharm* 2002; 59:364.
20. Spath P. *Hosp Peer Rev* 2003; 28:40.
21. Himmel W, Kron M, Hepe S, et al. *Family Practice* 1996; 13:247.
22. Grad R, Mallet L. *Can J Hosp Pharm* 1998; 51:23.
23. Chande VT, Exum T. *Pediatrics* 1994; 93:513.
24. Jones J, Clark W, Bradford J, et al. *J Emerg Med* 1988; 6:249.
25. Jones PK, Jones SL, Katz J. *Ann Emerg Med* 1990; 19:16.
26. Shesser R, Smith M, Adams S, et al. *Ann Emerg Med* 1986; 15:911.
27. Dudas V, Bookwalter T, Kerr KM, et al. *Am J Med* 2001; 111:26S.
28. Schneider SM, Gallery ME, Schafermeyer R, et al. *Ann Emerg Med* 2003; 42:167.
29. Clark K, Normile LB. *J Emerg Nurs* 2002; 28:489.
30. Svenson J, Besinger B, Stapczynski JS. *Am J Emerg Med* 1997; 15:654.
31. Joint Commission on Accreditation of Healthcare Organizations. Website found at www.jcaho.org. Accessed September 15, 2003.
32. Powell MF, Solomon DK, McEachen RA. *Am J Hosp Pharm* 1985; 42:831.
33. Whalen FJ. *Am J Hosp Pharm* 1981; 38:684.
34. Burda AM, Sigg T. *Am J Health-Sys Pharm* 2001; 58:2274.
35. Dart RC, Goldfrank LR, Chyka PA, et al. *Ann Emerg Med* 2000; 36:126.
36. The ACCP Clinical Practice Affairs Committee, Subcommittee B, 1998–1999. American College of Clinical Pharmacy. Practice guidelines for pharmacotherapy specialists. *Pharmacotherapy* 2000; 20:487.
37. American College of Clinical Pharmacy. Establishing and evaluating clinical pharmacy services in primary care. *Pharmacotherapy* 1994; 14:743.
38. Rudis MI, Brandl KM. Position paper on critical care pharmacy services. Society of Critical Care Medicine and American College of Clinical Pharmacy Task Force on Critical Care Pharmacy Services.[comment]. *Critical Care Medicine* 2000; 28:3746.
39. Kirk JK, Michael KA, Markowsky SJ, et al. *Pharmacotherapy* 1996; 16:723.
40. Lumsdon K, Hagland M. *Hosp & Health Networks* 1993; 67:34.
41. Shane R. *Am J Health-Sys Pharm* 1995; 52:1051.
42. Tidwell SL. *Prog Cardiovasc Nurs* 1993; 8:6.
43. Jahnke HK, Zadrozny D, Garrity T, et al. *J Emerg Nurs* 2003; 29:133.
44. Ng SM, Krishnaswamy P, Morissey R, et al. *Am J Cardiol* 2001; 88:611.
45. Shane R. *Top Hosp Pharm Manage* 1995; 14:55.
46. American Society of Health-System Pharmacists. *Am J Health-Sys Pharm* 2002; 59:282.
47. Greenberg MI, Jurgens SM, Gracely EJ. *J Emerg Med* 2002; 22:273.
48. Center for Disease Control and Prevention. Strategic National Stockpile. Website found at http://www.bt.cdc.gov/stockpile/. Accessed September 15, 2003.
49. Terriff CM, Tee AM. *Am J Health-Syst Pharm* 2001; 58:233.
50. Kozak RJ, Siegel S, Kuzma J. *Ann Emerg Med* 2003; 41:685.
51. Henretig FM, Mechem C, Jew R. *Ann Emerg Med* 2002; 40:405.
52. Teeter DS. *Am J Health-Sys Pharm* 2002; 59:928.
53. Avorn J, Soumerai SB. *N Engl J Med* 1983; 308:1457.
54. Solomon DH, Van Houten L, Glynn RJ, et al. *Arch Intern Med* 2001; 161:1897.
55. Swadron SP, Rudis MI, Azimian K, et al. *Acad Emerg Med* 2004; 11:244.
56. Spina SP, Dillon EC Jr. *Ann Pharmacother* 2003; 37:621.
57. Rudis MI, Touchette D, Swadron SP, et al. *Ann Emerg Med* 2004; 43:386.
58. Stone S, Rudis MI, Lee V, et al. *Ann Emerg Med* 2003.
59. Jain AL, Robertson GJ, Rudis MI. *Emerg Med Clin North Am* 2003; 21:1.
60. Zed PJ, Tisdale JE, Borzak S. *Arch Intern Med* 1999; 159:1849.
61. Carr R, Zed PJ. *Ann Pharmacother* 2002; 36:1727.
62. Clark K, Abu-Laban RB, Zed PJ, et al. *Can J Emerg Med* 2003; 5:49.
63. Yeung JK, Zed PJ. *Can J Emerg Med* 2002; 4:194.
64. Alagappan K, Grlic N, Steinberg M, et al. *Am J Med Qual* 2001; 16:17.
65. O'Connor J, Jeavons S. *J Adv Nurs* 2003; 41:53.
66. Sluiter JK, van der Beek AJ, Frings-Dresen MH. *Occup Environ Med* 2003; 60:373.
67. Williams S, Dale J, Glucksman E, et al. *BMJ* 1997; 314(7082):713.
68. Yang Y, Koh D, Ng V, et al. *J Occup Environ Med* 2001; 43:1011.
69. Marmar CR, Weiss DS, Metzler TJ, et al. *J Nerv Ment Dis* 1999; 187:15.
70. van Wormer K, Boes M. *Health & Social Work* 1997;22(2):87–92.
71. Neely KW, Spitzer WJ. *Prehospital & Disaster Medicine* 1997; 12:114.
72. Lipton H, Everly GS Jr. *Prehospital Emergency Care* 2002; 6:15.
73. Benedek DM, Holloway HC, Becker SM. *Emerg Med Clin North Am* 2002; 20:393.

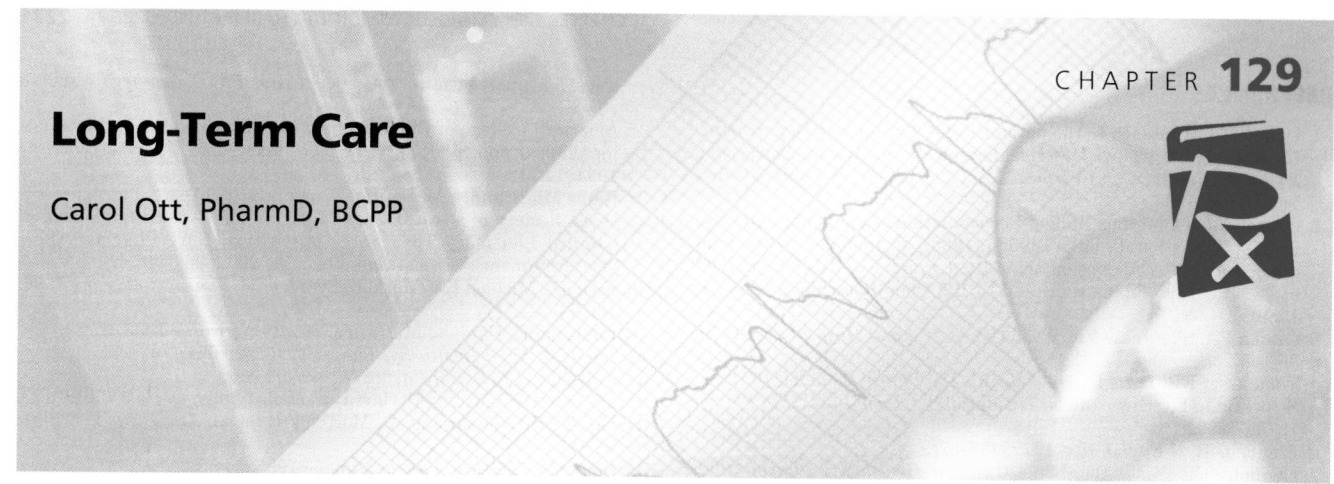

CHAPTER 129

Long-Term Care

Carol Ott, PharmD, BCPP

Long-term care has changed dramatically over the last 200 years. In the late 1700s, people who lived to old age were either taken care of by their children or were wealthy enough to afford in-home caretakers. Old-age homes and retirement communities began to appear in the 1800s. Pension and welfare systems were developed. In the 1930s, the Great Depression necessitated the Social Security Act of 1935 to create a national welfare system. For-profit homes were built in which state and Federal governments shared the cost of caring for the aged. Health care licensing systems were created by Hill-Burton in the 1940s. The 1950s and 1960s saw the government become the primary payor for nursing home care and costs began to escalate. Medicare and Medicaid were created in 1965 to provide government health insurance. Medicare and Medicaid payments to nursing facilities exploded, causing Medicare to restrict nursing home coverage. Decreased payments to nursing homes caused a diminished number of staff to care for a growing number of residents and the quality of nursing home care became a concern.[1] The Omnibus Budget Reconciliation Act of 1987 (OBRA 87) was enacted in part to address these quality-of-care concerns. OBRA 87 required that all nursing facilities certified by Medicare retain the services of a consultant pharmacist to ensure that all medication regimens provided to residents were periodically reviewed. The term *consultant pharmacist* generally refers to a pharmacist who practices in a long-term care setting to provide drug regimen review (DRR), medication storage and administration oversight, and staff and resident education.

Pharmacist involvement in long-term care activities grew as a result of these regulations, which include oversight of provision of medications to nursing facilities and consultant pharmacist duties. Pharmacists practicing in the field of geriatrics must not only be cognizant of these guidelines, but must also be able to manage patients with multiple disease states taking multiple medications. Nursing home care has been much improved with the enactment of OBRA '87 and its revision in 1999. While these regulations provide guidelines to medication management of the elderly, pharmacists must also be aware of the quality of life of the patient when recommending drug therapy interventions, including the complexity of the medication regimen, compliance issues, and side effect profiles of therapy.

POPULATION AND NURSING HOME CHARACTERISTICS

In 1950 there were approximately 12 million Americans aged 65 and older. That number is expected to approach 70 million by the year 2030.[2] Because of this, the need to address the is-

sues of long-term care becomes paramount. The impact of the growing elderly population has far-reaching effects on government and private finances, number and quality of nursing facility beds, and availability of home health care services. Health care systems will be providing care to a larger number of sicker patients, as the group of elderly over the age of 85 has increased >274% in the last 34 years. By the year 2050, nearly half of Americans will live to their 85th birthday and will comprise approximately 5% of the total US population.[3]

The male-female ratio continues to decline with age. In 1999, there were 100 women over the age of 85 compared to 49 men. Approximately 35% of women aged 65 to 74 were widowed, compared to 77% of women >85 years old. Older women had a higher poverty rate than older men—for those 65 to 74, 10.7% and 7.0%; 75 and over, 15.1% and 7.5%, respectively.[4] From 1994 to 1996, people aged 65 or older visited their physicians 11.4 times per year and accounted for more than 12 million patient discharges from non-Federal hospital stays. Patients >85 years old were twice as likely to be hospitalized than those aged 65 to 74.[2]

More than 1.5 million Americans resided in nursing homes in 1997. Approximately half of these residents were over the age of 85 and 75% of them were women.[2] In 1999, the number of nursing home residents had risen to 16.4 million in 18,000 nursing homes. Assistance with activities of daily living (ADLs) is the most common reason for admission to a nursing facility. These ADLs include bathing, dressing, toileting, and eating (Table 129-1). Often, residents are unable to follow a medication regimen, whether due to the complexity of the regimen itself or problems with remembering to take medications.

Nursing home care costs currently exceed $40,000 per resident per year. Medicare and Medicaid paid $51 million for nursing home care for residents >65 years old in 1995. This was greater than 70% of the total long-term care expenditures for Medicare/Medicaid in that year. Private long-term care insurance accounted for less than 1% of payments for nursing home care.[5] In 1998, total long-term care spending totaled >$117 billion, with Medicare paying 39%, Medicaid 17.8%, private insurance 7.4%, and 29.5% out-of-pocket payments. Most residents of nursing facilities receive Medicare, Medicaid, Veterans' Administration benefits, and/or use private insurance. Nearly 67% of nursing home residents received Medicaid in 1998.[6] A total of 33 million Americans received Medicare benefits in 1996.[2] Long-term care expenditures for older Americans with disabilities, including those receiving nursing home or community-based care, reached $123 billion in 2000, with more than 65% paid by the government.[7] The projected total long-term care costs (both institutional and community care) by all payors in 2020 is approximately $207 billion and in 2040 rises to $346 billion.[8]

Table 129-1. Characteristics of Nursing Homes

Total Number of Nursing Facilities		18000
Average Number of Beds/Facility		105
Average Occupancy Rate		87%
Private Pay/Day	Skilled Nursing	$146
	Intermediate Care	$114
	Residential	$101
Per Diem	Medicare	$213
	Medicaid	$105
Percentage of Residents with Assistance With ADLs	Bathing	94%
	Dressing	87%
	Toileting	56%
	Eating	47%

Data from National Center for Health Statistics. The National Nursing Home Survey: 1999 Summary Page. Available at: http://www.cdc.gov/nchs/products/pubs/pubd/series/sr13/160-151/sr_152.htm. Accessed March 5, 2003.

Definitions of Long-term Care Facilities

Table 129-2 provides current definitions of long-term care facilities used by the Centers for Medicare and Medicaid (CMS). "Skilled nursing facility" defines a facility that meets specific regulatory certification requirements set out by CMS to provide inpatient nursing care that does not meet the level of care required in a hospital setting. Previous terms for these facilities included *extended care facility, nursing facility, intermediate care facility,* and *skilled nursing home.* The certification requirements for CMS no longer differentiate between "skilled" and "intermediate" care. Intermediate care facilities/mental retardation exist to provide care for developmentally disabled individuals requiring care not meeting the level of skilled nursing or hospitalization.

GOVERNMENT AND PRIVATE PROGRAMS IMPACTING LONG-TERM CARE

There are many government and private certification programs that affect nursing facilities. Table 129-3 provides a selected list of these. Certification by government programs is required in all nursing facilities that care for residents receiving Medicare, Medicaid, and Veterans' Administration benefits. Payment for care-related services is based on the facility's ability to maintain a level of care set out by these government bodies. Accreditation by the Joint Commission on Accreditation of Healthcare Facilities (JCAHO) is voluntary. All of the above-mentioned agencies provide standards and regulations that facilities must comply with to maintain certification.

Legislation has also had a significant impact on long-term care, both in terms of financing health care for elders and improving quality of care in nursing facilities. The Social Security

Table 129-3. Selected Programs and Regulations Governing Long-Term Care

Centers for Medicare & Medicaid Services (CMS) (formerly HCFA, Health Care Financing Administration)

Health Insurance Portability and Accountability Act of 1996 (HIPAA)

Omnibus Budget Reconciliation Act of 1987, updated 1999 (OBRA 87)

Omnibus Budget Reconciliation Act of 1990 (OBRA 90)

Social Security Act of 1935 (SSA 1935)

The Joint Commission on Accreditation of Healthcare Facilities (JCAHO)

Veterans Health Administration (VHA)

Act of 1935, the Omnibus Budget Reconciliation Act of 1987 (revised 1999), the Omnibus Budget Reconciliation Act of 1990, the Health Insurance Portability and Accountability Act of 1996, and the Balanced Budget Act of 1997 are a few. Currently, there is considerable controversy over the proposed addition of a prescription drug benefit for Medicare beneficiaries.

The Social Security Act of 1935

The 1934 Committee on Economic Security met with the intention to produce a complete system of social insurance, to include workers' compensation, health insurance, disability insurance, old-age benefits, and survivors' benefits. Unfortunately, many of the health benefits proposed were not included in the January 1935 report to Congress, and it would take nearly three decades until all of the committee's visions were realized.[9] The United States Congress did enact the Social Security Act of 1935 (SSA), which created the Old-Age and Survivors Insurance (OASI) program. This provided retirement benefits to workers age 65 and older. The program became effective in 1937 and is financed by payroll tax paid by employees and employers. The Disability Insurance program was added to the SSA in 1956. In 2001, 39 million beneficiaries received benefit payments from the OASI, with total benefit payments of $372.3 billion. The number of OASI beneficiaries is projected to reach 72 million in 2030. In 2001, the estimated average monthly social security benefit payment was $874.[10] Revenues for Social Security are currently 14% less than expenditures and it is projected that Social Security will be depleted by 2030. At that time, revenues will only pay 70–75% benefits to beneficiaries.[11]

Medicare and Medicaid

The history of Medicare dates back to the enactment of Title 18 of the Social Security Act, "Health Insurance for the Aged" in 1965 (Table 129-4). This created Medicare Part A (Hospital Insurance) and Part B (Supplemental Medical Insurance). Benefits are payable to people >65 years old, Social Security

Table 129-2. Definitions of Long-Term Care Facilities

Skilled Nursing Facility (SNF)	(1) A facility (which meets specific regulatory certification requirements) which primarily provides inpatient skilled nursing care and related services to patients who require medical, nursing, or rehabilitative services but does not provide the level of care or treatment available in a hospital.
	(2) A nursing facility with the staff and equipment to give skilled nursing care and/or skilled rehabilitative services and other health-related services.
Intermediate Care Facility/Mental Retardation (ICF/MR)	A facility which primarily provides health-related care and services above the level of custodial care to mentally retarded individuals, but does not provide the level of care available in a hospital or skilled nursing facility.
Extended Care Services	An alternate name for "skilled nursing facility services"

Data from Centers for Medicare & Medicaid Services. The Glossary page. Available at: http://cms.hhs.gov/glossary. Accessed March 5, 2003.

Table 129-4. The History of Medicare

DATE	EVENT
1965	Title 18—"Health Insurance for the Aged" of the Social Security Act created Medicare. Part A—Hospital Insurance (HI) Part B—Supplemental Medical Insurance (SMI)
1972	Medicare expanded to include disabled persons who qualify for benefits under Disability Insurance program and certain individuals with end-stage renal disease.
1986	State and local government employees hired after March 31, 1986 and not covered under Social Security required to be covered by Medicare.
1997	The Balanced Budget Act of 1997 expanded delivery of health care under Medicare with the Medicare (+) Choice Program. (Medicare (+) Choice Program allows more types of health insurance plans, including managed care, to serve Medicare beneficiaries.)
1997	The Balanced Budget Act of 1997: home health services not associated with a hospital or skilled nursing facility stay for individuals enrolled in both HI and SMI were transferred from the HI program (Part A) to the SMI program (Part B) effective January 1998.
2000	Congress enacted the Benefits Improvement and Protection Act (BIPA) to increase payments to health insurance plans in an effort to stop plans from withdrawing from the Medicare (+) Choice Program.

Data from Facts From EBRI. August 2002 EBRI Fact Sheet. The Basics of Medicare Page. Available at: http://www.ebri.org/facts/0802fact.htm. Accessed March 5, 2003.

beneficiaries under age 65 with disabilities, and individuals needing renal dialysis or transplantation.[12] All Medicare providers are subject to Federal health care quality standards to qualify for payment. Because Medicare does not cover all needed services, the Balanced Budget Act of 1997 was enacted to expand delivery of health care under the Medicare (+) Choice program. Under this program, more types of health insurance plans, both private insurance and managed care, may provide services to Medicare beneficiaries. These private health insurance programs are referred to as "Medigap." The Centers for Medicare and Medicaid (CMS), formerly the Health Care Financing Administration (HCFA), is responsible for overseeing the administration of Medicare and Medicaid. Title 19 of the Social Security Act, "Grants to States for Medical Assistance Programs," was also enacted in 1965, creating Medicaid. Medicaid is a state program that provides medical services to individuals receiving state public assistance and augments hospital and nursing facility services that are mandated under Medicaid. The discretion for payment for services lies with the individual states.[12] States must cover certain persons who are poor, aged, blind, or disabled.[13] Currently, Medicare does not provide outpatient prescription drug benefits, while Medicaid will provide such benefits based on individual state drug programs and formularies.

Veterans' Health Administration

The Department of Veterans' Affairs provides many health care benefits to veterans of the United States Armed Services. These benefits vary based on many factors, including wartime service, service-connection of illness or injury, and whether or not the health care service was provided by a Veterans' Administration (VA) facility or provider.[14] A veteran who is a resident of a nursing home or is permanently housebound may be eligible for a benefit entitled "Aid and Attendance," which includes prescription medication. Veterans' Administration hospitals and services are available in every state. Veterans' Service Officers, who can be found in most areas, aid in the provision of multiple services to veterans. The Veterans' Millennium Health Care Act was signed into law on November 30, 1999 and will provide

increased access to long-term care, both in institutions and community-based care.[15]

The Omnibus Budget Reconciliation Act of 1987

The Omnibus Budget Reconciliation Act of 1987 or The Federal Nursing Home Reform Act was enacted in 1987 and took effect in 1990. This landmark legislation was brought about due to serious concerns about the quality of care in the nation's nursing facilities. Long-term care facilities utilizing Medicare and Medicaid funding must provide services that help each resident attain and maintain the highest practicable physical, mental, and psychosocial well-being.[16] Provisions are made in the OBRA 87' guidelines for quality of life, activities of daily living, resident assessment (MDS–Minimum Data Set), rights to remain in the nursing home, and freedom from unnecessary physical and chemical restraints. The impact of these regulations on pharmacy practice has been enormous. Requirements for dispensing pharmacy services, drug regimen review, and unnecessary psychoactive drugs have changed the practice of consultant pharmacy. These regulations were revised in 1999 to include selected Beer's criteria of inappropriate drugs in the elderly (Table 129-5). Prior to the revision, the unnecessary drug regulations primarily covered antipsychotics, anxiolytics, and sedative/hypnotics. The addition of the Beer's criteria to the regulations added other medications that may have detrimental side effects in the elderly or have little evidence of efficacy. Quality indicators have been developed based, in part, on OBRA 87. These include monitors of prevalence of depressive symptoms, use of psychoactive medications, and use of nine or more medications per resident.

The Omnibus Budget Reconciliation Act of 1990

The Omnibus Budget Reconciliation Act of 1990 requires that each state establish a system of drug use review (DUR) which would ensure that drugs used for Medicaid patients are appropriate, medically necessary, and not likely to result in adverse effects.[17] The prospective DUR process requires pharmacists to screen prescriptions for potential problems, offer to counsel patients about medications, maintain patient profiles, and document certain actions. One impact of OBRA 90 on long-term care is for nursing facilities with independent residential living areas. Residents in independent living facilities are generally required to take their own medications without significant intervention by the nursing staff. Pharmacies providing medications to these residents should have a mechanism in place to counsel these residents about their medications and provide documentation of this counseling.

The Health Insurance Portability and Accountability Act of 1996

The Health Insurance Portability and Accountability Act of 1996 (HIPAA) is a broad set of rules and procedures for protecting the privacy of patient health information. The finalized rules were released on August 9, 2002 and providers of health care must comply by April 14, 2003. Pharmacists and pharmacies, as providers, must take reasonable steps to limit the use or disclosure of private health information to the minimum necessary to accomplish the intended purpose of the use or disclosure. This does not apply to treatment activities, therefore, contacting a prescriber to verify the contents of a prescription is allowed without consent from the patient.[18] Nursing facilities must educate staff about HIPAA and the confidentiality of patient information. It is not acceptable to discuss patient information in an open nurses' station, hallway, cafeteria, or any

Table 129-5. Beers' Criteria

GENERIC	BRAND	HIGH SEVERITY?
Propoxyphene and combination products	Darvon Darvocet N-100	No
Indomethacin	Indocin	No
Phenylbutazone	Butazoladin	No
*Pentazocine	Talwin	Yes
Trimethobenzamide	Tigan	No
Methocarbamol	Robaxin	No
Carisoprodol	Soma	No
Oxybutynin	Ditropan	No
Chlorzoxazone	Paraflex	No
Metaxalone	Skelaxin	No
Cyclobenzaprine	Flexeril	No
*Flurazepam	Dalmane	Yes
*Amitriptyline	Elavil	Yes
*Doxepin	Sinequan	Yes
*Meprobamate	Equanil, Miltown	Yes (If recently started)
*Chlordiazepoxide	Librium	Yes
*Diazepam	Valium	Yes
*Disopyramide	Norpace	Yes
*Digoxin	Lanoxin	Yes (If recently started)
Dipyridamole	Persantine	No
*Methyldopa	Aldomet	Yes (If recently started)
Reserpine	Serpasil	No
*Chlorpropamide	Diabinese	Yes
*Dicyclomine	Bentyl	Yes
*Hyoscyamine	Levsin, Levsinex	Yes
*Propantheline	Pro-Banthine	Yes
*Belladonna alkaloids	Donnatal	Yes
*Clindinium/ chlordiazepoxide	Librax	Yes
Antihistamines	Several	No
Diphenhydramine	Benadryl	No
Ergot mesyloids	Hydergine	No
Iron supplements >325mg/day	Several	No
*Barbiturates	Several	Yes (If recently started)
*Meperidine	Demerol	Yes
*Ticlopidine	Ticlid	Yes

* Denotes inclusion in Tag#329, OBRA 1987 Guidance to Surveyors—Revised 1999
Data from Beers MH. *Arch Intern Med* 1997; 157:1531.

other public place. The HIPAA regulations provide for assessment of monetary sanctions for each HIPAA violation. The National Association of Chain Drug Stores (NACDS) and the American Pharmaceutical Association (APhA) have HIPAA implementation guidelines available.

The Joint Commission on Accreditation of Healthcare Facilities

The Joint Commission on Accreditation of Healthcare Facilities (JCAHO) has been providing accreditation to long-term care facilities for several years. JCAHO accreditation is not required for facility reimbursement for services by Medicare or Medicaid, but is encouraged by some private insurance plans. The goal of the Joint Commission is to improve the quality of health care. Sentinel events, which can include adverse drug reactions, must be reported to JCAHO by accredited facilities. Medication use standards are found primarily in the standards concerning care and treatment of residents (TX) in the JCAHO Standards for Long-Term Care.

Proposed Prescription Drug Benefit for Medicare Beneficiaries

Prescription drugs accounted for 1% of the total national health expenditure of $2.7 billion in 1960. That figure rose to 9.9% of $140.6 billion in 2001.[19] Medicare beneficiaries account for 15% of the US population, but incur 40% of out-of-pocket spending on prescription drugs. Nearly 75% of Medicare beneficiaries have prescription coverage from private health plans or retirement plans, but employment-based health plans are scaling back benefits for prescription drugs and increasing copayments. Medicare beneficiaries spent $87 billion on prescription drugs in 2002. The Congressional Budget Office estimates spending per Medicare beneficiary on outpatient prescription drugs to be $2439 in 2003 and $5816 in 2012. Individuals with Medicare benefits but no drug coverage had an average of 25 prescriptions filled in 1999. Those with drug coverage filled an average of 32 prescriptions. Medicare beneficiaries with Medicaid coverage received an average of 39 prescriptions. The need for a Medicare prescription drug benefit is enormous, but controversy exists as to how it should be provided. Of the proposals that have been issued, most include a deductible to be met before benefits commence. Others suggest a $1000 cap on prescription drug payments after the deductible is reached; and others a $4000 to $6000 stop loss after which Medicare would resume payments for prescription drugs. Questions of eligibility and percentage of individual state responsibilities have yet to be answered. The estimated cost of the benefit is between $200 billion and $500 billion per year between the years of 2005 and 2012.[20] One option that has been discussed is the use of a discount drug card. Many pharmacy organizations, including APhA (American Pharmacists Association), NACDS (National Association of Chain Drug Stores), and NCPA (National Community Pharmacists Association) have criticized this discount card as outside of the legislative authority of the Federal Government.[21] The concern of these organizations rests in the provision of appropriate pharmaceutical care as opposed to simply discounting prescription drugs without utilization review. A further concern for pharmacists is a reimbursement system that discounts beyond average wholesale price and without a reasonable dispensing fee. While the current controversy focuses on the community and outpatient pharmacy practice arena, many Medicare beneficiaries reside in long-term care facilities. While provision will likely be made to include these individuals in any prescription drug benefit, such provision will be complex due to the frequent duality of coverage by Medicaid and Medicare.

PHARMACY PRACTICE IN LONG-TERM CARE

Policies and Procedures

Policies and procedures for organizational aspects, medication orders, ordering and receiving medications from the pharmacy, medication storage in the nursing facility, disposal of medications, medication administration, and medication monitoring are required in long-term care facilities. Sample policy and procedure topics are provided in Table 129-6. The policy and procedure manual establishes guidelines and processes that define how pharmacy services are delivered to the facility. This manual should clearly define the scope of services of the pharmacy and responsibilities of both the nursing facility and the pharmacy. A multidisciplinary approach should be used in writing a policy and procedure manual to ensure that all disciplines involved in pharmacy services agree with and are able to easily use the manual. Most long-term care pharmacies provide services to several facilities and have a basic manual format that can be individualized to the needs of each facility. The requirements of federal and state laws governing pharmacy services in long-term care must be included in the

Table 129-6. Suggested Policy and Procedure Topics

Disposal of Medications and Medication-Related Supplies
Controlled Medications Disposal
Discharge Medications
Medication Destructionl
Returning Medications to Pharmacy
Syringe and Needle Disposal

Medication Administration
Controlled Medications
Enteral Tube Medications
Equipment and Supplies
General Guidelines
Infusion Therapy Products
Injectable Medications
Irrigation Solutions
Medication Administration By Route
Preparation of Emergency Medications
Reconstitution of Injectable Medications
Self-Administration of Medications

Medication Monitoring
Consultant Pharmacist Quarterly Report
Documentation and Communication of Consultant Pharmacist
    Recommendations
Drug Regimen Review
Medication Administration Monitoring - Med Pass Survey
Psychoactive Drug Monitoring
Quality Improvement
Standing Monitoring Orders for Routine Medication Monitoring

Medication Orders
Prescriber Medication Orders
Standing Orders
Stop Orders

Medication Storage
Bedside Medication Storage
Controlled Medication Storage
Infusion Therapy Product Storage
Medication Storage

Miscellaneous
Adverse Drug Reactions
Drug Product Problem Reporting
Drug Product Recalls
Investigational Medications
Medications Dispensed by Physicians
Medications Errors
Pass Medications
Syringe and Needle Inventory

Ordering and Receiving Medications from Pharmacy
Drug Information
Emergency Pharmacy Service and Kits
Floor Stock Medications
Infusion Therapy Product Labeling
Medication Labeling
Medication Packaging
Medications Brought in by Resident or Family
Ordering and Receiving Medications (Noncontract)
Ordering and Receiving Medications (Provider Pharmacy)
Pharmacy Hours and Delivery Schedule

Organizational
Noncontract Phamarcy
Provider Pharmacy
Consultant Pharmacist Provider Requirements
Infusion Therapy Produces Provider Requirements
Pharmaceutical Services Committee
Pharmacist/Provider Collaborative Practice Agreement

Data from D'Achille KM. Model Policy and Procedures for Pharmaceutical Care in the Long-Term Care Setting. ASCP, 1999.

manual. Table 129-7 provides a listing of relevant federal regulations and where each regulation may be found in the Centers for Medicare and Medicaid *Guidance to Surveyors*. Because of the changing environment of long-term care, the policy and procedure manual ideally should be reviewed and updated annually. The American Society of Consultant Pharmacists provides a reference entitled *Model Policy and Procedures for Pharmaceutical Care in the Long-Term Care Setting* that encompasses all topics required in nursing facilities.[22]

Drug Regimen Review

Drug regimen review (DRR) encompasses nearly all clinical activities of the consultant pharmacist. Each drug regimen must be reviewed at least monthly by the pharmacist when servicing a nursing facility. Reviews may be done quarterly in residential facilities and intermediate care facilities for the mentally retarded (ICFs/MR). Any irregularities found during the review must be reported to the attending physician and director of

Table 129-7. Relevant Regulations and Standards

REGULATION/STANDARDS	CMS REGULATION(S)	TAG #S	MDS SECTION	JCAHO STANDARD(S)
Pharmacy Provider	483.60(a)	F426		CC.3.1
	483.75(h)(1), (2)	F500		
Consultant Pharmacist	483.60(b)(1)–(3)	F427		TX.1
	483.20(b)(2)	F272	O	PE.2
Drug Regimen Review	483.60(c)(1), (2)	F428–30		PE.2
				TX.4
	483.25(l)(1)(i)–(vi)	F329	B-P	TX.4.1
Infusion Therapy Products				TX.2.4.2
Noncontract Pharmacy	483.60(a)	F426		CC.3.1
	483.75(h)(1), (2)	F500		
Medication Preparation and Documentation	483.60(a)	F426		CC.3.1
	483.25(m)(1), (2)	F332–3		TX.3
				TX.4.1
Parenteral Meds Preparation	483.25(k)(2)	F328	L4, P1, G, K, P	TX.2.4.2
Controlled Medications	483.60(b)(2)–(3)	F427		TX.2.10
Enteral Meds Preparation	483.25(k)(2)	F328	L4, P1, G, K, P	TX.2.4.2
Self-Adminsitration of Medications	483.10(n)	F176		TX.3.1
Freedom from Chemical Restraints	483.13(a)	F222	A, C, E, G, J, K, M	
Freedom from Unnecessary drugs	483.25(l)(1)(i)–(v)	F329		TX.4
Freedom from Antipsychotic drugs	483.25(l)(2)(i)	F330	B-P	
Gradual dosage Reduction of Antipsychotic drugs	483.25(1)(2)(ii)	F331		

CMS = Centers for Medicare & Medicaid Services; MDS = Minimum Data Set; JCAHO = The Joint Commission on Accreditation of Healthcare Facilities.

nursing of the facility. After the attending physician receives the consult written by the pharmacist, he/she must provide documentation of agreement or disagreement with the recommendations. The director of nursing can be provided a summary report of recommendations for review and follow up to ensure that all consults have received a response in a timely manner. Neither the director of nursing nor the physician is required to agree with the report or provide a rationale for acceptance or rejection of the recommendation.

Among the indicators that will be assessed by state and federal surveyors monitoring facilities for compliance with federal regulations is DRR. The number of DRRs performed per month will be compared to the average monthly facility census. If the number of reviews falls significantly short of patient census over several months, the facility may be found in noncompliance with regulations. The pharmacist should perform drug regimen reviews in the facility. Data sources necessary to perform appropriate drug regimen review may be found only in the resident chart and medication administration record.

The average number of prescriptions per resident in 1974 was 6.1. In general, this includes both routine and PRN (as needed) medications. The adequacy of DRR could be questioned if a significant number of residents take an average number of medications above this number. Current practice guidelines for many disease states common in the elderly call for use of multiple medications, which may cause an increase in the average number of medications per resident. Documentation by medicine, pharmacy, and nursing concerning reasons for use and efficacy are important in justifying continued use of medications. Adequacy of drug regimen review may also be questioned if the consultant pharmacist performs an excessive number of reviews on the same day. A total of 100 reviews performed on one day should be considered the maximum recommended in order to perform acceptable drug regimen review. The pharmacist performing reviews should determine the significance of any irregularity found. If an irregularity is found to be significant, the physician and/or nursing should be notified immediately and documentation should be provided of that communication to nursing and the attending physician. A signed and dated statement by the pharmacist may be provided for a nonsignificant irregularity to be responded to at a later time. The pharmacist is only responsible for documenting the irregularity and making a recommendation for resolution. It is then the responsibility of the facility to ensure communication to the attending physician. Irregularities that require nursing intervention should be reported to the director of nursing for resolution.

Examples of irregularities can include the following:

1. Multiple orders for the same drug by the same route
2. Drugs administered without regard to stop order policies
3. As needed (PRN) drug orders administered routinely for more than 30 days
4. Residents receiving three or more laxatives concurrently
5. Use of antipsychotics or antidepressants for less than 3 days
6. Concurrent use of two or more hypnotic drugs
7. Concurrent use of two or more antipsychotic drugs
8. Use of thyroid drugs without routine assessment of thyroid function (usually annual)
9. Use of a drug affecting blood pressure without a weekly recorded blood pressure
10. Use of anticoagulant therapy without assessment of clotting function at least monthly
11. Use of insulin or oral hypoglycemics without routine monitoring of blood sugar
12. Use of iron therapy without a red blood cell assessment
13. Use of urinary anti-infectives for chronic urinary tract infections if a urinalysis has not been performed at least once in the first 30 days of therapy
14. Use of three or more analgesics at the same time
15. Use of diuretics without determination of serum potassium within 30 days of initiation of therapy
16. Use of anticholinergic drug therapy with antipsychotic drugs without documented extrapyramidal side effects
17. Orders for drugs for which there is a known drug allergy
18. Inappropriate crushing of solid dosage forms that could result in resident discomfort or disruption of dosage form

The pharmacist should ensure that all medication orders have a corresponding diagnosis documented in the patient record. As needed (PRN) medication orders should include a reason for use in the order. The appropriate medication order includes the drug, dose, route of administration, frequency, and reason for use. Confusion in administration and documentation could result if a range of doses and frequency are given, for example 1 or 2 tablets every 4 to 6 hours. If an as needed (PRN) medication has not been given for greater than 30 to 60 days, a recommendation should be written for discontinuation of the medication. Routine laboratory monitoring should be ordered for appropriate medications. The pharmacist should ensure that the laboratory monitoring is ordered and that results are available in the patient record on a timely basis. Often, lab monitoring is ordered less frequently than would be found in an acute-care setting, for example, a potassium level may be appropriately obtained quarterly in the long-term care setting, but would be drawn much more frequently in a hospital. Significant drug-drug and drug-disease interactions should be identified. A consultant pharmacist should review a drug regimen for the above irregularities monthly, but may also choose to target a specific drug, disease, or laboratory value monthly. This may reduce the sometimes overwhelming nature of drug regimen review and provide focused data for drug use evaluation. The American Society of Consultant Pharmacists provides a reference entitled *Drug Regimen Review: A Process Guide for Pharmacists* that offers information regarding guidelines for appropriate drug regimen review.[23]

Unnecessary Drug Regulations, OBRA 87, Revised 1999

The Omnibus Budget Reconciliation Act of 1987 was enacted to improve the quality of care in the nation's nursing facilities. One of the most important issues addressed was that of unnecessary drugs, those medications that may be used as chemical restraints for difficult behavior problems. The concern was that many of these drugs were used to control residents for the convenience of staff. There is evidence that a substantial decrease in the use of antipsychotic drugs in nursing home residents resulted from the enactment of OBRA 87. According to one longitudinal study, there was a 26.7% reduction in antipsychotic drug use during a 30-month period from April 1, 1989 to September 30, 1991.[24]

The unnecessary drug regulations from OBRA 87 are presented in Table 129-8. These regulations require that each resident's drug regimen be free from unnecessary drugs. An unnecessary drug can include any medication that has an excessive dose, is duplicate therapy, or is used for an excessive duration. Monitoring of medication use is required, as is an adequate reason for use. Initially the unnecessary drug regulations focused on the use of antipsychotic medications. The regulation requires that facilities should not initiate antipsychotic drug therapy for any resident who is not already taking an antipsychotic when admitted to the facility unless the drug is being used for a specific documented condition with gradual dose reductions performed to ensure necessity of therapy. Environmental, medical, and behavioral interventions must be performed and documented as further justification of need for antipsychotic drug therapy. These interventions may include reducing nursing unit lighting at night, appropriate temperature regulation in resident rooms, assessment of pain, monitoring for fecal impaction and urinary tract infection, medication side effects, and behavioral care plans.

OBRA 87 also defined appropriate diagnoses for the use of antipsychotic medications in nursing facilities. Most of these diagnoses require symptoms of psychosis, whether schizophrenia, delusional disorder, psychotic mood disorders, or atypical

Table129-8. Unnecessary Drug Regulations OBRA 1987, Revised 1999

(1) Each Resident's drug regimen must be free from unnecessary drugs. An unnecessary drug is any drug when used:
  (Tag F329) (i) in excessive dose (including duplicate therapy); or
  (ii) for excessive duration; or
  (iii) without adequate monitoring; or
  (iv) without adequate indications for its use; or
  (v) in the presence of adverse consequences which indicate the dose should be reduced or discontinued; or
  (vi) any combinations of the reasons above.
(2) Antipsychotic drugs—Based on a comprehensive assessment of a resident, the facility must assure that:
  (Tag F330) (i) Residents who have not used antipsychotic drugs are not given these drugs unless antipsychotic drug therapy is necessary to treat a specific condition as diagnosed and documented in the clinical records; and
  (Tag F331) (ii) Residents who use antipsychotic drugs receive gradual dose reductions, and behavioral interventions, unless clinically contraindicated, in an effort to discontinue these drugs.

Data from Omnibus Budget Reconciliation Act OBRA 1987 (revised 1999) PL 100-203 Nursing home Reform Act; Guidance to Surveyors—Long Term Care Facilities; pp 114–128.

psychosis (Table 129-9). Residents with organic mental syndromes, including Alzheimer's dementia and vascular dementia, must have associated psychotic or agitated behaviors in order to justify the use of an antipsychotic. The guidelines also suggest that antipsychotics should not be used if specific behaviors are the only indication for use (see Table 129-9). Examples of such specific behaviors include wandering, indifference to surroundings, uncooperativeness, impaired memory, or agitated behaviors that do not present a danger to the resident or others. Residents receiving antipsychotics must be monitored for both efficacy of the medication and potential side effects. Efficacy monitoring would include observing for episodes of specific psychoses or agitated behaviors for which the medication is being used. Movement side effects (motor restlessness, tremors, involuntary movements of tongue or mouth, gait instability), anticholinergic side effects (constipation, dry mouth, urinary retention, blurred vision), and hypotension should be monitored. While there are no specific requirements for frequency of monitoring provided in the OBRA 87 regulations, episodes of behaviors and side effects are generally documented on every shift in most nursing facilities. Routine assessment of involuntary movements is also suggested. The AIMS (Abnormal Involuntary Movement Scale) and the DISCUS (Dyskinesia Identification System–Condensed Use Scale) are most often used for this purpose. Both scales require the resident to perform specific movements of the face, neck, and limbs to assess for possible long-term side effects of antipsychotic medication use. As these side effects are associated with longer-term use of therapy, the performance of these scales is suggested prior to initiation of antipsychotic use and every 3 to 6 months thereafter.

All psychoactive medications require monitoring of side effects and efficacy. This includes not only antipsychotics, but also anti-anxiety medications and sedative/hypnotics. Antidepressant medications are not included in the unnecessary drug regulations because of evidence that depression is underrecognized in the elderly population and any regulation of use of antidepressants may lead to reduced diagnosis and treatment. Many nursing facilities use one form to monitor all psychoactive medications and reduce required paperwork. Often, the provider pharmacy will furnish these forms preprinted with the resident and medication information. Med Pass, Incorporated (PO Box 750218, Dayton, Ohio, 45475-0218, 800-438-8361, sales@med-pass.com) has developed forms to aid in the monitoring of psychoactive medication use in the nursing facility. The American Society of Consultant Pharmacists also has a forms book available that contains examples of usable forms for this purpose.

Dosage reduction requirements of OBRA 87 also include all psychoactive medications (Table 129-10). Attempts at medication reduction should be performed at least twice in 1 year for short-acting benzodiazepines and antipsychotics and three times in 1 year for sedative/hypnotic medications before the further reduction or discontinuation of the drug can be deemed "clinically contraindicated." There are no specific requirements for the percent of reduction undertaken, but a 10% to 25% reduction at any one time can be suggested. This percent reduction will allow for evaluation of symptom emergence without causing a medication withdrawal reaction. Residents taking long-acting benzodiazepines for diagnoses other than a

Table 129-9. Appropriate Diagnosis for the Use of Antipsychotic Drugs

Acute psychotic episode	**Antipsychotics should not be used if one or more of the following is/are the only indication:**
Atypical psychosis	
Brief reactive psychosis	
Delusional disorder	
Huntington's disease	Agitated behaviors which do not represent danger to the resident or others
Organic Mental Syndromes (now called delirium, dementia, and amnestic and other cognitive disorders by DSM-IV) with associated psychotic and/or agitated behaviors	Anxiety
	Depression
	Fidgeting
	Impaired memory
	Indifference to surroundings
Psychotic mood disorders (including mania and depression with psychotic features)	Insomnia
	Nervousness
	Poor self care
	Restlessness
Schizoaffective disorder	Uncooperativeness
Schizophrenia	Unsociability
Schizophreniform disorder	Wandering
Tourette's disorder	

Data from Omnibus Budget Reconciliation Act OBRA 1987 (revised 1999) PL 100-203 Nursing Home Reform Act; Guidance to Surveyors—Long Term Care Facilities; pp 125–126.

Table 129-10. Unnecessary Drug Regulation-Required Dose Reduction (OBRA 87)

Long-Acting Benzodiazepine Drugs	Daily use <4 continuous months unless an attempt at a gradual dose reduction is unsuccessful (long-acting benzodiazepine use is appropriate only if short-acting benzodiazepine use has failed).
Short-Acting Benzodiazepine Drugs	A gradual dose reduction should be attempted at least twice in one year before one can conclude that a gradual dose reduction is clinically contraindicated.
Sedative/Hypnotic Drugs	A gradual dose reduction should be attempted at least three times within six months before one can conclude that a gradual dose reduction is clinically contraindicated.
Antipsychotic Drugs	A gradual dose reduction should be attempted twice in one year before one can conclude that gradual dose reduction is clinically contraindicated.

Data from Omnibus Budget Reconciliation Act OBRA 1987 (revised 1999) PL 100-203 Nursing Home Reform Act; Guidance to Surveyors—Long Term Care Facilities; pp 114–128.

neuromuscular disorder must also undergo a dosage reduction. Long-acting benzodiazepines should only be used when there is documented treatment failure with the use of a short-acting benzodiazepine. It is not sufficient for the physician to simply write an order "clinically contraindicated." There must be justification based on a clinical reason for use, psychiatric consultation, improvement in resident condition, and interdisciplinary monitoring. The exception to the requirement for "gradual dose reduction" is for those residents who have been diagnosed with a psychotic condition (schizophrenia, delusional disorder) taking an antipsychotic medication. However, it is still recommended that these residents undergo dose reduction as appropriate to their medical condition, as continued use of the drug may not be needed.

Recommended daily doses of psychoactive medications can also be found in the OBRA regulations (Table 129-11). At or

Table 129-11. Recommended Daily Doses of Psychoactive Drugs (OBRA87)

GENERIC	BRAND	DAILY ORAL DOSE
LONG-ACTING BENZODIAZEPINES		
Flurazepam	Dalmane	15 mg
Chlordiazepoxide	Librium	20 mg
Clorazepate	Tranxene	15 mg
Diazepam	Valium	5 mg
Clonazepam	Klonopin	1.5 mg
Quazepam	Doral	7.5 mg
Halazepam	Paxipam	40 mg
SHORT-ACTING BENZODIAZEPINES		
Lorazepam	Ativan	2 mg
Oxazepam	Serax	30 mg
Alprazolam	Xanax	0.75 mg
Estazolam	ProSom	0.5 mg
OTHER ANXIOLYTIC AND SEDATIVE DRUGS		
Diphenhydramine	Benadryl	50 mg
Hydroxyzine	Atarax, Vistaril	50 mg
Chloral Hydrate	Many Brands	750 mg
Temazepam	Restoril	7.5 mg
Triazolam	Halcion	0.125 mg
Zolpidem	Ambien	5 mg
ANTIPSYCHOTIC DRUGS		
Chlorpromazine	Thorazine	75 mg
Promazine	Sparine	150 mg
Triflupromazine	Vesprin	20 mg
Thioridazine	Mellaril	75 mg
Mesoridazine	Serentil	25 mg
Acetophenazine	Tindal	20 mg
Perphenazine	Trilafon	8 mg
Fluphenazine	Prolixin, Permitil	4 mg
Trifluoperazine	Stelazine	8 mg
Chlorprothixene	Taractan	75 mg
Thiothixene	Navane	7 mg
Haloperidol	Haldol	4 mg
Molindone	Moban	10 mg
Loxapine	Loxitane	10 mg
Clozapine	Clozaril	50 mg
Prochlorperazine	Compazine	10 mg
Risperidone	Risperdal	2 mg
Olanzapine	Zyprexa	10 mg
Quetiapine	Seroquel	200 mg

Daily oral doses represent those doses above which higher doses would need to be explained by the nursing facility.
Data from Omnibus Budget Reconciliation Act OBRA 1987 (revised 1999) PL 100-203 Nursing Home Reform Act; Guidance to Surveyors—Long Term Care Facilities; pp 117–121.

below these doses, geriatric patients will be less likely to suffer significant side effects. Use of doses above the recommendations will require explanation by the nursing facility, beyond the monitoring and dose reductions previously mentioned. Many nursing facilities provide this further documentation through the use of mental health consultation and multidisciplinary committees that monitor medication use and behavioral symptoms. Some of the medications listed in Table 129-11 were not available when the original regulations were written in 1987, but were added in 1999. Future revisions of the OBRA regulations will likely continue to provide updates to the recommended daily doses.

The 1999 revision of the OBRA 87 guidelines included use of medications other than psychoactive drugs that may be inappropriate in the elderly. This list of drugs and diagnoses/drug combinations was partially adapted from a paper entitled *Explicit Criteria for Determining Inappropriate Medication Use by the Elderly* by Mark H. Beers.[25] The list of inappropriate drugs found in the OBRA regulations are summarized in Table 129-5, along with the risk of severity of adverse events associated with use of each drug. The guidelines direct surveyors to assess resident use of these medications and ensure appropriate documentation of need for use. This documentation should provide adequate reason for use, justification for use of the drug over other options, and monitoring of drug efficacy and side effects. Inclusion in the list was determined based on efficacy, risk of side effects, and adverse effects on concomitant medical conditions.[25] For example, propoxyphene should be avoided in the elderly because it offers few advantages over acetaminophen in pain control and has significant neurologic and cardiotoxic side effects. Drugs with high anticholinergic side effects, such as amitriptyline, diphenhydramine, and dicyclomine, may cause constipation and urinary retention. Sedative/hypnotic medications should be avoided in residents with severe chronic obstructive pulmonary disease and sleep apnea. The reader is referred to the 1997 Beers article for further information regarding specific reasons for medication inappropriateness.

Medication Errors and Adverse Drug Reactions

Tags F332 and F333 of the OBRA guidelines define accepted rates of medication errors in a nursing facility and require that residents are free from significant medication errors (Table 129-12). The facility must monitor for medication errors and ensure an error rate of less than 5%. A medication error is defined as the administration of a drug that is not in accordance with: (1) the physician's order, (2) manufacturer's specifications, or (3) accepted professional standard. A significant medication error is one that causes the resident discomfort or jeopardizes his/her health or safety. Examples include: warfarin administered to a resident without a valid order; omission of a dose of an antibiotic; digoxin 0.25mg given when ordered dose is 0.125mg. The facility must have a policy and procedure in place for staff reporting of medication errors and the error rate should be reported to the Quality Assurance committee in the facility. It is suggested that the nursing facility monitor the occurrence of significant adverse drug reactions (ADR). An ADR is an unintended, undesirable, and unexpected effect of a prescribed medication or a medication error that results in: discontinuation of the drug or modification of the dose; initial or prolonged hospitalization; disability; treatment with further prescription medication; cognitive deterioration or impairment; or death. The JCAHO standards for long-term care TX.4.14 through TX.4.14.2 provide guidelines for the reporting and treatment of adverse drug reactions. 42 CFR 483.25(l) and 42 CFR 483.60(c)(2) of the CMS surveyor guidelines refer to adverse drug reactions. Surveyors for CMS will refer to the revised 1999 OBRA guidelines on unnecessary drugs when assessing for potential adverse drug reactions. If an ADR has occurred, the surveyors will review the resident chart for documentation of facility acknowledgment of

Table 129-12. Medication Error Regulation (OBRA87, Revised 1999)

The facility must ensure that:

(Tag F332) It is free of medication error rates of five percent or greater.

(Tag F333) Residents are free from any significant medication errors.

Medication Error: The observed preparation or administration of drugs or biologicals which is not in accordance with:

1. Physician's order
2. Manufacturer's specifications (not recommendations) regarding the preparation and administration of the drug or biological
3. Accepted professional standards and principles which apply to professionals providing services.

Medication Error Rate:

Medication Error Rate =

(Number of Errors Observed/Opportunities for Errors) × 100

A medication error rate of 5% or greater includes both significant and nonsignificant medication errors. It indicates that the facility may have systemic problems with its drug distribution system.

Significant and Nonsignificant Medication Errors:

Significant Medication Error—An error which causes the resident discomfort or jeopardizes his or her health or safety

*Determining Significance—The relative significance of medication errors is a matter of professional judgment.

1. Resident Condition
2. Drug Category
3. Frequency of Error

---

*Examples of significant and nonsignificant medication error may be found in OBRA 87 (revised 1999); Guidance to Surveyors—Long Term Care Facilities, Tag Number F333, pp 120–135.7.

Data from Omnibus Budget Reconciliation Act OBRA 1987 (revised 1999) PL 100-203 Nursing Home Reform Act; Guidance to Surveyors—Long Term Care Facilities; pp 129–131.

---

the adverse drug reaction and any treatment in response to the ADR. The MedWatch program of the Food and Drug Administration serves as a mechanism for reporting adverse drug reactions. If any of the above consequences result from an adverse drug reaction, a MedWatch report should be submitted. MedWatch forms may be downloaded at http://www.fda.gov/medwatch/ for use in submission. The FDA has recently added online submission of ADRs on this website.

Medication Pass Observation

Consultant pharmacists should monitor and make recommendations concerning medication administration passes on at least a quarterly basis. CMS surveyors observe medication administration as a part of the survey process for certification of the facility for Medicare/Medicaid. The objective of the med pass survey is to observe preparation and administration of medications in order to assess compliance with 42 CFR 483.25(m) (medication errors). The pharmacist should observe a minimum of 20 to 25 opportunities for error (both doses administered and doses ordered but not administered). The med passer should compare the medication label with the medication administration sheet to ensure that the drug, dose, and time are appropriate. The resident should be identified by the med passer to avoid administration to the wrong resident. In general, the med passer should adhere to the "5 rights"—right resident, right drug, right dose, right time, right route. Adequate hydration must be provided to the resident when administering medication. If medications are to be crushed for administration, ensure that the dosage form is suitable for crushing (ie, not sustained release or enteric coated). Medication carts should be locked when not in direct view of the medication passer to make certain that unauthorized individuals do not have access.

The acceptable medication error rate is less than 5% without any significant medication errors. A summary of this observation should be provided to the director of nursing and the Quality Assurance committee. As previously mentioned, The American Society of Consultant Pharmacists and Med Pass, Inc. can provide examples of medication pass observation worksheets and checklists.

The Minimum Data Set (MDS)

42 CFR 483.20 of The Omnibus Budget Reconciliation Act of 1987 requires that the facility conduct initial and periodic comprehensive assessment of each resident's functional capacity. This includes demographic information, community lifestyle and daily routine, cognitive patterns, communication, vision, mood and behavior patterns, psychosocial well-being, physical functioning, continence, disease diagnosis and health conditions, dental and nutritional status, skin conditions, activity pursuits, medications, special treatments and procedures, discharge potential, documentation of summary information obtained through resident assessment protocols (RAPs) and documentation of staff participating in the assessment. This assessment must be completed within 14 days of resident admission, quarterly, annually, and whenever there is a significant change in condition. The facility must use its state-approved resident assessment instrument. The facility must maintain 15 months of assessment data in the resident's clinical record that is readily available to all professional staff. The Resident Assessment Protocols (RAPs) are identified through responses to the individual sections of the MDS (triggers). These triggers identify residents who either have or are at risk for developing specific problems that require further evaluation. The RAPs provide the framework for individual resident care plans. Section O of the MDS involves medication use. Section O1 lists the number of medications the resident is taking (7-day look back), Section O2 is for new medications (90-day look back), Section O3 is injections (7-day look back), and Section O4 records the number of days that the resident received an antipsychotic, anxiolytic, antidepressant, hypnotic, or diuretic (7-day look back). Each medication should be coded based on the drug's pharmacological classification, not how it is being used. Doses are coded based on the number of days received, not the number of doses received. A PRN (as needed) medication is coded based on number of days given. Section U of the MDS is a list of medications that the resident has received in the last 7 days. This list includes the name of the medication and the dose ordered, the route of administration, the frequency of use, the amount administered (number of tablets/capsules), number of times a PRN medication was given, and the National Drug Code. The nursing facility likely will have a nurse serving as an "MDS Coordinator" to ensure that assessments are done on a timely basis. In general, the consultant pharmacist will not be asked by the facility to document on the MDS, but the pharmacist should be aware of the contents of the individual resident MDS for pertinent care issues and spot-check Section O for completion during drug regimen review. Updated information regarding the MDS can be found at http://cms.hhs.gov/medicaid/mds20.

Quality Indicators

The 1999 revision of the OBRA 87 regulations incorporated the use of quality indicators based on the MDS (Table 129-13). Five of the 24 indicators are derived from Section O. These are: (1) prevalence of symptoms of depression without antidepressant therapy; (2) prevalence of residents who take nine or more medications; (3) prevalence of antipsychotic use in the absence of psychotic or related conditions (high and low risk); (4) prevalence of antianxiety/hypnotic use; (5) prevalence of hypnotic use more than two times in last week. Consultant pharmacists need to be aware of these quality indicators and

Table 129-13. Quality Indicators Based on the Minimum Data Set (MDS)

ACCIDENTS	1. Incidence of new fractures
	2. Prevalence of falls
BEHAVIOR/ EMOTIONAL PATTERNS	3. Prevalence of behavioral symptoms affecting others (high risk and low risk)
	4. Prevalence of symptoms of depression
	5. Prevalence of symptoms of depression without antidepressant therapy
CLINICAL MANAGEMENT	6. Use of 9 or more different medications
COGNITIVE PATTERNS	7. Incidence of cognitive impairment
ELIMINATION/ INCONTINENCE	8. Prevalence of bladder or bowel incontinence (high risk and low risk)
	9. Prevalence of occasional or frequent bladder or bowel incontinence without a toileting plan
	10. Prevalence of indwelling catheter
	11. Prevalence of fecal impaction
INFECTION CONTROL	12. Prevalence of urinary tract infections
NUTRITION/ EATING	13. Prevalence of weight loss
	14. Prevalence of tube feeding
	15. Prevalence of dehydration
PHYSICAL FUNCTIONING	16. Prevalence of bedfast residents
	17. Incidence of decline in late loss ADLs (activities of daily living)
	18. Incidence of decline in ROM (range of motion)
PSYCHOTROPIC DRUG USE	19. Prevalence of antipsychotic use in the absence of psychotic or related conditions (high risk and low risk)
	20. Prevalence of antianxiety/hypnotic use
	21. Prevalence of hypnotic use more than two time in last week
QUALITY OF LIFE	22. Prevalence of daily physical restraints
	23. Prevalence of little or no activity
SKIN CARE	24. Prevalence of stage 1-4 pressure ulcers

Data from Center for Health Systems Research and Analysis. Quality indicators page. Available at: http://www.chsra.wisc.edu/CHSRA/Quality_Indicators/ toc.htm. Accessed March 6, 2003.

the facility performance on them. Quality indicators should be incorporated into the consultant pharmacist reports to the facility, along with an explanation of any deviation from the norm. If the facility has a high rate of residents taking more than nine medications or a high rate of use of antipsychotic medications in the absence of psychotic conditions, the facility will have to justify this to CMS surveyors. Consultant pharmacist drug regimen review recommendations and drug use evaluation may aid in providing justification. Prevalence of falls should be of interest to the consultant pharmacist when determining appropriateness of sedating drug therapy. Bowel and bladder incontinence and fecal impaction patterns may direct the consultant pharmacist to evaluate the facility's use of laxative medications. Prevalence of residents receiving tube feedings should prompt the consultant pharmacist to evaluate the drug regimen of those residents to ensure that all medications are suitable for tube administration and do not interact with tube feedings.

Interdisciplinary Health Care Teams

Interdisciplinary teams are defined as health care teams that have members from different disciplines; those members have interdependent, collaborative roles and meet to plan treatment and evaluate patient response.[26] Many disciplines can be involved in interdisciplinary care teams in long-term care (Table 129-14). While the MDS requires most of these disciplines to provide documentation on the resident assessment, care team meetings can aid the facility in integrating care such that the entire group is responsible for resident function and outcome. The interdisciplinary model works well in long-term care because the resident is being treated for chronic conditions, for which each discipline can contribute to a treatment plan with creative interventions that allow for the best possible functioning of the resident. Care plan meetings generally involve nursing, dietary, recreation, and social services. Pharmacy, respiratory therapy, physical therapy, and occupational therapy are consulted as needed based on the discussion in the care plan meeting. Ideally, these meetings would include the pharmacist, but most consultant pharmacists are responsible for many facilities and only spend a few days per month in each facility. One area in which a pharmacist may become more involved is behavioral care and treatment. There is a trend in nursing facilities toward developing a functional behavioral care committee that meets on a monthly or quarterly basis. This committee discusses residents with problem behaviors that are disruptive or dangerous to self and/or others. Disciplines represented include nursing, social services, recreation, psychology or psychiatry, medicine, and pharmacy. Because use of medications is often a large part of the discussion, having the pharmacist available to provide input regarding choice of drug therapy (or lack of effective drug therapy for the particular behavior), dosing, drug interactions and side effects, and regulatory requirements can optimize the resident outcome. Interdisciplinary care teams help to promote a level of respect for individual disciplines and the need for all in the care of residents in long-term care.

ETHICAL AND QUALITY OF LIFE CONSIDERATIONS

An individual's entitlement to the concern, respect, and protection of the community does not diminish with age.[27] This is considered to be the first principle of gerontology and is the principle which, if subscribed to by geriatric practitioners, can ease some of the ethical dilemmas that frequently arise. In this age of increasing technology, increasing cost of health care, and reduced number of individuals with comprehensive health care coverage, issues in the care of elderly patients are debated. Questions have been raised about the benefit of expenditures made in the last year of a patient's life by those who argue that medical resources should be rationed and given to those who can receive the most benefit in terms of longevity. The American Geriatric Society's policy on the allocation of health care resources points out that before any debate on rationing of medical resources can take place, practitioners should first focus efforts on unnecessary spending and waste in all areas of health care and not target a specific population, such as the elderly.[28] The general perception of nursing homes is that these facilities exist to provide comfort and care to geriatric patients in the end of life without going to extraordinary measures to prolong life. In reality, nursing homes are the end-of-life residences of many elderly individuals, and these facilities are expected to adhere to strict regulations regarding the rights of residents to health care.

CFR 42 483.10 of the Omnibus Budget Reconciliation Act encompasses resident rights. This regulation states that the resident has a right to a dignified existence, self-determination, and communication with and access to persons and services in-

Table 129-14. Multidisciplinary Approach to Resident Care

Pharmacy	Respiratory Therapy	Nursing
Medicine	Occupational Therapy	Dietary
Recreation	Social Services	Physical Therapy

side and outside the facility. Exercising these rights means that residents have autonomy and choice, to the maximum extent possible, about how they wish to live their everyday lives and receive care, subject to the facility's rules, as long as those rules do not violate a regulatory requirement.[29] Autonomy and self-determination in health care requires that health care practitioners have a respect for the individual and his/her right to decide what, if any, medical treatment is acceptable and appropriate. Practitioners can aid the person in this decision by providing clear and complete information about the benefits and risks of a particular treatment. While often difficult to ethically accept, those providing care to elderly nursing facility residents will encounter residents who refuse treatment. Documentation should be provided in the medical record concerning the counseling the resident received and a form of resident documentation of resident refusal. A resident should never be coerced into a treatment or made to feel that reprisals will result from refusal. While the responsibility for the outcome of the refusal of treatment lies with the resident, health care practitioners must continue to offer and provide optimal care regardless of the outcome. When a resident refuses treatment, the competency of the resident to make medical decisions can be called into question. Competency of an individual is a legal determination of ability to make decisions in one's best interest. Care must be taken by the health care team to recognize that the elderly are especially vulnerable to a transient lack of competency that has many causes, including medication side effects, delirium secondary to infection, and depression. Before pursuing a ruling on an individual's competency, the facility should ensure that all medical and psychiatric reasons for lack of decision-making abilities are ruled out. Often, a resident will be admitted to a facility with a durable power of attorney (POA) or health care representative/power of attorney (HCR/POA) already appointed. It is important to differentiate between these two terms. The durable POA is a surrogate appointed by the individual to handle his/her property and financial affairs. The HCR/POA is a person appointed by the individual to act in the individual's best interest in matters of health care should the individual be unable to do so. Either of these may be revoked by the individual as long as the person is deemed competent. If a resident does not have a HCR/POA and is deemed not to be competent to make medical decisions, the legal system will appoint a guardian for the resident. Guardianship proceedings often result from an urgent need for a responsible individual to make decisions.

The Federal Patient Self-Determination Act of 1990 was enacted in December 1991 in an attempt to offer patients the opportunity to make their wishes known prior to the need for a HCR/POA or guardian in the form of an advance directive. This Act requires all health facilities to maintain policies and procedures regarding written advance directives. Facilities must document whether or not a patient has an advance directive, but does not require that the facility prepare the document.[30] Advance directives essentially document the individual's wishes for health care should that individual become incapacitated. A patient may make statements about wishes for life-sustaining treatments, including cardiopulmonary resuscitation (CPR), mechanical ventilation, artificial hydration and nutrition, intravenous antibiotics, transportation to the hospital from the nursing facility for treatment of acute illness, and dialysis. These advance directives should be placed in a prominent place in the resident chart, along with the "code status" of the resident. The "code status" refers to the resident's wishes for CPR. Documentation must be made by the physician regarding "DNR" (do not resuscitate) or "full code" (CPR). The physician must talk to the resident or his/her agent prior to this documentation. The *living will* is another term used for advance directives.

The concept of *quality of life* is central to understanding decisions regarding what may or may not be in a resident's best interest. Quality of life is a nebulous term that is variably defined based on the circumstance. Quality of life is generally referred to as multidimensional, incorporating an individual's physical health and functioning, psychological health and functioning, social and role functioning, and perceptions of general well-being. Prolongation of life by life-sustaining measures does not ensure that the individual will continue to maintain a quality of life that is acceptable to him or her. Persons admitted to long-term care facilities are often facing considerable losses in terms of independence and previous lifestyle. They commonly have significant chronic medical conditions and receive multiple medications that may reduce their perceptions of a meaningful life. A resident may express to staff that he/she is not worth the time spent taking care of him/her and believe that no medical treatment can change the inevitable outcome of their demise. In these situations, the medical issues challenging a resident have little to do with the resident's well-being. The facility staff should make every effort to get to know a resident's likes and dislikes and activities enjoyed prior to admission. Residents often have roommates not of their choosing, are told when to eat and take medications, bathe based on a staff schedule, tolerate many individuals in a limited space, and cope with the fact that they live in an institution. It becomes more understandable that residents who are able to make their own medical decisions may choose not to pursue aggressive treatment when these factors are recognized. The practice of geriatrics, whether medicine, pharmacy, nursing, social services, or recreation, should always involve a cognizant effort on the part of the practitioner to recognize issues of quality of life.

GERIATRIC PHARMACOLOGY

There are many age-related changes in the pharmacokinetics of drugs that effect the geriatric patient's ability to appropriately process and eliminate medications. Table 129-15 provides a summary of these changes.

Absorption

Changes occurring in the gastrointestinal tract due to age can be expected to affect the absorption of drugs administered orally. The increased gastric pH that occurs secondary to gastric atrophy may alter drug ionization and solubility and decreased blood flow to the GI tract may decrease the rate and extent of drug absorption. Gastric atrophy also contributes to a decreased surface area for absorption. Decreases are seen in gastric emptying rate and intestinal motility. While most drugs are absorbed via passive transport, a few require active transport, which is reduced in the elderly, leading to a decreased bioavailability of the drug. Of more significance may be the decreased first-pass effect and hepatic extraction that is a function of aging, which may cause enhanced bioavailability of drugs that have a high first-pass effect. Absorption of drugs through the skin is poorly understood in geriatric patients. Evidence exists that while older patients may eventually attain serum levels transdermally similar to those of younger adults, the time to reach these levels may be longer.[31]

Distribution

The distribution of drugs in the body depends on factors such as blood flow, plasma protein stores, body fat, and total body water. Decreased cardiac output and tissue perfusion can lead to decreased renal and hepatic blood flow. A reduction in total body water causes a decrease in the volume of distribution of water-soluble drugs promoting increased plasma concentrations of these drugs. The elderly are more likely to have greater body fat and less lean body mass, which will increase the volume of distribution and terminal half-life of fat-soluble medications. The loading doses of some drugs may be affected by the altered volume of distribution caused by aging. For example, the loading dose of digoxin should be reduced in patients with

Table 129-15. Age-Related Pharmacokinetic Changes

PARAMETER	PHYSIOLOGIC CHANGES
Absorption	↓ active transport = ↓ bioavailability
	↓ first-pass effect = ↑ bioavailability
	↑ gastric pH
	↓ absorptive surface
	↓ splanchnic blood flow
	↓ gastrointestinal motility
	↓ gastric emptying rate
Distribution	↓ volume of distribution = ↑ plasma concentrations of water-soluble drugs
	↑ volume of distribution = ↑ t1/2 of fat-soluble drugs
	↑/↓ free fraction of highly plasma protein bound drugs
	↓ cardiac output
	↓ total body water
	↓ lean body mass
	↓ serum albumin
	↑ α_1-acid glycoprotein
	↑ body fat
	↓ tissue perfusion
Metabolism	↓ clearance = ↑ t1/2 for oxidatively metabolized drugs
	↓ clearance = ↑ t1/2 of drugs with high hepatic extration ratio
	↓ hepatic mass
	↓ hepatic blood flow
	↓ enzyme activity
Excretion	↓ clearance = ↑ t1/2 of renally eliminated drugs
	↓ renal blood flow
	↓ glomular filtration rate
	↓ tubular secretion
	↓ renal mass

renal dysfunction due to a reduction in volume of distribution and increased serum drug levels. Substantial changes may occur in serum albumin and α_1-acid glycoprotein. Nutritional deficiencies that include a lack of protein intake may cause a reduction in serum albumin. This can lead to a higher free fraction of drugs that are highly bound to albumin, such as phenytoin. When a routine serum level of phenytoin is drawn, a serum albumin should also be obtained to correct the phenytoin level for the reduced albumin. Other acidic drugs, such as naproxen and warfarin, may be affected by the serum albumin level. α_1-acid glycoprotein is increased in the plasma secondary to inflammation or cancer and can lead to enhanced levels of β-blockers, quinidine, and tricyclic antidepressants, causing a reduced free fraction of drug and reduced drug effects.[32]

Metabolism

The liver is responsible for the majority of drug metabolism, including Phase I (oxidative) and Phase II (conjugative) metabolism. It has been suggested that age-related declines in Phase I metabolism are likely due to age-related reduction in liver volume, rather than decreased enzymatic activity. Drugs that are metabolized by Phase I, including diazepam and theophylline, can be expected to have reduced clearance and increased half-life. Medications such as lorazepam and oxazepam, which undergo glucuronidation, are unaffected by age.[31] For this reason, use of short-acting benzodiazepines such as lorazepam and oxazepam are recommended over use of the longer-acting diazepam. Because of reduced blood flow to the liver, drugs that have a high hepatic extration ratio will have an increased plasma half-live and reduced clearance. While aging can cause a reduced enzymatic activity in the liver, elderly individuals who smoke may have liver induction of the P450 CYP1A2 enzyme. Drugs metabolized by CYP1A2 can be expected to have reduced plasma levels due to increased

metabolism. Some examples include amitriptyline, mirtazapine, clozapine, olanzapine, haloperidol, ondansetron, propranolol, theophylline, verapamil, and warfarin.

Elimination

Most drugs are primarily excreted renally. Aging is associated with reduction in renal mass. Glomerular filtration rate, tubular secretion, and renal blood flow are also reduced. The assumption is that most elderly individuals have declining renal function, but as many as one-third may have no renal impairment evident as measured by creatinine clearance. Although the estimation of the creatinine clearance is a useful tool in assessing renal function, it should only be used as a guide, as elderly patients often have a reduction in muscle mass, which is the primary source of serum creatinine. The most often used equation for estimating creatinine is the Cockcroft/Gualt equation:[33]

$$CrCl \text{ (males)} = \frac{(140 - \text{age in years}) \times (\text{total body weight in kg})}{72 \times SCr \text{ in mg/dl}}$$

For females, the result must be multiplied by 0.85.

ACE inhibitors, aminoglycosides, digoxin, furosemide, lithium, metformin, and vancomycin are examples of drugs whose elimination is impaired by age-related reductions in renal function. Digoxin and lithium have narrow therapeutic indices that require close monitoring of both drug serum levels and renal function in order to avoid significant side effects.

Altered Pharmacodynamics

Evidence exists that the elderly have an enhanced response to drug therapy. Many possible reasons for this have been suggested, including changes in number of receptors, changes in receptor affinity, postreceptor alterations, and age-related impairment of homeostatic mechanisms.[31] Elderly patients may have a greater response to opiates and benzodiazepines, causing an increase in analgesia and central nervous system side effects. They may be less responsive to β-blockers, either due to a reduction in the number of β receptors or alterations in receptor affinity for the drug. The anticoagulant effects of warfarin are enhanced in older individuals, leading to a greater risk of bleeding and a need for reduced and carefully monitored dosing. The elderly may have an increased sensitivity to drugs that affect dopamine. This includes metoclopramide, levodopa, dopamine agonists, and antipsychotics with significant dopamine-antagonist properties.[32]

DISEASE CONSIDERATIONS

In order to perform clinically guided drug regimen review, the pharmacist must have an understanding of common disease states that are likely to be present in the elderly population. Table 129-16 provides an overview of disease states by organ system. While it is beyond the scope of this chapter to provide in-depth discussion of each disease state, a brief overview of the disease and points relevant to the consultant pharmacist will be presented. Tables 129-17 and 129-18 provide useful websites for clinical guidelines for many disease states and information regarding the needs of geriatric patients. Table 129-19 lists selected geriatric care references that may aid the clinician in the treatment of the elderly.

Cardiovascular

Age-related changes in the cardiovascular system and reduced physical activity affect cardiovascular function in the elderly. A decrease in arterial elasticity contributes to an increase in afterload which causes an elevation in blood pressure. Left

Table 129-16. Common Geriatric Disease States

Blood Disorders	Esophageal Dysmotility
Anemia of Chronic Disease	Gallstones
Iron Deficiency Anemia	*Helicobacter pylori* Gastritis
Thrombocytopenia	Hiatal Hernia
Vitamin B12 Deficiency	Peptic Ulcer Disease
	Reflux Esophagitis
Bone/Rheumatologic	
Bone Fractures	**Neurologic**
Osteoarthritis	Alzheimer's Dementia
Osteoporosis	Essential Tremor
Paget's Disease	Parkinson's Disease
Rheumatoid Arthritis	Peripheral Neuropathies
	Stroke
Cardiovascular	Vascular Dementia
Atherosclerosis	
Cardiac Arrhythmias	**Ocular**
Coronary Artery Disease	Cataracts
Heart Failure	Glaucoma
Hyperlipidemia	
Hypertension	**Psychiatric**
Thromboembolism	Alcohol Abuse
Valvular Heart Disease	Anxiety
	Depression
Dermatological	Insomnia
Herpes Zoster	Late Life Psychosis
Psoriasis	
Rosacea	**Respiratory**
	Asthma
Endocrine	Chronic Obstructive
Diabetes Mellitus	Pulmonary Disease
Hyperthyroidism	Lung Cancer
Hypothyroidism	
	Urinary Tract
Gastroenterologic	Bacteriuria
Cholecystitis	Benign Prostatic Hyperplasia
Constipation	Diabetic Nephropathy
Diverticulitis	Renal Failure
Dysphagia	Urinary Incontinence

Table 129-18. Useful Web Sites

TITLE	WEB SITE
American Association of Retired Persons	www.aarp.com
American Pharmaceutical Association	www.aphanet.org
American Society of Consultant Pharmacists	www.ascp.com
American Society of Health System Pharmacists	www.ashp.com
Centers for Medicare & Medicaid	http://cms.hhs.gov
Cytochrome P450 Drug Interactions	http://medicine.iupui.edu/flockhart
ElderWeb	www.elderweb.com
Herbal Therapy	www.uiowa.edu/~idis/herballinks
Medscape	www.medscape.com
MedWatch	www.fda.gov/medwatch
National Institute on Aging	www.nia.hih.gov
Quality Indicators	www.chsra.wisc.edu
Veterans' Adminsitration	www.va.gov

be considered when there is a need for symptomatic control of heart failure and should be used along with an ACE inhibitor, diuretic, and beta-blocker.[35]

Atrial fibrillation (AF) is the most common cardiac arrhythmia seen in geriatric patients.

AF is often associated with structural heart disease and heart failure. It is a supraventricular tachycardia that occurs in isolation or in association with other arrhythmias. Patients with AF may have drug therapy for heart rate control, which allows the arrhythmia to continue, or for rhythm control. Restoration and maintenance of sinus rhythm will help to alleviate symptoms, prevent thromboembolism and reduce the risk of stroke. Drugs used to control heart rate are considered safer than those with an antiarrhythmic effect. Antiarrhythmics, such as amiodarine, propafenone, quinidine, digoxin, and sotalol may be used in an effort to convert AF to sinus rhythm. Digoxin, non-dihydropyridine calcium antagonists, and beta-blockers may be used for rate control in AF.[36] Anticoagulation with warfarin is recommended for all patients with atrial fibrillation to reduce the risk of thromboembolism and stroke. If a patient cannot tolerate warfarin, aspirin may be used, but is not as effective.

The Seventh Report of the Joint National Committee on Prevention, Detection, Evaluation, and Treatment of High Blood Pressure (Express, full report due Fall 2003) suggests that normal blood pressure is <120/80 mmHg. *Prehypertensive* is a new term used in the JNC VII and is defined at a blood pressure of 120–139/80–89 mmHg. Hypertension is divided into two stages. Stage 1 hypertension is a blood pressure of 140–159/90–99 mmHg, stage 2 hypertension is a blood pressure of >160/100 mmHg.[37] Initial drug choices for hypertension should include di-

ventricular diastolic filling is reduced and contraction and relaxation of the ventricle is prolonged, leading to heart failure.[34] Progressive heart failure becomes a vicious cycle of sympathetic response to decreased cardiac output causing tachycardia and left ventricular hypertrophy that further damages the heart muscle. Coronary artery disease, valvular heart disease, arrhythmias, and hyperlipidemia are common in the elderly.

Current guidelines for many of the cardiovascular diseases now include the use of several medications at one time to effectively treat these conditions. According to the ACC/AHA Practice Guidelines, patients with heart failure should receive a diuretic and an ACE inhibitor as maintenance therapy. Those who can tolerate a β-blocker should receive a low dose of metoprolol or carvedilol to reduce the increased heart rate that is a response to reduced cardiac output. Evidence suggests that spironolactone, as an aldosterone antagonist, may reduce the deleterious effects of aldosterone on the heart. Digoxin should

Table 129-17. Selected Clinical Guidelines Web Sites

TITLE	WEBSITE
Agency for Healthcare Research and Quality (AHRQ)	www.ahrq.gov/clinic/cpgonline.htm
American College of Cardiology	http://www.acc.org/clinical/statements.htm
American Medical Directors' Association (AMDA)	www.amda.com
CDC Prevention Guidelines	http://aepo-xdv-www.epo.cdc.gov/wonder/PrevGuid/prevguid.shtml
eGuidelines	http://www.eguidelines.co.uk
Healthlinks: Evidence-Based Practice and Guidelines	http://healthlinks.washington.edu/clinical/gidelines.html
National Guideline Clearinghouse (NGC)	http://www.guideline.gov.index.asp
National Heart, Lung, and Blood Institute	http://www.nhlbi.nih.gov/guidelines
National Library of Medicine	http://text.nlm.nih.gov
Primary Care Clinical Practice Guidelines	http://medicine.ucsf.edu/resources/guidelines
SUMSearch	http://SUMSearch.uthscsa.edu
Turning Research into Practice (TRIP)	www.tripdatabase.com

Table 129-19. Selected Geriatric Care References

Carstensen LL, et al. *The Practical Handbook of Clinical Gerontology*. Thousand Oaks, CA: Sage Publications, 1996.
Clark TR. *Nursing Home Survey Procedures and Interpretive Guidelines*. American Society of Consultant Pharmacists.
Dipiro JT, et al. *Pharmacotherapy: A Pathophysiologic Approach*, 5th edition. New York: McGraw-Hill, 2002.
Hazzard, WR, et al. *Principles of Geriatric Medicine and Gerontology*, 5th edition. New York: McGraw-Hill, 2003.
Kane RL, et al. *Essentials of Clinical Geriatrics*, 4th edition. New York: McGraw-Hill, 1999.
Koda-Kimble MA, et al. *Applied Therapeutics: The Clinical Use of Drugs*, 7th edition. Philadelphia: Lippincott Williams and Wilkins, 2001.
Semla TP, et al. *Geriatric Dosage Handbook*, 8th edition. American Pharmaceutical Association, 2003.
Tallis, RC, Fillit HM. *Brocklehurst's Textbook of Geriatric Medicine and Gerontology*, 6th edition. London: Churchill Livingstone and Elsevier Science Limited, 2003.

uretics and beta-blockers. These drug classes have been shown to reduce the morbidity and mortality associated with hypertension. ACE inhibitors may be a drug of first choice in patients with diabetes or heart failure, as these drugs may also have a renal protective effect. Patients having had a recent myocardial infarction should receive a beta-blocker to reduce the risk of subsequent MI. Diuretics and long-acting dihydropyridine calcium channel blockers are preferred for older persons with isolated systolic hypertension.[37] The JNC VII also suggests that most persons with significant hypertension will require two or more antihypertensives to control their condition.

The NCEP Guidelines for the treatment of hyperlipidemia suggest that drug therapy be initiated when the low-density lipoprotein cholesterol is >130 mg/dL. Drug therapy can include the *statins* (HMG-CoA reductase inhibitors), niacin, and bile acid sequestrants. If the patient is exhibiting hypertriglyceridemia, a *fibrate* such as gemfibrozil or fenofibrate may be used, but caution should be taken if gemfibrozil is to be used in combination with a statin as the risk for myalgias and rhabdomyolysis is increased.[38] Current evidence suggests that geriatric patients of any age may benefit from the use of a statin to reduce the risk of a cardiac event. Ezetimibe is a new medication for the treatment of hypercholesterolemia that is used in combination with dietary therapy or statins which inhibits the absorption of cholesterol in the small intestine.

Respiratory

Many residents of nursing facilities suffer from chronic obstructive pulmonary disease (COPD), often from smoking tobacco. The quality of life of patients with COPD changes dramatically based on their perceived ability to "catch their breath." Residents who use oxygen are often preoccupied with the oxygen availability in their tanks, the time of the next nebulizer treatment, and anxiety concerning the inability to breathe. Beta-agonists, such as albuterol, remain the mainstay of the treatment of COPD. Albuterol is a short-acting beta-agonist with an onset of action that can rapidly improve respiratory function. Side effects may include an increase in heart rate and anxiety, and reductions in serum potassium. Albuterol is often combined with ipratropium, an anticholinergic, which competitively inhibits cholinergic receptors producing bronchodilation. Long-acting beta-agonists, such as salmeterol, may be used; the patient should be aware that salmeterol should not be used as a "rescue" medication. Corticosteroids are often used in patients with COPD, either for acute exacerbations or long-term therapy when the individual progresses to more significant disease. Inhaled corticosteroids, including fluticasone and beclomethasone, are generally initiated after use of albuterol/ipratropium is not sufficient to control symptoms. Patients should be told to rinse the mouth after use of the inhaler to avoid drug-induced oral fungal infections. The anti-inflammatory efficacy of oral corticosteroids in COPD is not without a price. Diabetes mellitus, osteoporosis, psychological disturbance, and hypokalemia can result from the long-term use of corticosteroids.[39] Some studies have shown that patients receiving oral prednisone at a dose of >5mg/day for several months have a significant risk of osteporosis. Anxiety concerning shortness of breath is a significant problem for patients with COPD. Treatment of this anxiety can often improve the quality of life of the patient. Benzodiazepines, such as lorazepam, can be effective, but the lowest dose possible should be given to prevent respiratory depression.

Neurologic

Common neurologic disorders include Parkinson's disease, Alzheimer's disease, vascular dementia, stroke, and peripheral neuropathies. Stroke often occurs as a result of cardiovascular disease and hypertension. This event can be life-changing for the patient and can result in permanent disability or admission to an institution. Many stroke patients develop hemiparesis, or paralysis on one side of the body. Physical and occupational therapy can be instrumental in aiding these patients in a return to an acceptable quality of life. Antiplatelet therapy is often initiated after a stroke to prevent a recurrence, with aspirin being the most commonly used agent. Warfarin may be used as an alternative. Peripheral neuropathies often occur as a result of poorly controlled diabetes. Drug therapy can help to reduce the pain associated with the neuropathies, but often is only partially effective. Amitriptyline is a very effective medication for peripheral neuropathy, but its use is limited by anticholinergic side effects. Gabapentin has recently been approved for use in post-herpetic neuralgia and is used off-label for neuropathies.

Parkinson's disease results from a markedly decreased number of nigrostriatal dopamine neurons and from nigrostriatal dopamine loss. While primarily a disease of motor function, some patients can develop neuropsychological abnormalities and dementia later in the course of the disease. Anticholinergics, levodopa, and dopamine agonists are the mainstay of therapy for Parkinson's disease. Controversy exists over the optimal time to initiate levodopa due to concerns that dopamine, as a free radical, may cause more damage to the nigrostriatum. Strategic dosing of levodopa is important to minimize "wearing off" and "on-off" problems associated with levodopa therapy. Levodopa-carbidopa is available in regular and sustained release dosage forms to deal with these issues. COMT (catecholamine-O-methyltransferase) inhibitors may increase the amount of levodopa that crosses the blood-brain barrier by interfering with the metabolism of levodopa in the periphery. Tolcapone, the first COMT inhibitor released on the market, is associated with possible hepatotoxicity and guidelines exist for monitoring of liver function. Use of entacapone has largely replaced tolcapone due to a reduced risk of liver abnormalitites with entacapone. Parkinson's patients receiving drugs that boost dopamine in the brain are at risk for symptoms of psychosis, including hallucinations and delusions. Because use of dopaminergic agents is the most effective way to treat the movement problems associated with Parkinson's disease, many patients are resistant to discontinuing or reducing the dose of these drugs. Atypical antipsychotic agents such as quetiapine, risperidone, olanzapine, and clozapine may be used in low doses to minimize psychotic symptoms while not interfering with the need for elevated dopamine in the nigrostriatum.

Dementia is a common condition in nursing home residents. Alzheimer's dementia, Lewy body dementia, and vascular dementia are a few forms. Unfortunately, at this time, definitive diagnosis of Alzheimer's can only be accomplished at autopsy. It is a diagnosis of exclusion. When the individual with dementia is admitted to a nursing facility, he or she has generally declined enough in the course of the disease that control of behavioral symptoms and wandering are the greatest concerns. The acetylcholinesterase inhibitors (tacrine, donepezil, galantamine, and rivastigamine) are available as treatment for mild to moderate Alzheimer's dementia, but the goal of therapy with these agents should be to slow progression of the disease, not to improve cognition. Behavioral treatments for agitation in dementia include short-acting benzodiazepines, trazodone, and anticonvulsants, such as valproic acid and gabapentin. Antipsychotics may be used if documentation can be provided of psychotic symptoms.

Ocular

Visual disturbances secondary to hypertension and diabetes mellitus are common in the elderly population. Unfortunately, little treatment is available for these problems once they have arisen. Use of large-print books and books-on-tape can aid a visually impaired resident who enjoys reading. The resident room should be arranged simply so that the individual has a reduced risk of tripping or falling on furniture and other room items. Glaucoma is an ocular disorder that is characterized by changes in the optic nerve. Elevated intraocular pressure may be involved in the pathogenesis of glaucoma, but is no longer considered to be diagnostic for glaucoma.[40] The beta-blockers (timolol, bisoprolol) are considered to be first-line therapy for glaucoma. Other therapies include topical carbonic anhydrase inhibitors, prostaglandin analogues, and brimonidine. Pilocarpine, epinephrine, and apraclonidine are now considered second line agents in the treatment of glaucoma. The consultant pharmacist should ensure that these medications are appropriately administered such that optimal benefit is obtained, meaning that if a resident is receiving several different drops, the drops should be administered with enough time in between to allow for absorption in the eye.

Psychiatric

Recent evidence suggests that major depression is under-recognized in the elderly population, with the prevalence approaching 20% in females aged 65 to 80.[41] As has been previously mentioned, elderly individuals admitted to nursing facilities suffer life-changing losses in independence and self-esteem. As such, the symptoms of depression can manifest themselves in several ways in geriatric patients, including dementia, isolation, agitated behavior, weight loss, and psychosis. Antidepressants with high anticholinergic side effects should be avoided in the elderly patient. Sertraline, fluoxetine, citalopram, escitalopram, venlafaxine, and bupropion can be considered to be among the antidepressants of first choice for geriatric patients. Anxiety and insomnia often accompany the myriad of chronic diseases that may be present in the older patient. Treating the signs and symptoms of the chronic disease can in many cases alleviate this anxiety and insomnia, but if this is not effective, benzodiazepines, buspirone, and zolpidem can be helpful. If a patient has a diagnosis of sleep apnea, use of a sedative/hypnotic medication should be avoided, as well as the use of a benzodiazepine in a patient with a history of substance abuse.

Bone/Rheumatologic

Osteoporosis and related bone fractures occur frequently in the elderly. Most older persons will have some degree of bone loss related to lack of calcium intake and physical exercise. While osteoporosis has been associated in the female patient with the loss of estrogen after menopause, male patients who have an inadequate diet or take chronic oral corticosteroids may also be at risk. Current recommendations for adequate calcium intake are 1200 mg of calcium and 400–600 IU vitamin D per day. Single doses of calcium should not exceed 600 mg due to lack of absorption of calcium at higher doses. Calcium tablets should be taken with a meal to improve absorption and reduce the likelihood of gastrointestinal upset. Bisphosphonates, risedronate, and alendronate are adsorbed to bone and become a permanent part of the bone structure, preventing bone resorption. These drugs are indicated for the prevention and treatment of osteoporosis. Due to a risk of esophageal ulceration associated with these agents, the patient should take this medication on an empty stomach and remain in an upright position for 30 minutes after ingestion. Calcitonin is also available in injectable and intranasal form for the treatment of osteoporosis. The occurrence of a hip fracture in an elderly patient can cause significant morbidity and mortality. The consultant pharmacist should be aware of medications contained in a resident's drug regimen that could contribute to the risk of falls and act to minimize their use as much as possible.

Gastrointestinal

Swallowing difficulties can present a significant problem to the geriatric patient. A patient with dysphagia, often the result of a stroke, loses the ability to swallow due to lack of muscle control in the esophagus. Choking and aspiration pneumonia are common consequences of dysphagia, and residents with this problem will often require a mechanical soft or pureed diet and thickened liquids. Benzodiazepine anxiolytic medications can be associated with dysphagia secondary to muscle relaxant effects and should be considered when a resident develops dysphagia without signs or symptoms of stroke. This effect is not related to newly initiated drug therapy and may occur at any time during therapy. Patients with significant gastrointestinal complaints should be evaluated for *Helicobacter pylori* infection, a common cause of gastritis in the elderly. Testing for *H pylori* is relatively simple, and it is easily treated. The course of therapy often involves some combination of a macrolide antibiotic, amoxicillin, H2 antagonist or proton pump inhibitor, and/or bismuth subsalicylate in high doses for a 2-week course of therapy. Gastroesophageal reflux disease can be caused by lower esophageal sphincter relaxation associated with aging, exacerbated in those who smoke tobacco. Proton pump inhibitors and H2 antagonists are effective in treating this condition. NSAID-induced gastric ulcers can be a significant source of morbidity and mortality for the geriatric patient. Some evidence exists that COX 2 inhibitors (celecoxib, rofecoxib, valdecoxib) may exhibit a reduced risk of GI bleeding over traditional NSAIDs (nonsteroidal anti-inflammatory drugs). This may be due to a possible reduced deleterious effect of COX 2 inhibitors on the gastroprotective mucosal layer of the stomach as compared to NSAIDs. Constipation remains the most frequent gastrointestinal complaint in elderly individuals. Physiologically, these patients have a prolonged gastric emptying time and decreased gastric motility. Frequently, drug regimens containing multiple medications further effect gastric emptying and motility. Opiate analgesics, anticholinergics, antihistamines, tricyclic antidepressants, calcium channel blockers, NSAIDs, and iron and calcium supplements may all cause constipation. The surveyor guidelines of the OBRA 87 regulations require that documentation of necessary drug therapy be provided for use of three or more laxatives for a resident. Counseling of the resident and education of the facility staff may be necessary regarding appropriate expectations for bowel function and the use of laxatives.

Urinary Tract

Creatinine clearance decreases at the rate of approximately 0.75 ml/min/1.73 m^2 per year beginning in the fourth decade of life.[42] As has been previously mentioned, evaluation of renal function in the elderly using creatinine clearance can be problematic, as this equation is a function of serum creatinine, which is reduced in the elderly secondary to reduced muscle mass. A calculation of creatinine clearance should be made whenever possible for effective drug regimen review to assess the appropriateness of not only drug therapy, but also of dosing. Diabetic nephropathy is characterized by proteinuria of >300 mg/24 hr, an increase in blood pressure, and reduced glomular filtration rate. Microalbuminuria (proteinuria) is also an independent risk factor for myocardial infarction and stroke. ACE inhibitors and angiotensin receptor blockers have been shown to be beneficial in slowing the progression of renal disease in patients and should be considered in patients with progressive diabetic nephropathy.[43]

Benign prostatic hyperplasia is common is elderly males and causes significant distress related to urinary continence. The increased size of the prostate impedes urinary outflow due to a blockage of the bladder neck. Excessive α-adrenergic tone of the prostate may lead to contraction of the prostate gland around the urethra. α-blocking drugs such as terazosin and doxazosin are often used in the treatment of BPH. Finasteride, which blocks 5α-reductase and decreases serum dihydrotestosterone levels, is also effective. The patient taking these medications should be aware that clinical onset of drug action may take several weeks to months.

Endocrine

Much controversy currently exists regarding when to initiate treatment for hypothyroidism. Primary hypothyroidism is defined as an elevated TSH (thyroid stimulating hormone), and a low free T_4 level. Patients with a TSH between 6 and 10 μU per mL may be defined as having subclinical hypothyroidism and may be treated on the basis of documented signs and symptoms of hypothyroidism. These patients have a higher risk of developing overt hypothyroidism than those with a documented normal TSH. Levothyroxine is used as exogenous replacement therapy in patients with hypothyroidism. The TSH level may be used to monitor efficacy of levothyroxine replacement therapy, with the free T_4 obtained as necessary to substantiate TSH findings. When levothyroxine is initiated or the dose changed, a 6- to 8-week period should elapse before obtaining another TSH level. The dose initiation or change may not be reflected in the TSH level before this time.

Diabetes mellitus is a significant health problem in elderly patients. Dietary habits, obesity, and cigarette smoking can all contribute to an individual's risk of developing diabetes. It is especially troublesome in the long-term care environment to impress upon residents the need to comply with the recommended diet and exercise programs. Because quality of life is very important in the care of the elderly in the long-term care facility, often all that can be done is counseling and frequent fingerstick blood glucose measurements. The facility is responsible for providing an appropriate diet through the dietary department, but can often do little about food items brought into the facility by family members and friends. Continued monitoring and documentation of counseling is essential in ensuring that the facility is doing all that it can to provide optimal care to the resident.

Sulfonylureas, insulin, metformin, α-glucosidase inhibitors, and thiazolidinediones are all used in many different combinations in the treatment of diabetes in the older individual. Care must be taken in the use and monitoring of metformin due the risk of lactic acidosis in patients with low oxygen states, including heart failure, renal impairment, and respiratory dysfunction. The dose of metformin must be held prior to and after an intravenous dye procedure, as this procedure may lead to diminished renal function. There is some evidence the thiazolidinediones may be associated with changes in cardiovascular function, and this needs to be further studied before any definitive recommendation concerning their use may be made.

The appropriate use of hormone replacement therapy (HRT) in postmenopausal women is currently the cause of much debate. The results of the Women's Health Initiative study of the benefits and risks of combined estrogen and progestin therapy in women with an intact uterus were published in 2002. This arm of the study was stopped early because the risk of cardiovascular events, including coronary heart disease, stroke, and thromboembolic disease, and invasive breast cancer was greater than the beneficial effects of the therapy.[46] Data from the Women's Health Initiative study was further evaluated for the incidence of dementia and mild cognitive impairment in postmenopausal women (The Women's Health Initiative Memory Study). Women aged 65 years and older were more likely to develop dementia of any type if they had taken HRT. HRT did not prevent the development of mild cognitive impairment.[47] The Cache County Study examined the relationship between use of HRT and the risk of Alzheimer's disease in a group of elderly women with an average age of 73 years. The conclusion of this study was that prior use of HRT was associated with a decreased risk of Alzheimer's disease, but only if the use exceeded 10 years duration.[48] The American Heart Association has published recommendations for the use of HRT in the prevention of cardiovascular disease (CVD). These guidelines state that HRT should not be used for secondary prevention of CVD, and the decision to stop therapy in women who have been receiving long-term HRT should be based on noncoronary benefits of continued use and the patient preference.[49] Many clinical trials have shown a benefit of HRT in the reduction of bone fractures and colon cancer. The risks and benefits of the use of hormone replacement therapy must be weighed carefully for each individual patient.

Anemias

Iron deficiency anemia and anemia of chronic disease are often confused, and the laboratory evaluation of both may overlap. The consultant pharmacist should request several laboratory values in order to make this distinction: serum iron level, TIBC (total iron binding capacity), % saturation, ferritin. In both conditions, the serum iron level and percent saturation will be low. The difference lies in the values for TIBC and ferritin. In iron deficiency anemia, the TIBC will be elevated and the ferritin value low. In anemia of chronic disease, the TIBC will be low and the ferritin elevated. Most elderly patients with anemia suffer from anemia of chronic disease, for which iron therapy has no effect. Iron therapy serves to increase the ferritin level, ferritin being the stored form of iron. Adding additional iron to an already elevated ferritin level will not effectively treat the anemia. Iron supplementation can cause significant gastrointestinal distress and constipation. If supplementation is needed, the maximum recommended dose in the elderly is 325 mg/day.[44]

Pain Management

The appropriate management of pain is one of the biggest challenges facing practitioners in long-term care. The assumption by many elderly patients and practitioners is that pain is an inevitable consequence of aging and, as such, should simply be tolerated. Often, residents in long-term care facilities will not complain of pain and must be questioned by staff in order to adequately assess pain. Many hospitals and nursing facilities have begun to add pain assessment to monitoring of vital signs. Several pain scales are available that simplify the assessment process by allowing the resident to identify a face on a scale or give a number from 1 to 10 to quantify and qualify pain. Pain assessments should be performed on all nursing facility residents to provide a baseline by which to evaluate further complaints of pain.

The American Geriatrics Society has developed clinical practice guidelines for the management of chronic pain in older persons.[45] NSAIDs, acetaminophen, and opioid analgesics form the backbone of effective pain management. Risks and benefits of NSAID use in a particular elderly patient must be evaluated prior to initiation of drug therapy. Gastrointestinal bleeding is a problematic side effect of these drugs and use of H2-receptor antagonists and proton pump inhibitors is only partially effective in offsetting this effect. COX-2 inhibitors may provide the benefit of anti-inflammatory pain relief with a reduced risk of GI bleeding. Opioid analgesics are likely underused in the geriatric population because of fears of drug-dependency and addiction. This should not be a consideration in relieving pain in the end of life or in significant pain situations. Constipation, impaired consciousness, and hypoxia may result from the use of opioid analgesics and should be closely monitored. Codeine is metabolized by the P450 CYP2D6 isoenzyme system in the liver to an active form. Patients who also take P450 2D6 inhibitors (paroxetine, fluoxetine, cimetidine, quinidine) should receive another opioid analgesic, as the efficacy of codeine will be limited in these patients. Propoxyphene use should be avoided in geriatric patients, as the active metabolite, norpropoxyphene, is both cardio- and neurotoxic. There is also evidence that propoxyphene is no more effective than acetaminophen in pain relief. Acetaminophen can be found in many opioid combination products, and this should be accounted for in any further dosing of acetaminophen to ensure that the maximum daily intake of acetaminophen does not exceed 4 grams. Tramadol is an opiate analgesic that has a secondary mechanism of action thought to involve monoamines, including norepinephrine and serotonin. The dose of tramadol should not exceed 400 mg/day to avoid the risk of drug-induced seizures.

Adjuvant medications used in pain management include anticonvulsants (carbamazepine) and tricyclic antidepressants. Caution should be exercised in the use of tricyclic antidepressants in the elderly due to anticholinergic side effects that may produce confusion, constipation, and urinary retention. Recently, gabapentin has been approved for use in postherpetic neuralgia and is often used off-label for neuropathic pain. Gabapentin may also have an anxiolytic effect that may be beneficial for patients suffering from acute and chronic pain. Other anxiolytics, such as lorazepam and buspirone, may be considered for use in the management of pain.

REFERENCES

1. ElderWeb. The LTC Backwards and Forwards page. Available at : http://www.elderweb.com/history/. Accessed March 16, 2003.
2. National Center for Health Statistics. Health, United States, 1999 with Health and Aging Chartbook. Hyattsville, MD, 1999.
3. US Bureau of the Census. Sixty-five plus in the United States. Economics and Statistics Administration, US Department of Commerce. May 1995.
4. US Bureau of the Census. The Older Population in the United States. Economics and Statistics Administration, US Department of Commerce. March 1999.
5. US General Accounting Office. Long-term Care - Baby Boom Generation Presents Financing Challenges. Testimony Before the Special Committee on Aging, US Senate. March 9, 1998.
6. US General Accounting Office. Long-term Care Insurance–Better Information Critical to Prospective Purchasers. Testimony Before the Special Committee on Aging, US Senate. September 13, 2000.
7. Freedman VA, Martin LG, Schoeni RF. *JAMA* 2002; 288: 3137.
8. Congressional Budget Office. The Projections of Expenditures for Long-Term Care Services for the Elderly page. Available at: http://www.cbo.gov/. Accessed March 16, 2003.
9. Social Security Administration. 1934 Committee on Economic Security: Unpublished Report of the CES on Health Insurance page. Available at: http://www.ssa.gov/history/reports/cesmedical.html. Accessed March 16, 2003.
10. Employee Benefits Research Institute. The Facts From EBRI- The Basics of Social Security page. Available at: http://www.ebri.org/facts/0702fact.pdf. Accessed March 16, 2003.
11. US General Accounting Office. Social Security–Restoring Long-Term Solvency Will Require Difficult Choices. Testimony Before the Special Committee on Aging, US Senate. February 10, 1998.
12. Centers for Medicare and Medicaid. The Chapter 1–Program Background and Responsiblities page. Available at: http://cms.hhs.gov/manuals/pub07pdf/part-01.pdf. Accessed February 16, 2003.
13. US Department of Health and Human Services. The First 30 Years of Medicare and Medicaid. *JAMA* 1995; 274:262.
14. Department of Veterans Affairs. The Health Benefits and Services page. Available at: http://www.va.gov/health_benefits/. Accessed March 16, 2003.
15. US Congressional Budget Office. Budgetary Impact of H.R. 2116, the Veterans' Millennium Health Care Act page. Available at: http://www.cbo.gov/showdoc.cfm. Accessed March 16, 2003.
16. National Long-term Care Ombudsman Resource Center. The OBRA 87 Summary page. Available at: http://www.ltcombudsman.org/ombpublic/49_346_1023.cfm. Accessed March 16, 2003.
17. Brenner L. *American Druggist* 1992; (Dec):26.
18. Bishop SK, Winckler SC. *Journal of the American Pharmaceutical Association* 2002; 42:836.
19. Employee Benefits Research Institute. The Facts From EBRI–National Health Care Expenditures, 2001 page. Available at: http://www.ebri.org/facts/0203fact.html. Accessed March 16, 2003.
20. US Congressional Budget Office. The Issues in Designing a Prescription Drug Benefit for Medicare October 2002 page. Available at:' http://www.cbo.gov/showdoc.cfm. Accessed March 16, 2003.
21. American Pharmaceutical Association. The Statement of the American Pharmaceutical Association (APhA) Pharmacy Victorious in Suit Challenging Legality of Medicare Rx Discount Card Program page. Available at: http://www.aphanet.org/news/01_28_03%20drugcard%20Statement.htm. Accessed March 16, 2003.
22. D'Achille KM. *Model Policies & Procedures for Providing Pharmaceutical Care in the Long-Term Care Setting*. Alexandria, VA: American Society of Consultant Pharmacists, 1999.
23. ASCP. *Drug Regimen Review: A Process Guide for Pharmacists*. Alexandria, VA: American Society of Consultant Pharmacists, 1999.
24. Shorr RI, Fought RL, Ray WA. *JAMA* 1994; 271:358.
25. Beers MH. *Arch Intern Med* 1997; 157:1531.
26. Zeiss AM, Steffen AM. In: Carstensen LL, Edelstein BA, Dornbrand L, eds. *The Practical Handbook of Clinical Gerontology*. Thousand Oaks, CA: Sage Publications, 1996, Chap 19.
27. Harris J. In: Tallis RC, Fillit HM, eds. *Brocklehurst's Textbook of Geriatric Medicine and Gerontology*, 6th ed. London: Churchill Livingstone, 2003, Chap 24.
28. Pearlman RA. In: Hazzard WR, Bierman EL, Blass JP, et al. eds. *Principles of Geriatric Medicine and Gerontology*, 3rd ed. New York: McGraw-Hill, 1994, Chap 36.
29. Omnibus Budget Reconciliation Act OBRA 1987 PL 100-203 Nursing Home Reform Act. pp 2–3.
30. MedNotice-Constitutional Rights. The Federal Self-Determination Act of 1990 page. Available at: http://www.mednotice.com/rights.html. Accessed March 23, 2003.
31. Hanlon JT, Ruby CM, Guay D, et al, eds. *Pharmacotherapy: A Pathophysiologic Approaach*, 5th ed. New York: McGraw-Hill, 2002, Chap 7.
32. Guay DRP, Artz MB, Hanlon JT, et al. In: Tallis RC, Fillit HM, eds. *Brocklehurst's Textbook of Geriatric Medicine and Gerontology*, 6th ed. London: Churchill Livingstone, 2003, Chap 14.
33. Cockroft DW, Gault MH. *Nephron* 1976; 16:31.
34. Aronow WS. In: Tallis RC, Fillit HM, eds. *Brocklehurst's Textbook of Geriatric Medicine and Gerontology*, 6th ed. London: Churchill Livingstone, 2003, Chap 30.
35. Hunt SA. ACC/AHA Guidelines for the Evaluation and Management of Chronic Heart Failure in the Adult. *American College of Cardiology and American Heart Institute*. 2001.
36. Fuster V. *European Heart Journal* 2001; 22:1852.
37. Seventh Report of the Joint National Committee on Prevention, Detection, Evaluation, and Treatment of High Blood Pressure (JNC 7) Express. The NHLBI, JNC 7 Express page. Available at: http://www.nhlbi.nih.gov/guidelines/hypertention/jncintro.htm. Accessed May 29, 2003.
38. Pearlman BL. *Postgraduate Medicine* 2002; 112(2):13–26.
39. Singh JM, Palda VA, Stanbrook MB, et al. *Arch Intern Med* 2002; 162:2527.
40. Lesar TS. In: Dipiro JT, Talbert RL, Yee GC, et al, eds. *Pharmacotherapy: A Pathophysiologic Approach*, 6th ed. New York: McGraw-Hill, 2002, Chap 94.

41. Kando JC, Wells BG, Hayes PE. In: Dipiro JT, Talbert RL, Yee GC, et al, eds. *Pharmacotherapy: A Pathophysiologic Approach*, 6th ed. New York: McGraw-Hill, 2002, Chap 69.

42. Comstock TJ. In: Dipiro JT, Talbert RL, Yee GC, et al, eds. *Pharmacotherapy: A Pathophysiologic Approach*, 6th ed. New York: McGraw-Hill, 2002, Chap 42.

43. Lewis MJ, St. Peter WL, Kasiske BL. In: Dipiro JT, Talbert RL, Yee GC, et al, eds. *Pharmacotherapy: A Pathophysiologic Approach*, 6th ed. New York: McGraw-Hill, 2002, Chap 44.

44. Nayak LH, Tesfaye M, Winter RO. *Annals of Long-Term Care* 1999; 7(1):2.

45. AGS. The Management of Chronic Pain in Older Persons. *American Geriatrics Society* 1998.

46. Writing Group for the Women's Health Initiative Investigators. *JAMA* 2002; 288:321.

47. Shumaker SA, Legault C, Rapp SR, et al. *JAMA* 2003; 289:2651.

48. Zandi PP, Carlson MC, Plassman BL, et al. *JAMA* 2002; 288:2123.

49. Mosca L, Collins P, Herrington DM, et al. *Circulation* 2001; 104:499.

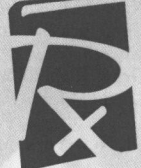

CHAPTER 130

Aseptic Processing for Home Infusion Pharmaceuticals

Hetty A Lima, RPh, FASHP

The provision of home care has existed since the turn of the last century, when societal concerns regarding immigration, industrialization, and infectious diseases spawned the need for visiting nurses. Early homecare services primarily consisted of midwife and nursing assistance for births, and the care of influenza and tuberculosis patients. This early form of home care paved the way for the development of alternate site healthcare. In the past, the term *home care* generally referred to community-based nursing services provided to patients in their homes. Today, the term has been expanded to include home/alternate site healthcare and encompasses: long-term care, and skilled nursing facilities, assisted living and subacute facilities, home care, diagnostic centers, outpatient clinics, ambulatory surgery, rehabilitation facilities, and emergency service markets.[1] The types of alternate site or home-care services are outlined in Table 130-1.

Since 1993, home health care has become the fastest growing segment of health care. In 1999, the US Supreme Court rendered a decision in *Olmstead v. L.C.*, affirming the Americans with Disabilities Act of 1990, which "increased pressure on federal and state programs to deliver advanced health care services to patients at home."[2]

Home infusion is an important component of the alternate site, home health care industry. Home infusion therapy provides therapies to a patient in either the home or alternate site care setting, and emerged as a result of significant changes that occurred in the delivery of health care in the United States. Home infusion therapy involves the prolonged and usually repeated injection of pharmaceutical products (eg, medications, nutrients, or other solutions) most often delivered intravenously, subcutaneously, intramuscularly, enterally, or epidurally. Commonly prescribed home infusion therapies include: antibiotics, chemotherapy, TPN, pain management, immune globulins, corticosteroids, inotropics, hydration, tocolytics, human growth hormone, blood clotting factors, colony-stimulating factors, steroids, other miscellaneous intravenous drugs as well as enteral nutrition.[1] According to the ASHP Guidelines Minimum Standard for Home Care Pharmacies,[3] a home care pharmacy is one that provides primarily, if not exclusively, home infusion products.

Infusion therapy always originates with a prescription from a physician who is overseeing the care of the patient and is designed to achieve physician-defined therapeutic endpoints. A home infusion provider must be a licensed pharmacy. Currently, there are approximately 4,000 pharmacies nationwide providing infusion therapy services. These pharmacies include: local, regional, and national organizations and can be independently owned or hospital-affiliated.[4] Home nursing services are often provided in conjunction with infusion therapy to ensure proper patient or caregiver training and education and to monitor the clinical care of the patient in the home; alternatively, home nursing services can also be provided by a qualified home health agency.

A more recent practice setting offshoot of home infusion pharmacy is the "specialty pharmacy." The most commonly accepted definition of specialty pharmacies are those that serve patients who have rare or chronic diseases with high-cost injectable, infusion, or biotech drugs.[5] Specialty pharmacy patients are generally harder to serve in that oftentimes specialty pharmacy products are often in short supply relative to mass-marketed pharmaceuticals and have more difficult delivery mechanisms (injectables). Oftentimes, the cost of the patient's specialty medication can exceed $10,000 per year. Examples of diseases managed by specialty pharmacies include: hemophilia, and related bleeding disorders, hepatitis, immune disorders, growth hormone deficiencies, multiple schlerosis, rheumatoid arthritis, and RSV.

Home infusion pharmacy services differ dramatically from most retail pharmacy operations. While retail pharmacies primarily dispense oral medications, infusion pharmacies must have the equipment necessary to safely prepare and store sterile parenteral products. This includes: laminar flow hoods to reduce the risk of microbial contamination, modified storage areas for certain drugs, and additional compounding equipment and supplies for mixing drugs.

The dramatic increase in the alternate site healthcare market has largely occurred due the nationwide effort to control health-care costs. During the 1980s, the US healthcare system underwent dramatic changes. In particular, with the introduction of the diagnosis-related groups (DRGs) as a cost-control measure, home care offered a cost-effective alternative following the post-acute hospital stage.[1] Driven by heightened emphasis on cost-effectiveness and cost-containment, technological advances have developed that enabled the safe and effective administration of IV therapies in the home.

Sterile Products in the Home

Because hospital stays have been dramatically reduced, injectable pharmaceuticals are increasingly administered to patients in the home (for both acute and chronic conditions), often by laypersons. The conditions of administration for parenteral products used in the home have introduced numerous concerns for pharmacists to be able to give reasonable assurance to patients that the products received and administered are safe and effective. Home infusion therapy has raised many issues requiring pharmacist's attention including: the use of many sterile products before quality control testing can be complete, potential exposure of the products to temperatures outside the desired storage range during shipping and/or delivery, and, in the home, administration by persons lacking professional

Table 130-1. Types of Alternate Site or Home-Care Services[1]

Pharmaceutical Includes high-tech infusion therapies, potential and oral medications, inhalation therapies, and clinical monitoring
Skilled Nursing Services
Semi-skilled Nursing Services
Custodial Care
Home Respiratory Therapy / Durable Medical Equipment
Hospice Care

skills, administration through devices that may not be adequately protected against contamination, and the lack of definitive evidence of stability for the 30- to 60-day shelf life often required.[6]

Given the realities of the conditions listed above, pharmacists must ensure that their aseptic technique for preparing and dispensing sterile products for home use is beyond reproach. Additionally, pharmacists must do all they can to influence the home-care environment so that the quality of their products will be maintained until the administration of the products to the patient is complete. It is the intent of this chapter to highlight those issues that are essential to ensuring proper aseptic technique is used for the preparation of safe and effective sterile home-care pharmaceuticals.

Aseptic technology is the application of a scientific understanding of the characteristics of viable microorganisms, applied in such a manner that the microorganisms are eliminated, with a high probability of success, from all of the process steps involved in compounding sterile pharmaceutical dosage forms. Regardless of where aseptic processing (compounding) is practiced on products prepared in an institutional setting, a home infusion pharmacy, or a pharmaceutical manufacturing facility, the principles are the same; only the practices differ. Practices will differ because of the nature of the product being produced, the size of the batch, the length of its projected shelf life, and the extent of the regulatory requirements involved. This chapter focuses on the distinctive practices of aseptic compounding applicable to sterile products used in the home. This practice is referred to as "home infusion pharmacy." Compounding is the preparation, mixing, assembling, packaging, and labeling of a drug or device as the result of a practitioner, patient, pharmacist (or Triad) relationship in the course of professional practice.[7]

The dispensing activities of home infusion pharmacies are licensed and regulated by their respective state boards of pharmacy, but there are no specific federal regulations governing these pharmacies, as is the case with the pharmaceutical industry.

Legal and Regulatory Oversight

Each home infusion pharmacy is governed by the State Board of Pharmacy laws for that particular state. While many states have adopted regulations that govern sterile products compounding, many have not. Currently, there is no principle authority on pharmacy compounding in the US. There are, however, health care accrediting organizations such as the Joint Commission on Accreditation of Healthcare Organizations (JCAHO) and the Accreditation Commission for Health Care, Inc. (ACHC), yet, neither organization addresses the specific needs of the home infusion or specialty pharmacy. Typically, these accreditations have become a vital prerequisite for doing business. Many third-party payers require home infusion organizations to be JCAHO or ACHC accredited for reimbursement to be rendered.[1]

Patient morbidity and mortality have resulted from incorrectly prepared or contaminated pharmacy-prepared sterile products. Patients receive sterile compounded products that have been stored for extended periods of time before use; and this allows for the growth of a pathological bioload of microorganisms.[8]

The FDA recently published a study that lends credence to its concerns regarding the under-regulated practice of pharmacy compounding. Regulators sampled 29 drugs from 12 pharmacies and found that more than one-third (10 of 29) failed either a drug assay or pyrogen test; nine out of ten drugs were subpotent, and one in ten was pyrogenic.[9] Tragic results of pharmacy compounding have reached the mass media in such outlets as the Associated Press and National Public Radio (NPR). A California-based compounding pharmacy extemporaneously prepared betamethasone in response to a national shortage. The drug was contaminated with *serratia* bacteria, and 38 people received spinal injections of contaminated betamethasone. Dozens of people were hospitalized and treated with antibiotics.[9] Mishaps such as this make a strong case for tighter control of compounded pharmaceuticals.

Other professional organizations have published guidelines on compounding and dispensing sterile products. The United States Pharmacopeia (USP) and the National Formulary and supplements all have legal implications for pharmacists.[11] The National Association of Boards of Pharmacy (NABP) has published less detailed model regulations for use by state boards of pharmacy[12] and the American Society of Parenteral and Enteral Nutrition (ASPEN) has published a special report on safe practices for parenteral nutrition products.[13]

In recent years, two other organizations have developed standards and technical assistance bulletins on the preparation of sterile products. The American Society of Health-Systems Pharmacists (ASHP) has published the *Technical Assistance Bulletin on Quality Assurance for Pharmacy-Prepared Sterile Products*[8] (ASHP-TAB), and the United States Pharmacopeia (USP) general chapter <1206>, *Sterile Drug Products for Home Use*[11], also provides guidance on compounding sterile pharmaceuticals.

The industrial perspective for the preparation of sterile injectable (parenteral) products is presented in Chapter 41 and is referenced when overlapping material is encountered. The reader is encouraged to read the entire chapter to glean applicable aseptic processing principles and practices. Expanded, highly relevant information also can be found in the chapter by Levchuk[14] and the book by Buchanan, McKinnon, Scheckelhoff, and Schneider.[15]

DISTINCTIVES OF ASEPTIC PROCESSING FOR HOME-CARE PHARMACEUTICALS (HCPS)

A reasonable distinction can be drawn between HCPs with a low risk of becoming contaminated under controlled aseptic processing conditions and those with a relatively high risk of such contamination occurring. The USP chapter defines these risks into two levels, low-risk and high-risk.[11] Detailed descriptions of these levels are given in the USP, and the reader should refer to the USP chapter for those details. Similarly, the ASHP has also classified risk levels, using three categories, the descriptions differing from those of the USP in relatively minor ways.[8]

The ASHP and USP guidelines contain valuable information for pharmacists involved in the preparation of sterile products for administration in either the hospital or home setting. However, each guideline contains unique information that is not contained in the other. All pharmacists who compound sterile products are encouraged to read both sets of guidelines and to determine the appropriate risk level of the sterile products that they prepare. As always, professional judgment should be exercised when applying these guidelines to specific pharmacy practice settings to ensure the highest level of product quality. A comparison of the ASHP and USP classifications and a discussion of the quality requirements for the preparation of pharmacy-prepared sterile products can be found in the articles by Avis[16] and Lima.[17]

Low-risk processing of HCPs normally consists of starting with sterile, commercially available pharmaceuticals, including large-volume injectables (LVIs), such as amino acids, high concentrated dextrose solutions, and sterile water for injection, small-volume injectables (SVIs), and sterile powders, packaged in sealed primary containers. Aseptic compounding of these products then occurs by combining, diluting, subdividing, or otherwise manipulating the products in a noncomplex manner to produce other products to meet the prescribed needs of one or at most, a small group of patients. The devices used to accomplish the manipulations are also sterile, clean, packaged, and disposable. These devices enable the manipulative transfers of liquids with limited exposure to the environment–a closed system. The primary requirement of this type of aseptic compounding is to maintain the sterility and freedom from contamination and the overall quality required of the HCPs when dispensed.

The risk of contamination increases if the HCPs are compounded using components that are not sterile, if the compounding is performed using open tanks or complex or multiple procedures, if an environmental exposure over a relatively long period of processing time is needed, or when a relatively long shelf life is anticipated. Such conditions meet the classification of *high risk*. The pharmacist should be trained to be able to differentiate the risk levels required for the preparation of a given HCP and designate the procedures to be used during for compounding.

Because most HCPs used in the home are not prepared from raw materials but from pharmaceutically manufactured products, and compounding manipulations generally consist of accurately measured liquid transfers, quality control testing requirements are fairly limited. However, the pharmacist is ultimately responsible for the final quality of all of the products dispensed, and confirmatory tests should be performed when appropriate. In such cases, adjustments must be made for sampling, for example, by preparing duplicate products so that one can be tested or by a planned program of sampling (for example, one out of a set of ten similar or identical product units will be tested).

Other distinctive characteristics of HCPs include: a relatively short shelf life of 30 to 60 days, rapid distribution by commercial transportation systems, and storage and administration to the patient by caregivers in the home. As stated previously, these dispensing activities fall under the oversight of the respective state boards of pharmacy and not of the Food and Drug Administration (FDA).

COMPOUNDING FACILITIES

Compounding facilities should be designed to provide adequate space for the work load anticipated and for the appropriate future expansion in work load. All too frequently, expansion space is not initially provided for in the compounding pharmacy and, as the service demands and compounding volume increases, the ability to maintain environmental and process control becomes compromised due to overcrowding.

The pharmacy compounding area must be designed to prevent the contamination of the HCPs during aseptic compounding. Therefore, the work area must be cleanable and sanitizable, with a minimum amount of particle shedding and crevices or other sites where dirt and microorganisms can accumulate. This means the compounding room must have structural surfaces of ceiling, walls, and floors, and work surfaces and storage surfaces that are smooth and resistant to cleaning and sanitizing. Stainless-steel work surfaces and epoxy-coated structural surfaces (or the like) are preferred because they generally meet

the required surface characteristics. Equipment and instruments must also meet these general requirements, as much as possible. Equipment with noncleanable, particle-shedding motors, gears, and other such structures should be contained, preferably in stainless-steel enclosures.

The arrangement of the compounding area should be planned for convenient work flow, with minimal crossover and controlled progression through barrier structures, doors, or pass-throughs from uncontrolled rooms (such as storerooms) to increasingly cleaner-controlled environments. The preceding environment serves as a buffer area to reduce the ingress of contaminants into the next area of a higher level of cleanliness.

The most critical work area, the area where the HCPs are compounded, is the Class 100 area (contains no more than 100 particles of 0.5 μm and larger per cubic foot) where the aseptic compounding manipulations will be performed. Compounding activity typically occurs on a laminar airflow workbench (LAFW), with an air stream cleaned by passage through a high-efficiency particulate air (HEPA) filter. The laminar flow air stream efficiently and continuously sweeps the work area with clean air at a velocity of 90 fpm ± 20%. For more details concerning air cleanliness classes, clean air operations, and laminar airflow, the reader is referred to Chapter 41.

An example of a medium-sized compounding pharmacy facility floor plan, taken from the USP,[11] is shown as Figure 130-1. Using this example, the compounding procedures followed for controlling the ingress of contamination may be illustrated as follows. The compounding supplies are brought from the storage room to the demarcation line on stainless steel or plastic carts. The supplies are then carefully removed from the primary packaging and are transferred to a cleaned and sanitized cleanroom cart. The cart is cleaned with filtered isopropyl alcohol (IPA). The supply items are then brought into the buffer room, with the cart wheels sanitized at the entryway.

Clean, sanitized supplies may be stored temporarily in the buffer room but, preferably, the needs for each compounding shift should be used directly from the cart. The supply cart(s) is positioned conveniently for use by the operator(s) (compounders) at the LAFW. At the end of each shift, or more

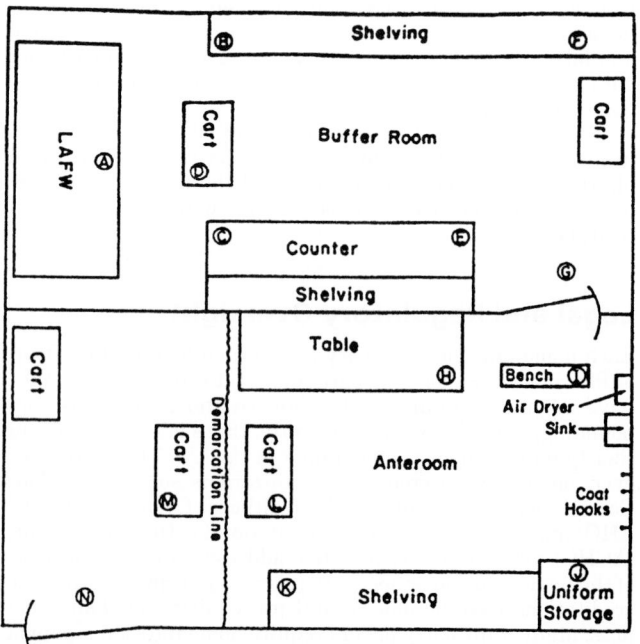

Figure 130-1. Example floor plan. Encircled letters are suggested environmental sampling sites. (From the USP 26-NF21. All rights reserved, © 2003. United States Pharmacopeia.)

frequently if needed, the operator should clean and sanitize the inside of the LAFW, other work surfaces, reorganize the work areas, and then remove the supply cart(s) from the buffer room, with any unused supplies. Assigned compounding personnel should remove trash and clean and sanitize the floors during the off-shift, following an established standard operating procedure (SOP).

The above example is given for illustrative purposes only. Compounding pharmacies and their operation will vary in accordance with the needs, design of facilities, and workload of the given home infusion pharmacy. Many hospitals and home infusion pharmacies have begun to use isolators for preparing HCPs. Isolators have been introduced to the US, but have been used for over two decades in England, Canada, and other European countries.[18,19] By design, the unit isolates the Class 100 critical area from its surrounding controlled area with sides of stainless steel, windows or of transparent plastic. By design, barrier isolators are more efficient than laminar flow hoods for aseptic compounding. When compared to a cleanroom, isolators are more economical to install and operate, require less space, are less costly to maintain, and ensure a clean environment in less time than what is typically required for cleanroom maintenance.[1]

The isolator's critical area is sterilized (not just sanitized) before use. Access for compounding personnel, also isolated from the critical area, is provided through glove ports or half-suits sealed in the walls. Sterile or externally sanitized supplies are introduced into the critical area through *pass-through* entry ports, the weakest link in the process if sanitization rather than sterilization is used. Reports indicate that contamination rates for HCPs compounded in isolators can be markedly reduced.

Environmental Control

Microorganisms and dust particles are ubiquitous to any workplace, even a traditional cleanroom. When microorganisms are suspended in air, they are most likely to gain entrance into an open container of drug product or onto any other exposed surface. Therefore, the objective of environmental control in a cleanroom is to minimize the presence of all contaminants insofar as possible, particularly those that are airborne. With aseptic compounding, it is particularly important to control microorganisms in the environment where products intended to be sterile are processed, because there is no final sterilization step at the end of the compounding process. Therefore, microorganisms must be prevented from reaching any critical site. As defined by the USP, a critical site is any opening providing a direct pathway between a sterile product and the environment or any surface coming in direct contact with the product and the environment.[11]

To prevent microorganisms from reaching a critical site, the critical environment should be sterile or as close to sterile as possible. Normally, the equipment of choice is a certified Class 100 LAFW. When effectively cleansed, sanitized, and operated, a Class 100 environment is attainable. Either a vertical or horizontal LAFW can be used for most HCP compounding unless the products are toxic or carcinogenic in nature. Then, only a vertical LAFW biocontainment cabinet should be used. The immediate compounding work surface should be nonpermeable and resistant to liquid cleaning and disinfecting agents. It should be made of polished stainless steel with coved seamless joints. In addition to frequent cleaning, a validated disinfectant should be used on all compounding and adjacent surfaces at least as frequently as at the end of each shift.[11] A valuable source of additional information about the use of disinfectants is a Parenteral Drug Association (PDA) Task Force report.[20] It should be noted that disinfectants can only be expected to supplement effective cleaning. They will not overcome inadequate cleaning and sanitizing and are not to be relied upon as sterilizing agents. Further, because of the risk of microbial resistance, it is good policy to rotate disinfectants at least every 6 months.

Although a certified Class 100 LAFW is effective in maintaining an aseptic environment, the laminar air flow is relatively gentle, and its overall efficiency is affected by its surroundings. Consequently, the LAFW should be surrounded with a buffer zone only slightly less environmentally controlled, as illustrated in Figure 130-1. All critical aseptic compounding should be performed within the Class 100 environment and operators should be well trained in aseptic compounding techniques. The buffer room should be a Class 10,000 cleanroom or better and should be used for the final decontamination of external surfaces of supplies before introducing them into the LAFW as well as for short-term storage of clean supplies to be used in the LAFW. The number of persons in the buffer room should always be limited to those properly authorized and trained in aseptic compounding procedures and limited to the number of individuals necessary to perform the required tasks.

The anteroom shown in Figure 130-1 is intended to be used for decontaminating supplies, equipment, and personnel prior to entrance into the buffer room. It is used to interrupt the potential flow of contaminants and microorganisms from the storage room into the buffer room, a very critical step in controlling potential contamination of HCPs. For example, in the anteroom, supplies would be removed from their shipping cartons, cleaned, and sanitized externally before placing them onto clean and sanitized carts for entry into the buffer room. The supply items would then be cleaned and sanitized externally again before placing them into the LAFW. Further, descriptive details of these control steps can be found in the USP.[11]

Environmental Monitoring

Monitoring the environmental cleanliness and microbial bioburden of the cleanroom provides the home infusion pharmacy with data that indicates how effectively compounding staff follow procedures for cleaning and maintaining the compounding environment.

An assessment of the level of control achieved and maintained in a clean room environment may be performed by measuring total particle counts (both viable and nonviable particles) in air samples of at least 10 ft^3, usually done by the use electronic samplers. The results are available instantly. Viable particle counts of the cleanroom are performed with one or more of methods, such as: settling plates, surface or contact plates, slit-to-agar samplers, or centrifugal samplers. However, the results are not available until after incubation, usually 48 hours. The incubation time is necessary to allow the microorganisms to multiply (grow) so that colonies become visible. The presence of microorganisms in the cleanroom are visually detected by the presence of a colony count which is expressed in 'colony-forming units' (cfus). The cfu serves as macro evidence that microbial bioburden exists in the cleanroom. However, it is not known whether or not each colony arose from a single or multiple microorganisms. A sufficiently large sample must be taken in order to detect microorganisms at least some of the time. This fact must be considered particularly in Class 100 compounding environments where the number of microorganisms is expected to be very low. In such situations, it may be necessary to sample a volume of 30 ft^3 or more. Additional details on environmental monitoring can be found in Chapter 41.

ENVIRONMENTAL MONITORING PROGRAM—An environmental monitoring program should be established for the compounding pharmacy to assist in the detection of out-of-control microbial limits. The environmental monitoring program also assesses if the appropriate level of cleanliness has been achieved and maintained in the cleanrooms. Using two or three of the sampling methods listed above, one selects the sites, frequency, and length of time (for volume monitoring) required to give adequate information concerning the level of microbial control being maintained. This is best determined by performing sampling at many sites daily for a minimum of two weeks, preferably confirmed by repeating the sampling six

Table 130-2. A Sample Dynamic Environmental Microbial-Monitoring Program

SITE	BASELINE cfu	LOW-RISK ACTION LEVEL	HIGH-RISK ACTION LEVEL
Settling Plates[a]			
A	0, 1	3	2
D	2, 3	6	4
E	4, 5	10	6
J	5	10	7
L	8	15	10
Contact Plates			
D	2, 3	6	4
E	4, 6	10	7
J	6	12	8
L	8	15	10
STA or Impaction Sampler[b]			
A	0, 1	3	2
E	5	10	7
H	8	15	10

[a] Based on 3-hr exposure, except 1 hr for "A." See Fig. 119.1 for site locations.
[b] Based on 10-ft³ samples.
Data from the USP23-AF18.

months later. As a minimum, at least the index finger of each operator should be rolled onto a contact plate. From the averaged data obtained, a selected, reduced number of sites should be chosen that, when monitored routinely, would best indicate whether or not appropriate environmental control is being maintained. Test sites should include both sites within the Class 100 environment as well as sites that could be expected to show the first sign of unacceptable increases in microbial levels if control is being lost.

A sample environmental sampling program based on the floor plan of Figure 130-1 is described in the USP,[11] and an example of a collected data set is listed in Table 130-2.[10] The USP chapter[11] provides practical information for establishing an environmental monitoring program as well as how to determine acceptable and out-of-limit environmental conditions. The example data for action levels (the cfu count signaling possible loss of control and requiring action to correct) for both low-risk and high-risk products are given with appropriately lower action levels when high-risk products are being processed. This is an example program for guidance and results should be adjusted for each home infusion pharmacy based upon baseline monitoring and trends. A program providing fewer data points, and still probably acceptable if all controls were in place, would be to use only settling and contact plates for testing.

A meaningful environmental monitoring program provides critical information that is essential for assuring that the risk of contamination of HCPs is under control and minimized. Without environmental monitoring data, the acceptability of aseptically prepared products as sterile is very uncertain. Extensive details concerning the development of a monitoring program and the methods used for its monitoring will be found in PDA Technical Report No. 13.[21] Although geared towards the pharmaceutical industry, the basic principles and methods of an environmental monitoring program are given, and their application to a home infusion pharmacy can be readily extracted.

COMPOUNDING DEVICES

Home infusion pharmacies rely heavily upon automated compounding devices for the aseptic preparation of sterile products. These compounding devices typically fall into two categories: those used for the preparation of intravenous total parenteral nutrition (TPN) solutions (total nutrient admixtures (TNAs)) or large-volume hydration solutions and those used for SVIs, such as antibiotics and medications for pain management. The SVI

devices are used to admix solutions into smaller drug-delivery systems, such as empty plastic bags, syringes, and other disposable elastomeric devices.

Home infusion pharmacy personnel must ensure that the equipment, apparatus, and devices used to compound sterile products are capable of consistently operating properly and within acceptable quantity tolerance limits as established by the device manufacturer. The pharmacy should have written policies and procedures for equipment calibration, annual maintenance, operational monitoring, and quality control procedures. Pharmacy personnel must document routine equipment maintenance and calibration checks and personnel should be qualified through both specific training and experience to use, in an expert manner, any of the equipment or devices required for preparing sterile products.

LARGE VOLUME INJECTABLE (LVI) COMPOUNDING DEVICES—LVI products can be compounded by using one or two basic methods: by gravity or by the use of an automated compounding device. Gravity compounding involves the manual aseptic transfer of sterile base solutions such as amino acids, dextrose, and lipid emulsion from one container to another using gravity-driven transfer. The remaining additives such as electrolytes, vitamins, and trace elements are also added manually with each additive transferred separately using a syringe. Gravity compounding involves low equipment costs, but has a high labor component. The risk of microbial contamination using the gravity method of compounding is higher due to the multiple manipulations made into the final container during the additive transfer process. Additionally, because each additive is added manually, the risk of touch contamination is greater.[22]

Most automated compounding devices used to prepare TPN and TNA liquids are electromechanical devices that measure opaque and transparent suspensions and solutions by gravimetric or volumetric methods. Some automated compounders can be used for the transfer of base solutions only, with the remaining additive components added manually versus other, more sophisticated automated compounders that can be used to compound the small volume additives and the base solutions.

Some automated compounding devices use calibrated gravimetric weighing to convert and monitor the actual volume dispensed. With volumetric compounders, base solutions are transferred from the source container to the final container using a rotary peristaltic pump. With each turn of the rotor, fluid is pulled from the source container and pushed into the final container. Often, these compounding devices are used as standalone instruments or they can be interfaced with a computer. TPN-compounding devices use a microprocessor system control, which provides the device with a measure of *self-test,* to ensure the integrity of the electrical control functions. The computer interfaced with these devices provides for the correct data transfer in an automated fashion consistent with standard pharmacy checking methods. The accuracy of the compounding unit is achieved through weighing the actual solution being delivered, converted by a specific gravity calculation to the required volume transferred. Thus, if any air is inadvertently transferred, it will not alter the accuracy of the compounded solution.[23]

Automated compounding devices have multiple channels for pumping the solutions of amino acids, dextrose, pooled electrolytes, and/or intravenous fat (lipid) emulsions into the final dispensing container or bag. TPN compounders do not normally use a sterilizing 0.22-micron filtration step as part of the admixture preparation process because of the resistance to flow induced by the filter and that because it is a closed system for dispensing sterile solutions. However, if an electrolyte pool is created for subsequent dispensing into individual TPN bags, the final solution should be filtered through a 0.22-μm filter prior to attaching the unit to the automated compounder. This step is included because the process is using an open system with a relatively long exposure of the solution to the environment. Further, this step eliminates any inadvertent microbiological and touch contamination introduced during the compounding process.

Table 130-3. Commonly Automated Pharmacy Compounding Devices Used to Prepare Home Infusion Products

AUTOMATED SYSTEM	MANUFACTURER	METHOD OF TRANSFER	NO. OF STATIONS	RANGE OF VOLUMES DELIVERED FROM EACH STATION	ADDITIONAL INFORMATION AVAILABLE FOR PN CALCULATIONS, QA CHECKS, & TRANSFER OF RX TO COMPOUNDER?
Nutrimix Macro	Abbott	Subtractive Gravimetric	4	10–4,000 mL	Yes
Nutrimix Micro	Abbott	Volumetric	10	—	Yes
Automix 3+3	Baxter	Additive Gravimetric	6	10–5,000 mL	Yes
Automix 3+3/AS	Baxter	Additive Gravimetric	6		
Micromix	Baxter	Additive Gravimetric	10	0.3–4,000 mL	Yes
Exacta-Mix	Baxa	Volumetric	6	1–9,990 mL	Yes
MicroMacro	Baxa	Volumetric	12	0.2–9.9 L	Yes
MicroMacro 23	Baxa	Volumetric	23		
HyperFormer	B. Braun	Volumetric	6	1–3,000 mL	No

Adapted from Chrai S, et al. *J Parenter Sci Technol* 1986; 10:104.

THE SOLUTION-COMPOUNDING PROCESS—Generally, in home infusion practice, pharmacy technicians perform the actual compounding of sterile products. The vast majority of states in the US allow technicians to compound sterile products under the direct supervision of a licensed pharmacist.

Prior to actually compounding an intravenous solution, the individual starting components should be selected by a technician and then checked by a pharmacist. This checking is performed to minimize any risk of selecting an incorrect product(s). These components are usually sterile, packaged, commercial IV products that have been subjected to quality control testing and release by the manufacturer. The external surfaces of the packages are then cleaned and sanitized, and the packages are brought into the cleanroom.

The operator should calibrate the automated compounder on a daily basis per the manufacturer's directions and recommendations. Usually, these calibration checks are documented in a QC log book and/or on a compounding (batch) record. The technician then connects the compounding device's transfer set to the device itself. Each different type of compounder has its own unique plastic solution-transfer set. Typically, these sets cannot be interchanged between the different compounding devices because the configurations are purposely different. The appropriate dispensing containers are then connected to the compounding device.

Next, the operator performing the compounding programs the device by entering the specific volumes of each of the different solutions, ie, amino acid, dextrose, electrolyte pool, and/or fat emulsion used into the device itself. The usual volume ranges for these liquids are from 10 to 5000 mL. The specific gravity of each of the respective solutions is then programmed into the compounding device's computer. Limits for specific gravities are usually 0.50 to 3.00 for each pump station, and specific solution specific gravities are provided by the pharmaceutical manufacturer.

Prior to actually starting the machine, operators should visually check the solution level in each of the stock solution containers to be sure there is an adequate supply and should ensure that the final product bag has been properly connected to the transfer set. Operators also should ensure that there are no kinks, clamped sites, or other obstructions in the tubing.

Immediately after the appropriate amounts of solutions have been transferred into the final dispensing container, the bag is removed from the compounder, air is expelled, and the bag is sealed. Bags are either crimped manually or with a device that uses radiofrequency waves to heat-seal the bags. The expected weight of the final TPN bag should have been calculated. The final compounded bags of product can then be weighed on a scale to provide a second gravimetric QC check for accuracy.

Some of the current compounding devices provide for as many as 23 different pump stations. Microcompounders allow for the accurate, aseptic dispensing of electrolytes for compounded TPN/TNA solutions with aliquot volumes as low as 0.2 mL.

Many nutritional compounding devices interface with software packages and simplify the formulation of TPN solutions, particularly by automating the complex calculations that help to minimize errors. Additionally, these instruments generate compounding records and prescription labels for the compounded product. Prescription labels can be generated in a variety of different formats, including providing a complete listing of all ingredients and quantities dispensed as well as a summary of clinical information, such as the total number of calories; amounts of proteins, carbohydrates, and fats; and solution osmolarity. Refer to Table 130-3 for a list of commonly used pharmacy compounding devices.

SMALL VOLUME INJECTABLE (SVI) COMPOUNDING DEVICES—In addition to nutritional compounding devices, home infusion pharmacies can also use compounders to prepare SVI solutions. These compounding devices are most frequently used for the pooling of electrolyte solutions and/or for reconstituting drugs over prolonged compounding operations. The solutions are dispensed into smaller drug-delivery systems such as plastic syringes, vials, disposable elastomeric pumps, cassettes, or empty bags.

Volume delivery for these types of compounding devices typically ranges from 0.01 to 9,999 mL.[24] Like the nutritional compounding devices, these compounders also employ brand-specific transfer sets. Prior to operation, the pump should be calibrated per the manufacturer's instructions. The operator then aseptically connects the transfer set to the compounding device's pump rotor. The transfer set is then primed and, using a universal spike adapter, is connected to a primary-source container. The operator then enters the desired pump volume(s) on a numeric keypad, and the solution is dispensed into the final container. Each unit is filled completely in one filling step, one unit at a time.

As the pump operates, it will deduct and record the delivered amount from the source-container volume. Once all the units have been filled, the transfer tubing is disconnected from the final unit, and any air remaining present is aspirated.

When filling specific drug-delivery systems, such as elastomeric devices, it is very important to adhere to the manufacturer's recommended speed setting. Because of the high pressures required to fill these devices accurately, transfer-set tubing wear can be quite high. Therefore, it is recommended that the transfer tubing set be examined after filling 50 units, for possible replacement.[24] Many of the SVI compounders have a memory recall function for storing dispensing information for subsequent compounding procedures.

Compounding Device Quality Control

As stated previously, TPN/TNA bags or small infusion drug delivery systems can be double-checked by weighing the final container or product to provide a second gravimetric check of the quantity of the final solution dispensed. Additionally, many compounding devices used in pharmacy practice come with some type of computerized bar-code verification system. Such systems clearly identify the different solutions used in the compounding process and prevent the compounding device from operating if an error has been made.

The refractive index (RI) also can be used to determine the accuracy of some compounded nutrient solutions. The RI serves as a gross predictor of compounding accuracy, for example, for dextrose solutions or dextrose containing solutions. The RI is the ratio of the normal velocity of light in air to the velocity in the solution being tested. The use of RI as a quality control test is particularly useful for neonatal and pediatric TPN solutions, for which accuracy of compounding is particularly important. The RI is based upon specific constants for dextrose and amino acids and their relationship to that of the final compounded TPN.[25]

PERSONNEL

Personnel are generally recognized as the principle source of contamination in a cleanroom because of the inherent shedding of both viable and nonviable particles from their body surfaces and clothing. Uniforms are worn to help contain these particles, but the personal hygiene and characteristic physical activities of each operator plays a critical role in the shedding of particles into the compounding environment. Therefore, training personnel to understand their personal characteristics and how to control their emission of particles while performing good aseptic practices (GAPs) is very critical.

GOWNING—Assuming good personal hygiene, the shedding of particles will increase as the level of the operator's activity increases. Because home infusion pharmacists and technicians will normally be standing or sitting at an LAFW, their level of activity will be moderate. However, they will be reaching into the critical work area and air currents may bounce from the front of their uniforms back into the critical work site,

and they will be exhaling toward the work area. Therefore, sterile gloves should be worn along with very clean, nonshedding gowns, face masks, and hair covers. Gowns should be long sleeved, snug-fitting at the wrist, closed front, and knee length. The frequent practice of wearing scrubs is questioned because of their normally high load of lint. Synthetic polymer gowns are preferred. Further, gowns should never be worn outside the buffer room; they should be captive to the cleanroom.

Sterile gloves should be worn, although these will quickly become contaminated from the surfaces of sanitized (not sterile) packages, LAFW surfaces, and other surfaces contacted. They should be resanitized frequently with sterile IPA. Face masks may be omitted if working at a VLAFW, and the transparent shield is always kept between the mouth and the critical work area. Shoe covers also should be worn to reduce tracking contamination onto the floor of the buffer room.

PRACTICING GOOD ASEPTIC TECHNIQUE—Pharmacists and technicians must be trained to understand their natural propensities for contaminating the environment and the impact their activities have on introducing that contamination into the HCP with which they are working. In general, the greatest concern is to prevent microbial contamination, but particulate matter and other physical and chemical contamination are also of concern. Therefore, operators must learn to practice good aseptic techniques (GAPs) automatically, to minimize the risk of contaminating the HCP that is being prepared. It is generally recognized that in the context of GAPs, the greatest risk of introducing contamination into a sterile product is through touch contamination by the operator. Therefore, special attention must be given to learning how to avoid this potential problem.

Space limitations do not permit detailed descriptions of practices that constitute GAPs, which are best learned by personal tutoring and practice. However, Avis has provided a list of key practices that should be followed,[16] and these are reproduced on Figure 130-2.

---

1. Practice good personal hygiene, be organized and level-headed.
2. Be healthy, without eczema or other skin rashes and free from allergies or other conditions causing sneezing and coughing.
3. Wash hands and arms thoroughly or disinfect with foamed alcohol.
4. Put on uniforms properly, avoiding contaminating the outside of the clean/sterile uniform components.
5. Replace a uniform or parts of a uniform that become contaminated while gowning or working.
6. Put on sterile latex gloves as the final gowning step.
7. Sanitize all internal surfaces of the LAFW (except the HEPA filter face) with an appropriate sanitizing agent, usually IPA.
8. Sanitize latex gloves (usually with IPA) as frequently as necessary while performing GAPs to maintain the aseptic condition of the outer surfaces.
9. Replace gloves with new sterile ones if they become punctured or torn.
10. Move with slow, smooth, gentle motions.
11. Do not talk unnecessarily.
12. Do not disrupt HEPA-filtered laminar air flow within the critical area.
13. Do not interpose arms or any other nonsterile object above a critical site in vertical laminar air flow (VLAF) or behind a critical site in horizontal laminar air flow (HLAF).
14. Do not spray or splash disinfectants where the liquid might enter a product container or reach other product contact sites.
15. Do not introduce any packages into the buffer room unless they have been adequately sanitized or sterilized externally.
16. Minimize in and out movement at the LAFW.
17. Arrange sterile supply items in the critical area so as not to interrupt the laminar air flow and to provide for efficient processing of the product(s).
18. Resanitize gloves with IPA after handling any package if the outside had uncertain sterility or surfaces such as switches of mixing pumps.
19. Cooperate with other operators and mutually assist in maintaining proper GAPs.
20. Pass through doorways, plastic curtains, or other passageways slowly and carefully to minimize the generation of wild, potentially contaminating air currents.
21. Do not leave open vials, tanks, or other critical sites exposed to the environment during breaks or other delays in operation.
22. Inspect all supply items before using and the finished product after preparation for evidence of defects.
23. Remove used supply items and clean/sanitize work area as needed.
24. Prepare and apply appropriate labels and complete documents away from the critical area or, preferably, pass product outside so that a second person can perform the paper work.
25. Remove used uniforms carefully to avoid distributing accumulated body contamination before exiting the gowning room.
26. Leave the HEPA filter blower operating all the time.

Figure 130-2. Key GAP practices. (From Avis KE. Assuring the quality of pharmacy-prepared sterile products. *Pharmaguide to Hospital Medicine* 1996: 9(2): 11–12. Copyright 1996, Lawrence DellaCorte Publications. All rights reserved.)

TRAINING

Because the potential for success in preparing a sterile HCP is so dependent upon the capability and reliability of the pharmacist or technician, the training and evaluation of such personnel must be given high priority. To be an effective practitioner of GAPs, the operator should understand the body of knowledge supporting such practices. Therefore, one of the objectives of aseptic compounding training is to transmit a basic level of knowledge (ie, the characteristics required of a sterile dosage form the reasons for the high standards of purity required for such products, quality control measures that apply, the facilities required and their operation, the environmental requirements for processing, the role of operators in performing GAPs. A brief summary of this body of knowledge is provided in this chapter, but other cited references should be consulted for more details.[7,11,15,16].

Methods

The most perfect body of knowledge retained only in the individual's mind will not result in reliable and proficient compounders. Compounding staff must be motivated to apply their knowledge of aseptic technique effectively. Therefore, didactic instruction must be coupled with experiential instruction, and both must be conveyed with enthusiasm and motivational examples.

ASEPTIC COMPOUNDING DIDACTIC INSTRUCTION—Intellectual knowledge can be acquired by formal lectures, through informal discussion methods, and or by one-on-one instruction. Each method has its own unique advantages and disadvantages. The formal lecture provides the most organized approach to transmitting the desired body of knowledge. All participants are ensured to have been exposed to the same information, but this does not guarantee that all individuals take in the same body of knowledge equally. Relatively large groups can be trained at one time and visual aids can be used effectively.

Informal discussion has the advantage of encouraging learning through active participation of the learner. However, it is more difficult to maintain organized control of the schedule of topics to be covered. The relevance to one's specific work needs usually can be implemented more effectively and the enhanced understanding of the student can be judged directly if the instruction is one-on-one. Because of the frequently small number of trainees, one-on-one aseptic technique training is commonplace. With such instruction, it is the responsibility of the instructor to give diligent attention to the risks of interruptions, inadequate preparation, and differences from instructor-to-instructor or from time-to-time in the quality of instructions given. When performed effectively, one-on-one instruction can be the most effective method for teaching sterile products compounding.

EXPERIENTIAL TRAINING—The ability to perform the GAPs required to prepare sterile HCPs safely, accurately, and elegantly is the objective of experiential training. Typically, this type of training should be given by an expert supervisor or designated trainer using mock sterile products (vials of sterile water vs. actual drug product) to establish the principles for the level of skill required of the learner. Subsequent practice to develop improved skills may be done under the tutelage of an experienced operator, with the supervisor continuing to provide oversight. Before being permitted to prepare actual sterile products for patient use, the trainee must be approved by the supervisor and successfully pass the compounding validation program. Retraining should be required whenever an operator fails compounding revalidation, when direct observation suggests the development of careless technique, or at least on an annual basis.

VALIDATION OF OPERATORS—Aseptic compounding validation may be defined as documented evidence that provides a high degree of assurance that a specific compounding process will consistently produce a product meeting its predetermined specifications and quality attributes.[7]

Before operators, pharmacists, or technicians may be permitted to prepare HCPs of any risk level for use by patients, they must demonstrate their basic knowledge and manipulative proficiency to prepare such products, that is, to be 'validated' to perform aseptic compounding. Greater expertise and proficiency is required for operators who will be responsible for the preparation of high-risk HCPs.

The following is an example of a compounding validation procedure that may be used for operators who have completed a basic training program and are certified by a supervisor as ready to be validated.

Sample Validation Program for Operators

The program consists of three portions, all three of which must be satisfactorily passed for the operator to be considered validated to compound HCPs. The program may be modified to meet the needs of a particular home infusion pharmacy, but the requirements should be at a level that will ensure proficiency of the operator. Revalidation should be required on an annual basis to ensure continued satisfactory performance.

TESTING FOR UNDERSTANDING—The pharmacist-in-charge or their designee shall administer a written or oral test consisting of at least 25 objective test items, most of which challenge the student's knowledge and understanding of aseptic technique. To successfully pass the test, a minimum of 23 items (92%) must be answered correctly.

OBSERVATION AND EVALUATION OF GAPS—Five different aseptic manipulations, representative of those that are routinely performed in the pharmacy, including at least one of the most complex methods, should be selected by the supervisor. The trainee is then required to perform these five procedures in accordance with the GAPs demonstrated in the training program, while being directly observed by the supervisor. Any observed deviations from GAPs shall be recorded. To pass this test no deviations from GAPs are permitted.

TRANSFER OF CULTURE MEDIUM—Using the most-complex type of HCP the trainee will be expected to prepare in actual practice, the trainee will prepare 20 of these simulated products in series, at one time, without the supervisor present. Sterile soybean casein digest (SCD) medium will be used in place of an actual drug product, otherwise the process will be simulated in all respects.

Post-compounding, the 20 *units* will be incubated at 30 to 35° C for up to 14 days and inspected for the development of any turbidity after 3 and 7 days. If any visible turbidity develops at any time during the incubation period in one or more of the containers, the test is terminated, and the trainee has failed the test. Turbidity indicates that at least one microorganism has gained entrance into the unit container and has grown, most likely due to a failure in GAP by the trainee.

If the trainee fails any portion of the example tests, retraining and retesting should be required. However, at the discretion of the supervisor, retraining and retesting may only be required for the failed portion(s) of the examination. Due to the tendency for even the best operators to gradually become less proficient over time, revalidation should be planned for all operators at least annually.

QUALITY-CONTROL REQUIREMENTS

The physical, chemical, and biological quality of an injectable product intended for administration to patients in the home must be of the highest quality attainable. This quality must be *built in* to the product in each step of the aseptic compounding process, that is, in the starting components, the design and operation of the compounding facilities, the control of the environment, and the qualifications of operators all contribute to the final quality of the product, either in a positive or negative manner. Therefore, the control of quality is a continuous process throughout the compounding of the product. Testing of the finished product can only confirm the quality built into the product during its preparation.

The home infusion pharmacy must develop written procedures to ensure the quality of each finished product, also called standard operating procedures (SOPs) or policies and procedures (P&Ps). SOPs then become the protocols to be followed meticulously to replicate established, reliable compounding procedures. These also become the basis for training new pharmacists or technicians.

In the aseptic processing of products intended for use by home patients, the starting components are typically clean, sterile, and quality-controlled; that is, they have been released as having met the pharmaceutical manufacturer's quality standards. Therefore, the challenge for the pharmacist is to maintain the final product free from the ingress of contaminants, particularly microorganisms and other foreign particles, during the process steps.

PRODUCT SIMULATION TESTING—Many HCPs contain ingredients that are nutrients for microorganisms. Even though other components of the product may inhibit growth, the ingress of even one microorganism during the aseptic compounding process may permit multiplication to occur with the reproduction of many microorganisms occurring within the product within a few hours. To prevent the development of such intolerable conditions, the compounding process must be controlled. Once a process is properly controlled, it can be validated as capable of producing the prescribed quality product. To evaluate the level of microbiological control achieved, a balanced culture medium (eg, soybean casein digest medium) may be substituted for the product during a simulation of the process, called a *media fill*. After incubation of the simulated product prepared, if no growth is observed in the culture medium by the 14th day, it can be concluded that no contaminating microorganisms were introduced during the process. This is the most rigorous biological evaluation of the process currently available for quality control. It is the most important test to be performed relative to the processing of HCPs and is the basis for validation of the aseptic process and the compounder's aseptic technique. Simulation testing should represent the range of compounding procedures typically encountered in the pharmacy, from simple transfers to the procedure with the most challenging manipulative complexity (eg, *worst case*).

FINAL PRODUCT RELEASE TESTING

Without question, the most critical quality-control focus is on the control of the aseptic compounding process for preparation of sterile products. Nevertheless, select product release testing should be performed, although modified because of the nature of the products, the very small lot sizes (often a single unit for a single patient), and their relatively short shelf life. There are four key categories of final product release testing: visual inspection, compounding accuracy, sterility testing, and pyrogen testing.

PHYSICAL INSPECTION—The simplest but practical and essential evaluation is physical (visual) inspection. All HCPs should be physically examined, that is, by critically looking at the product with a pharmaceutical assessment. The pharmacist should know if the color, clarity, and other appearance characteristics are appropriate. If there is any visible alteration from the expected, the pharmacist should be alerted to the possibility of some type of degradation, and an investigation should be performed. Furthermore, the USP requires that all final containers be inspected individually for the presence of visible particulate matter. If any particles are observed against either a white or black background, the container should be discarded.

COMPOUNDING ACCURACY—Compounding accuracy in the preparation of HCPs is normally considered to be the responsibility of the pharmacist-in-charge, using accurate measuring and compounding devices and appropriate, careful techniques. Established SOPs should require the measurements by one technician or pharmacist to be checked by a second pharmacist. For example, if syringes are used to measure a prescribed volume of a component, the syringe plunger should be drawn back to the measurement site used so that its accuracy can be determined by the pharmacist checker. As discussed previously, with automated mixing pumps the volume setting can be checked before it is moved for the next delivery. Electrolyte pool solutions used in PN, calculations should also be double checked.

STERILITY TESTING—As stated above, the best assurance of sterility of an HCP is through the evidence of validated aseptic compounding procedures. Compounding records verifying the sterility of the initial components of the product and of the devices used for preparing the HCP, the control of the Class 100 workspace and its buffer areas, and the qualifications of the operators, provide the greatest assurance that the final HCP is sterile. Therefore, a sterility test is not typically performed on a single or small lot of HCPs. However, a sterility test performed on a sample representative of a group of products prepared under essentially identical conditions (eg, the preparations of a single technician during a single work shift) may be appropriate. Operators must consider that the USP sterility test is a destructive test; that is, the test unit(s) is consumed in performing the test and would not be available for subsequent patient administration. Additionally, the test has practical limitations in that it requires a minimum incubation period of 7 days, during which most HCPs would already have been administered to the patient before test results would be known. Conversely, sterility testing should be performed on any lots of products made from nonsterile starting ingredients or when batches of HCPs are produced in open tanks, that is, when the product is exposed for a substantial period of time to the environment, often in a Class 1,000 or less clean room. The test requirements would be based upon the specifications for small lots of products as described in the USP[26] and adjusted for the small lot sizes.

Of the two test methods described by the USP, the membrane filtration technique is preferred. This method has the advantages that:

1. It concentrates small numbers of microorganisms and gives greater probability of recovery.
2. Large volumes of product can be filtered and thus tested.
3. The product is filtered away from any viable microorganisms, and any inhibitory effects from the product are minimized.

This method also provides a higher probability of detecting any viable microorganisms that may be present. The testing methods are described in the USP.[26] Because sterility testing and other analytical laboratory tests will not be performed in the pharmacy but in another facility, the pharmacist-in-charge is responsible for ensuring that the contracted testing laboratory is capable of performing all tests properly.

PYROGEN TESTING—The presence of pyrogens (the products of metabolism of microorganisms) normally is of little concern. But testing would be required under circumstances similar to the requirements for sterility testing. Detectable levels of pyrogens would normally occur only in the presence of a relatively high number of microorganisms; usually something that is not likely with most HCPs. However, pyrogen testing is a sensitive test and of particular value when microorganisms had been present in equipment or other areas of the compounding process even though they are dead at the time of testing. The *Bacterial Endotoxins Test,* the test method normally used, is described in Section <85> of the USP.[27]

EXPIRATION DATING—Although the shelf life of HCPs is normally not required to be more than 30 to 60 days, this dating is long enough given the nature of HCPs and the uncertain storage conditions that may occur during transportation and storage in the patient's home. Pharmacists must give careful consideration to the potential for sterile product degradation. A home infusion pharmacy usually does not have the capability of studying chemical drug degradation, nor is it possible, considering the many formulation variations that can occur with the prescribing privileges of physicians. Therefore, pharmacists are limited to the information that can be obtained from the drug's manufacturer, the pharmaceutical literature, and their professional judgment. Each of these sources, at best, can only provide the basis for a theoretical stability assessment. Only product-specific, experimentally determined stability data can provide a real determination of physical and chemical stability over time. The biological prediction of stability, that is, the likelihood of microorganisms growing in the product, can only be ensured by the level of reliability of the aseptic compounding methods used. Due to the nutrient nature of many HCPs and the inherent risk of even one microorganism gaining entrance into the product, the length of shelf life with uncertain conditions of storage should be conservatively limited.

For all HCPs, compounding documents should be available to provide a record of the product's complete processing history. These documents should refer to, and be founded upon, a complete set of SOPs that clearly describe the established procedures used to determine product stability and compounding methodology. The documented process history should be carefully reviewed for completeness, accuracy, and evidence of compliance with SOPs and other quality standards for the product before it is released for use in a patient.

LABELING

After a sterile product is prepared, it must be properly labeled to communicate the necessary information to ensure its appropriate use.[16] This is particularly true for product labels for sterile products used in the home environment, because of the following requirements:

- Labels must be understandable by a lay person, because the end user may be a patient, or family member.
- Labels should avoid medical abbreviations or potentially confusing terminology.
- Labels must give clear directions for administering the product via the prescribed method of administration. Instructions must be included for operating any infusion pump devices or other required administration techniques.
- Labels must be understandable by other health-care professionals, so that if the patient is treated at another site (eg, an emergency room) the correct administration of the drug can be continued.

Recognizing these requirements, the elements of a label for a home infusion pharmaceutical should include[15]:

- Prescription information-prescription number, date, and prescribing physician.
- Patient information—patient name and other identifying information, such as a patient number or address, if appropriate.
- Directions for use (eg, the time and frequency of administration, infusion rates, and pump settings) for the infusion device selected.
- Handling or storage requirements, including requirements for refrigeration and warming to room temperature before use, if applicable.
- Name and amount of drug present; if the admixture contains more than one dose, the label should indicate the amount of drug for one dose, the volume of the dose, and the total amount of drug and total volume present.
- Name and volume of the admixture solution.
- Expiration date under the recommended storage conditions; length of time product may be stored at room temperature, if appropriate.
- Initials of persons who prepared and checked the admixture.
- Auxiliary labels as appropriate.

Because home-care patients require significant detailed information about their products, many home infusion pharmacies choose to supplement the label with additional patient in-

formational materials. If an auxiliary label does not provide enough space, supplemental instruction sheets may be provided. It is the dispensing pharmacist's responsibility to ensure that all of the information needed by the patient or caregiver is provided.

If caregivers in the home must add ingredients to the HCP that are not stable for prolonged periods (such as insulin or vitamins), the product label should clearly indicate the amount and volume of each ingredient to be added just prior to infusion. Highlighting this information with a bright color, use of a separate additive label, or other techniques may be used to ensure that these additives are not omitted.

PARENTERAL NUTRIENT ADMIXTURES—Labeling of parenteral nutrient (PN) admixtures requires special attention. Total parenteral nutrition formulations are complex admixtures containing amino acids, dextrose, and lipids, as well as water, electrolytes, vitamins, and trace elements. PN labels are used by clinicians as a source of prescription information when patients are seen in outpatient settings or admitted to other sites of care. For this reason, PN formula information must be expressed in a manner that is clearly understandable not only by caregivers in the home, but also throughout the health-care system.

Currently, methods of macronutrient labeling vary widely among different organizations and sites of care. One of the most common ways of expressing nutrient quantities is as the final concentration of each ingredient, such as dextrose 25%. Calculations are required to determine the total nutrients included per day or per container. Other organizations label their parenteral nutrition formulations by specifying the volumes and initial concentrations before admixture of each ingredient (eg, 500 mL of 50% dextrose). Still other pharmacy's may label their PN formulas with the absolute quantity of each ingredient per preset volume of PN (eg, dextrose 250 g per liter), or home infusion organizations can also label PN formulas in terms of total quantities of each ingredient per day, such as dextrose 340 g per day. Electrolyte additives may be expressed in millimoles or milliequivalents per liter or per total volume. Unfortunately, this lack of labeling standardization causes confusion and the potential for errors, especially when patients are transferred between health-care environments.

Errors in managing the preparation of PN solutions can result in serious harm or even death for the patient. In fact, the misinterpretation of prescription labels has led to several serious patient incidents.[28] In one case, hospital personnel misinterpreted the dextrose content on the label of a home PN formulation, resulting in a pediatric patient's death.[28] The prescription label read *300 mL of 50% dextrose*. The hospital pharmacy misinterpreted this as a final concentration of dextrose 50%. The patient died after receiving the incorrect formulation for two days.

Another incident involved the misinterpretation of a label resulting in an iron overload with resultant liver toxicity in a child receiving PN with iron dextran.[29] The home PN label read iron dextran 1 mL, the intention being to use a 1 mg/mL iron dextran dilution prepared by the pharmacy. However, the solution was prepared with the undiluted 50 mg/mL concentration and not a 1 mg/mL solution, resulting in a 50-fold error in the dose that was administered.

As a result of these tragic events, the American Society of Parenteral and Enteral Nutrition (ASPEN) established the National Advisory Group (NAG) on Standards and Practice Guidelines for PN.[30] The purpose of this group was to identify problematic areas in PN therapy and to make recommendations and develop guidelines that fostered safer practices. Specific problem areas noted in the NAG included: nutrient requirements, labeling, compounding formulas, stability issues, filtering, and quality assurance. PN labeling was one of the areas identified by the group as problematic.

The NAG recommended that the macronutrient content of PN admixtures be labeled in grams per total volume and that other additives be labeled in total quantities per total volume[30]

This labeling method supports the use of a once-per-day nutrient admixture system, which is a cost-efficient method of PN compounding.[31] Organizations accustomed to labeling in other formats, such as amounts per liter, sometimes supplement the label with a second column indicating the latter information.

Auxiliary labels may also be useful to list other information such as individual concentrations of electrolytes in milliequivalents or millimoles, total and nonprotein calories per day, and the percentage of total and nonprotein calories provided as carbohydrate and fat.[30]

STORAGE IN THE PHARMACY

Monitoring the storage conditions in the pharmacy is necessary to ensure that sterile products retain their respective quality attributes. Controlled-temperature storage areas such as refrigerators and freezers should be monitored at least once daily, with results documented on a temperature log. Suitable temperature-recording devices include calibrated continuous recording devices (preferred) to a National Bureau of Standards (NBS) calibrated thermometer. Continuous recording devices should be minimally checked daily to confirm that the device is working properly and has not malfunctioned. Pharmacy staff should take care to avoid causing significant temperature aberrations, such as from holding refrigerator doors open too long or overloading the refrigerator.[11]

PACKAGING AND SHIPPING

The pharmacist's responsibility for ensuring the quality of sterile products used at home does not end when the product is dispensed from the pharmacy. Care must be taken that the handling of such products outside the pharmacy and at the site of administration ensures that the product maintains its original quality attributes, particularly sterility and stability. This requirement should be balanced with the need to deliver sterile products in a timely manner and at a frequency that minimizes delivery costs but avoids product waste because of changes in orders or expired shelf life of products.[15]

Transportation of the product to the site of administration must take place via a delivery or shipping system. In this chapter, delivery refers to the personal delivery of the sterile product by an employee of the home infusion organization (eg, the home care nurse who will administer the product, a delivery employee) while shipping refers to the use of a common carrier, or courier, such as a commercial package-handling service, or the mail. Each of these delivery methods has its unique challenges.

Delivery usually is assumed to be faster and more reliable than shipping. This can lead to a cavalier attitude about the need for properly packaging sterile products during delivery, because it is assumed that the product will be delivered to the home (or other administration site) within a short time. Oftentimes, long delivery routes, employee breaks and meals, or adverse traffic conditions can delay product delivery and adversely expose products to extremely hot or cold temperatures in the delivery van or nurse's car. Additionally, the shifting of packages during transportation can potentially lead to damaged products and/or hazardous spills.

Similarly, shipping products via a common carrier can also subject the product to extremes in temperatures and rough handling. When commercial air and truck carriers are used, the home infusion pharmacy is responsible for taking actions to ensure the quality of their services. Before using a commercial carrier, the pharmacy should confirm the carrier's capabilities for maintaining required delivery schedules, transit times, safe handling, and temperature control. The pharmacy should develop an effective system for monitoring the carrier's shipping performance. Some carriers provide electronic or telephone confirmation of delivery times. If this is not available, a review of delivery receipts or telephone follow-up calls with the patient or caregiver can be used to monitor the delivery timeliness of the carrier. Other important indicators to monitor include the condition of the products upon receipt and personnel courteousness.

Careful product packaging is essential to protect the integrity of the sterile products during shipping and delivery. Packaging materials should be selected to maintain required product temperature, minimize breakage, and to avoid leaks. Required components of product packaging includes: insulation for temperature control, cushioning to avoid product shifting and breakage, and a sealed leak-proof container to minimize the risk of leakage if a liquid product is damaged in transit.

INSULATION—Refrigerated sterile products for home use should be packaged in an insulated container to maintain temperatures within the USP recommended storage temperatures of 2° to 8°C. For personal deliveries, a sturdy reusable cooler is a cost-effective insulated container. For shipping, insulated containers, consisting of a Styrofoam inner liner with a cardboard outer box, are commercially available. A low-cost alternative involves placing a smaller cardboard box inside a larger cardboard box and filling the space between the boxes with Styrofoam packing peanuts. In either case, ice bricks or kool-it blocks are used inside the package to maintain product temperature. Tape should be used to completely seal box edges; this will also facilitate maintaining product temperature.

Even sterile products that do not require refrigerated storage may be labeled for storage at controlled room temperature (<85°F). In one study, the USP found that more than 90% of approximately 200 packages shipped from its Rockville, Maryland headquarters were exposed to unacceptably high temperatures during shipment. Temperature indicators in two-thirds of the packages registered spikes between 86° and 104°F at some point in transit.[31] Although ice bricks are not required, use of an insulated container for shipping or delivery, especially in the warm summer months, can help to avoid excessive heat.

CUSHIONING—Packaging materials such as Styrofoam packing peanuts, bubble wrap, Styrofoam wrap, or shredded or crumpled newspapers are useful to prevent damage due to product shifting. For best damage control, the box containing the product should be completely filled with the selected packaging material. Any free air spaces within the box increases the risk of product shifting, and contributes to decreased temperature control.

Packaging materials can also be used to avoid excessively cold product temperatures during transit. Avoid subjecting HCPs to freezing and extremely cold temperatures. Some protein-containing drug products can be denatured by freezing. Using a cardboard barrier to separate the drug product from the ice bricks can be helpful.

CONTAINERS—Within the package, the sterile drug product itself should be packaged in a primary container, usually made of glass or plastic that is designed to protect and contain the product. The primary container should minimize the risk of leaking, unless it is broken or otherwise damaged. Sometimes an outer wrap, in the form of a zip-lock plastic bag, is used to contain the liquid drug product in the event that the primary container is damaged and leakage occurs. The outer wrap is also useful to separate the drug product from food items when stored in the patient's refrigerator.

Chemotherapeutic drugs or other hazardous materials should be double bagged. Should an unexpected spill occur, hazardous spill kits should be available to use in containing and cleaning up the spill thus minimizing the hazard. When shipping hazardous materials, check both OSHA and local department of transportation (DOT) requirements for specific guidelines.

PACKAGE VALIDATION—Home infusion pharmacists should validate the packaging materials that they use to ensure that such materials maintain product temperatures within the acceptable range during shipping. The placement and number of ice bricks, product size and placement, air space within the package, insulation thickness, choice of packaging materials, expected ambient temperatures, and duration of shipping all influence the maintenance of the product's temperature.

Small, reusable computerized temperature probes are available for monitoring temperatures during normal shipping conditions. The temperature probe is placed as close as possible to the drug in the package to be evaluated. The product is then packaged and shipped or delivered via standard procedures. Upon receipt, the temperature probe should be returned to the pharmacy and the temperature data downloaded. The computerized probe records the temperatures experienced by the package during the entire delivery cycle. Ideally, the packaging system should maintain the product within the desired temperature range for the anticipated duration of shipment plus some additional margin of safety, in case the delivery is delayed.

Temperature indicators are also available. These indicators record a color change or other visual display of the maximum temperature experienced by the product during transit. Although these devices are not yet inexpensive enough for use with every shipment, they can be useful for initial validation and periodic retesting.

A less costly but less evaluative method of package evaluation involves post transit temperature checks. A thermometer is used to test the product temperature immediately upon product receipt, or the package is simply examined to assess whether the drug product is cold (but not frozen). Checking the temperature upon package receipt has limitations in that it gives an indication of the current temperature but does not reflect whether temperature fluctuations occurred during transit.

Designing a shipping package to meet both temperature and cost requirements will necessitate some experimental testing. Possible solutions for commonly encountered problems are listed in Table 130-4.

Evaluation and possibly redesigning the shipping package should be continued until a package is developed that adequately maintains the product within the desired temperature range for the anticipated duration of shipping. Once the package has been designed and the procedure for packing is complete and validated, the information should be put incorporated into a standard operating procedure (SOP) by home infusion pharmacy personnel. This SOP will ensure that packing techniques, configurations, and materials for groups of products with common storage characteristics will be standardized. Procedures also should be developed for products with unique storage conditions. Packaging should not vary from the established materials and procedure without retesting, as different packaging materials and configurations differ in their resistance to heat penetration or loss. Occasionally, shipments should be retested, especially whenever transit conditions vary, seasonal temperature changes occur, changes in transit times, or use of different packaging materials.

Table 130-4. Designing a Package for Shipping Refrigerated Sterile Products

POTENTIAL PROBLEMS	POSSIBLE SOLUTIONS
Temperature too cold (<2°)	• Fewer ice bricks • Cardboard barrier around product
Temperature too warm (>8°)	• Add more ice bricks • Use thicker insulation in box • Use more packaging materials to avoid air space in package
Temperature not maintained long enough for expected duration of shipment/delivery	• Add more ice bricks • Try larger ice bricks • Use a cardboard barrier around product plus more or larger ice bricks

STORAGE IN THE HOME

Sterile products must be stored under controlled conditions until the product is administered. Each drug product should be labeled to indicate its storage requirements and expiration date, including, if appropriate, the time of day beyond which the product should not be used.

Refrigerated products usually are stored in the patient's own refrigerator. The patient/caregiver should be trained to check the refrigerator temperature on a daily basis to ensure proper storage is maintained. If the patient does not have a refrigerator, alternative arrangements must be made. At one time it was common practice for the home infusion organization to provide patients with a refrigerator. In today's cost-conscious health care environment, other options, such as using a neighbor's refrigerator or storing the product with a visiting home health nurse, may be considered.

Unless otherwise indicated, sterile admixtures for home use should be refrigerated until the time of use. Even under ideal conditions, there is always some risk that microorganisms may gain entry into the sterile product. Therefore, HCPs should be stored at refrigerated temperatures to inhibit microbial growth, even if stability issues do not require such storage. There are a few exceptions including:

- Sterile products intended for administration promptly after compounding may be retained at room temperature. It should be noted that delivery time should be included when determining whether the product will be administered promptly; if in doubt, the product should be refrigerated during delivery.
- Reservoirs of medications, such as narcotic analgesics, intended for infusion over more than one day via an ambulatory infusion pump, should either be started promptly after preparation or be refrigerated until the start of infusion. Administration should be completed within seven days.
- Sterile products, such as 5-fluorouracil that should not be refrigerated after preparation should be used within 28 hours of preparation.[11]

The cumulative storage conditions experienced by a sterile product must also be considered. For example, products are commonly removed from the refrigerator and allowed to equilibrate to room temperature, only to be replaced in the refrigerator for later use, if not used as planned. The originally assigned expiration date may be invalidated by these circumstances. In this situation, the pharmacist must consider the cumulative effects of room-temperature storage when determining whether or not the product is stable for use. This may be fairly straightforward for products that have a well-accepted duration of stability at room temperature. For example, 24-hour stability at room temperature is the accepted limit for parenteral nutrition solutions, and 7 days at room temperature is the norm for multi-day infusion reservoirs containing narcotic analgesics. For other sterile products, the manufacturer, their product literature or other reputable source should be consulted for limits on room-temperature stability.

Product labeling should be used to explain requirements for storage and expiration dating. A separate information sheet should include instructions for proper storage, interpretation of expiration dating, and how to observe signs of unsuitability for use. Home-care products should be stored out of the reach of children and pets.

Home assessments should be performed to confirm compliance with appropriate drug storage conditions, cleanliness, separation of drugs from food items, avoidance of improper use or reuse of drugs or supplies, and proper disposal of drug waste. Home inventory quantities should be monitored as an indicator of compliance. If improperly stored, expired, or damaged products are found, the patient should be asked for consent to return or dispose of these items.[11]

Patients receiving sterile products in the home should be instructed about appropriate methods of waste disposal. Needles or other sharp objects should be placed in a commercially available sharps-disposal container, or alternatively, can be stored

130-5. Training Content for Administration of HCPs

- Inspection of products upon receipt for damage and temperature maintenance.
- Product storage requirements.
- Visual inspection before administration for leaks, cracks, particulates, precipitation, discoloration, oiling out, or other evidence of loss of product integrity.
- Label check to confirm right product, drug, dose, and administration time.
- Proper handwashing technique.
- Procedures for aseptic preparation of the product in a clean preparation area.
- Handling and set-up of infusion apparatus and supplies.
- Catheter care and maintenance.
- Clinical monitoring of the patient and the therapy.
- Emergency actions for common complications such as infection, catheter breakage or displacement, tubing disconnection, catheter occlusion, equipment battery change, or equipment malfunction.
- Emergency contact numbers and procedures.
- Proper waste disposal.

Data from USP 26-NF21.

in an impervious and sealable container (eg, empty coffee can.) The sharps container should be kept out of the reach of children. A process should be established for routine waste removal from the home. Options for sharps removal include having home infusion pharmacy personnel pick up the waste container, mailing the sharps container in a sealed package to an EPA-approved incineration facility, or having the patient or caregiver bring the sharps container to a health-care facility for disposal.

Most drug products are not hazardous, and empty containers, tubing, and the like may be disposed of with other household trash; however, local disposal requirements may be prescribed by the landfill where the waste will be sent. Additionally, special consideration to waste disposal must be given if the patient has a communicable disease such as HIV or hepatitis. Waste from hazardous products administered in the home, such as chemotherapy, should be stored in a separate area of the home and should be retrieved by the home infusion organization for incineration.

ADMINISTRATION

The individual or caregiver responsible for administering sterile products in the home must be properly trained. Basic training topics are listed in Table 130-5.

Certain methods of drug administration are unique to home care. These include: ambulatory infusion pumps, implantable infusion devices, and disposable infusion devices. All of these devices expose the sterile drug products to elevated temperatures (eg, body temperature) during administration. Reference data should be consulted to confirm that product stability will be maintained during storage and administration at these elevated temperatures during the intended period of administration.[11]

The home infusion pharmacist is ultimately responsible for compounding sterile products of acceptable strength, quality, and purity with appropriate packaging and labeling in accordance with good pharmacy practices, state pharmacy regula-

tions, official professional and compendial standards, and current scientific principles. Pharmacists practicing in the home infusion setting should continually expand their knowledge about aseptic compounding by participating in seminars, reviewing the professional literature, and consulting professional pharmacy trade organizations.

REFERENCES

1. Lima HA. *Pharmacy Practice News.* 1999; (July) 33.
2. Triller DM, Clause SL, Domarew C. *Am J Health-Syst Pharm.* 2002; 59:2356.
3. Am J Health-Syst Pharm. 1999; 56:629.
4. National Home Infusion Association (NHIA) White paper: Home infusion services, payment models, and operational costs. www. nhianet.org.
5. Burnell J. *Managed Healthcare Executive.* 2002; (Sept) 36.
6. Avis KE, Lima HA, McKinnon BT. In: Gennaro AR, ed. *Remington: The Science and Practice of Pharmacy.* 20th ed. Philadelphia: Lippincott, Williams & Wilkins, 2000.
7. International Academy of Compounding Pharmacists. The art and skill of pharmacy compounding. www.iacprx.org/about compounidng/index.html. Accessed 03/21/03.
8. *ASHP Technical Assistance Bulletin on Quality Assurance for Pharmacy-Prepared Sterile Products.* Bethesda, MD: American Society of Health-Systems Pharmacists, 1994–1995.
9. Subramaniam V, Sokol G, Zenger V, et al. Survey of drug products compounded by a group of community pharmacies: Findings from a food and drug administration study. Available online: www.fda.gov/cder/pharmacomp/communityPharmacy/default.htm.
10. Kastango ES, Bradshaw BD. *Infusion* 2003; 8:23.
11. Sterile drug products for home use. In: The United States Pharmacopeia (USP), 24th rev., and the National Formulary, 19th ed. Rockville, MD: The United States Pharmacopeial Convention, 1999:2130.
12. Model rules for sterile pharmaceuticals. Chicago: National Association of Boards of Pharmacy, 1993; 12.1.
13. National advisory group on standards and practice guidelines for parenteral nutrition. *J Parenter Enteral Nutr* 1998; 22:49.
14. Levchuk JW. In: Avis K et al eds: *Pharmaceutical Dosage Forms: Parenteral Medications,* ed 2, vol 1. New York: Dekker, 1992
15. Buchanan EC, et al. *Principles of Sterile Product Preparation.* Bethesda, MD: ASHP, 1995.
16. Avis KE. *Pharmaguide Hosp Med* 1996; 9(2): 1.
17. Lima HA. *Int J Pharmaceutical Compounding* 1999; 3:270.
18. Landry C, Bussieres JF, Lebel P, et al. *Am J Health-Syst Pharm* 2001; 58:1009.
19. Moussa M, Rahe H, Lo K. Int J Pharmaceutical Compounding 2003; 7:42.
20. Chrai S, et al. *J Parenter Sci Technol* 1986; 10:104.
21. *Tech Rpt 13.* Bethesda, MD: PDA, 1990.
22. Barber J, Stachnik J. Selection of parenteral nutrition compounding methods: Safety and efficiency considerations. An on-line continuing education course for nursing and allied health-care professionals. Available online: www.baxter.com/doctors/iv_therapies/education/iv_therapy_ce/pn_compounidng/html. Accessed 03/18/03.
23. Product specifications: Clintec Professional Services. Deerfield, IL: 1-800-422-2751.
24. Product specifications: Baxa Corporation. Englewood, CO; 1-800-567-2292.
25. Meyer GE, et al. Am J Health-Syst Pharm 1987; 44:1617.
26. USP 23, 8th suppl <71>. *Sterility Tests* 1998; 4297.
27. USP 23 <85>. *Bacterial Endotoxins Test* 1995; 1696.
28. Carey LC, Haffey M. *Home Care Highlights* 1995; 2: 7.
29. *Pharmacy Today.* Sept 1995.
30. Mirtallo JM, et al. *J Parenter Enteral Nutr* 1998; 22:49.
31. Mirtallo JM, et al. *Am J Health-Syst Pharm* 1986; 43:2205.
32. Conlan MF. *Drug Topics* 1998; (July):56.

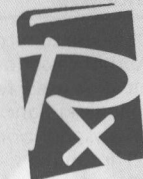

CHAPTER 131

The Pharmacist's Role in Substance Use Disorders

Lori A Wilken, PharmD, CDE, AE-C

Susan R Winkler, PharmD, BCPS

Ronnie A Weathermon, PharmD

Substance abuse and drug addiction permeate our society today, irrespective of one's socioeconomic status. Alcohol dependence is estimated to affect more than 7% of the adult population in the United States[1] and is responsible for 130,000 deaths annually.[2] Tobacco use is responsible for more than 440,000 deaths each year in the United States, and greater than 150 billion dollars is spent annually in direct and indirect costs attributable to smoking.[3] Over 70% of current smokers would like to quit; however, less than 3% of all smokers are able to successfully stop smoking each year.[4,5] Total direct and indirect costs associated with illicit drug use exceed $97.7 billion.[6] Even with these staggering numbers, substance use disorders are frequently overlooked as health care issues that pharmacists can impact.

As health care professionals, pharmacists are well positioned to take a major role in the disease management of substance use disorders and other comorbid conditions.[7] Pharmacists have knowledge of the pharmacology, pharmacokinetics, mechanisms of action, drug interactions, and adverse events associated with prescription medications and abused substances.[8] Therefore, taking an active responsibility in assessing patients and assuring the appropriate use of treatments for substance use is another opportunity in the ever-increasing role of the pharmacist.

Substance Use Disorders

Substance use disorders are a broad spectrum of behaviors related to the inappropriate use of legal or illegal products. These disorders encompass drug addiction, alcoholism, nicotine addiction, and inhalant abuse, to name a few. Addiction is defined as a disease process characterized by the continued use of a specific psychoactive substance, or the continuation of a particular behavior despite physical, psychological, or social harm. Patients exhibit addictive behavior usually due to dependence upon the substance. Dependence is classified as either physical or psychological. Physical dependence, a physiological state of adaptation to a specific psychoactive substance, is characterized by the emergence of withdrawal effects during abstinence, which may be relieved in total or in part by re-administration of the substance. Psychological dependence is a subjective sense of need for a specific psychoactive substance, either for its positive effects or to avoid negative effects associated with its abstinence. Consumption of the abused substance continues due to fear of withdrawal symptoms. Tables 131-1, 131-2, and 131-3 list common withdrawal symptoms associated with tobacco, alcohol, and opioid cessation.[1] Tolerance is defined as repeated exposure to the same dose of a psychoactive drug resulting in a diminished effect, so that higher dosages than usual are required to achieve a similar response. Tolerance commonly oc-

curs in alcohol, tobacco, and opioid abuse, causing the user to consume larger quantities of the substance to gain the same desired effect. Abstinence is defined as refraining from the use of the substance for a period of time, while a relapse is considered to occur when the individual resumes use of the substance after a period of abstinence. A lapse is considered to be a single episode of using the substance that does not lead to resuming continuous use of the substance.

Brief Interventions

Pharmacists are gaining increasing responsibility for direct patient care and are in an ideal position to provide brief interventions for substance use disorders. Usually, brief interventions are conducted in a primary care setting; however, these short dialogues with patients can take place in any setting where a pharmacist has an opportunity for one-on-one counseling with a patient (eg, retail, hospital, outpatient clinics). The purpose of a brief intervention is to reinforce behaviors toward abstinence in four or five successive patient interactions. Table 131-4 outlines a helpful strategy that can be used during brief counseling sessions known as the "5 A's." These consist of **A**sking, **A**dvising, **A**ssessing, **A**ssisting, and **A**rranging and can help the pharmacist focus each session and provide effective counseling within a short period of time.[9]

In general, such interventions begin with an assessment of the patient's substance use problem and a discussion of the potential health consequences with continued substance use. The pharmacist then offers advice on strategies to either cut down or abstain from use of the substance. Such strategies can include setting specific goals for reducing the number of alcoholic drinks consumed per day or cigarettes smoked per week and agreeing to written contracts that specify measures of progress toward changes in behavior.[10,11]

Recognizing the Addicted Patient

Identifying substance use in a patient should not be a challenge for the pharmacist. Asking a patient if he or she smokes, drinks alcohol, or uses other psychoactive substances should become as natural as asking a patient if he or she has any medication allergies. This information should be included in the demographic section of the patient's profile. Many patients will respect the confidentiality and privacy offered by their pharmacist; however, some patients may be dishonest in answering questions related to licit or illicit substance use, or they may become angry when questioned.

Table 131-1. Diagnostic Criteria for Nicotine Withdrawal

A. Daily use of nicotine for at least several weeks.
B. Abrupt cessation of nicotine use, or reduction in the amount of nicotine used, followed within 24 hours by four (or more) of the following signs:
   (1) dysphoric or depressed mood
   (2) insomnia
   (3) irritability, frustration, or anger
   (4) anxiety
   (5) difficulty concentrating
   (6) restlessness
   (7) decreased heart rate
   (8) increased appetite or weight gain.
C. The symptoms in Criterion B cause clinically significant distress or impairment in social, occupational, or other important areas of functioning.
D. The symptoms are not due to a general medical condition and are not better accounted for by another mental disorder.

From The American Psychiatric Association. *Diagnostic and Statistical Manual for Mental Disorders*, 4th ed, text revision. Washington DC: American Psychiatric Association, 2000.

Knowing as much information as possible about substance use is critical when dispensing prescription medications. Table 131-5 describes the various drug interactions with cigarette smoking. For example, smoking induces the cytochrome P-450 system in the liver causing drugs such as caffeine, clozapine, olanzapine, tacrine, and theophylline to be metabolized more quickly. Higher doses of these medications are required in smokers and dosage adjustments are necessary in patients that quit smoking. Tobacco use may also cause a pharmacodynamic interaction with medications such as benzodiazepines and beta-blockers, altering their expected response. Smokers may have less sedation and drowsiness with benzodiazepines and a decreased antihypertensive effect with beta-blockers.[12] This information may help motivate patients to make a smoking cessation attempt or remain abstinent. Disease states and medications that should automatically trigger the pharmacist to ask about the patient's smoking status are listed in Table 131-6. Common indicators that should prompt questioning regarding smoking status include prescribed medications for chronic obstructive pulmonary disease, asthma, diabetes, hypertension, and cholesterol lowering medications. Common interactions also occur between alcohol and prescription medica-

Table 131-2. Diagnostic Criteria for Substance Abuse

A. A maladaptive pattern of substance use leading to clinically significant impairment or distress, as manifested by one (or more) of the following, occurring within a 12-month period:
   (1) recurrent substance use resulting in failure to fulfill major role obligations at work, school, or home (eg, repeated absences or poor work performance related to substance use; substance-related absences, suspensions, or expulsions from school; neglect of children or household)
   (2) recurrent substance use in situations in which it is physically hazardous (eg, driving an automobile or operating a machine when impaired by substance use)
   (3) recurrent substance-related legal problems (eg, arrests for substance-related disorderly conduct)
   (4) continued substance use despite having persistent or recurrent social or interpersonal problems caused or exacerbated by the effects of the substance (eg, arguments with spouse about consequences of intoxication, physical fights).
B. The symptoms have never met the criteria for Substance Dependence for this class of substance.

From The American Psychiatric Association. *Diagnostic and Statistical Manual for Mental Disorders*, 4th ed, text revision. Washington DC: American Psychiatric Association, 2000.

Table 131-3. Diagnostic Criteria for Opiate Withdrawal

A. Either of the following:
   (1) cessation of (or reduction in) opioid use that has been heavy and prolonged (several weeks or longer)
   (2) administration of an opioid antagonist after a period of opioid use
B. Three (or more) of the following, developing within minutes to several days after criterion A:
   (1) dysphoric mood
   (2) nausea or vomiting
   (3) muscle aches
   (4) lacrimation or rhinorrhea
   (5) pupillary dilation, piloerection, or sweating
   (6) diarrhea
   (7) yawning
   (8) fever
   (9) insomnia.
C. The symptoms in Criterion B cause clinically significant distress or impairment in social, occupational, or other important areas of functioning.
D. The symptoms are not due to a general medical condition and are not better accounted for by another mental disorder.

From The American Psychiatric Association. *Diagnostic and Statistical Manual for Mental Disorders*, 4th ed, text revision. Washington DC: American Psychiatric Association, 2000.

tions. Interactions can be pharmacokinetic, as described above with cigarettes, or pharmacodynamic, often resulting in an additive effect with alcohol on the central nervous system. Pharmacokinetic interactions depend on the patient's level of drinking. With moderate alcohol consumption, competition occurs for the cytochrome P-450 metabolic pathway. Alcohol has a greater affinity for these enzymes, resulting in decreased metabolism of the medication and higher levels of it in the body. In chronic heavy drinkers, cytochrome P-450 activity is enhanced, resulting in potentially subtherapeutic levels of the medication.[13] Patients taking medications with sedative effects should be counseled on the additive sedation that can result when these products are taken in conjunction with alcohol.

Willingness to Change: The Transtheoretical Model

One of the most helpful concepts to understand when assisting a patient with a substance use disorder is the Transtheoretical Model for Change.[14] This model illustrates the process one goes through with *any* type of behavior change, whether it is quitting smoking or drinking alcohol, losing weight, or starting a new exercise regimen. Once the patient's readiness to change is determined, appropriate counseling may be more readily of-

Table 131-4. The "5 A's" for Brief Intervention

Ask about substance use	Identify and document substance abuse at every visit.
Advise to quit	In a clear, strong, and personalized manner urge user to quit.
Assess willingness to make a quit attempt	Is the substance abuser willing to make a quit attempt at this time?
Assist in quit attempt	For the patient willing to make a quit attempt, use counseling and pharmacotherapy to help him or her quit.
Arrange follow-up	Schedule follow-up contact, preferably within the first week after the quit date.

From Fiore MC, Bailey WC, Cohen SJ, et al. *Treating Tobacco Use and Dependence: Clinical Practice Guideline*. Rockville, MD: U.S. Department of Health and Human Services. Public Health Service, June 2000.

Table 131-5. Drug Interactions with Cigarette Smoking

DRUG	MECHANISM	COUNSELING COMMENT
Acetaminophen	Induction of CYP1A2	Patients may require less acetaminophen for pain relief if they quit smoking.
Caffeine	Induction of CYP1A2	Patients attempting abstinence may want to decrease their caffeine intake. Slower metabolism of caffeine causes insomnia, also a withdrawal symptom of nicotine.
Clozapine	Induction of CYP1A2	May require a lower dose once they stop smoking.
Diazepam	Unknown	Sedation may improve with abstinence. Smokers require higher doses.
Insulin	Increased catecholamines and cortisol; decreased subcutaneous absorption	Patients may be able to lower their insulin dose once they stop smoking.
Propoxyphene	Unknown	Pain may be controlled with lower doses after quitting smoking.
Propranolol	Increased release of catecholamines	Drug efficacy, blood pressure, and chest pain may improve with abstinence.
Tacrine	Induction of CYP1A2	Patients may require a lower dose once they stop smoking.
Theophylline	Induction of CYP1A2	The dosage of theophylline may need to be empirically lowered by one-third to one-fourth of the total daily dose once the patients stop smoking.
Tricyclic antidepressants	Increased hepatic metabolism	Patients may require a lower dose once they stop smoking.
Warfarin	Increased hepatic metabolism	Patients may require a lower dose once they stop smoking.

fered.[15] Recommending that a patient change a specific behavior before the decision to change has been made may lead to defensive behavior from the patient and frustration for the pharmacist.

The goal of the Transtheoretical Model for Change is to offer advice and motivation to move the patient forward to the next stage until the behavior change is imminent. The model is designed to be cyclical, meaning a patient may lapse or relapse and need counseling to restart the process. The patient may proceed completely or partially through the model of change several times before the behavior change becomes permanent.

The first stage of change is *precontemplation*. At this stage, a patient has not really thought about making a behavior change. The patient may appear defensive when asked about his/her substance use and whether stopping this use is in sight. Although the patient may not want to change at this stage, it is still very important to ask the patient about his/her habits and to offer advice to quit smoking or stop other substance use. Pharmacists and other health care providers need not get frustrated and surrender to a patient's lack of motivation at this stage. Repetition by asking the patient about their habits at this stage and counseling on the benefits of abstinence should continue at every visit until the patient is motivated to change.

For example, explaining the health risks of continuing to smoke may be used as a tactic to motivate a patient to quit smoking; however, this can sometimes backfire. Providing the patient with positive reasons to quit, such as decreased shortness of breath, monetary savings, possibly less medication in some instances, and a cleaner living environment, is more motivational than applying scare tactics. Saying a few words to the patient or providing a pamphlet with the benefits of stopping smoking may be enough to make the patient think about stopping smoking and motivate him/her to move forward to the next stage of quitting. Table 131-7 outlines some of the health benefits of stopping smoking.

Contemplation is the next stage of behavioral change. At this point, a patient is thinking about making a change, but has not yet identified a date or plan to do so. This stage is like a teeter-totter; the patient can move on to prepare for this change or fall back to not even considering it. Patients who are considering stopping smoking may be at this stage for some time before preparing for an actual quit date. Patients who use alcohol may continue to drink excessively for a long period of time without any immediate detrimental effects. They may realize that there is a problem, but think they have control over the situation and try to stop on their own, often with failure. Unfortunately, in those addicted to drugs or alcohol, it may take severe impairment before they fully understand the need for change.

Pharmacists, physicians, nurses, and other health care providers can have a positive impact on patients in the contemplation state. A few vital counseling tips can help make the difference between a patient's decision to change or continue their substance use. The goal is to motivate the patient to prepare for the change sooner rather than later. Sharing information on the benefits of abstinence from abused substances such as alcohol and tobacco, while providing different

Table 131-6. Cues for Smoking Cessation Counseling

MEDICATION OR DISEASE STATE	COMMENT
Antibiotics for otitis media	Exposure to second-hand smoke increases the incidence of ear infections in children.
Bisphosphonates and Calcium supplements	Cigarette smoke lowers a woman's estrogen level, making her more susceptible to bone fractures.
Diabetes	Heart disease is the most common cause for death in patients with diabetes. Smoking increases the risk of heart disease and may also contribute to insulin resistance.
Hyperlipidemia	Smoking lowers high-density lipoprotein (HDL) cholesterol.
Hypertension	Blood pressure is elevated after smoking due to vasoconstriction.
Inhalers	Smoking is the major cause of COPD. Smoking may also trigger asthma symptoms.
Mouth rinse for gingivitis	Smoking increases the incidence of gingivitis and tooth loss.
Oral contraceptives	Use of oral contraceptives and smoking increases the risk for stroke, myocardial infarction, and blood clots in women older than 35.
Prenatal vitamins	Smoking during pregnancy may cause congenital malformations and low birth weight.
Proton pump inhibitor or H$_2$ blockers	Smoking delays the healing of ulcers and worsens gastroesophageal reflux (GERD).

Table 131-7. Time Course of Health Benefits from Smoking Cessation

20 Minutes:	Blood pressure drops to normal. Pulse rate drops to normal. Body temperature of hands and feet increases to normal.
8 Hours:	Carbon monoxide blood level drops to normal. Oxygen blood level increases to normal.
24 Hours:	Chance of heart attack decreases.
48 Hours:	Nerve endings start regrowing. Ability to smell and taste is enhanced.
2 Weeks to 3 Months:	Circulation improves. Walking becomes easier. Lung function increases up to 30%.
1–9 Months:	Coughing, sinus congestion, fatigue, and shortness of breath decrease. Cilia regrow in lungs, increasing ability to handle mucus, clean the lungs, and reduce infection. Body's overall energy increases.
1 Year:	Excess risk of coronary heart disease is half that of a smoker.
5 Years:	Lung cancer death rate for average smoker (one pack a day) decreases by almost half. Stroke risk is reduced to that of a nonsmoker 5 to 15 years after quitting. Risk of cancer of the mouth, throat, and esophagus is half that of a continuing smoker.
10 Years:	Lung cancer death rate is similar to that of a nonsmoker. Pre-cancerous cells are replaced. Risk of cancer of the mouth, throat, esophagus, bladder, kidney, and pancreas decreases.
15 Years:	Risk of coronary heart disease is that of a nonsmoker.

From Cancer Facts and Figures, 1996, American Cancer Society.

methods to stop current behavior may motivate a patient to prepare for change.

Preparation is a vital stage for most patients to be successful with behavior change. For smokers, this stage usually occurs very close to the selected quit date. A few days to a month are often enough time for the patient to develop and practice their quit plan. Patients may move quickly from *preparation* to *action*, even without a complete quit plan. A few may be successful for the short-term, but may then relapse once an unplanned barrier is encountered. Therefore, assisting a patient with arranging and practicing a quit plan prior to the quit date may improve the success of the quit attempt. Support from friends, family, and coworkers is very important during both the preparation and action stage to ensure success.

Action is the stage in which the patient has changed their unwanted behavior from between 1 day and 6 months. This stage is often misinterpreted as the "end" of the cycle, because the patient has reached the goal of changing their behavior. Actually, this period of time requires the most counseling and encouragement in order to maintain the change. Smokers during this stage may be using medication and behavior modification techniques to stay abstinent. Despite medication and behavioral assistance, patients may still experience withdrawal. Contacting the patient on their quit date and seeing the patient in person one to two weeks after the quit date may prevent relapse. Congratulating the patient on quitting and offering assistance with any possible barriers the patient has encountered may help with continued abstinence. Encouraging the patient to remember his/her reasons for stopping smoking and the benefits he/she has noticed since the quit date are also important.

The *maintenance stage* begins after the patient has changed their unwanted behavior for 6 months. The patient will still need support and encouragement to maintain their behavior change. Congratulating the patient on continued abstinence and discussing the benefits he/she has experienced are important. Previous smokers may still have cravings for many years after their quit date. A reminder of the risks of returning to the substance use, the benefits of stopping, and the difficulty of making the change deters many from returning to their addiction. To prevent relapse, identify specific triggers and prepare the patient for these encounters. Encouraging a drinker to stay away from bars or restaurants that serve alcohol and to avoid hanging out with people they know will lead them to drink again may help prevent relapse.

Relapse can occur at any time. In smokers, it most commonly occurs within the first year after stopping. During the course of smoking cessation, most smokers make several quit attempts before being successful. All patients, regardless of whether they use alcohol, tobacco, or other drugs, should be encouraged to resume their efforts and to avoid treating this as a failure. Learning from each attempt at change may prevent relapse from occurring on the next attempt.

TOBACCO DEPENDENCE

Smoking History

Prior to obtaining a smoking history, baseline medical information should be obtained including the past and current medical history, current medication use, and alcohol and drug use. Baseline smoking information to be collected from a patient includes the number of cigarettes smoked in packs per day (ppd) (20 cigarettes = 1 pack), number of years smoked, number of previous quit attempts and methods used, reasons the patient wants to quit smoking, smoking triggers, barriers to successful quitting, and the reasons for any past relapses.

Trigger Planning

There are many behavioral and pharmacological strategies for smoking cessation depending on the patient's stage of change. If a patient is ready to quit, effective smoking cessation strategies must incorporate the "habit" and "withdrawal" components of tobacco addiction. Treatment must address withdrawal symptoms and cravings that are often responsible for relapse within the first few weeks, as well as the behavioral factors that often cause relapse later in the quit process.

Developing a quit plan involves a number of steps. If the patient is ready to quit, an important first step is to select a quit date. The selected date should not be too far in the future, but should give the patient enough time to prepare for that date. Ideally, the quit date should be set within the upcoming 1–2 weeks; however, for some patients it may be later than this. This date should be marked on a calendar, and friends and family should be informed of this important date. Prior to the quit date, smoking-related paraphernalia (eg, cigarettes, lighters, matches) should be thrown away.

Patients should be encouraged to critically evaluate their smoking habits prior to their quit date and identify their personal smoking triggers. This involves quantifying the number of cigarettes smoked per day, especially if the patient is unsure of the exact number and when he or she smokes. One method is to keep a "tally sheet" or a record of when, where, and why each cigarette was smoked for several days. This may also be useful in identifying an individual's smoking triggers. Triggers can be certain times, events, or people that produce an urge to smoke. Common triggers include after meals; when socializing; when drinking coffee, soda, or alcohol; and stress at work or stress from major life events. Each patient should identify his or her own specific triggers and write them down. The next step is to brainstorm and come up with a list of activities or actions that can be performed to deal with specific triggers. The idea is to have very specific activities already selected that can be utilized during a craving to overcome the desire to smoke and prevent a lapse or relapse. One counseling technique to assist with trigger planning is called the "4 D's." These include **D**elay, **D**o something else, **D**rink water, and **D**eep breathing. For example, those who like to smoke after meals may decide to brush their teeth or go for a walk instead. Those who like to smoke while driving can carry a water bottle, have a squeeze ball with them, or listen to relaxing music while in the car. Prior to quitting, patients who like to drink coffee in the morning can drink the coffee first and delay smoking their first cigarette by 30 minutes. Patients can also delay for 1–3 minutes when they are experiencing a craving. Each patient should identify several actions that will help manage his or her triggers and should actively engage in these activities during the quit process. It is also useful to review and examine past quit attempts and reasons for failure. Evaluating what was helpful and what factors caused the relapse can be important information to have for any subsequent quit attempts.

Individual Counseling

As a pharmacist, it is often difficult to determine exactly how to counsel a patient on stopping smoking. In the retail setting, the demands of dispensing prescriptions, answering telephones, and counseling patients on medications make it difficult to take time to discuss smoking cessation. In the hospital setting, this activity may not be viewed as a pharmacist's role at all; however, all health care professionals should take part in the effort to help patients stop smoking.

Every patient should be advised to quit smoking by every health care provider. A physician's advice alone improves abstinence rates compared to no intervention. Having a greater variety of health care providers involved in treatment for smoking cessation increases abstinence rates.[9] A 6-month study evaluating the efficacy of community pharmacists offering smoking cessation treatment found that brief counseling by a pharmacist along with nicotine replacement therapy is as effective as that same treatment offered by physicians and nurses. A combination of brief counseling by pharmacists, nicotine replacement therapy, and group counseling resulted in an abstinence rate at 6 months of 44%.[16]

Patients and health care providers have been led to believe that group sessions or self-help materials are the only effective means of helping a patient quit smoking. Actually, less than 10% of smokers will attend group sessions.[17] Therefore, if individual advice to quit is not offered, health care providers are missing 90% of smokers! The goal is to capture the individual's attention in the pharmacy, hospital, or clinic in order to motivate that patient to quit smoking.

Fear of defensive behavior from the patient, misunderstanding of the addiction by the pharmacist, and the pharmacist oftentimes never having smoked are perceived barriers to offering individual counseling. Pharmacists should not assume patients know and understand the health and life consequences of smoking. Providing the patient with individualized empathetic counseling may be motivating. Studies have shown that talking to the patient on an individual basis for just 3 minutes increases abstinence rates.[9] The "5 R's" provide a template for relaying an individualized approach to patients. These include **R**elevance, **R**isks, **R**ewards, **R**oadblocks, and **R**epetition and may motivate a patient to get ready to quit smoking. Table 131-8 lists the 5 R's. Also, with each encounter, the pharmacist gains new information and experience about medication efficacy, side effects, and trigger planning that can be applied to future patients.

Individual counseling offers the benefits of convenience, privacy, and individual attention. The time spent counseling is focused on the individual's specific needs. For example, if more time needs to be spent on behavioral modification, then this is possible. If the patient has special educational needs or requires close medication monitoring, then individual counseling is beneficial. Individual counseling has also been shown to achieve higher abstinence rates. As little as 10 minutes of counseling doubles the abstinence rate compared to no intervention at all.[9] Whether the patient returns for further instruction, uses self-help materials, or attends a group session, each patient should be asked and advised to quit smoking.

Group Counseling

Group sessions are able to offer group support, imitation, and competition. If the pharmacist has never smoked, sometimes it is difficult for the patient to believe that the pharmacist understands how difficult it is to quit smoking. This situation is avoided in a group setting as it allows patients to share experiences and questions with others in the group who are also going through the quitting process. The support from others makes quitting less lonely. Imitation of successful group members or competition within the group may also motivate patients to quit smoking.

Group sessions are difficult to conduct without some training or at least some planning. Establishing limitations and structure for the group alleviates unforeseen barriers to success. An enrollment process, including an application, can help create structure and identify a patient's willingness to participate. The application can also be used to collect a smoking history, determine if there are any learning or language barriers, and aid in coordinating dates and times for group sessions.

Including all patients that are at the same level of motivation is crucial. One or two participants who are not ready to quit

Table 131-8. The "5 R's" to Enhance Motivation to Quit Tobacco.

Relevance	Relate individualized factors (ie, current disease states, medications, family, cost) to how the patient will benefit from stopping smoking.
Risks	Patients may already know some risks to continuing to smoke. Examples: cancer, heart attack, and stroke. Also provide the patient with risks that relate personally to them. Examples: high blood pressure, increased shortness of breath, and bronchitis.
Rewards	Patients often enjoy smoking, so the rewards need to outweigh the benefits of continuing to smoke. Examples: saving money, improved smell and taste, healthier body, more time, freedom from the addiction, and improved self-esteem.
Roadblocks	Ask the patient what concerns or barriers they have to stopping and problem-solve with them ways to overcome these with this quit attempt. Examples: spouse smokes, weight concerns, fear of failure, stress, and other addictions.
Repetition	Do not give up on the patient! Continue to assist the patient until the patient quits smoking.

From Fiore MC, Bailey WC, Cohen SJ. Treating Tobacco Use and Dependence. Clinical Practice Guideline. Rockville, MD: U.S. Department of Health and Human Services, Public Health Service, June 2000.

smoking can shift the balance for other group members by offering excuses as to why now is not a good time to quit smoking. A simple question to ask on the application is "When do you see yourself stopping use of tobacco?" Include patients that answer similarly in the same group.

If the sessions will follow an agenda, a closed enrollment is beneficial. With a closed enrollment, all members of the group start and end at the same time. New members are not allowed into the group at different times needing to "catch up" to the others. This type of enrollment improves group cohesiveness and as each week passes, the group becomes more like a "family." This enrollment also ensures that the agenda for the meeting is met.

The group leader is as important as the participants. The group leader needs to facilitate the discussion for the meeting. Facilitating the meeting also means avoiding lecturing to the participants and ensuring that all participants have the opportunity to talk. This may mean going around the room asking for input or calling on participants. The facilitator should avoid allowing one person to dominate the group discussion.

Defining the optimal time frame and number of sessions for stopping smoking has been studied.[9] At least four group sessions significantly improves the quit rate. Meetings may be scheduled with half of the sessions preparing the participant to quit smoking and half occurring after the participant has stopped smoking to prevent relapse. Ideally, 31–90 minutes of counseling has been shown to increase abstinence rates. Sessions that are longer tend to lose the interest of the participant and do not improve the abstinence rate.[9]

Telephone Counseling

Telephone counseling has many benefits and is becoming more common as state-funded quit lines are being implemented across the country. Quit lines have been shown to double abstinence rates at one year in people who attempt to quit.[18] Quit lines offer the advantages of ease of use and availability, as many are staffed 24 hours per day, every day of the year. Pharmacists can save time and increase convenience for the patient with brief telephone contacts as a method of follow-up. This personalized, brief intervention can help maintain motivation to quit smoking and prevent relapse.

Cold Turkey/Tapering Method/Aversive Smoking

Cold turkey, aversive smoking, and tapering are alternative methods for smoking cessation that do not involve the use of medications during the quit process. The cold turkey method involves selecting a date and then quitting tobacco use on that date, while tapering or "cigarette fading" involves gradually cutting down on the number of cigarettes smoked per day or per week until cessation is reached. Cold turkey and tapering have not been shown to improve quit rates.[9] Smoking to the point of feeling ill is called aversive smoking. Rapid smoking and rapid puffing are aversive techniques that have been shown to double the quit rate compared to no intervention.[9] These techniques are not used frequently today due to the health risks associated with this type of smoking.

Medications for Smoking Cessation

Based on current guidelines, tobacco addiction is considered to be a chronic disease that often requires repeated interventions for success. Currently, first-line agents include bupropion SR (Zyban), nicotine gum, nicotine inhaler, nicotine nasal spray, and nicotine patches.[9] Nicotine lozenges have just been released and are not currently included in the guidelines; however, it is likely that they will also be considered as first-line agents. Every patient who is attempting to quit, except in special circum-

stances (ie, pregnancy, within 2 weeks post-myocardial infarction) should be offered at least one of these agents. When compared to placebo, each agent has been shown to approximately double the quit rate.[9] There are no guidelines to determine which of the first-line agents should be used in various situations; therefore, choice of first-line therapy is made based on a number of factors. These factors include the patient's smoking history and habits, past experience with any of the agents, co-existing medical conditions (ie, depression), contraindications to any of the agents, and patient and caregiver preference. Treatment can and should be individualized based on these factors. Prior to beginning a specific therapy, it is important for the patient to understand the proper use and dosing of that agent.

Combination therapy with two nicotine replacement products or with a nicotine replacement product and bupropion SR may improve the response rate in those trying to quit over that of single therapy.[19–22] Nicotine replacement therapy (NRT), if dosed according to the current guidelines, provides nicotine equivalent to smoking about 1 pack per day; therefore, in heavier smokers, withdrawal and cravings may still occur. One effective option is to use a nicotine replacement product on a scheduled basis and have available an additional agent that the patient can use when needed throughout the day. Effective combinations might include using a patch on a scheduled basis daily and adding an agent such as the nicotine gum, lozenge, or inhaler on an as needed basis. This provides additional nicotine replacement and may be especially useful for those patients who smoke greater than 1 ppd or who have failed monotherapy. Tables 131-9, 131-10, and 131-11 include dosing information on the first-line medications approved for smoking cessation.

Special Populations of Smokers

PSYCHIATRIC DISORDERS AND OTHER ADDICTIONS—Many psychiatric and substance abuse treatment programs have typically not addressed smoking as an addiction and, in the past, may have actually encouraged smoking. For example, until recently smoke-free AA meetings were not available and smoking at these meetings was commonplace. People with psychiatric disorders (ie, schizophrenia, depression, bipolar disorder, anxiety disorders) or other addictions (ie, alcohol, opiates) are estimated to be two to three times more likely to be tobacco dependent than the general population.[23] Biological, genetic, psychological, and social factors are all thought to play a role. In addition, patients may be managing medication side effects and disease symptoms by adjusting their smoking habits due to drug and disease state interactions.[24] Although few studies are available, the use of the first-line agents alone or in combination plus behavioral therapy may be effective in this subgroup of the population. In clinical practice, schizophrenic patients often have a difficult time quitting smoking and need a significant amount of follow-up and reinforcement. Patients with a history of depression who attempt to stop smoking risk a relapse of depression for the first 6 months after quitting.[25] For this reason, bupropion SR may be a good choice in these patients.

CARDIOVASCULAR DISEASE—Abstinence rates for cardiovascular patients at one year are greater than 50%, making this population one of the most motivated groups to quit smoking.[26] NRT and/or bupropion SR should be offered to these patients to ease withdrawal symptoms. Nicotine has sympathomimetic effects that increase blood pressure and heart rate and may cause coronary artery vasospasm. However, the amount of nicotine in NRT is much lower than the amount of nicotine in cigarettes. Studies have found that NRT does not cause myocardial infarction in the general population, nor does it exacerbate cardiovascular events in patients with pre-existing disease.[27, 28] Before using NRT, caution should be exercised in patients with a history of myocardial infarction, serious arrhythmias, or worsening angina within the past 2 weeks. A physician's monitoring and assessment of this type of patient is

Table 131-9. Nicotine Replacement Therapy: Transdermal Patches

	NICOTROL®	NICODERM CQ® GENERIC	PATIENT INSTRUCTIONS	POTENTIAL SIDE EFFECTS
Availability	5, 10, 15 mg OTC	7, 14, 21 mg OTC	Stop smoking. Peel the backing off the patch. Place the patch on a relatively hairless area between the neck and waist. Start wearing the patch the morning of the quit day and keep the patch on all day and night (remove 16 hour patch at bedtime and 24 hour patch at bedtime only with sleep disturbances). Change the patch daily, rotating it to a new site.	Local cutaneous reaction (erythema, pruritus, edema), headache, sleep disturbances (seen with 24 hour patch). Use cautiously in cardiovascular patients within 2 weeks post myocardial infarction, those with serious arrhythmias, and those with severe or worsening angina.
Patch Replacement Schedule	16 hours	16 or 24 hours		
Dosing Guidelines	15 mg × 6 weeks 10 mg × 2 weeks 5 mg × 2 weeks	>10 cigarettes/day: - 21 mg × 6 weeks - 14 mg × 2–4 weeks - 7 mg × 2–4 weeks <10 cigarettes/day, cardiovascular disease, or weigh <100 lbs. - 14 mg × 6 weeks - 7 mg × 2–4 weeks		

advised since these patients were excluded from most clinical trials. Bupropion SR has little effect on the cardiovascular system. Non-significant trends of increased blood pressure in patients treated with both bupropion SR and the nicotine replacement patch were seen in one study.[19]

PREGNANCY—Smoking during pregnancy has been shown to cause a number of adverse outcomes including spontaneous abortion, fetal growth retardation, preterm delivery, and sudden infant death syndrome.[29] Many women are motivated to quit smoking during pregnancy; however, there is little data available regarding the most efficacious method. Pregnant smokers should first be given extensive counseling on the benefits of stopping smoking and on behavioral techniques that may be beneficial. For heavier smokers unable to stop, NRT or bupropion SR may be an option.

SMOKELESS TOBACCO PRODUCTS/CIGARS—Advertisements promoting cigars and smokeless tobacco products, and possibly current restrictions on smoking in public places, have caused an increase in the use of these forms of tobacco. The use of cigars has increased 50% since 1993, primarily among males aged 18–24 years old. The rate of women smoking cigars has increased fivefold from 1990 to 1996.[30]

Cigar smoke is usually not purposefully inhaled, and the nicotine is absorbed through the buccal lining in the mouth. Cigars contain between 100 and 200 mg of nicotine, while most cigarettes contain about 8.4 mg of nicotine.[31] Only one-fourth of cigar smokers inhale; however, the lips, tongue, throat, and larynx of all cigar smokers are exposed to the carcinogens contained in cigars. The risk of lung cancer in cigar smokers who do not inhale is twice that of nonsmokers. The risk of oral, throat, and esophageal cancer is similar to that of cigarette smokers. Cigar smokers who inhale 5 cigars per day have about the same risk of lung cancer as a 1 pack per day cigarette smoker. Occasional cigar smokers are twice as likely as those who have never smoked cigars to start smoking cigarettes. Cigar smoking increases the risk of relapse in previous cigarette smokers.

Quitting cigar smoking decreases the risk of many cancers, chronic obstructive pulmonary disease, and coronary heart disease. Studies evaluating the effectiveness of pharmacotherapy to help regular cigar smokers are lacking.

Smokeless tobacco, also called spit tobacco, comes in two forms, snuff and chew tobacco. Snuff is available in sachets, moist, or dry. The user places a pinch or dip between the cheek and gum and the nicotine is absorbed through the buccal area. Dry snuff is the form more commonly available in Europe and is inhaled through the nose. Chew tobacco is available as loose leaf, plug, or twist form. The user of chew tobacco also places a "wad" in the cheek for buccal absorption.

Ninety-two percent of spit tobacco users are male. The use of these products tripled between 1972 and 1999.[32] Snuff or chew tobacco increases the risk of oral, pharynx, and esophageal cancer. Tobacco specific nitrosamines, formaldehyde, arsenic, polonium, and many other carcinogens are found in smokeless tobacco products. Increased blood pressure, cardiovascular disease, oral leukoplasia, and many dental complications are increased with smokeless tobacco use. Two to three times the amount of nicotine is absorbed in the buccal lining compared to cigarettes resulting in users of smokeless tobacco becoming highly addicted.

An oral examination with counseling, usually completed by a dentist, is an effective method to help smokeless tobacco users discontinue use.[33] Studies using nicotine replacement therapy and bupropion SR have conflicting results with long-term abstinence rates similar to placebo.[34–36] Smokeless tobacco users are likely to need aggressive therapy, possibly combination therapy and counseling with follow-up to maintain abstinence.

Monitoring

Blood pressure, pulse, weight, and carbon monoxide (CO) or a cotinine level should be assessed before medication is initiated and again after the quit date. CO is a poisonous gas that smokers inhale each time a cigarette is smoked. Carbon monoxide can be measured with the use of a small hand-held CO monitor which measures the amount of CO exhaled in parts per million (ppm). Some monitors can also convert the CO measurement to percentage of carboxyhemoglobin (% COHgb), which is the estimated amount of CO displacing oxygen on hemoglobin. Typically, cigarette smokers have CO levels between 15 and 40 ppm or between 3.0 and 7.0% COHgb. Cigar and pipe smokers may

Table 131-10. Nicotine Replacement Therapy

	GUM (NICORETTE)	ORAL INHALER (NICOTROL INHALER)	NASAL SPRAY (NICOTROL NS)	LOZENGE (COMMIT)
Availability	2 mg, 4 mg OTC Original, Orange, Mint	10 mg/cartridge Prescription only	10 mg/ml Prescription only	2mg, 4mg OTC
Dosing Schedule	2 mg: <25 cigarettes/day 4 mg: ≥ 25 cigarettes/day Begin with 1 piece every 1–2 hours for 6 weeks, then 1 piece every 2–4 hours for 3 weeks, then 1 piece every 4–8 hours for 3 weeks.	6–16 cartridges/day for the first 12 weeks Must use a minimum of 6 cartridges/day for the first 3–6 weeks (up to 12 weeks), then taper over 6–12 weeks.	1–2 sprays in each nostril/hour Gradually decrease rate over 6–8 weeks.	2mg: first cigarette >30 minutes after waking 4mg: first cigarette ≤30 minutes after waking Weeks 1 to 6: 1 lozenge every 1 to 2 hours (at least 9/day) Weeks 7 to 9: 1 lozenge every 2 to 4 hours Weeks 10 to 12: 1 lozenge every 4 to 8 hours
Dosing Guidelines	Stop smoking. Chew gum until a "tingling sensation" is felt. Place nicotine gum between cheek and gums ("Park") and leave gum there until tingling disappears. "Chew" and "park" gum for 1–2 hours, then use a new piece. Park in different areas.	Stop smoking. Individualize dosing to each patient. Short, shallow puffs minimize coughing and throat irritation. An open cartridge is good for one day. May take one week to adjust to side effects.	Stop smoking. Individualize dosing to each patient. Do not sniff, swallow, or inhale through the nose as the spray is administered.	Stop smoking. Suck on the lozenge until the taste becomes strong, then place the lozenge between the gum and cheek. Do not chew, bite, or swallow. When the taste fades, repeat the process until the lozenge is dissolved.
Duration of Therapy	12 weeks	18–24 weeks	12 weeks	12 weeks
Maximum Dose	2 mg: 30 pieces/day 4 mg: 20 pieces/day	16 cartridges/day	Do not exceed 10 sprays/hour or 80 sprays/day.	Do not exceed 20 lozenges/day.
Potential Side Effects	Jaw soreness, Hiccups, Nausea, Vomiting, Headache	Local irritation of throat and mouth, Coughing, Rhinitis	Hot/peppery sensation in nose and throat, Sneezing, Coughing, Watery eyes, Runny nose	Hiccups, Heartburn, Nausea
Comment	Avoid eating or drinking anything except water 15 minutes prior or after use of the gum to maximize absorption. If the gum is used properly, side effects will be minimized. The gum is difficult to use on a scheduled basis and patients may have withdrawal from lack of compliance. The original flavor tastes bad.	The inhaler mouthpiece looks like a plastic cigarette or cigarette filter. The cartridges contain nicotine that is absorbed in the buccal lining of the mouth when the patient puffs on the mouthpiece. Food and drink decrease the absorption of nicotine from the inhaler. Scheduled use is most efficacious.	The nasal spray has the fastest onset of action of the NRT products. Twenty percent of patients use the nasal spray at higher than recommended doses or for longer than recommended.	The lozenge has a mint flavor and is sugar-free. Scheduled use will enhance the efficacy of the lozenge.

have CO levels > 40 ppm, as these products emit high levels of CO. In clinical trials, a nonsmoker is often defined as having a CO < 10 ppm; however, in clinical practice, nonsmokers often achieve CO levels of 1 or 2 ppm. CO monitors with disposable mouthpieces are manufactured by *Bedfont* (Innovative Medical Marketing; T/A Bedfont Scientific, USA; 30 Jackson Road, Suite B-3; Medford, NJ 08055; 609-654-5561; Info@bedfontusa.com) and cost between $400 and $800. The CO monitor is a useful tool to provide the patient with immediate feedback regarding his or her smoking cessation efforts. However, if the patient is a light smoker, has severe restrictive or obstructive pulmonary disease, or has abstained from smoking for the past 8 hours, the reading may not be a true measurement of abstinence.

Cotinine is a metabolite of nicotine that can be measured in the blood, saliva, or urine. Cotinine can be detected in the serum for up to 7 days; however, if the patient is using nicotine replacement therapy, cotinine levels will remain elevated.[37] Cotinine measurements require laboratory analysis; therefore, they should be reserved for physician use in certain situations, especially prior to surgeries or procedures where the patient has committed to abstinence. Cotinine levels are often reported in research trials and are typically < 10 ng/mL for nonsmokers, but may be 300 ng/mL for a 1 ppd smoker.[38]

Relapse Prevention

Many potential barriers exist that may lead to relapse. Without a trigger plan, medication, and counseling, only 3–5% of patients who try to quit smoking are successful at 1 year.[39] For

Table 131-11. Bupropion SR (Zyban)

DOSAGE FORM	SUSTAINED-RELEASE TABLET DO NOT SPLIT OR CHEW TABLET.
Availability	150 mg Prescription only
Dosing Schedule	150 mg daily × 3 days; then 150 mg twice daily Space dosages 8 hours apart. Take last dose before 6 PM.
Dosing Guidelines	Initiate while patient is still smoking. Set quit date for 1–2 weeks after starting bupropion SR.
Duration of Therapy	7–12 weeks No clinical data to support use for more than 12 weeks.
Maximum Dose	300 mg daily
Potential Side Effects	Dry mouth (10%), Insomnia (30%), Dizziness (8%), Constipation (8%), Tremor (2%), Seizure (0.1%)*
Contraindications	History of seizures, bulimia, anorexia nervosa, or head trauma. Concomitant use of MAO inhibitors or Wellbutrin.

*Dose-dependent <= 300mg/day.

this reason, providing encouragement, motivation, congratulations, and assistance with barriers after the quit date and for at least 1 year is important. Asking the patient about previous quit attempts and causes for relapse may help in preparation for the current quit attempt. Common reasons for relapse include withdrawal symptoms, weight gain, and stress. Preparing the patient for these barriers before the quit date as part of the quit plan and then continuing the support after the quit date is important.

Withdrawal symptoms may be more intense or prolonged in some individuals. Using smoking cessation medications in combination or for longer periods of time may alleviate this cause of relapse. Educating the patient to be able to identify withdrawal symptoms (ie, cravings, irritability, trouble concentrating, insomnia) and to act quickly may help to prevent relapse. Before increasing or adding additional smoking cessation medications, an assessment should be made of whether current medications and trigger plans have been utilized appropriately.

Weight gain is a major barrier to stopping smoking, especially among women.[40] Smoking cessation usually results in less than a 10-pound weight gain over the first few months of abstinence for most patients. A small percentage of patients are at risk to gain more weight including those who smoke greater than 15 cigarettes per day, African Americans, and patients under the age of 55.[41] Women also tend to gain more weight than men. Reasons for the weight gain include decreased metabolism, improved taste and smell, and increased eating as a reward or to satisfy the hand-to-mouth habit.

It is important to be proactive with a patient that is concerned about weight gain or relapsed in the past due to weight gain. Patients need to be educated that it is likely that they will gain weight when they stop smoking, but this weight gain is a return to the weight they would have been had they never smoked. The health concern of gaining weight is negligible compared to continuing to smoke. A patient would have to gain 75 pounds before the risk of stopping smoking outweighs that of continuing to smoke.[42] Patients need to be counseled that stopping smoking is their primary concern. Starting a new exercise regimen or strict diet in addition may be too many habit and lifestyle changes at once and cause failure. However, clinical trials have shown that a diet and exercise program along with stopping smoking in patients concerned about weight gain may not be detrimental.[43,44]

Advise the patient to avoid substituting food for smoking cigarettes or rewarding the quit attempt with food. Counsel the patient to be smart about their food choices. Preparing healthy snacks such as carrot sticks, celery, broccoli spears, watermelon, and strawberries ahead of time helps the patient reach for these low-calorie snacks when cravings hit. Instead of eating, drinking a lot of water, keeping the hands busy, and staying active may alleviate unwanted pounds.

If weight gain is a concern that may prohibit the patient from stopping smoking, medications such as bupropion SR or nicotine gum should be considered. Studies using these medications have shown that patients maintain or lose weight while using the nicotine gum, bupropion SR, or the combination of bupropion SR and nicotine replacement therapy. However, this effect lasts only while the medications are being taken. After the medications are stopped, patients may then gain weight if they do not receive counseling on a healthy diet and exercise.

Moderate exercise may be beneficial to help with the decreased metabolic rate after stopping smoking and may also help relieve stress, which is often cited as a trigger. Preparing the stressed smoker with relaxation techniques and possible exercises can help avoid relapse during stressful situations. The pharmacist can suggest going for a walk during a lunch break or after meals, performing light weight lifting twice a week to relieve tension, practicing deep breathing to help in stressful situations, and listening to relaxing music. Guided imagery is another useful relaxation technique. This exercise involves taking a break at some point in the day and finding a quiet, relaxing place to sit. The patients then close their eyes and imagine themselves in a serene setting such as walking through a field of flowers or on the beach looking at a sunset. This exercise can be done alone, but also may be guided by another person. It takes some practice to become proficient, but it can be a very effective tool. To also help prevent relapse, the pharmacist should educate the patient that nicotine withdrawal can cause irritability and tension and should ensure that the patient has proper medication and support to help relieve these withdrawal symptoms.

Establishing Smoking Cessation Services

Smoking cessation services are usually very welcomed by patients and other health care providers. Receiving training to become a smoking cessation facilitator is beneficial in order to become skilled at helping smokers with behavioral modifications such as stress management and trigger planning. Training can also help with providing group education and marketing the service.

There are many resources including training programs, guidelines, web sites, and brochures available to initiate a smoking cessation service. The internet has a wealth of information for both the pharmacist and patient. Many patients enjoy the convenience of smoking cessation programs offered online. These programs should be supplemented with medication counseling and smoking cessation advice. Tables 131-12 and 131-13 provide details on available pharmacist and patient resources.

Marketing smoking cessation services is important. Marketing should include notifying local physician offices, dentists, and organizations such as the American Lung Association and American Cancer Society. Several days have been identified to help patients stop smoking including the "Great American Smoke-Out" and "World No Tobacco Day" that are ideal days to promote smoking cessation services and products. Posters for the "Great American Smoke-Out" and other special days are often provided by the sponsoring organizations free of charge. In outpatient settings, flyers detailing the smoking cessation program can be distributed with prescriptions. If the site of practice is hospital-based, consultations to provide smoking cessation counseling prior to discharge are very beneficial and are a highly needed service. Marketing this service to cardiovascular and pulmonary units would likely generate many consultations.

Table 131-12. Pharmacist's Resources for Establishing a Smoking Cessation Service

Treating Tobacco Use and Dependence. Clinical Practice Guideline.	www.surgeongeneral.gov	This thorough resource is a necessity for learning about effective behavioral and pharmacologic treatments.
Mayo Clinic	www.mayoclinic.org	Four-day nicotine dependence counselor training and program development seminar. CE for pharmacists is not offered.
American Lung Association	www2.lungusa.org/tobacco 1-800-LUNG-USA	Become a facilitator for the Freedom from Smoking program by calling a local ALA office. Sign on to the Freedom from Smoking online program and learn more about relaxation exercises and helpful suggestions to offer your patients. There is usually a fee to be trained as a facilitator and to purchase smoking cessation packets for the groups. After completing the training, a fee for providing Freedom from Smoking groups may be charged to participants.
Pamphlets and Brochures	American Cancer Society www.cancer.org 1-800-ACS-2345	Pamphlets and brochures are available on quitting smoking and smoking and pregnancy. Information about dip and a Spanish smoker's guide are available.
	Centers for Disease Control and Prevention www.cdc.gov/tobacco/	Pamphlets, fact sheets, advocacy groups, designated smoking cessation days, and statistics on smoking are available.

Offering educational books, brochures, or quit smoking paraphernalia (ie, water bottles, mints, car fresheners) and demonstrating smoking cessation medications (ie, nicotine inhaler) may make the program more attractive or marketable. Monitoring carbon monoxide, blood pressure, weight, and medication interactions may also add to the smoking cessation counseling.

Smoking cessation services are both rewarding and challenging. Waning commitment from patients highly addicted to nicotine, as well as lack of insurance coverage for medications, are barriers to this type of service. It is very rewarding helping a patient become smoke-free for good. Patients often do not realize how addicted to cigarettes they are until they quit. Reimbursement for smoking cessation is slowly gaining acceptance.

Table 131-13. Smoking Cessation Patient Resources

Special Days	New Year's Day	January 1st	Many smokers every year attempt to start the year without smoking.
	Tobacco Free Awareness Week	January 19th-25th	Encourages smokers who quit January 1st to continue to be successful. Also educates the public about the dangers of secondhand smoke and advocates smoke-free environments.
	Kick Butts Day	April 2nd	This day is for school children to stand up against tobacco.
	World No Tobacco Day	May 31st www.wntd.com	Global event to reduce tobacco dependence in individuals and to inform the public about the negative impact of tobacco use.
	Great American Smoke-Out	Third Thursday in November	Smokers are encouraged to throw away their cigarettes and not smoke for 24 hours.
Resources for Patients	Internet	www.Quitnet.com	This site offers an active chat room, expert counselors, quit plans, and information in Spanish.
		www.ffsonline.org American Lung Association	This site contains 7 modules including very nice worksheets on weight gain, relaxation exercises, and medications.
		www.smokeclinic.com	This site offers an individualized profile and 10 sessions to help a smoker quit for good. The smoke clinic contains a resource section for health care providers and the smoker. There is a $49.90 fee for using the program.
		www.smokefree.gov National Cancer Institute	Concise web site for steps to stopping smoking and instant messaging service where smokers can receive advice on stopping smoking.

Public Aid reimburses for all smoking cessation medications. Some insurers cover medications and group or individual meetings if the service is offered by an approved provider. This usually requires contacting the insurance company and submitting a description of the smoking cessation service to be provided. Requiring patients to pay for smoking cessation services enhances their commitment to quit smoking. However, many patients will provide the excuse that they cannot afford smoking cessation medications or services, yet they continue to pay $5 per pack of cigarettes.

Persistence with smoking cessation efforts from health care providers, with pharmacists being the most accessible, will lead to a more educated population willing to quit smoking.

ALCOHOL DEPENDENCE

Pharmacists in both retail and hospital settings face great challenges in dealing with patients who abuse alcohol. Since alcohol use is socially accepted throughout our society, patients tend to downplay warnings about the effects of alcohol consumption despite the potential adverse health consequences. Identifying patients who are dependent on alcohol is important because of the health effects and the potential for drug-alcohol interactions with over-the-counter (OTC) and prescription medications. Adverse consequences of drinking are not limited to alcoholics; even occasional drinkers can put themselves at risk if they consume alcohol in combination with other psychoactive or sedating agents. Disulfiram-like reactions can occur in select populations with even the slightest ingestion of alcohol. It is the role of the pharmacist to understand the mechanisms by which medications and alcohol interact and to provide appropriate interventions and counseling about risky drug-alcohol interactions when necessary.

The first step in dealing with the patient that consumes alcohol is to assess their drinking habits. Asking questions about alcohol use may elicit anger and suspicion in some patients, while others will be very honest and straightforward about their use. A pharmacist should be non-accusatory and assess each patient with caution and empathy. For example, questions about alcohol use posed to a lifelong non-drinker can be seen as rude and offensive. Alcoholics tend to underestimate how much they really drink. For example, a person who claims to consume six drinks a day may, in fact, consume as many as twelve drinks a day. Sometimes, a person with a heavy drinking problem will welcome questions related to their alcohol use. Embarrassed to seek assistance on their own, they may be looking for an avenue of help. As with any brief intervention, pharmacists should reinforce the importance of refraining from alcohol use during each encounter with the patient.

One quick method to assess alcohol abuse is the CAGE questionnaire. Physicians, nurses, or pharmacists can administer this brief intervention during any patient encounter. Table 131-14 lists the CAGE questions.[45] Item responses on the CAGE questionnaire are scored 0 or 1, with a higher score an indication of an alcohol problem. A total score of 2 or greater is considered clinically significant. The CAGE questions can be used in the clinical setting using informal phrasing. It has been demonstrated that they are most effective when used as part of a general health history and should not be preceded by questions about how much or how frequently the patient ingests alcohol.

Table 131-14. CAGE Questions

Cut down—Have you ever felt you should **c**ut down on your drinking?

Annoyed—Have people **a**nnoyed you by criticizing your drinking?

Guilty - Have you ever felt bad or **g**uilty about your drinking?

Eye opener—Have you ever had a drink first thing in the morning to steady your nerves or to get rid of a hangover (**e**ye opener)?

From Ewing JA. *JAMA* 1984; 252:1905. Copyright © 1984, *American Medical Association*. All rights reserved.

Table 131-15. Definition of a Standard Drink

	VOLUME (OUNCES)	ALCOHOL CONTENT (%)
Beer	12	4.5
Wine	5	12.9
Spirits	1.5	41.1

What is a Drink?

Table 131-15 shows the accepted beverage size and alcohol content for beer, wine, and distilled spirits.[46] This quantification of a standard drink should only serve as a general guide. The amount of alcohol consumed is difficult to quantify due to lack of standard measurements for a drink. The size of a drink depends on the type of alcohol consumed and the means in which it is delivered. For beer, wine coolers, and similar bottled and canned beverages, the drink size is consistent due to packaging.[46] For wine and distilled spirits, the size of the drink is dependent upon the person pouring the beverage. A drink consumed in the home may differ in size to one served at a bar or restaurant.

The alcohol content also varies within beverage classes. The standard alcohol content for the majority of beers consumed in the United States is 4.5%. However, some states have laws mandating lower alcohol levels. Light beer may have as low as 3.0% alcohol, whereas the microbrewery and specialty beers have an alcohol content greater than 9.0%.[46] Similar variations in alcohol content occur in the wine and distilled spirits categories. Distilled spirits have the largest variation, ranging from 30% to 94% alcohol by volume.

Alcohol Metabolism

Alcohol is a very small molecule and can be found almost everywhere within bodily fluids once it is consumed. Alcohol easily dissolves into water and does not concentrate in any one area within the body. Alcohol does not dissolve into fat tissues. Since females generally have a greater ratio of fat to body water than males, blood alcohol concentrations (BACs) tend to be higher when women drink equal amounts of alcohol compared to men. Every state in the United States has set legal limits for safe BACs for the operation of a non-commercial motor vehicle. Currently, BACs range from 0.08% to 0.10%. Although these standards define the legal limits, impaired driving can occur at much lower levels.[47]

Alcohol and Medications

Adverse reactions from alcohol can occur whether or not a person is a heavy drinker. Many OTC cough, cold, and oral hygiene products contain alcohol. Although the amount of alcohol in these products is usually less than 10%, certain populations may be very sensitive to these levels. A genetic variation in alcohol metabolism occurs primarily in people of Asian descent, although it occurs rarely in Caucasians as well. Consumption of even small amounts of alcohol in this population causes an unpleasant flushing reaction that includes hot flashes, facial flushing, nausea, and vomiting. This reaction occurs due to an inability of this subpopulation to completely metabolize acetaldehyde, a byproduct of alcohol metabolism in the liver. Thus, pharmacists should have a heightened awareness of this reaction and counsel patients taking these OTC products.

Several medications can produce a "disulfiram-like" reaction. This reaction blocks the oxidative metabolism of acetaldehyde causing acetaldehyde accumulation. People who consume alcohol with these medications or disulfiram will experience nausea and flushing from the acetaldehyde accumulation.[10] When alcohol is consumed in combination with disulfiram, the reaction may be so unpleasant that it prevents future episodes of alcohol ingestion in most patients. Thus, disulfiram is a medication used as aversive therapy in chronic drinkers. A list of common prescription medications that can precipitate this reaction are listed in Table 131-16. In patients with chronic medical conditions, this reaction can be serious, resulting in the dilation of blood vessels, a drop in blood pressure, and an increase in heart rate. A warning label should be placed on all prescriptions that have the potential to cause this "disulfiram-like" reaction.

Alcohol produces a sedative effect in the central nervous system (CNS). A misperception of many social drinkers is that alcohol can boost confidence and self-esteem. This brief feeling of confidence is a result of alcohol decreasing (depressing) inhibitions. As a person continues to ingest alcohol, they will experience impaired judgment, slowed reflexes, and fatigue. When alcohol is taken in combination with a sedating medication (prescription or OTC), the CNS depressive effect is synergistic, meaning that the combination of the two produces a greater amount of sedation than each one combined (ie, $1 + 1 = 3$). Labels on OTC medications generally have warnings about drinking alcohol due to this increased risk of sedation. Pharmacists should counsel patients not to combine alcohol with prescription or OTC products, especially if they are driving or operating heavy machinery.

Alcoholism as a Disease

Table 131-2 lists the DSM-IV-TR criteria for alcohol dependence.[1] Signs of alcohol dependence manifest both physiologically and socially. A person abusing alcohol will often develop tolerance, requiring larger amounts of intake over a long period of time. Withdrawal often occurs following a period of abstinence and drinking tends to happen more often out of fear of withdrawal. The patient recognizes that he/she should cut down on drinking, but individual efforts to control drinking often fail. The alcohol user will experience ever-increasing periods of time spent on drinking activities, while other important activities will fall by the wayside. Alcoholism affects all parts of a person's life, both at home and at their place of employment. Continued use can result in the loss of loved ones and unemployment.

Alcohol and drug use should be recognized and treated as a medical disease. Medically, alcoholism is a chronic, relapsing

Table 131-16. Medications That Cause Disulfiram-Like Reactions

TYPE OF MEDICATION	GENERIC NAME	BRAND NAME
Antibiotics	Cefoperazone	Cefobid
	Cefotetan	Cefotan
	Chloramphenicol	Various
	Griseofulvin	Fulvicin, Grifulvin, Grisactin
	Isoniazid	Nydrazid, Rifamate, Rifater
	Metronidazole	Flagyl
	Nitrofurantoin	Furadantin, Macrodantin
	Sulfamethoxazole	Bactrim, Septra
	Sulfisoxazole	Pediazole, Various
Cardiovascular Medications (Nitrates)	Isosorbide dinitrate	Dilatrate, Isordil, Sorbitrate
	Isosorbide mononitrate	Ismo, Imdur
	Nitroglycerin	Nitro-Bid, Nitrostat
Diabetes Medications (Sulfonylureas)	Chlorpropamide	Diabinese
	Glyburide	DiaBeta, Glynase, Micronase, Various
	Tolazamide	Tolinase, Various
	Tolbutamide	Orinase, Various

From Weathermon R, Crabb DW. *Alcohol Research & Health* 1999; 23:40.

disease with a biologic component, a genetic component, and a social component. Unfortunately, the stigma associated with substance abuse and the professionals who treat it serve as a barrier to providing patients much needed therapy. This stigma results in health care providers failing to properly recognize clinical clues or completely ignoring substance use altogether.[48]

Pharmacotherapy of Alcoholism

Currently, two FDA approved agents are available for the treatment of alcoholism: disulfiram and naltrexone. These agents are further categorized as aversive and anticraving medications.

AVERSIVE PHARMACOTHERAPY

Disulfiram (Antabuse) is the oldest pharmacologic agent used for the treatment of alcohol abuse. Used first in 1951, disulfiram is still dispensed as a deterrent against alcohol consumption. As discussed earlier, disulfiram blocks the oxidative metabolism of acetaldehyde, an intermediate by-product of alcohol, causing acetaldehyde accumulation. Thus, drinking alcohol within 12 hours of taking disulfiram produces a number of discomforting side effects. For example, within 5–15 minutes of consuming alcohol, disulfiram may cause facial flushing, followed by headache, tachycardia, hyperpnea (ie, deep, rapid breathing), and sweating. Severe nausea and vomiting can also occur and may lead to hypotension and dizziness. The intense reaction of alcohol and disulfiram is intended to serve as a deterrent to future consumption. Unfortunately, compliance with the medication limits the effectiveness and patients have learned to stop using disulfiram 1–2 days prior to a drinking episode. Experience demonstrates better abstinence rates when the patient is very motivated, or when spouses or treatment staff supervise disulfiram administration compared to when the patient self-administers the medication.

ANTICRAVING PHARMACOTHERAPY

NALTREXONE—Naltrexone is an opiate-receptor antagonist similar in structure to naloxone, which is used for opiate reversal. In contrast to disulfiram, concomitant use of naltrexone and alcohol does not cause detrimental side effects. In response to alcohol, endogenous opioids activate certain brain cells and induce some of the rewarding effects of alcohol. By blocking the actions of these endogenous opioids, naltrexone prevents alcohol from exerting these effects and may reduce the patient's desire to drink. However, naltrexone does not prevent the consumption of alcohol.[8] Initial studies of naltrexone demonstrated a reduction in the number of drinks, but it did not maintain a high level of abstinence. Newer clinical studies have not shown any benefit of naltrexone over placebo in delaying relapse to heavy drinking.[49]

ACAMPROSATE—Acamprosate has similar effects on alcohol craving as naltrexone, although it does not show any activity on opioid receptors.[50] Although the specific mechanism of action is unclear, acamprosate is thought to reduce cravings through binding to gaba-aminobutyric acid (GABA) receptors. Acamprosate also has serotonergic properties and activity as a noradrenergic antagonist.[51] In European trials, acamprosate demonstrated increased abstinence rates consistently when used as part of a multidisciplinary approach that included psychosocial or behavioral therapies. Subjects in one trial had a 43% abstinence rate after 48 weeks of acamprosate compared to a 21% abstinence rate in the control group.[52] The acamprosate treated subjects also stayed sober for a longer duration of time compared to the controls. In all trials, for those who did not quit drinking, acamprosate reduced the number of drinking days during the study period. Side effects for acamprosate were generally mild, with the most frequently reported side effect being diarrhea. Acamprosate has not yet met efficacy criteria held by the FDA and is still undergoing clinical trials in efforts to gain approval in the United States.

Alcohol Counseling

More than one alcohol treatment method is often necessary to promote abstinence and prevent relapse. Patients with alcohol disorders have better outcomes when they also participate in an organized treatment program. Whether this treatment program is mandated or voluntary, the alcoholic has an opportunity to interact with peers and professionals who are skilled and trained to help them through the recovery process. For example, the combination of pharmacotherapy and group counseling or Alcoholics Anonymous (AA) has been found to be more successful than treating alcoholism with pharmacotherapy alone.[53] Pharmacists should be able to refer patients to appropriate alcohol treatment centers, counseling groups, or AA organizations within their community. Alcohol counseling and treatment can be conducted in an inpatient or outpatient setting depending on the severity of the disease. There is no 'quick-fix' for a person in recovery, and any person entering treatment should realize that battling the disease of alcoholism is usually a life-long process.

Alcoholics Anonymous

AA is one of the first successful peer-based support programs developed outside of a clinical setting. AA is defined as "A fellowship of men and women who share their experience, strength, and hope with each other that they may solve their common problem and help others recover from alcoholism." The only requirement for membership is a desire to stop drinking. Two former alcohol abusers founded the association in 1935 and developed the "twelve-step" model of recovery. Since then, the twelve steps of AA have been adopted and utilized by people with all types of addictions and behavior problems (eg, Narcotics Anonymous, Overeaters Anonymous, and Gamblers Anonymous). Support groups such as Al-anon and Alateen have been developed for the friends and families of those in recovery. AA is now worldwide, and persons in recovery can find a meeting in almost every community. Information about AA and methods to locate AA meetings can be found at www.alcoholics-anonymous.org. For more information about Al-Anon/Alateen, call 1-888-4-AL-ANON (weekdays, 8 am to 6 pm EST) or visit the website, www.al-anon.alateen.org.

OPIATE ADDICTION

Pharmacists may have greater difficulty in detecting and intervening with patients addicted to narcotics or other illicit street drugs. Signs and symptoms of opiate addiction are as variable as the number of prescription and street drugs that are abused. A person who is 'high' on a narcotic may exhibit erratic behavior, or they may appear completely normal while experiencing a level of euphoria. Street drugs are constantly changing, and clandestine chemists often invent new delivery methods to streamline the drug supply chain.

Like tobacco and alcohol use disorders, the Transtheoretical Model for Change can be applied to those persons who are attempting to recover from opioid and illicit substance use; however, these substances provide a greater reward in the CNS, and it can be much harder to discontinue use without other interventions. Opioid withdrawal is often prolonged and painful, often resulting in clinically significant distress or impairment in social, occupational, or other important areas of functioning (see Table 131-3). Due to new treatment methods and novel drug therapies, pharmacists have a greater role in the treatment of opiate addiction.

Pharmacologic Treatment

METHADONE—Methadone maintenance and treatment programs exist throughout the United States. Methadone substitution is the preferred method of opioid maintenance and withdrawal for heroin addiction because of its long half-life and less profound sedation. Pharmacists have traditionally been responsible for the mixing and dispensing of daily doses of this Schedule II drug. Methadone substitution is highly regulated and requires strict documentation of the quantities and doses dispensed. Administering the correct dose of methadone is critical. Methadone is given orally in the smallest amount (generally 30 mg/day) that will prevent severe withdrawal signs, but not necessarily all signs. Higher doses may be required depending on the history of previous heroine abuse and tolerance. Higher doses should be given when physical signs of withdrawal are observed. Doses of 25–45 mg can produce unconsciousness if the person has not developed tolerance. After the appropriate dose has been established, it should be progressively reduced by not more than 20% each day.

BUPRENORPHINE SUBLINGUAL—Buprenorphine hydrochloride (Subutex) and buprenorphine hydrochloride plus naloxone hydrochloride (Suboxone) treat opiate dependence by preventing symptoms of withdrawal from heroin and other opiates. Administered sublingually, buprenorphine hydrochloride is intended for use at the beginning of treatment for opioid addiction. Naloxone in combination with sublingual buprenorphine is used for the maintenance period of treating opioid addiction. This combination is used to prohibit the abuse of intravenous buprenorphine.[54]

Buprenorphine sublingual formulations are the first narcotic drugs available for the treatment of opiate dependence that can be prescribed in a physician's office under the Drug Addiction Treatment Act (DATA) of 2000. Under this new law, medications for the treatment of opiate dependence that are subject to less restrictive controls than those of Schedule II can be prescribed in a doctor's office by specially trained physicians. This change is expected to provide patients greater access to needed treatment.

Role of the Pharmacist in Drug Abuse

Many pharmacists currently serve as specialists in addiction clinics and rehabilitation centers. Pharmacists' combined knowledge of medication therapy and the complex effects of illicit drugs make them a key resource in tailoring a patient's plan for recovery. As members of their community, hospital and retail pharmacists should create a list of substance abuse treatment resources, including the responsible contact person for each program or provider, and be able to refer individuals with addiction disorders for proper evaluation and treatment.

Curriculum Development

Education is the key to overcoming the many biases associated with addiction disorders. In the areas of assessment, intervention, and referral, pharmacists have the ability to assist in the early identification of individuals with addiction disorders by using standard screening instruments. Given this position, pharmacists should develop the skills needed to assume a greater role in substance abuse prevention, education, and treatment in organized health care settings and in the community. To achieve this, the professional pharmacy curriculum needs to address addiction disorders as it would other disease states. Pharmacists should be able to approach and treat substance abuse and addiction as they would any other chronic disease, without personal bias and judgment of the patient. Pharmacy curricula and continuing education programs need to aid in the development of communication skills so that pharmacists become confident in discussing substance use disorders with their patients.

In the area of treatment, pharmacists should be able to provide recommendations for the appropriate pharmacotherapeutic choices in individuals recovering from addiction disorders. Pharmacists can provide invaluable assistance in the development of treatment options for drug detoxification protocols used by health care providers. Pharmacists are aware of the different types of treatment modalities, their expected outcomes, and their cost-effectiveness. Pharmacists can also play an integral role in instructing drug abuse counselors and other health care professionals working in drug treatment programs on the pharmacology and mechanisms of action of abused substances and of medications used to treat substance use disorders.[7]

Finally, pharmacy school curricula should also focus on preventing the pharmacy candidate from developing problems with substance use. Pharmacy schools should develop policies to deal with and care for the student addict that are confidential and focus on aiding the student through a defined recovery process. Students should feel comfortable with their advisors and know that they are not alone; there is a place to turn when drug and alcohol problems develop during the education process.

The Addicted Pharmacist

Although health professionals have a similar rate of substance use disorders as the general population, patterns of abuse differ in this population. Health professionals tend to abuse alcohol and prescription drugs more often than illegal "street" drugs due to the accessibility of these substances. Pharmacists usually have stressful jobs where long hours and a great deal of responsibility are the norm (eg, ensuring the proper delivery of pharmaceutical care to patients).[55] Another reason for this problem of substance abuse is the pharmacist's close access to drugs and relatively comfortable income that allows easy access to alcohol and prescription drugs (ie, the "keys to the candy store" mentality).

Pharmacist Recovery Networks (PRNs) have been established in 47 states and are usually affiliated with state or local pharmacy organizations. PRNs serve as advocacy groups for pharmacists in all phases of recovery and often manage peers when they are going through recovery. Often, pharmacists who have been through the recovery process join the PRNs to give back and aid others in the profession who may need assistance; thus, new clients can draw upon the experience of those who have gone before them. PRNs meet on a regular basis as support groups and they also monitor laboratory testing for illicit drug use of those who are in the recovery process.

Clients are referred to a PRN by three methods. In the first scenario, a pharmacist will be ordered to enter into the PRN process by the state board of pharmacy. For example, a pharmacist who has been caught diverting medications or has been arrested for driving while intoxicated may have his/her license suspended and will be assigned to the PRN to undergo a supervised period of sobriety. Legal action may also be taken against the pharmacist depending on the nature of his/her offense. In most states, board of pharmacy meetings are public record, and the pharmacist runs the risk of his/her reputation being permanently scarred. The PRN is available to help the recovering pharmacist through this stressful period.

The second way in which a pharmacist can enter a PRN is through self-referral. This may occur after continued encouragement from friends, family, or peers. The pharmacist may also experience a close call, such as a medication error as a result of his/her impaired judgment, which may scare the pharmacist into joining the PRN. All activities of the self-referred client are kept confidential by the PRN and not reported to the board of pharmacy or the employer.

The final method of entry into a PRN is through an intervention. An intervention is a planned meeting involving the friends and family of the addicted pharmacist. A member of the PRN or an addiction specialist will coordinate this event. Interventions are designed to aid in getting the person into a recovery program immediately. Participants involved must be prepared for emotional outbursts, excuses, and physical struggles. The addicted pharmacist is often in denial about his/her problem and may have grandiose thoughts about overcoming the problem if given just one more chance. During the intervention, people close to the pharmacist will share ways in which the addiction has hurt them mentally and physically, and deficits in work performance may also be highlighted. These inequities are shared with love and compassion, and participants are trained not to lash out in anger. Interventions should not be attempted without careful planning and support from a trained expert.

Early intervention and referral into a recovery program is the key to assisting the addicted pharmacist. Many companies and hospitals have employee assistance programs that are confidential and covered through the employee's insurance plan. Every pharmacist should be familiar with his/her company's policies and procedures related to alcohol and drug addiction. All information related to the addiction disorder should remain confidential, and the employee should feel comfortable making inquiries without fear of being punished.

CONCLUSION

Substance use disorders range from ubiquitous tobacco use to illegal use of street drugs. The Transtheoretical Model for Change is a useful tool to help patients overcome their disease. Group therapy and individual counseling methods help to augment pharmacotherapeutic treatment methods for overcoming these disorders. Resources are available for individuals with tobacco, alcohol, or drug addictions. Pharmacists can play a vital role in detecting, intervening, and providing resources to patients who need assistance with recovery efforts. Help is also available through state support networks for pharmacists in need of help to overcome substance use disorders.

REFERENCES

1. The American Psychiatric Association. *Diagnostic and Statistical Manual for Mental Disorders*, 4th ed, text revision. Washington DC: American Psychiatric Association, 2000.
2. Inaba DS, Cohen WE, Holstein ME. *Uppers, Downers, All Arounders.* 3rd ed. Ashland, OR: CNS Publications, Inc., 1997.
3. Centers for Disease Control and Prevention. *MMWR* 2002; 51:300.
4. Centers for Disease Control and Prevention. *MMWR* 2002; 51:642.
5. Centers for Disease Control and Prevention. *MMWR* 2003; 52:303.
6. The National Institute on Drug Abuse, National Institutes of Health, U.S. Department of Health and Human Services. NIDA Info Facts: Costs to Society. January 31, 2003.
7. Holdford D, Kennedy DT, Bernadella P, et al. *Clin Therapeut* 1998; 20(2):328.
8. Dole EJ, Tommasello A. Recommendations for implementing effective substance abuse education in pharmacy practice. In: Haack MR, Adger H, eds. *Strategic Plan for Interdisciplinary Faculty Development: Arming the Nation's Health Professional Workforce for a New Approach to Substance Use Disorders.* Rhode Island: Association for Medical Education and Research in Substance Abuse, 2002: 263–271.
9. Fiore MC, Bailey WC, Cohen SJ, et al. Treating Tobacco Use and Dependence: Clinical Practice Guideline. Rockville, MD: U.S. Department of Health and Human Services, Public Health Service, June 2000.
10. Fuller RK, Hiller-Sturmhofel S. *Alcohol Research & Health* 1999; 23(2):69.
11. Rollnick S, Butler CC, Stott N. *Patient Education and Counseling* 1997; 31:191.
12. Zevin S, Benowitz NL. *Clin Pharmacokinet* 1999; 36:425.
13. Weathermon R, Crabb DW. *Alcohol Research & Health* 1999; 23:40.
14. DiClemente CC, Prochaska JO, Faithhurst SK, et al. *J Consult Clin Psychol* 1991; 59:295.
15. Pallonen UE, Leskinen L, Prochaska JO, et al. *Prev Med* 1994; 23:507.
16. Smith MD, McGhan WF, Laugher G. *American Pharmacy* 1995; NS35(8):20.
17. Henningfield JE, Schuh LM, Javik ME. Pathophysiology of tobacco dependence. In: Bloom FE, Kupfer DJ, eds. *Psychopharmacology:*

The Fourth Generation of Progress. New York: Raven Press, 1995:1715.

18. Zhu SH, Anderson CM, Tedeschi GJ, et al. *N Engl J Med* 2002; 347(14):1087.
19. Jorenby DE, Leischow SJ, Nides MA, et al. *N Engl J Med* 1999; 340:685.
20. Kornitzer M, Boutsen M, Dramaix M, et al. *Preventive Medicine* 1995; 24:41.
21. Blondal T, Gudmundsson LJ, Olafsdottir I, et al. *BMJ* 1999; 318(7179):285.
22. Bohadana A, Nilsson F, Rasmussen T, et al. *Arch Intern Med* 2000; 160(20):3128.
23. Breslau N, Johnson EO, Hiripi E, et al. *Arch Gen Psychiatry* 2001; 58:810.
24. Ziedonis DM, Williams JM. *Curr Opin Psychiatry* 2003; 16(3):305.
25. Glassman AH, Covey LS, Stetner F, et al. *Lancet* 2001; 357:1929.
26. DeBusk RF, Miller NH, Superko HR, et al. *Ann Intern Med* 1994; 120(9):721.
27. Kimmel SE, Berlin JA, Miles C, et al. *J Am Coll Cardiol* 2001; 37:1297.
28. Joseph AM, Norman SM, Ferry LH, et al. *N Engl J Med* 1996; 335:1792.
29. Dempsey DA, Benowitz NL. *Drug Safety* 2001; 24(4):277.
30. Gilpin EA, Pierce JP. *Am J Prev Med* 1999; 16(3):195.
31. Questions and Answers about Smokeless Tobacco and Cancer: Cancer Facts. October 1998. National Cancer Institute. Available from: (http://cis.nci.nih.gov/fact). Accessed 16 May 2002.
32. Substance Abuse and Mental Health Services Administration. (2003). *Results from the 2002 National Survey on Drug Use and Health: National Findings.* (Office of Applied Studies, NHSDA Series H-22, DHHS Publication No. SMA 03-3836). Rockville, MD.
33. Ebbert JO, Rowland LC, Montori VM, et al. *Addiction* 2003; 98:569.
34. Hatsukami D, Jensen J, Allen S, et al. *J Consult Clin Psychol* 1996; 64(1):153.
35. Howard-Pitney B, Killen JD, Fortmann SP. *Exp Clin Psychopharmacol* 1999; 7(4):362.
36. Glover ED, Glover PN, Sullivan CR, et al. *Am J Health Behav* 2002; 26(5):386.
37. Hurt RD, Dale LC, Offord KP, et al. *Clin Pharmacol Ther* 1993; 54:98.
38. Haley NJ, Axelrad CM, Tilton KA. *Am J Public Health* 1983; 73:1204.
39. Hughes JR, Gulliver SB, Fenwick JW, et al. *Health Psychol* 1992; 11:331.
40. Gritz ER, Klesges RC, Meyers AW. *Ann Behav Med* 1989; 11:144.
41. Williamson DF, Madans J, Anda RF, et al. *N Engl J Med* 1991; 324(11):739.
42. Grieger L. Nutritional tips for smoking cessation. Available from: (http://www.centerforhealthandwellnes.com). Accessed 7 March 2003.
43. Marcus BH, Albrecht AE, King TK, et al. *Arch Intern Med* 1999; 159:1229.
44. Danielsson T, Rossner S, Westin A. *BMJ* 1999; 319:490.
45. Ewing JA. *JAMA* 1984; 252:1905.
46. Dufour MC. *Alcohol Research & Health* 1999; 23:5.
47. Hingson RW, Heeren T, Winter MR. *Alcohol Research & Health* 1999; 23:31.
48. Chez RA, Andres RL, Chazotte C, et al. *Primary Care Update Ob/Gyns* 2001; 8:195.
49. Krystal JH, Cramer JA, Krol WF, et al. *N Engl J Med* 2001; 345:1734.
50. Wilde MI, Wagstaff AJ. *Drugs* 1997; 53:1038.
51. Littleton J. *Addiction* 1995; 90:1179.
52. Fiellin DA, O'Connor PG. *Am J Med* 2000; 108:227.
53. O'Malley SS. Strategies to maximize the efficacy of naltrexone for alcohol dependence. National Institute on Drug Abuse. NIH Publication No. 95-3899. 1995:53–64.
54. Suboxone®, Subutex® Package Insert. Reckitt Benckiser Pharmaceuticals, Inc. Richmond, VA. 2003.
55. ASHP Statement on the Pharmacist's Role in Substance Abuse Prevention, Education, and Assistance. *Am J Health-Syst Pharm* 2003; 60:1995.

CHAPTER 132

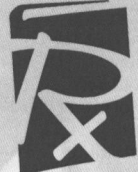

Complementary and Alternative Medical Health Care

Ara H DerMarderosian, PhD

June E Riedlinger, PharmD

Most people would agree that during the 20th century there have been more changes and improvements in medical science than in almost all of the preceding years of recorded history. The germ theory of the 20th century enabled the eradication of most microbial infections through the use of antibiotics and antiviral drugs. Numerous advances in medical technology have brought rapid and accurate analysis of specific invading organisms, the determination of the status of the blood and immunological systems, and the kinds and levels of drugs to administer to patients.

The new high-tech machines including x-rays, the CAT scan (*computerized axial tomography*), MRI (*magnetic resonance imaging*), ultrasound imaging, the PET scan (*positron emission tomography*) and others have allowed the location and diagnosis of most major cellular and body organ malfunctions, so that appropriate therapy can be undertaken. There have also been rapid advances in medicinal chemistry, natural product chemistry, computational chemistry, genomics, proteomics, etc. which have allowed for the synthesis of more compounds which might be useful as drugs and a better understanding of the mechanisms of action of these compounds.

The rapidly emerging field of biotechnology has spawned a bewildering array of bioengineered enzymes, peptides, hormones, and the like, which have allowed the replacement of normal body substances that maintain health.

Similarly, ways have been found to bolster and increase levels of newly recognized immunological factors that strengthen our infection defense mechanisms. Hence, it is easy to understand why modern conventional or orthodox medicine (allopathy) has generally held the upper hand of *efficacious* therapy in most advanced societies. However, in recent years it has appeared to have reached its limits in the minds of many individuals. More and more people expect perfect and complete results every time they seek medical help. When modern medicine fails, this attitude often leads to the search for help in alternative or complementary medicine, which appears to offer hope in a more holistic mode.

THE RISE OF ALTERNATIVE MEDICINE—The past few decades have generated a rapidly growing interest and popularity in alternative or complementary medicine because of its perceived, either potentially beneficial or pernicious effects on individual health or society.

Many reasons have been given for the resurgence of nontraditional or holistic medicine. Some have blamed a loss of faith in science (many people believe science has caused pollution, depletion of ozone, drug misuse, and iatrogenesis); others feel that confidence in orthodox medicine has eroded because it has failed to meet continuously rising medical expectations. Some feel that high-tech medicine does not care about or pay attention to the patient's belief system.

There is little doubt that rising costs of medical care have not helped promote efficient use of all the major advancements in medical technology or given better attention to the patient. Worldwide, it has been acknowledged that modern health care in the US has become an uncontrolled "monster" that is difficult, if not impossible, to contain. The political upheaval being caused by current health-care reforms in the US serves as an example.

Medical costs have risen over 15-fold in the past 40 years, and yet only a little over 40% of the people are served with adequate medical care. The current medical costs have been rising faster than inflation, and insurance costs have been unaffordable to many individuals and industries. Over 30 years ago, forecasters predicted that neither decreasing or increasing amounts of money spent on health would have any further effect on how long one could expect to live.

Some have said that we have reached a state of diminishing returns in modern medicine. The truth is that we have finally identified all the major disorders for which there is no easy cure. Many of these are the normal consequences of aging. There is little doubt that we will probably never fully conquer the old age–related disorders of bronchitis, arthritis, rheumatism, heart disease, back pain, high blood pressure, and many others. These degenerative chronic diseases of old age simply do not respond well, even to the most modern treatments.

Another problem that exists is the profit-driven motive to design drugs simply to capture a fraction of established markets. This has led to more and more "*me too*" drugs that do not really promise important therapeutic gains. Because of the great expense involved in developing totally new drugs with unique pharmacological properties, many drug companies have shied away from the efforts.

With all these problems in mind, it is easy to understand why complementary 2nd alternative medicine has been summoned to *fill the gap* not met by modern medicine.

Since the 1960s more and more Americans have turned to self-awareness and self-controlled medical treatments. *Wellness* as a concept and *prevention* as a mode of life have become standard thinking for a significant percentage of the American population. Our increased trade and relations with Asia and better communication with the traditional medical practices of Asia, Europe, Africa, and South America have opened new doors of treatment for all ills.

From the 1970s and 1980s up to 2000 and beyond numerous articles on alternative medicine have appeared in the literature. At least one author has given 92 alternative therapies ranging from acupressure (Shiatsu) to yoga. Over 50 books also have appeared under the titles of natural or nature's therapies.

Many of these alternative systems are complex and possess variable standards of qualification, training, and registration. Indeed, many within alternative medicine do not even agree on definitions for the numerous specialities let alone on standardization of treatment modalities. Generally, many of the theories on which alternative therapies are based are not in accord with current medical concepts. Nevertheless, many of these therapies have become popular and are in demand by the American public and should be understood by all health practitioners.

In 1990, the US population made an estimated 425 million visits to providers of nonconventional therapies at a cost of some $10 billion from their own pockets. Some of these therapies now are covered by health insurance, but many are not.

In November 1998, the *Journal of the American Medical Association (JAMA)* had as its major theme, alternative medicine. Statistics of the last few years have shown that 4 out of 10 Americans used alternative medical therapies in 1997. Further, the total visits to alternative medical practitioners increased by close to 50% from that in 1990 and in fact exceeded the patient visits for all US primary-care physicians. Monetarily, this population paid approximately $21.2 billion for services (an increase of 45%) provided by alternative medical practitioners. An updated survey by David M1. Eisenberg, MD, of Beth Israel Deaconess Medical Center in Boston, and his cohorts in 1997 showed that between 1990 and 1997, the prevalence of complementary/alternative medicine (CAM) increased by 25%, with the total number of visits increasing by 47% from an estimated 427 million in 1990 to 629 million in 1997. As mentioned above, the expenses for these services were about $21.2 billion, with $12.2 billion out-of-pocket, and exceeded the out-of-pocket expenses for *all hospitalizations* in 1997. This survey covered 16 CAM therapies, which included relaxation techniques, herbal medicine, massage, chiropractic, spiritual healing by others, megavitamins, self-help, imagery, commercial diet, folk, lifestyle diet, energy healing, homeopathy, hypnosis, biofeedback, and acupuncture.

Both the 1990 and 1997 surveys found that CAM was used most commonly for chronic conditions, which included back and neck problems, arthritis, headaches, and anxiety. An increase from 33.8% in 1990 to 42.1% in 1997 was seen in the use of at least 1 of the 16 CAM therapies. The largest increases were in the areas of use of herbal medicine, massage, megavitamins, self-help groups, folk remedies, energy healing, and homeopathy. Even though these data show increased use of CAM across the board, the level of patient disclosure of this to their physicians remained low at less than 40% in 1990 and 1997. Obviously, all health practitioners are concerned because at least 15 million Americans in 1997 took prescribed medications and herbal remedies concurrently. Since at least one in five patients who take prescription drugs also may take herbs, high-dose vitamins, and supplements, etc, investigators are concerned that millions of adults may be at risk for potential unintended herb or vitamin/drug interactions. They caution that the CAM market is continuing to grow, and that trend needs continuous monitoring based on scientific inquiry, clinical judgment, regulatory authority, and shared decision-making. They advise that the *don't ask* and *don't tell* approach to patient/physician communication must be discarded.

Further, interesting statistics from this study revealed that CAM was significantly more common among women (48.9%) than men (37.8) and less common among African-Americans (33.1%) than other racial groups (44.5%). Persons in the age range of 35 to 49 years reported higher rates of use (50.1%) than persons either older (39.1%) or younger (41.8%). CAM usage was higher among college-educated persons (50.6%) than persons with no college education (36.4%), and more common among those with annual incomes above $50,000 (48.1%) than those with lower incomes (42.6%). CAM usage was higher in the Western US (50.1%) than elsewhere in the US (42.1%). Surprisingly, the total out-of-pocket expenditures for CAM in 1997 (including professional service, herbals, vitamin diet products, books, and classes), were estimated conservatively to be about $27 billion. These studies also showed that 42% of all CAM use was attributable to the treatment of existing illness and/or health maintenance.

There is little doubt that all this concern led to Congress crafting legislation and establishing the National Center for

Complementary and Alternative Medicine (NCCAM) at the National Institutes of Health (NIH) in 1998. Congress empowered NCCAM to conduct basic and clinical research, train researchers and educate and communicate their findings to health professionals and the public, NCCAM leaders have stressed the importance at the dawn of the 21st century, of clarifying the lines between holism and reductionism. There is a strong desire to bring CAM into "integritive medicine" where the best of both philosophies are brought to bear in the medicine of the future. A few examples include studies into how accupuncture and meditation work and what lies behind the placebo effect. There is also the expectation of clarifying the basis for the effectiveness of selected herbal and nutritional supplements so that standardized preparations can be used with confidence for treating certain ailments.

During the latter part of the last decade (ca.1995–2004) there have been numerous programs and training courses on CAM in almost every medical, pharmacy, and nursing school in the US. While much relates to popular patient "pressure" for these treatments much also has related to their willingness to pay and to the increasing number of US insurance companies and managed-care organizations which also are willing to financially support unorthodox treatments.

In order to fully appreciate how quickly CAM has grown in the last decade, it is necessary to review the start with the Office of Alternative Medicine (OAM) in October of 1991 which led ultimately to NCCAM in 1998 and its continued growth up to 2004. Much of the history is covered in NCCAM's, Five Year Strategic Plan, 2001–2005, entitled, "Expanding Horizons of Healthcare." (Obtainable at their Web site: nccam.nih.gov). It is divided into 4 parts. Part I, The Case for Action, which covers advances in medical science in the 20th century, coupled with improvements, The Appeal of Nontraditional Approaches described Alternative Medical Systems, Mind-Body Interventions, Biologically based therapies, Energy therapies, CAM yesterday; Mainstream Healthcare Today, Resolving the Issue Responding to Public Demand.

Part II covers Future Directions including NCCAM's support of a broad portfolio of research, the clinical imperative. Contained in this part as well is, basic science research, NIH areas of emphasis, as well as collaboration and training, information and dissemination and integration topics.

Part III covers specifically NCCAM's Strategic Plan 2001–2005 which includes the confidence of Congress in authorizing NCCAM, their mission, their vision, the stakeholders, strategic areas, and specific goals. These goals include, investing in Research, training CAM investigators, expanding outreach programs, and facilitating the integration and the practice of responsible stewardship.

Part IV consists of several appendices consisting of major domains of CAM, important events in NCCAM history, a bio-

Table 132-1. Reasons for Popularity of Alternative/Complementary Medicine

Perceived and real limitations of allopathy.

Love (when it works) and hate (when it fails) relationships with *high-tech* medicine.

Lack of tender loving care. People complain about being seen as *problems* or interesting cases to solve rather than real persons.

Complaints of endless tests with ambiguous meanings.

Desire to be a partner in healing one's self.

Unhappy about being sent to various specialists.

Desire to have one physician who can treat whole person and not just a body part.

Desire to have a physician who listens, does not dictate therapies, and makes one a partner in recovery.

Desire to see the practitioner as a trusted friend and not an authority figure.

Desire to be empowered or given authority or trust over the manner of being healed and self-healing capabilities heeded.

graphical sketch of the director of NCCAM, the research and research training portfolio of NCCAM members, NCCAM outreach activities, evidence-based reviews, and the NCCAM Cancer Advisory Panel for CAM.

NCCAM also provides several publications on general information, consumer advisories, NCCAM fact sheets, cancer fact sheets, dietary supplements fact sheets, booklets and reports, and a newsletter.

DEFINITIONS—Table 132-1 provides a summary of reasons cited for why CAM has become popular in recent times. Table 132-2 provides criticisms and comments about CAM. Some organizations and health professionals have been against NCCAM since its inception. Sampon has in fact, published on the quackwatch web site a four page article on why NCCAM should be defunded (http://www.quackwatch.org/0.1quackeryrelatedtopics/nccam.html). He cites articles on the politics of CAM and gives his opinion on the waste of research dollars and the lack of proof of many CAM therapies. The Appendix provides a list of terms used in CAM as well as definitions for the numerous specialities. As with all listings of this sort there will be disagreements about reasons or definitions. However, these reasons and definitions should establish an understanding of the complex nature of the popularity and practice of complementary/alternative medical care.

The following practices in CAM are among the most popular in the US today. An attempt has been made to list and define all of these with minimal comments or judgments on efficacy, since there may be few hard data available. Most medical practitioners are aware that one out of three drugs or managements of disease may be successful regardless of true or known efficacy. It is with this thought that all practitioners should keep their minds open about all modalities of health care, as only time and science ultimately will show what is effective and what is not, in medicine. Studies & surveys on CAM in the U.S. reveal that 36% of adults are using some form of integrative medicine. If one includes megavitamin therapy and prayer specifically for health purposes, then the percentage of CAM users rises to 62%. Further, the surveys by NCCAM show that certain groups are more likely to use CAM and this includes more women than men, people of higher educational levels, people hospitalized in the past year, and former smokers. Generally, most practitioners have been in agreement that conventional medicine is best for the management of acute care.

Table 132-2. Comments and Criticisms about Complementary/Alternative Medicine

Many conventional practitioners and medical scientists believe these to be a modern form of quackery.
Some of the successes reported are *placebo* effects.
Most ailments treated successfully are self-limiting. Self-limiting disorders predominate in these areas of practice.
Many of the approaches lack scientific proof.
Relatively few studies are clinical, double-blind investigations.
Most references, books, and papers are not truly scientific publications, and many reports are anecdotal.

No attempt is made here to negate the necessity to handle emergencies in a hospital setting where all of the high-tech methods can usually solve severe traumatic medical problems. Conversely, many agree that numerous long-term health problems (aging, anxiety, arthritis, backaches, chronic pain, elevated blood pressure, headaches, ulcers, etc) often lend themselves to various complementary/alternative practices. Certainly, many of these can be treated less expensively and less invasively than with allopathy. The major caveat, of course, is that of providing care without causing harm or delay when allopathy clearly can do something that is efficacious. The ultimate choice must be made jointly by the patient and the practitioner, keeping in mind the limitations, advantages, and disadvantages of each medical practice.

Finally, it should be kept in mind that the preventative approach is of paramount importance in health. This is a major change in philosophy for the 21st century. More and more people have opted for the obvious and are protecting their future health with good nutrition, exercise, stress reduction, and cessation of smoking. Much of complementary and alternative medicine has moved in this direction or has practiced it for many years. Medical foods or *nutraceuticals* or functional foods also have been stressed recently and Tables 132-3 and 132-4 provide samples of foods and their contained active principles that may be preventative and curative for many medical problems, from appendicitis to ulcers.

For lack of a better place to cover an unusual "nutritional" or "food" product, it will be instructive to briefly mention shark cartilage because of its widespread continued promotion as a purported "cancer cure." In 1995 the annual world market for this and related products exceeded $30 million, although it has di-

Table 132-3. Examples of Foods with Purported Medical Properties

FOOD	CONSTITUENTS	PURPORTED MEDICAL PROPERTIES
Apple	Pectin, caffeic acid	Lowers cholesterol, blood pressure. Juice has antimicrobial, antidiarrheal properties. Possible protectant against cancer.
Banana and plantain	Fiber in unripe plantain, pectin	Prevents and heals ulcers, helps lower blood-cholesterol. Stimulates proliferation of cells in stomach lining and release of protective mucus.
Broccoli	Indoles, glucosinolates, dithiolthiones, carotenoids	Lowers risk of cancer.
Cabbage	Chlorophyll, dithiolthiones, flavonoids, indoles, isothiocyanates, phenolic caffeic & ferulic acids, vitamins E and C "growth factor" mucin-like substances	Lowers risk of colonic cancer, juice helps prevent and heal ulcers, stimulates immune system, kills microbes, is classed as desmutagen (cancer antagonist).
Chili pepper	Capsaicin, vitamin C	Increases mucous secretion in lung, acts as expectorant, alleviates chronic bronchitis and emphysema, decongestant, diminishes clot formation (fibrinolytic), topically effective analgesic used in cluster headaches, induces secretion of endorphin.
Spices, eg, cumin, cinnamon, ginger, mustard	Various active principles	Reduces cholesterol levels in animals.
Fenugreek	Various active principles, fiber	Helps control sugar levels in diabetics.

Table 132-4. Examples of Phytochemicals in Foods with Purported Medical Properties

PHYTOCHEMICALS	BOTANICAL SOURCE	PURPORTED PROPERTIES
Allicin, ajoene	Garlic	Stimulates biochemical pathways involving glutathione, which detoxifies foreign materials; intercepts activated car cinogensbefore they attach to DNA; inhibits prostaglandin E_2, which is linked to tumor promotion; has antimicrobial properties.
Flavonoids, phenolics, carotenoids, saponins, and triterpenoids	Citrus fruits	Enhance body's detoxification system; have antioxidant effects; regulate enzymes produced by cancer cells. Phenolics stimulate synthesis of glutathione, the body's detoxifier. Carotenoids quench damaging oxygen free radicals. Saponins and triterpenoids may block cell receptors for estrogen, which may protect against breast cancer. Inhibits prostaglandin E_2, which is linked to tumor promotion.
α-Linoleic acid, phenolic lignans	Flaxseed	These fatty acids diminish cholesterol formation; lignans have antiestrogenic activity, which may lower breast cancer risk. Inhibit prostaglandin E_2, which is linked to tumor promotion.
Glycyrrhizic acid, other related triterpenoids phenolics	Licorice	Antibiotic properties, phenolics inhibit key enzymes over-produced by cancer cells. Inhibit prostaglandin E_2, which is linked to tumor promotion.
Isoflavones	Soybeans	Inhibit activity of tyrosine kinases that are overproduced when normal cells are transformed into cancer cells.
Indoles, betacarbolenes	Cabbage-family members	Favor estrogen deactivation and excretion which minimizes tumor activation pathway.
Phenolic acids	Umbelliferous vegetables, eg, parsley, celery	Possible antiulcer properties.

minished in recent years for growing proof of lack of efficacy. At least two glycoproteins (sphyrnostatin 1 and 2) have been isolated from the cartilage of the hammerhead shark with early claims that these had strong antiangiogenic activity inhibiting tumor neovascularization. It was believed that this might be useful in human cancer therapy. Unfortunately, because macromolecules like this are not absorbed intestinally, high blood levels are not reached. To date, no controlled clinical studies have been published showing consistent significant efficacy for human cancer treatment. Preliminary results in a US trial showed 50% of cancer patients who took 100 mg of dried cartilage powder daily reported improvements in quality of life, appetite and relief of pain. However, later a more well documented study with sixty patients (various advanced cancers) showed no complete or even partial responses. These authors concluded that shark cartilage was inactive in advanced stage cancer and had no beneficial action in improving quallity of life.

All medical practices are beginning to pay a lot more attention to good and preventative aspects of nutrition as the US population ages and extends life well into the 70- to 90-year age potential.

Finally, it should be noted that money is now being spent in the academic and federal sectors to determine the veracity of alternative medicine as discussed earlier.

Temple University in Philadelphia developed a Center for Frontier Sciences for studying the mind/body connection as well as how electromagnetic fields may influence health. They also are looking into the potential of *soft* therapies in medicine, such as electroacupuncture and therapeutic touch. Almost all major universities have followed suit.

OAM AND NCCAM—Again in the latter part of 1992, in response to increasing public pressure, Congress established the Office of Alternative Medicine (OAM) within the Office of the Director of the National Institutes of Health (NIH) to facilitate the fair scientific evaluation of CAM and to establish an information clearinghouse. The OAM was designed primarily to encourage study and research in the many promising CAM approaches to determine which are potentially effective, safe, and economical as health-care practices. However with the passage of the fiscal year 1999 Omnibus appropriations bill, and the subsequent signing by the President on October 21, 1998, Congress established the National Center for

Complementary and Alternative Medicine (NCCAM). With stronger support and money the center has been devoted to the conduct and support of basic and applied research and training, and has disseminated information on CAM to health practitioners and the public. It also has been set up to carry out related programs that one hopes will continue to advance the investigation and application of CAM methods that prove to be efficacious.

This Act has the legislative reference bill number S 2440, section 601, and is summarized in the the web site http://altmed.od.nih.gov/nccam/. These references provide the details on the OAM change to NCCAM, their address, toll-free phone number and fax number, history, purpose, mission, program advisory council charter, fiscal year budget, program areas, extramural affairs (grants), 10 specialty research centers, research database evaluation program, NCAAM clearinghouse and media relations, international and professional liaison program, research development and investigation program, intramural research training program, and relations with other government agencies (eg, Agency for Health Care Policy and Research, Department of Defense, Food and Drug Administration (FDA), Health Care Financing Administration Agency, and the Centers for Disease Control and Prevention). The NCAAM also holds regular meetings with the FDA to seek its help in reevaluating current rules and regulations that govern research on the use of new devices, acupuncture needles, herbs, and homeopathic remedies. NCAAM also continues to keep in touch with most of the CAM organizations to provide them with new information regarding research support and development.

The Web site has a *What's New* section that provides a running update on new bills, grants, requests for applications, annual meetings, CAM citation index, and results of new research in CAM. Scientific exploration in CAM has become vigorous enough for Congress to raise the status of CAM from an *office* to a *national center*. It has given NCAAM the authority to fund its own research projects.

Certainly, the big jump in annual funding ($117,752,000 in FY 2004) will go a long way in helping prove its promises. With recent studies showing that at least two out of five Americans use an alternative therapy, it certainly behooves reductionist science to determine the real efficacy of holistic medicine.

THE DSHEA ACT OF 1994—The Dietary Supplement Health and Education Act of 1994 (DSHEA) was passed after substantial negotiations between members of the House and Senate and their staffs, including representatives from the dietary supplement industry. The Act is intended to enable consumers to make informed choices about nutrient supplements and subjects these products to the same general labeling requirements that apply to foods. Basically, the Act came about through enormous public pressure to maintain the *All-American* freedom of choice in self-nutrition and *medication*. The Act generated more calls, letters, and faxes of support than any previous bill.

For several decades the FDA regulated dietary supplements as foods, mainly to ensure that they were safe and wholesome and that labeling on them was true and not misleading. One focus to ensure safety was the FDA's regulation of the safety of all new ingredients, even those used in dietary supplements under the older 1958 Food Additive Amendments to the Federal Food, Drug, and Cosmetic Act (FD&C Act). With the passage of DSHEA, Congress amended the FD&C Act to add several newer provisions that apply directly to dietary supplements and their ingredients. Because of the new provisions, ingredients in dietary supplements are no longer subject to the premarket safety evaluations required of other new food ingredients or new uses of old food ingredients. Now they must meet the requirements of other safety provisions. The specific areas of coverage of the DSHEA include definition of dietary supplement, safety, literature, nutrition support statements, ingredient and nutrition information labeling, new dietary ingredients, good manufacturing practices (GMPs), Commission on Dietary Supplements; Office of Dietary Supplements; and effective date.

The DSHEA defines a dietary supplement as any product (besides tobacco) that contains a vitamin, mineral, herb, or amino acid that is intended as a supplement to the normal diet. No proof of safety is required for dietary supplements marketed prior to Oct 15, 1994, to remain on the market. They are considered safe unless they "present a significant or unreasonable risk of illness or injury under conditions of use recommended or suggested in labeling or, if no conditions of use are suggested or recommended in the labeling, under ordinary conditions of use." In contrast to over-the-counter (OTC) and ethical drugs for which manufacturers are required to prove safety and efficacy before marketing, the *grandfathered* dietary supplements are deemed safe unless proven unsafe by the FDA. So it is obvious that DSHEA regulates herbals (as well as other dietary supplements) more like foods than drugs. The Act does, however, grant the secretary of Health and Human Services emergency powers to withdraw a supplement from the market if it poses an imminent health hazard. This happened with ephedra in 2004.

Unique to the act is the labeling requirement that allows warnings and dosage recommendations as well as substantiated *structure or function* claims. Before this time, such labeling would cause the product to be *misbranded* and removed from the market. Now this labeling is allowed with specific limitations, *viz,* all claims must be accompanied by a conspicuous notice that they have not been evaluated by the FDA and in fact must state on the label "This product is not intended to diagnose, treat, cure or prevent any disease." The label must also contain the term *dietary supplement* and give each ingredient by name, quantity, total weight, and identity of any plant parts from which the botanical ingredient is derived.

All statements on the label must be truthful and not misleading. Any claim to conform to an official reference (eg, *United States Pharmacopeia*) must meet all the specifications or be deemed misbranded. The USP has begun to establish new monographs on dietary supplements. Also new is the ability to provide information representing a balanced view of the scientific information on the botanical along with its sale. This literature must be truthful, cannot promote a specific brand of the herbal, and must be displayed physically separate from the product. The burden of proof that the information is false or misleading lies with the FDA. Before this time, such literature was considered an extension of the label, and any implied clinical efficacy claims were the basis for judging the product *misbranded*. The law further states that these requirements "shall not apply to or restrict a retailer or wholesaler of dietary supplements in any way whatsoever in the sale of books or other publications as a part of the business of such retailer or wholesaler."

DSHEA further created a Commission of Dietary Supplement Labels to make recommendations for the regulation of all claims and statements, with forthcoming reports on a timely basis. In addition, DSHEA created the Office of Dietary Supplements within the NIH. This agency is entrusted with promoting the scientific study of the usefulness of dietary supplements. The head of this office is specified as the principal advisor on dietary supplements to the Secretary of Health and Human Services, the FDA Commissioner, and other federal officials. All health professionals should expect that both the FDA and the entire supplement industry will be active for many years to come in establishing new and continuously changing rules. In particular, pharmacists should keep abreast of all legal changes, to provide proper patient counseling and evaluate all health advertising claims that appear for herbals.

To completely cover all aspects of this Act would be difficult in this overview. However, the Act may be summarized as follows:

Definitions (eg, a dietary supplement may be a vitamin, mineral, herb or other botanical, an amino acid, a supplement that can increase total dietary intake, and a concentrate, metabolite, constituent, extract or combination of these ingredients).

Information on adulteration (eg, a product is unsafe if it presents a significant or unreasonable risk of illness or injury under the label's suggested conditions of use).

Statements on allowable claims (eg, claims a benefit related to a classical nutrient deficiency disease and discloses the prevalence of such diseases in the US).

Health claims (eg, a statement for a dietary supplement may not claim to diagnose, mitigate, treat, cure, or prevent a specific disease or class of diseases).

Labeling exemptions (eg, the Act adds a new paragraph to exempt from *labeling* a third-party publication used in connection with the sale of dietary supplements if it is not false or misleading and does not promote a particular brand).

Misbranding (eg, the Act is amended and deems a supplement misbranded unless it lists each ingredient, the quantity, and total quantity of ingredients in proprietary blends; unless it is identified as a *dietary supplement;* and if it comes from a plant and does not identify the part of the plant from which it is derived).

Adds new labeling requirements (eg, 1); the nutrient information shall first list those ingredients that are present in the product in a significant amount and for which a recommended daily requirement has been established (dietary ingredient not present in significant amounts do not have to be listed) and shall list any other ingredient present and identified as having no recommendation for daily consumption).

Data on good manufacturing practices (eg, authorizes the Secretary to issue regulations for GMPs for dietary supplements, including for expiration date labeling, but prohibits imposition of standards for which there is no current and generally available analytical methodology).

Establishes a Commission on Dietary Supplement Labeling (eg, establishes a seven-member Commission as an independent agency within the Executive Branch to conduct a study and issue a report making recommendations, within 2 years of enactment, to the White House and Congress on regulation of label claims for dietary supplements and legislation, if appropriate).

Provides regulations (eg, within 90 days of the issuance of the Commission's report, the Secretary shall publish in the *Federal Register* a notice of any recommendations made by the Commission for changes in regulations and shall include with such notice of proposal a rule making an opportunity for public comment).

Establishes an Office of Dietary Supplements (eg, to conduct and coordinate scientific research on the extent to which dietary supplements can limit or reduce various conditions, such as heart disease, cancer, birth defects, osteoporosis, etc, and collect and compile the results of such research).

Table 132-5. The Five Domains of Complementary and Alternative Medicine as Defined by NCCAM

1. Alternative Medical Systems, eg, homeopathic and naturapathic medicine, Oriental medicine, Ayurvedic medicine
2. Mind-body Interventions, eg, meditation, cognitive-behavioral therapy
3. Biologically Based Therapies, eg, dietary supplements, herbs
4. Manipulative and Body-Based Methods, eg, chiropathic, massage
5. Energy Therapies (2 types)
   5A. Biofield therapies, eg, Reiki, Therapeutic Touch, qi gong
   5B. Bioelectromagnetic-based therapies, eg, magnet therapies

The complete details of DSHEA may be obtained by writing to NCCAM or accessing various web sites, eg, http://vm. cfsan. da.gov/dms/dietsupp.html. Finally, in effect, the DSHEA has resulted in a deregulation of the supplement industry. Now, unlike food additives or drugs, supplements do not require FDA approval prior to marketing. It is the manufacturers alone who decide whether their products are effective and safe. If a problem arises, the burden of proof falls on the FDA to prove that the supplement poses an unreasonable risk and should be recalled from the market. As might be expected, the $4-billion-a year supplement industry will strongly oppose any stringent regulations. For example, there are proposals to create new regulatory categories for some supplements as *nutraceuticals*.

While generally understood to be foods with health-promoting qualities, they are not yet defined legally or scientifically. In perspective, supplements (pills, powders, or other typical medicinal dosage forms) really make up only a relatively small percentage of the $77 billion nutraceutical market. The largest percentage obviously relates to foods, snacks, and drinks that purport to satisfy the consumers' desire for health through foods. For example, complete liquid meals, originally intended for those too ill to eat regularly, are now marketed as nutritionally complete and convenient *instant* meals for persons with active lifestyles or too busy to prepare meals. Often these products contain all the protein, vitamins, and minerals (and other *healthful* ingredients) in easy-to-swallow form. Even ideal ingredients such as *energy inducers,* herbal phytochemicals, and antioxidants are added to foods for long-term healthful benefits. Consumers easily can find products such as orange juice with added calcium, or peanut butter fortified with all the essential vitamins and minerals.

DSHEA has allowed the food industry to market readily any food or ingredient currently being investigated in biochemical nutrition research. For the most part nutraceutical advocates are now urging the FDA to "lighten up" on its criteria on health claims so that manufacturers can make exclusive claims based on their own research even without being required to reveal their studies in public. There is already much disagreement on health claims, labeling matters, proof of efficacy, and safety regarding nutraceuticals. It will take several decades to resolve these issues as the battle between holistic approaches and reductionist science continues.

Of the numerous complementary/alternative procedures in existence, the most widely accepted are acupuncture, aromatherapy, bodywork, chiropractic, faith healing, herbalism, homeopathy, hypnosis, iridology, mind/body connection, naturopathy, and reflexology. Table 132-5 gives the five general categories of alternative medicine as defined by NCCAM.

ACUPUNCTURE

This has been a primary practice of the health-care system of China for at least 2500 years. The Chinese systematized acupuncture and were the first to include it in a medical book—*The Yellow Emperor's Classic of Internal Medicine* (written between 300 and 100 BCE). Acupuncture and Chinese medicine spread to Japan in the 6th century and to France in the 17th century. It got the attention of the American medical scene in 1972 when James Reston, a *New York Times* columnist who was covering President Nixon's visit to China, wrote about his appendectomy, which was performed with acupuncture instead of pharmaceutical anesthesia.

Most recently, the NIH issued a statement supporting the integration of acupuncture into Western medicine's therapeutic regimens for certain conditions. The 12-member panel of experts who weighed the evidence that supported these recommendations, concluded that there is *clear evidence* of acupuncture's efficacy for treating postoperative and chemotherapy nausea and vomiting, the nausea of pregnancy, and postoperative dental pain. For a number of other conditions, the panel concluded that acupuncture may be an effective adjunctive therapy. Specific conditions cited are addiction, stroke rehabilitation, headache, menstrual cramps, tennis elbow, fibromyalgia, low-back pain, carpal tunnel syndrome, and asthma.

The NIH panel of experts also explored what was known about the biological effects of acupuncture. Both human and animal studies were found to demonstrate that acupuncture can cause multiple biological responses. Some examples of these responses include release of opioid peptides during acupuncture and reversal of acupuncture-induced analgesic effects with naloxone administration, activation of the hypothalamus and the pituitary gland function, neurotransmitter and neurohormonal modulation, changes in the regulation of blood flow, and immune function alterations.

Questions regarding specificity of some of these biological changes have arisen because *sham* acupuncture point stimulation was found also sometimes to elicit biological effects. This makes research problematic, especially because nonspecific effects like the quality of the relationship between the clinician and the patient, trust, and expectations also are thought to account for a substantial proportion of acupuncture's effectiveness.

The system of healing for acupuncture is based on the fundamental concepts of Oriental medicine, which are strongly influenced by philosophical and metaphysical world views of Taoism, Confucianism, and Buddhism. The principle concepts of *yin* and *yang* harmony (balance of opposites), and the five phases or elements (represented by nature's elements: fire, earth, metal, water, and wood each of which correspond further to a color, emotion, Yin/Yang organ, sense organ, taste, season, tissue, sound, etc.) and the five substances (Qi, Jing, Shen, Blood, and Body Fluids are used to describe imbalances. Diagnostic procedures include physical examination similar to that in Western medicine but also include examination of pulse patterns in both wrists, tongue appearance, and abdominal and acupoint palpation. Often the practitioner will use herbal medicine, recommend exercise such as Qigong or Tai-Chi, and prescribe diets as adjuncts to acupuncture.

The therapeutic goal of acupuncture is to regulate the *Qi*, or *energy flow*, in the body through activating points on meridian pathways. Each meridian pathway is associated with specific organ systems that can be regulated by the stimulation of points on the skin surface or below. In classical Chinese texts at least 365 points are described, with a possible total of over 2000. In practice, a typical number of points a practitioner has in his or her repertory is 150. The acupuncturist may use needles, either inserted or held on the point, or may apply cupping, moxibustion, massage (*T'ui-na-Chinese, Shiatsu-Japanese),* or laser light to the point. Cupping involves inducing a vacuum in a small glass cup and immediately applying it to the skin surface at a meridian point. *Moxibustion* is a process in which small cones of the herb *Artemisia vulgaris L* (mugwort = *MOXA*) are placed on the needle or acupuncture point and then burned to produce a penetrating heat (thence removed before strong pain). Electrical stimulation also can be applied to inserted needles or to a meridian point directly for therapeutic effects.

Acupuncture needles are very fine (diameter, 0.12 to 0.34 mm) and may elicit a slight prick when inserted but do not, and should not, hurt once they are in place. The number of needles used in a treatment (usually 5 to 15), depth of needle insertion (usually 0.1 to 0.4 inches), diameter of needle used, and length of time the needle is kept in place vary in relation to the condition being treated. These parameters also will vary depending on the style (Chinese, Japanese, French) of acupuncture used; for instance, Japanese acupuncturists use finer needles more superficially. Finally, intradermal needles are used sometimes to engage a meridian point for longer periods of time.

Acupuncture needles have been made of bronze, gold, silver, copper, tin, and bamboo. Today, most acupuncturists use sterile, single-use, stainless-steel needles and are trained in *clean needle technique* guidelines and methods. The investigational label for acupuncture needles was removed in March 1996, when the FDA placed needles under Class 2 regulations, to ensure that reasonable safety would be maintained. A systematic review of the safety of acupuncture by Ernst and White (*American Journal of Medicine*, 2001), found the most common adverse events were needle pain (1–45%), tiredness (2–41%) and bleeding (0.03–38%). Uncommon side effects included a feeling of faintness or syncope (0–0.3% and phnemothorax was rare, occuring twice in nearly a quarter of a million treatments. Consumers who insure that their practitioner has adequate training and who use sterile disposable needles are unlikely to suffer adverse consequences from acupuncture treatments. Possible complications due to needle mishandling include organ puncture, infectious disease transmission, spinal cord injury, contact dermatitis, hematoma, and pain.

At least 300 programs are described nationally that use acupuncture, often combined with supportive counseling. Approximately 10,000 practitioners provide acupuncture to Americans today, of whom over 30% are MD or DO physicians. Licensing of acupuncturists varies from state to state and is designated by LAc, RAc, or CAc titles. It is obvious that anyone who wishes to be treated by acupuncture should be sure that the practitioner has attended an accredited acupuncture program (≥2 years), is licensed or registered in the state, or has passed the National Certification Commission for Acupuncture and Oriental Medicine examination for acupuncture. The American Association of Oriental Medicine has published a referral list of practitioners.

While the AMA has not officially sanctioned acupuncture, over 2000 of the US acupuncturists are MDs. Most feel it is difficult to understand and to accept the invisible energy-path or meridians theory of effectiveness. Many still claim a *placebo effect,* but even this has not held up to scientific testing. Some say that the distraction of the practice explained its efficacy. Most current research seems to indicate that the acupuncture stimulates the release of endorphins, enkephalins, and the natural anti-inflammatory agent, cortisol.

AROMATHERAPY

The basis of this form of therapy is aroma and the biochemical effects derived from the essential volatile oils of plant flowers and fruits. These fragrant extracts, when inhaled, allow patients to relax or bring about relief of pain. They also may induce a mild stimulation.

In most people, it is acknowledged that smell is undoubtedly the most acute of the five senses (at least 10,000 times more than any of the others). These volatile plant essential oils are inhaled and activate receptors in the nasal cavity. These, in turn, induce nerve impulses that travel rapidly from this olfactory bulb to the brain. The olfactory tract is connected directly to the limbic system, which is the control center in the brain for memory, emotions, and sexual arousal.

It has long been known that pleasant odors can mask offensive ones and that this perhaps was the basis for the use of incense in closed places wherever nonbathers congregated. In a like manner, almost all societies sought quiet refuge in pleasant odors and surroundings against the *smelly* world. Thus, in answer to the question "does aroma heal?", one can say that it will ease certain physical maladies such as headaches or colds as well as calm individuals who suffer from emotional irritability and nervousness. Recent studies show a usefulness in depression. The efficacy of aromatherapy in clinical situations has been tested widely in Europe.

Almost everyone acknowledges the powerful nudge of *smell memory* whenever their favorite food, perhaps originally from mother's kitchen, is sensed. Similarly, nearly everyone is repulsed by the odor of anything burning, probably a remnant of primitive instincts alerting one against potential danger.

In recent years, numerous studies have shown the usefulness of inhaled volatile oils to relieve bronchitis and sinusitis (eg, pine, thyme, peppermint, or eucalyptus), as a first-aid measure (eg, lavender for burns or tea tree for infections), and as massage oils to relax tense muscles (eg, rosemary or sage). The use of wintergreen oil is another example of a topically applied oil with a characteristic odor and aspirin-like analgesic qualities (viz Methyl Salicylate).

Aromatherapy long has been known and used in France, where René Gattefosse, a French chemist, coined the word in 1937. His personal experience of being healed after burning his hand and then plunging it into lavender oil to effect a cure led to its use in World War I to combat injuries. Today, many hospitals use essential oils to help relax patients and cleanse the air. Some have used aromas to help reduce the incidence of crime in subways, to increase worker productivity, and to increase students' concentration. World-wide research is being conducted to explain more fully how aromatherapy works, perhaps through the psychoneuroimmunology system, to promote both physical and emotional healing.

Aromatherapy encompasses a wide spectrum of use for essential oils, ranging from environmental fragrancing to body-mind therapy to internal medicine. In France, it is taught in medical schools; the oils are prescribed by a physician, prepared by a pharmacist, and taken internally. In many cases, essential oils (rosemary, mint) are incorporated into wellness programs because they are easy and pleasant to use and often mask malodorous facilities (eg, incontinence-related ammoniacal odors). Aromatherapy holds that pleasant aromas help maintain bodily balance and harmony and promote mental and emotional pleasantness. Most critics from allopathic medicine note the general lack of critical research on efficacy and the many unscientific pronouncements of its advocates. Even holistic practitioners fault aromatherapy because it promotes the use of the volatile oil and not the whole plant.

Finally, it should be cautioned that only very low doses or amounts of volatile oils are used in aromatherapy. Because they do represent the distilled essences of many pounds of flower parts and because they may contain pungent mixtures of terpenes, aldehydes, ketones, and esters, they are potentially powerful chemicals with pharmacological and toxicological effects. These should never be taken orally in a concentrated form. Several flavorful oils (wintergreen, cinnamon, mints) are used in highly diluted forms in mouthwashes, sprays, and the like for their topical antibacterial properties and refreshing taste.

There has recently been published a review summarizing all the randomized controlled trials (RCTs) testing the clinical efficacy of aromatherapy. It was found in twelve clinical trials, that six had no independent replication, and that six related to the relaxing qualities of various aromatic oils used topically in gentle massage. Those investigations suggest that aromatherapy massage does have a mild and transient anxiolytic effect. The authors concluded that while the effects are minimal, they may be of benefit for common patients by enhancing feelings of wellness. There have in recent years been several new tests and articles relating to aromatherapy.

AYURVEDIC MEDICINE

This system of medicine has its roots deep in the Indian philosophy of Asia. It emphasizes the use of a person's physical and mental abilities to reach harmony with the environment. The therapy here is composed of reaching a balance between diet, daily routine, and daily activities. Ayurveda literally means the *knowledge* or *science of life*. Many practice yoga (system or exercises) and meditation as part of Ayurveda. It has been described as an active or assertive program of prevention and can include a wide variety of things, including rising early in the morning, listening to parental advice, displaying consistent daily routine, basing exercise and activities on body type, drinking herbal teas, and having regular bowel movements.

There are many practices associated with Ayurvedic medicine including shirodara (pouring or dripping specially warm and prepared oils [eg, sesame oil] on the forehead for relief of tension and to bring on mental harmony); pulse reading (feeling for wave patterns, or *doshas*), which provides information on body types; taking histories on preference habits and dreams; physical exams of the body's *dhatus*, or tissues, and *srotases*, or passageways (exits of cleansing and elimination); cupping (using cups with a vacuum applied to the back) to lower blood pressure, increase circulation, or relieve muscle pain; sitting in a steam-filled sweatbox to cleanse the body; *panchakarma* (procedures to cleanse the body of accumulated wastes) using herbalized steam, oil massage, nasal flushing, laxatives, and medicated enemas.

Overall, Ayurveda is not a licensed practice in the US, but many health practitioners in related areas (nutritionists, chiropractors) do practice some aspects of it. At least several hundred physicians have trained in the US at Ayurvedic institutes. Basically, Ayurveda protects and sustains the body and does no harm. In India, physicians trained in this area complete a 5 1/2–year program of study, including a hospital residency.

Because Ayurvedic medicine uses nonstandard methods of diagnosis and treatment, conventional Western physicians often find it unsettling. However, those who have been trained in its practices (often Asian ethnic groups) use it to complement their conventional practices. Some have focused their criticism against the Maharishi ayurvedic system because of its perceived self-serving nature and great popularity in the US. Both traditional ayurvedic and Maharishi Ayurvedic therapies are being evaluated clinically at several localities, and one hopes time will reveal the good and bad aspects of the practices.

In 1999, an Ayurvedic college, The Center for Natural Medicine and Prevention, Maharishi University of Management, College of Maharishi Vedic Medicine in Fairfield, IA was granted a NIH/NCCAM Research Center Award to study cardiovascular disease and aging in African Americans. Ayurvedic medicine has been reviewed by the Agency for Healthcare Research and Quality (AHRQ) found on the NCCAM Website's health information page. According to AHRQ's review, the most common conditions for which studies of Ayurvedic therapies have been published were: diabetes mellitus, liver/hepatitis, infectious diseases, hypercholesterolemia, central nervous system disorders, (dementia/depression) and cardiovascular diseases. Herbal therapy was the most common subject published and no studies were found that tested Ayurvedic medicine as a whole system, and almost no studies were found on any other Ayurvedic modalities. The review found evidence to suggest that the single herbs *Coccinia indica,* holy basil, fenugreek, and *Gymnema sylvestre* and the herbal formulas Ayeesh-82 and D-400 have a glucose-lowering effect and deserve further study. For several other herbs, (*C. tamala, Eugenia jambolana* and *Momordica charantia*) less extensive evidence was found.

CHIROPRACTIC

As a result of searching for a uniform method of curing illness, Daniel David Palmer (1845–1913) devised a theory called chiropractic. A Greek word meaning laying of the hands. He based his treatment mainly on the manipulation of the spinal vertebrae. He, along with his son B.J., developed this treatment technique and started the first school in the world to teach chiropractic in Davenport, IA. As his practice gained a foothold, he refined the original basic theory that disease is caused by vertebra pressing on the spinal nerves. These blockages were referred to as subluxations, and he felt that dispatching these quick thrusts or adjustments would restore normal function to muscles, organs, joints, and other tissues.

Chiropractor physicians or practitioners take a complete medical history, perform an examination, and may take x-rays to find problems elated to what is called the vertebral subluxation complex. Attempts are made to locate muscle strength or weaknesses, extent of spinal mobility, skeletal deformities, or bad posture. Some practitioners attempt to evaluate the electrical activity of muscles and nerves, so that a baseline can be obtained to monitor any progress in treatments. If pathologies (fractures, tumors) are located, these are referred to appropriate allopathic practitioners.

The most common adjustment procedures are referred to as high-velocity, low force recoil thrust and/or rotational thrust. In the former procedure, the patient is placed in the prone position on a specially designed segmented table that can be raised or lowered so that the appropriate adjustments can be made. In the latter procedure, the patient is placed so that the upper body is twisted counter to the pelvis. Then, the spine is rotated to its normal limit while the chiropractor uses a short, fast thrust to the spine to realign it.

Today, many chiropractors fall into two groups, those who adhere strictly to Palmer's philosophy of adjustments to get rid of subluxations (straight chiropractors) or those who use the original technique coupled with exercises, treatments involving heat, and nutritional counseling (mixer chiropractors). Many of today's chiropractors treat neuromusculoskeletal ailments of the spine which include, but not limited to, lower back pain, sciatic pain, neck pain, headaches, shoulder pain, golfers and/or tennis elbow, wrist, hand, leg and foot pain.

While some orthodox allopathic practitioners doubt the claims of effectiveness, chiropractic devotees abound, usually swearing that regular medical practice provided no relief for their problems. At one time the AMA labeled chiropractic an unscientific cult, but now they are licensed in all 50 states and throughout Canada. In both countries, treatment is covered by many private health-insurance plans and all similar government agencies. During the 1970s up to the 2000s, chiropractic has moved from being considered unusual and dangerous to a place where it is accepted relatively well by both the lay and medical communities. It now ranks as the third largest primary-care profession in the Western world, with only medicine and dentistry exceeding it.

Some 60,000 licensed chiropractors and 16 accredited schools may be found in the US. They offer a four-year post-graduate curriculum covering much of what is given in the average medical school. Upon graduation, a Doctor of Chiropractic degree is earned. The scope of practice of chiropractic licensure in most states does not include surgery or the prescribing of medication. The basic philosophy of chiropractic is that the body has an innate ability to heal itself.

Numerous articles abound in the medical literature on the positive and negative aspects of chiropractic treatments. A 1996 systematic overview of conservative treatments for neck pain and headache failed to demonstrate convincingly that chiropractic is more effective than other interventions. Another meta-analysis of chiropractic for low back pain published in 1992 suggested that it is effective for acute low back pain. Yet another more recent and rigorous systematic review concluded that, "the available randomised clinical trials provided no convincing evidence of the effectiveness of chiropractic for acute or chronic low back pain." Nonetheless, a substantial number of studies have found chiropractic to be as effective as conventional therapy for various conditions. Certainly more research is indicated and the chiropractic profession is actively engaging in the research process.

HERBALISM

It is well known that herbs have been used in medicine by all cultures from the beginning of time. Almost every modern drug owes its origin to some medicinal plant. Of the numerous potent phytopharmaceuticals that have been used in US medicine, one can cite morphine (opium poppy), digitoxin (foxglove), diosgenin (Mexican yam), atropine (nightshade), colchicine (autumn crocus), quinine (cinchona trees), reserpine (Indian snakeroot), vincristine (periwinkle plant), podophyllin (mayapple), castor oil (castor-oil plant), anthraquinones (cascara), artemesinin (artemisia), taxol (Pacific yew), and the numerous antibiotics.

For centuries, right up to the 19th century, herbs were the major source of drugs and were kept in glass jars or as alcoholic extracts for long shelf-life or convenience of use. While they were put aside with the rapid advances in synthetic organic chemistry of the past 50 years, they still occupy an important place in medicine. For the most part, the reasons for their being left aside in the last 40 years included difficulty in identification and extraction, difficulty in patentability (in the US, products from nature cannot be patented), and abuses in the early 1900s when spurious plant mixtures were sold as cures for everything. [For the latter reason alone, plants have been considered quack cures by the medical establishment and the FDA and efforts in the US generally are aimed at keeping their use at a minimum.] There is little doubt that some reasons for this attitude exist, because modern medicine wishes that all herbals be standardized and show efficacy in the same way that single-entity synthetic drugs do. However, because of costs involved (up to several hundred million dollars) to do this, few companies have an incentive to produce drugs from natural products, patent problems notwithstanding.

So, currently, we are in an era when many herbals in the US (once standardized and common in pharmacies up to the 1960s) are now widely available in health-food stores and offered as *foods* with active ingredients not being appropriately standardized. With the upswing in consumer interest in CAM since the 1960s, high demand has been seen for these, to the extent that health foods and herbals have become a several billion dollar per year business. Part of this has been due to an international rise in the interest in herbals or because many countries never let them go as part of their traditional and cultural medical practices. Similarly, efforts of the NIH, through the cancer-screening program have uncovered numerous leads to potential drugs that currently are being used (eg, camptothecin, taxol).

Phytomedicinals (eg, garlic, ginkgo, ginger) from international traditions are being adopted for use by many Americans and presently are being investigated by medical researchers in the United States. However, Chinese, Ayurveda, and Tibetan herbalists, among others, usually use combinations of herbs in their prescriptions. Combinations of herbs are used by these herbalists because they believe that illness is attributed to an imbalance in the total person (including emotional and spiritual elements) and that an environment inhospitable to disease can be established by combining herbs with specific properties.

A Chinese herbalist would rarely, if ever, use one herb by itself and might include other ingredients such as zoological (eg, insects, reptiles) and mineral derivatives in their prescriptions. Chinese herbalists use four different categories of herbs in their prescriptions. The chief herb(s) support(s) the main therapeutic direction of the formula; the deputy herb(s) assist(s) the chief herb; the assistant or adjunctive herb(s) moderate(s) and support(s) the actions of the chief and deputy herbs; and the envoy herb(s) harmonize(s) and distribute(s) the actions of the other herbs. Chinese herbal medicine is based on a tradition that has developed over thousands of years. It stands as the most experienced of all the herbal *traditions*. Some English translations of Chinese herbal materia medicas and herbal therapeutics are available. While these can be useful to pharmacists, they are often difficult to interpret because plant activities and applications are given in Chinese medical terminology. For example,

herbs may be indicated for their Exterior-resolving, Heat-clearing, Qi-rectifying, or Blood-rectifying properties.

Practitioners of Chinese herbal medicine frequently use acupuncture with herbs, and herbs are taken for periods between acupuncture sessions. A formally trained practitioner would have a degree in Oriental medicine (OMD). Three states in the US, Nevada, New Mexico, and Texas require NCCAOM exams in acupuncture and Chinese herbology for acupuncture licensure (www.nccaom.org/states.html). This site also lists CA as having its own test but no mention is made of herbal medicine being required. Several companies are marketing Chinese herbal combinations in the US that have been derived from ancient recipes. One should be cautious about buying combination products from companies or stores that can not ensure that proper procurement or manufacturing procedures have been practiced in the preparation of the medicine, as there have been many reports in the medical literature of heavy-metal contamination, adulteration with prescription medications, and inclusion of misidentified plant materials.

Concomitantly, many of the crude forms of herbs have made it into this country via the various ethnic connections in the United States (eg, Japan and India on the West Coast and Mexico in the Southwest) and are being used in various cultural groups. So, while the use of herbs is moving rapidly to the mainstream, it behooves pharmacists and consumers to locate reliable information available in books and periodicals, in colleges of pharmacy (scientifically reliable), and in health-food stores (advocacy literature) with the view in mind that appropriate authors and articles in the valid scientific literature be stressed.

The powerful green wave of interest in phytopharmaceuticals (plant medicine) has prompted the FDA to develop labeling requirements for supplements, which include herbs, vitamins, minerals, and amino acids. The labeling requirements are found in the DSHEA, which was published first in September 1977. Under these regulations herbs will be considered dietary supplements, not food or drugs. After March 1999, all herbal products must be labeled with a *Supplement Facts* box. Many high-quality manufacturers of herbs began to include it on their products in 1998. The information on the product label includes nutrient content, health claims, and statements of nutritional support. Ingredients on the market as of October 1994 are *grandfathered*. New ingredients require submission of information to the FDA before marketing, but formal FDA approval is not required before marketing. The FDA published notice of proposed rulemaking for GMPs in February 1997 and will publish a final ruling upon thorough evaluation of the matter.

At least 60 to 100 other herbs that have been used for minor ailments are used in the US and elsewhere, eg, basil, thyme, rosemary, aloe, anise, boneset, buckthorn, cayenne pepper, chamomile, cranberry, echinacea, eucalyptus, evening primrose, feverfew, garlic, ginger, ginkgo, ginseng, goldenseal, hawthorn, juniper, licorice, milk thistle, peppermint, psyllium, senna, valerian, wintergreen, witch hazel, and yarrow. All of these have known active principles and a specific regulatory status in the US and other various countries, eg, GRAS, OTC, Commission E (Germany).

It also should be mentioned that perfectly acceptable non-pharmacologically active herbal teas have established themselves in the US popular drink marketplace. Where once we had only regular tea, there are now numerous varieties (with citrus flavors, cinnamon, fruit flavors), as well as mixtures of lemon tea, ginger tea, wintergreen, peppermint, blueberry, and many others.

As with Chinese medicine, one should be careful of sources, because different species may be used in different countries or may be adulterated accidently or purposefully.

As far as reliable dosage forms are concerned, tinctures (alcoholic extracts) and freeze-dried herbs are usually best. Dried (oven or sunlight) herbs sold in bulk, whole or powdered, or encapsulated forms may lose potency rapidly because of air oxidation.

Table 132-6. Selected Drug Interactions with Herbs

MEDICATION(S)	HERBS WITH POSSIBLE SYNERGISTIC OR ANTAGONISTIC EFFECTS
Anticoagulant and antiplatelet drugs	Alfalfa, astragalus, bilberry, evening primrose oil, garlic, ginger, ginkgo, ginseng, gugulipid, feverfew, scullcap
CNS stimulants	Guarana, kola, ephedra, St John's wort, yohimbe
CNS depressants	Hawthorn, skullcap, valerian
Antidepressants	Ginseng, ephedra, passion flower, St John's wort, yohimbe
Diabetes	Garlic, ginger, ginseng, hawthorn, ephedra, nettle
Hypertension	Devil's claw, ginseng, goldenseal, hawthorn, licorice, ephedra, squill, yohimbe

As far as dosage is concerned, one should start with the lowest recommended amount and work upward. Unless these herbs are standardized, there is little choice to obtain the active dose. Certainly, overdosing with herbs can have deleterious effects. One also should be careful of potential herb-drug interactions. These also can occur, so it is advisable to check with the experts (pharmacists, physicians, pharmacognosists, herbalists) before use. It is likewise imperative to monitor one's reactions, being careful to observe that desired effects are obtained and undesired effects (eg, rash) are avoided.

Many people in the US are turning to herbal medicine to treat their ills, and pharmacists are in a position that requires them to have resources to answer patients' questions and monitor for possible adverse effects. While no one reference is available that covers it all and information regarding drug interactions is especially lacking, there are some good resources available. See the *Bibliography* for suggestions for building a reference library on herbal medicine. The pharmacist has the opportunity to help build the database that is needed to use herbs safely. For many of the most popular herbs used by Americans today, some important drug interactions are known. See Table 132-6 for examples. Herbs without known drug interactions should be treated like any new prescription product that comes on to the market. Here too, pharmacists are called upon to participate in collection and management of drug interactions manifested. Unlike prescription drugs however, with herbal medicine, the patient is more likely to be taking herbs without the support of a conventional medical doctor. This puts the pharmacist in a more direct role with the patient in making sure that herbs taken with conventional prescription drugs are documented and monitored.

Regardless of the potential usefulness of herbal therapy, critics note the widespread availability of spurious data on them via advocacy literature. Even though the DSHEA Act of 1994 delimits OTC herbals from legally labeling them efficacious in treating diseases, much promotional literature is sold (books) or provided free as handouts alongside herbs, on or near the store shelves. Occasionally, dangerous herbs may be recommended, particularly in older books or references. Some *new age* publications promote herbs as having mystical or magical powers. Some also rightly point out that the rapid rise in herbal popularity has made it difficult to list them adequately for efficacy via the usual rigid pharmaceutical standards. Of course, the major reason for this is the cost (often millions of dollars) and lack of ability to patent natural products easily in the United States. Beyond this, it will always remain difficult to test the entire herbal product for the major active ingredient(s), which may take years to identify and characterize adequately. There are more reasons requiring adequately trained health personnel to advise patients on which herbs are safe and which may or may not be potentially useful for various health conditions.

Overall, in herbal therapy it is impossible to define the major active principle(s). Hence the clinical properties of these herbal products may not be known with certainty. This is because the herbs often contain several active components which may vary considerably from batch to batch of the herbal. It certainly is very expensive and time consuming to follow the conventional wisdom of isolation and assay directed identification of active compounds.

Several Asian traditions (eg, Chinese Traditional Medicine, Ayurvedic medicine, etc.) employ complex, often individualized mixtures of many (often 10–20) different herbs in each single prescription. Fortunately, most of the modern herbal products in the US consist of a single herb. Quite a few of these (eg, St. John's wort, *Ginkgo biloba*) have been subjected to a fair number of clinical studies. These have undergone fairly systematic reviews or meta-analyses. Obviously each herbal has to be evaluated on its own merit and experience in any traditional usage. One cannot simply state that all uses are justified, safe and consistently efficacious.

Several other herbal products have uncertain efficacy. A case in point is mistletoe (*Viscum album*) which has been recommended in Europe as a cancer treatment. Its popularity has prompted such use in Australia and in the US. Mistletoe proponents claim that it can arrest or delay tumor progression and improve quality of life. The lectins in the plant have been shown to possess antineoplastic activity. Unfortunately, a systematic review of all eleven controlled clinical trials demonstrated disappointing results. It was revealed that the average methodological quality of the primary studies was rather poor. While the results of most trials showed mistletoe to be favorable, the most vigorous one did not show good efficacy. To quote the authors, they "cannot recommend the use of mistletoe extracts in the treatment of cancer patients with an exception for patients involved in clinical trials." Since this study, several other new investigations have brought the overall conclusion that it is not effective for this purpose

Table 132-7 displays examples of herbal medicinal products for which systematic reviews and meta-analyses have been published. There are found in a text entitled Herbal medicine, a concise overview for professionals (Oxford Butterworth Heinemann Press, 2000.)

Finally, it should be remembered that herbs usually should be used for minor ills only. One should avoid self-medication for serious ailments or injuries. Certainly, the very young or old, pregnant or lactating women, and persons already on certain medications should not take herbal remedies without consulting with their physician.

Many ethnobotanical studies are continuing in the rain forests and elsewhere to ferret out any new potential leads to phytopharmaceuticals. Almost every plant or animal drug has dozens of potentially active constituents, and the potential pharmacological activity of each needs to be evaluated thoroughly. Several recent successes for newer medicines derived from plants via the FDA OTC and prescription drug development route are taxol, artemesinin, calanolide A, etoposide, and *Ginkgo biloba*. Hopefully, some of the CAM practices involving herbs will yield more phytopharmaceuticals in the near future.

HOMEOPATHY

Homeopathy is a system of medicine that has its own principles of practice and pharmacopoeia that differs from both phytopharmacy and conventional medicine. A homeopathic medication is often referred to as a "remedy", but herbalists may also use this term for herbal medications. Thus, the pharmacist must be careful when interpreting literature describing the use of botanical medications to distinguish if an herbal or homeopathic dosage form is being described. While it is difficult to define homeopathy specifically, because of cultural and historical perspectives, one may begin with a description provided by homeopaths:

Homeopathy is a therapeutic method. It clinically applies the Law of Similars (like cures like) and uses medically active substances at weak or infinitesimal doses.

Table 132-7. Examples of Herbal Medicinal Products for which Systematic Reviews and Meta-Analyses have been Published

COMMON NAME OF PLANT	INDICATION	EVIDENCE FOR EFFECTIVENESS
Aloe vera	Various	Poor
Artichoke	Hyperlipoproteinaemia	Poor
Feverfew	Prevention of migraine	Encouraging
Ginger	Nausea/vomiting	Encouraging
Ginkgo biloba	Dementia	Good
Ginkgo biloba	Intermittent claudication	Good
Ginkgo biloba	Tinnitus	Encouraging
Ginseng	Various	Poor
Horsechestnut	Chronic venous insufficiency	Good
Kava	Anxiety	Very good
Mistletoe	Cancer	Poor
Peppermint	Irritable bowel syndrome	Encouraging
St John's wort	Mild/moderate depression	Very good
Valerian	Insomnia	Encouraging

This assessment is based on an overview of systematic reviews. By Ernst (Year 2000)

Homeopaths believe that body is not reduced easily to the sum of its parts; therefore, they assess all the person's physical, mental, and emotional aspects in the course of finding the correct homeopathic medication.

The first basic principle, the *Law of Similars*, is that a substance that causes symptoms in a person may cure an illness that manifests those same symptoms. Hence, a homeopathic medication that mimics disease symptoms can be given to stimulate a person's body to fight against the symptoms depicted by the illness. The second basic principle *(Law of Infinitesimals)* and most controversial is the concept that the lower the concentration of a substance (derived from a botanical, animal, mineral source) in a properly manufactured homeopathic medication, the greater the effectiveness. However, for illnesses of a physical nature low potency (less diluted) homeopathic medications are used while more emotional or psychological-based conditions require the higher potency medications.

Further, even when so diluted that no more drug can be found, homeopaths believe that the preparation still is effective. The father of homeopathy, Hahnemann, taught his followers to use a single medicine at a time. However, in modern times, with the complexity of causes, eg, stress or cellular toxicities, many practitioners employ a pluralistic approach, termed *homeovitics*. Combinations of single homeopathic medications are also available for self-limiting illnesses, eg, colds and flu, seasonal allergies, headaches, and teething, etc., for which most people experience the same symptoms.

Generally, homeopaths found which drugs to prescribe through a process of placebo-controlled trials, which are referred to as *provings*. Guidelines for provings can be found in the current *Homeopathic Pharmacopoeia of the United States* (www.hpus.com/eligibil.html). These data are recorded in homeopathic materia medica texts and repertories. These books give symptoms and the drugs that have been observed to effect cures. For the most part, while these are guidelines, homeopaths emphasize individual uniqueness, and drug regimens must be tailored to individual needs.

Usually practitioners of homeopathy deal with such chronic disorders as allergies, arthritis, asthma, colitis, headaches, high blood pressure, and weight control. Certain deficiencies (anemia), hormonal imbalance, and some infections also are treated. Most practitioners of this field acknowledge the need for antibiotics for severe infections and the importance of conventional treatments for severe injuries or management of emergency situations.

Homeopathy is displaying a rebirth of popularity, even though for several decades it had been predicted that it would almost certainly disappear in the light of modern medicine. It is for this reason that pharmacists and other health professionals should be aware of the current status of this field. Finally, homeopathy is *not* herbal medicine even though both practices use botanical substances.

POPULARITY—Homeopathy reached its peak of popularity in the early 1900s. Today, there is a resurgence of the popularity of this old medical method. The FDA recently referred to a 100% increase in homeopathic drug products. Concern about this rapid influx of homeopathic drug products into the American marketplace led to the issuance in May 1988 of the FDA Compliance Policy Guide 7132.15 entitled *Conditions under Which Homeopathic Drug Products May Be Marketed.*

In December 1988, the Homeopathic Pharmacopoeia Convention of the United States (HPUS) issued the first volume of its *Homeopathic Pharmacopoeia Revision Service (HPRS)*. Along with its allopathic counterpart, the USP, the HPUS was adopted by Congress as an official compendium in 1938. Substances monographed in the HPUS are recognized as official drugs in the current FD&C Act and the *Code of Federal Regulations*. The HPUS updates manufacturing methods, provides guidelines for Rx-OTC status, and publishes monographs for all official homeopathic drug products. The 2000 year edition of the HPUS contains 1286 monographs of individual homeopathic medications.

Today, there are over 3000 recognized practitioners in the US whose practice is mostly homeopathic according to the National Center for Homeopathy in Alexandria, VA. Homeopathy has become a favorite of many dentists and veterinarians and is a integral part of naturopathic medical curriculums.

From 1994 to 1999, homeopathic drug sales were estimated to represent 0.26% of the US drug market and consumer sales increased by $30 million dollars. In the US, there are at least 40 schools although these programs are not yet recognized by the Department of Education as being accredited; however, the Council on Homeopathic Education is currently taking steps to establish professional standards of homeopathic education that will be submitted for accreditation status in the future. Currently, there are four homeopathic journals published in the US (*Homeopathy Today* [National Center for Homeopathy], the *Simillimum* [Homeopathic Academy of Naturopathic Physicians], *The American Homeopath* [North American Society of Homeopaths], *American Journal of Homeopathic Medicine* [American Institute of Homeopathy]).

In the health care systems of many countries around the world homeopathy plays a major role in their health care systems. In France, the Netherlands, Belgium, and Germany an estimated one third of conventional doctors use homeopathy or refer patients to a homeopath. Homeopaths are officially recognized in India and Germany and between 15% and 56% of the European population make use of homeopathy along with conventional treatment for a wide range of illnesses. The English royal family traditionally has been treated homeopathically and is one of its most famous proponents. In the United Kingdom homeopathy has been integrated within the national health care system for almost 50 years and currently has five homeopathy hospitals and a university offering a degree in homeopathy health sciences. In Russia, at least 20% of the medical care is homeopathic. Homeopathy also has a strong following Italy, and South America and traditionally has had a strong following in poorer countries. Because of homeopathy's strength and business success in foreign countries, there are many homeopathic pharmaceutical firms and homeopathic drug products coming into the US.

MODERN HISTORY—At the present time people in Europe (and to some extent here in the United States) who are disillusioned by allopathy have turned again to homeopathy. France and England show a remarkable upturn in homeopathy now under the relatively new umbrella of alternative or complementary medicine. Both French and English homeopaths have developed research centers for *in vitro* and clinical studies of homeopathic medicines. Doing research with homeopathy is complicated. One of the challenges involved with individualizing drug therapy is that many patients with the same chief complaint will required different drugs from a homeopath, based on the etiology and specific symptoms, as well as aspects of the patient's temperament. Therefore, an RCT, which tests a single homeopathic drug for a particular diagnostic category, is likely to fail because that drug will match the symptoms of only a small percentage of patients. In addition, the homeopathic drug must be administered in a potency and dosage schedule likely to be effective in that condition. The correct drug may have no apparent action if the potency is too low (given the individual needs or characteristics of a patient) or given too late to be effective.

Different approaches have been implemented to surmount this obstacle. One approach is to give patients a drug agreed on by two professional homeopaths, rather than a predetermined trial drug. A set of active and placebo drugs for each remedy likely to be effective for the disease state being tested is set up by a pharmacy who selects which agent a patient receives based on a randomization. Another approach involves performing the study on a diagnostic category for which a single homeopathic drug is likely to be effective in which patients are only accepted for the trial if their symptoms matched that of the remedy. Given the need to use the correct potency and dosage regimen for optimal therapeutic results, outcome research provides perhaps the most realistic evidence of homeopathy's effectiveness and reflects the results of homeopathy used in everyday practice by experienced homeopaths.

While there continue to be pro and con articles on the efficacy of homeopathy, two recent articles serve to summarize opposing reviews and difficulties in proof methodology. A meta-analysis of placebo-controlled trials in homeopathy (Linde K *et al,* 1997) reviewed 156 trials and identified 119 that met their inclusion criteria. At least 89 had adequate data for meta-analysis, and two sets of trials were used to assess reproducibility. The two reviewers assumed study quality using two scales and obtained data for information on clinical condition, homeopathy type, dilution, remedy, population, and outcomes. They found, after analysis, that their meta-analysis was *not* compatible with the hypothesis that the clinical effects of homeopathy are due completely to placebo. Further, however, they reported that they found insufficient evidence from their study that homeopathy is clearly efficacious for any single clinical condition. They recommend further research on homeopathy, particularly if it is rigorous and systematic.

A later review (Dean M, 1998) stated some objections to this study; it was felt that the meta-analysis may well have overestimated the positive effects of homeopathy and that the placebo question is not resolved. The authors suggested that different models are needed to answer different questions and that results would be more valid if based on a comprehensive literature search, appropriate classification of primary studies, clear discrimination between clinical effectiveness and placebo questions, more sound and transparent review methods, and a reliable and unconfounded clinical treatment model for testing the ultramolecular hypothesis.

A model for a possible mechanism of action of homeopathic medications is being researched with the premise that each original drug substance, when diluted and succussed in water, stimulates water's capacity to record patterns of energy shifts leading to the formation of a unique icelike crystalline structures in water called by various investigators as calthratos (Anagnostatos 1998) or I_E crystals (Lo and Bonavida 198). As more kinetic energy is added to the system by further succussions, more water molecules are attracted into the pattern, and more information is thus stored in the water. One research team (Anagnostatos 1998) used depolarization thermocurrent and differential scanning calorimetry measurements while another (Lo and Bonavida 1998) had used transmission electron micrography, fluorescence spectrophotometry, and ultraviolet (UV) spectroscopy to detect evidence of the crystalline structures identified. Using nuclear magnetic resonance (NMR) imaging, changes in potentized drug water have also been measured (Smith and Boricke, 1996).

The interested reader can find more detailed information on research discussed in this section and other models that are being investigated to explain a mechanism of action for homeopathic drugs in publications by Bellavite and Signorini and Gray, as well as on the National Center for Homeopathy Web site and the National Center for Complimentary and Alternative Medicine Web site at nccam.nih.gov/health/homeopathy/index.htm.

MEDICINES—Homeopathy uses a wide variety of pharmacologically active natural substances such as plants, animals, zoological specimens, and minerals in its repertoire. Most of these materials are used to prepare *Mother Tinctures* by maceration in alcohol according to conditions strictly defined by the HPUS. Using these tinctures as starting materials, they are subjected to successive dilutions according to the decimal or centesmal scale. Decimal dilutions are based on a 1:10 ratio represented by the Roman numeral X or D, and centesmal based on a 1:100 ratio by the Roman letter C. Hence, a 1X homeopathic dosage is a 10-fold dilution, 2X is a 100-fold dilution, 3X is a 1000-fold dilution, etc. The 1C represents a 100-fold dilution, 2C is a 10,000-fold dilution and 3C is a 1,000,000-fold dilution, etc. Most homeopathic over the counter remedies range from 6X and 6C to 30X and 30C. Professional homeopathic practitioners also use higher potencies of 200C, 1M (equal to 1000C) or higher M potencies in their practice. A dilution that Hahnemann developed in his later years (published in the 6th ed of the Organon), called LM, is made using a complicated procedure which uses trituration and succussion lending to a dilution factor of 1:50,000 of the final product which is commonly dispensed as a liquid. Currently, this potency is not found on the general market as OTC products. This potency is gaining popularity in the US as it allows the homeopathic practitioner to titrate the patient's dose more effectively than with X or C potencies.

It should be mentioned here that according to the laws of chemistry, there is a point at which a substance can be diluted so that no more original substance remains. The limit is referred to as Avogadro's number, which closely corresponds to the homeopathic dosage of 24X or 12 C (or one part in 10^{-24}). Even Hahnemann recognized that in all likelihood, extreme dilutions would not contain a single molecule of the original material. However, homeopaths believe that vigorous shaking (succussion) or pulverizing of a solution between dilutions releases into the solution or diluent a mysterious *essence* or *imprint* or *resonance* of the medicine as discussed previously. This message is purported to be of sufficient magnitude to stimulate the *vital force,* which mitigates illness. In the case of insoluble starting materials, the initial dilutions of the medicine are carried out by trituration (mixing and rubbing together in lactose).

While it is impossible to list all of the hundreds of homeopathic products available, it is instructive to list a few of the common drugs available and why they are used.

Arnica montana—A mountain herb widely used in homeopathic medications for bruises, sports injuries (soft tissue trauma), and aches, pains, and stiffness following excess physical activity.

Allium cepa—A product of the red onion, widely used in the treatment of colds, allergies, and hay fever. It also is suggested for patients who have congestive symptoms (nasal discharge, tearing eyes) in a warm room that improve in a cooler room.

Apis—A preparation made from whole crushed bees, used for inflammations accompanied by burning, stinging, and pain, such as in hives, insect bites, and tonsillitis, particularly when these maladies improve with cold compresses and are worsened by heat.

Arsenicum album—A product made from white arsenic and used for diarrhea or indigestion encountered during travel and for general food poisoning.

Atropa belladonna (Deadly nightshade)—A plant product used in homeopathy for a range of conditions including childhood fevers and throbbing headaches (with accompanying sensitivity to motion, noise, and light).

Rhus toxicodendron (Toxicondendron radicans)—A preparation made from the poison ivy plant, used homeopathically for sprains and strains of the arthritic type in which continued motion lessens the pain and improves range of motion.

Urtica urens—A medicine made from the stinging nettle plant and used for utricaria and pruritus aggravated by cold water.

Homeopathic products initially were once marketed exclusively through pharmacies; however, the current market is mostly in natural or health-food stores and pharmacies that specialize in natural products. This will probably change as pharmacies respond to their customers, and some studies may show effectiveness and safety of homeopathic drug products. A recent request to FDA for reports of adverse reactions to homeopathic drug products produced no substantiated reports. Recent studies and scientific articles in *Lancet, Nature*, the *British Medical Journal*, and other respected medical journals attest to the reliability and safety of homeopathically prepared substances in infinitesimal doses. However, controversy about their efficacy remains.

FDA ATTITUDES—As is well known in medicine, testimonials are easy to come by, but scientific proof is not. The FDA has long recognized homeopathic remedies as drugs, mainly as a way of controlling quality and use. The FDA has not subjected any of these remedies to premarket screenings for safety and effectiveness as with normal or conventional drugs. Homeopathic medications have NDC numbers listed on their packaging and can be designated as OTC or prescription drugs depending on the substance used and the indicated condition it treats.

DRUG SAFETY—Homeopathic drug products are well known for their safety. The current Homeopathic Pharmacopoeial Convention of the United States, which publishes *HPUS* and *HPRS,* has placed a high priority on ensuring the safety of official homeopathic drug products in the marketplace. Recent requests to the FDA for information on homeopathic drug products produced no confirmed reports of side effects or toxicity or adverse reactions regarding homeopathic drug products.

LABELING—Official homeopathic drug products must be identified properly on the label by using *HPUS* after the compendial name, eg, Arnica mont. 12X HPUS. The 12X indicates the potency or degree of dilution. Potencies are either indicated as numeral followed by an X, C, or D, etc. The number indicates the number of dilution steps taken to make the medicine, while the letters indicate the dilution scale used in the process.

OTC homeopathic drug products have no known side effects but must carry all of the customary warnings regarding pregnancy, nursing mothers, and tamper-evident features. Homeopathics are relieved of the obligation to bear an expiration date but otherwise must meet all provisions of the FDA and CFR, although many homeopathic manufacturers put expiration dates on their products. Homeopathics usually bear a legend which recommends that the consumer should discontinue use if the treated condition does not improve within a specified period of time or becomes worse. Homeopathics generally are marketed for conditions that are considered OTC by the FDA Scientific Advisory Panels. On single homeopathic products usually only 2 of the remedy's indications are listed and the consumer and pharmacist should be aware that prod-

uct has other indications as well. The pharmacist or consumer can check a materia medica to find all the indications of a particular homeopathic drug.

HOW HOMEOPATHY MAY WORK—Homeopathics possibly work by stimulating the body's own forces in the direction of cure. They are, therefore, most effective in children, when these forces are most active. Children's remedies are a most successful segment of the homeopathic drug market. One can safely advise a patient that there are no side effects or contraindications for OTC homeopathic drug products, especially if potencies of 12C or 24X are utilized.

Homeopathic drugs do not cover up or mask symptoms; they are claimed to stimulate the reactive processes of the body to overcome and correct the problem. Therefore, they may not provide instantaneous relief. While the patient may start to feel better in a short time, complete lasting relief may not occur for several days. Such relief may be lost by discarding a remedy as ineffective after a few hours. Generally, the longer a symptom has gone untreated, the longer it will take the homeopathic medicine to bring relief.

With a few exceptions, substances prepared according to the specifications of the HPUS, which are stored in a cool, dry place, out of direct sunlight and protected from contamination, retain their therapeutic effectiveness indefinitely.

If the patient fails to respond to an OTC homeopathic remedy in the stated period of time or if the symptoms worsen or new symptoms develop, the patient should discontinue use and seek the advice of a health professional.

HOMEOPATHIC PRESCRIBING—The homeopathic prescriber studies the patient *(takes the case)* in great detail. The aim is to know and treat the whole person, not just a single organ or set of symptoms. The patient's history is, by necessity, more detailed than that taken by an allopathic physician. After a careful consideration of the background and current symptoms, the prescriber usually is able to select the precise drug for the individual.

In some cases, when symptoms are acute (come on suddenly) and self-limiting, the patient can study a case to choose a single remedy or use a combination of three or four remedies that have been proved individually to apply to symptoms similar to those observed. The combination has the advantage of improving the probability of successful prescription; however, it is difficult to determine which individual remedy was responsible for clearing the symptoms. It should be remembered, though, that when the illness has persisted for years and has become chronic, it may take more time to achieve results and these cases are best treated by a experienced homeopath.

The homeopathic medical method is a specialty of many medical doctors, osteopaths, naturopaths, and other complementary and alternative practitioners. Four organizations in the US currently certify practitioners: The American Board of Homeotherapeutics, the Homeopathic Academy of Naturopathic Physicians (DHANP), the Council for Homeopathic Certification (CCH), and the National Board of Homeopathic Examiners (DNBHE). Certification ensures that the practitioner has had documented educational and experiential training and has passed a rigorous board examination. The National Center for Homeopathy has links to all the above organizations and a listing of practitioners on their web site which consumers and pharmacists can use to identify practitioners practicing in their area.

HOMEOPATHY AND ALTERNATIVE HEALTH PRACTICES IN MODERN MEDICINE—The main premise claimed for an increase in interest in homeopathy in the US is the recognition that diseases of the immune system have increased (eg, AIDS), the number of persons suffering from incurable viral conditions is increasing, bacterial infections are becoming resistant to commonly used antibiotics, allergies to foods and other common substances are becoming more prevalent, chronic disability is affecting persons more frequently at younger ages, and mental disease is affecting more and more persons.

There is also reference to futurists who believe that 21st century medicine will have both a *high-tech* and a *high-touch* component, with significantly greater reliance on self-care practices; wellness programs; therapeutic, nutritional, and fitness regimens; and other alternative or complementary practices. Also cited is a greater emphasis on more fully integrated concepts of how a person's psychological state affects various physiological processes. Homeopathy may fit some of these needs.

One major important facet of homeopathy is the extensive use of mineral, plant, and animal substances in therapy. An important scientific question should be one of testing whether high dilutions of these materials can in fact stimulate the immune system or the bodies vital force. While there have been a number of clinical trials in Europe, none have definitely shown a specific effect that can be duplicated under controlled conditions.

If homeopathy is to succeed scientifically, it needs verification. Thus far, it has survived on historical, and perhaps a placebo medicine, basis. There is ample evidence that numerous plant principles can stimulate the immune system. Seminal studies by Wagner and others have shown that there are multitudes of nonmicrobial compounds with potential homoeopathic immunostimulating activity in plants and fungi. He lists dozens of plants that contain immunostimulant alkaloids, terpenoids, phenols, quinones, lipids, lectins, polysaccharides, peptides, and proteins. Skeptics maintain the idea that a substance can cure by releasing energy, which puts homeopathy in the realm of metaphysics.

Another set of recent meta-analysis of 123 randomized or placebo-controlled investigations found that the clinical efficacy of homeopathy are not entirely due to placebo. This study has been criticized for pulling together data relating to all types of indications and remedies. Hence, it may important to assess defined disorders and remedies in order to see what evidence pro or con homeopathy emerges. One homeopathic product which has been studied more than any other is *Arnica montana*, often used for alleviating bruising and trauma. Two independent systematic reviews of all studies of homeopathic arnica gave no conclusive proof that it is clinically more effective than placebo. Similarly, studies of delayed-onset muscle soreness with homeopathic remedies produced no convincing evidence of any greater efficacy than placebo. Again in reviewing studies on alleviating asthma or headache via homeopathy means, there was no proven efficacy. Many homeopaths would claim that their approach can alleviate symptoms related to certain cancers and hence a role in supportive or fallestive care. Thus far, evidence in proving these claims is lacking.

On the brighter side, as discussed before, it is obvious that highly diluted homeopathic preparations are devoid of adverse side effects on drug interactions. However some homeopaths claim that about 20% of all patients may demonstrate an acute clinical deterioration (labelled "homeopathic aggravation") if the optimal remedy has been administered. This obviously is a safety issue for the higher doses remedies. There are also some homeopaths who advise their patients against vaccinations, which itself may be a hazard of neglect in certain situations.

HYDROTHERAPY

Hydrotherapy or balneotherapy or water treatments for medical purposes is probably as old as 'mankind'. As a matter of fact, hot water spas for pain relief (back pain, arthritis, injuries, etc.) were fairly common up to the last century. However, these practises declined in the Western world with the advent of hot showers, effective analgesics and the recent development of disposable "hotpacs" for muscular pain relief. Electric pads for back and arthritic pain have and continue to be used as well, although not strictly considered hydrotherapy but simply heat therapy for local pain relief and in low and upper circulation problems of various kinds. Because of lack of effectiveness over time, unwanted side-effects of drugs and recent interest in exercise coupled with heat hydrotherapy of various kinds has resurfaced in treating some conditions. These include osteoarthritis, rheumatoid arthritis, chronic heart failure, peripheral neuropathy, poor circulation, back pain, consipation, stress and anxiety control and pregnancy and labor. Overall, hydrotherapy does offer a rela-

tively safe and inexpensive and generally effective and useful alternative to the treatment of these and other related conditions. However, several articles have pointed out that the various methodological difficulties and lack of research funding, as well as great variation in types of medical conditions have precluded controlled trials to fully evaluate their true effectiveness.

Many studies which involved exercise regimens in hot-tubs or warm water pools, showed functional gains in patient's conditions. Others showed some possible dangers where some association was seen between the use of a hot tub or whirlpool during early pregnancy and the risk of miscarriage. Another study on the other hand, showed that hydrotherapy is a safe, nonpharmacological alternative for women to use during labor and delivery, infections from the use of commercial hot tubs have been reported. These also is considerable popular interest in colonic hydrotherapy, and one study in England concluded that it is practiced widely in the UK (as well as the US) with an estimated 5600 procedures carried out by different practitioners monthly. Many of these users appear to be well trained and a proportion have medical backgrounds. Clients who are frequently dissatisfied with orthodox medicine seem satisfied enough with the practice of colonic hydrotherapy to undergo regular purging by this method. Few serious effects were noted. Practitioners appear to do well financially in this practice.

HYPNOSIS

Hypnosis is a focused concentration somewhere between sleep or unconsciousness and awareness, usually brought on by a trained hypnotist. The hypnotized person shuts out distractions and pays strong attention to a particular object or subject, emotion, or memory. While once dismissed as quackery, hypnosis has gained new respect as a viable therapeutic modality for treating everything from fear to pain.

Although hypnosis is a current orthodox medicine, caution is still important, and one should have a proper diagnosis before submitting to it. It certainly does not make sense to use it as a possible coverup for some serious underlying medical problem. For this reason, the hypnotist should work with the primary physician, or the primary physician already has certified training in the discipline.

Many states now have local societies of clinical hypnosis. Among the strongest factors supporting hypnosis is the recognition that it can be a valuable adjunct to standard therapy. It has proved to be an excellent technique for managing chronic pain, particularly when standard treatment fails. However, it also is described as a coping mechanism and not a cure.

Hypnosis has proved able to allow persons to gain insight into their experience, which is completely separate from conscious awareness. Hence, it can be viewed as enabling unconscious awareness. It has been applied successfully to dealing with fear of flying, decreasing drug dependence for chronic pain, lowering dosages of analgesics and anesthetics, influencing the immune system, promoting healing, and regulating addictions.

A form of self-hypnosis referred to as *autogenic training* has been used by itself or in conjunction with biofeedback to induce relaxation in individuals. It has been in use for at least 60 years and was introduced by a German psychiatrist, Johannes Schultz. He studied how hypnosis affected the brain, nervous system, and the body and through experimentation was able to develop a series of exercises that led to the ability of patients to self-induce deep relaxation.

Considerable disagreement exists over how autogenic training works, but brain-wave changes and related physiological effects reveal that it somehow modifies the bodily response to acute stress. Perhaps it reduces stimuli from reaching regions of the brain under autonomic control. This form of self-hypnosis has been applied in helping to control anxieties, depression, allergies, and migraine headaches.

A recent review of the medical literature reveals numerous references to the application of hypnosis in several kinds of medical problems. Some of these include the potential usefulness of hypnosis for reducing hot flashes in breast cancer survivors, a systematic review of psychological therapies for nonulcer dsypepsia, psychological treatments for posttraumatic stress disorder, usefulness in treating nocturnal enuresis, management of labor pain during childbirth, reduction of procedural pain and distress in pediatric oncology, childhood habit cough, applying hypnosis in dermatology (eg, urticaria) general management in pain, usefulness in smoking cessation, and helping diminish anxiety and pain. Many of these articles are positive in nature but universally call for more clinically relevant studies. Admittedly, clinical double-blind cross-over studies involving hypnosis maybe difficult or impossible to conduct.

IRIDOLOGY

This is a system that attempts to correlate changes in the texture and color of the iris with various mental and physical illnesses. Practitioners further claim that iridology may identify dietary deficiencies and even locate accumulation of toxic substances in the body. The concept was devised by Ignatz von Peczely, a Hungarian physician of the 19th century. It was further developed by Bernard Jensen, an American chiropractor in the 1950s.

These practitioners divided the iris into six zones or concentric rings that they related to the body's systems. For example, the innermost zone related to the stomach, the next to the intestines, the third to the lymph and blood systems, the fourth to glands and organs, the fifth to skeleton and muscles, and the sixth to skin and elimination.

By attempting to *read* the degrees of light and darkness in the iris, clues could be obtained regarding a patient's health. While conventional medicine does examine the eyes for diagnostic reasons, the iridology procedures have not been widely accepted medically. Most orthodox physicians reject the theory that the iris can be used to give reliable and extensive information about the status of health or disease.

Relatively few legitimate medical articles exist on iridology based on a recent literature review. Almost all place this purported diagnostic procedure in the unproven category. One review by E. Ernst at the University of Exeter, UK., undertook a systematic review of all interpretable tests of the validity of iridology as a diagnostic tool and found it wanting. Three independent literature searches were performed to identify all blinded tests. The data were extracted in a predefined, standardized fashion. They found four case-control studies, the majority of which suggested that iridology is not a valid diagnostic method. They reported that patients and therapists should be discouraged from using this procedure. Several other studies have come to the same conclusions.

MANUAL HEALING— MASSAGE/BODYWORK

Manual healing is synonymous with the terms bodywork and massage. Therapeutic massage methods used by therapists today originate from Eastern and Western traditions. The Eastern traditions can be traced back to the folk medicine of China and the Ayurvedic medicine of India (1000 BCE). Western traditions can be traced back to Hippocrates, the ancient Greek physician, who wrote, "the physician must be experienced in many things, but most assuredly in rubbing. For rubbing can bind a joint that is too loose, and loose a joint that is too tight."

There are three main premises or paradigms that underlie these therapies, namely, relaxation, remediation, and holistic modifications. Relaxation is based on the well-documented human biological need for nonthreatening, nurturing touch, relaxing, pleasurable, sensual (not sexual), and stress-reducing. Remediation encompasses all of the hands-on healing approaches that seek the correction of dysfunction and alleviation of pain. Skills in assessment and evaluation of the patient's condition are applied to relaxation principles. The holistic paradigm considers

enhancing the body/mind/spirit's natural tendency to seek a higher order of functioning and well-being. Although these paradigms are distinct, they often overlap in practice. The massage/bodywork approaches can be divided into five categories:

1. Traditional massage.
2. Contemporary Western massage/bodywork.
3. Structural/functional/movement integration.
4. Oriental bodywork.
5. Energetic bodywork.

Before discussing specific examples of these practices, it is important to understand the regulatory systems that apply to massage/bodywork in the US. The Commission on Massage Therapy Accreditation (COMTA) sets the curriculum requirements for quality education and training of therapists. Minimum requirements include 500 hr of in-class supervised instruction; 100 hr of anatomy and physiology; 300 hr of massage theory, technique, and practice; 100 hr of instruction covering contraindications, business practice, history, ethics, and legalities; and successful completion of first aid and CPR training. In 1992, a national certification program for the broad range of massage/bodywork therapists was established. The National Certification Board for Therapeutic Massage and Bodywork (NCBTMB) awards this certification after the candidate passes the National Certification examination process.

The American Massage Therapy Association (AMTA) supported the creation of the NCBTMB and is the oldest and largest international member-driven organization representing the massage/bodywork therapy profession. It was founded in 1943 and in 1998 had nearly 24,000 members in over 20 different countries, with chapters in all 50 states, the District of Columbia, and the US Virgin Inlands. The COMTA was established to uphold AMTA's principles of ethics and professionalism in all phases of career training and professional development.

Government regulation of massage/bodywork varies widely from state to state; however, states are increasingly awarding licensure to practitioners who successfully complete a COMTA-accredited program and have attained National Certification from the NCBTMB.

A brief review of the current medical literature of the past few years reveals literally hundreds of articles dealing with the successful application of various types of massage in numerous medical conditions including muscle problems, body pain in the elderly, massage as an adjunct to analgesics in cancer treatment, asthma and allergy, dermatitis, labor pain, tennis elbow, depression, excessive exertion, and pediatric conditions. Few if any of these are done in clinical and double blind types of studies.

SPECIFIC THERAPEUTIC CATEGORIES

Traditional Massage

This is a form of bodywork that uses five basic strokes (effleurage/stroking, petrissage/kneading, friction, tapontemont/tapping, and vibration), developed by Johann Metzger of Amsterdam in the late 19th century. In the US this work was merged with Pehr Heinrik Ling along with several adjunct modalities to become the well-known *Swedish massage* of the 20th century. This massage primarily works on the soft tissue and more-superficial layers of the muscles and implements active and passive movements of the joints. It promotes deep relaxation, which reduces tension, stress, spasm, and pain; soothes injured muscles; and stimulates blood and lymphatic circulation.

Sports massage therapy uses Swedish massage techniques as a supplement to the athlete's warmup routine by enhancing circulation and reducing excess muscle and mental tension before competition. Postevent massage is geared toward reducing the trauma that occurs after the cessation of vigorous exercise and can help break up scar tissue and lessen fibrosis and adhesion that develops as a result of injury and immobilization.

The Touch Research Institute at the University of Miami School of Medicine has established formal review of studies supporting the positive effects of massage on anorexia, lower back pain, hypertension, migraine headache, multiple sclerosis, premenstrual symptoms, burns, infant health, and sleep disorders.

Contemporary Western Massage/Bodyworks

This system uses a wide variety of manipulative techniques. The approach is based on the Western sciences of neuromuscular massage, myofacial release, and positional release to relieve somatic pain or dysfunction. They are distinguished from the next category reviewed because emphasis is placed more on the patients' affected part(s) or symptoms rather than on the whole person. Myotherapy is an example of this kind of therapy. Myotherapy (Trigger Point Therapy) is a technique popularized by physical fitness and exercise expert Bonnie Prudden. It was developed by Dr. Janet Travell (Myotherapy, 2 vols.by Travell & Simons). Trigger points are tender or irritable spots in the muscles that produce pain in the body directly or indirectly (referred pain). Muscles pick up trigger points or become *armored* when the body encounters a traumatic event. The practitioner identifies trigger points by taking a detailed history of the patient's birth and early childhood experiences, accidents, operations, occupations, and other life incidents that might have caused physical/emotional distress. After the point(s) is (are) identified and located, pressure and massage are applied to the point and surrounding area, and the patient also is assigned stretching exercises to retrain the muscles. This therapy can be considered for patients who have recurrent pain from injuries in the past, and it can decrease or eliminate the need for analgesics.

Structural/Functional/Movement Integration Practitioners

These practitioners use a wide variety of manipulative techniques. Alexander Technique, Feldenkrais methods, Rubenfeld Synergy Method, Rosen method, and Trager Method feature movement to affect physiological structure and function along with education and awareness to change or enhance physiological functioning. Practices such as Rolfing use pressure or deep friction to alter the muscular and soft tissue structures. Breathing and emotional expression also are used to eliminate tension and change physiological functioning.

Frederick Matthias Alexander (a Shakespearean actor) developed his therapy by correcting periodic losses of his own voice. Experiments conducted by Frank Pierce Jones at Tufts University concluded that Alexander's methods effectively could interrupt or inhibit habitual and learned responses in body posture that interfere with proper body functioning. The practice restores poor or inhibited use of the body contributing to diseases including debilitating curvatures of the spine, rheumatism, arthritis, and a variety of GI and breathing disorders.

Moche Feldenkrais, a Russian-born Israeli physicist, like Alexander, developed his program by healing himself of a sports-related injury. He applied his experience of martial arts, physiology, anatomy, psychology, and neurology to develop two approaches: Awareness through Movement, which implements group awareness, and Functional Integration, which focuses on individualized hands-on touch and movement. The methods are useful for those who have limitations of movement brought on by stress, accidents, back problems, and other physically debilitating diseases. Performers and athletes use Feldenkrais to improve their level of performance and for enhanced personal growth.

The Ilana Rubenfeld (former musician and conductor) technique is a mixture of Alexander, Feldenkrais, and Gestalt psychotherapy. She combined gentle touch coupled with subtle movements and adjustments and emotional relaxation to achieve results. A caring presence that helps clients tap long-repressed memories and express deep feelings helps them release tensions and achieve physical comfort.

In the Rosen method, the practitioner focuses on gentle and deep pressure to relax the client. By paying attention to what is said and felt during the session, the practitioner helps the person deal with any repressed feelings and ultimately brings them relief.

The *light-touch* approach of Milton Trager, MD, in the Trager Psychophysical Integration Technique, pays attention to the subconscious roots of muscle weakness or tension. This school of thought believes that everyone develops mental and physical patterns that may limit movement or lead to pain and tension. Typical sessions include gentle, rhythmic rocking and other movements to teach the client that free movement and relaxation are possible and to promote a sensation of lightness, looseness, and well-being. Simple exercise *(mentastics)* performed at home helps clients to maintain good health through integrated and coordinated movements.

Bioenergetics was developed by psychiatrist Alexander Lowen, who was strongly influenced by Wilhelm Reich, MD, who coined the term *body armor*. The therapy is based on the idea that rigidity and tension in the body (body armor) leads to psychological problems or *vice versa*. Sessions involve a variety of positions that allow detection of tension areas. These then are relieved by a combination of talk therapy, deep breathing, massage, and bioenergetic exercises. When appropriate, the clients are allowed to kick, scream, strike objects, etc, to relieve tension. Hence, persons who react to life's various traumas by developing a tension pattern early in their lives, which leads to physical conditions such as ulcers, colitis, or arthritis, may be helped by this technique.

Rolfing, also called structural integration, was developed by Ida Rolf, who was a PhD biochemist from Columbia University. The technique involves applying deep, hands-on pressure to loosen the fascia (connective tissue surrounding and penetrating the muscles), thereby enabling the body to properly restructure itself. This intense and usually painful bodywork loosens the tightened muscles that serve to form a wall (armoring) protecting the patient from remembering painful life experiences. Some patients use Rolfing as an adjunct to psychotherapy, as a way to work with their bodies as well as their emotions.

Oriental Body Work

This comprises all the different styles of Oriental body work, originally developed throughout Asia. Shiatsu is an example of this kind of therapy. Reflexology is derived from oriental body work philosophy. Shiatsu, or Japanese acupressure, considers the client's symptoms as an expression of the condition of the whole person and focuses on relieving pain and discomfort by applying firm rhythmic pressure (usually with the fingers) on specific points along the meridians for 3 to 10 sec. Meridians are invisible channels of energy flow in the body, and the technique is designed to awaken the meridians. Once the proper energy flow is restored the body can function normally, and tensions and toxicities can be eliminated before they develop into illnesses. Acupressure massage techniques and practices also use rubbing, kneading, percussion, and vibration to improve circulation and to stimulate stale blood and lymph from tissues. Many books are available on self-acupressure techniques for the treatment of a variety of complaints. A popular item found in many stores today, including pharmacies, is a bracelet that fits over the acupressure points for the treatment of nausea.

Reflexology is an American refinement of Oriental wisdom. Dr William Fitzgerald first introduced the concept of Reflexology as Zone Therapy in 1913, and it was further refined in the 1940s by Eunice Ingham. The technique consists of stroking and applying gentle pressure to the feet (sometimes hands) to effect changes in other parts of the body, relax muscles, and stimulate the body's own natural ability to heal itself. Each part of the foot corresponds to different parts of the body. For example, the toes relate to the head and neck, the arch to the internal organs, the ball of the foot to the lungs and chest, and the heel to the pelvic area and sciatic nerve. Theoretically, reflexology stimulates sensory receptors in the nerve fibers of the foot, which produces energy (Indian *prana* or Chinese *qi*) that travels to the spinal cord from which it is dispersed throughout the nervous system. Other theories hold that the procedure relaxes the body and lessens any constricted blood vessels to improve circulation. Reflexology has been applied to the treatment of chronic conditions such as asthma, headaches/migraines, hypertension, constipation, sinus trouble, and stress/anxiety. Elaborate procedures by various practitioners are available, as well as self-reflexology or foot/hand massage.

Energetic Bodywork

This is represented by terms such as biofield, subtle energy, and energetic systems. These therapies help balance energy in the body and engender enhanced health and well-being. Therapeutic Touch and Reiki are well-known practices in America today. While many practitioners use these techniques free-standing, it is more common for therapists to incorporate this work into their massage or bodywork therapy. The idea behind energy work is that a life force flows through the body and psyche and can be redirected by various mind-body techniques. Therapeutic Touch, developed by Dolores Krieger, PhD, RN, and Dora Kunz is a contemporary application of many healing practices, such as visualization, laying on of hands, and aura therapy. With this method there is generally no physical contact between the client and practitioner. Therapists begin by entering a centered or calm state, then they place their hands 2 to 6 inches away from the client and with rhythmic and slow hand motions, detect blockages in the client's energy field. Once the blocked energy flow is detected, practitioners consciously direct or sensitively modulate human energies through their hands and balance any misalignment of the energy flow. The client may experience a range of experiences, from a discharge of previously suppressed emotions to a quiet, gentle sense of well-being. The technique primarily is known for its ability to relieve pain and reduce stress and anxiety. In Dr Krieger's latest book she also suggests that the practice may help reduce headache pain, calm crying babies, ease asthmatic breathing, reduce pain in postoperative patients, and reduce fever and inflammation.

Reiki is a Japanese word derived from *ray (divine wisdom)* and *ke (life force energy)*. The practice also is called Radiance Technique by the American International Reiki Association (AIRA), and this organization collects case studies to document uses and publishes a journal. According to Reiki philosophy, life-force energy is the essential source of direction and nourishment for the cells and organs of the body. Reiki practitioners can be trained to achieve proficiency at different levels. First-degree training or attunement is for physical healing, second degree is for mental healing, and higher levels (up to seven) allow the practitioner to heal at long distance. Imbalances in the living field of energy, or aura, are thought to be the cause of illness. As in Therapeutic Touch the practitioner does not make physical contact with the client. The therapist acts as a medium by channeling life-force energy through his or her hands at 12 positions on the body or within the aura of the client. Reiki proponents promote energy work as a complement to a long list of other traditional and modern health-care systems.

THE MIND-BODY CONNECTION

Almost all practitioners of medicine have acknowledged the importance of the mind and emotions in health. Only relatively recently, however, has research given us a glimpse of the possible mechanisms.

A whole new area of research has arisen that focuses on this, entitled psychoneuroimmunology (PNI). Basically, it is helping uncover the interconnecting neural pathways between the brain, and endocrine and immune systems. For the most part, it is accepted that molecular messages (hormones, etc) allow communication between cells of these organs. Their unique shape or chemical architecture determines their destination and function. They head toward another cell that has receptors (lock) uniquely shaped to accept them. As the agonist reaches the receptor, it binds with it and brings about a particular action.

Specifically, PNI researchers have located white blood cells that make hormones that fit receptors of certain brain cells. This may help the brain sense or detect infective organisms. The same biochemicals also may influence the mind by altering mood and behavior. Similarly, immune functions could be enhanced or depressed by variations in emotions. The major feature of understanding this process is the possibility that we may be able to gain conscious control over our own biochemistry. Already, it is accepted that people can deal with stress in constructive and even preventive ways.

Research has uncovered the fact that under long periods of stress, the adrenal glands increase the production of corticosteroids that are capable of depressing immune function. All of this can lead to a greater degree of vulnerability to illness. Many have learned how to mitigate these stress responses by using biofeedback, meditation, and related techniques.

Some investigators in PNI have speculated that because the brain and immune system possess a type of memory that can recall previous microbial encounters, it may be possible to tap into it as needed. Various procedures such as visualization, guided imagery, and self-hypnosis may allow this kind of conditioning.

In guided imagery, through suggestion or hypnosis, one is led to imagine a warrior leading an attack through the body to kill all of the diseased cells. There are over 15,000 cancer patients who have found solace in various free community wellness programs that have provided services that include new cancer therapies, seminars on nutrition, classes in guided imagery, and support groups. They provide no direct medical services, opting for the belief in fighting disease and freedom from stress through mental vigor and strength.

Some have thought that the well-known *placebo response* may be explained on this basis. Also, the widely recognized phenomenon of the *belief system* of the patient may play a part in the success or failure of medications, treatments, and other procedures used by health practitioners.

All of these may relate to PNI phenomena. All of these certainly recognize that heightened anxiety can lead to hypermotility in the intestine, ulcers, colitis, etc. Similarly, anger can raise blood pressure through the autonomic nervous system. Studies have revealed that depressed people are more vulnerable to physical ills than those who are not depressed.

Epidemiological data show that 5 years after a spouse dies, the death rates for widows and widowers are significantly greater than for those still married. Happily married women have a greater level of certain immune cells than unhappily married women. It has been shown that relaxation, exercise, and overall stress management can increase the number of T cells (up to 10%) in a group of men who have HIV.

A higher percentage of highly stressed than relaxed persons got sick when exposed to cold germs. This also may help to explain why laughter can mitigate an illness such as arthritis. It is part of the concept that positive thinking has medical power, as espoused by writers like Norman Cousins. Physicians in California such as Dr Dean Ornish have received grants from insurance companies to study how heart disease can be reversed through changes in diet and lifestyle (exercise, meditation, etc). Thus far, quite a good response has been elicited by these methods.

Many hospitals now are studying the relaxation response and Buddhist meditation to treat people with chronic pain, stress, and other related disorders. Similarly, transcendental meditation (TM) of the type espoused by Maharishi Mahesh Yogi has shown the ability to diminish stress and hypertension. Research in TM has demonstrated 56% lower hospitalization rates than normal for such treatments as reducing alcohol and drug abuse, diminishing muscle pain, and asthma attacks. Most major cities have programs (TM Centers) in leading hospitals.

In an overall summary of the strengths and weaknesses of mind/body therapies, one must keep in mind that while they generally may improve the quality of life and even prolong it, the right attitude cannot cure everything. Many people who have been taught that they can think themselves well may be prone to feeling like failures if the disease progresses. This can be a dreadful psychological burden. Nevertheless, sufficient successes, in many areas, promote the study and use of these methods.

NATUROPATHY

Natural therapies are the major modalities of general practitioners in the field of naturopathic medicine. There are three accredited colleges and a fourth which has candidate status in this discipline in the United States (Washington, Oregon, Arizona, Connecticut) today. Presently, 13 states (Alaska, Arizona, California, Connecticut, Hawaii, Kansas, Maine, Montana, New Hampshire, Oregon, Utah, Vermont, and Washington), as well as Washington DC, Puerto Rico, the Virgin Islands, and several Canadian provinces, license naturopaths. To obtain licensure, as a naturopathic physician (N.D.), the candidate must graduate from an accredited naturopathic college (4-5 year program) and pass a comprehensive physicians licensing examination (NPLEX). The scope of practice varies according to each state and some states (AZ, WA) even allow licensed naturopathic practitioners to prescribe allopathic medications with some restrictions.

Curricula in the graduate schools of naturopathy include medical training similar to MD's and OD's in the first two years. Botanical medicine, homeopathy, nutritional sciences, laboratory and clinical diagnosis, minor surgery, counseling, traditional Chinese medicine, and various aspects of physical medicine, eg, manipulative therapy, hydrotherapy, and physiotherapy are also included in the curriculum. Bastyr University also offers a program in Naturopathic Midwifery and this college as well as National College of Naturopathic Medicine and University of Bridgeport College of Naturopathic Medicine offers Master of Science in Acupuncture degree. The interested reader can find a chart comparing curricula of naturopathic medical schools with conventional schools of medicine on the American Association of Naturopathic Physicians web page. Generally, the NDs are trained as a primary care providers for all aspects of family health and wellness using diverse techniques that include modern and traditional scientific and empirical methods.

The dynamic philosophy of naturopathic medicine rests on six fundamental principles. The first involves the healing power of nature and a trust in the body's inherent wisdom to heal itself. Identifying and treating the causes of illness is a primary focal point and naturopaths are trained to look beyond the most apparent symptoms to find the underlying cause. Another important philosophy, one that naturopaths share with their allopathic medical colleagues, is to do no harm. Naturopaths strive to use the most natural, least invasive and toxic therapies in their management of patients. Naturopaths firmly believe that they are responsible for educating their patients to achieve and maintain health and spend considerable time to ensure this goal is met. Treating the whole person is a philosophy that allows the naturopath to view the body as an integrated whole in all its physical and spiritual dimensions. Finally, and most importantly, prevention of illness is the ultimate goal of every naturopath. With this philosophical base naturopathic physicians are unique in providing treatment and diagnosis that bridges both allopathic and natural medicine perspectives which combines scientific research with healing powers of nature.

Most allopaths criticize naturopathy as being overly vague with too much emphasis on nutritional counseling and untested herbal remedies. They simply feel that some of these modalities might be useful but really have not been subjected to modern scientific methods of experimentation and peer review. The naturopathic profession has recognized the need to answer these criticisms and over the past several years has increased their efforts to engage in science-based research. A review of NIH/NCCAM grants awarded in the last three years shows Bastyr University in particular has obtained several grants including most recently, a grant (North American Naturopathic Medical Research Consortium) to develop a research agenda for the naturopathic profession.

The American public continues to demonstrate a growing interest in preventing illness, and using more natural means to fight the illnesses they have developed. In the U.S. today there is perhaps no better-trained practitioner to meet his or her needs than a licensed naturopathic physician. The consumer and pharmacist should be cautious however because the term naturopathy is often used in association with practitioners who use natural healing methods and have not received the rigorous training of a licensed naturopathic physician. The consumer or pharmacist should check the credentials of a naturopathic physician before accepting treatment from them and can find listed practitioners in their area by checking the American Association of Naturopathic Physicians web site.

A brief review of the current literature through the Pubmed web site reveals a number of recent artistic dealing with naturopathy. These include its application in the treatment of menopausal symptoms, chronic facial pain, oncologists' and naturopath's nutrition beliefs and practices, the application of speleotherapy (the use of subterranean environments) as a therapeutic measure in the treatment of chronic obstructive airways diseases, various naturopathic procedures in German, Australia, and other countries, naturopathic applications in treating breast cancer, nutraceuticals in the management of cardiovascular diseases, cataract and naturopathic remedies, naturopathy applications in clinical practicing gynecology and obstetrics in Germany, the various naturopathic treatments for ear pain in children, the use of bioactive natural compounds for the treatment of gastrointestinal disorders, and a recent critical appraisal of naturopathy.

OZONE THERAPY

In recent years, various procedures for administering ozone have been promoted as treatments for cancer. So called, "optimal" techniques are applied via the exposure *ex vivo* of up to 300 mL of freshly drawn blood to a gas mixture of ozone and oxygen. This is followed by reinfusing this blood back into the patient. Various modes of action are claimed for support of ozone therapy in these treatments. For the most part, however, very few real rigorous clinical trials of the procedure exist. Among those which have been published, no good evidence of effect have been demonstrated. The proponents have played down any risks, yet some studies suggest serious complications, eg, hepatitis, and at least five fatalities have been reported. It is obvious that this procedure should be avoided until true safety and efficacy can been proven.

CONCLUSION: ATTITUDES AND CAVEATS

Some authors have listed over 50 common illnesses that may be alleviated by various natural therapies. Table 132-8 lists some of these along with their conventional treatments and alternative or complementary approaches to healing. But, before any of these are attempted, it is obviously important to obtain an accurate diagnosis of the problem by a qualified physician. Once this has been done, there should be an understanding of which method(s) may or may not really help, coupled with an involvement in the treatment selected. As discussed before, the belief-system of the patient is paramount in the success of most - management modalities. This is one of the major variables in any clinical double blind studies.

It is also imperative to know what constitutes an emergency problem, for which high-technology conventional medicine most likely will do the most good. These include moving-vehicle

Table 132-8. Various Illnesses and Treatment Options

ILLNESS	COMMON SENSE	CONVENTIONAL MEDICINE	ALTERNATIVE/COMPLEMENTARY MEDICINE
Acne	Keep face and hair clean. Use water-based cosmetics.	OTC agents, eg, benzoyl peroxide, tetracycline, isotretinoin.	Homeopathy, naturopathy, diet, shiatsu, vitamins and minerals
Allergies	Avoid allergic materials, *viz*, foods, plants, animals, drugs, dust, etc. Use air-conditioning dehumidifiers	Antihistamines, cromolyn sodium, steroids	Acupuncture, homeovitics, homeopathy, hypnotherapy, naturopathy, osteopathy, vitamins and minerals
Arthritis	Regular exercise. Warm baths	OTC acetaminophen, aspirin, ibuprofen	Acupuncture, bodywork, homeopathy, homeovitics, hypnotherapy, massage, naturopathy, yoga
Back pain	Practice good posture. Learn how to lift properly. Use firm seat with adequate back support. Rest	Exercises, corset or brace, surgery, drugs for pain relief and muscle relaxation.	Acupuncture, bodywork, chiropractic, homeopathy, massage, yoga
High blood pressure	Diet and exercise. Weight control. Low salt diet.	Antihypertensives (eg, beta-blockers, diuretics, calcium channel blockers)	Acupuncture, homeovitics, massage, naturopathy, shiatsu, yoga

accidents, shootings, explosions, severe trauma, burns, and broken bones and when heatstroke, poisoning, or related dramatic health-threatening events have occurred. Signs include difficult breathing, shortness of breath, severe wheezing, serious persistent diarrhea and/or vomiting, serious bleeding from any source, sudden strong pain in the chest or abdomen, rapid dizziness or vision impairment, loss of speech or slurred speech, and numbness or tingling in the extremities.

One should avoid self-diagnosis for any persistent problem. Often people try to treat bruises superficially when the real problem may be a broken bone. There are also warnings regarding adult's versus children's treatments. Healthy adults do have occasional diarrhea problems, but these can be serious for young children or the elderly, and appropriate treatments are needed. Similarly, pregnant and lactating women are more sensitive to drugs, herbals, certain foods, and certain alternative or complementary therapies. These all must be taken into account.

The Sep-Oct 1998 issue (updated periodically) of the *FDA Consumer* published an article entitled "An FDA Guide to Dietary Supplements," which provides background data on the 1994 DSHEA Act and FDA's current rules of regulation on these. Suggestions are provided for general safety and efficacy concerns; however, these are understandably incomplete because of the general lack of scientific knowledge about many of these products. Hence, it is important for consumers to do their homework on which CAM is appropriate, particularly in concert with an informed health professional. As mentioned earlier in this chapter, a number of important articles appeared during 1998–2004 that cover such areas as doubting the true existence of alternative medicine (Fontanarosa P *et al*); a national survey (US) focusing on the reasons for alternative medicine usage (Astin JA); *JAMA* publishing an entire issue on alternative medicine (Grady D); a new study on the growth of alternative medicine (Eisenberg D *et al*); and a review on cardiovascular herbs (Mashour N *et al*). There is little doubt that alternative medicine studies will continue unabated for some time yet, well into the next decade. A continued growing number of CAM sites on the Web has well attested to this fact and shows little sign of decreasing at this date.

Both conventional and alternative or complementary approaches to healing need to heed the following general guidelines:

Treat the whole person and not just the symptoms.
Promote preventative medicine, healthy lifestyle, and a wellness philosophy.
Gray areas in conventional medicine may be treated better by alternative or complementary medicine management.
Pay more attention to psychosocial and related disorders.
Give attention to personal factors and belief systems.

Most minor ailments are self-limiting. One out of three get relief in whatever they believe in.
Always be an active participant in the healing process (individual volition).
All natural products (plant- or animal-derived drugs) should be identified properly, standardized and analyzed, and appropriately dosed.
Both conventional and alternative or complementary medical practitioners should have open minds and cooperate in mutual research.

Finally, it is imperative that proper advice be given to patients seeking information on complementary and alternative medical therapies. Eisenberg (1998) has provided guidance on this matter by proposing a process for managing alternative therapy (after medical evaluation has been completed and conventional options have been offered), which includes a weekly plan coupled with patient monitoring over a 13-week time course. He also covers legal issues in alternative medicine (liability experience of alternative-care practitioners) and laws governing patient referral and delivery. Elion (1997) has published an article relating to the important issue of CAM and HIV infection. He concludes that the conventional scientific community harbors a significant prejudice against CAM, which limits the responsible evaluation of its safety and efficacy. His proposal here is focused on working toward an open scientific dialog that eventually will help solve such intractable disorders.

WEB SITES

[http://www.altmed.od.nih.gov/nccam]
HerbalGram [http://www.herbalgram.org/abcmission.html]
Herbnet [http://www.herbnet.con/associations.html]
Napralert [http://www.pmmp.uic.edu]
Herb Research Foundation [http://www.herbs.org]
Acupuncture [http://www.acupuncture.com]
Homeopathy [http://www.homeopathyhome.com]
Homeopathie Internationale, click on English icon on homepage [http://www.homeoint.org]
Homeopathic Educational Services [http://www.homeopathic.com]
http://onemedicine.com/aboutus/presummitsurvey.asp
http://www.chiro.org/alt.med_abstracts/index.shtml
http://www.mja.com.au/public/issues/170_02_15010/erns/ernst.html

ORGANIZATIONS

American Association of Oriental Medicine, Catasauqua, PA. Phone: 888-500-7999
American-International Reiki Association, 2201 Wilshire Boulevard, Suite 831, Santa Monica, CA 90403
American Massage Therapy Association, 820 Davis Street, Suite 100, Evanston, IL 60201

International Center for Reiki Training. Web site—http://www.reiki.org

National Certification Board for Therapeutic Massage and Bodywork, 8201 Greensboro Drive, Suite 300, McLean, VA 22102. Web site—http://www.ncbtmb.com

National Certification Commission for Acupuncture and Oriental Medicine, Washington, DC. Phone: 202-232-1404; Web site—http://www.nccaom.org

Touch Research Institute, University of Miami School of Medicine, Dept of Pediatrics, P.O. Box 016820, Miami, FL 33101. Web site—http://www.miami.edu/touch-research

National Center for Homeopathy, 801 N. Fairfax #306, Alexandria, VA 22314. Phone: 703-548-7790. Web site—http://www. homeopathic. org

American Association of Homeopathic Pharmacists, P.O. Box 80178, Valley forge, PA 19484. Phone: 610-735-5124. Web site—http://www.homeopathicpharmacy.org

American Association of Naturopathic Medical Colleges. Web site—http://www.aanmc.org

American Association of Naturopathic Physicians, 3201 New Mexico Avenue, NW Suite 350, Washington, DC 20016. Phone: 1-866-538-2267 (toll free). Web site—http://www.naturopathic.org.

BIBLIOGRAPHY

GENERAL

Anon. (Workshop on Alternative Medicine, Chantilly VA, Sep 14–16, 1992) *Alternative Medicine: Expanding Medical Horizon* [Rpt to NIH on Alternative System Practices in the US]. Washington, DC: US-GPO, 1992.

Astin JA. *JAMA* 1998; 279(19): 1548.

DerMarderosian A. *HerbalGram* 1991; 24: 30.

Dwjer J. *NY Med* 1993; 93(2): 105.

Eisenberg D, et al. *JAMA* 1998; 280(18): 1569.

Eisenberg DM. *N Engl J Med* 1993; 328(4): 246.

Elion R, et al. *Complement Altern Ther Prim Care* 1997; 24(4).

Fontanarosa P, et al. *JAMA* 1998; 280(8):1618-19.

Guiness A. *Family Guide to Natural Medicine.* Pleasantville, NY: Reader's Digest, 1993.

Grady D. *New York Times,* Nov 11: A21, 1998.

Hunter M. *Recent Results Cancer Res* 1991; 121: 293.

Israel R. *The Natural Pharmacy Product Guide.* Denver: Avery Publ, 1991.

Jonas WB. *JAMA* 1998; 280(18): 1616.

Kolcoba KY. *Adv Nurs Sci* 1992; 15(1): 1.

Korr IM. *J Am Osteopath Assoc* 1991: 161.

Myers SS, Benson H. *Behav Med* 1992; 18(1): 5.

Neafsey P. *Mech Ageing Dev* 1990; 51: 1.

Saline C. *Philadelphia Magazine,* May 1993, p 80.

Smolan R. *The Power to Heal. Ancient Arts and Modern Medicine.* New York: Prentice Hall, 1990.

Thacker HL, et al. *Cleve Clin J Med* 1999; 66(4): 213.

Kayne SB. *Complementary Therapies for Pharmacists.* London, UK: Pharmaceutical Press,2002.

Riedlinger J, Montagne M. *JMCP* 1997; 3(1):77–89.

Sampson W. Why NCCAM should be defunded (http://www.quackwatch.org/01quackeryrelatedtopics/nccam.htm l)

AROMATHERAPY

Buchbauer G, et al. *ACS Symp Ser* 1993; 525: 159.

Buckle J. *Crit Care Nurs* 1998; 18(5): 54.

Cawthorn A. *Complement Ther Nurs Midwifery* 1995; 1(4): 118.

de Groat AC, et al. *Contact Dermatitis* 1997; 36(2): 57.

Gattefosse R. *Gattefosse's Aromatherapy.* Essex, UK: CW Daniel Co, 1993.

Gibbons E. *Br J Theatre Nurs* 1998; 8(5): 34.

Haas M, Schnaubelt K. *Int J Aromather* 1993; 4(4): 13.

Howdyshell C. *Hosp J* 1998; 13(3): 69.

Lavabre M. *Aromatherapy Workbook.* Rochester, VT: Healing Arts Press, 1980.

Lis-Balchin M. *J R Soc Health* 1997; 117(5): 324.

Rose J, Earle S., ed. *The World of Aromatherapy.* Berkeley, CA: Frog Ltd, 1996.

Pacific Institute of Aromatherapy, PO Box 903, San Rafael, CA 94915.

Tisserand R. *The Essential Oil Safety Data Manual.* Sussex, England: Tisserand Aromatherapy Inst, 1990.

Welsh C. *Am J Hosp Palliat Care* 1987; 14(1): 42.

Cooke, B., Ernst, E. *Br J Gen Pract* 2000; 50; 493–496.

Tisserand R, Balacs T. *Essential Oil Safety.* Edinburg: Churchill Livingstone, 1995

Keville K. *Aromatherapy: Healing for the Body and Soul.* Lincolnwood, IL: Publications International Ltd., 1998.

MASSAGE

Barlow W. *The Alexader Technique.* New York: Knopf, 1973.

Bogusalawski M. *J Continu Educ Nurs* Oct 1979, p 9.

Bzdek V, Keller E. *Nurs Res* 1986; 35: 101.

Carter M. *Body Reflexology: Healing at Your Fingertips.* West Nyack, NY: Parker, 1986.

Feldendrais M. *Awareness Through Movement.* New York: Harper & Row, 1972. Reprint 1977.

Glick MS. *Intensive Care Nurs* 1986; 2(2):61.

Goats GC. *Br J Sports Med* 1994; 28(3): 153.

Krieger D. *Accepting Your Power to Heal: Personal Practice of Therapeutic Touch.* Santa Fe, NM: Bear, 1993.

Kunz K, Kunz B. *Hand and Foot Reflexology: A Self-Help Guide.* New York: Simon & Schuster, 1987.

Mannheimer JS. *J Rheumatol* 1987; 14(supp 15): 26.

Prudden B. *Myotherapy.* New York: Ballantine Books, 1987.

Ray B. *The Reiki Factor.* St Petersburg, FL: Radiance Association, 1988

Reid GW. *The Complete Book of Rolfing: Using the New Physical Therapy to Restructure Your Life.* New York: Drake, 1978.

Trager M, Guadagno C. *Trager Mentastics: Movement As a Way to Agelessness.* New York: Station Hill Press, 1987.

Hawes MC, Brooks WJ. *Stud Health Technol Inform* 2002; 91;365–368.

DeSousa A. Chatap G. *Presse Med* 33(12 Pt 1): 819–824.

Cassileth BR, Vickers AJ. *J Pain Symptom Manage* 2004; 28(3):244–249.

Balon JW, Mior SA. *Ann Allergy Asthma Immunol* 2004; 93(2 Suppl 1):S55–S60.

Crawford GH, Katz KA, Ellis E, et al. *Arch Dermatol* 2004; 140(8):991–996.

Spencer KM. *Midwifery Today Int Midwife* 2004; 70;11–13, 67.

Wang HL, Keck JF. *Pain Manag Nurs* 2004; 5(2):59–65.

Boisaubert B, Brousse C, Zaoui A, et al. *Ann Readapt Med Phys* 2004; 47(6):346–355.

Hinds T, McEwan I, Perkes J, et al. *Med Sci Sports Exerc* 2004; 36(8):1308–1313.

Hunt V, Randle J, Freshwater D. *Complement Ther Nurs Midwifery* 2004; 10(3):194–201.

Muller-Oerlinghausen B, Berg C, Scherer P, et al. *Dtsch Med Wochenschr* 2004; 129(24): 1363–1368.

Fellowes D, Barnes K, Wilkinson S. *Cochrane Database Syst Rev* 2004(2):CD002287.

NUTRITION/VITAMINS MEDICAL FOODS/NUTRACEUTICALS

Anon. *Dietary Supplement Health and Education Act (DSHEA),* 21 CFR 101.

Anon. *Food Label Use and Nutritional Education Survey.* Washington, DC: FDA Center for Food Safety & Nutrition, 1994.

Anon. *Nat Biotechnol* 1998; 16(1): 8.

Brower V. *Nat Biotechnol.* 1998; 16(8): 728.

Carper J. *Food Pharmacy.* New York: Bantam Books, 1991.

Chavance M, et al. *Int J Vitam Nutr Res* 1993; 63(1): 11.

DerMarderosian A. *Acta Hort* 1993; 332: 81.

Jack DB. *Mol Med Today* 1995; 1(3): 118.

Kien CL. *Curr Prob Pediatr* 1990; 20(7): 349.

Meydani S. *Nutr Rev* 1993; 51(4): 106.

Mindell E. *Earl Mindell's Vitamin Bible.* New York: Warner Books, 1991.

Ibid. Parent's Nutrition Bible. Carson CA: Hay House, 1992.

Ibid. Food as Medicine. New York: Simon & Schuster, 1994.

Ibid. Soy Miracle. New York: Simon & Schuster, 1995.

Mogadem M. *Am J Gastroenterol* 1990; 85(5): 510.

Sinclair S. *Altern Med Rev* 1999; 4(2): 86.

Williams MH. *Ont J Sport Nutr* 1994; 4(2): 120.

Holt S. *Alt Compl Ther* 1995; 1: 414–416.

Lee A, Langer R. *Science* 1983; 221: 1185–1187.

Mathews J. *J Natl Cancer Inst* 1993; 85: 1190–1191.

Miller DR, Anderson GT, Stark JJ, et al. *J Clin Oncol* 1998; 16: 3649–3655.

ACUPUNCTURE AND ORIENTAL MEDICINE

Anon. *Acupuncture. NIH Consensus Development Statement.* 1997; Nov 3–5;15(5).

Bareta JC. *Altern Ther Health Med* 1998; 4(1):22.

Bensky, D, Banolet R. *Chinese Herbal Medicines: Strategies and Formulas.* Seattle, WA: Eastland Press, 1992.

Cai W. *Am J Chin Med* 1992; 20(3–4): 331.

Cui M. *J Tradit Chin Med* 1992; 12(3): 211.

Hsu HY, *et al. Oriental Materia Medica: A Concise Guide.* Long Beach, CA: Oriental Healing Arts Institute, 1986.

Joshi YM. *J Assoc Physicians India* 1992; 40(3): 184.

Kaptchuk TJ. *The Web That Has No Weaver: Understanding Chinese Medicine.* New York: Congdon & Weed, 1983.

Klide AM. *Vet Clin North Am Small Anim Pract* 1992; 22(2): 374.

Maciocia G. *The Foundations of Chinese Medicine.* London: Churchill Livingstone. 1989.

Wu Dz. *Clin Neurol Neurosurg* 1990; 92(1): 13.

Ernst E, White AR. *Am J Med* 2001;110(6):481.

HYDROTHERAPY

Buchman DD. *The Complete Book of Water Therapy.* New York: Dutton, 1979.

Burke DT, *et al. Am J Phys Med Rehabil* 1998; 77(5): 394.

Kurabayashi H, *et al. Physiother Res Int* 1998; 3(4): 284.

Pagliaro P, *et al. J Electromyogr Kinesiol* 1999; 9(2): 141.

Tabacchi MH. *Altern Ther Health Med* 1998; Suppl: 1.

Zamparo P, *et al. Scand J Med Sci Sports* 1998; 8(4): 226.

Bender T, Karagulle Z, Balint GP, *et al. Rheumatol Int* 2004 (Jul 15).

Taffinder NJ, Tan E, Webb IG, *et al. Colorectal Dis* 2004; 6(4):258–260.

Chapuis C, Gardes S, Tasseau F. *Ann Readapt Med Phys* 2004; 47(5): 233–238.

Foley A, Halbert J, Hewitt T, *et al. Ann Rheum Dis* 2003; 62(12):1162–1167.

Alteneder RR, Hornbeck C. *AWHONN Lifelines* 2003; 7(5):445–449.

Hertz-Picciotto I, Howards PP. *Am J Epidemiol* 2003; 158(10):938–940.

Li DK, Janevic T, Odouli R, *et al. Am J Epidemiol* 2003; 158(10): 931–937.

Verhagen AP, Bierma-Zeinstra SM, Cardosa JR, et al. *Cochrane Database Syst Rev* 2003; 4:CD000518.

Taylor S. *Aust Crit Care* 2003; 16(3):111–115.

Barker KL, Dawes H, Hansford P, *et al. Arch Phys Med Rehab* 2003; 84(9):1319–1323.

Cider A, Schaufelberger M, Sunnerhagen KS, *et al. Eur J Heart Failure* 2003; 5(4):527–535.

Stringer M, Hanes L, *Online J Knowl Synth Nurs* 1999; 6(Jan 5):1.

CHIROPRACTIC/BODYWORK

Jordan A, *et al. Spine* 1998; 23(3):311.

Rogers RG. *J Manip Physio Ther* 1997; 20(2):80.

Boline PD, *et al. J Manip Physiol ther* 1995; 18(3):148

Bove G, *et al. JAMA* 1998; 280(18):1576

Nilsson N, *et al. J Manip Physiol Ther* 1997; 20(5):326.

Nelson CR, *et al: J Manip Physiol Ther* 1998; 21(8):511.

Adendelft WJ, *et al. J Manipulative Physiol Ther* 1992; 15(8): 487.

Bergmann TF. *J Manipulative Physiol Ther* 1992; 15(9): 591.

Cafarelli E, Flint F. *Sports Med* 1992; 14(1):

Caplan RL. *J Manipulative Physiol Ther* 1991; 14(1): 46.

Mootz RD, Cohen PA. *J Manipulative Physiol Ther* 1992; 15(7): 471.

Aker PD, Goss AR, Goldsmith CH, Peloso P. *BMJ* 1996; 313: 1291–1926.

Skekelli PG, Adams AH, Chassin MR *et al. Ann Intern Med,* 1992; 117: 590–598

Assendelft WJJ, Koer BW, van der Heiiden GIMG, Bowler I. *J Ther Physiol Ther* 1996;19: 499–507.

NATUROPATHY

American Association of Naturopathic Physicians, 2366 Eastlake Ave, East, Seattle, WA 98102.

Lohff B, *et al. Med Hypotheses* 1998; 51(2): 147.

Moore NG. *Altern Ther Health Med* 1998; 4(4): 25.

Mori K, *et al. J Naturopath Med* 1993; 4: 209.

Cramer EH, Jones P, Keenan NL, *et al. J Altern Complement Med* 2003; 9(4):529–538.

Kronenberg F, Fugh-Berman A. *Ann Intern Med* 2002; 137(10):805–813

Myers CD, White BA, Heft MW. *J Am Dent Assoc* 2002; 133(9):1189–1196.

Novak KL, Chapman GE. *Cancer Pract* 2001; 9(3):141–146.

Mills E, Hollyer T, Saranchuk R, *et al. BMC Med Educ* 2002; 2(1):2.

Beamon S, Falkenbach A, Fainburg G, *et al. Cochrane Database Syst Rev* 2001; (2):CD001741.

Buhring M. *Z Arztl Fortbild Qualitatssich* 1997; 91(7): 674–681.

Kraft K. *Versicherungsmedizin* 2004; 56(2):76–79.

Atwood KC 4th. *MedGenMed* 2004; 6(1):33.

Oppel L. Comment on: *Can Fam Physician* 2003; 49:1481–1487; Author reply: *Can Fam Physician* 2004; 50:223–224.

Fulop JA. *Naturopathic Integr Cancer Ther* 2003; 2(3):276–283.

Atwood KC 4th. *MedGenMed* 1003; 5(4):39.

Herman DD. *Am J Cardiovasc Drugs* 2002; 2(3):173–196.

Banks CN. *Clin Exp Ophthalmol* 2003; 31(6):546.

Cramer EH, Jones P, Keenan NL, *et al. J Altern Complement Med* 2003; 9(4):529–538.

Sarrell EM, Cohen HA, Kahan E. *Pediatrics* 2003; 111(5 Pt 1):e574–579.

Ghosh S, Playford RJ. *Clin Sci (Lond)* 2003; 104(6): 547–556.

OZONE THERAPY

Beck EG, Wasser G, Viebahn-Hänsler R. *Forsch Komplementärmed* 1998; 5: 61–75.

Bocci V. *Forsch Komplementärmed* 1996; 3: 25–33.

Kraft K, Stenkamp E, Vetter H. *Forsch Komplementärmed* 1995; 2: 352.

Diehm C, Rechsteiner HJ. *Wer heilt hat Recht?* Munich: Zuckschwerdt, 1987; 8–39.

Schmitt H. *Zur Ozontherapie.* Med dissertation. University of Marburg, 1982.

Gabriel C. *Lancet* 1996; 347: 541.

HOMEOPATHY

Dean M. *J Altern Complement Med* 1998; 4(4): 389–98.

Fisher P. *Complement Ther Nurs Midwifery* 1995; 1(6): 168.

Gaier H. *Thorsons Encyclopaedic Dictionary of Homeopathy.* London: Harper Collins, 1991.

Hill C, Doyuon F. *Rev Epidemiol Med Soc Sante Publique* 1990; 38(2): 139.

Vallance AK. *J Altern Complement Med* 1998; 4(1): 49.

Riedlinger J. The Academic Perspective on Homeopathy. Journal of the American Institute of Homeopathy. 2001;94(1):44–49.

Riedlinger J, Lennihan. Homeopathic Remedies, Chapter 48. In: Berardi RR. *Handbook of Nonprescription Drugs: An Integrative approach to Self-care,* 13th Ed. Washington, DC: American Pharmaceutical Association, 2002:1101.

Boiron T. Economic perspective on homeopathic pharmacy. Presented at the American Institute of Homeopathy, Homeopathy 2000 Rededication and Celebration. Washington, DC, June 21, 2000.

Jonas WB, Jacobs J. *Healing with Homeopathy: The Doctors' Guide.* New York: Warner Books, 1996:43.

Brinkhaus B, Schindler G, Lindner M, et al. Socioeconomic aspects of homeopathy as seen by decision-takers and service providers in the public health system. In: Ernst E, Hahn EG, eds. *Homeopathy: A Critical Appraisal.* Oxford, England: Butterworth Heinemann, 1998:221.

EECH. A survey of 10 countries where homeopathy is being practiced. The Committee for Foreign Affairs, Norwegian Homeopathic Association, March 1999. Available at: http://www.homeopathy-ecch.org/survey.html. Accessed May 14, 2003.

Belon P, Cumps J, Ennis M, et al. *Inflamm Res* 1999; 48:13:17–18.

Anagnostatos GS, Pissis P, Viras K, et al. Theory and experiments on high dilutions. In: Ernst E, Hahn EG, eds. *Homeopathy: A Critical Appraisal.* Oxford, England: Butterworth Heinemann, 1998: 221.

Lo S-Y, Bonavida B. Proceedings of the First International Symposium on Physical, Chemical and Biological Properties of Stable Water [I$_E$] Clusters. Singapore: World Scientific Publishing, 1998

Smith RB, Boericke GW. *J Am Inst Homeopathy.* 1996;61:197–212.

De Schepper L. *Hahnemann Revisited: A Textbook of Classical Homeopathy for the Professional.* Santa Fe, NM: Full of Life Publishing, 1999.

Kaplan B. *The Homeopathic Conversation The Art of Taking the Case.* London: Natural Medicine Press, 1992

Kayne S. *Homeopathic Pharmacy: An Introduction and Handbook.* Edinburgh: Churchill Kane; 1997.

Skinner S. *Homeopathy in Primary Care.* Gaithersburg, Md: Aspen Publications, 2001.

Vithoulkas G. *The Science of Homeopathy.* New York: Grove Weidenfeld, 1980.

Yasgur J. *Yasgur's Homeopathic Dictionary and Holistic Health Reference.* Greenville, Penn: Van Hoy Publishing, 1998.

Morrison R. *Desktop Companion to Physical Pathology.* Albany, Calif: Hahnemann Clinic Publishing; 1998.

Linde K, Clausius N, Ramirez C, *et al. Lancet* 1997; 350: 834–843

Ernst E, Pittler MH. *Arch Surg* 1998; 133:1187–1190

Lüdtke, R., Wilkins J, Klinische Wirksamkeitsstudien zu Arnica in homöopathischen Zuberetungen. In: Albrecht H, Frühwald M. editors Jahrbuch Band 5 (1998) Karl und Veronica Carstens-stiftung KVC Verlag Essen, 1999; 97–112

Ernst E, Barnes J. *Perfusion* 1998; 11:4–8

Lind K, Jobst KA. *Cochrane Library* 1998;1:1–7

Ernst E, *J Pain Symptom Manage* 1999; 18:353–357

HYPNOSIS

DePascalis V. *Int J Clin Exp Hypn* 1999; 47(2): 117.

Holroyd J. *Ibid* 1996; 44(1): 33. (Review)

Shaw AJ, *et al. Br Dent J* 1996; 180(1): 11. (Review)

Elkins G, Marcus J, Palamara L, *et al. Am J Clin Hypn* 2004; 47(1):29–42.

Soo S, Forman D, Delaney BC, *et al. Am J Gastroenterol* 2004; 99(9):1817–1822.

Robertson M, Humphreys L, Ray R. *J Psychiatr Pract* 2004; 10(2):106–118.

Blum NJ. *Urol Clin North Am* 2004; 31(3):499–507.

Huntley AL, Coon JT, Ernst E. *Am J Obstet Gynecol* 2004; 191(1):36–44.

Cyna AM, McAuliffe GL, Andrew MI. *Br J Anaesth* 2004; 93(4): 505–511.

Arias M. *Neurologia* 2004; 19(7):377–385.

Wild MR, Espie CA. *J Dev Behav Pediatr* 2004; 25(3):207–213.

Soo S, Moayyedi P, Deeks J, *et al. Cochrane Database Syst Rev* 2001; 4: CD002301.

Anbar RD, Hall HR. *J Pediatr* 2004; 144(2):213–217.

Weizman N, Heresco-Levy U, Lichtenberg P. *Harefuah* 2004; 143(1)42–46, 84–85.

Shenefelt PD. *Dermatol Nurs* 2003; 15(6):513–517.

Astin JA. *Clin J Pain* 2004; 20(1):27–32.

Marlow SP, Stoller JK. *Respir Care* 2003; 48(12):1238–1254.

Marcus J, Elkins G, Mott F. *Adv Mind Body Med* 2003; 19(2):24–27.

Mantle F. *Paediatr Nurs* 2003; 15(7):42–45.

Willemsen R. *Rev Belge Med Dent* 2003; 58(2):99–104.

Patterson DR, Jensen MP. *Psychol Bull* 2003; 129(4):495–521.

Buffet M. *Ann Dermatol Venereol* 2003; 130(Spec No 1):IS145–59.

IRIDOLOGY

Ernst E. *Forsch Komplementaremed* 1999; 6(1):7–9.

Bartholomew RE, Likely M. *Aust N Z J Public Health* 1999; 6(1):7–9.

Barrett B. *WMJ* 2001; 100(7):20–26.

Niggemann B, Gruber C. *Allergy* 2004; 59(8):806–808.

PHARMACOGNOSY AND HERBALISM

Bielory L, *et al. J Asthma* 1999; 36(1): 1. (Review)

Blumenthal M. *Popular Herbs in the U.S. Marketplace. Therapeutic Monographs.* (program 067-999-97-058-H04): ACPE, 1997.

Croom E, Walker L. *Drug Topics* Nov 6, 1995, p 84.

DerMardrosian A, Liberti L. *Natural Product Medicine.* Philadelphia: Stickley, 1988.

DerMardrosian A, ed. *The Review of Natural Products, Facts & Comparisons.* St Louis, 1995–present.

DerMardrosian A. *Pharm Hist* 1996; 38(1): 15.

DerMardrosian A. In *Medicinal Plants, Their Role in Health and Biodiversity.* Tomlinson T, Akerele O, eds. Philadelphia: University of Pennsylvania Press, 1998, p 177.

Duke J. *Handbook of Medicinal Herbs.* Boca Raton, FL: CRC Press, 1985.

Dwyer J, Rattray D, eds. *Magic and Medicine of Plants.* Pleasantville, NY: Reader's Digest, 1986.

Evans W. *Trease and Evans' Pharmacognosy,* ed 13. Philadelphia: Saunders, 1989.

Fugh-Berman A. *Prim Care* 1997; 24(4): 889.

Gillespie S. *Pharm Times* Dec 1997, p 53.

Gruber J, Der Marderosian A. *Lab Med* 1996; 27(3): 179.

Kapoor LD. *CRC Handbook of Ayurvedic Medicinal Plants.* Boca Raton, FL: CRC Press, 1990.

McGuffin M. *American Herbal Products Association's Botanical Safety Handbook.* New York: CRC Press, 1997.

Mindell E. *Herb Bible.* New York: Simon & Schuster, 1992.

Mills S, Bone K. *The Essential Guide to Herbal Safety.* St. Louis: Elsevier, 2005.

Murray M. *The Healing Power of Herbs.* Rocklin, CA: Prima Publ, 1995.

Robbers J, *et al. Pharmacognosy and Pharmacobiotechnology.* Philadelphia: Lea & Febiger, 1996.

Schultz N, *et al. Rational Phytotherapy, A Physicians's Guide to Herbal Medicine* (English edition), ed 3. Berlin: Springer Verlag, 1998.

Tyler VE. *Herbs of Choice: The Therapeutic Use of Phytomedicinals.* Binghamton, NY: Haworth Press, 1994.

Tyler VE, Foster S. *The Honest Herbal: A Sensible Guide to the Use of Herbs and Related Remedies,* ed 4. Binghamton, NY: Haworth Press, 1999.

Riedlinger JE, Tan P, Weidong L. *The Annals of Pharmacotherapy.* 2001;35:228–35.

Beuth, J. Clinical relevance of immunoactive mistetoe lectins-1, *Anti-Cancer Drugs,* 1997;8:853–855

Kleiinen, J. Knipschild, P. *Phytomedicine* 1994;1:255–260

Ernst, E. *Eur. J. Cancer* 2001 (in press)

Ernst, E. Herbal medicine A concise overview for professionals. Oxford: Butterworth Heinemann 2000

Bone, K. Standardized extracts - A balanced perspective *Herbalgram* 2001;53:50–55

Linde, K., *et al.* Systematic review of complementary therapies—an annotated bibliography. Part 2: Herbal medicine, BMC Complementary and Alternative Medicine (2001)1:5; http://www.biomedcentral.com/1472-6882/1/5

DEFINITIONS OF TERMS AND SPECIALITIES OF COMPLEMENTARY/ALTERNATIVE MEDICINE

Acupressure—The application of fingertip pressure on different parts of the body to treat specific symptoms or disorders.

Acupuncture—An ancient Chinese healing art that employs fine needles inserted at various locations (ca 2000) in the body to restore *the smooth flow of qi (energy).* Each location along a meridian is associated with specific organs, and every acupuncture point is considered to have a particular therapeutic effect.

Adaptogen—Agent (usually from plants such as ginseng) that helps or adapts the body or protects it from stress.

Allopathy—A system of medical treatment using remedies that produce effects upon the body differing from those produced by disease; now generally used to refer to standard or orthodox medical practice.

Alternative Medicine—Almost any form of therapy that is outside the purview of conventional modern medicine. Examples include homeopathy, chiropractic, and naturopathy. The name suggests a method other than the more conventional treatment.

Aromatherapy—The treatment of diseases through the use of various aromatic herbs, volatile oils, and similar preparations.

Ayurvedic Medicine—A system of medicine derived from an ancient Indian philosophy and the practice of which emphasizes the use of one's physical and mental abilities to achieve harmony with the environment. Therapy consists of maintaining a balance between diet, daily routine, and activities. Foods and herbs are used to modify these three basic life forces (doshas).

Belief-System—The belief or faith that the patient holds as his or her innermost cultural, spiritual, and psychological resource for healing. For modern man the healer may be a physician or priest, for Native Americans and Mexicans it is the *curandero* or *shaman,* for Alaskan Eskimos it is an *angakok,* and so forth. Each concept has its own specific practices that help the person with faith to be healed. The key to faith healing is belief. All healers must understand the patient-belief system, to achieve success in treating most disorders.

Bioenergetics—A combination of psychotherapy with bodywork (a wide range of massage-like therapies). It involves a combination of deep breathing, talk therapy, bioenergetic exercises, and massage to relieve tension and release confined emotions.

Chiropractic—A system of therapies based upon the theory that disease is caused by abnormal function of the nervous system. It attempts to restore normal function by manipulation and treatment of the structures of the body, especially those of the spinal column.

Colonic Irrigation—The flushing of the intestines with water or soapy solutions via a rectal enema for therapeutic, diagnostic, or nutritive purposes.

Complementary Medicine—This term often is used synonymously with alternative medicine. However, this name suggests that the procedures complement those that are considered to be conventional.

Faith Healing—The system or practice of treating disease by religious faith and prayer.

Folk Medicine—Therapy based on different cultures (eg, Indian folk medicine). It usually involves specific cultures, belief in chosen cures, and remedies based on plants, charms, and rituals unique to the specific folk culture.

Health Foods—Foods purported to be produced without the use of chemical fertilizers, herbicides, or pesticide sprays and sold without the addition of chemical additives (preservatives, fillers, artificial flavoring, or coloring agents). Many are claimed to be *natural* (ie, not containing added chemicals) and are purported to be healthier than the usual foods.

Herbs—Plants used for their medicinal, flavor, odor, or nutritive principles.

Holistic Medicine—Therapies that treat the whole person—mind and body—as opposed to just the part of the body where symptoms occur.

Homeopathy—A therapeutic method developed by Dr Samuel Hahnemann in the early 19th century. It clinically applies the law of Similar (like cures like) and uses medically active, potentized substances at weak or infinitesimal doses.

Homeovitics—A contemporary approach to homeopathy. It uses complex, pluralistic formulations in treating chronic diseases associated with toxicities by clearing, cellular detoxification, and regeneration.

Homeostasis—The maintenance of steady states (well or healthy states) in the organism by coordinated physiological processes.

Hypnosis—A state of altered consciousness, sleep, or trance induced artificially in a subject by means of verbal suggestion by the hypnotist or by the subject concentrating upon some object. The degree of hypnotic state may vary from mild, increased suggestibility to that comparable to surgical anesthesia.

Informed Skepticism—A stance in which one is kept informed about a new idea and doesn't necessarily believe it until it is proven scientifically.

Iridology—A diagnostic tool that purports to correlate changes in the color and texture of the iris with mental and physical disorders.

Macrobiotics—A branch of Zen philosophy that advocates a diet in which *Yin* (negative) and *Yang* (positive) foods are balanced to overcome disease and keep in good health. From the Greek roots *makros* (long) and *bios* (life). Certain foods are considered yin (eg, sugar or honey), while others are yang (eg, eggs or meat). Brown rice and other grains are in the middle, and diets are planned around these grains, with a balance of yin and yang foods accompanying them. Some food faddists have taken macrobiotics to an extreme, eliminating all foods except brown rice and thereby suffering nutritional deprivation.

Mind-Body Connection—Currently taken to refer to psychoneuroimmunology (PNI), the study of the connections between the brain and endocrine and immune neural pathway connections.

Naturopathy—Healing by the exclusive use of natural remedies (eg, light, heat, cold, water, vegetables, and fruits). No drugs or surgery are used.

Nutraceutical—The term used by some to promote health and healing through the use of foods as pharmaceuticals (eg, the increased consumption of garlic—allicin; ajoene—for antimicrobial, blood-thinning and cholesterol-lowering properties; or the cabbage-family members—indoles, beta-carbolenes—for anticancer properties, etc).

Natural—A method of healing or a product from natural sources used in medical treatment. A difficult term to define because it can mean different things to different people. See *Organic*.

Orthomolecular Medicine—The treatment or prevention of diseases by altering body concentrations of certain normally occurring substances (eg, vitamins) given in high doses.

Organic or Natural—In alternative medicine this usually means materials obtained from nature without the use of chemical fertilizers or pesticides.

Orthodox—Usually meaning the prevailing and most widely accepted procedures or medications.

Osteopathy—A school of healing that teaches that the body is a vital mechanical organism with coordinate and interdependent structural and functional integrity; the abnormality of either constitutes disease. It uses manipulation but also medicine, surgery, and other specialities.

Placebo Effect—A real physiological effect caused by an inactive drug.

Psychoneuroimmunology (PNI)—The newly emerging field of study that focuses on the series of neural pathways that interconnect the brain, endocrine, and immune systems. These pathways are felt to constitute a communications network between the mind and body that enables them to influence each other.

Quackery—The practice of medicine by a pretender to medical skill. Also referred to as a medical charlatan or quack.

Reflexology (Reflexotherapy)—Treatment by irritation of an area of the body distant from the lesion. It usually consists of using the hands to apply gentle pressure to the feet to ease pain, relieve tension, and restore energy. The term also can be applied to the technique of applying pressure to specific points on the hands and ears.

Risk/Benefit Ratio—Weighing the good effects of a drug or treatment against its bad effects.

Shamanism—In its potential medical applications, this term has been used to describe a way of achieving a kind of spiritual or emotional healing through the practice of ancient rituals (chanting, visualization, drumming). It has been used to treat pain, stress, anxiety, etc.

Shiatsu—A Japanese term for finger pressure or manual massage and pressure to stimulate and free energy pathways within the body.

Tea or Tisane—Any vegetable infusion or decoction used as a beverage.

Therapeutic Massage/Touch—A healing technique that combines traditional laying on of hands with certain Eastern theories of energy flow. It is based on the concept of unblocking *fields of energy* in the body to relieve pain or disease (backache, tension, headache).

Traditional Medicine—A term generally used to describe the native therapies of a certain region (eg, the traditional medicine of China) or the medical traditions of a particular culture.

Wellness—The concept of practicing all the things that keep one well. It involves maintaining good nutrition, exercise, stress-control, and good personal and familial social relationships.

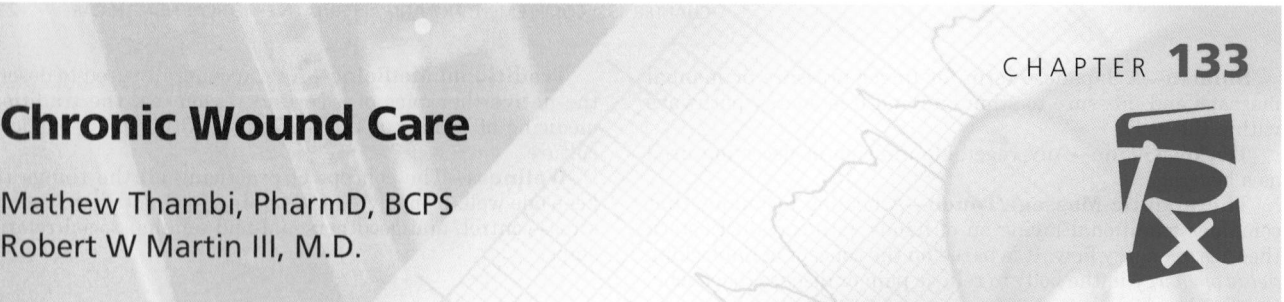

CHAPTER 133

Chronic Wound Care

Mathew Thambi, PharmD, BCPS
Robert W Martin III, M.D.

The prevention and care of wounds are pertinent aspects of caring for patients in diverse settings including the disabled elderly at home, non-ambulatory hospitalized patients, and those who have undergone surgery. Unfortunately, wound care is often neglected in health care, but remains a unique area in which pharmacists can play a vital role in a multidisciplinary approach. Pharmacists can aid in the selection of cost-effective topical and systemic therapies and dressings and help maintain the vigilance that is required for preventing and treating wounds.

The provision of wound care incurs an excessive burden to society, the health care system, and its patients. With respect to chronic skin ulcers, currently it is estimated that there are 1.7 million patients with pressure ulcers, over 1 million with venous ulcers, and 0.6 million with diabetic ulcers.[1,2] Each of these wounds requires a great deal of time and finances to change dressings, apply topical therapies, and provide in-patient surgical and medical therapy as needed. In 1995, the cost of caring for diabetic lower extremity ulcers to the Medicare system accounted for $1.5 billion.[1] Chronic wounds have also been shown to reduce significantly the quality of life in affected patients.[3,4] Despite these figures, there remains a need for increased attention to the subject of wound care by the medical literature and clinicians.[5]

ASSESSMENT

There are several types of wounds (Table 133-1). The most common chronic wounds include pressure, vascular, and diabetic ulcers. Acute wounds include those caused by surgery, trauma, and burns and are beyond the scope of this chapter. Each assessment of a wound should include etiology, location, size, depth, duration, characteristics of surrounding tissue, color, viability, characteristics of any drainage or exudate, pain, and temperature.[6] Follow-up assessments should be performed frequently and systematically to determine the effects of any efforts that have been made. A validated, standardized monitoring form should be used for this purpose rather than attempting to rely on memory or inconsistent descriptions in the patients' charts.[7] Two popular monitoring forms for pressure ulcers can be adapted to monitor other wounds as well. These are the Pressure Sore Status Tool (PSST) and the Pressure Ulcer Scale for Healing (PUSH).[8,9] Photographs of the wound adjacent to a ruler showing its size can also facilitate documentation of the wound healing process.

CHRONIC WOUND MANAGEMENT BY WOUND TYPE

Pressure Ulcers

Pressure ulcers were first described in 1593, by Fabricius Hildanus.[10] A pressure ulcer is an area of localized tissue destruction caused by the compression of the skin over a bony site for a prolonged duration. This compression interferes with tissue blood supply, leading to tissue anoxia and eventually cell death.[11] The incidence of pressure ulcers varies widely from 0.4% to 38.0% in hospitals to 2.2% to 23.9% in long-term care settings, each with an estimated cost of treatment of $500 to $40,000.[12] Pressure ulcers have also been associated with a four-fold increase in mortality in the geriatric population and can lead to pain, osteomyelitis, and sepsis.[13–15]

Because pressure ulcers are often considered preventable wounds, their development is increasingly used as an indicator of the quality of care that a patient receives from an institution.[12,16] Also, although sometimes unfair, the development or worsening of pressure ulcers can be viewed as neglect of the patient.[17] As a result, there is increased litigation related to failure to prevent the development or worsening of pressure ulcers.[18]

Pressure ulcers are classified according to the degree of tissue damage observed (Table 133-2) and can be first noticed in any of these stages. The tissue in the ulcer can range from viable tissue to nonviable or necrotic tissue.[11]

Pressure ulcers develop quickly in the presence of risk factors. Therefore, prevention is directed at avoiding, identifying, and reducing these factors as early as possible. Risk factors include immobility, incontinence, inadequate nutritional intake or absorption, reduced sensory perception, and diminished mental status. The Agency for Healthcare Research and Quality (AHRQ) recommends that a validated risk assessment tool, such as the Braden or Norton Scale, be used to encourage the routine, systematic assessment of these risks.[19]

The following have been adapted from the AHRQ guidelines for the prevention of pressure ulcers and should be implemented immediately in those with any risk factors.[7]

1. Any patient with a risk factor should undergo a daily systematic skin inspection with special attention to areas over bony prominences.
2. Frequent repositioning is a natural and an effective way of preventing pressure ulcers. Patients that are unable to reposition themselves adequately should be repositioned by nursing staff

Table 133-1. Types of Wounds

Traumatic	Autoimmune
Decubitus ulcers	Pyoderma gangrenosum
Self-induced ulcers	Crohn's disease of the skin
Lesch-Nyhan Syndorme	Hematologic
Factitial	Sickle cell disease
Vasuclar	Thalessemia
Venous	Infectious
Stasis ulcers	Bacterial
Postphlebitic syndrome	Erytrhasma
Arterovenous shunts	Malignant pyoderma
Arterial	Ecthyma gangrenosum
Large vessel	of *Pseudomonas* spp
Ateriosclerosis	Anthrax
obliterans	Tularemia
Thromoangitis	Blastomycosis-like
obliterans	pyoderma
Temporal arteritis	(staphylococcal)
Polyarteritis nodosum	Fungal/ Yeast
Small vessel	Blastomycosis
Raynauds	Sporotrichosis
phenomenon	Actinomycosis,
Vasculitis	Nnocardiosis
Wegener's disease	Candida Septicemia
Churg and Strauss	Viral
disease	Herpesvirus infection in
Atherosclerotic emboli	the immunosuppressed
Hypertensive ulcers	patient
Neuropathic ulcers	Protozoan infection
Diabetes (Mal perforans	Leishmaniasis
of the sole)	Amebiasis
Trigeminal Trophic	Mycobacterial infection
syndrome	(especially M. *marinum*)
Spinal cord lesions	Spider bite with necrosis
Neuropathies (variety	(especially brown
of causes)	recluse spider)
Neoplasm	Congenital/ Hereditary
Basal cell cancer	Prolidase deficiency
Squamous cell cancer/	Developmenta
Keratoacanthoma	(congenital) sinus
Melanoma	Aplasia cutis congenital
Cutaneous metastasis	Bart's syndrome
Cutaneous lymphoma	Focal dermal hypoplasia
	Panniculitis

every 2 hours. Physical rehabilitation is also an excellent method of promoting repositioning by the patients themselves.

3. Episodes of incontinence, perspiration, or wound drainage should be cleaned promptly due to the macerating effects of these wastes on healthy skin. Incontinence should also be treated appropriately and moisture absorbing adult diapers can be used to keep the skin dry. The patient's hygiene should be maintained with routine skin cleansing using a mild soap and minimal pressure.

4. Excessively dry skin should be treated with a moisturizer to prevent skin cracking.

5. A nutritional assessment of the patient's caloric, protein, and fat needs is required to help determine his/her risk of ulcer development.

6. To reduce the amount of friction and shear that occurs with movement, protective dressings, such as hydrocolloids, can be used on the elbows and heels. Oftentimes, when patients are sitting or have the heads of their beds elevated, they tend to slide slowly down their chair or bed. This sliding pulls at the skin and can lead to ulcer development. Maintaining the head of the bed as horizontal as possible will reduce these shear forces. Appropriate moving techniques that avoid dragging the patient across the bed linens will also reduce friction and shear injuries.

7. Pillows or foam can be used to relieve pressure on bony prominences from one another or from the bed. This is particularly important on the heels of immobile patients. A pillow under the lower leg can allow suspension of the heel. Foam heel protectors can also be used. For immobile patients at high risk, pressure reducing beds (eg, foam, air, gel, or water) should be used. Doughnut-type devices should not be used because evidence demonstrates that these are more likely to cause ulcers than prevent them.[20]

8. Spasticity, as it occurs in patients with spinal cord injury, causes shearing and increases the risk of pressure-ulcer development. Treatment includes administration of antispasmodics (eg, baclofen, benzodiazepines) to minimize spasms and decrease shearing.[11]

Once a pressure ulcer develops, the presence of necrotic tissue and infection must be managed as discussed under *General Treatment Considerations*. Preventive measures should also be continued to allow for healing of the pressure ulcer and to prevent the development of new pressure ulcers.

Vascular Ulcers

Vascular ulcers are divided into venous and arterial forms. Both forms occur primarily on the extremities, especially the legs.

VENOUS ULCERS

STASIS DERMATITIS/ STASIS ULCERS—Usually, venous ulcers develop over the inner ankle and are often associated with lower extremity edema that worsens with prolonged standing. They usually appear shallow, irregularly shaped, oozing, and bright red with granulation tissue. Unlike pressure and arterial ulcers, necrotic tissue is rarely present. In general, venous ulcers are much less painful than other types of ulcers but can vary widely in the degree of associated pain. The pathophysiology of these ulcers remains controversial but involves venous hypertension and dysfunction of venous valves.[21] This leads to an increased escape of fluid and various substances from capillaries into the interstitial space that eventually leads to tissue breakdown and ulcerations. Risk factors include the presence of obesity, edema, varicose veins, inactive or sedentary life-style, and a history of leg injury, phlebitis, or deep venous thrombosis. Reducing lower extremity edema is a mainstay of treating venous ulcers.[25]

The most noninvasive method of reducing edema is by supine leg elevation. The legs should be raised above the level of the heart several times a day for a total of 2 hours and during sleep. This relieves the swelling and venous hypertension that underlies the development and chronic nature of these ulcers. The time demands of this method make adherence difficult, especially in those patients with jobs that require prolonged periods of standing.[25]

Another option is compression therapy which is considered to be the standard of care for venous stasis ulcers by the United States Food and Drug Administration (FDA) because it has been shown to improve ulcer healing rates. Continued use after healing also prevents re-ulceration.[25] The methods of compres-

Table 133-2. Staging System and Nomenclature of Pressure Ulcers

STAGE	DEFINITION
I	The skin is intact but erythema, warmth, edema, induration, or hardness is present. In individuals with darker skin, erythema may present more discretely as subtle shades of red, blue, or purple.
II	The skin has been broken and may appear as an abrasion, blister, or shallow crater. Also referred to as a superficial ulcer.
III	There is a loss of skin at the wound site that may extend to, but not through, the fascia. This will appear as a deep crater.Also referred to as a partial-thickness ulcer.
IV	Full thickness skin loss with extensive destruction, tissue necrosis, or damage to muscle, bone, adipose, or supporting structures. Also referred to as a full-thickness ulcer.

Adapted from Bergsrtom N, Allman R, Alvarez OM, et al. Treatment of Pressure Ulcers. Clinical Practice Guideline, No. 15. AHRQ Publication No. 95-0652. Rockville, MD: U.S. Department of Health and Human Services, The Agency for Health Care Policy and Research; December 1994.

sion include inelastic, elastic, and sequential therapy.[27] The traditionally used inelastic bandage is the Unna boot, which is a type of cast. Before applying the boot, the local edema can be reduced by wrapping the foot in an elastic Ace bandage. When the swelling has been reduced as much as possible, layers of bandages are applied to the wound and foot. These bandages are moistened with zinc oxide and hardening compounds to harden the bandages into a cast or boot. As the edema begins to recur, the hard boot will compress the tissues at a pressure consistent with the degree of edema. The boot needs to be changed at least weekly or when drainage from the wound penetrates the boot. To keep the boot dry, patients will have to bathe rather than shower. So, if an Unna boot is to be used at home, it is important to determine whether the patient has a bath tub or shower stall. Elastic compression is achieved with elastic stockings that are applied like a sock or with bandages that are wrapped around the affected extremity. There are several types available that vary in size, area of coverage, and degree of compression. These should be washed and replaced as per the manufacturer instructions. Generally, sequential compression is used for prevention of deep vein thrombosis of the lower extremities. However, it is also used to reduce edema and heal chronic venous ulcers. It consists of a sleeve that is placed around the affected extremity that inflates in a sequential manner starting at the ankle and ending at the upper leg. Significant peripheral arterial disease is a contraindication to any type of compression therapy as this will worsen blood supply to already deficient tissues. Compression therapy can also exacerbate severe congestive heart failure by increasing preload pressures. Despite compression therapy, 30–60% of venous ulcers remain unhealed.[26–28]

An oral drug that has been studied for the treatment of venous ulcers is pentoxifylline. Pentoxifylline inhibits neutrophil adhesion, reduces the viscosity of blood by increasing the flexibility of erythrocytes, and has weak fibrinolytic activity. The largest randomized, placebo-controlled study to date included 200 subjects with "pure" venous ulcers that were confirmed to have venous disease without significant arterial disease.[29] Patients were treated until complete healing occurred or for 24 weeks, whichever happened first. The intervention consisted of pentoxifylline 400 mg by mouth three times daily or an identical placebo with both groups receiving compression therapy. Complete healing occurred in 64% of subjects receiving pentoxifylline and 53% of those receiving placebo. This difference was not statistically significant, but this could have been due to a lack of power.[30] Other, smaller trials yielded conflicting results. Therefore, a systematic review was performed to combine these results.[31] When only the outcome of "complete healing" was used, the relative risk of healing was significantly higher for the pentoxifylline treated group at 1.30 (CI 1.10–1.54). Side effects were uncommon and included gastrointestinal disturbances, dizziness, and headache. Pentoxifylline can be considered a safe and effective adjunct to compression therapy. Although cost-effectiveness studies are still required, its current role should be for chronic venous ulcers that fail to heal with compression therapy alone. The dose is 400 mg three times a day with meals. If gastrointestinal disturbances develop, the dose can be reduced to twice daily, although this may not be as effective. Pentoxifylline can increase levels of theophylline so theophylline levels should be closely monitored when these agents are taken together.[33]

ARTERIAL ULCERS, SMALL VESSEL ULCERS

ATHEROSCLEROSIS—Ischemic ulcers occur most often in elderly patients suffering from hyperlipidemia or diabetes mellitus. They are usually the result of atherosclerotic occlusion of arterial vessels in which cholesterol-containing plaques rupture and occlude vessels.[34] Even with excellent local care, frequently, an ischemic ulcer will not heal until surgical revascularization is accomplished.

Color duplex scanning of the arterial system or diagnostic arteriography may be necessary to define the underlying arterial abnormality. Angioplasty is the treatment of choice because bypass grafting in patients with ulcers carries an increased risk of wound or graft infection. For patients in whom angioplasty is not possible, some form of bypass operation, preferably using the saphenous vein, should be attempted.[35]

SMALL VESSEL VASCULITIS—The most common causes of vasculitic ulcers are rheumatoid arthritis, systemic lupus, and polyarteritis nodosa. The blood dyscrasias that most commonly lead to leg ulceration are sickle cell disease, thalassemia, thrombocythemia, and polycythemia rubra vera.[36]

HYPERTENSIVE ULCERS—Hypertensive ischemia due to high vascular resistance from arteriolar sclerosis results in interference with the compensatory relaxation that would normally occur distal to arterial narrowing resulting in poor tissue perfusion and subsequent ulcer formation. Clinically, a painful, lateral lower calf/ankle ulcer results in elderly women.[37]

Neuropathic Ulcers

DIABETIC FOOT ULCERS—Foot wounds are the most common cause of hospitalization for patients with diabetes.[38] A total of 15% of those with diabetes will develop a lower extremity ulcer at some time in their lives with 14–24% of them ultimately requiring an amputation.[39] Once diabetic foot ulcers develop, it can be very difficult for them to heal due to angiopathy, neuropathy, and immunopathy that frequently exist in these patients. Unfortunately, many of these ulcers progress toward the need for amputation. It is thought that relatively simple and inexpensive measures for ulcer prevention can reduce amputation rates by as much as 85%.[40]

As with pressure ulcers, it is important to determine first which diabetics are at higher risk for lower-extremity ulcers. Because foot ulcers precede most amputations in diabetics, the risk factors for foot ulcers are considered to be the same as those for leg amputations.[39,41]

The American Diabetes Association (ADA) stratifies patients with diabetes into high- and low-risk groups for diabetic foot ulcers. The presence of any of the following risk factors will place this patient type into the high risk group: loss of protective sensation (neuropathy), evidence of increased plantar pressure, limited joint mobility, peripheral vascular disease, current or past foot ulcer, bony deformity, or amputation. Those that are without any of these risk factors are classified as being at low risk. The ADA recommends that all patients with diabetes have a comprehensive annual examination of their feet along with extensive patient education. Those in the high-risk groups should be seen by a clinician every 3–6 months for the characteristic(s) that placed them at high risk.[39]

The following methods of preventing foot ulcers should be considered for all patients with diabetes.[39]

1. Lower extremity neuropathy is one of the most important predictors of ulcer formation and amputation.[42] Tight glycemic control has been shown to delay and reduce neuropathy significantly and should be attempted when appropriate.[43]
2. If neuropathy is present, plantar pressure should be reduced as much as possible with the use of shoes with cushioned soles or inserts and adequate room for the toes.
3. If bony deformities are present, such as bunions or Charcot foot, therapeutic footwear should be fitted by an expert.
4. Thickened, painful, mycotic, or ingrown toenails should be treated by a podiatrist.
5. Callus formation can increase plantar pressure and lead to ulcer formation. The use of shoes with cushioned soles or inserts can help prevent their formation. If significant calluses are present under the forefoot, debridement by a specialist can help relieve plantar pressure.
6. The risk of peripheral vascular disease can be reduced by the same methods of risk prevention as for cardiovascular disease (eg, smoking cessation, exercise, healthy diet, lipid management).

7. Patients with significant peripheral vascular disease should be seen by a vascular surgeon for possible medical, surgical, or radiographic intervention.
8. Skin should be kept supple with emollients, but these products should not be applied between the toes for fear of tissue breakdown.
9. Tinea pedis should be treated appropriately.
10. All patients should be educated on proper diabetic foot self-care (Table 133-3).

TRIGEMINAL TROPHIC SYNDROME—Trigeminal trophic syndrome is a rare complication of sensory denervation of the fifth cranial nerve caused by infarction, degeneration, tumor, or artificial destruction resulting in neurotrophic ulcerations of the nose and paranasal areas in elderly, mentally impaired women. Affected individuals usually have a prior history of trigeminal neuralgia and subsequent therapeutic intervention. There is a latent period of weeks to years between the initial trigeminal injury and the subsequent development of ulceration. The severity of the ulcer is directly proportional to the degree of analgesia in the corresponding area. Management is often unsuccessful. The use of protective devices, transcutaneous electrical stimulation, antibiotics, surgical repair, ipsilateral cervical sympathectomy, ionizing irradiation, analgesics, antihistamines, nerve blockade, iontophoresis have given variable results.[44,45]

Hematologic Ulcers

Patients with red blood cell membrane disorders or hemoglobinopathies (eg, sickle cell disease) have blood flow abnormalities due to erythrocyte sludging and resultant vascular occlusion and ulceration in 50–75% of patients with sickle cell disease.[46] Clinically, sickle cell leg ulcers occur as unilateral "punched out" medial malleoli ulceration in the second and third decades. Following healing of cutaneous ulcers, the tissue scarring impairs blood supply to the skin promoting ischemia, sickling, and recurrent ulceration with persistence for months to years. Management involves folate and zinc supplementation, hyperbaric oxygen therapy, or exchange transfusions.

Autoimmune Ulcers

PYODERMA GANGRENOSUM—Pyoderma gangrenosum is an autoimmune disease resulting in rapidly progressive ulcers. These begin as an innocuous pustule on a red base or as

Table 133-3. Patient Education on the Prevention of Diabetic Foot Ulcers

1. Understand that damage that can cause foot ulcers may not be felt.
2. Maintain good foot hygiene by washing feet daily and drying them well.
3. Trim toenails regularly and file rough edges.
4. Do not soak feet for prolonged periods of time. This can lead to maceration of skin and increase susceptibility to damage.
5. Use skin moisturizers to avoid dryness and cracking of the skin; however, moisturizers should not routinely be used between the toes.
6. Select well-fitted socks and shoes and inspect shoes for foreign objects or irregularities before placing them on.
7. Avoid foot trauma by wearing proper footwear at all times.
8. Do not attempt to warm feet in hot water or next to radiators or space heaters.
9. Inspect feet daily including the plantar aspects and between the toes. Those unable to examine the soles of their feet should be taught how to use a mirror to do this. If loss of vision is significant, inspect feet by touch or ideally, have a caregiver visually inspect them.
10. Consult medical care in the presence of maceration, fissures, erythema, or edema.

a red nodule rapidly (in a few days) enlarging to an ulcer with a liquefying center without eschar formation, a purple undermined boggy border, which may be covered by hemorrhagic blisters, and a peripheral red border. The lesions occur most commonly on the legs, although they may develop on virtually any part of the body. Approximately one-half of these patients will have an associated chronic inflammatory disease, such as rheumatoid arthritis, inflammatory bowel disease, chronic active hepatitis, sarcoid, a leukemia, myelofibrosis, or gammopathy. Systemic steroids are the mainstay of therapy and must be instituted rapidly and in very high doses. Other therapy that has been reported to be effective includes dapsone, cyclophosphamide, topical cromolyn sodium, minocycline intralesional steroids, clofazimine and cyclosporine.[47] Concomitant gentle debridement by daily whirlpool baths and silver sulfadiazine dressings are appropriate.

Congenital/Hereditary Syndromes with Ulceration of Skin

HYPOGONADISM—Hypogonadism secondary to pituitary abnormalities (ie, diabetes insipidus) or chromosomal defects (ie, Klinefelter's syndrome) has been associated with recurrent lower leg ulcerations.[48,49]

PROLIDASE DEFICIENCY—Prolidase deficiency is an autosomal recessive disease that results in distinct facial characteristics (ie, low hair line, frontal bossing, far apart eyes, narrow eyelid openings, tiny eyes, saddle nose, thick lips and high-arched palate), deafness, hyperextensible joints, protruding abdomen, mental retardation, short stature, and splenomegaly. Multiple, recurrent, chronic leg ulcers are a common finding. Prolidase deficiency should be suspected in patients who develop leg ulcerations at an early age and who have a family history of leg ulcers.[50]

LESCH-NYHAN SYNDROME—Lesch-Nyhan syndrome is a sex-linked recessive disorder characterized by aggressive self-mutilating behavior, apparent mental retardation, and spastic cerebral palsy. Following the eruption of teeth, the patients begin to bite themselves. Partial or total destruction of peri-oral tissues, particularly the lower lip, results. Partial or complete amputation of the fingers, nose, and tongue may also occur.[51] Decreased red blood cell hypoxanthine-guanine phosphoribosyltransferase activity confirms the diagnosis.

Neoplastic Ulcers

A variety of neoplasms can affect the skin. The possibility of malignancy, particularly in ulcers that do not heal after adequate treatment, should always be borne in mind. The most common malignancies are basal cell carcinoma, squamous cell carcinoma, and melanoma.[35] Although any site can be potentially affected, exposure of the extremities to the sun is commonly involved. The lesion presents as an asymptomatic ulcer with raised edges above the skin level. Pigmentation may indicate a melanoma. Raised pearly borders with overlying telangiectasias suggest basal cell carcinoma. A biopsy of the border of any non-healing ulcer should be obtained to rule out malignancy.

GENERAL TREATMENT CONSIDERATIONS

Although improving, evidence for therapies promoting wound healing or treating wound infections have been lacking. In 2001, the FDA Wound Healing Clinical Focus Group published "guidance" for future trials of new products in this field. An important aspect of this document was its description of appropriate outcomes for clinical trials. The document suggested that complete wound closure should be the primary endpoint of most clinical trials investigating a product's ability to improve wound healing.[52]

Wounds with Necrotic Tissue

For reasons beyond the scope of this chapter, the tissues within several types of wounds can begin to die. These include pressure, diabetic foot, and vascular ulcers along with surgical and traumatic wounds. Eventually, the necrotic tissue can dry into black, hard, mummified tissue, called *eschar*, or moisten into a yellow, gray, or green, malodorous, stringy tissue, called *slough*. The presence of this necrotic tissue impedes the clinician's ability to assess the wound and can hinder the healing process significantly. It also provides a medium for bacterial growth that can spread infection to healthy adjacent tissues of the skin, bone, and blood. Ideally, for healing to progress and infection to be prevented, this dead tissue should be removed from the wound bed without damaging the underlying healthy tissue. This process of removal is called debridement. Debridement is the mainstay of managing chronic pressure, diabetic foot, and arterial ulcers and many non-healing surgical and traumatic wounds.[53]

There are several methods of debridement: sharp, mechanical, enzymatic, and autolytic. Methods that selectively remove devitalized tissue without affecting healthy tissue are preferred over nonselective techniques. Other criteria for selection include the desired speed of debridement, degree of associated pain, quantity of exudate, presence of infection, and cost.[54]

Sharp debridement should be performed by an experienced clinician in accordance to state practice laws. Sharp debridement involves the use of a scalpel or scissors to remove necrotic tissue. It is the fastest method of debridement and the method of choice when there is an urgent need to remove a source of infection (eg, advancing cellulites, sepsis).[54] A drawback of sharp debridement is the significant degree of pain it can cause. The associated pain can also limit the amount of necrotic tissue that can be removed before the pain becomes unbearable. When planning sharp debridement, especially at the bedside, clinicians should administer pain medications and allow sufficient time for the onset of pain relief before debridement is attempted. An agent with a fast onset and time-honored effectiveness is intravenous morphine. Usually, its duration of action lasts long enough to cover the painful post-debridement period. The dose will depend on the patient's degree of pain, prior opiate use, and level of tolerance. Repeated doses should be given as needed during the procedure. Sharp debridement should be used with caution in patients who are receiving an anticoagulant or have hemophilia.

Mechanical debridement of devitalized tissue is performed with wet-to-dry dressings, whirlpool, or pulsed lavage. The wet-to-dry dressings consist of applying wet gauze primary dressings to the wound and securing it in place with a dry secondary dressing for about 8 hours. After this time, the dressings are pulled from the wound along with the tissue that has dried and adhered to it. This can be a very painful process for patients and premedication as described for sharp debridement is required unless significant loss of sensation is present. It may be tempting to wet the dressing before removal but this will defeat the purpose of the dressing because the tissue will no longer be removed along with the dressing. Whirlpool debridement involves submerging the wounded anatomy in a whirlpool bath. This method combines soaking, mechanical debridement (from the water pressure), and heat to loosen and remove the tissue. Further, the heat is thought to promote blood flow to the wound to improve healing and reduce infection. This method is nonselective, time-consuming, and may increase the risk of waterborne infections with *Pseudomonas aeruginosa*.[55] Pulsed lavage involves irrigating the wound with pressurized water from a variety of devices including irrigation syringes, squeeze bottles, and shower heads. The pressure should be between 4 and 15 psi to effectively remove devitalized tissue while minimizing harm

to healthy tissue.[19] All methods of mechanical debridement are nonselective and can remove healthy, healing tissue along with dead tissue. For this reason, these should be used only when attempting to remove infected tissue.

Enzymatic debriding ointments break down proteins, fibrin, elastin, and collagen within necrotic tissues. This helps to loosen and separate the devitalized tissue from the base of the wound for easier removal. This method is usually slower than sharp or mechanical debridement, but is selective for removing devitalized tissue. Enzymatic ointments can be applied as often as the dressing needs to be changed, generally once or twice a day.[56–58] When used for hard eschar, the eschar should be cross-hatched or scored with a scalpel before the agent is applied to allow deeper penetration of the enzymatic ointment. Despite this technique, enzymatic ointments do not work as well for hard eschar. The active ingredients of commercially available products in the US include papain, urea, and collagenase marketed in various combinations: papain and urea; papain, urea, and chlorophyllin; and collagenase (Table 133-4). For some products, chlorophyllin is added to reduce inflammation and odor. All of these agents, and even combination of agents, were developed in response to the great need for debriding agents during World War II with the first published study in 1940 by Glasser.[59,60] Unfortunately, no large, placebo-controlled clinical trials have been published on these agents to allow objective evaluation of their safety and effectiveness.[61] Patients should be warned that a transient burning sensation can occur with the application of these agents.

Autolytic debridement is a method of debridement that involves the application of an occlusive, moisture retentive dressing that takes advantage of the body's own enzymes to break down devitalized tissue. There are over 100 of these dressings available. To relieve confusion, these have been broadly subcategorized as transparent films, foams, hydrogels, hydrocolloids, alginates, and collagens (Table 133-5). Unfortunately, occlusive dressings are usually referred to in practice by their brand names, so it is important to know the brand names of each type used at one's institution (Table 133-6). These dressings keep wound fluid within the wound allowing the macrophages and neutrophils to digest necrotic tissue. In addition, these cover and protect the wound from bacteria and trauma. This tends to take the longest of the various methods of debridement. However, it is selective, non-invasive, painless, and less labor intensive than other methods. The dressing can also be left in place for several days as long as there is no leakage of wound fluid or infection. After the dressing is removed, the wound should be irrigated with normal saline to remove the liquefied, devitalized slough before the new dressing is applied. The disadvantages of this method include the time to achieve a clean wound, the associated foul odor, and unpleasant appearance of the slough when the dressing is removed. This malodorous slough is often mistaken as pus or infection, causing clinicians or patients sometimes to abandon this method prematurely. These dressings are also more expensive than traditional gauze dressings.

Some general considerations before selecting a dressing should be made as outlined by AHCPR guidelines. First, most wounds should be kept continuously moist. Wet-to-dry dressings with gauze are not considered moisture retaining dressings and

Table 133-4. Enzymatic Debriding Ointments

PRODUCTS	BRAND NAMES	COMPANY
Collagenase	Santyl	Smith & Nephew, Inc.
Papain-Urea	Accuzyme	Healthpoint
	Ethezyme	Ethex
	Kovia	Stratus Pharmaceuticals
Papain-Urea-Chlorophyllin	Panafil-Panafil-White	Healthpoint Healthpoint
	Ziox	Stratus Pharmaceuticals

Table 133-5. General Characteristics of Wound Dressing by Category

	GAUZE	HYDROGELS	POLYURETHANE FOAMS	HYDROCOLLOIDS	ALGINATES	TRANSPARENT FILMS	COLLAGENS
Properties	• Permeable • Use for wet-to-dry mechanical debridement • Absorbent	• Available as a gel or impregnated dressing or sheet • Primarily composed of water • Some types are absorptive • Semi-permeable • Semi-occlusive	• Permeable to vapor • Semi-occlusive	• Impermeable to vapor • Occlusive • Forms a moist gel as it absorbs exudate • Waterproof	• Forms a moist gel when in contact with the wound • Very absorbent	• One side is adhesive • Impermeable to liquid • Permeable to vapor	• Derived from animal sources
Indications	• Moderate to heavy drainage • Infected wounds • As secondary dressings • As packing for tunneled wounds or sinuses	• Dry wounds • Stage II to IV pressure ulcers • Wounds with exposed bone, muscle, or tendon	• Mild to moderate drainage • Stage I to IV pressure ulcers • Deep cavity wounds	• Thin hydrocolloids: dry to light drainage • Thick hydrocolloids: moderate to heavy drainage • Stage I to IV pressure ulcers	• Heavy drainage • Wounds with exposed bone or tendon	• Dry to mild drainage • Stage I pressure ulcers • Lacerations • As secondary dressings • Prophylaxis for areas of high friction / shear forces	• Heavy drainage • Stage IV ulcers
Advantages	• Can be used with infected wounds	• Keep dry wounds moist • Non-irritating upon removal	• Absorptive • Easy to apply and remove • Conforms to the contour of the anatomy	• Self-adhesive • Absorbent • Minimal irritation upon removal • Conforms to the contours of the anatomy	• Permeable • Non-occlusive • Highly absorbent • Conforms to the contours of the anatomy	• Allows visibility of the wound without removal • Reduces infection rates	• Promotes deposition of collagen and granulation tissue
Disadvantages	• Can damage healthy tissue and cause pain upon removal	• Most require secondary dressings	• Require secondary dressings	• Can only be used for smaller wounds in which one piece can cover	• Require secondary dressings to secure • Can be drying if low volume of drainage present	• Not absorbent • Have the potential of causing skin tears if removed improperly	• High cost • Current evidence does not show benefit over hydrocolloids for stage II and III pressure ulcers
Contraindications	• Do not use for healthy, granulating wounds • Wounds with exposed bone or tendon		• Wounds with exposed muscle, tendon, or bone		• Dry eschar	• Fragile skin	• Allergy to bovine products

Data from Lyder CH. Pressure ulcer prevention and management. *JAMA* 2003; 289(2):223; Wound Care Information Network. Available at: http://www.medicaledu.com. Accessed July 23, 2003; Helfman T, Ovington L, Falanga V. Occlusive dressing and wound healing. *Clin Dermatol* 1994;12:121; Fleck CA. Wound care dressings. *Extended Care Product News* 2002; 6;4–7.

Table 133-6. Trade Names of Occlusive Dressings

TRANSPARENT FILMS	COMPANY	HYDROCOLLOIDS	COMPANY
Acu-Derm	Acme United	CombiDerm ACD	Convatec
Bioclusive	Johnson & Johnson	Comfeel Ulcer Care Dressing	Coloplast Inc
Blister Film	Tyco Healthcare / Kendall	Cutinova Hydro	Beiersdorf Inc
CarraFilm	Carrington	Duoderm	Convatec
Hi / Moist Transparent	Catalina Biomedical	Exuderm	Medline
Omniderm	Doak	Hydrapad	Beiersdorf Inc
Opsite	Smith & Nephew United	Hydrocol	Bertek
Polyskin II	Tyco Healthcare / Kendall	Intact	Baxter Healthcare
SureSite	Medline Industries	Intrasite Wound Dressing	Smith & Nephew, Inc.
Tegaderm	3M	J & J Ulcer Dressing	Johnson & Johnson
Transite Exudate Transfer Film	Smith & Nephew United	Orahesive	Convatec
Transparent Adhesive	Baxter Healthcare	Replicare	Smith & Nephew
Uniflex	Smith & Nephew United	Restore Wound Care Dressing	Hollister Inc
Vari / Moist Modifiable	Catalina Biomedical	SignaDress Sterile	Convatec
Visi Derm II by Medline	WTS	Sween-A-Peel	Sween Corporation
		Tegasorb Ulcer Dressing	3M
FOAMS	**COMPANY**	Triad	Coloplast
Allevyn Hydrophilic Polymer	Smith & Nephew United	Ultec	Tyco Healthcare / Kendall
Biopatch	Beiersdorf	**CALCIUM ALGINATES**	**COMPANY**
Cutinova Plus Foam Gel Film	Beiersdorf	Algisite M	Smith & Nephew
Epi-Lock Synthetic	Calgon Vestal	Algosteril	Johnson & Johnson
Flexzan	Convatec	Curasorb	Tyco Healthcare / Kendall
Hydrasorb	Convatec	Fibracol Collagen	Johnson & Johnson
Lyofoam	Ferris	Kaltostat	Convatec
Mitraflex Dressing with Adhesive	Calgon Vestal	Sorbsan Absorbent	Dow B. Hickam
		Tegagen HI	3M
GELS AND HYDROGELS	**COMPANY**	Ultec Pro	Tyco Healthcare / Kendall
Biolex Wound Gel	Catalina Biomedical	**COLLAGENS**	**COMPANY**
Carrasyn	Carrington	Fibracol Plus	Johnson & Johnson
Carrington Wound Dressing Gel	Carrington	Promogran	Johnson & Johnson
Clearsite by NDM	WTS	**SILVER DRESSINGS**	**COMPANY**
Elasto-Gel	Southwest Tech	Arglaes Film and Powder	Medline Industries
Flexderm	Dow B. Hickam	SilvaSorb Sustained Release	
Intrasite Gel Hydrogel	Smith & Nephew	Super Absorbent	
Nu-Gel	Johnson & Johnson	Acticoat	Smith & Nephew
Replicare hydrocolloid	Smith & Nephew	**ODOR ABSORBERS**	**COMPANY**
Restore	Hollister	Actisorb Plus	Johnson & Johnson
Saf-Gel	Convatec	Carboflex	Convatec
2nd Skin Dressing	Spenso	Carbonet	Smith & Nephew
SoloSite	Smith & Nephew		
Tegagel	3M		
TenderWet	Medline Industries, Inc.		
TransiGel	Smith & Nephew		
Vigilon	Bard Home Health		

Data from Postsurgical wound care. U.S. Pharmacist Continuing Education. January, 2002; and Wound Care Information Network. Available at: http://www.medicaledu.com. Accessed July 23, 2003.

act by mechanical debridement rather than autolytic.[62] Second, studies do not demonstrate any significant differences among various non-gauze dressings in clinical outcomes.[19,63–65] Clinical judgment should be used to select them (see Table 133-5). Third, the dressing should keep the tissue surrounding the wound dry to avoid maceration. Wounds with excess exudate should be dressed with absorptive dressings to prevent "spilling over." Fourth, dressings should be easy to apply and should remain in place once applied. Fifth, wounds that track or tunnel into tissues causing cavities should be packed with dressings to avoid premature closure and abscess formation.[19]

If autolytic debridement is selected as a method of debridement, the specific dressing category should be based on the stage of the ulcer, amount of drainage (ie, exudate), presence of infection, and cost (see Table 133-5). For wounds that generate copious amounts of exudate, a highly absorbent dressing should be used including thick hydrocolloids or alginates. For mild to moderately draining wounds, hydrocolloid, hydrogel or foam dressings can be used. Dry or minimally draining, superficial wounds, can be dressed with transparent film or thin hydrocolloid dressings. For wounds that extend to underlying tissues, such as muscle, tendon, or bone, it is important to prevent desiccation of these tissues with a dressing, such as a hydrogel,

that will assuredly maintain a moist wound environment. Although collagen dressings are generally the most expensive type, they have not been proven to be superior. Each dressing is different and once a general category is selected, product information and cost of individual dressings within the selected category should be compared.

Another method of debridement is the application of sterile maggots, or *Lucilia sericata*, to the wound that will selectively digest necrotic tissue. Their benefits have been anecdotally published; it may be the fastest method of debridement after that of the scalpel. The main disadvantages are the high cost and the sensation felt by the movement of the maggots.[66,67]

Infection

All open wounds are colonized by bacteria from the surrounding environment. The presence of foul odor, purulence, or surrounding cellulitis are strong indicators of infection and should be treated with antibiotics. Appropriate systemic antibiotics should be used for immunocompromised or diabetic patients or patients that have cellulitis or systemic signs of infection (eg, fever, leukocytosis, tachycardia, hypotension). Otherwise, infections that are localized can be treated with topical antibiotics. In addition, infected wounds should be debrided of necrotic tissues that serve as reservoirs for bacterial growth. As described earlier, debridement can be accomplished by mechanical means except when associated with advancing cellulitis or sepsis when sharp debridement should be performed.

When obvious signs of infection are not present, the distinction between colonization and infection is difficult and controversial. Culturing swabs of an open wound is not recommended because this may represent superficial bacteria that are not invading the tissues. Also, the presence of slough in the wound can mimic that of purulent, infected tissue making it difficult to determine visually whether infection is present. To address this problem, recommendations are based on the principle that the greater the quantity of bacteria within the wound, the more likely the bacteria are to invade tissues and inhibit wound healing. The AHCPR recommends that if topical, broad-spectrum antibiotics (ie, silver sulfadiazine, triple antibiotic ointment) fail to reduce exudate or improve healing, quantitative cultures of a soft tissue biopsy should be performed. A quantitative culture with a bacterial count greater than 100,000 (10^5) organisms per gram of tissue (or mL of exudate) was defined as being sufficient enough to inhibit wound healing.[68] These wounds should probably be treated with systemic antibiotics. The AHCPR also recommends avoiding the use of topical antiseptics to reduce the bacterial burden of a wound due to the toxic effects of these substances on wound-healing cells.[19]

Nutrition

Nutrition plays a role in preventing wounds and healing existing wounds. A nutritional assessment, mentioned earlier in this textbook (ie, Chapter 107), should be performed routinely in patients that are at risk for wounds (eg, pressure ulcers, elective surgery) or who have existing wounds (eg, postoperative, traumatic, ulcers).

Malnutrition, as determined by nutritional parameters, is associated consistently with the development of pressure ulcers. These nutritional parameters include low body mass index,[69] recent weight loss,[70,71] reduced anthropometric measures, dehydration,[58] low prealbumin,[59] low albumin (<3.5),[72] reduced appetite,[73] lymphopenia (<1.50×10^9/L),[60] and low dietary intake.[74,75]

Supplemental nutrition consists of nutrient-rich fluids given orally, enterally, or parenterally in addition to meals (see Chapter 107 for further discussion). Because malnutrition is associated with pressure ulcer development, it is tempting to assume that providing supplemental nutrition to malnourished patients would reduce the rate of pressure ulcer development or improve their healing rates. However, the published randomized, clinical trials to date show no benefit of supplemental nutrition on the prevention or healing of wounds to balance the risks inherent to supplemental nutrition (reviewed elsewhere in this text).[76–82] It is unknown whether this is due to limited sample sizes of the studies or a lack of effect. It should be kept in mind that supplemental nutrition could even worsen wound care in incontinent patients by increasing urine and fecal output. These issues will remain until larger, well-randomized, comparative trials are conducted.

In the absence of firm evidence for or against supplemental nutrition, most clinicians will encourage and request assisted oral intake in nutritionally deficient patients. It is oftentimes possible to increase intake by determining from the patient and his/her family what foods the patient prefers. If these are not available at the institution, family members should be allowed to bring outside food to the patient. Also, dividing meals into smaller, more frequent schedules can allow better tolerance of them. In those who are unable to eat, supplemental nutritional should be based on the risks and benefits unrelated to wound care. The patient and family should be included in this decision.[83,84]

Growth Factors

Growth factors are proteins excreted from platelets, macrophages, fibroblasts, and endothelial cells that orchestrate a complex series of events involved in healing. There have been many attempts to synthesize these growth factors to promote healing.[85] The only approved growth factor to date, however, is becaplermin, a recombinant human platelet-derived growth factor BB (PDGF-BB). It was approved in December 1997 for the treatment of non-ischemic diabetic ulcers that extend into or past the subcutaneous tissue.[86] Becaplermin is thought to promote the chemotaxis and proliferation of cells involved in wound healing and the formation of granulation tissue. The largest study published to date of the approved strength of becaplermin for use on diabetic ulcers was a randomized, double-blind, placebo-controlled, clinical trial.[87] The primary end point was the proportion of subjects with complete wound healing within the 20-week treatment period. Patients were randomized to beclapermin 30 mcg/g, 100 mcg/g, or placebo with 127, 132, and 123 subjects in each arm, respectively. Treatment with the 100 mcg/g strength significantly improved the incidence of complete healing *versus* placebo (50% versus 35%). The incidence of complete healing with the 30 mcg/g formulation was similar to placebo. Becaplermin is non-irritating and undergoes negligible absorption so that side effects are similar to those of placebo. It is applied once a day, but should be removed gently with water after 12 hours. Any infection present should be treated to resolution before becaplermin is applied. The major disadvantages of this agent are that it must be stored in the refrigerator and it is very expensive. One 15 g tube currently costs $452.98 and will usually last approximately 2 weeks depending on the size of the wound.[88]

Pharmacy Involvement in Wound Care

As clinical pharmacists increasingly round with medical teams, they are able to see the daily management of chronic wounds as a part of the health care team. Many times when physicians and nurses apply topical creams and ointments to these wounds, they look toward the clinical pharmacist to determine the appropriate type and method of application. This will be most pharmacists' initial foray into the field of wound care. With knowledge of a field few are familiar with, a pharmacist can be increasingly relied upon for recommendations not only for topical creams and ointments but also for assessments, antibiotics, dressings, and other wound care products as well.

SUMMARY AND CONCLUSIONS

The focus of this review was on the most common types of chronic wounds: pressure, vascular, and diabetic ulcers. Many, less common types were also briefly reviewed. The prevention of these types of wounds varies with the type but the treatment will generally depend on the clinical presentation of the wound. The presence of necrotic tissue necessitates debridement to prevent infection and allow healing to progress. The methods of debridement include sharp, mechanical, enzymatic, and autolytic. The method chosen should be based on the need for selectivity, presence of infection, amount of associated pain, amount of drainage, available resources, and other patient specific factors. The distinction between infection and colonization is currently based on clinical signs and symptoms and colony counts. When infection is present, it should be treated appropriately. Despite an association between the development of wounds and poor wound healing with poor nutritional parameters, the role of supplemental nutrition remains unclear until further studies are done. Most clinicians, however, will prescribe supplemental nutrition to those with poor nutritional parameters if concern of poor wound healing or development of pressure ulcers exists. Growth factors show modest improvements in healing chronic wounds but at a significant cost.

REFERENCES

1. Kuhn B, Coulter S. *Nursing Econ* 1992; 10:353.
2. Limova M. *Dermatol Clin* 2002; 20:357.
3. Franks PJ, McCullagh L, Moffatt CJ. *Ostomy Wound Manage* 2003;49:26.
4. Lindholm C, Bjellerup M, Christensen OB, et al. *Acta Derm Venereol* 1993; 73:440.
5. Harding KG, Morris HL, Patel GK. *BMJ* 2002; 324:160.
6. Sussman C, Bates-Jensen BM, eds. *Wound Care: A Collaborative Practice Manual for Physical Therapists and Nurses*, 2nd ed. Geithersburg, MD: Aspen, 2001, Chap 4.
7. Bergstrom N, Allman RM, Carlson CE, et al. Clinical Practice Guideline, No. 3. AHRQ Publication No. 92-0047. Rockville, MD: U.S. Department of Health and Human Services, The Agency for Health Care Policy and Research; May 1992.
8. Bates-Jensen BM. *Adv Wound Care* 1997; 10:65.
9. Stotts NA, Rodeheaver GT, Thomas DR, et al. *J Gerontol* 2001; 56:M795.
10. Defloor T. *J Clin Nurs.* 1999; 8:206.
11. Ratliff CR. Rodeheaver GT. *Lippincott's Primary Care Practice* 1999; 3:242.
12. Lyder CH. *JAMA* 2003; 289:223.
13. Burd C, Langemo D, Olson B, et al. *J Gerontol Nurs* 1992; 18:29.
14. Bates-Jensen BM. *Ann Intern Med* 2001; 135:744.
15. Berlowitz DR, Brandeis GH, Anderson J, et al. *J Gerontol A Biol Sci Med Sci* 1997; 52(2):M106.
16. Lyder CH, Preston J, Grady N, et al. *Arch Intern Med* 2001; 161:1549.
17. Meehan M. *Ostomy Wound Manage* 2000; 46:46.
18. Bennett RG, O'Sullivan J, EdVito EM, et al. *J Am Geriatr Soc* 2000; 48:73.
19. Bergsrtom N, Allman R, Alvarez OM, et al. Clinical Practice Guideline, No. 15. AHRQ Publication No. 95-0652. Rockville, MD: U.S. Department of Health and Human Services, The Agency for Health Care Policy and Research; December 1994.
20. Crewe RA. *Care Sci Pract* 1987; 5:9.
21. London NJ. Donnelly. R. *BMJ* 2000; 320(7249):1589.
22. de Araujo T, Valencia I, Federman DG, et al. *Ann Intern Med* 2003; 138:326.
23. Falabella A, Falanga V. *Clin Plast Surg* 1998; 25:467.
24. Antonio JO. *Dermatol Surg* 1999; 11:880.
25. de Araujo T, Valencia I, Federman DG, Kirsner RS. *Ann Intern Med* 2003; 138:326.
26. Phillips TJ. *Dermatol Surg* 2001; 27:611.
27. Wiersema-Bryant LA, Kraimer BA. Management of edema. In: Sussman C, Bates-Jensen BM, eds. *Wound Care: A Collaborative Practice Manual for Physical Therapists and Nurses*, 2nd ed. Geithersburg, MD: Aspen, 2001, Chap 10.
28. Fletcher A, Cullum N, Sheldon TA. *BMJ* 1997; 315;576.
29. Dale JJ, Ruckley CV, Harper DR, et al. *BMJ* 1999; 319:875.
30. Dale JJ, Ruckley CV, Harper DR, et al. *BMJ* 1999; 319:875.
31. Jull A, Waters J, Arroll B. *Lancet* 2002; 359(9317):1550.
33. Trental [package insert]. King of Prussia, PA: Aventis Behring L.L.C., 2002.
34. Hallett JW, Greenwood LH, Robison JG. *Ann Surg* 1985; 202:647.
35. London NJM, Donnelly R. *BMJ* 2000; 320:1589.
36. Goode PS, Allman RM. *Med Clin North Am* 1989; 73:1511.
37. Duncan HJ, Farris IB. *J Vasc Surg* 1985; 2:581.
38. Calhoun Jh, Overgaard KA, Stevens CM, et al. *Adv Skin Wound Care* 2003: 31–45.
39. American Diabetes Association: Consensus Development Conference on Diabetic Foot Wound Care (Consensus Statement). *Diabetes Care* 1999; 22:1354.
40. Mayfield JA, Reiber GE, Sanders LJ, et al. *Diabetes Care* 1998; 21:2161.
41. Reiber GE, Pecoraro RE, Koepsell TD. *Ann Intern Med* 1992; 117:97.

42. Preventive foot care in people with diabetes. *Diabetes Care* 2003; 26(suppl 1):S78.
43. DCCT Research Group. *N Engl J Med* 1993; 329:977.
44. Arasi R, McKay M, Grist WJ. *Laryngoscope* 1998; 98:1330.
45. George AO. *Trop Doctor* 1990; 20:187.
46. Morgan AG. *J Trop Med Hyg* 1982; 85:205.
47. Sams WM. Inflammatory Ulcers. In: Sams Jr WM, Lynch PJ, eds. *Principles and Practic of Dermatology,* 2nd ed. New York: Churchill-Livingstone, 1996:917–921.
48. Monk BE, Pembroke AC. *Clin Exp Dermatol* 1983; 8:437.
49. Fuse H, Takahara M, Ito H, et al. *Urol Int* 1986; 41:235.
50. Bissonnette R Friedmann D, Giroux J-M et al. *J Am Acad Dermatol* 1993; 29:818.
51. Evans J, Sirikumara M, Gregory M. *Oral Surg Oral Med Oral Pathol* 1993; 76:437.
52. FDA Wound Healing Clinical Focus Group. Guidance for industry: Chronic cutaneous ulcer and burn wounds-developing products for treatment. Available at: http://www.fda.gov/cber/gdlns/ulcburn.htm. Accessed September 3, 2003.
53. Bates-Jensen BM. Management of necrotic tissue. In: Sussman C, Bates-Jensen BM, eds. *Wound Care: A Collaborative Practice Manual for Physical Therapists and Nurses*, 2nd ed. Gaithersburg, MD: Aspen, 2001, Chap 8.
54. Fleck C. *Wound Care* 2002; 82:4.
55. Sussman C. Whirlpool. In: Sussman C, Bates-Jensen BM, eds. *Wound Care: A Collaborative Practice Manual for Physical Therapists and Nurses*, 2nd ed. Gaithersburg, MD: Aspen, 2001, Chap 25.
56. Ziox [package insert]. Miami, FL: Stratus Pharmaceuticals, 2001.
57. Ethezyme and Ethezyme 830 [package insert]. St Louis, MO: Ethex Corp., 2001.
58. Santyl [package insert]. Largo, FL: Smith & Nephew, Inc., 2000.
59. Glasser SR. *Am J Surg* 1940; 40:320.
60. Klasen HJ. *Burns* 2000; 26:207.
61. Bolton L, Fattu A. *Clin Dermatol* 1994; 12:95.
62. Ovington LG. *Adv Skin Wound Care* 2002; 19:477.
63. Finnie A. *Br J Comm Nurs* 2002; 7(7):1.
64. Graumlich JF, Blough LS, McLaughlin RG, et al. *J Am Geriatr Soc* 2003; 51:147.
65. Lewis R, Whiting P, ter Riet G, et al. *Health Technol Assess* 2001; 5(14).
66. Thomas S, Jones M. *Nursing Standard* 2001; 15(22):59.
67. Sherman RA. *Wound Rep Reg* 2002; 10:208.
68. Robson MC, Stenberg BD, Heggers JP. *Clin Plast Surg* 1990: 17:485.
69. Casimiro C, Abelardo G, Luis U. *Nutrition* 2002; 18:408.
70. Guenter P, Malyszek R, Bliss DZ, et al. *Adv Skin Wound Care* 2000; 13(4 Pt 1):164.
71. Allman RM, Goode PS, Patrick MM, et al. *JAMA* 1995; 274(13):1014.
72. Anthony D, Reynolds T, Russell L. *J Adv Nurs* 2000; 32(2):359.
73. Perneger TV, Heliot C, Rae AC, et al. *Arch Intern Med* 1998;158(17):1940.
74. Bergstrom N, Braden B. *J Am Geriatr Soc* 1992; 40(8):747.
75. Thomas DR, Goode PS, Tarquine, et al. *J Am Geriatr Soc* 1996; 44(12):1435.
76. Myers SA, Takiguch S, Slavis S, et al. *Decubitus* 1990; 3(3):16.
77. Hartigrink HH, Wille J, Konig P, et al. *Clin Nutr* 1998; 17:287.
78. Mitchell SL, Kiely DK, Lipsitz LA. *Arch Intern Med* 1997; 157:327.
79. Henderson CT, Trumbore LS, Mobarhan S, et al. *J Am Coll Nutr* 1992; 11:309.
80. Myers SA, Takiguch S, Slavis S, et al. *Decubitus* 1990; 3(3):16.
81. Preshaw RM, Attisha RP, Hollingsworth WJ. *Can J Surg* 1979; 22:437.
82. Breslow RA, Hallfrisch J, Guy DG, et al. *J Am Geriatr Soc* 1993; 41:357.
83. Thomas DR. *Nutrition* 2001; 17:121.
84. Finucane TE, Christmas C, Travis K. *JAMA* 1999; 282:1365.
85. Lawrence WT, Diegelmann RF. *Clin Dermatol* 1994;12:157.
86. Weiman JT, Becaplermin Gel Studies Group. *Am J Surg* 1998; 176(Suppl 2A):74S.
87. Wieman TJ, Smiell JM, Su Y. *Diabetes Care* 1988; 21(5):822.
88. Drugstore.com. Available at: http://www.drugstore.com/pharmacy/prices/drugprice.asp?ndc=00045081015. Accessed September 8, 2003.

Table of Metric Doses with Approximate Apothecary Equivalents

These **approximate** dose equivalents represent the quantities usually prescribed, under identical conditions, by physicians using, respectively, the metric system and the apothecary system of weights and measures. Statements of quantity or strength in the labeling of drug products, when expressed in the metric and apothecary systems, shall utilize **exact** equivalents.

When prepared dosage forms such as tablets, capsules, etc, are prescribed in the metric system, the pharmacist may dispense the corresponding **approximate** equivalent in the apothecary system and vice versa, as indicated in the following table.

For the conversion of specific quantities in converting pharmaceutical formulas, use the **exact** equivalents. For prescription compounding, use the exact equivalents rounded to three significant figures.

Liquid Measure

Metric	Approximate Apothecary Equivalents	Metric	Approximate Apothecary Equivalents	Metric	Approximate Apothecary Equivalents
1000 mL	1 quart	10 mL	$2\frac{1}{2}$ fluid drams	0.5 mL	8 minims
750 mL	$1\frac{1}{2}$ pints	8 mL	2 fluid drams	0.3 mL	5 minims
500 mL	1 pint	5 mL	$1\frac{1}{4}$ fluid drams	0.25 mL	4 minims
250 mL	8 fluid ounces	4 mL	1 fluid dram	0.2 mL	3 minims
200 mL	7 fluid ounces	3 mL	45 minims	0.1 mL	$1\frac{1}{2}$ minims
100 mL	$3\frac{1}{2}$ fluid ounces	2 mL	30 minims	0.06 mL	1 minim
50 mL	$1\frac{3}{4}$ fluid ounces	1 mL	15 minims	0.05 mL	$\frac{3}{4}$ minim
30 mL	1 fluid ounce	0.75 mL	12 minims	0.03 mL	$\frac{1}{2}$ minim
15 mL	4 fluid drams	0.6 mL	10 minims		

Weight

Metric	Approximate Apothecary Equivalents	Metric	Approximate Apothecary Equivalents	Metric	Approximate Apothecary Equivalents
30 g	1 ounce	200 mg	3 grains	4 mg	$\frac{1}{15}$ grain
15 g	4 drams	150 mg	$2\frac{1}{2}$ grains	3 mg	$\frac{1}{20}$ grain
10 g	$2\frac{1}{2}$ drams	125 mg	2 grains	2 mg	$\frac{1}{30}$ grain
7.5 g	2 drams	100 mg	$1\frac{1}{2}$ grains	1.5 mg	$\frac{1}{40}$ grain
6 g	90 grains	75 mg	$1\frac{1}{4}$ grains	1.2 mg	$\frac{1}{50}$ grain
5 g	75 grains	60 mg	1 grain	1 mg	$\frac{1}{60}$ grain
4 g	60 grains (1 dram)	50 mg	$\frac{3}{4}$ grain	800 μg	$\frac{1}{80}$ grain
3 g	45 grains	40 mg	$\frac{2}{3}$ grain	600 μg	$\frac{1}{100}$ grain
2 g	30 grains ($\frac{1}{2}$ dram)	30 mg	$\frac{1}{2}$ grain	500 μg	$\frac{1}{120}$ grain
1.5 g	22 grains	25 mg	$\frac{3}{8}$ grain	400 μg	$\frac{1}{150}$ grain
1 g	15 grains	20 mg	$\frac{1}{3}$ grain	300 μg	$\frac{1}{200}$ grain
750 mg	12 grains	15 mg	$\frac{1}{4}$ grain	250 μg	$\frac{1}{250}$ grain
600 mg	10 grains	12 mg	$\frac{1}{5}$ grain	200 μg	$\frac{1}{300}$ grain
500 mg	$7\frac{1}{2}$ grains	10 mg	$\frac{1}{6}$ grain	150 μg	$\frac{1}{400}$ grain
400 mg	6 grains	8 mg	$\frac{1}{8}$ grain	120 μg	$\frac{1}{500}$ grain
300 mg	5 grains	6 mg	$\frac{1}{10}$ grain	100 μg	$\frac{1}{600}$ grain
250 mg	4 grains	5 mg	$\frac{1}{12}$ grain		

NOTE: A milliliter (mL) is the approximate equivalent of a cubic centimeter (cc).

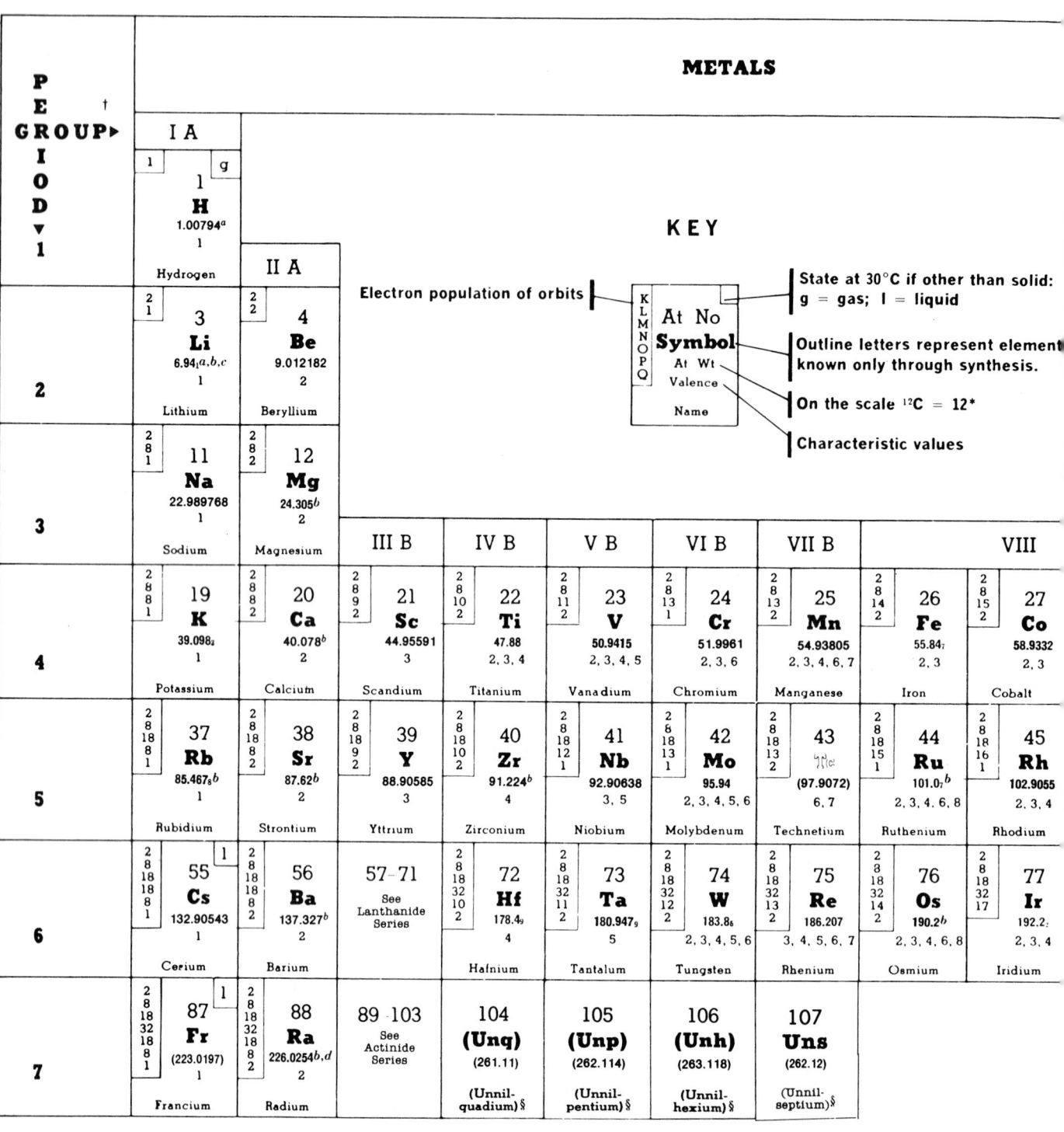

* Atomic weight is an alternative term for 'relative atomic mass of an element', A_r (E). The IUPAC values given here are scaled to A_r (^{12}C) = 12 and apply to elements as they exist in materials of terrestrial origin and to certain artificial elements. When used with due regard to the footnotes they are considered reliable to ± 1 in the last digit or ± 3 if that digit is subscript. Values in parentheses are for radioactive elements whose atomic weights cannot be quoted precisely without knowledge of the origin of the elements; the value given is the atomic mass number of the isotope of that element of longest known half-life.
† Beginning with Group III, authors differ in their presentation of the "A" and "B" groups of elements.
‡ Expected value from theoretical considerations. § Names and symbols provisionally suggested by IUPAC.

NON-METALS

INERT GASES

VII A | ZERO

1	g
1	
H	
1.00794[a]	
− 1	
Hydrogen	

2	g
2	
He	
4.002602[b]	
0	
Helium	

III A | IV A | V A | VI A

2 3 — **5 B** 10.811[a,c] 3 — Boron
2 4 — **6 C** 12.011[a] − 4; 2, 4 — Carbon
2 5 — **7 N** g 14.00674 − 3; 3, 5 — Nitrogen
2 6 — **8 O** g 15.9994[a] − 2 — Oxygen
2 7 — **9 F** g 18.9984032 − 1 — Fluorine
2 8 — **10 Ne** g 20.1797[c] 0 — Neon

2 8 3 — **13 Al** 26.981539 3 — Aluminum
2 8 4 — **14 Si** 28.0855 − 4; 4 — Silicon
2 8 5 — **15 P** 30.973762 − 3; 3, 5 — Phosphorus
2 8 6 — **16 S** 32.066[a] − 2; 2, 4, 6 — Sulfur
2 8 7 — **17 Cl** g 35.4527 − 1; 1, 3, 5, 7 — Chlorine
2 8 8 — **18 Ar** g 39.948[a,b] 0 — Argon

I B | II B

2 8 16 2 — **28 Ni** 58.69 2, 3 — Nickel
2 8 18 1 — **29 Cu** 63.546[a] 1, 2 — Copper
2 8 18 2 — **30 Zn** 65.39 2 — Zinc
2 8 18 3 — **31 Ga** 69.723 3 — Gallium
2 8 18 4 — **32 Ge** 72.61 4 — Germanium
2 8 18 5 — **33 As** 74.92159 − 3; 3, 5 — Arsenic
2 8 18 6 — **34 Se** 78.96 − 2; 4, 6 — Selenium
2 8 18 7 — **35 Br** 79.904 − 1; 1, 3, 5, 7 — Bromine
2 8 18 8 — **36 Kr** g 83.80[b,c] 0 — Krypton

2 8 18 18 — **46 Pd** 106.42[b] 2, 4 — Palladium
2 8 18 18 1 — **47 Ag** 107.8682[b] 1 — Silver
2 8 18 18 2 — **48 Cd** 112.411[b] 2 — Cadmium
2 8 18 18 3 — **49 In** 114.82[b] 3 — Indium
2 8 18 18 4 — **50 Sn** 118.71 2, 4 — Tin
2 8 18 18 5 — **51 Sb** 121.75 − 3; 3, 5 — Antimony
2 8 18 18 6 — **52 Te** 127.60[b] − 2; 4, 6 — Tellurium
2 8 18 18 7 — **53 I** 126.90447 − 1; 1, 3, 5, 7 — Iodine
2 8 18 18 8 — **54 Xe** g 131.29[b,c] 0 — Xenon

2 8 18 32 17 1 — **78 Pt** 195.08 2, 4 — Platinum
2 8 18 32 18 1 — **79 Au** 196.96654 1, 3 — Gold
2 8 18 32 18 2 — **80 Hg** 200.59 1, 2 — Mercury
2 8 18 32 18 3 — **81 Tl** 204.3833 1, 3 — Thallium
2 8 18 32 18 4 — **82 Pb** 207.2[a,b] 2, 4 — Lead
2 8 18 32 18 5 — **83 Bi** 208.980437 3, 5 — Bismuth
2 8 18 32 18 6 — **84 Po** (208.9824) 2, 4 — Polonium
2 8 18 32 18 7 — **85 At** (209.9871) 1, 3, 5, 7‡ — Astatine
2 8 18 32 18 8 — **86 Rn** g (222.0176) 0 — Radon

---

2 8 18 25 9 2 — **64 Gd** 157.25[b] 3 — Gadolinium
2 8 18 26 9 2 — **65 Tb** 158.92534 3, 4 — Terbium
2 8 18 28 8 2 — **66 Dy** 162.50 3 — Dysprosium
2 8 18 29 8 2 — **67 Ho** 164.93032 3 — Holmium
2 8 18 30 8 2 — **68 Er** 167.26 3 — Erbium
2 8 18 31 8 2 — **69 Tm** 168.93421 3 — Thulium
2 8 18 32 8 2 — **70 Yb** 173.04 2, 3 — Ytterbium
2 8 18 32 9 2 — **71 Lu** 174.967 3 — Lutetium

2 8 18 32 25 9 2 — **96 Cm** (247.0703) 3 — Curium
2 8 18 32 26 9 2 — **97 Bk** (247.0703) 3, 4 — Berkelium
2 8 18 32 27 9 2 — **98 Cf** (251.0796) 3 — Californium
2 8 18 32 28 9 2 — **99 Es** (252.083) 3‡ — Einsteinium
2 8 18 32 29 9 2 — **100 Fm** (257.0951) 3‡ — Fermium
2 8 18 32 30 9 2 — **101 Md** (258.10) 3‡ — Mendelevium
2 8 18 32 31 9 2 — **102 No** (259.1009) 3‡ — Nobelium
2 8 18 32 32 9 2 — **103 Lr** (262.11) 3‡ — Lawrencium

Element for which known variations in isotopic composition in normal terrestrial material prevent a more precise atomic weight being given; A_r (E) values should be applicable to any 'normal' material. [b]Element for which geological specimens are known in which the element has an anomalous isotopic composition, such that the difference between the atomic weight of the element in such specimens and that given in the table may exceed considerably the implied uncertainty. [c]Element for which substantial variations in A_r from the value given can occur in commercially available material because of inadvertent or undisclosed change of isotopic composition. [d]Element for which the value of A_r is that of the radioisotope of longest half-life.

Table of Logarithms

N	0	1	2	3	4	5	6	7	8	9		PP1	PP2	PP3	PP4	PP5	PP6	PP7	PP8	PP9
10	0000	0043	0086	0128	0170	0212	0253	0294	0334	0374		4	8	12	17	21	25	29	33	37
11	0414	0453	0492	0531	0569	0607	0645	0682	0719	0755		4	8	12	15	19	23	26	30	34
12	0792	0828	0864	0899	0934	0969	1004	1038	1072	1106		3	7	10	14	17	21	24	28	31
13	1139	1173	1206	1239	1271	1303	1335	1367	1399	1430		3	6	10	13	16	19	23	26	29
14	1461	1492	1523	1553	1584	1614	1644	1673	1703	1732		3	6	9	12	15	18	21	24	27
15	1761	1790	1818	1847	1875	1903	1931	1959	1987	2014		3	6	8	11	14	17	20	22	25
16	2041	2068	2095	2122	2148	2175	2201	2227	2253	2279		3	5	8	11	13	16	18	21	24
17	2304	2330	2355	2380	2405	2430	2455	2480	2504	2529		2	5	7	10	12	15	17	20	22
18	2553	2577	2601	2625	2648	2672	2695	2718	2742	2765		2	5	7	9	12	14	16	19	21
19	2788	2810	2833	2856	2878	2900	2923	2945	2967	2989		2	4	7	9	11	13	16	18	20
20	3010	3032	3054	3075	3096	3118	3139	3160	3181	3201		2	4	6	8	11	13	15	17	19
21	3222	3243	3263	3284	3304	3324	3345	3365	3385	3404		2	4	6	8	10	12	14	16	18
22	3424	3444	3464	3483	3502	3522	3541	3560	3579	3598		2	4	6	8	10	12	14	15	17
23	3617	3636	3655	3674	3692	3711	3729	3747	3766	3784		2	4	6	7	9	11	13	15	17
24	3802	3820	3838	3856	3874	3892	3909	3927	3945	3962		2	4	5	7	9	11	12	14	16
25	3979	3997	4014	4031	4048	4065	4082	4099	4116	4133		2	3	5	7	9	10	12	14	15
26	4150	4166	4183	4200	4216	4232	4249	4265	4281	4298		2	3	5	7	8	10	11	13	15
27	4314	4330	4346	4362	4378	4393	4409	4425	4440	4456		2	3	5	6	8	9	11	13	14
28	4472	4487	4502	4518	4533	4548	4564	4579	4594	4609		2	3	5	6	8	9	11	12	14
29	4624	4639	4654	4669	4683	4698	4713	4728	4742	4757		1	3	4	6	7	9	10	12	13
30	4771	4786	4800	4814	4829	4843	4857	4871	4886	4900		1	3	4	6	7	9	10	11	13
31	4914	4928	4942	4955	4969	4983	4997	5011	5024	5038		1	3	4	6	7	8	10	11	12
32	5051	5065	5079	5092	5105	5119	5132	5145	5159	5172		1	3	4	5	7	8	9	11	12
33	5185	5198	5211	5224	5237	5250	5263	5276	5289	5302		1	3	4	5	6	8	9	10	12
34	5315	5328	5340	5353	5366	5378	5391	5403	5416	5428		1	3	4	5	6	8	9	10	11
35	5441	5453	5465	5478	5490	5502	5514	5527	5539	5551		1	2	4	5	6	7	9	10	11
36	5563	5575	5587	5599	5611	5623	5635	5647	5658	5670		1	2	4	5	6	7	8	10	11
37	5682	5694	5705	5717	5729	5740	5752	5763	5775	5786		1	2	3	5	6	7	8	9	11
38	5798	5809	5821	5832	5843	5855	5866	5877	5888	5899		1	2	3	5	6	7	8	9	10
39	5911	5922	5933	5944	5955	5966	5977	5988	5999	6010		1	2	3	4	5	7	8	9	10
40	6021	6031	6042	6053	6064	6075	6085	6096	6107	6117		1	2	3	4	5	6	8	9	10
41	6128	6138	6149	6160	6170	6180	6191	6201	6212	6222		1	2	3	4	5	6	7	8	9
42	6232	6243	6253	6263	6274	6284	6294	6304	6314	6325		1	2	3	4	5	6	7	8	9
43	6335	6345	6355	6365	6375	6385	6395	6405	6415	6425		1	2	3	4	5	6	7	8	9
44	6435	6444	6454	6464	6474	6484	6493	6503	6513	6522		1	2	3	4	5	6	7	8	9
45	6532	6542	6551	6561	6571	6580	6590	6599	6609	6618		1	2	3	4	5	6	7	8	9
46	6628	6637	6646	6656	6665	6675	6684	6693	6702	6712		1	2	3	4	5	6	7	7	8
47	6721	6730	6739	6749	6758	6767	6776	6785	6794	6803		1	2	3	4	5	5	6	7	8
48	6812	6821	6830	6839	6848	6857	6866	6875	6884	6893		1	2	3	4	4	5	6	7	8
49	6902	6911	6920	6928	6937	6946	6955	6964	6972	6981		1	2	3	4	4	5	6	7	8
50	6990	6998	7007	7016	7024	7033	7042	7050	7059	7067		1	2	3	3	4	5	6	7	8
51	7076	7084	7093	7101	7110	7118	7126	7135	7143	7152		1	2	2	3	4	5	6	7	8
52	7160	7168	7177	7185	7193	7202	7210	7218	7226	7235		1	2	2	3	4	5	6	6	7
53	7243	7251	7259	7267	7275	7284	7292	7300	7308	7316		1	2	2	3	4	5	5	6	7
54	7324	7332	7340	7348	7356	7364	7372	7380	7388	7396		1	2	2	3	4	5	5	6	7

N	0	1	2	3	4	5	6	7	8	9		PP1	PP2	PP3	PP4	PP5	PP6	PP7	PP8	PP9
55	7404	7412	7419	7427	7435	7443	7451	7459	7466	7474		1	2	2	3	4	5	5	6	7
56	7482	7490	7497	7505	7513	7520	7528	7536	7543	7551		1	2	2	3	4	5	5	6	7
57	7559	7566	7574	7582	7589	7597	7604	7612	7619	7627		1	2	2	3	4	5	5	6	7
58	7634	7642	7649	7657	7664	7672	7679	7686	7694	7701		1	1	2	3	4	4	5	6	7
59	7709	7716	7723	7731	7738	7745	7752	7760	7767	7774		1	1	2	3	4	4	5	6	7
60	7782	7789	7796	7803	7810	7818	7825	7832	7839	7846		1	1	2	3	4	4	5	6	6
61	7853	7860	7868	7875	7882	7889	7896	7903	7910	7917		1	1	2	3	4	4	5	6	6
62	7924	7931	7938	7945	7952	7959	7966	7973	7980	7987		1	1	2	3	4	4	5	6	6
63	7993	8000	8007	8014	8021	8028	8035	8041	8048	8055		1	1	2	3	3	4	5	5	6
64	8062	8069	8075	8082	8089	8096	8102	8109	8116	8122		1	1	2	3	3	4	5	5	6
65	8129	8136	8142	8149	8156	8162	8169	8176	8182	8189		1	1	2	3	3	4	5	5	6
66	8195	8202	8209	8215	8222	8228	8235	8241	8248	8254		1	1	2	3	3	4	5	5	6
67	8261	8267	8274	8280	8287	8293	8299	8306	8312	8319		1	1	2	3	3	4	4	5	6
68	8325	8331	8338	8344	8351	8357	8363	8370	8376	8382		1	1	2	2	3	4	4	5	6
69	8388	8395	8401	8407	8414	8420	8426	8432	8439	8445		1	1	2	2	3	4	4	5	5
70	8451	8457	8463	8470	8476	8482	8488	8494	8500	8506		1	1	2	2	3	4	4	5	5
71	8513	8519	8525	8531	8537	8543	8549	8555	8561	8567		1	1	2	2	3	4	4	5	5
72	8573	8579	8585	8591	8597	8603	8609	8615	8621	8627		1	1	2	2	3	4	4	5	5
73	8633	8639	8645	8651	8657	8663	8669	8675	8681	8686		1	1	2	2	3	4	4	5	5
74	8692	8698	8704	8710	8716	8722	8727	8733	8739	8745		1	1	2	2	3	4	4	5	5
75	8751	8756	8762	8768	8774	8779	8785	8791	8797	8802		1	1	2	2	3	3	4	5	5
76	8808	8814	8820	8825	8831	8837	8842	8848	8854	8859		1	1	2	2	3	3	4	5	5
77	8865	8871	8876	8882	8887	8893	8899	8904	8910	8915		1	1	2	2	3	3	4	4	5
78	8921	8927	8932	8938	8943	8949	8954	8960	8965	8971		1	1	2	2	3	3	4	4	5
79	8976	8982	8987	8993	8998	9004	9009	9015	9020	9026		1	1	2	2	3	3	4	4	5
80	9031	9036	9042	9047	9053	9058	9063	9069	9074	9079		1	1	2	2	3	3	4	4	5
81	9085	9090	9096	9101	9106	9112	9117	9122	9128	9133		1	1	2	2	3	3	4	4	5
82	9138	9143	9149	9154	9159	9165	9170	9175	9180	9186		1	1	2	2	3	3	4	4	5
83	9191	9196	9201	9206	9212	9217	9222	9227	9232	9238		1	1	2	2	3	3	4	4	5
84	9243	9248	9253	9258	9263	9269	9274	9279	9284	9289		1	1	2	2	3	3	4	4	5
85	9294	9299	9304	9309	9315	9320	9325	9330	9335	9340		1	1	2	2	3	3	4	4	5
86	9345	9350	9355	9360	9365	9370	9375	9380	9385	9390		1	1	2	2	3	3	4	4	5
87	9395	9400	9405	9410	9415	9420	9425	9430	9435	9440		0	1	1	2	2	3	3	4	4
88	9445	9450	9455	9460	9465	9469	9474	9479	9484	9489		0	1	1	2	2	3	3	4	4
89	9494	9499	9504	9509	9513	9518	9523	9528	9533	9538		0	1	1	2	2	3	3	4	4
90	9542	9547	9552	9557	9562	9566	9571	9576	9581	9586		0	1	1	2	2	3	3	4	4
91	9590	9595	9600	9605	9609	9614	9619	9624	9628	9633		0	1	1	2	2	3	3	4	4
92	9638	9643	9647	9652	9657	9661	9666	9671	9675	9680		0	1	1	2	2	3	3	4	4
93	9685	9689	9694	9699	9703	9708	9713	9717	9722	9727		0	1	1	2	2	3	3	4	4
94	9731	9736	9741	9745	9750	9754	9759	9763	9768	9773		0	1	1	2	2	3	3	4	4
95	9777	9782	9786	9791	9795	9800	9805	9809	9814	9818		0	1	1	2	2	3	3	4	4
96	9823	9827	9832	9836	9841	9845	9850	9854	9859	9863		0	1	1	2	2	3	3	4	4
97	9868	9872	9877	9881	9886	9890	9894	9899	9903	9908		0	1	1	2	2	3	3	4	4
98	9912	9917	9921	9926	9930	9934	9939	9943	9948	9952		0	1	1	2	2	3	3	4	4
99	9956	9961	9965	9969	9974	9978	9983	9987	9991	9996		0	1	1	2	2	3	3	3	4

Glossary

A

AA   atomic absorption, Alcoholics Anonymous

AACP   American Association of Colleges of Pharmacy

AAFP   American Academy of Family Practice

AAGR   average annual growth

AAP   American Academy of Pediatrics

AAPCC   American Association of Poison Control Centers

AAPS   American Association of Pharmaceutical Scientists

AARP   American Association of Retired Persons

ABAT   American Board of Applied Toxicology

ABC   ATP binding casette

ABG   arterial blood gas

ABMS   American Board of Medical Specialties

ACA   American College of Apothecaries

ACD   acid-citrate-dextrose

ACE   angiotensin converting enzyme

ACEI   angiotensin converting enzyme inhibitor

ACCP   American College of Clinical Pharmacy, American College of Clinical Pharmacists

ACF   Administration for Children and Families

Ach   acetylcholine

ACh   acetylcholinesterase

ACHC   Accreditation Committee for Health Care

ACIP   American Committee on Immunization Practices, Immunization Practices Advisory Committee

ACP   American College of Physicians, acyl carrier protein

ACPE   Accreditation Council for Pharmaceutical Education

ACTH   corticotropin (adreno-corticotropic hormone)

AD   Alzheimer's disease, Alzheimer's dementia

ADA   American Dental Association, American Dietetic Association, adenosine deaminase, American Diabetes Association

ADCC   antibody-dependent cell-mediated cytotoxicity

ADE   adverse drug event, adverse drug experience

ADEPT   antibody directed enzyme prodrug therapy

ADH   antidiuretic hormone

ADL   activity of daily living

ADME   absorption, distribution, metabolism, and excretion

ADP   adenosine diphosphate

ADR   adverse drug reaction

AEC   Atomic Energy Commission

AERS   Adverse Event Reporting System

AES   Auger electron spectrometry

AF   atrial fibrillation

AFMS   Air Force Medical Service

AFP   α-1-fetoprotein

A/G   albumin-globulin ratio

AGD   agar gel diffusion

AHA   American Hospital Association, American Heart Association

AHCPR   Agency for Health Care Policy Research

AHF   antihemophilic factor

AHFS   American Hospital Formulary System

AHG   antihemophilic globulin

AHRQ   Agency for Healthcare Research and Quality

AI   adequate intake, aortic insufficiency

AIDS   acquired immunodeficiency syndrome

AIMS   abnormal involuntary movement scale

AIRA   American International Reiki Association

AL   allergy unit

ALARA   as low as reasonably achievable

ALF   American Liver Foundation

ALL   acute lymphoblastic leukemia

ALT   alanine aminotransferase

AMA   American Medical Association

AMC   Army Medical Center

AMCP   Academy of Managed Care Pharmacists

AMD   age-related macular degeneration

AMDA   American Medical Director's Association

AMI   acute myocardial infarction

AMTA   American Massage Therapy Association

ANA   antinuclear antibodies

ANC   acid neutralizing capacity

ANDA   abbreviated new drug application

ANF   atrial natriuretic factor

ANN   artificial neural network

ANOVA   analysis of variance

ANS   autonomic nervous system

AO   atomic orbital

AOA   American Osteopathic Association

AoA   Administration on Aging

APAP   acetaminophen

APC   antigen-presenting cell, ambulatory patient classification

APCI   atmospheric pressure chemical ionization

APHA   American Public Health Association

APhA   American Pharmacists Association

API   active pharmaceutical ingredient, atmospheric pressure ionization

APP   alternating pressure pad

APPM   Academy of Pharmacy Practice and Management

APRS   Academy of Pharmaceutical Research and Science

APSF   Anesthesia Patient Safety Foundation

APTT   activated partial thromboplastin time

ARB   angiotensin receptor blocker

ARDS   adult respiratory distress syndrome

ASA   acetylsalicylic acid, American Society for Anesthesia

ASCP   American Society of Consultant Pharmacists

ASHP   American Society of Health-System Pharmacists

ASNN   associate neural network

ASO   administrative service organization

ASP   Academy of Students of Pharmacy

ASPEN   American Society of Parenteral and Enteral Nutrition

ASRS   Aviation Safety and Reporting System

AST   aspartase aminotransferase

ATC   around-the-clock

ATCC   American *Type Culture Collection*

ATM   automated teller machine

ATN   acute tubular necrosis

ATP   adenosine triphosphate

ATPase   adenosine triphosphatase

ATSDR   Agency for Toxic Substances and Disease Registry

AUC   area under the curve

AV   atrioventricular

AZT   zidovudine

B

BAC   blood alcohol concentration

BAL   British anti-Lewisite, bioequivalent allergy unit

BBB   blood-brain barrier

BCE   before the Christian era

BCG   Bacillus Calmette Guerin

BCMA   Bar Code Medication Administration System

BCNP   Board Certified Nuclear Pharmacist

BCPS   Board Certified Pharmacotherapy Specialist

BCS   Biopharmaceutical Classification System

BET   bacterial endotoxin test

bFGF   basic fibroblast growth factor

BI   biological indicator

BIA   bacteria inhibition assay

BJA   Basic Journal Abstracts

BM   bowel movement

BMD   Bureau of Medical Devices, bone mineral density

BMI   body mass index

BMJ   British Medical Journal

BMS   between mean square

BMT   bone marrow transplantation

BOC   Board for Arthotists/Prosthetist Certification

BOP   Bureau of Prisons

BP   British Pharmacopeia

BPC   bulk pharmaceutical chemical

BPH   benign prostatic hypertrophy

BPS   Board of Pharmaceutical Specialties

BRH   Bureau of Radiologic Health

BSA   bovine serum albumin

BSC   Biomedical Service Corps

BSE   breast self-examination, bovine spongiform encephalopathy

BSS   between sum-of-squares, balanced salt solution

BUN   blood urea nitrogen

BWFI   bacteriostatic water for injection

C

CAD   coronary artery disease

CADD   computer-assisted drug design

CAGE   cut down, annoyed, guilty, eye opener

CAM   cell adhesion molecule, complimentary/alternative medicine

cAMP   cyclic adenosine monophosphate, cyclic adenosine-3′,5′-monophosphate

CARF   Commission on Accreditation of Rehab Facilities

CARTI   community-acquired respiratory tract infection

CAS   Chemical Abstracts Service, composite adherence score

CAT   cellulose acetate trimellitate, computer-aided tomography

CBAC   Chemical-Biological Activities

CBC   complete blood count

CBA   cost-benefit analysis

CBER   Center for Biologics Evaluation and Research

CCB   calcium channel blockers

CCD   countercurrent distribution

CCP   Council on Credentialing in Pharmacy

CCRF   Commissioned Corps Readiness Force

CD   circular dichroism

CDA   chiral derivatizing agent

CDC   Centers for Disease Control and Prevention

CDER   Center for Drug Evaluation and Research

CDM   certified disease management

CDRH   Center for Devices and Radiologic Health

CD-ROM   compact disk-read only memory

CE   capillary electrophoresis

CEA   carcinoembryonic antigen, cost-effectiveness analysis

CEC   capillary electrochromatography

CEO   chief executive officer

CEP   counterelectrophoresis

CF   complement fixation

CFC   chlorofluorocarbon

CFR   Code of Federal Regulations

CFSAN   Center for Food Safety and Applied Nutrition

CFTR   cystic fibrosis transmembrane regulator

CFU   colony-forming unit

CGD   chronic granulomatous disease

cGMP   cyclic guanosine-$3',5'$-monophosphate, current good manufacturing practice

CHAP   Commission on Health Accreditation Programs

CHD   coronary heart disease

CHF   congestive heart failure

CHO   Chinese hamster ovary

CI   confidence interval, chemical ionization

CIMS   chemical ionization mass spectrometry, chemical ionization mass spectroscopy

CIOMS   Council for International Organization of Medical Sciences

CIP   clean-in-place

CI-PDED   chlorine-selective pulsed discharge emission detector

CK   creatinine kinase

CLIA   Clinical Laboratory Improvement Amendments

CLL   chronic lymphoblastic leukemia

CLT   Central Limit Theorem

CMC   comprehensive medical chemistry, critical micelle concentration

CME   cystoid macular edema

CMI   cell-mediated immunity

CML   chronic myeloid leukemia

CMN   certificate of medical necessity

CMOP   Consolidated Mail Outpatient Pharmacies

CMRO$_2$ cerebral metabolic rate for oxygen

CMS   Centers for Medicare and Medicaid Services

CMV   cytomegalovirus

CN   Crigler-Najjar syndrome

CNS   central nervous system

CO   communication objective, carbon monoxide

COHgB   carboxyhemoglobin

COMTA   Commission on Massage Therapy Accreditation

CONSORT   Consolidated Standards of Reporting Trials

COPD   chronic obstructive pulmonary disease

COSTEP   Commissioned Officer Student Training and Externship Program

COSY   correlation spectroscopy

COX   cyclo-oxygenase

CPC   Council on Pharmacy and Chemistry, centrifugal partition chromatography

CPD   citrate-phosphate-dextrose

CPG   FDA's Compliance Policy Guide

CPI   consumer price index

CPMP   Committee for Proprietary Medicinal Products

CPOE   computerized physician order entry, computerized prescriber order entry

CPPDE   calcium pyrophosphate deposition disease

CPR   cardiopulmonary resuscitation

CPS   Compendium of Pharmaceutical Specialties

CPSC   Consumer Product Safety Commission

CPT   current procedural terms

CQI   continuous quality improvement

CREST   calcinosis, Reynaud's phenomenon, esophageal involvement, sclerodactyly, and telangiectasis

CRF   chronic renal failure

CRH   critical relative humidity, corticotropic releasing hormone

CRO   contract research organization

CRP   C-reactive protein

CRT   controlled-release tablet

CSA   Comprehensive Drug Abuse Prevention and Control Act of 1970, Controlled Substances Act

CSF   cerebrospinal fluid, colony stimulating factor

CSH   combat support hospitals

CSP   chiral stationary phase, compounding sterile preparations

CT   charge-transfer, compressed tablet, computerized tomography, computed tomography

CTL   cytotoxic T-lymphocyte

CTS   compressed tablet for solution

CTZ   chemoreceptor trigger zone

CUA   cost utility analysis

CV   coefficient of variation

CVD   cardiovascular disease

CVID   common variable immunodeficiency

CW   continuous wave

D

DEA   Drug Enforcement Administration

DAEA   diethylaminoethyl

D&C   drug and cosmetic

DATA   Drug Addiction Treatment Act

DBP   diastolic blood pressure

DC   direct current

DCBE   double contrast barium exam

DCCT   Diabetes Complications and Control Trial

DDMAC   FDA's Drug Marketing Advertising and Communications

DEA   Drug Enforcement Administration, Drug Enforcement Agency

DEET   diethyltoluamide

DF   degrees of freedom

DFV   daily food value

DHHS   Department of Health and Human Services

DI   diabetes insipidus

DIC   disseminated intravascular coagulation

DIP   desquamative interstitial pneumonitis

DIP   distal interphalangeal

DISCUS   dyskinesia identification system-condensed use scale

DJD   degenerative joint disease

DLBCL   diffuse large B-cell lymphoma

DLVO   Derjaguin-Landau-Verwey-Overbeek

DM   dermatomyositis

DMAA   Disease Management Association of America

DMSO   dimethyl sulfoxide

DMT   dimethyltryptamine

DNA   deoxyribonucleic acid

DNR   do not resuscitate

DOD   Department of Defense

DOT   directly observed treatment, Department of Transportation

DPCPTRA   Drug Price Competition and Patent Term Restoration Act

DPPC   dipalmitoylphosphatidylcholine

DPSV   differential pulse stripping voltammetry

DRE   drug response element, digital rectal examination

DRG   diagnosis-related group

DRI   dietary reference intake

DRP   drug-related problem

DRR   drug regimen review

DRV   daily reference value

DS   degree of substitution

DSC   differential scanning calorimetry

DSHEA   Dietary Supplement Health and Education Act

DSMB   Drug Safety and Monitoring Board

DSM   disease state management

DSMT   diabetes self-management training

DT   dispensing tablet

DTA   differential thermal analysis

DTAP   diphtheria and tetanus toxoids and acellular pertussis

DTAW   drug therapy assessment worksheet

DTP   diphtheria, tetaus and pertussis

DTPL   drug therapy problem list

DTwP   diphtheria and tetanus toxoids and whole-cell pertussis

DUE   drug utilization evaluation, drug usage evaluation

DUR   drug utilization review, drug use review

DV   daily value

DVA   Department of Veterans Affairs

DVD   digital video disk

DVT   deep venous thrombosis

DXA   dual energy x-ray absorptimometry

E

E&M   evaluation and management

EAR   estimated average requirement

EBM	evidence-based medicine	FAO	Food and Agriculture Organization	G-CSF	granulocyte colony-stimulating factor
EBV	Epstein-Barr virus	FBI	Federal Bureau of Investigation	GDEPT	gene-directed EPT
EC	ethics committee, effective concentration	FCT	film-coated tablet	GDP	gross domestic product
ECD	electron capture detector	F-D	force-displacement	GERD	gastroesophageal reflux disease
ECF	extracellular fluid	FDA	Food and Drug Administration	GFR	glomerular filtration rate
ECF-A	eosinophil chemotactic factor of anaphylaxis	FDAMA	FDA Modernization Act	GH	growth hormone
ECG	electrocardiogram	FD&C	Food, Drug and Cosmetic	GI	gastrointestinal
ECL	enterochromaffin-like	FDP	fibrinogen degradation products	GLC	gas-liquid chromatography
ECT	enteric-coated tablet	FEF	forced expiratory flow	GLP	good laboratory practice
ED	emergency department	FEPCA	Federal Environmental Pesticide Control Act	GLUT	glucose transporter
EDA	electron donor-acceptor			GMP	good manufacturing practice
ED$_{50}$	50% effective dose	FEV	forced expiratory volume	Gn-RH	gonadotropin-releasing hormone
EDI	electronic data interchange	FFA	free fatty acid	GN	glomerulonephritis
EDRF	endothelium-derived relaxing factor	FFT	fast Fourier transform	GNDF	glial cell line-derived neurotrophic factor
EDTA	ethylenediaminetetraacetic acid	FH	field hospital, familial hypercholesterolemia	GPCR	guanine nucleotide-coupled receptor
EDV	end diastolic volume	FHD	first human dose	GRAS	generally recognized as safe
EEG	electroencephalogram	FIA	flow injection analysis	GSC	gas-solid chromatography
EES	exfoliative erythroderma syndrome	FID	flame ionization detector, free induction decay	G6P	glucose 6-phosphate
EI	electron impact			G6PD	glucose 6-phosphate dehydrogenase
EIA	enzyme immunoassay	FIFRA	Federal Insecticide, Fungicide and Rodenticide Act	GVHD	graft vs host disease
EKG	electrocardiogram			GYN	gynecology
ELISA	enzyme-linked immunosorbent assay	FIR	far infrared		
ELS	evaporative light scattering	FLP	fragment length polymorphism	**H**	
ELSI	ethical, legal, and social implication	FMEA	failure mode and effects analysis	HA	hemagglutination
EM	electromagnetic, emergency medicine	FOBT	fecal occult blood test	HAA	hepatitis-associated antigen
EMIT	enzyme-mediated immunologic technique	FODA	fiber-optic Doppler anemometer	HAART	highly active antiretroviral therapy
EMS	error mean square	FPD	flame photometric detector	HACEK	haemophilus, actinobacillus, cardiobacterium, eikenella, kingella
EN	enteral nutrition	FPIA	fluorescence polarization immunoassay		
ENTOMA	Entomological Society of America	FRC	functional residual capacity	HACCP	hazard analysis and critical control point
ENZ-Aux	enzyme auxotroph bacterial assay	FSH	follicle-stimulating hormone	HBIG	hepatitis B immune globulin
EOF	electro-osmotic flow	FT	Fourier transformation	HBP	high blood pressure
EP	European Pharmacopeia	FTA	fluorescent treponemal antibody	HbS	hemoglobin S
EPA	Environmental Protection Agency	FTC	Federal Trade Commission	HBV	hepatitis B virus
EPMA	electron probe microanalysis	FT-IR	Fourier transform infrared spectrometry	HC	hydrocarbon
EPS	extrapyramidal symptom	FTMS	Fourier transform mass spectrometry	HCA	hierarchical cluster analysis
EPT	enzyme prodrug therapy	FT-NMR	Fourier transform nuclear magnetic resonance	HCFA	Health Care Financing Administration
Eq	equivalent, equation			HCFC	hydrochlorofluorocarbons
ERM	electrochemical relaxation measurements	FVC	forced vital capacity	HCG	human chorionic gonadotropin
ESCA	electron spectroscopy chemical analysis	**G**		HCM	health collaboration model
ESI	electrospray ionization	GABA	gamma-aminobutyric acid	HCP	home care pharmaceutical
E-Sign	Electronic Signatures in Global and National Commerce Act	GAD	generalized anxiety disorder	HCPCS	HCFA Common Procedure Coding System
ESR	electron spin resonance, erythrocyte sedimentation rate	GAO	General Accounting Office	HCPS	home-care pharmaceuticals
		GAP	good aseptic practice	HCR	health care representative
ESRD	end stage renal disease	GC	gas chromatography	HCTZ	hydrochlorothiazide
ET	enterostomal therapist	G-cells	gastrin-producing cells	HCV	hepatitis C virus
EU	endotoxin unit	GCP	Good Clinical Practices, Good Compounding Practices	HDL	high-density lipoprotein
F				HDPE	high-density polyethylene
FAA	Federal Aviation Administration	GC-MS	gas chromatography/mass spectrometry	HEDIS	health employer data and information set
FAB	fast-atom bombardment	GCP	Good Compounding Practices	HEPA	high-efficiency particulate air
				HepB	hepatitis B

HETP	height equivalent to a theoretical plate
HFA	hydrofluoroalkane
HFC	hydrofluorocarbons
HFMEA	health care failure modes and effects analysis
HGF	hyperglycemic factor
hGH	human growth hormone
HHS	Health and Human Services
Hib	*Haemophilus influenza* type b
HIC	hydrophobic interaction chromatography
HIMA	Health Industry Manufacturers Association
HIPAA	Health Insurance Portability and Accountability Act
HIV	human immunodeficiency virus
HLA	human leukocyte antigen
HLA-DR	human leukocyte antigen (locus) DR
HLB	hydrophile-lipophile balance
HLH	human luteinizing hormone
HME	home medical equipment
HMO	health maintenance organization
HOCA	high osmolality contrast agents
HOPE	Heart Outcomes Prevention Evaluation, Women's Health, Osteoporosis, Progestin, Estrogen Trial
HPDP	health promotion and disease prevention
HPA	hypothalamic-pituitary-adrenal
HPL	human placental lactogen
HPLC	high-performance liquid chromatography
HPLC/MS	high-performance liquid chromatography/mass spectrometry
HPRS	Homeopathic Pharmacopoeia Revision Service
HPUS	Homeopathic Pharmacopoeia of the United States
HPV	human papillomavirus
HRSA	Health Resource and Services Administration
HRT	hormone replacement therapy
HSA	human serum albumin
HSAB	hard and soft acid-base
HSV	herpes simplex virus
HT	hypodermic tablet
HTS	high-throughput screen
HUS	hemolytic-uremic syndrome
HVAC	heating, ventilating, and air conditioning
HWD	hot wire detector

I

I	electric current
IBD	inflammatory bowel disease
IBW	ideal body weight
IC	ion chromatography
ICD	International Classification of Diseases
ICF	intracellular fluid, intermediate care facility
ICH	International Committee on Harmonization
ICP	inductively coupled argon plasma, intercostals position
ICR	ion cyclotron resonance
ICSH	interstitial cell-stimulating hormone
ICU	intensive care unit
ID	intradermal
IDDM	insulin dependent diabetes mellitus
IDIS	Iowa Drug Information Service
IDU	injection drug user
IEC	institution ethics committee
IFN	interferon
Ig	immunoglobulin
IGIM	immune globulin intramuscular
IGIV	immune globulin intravenous
IGT	impaired glucose tolerance
IHD	ischemic heart disease
IHGFC	International Human Genome Sequencing Consortium
IHI	Institute for Healthcare Improvement
IHS	Indian Health Service
IL	interleukin
ILP	inductive logic programming
IM	intramuscular
IMA	Individual Mobilization Augmentee
IN	intranasal
INADEQUATE	incredible natural abundance double quantum transition experiment
IND	Investigational New Drug
INEPT	insensitive nucleus enhancement by polarization transfer
INN	International Nonproprietary Names
INR	International Normalized Ratio
IOL	intraocular lens
IOM	Institute of Medicine
IOP	intraocular pressure
IPA	International Pharmaceutical Abstracts, isopropyl alcohol
IPE	introductory practice experiences
IPM	integrated pest management
IPV	inactivated polio virus
IR	infrared
IRB	institutional review board
IRR	Individual Ready Reserve
IS	information sciences
ISE	ion-sensitive electrode
ISF	interstitial fluid
ISI	Institute for Scientific Information
ISMP	Institute for Safe Medication Practices
ISO	International Standardization Organization
ISP	internet service provider
ISPE	International Society for Pharmaceutical Engineering
ISS	ion-scattering spectroscopy
ITA	intention to treat analysis
ITP	idiopathic thrombocytopenic purpura, immune thrombocytopenia purpura
IUD	intra-uterine device
IUPAC	International Union of Pure and Applied Chemistry
IV	intravenous
IVD	*in-vitro* diagnostic
IVF	intravascular fluid
IVIV	*in vitro—in vivo*

J

JAMA	Journal of the American Medical Association
JCAH	Joint Commission on Accreditation of Hospitals
JCAHO	Joint Commission on Accreditation of Healthcare Organizations
JNC	Joint National Committee
JP	Japanese Pharmacopeia

K

KS	ketosteroid, Kaposi's sarcoma
kGy	kilogray
KVO	keeping the vein open

L

LAFW	laminar airflow workbench
LAIV	live attenuated influenza vaccine
LAL	limulus amebocyte lysate
LC	liquid chromatography
LC-FTIR	liquid chromatography-Fourier transform infrared
LC-MS	liquid chromatography
LCST	lower critical solution temperature
LDL	low-density lipoprotein
LDPE	low-density polyethylene
LED	light-emitting diode
LF	laminar flow
LH	luteinizing hormone
LLDPE	linear low-density polyethylene
LLE	liquid-liquid extraction
LOCA	lower osmolality contrast agents
LPL	lipoprotein lipase gene
L/S	least square, lecithin to sphingomyelin ratio
LSD	lysergic acid diethylamide
LT	leukotriene
LTCF	long term care facility
LTH	luteotropin
LVEDP	left ventricular end diastolic pressure
LVI	large-volume injection
LVP	large-volume parenteral

M

MAb	monoclonal antibody
MAC	maximum allowable cost, minimum alveolar concentration
MALDI	matrix-assisted laser desorption ionization
MALT	mucosa-associated lymphoid tissue
MAOI	monoamine oxidase inhibitor
MAP	maximum *a posteriori*
MAS	magic angle spinning
MASH	mobile army surgical hospital
MAT	mean absorption time
MAUT	multi-atribute utility theory
MBC	minimum bactericidal concentration
MBNQ	Malcolm Baldrige National Quality Program
MCH	mean corpuscular hemoglobin
MCHC	mean corpuscular hemoglobin concentration
MCO	managed care organization
MCP	metacarpophalangeal
MCT	multiple compressed tablet
MCV	mean corpuscular volume
MDI	metered-dose inhaler
MDR	multidrug resistance
MDS	minimum data set
MEC	minimum effective concentration
MECC	micellar electrokinetic capillary chromatography
MedDRA	Medical Dictionary for Drug Regulatory Affairs
MEKC	micellar electrokinetic chromatography
MEMS	medication event monitoring system
mEq	milliequivalent
MER	medication errors reporting
MERP	medication error reduction program
MHHP	Minnesota Hospital and Healthcare Partnership
MHC	major histocompatibility complex
Mho	reciprocal ohm
MI	mitral insufficiency, myocardial infarction
MIA	metabolite bacterial inhibition assay
MIC	minimum inhibitory concentration
MIL-STD	military standard
MKT	mean kinetic temperature
MLV	multilamellar vesicle
MMR	measles, mumps, and rubella
MMWR	Morbidity and Mortality Weekly Report
MNT	medical nutrition therapy
MO	molecular orbital
MPBR	master production batch record
MPD	minimum pyrogenic dose
MPJE	Multistate Pharmacy Jurisprudence Exam
MQ-NMR	multiple quantum technique nuclear magnetic resonance
MR	mental retardation, mentally retarded
MRC	medical research council
MRFIT	Multiple Risk Factor Intervention Trial
MRI	magnetic resonance imaging
MRIP	Model Rules for Institutional Pharmacy
mRNA	messenger RNA
MRS	magnetic resonance spectroscopy
MRT	mean residence time
MS	mass spectrometry, mass spectroscopy, multiple sclerosis, mitral stenosis
MSC	Medical Service Corps
MSD	mass spectral detector
MS/MS	mass spectrometry/mass spectrometry
MSPPA	Model State Pharmacy Practice Act
MSUD	maple syrup urine disease
MTC	minimum toxic concentration
MTP	metatarsophalangeal
MTT	mean transit time
MTX	methotrexate
MUE	medication-use evaluation
MW	molecular weight
MWQ	minimum weighable quantity

N

NABP	National Association of Boards of Pharmacy
NACDS	National Association of Chain Drug Stores
NADPH	nicotinamide-adenine-dinucleotide phosphate
NAG	ASPEN's National Advisory Group
NAMS	North American Menopause Society
NARD	National Association of Retail Druggists
NASA	National Aeronautics and Space Administration
NASHP	National Academy for State Health Policy
NCBTMB	National Certification Board for Therapeutic Massage and Bodywork

NCCAM	National Center for Complimentary and Alternative Medicine	NPLEX	Naturopathic Physician Licensing Examination
NCCAOM	National Center for Complimentary and Alternative Oriental Medicine	NPN	nonprotein nitrogen
		NPR	National Public Radio
		NPSF	National Patient Safety Foundation
NCCLS	National Committee for Clinical Laboratory Standards	NPSG	National Patient Safety Goals
NCC MERP	National Coordinating Council for Medication Error Reporting and Prevention	NQF	National Quality Forum
		NQMC	National Quality Measures Clearinghouse
		NRC	Nuclear Regulatory Committee, Nuclear Regulatory Commission
NCE	new chemical entity		
NCEP	National Cholesterol Education Program	NRT	nicotine-replacement therapy
NCF-A	neutrophil chemotactic factor of anaphylaxis	NSABP	National Surgical Adjuvant Breast and Bowel Project
NCHC	National Coalition on Health Care	NSAID	nonsteroidal anti-inflammatory drug
NCI	negative-ion chemical ionization, National Cancer Institute	NSF	National Science Foundation
NCPA	National Community Pharmacists Association	NTI	narrow therapeutic index

O

OA	"open access," osteoarthritis
OAM	Office of Alternate Medicine
OASI	Old-Age and Survivors Insurance
OB	obstetrics
OBDIV	operational division
OBRA	Omnibus Budget Reconciliation Act
OCD	obsessive-compulsive disorder
OCP	oral contraceptive pill
OD	outside diameter
ODT	orally disintegrating tablet
OEF	Operation Enduring Freedom
OIF	Operation Iraqi Freedom
OLV	oligolamellar vesicles
OMD	Oriental medicine degree
OPV	oral polio vaccine
OR	operating room
ORD	optical rotatory dispersion
OSHA	Occupational Safety and Health Administration
OT	old tuberculin
OTC	over-the-counter, ornithine transcarbamylase
O/W	oil-in-water

P

PAD	premature atrial depolarization
PADE	potential adverse drug event
PAGE	polyacrylamide gel electrophoresis
P&P	policies and procedures
P&T	pharmacy and therapeutics
PANSS	positive and negative syndrome scale
PAO	peak acid output
PAW	pulmonary arterial wedge
Pb	phenobarbital

NCPDP	National Council for Prescription Drug Programs
NCPIE	National Council on Patient Information and Education
NCPS	National Center for Patient Safety
NCQA	National Committee for Quality Assurance
NDA	New Drug Application
NDC	National Drug Code
NDMS	National Disaster Medical System
NEPM	non-parametric population modeling
NGC	National Guideline Clearinghouse
NHANES	National Health and Nutrition Examination Survey
NHGRI	National Human Genome Research Institute
NIDA	National Institute on Drug Abuse
NIDDM	non-insulin dependent diabetes mellitus
NIH	National Institutes of Health
NIMH	National Institute for Mental Health
NIOSH	National Institute for Occupational Safety and Health
NIR	near infrared
NISPC	National Institute for Standards in Pharmacist Credentialing
NIST	National Institute of Standards and Technology
NKC	natural killer cell
NMR	nuclear magnetic resonance
NOE	nuclear Overhauser effect
NPD	nitrogen phosphorus detector
NPH	neutral protamine Hagedorn

PBE	proton-balance equation
PBI	protein-bound iodine
PBM	pharmacy benefit management, pharmacy benefit manager
PBP	penicillin-binding protein
PBR	production batch record
PC	personal computer, percutaneous
PCA	patient-controlled analgesia, principal component analysis
PCCF	pharmacist care claim form
PCP	phencyclidine, *pneumocystis carinii* pneumonia
PCR	polymerase chain reaction
PCV	pneumococcal conjugate vaccine
PDA	Parenteral Drug Association, personal digital assistant
PDCA	Plan-Do-Check-Act
PDGF	platelet-derived growth factor
PDMA	Prescription Drug Marketing Act
PDR	Physicians' Desk Reference
PDSA	Plan-Do-Study Act
PDUFA	Prescription Drug User Fee Act
PE	pulmonary embolism
PEG	polyethylene glycol, percutaneous endoscopic gastrostomy
PEPI	Postmenopausal Estrogen/Progestin Interventions
PEPT1	plasma membrane peptide transporter
PET	positron emission tomography, positron emission test
PFG	pulsed field gradients
PFM	peak flow meter
PFR	peak flow rate
PGDB	Prevention Guidelines Database
PGE	prostaglandin E
PHI	personal health information, protected health information
PhRMA	Pharmaceutical Research and Manufacturers Association
PHS	US Public Health Service
PHSA	Public Health Service Act
PICVI	plasma impulse chemical vapor deposition
PID	photo-ionization detector, pelvic inflammatory disease
PIP	proximal interphalangeal
PIT	phase inversion temperature
PKC	protein kinase C
PKU	phenylketonuria
PL	Public Law
PLAN	Pharmacists' Learning Assistance Network

PLC	programmable logic controllers, phospholipase C
PLM	polarized light microscopy
PM	polymyositis
PMA	Pharmaceutical Manufacturers Association
PMMA	polymethylmethacrylate, (methacrylic acid)
PMN	polymorphonuclear leukocyte
PMS	post-marketing surveillance
PN	parenteral nutrition
PND	paroxysmal nocturnal dyspnea
PNI	psychoneuroimmunology
PNS	peripheral nervous system
PNSU	probability of nonsterile unit
PNU	protein nitrogen unit
POA	durable power of attorney
POC	point-of-care
POMR	problem-oriented medical record
POST	Polymer Science and Technology
PP	protein precipitation
PPA	phenylpropanolamine
PPAC	pharmacy practice activity classification
PPD	purified protein derivative
PPI	proton pump inhibitor, patient package insert
PPLO	pleuropneumonia-like organism
ppm	parts per million
PPO	preferred provider organization, poly(propylene oxide)
PPPA	Poison Prevention Packaging Act
PPS	professional pharmacy services
Prl	prolactin
PRN	as needed, Pharmacist Recovery Network
PRO	professional review organization
PSA	prostate specific antigen
PSC	Program Support Center, pluripotent stem cell
PSE	porto-systemic encephalopathy
PSIT	Pennsylvania Smell Identification Test
PSP	phenolsulfonthalein
PSST	pressure sore status tool
PST	pocket smell test
PSVT	paroxysmal supraventricular tachycardia
PT	prothrombin time
PTA	plasma thromboplastin antecedent
PTC	plasma thromboplastin component
PTCB	Pharmacy Technician Certification Board
PTFE	polytetrafluoroethylene
PTH	parathyroid hormone
PT/INR	prothrombin time/international normalized ratio

PTSD — post-traumatic stress disorder

PTT — partial thromboplastin time

P2C2 — professionals and patients for customized care

PUSH — pressure ulcer scale for healing

PVC — premature ventricular contraction

PVD — premature ventricular depolarization

PVP — polyvinylpyrrolidone

PWDT — pharmacist's workup of drug therapy

Q

Q — coulomb

QA — quality assurance

QALY — quality-adjusted life years

QC — quality control

QOL — quality of life

R

RA — rheumatoid arthritis

RAM — random access memory

R&D — research and development

RAP — resident assessment protocol

RBC — red blood cell

RBRVS — resource-based relative value scale

RCA — root cause analysis

RCC — renal cell carcinoma

RCT — randomized controlled trial

RDA — recommended daily allowance, recommended dietary allowance

rDNA — recombinant DNA

RDI — reference daily intake

REM — rapid eye movement

RES — reticuloendothelial system

RF — rheumatoid factor

RFLP — restriction fragment length polymorphism

RH — relative humidity

Rh — rhesus blood factor/group

rhGM — recombinant granulocyte-macrophage

RI — refractive index

RIA — radioimmunoassay

RIBA — recombinant immunoblot assay

RMP — risk management program

RNA — ribonucleic acid

RNAi — RNA interference

RNase — ribonuclease

RO — reverse osmosis

ROI — return on investment

rPA — recombinant plasminogen activator

RPC — reverse-phase chromatography

RPN — risk priority number

RPR — rapid plasma reagin

RPS — Remington's Pharmaceutical Sciences

RSD — relative standard deviation

RSE — reference standard endotoxin

RSV — respiratory syncytial virus

RV — residual volume

RVU — relative value unit

Rx — prescription

S

SA — sinoatrial

SAD — sunlight affective disorder

SADR — suspected adverse drug reaction

SAE — serious adverse event

SAL — sterility assurance level

SAMHSA — Substance Abuse and Mental Health Services

SAP — sterility assurance probability

SARA — Superfund Amendment and Reauthorization Act

SARS — severe acute respiratory syndrome

SBP — systolic blood pressure

SC — subcutaneous

SCD — soybean casein digest

SCID — severe combined immunodeficiency

SCOT — support-coated open tubular

SCT — sugar-coated tablet

SD — standard deviation

SDO — standards development organization

SDS — special delivery system

SEC — size-exclusion chromatography, soft elastic capsule

SERM — selective estrogen-receptor modulator

SFC — supercritical fluid chromatography

SI — International System of Units

SIADH — syndrome of inappropriate antidiuretic hormone secretion

SIDS — sudden infant death syndrome

SIMS — secondary ion mass spectrometry

siRNA — small interfering RNA

SLE — systemic lupus erythematosus

SMBGP — self-monitoring blood glucose product

SMILES — Simplified Molecular Line Entry Specification

SMU EC — Safe Medication Use Expert Committee

SNDA — supplemental new drug application

SNP — single nucleotide polymorphism

SOAP — subjective, objective, assessment, and plan

SOP — standard operating procedure

SPE — solid phase extraction

SPF — sun protective factor

SRM — selected reaction monitoring

SSA — Social Security Act

SSRI — selective serotonin reuptake inhibitor

STA — slit-to-agar

STD — sexually transmitted disease

STH — somatotrophic hormone

STP — standard temperature and pressure

SUPAC — scale-up and post-approval changes

SUV — small unilamellar vesicles

SVI — small-volume injection

SVM — support vector machine

SVP — small-volume parenteral

SWI — sterile water for injection

SWOT — strengths, weaknesses, opportunities, and threats

T

T_3 — triiodothyronine

T_4 — thyroxine

TAP — total available pool

TB — tuberculosis

TBG — thyroxine-binding globulin

TBPA — thyroxine-binding prealbumin

TC — total cholesterol

TCD — thermal conductivity conductor

TCGF — T-cell growth factor

TCR — T-cell receptor

TD — toxicodynamic, tetanus and diphtheria

TDD — telecommunication device for the deaf

TDDS — transdermal drug-delivery system

TESS — toxic exposure and surveillance system

TG — triglyceride

TGA — thermogravimetric analysis

TH — T helper

TIA — transient ischemic attack

TIBC — total iron binding capacity

TIV — trivalent inactivated influenza vaccine

TK — toxicokinetic

TLC — thin-layer chromatography, therapeutic life-style change

TM — transcendental meditation

TMA — thermomechanical analysis

TMP-SMZ — trimethoprim-sulfamethoxazole

TNA — total nutrient admixture

TNF — tissue necrosis factor

TOC — total organic carbon

TOPS — Take Off Pounds Sensibly

tPA — tissue plasminogen activator

TPC — total pharmacy care

TPN — total parenteral nutrition

TPO — treatment, payment and health care operations

TPU — Troop Program Unit

TPQ — total product quality

TQM — total quality management

TRH — thyrotropin-releasing hormone

TRIP — turning research into practice

T.R.U.E. — thin-layer rapid use epicutaneous

TS — test solution

TSD — thermionic specific detector

TSH — thyroid-stimulating hormone

TT — tablet triturate

TTP — thrombotic thrombocytopenic purpura

TV — tidal volume

2D-NMR — two-dimensional nuclear magnetic resonance

U

UCC — Uniform Commercial Code

UCR — usual, customary and reasonable

UL — tolerable upper intake level

ULV — unilamellar vesicles, ultralow-volume

UPIN — unique provider identification number

URI — upper respiratory infection

URL — Uniform Resource Locater

USAF — United States Air Force

USAN — United States Adopted Names

U.S.C. — United States Code

USDA — United States Department of Agriculture

USNS — United States Naval Ship

USP — United States Pharmacopeia

USP DI — USP Drug Information

USP/NF — United States Pharmacopeia/National Formulary

USPSTF — United States Preventive Services Task Force

UTI — urinary tract infection

UV — ultraviolet

V

V — volt

VA — Veterans Affairs

VC — vital capacity

VDRL — Venereal Disease Research Laboratory

VEGF — vascular endothelial growth factor

VHA — Veterans Health Administration

VIP — vasoactive intestinal polypeptide

VIPPS — verified internet pharmacy practice sites

Vis — visible

VLCD — very low calorie diet

VLDL — very low-density lipoprotein

VOC — volatile organic compound

VTE — venous thromboembolism

VNTR — variable number of tandem repeats

v/v	percent volume in volume	WAVE	Women's Angiographic Vitamin and Estrogen	WIC	Special Supplemental Program for Women, Infants, and Children	XML	extensible markup language
VWD	von Willebrand's disease	WBC	white blood cell	W/O	water-in-oil	XRD	X-ray diffraction
VWF	von Willebrand factor	WCOT	wall-coated open tubular	w/v	percent weight in volume	XRPD	X-ray powder diffraction
		WFI	water for injection				
W		WHA	World Health Assembly	w/w	percent weight in weight	**Y**	
W	watt					**Z**	
WA	wide awake	WHIMS	Women's Health Initiative Memory Study	**X**		Z	atomic number
WAP	wireless application protocol					ZE	Zollinger-Ellison syndrome
WAS	Wiskott-Aldrich syndrome	WHO	World Health Organization	X-LA	X-linked agammaglobulinemia	ZSR	zeta sedimentation ratio

Index